MANIFESTATIONS
OF DISEASE
IN THE NEONATE

Large Animal
INTERNAL MEDICINE

To study the phenomena of disease without books
is to sail an uncharted sea, while to study books
without patients is not to go to sea at all.

SIR WILLIAM OSLER

THIRD EDITION

Large Animal INTERNAL MEDICINE

BRADFORD P. SMITH
DVM, Diplomate ACVIM

Professor
Department of Medicine
and Epidemiology

Director
Veterinary Medical Teaching Hospital
School of Veterinary Medicine
Associate Dean for
Clinical Programs

University of California
Davis, California

with 471 illustrations

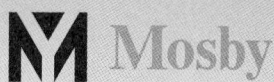 Mosby

An Affiliate of Elsevier Science

St. Louis   London   Philadelphia   Sydney   Toronto

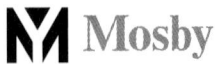

An Affiliate of Elsevier

Publishing Director: **John A. Schrefer**
Editorial Manager: **Linda Duncan**
Senior Developmental Editor: **Teri Merchant**
Project Manager: **John Rogers**
Project Specialist: **Beth Hayes**
Designer: **Teresa Breckwoldt**

THIRD EDITION

NOTICE
Pharmacology is an ever-changing field. Standard safety precautions must be followed, but as new research and clinical experience broaden our knowledge, changes in treatment and drug therapy may become necessary or appropriate. Readers are advised to check the most current product information provided by the manufacturer of each drug to be administered to verify the recommended dose, the method and duration of administration, and contraindications. It is the responsibility of the treating veterinarian, relying on experience and knowledge of the patient, to determine dosages and the best treatment for each individual patient. Neither the publisher nor the editor assumes any liability for any injury and/or damage to persons or property arising from this publication.

Mosby, Inc.
An Affiliate of Elsevier
11830 Westline Industrial Drive
St. Louis, Missouri 63146

Printed in the United States of America

Library of Congress Cataloging in Publication Data

Large animal internal medicine: diseases of horses, cattle, sheep, and goats / [edited by] Bradford P. Smith.—3rd ed.
    p.   ; cm.
  Includes bibliographical references and index.
  ISBN 0-323-00946-8
  1. Veterinary internal medicine. I. Smith, Bradford P.
  [DNLM: 1. Veterinary Medicine. 2. Animal Diseases. 3. Diagnosis, Differential.
SF 745 L322 2002]
SF745 .L37 2002
636.089'6—dc21

2001030758

04 05 06 TG/KPT 9 8 7 6 5 4 3

Consulting Editors

Trevor R. Ames, MS, DVM, DIPL ACVIM

John C. Baker, DVM, PHD, DIPL ACVIM

Terry L. Blanchard, DVM, MS, DIPL ACT

Gordon W. Brumbaugh, DVM, PHD, DIPL ACVIM

T. Douglas Byars, DVM, DIPL ACVIM, ACVECC

Gary P. Carlson, DVM, PHD, DIPL ACVIM, ACVP

Stan W. Casteel, DVM, PHD, DIPL ABVT

Rick Corbett, BSc, MSc, PAg

Victor Cortese, DVM, PHD, DIPL ABVP (DAIRY)

James S. Cullor, DVM, PHD

Thomas J. Divers, DVM, DIPL ACVIM, ACVECC

Lorraine Doepel, BSc

Noël O. Dybdal, DVM, PHD, DIPL ACVIM

Nancy E. East, MS, DVM, MPVM

Anne G. Evans, DVM, MBA, DIPL ACVD

Susan L. Ewart, DVM, PHD, DIPL ACVIM

Francis D. Galey, DVM, PHD, DIPL ABVT

A. J. Heinrichs, MS, PHD

Melissa T. Hines, DVM, PHD, DIPL ACVIM

David R. Hodgson, BvSc, PHD, DIPL ACVIM, FACSM

R. Neil Hooper, DVM, MS, DIPL ACVS

John K. House, BVMS, PHD, DIPL ACVIM

Janet K. Johnston, DVM, DIPL ACVIM

Vernon C. Langston, DVM, PHD, DIPL AVCP

Jeanne Lofstedt, BVSc, MS, DIPL ACVIM

John Maas, MS, DVM, DIPL ACVN, ACVIM

Sheila M. McGuirk, DVM, PHD, DIPL ACVIM

Cecil P. Moore, DVM, MS, DIPL ACVO

James N. Moore, DVM, PHD, DIPL ACVS

Debra Deem Morris, MS, DVM, DIPL ACVIM

Michael J. Murray, DVM, MS, DIPL ACVIM

Steven M. Parish, DVM, DIPL ACVIM

Erwin G. Pearson, DVM, MS, DIPL ACVIM

Virginia B. Reef, DVM, DIPL ACVIM

Joan Dean Rowe, DVM, MPVM, PHD

George Saperstein, DVM

Harold C. Schott II, DVM, PHD, DIPL ACVIM

Brad Seguin, DVM, PHD, DIPL ACT

Mary O. Smith, BVM&S, PHD, MRCVS, DIPL ACVIM (NEUROLOGY)

Susan M. Stover, DVM, PHD, DIPL ACVS

Raymond W. Sweeney, VMD, DIPL ACVIM

Ronald L. Terra, DVM, MS, DIPL ABVP

Mats H.T. Troedsson, DVM, PHD, DIPL ACT

James R. Turk, DVM, PHD, DIPL ACVP

Jeff W. Tyler, DVM, MPVM, PHD, DIPL ACVIM

Christine A. Uhlinger, VMD, MPH, DIPL ABVP

Wendy E. Vaala, VMD, DIPL ACVIM

Stephanie J. Valberg, DVM, PHD, DIPL ACVIM

David C. Van Metre, DVM, DIPL ACVIM

Dickson D. Varner, DVM, DIPL ACT

Maurice E. White, DVM, DIPL ACVIM, ABVP

Stephen D. White, DVM, DIPL ACVD

Susan L. White, DVM, MS, DIPL ACVIM

Jami L. Whiting, DVM

Pamela A. Wilkins, DVM, PHD, DIPL ACVIM

W. David Wilson, BVMS, MS, MRCVS

Contributors

Monica R. Aleman, MVZ, DIPL ACVIM
Comparative Pathology
Department of Surgical and Radiological Sciences
School of Veterinary Medicine
University of California, Davis, California

Trevor R. Ames, DVM, MS, DIPL ACVIM
Chair and Professor
Department of Clinical and Population Medicine
College of Veterinary Medicine
University of Minnesota, St. Paul, Minnesota

Jane E. Axon, BVSc, MACVSc
Lecturer, Large Animal Medicine
New Bolton Center
School of Veterinary Medicine
University of Pennsylvania, Kennett Square, Pennsylvania

John C. Baker, DVM, PHD, DIPL ACVIM
Associate Dean for Research and Graduate Studies
Professor, Department of Large Animal Clinical Services
College of Veterinary Medicine
Michigan State University, East Lansing, Michigan

George M. Barrington, DVM, PHD, DIPL ACVIM
Assistant Professor, Department of Veterinary Clinical Sciences
College of Veterinary Medicine
Washington State University, Pullman, Washington

Jill Beech, VMD, DIPL ACVIM
Chief of Reproduction, Department of Clinical Sciences
New Bolton Center
College of Veterinary Medicine
University of Pennsylvania, Kennett Square, Pennsylvania

Steven L. Berry, DVM, MPVM
Extension Dairy Management and Health Specialist
Department of Animal Science
School of Veterinary Medicine
University of California, Davis, California

Christine F. Berthelin-Baker, DVM, DIPL ACVIM (NEUROLOGY)
Neuropathology Unit, Central Veterinary Laboratory
New Haw, Addlestone, Surrey, England

Jill McClure Blackmer, DVM, MS, DIPL ACVIM, ABVP
Professor of Equine Medicine
Department of Veterinary Clinical Sciences
School of Veterinary Medicine
Louisiana State University, Baton Rouge, Louisiana

John T. Blackwelder, MS, DVM
College of Veterinary Medicine
North Carolina State University, Raleigh, North Carolina

Terry L. Blanchard, DVM, MS, DIPL ACT
Professor of Large Animal Medicine and Surgery
College of Veterinary Medicine
Texas A & M University, College Station, Texas

Anthony T. Blikslager, DVM, PHD, DIPL ACVS
Assistant Professor, Equine Surgery
Department of Clinical Sciences
College of Veterinary Medicine
North Carolina State University, Raleigh, North Carolina

Richard A. Bowen, DVM, PHD
Associate Professor, Department of Physiology
College of Veterinary Medicine and Biomedical Sciences
Colorado State University, Fort Collins, Colorado

James P. Brendemuehl, DVM, PHD, DIPL ACT
Assistant Professor, Veterinary Teaching Hospital
College of Veterinary Medicine
Oregon State University, Corvallis, Oregon

Gordon W. Brumbaugh, DVM, PHD, DIPL ACVIM
Associate Professor, Veterinary Physiology and Pharmacology
College of Veterinary Medicine
Texas A & M University, College Station, Texas

T. Douglas Byars, DVM, DIPL ACVIM, ACVECC
Director, Equine Internal Medicine
Hagyard-Davidson-McGee Associates
Lexington, Kentucky

Gary P. Carlson, DVM, PHD, DIPL ACVIM, ACVP
Professor and Chairman, Department of Medicine and Epidemiology
School of Veterinary Medicine
University of California, Davis, California

Elizabeth Ann Carr, DVM, PHD, DIPL ACVIM
Assistant Professor, Equine Medicine
Department of Large Animal Clinical Sciences
College of Veterinary Medicine
Michigan State University, East Lansing, Michigan

Stan W. Casteel, DVM, PHD, DIPL ABVT
Professor of Toxicology, Veterinary Medical Diagnostic Laboratory
College of Veterinary Medicine
University of Missouri, Columbia, Missouri

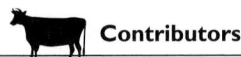
Harry Michael Chaddock, DVM
Division Director and State Veterinarian
Michigan Department of Agriculture
Animal Industry Division, Lansing, Michigan

Erin S. Champagne, DVM, DIPL ACVO
Clinical Assistant Professor
Department of Veterinary Medicine and Surgery
College of Veterinary Medicine
University of Missouri, Columbia, Missouri

Noah D. Cohen, VMD, MPH, PHD, DIPL ACVIM
Associate Professor
Department of Large Animal Medicine and Surgery
College of Veterinary Medicine
Texas A & M University, College Station, Texas

Anthony W. Confer, DVM, MS, PHD, DIPL ACVP
Associate Dean for Research for Graduate Education and
Professor and Endowed Chair for Food Animal Research
College of Veterinary Medicine
Oklahoma State University, Stillwater, Oklahoma

Vanessa L. Cook, MA, VETMB, MS, MRCVS, DIPL ACVS
Lecturer, Large Animal Emergency Surgery
College of Veterinary Medicine
Cornell University, Ithaca, New York

Rick Corbett, BSC, MSC, PAG
Provincial Dairy Nutritionist
Alberta Agriculture, Food and Rural Development
Edmonton, Alberta, Canada

Kevin T.T. Corley, BSC, BVM&S, PHD, MRCVS
Lecturer in Equine Medicine and Critical Care
Royal Veterinary College
University of London
North Mymms, Herts., United Kingdom

Victor Cortese, DVM, PHD, DIPL ABVP (DAIRY)
Pfizer Animal Health, Exton, Pennsylvania

James S. Cullor, DVM, PHD
Professor, Department of Pathology, Microbiology, and Immunology
School of Veterinary Medicine
University of California, Davis, California

Robin M. Dabareiner, DVM, PHD, DIPL ACVS
Assistant Professor of Lameness
College of Veterinary Medicine
Texas A & M University, College Station, Texas

Andrew J. Dart, BVSC, DVCS, MACVSC, DIPL ACVS, ECVS
Senior Registrar
University of Sydney, New South Wales, Australia

Eric W. Davis, DVM, MS, DIPL ACVIM, ACVS
Department of Large Animal Clinical Sciences
College of Veterinary Medicine
University of Tennessee, Knoxville, Tennessee

Fabio Del Piero, DVM, DIPL ACVP
Assistant Professor of Pathology
Department of Pathobiology and Clinical Studies
New Bolton Center
School of Veterinary Medicine
University of Pennsylvania, Kennett Square, Pennsylvania

Joseph Di Pietro, DVM, MS
Dean, College of Veterinary Medicine
University of Florida, Gainesville, Florida

Thomas J. Divers, DVM, DIPL ACVIM, ACVECC
Professor, Large Animal Medicine
College of Veterinary Medicine
Cornell University, Ithaca, New York

Lorraine Doepel, BSC
University of Alberta, Edmonton, Alberta, Canada

Brett Dolente, VMD
Lecturer, Section of Medicine
New Bolton Center
School of Veterinary Medicine
University of Pennsylvania, Kennett Square, Pennsylvania

Maarten Drost, DVM, DIPL ACT
Professor, Department of Large Animal Clinical Sciences
College of Veterinary Medicine
University of Florida, Gainesville, Florida

Gerald E. Duhamel, DMV, PHD, DIPL ACVP
Professor, Department of Veterinary and Biomedical Sciences
University of Nebraska, Lincoln, Nebraska

Noël O. Dybdal, DVM, PHD, DIPL ACVIM
Genentech, Inc, South San Francisco, California

Joan Dziezyc, DVM, DIPL ACVO
Associate Professor
Department of Small Animal Medicine and Surgery
College of Veterinary Medicine
Texas A & M University, College Station, Texas

Jack Easley, DVM, MS, DIPL ABVP (EQUINE)
Private Equine Practitioner
Equine Veterinary Practice, Shelbyville, Kentucky

Nancy E. East, DVM, MPVM
Associate Professor (retired),
Department of Medicine and Epidemiology
School of Veterinary Medicine
University of California, Davis, California

Anita J. Edmondson, BVM&S, MPVM, MRCVS
Staff Veterinarian, Aimal Health and Food Safety Services
California Department of Food and Agriculture
Sacramento, California

John A. Ellis, DVM, PHD, DIPL ACVP, ACVM
Professor, Department of Veterinary Microbioloby
Western College of Veterinary Medicine
University of Saskatchewn, Saskatoon, Saskatchewan, Canada

Robert V. English, DVM, PHD
Animal Eye Care, Cary, North Carolina

Anne G. Evans, DVM, MBA, DIPL ACVD
Consultant/Analyst, Evans Associates, La Jolla, California

James F. Evermann, MS, PHD
Professor, Infectious Diseases
Department of Veterinary Clinical Sciences and Diagnostic Laboratory
College of Veterinary Medicine
Washington State University, Pullman, Washington

Susan L. Ewart, DVM, PHD, DIPL ACVIM
Associate Professor, Large Animal Clinical Sciences
College of Veterinary Medicine
Michigan State University, East Lansing, Michigan

Gilles Fecteau, DMV, DIPL ACVIM
Associate Professor, Université Montréal
St. Hyacinthe, Quebec, Canada

Andrew T. Fischer, Jr., DVM, DIPL ACVS
Chino Valley Equine Hospital, Chino, California

Sherrill A. Fleming, DVM, DIPL ABVP (FOOD ANIMAL), ACVIM
Associate Professor, Food Animal Medicine
College of Veterinary Medicine
Mississippi State University, Mississippi State, Mississippi

Robert W. Fulton, DVM, PhD, DIPL ACVM
Professor of Virology, Department of Veterinary Pathobiology
College of Veterinary Medicine
Oklahoma State University, Stillwater, Oklahoma

Francis D. Galey, DVM, PhD, DIPL ABVT
Director, Wyoming State Veterinary Laboratory
Head, Department of Veterinary Sciences
University of Wyoming, Laramie, Wyoming

Franklyn Garry, DVM, MS, DIPL ACVIM
Professor, Department of Clinical Sciences
College of Veterinary Medicine and Biomedical Sciences
Colorado State University, Fort Collins, Colorado

Lisle W. George, DVM, PhD, DIPL ACVIM
Professor, Department of Medicine and Epidemiology
School of Veterinary Medicine
University of California, Davis, California

Terry C. Gerros, DVM, DIPL ACVIM
Hood River Veterinary Hospital, Hood River, Oregon

Carol L. Gillis, DVM, PhD
Equine Ultrasound Consultant, Vacaville, California

Mary Belle Glaze, DVM, MS, DIPL ACVO
Associate Professor of Veterinary Ophthalmology
Veterinary Clinical Sciences
School of Veterinary Medicine
Louisiana State University, Baton Rouge, Louisiana

David P. Gnad, DVM
Assistant Professor, Department of Clinical Sciences
College of Veterinary Medicine
Kansas State University, Manhattan, Kansas

Daniel H. Gould, DVM, PhD, DIPL ACVP
Professor of Pathology, Department of Pathology
College of Veterinary Medicine and Biomedical Sciences
Colorado State University, Fort Collins, Colorado

Dan Grooms, DVM, PhD, DIPL ACVIM
Assistant Professor, Department of Large Animal Clinical Sciences
College of Veterinary Medicine
Michigan State University, East Lansing, Michigan

Charles Guard, DVM, PhD
Associate Professor
Population Medicine and Diagnostic Science
College of Veterinary Medicine
Cornell University, Ithaca, New York

Spring K. Halland, DVM
Department of Large Animal Medicine
Veterinary Medical Teaching Hospital
School of Veterinary Medicine
University of California, Davis, California

Kevin K. Haussler, DVM, DC, PhD
Lecturer, Department of Biomedical Sciences
College of Veterinary Medicine
Cornell University, Ithaca, New York

A.J. Heinrichs, MS, PhD
Professor, Dairy and Animal Science
The Pennsylvania State University
University Park, Pennsylvania

Nancy L. Hesters, DVM, MBA
Randleman, North Carolina

Melissa T. Hines, DVM, PhD, DIPL ACVIM
Assistant Professor, Veterinary Teaching Hospital
College of Veterinary Medicine
Washington State University, Pullman, Washington

H.F. Hintz, PhD
Professor, Animal Nutrition
Cornell University, Ithaca, New York

Dwight C. Hirsh, DVM, PhD
Professor of Microbiology
Chief, Microbiology Service
Veterinary Medical Teaching Hospital
School of Veterinary Medicine
University of California, Davis, California

Charles A. Hjerpe, DVM
Professor Emeritus
School of Veterinary Medicine
University of California, Davis, California

David R. Hodgson, DVM, PhD, DIPL ACVIM, FACSM
Professor of Large Animal Medicine and Director,
University Veterinary Centre, Camden
Faculty of Veterinary Science, University of Sydney
Camden, New South Wales, Australia

Patricia A. Hogan, VMD
New Jersey Equine Clinic, Clarksburg, New Jersey

Clifford M. Honnas, DVM, DIPL ACVS
Associate Professor
Equine Orthopedic Surgery and Lameness
Large Animal Clinic
College of Veterinary Medicine
Texas A & M University, College Station, Texas

R. Neil Hooper, DVM, MS, DIPL ACVS
Associate Professor of Surgery
Department of Large Animal Medicine and Surgery
College of Veterinary Medicine
Texas A & M University, College Station, Texas

John K. House, BVMS, PhD, DIPL ACVIM
Assistant Clinical Professor
Food Animal Medicine and Surgery
School of Veterinary Medicine
University of California, Davis, California

Elaine Hunt, DVM, DIPL ACVIM
Associate Professor, Food Animal Medicine
College of Veterinary Medicine
North Carolina State Universtiy, Raleigh, North Carolina

Janet K. Johnston, DVM, DIPL ACVIM
Department of Clinical Studies
New Bolton Center
School of Veterinary Medicine
University of Pennsylvania, Kennett Square, Pennsylvania

Robert L. Jones, DVM, PhD, DIPL ACVM
Professor, Department of Microbiology
College of Veterinary Medicine and Biomedical Sciences
Colorado State University, Fort Collins, Colorado

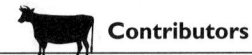
Samuel L. Jones, DVM, PhD, Dipl ACVIM
Assistant Professor of Equine Medicine
College of Veterinary Medicine
North Carolina State University, Raleigh, North Carolina

Carter E. Judy, DVM
Resident III, Equine Surgery
Veterinary Medical Teaching Hospital
School of Veterinary Medicine
University of California, Davis, California

Steven G. Kamerling, RPh, PhD
Senior Scientist, Discovery Research
Pharmacia Animal Health, Kalamazoo, Michigan

Andris J. Kaneps, DVM, PhD, Dipl ACVS
Assistant Professor of Equine Orthopedics
College of Veterinary Medicine
The Ohio State University, Columbus, Ohio

Vernon C. Langston, DVM, PhD, Dipl ACVCP
Associate Professor of Clinical Pharmacology
College of Veterinary Medicine
Mississippi State University, Mississippi State, Mississippi

Richard A. LeCouteur BVSc, PhD, Dipl ACVIM (Neurology)
Professor of Neurology and Neurosurgery
Department of Surgical and Radiological Sciences
School of Veterinary Medicine
University of California, Davis, California

Guy D. Lester, BVMS, PhD, Dipl ACVIM
Associate Professor, Large Animal Medicine
College of Veterinary Medicine
University of Florida, Gainesville, Florida

Stuart Lincoln, DVM, PhD, Dipl ACVP
Professor Emeritus, Caine Veterinary Teaching Center
University of Idaho, Caldwell, Idaho

Robert L. Linford, DVM, PhD, Dipl ACVS
Associate Professor, Equine Surgery and Medicine
College of Veterinary Medicine
Mississippi State University, Mississippi State, Mississippi

Michael A. Livesay, BVMS, Dipl ACVS
Cinder Hill Equine Veterinary Clinic
Horsted Keynes, Haywards Heath
West Sussex, United Kingdom

K.C. Kent Lloyd, DVM, PhD
Associate Professor, Veterinary Anatomy, Physiology, and Cell Biology
Center for Comparative Medicine
School of Veterinary Medicine
University of California, Davis, California

Jeanne Lofstedt, BVSc, MS, Dipl ACVIM
Associate Dean, Academic Affairs
Professor, Department of Health Management
Atlantic Veterinary College
University of Prince Edward Island
Charlottetown, Prince Edward Island, Canada

Guy H. Loneragan, BVSc (Hons), MS
Integrated Livestock Management
Department of Clinical Sciences
College of Veterinary Medicine and Biomedical Sciences
Colorado State University, Fort Collins, Colorado

John Maas, DVM, MS, Dipl ACVN, ACVIM
Extension Veterinarian
School of Veterinary Medicine
University of California, Davis, California

Melinda H. MacDonald, DVM, PhD, Dipl ACVS
Assistant Professor Equine Surgery
Department of Surgical and Radiological Sciences
School of Veterinary Medicine
University of California, Davis, California

Robert J. MacKay, BVSc, PhD, Dipl ACVIM
Professor, Large Animail Medicine
Department of Large Animal Clinical Sciences
College of Veterinary Medicine
University of Florida, Gainesville, Florida

John E. Madigan, DVM, MS, Dipl ACVIM
Professor, Department of Medicine and Epidemiology
School of Veterinary Medicine
University of California, Davis, California

K. Gary Magdesian, DVM, Dipl ACVECC
Lecturer, Equine Medicine and Emergency/Critical Care
Veterinary Medical Teaching Hospital
School of Veterinary Medicine
University of California, Davis, California

David J. Maggs, BVSc (Hons), Dipl ACVO
Assistant Professor
Department of Surgical and Radiological Sciences
College of Veterinary Medicine
University of California, Davis, California

John B. Malone, DVM, PhD
Professor, Veterinary Parasitology
Pathobiological Sciences
School of Veterinary Medicine
Louisiana State University, Baton Rouge, Louisiana

Peggy Sue Marsh, DVM
Lecturer, Equine Medicine
Department of Large Animal Medicine and Surgery
College of Veterinary Medicine
Texas A & M University, College Station, Texas

Patrick M. McCue, DVM, PhD, Dipl ACT
Associate Professor, Department of Clinical Sciences
College of Veterinary Medicine and Biomedical Sciences
Colorado State University, Fort Collins, Colorado

Laurie A. McDuffee, DVM, PhD, Dipl ACVS
Assistant Professor, Department of Health Management
Atlantic Veterinary College
University of Prince Edward Island
Charlottetown, Prince Edward Island, Canada

Sheila M. McGuirk, DVM, PhD, Dipl ACVIM
Professor, Department of Medical Sciences
School of Veterinary Medicine
University of Wisconsin, Madison, Wisconsin

Dennis M. Meagher, DVM, MS, PhD, Dipl ACVS
Professor Emeritus, Department of Surgical and Radiological Sciences
School of Veterinary Medicine
University of California, Davis, California

Nat T. Messer IV, DVM, Dipl ABVP
Associate Professor, Department of Veterinary Medicine and Surgery
College of Veterinary Medicine
University of Missouri, Columbia, Missouri

Paul G.E. Michelsen, MS, DVM
Mendocino Equine Clinic, Potter Valley, California

Nicholas J. Millichamp, BVetMed, PhD, MRCVS, Dipl ACVO
Associate Professor
College of Veterinary Medicine
Texas A & M University, College Station, Texas

Cecil P. Moore, DVM, MS, Dipl ACVO
Professor and Chairman
Department of Veterinary Medicine and Surgery
Director, Veterinary Medical Teaching Hospital
College of Veterinary Medicine
University of Missouri, Columbia, Missouri

James N. Moore, DVM, PhD, Dipl ACVS
Professor and Head, Department of Large Animal Medicine
College of Veterinary Medicine
University of Georgia, Athens, Georgia

Debra Deem Morris, DVM, MS, Dipl ACVIM
North Jersey Animal Hospital, Wayne, New Jersey

Derek A. Mosier, DVM, PhD, Dipl ACVP
Professor of Pathology
Department of Diagnostic Medicine/Pathobiology
College of Veterinary Medicine
Kansas State University, Manhattan, Kansas

Michael Murphy, DVM, PhD, Dipl ABVT
Associate Professor, Veterinary Diagnostic Medicine
College of Veterinary Medicine
University of Minnesota, St. Paul, Minnesota

Michael J. Murray, DVM, MS, Dipl ACVIM
Professor and Adelaide C. Riggs Chair in Equine Medicine
Marion duPont Scott Equine Medical Center
Virginia-Maryland Regional College of Veterinary Medicine
Virginia Tech, Blacksburg, Virginia

Mark P. Nasisse, DVM, Dipl ACVO
Veterinary Eye Specialists of the Carolinas
Greensboro, North Carolina

Jonathan M. Naylor, BSc, BVSc, PhD, Dipl ACVIM, ACVN
Professor, Department of Large Animal Clinical Sciences
Western College of Veterinary Medicine
University of Saskachewan, Saskatoon, Saskatchewan, Canada

James A. Orsini, DVM, Dipl ACVS
Associate Professor of Surgery
New Bolton Center
School of Veterinary Medicine
University of Pennsylvania, Kennett Square, Pennsylvania

Guy H. Palmer DVM, PhD, Dipl ACVP
Professor of Microbiology and Pathology
College of Veterinary Medicine
Washington State University, Pullman, Washington

Mary Rose Paradis, DVM, MS, Dipl ACVIM
Associate Professor, Large Animal Medicine
School of Veterinary Medicine
Tufts University, North Grafton, Massachusetts

Steven M. Parish, DVM, Dipl ACVIM
Professor, Large Animal Internal Medicine
Veterinary Teaching Hospital
College of Veterinary Medicine
Washington State University Pullman, Washington

John R. Pascoe, BVSc, PhD, Dipl ACVS
Professor, Veterinary Medicine
School of Veterinary Medicine
University of California, Davis, California

Erwin G. Pearson, DVM, MS, Dipl ACVIM
Professor, Large Animal Medicine
College of Veterinary Medicine
Oregon State University, Corvallis, Oregon

Arlena B. Pipkin, DMV
Bakersfield, California

Konnie H. Plumlee, DVM, MS, Dipl ABVT, ACVIM
Veterinary Toxicologist, Arkansas Diagnostic Laboratory
Livestock and Poultry Commission, Little Rock, Arkansas

Kimberly D. Rager, DVM
Resident II, Large Animal Internal Medicine
Food Animal Emphasis
Veterinary Medical Teaching Hospital
School of Veterinary Medicine
University of California, Davis, California

Virginia B. Reef, DVM, Dipl ACVIM
Professor of Medicine, Widener Hospital
Director of Large Animal Cardiology and Ultrasonography
Chief, Section of Sports Medicine & Imaging
New Bolton Center
School of Veterinary Medicine
University of Pennsylvania, Kennett Square, Pennsylvania

Craig R. Reinemeyer, DVM, PhD
President, East Tennessee Clinical Research, Inc.
Knoxville, Tennessee

David G. Renter, DVM
Food Animal Health and Management Center
College of Veterinary Medicine
Kansas State University, Manhattan, Kansas

James Paul Reynolds, DVM, MPVM
Chief, Dairy Production Medicine
Veterinary Medicine Teaching and Research Center
School of Veterinary Medicine
University of California, Davis, California

Steven M. Roberts, DVM, MS, Dipl ACVO
Animal Eye Center, Loveland, Colorado

Joan Dean Rowe, DVM, MPVM, PhD
Associate Professor, Department of Population Health and
    Reproduction
School of Veterinary Medicine
University of California, Davis, California

Bonnie R. Rush, DVM, MS, Dipl ACVIM
Associate Professor, Department of Clinical Sciences
College of Veterinary Medicine
Kansas State University, Manhattan, Kansas

Guy St. Jean, DMV, MS, Dipl ACVS
Professor of Surgery and Head
Department of Veterinary Clinical Sciences
School of Veterinary Medicine
Ross University, Basseterre, St. Kitts, West Indies

George Saperstein, DVM
Chair, Department of Environmental and Population Health
School of Veterinary Medicine
Tufts University, North Grafton, Massachusetts

William J.A. Saville, DVM, PhD, Dipl ACVIM
Assistant Professor, Epidemiologist/Large Animal Internist
College of Veterinary Medicine
The Ohio State University, Columbus, Ohio

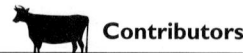
John W. Schlipf, Jr., DVM, MS, DIPL ACVIM
Assistant Professor, Large Animal Internal Medicine
Veterinary Teaching Hospital
College of Veterinary Medicine
Oregon State University, Corvallis, Oregon

Harold C. Schott II, DVM, PHD, DIPL ACVIM
Associate Professor, Equine Medicine
Department of Large Animal Clinical Sciences
College of Veterinary Medicine
Michigan State University, East Lansing, Michigan

Loren G. Schultz, DVM
Department of Clinical Sciences
College of Veterinary Medicine
Kansas State University, Manhattan, Kansas

Brad Seguin, DVM, MS, PHD, DIPL ACT
Professor, Department of Clinical and Population Sciences
College of Veterinary Medicine
University of Minnesota, St. Paul, Minnesota

Debra C. Sellon, DVM, PHD, DIPL ACVIM
Associate Professor, Equine Medicine
College of Veterinary Medicine
Washington State University, Pullman, Washington

Nathan M Slovis, DVM, DIPL ACVIM
Internist, Hagyard-Davidson-McGee Associates
Lexington, Kentucky

Bradford P. Smith, DVM, DIPL ACVIM
Professor, Department of Medicine and Epidemiology
Director, Veterinary Medical Teaching Hospital
Associate Dean, Clinical Programs
School of Veterinary Medicine
University of California, Davis, California

John Andrew Smith, DVM, MS, MAM, DIPL ACVIM
(LARGE ANIMAL), ACPV
Director of Health and Hatchery Services
Fieldale Farms Corporation, Baldwin, Georgia

Mary O. Smith, BVM&S, PHD, DIPL ACVIM (NEUROLOGY)
Associate Professor, Department of Clinical Sciences
College of Veterinary Medicine and Biomedical Sciences
Colorado State University, Fort Collins, Colorado

Joseph Hoyt (Joe) Snyder, DVM
Owner/Practitioner Myrtle Veterinary Hospital
Myrtle Point, Oregon

Stanley P. Snyder, DVM, PHD, DIPL ACVP
Professor of Pathology, Veterinary Diagnostic Laboratory
College of Veterinary Medicine
Oregon State University, Corvallis, Oregon

J. Glenn Songer, PHD
Professor
Department of Veterinary Science and Microbiology
University of Arizona, Tucson, Arizona

Sharon J. Spier, DVM, PHD, DIPL ACVIM
Associate Professor, Department of Medicine and Epidemiology
School of Veterinary Medicine
University of California, Davis, California

†Anthony A. Stannard, DVM, PHD, DIPL ACVD
Professor and Chair, Department of Medicine
School of Veterinary Medicine
University of California, Davis, California

Susan M. Stover, DVM, PHD, DIPL ACVS
Professor, Department of Anatomy, Physiology, and Cell Biology
School of Veterinary Medicine
University of California, Davis, California

George M. Strain, PHD
Interim Vice Chancellor for Research and
Graduate Dean, Office of Research and Graduate Studies
Professor of Neuroscience
Department of Comparative Biomedical Sciences
School of Veterinary Medicine
Louisiana State University, Baton Rouge, Louisiana

Corinne R. Sweeney, DVM, DIPL ACVIM
Professor of Medicine, Department of Clinical Studies
New Bolton Center
School of Veterinary Medicine
University of Pennsylvania, Kennett Square, Pennsylvania

Raymond W. Sweeney, VMD, DIPL ACVIM
Associate Professor of Medicine
School of Veterinary Medicine
University of Pennsylvania, Kennett Square, Pennsylvania

Ronald L. Terra, DVM, MS, DIPL ABVP
Lander Veterinary Clinic, Inc., Turlock, California

Philip G.A. Thomas, PHD, DIPL ACT
West Chermside Veterinary Hospital
Stafford Heights, Queensland, Australia

Mark C. Thurmond, DVM, PHD
Professor, Department of Medicine and Epidemiology
School of Veterinary Medicine
University of California, Davis, California

Mats H.T. Troedsson, DVM, PHD, DIPL ACT
Associate Professor, Equine Reproduction
Department of Clinical and Population Sciences
College of Veterinary Medicine
University of Minnesota, St. Paul, Minnesota

James R. Turk, DVM, PHD, DIPL ACVP
Associate Professor, Department of Veterinary Pathobiology
College of Veterinary Medicine
University of Missouri, Columbia, Missouri

Jeff W. Tyler, DVM, MPVM, PHD, DIPL ACVIM
Associate Professor, Department of Veterinary Medicine and Surgery
College of Veterinary Medicine
University of Missouri, Columbia, Missouri

Christine A. Uhlinger, VMD, MPH, DIPL ABVP
Brandywine Equine Clinic, Cary, North Carolina

Wendy E. Vaala, VMD, DIPL ACVIM
Mid Atlantic Equine Medical Center, Ringoes, New Jersey

Stephanie J. Valberg, DVM, PHD, DIPL ACVIM
Associate Professor, Department of Clinical and Population Sciences
College of Veterinary Medicine
University of Minnesota, St. Paul, Minnesota

†Deceased.

Steven D. Van Camp, DVM, DIPL ACT
Associate Professor of Theriogenology (Retired)
College of Veterinary Medicine
North Carolina State University, Raleigh, North Carolina

David C. Van Metre, DVM, DIPL ACVIM
Assistant Professor, Department of Clinical Sciences
College of Veterinary Medicine and Biomedical Sciences
Colorado State University, Fort Collins, Colorado

Dickson D. Varner, DVM, DIPL ACT
Professor and Chief of Theriogenology
Department of Large Animal Medicine and Surgery
Texas A & M University, College Station, Texas

Pamela Von Matthiessen, DVM, MD, DIPL ACVS
Department of Internal Medicine
Kettering Medical Center, Dayton, Ohio

Kristina R. Vygantas, DVM
Resident in Ophthalmology
College of Veterinary Medicine
Auburn University, Auburn, Alabama

Angeline E. Warner, DVM, DSc, DIPL ACVIM
Associate Director for Clinical Care
Animal Resources and Comparative Medicine
Harvard Medical School, Boston, Massachusetts

Jeffrey P. Watkins, DVM, MS, DIPL ACVS
Professor and Chief of Surgery
Department of Large Animal Medicine and Surgery
College of Veterinary Medicine
Texas A & M University, College Station, Texas

Johanna L. Watson, DVM, PHD, DIPL ACVIM
Assistant Clinical Professor of Medicine
Department of Medicine and Epidemiology
School of Veterinary Medicine
University of California, Davis, California

Eugene C. White, DVM
Assistant Professor
Department of Environmental and Population Health
School of Veterinary Medicine
Tufts University, North Grafton, Massachusetts

Maurice E. White, DVM, DIPL ACVIM, ABPV
Professor, Department of Clinical Sciences
New York State University College of Veterinary Medicine
Cornell University, Ithaca, New York

Nathaniel A. White II, DVM, MS, DIPL ACVS
Theodora Ayer Randolph Professor of Surgery
Marion duPont Scott Equine Medical Center
Virginia Maryland Regional College of Veterinary Medicine
Virginia Tech, Blacksburg, Virginia

Stephen D. White, DVM, DIPL ACVD
Professor, Department of Medicine and Epidemiology
School of Veterinary Medicine
University of California, Davis, California

Susan L. White, DVM, MS, DIPL ACVIM
Professor, Department of Large Animal Medicine
College of Veterinary Medicine
University of Georgia, Athens, Georgia

Jami L. Whiting, DVM
Dubai Equine Hospital
Dubai, United Arab Emirates

R. David Whitley, DVM, MS, DIPL ACVO
Professor of Ophthalmology
Department of Clinical Sciences
College of Veterinary Medicine
Auburn University, Auburn, Alabama

Robert H. Whitlock, DVM, PHD, DIPL ACVIM
Associate Professor of Medicine
Department of Clinical Studies
New Bolton Center
School of Veterinary Medicine
University of Pennsylvania, Kennett Square, Pennsylvania

Steven E. Wikse, DVM, DIPL ACVP
Associate Professor
Department of Large Animal Medicine and Surgery
College of Veterinary Medicine
Texas A & M University, College Station, Texas

Pamela A. Wilkins, DVM, PHD, DIPL ACVIM
Assistant Professor, Large Animal Medicine
New Bolton Center
School of Veterinary Medicine
University of Pennsylvania, Kennett Square, Pennsylvania

W. David Wilson, BVMS, MS, MRCVS
Associate Professor
Department of Veterinary Medicine and Epidemiology
School of Veterinary Medicine
University of California, Davis, California

Anne M. Zajac, DVM, PHD
Associate Professor
Department of Biomedical Sciences and Pathobiology
Virginia-Maryland Regional College of Veterinary Medicine
Blacksburg, Virginia

Jerry L. Zaugg, DVM, PHD
Professor, Caine Veterinary Teaching Center
University of Idaho, Caldwell, Idaho

Steven C. Zicker, DVM, PHD, DIPL ACVIM, ACVN
Science and Technology Center
Hill's Pet Nutrition, Inc, Topeka, Kansas

Preface

CONTENT

Large Animal Internal Medicine is an encyclopedic volume for the large-animal veterinarian working with horses, cattle, sheep, or goats. Using the same format as the second edition, this edition provides the most current information available. This edition contains more than 450 illustrations. The neonatal section has once again been strengthened by the addition of an outstanding new author. The chapters on neurology, the alimentary tract, and parasites have been significantly revised, and the chapter on vaccinations has been rewritten and improved.

PROBLEM-ORIENTED APPROACH TO DISEASE DIAGNOSIS

The catch-22 of most textbooks is that the clinician must know the diagnosis to locate and read about a specific disease. *Large Animal Internal Medicine* is a multiauthored text that allows the clinician to use the problem-oriented approach to the diagnosis of diseases of horses, cattle, sheep, and goats. Over 130 clinical signs or manifestations of disease are discussed. They are listed alphabetically on pp. 25 and 26; this list can be used to locate a particular manifestation of disease. These same manifestations are listed by organ system at the beginning of Chapters 3 to 14. A favorite feature of the first and second editions is the differential diagnosis boxes. We have retained these invaluable diagnostic tools in this edition. Throughout Part Two, complete lists of common, less common, and uncommon diseases associated with manifestations or signs of disease are given in these easy-to-find boxes (see pp. xix to xx for examples). The clinician is given an approach to each manifestation of disease and a method to work toward a diagnosis. The pathophysiology of that particular manifestation of disease is concisely summarized. Even if a final diagnosis is not reached, the animal with diarrhea, cough, or other problem can be treated symptomatically, a practice that is commonly used in the everyday world.

Similarly, abnormalities in laboratory test results are discussed, and complete lists of diseases associated with a given laboratory abnormality are found in easy-to-read boxes (see p. xxi for an example). Interpretation of abnormalities in clinical chemistry, hematology, blood proteins, and clotting tests is made easy. For example, if the problem is an elevated serum calcium, the causes of hypercalcemia are discussed concisely, and lists of diseases are given. The clinician can then proceed to a rational approach to the particular laboratory abnormality. Many readers have found the table for conversion from "American" units to SI units extremely useful.

ORGANIZATION

The basic organization has not changed from the second edition. The book is divided into seven parts:
- PART ONE: History, Physical Examination, and Medical Records
- PART TWO: Manifestations of Disease
- PART THREE: Disorders and Management of the Neonate
- PART FOUR: Collection of Samples and Interpretation of Laboratory Tests
- PART FIVE: Disorders of the Organ Systems
- PART SIX: Preventive and Therapeutic Strategies
- PART SEVEN: Congenital, Hereditary, Immunologic, and Toxic Disorders

A detailed discussion of each disease is contained in Parts Five, Six, and Seven of *Large Animal Internal Medicine*. Once the reader has a list of diseases that fit the current problem, specific diseases can be found in these final sections of the book. The organization is that of a traditional disease-oriented text:
- Definition and Etiology
- Clinical Signs and Differential Diagnosis
- Clinical Pathology
- Pathophysiology
- Epidemiology
- Necropsy Findings
- Treatment and Prognosis
- Prevention and Control

Part Five is organized according to body system and includes internal medicine approaches. Diagnostic tests used in that system are delineated, including: ultrasound, endoscopy, radiography, thermography, computed tomography, magnetic resonance imaging, sample collection techniques, electrocardiography, cerebrospinal fluid collection, and biopsy of organs. Numerous illustrations include photographs, ultrasound images, radiographs, electrocardiogram tracings, and endoscopic views. These chapters are written by experts in the field of large animal internal medicine and give details of the most up-to-date treatments available. *Large Animal Internal Medicine* complements existing texts dealing with current therapy.

A neonatal disease section (Part Three), organized by presenting problem, discusses everything from diarrhea to septicemia of foals, calves, lambs, and kids. To aid the clinician in arriving at the proper diagnosis, lists of diseases are given for each manifestation of neonatal disease and are presented in Chapter 20. In addition, there are complete lists of all congenital abnormalities of horses and ruminants and the causes of each (Chapters 47 and 48), including whether the condition is believed to be hereditary. Differences in approach to diagnosis or treatment of neonates and adult animals are thoroughly cross-referenced throughout the text.

Preventive and Therapeutic Strategies, Part Six, includes chapters with practical information on antimicrobial therapy, disinfectants, vaccines and vaccination programs, and parasite control programs. Chapter 46 deals with nutrition of the sick animal and gives formulas for both enteral and parenteral support.

POPULAR FEATURES RETAINED

COLOR INSERT. Chapter 37, Diseases of the Eye, contains color plates of ophthalmologic conditions that are best seen in full color.

PRINTED ENDPAPERS. The printed endpapers found in the front and back of the text provide information that is referred to frequently:

Manifestations of Disease
Manifestations of Disease in the Neonate
Clinical Chemistry: Normal Range for Large Animals
Normal Values for Erythron Data in Ruminants and the Horse
Normal Values for Leukogram Data (Adult Animals)
Normal Values for Hemostatic Data in Ruminants and the Horse

NEW TO THIS EDITION

COLOR PLATES. Twelve new color plates give endoscopic views of equine alimentary tract disorders.

NEW TOPICS. The range of new topics is extraordinary. Every chapter has been thoroughly updated. A sampling of new topics includes the slap test for assessing laryngeal adductor reflexes, blood pressure ranges, Hendra virus, breath tests as a diagnostic tool, new agents for preventing and treating ulcers, West Nile virus, equine motor neuron disorder, legal aspects of treatments for mastitis, treatment of hypophosphatemia, effects of bovine somatotropin, polysaccharide storage myopathy, mitochondrial myopathy, glycogen branching enzyme deficiency, equine coital exanthema, effects of certain drugs on the fetus, milbemycins as anthelmintics, *Neospora caninum* as a cause of congenital defects, new genetic diseases of horses, new tests for *Clostridium difficile*, and new findings on bovine viral diarrhea infection.

INDEX

As a reference, a book is only as good as its index. The index of *Large Animal Internal Medicine* is thorough and extensive, making it easy to use to find the answer to any question you may have. The initial page number given is the primary listing.

ACKNOWLEDGMENTS

Many people worked hard to make *Large Animal Internal Medicine* the quality text that it is. One hundred eighty two authors contributed in their area of expertise. Special thanks to Linda Duncan, Teri Merchant, Beth Hayes, and all the others at Mosby/Harcourt who worked so hard on this project.

The motivation for undertaking *Large Animal Internal Medicine* came, in large part, from having been influenced in my professional career by many teachers and colleagues with high standards. My gratitude to them and respect for them runs deep.

Finally, I would like to acknowledge the support and encouragement of my terrific family: Yibi, Chris, Alex, and Bonnie.

BRADFORD P. SMITH
Davis, California

Causes of Diarrhea in the Horse (Except Neonate; See Chapter 20 for Neonate)

COMMON CAUSES
Colitis/typhlitis
Salmonellosis
Enteritis, unknown etiology
Potomac fever (equine monocytic ehrlichiosis)
Endotoxemia/gram-negative sepsis
Overfeeding or sudden change in diet
Clostridium difficile

LESS COMMON CAUSES
Parasites, worms
Eosinophilic gastroenteritis
Renal failure, uremia
Necrotizing enterocolitis
Heart failure
Enterotoxemia
Campylobacter jejuni
Intestinal lymphosarcoma
Cathartic/laxatives
Parasympathomimetics
Chronic granulomatous bowel disease
Proximal enteritis
Peritonitis
Intussusception
Sand, gravel, or enterolith in gut lumen
Gut stenosis

LESS COMMON CAUSES—cont'd
Antibiotic use
Rhodococcus (Corynebacterium) equi gut infection
Cryptosporidiosis
Giardiasis
Toxins or poisonous plants (see box that follows)

UNCOMMON CAUSES
Hepatic failure
Cholelithiasis
Vascular aneurysm
Combined immunodeficiency
Agammaglobulinemia
Lactose intolerance
Colorectal polyps
Anaphylaxis
Vitamin A deficiency
Tularemia
Snake bite, insect or spider sting
Histoplasmosis
Hydroallantois
Hyperlipidemia
Internal abdominal abscess
Pheochromocytoma
Viral arteritis
Besnoitiosis (globidiosis) (exotic)

Toxic Causes of Diarrhea in the Horse

Phenylbutazone toxicity
Blister beetle toxicity (cantharidin)
Salt poisoning
Selenium toxicity
Slaframine toxicity (slobber factor)
Amitraz toxicity
Propylene glycol toxicity
Dioctyl sodium sulfosuccinate (DSS) toxicity
Sulfur toxicity
Phosphorus toxicity
Nicotine (black leaf 40) toxicity
Reserpine toxicity
Arsenic toxicity
Mercury toxicity
Monensin, lasalocid, or salinomycin toxicity
Organophosphate toxicity

PLANT TOXINS
Oleander poisoning
Japanese yew *(Taxus cuspidata)* poisoning
Castor bean poisoning
Avocado poisoning
Thorn apple *(Datura stramonium)* toxicity
Potato poisoning
Heath (Ericaceae) poisoning
Algae poisoning
Acorn or oak poisoning
Hypericum (St. John's wort, Klamath weed) poisoning
Agrostemma githago (corn cockle) poisoning
Mycotoxicosis
Pimela poisoning (St. George disease) (exotic)
Grass sickness (exotic)

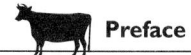

Causes of Diarrhea in Ruminants (Except Neonate; See Chapter 20 for Neonate)

COMMON CAUSES
Parasitism, worms
Coccidiosis
Salmonellosis
Colitis/typhlitis
Enteritis, unknown etiology
Indigestion (spoiled feed, overfeeding, or sudden change)
Displaced abomasum (B)
Abomasal torsion (B)
Peritonitis
Intussusception
Sepsis/toxemia
Johne's disease
Enterotoxemia
Grain overload
Bovine viral diarrhea (BVD) (B)
Winter dysentery (B)
Liver failure
Malignant catarrhal fever (MCF) (B)
Molybdenosis/copper deficiency
Heart failure
Uremia, renal failure
Rompun, following large doses
Cathartic/laxatives
Parasympathomimetics
Toxins or poisonous plants (see following box)

LESS COMMON CAUSES
Amyloidosis
Giardiasis
Intestinal obstruction, partial
Intestinal neoplasia
Traumatic reticuloperitonitis (hardware)
Vagal indigestion
Selenium deficiency (White muscle disease)

LESS COMMON CAUSES—cont'd
Cecal dilation (B)
Liver abscess
Brisket disease (high altitude disease) (B)
Sarcocystosis (B)
Bluetongue
Bovine leukosis (BLV) (B)

UNCOMMON CAUSES
Fat necrosis (B)
Abomasal impaction
Duodenal ulcers
Systemic candidiasis
Vitamin A deficiency
Volvulus, root of mesentery
Water intoxication (B)
Cholelithiasis
Cobalt deficiency
Zinc deficiency (baldy calf) (B)
Hydrops allantois (B)
Lethal trait A 46, keratogenesis imperfecta
    (parakeratosis) (B)
Zygomycosis, mucormycosis
Pregnancy toxemia
Bacillary hemoglobinuria
Rumen flukes, paramphistomosis
Pancreatic adenocarcinoma
Bee or wasp sting
Pseudorabies
Rift Valley fever (exotic)
Rinderpest (exotic)
Schistosomiasis (exotic)
Theileriosis (East Coast fever) (exotic)
Wesselsbron disease (exotic) (B,O)
Heartwater (exotic)

B, Bovine; *O*, ovine.

Toxic Causes of Diarrhea in Ruminants

Arsenic poisoning
Sulfur poisoning
Salt poisoning
Propylene glycol
Levamisole
Monensin
Polybrominated biphenyl
Sodium bicarbonate
Aflatoxin
Herbicide
Zinc
Phosphorus toxicity
Nicotine (black leaf 40) toxicity
Copper
Chlorpyrifos (dursban)
Phosphate fertilizer
Lincomycin
Trichothecene (T-2 toxin)

PLANT TOXINS
Oak (acorn poisoning)
Caddia (coffee weed)

PLANT TOXINS—cont'd
Selenium accumulators
Slaframine (blackpatch diseased legumes, slobber factor)
Mycotoxicoses
Helenium (sneezeweed, bitterweed)
Solanum (nightshade)
Pyrrolizidine alkaloid (senecio, crotalaria, amsinkia)
Brassica (mustards, crucifers, cress)
Oleander poisoning
Japanese yew (*Taxus cuspidata*) poisoning
Whitehead (*Sphenosciadium capitellatum*)
Pokeweed (*Phytolacca americana L*)
Mushroom
Inkweed (*Drymaria pachyphylla*)
Tung tree (aleurites)
Chinese tallow tree
Kalanchoe (crassulaceae)
Sesbania (rattlebox)
Gutierrezia (broomweed, snakeweed)
Hypericum (St. John's-wort; Klamath weed) poisoning
Agrostemma githago (corn cockle) poisoning

Causes of Elevations in Serum Enzymes

ELEVATION OF SDH
Common Causes
Acute liver failure
Liver abscess
Secondary to damaged bowel
Strangulating intestinal lesion
Acute toxic enteritis
Chronic liver failure

Less Common Causes
Acute and severe anemia
General anesthesia
Anoxia

ELEVATION OF GGT
Common Causes
Acute liver failure
Chronic liver failure
Pyrrolizidine alkaloid toxicity
Aflatoxicosis
Cholangiohepatitis
Cholelithiasis
Liver flukes

Uncommon Causes
Higher normal range in young animals
Fatty liver

ELEVATION OF AP
Common Causes
Acute liver failure
Chronic liver failure
Pyrrolizidine alkaloid toxicity
Cholangiohepatitis
Cholelithiasis
Liver flukes

Uncommon Causes
Higher normal range in young animals
Fatty liver

ELEVATION OF CPK
Common Causes
Exertional rhabdomyolysis (azoturia, myositis, tying-up)
Nutritional myodegeneration (selenium, vitamin E deficiency)
Postendurance ride multisystemic disorder
Alert downer cow syndrome (muscle crush syndrome)
Malignant hyperthermia
Malignant edema
Prolonged recumbency with inability to rise

Uncommon Causes
Normal postexercise or postshipping modest increase
Acute cardiomyopathy
Purpura hemorrhagica
Equine influenza
Sarcosporidiosis
Local irritation from intramuscular injections

ELEVATION OF LDH
Common Causes
MUSCLE DISEASE
Exertional rhabdomyolysis (azoturia, myositis, tying-up)
Nutritional myodegeneration (selenium, vitamin E deficiency)
Postendurance ride multisystemic disorder
Alert downer cow syndrome (muscle crush syndrome)
Malignant hyperthermia
Malignant edema

LIVER DISEASE
Acute liver failure
Chronic liver failure
Cholangiohepatitis
Cholelithiasis

IN VITRO HEMOLYSIS

Uncommon Causes
Hemolytic anemia
Acute cardiomyopathy
Purpura hemorrhagica
Equine influenza
Sarcosporidiosis
Local irritation from intramuscular injections
Fatty liver

ELEVATION OF AST (SGOT)
Common Causes
MUSCLE DISEASE
Exertional rhabdomyolysis (azoturia, myositis, tying-up)
Nutritional myodegeneration (selenium, vitamin E deficiency)
Postendurance ride multisystemic disorder
Alert downer cow syndrome
Malignant hyperthermia
Malignant edema

LIVER DISEASE
Acute liver failure
Chronic liver failure
Cholangiohepatitis
Cholelithiasis
Liver flukes

IN VITRO HEMOLYSIS

Uncommon Causes
Hemolytic anemia
Acute cardiomyopathy
Purpura hemorrhagica
Equine influenza
Sarcosporidiosis
Local irritation from intramuscular injections
Fatty liver

The Use of the
CONSULTANT Diagnostic Database
for Development of This Textbook

MAURICE E. WHITE

The writing of *Large Animal Internal Medicine* was facilitated by CONSULTANT, an online diagnostic system.[1-5] CONSULTANT is a database that contains information on the diseases described in the veterinary literature: 1163 diseases of cattle, 1126 of horses, 768 of sheep, 625 of goats, 606 of swine, 1422 of dogs, 966 of cats, and 321 of birds at the time this is being written. For each disease there are a brief description, references, Web links, and the clinical signs that might be seen. Information in the database is updated daily on the basis of review of the periodical literature in the Flower-Sprecher Veterinary Library at Cornell University. CONSULTANT is available on the World Wide Web at http://www.vet.cornell.edu/consultant/consult.asp; it receives more than a million hits per year from over 200,000 users, and its use is steadily rising.

Two characteristics of CONSULTANT are the keys to its use for this textbook. One is that it is extremely current; online editing is rapid, and information from the literature appears in the database quickly, usually within a few days of publication. This rapid updating, combined with the large number of sources of information, allows CONSULTANT to contain a breadth of up-to-date information that is difficult to find elsewhere. The second important factor is the ability of the user to enter a clinical sign or signs (e.g., cough, colic, abortion) for a given species and be given a list of the diseases for which that sign or signs have been reported and information on each of them.

How was CONSULTANT used for development of *Large Animal Internal Medicine*? Much of this textbook is organized by clinical signs. CONSULTANT provided a broad overview of possible causes for clinical problems that the authors were encouraged to incorporate into their lists of differential diagnoses. In particular, the large amount and simplicity of retrieval of information in CONSULTANT allowed easy access to poisonings, rare diseases, or diseases exotic to North America, which would have been difficult to find in a standard literature review. Contributors were encouraged to compress, rank, and add to the CONSULTANT-generated lists on the basis of clinical experience. The use of the database in this fashion gave authors rapid access to information that helped them organize sign-based chapters.

CONSULTANT and this textbook are symbiotic. The database can be thought of as a consultant generalist that "knows" a little about almost every disease in veterinary medicine and is up-to-date. Despite that, it remains merely a tool for the clinician who uses it. For example, there are dozens of causes of epistaxis in the horse, and it is simple to get a complete list of them and other information from CONSULTANT. But the clinician must then decide which causes to pursue in an individual patient, in what order, by what means, at what cost, and to what treatment or prognostic end. When tough decisions must be made, expert opinions such as those found in this book are of great help.

While the future will include online textbooks, and CONSULTANT itself contains many links that represent the early outline of such a text, the printed word can still be an efficient way to capture knowledge. Cooperation such as that between CONSULTANT and Large Animal Internal Medicine allows the practitioner and student to benefit from the linkage between the tireless memory and ease of retrieval of the computer and the convenience of expert knowledge in book form.

REFERENCES

1. White ME: Computer-assisted diagnosis; experience with the CONSULTANT program, *J Am Vet Med Assoc* 187:475-476, 1985.
2. White ME: An analysis of journal citation frequency in the CONSULTANT database for computer-assisted diagnosis, *J Am Vet Med Assoc* 190:1098-1101, 1987.
3. White ME: Names and codes of the diseases and clinical signs of dogs, cats, horses, cattle, sheep, goats and swine from the CONSULTANT diagnostic database, *Cornell Vet* 77(suppl 10):1-165, 1987.
4. White ME, Lewkowicz J: The CONSULTANT database for computer-assisted diagnosis and information management in veterinary medicine, *Automedica* 8:135-140, 1987.
5. Viera A: CONSULTANT on the WorldWide Web, reducing information isolation of veterinary practitioners, *Association for Veterinary Informatics Newsletter*, 1997. Available from http://netvet.wustl.edu/org/avi/newsletter/avi9706.htm#_Toc406575088.

Contents

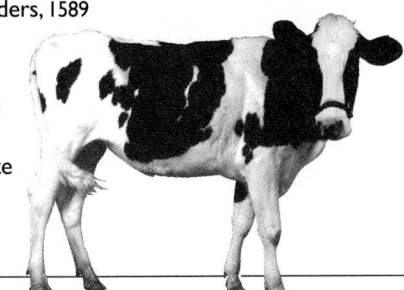

Detailed Contents

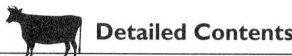

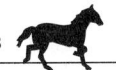

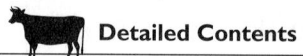

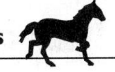
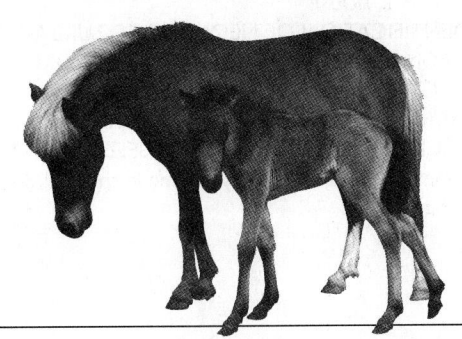

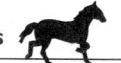

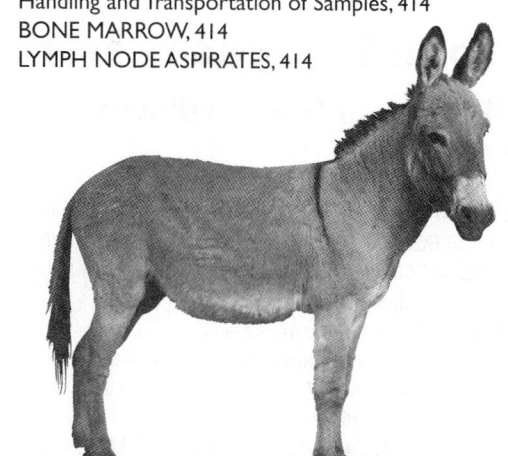

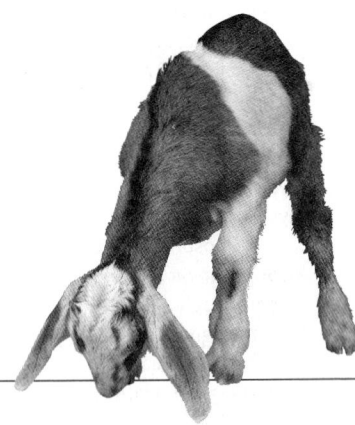

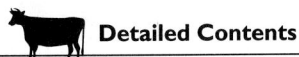

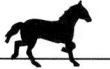

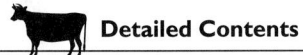

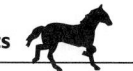

33 Diseases of the Nervous System, 873

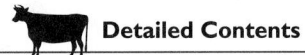

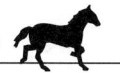

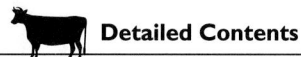

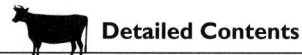
38 Diseases of the Skin, 1200

Consulting Editor: STEPHEN D. WHITE

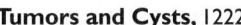

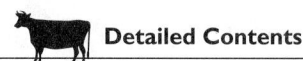

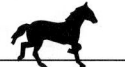

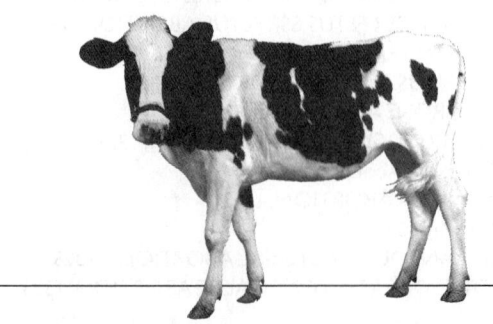

46 Nutrition of the Sick Animal: Preventive and Therapeutic Strategies, 1458

PART SEVEN
CONGENITAL, HEREDITARY, IMMUNOLOGIC, AND TOXIC DISORDERS, 1463

47 Congenital Defects and Hereditary Disorder in Ruminants, 1465

48 Congenital Defects and Hereditary Diseases in the Horse, 1556

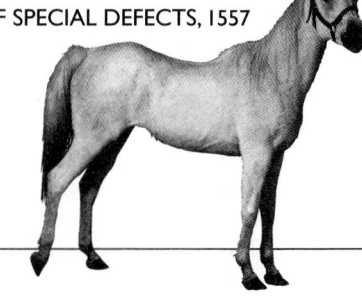

Large Animal
INTERNAL
MEDICINE

HISTORY, PHYSICAL EXAMINATION, AND MEDICAL RECORDS

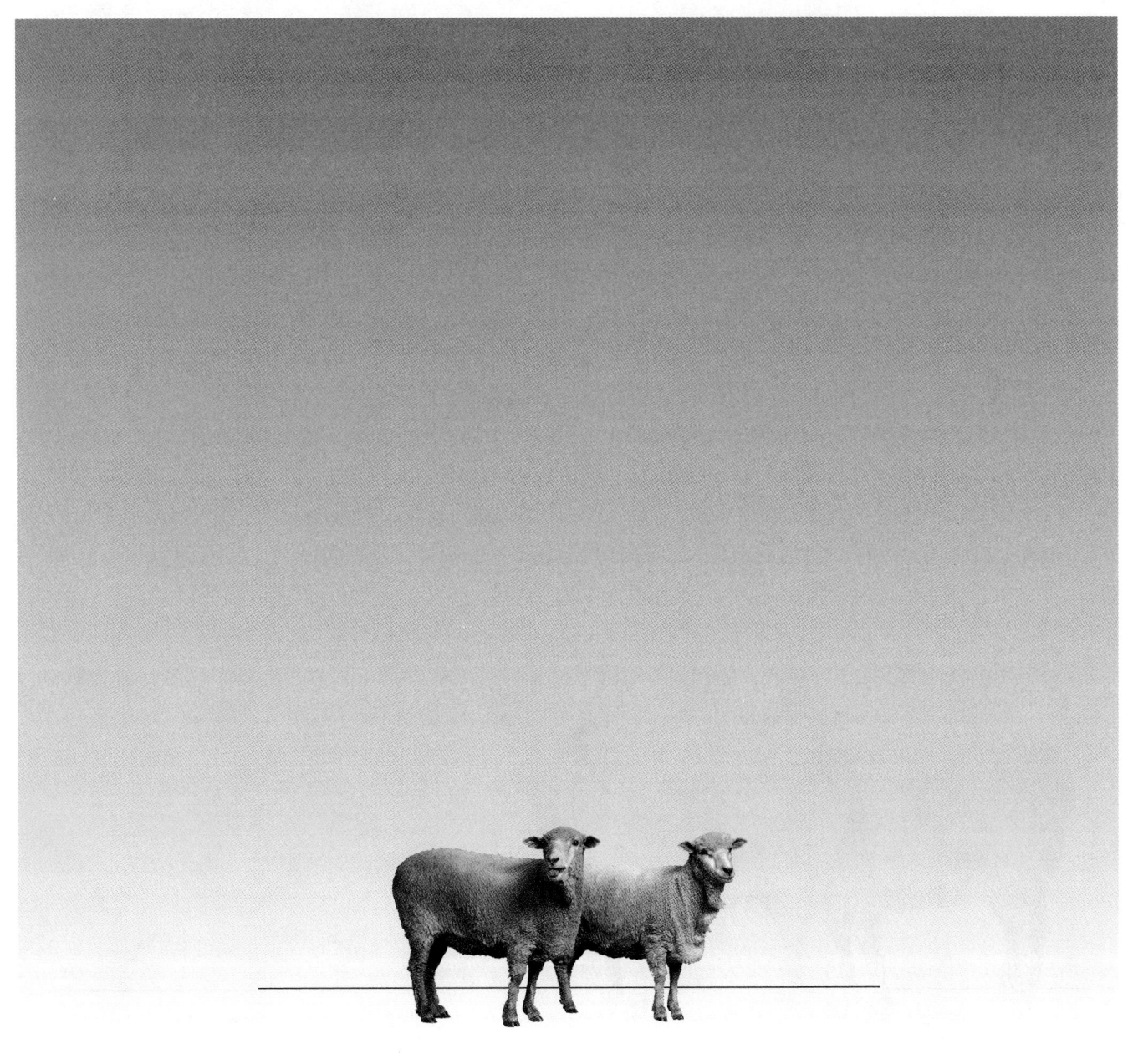

Ruminant History, Physical Examination, and Records

RONALD L. TERRA

OBTAINING THE HISTORY

The initial and often the most important step in the diagnostic approach to the sick ruminant is the physical examination. Throughout this process an anamnesis is obtained by asking questions of the owner/manager during the examination of the animal. The examiner should obtain the signalment either by observation or by questioning the owner. The information that one wishes to obtain while taking the history is that which is related to the chief, or presenting, complaint, that is, the complaint, the duration, whether the onset was gradual or sudden, and any associated signs that have been noted. For females, one must know when the last parturition occurred and for dairy cows, what the production parameters were in the previous lactation. With dairy cows, a drop in milk production is often the only sign noted by the owner. Weight can either be approximated or determined exactly if facilities exist to do so. What and how the animal is fed are questions to be asked. Does the animal refuse any or all of the feed offered? Is there more than one ration or feeding regimen for this particular operation? If so, are these same signs noted in animals exposed to different feeding practices? The examiner also obtains vaccination and worming history and inquires about pasture or housing practices to determine the influence that management factors have on the incidence of the disease. Previous diseases noted in the herd, therapeutic regimens used, and resolution of these previous problems are pertinent aspects. Finally, the examiner should note the treatment history of the patient. An example of a history questionnaire that can be used for ruminants is included (Fig. 1-1). Specific problems that are noted in the history or physical examination can be looked up on p. 25, and lists of differential diagnoses considered.

EXAMINATION

A complete examination should always be performed even though the presenting complaint is easily recognizable. The physical examination provides the veterinarian with information that is used to assess the health status of the patient. This information, combined with that obtained while taking the history, enables the practitioner to determine which specific signs of disease are present and often to localize the disease process to specific organ systems. It also helps to determine which ancillary diagnostic tests must be performed. Additional information gathered during the examination may reveal disorders other than the presenting complaint that warrant further attention and may have a profound influence on the prognosis of the case. Realistically, economic and time constraints preclude full examinations in some cases. In these situations the veterinarian must be familiar enough with the complete physical examination to know which aspects can be excluded and which should be performed.

A systematic approach to the animal must be developed and used on every physical examination. The first step is to form an initial overall impression by observing the animal from a distance. The animal is then restrained and examined topographically, beginning on one side, moving to the other, and then evaluating the rear and finally the head and neck. Thus individual organs and systems are examined completely, although disjointedly, and the information gained is correlated to form the complete diagnosis.

Visual Examination

As observations are made and a physical examination performed, it is important to follow a systematic approach and to

VETERINARY MEDICAL TEACHING HOSPITAL

FOOD ANIMAL

INITIAL ENCOUNTER HISTORY

PATIENT ID: _____ REFERRAL: ☐ YES   ☐ NO   ☐ DON'T KNOW

REFERRING VETERINARIAN: _____

OWNER: _____

PATIENT NAME OR TAG NUMBER: _____

DATE OF BIRTH: ___/___/___

SPECIE: _____   BREED: _____   SEX: _____   WEIGHT (Kg): _____

DATE OF ENTRY: ___/___/___   ☐ AMBULATORY ☐ IN-HOUSE   DURATION OF PRESENT PROBLEM (days): _____

PRESENTING COMPLAINT _____

FEED: ☐ IRRIGATED PASTURE   ☐ NATIVE DRYLAND PASTURE   ☐ ALFALFA HAY/CUBES   ☐ OAT GRASS/HAY   ☐ SUDAN HAY

☐ SILAGE/HAYLAGE   ☐ COMPLT MILLED RATION   ☐ ALMOND HULLS   ☐ GREEN CHOP   ☐ GRAIN

☐ MILK   ☐ TRACE MINERAL SALT   ☐ OTHER

HOUSING: ☐ FEEDLOT   ☐ DAIRYLOT/PEN   ☐ CALF PEN   ☐ IRRIGATED PASTURE   ☐ NATURAL DRYLAND PASTURE   ☐ OTHER

VACCINE: ☐ PASTEURELLA   ☐ CLOSTRIDIUM (2-7) ☐ SALMONELLA   ☐ BLUE TONGUE   ☐ E. COLI   ☐ IBR

☐ TETANUS   ☐ HEMOPHILUS   ☐ ANAPLASMOSIS   ☐ CHLAMYDIA   ☐ ROTA-CORONA   ☐ LEPTO (1-5)

☐ BRUCELLA   ☐ BVD   ☐ VIBRIO   ☐ PI3   ☐ OTHER

WORMING DATES: ___/___/___   WORMERS: _____   _____   _____

___/___/___   _____   _____   _____

___/___/___   _____   _____   _____

MILK PRODUCTION PER PREVIOUS 305 DAY LACTATION (lbs): _____   MOST RECENT PARTURITION: ___/___/___

DECREASED MILK PRODUCTION: ☐ SUDDEN ONSET   ☐ GRADUAL ONSET   ☐ UNK ONSET   ☐ NO CHANGE

DECREASED FEED INTAKE: ☐ SUDDEN ONSET   ☐ GRADUAL ONSET   ☐ UNK ONSET   ☐ NO CHANGE

PREVIOUS ILLNESSES: _____

OTHERS IN HERD WITH DIARRHEA: ☐ YES ☐ NO ☐ UNK   OTHERS IN HERD WITH WEIGHT LOSS: ☐ YES ☐ NO ☐ UNK

OTHER IN HERD WITH BREATHING DIFFICULTY: ☐ YES ☐ NO ☐ UNK

DEATHS IN HERD: _____   ANIMALS IN HERD: _____   ANIMALS AT RISK: _____

PAST TREATMENTS, ADDITIONAL HISTORY: _____

D1903 (1/84)

FIG. 1-1 ■ Example of an initial encounter history form for use in ruminants.

record findings. A check-off format form has been found to be extremely useful (Fig. 1-2). While observing the animal from a distance, the examiner should assess its posture, gait, behavior, and physical condition. Observation of the other members of the flock or herd helps to differentiate normal from abnormal characteristics under each particular management system because normal may vary from farm to farm and what is considered "normal" for a farm by the owner herdsman might actually be abnormal; this information is valuable for assessing the incidence of a disease or disorder that is caused by manage-

VETERINARY MEDICAL TEACHING HOSPITAL

FOOD ANIMAL

PHYSICAL EXAM DATA

Circle Choice if abnormal

i.e. Ears: ☐ warm ☒ cold

PATIENT ID: _____   **PHYSICAL EXAM:** DATE: ___/___/___

AGE (Estimate to nearest year):_____ **WEIGHT (kg):**_____ **GENERAL BODY CONDITION:** ☐EMACIATED ☐THIN ☐NORMAL FOR USE (GOOD) ☐OVERWEIGHT

GENERAL ATTITUDE: ☐ NORMAL ☐ DEPRESSED ☐ SOMNOLENT/COMATOSE ☐ HYPERAESTHETIC ☐ CONVULSING ☐ RECUMBENT

LATERAL BODY SHAPE: ☐ NORMAL ☐ ARCHED ☐ GAUNT ☐ SWAY BACK **POSTERIOR SHAPE:** ☐ NORMAL ☐ APPLE ☐ PEAR ☐ PAPPLE

GAIT: ☐ NORMAL ☐ LAME ☐ STIFF ☐ PARESIS ☐ PARALYSIS ☐ SOLE ABSCESS ☐ SEPTIC ARTHRITIS ☐ FRACTURE ☐ JOINT INJURY

☐`FOOT ROT ☐ OTHER   **GAIT ABNORMALITY LOCATION:** _____

HYDRATION: ☐ NORMAL ☐ SLT/MILD DEHY ☐ MOD DEHY ☐ SEVERE DEHY

SKIN: ☐ NORMAL ☐ RINGWORM ☐ DERMATITIS ☐ PARASITES ☐ OTHER

TPR'S (Use additional page if necessary)

DATE: ___/___/___ TEMP: _____ H.R.: _____ RESP: _____   DATE: ___/___/___ TEMP: _____ H.R.: _____ RESP: _____

DATE: ___/___/___ TEMP: _____ H.R.: _____ RESP: _____   DATE: ___/___/___ TEMP: _____ H.R.: _____ RESP: _____

CRANIAL NERVES: ☐ NORMAL ☐ HEAD TILT ☐ NYSTAGMUS ☐ FACIAL PARALYSIS ☐ STRABISMUS ☐ WEAK JAW/TONGUE

☐ PHARYNGEAL PARESIS

EARS: ☐ WARM ☐ COLD   **SCLERA AND VESSELS:** ☐ NORMAL ☐ PALE ☐ INJECTED ☐ ICTERIC

EYES: ☐ NORMAL ☐ KERATITIS ☐ CONJUCTIVITIS ☐ UVEITIS ☐ TUMOR ☐ MIOSIS ☐ MYDRIASIS ☐ ABSENT MENACE ☐ BLIND(L)

☐ BLIND (R) ☐ TEARING ☐ OTHER

NOSE: ☐CLEAN ☐DIRTY ☐DRY ☐MOIST ☐SCALY ☐MUCOPURULENT DISCHG. ☐SEROUS/MUCOID DISCHG. ☐BLOODY DISCHG. ☐OTHER

MOUTH/TONGUE: ☐ NORMAL ☐ FIRM MASSES ☐ ULCERS/EROSIONS ☐ VESICLES ☐ PALE MUC MEMB ☐ CYANOTIC MUC MEMB

☐ EXCESSIVE SALIVATION   ☐ ICTERIC MUC. MEMBRANES

LYMPH NODES: ☐ NORMAL ☐ ENLARGED   **HEART SOUNDS:** ☐ NORMAL ☐ MUFFLED/SPLASHY ☐ MURMUR ☐ OTHER

JUGULAR VEINS: ☐ NORMAL ☐ DISTENDED ☐ PULSE ☐ PHLEBITIS   **MAMMARY VEIN:** ☐ NORMAL ☐ PULSE

SUBMANDIBULAR/BRISKET EDEMA: ☐ PRESENT ☐ ABSENT   **DYSPNEA:** ☐ YES ☐ NO

COUGH: ☐ NONE ☐ MILD/OCCASIONAL ☐ MARKED   **BREATH:** ☐ NORMAL ☐ FOUL ☐ ACETONE

BREATHING SOUNDS (AUSCULTATION): ☐ NORMAL ☐ EXPIRATORY HARSHNESS ☐ CRACKLES/WHEEZES ☐ DULL VENTRALLY

☐ INSPIRATORY DYSPNEA/NOISE

PERCUSSION OF CHEST: ☐ NORMAL ☐ DULL VENTRALLY ☐ OTHER

RUMEN CONTRACTIONS/MIN: _____   **STRENGTH OF CONTRACTIONS:** ☐ NONE ☐ WEAK (SECONDARY) ☐ MODERATE ☐ NORMAL (STRONG)

NATURE OF RUMEN CONTENTS: ☐ GAS ☐ FLUID ☐ DOUGHY (NORMAL) ☐ EMPTY ☐ IMPACTED   **RUMEN pH** (If contents not doughy): _____

XIPHOID PAIN RESPONSE: ☐ NEGATIVE ☐ EQUIVOCAL ☐ POS GRUNT

PINGS: ☐ NONE ☐ RUMEN ☐ ABOMASM LT ☐ ABOMASM RT ☐ SPIRAL COLON ☐ CECUM

FECES: ☐ NORMAL ☐ WATERY ☐ MELENA ☐ CONSTIPATED ☐ BLOODY ☐ MUCUS/FIBRIN ☐ OTHER

MAMMARY GLAND: ☐ LACT NORMAL ☐ NONLACT NORMAL ☐ CLINICAL MASTITIS/ABSCESS ☐ CMT POSITIVE/SUBCLINICAL MASTITIS ☐ OTHER

RECTAL EXAM: ☐ NO ABNORMALITIES ☐ ABNORMALITIES (EXPLAIN): _____

UTERUS (Px = months preg): ☐ NORMAL NONPREG ☐ P1 ☐ P2 ☐ P3 ☐ P4 ☐ P5 ☐ P6 ☐ P7 ☐ P8 ☐ P9 ☐ RETAINED PLACENTA

☐ PYOMETRA ☐ METRITIS ☐ OTHER

PREGNANCY TEST BY: ☐ RECTAL PALPATION ☐ ULTRASOUND ☐ ABDOMINAL BALLOTTEMENT

URINE: ☐ NORMAL GROSS APPEARANCE ☐ CLOUDY ☐ BLOODY ☐ CLOUDY & BLOODY ☐ KETONE NEG ☐ KETONE POS ☐ PROTEIN NEG

☐ PROTEIN POS ☐ GLUCOSE NEG ☐ GLUCOSE POS ☐ OTHER

URINE pH: _____   **FEMALE GENITALIA:** ☐ NORMAL ☐ VAGINITIS ☐ VAGINAL TEAR ☐ R-V TEAR ☐ CERVICITIS ☐ PROLAPSED VAGINA

☐ OTHER

MALE GENITALIA: ☐ NORMAL ☐ CASTRATED ☐ ORCHITIS ☐ EPIDIDYMITIS ☐ PREPUTIAL ABSCESS/CELLULITIS ☐ PENILE HEMATOMA

☐ HYPOPLASTIC/ATROPHIC ☐ OTHER

OTHER ABNORMAL FINDINGS: _____

CLINICIAN: _____   **STUDENT:** _____

D1901 (1/84)

FIG. I-2 ▓ Example of a data sheet for the recording of the pertinent findings from the physical examination.

ment. As more animals in more herds are observed, a background of knowledge is gained that allows the practitioner to assess these management deficiencies more reliably.

The general appearance and conformation of the animal are included in determining posture. These are assessed in light of the age and breed of the patient. Determining abnormalities in posture can be difficult; however, noting these subtle changes can contribute greatly to the diagnosis of a disease process. Conformation is recognized by looking at the overall size and shape with particular regard to height, width, and relationship of the head, neck, and legs to the trunk. The general appearance of the patient in light of overall conformation can then be assessed. Is the young, growing animal within breed standards for size and weight? (See Chapters 9 and 13.) The condition of the hair coat and presence of external parasites can be noted during the physical examination (e.g., frank hair loss, as seen in louse infestation, or dander and scruffiness of the hair coat, as seen in chronic debilitating diseases).

Observe the animal for signs of abdominal splinting or arching of the back, as can be seen with peritonitis. This posture can also be noted with other disease processes when these produce pain in the ventral abdomen. Lateral curvature of the spine could indicate a congenital defect or a chronic spinal lesion nature. Carrying the tail up away from the body is seen with conditions resulting in pain or irritation in the perineal region, vagina, or rectum. Standing with all four legs in the classic "saw-horse" stance with the neck and tail held erect is typical of tetanus. Abduction of the elbows is seen in disorders that cause thoracic pain. Lameness can be noted by observing unwillingness to bear weight fully on the affected limb, either while standing or walking. Loss of extensor or flexor capabilities of the joints is seen in nerve paralysis or paresis; it can also be caused by tendon and/or joint contractures, in which case joints are rigid. Walking as if all four feet are sore may indicate laminitis. With bright and alert recumbent animals, a thorough examination to rule out fractures or severe joint trauma is essential. Once these are ruled out, inability to stand may be indicative of generalized muscular paresis or paralysis. These can be of a primary nature, as is seen with lesions within the spinal column causing cord compression, or secondary to mineral or electrolyte deficiencies (i.e., hypocalcemia, hypomagnesemia, or hypokalemia).

To be able to judge the behavior of the animal as being normal or abnormal, the observer must call on a large amount of experience. Observing the animal from a distance allows assessment of eating and drinking behavior, as well as assessment of the subject as it is ruminating, urinating, and defecating. How the animal gets up or lies down and how it ambulates are important. Signs indicative of estrus or signs commonly seen with calving might be considered normal or abnormal, given the history and behavior of the animal during these events. Observing the patient during the milking process may also be beneficial. The influence of the manager on animal behavior is very important, as is the overall temperament of the particular breed or herd in question. Normal animals react to the approach of a human being by moving away; however, those that have had extensive contact with people may be more inquisitive. Within a herd one can note animals that are more tolerant than others, more stubborn, more restless, and more anxious. These traits are not necessarily abnormal and need to be differentiated from behavior that would be considered secondary to disease. In general, one must determine whether the behavior is one of a depressed or apathetic animal or of a hyperexcitable or frenzied animal.

Nutritional status and physical condition are assessed by means of observation and palpation. Special attention is paid to the dewlap, the spinous processes of the thoracic and lumbar vertebrae, the shoulder area, and the area around the tailhead. Determination of body condition will then result in a classification of the animal as being anywhere from severely emaciated or cachectic to extremely overconditioned or fat (see Chapters 9 and 13 for body scores). Next it must be determined whether the condition is of a primary or nutritional nature or the result of disease. Disease processes can influence or be influenced by the animal's body condition. Extremely thin animals are seen in primary undernutrition and also with chronic disease. Females carrying multiple fetuses and lactat-

ing animals with metabolic abnormalities secondary to abomasal displacements would also show signs of weight loss. Overconditioned animals are at greater risk for a wide variety of disorders primarily related to the accumulation of fat in the liver and excessive fat storage in the omentum.

Physical Examination

With the animal properly restrained, the physical examination can now progress to specific palpation, auscultation, and percussion. Obtaining a sample of urine for urinalysis is of great value if incorporated into the physical examination; it is easy to perform with the use of dipsticks such as N-multistix. Stroking the perineal region can aid in eliciting urination in the bovine; however, even this is futile if the animal is apprehensive. Consequently, it is recommended to do this first, while the patient is still fairly relaxed. In the male, elicitation of urination is slightly more difficult and requires massaging of the preputial orifice. Another method is to wash the outside of the prepuce with warm water, but this is less successful. In the female sheep and goat stroking the perineal area can be attempted, but positive results are rarely achieved. A method that is more reliable but that causes the animal much greater stress is to prevent it from breathing until urination is stimulated. In male or castrated male sheep and goats, gentle massage of the prepuce sometimes results in urination. If that fails, the breath-holding technique can be used. It is recommended that this not be attempted on patients that are severely compromised because of any disease process. (See Chapter 22 for further information on interpretation of the urinalysis.)

Body temperature is then measured with a rectal thermometer. Normal values for each species are given in Table 1-1. There are no absolute values, and the upper and lower limits should be adjusted as necessary to account for ambient temperature and housing. For example, if the ambient temperature is greater than 37.5° C (100° F), a body temperature of 39.5° C (103° F) may still be considered normal for the adult bovine, especially if the animal is not allowed access to shade. When body temperatures approach 41° C (106° F), as a result of very high ambient temperatures, heat stroke may occur. Keep in mind that the animal tries to maintain its body temperature within these normal limits, and marked deviation from the norm would be indicative of a disease process. A markedly elevated temperature is seen in acute, severe inflammatory processes. Pathologic lowering of the body temperature is seen in disorders that cause an inhibition of metabolism such as postparturient paresis, neonatal hypoglycemia, the end stages of a chronic disease, or severe septicemia resulting from gram-negative bacteria. There is a normal diurnal variation in body temperature of as much as 0.5° to 1° C. In the female there can also be a slight increase in

TABLE 1-1

Normal Values for Temperature in the Ruminant[1-3]

Animal	Degrees Celsius	Degrees Farenheit
Cattle		
Adult	38-39	100.5-102.5
Calf	39-40.5	101.5-103
Sheep		
Adult	39-40	102-103.5
Lamb	39.5-40.5	102.5-104
Goat		
Adult	38.5-39.5	101.5-103.5
Kid	39-40.5	102-104

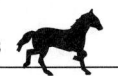

temperature in the days preceding estrus. Neonates are poor thermoregulators and often have a normal body temperature of 0.5° to 1° C higher than adults.

In the evaluation of the thoracic and abdominal cavities, the initial step is the ballottement of the abdomen on the right side. An increase in fluid being sequestered intraabdominally could be related to some degree of intestinal or ruminal stasis or associated with an increase in peritoneal fluid, as with peritonitis or ruptured bladder. Ballottement can also reveal whether any firm masses such as a fetus, impacted abomasum, abscess, or tumor are located in the abdomen. In goats the abdominal fat pad is quite prominent and tends to obscure any significant finding on ballottement. Deep palpation of the paralumbar fossa can sometimes reveal masses in this region, including lymphomas, fat necrosis, or abscesses. In goats, lambs, and calves, two hands are used to deeply palpate the abdomen; the normal freely movable left kidney is usually readily palpable. On the right side an enlarged or painful liver or kidney can be noted. Palpation of an abnormal swelling or firmness, especially with the elicitation of pain, indicates a problem that must be further evaluated.

The spinal column and ribcage are then palpated; the presence of fractures, the enlargements of the costochondral junctions, or the elicitation of pain are noted. Enlargements or fractures of the costochondral junction are commonly seen in young animals with deficiencies of calcium, copper, or vitamin D.

Auscultation with concurrent percussion by snapping the finger against the thoracic and abdominal walls is the next procedure. Gas trapped within abdominal viscera elicits a "pinging" sound that can be heard with the stethoscope. Localization of these gas pings to certain areas within the abdomen is helpful in determining which alimentary structure is involved (Figs. 1-3 to 1-5). If the cecum is enlarged and gas filled, an abdominal ping results, which can extend caudally to the tuber coxae and cranially through the paralumbar fossa and under the ribcage on the right side (see Fig. 1-3). The diameter of this area can be variable and range from 6 inches (15 cm) in a cecal displacement to 3 feet (1 m) horizontally in cecal torsions. Spiral colon pings are generally localized to the right dorsocranial paralumbar fossa and rarely extend farther forward than the tenth intercostal space. They tend to be round areas 10 inches (25 cm) or less in diameter centered high under the last rib (see Fig. 1-3) and are commonly found in sick cattle that are anorectic. These pings have no specific diagnostic significance. Gas pings associated with a right-sided displacement or torsion of the abomasum can extend as far cranially as the ninth intercostal space and caudally into the paralumbar fossa (see Fig. 1-4). The diameter of displacements is usually 18 inches (45 cm) whereas that of torsions can be up to 3 feet (1 m). In cases of abomasal volvulus, the animal is usually exhibiting other systemic signs such as increased heart rate, dehydration, depression, scleral injection, and mild colic. In simple right-sided displacements or dilations of the abomasum, the only significant finding may be the small gas ping localized to the abomasum in a cow with depressed appetite and decreased milk production.

On the left side, gas pings can be noted as originating from the rumen, the peritoneum, or a left displaced abomasum (LDA). The auscultation of a gas ping that is primarily localized to the dorsal aspect of the paralumbar fossa and auscultable on both sides of the spinal column would be indicative of a pneumoperitoneum. The extent of these pings can be from the thoracolumbar junction caudally to the retroperitoneal space. Pings associated with ruminal tympany occupy the whole of the paralumbar fossa, can extend dorsally to the spinal column, but generally do not extend over to the right side (see Fig. 1-5). LDA results in a gas ping that is localized, easily outlined, and approximately 12 to 18 inches (30 to 45 cm) in diameter. Caudal extent of the displacement is generally the thirteenth rib; however, it can extend into the paralumbar fossa, in which case the outline of the abomasum can be easily palpated. The LDA should ping over the eleventh rib on a line from the hip to the elbow (see Fig. 1-5). Rumen gas associated with a left-sided ping will rarely ping at this location. Identification of a fluid line within the displacement can aid in diagnosis and is accomplished by ballotting the left paralumbar fossa while auscultating the area of the gas ping concurrently, a process known as succussion. LDA often gives a pitch that changes in tone as it is

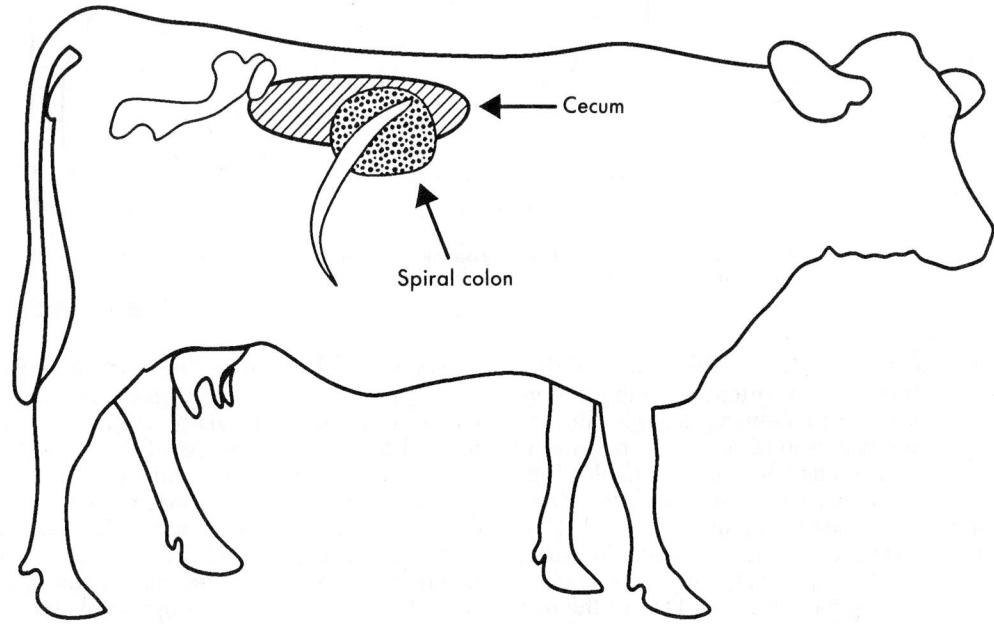

FIG. I-3 ■ Schematic representation of areas of gas pings elicited by percussion of the cecum and spiral colon.

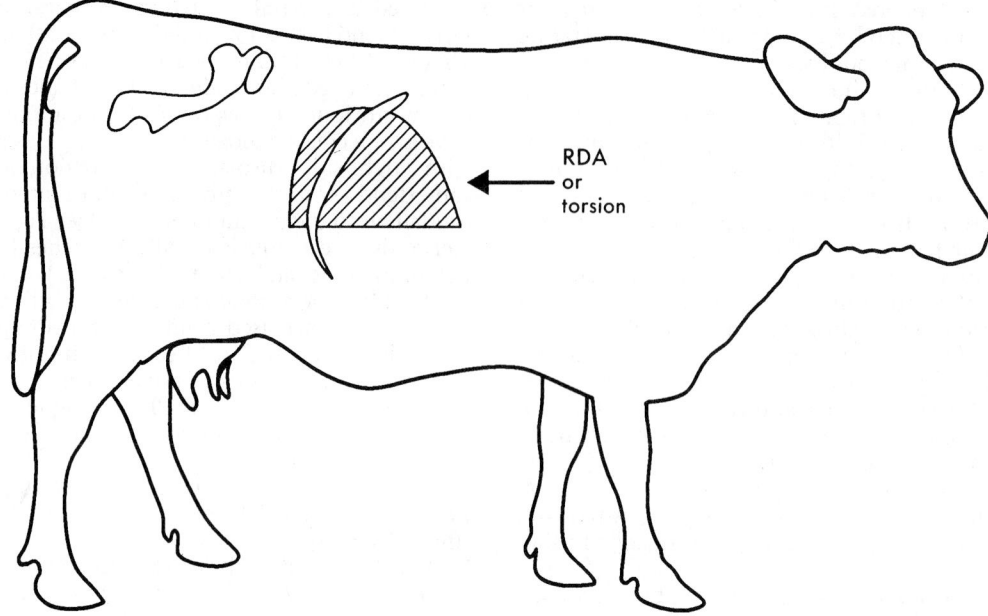

FIG. 1-4 ▪ Schematic representation of the area of the gas ping percussed in association with a right displaced abomasum *(RDA)* or abomasal torsion.

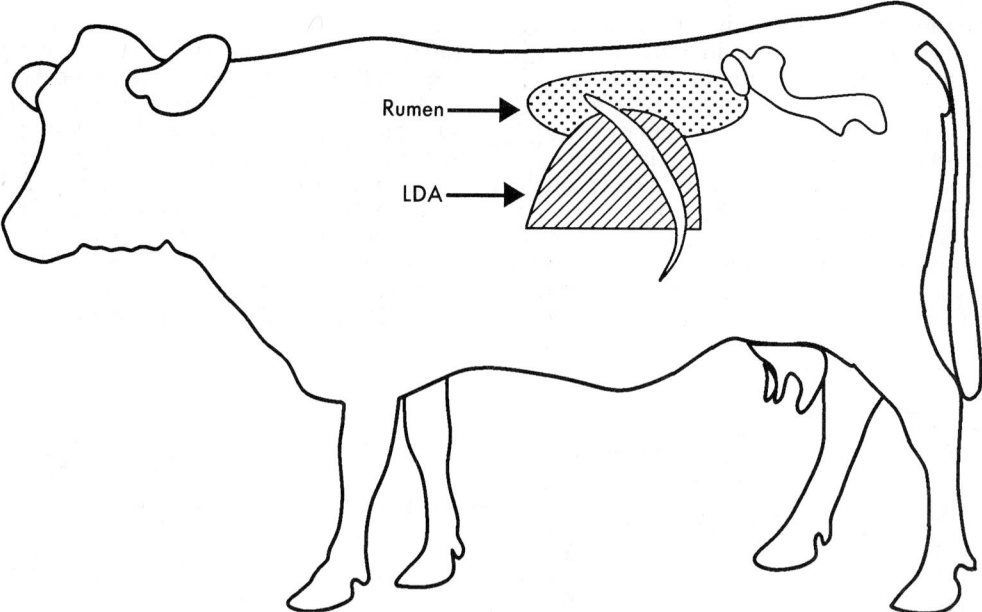

FIG. 1-5 ▪ Schematic representation of the area of the gas ping percussed in association with a left displaced abomasum *(LDA)* or gas ping in the rumen.

percussed, as a result of movement of the rumen behind the abomasum. Often with LDA, intermittent gas bubbling or "toilet flushing" sounds are heard. Rumen gas can be further differentiated from gas trapped in an LDA by rectal palpation of, and passage of a stomach tube into, the rumen; blowing into the rumen yields obviously auscultable sounds unless an LDA is present, in which case the sounds are muffled as the practitioner listens over the area of the ping. Performing a rumen or abomasal tap, the Liptac test, can further differentiate whether the ping originates from an LDA or the rumen. Fluid collected from an LDA would have a pH of less than 4 whereas that of the rumen should be 6 or higher.

The rumen is examined by both auscultation and palpation. It should have a doughy texture with a small gas cap in its dorsal regions and usually is not distended above a plane formed by the lateral aspect of the last rib. Increased accumulation of gas within the rumen would be seen with acute primary frothy bloat and also with free gas bloat. The rumen contractions should be counted, observed, and auscultated. Normally, primary ruminal contractions occur one and one-half to three times a minute, and the force of the contraction should displace the lateral body wall at least 1/2 to 1 inch (1 to 2 cm). When auscultated, the ruminal contraction sounds like a dull roar that starts quietly, rises to a peak, and dies

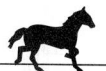

TABLE 1-2

Normal Resting Heart Rates (Beats/Min) for Adult and Young (<30 Days of Age) Ruminants[1-3]

Animal	Average	Range
Cattle		
Adult	60	40-80
Calf	120	100-140
Sheep		
Adult	75	60-120
Lamb	140	120-160
Goat		
Adult	85	70-110
Kid	140	120-160

TABLE 1-3

Normal Resting Respiratory Rates (Breaths/Min) for Adult and Young Ruminants[1-3]

Animal	Average	Range
Cattle		
Adult	24	12-36
Calf	48	30-60
Sheep		
Adult	36	12-72
Lamb	50	30-70
Goat		
Adult	28	15-40
Kid	50	40-65

away. Hypocalcemia and peritonitis are examples of disorders that result in weak or absent ruminal contractions. Hypermotility is rarely seen but can occur and has been described in association with vagal indigestion.

The cardiac region of the thorax is auscultated next. Heart rate and rhythm are determined at this time. Rate varies among species, and age differences within species are noted. In general, older or larger animals have a slower heart rate. Table 1-2 lists the ranges of heart rate that are considered normal for the ruminant species, depending on age. Tachycardia can be seen in animals that have been stressed or excited, as in the process of restraint. However, with time the rate should return to within a more normal range. Any deviation from the normal heart rate in a quiet, relaxed animal implies a general disturbance of the normal health of the animal. Increased heart rate can be seen with fever, inflammation, pain, hypocalcemia, or metabolic disturbances that result in hypovolemia. Bradycardia is seen with conduction disorders within the heart muscle and with some metabolic disorders (uremia, hypokalemia). The most common causes of arrhythmias are atrial fibrillation in adult cattle and hyperkalemia in diarrhetic neonates. Location and intensity of the heart sounds are also important to note, because muffling or displacement of the sounds can indicate space-occupying lesions within the thorax, pericardium, or mediastinum. With pericardial effusion the heart sounds are initially dull but develop splashy washing machine sounds as a gas-fluid interface develops. This often takes weeks. Normally the heart occupies a space on the ventral thorax between the third and sixth ribs. Most of the heart mass is located on the left side of the chest; thus the heart sounds should be louder on that side. However, if the heart is muffled on the left side and louder than normal on the right, one should consider the possibility of inflammation of the pericardium or lung lobes on the left side of the chest. Displacements of the heart sounds caudally are an indication of a space-occupying lesion in the anterior thorax or mediastinum, such as an abscess or neoplasm. Cranial displacements of the heart sounds would be noted with distention of the rumenoreticulum, eventration of abdominal viscera into the thorax through a diaphragmatic hernia, or other space-occupying lesions as noted above. If any murmurs are noted on auscultation, an attempt should be made to localize the murmur to a specific heart valve. While auscultating the heart, the pulse should also be palpated. The easiest point to find a pulse while the heart is being auscultated is at the external maxillary artery. Pulse deficits in conjunction with an increase in heart rate are seen in arterial fibrillation and premature ventricular contractions. The heart rhythm is also noted. Dropped beats, gallop rhythm, and sinus arrhythmias should be compared with other clinical signs to determine importance.

The prefemoral and prescapular lymph nodes are palpated. Enlargements would be seen with inflammatory processes occurring in the regions that they drain. The skin is then palpated, starting along the top line and moving down over the abdominal and chest walls to the ventral midline. The presence of subcutaneous gas or edema is noted, as is any elicitation of pain. Emphysema can have iatrogenic causes (i.e., be secondary to abdominal surgery) or result from pulmonary alveolar rupture, gas gangrene, or puncture wounds. Edema, if noted, is usually ventral and is the result of lowered plasma oncotic pressure or increased venous pressure. Right-sided heart failure as seen in traumatic reticulopericarditis, pericarditis, mediastinal masses, or severe pulmonary disease results in increased venous pressure. If this is the case, a distention of the jugular veins with jugular pulse should also be evident. Protein-losing enteropathies or nephropathies are causes of lowered oncotic pressure, as is liver failure, which results in a lack of synthesis of plasma proteins. Fluid and gas from subcutaneous injection of large volumes of medications such as calcium gluconate can sometimes be confusing.

The thorax is then auscultated and percussed. Respiratory rate (Table 1-3) and pattern are determined at this time, and the lungs are auscultated. If increased inspiratory or expiratory effort is noted, it should be correlated with auscultatory and percussive findings in an effort to determine lung pathology. Normal ruminant lung sounds vary greatly among species. In calves, sheep, and goats the relatively thin chest wall allows one to hear inspiratory sounds ventrally and over the large airways whereas expiratory sounds are minimal (except in sheep, where they are frequently audible because of the large amount of mucus in sheep airways). In larger cattle, only very faint inspiratory sounds are normally heard. Lung sounds can be classified as normal or harsh (tubular) or as wheezes or crackles. These sounds can vary over the different areas of the thorax or can be found singularly over the entire lung field. Significant pulmonary pathology may be present in ruminants *without* any auscultable abnormalities. Total absence of lung sounds ventrally indicates pleural effusion or pulmonary abscessation with loss of airways. When ventral consolidation of the lung occurs, airway sounds are transmitted well and easily heard ventrally as pipestem sounds similar to those heard over the trachea whereas percussion reveals a marked increase in ventral lung density. The trachea should also be auscultated. Inspiratory dyspnea and stridor are usually the result of extrathoracic obstructions to airflow (nose, pharynx, larynx, extrathoracic trachea). Pneumothorax can also result in loss of auscultable airway sounds, which may be absent dorsally or entirely over the entire side if the lung has collapsed completely.

Placing the middle finger in the intercostal space and slapping the finger with the opposite hand, or by using a tablespoon and rubber hammer accomplish percussion of the chest wall to determine the ventral lung border. Percussion is most useful in goats and calves. In sheep the wool precludes effective use of the technique, and in adult cattle the chest wall is often too thick to effectively evaluate changes in percussion tones. The chest is percussed in a dorsal-to-ventral direction, moving caudal to cranial on the chest wall. A change in resonance is noted when the ventral border is reached; a line demarcating this change in resonance is the junction of the diaphragm to the thoracic wall. In the ruminant this line should be described by joining a point at the junction of the eleventh rib and the epaxial musculature dorsally to a point at the middle of the ninth rib, and then cranially to the point of the olecranon. The cranioventral portion of the percussed thorax is dull because of the heart field (about 3 inches [7.5 cm] above the olecranon in adult cattle; 1 to 2 inches [2.5 to 5 cm] in calves, sheep, and goats). Finding an increased area of dullness in the cranioventral lung field associated with harsh lung sounds would be an indication of lung consolidation as seen in *Pasteurella* pneumonia. Pulmonary emphysema (atypical interstitial pneumonia) should be considered when the lung field is larger than expected, the animal is dyspneic, and airway sounds are minimal. A ventral border that is markedly elevated and in a straight line could be an indication of pleural effusion. In this case auscultation would reveal decreased lung sounds ventrally and possibly the presence of pleural friction rubs. Acoustic percussion of the lung field can only extend into the chest to a depth of 2 to 2½ inches (5 to 6 cm). Lesions within the thoracic cavity lying deeper than this cannot be percussed.

The next step in the physical examination is to detect evidence of pain in the ventral portion of the abdomen and thorax. This can be accomplished through the use of the withers pinch test or by ballottement of the xiphoid region. The withers pinch test involves auscultating the trachea while the withers are simultaneously squeezed and pushed ventrally. Painful lesions result in the ruminant resisting normal ventral movement of the spine and/or emitting a grunt or holding its breath when this test is performed. Ballottement of the xiphoid is also done while the trachea is auscultated. The xiphoid region is pushed with a knee or struck with a closed fist, and an elicitation of a grunt would indicate pain in this region. The examiner can then ballotte the remainder of the ventral abdomen and thorax to classify the lesion as localized or diffuse. If localized, the region affected should be identified. It should be noted that the animal may kick the examiner during the xiphoid ballottement test; thus proper precautions should be taken.

The subcutaneous abdominal veins are assessed next and palpated along their length for the presence of thickened walls, distention, or pulses. Distention and pulses may be abnormal if they correlate with other clinical evidence of right-sided heart failure. Thickening of the wall or evidence of thrombosis would often be seen as a consequence of faulty intravenous injection of irritating substances, or of injuries that result in hematomas or abscesses.

If the animal is lame or has postural abnormalities, the feet and legs are palpated next. If the animal is uncooperative, it may be necessary to sedate and/or cast it. If sedation is necessary, it should be performed at the end of the physical examination. Care should be exercised for obvious reasons. The examination consists of comparing one foreleg with the other and then comparing both with the expected norm. The same procedure is followed for the hind legs. Abnormalities in the shape of the claw may be hereditary or caused by nutritional deficiencies, poor leg conformation, poor housing, or as a sequela to laminitis. The coronary bands should be palpated for evidence of pain or increased heat. An attempt should be made to pick up all four feet individually and observe the soles and interdigital regions for necrotic areas, areas of bruising or swelling, draining tracts, or presence of foreign bodies. The fetlock, carpal and tarsal, stifle, and elbow joints are all easily accessible and should be examined for swelling, tenderness, edema, heat, instability, and crepitation. Each joint should be tested over its full range of motion, and any elicitation of pain should be noted. Physical findings should be consolidated into a decision as to whether the joint problems are infectious or traumatic. Sheep or goats with acute polyarthritis most commonly have mycoplasma or chlamydial infection. Chronic joint pain in goats (often with soft-tissue thickening and enlargement caused by synovitis) is frequently attributable to caprine arthritis encephalomyelitis. Conformation of the legs should be analyzed because this could contribute to a joint or foot problem. The pelvic girdle does not lend itself to extensive examination; however, one can note symmetry or asymmetry and further evaluate during the rectal examination. Fractures of the tuber coxae, subluxation of the sacroiliac junction, acetabular fractures, fractures of the head or neck of the femur, and dislocation of the coxofemoral joint may all be diagnosed by evidence gained during palpation and observation of the pelvic area. The dislocated or fractured limb is frequently shorter than the normal opposite limb. The tail can also be examined for evidence of fractures, paresis, or paralysis.

The perineal region is examined by noting the external condition of the genitals and rectum. Anal sphincter tone can be assessed, and the presence of vaginal discharge can be noted. In males the testicles, spermatic cord, and epididymis should be palpated for the presence of nodules or areas of fibrosis. The testicular circumference can be measured and compared to what is expected for age and breed. These measurements are noted in Tables 1-4 and 1-5. The perineal part of the penis can be palpated for the presence of hematoma or swelling and pain (cellulitis or abscess). In the female the supramammary lymph nodes can be felt at the attachment of the udder to the perineum. Enlargement of these nodes occurs with mastitis or lymphosarcoma. The udder is palpated for the presence of fibrotic areas, commonly seen secondary to staphylococcal mastitis or associated with *Actinomyces pyogenes* abscesses. The presence of a swollen quarter

---

TABLE 1-4

Expected Values for the Scrotal Circumference of the Bull at Different Ages[4]

Age (Months)	Scrotal Circumference (cm)
12-14	30-34
15-20	31-36
21-30	32-38
>31	34-39

TABLE 1-5

Expected Values for the Scrotal Circumference of the Ram at Different Body Weights[5]

Body Weight (kg)	Scrotal Circumference (cm)
<45	23-27
45-70	27-33
70-90	30-36
90-115	31-37
115-135	33-38
135-160	36-40

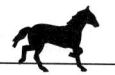

or quarters with pain and heat may be associated with mastitis caused by gram-negative bacteria. Cold damp areas of skin on the udder that are discolored, necrotic, and possibly sloughing are evidence of gangrenous mastitis. In lactating animals milk should be present in each quarter, and some of this milk should be expressed for examination. The milk should be of normal color and consistency and should not have any appreciable smell. The presence of leukocytic flakes or clots (garget) is an indication that the udder is mounting an inflammatory response. This response can be measured qualitatively by using the California Mastitis Test (CMT). One should also collect individual quarter samples from those quarters showing garget or those that test positive on the CMT for bacterial culture and sensitivity.

The next step is to evaluate the head and neck regions. The head should be symmetric in appearance, and any asymmetry should be evaluated to determine whether the deviation is caused by a neuromuscular or a skeletal defect. Facial nerve paralysis results in one type of asymmetry whereas a frontal sinusitis with concurrent displacement of the frontal bone appears differently. Discharges from the eyes, ears, nose, or mouth are noted and correlated with other physical findings. The oral cavity is examined by grasping the tongue with the hand and extending it out through the interdental space. Muscular tone of the tongue is evaluated at this time. The normal animal will resist extraction of the tongue and will quickly retract the tongue into the oral cavity when released. Increased ease of extraction and delayed retraction would be indicative of diseases resulting in flaccid paralysis or paresis of skeletal muscle, such as seen in botulism, for example. The tongue and oral mucosa are examined for the presence of erosions, ulcerations, foreign bodies, or areas of necrosis. The dental arcade is evaluated for age of animal, absence of teeth, loose teeth, or necrotizing gingivitis. The color of the mucous membranes is noted. Icterus, pallor, hyperemia, cyanosis, excessive reddening, or brown "mud-colored" mucous membranes can all be noted, depending on the underlying disorder. Mucous membrane color is best evaluated in the eyes and/or vulva because of the presence of pigments in the oral mucosa of many ruminants. The smell of the breath is noted and, if fetid, might be an indication of a retropharyngeal abscess caused by trauma, lung abscess, or gangrenous pneumonia. If the breath is foul, deep palpation within the oral cavity for an abscess or necrotic area is indicated.

The mucous membranes of the nares are examined, and erosions and ulcerations are noted. Nasal discharges can be an indication of a pulmonic problem but can also be seen with a sinusitis. Generally bilateral discharge is most commonly associated with pneumonia, and a unilateral discharge is more an indication of a sinus problem. However, percussion of the sinuses is necessary to fully evaluate the presence of a discharge. Normal sinuses percuss with a hollow sound, much like that of a hollow tree, and dullness on percussion might indicate sinusitis, sinus cyst, or other fluid or mass in the sinus.

The eyes are examined next. The sclera and mucous membranes are evaluated in much the same manner as the oral and nasal mucous membranes. The corneas are examined for the presence of opacities, discolorations, ulcerations, and lacerations. The position and size of the corneal opacities or ulcerations can be helpful in determining the etiology. Foreign bodies such as plant awns and seeds beneath the third eyelid often cause opacity of the medial aspect of the cornea. Infectious bovine keratoconjunctivitis (pinkeye) is usually localized to the central cornea and causes severe corneal ulceration. When the mucosal diseases cause corneal opacities, they generally do so at the junction of the cornea and sclera and usually do not ulcerate the cornea. The anterior chamber should be examined for the presence of hyphema or hy-

popyon. These can sometimes be seen in animals with severe bacteremia, especially in neonates with failure of passive transfer. The animal should be evaluated for the presence of a menace reflex (absent in normal neonates for up to 2 weeks), and the pupillary light responses should be observed. Nystagmus and strabismus should be characterized, if present, because the direction is important in localizing the lesion. Nystagmus or strabismus or deficits noted in the pupillary light reflex or menace reflex are indicative of underlying neurologic or ophthalmologic disease.

The ears should be palpated and evaluated as to their temperature and the presence of skin lesions. They should be warm to the touch. Ears that are cold are an indication that there is decreased blood flow to the periphery, as seen in hypocalcemic states, with decreased cardiac output, or severe toxic states caused by peripheral vasoconstriction. The presence of small crusty areas or erosions of the skin of the pinna is seen in some of the mucosal diseases such as bluetongue or bovine virus diarrhea. In sheep with acute bluetongue, edema of the face and ears sometimes occurs. If aural discharge or head tilt is present, the ear canal should be examined grossly and with the use of an otoscope for the presence of foreign body or parasites. Purulent discharge can be noted and would be an indication of otitis externa. Noting that the eardrum has ruptured along with the purulent discharge would be diagnostic of otitis media (and possibly otitis interna). Animals that have suffered trauma to the laryngeal or throat latch region and have a basisphenoid fracture can present with bloody discharge from the aural canal. Correlation of the otoscopic findings with other clinical findings would be necessary to arrive at a definitive diagnosis.

The palpable lymph nodes of the head and neck include the parotid, the submandibular, and the deep retropharyngeal. The deep retropharyngeals can be palpated externally, if enlarged, in the sheep, goat, or calf. They can be examined in the adult bovine by extending the hand through the mouth and palpating the pharynx. By keeping the animal's mouth open with one hand and guiding the other hand along the dorsum of the tongue to its base, the examiner can then extend the hand aboral into the pharynx. Enlargements of the deep retropharyngeals, abscesses, or other masses can then be palpated. The most common causes of masses or abscesses in the pharyngeal region are infectious or iatrogenic (e.g., secondary to trauma from a balling gun, paste wormer gun, or other instrument). The submandibular nodes are located in the intermandibular space and are identified by slipping the skin and underlying tissue through the fingers. These nodes are oval and about the size of a walnut, or 1 to 2 inches in diameter ($2\frac{1}{2}$ to 5 cm). The parotid lymph nodes are almond shaped and are located just caudal to the ramus of the mandible and about 4 inches (10 cm) ventral to the ear.

The skin of the neck is palpated, with attention paid to the presence of abscesses, lacerations, or other lesions. Skin turgor can be assessed by tenting the skin and measuring the time taken for the skin to return to normal shape. This is used to determine the state of hydration. In normal, hydrated animals the skin returns to normal position within 1 second. Using other factors such as sunken eyes, dryness of mucous membranes, abnormal heart rate, and degree of illness, an estimation of percent dehydration is made. Dehydration is first noted clinically when the animal is about 5% dehydrated, and death occurs at 12% to 15% dehydration.

The larynx should be palpated for enlargement and the presence of pain. The trachea should also be palpated for the presence of fractured tracheal rings, collapsed areas, and the presence of pain on palpation. The jugular veins are examined for the presence of distention and pulses. Thrombosed veins should also be noted because this condition may alter the desired course of therapy and often prevents placement of

LANDER VETERINARY CLINIC, INC

2930 Lander Avenue
Turlock, California 95830

Telephone (209) 634-5801
Fax (209) 634-2228

DIAGNOSTIC AND TREATMENT SHEET

FARM OWNER _____   DATE _____

ANIMAL ID NUMBER _____   PRODUCTION CLASS _____
                                       LACTATING COW/DRY COW/HEIFER/CALF/BULL

PHYSICAL EXAM

TEMPERATURE	NORMAL	FEVER	HYPOTHERMIA		
RUMEN MOTILITY	NORMAL	WEAK	ABSENT	BLOAT	COLLAPSED
ABDOMINAL PINGS/SPLASHES/PAIN	NORMAL	ABNORMAL	LDA/RDA/RTA	GRUNT	DIARRHEA
RECTAL PALPATION FINDINGS	NORMAL	ABNORMAL	DISTENDED BOWEL	KIDNEY	OTHER
MANURE	NORMAL	DIARRHEA	SCANT/NEG	FIRM	BLOOD/FIBRIN
URINE	NORMAL	KETONES	+ ++ +++	BLOOD/PUS	
REPRODUCTIVE TRACT	NORMAL	PREGNANT	METRITIS	PERIMETRITIS	ADHESIONS
LUNGS	NORMAL	PNEUMONIA	EMPHYSEMA	PLEURITIS	CHRONIC
HEART SOUNDS/RHYTHM	NORMAL	MURMUR	ARRHYTHMIA	SPLASHING	MUFFLED
LYMPH NODES/CNS	NORMAL	ENLARGED	DOWN COW	CNS SIGNS	
MAMMARY GLANDS	NORMAL	MASTITIS	TEAT ABNORMALITY		
EYES/MOUTH/MUCOUS MEMBRANES	NORMAL	ABNORMAL	PALE/JAUNDICE	SQUAMOUS CELL	LUMPY JAW
LIMBS/BODY EXTERIOR	NORMAL	ABNORMAL	SKIN LESIONS	LAMENESS	INJURY

Diagnosis 1. _____ 2. _____ 3. _____

treatment

IV FLUIDS	CALCIUM	DEXTROSE	7.2% NA CL	K CL	ELECTROLYTES	PHOSPHAID
ANTIINFLAMMATORY	DEXAMETHASONE	PREDEF 2X	BANAMINE	PHENYLBUT	ASPIRIN	SOLUDELTA
ANTIBIOTICS	OXYTETRACYCLINE	ALBON	PENICILLIN G	POLYFLEX	NAXCEL	TRIBRISSEN
RUMENATORICS	LAXATIVE BOLUS	EPSOM SALTS	CHARCOAL	MINERAL OIL	NUTRADRENCH	NA HCO3
VITAMINS/MINERALS	MULTI B	B 12	D PANTHENOL	VIT E/SE	ORAL KCL	ORAL PO4
ANALGESICS	TORBUGESIC	VALIUM	EPIDURAL	SEDATION		
LONG ACTING ANTIBIOTICS	LA 200	MICOTIL	NUFLOR	LS 50	ERYTHROMYCIN	LA SULFA
HORMONES	OXYTOCIN	GNRH	LUTALYSE	ECP		
OTHER	EQUIPOISE	NA IODIDE	IU OXYTET BOL			

SURGERY   LDA ☐   RDA ☐   EXPLORATORY ☐   C-SECTION ☐   OTHER ☐ _____

FOLLOW-UP THERAPY   PROGNOSIS   EXC ☐   good ☐   fair ☐   poor ☐

1. _____

2. _____

3. _____

4. _____

WITHDRAWAL INFORMATION

DRUG _____   MILK _____   SLAUGHTER _____

DOCTOR: _____

FIG. 1-6 ■ Example of a diagnostic and treatment sheet. (Courtesy Lander Veterinary Clinic, Inc., Turlock, Calif.)

a catheter. The venous stasis test is performed on the jugular by holding off the vein in the midcervical region. Normally the vessel fills above the point of occlusion and remains collapsed below. With restricted venous blood flow, as seen in cases of right heart failure, a positive stasis test can result. In these cases the vessel below the occluded point fails to collapse or takes a prolonged time to do so, and a jugular pulse is frequently present.

The final step in the physical examination is rectal palpation. This cannot be accomplished in small ruminants, so this section is directed primarily toward the bovine. The pelvic area is evaluated for the presence of retroperitoneal abscesses or fractures of the pelvic bones. The left kidney can be palpated for overall size and shape, which is normally lobulated in cattle, and the kidney can be gently squeezed to determine if pain is evident. The rumen should be palpated, and findings compared with those noted on percussion and auscultation. If there is any evidence of intraabdominal gas pings, an attempt should be made to palpate the suspected organ. This can provide information that may be helpful in determining therapeutic or diagnostic directions. The rectal palpation can reveal the presence of masses that were not palpable externally, such as fat necrosis or tumors. Adhesions and evidence of peritonitis can also be palpated rectally, and attempts should be made to localize them to a specific area of the abdomen to establish potential etiology. The preiliac (or internal iliac) lymph nodes are located by sweeping the hand along the craniodorsal face of the ilium. These nodes normally have the size and shape of a walnut. Enlargements are noted with lymphosarcoma, peritonitis, and severe limb inflammation. The lymph nodes of the aortic bifurcation are very small and not easily palpated. Their ability to be palpated would be evidence of abnormal enlargement. Palpation of the genital tract is directed toward establishing size, shape, and presence of abnormalities. These contents could be normal, as with a pregnant animal bearing a fetus, or abnormal, as seen with a pyometra. If it is determined that a cow is not pregnant, the ovaries and oviducts should be palpated for structures and abnormalities. In the bull, particular attention should be paid to the prostate, seminal vesicles, and bulbourethral gland.

MEDICAL RECORD

The information gathered by means of the physical examination (see Fig. 1-2) is compiled and correlated with the data obtained during the history (see Fig. 1-1). A problem list should be formulated through the physical examination and anamnesis, leading to the development of a specific diagnostic plan, diagnostic ruleouts, and a proposed course of therapy (Fig. 1-6). Prognosis can also be assessed with the information now in the examiner's hands. Accurate recording of the abnormalities noted during the examination should become part of the medical record and can prove valuable in following the course of the case. In addition, with each complete and accurate physical examination performed, the practitioner becomes more skilled in the procedure, adapting it to fit his or her needs, and using his or her time more efficiently. With the numbers of diagnostic tests available to the profession today, the information gained from the physical examination will allow the examiner to pick the tests that are specific for those disorders suspected, which saves the practitioner time and the client money.

DIAGNOSTIC TESTS THAT CAN BE APPLIED IN THE FIELD

There are laboratory procedures that can be performed in the field, the results of which would prove beneficial in the development of a diagnostic plan. These include the CMT, par-

tial urinalysis (dipsticks), ruminal pH determination, and milk or blood progesterone tests. Additionally, some serum chemistries can be performed at cow-side with the use of the I-stat.*

The CMT is a simple procedure that aids in the detection of clinical or subclinical mastitis (see Chapter 36). This procedure is done routinely during all physical examinations of lactating cows. Partial urinalysis is accomplished by collecting the urine and using any one of a number of urine dipsticks that can be commercially obtained. With a suspected case of lactic acidosis, a rumen sample can be collected through the stomach tube, and rumen pH can be determined. Most drugstores carry pH paper that can be used for this procedure. Be certain that the paper has a standard range, since there are papers that are specific for the acidic or the alkaline range. A rumen pH below 5.0 would be indicative of lactic acidosis. Numerous cow-side progesterone assays that use either milk or blood as substrate have recently been developed. These can be relatively easy to use and interpret or they can be difficult, so discretion should be used when making initial purchases. These ancillary diagnostic procedures are explained in greater detail later in this text.

INSURANCE, INTERSTATE, AND PREPURCHASE HEALTH EXAMINATIONS

The complete physical examination as described above is necessary for a proper prepurchase or insurance examination. For insurance purposes a more complete accounting of the examination must be done. This means that all findings, whether normal or abnormal, have to be recorded. A specific form is generally provided by the insuring agent, and this should be used. Potential for future legal action also exists whenever an animal is insured; therefore it is in the practitioner's best interest to complete the insurance form accurately.

The prepurchase examination is similar to the insurance examination. The physical examination form (see Fig. 1-2) can be used to record findings. The prepurchase examination could be performed on the highly pedigreed female who is being consigned to sale, but it is more often performed on the male scheduled for use as an artificial insemination stud. Occasionally one could be asked to examine an animal under consideration for purchase. Experience indicates that the veterinarian should be employed by the potential buyer in these cases. This arrangement avoids any potential accusations of conflict of interest on the part of the examining veterinarian. A complete blood count and a chemistry panel should be run. Generally it is prudent to certify that the animal is healthy and to test for tuberculosis, brucellosis, and bovine leukosis (using agar gel immunodiffusion). Additional laboratory tests for anaplasmosis and bluetongue may be indicated. Often an animal being consigned to sale or one going into artificial insemination service is required to meet federal regulations for interstate shipment. This information can be obtained from the federal veterinarian in charge in your area or from the office of the state veterinarian in the state of destination.

A problem arises when the number of animals submitted for interstate health examination is large. Economic and time constraints usually preclude complete examination of all the animals presented. At such times the visual examination described earlier can prove helpful in determining which animals are to be singled out for the more complete physical examination. The examination of individuals is less complete than for prepurchase or insurance examinations, because

---

*i-Stat Serum Chemistry Analyzer, i-Stat Corp., Princeton, NJ 08540; distributed by Heska Corp., 1801-A Airport Road, Waukesha WI 53188.

such factors as fertility are not at issue when filling out an interstate health certificate. Choosing animals with abnormalities in behavior, physical condition, gait, or posture allows the practitioner to concentrate on those that have the most potential to be diseased. Also, one can be fairly confident that, if all the animals appear normal on the general examination, they are healthy and would be suitable for interstate shipment as long as the results of the intradermal tuberculosis test and required serologic tests prove negative. To sign an interstate health certificate, a veterinarian must be accredited and licensed in a state. It is essential that a veterinarian signing an interstate health certificate have examined the livestock sufficiently and diligently enough to be confident that no infectious or contagious diseases are present in the con-signed group. A call should be placed to the office of the state veterinarian in the state of destination to be sure that all current requirements are fulfilled before shipment is scheduled.

REFERENCES

1. Stöber M: General examination. In Rosenberger G: *Clinical examination of cattle*, ed 2, Philadelphia, 1979, WB Saunders, pp 73-75.
2. Anonymous: Clinical values and procedures. In Fraser CM: *Merck veterinary manual*, ed 6, Rahway, NJ, 1986, Merck, p 910.
3. East NE: Personal communication, 1982, University of California, Davis, Calif.
4. Chenoweth PJ, Ball L: Breeding soundness evaluation in bulls. In Morrow DA: *Current therapy in theriogenology*, Philadelphia, 1980, WB Saunders, pp 330-339.
5. Braun WF, Thompson JM, Ross CV: Ram scrotal circumference measurements, *Theriogenology* 13:221, 1980.

Equine History, Physical Examination, and Records

T. DOUGLAS BYARS

JAMI L. WHITING

The ideal purposes of the physical examination are to determine what or if a problem exists. The results should establish a diagnostic plan, prepare a therapeutic approach, and develop a prognosis.

The nature of an internal medicine problem does not always allow for each objective of the physical examination to spontaneously or quickly generate either a diagnosis or prognosis. More realistically, the examination process dictates the specific laboratory tests or procedures to be performed that support the diagnostic or therapeutic effort. The clinician's self-disciplines regarding the extent of the physical examination should be guided by experience, efficiency of time, and the ancillary diagnostic aids that are available. A complete and extensive examination for each patient may not always be practical, especially in busy private or academic practice situations. In these cases, the clinician should provide for the client's concerns by an expedient history and a pertinent physical examination process that addresses the client's complaint (e.g., a rectal examination is not required for an evaluation of a pneumonia).

PHYSICAL EXAMINATION RECORD

Preparation for the initial contact time with the client and patient should begin with a system of record keeping. Ambulatory records will usually be more flexible than "in-house" hospital admission forms. Both field and clinic forms should include designated spaces for the client or agent's address and phone number. An area for the complete signalment (name, sex, breed, color, age), including an estimated weight should be provided. If the patient is unnamed (as with foals), it should be listed in the dam's name with the year of birth (e.g., Curious '00). The sire's name should not be used because more than one foal per year would be expected from a stallion's crop. Whenever surrogate mares produce multiple foals from a single embryo transfer dam, a new system of naming/identification will have to be incorporated.

(Fig. 2-1 is a sample admission form with the history and physical examination sections included.)

EQUINE INSURANCE

If the animal is insured, this should be documented, preferably with the insurer's telephone number. It is the client's, or their agent's, responsibility to notify the insurance company representative whenever an animal insured for full mortality contracts an illness requiring a veterinary examination. If the patient is insured, it is considered a professional courtesy for the veterinarian to also communicate directly with the insurance company, especially with a life-threatening illness. Also, permission from the insurance company is required whenever a general anesthetic, surgical procedure, or euthanasia is to be performed. Whenever euthanasia is requested, the insurance company may require a second opinion from an adjusting veterinarian. If a direct representative from the insurance company cannot be contacted immediately, the clinician must exercise professional judgment in assuming the responsibility for a humane or critical decision. The client or agent should be in agreement with the decision, and all communications and pertinent data should be documented in the medical record. If a necropsy is to be performed, it should preferably be in the presence of another veterinarian from a different practice. Table 2-1 is an abbreviated list of the types of equine insurance offered.[1]

HISTORY

The medical history should be directed to the clinical problem. The "herd health" of the stable or farm is briefly depicted by the vaccination and parasite control program. The diet should be determined, including the grazing environment, stalled or housing schedule, and the medical problems concerning other animals on the premises that may coincide with a group incidence of the client complaint. The existence and the type of insurance on the patient should be noted.

15

HAGYARD-DAVIDSON-McGEE ASSOCIATES, P.S.C.
VETERINARIANS

PATIENT MEDICAL RECORD

ADMITTED		DISCHARGED	DIED	EUTHANIZED		ADMITTING CLINICIAN:
DATE: / / TIME:	☐ AM ☐ PM	DATE: / /		TIME:	☐ AM ☐ PM	

PATIENT NAME: AGE: SEX: BREED: COLOR:

FARM/TRAINER:	REFERRING VETERINARIAN:
☐ INPATIENT ☐ OUTPATIENT ☐ ICU ☐ BARN ☐ ISOLATION ☐ A/C ☐ NEURO	PRESENTING COMPLAINTS:

HISTORY   VACC. ☐   PARASITE CONTROL ☐   DIET: HAY _____   GRAIN _____   TELEPHONE RE-CHECK ☐   TIME

PHYSICAL EXAMINATION:

(1) GEN	☐ N ☐ ABN ☐ NE	(2) INTEG	☐ N ☐ ABN ☐ NE	(3) MUC/SKEL.	☐ N ☐ ABN ☐ NE	(4) CIRC	☐ N ☐ ABN ☐ NE	(5) RESP	☐ N ☐ ABN ☐ NE	(6) DIG	☐ N ☐ ABN ☐ NE
(7) GU	☐ N ☐ ABN ☐ NE	(8) EYES	☐ N ☐ ABN ☐ NE	(9) NEURO	☐ N ☐ ABN ☐ NE	(10) LYMPH	☐ N ☐ ABN ☐ NE	T _____ P _____ R _____ WT _____			

DESCRIBE ABNORMAL (USE NUMBERS ABOVE)

MASTER PROBLEM LIST:

FINAL DIAGNOSIS:

Continued

FIG. 2-1   Example of a history and physical examination form that can be used in equine practice.

HAGYARD-DAVIDSON-MCGEE ASSOCIATES, P.S.C.

Patient History and Billing Information

Note: The following information MUST be completed prior to or within 24 hours of admission of the patient. Any information not applicable should be marked "N/A".

Date Admitted: _____   Has Horse previously been a patient of HDM? ☐ ☐   Date? _____
                                                                                   Yes No

A) Patient Name: _____

                  Age: _____   Sex: _____   Breed: _____   Color: _____

                  Is Patient Insured? ☐ ☐   Insurance Carrier: _____   Policy Type: ☐ ☐
                                   Yes No   (check which applies) Mortality Medical

B) Farm Name (where horse resides): _____

                  Farm Manager/Trainer/Agent: _____

                  Address: _____
                              Street   City   State   Zip
                  Telephone: _____
                  (& area code)   Daytime   Evening   Fax

C) Owner Name (party responsible for bill): _____

                  Address: _____
                              Street   City   State   Zip
                  Telephone: _____
                  (& area code)   Daytime   Evening   Fax

D) Referring Veterinarian: _____

                  Telephone: _____
                  (& area code)   Daytime   Evening   Fax

E) Who should HDM communicate with regarding status of the patient? _____

F) Patient History (include any medications): _____

_____

_____

_____

G) Agreement for Treatment and Payment of HDM Charges:

        I hereby authorize HDM to perform any surgical procedure(s) or reasonably necessary emergency treatment ("Services) which it deems reasonably necessary for the patient's survival, well being, or usefulness and I agree that the Owner of the patient and <u>I, individually, will be jointly and severally obligated to pay all charges rendered by HDM</u> relating to the Services and care of the patient.

        _____   _____
                  Signature of Owner/Agent   Date Signed

      For Office Use Only: _____   _____   _____
                                 Received By   Date Received   Account #

FIG. 2-1, cont'd ▓ For legend see opposite page.

TABLE 2-1

Equine Insurance

Type of Insurance*		Role of Attending Veterinarian
Perils	Covers mortality claims for shipping accidents, fire, and natural disasters such as lightning	Inform clients of responsibility to inform insurance company
Mortality†	Covers mortality claims for all life-threatening conditions (e.g., colics)	Inform clients of responsibility to inform insurance company of any anesthetic, surgical needs, or euthanasia
Use	Covers a loss in intended use (e.g., racing, fertility)	Inform clients of responsibility to inform insurance company of any anesthetic, surgical needs, or euthanasia

*The client is responsible for the costs of veterinary care and treatment unless a medical/surgical policy exists.
†Fetal mortality insurance covers unborn foals, usually until 24 hours after birth.

In dealing with neonates, the reproductive and foaling history of the mare is important in establishing an early diagnosis. Any compromises to the mare's gestation, foaling, placental abnormalities, or lactation should be questioned; and any problems during previous pregnancies are considered to be important pertinent historical data.

The determination of medication use before hospitalization will aid in determining if "masking" agents have been used. Analgesics such as flunixin meglumine can mask signs of pain or colic and can alter interpretation of the severity the horse's condition on arrival. The failure of previous medical treatments can aid in the initial selection of more appropriate therapeutic planning. Tranquilizers or sedatives are frequently used for vanning and shipping purposes. These drugs can cause the false clinical signs of lethargy, weakness, and ataxia. In many instances, a van driver or hauler is unaware of medication use or the patient's problem.

The patient's individual problems should be determined according to such factors as clinical history of onset, feed and water consumption, fevers, and decrease in performance. In essence, the clinician must effectively "zero in" on the problems at hand.

PHYSICAL EXAMINATION

The extent of the physical examination will be subject to the environment where the examination is conducted (field vs. hospital), the equipment available, and the ancillary personnel for restraint and procedural purposes. In a hospital setting, the clinician should have available or have access to as much as possible of the equipment list in Box 2-1. The physical examination sheet should provide a systematic list of the organ systems being evaluated (see Fig. 2-1). The vital signs (temperature, pulse, and respiratory rate) should be documented in the "calm" animal, if possible. Abnormal findings are described in an appropriate space provided, usually below the body systems checklist. Using the same numeral for each body system throughout the examination process and in problem identification is useful for future caseload recall, especially if a computer is used and codes can be applied to clinical findings and diagnosis. At the completion of the physical examination, the major problems identified are listed, and appropriate laboratory tests can be requested. The final diagnosis is seldom filled out at the time of the initial examination. The final diagnosis represents the final assessment and should be filled in at the appropriate time (e.g., hospital discharge).

A general evaluation of the equine patient should be made from afar. The initial observations of body weight, posture, weakness, lethargy, incoordination, lameness, and musculoskeletal asymmetry are more easily observed from a slight distance away from the patient.

BOX 2-1

Recommended Examination Room Equipment and Ancillary Services

EXAMINATION ROOM EQUIPMENT
Records (examination sheet and request forms)
Thermometer
Clock with second hand
Stethoscope
Twitch
Rectal sleeves and lubricant
Nasogastric tube
Hoof knife and testers
Ophthalmoscope
Otoscope
Endoscope
Electrocardiogram (ECG) machine
Ultrasound (linear or sector scanner)*
Sphygmomanometer and Doppler (tail or limb)

ANCILLARY SERVICES
Radiology services
Ultrasound consultation
Laboratory services

*The ultrasound service is more appropriately located in the examination room rather than as a consultation service.

The integumentary system can usually be quickly evaluated as to the type, distribution, number of lesions, and site-layer of involvement (e.g., 3 × 6 × 2 cm raised, nodular, nonpainful mass involving the cutis and subcutis). Such a lesion is readily available for superficial evaluation. However, subtle lesions of petechia and ecchymosis cannot be visualized in the integument, because the hair coat and pigment hide the obvious lesions seen in other species such as purpura of nonpigmented humans and pigs. In these instances, the mucous membranes must be examined as an extension of the integumentary system. If obvious multiple lesions of the skin are present, it usually expedites documentation by drawing a picture of a horse and inserting the data base distribution in the drawing, including both sides of the horse (see Skin Disease Examination, Chapter 11). Gross generalized distortions (e.g., anasarca) may be viewed as lesions of possibly more than one body system (integument and circulatory).

For the internist, evaluation of the musculoskeletal system usually involves a cursory examination of the site and appearance of the disease processes. Lamenesses are more commonly evaluated by clinicians familiar with diagnostic nerve blocks, arthrocentesis methods (e.g., septic arthritis in foals), and radiographic findings. If laminitis is present, the clini-

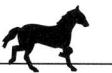

cian should be able to add to the clinical prognosis by Obel grading (1 to 4) and palpation of the coronary bands for the determination of the "sinker" syndrome (distal phalangeal displacement).[2]

Evaluation of the circulatory system starts with a heart rate, rhythm, and any presence of murmurs. Mucous membrane color, capillary refill time, scleral injection, palpable changes in the temperature of the ears and extremities, jugular pulsation, and pitting subcutaneous edema are the most common obvious circulatory physical examination parameters. The heart should be auscultated bilaterally, and murmurs graded (I-VI or I-V) and described as to the valvular site and phase of the cardiac cycle. Arrhythmias usually involve an ECG request, except with the common findings such as type II heart blocks in clinically asymptomatic horses. Type II heart block in normal horses can usually be obliterated by exciting the horse by a threatening gesture. In addition to ECG requests, transcutaneous ultrasound examination of the heart and pericardium and transrectal evaluation of the caudal aorta and iliacs for intraabdominal thrombotic lesions can be used.[3,4] If procedural assessments of blood pressure are needed, a manometer for central venous pressure, or a sphygmomanometer with Doppler ultrasound are used on the base of the tail in adults and the tail or inside radius (forearm) in foals.[5]

The respiratory system is similar to the circulatory system in that the rate and mucous membrane color are important assessments. Respiratory effort and the phase of increased work should be assessed (e.g., heaves). Auscultation should be of both the upper (larynx and trachea) and lower airways. Nasal airflow can be determined by wetting the hands and holding them gently over the nostrils so that both intensity and equality of air movement can be assessed. Smelling the breath for fetid or necrotic odors (ozena) is similarly important, and endoscopic evaluation of the upper airways should be an adjunct to abnormal clinical findings. A penlight can be used to visualize the internal nares (septal mucosa). Percussion of the sinuses should be performed for detection of dullness, suggesting sinusitis or the presence of fluid within the sinus cavity.

The interpretation of lung sounds have been described elsewhere,[6] and the clinician should make an effort to auscultate regions of the thorax bilaterally and document findings as to the location or absence of sounds and the phase of respirations involved.

Percussion is a reliable clinical tool and should be performed in suspected abscess, tumor, or pleural effusion cases. A pleximeter and tablespoon are the only tools required, although some clinicians are adept at direct finger percussion of the chest. In foals, percussion can be performed by placing a stethoscope on one side of the chest and reaching over the back of the foal to manually percuss the opposite side. Fractured ribs may be recognized in the neonatal foal as palpable asymmetry or a bony crepitus ("clicks").

Ultrasound has revolutionized the clinical evaluation of the thoracic cavity. Subtle pneumonia, abscess, and pleural effusion represent rapid and definitive objective findings.[3] Unfortunately, the familiarity of clinicians in thoracic interpretation is directly related to access and frequency of ultrasound use. The presence of an ultrasound machine should be as readily available as an endoscope. Ultrasound may, in fact, obviate the need for chest radiographs in numerous cases, thereby increasing efficiency and decreasing client costs.

The gastrointestinal system is usually examined by bilateral auscultation of intestinal sounds if a clinical complaint involving the abdomen is present. In addition, the abdomen should be auscultated ventrally for sounds similar to "ocean waves" or sand pouring on itself, indicative of the presence of sand within the gastrointestinal tract.[7] In cases where the gastrointestinal tract is the site of the primary lesion, checking for gastric reflux and rectal examinations[8] may become an examination necessity. Clinicians should strive to become adept at rectal palpation and regard the procedure as a premier diagnostic skill while respecting the risks involved for the patient and veterinarian. The patient should be observed eating or drinking whenever dysphagia is suspected. Nasogastric intubation is useful in evaluating dysphagia and esophageal blockage (choke) and determining the presence or absence of gastric reflux. Ultrasound evaluation of the abdomen may quickly reveal peritonitis, uroperitoneum, hemorrhage, ascites, or abdominal masses. In adults, the latter lesions usually can be scanned transrectally if the operator has been able to manually palpate the mass lesion. The use of long endoscopes (e.g., 2-3 m) are valuable in the visual assessment of the esophagus and stomach with lesions such as gastric ulceration. For a diagnostic endoscopic examination of the stomach, it is recommended that the patient be held off feed for at least 12 hours to allow complete visualization of the stomach.[9]

The urogenital system can be examined by manual palpation, rectal palpation, vaginoscopic (speculum examination) viewing, endoscopic viewing, and ultrasound. Catheterized samples should be obtained (e.g., cultures, urinalysis) before any contaminating invasive procedures are performed and prior to initiating fluid therapy. Sphincter tone may be subjectively or objectively assessed in horses with urinary incontinence or stranguria.

The eyes can be examined by a rapid visual assessment using a penlight. The cornea and cranial and caudal lens capsules can be evaluated by horizontally moving the penlight and noting the crossing light reflexes. Pupillary constriction to light and the "menace" response should be observed, although these reflexes may be significantly slower in the neonate. An ophthalmoscopic retinal examination should be performed whenever the eyes represent the primary complaint, and fluorescein dye strips used for the detection of corneal ulcers. Blindfolding of one eye at a time may aid in the assessment of unilateral blindness and should be conducted in a safe area with "blunt" devices contrived as an obstacle course.

The neurologic system examination should involve a consistent procedure for all cases with nervous system disorders (see Nervous System Examination, Chapters 8 and 33). The patient's attitude, posture, and head carriage should be assessed from afar. The cranial nerves should be evaluated, followed by examination of the spinal reflexes and tail tone. Sensory deficits should be noted at this time. Postural responses (e.g., placement, hemi-hopping, sway) can then be assessed before observing the patient in locomotion. Notes regarding symmetry, asymmetry, ambulation, muscle atrophy, and upper and lower motor neuron deficits should be documented to aid in determining the sites for any additional ancillary tests such as radiographs. Blindfolding should be conducted in a safe area, especially for patients with vestibular disease. An area of incline is useful for exacerbating the locomotor deficits, especially when the horse is led with the head elevated.

The lymphatic system is usually evaluated merely by recording any obvious lymphadenopathy. This can be regional or local (as in strangles) or generalized (cutaneous lymphosarcoma) and may be appreciated on rectal examination. Lymphangitis or the presence of edema should also be noted.

Once a patient has been admitted to the clinic or hospital, other records should be used for monitoring and assessing the patient (Figs. 2-2 to 2-4).

HAGYARD-DAVIDSON-MCGEE ASSOCIATES, P.S.C.
VETERINARIANS

PROGRESS NOTES

DATE/TIME

PATIENT _____

T	
P	
R	
A	
BM	
T	
P	
R	
A	
BM	
T	
P	
R	
A	
BM	
T	
P	
R	
A	
BM	
T	
P	
R	
A	
BM	
T	
P	
R	
A	
BM	

FIG. 2-2 ▮▮ Example of progress notes form. *A,* Mental attitude; *BM,* bowel movement; *P,* pulse; *R,* respiratory rate and character; *T,* temperature.

						COLOR	GI MOTILITY			LUNGS		

HAGYARD-DAVIDSON-McGEE ASSOCIATES, P.S.C.

INTENSIVE CARE FLOW SHEET

PATIENT:

DATE/TIME	T	P	R	CRT	COLOR MUC. MEM.	GI MOTILITY LT. RT.	FECES	LUNGS LT. RT.	TREATMENT/COMMENTS

FIG. 2-3 ▦ Example of an intensive care flow sheet used in equine practice. *CRT,* Capillary refill time; *P,* pulse; *R,* respiratory rate; *T,* temperature.

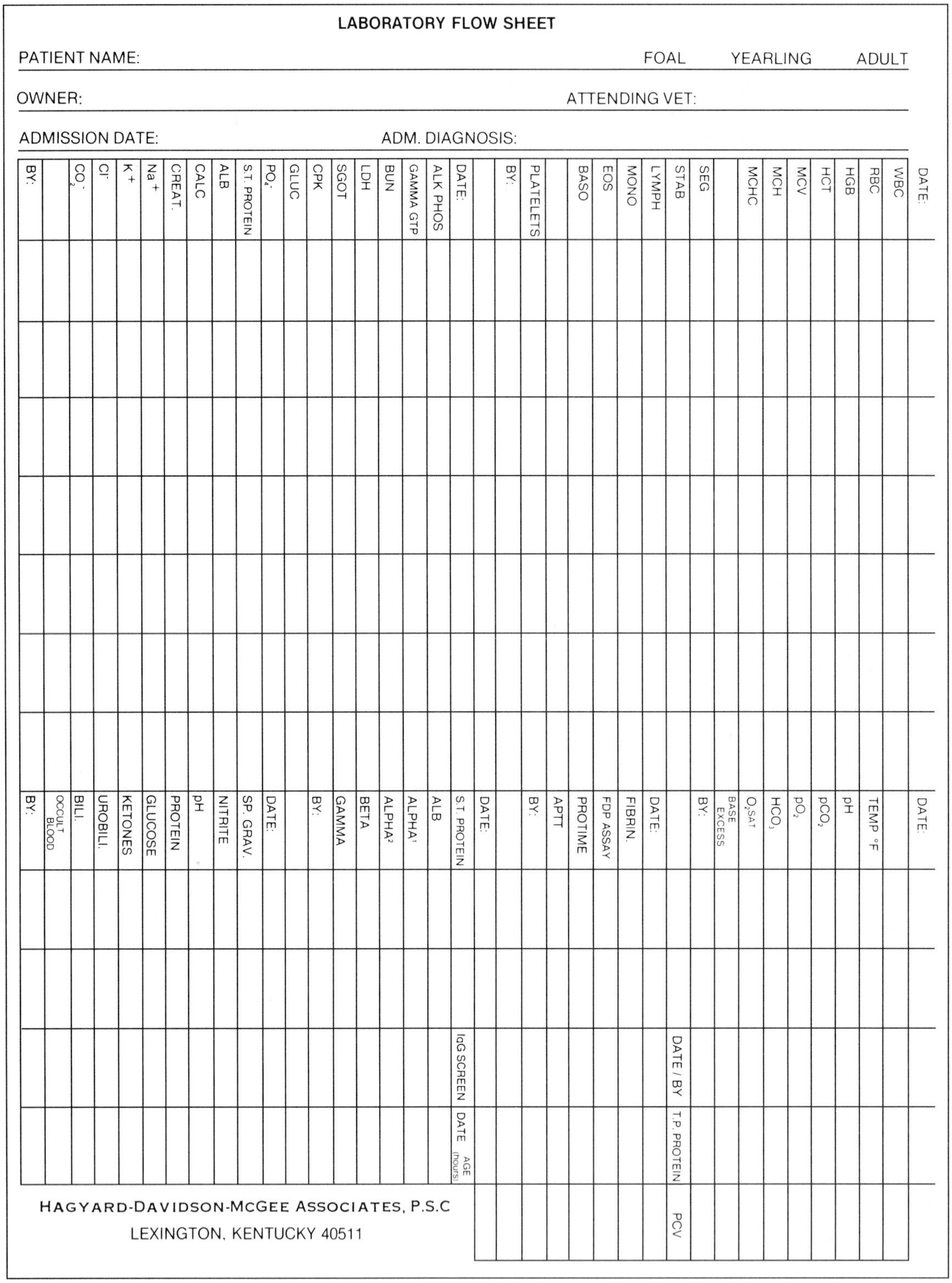

LABORATORY FLOW SHEET

PATIENT NAME: FOAL   YEARLING   ADULT

OWNER: ATTENDING VET:

ADMISSION DATE: ADM. DIAGNOSIS:

Column labels (first block): BY:, CO₂, Cl⁻, K⁺, Na⁺, CREAT., CALC, ALB, S.T. PROTEIN, PO₄, GLUC, CPK, SGOT, LDH, BUN, GAMMA GTP, ALK PHOS, DATE:

Column labels (second block): BY:, PLATELETS, BASO, EOS, MONO, LYMPH, STAB, SEG, MCHC, MCH, MCV, HCT, HGB, RBC, WBC, DATE:

Lower-left block labels: BY:, OCCULT BLOOD, BILI., UROBILI., KETONES, GLUCOSE, PROTEIN, pH, NITRITE, SP. GRAV., DATE:

Lower-middle block labels: BY:, GAMMA, BETA, ALPHA², ALPHA¹, ALB, S.T. PROTEIN, DATE:

Block labels: BY:, APTT, PROTIME, FDP ASSAY, FIBRIN, DATE:

Block labels: BY:, BASE EXCESS, O₂ SAT, HCO₃, pO₂, pCO₂, pH, TEMP °F, DATE:

IgG SCREEN, DATE, AGE (hours)

DATE / BY, T.P. PROTEIN, PCV

HAGYARD-DAVIDSON-McGEE ASSOCIATES, P.S.C
LEXINGTON, KENTUCKY 40511

FIG. 2-4 ■ Example of a laboratory results flow sheet used in equine practice to record serial test results on a single sheet to enable visualization of trends.

Use of Ancillary Equipment in the Examination Procedure

Advancing technologies are allowing the practitioner or clinician to add to or replace many physical examination procedures with techniques capable of providing diagnostic information or direct therapeutic intervention. Ultrasound of the chest for the definitive diagnosis of a pleural effusion is an example of an objective procedure that may obviate much of the traditional physical examination procedures used for the clinical diagnosis of pleuropneumonia (e.g., auscultation, percussion, ballottement). For diagnostic equipment to be used in this capacity, it should be available in the physical examination area.

The size of equipment is a determining factor in whether or not a diagnostic tool is suitable for the examination area.

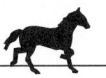

For example, equipment such as computerized axial tomography scanners and scintigraphy units do not currently fit into the space available in most hospital physical plants. Large, modular ultrasound machines can be cumbersome in small areas, although units available for field reproductive use (linear or sector scanners) are appropriate for any area, including vehicle transport. The choice of ultrasound equipment is an individual decision based on need, budget, and available units. Security should also be a consideration in stocking an examination area with equipment and medications. The clinical examination areas of most facilities tend to be high-traffic regions; this may be a primary reason for not stocking certain pieces of equipment in both university practices and private facilities.

MEDICAL RECORD

In 1968 Lawrence Weed[10] published on the use of the problem-oriented medical record. This system of record keeping emphasized the justifications for daily decision making during hospitalization. Problems are defined by the history, physical examination, and laboratory findings. Daily, and more frequently for intensive care unit patients, *subjective* findings are documented (e.g., appetite, attitude), and *objective* data recorded (e.g., heart rate, temperature). This information is then *assessed* by the clinician (e.g., patient is febrile), and a *plan* derived based on the assessment (e.g., resubmit laboratory tests, change antibiotic medications). The abbreviated form of this medical record is SOAP and is applied to each problem identified. Although the system encourages medical judgment and accountability, it more directly serves as a teaching tool within institutions by which the student's clinical thinking can be evaluated by the in-charge clinician. In private practices, the method of record keeping is more flexible and tends to document vital information that primarily serves as an accounting of services and provides a medical-legal record. Unfortunately, many medical records function only as an invoice and do not record medical information regarding the patient. This is more often true of ambulatory records but can be found in certain hospital practices. Whichever system is used, the responsible medical record should provide medical information, justification for charges, and a protection from liability. A thorough medical record further allows for the retrieval of retrospective information. The accumulation of data is beneficial to the communication of clinical caseload experiences to other clinicians for the benefit of their patients.

Medical Record Filing

Two major systems exist, numeric and name filing. Numeric systems offer consistency of the record and avoid the confusion of patients with similar names. The latter problem of name similarity is primarily confined to the nonregistered breeds of horses. Breed registration requires name approval to avoid duplication, among other undesirable designations.

Again, for record keeping purposes, clinics or ambulatory records for unnamed young horses are best designated by their dam's name and the foal's year of birth (e.g., Curious '00), and filed by month and year of examination. A "master" admission log should be maintained for record retrieval purposes, especially when a patient has been seen on multiple occasions. Color coding, along with numbering of the file folders, may be helpful in record retrieval. Computers offer the advantage that records can be retrieved by any one of a number of recall parameters (e.g., problem, client).

Record Keeping for Special Purposes

The Drug Enforcement Administration (DEA) requires veterinary practices to maintain detailed inventory records for scheduled drugs. Drug inventory and use must be documented in a record book kept accessible to the area contained behind two locks where the scheduled drugs are stored. Records must be documented to either a clinic area where a minimal volume of drug can be kept (e.g., a single vial of diazepam), or for patient use. Use should identify the patient, volume used, date, and the authorized person who obtained the drug. The drug use should be further documented in the patient medical record so as to account for the volume having been depleted from the inventory. A monthly or bimonthly accounting suitable for inspection should be conducted from the storage inventory and patient files to accurately account for scheduled drug use. This same accounting and inventory system applies to ambulatory vehicles.

Occupational Safety and Health Administration (OSHA) records are comparative to the DEA ongoing inventory and use records and are stringent in terms of compliance with OSHA regulations.[11] Documentation regarding safety procedures (e.g., fire safety inspections) are required following an initial inspection for labeling and safety protocol. Upgrading of Material Safety Data Sheets (MSDS) is a further requirement and should comply with current standards.

REFERENCES

1. Byars TD, Dixon T: Equine insurance, *The compendium* 15:614-625, 1993.
2. Baxter GM: Equine laminitis caused by distal displacement of the distal phalanx: 12 cases (1976-1985), *J Am Vet Med Assoc* 189:3, 326-329, 1986.
3. Rantanen NW: Diagnostic ultrasound, *Vet Clin North Am* 2:1, 1986.
4. Reef VB et al: Use of ultrasonography for the detection of aortic-iliac thrombosis in horses, *J Am Vet Med Assoc* 190:3, 286-288, 1985.
5. Franco RM et al: Study of arterial blood pressure in newborn foals using an electronic sphygmomanometer, *Equine Vet J* 18:6, 475-478, 1986.
6. Roudebush P: Lung sounds, *J Am Vet Med Assoc* 181:2, 122-126, 1982.
7. White NA: Examination and diagnosis of the acute abdomen. In White NA, ed: *The equine acute abdomen*, Philadelphia, 1990, Lea & Febiger, p 116.
8. Byars TD, George LW: A teaching method for rectal palpation in the horse, *J Vet Med Educ*, Spring 1980.
9. White NA: Examination and diagnosis of the acute abdomen. In White NA, ed: *The equine acute abdomen*, Philadelphia, 1990, Lea & Febiger, p 134.
10. Weed LL: Medical records that guide and teach, *N Engl J Med* 278:593, 1968.
11. Seibert PJ: Complying with the Hazard Communications Standard, *J Am Vet Med Assoc* 204:4, 531-533, 1994.

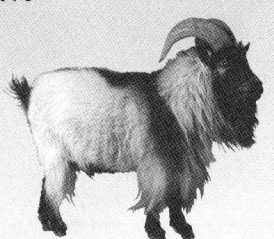

*See Chapter 20, p. 319, for neonatal manifestations of disease.

Continued

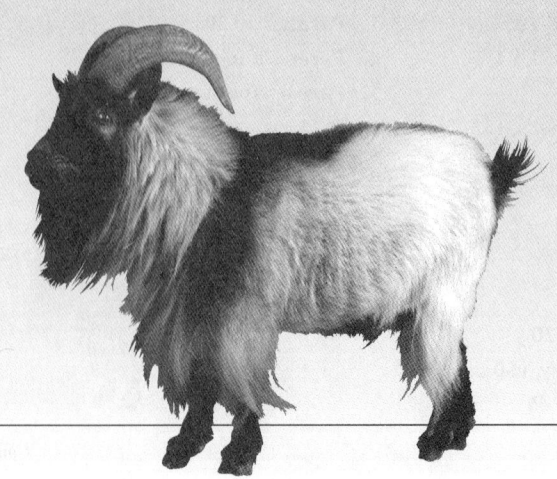

Pain

JAMES N. MOORE
Consulting Editor

MAJOR CLINICAL SIGNS/PROBLEMS ENCOUNTERED

Abdominal pain, 31
    Tail swishing
    Bruxism (teeth grinding)
    Pawing
    Stamping the feet
    Stretching
    Looking at the abdomen
    Kicking at the abdomen
    Lying down
    Treading the hind feet
    Splinting
    Elevated heart and respiratory rates
    Sweating
    Rolling
    Grunting
    Decreased milk production
    Ketosis
    Anorexia
    Depression

Chest pain, 32
    Reduced movement
    Rapid, shallow respiration
    Splinting of the thorax
    Grunting
    Abduction of the elbows
    Weight loss
    Hemoptysis

Pain in the extremities, 33
    Reluctance to move
    Abnormal gait
    Swelling
    Skin abrasions/lacerations
    Weight loss
    Decubital sores
    Exudation

Back/neck pain, 34
    Reluctance to move
    Reluctance to bend neck
    Pain on palpation
    Reduced performance
    Recumbency
    Straining

Pain on urination, 34
    Straining
    Prolonged urination/dripping urine
    Grunting
    Restlessness
    Estrus behavior
    Arching of the back
    Kicking at abdomen
    Tail switching
    Treading
    Recumbency
    Discharge

ANATOMIC AND PHYSIOLOGIC BASIS OF PAIN

What Is Pain?

STEVEN G. KAMERLING
JAMES N. MOORE

The International Association for the Study of Pain (IASP) describes pain as an unpleasant sensory and emotional experience associated with actual or imminent tissue damage.[1] However, this definition continues to be debated. Although most agree that pain is "perceived" by organisms with a nervous system, the degree of "suffering" experienced by various animals is controversial. In human medicine many feel that pain must be defined in the context of intelligence, consciousness, and the memory of painful experiences. However, pain reactions are readily recognizable in large animals and are clearly "remembered" by animals that have experienced them. Perhaps what differentiates humans and other animals is the complexity and manner in which pain is expressed. In verbally competent humans, linguistically reported pain is the gold standard. In human neonates and animals, pain reactions or behaviors become paramount. Despite phylogenetic differences among members of the animal kingdom, it is incumbent upon the veterinary practitioner to presume that large animals perceive, react to, and suffer from painful stimuli and experiences.

Nociceptors and Nociception

The IASP definition of pain highlights two important aspects of pain, namely a sensory discriminative component and an emotional, or affective, component. The sensory component of pain is often referred to as nociception, or the sensory reception of noxious or injurious stimuli by nociceptors. Nociceptors are sensory neurons with free, unmyelinated nerve endings. They respond selectively to noxious stimuli but cannot be characterized based purely on histology. The three main functional types of nociceptors are mechanical, thermal, and chemical. Anatomically they are classified as A-delta or C-polymodal. A-delta nociceptors are unimodal, high-threshold, small-diameter, myelinated fibers that respond to deforming mechanical stimuli such as tissue compression. They typically do not respond to excessive temperatures or chemicals unless sensitized. C-polymodal nociceptors are small-diameter, unmyelinated, slowly conducting fibers that respond to chemical, thermal, and mechanical extremes. Thermal nociceptors, typically found in skin, respond to temperatures in excess of 45° C. For example, we have observed that radiant heat sufficient to raise the temperature of the skin over the withers (44° to 50° C) elicits the protective twitch reflex within 5 seconds. Chemical nociceptors respond to noxious chemicals (e.g., caustics, acids, bases, hypertonic solutions) or inflammatory mediators (e.g., prostaglandins, bradykinin). Nociceptors exist in muscles, the skin, the periosteum, most internal organs, the tooth pulp, the cornea, and the meninges. With the exception of the meninges (i.e., headache), "pain" in these tissues can be readily recognized.

Nociceptors serve to warn an animal of imminent or ongoing tissue injury. This warning typically elicits protective reflexes, such as the skin twitch reflex described above. Such nociceptive reflexes attempt to separate the animal from the noxious stimulus. The limb withdrawal reflex after the application of a hoof tester can be used as a measure of pain threshold in horses.[2] Pain threshold can be defined as the stimulus intensity (e.g., temperature, pressure) that is sufficient to elicit a behavioral pain response. We have observed that nonsteroidal antiinflammatory analgesics (NSAIDs) increase the amount of hoof compression tolerated by laminitic horses.[3] We have also observed that opioid analgesics lengthen the time required to produce the limb withdrawal and skin twitch reflexes in horses exposed to noxious heat.[4] Because these analgesics act preferentially on nociceptors and their peripheral and central pathways, these reflexes represent true "pain responses" by the horse. Clearly, such reflexes are critical in protecting horses from hostile environmental insults.

Inflammatory Pain and Hyperalgesia

The reflexes discussed above signal imminent tissue injury; but what happens when tissues are histopathologically damaged? The sensitivity of damaged tissues (especially skin) to pain and other stimuli differs from that of normal intact tissue. The first phenomenon to be observed in injured tissue is allodynia. Allodynia refers to the production of pain by a stimulus that previously was nonpainful. For example, lightly probing the withers of a horse does not usually elicit a response. However, we have observed that gently stroking the same site in horses with severe dermatophylosis can elicit a vigorous, attention-getting twitch response. This is an example of allodynia. The second phenomenon is hyperalgesia.

Hyperalgesia occurs when previously painful stimuli produce pain of greater magnitude, duration, or area. Osteoarthritis is a condition associated with inflammatory hyperalgesia, in which weight bearing on already painful joints results in greater pain. Nonsteroidal antiinflammatory drugs are particularly effective in reducing hyperalgesia, but have little effect on pain sensitivity in healthy tissue.

The phenomenon of hyperalgesia is a subject of considerable study. Current theories suggest that persistent tissue injury is mediated by numerous endogenous chemicals, which can change both the peripheral and central nervous systems. Peripheral hyperalgesia occurs at the site of injury. It is mediated by the release of arachidonic acid and its ultimate conversion to prostaglandins (mainly PGE_2) and leukotrienes (mainly LTB_4 products). Together with bradykinin and histamine, nociceptors are rendered hyperresponsive to noxious stimuli. Serotonin from platelets and mast cells, and interleukin (IL) 1, IL8, and tumor necrosis factor from immune cells contribute. Retrograde release of substance P and calcitonin gene–related peptide from neighboring nociceptors amplify the hyperalgesia. The sympathetic nervous system appears to be involved in hyperalgesia, as norepinephrine, released from sympathetic efferents, provides additional amplification. In fact, sympathectomies have been used to minimize certain types of intractable pain.

More recently adenosine (and other ATP products) and the excitatory amino acid glutamate have been implicated in the pain amplification cascade. The short-lived gaseous neurotransmitter, nitric oxide, is produced at inflammatory sites and by pain neurons in the central nervous system. Nitric oxide is formed by the action of the enzyme, nitric oxide synthase, on L-arginine. In fact, nitric oxide synthase inhibitors (e.g., L-NAME) reduce inflammatory pain in several laboratory animal species. Nerve growth factor has also been recognized as contributing to hyperalgesia. As research in this area grows, new mediators are likely to be identified. A number of these mediators appear to exist in horses and other species. Currently, they are targets for pharmacologic intervention in the pain process.[5]

Hyperalgesia also appears to occur centrally within the spinal cord, mirroring the peripheral event. Many of the same transmitter substances released peripherally by the nociceptor are released in the spinal cord. Persistent tissue damage triggers the release of substance P, and glutamate/aspartate from the intraspinal terminals of the nociceptors, activating NK-1 and NMDA/AMPA receptors, respectively. These powerful excitatory transmitters appear to lower the response thresholds of second-order dorsal horn neurons. This process appears to mediate both allodynia and hyperalgesia and is often referred to as secondary or central hyperalgesia. In fact, recent evidence suggests that prostaglandins are also released into the spinal cord from peripherally activated nociceptors. Therefore aspirin-like NSAIDs, which inhibit prostaglandin synthesis, may act at the site of injury and centrally to relieve inflammatory pain. Lastly, persistent tissue inflammation may recruit previously inactive neurons or silent nociceptors, which are quiescent in normal tissue. These nociceptors may further enhance the excitability of the spinal cord to peripheral pain.

The prevention of secondary hyperalgesia is of great interest in human and veterinary medicine. It has been proposed that if the barrage of sensory impulses from damaged tissue can be prevented from influencing the spinal cord, less central hyperalgesia should occur. This has been supported by a growing number of studies. For example, intraspinal administration of local anesthetics and opiates to animals before surgery results in less postoperative pain than if the same drugs are administered postoperatively. Thus the preemptive use of analgesics and anesthetics may reduce postoperative pain and improve recovery. The relatively common procedure of lumbar puncture should lend itself well to preemptive

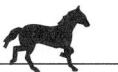

analgesic therapy in horses and other large animals. From these approaches, it has been suggested that the developing nervous system remembers pain. Stated another way, pain changes the nervous system. Consequently, the long-term impact of surgery-induced pain should perhaps be reexamined.

Pain Transmission Within the Central Nervous System

The simplest pain responses are unconscious motor reflexes. These reflexes are segmentally controlled within the spinal cord and do not require conscious intervention. In fact, animals whose spinal cords have been severed can still demonstrate withdrawal reflexes below the level of transection. Such reflexes normally serve to protect animals from injury.

Noxious stimuli are initially transduced by A-delta and C-nociceptors, which then synapse with spinal cord dorsal horn neurons in several of the layers or laminae. Lamina I (i.e., the marginal zone), the most superficially located layer, receives A-delta and C fibers that carry pain and temperature information. Lamina II (i.e., the substantia gelatinosa) consists mostly of interneurons that integrate information from A-delta and C-fibers from Lissauer's tract. Warmth, cold, and pain are integrated and modulated in laminae III and IV. Lamina V and VI neurons are critical in pain processing and modulation. They receive information primarily from thermosensitive and mechanosensitive nociceptors and may project directly to the thalamus and brain. They also receive input from descending brainstem pathways capable of modulating pain signals.[6] The relatively superficial location of the pain pathways in the spinal cord helps explain the rapid and selective analgesia achieved after intrathecal administration of local anesthetics in horses.

The dorsal column pathway and spinothalamic tract are involved in conveying pain signals from the spinal cord to the brainstem or brain. There are species differences in the roles of each of these pathways. For example, the spinothalamic tract is more important in pain transmission in primates than nonprimates. The dorsal column–medial lemniscus pathway carries information about pain, touch, and pressure. It is unique in that some nociceptors travel directly to the brainstem via this pathway, resulting in rapid contact between periphery and brain. The brainstem plays a key role in the autonomic responses to pain (see below). Cells from the medial lemniscus synapse with the intralaminar nuclei of the thalamus. The spinothalamic tract carries information about pain, temperature, and to some extent, touch. However, spinothalamic tract cells originate mainly in lamina V and do not synapse with the brainstem. Instead they innervate the ventral posterior and other nuclei of the thalamus. The trigeminal nerve contains nociceptors that convey temperature and pain information from the face, jaw, teeth, tongue, and lips. These trigeminal nociceptors synapse with the nucleus of the spinal tract (similar to the spinothalamic tract) and go on to form the trigeminothalamic tract. This is a particularly important pathway in horses considering that orofacial pain, applied through a bit, is employed to command attention and control motor behavior. The spinothalamic tract pathways appear to play an important, albeit not exclusive, role in chronic burning pain states especially involving the polymodal nociceptors. Overall, it is generally believed that the lateral thalamus is involved in the discriminative sensory component of pain, while the medial thalamus mediates the emotional and motivational aspects of pain.[7]

Processing of pain in cortical sites may to some extent underlie species differences in the experience and expression of pain. Clearly, the relative size and complexity of the cerebral cortex differs among animals. Modern functional imaging studies show that painful stimuli activate subcortical regions such as the periaqueductal gray, the hypothalamus, the amygdala, and the cerebellum. However, pain stimuli selectively activate cortical sites such as the insular and cingulate cortices, which receive input from the thalamus. Interestingly, the frontal and cingulate cortices of the cerebrum seem to be necessary for experiencing suffering. Early human studies have indicated that patients receiving frontal lobotomies were able to describe a painful stimulus but not be concerned about it.[7,8]

Types of Physical Pain

Pain has often been categorized as superficial, deep somatic, and visceral. Cutaneous or superficial pain tends to be definitive, well localized, constant, and may follow the distribution of somatic nerves. Deep somatic and visceral pain tends to be diffuse, dull, poorly localized, periodic, and elicits more pronounced autonomic changes. Visceral pain may also be referred to other deep or cutaneous sites.

It may be more relevant for the practitioner to identify pain in terms of its site of origin. Visceral, musculoskeletal, and cutaneous pain are perhaps the most recognizable in large animals. Rapid distention, ischemia, pulling on the root of the mesentery, or high luminal pressures of any portion of the hollow viscus elicits pain behavior in horses and cattle. This is most rapidly characterized by biting, looking at, or kicking at the abdomen or thorax and probably reflects an attempt to remove the painful stimulus from the referred site. Dorsolateral rolling, whole body hyperextension, and groaning can be observed in horses with severe intestinal colic. Muscle pain can be induced by strenuous exercise, trauma, or sustained contraction. Alterations in weight bearing, abnormal body postures, and lameness and tenderness upon palpation are the most recognizable signs. Severe rhabdomyolysis ("tying up") certainly initiates dramatic changes in muscle tension. Joint pain accompanies acute traumatic, infectious, and degenerative arthritis. It is associated with decreased range of motion, hypoactivity, and lameness. Cutaneous pain usually results from traumatic skin injury, bite wounds, or infections. Typically these sites of injury may be guarded, scratched, or licked. Exaggerated withdrawal or evasive reflexes may occur in an attempt to remove the noxious stimulus. Corneal pain can be elicited by chemical, thermal, or mechanical stimuli and is often accompanied by increased tear production and blinking. Dental pain, perhaps the only sensation in teeth, is difficult to detect in large animals, but has been associated with head tossing, jaw opening, or mandibular activation. Whereas headache pain is of considerable concern in human medicine, there have been no systematic attempts to identify or characterize this phenomenon in large animals.

Autonomic and Emotional (Affective) Components of Pain

The affective, or emotional, responses to painful stimuli seem to vary widely among the animal kingdom and within a species. As alluded to above, the neuroanatomic correlates of emotional pain involve higher brain functions and add another dimension to simple reflex responses. Humans experiencing pain often use terms such as exhausting, terrifying, sickening, cruel, and vicious. Changes in facial expression, body posture, and gestures signaling disgust, fear, and anger have also been described.[9] These expressions serve to alert others to an individual's condition of pain. Some of these human "emotions" may have large-animal counterparts. In addition to site-related motor responses, changes in temperament have been described.[10] Animals showing aggression in the form of kicking, biting, striking, head butting, teeth grinding, fighting, and escaping may be in pain. Grunting, moaning, or squealing may be heard. On the other hand, some individuals may appear docile and defeated. Changes in facial expression such as dull eyes; drooping eyelids, ears, and head; excessive tears; and hyperresponsiveness to light or sound may be observed. Thus animals and humans may share the fear-, anxiety-, and anger-associated expressions of pain.

Along with the expression of pain behaviors, autonomic disturbances in homeostasis occur. It is worth noting that some nociceptive dorsal horn neurons synapse with the pontine and midbrain reticular formation, the lateral periaqueductal gray (PAG), the ventral medulla, and the hypothalamus. Nociceptive activation of the ventral medulla results in increases in heart and respiratory rates and blood pressure. Activation of the hypothalamus results in the release of vasopressin and ACTH, which affect hemodynamics and blood glucose. Stimulation of the reticular formation results in enhanced vigilance and attention. Activation of the PAG results in recruitment of an endogenous, descending pain suppression system (see endogenous pain suppression below), which "attempts" to modulate the intensity of painful stimuli at the level of the spinal cord. These gross autonomic and metabolic responses contribute to the aversive and arousal nature of the painful experience.

In addition to its aversive quality, pain can motivate and be learned and avoided by animals. The application of acute pain is used universally to control equine behavior. The use of a bit to coerce movement, the application of a whip to increase racing performance, the employment of a twitch for restraint, and sole "soring" to increase gait animation serve as examples. There is little doubt that the average horse learns and remembers the aversiveness of these stimuli and "works" to avoid them. However, acute pain (e.g., kicking, biting) is inflicted conspecifically to establish social and reproductive dominance within a herd. Pain can also be used to subdue adversarial predators. Past experiences can profoundly influence the affective response to pain. Factors such as anticipation, anxiety, and fear can negatively influence future pain response. Horses who appear "head shy" from years of abuse have learned, all too well, how to detect and avoid imminent tissue injury.

PATHOPHYSIOLOGIC EFFECTS OF PAIN

Acute Pain

Pain of short duration alerts animals to potential injury and is adaptive for survival. It is also a signal to "disuse" injured tissue to promote healing and rest. It usually elicits quick behavioral action and resolves without a significant disruption in homeostasis. Acute pain may be caused by environmental stimuli, trauma, surgery, acute medical conditions, or normal physiologic processes (e.g., parturition). A common constellation of signs may be seen in large animals. Neurologic signs include behavioral excitement, confusion, tremors, rigidity, twitching, hyperreflexia, and ataxia or immobility, paralysis, and inertia. Cardiorespiratory signs include hypertension, tachycardia, vasospasm, venous stasis, and tachypnea. Gastrointestinal hypomotility or hypermotility, urinary retention, sweating, and hyperthermia may also occur. Acute pain of a more debilitating nature may produce more profound changes in posture, temperament, and locomotion. Head and neck ptosis, rolling on the ground, hyperextension or hyperflexion of the body and neck, widened stance, and prolonged sternal or lateral recumbency may be observed. A spectrum of emotional reactions (see above) from aggressiveness, anxiety, self-mutilation, and vocalization (moaning, grunting) to marked depression may occur. Specific lamenesses and weight-bearing deficits may accompany more specific musculoskeletal insults.[10]

Chronic Pain

Fortunately, most acute pain resolves and homeostasis is restored. However, extensive tissue injury or disease may result in pain that persists for days or weeks. Such pain is often associated with inflammation and accompanying allodynia and hyperalgesia. Pain states that persist for months, even after healing has occurred, are classified as chronic. Chronic pain often includes a continuation of the acute manifestations described above. However, more global, systemic changes emerge as unabated pain continues.

Chronic pain can be best assessed by noting changes in eating, sleeping, social behavior, reproductive activity, personality, growth and performance, body position, activity level, and certain physiologic signs. Chronic unrelieved pain may result in depression, inappetence, weight loss, and reduced growth or milk production (e.g., in cows or goats). Musculoskeletal pain may actually impair mobility and prevent normal social competition for food, contributing to further weight loss. Disruption in sleep-wake cycles may add to the overall debility. Psychologic alterations expressed as personality changes toward an owner or cohort may emerge along with a positional change in the herd hierarchy. Conspecific grooming and other social interactions may decline as well. Signs of psychomotor stress may develop including trembling and rigidity, as well as stereotypies such as pacing, head shaking, pawing, scratching, and stall walking.

The persistent disruption in homeostasis may have serious long-term consequences. Increased release of cortisol, catecholamines, and renin are associated with pain and other forms of distress. These hormonal responses can impair normal cardiovascular function and may contribute to hypertension. In fact, acute changes in plasma concentrations of cortisol, catecholamines, glucagon, blood glucose, insulin, β-endorphin, lactate, and growth hormone have been used as indirect measures of pain. Depending upon the site of pain or injury, prolonged recumbency in large animals can result in pulmonary congestion, hypoxia, pneumonia, and altered thermoregulation. There are also some data to suggest that chronic pain may be immunosuppressive.

Although the use of analgesics for pain relief is not discussed in this chapter, it is worth noting that analgesics can be used to diagnose pain. Opiates elevate the nociceptive threshold by preferentially inhibiting dorsal horn neurons in pain reflex pathways. This in part explains their ability to dull pain sensations. This occurs without altering other sensory modalities (e.g., touch, pressure). Opiates also activate (1) descending brainstem inhibitory pathways, which alter spinal pain transmission, and (2) ascending pathways to the nucleus accumbens, amygdala, frontal cortex, striatum, thalamus, hypothalamus, and ventral hippocampus.[11] These latter sites are intimately associated with emotionality and the affective and autonomic responses to pain. Therefore relief of the above behavioral signs and symptoms by opioids is indirect evidence that pain contributed to their expression.

Are Animal and Human Pain Equivalent?

Whether nonhuman animals feel pain the way humans do continues to be debated, along with the need for analgesics. Arguments favoring a difference include the following:
- The relative speed with which animals recover from major surgery
- Stoicism in the face of severe injury
- Anatomic differences in pain pathways
- Lesser-developed cortices in nonhuman animals
- Unusual responses to some analgesic drugs

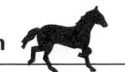

Arguments favoring a similarity include the following:
- The hypothesis that stoicism is adaptive and reflects a difference in pain expression rather than perception
- Acute and chronic pain symptoms and sequelae are similar
- Autonomic and endocrine responses to pain are similar
- The same chemical, thermal, and mechanical stimuli elicit pain in both humans and animals
- The same pain-mediating neurotransmitters and modulators are found in humans and animals
- There is qualitative similarity in the neuroanatomic pain pathways
- Surgical procedures (e.g., auricular, thoracotomy) and diseases (e.g., arthritis, pancreatitis, colic) that are painful to humans are also painful to animals
- Opioids are universally analgesic

Although these arguments persist, many large-animal practitioners avoid the use of analgesics because they mask symptoms and impair the diagnosis of underlying disease. Drugs such as NSAIDs may also produce serious side effects such as gastric/abomasal ulcers. On the other hand, public and regulatory agencies are insisting on the recognition, avoidance, and treatment of animal pain whenever possible.

Endogenous Pain Suppression

The expression of pain seems to differ widely across and within animal species. Some animals (and humans) cry out at the slightest provocation, whereas others seem to endure traumatic insult interminably. Most veterinary practitioners have had the misfortune of observing a horse finish or perhaps win a race, undeterred, on a fractured cannon bone. One may ask how this occurs. There is growing neurochemical and neuroanatomic evidence for the existence of an endogenous pain suppression system with segmental and suprasegmental components.

The segmental component is thought to exist within the dorsal horn of the spinal cord. It is probably this system that we activate when we lightly but vigorously rub a recently acquired bruise for pain relief. Similarly, the licking or light rubbing of a fresh wound by an animal would represent the corollary process. The light touch/vibration stimulates larger-diameter, A-beta mechanoceptive afferents at or near the site of injury. At the same time, A-delta and C-fibers are transmitting nociceptive signals from the injured site. These fibers somatotopically converge on a common spinothalamic tract (ST) cell. However, the A-beta fiber is thought to activate an inhibitory interneuron en route to the ST cell. Thus the large fiber damps down or closes the gate to pain signals delivered by the neighboring nociceptor. This formed the basis of the Gate Control Theory of Pain by Melzack and Wall.[12] This theory has also been advocated to explain the operation of transcutaneous electrical nerve stimulation (TENS) devices. These devices deliver nonnoxious electrical stimuli to the skin via electrodes placed at or near injured or inflamed sites. The DC electrical current activates mainly large-diameter, cutaneous, low-threshold mechanoceptors, which damp down nociceptor input from converging dermatomes. Variations in impulse magnitude, shape, frequency, and duration are selected to maximize this effect. TENS devices are used routinely in human medicine and by racetrack practitioners to reduce inflammatory pain.

For function in the face of severe pain and distress, certain endogenous coping mechanisms exist that modulate the intensity and quality of pain. The best understood of these is the descending pain suppression system. This system consists of a family of descending neurons from the hypothalamus, midbrain periaqueductal gray (PAG), rostral ventromedial medulla (RVM), and dorsolateral pontine tegmentum (DLPT). These pathways form a cascading neuronal circuit that ultimately influences activity in pain-sensitive spinothalamic tract cells in the spinal cord dorsal horn. The neuronal components of this descending system are activated by pain and other stressful stimuli.[11]

The command center of the system is the PAG. The PAG contains both opiate receptors and enkephalins. Enkephalins are small, short-acting peptides that bind to opiate receptors and mimic the actions of morphine. In fact, the name is derived from the term *en*dogenous *cephalic* peptide. Activation of or the application of morphine or enkephalin into the PAG activates the RVM. The RVM then releases serotonin from its terminals in the spinal cord dorsal horn. Serotonin is an indoleamine neurotransmitter involved in the control of mood, vigilance, sleep, and pain threshold. Once released into the spinal cord, serotonin activates specific dorsal horn interneurons that contain enkephalin. The enkephalins then act on opioid receptors located on pain-responsive neurons in the spinal cord. Stimulation of these opioid receptors inhibits the pain-responsive cells, rendering them less excitable by nociceptive signals from the periphery. The PAG also activates the DLPT, which sends its norepinephrine-releasing neurons to the dorsal horn as well. The norepinephrine acts on α_2-receptors also located on pain-sensitive neurons, inhibiting them. Thus three separate neurotransmitter systems play a role in endogenous pain modulation—serotonin, enkephalin, and norepinephrine. Activation of these systems ultimately results in inhibition of pain reflexes and pain sensations (i.e., analgesia).[11] This profound mechanism not only explains how pain can induce endogenous analgesia, but also how intrathecal and systemically administered morphine and xylazine relieve pain.

Another important morphine-like peptide involved in the production of endogenous analgesia is β-endorphin. It is now well known that pain, parturition, exercise-stress, acupuncture, and surgery increase circulating levels of this pituitary hormone along with adrenocorticotropic hormone (ACTH). It can be detected in plasma and cerebrospinal fluid. It is larger and longer-acting than enkephalin, and also binds to opioid receptors. It produces analgesia when administered and its effects can be blocked by the opioid antagonist naloxone. Endorphins have been identified in the horse. Endorphins are involved in regulating pain threshold in horses, as they follow the same diurnal rhythm.[13] Plasma concentrations of endorphins and pain threshold also appear to increase following strenuous exercise in thoroughbreds.[14] Endogenous opioids are also found in the gastrointestinal tract and are thought to modulate muscle tone and possibly sensation. We believe that this system is operative in the horse, as we have observed colic pain and diarrhea in horses receiving the opioid antagonist naloxone.[15]

Approach to Diagnosis of Abdominal Pain

Diseases characterized by abdominal pain occur commonly in horses and ruminants. In most instances the painful stimuli originate secondary to an intestinal obstruction or malposition (Boxes 3-1 and 3-2). In male or castrated male sheep and goats, the most common cause of abdominal pain is urolithiasis. When the pain is intestinal in origin, there may be distention of the intestinal wall with gas or ingesta, increased tension on the mesentery, or ischemia of the intestine. The clinical signs exhibited by the animal depend on the species, the age of the particular animal, and the severity of the underlying cause. The presence of abdominal pain may be characterized by outward clinical signs ranging from mild depression to repeated pawing or stamping of the feet to violent behavior. For example, in the horse many problems can cause abdominal pain, ranging from distention of the cecum with gas to simple obstruction of the intestinal lumen with ingesta to severe strangulation obstructions (see Colic, Chapter 7). Consequently,

BOX 3-1

Causes of Abdominal Pain in the Horse

COMMON CAUSES
Accumulation of gas
Intestinal obstruction
Intestinal muscle spasm (cramps)
Gastric ulcers (foal)
Meconium impaction (neonate)
Parturition

LESS COMMON CAUSES
Colitis/enteritis
Colonic displacements
Colonic volvulus
Ileal impaction
Ileus
Intestinal foreign body (sand, enterolith, phytobezoar)
Irritant cathartics
Parasympathomimetic drugs
Peritonitis
Proximal enteritis (duodenitis-jejunitis)
Small intestinal strangulation obstructions
Thromboembolism
Uroperitoneum (ruptured bladder in newborn)
Uterine torsion

UNCOMMON CAUSES
Acute hepatitis
Acute toxic enteritis
Ascarid impaction
Botulism
Cantharidin toxicity
Cholelithiasis
Rhodococcus (Corynebacterium) equi mesenteric abscess
Equine viral arteritis
Gastric dilation (cribbing, wind sucking)
Hernias (diaphragmatic, umbilical, other)
Intraabdominal adhesions
Intussusception
Malignant mesothelioma
Mesenteric abscess *(Streptococcus equi, Streptococcus zooepidemicus)*
Necrotizing enterocolitis (foals)
Neoplasia
Pedunculated lipoma
Plant poisonings
Potomac horse fever
Psychogenic colic
Rectal tear
Stenosis or stricture of bowel
Tetanus
Urolithiasis

BOX 3-2

Causes of Abdominal Pain in Ruminants

COMMON CAUSES
Abomasal gas (calf)
Abomasal volvulus
Abomasal ulcer
Accumulation of gas (bloat)
Cecal displacement/torsion
Intestinal torsion/volvulus
Intussusception
Peritonitis
Traumatic reticuloperitonitis
Urolithiasis
Uterine tear with peritonitis/adhesions
Vagus indigestion

LESS COMMON CAUSES
Abomasal displacement
Abomasal impaction
Atresia coli (neonate)
Cholelithiasis
Cystitis/pyelonephritis
Enterotoxemia
Enterotoxigenic colibacillosis (neonate)
Fat necrosis with intestinal obstruction
Ileus
Intestinal adhesions
Rumenitis
Thrombophlebitis
Uterine torsion

UNCOMMON CAUSES
Hepatitis/liver abscess
Intestinal neoplasia
Plant poisonings

Abdominal pain caused by liver disease is uncommon; however, it can occur in cases of severe hepatic lipidosis (especially in ponies and miniature horses). In horses with cholelithiasis, intermittent abdominal pain is the most common clinical sign, presumably resulting from bile duct distention.[16]

Approach to Diagnosis of Chest Pain

Generally pain associated with conditions involving the pleural cavity is severe. The painful stimuli usually originate from the inflamed parietal pleura because few nociceptors are present in the visceral pleura. Because of the primary involvement of the parietal pleura, the pain is referred to a site directly overlying the thoracic wall. Consequently, if the focus of inflammation is relatively well localized, as occurs with traumatic reticuloperitonitis-pericarditis, sensitivity to externally applied pressure may be restricted to one area of the chest wall (Box 3-3). If, however, the inflammation is generalized as in equine pleuropneumonia, pain may be elicited by applying digital pressure over several sites. Similarly, because movement of the inflamed tissue accentuates the production of painful impulses, the animal remains stationary and is reluctant to lie down; the elbows are abducted; the chest wall is splinted; and the respiratory excursions are shallow, rapid, and accompanied by grunting. It is common that the severity of pain is reduced as the volume of pleural effusion increases.

Chest pain may also develop acutely as a result of pulmonary arterial thromboembolism in cattle (Box 3-4). Pre-

the clinical signs exhibited by the horse may range from repeated pawing with a front foot and turning around to look at the abdominal region to uncontrollable rolling and thrashing. Although the severity of the clinical signs exhibited by the horse tends to correlate with the severity of the underlying problem, exceptions to this rule occur commonly. Thus the importance of performing a thorough physical examination in these instances cannot be overstated. Finally, the age of the animal must be considered in light of the clinical signs manifested. For example, the foal frequently swishes its tail from side to side and rolls up onto its back as part of its characteristic response to the presence of abdominal pain. In addition, bruxism is not an uncommon manifestation of pain in foals.

BOX 3-3

Causes of Chest Pain in the Horse

COMMON CAUSES
Lung abscess
Pleuritis
Pleuropneumonia
Pneumonia

LESS COMMON CAUSES
Choke
Fractured ribs
Mediastinal masses (abscess, tumor)
Neoplasia
Osteomyelitis
Ruptured esophagus
White muscle disease (rhabdomyolysis, tying up)

BOX 3-4

Causes of Chest Pain in Ruminants

COMMON CAUSES
Pleuropneumonia
Pneumonia
Shipping fever complex
Thrombosis of the caudal vena cava
Traumatic reticuloperitonitis-pericarditis

LESS COMMON CAUSES
Acute bovine emphysema (atypical interstitial
    pneumonia)
Choke
Fractured ribs
Mediastinal masses (abscess, tumor)
Osteomyelitis
Pleuritis
Ruptured esophagus

BOX 3-5

Causes of Pain in Extremities of the Horse

COMMON CAUSES
Degenerative joint disease
Hoof wall defects
Improper trimming/shoeing
Lacerations
Ligamentous strain (sprain)
Navicular disease
Sole abscesses and bruises
Synovitis

LESS COMMON CAUSES
Bucked shins
Cellulitis/abscess
Epiphysitis
Flexural deformities (contracted tendons)
Fractures
Desmitis
Laminitis
Osteomyelitis
Osteochondrosis
Septic arthritis/physitis
Tenosynovitis

UNCOMMON CAUSES
Keratoma
Neoplasia
Purpura hemorrhagica
Toxins
Ulcerative lymphangitis
Upward fixation of the patella
White muscle disease (rhabdomyolysis, tying up)

sumably the acute development of pulmonic ischemia in such instances causes the local generation and release of several proinflammatory substances. Most of these problems occur secondary to thrombosis of the caudal vena cava.

Although less dramatic than that accompanying either pleuropneumonia or thromboembolism, pain also accompanies pneumonia and pulmonary contusions. The pain associated with pneumonia occurs secondary to pleural irritation and is only well localized if the parietal pleura is involved. Because the pain appears to be most evident during forced respiratory excursions, splinting of the thorax is common. Chest pain may also occur secondary to traumatic incidents. Although fractured ribs occur rarely in horses and ruminants, they must be given some consideration in an animal exhibiting clinical signs of chest pain. Fractured ribs occur more commonly in neonatal foals during birth and may result in respiratory distress. Clearly the force required to fracture a rib will cause severe bruising/inflammation of the underlying pleura.

Approach to Diagnosis of Pain in the Extremities

Although the reflex contraction of flexor muscles occurs with all types of pain, this reflex is most evident when there is

pain in the extremities. Thus, as a result of a painful stimulus and to minimize the continued stimulation of the nociceptors in the affected area, the animal alters its stance or gait to protect the source of pain. Therefore it is vital that the animal be inspected initially from a distance to determine which limb is involved. It may be necessary to move the animal either at a walk or faster gait to identify the affected limb. It is important for the clinician to recognize that (1) the painful impulses may originate from several tissues in the extremity, including the skin, joint, periosteum, muscle, or the sensitive laminae of the distal phalanx; and (2) there may be several factors contributing to the source of the pain. These factors may represent a particular conformational, breed, or familial predisposition toward development of the condition, the effects of nutritional imbalances on the development/stability of either bone or soft tissue, the effects of the use/performance of the animal, the possible involvement of infectious agents, and the effects of trauma (Boxes 3-5 and 3-6).

Careful palpation of both the soft tissues and bones of the limbs must be performed to identify sources of inflammation or pain. Furthermore, the responses, if any, to flexion and extension of the joints must be evaluated, and the examination performed in a systematic manner. It may be necessary to inject a local anesthetic over a sensory nerve or into a synovial structure (joint, tendon sheath, bursa) to prevent the conduction of pain impulses to the central nervous system. The judicious use of local anesthesia combined with a careful physical examination should allow the affected site to be identified. On the basis of this information, the clinician can then make efficient use of other diagnostic aids

BOX 3-6

Causes of Pain in Extremities of Ruminants

COMMON CAUSES
Degenerative arthritis
Foot rot
Interdigital fibroma
Lacerations and foreign bodies
Laminitis (horizontal fissures of hoof wall)
Sole abscess
Sole bruise; puncture wounds
Sole ulcers
Traumatic gonitis
Vertical fissure of hoof wall (sand crack)

LESS COMMON CAUSES
Caprine arthritis encephalomyelitis (C)
Chlamydial polyarthritis (O, C)
Coxofemoral luxation
Digital tenosynovitis
Mycoplasma polyarthritis (O, C)
Rupture of cranial cruciate ligament
Septic arthritis
Septic navicular bursitis
Upward fixation of the patellar

UNCOMMON CAUSES
Bone/physeal abscess
Bicipital bursitis
Fescue foot
Fractures
Neoplasia
Peripheral nerve paralyses
Sacroiliac luxation
Toxins and plant poisonings

C, Caprine; O, ovine.

BOX 3-7

Causes of Neck/Back Pain in the Horse

COMMON CAUSES
Exertional rhabdomyolysis
Fractures of dorsal spinous processes
Ligamentous strain
Muscular damage
Overriding dorsal spinous processes
Thrombophlebitis

LESS COMMON CAUSES
Fracture of the cervical vertebrae
Meningitis
Ossifying spondylosis
Postanesthetic myopathy
Tetanus

UNCOMMON CAUSES
Clostridial myopathy
Congenital defects
Renal pain (acute pyelonephritis, renal calculus)
White muscle disease

BOX 3-8

Causes of Pain in the Neck/Back in Ruminants

COMMON CAUSES
Meningitis
Muscle injury
Tuber coxae fractures
Urolithiasis
Vertebral/sacral fractures
White muscle disease
Vertebral/spinal abscess

LESS COMMON CAUSES
Bladder calculus
Clostridial myopathy
Pharyngeal abscess
Renal pain (acute pyelonephritis or renal calculus)
Ruptured/ulcerated esophagus
Sacroiliac subluxation
Tetanus
Thrombophlebitis
Vertebral neoplasia

(radiography, synovial fluid analysis, scintigraphy, ultrasonography) to determine the underlying cause of the pain and direct therapy accordingly.

Approach to Diagnosis of Back/Neck Pain

The association between pain arising from either the back or the neck and irritation of spinal nerve roots has not been as well established in large animal species as it has in small animals or people. However, there is considerable evidence that muscle damage, ligamentous strain, sacroiliac strain, and either fracture or overriding of the dorsal spinous processes of the thoracic vertebrae cause varying degrees of back pain in horses.[17,18] Attention must be given to the detection and treatment of exertional rhabdomyolysis in horses and postanesthetic myopathy in horses and cattle (Boxes 3-7 and 3-8). Each of these conditions is characterized by painful impulses originating from ischemic or damaged muscle. Similarly, the development of nutritional myopathy associated with selenium deficiency must be considered in horses and ruminants in certain areas of the country. All large animals are susceptible to traumatic incidents that may result in fracture of either cervical or sacral vertebrae. Horses occasionally rear up and fall over backward, fracturing the sacrum or dorsal processes of the thoracic vertebrae. Cattle fracture the pelvis or develop sacroiliac luxations when they slip on concrete floors, often when mounting is occurring during estrus.

Neck pain is frequently manifested by splinting and unwillingness to eat from the ground or assume any but the most benign neck position. Trauma is the most common cause, but meningitis may also cause severe neck pain.

Approach to Diagnosis of Pain on Urination

Although the term dysuria means difficult urination, its use has become synonymous with pain on urination. The painful impulses may arise from distention of the wall of the urethra, bladder, pelvis of the kidney, or irritation or spasm of the urethra. The most common causes of dysuria are inflammatory or obstructive conditions involving the urethra (Boxes 3-9 and 3-10). Thus care must be exercised to identify uroliths, strictures, urethritis, vaginitis, neoplasia, or fractures involving the pelvic bones. Because urethritis may coexist with other inflammatory conditions involving the urinary tract (e.g., cysti-

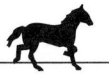

BOX 3-9

Causes of Pain on Urination in the Horse

COMMON CAUSES
Bladder calculus
Ruptured bladder
Less common causes
Cystitis
Neoplasia
Urethritis
Urethral calculi
Vaginitis

UNCOMMON CAUSES
Pelvic fracture
Urethral strictures

BOX 3-10

Causes of Pain on Urination in Ruminants

COMMON CAUSE
Urolithiasis

LESS COMMON CAUSES
Cystitis
Prolapsed prepuce
Pyelonephritis
Preputial injury/infection
Vaginitis

---

tis, pyelonephritis), the diagnostic plan should include physical and laboratory assessments of the kidneys, ureters, and bladder. Urine should be collected for urinalysis, culture, and sensitivity. A rectal examination should be performed to detect vesical calculi, tumors, and alterations in the architecture of the kidneys or the size of the ureters. Because the severity of pain can resemble that associated with acute abdominal obstruction, the physical examination must be thorough.

Urolithiasis occurs more commonly in ruminants than in horses. Of the ruminants, young feedlot steers less than 18 months of age and male sheep and goats (intact or castrated) appear to be at the highest risk. There is an association between sorghum feeds, diets high in magnesium, and the development of the condition. In horses, urinary calculi occur most commonly in geldings, and straining to urinate is the most common clinical sign. Rectal examination of the blad-

der, endoscopic examination of the urethra, and urinalysis are important aspects of the diagnostic plan. Most calculi in horses are rough, calcium carbonate stones, whereas most calculi in ruminants are magnesium ammonium phosphate, calcium phosphate, carbonate, or silicate in composition (see Chapter 32). Rupture of the bladder, the urethra, or occasionally the ureter may occur secondary to the obstruction.

Straining to urinate is a common clinical sign in newborn foals with a ruptured bladder. This condition generally occurs after the first 24 hours of life, occurs most commonly in males, and involves the dorsal aspect of the bladder. Presumably the rupture occurs during parturition. The diagnosis is facilitated by comparison of creatinine concentration in the blood and peritoneal fluid and by determination of serum electrolyte status. Most foals with the condition are hyperkalemic, hyponatremic, and hypochloremic.

REFERENCES

1. Anand KJS et al: Consciousness, behavior, and clinical impact of the definition of pain, *Pain Forum* 8:64-73, 1995.
2. Kamerling SG, Karns PA, Bagwell CA: Quantification of equine hoof lameness using a calibrated electronic hoof tester, *Proc Am Assoc Equine Pract* 9:307, 1988.
3. Owens JG et al: Effects of ketoprofen and phenylbutazone on chronic hoof pain and lameness in the horse, *Equine Vet J* 27:296-300, 1995.
4. Kamerling SG et al: Dose-related effects of fentanyl on nociception, behavior and autonomic responses in the horse, *Gen Pharmacol* 16:253-258, 1985.
5. Bevan S: Nociceptive peripheral neurons: cellular properties. In Wall PD, Melzack R, eds: *Textbook of pain*, London, 1999, Churchill Livingstone, pp 85-103.
6. Jessell TM, Kelly DD: Pain and analgesia. In Kandel ER et al, eds: *Principles of neural science*, New York, 1991, Elsevier, pp 385-399.
7. Craig AD, Dostrovsky JO: Medulla to thalamus. In Wall PD, Melzack R, eds: *Textbook of pain*, London, 1999, Churchill Livingstone, pp 183-214.
8. Yaksh TL: Central pharmacology of nociceptive transmission. In Wall PD, Melzack R, eds: *Textbook of pain*, London, 1999, Churchill Livingstone, pp 253-308.
9. Craig KD: Emotions and psychobiology. In Wall PD, Melzack R, eds: *Textbook of pain*, London, 1999, Churchill Livingstone, pp 331-344.
10. Short CE: Pain in animals. In Wall PD, Melzack R, eds: *Textbook of pain*, London, 1999, Churchill Livingstone, pp 1007-1016.
11. Fields HL, Basbaum A: Central nervous system mechanisms of pain modulation. In Wall PD, Melzack R, eds: *Textbook of pain*, London, 1999, Churchill Livingstone, pp 309-330.
12. Melzack R, Wall PD: Pain mechanisms: a new theory, *Science* 150:971-999, 1965.
13. Hamra JG et al: Diurnal variation in plasma beta-endorphin levels and experimental pain thresholds in the horse, *Life Sci* 53:121-129, 1993.
14. Hamra JG, Kamerling SG, Bagwell CA: Endorphin and exercise-induced analgesia in performance horses. In Tobin T et al, eds: *Proceedings of the Seventh International Conference Racing Analysts and Veterinarians*, Louisville, Ky, pp 471-480, 1988.
15. Kamerling SG, Hamra JG, Bagwell CA: Naloxone-induced abdominal distress in the horse, *Equine Vet J* 22:241-243, 1990.
16. Johnston JK et al: Cholelithiasis in horses: ten cases (1982-1986), *J Am Vet Med Assoc* 194:405-409, 1989.
17. Jeffcott LB: Diagnosis of back pain in the horse, *Compend Cont Educ (Pract Vet)* 3:S134-S143, 1981.
18. Martin BB, Klide AM: Use of acupuncture for the treatment of chronic back pain in horses: stimulation of acupuncture points with saline solution injections, *J Am Vet Med Assoc* 190:1177, 1987.

Alterations in Body Temperature

SUSAN L. WHITE

MAJOR CLINICAL SIGNS/PROBLEMS ENCOUNTERED

CONTROL OF BODY TEMPERATURE

Mammalian species maintain core body temperature within a narrow range despite extremes in environmental conditions. Core body temperature is not constant but exhibits diurnal variation. The normal range of temperature for individuals within a species may vary by as much as 1° C (2° F).

Maintenance of body temperature is under neuronal control in a negative feedback system. Warm- and cold-sensitive neurons within the hypothalamus sense existing core body temperature. Integrative structures located in the preoptic region of the anterior hypothalamus (POAH) that act similarly to a thermostat with a desired "set" point recognize temperatures as either too low or too high and activate both behavioral and autonomic effector responses to either lose or gain heat[1] (Fig. 4-1).

Heat production occurs primarily from muscle activity, which can be varied according to need. Muscle activity may range from inapparent contractions to generalized shivering. Digestion of food also contributes significantly to total body heat and may be clinically important as a means of heat production in ruminants both in low environmental temperatures and in high temperatures when the threshold for heat stroke may be lowered. Heat conservation occurs from adrenergic autonomic stimuli to decrease peripheral circulation and cause piloerection. Behavioral means of heat conservation include adopting a "huddled" posture, group aggregation, and seeking a sheltered environment.

Heat loss occurs from conduction, convection, and radiation from body surfaces and by evaporation. Sympathetic vasodilation of cutaneous vessels contributes to surface cooling. As ambient temperature rises, evaporative heat loss becomes more important. In ruminants evaporative heat loss is confined to the respiratory system; respiratory rate increases concurrently with temperature. In horses sweating aids evaporative heat loss. Behavioral responses that contribute to heat loss include seeking shade and wind currents, and wading into water.

CONDITIONS OF INCREASED BODY TEMPERATURE

Body temperature disorders in which the core body temperature set point is unaltered can occur from increased heat production, absorption of heat, or impairment of heat loss. Central nervous system disorders that disturb the hypothalamic regulatory center as well as certain drugs and metabolic disorders may also cause temperature changes. Phenothiazine tranquilizers are a recognized cause of loss of ability to control body temperature. Erythromycin may induce hyperthermia during hot weather, particularily in foals.[2] Hyperkalemic periodic paralysis has also been associated with episodes of hyperthermia.[3]

Exercise

During sustained exercise, heat production may exceed the ability of heat loss mechanisms, leading to a stable increase in core body temperature proportional to the intensity and du-

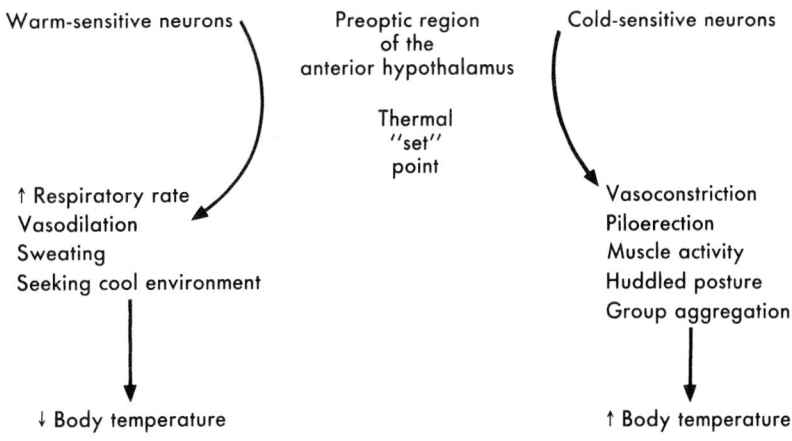

FIG. 4-1 ▉ Regulation of body temperature.

ration of exercise. The elevation in temperature often persists for several hours following exercise but returns to normal with rest as heat loss mechanisms remain activated. Body temperatures during exercise greater than 2° C (4° F) above normal, especially if reached early in exercise, are usually the result of severe environmental conditions and/or failure in heat loss mechanisms. Peripheral cooling to augment heat loss should be used to lower body temperature as increases in temperature caused by exercise are unaffected by antipyretic drugs.[1,4-6]

The intense muscular activity associated with generalized tonic clonic seizures may, like vigorous exercise, cause a rise in body temperature. If central heat regulatory systems are unaffected by the disease process, body temperature returns to normal no longer than 48 hours after the last seizure. Elevated temperatures that persist for longer periods should prompt investigation into other causes for the increased temperature.[7]

Malignant Hyperthermia

Malignant hyperthermia consists of a group of inherited skeletal muscle calcium metabolism disorders in which a hypermetabolic state of muscle is induced by the administration of halogenated inhalation anesthetics, depolarizing skeletal muscle relaxants, or, occasionally, local anesthetics. Rapid increase in core body temperature, skeletal muscle rigidity, tachycardia, metabolic acidosis, and muscle necrosis may lead to death. Although malignant hyperthermia is most common in humans and pigs, it has been reported in horses.[8-10]

Ergopeptine Alkaloid Toxicosis

Tall fescue infected with the endophyte *Neotyphodium coenophidium* contains vasoactive ergopeptine alkaloids that cause vasoconstriction and reduced blood flow to the skin of ruminants. These alkaloids also induce bronchoconstriction and pulmonary vasoconstriction, which further compromises ruminants' ability to lose heat, especially during hot environmental conditions. Affected animals have a poor appetite and other indications of poor performance recognized as part of the syndrome of fescue toxicosis or "summer slump."[11] A related endophyte infesting perennial ryegrass has been found to produce a similar hyperthermic condition in the western United States.[12] *Claviceps purpurea* infestations of either annual or perennial ryegrass also have been reported to produce a similar hyperthermic syndrome, which may lead to heat prostration and death when ambient temperatures are high.[13,14] Cattle affected by any of the above ergopeptine alkaloids have few to no clinical signs when environmental conditions are cool and heat loss mechanisms

are not challenged. It is not yet known, however, if all of the effects of the alkaloids are peripheral or if they may also act within the central nervous system.[11]

Heat Stroke

When animals are exposed to high ambient temperatures, intense solar radiation, and/or high humidity such that heat load increases at a rate faster than heat can be dissipated, heat stroke may develop. Heat stroke is more common in ruminants because of their inability to sweat and thus their diminished evaporative ability for heat loss. Sheep with fleece and large dense cattle are especially prone to heat stroke when denied access to shade or adequate water or when physical activity is imposed on them. Rectal temperatures will often exceed 41.5° C (107° F), and central body temperature may exceed 44.5° C (112° F). Horses continuously exercised in high heat and humidity may also develop heat stroke. Evaporative heat loss by sweating is the most important means of heat loss as metabolic heat production increases during exercise, especially as ambient temperature and humidity increase. Efficiency of evaporative heat loss diminishes when temperature and humidity are high and there is a significant radiation component resulting from strong sunshine.[15] Horses' susceptibility to heat stroke is enhanced if dehydration and electrolyte imbalances occur because of large losses of sweat (see Exhausted horse syndrome).

As rectal temperature increases above 41.5° C (107° F), the homeostatic mechanisms of temperature regulation fail; peripheral vasoconstriction, decreased blood pressure, and decreased cardiac output occur. The animals are lethargic and have weak flaccid muscles; prostration and shock occur rapidly. Disseminated intravascular coagulation, liver damage, renal failure, and myocardial necrosis are frequent complications.

Anhidrosis

As many as 25% of racing horses in hot, humid environments lose their ability to sweat and subsequently suffer from hyperthermia as a result of impairment of heat loss.[16] Although many of these horses are shipped to hot environments from more temperate regions, horses indigenous to hot, humid areas that perform less rigorously or not at all may also develop anhidrosis.[17] In addition to hyperthermia, clinical signs are poor performance, total or partial loss of ability to sweat, increased respiratory rates 3 to 5 times normal, and dry thin hair coats with areas of alopecia (see also Anhidrosis, Chapter 39).

BOX 4-1

Drugs Associated With Fever

FREQUENTLY
Penicillins
Sulfonamides
Erythromycin
Antihistamines
Procainamide
Quinidine
Amphotericin B

OCCASIONALLY
Cephalosporins
Cimetidine
Iodides
Rifampin
Levamisole
Furazolidone

RARELY
Chloramphenicol
Tetracyclines
Others

Modified from Lipsky BA, Hirschmann JV: Drug fever, *JAMA* 234:851-854.

BOX 4-2

Toxins Associated With Fever in the Horse

Blister beetle (cantharidin)
Selenium
Arsenic
Mercury
Chlorinated hydrocarbons
Dinitrophenol
Propylene glycol
Trichloroethylene-extracted feed
Mycotoxicosis

PLANT TOXINS
Pyrrolizidine alkaloid–containing plants, algae
Algae
Castor bean (*Ricinus* spp.)
Water hemlock (*Cicuta* spp.)
Jimson weed (*Datura* stramonium)

BOX 4-3

Toxins Associated With Fever in Ruminants

Arsenic
Selenium
Mercury
Zinc
Crude oil, kerosene, coal oil
Organochlorine, chlorinated hydrocarbons
Iodine
Paraquat
Dinitrophenol
Propylene glycol
Trichloroethylene-extracted feeds
Halothane toxicity (C)

PLANT TOXINS
Fescue toxicosis (B)
Ergot
Pyrrolizidine alkaloid–containing plants
Algae
Brassica spp. (mustards, crucifers, cress)
Bracken fern
Castor bean
Water hemlock
Milkweed (*Asclepias* spp.) (B, O)
Buttercup (*Calthapalustris* and *Ranunculus* spp.) (O)
Rhododendron (C, O)
Gossypol toxicity (B)
Jimson weed (*Datura stramonium*)

B, Bovine; *C*, caprine; *O*, ovine.

---

and extreme rises in body temperature.[19] Chronic or low-level exposure of these compounds may present clinically as hyperthermia.

FEVER

True fever differs from other hyperthermic states in that the desired core body temperature or set point is elevated. This new, higher set point is vigorously defended by the same mechanisms that maintain body temperature in health. Initiation of the febrile state can occur by a variety of infectious, inflammatory, immunologic, neoplastic, or traumatic conditions that cause the production of multifunctional pyrogenic cytokines by a wide variety of cells, but primarily by fixed or circulating monocytes and macrophages (Fig. 4-2). Currently at least 9 cytokines have been shown to induce the febrile response in man and animals. Of these cytokines, interleukin 1 (IL-1α, IL-1β) and tumor necrosis factor alpha (TNF-α) are the most potent. Each of these cytokines induce each other and stimulate the production of other pyrogenic cytokines (IL-6, interferon [IFN-α, IFN-β, IFN-γ], ciliary neurotropic factor, and IL-11) that signal cells through a common receptor (glycoprotein 130). Pyrogenic cytokines reach the POAH via the circulation and interact with the endothelium of the capillaries of the circumventricular vascular organs.[1,20,21]

The exact mechanism of action of pyrogenic cytokines in the central nervous system is unknown. The production of arachidonic acid and its metabolism to prostaglandin E_2 (PGE$_2$), particularly by the cyclooxygenase 2 pathway, is clearly important because cyclooxygenase inhibitors, and specifically COX2 inhibitors, effectively reduce the febrile temperature to normal, but have no effect on normal body temperature.[1,21,22] PGE$_2$ is thought to initiate neuronal signaling by producing a cascade of changes in cyclic neu-

---

Diseases of the Nervous System

Central nervous system disorders that damage areas of the hypothalamus associated with temperature regulation may lead to either decreases or increases in body temperature, although hypothermia is most common. Hemorrhage, space-occupying masses (abscesses, tumors), infectious or inflammatory diseases, or degenerative disorders have all been implicated in hyperthermia. Central hyperthermia is usually characterized by lack of diurnal variation, absence of sweating, resistance to antipyretic drugs, and excessive response to external cooling.[1,18]

Certain toxins and drugs may act to increase body temperature by an increase in metabolic work (Boxes 4-1 to 4-3). Chlorophenols and nitrophenols, used as herbicides and wood preservatives, cause uncoupling of oxidative phosphorylation within mitochondria and lead to rapid

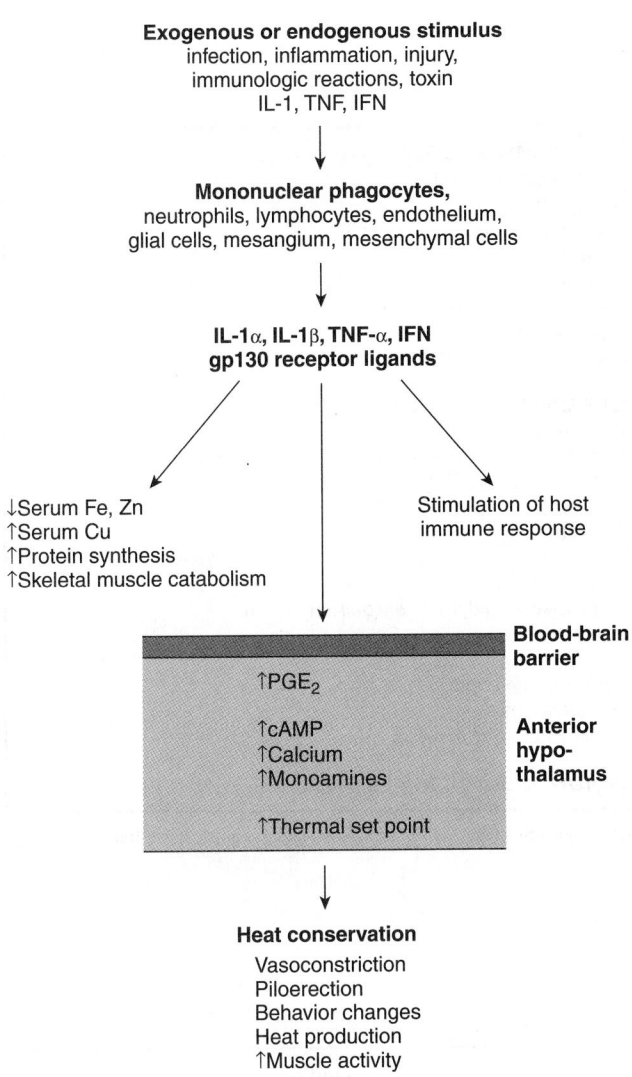

Exogenous or endogenous stimulus
infection, inflammation, injury,
immunologic reactions, toxin
IL-1, TNF, IFN

Mononuclear phagocytes,
neutrophils, lymphocytes, endothelium,
glial cells, mesangium, mesenchymal cells

**IL-1α, IL-1β, TNF-α, IFN
gp130 receptor ligands**

↓Serum Fe, Zn
↑Serum Cu
↑Protein synthesis
↑Skeletal muscle catabolism

Stimulation of host
immune response

**Blood-brain
barrier**

↑PGE$_2$

↑cAMP
↑Calcium
↑Monoamines

**Anterior
hypo-
thalamus**

↑Thermal set point

Heat conservation
Vasoconstriction
Piloerection
Behavior changes
Heat production
↑Muscle activity

FIG. 4-2 Pathogenesis of fever.

cleotides, calcium, and neurotransmitters, changes that result in a higher set point within the hypothalmic thermoregulatory center (see Fig 4-2).[21,22]

In addition to a rise in body temperature, the febrile state is accompanied by a variety of metabolic, hematologic, and immunologic changes. IL-6 and IL-11, induced by IL-1α, IL-1β, and TNF-α, induce the synthesis of fibrinogen, C-reactive protein, haptoglobin, ceruloplasmin, and certain macroglobulins, known collectively as acute phase proteins, by hepatocytes. In addition, these cytokines mediate the accompanying hypoferremia, hypozincemia, and hypercupremia of the acute phase response. Pyrogenic cytokines stimulate the activation and proliferation of T-lymphocytes and of antibody-producing B lymphocytes, which in turn produce additional cytokines that both enhance and inhibit further production of pyrogenic cytokines.[20,21]

Pyrogenic cytokines, particularily IL-1 and TNF-α, cause membrane perturbation in a variety of body tissues, with a resultant increase in phospholipases and the production of arachidonic acid. Subsequent production of mediators depends on the metabolic pathways for arachidonic acid in the target tissue. Prostaglandins induced by pyrogenic cytokines have been shown to stimulate the muscle catabolism associated with fever and to induce collagenase synthesis from synovial cells.[23] These processes contribute to the muscle and

joint pain associated with fevers that are relieved by cyclooxygenase inhibitors. Lymphocyte and granulocyte response to IL-1 has been shown to be blocked by inhibitors of lipoxygenase but unaffected by indomethacin.[20] Local tissue responses to IL-1β and TNF-α may stimulate afferent neural impulses that are responsible for many of the behavioral changes (increased sleep, decreased appetite, and loss of social behavior) associated with fever. Transection of the visceral vagal afferents has been shown to attenuate febrile behavorial responses, but not the temperature elevation, to intraperitoneal LPS injection in rats.[24]

Physiologic control of the febrile response is multifactorial and prevents extreme elevations in body temperature, which are incompatible with life in most instances. TNF-α inhibits further production of itself. IL-1 and other inhibitory cytokines stimulate the production of IL-1 receptor agonist, which prevents further binding of IL-1. In addition, one of the receptors on cell surfaces for IL-1 (type II receptor) does not result in cell signaling, and is thought to serve as a "decoy" receptor to decrease the concentration of IL-1.[1,25] IL-10, induced by pyrogenic cytokines, inhibits both IL-1 and TNF production.[26] Circulating pyrogenic cytokines may be bound to carrier molecules that reduce or prevent the interaction with receptors. For example, IL-1β has been shown to bind to α_2-macroglobulin, a protein increased during the acute phase reponse.[1] Within the brain both arginine vasopressin (AVP) and alpha melanocyte-stimulating hormone (αMSH) act as potent antipyretic agents. Receptors for AVP, which acts as a neurotransmitter within the brain, are found lateral to the PAOH and decrease fever in both natural and experimentally induced fever whereas injection of AVP receptor antagonist elevates fever and delays defervescence.[27] αMSH binds to local melanocortin receptors within the brain and on cell receptors of immune cells to decrease fever and inflammation. When administered systemically to humans, αMSH is 20,000 times more potent on a molar basis than acetaminophen in decreasing fever from endogenous pyrogens.[28]

In summary, the occurrence of fever during disease results from a complex interaction of multiple cytokines that act locally (site of tissue injury), systemically (in the circulation), and in the POAH of the brain and affect the immune, endocrine, and nervous systems.

Beneficial Effects of Fever

Body temperatures in pyrogenic cytokine-mediated fevers, in contrast to hyperthermic states, rarely exceed 2.5° C (5° F) above normal. Although the severity of some viral infections is decreased at these temperatures, most pathogens are not affected by a modest rise in temperature. Studies on bacterial infections in fish, lizards, rabbits, and humans, however, have shown an increase in survival correlated with the presence of fever.[29] Consequently, enhanced host defenses are the most likely mechanism for the beneficial effect of fever. Increased lymphocytic proliferative responses to mitogens, enhancement of B cells, and increased activity of interferon have all been correlated with fever. Activity of IL-1 and other pyrogenic cytokines is also increased at temperatures obtained during fever.[1,21]

One well-studied effect of fever on bacterial proliferation is the effect of hypoferremia. Bacteria, which require iron for multiplication, are inhibited by the reduced availability of iron during the acute-phase reaction. This response is augmented by the increased susceptibility of bacteria to low iron at higher temperatures.[30] Certain neoplastic cells are inhibited during fever, although it is yet unclear how much is caused by direct inhibition of neoplastic cell division or how much results from augmentation of immune responses.

BOX 4-4

Infectious Causes of Fever in the Horse

COMMON CAUSES
Upper respiratory viral diseases
Strangles, *Streptococcus equi*
Pneumonia, bacterial or viral
Pleuropneumonia
Gastrointestinal parasitic infections
Enteritis of unknown causes
Salmonellosis
Equine monocytic ehrlichiosis (Potomac horse fever)
Proximal duodenitis-jejunitis
Rotavirus diarrhea (foals)
Endotoxemia from gastrointestinal disorders
Septicemia, septic arthritis, osteomyelitis (foals)
Urachal abscess (foals)
Metritis
Peritonitis
Tetanus
Traumatic tenosynovitis, cellulitis
Localized occult abscesses (thorax, abdomen, upper respiratory system)
Tumors (see Box 4-6)

LESS COMMON CAUSES
Equine encephalomyelitis (EEE, WEE, VEE)
Osteomyelitis (adults)
Vesicular stomatitis

LESS COMMON CAUSES—cont'd
Tyzzer's disease (foals)
Malignant edema
Bacterial endocarditis
Mastitis
Pyelonephritis
Equine infectious anemia
Equine viral arteritis
Otitis media and interna

UNCOMMON CAUSES
Pericarditis
Systemic or pneumonic aspergillosis, candidiasis
Pneumocystis carinii (CID foals)
Brucellosis
Tularemia
Anthrax
Rabies
Lyme disease *(Borrelia burgdorferi)*
Nocardiosis
Coccidioidomycosis
Babesiosis, piroplasmosis
Toxoplasmosis
Other infectious diseases

IMMUNOLOGIC CAUSES (see Box 4-8)

CID, Combined immunodeficiency; *EEE,* eastern equine encephalitis; *WEE,* western equine encephalitis; *VEE,* Venezuelan equine encephalitis.

BOX 4-5

Infectious Causes of Fever in Ruminants

COMMON CAUSES
Mastitis
Metritis
Pneumonia: viral, mycoplasma, bacterial
Traumatic reticuloperitonitis (B)
Leptospirosis
Septicemia, osteomyelitis, infectious arthritis, omphalophlebitis (neonates)
Toxemia from gastrointestinal disorders
Enteritis
Abscesses
Pharyngeal trauma
Internal lymph nodes (C, O)
Verminous pneumonia (B)
Listeriosis
Bovine viral diarrhea (BVD), mucosal disease (B)
Otitis media, interna
Balanoposthitis (O)
Clostridial infections
Blackleg *(Clostridium chauvoei)*
Clostridium perfringens types D, A (C, O)
Anaplasmosis
Contagious ecthyma (C, O)
Haemophilus somnus infection (thromboembolic meningoencephalomyelitis)
Mycoplasma spp. arthritis, septicemia (C)

LESS COMMON CAUSES
Endocarditis
Pericarditis (B)
Bluetongue (O)

LESS COMMON CAUSES—cont'd
Tetanus
Vesicular stomatitis
Malignant catarrhal fever (B)
Verminous pneumonia (C, O)
Cystitis, pyelonephritis
Epididymitis (C, O)
Chlamydial abortion (O)
Enzootic abortion (C, O)
Epizootic abortion (B)
Caprine arthritis encephalomyelitis (C)
Hoof abscess, foot rot

UNCOMMON CAUSES
Neoplasms (see Box 4-7)
Rabies
Infectious necrotic hepatitis *(Clostridium novyi)*
Sarcocystosis (B)
Tuberculosis (B)
Systemic candidiasis, aspergillosis
Eperythrozoonosis
Brainstem, pituitary abscess
Systemic toxoplasmosis (C, O)
Tularemia
Pseudorabies
Brucellosis
Ovine progressive pneumonia
Chlamydial sporadic bovine encephalomyelitis
Other infectious diseases

IMMUNOLOGIC CAUSES (see Box 4-9)

B, Bovine; *C,* caprine; *O,* ovine.

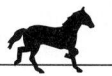

Adverse Effects of Fever

The beneficial effects of fever during bacterial infections in rabbits have been shown to reverse at temperatures greater than 3° C (5° F) above normal. Catabolic metabolic processes during fever are markedly different from the catabolism of starvation. Protein loss occurs four times as rapidly in individuals with infectious or inflammatory diseases compared with starvation-adapted individuals. Ketonemia is inhibited, resulting in the oxidation of large amounts of muscle-derived amino acids for energy. This cytokine-driven catabolism, combined with the decreased feeding behavior that accompanies fever, variable anorexia (even if feed is provided), and increased metabolic rate at higher temperatures, can result in rapid and severe muscle wasting, weakness, and atrophy. In humans, high fevers frequently cause seizures, especially in children,[18] but this is rare in animals, unless temperatures reach 42° C (108° F) in neonates. Prolonged high fevers in debilitated animals may lead to failure of the cardiovascular system.

Fever is one of the earliest and most prominent manifestations of the acute-phase reaction. Veterinarians have used the clinical thermometer to aid in diagnosis and monitor the progress of illness in animals since 1770. With the increased knowledge of the pathogenesis of fever has come a better appreciation of the diverse etiologies of the febrile state. In ruminants and horses, however, infectious disease remains the most common reason for fever (Boxes 4-4 and 4-5). Careful evaluation for the presence of infectious disease is always indicated, especially when the onset of a fever is abrupt; is greater than 39.4° C (103° F); and is accompanied by depression, variable loss of appetite, serous nasal exudate, epiphora, enlargement of lymph nodes, or diarrhea and a decreased or increased leukocyte count. Other causes of fever are neoplasia (Boxes 4-6 and 4-7), immune-mediated diseases (Boxes 4-8 and 4-9),

---

BOX 4-6

Neoplastic Causes of Fever in the Horse

COMMON CAUSES
Metastatic melanoma
Lymphosarcoma
Squamous cell carcinoma
Fibrosarcoma

LESS COMMON CAUSES
Granulosa cell tumor in mares
Undifferentiated reticuloendothelial cell sarcoma
Adenocarcinoma
Myeloproliferative diseases

UNCOMMON CAUSES
Hemangiosarcoma
Mesothelioma
Pheochromocytoma
Osteosarcoma
Myeloma of the gastrointestinal tract

BOX 4-7

Neoplastic Causes of Fever in Ruminants

COMMON CAUSES
Bovine leukosis (B)
Lymphosarcoma
Squamous cell carcinoma

LESS COMMON CAUSES
Adenocarcinoma
Metastatic melanoma (C)

LESS COMMON CAUSES—cont'd
Liver neoplasia
Mesothelioma

UNCOMMON CAUSES
Skeletal neoplasia
Malignant neuroblastoma

B, Bovine; C, caprine.

BOX 4-8

Immunologic Causes of Fever in the Horse

COMMON CAUSES
Purpura hemorrhagica
Urticaria
Drug-induced fever

LESS COMMON CAUSES
Immune-mediated hemolytic anemia, thrombocytopenia
Combined immunodeficiency of foals
IgM deficiency

LESS COMMON CAUSES—cont'd
Pemphigus foliaceus
Chronic necrotizing vasculitis
Neonatal isoerythrolysis

UNCOMMON CAUSES
Connective tissue disorders, rheumatoid arthritis
Transient agammaglobulinemia of foals
Bullous pemphigoid

BOX 4-9

Immunologic Causes of Fever in Ruminants

COMMON CAUSES
Drug allergies
Urticaria (milk allergy in cattle)

LESS COMMON CAUSES
Neonatal isoerythrolysis (B)

UNCOMMON CAUSES
Pemphigus foliaceus (C)

B, Bovine; *C,* caprine.

BOX 4-10

Noninfectious Inflammatory and Miscellaneous Causes of Fever in the Horse

Hepatic disorders
  Hyperlipidemia, equine hepatic lipidosis
  Acute hepatic necrosis (Theiler's disease)
  Chronic active hepatitis
  Cholelithiasis
Hyperkalemic periodic paralysis
Foreign bodies
  Nasal, oral, pharyngeal, tracheal, bronchial
Thrombophlebitis
Ocular trauma
Recurrent uveitis
Burns, smoke inhalation
Snakebite
Acute renal failure

BOX 4-11

Noninfectious Inflammatory and Miscellaneous Causes of Fever in the Ruminant

Phlebitis, thrombophlebitis
Salt toxicity, water deprivation
Acute bovine pulmonary emphysema
Fat necrosis (B)
Burn, smoke inhalation
Ocular trauma
Snakebite
Acute renal failure
Primary photosensitization
Cholelithiasis (B)
Postparturient hemoglobinuria (B)

B, Bovine.

---

noninfectious inflammation (Boxes 4-10 and 4-11), and certain drugs.

FEVERS OF UNKNOWN ORIGIN

Most febrile illnesses encountered in large animal practice are caused by infectious diseases that are readily diagnosed by careful evaluation of history and physical examination or

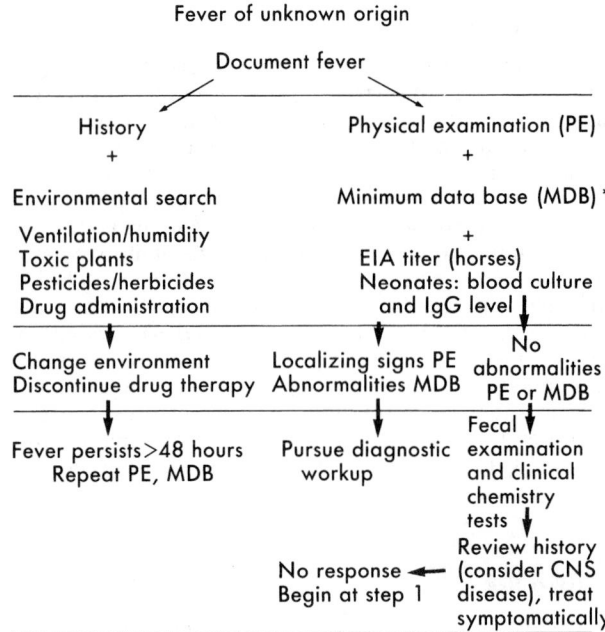

FIG. 4-3 ▮ Approach to fever of unknown origin (FUO). *CNS,* Central nervous system.

are of short duration, run their course, and progress to complete recovery within 2 weeks without a specific etiologic diagnosis having been made. Some febrile conditions, however, continue for weeks or months, accompanied only by nonspecific signs of depression, variable anorexia, and weight loss, while the diagnosis remains obscure. Patients with prolonged febrile episodes of 3 weeks duration or longer in which a diagnosis has not been made after a week of routine diagnostic efforts are considered to have fever of unknown origin (FUO). Most cases of FUO are caused by common diseases with an unusual presentation; an ordered, problem-oriented approach to diagnosis will render a diagnosis in 90% of cases.[30,31] The following steps are suggested (Fig. 4-3).

Document Fever

A temperature chart consisting of at least twice-daily determination of rectal temperature should be completed to characterize the fever pattern. *Intermittent fevers* are characterized by diurnal variation in which a peak elevation of temperature of greater than 0.75° C (1.5° F) occurs, followed by a decline in temperature, which in some patients falls within the normal range. Most intermittent fevers peak in late afternoon or evening, with the lowest temperatures occurring in the morning; but approximately 10% of the cases will have a reverse pattern. Intermittent fever is most commonly associated with pyrogenic infections, although it may occur in neoplasia, especially if tissue necrosis and inflammation are concurrent. *Remittent fevers* are characterized by a period of days in which elevated temperatures occur, followed by several days of normal temperature, only to have the cycle repeat again. Brucellosis in ruminants, equine infectious anemia (EIA) in horses, and blood-borne protozoal diseases such as babesiosis may exhibit this type of pattern. *Sustained fevers* are characterized by a consistently raised temperature without variation and appear as a "flat line" on a temperature chart. Fevers caused by drug administration and certain toxins may be of this type,

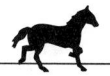

especially if the patient does not exhibit any other signs of illness.[18] Any pharmacologic agents being administered to the patient should be discontinued. Defervescence of fever from drug administration should occur in 48 hours.

Consideration of Epidemiology

Repeated efforts to obtain a complete history in chronologic order of development of clinical signs may be necessary to extract all the information pertaining to the individual animal. A knowledge of forage available, presence of nutrient deficiencies and excesses, toxic plants, infectious organisms indigenous to the area, as well as the threat of exotic diseases is necessary for the present and past geographic environment of the animal.

Physical Examination

A physical examination (see Chapters 1 and 2) should be carefully performed to evaluate all body systems as thoroughly as possible and repeated as often as practical, because it is unusual for a disease to cause a prolonged fever without the occurrence of some physical signs. Examination should include:

1. Horses
   a. Complete visual or manual oral examination; endoscopic examination of upper airway structures and of the trachea and bronchi (if length of the endoscope allows)
   b. Thorough auscultation of cardiopulmonary system at rest, with rebreathing bag, and following exercise; evaluation of peripheral perfusion before and after exercise
   c. Palpation of external lymph nodes, ballottement, and deep palpation of external abdomen for pain
   d. Rectal examination
   e. Fecal odor, consistency, volume and frequency of defecation
   f. Evaluation of external genitalia and mammary gland
   g. Evaluation of musculoskeletal conformation and gait analysis for lameness
2. Ruminants
   a. Complete visual or manual oral examination
   b. Thorough auscultation of cardiopulmonary system, evaluation of peripheral perfusion
   c. Palpation of all external lymph nodes
   d. Rate and quality of rumen contractions, abdominal ping, and ballottement for pain
   e. Fecal color, consistency, volume, frequency of defecation
   f. Complete udder examination and milk evaluation of lactating females
   g. Testicular and penile palpation of males
   h. Complete rectal examination (cattle)
   i. Evaluation of musculoskeletal conformation and gait analysis for lameness

Diagnostic Aids (Table 4-1)

All cases of FUO should have a laboratory database consisting of a complete blood count (CBC), urinalysis, and biochemical profile. The CBC should include morphology of red blood cells and white blood cells (WBCs), WBC differential, and fibrinogen determination. Chronic inflammatory disease produces characteristic changes in the CBC (see Chapters 24 to 26), and morphologic evaluation of the blood smear may reveal bloodborne parasites. Serum protein and albumin determinations characterize either hypoproteinemia or hyperproteinemia. Serum protein electrophoresis and immunoelectrophoresis fur-

ther classify deficiencies or increased production of proteins. Serum enzyme determinations and bile acid concentration for liver evaluation are also warranted.

Because much of the abdomen is unavailable to rectal palpation, abdominocentesis and evaluation of peritoneal fluid for protein, cellularity, and cell morphology are justified. Peritoneal fluid is obtained more consistently in horses than in ruminants with abdominal disease because of the presence of the greater omentum and the fact that fibrinous adhesions form rapidly in ruminants with inflammatory abdominal disease. Peritoneal fluid evaluation is usually most helpful in inflammatory diseases, but it may be diagnostic in some cases of abdominal neoplasia. Bacterial culture and sensitivity of peritoneal fluid are indicated in inflammatory diseases when WBCs show degenerative or toxic changes, but are rarely positive unless gross bowel contamination has occurred.

Blood cultures are best used after characterization of a remittent fever and evidence of pyogenic inflammatory disease from the laboratory database. Any antimicrobial therapy should be discontinued 48 to 72 hours before sampling. Three to five samples should be collected at least 45 minutes apart and are best taken directly into culture media. Sampling just before and during a temperature rise is more likely to yield positive results than sampling at the temperature peak and decline.

Single serologic determinations usually are of value only in those diseases in which one positive titer is significant and when the disease is characterized by persistent infection such as in EIA, brucellosis, or Johne's disease. In many instances, vaccination history and/or accompanying clinical signs must be correlated with titer determinations. Paired samples for toxoplasmosis, babesiosis, and various mycotic diseases (especially coccidioidomycosis) are indicated when the diagnosis remains obscure. Virus isolation, particularly in persistent bovine viral diarrhea (BVD)–infected cattle, may be helpful.

Evidence of gastrointestinal protein loss, chronic diarrhea, or persistent melena warrants several fecal or rectal biopsy cultures for salmonella in horses and calves, whereas such signs in adult dairy cattle also warrant ruling out bovine leukosis as the cause.

Also helpful are biopsies of enlarged lymph nodes, accessible abdominal masses, and the liver and kidney when laboratory data indicate abnormalities. Liver biopsies should be cultured and evaluated histologically because bacterial cholangiohepatitis can be a cause of FUO.

Radiographic evaluation, particularly of the thorax, should be performed in horses and small ruminants and is often possible in dairy cattle. Ultrasonographic examination of the heart may definitively diagnose cardiac abnormalities and provide more complete scrutiny of other organs in the thorax and abdomen. Ultrasonographic examination also aids in percutaneous biopsy of abdominal structures and may help make the decision for exploratory laparotomy.

Exploratory laparotomy without direct evidence of abdominal disease should be performed only in patients that are becoming progressively debilitated and in whom all other avenues of diagnosis have been exhausted. Blind exploratory laparotomies usually do not contribute to diagnosis, are costly, and are not without risk. Exploratory laparotomy is used for diagnostic purposes more routinely in ruminants than in horses.

The use of therapeutic trials of antimicrobials in FUO should be restricted to those cases in which strong evidence of a bacterial infection exists. The therapeutic regimen should be as specific as possible and administered for a predetermined amount of time. Inappropriate use of broad-spectrum antimicrobials for all febrile diseases contributes to interference in accurate diagnosis.

TABLE 4-1

Fever of Unknown Origin: Diagnostic Procedures

Procedure	Indications
Abdominocentesis	Abdominal pain
	Abnormal rectal examination (e.g., mass)
	Fluid wave on ballottement
Biopsy	Enlarged lymph nodes or other mass found
	Abnormal renal or liver function tests
	Vesicular or ulcerative skin lesions
Blood culture	Intermittent fever, especially neonate with failure of passive transfer
	Neutropenia or neutrophilia $\pm$ bands
	Increased fibrinogen
	Cardiac murmurs (bacterial endocarditis)
Radiography	Any musculoskeletal pain, heat, swelling
	Thorax, see Transtracheal aspirate
Synovial fluid aspirate	Joint effusion, heat, pain
Thoracocentesis	Abnormal percussion of chest
	Fluid line thoracic radiographs
Transtracheal aspirate	Persistent cough or nasal exudate with normal upper respiratory tract
	Abnormal auscultation/percussion of thorax
	Persistent increased respiratory rate
	Exercise intolerance with normal cardiovascular system
Immunodiagnostic screening	
Serum protein electrophoresis	Abnormal serum protein
Serum protein immunoelectrophoresis	Hypergammaglobulinemia
	Hypogammaglobulinemia (horses)
Direct Coombs' test	Hemolytic anemia
	RBC autoagglutination
Skin biopsy direct immunofluorescence	Vasculitis, purpura
	Vesicular or ulcerative skin lesions
Antinuclear antibody	Multiple noninfectious arthritis
ECG	Dysrhythmia, congestive heart failure
Bone marrow aspiration	Anemia
	Thrombocytopenia
Gastrointestinal absorptive tests (horse)	Hypoproteinemia with normal kidney, liver
Serology	Persistent undiagnosed disease
Exploratory laparotomy	Abnormal rectal examination
	Chronic abdominal pain
	Abnormal peritoneal fluid
Ultrasonography	Cardiac murmurs, arrhythmias
	Abnormal liver or kidney function tests
	Abdominal mass
	Suspect fluid in thorax, pericardium, abdomen

HYPOTHERMIA

Decreases in body temperature may occur when environmental stresses (cold, wet, wind) overwhelm the body's capability of heat production (especially when weakened from disease), when central nervous system disease has resulted in damage to the regulatory centers within the hypothalamus, or when adrenergic or sympathetic effector systems have been damaged. Newborns, cachectic, and very aged animals are most susceptible to heat loss caused by cold exposure (see Weak calf syndrome, Chapter 20, for nutritional implications). Concurrent signs of septic disease in hypothermic animals signify a guarded prognosis because the body's defense mechanisms are often overwhelmed when core body temperature declines.[32] Severely hypothermic animals (core body temperature <30° C) are profoundly depressed and have marked reduction in ventilation, absence of muscle activity, and decreased reflexes. Decreased intravascular volume and depressed cardiac function lead to hypoxia, acidemia, and cardiac dysrhythmias. Newborns are often hypoglycemic and have potassium imbalances. These animals should be warmed by protecting them from wind or drafts, drying them, and providing a microenvironment of high ambient temperature. Applying thermal blankets and housing them in an insulated stall, with or without supplemental heat, are superior to direct external heat from heat lamps or other sources. Direct external heat without environmental control causes cutaneous vasodilation, often exacerbates central hypothermia, and contributes to cardiovascular compromise.

Animals with severe hypothermia should be warmed gradually over 24 hours, with careful monitoring of body temperature and the cardiovascular system. Maintenance of adequate systemic perfusion is the most important means of preventing cardiac failure.[33] Acidosis and potassium imbalances are common and may fluctuate rapidly. Consequently, repeated measurements, especially when a patient's clinical condition worsens in the process of warming, are often necessary. Appropriate crystalloid fluids, warmed to body temperature, are usually necessary throughout the warming process. Evaluation of blood glucose and concurrent dextrose therapy, especially in neonates, should also be performed.

Warmed, humidified oxygen therapy both as an aid in treatment of hypoxia and as a means of warming is helpful.

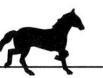

Gastric (rumen) or rectal lavage with warmed fluids may also be used. However, care should be taken in rapid rewarming because an imbalance in the basal metabolic rate (which is temperature dependent) and systemic perfusion may result in life-threatening cardiac dysrhythmias and worsening of metabolic acidosis and hypoxia. In many instances, adverse metabolic effects of disease are slowed at low body temperatures and, as body temperature elevates, signs of systemic disease become apparent. In hypothermic animals in shock, particularly neonates, severe anoxic changes in the bowel wall may result in severe diarrhea, sloughing of mucosa, or clostridial growth in the bowel.

REFERENCES

1. Dinarello CA: Thermoregulation and the pathogenesis of fever, *Infec Dis Clin North Am* 10:433-450, 1996.
2. Traub-Dargatz J: Hyperthermia syndrome in foals, *Equine Dis Q* 3:3-4, 1994.
3. Cornick JL, Seahorn TL, Hartsfield SM: Hyperthermia during isoflurane anaesthesia in a horse with suspected hyperkalaemic periodic paralysis, *Equine Vet J* 26:511-514, 1994.
4. Johnson SC, Ruhling RO: Aspirin in exercise-induced hyperthermia: evidence for and against its role, *Sports Med* 2:1-7, 1985.
5. Williamson LH et al: Comparison of two post exercise cooling methods. In Robinson NE, ed: *Equine exercise physiology 4*, Newmarket, UK, 1994, Equine Veterinary Journal, pp 337-342.
6. Kohn CW, Hinchcliff KW, McKeever KH: Total body washing with cool water facilitates heat dissipation in horses exercised in hot, humid conditions, *Am J Vet Res* 60:299-305, 1999.
7. Wachtel RJ, Steele GH, Day JA: The natural history of fever following seizure, *Arch Intern Med* 147:1153-1155, 1987.
8. Smyth GB: Spinal cord decompression and stabilisation of a comminuted axis fracture complicated by intraoperative malignant hyperthermia like reaction in a filly, *Aust Equine Vet* 10:133-136, 1992.
9. Waldron-Mease E et al: Malignant hyperthermia in a halothane-anesthetized horse, *J Am Vet Med Assoc* 179:896-898, 1981.
10. Manley SV, Kelly AB, Hodgson D: Malignant hyperthermia-like reactions in three anesthetized horses, *J Am Vet Med Assoc* 183:85-89, 1983.
11. Oliver JW: Physiologic manifestations of endophyte toxicosis in ruminant and laboratory species. In Bacon CH, Hill NS, eds: *Neotyphodium/grass interactions*, New York, 1997, Plenum Press, pp 311-346.
12. Wilson AD, Gay CC, Franson SC: An *Acromonium* endophyte of *Lolium perenne* associated with hyperthermia of cattle in Pacific County, Washington, *Plant Dis* 76:212, 1992.
13. Jessep TM et al: Bovine idiopathic hyperthermia, *Aust Vet J* 64:353-354, 1987.
14. Peet RL, McCarthy MR, Barbetti MJ: Hyperthermia and death in feedlot cattle associated with the ingestion of *Claviceps purpurea*, *Aust Vet J* 68:121, 1991.
15. Schroter RC, Marlin DJ: An index of the environmental thermal load imposed on horses and riders by hot weather conditions, *Equine Vet J Suppl* 20:16-22,1995.
16. Warner AE, Mayhew IG: Equine anhidrosis: a survey of affected horses in Florida, *J Am Vet Med Assoc* 180:627-629, 1982.
17. Mayhew IG, Ferguson HO: Clinical, clinicopathological, and epidemiological features of anhidrosis in central Florida thoroughbred horses, *J Vet Intern Med* 1:136-141, 1987.
18. Petersdorf RG, Root RK: Alterations in body temperature. In Braunwald E et al, eds: *Harrison's principles of internal medicine*, ed 11, New York, 1987, McGraw-Hill.
19. Hatch RC: Veterinary toxicology. In Booth NH, McDonald LE, eds: *Veterinary pharmacology and therapeutics*, ed 5, Ames, Iowa 1982, Iowa State University Press, pp 927-1064.
20. Kluger MJ: Fever: role of pyrogens and cryogens, *Physiol Rev* 71:93-126, 1991.
21. Mackowiak PA et al: Concepts of fever: recent advances and lingering dogma, *Clin Infect Dis* 25:119-138, 1997.
22. Coceani F, Akarsu ES: Prostaglandin E_2 in the pathogenesis of fever: an update, *Ann NY Acad Sci* 856:76-82, 1998.
23. Harris RL et al: Manifestations of sepsis, *Arch Intern Med* 147:1895-1906, 1987.
24. Luheshi GN: Cytokines and fever: mechanisms and sites of action, *Ann NY Acad Sci* 856:83-89, 1998.
25. Zetterstrom M et al: Delineation of the proinflammatory cytokine cascade in fever induction, *Ann NY Acad Sci* 856:48-61, 1998.
26. Leon LR, Kozak W, Kluger MJ: Role of IL-10 in inflammation, *Ann NY Acad Sci* 856:69-75,1998.
27. Pittman QJ et al: Vassopressin-induced antipyresis, *Ann NY Acad Sci* 856:53-61, 1998.
28. Catania A, Lipton JM: Peptide modulation of fever and inflammation within the brain, *Ann NY Acad Sci* 856:62-68, 1998.
29. Weinstein MP et al: Spontaneous bacterial peritonitis: a review of 28 cases with emphasis on improved survival and factors influencing prognosis, *Am J Med* 64:592-598, 1978.
30. van Miert ASJPAM: Fever and associated clinical haematologic and blood biochemical changes in the goat and other animal species, *Vet Q* 7:200-216, 1985.
31. Mair TS, Taylor FGR, Pinsent PJN: Fever of unknown origin in the horse: a review of 63 cases, *Equine Vet J* 21:260-265, 1989.
32. Normal DC, Grahn D, Yoshikama TT: Fever and aging, *J Am Geriatr Soc* 33:859-863, 1985.
33. Moss JF et al: A model for the treatment of accidental severe hypothermia, *J Trauma* 26:68-74, 1986.

CHAPTER
5

Alterations in Respiratory Function

W. DAVID WILSON

JEANNE LOFSTEDT

Consulting Editors

MAJOR CLINICAL SIGNS/PROBLEMS ENCOUNTERED

COUGH

Definition

Coughing, a normal and important respiratory defense mechanism, is the sudden, forceful, noisy expulsion of air through the glottis to clear mucus, particles, and other material from the tracheobronchial tree and glottis.

Pathophysiology

The mucociliary escalator and the cough reflex are the major protective mechanisms that function together to remove material from the respiratory tract.[1,2] Particles trapped in mucus are carried toward the trachea by continuous waves of ciliary motion that start at the level of the terminal bronchioles. Coughing may effectively empty the tracheobronchial tree of secretions proximal to the level of the segmental bronchi.[3]

Coughing is an involuntary reflex that can also be suppressed or initiated voluntarily.[2,3] The reflex pathway involves sensory receptors of nerve fibers that extend between epithelial cells and ramify throughout the tracheobronchial tree from the level of the larynx to the respiratory bronchioles.[4,5] These receptors, many of which are probably irritant receptors, are particularly numerous in the trachea and bronchi,

especially around the hilus of the lung and at the bifurcation of bronchi.[1,4] Other receptors that can stimulate coughing are found in the lung parenchyma and pleura and in other locations. Irritant receptors are stimulated by mechanical deformation such as that induced by pinching the trachea or by bronchoconstriction, by chemically inert dusts such as carbon, by pollutant gases such as ammonia, by inflammatory conditions, and by chemical mediators such as histamine (Boxes 5-1 and 5-2).[2,4] Sensitivity to mechanical stimulation varies along the airway, and in horses the upper airway cough receptors appear to be less active than in many other species.[6] For example, a stomach tube inadvertently passed into the trachea frequently does not induce coughing until it reaches the bifurcation. Similarly, endoscopic examination often reveals a large pool of exudate in the trachea of horses with little or no history of coughing.[6] Foals with *Rhodococcus equi* pneumonia often have a tracheal rattle, reflecting accumulation of tenacious exudate in the trachea, but may not cough. Repeated stimulation of irritant receptors over several hours does not appear to diminish sensitivity but may lead to changes in threshold.[4]

In addition to initiating the cough reflex, stimulation of irritant receptors in large airways causes reflex bronchoconstriction through the parasympathetic nervous system.[4] Stim-

---

BOX 5-1

Causes of Coughing in the Horse

COMMON CAUSES
Equine influenza A2 virus
Equine herpesvirus types 1 and 4 (EHV-1, EHV-4)
Other viruses (rhinovirus types 1, 2, 3; reovirus)
Bacterial pneumonia
Bacterial pleuropneumonia, pleuritis
Chronic obstructive pulmonary disease (COPD)
Mechanical causes (e.g., nonspecific dust irritation)
Pharyngitis (acute; chronic pharyngeal lymphoid hyperplasia)
Postviral hyperreactive airways

LESS COMMON CAUSES
Strangles (*Streptococcus equi* infection)
Equine viral arteritis
Parascaris equorum migration
Pharyngeal paresis
Guttural pouch empyema
Guttural pouch mycosis
Pharyngeal, laryngeal trauma or surgery
Postsurgical aspiration (e.g., after laryngeal prosthesis surgery)
Epiglottal entrapment
Subepiglottal cyst or abscess
Chondritis, chondromas of the arytenoid cartilages
Retropharyngeal abscess
Tracheal collapse (including scabbard trachea in ponies)
Tracheal stenosis, stricture
Choke, esophageal obstruction
Aspiration pneumonia (foreign bodies, feed material)
Inhalation pneumonia (smoke, thermal injury, noxious gases)
Lungworm infection (*Dictyocaulus arnfieldi*)
Pulmonary abscessation
Exercise-induced pulmonary hemorrhage (EIPH)
Pulmonary edema (smoke inhalation, acute renal failure, overhydration, septicemia, anaphylaxis)
Summer pasture–associated obstructive airway disease (SPOAD)
Left heart failure
Congestive cardiac failure
Neonatal septicemia

UNCOMMON CAUSES
Tuberculosis
Pneumoconiosis or silicosis; other interstitial pneumonias
Eosinophilic interstitial pneumonia
Nocardiosis
Coccidioidomycosis
Chlamydia psittaci pneumonia

UNCOMMON CAUSES—cont'd
Mycoplasma spp. pleuritis
Tularemia
Pulmonary hydatidosis
Tracheal perforation or rupture
Cryptococcosis
Dorsal displacement of the soft palate (laryngopalatal dislocation)
Rostral displacement of the palatopharyngeal arch
Idiopathic laryngeal hemiplegia
Guttural pouch neoplasia
Rectus capitis ventralis muscle rupture
Adenovirus infection
Pneumocystis carinii pneumonia
Esophageal ectasia, dysfunction, stricture, perforation; esophagitis
Megaesophagus
Progressive ethmoidal hematoma
Nasal or paranasal sinus neoplasia
Fistula (pharyngeal, esophageal, esophagobronchial, esophagotracheal, bronchobiliary)
Foreign body (nasal, pharyngeal, laryngeal, tracheal, bronchial)
Infarctive lobar pneumonia
Bronchopleural fistula
Pleural mesothelioma
Pneumothorax
Pulmonary tumor, primary or metastatic
Lymphosarcoma, lymphoma, leukemia
Pulmonary aspergillosis
Phycomycosis, pythiosis
Plant awn stomatitis
Anaphylaxis or acute drug reaction
Atrial fibrillation
Tetralogy of Fallot
Cor pulmonale
Endocarditis
Ruptured mitral chordae tendinae
Melioidosis, *Pseudomonas pseudomallei* (exotic)
Glanders (exotic)
African horse sickness (exotic)

TOXIC CAUSES
Crofton weed (*Eupatorium adenophorum*)
α-Naphthyl thiourea (ANTU)
Pentachlorophenol
Organophosphate
Carbamate

---

ulation of nerve endings in smaller airways does not directly initiate coughing but does cause bronchoconstriction, which may initiate coughing indirectly.[4] The role of bronchoconstriction in the induction of coughing is supported by studies in asthmatic people that have shown that coughing can be prevented by aerosol administration of salbutamol (a bronchodilator) or of local anesthetics or chromolyn sodium.[7,8] This suggests that mediator release (blocked by chromolyn) causes bronchoconstriction (blocked by bronchodilators), which stimulates irritant receptors (blocked by local anesthetics) and causes coughing.[4] Much of the airflow obstruction in horses with chronic obstructive pulmonary disease (COPD) appears to be mediated through these pathways and in many cases can be eliminated with atropine, a parasympatholytic bronchodilator.[4]

Myelinated afferent fibers from receptors in the pharynx, larynx, trachea, and bronchi pass in the glossopharyngeal, vagal and, to a lesser extent, the trigeminal and phrenic nerves to the cough center in the medulla oblongata.[1,3,5] Efferent fibers pass in the vagal, phrenic, and other spinal nerves to supply the muscles of the larynx, tracheobronchial tree, diaphragm, intercostal muscles and abdominal muscles.[1,5]

Mechanics of Coughing

The mechanical events that produce coughing occur during four phases: inspiration, compression, expression, and relaxation.[2-4] These four phases are necessary to create the decreased airway cross-sectional area and high airflow rates needed for an effective cough. Coughing is a maximum

BOX 5-2

Causes of Coughing in Ruminants

COMMON CAUSES

*Mannheimia hemolytica** or *Pasteurella multocida* pneumonia (includes shipping fever and enzootic calf pneumonia)
Haemophilus somnus pneumonia (B)
Lungworm infection, verminous pneumonia
Atypical interstitial pneumonia (B)
Chronic bacterial pneumonia with abscessation or consolidation (*Arcanobacterium pyogenes** and other bacteria)
Infectious bovine rhinotracheitis (IBR; BHV-1) (B, C)
Bovine respiratory syncytial virus (B)
Parainfluenza virus type 3
Mycoplasma spp. pneumonia
Caprine *Mycoplasma mycoides* subsp. *mycoides* infection (C)
Caprine arthritis-encephalomyelitis (CAE) pneumonia (C)
Necrotic laryngitis, calf diphtheria (B, O)
Abscess (oral, lingual, retropharyngeal, pharyngeal, laryngeal)
Trauma (pharyngeal, laryngeal, tracheal, bronchial, chest wall)
Esophageal obstruction, foreign body choke
Septicemia (neonates)

LESS COMMON CAUSES

Bovine rhinovirus (B)
Bovine adenovirus (B)
Bovine malignant catarrhal fever (B)
Bovine virus diarrhea (BVD-MD) (B)
Herpesvirus DN-599 (B)
Bovine herpesvirus type 4 (BHV-4) (B)
Bovine coronavirus (B)
Pulmonary adenomatosis (Jaagsiekte) (O)
Ovine adenovirus (O)
Caprine respiratory syncytial virus (C)
Ovine progressive pneumonia and arthritis, Maedi (O)
Aspiration, foreign body pneumonia
Foreign body (pharyngeal, laryngeal, tracheal, bronchial, pulmonary)
Inhalation pneumonia (smoke, noxious gases, thermal injury)
Pulmonary embolus from posterior vena cava thrombosis (B)
Anaphylaxis or adverse drug reaction
Reaction to death of parasites after anthelmintic treatment (B)
Milk allergy in cows (B)
Farmer's lung disease (hypersensitivity to *Faenia rectivirgula* and other mold spores) (B)
Pleuritis, pleural effusion
Pneumothorax
Diffuse fibrosing alveolitis (B)
Left heart failure (left atrioventricular [mitral] insufficiency, pericarditis, congenital cardiac defects, other causes)

LESS COMMON CAUSES—cont'd

High altitude disease (B)
Enzootic bovine leukosis (B)
Chlamydia psittaci pneumonia

UNCOMMON CAUSES

Diaphragmatic hernia
Pleural mesothelioma (B, C)
Sarcocystosis (B)
Sporadic bovine leukosis, thymic lymphosarcoma (B)
Tuberculosis
Tularemia (O)
Tracheal actinomycosis
Tracheal collapse, stricture, stenosis
Phycomycosis, pythiosis (B)
Pulmonary aspergillosis
Rhinosporidiosis
Zygomycosis, mucormycosis (B)
Pulmonary listeriosis (B)
Pneumocystis carinii pneumonia
Cor pulmonale (C)
Neoplasia (nasopharyngeal, oropharyngeal, pulmonary)
Postpartum hemolytic-uremic syndrome (B)
Esophageal rupture, laceration, ulceration, megaesophagus, hiatal hernia
Neoplasia, skeletal (B, O)
Buss disease, chlamydial sporadic bovine encephalomyelitis (B)
Winter dysentery (B)
Ascaris suum migration in calves (B)
Rinderpest (exotic)
Theileriosis, East Coast fever (exotic)
Melioidosis, *Pseudomonas pseudomallei* (exotic)
Contagious bovine pleuropneumonia (exotic) (B)
African bovine malignant catarrhal fever (exotic) (B)
Virulent sheep and goat pox (exotic) (O, C)
Peste des petits ruminants (exotic) (O, C)
Contagious caprine pleuropneumonia (exotic) (C)
Viral dermatitis of goats (exotic) (C)
Ibaraki disease (exotic) (B)

TOXIC CAUSES

Organophosphate, carbamate
Mercury (B)
Iodine (B, O)
Insect fogger (B)
Levamisole (O, C)
Nitrogen dioxide (B)
Hairy vetch (*Vicia villosa*) (B)
Sneezeweed (*Helenium* spp.)
Aflatoxicosis (C)

B, Bovine; *C,* caprine; *O,* ovine.
*Formerly named *Pasteurella hemolytica.*
**Formerly named *Actinomyces pyogenes.*

expiratory flow maneuver that begins with deep inhalation to expand lung volume, increase elastic recoil, and dilate the airways through the pulling effect (tethering) of surrounding lung tissue.[9] Closure of the glottis is followed by forced expiratory efforts involving the rib cage, abdomen, and diaphragm, which increase pressure in the abdominal, pleural, and alveolar spaces to over 500 mm Hg.[4] The glottis then opens suddenly, allowing the elevated alveolar pressure to rapidly accelerate gas flow from the respiratory tree.[2,4,9] This high-velocity gas stream shears exudate from the airway walls and lumen and carries it to the oropharynx, from which

point it is swallowed or expectorated.[9] Airflow stops before the animal has exhaled to residual volume because the glottis closes or the driving force provided by the muscles abates.[4] The characteristic sound of coughing is produced by tissue and gas vibration in the airway.[4]

During forced expiration such as occurs with coughing, the increased pleural pressure is transmitted to the intrathoracic airways and alveoli. Intraalveolar pressure exceeds pleural pressure by an amount equal to the elastic recoil pressure of the lung.[4,9] A pressure gradient thus exists between the alveoli and atmospheric pressure at the nostrils and

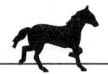

mouth. At a point in the airways known as the equal pressure point (EPP), the pressure in the airway lumen equals the pleural pressure because the elastic recoil pressure has been dissipated.[2-4,9] In the intrathoracic airways rostral to this point, the intralumenal pressure is lower than the pleural pressure; thus a transmural pressure gradient exists, which tends to cause the airways to be dynamically compressed or collapsed.[2,4,9] The location of the EPP is determined by the elastic recoil pressure, and thus indirectly by lung volume, and by the frictional resistance to flow in the airways between the alveoli and the EPP.[4] At high lung volumes, elastic recoil pressure is high, resistance in peripheral airways is low, and the EPP is probably located in the larger intrathoracic airways, which have cartilaginous support for their walls.[4] As lung volume decreases, elastic recoil force decreases, airway resistance increases, and the EPP moves more peripherally, subjecting lower and less well-supported parts of the tracheobronchial tree to dynamic compression.[3,4,9] Dynamic compression reduces the cross-sectional area of intrathoracic airways and thus increases the velocity of airflow through the narrowed segment.[4] These spikes of accelerated airflow promote more effective shearing of mucus and debris from the airway wall and lumen during coughing.[9]

Dynamic compression also increases the resistance to airflow.[4] Once dynamic compression of peripheral (smaller) airways occurs, further increases in expiratory effort cause greater narrowing of the airway; thus the flow rate that can be generated at a given lung volume does not increase beyond a certain maximum point (maximum expiratory flow).[4] Maximum expiratory flow decreases progressively as the animal exhales because lung volume declines. Thus coughing beginning at high lung volumes achieves the highest airflows.[4] However, only the larger intrathoracic airways are compressed and subjected to these spikes of higher airflow velocity.[2,4,9] As lung volume falls or if cough is initiated at lower lung volumes, smaller airways are dynamically compressed and cleared of mucus.[2,3,9] The effectiveness of coughing can thus be improved by repeating it several times in succession, either in a progression from high to low lung volume during the same breath or by inhaling between each breath.[4]

Because maximum airflows are lower in smaller airways, coughing is probably less effective in clearing material from the smaller airways than from the larger ones.[4] In the alveolar regions of the lung, gas flows are too slow for coughing to be an effective means of clearance.[9] In addition, because only intrathoracic airways are dynamically compressed and subjected to these spikes of higher flow velocity during forced expiration, the extrathoracic trachea should be less effectively cleared by coughing.[4] However, horses and other animals with long necks do not seem to have great difficulty in clearing their airways, although they do lower their heads and straighten their airways during coughing to assist the clearance process.

With diseases such as COPD that cause narrowing of the airway lumen, the increased resistance to airflow, especially in peripheral airways, causes the EPP to move more peripherally toward the alveoli, resulting in a reduction in the maximum expiratory flow rate.[2,4] In this situation the effectiveness of coughing in clearing the airways is reduced. Thus bronchodilation may greatly improve the effectiveness of coughing in patients with COPD.[4]

Of the many causes of coughing in large animals, viral infections such as equine influenza and infectious bovine rhinotracheitis (IBR) are particularly important, because they cause outbreaks of respiratory disease that have acute onset of coughing as a prominent feature and that are frequently associated with persistence of coughing for prolonged periods after signs of acute disease have abated. These features of viral infections reflect the decreased effectiveness of mucociliary clearance resulting from virus-induced injury to ciliated epithelial cells, together with exposure and sensitization of irritant airway receptors that leads to persistent bronchial hyperreactivity.[4,10] Affected individuals show bronchoconstriction and coughing in response to mildly irritating stimuli such as dust, stable pollutants, cold air, dry air, and exercise that would not normally cause coughing. Coughing subsides only when the airway epithelium has healed, which takes approximately 7 weeks.[4]

The role of mucus in coughing is not clear.[4] Fluid flushed over the tracheobronchial epithelium stimulates irritant receptors, particularly if the fluid is hypertonic or hypotonic.[7,8,11] Coughing is also stimulated by fluid that lacks permeant anions (i.e., anions that have a hydrated size and membrane-penetrating characteristics similar to the chloride anion).[12] Excessive accumulation of mucus in the airways may mechanically stimulate irritant receptors and cause coughing.[4] However, mucus may have a protective effect by coating the epithelium with a layer that separates the receptors from the irritants.[4]

Coughing is a prominent feature of cardiac disease in many species, although cardiac diseases are not often encountered in large domestic animals. Failure of the left heart as a result of congenital defects, valvular stenosis or incompetence, conduction disturbances, myocardial disorders, or restrictive pericardial disease causes an increase in pressure in the pulmonary venous return from the lung. This results in transudation of fluid from the pulmonary capillaries into the pulmonary parenchyma and airspaces (cardiogenic pulmonary edema) and causes swelling of the mucosal lining of small airways.[2] These changes stimulate cough receptors and initiate the cough reflex. Coughing that occurs secondary to cardiac disease is usually chronic, although acute-onset coughing may be observed with ruptured mitral chordae tendinae and bacterial endocarditis.[13]

Approach to Diagnosis of Coughing

HISTORY. The history should include questioning relative to the patient, the cough, the environment, and management. The *age* of the affected animal is important because many conditions have a marked age incidence. For example, *R. equi* pneumonia occurs primarily in foals younger than 6 months of age, equine herpesvirus type 4 predominantly affects weanling and yearling horses, atypical interstitial pneumonia (fog fever) affects predominantly pastured adult cattle, and COPD affects primarily mature stabled horses. The *use of the horse;* its state of fitness; the presence of vices such as crib biting; and any *history of contact with other horses* at shows, events, sales, racetracks, or breeding farms should be determined.

Recent stressors such as transportation, surgery, strenuous activity, or weaning should be determined, because these are known risk factors for conditions such as pneumonia and pleuropneumonia. The duration of ownership of the animal, its previous health, and the geographic location of origin, if it was recently purchased, may help identify regional diseases not normally seen in the area (e.g., systemic mycosis, lungworms, or silicosis in horses) or indicate the degree of stress likely to have been recently experienced. For recently purchased feedlot cattle and sheep, it should be determined if the animals were preconditioned before sale, their place of origin, the number of sale yards through which they have passed, and the duration of transportation.

When evaluating for potentially contagious diseases or those related to common environmental conditions, the vaccination status of the affected animal and herdmates and the presence of similar clinical signs in other in-contact animals sharing common facilities or common airspaces should be determined. In nursing animals the vaccination status of the dam is important. A history of other signs such as anorexia, nasal discharge, weight loss, exercise intolerance, stridor, lymphadenopathy, facial swelling, diarrhea, colic, and edema may provide important clues to the cause of the current problem. Weight loss occurs in many acute and chronic diseases, both infectious and noninfectious. Anorexia may indicate that the animal feels too systemically sick to eat, that it has a sore throat, or that it is devoting so much effort to breathing that it will not eat.

Environmental considerations such as the introduction of new animals into the environment or the return of animals from shows, sales, training centers, or breeding farms should increase the suspicion of infectious viral or bacterial diseases such as IBR in cattle or influenza in horses. For diseases such as *R. equi* pneumonia in foals, it is useful to know if similar cases have been seen on the premises in the past. The type of housing or pasturing facilities should be evaluated, particularly with regard to airspace, ventilation, sanitation, stocking density, dust, shade, and shelter. Equine stabling facilities that have enclosed barns, particularly when the stalls face a central arena or are located under a hay storage loft, promote the spread of contagious agents and almost invariably increase the concentration of dust, mold spores, and noxious gases such as ammonia and tractor exhaust fumes in the environment. The type of feed and bedding, storage facilities, and feeding arrangements should be evaluated, especially in chronically coughing horses suspected of having allergic lung disease. Quantitative measures of ventilation and environmental quality can be made and can prove helpful in case management and in monitoring the effectiveness of measures to reduce environmental dust and other pollutants.[14]

A history of recent access to lush green pastures is frequently obtained in cattle with atypical interstitial pneumonia (fog fever). The quality of the feed should be evaluated visually and by smell, particularly with regard to the presence of mold spores. General management, pasture management, and parasite control measures should also be evaluated, especially if lungworm infection is suspected. Horses with lungworm infection almost invariably have a history of current or previous cograzing with donkeys. The season and seasonal incidence of recurrence of the coughing can provide useful clues (e.g., marked seasonal worsening of signs in the late autumn when horses are stabled suggests chronic allergic respiratory disease). The history should also include the nature of previous treatments and the response.

Important historic factors about the cough include the time and speed of onset; frequency; duration (chronic if longer than 1 month); relation to feeding, housing, or weather; relation to exercise and timing during exercise; improvement, deterioration, or other change since onset; and the presence of and similarity to previous episodes of coughing or respiratory disease. Many coughs are exacerbated by exercise because exercise places greater stress on the respiratory tract. The resulting rapid airflow improves mobilization of secretions and irritates the airway directly. Coughs that occur during eating suggest sensitivity to molds or pollens in feed, inflammatory conditions of the larynx or pharyngeal region, or laryngeal or pharyngeal problems, including complications of surgery, that interfere with swallowing or guarding of the lower airway. The effort required to cough and associated pain may also give clues to the cause of the cough.

The character of the cough should be evaluated, because certain features of a cough tend to point toward its origin and possible causes but are by no means pathognomonic for either. Coughs originating in the upper airway are usually of acute onset, loud, harsh, coarse, dry, hacking, and nonproductive in character. Painful upper airway conditions such as acute pharyngitis, strangles, or necrotizing laryngitis can make the cough more muted. Lower airway coughs are usually soft, deep, and productive (mucus, pus) and tend to be more persistant than coughs originating in the upper airway. However, chest pain frequently attenuates coughing in horses with pleuropneumonia. In horses the fixed intranarial position of the larynx usually precludes coughing up sputum into the mouth; thus the productive nature of coughing is difficult to assess. Excess mucus or exudate that is coughed up into the pharynx is usually swallowed; thus a cough can be productive without evidence of a nasal discharge. Swallowing efforts that follow a cough generally indicate that the cough is productive.

PHYSICAL EXAMINATION. The extent of the physical examination varies with the information already gained and the severity of the problem. It should include both distant and close evaluation of the patient and the environment. In addition to a detailed examination of the respiratory and cardiovascular systems, a general physical examination should be completed so that diseases in other systems can be detected and systemic manifestations of cardiopulmonary disease can be evaluated. The attitude of the animal, the respiratory rate and character, the presence of excessive intercostal or abdominal respiratory effort or of a "heave line" or "barrel chest," the presence and nature of respiratory distress or stridor at rest, and the presence and character of any nasal and ocular discharge should be noted before the animal is restrained. The following should then be determined: (1) rectal temperature, pulse rate, pulse rhythm and character, mucous membrane color, and capillary refill time; (2) symmetry of airflow from each nostril; (3) odor from the nose and mouth; (4) facial symmetry and swelling; (5) resonance or painful response on percussion of the maxillary and frontal sinuses; (6) enlargement of submandibular, parotid, retropharyngeal, and other regional lymph nodes; (7) enlargement of the parotid salivary glands or thyroid gland; (8) swelling, pain, or palpable abnormalities in the retropharyngeal region; (9) palpable swelling or flattening of the cervical trachea; and (10) masses at the thoracic inlet and palpable turbulence such as a tracheal rattle in the extrathoracic airway. The oral cavity should also be examined. If spontaneous coughing is not heard during the physical examination, a cough should be induced after auscultation of the airways by pinching the larynx or trachea, and it should be ascertained whether the induced cough sounds like the animal's spontaneous cough. Pinching of the trachea generally causes normal animals to cough once or twice, whereas it often induces paroxysmal coughing in animals with lower airway disease. The laryngeal or tracheal cough reflexes show increased sensitivity in most infective and inflammatory airway diseases.[13]

The larynx, trachea, lungs, and heart on both sides of the chest should be carefully *ausculted* in a quiet environment with the animal at rest and after the rate and depth of respiration have been increased by application of a rebreathing bag, by temporary occlusion of the nostrils, or by light exercise (see Cyanosis, p. 70). This permits detection of turbulent airflow, increased or decreased bronchovesicular sounds, wheezes, crackles, pleural friction rubs, or pleural fluid splashes, all of which indicate disease of the airways, pulmonary parenchyma, or pleura. Wheezes and crackles reflect airway narrowing and dynamic airway collapse, respectively, and are both evidence of small airway disease.[13] A small or medium-size plastic trash bag makes an adequate rebreathing bag; a plastic rectal sleeve is satisfactory for foals or calves if the opening is stretched so that it does not occlude the nostrils. The response to application of a rebreathing bag should also be noted. Most horses tolerate this procedure well and breathe more deeply, whereas animals with chest pain often do not. Normal horses do not cough when the bag is applied unless they have been eating recently, whereas horses with airway irritation caused by pneumonia or other conditions often cough paroxysmally in response to application of a re-

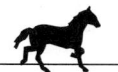

breathing bag. The time taken to regain the normal respiratory rate and character after removal of the bag provides a reasonable crude indicator of ventilatory reserve. Normal animals recover quickly, within a few breaths, whereas respiration may be altered for several minutes in animals with significant lung disease.

The chest wall should be *palpated* to detect pleural friction rubs or lesions such as rib fractures, and the symmetry of chest expansion should be determined. Unilateral chest pain (pleurodynia) often reduces chest excursion on the affected side. Both sides of the chest should be *percussed* systematically to detect changes in resonance and chest pain. The caudoventral percussion border in the normal horse traces from the level of the tuber coxae at the seventeenth intercostal space (the horse normally has 18 pairs of ribs) to the level of the tuber ischii at the fifteenth intercostal space to midthorax at the thirteenth intercostal space to the level of the point of shoulder at the eleventh intercostal space; it continues as a curving line to a point 1 to 3 inches above the olecranon. The normal caudoventral percussion boundary in cattle and small ruminants traces from the eleventh intercostal space at the level of the lateral edge of the epaxial musculature to the ninth rib at a level halfway between the costochondral junction and the lateral edge of the epaxial musculature to the fifth rib at the olecranon (cattle, goats, and sheep normally have 13 pairs of ribs). Percussion is an important diagnostic tool in all large animals, but it is most useful in foals, calves, and goats. The precise percussion boundaries, degree of resonance, and auscultation findings are influenced by age, size, body condition, fitness, and hair coat, as well as by disease processes; a gas-filled abdominal viscus can also confuse interpretation. Hyporesonance (dullness) may indicate pulmonary consolidation, large mass lesions, cardiomegaly, pleural effusion, or other pleural disease. Free pleural fluid usually causes an abrupt change from normal resonance above a horizontal fluid line to hyporesonance below this line. Hyperinflation or pneumothorax may cause hyperresonance with or without expansion of the normal percussion boundaries. A painful response to percussion may indicate pleuritis or some other inflammatory process involving the parietal pleura.

In cattle the presence of thoracic or cranial abdominal pain should be ascertained by application of upward pressure to the xiphoid area with the knee or by application of downward pressure with both hands just caudal to the withers. Animals with cranial abdominal or thoracic pain resist these maneuvers and may make an audible or auscultable grunting noise. Signs such as jugular distention or pulsation (or both) and peripheral edema, which may indicate heart failure, should be noted; and the heart should be ausculted to detect murmurs, dysrhythmias, muffling of heart sounds, or other abnormalities that would indicate the need for further cardiovascular diagnostic procedures.

COMPLETE BLOOD COUNT. A complete blood count, including fibrinogen concentration, usually reveals nonspecific findings but may be useful in the evaluation of cases in which primary or secondary inflammatory conditions are suspected and in conditions such as pulmonary thromboembolism secondary to caudal vena cava thrombosis in cattle and guttural pouch mycosis in horses in which blood-loss anemia is likely to be a complicating problem. Acute viral infections often induce a transient anemia and leukopenia, predominantly lymphopenia, followed by a monocytosis during recovery. Neutrophilia and hyperfibrinogenemia are features of many inflammatory conditions but are usually most marked when bacterial infection is involved. Some parasitic diseases (e.g., lungworm infection in cattle) may induce eosinophilia, as may allergic conditions, but eosinophilia is not a common feature of either lungworm infection or allergic COPD in the horse.

NASOPHARYNGEAL SWABBING. Nasopharyngeal swabbing and direct cytologic examination and culture are indicated for confirmation of viral or bacterial infections that involve the upper airway. Because a large number of bacteria normally inhabit the nasopharynx, only the presence of *Streptococcus equi* or some other pathogen not considered part of the resident flora can be considered significant. When clinical signs suggest a viral respiratory infection, especially when an outbreak of coughing occurs in several animals, *virus identification or isolation (or both)* from nasopharyngeal swabs and/or tracheal wash samples collected during the acute phase of the disease and *viral serologic tests* on acute and convalescent serum samples are indicated. Under these circumstances, sampling as many of the most severely affected, often younger, animals as early as possible in the disease course maximizes the chances of establishing an etiologic diagnosis. Large absorbent swabs* should be used for nasopharyngeal swabbing. The end of the swab should be placed in a viral transport medium for dispatch to the diagnostic laboratory, which should be notified in advance that samples will be submitted. Antigen-capture enzyme-linked immunosorbent assay (ELISA) tests† and polymerase chain reaction (PCR) tests are now available for testing of nasopharyngeal swabs and other samples to confirm a diagnosis of viral infection. These rapid-screening tests are sensitive, less cumbersome to perform than virus isolation, do not require such stringent conditions for handling and transporting samples, and provide results sufficiently quickly that specific control measures can be implemented. However, they do not yield an isolate that can be used to monitor genetic and antigenic evolution of the viral agent. Serologic testing often provides only retrospective information, but it can prove very helpful in the formulation of future control measures, including vaccination. The larger the number of animals tested, the more informative are the results of serologic testing in a herd or flock. Serologic testing is also indicated when pneumonia caused by *Coccidioides immitis* or other fungal agents is suspected.

ENDOSCOPIC EXAMINATION. Endoscopic examination of the nasal passages, conchae (turbinates), pharynx, larynx, and trachea allows the presence, nature, and source of exudates and the presence of anatomic or functional abnormalities or mass lesions to be noted. Endoscopic examination of the upper airway should be performed without the use of sedatives or tranquilizers if possible because these alter the tone and function of the muscles supporting laryngeal and pharyngeal anatomy and function and confuse interpretation of endoscopic findings. In the horse the interior of the guttural pouches may be examined by advancing the endoscope through the pharyngeal openings of each guttural pouch using a guide wire such as a closed biopsy instrument passed through the biopsy channel of the endoscope and into the pouch. Most coughing horses have lower airway disease, which is reflected in accumulation of endoscopically visible exudate in the horizontal trachea, particularly after exercise. Lungworm larvae may be grossly visible in the trachea of horses with lungworm infection. Deeper bronchoscopic examination is necessary to determine whether exudate is a reflection of diffuse airway disease or whether it arises from a specific area of the lung, such as would occur with a pulmonary abscess or a foreign body lodged in a bronchus. Sedation may or may not be needed to permit endoscopic examination of the extrathoracic airways in the standing horse. Sedation with xylazine or detomidine supplemented with

---

*Fox 16-inch Procto Swabs, Allegiance Healthcare, Hayward, CA.
†For example, influenza Directigen Flu A test, Becton-Dickinson, Franklin Lakes, NJ.

butorphanol is recommended to facilitate bronchoscopy and to dampen the cough reflex, as is spraying of the carina and bronchial branches with 2% lidocaine via the biopsy channel of the endoscope to reduce coughing during the procedure. Tracheobronchial aspiration and bronchoalveolar lavage can be performed by introduction of appropriate catheters via the biopsy channel of the endoscope.

TRACHEAL ASPIRATION. Tracheal aspiration with cytologic studies and quantitative or semiquantitative aerobic and anaerobic culture of collected samples is indicated in the evaluation of patients suspected of having disease of the lungs or pleura, particularly if an infectious etiology is likely. Tracheal wash samples collected using the percutaneous transtracheal technique are preferred for bacterial culture, but collection of samples via an endoscope using double-sheathed catheters is acceptable and less subject to complications. If tracheal aspiration is to be performed percutaneously, the procedure should precede endoscopic examination of the lower airways to avoid contamination. Cultures may fail to reveal the primary bacterial pathogen, especially in cases treated with antibiotics. The diagnostic value of tracheal wash samples can be improved by discontinuing antibiotic therapy for at least 24 hours before collecting samples, rapid processing of samples, use of antibiotic removal devices and selective culture media and, if necessary, repeat sampling. Culture results should be evaluated in relation to the clinical signs, clinical experience (especially on the farm of origin of the patient), results of cytologic evaluation, and response to treatment.

BRONCHOALVEOLAR LAVAGE. Samples collected by bronchoalveolar lavage (BAL) are less useful than those collected by tracheal aspiration for evaluating infectious lower airway diseases and focal pulmonary conditions because the technique samples secretions from only a limited area of the caudodorsal lung and is subject to contamination during collection. However, BAL yields better samples for cytologic assessment and is therefore preferred for evaluation of patients with generalized, noninfectious lower airway diseases such as COPD or silicosis. BAL samples can be collected under endoscopic guidance by means of catheters introduced through the biopsy channel of a suitable endoscope (less than 9 mm in diameter and longer than 180 cm) or by using commercially available BAL tubes. The advantage of collection via endoscopy is that specific areas of the lung can be sampled, although gaining access to the cranial lung lobes is difficult with any method.

Neutrophils are usually the predominant cell type in BAL fluid or tracheal washes of horses with COPD and in animals with bacterial infections. The neutrophils usually show degenerative changes when significant bacterial infection is present. Large numbers of eosinophils are a feature of parasitic infections such as lungworms, some allergic conditions, and infiltrative eosinophilic interstitial pneumonia. The presence of hemosiderin-laden macrophages is an indication of recent pulmonary hemorrhage, and finding refractile intracytoplasmic granules in macrophages or giant cells should raise the suspicion of silicosis, especially in animals showing radiographic evidence of marked pulmonary interstitial disease. Noting the presence, number, location (intracellular or extracellular), and Gram stain characteristics of bacteria permits a reasoned selection of antibiotic treatment while awaiting the results of culture and susceptibility tests.

ULTRASOUND EXAMINATION. Ultrasound examination of the chest is indicated to evaluate for and determine the extent of pleural effusion, pleural roughening, pleural fibrin deposits, gas echoes in pleural fluid, pleural adhesions, and pulmonary lesions such as consolidation, atelectasis, or abscessation in animals with lesions in contact with the pleural surface or in animals in which sufficient pleural fluid has ac-

cumulated to allow evaluation of the underlying lung. Ultrasound also can be useful for examining externally visible lesions such as possible retropharyngeal abscesses that may be impinging on the airway and causing coughing.

BLOOD GAS ANALYSIS. Blood gas analysis on arterial blood to determine oxygen (O_2) and carbon dioxide (CO_2) tensions is indicated in the evaluation and monitoring of patients in which a history or clinical signs of coughing are accompanied by signs of respiratory distress or cyanosis (see Respiratory Distress, p. 64, and Cyanosis, p. 70).

THORACOCENTESIS. Thoracocentesis with culture and cytologic examination of collected samples is indicated in animals with clinical or ultrasonographic evidence of effusive pleural disease. Determination of the pH, glucose level, and lactate dehydrogenase (LDH) concentration in pleural fluid collected into a heparinized tube or syringe helps differentiate septic from nonseptic effusions while awaiting culture results.[15] The best site for collecting pleural fluid can be confirmed by ultrasonography after auscultation and percussion of the chest. The sixth or seventh intercostal spaces at the level of the costochondral junction are commonly used sites in horses and cattle. The thorax should be penetrated in the part of the intercostal space immediately adjacent to the cranial border of the rib to avoid the intercostal vessels and nerves.

PLEUROSCOPY. Pleuroscopy is a more invasive procedure with limited indications that include investigation of chronic pleural diseases such as abscesses, pleural adhesions, and possible primary or metastatic pulmonary or pleural neoplasia such as lymphosarcoma, gastric squamous cell carcinoma, or mesothelioma.

FECAL EXAMINATION. Fecal examination using the Baermann technique to detect lungworm larvae is indicated in ruminants suspected of having a lungworm infection. Because lungworm infections in the horse rarely become patent, larvae are not usually demonstrable by fecal examination. Pulmonary signs related to *Parascaris equorum* infection in foals occur during the prepatent (migratory) period, thus the fecal flotation test for ascarid eggs often yields a negative result despite significant parasitic infection.

RADIOGRAPHIC EXAMINATION. Radiography of the chest is indicated in patients suspected of having lower airway disease to determine the presence, severity, and pattern of disease changes involving the lungs, pleura, and mediastinum. Four overlapping lateral projections usually are required to evaluate the whole lung field in an adult horse. Because ventrodorsal projections are possible only in young foals, lateral projections from each side may be necessary to lateralize lesions within the chest. Radiographs of the lungs are particularly useful for determining the prognosis and for monitoring the response to therapy of pulmonary diseases such as bacterial pneumonia and lung abscesses. The cardiac silhouette and the pattern and caliber of the aorta, vena cava, pulmonary artery, pulmonary veins, and other vessels should be evaluated for evidence of cardiac failure and pulmonary vascular disease. Radiographs of the pharynx, retropharyngeal area (including guttural pouches in the horse), larynx, and proximal trachea are indicated in some cases to confirm problems not definitively diagnosed by clinical examination and endoscopy.

NUCLEAR SCINTIGRAPHY. Nuclear scintigraphy using aerosolized [99m]technetium-labeled diethylenetriaminepentaacetic acid (DPTA) and intravenously injected [99m]technetium-labeled microaggregated albumin particles has recently been used to determine patterns of pulmonary ventilation, perfusion, and ventilation/perfusion ratios.[16,17] This technique requires special equipment and personnel but provides an objective assessment of pulmonary function and gas exchange capability.[17]

BIOPSY. Biopsy, with histologic evaluation of samples, is indicated to diagnose certain mass lesions such as neoplasms, cysts, polyps, fungal granulomas, or foreign body granulomas in or surrounding the airway. Masses in the airway can be biopsied through the biopsy channel of fiberoptic or video endoscopes, but these samples inevitably are small. Biopsies can also be collected at the time of exploratory or corrective surgery from lesions in the upper airway. Lung biopsies can be collected blindly, using Tru-Cut, Biopty, or similar instruments, preferably from the peripheral areas of the lung to reduce the likelihood of serious hemorrhage (see Chapter 29). Focal lesions should be visualized ultrasonographically or radiographically before or during the biopsy procedure. Lung biopsy is most useful for diagnosing diffuse nonseptic conditions such as pneumoconiosis. The inherent risks associated with the procedure indicate that percutaneous lung biopsy should be reserved for circumstances in which the animal is not showing signs of marked respiratory distress, uncontrollable coughing, or bleeding disorders and a high likelihood exists that the procedure will yield significant diagnostic information. Open lung biopsy is rarely indicated.

IMMUNOGLOBULIN DETERMINATIONS. Quantitative immunoglobulin determinations and possibly other *immune function tests* may be indicated in animals, especially young ones, with chronic or recurrent respiratory tract infections or other indications of immune compromise.

INTRADERMAL ALLERGEN SKIN TESTING. Intradermal allergen skin testing, a *radioallergosorbent test (RAST) for IgE on serum,* or *inhaled challenge* have been used to evaluate animals suspected of having allergic respiratory disease. Coughing horses with COPD that show exacerbation of signs in certain environments or with certain feeding practices are considered candidates for testing. The results of intradermal allergen tests often do not prove useful because many normal horses show sensitivity to mold spores, and there is limited correlation between the dermal and pulmonary reactivities to mold antigens.[10] However, a number of horses with COPD have been hyposensitized successfully using allergens selected on the basis of allergen skin testing or RAST. The crude trial and error approach of adding or removing potential allergens from the environment is sometimes very helpful diagnostically and therapeutically in COPD cases in which an allergic etiology is suspected. Feeding of pellets instead of hay and using shredded paper, peat moss, or wood shavings instead of straw bedding are common examples of this approach (see the section on COPD in Chapter 29).

PULMONARY FUNCTION TESTING. Pulmonary function testing and evaluation of airway dynamics during exercise currently are largely research techniques, but they could prove extremely useful in clinical evaluation of horses in the future (see Chapter 29). Test results indicate physiologic abnormalities rather than identify specific etiologic agents or pathologic lesions. Some indications for pulmonary function testing might include the following:

- To evaluate horses with a history of poor performance or exercise intolerance but no other detectable abnormalities
- To assess the degree of functional impairment in horses with known evidence of respiratory disease
- To determine if a horse has recovered from a diagnosed respiratory disorder and can be returned to training
- To rule out functional pulmonary abnormalities in horses with upper airway conditions amenable to surgical correction
- To objectively assess the efficacy of therapeutic regimens

BRONCHODILATOR RESPONSE TESTING. Bronchodilator response testing involves determining the response of measured pulmonary functions and pleural pressures to bronchodilator drugs such as isoproterenol, atropine, clen-buterol, or pirbuterol, administered parenterally or by aerosol. Results are often helpful in determining the pathogenesis of COPD and the likely response to bronchodilator therapy. In the field setting, useful information can be gained by assessing the response of respiratory rate, respiratory character, and lung sounds to intravenous (IV) administration of a low dose of atropine (5 to 7 mg/450-kg horse). This test can be made more objective by measuring pleural pressures using a Ventigraph recorder* attached to an esophageal catheter.[10]

DIFFERENTIAL DIAGNOSIS OF COUGHING. The differential diagnosis of coughing can be enhanced by arbitrarily categorizing it on the basis of *duration of signs* into acute or chronic (more than 1 month) and by the *presence or absence of fever.*[18] It should be kept in mind that some acute coughs become chronic and, conversely, that conditions that cause chronic coughing may be seen early in the disease course. Conditions typically associated with *acute coughing* include viral, bacterial, and parasitic infections of the upper and lower respiratory tract; acute allergic reactions or acute toxic injury to the lung such as in atypical interstitial pneumonia (fog fever) of cattle; foreign bodies; choke; injuries to the larynx, trachea, or chest; pharyngeal or laryngeal dysfunction secondary to neurologic disorders or surgery; aspiration of food material or foreign bodies; smoke inhalation; and compressive upper airway lesions such as retropharyngeal abscesses or necrotic laryngitis. In most instances, outbreaks of sudden-onset coughing in groups of animals are the result of viral infection involving the upper and lower respiratory tract.[6,13]

Conditions typically associated with *chronic coughing* include chronic bacterial pneumonia; pulmonary abscess; chronic pleuritis; chronic allergic pulmonary diseases such as COPD in horses and farmer's lung disease in cattle; postviral bronchial hyperreactivity, chronic viral respiratory disease such as ovine progressive pneumonia and caprine arthritis-encephalomyelitis pneumonia; irritant airway disease caused by environmental irritants such as dust; lungworm infections, particularly in horses and small ruminants; functional or anatomic problems in the pharynx or larynx that interfere with guarding of the airway, including postsurgical problems; heart failure resulting in pulmonary edema; tumors or polyps in the upper airway or lung; mycotic infections of the upper airway, lung, or pleura; chronic guttural pouch infections in horses; tracheal collapse, especially in ponies; chronic interstitial disease such as pneumoconiosis caused by inhalation of particulate material; and so-called nuisance coughs. Nuisance coughs are common in horses, especially at the beginning of exercise, which emphasizes the fact that coughing is a normal airway protective mechanism and not always evidence of overt disease. Nuisance coughs tend to bother the owner more than the horse and can result from habit; vices such as crib biting, wind sucking, or greedy eating; and environmental factors such as dust, ammonia, and cold air. Some of these nuisance coughs are correctable by modifying the stabling or work environment.

Cough with fever usually indicates a primary infectious cause or a secondary infection superimposed on a noninfectious cause.[18] Fever is a typical but not an invariable feature of aspiration pneumonia, bacterial pneumonia, pulmonary abscess, viral respiratory tract infection, strangles, fungal pneumonia, pleuropneumonia (bacterial, viral, or mycoplasmal), acute bronchointerstitial pneumonia, and thoracic neoplasia.[18]

Cough without fever is typically found in COPD, abnormalities of the larynx or pharynx, parasitic pneumonia, exercise-induced pulmonary hemorrhage (EIPH), tracheobronchial

---

*Boehringer Ingelheim, Vet Medica, Inc, St Joseph, Mo.

foreign body, tracheal collapse, and airway-oriented neoplasia (e.g., bronchial carcinoma).[18] Horses with chronic interstitial pneumonia such as silicosis or granulomatous pneumonia are usually afebrile but may have mild to moderate fever.[18]

REFERENCES

1. Weinberger SE: *Principles of pulmonary medicine*, Philadelphia, 1986, WB Saunders, pp 22-30.
2. Pierce JA: Cough. In Blacklow RS, ed: *Signs and symptoms: applied pathologic physiology and clinical interpretation*, ed 6, Philadelphia, 1970, JB Lippincott, pp 317-330.
3. Muran O: Cough. In Glauser FL, ed: *Signs and symptoms in pulmonary medicine*, Philadelphia, 1983, JB Lippincott, pp 12-19.
4. Robinson NE: Pathophysiology of coughing, *Proc Am Assoc Equine Pract* 32:291-298, 1986.
5. Cornelius LM: Coughing. In Lorenz MD, Cornelius LM, eds: *Small animal medical diagnosis*, Philadelphia, 1987, JB Lippincott, pp 207-214.
6. Brown CM: Coughing and labored breathing. In Brown CM, ed: *Problems in equine medicine*, Philadelphia, 1989, Lea & Febiger, pp 81-96.
7. Pounsford JC, Birch MJ, Saunders KB: Effect of bronchodilators on the cough response to inhaled citric acid in normal and asthmatic subjects, *Thorax* 49:662-667, 1985.
8. Sheppard D et al: Mechanism of cough and bronchoconstriction induced by distilled water aerosol, *Am Rev Respir Dis* 127:691-694, 1983.
9. Amis TC: Clinical respiratory physiology. In Kirk RW, ed: *Current veterinary therapy. VIII, Small animal practice*, Philadelphia, 1983, WB Saunders, pp 191-201.
10. McGorum B: Differential diagnosis of chronic coughing in the horse, *In Pract* 16:55-60, 1994.
11. Widdicombe JG: Respiratory reflexes and defense. In Brain JD, Proctor DF, Reid LM, eds: *Respiratory defense mechanisms*, II, New York, 1977, Marcel Dekker, pp 593-630.
12. Eschenbacher WL, Bousey HA, Sheppard D: Alterations in osmolarity of inhaled aerosols causes bronchoconstriction and cough, but absence of a permeant anion causes cough alone, *Am Rev Respir Dis* 129:211-215, 1984.
13. Mair T: Differential diagnosis and treatment of acute onset coughing in the horse, *In Pract* 16:154-162, 1994.
14. Clark AF: Air hygiene and equine respiratory disease, *In Pract* 9:196-204, 1987.
15. Brumbaugh GW, Benson PA: Partial pressures of oxygen and carbon dioxide, pH, and concentrations of bicarbonate, lactate, and glucose in pleural fluid from horses, *Am J Vet Res* 51:1032-1037, 1990.
16. O'Callaghan MW et al: Exercise-induced pulmonary hemorrhage in the horse: results of a detailed clinical, postmortem, and imaging study. VII. Ventilation/perfusion scintigraphy in horses with EIPH, *Equine Vet J* 19:423-427, 1987.
17. Hinchcliff KW, Byrne BA: Clinical examination of the respiratory system, *Vet Clin North Am (Equine Pract)* 7:1-26, 1991.
18. Wilson WD: Coughing. In Brown CM, ed: *5-Minute veterinary consult: equine*. In Press, 2001.

NASAL DISCHARGE

Definition

Nasal discharge, which is any nongaseous material that exits the respiratory tract through the external nares, is described according to its *physical characteristics* (serous, mucoid, purulent, hemorrhagic [sanguinous], a combination of these types, or feed material), *acuteness of onset* (sudden or insidious), *origin* (unilateral or bilateral); *volume* (profuse or scant), and *association with activity* (spontaneous or intermittent).[19-21]

Pathophysiology

NORMAL NASAL SECRETIONS. The ciliated, pseudostratified columnar epithelium lining the respiratory tract from the nasal passages to the level of the respiratory bronchioles contains serous, mucous, and mixed tubuloalveolar glands in its lamina propria.[19] Goblet cells are present in large numbers throughout the nasal cavity and are present in the airway mucosa to the level of secondary and tertiary bronchi.[19] The secretions of these glands and goblet cells and the fluid transudated from serum together serve to warm and humidify inspired air, trap particulate matter, protect the respiratory

epithelium from desiccation and infection, and provide the serous-mucous bilayer necessary for effective ciliary function.[22,23] The tracheobronchial fluid that constitutes the mucous blanket in the lower parts of the respiratory tract contains exfoliated epithelial cells, alveolar macrophages, and other mononuclear cells, glycoproteins, bacteriostatic proteins (primarily lysozyme), lactoferrin, secretory IgA, IgG, IgM, and serum proteins (primarily albumin).[22,23] The cilia lining the pseudostratified columnar epithelium beat in coordinated waves to carry mucus, trapped particles, and cells from the lower respiratory tract to the nasopharynx. Material cleared from the tracheobronchial tree is normally swallowed upon reaching the pharynx but may appear at the external nares as nasal discharge.[23]

Serous nasal secretions in normal animals are responsible for the moist appearance of the ventral portion of the external nares. In cattle normal nasal secretions are more voluminous and more mucoid compared with other large animal species. Healthy cattle keep their external nares clean through licking. Cattle that are systemically ill or otherwise debilitated often neglect to do this, and as a result mucoid secretions accumulate and crust around the external nares. On the other hand, a buildup of nasal discharge in cattle with respiratory disease can be removed by frequent nose licking, masking the presence of disease.

Lacrimal secretions also drain into the nasal passages through the nasolacrimal ducts and may appear at the external nares as a thin, watery, clear, nonviscous discharge, particularly in animals with conjunctival irritation or ocular inflammatory diseases that stimulate excessive lacrimation.[20]

ABNORMAL NASAL SECRETIONS. Inflammatory conditions involving the nasal cavity stimulate increased production of glandular secretions.[23] These secretions initially are serous but later become mucoid and purulent as secondary bacterial invasion induces an influx of neutrophils.[19] Serous nasal discharge generally indicates disease conditions affecting the nasal passages or upper respiratory tract.

Inflammation, irritation, and other pathologic states affecting the trachea and bronchi increase the production of mucous and serous secretions in the tracheobronchial tree[23] (Boxes 5-3 and 5-4). Initially the accompanying nasal discharge is mucoid (clear, colorless, thin, and elastic in consistency), but with chronicity and secondary bacterial invasion, neutrophils and other inflammatory cells accumulate in the tracheobronchial secretions and the nasal discharge becomes purulent, progressing from cloudy to opaque and then to viscous with a whitish cream color (Boxes 5-5 and 5-6).

Conditions such as chronic bronchitis and chronic obstructive pulmonary disease cause goblet cell hyperplasia and increased mucus production, which may be reflected as a discharge at the external nares, depending on the efficiency with which the animal swallows these secretions. In some cases nasal discharge is evident only early in the morning or after a period of recumbency because in these situations secretions accumulate in the trachea and pharynx, drain into the nasal passages, and exit from the nares.

Hemorrhagic (sanguinous) nasal discharge, or epistaxis, occurs secondary to trauma, coagulopathies, and erosive or invasive conditions that insult the richly vascular nasal mucosa or secondary to conditions that invade regional blood vessels such as occurs when the internal carotid artery is eroded by a mycotic plaque in horses with guttural pouch mycosis. Pulmonary disorders such as infarctive pneumonia in horses and pulmonary thromboembolism secondary to posterior vena cava thrombosis in cattle may also induce epistaxis (see Epistaxis, p. 60).[19-21]

Foul odor (ozena) accompanying nasal discharge suggests an anaerobic infection, a necrotizing condition (e.g., fungal infection, neoplasia, turbinate necrosis, or necrotizing pneu-

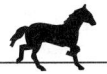

BOX 5-3

Causes of Serous and Mucoid Nasal Discharge in the Horse

COMMON CAUSES

Influenza
Equine herpesvirus types 1 and 4 (EHV-1, EHV-4)
Rhinovirus
Other viruses (e.g., adenovirus, reovirus, EHV-2)
Pharyngitis, chronic pharyngeal lymphoid hyperplasia
Nasal or paranasal sinus infection, cysts, polyps, tumors
Early bacterial pneumonia or pleuritis
Early strangles (*Streptococcus equi* infection)
Guttural pouch infection, mycosis
Overflow of nasolacrimal ducts
Chronic obstructive pulmonary disease (COPD)

LESS COMMON CAUSES

Equine viral arteritis
Burn (thermal, chemical)
Anaphylaxis or acute drug reaction
Aspiration or foreign body pneumonia, smoke inhalation
Foreign body (nasal, pharyngeal, guttural pouch, tracheal, or bronchial)
Summer pasture–associated obstructive airway disease (SPOAD)

UNCOMMON CAUSES

Nasal fungal infection (rhinophycomycosis), aspergillosis
Nasal amyloidosis
Coccidioidomycosis
Restrictive pulmonary disease, pneumoconiosis
Trauma to the skull or upper airway
Tuberculosis

UNCOMMON CAUSES—cont'd

Tularemia
Guttural pouch neoplasia
Chlamydia psittaci pneumonia
Nocardiosis
Cryptococcosis
Fungal granuloma, maduromycosis, rhinosporidiosis, mycetoma, pythiosis
Lungworm infection (*Dictyocaulus arnfieldi*)
Ascarid migration
Cyst (pharyngeal, subepiglottal)
Progressive ethmoidal hematoma
Lymphosarcoma, lymphoma, leukemia
Halicephalobus (Micronema) deletrix granuloma
Pulmonary edema
Pulmonary aspergillosis
Stachybotryotoxicosis
Trichloroethylene-extracted feed toxicity
Pentachlorophenol toxicity
Organophosphate, carbamate toxicity
Ammonia toxicity
St. George disease (*Pimelea* spp. poisoning) (exotic)
Trypanosoma evansi, Surra (exotic)
Trypanosoma equinum, Mal de Caderas (exotic)
Trypanosoma hippicum, Murrina de Caderas (exotic)
Besnoitiosis, globidiosis (exotic)
African horse sickness (exotic)
Getahvirus (exotic)
Glanders (exotic)
Louping ill (exotic)

---

monia), foreign body, or communication between the oral and nasal cavities (e.g., maxillary sinusitis secondary to a patent infundibulum in the horse).[21]

Food or water may drain from the external nares when there is communication between the oral and nasal cavities (e.g., cleft palate); in association with swallowing disorders (e.g., pharyngeal paresis secondary to botulism, cranial nerve damage secondary to guttural pouch mycosis in the horse); or in cases of obstructive dysphagia (e.g., severe pharyngitis, guttural pouch enlargement in horses, retropharyngeal abscesses, esophageal obstruction, obstructions of the gastrointestinal tract that lead to regurgitation of food from the stomach).[19-21] The respiratory position of the epiglottis dorsal to the soft palate in the horse means that except in cases of laryngopalatal dislocation, food regurgitated from the digestive tract enters the nasopharynx and appears at the external nares rather than at the mouth (see Regurgitation and Vomiting, Chapter 7).

Chronic nasal discharges often cause scalding in the area ventral to the external nares.[20] Mucoid and purulent nasal discharges tend to dry and crust as an admixture with environmental dust and dirt around the external nares. In all large animal species but particularly in sheep and goats, tenacious exudates may obstruct the nasal passages and induce a snuffling noise. Horses with profuse nasal discharge often rub the nose on the dorsum of the front fetlock and cannon regions. During the physical examination these areas should be inspected for mucoid exudate, dried crusts, or swarms of flies.

ACUTENESS OF ONSET. Sudden-onset nasal discharge usually is associated with acute infection, trauma, or esophageal obstruction, whereas nasal discharge of insidious onset generally accompanies chronic infection, neoplasia, or a progressive neurologic disease that causes dysphagia.[24]

ORIGIN OF NASAL SECRETIONS. Unilateral nasal discharge generally originates from structures located rostral to the caudal end of the nasal septum. Bilateral nasal discharge results from disease processes affecting structures caudal to the caudal end of the nasal septum or from conditions involving the nasal passages or paranasal sinuses bilaterally.[20,21] A discharge that appears from one nostril on some days and from the opposite nostril on others generally indicates a lesion or disease process caudal to the nasal septum.[21] The paired guttural pouches of the horse drain separately through ostia located dorsolaterally in the wall of the nasopharynx. Exudate draining from the guttural pouches may appear unilaterally at the ipsilateral nostril if the volume of drainage is small, but moderate to profuse guttural pouch drainage appears as a bilateral nasal discharge.[21]

VOLUME OF NASAL SECRETIONS. The volume of nasal discharge frequently increases when the head is lowered, regardless of the source of the discharge, because of pooling of exudate in the trachea, pharynx, or nasal passages. However, the appearance of profuse, unilateral, purulent nasal discharge when the head is lowered generally indicates sinus empyema, and profuse bilateral nasal discharge under these circumstances suggests guttural pouch empyema.[20] This is attributed to accumulation of large volumes of exudate in the sinus cavities or guttural pouches when the head is elevated and to the fact that the ostia through which these structures drain are not located on the most dependent aspect of these cavities; thus significant drainage can occur only when the head is lowered. Nasal discharge observed only after exercise suggests an origin in the lower respiratory tract.[25]

BOX 5-4

Causes of Serous or Mucoid Nasal Discharge in Ruminants

COMMON CAUSES

Debilitating illnesses that reduce lingual nose cleaning in
cattle (B)
Mannheimia hemolytica or *Pasteurella multocida* pneumonia
(includes shipping fever and enzootic calf pneumonia)
Haemophilus somnus pneumonia (B)
Nose bots *(Oestrus ovis)* (O, C)
Lungworm infection, verminous pneumonia
Atypical interstitial pneumonia (B)
Infectious bovine rhinotracheitis (IBR; BHV-1) (B, C)
Bovine respiratory syncytial virus (B)
Parainfluenza virus type 3
Mycoplasma spp. pneumonia
Caprine *Mycoplasma mycoides* subsp. *mycoides* infection (C)
Caprine arthritis-encephalomyelitis (CAE) pneumonia (C)
Early bacterial pneumonia
Trauma (nasal, oral, pharyngeal, laryngeal, tracheal,
bronchial, chest wall)
Abscess (oral, pharyngeal, retropharyngeal)
Esophageal obstruction, foreign body, choke
Septicemia (neonates)

LESS COMMON CAUSES

Paranasal sinus infection
Foreign body (oral, pharyngeal, laryngeal, tracheal, bronchial,
pulmonary)
Aspiration, foreign body pneumonia
Ovine progressive pneumonia and arthritis, Maedi (O)
Bluetongue
Bovine virus diarrhea (BVD-MD) (B)
Ovine adenovirus (O)
Caprine respiratory syncytial virus (C)
Bovine rhinovirus (B)
Bovine adenovirus (B)
Bovine malignant catarrhal fever, early (B)
Herpesvirus DN-599 (B)
Bovine herpesvirus type 4 (BHV-4) (B)
Pulmonary adenomatosis (Jaagsiekte) (O)
Inhalation pneumonia, smoke, noxious gases
Anaphylaxis or adverse drug reaction
Milk allergy in cows (B)
Farmer's lung disease (hypersensitivity to *Faenia rectivirgula*,
Aspergillus fumigatus, and other mold spores) (B)
Chlamydia psittaci pneumonia
Burns (thermal, chemical)
Vagal indigestion, abomasal impaction
Nasal adenoma, adenopapilloma, adenocarcinoma, polyp
(O, C)

UNCOMMON CAUSES

Familial allergic rhinitis (B)
Bovine nasal granuloma, atopic rhinitis, summer snuffles (B)
Fungal granuloma, maduromycosis, mycetoma,
rhinosporidiosis
Nasal actinobacillosis (B)
Sarcocystosis (B)
Tularemia (O)
Phycomycosis, pythiosis (B)
Pulmonary aspergillosis
Bronchobiliary fistula (yellow froth) (B)
Zygomycosis, mucormycosis (B)

UNCOMMON CAUSES—cont'd

Pneumocystis carinii pneumonia
Neoplasia (nasal, paranasal sinus, pharyngeal, pulmonary)
Buss disease chlamydial sporadic bovine encephalomyelitis
(B)
Winter dysentery (B)
Immune deficiency states
Pregnancy toxemia (B)
Border disease (hairy shaker) (O, C)
Lymphosarcoma
Johne's disease
Listeriosis (C)
Tetanus
Rinderpest (exotic)
Theileriosis, East Coast fever (exotic)
Contagious bovine pleuropneumonia (exotic) (B)
African bovine malignant catarrhal fever, early (exotic) (B)
Virulent sheep and goat pox (exotic) (O, C)
Peste des petits ruminants (exotic) (O, C)
Contagious caprine pleuropneumonia (exotic) (C)
Rift Valley fever (exotic)
St. George disease (*Pimelea* spp. poisoning) (exotic)
Trypanosoma evansi, Surra (exotic) (B)
Trypanosomiasis, Nagana (exotic)
Jembrana disease (exotic) (B)
Sweating sickness (exotic) (B, O)
Cestrum poisoning (exotic)
Stinkweed poisoning (exotic) (B)
Endemic ethmoid carcinoma (exotic) (B)
Ephemeral fever (exotic) (B)
Lumpy skin disease (exotic) (B)
Nasal schistosomiasis (exotic)
Besnoitiosis, globidiosis (exotic)
Louping ill (exotic)
Theilezia rhodensis (exotic)
Cotyledon spp. poisoning, Krimpsiekte (exotic) (O, C)
Gedoelstia hasleri nasal bots (exotic) (O, C)
Nairobi sheep disease (exotic) (O, C)
Schistosoma nasale (exotic) (B)

TOXIC CAUSES

Organophosphate or carbamate
Mercury (B)
Iodine (B, O)
Ammonia
Sodium hydroxide (caustic soda)
Trichloroethylene-extracted feed (B, O)
Formaldehyde irritation
Oxalate (B, O)
Thallium (O)
Furazolidone
Hairy vetch *(Vicia villosa)* (B)
Ergot *(Claviceps purpura)*
Sneezeweed (*Helenium* spp.)
Aflatoxicosis (C)
Rubber weed (*Hymenoxys* spp.)
Acorn, oak (B, O)
Perennial broomweed (*Gutierrezia* spp.)
Chinese tallow (*Sapium sebiferum*) (B)
Stachybotryotoxicosis
Slender ice plant (*Mesembryanthenum nodiflorum*)

B, Bovine; C, caprine; O, ovine.

BOX 5-5

Causes of Purulent Nasal Discharge in the Horse

COMMON CAUSES
Postviral bacterial infection of the respiratory tract
Strangles (*Streptococcus equi* infection)
Bacterial rhinitis
Pharyngitis
Bacterial pneumonia
Bacterial pleuritis or pleuropneumonia
Guttural pouch empyema or chondroids
Guttural pouch mycosis
Lung abscess
Pharyngeal, retropharyngeal abscess
Paranasal sinus infection, cyst, tumor (unilateral discharge)
Fungal rhinitis (rhinophycomycosis), nasal granuloma, nasal aspergillosis (unilateral discharge)
Nasal foreign body (unilateral discharge)
Conchal necrosis (unilateral discharge)
Progressive ethmoidal hematoma (unilateral discharge)
Nasal tumor, polyp, cyst (unilateral discharge)
Trauma (nasal, skull, upper airway) (unilateral or bilateral discharge)

LESS COMMON CAUSES
Burn (thermal, chemical)
Aspiration or foreign body pneumonia, smoke inhalation
Foreign body (pharyngeal, guttural pouch, tracheal, bronchial)

LESS COMMON CAUSES—cont'd
Esophageal obstruction, choke, stricture, ectasia, megaesophagus
Neurologic deficits affecting swallowing

UNCOMMON CAUSES
Coccidioidomycosis
Tuberculosis
Tularemia
Guttural pouch neoplasia
Chlamydia psittaci pneumonia
Nocardiosis
Cryptococcosis
Fungal granuloma, maduromycosis, rhinosporidiosis, mycetoma, pythiosis
Ascarid migration
Lymphosarcoma, lymphoma, leukemia
Halicephalobus (Micronema) deletrix granulomas
Pulmonary aspergillosis
Pneumocystis carinii pneumonia
Ammonia toxicity
Trypanosoma evansi, Surra (exotic)
Besnoitiosis, globidiosis (exotic)
African horse sickness (exotic)
Glanders (exotic)
Melioidosis, *Pseudomonas pseudomallei* (exotic)

BOX 5-6

Causes of Purulent Nasal Discharge in Ruminants

COMMON CAUSES
Debilitating illnesses that reduce lingual nose cleaning in cattle
Postviral bacterial infection of the respiratory tract
Mannheimia hemolytica or *Pasteurella multocida* pneumonia
Haemophilus somnus pneumonia (B)
Necrotic laryngitis, calf diphtheria (B)
Lungworm infection, verminous pneumonia
Mycoplasma spp. pneumonia
Caprine *Mycoplasma mycoides* subsp. *mycoides* infection (C)
Chronic bacterial pneumonia with consolidation or abscessation (*Arcanobacterium pyogenes* and other bacteria)
Esophageal obstruction, foreign body, choke
Nose bots *(Oestrus ovis)* (O, C)
Trauma (nasal, oral, pharyngeal, laryngeal, tracheal, bronchial, chest wall)
Abscess (oral, pharyngeal, retropharyngeal)
Septicemia (neonates)

LESS COMMON CAUSES
Foreign body (oral, pharyngeal, laryngeal, tracheal, bronchial, pulmonary)
Aspiration, foreign body pneumonia
Paranasal sinus infection
Pulmonary embolism from posterior vena cava thrombosis (B)
Ovine progressive pneumonia and arthritis, Maedi (O)
Bovine malignant catarrhal fever (B)
Bluetongue

LESS COMMON CAUSES—cont'd
Pulmonary adenomatosis (Jaagsiekte) (O)
Inhalation pneumonia, smoke, noxious gases
Chlamydia psittaci pneumonia
Burns (thermal, chemical)
Vagal indigestion, abomasal impaction
Nasal adenoma, adenopapilloma, adenocarcinoma, polyp (O, C)

UNCOMMON CAUSES
Ovine nasal granuloma, atopic rhinitis, summer snuffles (B)
Fungal granuloma, maduromycosis, mycetoma, rhinosporidiosis
Nasal actinobacillosis (B)
Bovine salmonellosis (B)
Sarcocystosis (B)
Tularemia (O)
Tuberculosis
Phycomycosis, pythiosis (B)
Pulmonary aspergillosis
Bronchobiliary fistula (yellow froth) (B)
Zygomycosis, mucormycosis (B)
Pneumocystis carinii pneumonia
Neoplasia (nasal, paranasal sinus, pharyngeal, pulmonary)
Immune deficiency states
Lymphosarcoma

TOXIC AND EXOTIC CAUSES
See Box 5-4, p. 56.

B, Bovine; *C,* caprine; *O,* ovine.

Approach to Diagnosis of Nasal Discharge

Because many conditions, particularly those involving the lower respiratory tract, are associated with both nasal discharge and cough, the diagnostic approach used for large animal patients presented for evaluation of nasal discharge is similar to that used to for large animals presented for evaluation of cough (see Cough, p. 46). Only those components of the history and diagnostic evaluation that differ substantially from those used in patients with cough are described in depth in this section.

HISTORY. The patient history should include information about the rapidity of onset and duration of nasal discharge; whether the discharge is consistently unilateral, consistently bilateral, or intermittently bilateral; and the volume, color, consistency, and odor of the discharge.

The association of discharge with certain activities such as initiation of exercise, when the animal is first disturbed in the morning, or when it is eating with its head lowered, can provide useful clues to the origin or etiology. It should be determined if the animal is showing signs of respiratory disease (e.g., cough, respiratory distress, or exercise intolerance), dental disease (e.g., quidding or slow eating), or systemic disease (e.g., weight loss, depression, anorexia, fever, or lymphadenopathy).

It should also be determined if in-contact animals have exhibited nasal discharge or other signs of respiratory disease. The vaccination status of affected and in-contact animals should be ascertained. Recent stressors such as transportation, surgery, or weaning should be noted, and a history of contact with other animals at sales, shows, or other events should be established. Environmental quality and the overall management of the affected animal and the herd should be assessed (see Cough, p. 46). Progression or improvement in the signs, attempted therapy, and response to current or previous treatments should also be ascertained.

PHYSICAL EXAMINATION. Physical examination of an animal showing nasal discharge should include inspection from a distance and close examination using *auscultation, palpation,* and *percussion* techniques (see Physical Examination, p. 50, and Cough, p. 46).

The character and volume of the nasal discharge should be noted. Particular attention should be paid to whether:
- The nasal discharge is unilateral or bilateral
- The airflow from both nostrils is symmetric
- Odor emanates from the oral or nasal cavity
- Facial asymmetry is present
- A painful response is elicited on percussion of the maxillary and frontal sinuses
- Enlargement of submandibular, parotid, retropharyngeal, or other regional lymph nodes is present
- Palpable turbulence, such as a tracheal rattle, is present

The depth and symmetry of chest expansion should be assessed, and the rostral end of both nasal passages should be illuminated with a penlight and examined carefully.

A thorough *oral examination,* which should include probing of the occlusal surfaces of the maxillary cheek teeth with a fine dental pick, is important, especially in horses with a unilateral malodorous nasal discharge. Particular attention should be paid to detecting erosive periodontal disease, cracked or broken maxillary cheek teeth, and patent infundibulae. Because the roots of the third through the sixth maxillary cheek teeth in the horse are contained within the maxillary sinus, infection of these teeth frequently leads to sinus empyema with drainage from the nasomaxillary opening into the middle nasal meatus and ultimately to a unilateral nasal discharge. In cattle the oral examination should include palpation of the base of the tongue, the oropharynx and, if possible, the larynx to detect mass lesions or swelling of the tongue.

Further diagnostic evaluation of nasal discharge may include a complete blood count with determination of the fibrinogen concentration, a serum biochemistry profile, endoscopy of the upper and lower airways and the esophagus, nasal or nasopharyngeal swabbing for virus isolation, virus serologic testing, tracheal aspiration, bronchoalveolar lavage, ultrasonography, thoracocentesis, radiography, blood gas analysis, nuclear scintigraphy, fecal examination, pulmonary function testing, and lung biopsy. For further information on diagnostic procedures not discussed below, see Cough, p. 46.

ENDOSCOPIC EXAMINATION. Endoscopic examination of the upper and lower airways is a useful ancillary diagnostic procedure in all animals with nasal discharge. The nasal passages; the conchae (turbinates), including the ethmoidal conchae; the nasal septum; and the pharynx, larynx, and trachea should be examined through both nostrils. The presence, nature, and origin of exudates and the presence of anatomic or functional abnormalities or mass lesions should be noted. Although it is not possible to introduce an endoscope into the paranasal sinuses, drainage from the sinuses may be detected by examining the middle meatus.[21] Examination of the middle meatus area may also reveal turbinate necrosis or mass lesions (e.g., tumors, fungal granulomas, nasal foreign bodies). Lesions such as progressive hematomas (expanding mass lesions of variable size on the ethmoid turbinates) can be visualized by advancing the endoscope slightly, after deflecting its tip dorsally, from a position in the caudal part of the ventral meatus just rostral to the choana. In the horse the pharyngeal openings of the guttural pouches, which are located dorsolaterally on the wall of the pharynx, should be inspected for drainage. The interior of the guttural pouches can be examined for exudate, arterial aneurysms, mycotic plaques, and other proliferative lesions by advancing the endoscope through the pharyngeal openings of each guttural pouch.

Bronchoscopic examination may prove useful for identifying the bronchus of origin of pulmonary exudates and for facilitating appropriate bronchoalveolar lavage. In horses with intermittent bilateral nasal discharge, it may be helpful to repeat the endoscopic examination after exercise, which often mobilizes secretions from the lower respiratory tract and causes them to pool in the horizontal trachea. Endoscopic examination of the esophagus is indicated in patients with a history of dysphagia or return of ingesta through the nose (Boxes 5-7 and 5-8).

RADIOGRAPHY. Radiography with lateral, dorsoventral, and oblique radiographic projections of the nasal passages, paranasal sinuses, pharynx, retropharyngeal area (including guttural pouches in the horse), larynx, and proximal trachea is indicated to confirm problems identified by clinical examination and endoscopy and to identify conditions not recognized by other diagnostic techniques. The demonstration of increases in tissue density, fluid lines, bony lysis or proliferation, distortion of normal architecture, or changes around tooth roots assists in the diagnosis and localization of disorders of the nasal passages, conchae, and paranasal sinuses. Space-occupying lesions in the oropharynx, nasopharynx, or larynx may also be demonstrated by radiographic examination of these areas. The presence of fluid lines, soft tissue densities, or thickening of the floor of the guttural pouches helps differentiate guttural pouch diseases (e.g., empyema) from other space-occupying lesions (e.g., abscesses) in the retropharyngeal region. Contrast radiographic studies such as barium swallows are indicated to evaluate aspiration during swallowing in horses suspected of having pharyngeal paresis. Carotid angiography under general anesthesia has been used to demonstrate aneurysms in the internal carotid artery of horses with guttural pouch

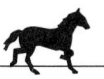

BOX 5-7

Causes of Ingesta in Nasal Discharge in the Horse

COMMON CAUSES
Esophageal obstruction, choke
Cleft palate, palatal hypoplasia (neonate)
Pharyngitis
Strangles (*Streptococcus equi* infection)
Dorsal displacement of the soft palate
Guttural pouch infection, mycosis, neoplasia
Glossopharyngeal nerve damage
Botulism, shaker foal
Retropharyngeal abscess

LESS COMMON CAUSES
Complications of laryngeal surgery
Laryngeal web defect
Epiglottal entrapment, subepiglottal abscess or cyst
Tetanus
Fistula (pharyngeal, esophageal, esophagobronchial, esophagotracheal)
Esophageal stricture, ectasia, diverticulum, megaesophagus, ulcer, rupture
Gastric, duodenal ulceration (foals)

LESS COMMON CAUSES—cont'd
Gastric dilation, rupture
Proximal enteritis, jejunitis
Small intestinal obstruction
Rabies
Other neurologic deficits affecting swallowing

UNCOMMON CAUSES
Persistent right aortic arch, vascular ring anomaly
Gastric tumor
Gastric stenosis
Rostral displacement of the palatopharyngeal arch
Hypoplasia of the soft palate
White muscle disease, nutritional myodegeneration
Rectus capitis ventralis muscle rupture
Lymphosarcoma, lymphoma, leukemia
Oleander poisoning
White snakeroot (tremetol) poisoning
Lead toxicity
Grass sickness (exotic)

BOX 5-8

Causes of Ingesta in Nasal Discharge in Ruminants

COMMON CAUSES
Esophageal obstruction, foreign body, choke
Pharyngeal, retropharyngeal abscess
Pharyngeal trauma, foreign body
Megaesophagus (B, C)

LESS COMMON CAUSES
Rhododendron poisoning (O)
Diaphragmatic hernia
Water deprivation, salt toxicity (B, O)
Ruptured or lacerated esophagus
Tetanus
Cleft hard or soft palate
Glossopharyngeal nerve damage

UNCOMMON CAUSES
Neoplasia of the esophagus or rumen (B)
Persistent right aortic arch, vascular ring anomaly (B, O)
Listeriosis
Bronchobiliary fistula (yellow froth) (B)
Congenital defects of Kodiak Island calves (B)
Oleander poisoning
White snakeroot (tremetol) poisoning (B, O)
Crude oil toxicity (B)
Geigeria spp. poisoning
Sneezeweed (*Helenium* spp.) poisoning
Rubberweed (*Hymenoxys* spp.) poisoning

B, Bovine; *C*, caprine; *O*, ovine.

---

mycosis.[26] Thoracic radiographs are indicated in patients suspected of having pulmonary, mediastinal, or pleural disease to determine the presence, pattern, and severity of radiographic changes.

COMPUTED TOMOGRAPHY SCANNING. Computed tomography (CT) scanning with horses positioned in dorsal recumbency under general anesthesia has recently been used with great success to more accurately define the location, nature, and extent of lesions involving the nasal passages and paranasal sinuses. The technique has proved particularly useful for evaluating mass lesions and the roots of the cheek teeth.

ULTRASOUND EXAMINATION. Ultrasound examination of externally visible lesions such as possible retropharyngeal abscesses or distended guttural pouches assists in characterization of lesions and collection of samples by aspiration or biopsy. Thoracic ultrasound is indicated when lower airway, pleural, or cardiac disease is the suspected cause of nasal discharge.

PERCUTANEOUS ASPIRATION. Percutaneous aspiration, either blindly or with the assistance of ultrasound, followed by cytology and culture of aspirated material, is useful in the evaluation of masses such as submandibular or retropharyngeal abscesses that are also causing a nasal discharge.

CENTESIS. Centesis of affected paranasal sinuses helps localize the source of exudates and provides samples for cytologic examination and culture in patients with chronic unilateral nasal discharge in which sinus percussion or radiographic examination (or both) suggests the presence of a sinus lesion. In the horse either the rostral or caudal maxillary sinus can be entered first, depending on which is suspected to be involved. If no exudate can be aspirated, either directly or after lavaging the sinus, and if increased purulent drainage from the ipsilateral nostril is not accomplished during lavage, the other maxillary sinus cavity is entered and the procedure repeated. If the aspirated material is not malodorous and if there is no evidence of dental disease, there is a reasonable likelihood that primary (nondental) sinusitis is present. In the horse the rostral maxillary sinus can be entered at a site 1 to 2 cm dorsal and 2 to 3 cm caudal to the rostral end of the facial crest. The caudal maxillary sinus is entered at a point midway between the medial canthus of the eye and the facial crest. After shaving and surgical preparation of the skin and subcutaneous placement of a small volume of local anesthetic, a stab incision is created through the skin and extended down to the periosteum. A small hole is then drilled through the bone with a Steinmann pin in a hand-held chuck or a 14-gauge needle. A 14-gauge cannula is introduced into the sinus and, if necessary, a No. 5 French catheter can be inserted through the cannula to facilitate sample collection and lavage (see Diseases of the Paranasal Sinuses, Chapter 29).

CATHETERIZATION. Catheterization of the guttural pouches via the pharyngeal orifice, either blindly or under endoscopic guidance, followed by aspiration, culture, and cytologic examination of aspirated contents is helpful in the evaluation of horses with chronic purulent nasal discharge in which guttural pouch empyema is suspected or has been confirmed by radiographic or endoscopic examination. In horses with large accumulations of fluid exudate, voluminous drainage of pus both through and around the catheter may occur when the pouch is first catheterized. In horses with chronic guttural pouch infections accompanied by tenacious or inspissated exudate, lavage with 250 to 400 ml of sterile saline or Ringer's solution facilitates sample collection.

REFERENCES

19. Lappin LR: Sneezing and nasal discharge. In Lorenz MD, Cornelius LM, eds: *Small animal medical diagnosis,* Philadelphia, 1987, JB Lippincott, pp 231-240.
20. Kelly WR: Nasal discharge. In Kelly WR, ed: *Veterinary clinical diagnosis,* ed 3, London, 1984, Ballière Tindall, pp 110-111.
21. Greet T: Differential diagnosis of nasal discharge in the horse, *In Practice* 8:49-57, 1986.
22. Amis TC: Clinical respiratory physiology. In Kirk RW, ed: *Current veterinary therapy. VIII, Small animal practice,* Philadelphia, 1984, WB Saunders, pp 191-201.
23. Thompson JA, Muren O: Sputum production. In Glauser FL, ed: *Signs and symptoms in pulmonary medicine,* Philadelphia, 1983, JB Lippincott, pp 20-27.
24. Brown CM: Purulent nasal discharge. In Brown CM, ed: *Problems in equine medicine,* Philadelphia, 1989, Lea & Febiger, pp 97-106.
25. Webbon PM: Pulmonary and pleural disease in the horse. In Hickman J, ed: *Equine surgery and medicine,* vol 2, London, 1986, Harcourt Brace Jovanovich, pp 283-314.
26. Colles CM, Cook WR: Carotid and cerebral angiography in the horse, *Vet Rec* 113:483-489, 1983.

EPISTAXIS AND HEMOPTYSIS

Definition

Epistaxis is defined as the presence of blood at the external nares[27]; the amount of blood at the nostrils can range from small flecks incorporated in serous nasal discharge to large volumes flowing freely from both nostrils. The coughing up of blood is called hemoptysis.[28]

Pathophysiology

Blood at the external nares originates from one or more of the following structures: nasal cavity, paranasal sinuses, gut-

tural pouch (auditory tube diverticulum), oral cavity, pharynx, larynx, trachea, or lungs.[27] These respiratory structures may be affected by a primary disease process or may be one of many mucosal surfaces involved in a bleeding diathesis (Boxes 5-9 and 5-10). The actual disease condition, affected structure, and the large animal species involved determines whether epistaxis is profuse or scant, unilateral or bilateral, induced by exercise, accompanied by hemoptysis, and/or associated with concurrent abnormal nasal discharge.

NASAL CAVITY OR PARANASAL SINUS PATHOLOGIC CONDITIONS. Epistaxis associated with diseased respiratory tract structures rostral to the caudal border of the nasal septum (e.g., nasal cavity, paranasal sinuses) usually is unilateral and appears spontaneously (i.e, occurs without exertion or lowering of the head). However, with profuse hemorrhage from these sites, blood may drain caudally, accumulate in the pharynx, and exit from both nostrils.

Nasal cavity structures are highly vascular and prone to injury. Bleeding can be caused by foreign bodies, fungal granulomas, or neoplasms that invade the nasal cavity; epistaxis associated with these lesions is commonly unilateral, scant, and evident only intermittently. Trauma induced by passage of a nasogastric tube or endoscope is the most common cause of profuse hemorrhage of nasal origin in horses.[27] Erosive diseases that affect the paranasal sinuses of horses (e.g., progressive ethmoidal hematoma)[27] or sheep (endemic nasal adenocarcinoma)[29] commonly cause a unilateral, serosanguinous nasal discharge preceded or accompanied by mucopurulent discharge. In the case of sinusitis the exudate often is malodorous, particularly when the process occurs secondary to dental disease. Epistaxis resulting from fractures of the nasal bones or skull can be scant or profuse, depending on the extent of the fracture.

PATHOLOGIC CONDITIONS OF THE GUTTURAL POUCHES OF THE HORSE. Spontaneous epistaxis that occurs at rest in a mature horse warrants consideration of the guttural pouch as the source of hemorrhage.[30] In the case of guttural pouch mycosis, epistaxis is caused by fungal erosion of the internal carotid artery in the roof of the medial compartment of the guttural pouch.[30-32] The horse initially experiences several episodes of minor hemorrhage characterized by a small amount of fresh blood at the external nares; this may be preceded by a unilateral catarrhal nasal discharge and followed by a seromucous nasal discharge. Ultimately, massive arterial bleeding associated with erosion of the internal carotid artery manifests as large volumes of blood gushing from both nostrils.[31] Epistaxis caused by bleeding from the guttural pouch is most pronounced on the ipsilateral side, but nasal bleeding is usually bilateral in this condition, especially if hemorrhage is profuse, because the nasopharynx drains into both nasal passages.[32]

PULMONARY PATHOLOGIC CONDITIONS. In horses pulmonary hemorrhage manifests as bilateral epistaxis, most often during or immediately after strenuous exercise.[27] However, in many cases of pulmonary hemorrhage, epistaxis may not be observed because blood originating from the lungs is swallowed when it reaches the pharynx. Hemoptysis, the hallmark of pulmonary hemorrhage in cattle, is rarely observed in horses because the laryngopalatal articulation of the horse fixes the larynx in an intranarial position and generally prevents blood flow from the nasopharynx to the oropharynx and mouth. In contrast to humans and other animal species, where foaming of blood exiting the nares suggests pulmonary hemorrhage, foaming of the blood is rarely encountered in horses with pulmonary hemorrhage because the horizontal position of the major bronchi allows blood to pool and flow freely without having to be coughed up.

BOX 5-9

Causes of Epistaxis in the Horse

COMMON CAUSES
Exercise-induced pulmonary hemorrhage (EIPH)
Guttural pouch mycosis
Progressive ethmoidal hematoma
Nasal trauma
Pharyngeal or retropharyngeal trauma or abscess
Nasal polyps
Tumors (nose, paranasal sinuses)
Foreign body (nasal, pharyngeal, laryngeal, tracheal, bronchial)
Purpura hemorrhagica

LESS COMMON CAUSES
Pleuropneumonia
Infarctive lobar pneumonia
Pulmonary neoplasia
Fungal granuloma (maduromycosis, aspergillosis, rhinosporidiosis, mycetoma)
Cryptococcal rhinitis
Coccidioidomycosis
Guttural pouch empyema
Guttural pouch neoplasia
Guttural pouch foreign body
Vesicular stomatitis
Atrial fibrillation
Idiopathic thrombocytopenic purpura
Immune-mediated thrombocytopenia
Lymphosarcoma
Myeloproliferative disease
Disseminated intravascular coagulation (DIC)
Toxic hepatic failure

LESS COMMON CAUSES—cont'd
Multiple clotting defects (foals)
Equine infectious anemia (EIA)
Skull fracture
Gunshot
Pharyngeal lymphoid hyperplasia

UNCOMMON CAUSES
Nasal amyloidosis
Rectus capitis ventralis rupture
Black's disease (Clostridium novyi)
Snakebite
Retrobulbar neoplasia
Chronic hepatitis or cholangitis
Acute renal failure
Cardiac neoplasia
Laryngeal hemiplegia
Phycomycosis, pythiosis, zygomycosis
Thrombasthenia-like syndrome
Besnoitiosis, globidiosis (exotic)
Dacryohemorrhea (exotic)

TOXIC CAUSES
Arsenic
Warfarin or dicoumarol
Stachybotryotoxicosis (Stachybotrys spp.)
Plant toxins
Moldy sweet clover (Melilotus alba)
Pyrrolizidine alkaloid (e.g., common groundsel [Senecio vulgaris], fiddleneck [Amsinckia spp.], tansy ragwort [Senecio jacobeae])

BOX 5-10

Causes of Epistaxis in Ruminants

COMMON CAUSES
Pharyngeal or retropharyngeal trauma or abscess
Lung embolus from caudal vena cava thrombosis (CVCT) (B)
Infection of paranasal sinuses
Nasal trauma
Foreign body (nasal, pharyngeal, laryngeal, tracheal, bronchial)
Nasal bots (Oestrus ovis) (C, O)
Nasal adenoma, adenopapilloma, adenocarcinoma (C, O)
Dehorning of adult animals (B)

LESS COMMON CAUSES
Nasal granuloma, atopic rhinitis (B)
Fungal granuloma (maduromycosis, rhinosporidiosis, mycetoma) (B, C)
Neoplasia (nose, paranasal sinuses)
Skull fracture
Gunshot injury
Bluetongue (O)
Vesicular stomatitis
Bovine virus diarrhea (BVD-MD) (B)
Malignant catarrhal fever (B)
Infectious bovine rhinotracheitis (IBR; BHV-1) (B)

UNCOMMON CAUSES
Black's disease (Clostridium novyi) (B, O)
Acute anthrax (Bacillus anthracis)
Bacillary hemoglobinuria (Clostridium hemolyticum) (B, O)
Snakebite
Acute renal failure
Endocarditis

UNCOMMON CAUSES—cont'd
Liver fluke disease
Pulmonary neoplasia
Pasteurella pneumonia or septicemia (C, O)
Xylazine-induced pulmonary edema (O)
Idiopathic granulocytopenia or thrombocytopenia (B)
Hemophilia A (factor VIII deficiency) (B)
Factor XI deficiency (B)
Hereditary platelet aggregating disorder in Simmentals (B)
Cardiomyopathy in polled Hereford calves (B)
Trypanosomiasis (exotic) (B, O)
Ondiri disease (exotic) (B, O)
Besnoitiosis, globidiosis (exotic) (B, O)
Endemic ethmoid carcinoma (exotic) (B)
Gedoelstia hasleri nasal bots (exotic) (O, C)
Nairobi sheep disease (exotic) (O, C)
Leech infestation (hirudiniasis) (exotic)

TOXIC CAUSES
Mercury
Arsenic
Warfarin, diphacinone
Furozolidone
Trichlorethylene-extracted feed
Oak (acorn poisoning)
Bracken fern (Pteridium aquilina)
Moldy sweet clover (Melilotus alba)
Phytogenous selenium poisoning (e.g., Astragalus spp.)
Oxalate poisoning (e.g., Halogen spp., Sarcobatus spp.)
Stachybotryotoxicosis (Stachybotrys spp.)
Mycotoxicosis

B, Bovine; C, caprine; O, ovine.

Exercise-induced pulmonary hemorrhage (EIPH), a syndrome experienced by 40% to 75% of racing horses, is characterized by hemorrhage into the tracheobronchial tree during competitive exercise.[27] Although pulmonary hemorrhage can be identified by endoscopic examination of the trachea immediately after exercise in these horses, EIPH manifests as frank epistaxis at the external nares in only a small percentage of cases.[33] Bleeding at the nares may range from a slight orange-tinged serous nasal discharge to a constant trickle of fresh blood that persists for several hours after exercise.[27] The current thinking is that a combination of racing stress (marked pulmonary hypertension and increased blood viscosity) and local small airway disease probably is involved in the development of EIPH.[34] The exact source of hemorrhage in horses with EIPH has not been identified, but it is known that affected horses have proliferation of the bronchial arterial blood supply to the lungs.[35] Fatal massive epistaxis, an infrequent sequela to exercise, has been attributed to tearing of the lung in association with pleural adhesions or focal shear stress.[36] Other less common causes of postexercise pulmonary hemorrhage in horses include pulmonary abscesses or pleuropneumonia with pulmonary infarction; in these cases the odor of the breath may be fetid, and hemorrhage may occur spontaneously (without exercise), which aids in the differentiation of these conditions from EIPH.[27,37]

Caudal vena cava thrombosis (CVCT) (also known as pulmonary embolic aneurysm or pulmonary thromboembolism) is the disease most likely to be associated with epistaxis and hemoptysis in cattle (Box 5-11).[38] This sporadic, fatal condition of feedlot cattle is the result of a four-step sequence of events that culminates with the rupture of a pulmonary artery aneurysm into a bronchus. Initially, affected cattle exhibit tachypnea, lethargy, painful cough, melena, and anemia. Terminally the disease is characterized by discharge of bright, foamy red blood from the nose and mouth, severe respiratory distress, and widespread pulmonary crackles.[38]

Pulmonary edema present in the terminal stages of left heart failure may also be responsible for bilateral serosanguinous discharge at the external nares of large animals.[27]

PATHOLOGIC CONDITIONS OF THE ORAL CAVITY, PHARYNX, OR LARYNX. Less often, epistaxis can result from bleeding from lesions in the oral cavity, pharynx, or larynx. Examples include oral cavity erosions associated with infectious diseases (e.g., mucosal form of bovine virus diarrhea infection in cattle, or bluetongue in sheep); erosions associated with epiglottic entrapment in horses; foreign bodies wedged in the mouth or pharynx of large animals; and pharyngeal or retropharyngeal trauma caused by a "balling gun."

BLEEDING DIATHESIS. A number of inherited and acquired coagulation disorders of large animals manifest as epistaxis.[39] Inherited clotting factor deficiencies (usually deficiencies of factors VIII, IX, or XI) or acquired factor deficiencies (those caused by warfarin, sweet clover toxicosis, or advanced liver disease) cause bleeding from large vessels. In addition to epistaxis, subcutaneous hematomas, hemarthrosis, melena, hematuria, and prolonged bleeding from sites of injury may be observed. With conditions causing vasculitis (e.g., equine purpura hemorrhagica, equine viral arteritis), small vessel bleeding occurs. Vasculitis is characterized by mucous membrane petechiae and ecchymoses and demarcated areas of skin edema. Nasal mucous membrane petechiae associated with vasculitis may manifest as epistaxis. Similarly, thrombocytopenia (e.g., immune-mediated thrombocytopenia in horses, bracken fern toxicosis in cattle) is characterized by mucous membrane petechiae and occasionally epistaxis. In rare cases disseminated intravascular coagulation (DIC) in large animals manifests as a consumptive coagulopathy with bleeding from mucous membranes and blood at the external nares.

Approach to Diagnosis of Epistaxis and Hemoptysis

HISTORY. History taking should closely follow that described for animals with nasal discharge and should include duration of ownership, time of first appearance of blood at the nares, number of times the animal has bled, volume and color of blood, presence of blood at one or both nostrils, association of epistaxis with exercise, swallowing motions or cough after exercise, concurrent hemoptysis, other signs of respiratory tract disease (e.g., stridor, cough, nasal discharge, respiratory distress), evidence of central nervous system involvement (e.g., feed particles at the nares, drooping of the lip or ear), possibility of recent trauma (e.g., nasogastric intubation or head injury), and exposure to toxic plants (e.g., bracken fern or sweet clover).

PHYSICAL EXAMINATION. A complete physical examination should be performed to detect abnormalities indicative of systemic disease or disease affecting other body systems. This examination should include assessment of the attitude of the animal; determination of rectal temperature, pulse rate, and respiratory rate and character; evaluation of mucous membranes for color and petechiae; inspection of the animal to detect hematomas or prolonged bleeding from sites of injury; and neurologic examination to detect neurologic dysfunction (e.g., dysphagia, Horner's syndrome, facial paralysis, head tilt, or nystagmus), which may accompany guttural pouch mycosis.

EVALUATION OF THE HEAD AND RESPIRATORY SYSTEM. A complete evaluation of the head and respiratory system should also be carried out. The nasal bones and flat bones overlying the maxillary and frontal sinuses should be examined for asymmetry or deformation; the eyes should be evaluated for exophthalmos or epiphora; the nasal mucosae should be inspected with a light source to demonstrate erosive, ulcerative, or mass lesions; and the sinuses should be percussed to detect altered resonance or pain. On continuing the examination, the following should be evaluated: symmetry and amount of airflow through the nostrils and the effect of occluding each nostril independently; odor at the nose or mouth; presence of stridor; and the effect of applying pressure to the larynx or trachea. The oral cavity should be carefully inspected in animals in which epistaxis is accompanied by a necrotic breath odor. Special attention should be paid to the maxillary cheek teeth of horses and the base of the tongue and the oropharynx of all large animals. Structures in the external pharyngeal region (mandibular lymph nodes, Viborg's triangle, retropharyngeal lymph nodes, parotid salivary gland) should be observed and palpated for swelling, heat, or pain, and the trachea should be observed and palpated where exposed to detect any abnormalities. The larynx, trachea, and lungs should be carefully ausculted at rest and after application of a rebreathing bag for abnormally loud

---

BOX 5-11

Causes of Hemoptysis in Ruminants

Caudal vena cava thrombosis (CVCT)
Aspiration pneumonia
Pharyngeal or retropharyngeal abscess or trauma
Thoracic trauma (fractured ribs or sternum)
Foreign body (nasal, oropharyngeal, tracheal, bronchial)
Pulmonary aspergillosis

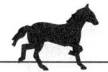

breath sounds, crackles, or wheezes, which may implicate pulmonary disease as the cause of epistaxis. Careful cardiac auscultation should be carried out to detect murmurs or dysrhythmias, which may be associated with left heart failure and pulmonary edema. The chest wall should be palpated to detect rib fractures or pleural friction rubs, and the thorax should be percussed bilaterally to demonstrate large mass lesions, pleural effusion, or pleurodynia.

COMPLETE BLOOD COUNT. A complete blood count and assessment of fibrinogen concentration can be useful in the evaluation of animals with primary or secondary inflammatory conditions or those that have developed blood loss anemia as a sequela to epistaxis (e.g., horses with guttural pouch mycosis or cattle with pulmonary thromboembolism secondary to CVCT). The degree of anemia may give an indication of the severity and chronicity of the bleeding or, in cases of bracken fern poisoning, of the degree of bone marrow suppression.

PROFILE. A clotting profile should be performed (platelet count, prothrombin time [PT], activated partial thromboplastin time [APTT], concentration of fibrin degradation products [FDPs] and plasma antithrombin III) if petechiae of mucous membranes or a tendency to bleed was noted on the general physical examination or if the history suggests exposure to sweet clover, warfarin, or bracken fern.

BIOCHEMISTRY PROFILE. A biochemistry profile should be performed to detect disease processes in organ systems other than the lungs (e.g., increased liver enzyme activity in cattle with hemoptysis secondary to CVCT or animals with liver failure causing secondary clotting factor deficiency).

OCCULT BLOOD. Feces should be tested for occult blood. Positive results may suggest swallowing of blood originating from the lungs or pharynx or gastrointestinal bleeding.

ENDOSCOPIC EVALUATION. Endoscopic evaluation using a fiberoptic or video endoscope is a useful diagnostic aid in cases of epistaxis. The nasal passages, nasomaxillary aperture in the middle meatus, turbinates (conchae), nasal septum, pharynx, guttural pouches, larynx, and tracheobronchial tree should be systematically evaluated through both nostrils at rest and after exercise to determine the presence, nature, and source of blood and the anatomic or mass lesion responsible for the bleeding. Care should be taken when endoscopy is performed in horses with guttural pouch mycosis, because dislodging a clot of blood in the affected guttural pouch may result in fatal hemorrhage.[40] Similarly, the stress of endoscopy may prove fatal to cattle with pulmonary thromboembolism secondary to CVCT. If EIPH is suspected, endoscopy should be performed 30 to 120 minutes after strenuous exercise to allow time for the mucociliary escalator to transport blood to where it can be visualized[33]; this blood may persist from 6 hours to 4 days after exercise, depending on the severity of pulmonary hemorrhage. It is important to remember that EIPH may not be repeatable. In one study only 33% of thoroughbred racehorses tested positive for EIPH on all subsequent endoscopic examinations after breezing.[41] Biopsy (with histologic evaluation and possibly culture of samples) is indicated when granulomas, polyps, erosions, or mass lesions are visualized through the endoscope.

ASPIRATION, LAVAGE, AND THORACOCENTESIS. Percutaneous transtracheal aspiration or endoscopic tracheal aspiration, bronchoalveolar lavage (BAL), or thoracocentesis with cytologic studies and culture of collected samples are indicated when pulmonary or pleural diseases are thought to be responsible for hemorrhage into the respiratory tract. BAL is a technique best suited to evaluation of diffuse lung disease; BAL fluid analysis can yield a normal result in horses with focal lung disease (e.g., pulmonary abscess, pneumonia or pleuropneumonia) because lavage fluid is instilled into a

limited region of the lung.[42] Quantitative culture techniques should be used for samples obtained via BAL because contamination by nasopharyngeal organisms can occur.[43] Although there is a poor correlation between cytologic findings in tracheal wash fluid and histopathologic changes in the lungs of individual horses, increased cell counts with degenerative neutrophils and large numbers of intracellular and extracellular bacteria suggest a diagnosis of bronchopneumonia.[44] Percutaneously obtained tracheal wash samples are usually not contaminated by oropharyngeal organisms and can be submitted for culture[43]; transendoscopically obtained samples may be contaminated with *Pseudomonas* spp. and anaerobic bacteria despite the use of guarded tracheal swabs.[45] The presence of hemosiderophages in tracheobronchial aspirates or BAL fluid is generally considered indicative of previous pulmonary hemorrhage[33]; however, mucopolysaccharides engulfed by alveolar macrophages can bind plasma iron in the absence of pulmonary hemorrhage to form an iron pigment resembling hemosiderin.[46]

RADIOGRAPHIC EXAMINATION. Radiographic examination of the nasal passages, paranasal sinuses, pharynx, retropharyngeal region (including the guttural pouches), larynx, and trachea is indicated if the source of nasal bleeding cannot be definitively diagnosed through physical examination and endoscopy. The nasal passages, turbinates, and paranasal sinuses should be evaluated for fluid lines, cystic structures, bony lysis or proliferation, distortion of normal architecture, or changes in the tooth roots. Space-occupying lesions in the pharynx and larynx may also be demonstrated by radiographic examination. Demonstration of a fluid-air interface in the guttural pouch may indicate guttural pouch hemorrhage or guttural pouch empyema.[27] New bone formation and sclerosis at the junction of the stylohyoid bone with the petrous temporal bone may accompany mycotic infections of the guttural pouch.[27] Thoracic radiographs using four overlapping lateral views in adult horses and cattle and lateral and ventrodorsal views in immature animals and small ruminants aids in identification and definition of diseases affecting the lungs, pleurae, and mediastinum.[43]

ULTRASOUND EXAMINATION. Ultrasound examination is used as an adjunct to thoracic radiology in animals suspected of having pleural effusion[43]; this procedure allows the examiner to determine the extent of the effusion and the presence of fibrin deposits or pleural adhesions. Pulmonary consolidation, atelectasis, infarction, and abscessation can also be demonstrated with this technique if these lesions are contiguous with the pleural surface.[43] Ultrasound examination of externally visible swellings such as enlarged retropharyngeal lymph nodes or distended guttural pouches may provide additional diagnostic information and assist with appropriate placement of needles or biopsy instruments for sample collection.

PARACENTESIS. Paracentesis of the *maxillary sinus*[43] can be performed if percussion and inspection indicate that a lesion in the maxillary sinus may be the cause of epistaxis. Using sedation and analgesia, a small hole is trephined into the maxillary sinus with a Steinmann pin or 14-gauge needle; sinus contents can then be aspirated and submitted for cytologic and bacteriologic examination (See Nasal Discharge, p. 54).

PLEUROSCOPIC EXAMINATION. Pleuroscopic examination[47] can be performed in a standing, sedated patient using a sterile rigid or fiberoptic endoscope. This procedure is indicated for patients in which large intrathoracic masses and adhesions were demonstrated by thoracic radiology and ultrasonography. Pleuroscopy allows direct visualization of affected structures and provides an opportunity to biopsy masses or aspirate fluid. Pleuroscopy is a procedure fraught with complications (e.g., pneumothorax, lung lacerations, infection) and should be reserved for cases in which less invasive procedures have failed to adequately diagnose the condition.[43]

In some teaching and research institutions *ventilation* and *perfusion ratios* can be measured in horses using nuclear scintigraphic techniques. A study of horses with EIPH demonstrated both ventilation and perfusion deficits in the dorsocaudal lung field that corresponded to the area in which EIPH lesions were detected at postmortem.[48]

REFERENCES

27. O'Callaghan MW: Bleeding from the nose. In Brown CM, ed: *Problems in equine medicine*, Philadelphia, 1989, Lea & Febiger, pp 107-121.
28. Cornelius LM: Hemoptysis. In Lorenz MD, Cornelius LM, eds: *Small animal medical diagnosis*, Philadelphia, 1987, JB Lippincott, pp 224-226.
29. Rings MD, Rojko J: Naturally occurring nasal obstructions in 11 sheep, *Cornell Vet* 75:269-276, 1985.
30. Greet TRC: Outcome of treatment in 35 cases of guttural pouch mycosis, *Equine Vet J* 19:483-487, 1987.
31. Freeman DE: Diagnosis and treatment of diseases of the guttural pouch, *Compend Cont Educ Pract Vet* 11:S3-S11, 1980.
32. Cook WR: The clinical features of guttural pouch mycosis in the horse, *Vet Rec* 83:336-345, 1968.
33. Sweeney CR: Exercise-induced pulmonary hemorrhage, *Vet Clin North Am (Equine Pract)* 7:93-104, 1991.
34. Smith JD et al: Exercise-induced pulmonary hemorrhage findings. I, *Equine Pract* 14:19-25, 1992.
35. O'Callaghan MW et al: Exercise-induced pulmonary hemorrhage in the horse: results of a detailed clinical, postmortem and imaging study. III, Subgross findings in lungs subjected to latex perfusions of the bronchial and pulmonary arteries, *Equine Vet J* 19:394-404, 1987.
36. Gunson DE, Sweeney CR, Soma LR: Sudden death attributable to exercise-induced pulmonary hemorrhage in racehorses: nine cases (1981-1983), *J Am Vet Med Assoc* 193:102-106, 1988.
37. Carr EA et al: Acute hemorrhagic pulmonary infarction and necrotizing pneumonia in horses: 21 cases (1967-1993), *J Am Vet Med Assoc* 210:1774-1778, 1997.
38. Wikse SE: Feedlot cattle pneumonias, *Vet Clin North Am (Food Anim Pract)* 1:289-310, 1985.
39. Morris DD: Diseases associated with blood loss and hemostatic dysfunction. In Smith BP, ed: *Large animal internal medicine*, St Louis, 1990, Mosby, pp 1069-1084.
40. Hawkins DL: Diseases of the guttural pouches. In Robinson NE, ed: *Current therapy in equine medicine 3*, Philadelphia, 1992, WB Saunders, pp 275-280.
41. Pascoe JR et al: Exercise-induced pulmonary hemorrhage in racing thoroughbreds: a preliminary study, *Am J Vet Res* 24:703-707, 1981.
42. Rossier Y, Sweeney CR, Ziemer EL: Bronchoalveolar lavage fluid cytologic findings in horses with pneumonia or pleuropneumonia, *J Am Vet Med Assoc* 198:1001-1004, 1991.
43. Hinchcliff KW, Byrne BB: Clinical examination of the respiratory system, *Vet Clin North Am (Equine Pract)* 7:1-26, 1991.
44. Beech J: Cytology of tracheobronchial aspirates in horses, *Vet Pathol* 12:157-164, 1975.
45. Sweeney CR, Sweeney RW, Benson SE: Comparison of bacteria isolated from specimens obtained by use of endoscopic guarded tracheal swabbing and percutaneous tracheal aspiration in horses, *J Am Vet Med Assoc* 195:1225-1232, 1989.
46. Roszel JF et al: Siderophages in pulmonary cytology specimens from racing and nonracing horses, *Proc Am Assoc Equine Pract* 33:321-329, 1987.
47. Mansmann RA, Bernard-Strother S: Pleuroscopy in horses, *Mod Vet Pract* 66:9-17, 1985.
48. O'Callaghan MW et al: Exercise-induced pulmonary hemorrhage in the horse: results of a detailed clinical, postmortem and imaging study. VII, Ventilation/perfusion scintigraphy in horses with EIPH, *Equine Vet J* 19:423-427, 1987.

RESPIRATORY DISTRESS (DYSPNEA)

Definition

Respiratory distress indicates an inappropriate degree of effort to breathe based on an assessment of respiratory rate, rhythm, and character.[49,50]

Respiratory distress is a clinical sign that implies labored breathing, whereas dyspnea is a symptom that describes the subjective feeling of difficult, uncomfortable, or unpleasant breathing (shortness of breath) in human patients.[49-51] As such the term dyspnea is not strictly applicable to animal patients, although it is widely used by veterinarians to describe respiratory distress.

Manifestations of respiratory distress include elevated respiratory rate (Tachypnea, see p. 69), extended head and neck position, mouth breathing (ruminants), nostril flaring (horses, sheep, and goats), exaggerated intercostal or abdominal effort (or both), a double expiratory lift and a "heave line" (expiratory respiratory distress), abducted elbows, stridor, anxious expression, and inactivity. Animals in severe respiratory distress may show cyanosis (see p. 64) and (especially those with severe obstructive pulmonary disease) may exert so much effort to breathe that the whole body rocks, the anus pumps in and out, and the animal does not move or eat because this diverts its energies from respiration.[50]

Pathophysiology

Normal respiratory rate and character are maintained by central and peripheral monitoring of blood gas and acid-base status, with resulting reflex adjustments that maintain carbon dioxide (CO_2), oxygen (O_2), and the blood hydrogen ion concentration (pH) within a narrow range.[52] Respiratory distress may occur for the following reasons[53]:

- Inadequate oxygenation of blood (i.e., a need for additional oxygen)
- Compensation for metabolic acidosis
- Excessive environmental heat
- Disorders that damage the central nervous system respiratory centers in the medulla (e.g., head trauma, inflammation, mass lesions) if they disrupt the control of breathing
- Disorders that cause dysfunction of motor nerves or weakness of respiratory muscles (e.g., polyradiculoneuritis, myasthenia gravis, or diaphragmatic paralysis)
- Painful conditions involving the respiratory sensory nerves, muscles, pleura, and ribs (e.g., chest trauma, pleural infection, or neoplasia)

Inadequate oxygenation of blood leads to arterial hypoxemia (low partial pressure of oxygen in arterial blood [Pa_{O_2}]). This can be caused by a low partial pressure of inspired oxygen (PI_{O_2}), such as occurs at high altitude; by disorders that interrupt the transfer of oxygen from the environment to the blood (e.g., upper and lower airway obstruction, pulmonary disease associated with alveolar flooding or collapse, and pulmonary or intracardiac right-to-left shunting of blood); or by a decrease in the oxygen-carrying capacity of the blood, such as occurs in anemia, methemoglobinemia, and carboxyhemaglobinemia.[53] Primary or secondary disease conditions that affect the respiratory and cardiovascular systems induce arterial hypoxemia by causing alveolar hypoventilation, ventilation-perfusion mismatch, diffusion limitation, right-to-left shunting of blood, or combinations of these abnormalities (see Cyanosis, p. 70).[49,53]

Compensation for metabolic acidosis involves "blowing off" carbon dioxide, which may increase both the rate and depth of respiration.[53] The resulting hyperventilation causes a decline in the partial pressure of arterial carbon dioxide (Pa_{CO_2}) in the face of clinical signs of respiratory distress.

Animals dissipate a considerable amount of heat through the respiratory tract. In ruminants, but not in horses, heat dissipation is further aided by the animals' ability to mouth breathe and pant to increase evaporative cooling of blood passing through the tongue and other structures in the oral cavity and oropharynx. The need to dissipate heat is the mechanism through which excessively hot environmental temperatures induce labored breathing (Boxes 5-12 and 5-13). Apparent respiratory distress also occurs when the weather is not excessively hot but the temperature has risen rapidly, such as occurs when cattle in cold climates are brought indoors in the winter. When the environmental temperature has been consistently low,

Text continued on p. 68

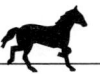

BOX 5-12

Causes of Respiratory Distress in the Horse

COMMON RESPIRATORY CAUSES
Bacterial pneumonia
Pleuropneumonia, pleuritis
Pleuropneumonia
Pulmonary abscessation
Chronic obstructive pulmonary disease (housing or pasture associated)
Strangles (*Streptococcus equi* infection)
Viral pneumonia (influenza, adenovirus, equine viral arteritis, others)
Equine herepesvirus types 1 and 4 (EHV-1, EHV-4)
Aspiration pneumonia
Prematurity, dysmaturity, immaturity (foals)
Neonatal septicemia (foals)
Pharyngeal, retropharyngeal abscess or trauma

COMMON NONRESPIRATORY CAUSES
Cardiac disease (e.g., congestive cardiac failure, mitral insufficiency, other cardiac diseases)
Shock (septic, cardiogenic, hypovolemic, acute blood loss)
Endotoxemia
Anemia (e.g., neonatal isoerythrolysis, autoimmune hemolytic anemia, blood loss, other causes of acute anemia)
Pain (e.g., abdominal crisis, laminitis, myopathy, fracture, other lameness)
Hyperthermia (e.g., fever, postexhaustion syndrome, anhidrosis, heat stroke, erythromycin associated)

LESS COMMON RESPIRATORY CAUSES
Epiglottic entrapment with secondary infection or granulation
Arytenoid chondritis
Guttural pouch empyema, tympany, mycosis, neoplasia
Progressive ethmoid hematoma
Nasal polyps
Pharyngeal, subepiglottic cysts
Fungal rhinitis, cryptococcal rhinitis, equine nasal granuloma, nasal aspergillosis, rhinosporidiosis, rhinophycomycosis, maduromycosis, mycetoma
Cleft palate
Laryngeal or hyoid trauma, fractured laryngeal cartilages, laryngeal granuloma or scar
Paranasal sinus infection, cyst, trauma, tumor
Nasal trauma, nasal neoplasia
Foreign body (nasal, pharyngeal, laryngeal, tracheal, bronchial)
Exercise-induced pulmonary hemorrhage (EIPH)
Parasitic pneumonia (*Dictyocaulus arnfieldi*)
Coccidioidomycosis, cryptococcosis, mycotic pneumonia
Inhalation pneumonia, smoke inhalation, drowning, water inhalation
Hyaline membrane disease (foals)
Acute bronchointerstitial pneumonia
Neonatal maladjustment syndrome
Fractured ribs or sternum, thoracic trauma
Pneumothorax
Diaphragmatic hernia
Mediastinal abscess

LESS COMMON NONRESPIRATORY CAUSES
Purpura hemorrhagica
Blood or plasma transfusion reaction
Complications of fluid therapy
Anaphylaxis
Intracarotid injection
Acidosis
Gastric distention (e.g., as in small intestinal obstruction)
Pulmonary edema

LESS COMMON NONRESPIRATORY CAUSES—cont'd
Malignant hyperthermia
Cardiovascular anomalies (ventricular septal defect, patent ductus arteriosus, tetralogy of Fallot, common ventricle, other anomalies)
Endocarditis
Pericarditis
Cardiac dysrhythmias (atrial fibrillation, heart block, ventricular premature beats, ventricular tachycardia, ventricular fibrillation)
Ruptured mitral chordae tendinae
Mitral insufficiency or stenosis
Clostridial infections (e.g., tetanus, malignant edema, injection abscess)
Procaine penicillin G reaction or intravascular administration
Hyperkalemic periodic paralysis (HYPP)

UNCOMMON RESPIRATORY CAUSES
Stenotic external nares
Cutaneous, nasal amyloidosis
Cutaneous, nasal habronemiasis (summer sore)
Failure of closure of the false nostril
Abnormalities of the nasal septum
Choanal (posterior nares) atresia or stenosis (foals)
Nasopharyngeal cicatrix
Laryngopalatal dislocation (dorsal displacement of soft palate), soft palate hypoplasia
Rostral displacement of the palatopharyngeal folds
Pharyngeal hematoma
Laryngeal paralysis
Fistula (pharyngeal, esophageal, esophagobronchial, esophagotracheal)
Chondroma of the arytenoid cartilage
Laryngeal spasm
Hypertrophic ossification of the laryngeal cartilages, laryngeal chondropathy
Neoplasia of the upper airway
Tracheal stenosis, stricture, collapse, rupture
Phycomycosis, pythiosis
Pneumoconiosis (e.g., silicosis)
Interstitial pneumonia (restrictive pulmonary disease)
Pulmonary thromboembolism
Pneumocystis carinii pneumonia
Pulmonary lobar hypertrophy (foals)
Infarctive lobar pneumonia
Chlamydia psittaci pneumonia
Pulmonary nocardiosis
Pulmonary tuberculosis
Pulmonary aspergillosis
Besnoitiosis (*Besnoitia besnoiti* and *Besnoitia jellisoni*)
Pulmonary neoplasia (primary or metastatic)
Pleural neoplasia (mesothelioma, lymphosarcoma)
Embryonic cyst (mediastinal, branchial, cervical, thyroglossal duct)
Morbillivirus infection (exotic)

UNCOMMON NONRESPIRATORY CAUSES
Nutritional myodegeneration
Lactation tetany (eclampsia)
Hydroallantois or hydramnios
Methemoglobin reductase deficiency
Hemophilia A (factor VIII deficiency)
Acute hepatic insufficiency
Electrocution
Cor pulmonale
Neoplasia (all systems)
Snake or insect bite

Continued

BOX 5-12

Causes of Respiratory Distress in the Horse—cont'd

UNCOMMON NONRESPIRATORY CAUSES—cont'd
Aortoileofemoral thrombosis
Equine motor neuron disease
Cholesteremic granuloma

TOXIC CAUSES
Vitamin D
Lead
Organophosphate-associated laryngeal paralysis
Monensin, lasolacid, salinomycin
Propylene glycol
Iron
Dinitrophenol
Selenium
Bromide
Sodium fluoroacetate
Strychnine
Ammonia
Theobromine, chocolate

TOXIC CAUSES—cont'd
Cantharidin (blister beetle)
α-Naphthyl thiourea (ANTU)
Red maple *(Acer rubrum)*
Water hemlock *(Cicuta* spp.)
Oleander *(Nerium oleander)*
Japanese yew *(Taxus cuspidata)*
Larkspur *(Delphinium* spp.)
Ryegrass *(Lolium* spp.)
White snakeroot *(Eupatorium rugosum)*
Crofton weed *(Eupatorium adenophorum)*
Pyrrolizidine alkaloid
Locoweeds *(Astragalus* spp., *Oxytropis* spp.)
Avocado *(Persea americana)*
Hoary alyssum *(Bertonea incana)*
Coffee senna seed *(Cassia occidentalis)*
Rubber vine *(Cryptostegia grandiflora)*
Birdsville disease *(Indigofera* spp.) (exotic)
Tachyandra paralysis (exotic)

BOX 5-13

Causes of Respiratory Distress in Ruminants

COMMON RESPIRATORY CAUSES
Mannheimia hemolytica or *Pasteurella multocida* pneumonia
(includes shipping fever and enzootic calf pneumonia)
Bacterial pneumonia with consolidation or abscessation
(Arcanobacterium and other bacteria)
Haemophilus somnus pneumonia (B)
Visceral caseous lymphadenitis *(Corynebacterium pseudotuber-culosis)* (O, C)
Aspiration or foreign body pneumonia (especially after hypocalcemia)
Necrotic laryngitis *(Fusobacterium necrophorum)* (B, O)
Infectious bovine rhinotracheitis virus (IBR; BHV-1) (B)
Respiratory syncytial virus
Ovine progressive pneumonia virus (O)
Mycoplasma mycoides subsp. *mycoides, Mycoplasma agalactiae,*
other *Mycoplasma* spp. (C)
Mycoplasma ovipneumoniae (O)
Parasitic pneumonia *(Dictyocaulus viviparus* [B], *Dictyocaulus filaria* [O, C], *Müllerius capillaris* [O, C], *Protostrongylus rufescens* [O, C])
Bovine atypical interstitial pneumonia (B)
Acute bovine pulmonary edema and emphysema (B)
Farmer's lung disease *(Faenia rectivirgula* hypersensitivity pneumonitis) (B)

COMMON NONRESPIRATORY CAUSES
Hyperthermia (fever, heat stroke, rapid rise in ambient temperature, other)
Pain (abdominal crisis, urethral calculi, traumatic reticuloperitonitis, other)
Distended abdominal viscus
Acidosis (ruminal lactic acidosis, pregnancy toxemia, other)
Electrolyte aberrations (hypocalcemia, hypomagnesemia, other)
Hypovolemic, cardiac, or septic shock
Fluid or electrolyte loss (acute diarrhea, gastrointestinal obstruction, other)
Endotoxemia (coliform mastitis, metritis, enteritis, salmonellosis, septicemia, other)

COMMON NONRESPIRATORY CAUSES—cont'd
Neonatal septicemia
Anemia (iron deficiency, postparturient hemoglobinuria, hemolytic, anaplasmosis, eperythrozoonosis, other)
White muscle disease (nutritional myodegeneration)
Anaphylaxis or allergy, milk allergy

LESS COMMON RESPIRATORY CAUSES
Pulmonary embolus from posterior vena cava thrombosis (B)
Parainfluenza virus type 3
Adenovirus (B, O)
Nasal trauma
Tumors of the nose, paranasal sinuses, oral cavity
Nasal granulomas (fungal granuloma, atopic rhinitis)
Congenital cystic nasal conchae
Nose bots *(Oestrus ovis)*
Sinusitis (maxillary, frontal, postdehorning)
Laryngeal trauma or abscess
Trauma (oral, pharyngeal, retropharyngeal), abscess, hematoma
Tracheal stenosis, collapse, stricture
Bovine rhinovirus (B)
Bovine malignant catarrhal fever (B)
Bovine herpesvirus DN-599 (B)
Ascaris suum migration (calves) (B)
Thoracic trauma, rib fracture
Pneumothorax
Pleuritis or pleural effusion
Caprine arthritis-encephalitis (CAE) pneumonia (C)
Sheep pulmonary adenomatosis virus (Jaagsiekte) (O)
Smoke inhalation
Foreign body (nasal, oral, pharyngeal, laryngeal, tracheal, bronchial)
Caprine herpesvirus (C)
Bluetongue
Peste des petits ruminants (C, O) (exotic)

B, Bovine; *C,* caprine; *O,* ovine.

Continued

BOX 5-13

Causes of Respiratory Distress in Ruminants—cont'd

LESS COMMON NONRESPIRATORY CAUSES
Congenital cardiac anomalies (ventricular septal defect, tetralogy of Fallot, patent ductus arteriosus, transposition of the great vessels, other anomalies)
Acquired cardiac failure (bacterial endocarditis, valvular incompetence, valvular stenosis, cardiomyopathy, pericarditis, other causes)
Central nervous system disease (trauma, meningoencephalitis, encephalomalacia, abscess, louping ill, pseudorabies, other causes)
Esophageal obstruction, foreign body, laceration, rupture, megaesophagus
Clostridial diseases (Black's disease, enterotoxemia, tetanus, blackleg, bacillary hemoglobinuria, others)
Anthrax
Complications of fluid therapy (pulmonary edema)
Water deprivation (salt poisoning) (B)
Blood transfusion reaction
Anaphylaxis
Burn, thermal injury, electrocution
Systemic toxoplasmosis (C, O)
Tick paralysis (C, O)
Bladder rupture
Bee or wasp sting, snakebite
Photosensitization

UNCOMMON RESPIRATORY CAUSES
Actinobacillosis (wooden tongue)
Actinomycosis (lumpy jaw)
Diaphragmatic hernia
Pleural mesothelioma
Pneumocystis carinii pneumonia
Pulmonary aspergillosis
Pulmonary neoplasia
Pulmonary tuberculosis
Chlamydia psittaci pneumonia
Cyst (branchial, cervical, salivary, thyroglossal duct)
Bronchobiliary fistula
Contagious bovine pleuropneumonia (exotic) (B)
Endemic ethmoid carcinoma (exotic) (B)
Theileria annulata and *Theileria hirci* (exotic) (B)
Heartwater (*Cowdria ruminatum*) (exotic)

UNCOMMON NONRESPIRATORY CAUSES
Retrobulbar neoplasia (B)
Enzootic bovine leukosis (B)
Thymic lymphosarcoma or thymoma
Calf lymphosarcoma (B)
Adult multicentric lymphosarcoma (B)
Embryonal mediastinal cyst
Dwarfism (B)
Botulism
Vesicular stomatitis
High altitude (brisket) disease, cor pulmonale (B, C)
Procaine penicillin G reaction or intravascular administration
Liver disease (infectious, toxic, parasitic, other)
Border disease (hairy shaker) (C, O)

TOXIC CAUSES
Sodium fluoroacetate
Strychnine
Sulphur (B, O)
Propylene glycol (B)
Oxalate, ethylene glycol (B, O)
Urea or nonprotein nitrogen

TOXIC CAUSES—cont'd
Potassium (B)
Nitrates
Bromide (B,C)
Lead
Mercury (C)
Iron (B, C)
Selenium
Arsenic
Organophosphate or carbamate
Organochlorine or chlorinated hydrocarbon
Permethrin
Gossypol
Ergot (*Claviceps purpura*)
Phosphate fertilizer (B, O)
Vitamin D_3 (B)
Warfarin, dicoumarol, diphacinone
Metaldehyde
Formaldehyde
Ammonia
Hydrogen sulfide
Monensin, salinomycin
Dinitrophenol (B, O)
Copper (acute oral toxicity)
Insect fogger pneumonitis (B)
Aflatoxicosis (C)
Levamisole (C, O)
Polychlorinated biphenyl (PCB) (B)
Xylazine-induced pulmonary edema (O)
Carbolic dips (O)
Cyanogenic plants (arrow grass, Johnson grass, common sorghum, sudan grass, chokecherry, acacia, other plants)
Avocado (*Persia americana*)
Moldy sweet clover (*Melilotus* spp.)
Moldy sweet potato (*Ipomoea batatas*) (B)
Brassica spp.
Ryegrass (*Lolium* spp.) (B, O)
Larkspur (*Delphinium* spp.)
Japanese yew (*Taxus cuspidata*)
Hairy vetch (*Vichia villosa*) (B)
Whitehead (*Sphenosciadium capitellatum*) (B)
White snakeroot (*Eupatorium rugosum*) (B, O)
Chinese tallow (*Sapium sebiferum*) (B)
Purple mint (*Perilla frutescens*) (B)
Oleander (*Nerium oleander*)
Nightshade (*Solanum* spp.) (B)
Cocklebur (*Xanthium* spp.) (B, O)
Locoweeds (*Astragalus* spp., *Oxytropis,* spp.) (B, O)
Foxglove (*Digitalis purpurea*) (B)
Water hemlock (*Cicuta* spp.)
Milkweed (*Asclepias* spp.) (B, O)
Hepatotoxic plants (*Senecio* spp., *Amsinckia* spp., others containing pyrrolizidine alkaloid)
Fescue summer poisoning (B)
Rubberweed (*Hymenoxys* spp.)
Sneezeweed (*Helenium autumnale*)
False hellebore (*Veratrum* spp.) (B, O)
Rhododendron (*Andromeda* spp.) (B, O)
Algae
Lupines (*Lupinus* spp.) (B, O)
Prickly paddy melon (*Cucumis myriocarpus*)

NOTE: Respiratory distress is a sign associated with toxicity caused by a large number of plant species. Not all have been listed here.

cattle in feedlots may also experience respiratory distress if the temperature suddenly rises to 4.4° to 10° C (40° to 50° F).

Observation of the nature of the respiratory distress may give important clues as to the functional characterization, and perhaps etiology, of the underlying disease process. Obstructive diseases involving the intrathoracic airways (e.g., COPD in horses and farmer's lung in cattle) are more likely to cause flow limitation during expiration because of dynamic airway collapse (see Cough, p. 46).[49,54,55] This results in expiratory respiratory distress and a pattern of respiration in which the expiratory phase occupies an increased proportion of the respiratory cycle as the patient attempts to expel air from the lungs.[49] In the extrathoracic airways, dynamic collapse occurs during inspiration because intraluminal pressures are subatmospheric at this time.[49,54,55] Therefore patients with upper airway obstructions, especially of the non-fixed type (e.g., laryngeal hemiplegia), generally show inspiratory respiratory distress and have a prolonged inspiratory phase.[49,54] Fixed airway obstructions of either the upper or lower airway (e.g., intraluminal mass, bronchoconstriction) are present during both phases of respiration and may lead to both inspiratory and expiratory distress.[49] However, the distress is likely to be accentuated during a particular phase of respiration, depending on the anatomic site of the obstruction (i.e., fixed upper airway obstructions cause more distress during inspiration, and fixed lower airway obstructions cause more distress during expiration). Restrictive diseases (e.g., pleural effusion, pneumoconiosis) inhibit expansion of the lungs and therefore generally lead to inspiratory respiratory distress.[49] An animal with restrictive disease must perform more respiratory work than normal to expand its lungs, and a common strategy for maintaining adequate ventilation is to increase the respiratory rate and lower the tidal volume (i.e., rapid, shallow breathing).[49] Animals with obstructive diseases generally have a normal or even increased tidal volume.[49]

In many instances, respiratory distress is not apparent at rest but occurs in association with exercise. Under these circumstances the animal's capacity to exercise is impaired, and the owner may complain of exercise intolerance (see Exercise Intolerance and Poor Performance in Horses, p. 81).

Approach to Diagnosis of Respiratory Distress

HISTORY. After ruling out environmental causes of respiratory distress (e.g., heat stress, high humidity, moving from outside into a heated barn in the winter, handling stress, or relocation to high altitude) and attending to the immediate needs of the patient, a careful history should be taken that includes the following factors: time and speed of onset of the clinical signs of respiratory distress; progression of clinical signs; whether this is the first episode of respiratory distress or whether the animal is subject to recurrent attacks; whether signs are present at rest or only after exercise; the relationship of signs to environmental conditions and the response to environmental change; recent administration of pharmacologic or biologic agents; the presence of an audible respiratory noise; or other signs of respiratory tract, oropharyngeal, or neurologic disease (e.g., nasal discharge, cough, dysphagia, facial paralysis, or retropharyngeal swelling). A history of recent trauma or exposure to potentially toxic substances, such as lead-containing paints, nitrate-accumulating plants or urea (ruminants), or carbon monoxide, should be elicited. The animal's appetite and attitude and signs of disease (e.g., diarrhea) in other systems should be determined. In neonates the circumstances surrounding gestation and parturition should be ascertained, because prematurity, dysmaturity, congenital infection, birth trauma (e.g., rib fracture) related to dystocia, prolonged parturition, and aspiration of amniotic fluid and

meconium are all important causes of respiratory distress. However, it should be noted that tachypnea, with respiratory rates of 60 to 80 breaths/min, is normal in foals during the first 30 minutes after birth as they "blow off" carbon dioxide (see Disorders and Management of the Neonate, Chapters 15 to 20).

PHYSICAL EXAMINATION. The physical examination should follow the same general approach as that described for cough. In particular, the following should be determined: rectal temperature, pulse rate, respiratory rate and character; regularity and pattern of breathing; presence of excessive intercostal or abdominal respiratory effort; synchrony and symmetry of chest excursion; presence of a "heave line"; presence or absence of stridor at rest (the examiner listens at the nostrils); symmetry of airflow from each nostril; effect of occlusion of each nostril independently; odor from the nose or mouth (or both); presence and character of nasal discharge; swelling around the external nares, inside the nasal passages, or inside the false nostril; facial symmetry and swelling; ocular discharge; resonance or painful response on percussion of the maxillary and frontal sinuses; palpable abnormalities of the mandibles and hyoid apparatus; enlargement of submandibular, parotid, retropharyngeal, and other regional lymph nodes; enlargement of the parotid salivary glands or thyroid gland; swelling, pain, or palpable abnormalities in the retropharyngeal region; a palpable, left-sided pit on the dorsal surface of the larynx; accentuation of stridor, induction of a cough, or evidence of pain on application of pressure to the larynx and trachea; palpable swelling or flattening of the cervical trachea; masses at the thoracic inlet; and palpable turbulence in the extrathoracic airway.

The mucous membranes should be examined carefully for cyanosis, pallor, cherry red color, hemorrhages, congestion, or injection. The capillary refill time should be determined, and the peripheral pulse rate, rhythm, and character should be assessed. Other signs of heart failure (e.g., jugular distention or pulsation and peripheral edema) and signs of dehydration (e.g., delayed jugular filling, dry mucous membranes, and altered skin turgor) should be noted. The larynx, trachea, and lungs should be carefully *ausculted* at rest and after the rate and depth of respiration have been increased, if it is safe to do so, by application of a rebreathing bag, by occlusion of the nostrils, or by exercising the animal, so that turbulent airflow and abnormal lung sounds may be detected. The heart should be auscultated to detect murmurs, cardiac dysrhythmias, muffling of heart sounds, or other abnormalities. The chest wall should be carefully *palpated* to detect rib fractures and other lesions; and both sides of the chest should be *percussed* to detect large mass lesions, lung consolidation, pleural effusion, hyperinflation, or a painful response, which may indicate pleuritis. A thorough oral examination is important, and in cattle this should include palpation of the base of the tongue, the oropharynx and, if possible, the larynx (see Nasal Discharge, p. 54).

A general physical examination should be completed so that diseases in systems other than the cardiovascular and respiratory systems (e.g., respiratory distress in cattle secondary to ruminal bloat and respiratory distress secondary to central nervous system trauma or severe metabolic acidosis) can be detected. Attempts should also be made to identify conditions that may cause severe acid-base disturbances and hemoconcentration (e.g., diarrhea, renal disease), pain (e.g., laminitis or trauma), or hyperthermia (e.g., infectious conditions or heat stroke).

Further diagnostic evaluation of respiratory distress may include a complete blood count with fibrinogen concentration; blood gas analysis; serum biochemistry determinations; endoscopy of the upper and lower airways and esophagus;

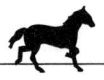

nasal or nasopharyngeal swabbing or scraping; virus identification, isolation, and serologic testing; bronchodilator response testing; tracheal aspiration; bronchoalveolar lavage; ultrasound examination of the chest and of suspected mass lesions that impinge on the upper airway; thoracocentesis; radiography of the nasal passages, paranasal sinuses, pharynx, guttural pouches, larynx, trachea, and chest; fecal examination for lungworms and other parasites; CT scanning of the upper airway; nuclear scintigraphy; pulmonary function testing; and biopsy of externally visible or palpable lesions or those identified by ultrasound, endoscopy, or radiography as described for the evaluation of cough and nasal discharge (see Cough, p. 46, and Nasal Discharge, p. 54).

COMPLETE BLOOD COUNT. A complete blood count, including fibrinogen and plasma protein concentrations, helps evaluate the role of hemoconcentration, anemia, or leukocytosis and hyperfibrinogenemia, which may accompany pneumonia and other inflammatory conditions.

ENDOSCOPIC EXAMINATION. Endoscopic examination of the upper and lower airways using fiberoptic or video endoscopes is particularly helpful in evaluating patients suspected of having obstructive disease[56] (see Cough, p. 46, Nasal Discharge, p. 54, and Stridor, p. 76). Endoscopic examination of the esophagus is indicated in patients with a history of bloat, dysphagia, or return of ingesta through the nose in addition to respiratory distress (see Nasal Discharge, p. 54, and Stridor, p. 76).

BLOOD GAS ANALYSIS. Blood gas analysis and acid-base determinations on arterial blood should be performed to determine O_2 and CO_2 tensions so that the contribution of hypoxemia or acidosis to the signs of respiratory distress can be ascertained. The normal PaO_2 for the horse is 83.6 ± 1.7 mm Hg, and the normal $PaCO_2$ is 42.2 ± 0.8 mm Hg.[57] Hypoxemia is defined as a PaO_2 below 80 mm Hg.[57] Cyanosis is usually not evident until the PaO_2 is much lower than this (usually below 40 mm Hg).[57] Hypercarbia, or hypercapnia, refers to an increased $PaCO_2$ (above 44 mm Hg).[57] Because CO_2 diffuses very readily, considerable ventilatory dysfunction can occur before the $PaCO_2$ rises; therefore severe hypoxemia can occur with a normal $PaCO_2$. Because venous blood samples reflect tissue metabolism, they are not considered adequate for evaluating pulmonary function. However, a partial pressure of carbon dioxide in venous blood ($PvCO_2$) above 60 mm Hg usually reflects arterial hypercapnia, and a partial pressure of oxygen in venous blood (PvO_2) below 20 mm Hg usually indicates arterial hypoxemia.[58]

INSUFFLATION OF 100% OXYGEN. Insufflation of 100% oxygen causes a significant increase in PaO_2 if hypoxemia is caused by hypoventilation or ventilation-perfusion mismatch, whereas little or no improvement in PaO_2 occurs if hypoxemia is caused by anatomic or physiologic right-to-left shunting.[49] Blood samples should be evaluated for abnormal hemoglobin (e.g., methemoglobin) and also if exposure to nitrates or similar toxins is suspected (see Cyanosis, p. 70).

RADIOGRAPHIC EXAMINATION. Radiographic examination of the nasal passages, pharynx, larynx, and trachea permits detection and evaluation of obstructive lesions in the upper airway, especially if tachypnea is accompanied by inspiratory stridor, asymmetric nasal airflow, or other evidence of upper airway obstruction.

Radiographic examination of the trachea and thorax should include end-inspiratory phase radiographs to facilitate identification of pulmonary lesions and disorders such as dynamic collapse of the trachea that are visible only on inspiratory phase radiographs. Chest radiographs help detect evidence of pneumonia, pleural effusion, pneumothorax, cardiomegaly, and mediastinal lesions. The cardiac silhouette

and the pattern and caliber of the aorta, vena cava, pulmonary artery, pulmonary veins, and other vessels should also be evaluated for evidence of cardiac failure and pulmonary vascular disease. *Contrast angiography* and other diagnostic procedures, such as *echocardiography, electrocardiography,* and *hemodynamic (pressure and flow) studies,* may be indicated in patients with respiratory distress that has occurred secondary to cardiovascular disease.

ULTRASOUND EXAMINATION. Ultrasound examination of the thorax is performed to detect pleural inflammation and effusion, pulmonary consolidation, pulmonary abscessation, and cardiac anomalies if the clinical examination suggests that pulmonary, pleural, or cardiac disease is the cause of the signs of respiratory distress.

REFERENCES

49. Amis TC: Clinical respiratory physiology. In Kirk RW, ed: *Current veterinary therapy. VIII, Small animal practice,* Philadelphia, 1983, WB Saunders, pp 191-201.
50. Kelly WR: Respiration. In Kelly WR, ed: *Veterinary clinical diagnosis,* ed 3, London, 1984, Ballière Tindall, pp 39-46.
51. Weinberger SE: Presentation of the patient with pulmonary disease. In Weinberger SE, ed: *Principles of pulmonary medicine,* Philadelphia, 1986, WB Saunders, pp 22-30.
52. Brown CM: Coughing and labored breathing. In Brown CM, ed: *Problems in equine medicine,* Philadelphia, 1989, Lea & Febiger, pp 81-96.
53. Cornelius LM: Dyspnea. In Lorenz MD, Cornelius LM, eds: *Small animal medical diagnosis,* Philadelphia, 1987, JB Lippincott, pp 215-223.
54. Robinson NE: Functional abnormalities caused by upper airway obstruction and heaves: their relationship to the etiology of epistaxis, *Vet Clin North Am (Large Anim Pract)* 1:17-34, 1979.
55. Robinson NE, Sorenson PR: Pathophysiology of airway obstruction in the horse: a review, *J Am Vet Med Assoc* 172:299-303, 1978.
56. Haynes PF: Exercise intolerance and noise production, *Proc Am Assoc Equine Pract* 27:43-47, 1981.
57. Willoughby RA, McDonnell WN: Pulmonary function testing in horses, *Vet Clin North Am (Large Anim Pract)* 1:171-196, 1979.
58. Kosch PC et al: Developments in management of the newborn foal in respiratory distress. I, Evaluation, *Equine Vet J* 16:312-318, 1984.

TACHYPNEA

Definition

Tachypnea is the term used to describe an increase in the respiratory rate; the term hyperpnea is used when both the rate and depth of respiration have increased.

The respiratory rate, which is assessed by counting rib or nostril movements or by thoracic or tracheal auscultation, is best determined before the patient is disturbed or restrained. Under average conditions of temperature and humidity, acceptable ranges for the respiratory rate in normal adult animals are: cattle, 10 to 30 breaths/min; horses, 8 to 15 breaths/min; sheep and pigs, 10 to 20 breaths/min; and goats, 25 to 35 breaths/min. Resting respiratory rates in young animals are higher than those in adults. A neonatal foal has a resting respiratory rate of 60 to 80 breaths/min during the first 30 minutes of life, a rate that later falls to 20 to 40 breaths/min. A young calf has a respiratory rate of 20 to 50 breaths/min by 30 minutes of age.

Pathophysiology

Respiratory rate, depth, and rhythmicity are regulated by respiratory centers in the brainstem. Central chemoreceptors responding to increased levels of CO_2 (decreased cerebrospinal fluid pH) and peripheral chemoreceptors (carotid and aortic bodies) responding to hypoxemia (PaO_2 below 60 mm Hg), increases in $PaCO_2$, and decreases in pH initiate increases in the respiratory rate. Mechanoreceptors in the lungs and joints also influence ventilation. Lung inflation stimulates stretch receptors in the airways, which decreases the inspiratory effort, whereas mechanoreceptors in the joints are thought to

---

BOX 5-14

Causes of Tachypnea in the Horse*

COMMON RESPIRATORY CAUSES
Bacterial pneumonia
Pleuropneumonia, pleuritis
Pulmonary abscessation
Chronic obstructive pulmonary disease (COPD)
Viral pneumonia (equine influenza, adenovirus, equine viral arteritis, others)
Equine herpesvirus types 1 and 4 (EHV-1, EHV-4)
Aspiration pneumonia
Prematurity, dysmaturity, or immaturity (foals)

COMMON NONRESPIRATORY CAUSES
Hyperthermia (fever, postexhaustion syndrome, heat stroke, anhidrosis, other)
Pain (abdominal crisis, laminitis, exertional myopathy, other)
Acidosis (acute enterocolitis, urinary bladder rupture, renal tubular acidosis, other)
Anaphylaxis
Blood transfusion reaction
Shock (hypovolemic, cardiac, septic)
Anemia (neonatal isoerythrolysis, blood loss, hemolytic anemia, iron deficiency, bone marrow suppression, ruptured middle uterine artery, other)
Cardiac disease (ruptured mitral chordae tendinae, ventricular septal defect, endocarditis, other)
Gastric dilation

LESS COMMON RESPIRATORY CAUSES
Smoke inhalation pneumonia
Parasitic pneumonia (*Dictyocaulus arnfieldi*)

LESS COMMON RESPIRATORY CAUSES—cont'd
Stenotic nares, choanal atresia
Nasal septum abnormalities
Neoplasia (nose, paranasal sinuses)
Fungal granuloma
Nasopharyngeal cicatrix
Paranasal sinus infection
Dorsal displacement of the soft palate
Pharyngeal or retropharyngeal abscess or trauma
Epiglottic entrapment
Chondroma of arytenoid cartilage
Guttural pouch empyema
Tracheal stenosis, collapse, stricture
Foreign body (nasal, nasopharyngeal, laryngeal, tracheal, bronchial)
Diaphragmatic hernia
Pneumothorax
Thoracic trauma

LESS COMMON NONRESPIRATORY CAUSES
Anaphylaxis
Air embolism
Intracarotid injections
Fluid therapy complications
Tetanus (*Clostridium tetani*)
Malignant edema (*Clostridium septicum*)
Malignant hyperthermia
Meningoencephalitis
Anemia (piroplasmosis, iron deficiency, hemolytic blood loss, other)

*All causes of respiratory distress (pp. 65-66) are also causes of tachypnea.

---

be partly responsible for the increases in ventilation that occur during exercise. Pulmonary chemoreceptors that influence the respiratory cycle include irritant receptors in the airways, which are stimulated by dust and histamine, and J receptors, which apparently detect levels of interstitial fluid and are thought to be responsible for the respiratory pattern observed in animals with pulmonary edema.

Tachypnea is classified as physiologic when it occurs in the absence of underlying disease and as pathologic when it is a manifestation of respiratory distress. Physiologic tachypnea is associated with pain, exertion, heat, fever, anxiety, and other stresses (Boxes 5-14 and 5-15). Factors predisposing to pathologic tachypnea are the same as those that cause respiratory distress: inadequate oxygenation of the blood (i.e., a need for additional oxygen); compensation for metabolic acidosis; excessive environmental heat; disorders that damage the central nervous system respiratory centers in the medulla (e.g., head trauma, inflammation, mass lesions) if they disrupt the control of breathing; disorders that cause dysfunction of motor nerves and/or weakness of respiratory muscles (e.g., botulism, myasthenia gravis, or diaphragmatic paralysis); and painful conditions involving the respiratory sensory nerves, muscles, pleurae, and ribs (e.g., chest trauma, pleural infection, or neoplasia)[59] (see Respiratory Distress, p. 64).

Approach to Diagnosis of Tachypnea

Because tachypnea is a manifestation of respiratory distress, the approach used for evaluating patients with tachypnea is the same as that used for evaluation of respiratory distress (see p. 68).

REFERENCE
59. Cornelius LM: Dyspnea. In Lorenz MD, Cornelius LM, eds: *Small animal medical diagnosis*, Philadelphia, 1987, JB Lippincott, pp 196-203.

CYANOSIS

Definition

Cyanosis is the bluish discoloration of skin, conjunctivae, and visible mucous membranes that results from an increase in the absolute amount of reduced hemoglobin in the blood.[60]

Pathophysiology

Oxygen is carried in blood in two forms, dissolved and in combination with hemoglobin (Hb). The amount of dissolved oxygen present in arterial blood is relatively small and is proportional to the PaO_2. Oxygen transport to tissues is facilitated by the ability of hemoglobin in erythrocytes to combine in a reversible manner with oxygen. When erythrocytes pass through the pulmonary circulation, oxygen binds to hemoglobin, forming oxyhemoglobin (HbO_2). As oxyhemoglobin passes through systemic capillaries, oxygen diffuses into tissues, and hemoglobin is once again formed.

The Bohr effect describes the ability of hemoglobin to bind to a number of different ligands (CO_2, H^+ and 2,3-diphosphoglycerate [2,3-DPG]), which results in modification of hemoglobin's affinity for oxygen. When tissue pH decreases, hemoglobin acts as a buffer and binds excess H^+, which decreases its affinity for oxygen. When the CO_2 con-

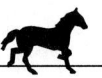

BOX 5-14

Causes of Tachypnea in the Horse—cont'd

LESS COMMON NONRESPIRATORY CAUSES—cont'd
Cardiovascular anomalies (tetralogy of Fallot, tricuspid insufficiency, atrial septal defect, hypoplastic left heart, transposition of great vessels, persistent right aortic arch, patent ductus arteriosus)
Cor pulmonale
Pericarditis
Atrial fibrillation
Ventricular tachycardia, fibrillation, flutter

UNCOMMON RESPIRATORY CAUSES
Pulmonary lobar hypertrophy
Branchial or thyroglossal duct cyst
Tracheal rupture
Fracture of laryngeal cartilage
Fracture of hyoid bone
Cutaneous or nasal amyloidosis
Pulmonary tuberculosis
Pulmonary nocardiosis
Pneumocystis carinii pneumonia

UNCOMMON NONRESPIRATORY CAUSES
Lactation tetany
Hydroallantois or hydrops
Nutritional myodegeneration (foals)
Methemoglobin reductase deficiency
Acute hepatic insufficiency
Electrocution
Cardiac neoplasia
Embryonal mediastinal cyst

TOXIC CAUSES
α-Naphthyl thiourea (ANTU)
Arsenic
Bromide
Sodium fluoroacetate
Cantharidin (blister beetle)
Ammonia
Amitraz
Propylene glycol
Dioctyl sodium sulfosuccinate
Iron
Selenium
Metaldehyde
Organophosphate
Organochlorine, chlorinated hydrocarbon
Phenothiazine
Potassium
Larkspur (*Delphinium* spp.)
Japanese yew *(Taxus cuspidata)*
White snakeroot *(Eupatorium rugosum)*
Water hemlock *(Cicuta* spp.)
Jimson weed *(Datura stramonium)*
Potato *(Solanum tuberosum)*
Cyanogenic plants
Onion (*Allium* spp.)
Red maple *(Acer rubrum)*

BOX 5-15

Causes of Tachypnea in Ruminants

COMMON RESPIRATORY CAUSES
Mannheimia hemolytica or *Pasteurella multocida* pneumonia (includes shipping fever and enzootic calf pneumonia)
Haemophilus somnus pneumonia (B)
Visceral caseous lymphadenitis (*Corynebacterium pseudotuberculosis*) (C, O)
Chronic bacterial pneumonia with consolidation or abscessation (*Arcanobacterium pyogenes* and other bacteria)
Necrotic laryngitis *(Fusobacterium necrophorum)* (B)
Pulmonary embolus from posterior vena cava thrombosis (B)
Respiratory syncytial virus
Parainfluenza type 3 virus
Adenovirus (B, O)
Infectious bovine rhinotracheitis virus (IBR; BHV-1) (B)
Ovine progressive pneumonia virus (O)
Mycoplasma spp.
Caprine *Mycoplasma mycoides* subsp. *mycoides* infection
Mycoplasma ovipneumoniae (O)
Parasitic pneumonia (*Dictyocaulus viviparus* [B]; *Dictyocaulus filaria* [O, C]; *Müllerius capillaris* [O, C]; *Protostrongylus rufescens* [O, C])
Bovine atypical interstitial pneumonia (B)
Acute pulmonary edema and emphysema (B)
Farmer's lung (*Faenia rectivirgula* hypersensitivity pneumonitis) (B)
Aspiration or foreign body pneumonia

COMMON NONRESPIRATORY CAUSES
Hyperthermia (fever, heat stroke, rapid rise in ambient temperature, other)
Pain (abdominal crisis, urethral calculi, traumatic reticuloperitonitis, musculoskeletal injury, other)
Acidosis (ruminal lactic acidosis, pregnancy toxemia, other)
Electrolyte aberrations (hypocalcemia, hypomagnesemia, other)
Shock (hypovolemic, cardiac, septic)
Anemia (iron deficiency, postparturient hemoglobinuria, blood loss, other)
Distended abdominal viscus (ruminal bloat, other)
Anaphylaxis
Blood transfusion reaction
White muscle disease

LESS COMMON RESPIRATORY CAUSES
Nasal trauma
Tumors of the nose and paranasal sinuses
Nasal granulomas (fungal granuloma, atopic rhinitis)
Congenital cystic nasal conchae
Laryngeal trauma, abscess
Tracheal stenosis, collapse, stricture
Bovine rhinovirus (B)
Bovine malignant catarrhal fever (B)
Ascaris suum migration (calves) (B)

B, Bovine; C, caprine; O, ovine.

Continued

BOX 5-15

Causes of Tachypnea in Ruminants—cont'd

LESS COMMON RESPIRATORY CAUSES—cont'd
Thoracic trauma, other causes of chest pain
Pneumothorax
Diaphragmatic hernia
Pleuritis or pleural effusion
Caprine arthritis-encephalitis (CAE) pneumonia (C)
Sheep pulmonary adenomatosis virus pneumonia (O)

LESS COMMON NONRESPIRATORY CAUSES
Cardiac anomalies (ventricular septal defect, tetralogy
    of Fallot, other)
Endocarditis
Pericarditis
Central nervous system disease (meningoencephalitis,
    polioencephalomalacia, other)
Esophageal obstruction or foreign body
Clostridial diseases (Black's disease, enterotoxemia, tetanus)
Anaphylaxis

UNCOMMON RESPIRATORY CAUSES
Pleural mesothelioma
Pneumocystis carinii pneumonia
Pulmonary aspergillosis
Pulmonary neoplasia
Cyst (branchial, cervical, thyroglossal duct) (B)
Bronchobiliary fistula
Contagious bovine pleuropneumonia (exotic) (B)
Endemic ethmoid carcinoma (exotic) (B)

UNCOMMON NONRESPIRATORY CAUSES
Bluetongue (B, O)
Thymic lymphosarcoma (B)

UNCOMMON NONRESPIRATORY CAUSES—cont'd
Retrobulbar neoplasia (B)
Calf lymphosarcoma (B)
Adult multicentric lymphosarcoma (B)
Embryonal mediastinal cyst
Dwarfism (B)
Anthrax

TOXIC CAUSES
Sodium fluoroacetate
Strychnine
Sulphur
Propylene glycol
Urea or nonprotein nitrogen
Water deprivation or salt toxicity
Potassium
Nitrates
Bromide
Iron
Selenium
Organophosphate
Organochlorine or chlorinated hydrocarbon
Larkspur (*Delphinium* spp.)
Japanese yew (*Taxus cuspidata*)
Sneezeweed (*Helenium autumnale*)
Hairy vetch (*Vichia villosa*)
Whitehead (*Sphenosciadium capitellatum*)
White snakeroot (*Eupatorium rugosum*)

NOTE: Tachypnea is a rather nonspecific sign and is associated with toxicity caused by a large number of plant species; only a few are listed above. See also Box 5-13, p. 67.

B, Bovine; *C,* caprine; *O,* ovine.

---

centration increases, some CO_2 is converted to bicarbonate and the remainder is bound to hemoglobin to form carbaminohemoglobin; this also decreases the affinity of hemoglobin for oxygen. Therefore the net effect of a decreased blood pH and increased blood CO_2 concentration is unloading of oxygen to the tissues. Conversely, as the CO_2 concentration in the pulmonary capillaries decreases and blood pH rises, the affinity of hemoglobin for oxygen increases; thus the net effect of elevated blood pH in pulmonary capillaries is increased uptake of oxygen by hemoglobin.

The affinity of hemoglobin for oxygen is also influenced by the concentration of 2,3-DPG, a metabolic intermediate of the Rappaport-Lubering shunt involved in erythrocyte glycolysis. An increase in the 2,3-DPG concentration may occur in association with chronic hypoxemia (high altitude, chronic lung disease), anemia, chronic alkalosis, phosphate retention, and red cell pyruvate kinase deficiency. When the 2,3-DPG concentration is increased, the affinity of hemoglobin for oxygen is decreased, resulting in improved unloading of oxygen to peripheral tissues. Conversely, a decreased 2,3-DPG level results in an increased affinity of hemoglobin for oxygen. A decrease in the 2,3-DPG concentration may occur in stored blood, in association with chronic acidosis, and with hypophosphatemia.

Cyanosis develops when the oxygen saturation of hemoglobin is below 80%. With a normal oxygen-hemoglobin dissociation curve, the PaO_2 usually is below 40 mm Hg before cyanosis is noted in the patient.[61] The hemoglobin concentration of blood must be near normal for cyanosis to be clinically evident[62]; therefore patients with severe anemia and concomitant marked arterial oxygen desaturation may not show cyanosis. In contrast, patients with marked polycythemia may be cyanotic at a higher arterial oxygen saturation than patients with normal hematocrit values.

Classification

Cyanosis can be classified as either *peripheral* or *central*.

PERIPHERAL CYANOSIS. Peripheral cyanosis is caused by slowing of blood flow to an area, resulting in abnormally increased extraction of oxygen from normally saturated arterial blood. Decreased blood flow through the peripheral capillary bed may be caused by vasoconstriction of superficial vessels, obstruction of arteries or veins, or low cardiac output. Peripheral cyanosis is observed in the extremities, nose, and ears and usually is not associated with cyanosis of mucous membranes. Peripheral cyanosis is rarely recognized in large domestic animals because of their skin pigmentation and hair cover.

CENTRAL CYANOSIS. Central cyanosis results from either inadequate oxygenation of arterial blood or from the presence of an abnormal hemoglobin derivative and is characterized by cyanosis of mucous membranes (Table 5-1). Causes of inadequate oxygenation of arterial blood are respiratory diseases or congenital cardiac anomalies that cause right-to-left shunting (Boxes 5-16 and 5-17). Acquired abnormalities of hemoglobin function can be induced by a number of chemicals. Exposure to these chemicals results in the formation of methemoglobin or sulfhemoglobin, neither of which is capable of binding oxygen. Nitrites and nitrates are powerful reducing agents that produce methemoglobine-

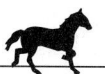

BOX 5-16

Causes of Central Cyanosis in the Horse

COMMON CAUSES

Bacterial pneumonia, pleuritis, pulmonary abscessation
  (*Rhodococcus equi, Streptococcus* spp., other bacteria)
Chronic obstructive pulmonary disease (COPD)
Aspiration pneumonia
Viral pneumonia (equine influenza, adenovirus, other viruses)
Equine herpesvirus types 1 and 4 (EHV-1, EHV-4)
Acute bronchointerstitial pneumonia
Prematurity, dysmaturity, immaturity (foals)
Ventricular septal defect with pulmonary hypertension
Tetralogy of Fallot
Toxic methemoglobinemia
Anaphylaxis
Shock (hypovolemic, cardiac, septic)

LESS COMMON CAUSES

Stenotic nares or choanal atresia
Neoplasia (nose, paranasal sinuses)
Nasal granuloma
Nasopharyngeal cicatrix
Tracheal stenosis, collapse, stricture
Tracheal rupture or perforation
Diaphragmatic hernia
Pneumothorax
Pulmonary edema
Smoke inhalation pneumonia
Pneumoconiosis interstitial pneumonia
Atrial septal defect with pulmonary hypertension

UNCOMMON CAUSES

Pulmonary lobar hypertrophy (foals)
Embryonal mediastinal cyst

UNCOMMON CAUSES—cont'd

Pulmonary tuberculosis, nocardiosis
Pneumocystis carinii pneumonia
Air embolism
Pulmonary neoplasia
Transposition of great vessels
Tricuspid atresia
Aortic, pulmonary artery rupture
Interruption of aortic arch
Common ventricle with separate pulmonary outflow
  chamber
Multiple cardiac anomalies
Methemoglobin reductase deficiency
Lactation tetany
Clostridial diseases
Malignant hyperthermia

TOXIC CAUSES

Sulfur, hydrogen sulfide
α-Naphthyl thiourea (ANTU)
Chlorinated hydrocarbon
Organophosphate, carbamate
Red maple (*Acer rubrum*) *
Redroot pigweed (*Amaranthus retroflexus*) *
Sudan grass (*Sorghum vulgare var sudanensis*) *
Mintweed (*Salvia reflexa*) *
Lamb's-quarter (*Chenopodium album*) *
Variegated thistle (*Silybum marianum*) *
Winged thistle (*Carduus tenuiflorus*) *

*Nitrate accumulator, which causes methemoglobinemia.

TABLE 5-1

Pathophysiologic Classification of Central Cyanosis and Examples of Associated Conditions

Classification	Associated Condition

Decreased arterial oxygen saturation	Respiratory disease
	  Ventilation-perfusion mismatch
	  Alveolar hypoventilation
	  Impaired oxygen diffusion
	  Pulmonary arteriovenous shunting
	Cardiac disease
	  Cardiac anomalies that cause right-to-left shunting (e.g., tetralogy of Fallot)

Abnormal hemoglobin derivative	Methemoglobinemia Sulfhemoglobinemia

mia by directly oxidizing hemoglobin to methemoglobin. Nitrate poisoning is most commonly associated with the incorporation of nitrate-accumulating plants (e.g., pigweed [*Amaranthus retroflexus*], lamb's-quarter [*Chenopodium album*], and mintweed [*Salvia reflexa*]) in livestock forage. Nitrate intoxication usually is seen only in ruminants because rumen microorganisms reduce nitrate to the more toxic nitrite ion. Congenital defects in hemoglobin function have been reported in humans and may occur in large domestic animals. Examples of such defects are nicotinamide adenine dinu-

cleotide methemoglobin reductase deficiency and familial methemoglobinemia.

Conditions That Predispose to Hypoxemia and Central Cyanosis

The remainder of this section is confined to the discussion of respiratory conditions and cardiovascular anomalies that predispose to hypoxemia and central cyanosis. Impaired pulmonary function may cause hypoxemia and, in some circumstances, cyanosis. Mechanisms by which hypoxemia of pulmonary origin can arise include alveolar hypoventilation, reduced gas transfer or diffusion across the blood-gas barrier, ventilation-perfusion mismatch, pulmonary arteriovenous shunt, or a combination of these factors.[60,62] An additional cause of hypoxemia is the decrease in the partial pressure of alveolar oxygen that occurs at high altitudes.

ALVEOLAR HYPOVENTILATION. Alveolar hypoventilation is defined as a reduced volume of inspired air reaching the alveoli per unit time. Alveolar hypoventilation is always associated with an increased $PaCO_2$. Conditions associated with alveolar hypoventilation are drug-induced respiratory depression (morphine, barbiturates), brainstem disease (encephalitis, trauma, hemorrhage, neoplasia), and transection of the cervical spinal cord. All these conditions prevent proper generation and transmission of signals from the respiratory center to respiratory muscles. Other possible causes of alveolar hypoventilation are abnormal respiratory muscle function (diaphragmatic hernia, botulism), thoracic cage abnormalities (rib fracture), increased airway resistance (e.g.,

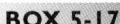

BOX 5-17

Causes of Central Cyanosis in Ruminants

COMMON CAUSES
Bacterial pneumonia, pulmonary abscessation (*Mannheimia hemolytica, Arcanobacterium pyogenes, Pasteurella multocida, Corynebacterium pseudotuberculosis* [O, C], other bacteria)
Viral pneumonia (respiratory syncytial virus [B], ovine progressive pneumonia [O], caprine arthritis-encephalomyelitis [C], other viruses)
Parasitic pneumonia (*Dictyocaulus viviparus* [B], *Dictyocaulus filaria* [O, C])
Aspiration pneumonia
Acute bovine pulmonary edema and emphysema (B)
Pulmonary edema
Ventricular septal defect with pulmonary hypertension
Tetralogy of Fallot
Toxic methemoglobinemia
Anaphylaxis
Shock (hypovolemic, cardiac, septic)
Rumen bloat

LESS COMMON CAUSES
Obstruction of nasal passages or paranasal sinuses (neoplasm, granuloma, abscess, other)
Laryngeal abscess
Tracheal stenosis, collapse, stricture
Tracheal rupture, perforation
Diaphragmatic hernia
Prematurity, dysmaturity, immaturity
Inhalation pneumonia (smoke)
Pneumothorax
Hemothorax
Pulmonary contusion
Ventricular septal defect with pulmonic stenosis
Postparturient hemoglobinuria
Clostridial diseases (e.g., malignant edema, blackleg, tetanus)
Bluetongue (O)
Obstructive urolithias, ruptured urethra

UNCOMMON CAUSES
Pleural mesothelioma (B)
Water inhalation (drowning)

UNCOMMON CAUSES—cont'd
Pulmonary adenomatosis (O)
Transposition of great vessels
Double-outlet right ventricle
Common ventricle with separate pulmonary outflow chamber
Acute anthrax
White liver disease (exotic) (O)
Sweating sickness (exotic) (B, O)

TOXIC CAUSES
Strychnine
Arsenic
Metaldehyde
Hydrogen sulfide
Organochlorine, chlorinated hydrocarbon
Organophosphate, carbamate
Acute selenium toxicosis
Nitrate, nitrite
Perennial broomweed (*Gutierrezia microcephala*)
Oleander (*Nerium oleander*)
Whitehead (*Sphenoscadium capitellatum*)
Milkweed (*Asclepias* spp.) (O)
Rhododendron (*Andromeda* spp.)
Fireweed (*Kochia scoparia*)
Canary grass (*Phalaris* spp.)
Kikuyu poisoning (exotic) (B, O)
Albizia poisoning (exotic) (B, O)
Euphorbia, sarcostemma poisoning (exotic) (B, O)
Acacia poisoning (exotic) (B, O)
Wild onion (*Allium validum*)* [O]
Variegated thistle (*Silybum marianum*)*
Redroot pigweed (*Amaranthus retroflexus*)
Sudan grass (*Sorghum vulgare var sudanensis*)*
Winged thistle (*Carduus terviflorus*)*
Mintweed (*Salvia reflexia*)*
Lamb's-quarter (*Chenopodium album*)*
Many pasture grasses fed during optimum growth conditions*
Locoweeds (*Astragalus* spp., *Oxytropis* spp.)*

B, Bovine; C, caprine; O, ovine.
*Nitrate accumulator, which causes methemoglobinemia.

---

stenotic nares, laryngeal stricture or paresis, foreign body obstruction, bronchitis, bronchiectasis), and pleural space disease (inflammatory or neoplastic effusions, pneumothorax, hydrothorax, chylothorax, pyothorax, hemothorax).

IMPAIRED DIFFUSION. Impaired diffusion, a second cause of hypoxemia, results from an increase in the blood-gas barrier. Equilibrium between alveolar oxygen and pulmonary blood oxygen is not reached because of the increased barriers through which oxygen must pass to reach hemoglobin. Because carbon dioxide diffuses more readily than oxygen, the $Paco_2$ usually is not increased in conditions that cause impaired diffusion. In fact, the $Paco_2$ may actually be reduced because of hyperventilation stimulated by hypoxemia. Conditions that may result in impaired diffusion are pneumonia, pulmonary edema, atelectasis, pulmonary contusions, and pulmonary neoplasms.

VENTILATION-PERFUSION MISMATCH. Ventilation-perfusion mismatch occurs eventually in all generalized pulmonary diseases and is the predominant mechanism by which hypoxemia develops in respiratory conditions. Overall gas exchange is impaired by uneven ventilation and blood flow. Lung areas that are overperfused in relation to ventilation (low ventilation/perfusion ratio) contribute disproportionate amounts of blood with a low Pao_2 to the systemic circulation. Examples of respiratory diseases that can result in a low ventilation/perfusion ratio include bronchitis, bronchoconstriction, airway closure, pulmonary atelectasis or consolidation, and local restriction of lung movement. In the case of pulmonary embolization or decreased pulmonary arterial pressure, ventilation may exceed perfusion (high ventilation/perfusion ratio) and result in pathologic dead space. Pulmonary mechanisms can partly compensate for ventilation-perfusion inequalities. Alveolar hypoxia may lead to reflex pulmonary arterial constriction, which redirects blood flow to alveoli that are adequately ventilated. Airway hypocapnia can stimulate bronchoconstriction, resulting in redirection of airflow to better-perfused alveoli.

SHUNTING. Shunting is defined as any mechanism by which blood that has not passed through ventilated areas of the lung is added to arteries of the systemic circulation. The

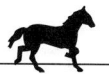

term *venous admixture* is used to describe venous blood that passes through the lungs without being properly oxygenated. Animals with venous admixture often hyperventilate and thus have normocapnia or hypocapnia in association with hypoxemia. The most common cause of shunting is congenital heart disease, which allows unoxygenated blood from the right heart to pass directly into the left heart without passing through the pulmonary circulation. Intrapulmonary anatomic shunts can result from pulmonary artery to pulmonary venous fistulas or severe lung lobe consolidation, in which a large part of the lung is ventilated but not perfused. Cyanosis or hypoxemia unresponsive to oxygen therapy suggests the presence of such congenital cardiac anomalies or intrapulmonary shunts.[63] Examples of the more common cyanotic congenital cardiac defects are tetralogy of Fallot, truncus arteriosus, transposition of the great arteries, tricuspid atresia, and hypoplastic left heart syndrome.[61,63] Aside from congenital defects, reversion to fetal circulation should be considered in any critically ill neonatal animal with hypoxemia that is unresponsive to oxygen insufflation.[63]

Approach to Diagnosis of Cyanosis

HISTORY. The history should include questions about the duration of the cyanosis (e.g., cyanosis that has been present since birth or an early age may indicate congenital heart disease with right-to-left shunting); possible exposure to toxic plants or chemicals that may result in production of abnormal types of hemoglobin; evidence of an abnormal respiratory pattern (respiratory distress, inspiratory stridor, cough); and signs of episodic weakness or syncope that may be consistent with congenital cardiac anomalies or severe upper airway obstruction (e.g., tracheal collapse or severe laryngeal edema associated with necrotic laryngitis in calves).

PHYSICAL EXAMINATION. The physical examination should include *inspection* to detect abnormalities in the respiratory pattern (e.g., tachypnea, respiratory distress, or stridor). Careful *auscultation* of the larynx, trachea, and lungs is also imperative. A rebreathing bag (8-L capacity for adult horses and cattle, 1- to 2-L capacity for calves, foals, and small ruminants) causes a temporary buildup of CO_2, stimulates the respiratory center, and prompts deep breaths when the animal is again allowed to inspire room air. Loud breath sounds, pulmonary crackles and wheezes, or pleural friction rubs may suggest that cyanosis is associated with a pathologic respiratory condition. Loud cardiac murmurs accompanied by precordial thrills point to congenital heart disease as the cause of cyanosis.

Palpation and *percussion* of the chest are also important examination procedures in an animal with cyanosis. Chest palpation may reveal pleural friction rubs or the pain and crepitus associated with rib fractures. Increased resonance on percussion may indicate pneumothorax, whereas decreased resonance suggests pulmonary congestion or consolidation, pleural effusion, or a space-occupying lesion in the thorax.

ENDOSCOPIC EXAMINATION. An endoscopic examination should be performed if upper airway obstruction or malformation is suspected.

RADIOGRAPHIC EXAMINATION. Radiographs of the upper respiratory tract and thorax can be used to further characterize a pathologic respiratory condition. Abnormalities that may be detected include space-occupying lesions in the oropharynx, nasopharynx, or larynx; tracheal compression or collapse; enlargement or distortion of the cardiac silhouette; pulmonary consolidation; pneumothorax; pleural effusion; or pulmonary abscessation.

ULTRASOUND EXAMINATION. Ultrasound examination of the chest and heart is indicated to characterize cardiac anomalies and to detect the presence and determine the extent of pleural effusion, pulmonary consolidation, and pulmonary abscessation.

ARTERIAL BLOOD GAS ANALYSIS. Arterial blood gas analysis is indicated to determine O_2 and CO_2 tension. In foals and calves arterial samples usually are obtained from the great metatarsal artery or the brachial artery as it crosses the medial aspect of the foreleg.[64] The auricular artery is also convenient in calves. The femoral artery can be used in neonates but is less convenient because it has a tendency to roll. The facial artery can be used in adult horses, and the auricular or coccygeal artery can be used in mature ruminants.[65] During the sampling process the patient should be quiet and not struggling, which can decrease the $PaCO_2$.[66] Local subcutaneous infiltration of 2% lidocaine without epinephrine over the artery being sampled minimizes needless struggling and facilitates sample collection. A heparinized syringe and a 22- to 26-gauge needle can be used. Any air bubbles should be removed after sample collection and the needle properly sealed. If the sample is kept on ice, the pH will remain unchanged for $3^1/_2$ hours and the blood gases for 6 hours.[67] The animal's temperature should be recorded at the time of sample collection so that it can be used in the calculation of actual blood gas concentrations. Hypoxemia is defined as a PaO_2 below 60 mm Hg.[66] Cyanosis is usually not evident until the PaO_2 is below 40 mm Hg. Hypercarbia, or hypercapnia, refers to an increased $PaCO_2$ (above 50 mm Hg).[66] Because CO_2 diffuses readily, considerable ventilatory dysfunction can occur before the $PaCO_2$ rises; therefore severe hypoxemia can occur with a normal $PaCO_2$. An elevated $PaCO_2$ generally indicates that hypoventilation or a severe pulmonary pathologic condition is present. Venous blood samples reflect tissue metabolism and usually are not considered useful for evaluating pulmonary function. However, a $PvCO_2$ above 60 mm Hg generally indicates arterial hypercapnia, and a PvO_2 below 20 mm Hg indicates arterial hypoxemia.[64] Measuring the PaO_2 5 minutes after *insufflation of 100% oxygen* can help in determining if significant right-to-left shunting is present. In full-term neonates and adults the PaO_2 should exceed 200 mm Hg after 5 minutes of oxygen administration.[66] Continued cyanosis and inability to raise the PaO_2 above 100 mm Hg are highly suggestive of a right-to-left shunt.

COMPLETE BLOOD COUNT. A complete blood count should be performed to determine if polycythemia or inflammatory leukogram is present. Polycythemia may develop secondary to chronic hypoxemia associated with long-standing pulmonary disease or right-to-left shunting. An inflammatory leukogram would be consistent with a diagnosis of bacterial or aspiration pneumonia or other inflammatory respiratory condition.

HEPARINIZED BLOOD. A sample of heparinized blood should be shaken gently in the air for 15 minutes. Reduced hemoglobin (cardiovascular or respiratory disease) turns red on exposure to air, whereas methemoglobin remains chocolate brown after shaking.

SPECTROSCOPIC EXAMINATION. A spectroscopic examination should be performed to determine if methemoglobin is present. Methemoglobin is stable in refrigerated heparinized blood for only a few hours. To preserve methemoglobin, one part of blood can be mixed with 20 parts of phosphate buffer (pH 6.6) or diluted 1:20 in distilled water. These diluted samples can be refrigerated or frozen until they are analyzed.

REFERENCES

60. Krotje LT: Cyanosis: physiology and pathogenesis, *Compend Cont Educ Pract Vet* 9:271-278, 1987.
61. Lombard CW: Cardiovascular diseases. In Koterba AM, Drummond WH, Kosch PC, eds: *Equine clinical neonatology*, Philadelphia, 1990, Lea & Febiger, pp 240-261.
62. Calvert CA: Cyanosis. In Lorenz MD, Cornelius LM, eds: *Small animal medicine diagnosis*, Philadelphia, 1987, JB Lippincott, pp 196-203.

63. Bernard WV, Reimer JM: Examination of the foal, *Vet Clin North Am (Equine Pract)* 10:37-66, 1994.
64. Koterba AM: Respiratory disease: approach to diagnosis. In Koterba AM, Drummond WH, Kosch PC, eds: *Equine clinical neonatology*, Philadelphia, 1990, Lea & Febiger, pp 153-176.
65. Pringle JK: Ancillary testing for the ruminant respiratory system, *Vet Clin North Am (Food Anim Pract)* 8:243-256, 1992.
66. Beech J: Respiratory problems in foals, *Vet Clin North Am (Equine Pract)* 1:131-149, 1985.
67. Kosch PC, Koterba AM, Coons TJ: Development and management of the newborn foal in respiratory distress. I, Evaluation, *Equine Vet J* 16:212-218, 1984.

ABNORMAL RESPIRATORY NOISE (STRIDOR)

Definition

Stridor is an abnormal, intense respiratory sound (wheeze) that is audible without the use of a stethoscope. The sound usually is generated in the upper airway and is most often heard during inspiration.

Pathophysiology

The extrathoracic airway of the horse consists of segments that are relatively rigid (e.g., the nasal fossa and extrathoracic trachea) and others (e.g., the nostrils, soft palate, and larynx) that are not only elastic but also have valvelike actions that are further capable of modifying the cross-sectional area and therefore resistance to airflow.[68,69] Pressures in the extrathoracic airways are subatmospheric during inspiration,[68-70] which causes the less rigidly supported parts of the upper airway to narrow (dynamic collapse) during inspiration.[68-73] A major function of the upper airway muscles and other supporting structures is to prevent this dynamic collapse during periods of high inspiratory gas flow.[68] Disease in these structures or a more rostral obstructing lesion that causes a greater negative pressure during inspiration may make them incapable of resisting axial displacement.[68,70] The increased resistance to flow induced by static or dynamic obstructions increases the driving pressure and therefore the work needed to move a given volume of air.[69]

Approximately 80% of the total airway resistance to gas flow at rest and during exercise is located in the upper airway rostral to the thoracic inlet.[70] Nasal resistance, most of which is caused by resistance just within the external nares, comprises more than 50% of the total upper airway resistance in the horse.[71,72] In most species, including ruminants, this resistance can be bypassed by mouth breathing to accommodate the high airflow rates that accompany strenuous exercise. The horse, in contrast, is limited to nasal breathing even during exercise,[70-72,74] because the larynx is firmly maintained in an intranarial position by the tight seal formed around it by the muscular palatopharyngeal ring (intrapharyngeal osteum) except during swallowing.[74,75] Therefore mechanisms other than mouth breathing are needed to reduce the energy cost of breathing in the horse.[68,71,74] These mechanisms include dilation of the distensible external nares by actively pulling the alar folds laterally, vasoconstriction in the erectile nasal vascular tissues to reduce congestion in the nasal mucosa, straightening of the respiratory tract, and dilation of the larynx by abduction of the vocal folds.[68-71,73,74,76,77]

The horse is capable of generating very high respiratory rates during fast exercise. This is accomplished at the canter and gallop, but not at the trot, by locking respiration to locomotion so that the horse takes one breath for each stride.[75,78-80] Exhalation occurs each time the lead forelimb strikes the ground.[74,75,78] The horse can swallow during fast galloping exercise; the entire process is completed in exactly a two-stride sequence.[75,81]

At all levels of the respiratory tract, respiratory sounds are thought to result from vibrations in tissue and sudden changes in the pressure of gas moving in the airway lumen.[70,75] Airflow in the normal respiratory tract at rest occurs in a laminar fashion (i.e., the air closest to the wall of the airway is almost stationary, whereas succeeding layers toward the center of the lumen move progressively more rapidly).[75] Respiration in normal horses and in ruminants at rest does not generate easily audible sounds.

High rates of gas flow and airway narrowing increase both the tendency for dynamic collapse and the degree of turbulence and genesis of sounds. Very high peak flow rates of 125 ml/sec/kg have been reported in galloping horses.[80] At exercise, significant sound frequencies are generated and can be detected using sound spectrography or radiostethoscopes, although most of these sounds are of frequencies and amplitudes not detectable by the human ear.[82,83] Deformities in the wall and masses in the lumen of the airway cause airway narrowing and further disturbances in laminar flow, resulting in more severe turbulence and sudden changes in the pressure of moving gas, which may generate audible sounds.[75] High airflow rates are necessary to induce most audible stridors, therefore examination of the horse at exercise is an essential part of the physical examination.[74,75]

Stridor is best heard during inspiration in most cases because the usual source of origin, the upper airway, is subject to dynamic narrowing during the inspiratory phase of the respiratory cycle.[68,71,72] In particular, nonfixed obstructions, such as the paretic vocal folds of horses with idiopathic laryngeal hemiplegia (ILH), only cause obstruction to airflow and turbulence when dynamically drawn into the airway by the high inspiratory airflow rates that accompany fast exercise. Other obstructions such as arytenoid chondritis are fixed and obstruct airflow during both inspiration and expiration, which frequently results in audible stridor during both phases of respiration.

The pharynx is the site of greatest airway angulation as a result of flexion of the atlantooccipital joint. At rest the horse's head is usually held at about 50 degrees to the horizontal plane.[75] At the gallop the horse extends its head and neck and thus straightens the pharyngeal airway.[75] This maneuver also stretches and straightens the trachea, making it less compliant and less subject to dynamic narrowing during inspiration.[71] When ridden at a collected canter, the horse is forced to flex its poll so that its face is nearly vertical, thereby increasing the angulation of the pharyngeal airway and the obstruction to gas flow at this point.[75] Therefore abnormal respiratory sounds originating in the pharyngeal region are often more easily heard when the horse is ridden at a collected canter than when it is exercised at a full, extended gallop.[74,75]

Because food animals are not normally expected to perform fast exercise, signs of stridor are usually present at rest when they are presented to veterinarians for examination. Stridor in resting animals usually indicates moderate to severe upper airway obstruction of a fixed nature. In ruminants the epiglottis is relatively short and blunt, and the palatopharyngeal ring allows the laryngopalatal dislocation necessary for mouth breathing. In conditions that give rise to respiratory distress and mouth breathing, the turbulence produced is often sufficient to induce abnormal (grunting) expiratory sounds, which may be classified as expiratory stridor. The external nares of cattle are much less compliant than those of sheep, goats, and horses, which prevents dynamic collapse during inspiration; thus conditions such as paresis of the nares that cause stridor in sheep, goats, and horses do not cause stridor in cattle (Boxes 5-18 and 5-19).

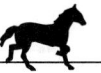

BOX 5-18

Causes of Stridor in the Horse

COMMON CAUSES
Idiopathic laryngeal hemiplegia (ILH, roaring)
Dorsal displacement of the soft palate (laryngopalatal
    dislocation)
Epiglottic entrapment
Retropharyngeal abscess
Strangles (*Streptococcus equi* infection)
Guttural pouch empyema
Chronic pharyngeal lymphoid hyperplasia
Arytenoid chondritis
Guttural pouch mycosis
Laxity of the alar cartilage

LESS COMMON CAUSES
Arytenoid chondroma, chondropathy
Pharyngeal paresis
Botulism, shaker foal
Dynamic collapse of the pharynx
Subepiglottal, pharyngeal cyst
Subepiglottal abscess
Epiglottal retroversion
Guttural pouch tympany
Guttural pouch neoplasia
Rostral displacement of the palatopharyngeal arch
Nasal fungal infection (e.g., aspergillosis, rhinophycomycosis)
Nasal polyp
Nasal foreign body
Nasal trauma
Nasal tumor
Nasopharyngeal cicatrix
Progressive ethmoidal hematoma
Sinusitis (sinus empyema)
Sinus cyst
Sinus tumor
Atheroma
Laryngeal trauma
Tracheal collapse (scabbard trachea)
Tracheal stricture, stenosis
Tracheal chondroma
Tracheal rupture, perforation
Stenotic nares
Laryngeal edema
Purpura hemorrhagica
Anaphylaxis or acute drug reaction
Chronic lead poisoning
Choanal (posterior nares) atresia, hypoplasia (foals)

LESS COMMON CAUSES—cont'd
Fracture of laryngeal cartilages
Laryngeal granuloma, scar tissue
Equine influenza
Exercise-induced pulmonary hemorrhage (EIPH)
Jugular thrombosis
Hyperkalemic periodic paralysis (HYPP)

UNCOMMON CAUSES
Amyloidosis (cutaneous, nasal)
Lymphosarcoma, lymphoma
Bee or wasp sting
Snakebite
Thyroid adenoma, adenocarcinoma
Vesicular stomatitis
Retrobulbar neoplasia
Dystrophic myodegeneration (white muscle disease)
Neoplasia (oral, mandibular, maxillary, laryngeal, pharyngeal,
    tracheal)
Coccidioidomycosis
Inhalation pneumonia, smoke inhalation
Burns (thermal, chemical)
Congestive cardiac failure
Cutaneous habronemiasis
Unilateral ventral displacement of the roof of the nasopharynx
Epiglottiditis
Hyoid bone injuries
Fungal granuloma, maduromycosis, rhinosporidiosis, myce-
    toma, cryptococcal rhinitis, equine nasal granuloma
Goiter
Hypertrophic ossification of the laryngeal cartilages
Abnormalities of the nasal septum
Intramural esophageal cyst
Foreign body (nasal, pharyngeal, laryngeal, tracheal,
    bronchial)
Hyperparathyroidism
Phycomycosis, pythiosis
Anaerobic abscesses (e.g., *Clostridium perfringens*)
Besnoitiosis, globidiosis (exotic)
Glanders (exotic)

TOXIC CAUSES
Organophosphate-induced laryngeal paralysis
Lead-induced laryngeal paresis
Reserpine

BOX 5-19

Causes of Stridor in Ruminants

COMMON CAUSES
Necrotic laryngitis (calf diphtheria) (B, O)
Abscess (pharyngeal, laryngeal, retropharyngeal, oral)
Nose bots (*Oestrus ovis*) (C, O)
Caseous lymphadenitis (*Corynebacterium pseudotuberculosis*)
    (C, O)
Actinobacillosis (wooden tongue, nasal actinobacillosis)
Nasal adenocarcinoma, adenoma, adenopapilloma, polyp
    (C, O)
Trauma (oral, nasal, pharyngeal, laryngeal, tracheal)
Anaphylaxis or drug reaction

COMMON CAUSES—cont'd
Sinusitis
Foreign body (nasal, oral, pharyngeal, laryngeal, tracheal,
    bronchial)

LESS COMMON CAUSES
Actinomycosis (lumpy jaw)
Tracheal stenosis, collapse, stricture
Bovine leukosis (enzootic adult lymphosarcoma) (B)
Sporadic bovine leukosis (adult multicentric lymphosar-
    coma) (B)

B, Bovine; *C*, caprine; *O*, ovine.

Continued

BOX 5-19

Causes of Stridor in Ruminants—cont'd

LESS COMMON CAUSES—cont'd
Thymic lymphosarcoma (juvenile) (B)
Mannheimia hemolytica or *Pasteurella multocida* pneumonia
   (includes shipping fever and enzootic calf pneumonia)
Infectious bovine rhinotracheitis (IBR; BHV-1) (B)
Atypical interstitial pneumonia (B)
Malignant catarrhal fever (B)
Vesicular stomatitis
Clostridial infection of the head (O)
Pulmonary embolism from posterior vena cava
   thrombosis (B)
Snakebite
Bee or wasp sting
Bovine nasal granuloma, atopic rhinitis (summer
   nuffles) (B)
Honker syndrome in feedlot cattle (B)
Neoplasia (nasal, paranasal sinus, oral, pharyngeal, laryngeal,
   tracheal, maxillary, mandibular, retrobulbar)
Congenital abnormalities
Inhalation pneumonia, smoke inhalation

UNCOMMON CAUSES
Tuberculosis (B)
Congenital cystic nasal conchae (B)
Choanal atresia (O)
Salivary cyst, mucocele, ranula, trauma (C)
Photosensitization in Southdown and Corriedale sheep (O)
Fungal granuloma, maduromycosis, rhinosporidiosis, myce-
   toma (B, C)
Phycomycosis, pythiosis (B)
Goiter, iodine deficiency
Hyperparathyroidism (B, C)
Enzootic ataxia, swayback (C, O)
Besnoitiosis, globidiosis (exotic)
Endemic ethmoid hematoma (exotic) (B)
African bovine malignant catarrhal fever (exotic) (B)
Lumpy skin disease (exotic) (B)
Nasal schistosomiasis (exotic)
Virulent sheep and goat pox (exotic) (C, O)
Peste des petits ruminants (exotic) (C, O)
Gedoelstia hasleri nasal bots (exotic) (C, O)

B, Bovine; *C,* caprine; *O,* ovine.

Approach to Diagnosis of Stridor

HISTORY. The procedure for taking a history should follow that used in the evaluation of cough and nasal discharge (see Cough, p. 46, and Nasal Discharge, p. 54). The history should also include the duration of ownership; time of onset of the clinical signs of stridor; progression of clinical signs; presence or absence of the noise at rest; relation of noise to fitness; relation of noise to speed, duration, and direction of work; relation of noise to head position during work; association of noise with poor performance or exercise intolerance; and other signs of respiratory tract, oropharyngeal, or neurologic disease (e.g., nasal discharge, cough, dysphagia, or retropharyngeal swelling).

PHYSICAL EXAMINATION. A physical examination of the entire respiratory tract at rest should be performed as described for cough (see p. 64) and respiratory distress (see p. 46). In addition, the presence or absence of stridor at rest should be ascertained by listening at the nostrils, and digital pressure should be applied to the retropharyngeal region and to the larynx during palpation of these areas to evaluate whether stridor or pain (or both) can be easily induced or exacerbated. The dorsal surface of the larynx should be palpated with the fingertips with the horse relaxed and its head and neck in an extended position. This permits comparison of the prominence of the muscular process of the arytenoid cartilages and the thickness of the cricoarytenoideus dorsalis (CAD) muscle, both of which are affected in horses with atrophy of the CAD in association with ILH. Air turbulence, flattening, swelling, and pain should be assessed during palpation of the extrathoracic airway. The larynx, trachea, and lungs should be carefully *ausculted,* and the chest should be *percussed.* A thorough oral examination should be completed, particularly in ruminants; in cattle this should include palpation of the base of the tongue, the oropharynx, and, if possible, the larynx through the oral cavity.

FIELD EXERCISE TESTING.[75] In performance horses most examinations are carried out because the horse makes a noise only when worked, because of exercise intolerance or poor performance, or as part of a prepurchase examination. Unless a high-speed treadmill is available, the exercise testing should be completed under saddle with a competent rider, preferably with an intensity of work that matches the horse's normal activity.[70,74] It is less satisfactory but often necessary to work the horse on a lunge line, in which case it should be lunged in both directions.[74]

The horse should be worked in a circle about 30 yards in diameter so that it passes close to the observer on each circuit.[75] The observer should first identify the expiratory sound by its association with locomotion and then try to fit abnormal sounds into this base rhythm. At fast speed respiration is very rapid; thus the observer should not stand too far away from the horse because the slow speed at which sound is transmitted confuses interpretation of whether the sound is inspiratory or expiratory.[75,81] In cold weather the visibility of exhaled breath aids interpretation. It is important to ride the horse in both directions because an abnormal sound is frequently heard more clearly when the horse is exercising in one direction rather than the other.[74] If the presence or character of a respiratory noise remains in doubt after the horse has been exercised in a circle at a collected canter, the horse should be galloped until it is blowing hard and then ridden past the observer at a fast gallop.[74]

A satisfactory exercise test should include at least 5 minutes of work at the canter, after which the horse should immediately be brought over to the observer so that the character and sequence of abnormal sounds that persist can be determined. All horses that have been worked adequately make a loud expiratory blowing sound at this time. Turbulence of airflow in the larynx may be audible with a stethoscope.[75] Inducing adduction of the vocal fold, particularly on the right side, by application of gentle pressure in a rostromedial direction to the muscular process of the arytenoid cartilage often accentuates an inspiratory noise in horses with laryngeal hemiplegia. Noises originating from unilateral lesions in the nasal passages are easily localized because the sound can be eliminated by alternately blocking off airflow through each nostril with the hand. Temporary occlusion of both nostrils simultaneously may provoke laryngopalatal dislocation and a loud gurgling sound in a susceptible horse.[74,75] The presence of nasal discharge or blood at the nostrils should be noted, and the time required for the heart and respiratory rates to return to preexercise values should be interpreted in light of the severity of the exercise test.[74]

INTERPRETATION OF ABNORMAL SOUNDS. A normal horse makes no audible respiratory sound at rest and when exercised at a canter or slow gallop makes only a blowing expiratory sound.[70,74,75] In unfit horses, particularly overweight ones, an inspiratory sound is also frequently audible. This sound can be quite loud, and it may be difficult to differentiate from sounds caused by abnormalities of the respiratory tract.[73,74] Thus evaluation of the horse's "wind" is best carried out when the horse is in fit condition for its intended use. It takes at least 1 month for an older horse that has been turned out to pasture to regain a satisfactory level of fitness to perform a meaningful wind examination. Many normal horses produce a harsh expiratory "high blowing sound" of variable pitch, which results from resonance in the cavity of the false nostril during expiration.[74,75,81] If the source of the stridor remains in doubt, temporary suturing of the alar fold dorsal to the nostril can help localize noises suspected of being caused by vibration of the alar fold.

Horses with ILH make a rather characteristic biphasic sound, the inspiratory sound occurring between successive expiratory sounds. The pitch of the sound can vary from a whistle to a deep roar, the lower-pitched note giving rise to the so-called sawing wood sounds.[75] Sonographic and spectrographic analysis of the sounds produced by "roarers" indicates that the range of sound frequencies generated by these horses is the same as that produced by normal horses.[82,83] However, horses that make an audible whistle generate an intense band of frequencies centered on 1.9 kHz that are thought to result from amplification by the still-patent lateral ventricle of the frequency generated by vibration of the incompletely abducted left vocal fold.[83] In a normal horse the left vocal fold is fully abducted and the cavity of the lateral ventricle is thus obliterated during strenuous exercise.[77]

The sounds generated by horses with laryngeal chondritis, severe proliferative pharyngeal lymphoid hyperplasia, epiglottic entrapment, and tracheal stenosis can be very similar to those caused by ILH.[74,75] Laryngopalatal dislocation (dorsal displacement of the soft palate) gives rise to a transient, vibrant, gurgling sound.[72,74,75] In many instances a severe exercise test is required to induce this condition; thus this sound may be heard only during a race.[70,74,75] It is thought that the condition may occur when pharyngeal stimulation causes swallowing during fast exercise.[75] Instead of the horse completing the process and returning the larynx to an intranarial position, the larynx remains in the oropharynx, with the epiglottis beneath the soft palate. At the subsequent inspiration the palatopharyngeal arch tends to be drawn into the rima glottis, and at expiration it is driven toward the roof of the pharynx by the air stream. The palatopharyngeal arch acts as an airway obstruction, and the tissue vibration and resulting turbulence generate a sound of varying pitch and intensity, often described as gurgling followed by swallowing.[75] The horse often slows suddenly or stops when this event occurs, and the jockey often reports that the horse stopped after "choking" or "swallowing its tongue." If repeated swallowing is successful in relocating the normal laryngopalatal respiratory arrangement, the horse often continues to race after slowing or stopping.[70]

Gross obstruction of the airway by pressure from pus-filled guttural pouches, retropharyngeal abscesses, large subepiglottal cysts or abscesses, or large proliferative lesions (e.g., laryngeal tumors) produces loud, stertorous breathing (snoring) often heard at rest and readily so with exercise; both inspiratory and expiratory sounds are clearly audible.[75]

In a normal horse the pattern of respiratory sounds is regular and synchronized with the pace of the exercise. Laryngeal irritation caused by exudate from the upper or lower airway, pharyngeal lymphoid hyperplasia, or other inflammatory or space-occupying conditions causes the horse to swallow more frequently during exercise, which generates an irregular pattern of respiratory sounds characterized at the canter and gallop by a respiratory cycle of double the normal length.[75,81]

Interpretation of stridor in yearlings presented for sale is difficult because these animals are rarely fit and it is usually possible to exercise them only at a canter on a lunge line. It has been shown that resentment of restraint under such circumstances can significantly alter the linking of locomotion and respiration, which complicates recognition of the respiratory phasing of noise production.[77] In addition, there is not always a close correlation between noise production, endoscopically visible abnormalities, and signs of exercise intolerance even in fit adult horses.[70,74]

ENDOSCOPIC EXAMINATION. Endoscopic examination of the upper airway is the most useful diagnostic procedure for investigating stridor. The examination should be performed at rest before exercise, again immediately after exercise or, if possible, during exercise on a high-speed treadmill. Endoscopic examination immediately after cessation of exercise is less satisfactory than endoscopy during treadmill exercise because dynamic collapse of the rima glottis terminates rapidly on cessation of exercise. Because sedatives and tranquilizers may alter the tone and function of the muscles supporting laryngeal and pharyngeal anatomy and function, endoscopic examination should be performed without chemical restraint whenever possible.[70] The nasal passages, conchae (turbinates) (including the ethmoidal concha), nasal septum, pharynx, larynx, and trachea should be examined through both nostrils so that the presence, nature, and source of exudates and the presence of anatomic or functional abnormalities or mass lesions can be determined. If problems are suspected in the guttural pouches, the interior of these structures should be examined for exudate, proliferative lesions, or arterial aneurysms by advancing the endoscope through the pharyngeal openings. Because the larynx is viewed slightly obliquely when examined from the left or right ventral meatus, an apparently asymmetric larynx should be viewed through both nostrils.[70,74]

Interpretation of the findings of the endoscopic examination of the pharynx and larynx is by no means straightforward. The results can be influenced by the day the examination was done, the use of sedation, the side through which the endoscope is passed, and the observer's interpretation.[84] The appearance of laryngeal symmetry or asymmetry in resting horses varies considerably and therefore is of limited clinical usefulness unless complete hemiparalysis is present. Many horses have asynchronous or asymmetric laryngeal movement at rest but not during exercise, whereas other horses have a normal-appearing larynx at rest but suffer dynamic collapse during exercise. Interpretation of findings is improved by use of an objective grading system, which includes assessment of the ratio of the areas of the left and right half of the rima glottis and by correlating findings at rest with those observed on video endoscopy performed during maximal exercise.[84] For evaluation of the larynx at rest, full abduction of the vocal folds should be induced by exercise or by temporary occlusion of the nostrils.[74] Contralateral adductory laryngeal movement should be stimulated by slapping the horse just behind the withers (slap test).[85] To induce the horse to swallow, the tip of the epiglottis should be touched with the endoscope, or water should be flushed through the endoscope. These maneuvers help to establish whether movement of the arytenoid cartilages is synchronous and symmetric and increase the predictive value of endoscopic observations, allowing laryngeal function to be graded as follows[84]:

Grade 1: Synchronous, full adduction and abduction of the left and right arytenoid cartilages (considered normal).

Grade 2: Asynchronous movement (e.g., hesitation, fluttering, adductor weakness) of the left arytenoid cartilage during any phase of respiration but full abduction of the left arytenoid cartilage, inducible by nasal occlusion or swallowing. Grade 2 findings are considered a normal variation and are not usually associated with dynamic airway collapse during exercise.

Grade 3: Asynchronous movement of the left arytenoid cartilage but full abduction is not inducible by nasal occlusion or induction of swallowing. The true functional significance of grade 3 findings can be determined only by performing endoscopic examination during maximal exercise on a high-speed treadmill, a procedure that has led to subclassification of grade 3 findings.[86] Some grade 3 horses (*grade 3A*) are able to achieve full abduction during exercise, whereas others maintain a partly abducted position similar to the resting position (*grade 3B*) or experience dynamic collapse (*grade 3C*).[86]

Grade 4: Marked asymmetry of the larynx at rest and no substantial movement of the left arytenoid cartilage during any phase of respiration. These horses have complete left laryngeal hemiplegia, are true "roarers," and consistently experience dynamic collapse on inspiration during strenuous exercise.[84]

Performing an endoscopic examination during maximal exercise on a high-speed treadmill makes it possible for a stationary observer to gain a good dynamic appreciation of the significance of upper airway abnormalities (i.e., dynamic endoscopy)[86-90] (see Exercise Intolerance and Poor Performance in Horses, p. 81). Dynamic changes in airway lumen diameter occur quickly during treadmill endoscopy and may be difficult to visualize. Therefore the endoscopic examination should be videotaped for later playback in slow motion and freeze-frame.[90] It is important to exercise horses maximally and to exhaustion (inability to keep up with the treadmill), because some abnormalities are only apparent at maximal exercise toward the end of a race when pharyngeal or laryngeal muscles become fatigued and are no longer able to resist the transmural pressure gradient, which tends to induce dynamic collapse of the upper airway during inspiration.[86-90] Endoscopic identification of an upper respiratory tract abnormality in a resting horse does not necessarily mean that it is inducing a problem during exercise and, conversely, the absence of an upper respiratory tract abnormality at rest does not rule out the possibility of intermittent airway obstruction during strenuous exercise. For example, dorsal displacement of the soft palate, epiglottic entrapment, dorsal displacement of the epiglottis, dynamic collapse of the left arytenoid cartilage or vocal fold (or both), and unilateral or bilateral ventral displacement of the roof of the pharynx (dynamic pharyngeal collapse) have been observed during treadmill exercise in horses with an endoscopically normal upper airway at rest.[86-90]

RADIOGRAPHIC EXAMINATION. Radiographic examination of the nasal passages, paranasal sinuses, pharynx, retropharyngeal area (including guttural pouches), larynx, and proximal trachea is indicated to confirm anatomic or functional problems or space-occupying lesions not definitively diagnosed by clinical examination and endoscopy (see Nasal Discharge, p. 54, and Respiratory Distress, p. 64). Radiography is particularly useful for visualizing subepiglottic masses such as cysts or abscesses and for evaluating the epiglottis of the horse when it is obscured from endoscopic view by dorsal displacement of the soft palate or other space-occupying lesions. An accurate assessment of epiglottic length can also be made from standardized true lateral radiographs of the larynx by measuring the distance from the body of the thyroid cartilage to the tip of the epiglottis (thyroepiglottic length).[91] The mean ± SD thyroepiglottic length in normal thoroughbred horses is reported to be 8.76 ±

0.44 cm.[91] Significantly shortened thyroepiglottic lengths have been recorded in thoroughbred horses with dorsal displacement of the soft palate (laryngopalatal dislocation) and in those with entrapment of the epiglottis in the aryepiglottic folds.[91] Tracheal diseases such as chondroma or dynamic collapse may be visualized on radiographs of the trachea, particularly those made during the inspiratory phase.

ULTRASOUND EXAMINATION. Ultrasound examination of externally visible lesions such as possible retropharyngeal abscesses that may be impinging on the airway help to characterize lesions and assist in the collection of samples by aspiration or biopsy.

BIOPSY. Biopsy and histologic evaluation of samples are indicated to diagnose certain mass lesions such as neoplasms, cysts, polyps, fungal granulomas, or foreign body granulomas in or surrounding the airway. Masses in the airway can be biopsied through the biopsy channel of fiberoptic or video endoscopes, but these samples inevitably are small. Larger samples can be collected from lesions in the nares, nasal diverticulum, and nasal passages using uterine biopsy forceps or curettes. Hemorrhage usually accompanies such procedures. Biopsies can also be collected at the time of exploratory or corrective surgery from lesions in the nasal passages, pharynx, larynx, and guttural pouches. Lesions such as habronemiasis involving the external nares and lesions in other accessible areas such as the parotid salivary gland can be biopsied percutaneously using Tru-Cut or similar instruments.

ASPIRATION. Aspiration, either blindly or with the assistance of ultrasound, followed by cytologic examination and culture of aspirated material is useful in the evaluation of masses such as retropharyngeal abscesses that are causing stridor by impinging on the upper airway.

SWABBING OR SCRAPING. Nasal or nasopharyngeal swabbing or scraping followed by direct cytologic examination and culture is indicated for confirmation of nasal fungal infection and bacterial infections of the upper airway (e.g., strangles).

COMPLETE BLOOD COUNT. A complete blood count, including fibrinogen concentration, can be useful in evaluating patients suspected of having a primary or secondary inflammatory condition or conditions such as ethmoidal hematoma and guttural pouch mycosis in which blood-loss anemia is likely to be a complicating problem.

ASPIRATION, LAVAGE, OR THORACOCENTESIS. Transtracheal aspiration, bronchoalveolar lavage, and/or thoracocentesis with cytologic examination and culture of collected samples is indicated in the evaluation of patients suspected of having disease of the lungs or pleura.

REFERENCES
68. Robinson NE: Functional abnormalities caused by upper airway obstruction and heaves: their relationship to the etiology of epistaxis, *Vet Clin North Am (Large Anim Pract)* 1:17-34, 1979.
69. Pascoe JR: Upper airway flow dynamics. In Robinson NE, ed: *Current therapy in equine medicine 3,* Philadelphia, 1992, WB Saunders, pp 291-294.
70. Haynes PF: Exercise intolerance and noise production, *Proc Am Assoc Equine Pract* 27:43-47, 1981.
71. Art T, Serteyn D, Lekeux P: Effect of exercise on the partitioning of equine respiratory resistance, *Equine Vet J* 20:268-273, 1988.
72. Robinson NE, Sorenson PR: Pathophysiology of airway obstruction in the horse: a review, *J Am Vet Med Assoc* 172:299-303, 1978.
73. Derksen FJ et al: Effect of laryngeal hemiplegia and laryngoplasty on airway flow mechanics in exercising horses, *Am J Vet Res* 47:16-20, 1986.
74. Greet TRC: The respiratory tract. In Hickman J, ed: *Equine surgery and medicine,* vol 1, London, 1985, Academic Press, pp 247-296.
75. Gerring EL: Differential diagnosis of equine respiratory noises, *In Practice* 7:109-117, 1985.
76. Cook WR: Clinical observations on the anatomy and physiology of the equine upper respiratory tract, *Vet Rec* 79:440-446, 1966.
77. Cook WR: Some observations on form and function of the equine upper airway in health and disease. II, Larynx, *Proc Am Assoc Equine Pract* 27:393-451, 1981.

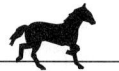

78. Attenburrow DP: Time relationship between the respiratory cycle and limb cycle in the horse, *Equine Vet J* 14:69-72, 1982.

79. Attenburrow DP: Respiration and locomotion. In Snow DH, Persson SGB, Rose RJ, eds: *Equine exercise physiology*, Cambridge, 1983, Granta Editions, pp 17-26.

80. Hörnicke H, Meixner R, Pollmann U: Respiration in exercising horses. In Snow DH, Persson SGB, Rose RJ, eds: *Equine exercise physiology*, Cambridge, 1983, Granta Editions, pp 7-16.

81. Attenburrow DP: Respiratory sounds recorded by radiostethoscope from normal horses at exercise, *Equine Vet J* 10:176-179, 1978.

82. Barnes GRG et al: Sound spectrography in the diagnosis of equine respiratory disorders: a preliminary report, *N Z Vet J* 27:145-146, 1979.

83. Attenburrow DP: Resonant frequency of the lateral ventricle and saccule and "whistling." In Snow DH, Persson SGB, Rose RJ, eds: *Equine exercise physiology*, Cambridge, 1983, Granta Editions, pp 27-32.

84. Hackett RP et al: The reliability of endoscopic examination in assessment of arytenoid cartilage movement in horses. I, Subjective and objective laryngeal evaluation, *Vet Surg* 20:174-179, 1991.

85. Greet TRC et al: The slap test for laryngeal adductory function in horses with suspected cervical spinal cord damage, *Equine Vet J* 12:127-131, 1980.

86. Hammer EJ et al: Videoendoscopic assessment of dynamic laryngeal function during exercise in horses with grade 3 left laryngeal hemiparesis at rest: 26 cases (1992-1995), *J Am Vet Med Assoc* 212:399-403, 1998.

87. Morris E: Dynamic endoscopy of the upper airway. In Robinson NE, ed: *Current therapy in equine medicine 3*, Philadelphia, 1992, WB Saunders, pp 774-776.

88. Morris EA, Seeherman HJ: Clinical evaluation of poor performance in the racehorse: the results of 275 evaluations, *Equine Vet J* 23:169-174, 1991.

89. Ducharme NG: Dynamic pharyngeal collapse. In Robinson NE, ed: *Current therapy in equine medicine 3*, Philadelphia, 1992, WB Saunders, pp 283-285.

90. Martin BB et al: Causes of poor performance of horses during training, racing, or showing: 348 cases (1992-1996), *J Am Vet Med Assoc* 216:554-558, 2000.

91. Linford RL et al: Radiographic assessment of epiglottic length and pharyngeal and laryngeal diameters in the thoroughbred, *Am J Vet Res* 44:1660-1666, 1983.

EXERCISE INTOLERANCE AND POOR PERFORMANCE IN HORSES

STEPHANIE J. VALBERG
W. DAVID WILSON

The popularity of performance horses has broadened our perspective on health beyond the conventional diagnosis of health or disease in a horse at rest. Sports medicine defines equine health as the optimum function of all body systems during the expected level of performance. Because many body systems function at only a small fraction of their maximum capacity in a resting athlete, a clearer understanding of exercise responses in the horse and new methods of evaluating horses during exercise are needed.

Exercise Responses

As horses accelerate during exercise, motor units within active muscles fire in a coordinated fashion to produce the power necessary to drive the animal forward. Initially slow-twitch type 1 muscle fibers are recruited, followed at increasing speed by recruitment of oxidative fast-twitch type 2A fibers and finally by the fastest and most powerful muscle fibers, type 2B. The increased demand for adenosine triphosphate (ATP) to support muscle contractions during exercise can be met initially by small intracellular stores of creatine phosphate, but within seconds oxidative or glycolytic metabolism (or both) is activated. At submaximum speeds the major factors contributing to fatigue are total depletion of fuel reserves (glycogen), fluid and electrolyte losses, and hyperthermia.[92] Training increases the oxidative and endurance capacity of skeletal muscle by increasing the volume of mitochondria and the capillary density surrounding muscle fibers.[93] This delays the onset of fatigue by increasing the availability and metabolism of plasma free fatty acids and glucose, thus sparing muscle glycogen.

When a horse accelerates toward a maximum speed, a peak in the total amount of oxygen consumed is realized (VO_{2max}). Additional energy to produce speeds beyond VO_{2max} must be supplied by anaerobic glycolysis with lactic acidosis as a consequence. The term anaerobic threshold has been used to describe the speed at which this exponential rise in lactate begins to occur. Fatigue with maximum (fast) exercise occurs when muscle pH falls so low that glycolysis and excitation contraction coupling are inhibited and muscle ATP concentrations fall.[94,95] Muscle glycogen stores are not a limiting factor with maximum exercise.[96] Training over time increases the mitochondrial volume and the ratio of type 2A to type 2B muscle fibers.[93,97] As a result, the onset of anaerobic metabolism is delayed until a higher speed is reached, and horses are able to maintain a higher speed over a given distance.

The cardiovascular system plays a central role in the oxygenation of blood by the lungs, in the delivery of oxygen and other energy substrates to exercising muscles, and in the removal of metabolic products from those muscles. Cardiac output increases with exercise in horses, largely as a function of an increase in heart rate.[98] As exercise begins, the heart rate quickly increases and then reaches a steady state within minutes at a submaximum speed. With increasing exercise intensity the heart rate shows a linear relationship with speed up to a maximum rate of 210 to 230 beats/min. The mean systemic arterial pressure does not change with submaximum exercise but rises with maximum exercise. Mean pulmonary arterial pressures increase with speed as the heart rate increases, reaching remarkably high levels that are four times resting values.[99] The oxygen-carrying capacity of the blood also rises with increasing speed through splenic contraction and a more than 50% increase in blood hemoglobin.[100] The increase in blood viscosity that occurs with splenic contraction is believed to contribute to the increase in blood pressure with exercise. Among the adaptive cardiovascular responses to training are a lowered heart rate and blood pressure at the same exercise intensity[101]; increased red cell volume[100]; and increased capillarization of muscle.[93]

After an initial abrupt rise, the respiratory rate increases linearly with the speed of trotting until at a canter or gallop, respiration is linked to stride frequency on a 1:1 basis.[102,103] This leaves less time available for completing a respiratory cycle at faster speeds. To counter this, inspiratory and expiratory airflow velocities must increase to maintain or increase minute volume. As airflow rates increase, increased turbulence and an increased tendency for dynamic narrowing of the airways causes an increased resistance to flow and increases the work (energy cost) of breathing.[104,105] A finite maximum flow rate is eventually achieved, beyond which the expiratory muscles and the physical characteristics of the respiratory tract do not permit further increases in flow rate.[104] In addition, a maximum stride frequency is reached, restricting the maximum respiratory rate to 140 to 150 breaths/min.[102,103] It has been suggested that beyond the finite maximum flow rate, the animal is forced to hypoventilate, which may result in arterial hypoxemia during fast exercise.[106] The limitation placed on oxygen diffusion by blood hyperviscosity and the short transit time of blood through the pulmonary capillary bed at rapid heart rates also likely contribute to arterial hypoxemia.[107] The arterial hypoxemia and incomplete saturation of hemoglobin that occur during strenuous exercise do not necessarily limit delivery of oxygen to the tissues, however, because the decline in blood oxygen tension is offset by the increase in the total blood hemoglobin oxygen content resulting from splenic contraction. This fact, together with the horse's ability to sustain at least a sixfold increase in cardiac output between rest and the point of maximum oxygen uptake (VO_{2max})[108] are the major factors that contribute to the enormous aerobic capacity of the horse.

In contrast to the muscular and cardiovascular systems, the respiratory system shows little adaptation to training. Whether the apparent inability of the equine respiratory system either to adjust to training[109] or to compensate fully for the increased flow demands of heavy exercise limits athletic performance remains to be proven. However, it is likely that the maximally exercising horse is operating near the upper limit of ventilation and that even slight degrees of respiratory disease profoundly affect oxygen uptake and performance.[110] Any condition that causes increased resistance to airflow, decreased minute volume, decreased diffusion of gases, ventilation-perfusion mismatch, shunt, or increased oxygen cost of breathing constitutes a respiratory cause of exercise intolerance.

Approach to Diagnosis of Exercise Intolerance and Poor Performance

Top athletes arise from both a genetic background that emphasizes athletic ability and environmental influences that capitalize on this inherent potential. A coordinated, energy-efficient gait, muscular power and endurance, a large capacity for oxygen transport, and several intangible factors, such as the horse's mental toughness and competitive spirit and the rider's skill, all contribute to successful performance. *Poor performance* most often results from inadequate training, a lack of genetic potential, or both or from a congenital or acquired dysfunction of the locomotor, cardiovascular, or respiratory systems. The term exercise intolerance is often used to describe this inability to perform up to an expected or previously attained intensity of exercise.

HISTORY. An accurate history is a fundamental part of the evaluation of exercise intolerance and should include the age, breed, and use of the horse and the training and feeding programs. The onset (time and rapidity) of the problem, previous performance history, the activity level at which signs are observed, whether the horse performs well at first and then suffers tailing off of performance (no stamina), or whether performance is poor throughout the work period should be ascertained. If performance drops off during work, it should be established whether it is associated with the onset of other signs such as stridor. Coughing, respiratory distress, stridor, or excessive sweating associated with stress or exercise should be noted. It should be ascertained whether the affected horse or in-contact horses have recently shown signs of respiratory disease, especially viral infections, and whether other horses are perceived to be performing poorly. It should be determined if the horse has shown lameness, gait abnormalities, or bitting problems. Any medications or other treatments that have been used and their effects should be noted.

In particular, it is important to distinguish from the history between horses that have never been able to perform satisfactorily and horses that suddenly or gradually show a reduction in the level of performance on a background of satisfactory performance. The first scenario suggests a lack of genetic potential, congenital abnormalities, or inadequate training. Some horses do not have the genetic background to perform the expected work (e.g., racing quarter horses rarely make good endurance horses, and thoroughbreds from sprinting families rarely excel at distances of more than $1\frac{1}{4}$ miles).

CLINICAL EXAMINATION. Overt clinical diseases that cause exercise intolerance at moderate speeds usually can be diagnosed with a good history, physical examination, and selected ancillary diagnostic techniques. The diagnostic procedures and specific diseases that can be identified at rest are detailed in subsequent chapters in this book (particularly

Chapters 28, 29, 35, 36, and 40). Problems that are subclinical at rest provide a greater diagnostic challenge. When testing procedures at rest fail to identify the cause of exercise intolerance, various types of ancillary diagnostic procedures including exercise tests may be used to further define the problem. Because the respiratory, cardiovascular, musculoskeletal, and hematopoietic systems are all important for competitive performance and because diseases in these systems are the most likely causes of exercise intolerance, these systems should receive particular attention in the detailed clinical examination of the horse at rest.

HEMATOLOGIC ASSESSMENT. Hematologic tests have historically been popular in the evaluation of fitness and performance because they are easy to perform and because of the important role of hemoglobin in oxygen transport.[111,112] Routine hematologic evaluation may be useful in monitoring the general health status and perhaps fitness of horses if the conditions of collection, particularly in relation to time of day and exercise, can be carefully controlled and if attention is paid to horses that become excited before or during sample collection.

Anemia can result in a decreased oxygen-carrying capacity during exercise. Veterinarians traditionally have regarded resting hematocrits below 35% as abnormal and likely to cause suboptimum racing performance, but values lower than this have been found in normal thoroughbred racehorses.[113] Endurance horses and eventing horses usually have resting hematocrit values that are lower than those of racehorses.[113] However, the fact that a significant proportion of equine red blood cells and hemoglobin are contained in the splenic reserve makes interpretation of resting values for these parameters difficult (inaccurate). There is no correlation between the resting level of hemoglobin and the total body hemoglobin or red cell mass.[100,113] Consequently, even though total body hemoglobin does increase in response to training and may correlate with performance, this cannot be determined from a resting blood sample. Measurement of the total hemoglobin or total red cell mass requires collection of a blood sample after strenuous exercise or after administration of epinephrine to mobilize the red cell reserve and the determination of plasma volume using a technique such as Evans blue dye dilution.[59] These techniques have been used to document red cell hypervolemia in poorly performing, overtrained standardbreds.[100]

Some veterinarians use the resting leukocyte count to monitor fitness, and particularly overtraining, in performance horses.[113] Decreases in the neutrophil/lymphocyte (N/L) ratio have been used to indicate overtraining (training off or adrenal exhaustion). However, the N/L ratio varies in individual horses, depending on when it is determined in relation to the timing and type of exercise, and on factors such as age, stress, and disease. Reliable evidence indicates that the N/L ratio is not a good predictor of adrenal status.[114] Indeed, adrenal function in horses with "adrenal exhaustion syndrome" remains to be accurately characterized on the basis of reproducible function tests.

SERUM BIOCHEMICAL PROFILES. Biochemistry profiles are commonly used to monitor performance horses and to evaluate those with performance problems. These profiles are useful, but interpretation must take into account that when a large number of measurements are performed, there is a high statistical probability that one or two results will be outside the normal range (95% confidence).[113] If only one or two results on a profile are slightly abnormal, the tests are best repeated on a second sample before the true significance of the result is ascribed. Biochemistry profiles are most useful in detecting horses with subclinical muscle problems (either primary exertional rhabdomyolysis or muscular problems secondary to skeletal problems), liver dis-

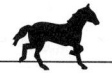

eases, renal diseases, and gross disturbances in electrolyte and acid-base regulation. Biochemical profiles usually include aspartate aminotransferase (AST), creatine kinase (CK), lactate dehydrogenase (LDH), alkaline phosphatase (AP), γ-glutamyltransferase (GGT), sorbitol dehydrogenase (SDH), blood urea nitrogen (BUN), creatinine, sodium (Na), potassium (K), chloride (Cl), bicarbonate, phosphate, calcium (Ca), magnesium (Mg), glucose, and other parameters that are of variable clinical relevance. Studies of horses during training have failed to show any correlation between resting or exercising values for these parameters and fitness.[113]

EVALUATION OF THE RESPIRATORY TRACT. Standard parameters of a routine examination including rectal temperature, respiratory rate, respiratory character, mucous membrane color, and capillary refill time should be carefully evaluated at rest. The presence of nasal discharge, cough, edema, jugular distention or pulsation, or other signs suggesting local or systemic disease should be noted. The larynx, muscular process of the arytenoid cartilages, retropharyngeal area, and trachea should be palpated for size and symmetry. The heart and lungs should be carefully ausculted and percussed at rest, and auscultation of the lungs should be repeated as the horse is induced to breathe more deeply by application of a rebreathing bag. When stridor is part of the history, the upper respiratory tract should receive particular attention in the diagnostic evaluation. Not only must the character of the noise be determined, but the extent of work the patient can tolerate before exhibiting diminished performance must be established, because this helps in the interpretation of abnormalities seen on the endoscopic examination (see Stridor, p. 70). Often the onset and intensity of the stridor coincides with a decrease in work capacity that is typical of certain obstructive airway diseases. Endoscopy, including treadmill endoscopy if facilities permit, and radiography form an important part of the diagnostic evaluation of horses with upper airway abnormalities[115] (see Respiratory Distress, p. 64, and Stridor, p. 76). The most common abnormalities of the upper airway that cause poor performance include dorsal displacement of the soft palate, dynamic pharyngeal collapse, dynamic collapse of the left arytenoid cartilage in association with ILH, epiglottic entrapment, pharyngitis, and collapse of the alar folds.[116,117] Diminished performance in horses with mild or subclinical viral infection is probably mediated at least partly by abnormalities in the respiratory tract.[118] If no abnormalities are detected at rest, functional disturbances of airflow may occur during maximum exercise, and these disorders can best be identified by examining the upper airway using video endoscopy during treadmill exercise. The use of Velcro to attach the endoscope to the halter after insertion of the tip of the endoscope to the depth of the guttural pouch openings decreases the blurring of the image that occurs during exercise. Slow-motion playback must be used because many abnormalities occur rapidly with each respiratory cycle. In particular, dorsal displacement of the soft palate and the extent of dynamic laryngeal obstruction with ILH can be more fully evaluated with treadmill exercise tests.[115-117] The presence of inspiratory or expiratory obstruction can be further evaluated during treadmill exercise by introducing transducers via the nostrils to measure airway pressures at the level of the pharynx and trachea.[115,117] During a treadmill exercise test, samples for blood gas analysis can be drawn from extension tubing connected to an 18-gauge, 2-inch catheter inserted into the transverse facial artery.

Further diagnostic evaluation of the lower airways is indicated in horses with an abnormal respiratory rate or character, cough, nasal discharge, abnormal lung sounds, prolonged recovery after application of a rebreathing bag, or a history of EIPH, cough, or respiratory distress with exercise. Horses in which excess mucus or exudate can be demonstrated in the trachea during endoscopy performed after exercise are also candidates for further evaluation. Applicable tests include a complete blood count, tracheal wash or bronchoalveolar lavage, endoscopy, radiography, and ultrasound examination (see Cough, p. 46, and Stridor, p. 76). Tracheal wash samples collected after exercise are more likely to identify lower airway disease than those collected before exercise.[119] Respiratory viral infection, EIPH, bronchiolitis, reactive airway disease, recurrent airway obstruction, and COPD are all conditions that may not be apparent at rest but that constitute significant causes of exercise intolerance.

EVALUATION OF THE CARDIOVASCULAR SYSTEM. A full evaluation of the mucous membranes, capillary refill time, pulse rate, pulse character and rhythm, heart rate and rhythm, and auscultatory findings is an important part of the evaluation of the performance horse. Failure to maintain cardiac output because of an inability to regulate either heart rate or stroke volume is the mechanism through which cardiac diseases induce exercise intolerance. Many cardiac dysrhythmias and valvular dysfunctions are readily apparent on auscultation of the resting horse. However, the contribution of mild abnormalities to exercise intolerance may require exercise testing. In addition, some arrhythmias and valvular or myocardial dysfunctions can be detected only during or shortly after exercise. Thus resting and exercising electrocardiography (ECG) and echocardiography before and immediately after exercise are indicated.[115,117] The heart rate can be monitored during exercise using either telemetric ECG or commercial heart rate monitors. Electrocardiograms provide the additional benefit of evaluating both heart rate and rhythm. Supraventricular tachyarrhythmias, the most important of which is atrial fibrillation (AF) in horses, can lead to heart rates exceeding 240 beats/min at submaximum exercise.[120] Under these circumstances, cardiac output may be limited by the decreased time available for diastolic perfusion of the myocardium; the absence of atrial contraction; and the reduced time for passive ventricular filling, leading to reduced stroke volume. Many horses with AF maintain efficient circulation at rest and during light exercise but are intolerant to strenuous exercise because they are unable to increase cardiac output sufficiently at rapid heart rates.[121] Some horses show transient paroxysmal atrial fibrillation during exercise but not at rest.[81] These are often easiest to observe in ECG tracings obtained within 60 seconds after an exercise test. Conversion to sinus rhythm, either spontaneously or with quinidine sulfate, usually leads to a return to normal performance in horses with atrial fibrillation.[122,123] The ability to maintain cardiac output can be compromised by other cardiac arrhythmias such as ventricular tachycardia and ventricular premature depolarization.[117,124] The frequency of premature depolarization can increase with exercise, and the timing of resultant abnormal extra systoles can reduce cardiac output even at submaximum heart rates.[124] Intraatrial block, second-degree AV block, and intraventricular block have also been documented in exercise-intolerant, poorly performing horses.[125,126] Horses with cardiac arrhythmias may show abnormal elevations in lactate concentration in response to exercise, indicating a lowered anaerobic threshold, which contributes to exercise intolerance.[101]

Electrocardiography is believed by some veterinarians to be of value in identifying myocarditis. T wave abnormalities (positive and peaked T waves, in contrast to the normal diphasic T waves) in multiple leads on the resting ECG traces have been found in a high percentage of horses with a history of fading during the final portion of a race.[125] T waves are highly labile, affected by training status, and the mechanism by which abnormal T waves are generated is uncertain. However, T wave changes have been identified in some horses with myocarditis confirmed at necropsy.[113,126,127]

Myocarditis may be more definitively documented by evaluating the distribution of serum isoenzymes of LDH or CK. Although total LDH concentrations in serum are often normal, with myocarditis the percentage of the LDH_1 isoenzyme may be elevated.[128] A positive correlation has been demonstrated between heart size and racing performance.[126] ECG has been used to assess performance potential by heart score measurement. The heart score represents the mean QRS duration in leads 1, 2, and 3 expressed in milliseconds and has been strongly correlated with heart weight and prize money won by racehorses.[113,126] The physiologic basis for heart score remains in dispute, and expertise is required to standardize leads and measure QRS complexes.

An *echocardiogram* provides essential information in many cases that have clinical evidence of valvular or myocardial dysfunction. The pericardium, the size of the heart chambers, the presence of congenital defects, the function of valvular leaflets and myocardial contractility all can be assessed (see Chapter 28). Decreased myocardial contractility, regurgitant leaks caused by valvular incompetence, left-to-right shunts, and increases in afterload, such as occurs in aortic stenosis, result in systolic dysfunction and a drop in cardiac output.[129] A pulsed, continuous, or color flow Doppler technique may be necessary to determine the size and significance of any disturbances to flow. Cardiac conditions such as effusive pericarditis and myocardial fibrosis and peripheral vascular conditions that inhibit venous return may interfere with ventricular filling during diastole, resulting in decreased end-diastolic volume, stroke volume, and cardiac output.[129] Measurement of fractional shortening before and immediately after treadmill exercise, when pulse rates are above 100 beats/min, permits documentation of resting and exercise-induced myocardial dysfunction.[117] Contrast angiographic studies may be indicated if congenital or acquired cardiac outflow problems are suspected. Nuclear angiocardiography is also useful for evaluating myocardial contractility, cardiac chamber enlargement, outflow problems, and other abnormalities. Hemodynamic studies, which measure pulmonary capillary wedge pressure, pulmonary driving pressure, and pressure in the right heart and pulmonary artery, have proven useful in detecting early cardiac and pulmonary failure in poorly performing trotting horses. These studies involve the introduction of flow directional balloon-tipped catheters through the jugular vein into awake horses.[128]

EVALUATION OF THE SKELETAL SYSTEM. A lameness examination, including appropriate flexion tests and other stress tests, should be completed to help rule out musculoskeletal problems. If lameness is observed, appropriate diagnostic nerve blocks, radiographs, scintigraphy, rectal examination of the bony pelvis and aortoileofemoral arterial pulses, or ultrasound examination are indicated to help localize the lameness and determine its cause, significance, and prognosis. Some lameness problems that are only evident at high speed may best be evaluated using treadmill exercise. For example, aortoileofemoral thrombosis reduces peripheral perfusion but often causes only progressive hindlimb lameness with exercise. Foot balance should be carefully assessed at rest and, if possible, during exercise, because gait changes and subtle lameness related to foot imbalance can adversely affect performance. Dynamic evaluation of hoof balance can be accomplished by examining videotapes recorded from behind the horse while it is exercising on a high-speed treadmill or by trotting the horse over force plates embedded in a firm level surface.[130]

Subtle lameness can increase the metabolic cost of locomotion by inducing changes in gait and coordination, which accelerate the onset of fatigue. In the same fashion, some horses may have an inefficient gait that reduces their performance capacity. Video imaging systems and gait analysis may play an increasingly important role in identifying these individuals in the future.

EVALUATION OF THE MUSCULAR SYSTEM. Primary skeletal muscular limitations on performance may occur as the result of painful conditions such as exertional rhabdomyolysis. Measurement of serum AST and CK after an exercise test are most useful in detecting horses with chronic or subclinical forms of exertional rhabdomyolysis. Serum muscle enzyme concentrations are measured in blood samples collected before exercise and again 4 to 6 hours after completion of exercise. In the past it has been recommended that the exercise test be conducted at a speed and duration of exercise similar to that expected of the horse in competition. However, it has been shown that a 15- to 30-minute test at a slow trot is sufficient to produce abnormal elevations in serum CK (more than twofold to threefold) in susceptible horses.[131] Standardbred and thoroughbred horses with histories of recent episodes of recurrent exertional rhabdomyolysis and horses with polysaccharide storage myopathy often show a greater than twofold increase over normal resting values in response to an exercise test.[131]

Muscle biopsy is a relatively simple procedure that can prove useful for characterizing the nature of an identified exertional myopathy. However, the procedure is not widely used in the diagnostic assessment of poor performance because the evaluation of samples requires considerable histochemical expertise. Percutaneous techniques using a 6-mm-diameter needle* and local anesthetic are routinely used. The middle gluteal muscle is most often biopsied because it is relatively accessible and active at all intensities of exercise.[93,97,132] In adult horses a biopsy is collected at a depth of $2^{1}/_{2}$ to 3 inches from a site 8 inches from the tuber coxae along a straight line connecting the point of the tuber coxae with the base of the tail. Open surgical biopsies are most easily obtained from the semimembranosus or semitendinosus muscle at a site approximately 3 inches below the tuber ischii. After the skin has been shaved and aseptically prepared, lidocaine is injected under the skin. A 2-inch-long incision is made through the skin and fascia, and two parallel incisions, 1-inch long and $^{1}/_{2}$ inch apart, are made vertically in the muscle. The muscle is grasped in one place, to prevent handling artifacts, and the biopsy is first transected proximally, freed to a depth of $^{1}/_{4}$ inch, and then transected distally. Muscle samples should be frozen in isopentane that has first been chilled in liquid nitrogen. Commonly used histologic and histochemical stains include adenosine triphosphatase (ATPase) after alkaline and acid preincubations, nicotinamide dinucleotide diaphorase (NADH), periodic acid–Schiff (PAS), and hematoxylin and eosin.

An estimate of the state of training can be made by determining the percentage of type 1, type 2A and type 2B muscle fibers as well as the oxidative capacity of skeletal muscle in these small muscle samples. In general, horses suited for short distance, fast exercise have a greater proportion of fast-twitch fibers in the middle gluteal muscles than horses suited for longer distance events, which have a higher proportion of slow-twitch type 1 fibers.[132] The proportion of type 1 to type 2 fibers is thought to be genetically based and cannot be manipulated to a great extent by training, whereas age and training increase the proportion of oxidative fast-twitch type 2A fibers relative to type 2B fibers.[93,97,131] Histochemical assessment of NADH staining or quantitative measurement of enzymes such as citrate synthase in biopsy samples frozen rapidly in liquid nitrogen may provide a guide to the state of aerobic fitness.[129] The use of muscle

---

*Bergstrom biopsy needle, Mortenson, Copenhagen, Denmark.

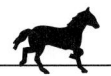

biopsies in horses with poor performance has also aided in the identification of oxidative enzyme defects in Arabian horses and glycogen storage disorders in quarter horses that can markedly affect performance.[132,133]

Standardized Exercise Testing

Exercise intolerance is ultimately a neuromuscular phenomenon resulting from extreme metabolic stress at the level of the muscle fibers.[94] Under many circumstances premature muscle fatigue occurs secondary to disorders that affect oxygen transport (cardiopulmonary systems) or mechanical efficiency (lameness) (Box 5-20). Standardized treadmill exercise tests are often required to assess the function of these systems at high speeds to determine the primary cause of poor performance and to measure the metabolic response of

skeletal muscle relative to work intensity. In a substantial number of cases, poor performance results from related or unrelated disorders in more than one body system, such as dynamic airway obstruction and cardiac dysrhythmia in the same horse.[117]

TREADMILL TESTS. Horses often need to be acclimated to a treadmill before representative exercise testing can be performed. Standardbred horses are typically exercised while wearing their usual racing tack, whereas horses of other breeds are typically exercised in a halter or bridle with a lead rope attached to each side. Most horses exercise comfortably on a treadmill after two to four training sessions at speeds that include all gaits to be tested. Breaking into a canter is an important skill to train horses to perform on the treadmill. During one of the training sessions, endoscopy of the upper airway can be performed to evaluate upper airway function

---

BOX 5-20

Causes of Exercise Intolerance That Are Inapparent at Rest

RESPIRATORY CAUSES
Obstructive Upper Airway Diseases
Common Causes
Laryngopalatal dislocation (dorsal displacement of the soft palate)
Dynamic pharyngeal collapse
Dynamic collapse of the left arytenoid cartilage in association with idiopathic laryngeal hemiplegia
Chronic pharyngeal lymphoid hyperplasia
Epiglottic entrapment
Axial deviation of the aryepiglottic folds
Arytenoid chondritis
Paranasal sinus empyema
Paranasal sinus cysts
Guttural pouch infections

Uncommon Causes
Dynamic collapse of the alar folds
Nasal polyps
Progressive ethmoid hematoma
Subepiglottic cysts
Epiglottic retroversion
Chondroma of the arytenoid cartilages
Fractured laryngeal cartilages
Nasopharyngeal cicatrix

Congenital
Choanal (posterior nares) atresia or stenosis
Excessive alar folds
Stenotic nares
Abnormalities of the nasal septum
Rostral displacement of the palatopharyngeal arch
Tracheal stenosis, stricture, collapse

Lower Airway Diseases
Common Causes
Exercise-induced pulmonary hemorrhage (EIPH)
Recurrent airway obstruction (RAO or COPD)
Equine herpesvirus types 1 and 4 (EHV-1 and EHV-4)
Other viral infections (influenza, rhinovirus, adenovirus, reovirus)
Inflammatory lower airway disease
Bacterial pneumonia
Pleuropneumonia, pleuritis

Uncommon Causes
Pulmonary abscess
Pneumoconiosis (e.g., silicosis)

RESPIRATORY CAUSES—cont'd
Lower Airway Diseases—cont'd
Uncommon Causes—cont'd
Interstitial pneumonia
Diaphragmatic hernia

CARDIOVASCULAR CAUSES
Common Causes
Atrial fibrillation
Ventricular premature contractions
Ventricular tachycardia
Mitral insufficiency
Aortic insufficiency
Resting or exercise-induced myocardial dysfunction and reduced fractional shortening
Pericarditis
Aortoileofemoral arteriosclerosis or thrombosis

Uncommon Causes
Ventricular septal defects
Monensin toxicity
Heart block (intraatrial, second- and third-degree atrioventricular and intraventricular)
Endocarditis
Congestive cardiac failure
Ruptured chordae tendinea
Cor pulmonale
Congenital defects

MUSCULOSKELETAL CAUSES
Exertional rhabdomyolysis
Lameness involving limbs, sacroiliac joint, back
Focal muscle strain

METABOLIC AND SYSTEMIC CAUSES
Anemia
Fluid and electrolyte imbalances
Anhydrosis
Heat exhaustion
Neoplasia
Liver disease (pyrrolizidine alkaloid)

GENERAL CAUSES
Obesity
Poorly trained horse
Poor genetic potential
Administration of illicit medications (doping)

during maximal speeds. Two types of standardized exercise tests can be used: a high-speed test, in which horses are accelerated to maximal speed for their normal racing distance, or an incremental test, in which speed is increased every 1 or 2 minutes until fatigue is reached. The incremental exercise test is used most commonly because it includes both submaximal and maximal intensities and is readily reproducible. Many exercise tests are performed with the treadmill set at a 10% slope to minimize the possibility of injury at top speeds and to ensure that maximum exercise intensity is reached.

A number of measurements are possible during treadmill exercise testing. In its simplest form, the heart rate can be monitored at each intensity of exercise using a heart rate monitor, although recording of an ECG during exercise provides additional information about exercise-associated dysrhythmias.[117] Blood samples can also be drawn from a jugular catheter during the final 15 seconds at each speed. A linear relationship between heart rate and speed is expected, with a plateau forming at the maximum heart rate. The maximum heart rate does not change with training, but the speed at which the maximum heart rate is reached should increase with training. As an alternative, a linear regression can be used to determine the horse's speed at a heart rate of 200 beats/min (V_{200}). V_{200} is close to the anaerobic threshold, may predict aerobic capacity, increases with increasing fitness, and has a high individual predictability that allows for early and valid detection of clinical disorders that limit performance.[101,113,134] The speed at which horses reach a maximum heart rate has been proposed as a better measure than V_{200} because it is an absolute rather than a relative measure; however, measurement of maximum heart rate requires a more strenuous exercise test. Parameters such as the velocity at which the whole blood lactate value reaches 4 mmol/L (V_{LA4}) and the heart rate at which blood lactate reaches 4 mmol/L (HR_{LA4}) can be calculated to evaluate the anaerobic threshold.[101,134] The rate of lactate accumulation may also provide valuable information.

Lactate concentrations can be determined in either whole blood or plasma. Recent studies suggest whole blood lactate may provide a more accurate reflection of lactate accumulation than plasma lactate,[135] because red blood cells actively take up lactate and buffer it, and the type and number of red blood cell lactate transporters differ markedly among horses.

The value of V_{200}, V_{LA4}, HR_{LA4}, and other parameters is that they provide standards against which improvement or deterioration in fitness can be assessed and individual horses can be objectively compared.[101,113,134] Hematocrits can also be easily determined from blood samples obtained at each speed to provide a rough estimate of the number of circulating red blood cells. Blood samples drawn before and 4 hours after exercise for measurement of CK concentration can be used to screen for subclinical exertional rhabdomyolysis.

Further evaluation of the oxygen transport system can be obtained in laboratories where the sophisticated open-flow gas-collection system necessary to measure oxygen consumption ($\dot{V}O_2$) is available. During the incremental exercise test, a plateau in oxygen consumption eventually is reached, representing maximum oxygen uptake. $\dot{V}O_2$ can be used at submaximum speeds to calculate the oxygen cost of locomotion, and $\dot{V}O_{2max}$, a key indicator of aerobic capacity, can be determined. The cardiopulmonary system can be further evaluated during exercise by measuring arterial blood gases from the transverse facial artery using an 18-gauge indwelling catheter.[134] An accurate measure of the total red blood cell volume in a horse can be determined using an Evans blue dye dilution technique immediately after maximal exercise.

FIELD TESTS. Standardization of field exercise tests is very difficult because weather, track conditions, and other factors influence the amount of work performed. The simplest form of exercise test involves timing a horse exercising maximally over a fixed distance and evaluating heart rate recovery rates. Additional information can be obtained by measuring heart rate during exercise using a cardiotachometer.[113] As fitness improves, the heart rate for a given speed of exercise should be lower. Incremental field exercise tests have been used most successfully in standardbred horses in which the heart rate and blood lactates were measured after several heats at predetermined increases in pace. At speeds above 450 m/min, lactate begins to accumulate in the blood during exercise; the precise kinetics of accumulation depends on the horse's fitness and exercise capacity. Fitness responses include a lower heart rate and lactate concentration for the same exercise speed. The value of these measurements is only as good as the standardization of the testing procedures used.

REFERENCES

92. Snow DH et al: Alterations in blood, sweat, urine and muscle composition during prolonged exercise in the horse, *Vet Rec* 110:371-384, 1982.
93. Henckel P: Training- and growth-induced changes in the middle gluteal muscle of young standardbred trotters, *Equine Vet J* 14:134-140, 1983.
94. Harris RC: Muscle fatigue: the other side of the performance coin, *Equine Vet J* 17:409-411, 1985.
95. Sewel DA, Harris RC: Adenine dinucleotide degradation in the thoroughbred horse with increasing exercise duration, *J Appl Physiol* 65:271-277, 1992.
96. Valberg S: Metabolic responses to racing and fiber properties of skeletal muscle in standardbred and thoroughbred horses, *J Equine Vet Sci* 7:6-12, 1987.
97. Lindholm A et al: Muscle histochemistry and biochemistry of thoroughbred horses during growth and training. In Snow DH, Persson SGB, Rose RJ, eds: *Equine exercise physiology*, Cambridge, 1983, Granta Editions, pp 211-217.
98. Evans DL: Cardiovascular adaptations to exercise and training, *Vet Clin North Am (Equine Pract)* 1:513-531, 1985.
99. Erickson BK et al: Pulmonary artery and aortic pressure changes during high intensity treadmill exercise in the horse: effect of furosemide and phentolamine, *Equine Vet J* 24:215, 1992.
100. Persson SGB: On blood volume and working capacity in horses, *Acta Vet Scand Suppl* 19:1-189, 1967.
101. Persson SGB: Evaluation of exercise tolerance and fitness in the performance horse. In Snow DH, Persson SGB, Rose RJ, eds: *Equine exercise physiology*, Cambridge, 1983 Granta Editions, pp 441-457.
102. Attenburrow DP: Time relationship between the respiratory cycle and limb cycle in the horse, *Equine Vet J* 14:69-72, 1982.
103. Hörnicke H, Meixner R, Pollmann U: Respiration in exercising horses. In Snow DH, Persson SGB, Rose RJ, eds: *Equine exercise physiology*, Cambridge, 1983, Granta Editions, pp 7-16.
104. Art T, Serteyn D, Lekeux P: Effect of exercise on the partitioning of equine respiratory resistance, *Equine Vet J* 20:268-273, 1988.
105. Haynes PF: Exercise intolerance and noise production, *Proc Am Assoc Equine Pract* 27:43-47, 1981.
106. Bayly WM et al: The effects of maximal exercise on acid-base balance and arterial blood gas tension in thoroughbred horses. In Snow DH, Persson SGB, Rose RJ, eds: *Equine exercise physiology*, Cambridge, 1983, Granta Editions, pp 400-407.
107. Dempsey JA, Hanson P, Henderson K: Exercise-induced hypoxaemia in healthy human subjects at sea level, *J Physiol (Lond)* 355:161-175, 1984.
108. Thornton J et al: Effects of training and detraining on oxygen uptake, cardiac output, blood gas tensions, pH, and lactate concentrations during and after exercise in the horse. In Snow DH, Persson SGB, Rose RJ, eds: *Equine exercise physiology*, Cambridge, 1983, Granta Editions, pp 470-486.
109. Rose RJ, Evans DL: Cardiovascular and respiratory function in the athletic horse. In Gillespie JR, Robinson HE, eds: *Equine exercise physiology 2*, Davis, Calif, 1987, ICEEP Publications, pp 1-24.
110. Hillidge CJ: What limits equine performance? *Equine Vet J* 20:238-241, 1988.
111. Steel JD, Whitlock LE: Observations on the haematology of thoroughbred and standardbred horses in training and racing, *Aust Vet J* 36:136-143, 1960.
112. Sykes PE: Biochemistry as an aid in equine track practice, *Proc Am Assoc Equine Pract* 12:283-290, 1966.
113. Rose RJ: Poor performance syndrome: investigation and diagnostic techniques. In Robinson NE, ed: *Current therapy in equine medicine*, ed 2, Philadelphia, 1987, WB Saunders, pp 469-474.

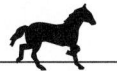

114. Rossdale PD, Burguez PN, Cash RSG: Changes in blood neutrophil/lymphocyte ratio related to adrenocortical function in the horse, *Equine Vet J* 14:293-298, 1982.
115. Parente EJ: Testing methods for exercise intolerance in horses, *Vet Clin North Am* 12:421-434, 1996.
116. Morris EA, Seeherman HJ: Clinical evaluation of poor performance in the racehorse: the results of 275 evaluations, *Equine Vet J* 23:169-174, 1991.
117. Martin BB et al: Causes of poor performance of horses during training, racing, or showing: 348 cases (1992-1996), *J Am Vet Med Assoc* 216:554-558, 2000.
118. Mumford JA, Rossdale PD: Virus and its relationship to "poor performance" syndrome, *Equine Vet J* 12:3-9, 1980.
119. Martin BB, Beech J, Parente EJ: Cytologic examination of specimens obtained by means of tracheal washes performed before and after high-speed treadmill exercise in horses with a history of poor performance, *J Am Vet Med Assoc* 214:673-677, 1999.
120. Deegen E, Buntenkötter S: Behaviour of the heart rate of horses with auricular fibrillation during exercise and after treatment, *Equine Vet J* 8:26-29, 1976.
121. Deem DA, Fregin GF: Atrial fibrillation in horses: a review of 106 clinical cases with consideration of prevalence, clinical signs, and prognosis, *J Am Vet Med Assoc* 180:261-265, 1982.
122. Holmes JR: Cardiac arrhythmias on the racecourse. In Gillespie JR, Robinson HE, eds: *Equine exercise physiology 2*, Davis, Calif, 1987, ICEEP Publications, pp 781-785.
123. Rose RJ, Davis PD: Treatment of atrial fibrillation in three racehorses, *Equine Vet J* 9:68-71, 1977.
124. Holmes JR, Alps BJ: The effect of exercise on rhythm irregularities in the horse, *Vet Rec* 78:672-683, 1966.
125. Stewart JH et al: A comparison of electrocardiographic findings in racehorses presented either for routine examination or poor racing performance. In Snow DH, Persson SGB, Rose RJ, eds: *Equine exercise physiology*, Cambridge, 1983, Granta Editions, pp 135-143.
126. Steel JD: *Studies on the electrocardiogram of the racehorse*, Sydney, 1963, Australasian Medical Publishing.
127. Persson SGB, Forssberg P: Exercise tolerance in standardbred trotters with T-wave abnormalities in the electrocardiogram. In Gillespie JR, Robinson HE, eds: *Equine exercise physiology 2*, Davis, Calif, 1987, ICEEP Publications, pp 772-780.
128. Nuytten J et al: Heart failure in horses: hemodynamic monitoring and determination of LDH_1 concentration, *J Equine Vet Sci* 8:214-216, 1988.
129. Kittleson M: Pathophysiology and treatment of heart failure. In Tilley LP, Owens JM, eds: *Manual of small animal cardiology*, New York, 1985, Churchill Livingstone, pp 307-332.
130. Seeherman H: The use of high-speed treadmills for lameness and hoof balance evaluations in the horse, *Vet Clin North Am (Equine Pract)* 7:271-195, 1991.
131. Snow DH, Valberg SJ: Muscle anatomy, physiology and adaptations to exercise and training. In Hodgson DH, Rose RJ, eds: *The athletic horse*, Philadelphia, 1994, WB Saunders, pp 145-179.
132. Valberg SJ et al: Exertional rhabdomyolysis in quarter horses and thoroughbreds: one syndrome, multiple etiologies, *Equine Vet J Suppl* 30:533-538, 1999.
133. Valberg S et al: Skeletal muscle mitochondrial myopathy as a cause of exercise intolerance in a horse, *Muscle and Nerve* 17:305-312, 1994.
134. Rose RJ, Hodgson DH: Clinical exercise testing. In Hodgson DH, Rose RJ, eds: *The athletic horse*, Philadelphia, 1994, WB Saunders, pp 245-258.
135. Vaihkonen LK, Hyyppa S, Poso AR: Factors affecting accumulation of lactate in red blood cells, *Equine Vet J Suppl* 30:443-447, 1999.

Alterations in Cardiovascular and Hemolymphatic Systems

SHEILA M. McGUIRK

VIRGINIA B. REEF

MAJOR CLINICAL SIGNS/PROBLEMS ENCOUNTERED

PERIPHERAL EDEMA/PLEURAL EFFUSION/ASCITES

Edema is an abnormal accumulation of extracellular fluid in the interstitial spaces of the tissues or in body cavities and it can be generalized or localized. If the fluid accumulation occurs in the pleural cavity, it is referred to as pleural effusion or hydrothorax; if the fluid accumulation is in the abdominal cavity, it is referred to as ascites.

Fluid accumulates more easily in those parts of the body where the connective tissue structure is relatively loose. The accumulated fluid tends to gravitate to the dependent areas of the body. In the cow, generalized edema is detected externally by swelling of the submandibular tissue, brisket, ventral abdomen, and occasionally the limbs. External manifestation of generalized edema in the horse is frequently in the pectoral region between the front limbs, along the ventral abdomen, on the prepuce in stallions and geldings, on the limbs, and sometimes on the head. Stocking up, or limb edema restricted to the lower limbs, is commonly detected in stabled horses with no underlying disease. Large amounts of fluid may accumulate before clinical signs become evident. External evidence of pulmonary edema (i.e., a frothy, possibly blood-tinged fluid in the nares or expectorated) is rarely detected in large animals. There are numerous causes of edema, including congestive heart failure (CHF) (Boxes 6-1 and 6-2). Edema is a late sign of CHF; other subtle signs of failure may be present before edema appears.

Mechanisms of Edema

Edema is caused by an alteration in the equilibrium between capillary permeability and the forces that govern fluid movements at the capillary level. These forces are:
1. Intravascular hydrostatic pressure
2. Interstitial fluid hydrostatic pressure, which exerts a counterpressure to keep fluid within the capillary

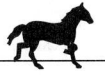

BOX 6-1

Causes of Peripheral Edema/Pleural Effusion/ Ascites in the Horse

COMMON CAUSES
Chronic heart failure
Mitral or tricuspid valve regurgitation
Aortic valve insufficiency
Vegetative endocarditis
Congenital heart defects
Cardiomyopathy
Vitamin E/selenium deficiency
Pericarditis
Pleuritis
Neoplasia: lymphosarcoma
Hypoproteinemia
Liver disease
Gastrointestinal malabsorption: inflammatory bowel disease, neoplasia, parasitism
Peritoneal or pleural effusion
Vasculitis
Equine infectious anemia
Purpura hemorrhagica
Equine ehrlichiosis
Equine viral arteritis
Thrombophlebitis
Lymphatic obstruction
Ulcerative lymphangitis
Lymphadenitis (*Corynebacterium pseudotuberculosis* abscesses)
Trauma

UNCOMMON CAUSES
Heart base tumor other than lymphosarcoma
Neoplasia: plasma cell myeloma, squamous cell carcinoma, fibrosarcoma
Starvation
Kidney disease: glomerulonephritis, amyloidosis
Monensin toxicity
Copper deficiency
Counterirritant application
Hemodilution
Pregnancy
Ruptured bladder
Cassia oxidentalis toxicity

BOX 6-2

Causes of Peripheral Edema/Pleural Effusion/ Ascites in Ruminants

COMMON CAUSES
Chronic heart failure
Mitral or tricuspid valve regurgitation
Vegetative endocarditis
High-altitude disease (Brisket disease)
Congenital heart defects
Cor pulmonale
Vitamin E/selenium deficiency
Pericarditis (traumatic reticulopericarditis)
Pleuritis
Heart base tumor; lymphosarcoma
Hypoproteinemia
Liver disease
Kidney disease: amyloidosis, glomerulonephritis
Gastrointestinal malabsorption: lymphosarcoma, Johne's disease, parasitism
Peritoneal or pleural effusion
Lymphatic obstruction (*Corynebacterium pseudotuberculosis*, lymphosarcoma)
Thrombophlebitis
Urolithiasis: ruptured urethra or bladder

UNCOMMON CAUSES
Cardiomyopathy
Starvation
Hemodilution
Monensin toxicity
Lasalocid toxicity
Copper deficiency
Infectious myocarditis
Vasculitis
Trauma
Pregnancy
Caudal vena caval thrombosis
Ehrlichiosis
Gossypol toxicity
Cassia occidentalis
Phalaris spp. toxicity
Oxytropis sericea (locoweed) toxicity

---

3. Intravascular colloid oncotic pressure exerted by plasma proteins, which favors the resorption of interstitial fluid; the major determinant of colloid osmotic pressure of the capillary is albumin
4. Interstitial fluid colloid osmotic pressure exerted by some proteins in the interstitial fluid, which resists resorption of fluid from the interstitial space
5. Vascular surface area capable of fluid transport
6. Vascular permeability to proteins and water

Activation of complement along with liberation of cytotoxic agents such as oxygen radicals, leukotrienes, hydrogen peroxide, platelet-activating factor, and lysosomal enzymes contribute to the endothelial and epithelial damage, causing permeability edema. Subsequent increase in colloid osmotic pressure causes fluid accumulation in the interstitial space. The most common causes of increased capillary permeability are trauma, infection, endotoxemia, and hypersensitivity (allergic) vasculitis. Topical administration of counterirritants can also cause local increase in capillary permeability. Equine purpura hemorrhagica, the most common vasculitic disease in horses, may in its mildest form have symptoms of mucosal petechiae and plaques of edema or in severe cases serum exudation from and necrosis of skin surfaces.

Increased hydrostatic pressure can cause either localized or generalized edema. In horses and ruminants the most common causes of increased hydrostatic pressure are CHF, venous thrombosis, liver disease causing obstruction of the portal venous system, lymphadenopathy, a mediastinal mass, compression bandages, limb immobilization, or topical administration of counterirritants. Congestive heart failure occurs when there is concomitant pulmonary and systemic vascular congestion. The compensatory salt and water retention increases ventricular diastolic, venous, and capillary pressures, which can result in the formation of generalized edema. Arteriolar vasodilation, caused by release of tissue mediators of inflammation or increased venous pressure resulting from obstruction to venous outflow, can also elevate capillary hydrostatic pressure and result in edema formation.

When the plasma protein concentration decreases from normal to values less than 5 g/dl or albumin concentration is less than 1.5 g/dl, generalized edema may occur. Hypoproteinemia can result from (1) decreased production of plasma proteins with starvation, liver disease, or severe heart failure, or (2) augmented loss of plasma proteins resulting from kidney disease, protein-losing enteropathies (Johne's disease, chronic inflammatory bowel disease), peritonitis, or pleuritis. Hemodilution as a result of overzealous administration of fluids or decreased elimination of fluid can cause edema. Failure to excrete adequate water to maintain fluid balance can result from decreased glomerular filtration as a result of kidney disease or heart failure.

Increased tissue colloid osmotic pressure is rarely a cause of edema in horses and ruminants. Interstitial fluid has a lower plasma protein concentration than plasma. When capillary permeability is increased or when abnormal protein-like material is present in the interstitial space, edema can develop by this mechanism. The latter may occur with infection or after administration of topical counterirritants.

Lymphedema occurs when lymphatics are absent or obstructed. Congenital absence of lymphatics is extremely rare. Obstruction to lymphatic drainage can be caused by tumor, local inflammation (lymphangitis or lymphadenitis), or elevated central venous pressure as in heart failure.

Approach to Diagnosis of Peripheral Edema/Pleural Effusion/Ascites

1. Take history. Note especially history of deworming program, diet, and vitamin or mineral supplements. Determine onset, progression, and duration of the problem and whether other animals are affected. Ask about history of fever, signs of respiratory disease or difficulty, appetite, consistency of feces, or previous medications. Establish the function of the animal and whether there have been changes in performance capability. Compare growth and activity level to that of peers.
2. Perform a physical examination and record vital signs. Determine whether edema is localized or generalized. Palpate external lymph nodes. Palpate edematous areas to determine whether there is heat, pain, or fluid exudation. Edema is typically cool, nonpainful, and pitting, leaving an indentation when a finger is pushed against it. Carefully auscultate heart and lungs. Note abnormalities in cardiac rhythm, murmurs, or other sounds associated with the cardiac cycle. Palpate a peripheral pulse; observe mucous membranes for color, capillary refill time, and petechiae. Observe the jugular vein for distention and pulsations. Evaluate peripheral veins, including the mammary vein, for distention and pulsations. Perform a rectal examination to determine whether internal lymph nodes are enlarged.
3. Obtain blood for the following:
   a. CBC (includes fibrinogen and plasma protein concentration)
   b. Selenium concentrations if cardiomyopathy suspected
   c. *Ehrlichia equi* morula in granulocytes or *Ehrlichia* DNA by polymerase chain reaction if edema, petechial hemorrhages, fever, icterus, or muscle stiffness is present
4. Test serum for the following:
   a. Albumin and globulin concentrations
   b. Muscle enzyme (creatine kinase [CK], including creatine kinase, myocardial bound [CK-MB] [isoenzyme]; cardiac troponin I [cTnI]; and aspartate aminotransferase [AST]) concentrations
   c. Liver enzyme concentrations and liver function (AST, SDH, alkaline phosphatase, γ-glutamyltransferase [GGT], bilirubin, and bile acid concentrations); values may be elevated in congestive heart failure (CHF)
   d. Test for kidney function as follows: serum urea nitrogen (SUN) and creatinine concentrations, serum electrolyte (Ca, P, Na, K, Cl) concentrations, fractional ex-

cretion of electrolytes (see Chapter 22 for method), urinalysis; serum concentrations of Na may be decreased, and SUN may also be elevated in chronic heart failure
   e. Check for antibodies to equine infectious anemia virus by agar gel immunodiffusion or Coggins' test
   f. Determine titers to equine viral arteritis by serum neutralization if there is ocular inflammation, nasal discharge, abortion, or fever with edema
   g. *E. equi* antibodies as demonstrated by immunofluorescence if physical examination reveals icterus and fever with edema
   h. Vitamin E levels if cardiomyopathy suspected
5. Record an ECG to rule out an arrhythmia or conduction disturbance (see Chapter 30); if abnormalities of the ECG are noted, an echocardiogram should be performed.
6. Perform Doppler echocardiography if there is a cardiac murmur that is not localized to the left heart base, that radiates, is greater than 3/6 intensity or is of significant duration
7. Analyze fluid to rule out peritonitis, pleuritis, and pericarditis; if physical examination and CBC findings are compatible, examine:
   a. Pleural fluid
   b. Pericardial fluid
   c. Peritoneal fluid
8. Isolate virus from nasopharyngeal swabs, buffy coat, or semen for equine viral arteritis if clinical signs are compatible.
9. Oral D-xylose or glucose absorption test should be done in horses if there is hypoproteinemia and if starvation, renal disease, hepatic disease, pleuritis, peritonitis, infectious gastrointestinal disease, and hemodilution have been ruled out; these tests are not useful in ruminants unless intraabomasal instillation of D-xylose or glucose is accomplished.

CARDIAC ARRHYTHMIAS

Cardiac arrhythmias are abnormalities in the normal heart rate, rhythm, or conduction pattern. Arrhythmias result from abnormalities of impulse generation or impulse conduction or a combination of both. In the normal heart the impulse is generated in the sinus node because it has the highest rate of spontaneous depolarization. There is variability in reported normal range for heart rate in the large adult animal species, but there is general acceptance for the following ranges:

Horses: 26 to 50 beats/min; 60 to 80 beats/min in foals
Cattle: 49 to 84 beats/min
Sheep and goats: 70 to 90 beats/min

Generally rates within these specified ranges result in atrial contraction, followed shortly by ventricular contraction.

Arrhythmias are more common in horses than in other domestic animal species. As many as 25% of horses that have no other signs of heart disease have cardiac arrhythmias during routine examination or electrocardiography.[1] During continuous 24-hour electrocardiography, 44% of normal horses had second-degree atrioventricular (AV) block, 10% had sinus arrhythmia, 3% had sinoatrial block, 27% had occasional supraventricular extrasystoles, and 15% had occasional ventricular arrhythmias.[2] Cardiac arrhythmias may be present in 40% of horses that have other signs of cardiac disease.[1] Unlike other species, the horse has arrhythmias at rest that are considered benign or functional. Benign, physiologic, or functional arrhythmias are usually bradyarrhythmias and are thought to be the result of increased vagal tone. These arrhythmias disappear at high heart rates (exercise or excitement) or with the administration of atropine (0.02 to 0.05 mg/kg subcutaneously [SC] or intramuscularly [IM]) or glycopyrrolate (0.003 to

0.006 mg/kg SC or IM). Some examples of benign or functional arrhythmias are as follows:

- Second-degree AV block
- Sinus arrhythmia
- Sinus bradycardia
- Sinoatrial (SA) block
- SA arrest

Other arrhythmias are usually considered to be pathologic, even if there are no other overt signs of cardiac disease. Some examples of pathologic arrhythmias are:

- Atrial fibrillation
- Atrial and ventricular premature depolarizations
- Supraventricular or ventricular tachycardia
- Third-degree (complete) AV block

The most effective method of identifying the specific arrhythmia is by performing an electrocardiogram (ECG). Arrhythmias that are transient or intermittent may not be detected with resting electrocardiography. Radiotelemetry or continuous 24-hour ECG recordings are useful to characterize the type, frequency, and severity of arrhythmias. Exercising electrocardiography may identify arrhythmias that are absent or clinically insignificant at rest, but that may impair performance.

In general, cattle do not have benign arrhythmias like horses, but they are frequently found to have sinus bradycardia and sinus arrhythmia associated with lack of feed intake. These arrhythmias were previously thought to be abnormal and associated with vagal indigestion but have been shown to occur in normal cattle held off feed for 12 to 48 hours.[3] Cattle with gastrointestinal disease seem to have increased susceptibility to cardiac arrhythmias, especially atrial premature depolarizations and fibrillation. Although the reason for the susceptibility is not established, abnormal electrolyte concentrations, acid-base disturbances, and aberrations in autonomic nervous system balance have been proposed.[4,5] Sinus arrhythmia in goats is considered to be a benign arrhythmia and is present in many normal animals.

Mechanisms of Cardiac Arrhythmias

Arrhythmias result from abnormalities of impulse generation or impulse conduction or a combination of both. A variety of mechanisms can cause abnormal impulse generation or conduction (Boxes 6-3 and 6-4). Abnormal impulse generation occurs because of localized changes in ionic currents that flow across the membranes of single cells or groups of cells. Abnormal impulse generation can be seen as automaticity (normal and abnormal) or triggered activity.

Automaticity, the ability to initiate action potentials spontaneously, is a property of cells in the sinus node, some parts of the atria, the AV junction, and the His-Purkinje system. Cardiac disease can be responsible for the development of automaticity in cells that normally do not have this property. Normal automaticity develops when the membrane potential slowly falls (i.e., becomes less negative) during diastole. When the membrane reaches its threshold potential, an impulse is initiated. The most common clinical arrhythmias that are thought to be caused by the automaticity mechanism are sinus tachycardia and sinus bradycardia, which are the result of alterations in autonomic nervous system tone. Enhanced automaticity in another area of the heart that is capable of automaticity (spontaneous depolarization) may be responsible for atrial or ventricular premature beats. It is not clear what clinical arrhythmias are caused by triggered activity.

Under certain circumstances, conduction abnormalities allow a propagating impulse, which has already excited the heart, to persist and reexcite the atria or ventricles after the end of the refractory period. This can occur in an ordered or random fashion. Random reentry occurs over reentrant pathways that continuously change in size and location with time

whereas ordered reentry occurs over a relatively fixed reentrant pathway. Impulse propagation may be slow enough that reentrant circuits can be established in very small areas of myocardium. In large animals the size of the myocardial circuit is large enough that relatively mild alterations in impulse propagation may make reentry feasible and may account for the relatively greater frequency of arrhythmias in these species. Although it is not possible to precisely define the mechanism of clinical arrhythmias, it is believed that atrial and ventricular fibrillation may be caused by random reentry.

Under clinical conditions, cardiac arrhythmias may be associated with disturbances in electrolyte concentrations, especially potassium and calcium, in acid-base balance, and in autonomic nervous system balance. These conditions can precipitate cellular changes conducive to the development of arrhythmias by any of the above mechanisms.

Approach to Diagnosis of Cardiac Arrhythmias

It is important to distinguish between abnormal arrhythmias that are primary and those that are secondary. Most abnormal

---

BOX 6-3

Causes of Cardiac Arrhythmias in the Horse

COMMON CAUSES
Excitement
Fever
Toxemia
Colic
Electrolyte abnormalities
Congenital defects
Myocarditis
Valvular disease

UNCOMMON CAUSES
Pericarditis
Cardiomyopathy
Cardiac or heart base tumor
Aortic root rupture
Aortic-cardiac fistula

BOX 6-4

Causes of Cardiac Arrhythmias in Ruminants

COMMON CAUSES
Gastrointestinal disease
Lymphosarcoma
Valvular heart disease
Myocardial diseases
Brisket disease
Pericarditis
Cor pulmonale caused by pulmonary hypertension
Excitement
Foot rot
Fever
Toxemia
Electrolyte abnormalities
Myocarditis

UNCOMMON CAUSES
Cardiomyopathy

arrhythmias of horses and cattle are tachyarrhythmias. Primary arrhythmias are caused by pathologic conditions of the heart (myocarditis, valvular disease, conduction system abnormalities, and pericarditis). Secondary arrhythmias develop in the absence of heart disease and can be caused by excitement, fever, electrolyte imbalances, gastrointestinal disturbances, or toxemia. The treatment and prognosis for the two types of arrhythmias can be very different, and examination and laboratory tests are used to assist in making the distinction.

1. Take history. Determine the diet, feed additives, or medication (including furosemide or other prerace medications); note whether there has been exercise intolerance, syncope, fever, coughing, or edema; inquire about gastrointestinal problems, diarrhea, or colic; inquire about access to cattle or chicken feed and about previous respiratory tract infections in this animal or stablemates.

2. Perform a physical examination to determine whether there is primary cardiac disease. Record vital signs to determine whether this is a bradyarrhythmia or tachyarrhythmia. Careful auscultation should note which heart sounds are present and characterize the arrhythmia. There may be irregularities in the basic rhythm, added sounds, or long pauses; classification of heart rate by regularity of rhythm can distinguish one arrhythmia from another (see Chapter 28). Note whether a pulse deficit is present by simultaneous auscultation and palpation of the peripheral arterial pulse; note the strength of the peripheral arterial pulse; observe the jugular vein for pulsations and distention; examine peripheral veins for distention; and examine mucous membrane color and capillary refill time. Careful auscultation of the lungs with and without a rebreathing bag should be performed.

3. Record an ECG. The base-apex lead can be used to screen for arrhythmias; it is attached using a positive, negative, and ground lead as follows:
   a. Positive lead is attached to skin over the left fifth intercostal space at the point of maximal intensity (PMI) of the apex beat; using lead I, this is the left arm electrode; using lead II or lead III, it is the left leg electrode.
   b. Negative lead is attached to the skin of the right jugular furrow two thirds of the distance from the ramus of the mandible to the thoracic inlet; using lead I or lead II, this is the right arm; using lead III, it is the left arm. ECG interpretation is discussed in Chapter 28.

4. If there is a cardiac murmur, perform an echocardiogram. Look for evidence of myocardial failure, chamber dilation, tumor, endocarditis, congenital defects, or pericardial effusion.

5. Obtain feed for analysis if ionophore (monensin, lasalocid) exposure is suspected.

6. Obtain blood for the following:
   a. CBC
   b. Selenium concentrations if cardiomyopathy suspected
   c. Blood gas determinations and acid-base status

7. Test serum for the following:
   a. Electrolyte (Na, K, Cl, Ca, Mg, P) concentrations
   b. Vitamin E (α-tocopherol) concentration
   c. Cardiac isoenzyme determinations of CK (CK-MB) and cardiac troponin-I (cTnI)[6] if myocarditis or myocardial necrosis is suspected

8. Test urine for the following:
   a. Electrolyte (Na, K, Cl) concentrations
   b. Creatinine determination

9. Calculate fractional excretion of potassium in the urine. This will be variable, depending on the diet, but a low value indicates the need for supplementation.

10. Treat the arrhythmia if:
   a. Patient is hemodynamically unstable (e.g., poor cardiac output, weak peripheral pulses, cold extremities, syncopal).
   b. There is ventricular tachycardia with a rapid rate (heart rate >100 beats/min for horses and >120 beats/min for cows).
   c. There are multifocal ventricular ectopic beats.
   d. A QRS is detected in the preceding T wave (R on T).
   e. There are more than 15 extra systoles per minute.
   f. There is advanced second-degree or complete (third-degree) AV block.
   g. The primary problem is cured or the condition is stabilized, and the patient is symptomatic with the cardiac arrhythmia.

REFERENCES

1. Detweiler DK, Patterson DF: The cardiovascular system. In Catcott EJ, and Smithcors JF, eds: *Equine medicine and surgery*, ed 2, Santa Barbara, Calif, 1982, American Veterinary Publications, pp. 645-704.
2. Reef VB: Frequency of cardiac arrhythmias and their significance in normal horses, *Proc Am Coll Vet Intern Med* 7:506, 1989.
3. McGuirk SM, Bednarski RM: Bradycardia associated with fasting in cattle, *Proc Fourth Ann Vet Med Forum* 2:10-29 to 10-31, 1986.
4. Goetz LK, Voros HS, and Lattmann: Respiratory mechanics and ECG findings in experimentally induced metabolic alkalosis in adult cattle, *Dtsch Tierarztl Wschr* 91:307-313, 1984.
5. McGuirk SM et al: Atrial fibrillation in cows: clinical findings and therapeutic considerations, *J Am Vet Med Assoc* 182:1380-1386, 1983.
6. O'Brien PJ, Landt Y, Landenson JH: Differential reactivity of cardiac and skeletal muscle from various species in a cardiac troponin I immunoassay, *Clin Chem* 43:2333-2338, 1997.

CARDIAC MURMURS

Throughout the cardiovascular system blood has a laminar or streamline flow, except in the heart and sometimes in the aorta. Occasionally conditions occur that cause turbulent flow that is sufficient to cause resonance in adjacent structures. This resonance may be heard as a murmur when a critical level of turbulence is reached (Boxes 6-5 and 6-6). The factors that determine whether blood flow is laminar or turbulent are related by the Reynolds number, which is the ratio of the inertial to viscous forces. When the Reynolds number exceeds a critical value (about 2000 in large vessels), turbulence occurs. Increased flow velocity or reduced blood viscosity (e.g., anemia) predisposes to murmur development. The characteristics of the murmur depend on the velocity of the blood flow and the nature of the structures that are caused to vibrate.

It is useful to characterize murmurs with regard to location in the cardiac cycle (systolic, diastolic, or continuous), timing in the cardiac cycle (early, mid, late, holo-), intensity (loudness), shape or frequency, PMI, and radiation of the murmur. Systolic murmurs occur anytime between the first and second heart sound. Diastolic murmurs occur between the second and first heart sounds. Continuous murmurs occur throughout the cardiac cycle (Fig. 6-1). The intensity of murmurs is frequently graded a scale of 1 to 6[7]:

■ *Grade 1* is a soft murmur, heard only after minutes of careful listening.
■ *Grade 2* is a soft murmur that is heard immediately on auscultation.
■ *Grade 3* is a murmur of moderate intensity.
■ *Grade 4* is a loud murmur associated with a palpable thrill.
■ *Grade 5* is a loud murmur, which is not heard when the stethoscope is removed from the chest wall.
■ *Grade 6* is a loud murmur, which is audible with the entire stethoscope chest piece held away from the chest wall.

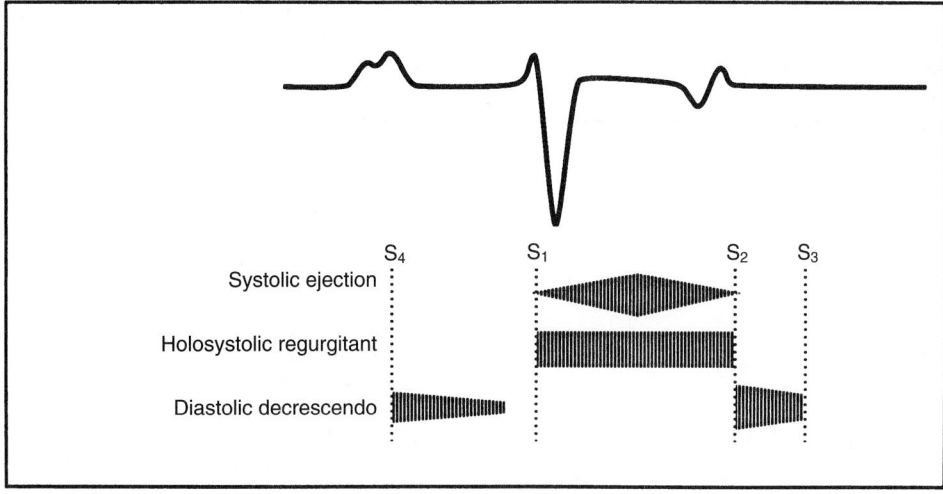

FIG. 6-1 ▓ Phonocardiographic characteristics of systolic ejection, holosystolic (pansystolic) regurgitant, and diastolic decrescendo cardiac murmurs.

BOX 6-5

Causes of Cardiac Murmurs in the Horse

COMMON CAUSES	**COMMON CAUSES—cont'd**
Anemia	Congenital defects
Excitement	Myocarditis
Fever	
Functional	**UNCOMMON CAUSE**
Exercise	Cardiomyopathy
Valvular disease: degenerative, infective, dilation	Pericarditis

---

BOX 6-6

Causes of Cardiac Murmurs in Ruminants

COMMON CAUSES	**COMMON CAUSES—cont'd**
Anemia	Lymphosarcoma
Excitement	Pericarditis (usually traumatic reticulopericarditis)
Fever	
Functional	**UNCOMMON CAUSES**
Valvular disease: infective, degenerative, dilation	Cardiomyopathy
Congenital defects	Myocarditis

The PMI of a murmur usually corresponds to the location of one of the heart valves. Murmurs associated with the mitral valve will frequently be heard best in the left fifth intercostal space just dorsal to the level of the elbow. These murmurs usually radiate dorsally or toward the aortic valve area. Pulmonic valve and aortic valve murmurs are best heard at the base of the heart. To access this area, the hand is moved under the left triceps muscle to the third and fourth intercostal spaces just below the level of the shoulder. Aortic valve murmurs are located just dorsal and caudal to the pulmonic valve. Murmurs associated with the tricuspid valve are frequently located in the right third or fourth intercostal space between the shoulder and elbow.

Most systolic murmurs fall into one of two categories: ejection or regurgitant (see Fig. 6-1). Systolic ejection murmurs are caused by obstructed, increased, or turbulent blood flow across normal or damaged semilunar valves. Valvular obstruction is rare in large animals but functional ejection murmurs are commonly found in healthy horses. The PMI of the functional murmur is typically at the pulmonic or aortic valve or just dorsal to them over the great vessels. It is crescendo-decrescendo murmur that is audible early to mid-systole. The diagnostic considerations for systolic ejection murmurs are given in Box 6-7. The innocent or functional murmur may be distinguished from a pathologic murmur by being of lower and variable intensity, peaking in early-to-mid systole, ending well before the second heart sound, and having no radiation. The physiologic systolic ejection murmur may disappear or become louder following exercise. Diagnostic considerations for systolic regurgitant murmurs are listed in Box 6-7.

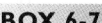

BOX 6-7

Possible Causes of Ejection and Regurgitant Systolic Cardiac Murmurs

EJECTION
Innocent
Anemia
Fevert
Aortic stenosis
Pulmonic stenosis
Atrial septal defect
Ventricular septal defect
Tetralogy of Fallot

REGURGITANT
Mitral valve regurgitation
Tricuspid valve regurgitation
Ventricular septal defect
Tetralogy of Fallot

3. Obtain blood for CBC (includes fibrinogen and total plasma protein concentration).
4. Test serum for the following:
   a. Electrolyte concentrations
   b. Bovine leukosis virus (BLV) agar gel immunodiffusion test AGID status (cows)
   c. Cardiac isoenzyme determinations of CK (CK-MB) and cardiac troponin-I (cTnI)[6] if myocarditis or myocardial necrosis is suspected
5. Record an ECG.
6. Perform a phonocardiogram to confirm timing and shape of murmur.
7. Perform an echocardiogram to look for valve abnormalities, congenital defects, and chamber enlargement and wall motion abnormalities; use color flow Doppler echocardiography to estimate the severity of the jet associated with a shunt, valvular regurgitation, or stenosis (rare); Doppler and contrast echocardiography can be used for examination of congenital defects and some valvular insufficiencies.
8. Take radiographs to find evidence of pulmonary edema or pleural effusion.
9. Cardiac catheterization for pressures, oximetry, or angiocardiography may complement data obtained noninvasively with Doppler echocardiography.

REFERENCES

7. Freeman AR, Levine SA: The clinical significance of the systolic murmur: a study of 1000 consecutive "noncardiac" cases, *Ann Intern Med* 6:1371-1376, 1933.
8. Reef VB: Cardiovascular disease in the equine neonate, *Vet Clin North Am (Equine Pract)* 1:117-129, 1985.

MUFFLED HEART SOUNDS

Auscultation of heart sounds requires that the vibrations generated by the heart be transmitted through the tissues of the thorax to the outer chest wall with sufficient amplitude to be heard. Blood transmits sound very well, whereas lung tissue strongly attenuates sound waves. The chest wall itself causes attenuation of the sound that is most significant at the interface between bone and muscle. Therefore physical factors in a normal patient, such as a large, thick chest or obesity, can cause heart sounds to be muffled. If the environment for auscultation is conducive to hearing heart sounds, other factors such as stethoscope quality may cause muffling of heart sounds in a normal patient. One should strive to have a stethoscope with comfortably fitting earpieces, thicker and shorter tubing, a rigid diaphragm to hear S_1, S_2, and higher-frequency sounds, and a bell piece for auscultation of S_3, S_4, low-frequency sounds and murmurs.

Heart sounds are muffled primarily because of displacement of the heart from the thoracic wall by fluid (pericardial effusion), a soft tissue mass (abscess or tumor), or air (pneumothorax, pneumomediastinum, or emphysema) (Boxes 6-8 and 6-9). Rarely is muffling of heart sounds attributed to weak cardiac contractions alone, although this may be a finding in recumbent cows with marked hypocalcemia.

Regurgitant murmurs typically begin with AV valve closure and end after pulmonic and aortic valve closure, making the second heart sound inaudible. They can be variable in duration, however, and occur early, mid-, or late systole or can be pansystolic or holosystolic. Location of the PMI and the direction of radiation of the systolic murmur distinguish mitral or tricuspid valve regurgitation from a VSD. Systolic clicks are rare in horses and cattle but may indicate abnormalities of the chordae tendineae, AV valve prolapse, or dilation of the aorta.

Diastolic murmurs can occur between S_4 and S_1 (atrial systolic murmurs), between S_2 and S_3 (ventricular filling murmurs), or from S_2 to S_1 (aortic insufficiency). Both the atrial systolic and ventricular filling murmurs are usually functional, can be heard over left or right hemithorax, and can vary in intensity. The aortic valve regurgitation murmur is typically a decrescendo murmur with its PMI over the aortic valve that begins immediately after S_2 (see Fig. 6-1). Some aortic regurgitation murmurs can be harsh or musical, associated with high-frequency vibrations of an aortic valve leaflet, and they may be audible over the right thorax.

Continuous murmurs are uncommon in horses and ruminants. Patent ductus arteriosus, a finding in normal foals for a short time after delivery, can be heard in the left third intercostal space. This murmur can be continuous but is more frequently systolic.[8] A continuous "washing machine" murmur, which is most easily heard over the left cardiac area, is associated with traumatic pericarditis in cattle and is caused by the accumulation of fluid, gas, and fibrin within the pericardium. Acquired systolic and diastolic murmurs in adult horses or cattle are usually the result of separate murmurs.

Approach to Diagnosis of Cardiac Murmurs

1. Take a history. Note the age, onset, duration, and progression of the condition. Determine exercise capability, growth, and attitude; inquire about previous fever, illness, or medications.
2. Perform a physical examination. Record vital signs. Determine timing, duration, intensity, location of PMI, shape, and radiation of murmur. Palpate peripheral arterial pulse and observe jugular vein for distention and pulsations. Carefully auscultate the lungs at rest and during deep inspiration.

Approach to Diagnosis of Muffled Heart Sounds

1. Take a history. Inquire about any change in attitude, appetite, diet, or posture; determine whether a magnet has been administered to cattle; note any history of fever, weight loss, respiratory disease, colic, or diseases of other body systems and the deworming history; determine whether cattle are known to be BLV positive.
2. Perform a physical examination and determine vital signs. Carefully auscultate the lungs to establish whether there is ventral dullness or whether there is evidence of increased

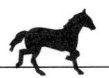

Causes of Muffled Heart Sounds in the Horse

COMMON CAUSES
Obesity
Large or thick chest wall
Pericarditis
Neoplasia: lymphosarcoma
Abscess
Chronic heart failure

UNCOMMON CAUSES
Pulmonary emphysema
Pneumothorax
Neoplasia: squamous cell carcinoma, fibrosarcoma

Causes of Muffled Heart Sounds in Ruminants

COMMON CAUSES
Obesity
Large or thick chest wall
Pericarditis (traumatic reticulopericarditis)
Neoplasia: lymphosarcoma
Abscess
Chronic heart failure
Emphysema

UNCOMMON CAUSE
Pneumothorax

---

or added sounds from pulmonary parenchyma compression; carefully auscultate the heart for pericardial friction rubs; determine whether there are signs of CHF (jugular venous distention, peripheral edema); percuss the thorax to determine whether there is emphysema, pleural fluid, or pneumothorax; note that pleural fluid in the absence of pericardial effusion causes radiating heart sounds but absence of airway sounds; determine whether there is thoracic and/or abdominal pain; in cattle, check for presence of a reticular magnet using a compass or stud finder.

3. Obtain blood for the following:
   a. CBC
   b. Fibrinogen concentration
   c. Plasma or serum protein concentration
   d. Liver enzymes and tests for liver function (AST, SDH, alkaline phosphatase, GGT, bilirubin, and bile salt concentration)
   e. Tests for kidney function (urinalysis, creatinine, blood urea nitrogen [BUN], Na, K, Cl, P concentrations and fractional excretion of Na, Cl, P)
4. Test serum for BLV serology and for equine influenza, viral arteritis, and herpes virus.
5. Take radiographs of the thorax to determine whether there is pulmonary parenchymal and/or pleural or pericardial disease.
6. Perform an ECG and thoracic ultrasound examination to determine if there is pericardial or pleural fluid, a cardiac mass, or a mass in the cranial mediastinum compressing the heart. Determine the location and type of fluid present.
7. Analyze pericardial or pleural fluid and perform culture and sensitivity testing if indicated.

CARDIOVASCULAR EXERCISE INTOLERANCE/WEAKNESS/SYNCOPE

Exercise intolerance, weakness, or syncope can be clinical signs associated with disease in many body systems. Exercise intolerance can be manifested as sudden deceleration or stopping, failure to perform at an expected level, a sudden change in the level of performance or production, lowered enthusiasm for work, cough on exertion, evidence of respiratory distress, or excessive sweating. Weakness can be manifested as recumbency, difficulty in rising from recumbency, muscle tremors or fasciculations, reluctance to move, or toe dragging. Syncope is a sudden collapse and loss of consciousness (fainting).

Mechanisms of Cardiovascular Exercise Intolerance/Weakness/Syncope

The clinical signs of exercise intolerance, syncope, or weakness can be caused by cardiovascular disease (Boxes 6-10 and 6-11). They are the result of failure to maintain cardiac output, caused by inability to regulate either heart rate or stroke volume. A normal horse increases cardiac output at submaximum heart rates (less than 210 beats/min in horses) primarily by tachycardia. At maximum heart rates (approximately 210 to 240 beats/min in horses), subsequent increments in cardiac output occur by increased stroke volume.[9] The maximum heart rate for cattle and small ruminants has not been published.

Supraventricular cardiac arrhythmias, primarily atrial fibrillation in horses, can lead to heart rates greater than 240 beats/min with submaximum exercise.[10,11] Heart rates exceeding the maximum rate may limit cardiac output by decreasing the time for diastolic perfusion of the myocardium or by limiting stroke volume because the short diastolic intervals leave inadequate time for ventricular filling. The ability to maintain cardiac output can also be compromised by other cardiac arrhythmias such as ventricular premature systoles. The frequency of extrasystoles can increase with exercise, and the timing of the abnormal beats can reduce cardiac output even at submaximum heart rates.[12] Horses with cardiac arrhythmias can have abnormal elevations in lactate concentration in response to exercise, indicating a lower anaerobic threshold and leading to exercise intolerance.[13,14]

Cardiac output maintenance may also be compromised in animals by diseases affecting myocardial contractility or diseases that result in increased end-systolic volume despite a submaximum heart rate.[15] Diseases that result in decreased venous return (peripheral vascular disease) can also reduce cardiac output and cause signs of exercise intolerance, weakness, or syncope.

Exercise intolerance or weakness can also be caused by painful peripheral vascular conditions or conditions causing peripheral hypoxia or lactic acid accumulation. In horses such conditions may exist with aortic-iliac thrombosis. Sudden episodes of weakness and collapse without change in consciousness are associated with hyperkalemic period paralysis in horses (see Chapter 40).

Syncope may be associated with epilepsy or other CNS disturbance. If cardiovascular and pulmonary function appear normal, the nervous system should be examined in detail (see Chapter 33). Frequently, collapse during exercise indicates of cardiovascular disease; collapse at rest indicates a noncardiovascular disease.

10. Amada A et al: Atrial fibrillation in the horse: clinical and histopatho-logical studies of two cases, *Exp Rep Equine Health Lab* 11:51-69, 1974.
11. Deegen E, Buntenkotter S: Behaviour of the heart rate of horses with au-ricular fibrillation during exercise and after treatment, *Equine Vet J* 8:26-19, 1976.
12. Holmes JR, Alps BJ: The effect of exercise on rhythm irregularities in the horse, *Vet Rec* 78:672-683,1966.
13. Maier-Bock H, Ehrlein H-J: Heart rate during a defined exercise test in horses with heart and lung diseases, *Equine Vet J* 10:235-242, 1978.
14. Persson SGB: Analysis of fitness and state of training. In Snow DH, Pers-son SGB, Rose RJ, eds: *Equine exercise physiology*, Cambridge, England, 1983, Granta Editions.
15. Miller RJ, Holmes JR: Effect of cardiac arrhythmia on left ventricular and aortic blood pressure parameters in the horse, *Res Vet Sci* 35:190-199, 1983.

BOX 6-10

Causes of Exercise Intolerance/Weakness/Syncope in the Horse*

COMMON CAUSES
Myocardial disease
Cardiac arrhythmias
Aortic or pulmonary artery rupture
Aortic-iliac-femoral arteriosclerosis or thrombosis
Congenital heart defects
Chronic heart failure
Pericardial disease
Hyperkalemic periodic paralysis
Central nervous system disturbances resulting in loss of consciousness

*See Chapter 5 for additional noncardiac causes.

BOX 6-11

Causes of Exercise Intolerance/Weakness/Syncope in Ruminants*

COMMON CAUSES
Myocardial disease
Cardiac arrhythmias
Congenital heart defects
Chronic heart failure

*See Chapter 5 for additional noncardiac causes.

Approach to Diagnosis of Exercise Intolerance/Weakness/Syncope

1. Take history. Establish onset of problem, previous perfor-mance history, and activity level when clinical signs are observed. Determine whether there is coughing, dyspnea, or excessive sweating associated with stress or exercise.
2. Perform a physical examination and record vital signs to determine whether lameness or respiratory or neurologic disease is the cause of these clinical signs. Of particular importance are heart rate at rest, peripheral arterial pulse characteristics, presence of pulse deficits, mucous mem-brane color, and appearance of jugular venous pulses. Lungs should be auscultated for evidence of pulmonary edema or pleural effusion. The chest should be percussed. Rectal examination should be performed to evaluate aor-toiliac arterial pulses; metatarsal artery pulses and saphe-nous vein refill should be evaluated.
3. Record an ECG at rest, during exercise (preferably with ra-diotelemetry), and after exercise, if it is safe for the animal to exercise. Perform a continuous 24-hour ECG to evalu-ate frequency of arrhythmias.
4. Perform a stress echocardiogram before and after exercise to evaluate size of heart chambers, to look for congenital defects or acquired valvular heart disease, and to evaluate myocardial contractility and ventricular wall motion.
5. Perform an exercise test to measure a parameter of lactic acid concentration (i.e., lactic acid accumulation after ex-ercise test, lactic acid concentration at defined velocity of exercise, or velocity of exercise at a defined lactic acid con-centration), arterial blood gas concentrations, preexercise and postexercise CK levels, cTnI, and exercise endoscopy to make an upper airway evaluation.

REFERENCES
9. Evans EL: Cardiovascular adaptations to exercise and training, *Vet Clin North Am (Equine Pract)* 1:513-531, 1985.

VENOUS DISTENTION/PULSATIONS

The jugular venous pulsations observed in the neck are pri-marily a reflection of right atrial and right ventricular activity. There may be some small contribution from carotid arterial impact.[16] The jugular venous pulse reflects the right atrial or central venous pressure, which is influenced by blood vol-ume, right ventricular cardiac output, and right atrial con-tractility (Boxes 6-12 and 6-13). Jugular venous pulsations are observed in normal animals, but the pulse seldom radi-ates more than one third of the distance from the thoracic inlet to the ramus of the mandible when the head is held in a normal, upright position.

Mechanisms of Venous Distention/Pulsations

The normal jugular venous pulse consists of three positive and two negative deflections (Fig. 6-2). The first and domi-nant positive wave is the A wave, produced by atrial contrac-tion. During atrial relaxation the pressure declines until ven-tricular systole. The second positive deflection is the C wave, which is produced by the bulging of the tricuspid valve leaflets into the right atrium during early (isovolumetric) right ventricular systole. Carotid arterial impact on the jugu-lar vein may also contribute to the C wave.[16] As the ventricle contracts, the plane of the tricuspid valve is pulled toward the apex of the heart and the atrial pressure declines, producing the X descent. The X descent is terminated by the V wave, which is associated with venous return, subsequent atrial fill-ing, and a closed tricuspid valve. At the end of ventricular sys-tole, the atrial pressure falls again as a result of tricuspid valve opening and rapid right ventricular filling. This is called the Y descent. The Y descent is terminated as the pressure gradu-ally rises with right heart filling.

Abnormal pulsations occur with increased resistance to right ventricular filling, regardless of the cause. Distention and pulsations in the jugular vein are usually associated with an elevated right ventricular pressure, such as occurs in right heart failure, constrictive pericarditis or, more rarely, in car-diomyopathy. Prominent jugular pulsations are noted with tricuspid valve regurgitation and certain cardiac arrhythmias, especially those arrhythmias associated with atrial contrac-tion against a closed AV valve. The carotid arterial pulse can mimic venous jugular venous pulsations. To distinguish among the causes of jugular venous pulsations, lightly com-press but do not occlude the jugular vein at the thoracic inlet. The jugular vein will distend enough to eliminate carotid ar-terial pulsations. If pulsations are still present, tricuspid valve regurgitation, atrial arrhythmias, or right heart failure should be considered. If the jugular vein is compressed near the ra-mus of the mandible and massaged toward the thoracic inlet, refilling is indicative of tricuspid valve regurgitation. Jugular venous distention without pulsations can occur with com-pression of the cranial vena cava from a cranial thoracic or mediastinal mass or from occlusion of the jugular vein with a thrombus.

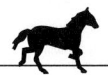

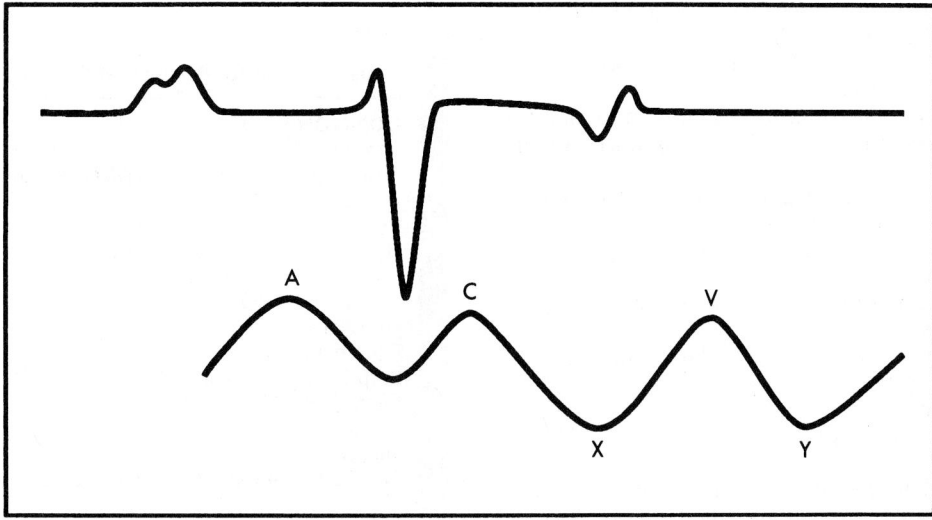

FIG. 6-2 ▓▓ Schematic illustration of a venous (jugular or atrial) pressure curve and its relationship to events of the electrocardiogram. *A,* Positive wave produced by atrial contraction; *C,* second positive deflection caused by bulging of the tricuspid valve during isovolumetric systole; *X,* first negative wave produced by the plane of the AV valve being pulled toward the apex of the heart during systole; *V,* positive pressure wave caused by venous return; *Y,* negative wave produced by AV valve opening.

BOX 6-12

Causes of Jugular Venous Distention/Pulsation in the Horse

COMMON CAUSES	UNCOMMON CAUSES
Right heart failure	Monensin toxicity
Chronic heart failure	Pericarditis
Cardiomyopathy	Myocarditis
Atrial fibrillation	Squamous cell carcinoma
Tricuspid insufficiency	Fibrosarcoma
Cranial mediastinal mass	Cor pulmonale
Lymphosarcoma	Chronic obstructive pulmonary disease
Abscess	Overhydration
Jugular venous phlebitis/thrombosis	

BOX 6-13

Causes of Jugular Venous Distention/Pulsation in Ruminants

COMMON CAUSES	COMMON CAUSES—cont'd
Right heart failure	Heart base tumor: lymphosarcoma
Chronic heart failure	Heart base abscess
Vitamin E/selenium deficiency (white muscle disease)	Cor pulmonale caused by chronic pneumonia
Cardiomyopathy	Brisket disease
Tricuspid insufficiency	
Monensin toxicity	**UNCOMMON CAUSES**
Pericarditis	Overhydration
Jugular venous phlebitis/thrombosis	Cranial mediastinal mass

Approach to Diagnosis of Venous Distention/Pulsations

1. Take history. Note especially history of respiratory disease, exposure to high altitude and locoweed or ingestion of potential cardiotoxins. Determine whether other animals have been similarly affected, whether the BLV status of affected cattle is known, or whether a magnet has been administered.

2. Perform a physical examination. Determine whether there is tachypnea or tachycardia. Carefully auscultate for abnormal heart sounds, rhythm, or intensity of sounds; note whether jugular veins are patent. Look for jugular venous pulsations as described above.

3. Obtain blood for the following:
   a. CBC
   b. Fibrinogen concentration
   c. Total protein concentration

d. BLV status (bovine) and serology for equine influenza, viral arteritis, and herpes virus

e. Vitamin E (serum) and selenium concentrations if cardiomyopathy suspected

4. Take radiographs of the thorax and abdomen to establish whether there is respiratory disease, a magnet, or a penetrating foreign body.

5. Record an ECG when there is an arrhythmia to look for atrial premature depolarizations.

6. Perform an echocardiogram to examine the following:
   a. Right ventricular size and function
   b. Right atrium for abnormal size or structures
   c. Tricuspid valve
   d. Pulmonary artery to check for dilation indicative of pulmonary hypertension
   e. Left atrial size
   f. Left ventricular function
   g. Pericardium
   h. Interventricular septal thickness and motion

7. Perform ultrasound examination of the cranial thorax and cranial mediastinum.

8. Jugular venous catheterization may be useful to determine right atrial (central venous), right ventricular, and pulmonary arterial pressures.

PAINFUL PERIPHERAL SWELLINGS

Close inspection of the skin and extremities of patients can reveal evidence of peripheral vascular or lymphatic system disease. These diseases can be manifested by diffuse swelling, localized swelling (papules, nodules, macules, or wheals), or subcutaneous edema of the extremities. Frequently there is necrosis, ulceration of the skin, and exudation as the disease progresses. Animals may be lame or dyspneic, have heat in the involved area, or exhibit a painful response to palpation of the area (Boxes 6-14 and 6-15). Differentiate from nonpainful peripheral edema.

Approach to Diagnosis of Painful Peripheral Swellings

1. Take history. Establish whether there is a history of a wound or trauma to the area or previous drainage; inquire about previous infections, particularly those referable to the respiratory system, in this animal or others; determine vaccination, deworming, and drug administration history.

2. Perform a physical examination. Determine vital signs. Note whether animal is febrile; examine extremities for wounds, dilated lymphatic channels, ulcers, focal swellings, and edema; determine the temperature and sensitivity of the swollen area; examine mucous membranes for color and presence of hemorrhages; perform a rectal examination and palpate aortic quadrifurcation in horses for vessel size, firmness, pain, fremitus, and strength of pulse; evaluate these vessels before and after exercise, if indicated.

3. Obtain blood for the following:
   a. CBC (includes examination of red blood cells, neutrophils, and eosinophils for inclusion bodies or morula and determination of platelet count)
   b. Fibrinogen concentration
   c. Total protein concentration
   d. Coombs or direct immunofluorescence test
   e. Appropriate tests for equine ehrlichiosis (IFA), piroplasmosis (CF), or viral arteritis (SN), if indicated

4. Take radiographs of swollen extremities, if appropriate.

5. Perform an ultrasound examination of the swelling, if appropriate.

6. Obtain Gram stain, and bacterial and fungal culture of ulcerated area or exudate.

7. Perform a biopsy of granulomas if appropriate.

8. Analyze and culture fluid obtained from dilated lymphatic channels or localized edematous areas.

9. Analyze urine to look for hemoglobinuria or hematuria.

10. Test feces for fecal occult blood.

ENLARGED LYMPH NODES

Diffuse or single lymph node enlargement occurs with infectious (bacterial, viral, fungal), neoplasia, and, rarely, immune-mediated causes in large animals (Boxes 6-16 and

---

BOX 6-14

Causes of Painful Peripheral Swellings in the Horse

COMMON CAUSES
Thrombophlebitis
Abscess (*Corynebacterium pseudotuberculosis* in western United States)
Cellulitis
Hypersensitivity vasculitis (complicated by skin necrosis and secondary infection)
Equine viral arteritis
Ehrlichia equi
Equine infectious anemia
Purpura hemorrhagica
Clostridium spp. myositis
Insect bite
Snakebite
Application of topical counterirritants, firing, or soring

UNCOMMON CAUSES
Frostbite
Piroplasmosis
Ulcerative lymphangitis
Epizootic lymphangitis
Glanders
Sporotrichosis
Immune vasculitis
Aortoiliac thrombosis
Sporadic lymphangitis
Congenital lymph node and lymphatic dysgenesis

BOX 6-15

Causes of Painful Peripheral Swellings in Ruminants

COMMON CAUSES
Thrombophlebitis
Abscess
Clostridial myositis
Malignant edema
Blackleg
Fescue foot
Ergotism
Cellulitis (injection site or wound)
Insect bite
Snakebite
Frostbite

UNCOMMON CAUSES
Disseminated hemangiosarcoma
Ehrlichiosis

Causes of Enlarged Lymph Nodes in the Horse

COMMON CAUSES
Strangles
Lymphosarcoma
Upper respiratory infection
Corynebacterium pseudotuberculosis lymphadenitis

UNCOMMON CAUSES
Ulcerative lymphangitis
Epizootic lymphangitis
Sporadic lymphangitis
Glanders
Plasma cell myeloma
Tuberculosis
Hemolytic uremic–like syndrome

Causes of Enlarged Lymph Nodes in Ruminants

COMMON CAUSES
Caseous lymphadenitis *(Corynebacterium pseudotuberculosis)*
Lymphosarcoma (including bovine leukosis virus)
Abscess/cellulitis of area drained

UNCOMMON CAUSES
Tuberculosis
Sporadic bovine encephalomyelitis
Malignant catarrhal fever

6-17). Lymphadenopathy may cause obstruction to lymphatic drainage, leading to peripheral edema, pleural effusion, or ascites. The peripheral lymph nodes that are most readily accessible for examination are the submandibular (horses), superficial cervical (ruminants), and superficial inguinal (ruminants) lymph nodes. When there is generalized lymphadenopathy, internal lymph nodes may be enlarged, causing clinical signs such as dyspnea, esophageal obstruction, diarrhea, or other signs of organ dysfunction.

Approach to Diagnosis of Enlarged Lymph Nodes

1. Take history. Note especially history of weight loss, inappetance, depression, lethargy, or lymph node enlargement; inquire about previous illness or wounds; for cattle, determine whether there is a history of lymphosarcoma in the family or herd and whether the cow has a positive BLV test; for sheep and goats, determine whether there is a history of *Corynebacterium pseudotuberculosis* abscesses in the flock/herd.
2. Perform physical examination. Determine vital signs. Examine peripheral lymph nodes or other swellings, and perform a rectal examination to palpate accessible internal lymph nodes, and when appropriate, examine the uterus in cattle; check mucous membranes for pallor or icterus; determine whether there is jugular venous distention or pulsations or whether there is evidence of pleural or pericardial effusion or ascites.

3. Obtain blood for the following:
    a. CBC to examine for anemia or leukemic changes. Note inclusions, morula, or abnormal appearance of cells.
    b. Serum chemistry profile to determine if there are signs of other organ dysfunction (e.g., gastrointestinal [hypoproteinemia], liver, or kidney)
4. Test feces for occult blood, if indicated.
5. Perform ultrasonographic examination of the lymph node or swelling.
6. Obtain lymph node or swelling aspirate and biopsy for culture and histopathologic examination.
7. Obtain a bone marrow sample for cytologic examination.

ABNORMAL PERIPHERAL PULSE

Palpation of the arterial pulse is an important aspect of the examination of the patient with cardiovascular disease. Arterial pulse strength and contour (how fast pressure rises and falls) are the objectives of the examination and are determined by the cardiac output, heart rate, and vascular impedance. The arterial pressure pulse begins with the opening of the aortic valve and ventricular ejection and rises rapidly in early systole. The pulse pressure reaches a peak and then declines as ventricular ejection slows. During isovolumic relaxation (before AV valve opening), there is a transient reversal of flow in the arterial system, and an incisura or dicrotic notch (Fig. 6-3) is inscribed on the descending limb of the pressure curve. Following the incisura, there is a small positive wave that is attributed to elastic recoil of the aorta and the aortic valve and the summation of reflected waves from more distal arteries.[15] After the positive wave, the pulse pressure declines because there is peripheral runoff of blood in diastole. The incisura and secondary positive wave are not usually palpable. Palpation of peripheral arteries (facial, transverse facial, and digital arteries in the horse and median and coccygeal arteries in ruminants) normally reveals a smooth, rapid upstroke, dome-shaped summit, and a downstroke that is slightly more prolonged than the upstroke.

Pressure values and pulse wave configurations are altered as the pressure waves are transmitted through the peripheral arterial tree. With increasing distance from the heart, the dicrotic notch and second positive wave disappear, the systolic pressure gets higher (loss of distensibility in the distal arteries and summation of reflected pulse waves from the distal vascular bed), and the diastolic pressure gets lower. The difference between the systolic and diastolic pressure determines pulse pressure and can be evaluated by an impression of pulse strength. Pulse pressure increases as one moves to more peripheral arterial sites. The mean arterial pressure changes very little but decreases slightly as one moves downstream in the arterial system from the pressure source. Systolic blood pressure, as measured indirectly at the tail or on a limb, is higher than that measured in the ascending aorta. In smaller arterial beds (e.g., arteries of the ear), the pulse wave is gradually dampened and pulsatile characteristics are lost on the capillaries and small veins.

Mechanisms of Abnormal Peripheral Pulse

Hyperkinetic arterial pulses occur in patients with increased cardiac output (e.g., fever, exercise, excitement), increased stroke volume, or bradycardia (Boxes 6-18 and 6-19). It may also occur when there is rapid runoff of blood in the arterial system, as occurs with aortic valve regurgitation, patent ductus arteriosus, or aortic cardiac fistulas. In aortic valve regurgitation the rapidly rising, hyperdynamic pulse is caused by increased stroke volume (regurgitated blood in the left ventricle), followed by a rapid runoff of pressure later in systole as a result of regurgitation (see Fig. 6-3).

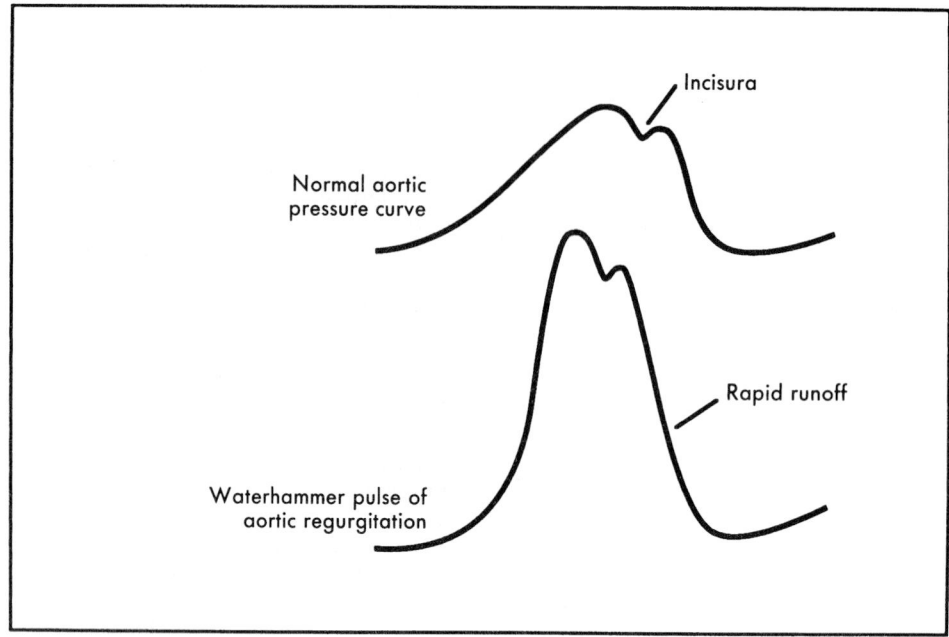

FIG. 6-3 ▌ Schematic illustration of the normal arterial pressure pulse. The incisura that occurs during the descending limb is caused by a transient reversal in flow during isovolumic relaxation. Compared with the normal arterial pressure pulse, the waterhammer pulse of aortic regurgitation builds rapidly and has a rapid runoff.

BOX 6-18

Causes of Abnormal Peripheral Pulse in the Horse

COMMON CAUSES
Dehydration
Shock
Toxemia
Congestive heart failure
Electrolyte imbalances
Acid-base disorders
Hypertension
Hypotension
Exercise

COMMON CAUSES—cont'd
Fever
Laminitis
Aortic insufficiency
Cardiac arrhythmias

UNCOMMON CAUSE
Peripheral arteriovenous shunt
Patent ductus arteriosus

BOX 6-19

Causes of Abnormal Peripheral Pulse in Ruminants

COMMON CAUSES
Dehydration
Shock
Toxemia
Congestive heart failure
Electrolyte imbalances
Acid-base disorders
Fever
Cardiac arrhythmias

UNCOMMON CAUSES
Patent ductus arteriosus
Aortic insufficiency
Peripheral arteriovenous shunt

Hypokinetic pulses are present in patients with diminished stroke volume caused by hypovolemia, left ventricular failure, or, rarely, in large animals, mitral or aortic valve stenosis.

Abnormal peripheral pulses are detected in patients with cardiac arrhythmias. With premature ventricular contractions

(PVCs), the compensatory pause that occurs after the PVC allows a longer period of time for ventricular filling, which results in a greater end-diastolic volume, increased contractile force, and a stronger pulse in the beat following the PVC. The strength of the peripheral pulse is variable in arrhythmias such as atrial fibrillation because the irregular rhythm is as-

sociated with variable time for ventricular filling. Certain arrhythmias, particularly tachyarrhythmias, allow inadequate ventricular filling to generate a peripheral arterial pulse, and a pulse deficit is palpated.

Approach to Diagnosis of Abnormal Peripheral Pulse

1. Take history. Note changes in appetite, attitude, milk production, or ability to exercise; determine whether there have been signs of previous illness and duration and progression of the problem.
2. Perform a physical examination. Determine vital signs. Note whether there is a cardiac arrhythmia, murmur, or other evidence of heart disease (e.g., jugular venous distention or pulsation, edema). Palpate the pulse in multiple sites and bilaterally to rule out occlusive arterial disease; check patient's hydration.
3. Obtain blood for the following:
   a. CBC—look for evidence of toxemia or anemia
   b. Blood gases to determine acid-base balance
   c. Electrolyte concentration, especially Ca and K
4. Record an ECG to characterize any arrhythmia.
5. Determine blood pressure. The site for indirect blood pressure measurement in the standing animal is the tail over the coccygeal artery; a limb can be used in a recumbent animal. Take the mean of several (minimum of three) readings in which the blood pressure cuff is gradually inflated and deflated at approximately 2 to 4 mm Hg/sec; values obtained should be corrected for the difference in height between the site measured and the heart, which is considered to be at the level of the shoulder; the difference in height (centimeters) between the heart and the site of pressure measurement is multiplied by 0.77 (constant used to convert centimeters of blood to millimeters of mercury). In standing horses approximately 27 mm Hg is added to the indirectly measured coccygeal artery pressure to give the corrected value[17]; no correction factor is needed if the measurement is made in a recumbent animal. An appropriately sized blood pressure cuff is considered to be one fourth of the tail circumference[18]; in horses a 4.5- to 5.6-cm cuff has been recommended for electronic oscillometric devices, and a 10.6-cm cuff for ultrasonic flowmeters.[17] Values for normal horses by blood flow detection methods are 79/49 to 145/106 mm Hg (uncorrected for the height of the tail).[16]

   Blood pressure can be evaluated by Doppler or measurements can be recorded by direct cardiac catheterization (see Chapter 28).
6. Perform an echocardiogram to evaluate size of chambers, myocardial function, presence of valvular or pericardial disease, or congenital defects.

REFERENCES

16. O'Rourke RA: Physical examination of the arteries and veins (including blood pressure determination). In Hurst JW, editor: *The heart*, ed 6, vol 1, New York, 1986, McGraw-Hill, pp 138-156.
17. Parry BW: Practical assessment of the circulatory status of equine colic cases, *Compend Cont Educ Pract Vet* 8:S236-S246, 1986.
18. Fregin GF: The cardiovascular system. In Mansmann RA, McAllister ES, eds: *Equine medicine and surgery*, Santa Barbara, Calif, 1982, American Veterinary Publications, pp 645-704.

Alterations in Alimentary and Hepatic Function

BRADFORD P. SMITH

K. GARY MAGDESIAN

MAJOR CLINICAL SIGNS/PROBLEMS ENCOUNTERED

Diarrhea, 102
Colic (abdominal pain), 108
Melena, 111
Blood, fibrin, and/or mucus in feces (dysentery), 112
Abdominal distention/constipation, 113

Regurgitation/vomiting, 114
Dysphagia, 116
Oral vesicles, erosions, ulcers, or growths, 118
Dental abnormalities, 119
Icterus (jaundice), 120

DIARRHEA

K. GARY MAGDESIAN
BRADFORD P. SMITH

Diarrhea is defined as an increase in the frequency, fluidity, or volume of bowel movements. Diarrhea may be a sign of a primary bowel disease or a nonspecific response to sepsis, toxemia, or disease of another organ system.

Under normal circumstances a large volume of essentially isotonic fluid enters the proximal bowel daily. Most of this fluid is resorbed, and only a small percentage is passed with the feces. The fluid comes from dietary intake and from endogenous secretions of the upper digestive tract. The total daily volume exchanged exceeds that of the animal's total extracellular fluid volume. Normally absorption just exceeds secretion; therefore very small changes in rate of absorption or secretion can result in diarrhea. In the horse most water resorption occurs in the cecum and large colon, and diarrhea in the horse usually involves some abnormality in the lumen or wall of the large bowel.

Normal fecal color is tan, brown, or greenish, depending on diet. The adult horse normally produces 11 to 13 kg of fecal material per day (20 to 28 g/kg of body weight per day) while on a diet of grass hay and 3 lb of oats.[1] Fecal output was as high as 20 kg/day in horses fed a mixture of alfalfa and orchard grass ad libitum.[2] Horses with chronic watery diarrhea can produce up to 214 g/kg of body weight per day,[1] which is over 90 L of diarrhea in a 450-kg horse. Cattle normally produce 15 to 28 kg of feces per day with a water content of about 75% to 85% on a diet of grass hay.[3] Fluidity of cattle feces can increase markedly in animals on lush green feed. Sheep and goat feces contain only 50% to 60% water.[3] Fluid feces in the cow and unformed feces in the horse, goat, and sheep are very nonspecific signs that often accompany sepsis or illness other than a primary gastrointestinal disease.

Animals with chronic diarrhea rarely develop severe dehydration because they compensate for increased fecal water losses by increasing water consumption by an equivalent amount. Normal water consumption in the horse on a hay diet in a mild ambient temperature environment is about 24 to 30 L/day whereas cattle consume 30 to 60 L/day based on 10 kg of dry matter feed intake. Water and feed intake do not increase linearly with increasing body size, but by multiplying body weight in kilograms by the 0.75 power ($BW_{kg}^{0.75}$) times a base factor (about 200 ml for water). Thus a 500-kg horse requires 21 liters of water. The effect of temperature on water intake is dramatic and is not linear; as ambient temperatures rise close to 37° C (98° F), water intake per kilogram of dry matter increases much more rapidly than at lower temperatures. Exercise and loss through sweat, particularly in the horse, can dramatically increase salt and water requirements.

Mechanisms of Diarrhea (Box 7-1)

The following five major mechanisms produce diarrhea:

- Decreased or damaged absorptive surface area (malabsorption)
- Increased numbers of osmotically active particles within the intestinal lumen
- Increased volume of secretion of solutes and water
- Abnormal intestinal motility resulting in decreased transit time
- Increased blood-to-lumen pressure as in heart failure or acute or chronic inflammatory bowel diseases

The common net result is an increase in fecal water.

Decreased surface area is mainly a result of villus blunting (atrophy) and/or microvillus damage in the small intestine, which lead to malabsorption. Both occur to some degree with most enteric diseases, and regeneration of surface area from crypt cells with healing is accompanied by a gradual decrease in volume of diarrhea. Diseases in which this is a major mechanism include neonatal diseases such as rotavirus and coronavirus enteric disease,[4] cryptosporidiosis, acute inflammatory disease such as salmonellosis, and chronic diseases such as Johne's disease and other granulomatous bowel diseases. The finding of villus atrophy is so nonspecific that it is not diagnostic in itself. It can even occur in advanced cases of secondary copper deficiency (molybdenosis) with diarrhea. Loss of villus epithelial cells can result in maldigestion because these cells produce important enzymes such as lactase. Many neonates with diarrhea have a temporary lactose intolerance as a result.

Inflammation can be accompanied by increased mucus production and increases in membrane pore size through which tissue fluids and serum proteins leak into the lumen. This is associated with increased capillary and lymphatic hydraulic pressures. Whether acute *(Salmonella)* or chronic (Johne's), inflammatory bowel diseases are protein-losing enteropathies. Low plasma proteins, particularly low albumin, are often found (unless dehydration is present). Bowel inflammation often results in transudation and exudation of serum proteins, blood, and/or mucus, resulting in dysentery (bloody diarrhea). In addition to salmonellosis, dysentery may also commonly be seen with enterotoxemia caused by *Clostridium perfringens* type A, B, or C, *Clostridium difficile*, by attaching effacing *Escherichia coli*, *Campylobacter jejuni*, coccidiosis, malignant catarrhal fever (MCF), arsenic toxicity, and oak toxicity. Inflammation results in malabsorption, maldigestion, osmotic effects, and, in acute disease, changes in intestinal motility. Because most water absorption in the horse occurs in the cecum and colon, inflammatory typhlitis and colitis are the major causes of diarrhea (Boxes 7-2 and 7-3).

Irritation of the bowel with a foreign body such as sand may result in either low-grade recurrent colic or diarrhea. Weight loss may also be evident with a large amount of sand. Sand accumulation in the large bowel of the horse may be suspected when there is evidence of a significant amount of sand in the feces. Irritation probably causes diarrhea through creation of an inflammatory response and altered motility.

Osmotic diarrhea results from any disease causing maldigestion and/or malabsorption. Any osmotically active solute can produce diarrhea in normal animals if given in quantities sufficient to surpass the intestinal capacity for digestion or absorption. Disaccharides are natural examples. Osmotic cathartics such as dioctyl sodium sulfosuccinate (DSS) hold water in the intestine and act as fecal softeners. Magnesium phosphates and sulfates and other divalent and trivalent cations and anions are poorly absorbed and thus are effective laxatives and cathartics.

Osmotic diarrhea can be associated with ingestion of osmotically active poorly absorbed solutes, overloading of the

---

BOX 7-1

Mechanisms of Diarrhea

Malabsorption (villus atrophy)
Osmotic overload
Secretory
Abnormal motility
Increased blood-to-lumen hydraulic pressure

BOX 7-2

Causes of Diarrhea in the Horse (Except Neonate; See Chapter 20 for Neonate)

COMMON CAUSES
Colitis/typhlitis
Salmonellosis
Enteritis, unknown etiology
Potomac fever (equine monocytic ehrlichiosis)
Endotoxemia/gram-negative sepsis
Overfeeding or sudden change in diet
Clostridium difficile

LESS COMMON CAUSES
Eosinophilic gastroenteritis
Renal failure, uremia
Necrotizing enterocolitis
Heart failure
Enterotoxemia
Campylobacter jejuni
Intestinal lymphosarcoma
Cathartics/laxatives
Parasympathomimetics
Chronic granulomatous bowel disease
Proximal enteritis
Peritonitis
Intussusception
Sand, gravel, or enterolith in gut lumen
Gut stenosis
Antibiotic use
Rhodococcus (Corynebacterium) equi gut infection (mainly foals)
Cryptosporidiosis (mainly foals)
Giardiasis (mainly foals)
Toxins or poisonous plants (see Box 7-3)

UNCOMMON CAUSES
Hepatic failure
Cholelithiasis
Vascular aneurysm
Combined immunodeficiency
Agammaglobulinemia
Lactose intolerance
Colorectal polyps
Anaphylaxis
Vitamin A deficiency
Tularemia
Snake bite, insect or spider sting or bite
Histoplasmosis
Hydroallantois
Hyperlipidemia
Internal abdominal abscess
Pheochromocytoma
Viral arteritis
Besnoitiosis (globidiosis) (exotic)

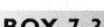
---

intestine with carbohydrates or lipids beyond the amount that can be digested and absorbed, sudden dietary changes resulting in marked shifts in gut flora and resulting bacterial action on ingested substrate (e.g., grain overload), or from bowel disease in which surface area is diminished or digestion interfered with in some manner. Lactase deficiency, secondary to rotavirus or *Clostridium difficile* infections, may result in osmotic diarrhea in foals.[5] These result in increased concentrations of undigested and/or unabsorbed nutrients entering the lower bowel, increased bacterial fermentation, and an increase in the concentration of osmotically active particles. Unfavorable electrochemical gradients prevent resorption. Mucosal digestive enzyme levels are often decreased with any disease involving the small intestine, resulting in maldigestion. When osmotic diarrhea is suspected in mature animals, dietary modification to basic roughage should be tried as part of the nonspecific therapy. Sodium and potassium are normally present in roughly equal amounts in feces and (with a little ammonium) make up the vast majority of cations in the feces. Concentrations of sodium and potassium in feces and osmotically active nonelectrolytes influence fecal water. Large amounts of osmotically active nonelectrolytes may cause osmotic diarrhea. In general, osmotic diarrheas diminish when the animal is fasted. When the offending substance is reintroduced, diarrhea occurs.

Secretory diarrheas are most important in neonates[4] (enteropathogenic *E. coli*), but many strains of *Salmonella* associated with colitis in large animals may produce enterotoxins that stimulate secretion. Enterotoxins act by stimulating cyclic AMP or other messengers to promote secretion of chloride, sodium, and other electrolytes into the gut lumen. Water is carried with these electrolytes and osmotically retained. The hallmark of secretory diarrheas is the large volume of feces produced.

Examples of secretory diarrheas are enterotoxigenic *E. coli* and many strains of *Salmonella* and *C. perfringens. Salmonella* and other invasive organisms produce inflammation that may induce prostaglandin-mediated secretion as well. Secretion may occur with viral diarrhea by a different mechanism, as damaged mature (absorbing) villus cells are replaced by immature (secreting) crypt cells.[6]

Decreased intestinal transit time associated with increased peristalsis and/or decreased segmentation appears to occur in many bowel diseases because of bowel irritation. *Peritonitis* is a major cause of bowel inflammation and should always be explored as a contributing cause of diarrhea, especially when fecal output volume is scant. Abnormal motor patterns have been demonstrated to occur with many infectious diarrheas and may be a bowel response to irritation and/or increased intraluminal volume. Elimination of gut contents thus appears to be a normal gut defense mechanism against infection and probably should not be pharmacologically alleviated in acute infectious diarrheas. Primary motility disorders of animals are not well recognized; diarrhea associated with nervous or excited animals may be the best example of this type. In general, fecal volume associated with motility disorders is not great.

Increased hydraulic pressures from the blood to lumen also decrease net absorption of fluid. These can result from decreased oncotic pressure (hypoalbuminemia), increased capillary hydrostatic pressure (heart failure or portal hypertension as with liver disease), or decreased lymphatic drainage associated with inflamed or blocked lymph vessels or nodes (lymphosarcoma). These mechanisms are most commonly associated with chronic diarrhea, but acute inflammation can also result in diarrhea associated with this mechanism.

Two or more of these mechanisms are probably at work in most diarrheal diseases. Therapy of diarrhea is therefore nonspecific, except when the actual causative agent can be identified. Diagnosis of a specific causative agent is most important when diarrhea is caused by an infectious agent, so that appropriate therapeutic steps can be taken before chronicity develops, spread of disease can be prevented, and an accurate prognosis can be made.

In mature horses, small intestinal diseases such as granulomatous bowel disease or duodenitis/proximal jejunitis (anterior enteritis) may not be associated with diarrhea, and diseases of the stomach almost never cause diarrhea. Most significant diarrheal disease in horses involves the large colon because this is the principal site of water absorption. The exception to this is the neonatal foal, in which primarily small intestinal diseases such as rotavirus infection and cryptosporidiosis may cause severe diarrhea.

The frequency of defecation is usually increased when diarrhea is present and is most frequent when the colon and/or rectum are irritated. When these areas are involved, *tenesmus* (straining) may result. Tenesmus can also occur with hepatic failure in ruminants and in horses and ruminants with rectal tears or strictures, vaginitis, retained placenta, dystocia, intussusception, urolithiasis, rabies, and diseases involving the nervous system when there is retention of feces or urine. Severe rectal irritation can lead to straining and rectal prolapse.

In ruminants, abnormalities such as grain overload (toxic indigestion) resulting in ruminal osmotic changes can produce diarrhea, as can changes in abomasal pH such as occur with type II ostertagiasis. Diarrhea in ruminants is frequently caused by forestomach problems (Boxes 7-4 and 7-5). The colon and remainder of the distal bowel are involved in

BOX 7-4

Causes of Diarrhea in Ruminants (Except Neonate; see Chapter 20 for Neonate)

COMMON CAUSES
Parasitism, worms
Coccidiosis
Salmonellosis
Colitis/typhlitis
Enteritis, unknown etiology
Indigestion (spoiled feed, overfeeding, or sudden change)
Displaced abomasum (B)
Abomasal torsion (B)
Peritonitis
Intussusception
Sepsis/toxemia
Johne's disease
Enterotoxemia
Grain overload (rumen acidosis)
Bovine viral diarrhea (B)
Winter dysentery (B)
Liver failure
Malignant catarrhal fever (B)
Molybdenosis/copper deficiency
Heart failure
Uremia, renal failure
Rompun, following large doses
Cathartic/laxatives
Parasympathomimetics
Toxins or poisonous plants (see Box 7-5)

LESS COMMON CAUSES
Amyloidosis
Giardiasis (mainly calves)
Intestinal obstruction, partial
Intestinal neoplasia
Traumatic reticuloperitonitis (hardware)
Vagal indigestion
Selenium deficiency (White muscle disease)

LESS COMMON CAUSES—cont'd
Cecal dilation (B)
Liver abscess
Brisket disease (high-altitude disease) (B)
Sarcocystosis (B)
Bluetongue (O)
Bovine leukosis (BLV) (B)

UNCOMMON CAUSES
Fat necrosis (B)
Abomasal impaction
Duodenal ulcers
Systemic candidiasis
Vitamin A deficiency
Volvulus, root of mesentery
Water intoxication (B)
Cholelithiasis
Cobalt deficiency
Zinc deficiency (baldy calf) (B)
Hydrops allantois (B)
Lethal trait A 46, keratogenesis imperfecta (parakeratosis) (B)
Zygomycosis, mucormycosis
Pregnancy toxemia
Bacillary hemoglobinuria
Rumen flukes, paramphistomosis
Pancreatic adenocarcinoma
Bee or wasp sting
Pseudorabies
Rift Valley fever (exotic)
Rinderpest (exotic)
Schistosomiasis (exotic)
Theileriosis (East Coast fever) (exotic)
Wesselsbron disease (exotic) (B, O)
Heartwater (exotic)

B, Bovine; *O*, ovine.

BOX 7-5

Toxic Causes of Diarrhea in Ruminants

Arsenic poisoning
Sulfur poisoning
Salt poisoning
Propylene glycol
Levamisole
Monensin
Polybrominated biphenyl
Sodium bicarbonate
Aflatoxin
Herbicide
Zinc
Phosphorus toxicity
Nicotine (black leaf 40) toxicity
Copper
Chlorpyrifos (dursban)
Phosphate fertilizer
Lincomycin
Trichothecene (T-2 toxin)
Plant toxins
Oak (acorn poisoning)
Caddia (coffee weed)

Selenium accumulators
Slaframine (blackpatch diseased legumes, slobber factor)
Mycotoxicoses
Helenium (sneezeweed, bitterweed)
Solanum (nightshade)
Pyrrolizidine alkaloid (*Senecio, Crotalaria, Amsinckia* spp)
Brassica (mustards, crucifers, cress)
Oleander poisoning
Japanese yew *(Taxus cuspidata)* poisoning
Whitehead *(Sphenosciadium capitellatum)*
Pokeweed *(Phytolacca americana L)*
Mushroom
Inkweed *(Drymaria pachyphylla)*
Tung tree (aleurites)
Chinese tallow tree
Kalanchoe (crassulaceae)
Fungal toxicity
Sesbania (rattlebox)
Gutierrezia (broomweed, snakeweed)
Hypericum (St. John's wort; Klamath weed) poisoning
Agrostemma githago (corn cockle) poisoning

diseases such as salmonellosis. Gram-negative infections and resulting endotoxemia, found in conditions such as coliform mastitis and septic metritis, are relatively common causes of nonspecific diarrhea. Diarrhea may be (1) a manifestation of a primary disease (bovine viral diarrhea; Johne's; *Clostridium difficile*), (2) one of the signs of a generalized disease (MCF, uremia), or (3) secondary to toxemia (coliform mastitis, septic metritis).

Nonspecific Fluid Therapy for Diarrhea

Dehydration, electrolyte losses, and acid-base abnormalities can occur rapidly when diarrhea is present. Symptomatic treatment to correct these problems is an important component of nonspecific therapy in animals with diarrhea. Very often the cause of diarrhea remains undetermined, yet symptomatic correction of dehydration and acid-base and electrolyte abnormalities can result in a return to normal function, particularly if the diarrhea is acute and severe. Fluids and electrolytes can be given orally or parenterally. Oral fluids can be given rapidly and inexpensively. Oral fluids should be isotonic or hypotonic. The degree of dehydration should be estimated as a percentage of body weight. Mild dehydration is usually considered less than 5%; moderate, 5% to 8%; and severe, over 8%. Thus a severely dehydrated 450-kg patient with an estimated 10% dehydration (weakness, cold extremities, sunken eyes, decreased urine output, decreased elastic skin rebound, weak pulse, rapid heart rate) requires 45 L of fluids.

The best way to determine electrolyte needs is to take a plasma or serum sample before initiating fluid therapy. Electrolyte requirements can be estimated; with diarrhea, mixed water and electrolyte losses occur, so that sodium-containing fluids are usually required to replace lost sodium and improve blood volume (see also Chapter 22, section on fluid and electrolyte balance). Unless the acid-base status can be measured, the safest sodium-containing fluids are balanced polyionic fluids such as Ringer's or lactated Ringer's solution. Normal saline is a satisfactory alternative in most cases, but the relatively high concentration of chloride ions in saline can aggravate a preexisting metabolic acidosis unless hypochloremia is also present. In general, it is best not to include gram quantities of sodium bicarbonate in fluids unless there is good evidence that a severe metabolic acidosis exists. Flow rates for administering isotonic intravenous fluids should be kept as slow as possible to avoid fluid overload, pulmonary edema, and excessive diuresis. When the patient is shocky, flow rates close to 20 ml/kg/hr may be required, but in general rates below 10 ml/kg/hr are desirable. Hypertonic saline (7% NaCl) may be given rapidly IV at a dose of 4 to 5 ml/kg. See Diarrhea, Chapter 20, and fluid and electrolyte balance, Chapter 22 for more details on fluids and acid-base balance.

Approach to Diagnosis of Diarrhea in the Horse (for Neonates, see Chapter 20)

1. Take history. Especially note change in diet, deworming program, and whether diarrhea is acute or chronic. Note appetite, whether animal is drinking an adequate volume of water, and whether salt is available. Note whether it is a single or multiple case, if there are intercurrent diseases, or if other medications or exposure to toxins are involved. Most antibiotics have been associated with diarrhea in horses, but especially lincomycin, tetracyclines, and erythromycin. Antimicrobials should be discontinued if diarrhea developed during the time of their use. Most bacterial and protozoal agents rely on altered intestinal microflora to proliferate in the gut and cause diarrhea. Note whether nonsteroidal antiinflammatory agents were used before the development of diarrhea. Many causes of diarrhea can be eliminated from consideration on the basis of history.

2. Perform physical examination. Take vital signs (often normal in chronic cases). Perform rectal examination unless an infectious contagious agent is suspected. Note weight loss. Systemic signs of toxemia or dehydration often accompany acute colitis, salmonellosis, equine monocytic ehrlichiosis (Potomac fever), clostridiosis, and many other acute diseases.

3. Examine feces. Perform gross inspection; note whether blood or fibrin is present (see list of causes of dysentery).
    a. Perform microscopic examination for ova and protozoa, especially for chronic cases. Perform Gram stain of feces. A predominance of gram-positive rods may indicate an anaerobic overgrowth such as occurs with *C. difficile* infections.
    b. Multiple cultures for *Salmonella, C. difficile* and *Campylobacter* if onset is acute, if animal is febrile, or if feces contains fibrin and mucus. A commercial polymerase chain reaction (PCR) test can be utilized to evaluate for salmonellosis.[7] An evaluation for *C. difficile* should be made if the diarrhea is temporally associated with antibiotic administration. Cultures should be performed on selective media (cycloserine-cefoxitin-fructose agar). Several ELISA kits are available for identification of toxin A (enterotoxin) and B (cytotoxin) in feces. A stool cytotoxin cell culture is available for toxin B.[8,9]
    c. Fecal occult blood (if positive, see list of causes of melena and blood in feces, pp. 112 and 113).
    d. Fecal osmolality, sodium, and potassium concentrations (optional). Electrolyte concentration in feces is roughly twice the sodium plus potassium. When this value is much lower than the measured osmolality of the feces, the difference is caused by osmotically active nonelectrolytes, and osmotic diarrhea is confirmed.
    e. Check for sand by placing some feces in a bucket of water, mixing thoroughly, and decanting the water. If a radiographic unit with the appropriate power capability is available, abdominal radiographs can be taken to detect the presence and amount of sand.
    f. A PCR test is available for detection of *Lawsonia intracellularis*-like organisms in weanlings with diarrhea, weight loss, and hypoalbuminemia.[10]
    g. *Rhodococcus equi* can cause diarrhea in 1- to 6-month-old foals. Diagnostic tests include cultures of transtracheal aspirates, abdominal fluid cytology and culture, abdominal ultrasonography, and PCR techniques on a limited availability.[11]
    h. If all other cultures are negative and an infectious cause of diarrhea is suspected, the feces should be cultured for *Aeromonas* sp. and *Clostridium perfringens*.[12] A positive culture for *C. perfringens* should be coupled with an evaluation for the presence of toxin genes to confirm pathogenicity, as the organism may be cultured as part of the normal flora. Recent reports implicate a novel β-2 toxin-producing *C. perfringens* as a potential pathogen in colitis of adult horses.[13]

4. Obtain blood for the following:
    a. CBC (includes fibrinogen and plasma proteins). Increased fibrinogen indicates inflammation. Decreased proteins indicate protein-losing enteropathy. Thrombocytopenia may indicate a coagulopathy. Neutropenia with or without a toxic, left shift is often present with infectious and inflammatory causes of acute colitis, indicating a systemic inflammatory response syndrome. An elevated packed cell volume (PCV) and

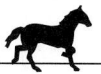

red cell mass is often present, indicating hemoconcentration and splenic contraction in horses.

b. Acid-base values if acute and dehydrated or toxic. Although acid-base values are not of much use diagnostically, they allow for initiation of proper nonspecific supportive therapy. S/Pecial Chem Micro CO_2 device described previously or blood gases can be used.

5. Test serum for the following:
   a. Electrolytes (Na, K, Cl) (nonspecific).
   b. BUN—prerenal azotemia is common as a result of dehydration; check again after rehydration. Serum chemistries should be evaluated for liver and other organ disease.
   c. Albumin/globulin values; hypoalbuminemia is seen with chronic protein-losing enteropathies such as granulomatous bowel disease, with phenylbutazone toxicity, and with acute colitis conditions.
   d. Specific IgA, IgM, and IgG levels; immunodeficient individuals may have chronic diarrhea. Elevated globulins may indicate the presence of chronic disease.
   e. Paired sera for *Ehrlichia risticii* titer following acute diarrhea with fever. PCR techniques can be used to identify the agent in whole blood samples.
   f. Clotting times (PT/PTT or ACT) should be monitored as indicators of coagulopathies such as disseminated intravascular coagulation (DIC). Antithrombin III levels can be monitored for the risk of thromboses.

6. Perform paracentesis. Cytology, protein, and fibrinogen values for chronic cases to rule out peritonitis, tumors, and mesenteric abscess.

7. Perform function and absorption tests.
   a. Oral glucose or xylose small intestine absorption tests (see Chapter 30) for chronic cases, particularly if a high index of suspicion exists because of hypoalbuminemia. If tests indicate malabsorption, either biopsy the gut (or rectum) or assess response to treatment for 60 days following larvicidal anthelmintic dose.
   b. Perform liver function tests such as sodium sulfobromophthalein (BSP) half-time or serum bile acid levels if liver is suspected as a result of elevated liver enzyme levels and/or hypoalbuminemia. Liver enzymes are elevated in most cases of enterocolitis and in these cases do not indicate primary liver disease (see Chapter 31).

8. Examine tissue.
   a. Rectal or intestinal biopsy for microscopic examination and fluorescent antibody for immune-mediated diseases (also culture for *Salmonella*). Rectal histopathology is particularly useful in horses with hypoalbuminemia or weight loss.[14]
   b. Liver biopsy if indication of involvement in chronic cases.

9. Toxicology.
   a. Blood lead, liver lead, and liver arsenic concentrations can be measured if toxicity is suspected.[15]
   b. High-pressure liquid chromatography or gas-chromatography-mass spectrometry can be used to detect cantharidin (blister beetle toxin) in urine or gastrointestinal contents.[16]
   c. Urine and gastrointestinal contents can be evaluated for the presence of oleandrin using thin layer chromatography. Oleander toxicity should be suspected in animals with diarrhea, arrhythmias, and renal disease.[17]

10. Evaluate response to treatment with undiagnosed *chronic* diarrhea.
   a. Alter diet to simple grass hay. Alternatively, a pelleted diet can be tried, especially if right dorsal colitis is sus-

pected. Psyllium mucilloid, at 4 oz, and 1 to 2 cups of corn oil can be added to the daily diets of horses with right dorsal colitis.[18,19]

b. Stop nonsteroidal drugs such as phenylbutazone if toxicity is possible cause.

c. If no protozoa are seen in fecal sample, attempt transfaunation with colon or cecum contents from normal animal (if not available, use feces).

d. Attempt to classify into type by rectal biopsy; many changes are nonspecific.
   (1) Fibrosis and inflammatory changes point to a poor prognosis. Administer potentiated sulfas (5 mg/kg trimethoprim tid is therapeutic dose) and iodochlorhydroxyquin (Rheaform 10 g/450 kg horse/day) for 2 weeks.
   (2) Mononuclear cell infiltrate. Administer 20 to 30 mg dexamethasone (Azium) per day, tapering down to 10 mg in 1 week; if response is favorable, continue with 600 to 800 mg prednisolone PO per day, taper over 2 months.
   (3) Eosinophilic infiltrate. Administer larvicidal anthelminthic dose plus corticosteroids as above.

e. Transfusion with plasma (1 to 2 ml/kg) in young horses 2 to 12 months of age that may need some additional serum factor to suppress diarrhea. Synthetic colloids, such as hetastarch, can be used in animals with reduced colloid osmotic pressure (hypoalbuminemia), especially if edema is present. Hetastarch has been used at 10 ml/kg.[20]

f. Horses with Potomac fever often respond favorably to systemic treatment with tetracycline.

g. Metronidazole (15 mg/kg PO tid) can be used empirically, especially if an anaerobic overgrowth is suspected, or when the diarrhea is secondary to antibiotic use.[21]

Approach to Diagnosis of Diarrhea in Ruminants (for Neonates, see Chapter 20)

1. Take history. Especially note diet, appetite, previous deworming and vaccinations, and whether it is an individual or herd problem. In animals less than 1 year of age coccidia, ostertagia, or other helminths should be strongly considered. Determine if onset is acute or chronic. If chronic, first consider diseases such as parasitism, Johne's, copper deficiency (molybdenosis), selenium deficiency, liver failure, and other diseases of individual cows such as bovine leukosis virus (BLV), amyloidosis, heart failure, or uremia.

2. Perform physical examination. Especially note weight loss, fever, systemic signs, rumen activity, and oral lesions. Perform rectal examination. In most acute-onset diseases, vital signs are abnormal and systemic involvement or oral lesions (especially with BVD) may be obvious.

3. Examine feces.
   a. Gross inspection.
   b. Microscopic examination for ova and parasites.
   c. Culture for *Salmonella* if animal is febrile or feces are inflammatory appearing (fibrin/mucus).
   d. Check for fecal occult blood.
   e. Culture of *Mycobacterium paratuberculosis* if weight loss is a problem (especially if a herd problem in animals over 2 years of age).

4. Take rectal scrapings of mucus.
   a. Make thin smear on slide for acid-fast staining for Johne's. Examine under oil immersion lens.

5. Obtain blood for the following:
   a. Plasma proteins.
   b. Fibrinogen.

BOX 7-6

Gastrointestinal Causes of Colic in the Horse

COMMON CAUSES
Accumulation of intestinal, cecal, or colonic gas
Hypermotility and intestinal spasms
Feed impaction, constipation
Meconium impaction (newborn)
Gastric ulcers (foal)

LESS COMMON CAUSES
Thromboembolism
Intestinal foreign body (sand; enterolith; phytobezoar)
Volvulus of small intestine
Pedunculated lipoma with bowel strangulation
Hernia, inguinal, epiploic, umbilical, diaphragmatic
Nephrosplenic ligament bowel entrapment
Ascarid impaction
Massive strongyle infection
Gastric dilation
Anterior enteritis (duodenitis/proximal jejunitis)
Enteritis, impending or active
Peritonitis
Parasympathomimetic drugs
Irritant cathartics
Necrotizing enterocolitis
Psychogenic colic
Rectal tear
Volvulus or displacement of large bowel
Rupture of stomach or intestine
Ileus
Intussusception

UNCOMMON CAUSES
Abdominal adhesions
Intramural hematomas of stomach or intestine
Stenosis or stricture of bowel lumen

UNCOMMON CAUSES—cont'd
Botulism
Tetanus
Potomac fever
Exhaustion
Anaphylaxis
Rhodococcus equi (Corynebacterium) gut abscesses
Cribbing or wind sucking
Abdominal fibroma
Segmental ischemic necrosis following mesocolic tearing
Equine viral arteritis
Anthrax with bleeding
Malignant edema (*Clostridium* spp.)
Malignant mesothelioma
Gastric or intestinal tumor
Atropine
Vitamin K_3 deficiency (moldy sweet clover)

TOXINS
(See also toxins listed under Diarrhea)
Cantharidin toxicity
Dioxin
Trichloroethylene-extracted feed toxicity
Warfarin (dicumarol)
Herbicides
Lead
Nitrophenyl urea (vacor)
Phenylbutazone or other nonsteroidal antiinflammatory drugs
Poison plants (many of those that produce diarrhea also produce colic; see plant toxins listed under Diarrhea)
African horse sickness (exotic)
Grass sickness (exotic)

---

c. In acute cases, electrolytes and acid-base status.
d. If a herd problem, copper and selenium status.
6. Test serum for the following:
a. BUN.
b. Liver enzymes (γ-glutamyltransferase [GGT] and sorbitol dehydrogenase [SDH]).
c. Albumin/globulin values.
d. AGID for BLV (single animals); request gp51 and p24 antibody status.
e. If Johne's suspected, perform ELISA test.
7. Perform paracentesis. Paracentesis rules out gross peritonitis, but many false-negatives are possible as a result of focal or fibrinous peritonitis.
8. Perform urinalysis for protein to rule out consideration of amyloidosis or other multisystemic immune-mediated disease. Because ruminants normally have a urine pH of 8 or higher, most dipstick tests will give a trace or a 1+ positive reading for urine protein even when the animal/urine is normal.
9. Examine tissue.
a. Rectal, intestinal, or mesenteric lymph node biopsy for acid-fast stain for Johne's, for culture for *Salmonella*, and for presence of lymphosarcoma.
10. Feed analysis (herd problem only).
a. Copper, molybdenum, and selenium.
b. Toxins suspected (e.g., mercury, arsenic).
11. Tap abomasum for increased pH; rule out type II ostertagiasis.

12. Necropsy (herd problem only).
a. Pick severely affected individual to examine thoroughly.

COLIC

K. GARY MAGDESIAN
BRADFORD P. SMITH

Colic is defined as the manifestation of visceral abdominal pain. Colic may be the result of nongastrointestinal pain, such as urinary tract obstruction (Boxes 7-6 and 7-7). This section discusses colic of gastrointestinal origin. Pain may be acute, chronic, or recurrent. Gas distention or recognizable organic problems such as displacements are most frequently associated with acute colic. Five basic causes in large animals are as follows:
1. Distention of gut with fluid, gas, or ingesta
2. Pulling on the root of the mesentery
3. Ischemia or infarction
4. Deep ulcers in the stomach or bowel
5. Peritoneal pain (peritonitis)
The horse exhibits colic frequently, because it appears to have a low threshold to pain and is frequently beset by minor digestive disturbances that result in a distended bowel. Signs of colic in the horse include restlessness, lying down and getting up, groaning, grunting, rolling, sweating, kicking at the abdomen, or suddenly dropping to the ground in pain. Anorexia and depression often accompany these signs. Horses also have an increased heart rate with weak pulse

BOX 7-7

Causes of Colic in Ruminants

COMMON CAUSES
Increased intestinal gas
Intussusception
Torsion or volvulus of the mesenteric root
Peritonitis
Intestinal foreign body/obstruction
Urolithiasis
Ruptured bladder
Acute pyelonephritis
Abomasal torsion
Abomasal ulcer
Cecal dilation/volvulus
Severe bloat

LESS COMMON CAUSES
Cystitis/urinary tract disease
Abomasal bloat (neonates)
Uterine torsion or rupture
Hernia
Parturition, impending
Hypermotility and spasms of gut
Feed impaction
Right displaced abomasum
Acute traumatic reticulitis, abomasitis, or duodenitis
Acute liver disease
Vagal indigestion
Atresia coli (neonates)

UNCOMMON CAUSES
Rabies
Rectal tear

UNCOMMON CAUSES—cont'd
Rectal prolapse
Grain overload
Water intoxication
Winter dysentery
Ovarian abscess
Fat necrosis
Cholelithiasis
Intestinal adhesions
Enterotoxemia
Ileus
Intestinal strangulation
Inversion of uterine horn
Malignant edema
Malignant mesothelioma
Ruptured uterine artery
Intestinal neoplasia
Aortic, iliac, or femoral thrombosis
Anaphylaxis
Renal cysts
Ruptured prepubic tendon
Vaginal laceration
Torsion of descending colon
Rinderpest (exotic)

TOXINS
Plant poisonings (many of those that cause diarrhea also produce colic; see plant toxins listed under Diarrhea)

---

quality and develop prolonged capillary refill time, cold extremities, and bright red (vasodilatory phase) followed by dark (vasoconstrictive phase) mucous membranes if the problem is severe and affects cardiovascular integrity.

Evidence of shock is usually present only when the disease condition is severe and involves infarctive disease (volvulus, torsion, thromboembolism) or advanced visceral distention (extreme flatulence, impaction, or dilation). Foreign bodies such as sand or enteroliths in the large colon may result in *low-grade recurrent colic*. When an enterolith is passed into the transverse colon where it obstructs the bowel, *signs of complete obstruction* and acute colic ensue. These signs are manifestations of visceral pain, mediated by the sympathetic nervous system. External palpation and pushing on the abdomen does not usually elicit pain unless the affected inflamed or dilated viscus is contacted.

In contrast, parietal pain associated with *peritonitis* usually is responsive to external palpation. Whereas the animal with visceral pain is showing active signs of colic, the animal with parietal pain is usually reluctant to move and has a splinted abdomen. Acute peritonitis occurs within minutes following rupture of the stomach or perforation of an ulcer as a result of immediate irritation of serosal surfaces by the acid contents whereas with rupture of the colon or rectum it may take 12 hours or more before peritonitis is clinically apparent.

Ruminants exhibit colic less frequently than horses, probably because of a higher threshold to pain and because dietary shifts principally affect the rumen; thus intestinal gas pains occur less frequently. Colic with visceral pain (including urinary tract) is manifested by grinding the teeth (odontoprisis or bruxism), grunting/groaning, treading with the hind feet, kicking at the abdomen, restlessness, repeatedly lying down and getting up, and anorexia and depression. With parietal pain caused by peritonitis, ruminants demonstrate abdominal pain by arching the back, splinting, and exhibiting pain on deep palpation of the area. These signs are seen most commonly with traumatic reticuloperitonitis and abomasal ulcers; rarely are these diseases associated with the colic signs described above.

Diagnosis and Management of Colic in the Horse

1. Take history. Because colic is a common problem in horses, mild to moderate degrees of abdominal pain are often initially treated symptomatically with analgesics and/or laxatives before major diagnostic efforts are undertaken. Most colic of mild to moderate severity responds favorably to symptomatic treatment. In general, severe pain or pain that is unresponsive to analgesics indicates a more serious condition for which more aggressive medical management or surgical correction may be indicated.

   Recurrent mild-to-moderate colic *may* be an indication of a more serious problem such as bowel entrapment or displacement thromboembolism, internal abscess, enterolith, sand or other foreign body, tumor, gastric ulcer, hypobiotic cyathostomiasis, *S. vulgaris* larval migration, heavy burden of ascarids, abdominal adhesions, strictured bowel, or urinary tract disease.

2. Perform physical examination. Intestinal causes of colic can often be differentiated from colic associated with other organ systems (Box 7-8) by physical examination

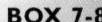

BOX 7-8

Extraintestinal Causes of Colic in the Horse

COMMON CAUSES
Mesenteric abscess
Ovarian tumor, abscess, or hematoma
Parturition
Acute hepatitis (massive necrosis) or hepatic lipidosis
Diaphragmatic hernia
Ruptured bladder (foal)
Uterine torsion

LESS COMMON CAUSES
Urinary tract or renal disease, including urolithiasis
Pleuritis or pericarditis (referred pain)
Retained placenta
Uterine rupture or retroflexion
Spermatic cord thrombosis or torsion

UNCOMMON CAUSES
Perirectal abscess
Pheochromocytoma
Purpura hemorrhagica
Biliary atresia
Vaginal or vulvar tear
Cholelithiasis
White muscle disease
Rabies
Rupture of prepubic tendon
Splenitis, splenic abscess, splenomegaly
Cauda equina neuritis with retention of feces or urine

---

findings. Although extraintestinal origins of acute colic are relatively uncommon in the horse, they include mainly abdominal abscesses, tumors, cholelithiasis or cholestatic disease, and genitourinary tract disease and tend to be recurrent. It is important to note the presence or absence of normal intestinal borborygmi and whether or not feces are being passed in determining whether the problem is extraintestinal. Careful auscultation of the thorax should be performed to evaluate for the presence of diaphragmatic hernias or pleural disease. The testicles should be palpated on all stallions to screen for scrotal hernias or testicular torsions. Rectal examination findings often help to determine anatomic location within gut or other site. Abdominal tumors, abscesses, and other masses may be palpable. Although mild to moderate chronic intermittent colic may be of extraintestinal or intestinal origin, most cases of severe unremitting colic indicate gut involvement, often with anatomic displacement.

3. Use ultrasound and radiology. Ultrasound may help in locating masses, adhesions, or enlarged liver. It may also be helpful in the diagnosis of gastrointestinal disease, including nephrosplenic entrapment of the large colon and small intestinal distention. Ultrasound can be particularly useful in foals and small ruminants because of their size. Radiology can also be useful in detecting enteroliths or sand in adult horses and in some gastrointestinal conditions of foals. Rarely is radiology useful in diagnosing the cause of colic in ruminants, except for urethrographs in sheep and goats to locate a urethral stone.

4. Examine feces. Gross examination of feces should be performed. The presence of sand can often be detected by mixing feces with water in a bucket, then pouring off the water and looking for sediment.

   If no feces are passed, a more serious condition is usually indicated, particularly if intestinal sounds are absent.

5. Use laboratory aids. Laboratory aids of immediate benefit in diagnosis and management include PCV and plasma proteins to aid in assessing hydration and vascular integrity and a paracentesis to evaluate abdominal fluid grossly and microscopically. Pain and excitement alone can elevate the PCV, but there is a correlation of elevated PCV (>55%) in colics with nonsurvival. Plasma proteins are not elevated unless blood volume is decreased through shifts in compartmental distribution of body fluids. In colic cases these fluid shifts usually mean that an increased and abnormal amount of extracellular fluid is in the gut lumen, a "third space" where it is of little use in maintaining blood volume.

   Abdominal fluid is normally present in small volume (a few drops to 50 ml); is clear and colorless to yellow; and has a total protein below 2.5 g/dl, specific gravity less than 1.015, little or no fibrinogen (<100 mg/dl), and fewer than 10,000 WBC/μl. Elevations in these parameters or increased numbers of neutrophils in peritoneal fluid often indicate inflammation on serosal surfaces. Comparisons of abdominal fluid glucose to serum glucose (greater than 50 mg/dl difference is abnormal), evaluation of abdominal fluid pH, and LDH concentrations can aid in the diagnosis of septic peritonitis.[22] Grossly, fluid changes to cloudy yellow, then to blood-tinged with fibrin clots, and finally to black in color as bowel necrosis and hemolysis of extravasated red blood cells (RBCs) occur. Elevated levels of peritoneal fluid protein are consistently found in anterior enteritis (duodenitis/proximal jejunitis) and provide a useful differential aid, although this finding is also common in cantharidin poisoning. Elevated protein levels are present in peritonitis but accompanied in these cases by elevated numbers of neutrophils. If peritoneal fluid is grossly contaminated with feed material, rupture of a viscus should be considered. Another peritoneal tap in a different location should be undertaken if the possibility of bowel penetration during paracentesis cannot be ruled out. It is not necessary to have abnormal peritoneal fluid before consideration of surgical correction of colic is contemplated.

   Many chemical analyses (i.e., lactate) of blood or peritoneal fluid have been recommended as an aid in prognosis and gauging severity of tissue damage. Plasma fibrinogen, as well as peripheral leukocyte counts, can aid in the differentiation of enterocolitis or anterior enteritis from strangulating lesions. Serum electrolyte concentrations and acid-base status are important from a therapeutic standpoint. Serum biochemistries, including liver enzymes and creatinine and BUN are important in evaluating for liver and renal compromise. Hyperglobulinemia may be indicative of chronic disease.

6. Evaluate response to treatment. The approach to diagnosis of colic signs is often tied in with management because if the animal's pain cannot be alleviated, surgical intervention and specific diagnosis of displacements, internal hernias, masses, and adhesions are the next step. The initial diagnosis especially considers the history of deworming and feeding. The findings of the physical examination, including rectal examination and evaluating degree of pain, determine whether additional laboratory workup is indicated. In many cases with mild to moderate pain and no evidence of shock, standard treatment is parenteral administration of an analgesic agent (see Chapter 3) and oral administration of a mild laxative such as DSS (approximately 1 ml/kg of 5% DSS) or mineral oil (4 L). When a nasogastric tube is passed, the stomach should be checked for reflux and decompressed as needed. The pH of the gastric reflux may indicate primary gastric dilation if acidic, or small intestinal blockage or ileus if alkaline.

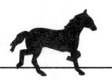

Dark brown, foul-smelling, and alkaline reflux is often associated with anterior enteritis (duodenitis/proximal jejunitis). If a significant amount of reflux is present, oral medications should be withheld. If cardiovascular function is impaired (poor mucous membrane color and capillary refill, weak pulse, cold extremities, impending shock), sodium-containing fluids should be given intravenously at a rate of 3 to 10 L/hr to a 450-kg horse.

Large amounts of painful gas auscultable in the right flank can be tapped and drawn off, although the risk for peritonitis should be considered. The cecum is trocarized, using a 14- to 16-gauge 6-inch needle inserted through aseptically prepared skin. The principles of colic management include (1) control of pain, (2) relief of distention, (3) relief of obstruction, and (4) control of shock.

7. Perform exploratory surgery. In making a decision concerning management of colic, it is important to separate impending enteritis and peritonitis from bowel disease requiring surgical intervention. Anterior or proximal enteritis can result in prolonged moderate pain and requires constant or frequently repeated analgesic administration and gastric decompression of the foul-smelling, dark reddish-to-brownish stomach contents. However, pain often subsides, and is replaced with depression, after gastric decompression in horses with anterior enteritis, whereas horses with strangulating lesions often remain in pain. The presence of fever or decreased total white blood cell (WBC) count (with neutropenia) may be indications of impending or ongoing enteritis, in which case surgery may be contraindicated. *Surgery is indicated in the following situations:*
   a. Pain is severe and intractable.
   b. Pulse is weak and rate is rising over 70 beats/min.
   c. Perfusion is poor, as evidenced by cold extremities, mucous membranes are off color, and capillary refill is poor.
   d. No gut sounds are auscultated (a lack of fecal production).
   e. Bowel is markedly distended.
   f. Large volumes of yellowish alkaline gastric reflux are present.
   g. Abdominocentesis indicates damaged bowel (blood tinged, increased protein, increased WBCs).
   Surgery may be contraindicated in the following situations:
   a. Fever.
   b. Neutropenia or marked neutrophilia.
   c. Severe icterus or marked enzyme abnormalities indicating primary liver disease.
   d. Foul-smelling, brownish-red gastric reflux characteristic of proximal enteritis (duodenitis/jejunitis).
   e. Evidence of an extraintestinal cause not amenable to surgical correction.
   f. Colitis or diarrhea.

Diagnosis and Management of Colic in Ruminants

1. Take history. Colic in neonates is most often associated with increased abomasal or intestinal gas and is discussed in Chapter 20. Perforating ulcers are not uncommon as a cause of colic in calves 1 to 6 months of age.

   It should be determined whether the onset of colic was acute or chronically recurrent. Few diseases cause recurrent colic in ruminants. Urolithiasis is probably the most common cause of colic in male or neutered male goats and sheep and occurs under varied dietary and environmental conditions. Urolithiasis in cattle occurs most frequently in bulls or steers eating high-grain diets, but silicate stones can occur in very young animals and animals on pasture diet.

2. Perform a physical examination. Take vital signs; with torsion or severe peritonitis, shock signs such as rapid heart

rate (>90 beats/min), cold extremities, and weakness may be seen. Tympany can be detected by simultaneous auscultation and percussion. Such causes of colic as cecal dilation, bloat, free gas in the peritoneal cavity, and severe abomasal dilation can be diagnosed in this way (see Figs. 1-3 to 1-5). Rectal examination detects such abnormalities as gas in the cecum, uterine abnormalities, urinary tract disease, and intussusception. Observe animal urinating to rule out obstructive urolithiasis.

3. Examine feces. Observe grossly; intussusception usually has scant dark red (almost black) feces. Scant feces are seen with cecal dilation or displacement.

4. Check preputial hairs and urethral process for sediment and stones. Grit on the preputial hairs is often associated with urolithiasis. Observe animal urinating and check urine for abnormalities. Rule out pyelonephritis.

   Radiology and ultrasound can be useful in sheep and goats when urolithiasis is a consideration. Ultrasound can detect a distended bladder, and stones may sometimes be detected. Radiology (lateral view) may detect a stone in the urethra or stones in the bladder. A contrast urethrogram may also be diagnostic.

5. Perform paracentesis to look for peritonitis caused by perforated abomasal ulcer, serosal devitalization, intussusception, or ruptured bladder. Interpret as above for horses, except that normal peritoneal fluid protein concentration can go as high as 5 g/dl in ruminants.

6. Other laboratory aids such as CBC and clinical chemistries are seldom diagnostic in ruminant colic. If grossly abnormal, they may be grounds for formulating a poor prognosis. Intussusception may be associated with neutrophilia (as well as dark feces and colic) in some cases.

7. Symptomatic treatment of colic includes analgesics and, if heart rate is over 90 beats/min, intravenous fluid therapy with a sodium-containing fluid. Take blood sample for electrolytes and acid-base status before initiating fluid therapy. The S/Pecial Chem Micro CO_2 apparatus or blood gas analysis can provide rapid assessment of metabolic acid-base status.

8. Surgical exploration is indicated if colic is persistent, abdominal distention occurs, the heart rate is over 100 beats/min, feces are scant (especially those that are dark red and indicative of intussusception), there are pings indicating abomasal or cecal displacement or torsion, or the peritoneal fluid indicates bowel devitalization (blood-tinged fluid with elevated protein and WBCs). If surgical exploration is indicated, an important consideration is whether the animal will remain standing under local anesthesia during surgery. It is often best to perform abdominal surgery on animals with colic in left lateral or dorsal recumbency, aided by sedation and restraint, to avoid sudden collapse when painful surgical manipulations are performed. If the left lateral position is selected, use padding to raise the hip and shoulder so that the abdominal viscera can sit in a depression.

MELENA
BRADFORD P. SMITH

Melena (dark, tarry feces) is caused by blood in the lumen of the stomach or proximal intestinal tract, resulting in black (digested) blood appearing in the feces (Boxes 7-9 and 7-10). Usually blood is a result of a bleeding ulcer in the stomach or abomasum but may also result from ingestion, oral or pharyngeal bleeding, or coughing up blood that is then swallowed. In ruminants, dark red feces from an intussusception are the main differential to be considered. Blood must stay in the intestinal tract for hours before the hemoglobin is altered and turns black. Small amounts of hemoglobin can be

---

BOX 7-9

Causes of Melena in the Horse

COMMON CAUSES
Gastric or duodenal ulcer
Gastric squamous cell carcinoma
Coughing up and swallowing blood

LESS COMMON CAUSES
Phenylbutazone toxicity (nonsteroidal antiinflammatory
    drugs)
Purpura hemorrhagica
Gastroenteritis with bleeding
Warfarin toxicity or other coagulation disorder
Colonic hematomas
Disseminated intravascular coagulation with mucosal
    hemorrhage
Anterior or proximal enteritis (duodenitis/proximal
    jejunitis)
Arsenic toxicity

UNCOMMON CAUSES
Lupus erythematosus
Factor VIII deficiency, hemophilia A
Histoplasmosis

BOX 7-10

Causes of Melena in Ruminants

COMMON CAUSES
Abomasal ulcer
Intussusception

LESS COMMON CAUSES
Lung abscess with ruptured blood vessel
Oak toxicity
Coccidiosis
Gastroenteritis with bleeding
Arsenic toxicity
Postpartum (ingestion of blood)
Intestinal parasites
Toxicity from nonsteroidal antiinflammatory drugs
Abomasal torsion or volvulus

UNCOMMON CAUSES
Duodenal ulcers
Hemophilia A, factor VIII deficiency
Bacillary hemoglobinuria
Sulphur toxicity
Warfarin poisoning or other coagulation disorder
Narthecium asiaticum maxim poisoning (exotic)

---

detected by using one of the tests for occult blood. In general, fairly large volumes of blood (1 to 2 L) are required to produce a positive fecal occult blood test in the horse.* A 24- to 48-hour time period is needed for orally administered blood to reach the rectum in the horse. In ruminants, smaller

*Carlson G: Personal communication, 1990.

volumes of blood are needed to produce a positive fecal occult test, and a faster transit time is expected.

In approaching a diagnosis, rule out pulmonary, oral, or pharyngeal bleeding. Bleeding of gastrointestinal origin can be determined to be caused by mucosal disease or full-thickness bowel disease (such as an intussusception or neoplasia) by examining peritoneal fluid for abnormalities. Abnormalities in peritoneal fluid are usually present in the case of serosal involvement. Bleeding abomasal ulcers are probably the leading cause of melena in ruminants. They can be silent except for the dark feces and weakness if severe anemia develops. In older horses, gastric squamous cell carcinoma is a frequent cause of gastric hemorrhage. Significant bleeding is much less common in foals and calves with gastric ulcers, and melena is rare in foals and calves with gastric ulcers.

Consideration should be given to whether or not the melena is the result of clotting abnormalities associated with such diseases as disseminated intravascular coagulation (DIC) or warfarin poisoning. In cattle with colic and dark red-to-black feces, intussusception should be considered likely.

When severe anemia develops, there is evidence of blood loss because the decrease in PCV and RBCs is accompanied by a decrease in plasma proteins. Nonspecific therapy for melena consists principally of blood transfusions in life-threatening cases. Sudden, massive gastric or abomasal bleeding may result in anemia and collapse before melena has appeared.

In the foal, gastric ulcers may be treated with histamine 2 (H_2) blockers such as ranitidine or cimetidine. These drugs are probably less effective in ruminants. Their benefit in ruminants with abomasal ulcers is not well understood at present. New drugs such as the hydrogen pump blocker omeprazole are useful and potent gastric pH effectors. Therapy with protectants such as sucralfate (which coats the ulcer) is a viable and clinically useful therapy in the horse. In ruminants, orally administered protectants and antacids are so diluted by the time they reach the abomasum that they are probably of limited benefit.

BLOOD, FIBRIN, AND/OR MUCUS IN FECES (DYSENTERY)

BRADFORD P. SMITH

Bloody diarrhea is termed *dysentery*. Fresh blood or clots in the feces is termed *hematochezia* and is the result of bleeding into the distal intestinal tract. Occasionally blood from the female reproductive tract may appear in or on the feces. Fibrin indicates severe inflammatory bowel disease. Fibrin appears as casts, chunks of yellow-gray material, or mucosa-like sheets. Mucus in feces increases with inflammatory bowel diseases such as salmonellosis. It is often seen when fecal volume is small in animals that are anorectic, in which case the feces are often coated with mucus. This mucus coating can become very obvious in the horse and is not a sign of bowel disease in this case.

Frank blood in feces without diarrhea and other evidence of gastrointestinal dysfunction or systemic illness may be a result of a bleeding disorder, a traumatic foreign body, rectal examination trauma, sadistic rectal trauma, or rectal trauma in a mare from a stallion penetrating the rectum (Boxes 7-11 and 7-12). Many of the diseases listed as causes of melena may also result in gastrointestinal hemorrhage and are therefore listed in both places. If the bleeding is in the distal gastrointestinal tract, fresh blood may be seen in the feces. With diseases midway down the tract, such as intussusception, fecal material is dark red and may appear black until a sample is examined closely and spread on a white surface.

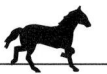

BOX 7-11

Causes of Blood, Fibrin, or Mucus in Feces of the Horse

COMMON CAUSES
Foreign body
Rectal tear/trauma
Intussusception
Blister beetle (cantharidin) toxicity
Colitis, unknown etiology
Salmonellosis

LESS COMMON CAUSES
Purpura hemorrhagica
Small strongyle infection (cyathostomiasis)
Colorectal polyps
Eosinophilic gastroenteritis
Acorn or oak poisoning
Arsenic toxicity
Organophosphate toxicity
Warfarin poisoning or other coagulation disorder
Mycotoxicoses
Besnoitiosis (globidiosis) (exotic)

BOX 7-12

Causes of Blood, Fibrin, or Mucus in Feces of Ruminants

COMMON CAUSES
Foreign body
Intussusception
Coccidiosis
Salmonellosis

LESS COMMON CAUSES
Rectal tear or trauma
Rectal examination trauma
Volvulus, root of mesentery
Malignant catarrhal fever
Enterotoxemia
Bovine viral diarrhea
Arsenic toxicity
Abomasal torsion
Warfarin poisoning or other coagulation disorder
Castor bean *(Ricinus)* poisoning
Tung tree poisoning (aleurites)
Solanum (nightshade, potato) poisoning
Sesbania (rattlebox) poisoning
Bracken fern

BOX 7-13

Causes of Abdominal Distention/Constipation in the Horse

COMMON CAUSES
Ileus
Intestinal foreign body such as enterolith (see Colic)
Peritonitis
Intestinal obstruction, impaction, or gas (see Colic)
Necrotizing enterocolitis (foals)
Torsion or volvulus of gut (see Colic)
Sudden decrease in exercise

LESS COMMON CAUSES
Pregnancy
Pelvic mass (abscess, tumor)
Cecal tympany (see Colic)
Hernia, obstructive (see Colic)
Intussusception (see Colic)

UNCOMMON CAUSES
Anticholinergics
Opiates
Intrinsic colonic nerve dysfunction
Anorectal pain
Perineal hernia
Hypokalemia
Tetanus
Hypocalcemic tetany
Intramural hematomas on gut
Propylene glycol toxicity
Grass sickness (exotic)

ABDOMINAL DISTENTION/CONSTIPATION

BRADFORD P. SMITH

Abdominal distention may be caused by feed, fluid, gas, feces, or a neoplasm (Boxes 7-13 and 7-14). Pregnancy or extreme obesity may also result in an enlarged abdomen. The physical examination should determine which of these is the most likely cause. Often in ruminants the distention can be seen as primarily left sided, right sided, or bilateral. For example, bloat in ruminants results in a characteristic high left-sided gas distention. It may be primary or associated with vagal indigestion, tetanus, or hypocalcemia. With vagal indigestion the rumen becomes enlarged and fluid-filled, often giving a pear shape to the abdomen as it is viewed from the rear, or a pear shape on the right and an apple shape on the left (papple shape) if some degree of bloat is also present. Hypocalcemia and hypokalemia contribute to ileus and may result in constipation and abdominal enlargement. In sheep, abomasal impaction and enlargement associated with abomasal emptying defects can result in an enlarged abdomen with decreased food intake. When a mass (most commonly an abscess, a tumor, or a fat necrosis [cattle only]) obstructs fecal passage, abdominal enlargement can become severe. With obstructive disease, some degree of colic is almost always present. Ruptured bladder results in a large fluid-filled abdomen, but constipation is not an obvious sign.

The most common causes of decreased fecal output in ruminants and horses are decreased feed intake and dehydration. In these cases, the animal will appear gaunt or have a relatively empty abdomen or rumen. Horse feces in cases of prolonged transit are often covered with a layer of tenacious, thick, yellow mucus. When a functional obstruction (ileus, vagal indigestion) or physical obstruction (impaction, foreign body, displaced intestine, fat necrosis) occurs as a cause of constipation, the abdomen is more likely to appear normally full or to become distended. Rectal examination is of great help in determining whether a mass or an obstruction exists because loops of distended small bowel can sometimes be palpated in the latter case.

Radiographs and ultrasound may be valuable to help determine the cause of abdominal distention in foals, calves,

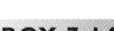

BOX 7-14

Causes of Abdominal Distention/Constipation in Ruminants

COMMON CAUSES
Pregnancy
Obesity
Vagal indigestion
Grain overload
Bloat
Ileus
Cecal volvulus/dilation with ileus
Peritonitis, traumatic or other cause
Fat necrosis involving rectum or colon
Ruptured bladder (uroperitoneum)
Intestinal obstruction
Pelvic mass (abscess, tumor)
Hypocalcemia
Omasal obstruction/foreign body

LESS COMMON CAUSES
Anticholinergics
Intussusception
Abomasal volvulus
Abomasal impaction
Tetanus
Abomasal bloat (calf)
Necrotizing enterocolitis (calf)

UNCOMMON CAUSES
Hydrops
Ascites
Torsion of descending colon
Internal herniation, especially diaphragmatic hernia involving reticulum
Displacement of intestine to left of rumen
Stenosis of duodenum
Adhesions of intestine
Bovine leukosis
Intestinal volvulus
Atresia of anus, colon, rectum or intestine
Abomasal adenocarcinoma
Omental bursitis
Perforated abomasal ulcer
Zinc toxicity
Crude oil toxicity
Diesel fuel toxicity
Propylene glycol toxicity
Larkspur poisoning

and small ruminants. Increased gastrointestinal gas may result in abdominal distention. Abomasal bloat and necrotizing enterocolitis in young animals may best be confirmed with lateral abdominal radiographs.

Dehydration may also result in dry feces but not in abdominal enlargement. When constipation is present and feces are drier than normal, rehydration and correction of hypocalcemia, hypokalemia, and any existing acid-base abnormalities are important parts of correction of the constipation. Other nonspecific therapies for functional constipation include laxatives, cathartics, and cholinergic drugs. When treating constipation, which is usually a secondary problem, it is important to simultaneously attempt to diagnose the primary disease.

In ruminants, when abdominal distention involves the rumen or is caused by pregnancy or obesity, colic is absent. When abdominal distention is the result of obstruction from the pylorus distal, colic is usually present. Abdominal distention and constipation are frequently accompanied by colic in the horse, regardless of anatomic site involved (review the approach to colic).

REGURGITATION/VOMITING
BRADFORD P. SMITH

Regurgitation is the reflux of esophageal, gastric, or rumen contents into the mouth or nose. This may be caused by malfunction of the esophagus or in ruminants as part of the normal physiology for rechewing ingested plant fiber (Boxes 7-15 and 7-16). Vomiting is a coordinated, centrally (medulla) mediated event, usually preceded by nausea (inappetence), increased salivation, or retching. In vomiting the abdominal musculature contracts, the diaphragm is pushed caudally, and the cardia relaxes. The medullary vomiting center can be stimulated by visceral afferent stimuli or through the chemoreceptor trigger zone. Most toxins and drugs that cause vomiting act by directly affecting the chemoreceptor trigger zone. Other than with toxins, most cases of feed returning to the mouth in large animals are examples of regurgitation rather than true vomiting. Vomiting is unusual in both ruminants and horses.

Although regurgitation is a normal phenomenon in ruminants, it is unusual to find excessive regurgitation as a sign of disease. Physical blockage of rumenoreticular outflow by a foreign body, warts, granulomas, or diaphragmatic hernia can cause rumen distention and excessive regurgitation following eating. An esophageal foreign body can cause irritation and result in regurgitation. Animals with facial paralysis may drool feed and saliva on the affected side; this should be differentiated from animals with excessive or abnormal regurgitation. Vomiting or forced regurgitation in ruminants is rare and is seen principally with the toxins listed.

Horses have such a marked tone at the cardiac sphincter that vomiting occurs only when extreme intragastric pressures develop, usually in small intestinal obstructive diseases or proximal enteritis. Vomiting in the horse thus often occurs with gastric rupture or terminally with shock. Stomach contents are usually pH 5.0 or below. Because it is a terminal event, vomiting in the horse is often grounds for rendering a poor prognosis. Abdominocentesis should be performed on a horse following vomiting to rule out gastric rupture. To avoid this sequence of events, decompression using a nasogastric tube should be performed in any horse with evidence of gastric distention (see approach to colic). Regurgitation and vomiting in horses most commonly occurs from the nose rather than into the mouth, because of the anatomy of the soft palate. With choke (esophageal obstruction), esophageal regurgitation from the nares consists of mixed feed and saliva.

In foals a few weeks to several months of age, milk returning from the nares is often associated with gastric ulceration, along with signs of colic, lying in dorsal recumbency, hypersalivation, and champing movements of the mouth. In advanced cases with duodenal ulcers, pyloric outflow can be obstructed by scarring, resulting in more pronounced signs. Foals 1 to 6 months of age are most susceptible to gastric ulceration.

Occasionally neonatal foals without cleft palate will have some mild degree of dysphagia with milk regurgitation from the nose for the first 24 to 48 hours of life, which spontaneously corrects. The cause of this is unknown, but would appear to be a failure of normal swallowing events to be sufficiently strong or coordinated in the newborn. The major ruleout in these cases is cleft palate.

Approach to Diagnosis of Regurgitation/Vomiting

Evaluation of regurgitation/vomiting should include a history to determine possible exposure to toxins or poison

BOX 7-15

Causes of Regurgitation/Vomiting in the Horse

COMMON CAUSES
Choke
Damaged esophagus, foreign body, or diverticulum
Foreign body in pharynx, trachea, or nose
Guttural pouch infection and pharyngeal paresis with nerve
    involvement
Gastric dilation
Gastric rupture

LESS COMMON CAUSES
Snake bite
Tetanus
Tick paralysis
Anterior enteritis (duodenitis/proximal jejunitis)
Gastric stenosis, ulcers
Hydrocephalus, meningitis, encephalitis
CNS trauma
Polyneuritis
Peritonitis
Persistent right aortic arch
Grass sickness (exotic)

TOXINS
Phosphorus
α-Naphthylthiourea (ANTU)
Cyanide
Herbicides
Arsenic
Lead
Nitrophenyl urea (vacor)
Organochlorine

PLANT TOXINS
Oleander
Castor bean
Death camas (*Zigandenus* spp.)
Algae
Heath (Ericaceae)

BOX 7-16

Causes of Regurgitation/Vomiting in Ruminants

COMMON CAUSES
Esophageal trauma or foreign body
Oral/pharyngeal foreign body, abscess, or trauma
Salt toxicity (water deprivation-access)
Tumor, papilloma, or other mass in rumen or esophagus
Toxins and poisonous plants

LESS COMMON CAUSES
Megaesophagus
Hiatal or diaphragmatic hernia
Esophageal diverticulum
Esophageal reaction to *Hypoderma lineatum* (B)
Hydrocephalus
Meningitis, meningoencephalitis
Central nervous system trauma

UNCOMMON CAUSES
Intestinal neoplasia
Traumatic reticulitis
Tick paralysis
Tetanus
Bluetongue (O)
Peritonitis
Persistent right aortic arch
Pseudorabies
Rift Valley fever (exotic)

TOXINS
Methanol or ethanol
Acute oral copper
Phosphorus

TOXINS—cont'd
Arsenic
Nitrates
Crude oil
Diesel fuel
Snake bite

PLANT TOXINS
Solanum spp.
Melia (chinaberry)
Larkspur *(Delphinium)*
Cyanogenic plants
Nitrate accumulators
Death camas (*Zigandenus* spp.)
Castor bean
Oleander
Cocklebur
Tremorgenic toxins
Heath (Ericaceae)
Helenium (sneezeweed, bitterweed)
Hymenoxys (rubberweed, bitterweed)
Veratrum (hellabore)
Amianthium (stagger grass)
Haplopapus (burroweed)
Psilostrophe (paper flowers) (O)
Agrostemma githago (corn cockle)
Kalmia (laurel)
Kikuyu (exotic)
Ibaraki disease (exotic)
Geigeria (exotic)
Yellow-wood (exotic)

B, Bovine; *O*, ovine.

plants, which is most likely when multiple animals are affected. Age of the animal limits some considerations; young animals are more prone to meningitis and central nervous system (CNS) trauma, and congenital problems such as esophageal diverticula and persistent right aortic arch are only found in neonates and may not be manifest as choke or regurgitation until solid food intake is increased.

The physical examination can determine whether the problem is vomiting or regurgitation. In ruminants, regurgitation often occurs as a result of distention and overfilling of the rumen, resulting in an obviously distended abdomen. Painful pharyngeal lesions can also cause pharyngeal paresis, which results in gagging and regurgitating. In horses the most common causes of feed coming from the nares are spontaneous choke and pharyngeal paresis associated with guttural pouch lesions (see section on dysphagia).

Physical examination should also include passing a stomach tube to determine whether any impedance to passage of ingesta is present (Box 7-17). Endoscopy is useful to visualize esophageal defects. Many endoscopes currently in use are not long enough to reach the stomach of the adult horse. Endoscopy of the rumen is rarely diagnostic, because it is almost impossible to empty it adequately to allow for visualization of a lesion. Ultrasound of the cervical esophagus may also be useful.

In horses and small ruminants radiography, particularly barium contrast studies, can be useful in detecting esophageal abnormalities. In foals, prolonged gastric emptying time may be diagnosed from contrast studies. Normal emptying and movement of contrast into small bowel occurs in less than 2 hours and reaches the large bowel by 3 hours. Radiography may also be useful in detecting diaphragmatic hernia.

The most significant complications of regurgitation/ vomiting include aspiration pneumonia, dehydration, and electrolyte imbalances. The marked hypochloremic alkalosis common to most monogastrics is rare in horses and occurs in ruminants mainly with internal vomiting (one type of vagal indigestion) associated with reflux of abomasal contents back into the rumen.

Vomiting, like diarrhea, is often an attempt by the body to rid itself of a noxious or toxic substance. Antiemetics are therefore rarely indicated in vomiting of central origin and rarely effective in regurgitation in large animals.

DYSPHAGIA (INCLUDING FEED FROM NARES AND EXCESSIVE SALIVATION)

BRADFORD P. SMTH

Dysphagia is used here to define abnormalities of prehension, mastication, or swallowing. It is associated with diseases of the mouth, lips, pharynx, esophagus, mandible, or masseter muscles or, in the case of neurologic problems, with central or peripheral lesions resulting in malfunction in these

areas. Diseases resulting in erosions, ulcers, swellings, crusts, or growths in or on the lips, mouth, or pharynx are discussed under a separate heading. Painful causes of dysphagia, such as dental problems, require differentiation from oral lesions such as ulcers as a cause of pain resulting in dysphagia.

The causes of dysphagia can be divided into three categories: (1) pain induced, (2) neurologic, and (3) obstructive (Boxes 7-18 and 7-19). A fourth category is mechanical interference with prehension and swallowing, but this usually appears similar to painful lesions in its manifestation. Particularly in horses, worn, missing, capped, abscessed, overgrown, or broken teeth often result in mechanical interference with chewing, resulting in half-chewed feed being dropped from the mouth (quidding). Observation of the animal as it attempts to eat and a good physical examination, including oral inspection and passage of a stomach tube to rule out choke, are essential in determining the cause of dysphagia. Use of a fiberoptic endoscope to visualize the pharynx, guttural pouches, and esophagus may be helpful. Plain film radiographs and barium swallows may also be indicated to see functional abnormalities in pharynx and esophagus during swallowing and to rule out fractures of the hyoid or mandible. Ultrasound should also be employed.

Pain is probably the most frequent cause of dysphagia in ruminants and horses. Oral lesions, oral foreign bodies, and poor teeth result in decreased feed intake, increased salivation, and often in dropping feed from the mouth while attempting to chew. Dental problems are relatively common in sheep and goats. In cattle, pharyngeal injuries from balling guns and paste wormers can result in severe pharyngeal cellulitis, which is manifested by an extended head, ptyalism, foul breath, and a painful, externally palpable, pharyngeal swelling. Mandibular fractures must be ruled out by careful examination, because even nondisplaced unilateral mandibular fractures can result in weak jaw tone, reluctance to eat, and drooling

When dysphagia is associated with loss of large amounts of saliva, metabolic acid-base and electrolyte disorders may develop. Cattle and sheep have saliva high in sodium (136 to 201 mEq/L) and bicarbonate (108 mEq/L) with potassium and chloride values in the 14- to 15-mEq/L range.[23,24] As a result, losses of large amounts of saliva can result in hypovolemia and severe metabolic acidosis. In contrast, horses have relatively high levels of salivary chloride (48 to 82 mEq/L) with relatively low salivary bicarbonate (44 to 52 mEq/L). Equine salivary potassium is 14 to 18 mEq/L, and sodium 54 to 90 mEq/L.[25,26] As a result, horses with esophageal fistulas that lost saliva had a transient metabolic alkalosis.[25]

In the horse a common cause of acute dysphagia is choke (esophageal obstruction), followed in frequency by pharyngeal paresis (neurologic) resulting from lesions in the guttural pouch that affect the pharyngeal nerves. Feed coming from the nose is the most obvious sign of both of these conditions. In choked horses, as a result of the length and position of the soft palate, feed comes mainly from the nares rather than coming back into the mouth. Choke and other obstructive diseases can be easily identified by using a nasogastric tube, whereas pharyngeal paresis may be associated with a number of neurologic or neuromuscular conditions, such as botulism or guttural pouch mycosis, which require careful differentiation. The most frequent serious problem associated with choke or pharyngeal paresis is inhalation (aspiration, foreign body) pneumonia. Mineral oil or other material that is particularly damaging if it gains entry into the lung should never be used in choke for this reason. In any animal with dysphagia, care must be taken to prevent aspiration pneumonia and to evaluate the thorax periodically.

Animals with facial paralysis often drool from the affected side and may pack feed into the cheek on the affected side.

BOX 7-18

Causes of Dysphagia in the Horse

PAIN

Tooth root abscess or periodontal disease
Worn, missing, capped, overgrown or broken teeth
Foreign body in mouth, pharynx, nose
Oral vesicles, erosions, ulcers, or growths
Pharyngeal abscess, cellulitis, trauma, fistula, or neoplasia
Esophageal choke, trauma
Strangles
Rupture of rectus capitus ventralis muscle
Snake bite
Oral, mandibular, or maxillary fracture, neoplasia, or
    granulomas
White muscle disease
Epiglottiditis, epiglottic cysts
Trauma or excessive traction to tongue
Hyoid bone injury
Nasal mass (granuloma)

OBSTRUCTION

Pharyngeal abscess, cellulitis, trauma, fistula, or neoplasia
Esophageal choke, trauma, megaesophagus
Strangles
Rostral displacement of palatopharyngeal arch
Damaged or abnormal esophagus
Cleft palate
Dorsal displacement of soft palate
Epiglottiditis, epiglottic cysts
Nasal mass (granuloma)
Lymphosarcoma
Purpura hemorrhagica

NEUROLOGIC, NEUROMUSCULAR

Yellow star thistle (Nigropallidal encephalomalacia)
Guttural pouch mycosis, infection, or tympany
Megaesophagus
Botulism
Lead toxicity
Rabies
Snake bite
Tetanus
Tick paralysis
Encephalitis, meningitis
Encephalopathy, hepatic
White muscle disease
Cerebrospinal nematodiasis
Electrocution
Transit or lactation tetany
Lymphosarcoma
Myeloproliferative disease
Myotonia
Otitis interna and media
Pontomedullary, brainstem neoplasia, pituitary abscess,
    trauma, neoplasm
Postanesthetic myasthenia
Herbicide toxicity
White snakeroot (tremetol) toxicity
Moldy corn poisoning
Locoweed (Astragalus, Oxytropis) toxicity
West Nile fever
Borna disease, Near East encephalitis (exotic)
Grass sickness (exotic)

BOX 7-19

Causes of Dysphagia in Ruminants

PAIN

Oral vesicles, erosions, ulcers, growths (see following section)
Foreign body
Pharyngeal abscesses/cellulitis or tumor
Traumatic or irritant stomatitis
Snake bite
White muscle disease
Actinobacillosis
Actinomycosis
Worn, missing, overgrown or broken teeth
Periodontal disease or tooth root abscesses
Oral, maxillary, or mandibular neoplasia
Fractured mandible or maxilla
Stomatitis
Necrotic laryngitis (calf diphtheria)
Ruptured or damaged esophagus

OBSTRUCTION

Foreign body
Pharyngeal abscess/cellulitis or tumor
Choke
Snake bite
Actinobacillosis
Oral, maxillary, or mandibular neoplasia
Megaesophagus
Hiatal or diaphragmatic hernia
Cleft palate
Bovine leukosis

NEUROMUSCULAR

Listeriosis
Rabies

NEUROMUSCULAR—cont'd

Tetanus
Botulism
Tick paralysis
Encephalitis, encephalopathy
Brain abscess
White muscle disease
Megaesophagus
Paresis of masseter muscles (mandibular branch of
    trigeminal)
Bovine leukosis
GM 1 Gangliosidosis in Freisian cattle
Meningitis
Encephalitis or encephalopathy
Atlantoaxial subluxation or occipitoatlantoaxial
    malformation
Hypocalcemia
Otitis media and interna
Pontomedullary brainstem neoplasia, trauma, infection,
    inflammation
Pituitary abscess
Pseudorabies
White snakeroot (tremetol) poisoning
Fireweed (Kochia scoparia) poisoning
Locoweed (Astragalus, Oxytropis) poisoning
Mercury poisoning
Kikuyu poisoning (exotic)
Ibaraki disease (exotic) (B)
Geigeria poisoning (exotic)
Ephemeral fever (exotic) (B)

B, Bovine.

BOX 7-20

Conditions Accompanied by Oral Vesicles, Erosions, Ulcers, or Growths in the Horse

COMMON CAUSES
Vesicular stomatitis
Phenylbutazone toxicity
Yellow bristle grass (*Setaria lutescens* or *Setaria glauca*) ulcers
Other plant awn stomatitis
Oral foreign body

LESS COMMON CAUSES
Irritant or caustic chemical stomatitis
Periodontal gingivitis
Blister beetle (cantharidin) toxicity
Uremia

BOX 7-21

Conditions Accompanied by Oral Vesicles, Erosions, Ulcers, or Growths in Ruminants

COMMON CAUSES
Vesicular stomatitis
Bluetongue (O)
Contagious ecthyma (Orf virus) (O, C)
Bovine viral diarrhea/mucosal disease (B)
Bovine papular stomatitis (B)
Traumatic or irritant stomatitis
Bristle grass (*Setaria lutescens* or *Setaria glauca*) ulcers
Other plant awn stomatitis
Oral foreign body
Actinobacillosis (woody tongue)

LESS COMMON CAUSES
Actinomycosis (lumpy jaw)
Cheek abscess
Periodontal gingivitis
Oak or acorn toxicity
Malignant catarrhal fever (B)
Irritant or caustic chemicals

UNCOMMON CAUSES
Caprine herpes virus (C)
Necrotic stomatitis

UNCOMMON CAUSES—cont'd
Epidermolysis bullosa
Familial acantholysis (B)
Oral neoplasia
Epitheliogenesis imperfecta
Hereditary zinc deficiency (baldy calf) (B)
Electrical injury
Bovine herpes 2 mammillitis (B)
Elaeophorosis (O)
Chlorinated naphthalene toxicity (B)
Thallium toxicity (O)
Giant hogweed (*Heracleum mantegazzianum)* toxicity
Lead toxicity
Mycotoxicoses
Ibaraki disease (exotic) (B)
Lumpy skin disease (exotic) (B)
Sweating sickness (exotic) (B)
Sheep and goat pox (exotic) (O, C)
Peste des petits ruminants (exotic) (O,C)

B, Bovine; *C*, caprine; *O*, ovine.

Listeriosis in ruminants is frequently associated with facial paralysis. In horses facial paralysis is usually caused by halter trauma or a blow to the head.

ORAL VESICLES, EROSIONS, ULCERS, OR GROWTHS

BRADFORD P. SMITH

Oral lesions are found with many conditions (Boxes 7-20 and 7-21). In general, they result in some degree of dysphagia or reluctance to eat because of pain. The lesions include vesicles, erosions, ulcers, crusts, or growths in or on the lips, tongue, gums, palate, or pharynx. Oral lesions are often associated with champing and increased amounts of saliva being observed on the lips or running from the mouth. When the volume of saliva is increased, the condition is called ptyalism, and the animal may be observed swallowing repeatedly. Pseudoptyalism refers to a normal volume of saliva that, because it is not swallowed, is visible to the observer, and may be confused with dysphagia (see previous section).

The approach to determining the cause of oral lesions is based on first determining whether the cause is likely to be an infectious disease (Table 7-1). Essentially all these infectious diseases are associated with a fever, although it is short-lived and moderate in the case of bovine papular stomatitis. Papular stomatitis rarely causes illness and is usually an incidental finding in calves with a different clinical problem. Most of the infectious diseases are associated with additional lesions or symptoms. They can be conveniently grouped into those causing diarrhea and those not usually associated with diarrhea. Of those not associated with diarrhea in North America, vesicular stomatitis (VS) is most common in cattle and horses, bluetongue in sheep, and contagious ecthyma (CE) in sheep and goats. CE can be readily differentiated from bluetongue because it involves primarily lips and gums and is proliferative, whereas bluetongue involves the tongue and dental pad most severely, is erosive, and is associated with other signs of generalized vasculitis. Laboratory diagnosis in acute cases of VS is done by working with state and federal veterinarians. Because VS is highly contagious and similar in clinical appearance to foot-and-mouth disease, quarantine and proper diagnosis are essential. Bluetongue is diagnosed by serology (AGID) and virus isolation. CE can be diagnosed serologically, by fluorescent antibody on the impression smear or biopsy of a lesion, and by isolation. Asymptomatic seroconversion to bluetongue is common where *Culicoides*

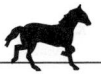

TABLE 7-1

Infectious Diseases Associated With Oral Lesions in Cattle, Sheep, Goats, and Horses

Disease	Natural Species	Oral Lesions	Other Lesions
Vesicular stomatitis (VS)	Cattle Horse Sheep (rare)	Vesicles for short time, then large ulcers; tongue usually severely involved	Teats and feet may be involved
Bluetongue	Sheep Goat (rare) Cattle (rare)	Large oral ulcers; dental pad and tongue most affected; generalized vasculitis	Coronitis, muscle degeneration, lameness, pulmonary edema, edema of face and ears
Contagious ecthyma (Orf, CE)*	Sheep Goat	Proliferative scabby lesion on lips to fleshy growth on gums	Occasionally on teats of nursing dams
Bovine papular stomatitis*	Cattle	Round, dark red, raised papules on muzzle and on hard palate	Occasionally in esophagus
Foot-and-mouth (exotic)	Cattle Sheep Goats	Vesicles for short time, then large ulcers	Teats and coronary bands often involved
Bovine viral diarrhea/ mucosal disease (BVD/MD)	Cattle	Ulcers in mouth, particularly on hard palate; erosive stomatitis	May have skin lesions; a few have corneal edema or enlarged lymph nodes; pneumonia and lesions in esophagus and gastrointestinal tract common; severe diarrhea
Malignant catarrhal fever (MCF)	Cattle	Erosive stomatitis with ulcers; generalized vasculitis	Purulent nasal discharge, corneal edema, enlarged lymph nodes, ± cracking skin, ± central nervous system signs; severe diarrhea; high fever
Rinderpest (exotic)	Cattle Sheep Goat	Erosive stomatitis	Blepharospasm, severe intestinal involvement, and diarrhea
Alimentary form of infectious bovine rhinotracheitis (IBR) in calves	Cattle	Gray pinpoint pustules on soft palate and occasionally in nares; minimal oral lesions	Rhinotracheitis, conjunctivitis, pneumonia

*Infectious to humans.

vectors are active. Congenital defects can result from bluetongue infection of the fetus in sheep, goats, and cattle.

The two most common North American infectious diseases associated with oral lesions and diarrhea in cattle are bovine virus diarrhea/mucosal disease (BVD/MD) and malignant catarrhal fever (MCF). MCF can usually be differentiated because it most commonly occurs sporadically in single animals and has signs of generalized vasculitis such as bilateral corneal opacity, mucopurulent nasal discharge, enlarged lymph nodes, and very high fever. Dysentery is common in MCF, and some animals exhibit CNS signs or have thickened and cracking skin. Laboratory diagnosis in acute cases of BVD involves fluorescent antibody testing of slides made from lesion swabs, buffy coat, or tissue. Virus isolation from swabs, serum, or buffy coat and a rise in serum titer from acute to convalescent samples are also diagnostic. Asymptomatic seroconversion is also common, and infection of the fetus may result in congenital anomalies, including cerebellar hypoplasia in cattle.

In animals without fever and other signs of systemic involvement, irritants and caustic chemicals should be considered as possible causes of oral lesions. Horses and young calves are susceptible to severe ulceration when consuming hay contaminated with yellow bristle grass, which is armed with barbed bristles.[27] Horses sometimes develop gingivitis or oral ulcers associated with dry plant awns called foxtails, which become embedded into the gums around teeth. Foals and ponies are most susceptible to phenylbutazone toxicity, which can produce oral ulceration. In cattle the surface of masses produced by actinobacillosis and actinomycosis

sometimes ulcerate. Many cattle without significant disease have one or more small ulcers of traumatic origin from plant awns on the hard palate and in the cleft (sulcus lingualis) where the base and shaft of the tongue meet.

DENTAL ABNORMALITIES

BRADFORD P. SMITH

Chronic fluorosis is a cause of a variety of dental abnormalities in young animals with developing teeth (Boxes 7-22 and 7-23). Although cattle are most frequently involved, all large animals are susceptible. The teeth may appear mottled, striated, chalky, hypoplastic, or have defective calcification. In severe cases, teeth may be yellow, brown, or black and have multiple caries. Animals of any age may also develop bone lesions associated with chronic fluorosis.

Porphyria is a rare congenital condition of cattle transmitted by a simple autosomal-recessive gene. The teeth often appear pink because of the presence of porphyrins and fluoresce pink, purple, or red when exposed to ultraviolet light. Affected calves often develop photosensitization and anemia. This condition must be differentiated from superficial staining caused by ingestion of black walnut hulls or other compounds with staining properties.

Excessive or uneven wear or loss of teeth is often seen in horses and ruminants as they age. Tooth wear, particularly of incisors, is more rapid in animals on sandy range. Periodontal disease can cause premature loss of teeth (broken mouth) and tends to be most common in sheep in some geographic areas; the cause for this is unknown.[28]

BOX 7-22

Causes of Dental Cavities, Abnormalities of Tooth Color, and Loose Teeth in the Horse

Periodontal disease
Chronic fluoride toxicity
Dental decay
Fractured teeth
Osteomalacia, osteodystrophy
Halicephalobus (Micronema) deletrix granulomas of mandible or maxilla
Skeletal neoplasia of mandible or maxilla
Hyperparathyroidism
Tooth root abscess with osteomyelitis, secondary to open infundibulum
Ameloblastoma (odontoma)
Dental stain (black walnut hull ingestion or other compound)

BOX 7-23

Causes of Dental Cavities, Abnormalities of Tooth Color, and Loose Teeth in Ruminants

Chronic fluoride toxicity
Bovine erythropoietic porphyria
Fractured teeth
Osteogenesis imperfecta in Friesians
Osteomalacia, osteodystrophy
Actinomycosis
Skeletal neoplasia of mandible or maxilla
Lymphosarcoma (goat and sheep)
Periodontal disease
Broken mouth (old worn teeth)
Tooth root abscess with osteomyelitis
Ingestion of black walnut hulls or other dental stain

BOX 7-24

Causes of Icterus in the Horse

LIVER
Common Causes
Pyrrolizidine alkaloid toxicity
Serum-associated hepatitis
Acute hepatitis
Chronic active hepatitis
Cholangitis or cholangiohepatitis
Bile stones, other biliary obstruction
Fasting hyperbilirubinemia

Less Common Causes
Aflatoxicosis with liver failure
Tyzzer's disease (foals)
Hepatic lipidosis
Hepatic abscess

Uncommon Causes
Black disease (infectious necrotic hepatitis)
Hemangioma, hemangiosarcoma, angiosarcoma
Cardiac neoplasm
Viral arteritis
Gastric or duodenal ulcers
Severe ascarid infection
Lymphosarcoma

HEMOLYTIC ANEMIA
Common Causes
Immune-mediated hemolytic anemia
Ehrlichiosis *(Ehrlichia equi)*
Neonatal isoerythrolysis

Less Common Causes
Piroplasmosis (babesiosis)
Snake bite
Blood transfusion
Erythrocytosis

Uncommon Causes
Equine viral arteritis
Leptospirosis
Bee or wasp sting
Sulfur toxicity
Trichloroethylene-extracted feed
Iron toxicity
Phosphorus toxicity
Herbicide toxicity
Phenothiazine toxicity
White snakeroot poisoning (tremetol)
Onions
Red maple *(Acer rubrum)*
Pentachlorophenol toxicity
Oak toxicity
Mycotoxicosis
Surra, *Trypanosoma evansi* (exotic)
Mal de caderas, *Trypanosoma equinum* (exotic)
Murrina de caderas, *Trypanosoma hippicum* (exotic)

The most common dental disease in horses has been described as periodontal disease.[29] In horses fractured teeth or teeth with a small tract into the root through an open infundibulum often result in tooth root abscesses. This dental decay is a result of hypoplasia of the cementum of the enamel lakes and occurs most frequently in the second and third lower cheek teeth and third and fourth upper cheek teeth.[30] These can cause sinusitis and foul-smelling unilateral nasal discharge if upper cheek teeth are involved or draining tracts to the exterior skin surface if lower cheek teeth are involved.

Most of the other causes of dental abnormalities listed here are bone abnormalities that cause secondary loss of teeth. See Chapter 30 for more details.

ICTERUS (JAUNDICE)
BRADFORD P. SMITH

Icterus and *jaundice* are synonymous terms referring to the expression of a yellow coloration in the sclera and mucous membranes resulting from increased amounts of bilirubin in tissues and increased serum bilirubin levels (Boxes 7-24 and 7-25). Bilirubin especially stains elastic tissues and is thus most visible in the sclera and vulva. Icterus usually indicates *decreased excretion* of bilirubin with liver or biliary tract diseases or *increased production* of bilirubin with hemolytic anemia.

The accumulation of conjugated bilirubin results in more pronounced jaundice than does a similar amount of unconjugated bilirubin, with the result that the most pronounced jaundice is usually seen with hepatic or biliary obstructive dis-

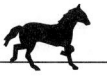

BOX 7-25

Causes of Icterus in Ruminants

LIVER
Common Causes
Pyrrolizidine alkaloid toxicity
Aflatoxicosis
Fat cow syndrome (fatty liver)

Less Common Causes
Acute hepatitis
Liver flukes
Infectious necrotic hepatitis (black disease)
Liver abscess
Cholangiohepatitis

Uncommon Causes
Sarcocystosis
Hepatic neoplasia
Ruptured gallbladder
Cholelithiasis
Biliary obstruction
Nolina (beargrass) toxicity
Lantana toxicity
Agave toxicity
Wesselbron disease (exotic) (B, O)

HEMOLYTIC ANEMIA
Common Causes
Leptospirosis
Anaplasmosis
Bacillary hemoglobinuria *(Clostridium hemolyticum)*
Piroplasmosis, babesiosis (exotic)

Less Common Causes
Snake bite
Immune-mediated hemolytic anemia
Transfusion reaction
Postparturient hemolytic anemia
Copper toxicity (especially sheep)
Neonatal isoerythrolysis
Yellow lamb disease *(Clostridium perfringens* type A) (O)

Uncommon Causes
Anaplasma ovis
Eperythrozoonosis
Bee or wasp sting
Brassica sp. toxicity
Trichloroethylene extracted feed toxicity
Iron toxicity
Onion poisoning
Zinc poisoning
Phosphorus poisoning
Mercury poisoning
Fireweed *(Kochia scoparia)* poisoning
Mycotic lupinosis
Mycosporum poisoning
Theileriosis (East Coast fever) (exotic)

B, Bovine; *O,* ovine.

minants also experience a rise in plasma unconjugated bilirubin, often to a level between 0.5 and 2.0 mg/dl.

In determining the cause of icterus, laboratory tests, including PCV, RBC count, and the liver enzymes sorbitol dehydrogenase (SDH) and γ-glutamyltransferase (GGT), should be determined. In horses, alkaline phosphatase (AP) may also be useful, although it is not liver specific.

When active hepatocellular damage is occurring, SDH, which is liver specific, and aspartate aminotransferase (AST [SGOT]), which is not liver specific, are found in serum in elevated levels. GGT and AP are more indicative of biliary tract disease or proliferation and tend to rise more slowly but also to remain elevated for a longer period than SDH, which has a short half-life. Elevated levels of GGT or AP are often associated with chronic liver disease, cholangitis, cholelithiasis, or liver flukes. *It is possible to have liver disease without icterus.* Production and elimination of bilirubin are often equal in chronic liver disease, but acute liver disease or liver failure is usually associated with icterus. Although liver function tests such as BSP half-time can be run to determine the extent of liver damage, in most cases a liver biopsy must be taken for histopathologic examination to make a specific etiologic diagnosis of the cause of liver disease.

Liver abscesses rarely result in icterus because they rarely damage a sufficient percentage of liver to impair bilirubin clearance. They do cause multifocal hepatic damage and therefore are often associated with increased levels of SDH and AST when in the acute stages of formation.

Hemolytic anemia is characterized by destruction of RBCs either intravascularly or in the reticuloendothelial organs. This increased destruction results in production of bilirubin more rapidly than it can be removed by the liver, resulting in icterus. The specific cause of hemolytic anemia may sometimes be evident, as when autoagglutination is seen (autoimmune hemolytic anemia), anaplasma bodies are visible in stained RBCs of cattle, or *Ehrlichia equi* blue cytoplasmic inclusion bodies are seen in stained neutrophils.

In sheep, the most common cause of severe icterus is copper toxicity.

REFERENCES
1. Merritt AM et al: Plasma clearance of (^{51}Cr) albumin into the intestinal tract of normal and chronically diarrheal horses, *Am J Vet Res* 38:1769-1774, 1977.
2. Holland JL et al: Calculation of fecal kinetics in horses fed hay or hay and concentrate, *J Anim Sci* 76:1937-1944, 1998.
3. Church DC: *Digestive physiology and nutrition of ruminants,* ed 2, Corvallis, Ore, 1979, O&B Books.
4. Moon HW: Mechanisms in the pathogenesis of diarrhea, *J Am Vet Med Assoc* 172:443-448, 1978.
5. Weese JS, Parsons DA, Staempfli HR: Association of *Clostridium difficile* with enterocolitis and lactose intolerance in a foal, *J Am Vet Med Assoc* 214:229-232, 1999.
6. Ulshen MH: Diarrhea and steatorrhea. In Hoeckelman RA, ed: *Primary pediatric care,* St Louis, 1987, Mosby, pp 905-916.
7. Cohen ND, Divers TJ: Acute colitis in horses. I. Assessment, *Compend Cont Educ (Pract Vet)* 20:92-98, 1998.
8. Magdesian KG, Madigan JE, Hirsh DC, et al: *Clostridium difficile* and horses: a review, *Rev Med Microbiol* 8:S46-S48, 1997.
9. Donaldson MT, Palmer JE: Prevalence of *Clostridium perfringens* enterotoxin and *Clostridium difficile* toxin A in feces of horses with diarrhea and colic, *J Am Vet Med Assoc* 215:358-361, 1999.
10. Brees DJ et al: *Lawsonia intracellularis*-like organism infection in a miniature foal, *J Am Vet Med Assoc* 215:511-514, 1999.
11. Soedarmant I et al: Pheno- and genotyping of *Rhodococcus equi* isolated from faeces of healthy horses and cattle, *Res Vet Sci* 64:181-185, 1998.
12. Hathcock TL et al: The prevalence of *Aeromonas* sp in feces of horses with diarrhea, *J Vet Intern Med* 13:357-360, 1999.
13. Herholz C et al: Prevalence of β-2 toxigenic *Clostridium perfringens* in horses with intestinal disorders, *J Clin Micro* 37:358-361, 1999.
14. Pearson EG, Heidel JR: Colonic and rectal biopsy as a diagnostic aid in horses, *Compend Cont Educ (Pract Vet)* 20:1354-1359, 1998.
15. Pace LW et al: Acute arsenic toxicosis in five horses, *Vet Path* 34:160-164, 1997.

ease. Laboratory examination of serum for relative amounts of unconjugated (indirect reacting) and conjugated (direct reacting) bilirubin is essential in determining the cause of the icterus. Generally, mainly unconjugated bilirubin levels are elevated with hemolytic anemia. Anorectic horses may have a plasma unconjugated bilirubin of 5 or 6 mg/dl without any evidence of hemolytic anemia or liver disease. Anorectic ru-

16. Guglick MA, Macallistar CG, Panciera R: Equine cantharidiasis, *Compend Cont Ed (Pract Vet)* 18:77-83, 1996.
17. Galey FD et al: Diagnosis of oleander poisoning in livestock, *J Vet Diagn Invest* 8:358-364, 1996.
18. Bueno AC, Seahorn TL, Moore RM: Diagnosis and treatment of right dorsal colitis in horses, *Compend Cont Educ (Pract Vet)* 22:173-181, 2000.
19. Cohen ND, Mealey RH, Carter GK: The recognition and medical management of right dorsal colitis in horses, *Vet Med* 90:687-692, 1995.
20. Jones PA, Tomasic M, Gentry PA: Oncotic, hemodilutional and hemostatic effects of isotonic saline and hydroxyethyl starch solutions in clinically normal ponies, *Am J Vet Res* 58:541-548, 1997
21. McGorum BC, Dixon DG, Smith GE: Use of metronidazole in equine acute idiopathic toxaemic colitis, *Vet Rec* 142:635-638, 1998.
22. Van Hoogmoed L et al: Evaluation of peritoneal fluid pH, glucose concentration, and lactate dehydrogenase activity for detection of septic peritonitis in horses, *J Am Vet Med Assoc* 214:1032-1036, 1999.
23. McDougall EI: Studies on ruminant saliva. I. The composition and output of sheep's saliva, *Biochem J* 43:99-109, 1948.
24. Phillipson AT, Mangan JL: Bloat in cattle. XVI. Bovine saliva: the chemical composition of the parotid, submaxillary and residual secretions, *N Z J Agri Res* 2:990-1001, 1959.
25. Stick JM, Robinson NE, Krehbiel, JD: Acid-base and electrolyte alterations associated with salivary loss in the pony, *Am J Vet Res* 42:733-737, 1981.
26. Alexander F: A study of parotid salivation in the horse, *J Physiol* 184:646-656, 1966.
27. Bankowski RA, Wichmann RW, Stuart EE: Stomatitis of cattle and horses due to yellow bristle grass *(Setaria lutescens)*, *J Am Vet Med Assoc* 129:149-155, 1956.
28. Andrews AH: Acquired diseases of the teeth and mouth in ruminants. In Harvey CE, ed: *Veterinary dentistry*, Philadelphia, 1985, WB Saunders, pp 256-271.
29. Baker GJ: Oral examination and diagnosis: management of oral diseases. In Harvey CE, ed: *Veterinary dentistry*, Philadelphia, 1985, WB Saunders, pp 217-228.
30. Baker GJ: Dental disorders in the horse, *Compend Cont Educ (Pract Vet)* 4:S507-S515, 1982.

Localization and Differentiation of Neurologic Diseases

MARY O. SMITH

Consulting Editor

MAJOR CLINICAL SIGNS/PROBLEMS ENCOUNTERED

TERMINOLOGY AND DESCRIPTION OF CLINICAL SIGNS OF NEUROLOGIC DISEASE (TABLE 8-1)

**Telencephalon (cerebrum, basal ganglia)
    and diencephalon (thalamus)**
  Changes in behavior
  Changes in the level of consciousness
  Dullness (depression)
  Stupor
  Coma
  Excitement, mania
  Seizures (convulsions)
  Narcolepsy
  Vision disturbance
  Blindness in both visual fields (amaurosis)
  Blindness in the contralateral visual field (hemianopsia)

Menace reflex deficit
Change in pupil size: small to pinpoint pupils
Circling (towards the side of the lesion)
Head turn (towards the side of the lesion)
Gait usually normal
Abnormal postural reactions (contralateral)
Decreased or absent conscious proprioception
Obvious ataxia, paresis (weakness), or paralysis are rare
Abnormal spinal reflexes
Hyperreflexia
Altered muscle tone
Spasticity

Urinary incontinence (upper motor neuron)
Tremors
Mesencephalon (midbrain)
Changes in the level of consciousness
Dullness (depression)
Stupor
Coma
Narcolepsy
Abnormal posture
Opisthotonos
Decerebrate posture
Abnormal visual or ocular function
Blindness in both visual fields (amaurosis)
Blindness in the contralateral visual field (hemianopsia)
Change in pupil size
    Small pupils in early/mild lesions
    Dilated, nonresponsive pupils in severe lesions
Menace reflex deficit (contralateral)
Anisocoria (asymmetric lesions)
Circling (toward side of lesion—ipsiversive)
Head turn (toward side of lesion—ipsiversive)
Abnormalities of gait (contralateral to lesion)
Decreased or absent conscious proprioception
Ataxia
Paresis (weakness)
Paralysis
Abnormal spinal reflexes
Hyperreflexia
Altered muscle tone
Spasticity
Urinary incontinence (upper motor neuron)
Metencephalon (pons, cerebellum)
Abnormal posture
Head tilt
Decerebellate posture
Circling (usually away from side of lesion)
Head turn (usually away from side of lesion)
Nystagmus (variable)
Abnormalities of gait
Ataxia
Hypermetria or dysmetria
Abnormal spinal reflexes (occasional)
Hyperreflexia
Altered muscle tone
Contralateral spasticity
Ipsilateral hypotonus
Urinary incontinence (upper motor neuron) (rare)
Medulla oblongata
Changes in the level of consciousness
Dullness (depression)
Abnormal posture
Head tilt (toward side of lesion—ipsiversive)
Circling (toward side of lesion—ipsiversive)
Head turn (toward side of lesion)
Strabismus
Nystagmus—spontaneous, abnormal
Dysphagia
Facial anesthesia, analgesia
Facial paresis/paralysis
Menace reflex deficit
Jaw weakness
Roaring, snoring, dysphonia
Tongue weakness, deviation, or paralysis
Abnormalities of gait—ipsilateral
Decreased or absent conscious proprioception
Ataxia
Paresis (weakness)
Paralysis

Abnormal spinal reflexes
Hyperreflexia
Altered muscle tone
Normal to increased muscle tone
Urinary incontinence (upper motor neuron)
Spinal cord C1-C5
Abnormalities of gait in thoracic and pelvic limbs—ipsilateral
Decreased or absent conscious proprioception
Ataxia
Paresis (weakness)
Paralysis
Abnormal spinal reflexes—ipsilateral
Hyperreflexia in both thoracic and pelvic limbs
Decreased to absent caudal cervical and auricular reflexes
Decreased to absent slap test (horses)
Altered muscle tone
Normal to increased muscle tone
Urinary incontinence (upper motor neuron)
Spinal cord C6-T2
Abnormalities of gait in thoracic and pelvic limbs—ipsilateral
Decreased or absent conscious proprioception
Ataxia
Paresis (weakness)
Paralysis
Abnormal spinal reflexes—ipsilateral
Hyporeflexia in thoracic limbs
Hyperreflexia in pelvic limbs
Decreased to absent caudal cervical and auricular reflexes
Decreased to absent slap test (horses)
Absent panniculus reflex
Horner's syndrome (ipsilateral)
Altered muscle tone
Decreased muscle tone in thoracic limbs
Normal to increased muscle tone in pelvic limbs
Urinary incontinence (upper motor neuron)
Spinal cord T3-L2
Abnormalities of gait in pelvic limbs only—ipsilateral
Decreased or absent conscious proprioception
Ataxia
Paresis (weakness)
Paralysis
Abnormal spinal reflexes—ipsilateral
Hyperreflexia in pelvic limbs only
Decreased panniculus reflex caudal to lesion
Altered muscle tone—ipsilateral
Normal to increased muscle tone in pelvic limbs
Urinary incontinence (upper motor neuron)
Spinal cord L3-S3
Abnormalities of gait in pelvic limbs only—ipsilateral
Decreased or absent conscious proprioception
Ataxia
Paresis (weakness)
Paralysis
Abnormal spinal reflexes—ipsilateral
Hyporeflexia in pelvic limbs only
Altered muscle tone
Decreased muscle tone in pelvic limbs
Flaccidity of the tail
Urinary incontinence (lower motor neuron)
Fecal incontinence (lower motor neuron)
Peripheral nerve and muscle
Abnormalities of gait
Paresis to paralysis in 1 to 4 limbs
Decreased or absent conscious proprioception
Ataxia
Paresis (weakness)
Paralysis

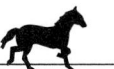

Abnormal spinal reflexes—ipsilateral
Hyporeflexia in 1 to 4 limbs
Altered muscle tone
Decreased muscle tone in 1 to 4 limbs

Muscle atrophy in 1 to 4 limbs
Flaccidity of the tail
Urinary incontinence (lower motor neuron)
Fecal incontinence (lower motor neuron)

TABLE 8-1

Localization of Central Nervous System (CNS) Lesions According to Major Signs Encountered

Symptom/Problem Encountered	Usual Lesion Location
CHANGES IN GAIT AND LOCOMOTION	
Ataxia	Nonspecific; any area of the CNS
Conscious proprioceptive deficit Knuckling Abduction/adduction Abnormal postural placement	Nonspecific; any area of CNS except cerebellum
Hypermetria	Cerebellum, cerebellar peduncles, spinocerebellar tracts
Circling, or falling to one side	Basal ganglia, cortex, vestibular nuclei, cerebellum
Paraplegia/hemiplegia	Nonspecific
CHANGES IN SENSORIUM AND BEHAVIOR	
Coma or semicoma	Brainstem, thalamus, cortex
Depression	Brainstem, thalamus, cortex
Convulsions	Brainstem, thalamus, cortex
Head pressing, propulsive walking	Cortex (frontal lobe), limbic system
Aggression/rage	Limbic system, frontal lobe, amygdala
Inappropriate sexuality	Limbic system
Hyperphagia/hypophagia	Hypothalamus
Diabetes insipidus	Hypothalamus
Head shaking	Unknown, probably peripheral neuropathy
CHANGES IN HEAD POSTURE	
Stiff neck	Meninges, cervical spine
Head tilt	Thalamus, cerebral cortex, medulla, cerebellum
Head tremor	Cerebellum, basal ganglia
Opisthotonos	Cerebellum (rostral vermis), rostral brainstem, cerebrum, cranial nerve VIII
CRANIAL NERVE DYSFUNCTION	
Amaurosis	Cortex, internal capsule, optic chiasm, optic nerve, eye
Anisocoria	Cervical spine, vagosympathetic trunk, mesencephalon (oculomotor nerve nucleus), cranial cervical ganglion, ciliary ganglion, oculomotor nerve
Mydriasis	Oculomotor nerve, brainstem (mesencephalon), eye
Miosis	Vagosympathetic trunk, ciliary ganglia, tectum, brainstem, cervical spinal cord
Ptosis	Facial nerve, vagosympathetic trunk, ciliary ganglion, tectum, brainstem, cervical spinal cord
Strabismus	
Ventrolateral	Cerebellum, vestibular nucleus, oculomotor nerve
Dorsomedial	Trochlear nerve
Medial	Abducent nerve
Nystagmus	
Horizontal	Nerve VII (peripheral)
Vertical/rotatory	Vestibular nuclei, peripheral vestibular receptor, cerebellum, vestibulocochlear nerve
Jaw drop	Metencephalon, trigeminal motor nucleus, trigeminal nerve
Flaccid tongue	Medulla, hypoglossal nerve, hypoglossal nucleus, tongue muscle
Facial paralysis	Medulla, facial nerve, facial muscles
Facial analgesia	Trigeminal nerve (sensory component)
Dry eye	Cranial nerve VII before entering petrous temporal bone
CHANGES IN REFLEXES	
Patellar	L4-L6 spinal cord, femoral nerve, quadriceps femoris muscle
Flexors (forelimbs)	C-5-T2 spinal cord segments, radial, ulnar, musculocutaneous and median nerves, and innervated muscles
Flexors (rear limbs)	L6-S2 spinal cord segments (hindlimbs), femoral, ischiatic, peroneal, and tibial nerves, also flexor and extensor muscles of the limbs
Triceps	C6-T1 spinal cord segments, radial nerve, triceps mucle
Panniculus	C8 spinal cord segment, thoracordorsal nerve, dorsal column of thoracic spinal cord
Anal	S1-S5 sacral spinal cord segments, pudendal nerve
Ear twitch	Dorsal columns of C1-C3 spinal cord segments; facial nerve, facial nucleus, muscles of ear
Dysuria (dribbling urine)	Spinal cord, pons, pelvic nerves, bladder wall

The clinical signs of neurologic disease depend on the location of the disease process within the nervous system. Widely varying disease entities may produce similar or identical clinical signs. Seizures, for example, may be the result of metabolic, toxic, traumatic, neoplastic, or other etiologies. Definitive diagnosis of neurologic disease therefore cannot be made on the basis of clinical signs alone. Localization of lesions within the nervous system, however, is the first and key step in developing a differential diagnosis list, and a rational diagnostic and therapeutic plan for any animal presenting with signs of neurologic disease. Lesions are localized with the help of the neurologic examination. In this chapter the clinical signs of neurologic disease and the methods and interpretation of the neurologic examination are described. Fortunately for the veterinarian, the clinical anatomy and the functions of the nervous systems of the various domestic animal species are almost identical. Thus the clinical signs of neurologic lesions are, for the most part, similar in all these species.

DIAGNOSIS OF NEUROLOGIC DISEASES

Signalment

MARY O. SMITH
LISLE W. GEORGE

The species, breed, age, and pedigree of an animal are important considerations in the differential diagnosis of neurologic disease. Many diseases are species-specific, particularly in the case of infectious and genetic diseases. Equine protozoal myeloencephalitis, for example, would not be a differential diagnosis in the case of cattle with signs of neurologic disease. Other infectious diseases, such as rabies virus infection, can affect many species. In yet other cases, all species may be affected but may show varying susceptibility to the disease. Such is the case with tetanus caused by *Clostridium tetani* exotoxin: horses and small ruminants appear to have significantly greater susceptibility to the disease than do cattle. Some diseases are not only species-specific, but also have higher incidence in certain breeds of that species. An example of this is equine degenerative myeloencephalopathy, which has been reported in several breeds of horses, but has an increased incidence in some breeds, such as the Appaloosa.[1] Examples of the numerous other breed-related neurologic diseases of large animals include cerebellar abiotrophy (Arabian foals), progressive ataxia (Charolais), demyelinating myelopathy (Limousins), neuraxial edema (polled Herefords), hydrocephalus (horned Herefords and shorthorns), epileptic seizures and weaver syndrome (Brown Swiss cattle), ceroid lipofuscinosis (Hampshire sheep), cerebellar abiotrophy, GM1 gangliosidosis (Holsteins), and many others.[2-9] Atlantoaxial malformations most commonly occur in Arabian foals and Holstein calves, but are not seen exclusively in those breeds.[10,11]

Disease susceptibility also may be linked to age. Acute lead poisoning, for example, occurs most commonly in calves, whereas adult cattle tend to develop the subacute form of the disease.[12] Some diseases are found in the neonate at birth. A large number of congenital disorders of the central nervous system (CNS) can affect domestic livestock. These diseases have a variable clinical course, depending on the nature of the disorder. Inborn errors of myelin metabolism worsen with age, whereas other developmental conditions may remain stable throughout the animal's life.[13-18] Examples of these disorders are listed in Chapters 47 and 48.

A knowledge of the most likely disease entities to occur within individual animals or groups of animals of particular species, breeds, and ages therefore can greatly assist the clinician in arriving at a list of likely differential diagnoses and formulating a rational diagnostic and therapeutic plan.

History

Many disorders of the CNS produce characteristic patterns of onset and progression, which can have diagnostic importance. Some CNS diseases occur acutely, developing the full range of clinical signs within hours. If the disease is not fatal, the signs either stabilize by 24 hours and remain constant thereafter or improve. Diseases that may display this clinical course include traumatic injuries, and some types of toxic, infectious, and metabolic diseases. Diseases with degenerative, viral, or neoplastic etiologies may develop more slowly, requiring days to weeks before the full extent of clinical signs is apparent.[2,19,20]

Diet

The diet of patients with neurologic disease should be evaluated[21-27] (Table 8-2). Common deficiencies of livestock include vitamins A and E, copper, selenium, and magnesium. Vitamin A deficiency occurs in feedlot animals that have no access to green plants; affected cattle become blind and develop seizures. Equine motor neuron disease is seen in horses that are housed without access to pasture and whose diet is deficient in vitamin E.[28] Copper deficiency occurs in ruminants pastured in areas with shale or volcanic soils, which are either deficient in copper or contain high concentrations of molybdenum and sulfur (secondary copper deficiency). The deficiency produces demyelination of the spinal cord in lambs or kids and pathologic fractures of the lumbar spine of rapidly growing calves. Dietary deficiency of calcium in rapidly growing weaned calves also results in vertebral and long bone fractures. Although dietary deficiencies of vital nutrients are commonly associated with the development of neurologic diseases, oversupplementation of certain nutrients also may produce neurologic disorders. Overfeeding of calcium, protein, and energy to horses, for instance, has been linked to the development of cervical vertebral instability and stenosis (wobbler syndrome) in horses.

Environment

Examination of the patient's environment may provide valuable information about the cause of CNS disease. Outbreaks of botulism and listeriosis have been associated with ingestion of rotting vegetation around haystacks, silos, or feed bunks.[29,30] Plant poisonings are common in livestock and identification of neurotoxic plants is important whenever multiple animals are simultaneously affected[30-32] (Table 8-3). Clinical signs of plant poisonings are variable and may include ataxia, hypermetria, head tremors, convulsions, paralysis, coma, or sudden death. Nonplant neurointoxicants of livestock include lead, ethylene glycol, organic mercurials, chlorinated hydrocarbons, organophosphates, salt, sulfur, petroleum distillates, and many others. Dose of the neurointoxicant may be important, with different clinical signs appearing depending on the level of exposure to the intoxicant. Ingestion of high concentrations of organophosphates or carbamates inhibits cholinesterase and produces signs of parasympathetic and neuromuscular activation, including marked ataxia, coma, muscle tremors, salivation, and miotic pupils. When low doses of organophosphates are ingested chronically, however, the result is an axonopathy of spinal cord and medullary neurons. The clinical signs that result are predominantly those of hind limb paresis and ataxia, which may progress to tetraparesis and recumbency.[33] Ingestion of petroleum distillates by cattle (motor oil, gasoline, kerosene) can induce narcosis. Some petroleum distillates also may contain toxic concentrations of lead. Other sources of lead include paints, batteries, waste dumps, and smelters. Thera-

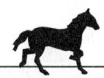

TABLE 8-2

Dietary Deficiencies Associated With Neurologic Disorders of Livestock

Dietary Deficiency	Disease Produced	Neurologic Sign
Copper	Demyelination, pathologic fractures of vertebrae	Ataxia, recumbency
Vitamin E	Demyelination	Ataxia, recumbency
Vitamin A	Encephalopathy	Convulsions, blindness
Magnesium	Grass tetany/transport tetany/milk tremors	Convulsions, tremors, ataxia
Potassium	Weakness	Postpartum recumbency
Calcium/phosphorus	Milk fever, pathologic vertebral fractures, tetany	Weakness, ataxia, recumbency, tetany
Vitamin E/selenium	Nutritional myodegeneration	Weakness, ataxia, recumbency, acute death

TABLE 8-3

Poisonous Plants Producing Neurologic Signs (Also See Chapter 50)

Plant Poisoning	Clinical Signs
Bermuda grass (*Cynodon dactylon*)	Ataxia, head tremors, truncal ataxia, spasms recumbency
Water hemlock (*Cicuta maculata*)	Tremors, vomiting, ataxia, sudden death, convulsions, odontoprisis, pupillary dilation, abortions, bloat
Poison hemlock (*Conium maculatum*)	Tremors, vomiting, ataxia, sudden death, abortions, pupillary dilation, bradycardia, coma
Blue green algae (*Aphanizomenon, Anabaena flos aquae*)	Sudden death, tremors, salivation, miosis, bradycardia
Laburnum (*Laburnum anagyroides*)	Excitement, incoordination, convulsions, death
Milkweed (*Aesclepias* spp.)	Tremors, salivation, ataxia
Larkspur (*Delphinium*)	Ataxia, collapse, recumbency, inability to lift head, tremors of face, flank, and hip; vomiting
Ryegrass ergot (*Claviceps paspali*)	Ataxia, head tremors, truncal ataxia, spasms, recumbency
Tobacco (*Nicotiana* spp.)	Tremors, salivation, ataxia, convulsions, birth defects
Nightshades (*Atropa* spp., *Solanum* spp.)	Tremors, ataxia, recumbency, convulsions
Monkshood (*Aconitum*)	Restlessness, salivation, paresthesia, irregular heartbeat, recumbency, coma
Locoweed (*Astragalus* spp.)	Ataxia, weight loss, recumbency, hyperesthesia
White snakeroot (*Eupatorium rugosum*)	Tremors, salivation, convulsions
Rayless goldenrod (*Haplopappus heterophyllus*)	Lassitude, depression, arched back, stiff-legged gait, tremors, weakness, collapse
Bracken fern (*Pteridium aquilinum*)	Ataxia, weight loss, strip sweating (horses only)
Horse tail (*Equisetum arvensii*)	Ataxia, weight loss, strip sweating (horses only)
Yellow star thistle (*Centaurea solstitialis*)	Facial rigidity, lack of prehension, ataxia, depression (horses only)
Tansy ragwort (*Senecio jacobea*) and Groundsel (*Senecio vulgaris*)	Ataxia, depression, somnolence, excitability, head pressing (hepatic encephalopathy)
Fiddleneck (*Amsinckia intermedia*)	Ataxia, depression, somnolence, excitability, head pressing (hepatic encephalopathy)
Rattlebox (*Crotolaria spectabilis*)	Ataxia, depression, somnolence, excitability, head pressing (hepatic encephalopathy)
Death camus (*Zigadenus* spp.)	Trembling, uncontrolled running, recumbency, opisthotonos, convulsions, vomiting, salivation
Dutchman's breeches (*Dicentra*)	Trembling, uncontrolled running, recumbency, opisthotonos
Buckeye (*Aesculus* spp.)	Incoordination, twitching, sluggishness
Rape (*Brassica napus*)	Blindness, ataxia, aggressiveness
Cheesewood (*Malva*)	Tremors, worsened by forced exercise
Lupine (*Lupinus*)	Tremors, hyperexcitability, depression

peutic and dietary interventions also may result in toxicoses when improperly administered. Overtreatment of cattle with nitrofurazone or propylene glycol produces profound ataxia, depression, and coma. Ingestion of ammonia or ammoniated feedstuff produces hyperesthesia, excitability, coma, and convulsions. High concentrations of salt in drinking water or, more commonly, lack of fresh water or interruption of the water supply followed by unlimited access to water, can result in laminar necrosis of the cerebral cortex or eosinophilic meningitis.[34] The clinical signs are those of cerebral dysfunction, including blindness, dullness, seizures, coma, and death. Although this syndrome has been reported in cattle and sheep,[35,36] pigs seem to be particularly susceptible.

Geographic area also may be important in the differential diagnosis of neurologic disease. Certain infectious diseases may be more common in particular areas of the country or even regions within a single state, where the conditions for disease vectors are optimal.[37] The travel history of the animal must be considered, as well as the animal's location at the time clinical signs appeared. Travel also may result in increased contact with other animals and greater risk of exposure to infectious diseases. Recent movement of animals onto premises may be important with respect to the likelihood of infectious diseases such as equine herpesvirus-1 and equine infectious anemia.

Vaccination and Infectious Disease History

When a neurologic problem is evaluated, the vaccination history and previous herd or individual disease problems should be noted. Some vaccines are highly protective, whereas others are less so. Examples of effective vaccines include focal symmetric encephalomalacia (enterotoxemia caused by *Clostridium perfringens* type D), rabies, and tetanus. Some outbreaks of herpes myelitis in horses have even been attributed to administration of certain poorly attenuated modified live virus vaccines (no longer available). Neurologic disease may be a secondary complication of disease in another organ system. Foals and calves with severe diarrhea, for example, may convulse secondary to hypokalemia, hypernatremia, or hypoglycemia. Preexisting diseases or clinical syndromes should be determined. For example, outbreaks of the CNS form of equine herpesvirus I are often preceded by respiratory disease or abortions in herdmates. Thromboembolic meningoencephalitis of cattle often follows an outbreak of respiratory disease within the herd. Historical evidence of limited colostral intake may be important in the diagnosis of bacterial meningitis of neonates. Bloody diarrhea often precedes the onset of nervous coccidiosis of calves.

Gestational Stage

Hypomagnesemia, eclampsia (hypocalcemia), and nervous ketosis are common causes of convulsions and tremors in adult livestock. These diseases usually occur between the end of the last trimester and the first 2 months following parturition.

NERVOUS SYSTEM EXAMINATION

General Comments

A thorough physical examination should always precede or be performed concurrently with the neurologic examination. Physical examination may reveal evidence of systemic disease that underlies the neurologic problem, such as icterus in animals with liver disease resulting in hepatic encephalopathy, unthriftiness in animals on poor diets, or traumatic injuries. In some instances, disease of organ systems other than the nervous system may take precedence for diagnosis and treatment. Such may be the case with animals in shock or suffering from other life-threatening cardiovascular or respiratory disturbances. A common practice is to perform a general physical examination followed by a neurologic examination, but many aspects of nervous system function, such as assessment of mental status and cranial nerve examination, may be carried out during the physical examination.

The neurologic examination should be carried out in a systematic fashion. The exact order of the examination is not important in itself, but procedures that may cause discomfort or pain, such as palpation of the spine, should be left until last. A common system used by many neurologists is to start at the head and progress caudally to the tail. This system is very useful in small animals, but may be less so in large animals. Because large animals are less amenable to handling than the typical cat or dog, an alternative system for the neurologic examination is to begin with procedures that require minimal handling of the animal, such as observation of mental status, posture, and gait, and proceed to those that require greater manipulation: examination of the cranial nerves, assessment of spinal reflexes, and so on. The latter is the system that is described below. Each individual should develop a system that is effective for him or her, bearing in mind that one goal of the neurologic examination is to induce as little stress in the animal as possible because stress may alter the results of the examination.

Neurologic examination alone rarely leads to definitive diagnosis, but rather helps to answer the questions: Does the animal have neurologic disease? and What is the location of the neurologic lesion? Once these two questions are answered a list of differential diagnoses can be made in light of other information such as the signalment of the animal and the history of the current problem. The diagnostic plan is based on the location of the lesion and the most likely differential diagnoses.

Mentation and Behavior

Initial examination should be done from a distance. The examiner observes the animal's mental state and whether its responses to its surroundings are appropriate. This is done ideally in the animal's usual environment, where it would be expected to be most calm. When this is not possible, the influence of factors such as the stress and excitement of previous travel, and the animal's natural fear of unfamiliar surroundings, sounds, and smells must be taken into account. The reports from the animal's usual handler may be informative, if he or she is a good observer and has an understanding of normal behavior in animals. Compare the patient's interaction with its environment to a summary of its previous behavior and to the activities of the herdmates. Normal animals respond to mild stimulation. Most normal animals actively seek food when offered but vigorously avoid needle pricks. All livestock should recognize and fear strangers and should show awareness of the examiner's position. Normal animals change the posture of the head, ears, and eyes as the examiner moves. Depending on previous conditioning, normal behavior may include cautionary moves, avoidance, belligerence, or affection. Animals with decreased mental awareness (obtunded, dull, depressed) have reduced responses that may include lassitude, lack of recognition, unwillingness to rise or lift the head from the ground, head pressing, propulsive walking, lack of appetite, drooped ears, convulsions, stupor, or coma (Fig. 8-1). Hyperexcitability, rage, mania, or frantic motor activities are suggestive of a lesion of the limbic system, an assembly of connected groups of neurons (nuclei) and neuronal tracts in the cerebrum, thalamus, hypothalamus, and midbrain that is involved in

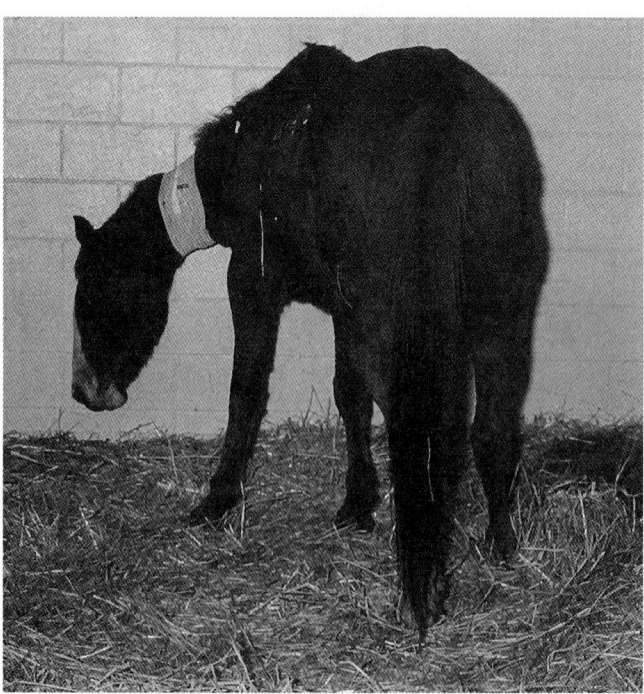

FIG. 8-1 ▌ Dull mentation in a horse with cerebral toxicosis caused by sage toxicity (*Salvia* sp.).

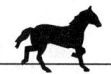

emotional responses and patterns of behavior. Such animals may strike or kick at inappropriate times, demolish their stall, bellow, show belligerence, or, if recumbent, struggle violently. The age, species, previous management system, and even the breed of animal are important considerations in the assessment of behavior. Bulls and stallions exhibit very different behavior from steers and geldings. Beef cattle behave differently from dairy cattle. Animals that are handled regularly show fewer and milder fearful or aggressive responses than do animals that are rarely handled.

Changes in mental status are a consequence of disease affecting either the cerebrum or the ascending reticular activating system (ARAS). The cerebral cortex is the "seat of consciousness"; conscious perception of both external stimuli (e.g., vision, hearing, touch) and internal stimuli (e.g., abdominal pain) depends on the integrity of the cerebral cortex. Both primary intracranial diseases (e.g., encephalitis, traumatic injury) and extracranial diseases (e.g., metabolic derangements, toxicities) can alter the functions of the cerebral cortex.

The ARAS is composed of a number of neuronal pathways that lie centrally within the brainstem (medulla oblongata, midbrain, and thalamus). The ARAS receives collateral input from all sensory information reaching the brain, which it conveys ultimately to the cerebral cortex, where it reaches the level of consciousness. The ARAS is important in maintaining the animal's level of consciousness and arousal. The relationship between the cerebral cortex and the ARAS is sometimes described as follows: the cerebral cortex determines the content of consciousness and the ARAS determines the level of consciousness. Diseases affecting the ARAS tend to produce more profound depression of consciousness, such as coma, than do those affecting the cerebral cortex itself, although this is not an absolute rule. Lesions of the ARAS occur commonly within the midbrain segment of this system, so that other signs of midbrain disease, such as pupillary dilation and loss of the oculocephalic reflexes (see below), are often observed in animals with lesions of the ARAS.

A seizure (convulsion, ictus) is a manifestation of cerebral cortex dysfunction characterized by loss of consciousness or involuntary motor activities. Seizures may be generalized or focal (partial). The terms *grand mal* and *petit mal* often are used to mean generalized seizure and focal seizures, although the use of these terms is incorrect in veterinary medicine. Generalized seizures are characterized by complete loss of consciousness and variable degrees of involuntary motor activity, which may include flailing of the limbs, vocalization, salivation, vomiting, elimination of feces and urine, and nystagmus. Focal seizures are characterized by localized involuntary movements with or without obvious alterations of consciousness. Alternatively, focal seizures may result in episodes of abnormal or bizarre behavior, or momentary lapses of consciousness without collapse or significant motor activity. A third form of seizure is focal with secondary generalization. The onset of the seizure is focal, but seizure activity subsequently spreads throughout the cerebral cortex, resulting in a generalized seizure. Animals with this form of seizure activity exhibit initial focal signs, such as head turning, bellowing, focal tremors, and so on, followed by loss of consciousness and generalized signs of involuntary motor activity, as described above. In most animals with focal seizures, with or without secondary generalization, the outward manifestation of the seizure is always the same. Seizures may be preceded by an aura, a period in which the animal exhibits anxiety or restless behavior shortly before the onset of the seizure itself. In most cases of seizures in animals, however, an aura is not observed. A postictal phase, a period of time subsequent to the seizure during which the animal exhibits abnormal behavior such as lethargy, restlessness, or anxiety, is usual after seizures in most animals. The postictal phase usually lasts a few minutes to hours, but may be as long as several days. The postictal phase may be the only stage of the seizure observed by the animal's handler. Thus any animal with a history of episodes of abnormal behavior should be suspected of having seizures. The typical history is that the animal is found in a dull or excited state, without the handler observing the onset of this change of behavior. Additional supporting evidence includes physical injuries such as scrapes and cuts that may have been incurred during the seizure itself.

Abnormalities of cerebral cortex dysfunction are the ultimate cause of seizure activity. During a seizure small or large groups of neurons in the cerebral cortex exhibit spontaneous electrical activity resulting in the clinical manifestations of focal or generalized seizures. Whereas neurons in the cerebral cortex ultimately become involved, abnormal electrical activity can begin elsewhere in the brain, such as in the brainstem, with subsequent spread of this activity to the cerebrum. Causes of seizures are legion, including alterations in the neuronal environment resulting from metabolic disturbances or toxicities, and the effects of structural brain diseases such as traumatic injuries, neoplasia, and inflammatory conditions. Diagnosis of seizures and other states of altered mentation must include a thorough physical examination and screening for metabolic diseases such as electrolyte imbalances and hepatic or renal failure.

Abnormalities in the neurologic examination found during the time between seizures (interictal period) supports a diagnosis of primary brain disease, and is an indication for diagnostic procedures such as cerebrospinal fluid tap. Some toxins cause systemic signs as well as seizures, such as neuromuscular involvement (tremors, weakness) or parenchymal organ failure (icterus, uremia). Such signs, combined with a good clinical history and complete examination of the animal's environment, will help to direct specific toxicologic screening tests.

Narcolepsy is a condition wherein the normal mechanisms of sleep are disturbed. Although sudden onset of REM sleep is one manifestation of narcolepsy, the acute onset of cataplexy—complete paralysis of striated muscles—usually is a more prominent clinical feature. Animals may be observed to suddenly collapse to the ground or to buckle at the knees. Cardiac and respiratory muscles are not affected. Narcoleptic attacks may be difficult to distinguish from seizures, but are not accompanied by the involuntary motor activity that characterizes most generalized seizures. In some cases owners observe traumatic injuries to the head, face, and limbs, without observing the cataplectic attacks that cause the trauma. Narcolepsy has been reported both in cattle and horses.[38-40]

Gait

Gait should be evaluated by moving the animal in a straight line, then in a tight circle, and over obstructions. Quadrupeds begin walking by protracting the rear limb, followed by the forelimb of the same side, then the opposite rear limb, and finally the opposite forelimb. Gait on a level surface requires integrity of the musculature, motor and sensory components of the peripheral nerves, local spinal reflexes, ascending and descending pathways in the spinal cord, and centers within the brainstem. Dysfunction of any of these areas results in an animal with mild to severe proprioceptive disturbances when standing or walking, which are exacerbated by turning the animal in a circle or stepping it on and off a curb. Animals with cerebral disease usually are able to perform simple motor activities such as walking along a straight path without obvious deficits, but exhibit decreased proprioception when they are required to perform complex motor activities, such as walking on slopes or negotiating obstacles such as curbs or ground poles. Performance of such complex maneuvers requires coordination of proprioception and motor activities within the cerebral cortex, basal ganglia, and other CNS centers. Further information about conscious proprioception can be gained by walking and then trotting the patient, or walking or trotting the patient briskly and then stopping suddenly. While a helper is walking the animal in a straight line on a level surface, the examiner should take hold of the tail and pull the animal sharply to one side. The normal animal will move toward the pull, but should not stumble or fall. If the tension on the tail is maintained, strength can be assessed. Animals with lesions anywhere within the ascending or descending pathways controlling gait may show decreased proprioception in the form of stumbling, tripping, or crossing the limbs or may be weak. This maneuver also is useful for assessing the symmetry of a lesion.

Proprioception is the sense of position in space. Receptors lie in the skin, joints, and muscles. Ascending pathways run mainly in the dorsal funiculus of the spinal cord, relaying information to centers in the brainstem and cerebral cortex. Descending pathways involved in proprioception are largely similar to those that control gait. The vestibular system and pathways in the spinal cord to and from the vestibular centers in the medulla oblongata and cerebellum also help to control proprioception. Abnormalities of proprioception include knuckling, stumbling, adduction or abduction of the limbs, circumduction, or interference between limbs (Fig. 8-2). Animals with proprioceptive deficits often slap down the feet hard, rather like the gait of a person walking down stairs in the dark, unsure of where the next step is. Walking the animal off a curb or step exaggerates this appearance. When spun in a tight circle, normal animals lift the inside forefoot as the weight shifts. The outside rear leg is put down within a line demarcated by the lateral margin of the trunk. When spun in a tight circle, patients with abnormal proprioception may pivot on the inner forefoot rather than lifting it and replacing it into a normal position. The outside foot may circumduct widely, knuckle, or buckle, and the inside foot may step on the outside foot. Animals with abnormal proprioception worsen when they are required to climb hills, lift the foot over a curb, or are walked with the head elevated. The gait of noncompliant cattle may be assessed by observation of maneuvers through corrals, alleys, or a squeeze chute.

Both strength and proprioceptive function can be tested further by having the animal back up. The normal subject should be able to do so in a smooth, coordinated fashion. Animals with lesions of either the ascending or descending motor pathways may exhibit abnormalities such as foot dragging and weakness, sometimes to the point of "dog-sitting." Otherwise cooperative animals may be reluctant to back and will try avoidance maneuvers such as circling to one side or the other in order to not have to move straight backwards. Such tactics should raise the index of suspicion of a neurologic deficit. Care should be taken when backing an animal with severe neurologic deficits because some animals could fall backward during the procedure. Animals that are uncooperative or that have been little handled may exhibit reluctance to back that is not caused by neurologic disease. Observing the patient's general level of cooperation and having a good history will help the examiner determine whether the problem is caused by neurologic disease or is the result of the animal's lack of compliance.

Cerebellar disease causes generalized ataxia with a rolling, drunken gait. Protraction of the limbs is delayed and limb movements are exaggerated, a condition known as hypermetria. This is often accompanied by opisthotonos, which is a hyperextension of the head and neck, and intention tremor,

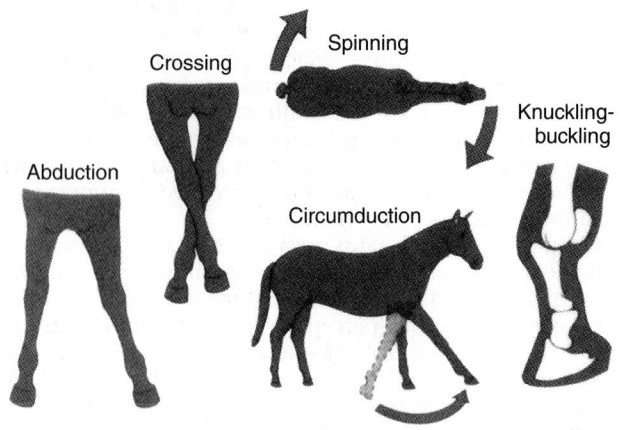

HORSE PROPRIOCEPTIVE DEFICITS

FIG. 8-2 ▓ Examples of conscious proprioceptive deficits in a horse. The signs of proprioceptive deficits in ruminants are similar.

most easily observed in the head. Purposeful movements, such as reaching out to take food, exaggerate intention tremor, and muscular relaxation, as in a recumbent animal, eliminates it.

Spontaneous circling is seen in diseases of the vestibular system, midbrain, and cerebrum. Circling varies from a mild tendency to circle in one direction to tight and compulsive circling, seen particularly in midbrain disease. Circling occurs towards the side of the lesion, except in paradoxical vestibular disease (caused by lesions in the vestibular components of the cerebellum), in which the animal circles away from the side of the lesion. Localization of the neurologic lesion in animals that circle is made on the basis of other neurologic abnormalities, such as the state of consciousness, the presence of proprioceptive deficits, and the presence of signs such as head tilt, spontaneous nystagmus, seizures, or abnormal ocular function.

Conscious Proprioception and Postural Reactions

The integrity of conscious proprioceptive pathways may be tested by means of the postural reactions. Normal large animals stand at rest with the limbs in line with the abaxial boundaries of the trunk. When the limbs are moved, normal animals do not permit the limbs to be placed outside of the body axis or across midline. After placement of the limbs in an abnormal position, the neurologically intact animal returns to a normal stance within a few seconds. Animals with conscious proprioceptive deficits allow the limb to remain in the abnormal position for longer than the usual period of time. This can vary from slightly slowed replacement of the limb into a normal position, to animals that do not try to replace the limb at all. The examiner should cross one of the animal's limbs over the opposite limb, or abduct one limb; the normal response is for the limb to be placed back into the resting position. Normal animals often strongly resist attempts to place the limbs in abnormal positions. Animals with proprioceptive deficits may spontaneously place the limbs in abnormal positions: excessively adducted, abducted, or even crossed. Abnormalities of proprioception alone are poorly localizing signs, although a couple of generalities may be stated. Unilateral lesions rostral to the medulla oblongata produce mild to moderate proprioceptive and postural deficits in the contralateral limbs. Unilateral lesions in the medulla oblongata or spinal cord produce more severe proprioceptive and postural deficits in the ipsilateral limbs. Lesions in the cerebellum very rarely result in deficits in postural reactions and conscious proprioception.

Additional postural reactions, such as hopping and hemiwalking, can be tested in small ruminants, calves, and some foals. Hopping is tested in the forelimbs by lifting the rear limbs a few inches off the ground by means of a hand and arm placed around the abdomen, flexing one forelimb slightly, and moving the animal away from the side of the flexed forelimb, so that it has to hop laterally on the forelimb still in contact with the ground. It is easiest if the examiner stands in one place and turns clockwise when testing the animal's right forelimb and counterclockwise when testing the left forelimb. Hopping in the rear limbs can be tested similarly, supporting both forelimbs off the ground with an arm around the chest. Hemiwalking is tested by supporting both limbs on one side of the body in a slightly flexed position and pushing the animal toward the opposite side so that it must walk laterally on the two limbs still in contact with the ground. Both hopping and hemiwalking should be done with care not to push the patient over. Hopping and hemiwalking involve the same ascending and descending motor tracts involved in regular gait, but also require integrity of the cerebral cortex. These maneuvers are abnormal on the ipsilateral side in animals with lesions in the skeletal muscles, peripheral nerves, spinal cord, and medulla oblongata and on the contralateral side in animals with lesions in the midbrain, thalamus, or cerebrum. Animals with cerebral lesions have normal gait on a level surface, but marked deficits in hemiwalking and hopping.

Abnormalities of Posture and the Righting Response

Posture refers to the position of the body and head in space, with relationship to gravity and to each other. Animals adopt slightly different postures when on a sloped surface or an uneven surface compared with posture on a level surface. However, sustained postures such as head tilt (Fig. 8-3), in which one ear is closer to the ground than the other, or head turn (Fig. 8-4), where the muzzle is turned back toward the trunk are abnormal. Circling often accompanies head tilt and head turn, and all tend to be towards the direction of the lesion. The exception to this rule occurs in paradoxical vestibular syndrome as a result of involvement of the cerebellar components of the vestibular system, in which head tilt and circling occur in the direction away from the side of the lesion. When proprioceptive deficits accompany circling they are ipsilateral when the lesion is in the medulla oblongata and contralateral when the lesion lies in the cerebrum, thalamus, or midbrain. Head tilt, head turn, and circling reflect the presence of lesions that are unilateral within the neuraxis or are asymmetric.

The righting response is most easily tested in small ruminants and in recumbent large animals (Fig. 8-5). The response is initiated by receptors in the eyes and vestibular labyrinths and by proprioceptive receptors in the joints, tendons, and muscles. Information regarding limb position and balance is relayed ultimately to the cerebral cortex. Descending impulses are initiated in the motor cortex and relayed via the brainstem and spinal cord to the appendicular musculature. The normal response to stimulation is to lift the head, assume sternal recumbency, and to rise. The normal horse rises on the forelimbs first, whereas the normal ruminant rises on the rear limbs first. Animals that are reluctant to rise but do so normally after sufficient stimulation may have a disease of the cerebral cortex or the thalamus. Animals that are in lateral recumbency and unable to lift the head from

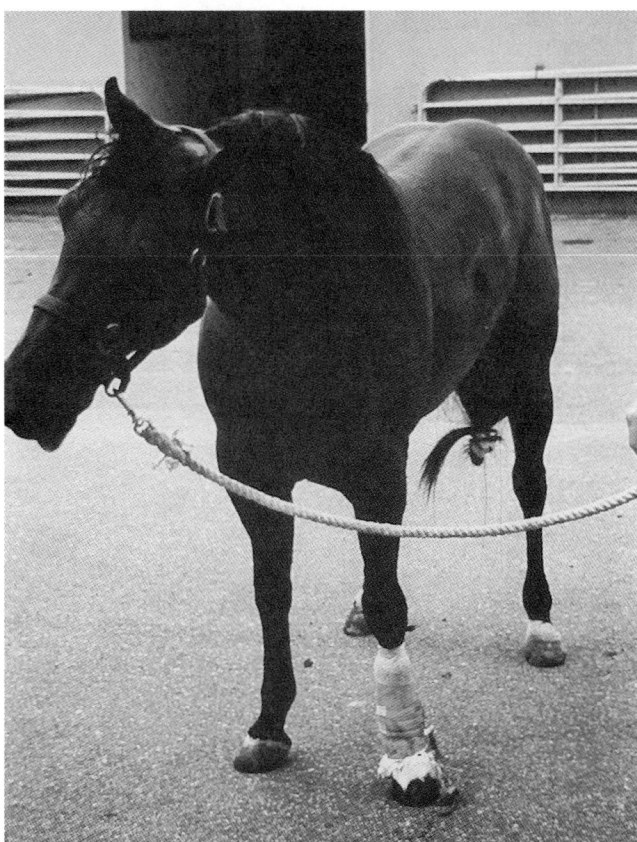

FIG. 8-3 ▐▐ Head tilt caused by vestibular dysfunction in a horse that sustained head trauma.

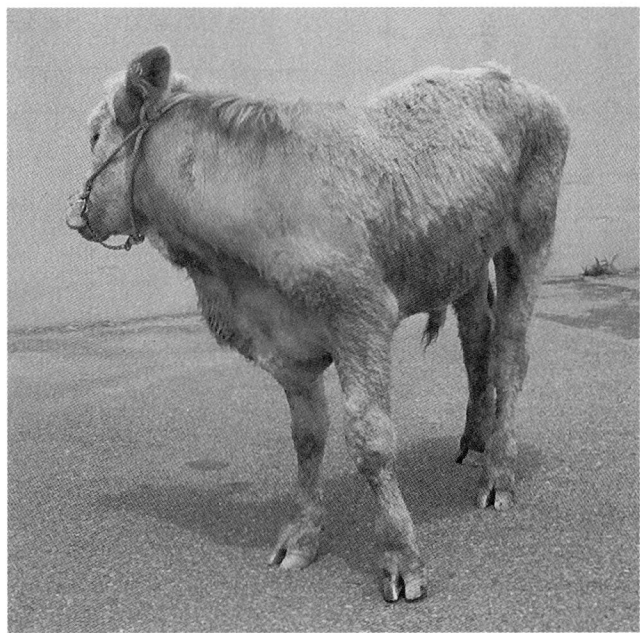

FIG. 8-4 ▐▐ Head turn in a steer with polioencephalomalacia.

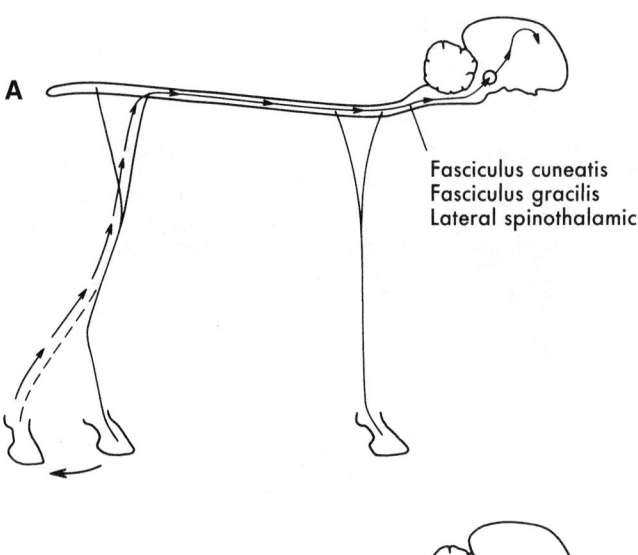

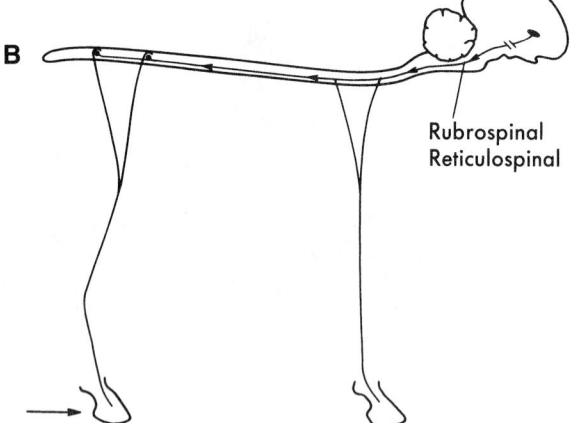

FIG. 8-5 ▓ **A,** Afferent pathways responsible for providing proprioceptive information to the brainstem and higher centers. **B,** Efferent pathways responsible for providing motor activities to the motor neurons.

the ground may have lesions in the peripheral or brainstem vestibular centers, or in the cervical spinal cord proximal to the C4 spinal cord segment. Unilateral lesions in this area result in an inability to lift the head from the ground when the lesion side is up. When the lesion side is down, the animal can raise the head slightly. Animals with incomplete lesions of the cervicothoracic spinal cord (C7 to T1 spinal cord segments) are able to lift the head and neck but may remain recumbent. Animals with lesions of the thoracolumbar and lumbosacral spinal cord (T3 to S3 spinal cord segments) usually can lift the head and neck, arise on the forelimbs, and assume a dog-sitting position when stimulated.

Spinal Reflexes

The spinal reflexes are stereotyped responses to specific stimuli. They include the myotactic or tendon reflexes, the panniculus or cutaneous reflex, the perineal reflex, and several others. As their name implies, spinal reflexes depend on the integrity of local spinal cord segments, as well as the peripheral nerves, neuromuscular junctions, and muscles. Lesions in the spinal cord that are located rostral to the spinal origin of the peripheral nerves to the limbs being tested result in normal to increased spinal reflexes, and are commonly referred to as upper motor neuron lesions. Lesions in the spinal cord segments at the level of the reflex arc, or in the periph-

eral nerves, neuromuscular junctions, or muscles, result in decreased spinal reflexes and are commonly referred to as lower motor neuron lesions.

It is appropriate at this point to define the terms *upper motor neuron* and *lower motor neuron.* Upper motor neurons (UMN) are nerve cells whose cell bodies lie within the brain and whose axons terminate at synapses within the brain or in the spinal cord. Disease affecting upper motor neurons results in normal to increased spinal reflexes, as well as ataxia, variable severity of weakness, and sometimes increased muscle tone (spasticity). The nerve cell bodies of lower motor neurons (LMN) lie in the nuclei of cranial nerves in the brainstem, or within the ventral horn gray matter of the spinal cord. Their axons project beyond the central nervous system, course within the peripheral or cranial nerves, and terminate at neuromuscular junctions. Disease affecting lower motor neurons results in decreased spinal reflexes, ataxia, moderate to severe weakness, decreased muscle tone, and rapid, pronounced atrophy of the denervated muscles.

Myotactic Reflexes

Myotactic or tendon reflexes are tested by sharply striking the tendon of a specific muscle (or sometimes the muscle itself) and evaluating the strength of the reflex contraction. The ascending component of the reflex arc involves the muscle spindles, which are stretch detectors, sensory fibers in the peripheral nerve, the dorsal nerve root and its ganglion, and the central projection of the sensory nerve fiber onto the ventral horn cell in the same spinal cord segment (Fig. 8-6). The descending component of the reflex arc involves the ventral horn cell (LMN), the ventral nerve root, the motor fibers in the peripheral nerve, the neuromuscular junction, and the myofibers in the muscle being tested. Lesions in either the ascending or descending components of the reflex arc result in a decreased to absent myotactic reflex. Lesions in the spinal cord above the level of the reflex arc and lesions of the brain result in a normal to increased myotactic reflex.

The myotactic reflexes can be tested only in the recumbent animal, thus are able to be examined only in a limited number of large animal patients. These reflexes should be tested only in the limbs that are uppermost when the animal is lying on one side. The animal must be turned over to test the limbs on the opposite side. These reflex responses are more subtle than in small animals and may not be elicited in some normal patients. The reflex responses are assigned a qualitative clinical score. One common classification is as follows:

0—No reflex activity
1—Hypoactive
2—Normal
3—Hyperactive
4—Hyperactive and clonic

Clonus is a phenomenon observed with severe UMN lesions; the response of the muscle being tested is rapid, repeated contractions rather than a single contraction. The innervation of the limbs is shown in Tables 8-4 and 8-5.

FORELIMB MYOTACTIC REFLEXES

Triceps Reflex. Hold limb moderately flexed at the elbow and percuss the triceps tendon just above the olecranon using a heavy instrument, such as a balling gun. In smaller subjects a rubber pleximeter can be used, as is done in cats and dogs. The normal response is a contraction of the triceps muscle, leading to retraction of the upper limb and extension of the elbow. The triceps reflex measures the integrity of the radial nerve and the C7 to T1 spinal segments.

Biceps Reflex. Hold the limb moderately extended at the elbow and place the supporting hand over the attachment of the biceps muscle on the anteromedial aspect of the limb at the level of the elbow joint. Percuss the biceps tendon or the

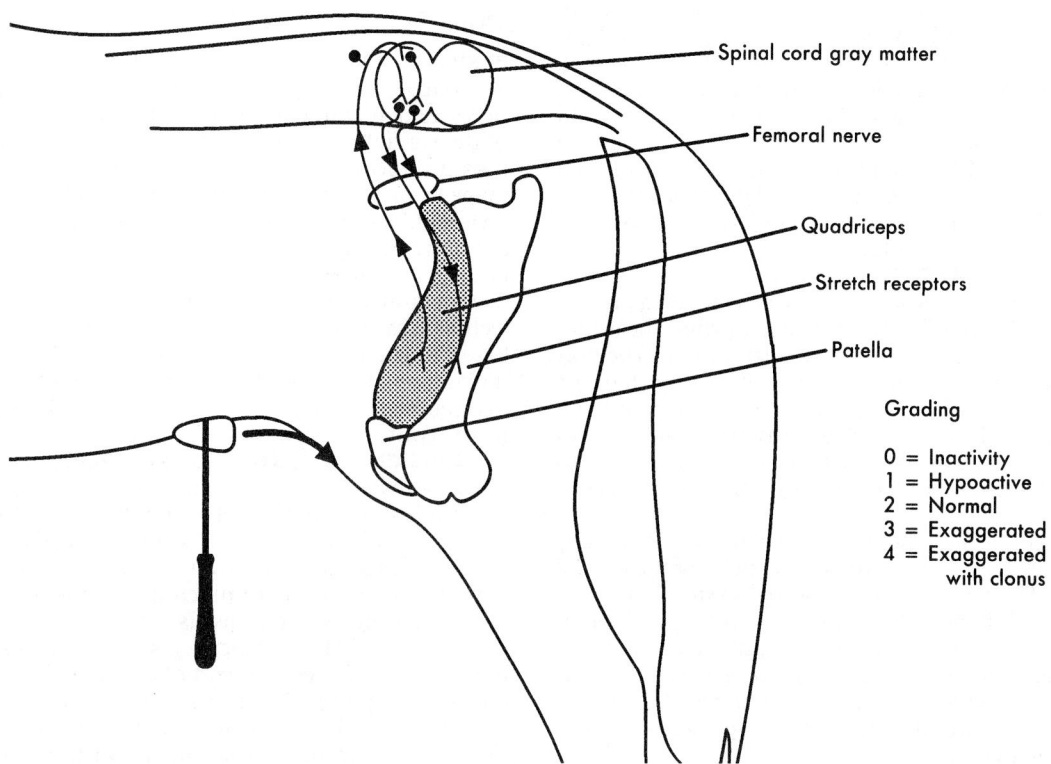

- Spinal cord gray matter
- Femoral nerve
- Quadriceps
- Stretch receptors
- Patella

Grading

0 = Inactivity
1 = Hypoactive
2 = Normal
3 = Exaggerated
4 = Exaggerated
    with clonus

FIG. 8-6 ▇ Pathways governing patellar tendon reflex.

TABLE 8-4

Innervation of the Forelimbs of Large Animals

Spinal Cord Segment	Peripheral Nerve	Muscle(s)
C7	Suprascapular	Supraspinatus, infraspinatus
C6, C7	Subscapular	Subscapularis
C7, C8, T1	Pectoral	Subscapularis, pectoral muscles
C6*, C7, C8	Musculocutaneous	Biceps brachii, coracobrachialis, brachialis
C8, T1, T2	Median	Flexor carpi radialis, deep digital flexor, superficial digital flexor
C8*, T1, T2	Ulnar	Flexor carpi ulnaris, deep digital flexor, superficial digital flexor
C7, C8, T1	Radial	Triceps, extensor carpi radialis, ulnaris lateralis, lateral and common digital extensors
C6†, C7, C8	Axillary	Deltoideus, teres minor, subscapularis, cleidobrachialis
C7, C8	Long thoracic	Serratus ventralis
C8, T1, T2†	Thoracodorsal	Latissimus dorsi
C8, T1, T2	Lateral thoracic	Panniculus

*Contributes innervation in the ruminant only.
†Contributes innervation in the horse only.

TABLE 8-5

Innervation of the Hindlimbs of Large Animals

Spinal Cord Segment	Peripheral Nerve	Muscle(s)
L3†, L4, L5, L6*	Femoral	Quadriceps
L5†, L6, S1	Cranial gluteal	Gluteals, tensor fascia latae
S1, S2, S3, S4, S5†	Caudal gluteal, pudendal	Biceps femoris, middle and superficial gluteals
L5†, L6, S1, S2	Ischiatic, fibular	Lateral digital extensor, long digital extensor, short digital extensor, cranial tibial
L5†, L6, S1, S2	Tibial	Gastrocnemius, popliteus, superficial and deep digital flexor, interosseus
L5†, L6, S1, S2	Pudendal	Retractor penis
S3-Cd5	Caudal rectal	Rectum, anal sphincter, bladder

*Contributes innervation in the ruminant only.
†Contributes innervation in the horse only.

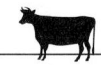

taut biceps muscle with a heavy instrument. Contraction of the muscle may be perceived visually or by palpation. A slight flexion of the elbow and extension of the carpus is normal. The test measures the function of the musculocutaneous nerve and spinal cord segments C6 to C8 in ruminants and C7 and C8 in horses.

Lesions rostral to C6 result in general hyperreflexia of both forelimbs and hindlimbs. Lesions located in spinal segments C5 to T2 result in hyporeflexia to areflexia of the forelimbs and hyperreflexia of the hindlimbs.

REAR LIMB MYOTACTIC REFLEXES

Patellar (Quadriceps) Reflex. Flex the stifle moderately and sharply percuss the middle patellar ligament with a heavy instrument, or a rubber pleximeter in smaller subjects. The normal reflex is a sharp contraction of the quadriceps femoris muscle resulting in extension of the stifle and a forward jerk of the lower limb. The patellar reflex measures the function of the femoral nerve, the quadriceps femoris muscle, and L3 to L5 and L4 to L6 spinal cord segments in the horse and cow, respectively.

Cranial Tibial Reflex. The cranial tibial reflex is elicited by flexing the hock and sharply striking the belly of the cranial tibial muscle. The reflex consists of a slight extension of the digit. The cranial tibial reflex is mediated through the peroneal and sciatic nerves and spinal cord segments L5 to S2 or L6 to S2 in the horse and the ruminant, respectively. Lesions of the spinal cord anterior to L3 segments result in hyperreflexia whereas lesions of L3 to L6 spinal segments result in hyporeflexia or areflexia.

The reflex part of the test measures the function of the peroneal, tibial, and sciatic nerves and the function of L6 to S2 spinal segments. The peroneal nerve supplies cutaneous innervation to the dorsolateral aspect of the limb. The tibial nerve supplies innervation to the caudomedial and dorsomedial aspect of the limb.

Flexor Reflexes

The flexor reflexes are performed in the recumbent large animal. A painful stimulus is applied to the uppermost foot. The normal reflex consists of two phases: (1) a rapid limb flexion, and (2) a slower conscious perception of the stimulus, characterized by attempts to assume sternal recumbency, vocalization, ear and eye movements, violent kicking, etc. The forelimb flexor reflex tests the integrity of the axillary, median, and musculocutaneous nerves and spinal cord segments C5 through T2, as well as the flexor muscles of the limb. The hindlimb flexor reflex is mediated by means of the sciatic, peroneal, and tibial nerves and the hindlimb flexor muscles.

Spinal cord and peripheral nerve lesions may be localized further by testing the integrity of the sensory innervation of the skin of the limbs. Areas of decreased or absent cutaneous sensation reflect lesions of the peripheral nerves innervating those regions of the skin or of the spinal cord segments in which those sensory nerves terminate. The skin over the trunk and much of the limbs is innervated by more than one peripheral nerve. Some areas of the limbs derive sensory innervation from a single peripheral nerve. These areas are termed the autonomous zones for those peripheral nerves. Damage to a peripheral nerve innervating the skin of a limb therefore will result in decreased to absent cutaneous sensation in the autonomous zone for that nerve. This information can be used to localize lesions. Decrease or loss of sensation to an entire limb, or to limbs on both sides of the body suggest a lesion affecting several local spinal cord segments, or a transverse spinal cord lesion rostral to the affected limbs.

Other Spinal Reflexes

PERINEAL REFLEX. The perineal reflex is elicited by pinching the mucocutaneous junction of the anus. The normal reflex includes tightening of the sphincter muscle and contraction of the ventral tail muscles. Conscious sensation of the stimulus produces avoidance or protective responses that may range from a slight movement of the rear limbs and pelvis to a violent kick. The reflex is mediated by the internal pudendal nerve and spinal cord segments S1 to S5. Lesions in the nerve or in the sacral spinal cord result in a dilated, atonic rectal sphincter that fails to respond to noxious stimuli, as well as fecal impaction in the rectum and a dilated urinary bladder. The bladder is full of urine and dribbles whenever digital pressure is applied through the rectum or vagina. The perineum remains wet and may become irritated ("scalded") by the continuous overflow of urine.

PANNICULUS (CUTANEOUS) REFLEX. The panniculus reflex is a wrinkling or flinching of the skin over the trunk when it is stimulated by light touch or by pinching. The skin over the caudal flank usually is the most sensitive. Run the tip of a closed hemostat over the skin, tap the skin lightly with the hemostat tip, or pinch the skin lightly with the hemostat. The normal response is a skin twitch, together with a conscious avoidance maneuver, such as moving away from the stimulus. The afferent part of the panniculus reflex is mediated through the dorsal nerve rootlets and the segmental spinal nerves that are distributed to the stimulated area. These ascend in the dorsal funiculi of the spinal cord and synapse on the efferent neurons in spinal segments C8 to T1 in ruminants and C8 to T2 in horses. The axons exit the ventral rootlet and form the thoracodorsal nerve, which innervates the cutaneous trunci muscle. The degree of reflex responsiveness varies among the large animal species. Sheep, goats, and English breeds of cattle possess a poor panniculus reflex. Horses and Zebu cattle have a well-developed reflex.

CERVICAL REFLEXES. Two reflexes have been described in the cervical area of the horse.[41] The cervical reflex is similar to the panniculus reflex. Tapping or pinching the skin of the caudal half of the cervical region results in a local skin twitch. The pathway is believed to involve the cervical segmental spinal nerves and the local spinal cord segments.

The cervicoauricular reflex is elicited in horses by covering the eye and lightly tapping the skin over vertebrae C1 to C3. In normal horses the ear reflexively twitches cranially and ventrally as the skin is stimulated. This test measures the integrity of the dorsal funiculi of C1 to C3 spinal cord segments and the facial nerve in the medulla oblongata. The diagnostic usefulness of the test in ruminants is unknown.

Both these reflexes are variable and are not always found in normal animals. Increased experience of the examiner, however, seems to be associated with increased reliability of these reflexes. Both reflexes may be abnormal in animals with lesions affecting the cervical spinal cord, such as equine wobbler syndrome. The cervicoauricular reflex also may be decreased or absent in animals with caudal brainstem lesions, involving the facial nerve, or with peripheral facial nerve lesions.

"SLAP" TEST (LARYNGEAL ADDUCTOR REFLEX). A sharp slap applied in the saddle region on one side of a horse's thorax results in adduction of the vocal folds of the larynx on the opposite side.[42] This reflex can be palpated as a contraction of the cricoarytenoideus dorsalis muscle. Standing on one side of the animal the examiner curls his or her fingers around the dorsal aspect of the larynx on the opposite side. A slap is applied to the saddle region on the side on which the examiner is standing. The response is palpated as a small movement under the fingertips over the cricoarytenoideus dorsalis muscle on the opposite side of the larynx.

It is often useful to have a helper apply the slap rather than to have the examiner do so. The pathway for the reflex is only partially understood. Sensory information from the skin is relayed to the spinal cord in the segmental spinal nerves. The ascending information then crosses the spinal cord and runs rostrally in a contralateral pathway to the origin of the vagus nerve in the nucleus ambiguus in the medulla oblongata. Descending output from the nucleus ambiguus runs in the cervical vagosympathetic trunk, and thence to the recurrent laryngeal nerve, which branches from the vagus in the cranial thorax. The recurrent laryngeal nerve runs rostrally alongside the trachea to the larynx. Thus the pathway for this reflex is almost entirely contralateral to the side on which the stimulus (the slap) is applied. Abnormalities in the laryngeal adductor response are seen in animals that have lesions of the cervical spinal cord, but also in those with caudal brainstem lesions, vagus nerve lesions, and lesions of the recurrent laryngeal nerve ("roarers"). Interpretation of the results of this test depends somewhat on the experience of the examiner. Presence of the response bilaterally is normal. Unilateral absence of the response suggests a lesion in one of the structures described above. Bilateral absence of the response is harder to interpret because it may be the result of a bilateral lesion, or the result of inability to palpate the cricoarytenoid contraction in a large or heavily muscled horse. The laryngeal adduction elicited in this test also can be observed using an endoscope. The laryngeal adductor response tends to fatigue, so it may disappear if tested repeatedly over a short period.

Muscle Mass and Tone

Normal mass and tone of the musculature depends on an intact nerve supply. Primary diseases of muscle and loss of use of a limb secondary to orthopedic disease are often associated with mild to moderate muscle atrophy that develops over weeks to months. Atrophy caused by denervation, however, is more severe and rapid in onset. Visible loss of mass of specific muscles or groups of muscles is most likely caused by damage to the nerve supply to those muscles, either by direct injury to peripheral nerves or injury to the origins of those nerves in the ventral horn gray matter of the spinal cord (Fig. 8-7). Knowledge of the central origins of the nerves to the limbs and the course of those nerves in the periphery can be used to specifically localize neurologic lesions (see Tables 8-4 and 8-5). Electromyography and nerve conduction testing can further be used to help identify muscle denervation and peripheral neuropathies (Chapter 33). Regeneration of peripheral nerves after an acute insult can occur. Regeneration is accomplished by outgrowths of axonal buds from the proximal stump. The buds either grow along previous peripheral nerve rootlets or generate new neural pathways in concert with proliferation of myelin precursor cells. The rate of growth of the axonal buds has been estimated to be approximately 1 to 4 mm/day.[43]

Muscle tone can be evaluated in the recumbent animal by passively flexing the limbs. Evaluation is not accurate in the standing animal or in animals supported in slings because of resistance from taut bands of connective tissue. In normal animals repeated flexion is accompanied by an increase in the tone in the flexed limb. The limbs of animals with a lower motor neuron deficit remain flaccid. Small ruminants tend to show a greater relative amount of extensor tone in the limbs than do cattle or horses. Evaluation of the test must be conservative because some severely obtunded large animals display generalized hypotonia, even though the lower motor neurons are functional. The cause of the hypotonia is unknown.

The tone of the forelimbs is controlled through spinal cord segments C6 to T1 and the radial, musculocutaneous,

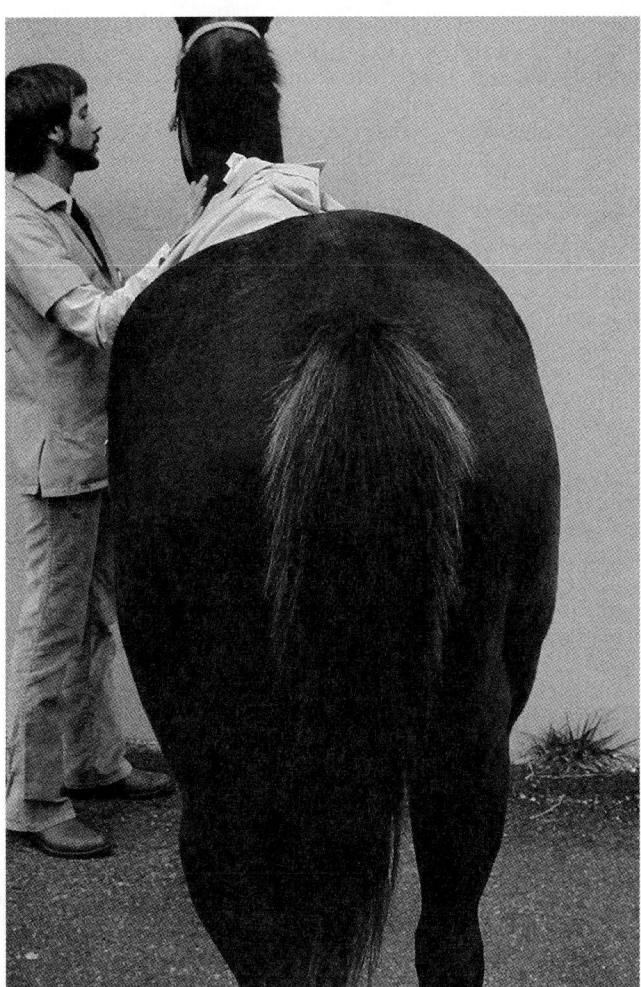

FIG. 8-7 ▮ Muscle atrophy in the gluteal muscles in a horse with equine protozoal myelonencephalitis.

median, ulnar, axillary, and long thoracic nerves. The motor tone of the rear limbs is controlled through spinal cord segments L3 to S2 and the femoral, cranial and caudal gluteal, and sciatic nerves. The lower motor neurons to the anus originate in spinal cord segments S1 to S5, via the pudendal nerve. The tail is innervated by the coccygeal segmental spinal nerves.

Examination of Cranial Nerves

CRANIAL NERVE I—OLFACTORY NERVE. Reliable and specific testing of the sense of smell is difficult in animals. Large animals require an intact sense of smell to eat properly, so it can be inferred that animals with good appetites possess adequate sense of smell. Having an animal track food moved from side to side in front of the nose may be helpful. Ensure that the food has an appealing odor. Irritating substances such as ammonia should not be used for evaluation of olfactory nerve function; such compounds stimulate nociceptors in the nasal mucosa, which are the dendrites of the maxillary nerve (CN V), rather than stimulating olfactory receptors innervated by the olfactory nerve. Loss of the sense of smell is more likely to be caused by disease within the nasal passages than by a primary neurologic disease.

CRANIAL NERVE II—OPTIC NERVE. Vision is the function of cranial nerve II, the optic nerve. Observing the animal's response to its environment provides a good initial assessment. Does it respond to visual cues, such as movement, or does it walk into objects? Noise may cause the animal to turn its head toward the sound, so the observer must be careful to distinguish such responses from those made in response to visual cues. A maze can be set up using straw bales or other objects and the animal gently driven through the maze. Normal animals will avoid colliding with objects. Animals that are severely obtunded, however, may walk into objects even when they can see. Thorough evaluation of the complete neurologic examination is necessary to distinguish this from true blindness.

The menace response measures the integrity of the entire visual pathway. The ascending pathway runs from the retina via the optic nerves, midbrain, and internal capsule to the visual areas in the occipital lobe of the cerebrum. Information from the visual cortex is processed and relayed to the motor cortex. The descending pathway of the menace response runs from the motor cortex via the pons to the nucleus of the facial nerve in the medulla oblongata and thence via the facial nerve to the orbicularis oculi muscle. Input to this motor pathway also arises from the cerebellum. The menace test is performed by rapidly advancing the hand toward the eye and observing a reflex closure of the eyelids. In addition to the closure of the eyelids, some animals display a generalized avoidance response characterized by coordinated movement of the head and neck away from the stimulus. The opposite eye may be covered to ensure that only one eye is being stimulated. Care must be taken not to touch the face or eyelashes. Many authors warn that air currents generated by rapid movement of the hand toward the face can elicit the response even in blind animals, but this has not been our experience. The menacing gesture is directed first at the nasal and then at the temporal parts of the visual field. Blindness in one visual field is termed *hemianopsia*. The menace response measures the integrity of the retina, optic nerve, optic chiasm, midbrain, internal capsule, and occipital cortex. There is approximately 90% crossing over of optic nerve fibers in the optic chiasm of livestock. Animals with a postchiasmal lesion in the internal capsule, midbrain, or occipital lobe will show hemianopsia in the contralateral visual field. In practical terms, lesions central to the optic chiasm cause loss of vision in the opposite eye, with apparently normal vision in the ipsilateral eye.

Menace deficit may be the result of facial nerve paralysis. In such cases the animal does not blink, but shows avoidance of the stimulus by pulling the head away. Facial nerve deficits will be apparent in these animals by their inability to close the eyelids under any circumstances, and by other signs such as facial drooping on the same side. Animals with cerebellar disease also may display a menace deficit, yet possess normal vision. The precise pathway by which the cerebellum influences the menace reflex is not known, but interruption of this pathway is thought to disrupt upper motor neuron control of the facial nerve, which becomes dysfunctional. Menace deficits resulting from facial nerve or cerebellar disease may be differentiated from deficits in other areas by maze testing. Animals with cerebellar or facial nerve disease retain visual acuity and maneuver through the course successfully. The maze test measures the patient's ability to identify and avoid obstacles. In addition to the optic pathways, the test measures the integrative pathways in the frontal and parietal lobes of the brain, the motor neurons, and the proprioceptive pathways (Table 8-6). Myasthenic diseases (e.g., botulism, hypocalcemia, or hypomagnesemia) result in bilaterally decreased menace and palpebral responses, but do not produce blindness.

The pupillary light reflex measures the integrity of the retina, optic nerves, optic chiasm, pretectal and oculomotor nuclei in the midbrain, oculomotor nerve, ciliary ganglia, and constrictor pupillae muscle. The test is performed by shining a bright light into each eye, and observing constriction of the pupil in the ipsilateral eye (direct response) and the contralateral eye (indirect response). Reducing the ambient light level may facilitate this test by causing the pupils to dilate. The reflex in large animals is considerably slower than observed in cats and dogs. The effects on the pupillary light reflex of lesions at various levels along the visual pathway are shown in Table 8-6.

Unilateral lesions of the cerebral cortex result in blindness of the opposite eye. The pupillary light reflexes usually are normal. If the cortical disease is accompanied by increased intracranial pressure, the oculomotor nerve or nucleus may become dysfunctional because of ischemia, resulting in ipsilateral mydriasis.

CRANIAL NERVES III, IV, AND VI—OCULOMOTOR, TROCHLEAR, AND ABDUCENT. The position of the globe in the orbit is governed by the activity of the oculomotor, trochlear, and abducent nerves. Dysfunctions of these nerves result in deviation of the globe that is constant in all head positions. Loss of oculomotor nerve function results in a ventrolateral strabismus. Trochlear nerve dysfunction results in rotation of the dorsal aspect of the globe away from the midline (dorsomedial strabismus). In large animals that have horizontal pupils, trochlear nerve lesions cause deviation of the pupil such that the medial aspect of the pupil is dorsal to the lateral aspect. The trochlear nerve crosses the midline twice in the area of the midbrain before exiting the cranial vault. Therefore unilateral lesions could result in contralateral or ipsilateral strabismus, depending on the location of the lesion within the brainstem. Lesions of the trochlear nerve are, in our experience, extremely rare. Loss of abducent

TABLE 8-6

Guide to Neuroophthalmologic Lesion Location

Lesion Location	Menace Response		Pupillary Light Response		Maze Test
	Ipsilateral	Bilateral	Ipsilateral	Bilateral	
Unilateral retina, optic nerve	Absent	Present	Normal	Normal	Abnormal
Bilateral retina, optic nerve, optic chiasm	Absent	Absent	Fixed	Fixed	Abnormal
Unilateral oculomotor nerve	Absent	Present	Dilated nonresponsive	Normal	Normal
Unilateral occipital cortex	Present	Absent	Normal*	Normal*	Abnormal
Bilateral occipital cortex	Absent	Absent	Normal	Normal	Abnormal
Bilateral vagosympathetic trunk	Present	Present	Miotic	Normal	Normal
Bilateral cerebellar cortex	Absent	Absent	Normal	Normal	Normal†

*Assuming that no cortical swelling has occurred.
†Animals walk abnormally, but recognize and generally avoid obstacles.

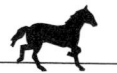

nerve function results in medial strabismus with inability to retract the globe, which is best demonstrated by restraining the head of the patient, opening the palpebral fissure, and touching the cornea. The normal reflex is a retraction of the globe with protrusion of the third eyelid.

Function of the oculomotor, trochlear, and abducent nerves also is observed when testing the oculocephalic reflexes. When the head is turned from side to side a horizontal nystagmus is observed, with the fast phase of the nystagmus in the direction of the head movement. The sensory receptors for this reflex lie within the semicircular canals of the inner ear, and they detect angular acceleration of the head. Input from the semicircular canals is transferred to the vestibular centers in the medulla oblongata and the cerebellum, and thence via the medial longitudinal fasciculus and reticular formation to the nuclei of cranial nerves III, IV, and VI. Lesions of the peripheral or central components of the vestibular system therefore also can result in abnormal eye position (strabismus) and movement (nystagmus), described in more detail below. In such cases, however, the strabismus changes when the head and neck are moved, in contrast to the constant deviation of the globe seen with direct lesions to the oculomotor, trochlear, and abducent nerves. Vestibular dysfunction also results in spontaneous nystagmus, which can be used to differentiate these conditions from dysfunctions of nerves III, IV, and VI.

CRANIAL NERVE V—TRIGEMINAL NERVE. The trigeminal nerve is sensory to the face and motor to the muscles of mastication. The sensory functions of the trigeminal nerve are tested by lightly stimulating the face using the tip of a closed hemostat. In animals that are head-shy, the examiner can use his or her fingers to stimulate the skin of the face. The forehead is innervated by the ophthalmic branch of the nerve, the upper jaw and muzzle by the maxillary branch, and the lower jaw by the mandibular branch. Each area should be tested specifically. The normal response is one of avoidance using neck, facial, and appendicular musculature; the animal usually pulls the head away and blinks simultaneously. Some areas such as the cheeks, forehead, and chin are normally less sensitive whereas the periorbital region, the nasal planum, and the lips are very sensitive. The test evaluates the function of the sensory part of the trigeminal nerve, the trigeminal ganglion, the nucleus and spinal tract of the trigeminal nerve, the pontine sensory tract nucleus of CN V, the thalamus, the sensorimotor cortex, and the motor neurons of the head, which innervate the muscles of facial expression and run in the facial nerve (cranial nerve VII). After the trigeminal nerve enters the lateral aspect of the medulla, axons both ascend and descend through the medulla as the spinal tract of the trigeminal nerve. Ascending information ultimately reaches the sensorimotor cortex, where it is consciously perceived. Descending information projects to the nucleus of the facial nerve in the medulla and also into the first cervical spinal segment. Unilateral loss of facial sensation most commonly results from damage to the peripheral portion of the trigeminal nerve, the trigeminal ganglion in the petrosal bone of the skull, or the contralateral cerebral cortex. Lesions affecting the spinal tract of the trigeminal nerve in the medulla and midbrain would likely be fatal, because they also would affect adjacent respiratory and cardiovascular centers in the brainstem. Patients with bilateral facial hypoesthesia probably have bilateral cerebral cortex disease.

The palpebral reflex is performed by lightly touching the periorbital area and observing a brisk closure of the eyelids. This reflex measures the sensory function of the trigeminal nerve and the motor function of the facial nerve and orbicularis oculi muscle. Simultaneous loss of the menace response and the palpebral reflex suggests a lesion in the facial nerve or the orbicularis oculi muscle. Loss of the palpebral reflex with

normal menace responses suggests a lesion in the trigeminal nerve or ganglion. Loss of menace response with preservation of the palpebral reflex indicates occipital cerebrocortical dysfunction (cortical blindness) or a cerebellar lesion.

The jaw should be opened to assess the strength of the masticatory muscles. This measures both the sensory (proprioceptive) fibers of the trigeminal nerve and the motor component of the nerve. Bilateral lesions of the motor component of the trigeminal nerve result in a dropped jaw. Affected animals may protrude the tongue but can retract it normally when stimulated. Animals with dropped jaws may drool saliva because they cannot trap it within the oral cavity. Unilateral lesions of the trigeminal nerve produce asymmetric jaw closure, with a slight gap between the occlusal surfaces of the teeth on the affected side; these signs, however, are not readily apparent.

CRANIAL NERVE VII—FACIAL NERVE. The motor nucleus of CN VII originates in the middle and ventral part of the medulla oblongata. The motor fibers are distributed to muscles of facial expression. Just as the motor fibers are exiting from the lateral aspect of the brainstem they merge with axons from the parasympathetic facial nucleus. These fibers innervate the lacrimal and salivary glands. They separate from the motor component of the facial nerve as it traverses the petrous temporal bone. Lesions of CN VII located between the brainstem and the petrous temporal bone usually result in "dry eye." More distal lesions, however, have no effect on tear production. The tone of the facial musculature is examined by palpation of the ears, lips, eyelids, and muzzle. Clinical signs of facial nerve dysfunction include drooped ear and lips, drooling saliva, and retention of food in the cheek pouch on the denervated side (Fig. 8-8). Closure of the eyelids is weak in partial facial nerve lesions and absent in severe lesions. Despite this, there is slight drooping of the upper eyelid (ptosis) because of paralysis of the frontalis muscle, which contributes to eyelid retraction. In species with a soft muzzle (e.g., horses, sheep, and goats), there is a marked deviation of the filtrum after a unilateral loss of facial nerve function. The filtrum of affected cattle is not deviated because of the large amount of fibrous tissue in the planum nasale. In chronic facial paralysis the face may be deviated toward the affected side because of atrophy and contracture of the denervated musculature of the face.

CRANIAL NERVE VIII—VESTIBULOCOCHLEAR NERVE
Vestibular System. The function of the vestibular system, which comprises the sensory structures in the inner ear (semicircular canals, utriculus, saccule), the vestibular portion of cranial nerve VIII, and the central components of the vestibular system in the medulla oblongata and cerebellum, is tested by assessment of the gait, extensor tone, head posture, and eye movements. Signs of vestibular dysfunction include a staggering gait, circling, falling, rolling, head tilt, and spontaneous nystagmus. Signs can be classified as peripheral, central, or paradoxical in type. Lesions affecting the inner ear or cranial nerve VIII result in signs of peripheral vestibular disease, lesions affecting vestibular structures in the medulla oblongata result in central vestibular signs, and lesions affecting vestibular structures in the cerebellum result in paradoxical vestibular signs. Blindfolding affected patients results in a worsening of clinical signs because of elimination of compensatory mechanisms from optic centers. Recumbent animals with vestibular lesions tend to lie with the side of the vestibular lesion downward. When turned, these animals spontaneously rotate back to the lesion-down position and may strongly resist attempts to turn them over. Animals with unilateral vestibular disorders may have a ventral strabismus in the ipsilateral eye and a dorsal strabismus in the contralateral eye. This sign is seen with either central or peripheral vestibular lesions. Assessment of strabismus should be

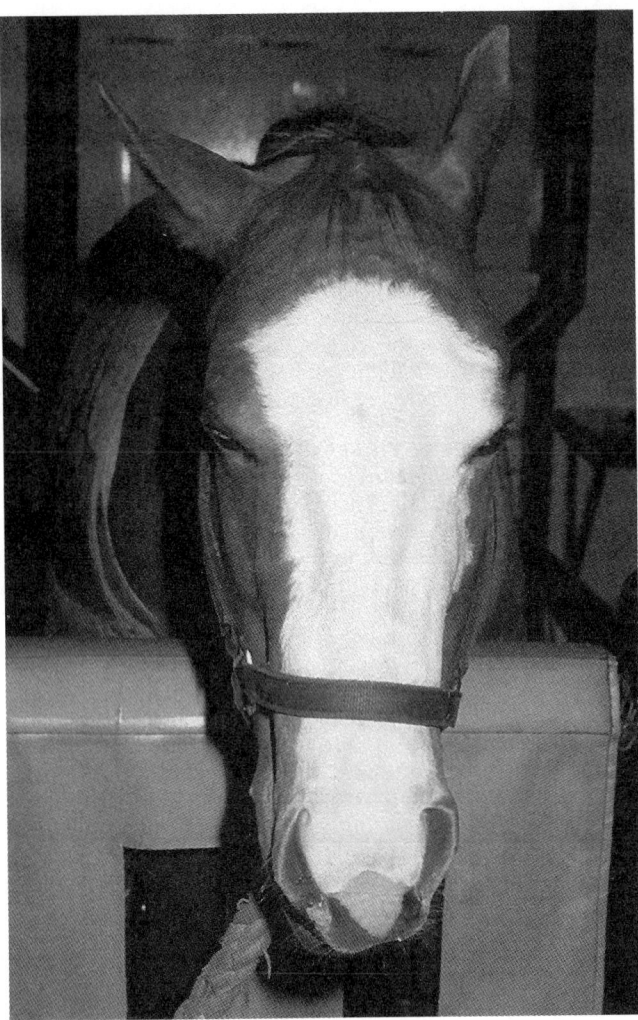

FIG. 8-8 ■ Acute right facial paralysis in a horse with guttural pouch mycosis. Note the drooped right ear and deviation of the muzzle toward the left side.

performed on the standing animal with the head held in normal posture. All species of livestock keep the eyes centered in the orbit when the head is in the neutral position. Cattle and sheep keep the optic plane parallel to the ground when the head is moved. This results in a positional ventrolateral strabismus of the right eye when the head is rotated to the left, and vice versa, and a ventral strabismus when the head is raised. In contrast, the normal horse and goat maintain the eye in the center of the palpebral fissure in all head positions.

Bilateral, symmetrical lesions of the vestibular system do not produce head tilt, nystagmus, or strabismus. Affected animals are reluctant to move. They stand with a base-wide posture, with the head held low, and fall easily when forced to move.

CRANIAL NERVES IX, X, AND XI—GLOSSOPHARYN-GEAL, VAGUS, AND SPINAL ACCESSORY NERVES. Cranial nerves IX, X, and XI originate in the nucleus ambiguus, a column of motor neurons that extends from the middle to the caudal medulla oblongata, located in a ventrolateral position. They are motor to the muscles of the neck, pharynx, and palate. The vagus nerve contains efferent fibers that stimulate the secretions of glands of the visceral and respiratory mucosa and control forestomach motility in ruminants. The glossopharyngeal and accessory nerves carry afferent fibers

from the mucosa of the tongue, larynx, and pharynx. The signs of glossopharyngeal and vagus nerve dysfunction include dysphonia (roaring, snoring), dysphagia, and regurgitation. Animals with pharyngeal paralysis regurgitate food from the nose. Roaring is a characteristic stertorous sound emanating from the larynx. The abnormal sound can be increased by exercise. Functional examination of these nerves should include auscultation of the larynx for stertorous airway sounds, observation of the animal as it swallows, passage of a nasogastric tube to evaluate deglutition, endoscopic examination to evaluate pharyngeal and laryngeal activity, and palpation of the cricoarytenoideus dorsalis muscle for atrophy. The slap test, described above, is a test for function of the vagal innervation of the larynx. Specific descriptions of the endoscopic appearance of pharyngeal paralysis and roaring are presented elsewhere (see Chapter 29).

Signs of spinal accessory nerve dysfunction are extremely rare and include atrophy of the trapezius, sternocephalicus, and brachiocephalicus muscles.

SYMPATHETIC INNERVATION OF THE HEAD— HORNER'S SYNDROME

Preganglionic sympathetic fibers that innervate structures of the head originate from the first three thoracic spinal cord segments. These fibers emerge with the origins of the nerves that form the brachial plexus. They ascend the neck in the peripheral vagosympathetic trunk to the cranial cervical ganglion under the tympanic bulla, where they synapse with postganglionic sympathetic fibers. The postganglionic fibers are distributed to the smooth muscles of the head through the ciliary nerves, passing through the petrous temporal bone area. Lesions anywhere along the course of the preganglionic or postganglionic sympathetic nerves, in spinal cord segments T1-T3 or, rarely, in the upper motor neuron component of the sympathetic pathway in the cervical spinal cord or brainstem (tectotegmentospinal tract), cause a characteristic constellation of clinical signs known as Horner's syndrome. Signs include miosis, enophthalmia, ptosis, and increased warmth on the ipsilateral side of the face. In cattle there is a loss of sweating on the ipsilateral side of the planum nasale, whereas in horses there is excessive sweating on the affected side. The enophthalmia is caused by paralysis of the periorbital smooth muscle that normally pulls the globe toward the surface of the orbit. The relaxation of the periorbita results in the sinking of the globe. Miosis is produced by the lack of pupillary dilation in response to normal sympathetic activity.

Diseases that produce Horner's syndrome in large animals include compressive lesions of the gray matter in the T1 to T3 spinal segments, neoplasms (lymphosarcoma, melanoma, or neurofibroma), mediastinal or thoracic abscesses, abscesses in the cervical sympathetic trunk, esophageal perforations, guttural pouch mycosis, otitis media/interna, and retrobulbar abscesses. Transient Horner's syndrome may occur after intravenous injection of xylazine. Preganglionic and postganglionic denervation may be differentiated by instillation of 1:1000 epinephrine (0.1 ml) into the eye with the miotic pupil. Pupillary dilation occurs by 20 to 40 minutes in eyes with postganglionic and preganglionic lesions, respectively. Lesions of the mesencephalon (brainstem) at the level of the rostral colliculus may produce miotic pupils without other signs of Horner's syndrome. This is a common sign in cattle with polioencephalomalacia and lead poisoning.

CRANIAL NERVE XII—HYPOGLOSSAL NERVE. The hypoglossal nerve supplies motor impulses to the muscles of the tongue and the geniohyoideus muscle. The cell body of the nerve is located in the dorsomedial aspect of the caudal medulla oblongata. Hypoglossal nerve function is tested by pulling the tongue out of the mouth. Normal animals should have forceful resistance to passive manipulation of the

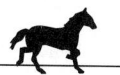

tongue. Lesions of the hypoglossal nerve result in flaccidity of the tongue. With unilateral lesions, the tongue falls out of the mouth toward the side of the lesion. Chronic lesions of the hypoglossal nerve result in deviation of the tongue towards the side of the lesion, because of muscular atrophy and contracture on the affected side.

Other Aspects of Physical Examination of the Patient With Neurologic Disease

Diagnosis of a neurologic disease can often be facilitated by the observation of physical abnormalities in other systems. When examining animals with a chronic ataxia or tetraparesis, the head, neck, and back should be gently manipulated while palpating the spine for crepitation or swelling. This finding could indicate the presence of fracture, malformation, or luxation of one or more cervical vertebrae, or vertebral osteomyelitis. Do not manipulate the neck whenever there is evidence of acute cervical vertebral trauma. Swelling, bruising, or hair loss on the skin around the head or bleeding from the ears or nose could signify cranial trauma. Hair loss and dermatitis around the perineum may indicate urinary incontinence. In neonates, a hairless patch over the dorsum of the spine could indicate a meningomyelocele. Displacement of the sacrum could indicate sacroiliac luxation. Crepitation over coxofemoral or stifle joints of recumbent cattle could indicate a luxation or fracture. If luxation of the coxofemoral joint is suspected, the animal should be rolled on its back, and the length of the two pelvic limbs should be compared while the legs are held in extension. A pelvic examination should be performed in all large animals to detect displacement of the hip joint into the obturator foramen or fractures through the shaft of the ilium. All joints should be passively manipulated to detect dislocations or fractures. The heart should be ausculted for murmurs that could suggest left-sided endocarditis because such lesions can shower bacteria into the meninges. Odors on the breath such as ammonia, ketones, or petroleum distillates could provide clues about possible toxic etiologies. Identification of concurrent bronchopneumonia may indicate the possibility of thromboembolic meningoencephalitis in cattle or herpesvirus myelitis in horses. The ocular fundus should be examined ophthalmoscopically to detect retinal hemorrhages (trauma), papilledema (increased intracranial pressure), or vasculitis.

Examination of the Neonate

Most of the physical diagnostic techniques described in the preceding paragraph for the adult may be applied in examination of the neonate. Most spinal reflexes of livestock are well developed after birth. In the normal foal under 3 weeks of age, the limbs are hypertonic and hyperreflexic, with occasional myoclonus occurring after percussion of the patellar or triceps tendons. This hyperreflexia is most pronounced in the rear limbs. A lack of menace response for up to 2 weeks after delivery has also been observed. Nevertheless, foals are visual and aware of their surroundings almost immediately after birth. When restrained, the newborn foal relaxes into a trancelike state, periodically awakening and struggling violently before becoming passive again.

The results of daily examinations of 10 normal calves indicated that the spinal reflexes were present by 24 hours after birth. Most cortical responses were developed by 3 weeks of age. Bottle-reared calves aggressively attempt to suckle while being examined, including vigorously butting of the handler with the head. Beef calves attempt to escape restraint and do not attempt to suckle. See Chapters 15 to 20 for more details on neonates.

LOCALIZATION OF CENTRAL NERVOUS SYSTEM LESIONS

Localization of a CNS lesion on the basis of clinical signs is vital because many specific diseases are restricted to particular regions of the CNS. Thus localization of a CNS lesion facilitates both differential diagnosis and specific diagnosis of the disorder. Ancillary diagnostic testing is determined both by the likely differential diagnoses and by the location of the lesion within the nervous system. Once the clinician has located the anatomic site of a neurologic lesion, a list of rule-out diagnoses may be formulated. Additional tests, including cerebrospinal fluid (CSF) analysis, radiography, serology, electroencephalography, and myelography, can be performed to further characterize the disease.

Lesions can be localized to one of seven regions of the CNS: cerebral cortex and thalamus, midbrain, cerebellum, medulla oblongata, spinal cord, peripheral nerve (either cranial nerves or spinal nerves), or muscle. Further localization to specific areas of these larger structures often can be determined after the neurologic examination.

LOCALIZATION OF NEUROLOGIC DISEASES BY MAJOR CLINICAL SIGNS

Abnormal Mentation and Behavior and Seizures

Decreased mental alertness (dullness, obtundation, depression, stupor, coma) is the most common change seen in mental status in animals with neurologic disease, although increased responsiveness to external stimuli (anxiety, mania, aggression) sometimes can be the result of nervous system dysfunction. Altered mentation results from changes in the cerebrum, thalamus, or ascending reticular activating system (ARAS). Diseases affecting the ARAS tend to produce severe changes in mentation (stupor, coma), whereas those affecting the cerebrum or thalamus tend to produce a wider range of clinical signs, from mild dullness to coma. In order of worsening severity, decreased mental status in animals can be categorized as follows.

DULL, DEPRESSED, MILDLY TO MODERATELY OBTUNDED. Animals have decreased responsiveness to their surroundings, may ignore visual and auditory stimuli, may stop interacting with herdmates, and may be inappetent.

SEVERE DEPRESSION/OBTUNDATION. Animals are ambulatory, but sometimes appear to be blind and walk into objects. They will respond only to fairly strong stimuli such as very loud noises and vigorous handling.

STUPOR. The animal appears asleep, and will respond only to very vigorous and painful stimuli. Responses even to these stimuli are blunted.

COMA. The animal appears asleep and will not respond even to the most painful stimuli. Animals in coma are recumbent. They may adopt abnormal posture, particularly decerebrate posturing (opisthotonos, all four limbs rigidly extended), and may have other abnormal signs such as loss of the oculocephalic and pupillary light reflexes.

MANIA, ANXIETY. Animals that exhibit abnormally heightened reactions and responses vary widely in the severity of their signs, from mildly overreactive, to bellowing, rearing, and attacking people, animals, or objects around them.

SEIZURES, COLLAPSE. Episodic abnormalities in behavior or consciousness usually are the result of seizure activity, narcolepsy/cataplexy, or syncopal attacks caused by cardiovascular or respiratory dysfunction. Intermittent toxicities, or fluctuating metabolic abnormalities, such as occasionally occurs with hepatic encephalopathy, also may cause episodic changes in mentation and behavior. Animals with a history of episodic collapse should undergo a very thorough physical examination to determine whether disease of the cardiovascular system (e.g., cardiac arrhythmias, intermittent hemorrhage) or respiratory system (e.g., laryngeal paralysis) is present. Animals that have seizures usually have a period of abnormal behavior after the seizure (postictal phase of the seizure) whereas those with narcolepsy/cataplexy or nonneurologic causes of collapse usually do not. Seizures and narcolepsy/cataplexy are discussed in more detail below.

Signs of cerebral and thalamic disease are variable in severity and are difficult to distinguish from one another clinically. The thalamus and cerebrum can be thought of as a functional unit, to some extent, because the thalamus is the relay center via which sensory information from the periphery reaches the cerebrum, and through which motor impulses from the cerebrum are transmitted to the brainstem motor centers. Diffuse cerebral disease often results from metabolic, toxic, or infectious diseases. Increased intracranial pressure, the consequence of early acquired hydrocephalus, mass lesions within the cranial vault, inflammatory diseases, or cerebral edema, tends to produce signs of diffuse cerebral disease, which can range from mild to severe. Mild to moderate cerebral dysfunction usually results in an animal with decreased mental awareness, or, more rarely, one that is excited and overreactive. Diffuse disease does not result in circling, and gait on a level surface may appear normal, or almost so. Gait is abnormal, however, when the animal is challenged to ascend or descend slopes, step over objects on the ground, step onto and off curbs, circle, or back. Both ataxia and paresis become apparent, although the former usually is more obvious. Postural and proprioceptive reflexes and reactions similarly are abnormal. When walking at normal speed on a level surface, local reflexes in the spinal cord and regulatory information from the red and reticular nuclei in the brainstem control simple gait patterns. Movements that require visual input or complex limb and body integration of movements are initiated in motor centers of the cerebral cortex. The combination of normal gait on a level surface with obvious proprioceptive and postural deficits should immediately alert the examiner to the likelihood of cerebral or thalamic disease.

Response to visual stimuli, such as an open hand directed towards the face, may be decreased or absent because of involvement of the visual pathways in the cerebral cortex or the internal capsule (see Blindness, below). Pupillary light reflexes and oculocephalic reflexes tend to remain normal in animals with cerebral disease, except in the most severe cases. Response to all sensory input to the cerebrum often is decreased, but this is most obvious in the head, where the facial reflex (twitching of the facial skin and superficial musculature in response to tactile stimuli) and the palpebral reflex are decreased to varying degrees. It is common to mistake this for the presence of a second lesion, affecting the trigeminal nerve, facial nerve, or both, but such lesions need not be present to account for these clinical signs. In trigeminal or facial nerve lesions the clinical deficits tend to be more severe than when cerebrocortical disease is present, and mental status is normal when the cranial nerve lesions are peripheral in location. Horses with severe cerebrocortical lesions may fail to retract the tongue after it is pulled from the mouth, but can do so when stimulated vigorously. Animals with lesions of the hypoglossal nerve may not be able to retract the tongue at all, or the tongue may be very weak.

The hypothalamus regulates primitive functions such as eating, drinking, and cardiovascular and sexual function. Lesions of the hypothalamus may cause behavioral changes ranging from profound depression, rage, and inappropriate sexual activities, to unusual affection, as well as polydipsia, polyuria, bradycardia, and abnormal appetite (pica).

Seizures are the physical manifestations of spontaneous paroxysmal electrical activity in the brain. Although a focus of abnormal activity may originate in the thalamus or elsewhere in the brainstem, spread of this activity to the cerebral cortex results in the observable seizure activity. When the seizure activity is limited to a small area of the cerebral cortex the seizure that results is focal in type, resulting only in localized abnormal motor activity, such as muscular twitching in the face or in one limb, or episodes of abnormal behavior. More commonly the seizure is generalized, or starts focally and becomes generalized to the entire cerebral cortex. Generalized seizures cause loss of consciousness, collapse, and generalized tonic-clonic motor activity. The presence of seizures necessitates a localization of the neurologic lesion to the cerebrum, but the initiating cause may lie elsewhere in the brain, or even be extracranial in origin. Epilepsy is a term that means repeated seizures of any cause, although it is often used to indicate seizures of unknown etiology. The nature of the seizure, whether focal or generalized, is not a reliable indicator of the underlying cause. Congenital or idiopathic epilepsy, such as benign epilepsy of Arabian foals, causes generalized seizures. Partial or focal seizures indicate an acquired etiology. Animals with seizures should undergo a complete physical examination, together with diagnostic testing for suspected toxins and underlying metabolic diseases, as well as a thorough neurologic examination to localize any interictal neurologic signs. Further diagnostics, such as cerebrospinal fluid analysis, are performed as indicated after this initial workup.

When cerebral and thalamic disease is lateralized or asymmetric in severity, asymmetry of clinical signs becomes apparent. Circling occurs often, ranging from a tendency to drift toward one side, to obvious and persistent circling. Circling caused by forebrain disease remains more a tendency to circle rather than compulsive circling, which occurs in midbrain disease. In more severe cases it usually is possible to stop the animal from circling, although it may be very reluctant to turn in the opposite direction. Proprioceptive and postural reaction deficits are present in the limbs on the side of the body opposite to the lesion (contralateral), and vary in severity with the severity of the underlying neurologic disease. A head turn towards the side of the lesion (ipsilateral) may be present, but head tilt is not found. The absence of signs such as head tilt, nystagmus, and strabismus, together with the presence of contralateral proprioceptive and postural reaction deficits, distinguishes forebrain lesions from those affecting the vestibular system. In the latter, head tilt, nystagmus, and/or strabismus usually are present, and proprioceptive and postural reaction deficits either are absent (peripheral vestibular disease) or are present ipsilateral to the lesion (central vestibular disease, see below).

Specific diseases associated with the cerebrum of ruminants and horses are given in Tables 8-7 and 8-8, respectively.

Diseases that are restricted to the thalamus are rare in domestic animals. Most lesions affecting the thalamus alone result from infarctions or parasitic migration through the CNS. The thalamus may be involved in multifocal nervous system disease, such as occurs with infectious diseases. The clinical signs of thalamic disease are, for the most part, similar to signs of ipsilateral cerebral dysfunction.

Blindness and Ocular Abnormalities

Blindness may be the result of lesions in the eye, optic nerve, optic chiasm, or the central projections of the visual pathways. Animals presented with the complaint of blindness should receive a thorough ophthalmologic examination to determine whether primary ocular disease is the cause of the problem (see Chapter 37). Sophisticated diagnostics such as electroretinography (ERG) may be indicated in some ani-

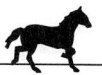

TABLE 8-7

Diseases of Ruminants That May Produce Cortical/Thalamic Signs

Disease	Predominant Clinical Signs	Species Affected
Rabies	Depression, excitement, aggressiveness, hyperesthesia, analgesia, anesthesia, proprioceptive deficits, recumbency, propulsive walking, head-pressing, tenesmus, hypersexuality, and salivation	Cow, sheep, goat
Trauma/hematoma/brain edema	Depression, somnolence, blindness, ataxia, proprioceptive deficits, opisthotonos, facial anesthesia, weak tongue, convulsions, anisocoria (late), head tilt, head-pressing, blood from ears or nose, decerebrate rigidity	Cow, sheep, goat
Polioencephalomalacia	Depression, somnolence, blindness, ataxia, proprioceptive deficits, facial anesthesia, weak tongue, anisocoria (late), head-pressing, opisthotonos, convulsions, odontoprisis, decerebrate rigidity	Cow, sheep, goat
Sulfur poisoning	Depression, somnolence, blindness, ataxia, proprioceptive deficits, facial anesthesia, weak tongue, anisocoria (late), head-pressing, opisthotonos, convulsions, odontoprisis, decerebrate rigidity	Cow, sheep, goat
Lead poisoning	Depression, somnolence, blindness, ataxia, proprioceptive deficits, facial anesthesia, weak tongue, anisocoria (late), head-pressing, opisthotonos, odontoprisis, convulsions, decerebrate rigidity	Cow, sheep, goat
Salt poisoning	Depression, somnolence, blindness, ataxia, proprioceptive deficits, opisthotonos, facial anesthesia, weak tongue, convulsions, anisocoria (late), head tilt, head-pressing, decerebrate rigidity	Cow, sheep, goat
Scrapie	Chewing, licking, wool break, depression, weight loss, ataxia, reduced menace, hypertonicity, hyperreflexia, proprioceptive deficit, recumbency, coma	Sheep, goat
Bovine spongiform encephalopathy	Aggression, weight loss, milk production, ataxia, proprioceptive deficit, recumbency, coma	Cow
Border disease	Ataxia, tremors, bunny-hopping	Sheep, goat
Vitamin A deficiency	Depression, somnolence, blindness with fixed pupils, ataxia, proprioceptive deficits, facial anesthesia, weak tongue, head-pressing, opisthotonos, convulsions, odontoprisis, decerebrate rigidity	Cow, sheep, goat
Brain abscess/meningitis	Recumbency, opisthotonos, blindness, hyperesthesia, stiff neck, proprioceptive deficit, ataxia, head-pressing, depression, coma	Cow, sheep, goat
Plant poisonings	Convulsions, blindness, ataxia, propulsive walking, head-pressing, odontoprisis, hyperexcitability, salivation, proprioceptive deficit, sudden death, vomiting, fetal malformations	Cow, sheep, goat
Nitrofurazone toxicosis	Hyperirritability, propulsive running, muscular tremors, blindness, convulsions	Cow
Grass staggers	Tremor, ataxia that worsens with excitement/exercise	Cow, sheep, goat
Pseudorabies	Depression, ataxia, hyperesthesia, paresthesia, aggressiveness, fear, head-pressing, propulsive walking, hypersexuality, salivation, coma, convulsions, recumbency, conscious proprioceptive deficit	Cow, sheep, goat
Malignant catarrhal fever	Aggression, rage, proprioceptive deficit, depression, head-pressing, blindness, nystagmus, bellowing, mucosal and skin erosions, lymphadenopathy, diarrhea	Cow
Caprine arthritis encephalitis	Depression, ataxia, head-pressing, convulsions, coma	Goat
Maedi-visna	Depression, ataxia, head-pressing, convulsions, coma	Sheep
Sarcocystis spp.	Seizures, blindness, opisthotonos, nystagmus, ataxia, muscular weakness, tremors, hyperexcitability, hypersalivation, recumbency	Cow
Brain tumor	Depression, facial paresis or paralysis, facial anesthesia or analgesia, head tilt, strabismus, nystagmus, loss of menace, hypermetria, ataxia	Cow
Sporadic bovine encephalomyelitis	Blindness, circling, ataxia, proprioceptive deficits, pleural friction rubs, pericardial friction rubs, abdominal tenderness	Cow
Urea poisoning	Muscle tremor, bloat, salivation, incoordination, struggling, ataxia, proprioceptive deficit, recumbency, bellowing, coma, convulsion	Cow
Ammoniated feed toxicosis	Trembling, fear, uncontrolled running, crashing through objects, coma, convulsion	Cow
Diplodiosis	Blindness, ataxia, depression, recumbency, convulsions, hyperesthesia	Cow
Ceroid lipofuscinosis	Blindness, ataxia, weight loss, coma, convulsion	Cow
Hydrocephalus/hydranencephaly/ microcephaly/anencephaly	Blindness, ataxia, proprioceptive deficit, ventrolateral strabismus, failure to suckle, dysphonia	Cow, sheep, goat
Citrullinemia	Recumbency, coma, convulsions, death by 4 days of age	Cow
Globoid cell leukodystrophy	Ataxia, proprioceptive deficits, hyperreflexia, depression, coma	Sheep
Infectious bovine rhinotracheitis	Fever, bellowing, coma, convulsions, somnolence, hyperexcitability, hyperesthesia, proprioceptive deficit, recumbency	Cow
Insecticide poisoning (organophosphate carbamate)	Salivation, vaginal discharge, diarrhea, tremors, coma, convulsion, diarrhea, proprioceptive deficit, recumbency	Cow, sheep, goat
Organochlorine poisoning	Tremors, hyperesthesia, recumbency, coma, convulsions	Cow, sheep, goat
Propylene glycol poisoning	Depression, bloat, ataxia, recumbency, proprioceptive deficit	Cow, sheep, goat

Continued

TABLE 8-7

Diseases of Ruminants That May Produce Cortical/Thalamic Signs—cont'd

Disease	Predominant Clinical Signs	Species Affected
Ethylene glycol poisoning	Depression, somnolence, blindness, ataxia, proprioceptive deficits, facial anesthesia, weak tongue, head-pressing, opisthotonos, convulsions, odontoprisis, decerebrate rigidity	Cow, sheep, goat
Nitrofurazone poisoning	Depression, proprioceptive deficit, recumbency, convulsion, coma	Cow, sheep, goat
Hypocalcemia	Cow, doe: weakness, ataxia, inappetence, bloat, proprioceptive deficit, cool extremities, weak pulse, bizarre head posture, dysuriat	Cow, goat
	Ewe: rigidity, tremors, hyperesthesia, convulsions, rapid, irregular breathing, odontoprisis	Sheep
Hypomagnesemia	Stiffness, hyperexcitability, recumbency, ataxia, proprioceptive deficit, muscle tremors	Cow
Nervous ketosis	Aggressiveness, tremors, ataxia, paresthesia, recumbency, proprioceptive deficit, hyperesthesia, bellowing	Cow
Hypoglycemia	Coma, semicoma, convulsions, blindness, hyperesthesia, cold extremities	Cow, sheep, goat
Nervous coccidiosis	Diarrhea, recumbency, depression, somnolence, blindness, proprioceptive deficit, propulsive walking, head-pressing	Cow
Hepatic encephalopathy	Hyperexcitability, aggression, rage, odontoprisis, ataxia, proprioceptive deficit, head-pressing, coma, convulsions, semicoma, blindness, tenesmus, rectal prolapse	Cow, sheep, goat
Idiopathic epilepsy	Intermittent psychomotor seizures	Cow, goat
Narcolepsy	Sleep state, recumbency, loss of consciousness, loss of motor activity, rapid eye movement	Cow
Propylene glycol toxicosis	Ataxia, depression, bloat, characteristic garliclike odor	Cow, sheep, goat
Coenuris cerebralis	Blindness, circling, ataxia, conscious proprioceptive deficit, head tilt, recumbency, coma, convulsions	Sheep
Theileriosis (central nervous system form, exotic)	Depression, hypersensitivity, ataxia, circling, paralysis, and convulsions	Cow
Babesiosis (exotic)	Odontoprisis, ataxia, conscious proprioceptive deficits, coma, convulsions	Cow
Louping ill (exotic)	Fever, anorexia, depression, constipation, muscular tremors, head tremors, hypermetria, ataxia, proprioceptive deficits, hyperexcitability, incoordination, rabbit hopping gait, recumbency, convulsions, coma	Sheep, cow
Borna disease (exotic)	Head tremors, hyperesthesia, ataxia, anorexia, propulsive walking, coma, convulsions	Cow, sheep, goat
Sarcocystis	Fever, weight loss, tremors, weakness, diarrhea, loss of hair on the tail switch, abortions	Cow
Heartwater (exotic)	Hyperesthesia, behavioral changes, muscular fasciculations, hypermetria, ataxia, conscious proprioceptive deficits, head-pressing	Cow, sheep, goat
Trypanosomiasis (exotic)	Ataxia, conscious proprioceptive deficit, somnolence, circling, head-pressing	Cow

mals. When no ocular disease can be found to account for blindness, a lesion in the nervous system is likely to be responsible. Observation of the animal's ability to negotiate its environment, particularly in unfamiliar surroundings, and eliciting the menace reflex are the primary methods of determining visual function. Further testing can be performed by setting up a maze of objects for the animal to negotiate, by utilizing different light levels and assessing vision in bright versus dim light, and by blindfolding each eye in turn when unilateral deficits are suspected. Eighty percent to 90% of optic nerve fibers (axons of retinal ganglion cells) cross to the opposite side of the brain in the optic chiasm of ungulates; thus central representation of vision in these species is predominantly contralateral. Fibers that remain uncrossed originate from the temporal aspect of the retina. Lesions in the visual apparatus distal to the optic chiasm (i.e., lesions of the globe, the retina, or the optic nerve) produce ipsilateral visual deficits. Lesions proximal to the optic chiasm produce lesions in the opposite visual field (contralateral hemianopsia). The discussion below refers to severe or complete lesions, because these are most easily understood and described. Partial lesions will produce similar but milder signs, for example, reduced visual acuity rather than complete blindness. Absent or re-

duced menace reflex also can be caused by lesions of the facial nerve (CN VII), the cerebellum, or the cerebrum. Animals with facial nerve lesions can see, but cannot blink even when the canthi of the eye are touched. Animals with cerebellar disease can see and can blink in response to the examiner touching the periorbital area. Cerebellar disease causes additional signs such as intention tremor, hypermetria, and ataxia. Animals with moderate to severe cerebral disease usually will blink in response to tactile stimulation of the face and periorbital area, but appear to have decreased vision and may have a reduced to absent menace reflex (see above). Localization of lesions causing blindness is summarized in Table 8-6.

Pupil size and movement of the globes are mediated via cranial nerves II, IV, VI, and the sympathetic innervation of the eye. Clinical signs of diseases affecting these nerves are described in the sections on cranial nerves and Horner's syndrome.

Circling

Circling can be a manifestation of lateralized disease in several regions of the brain: the cerebrum and thalamus, the midbrain, or the medulla oblongata. Circling associated

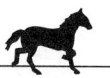

TABLE 8-8

Diseases of the Horse That Produce Cortical Disease

Disease	Predominant Clinical Signs
Hepatoencephalopathy	Aggression, rage, hyperexcitability, odontoprisis, ataxia, proprioceptive deficit, head pressing, convulsions, coma, semicoma, blindness, fear, red urine (hemolysis), icterus
Parasitic migration	Head tilt, hyperexcitability, odontoprisis, ataxia, proprioceptive deficit, head pressing, circling, coma, semicoma, blindness, anisocoria, convulsion, tongue dystonia
Rabies	Recumbency, ataxia, proprioceptive deficit, aggression, depression, coma, semicoma, head pressing, circling, propulsive walking, mydriasis, tenesmus, fear, continual chewing
Leukoencephalomalacia	Recumbency, ataxia, proprioceptive deficit, aggression, depression, coma, semicoma, head pressing, circling, propulsive walking, mydriasis, tenesmus, fear, continual chewing
Brain abscess/meningitis	Head pressing, blindness, conscious proprioceptive deficit, ataxia, circling, depression, convulsions, hyperexcitability, stiff neck, rigid legs, fever, propulsive walking
Brain tumor	Depression, facial paresis or paralysis, facial anesthesia or analgesia, head tilt, strabismus, nystagmus, loss of menace, hypermetria, ataxia
Trauma/hematoma	Head pressing, blindness, conscious proprioceptive deficit, ataxia, circling, depression, convulsions, hyperexcitability, stiff neck, rigid legs, fever, propulsive walking, blood from ear or nose

Viral encephalomyelitis
    Eastern equine encephalomyelitis
    Near Eastern encephalitis
    Venezuelan equine encephalomyelitis
    Western equine encephalomyelitis
    Equine herpesvirus-1
    West Nile virus
    Borna
	Head pressing, blindness, conscious proprioceptive deficit, ataxia, circling, depression, coma, convulsions, recumbency, hyperexcitability, stiff neck, rigid legs, fever, propulsive walking

Equine protozoal myeloencephalitis	Seizures, head tilt, facial paralysis, circling, nystagmus, dysphagia, facial paralysis, blindness, ataxia, paresis, hyporeflexia, hyperreflexia
Hydrocephalus	Coma, semicoma, blindness, somnolence, head pressing, dysphonia, ataxia, conscious proprioceptive deficit, weak tongue
Idiopathic epilepsy	Intermittent psychomotor seizures, normal interictal periods
Narcolepsy	Intermittent sleeplike states with stress, normal between attacks

with cerebral disease is toward the side of the lesion (ipsiversive), and is thought to result from lesions affecting the deep structures of the cerebrum or thalamic components, rather than the cerebral cortex. Animals that circle secondary to cerebral disease often have a head turn toward the side of the lesion, in addition to the circling. Whereas gait may appear normal on a level surface, affected animals have proprioceptive and postural reaction deficits on the side of the body contralateral to the lesion. Head tilt and spontaneous nystagmus are not present. Physiologic nystagmus (the oculocephalic reflex) is normal when the examiner turns the animal's head from side to side. The severity of circling seen with lateralized cerebral disease is variable, from a subtle tendency to marked circling.

Disease affecting solely or predominantly one side of the midbrain also results in circling. The circling is ipsiversive, occurs without manifestations of head tilt or spontaneous nystagmus, and is accompanied by contralateral proprioceptive and postural reaction deficits. Circling in midbrain disease is compulsive, in contrast to that seen in cerebral disease or vestibular disease. In both cerebral and midbrain disease the animal's level of consciousness usually is decreased, more severely with midbrain than cerebral disease. Midbrain lesions also may cause abnormalities of the oculocephalic and pupillary light reflexes because of the involvement of the somatic and parasympathetic nuclei of the oculomotor nerve (CN III) and the medial longitudinal fasciculus. The medial longitudinal fasciculus relays sensory information from vestibular centers in the medulla oblongata to the nuclei of cranial nerves III, IV, and VI.

Severe midbrain disease results in decerebrate posture: the animal is unconscious and in opisthotonus (extreme extension of the head and neck) with extensor rigidity of all four limbs. Severe midbrain disease may be the result of traumatic injuries, infectious diseases, and particularly is a consequence of increased intracranial pressure from a variety of causes. When intracranial pressure is increased above normal there is a tendency for the occipital lobes of the cerebrum to be herniated caudally, under the tentorium cerebelli. This results in compression of the midbrain and may be fatal. The presence of decerebrate rigidity warrants a very grave prognosis and the need for immediate and aggressive treatment with agents that decrease intracranial pressure (intravenous mannitol, DMSO, and other diuretics).

Head Tilt and Nystagmus

The presence of a head tilt, wherein one ear is held closer to the ground than the other, indicates disease of the vestibular system. Head tilt usually is accompanied by spontaneous (abnormal) nystagmus and a variety of other clinical signs. Vestibular disease can be classified as peripheral or central. Peripheral vestibular disease occurs when lesions of the vestibular apparatus of the inner ear (utricle, saccule, semicircular canals) are present, or when there is abnormality of the peripheral portion of the vestibulocochlear nerve (CN VIII). Animals with peripheral vestibular lesions have normal mentation but may be extremely disoriented, making assessment of mentation difficult. The head tilt in peripheral vestibular disease is toward the side of the lesion. The vestibular system is involved in the maintenance of normal posture. Unilateral peripheral vestibular dysfunction causes decreased extensor tone in the limbs ipsilateral to the lesion and increased extensor tone in the contralateral limbs, resulting in the clinical signs of leaning, falling, and rolling toward the affected side. Proprioception and postural reactions are normal in peripheral vestibular disease, although they may be hard to evaluate in severe cases and in larger animals.

Peripheral vestibular lesions produce a horizontal or rotatory nystagmus, with the fast phase directed away from the side of the lesion. The direction of the nystagmus in relation to the rest of the head is unchanged no matter what the position of the head. Physiologic nystagmus may be absent in severe cases but more often it is decreased, particularly when the head is turned toward the side of the lesion. The facial nerve runs in proximity to the petrous temporal bone, and facial paralysis may be present in animals with peripheral vestibular disease when the facial nerve also is damaged by the underlying etiology, such as may occur in traumatic injuries or severe otitis media/interna. Similarly, involvement of the postganglionic sympathetic nerve to the eye as it courses through the petrous temporal bone results in an ipsilateral Horner's syndrome (ptosis, miosis, enophthalmos, facial sweating in horses, reduced sweating on the nasal planum in cattle).

Lesions within the vestibular centers in the medulla oblongata and cerebellum also cause vestibular dysfunction. Central vestibular disease may produce clinical signs similar to peripheral vestibular lesions, but can be distinguished from the latter by a number of features. Head tilt in central vestibular disease usually is toward the side of the lesion, but may be in the opposite direction when the underlying disease involves the cerebellum (paradoxical vestibular syndrome). Similarly, nystagmus may be identical to that seen in peripheral vestibular disease, but also may be vertical, diagonal, different in each eye (disconjugate nystagmus), may change in direction when the position of the head is changed (positional nystagmus), or may be horizontal or rotatory with the fast phase toward the side of the lesion (paradoxical vestibular syndrome). Signs of involvement of the motor and sensory tracts to the limbs as they course through the medulla usually accompany central vestibular disease. Proprioceptive and postural reaction deficits are present in the ipsilateral limbs, together with mild hyperreflexia. The nuclei of cranial nerves V to XII also may be affected by diseases that cause central vestibular lesions. Signs of cranial nerve dysfunction accompanying vestibular abnormalities, other than that of the facial nerve alone, indicate central vestibular disease. Horner's syndrome, however, is not seen in conjunction with central vestibular disease. Decreased mentation often occurs in animals with central vestibular disease, in contrast to the normal mental status of animals with peripheral vestibular lesions.

Animals with either peripheral or central vestibular lesions tend to lean against the walls and may fall when forced to perform a complex motor maneuver. They may adopt recumbency with the lesion side directed down and have poor righting responses, particularly from lesion-side-down recumbency. When positioned so that the lesion side is directed up, they often will roll to a lesion-down position. Blindfolding the patient eliminates visual compensatory mechanisms and therefore increases the severity of the clinical signs. Blindfolding may help in the detection of subtle lesions, but should be done with caution, because it may result in falling. Animals with vestibular disease occasionally may have slight ventral strabismus in the ipsilateral eye and slight dorsal strabismus in the contralateral eye. This strabismus can be differentiated from the ventrolateral strabismus seen with lesions of the oculomotor nerve because the strabismus accompanying vestibular lesions is mild and changes or disappears when the head position is changed. The strabismus in animals with paralysis of the oculomotor nerve does not change as the head position is altered. In the cow and sheep, evaluation of globe position must be conducted with the head held in normal position because these animals rotate the globe downward when the head and neck are extended. Conversely, the globe is maintained in the center of the palpebral fissure at all head positions in the horse and the goat.

Animals with bilateral vestibular lesions do not have head tilt or nystagmus. The animal stands with the legs base-wide and may fall to either side when the head position is rapidly altered. Affected animals may show a coarse side-to-side head tremor. Bilateral vestibular lesions usually are peripheral in type, and are rarely encountered in clinical practice. Central lesions extensive enough to cause bilateral vestibular disease are likely to be fatal.

Incoordination, Hypermetria, Dysmetria, and Intention Tremor

Clinical signs that occur in animals with cerebellar disorders include hypermetria, intention tremor, and truncal ataxia (excessive body sway during movement along a straight path). Conscious proprioceptive fibers do not pass through the cerebellum. Consequently, postural placement of the limbs is normal. Animals with cerebellar disease move the limbs with excessive rate, range, and force. There is a slight delay in lifting the limb from the ground. At the peak of protraction, the limbs are lifted too high and too far anteriorly. The legs then hit the ground with excessive force. When the animal is turned, the legs circumduct. The animal may violently thrust the outside rear limb backward and laterally when turned. The forelimbs and the hindlimbs occasionally collide during the turn (interference). At rest, the animal stands with the legs abducted, in a base-wide stance. This is not a conscious proprioceptive deficit, however, because the animal consciously returns the limbs to the base-wide posture if the leg position is manually corrected. There is intention tremor, most marked in the head. When the animal attempts to reposition the head, it overshoots the intended position, corrects, and then overshoots again. The sequence of overcompensation and overcorrection results in a coarse oscillation. The head tremor is most conspicuous when the animal is alert, especially when eating. Intention tremor disappears when the animal is recumbent and the musculature is relaxed. In animals with cerebellar disorders, the extensor muscles of the limbs may be hypertonic, and spinal reflexes occasionally are exaggerated. Foals with cerebellar disease fall backward. This does not usually occur in ruminants. Lesions of the rostral cerebellar vermis can result in opisthotonos. Animals with cerebellar cortical disease may lack a menace response but retain their vision and can negotiate around obstacles. The reason for the menace deficit is unclear, but it is thought to result from disruption of efferent pathways emanating from the occipital (visual) cortex and passing through the cerebellar cortex to the motor nucleus of the facial nerve. Animals with pure cerebellar dysfunction remain bright, alert, and responsive to external stimuli. Animals with very severe lesions of the cerebellum may be recumbent and unable to rise, with decerebellate posture. This posture is characterized by opisthotonos and forelimb extensor rigidity, with normal or flexed hindlimbs. Unlike decerebrate rigidity, animals in decerebellate rigidity have normal mentation and a good prognosis if the underlying disease is not progressive. Cerebellar disease is often bilaterally symmetrical, but lateralized lesions cause signs on the ipsilateral side of the body. Diseases that cause spasticity or tremors in livestock are listed in Table 8-9.

Involvement of the vestibular components of the cerebellum (caudal cerebellar peduncle, flocculonodular lobe, and fastigial nucleus) results in signs of paradoxical vestibular syndrome, described above.

Abnormalities of Cranial Nerve Function

The normal functions of the cranial nerves are described above, in the discussion of the neurologic examination. Cranial nerve dysfunction may be central or peripheral in type, depending on whether the neurologic lesion lies within the central com-

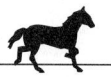

TABLE 8-9

Diseases of Spasticity or Tremors in Horses and Ruminants

Disease	Clinical Manifestations	Species Affected

Cerebellar hypoplasia
    Bovine viral diarrhea
    Bluetongue
    Akabane
    Border disease
    Wesselbron disease
    Hereditary
	Intentional head tremor, base-wide stance, hypermetria, hypertonia, hyperreflexia, truncal ataxia, menace deficit, opisthotonos	Cattle, sheep, goats

Cerebellar abiotrophy	Intentional head tremor, base-wide stance, hypermetria, hypertonia, hyperreflexia, truncal ataxia, menace deficit, opisthotonos	Cattle, horses
Daft lambs	Recumbency, hypertonicity, hyperreflexia, deafness, intentional head tremors, hypermetria	Sheep

Grass staggers
    Bermuda
    Kikiyu
    Rye grass
    Mycotic tremorgens
    Canary
    Dallis
	Hypermetria, hyperreflexia, truncal ataxia, head tremors, base-wide stance, recumbency, ptyalism, hyperexcitability, hyperesthesia	Cattle, sheep, goats

Hypomagnesemia	Hypermetria, hyperreflexia, truncal ataxia, recumbency, hyperesthesia, menace deficit, opisthotonos, aggressiveness, hypertonia	Cattle, horses
Lysosomal storage disease	Intentional head tremor, base-wide stance, hypermetria, hypertonia, hyperreflexia, truncal ataxia, menace deficit, opisthotonos, blindness, aggressiveness	Cattle, goat
Locoism and *Swainsonia* poisoning	Ataxia, conscious proprioceptive deficit, depression, intentional head tremor, loss of herd instinct, maniacal behavior, flaccidity of the nose and lips, base-wide stance	All species
Hereditary neuraxial edema	Recumbency, head tremor, good appetite, hyperesthesia, nystagmus, strabismus, muscular fasciculations	Cattle
Bovine familial convulsions and ataxia	Tetaniform seizures, ataxia, hypermetria, hyperreflexia, head tremors, truncal ataxia	Cattle
Maple syrup urine disease	Depression, recumbency, opisthotonos, stimulus-induced tetanic spasms, convulsions, generalized decrease of spinal reflexes	Cattle
Solanum dimidiatum	Head tremors, hypermetria, hypertonia, hyperesthesia, weight loss, opisthotonos, recumbency, and convulsions	Cattle

ponents of the cranial nerves within the brain or in the peripheral portions of the nerves. Clinical signs of cranial nerve dysfunction are ipsilateral to the lesions that cause them.

BLINDNESS, STRABISMUS, OCULAR PARESIS OR PARALYSIS, ABNORMALITIES OF PUPIL SIZE OR PUPILLARY LIGHT REFLEXES. Lesions involving cranial nerves II, III, IV, and VI are described above, in the discussion of blindness and other visual dysfunctions.

FACIAL HYPOESTHESIA OR ANALGESIA, DROPPED JAW. Loss of or decrease in sensory perception on the face, including the inside of the mouth, the nasal planum, the cornea, and the lower jaw area is the result of lesions of the trigeminal nerve. It is important to distinguish this from the signs of contralateral cerebral disease or facial nerve paralysis. In the former case conscious perception of the stimulus is decreased, but animals will respond to vigorous or painful stimuli and usually will blink in response to corneal stimulation. Animals with cerebral disease have decreased mental alertness and may have other signs of cerebral disease, such as seizures, circling, or contralateral hemiparesis. Facial nerve lesions result in an inability to move the muscles of facial expression or blink on the affected side, but animals will avoid stimulation of the face by pulling away the head and neck in a coordinated fashion. Unilateral loss of facial sensation most commonly results from damage to the peripheral portion of the trigeminal nerve, the trigeminal ganglion in the petrosal bone of the skull. Bilateral facial hypoesthesia is most likely caused by cerebral disease rather than trigeminal nerve disease. The mandibular branch of the trigeminal nerve also carries motor innervation to the muscles of mastication from the pontine motor nucleus of the trigeminal nerve. Bilateral in-

volvement of the motor component of the nerve results in a dropped jaw and inability to prehend and chew food, together with drooling saliva. The muscles of mastication atrophy, most obvious in the masseter and temporalis muscles. Unilateral disease causes atrophy of the denervated muscles, and mild jaw weakness may be appreciated, but the animal can still eat and close the jaw. The most important differential diagnosis for dropped jaw is rabies. A careful history must be taken, to elucidate the risk of exposure to this disease, as well as whether the animal has been vaccinated. Central lesions in the trigeminal nerve also may involve adjacent structures in the brainstem, such as the facial nerve, the vestibular system, and the long sensory and motor tracts to the limbs.

FACIAL PARESIS OR PARALYSIS. Lesions of the facial nerve result in ipsilateral atonia or hypotonia of the facial muscles. The clinical signs of facial nerve paralysis in all large animals include ptosis, dropped ear, and absence of the menace response and palpebral reflex. There is accumulation of food in the cheek pouch and commissure of the lips on the ipsilateral side. Affected animals frequently drool saliva from the lip commissure on the affected side. The animal is unable to open the nostril on the affected side during inspiration. The muzzle of the horse, goat, and sheep deviates away from the direction of the neurologic lesion. Deviation of the muzzle is not seen in cattle because of the normal rigidity of the planum nasale. If the neurologic lesion is located between the medulla oblongata and the skull, the ipsilateral eye may be dry because of loss of innervation from the parasympathetic nucleus of CN VII. Lesions of the central components of the facial nerve in the medulla oblongata also destroy proprioceptive tracts and reticular system neurons, resulting in conscious proprioceptive deficits and, sometimes, decreased mentation. Lesions of the peripheral component of CN VII result in facial atonia or hypotonia, but do not produce depression or conscious proprioceptive deficits.

HEAD TILT, SPONTANEOUS NYSTAGMUS, DEAFNESS.
Lesions involving cranial nerve VIII, the vestibulocochlear nerve, produce signs of vestibular dysfunction, as described previously. Deafness also may be a consequence of vestibulocochlear nerve disease. Bilateral deafness has been reported in Paint horses, where it may be a heritable defect associated with the gene for white coat color, similarly to the situation that exists in a number of breeds of dog with white or merle coat color.[44] Deafness also can result from severe aural disease. Although bilateral deafness is fairly easy to recognize clinically, unilateral deafness may be less obvious. Inability to localize sound occurs when animals have unilateral deafness and may be suspected when animals alert to sound but do not turn toward the sound. Auditory evoked potentials can be used to determine integrity of the auditory pathway in the inner ear and medulla oblongata.

DYSPHAGIA, DYSPHONIA, STERTOROUS BREATHING.
Lesions in the nucleus ambiguus (CNs IX, X, and XI) produce dysphonia, inspiratory dyspnea, dysphagia, and neurogenic atrophy of the trapezius, sternocephalicus, and brachiocephalicus muscles. The inspiratory dyspnea is characterized by roaring and snoring. Roaring is a stertor that is made during peak inspiratory flow. It is caused by paralysis of the cricoarytenoideus dorsalis muscle, resulting in a failure to abduct the vocal folds during inspiration. Additional evidence of paralysis of CNs IX to XI may be obtained by endoscopic examination of the pharynx. Other signs of paralysis of CNs IX to XI include failure to abduct the vocal folds, collapse of the pharynx, dorsal displacement of the soft palate, and inability to swallow a nasogastric tube. Lesions in the peripheral parts of the glossopharyngeal, vagus, and accessory spinal nerves produce similar laryngeal signs but may be differentiated from centrally located lesions by attitude, appetite, and conscious proprioceptive responses. Animals with peripheral nerve deficits remain alert and appetent and do not show conscious proprioceptive deficits, whereas animals with centrally

TABLE 8-10

Clinical Signs of Cranial Nerve Dysfunction

Cranial Nerve	Central Origin or Projection	Clinical Signs of Dysfunction	Comments
I—Olfactory	Olfactory bulb, limbic system (behavior and emotion centers), cerebral cortex	Loss of sense of smell (anosmia)	Olfactory nerve lesions are rare and difficult to detect clinically.
II—Optic	Optic chiasm, optic tract, lateral geniculate nucleus, optic radiation, occipital cortex	Blindness	See text for additional comments (Blindness).
III—Oculomotor	Midbrain somatic and parasympathetic nuclei	Ventrolateral strabismus, ptosis (somatic component); dilated, nonresponsive pupil (parasympathetic component)	
IV—Trochlear	Midbrain	Dorsomedial strabismus	Trochlear nerve lesions are rare and usually accompanied by other signs of midbrain dysfunction.
V —Trigeminal	Pons (motor nucleus), medulla and rostral cervical spinal cord (sensory tract)	Dropped jaw in bilateral motor paralysis; decrease or loss of sensation to most of the structures of the head and face in sensory nerve disease	Rabies is an important differential diagnosis in animals with a dropped jaw.
VI—Abducent	Rostral medulla oblongata	Medial strabismus (paralysis of the lateral rectus muscle)	
VII—Facial	Medulla oblongata (rostral to middle); motor, sensory, and parasympathetic components	Facial paresis to paralysis (motor component); loss of sense of taste to rostral two thirds of the tongue, loss of sensation on medial aspect of the pinna (sensory components); decreased tear production (dry eye) and decreased salivation (parasympathetic components)	The facial nerve is particularly susceptible to damage in its peripheral course because of its proximity to the middle ear and to the guttural pouch in horses, and its superficial location on the face.
VIII—Vestibulocochlear	Medulla oblongata (middle)	Decreased hearing or deafness; vestibular signs (head tilt, nystagmus, falling, rolling)	See description of vestibular disease in text.
IX, X, XI—Glossopharyngeal, vagus, accessory	Medulla oblongata (nucleus ambiguus in middle to caudal medulla and rostral cervical spinal cord)	Dysphagia (IX and X), laryngeal paresis to paralysis (X), atrophy of sternocephalicus, brachiocephalicus, and trapezius muscles (XII)	Rabies is an important differential diagnosis in animals with dysphagia or choke.
XII—Hypoglossal	Medulla oblongata (middle to caudal)	Paresis to paralysis of the tongue	Acute unilateral lesions result in the tongue being deviated away from the side of the lesion. In chronic disease atrophy and contracture of the affected side of the tongue results in deviation toward the affected side.

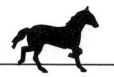

located lesions may be depressed and inappetent and may have proprioceptive and postural deficits. Animals with bilateral lesions in the peripheral nerves are unable to open the glottis during inspiration and become cyanotic. Peripheral lesions of the accessory nerve that have been present for longer than 1 month may produce neurogenic atrophy of the trapezius, brachiocephalicus, and sternocephalicus muscles. This is frequently accompanied by aspiration pneumonia. Lesions of the visceral efferent component of CN X in ruminants produce vagal indigestion, which is characterized by rumenal distention with fluid, rumenal tympany, abomasal stasis, and sometimes a hypochloremic, hypokalemic metabolic alkalosis. This is an important disease of the ruminant gastrointestinal tract. Hypoglossal nerve lesions produce a weak or flaccid tongue. In animals with unilateral lesions, the tongue falls toward the same side as the lesion and is flaccid when it is manually extended from the mouth. After prolonged denervation (1 month or more) the ipsilateral side of the tongue atrophies. Horses with lesions in the sensorimotor cortex may also fail to retract the tongue normally; however, the tongue tone is variable, and the animal can retract it if it receives sufficient stimulation. In comparison, the tongue tone is consistently weak in cases of hypoglossal paralysis.

Signs of cranial nerve dysfunction, together with the central origins or projections of the nerves are summarized in Table 8-10. Diseases that involve the brainstem and cranial nerves are summarized in Table 8-11.

Lesions of the medulla oblongata can produce severe depression, somnolence, or coma as a result of ARAS dysfunction in addition to signs of vestibular dysfunction and functional deficits in cranial nerves V to XII. Other clinical signs of medullary lesions include ipsilateral paresis and conscious proprioceptive deficits as a result of dysfunction in the rubrospinal, reticulospinal, spinothalamic, and spinocerebellar pathways. The spinal reflexes of the ipsilateral limbs are exaggerated and the extensor muscle tone is increased. Further details are given in the discussion of quadriparesis and hemiparesis below.

Measurement of Brainstem Function Using Auditory Evoked Potentials

The integrity of the vestibulocochlear apparatus can be examined using brainstem auditory evoked potentials.[45-47] This method examines the averaged waveform that is generated after an auditory click in the ear. The individual signals from

TABLE 8-11

Diseases of the Brainstem and Cranial Nerves

Disease	Location	Clinical Signs and Laboratory Findings
Viral encephalomyelitis, rabies, malignant catarrhal fever (cattle only)	Multifocal brainstem, particularly medulla oblongata	Head tilt, nystagmus, circling, ataxia, proprioceptive deficit, tongue paralysis, anisocoria, dilated nonresponsive pupils, strabismus, paralyzed tongue, dysphonia, dysphagia, plus cortical signs (rage, fright, fear, convulsions); CSF may show pleocytosis (mainly mononuclear cells); high protein
Listeriosis (cattle)	Multifocal brainstem, particularly basal ganglia, metencephalon, and medulla oblongata	Circling, head tilt, facial paralysis, roaring, snoring, dysphagia, depression, coma, convulsions, ataxia, proprioceptive deficit, CSF shows pleocytosis (mainly mononuclear), and increased protein
Thromboembolic meningoencephalomyelitis (cattle)	Multifocal brainstem and cortex	Circling, nystagmus, head tilt, strabismus, tongue paralysis, dysphagia, facial paralysis, coma, convulsions, depression, xanthochromic CSF with increased neutrophils
Peripheral vestibular disease	Petrous temporal bone, membranous labyrinths, vestibulocochlear nerve, also associated with facial nerve paralysis	Head tilt, circling, or leaning toward lesion side, ventrolateral strabismus on ipsilateral side, dorsomedial strabismus on contralateral side, nystagmus (usually horizontal and constant)
Verminous migration	Multifocal brainstem, most commonly thalamus, diencephalon	Circling, nystagmus, head tilt, strabismus, tongue paralysis, facial paralysis, depression, coma, convulsions, depression, proprioceptive deficit, bradycardia, salivation, head pressing, hemianopsia; high protein and increased WBCs in CSF

Space-occupying mass
  Tumor
  Abscess
	Cerebellopontine angle; cranial nerves 5, 7, and 8	Head tilt, strabismus, proprioceptive deficit, facial analgesia, jaw drop, depression, coma, strabismus, nystagmus, hyperreflexia, hypertonia, falling or circling toward affected side, blindness on contralateral side, tongue paralysis, hemianopsia, bradycardia, coma, convulsion

Horner's syndrome	C8 to T1 motor neurons (gray matter), spinal roots, vagosympathetic trunk, sympathetic tracts of spinal cord, periorbita	Miosis, enophthalmos, lack of nasal sweat (cattle only), ipsilateral facial swelling (horses only)
Guttural pouch mycosis (horses)	Guttural pouch	Dysphagia, head shyness, head shaking, roaring, dysphonia, protrusion of the tongue from the mouth, epistaxis, head tilt, nystagmus, facial sweating, shivering, Horner's syndrome, colic, facial paralysis

CSF, Cerebrospinal fluid; *WBCs*, white blood cells.

a single click stimulus are small and therefore must be amplified by repeating the stimulus (30 to 100 dB, 10 Hz) between 30 and 1000 times and recording the voltage difference between two electrodes placed on the head. The recording electrode is usually placed over the petrous temporal bone, and the reference electrode at the vertex, or elsewhere on the head. The technique of signal averaging is used to eliminate background electrical activity and enhance the specific waveforms generated by the auditory impulse. The response usually is measured for 10 ms after the stimulus is applied. Ablation of the entire cochlear apparatus and vestibular nerve, as might occur with otitis interna, would result in a loss or attenuation of waveform activity after the click stimulus. Injury to the brainstem vestibular nuclei would result in a loss of waves II through VI. Damage to the trapezoid body (pons), lateral lemniscus, caudal colliculus, and medial geniculate body would result in a loss of waveforms III through VI, respectively. Increased latency between the peaks is usually associated with toxic or degenerative diseases of the CNS.

Paresis and Ataxia in Two or Four Limbs

Quadriparesis and hemiparesis are seen with lesions affecting the mid- to caudal brainstem (midbrain, medulla oblongata) or the cervical spinal cord (C1-T2 spinal cord segments). Quadriparesis also can be seen in generalized peripheral nerve or muscle disease, discussed below. Paraparesis results from disease affecting the spinal cord between segments T3 and L2, or the peripheral nerves to the hindlimbs. Disease of the cerebrum and thalamus does not produce appreciable paresis and ataxia when the animal is walking in a straight line on a level surface, but these signs become apparent in the limbs contralateral to the lesion when the animal is asked to circle, back, step over obstacles, or walk on a slope. Localization of the lesion when signs of paresis and ataxia are present depends on the assessment of muscle mass and tone, spinal reflexes, and evaluation of brainstem function, as determined by the presence or absence of signs such as altered mentation, cranial nerve deficits, or vestibular dysfunction.

Quadriparesis and ataxia with normal muscle mass and tone and normal to increased spinal reflexes indicate a lesion in the brainstem or in spinal cord segments C1-C5. Presence of clinical signs of brain disease will facilitate localization of the lesion to an intracranial site, as described above. Lesions in the midbrain cause contralateral postural and proprioceptive deficits, whereas those in the medulla oblongata cause ipsilateral signs. Cerebellar disease causes a truncal ataxia, without significant loss of proprioceptive or postural functions, and with no or mild hyperreflexia of the limbs. Lesions of the thalamus and cerebrum cause minimal to no paresis or ataxia when the animal is gaited on a level surface, but contralateral proprioceptive and postural reaction deficits are present. Altered mentation and other signs of cerebral or thalamic disease are expected, such as circling or cortical blindness. Animals with spinal cord disease have normal mentation. The clinical signs shown by such patients depend on the location of the lesion and the relative amount of damage to gray (cell bodies) and white (myelinated spinal cord tracts) matter. Loss of white matter results in sensory loss whereas gray matter damage produces lower motor neuron deficits. The sensory losses are either proprioceptive responses or cutaneous sensory deficits. White matter is usually more susceptible to pressure changes than gray matter so proprioceptive deficits are consistently observed during the first stages of spinal cord disease. Spinal cord diseases may be localized to one of the following five regions: high cervical (C1 to C5), cervicothoracic (C6 to T2), thoracolumbar (T3

to L2), lumbosacral (L3 to S2), and sacrococcygeal (S3 to Cd5) regions. Tables 8-4 and 8-5 list the peripheral nerves and the spinal segments that innervate them.

Cervical Spinal Cord

Animals with incomplete section of the cervical region of the spinal cord display hemiparesis or tetraparesis. The clinical signs include knuckling, stumbling, failure to lift the inside feet when turned in a tight circle, interference, hypermetria, abnormal postural placement responses, crossing over midline when turned, and excessive truncal sway. Animals with more severe lesions of the cervical spinal cord become recumbent and are unable to lift the head from the ground. There is an asymmetric righting response in animals with unilateral lesions. They can raise the head and neck to a variable distance only when lying with the lesion side facing down. Muscle tone and spinal reflexes in the limbs of recumbent animals are exaggerated. The urinary bladder is distended. The animals have difficulty urinating, and afterward the bladder contains a large amount of urine. Animals with complete spinal cord transection anterior to C6 die suddenly as a result of paralysis of the intercostal muscles and the diaphragm.

Lesions between C6 and T2 spinal segments (brachial intumescence) result in conscious proprioceptive deficits in all four limbs and tetraparesis or tetraplegia. There is hypotonia and hyporeflexia of the forelimbs and hypertonia and hyperreflexia of the hindlimbs. Unilateral lesions result in ipsilateral signs. Lesions of C6 to T2 segments involving white but not gray matter do not produce forelimb hypotonia. Conscious perception of painful stimuli may be depressed in all limbs. Flexor reflexes in the forelimbs may be depressed but are normal in the hindlimbs. The righting responses of the head and neck are normal. Urination is difficult, and the urinary bladder is distended and has a large residual volume. After 1 month or more, lesions of the gray matter of the spinal cord or the peripheral nerves may result in neurogenic atrophy of one or more muscle groups of the forelimbs. Gray matter lesions of T1 to T3 spinal segments may result in Horner's syndrome, which is characterized by miosis, enophthalmos, and ptosis in all species. Unilateral facial sweating occurs in horses; lack of sweating on the planum nasale occurs in cattle. Differentiation of high (C1-C5) and low (C6-T2) cervical spinal cord lesions may be difficult in horses, especially when signs are fairly mild.

Lesions of the thoracolumbar region (T3 to L3) result in normal activity of the forelimbs and proprioceptive deficits in the hindlimbs. These deficits are similar to those described above for the cervical areas and include ataxia, knuckling, stumbling, abduction, adduction, interference, excessive truncal sway, and failure to lift the inside foot when pivoted in a tight turn. With complete lesions, the animal becomes recumbent but intermittently assumes a dog-sitting position, with the forelimbs extended and weight bearing and the hindlimbs flexed. Muscle tone and spinal reflexes are exaggerated in the hindlimbs. The urinary bladder is distended, and residual volume is large. The tone of the urethral sphincter is normal. Young animals with severe spinal cord lesions between T2 and L2 display transient hypertonia of the forelimbs (Schiff-Sherrington syndrome). This condition is caused by interference with inhibitory fibers ascending from the lumbar segments in the dorsal funiculi to the lower motor neurons of the forelimbs.[48] These fibers synapse on the neurons of the brachial intumescence. Hypertonia from this deficit may be differentiated from cervical cord lesions by the lack of conscious proprioceptive deficits in the forelimbs of animals with thoracolumbar lesions.

The lumbosacral region (L3 to S2) of the spinal cord contains lower motor neuron efferents and general propriocep-

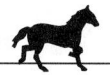

tive afferents to the pelvic limbs. Lesions in this area result in paraparesis or paraplegia. Affected animals show ataxia and conscious proprioceptive deficits of the hindlimbs. Patients with complete spinal cord lesions of L3 to S2 have flaccid paraplegia, which is accompanied by hyporeflexia or areflexia in the hindlimbs. With prolonged denervation, neurogenic atrophy of the hindlimb musculature occurs. Lesions located between L3 and L6 spinal cord segments result in urinary bladder distention and maintenance of a large residual volume. The sphincter tone is intact, but urine is not voided unless the intravesicular pressure exceeds that of the sphincter. These animals usually have contact dermatitis of the perineum and preputial area because of urine scalding.

Lesions located around S1 and S2 segments result in bladder distention and flaccidity. Urine may drip continuously from the urethral orifice. The rate of flow may be increased by manually pressing on the bladder during a rectal examination. Lesions of the sacrococcygeal (S3 to Cd5) region (cauda equina) produce flaccidity of the tail and anus and, in males, paraphimosis. Lesions in this area also result in desensitization of the tail, penis, vulva, anus, and perineum. The urethral sphincter is dilated, and urine constantly drips from the urethral orifice. The animal does not evacuate the bladder and is unable to defecate, resulting in a large dilated urinary bladder and distention of the rectum with feces. If the entire neurologic lesion is located caudal to S3, ataxia or conscious proprioceptive deficit is not present. The combination of flaccidity of the tail and anus, and the constant urine leakage produces contact dermatitis of the perineum and hindlimbs. Perineal scalding is characteristic of lesions of the cauda equina. Specific diseases of the spinal cord, peripheral nerves, or motor end plate are listed in Table 8-12.

TABLE 8-12

Diseases of the Spinal Cord, Peripheral Nerve, and Motor End Plate of Large Animals

Disease	Signs	Species Affected
Occipitoatlantoaxial malformation	Ataxia, spasticity, hyperreflexia, crepitation or pain with neck flexion, head tilt, torticollis, proprioceptive deficit, visible swelling or asymmetry	Cow, horse
Fractures/dislocations	Tetraparesis, tetraplegia, paraparesis, paraplegia, hyperreflexia, stiff neck, recumbency, proprioceptive deficit, acute death, crepitation pain, or swelling	All species
Cervical spinal abscesses	Tetraparesis, tetraplegia, paraparesis, paraplegia, recumbency, stiff neck, proprioceptive deficit, acute death, crepitation or pain, swelling	All species
Myelopathy	Tetraparesis, tetraplegia, paraparesis, paraplegia, recumbency, proprioceptive deficit	Horse
Cervical stenotic myelopathy	Tetraparesis, tetraplegia, paraparesis, paraplegia, recumbency, stiff neck, proprioceptive deficit, strip sweating	Horse
Cervical vertebral instability	Tetraparesis, tetraplegia, paraparesis, paraplegia, recumbency, stiff neck, proprioceptive deficit, acute death, crepitation, or pain	Horse
Spinal tumor (lymphosarcoma, neurofibroma)	Tetraparesis, tetraplegia, paraparesis, paraplegia, recumbency, proprioceptive deficit	All species
Equine rhinopneumonitis	Tetraparesis, tetraplegia, paraparesis, paraplegia, recumbency, proprioceptive deficit, flaccid anus, flaccid tail, dysuria, distended bladder, impacted rectum, urine scalding	Horse
Copper deficiency	Tetraparesis, tetraplegia, paraparesis, paraplegia, recumbency, proprioceptive deficit	Sheep, goat
Cauda equina neuritis	Pruritis in the perineum, hair loss in perineum, analgesia in the perineum, flaccid tail, flaccid anus, paraphimosis, dysuria, facial palsy, head tilt, leaning, nystagmus	Horse
Ischemic myelopathy (fibrocartilaginous embolism)	Paraplegia, tetraplegia, flaccid tail, flaccid anus, areflexia at site of lesion, hyperreflexia distal to site of lesion, proprioceptive deficit	Horse, sheep
Caprine arthritis encephalitis virus	Tetraparesis, tetraplegia, paraparesis, paraplegia, recumbency, proprioceptive deficit	Goat
Segmental myelitis	Tetraparesis, tetraplegia, paraparesis, paraplegia, recumbency, stiff neck, proprioceptive deficit, strip sweating, hyporeflexia, areflexia, lower motor neuron deficit, facial nerve paralysis, jaw drop	Horse
Developmental defects (spina bifida, Arnold-Chiari syndrome, syringomyelia, hemivertebrae, spinal cysts)	Paraplegia, paraparesis, tetraplegia, tetraparesis, hypotonia, atonia, neurogenic atrophy, torticollis, scoliosis, kyphoscoliosis, misshapen tail, absence of skin over dorsal midline	All species
Verminous migration	Tetraparesis, tetraplegia, paraparesis, paraplegia, recumbency, proprioceptive deficit, head tilt, hyporeflexia, areflexia, hyperreflexia, hypertonia, hypotonia	All species
Tetanus	Stiffness, normal reflexes, flashing third eyelid, trismus, bloat, convulsions, coma, raised tail head	All species
Botulism	Flaccidity, ataxia, dysphagia, hyporeflexia, pupillary dilation, facial hypotonia, flaccid tail, flaccid anus	All species
Progressive ataxia	Ataxia, conscious proprioceptive deficit, recumbency	Charolais cattle
Locoism	Ataxia, conscious proprioceptive deficit, recumbency, bizarre behavior	All species
Dying back axonopathies	Hypermetria, hyperreflexia, proprioceptive deficit, flaccid tail, anus, fecal and urine retention, urine scalding, recumbency	All species
Elso heel (spastic paresis)	Affected hindlimb is hyperextended and swings in pendulum fashion, tail head is elevated	Cow
Spastic syndrome (crampy)	Episodic hyperextension of the hindlimb, extension of the limb behind the cow, head and neck extension	Cow
Peripheral nerve injuries	Areflexia, hypotonia, hyporeflexia, atonia, anesthesia, analgesia of a specific area of limbs or trunk, inability to support weight, normal function of limbs distal to denervated site	All species

Continued

TABLE 8-12

Diseases of the Spinal Cord, Peripheral Nerve, and Motor End Plate of Large Animals—cont'd

Disease	Signs	Species Affected
Ionophore toxicosis (salinomycin, lasalocid, monensin)	Tetraparesis, tetraplegia, ataxia, conscious proprioceptive deficit, colic, cardiac dysrhythmia, sudden death	All species
Periodic hyperkalemia	Episodic tremors, weakness, spasticity during episodes, recumbency	Horses, cow
Myotonia congenita	Episodic weakness, spasticity during episodes	All species
Bromide intoxication	Weakness, ataxia, stumbling, proprioceptive deficit, closed eyelids, drooped head and neck, paraphimosis	Horse
Coyotillo poisoning	Progressive weakness, hypermetria, areflexia	Goat
Humpy back/Coonabaran disease	Arched back, ataxia, conscious proprioceptive deficit, hindlimb stiffness, recumbency	Sheep
Neosporosis	Recumbency, ataxia, conscious proprioceptive deficit, neurogenic atrophy	Calf
Cycad palm poisoning	Posterior paresis, conscious proprioceptive deficit, elevated tail head, paraparesis, paraplegia	Cow
Acquired torticollis	Abnormally positioned head and neck	All species
Sorghum toxicosis	Ataxia, paraparesis, paraplegia, rabbit-hopping gait, proprioceptive deficit, recumbency, weight loss	Horse, cow
Stringhalt	Normal at rest, involuntary hyperflexion of the hock and stifle	Horse
Tick paralysis	Progressive generalized paresis, ataxia, recumbency, flaccid tail, flaccid anus, weak facial muscles	All species

Muscle Atrophy, Reduced Muscle Tone, Flaccid Paresis, Focal Analgesia

Clinical signs of reduced muscle tone, muscle atrophy, and flaccid paresis indicate peripheral nerve, muscle, or neuromuscular diseases. Signs may be localized to a single limb, as in the case of traumatic peripheral nerve injury; generalized, as in botulism and many myopathies; or multifocal, as in equine protozoal myelonencephalitis and other diseases that attack multiple areas of the CNS, destroying the ventral horn gray matter of the spinal cord, or nuclei of cranial nerves in the brainstem. Details of neuromuscular diseases and the use of ancillary diagnostic testing to localize peripheral nerve, muscle, and neuromuscular disease is described in Chapter 33.

Peripheral nerve lesions, whether of the central components of the nerves in the spinal cord and brainstem, or along their peripheral course in the limbs and head, also can result in focal hypalgesia or anesthesia. Knowledge of the autonomous zones for the peripheral nerves innervating the limbs can be used to localize such peripheral nerve lesions.[49,50]

Urinary Incontinence and Urine Retention

The clinical signs of urinary bladder denervation are variable and depend on the lesion location. Lesions of the sacral segments of the spinal cord produce a flaccid bladder, which distends with a large residual volume. Spontaneous urine leakage occurs continuously from the urethra. Additional urine flow occurs when the abdominal pressure is increased. The urethral sphincter is dilated and atonic. Lesions of the brainstem or spinal cord anterior to S1 produce reflex dyssynergia, a disturbance in coordination of micturition, wherein the facilitatory influence of the bladder stretch receptor (afferents) maintains tonic activity on the efferents of the urethral sphincter. The lack of inhibition of these reflexes from the upper motor neuron pathways produces hypertonicity of the urethral sphincters and results in an impediment to urine flow. There is a high intravesicular pressure and a large postvoiding urine volume. The urine escapes paroxysmally only when the intravesicular pressure exceeds the sphincter pressure. After approximately 1 month of denervation, local spinal reflexes between the sacral afferent and efferent neu-

rons develop in the S1 to S5 segments, and incomplete voiding occurs. In these cases the residual volume remains large, and the normal urination posture is not attained.

REFERENCES

1. Blythe L, Hultgren B, Craig A: Clinical, viral, and genetic evaluation of equine degenerative myeloencephalopathy in a family of Appaloosas, *J Am Vet Med Assoc* 198:1008, 1991.
2. Jolly R, Hartley W: Storage disease in domestic animals, *Aust Vet J* 53:1-8, 1977.
3. Cho D, Liepold H: Cerebellar cortical atrophy in a Charolais calf, *Vet Pathol* 15:264-266, 1978.
4. White M, Whitlock R, DeLahunta A: A cerebellar abiotrophy of calves, *Cornell Vet* 65:476-491, 1975.
5. Stuart LD, Liepold HW: Lesions in bovine progressive degenerative myeloencephalopathy ("weaver") of Brown Swiss cattle, *Vet Pathol* 2:13-23, 1985.
6. Palmer A, Blakemore W: Progressive ataxia of Charolais cattle associated with a myelin disorder, *Vet Rec* 91:592-594, 1972.
7. Duffell S: Neuraxial oedema of Hereford calves with and without hypomyelinogenesis, *Vet Rec* 118:95-98, 1986.
8. Atkeson F, Ibsen H, Eldridge F: Inheritance of an epileptic type character in Brown Swiss cattle, *J Hered* 35:45-48, 1944.
9. Axthelm M et al: Hereditary internal hydrocephalus of horned Hereford cattle, *Ann Proc Am Assoc Vet Lab Diag* 23:115-126, 1980.
10. Watson A, Mayhew I: Familial congenital occipitoatlantoaxial malformation (OAAM) in the Arabian horse, *Spine* 334-339, vol. 11, 1986.
11. Watson A, Wilson J, Cooley A: Occipito-atlanto-axial malformation with atlanto-axial subluxation in an ataxic calf, *J Am Vet Med Assoc* 187:740-742, 1985.
12. Little PJ, Sorensen DK: Bovine polioencephalomalacia, infectious thromboembolis meningoencephalitis, and acute lead poisoning in feedlot cattle, *J Am Vet Med Assoc* 155:1892-1903, 1969.
13. Young S, Cordy D: An ovine fetal encephalopathy caused by bluetongue vaccine virus, *J Neuropathol Exp Neurol* 23:635-659, 1964.
14. Schultz G, DeLay P: Losses in newborn lambs with bluetongue vaccination of pregnant ewes, *J Am Vet Med Assoc* 127:224-228, 1955.
15. Luedke A, Jochim M, Jones R: Bluetongue in cattle: effects of Culicoides varipennis transmitted bluetongue virus on pregnant heifers and their calves, *Am J Vet Res* 38:1687-1695, 1977.
16. Richardson C, Hebert C, Done J: Experimental border disease in sheep: dose-response effect, *Br Vet J* 202-208, 1976.
17. Potts B et al: Viral persistence and abnormalities of the central nervous system after congenital infection of sheep with border disease virus, *J Infect Dis* 151:337-343, 1985.
18. Kurogi H et al: Congenital abnormalities in newborn calves after inoculation of pregnant cows with akabane virus, *Infect Immunol* 17:338-343, 1977.
19. Guard C, Rebhun W, Perdrizet J: Cranial tumors in aged cattle causing Horner's syndrome and exophthalmos, *Cornell Vet* 74:361-365, 1984.

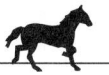

20. Lampert P, Gajdusek C, Gibbs C: Subacute spongiform virus encephalopathies, *Am J Pathol* 68:626-646, 1972.
21. Mayhew I, DeLahunta A, Whitlock R: Spinal cord disease in the horse, *Cornell Vet* 68 (suppl 6):24-35, 1978.
22. Fraser H, Palmer A: Equine incoordination and wobbler disease of young horses, *Vet Rec* 80:338-355, 1967.
23. Wagner P et al: A study of the heritability of cervical vertebral malformations in horses, *Proceedings of the Thirty-Sixth Annual Convention of the American Association of Equine Practitioners*, 1986, pp 43-59.
24. Day J, Mantle P: Tremorgenic forage and rye grass stages, *Vet Rec* 106:463-464, 1980.
25. Mayhew I et al: Equine degenerative myeloencephalopathy: a vitamin E deficiency that may be familial, *J Vet Intern Med* 1:45-50, 1987.
26. Divers T et al: Blindness and convulsions associated with vitamin A deficiency in feedlot steers, *J Am Vet Med Assoc* 189:1579-1582, 1986.
27. Suttle W, Field A, Barlow R: Experimental copper deficiency in sheep, *J Comp Pathol* 80:151-162, 1970.
28. Divers T, Mohammed H, Cummings J: Equine motor neuron disease, *Vet Clin North Am Equine Pract* 13:97-105, 1997.
29. Killinger A, Mansfield M: Epizootiology of listeric infection of sheep, *J Am Vet Med Assoc* 157:1318-1324, 1970.
30. Kingsbury J: *Poisonous plants of the United States and Canada*, Englewood Cliffs, NJ, 1964, Prentice-Hall.
31. Cordy D: Nigropallidal encephalomalacia in horses associated with ingestion of yellow star thistle, *J Neuropathol Exp Neurol* 13:330-342, 1954.
32. Obel A: Studies on grass disease: the morphological picture with reference to the vegetative nervous system, *J Comp Pathol* 65:334-339, 1961.
33. Nicholson S: Bovine posterior paralysis due to organophosphate poisoning, *J Am Vet Med Assoc* 165:280-281, 1974.
34. Smith D: Poisoning by sodium salt: a cause of eosinophilic meningoencephalitis in swine, *Am J Vet Res* 18:825-850, 1957.
35. Pardovan D: Polioencephalomalacia associated with water deprivation in cattle, *Cornell Vet* 70:153-159, 1980.
36. Scarratt W, Collins T, Sponenberg D: Water deprivation-sodium chloride intoxication in a group of feeder lambs, *J Am Vet Med Assoc* 186:977-978, 1985.
37. Blythe L et al: Prevalence of serum antibodies to Sarcocystis neurona in horses residing in Oregon, *J Am Vet Med Assoc* 210:525-527, 1997.
38. Sweeney C et al: Narcolepsy in a horse, *J Am Vet Med Assoc* 183:126-128, 1983.
39. Strain G et al: Narcolepsy in a Brahman bull, *J Am Vet Med Assoc* 185:538-541, 1984.
40. Hines MT, Schott HC, Byrne BA: Adult-onset narcolepsy in the horse, *Proceedings of the Thirty-Ninth Annual Convention of the American Association of Equine Practitioners*, 1993, pp 289-296.
41. Rooney J: Two cervical reflexes in the horse, *J Am Vet Med Assoc* 162:117-118, 1973.
42. Greet T et al: The slap test for laryngeal adductory function in horses with suspected cervical spinal cord damage, *Equine Vet J* 12:127-131, 1980.
43. De Lahunta A: *Veterinary neuroanatomy and clinical neurology*, Philadelphia, 1983, WB Saunders.
44. Burns G: Personal Communication, 1995.
45. Strain G et al: Brainstem auditory evoked potential measurements in Holstein cows, *J Vet Intern Med* 3:144-1448, 1989.
46. Mayhew I, Washbourne J: A method of assessing auditory and brainstem function in horses, *Br Vet J* 146:509-518, 1990.
47. Mayhew I, Washbourne J: Short latency auditory evoked potentials recorded from non-anesthetized thoroughbred horses, *Br Vet J* 148:315-327, 1992.
48. Chiapetta C, Baker J, Feeney D: Sacral fracture, extensor hypertonia of thoracic limbs and paralysis of the pelvic limbs (Schiff-Sherrington syndrome) in an Arabian foal, *J Am Vet Med Assoc* 186:387-388, 1985.
49. Hines MT, Schott HC, Byrne BA: Adult onset narcolepsy in horses, *Proceedings of the Thirty-Eighth Annual Convention of the American Association of Equine Practitioners*, 1993, pp 289-296.
50. Lunn DP et al: Familial occurrence of narcolepsy in miniature horses, *Equine Vet J* 25: 483-487, 1993.

Alterations in Body Weight or Size

JOHN MAAS

MAJOR CLINICAL SIGNS/PROBLEMS ENCOUNTERED

Decreased growth/decreased weight gain, 152
Weight loss, 160

Obesity, 168
Pica, 170

DECREASED GROWTH/DECREASED WEIGHT GAIN

Slowed growth and below-normal weight gain usually happen at the same time, although occasionally they develop separately. By definition a decrease in growth and weight gain is limited to the growing animal; similar pathogenic mechanisms cause weight loss or an emaciated condition in an adult patient. This arbitrary division allows the clinician to consider possible causes that are more or less common for a given age-group.

Potential growth/weight gain is genetically determined. It differs according to species, breed, and sex, and marked differences in potential growth exist within a breed. The potential for growth is greater in the offspring of multiparous females than in those from primiparous females. The normal or minimum growth/weight gain rates for common breeds of the various species are outlined in the section on assessment of growth/weight gains.

Mechanisms of Decreased Growth/Weight Gain

Major pathogenic mechanisms that result in decreased growth/weight gain include the following:
- Inadequate dietary intake of essential nutrients
- Concurrent toxicosis
- Genetic errors in metabolism or physiologic function

- Parasitism
- Infections or inflammatory processes
- Multiple etiologies and environmental causes

Boxes 9-1 and 9-2 list many of the possible causes of decreased growth/weight gain. Many disease conditions can adversely affect growth by more than one of the following mechanisms:

Inadequate intake of one or more essential nutrients is an important cause of decreased growth. A decrease in quantity *and* quality of feed energy and protein is commonly seen. Diets low in digestible energy or protein, or both, reduce total daily intake (see Table 9-4) because of the increased turnover time ($T_{1/2}$) in the gastrointestinal tract and subsequent decreased throughput. This compounds the problems caused by an inadequate intake of digestible nutrients. Protein-calorie malnutrition (PCM) is the most common clinical cause of decreased growth/weight gain in young animals. It is characterized by smaller size and lower weight than the normal minimums for age, breed, and sex. Diets that lack any of the other essential nutrients (fatty acids, minerals, vitamins, or trace minerals) can also cause decreased growth. Patients growing slowly as a result of inadequate diets often have normal or increased appetites until they are terminally ill, and physical findings and clinicopathologic data often are within the normal range until the disease process is well advanced. Inadequate intake of di-

BOX 9-1

Causes of Decreased Growth/Weight Gain in the Horse

COMMON CAUSES
Protein-calorie malnutrition (PCM)
Parasitism (worms, bots)
Bacterial pneumonia, lung abscessation
Pleuropneumonia, pleuritis
Gastric ulcers
Lameness (e.g., osteomyelitis, arthritis)
Prematurity, dysmaturity
Salmonellosis
Diarrhea, unknown etiology

LESS COMMON CAUSES
Esophageal stricture, megaesophagus
Peritonitis
Cardiac/great vessel anomalies
Jaw pain (arthritis, fracture, dental abnormality)
Cryptosporidiosis
Selenium deficiency
Copper deficiency
Vitamin A deficiency
Vitamin D deficiency

LESS COMMON CAUSES—cont'd
Thiamine deficiency
Phosphorus deficiency
Osteodystrophy, osteomyelitis
Inhalation pneumonia
Lead toxicity
Goiter
Generalized steatitis
Rotavirus infection (foals)
Wound myiasis

UNCOMMON CAUSES
Gonadal dysgenesis, intersex (XO, XXY)
Ammonia toxicity
Sarcocystosis
Fluorosis
Renal hypoplasia
Hydrocephalus
Myeloproliferative disease
Biliary atresia
Hepatic portosystemic shunt

BOX 9-2

Causes of Decreased Growth/Weight Gain in Ruminants

COMMON CAUSES
Protein-calorie malnutrition (PCM)
Pasteurella, Haemophilus pneumonia
Ostertagiasis I and II
Coccidiosis
Parasitism (flukes, gastrointestinal worms, lungworms)
Salmonellosis
Bovine virus diarrhea
Hepatic abscessation, liver disease
Rotavirus infection
Diarrhea, undifferentiated
Lameness (footrot, laminitis, foot warts, osteomyelitis)
Cryptosporidiosis
Enterotoxigenic *Escherichia coli*
Coronavirus
Selenium deficiency
Copper deficiency
Sarcoptic mange

LESS COMMON CAUSES
Johne's disease
Cardiac/great vessel anomalies
Hydrocephalus
Myiasis
Ammonia (urea) toxicity
Goiter
Eperythrozoonosis
Arthrogryposis
Thiamine deficiency
Cobalt deficiency
Urachal/bladder abscess
Peritonitis
Pharyngeal abscess, injury
Giardiasis
Osteodystrophy, rickets
Neonatal isoerythrolysis
Immune-mediated anemia
Zinc deficiency
Vitamin A deficiency
Adenovirus infection
Tick infestation
Sarcocystosis
Abomasal ulcers

UNCOMMON CAUSES
Gonadal dysgenesis, intersex
Brisket disease
Epidermolysis bullosa
Phosphorus deficiency
Osteogenesis imperfecta in Friesians
Calf lymphosarcoma
Granulocytopathy
Congenital porphyria
Hypersensitivity to soy protein
Bacteroides fragilis diarrhea
α-Mannosidosis
Generalized glycogenosis
Zygomycosis
Mucormycosis
Omental bursitis
Schistosomiasis (exotic)
Trypanosomiasis (exotic)
Hyena disease (exotic)
Lethal skin defects in Japanese black cattle (exotic)
Babesiosis (exotic)

TOXINS
Pyrrolizidine alkaloid toxicosis
Herbicide toxicity
Zinc toxicity
Fluorosis
Selenium toxicity
Aflatoxicosis
Ergotism
Iodine toxicity

PLANT TOXINS
Cassia sp.
Bracken fern
Fescue toxicity
Leucaena leucocephala
Oxalate toxicity

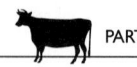

gestible energy and protein (or essential fatty acids in the neonate primarily adapted to a milk diet) results in inadequate levels of amino acids, fats, and carbohydrates for normal metabolism and growth.

Deficiencies of minerals (calcium, phosphorus, and magnesium) result in improper skeletal formation. Deficiencies in other minerals (e.g., sodium, chloride, potassium), trace minerals (e.g., copper, zinc, manganese), and vitamins (e.g., A, D, E, thiamine) cause biochemical dysfunctions that lead to inefficient metabolism and growth.

Toxicities usually result in decreased weight gain by interfering with metabolic pathways (i.e., ammonia toxicity), by causing loss of body reserves (i.e., bracken fern toxicity) or anorexia, or by means of a combination of mechanisms. The pathogenic mechanisms of many toxins are not yet known.

Genetic diseases (α-mannosidosis, dwarfism) result in decreased growth through generalized errors in the genetic code or interference with strategic reactions in one or more metabolic pathways. Congenital malformations (tetralogy of Fallot) create physiologic inefficiencies that require energy beyond the body's ability to supply it.

Parasitism results in decreased growth/weight gain by the following:

■ Increasing nutrient requirements
■ Increasing nutrient losses
■ Decreasing nutrient absorption

The animal's metabolic rate and nutrient requirements may increase as a result of inflammatory reactions that arise secondary to parasitism and certain products of parasite metabolism.

Infections or inflammatory processes can result in decreased growth/weight gain by a variety of mechanisms, alone or in combination. The decrease in growth can be of short duration with recovery and compensatory gain (cryptosporidiosis) or long term (chronic bronchopneumonia). Infections or inflammatory processes can also result in the following:

■ Malabsorption of nutrients (chronic salmonellosis, acute rotavirus diarrhea)
■ Anorexia (pharyngeal abscesses)
■ Increased nitrogen turnover
■ Direct protein losses (salmonellosis)
■ Increased energy or protein requirements secondary to inflammation

Environmental factors such as extreme heat, cold, or humidity result in decreased growth/weight gain. Combined etiologic causes are common (e.g., calves with PCM housed in poorly ventilated or overly humid conditions become much more susceptible to infectious pneumonia).

Approach to Diagnosis of Decreased Growth/Weight Gain in the Horse

1. Take a history. Obtain an *accurate* dietary history. Include amounts (weight) of each feedstuff fed per day. Inspect all forages and concentrates for quality, signs of spoilage, abnormal color or odor, and quantity on hand. Carefully note any changes in the feeding program. Has the patient been weaned from a milk diet recently? Determine the patient's age and, if the patient is a foal, the weight and condition of the mare. Note any environmental factors that might increase dietary requirements or decrease dietary intake and examine the environment for possible toxic substances. Check for signs or a history of a previous infectious disease (e.g., diarrhea, cough, pyrexia). Determine the deworming history.

2. Perform a physical examination. Is the patient small, thin, or underweight according to weight charts (Table 9-1, Figs. 9-1 and 9-2)? Carefully note any signs of infectious disease.

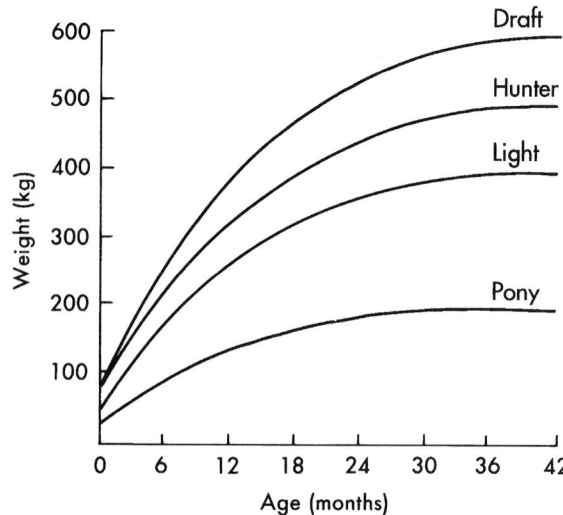

FIG. 9-1 ■ Estimated weight gain of horses of various mature body weights. (Modified from National Research Council: *Nutrient requirements of horses,* Washington, DC, 1978, National Academy of Sciences, NRC.)

TABLE 9-1

Weight as a Percentage of Mature Body Weight in Horses

Age (Months)	Ponies[4] (%)	Light Horses[1-3,5] (%)	Draft Horses (%)
6	55	46	40
12	75	67	57
18	84	80	75

3. Examine the feces. Perform a microscopic examination for parasite ova after flotation. Perform a fecal occult blood test; if the result is positive, see the section on melena in Chapter 7. If diarrhea is present, see the section on diarrhea in Chapter 7.

4. Analyze the blood. Do a complete blood count (CBC), including plasma protein and fibrinogen. Examine the results closely for signs of an inflammatory process. Calculate the erythrocytic indices if anemia is present and characterize the anemia.

5. Perform serum chemistry analyses. The albumin level is usually within normal limits in PCM until the condition is terminal. It is lower in neonates than adults (approximately 1 g/dl less) and increases to normal adult concentration by approximately 6 months of age. The globulin concentration may be increased with chronic inflammation, and the albumin/globulin ratio may be decreased. The glucose concentration is usually normal, although it may be decreased near death or elevated as a result of stress (glucocorticoid influence). Other serum chemistry abnormalities may indicate a primary disease condition. Decreased growth is common secondary to another disease condition.

6. Analyze the diet. Is feedstuff quality adequate to allow sufficient intake? Does the patient have a normal or increased appetite? The diet should supply digestible energy and protein in amounts adequate for maintenance and growth. Young horses require adequate levels of essential

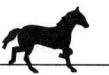

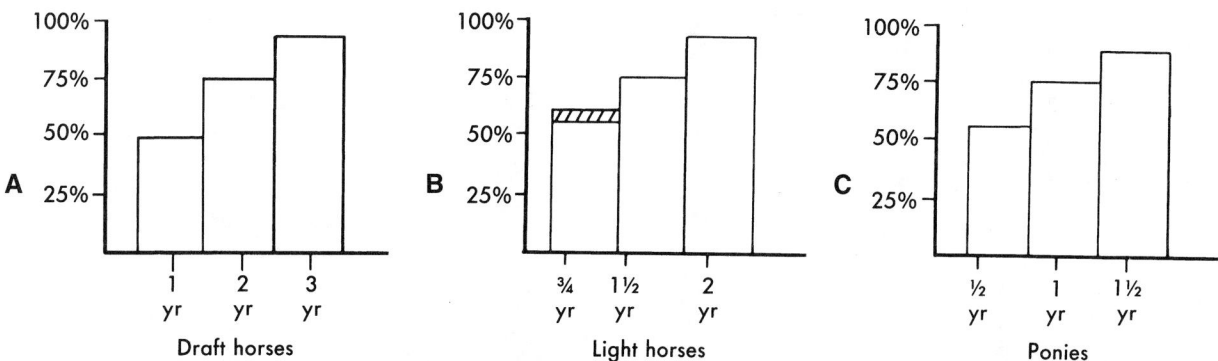

FIG. 9-2 ▓ A to C, Body weight as a percentage of mature body weight for horses at a given age. (A Modified from Crampton WW: *J Agricul Hort* 26:172, 1923; **B** modified from Lewis LD: *Feeding and care of the horse,* Philadelphia, 1982, Lea & Febiger; **C** modified from Hintz HF: *Factors affecting the growth rate of horses,* Horse Short Course Proceedings, Texas A & M Animal Agriculture Conference, 1979, College Station, Texas.)

TABLE 9-2

Daily Nutrient Requirements for Growth in Equines of Various Mature Body Weights

Mature Body Weight (kg/lb)	Category	Weight		Daily Gain		Digestible Energy (Mcal)	Total Digestible Nutrients (kg)	Crude Protein (kg)	Calcium (g)	Phosphorus (g)
		kg	lb	kg	lb					
Ponies 200 kg (440 lb)	Nursing foal (3 months of age)	60	132	0.7	1.54	7.35	1.67	0.41	18	11
	Weanling (6 months of age)	95	209	0.5	1.1	8.8	2	0.47	19	14
	Yearling (12 months of age)	140	308	0.2	0.44	8.15	1.85	0.35	12	9
Horses 400 kg (880 lb)	Nursing foal (3 months of age)	125	275	1	2.2	11.51	2.62	0.65	27	17
	Weanling (6 months of age)	185	407	0.65	1.43	13.03	2.96	0.66	27	20
	Yearling (12 months of age)	265	583	0.4	0.88	13.8	3.14	0.6	24	17
Horses 500 kg (1100 lb)	Nursing foal (3 months of age)	155	341	1.2	2.64	13.66	3.1	0.75	33	20
	Weanling (6 months of age)	230	506	0.8	1.76	15.6	3.55	0.79	34	25
	Yearling (12 months of age)	325	715	0.55	1.21	16.81	3.82	0.76	31	22
Horses 600 kg (1320 lb)	Nursing foal (3 months of age)	170	374	1.4	3.08	15.05	3.42	0.84	36	23
	Weanling (6 months of age)	265	583	0.85	1.87	16.92	3.85	0.86	37	27
	Yearling (12 months of age)	385	847	0.6	1.32	18.85	4.28	0.9	35	25

Modified from National Research Council (NRC): *Nutritional requirements of horses,* Washington, DC, 1978, National Academy of Sciences, NRC.

amino acids for growth, with lysine being the first limiting amino acid in the equine. Weanlings require 0.6% to 0.7% and yearlings require 0.4% lysine in their diets. Soybean meal and alfalfa hay contain 3.3% and 0.9% lysine, respectively. If the dietary history indicates that nutrients for maintenance and growth have been steadily consumed, the search for a primary condition should resume. Nutrient requirements for maintenance and growth of horses are summarized in Tables 9-2 and 9-3.

7. Perform function tests. Oral glucose and D-xylose absorption tests (see Chapter 30) can be performed to assess carbohydrate absorption. Normal serum albumin concen-

trations are helpful in assessing protein absorption, and the presence of normal serum concentrations of direct bilirubin indicates probable normal fat absorption.

Approach to Diagnosis of Decreased Growth/Weight Gain in Ruminants

1. Take a history. Identify the problem as acute, subacute, or chronic. Obtain an accurate dietary history, including diet information when a milk diet is being fed (birth to 2 or 3 months of age). Note age and condition of dam if patient was suckled before weaning. An accurate

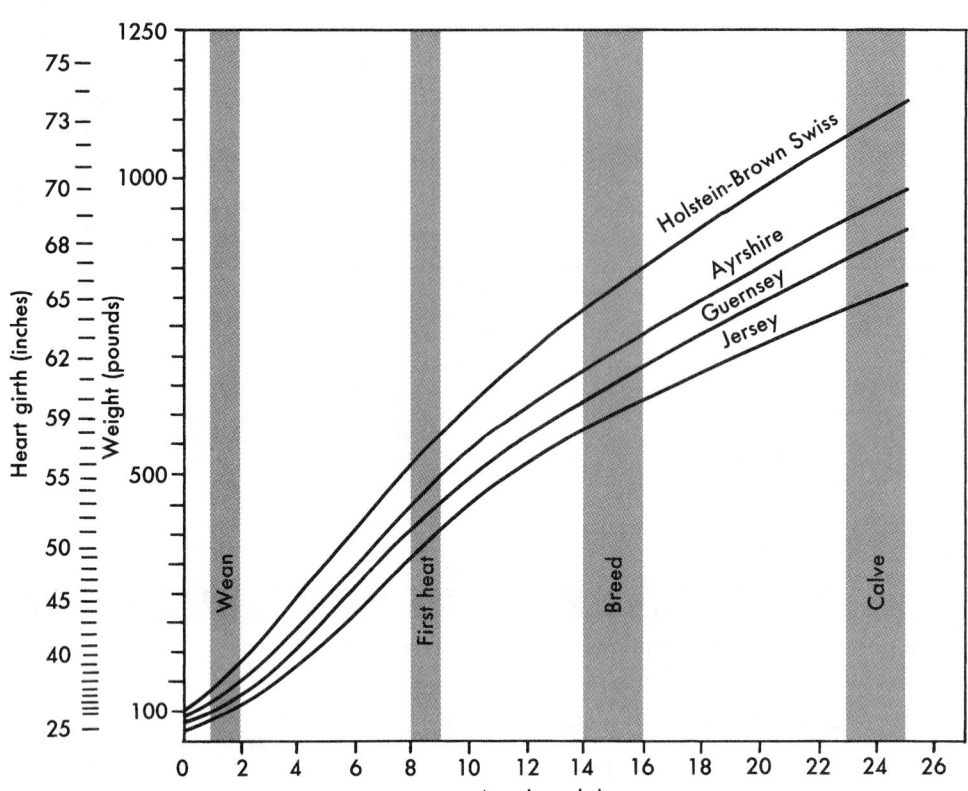

FIG. 9-3 ▓ Minimum growth curve for dairy heifers. (From Sniffen CJ: *Feed Management* 35:37, 1984.)

TABLE 9-3

Daily Nutrient Requirements of Horses and Ponies of Mature Body Weight

Category	Digestible Energy (Mcal)	Total Digestible Nutrients (kg)	Crude Protein (kg)	Calcium (g)	Phosphorus (g)
MATURE HORSES, 500 kg OF MATURE BODY WEIGHT					
Maintenance	16.4	3.73	0.63	23	14
Mares, last 90 days of gestation	18.4	4.17	0.75	34	23
Lactation, first 3 months	28.3	6.43	1.36	34	28
MATURE PONIES, 200 kg OF MATURE BODY WEIGHT					
Maintenance	8.24	1.9	0.32	9	6
Mares, last 90 days of gestation	9.23	2.1	0.39	14	9
Lactation, first 3 months	14.58	3.31	0.71	24	16

Modified from National Research Council (NRC): *Nutrient requirements of horses,* Washington, DC, 1978, National Academy of Sciences, NRC.

postweaning dietary history is essential. Suckled animals are developed ruminants at weaning, but hand-reared animals (dairy calves, bummer lambs, and dairy kids) are usually not fully developed ruminants at the time they are weaned from milk. Inspect all forages and concentrates for quality, signs of spoilage, or abnormal color or odor. Because ruminants are often fed in groups, note whether all animals have adequate space to eat simultaneously. Determine the patient's age and weight. Check for signs or a history of previous infectious disease. Determine parasite control procedures. Examine the environment, including feed preparation areas and equipment, for possible toxic substances (e.g., zinc from galvanized buckets).

2. Perform a physical examination. Check the patient against age and weight charts (Figs. 9-3 through 9-6). Carefully note any signs of infectious or parasitic disease.
3. Examine the feces. Perform flotation, sedimentation, and Baermann's procedures to detect patent parasitic infestation. Perform a fecal occult blood test; if the result is positive or if there is evidence of diarrhea, see the section on melena or diarrhea in Chapter 7.
4. Analyze the blood. Perform a CBC, including plasma protein and fibrinogen. Calculate the erythrocytic indices and document and characterize the anemia if present. If a herd problem exists in a selenium-deficient region, measure the whole blood selenium concentration or glutathione peroxidase activity.

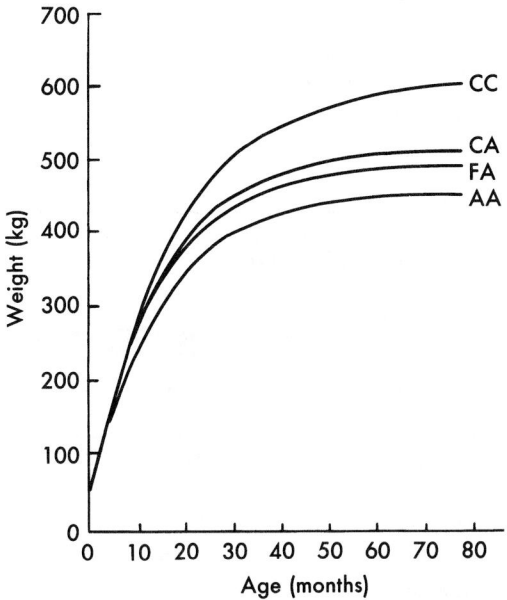

FIG. 9-4 ▦ Estimated growth curves for beef cows of various breeds. *AA*, Angus; *CC*, Charolais; *CA*, Charolais × Angus; *FA*, Holstein × Angus. (Modified from Nadarajah K, Marlowe TJ, Notter DR: *J Anim Sci* 59:965, 1984.)

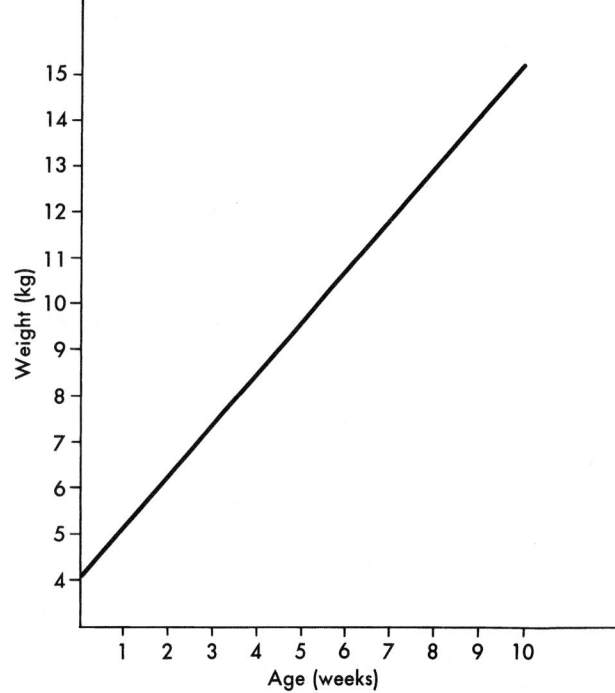

FIG. 9-6 ▦ Growth curve for young goats. (Modified from Morand-Fehr P, Hervien P Bas, Sauvant D: *Proc Third Int Conf Goat Prod Dis* 3:96-103, 1982.)

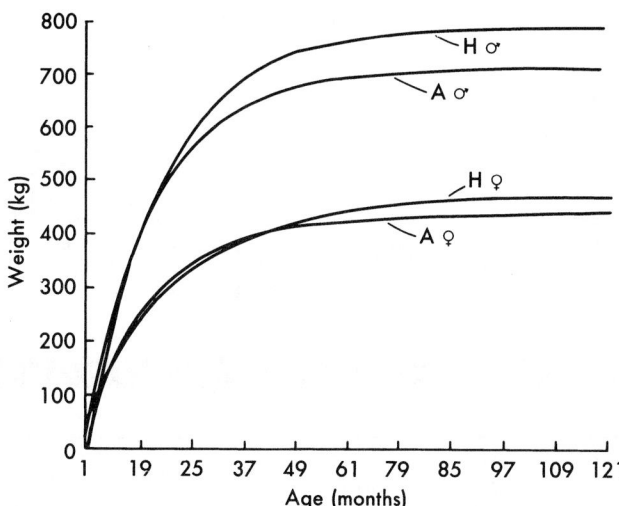

FIG. 9-5 ▦ Mean growth curves of Angus (*A*) and Hereford (*H*) males (♂) and females (♀). (Modified from Brown JE, Brown CJ, Butts WT: *J Anim Sci* 34:525, 1972.)

TABLE 9-4

Maximum Dry Matter Intake (DMI) Related to Forage Quality for Cattle

Forage Quality	Maximum DMI/Day (% Body Weight)	Maximum DMI for 500 kg/Cow/Day (kg)
POOR Oat straw Corn stover	1-1.5	5-7.5
AVERAGE Meadow grass hay	2	10
EXCELLENT Alfalfa hay (25% crude fiber) Corn silage	2.5	12.5

From Maas J: *Vet Clin North Am* 3:634, 1987.

5. Perform serum chemistry analyses. Serum albumin is decreased late in PCM. Albumin is normally lower in neonates (approximately 1 g/dl less) than in adults. The blood urea nitrogen (BUN) level is often low in ruminants as a result of urea recycling through saliva. Total serum calcium may be decreased with hypoalbuminemia (ionized serum calcium remains normal), anorexia, or hypocalcemic syndromes (milk fever). Serum phosphorus may be increased during severe starvation or decreased with anorexia.

Hypophosphatemia may be the result of dietary deficiency or *Brassica* feeding, or it may be associated with copper deficiency. Measure serum (plasma) copper if a herd problem exists in a copper-deficient region (or a region with excess molybdenum or sulfate or both). Copper (serum or plasma) concentrations below 0.5 μg/ml (ppm) indicate deficiency. Liver copper levels are even more indicative of status. Serum glucose may be increased with stress or decreased or normal near death.

6. Analyze the diet. Note if the quality is adequate to allow sufficient intake in developed ruminants (Table 9-4). If anorexia is present, look for more specific signs. If the patient is being fed a milk diet, check dietary requirements (Tables 9-5 and 9-6). If the diet supplies adequate nutrients for maintenance and growth, consider decreased growth/weight gain to be caused by a primary disease condition.

Compare nutrient intake to requirements for maintenance and growth of the various ruminant species (Tables 9-5 through 9-11).

TABLE 9-5

Daily Energy and Protein Requirements for 50-kg Calves on a Milk Diet

Digestible Energy Requirements		Digestible Protein Requirements	
Maintenance	45-55 kcal/kg body weight	Maintenance	0.5 g/kg body weight
Gain	300 kcal/100 g gain in body weight*	Gain	22 g/100 g of weight gain†
0.5 kg daily gain	1500 kcal		
1 kg daily gain	3000 kcal		

*A 50-kg calf gaining 0.75 kg/day would have a daily energy requirement of 5000 kcal of digestible energy (2750 kcal maintenance + 2250 kcal/0.75 kg of gain).
†A 50-kg calf gaining 0.75 kg/day would have a daily protein requirement of 190 g of digestible protein (25 g of maintenance + 165 g of gain).

TABLE 9-6

Net Energy (NE) Requirements of Young Lambs on Milk-Replacer Diets*

Average Daily Gain (g)	Body Weight in Kilograms (Pounds)				
	5 (11)	7.5 (16.5)	10 (22)	12.5 (27.6)	15 (33)
	NE_m required, kcal/day				
	359	487	603	712	817
	NE_g required, kcal/day				
100	127	172	214	253	290
150	193	262	325	383	440
200	261	353	438	518	594
250	330	447	555	655	751
300	401	543	674	796	913
350	473	641	796	940	1078
400	547	742	921	1088	1247

From Chiou PWS, Jordan RM: *J Anim Sci* 37:581-587, 1973.
NE_m, Net energy of maintenance; NE_g, net energy of gain.
*Protein requirements for young lambs on a milk-replacer diet are approximately 20 g, 40 g, and 60 g for weight gains of 0, 100, and 200 g/day, respectively.

TABLE 9-7

Net Energy (NE) Requirements for Growth of Beef Cattle (Mcal/day)

Daily Gain (kg)	Body Weight in Kilograms/ (NE_m Required)			
	150 (3.3)	200 (4.1)	250 (4.89)	300 (5.55)
Medium-frame steer calves	NE_g required			
0.4	0.87	1.08	1.28	1.47
0.8	1.87	2.32	2.74	3.14
1	2.39	2.96	3.5	4.02
Large-frame bull calves and compensating large-frame yearling steers				
0.4	0.69	0.85	1.01	1.15
0.8	1.47	1.82	2.15	2.47
1	1.87	2.32	2.75	3.15
Medium-frame heifer calves				
0.4	1.05	1.31	1.55	1.77
0.8	2.29	2.84	3.36	3.85
1	2.94	3.65	4.31	4.94

Modified from National Research Council (NRC): *Nutrient requirements of beef cattle*, Washington, DC, 1984, National Academy of Sciences, NRC.
NE_m, Net energy of maintenance; NE_g, net energy of gain.

TABLE 9-8

Daily Nutrient Requirements for Growth of Dairy Calves

Body Weight (kg)	(lb)	Breed	Age (Weeks)	Daily Gain (kg)	Digestible Energy (Mcal)	Total Digestible Nutrients (kg)	Crude Protein (g)	Calcium (g)	Phosphorus (g)
HEIFERS AND BULLS FED ONLY MILK									
25	55	Small	1	0.3	2.38	0.54	111	6	4
30	66	Small	3	0.35	2.77	0.63	128	7	4
42	92.4	Large	1	0.4	3.31	0.75	148	8	5
50	110	Large	3	0.5	4.01	0.91	180	9	6
GROWING HEIFERS AND BULLS FED MIXED DIETS									
50	110	Large	3	0.5	5.42	1.23	198	10	6
GROWING DAIRY HEIFERS									
100	220	Small	26	0.5	8.35	1.89	360	16	6
200	440	Small	54	0.5	14.06	3.19	586	20	13
300	660	Small	83	0.5	18.74	4.25	746	23	17
GROWING DAIRY BULLS									
100	220	Small	26	0.5	8.35	1.89	361	16	8
200	440	Large	24	0.5	13.66	3.1	602	20	13
300	660	Large	38	0.5	18.56	4.21	777	24	18

Modified from National Research Council (NRC): *Nutrient requirements of dairy cattle*, Washington, DC, 1978, National Academy of Sciences, NRC.

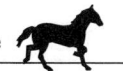

TABLE 9-9

Protein Requirements for Growth of Beef Cattle (g/day)

Daily Gain (kg)	Body Weight in Kilograms			
	150	200	250	300
MEDIUM-FRAME STEER CALVES				
0.4	428	482	532	580
0.8	575	621	664	704
1	642	682	720	755
LARGE-FRAME CALVES AND COMPENSATING LARGE-FRAME YEARLING STEERS				
0.4	438	494	547	597
0.8	597	649	697	741
1	673	721	765	807
MEDIUM-FRAME HEIFER CALVES				
0.4	409	459	505	549
0.8	537	574	608	640
1	562	583	603	621

Modified from National Research Council (NRC): *Nutrient requirements of beef cattle*, Washington DC, 1984, National Academy of Sciences, NRC.

TABLE 9-10

Calcium (Ca) and Phosphorus (P) Requirements for Growth of Beef Cattle (g/day)

Daily Gain (kg)	Mineral	Body Weight in Kilograms			
		150	200	250	300
MEDIUM-FRAME STEER CALVES					
0.4	Ca	16	17	17	18
	P	9	10	12	13
0.8	Ca	27	26	25	25
	P	12	13	14	15
1	Ca	32	31	29	29
	P	14	15	16	16
LARGE-FRAME BULL CALVES AND COMPENSATING LARGE-FRAME YEARLING STEERS					
0.4	Ca	17	18	19	19
	P	9	11	22	13
0.8	Ca	28	28	28	28
	P	13	14	15	16
1	Ca	34	34	33	33
	P	15	16	17	18
MEDIUM-FRAME HEIFER CALVES					
0.4	Ca	15	16	16	17
	P	9	10	11	12
0.8	Ca	25	23	23	22
	P	12	12	13	14
1	Ca	29	27	26	24
	P	13	14	14	15

Modified from National Research Council (NRC): *Nutrient requirements of beef cattle*, Washington, DC, 1984, National Academy of Sciences, NRC.

TABLE 9-11

Nutrient Requirements for Growth in Sheep of Various Mature Body Weights

Category	Body Weight		Daily Gain		Metabolizable Energy (Mcal)	Total Digestible Nutrients (kg)	Crude Protein (g)	Calcium (g)	Phosphorus (g)
	kg	lb	kg	lb					
Replacement ewe lambs	30	66	0.23	0.5	2.8	0.78	185	6.4	2.6
	40	88	0.18	0.4	3.3	0.91	176	5.9	2.6
	50	110	0.12	0.26	3.2	0.88	136	4.8	2.4
	60	132	0.1	0.22	3.2	0.88	134	4.5	2.5
Replacement ram lambs	40	88	0.33	0.73	5	1.1	243	7.8	3.7
	60	132	0.32	0.7	6.7	1.5	263	8.4	4.2
	80	176	0.29	0.64	7.8	1.8	268	8.5	4.6
	100	220	0.25	0.55	8.4	1.9	264	8.2	4.8
Finishing lambs (4-7 months)	30	66	0.29	0.65	3.4	0.94	191	6.6	3.2
	40	88	0.27	0.6	4.4	1.22	185	6.6	3.3
	50	110	0.2	0.45	4.4	1.23	160	5.6	3
Early weaned lambs— moderate growth	10	22	0.2	0.44	1.4	0.4	127	4	1.9
	20	44	0.25	0.55	2.9	0.8	167	5.4	2.5
	30	66	0.3	0.66	3.6	1	191	6.7	3.2

Modified from National Research Council (NRC): *Nutritional requirements of sheep*, Washington, DC, 1978, National Academy of Sciences, NRC.

REFERENCES

1. Budzynski M et al: Growth in halfbred horses, *Roczniki Nauk Roln B* 93:21, 1961.
2. Cunningham K, Fowler S: A study of growth in quarter horses, *La Agr Exp Stn Bull*, p 546, 1961.
3. Hintz HF: A review of recent studies on the growth of horses, *Calif Vet*, March 1979, p 17.
4. Jordan RM: Growth pattern in ponies, *Proc Fifth Equine Nutr Physiol Symp* 5:63, 1977.
5. Reed KF, Dunn NK: Growth of the Arabian horse, *Proc Fifth Equine Nutr Physiol Symp* 5:99, 1977.

WEIGHT LOSS

The clinical problem of weight loss suggests that a patient or group of patients has lost weight over a known period of time. It may also suggest that the patient has reached a subnormal adult weight and size (see section on decreased growth/decreased weight gain, above). Two physiologic conditions commonly accompanied by mild to moderate weight loss are (1) the early stages of lactation and (2) a high level of exercise-related performance. Late pregnancy can be associated with decreased body condition without actual weight loss. This deterioration of body condition may be mild and within normal limits or severe and a threat to the health of the dam and the neonate.

Weight loss is most commonly associated with one or more of the following circumstances (other causes are listed in Boxes 9-3 and 9-4):
- Anorexia
- Increased nutrient demands
- PCM

Anorexia usually occurs secondary to a primary disease. Increased nutrient requirements can be associated with physiologic conditions (e.g., cold weather, exercise, pregnancy, lactation) or pathologic processes (e.g., sepsis, trauma, parasitism, burns). Inadequate feed quality (see Table 9-4) or

---

BOX 9-3

Causes of Weight Loss in the Horse

COMMON CAUSES
Protein-calorie malnutrition (PCM)
Pyrrolizidine alkaloid hepatotoxicity
Sand colic/impaction
Streptococcus equi (strangles, pneumonia abscessation)
Wound myiasis
Parasitism
Pneumonia/lung abscesses
Pleuritis
Chronic obstructive pulmonary disease
Chronic renal failure
Acute renal failure
Combined immunodeficiency disease in foals
Cribbing, wind sucking
Rhodococcus equi infection
Strongylus vulgaris thromboembolism
Pituitary adenoma
Squamous cell carcinoma of the stomach
Neoplasia
Dental, jaw abnormalities
Obstruction of the small colon
Gastric/duodenal ulcers
Infectious arthritis
Peritonitis
Internal abdominal abscess

LESS COMMON CAUSES
Toxic hepatopathy
Chronic hepatitis
Urolithiasis
Spinal abscessation
Osteomyelitis
Tuberculosis
Vesicular stomatitis
Glomerulonephritis
Cardiac/great vessel anomalies
Congestive heart failure
Endocarditis, pericarditis
Nocardiosis
Esophageal abnormalities
Agammaglobulinemia
Anhidrosis
Idiopathic diarrhea
Gastric impaction

LESS COMMON CAUSES—cont'd
Paranasal sinus infection
Splenic rupture, abscess
Granulosa cell tumor
Hyperlipemia
Giardiasis
Lymphoma, lymphosarcoma
Eosinophilic enteritis
Granulomatous enteritis
Guttural pouch infection
Oral foreign body
Purpura hemorrhagica
Pyelonephritis
Malignant melanoma
Coccidioidomycosis
Theiler's disease
Cryptococcosis
Cryptosporidiosis (foals)
Panniculitis
Aflatoxicosis
Equine adenovirus
Babesiosis
Equine viral arteritis
Equine infectious anemia

UNCOMMON CAUSES
Rabies
Nigropallidal encephalomalacia
Rectus capitus ventralis muscle rupture
Renal neoplasia
Seborrhea
IgM-deficiency (foals)
Skeletal/vertebral neoplasia
Botulism
Equine motor neuron disease
Testicular neoplasia
Mammary carcinoma
Tularemia
Vitamin A deficiency
Nutritional myodegeneration
Brucellosis
Phosphorus deficiency
Rotavirus infection (foals)
Renal tubular acidosis

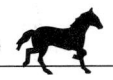

quantity commonly results in PCM of varying degrees. Weight loss can also occur with deficiency of essential micronutrients such as copper, cobalt (vitamin B_{12}), or vitamin A.

Mechanisms of Weight Loss

Anorexia is the loss of appetite or lack of desire for food; it may be complete or partial. It is a primary mechanism for weight loss of short or intermediate duration. In domestic species, anorexia is invariably associated with a primary disease condition. It must be differentiated from dysphagia by observation. The distinction between the conditions that cause anorexia and those that control hunger and satiety is not clear; however, many diseases that cause anorexia have in common dehydration, electrolyte imbalances, and/or acid-base disorders.

Weight loss results from decreased nutrient intake. When partial anorexia occurs over a long period, the weight loss may be subtle and go unrecognized, whereas acute, complete anorexia results in a more dramatic weight loss. Thus anorexia results in a secondary or conditional state of PCM.

In addition to causing anorexia, many disease processes cause an increase in the nutrient requirements for basal metabolism. Nutrient requirements for maintenance, growth, pregnancy, lactation, and exercise have been well defined for the various species. Nutrient requirements in disease have barely been examined, and most of the research has been done on laboratory animals and humans. In human patients, published estimates indicate that requirements for energy and protein increase approximately 10% after elective surgery, 20% with fractures, 30% to 60% with severe infection or sepsis, 40% with peritonitis, and 50% to 110% with major burns.[6,7] Extrapolation of these data directly to equine and ruminant patients is probably not possible; however, the figures do indicate the degree of change in nutrient requirements as a result of disease. The

---

BOX 9-3

Causes of Weight Loss in the Horse—cont'd

UNCOMMON CAUSES—cont'd
Liver fluke
Prognathia, brachygnathia
Portal vein shunt
Enzootic cystitis
Polycystic disease
Aortic aneurysm
Colonic fistula
Autoimmune anemia/thrombocytopenia
Hyperparathyroidism
Systemic granulomatous inflammation
Bullous pemphigoid
Urinary bladder neoplasia
Lupus erythematosus
Cholelithiasis
Erythrocytosis
Fluorosis
Basophilic enterocolitis
Micronema deletrix infection of the central nervous
    system
Horsefly-deerfly infestation
Ovarian adenoma
Eosinophilic dermatitis
Diabetes mellitus
Pancreatic neoplasia
Esophageal mucosal disease
Exuberant granulation tissue of the stomach
Fungal granuloma
Steatitis
Goiter
Multiple cartilaginous exostoses
Histoplasmosis
Malignant mesothelioma
Micropolyspora faeni hypersensitivity pneumonitis
Atrial fibrillation
Ileal hypertrophy
Myeloproliferative disease
Cauda equina neuritis
Otitis media, interna
Pemphigus foliaceous
Pheochromocytoma
Phycomycosis
Pleural mesothelioma
Pneumocystis carinii pneumonia

UNCOMMON CAUSES—cont'd
Pulmonary aspergillosis
Pulmonary neoplasia
Pyloric stenosis
Trypanosoma evansi infection (exotic)
Trombiculiasis (exotic)
Nagana (exotic)
Pseudomonas pseudomallei infection (exotic)
Uasin Gishu skin disease (exotic)
Besnoitiosis (exotic)
Dourine (exotic)
Glanders (exotic)
Grass sickness (exotic)
Louping ill (exotic)
Trypanosoma equinum infection (exotic)
Trypanosoma hippicum infection (exotic)
Stachybotryotoxicosis (exotic)

TOXINS
Dioxin
Vitamin D calcinosis
Zinc
4-Aminopyridine
Selenium
Vitamin K_3
Pentachlorophenol
Arsenic
Mercury
Phenylbutazone/flunixin and other nonsteroidal antiinflam-
    matory drugs
Aflatoxicosis

PLANT TOXINS
Yellow star thistle
Red maple leaf
White snakeroot (tremetol)
Plant calcinosis
Thornapple
Crofton weed
Pimela (exotic)
Swainsonia (exotic)
Birdsville disease (exotic)
Pachysandra paralysis (exotic)

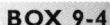

BOX 9-4

Causes of Weight Loss in Ruminants

COMMON CAUSES
Proteint-calorie malnutrition (PCM)
Bacterial pneumonia, pulmonary abscessation
Parasitism (lungworms, gastrointestinal parasites)
Johne's disease (paratuberculosis)
Bovine leukosis
Peritonitis
Ruminal lactic acidosis
Urolithiasis
Pyrrolizidine alkaloid toxicity
Displaced abomasum
Hepatic abscess
Abomasal ulcer
Rotavirus diarrhea
Coronavirus diarrhea
Sarcoptic mange
Footrot
Pedal osteomyelitis
Sole abscess
Traumatic reticuloperitonitis, pericarditis
Ketosis
Vagal indigestion
Winter dysentery (B)
Salmonellosis
Fat necrosis (B)
Actinobacillosis
Actinomycosis
Pharyngeal, retropharyngeal abscess
Pyelonephritis, cystitis
Selenium deficiency
Bovine virus diarrhea (B)
Coccidiosis
Copper deficiency
Dental abnormalities
Enterotoxigenic colibacillosis
Agammaglobulinemia (failure of passive transfer) in
  neonates
Fescue toxicity (B)
Anaplasmosis (B)
Septic arthritis
Infectious bovine rhinotracheitis (B)
Intussusception
Leptospirosis
Mastitis, coliform or staphylococcal
Lice/ked infestation
Hepatic abscess
Liver fluke infestation
Pasteurellosis, septicemic
Pregnancy toxemia

COMMON CAUSES—cont'd
Bluetongue (O)
Cryptosporidiosis
Mammary abscess
Wound myiasis
Diarrhea, unknown etiology

LESS COMMON CAUSES
Rabies
Sarcocystosis (B)
Sodium chloride deficiency
Cardiac/great vessel anomalies
Thymic lymphosarcoma (B)
Tuberculosis
Ulcerative stomatitis
Vesicular stomatitis
Salt toxicity, water deprivation
Psoroptic mange
Postparturient hemoglobinuria
Malignant catarrhal fever
Aspiration pneumonia
Brisket disease
Neoplasia
Omasal impaction
Abomasal impaction
Listeriosis
Pleuritis
Renal amyloidosis
Acute renal failure
Hydronephrosis, urachal abscess, bladder abscess
Dermatophilosis
Glomerulonephritis
Thiamine deficiency
Fluorosis
Esophageal malfunctions
Cobalt deficiency
Coneurosis (gid)
Congenital porphyria
Endocarditis
Aflatoxicosis
Eperythrozoonosis
Mandible, maxilla fracture
Goiter
Lingual injury, abscess
Vena caval thrombosis
Colonic obstruction
Otitis media, externa
Papular stomatitis (B)
Micropolyspora faeni hypersensitivity pneumonitis

B, Bovine; *O*, ovine.

---

stress of many disease processes enhances the activity of the sympathetic nervous system, resulting in increased epinephrine release, impaired insulin release, and enhanced glucagon secretion. These events lead to a relative decrease in insulin, resulting in hyperglycemia caused by enhanced glycogenolysis and gluconeogenesis. Increased catecholamines are also associated with increased release of fatty acids. The elevation of corticosteroid levels probably contributes to the increased protein breakdown observed in stress. The net effect is inefficient metabolic activity and increased nutrient requirements. Weight loss occurs when nutrients are not supplied.

In conditions such as burns, peritonitis, pleuritis, or granulomatous bowel disease, nutrients (particularly proteins) are lost. In many disease conditions, concurrent anorexia and increased nutrient requirements greatly increase the risk of PCM and weight loss. Certain conditions, such as Johne's disease in ruminants and granulomatous enteritis in horses, are also associated with a malabsorption or malassimilation syndrome. In these types of diseases, nutrients are not efficiently digested and absorbed; anorexia may be absent, and dietary intake may appear normal, but weight loss still occurs.

A common cause of weight loss in domestic animals is

BOX 9-4

Causes of Weight Loss in Ruminants—cont'd

LESS COMMON CAUSES—cont'd
Loss of teeth, periodontal disease
Sinusitis

UNCOMMON CAUSES
Buss disease (transmissible serositis) (B)
Neoplasia (other than bovine leukemia virus)
Systemic candidiasis
Local and systemic mycoses
Mycoplasma arthritis
Ulcerative posthitis, vulvitis (B)
Polycythemia (B)
Phosphorus deficiency
Vitamin A deficiency
Zinc deficiency
Meuse-Rhine-Yssel muscular dystrophy (B)
Epidermolysis bullosa (B, O)
Familial acantholysis
Portal vein anomaly
Granulocytopathy
Pulmonary listeriosis
Cholelithiasis
Bronchobiliary fistula (B)
Hypersensitivity to soy/milk replacer
Diabetes mellitus
Idiopathic granulocytopia/thrombocytopenia
Endocardial fibroelastosis (B)
α-Mannosidosis (B)
Fungal granuloma
Generalized glycogenosis (B)
GMI gangliosidosis
Hereditary zinc deficiency (B)
Lethal trait A-46, keratogenesis imperfecta (B)
Omental bursitis (B)
East Coast fever (theileriosis) (exotic)
Tick-borne fever (exotic)
Idiopathic sporadic bovine encephalomyelitis
  (exotic) (B)
Surra (exotic) (B)
Trypanosomiasis (exotic)
Melioidosis, *Pseudomonas pseudomallei* (exotic)
Petechial fever (exotic) (B)
Besnoitiosis (exotic)
Ibaraki disease (exotic) (B)
Turning sickness (exotic) (B)
Contagious pleuropneumonia (exotic) (B)
Schistosomiasis (exotic)
Louping ill (exotic)
Foot-and-mouth disease (exotic)

UNCOMMON CAUSES—cont'd
Lethal skin defects in Japanese black cattle (exotic)
Echinococcosis (exotic)
Endemic ethmoid carcinoma (exotic)
African bovine malignant catarrhal fever (exotic)
Idiopathic storage disease in cattle (exotic)
Babesiosis (exotic)

TOXINS
Selenium
Trichothecene (T-2)
Vitamin D_3
Diesel fuel
Polybrominated biphenyls
Cobalt
Herbicides
Zinc
Furazolidone
4-Aminopyridine
Chlorpyrifos
Toxins associated with crude oil, kerosene
Ergotism
Arsenic
Lead
Mercury
Ethylene glycol
Stachybotryotoxicosis (exotic)

PLANT TOXINS
Gossypol (cottonseed)
Helenium, sneezeweed
Acorn, oak
Bracken fern
Perennial broomweed (*Gutierezzia*)
Cocklebur
Hairy vetch (*Vicia villosa*)
White snakeroot (tremetol)
Mushroom
Tung tree
Fireweed ((*Kochia scoparia*))
Locoweed (*Oxytropis, Astragalus*)
Phalaris sp.
Bermuda grass
Pimela sp. (exotic)
Geigeria sp. (exotic)
Cestrum sp. (exotic)
Yellow wood (exotic)
Leucaena leucocephala sp. (exotic)

parasitism. The mechanisms by which parasite infestation can result in weight loss include:

- Loss of body fluids and tissues, resulting in increased nutrient requirements
- Competition for nutrients in the gastrointestinal tract
- Malassimilation and malabsorption
- Inflammation, causing increased nutrient requirements
- Anorexia (in advanced stages of the disease process)
- Micronutrient deficiencies
- Organ or vascular damage from migrating parasite larvae

PCM continues to be a persistent problem in domestic an-imals. The lack of major nutrients obviously results in weight loss. PCM and associated weight loss can occur through several mechanisms. The most direct cause is inadequate availability of feed to meet dietary requirements. This can occur as frank underfeeding of all animals or as a consequence of inadequate feeding facilities that create competition among animals for available feed. The latter circumstance occurs most dramatically when animals of varying ages are mixed; the younger animals with the highest requirements are often pushed away by older, dominant individuals.

The quality of the diet, particularly forages such as hay, also can be an important factor. Table 9-4 lists guidelines for estimating the maximum daily intake by cattle. It is evident that as forage quality (digestibility) decreases, maximum daily intake decreases because of the longer time feed stays in the rumen until it is small enough to pass through the reticuloomasal orifice. Maximum dry matter intake (DMI) as a percentage of body weight is somewhat higher in small ruminants than in cattle. However, the energy requirement per kilogram of body weight is higher in small ruminants than in cattle. Similar estimates for maximum DMI in horses related to forage quality are not available. Horses do not have a pregastric fermentation organ (rumen) and can ingest slightly more of the same quality forage than cattle. Thus the quality of feed, particularly the forage, determines the maximum intake of nutrients. Low-quality forages are often the cause of PCM, even when unlimited quantity is available.

Environmental factors can have a major influence on nutrient requirements and the subsequent risk of PCM and weight loss. The most important environmental factor is the ambient temperature. Nutrient requirements for maintenance change with a decreasing ambient temperature as follows:

- *Beef cattle:* 1% increase in maintenance energy requirements (total digestible nutrients [TDN], net energy of maintenance [NE_m], digestible energy [DE], and metabolizable energy [ME]) for each 1° C drop below 20° C (68° F)
- *Dairy cattle (lactating):* 25% increase in energy requirements (TDN, net energy of lactation [NE_L]) as ambient temperature drops from 20° C (68° F) to −10° C (14° F)
- *Sheep with 10-cm wool:* 1% increase in energy requirements (TDN, ME, DE) for each 1° C drop below lower critical temperature (approximately −10° C)

The changes for horses are probably similar to those for beef cattle, but the effects of multiple changes in environmental conditions (e.g., temperature, wind, rain) are difficult to predict. As nutrient requirements increase, the dietary intake must also increase to prevent weight loss as a result of PCM.

Deficiencies of micronutrients often result in inefficiencies in basic biochemical pathways. These inefficiencies, if marked, can be associated with weight loss. Genetic errors in metabolism can cause similar disturbances, but these are usually manifest as decreased growth in young animals.

Approach to Diagnosis of Weight Loss in the Horse

1. Take a history. Question the caretaker closely about any additional signs such as diarrhea, coughing, dysphagia, or polyuria. Weight loss is often suspected but not documented in the initial complaint or history. Acute weight loss of 5% to 10% is quite significant; therefore it is important to quantitate weight loss or any decline in body condition. The presence of these signs in the history may indicate that a primary disease is involved. Obtain an *accurate* dietary history, particularly when additional signs might indicate that a primary disease is *absent*. Inspect all forages and concentrates for quality, signs of spoilage, abnormal color or odor, and quantity on hand. If horses are fed in a group, does the system allow for adequate consumption by all animals? Has the feeding program been changed in relation to the onset of weight loss? The history should include the *weight* (amount) of each feedstuff fed and consumed per day. Determine if the patient is anorexic. Determine the deworming history. If possible, determine the nutrient analysis of the feedstuffs being fed. Examine the environment for possible toxic substances.
2. Perform a physical examination. Examine the patient closely for signs of concurrent disease (e.g., diarrhea, pyrexia, dysphagia, abnormal dentition, melena, icterus, dyspnea, tachycardia). Is the patient able to prehend, masticate, and swallow food normally? Is the animal hungry? Weigh the patient (or use a heart girth tape) and note the body condition (see Table 9-21).
3. Analyze the diet. Is the feed quality adequate to allow sufficient intake? Does the patient have a normal or increased appetite? Is anorexia present? Use the flow sheet in Fig. 9-7 to aid decision making. Compare the nutrient intake from the diet with nutrient requirements (see Table 9-3). Include pertinent environmental and management factors. If the dietary history indicates that adequate nutri-

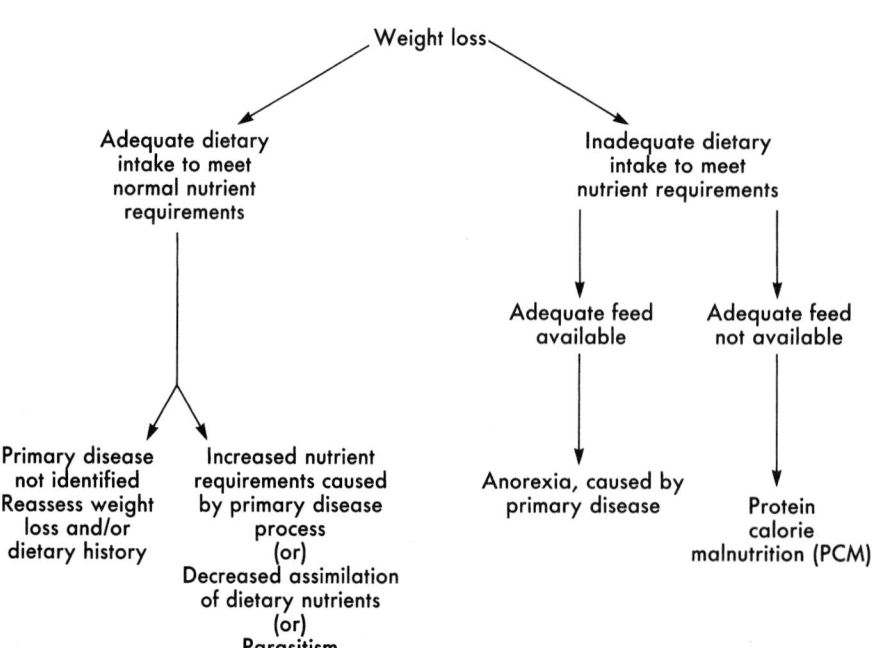

FIG. 9-7 ▮▮ Flow sheet for classifying conditions associated with weight loss.

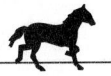

ents for maintenance and performance have been steadily consumed, the search for a primary condition should resume.

4. Examine the feces. Perform a microscopic examination for parasite ova after flotation. Perform a fecal occult blood test; if the result is positive, see the section on melena in Chapter 7. If diarrhea is present, see the section on diarrhea in Chapter 7.

5. Analyze the blood. Perform a CBC, including plasma protein and fibrinogen. Examine the results closely for indication of an inflammatory process (e.g., leukocytosis, neutrophilia, leukopenia, hyperfibrinogenemia, decreased plasma protein/fibrinogen ratio [below 10]). Calculate the erythrocytic indices for characterization of anemia if present.

6. Perform serum chemistry analyses. The serum albumin half-life is approximately 19 days in horses. Hypoalbuminemia is associated with internal abscessation, PCM, liver disease, renal disease, and granulomatous bowel disease, among other conditions. Albumin is often within normal limits in PCM until the patient is near death. Globulin (particularly γ-globulins) may be increased with inflammation, and the albumin/globulin ratio may be decreased. The glucose concentration is usually normal or elevated as a result of stress. Hyperlipidemia (triglycerides 100 to 500 mg/dl) is associated with anorexia or pituitary tumors. Hyperlipemia (triglycerides above 500 mg/dl) is a serious condition associated with anorexia and often azotemia in horses and ponies under severe physiologic stress (PCM and lactation). Unconjugated bilirubin levels can rise to 6 or 7 mg/dl with anorexia or decreased food intake. An elevated γ-glutamyltransferase (GGT) (above 25 IU/L) may indicate hepatic or pancreatic disease.

7. Perform function tests. Oral glucose and D-xylose absorption tests (see Chapter 30) can be performed to assess carbohydrate absorption. Measurable serum concentrations of direct (conjugated) bilirubin indicate probable normal fat absorption.

Approach to Diagnosis of Weight Loss in Ruminants

1. Take history. Question the caretaker closely about any additional signs that might indicate a primary disease (e.g., diarrhea, coughing, dysphagia, polyuria, depression, agalactia). Note if body condition is less than desired. Quantitate the weight loss or body condition score if possible. Acute weight loss of 5% to 10% is quite significant. Carefully note the production level (e.g., pregnancy [single, twins, triplets], lactation [level of milk production]). Obtain an *accurate* dietary history, particularly when signs of a primary disease are absent. Inspect all forages, concentrates, and feed additives for quality, signs of spoilage, abnormal color or odor, and quantity on hand. Be sure the feeding system allows for adequate consumption by all animals and that competition for feedstuffs does not occur. Check to see if the feeding program was changed before the onset of observed weight loss or loss of body condition. The history should include the *weight* of each feedstuff and supplement fed and consumed per day. The maximum DMI can be estimated according to feed quality for cattle (see Table 9-4). Determine the parasite control program. Determine or estimate the nutrient analysis of the feedstuffs being fed. Examine the environment for possible toxic plants or substances.

2. Perform a physical examination. Examine patients carefully for signs of concurrent disease (e.g., diarrhea, decreased rumen motility, pyrexia, dysphagia, abnormal dentition, melena, icterus, mastitis, metritis, dyspnea, tachycardia). Is the patient hungry? Weigh the patient (or use a heart-girth measurement) and note the body condition score (see Tables 9-18 through 9-20). Observe the patient for signs of muscle wasting and the presence or absence of subcutaneous fat. Test the milk with nitroprusside powder (a positive reaction indicates an acetoacetate concentrate above 5 mg/dl and is diagnostic of ketonlactia and ketonemia). Measure the rumen pH (pH above 7 is indicative of anorexia). Examine the skin for evidence of lice or keds.

3. Analyze the diet. Is the feed quality adequate to allow sufficient intake of nutrients (see Table 9-4)? Determine if the patient or patients have a normal appetite. Is anorexia present? Compare the nutrient intake from the diet with the requirements for the appropriate species (Tables 9-12 through 9-17). Consider any important environmental and management factors. If the dietary history and analysis indicate that adequate nutrients have been steadily consumed, the search for a primary cause for the weight loss should be resumed.

TABLE 9-12

Daily Nutrient Requirements for Dairy Cattle

Body Weight (kg)	Body Weight (lb)	NE$_L$ (Mcal)	Total Digestible Nutrients (kg)	Crude Protein (g)	Calcium (g)	Phosphorus (g)
MAINTENANCE OF MATURE LACTATING COWS						
400	880	7.16	3.15	373	15	13
500	1100	8.46	3.72	432	18	15
600	1320	9.7	4.27	489	21	17
650	1430	10.3	4.53	515	22	18
700	1540	10.89	4.79	542	24	19
MAINTENANCE PLUS LAST 2 MONTHS OF GESTATION OF MATURE DRY COWS						
400	880	9.3	4.1	702	26	18
500	1100	11	4.84	821	31	22
600	1320	12.61	5.55	931	37	26
650	1430	13.39	5.9	984	39	28
700	1540	14.15	6.23	1035	42	30

Modified from National Research Council (NRC): *Nutrient requirements of dairy cattle,* Washington, DC, 1978, National Academy of Sciences, NRC.
NE$_L$, Net energy of lactation.

TABLE 9-13

Daily Nutrient Requirements for Lactating Dairy Cows at Various Production Levels

Daily Milk Production (3.5% Butterfat)		NE$_L$ (Mcal)	Total Digestible Nutrients (kg)	Crude Protein (kg)	Calcium (g)	Phosphorus (g)
(kg)	(lb)					
400 kg OF BODY WEIGHT						
20	44	21	9.23	2	67	48
30	66	28	12.27	2.83	96	66
40	88	34.80	15.31	3.65	116	83
500 kg OF BODY WEIGHT						
20	44	22.26	9.80	2.07	70	50
30	66	29	12.84	2.9	96	68
40	88	36	15.88	3.71	119	85
600 kg OF BODY WEIGHT						
20	44	23.5	10.35	2.2	73	52
30	66	30.4	13.39	2.95	99	70
40	88	37.3	16.43	3.77	125	87
700 kg OF BODY WEIGHT						
20	44	24.69	10.87	2.2	59	54
30	66	31.59	13.91	3	77	72
40	88	38.49	16.95	3.82	94	89

Modified from National Research Council (NRC): *Nutrient requirements of dairy cattle,* Washington, DC, 1978, National Academy of Sciences, NRC.
NE$_L$, Net energy of lactation.

Table 9-14

Daily Nutrient Requirements for Mature Beef Cows

Reproductive Status	Daily Gain (kg)	Total Digestible Nutrients (kg)	Crude Protein (kg)	Calcium (g)	Phosphorus (g)
MATURE 500-kg (1100 lb) BEEF COW					
Nonpregnant/maintenance	0	4.3	0.63	17	17
Pregnant, third trimester	0.4*	5.1	0.73	25	20
Lactating, 20 lb milk/per day	0	6.6	1.18	38	27
MATURE 600-kg (1320 lb) BEEF COW					
Nonpregnant/maintenance	0	4.9	0.69	20	20
Pregnant, third trimester	0.4*	5.7	0.83	28	23
Lactating, 20 lb milk/per day	0	7.5	1.35	43	31

Modified from National Research Council (NRC): *Nutrient requirements of beef cattle,* Washington, DC, 1984, National Academy of Sciences, NRC.
*This gain represents only the growth of the fetus.

TABLE 9-15

Daily Nutrient Requirements for Bulls: Maintenance and Regaining Body Condition

Weight (kg)	Daily Gain		Total Digestible Nutrients (kg)	Crude Protein (kg)	Calcium (g)	Phosphorus (g)
	(kg)	(lb)				
650	0.6	1.3	7.4	0.96	27	24
700	0.6	1.3	7.8	1	29	26
800	0*	0	6.3	0.88	27	27
800	0.2	0.4	7.1	0.96	27	27

Modified from National Research Council (NRC): *Nutrient requirements of beef cattle,* Washington, DC, 1984, National Academy of Sciences, NRC.
*Maintenance only, no gain.

TABLE 9-16

Daily Nutrient Requirements of Sheep

Body Weight		Weight Change/ Day		Digestible Energy (Mcal)	Total Digestible Nutrients (kg)	Crude Protein (g)	Calcium (g)	Phosphorus (g)
(kg)	(lb)	(g)	(lb)					
EWES, MAINTENANCE, MODERATE CONDITION								
60	132	10	0.02	2.7	0.61	104	2.3	2.1
80	176	10	0.02	3.2	0.72	122	2.7	2.8
90	198	10	0.02	3.4	0.78	131	2.9	3.1
EWES, FLUSHLING—2 WEEKS PREBREEDING AND FIRST 3 WEEKS OF BREEDING								
60	132	100	0.22	4.4	1	157	5.5	2.9
80	176	100	0.22	4.9	1.12	171	5.9	3.6
90	198	100	0.22	5.1	1.18	177	6.1	3.9
EWES, NONLACTATING, FIRST 15 WEEKS OF GESTATION								
60	132	30	0.07	3.2	0.72	121	3.2	2.5
80	176	30	0.07	3.6	0.82	139	3.8	3.3
90	198	30	0.07	3.8	0.87	148	4.1	3.6
EWES, LAST 4 WEEKS GESTATION (130%-150% LAMBING RATE EXPECTED) OR LAST 4-6 WEEKS LACTATION SUCKLING SINGLES								
60	132	180 (45)	0.4 (0.1)	4.4	1	184	6	5.2
80	176	180 (45)	0.4 (0.1)	4.9	1.12	202	6.3	6.1
90	198	180 (45)	0.4 (0.1)	5.1	1.18	212	6.4	6.5
EWES LAST 4 WEEKS OF GESTATION (180%-225% LAMBING RATE EXPECTED)								
60	132	225	0.5	5.1	1.17	205	6.9	4
80	176	225	0.5	5.7	1.3	223	8.3	5.1
90	198	225	0.5	6	1.37	232	8.9	5.7
EWES, FIRST 6-8 WEEKS LACTATION SUCKLING SINGLES OR LAST 4-6 WEEKS LACTATION SUCKLING TWINS								
60	132	−25	−0.06	6.6	1.5	319	9.1	6.6
80	176	−25	−0.06	7.4	1.69	344	9.5	7.4
90	198	−25	−0.06	7.6	1.75	353	9.6	7.8
EWES, FIRST 6-8 WEEKS LACTATION SUCKLING TWINS								
60	132	−60	−0.13	7.4	1.69	405	10.7	7.7
80	176	−60	−0.13	8.6	1.95	435	11.2	8.6
90	198	−60	−0.13	9.2	2.08	450	11.4	9
REPLACEMENT EWE LAMBS								
30	66	227	0.5	3.4	0.78	185	6.4	2.6
40	88	182	0.4	4	0.91	176	5.9	2.6
50	110	120	0.26	3.9	0.88	136	4.8	2.4
60	132	100	0.22	3.9	0.88	134	4.5	2.5
REPLACEMENT RAM LAMBS								
40	88	330	0.73	5	1.1	243	7.8	3.7
60	132	320	0.7	6.7	1.5	263	8.4	4.2
80	176	290	0.64	7.8	1.8	268	8.5	4.6
100	220	250	0.55	8.4	1.9	264	8.2	4.8
LAMBS FINISHING—4-7 MONTHS OLD								
30	66	295	0.65	4.1	0.94	191	6.6	3.2
40	88	275	0.6	5.4	1.22	185	6.6	3.3
50	110	205	0.45	5.4	1.23	160	5.6	3
EARLY WEANED LAMBS—MODERATE GROWTH POTENTIAL								
10	22	200	0.44	1.8	0.4	127	4	1.9
20	44	250	0.55	3.5	0.8	167	5.4	2.5
30	66	300	0.66	4.4	1	191	6.7	3.2

Modified from National Research Council (NRC): *Nutrient requirements of sheep,* Washington, DC, 1985, National Academy of Sciences, NRC.

TABLE 9-17

Daily Nutrient Requirements of Goats

Body Weight kg	lb	Digestible Energy (Mcal)	Total Digestible Nutrients (g)	Crude Protein (g)	Calcium (g)	Phosphorus (g)
MAINTENANCE, STABLE FEEDING CONDITIONS, MINIMAL ACTIVITY						
30	66	1.59	362	51	2	1.4
60	132	2.68	608	86	3	2.1
90	198	3.68	824	116	4	2.8
MAINTENANCE PLUS LATE PREGNANCY						
30	66	3.33	759	133	4	3.8
60	132	4.42	1005	168	5	3.5
90	198	5.37	1221	198	6	4.2
LACTATION, 4% FAT MILK AND 5-kg MILK PRODUCTION PER DAY						
30	66	9.24	2092	411	17	11.9
60	132	10.33	2338	446	18	12.6
90	198	11.28	2554	476	19	13.3

Modified from National Research Council (NRC): *Nutrient requirements of goats,* Washington, DC, 1981, National Academy of Sciences, NRC.

4. Examine the feces. Perform flotation, sedimentation, and Baermann's procedures to detect patent parasitic infestations. If the feces test positive for occult blood or are very dark, see the section on melena in Chapter 7. If there is evidence of or apparent diarrhea, see the section on diarrhea in Chapter 7.

5. Analyze the blood. Perform a CBC, including plasma protein and fibrinogen. Interpret for evidence of inflammation. Calculate the erythrocytic indices and characterize the anemia if present. Analyze for blood selenium concentration or glutathione peroxidase activity if a herd problem of weight loss exists in a selenium-deficient region.

6. Perform serum chemistry analyses. The serum albumin half-life is approximately $16^{1}/_{2}$ days in cattle and 14 days in sheep and goats. Hypoalbuminemia is associated with internal abscessation, PCM, liver disease, renal disease, and Johne's disease, among other conditions. In the first two of these conditions, albumin is often normal until the patient is near death, whereas with protein-losing renal or gut disease or with failure to make albumin in severe hepatic disease, hypoalbuminemia is often seen by the time noticeable weight loss occurs. Globulins, particularly γ-globulins, may be increased with inflammation, and the albumin/globulin ratio may be decreased. The serum glucose concentration is usually not helpful in determining the cause or causes of weight loss. An elevated serum GGT (above 25 IU/L) may indicate hepatic disease or, in rare cases, pancreatic disease. Serum BUN is often low with PCM in ruminants because of salivary urea recycling. Serum (total) calcium may be decreased with hypoalbuminemia, anorexia, or hypocalcemic syndromes. Serum phosphorus may be increased during severe starvation or Johne's disease or decreased with anorexia. The serum (plasma) copper concentration may be decreased if a herd problem of copper deficiency exists. Weight loss is particularly associated with copper deficiency when diarrhea is present in a region known to be copper deficient or in a region with excess dietary molybdenum or sulfates or both. A low serum copper concentration (below 0.5 mg/ml or ppm) indicates deficiency. Ketonlactia (above 5 mg/dl), indicated by a positive reaction (blue or purple) of milk with nitroprusside, may be associated with anorexia in ketosis or other conditions. Plasma β-hydroxybutyrate (BHB) concentrations have been reported to be a useful tool in diagnosing *inadequate caloric intake* in pregnant sheep.[8] Plasma BHB concentrations should be less than 0.8 mmol/L in pregnant ewes not being underfed.[8]

7. Pathologic findings. Ruminants with PCM exhibit serous atrophy of fat in the coronary grooves of the heart and bone marrow at necropsy. Subcutaneous, abdominal, and perirenal fat are not present.

OBESITY

Mechanisms of Obesity

Obesity is a common problem in domestic species. Obese patients (especially ruminants) are at particular risk for reproductive failure or metabolic disease late in pregnancy or during lactation.

The mechanism of obesity is invariably an intake of total dietary energy above that needed for maintenance and production or exercise over a long period. Obesity occurs most commonly in stabled horses fed concentrates (grain) or horses and ponies on lush pasture. Purebred or pet sheep and goats (particularly wethers) tend to be overfed. In dairy cattle, obesity occurs when cattle are fed well above requirements for maintenance and actual milk production for long periods. Poor reproductive performance is often associated with the initiation of obesity and is also a common sequela to obesity. Feeding for high milk production for lengthy periods in production groups predisposes infertile cows to become fat cows. Dry cows with access to high-energy diets are also predisposed to fat cow syndrome (see Chapter 31). Obese horses and ponies that are rapidly losing weight or anorexic are particularly susceptible to hyperlipidemia and hyperlipemia.

Diagnosis of Obesity in Horses and Ruminants

Diagnosis is obvious; it is made by physical examination. The clinical signs of fat cow syndrome (fatty liver) and its diagnosis and treatment are described in Chapter 31. Clinical descriptions of obesity are straightforward (Tables 9-18 to 9-21) and require minimum interpretation.

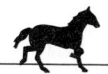

TABLE 9-18

Body Conditioning Scoring System for Beef Cattle

Group	Score	Definition
Thin condition	1	Emaciated Cow is extremely emaciated with no detectable fat over spinous processes, transverse processes, hipbones, or ribs. Tailhead and ribs project quite prominently.
	2	Poor Cow still appears somewhat emaciated, but tailhead and ribs are less prominent. Individual spinous processes are still rather sharp to the touch, but some tissue exists along spine.
	3	Thin Ribs are still individually identifiable but not quite as sharp to the touch. There is obvious palpable fat along spine and over tailhead and some tissue cover over dorsal part of ribs.
Borderline condition	4	Borderline Individual ribs are no longer visually obvious. Spinous processes can be identified individually on palpation but feel rounded rather than sharp. There is some fat cover over ribs, transverse processes, and hipbones.
Optimum moderate condition	5	Moderate Cow has generally good overall appearance. On palpation, fat cover over ribs feels spongy, and areas on either side of tailhead now have palpable fat cover.
	6	High moderate Firm pressure must be applied to feel spinous processes. High degree of fat cover is palpable over ribs and around tailhead.
	7	Good Cow appears fleshy and obviously carries considerable fat. There is a very spongy fat cover over ribs and over and around tailhead. "Rounds" or "pones" of fat are beginning to be obvious. There is some fat around vulva and in crotch.
Fat condition	8	Fat Cow is very fleshy and overconditioned. Spinous processes are almost impossible to palpate. There are large fat deposits over ribs, around tailhead, and below vulva. "Rounds" or "pones" of fat are obvious.
	9	Extremely fat Cow is obviously extremely wasty and patchy and looks blocky. Tailhead and hips are buried in fatty tissue, and "rounds" or "pones" of fat protrude. Bone structure is no longer visible and barely palpable. Animal's mobility may even be impaired by large fatty deposits.

From Spitzer JC: Influences of nutrition on reproduction in beef cattle. In Morrow DA, ed: *Current therapy in theriogenology*, Philadelphia, 1986, WB Saunders.

TABLE 9-19

Body Conditioning Scoring System for Dairy Cattle

Score	Description
1	Individual spinous processes have limited flesh covering and are prominent; the ends are sharp to the touch, and together the processes form a definite overhanging shelf effect to the loin region. Individual vertebrae of the chine, loin, and rump regions are prominent and distinct. Hooks and pin bones are sharp with negligible flesh covering, and severe depressions between hooks and pin bones are noted. The area below the tailhead and between the pin bones is severely depressed, causing the bone structure of the area to appear extremely sharp.
2	Individual spinous processes are visually discernible but not prominent. The ends of processes are sharp to the touch, although they have greater flesh covering, and the processes do not have a distinct overhanging shelf effect. Individual vertebrae of chine, loin, and rump regions are not visually distinct but are readily distinguishable by palpation. Hooks and pin bones are prominent, but the depression between them is less severe. The area below the tailhead and between the pin bones is depressed, but the bone structure is not devoid of flesh covering.
3	Spinous processes are discernible by applying slight pressure. Together the processes appear smooth, and the overhanging shelf effect is not noticeable. Vertebrae of the chine, loin, and rump regions appear as rounded ridges, and hooks and pin bones are rounded and smooth. The area between the pin bones and around the tailhead appears smooth, with no sign of fat deposition.
4	Individual spinous processes can be distinguished only by firm palpation, and together the processes appear flat or rounded with no overhanging shelf effect. The ridge formed by the vertebral column of the chine region is rounded and smooth, but loin and rump regions appear flat. Hooks are rounded, and the span between the hooks and pin bones is rounded, with evidence of subcutaneous fat deposition.
5	Bone structure of the vertebral column, spinous processes, hooks, and pin bones is not visually apparent, and evidence of subcutaneous fat deposition is prominent. The tailhead appears to be buried in fatty tissue.

From Wildman EE et al: *J Dairy Sci* 65:495-501, 1982.

TABLE 9-20

Body Condition Scoring System for Sheep

Score	Description
0	Animal is extremely emaciated and at the point of death. No muscular or fatty tissue can be detected between the skin and the bone.
1	The spinous processes are prominent and sharp. The transverse processes are also sharp; the fingers pass easily under the ends, and it is possible to feel between each process. The eye muscle areas are shallow with no fat cover.
2	The spinous processes still feel prominent but also smooth, and individual processes can be felt only as fine corrugations. The transverse processes are smooth and rounded, and the fingers can be passed under the ends with a little pressure. The eye muscle areas are of moderate depth but have little fat cover.
3	The spinous processes are detected only as small elevations; they are smooth and rounded, and individual bones can be felt only with pressure. The transverse processes are smooth and well covered, and firm pressure is required to feel over the ends. The eye muscle areas are full and have a moderate degree of fat cover.
4	With pressure the spinous processes can just be detected as a hard line between the fat-covered muscle areas. The ends of the transverse processes cannot be felt. The eye muscle areas are full and have a thick covering of fat.
5	The spinous processes cannot be detected even with firm pressure, and there is a depression between the layers of fat where the spinous processes would normally be felt. The transverse processes cannot be detected. The eye muscle areas are very full and have a very thick fat cover. Large deposits of fat may be seen over the rump and tail.

From Russel A: *Practice* 6:91, 1984.

TABLE 9-21

Body Condition Scoring System for Horses

Score	Description
1	Poor. Animal is extremely emaciated. Spinous processes, ribs, tailhead, tuber coxae, and tuber ischii project prominently. Bone structure of the withers, shoulders, and neck is noticeable. No fatty tissue can be felt.
2	Very thin. Animal is emaciated. There is a slight fat covering over the base of the spinous processes; the transverse processes of the lumbar vertebrae feel rounded. Spinous processes, ribs, tailhead, tuber coxae, and tuber ischii are prominent. Bone structure of the withers, shoulders, and neck is faintly discernible.
3	Thin. Fat buildup is present about halfway on the spinous processes; the transverse processes cannot be felt. There is a slight fat cover over the ribs. Spinous processes and ribs are easily discernible. Tailhead is prominent, but individual vertebrae cannot be visually identified. Tuber coxae appear rounded but are easily discernible; tuber ischii are not distinguishable. Bone structure of the withers, shoulders, and neck is accentuated.
4	Moderately thin. Negative crease can be seen along the back. Faint outline of ribs is discernible. Tailhead prominence depends on conformation; fat can be felt around tailhead. Tuber coxae are not discernible. Withers, shoulders, and neck are not obviously thin.
5	Moderate. Back is level. Ribs cannot be visually distinguished but can be felt easily. Fat around tailhead is somewhat spongy. Withers appear rounded over spinous processes, and shoulders and neck blend smoothly into the body.
6	Moderately fleshy. Slight crease may be seen down the back. Fat over ribs is spongy, and fat around tailhead is soft. Fat is beginning to be deposited along withers, behind shoulders, and along neck.
7	Fleshy. Crease may be seen down the back. Individual ribs can be felt, but there is noticeable filling of fat between ribs. Fat around tailhead is soft. Fat is deposited along withers, behind shoulders, and along neck.
8	Fat. Crease is seen down the back. Ribs are difficult to feel. Fat around tailhead is very soft. Areas along withers and behind shoulders are filled with fat, and neck is noticeably thickened. Fat is deposited along inner thighs.
9	Extremely fat. Obvious crease is seen down the back. Patchy fat appears over ribs. Bulging fat is seen around tailhead along withers, behind shoulders, and along neck. Fat along inner thighs may cause thighs to rub together. Flank is filled with fat.

From Henneke GD et al: *Equine Vet J* 15:371-372, 1983.

PICA

Pica is defined as a depraved or abnormal appetite. It is usually associated with animals that chew or eat wood (fences, trees, buildings), dirt, bones, or other inanimate objects not usually considered feedstuffs. The mechanism or mechanisms of pica are not yet understood. Pica has been associated with PCM, parasitism, and obesity and with deficiencies of phosphorus, salt, protein (kwashiorkor), and micronutrients. Diagnosis is by observation or history or both. The main emphasis must be placed on identification of the primary problem. Pica must be differentiated from abnormal behavior associated with certain central nervous system diseases.

REFERENCES

6. Kinney JM: The application of indirect calorimetry to clinical studies. In Kinney JM, ed: *Assessment of energy metabolism in health and disease*, Columbus, Ohio, 1980, Ross Laboratories.
7. Long CL et al: Metabolic response to injury and illness: estimation of energy and protein needs from indirect calorimetry and nitrogen balance, *J Enter Parenter Nutr* 3:452-456, 1979.
8. Russel A: Nutrition of the pregnant ewe, *Practice* 7:23, 1985; *Vet Rec (Practice* 7:23, suppl)116:29, 1985.

Alterations in Urinary Function

THOMAS J. DIVERS

DAVID C. Van METRE

Consulting Editors

MAJOR CLINICAL SIGNS/PROBLEMS ENCOUNTERED

DYSURIA AND STRANGURIA

Dysuria is difficult or painful urination; stranguria is slow and painful urination. Because these two clinical signs are often difficult to distinguish in large animal medicine, they are considered together in this section. Dysuria and stranguria usually are caused by (1) urethral obstruction; (2) inflammation of the urethra, the bladder, or both; or (3) neurologic conditions that prevent normal emptying of the bladder. In foals and calves these two conditions may also develop as a consequence of urachal abscesses, which prevent normal bladder emptying.

The horse voids urine very actively and forcefully. Both male and female adult horses normally may groan and strain on urination. This should not be misinterpreted as dysuria or stranguria. In other large animal species, urination is more passive, and straining or groaning normally is not observed. Conditions in which a horse may appear to have dysuria include lower urinary tract disease, abdominal pain, peritonitis, severe musculoskeletal disease, or neurologic disease. With any of these conditions, the horse may attempt to posture and urinate but may not be able to increase intraabdominal pressure sufficiently to allow complete voiding.

In the horse both dysuria and stranguria may manifest as straining, urination of shorter duration than normal, or frequent attempts to urinate that produce only small amounts of urine (pollakiuria). The urine may be discolored; for example, some diseases that cause dysuria or stranguria also cause hematuria. Normal adult horse urine is very cloudy because it contains large quantities of calcium carbonate crystals and mucus.

Dysuria or stranguria in large animal species may be confused with tenesmus. This is most frequently a dilemma in neonatal foals with a ruptured bladder or meconium impaction. However, with tenesmus the rear feet of the foal are positioned slightly more anterior than with stranguria or dysuria.

The clinical signs of dysuria and stranguria in ruminants may be similar to those in horses, except that urine dribbling is more common in male sheep and goats with calculi. Vocalization is associated with dysuria in male goats with urethral obstruction. The animal may show intermittent forceful

BOX 10-1

Causes of Dysuria, Stranguria, and Urinary Incontinence in the Horse

Urethral calculi
Urethral injury
Cystic calculi
Hemorrhage into the urinary tract
Penile or preputial trauma or swelling
Vaginal or urethral trauma or swelling (especially after foaling)
Cantharidin toxicosis
Bladder neoplasia
Habronemiasis
Urethritis
Smegma accumulation
Cystitis
Ruptured bladder
Equine neonatal maladjustment
Ruptured ureter
Herpes myelitis
Sorghum cystitis
Rabies
Estrogen-responsive dysuria
Ectopic ureter
Prolapsed bladder (after foaling)
Severe spinal cord disease
Recumbency
Myositis
Laminitis
Vertebral body infection or fracture
Pelvic fracture
Vertebral spondylitis
Colic
Peritonitis

BOX 10-2

Causes of Dysuria and Stranguria in Ruminants

CATTLE
Urethral calculi
Hemorrhage into the urinary tract
Urethral injury secondary to calving or breeding
Penile or preputial injury
Cystitis
Rabies
Pelvic bladder
Urachal abscess
Sacral fracture
Extradural lymphosarcoma in the vertebral canal
Spinal cord trauma or pressure
Bladder neoplasia
Prolapsed bladder (accompanying vaginal prolapse)
Congenital urethral disorders (stricture, dilation, ectopia)

GOATS AND SHEEP
Urethral calculi
Cystitis
Injury to urethra or swelling around urethra
Spinal cord trauma or compression
Ulcerative posthitis

contraction of abdominal muscles, seen as "heaving" of flanks. Urine scalding of the perineal region or rear legs may be noted in either ruminants or horses with dysuria or stranguria. Intermittent prolapse of the prepuce may be another clinical sign of dysuria and stranguria in males.

Approach to Diagnosis of Dysuria and Stranguria

Obtaining a complete history is most important if the cause of the stranguria or dysuria is to be determined (Boxes 10-1 and 10-2). For example, urethral calculi should be suspected immediately in a sheep or goat with dysuria that was castrated at an early age and in castrated feedlot sheep and cattle fed high-grain diets. A history of more than one horse showing clinical signs of spinal cord disease and respiratory disease, along with stranguria, should immediately lead the practitioner to consider herpes myelitis as the most likely cause. A history of dysuria, stranguria, or both developing after parturition usually indicates an injury to the lower urinary tract. After the history has been taken, the urinary tract should be examined. If possible the animal should be observed urinating and a sample of urine collected to determine the presence of inflammatory cells, blood, or excessive crystals. The male's preputial hairs or the female's perineal region should be closely inspected for the presence of crystals. In ruminants with urethral or cystic calculi, crystals sometimes can be found at these locations. In the male the area of the urethra should be palpated percutaneously. Swelling, pain, or abnormal urethral pulsations may be detected by palpation. Marked swelling and pain along the ventral body wall in a

bull or steer with dysuria or stranguria strongly suggests a urethral rupture, which usually occurs in the sigmoid flexure area. The urethral orifice can be visualized in most males; if urethral calculi are suspected in a male sheep or goat, an attempt should be made to exteriorize the penis and examine the most distal part of the urethra. This procedure often requires sedation and an epidural block. Continued evidence of pain, dysuria, or stranguria after relief of a blockage usually indicates cystitis, urethritis, or another calculus in the urethra.

A transabdominal ultrasound examination is an important diagnostic procedure that can be used to detect bladder distention or rupture, uroperitoneum, bladder masses, and abnormalities of the umbilical structures. A 5-MHz sector or linear ray probe or a 7.5-MHz linear probe are most commonly used in either the standing or laterally recumbent position for visualization of these structures.

If swelling or pain is found on palpation of the most distal part of the equine penis, it may be necessary to tranquilize the horse so that this area can be examined more closely. If a small amount of blood is observed in the postejaculate fluid of a horse, the area around the urethral orifice should be inspected closely for habronemiasis, neoplasia, or both. If these are not found, endoscopy can be used to detect abnormalities in the urethra such as rupture of the corpus spongiosum.[1] An endoscope less than 10 mm in diameter and 1 m long or longer should be used for this examination.

Rectal or abdominal palpation to determine the size of the bladder should be performed when dysuria and stranguria are present. In small ruminants a distended bladder usually can be palpated by simultaneously placing one hand on each side of the caudal ventral abdomen. If the bladder has been ruptured, it will be difficult to identify by palpation but ascites can be detected. To confirm uroperitoneum, a sample of peritoneal fluid should be obtained for measurement of the creatinine concentration, which should then be compared to the serum creatinine concentration. The creatinine concentration of peritoneal fluid is twice as high or higher than the serum creatinine value in animals with uroperitoneum.[2,3] A potassium level above 10 mEq/L in peritoneal fluid also indicates urine in the peritoneal cavity.[4] Distention of the bladder may occur as a result of urethral obstruction or because of a neurologic condition that prevents normal emptying of the bladder. In the horse, bladder distention may also be found with abdominal pain or musculoskeletal disease (e.g., back pain or neurologic disease that causes severe paresis). These systems should be evaluated when no primary disease is found in the urinary system. Horses recumbent from any cause may also develop a severely distended bladder. A careful rectal examination of the bladder and the proximal urethra of the horse might allow identification of a urethral or cystic calculi. Most cystic calculi in the horse are singular and located in the trigone of the bladder. Cystic calculi can be missed during rectal palpation if the arm is placed too far in the rectum or if the bladder has sufficient urine to prevent palpation of the stone. Most bladder stones in the horse are best palpated with only the hand and wrist in the rectum. If there is a large amount of urine in the bladder, a transrectal ultrasound examination using a linear probe may allow easy visualization of the stone. Sabulous calculi may be found in horses with urinary incontinence and on rectal examination may give the impression of a bladder tumor or large stone.[5] Affected horses usually have incontinence and dysuria. Urethral calculi are most commonly lodged just below the anus in horses. In some horses these can be felt when palpating the perineal area. Urethral stones can also be confirmed by ultrasound (7.5 MHz) (Fig. 10-1) or by urethroscopic examination. If the horse is sufficiently sedated for the urethroscopic examination, the stone occasionally may be pushed back into the bladder during the examination. If a urinary calculus is detected in the horse, an ultrasound examination of the entire urinary tract should be performed, because some horses with cystic calculi may have other stones in one or both kidneys.

If a neurologic disease is causing primary bladder dysfunction, an attempt should be made to determine whether the primary lesion is affecting the detrusor muscle (which provides bladder contraction) or the urethral sphincter muscles of the bladder. This determination is often helpful in localizing the lesion and is important when selecting treatment. If innervation to the detrusor muscle is affected and the urethral pressure is either normal or increased, the animal will have dysuria, and on rectal palpation the bladder will be moderately to severely distended. The neurologic signs that affect the rear limbs of such patients are more commonly those of upper motor neuron disease, and the term "upper motor neuron bladder" may be used to describe the dysuria (e.g., herpes myelitis). The animal frequently postures and strains to urinate but voids only a small amount of urine. If a neurologic condition has affected sacral nerves that supply the urethral sphincter muscle, a "lower motor neuron bladder" is present, and urinary incontinence is the predominant clinical sign (e.g., cauda equina neuritis in horses or lymphoma in cattle). In a horse with dysuria and lower motor neuron (LMN) dysfunction, the bladder usually is moderately to severely distended and urine can be expressed easily if pressure is applied to the bladder during rectal examination. With LMN dysfunction urine may also be voided as the animal walks. Other neurologic signs involving the sacral and coccygeal nerves often are apparent, such as decreased tail and anal tone. Ataxia of the rear limbs may or may not be present with an LMN bladder. Urethral and bladder pressure profiles can be determined to better assess the location of the lesion.[6-8]

Estrogen-responsive incontinence has been reported but is rare in the horse.[9] If dysuria, incontinence, or stranguria are believed to be caused by an inflammatory disease of the urethra or bladder, the absence or presence of sepsis should be determined. This can be done by collecting a midstream or catheterized urine sample (or both) and quantitating the

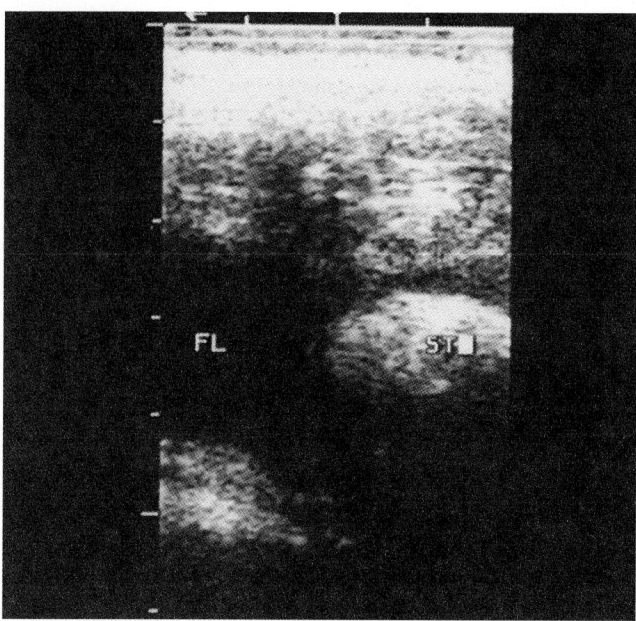

FIG. 10-1 Transcutaneous sonogram (7.5 MHz) of the perineal region of an adult male horse demonstrating a urethral calculus *(ST)* with fluid accumulation *(FL)* in the more proximal urethra.

number of white blood cells and bacteria in the urine. Evaluation of both a catheterized and midstream-voided sample should help determine the location of the inflammatory disease. Quantitative cultures of the samples should be performed soon after collection. Animals with lower urinary tract infections usually have 10,000 or more organisms per milliliter of urine.[10] Normal male and female horses have less than 20,000 colony-forming units (CFU) per milliliter of urine on a free catch sample and less than 500 CFU/ml on a catheterized sample. Female horses show greater contamination by free catch than male horses.[11] In the adult horse endoscopic examination of both the urethra and the bladder can be performed easily and may reveal the specific site of inflammatory disease, obstruction, or both.[12] Endoscopy can be useful for examining the urethra, bladder mucosa, and ureteral opening. In males the small urethral diameter and greater length requires an endoscope 1 m or longer and 10 mm or less in diameter. In most horses the bladder can be visualized with a 1.2-m scope, although a longer scope may be required for some. Ultrasound examination per rectum is helpful in detecting cystic calculi concretions and ureteral calculi that may be associated with the urinary tract infection.

An accumulation of smegma, composed of mucus and cellular debris, may cause preputial swelling and dysuria in adult male horses. The smegma usually can be found as a hard, waxy mass in the urethral diverticulum. Prepucial swelling without pain or discharge may be caused by a peripheral cushingoid syndrome.[13]

Few disorders in large animals cause urinary incontinence without stranguria or dysuria. Ectopic ureter or ureters should be considered in young animals with persistent urinary incontinence. Vaginoscopic or cystoscopic examination or both usually are the most helpful procedures in confirming the diagnosis. Locating the opening of the ectopic ureter can be difficult.

HEMATURIA

Hematuria is defined as blood in the urine. It may appear as gross blood clots passed at the beginning, during, or at the

---

BOX 10-3

Causes of Hematuria in the Horse

URETHRA
Habronemiasis
Calculi
Idiopathic in males (proximal dorsal urethral
  hemorrhage)
Urethritis
Neoplasia (most commonly squamous cell carcinoma)
Trauma

BLADDER
Calculi
Cystitis
Neoplasia
Amorphous debris
Bleeding diathesis (e.g., warfarin)
Blister beetle

KIDNEY
Calculi
Trauma
Nephritis
Leptospirosis
Vascular anomaly
Parasite migration (*Halicephalobus* spp.)
Neoplasia
Vasculitis
Glomerulopathy
Papillary necrosis
Blister beetle
Idiopathic
Exercise

BOX 10-4

Causes of Hematuria in Ruminants

URETHRA
Calculi
Trauma
Urethritis
Papilloma

BLADDER
Bracken fern or other bleeding diathesis
Papilloma or neoplasia
Calculi
Cystitis
Polyps

KIDNEY
Pyelonephritis
Trauma
Infarction
Malignant catarrhal fever
Severe endotoxic shock
Leptospirosis

---

end of urination or as a more uniform red discoloration throughout urination without clots. If large clots are present, obstruction of the urinary tract may occur, resulting in stranguria and dysuria.

Approach to Diagnosis of Hematuria

The history is an important part of the diagnostic approach; it should include the animal's age, the duration of the hematuria, and the time during urination that hematuria is most pronounced (Boxes 10-3 and 10-4). For example, a horse that is seen to have hematuria after exercise should be suspected of having cystic calculi or, less commonly, renal calculi, although hematuria may be seen briefly in normal horses after high-intensity exercise. Lesions of the urethra most often produce hematuria at the beginning of urination, although in a horse with proximal urethral disease (rupture of the corpus spongiosum), this hemorrhage may be seen only at the end of urination.[1,14] Hematuria that originates from the bladder is most likely to be seen at the end of urination or certainly would be more pronounced at that time. Hemorrhage originating from the upper urinary tract would likely be more pronounced at the end of urination but might be seen throughout urination. If the urine discoloration appears uniform throughout urination and no clots are obvious, the practitioner first must make sure that the discoloration is hematuria and not hemoglobinuria, bilirubinuria, or myoglobinuria. This can be accomplished easily by examining urine sediment for cell types and the presence of crystals. Dipstick evaluation of the urine, along with assessment of the patient's packed cell volume, the plasma protein, and the color of the plasma and mucous membranes, should also be performed. If hematuria is confirmed, a physical examination of the urinary system should proceed to confirm the site of the hema-

turia. This process includes examination of the urethra and rectal palpation of the bladder, the ureters, and the left kidney in horses and cows. Additional diagnostic steps (e.g., endoscopy, ultrasound) may be required in a few cases to determine the origin of the hematuria.

If hematuria is believed to originate from the urethra, tranquilization and examination of the most distal urethral opening, along with endoscopic examination of the urethra, may identify the lesion (as mentioned above, in male horses endoscopic examination requires an endoscope less than 10 mm in diameter and 1 m long or longer). It is not uncommon for geldings and stallions to have hematuria associated with a lesion in the most proximal urethra.[1,14] Endoscopic and ultrasound examination of the bladder of either males or females may help identify the origin of the hematuria. Hematuria that originates from the bladder often can be diagnosed by rectal palpation because causes such as cystic calculi or neoplasia of the bladder are readily palpated. More discrete lesions may need to be identified by endoscopic examination. If there is no hemorrhage from the bladder wall, the openings of the ureters and the color of the urine coming from both of them should be visualized during the endoscopic examination. This is best performed after suctioning urine from the bladder and then distending the bladder with air, taking care that bubbling of the urine does not occur. The ureteral opening can be seen dorsally as the scope is first introduced into the bladder. The two openings can be visualized simultaneously by passing the scope farther into the bladder and retroflexing the scope caudally until the entire trigone area is visualized. If the discoloration is coming from a ureteral opening, the next diagnostic step is ultrasound examination of either the right or left kidney.

The urine of a small number of horses may cause a reddish discoloration in the snow, causing unnecessary alarm to owners. This is thought to be caused by a particular pigment in the urine of those few horses.[15] Their urine will appear normal until it contacts the snow.

PYURIA

Pyuria is defined as purulent debris in the urine. This may be either a gross or a microscopic observation. Dysuria, stranguria, pollakiuria, crystalluria, urine scalding of the perineum, or even hematuria may accompany the pyuria. A fever may or may not be present, but if the pyuria originates from the upper urinary tract, the animal often may be systemically ill. The pyuria may be a result of an inflammatory or a septic disease (or both) or of a nonseptic inflammatory disease. If the sepsis is caused by a bacterial infection, bacteriuria is present. Most urinary tract infections in horses and cows are a result of ascending infection. Predisposing factors such as injury to the urethra or neurologic dysfunction are associated with urinary tract infections. The pathogenic organisms most often are gram-negative bacteria with fimbrial adhesions that allow attachment to the uroepithelium. Gram-positive bacteria such as *Staphylococcus, Corynebacterium,* and *Streptococcus* organisms may also cause urinary tract infections. Neonatal foals treated with antibiotics commonly develop *Candida* cystitis.[16]

The initial approach to the diagnosis of pyuria should be to determine the location or origin of the pyuria, the etiology, and any predisposing causes. In females it is especially important to examine the reproductive tract to confirm that it is not the source of the pyuria. Inflammatory diseases of the urethra that cause pyuria usually have obvious clinical signs of dysuria but minimal systemic effects. With inflammatory or septic diseases of the bladder, dysuria may not be as pronounced as with urethral lesions, but it is present in most cases. Low-grade fever may be present with cystitis, but the animal rarely appears to be systemically ill. Pyuria that originates from the upper urinary tract may cause minimum signs of dysuria, but clinical signs of systemic illness are more likely with upper urinary tract infection than with lower urinary tract infection. Pyuria can be confirmed as originating from the urethra by the history, percutaneous palpation of the urethra, and endoscopic examination of the urethra. A culture of the most inflamed area of the urethra, using a uterine culturette, should be performed if a septic process is suspected. If this cannot be accomplished, a urine sample collected at the beginning of urination should be cultured. Interpretation of these cultures may be difficult, because bacteria can be cultured from this area in normal animals.

Cystitis is any inflammatory disease of the bladder, and it can be septic or nonseptic in origin. The history should be taken, and a complete examination of the entire urinary tract, including rectal palpation or percutaneous abdominal palpation of the bladder in small ruminants, should be performed if cystitis is suspected. The determination of a thickened bladder on rectal examination is often a subjective finding. Cytologic examination and quantitative culture of a midstream-voided urine sample or preferably a catheterized urine sample are important in determining the presence of cystitis and identifying any etiologic agents. Predisposing factors such as calculi or neurologic diseases should always be considered. To be labeled pyuria a midstream-voided or catheterized sample should have eight or more white blood cells per high-power microscopic field, and in septic cystitis the guideline is 10,000 or more organisms per milliliter of urine.[10]

Pyuria that originates from the upper urinary tract can be determined by the history, clinical and ultrasound examinations, and evidence of systemic illness. The rectal examination may reveal enlargement of one or both ureters and possibly an enlargement or abnormal shape (or both) of the left kidney. The right kidney occasionally can be palpated per rectum in the horse or cow if the kidney is grossly enlarged. Although cytologic examination of the urine may indicate pyuria, sepsis may not always be apparent with upper urinary tract infections. This may be especially true if the sepsis originates from a nephrolith. If *Leptospira interrogans pomona* is suspected as a cause of pyuria, urine sediment should be placed on a microscope slide, air dried, and examined by fluorescent antibody for *Leptospira* antigen.[17] An ultrasound ex-

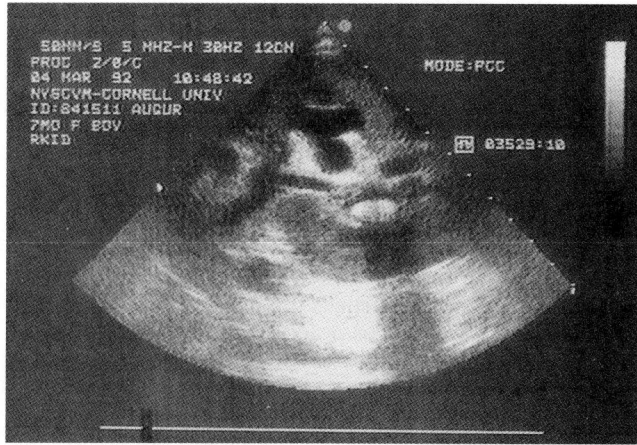

FIG. 10-2 ■ Nephrolith with an easily visible acoustic shadow in a calf; urine tests showed more than 100,000 *Actinomyces pyogenes* organisms per milliliter of urine.

amination of both kidneys and ureters should be performed in all horses with evidence of upper urinary tract infection.[18,19] The presence of renal calculi in animals with upper urinary tract infections makes successful medical treatment unlikely. Ultrasound examination of the kidneys may also be helpful in cows with chronic pyelonephritis[20] (Fig. 10-2) and in small ruminants with urethral obstruction. The technique for ultrasound examination of the right kidney in cows is described.[21] Ultrasound examination of the left kidney in the cow and horse may also be performed per rectum.[20]

UREMIA

Uremia is caused by the presence of excessive urinary constituents in the blood and their systemic toxic effect. Much effort has been expended in trying to identify uremic toxins in the blood, and it seems most plausible that several toxins are associated with the uremic process, including urea, parathyroid hormone, guanidino, and phosphorus.[22,23] The predominant clinical signs of uremia seen in large animals are depression and anorexia. Seizures or encephalopathy or both associated with cerebral edema and the microscopic appearance of Alzheimer type II cells may occur in some cases with severe uremic episodes.[24,25] Weight loss, oral erosions, gastrointestinal ulcers, polyuria, polydipsia, melena, diarrhea, and accumulation of excessive dental tarter are other noticeable effects. Coagulopathy, platelet dysfunction, or both are not unusual. Uremia may be the result of either acute or chronic renal failure.

Anatomic and Physiologic Considerations

A knowledge of the structure and function of the nephron is important for understanding the pathophysiology of renal diseases. For this discussion, it is convenient to divide the nephron into three structural components: the glomerulus, the tubules, and the microvasculature.

GLOMERULUS. The glomerulus filters plasma, allowing the transfer of certain plasma components across the glomerular membrane into Bowman's space. The "glomerular filtration apparatus" can be simplistically divided into three structures, the outermost being the fenestrated endothelial cells of the glomerular capillaries. The fenestrations, or gaps, between the endothelial cells are approximately 70 to 100 nm wide.[26] Immediately beneath the fenestrated endothelium lies the glomerular basement membrane, which in human beings is approximately 320 nm thick.[26] Incorporated into this membrane are polyanionic proteoglycans, such as heparin sulfate, that provide a dense concentration of negative charge and repel anionic plasma proteins.

Visceral epithelial cells, or podocytes, form the innermost layer of the filtration apparatus. These cells have interdigitating "foot processes," or cellular extensions that form a meshlike layer perforated with 20- to 30-nm-wide filtration slits.[26] These three layers combine to form a filtration barrier for many plasma macromolecules. Molecular size and net molecular charge determine which macromolecules can traverse the filtration membrane. With normal glomerular function, the final ultrafiltrate that enters the nephron lumen is virtually free of plasma macromolecules of molecular weight greater than approximately 65,000 Daltons or of a molecular diameter greater than approximately 3.5 nm.[26] Thus albumin, many coagulant and anticoagulant factors (such as antithrombin III), complement factors, and immunoglobulins are not normally transferred from plasma into the nephron lumen. Disruption of any of these components of the filtration apparatus can result in loss of this vital discriminatory capability, leading to consequences such as poor plasma oncotic pressure from albumin loss in the urine. Finally, the mesangium, or mesangial matrix, provides internal structural support for the glomerulus and its capillary tuft. Mesangial cells, through their contractile properties and ability to respond to neurohormonal agents, contribute to regulation of intraglomerular blood flow.[26] These cells also can ingest macromolecules retained in the glomerulus during filtration. With glomerular injury, alterations in permeability and hydrostatic pressure in the glomerulus may cause retention of large numbers of plasma macromolecules in the glomerulus. Mesangial cell proliferation is thought to occur in response to this event, and the mesangial cells may phagocytize these retained substances.[26] As the cell number and matrix content of the mesangium increases, the delicate structure of the glomerulus is disrupted, further impairing glomerular function.

TUBULES. Renal tubular cells, particularly those of the proximal convoluted tubule and ascending limb of Henle, are very metabolically active. Numerous mitochondria are found in these cells, because many resorptive and secretory mechanisms require adenosine triphosphate to move ions and organic molecules against charge or chemical gradients, or both. The high oxidative capacity of these cells makes them very prone to hypoxic injury.[26] In addition, the proximal location in the nephron exposes them to higher concentrations of certain toxic compounds that might be resorbed from the tubular filtrate.[26] Therefore disease states, toxic substances, or pharmacologic agents that reduce oxygen delivery to tubular cells (e.g., hypovolemic shock) or that directly injure these cells (e.g., aminoglycosides) may result in impairment or loss of concentrating ability, waste excretion, acid-base regulation, and electrolyte balance. Another clinically relevant characteristic of these cells is their ability to replace, by mitosis, dead or senescent tubular epithelium. However, effective replacement of tubular epithelial cells requires an intact *epithelial basement membrane*. Toxic, hypoxic, infectious, or inflammatory conditions that result in destruction of this basement membrane in a sufficient number of nephrons would limit recovery from renal injury, making the status of the basement membrane an important prognostic criterion in ultrastructural evaluation of biopsy specimens.

MICROVASCULATURE. Not only is blood flow through the vessels surrounding the nephron vital for tubular cell health, both the renal endocrine responses to changes in blood pressure and renal handling of solute are highly dependent on normal renal perfusion and vasomotor control. Blood flow distribution in the kidney is highly influenced by intrarenal production of vasoactive prostaglandins.[26] These prostaglandins are particularly vital for protective redistribution of blood flow during the kidney's adaptation to relatively low blood flow states (e.g., dehydration or shock). Nonsteroidal antiinflammatory drugs (NSAIDs) may temporarily diminish or even eliminate intrarenal prostaglandin synthesis; if such drugs are administered to a volume-depleted patient, and especially if they are administered repetitively, serious impairment of renal function may result from ischemic damage to tubular cells. Prostaglandins appear to redirect blood flow to the deeper areas of the cortex and medulla during low blood flow states.[27] As a result, necrosis and hemorrhage in the renal papillae are common lesions in NSAID nephrotoxicosis. A more insidious form of NSAID toxicosis occurs when these drugs are administered concurrently with other potentially nephrotoxic agents. NSAIDs have been documented as augmenting aminoglycoside nephrotoxicosis in humans[28] and are suspected of doing the same in large animals.[29] This augmentation of aminoglycoside nephrotoxicosis may be due in part to NSAID-induced changes in renal hemodynamics, with impaired tubular cell metabolism being a critical factor.[28]

PATHOPHYSIOLOGY OF ACUTE RENAL FAILURE

Acute renal failure is characterized by a sudden decline in the glomerular filtration rate (GFR), tubular dysfunction, and concurrent development of uremia. Renal failure may result from complete loss of function of a large number of nephrons, partial loss of function of most nephrons, or any combination thereof. Remaining functional nephrons may undergo hypertrophy, a concomitant lowering of arteriolar resistance, and an increase in glomerular plasma flow.[30] The predominant pathophysiologic mechanisms that cause renal failure in large animals are injury to the renal tubular epithelium and changes in intrarenal hemodynamics.[31] The filtration rate may be further diminished in certain diseases by a reduction in hydraulic permeability of the glomerular basement membrane. In acute renal failure, the alterations in intrarenal hemodynamics with decreased glomerular hydrostatic pressure include a reduction in renal perfusion pressure (i.e., shock), constriction of afferent arterioles, efferent arteriolar dilation, constriction of both arterioles with greater constriction of the afferent arteriole, endothelial cell swelling, fibrin occlusion of renal vasculature, and/or other mechanisms of change in renal blood flow.[31] A variety of mediators, including angiotensin; thromboxane; vasopressin; adrenergic hormones; adenosine; endothelin and its dilator antagonist, endothelium-dependent relaxing factor; lipopolysaccharide (LPS); tumor necrosis factor (TNF); and other cytokines may be involved in the dysfunction process.[31-33] Decreased glomerular hydrostatic pressure may also occur in any individual nephron as a reflex mechanism that occurs secondary to tubular obstruction.[34] With ischemic renal injury the renal epithelium is damaged, especially the highly metabolic epithelial cells of the proximal tubules. The proximal tubules also are more susceptible to toxic injury than the more distal aspects of the nephron because most toxins are resorbed in highest concentrations in the proximal convoluted tubule cells. Ischemic or toxic injury to these cells causes cellular hypoxia, free radical production, organelle destruction, and cell death. The death of renal tubular epithelial cells results in obstructing debris and cast development in the tubular lumen. A retrograde flow of uremic toxins may then develop, which accounts for a further decline in "effective" GFR. These tubular and vascular factors are probably interdependent in acute renal failure.

The causes of acute renal failure can be somewhat simplistically divided into acute inflammation or obstruction (or

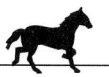

both), hemodynamic changes, toxic tubular nephrosis, and immunologic disorders (Boxes 10-5 and 10-6). Any condition that predisposes the patient to marked hypotension, the release of endogenous pressor agents, or both has the potential to initiate hemodynamically mediated acute renal failure. Systemic hypotension and/or afferent arteriole constriction or afferent-efferent arteriolar pressure imbalance, along with tubular obstruction, cause the decrease in renal perfusion. Endotoxemia, complement-mediated coagulopathies, and/or severe systemic hypotension often are involved in hemodynamically mediated acute renal failure in large animals.[31,33] The initial renal dysfunction caused by most nephrotoxins is the result of tubular swelling and necrosis of proximal cortical tubular cells. The mechanisms of the tubular epithelial disease may be lysosomal dysfunction, mitochondrial dysfunction, or abnormal protein synthesis, resulting in epithelial swelling, tubular obstruction, or both.[35]

Although not documented in large animals, immunologic reactions to certain drugs may be a cause of nephrosis. Immunologically mediated diseases possibly could cause either acute interstitial nephritis or acute glomerulonephritis.

The diagnosis of acute renal failure usually can be made from the history, physical examination, measurement of serum chemistries, and urinalysis. If a large animal is in acute renal failure, azotemia (elevated creatinine and urea nitrogen) would be present concurrently with a urine specific gravity below 1.021.[31,36] With acute renal failure, the urine is not always isosthenuric. The fractional excretion of sodium and urine γ-glutamyltransferase/creatinine ratio will be increased, but their measurements are unlikely to provide important additional information. The normal serum creatinine concentration may vary considerably by age and breed (e.g., heavily muscled quarter horses may normally have a value of nearly 2 mg/ml). Newborn foals occasionally may have a serum

---

BOX 10-5

Causes of Acute Renal Failure in Horses

HEMODYNAMIC CAUSES
Severe hypovolemia (e.g., colitis)
Septic shock
Hemorrhagic shock
Heart failure
Coagulopathies
Adverse drug reaction
Pigment nephropathy

TOXIC NEPHROSIS
Aminoglycosides
Tetracycline
Vitamin D
Mercury

TOXIC NEPHROSIS—cont'd
Nonsteroidal antiinflammatory drugs
Amphotericin
Pigment nephropathy

IMMUNOLOGIC CAUSES
Drug-induced interstitial nephritis
Glomerulopathy

SEPTIC CAUSES
Actinobacillus
Leptospira spp.
Pyelonephritis

BOX 10-6

Causes of Acute Renal Failure in Ruminants

HEMODYNAMIC CAUSES
Renal vein thrombosis
Bloat (severe)
Shock (hypovolemic or septic)
Heart failure

TOXIC PLANTS
Oak or acorn (*Quercus* spp.)
Halogeton glomerulatus
Sarcobatus vermiculatus (greasewood)
Oxalis spp. (soursob)
Amaranthus spp. (pigweed)
Kochia spp.
Rumex spp. (sorrel, dock)
Chenopodium album (lamb's-quarter)
Rheum rhaponticum (rhubarb)
Salsola pestifer (Russian thistle)
Lantana camara
Isotropis spp.

DRUGS
Aminoglycoside antibiotics
Sulfonamides
Oxytetracycline
Monensin

CHEMICALS
Arsenic
Mercury
Ethylene glycol
Gasohol by-products
Paraquat
Chlorinated hydrocarbons
Sodium fluoride
Copper

ENDOGENOUS PROTEINS
Hemoglobin
Myoglobin

MYCOTOXINS
Ochratoxin
Citrinin

SEPTIC CAUSES
Pyelonephritis
Infarction and renal necrosis
Septic mastitis
Septic metritis

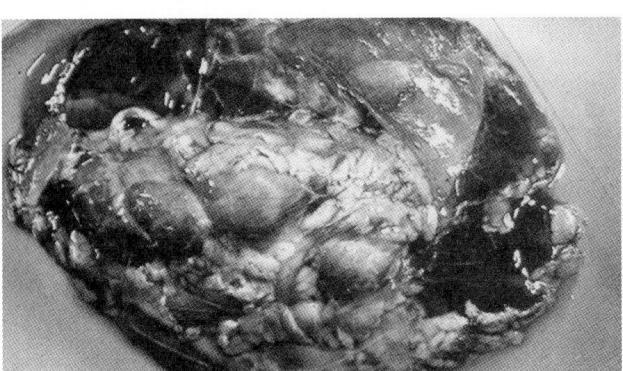

FIG. 10-3 ■ Perineal edema in a calf with acute renal failure caused by acorn toxicosis.

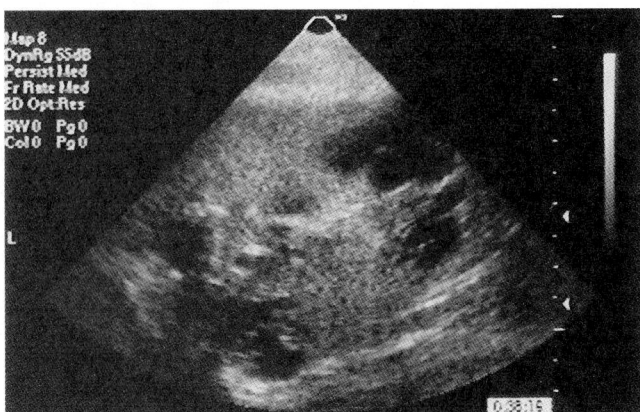

FIG. 10-5 ■ Chronic renal failure in a 14-year-old donkey. Multiple cysts (probably acquired) and increased echogenicity of the renal parenchyma can be seen; normal corticomedullary separation is absent.

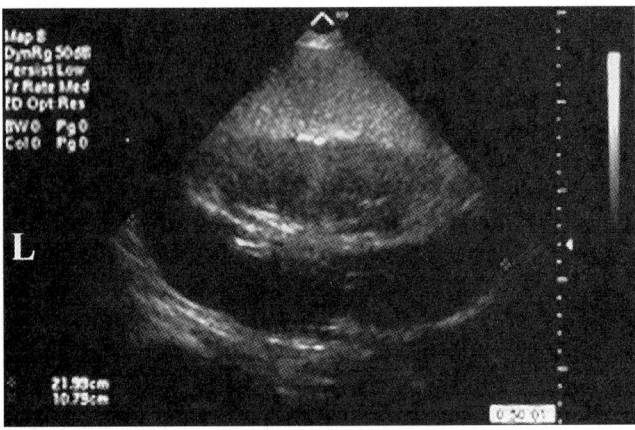

FIG. 10-4 ■ Renomegaly in a standardbred racehorse with myoglobinuric acute renal failure. The serum creatinine was 13.9 mg/dl at the time of the ultrasound. The horse recovered completely.

creatinine value of 6 mg/dl or higher at birth without abnormal renal function. The elevation indicates placental dysfunction, and these foals have a higher incidence of neonatal maladjustment syndrome. The GFR and renal plasma flow in newborn, healthy foals are similar to values reported for mature horses.[37] Cytologic examination of the urine may be helpful with inflammatory causes of acute renal failure.[17] Rectal palpation and ultrasound examination may be helpful in the diagnosis of obstructive causes of acute renal failure and oliguric acute renal failure.[18-20] Markedly swollen or edematous kidneys may be detected with acute oliguric/anuric renal failure (Fig. 10-3). This generally is a poor prognostic finding, but some animals recover (Fig. 10-4).

PATHOPHYSIOLOGY OF CHRONIC RENAL FAILURE

Chronic renal failure is the result of a slow, progressive loss of nephron function or population or both. This continued loss of nephrons results in a decrease in functional mass. Failure occurs when enough nephrons are lost or their function is sufficiently decreased to affect body condition and function. With either acute or chronic renal failure, more than two thirds of the nephron function must be lost for clinical effects to be noted. Regardless of the initial tubulointerstitial lesion, the histologic end result is often the same; that is, an increase

in extracellular matrix (ECM) and glomerulosclerosis.[38] Many factors have been determined to cause the morphologic or functional changes in nephrons that result in chronic renal failure, including systemic hypertension, cytokines and growth factors, calcium and phosphorus deposition, lipid abnormalities, and intrarenal vascular changes.[30,39-44] Compensatory changes in the intrarenal hemodynamics of the remaining functional nephrons are also responsible for progressive loss of nephrons. Afferent arteriolar tone decreases more than efferent arteriolar tone in the remaining nephrons, and hydraulic pressure in the glomerular capillaries rises, increasing the amount of filtrate and often causing proteinuria in those nephrons. Increased protein in the luminal fluid causes increased reabsorption of filtered protein, which can contribute substantially to renal interstitial injury by activating intracellular events, including up-regulation of vasoactive and inflammatory genes.[30] The process at first is helpful to the patient with renal failure, but ultimately it is detrimental.[30] The degree of proteinuria may be involved in the progressive glomerulosclerosis, which occurs in chronic renal failure.[39] In large animals, as in other species, the degree of proteinuria and the type and degree of the initial insult may be directly associated with the speed at which the disease progresses. Chronic renal failure in large animals usually is the result of progressive glomerular disease that may be immunologically mediated or of tubulointerstitial disease caused by unreversed or progressive nephrotoxic, hemodynamic, obstructive, or septic causes.[45] Chronic renal failure may also have a congenital cause, such as renal dysplasia or polycystic renal disease[46] (Fig. 10-5).

The diagnosis of renal failure is based on the history, physical examination, and laboratory findings of azotemia with isosthenuria (Boxes 10-7 and 10-8). With chronic renal failure the urine specific gravity usually is in the isosthenuric range (1.008 to 1.014).[45] If the serum creatinine is only in the high normal range, other tests may be used to estimate the GFR. These include endogenous 24-hour urinary creatinine clearance[47] and blood clearance of ^{99m}technetium (^{99m}Tc)-labeled diethylenetriamine penta-acetic acid (DPTA).[48] The 24-hour urinary creatinine clearance test is easily performed on male horses with a normal value of 1.877 ± 0.45 ml/min/kg, but it is more difficult with females.[47] Furthermore, urinary creatinine clearance is more variable than plasma creatinine and is often a less reliable guide to GFR than plasma creatinine.[49] ^{99m}Tc-DTPA is a vascular agent that quickly equilibrates with the extracellular fluid space. It accumulates in the kidney by glomerular filtration with no tubular absorption or secretion.[48] The ^{99m}Tc-DTPA clearance test can be easily performed on both male and female horses using 4 to 6 MCi for injec-

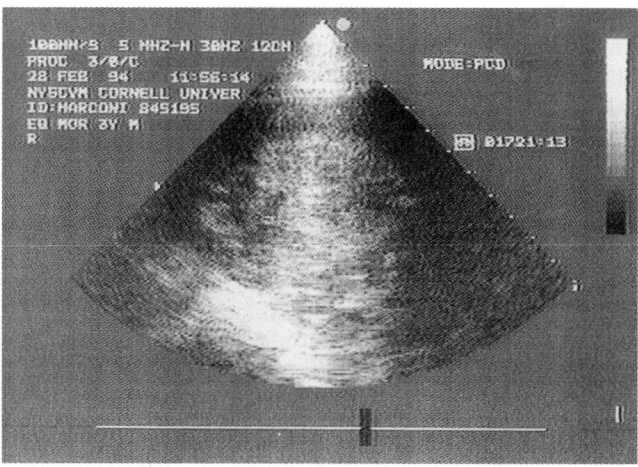

FIG. 10-6 ▓ Sonogram (5 MHz) of the right kidney of a 3-year-old Morgan stallion with chronic interstitial fibrosis and renal failure.

BOX 10-7

Causes of Chronic Renal Failure in the Horse

TUBULOINTERSTITIAL CAUSES
Any of the vascular, septic, or toxic causes of acute renal failure
Chronic or intermittent obstruction (especially of the ureters)
Chronic pyelonephritis
Granulomatous infiltration
Neoplasia
Nonsteroidal antiinflammatory–induced papillary necrosis
Renal dysplasia
Polycystic disease

GLOMERULAR CAUSES
Renal hypoplasia
Amyloidosis
Glomerulosclerosis (unknown cause)
Glomerulonephritis (immune mediated)

BOX 10-8

Causes of Chronic Renal Failure in Ruminants

TUBULOINTERSTITIAL CAUSES
Any of the vascular, toxic, or septic causes of acute renal failure
Chronic obstruction (urolithiasis)
Chronic pyelonephritis

GLOMERULAR CAUSES
Glomerulonephritis (rare) except for Finnish Landrace lambs
Amyloidosis

---

tion, with samples collected from the opposite jugular vein at 5, 15, 30, 45, 60, 90, 120 and 180 minutes.[50] The published values for GFR using this technique are 1.79 ml/min/kg and 1.47 ml/min/kg with a standard deviation of ± 0.49 and ± 0.27, respectively.[48,50,51] Ultrasound examination of the kidneys is most useful in chronic renal failure because cysts showing increased echogenicity (e.g., fibrotic cysts) (Fig. 10-6), nephroliths, or both may accompany this condition. Smaller than normal kidney size and inability to distinguish normal renal architecture are common findings with CRF. Biopsy would be useful in confirming the fibrosis and in some cases may provide helpful information on causative factors.[52]

POLYURIA

Polyuria can be defined as the passage of abnormally large amounts of urine. This may be a normal response when excessive fluid, electrolytes, or both are presented to the tubules of a healthy kidney. It may also occur with renal failure when tubular function is impaired or when enough individual nephrons have been lost that the remaining ones are presented with excess fluid and/or solute. Polyuria is also present in central or neurogenic diabetes insipidus (caused by insufficient secretion of antidiuretic hormone [ADH]), nephrogenic diabetes insipidus (caused by diminished effect of ADH on receptors in the kidney), renal medullary washout (caused by an insufficient interstitial concentration gradient), excessive drinking (polydipsia), pyelitis, liver failure, fluid administration, and certain electrolyte abnormalities; and it may occur after urinary tract obstructions have been relieved.

Evaluation of an animal with polyuria should begin with an inquiry about any history of recent disease, drug administration, or known laboratory evidence of renal disease (Box 10-9). After completion of the history and a review of the patient's medical records, the initial diagnostic step is to collect a urine sample to measure the osmolality or specific gravity (UspG). If the osmolality is close to the isosthenuric range and the concentration remains similar to the plasma concentration regardless of the patient's fluid volume status (UspG of 1.008 to 1.014), primary renal disease should be considered as a cause of the polyuria. Determination of the GFR would be indicated. If the basic measurements of the GFR (e.g., serum creatinine, radionuclide clearance studies and/or 12- or 24-hour urinary creatinine clearance) are not abnormal, a water deprivation test may be needed to determine the tubules' ability to concentrate urine. This test should be performed with caution, because prerenal factors that will develop may exacerbate a preexisting renal disease.

As an alternative to the water deprivation test in identifying tubular disease and dysfunction as the cause of polyuria, the fractional excretion of sodium in the urine can be measured. This test is performed on simultaneously collected urine and serum samples by measuring the creatinine and sodium in both the serum and the urine. The fractional excretion $F_{ex}\%$ of sodium is then determined by the formula

$$F_{ex}\% = \frac{[Na_u]}{[Na_p]} \div \frac{[Cr_u]}{[Cr_p]} \times 100$$

where Na_u is the urine sodium concentration, Na_p is the plasma creatinine concentration, Cr_u is the urine creatinine concentration, and Cr_p is the plasma creatinine concentration. A fractional sodium excretion value above 1% in adult large animals is highly suggestive of primary tubular disease or sodium toxicity.[53,54]

If the UspG or osmolality is less than that of the plasma (approximately 1.007), diabetes insipidus, polydipsia, and renal medullary washout should be considered. Diabetes insipidus, although rare, has been reported in the horse and may be the result of inadequate secretion of vasopressin (neurogenic diabetes insipidus) or inadequate response to vasopressin in the kidney (nephrogenic diabetes insipidus).[55] Inappropriate response to vasopressin in the kidney may be a result of receptor abnormalities or improper interstitial fluid concentration, which may occur with abnormally low concentrations of chloride, urea, or potassium. Foals occa-

---

BOX 10-9

Causes of Polyuria in Horses and Food Animals*

Acute renal failure
Chronic renal failure
Pyelitis
Hyperglycemia
Diabetes mellitus
Psychogenic water intoxication (horses)
Steroid administration
Cushing's disease
Fluid administration
Diuretic administration
Salt deficiency
Salt toxicity
Diabetes insipidus
Severe deficiencies of chloride, potassium, or urea

---

*Foals and lactating dairy cattle normally have a very low urine specific gravity, which is not considered polyuria.

sionally may have inappropriately high vasopressin responses, resulting in hyponatremia.

URACHAL LEAKAGE OF URINE

The clinical signs of incomplete urachal closure in newborn animals are visible dripping of urine from the ventral abdomen, swelling of the umbilical area, or both. Signs are normally noted soon after birth but may occur at any time during the first several weeks of life. The primary diagnostic approach to urachal disease in newborn animals is to determine if the improper closure is due to a septic, inflammatory disease or a less serious incomplete closure. If incomplete closure first develops after the animal is several days of age, infection of the urachus should be strongly considered. The determination of infection can usually be made by consideration of the history (i.e., inadequate colostrum administration and clinical findings of fever or pain, heat, or exudate at the site of the urachus). If findings indicate infection, percutaneous palpation and ultrasonography may determine the extent of the infection.[56] This determination is important in deciding between medical and surgical therapy. Surgical removal of a deep abscess of the urachus or umbilical vessels (or both) is often the treatment of choice. Pollakiuria and dysuria may occur in older foals and calves with a urachal abscess.[57,58]

CRYSTALLURIA

Crystalluria is defined as the presence of crystals in the urine. These may occur microscopically, in which case no clinical signs may be observed. However, they may be an indication of a more severe problem such as renal failure or urinary tract infection. Crystals may also form on the preputial hairs and may be seen grossly. If they are observed, the likelihood of a urinary tract infection or the possibility of obstruction, or both, should be considered. If the crystals congregate into a large mass in the urinary tract, they may obstruct the renal pelvis, the ureter, the urethral opening, or the urethra. Smaller, more microscopic formations may obstruct individual nephrons. If the obstruction affects the urethra, clinical signs are usually pronounced. Swelling at the site of the urethral blockage may be palpated in some cases or, if urethral rupture has occurred, gross swelling becomes obvious. Obstruction of the urethral opening at the neck of the bladder, commonly associated with larger stones or clusters of stones, usually results in abdominal discomfort, stranguria, hema-

turia, and dysuria. Rupture of the bladder with abdominal enlargement and uroperitoneum can occur from urethral obstruction or obstruction at the neck of the bladder. Intermittent or persistent obstruction of one ureter causes hydronephrosis and renal disease but may not produce any obvious clinical signs. If both ureters are persistently or intermittently obstructed, renal failure eventually develops. A clinical examination, including rectal and ultrasound examination, is valuable in determining the number of calculi, the location of the calculi, and other pathologic conditions of the urinary system.[18]

If crystalluria and pyuria are found in the same patient, crystalluria could be a predisposing cause of the urinary tract infection or it may be the result of the urinary tract infection. Affected animals may exhibit urine scalding in addition to pyuria, dysuria, and stranguria. Infections of the upper urinary tract often produce signs of systemic illness. The approach to urinary tract infections is discussed in the section on pyuria, p. 174-175.

The location of initial formation of the calculi is not clear in all cases; certainly some calculi originate in the renal tubules. Stone formation in the kidney may be predisposed by a local nidus such as tubular epithelial or renal crest sloughing. Abnormal secretion or solubility of electrolytes (e.g., calcium), or both, along with decreased urine flow, may be involved in the development of renal calculi. Changes in the pH of the urine may also affect the solubility of crystalloids. The effect that dietary imbalances may have on the formation of urinary calculi can be evaluated by determining the mineral content of the calculus and the ration composition and by consideration of fluid intake.[59]

The diagnostic approach to crystalluria is to determine why the crystalluria is present and whether an obstruction exists. If urinary obstruction is present, surgery is needed in most cases. With persistent or intermittent obstruction of the ureter or renal pelvis, chronic renal failure may already exist, which would most likely exclude any surgical correction.

DIAGNOSTIC VALUE OF URINE DIPSTICK EXAMINATION IN LARGE ANIMALS

A simple reagent strip "dipstick" urinalysis is often helpful in large animal practice. Reagent strip examination of the urine should be routinely used for sick cows because of the ease of urine collection. The pH of the urine in herbivores should be alkaline (over 7.4). An acidic pH suggests anorexia and hypokalemia or systemic acidosis (e.g., ruminal acidosis). However, acidic urine is not uncommon in volume-depleted, hypokalemic, hypochloremic cattle with systemic alkalosis (paradoxic aciduria).[60] A strong alkaline reaction in a depressed, anorexic and acidotic horse should arouse the suspicion of renal tubular acidosis.[61] Horses with type II renal tubular acidosis (RTA) have low fractional excretion of potassium and normal fractional excretion of sodium, whereas horses with type I RTA have high fractional excretion of sodium and normal fractional excretion of potassium.[62]

The urine protein reading is most commonly a trace amount to +1 in herbivores because of the alkaline pH. A strong urine protein reaction indicates severe glomerular protein leakage or, more commonly, hemorrhage, hemolysis, or myoglobinuria. The degree of proteinuria may have to be further evaluated by quantitative laboratory testing and determining urinary protein/creatinine ratio because some large animals have a strong reaction to the dipstick, but quantitative determination is normal. A positive blood reaction can occur with hemoglobinuria, myoglobinuria, hematuria, or contamination of the urine with reproductive or fecal blood. The test result is often positive with acute renal failure in large animals. A positive ketone reaction is rare in the horse but may occur with hyperlipidemia. In dairy cattle a strong reaction suggests primary ketosis, whereas a weaker reaction reflects secondary ketosis, such as is commonly seen with abomasal displacement. A positive reaction for bilirubin is rare in cattle; in horses it usually indicates liver disease, although false-positive results do occur. The urobilinogen reaction has little practical use in large animals.

Glycosuria can occur with stress (especially in horses), previous glucose therapy, Cushing's disease, rabies, enterotoxemia, renal disease, and a variety of metabolic disturbances (e.g., diabetes mellitus, hyperammonemia) or from xylazine administration in cattle. Extremely high readings may be found in very sick cattle just before death.

REFERENCES

1. Schumacher J et al: Urethral defects in geldings with hematuria and stallions with hemospermia, *Vet Surg* 24:250-254, 1995.
2. Richardson DW, Kohn CW: Uroperitoneum in the foal, *J Am Vet Med Assoc* 182:267-271, 1983.
3. Sockett D, Knight AP: Metabolic changes associated with obstructive urolithiasis in cattle, *Compend Cont Educ* 6:S311-S315, 1984.
4. VanMetre DC, Smith BP: Clinical management of urolithiasis in small ruminants, *Proceedings of the Ninth Annual Forum, American College of Veterinary Internal Medicine*, New Orleans, 1991.
5. Holt PE, Mair TS: Ten cases of bladder paralysis associated with sabulous urolithiasis in horses, *Vet Rec* 127:108-110, 1990.
6. Clarke ES et al: Cystometrography and urethral pressure profiles in healthy horses and pony mares, *Am J Vet Res* 58:552-555, 1987.
7. Kay AD, Lavoie FP: Urethral pressure profilometry in mares, *J Am Vet Med Assoc* 191:212-216, 1987.
8. Ronen N: Measurement of urethral pressure profiles in the male horse, *Equine Vet J* 26:55-59, 1994.
9. Madison JB: Estrogen-responsive urinary incontinence in an aged pony mare, *Compend Cont Educ* 6:S390-S392, 1984.
10. Stamm WE: Measurement of pyuria and its relation to bacteriuria, *Am J Med* 28:53-58, 1983.
11. MacLeay JM, Kohn CW: Results of quantitative cultures of urine by free catch and catheterization from healthy adult horses, *J Vet Intern Med* 12:76-78, 1998.
12. Sullins KE, Traub-Dargatz JL: Endoscopic anatomy of the equine urinary tract, *Compend Cont Educ (Pract Vet)* 6:S663-668, 1984.
13. Johnson PJ, Ganjam VK: Laminitis, hypothyroidism and obesity: a peripheral cushingoid syndrome in horses? *Proceedings of the Seventeenth Annual American College of Veterinary Medicine Forum*, Chicago, 1999.
14. Lloyd KC et al: Ulceration in the proximal portion of the urethra as a cause of hematuria in horses: four cases (1978-1985), *J Am Vet Med Assoc* 194:1324-1326, 1989.
15. Coffman JR: *Equine clinical pathology and pathophysiology*, Bonner Springs, Kan, 1981, Veterinary Medicine Publishing.
16. Jose-Cunilleras E, Hinchcliff KW: Renal pharmacology, *Vet Clin North Am* 15:647-659, 1999.
17. Divers TJ, Byars TD, Shin SJ: Renal dysfunction associated with infection of *Leptospira interrogans* in a horse, *J Am Vet Med Assoc* 201:1391-1392, 1992.
18. Ehnen SJ et al: Obstructive nephrolithiasis and ureterolithiasis associated with chronic renal failure in horses, *J Am Vet Med Assoc* 197:249-253, 1990.
19. Woolridge AA et al: Chronic renal failure associated with nephrolithiasis, ureterolithiasis, and renal dysplasia in a 2-year-old quarter horse gelding, *Vet Radiol Ultrasound* 40:361-364, 1999.
20. Divers TJ, Reef VB, Roby KA: Nephrolithiasis resulting in intermittent ureteral obstruction in a cow, *Cornell Vet* 2:143-149, 1989.
21. Braun U: Ultrasonographic examination of the right kidneys in cows, *Am J Vet Res* 52:1933-1939, 1991.
22. Ringoir S, VanHolder R, Massey SG: *Uremic toxins*, New York, 1986, Plenum Press.
23. Tanaka A et al: Plasma, urinary, and erythrocyte concentrations of guanidino compounds in patients with chronic renal failure, *Ren Fail* 21:499-514, 1999.
24. Bouchard PR et al: Uremic encephalopathy in a horse, *Vet Pathol* 31:111-115, 1994.
25. Summers BA, Smith CA: Renal encephalopathy in a cow, *Cornell Vet* 75:524-530, 1985.
26. Cotran RS, Kumar V, Collins T: The kidney. In Cotran RS, Kumar V, Collins T, eds: *Robbins' pathologic basis of disease*, ed 4, Philadelphia, 1989, WB Saunders.
27. Boothe DM: Prostaglandins: physiology and clinical implications, *Compend Cont Educ (Pract Vet)* 6:1010-1020, 1984.
28. Assael BM et al: Prostaglandins and aminoglycoside nephrotoxicity, *Toxicol Appl Pharmacol* 78:386-394, 1985.
29. Hinchcliff KW, Shaftoe S, Dubielzig RR: Gentamicin-induced nephrotoxicosis in a cow, *J Am Vet Med Assoc* 192:923-925, 1988.
30. Remuzzi G, Bertani T: Pathophysiology of progressive nephropathies, *N Engl J Med* 339:1448-1455, 1998.
31. Divers TJ et al: Acute renal failure in six horses resulting from hemodynamic causes, *Equine Vet J* 19:178-183, 1987.
32. Guignard J-P et al: Acute renal failure, *Crit Care Med* 21:S349-S351, 1993.
33. Messmer UK, Briner VA, Pfeilschifter J: Tumor necrosis factor-alpha and lipopolysaccharide induce apoptotic cell death in bovine glomerular endothelial cells, *Kidney Int* 55:2322-2337, 1999.
34. Tannere GA: Nephron obstruction and tubuloglomerular feedback, *Kidney Int* 22:213-228, 1982.
35. Houghton DC et al: Chronic gentamicin nephrotoxicity: continued tubular injury with preserved glomerular filtration function, *Am J Pathol* 123:183-194, 1986.
36. Divers TJ et al: Acute renal disorders in cattle: a retrospective study of 22 cases, *J Am Vet Med Assoc* 181:694-699, 1982.
37. Holdstock NB, Ousey JC, Rossdale PD: Glomerular filtration rate, effective renal plasma flow, blood pressure, and pulse rate in the equine neonate during the first 10 days postpartum, *Equine Vet J* 30:335-343, 1998.
38. Drukker A: The progression of chronic renal disease: immunological, nutritional, and intrinsic renal mechanisms, *Isr J Med Sci* 33:739-743, 1997.
39. Cappeli P et al: Lipids in the progression of chronic renal failure, *Nephron* 62:31-35, 1992.
40. Klahr S, Schraner G, Ichikawa I: The progression of renal disease, *N Engl J Med* 318:1657-1666, 1988.
41. Johnston CI et al: Mechanism of progression of renal disease: current hemodynamic concepts, *J Hypertens Suppl* 16:S3-S7, 1998.
42. Savin M: Chronic renal insufficiency: (1) adaptation of nephron function in chronic renal insufficiency and (2) progression of chronic renal insufficiency, *Srp Arh Celok Lek* 126:261-270, 1998.
43. Baud L, Fouqueray B, Bellocq A: Inflammatory mechanisms of renal fibrosis: glomerulonephritis, *Bull Acad Natl Med* 183:23-31, 1999.
44. Vleming LJ, Bruijn JA, van Es LA: The pathogenesis of progressive renal failure, *Neth J Med* 54:114-128, 1999.
45. Divers TJ: Chronic renal failure in horses, *Compend Cont Educ* 5:S310-S317, 1983.
46. Ramierz S et al: Ultrasound-assisted diagnosis of renal dysplasia in a 3-month-old quarter horse colt. *Vet Radiol Ultrasound* 39:143-146, 1998.
47. Morris DD, Divers TJ, Whitlock RH: Renal clearance and fractional excretion of electrolytes over a 24-hour period, *Am J Vet Res* 45:2431-2436, 1984.
48. Matthews HK et al: Comparison of standard and radionuclide methods for measurement of glomerular filtration rate and effective renal blood flow in female horses, *Am J Vet Res* 53:1612-1616, 1992.
49. Walser M: Assessing renal function from creatinine measurements in adults with chronic renal failure, *Am J Kidney Dis* 32:23-31, 1998.
50. Daniel GB et al: Renal nuclear medicine: a review, *Vet Radiol Ultrasound* 40:572-587, 1999.
51. Walsh DM, Royal HD: Evaluation of a single injection of ^{99m}Tc-labeled diethylenetriaminepentaacetic acid for measuring glomerular filtration rate in horses, *Am J Vet Res* 53:776-780, 1992.
52. Divers TJ: Assessment of the urinary system, *Vet Clin North Am (Food Am Pract)* 8:373-382, 1992.
53. Olson WG et al: Assessment of sodium deficiency and polyuria/polydipsia in dairy cows, *Bov Pract* 24:126-133, 1989.
54. Grossman BS et al: Urinary indices for differentiation of prerenal azotemia and renal azotemia in horses, *J Am Vet Med Assoc* 180:284-288, 1982.
55. Schott HC II et al: Nephrogenic diabetes insipidus in sibling colts, *J Vet Intern Med* 7:68-72, 1993.
56. Reef VB et al: Clinical, ultrasonographic, and surgical findings in foals with umbilical remnant infections, *J Am Vet Med Assoc* 195:69-72, 1989.
57. Trent AM, Smith DF: Pollakiuria due to urachal abscesses in two heifers, *J Am Vet Med Assoc* 184:984-986, 1984.
58. Dean PW, Robertson JT: Urachal remnant as a cause of pollakiuria and dysuria in a filly, *J Am Vet Med Assoc* 192:375-376, 1988.
59. Petersson KH et al: Influence of magnesium, water, and sodium chloride on urolithiasis in veal calves, *J Dairy Sci* 71:3369-3377, 1988.
60. Gingerich DA, Murdick PW: Paradoxic aciduria in bovine metabolic alkalosis, *J Am Vet Med Assoc* 166:227, 1975.
61. Ziemer EL et al: Clinical features of treatment of renal tubular acidosis in two horses, *J Am Vet Med Assoc* 190:294-296, 1987.
62. MacLeay JM, Wilson JH: Type II renal tubular acidosis and ventricular tachycardia in a horse, *J Am Vet Med Assoc* 212:1597-1599, 1988.

Alterations in the Skin

STEPHEN D. WHITE

ANNE G. EVANS

MAJOR CLINICAL SIGNS/PROBLEMS ENCOUNTERED

GENERAL APPROACH TO DIAGNOSIS OF DISEASES THAT CAUSE CHANGES IN THE SKIN

Dermatologic diseases are often a frustrating aspect of large animal practice because skin problems arising from different causes may have a similar clinical appearance (Tables 11-1 and 11-2). To manage skin problems successfully, the practitioner must use a systematic approach to arrive at an accurate diagnosis by obtaining a complete history, performing a thorough physical examination and, when appropriate, using one or more simple diagnostic techniques.[1] The following sections discuss the materials and methods necessary to perform techniques commonly used to diagnose large animal skin disease.

History

To obtain a meaningful differential diagnosis, all the questions listed on the sample history form (Fig. 11-1) should be answered. Often it is helpful to repeat the questions to the owners at a later time or to give them a history form to complete at their leisure, which allows greater opportunity to remember details relevant to the skin disease. The goals should be to determine the initial features of the skin disease, how the problem has progressed, and what factors have influenced its progression to the present state.

Physical Examination

The diagrams and terms listed on the sample form (Fig. 11-2) may serve as a useful guide for recording the physical find-

ings. First, the animal's overall condition should be assessed. A general physical examination should be performed to determine if the disease process is limited to the skin or if systemic signs of disease are also present. Attention next should be focused on the skin and hair coat. The distribution of the lesions should be noted, as well as any particular body areas that are affected. The size and morphology of the individual lesions should be characterized; that is, whether all the lesions have the same morphology or several different types are present (e.g., papules, nodules, wheals, patches of alopecia). The mucous membranes should be examined and the skin surface palpated to determine features not readily noted visually (e.g., crusts beneath the hair, dryness, ability to epilate hairs, presence of peripheral lymphadenopathy).

The practitioner's goal should be to describe accurately the animal's clinical appearance to someone who has never seen it and, more important, to provide a written record for future reference.

Diagnostic Techniques

For most of the techniques that follow, a good-quality microscope equipped with ×4, ×10, ×40, and ×100 objectives is recommended.

SKIN SCRAPINGS. Skin scrapings are used primarily to demonstrate microscopic ectoparasites, specifically mites. Scraping is a quick, simple, inexpensive diagnostic technique that is more useful in ruminants than horses because equine mite infestations are relatively uncommon. The materials needed to perform a skin scraping are a sterile container, mineral oil, a No. 10 scalpel blade, glass slides, and coverslips. If

Text continued on p. 194

Table 11-1

Disorders that Cause Clinical Signs of Skin Disease in the Horse

Disorder	Clinical Sign								
	Pruritus*†	Nodules, Tumors, Swellings*†	Ulcerations and Erosions†	Papules, Pustules, Vesicles†	Scaling and Crusting†	Abnormal Coat Length/ Density	Abnormal Pigmentation	Can Be Associated With Systemic Disease	Exotic
Nutritional									
Protein-calorie starvation					+	∨		†	
Endocrine									
Hyperadrenocorticism	+				+	∧		+	
Autoimmune									
Pemphigus foliaceus			+	†	†	∨			
Bullous pemphigoid			+	+					
Hypersensitivities									
Urticaria (hives)	+	†			+				
Anaphylaxis	+	+							
Vasculitis			†		†	∨		+	
Dietary hypersensitivity	+				+			+	
Drug eruption	+	+	+	+	+			+	
Erythema multiforme	+	+		+	+			+	
Dermatographism		+							
Contact dermatitis									
Irritant (nonallergic)	+		†	†	†				
Allergic	+		+	+	+				
Bacterial									
Dermatophilosis (rain scald)	+		+		†	∨		+	
Cellulitis			+					+	
Ulcerative lymphangitis			+						
Corynebacterium pseudotuberculosis		†	+					+	
Corynebacterium equi (rare)		+	+					+	
Streptococcus spp. (rare)		†	+					+	
Strangles (*Streptococcus equi*)		+	+					†	
Botryomycosis (*Staphylococcus aureus*)		+	+						
Folliculitis/furunculosis									
Grease heal/scratches			+	+	†				
Staphylococcus organisms, coagulase positive		+	+	†	+				
C. pseudotuberculosis		+	+	+	+				
Staphylococcus organisms, coagulase negative		+	+	+	+				
Bacillus spp. (occasionally)		+	+	+	+				
C. equi (rare)		+	+	+	+				
Impetigo		+							
Nocardiosis		+							
Actinobacillosis									

From White ME, Lewkowicz JM: Consultant. Diagnosis/sign search package, Version 1.1 NYSCVM, Ithaca, NY, 1995, Cornell University.

+, Diseases manifesting the indicated symptom *some or all of the time*; >, increased coat length/density or pigmentation; <, decreased coat length/density or pigmentation; †, >, <, disorders most commonly diagnosed manifesting indicated symptom.

*Diseases associated with these signs may secondarily form ulcerations and erosions.

†Diseases associated with these signs may secondarily cause alopecia.

Continued

Table 11-1

Disorders that Cause Clinical Signs of Skin Disease in the Horse—cont'd

Disorder	Clinical Sign								
	Pruritus*†	Nodules, Tumors, Swellings*†	Ulcerations and Erosions†	Papules, Pustules, Vesicles†	Scaling and Crusting†	Abnormal Coat Length/Density	Abnormal Pigmentation	Can Be Associated With Systemic Disease	Exotic
Bacterial—cont'd									
Actinomycosis		+							
Fistulous withers/poll evil (*Brucella* spp. +/− *Actinomyces*)		+							
Tuberculosis		+	+					+	
Anthrax		+						+	+
Glanders (*Pseudomonas mallei*)		+						+	+
Melioidosis (*Pseudomonas pseudomallei*)		+						+	
Fungal									
Superficial									
Dermatophytosis	+	+		+		∨			
Piedra					+	∨			
Intermediate									
Sporotrichosis		+							
Aspergillosis		+							
Phycomycosis		+							
Phaeohyphomycosis		+							
Mycetoma		+							
Rhinosporidiosis		+							
Chromomycosis		+							
Maduromycosis		+							
Histoplasmosis (*Histoplasma farciminosus*)		+						+	+
Deep									
Coccidioidomycosis		+	+	+				+	
Blastomycosis (North American)		+	+	+				+	
Viral									
Papillomatosis		+		+					
Coital exanthema (EHV-3)				+					
Vesicular stomatitis				+				+	
Parasitic									
Pediculosis (lice)	+				+				
Acariases									
Trombiculidiasis	+			+	+				
Chorioptic mange	+			+	+				
Demodecitic mange	+			+	+	∨	∨		
Psoroptic mange	+			+	+				+
Sarcoptic mange	+			+	+				+

Pyemotes (straw itch mite)
Flying insects
  Culicoides hypersensitivity
  Stomoxys calcitrans (stable fly)
  Tabanidae
    Tabanus, Hybomitra spp. (horse fly)
    Chrysops sp. (deer fly)
  Simulidae spp. (blackflies, buffalo gnats)
  Lyperosia (Haematobia) irritans
  Musca spp.
  Mosquitos
  Bee/wasp stings
Oxyuris equi (pinworms)
Cutaneous onchocerciasis
Cutaneous habronemiasis
Hypoderma sp. (warbles)
Myiasis
Spider bites
Fleas
Ticks
Environmental
  Burns
    Thermal
    Chemical
    Frictional
  Ultraviolet
  Frostbite
  Photosensitization
Toxic
  Chemical toxicities
    Iodine
    Selenium (alkali disease)
    Thallium
    Trichlorethylene-extracted feed
    Pentachlorophenol
    Polybrominated biphenyl
    Chlorinated naphthalene
  Plant toxicities
    Pyrrolizidine alkaloid
    Hairy vetch
Neoplasia
  Tumors of epithelial origin
    Papillomas
    Squamous cell carcinoma
    Epidermoid cyst
    Dermoid cyst
    Basal cell carcinoma
    Adenoma/adenocarcinoma
  Tumors of mesenchymal origin
    Equine sarcoid
    Fibroma/fibrosarcoma
    Neuroma
    Schwannoma

From White ME, Lewkowicz JM: Consultant. Diagnosis/sign search package, Version 1.1 NYSCVM, Ithaca, NY, 1995, Cornell University.

Table 11-1

Disorders that Cause Clinical Signs of Skin Disease in the Horse—cont'd

Disorder	Pruritus*†	Nodules, Tumors, Swellings*†	Ulcerations and Erosions†	Papules, Pustules, Vesicles†	Scaling and Crusting†	Abnormal Coat Length/Density	Abnormal Pigmentation	Can Be Associated With Systemic Disease	Exotic
Neoplasia—cont'd									
Tumors of mesenchymal origin—cont'd									
Lipoma/liposarcoma		+							
Hemangioma		+							+
Round cell tumors									
Melanoma		†						∨	
Cutaneous lymphosarcoma		†						+	
Mastocytoma		†							
Histiocytoma		+							
Genetic/congenital defects									
Black hair follicle dystrophy							∨		
Nevi		+							
Temporal teratoma (dentigerous cyst)		+							
Epitheliogenesis imperfecta			+					∨	+
Hyperelastosis cutis			+					∨	
Arabian fading syndrome									
Albinism									
Diseases of uncertain etiology									
Nodular necrobiosis		†						∨	
Aural plaques		+			†				
Cutaneous amyloidosis		+		+			∨		+
Generalized granulomatous disease		+		+	†				†

Anhidrosis (dry coat)
Seborrhea, primary
Mane and tail
Cannon keratosis
Linear keratosis
Generalized
Variegated, reticulated leukotrichia
Vitiligo (equine leukoderma)
Hyperesthetic leukotrichia
Unilateral papular equine dermatitis
Alopecia areata
Angioneurotic, idiopathic edema
Other
Hematoma/seroma
Exuberant granulation tissue
Subcutaneous foreign body
Trauma
Excoriations
Lacerations
Mechanical abrasions
Pressure necrosis (sores, galls)
Bursitis of the elbow (capped elbow)
Calcaneal bursitis (capped hock)
Calcinosis circumscripta
Scarring, postinflammatory
Telogen effluvium

From White ME, Lewkowicz JM: Consultant. Diagnosis/sign search package, Version 1.1 NYSCVM, Ithaca, NY, 1995, Cornell University.

Table 11-2

Disorders that Cause Clinical Signs of Skin Disease in Ruminants

Disorder	Pruritus*†	Nodules, Tumors, Swellings*†	Ulcerations and Erosions†	Papules, Pustules, Vesicles†	Scaling and Crusting†	Abnormal Coat Length/Density	Abnormal Pigmentation	Can Be Associated With Systemic Disease	Exotic
Nutritional									
Protein-calorie starvation					+	✓		+	
Zinc deficiency					+	✓		+	
Copper deficiency					+	✓	✓	+	
Iodine deficiency						✓		+	
Vitamin A deficiency					+	✓		+	
Vitamin E/selenium deficiency						✓		+	
Vitamin C–responsive dermatosis (B)						✓		+	
Autoimmune									
Pemphigus foliaceus (C)	+		+	+	+				
Hypersensitivities									
Urticaria (hives)	+	+			+			+	
Anaphylaxis	+	+						+	
Milk allergy (B)	+	+						+	
Drug eruption	+	+	+	+	+	✓			
Contact dermatitis									
Irritant (nonallergic)	+		+	+	+				
Allergic	+		+	+	+				
Bacterial									
Dermatophilosis (rain scald)	+		+		+	✓			
Foot rot			+						
Ulcerative posthitis/vulvitis			+		+				
Impetigo			+	+	+				
Mammary pustular dermatitis				+					
Staphylococcal (B)			+	+	+				
Actinobacillosis (O)			+	+	+				
Folliculitis/furunculosis									
Pseudomonas spp.		+	+	+	+				
Staphylococcus spp.		+	+	+	+				
Corynebacterium spp.		+	+	+	+				
Caseous lymphadenitis		+						+	
Corynebacterium pseudotuberculosis, C. ovis (O,C)									
Ulcerative lymphangitis		+							
C. pseudotuberculosis (B)								+	
Cellulitis (*Clostridia* spp.)			+						
Abscesses (*C. pseudotuberculosis*)		+	+						
Botryomycosis (*Pseudomonas* spp.) (B)		+							
Actinobacillosis		+						+	
Actinomycosis (B)		+	+						
Nocardiosis		+						+	
Tuberculosis								+	
Anthrax		+						+	
Bovine farcy (*Nocardia farcinica*)								+	+
Melioidosis (*Pseudomonas pseudomallei*)		+						+	+

Fungal
Superficial
Dermatophytosis
Candidiasis (B)
Tinea versicolor (C)
Intermediate
Sporotrichosis (B)
Phycomycosis
Phaeohyphomycosis (B)
Mycetoma
Rhinosporidiosis (B)
Chromomycosis (B)
Maduromycosis
Systemic
Aspergillosis (B)

Viral
Contagious ecthema (Orf) (O,C)
Fibropapillomatosis and papillomatosis
Pseudorabies
Scrapie (O,C)
Pseudocowpox (B)
Ulcerative dermatosis (O)
Infectious bovine rhinotracheitis (B)
Bovine herpes mammillitis (BHV-2) (B)
Mammary pustular dermatitis (BHV-3)
Caprine herpes virus (C)
Bovine virus diarrhea (B)
Bluetongue
Bovine papular stomatitis (B)
Vesicular stomatitis (B)
Malignant catarrhal fever (B)
Foot and mouth disease
Cowpox (B)
Lumpy skin disease (Knopvelsiekte) (B)
Pseudolumpy skin disease (B)

Parasitic
Pediculosis (lice)
Hypoderma sp. (warbles)
Acariases
Chorioptic mange
Psoroptic mange
Trombiculidiasis
Demodectic mange
Sarcoptic mange
Psorergatic mange (B,O)
Pyemotes (straw itch mite)

Continued

From White ME, Lewkowicz JM: Consultant. Diagnosis/sign search package, Version 1.1. NYSCVM, Ithaca, NY, 1995, Cornell University.
B, Bovine; *C*, caprine; *O*, ovine.
+, Diseases manifesting the indicated symptom *some or all of the time*; >, increased coat length/density or pigmentation; <, decreased coat length/density or pigmentation; †, >, <, disorders most commonly diagnosed manifesting indicated symptom.
*Diseases associated with these signs may secondarily form ulcerations and erosions.
†Diseases associated with these signs may secondarily cause alopecia.

Table 11-2

Disorders that Cause Clinical Signs of Skin Disease in Ruminants—cont'd

Disorder	Pruritus*†	Nodules, Tumors, Swellings*†	Ulcerations and Erosions†	Papules, Pustules, Vesicles†	Scaling and Crusting†	Abnormal Coat Length/Density	Abnormal Pigmentation	Can Be Associated With Systemic Disease	Exotic
Parasitic—cont'd									
Flying insects									
Musca spp.	+		+	+	+				
Lyperosia (Haematobia) irritans	+		+	+	+				
Stomoxys calcitrans (stable fly)	+		+	+	+				
Tabanidae									
Tabanus, Hybomitra spp. (horsefly)	+		+	+	+				
Chrysops sp. (deer fly)	+		+	+	+				
Culicoides hypersensitivity	+								
Simulidae (blackflies, buffalo gnats)	+		+	+	+				
Hydrotaea irritans (O)	+		+	+	+				+
Mosquitos	+			+	+				
Bee/wasp stings	+	+							
Malophagus ovinus (sheep keds) (O,C)	+		+	+	+				
Myiasis		+							
Fleas	+			+	+				
Ticks	+	+		+					
Stephanofilariasis (B)			+		+	V			
Elaeophorosis (O,C)			+		+	V			
Parelaphostrongylosis (O,C)			+			V			
Pelodera strongyloides			+		+	V			
Parafilaria bovicola (B)		+			+			+	+
Theileriasis (East Coast fever)		+						+	+
Environmental									
Burns									
Thermal			+	+	+				
Chemical			+	+	+				
Frictional			+		+				
Ultraviolet			+						
Frostbite			+		+			+	
Photosensitization		+	+	+	+	V		+	
Toxic									
Chemical toxicities									
Molybdenum				+		V	V	+	
Selenium				+		V		+	
Iodine					+			+	
Polybrominated biphenyl					+			+	
Chlorinated naphthalene								+	
Trichlorethylene-extracted feed								+	
Dicoumarol (warfarin)				+				+	
Thallium			+					+	
Plant toxicities									
Pyrrolizidine alkaloid					+	V		+	
Perennial broomweed					+	V		+	
Kochia scoparia				+				+	

Potato dermatitis
Ergotism
Fescue foot
Moldy sweet clover
Mycotoxic lupinosis
Neoplasia
Tumors of epithelial origin
Papillomas
Squamous cell carcinoma
Epidermal inclusion cysts (B,O)
Dermoid cysts (B,O)
Tumors of mesenchymal origin
Fibroma/fibrosarcoma
Neurofibroma (B)
Lipoma (B)
Hemangioma (B)
Round cell tumors
Melanoma (B)
Mastocytoma (B)
Cutaneous lymphosarcoma
Genetic/congenital defects
Wattles (C)
Nevi
Epitheliogenesis imperfecta
Hyperelastosis cutis (B,O)
Familial acantholysis (B)
Epidermolysis bullosa (B,O)
Congenital icthyosis (B)
Bovine inherited parakeratosis
Excessive cranial thymic tissue (C)
Congenital tumors
Congenital hypotrichosis
Border disease (hairy shaker) (O)
Hypertrichosis (European Friesians) (B)
Albinism (B)
Oculocutaneous hypopigmentation (angus)
Chediak-Higashi syndrome (B)
Other
Trauma
Excoriations
Lacerations
Mechanical abrasions
Scarring, postinflammatory
Pressure necrosis
Hematoma/seroma
Hygroma (callus, bursitis)
Sterile eosinophilic folliculitis (B)
Telogen effluvium
White liver disease (B,O)

From White ME, Lewkowicz JM: Consultant. Diagnosis/sign search package, Version 1.1. NYSCVM, Ithaca, NY, 1995, Cornell University.

DERMATOLOGY HISTORY FORM

Owner_____Date_____

Animal's name_____Case #_____

Age of animal_____

Age when purchased_____Age when skin problem started_____

Where on the body did the problem start?_____

What did the skin problem look like initially?_____

How has it spread or changed?_____

What season did the problem start?_____

Is the problem seasonal or year round?_____

If seasonal, what seasons is the disease present?_____

Does the animal itch?_____If so, where?_____

Do any animals contacting the affected animal have skin problems?_____

Do any people in contact with the animal have skin problems?_____

Is fly control used?_____If so, describe_____

_____

Do any relatives of this animal have skin problems?_____If yes, explain_____

_____

List injectable, oral, or topical medications that have been used before and after onset of the disorder_____

_____

_____

Which medications were of benefit?_____

_____

Which medications aggravated the condition?_____

_____

Describe the environment where the animal is kept, including bedding_____

_____

_____

_____

What is the animal fed?_____

_____

Any additional information you feel is relevant to the skin disease_____

_____

_____

FIG. 11-1 ▦ Sample dermatologic history form.

DERMATOLOGY PHYSICAL EXAMINATION FORM

Date_____

Distribution of lesions:

_____

_____

_____

Primary lesions (circle):

Macule	Patch	Papule
Pustule	Vesicle	Bulla
Wheal	Nodule	Tumor

Secondary lesions (circle):

Scale	Erosion	Excoriation
Fissure	Ulcer	Lichenification
Erythema	Alopecia	Hyperpigmentation
Crust	Comedone	

Pruritus_____Epilation_____

Skin thickness_____Skin tone_____

Hair coat_____External parasites_____

Diagnostic workup:

Skin scrapings_____

KOH preparation_____

Dermatophyte culture_____

Acetate tape prep_____

Dermatophilus prep _____

Histopathology_____

Immunofluorescence_____

Microfilarial prep_____

Bacterial culture & sensitivity_____

Differential diagnosis:_____

Initial therapy:_____

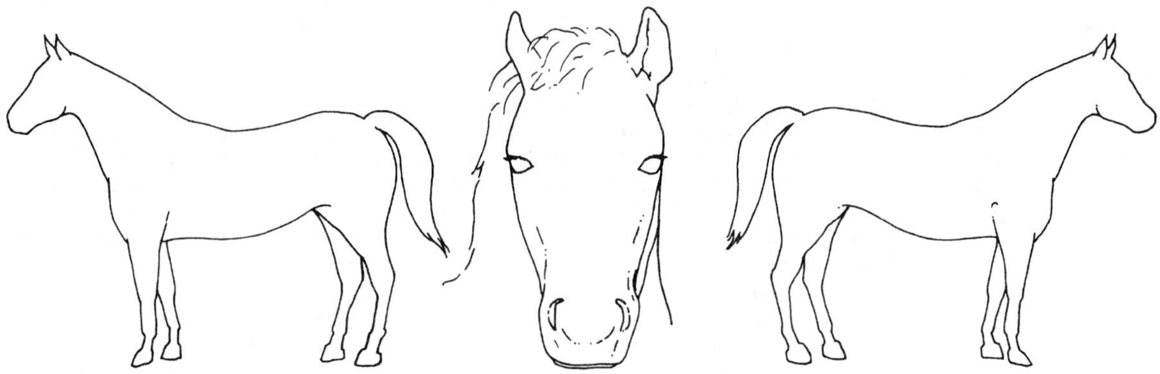

FIG. II-2 ▓ Sample dermatologic physical examination form.

the region to be sampled has hair (e.g., a fetlock), the hair should be lightly clipped before scraping. Multiple superficial scrapings that cover large surface areas should be performed, as well as several scrapings covering a small area that are deep enough to create capillary oozing. The collected material should be placed in a container until it can be examined microscopically. Some of the sample can then be placed on a glass slide and finely dispersed in enough mineral oil to provide a confluent layer without air bubbles beneath a coverslip. The slide should be scanned systematically with the ×10 objective. If something of significance is noted, the ×40 objective can be used to examine the specimen in more detail.

DERMATOPHYTE CULTURE. The materials necessary to perform a dermatophyte culture include dermatophyte test medium, 70% isopropyl alcohol, mosquito forceps, a No. 10 scalpel blade, and sterile empty containers such as evacuated blood collection tubes. The forceps and each lesion to be sampled should be wiped gently with isopropyl alcohol to remove as many bacterial and saprophytic contaminants as possible and allowed to dry. Multiple small, scaling, and lightly crusted lesions should be sampled; the samples should be stored in individual containers until they can be cultured and then preferably should be plated separately. Broken hairs, scales, and crusts from the periphery of the lesions are collected (because dermatophytes cause peripherally expanding lesions). A blade may be useful for scraping scales and debris from the skin surface. The forceps are used to pluck broken hairs.

The samples should be removed from the containers with a sterile forceps in a clean working area and gently pressed onto, but not buried beneath, the culture medium. The top of the culture dish or vial should be loosely replaced to allow sufficient ventilation for the culture to grow. Most dermatophytes grow at room temperature, except for some strains of *Tricophyton verrucosum*, which requires incubation at 37° C (98.6° F). The colony usually first appears in 5 to 7 days, although all cultures should be allowed to incubate for 3 weeks before a negative result is declared.

Dermatophyte test medium is an amber-colored Sabouraud's dextrose agar containing phenol red, a pH indicator, and several antibacterial and antifungal agents to inhibit growth of contaminant organisms. Dermatophytes preferentially use the protein in the medium as they begin to grow, producing alkaline metabolites that cause the medium to turn red. The dermatophyte colony is typically a white to beige, powdery to fluffy growth; the colonies are never dark colored. Most saprophytic (contaminant) fungi metabolize the carbohydrates first, producing acidic metabolites that do not change the color of the medium. It should be stressed that after the carbohydrate source has been depleted, saprophytes use the proteins and produce a red color change.

Positive identification of a dermatophyte would be made in most instances if a white to beige, powdery to fluffy colony began to appear on the medium at the same time or within 24 hours of the appearance of a red color change in the medium (Fig. 11-3). An infrequently encountered exception to this rule is growth of the saprophyte *Scopulariopsis brevicaulis*, a tan to light brown, smooth or mealy colony that produces a concurrent red color change in the medium. A dermatophyte could be ruled out under the following circumstances of culture growth: (1) growth of either a light- or dark-colored colony without a concurrent red color change in the medium, (2) growth of a black- or green-colored colony despite a concurrent red color change in the medium, or (3) growth of a mucoid colony despite a concurrent red color change in the medium.

It is essential to check the cultures daily to determine if the red color change and colony growth occur nearly simultaneously. The presence of a light-colored colony on an entirely red medium could be a saprophyte that has grown long

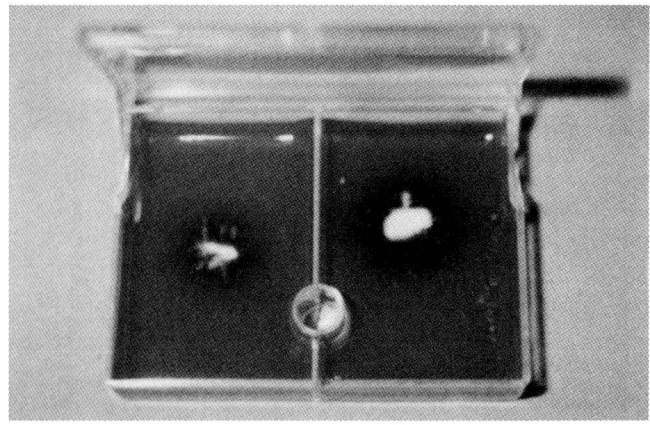

FIG. 11-3 ■ Positive result on dermatophyte culture. Growth of light-colored colony and simultaneous red color change are shown on dermatophyte test medium (right half of culture plate). Growth of dermatophyte on rapid-sporulating medium is shown on left half of culture plate.

enough to deplete the carbohydrate source and begun to use the proteins. If any doubt exists about the type of colony growth, the sample should be submitted to a diagnostic laboratory for specific identification.

POTASSIUM HYDROXIDE (KOH) PREPARATION. A potassium hydroxide (KOH) preparation may permit immediate diagnosis of dermatophytosis, but it takes practice to recognize the diagnostic features of a positive result with a KOH preparation, and a negative result does not rule out a diagnosis of dermatophytosis. If a KOH preparation yields a negative result, a dermatophyte culture still should be performed to obtain a definitive diagnosis.

The materials necessary to perform a KOH preparation include mosquito forceps, a No. 10 scalpel blade, a sterile empty container, glass microscope slides, coverslips, a Bunsen burner, and clearing solution. As with a dermatophyte culture, it is important to sample several lesions to increase the chances of obtaining a diagnostic sample. Hairs and scales are collected from the periphery of the lesions with the mosquito forceps and the scalpel blade. The samples are stored in the sterile container until a microscopic examination can be performed. A drop of the clearing solution is placed on a glass slide, hairs and scales are added to the solution, and a coverslip is placed over the material. The slide should be scanned systematically with the ×10 objective for abnormal-appearing hairs with a fuzzy internal structure. If these features are noted, a higher powered objective should be used for more detailed examination. A positive result with a KOH preparation demonstrates hyphae, which usually are uniform in width and septate. Beadlike chains of arthroconidia may be seen as well (Fig. 11-4).

The purpose of the clearing solution is to dissolve the hard keratin and bleach the melanin of the hair shaft so that the fungal hyphae and arthroconidia can be identified more readily. Care should be taken not to spill any clearing solution on the microscope because it can damage the lenses. Several types of clearing solutions are available. If 15% KOH is used, the slide should be heated for 15 to 20 seconds to facilitate clearing before examination. As an alternative, the preparation can be allowed to stand at room temperature for 30 minutes before viewing. A quicker method of clearing involves using a KOH–dimethyl sulfoxide (DMSO) solution*

---

*Dermassay Clearing Solution, Pitman Moore, Washington Crossing, NJ 97882.

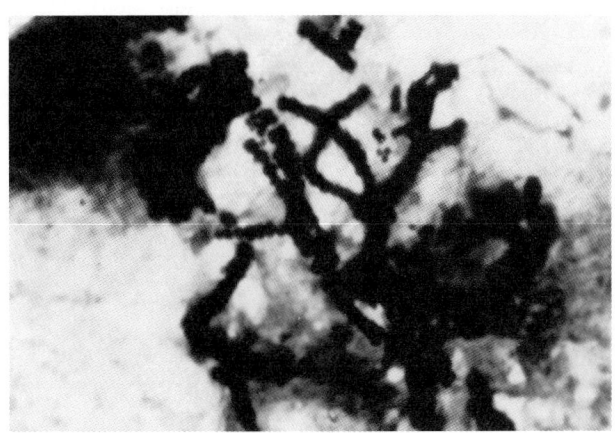

FIG. 11-4 ▓ Positive result on potassium hydroxide (KOH) preparation. Note the small, spherical fungal elements (arthroconidia) on the hair shaft.

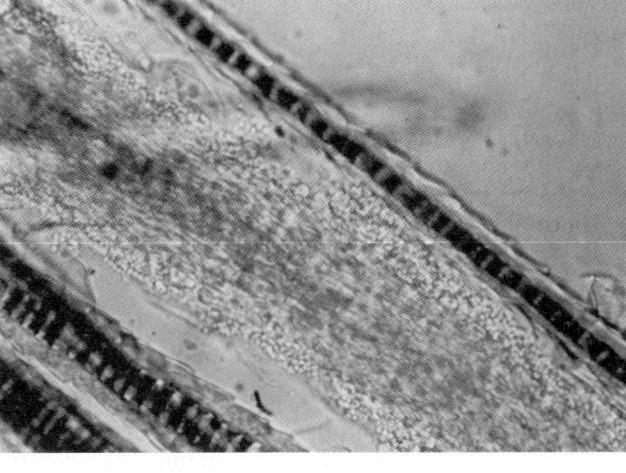

FIG. 11-5 ▓ Positive result on *Dermatophilus* preparation. *Dermatophilus congolensis* is a large, gram positive, filamentous bacterium that divides horizontally and longitudinally, forming parallel rows of cocci (zoospores) that are commonly described as "railroad tracks."

that permits immediate examination, although the specimen must be examined within 30 minutes of preparation or it will overclear.

Examination of KOH preparations requires considerable experience, because fungal elements may be easily overlooked (false-negative result) and numerous artifacts such as fibers, cholesterol crystals, or oil droplets may be mistaken for fungal elements (false-positive result). It is always advisable to perform a dermatophyte culture in conjunction with a KOH preparation.

ACETATE TAPE PREPARATION. Acetate tape preparations are used primarily to diagnose infection with *Oxyuris equi*, although they may also be used to diagnose *Chorioptes* spp. The materials required to perform an acetate tape preparation include acetate (nonfrosted) tape, mineral oil, and glass microscope slides. A piece of the tape is pressed over several areas in the anal and perianal region when looking for *O. equi* or over an affected region that has been lightly clipped when looking for *Chorioptes* spp. The tape is then placed with the adhesive side down on a glass slide liberally coated with mineral oil. The purpose of the oil is to help clear the debris and facilitate examination of the preparation for parasites. The preparation is scanned with the ×10 objective for organisms.

DERMATOPHILUS **PREPARATION.** This test is used as an aid in identification of *Dermatophilus congolensis*. Crusts should be removed from the patient and the excess hair carefully trimmed from the crusts with a small pair of scissors. The crusts are minced with the scissors and mixed with several drops of saline on a glass slide. After the crusts have softened in the saline for several minutes, they should be crushed with the tip of an applicator stick. The excess debris is removed, and the slide is allowed to air dry. The slide should then be heat fixed; stained with Gram, Giemsa, or Wright stain; and examined for the characteristic bacteria. *D. congolensis* organisms are gram-positive, branching, filamentous bacteria that divide horizontally and longitudinally, forming parallel rows of cocci (zoospores) that commonly are described as resembling "railroad tracks" (Fig. 11-5).

CYTOLOGIC STUDIES. Cytologic studies are of value when dealing with pustules, vesicles, nodules, tumors, or swellings. They can quickly indicate the presence or absence of infectious organisms and provide a rough assessment of the spectrum of cell types present in a lesion (e.g., neoplastic, acantholytic, or inflammatory). The surface of the lesion should be gently shaved (if necessary), wiped with an antiseptic solution, and dried with a sterile gauze pad. Particular

care must be taken not to rupture fragile pustules and vesicles. Cytologic evaluation of pustules and vesicles is best accomplished by gently opening an intact lesion with the tip of a sterile No. 15 scalpel blade and smearing the contents on the surface of a glass slide. The slide should be allowed to air dry. It should be heat fixed, stained with Gram, Giemsa, or Wright stain, and examined. Nodules, tumors, and swellings are best evaluated by fine-needle aspiration. A 25- or 22-gauge needle on a 12-ml syringe is introduced into the mass, and negative pressure is applied. Several passes through the mass at different angles should be performed. After negative pressure has been released, the needle is removed from the mass. The needle is then removed from the syringe, the syringe is filled with air, and the needle is reattached. The contents of the needle are pushed out onto glass slides, which are subsequently dried, fixed, and stained as outlined previously.

BIOPSY FOR ROUTINE HISTOPATHOLOGIC EXAMINATION. The following materials are needed to perform a skin biopsy:
- 6-mm and 4-mm biopsy punches
- No. 15 scalpel blade
- Sharp scissors
- Adson forceps
- Needle holders
- No. 2-0 or 3-0 nonabsorbable suture
- 2% lidocaine
- 3-ml syringe with a 22- to 25-gauge needle
- Tongue depressor or cardboard
- Gauze
- 10% buffered formalin

It is important not to surgically prepare a lesion that is going to be biopsied for histopathologic examination. Shaving and scrubbing remove crusts and epithelial tissue that may be important in reaching a diagnosis. Cutaneous infections caused by biopsies taken in this manner are extremely uncommon.

Local anesthesia is sufficient for obtaining most skin biopsies. A 22- to 25-gauge needle is inserted at the margin of the lesion until the bevel is buried in the subcutaneous tissue beneath the lesion. The 2% lidocaine (0.5 to 1 ml) is injected, allowing 1 to 2 minutes for the anesthetic to take effect. Infiltration of the dermal or epidermal tissue with lidocaine should be avoided because this causes artifactual changes in the specimen.

Four techniques can be used to biopsy skin: the excisional, wedge, punch, or elliptic technique. When the lesion to be

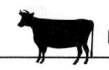

sampled is a single nodule, the ideal biopsy technique is excisional because the lesion can be eliminated at the same time the histologic diagnosis is made. If the lesion is a tumor and too large to be excised, a generous wedge biopsy should be performed, which ideally extends from the margin to the center and for the full depth of the lesion.

Most lesions can be sampled with a 6-mm biopsy punch. A disposable biopsy punch* usually can be used to obtain two to three biopsies before its edge is dulled and it must be discarded. The punch is placed directly over the lesion and rotated in a continuous circular motion while pressure is applied until the blade of the punch is in the subcutaneous tissue. If the punch has cut to a sufficient depth, when it is removed the tissue sample is free of the adjacent dermis and remains only loosely attached to the underlying subcutaneous tissue by a thread of connective tissue. A small pair of Adson forceps is used to gently grasp the subcutaneous part of the biopsy and elevate it from the surrounding tissue. The specimen is then cut free with a pair of sharp scissors. It is important to avoid handling the epidermal and dermal part of the sample during this procedure to minimize artifactual changes in the tissue sample. The sample is gently blotted to remove any surface hemorrhage and immediately placed in 10% buffered formalin for fixation. The site from which the sample was taken may then be cleaned with an antiseptic solution and closed with either two simple interrupted sutures or a cruciate stitch using No. 2-0 or 3-0 nonabsorbable sutures.

Although punch biopsies are convenient and easy to use, they are not appropriate for vesicular, bullous, and ulcerative lesions. For these lesions the method of choice is a surgical elliptical biopsy. The biopsy of vesicular and bullous lesions should encompass the entire lesion. Biopsy of samples of ulcerations should include abnormal tissue, the leading edge of the lesion, and normal tissue. Because an ulcer lacks epithelial tissue, the leading edge where epithelium remains may be the most rewarding in providing a histologic diagnosis. Thus the skin is biopsied so that the long axis of the ellipse crosses perpendicular to the leading edge of the ulcer (Fig. 11-6). It is important to mount surgical elliptical biopsies before placing them in formalin or they will curl during fixation, resulting in distortion of the histologic features during sectioning. To mount the specimen, the subcutaneous surface is placed on a small piece of tongue depressor or cardboard while gentle pressure is applied to the tissue so that it adheres to the surface.

Ideally biopsy specimens should be submitted to a veterinary histopathologist with a special interest and training in dermatopathology. Submission of adequately biopsied specimens of properly chosen lesions is the clinician's responsibility. To further increase the chances of securing clinically valuable information from the biopsy samples, the clinician must also provide the pathologist with a concise history of the skin problem, physical findings, a description of the morphology and location of the lesions, and a list of differentials for diagnosis. When the suspected clinical diagnoses are provided, the pathologist's efforts can be directed specifically toward confirming or ruling out those diagnoses.

BIOPSY FOR DIRECT IMMUNOFLUORESCENCE TESTING. The biopsy for direct immunofluorescence test can be used as an adjunct to conventional histologic testing when the clinician suspects that the patient has an immune-mediated skin disease. The materials and the technique for biopsy for immunofluorescence are essentially identical to those for a routine histologic examination except that the medium used for tissue fixation is Michel's fixative, which can be provided by most veterinary diagnostic laboratories. Administration of

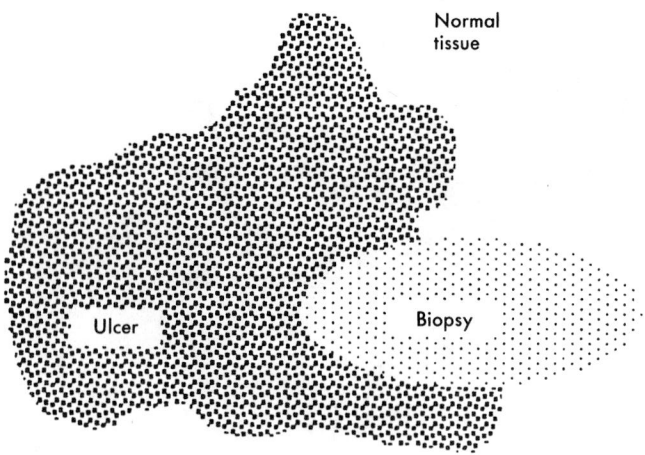

FIG. 11-6 ▓ An ulcerative lesion should be biopsied in an elliptical fashion, using a No. 15 scalpel blade, so that the long axis of the ellipse crosses perpendicular to the leading edge of the lesion.

corticosteroid medications within 3 weeks of testing may be associated with false-negative test results. It is advisable to bisect biopsy samples along their long axis, submitting half for direct immunofluorescence and half for histopathologic examination. As an alternative, immunochemistry testing using immunoperoxidase techniques may be performed on the paraffin block prepared for the histopathologic study (i.e., the formalinized tissue section).

MICROFILARIAL PREPARATION. The microfilarial preparation technique is applicable to the diagnosis of cutaneous onchocerciasis in horses, stephanofilariasis in cattle, and elaeophorosis and parelaphostrongylosis of sheep and goats. After selecting the lesion to be sampled, a 6-mm punch biopsy is used to obtain the tissue sample in the same manner as for the histopathologic biopsy. The tissue should be split and half preserved in 10% buffered formalin for routine histologic studies. The other half is placed on a dampened gauze sponge in a tightly closed container until the preparation can be performed. A small piece of the tissue that includes the dermis is placed on a glass slide and minced with a razor blade; a few drops of nonbacteriostatic saline are added. Bacteriostatic saline, which kills the microfilaria and thus makes their identification more difficult, should not be used. The specimen is incubated at room temperature for 15 minutes. The slide is then scanned with the ×4 objective along the margins of the tissue debris while the clinician searches for indication of motion in the saline. If the characteristic whiplash movement of the parasite is noted, a higher-powered objective should be used. If the preparation result is negative, a small amount of water is added to a petri dish, the glass slide is rested on two wooden sticks above the water, and the cover is replaced on the dish. The preparation should be incubated for several hours or overnight and reexamined. The petri dish helps prevent the sample from drying out.

BACTERIAL CULTURE. A large number of nonpathogenic bacteria are present on the surface of the skin of horses and ruminants. Therefore, to prevent culture contamination by surface bacteria, the lesions should be gently shaved, washed with an antiseptic soap, and dried with a sterile gauze pad. Ulcerative lesions should not be cultured because any bacteria isolated are more likely to be opportunistic rather than primary pathogens. If the lesions are fluctuant, the overlying skin can be opened gently with a No. 15 blade and some of the contents of the lesion transferred with the blade to the tip of a sterile culture swab. It is advisable to avoid placing the swabs directly on the skin surface, particularly when sam-

---

*Baker's Biopsy Punch, Chester A. Baker Laboratories, 50 NW 176th St., Miami, FL 33169.

pling small lesions, because nonpathogenic bacteria from the skin surface can be inadvertently cultured.

Nodules and tumors should be cultured by aseptically excising the lesion or by obtaining a generous wedge of the tissue. As described above, the clinician initially performs a sterile surface preparation of the skin to remove surface contaminants, and a perilesional injection of 2% lidocaine is used to anesthetize the tissue. The sample is placed in a transport medium and sent to a microbiology laboratory for culture. When pyoderma is suspected as the cause of a papular eruption, it is advisable to obtain a sterile, 6-mm punch biopsy of skin to submit for bacterial culture.

SUBCUTANEOUS AND DEEP FUNGAL CULTURE. Subcutaneous and deep fungal cultures should be performed on nodules, tumors, or swellings. The technique is identical to that described for bacterial culture of these lesions.

REFERENCE

1. Evans AE, Stannard AA: Diagnostic approach to equine skin disease, *Compend Cont Educ (Pract Vet)* 8:652-661, 1986.

PRURITUS

Definition

Pruritus is an unpleasant sensation that provokes the desire to scratch. It is designated a primary cutaneous sensation, along with heat, cold, pain, and touch. There are two broad categories of pruritus. Physiologic, or spontaneous, itch refers to a sharp, well-defined, pruritic sensation that is sufficiently intense to prompt scratching but that does not result in significant irritation of the skin; this is a frequent daily occurrence in normal individuals. Pathologic itch is the less well-defined pruritus that occurs in a variety of primary and secondary skin disorders and in systemic diseases. It is an intense cutaneous discomfort that provokes vigorous scratching.[2]

Mechanisms of Pruritus

Pruritus is a distinct sensory quality transmitted from an arborizing network of nerve endings situated at or near the dermoepidermal junction. The sensation is carried to the spinal cord through small, unmyelinated C fibers. The fibers enter the dorsal root of the spinal cord and ascend in the ventrolateral spinothalamic tract through the posterior ventral nucleus of the thalamus to the sensory cortex. The pruritic sensation may be modified in the sensory cortex by emotional factors or competing stimuli.[3,4]

Many physical and chemical stimuli can evoke pruritus, and many substances have been implicated as mediating pruritus in humans. Examples of these mediators, which are assumed to have importance in domestic animals as well, include the following[4]:

- *Histamine.* Histamine has been regarded as the classic mediator of pruritus. Histamine is present in mast cells in the dermis and in blood basophils. An intradermal injection of histamine produces pruritus within 20 to 50 seconds. Because many pruritic disorders respond poorly to antihistamines given either therapeutically or prophylactically, histamine is not believed to be the primary mediator of pruritus.
- *Endopeptidases.* Mucunain, from the plant *Mucuna pruriens,* was the first endopeptidase to be demonstrated. It produces pruritus without any objective signs of erythema or urticaria. Other endopeptidases that have since been reported to induce pruritus include trypsin, papain, and kalikrein. Bradykinin has also been implicated, though it may produce pruritus primarily by activating histamine release.
- *Prostaglandins (E series and endoperoxidases).* Prostaglandins induce pruritus by potentiating the release of proteases

from keratinocytes and leukocytes and by lowering the threshold and increasing the duration of histamine-induced pruritus.
- *Endogenous opioid peptides.* Injection of morphine into the medulla and cerebral cisterns of animal species has been shown to elicit pruritus. The opiate antagonist naloxone hydrochloride has an attenuating effect on the histamine-induced component of pruritus.
- *Substance P.* Substance P is a neurotransmitter found in the central and peripheral nervous systems. When introduced intradermally, it elicits a pruritic response.

Many factors can potentiate existing pruritus. Neurologic factors such as boredom and tiredness can potentiate a pathologic itch and possibly transform a physiologic itch into a pathologic itch. Local axonal reflexes can potentiate pruritus; that is, if a second stimulus is applied to an area close to one that is pruritic, the second stimulus, irrespective of its type, is perceived as an itch. In addition, skin with chronic dermatitis has limited perception of stimuli, and any stimulus applied to the affected region may be perceived as either a burning sensation or an itch. This phenomenon is known as "conversion itch." Secondary bacterial infections, vasodilation, and inflammation result in a local increase in proteases that potentiate pruritus.[3]

Pruritus can be diminished by several nonpharmacologic mechanisms, the most common being application of competing stimuli. Pruritus is a minor sensation compared with the other primary sensations of heat, cold, touch, and pain; thus local application of a competing stimuli to a pruritic area often suppresses the pruritic sensation. Scratching is an example of a competing stimuli. Scratching may relieve pruritus by disturbing the rhythm of afferent impulses traveling toward the central nervous system. An alternative theory is that scratching may cause transient damage to nerve fibers that convey the pruritic sensation. Unfortunately the effect is short-lived because the epidermal damage induced by scratching causes the release of epidermal proteases that may later increase the degree of pruritus. Centrally acting factors such as diversions or distractions can also diminish the perception of pruritus by providing competing stimuli directly to the cortex rather than locally to the skin.[3]

Approach to Diagnosis of Pruritus

Pruritus is the most common sign of cutaneous disease. It may represent a manifestation of a systemic disease, a hypersensitivity reaction, or a primary skin disease. Because pruritus may be a feature of a more generalized disease process, it is important to take the patient's general health into account. Is disease truly limited to the skin, or are other organ systems involved and, if so, which organ systems are affected? Hypersensitivity reactions, which are commonly pruritic, may or may not be limited to the skin. For example, anaphylaxis is a life-threatening hypersensitivity reaction that may manifest as pruritus in its early stages. Pruritic diseases that are limited to the skin encompass a wide spectrum of dermatology, including immune-mediated diseases such as pemphigus foliaceus; infectious diseases, including those caused by bacteria, viruses, fungi, and parasites; direct irritation by chemicals; and photoactivated dermatoses. It is helpful to formulate a differential diagnosis by considering each of these broad categories of diseases and using historic information, other cutaneous signs, and appropriate diagnostic tests to narrow the list of differential diagnoses.

The following steps are a guide to the diagnosis of pruritus in the horse and ruminant:

1. History (see Fig. 11-1). Pay particular attention to whether the pruritus is a seasonal or year-round condition. A seasonally recurrent pruritic disease tends to suggest either a seasonal allergen as the etiology (e.g., pollens)

or, more likely, a seasonal parasite. Lice are a bigger problem in the winter, trombiculidiasis tends to occur in the late summer and early fall, and most of the flying insects are present in the spring, summer, and early fall. Determine the level of fly exposure for the animal that is pruritic in the warmer months.

a. Determine if the pruritus is generalized or localized, and if localized, what areas of the body are affected. Certain parasites tend to create pruritus in very specific areas of the body. Photoactivated dermatoses are limited to the white-haired regions.

b. Determine if contact animals of the same and different species are affected or unaffected. A group of pruritic animals is more likely to have a contagious problem (e.g., bacterial [dermatophilosis], fungal [dermatophytosis], parasitic, or viral). A single pruritic animal among a group of unaffected animals is more likely to be experiencing a hypersensitivity reaction (drug, food, or inhalant).

c. Determine what topical and systemic medications were given to the patient both before and after the onset of the problem. Medications given before onset may be the cause of the pruritus, and those given after onset may interfere with the results of diagnostic tests.

2. Physical examination (see Fig. 11-2). In particular note the following:

a. If all the cutaneous lesions can be attributed to self-trauma or if other primary cutaneous changes are present (e.g., wheals, nodules, pigmentary changes) that may help to narrow the differential diagnosis.

b. If contact animals show evidence of disease.

c. Which areas of the body are affected and which are spared.

d. The number of flying insects, if the patient is examined in its home environment.

e. If, upon close inspection, the coat shows evidence of small but grossly visible parasites such as lice or their eggs.

3. Skin scrapings
4. Acetate tape preparations
5. Dermatophyte culture and KOH preparation
6. *Dermatophilus* preparation
7. Microfilarial preparation
8. Biopsy for routine histopathologic examination
9. Biopsy for direct immunofluorescence testing
10. Bacterial culture and sensitivity
11. Hypoallergenic test diets (see Chapter 40)
12. Intradermal skin testing (see Chapter 40)

REFERENCES

2. Moschella SL, Hurley HJ: *Dermatology*, ed 2, Philadelphia, 1985, WB Saunders.
3. Halliwell REW: Pathogenesis and treatment of pruritus, *J Am Vet Med Assoc* 164:793-796, 1974.
4. Martin J: Pruritus, *Int J Dermatol* 24:634-639, 1985.

NODULES, TUMORS, AND SWELLINGS

Definition

A nodule is a circumscribed, solid elevation larger than 1 cm in diameter that does not deform when palpated. Nodules extend into the deeper layers of the skin and are usually the result of cellular infiltrates in the dermis or subcutis. "Tumor" is a vague term that usually refers to a neoplastic, nodular enlargement of the skin or subcutaneous tissue.[5,6] The term "tumor" is most commonly used to describe very large nodular neoplasms. In addition to nodules and tumors, swellings include elevated lesions that pit with pressure (wheals) and fluctuant lesions (cysts and abscesses).

Mechanisms of Nodule, Tumor, and Swelling Formation

Nodular lesions can be subdivided into inflammatory and neoplastic lesions. Inflammatory nodules are composed of a massive mixed cellular infiltrate involving the dermis, the subcutis, or both. The inflammatory infiltrate may contain variable numbers of neutrophils, histiocytes, lymphocytes, plasma cells, and eosinophils. Cellular infiltration usually is stimulated by the presence of foreign material, and the nature of that material influences the composition of the inflammatory infiltrate. The foreign material may be infectious (bacteria or fungi) or noninfectious (fibrin, crystalline material, or other inert substances). Grossly visible nodules develop as the masses of inflammatory cells accumulate in the tissues to phagocytize or wall off the foreign material. The presence of the inflammatory cells may stimulate the formation of scar tissue. As the lesion enlarges, the dermis and subcutis are obliterated by the inflammatory infiltrate and the overlying epidermis may become atrophic, resulting in ulceration of the nodule's surface.

Most cutaneous and subcutaneous neoplasms form nodular lesions. Cutaneous and subcutaneous neoplasms may be either primary (arising directly from a cell type of the epidermis, dermis, or subcutis) or secondary (metastasizing from a distant tissue of origin). Cytologically and histologically neoplasms are composed of a uniform population of pleomorphic cells that demonstrate varying degrees of atypia. The cellular characteristics of an individual neoplasm depend on the cell type of origin and the degree of differentiation of that cell type. Neoplasms often stimulate a secondary inflammatory reaction, resulting in a mixed population of nonneoplastic cells that surrounds or is dispersed throughout the population of neoplastic cells.

Swellings include solid lesions, such as nodules and tumors, as well as wheals, cysts, and abscesses. Wheals (hives, urticaria) are transient, localized, inflammatory lesions caused by a vascular reaction in the dermis in which vasodilation results in erythema and fluid transudation. The fluid is not compartmentalized but dispersed evenly throughout the dermal tissue.[7] The result is an elevated lesion that, unlike a nodule, pits with pressure and dissipates within minutes to hours as the fluid is resorbed. Typically a sparse, perivascular infiltrate that is usually lymphocytic is seen, although the infiltrate may be dense and intermingled with eosinophils.[8] Wheals are usually well-circumscribed lesions. With confluence they may assume geometric shapes.

A cyst (Latin for *sac*) is an epithelium-lined cavity containing fluid or semisolid material.[5] It is an elevated, smooth, well-circumscribed, fluctuant mass. Cutaneous cysts usually are lined by adnexal epithelium (hair follicle, sebaceous or apocrine epithelium) and are filled with cornified cellular debris and sebaceous or apocrine secretions.

An abscess is a localized, fluid-filled, fluctuant lesion; if large enough, it may be balloted. It results from a dermal or subcutaneous accumulation of the debris of dead cells and tissue elements liquefied by the proteolytic and histolytic enzymes elaborated by polymorphonuclear cells (e.g., pus). Abscesses most commonly result from localized infection, although they can be sterile.

Approach to Diagnosis of Nodules, Tumors, and Swellings

Nodules, tumors, and swellings may arise from a variety of cutaneous disorders and, in rare cases, as a sign of a systemic disease. The major categories of diseases that should be considered when forming a differential diagnosis include hypersensitivity reactions, infectious diseases, sterile inflammatory diseases, and neoplasia. The primary systemic diseases that should be considered are lymphosarcoma, amyloidosis, and anaphylaxis.

The following steps are a guide to the diagnosis of nodules, tumors, and swellings in the horse and ruminants:
1. History (see Fig. 11-1). Pay particular attention to:
   a. Signalment. Older animals, particularly gray horses that are predisposed to melanomas, are at greater risk for cutaneous neoplasia. However, this condition is not necessarily restricted to older animals; equine sarcoids are frequently recognized in horses as young as 3 years of age.
   b. Temporal course of development. Rapid onset of the lesion or lesions might suggest a hypersensitivity reaction. If only a single lesion is present, hypersensitivity to an insect or spider bite should be considered. Rapid onset of generalized lesions such as wheals suggests a differential diagnosis of drug, flying insect, food, or inhalant allergies.
   c. A recent history of systemic disease, which might suggest that the lesion is a bacterial abscess.
2. Physical examination (see Fig. 11-2). In particular:
   a. Determine by palpation if the cutaneous lesions are nodules, tumors, or swellings.
   b. Inspect the lesion or lesions closely for evidence of cutaneous parasitism (ticks, breathing pores associated with *Hypoderma* larvae, yellow granules associated with cutaneous habronemiasis).
   c. Determine if the lesions are painful or pruritic (e.g., evidence of excoriations).
3. Fine-needle aspirate for cytologic studies
4. Biopsy for histopathologic examination
5. Bacterial culture and sensitivity
6. Subcutaneous and deep fungal cultures
7. Dermatophyte culture and KOH preparation

REFERENCES
5. Ackerman AB: *Histologic diagnosis of inflammatory skin diseases: a method by pattern analysis,* London, 1978, Lea & Febiger.
6. Muller GH, Kirk RW, Scott DW: *Small animal dermatology,* ed 3, Philadelphia, 1983, WB Saunders.
7. Moschella SL, Hury HJ: *Dermatology,* ed 2, Philadelphia, 1985, WB Saunders.
8. Lever WF: *Histopathology of the skin,* ed 6, Philadelphia, 1983, JB Lippincott.

ULCERATIONS AND EROSIONS

Definition

An ulcer is a cutaneous defect that results from a complete loss of the epidermis and usually part of the underlying dermis. Ulcers often heal with scarring that is caused by destruction of dermal collagen. An erosion is a cutaneous defect that results from a partial loss of the epidermis that does not penetrate beneath the basal laminar zone. Because an erosion does not involve the dermis, it heals without leaving a scar.[9] Because the epidermis is a cutaneous barrier to invading microorganisms, ulcers and erosions often are secondarily infected.

Mechanisms of Ulcer and Erosion Formation

Ulcers and erosions are secondary lesions. Primary lesions develop spontaneously and are a direct reflection of underlying disease. Secondary lesions evolve from primary lesions or are artifacts induced by excoriation or external trauma. Primary lesions that may lead to the formation of ulcers and erosions include fluid-filled lesions such as pustules and vesicles. Rupture of these fragile lesions results in epidermal destruction and erosion or ulcer formation. Swellings such as abscesses and cysts may also rupture, resulting in ulceration,

but these primary lesions are more stable and often remain intact. Nodules and tumors may become secondarily eroded or ulcerated. As the nodule or tumor enlarges, the mass exerts pressure on the overlying epidermis, leading to epidermal atrophy and ultimately a break in epidermal confluence, resulting in ulceration and erosion. The most common cause of ulceration and erosion is pruritus, which induces excoriation and hence epidermal destruction. Ulcers and erosions may also result from external trauma, such as epidermal destruction arising from mechanical, thermal, or chemical causes.

Approach to Diagnosis of Ulcerations and Erosions

To diagnose the cause of an ulcer or erosion, the clinician must first determine the primary lesion that resulted in ulceration and erosion. Ulcers and erosions that occur secondary to pustules and vesicles, to swellings such as abscesses and cysts, to nodules and tumors, to pruritus, and to external trauma must be differentiated. The list of differential diagnoses relevant to each of these groups of primary lesions is then considered.

The following steps are a guide to the diagnosis of ulcerations and erosions in the horse and ruminants:
1. History (see Fig. 11-2)
   a. Determine if the animal is pruritic.
   b. Determine if the animal has been subjected to external trauma (mechanical, thermal, or chemical).
   c. Determine what topical and systemic medications have been given to or used on the patient before the onset of the problem. Use of certain topical agents may suggest a diagnosis of contact dermatitis, whereas administration of systemic medications may suggest that the etiology is a drug hypersensitivity.
2. Physical examination (see Fig. 11-2)
   a. Examine the oral cavity and mucocutaneous junctions for lesions. Oral or mucocutaneous lesions (or both) in the horse might suggest a diagnosis of bullous pemphigoid. In a ruminant these lesions often are seen with viral infections (see oral ulcerations and erosions in Chapter 7).
   b. Look for evidence of excoriation, suggesting that the ulcerations and erosions have occurred secondary to pruritus.
   c. Look for evidence of primary lesions such as pustules, vesicles, nodules, tumors, or swellings, which may have preceded the ulcerations and erosions.
3. Biopsy for routine histopathologic examination
4. Biopsy for direct immunofluorescence testing

REFERENCE
9. Ackerman AB: *Histologic diagnosis of inflammatory skin diseases: a method by pattern analysis,* London, 1978, Lea & Febiger.

PAPULES, PUSTULES, AND VESICLES

Definition

A papule is a solid, circumscribed, elevated lesion up to 1 cm in diameter. Papules are essentially small nodules that do not extend beneath the dermis. A pustule is a fluctuant, circumscribed, elevated accumulation of pus (inflammatory cells and necrotic debris) up to 1 cm in diameter (e.g., a small abscess). Pustules are frequently associated with infectious diseases, although a pustule can be sterile. A vesicle is a fluid-filled, acellular, circumscribed, elevated lesion up to 1 cm in diameter. A bulla is a vesicle that is larger than 1 cm in diameter. All these lesions can be either follicular or nonfollicular in orientation, depending on the underlying etiology. Pustules and vesicles are rarely seen clinically because of their fragility and hence their susceptibility to rupture. Because papules are solid lesions, they are more stable and therefore more commonly encountered.[10,11]

Mechanisms of Papule, Pustule, and Vesicle Formation

Papules usually form as a result of an infiltrate in the dermis, which can be either cellular or noncellular. Cellular infiltrates may include inflammatory or neoplastic cells, although neoplastic papular lesions are relatively uncommon in large animals. Inflammatory infiltrates may be mixed, containing variable numbers of neutrophils, histiocytes, lymphocytes, plasma cells, and eosinophils, or one cell type may predominate. The composition of the inflammatory cells is influenced by the underlying cause of the papule, and the possible etiologies are extensive. Neoplastic papular cellular infiltrates usually are primary (arising from a cell type of the epidermis or dermis) or, less commonly, secondary (metastasizing from a distant tissue of origin). Cytologically and histologically neoplastic infiltrates are composed of a uniform population of pleomorphic cells that demonstrate varying degrees of atypia. The cellular characteristics depend on the cell type of origin and the degree of differentiation of that cell type. A secondary inflammatory infiltrate may be present, resulting in a mixed population of neoplastic and nonneoplastic cells. Noncellular papular infiltrates include substances such as edema fluid, amyloid, and proliferative collagen. Epidermal hypertrophy may contribute to or be the sole cause of papule formation.

Pustules form as the result of an intraepidermal, subcorneal or, less commonly, subepidermal accumulation of inflammatory cells. Infiltration of inflammatory cells, particularly polymorphonuclear leukocytes, leads to the release of proteolytic enzymes that liquefy tissue elements and result in the formation of a fluctuant lesion. Eosinophils, acanthocytes, and infectious organisms may also be noted in a pustule, depending on the underlying etiology. The stimulus leading to pustule formation is most commonly infectious, although pustules can result from noninfectious etiologies such as hypersensitivity reactions and autoimmune disease.

Vesicles form either at the dermoepidermal junction (subepidermal) or in the epidermis (intraepidermal) as a result of destruction of the basement membrane zone or confluence of intercellular edema (spongiosis). Clinically the two types of vesicles are indistinguishable. Vesicles form as the result of some viral diseases, during severe inflammatory reactions (allergic contact dermatitis), or with cutaneous physical damage (mechanical, chemical, or thermal).[10] In pemphigus foliaceus autoantibodies bind to desmogleins (transmembrane proteins), causing disruption of intraepidermal cellular attachments. The result is intraepidermal cleft formation that leads to vesiculation. In bullous pemphigoid complement-activating antibodies bind to antigens in the basement membrane zone, causing degranulation of mast cells, chemotaxis of neutrophils and eosinophils, and release of tissue-destructive enzymes that injure the basement membrane zone. The result is loss of dermoepidermal adherence and vesicle formation.[12] Vesicles are transient, fragile lesions and therefore are rarely recognized clinically. If they are not destroyed by surface trauma, rapid infiltration by inflammatory cells transforms a vesicle into a pustule.

Approach to Diagnosis of Papules, Pustules, and Vesicles

Although papules, pustules, and vesicles may look somewhat similar on a cursory physical examination, the clinician must differentiate among the three and determine which of the lesions are present. The differential diagnoses relevant to papules, pustules, and vesicles are not necessarily the same. In all cases it is important to determine if disease is limited to the skin or if the patient's general health is compromised as well.

Papular lesions have the most extensive differential diagnoses:

1. Hypersensitivity reactions. Parasitic hypersensitivities are the most common (*Culicoides* hypersensitivity), although food and drug hypersensitivities should also be considered. Most hypersensitivity reactions are pruritic.
2. Parasites. Some species simply irritate the skin with their bites (*Lyperosia [Haematobia] irritans*) without inducing a hypersensitivity reaction.
3. Infectious diseases (bacterial, fungal, and viral). Typically papules caused by infections have a follicular orientation.
4. Certain neoplastic diseases (papillomas or sarcoids).
5. Uncommon causes, including autoimmune diseases, such as pemphigus foliaceus, and diseases of uncertain etiology, such as generalized granulomatous disease. In both of these the signs of systemic disease usually are present.

Pustules are most commonly associated with bacterial infections, although fungi and, in rare cases, parasites (*Demodex* spp.) can cause pustule formation. Sterile pustular diseases are less frequently seen (drug eruptions, sterile eosinophilic folliculitis of cattle) but should be included in the differential diagnoses. Any disease that forms vesicles as a primary lesion is likely to form pustules secondarily. Vesicles are rapidly infiltrated by inflammatory cells and transformed into pustules. Diseases commonly associated with vesicles include viral diseases of ruminants, autoimmune diseases, contact dermatoses, and burns.

The following steps are a guide to the diagnosis of papules, pustules, and vesicles in the horse and ruminants:

1. History (see Fig. 11-1)
   a. In particular, determine whether the lesions are pruritic, painful, or asymptomatic.
   b. Determine if contact animals of the same and different species are affected or unaffected. If contact animals are affected, a contagious problem should be considered: fungal (dermatophytosis), bacterial (dermatophilosis), viral (contagious ecthyma), or parasitic (*Culicoides* hypersensitivity).
   c. Trace the temporal course of development. Rapid onset of lesions might suggest a hypersensitivity reaction.
   d. Check for seasonality. A seasonal problem suggests a parasitic cause. Lice are a problem in the winter, trombiculidiasis tends to occur in the fall, and most of the flying insects are present in the spring, summer, and early fall.
   e. Determine what topical and systemic medications have been given to or used on the patient before the onset of the problem. Use of certain topical agents may suggest a diagnosis of contact dermatitis, whereas administration of systemic medications may suggest that the etiology is a drug hypersensitivity.
   f. Determine if the animal has been subjected to external trauma (thermal or chemical).
2. Perform a physical examination (see Fig. 11-2)
   a. Gently palpate the lesions to determine if they are solid (papules) or fluctuant (pustules or vesicles).
   b. Note if the lesions have a follicular orientation, suggesting an infectious etiology.
   c. Check for lesions involving the oral cavity and mucocutaneous junctions.
   d. Look for evidence of excoriation, suggesting that pruritus is a feature of the disease.
   e. Inspect the coat closely for small but grossly visible parasites such as lice or their eggs.
   f. Inspect contact animals for evidence of disease.

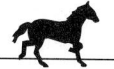

3. Skin scrapings of papular lesions
4. Cytologic studies
5. Dermatophyte culture and KOH preparation
6. *Dermatophilus* preparation
7. Bacterial culture and sensitivity
8. Microfilarial preparation
9. Biopsy for routine histopathologic examination
10. Biopsy for direct immunofluorescence testing

REFERENCES

10. Ackerman AB: *Histologic diagnosis of inflammatory skin diseases: a method by pattern analysis,* London, 1978, Lea & Febiger.
11. Muller GH, Kirk RW, Scott DW: *Small animal dermatology,* ed 3, Philadelphia, 1983, WB Saunders.
12. Sams WM, Gamon WR: Mechanism of lesion production in pemphigus and pemphigoid, *J Am Acad Dermatol* 6:431, 1982.

SCALING AND CRUSTING

Definition

Scale is a visible accumulation of fragments of the horny layer of the skin (stratum corneum); it represents the final product of epidermal keratinization. Histologically scale is recognized as hyperkeratosis and can be subdivided into parakeratosis (cornification with nuclear retention) or orthokeratosis (cornification without nuclear retention). In some conditions parakeratosis and orthokeratosis may be present together. Grossly the scale varies in appearance. The color may be white, silver, yellow, brown, or gray. The consistency may be branny, powdery, flaky, coarse, greasy, or dry. Scale can be either loose or adherent to the skin or hair shafts.

Crusts are dried exudate that adheres to the skin surface and hair. They often cover erosions or ulcerations. Heaped-up crusts are referred to as vegetations. Crusts are composed of variable amounts of serum, cells (leukocytes, erythrocytes, keratinocytes), fibrin, infectious agents (bacteria and fungi), dirt, and medications. On the basis of their histologic composition, crusts may be subdivided into cellular, serocellular, serous, and hemorrhagic types.[13,14]

Mechanisms of Scale and Crust Formation

Scale results from increased desquamation (exfoliation) of the stratum corneum. Exfoliation is the final stage of keratinization, the process by which the permanent population of cells of the basal layer of the epidermis divides, undergoes specific patterns of differentiation, and progresses toward the surface, where it is shed.[15] Excessive exfoliation and scale formation occur when the rate of keratinization is accelerated; when trauma to the surface of the epidermis (chemical, mechanical, or thermal) loosens the stratum corneum; or when the epidermal intercellular cementing material is destroyed, resulting in loss of cohesion between epidermal cells.

Because crusts are composed primarily of serum and cells, their presence on the skin surface implies that vascular and epidermal permeability have increased to permit their formation. Serum and inflammatory cells are released into the tissues from the dermal vasculature and then cross the epidermis to the skin surface either through breaks in the continuity of the epidermis (erosions or ulcerations) or by permeating between the intercellular spaces. The exudate dries on the skin surface, in combination with any medication or dirt that was already present on the hair or skin, to form the visible crust. Desquamating keratinocytes (fragments of stratum corneum or acanthocytes) may be swept up in the exudate and become part of the crusts. Bacteria frequently invade crusts after they have formed and will be noted on histologic examination, even though they may not be a factor

in the pathogenesis. Fungal organisms, when present, are more likely to be significant to the pathogenesis of the crust formation.

Approach to Diagnosis of Scaling and Crusting

The most important factor in determining the underlying cause of scale or crust formation in either a horse or ruminant is to determine if the patient is pruritic and if some or all of the lesions are induced by self-trauma. If pruritus is a feature, the approach to diagnosis of pruritus should be used because all pruritic diseases can cause scale and crust formation. If the patient is not pruritic, the most important differential diagnoses to consider include infectious diseases (particularly dermatophilosis and dermatophytosis), nutritional disorders, toxicities, autoimmune disease (pemphigus foliaceus), endocrinopathies (equine hyperadrenocorticism), cutaneous filariasis, photosensitization, irritant contact reactions or burns, and diseases of uncertain etiology (equine: generalized granulomatous disease, anhidrosis, aural plaques, reticulated leukotrichia, and primary seborrhea). Viral diseases are important nonpruritic causes of scaling and crusting in ruminants, although usually associated ulceration and erosion with involvement of the oral cavity and mucocutaneous regions is seen.

The following steps are a guide to the diagnosis of scaling and crusting in the horse and ruminants:

1. History (see Fig. 11-1)
   a. In particular, determine if the patient is pruritic.
   b. Determine if contact animals of the same or different species are affected. If they are, a contagious problem should be considered: fungal (dermatophytosis), bacterial (dermatophilosis), viral, or parasitic.
   c. Check for seasonality. A seasonal problem suggests a parasitic cause. Lice are a problem in winter, trombiculidiasis tends to occur in the fall, and most of the flying insects are present in the spring, summer, and early fall. Most parasitic dermatoses are also pruritic.
   d. Determine what medications have been given systemically or applied to the patient. Use of certain topical agents may suggest a diagnosis of contact dermatitis, whereas administration of systemic medications may suggest that the etiology is a drug hypersensitivity.
2. Physical examination (see Fig. 11-2)
   a. Look for evidence of excoriation, suggesting that pruritus is a feature.
   b. Inspect the coat closely for small but grossly visible parasites such as lice or their eggs.
   c. Inspect contact animals for evidence of disease, suggesting a contagious etiology.
3. Skin scrapings
4. Acetate tape preparations
5. Dermatophyte culture and KOH preparation
6. *Dermatophilus* preparation
7. Biopsy for routine histopathologic examination (careful histologic examination of scale and crusts is essential to the search for the underlying cause of their formation)
8. Microfilarial preparation
9. Biopsy for direct immunofluorescence testing
10. Bacterial culture and sensitivity

REFERENCES

13. Ackerman AB: *Histologic diagnosis of inflammatory skin diseases: a method by pattern analysis,* 1978, Lea & Febiger.
14. Muller GH, Kirk RW, Scott DW: *Small animal dermatology,* ed 3, Philadelphia, 1983, WB Saunders.
15. Montagna W, Parakkal PF: *The structure and function of the skin,* ed 3, New York, 1974, Academic Press.

ABNORMAL COAT LENGTH AND DENSITY

Definition

Abnormalities in coat length and density can be subdivided into decreased coat length and density (alopecia, hypotrichosis) and increased coat length and density (hirsutism, hypertrichosis). Hirsutism, or excessive body hair, is far less common than alopecia, which is an absence of hair from areas where hair is normally present. Alopecias are usually classified as scarring (cicatricial) or nonscarring (noncicatricial). In cicatricial alopecias the hair follicles are destroyed, and hair loss is permanent because neogenesis of the hair follicle does not occur in an adult. In nonscarring alopecias the hair follicles are retained; therefore the potential for regrowth remains.[16] Both alopecia and hirsutism may be complete or partial, diffuse or focal, congenital or acquired.

Mechanisms of Development of Abnormal Coat Length and Density

A basic understanding of the dynamics of hair structure and development is essential to an understanding of the mechanisms associated with pathologic changes in coat length and density.

The hair follicle and the sebaceous and apocrine glands are epidermal appendages. The hair follicle forms during fetal development as a downgrowth of epidermal cells toward a group of mesenchymal cells that ultimately become the dermal papillae. The sebaceous and apocrine glands begin as buds of epithelium from the sides of the developing hair follicle.

Hair is composed of keratin and is the product of the hair follicle. The hair shaft is the part of the hair that emerges from the skin surface. The hair root is the part of the hair in the follicle. The hair bulb is a knob of epidermal cells that attaches the follicle to the dermal papilla. The hair follicle and shaft each have distinct layers. There are two types of hair follicles: simple and compound. A simple hair follicle produces a single hair. A compound hair follicle produces multiple hairs with bundles of hairs sharing a common skin opening and a single follicle down to the level of the sebaceous gland. Below the sebaceous gland the follicle branches so that each hair has its own hair bulb. Horses and cattle have only simple follicles. Goats and sheep have a mixture of simple and compound hair follicles (Fig. 11-7).

The normal hair growth cycle is divided into three repeating stages: anagen, catagen, and telogen, with the size and shape of the follicle changing during each stage (Fig. 11-8). The amount of time a follicle spends in each phase varies with the species, breed, individual, and body region. In addition, it is influenced by factors such as photoperiod, stress, and disease. Anagen is the active phase of hair growth. Catagen is the transition stage from the growing to the resting state. Catagen is short, and the hair quickly enters the telogen phase, in which hair growth stops. As the follicle reenters anagen, a new hair grows up beside the old and dislodges it. The signal that stimulates progression from telogen to anagen is unknown.[17]

Coat abnormalities may result from a multitude of endogenous and exogenous factors that can modify the normal pattern of hair growth and development.

The length, density, and texture of the coat of a normal animal are determined genetically, and a variety of hereditary defects result in coat abnormalities. These defects may cause changes in hair length, density, or quality. Coat quality may be abnormal at birth or may become apparent sometime before 6 months of age. A given defect may alter the number of follicles present in the skin, or the number of follicles present may be normal, but there may be genetic alterations in the way the hair is produced. Altered hair production may manifest as an increased or a decreased growth rate or as structural deformities that result in weak hair shafts that break easily.

Nutritional imbalances can affect growth and maintenance of the coat in various ways, depending on the species. Nutritional deficiencies may result in a shift of greater numbers of follicles into telogen, thus increasing shedding. Dietary carbohydrate and protein deficiencies reduce the length, diameter, and strength of hair. Reinforcing the diet with carbohydrate and protein releases protein for keratin formation, provides energy to use protein, and maintains mitotic activity in the hair matrix. Fatty acid deficiencies affect lipid production in the skin, leading to a dry coat with increased fragility. A variety of vitamin and mineral deficiencies may also result in poor hair growth or quality.

Inflammatory skin diseases frequently result in hair loss. Infectious inflammatory processes such as dermatophytosis and pyoderma are usually directed specifically at the hair or hair follicle. Inflammatory processes directed elsewhere may still affect the hair follicle by sweeping it up as an "innocent bystander."

Hormonal effects on hair growth are complex. Thyroid hormones, corticosteroids, sex hormones, melanocyte-stimulating hormone (MSH), adrenocorticotropic hormone (ACTH), growth hormone, and prolactin all affect hair growth. The effect of a single hormone may be modified in the presence of other hormones, and the importance or effect of any one hormone on hair growth may differ from species to species. Hormonal variations affect the hair coat quality and length by altering the period of time that hair follicles spend in any given part of the cycle, by influencing the rate of hair growth, and by inducing follicular atrophy. External factors such as changes in the photoperiod influence hair growth by altering hormonal levels.[17,18]

Trauma to the skin is a frequent secondary cause of hair loss. Self-trauma induced by pruritus is the most common cause of alopecia. Hairs may be lost either from trauma to the hair shaft, resulting in breakage, or from trauma to the dermis, resulting in destruction of the hair follicle. In the former case, the hair regrows once the source of trauma has been removed. In the latter case, hair loss is permanent.

A variety of factors can result in hair loss by causing an abrupt shift of hairs into the telogen phase. Recognized causes of telogen effluvium include stress from high fever or severe illness and parturition.[18]

Approach to Diagnosis of Abnormal Coat Length and Density

The differential diagnosis of abnormalities resulting in increased coat and length density is relatively limited and does not provide much of a diagnostic dilemma for the clinician. In the horse increased coat length and density is an acquired abnormality associated with equine hyperadrenocorticism. In ruminants all the defects are congenital and are either the result of an in utero infection (border disease) or a breed-specific hereditary defect.

The diagnostic approach to decreased coat length and density is not so simple because the differential to be considered is extensive. The initial step is to determine if the alopecia is congenital, implying a hereditary defect, or acquired. If the abnormality is acquired, the clinician must determine if it is a primary alopecia or secondary to another cutaneous abnormality such as pruritus or ulceration. If alopecia is the result of another primary cutaneous abnormality, the clinician should focus on the differential associated with that primary abnormality. Finally, to help provide a prognosis for hair regrowth, the clinician must biopsy to determine if the alopecia is scarring (cicatricial) or nonscarring (noncicatricial). Irrespective of the underlying cause and its resolution, hair will not regrow with a cicatricial alopecia

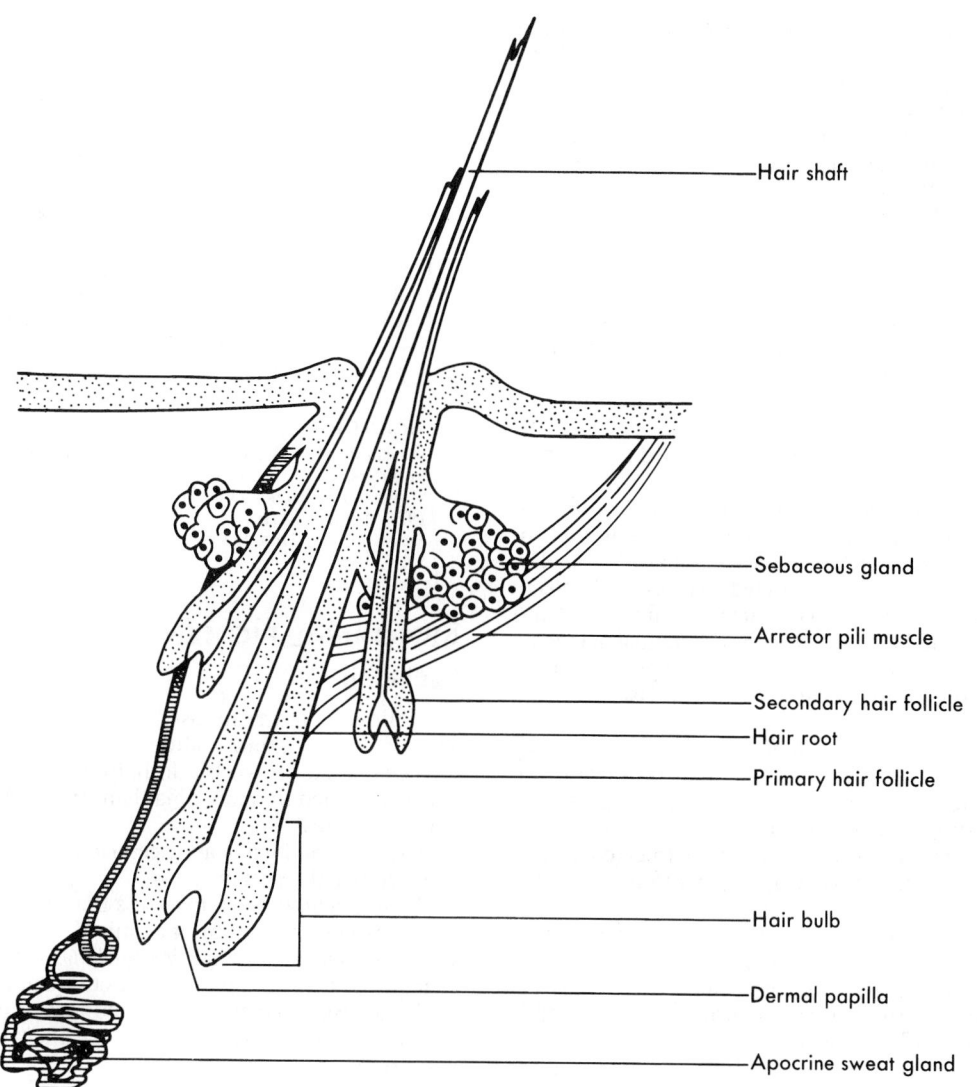

Hair shaft

Sebaceous gland

Arrector pili muscle

Secondary hair follicle

Hair root

Primary hair follicle

Hair bulb

Dermal papilla

Apocrine sweat gland

FIG. 11-7 ▓ Longitudinal section of a compound hair follicle.

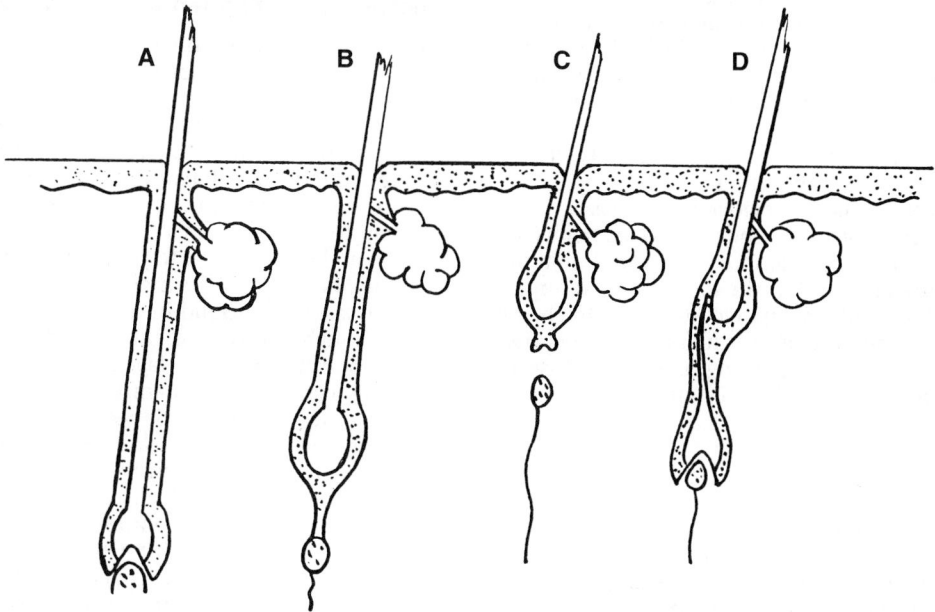

FIG. 11-8 ▓ Stages of the hair growth cycle. **A,** Anagen. **B,** Catagen. **C,** Telogen. **D,** Early anagen.

because by definition the hair follicle has been destroyed. In a noncicatricial alopecia the potential for hair regrowth remains as long as the underlying cause for hair loss can be identified and resolved.

The following steps are a guide to the diagnosis of decreased coat length and density in the horse and ruminants:
1. History (see Fig. 11-1)
   a. Determine whether the lesions are congenital or acquired. If they are congenital, determine if any relatives are affected and if the lesions have progressed since birth.
   b. If the alopecia is acquired, determine if the animal is pruritic and if other cutaneous lesions in addition to alopecia have been observed.
   c. Determine if the animal's diet is nutritionally complete.
   d. Determine if the animal has been exposed to any toxic substances.
   e. Determine if contact animals of the same or different species are affected. If contact animals are affected, a contagious problem such as dermatophytosis or dermatophilosis should be considered. Because feed and environment are also shared, dietary deficiencies and toxicities should be included in the differential diagnosis.
   f. Determine what medications have been given systemically or applied topically to the patient. Use of certain topical agents, along with a history of an inflammatory stage preceding or coincident with the alopecia, may suggest a diagnosis of contact dermatitis. Administration of systemic medications may suggest that the etiology is a drug hypersensitivity.
   g. Determine if the animal has been subjected to any stresses that might provoke a telogen effluvium.
2. Physical examination (see Fig. 11-2)
   a. Check for evidence of disease in organ systems other than the skin. Does the animal appear thin and malnourished, suggesting hair loss related to a dietary deficiency? Is it febrile or suffering from a severe systemic disease, suggesting a telogen effluvium?
   b. Can the hairs be epilated readily from the coat? If not, hair loss may be caused by trauma (self-induced or external). If so, underlying nutritional, hormonal, or stress-related causes of alopecia are more likely.
   c. Look for evidence of excoriation, suggesting that self-trauma is the cause of the hair loss.
   d. Determine whether the lesions are generalized or localized, either to particular areas of the body or to certain hair colors (e.g., black hair follicle dystrophy of Appaloosas). Note if the hair loss has a symmetric pattern.
   e. Inspect the coat closely for small but grossly visible parasites such as lice or their eggs.
   f. Inspect contact animals for evidence of disease.
3. Microscopic examination of the ends of affected hairs (Are the ends of the hairs sharply blunted, suggesting that the hair shaft has broken and that the hair loss is traumatically induced? If the ends are tapered, it is more likely the hairs are being lost because of follicular atrophy, because follicles are shifting into the telogen phase, or because an inflammatory process is affecting the hair root.)
4. Skin scrapings
5. Acetate tape preparations
6. Dermatophyte culture and KOH preparation
7. Microfilarial preparation
8. Biopsy for routine histopathologic examination (Sagittal sections should be evaluated to determine the proportion of hairs in the anagen, catagen, and telogen phases; for the presence or absence of inflammation and infectious organisms; and for evidence of scarring, which suggests a poor prognosis for hair regrowth. Cross-sections of the biopsy specimen should be evaluated in noninflammatory alopecias to determine the number of hair follicles present per given area.)

The following steps are a guide to the diagnosis of increased coat length and density in the horse and ruminants:
1. Horses demonstrating increased coat length and density should be evaluated with appropriate laboratory tests for hyperadrenocorticism.
2. Lambs with increased coat length and density should be evaluated for evidence of border disease.
3. Cattle with increased coat length and density probably have hereditary hypertrichosis.

REFERENCES

16. Moschella SL, Hurley HJ: *Dermatology*, ed 2, Philadelphia, 1985, WB Saunders.
17. Montagna W, Parakkal PF: *The structure and function of the skin*, New York, 1974, Academic Press.
18. Fadok VA: The dynamics of hair growth and development, *Dermatol Rep* 4:4-6, 1985.

ABNORMAL PIGMENTATION

Definition

The following terms are used when discussing pigmentation and pigmentary abnormalities.
- *Melanin* is a brown-black, light-absorbing, insoluble pigment formed in many organisms by specialized cells called melanocytes.
- *Hyperpigmentation* is an excessive tissue deposition of pigment, usually melanin.
- *Hypopigmentation* refers to less than normal pigmentation and can be congenital or acquired.
- *Leukoderma (acroderma, hypomelanosis)* is a partial or total acquired loss of melanin pigment from the skin. The term *vitiligo* also refers to an acquired loss of melanin from the skin but is often reserved for a specific type of leukoderma found in humans.
- *Leukotrichia (acromotrichia)* is an acquired loss of pigment from the hair.
- *Albinism* is a congenital lack of pigment in all tissues.

Mechanisms of Pigmentation Abnormalities

Cutaneous pigmentation results from the interaction of melanocytes and keratinocytes. The degree of "baseline" pigmentation observed in an animal is genetically controlled. Melanocytes are presumed to be of neural crest origin and to migrate from this site during embryologic development. They are present in nearly all tissues but occur in the highest numbers in the epidermis, mucous membrane epithelium, dermis, hair follicles, leptomeninges, uveal tract, and retina. Epidermal melanocytes are found in the basal cell layer, and each melanocyte supplies melanin to 10 to 40 keratinocytes. Melanin is usually found in the deeper layers of the epidermis, although darkly pigmented animals may have melanin throughout the epidermal layers.

Melanocytes produce membrane-bound organelles called melanosomes that fuse with vesicles containing the enzyme tyrosinase. Melanin, a black-brown pigment, is produced from tyrosine in the presence of tyrosinase and copper. It is deposited on the protein matrix in the melanosomes. Once melanosomes are fully melanized, they disperse to the periphery of the dendrites of the epidermal melanocytes, and the dendritic tips are phagocytized by keratinocytes. Melanin is also synthesized and transferred to cells of the hair shaft during the anagen phase.[19,20]

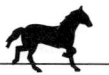

In general, mechanisms associated with pathologic pigmentary disturbances in large animals are poorly understood. Hyperpigmentation results from increased amounts of melanin in the epidermis or dermis or both. The melanin may be present in melanocytes, keratinocytes, or melanophages (dermal histiocytes that have phagocytized melanin pigment). Hyperpigmentation is an uncommon problem in horses because most normally have darkly pigmented skin. Factors that promote pigmentation in human beings include hormonal influences, ultraviolet light (UVL), inflammation, and friction, but the influence of these factors in altering the normal pigmentation of large animals is unclear. Hyperpigmentation is reversible. With removal of the pigment-promoting stimulus, it tends to decline over time to the baseline level.

Melanocyte-stimulating hormone (melanotropin) is among the hormones shown in experimental situations to stimulate hyperpigmentation. MSH acts by affecting the levels of cyclic adenosine monophosphate (cAMP), resulting in increased tyrosinase activity. MSH also causes increased dispersion of melanosomes into melanocyte dendritic processes, where they are phagocytized by keratinocytes. Increased levels of ACTH in human beings, such as occurs in pituitary hyperadrenocorticism and primary hypoadrenocorticism, results in hyperpigmentation. Hyperpigmentation is also noted with increased levels of estrogens, progesterones, and androgens, although the mode of action of these hormones on melanocytes is not known.

The role of UVL on the pigmentary system is evident in humans and may also be a factor in stimulating pigment synthesis in large animals. UVB (290 to 320 nm), the major influence, causes increased tyrosinase activity that leads to increased pigment formation, an increase in the number of melanosomes, and increased transfer from melanocytic dendrites to keratinocytes.

Inflammation from a variety of causes and persistent cutaneous trauma from friction induce hyperpigmentation. Stimuli that have been shown to result in hyperpigmentation in human beings and that may be factors in large animals include physical cutaneous damage (trauma, friction), chemicals (primary irritants, allergic sensitizers, photosensitizers), infectious agents, and nutritional disturbances.[19,20] The mechanism of inflammatory-induced hyperpigmentation may be related to the production of prostaglandins from arachidonic acid.

Hypopigmentation is the result of a decreased amount of melanin in the epidermis or dermis (or both) and may be congenital or acquired. Possible mechanisms include decreased melanin production (defects in melanocyte migration during embryogenesis or disorders of melanin synthesis), decreased dispersion of melanin granules (defective transfer of melanin to keratinocytes), and increased loss of melanin (accelerated desquamation of epidermal melanin, epidermal pigment loss caused by disruption of the basement membrane with resultant pigment incontinence, or immunologic destruction of melanin or melanocytes).[19]

Several congenital genetic abnormalities that result in partial or total hypopigmentation have been identified in large animals. Albinism is a recessive condition in which a normal complement of melanocytes is present but a biochemical defect results in lack of ability to synthesize tyrosinase, so that melanin is not produced. There is complete lack of melanin in all tissues in a true albino. Pseudoalbinism, in which there is ocular pigmentation, is more common. Other genetic disorders include abnormal melanosome production and abnormalities in melanocyte development and migration from the neural crest (piebaldism).[19-21]

Acquired hypopigmentation (leukoderma) may be caused by several factors, including genetic abnormalities, trauma, inflammation, dietary imbalances, hormonal influences, and immunologic disorders. In some cases acquired hypopigmentation is idiopathic.[19] Juvenile Arabian leukoderma appears to have a genetic basis because of the predilection for the Arabian breed and the occurrence of the disease in young animals.[22] Trauma and inflammation are the most common factors associated with depigmentation, particularly in the horse. The intensity of the inflammatory reaction may bear little relation to the degree of postinflammatory leukoderma.[19] Dietary abnormalities, particularly molybdenum toxicity and copper deficiency, are associated with faded or washed out coat color in food animals.[21] Severe protein deficiency, such as occurs in kwashiorkor in humans, can lead to deficient melanin pigmentation.[19] Melatonin is a hormone produced by the pineal gland that antagonizes MSH, thus causing decreased pigmentation, although an association with pathologic hypopigmentation in large animals has not been documented. Immunologic destruction of melanocytes has been documented in humans and is suspected of being a factor in acquired hypopigmentation in the dog but has not yet been documented in large animals.[19,23] Idiopathic leukodermas are noted in all species.

Leukotrichia is the result of decreased amounts of melanin in the hair shaft. In most cases the pathogenesis is speculative, and the actual factors are unknown. Melanocytes in the hair bulbs can be affected independently of melanocytes in the epidermis, and leukotrichia without a coexistent leukoderma is common. Leukoderma, however, is usually accompanied by leukotrichia; thus, when seen in combination, the pathogenesis of the two syndromes is the same. Several leukotrichias that occur independently of leukoderma appear to be genetically induced because of breed predilections (e.g., reticulated leukotrichia of quarter horses and spotted leukotrichia of Arabians). In addition, a viral infection is suspected as one of the causes of hyperesthetic leukotrichia of horses.[22]

Approach to Diagnosis of Pigmentation Abnormalities

The initial approach to diagnosis of pigmentary abnormalities is to determine whether the defect is congenital or acquired. Congenital pigmentary abnormalities are almost always caused by a genetic defect, whereas acquired abnormalities most commonly do not have a hereditary basis, although there are exceptions. If the abnormality is acquired, the clinician must determine if it is a primary pigmentary abnormality or if it is associated with some other pathologic change such as inflammation or trauma. If associated changes are a feature of the disease, differential diagnosis should focus on the initial pathologic changes.

The following steps are a guide to the diagnosis of pigmentation abnormalities in the horse and ruminants:
1. History (see Fig. 11-1)
   a. If the pigmentary change is congenital, determine if related animals are affected and if the lesions have progressed or regressed since birth. Take note of the patient's signalment and determine if that breed has been documented to have congenital pigmentary abnormalities.
   b. If the pigmentary change is acquired, determine if the animal has been subjected to cutaneous trauma, which could result in posttraumatic pigmentary change. Determine if other cutaneous lesions in addition to the pigmentary changes have been observed (e.g., inflammation, ulceration).
   c. Determine if the animal's diet is nutritionally complete and balanced.
   d. Determine if the animal has been exposed to any toxic substances.
   e. Determine if contact animals of the same or different species are affected. Because feed and environment are shared, if contact animals are affected, dietary imbal-

ances and toxicities should be included in the differential diagnosis.

    f. If the affected animal is a horse, determine what parasiticidal agents have been administered and if they are effective for microfilaria of *Onchocerca cervicalis*.

2. Physical examination (see Fig. 11-2)

    a. Check for evidence of disease in organ systems other than the skin. Does the animal appear thin and malnourished, suggesting a pigmentary change secondary to a dietary deficiency or toxicity?

    b. If the patient's problem is hypopigmentation, examine the coat closely to determine if leukoderma, leukotrichia, or both are present.

    c. Look for evidence of other cutaneous lesions (inflammation, ulceration) that could result in postinflammatory pigmentary changes.

3. Microfilarial preparation

4. Biopsy for routine histopathologic examination (Affected, unaffected, and marginally affected areas should all be biopsied and labeled appropriately for histologic comparison.)

REFERENCES

19. Moschella SL, Hurley HJ: *Dermatology,* ed 2, Philadelphia, 1985, WB Saunders.
20. Montagna W, Parakkal PF: *The structure and function of the skin,* New York, 1974, Academic Press.
21. Blood DC, Radostits OM, Henderson JA: *Veterinary medicine,* ed 6, London, 1983, Baillière Tindall.
22. Stannard AA: *Modern veterinary practice seminars: equine dermatology,* Santa Barbara, Calif, Oct 1 and 2, 1984.
23. Muller GH, Kirk RW, Scott DW: *Small animal dermatology,* ed 3, Philadelphia, 1983, WB Saunders.

Alterations in Sexual Function

MATS H.T. TROEDSSON

Consulting Editor

MAJOR CLINICAL SIGNS/PROBLEMS ENCOUNTERED

ALTERATIONS IN MALE SEXUAL FUNCTION

PATRICK M. McCUE

To be a satisfactory breeder under natural service conditions, the stallion or male ruminant must have (1) normal genital organs, (2) the libido necessary to tease females and gain an erection, (3) the physical ability to mount and intromit the penis into the female's vagina, and (4) an adequate number of normal spermatozoa in each ejaculate. Digression from normal sexual function in males usually is recognized clinically by changes in sexual behavior, abnormalities or diseases of the genital organs, or a decreased pregnancy rate in dams bred.

MECHANISMS OF ALTERED MALE SEXUAL FUNCTION

Sexual function may be altered by any of four major mechanisms: general physical abnormalities, abnormalities of the genital organs, decreased libido, or poor semen quality (Boxes 12-1 and 12-2).

The male must be mobile enough, especially in a pasture breeding program, to locate, tease, mount, and breed estral females successfully. Musculoskeletal abnormalities may limit reproductive ability or desire. Hindlimb conformation defects and back problems in bulls and rams, degenerative joint disease involving the hock in stallions, and foot problems in rams are examples of conditions that may cause enough discomfort to interfere with the normal breeding process or prevent normal mobility, impairing reproductive performance.[1-3]

Congenital or acquired abnormalities of the genital organs, including the penis, prepuce, scrotum, testicles, spermatic cords, or accessory sex glands, can lead to altered sexual function or infertility. Congenital abnormalities such as persistent penile frenulum and penile deviations in bulls may prevent normal intromission.[4] Acquired lesions such as a penile hematoma caused by rupture of the tunica albuginea of bulls at time of service may limit sexual function by causing paraphimosis, adhesions, or sensory nerve damage.[5]

Libido is an essential component of breeding performance but may be difficult to measure during a breeding soundness examination. Libido has been demonstrated to be an inherited behavioral trait in bulls.[6]

Semen volume, the concentration of spermatozoa, the percentage of progressive motility, and the percentage of morphologically normal spermatozoa are semen parameters

---

BOX 12-1

Causes of Altered Sexual Function in Stallions

ABNORMALITIES OF THE PENIS
Balanoposthitis
Paraphimosis
Phimosis
Trauma
Hematoma, seroma
Abscess
Urolithiasis
Equine coital exanthema
Tumor (squamous cell carcinoma)
Cutaneous habronemiasis (equine summer sores)
Improper use of stallion rings

ABNORMALITIES OF THE PREPUCE
Trauma
Foreign body
Preputial stenosis
Balanoposthitis
Tumor (squamous cell carcinoma, sarcoid)
Hematoma
Abscess
Cutaneous habronemiasis
Varicosities of the preputial vein
Equine viral arteritis

ABNORMALITIES OF THE TESTICLES, SPERMATIC CORD, AND SCROTUM
Testicular hypoplasia, atrophy
Testicular degeneration
Segmental aplasia
Testicular, scrotal neoplasia
Thrombosis of the spermatic cord
Torsion of the spermatic cord
Orchitis, epididymitis
Sperm, parasitic granuloma
Trauma
Hematoma, hematocele
Inguinal, scrotal hernia
Androgen, anabolic steroid effects
Cryptorchidism
Pseudohermaphrodism
Actinomycosis
Chemical irritation of the scrotum
Equine viral arteritis

LACK OF LIBIDO
Malnutrition, protein-calorie starvation
Testicular neoplasia

LACK OF LIBIDO—cont'd
Lameness
Trauma, foreign body of the prepuce
Overuse
Equine coital exanthema
Iodine deficiency
Penile trauma, hematoma, abscess
Psychologic impotence

INFERTILITY
Segmental aplasia of the reproductive tract
Vesicular gland adenitis
Malnutrition, protein-calorie starvation
Testicular degeneration
Testicular hypoplasia, atrophy
Testicular neoplasia
Thrombosis of the spermatic cord
Torsion of the spermatic cord
Urolithiasis
Vitamin A deficiency
Hemospermia
Lameness
Iatrogenic causes, including artificial insemination–associated infertility
Bacterial contamination of the semen
Brucellosis
Trauma, foreign body of the prepuce
Balanoposthitis
Paraphimosis
Orchitis, epididymitis
Sperm, parasitic granuloma
Androgen, anabolic steroid use
Testicular trauma, hematoma, hematocele
Chromosomal abnormalities
Hermaphrodism, pseudohermaphrodism
Cryptorchidism
Ejaculation failure
Frostbite
Abnormalities of spermatogenesis
Sperm storage dysfunction
Iodine deficiency
Heat stress, heat stroke
Inguinal, scrotal hernia
Psychologic impotence

---

measured during a breeding soundness examination. Abnormalities of semen quality associated with decreased fertility in bulls include spermatozoa morphology and, to a lesser degree, motility.[2,4]

Approach to Diagnosis of Altered Male Sexual Function

A complete breeding soundness examination and history should be obtained, including vaccinations, number of females bred each year, conception rates, breeding methods (natural service or artificial insemination), and results of previous breeding soundness examinations (Box 12-3). The animal should be given a general physical examination. Hindlimb conformation, the presence of degenerative joint disease, laminitis, foot abscesses, abnormal foot wear, interdigital fibromas (bulls), foot rot (rams), and caprine arthritis-encephalitis (CAE) (bucks) should be noted. An ophthalmologic examination should be done to ensure that the animal has adequate vision and that no significant pathologic condition is present. Range animals showing weight loss and a decline in reproductive performance should be given an oral examination, and the parasite control program should be evaluated.

The external genital organs should be examined carefully. The penis of the stallion is easiest to examine after an erection is obtained by teasing to an estral female. In ruminants

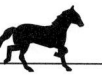

BOX 12-2

Causes of Altered Male Sexual Function in Ruminants

ABNORMALITIES OF THE PENIS
Penile deviation (B)
Balanoposthitis
Paraphimosis
Phimosis
Penile-preputial adhesions (B)
Penile hair ring (B)
Penile trauma, hematoma, abscess
Urethral calculi
Ruptured urethra
Persistent penile frenulum (B)
Papillomatosis
Infectious bovine pustular vulvovaginitis (B)
Herpes vulvovaginitis (C)
Ovine ulcerative dermatosis (O)

ABNORMALITIES OF THE PREPUCE
Abscess, cellulitis
Balanoposthitis
Trauma
Foreign body
Preputial stenosis
Prolapsed prepuce
Ulcerative posthitis (pizzle rot)
Ovine ulcerative dermatosis (O)

ABNORMALITIES OF THE TESTICLES, SPERMATIC CORDS, AND SCROTUM
Scrotal abscess (O)
Orchitis, epididymitis
Segmental granuloma, spermatocele
Testicular degeneration
Testicular hypoplasia, atrophy
Varicocele
Zinc deficiency
Testicular tumors
Brucellosis (B, O)
Testicular trauma, hematoma, hematocele
Inguinal, scrotal hernia
Cryptorchidism
Actinomycosis
Intersex in polled goats (C)
Pseudohermaphrodism (C)
Progressive degenerative myeloencephalopathy of Brown
    Swiss cattle (B)

LACK OF LIBIDO
Malnutrition, protein-calorie starvation
Ulcerative posthitis
Vertebral osteophytosis, spondylosis (B)
Zinc deficiency
Lameness
Trauma, foreign body of the prepuce
Prolapsed prepuce (B, O)
Loss of penile sensation (B)
Penile hair ring (B)
Corpus cavernosum vascular shunts (B)
Iodine deficiency
Psychologic impotence
Penile trauma, hematoma, abscess
Persistent penile frenulum (B)
Epididymitis, orchitis (O, C)
Intersex in polled goats (C)
Progressive degenerative myeloencephalopathy of Brown
    Swiss cattle (B)

LACK OF LIBIDO—cont'd
Obesity
Spondylosis (B)

INFERTILITY
Testicular degeneration
Orchitis, epididymitis
Trauma, foreign body of the prepuce
Paraphimosis
Heat stress, heat stroke
Penile trauma, hematoma, abscess
Segmental aplasia
Vesicular gland adenitis
Sperm granuloma, spermatocele
Malnutrition, protein-calorie starvation
Testicular hypoplasia, atrophy
Ulcerative posthitis (pizzle rot)
Urolithiasis
Varicocele
Vitamin A deficiency
Zinc deficiency
Manganese deficiency
Iodine deficiency
Hemospermia
Lameness
Iatrogenic, including artificial insemination–associated
    infertility
Balanoposthitis
Testicular trauma, hematoma, hematocele
Cryptorchidism
Dermatophilosis
Frostbite
Inguinal, scrotal hernia
Psychologic impotence
Hermaphrodism, pseudohermaphrodism
Short retractor penis muscle in Dutch Friesian bulls (B)
Abscess of scrotum (O)
Prolapsed prepuce (B, O)
Penile deviation (B)
Penile-preputial adhesions (B)
Vertebral osteophytosis, spondylosis (B)
Testicular tumors (B, O)
Bulls co-twin with freemartins (B)
Progressive degenerative myeloencephalopathy of Brown
    Swiss cattle (B)
Infectious bovine rhinotracheitis–contaminated semen (B)
Infectious bovine rhinotracheitis–associated dermatitis (B)
Bovine virus diarrhea–contaminated semen (B)
Chromosomal abnormalities (B, O)
Loss of penile sensation (B)
Penile hair ring (B)
Bovine herpesvirus type 1
Corpus cavernosum vascular shunt (B)
Urethral fistula (B)
Cold weather–associated infertility (B)
Papillomatosis, warts (B)
Abnormalities of spermatogenesis
Micropenis, penile hypoplasia (B)
Persistent penile frenulum (B)
Ovine ulcerative dermatosis (O)
Congenital phimosis (O)
Overuse
Chorioptic mange (O, C)
Hexachlorophene toxicity
Gynecomastia (C)

B, Bovine; *C,* caprine; *O,* ovine.

**Outline of a Breeding Soundness Examination
for Diagnosis of Male Infertility**

1. Species, breed
2. Age
3. Month of evaluation
4. Breeding history
5. Physical examination
   a. General
   b. External genital organs
      (1) Penis
      (2) Prepuce
      (3) Testes
      (4) Scrotum
      (5) Epididymides
6. Libido
7. Mating ability
8. Semen evaluation
   a. Motility
   b. Concentration
   c. Morphology
   d. Volume
9. Microbiologic culture
10. Serologic tests

manual palpation of the penis per rectum or by use of an electroejaculator is suitable in many cases. The penis should be normal in size and shape and free of lesions. In bulls, deviations or other abnormal configurations such as corkscrew penis may occur with use of an electroejaculator and therefore cannot be considered abnormal.[5] Rams and bucks should be carefully examined for abnormalities of the urethral process, including the presence of calculi.[8] The lesions most often observed on the penis of stallions are squamous cell carcinoma and cutaneous habronemiasis.[9,10]

The prepuce should also be examined for lesions. Strictures of the preputial orifice may increase the risk of phimosis or paraphimosis. Bulls of the *Bos indicus* breeds often have a pendulous prepuce that is predisposed to traumatic injury, abscessation, stricture formation, and eversion.[5,11] Ulcerative posthitis (pizzle rot) caused by *Corynebacterium renale* in rams on a high-protein diet is the most common lesion of the prepuce in rams.[12]

The scrotum, testicles, and spermatic cords should be examined for size, consistency, symmetry, and presence of lesions. Two scrotal testicles should be present, each smooth, resilient on palpation, and freely movable. The scrotal circumference should be measured in ruminants and the scrotal width measured in stallions. These measurements are correlated with the amount of testicular parenchyma and therefore the capacity to produce spermatozoa. Mature stallions should have a scrotal width of at least 8 cm. Yearling beef bulls should have a scrotal circumference of 30 cm or more, depending on the animal's age and breed.[7] The epididymides should be palpated for position, size, and presence of lesions. The most common palpable abnormality in rams is epididymitis caused by infection with *Brucella ovis*, *Actinobacillus seminis*, or *Histophilus ovis*.[8,12,13] A definitive diagnosis is obtained by isolation of bacterial organisms in the semen and serologic testing.

Diseases of the accessory sex glands are diagnosed most frequently in bulls. Vesicular gland adenitis is clinically recognized by the presence of leukocytes in the semen and enlargement, induration, and loss of lobulation noted during palpation and ultrasonographic examination of the glands per rectum.[14,15]

Libido and the ability to mate should be assessed after the physical examination. The male should be teased to a female in estrus. Interest in and interactions with the female and ability to gain an erection, mount, intromit the penis into the vagina (or into an artificial vagina), and ejaculate are noted. Libido and mating ability cannot be evaluated when using an electroejaculator to collect semen from ruminants.

The evaluation of semen quality is a major part of the breeding soundness examination. Semen from stallions is collected into an artificial vagina. Semen from ruminants may be collected into an artificial vagina or obtained by use of an electroejaculator. Semen collected by electroejaculation usually has a higher volume and a lower concentration of spermatozoa than semen collected by an artificial vagina. Semen quality in ruminants is scored primarily on the basis of motility and morphology.[7] Evaluation of semen from stallions should include determination of motility, concentration, morphology, and volume. The motility of the spermatozoa should be evaluated microscopically on raw and extended semen immediately after collection. Concentration can be measured by use of a hemocytometer or a calibrated spectrophotometer. Morphology can be evaluated microscopically, using stained semen samples (e.g., eosin-nigrosin stain) or preferably phase-contrast microscopy. Computer-assisted semen analysis (CASA) exists but is not routinely available because of its expense. Most stallions are evaluated by the collection of two ejaculates 1 hour apart. The total number of progressively motile, morphologically normal spermatozoa in the second ejaculate is most critically evaluated. Occasionally ejaculates from stallions are collected once daily for 5 to 10 days to more fully evaluate potential fertility.[16]

The age of the stallion or male ruminant being evaluated for potential fertility may influence the semen parameters, measurements of the testicular size, mating ability, and libido. Puberty is attained in the male equine at 18 months, in the bull at 9 to 12 months, and in the ram and buck at 7 to 8 months.[17] Semen parameters and testicular size continue to increase until sexual maturity is reached. The season of the year in which the fertility evaluation is done may affect semen parameters in the stallion, ram, and buck.

Microbiologic samples should be routinely collected when evaluating infertility in the stallion and when evaluating high-risk populations of bulls. Smegma samples should be collected from the prepuce of bulls and cultured for *Trichomonas foetus* and *Campylobacter fetus*. Swabs from the preejaculate and postejaculate urethra, semen, and fossa glandis of stallions should be cultured for potentially pathogenic bacterial organisms, especially *Taylorella equigenitalis*, *Pseudomonas aeruginosa*, and *Klebsiella pneumoniae*.[9] The semen of rams should be cultured for *B. ovis*, *A. seminis*, and *H. ovis*.[8,12,13]

It must be emphasized that the breeding soundness examination is a measure of potential fertility.[18] True fertility can only be determined by the results of breeding trials or by conception and live birthrates in dams bred.

REFERENCES

1. Slusher SH: Infertility and diseases of the reproductive tract of stallions. In Youngquist RS, ed: *Current therapy in large animal theriogenology*, Philadelphia, 1997, WB Saunders.
2. Barth AD: Evaluation of potential breeding soundness of the bull. In Youngquist RS, ed: *Current therapy in large animal theriogenology*, Philadelphia, 1997, WB Saunders.
3. Kimberling CV, Marsh DJ: Breeding soundness evaluation and surgical sterilization of the ram. In Youngquist RS, ed: *Current therapy in large animal theriogenology*, Philadelphia, 1997, WB Saunders.
4. Hopkins FM: Diseases of the reproductive system of the bull. In Youngquist RS, ed: *Current therapy in large animal theriogenology*, Philadelphia, 1997, WB Saunders.

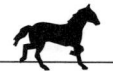

5. Ott RS: Breeding soundness examination of bulls. In Morrow DA, ed: *Current therapy in theriogenology: diagnosis, treatment, and prevention of reproductive diseases in small and large animals*, ed 2, Philadelphia, 1986, WB Saunders.

6. Chenoweth PJ: Libido testing. In Morrow DA, ed: *Current therapy in theriogenology: diagnosis, treatment, and prevention of reproductive diseases in small and large animals*, ed 2, Philadelphia, 1986, WB Saunders.

7. Chenoweth PJ, Spitzer JC, Hopkins FM: A new bull breeding soundness evaluation form, *Proc Soc Theriogenol*, 1992, pp 63-70.

8. Ott RS, Memom MA: *Sheep and goat manual*, vol 10, Hastings, Neb, 1980, Society for Theriogenology.

9. Kenney RM et al: *Clinical fertility evaluation of the stallion*, Hastings, Neb, 1983, Society for Theriogenology.

10. Blanchard TL: Stallion genital tract pathology, *Proc Soc Theriogenol*, 1987, pp 88-117.

11. Memom MA et al: Preputial injuries in beef bulls: 172 cases (1980-1985), *J Am Vet Med Assoc* 193:481-485, 1988.

12. Bruere AN: Examination of the ram for breeding soundness. In Morrow DA, ed: *Current therapy in theriogenology: diagnosis, treatment, and prevention of reproductive diseases in small and large animals*, ed 2, Philadelphia, 1986, WB Saunders.

13. Walker RL et al: Association of age of ram with distribution of epididymal lesions and etiologic agent, *J Am Vet Med Assoc* 188:393-396, 1986.

14. Linhart RD, Parker WG: Seminal vesiculitis in bulls, *Comp Cont Educ (Pract Vet)* 10:1428-1448, 1988.

15. Malmgren L, Sussemilch B-I: Ultrasonography as a diagnostic tool in a stallion with seminal vesiculitis: a case report, *Theriogenology* 37:935-938, 1992.

16. Love CC: Examination of the male reproductive tract: evaluation of potential breeding soundness. In Youngquist RS, ed: *Current therapy in large animal theriogenology*, Philadelphia, 1997, WB Saunders.

17. Roberts SJ: *Veterinary obstetrics and genital diseases (theriogenology)*, ed 3, North Pomfret, Vt, 1986, SJ Roberts.

18. Ott RS: Current thinking on breeding soundness examination of bulls, *Proc Soc Theriogenol*, 1987, pp 14-31.

CYCLIC IRREGULARITY

STEVEN D. Van CAMP

Cyclic irregularity refers to an abnormal interval from the first day of estrus until the first day of the subsequent estrus. The alteration in the cycle length may occur during estrus or during the interestrous interval. Irregular cycles may be related to erroneous estrous detection, seasonal transitions, corpus luteum life span alterations, ovulation derangements, embryo or fetal wastage, or behavioral aberrations. In some cases the cause of the cyclic irregularity is unknown.

Inaccurate heat detection may appear as irregular cycles. Missed heats should be expected if the heat intervals approximate multiples of the normal cycle length (e.g., 42 or 63 days in the cow or mare). Silent heats (no clinical signs of estrus) were found to occur less often than suspected when cows were observed 24 hours a day, although silent heats do sometimes occur. The first ovulation of the season (ewe and doe) and the initial postpartum ovulation in cows usually are silent. Substrum, weak, or short heats occur more commonly in the early postpartum period in the cow and may be due to insufficient progesterone priming of the behavior center for optimum expression of estrus.[19] Vaginal or urinary tract disease may cause frequent urination, which may be misinterpreted as estrus in mares.

Artificial insemination records may indicate that breedings are grouped so that two or more cows are bred the same day. This may indicate a failure to determine which animal is actually in heat. Short cycles may also indicate a lack of discrimination between the riding cow and the cow in standing heat. This type of error in estrous detection often results in the same cows being rebred within 3 days.

Anestrus is a particularly important type of cyclic irregularity with several causes. It is dealt with in a separate section of this chapter.

Nymphomania, a state of persistent or frequent heats, is the antithesis of anestrus. Many mares thought to be nymphomaniacal are actually exhibiting some degree of vir-ilism. Frequently their ovaries are small and firm and appear inactive. These mares may actually be aggressive toward the stallion instead of receptive.[20] The cause of this condition is unknown. Because frequent urination is associated with estrus in the mare, urine poolers, or mares with ectopic ureters or urethral anomalies are often mistaken for nymphomaniacs. Furthermore, nymphomania must be differentiated from behavioral abnormalities in a mare that is angry or upset. These temperamental mares frequently squirt urine and wink in association with tail wringing when forced to perform. Passive acceptance of the male, as can be seen in gonadal dysgenesis mares, can be mistaken for nymphomania. Mares with these chromosomal aberrations may accept service by the male, but they do not show the characteristic signs of estrous behavior in his presence. Nymphomania may be seen in cases of hormone-secreting ovarian tumors. Nymphomania also may indicate an ovulatory anomaly. Nymphomania in cows and goats is most often associated with ovarian follicular cysts. In ruminants, luteinized cysts, which cause anestrus, are more common.

MECHANISMS OF IRREGULAR CYCLES

Cyclic derangements occur either during estrus or in the interestrous interval. A delay in follicular maturation or ovulation may result in a prolonged proestrus or persistent estrus. This is seen in mares entering or leaving the physiologic breeding season in the transition from or to winter anestrus. It is likely the result of changing patterns of hypothalamic releasing factor and pituitary gonadotropin secretion.[21] Ovarian insensitivity to these substances may also play a role. The tubular tract may be insensitive to the ovarian hormones and may be atypical for the structures present on the ovaries.[22] This may be due to a lack of priming effect of progesterone on the tract. The estral behavior and ovarian structures may not correlate in these mares. They may have large follicles without heat or may show heat without large follicles being present. This may be due to changes in the central nervous system's response to the sex steroids during the transition season.

Failure of ovulation can result in prolonged estrus. Mares frequently form persistent follicles during the transitional seasons. These usually regress with time and are not a long-term cause of infertility.[23] Ovulation failure can result in the development of follicular cysts and frequent or persistent heats in cattle.[24]

Other ovulation irregularities include delayed ovulation and premature ovulation. Delayed ovulation rarely occurs in animals. What may appear to be delayed ovulation is often erroneous heat detection or premature breeding. Similarly, premature ovulation is often misdiagnosed because of inaccurate heat detection. Premature ovulation may be suspected in heat-stressed animals that only show heat for short periods at the peak of estrus, or during the cool of the night.[25]

The mare seems to have a unique type of ovulation anomaly. After having one or more normal cycles, mares may spontaneously have a fertile, diestrous ovulation without signs of estrus. If the new corpus luteum develops after day 10 of diestrus, it has not had time to mature and become sensitive to prostaglandin-induced lysis. Thus the mare skips the next expected estrus and has a prolonged diestrus.[23]

The corpus luteum controls the length of diestrus and the interestrous interval in cycling animals. Premature lysis of the corpus luteum results in a short interestrous interval. If prostaglandin-induced lysis of the corpus luteum is prevented, the corpus luteum persists and a prolonged diestrus results.

Irritation or inflammation of the endometrium may cause premature release of prostaglandin and lysis of the mature corpus luteum, resulting in a short interestrous interval.

Irritation of the endometrium late in diestrus may interfere with the action of prostaglandin on the mature corpus luteum, leading to a prolonged diestrus. Intrauterine therapy with irritating solutions may alter the interestrous interval, depending on when they are administered in the cycle. Treatment between 4 and 10 days after ovulation causes a short cycle in the cow. Intrauterine treatment late in diestrus, 15 to 17 days after ovulation, results in a prolonged cycle, presumably because of a disruption of the synthesis or release of prostaglandin. In both cases the mare comes into heat 7 to 10 days after treatment.[26] Inadvertent intrauterine insemination during diestrus may induce a heat similar to that induced by infusion of other irritating solutions. Thus a split heat or short cycle may be seen.

Prolonged diestrus must be differentiated from early embryonic or fetal death. If embryonic death occurs after the time of maternal recognition of pregnancy (see the section Repeat Breeder), the next heat is skipped and the female returns to heat after a prolonged diestrus. This may last several months in the mare if the fetus is lost after the endometrial cups begin secreting equine chorionic gonadotropin (see the section, Anestrus).

Diseases that cause endometritis may cause cyclic irregularity by two mechanisms. Endometritis results in premature lysis of the corpus luteum, leading to a short cycle. Endometritis also may result in early embryonic death, which may culminate in a prolonged diestrus. Some viral agents, including some modified live vaccine strains, may attack the ovary and corpus luteum directly. The resulting oophoritis can lead to necrosis of the corpus luteum; therefore vaccination around the time of breeding is contraindicated.[27-29]

These agents may also cause embryonic death, leading to apparent cyclic irregularity.[29-31]

Approach to Diagnosis of Irregular Cycles

Clinical evaluation of a case of cyclic irregularity requires a detailed reproductive history, more so than many other reproductive problems. Examination of breeding records is essential. In dairy cows, errors in estrous detection are indicated when (1) more than 10% of the interestrous intervals are between 3 to 17 days or 25 to 35 days long; (2) more than 5% of the cows have two artificial inseminations within 3 days; or (3) cows are calving early or are further in gestation than predicted from the last breeding when examined for pregnancy. Seventy percent of cows should have an interestrous interval of less than 30 days, and 60% should be in the range of 18 to 24 days. The ratio of 18-to-24-day cycles to 38-to-46-day cycles should be 5:1. Evaluation of heat detection methods is important when dealing with a hand mating or artificial insemination program. Discussing the owner's understanding of the normal reproductive physiology of the species often is enlightening, and client education may be required. Observation of the teasing behavior of the animal is helpful, and examination of the reproductive tract should provide valuable information. Ancillary procedures such as ultrasonography, uterine culture, cytologic studies, and endometrial biopsy are often needed. Prediction of estrus through rectal examination or determination of the progesterone concentration (or both) may help. Progesterone determination on a sample collected at the time of insemination can be useful in evaluating the accuracy of heat detection. With ruminants, it may be wise to suggest the use of a teaser, or marker male. Heat detection aids (e.g., Kmar patches, tail chalk) are effective if applied properly and observed regularly. Serologic and microbiologic evaluation for the diseases known to cause endometritis or early embryonic death may need to be done if the source of the problem has not been determined.

Problems with cyclic irregularity can be difficult to decipher (Boxes 12-4 and 12-5). Management plays a large part, and it often is difficult to convince the client of this.

BOX 12-4

Causes of Cyclic Irregularity in the Mare

COMMON CAUSES
Transition season
Erroneous heat detection
Diestrus ovulation
Intrauterine therapy
Diestral endometrial biopsy
Pneumovagina
Endometritis
Pubertal cycles
Early embryonic death
Spontaneous corpus luteum prolongation
Endophyte-infested fescue
Cervical dilation

LESS COMMON CAUSES
Urovagina
Rectovaginal fistula
Ovarian tumors
Pyometra
Persistent follicles
Split heats
Endotoxemia
Hemorrhagic anovulatory follicles
Old age

UNCOMMON CAUSES
Contagious equine metritis
Corpus luteum inadequacy
Anabolic steroids
Progesterone therapy
Phosphorus deficiency
Sex chromosome anomalies

BOX 12-5

Causes of Cyclic Irregularity in Ruminants

COMMON CAUSES
Erroneous heat detection
Endometritis
Intrauterine therapy
Cystic ovaries
Heat stress
Leptospirosis
Infectious bovine rhinotracheitis (IBR) (B)
Bovine virus diarrhea (BVD) (B)
Campylobacteriosis
Trichomoniasis
Embryonic death after maternal recognition of pregnancy

UNCOMMON CAUSES
IBR- or BVD-infected semen
Bluetongue-infected semen
Zearalenone toxicity
Ovarian neoplasia
Corpus luteum inadequacy
Copper deficiency (O, C)
Molybdenum deficiency (O, C)
Iodine deficiency
Phytoestrogen toxicity

B, Bovine; *C,* caprine; *O,* ovine.

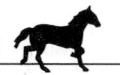

REFERENCES

19. Roberts SJ: *Veterinary obstetrics and genital diseases (theriogenology)*, ed 3, North Pomfret, Vt, 1986, SJ Roberts, pp 495-511.
20. Roberts SJ: *Veterinary obstetrics and genital diseases (theriogenology)*, ed 3, North Pomfret, Vt, 1986, SJ Roberts, pp 593-598.
21. Adams GP, Bosu WTK: Reproductive physiology of the nonpregnant mare: an overview and update, *Vet Clin North Am (Equine Reprod)* 2:161-176, 1988.
22. Kenney RM: Cyclic and pathologic changes of the mare endometrium as detected by biopsy, with a note on early embryonic death, *J Am Vet Med Assoc* 172:241-262, 1978.
23. Neely DP: Reproductive endocrinology and fertility in the mare. In Neely DP, Liu IKM, Hilman RB, eds: *Equine reproduction*, Princeton Junction, NJ, 1983, Veterinary Learning Systems.
24. Roberts SJ: *Veterinary obstetrics and genital diseases (theriogenology)*, ed 3, North Pomfret, Vt, SJ Roberts, pp 478-494.
25. Drost M, Thatcher WW: Heat stress in dairy cows, *Vet Clin North Am (Bovine Reprod)* 3:609-618, 1987.
26. Seguin B: Altering estrous cycles in the cow by intrauterine infusion. In Morrow DA, ed: *Current therapy in theriogenolgy*, Philadelphia, 1980, WB Saunders.
27. Sentongo YK, Johnson RH, Smith JR: Association of bovine viral diarrhoea–mucosal disease virus with ovaritis in cattle, *Aust Vet J* 56:272-273, 1980.
28. Van Der Maaten MJ, Miller JM, Whetstone CA: Ovarian lesions induced in heifers by intravenous inoculation with modified-live infectious bovine rhinotracheitis virus on the day after breeding, *Am J Vet Res* 46:1996-1999, 1985.
29. Miller JM, Van Der Maaten MJ: Experimentally induced infectious bovine rhinotracheitis virus infection during early pregnancy: effect on the bovine corpus luteum and conceptus, *Am J Vet Res* 47:223-228, 1986.
30. Chaing BC et al: The effect of infectious bovine rhinotracheitis vaccine on reproductive efficiency in cattle vaccinated during estrus, *Theriogenology* 33:1113-1120, 1990.
31. McGowan MR et al: Increased reproductive losses in cattle infected with bovine pestivirus around the time of insemination, *Vet Rec* 133:39-43, 1993.

ANESTRUS

STEVEN D. Van CAMP

Anestrus, the lack of estrus, is a sign, not a disease. It may be a normal physiologic phenomenon, a sign of disease, or an indication of inefficient heat detection. In adult animals, pregnancy is the most common cause of anestrus and should be ruled out before proceeding with diagnostic tests. Other etiologies are those associated with an active corpus luteum and elevated progesterone levels, and those associated with low progesterone levels and the absence of an active corpus luteum.[32] Sequential ovarian palpations or determinations of the progesterone concentration can be helpful in determining the cause (Boxes 12-6 and 12-7).

BOX 12-6

Causes of Anestrus in the Mare

COMMON CAUSES
Season (fall, winter)
Poor heat detection
Corpus luteum persistence
Diestrus ovulation
Pregnancy
Early embryonic death after recognition of pregnancy
Fetal death after endometrial cup formation
Psychologic impediments
Maternal behavior

LESS COMMON CAUSES
Ovarian tumors
Pituitary tumors
Pyometra
Weight loss

LESS COMMON CAUSES—cont'd
Chronic disease
Lactation
Old age

UNCOMMON CAUSES
Gonadal dysgenesis
Intersex conditions
Progesterone therapy
Nonsteroidal antiinflammatory drugs (NSAIDs)
Phosphorus deficiency
Ovarian hypoplasia
Anabolic steroids
Zearalenone toxicity
Chromosomal abnormalities

BOX 12-7

Causes of Anestrus in Ruminants

COMMON CAUSES
Season (C, O)
Pregnancy
Poor heat detection
Luteal cysts (B, C)
Pyometra
Poor nutrition, energy
Heat stress
Foot and leg problems
Poor footing (B)
Nursing beef cows and ewes (B, O)
Lactation (O)
Freemartinism (B, C)
Intersex conditions (C)
Postpartum period
Heavy lactation

COMMON CAUSES—cont'd
Primiparity
Periparturient disease

LESS COMMON CAUSES
Mucometra
Hydrometra
Macerated fetus
Mummified fetus
Trichomoniasis pyometra
Anaplasmosis
Johne's disease
Caprine arthritis-encephalitis (C)
Pseudopregnancy (C)
Insufficient number of cycling herd mates

B, Bovine; *C*, caprine; *O*, ovine.

Continued

MECHANISMS OF ANESTRUS

The following mechanisms can cause anestrus:

1. *Inadequate heat detection.* In nonpregnant, hand-bred, or artificially inseminated animals, the intensity of estrous behavior may be diminished by environmental factors such as high ambient temperature and humidity or poor footing in the paddock. Clinical disease, such as musculoskeletal pain, may also prevent the normal expression of estral behavior. Too few cycling herd mates may limit the ability to detect cows in heat.

2. *Psychologic problems.* Nervous mares, mares with foals, or dominant, fat, or phlegmatic mares experiencing normal estrous cycles may be reluctant to show estrus. Vigorous teasing with an aggressive stallion may be necessary to elicit estrous behavior in these animals.[33] Sequential ovarian palpations or determinations of the progesterone concentration (or both) may be useful for predicting the next estrous period.

3. *Energy deficiency.* Inadequate prepartum nutrition or insufficient energy in the ration during lactation in dairy cattle and in postpartum beef cattle nursing a calf can delay the return to estrus after parturition.[34]

4. *Photoperiod.* Photoperiod plays an important role in the cyclic patterns of seasonal breeders such as the mare, ewe, and doe. The mare is a long-day breeder and has a normal anestrus period during the late fall and winter months. The ewe and doe are short-day breeders and are normally anestrus in the spring and early summer, although breed variations occur.[35] Some sheep and goats near the equator have cycles throughout the year, presumably because of the consistency of the photoperiod.[36] The cow is not considered a seasonal breeder, but an increased photoperiod (18 hours of light to 6 hours of dark) has been shown to shorten postpartum anestrus in winter-calving beef cows.

5. *Hypothalamic or pituitary suppression or lack of stimulation.* Poor nutrition, heavy lactation, periparturient disease, hormone-secreting ovarian tumors, weight loss, or inanition associated with chronic disease may prevent stimulation of the pituitary by gonadotropin-releasing hormone from the hypothalamus.[33] Thus the pituitary does not release enough follicle-stimulating hormone (FSH) and luteinizing hormone (LH) for folliculogenesis, estrogen production, and ovulation by the ovaries. The inactive ovaries produce inadequate estrogen to cause behavioral estrus.

6. *Congenital or hereditary anomalies, including freemartinism in the cow and doe, intersex conditions that occur in polled goats, and gonadal dysgenesis in the mare.* The ovaries of these animals are unable to respond to FSH and LH stimulation from the pituitary. These animals frequently have rudimentary or hypoplastic ovaries and never display estrus.[37]

7. *Abnormal progesterone levels.* Inadequate progesterone exposure of the pituitary or hypothalamus before the first cycle of the season (ewe and doe) or the first postpartum estrus (cow) usually results in a silent heat.[34,38] On the other hand, suppression of the pituitary, the hypothalamus, or both by a high progesterone level can result in ovarian acyclicity or masking of behavioral estrus, or both.

8. *Retained or persistent corpora lutea.* These can occur spontaneously in the mare without evidence of a uterine pathologic condition. The mare is disposed to diestrous ovulations without estrus and the formation of corpora lutea that mask the next expected estrus. These previously cycling mares often demonstrate anestrus of several months' duration during the breeding season.[37] Persistent corpora lutea in the mare may also occur after fetal death while the endometrial cups are still producing equine chorionic gonadotropin. These mares often undergo a 1- to 4-month anestrus period. Corpus luteum persistence and anestrus can occur when the production or release of the luteolysin prostaglandin $F_{2\alpha}$ ($PGF_{2\alpha}$) is prevented. Segmental aplasia of a major portion of a uterine horn may prevent $PGF_{2\alpha}$ from acting on the ipsilateral ovary of the ruminant and result in corpus luteum persistence.[32]

9. *Fluid, foreign bodies, or pathologic material in the uterine lumen.* Mucometra, hydrometra, and pyometra prevent the release of $PGF_{2\alpha}$ in ruminants.[32] Thus the corpus luteum persists and results in anestrus. Pyometra in the mare may result in anestrus if the endometrial damage is severe enough to prevent production of $PGF_{2\alpha}$.[37] The presence of a mummified or macerated fetus in the ruminant uterus prevents release of $PGF_{2\alpha}$ and results in anestrus.[32]

Approach to Diagnosis of Anestrus

Knowledge of the reproductive physiology of the species involved is essential to understanding the cause of anestrus. Determining the cause of anestrus relies on an in-depth general and reproductive history, a thorough physical examination, and evaluation of the estrus detection programs involved. Pregnancy must be ruled out when dealing with any case of anestrus. In dairies using Dairy Herd Improvement Association (DHIA) records, inadequate heat detection must be suspected if the cows are determined to be cycling by palpation or progesterone tests but fewer than 50% of the possible estrus periods are detected; fewer than 70% of the cows are seen to be in heat by 60 days postpartum; and the average number of days to first service is over 80. The reproductive tract of the nonpregnant anestrus animal must be evaluated for any pathologic condition that might prevent estrus. The uterus of the ruminant should be evaluated for the presence

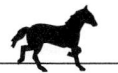

of fluid, a macerated or mummified fetus, or a foreign body. Ultrasonography or radiology may aid the diagnosis of these conditions in small ruminants. The ovaries should be evaluated for luteal cysts (ruminants) or neoplasia. Ultrasonography and hormone concentration determination are often helpful if rectal palpation of the ovaries is impossible. If the ovaries appear to be normal in size, an attempt should be made to determine the presence of a functional corpus luteum producing progesterone. On-site milk or serum progesterone test kits are available for mares and ruminants. Sequential tests at weekly intervals may prove helpful in eliminating inadequate estrus detection as the source of the complaint of anestrus.

Some of the DHIA reproductive parameters can be used to assess the efficiency of estrous detection. The percentage of cows in heat by 60 days after parturition, the percentage of cows bred by 90 days after parturition, and the average number of days to first breeding can be used to evaluate the accuracy of heat detection if most cows have been determined to have normal, cycling reproductive tracts.[39] In addition, a 24-day heat detection trial can be conducted. Of the nonpregnant, cycling cows, 80% to 85% should be found to be in heat within a 24-day period if estrous detection is adequate.

Anestrus is a frequent reproductive complaint. Often a number of causes are involved in a herd problem. The two most important causes of anestrus in a herd are poor estrous detection and inadequate nutrition. Concurrent, nonreproductive disease must be kept in mind when an individual anestric animal is examined.

REFERENCES

32. Roberts SJ: *Veterinary obstetrics and genital diseases (theriogenology)*, ed 3, North Pomfret, Vt, 1986, SJ Roberts, pp 495-512.
33. Roberts SJ: *Veterinary obstetrics and genital diseases (theriogenology)*, ed 3, North Pomfret, Vt, 1986, SJ Roberts, p 595.
34. Hopkins SM: Bovine anestrus. In Morrow DA, ed: *Current therapy in theriogenology: diagnosis, treatment, and prevention of reproductive diseases in small and large animals*, ed 2, Philadelphia, 1986, WB Saunders.
35. Ward WR: The breeding season and estrous cycle. In Morrow DA, ed: *Current therapy in theriogenology: diagnosis, treatment, and prevention of reproductive diseases in small and large animals*, ed 2, Philadelphia, 1986, WB Saunders.
36. Smith MC: The reproductive anatomy and physiology of the female goat. In Morrow DA, ed: *Current therapy in theriogenology: diagnosis, treatment, and prevention of reproductive diseases in small and large animals*, ed 2, Philadelphia, 1986, WB Saunders.
37. Neely DP: Evaluation and therapy of genital disease in the mare. In Neely DP, Liu IKM, Hilman RB, eds: *Equine reproduction*, Princeton Junction, NJ, 1983, Veterinary Learning Systems.
38. Roberts SJ: *Veterinary obstetrics and genital diseases (theriogenology)*, ed 3, North Pomfret, Vt, 1986, SJ Roberts, pp 654-656.
39. Grunsenmeyer D: Evaluating dairy herd reproduction status using DHI records, 1983, *Western Regional Extension Bulletin* No. 67, US Department of Agriculture.

REPEAT BREEDER

STEVEN D. Van CAMP

Managing repeat breeders is often frustrating and expensive. The repeat breeder is an animal that has been bred during three or more successive heat periods without being diagnosed pregnant.[40] An incidence of 10% to 15% repeat breeders is considered acceptable for dairies.[41] The incidence increases with the herd size and the level of milk production and with the use of artificial insemination.[42] This may be an even greater problem in the horse because 5% to 8% of mares lose their pregnancy in the first 4 months of gestation.[42] The use of ultrasonography and embryo collection indicates that the incidence of early embryonic death in the mare is likely even higher.[43]

BOX 12-8

Causes of Repeat Breeding in the Mare

COMMON CAUSES
Transition season
Endometritis
Poor timing of artificial insemination
Pneumovagina
Metritis
Endometrial fibrosis
Poor heat detection
Ovulation failure
Twins
Uterine lymphatic lacunae
Endometrial cysts
Early foal heat breeding
Poor uterine clearance
Ventral uterine sacculation
Endophyte-infested fescue

LESS COMMON CAUSES
Urovagina
Rectovaginal fistula
Malnutrition
Pyometra
Heat stress
Poor semen quality
Old age

UNCOMMON CAUSES
Salpingitis
Hydrosalpinx
Oviductal adhesions
Oophoritis
Uterine neoplasia
Cervical neoplasia
Ovarian neoplasia
Parovarian cysts
Contagious equine metritis
Iodine deficiency
True hypothyroidism
Phosphorus deficiency
Zearalenone toxicity
Intersexuality
Gonadal dysgenesis, sex reversal, trisomy
Other karyotype abnormalities
Teratogenic factors
Vitamin A deficiency
Cervical trauma
Luteal insufficiency

The etiologies of repeat breeding are numerous and are related to male, female, and management factors (Boxes 12-8 and 12-9). The pathogenesis of repeat breeding involves either a failure of fertilization or early embryonic death (EED).[41] Some etiologies, such as heat stress in the herd, may involve both mechanisms. Fertilization rates are normal in heat-stressed cows that are bred artificially, but heat stress increases the rate of EED. Heat stress can cause failure of fertilization by affecting spermatogenesis in males used in a natural breeding program.[44] When dealing with an individual repeat breeder, it is often wise to begin with the female. When several females are affected, the male should be eliminated as a source of the problem before proceeding. Management errors may be related to either male or female factors.

In natural breeding operations using highly fertile males, EED is more likely than failure of fertilization to be a cause of

---

BOX 12-9

Causes of Repeat Breeding in Ruminants

COMMON CAUSES	UNCOMMON CAUSES
Heat detection	Johne's disease
Poor timing of artificial insemination	Tuberculosis
Poor artificial insemination technique	Vitamin A deficiency
Malnutrition	Zinc deficiency
Follicular cysts	Manganese deficiency
Endometritis	Cobalt deficiency
Heat stress	Copper deficiency
Trichomoniasis	Molybdenum toxicity
Campylobacteriosis	Selenium toxicity
Leptospirosis	Iodine deficiency
Inadequate uterine involution	Iodine toxicity (B, O)
	Oophoritis
LESS COMMON CAUSES	Fat necrosis (B)
Poor semen quality	*Brasilia* toxicity
Inadequate male power (not enough males)	Ovarian tumors
Infectious bovine rhinotracheitis (IBR) (B)	Progressive degenerative myeloencephalopathy of Brown
Bovine virus diarrhea (BVD) (B)	Swiss cattle (B)
Bluetongue	Polybrominated biphenyl toxicity (B)
Brucellosis	Phytoestrogen toxicity (B, O)
Anaplasmosis	Hydrosalpinx
Toxoplasmosis (C, O)	Salpingitis
Border disease (C, O)	Cervical anomalies and cysts
Selenium deficiency	Chromosomal abnormalities (1/29 or 14/20 centric fusions)
Phosphorus deficiency	Fluoride toxicosis
Ureaplasmosis	Segmental aplasia
Urine pooling	Uridine monophosphate synthase deficiency
Pneumovagina, pneumouterus	Delayed ovulation
Oviductal bursal adhesions	Schistosomiasis (exotic)
Segmental aplasia	Tick-borne fever (exotic)
Rectovaginal fistula	Epivag (exotic)
Parovarian cysts	*Leucaena leucocephala* (exotic)
Zearalenone toxicity (B, O)	Besnoitiosis (exotic)
Fescue toxicity	Maedi, Visna (exotic)
Uterine tumors	Lumpy skin disease (exotic)
Defective embryos	Onion grass toxicity (exotic)
Dietary protein toxicity	

B, Bovine; *C,* caprine; *O,* ovine.

---

infertility.[41,43] However, this may not be true when artificial insemination or marginally fertile males are used. The interval between heats may help distinguish between EED and failure of fertilization. Failure of fertilization usually does not affect the interestrous interval. However, EED may prolong the interestrous interval if the fetal wastage occurs after the time of maternal recognition of pregnancy. Maternal recognition of pregnancy occurs at approximately days 15 to 17 after estrus in the cow, days 11 to 14 in the mare, and days 12 to 13 in the ewe.[45] Animals experiencing EED after pregnancy recognition often have interestrous intervals corresponding to multiples of a normal cycle length.

Approach to Diagnosis

Clinical differentiation of EED from failure of fertilization is difficult. In addition to evaluation of heat detection and breeding techniques, it is important to obtain a detailed history. When dealing with a herd problem, the clinician begins by evaluating the male or males used or assesses the semen quality and techniques used for artificial insemination. When dealing with an individual repeat breeder, evaluation of the female is the first step.

Evaluation of the male should include evaluation of the animal's physical condition, including the genitalia. The quality of the semen should be checked. The male's libido and ability to mount should be determined by observation or through historic information. Examination of the male for venereally transmitted diseases, such as trichomoniasis and campylobacteriosis in the bull and contagious equine metritis in the stallion, may be warranted if other factors are ruled out. When dealing with an artificial insemination program, the semen quality should be evaluated and the thawing, transporting, timing, and deposition techniques should be evaluated.

Errors in heat detection and the timing of breeding are major management causes of repeat breeding. Discussing and observing the methods used to determine when an animal should be bred is important in dealing with both the individual animal and the herd. Milk or serum progesterone determinations at the time of breeding have proved helpful in determining the accuracy of heat detection and timing of insemination. In some dairies 40% to 50% of the cows are bred at the wrong time.

Examination of the female or females should begin with evaluation of the body condition. Poor nutrition has been associated with repeat breeding.[46] The reproductive examination should include evaluation of the vulva, vagina, cervix, uterus, oviducts, and ovaries. Poor vulvar conformation may lead to pneumovagina and endometritis, resulting in EED.

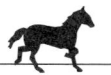

The spermicidal effect of urine may cause failure of fertilization in the mare or cow that pools urine in the vagina. Cervical canal occlusion can prevent fertilization. An abnormal uterine environment may also lead to repeat breeding. Large volumes of pus and debris associated with a postpartum metritis may cause failure of fertilization because of its effect on sperm. Endometritis with minimal intraluminal pus rarely causes failure of fertilization but often results in EED. Unlike ruminants, the mare may continue to display estrus while experiencing a pyometra. The volume of pus present in the uterus is likely to cause failure of fertilization. Hydrosalpinx or salpingitis may lead to failure of fertilization by blocking sperm or ovum passage. Ovulation abnormalities such as delayed ovulation or ovarian cyst formation may result in failure of fertilization. Whenever possible, including a uterine culture, cytologic smear, and endometrial biopsy as part of the examination is likely to help determine the cause of the infertility.

Differentiation of EED from failure of fertilization in repeat breeders has been facilitated by the use of embryo flushing techniques and ultrasonography. Collection of unfertilized ova indicates failure of fertilization; collection of degenerating embryos indicates very early embryonic death. In ruminants, failure to collect ova or embryos may indicate oviductal blockage resulting in failure of fertilization. This is not the case for mares because they usually retain unfertilized ova in the oviducts.

Ultrasonic determination of pregnancy in the mare and cow have made very early detection of pregnancy possible. Loss of an embryo after detecting it with ultrasound at 10 days of gestation confirms EED. Pregnancy wastage can be confirmed later in gestation with sequential rectal palpations of the reproductive tract or ultrasonic evaluation. Hormone assays are also helpful for confirming embryo or fetal loss.

An assay for equine chorionic gonadotropin (ECG), previously called pregnant mare serum gonadotropin (PMSG), can be used to determine if a mare was pregnant long enough to stimulate formation of the endometrial cups and ECG production. ECG can be detected at about 40 days of gestation with these kits. The endometrial cups continue to produce ECG until 120 to 150 days of gestation even if the fetus dies. Therefore ECG can be used to confirm EED but not failure of fertilization. Progesterone determination cannot be used to confirm pregnancy in the mare or ruminants. However, it can be used to confirm nonpregnancy if the progesterone level is low early in the expected gestation. A bovine early conception factor test can be used to confirm fertilization, but it does not rule out EED later.

The fetally derived hormone-metabolite estrone sulfate has been used to determine the presence of a live fetus. It is detectable in the serum or urine of the dam if the fetus is alive after 45 days of gestation in the doe, 70 days of gestation in the ewe, 100 days of gestation in the mare, and 120 days of gestation in the cow.[47,48] Thus a decline in estrone sulfate indicates death of the fetus. Estrone sulfate is probably most helpful in confirming fetal loss in the doe and ewe because other techniques are available in the larger species.

Infertility associated with repeat breeding is a perplexing clinical problem. The economics involved often do not warrant pursuing the etiology. If the etiology is determined, therapy often is unrewarding.

Boxes 12-8 and 12-9 list the causes of repeat breeding the in mare and ruminants. The causes have been divided into expected frequencies of occurrence.

REFERENCES
40. Zemjanis R: "Repeat breeding" or conception failure in cattle. In *Current veterinary therapy in theriogenology*, Philadelphia, 1980, WB Saunders.
41. Roberts SJ: *Veterinary obstetrics and genital diseases (theriogenology)*, ed 3, North Pomfret, Vt, 1986, SJ Roberts, pp 559-569.
42. Roberts SJ: *Veterinary obstetrics and genital diseases (theriogenology)*, ed 3, North Pomfret, Vt, 1986, SJ Roberts, pp 625-627.
43. Ball B: Embryonic loss in mares, *Vet Clin North Am (Equine Pract)* 4:263-290, 1988.
44. Drost M, Thatcher WW: Heat stress in dairy cows, *Vet Clin North Am (Bovine Reprod)* 3:609-618, 1987.
45. Roberts SJ: *Veterinary obstetrics and genital diseases (theriogenology)*, ed 3, North Pomfret, Vt, 1986, SJ Roberts, pp 107-110.
46. Hopkins SM: Bovine anestrus. In Morrow DA, ed: *Current therapy in theriogenology: diagnosis, treatment, and prevention of reproductive diseases in small and large animals*, ed 2, Philadelphia, 1986, WB Saunders.
47. Nachreiner RF: Laboratory endocrine diagnostic procedures in theriogenology. In Morrow DA, ed: *Current therapy in theriogenology: diagnosis, treatment, and prevention of reproductive diseases in small and large animals*, ed 2, Philadelphia, 1986, WB Saunders.
48. Tsang CPW: Plasma levels of estrone sulfate, free estrogens, and progesterone in the pregnant ewe throughout gestation, *Theriogenology* 10:97-111, 1978.

PREGNANCY LOSS

PATRICK M. McCUE
MATS H.T. TROEDSSON

Pregnancy loss refers to the failure of a conceptus to be maintained successfully to term. Pregnancy loss may be classified as early embryonic death (EED), abortion, or stillbirth, depending on the gestational stage when the pregnancy loss occurred. EED refers to the death of a conceptus before organogenesis is complete (approximately 55 days in horses, 45 days in cattle, and 34 days in sheep).[49] Abortion refers to pregnancy loss after the completion of organogenesis. Stillbirth refers to the delivery of a nonviable fetus at or near term.

EARLY EMBRYONIC DEATH

The exact incidence of EED in any species is difficult to determine, because most losses occur before pregnancy can be routinely diagnosed. Embryonic death early in pregnancy usually results in reabsorption of the embryonic tissues and fluids. Consequently, EED cannot be distinguished from failure of fertilization in most instances. However, despite the lack of clinical evidence, EED probably accounts for the largest percentage of reproductive wastage in large animals. The incidence of EED has been estimated at 5% to 24% in mares,[50] 30% to 35% in cows,[51] and 20% to 30% in ewes.[52] The rate of EED is much higher in subfertile or repeat breeder females and in older females.

Loss of the embryo before maternal endocrine recognition of the pregnancy (i.e., days 14 to 16 in the mare, days 15 to 17 in the cow, and day 12 in the ewe and doe) results in return to estrus at the normal time. Embryonic loss after this critical period may result in persistence of the corpus luteum in horses, pseudopregnancy in goats, or irregular returns to estrus in cattle.

Chromosomal and genetic defects of the oocyte, sperm, or embryo; a poor oviductal or uterine environment; endocrine dysfunction; and maternal stress are all considered important factors in the pathogenesis of EED.[50,53] Infectious agents such as *Trichomonas foetus* and *Campylobacter fetus* ssp. *venerealis* in cattle[53] and *Streptococcus zooepidemicus* and other bacteria in horses[54] can cause EED. Endogenous release of $PGF_{2\alpha}$ during the corpus luteum–dependent stage of gestation may result in luteolysis and subsequent embryonic loss or abortion in any large animal species. Luteal insufficiency associated with low plasma progesterone concentrations has been suggested as a possible cause of EED in horses, cattle, and sheep, although scientific evidence is limited.[51,55]

ABORTION

The rate of abortion after pregnancy diagnosis at 60 days of gestation has been estimated to be approximately 10% in horses[56] and 3% to 4% in cattle.[57] Fetal death may result in abortion (expulsion of the fetus from the uterus) or retention of the fetus in the uterine lumen, with subsequent fetal maceration or mummification. In animals with a corpus luteum–dependent pregnancy for all or most of gestation (cows, goats, llamas), death of the fetus usually results in the abortion of an autolyzed fetus because of a delay between the time of fetal death and lysis of the corpus luteum. In species that do not depend on a corpus luteum for maintenance of pregnancy for most of gestation (i.e., mares and ewes), fetal death causes an immediate decrease in placental progesterone production and rapid expulsion of a relatively nonautolyzed fetus. Mummification is characterized by fluid reabsorption from a fetus retained in a sterile uterine environment. Fetal mummification is most common in multiparous species with a corpus luteum–dependent pregnancy (i.e., sows) and is rare in uniparous species that are corpus luteum independent for most of gestation (i.e., mares). Maceration refers to the degenerative changes that occur in a fetus after retention in a nonsterile uterine environment. Fetal maceration may be associated with significant maternal endometrial damage.

HORSES. Equine abortions may be characterized as infectious or noninfectious in origin. Most equine abortions occur secondary to placental dysfunction. One of the most commonly diagnosed infectious cause of abortion in horses is equine herpesvirus type 1 (EHV-1).[56] Abortion caused by EHV-1 usually occurs after 7 months of gestation and accounts for 10% to 15% of all diagnosed equine abortions. *Nocardioform actinomycete*, a filamentous, branching bacillus, has recently been identified as a significant cause of chronic placentitis and subsequent late-term abortion, stillbirth, and premature birth.[58] *Leptospira* spp. have also been recently identified as a significant cause of equine abortion in Kentucky.[59] Bacterial and fungal abortions in mares are primarily caused by infections that ascend through the cervix, causing placentitis and subsequent fetal infection. The bacterial organisms most commonly cultured from aborted fetuses include *Streptococcus* spp., *Escherichia coli*, *Pseudomonas* spp., *Klebsiella* spp., and *Staphylococcus* spp. The most frequently recovered fungi are *Aspergillus* spp.

The most common noninfectious cause of equine abortion is twin pregnancy.[56] Inability of the uterus to support two fetuses to term because of insufficient placental support may result in abortion at any stage of gestation but is most common after 7 months. Early diagnosis of the pregnancy using ultrasonography allows for highly successful manual reduction of one twin if done before day 25 of pregnancy. This technique has significantly reduced the incidence of abortion caused by twin pregnancies.

RUMINANTS. Infectious bovine rhinotracheitis–infectious pustular vulvovaginitis (IBR-IPV) virus and bovine virus diarrhea–mucosal disease (BVD-MD) virus are two of the most common viral causes of abortion in cattle.[60] Bacterial abortions caused by *Brucella abortus*, *Actinomyces pyogenes*, *Bacillus* spp., *Listeria monocytogenes*, *Escherichia coli*, *Leptospira* spp., and *Pasteurella haemolytica* and fungal abortions caused by *Aspergillus* spp. and *Mucor* spp. usually result from hematogenous spread and localization in the placenta.[61] Protozoal abortion, caused by *Neospora* organisms, has recently been recognized as a significant cause of abortion in cattle worldwide.[62] Epizootic bovine abortion (EBA) is a common cause of third trimester abortion in susceptible heifers and cows inhabiting the foothills of the Sierra Nevada mountain range of California, Nevada, and Oregon.[63] The vector for EBA is the argasid tick *(Ornithodoros coriaceus)*, but the etiologic agent has not been identified.

Campylobacteriosis (vibriosis) caused by *Campylobacter fetus* and *Campylobacter fetus* ssp. *jejuni*, and enzootic abortion of ewes caused by *Chlamydia psittaci* are the most common infectious causes of abortion in sheep.[64] They are characterized by abortion in the last 4 to 6 weeks of gestation, premature births, stillbirths, and birth of weak, infected lambs. *C. psittaci* is also the most common cause of infectious abortion in goats in the United States.[65]

Noninfectious causes of large animal abortion include genetic or chromosomal factors, maternal stress, inadequate nutrition, vitamin or mineral deficiencies, ingestion of poisonous plants or other toxins, hormonal factors, environmental factors, physical factors, and certain medications.

Approach to Diagnosis of Abortion

A definitive diagnosis is reached in 20% to 40% of bovine abortions,[49] 50% to 60% of equine abortions,[56] and 30% to 40% of sheep abortions.[66] The generally low diagnostic success is due to the complexity of the condition (Boxes 12-10 and 12-11). Abortion involves disease in the maternal, placental, and fetal compartments individually or together, and all these compartments have to be examined thoroughly. In addition, a "triad" of determinants for animal disease has to be considered: (1) the presence of a pathogenic organism, (2) the environment in which a host lives, and (3) the susceptibility of the host to the disease.[67] To enhance diagnostic success, information and samples must be collected from the fetus, placenta, dam, and herd. A thorough history should be obtained, including the gestational age of the fetus; reproductive, medical, and vaccination history of the dam and other individuals in the herd; previous abortions and diagnoses; new arrivals to the herd and contacts of the animal with other herds; potential causes of maternal stress; possible access to toxins and poisonous plants; and sources of water and nutrition.

A physical examination that includes all body systems should be performed on the dam. Samples should be collected from the vagina, uterus, or both for culture and cytologic studies. Examination of the reproductive system should include palpation or ultrasonography of the reproductive tract per rectum, speculum examination of the vagina, and digital examination of the cervix. Paired serum samples from the dam and other females in the herd (10 animals or 10% of the herd, whichever is greater) may also help demonstrate an immunologic response to an infectious agent. Maternal serologic testing is generally most useful if paired samples are submitted, combined with accurate information about the animal's vaccination history. However, postabortion titers from cows that aborted can be compared to titers from nonaffected cows in the herd at a similar stage of lactation. Demonstration of a fourfold rise in titer between acute and convalescent serum samples suggests recent exposure to an agent, but the presence of antibodies does not necessarily indicate that the agent caused the abortion. An exception can be made for brucellosis and leptospirosis, for which a high titer from a single sample can be diagnostic.

For optimal diagnostic efficiency, the entire aborted fetus and placenta should be submitted to a diagnostic laboratory for necropsy. If this cannot be done, a prompt necropsy should be performed, and collections of fetal, placental, and maternal samples should be submitted to a diagnostic laboratory (Table 12-1).

A systematic necropsy must be performed on the aborted fetus. Fetal age and development may be assessed by mea-

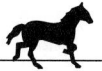

BOX 12-10

Causes of Pregnancy Loss in the Mare

COMMON CAUSES

Impaired oviductal and uterine environment (EED)
Chronic endometritis (EED/Ab)
Embryonic defects (EED)
Endometrial fibrosis (EED/Ab)
Twinning (Ab)
Equine herpesvirus type 1 (EHV-1) (Ab)
Bacterial placentitis (*Streptococcus* spp., *Escherichia coli*, *Pseudomonas* spp., *Klebsiella* spp., *Staphylococcus* spp) (Ab)
Fungal placentitis (Ab)

LESS COMMON CAUSES

Endotoxemia (EED/Ab)
Leptospirosis (Ab)
Umbilical cord abnormalities (Ab)
Fetal anomalies (Ab)
Maternal stress, other disease (EED/Ab)
Chromosomal abnormalities (Ab/EED)
Fescue toxicity (EED/Ab)
Advanced maternal age (EED)
Equine viral arteritis (Ab)
Equine infectious anemia (Ab)
Uterine torsion (Ab)
Endocrine factors (EED)
Malnutrition (EED/Ab)
Drug-induced causes (EED/Ab)
Premature separation of the placenta (Ab)
Fetal asphyxia (Ab)
Placental insufficiency (Ab)

UNCOMMON CAUSES

Ehrlichia risticii (Potomac horse fever) (Ab)
Uterine body pregnancy (Ab)
Endometrial adhesions (EED)
Taylorella equigenitalis (contagious equine metritis) (EED)
Uterine lymphatic lacunae, cysts (EED/Ab)
Hyperlipemia (Ab)
Lymphosarcoma (Ab)
Iatrogenic causes (EED/Ab)
Fetal diarrhea syndrome (Ab)
Ergot toxicity (EED/Ab)
Brucellosis (Ab)
Mycobacterium infection (Ab)
Corynebacterium pseudotuberculosis (Ab)
Rhodococcus equi (Ab)
Mycoplasma infection (Ab)
Coccidioidomycosis (Ab)
Histoplasmosis (Ab)
Babesiosis (Ab)
Vitamin A deficiency (Ab)
Iodine deficiency (EED/Ab)
Granulosa theca cell tumors (Ab)
Cryptococcosis (Ab)
Sorghum, Sudan grass (Ab)
Locoweed (*Astragalus* spp.)
Hoary alyssum poisoning (Ab)
Salmonella abortus equi (Ab)

Ab, Abortion; *EED,* early embryonic death.

BOX 12-11

Causes of Pregnancy Loss in Ruminants

COMMON CAUSES

Campylobacter infection (B: EED; O, C: Ab)
Epizootic bovine abortion (B: Ab)
Actinomyces pyogenes (B: Ab)
Bacillus spp. (B: Ab)
Bovine protozoal abortion (*Neospora* spp.) (B, C: Ab)
Infectious bovine rhinotracheitis–infectious pustular vulvovaginitis (IBR-IPV) virus (B: EED/Ab)
Leptospirosis (B, O, C: Ab)
Trichomoniasis (B: EED/Ab)
Brucellosis (B, O, C: Ab)
Bovine virus diarrhea (BVD) (B: EED/Ab)
Toxoplasmosis (O, C: EED/Ab)
Border disease (O, C: EED/Ab)
Chlamydiosis (O, C: Ab)
Embryonic defects (B, O, C: EED)
Bacterial abortion (B, O, C: Ab)

LESS COMMON CAUSES

Twinning (B: Ab)
Prenatal asphyxia (B, O, C: Ab)
Akabane virus (B, O, C: Ab)
Q fever (*Coxiella burnetii*) (O, C: Ab)
Mycotoxicosis (B, O, C: Ab)
Anaplasmosis (B, O, C: Ab)

LESS COMMON CAUSES—cont'd

Ureaplasma infection (B, O: EED/Ab)
Mycoplasma infection (B, C: Ab)
Chromosomal abnormalities (B, O, C: EED/Ab)
Malnutrition, protein-calorie starvation (B, O, C: EED/Ab)
Bluetongue (B, O: EED/Ab)
Haemophilus somnus (B: Ab)
Tuberculosis (B: Ab)
Uterine torsion (B: Ab)
Water deprivation–salt toxicity (B, O, C: Ab)
Selenium deficiency (B, O, C: Ab)
Mycotic, fungal abortion (B, O, C: Ab)
Salmonellosis (B, O, C: EED/Ab)
Nitrate-nitrite poisoning (B, O: Ab)
Drug-induced causes (B, O, C: EED/Ab)
Endotoxemia (B, O, C: EED/Ab)
Cache Valley virus (B, O: EED/Ab)
Maternal stress (O, C: Ab)
Pregnancy toxemia (O, C: Ab)
Umbilical cord, placental abnormalities (B, O, C: Ab)
Fetal anomalies (B, O, C: Ab)
Deficiency of uridine monophosphate synthase (DUMPS) (B: EED)
Listeria (B, O, C: Ab)

Ab, Abortion; *B,* bovine; *C,* caprine; *EED,* early embryonic death, *O,* ovine.

Continued

BOX 12-11

Causes of Pregnancy Loss in Ruminants—cont'd

UNCOMMON CAUSES	UNCOMMON CAUSES—cont'd
Pine needle poisoning (B: Ab)	Lead toxicity (B, O: EED/Ab)
Chlorinated naphthalene toxicity (B: Ab)	Liver fluke disease (B, O, C: Ab)
Osteopetrosis (B: Ab)	Locoweed (*Astragalus, Oxytropis* spp.) (B, O, C: EED/Ab)
Lathyrus poisoning (B, O, C: Ab)	Ryegrass poisoning (B,O: Ab)
Cobalt deficiency (B: EED/Ab)	*Sarcocystis* infection (B, O, C: Ab)
Yersinia pseudotuberculosis (B, O, C: Ab)	*Veratrum* poisoning (O, C: EED/Ab)
Death camas (*Zigandenus* sp.) (O: Ab)	Vitamin A deficiency (B, O, C: Ab)
Foxglove (B: Ab)	Polybrominated biphenyl toxicity (B: EED/Ab)
Phosphate fertilizer toxicity (O: Ab)	Broomweed (*Gutierrezia* spp.) (B, O, C: Ab)
α-Mannosidosis (B, O, C: Ab)	Bacillary hemoglobinuria (B, O: Ab)
Ergot toxicity (B, O: EED/Ab)	*Tetraglymia glabrata* (O: Ab)
Iodine deficiency (O, C: EED/Ab)	Copper deficiency (O, C: Ab)
Hydrops fetalis (B, O: Ab)	Caprine herpesvirus infection (C: Ab)
Iatrogenic causes (B, O, C: EED/Ab)	Habitual abortion in Angora goats (C: Ab)

Ab, Abortion; *B*, bovine; *C*, caprine; *EED*, early embryonic death, *O*, ovine.

TABLE 12-1

Tissue Samples to Be Submitted for Diagnosis of the Cause of Abortion

Source	Preservation Method	
	Chilled or Frozen	**Fixed***
Aborted fetus	Lung, liver, kidney, spleen, thymus, skeletal muscle, heart, heart blood, abomasum and stomach contents	Lung, liver, kidney, spleen, thymus, skeletal muscle (diaphragm), heart, adrenal gland, lymph node, brain
Placenta	Allantochorion (ruminants: cotyledons and intercotyledonary areas), allantoamnion, amniotic fluid, cord blood	Allantochorion (ruminants: cotyledons and intercotyledonary areas), allantoamnion
Dam/herd	Paired serum samples, vaginal or uterine swabs	

*10% Formalin or Bouin fixative should be used.

suring crown-rump length, hair patterns, and color. Meconium staining of the skin suggests uterine fetal distress. The condition of the fetus, including the degree of autolysis, should be noted. A careful examination for fetal anomalies (e.g., cerebellar hypoplasia, hydrocephalus, cleft palate, cardiac anomalies) should be performed. Histopathologic samples should be immersed in a volume of 10% buffered formalin (or Bouin fixative) equivalent to 10 times the volume of tissue. Samples for culture, virus isolation, and fluorescent antibody tests should be submitted on ice in separate sterile containers. A sample of abomasum and stomach contents should be aseptically collected for culture. Fetal heart blood or thoracic fluid may be collected for serologic evaluation. A late-term fetus is immunologically competent, and high titers may indicate activity of a pathogenic agent. Serologic testing of fetal fluids can be useful both in detecting a nonspecific active fetal immune response (total IgG) and for titers against a specific antigen.

The fetal membranes should be examined for size, weight, degree of autolysis, condition, and completeness. Samples of placental tissue, especially areas with lesions, should be collected for histologic examination, impression smears, bacterial culture, virus isolation, and fluorescent antibody tests. The equine placenta should be examined for integrity, lesions, and distribution of chorionic villi. The normal equine placenta is everted after expulsion with the allantoic surface presented outward and chorioallantois ruptured at the site of the cervical star. Blood should be collected from the free end of the cord.

The allantoic surface should be examined for abnormalities such as multiple allantoic pouches that may indicate compromised fetal circulation.[68] The chorionic surface of the placenta should be examined for lesions and distribution of chorionic villi. Areas of avillous chorion are normally observed in association with the cervical star, narrow folds over large vessels, and areas opposing endometrial cups. Absence of chorionic villi over a circumscribed area is characteristic of twins and represents the region where two placentas were in contact. The region of the placenta adjacent to the cervix should be examined for loss of chorionic villi and the presence of inflammatory exudate, a hallmark of ascending infection.

The cotyledons and intercotyledonary spaces of the ruminant placenta should be carefully examined for lesions. Autolytic changes of the placenta may be difficult to interpret. Some normal features of the bovine placenta must be kept in mind.[57] Amniotic plaques are present on the inner surface of the amnion and on the umbilical cord. They are most prominent at 3 to 7 months of gestation. Necrotic areas of the chorioallantois in the tips of the uterine horns are also normal and caused by insufficient vascularization to that area. Mineralization of the placenta is normal during the first months of gestation but may reflect placental injury associated with infection at the end of gestation.

All aborted fetuses and placental tissues should be handled with care, and tissues not submitted to a diagnostic laboratory should be burned or buried. Dams that have aborted should be isolated from the remainder of the herd.

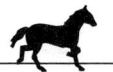

REFERENCES

49. Roberts SJ: *Veterinary obstetrics and genital diseases (theriogenology)*, ed 3, North Pomfret, Vt, 1986, SJ Roberts, pp 38-50; 162.
50. Ball BA: In McKinnon AO, Voss JL, eds: *Equine reproduction*, Philadelphia, 1993, Lea & Febiger.
51. Peters AR, Ball PJH: *Reproduction in cattle*, ed 2, Oxford, 1995, Blackwell Science.
52. Nancarrow CD: Embryonic mortality in the ewe and doe. In Zavy MT, Geisert RD, eds: *Embryonic mortality in domestic species*, Ann Arbor, Mich, 1994, CRC Press.
53. Bondurant RH: Influence of infectious diseases on reproduction. In Cupps PT, ed: *Reproduction in domestic animals*, ed 4, New York, 1991, Academic Press pp 637-656.
54. Pycock JF: Breeding management of the problem mare. In Samper JC, ed: *Equine breeding management and artificial insemination*, Philadelphia, 2000, WB Saunders.
55. Ball BA, Daels PF: Early pregnancy loss in mares: applications for progestin therapy. In Robinson NE, ed: *Current therapy in equine medicine*, Philadelphia, 1997, WB Saunders.
56. Acland HM: Abortion in mares. In McKinnon AO, Voss JL, eds: *Equine reproduction*, Philadelphia, 1993, Lea & Febiger.
57. Miller RB: Bovine abortion. In Morrow DA, ed: *Current therapy in theriogenology: diagnosis, treatment, and prevention of reproductive diseases in small and large animals*, ed 2, Philadelphia, 1986, WB Saunders.
58. Hong CB et al: Etiology and pathology of equine placentitis, *J Vet Diagn Invest* 5:56-63, 1993.
59. Donahue JM et al: Diagnosis and prevalence of *Leptospira* infection in aborted and stillborn horses, *J Vet Diagn Invest* 3:148-151, 1991.
60. Kirkebride CA: *Laboratory diagnosis of abortion in food animals*, Madison, Wis, 1984, American Association of Veterinary Laboratory Diagnosticians.
61. Yaeger M, Holler CD: Bacterial causes of bovine infertility and abortion. In Youngquist RS, ed: *Current therapy in large animal theriogenology*, Philadelphia, 1997, WB Saunders.
62. Abbitt B: Protozoal abortion in cattle. In Youngquist RS, ed: *Current therapy in large animal theriogenology*, Philadelphia, 1997, WB Saunders.
63. BonDurant RH, Anderson ML: Epizootic bovine abortion. In Youngquist RS, ed: *Current therapy in large animal theriogenology*, Philadelphia, 1997, WB Saunders.
64. East NE: Pregnancy diagnosis, abortions, and periparturient diseases: symposium on sheep and goat medicine, *Vet Clin North Am (Large Anim Pract)* 5:601-618, 1983.
65. East NE: Chlamydiosis. In Morrow DA, ed: *Current therapy in theriogenology: diagnosis, treatment, and prevention of reproductive diseases in small and large animals*, ed 2, Philadelphia, 1986, WB Saunders.
66. Menzies PI, Miller R: Abortion in sheep: diagnosis and control. In Youngquist RS, ed: *Current therapy in large animal theriogenology*, Philadelphia, 1997, WB Saunders.
67. Schwabe CW, Rieman HP, Franti CE: *Epidemiology in veterinary practice*, Philadelphia, 1977, Lea & Febiger.
68. Miller RB: Evaluation of the equine and bovine placenta: lesions vs non-lesions, *Proc Soc Theriogenol*, 1993, pp 39-44.

FESCUE TOXICOSIS

JAMES P. BRENDEMUEHL

Tall fescue (*Festuca arundinacea* Schreb.) is a cool-season, seed-propagated, perennial grass that is grown in many regions of the United States. It is traditionally recognized to be the most widely grown pasture grass in the humid areas of the southeastern and northwestern United States. Recent surveys have demonstrated endophyte-infected forage in more than half of all forage samples tested in all geographic areas of the United States.[69,70] An endophytic fungus, *Neotyphodium coenophialum*, has been shown to be widely spread wherever tall fescue is grown.[70] Undesirable signs in animals grazing tall fescue have been associated with the presence of the asymptomatic fungal endophyte (also see Chapter 50).

CLINICAL MANIFESTATIONS OF FESCUE TOXICOSIS

Agalactia or hypogalactia is the most commonly reported clinical sign in mares grazing endophyte-infected fescue.[71,72] Mares grazing endophyte-infected fescue show significantly lower prolactin concentrations than mares grazing endophyte-free forage. Hypoprolactinemia associated with endophyte ingestion would inhibit normal mammary development in the prepartum period. Prolactin concentrations increase in the immediate prepartum period in the mare and return to baseline levels several weeks postpartum. Episodic increases in prolactin associated with nursing by the foal suggest the requirement of prolactin to maintain lactogenesis.[73] Suppression of prolactin by ergopeptines during the prepartum period in the cow reduced milk yields but had no effect after lactogenesis had been established. Therefore it appears that the endophyte reduces milk yield postpartum because of reduced intake.

Calving rates are decreased by the presence of endophyte in tall fescue.[74] Ewes grazing endophyte-infected fescue demonstrated a prolonged interval to conception after introduction of the ram compared to ewes on endophyte-free pasture.[75] Necropsy results and time to return to estrus indicated embryonic mortality as a cause. Mares grazing endophyte-infected fescue demonstrated increased embryonic loss rates, prolonged luteal function, and decreased per-cycle pregnancy rates compared to mares grazing endophyte-free pastures.[76]

Puberty in heifers is delayed by grazing endophyte-infected tall fescue. Progesterone concentrations were additionally decreased in heifers grazing endophyte-infected fescue, indicating luteal function was impaired.[77] Altered luteal function caused by endophyte exposure could possibly affect cyclicity and reduce pregnancy maintenance.

Mares grazing endophyte-infected tall fescue demonstrate a significant incidence of prolonged gestation, agalactia, dystocia, poor foal viability, and retained and thickened placentas.[71,78] Foals born to mares grazing endophyte-infected tall fescue are typically weak at birth with characteristic signs of dysmaturity, including overgrown hooves, irregular dental eruption, lanugo, and flexor laxity. Foal weights are significantly greater in endophyte-exposed mares despite reduced muscle mass. At birth, concentrations of triiodothyronine, progestagens, adrenocorticotropic hormone, and cortisol were significantly lower in foals from mares grazing endophyte-infected fescue.[79]

Endocrine alterations in pregnant mares grazing endophyte-infected fescue are a depression in prolactin,[71,72,79,83] thyroxine,[80] progestogens,[71,79,83] and relaxin.[81] Progesterone concentrations did not differ in mares that experienced early embryonic death, indicating an effect of the endophyte other than impaired luteal function.[76] Total progestogen concentrations were reduced with endophyte exposure of pregnant mares only after day 300 of gestation.[82] Short-term exposure of late-gestation mares to endophyte-infected fescue results in significant decreases in prolactin and progestogens.[82] At birth, concentrations of total progestogens were significantly reduced in mare jugular, foal jugular, and umbilical artery plasma, indicating reduced fetal and placental progestogen synthesis.[79]

Placental alterations in mares associated with consuming endophyte-infected fescue include premature separation of the allantochorion, increased allantochorion weight and thickness, and retained placenta.[71,78,83] Transabdominal ultrasonography demonstrated a significant increase in uteroplacental thickness in endophyte-infected mares. However, this was not observed until an average of 8 hours before the onset of labor.[84] Premature separation of the allantochorion was detected in conjunction with the increase in placental thickness. Histologic evaluation of the allantochorion revealed a significant increase in the splanchnic mesoderm caused by edema.

Approach to Diagnosis of Fescue Toxicosis

Definitive diagnosis of fescue toxicosis involves identification of the causative endophytic fungus in forage or seed samples by microscopic examination (Boxes 12-12 and 12-13). Ergopeptine concentrations may additionally be determined by high-pressure liquid chromatography analysis or specific enzyme-linked immunosorbent assay (ELISA). A presumptive diagnosis of fescue toxicosis can be made in cattle based on expression of the characteristic clinical signs of hyperthermia, excessive salivation, long, rough hair coat, necrosis of the tail and ear tips, and fat necrosis in association with consuming fescue forage. Hypoprolactinemia is supportive of the diagnosis, but the assay is not commercially available.

A presumptive diagnosis of fescue toxicity in the pregnant mare is based on the observation of failure of normal mammary development for gestational stage. Prolongation of gestation is commonly reported as well. An accurate breeding history should include dates of breeding, dates of confirmed pregnancy diagnosis, and absence of parturition at the antic-ipated time. A history of recent exposure to fescue pasture or hay is supportive. In tall fescue–endemic areas, pastures that contain tall fescue grass should be considered infected with the endophyte unless specific testing has confirmed otherwise. Determination of total plasma progestogen concentrations is a sensitive indicator of endophyte exposure after 300 days of gestation.[82]

Management of a mare suspected of endophyte exposure should consist of removing the mare from the suspected pasture or hay source and maintaining the mare in a stall or dry lot under close observation. High-quality hay, preferably legume, should be provided. Because of the increased incidence of dystocia in mares grazing endophyte-infected tall fescue, close monitoring of the mare and attendance at parturition is critical to minimize risk to the mare and loss of the foal. Removal of mares from infected fescue by day 300 of gestation has been demonstrated to alleviate the toxic effects on the mare and foal. Removal after day 300 carries an increased risk of prolonged gestation, agalactia, dystocia, and neonatal death. Induction of parturition is not recommended because of the high incidence of fetal dysmaturity, fetal oversize, and failure of pelvic relaxation associated with endophyte exposure. Elective cesarean section deliveries of postdate gestation mares have resulted in significantly higher foal survival rates than spontaneous deliveries.

Where removal of pregnant mares from infected fescue is not practical or mares are inadvertently grazed on endophyte-infected fescue beyond the recommended stage of gestation for removal, pharmacologic intervention is warranted. Several DA_2 dopamine receptor antagonists; perphenazine,[85] fluphenazine,[81] domperidone [86] and the dopamine depletor, reserpine,[87] have been investigated prophylactically to prevent or therapeutically to treat clinical fescue toxicosis. Perphenazine[85] and fluphenazine[81] have demonstrated mixed success in preventing toxicosis in restricted clinical trials. Reserpine [87] was ineffective in preventing prepartum agalactia and prolonged gestation but was sufficient to resolve postpartum agalactia. Domperidone[88] has demonstrated efficacy in both the prevention and treatment of clinical fescue toxicosis in clinical trials involving large numbers of mares in numerous locations.

BOX 12-12

Manifestations of Fescue Toxicity in the Mare

Agalactia, hypogalactia
Hypoprolactinemia
Decreased relaxin prepartum
Prolonged gestation
Early embryonic death
Cyclic irregularity
Dystocia
Premature allantochorion separation
Allantochorion edema
Increased placental weight
Retained placenta
Corpus luteum persistence
Decreased pregnancy rates
Decreased total progestagens prepartum
Poor neonatal viability
Reduced colostral immunoglobulin G (IgG) absorption
Neonatal hypoadrenalism
Neonatal hypopituitarism
Neonatal hypothyroidism
Fetal oversize
Hirsutism
Hyperhidrosis

BOX 12-13

Manifestations of Fescue Toxicity in Ruminants

Agalactia, hypogalactia
Reduced calf birth weight
Hypoprolactinemia
Reduced serum cholesterol
Reduced conception rates
Reduced pregnancy rates
Early embryonic death
Cyclic irregularity
Delayed return to cyclicity postpartum
Dystocia
Hyperthermia
Hyperpnea
Hirsutism
Reduced weight gain
Photosensitization
Necrosis of the digits
Necrosis of the ears and tail
Fat necrosis

REFERENCES

69. McCluskey B et al: Survey of endophyte infection and its associated toxin in pastures grazed by horses, *Proc Am Assoc Equine Pract* 45:213-216, 1999.
70. Shelby RA, Dalrymple LW: Incidence and distribution of tall fescue endophyte in the United States, *Plant Disease* 71:783-786, 1987.
71. Garret LW et al: Reproductive problems of pregnant mares grazing endophyte-infected fescue pastures, *J Anim Sci* 51(suppl 1):237, 1980.
72. Boosinger TR et al: Prolonged gestation, decreased triiodothyronine, and thyroid gland histomorphology in newborn foals from mares grazing *Acremonium coenophialum*–infected fescue pasture, *Am J Vet Res* 56:66-69, 1995.
73. Worthy K et al: Plasma prolactin concentrations and cyclic activity in pony mares during parturition and early lactation, *J Reprod Fertil* 77:569-574, 1986.
74. Gay N et al: Effects of endophyte-infected tall fescue on beef cow-calf performance, *Appl Agric Res* 3:182-186, 1988.
75. Bond J et al: Reproductive performance and lamb weights for ewes grazing endophyte-infected tall fescue, *Nutr Rep Int* 37:1099-1115, 1988.
76. Brendemuehl JP et al: Influence of endophyte-infected tall fescue on cyclicity, pregnancy rate, and early embryonic loss in the mare, *Theriogenology* 42:489-500, 1990.
77. Schmidt SP et al: Fescue fungus suppresses growth and reproduction in replacement beef heifers, *Highlights Agric Res* 33:150-151, 1986.
78. Putnam MR et al: Effects of the fungal endophyte *Acremonium coenophialum* in fescue on pregnant mares and foal viability, *Am J Vet Res* 52:2071-2074, 1991.
79. Brendemuehl JP et al: Plasma progesterone, triiodothyronine, and cortisol concentrations in postdate gestation foals exposed in utero to tall fescue endophyte *Acremonium coenophialum*, *Biol Reprod Monograph Series 1: Equine Reprod* 6:53-59, 1995.
80. Tompson FN et al: Thyroidal and prolactin secretion in agalactic mares, *Theriogenology* 25:575-580, 1986.

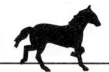

81. Ryan P et al: Effects of fescue toxicoses and fluphenazine on relaxin concentrations in pregnant pony mares, *Proc Am Assoc Equine Pract* 44:60-61, 1998.
82. Brendemuehl JP et al: Effects of short-term exposure to and removal from the fescue endophyte *Acremonium coenophialum* at 300 days of gestation on pregnant mares and foal viability, *Biol Reprod Monograph Series 1: Equine Reprod* 6:61-67, 1995.
83. McCann JS et al: Influence of endophyte-infected tall fescue on serum prolactin and progesterone in pregnant mares, *J Anim Sci* 70:217-223, 1992.
84. Brendemuehl JP et al: Ultrasonographic and histomorphometric evaluation of the allantochorion of pregnant mares grazing tall fescue infected with the endophyte *Acremonium coenophialum*, *Am J Vet Res* 2000 (in press).
85. Ireland FA et al: Effects of bromocriptine and perphenazine on prolactin and progesterone concentrations in pony mares during late gestation, *J Reprod Fertil* 92:179-186, 1991.
86. Redmond LM et al: Efficacy of domperidone and sulpiride as treatments for fescue toxicoses in horses, *Am J Vet Res* 55:722-729, 1994.
87. Evans TJ et al: A comparison of the relative effectiveness of domperidone and reserpine in treating equine fescue toxicoses, *Proc Am Assoc Equine Pract* 45:207-209, 1999.
88. Cross DL et al: Clinical effects of domperidone on fescue toxicoses in pregnant mares, *Proc Am Assoc Equine Pract* 45:203-206, 1999.

PROLONGED GESTATION

MICHAEL S. SPENSLEY

Many factors influence the duration of gestation in horses and ruminants. Normal variations in length of gestation have been attributed to genetic, nutritional, and environmental factors.[89,90] The species, breed, and sex of the fetus, ambient temperature, and length of photoperiod are among factors that, within normal variations, affect the duration of gestation.[89-92] The duration of pregnancy in thoroughbred mares ranges from 310 to 374 days,[92] in dairy cows from 275 to 292 days, in beef cows from 271 to 310 days, in ewes from 143 to155 days, and in does from 146 to 155 days.[93] Prolonged gestation periods are those that exceed the normal gestational variation attributable to genetic, nutritional, and environmental factors. In pathologic prolonged gestation there is an impediment to the mechanisms that terminate gestation and initiate parturition. Pathologically prolonged gestation has been attributed to genetic, infectious, and toxic factors.[94]

Of the several forms of prolonged gestation with genetic causes in cattle, the best described forms have been observed in Guernsey and Holstein cattle.[90,91,94,95] In each the fetus fails to initiate parturition at term because of fetal adrenal hypoplasia. Prolonged gestation, from 3 weeks to 3 months beyond normal term, has been observed in a number of dairy cattle breeds.[96] Graves, Hansel, and Krook[95] described a Holstein fetus of 441 days' gestation in which the pituitary pars distalis was aplastic and the adrenal and thyroid glands were severely hypoplastic. Two different types of fetuses have been associated with prolonged gestation in cattle.[89] In the first type, fetuses had a large skeleton and excessive growth of epidermal organ structures such as hair and hooves but no obvious deformities. The second type of fetus was mature or immature and exhibited cranial and central nervous system anomalies; growth ceased at about 7 months of gestation. Both types of calves had hypoplastic or absent adrenal glands. These anomalies have been observed to be inherited as an autosomal recessive trait.[90,94]

Several infectious agents have been incriminated in prolonged gestation in ruminants. Bluetongue virus, bovine diarrhea virus, and border disease virus may cause severe cerebral lesions in the fetus, resulting in the absence of a hypothalamus and pituitary stalk. Again, by virtue of the lack of adrenocorticotropic hormone, the sequence of events necessary for parturition does not occur.[94]

Veratrum californicum contains the teratogenic agent cyclopamine. When pregnant ewes ingest cyclopamine on the fourteenth day of gestation, their fetuses lack a pituitary gland or have a malformed hypothalamic stalk. These defects result in prolonged gestation by virtue of secondary adrenal hypoplasia.[94]

Prolonged gestation in mares has been cited as an indication for induction of parturition.[97,98] However, the clinical significance of prolonged gestation in mares is undetermined because there is no apparent correlation between duration of gestation and readiness for birth. Dysmature neonatal foals have resulted from gestations of normal and longer than normal durations; alternatively, 399 days' gestation resulted in births of normal twin foals.[99] Prolonged gestation in the mare has not generally been associated with excessively large foals and dystocia.[100] Therefore, in the absence of clinical signs that warrant induction of parturition in a high-risk pregnancy and the fulfillment of criteria for induced parturition, there is no reason to perform elective parturition induction in mares in which gestation is prolonged.

Approach to Diagnosis of Prolonged Gestation

Approach to the diagnosis of prolonged gestation in mares and ruminants is essentially similar (Boxes 12-14 and 12-15). If the client is concerned about what is apparently prolonged gestation in an otherwise normal dam, an accurate breeding history should be obtained. Because no pathognomonic clinical or laboratory findings are associated with prolonged gestation, the diagnosis is predicated on the history and a general physical examination of the dam. The overall condition of the dam should be determined. In addition to the reproductive history, exposure to infectious agents and toxic plants should be determined. The most important anamnestic factors are breeding dates, dates of confirmed pregnancy examinations, and absence of parturition at the expected time.

BOX 12-14

Causes of Prolonged Gestation in the Mare

Fescue toxicity
Fetal mummification
Delayed embryonic development

BOX 12-15

Causes of Prolonged Gestation in Ruminants

Fetal mummification
Fetal hypothalamic-hypophysial-adrenal axis disorder
Autosomal recessive genetic disorder affecting Holstein and Guernsey cattle (B)
Vitamin A deficiency (B)
Veratrum album toxicity (B)
Veratrum californicum toxicity (cyclopamine) (O)
High environmental temperature (B)
Fescue toxicity
Hydrops amnii (B, O)
Bluetongue (B, O)
Bovine viral diarrhea (B)
Border disease (O)
Salsola tuberculata toxicity (Grootlamsiekte [exotic]) (O)
Akabane virus (exotic) (B, O)

B, Bovine; *O*, ovine; *C*, caprine.

The reproductive tract should be examined for the gravid uterus and evidence, although tenuous, of the term or near-term fetus. Diagnostic ultrasonography can be incorporated into the workup to enhance the assessment of viability and fetal well-being by determination of fetal heart rates, fetal size and movement, uteroplacental thickness, and estimation of allantoic fluid volume.[101-103] Parturition should not be induced unless the objective is fetal survival in the face of a high-risk pregnancy.[103] Otherwise, the mare should be examined and, if appropriate, the owner assured that the gestation is probably normal and that patience will likely result in a normal foal with adequate colostrum and passive immunity.[104]

REFERENCES

89. Holm LW: Prolonged pregnancy. In Brandly CA, Cornelius CC, eds: *Advances in veterinary science*, vol 2, New York, 1967, Academic Press.
90. Drost M: Role of the fetus in prolonged gestation in the cow, *Proc Soc Theriogenol*, 1979, pp 132-138.
91. Roberts SJ: *Veterinary obstetrics and genital diseases (theriogenology)*, ed 3, North Pomfret, Vt, 1986, SJ Roberts.
92. Rossdale PD, Ricketts SW: *The practice of equine stud medicine*, London, 1974, Ballière Tindall.
93. Smith MC: Clinical reproductive anatomy and physiology of the doe. In Youngquist RS, ed: *Current therapy in large animal theriogenology*, Philadelphia, 1997, WB Saunders.
94. Osburn BI, Kennedy PC: Abortion and prenatal disease. In Howard JL, ed: *Current veterinary therapy 3: food animal practice*, Philadelphia, 1981, WB Saunders.
95. Graves TK, Hansel W, Krook L: Prolonged gestation in a Holstein cow: adenohypophyseal aplasia and skeletal pathology in the offspring, *Cornell Vet* 81:277-294, 1991.
96. Callahan CJ et al: Prolonged gestation in a Holstein-Friesian cow: clinical and reproductive steroid studies, *Cornell Vet* 59:370-387, 1969.
97. Hillman RB: Induction of parturition. In Robinson NE, ed: *Current therapy in equine medicine*, ed 2, Philadelphia, 1987, WB Saunders.
98. Carleton CL, Threlfall WR: Induction of parturition in the mare. In Morrow DA, ed: *Current therapy in theriogenology 2: diagnosis, treatment, and prevention of reproductive diseases in small and large animals*, Philadelphia, 1986, WB Saunders.
99. Vandeplaassche MM: Obstetrician's view of the physiology of equine parturition and dystocia, *Equine Vet J* 12:45-49, 1980.
100. Vandeplaassche MM: Prepartum complications and dystocia. In Robinson NE, ed: *Current therapy in equine medicine*, ed 2, Philadelphia, 1987, WB Saunders.
101. Adams-Brendemuehl C, Pipers FS: Antepartum evaluations of the equine fetus, *J Reprod Fertil* 35(suppl):565-573, 1987.
102. Adams-Brendemuehl C: Fetal assessment. In Koterba AM, Drummond WH, Kosch PC, eds: *Equine clinical neonatology*, Philadelphia, 1990, Lea & Febiger.
103. Sanstchi EM et al: Evaluation of equine high-risk pregnancy, *Compend Cont Educ Pract Vet* 16:80-87, 1994.
104. Lofstedt RM: Miscellaneous diseases of pregnancy and parturition. In McKinnon AO, Voss JL, eds: *Equine reproduction*, Philadelphia, 1993, Lea & Febiger.

DYSTOCIA

MICHAEL S. SPENSLEY
MATS H.T. TROEDSSON

Dystocia is defined as difficult parturition; it may be a sign of either maternal or fetal conditions that impede fetal passage through the birth canal.[105] Dystocia in mares and ruminants is more likely to be attributable to fetal causes such as malpresentation, malposition, and malposture than to maternal conditions[105,106] (Boxes 12-16 and 12-17). The overall incidence of dystocia and incidences of types of dystocia vary among the species and breeds within a species.[107] Cattle, especially first-calving heifers and larger breeds, are more commonly affected by dystocia; the overall incidence of bovine dystocia ranges from 3% to 25%.[105] The incidence of dystocia among thoroughbred mares is 4%,[106] and in does, 3% to 5%.[108] The incidence of dystocia is generally greater in sheep than in goats.[109] Dystocia represents an emergency situation that commands prompt resolution to afford the optimum

---

BOX 12-16

Causes of Dystocia in the Mare

COMMON CAUSES
Malpresentation
Malposition
Malposture
Abortion
Arthrogryposis
Twinning

LESS COMMON CAUSES
Fescue toxicity
Preterm parturition
Torticollis
Vaginal, vulvar obstructions (hematoma, callus, abscess, tumor)
Pelvic injury, fracture

UNCOMMON CAUSES
Fetopelvic disproportion
Congenital defects
Hydrocephalus
Uterine dorsoretroflexion
Uterine torsion
Hydrops of fetal membranes
Rupture of prepubic tendon
Fetal mummification, maceration
Vaginal prolapse
Abdominal, inguinal hernia
Uterine inertia
Induction of parturition
Premature separation of chorioallantois from endometrium
Uterine laceration

---

prognosis for dam and fetus. Reposition, traction, fetotomy, and cesarean section are the obstetric procedures available for the management of dystocia.[110] The economics of large animal practice often play a significant role in determining which course to pursue in resolving dystocia. The lives of the dam and the fetus may be at risk. Although the objective should be the survival of both, unless otherwise advised by the owner and if conditions are not prohibitive, the well-being of the dam and her reproductive potential should have priority over the fetus.

Although parturition has been divided into three distinct stages for descriptive purposes, the stages overlap clinically, and normal parturition is observed as a continuous process.[106] The equine fetus is lying in a ventral or ventrolateral position with head and fore limbs flexed during late gestation.[111] During the first stage of parturition the fetus plays an active role, along with myometrial contractions, in assuming correct extremity posture as it positions itself for delivery through the birth canal. The second stage of parturition commences with rupture of the chorioallantois and culminates in delivery of the fetus. Myometrial contractions continue during third-stage parturition, which ends with the expulsion of the placenta. In the mare parturition is a forceful, explosive act. The time between rupture of the chorioallantoic membrane and delivery of the fetus is normally about 20 minutes.[105] Separation of the fetal membranes from the endometrium may occur within 1 to 2 hours after the second stage of parturition commences; therefore the retained fetus must be delivered quickly or it will asphyxiate. Fetal expul-

BOX 12-17

Causes of Dystocia in Ruminants

COMMON CAUSES
Fetopelvic disproportion (B, common; C, O, uncommon)
Malpresentation
Malposition
Malposture
Twins, triplets (B)
Uterine torsion
Periparturient hypocalcemia (B)
Failure of cervix to dilate (B, O; rare in C)
Lymphedema

LESS COMMON CAUSES
Preterm parturition
Abortion
Congenital defects (fetal monsters)
Hydrops of fetal membranes (B, O)
Emphysematous fetus
Hydrocephalus (more common in B than O, C)
Extremity ankylosis (more common in B than O, C)
Breeding immature, young, small for age females
Obesity (B)
Pregnancy toxemia (O, C)
Uterine inertia
Fetal mummification, maceration
Uterine, cervical, vaginal obstruction
Retained fetus
Pelvic fracture
Vaginal prolapse

UNCOMMON CAUSES
Phytoestrogen toxicity (B, O)
Rectovaginal constriction of Jersey cattle (B)
Uterine rupture
Abdominal, inguinal hernias
Lipomatosis (B)
Lupine poisoning, arthrogryposis (B)
Polybrominated biphenyl toxicity
Bovine fetal tumors
Rupture of prepubic tendon (B)
Hereditary edema, lymphedema in Ayrshire calves
Prolonged gestation (B, O)
Chlorinated naphthalene toxicity

B, Bovine; C, caprine; O, ovine.

sion in the ruminant is not quite as explosive as in the mare; second-stage parturition in the bovine usually requires ½ hour to 4 hours.[105] Ewes and does require a range of ½ hour to 2 hours to complete the second stage, or slightly longer if twins or triplets are present.[105] Primiparous animals generally require a longer time to expel the fetus than do multiparous dams.

Dystocia in large animals is often accompanied by forceful straining. The dam may attempt to lie down and stand repeatedly. This is characteristic of dams with dystocia that is caused by fetopelvic disproportion, malposture, or fetal impaction. Alternatively, the dam may stand quietly with minimal or no straining, as in cases of uterine inertia, uterine rupture, or exhaustion associated with prolonged dystocia of any cause. Whatever the presentation of the dam, the attending veterinarian must be prepared for unexpected behavior when attempting to perform obstetric examinations and procedures. The dam, fetus, attendants, and veterinarians must be protected from injury. The dam should be placed in open-ended stocks with movable sides or a straw-bedded box stall. During obstetric examination and manipulation, mares and cows may attempt to get up and lie down, or they may suddenly collapse. Such sudden movements may injure the dam and veterinarian if rigid, closed-end stocks are used. Minimum physical restraint should be used; however, restraint should be sufficient to permit completion of the obstetric examination and procedures with efficiency and safety. Adequate physical restraint may be achieved in the mare with a twitch or a lip chain. Little is known about the pharmacokinetics of drugs in pregnant domestic animals. Accordingly, it must be assumed that sedative and anesthetic drugs will depress neonatal and fetal functions at least as much as those of the mare. The effects on myometrial activity of drugs administered to dams experiencing dystocia must also be considered. Acepromazine has little effect on the fetus and is generally considered safe for use in the pregnant mare. However, acepromazine was shown to have a suppressive effect on myometrial activity in cycling mares.[112] Xylazine causes significant fetal cardiovascular compromise in horses and has been reported to stimulate myometrial activity in cows and mares.[112-114] The fetal and myometrial effects of detomidine are similar but of longer duration compared with those of xylazine.[112,113] The effects of detomidine on myoelectrical activity in the uteri of cows and mares treated during the last trimester of pregnancy were dose dependent.[115,116]

As equipment is being organized and the process of evaluating the dam begins, a pertinent reproductive history should be obtained, including the dam's age, her previous breeding history, and the outcomes of previous pregnancies (i.e., abortion, normal parturition, dystocia). Her present gestational status should be determined; has parturition commenced at term or is it a preterm or postterm delivery? Her udder should be examined to determine the stage of development. Information about the progress of the current parturition should be obtained. The time since rupture of the chorioallantoic membrane, the duration and intensity of labor, whether fetal membranes or parts have appeared at the vulva, and previous attempts to assist in delivery should be noted. If the dam is recumbent, the veterinarian should determine if she has attempted to or been able to rise. Although a complete examination of the dam is optimum, it should be postponed until after the delivery of the fetus. However, in obtaining the dam's reproductive history, questions about her current physical condition should be included. Such predisposing factors as recent weight loss, systemic disease, and trauma should be considered. She should be assessed for signs of hemorrhage, dehydration, and shock.

After the tail has been wrapped, the perineal area should be thoroughly and gently washed and rinsed. Examination of the dam's reproductive tract may cause some discomfort or pain. Temperance regarding analgesia and sedation must be practiced. Caudal epidural anesthesia (4 to 8 ml of 2% lidocaine or other anesthetic) is often an excellent means of facilitating examination and resolution of dystocia and at the same time minimizing trauma to the dam, fetus, and operator. Lidocaine epidural anesthesia may cause hindlimb weakness and ataxia. Safe and effective analgesia can also be induced by epidural administration of xylazine (0.17 mg/kg diluted in 10 ml physiologic saline). A combination of lidocaine (0.22 mg/kg) and xylazine (0.17 mg/kg) resulted in an onset of analgesia within a few minutes and a duration of over 5½ hours.[117] Although vaginal sensitivity and the Ferguson reflex both are reduced by epidural anesthesia, myometrial contractions and abdominal press are not totally eliminated. Great care must be taken during the examination of the genitalia and fetus. In addition to the viability of fetus and dam, the dam's future reproductive potential is at risk and must be preserved. The vulva, vestibule, vagina, and cervix should be carefully examined. The location of the fetus in the birth canal, as well as its viability, presentation, position, and posture, should be determined. Schuijt and Ball[118] described a procedure to manually dilate the bovine birth canal before forced extraction is attempted. In the management of dystocia in any species, forced extraction should proceed only after maximal dilation of the caudal reproductive tract in order to minimize the potential for injuries to the dam during parturition (i.e., cervical, vaginal, and vulvar lacerations, hematomas, postparturient vaginal necrosis and obturator, perineal and gluteal paralyses).[105,119] Mares are especially susceptible to cervical lacerations, which may have detrimental consequences on the dam's future reproductive performance. Slow traction with continuous palpation of cervical stretching by the attending obstetrician is therefore recommended in equine dystocias.

The integrity of the birth canal, fluids, and fetal membranes serves as an indicator of the length of time the dystocia has persisted and the well-being of the fetus. Generous lubrication is required in all cases of dystocia and should be applied continuously during the management of dystocia to prevent damage to the dam's birth canal. Lubricating preparations consisting of methyl cellulose are superior to those consisting of mineral oil or soaps. Several liters of lubricants should be infused into the bovine and equine uterus by the use of a nasogastric tube.

Traction or forced extraction can usually be successfully implemented after correction of malpresentation, malposition, or malposture. In equine dystocia, if the foal is still alive and dystocia cannot be relieved quickly (20 minutes) or if it is determined that extensive manipulation will be required, general anesthesia may be induced. Because of the length of the extremities of the foal, mutation is more difficult in the mare than in the cow, and requires extensive repulsion to provide adequate room for manipulation. Examination and manipulation can be greatly facilitated by elevating the mare's hindquarters, enabling the fetus and viscera to recede cranially into the mare's abdominal cavity, thereby allowing more room for the operator.[120] If a nonviable fetus cannot be delivered by traction or forced extraction or if the owner is unwilling to select cesarean section, fetotomy can be performed.[110,120] Beyond the delivery of the nonviable fetus, fetotomy is indicated to save the mare and her subsequent fertility.[110] The advantages of fetotomy include avoiding major abdominal surgery (cesarean section) and its complications and preserving the birth canal because excessively large parts are not forced through it.[105,119-121] At the same time, the primary disadvantage of fetotomy, particularly if not properly performed by an experienced obstetrician, is trauma to the birth canal by instruments, wire, or bone.[105] The indications, equipment, procedures, and complications of fetotomy have been reviewed in several publications.[105,110,119-121]

Cesarean section is indicated for a dam with dystocia when attempts to deliver the fetus by reposition, traction, and fetotomy are unsuccessful or contraindicated, and continued attempts may compromise the fetus, the dam, or her subsequent fertility.[105,107,109,122-129] Cesarean section may be the only rational procedure for delivery of some fetuses (i.e., emphysematous fetuses, deformed fetuses, and bicornuate fetuses). In addition, high-risk pregnancies caused by maternal conditions can be effectively and efficiently managed by cesarean section.[125] The specific indications, procedures, and complications of cesarean section have been reviewed in a number of publications.[105,107,122-129]

Management of a case of dystocia is not complete until a systematic examination, focusing on the dam's reproductive tract, has been conducted. Complications during dystocia involving the reproductive tract and other body systems can affect the outcome of the case.[105,130-132] As much as possible, examination of the dam's reproductive tract should rule out the presence of another fetus in the uterus or abdominal cavity.[105] The most common reproductive injuries incurred by dams during parturition include cervical, vaginal, and vulvar lacerations, hematomas, postparturient vaginal necrosis, and uterine hemorrhage.[119,132,133] Gastrointestinal complications, such as constipation associated with unwillingness to defecate, postpartum perineal inflammation, and bruising or rupture of entrapped or compressed segments of the gastrointestinal tract, can follow parturition in the mare.[132] Musculoskeletal and neurologic complications have been reported after parturition in cows and mares.[105] Retained placenta, delayed uterine involution, metritis, and laminitis may result from normal parturition but are more likely sequelae of dystocia.[105,132,134]

The signs associated with normal progression of each of the stages of parturition must be explained carefully to clients and farm managers. It is only through understanding the clinical signs associated with events of normal parturition that clients become proficient at recognizing abnormal events and know when to seek professional assistance.

REFERENCES

105. Roberts SJ: *Veterinary obstetrics and genital diseases (theriogenology)*, ed 3, North Pomfret, Vt, 1986, SJ Roberts.
106. Rossdale PD, Ricketts SW: *Equine stud farm medicine*, ed 2, Philadelphia, 1980, Lea & Febiger.
107. Arthur GH, Noakes DE, Pearson H: *Veterinary reproduction and obstetrics (theriogenology)*, ed 5, London, 1982, Baillière Tindall.
108. Brown W: Parturition and dystocia in the goat. In Youngquist RS, ed: *Current therapy in large animal theriogenology*, Philadelphia, 1997, WB Saunders.
109. East NE: Pregnancy toxemia, abortions, and periparturient diseases: symposium on sheep and goat medicine, *Vet Clin North Am (Large Anim Pract)* 5:601-618, 1983.
110. Vandeplaasche MM: Dystocia. In McKinnon AO, Voss JL, eds: *Equine reproduction*, Philadelphia, 1993, Lea & Febiger.
111. Jeffcott LB, Rossdale PD: A radiographic study of the foetus in late pregnancy and during foaling, *J Reprod Fertil* 27(suppl):563, 1979.
112. Gibbs HM, Troedsson MHT: The effect of acepromazine, detomidine, and xylazine on myometrial activity in the mare, *Biol Reprod Monograph Series 1: Equine Reprod* 6:299-304, 1995.
113. LeBlanc MM, Norman WM: Sedation and anesthesia of the mare during obstetric manipulation, *Proc Am Assoc Am Pract* 38:619-622, 1992.
114. Gilbert RO, Schwark WS: Pharmacologic consideration in the management of peripartum conditions in the cow, *Vet Clin North Am (Food Anim Pract)* 8:29-56, 1992.
115. Jedruch J, Gajewski Z: The effect of detomidine hydrochloride (Dormosedan) on the electrical activity of the uterus in cows, *Acta Vet Scand* 82(suppl):189-192, 1986.
116. Jedruch J, Gajewski Z: The effect of detomidine hydrochloride (Dormosedan) on the electrical activity of the uterus in pregnant mares, *Acta Vet Scand* 30:307-311, 1986.
117. Grubb TL, Reibold TW, Huber MJ: Comparison of lidocaine, xylazine, and xylazine/lidocaine for caudal epidural analgesia in horses, *J Am Vet Med Assoc* 201:1187-1190, 1992.
118. Schuijt G, Ball L: Delivery by forced extraction and other aspects of bovine obstetrics. In Morrow DA, ed: *Current therapy in theriogenology: diagnosis, treatment, and prevention of reproductive diseases in small and large animals*, ed 2, Philadelphia, 1986, WB Saunders.
119. Mortimer RG, Toombs RE: Abnormal bovine parturition: obstetrics and fetotomy, *Vet Clin North Am (Food Anim Pract)* 9:323-341, 1993.
120. Blanchard TL et al: Management of dystocia in mares: examination, obstetrical equipment, and vaginal delivery, *Compend Cont Educ Pract Vet* 11:745-753, 1989.
121. Bierschwal CJ, de Bois CHW: *The technique of fetotomy in large animals*, Bonner Springs, Kan, 1972, VM Publishing.
122. Hudson RS: Genital surgery of the cow. In Morrow DA, ed: *Current therapy in theriogenology: diagnosis, treatment, and prevention of reproductive diseases in small and large animals*, ed 2, Philadelphia, 1986, WB Saunders.
123. Campbell ME, Fubini SL: Indications and surgical approaches for cesarean section in cattle, *Compend Cont Educ Pract Vet* 12:285-292, 1990.
124. Taylor TS et al: Management of dystocia in mares: uterine torsion and cesarean section, *Compend Cont Educ Pract Vet* 11:1265-1273, 1989.
125. Santschi EM et al: Evaluation of equine high-risk pregnancy, *Compend Cont Educ Pract Vet* 16:80-87, 1994.
126. Vandeplaasche MM: Obstetrician's view of the physiology of equine parturition and dystocia, *Equine Vet J* 12:45-49, 1980.
127. Vandeplaasche MM et al: Cesarean section in the mare, *Proc Am Assoc Equine Pract* 23:75-80, 1977.
128. Stashak TS, Vandeplaasche MM: Cesarean section. In McKinnon AO, Voss JL, eds: *Equine reproduction*, Philadelphia, 1993, Lea & Febiger.

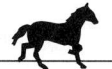

129. Juzwiak JS et al: Cesarean section in 19 mares: results and postoperative fertility, *Vet Surg* 191:50-52, 1990.
130. Kersting K: Postpartum care of cow and calf. In Youngquist RS, ed: *Current therapy in large animal theriogenology*, Philadelphia, 1997, WB Saunders.
131. Vandeplaasche MM: Prepartum complications and dystocia. In Robinson NE, ed: *Current therapy in equine medicine*, ed 2, Philadelphia, 1987, WB Saunders.
132. Zent WW: Postpartum complications. In Robinson NE, ed: *Current therapy in equine medicine*, ed 2, Philadelphia, 1987, WB Saunders.
133. Lofstedt RM: Miscellaneous diseases of pregnancy and parturition. In McKinnon AO, Voss JL, eds: *Equine reproduction*, Philadelphia, 1993, Lea & Febiger.
134. Blanchard TL et al: Management of dystocia in mares: retained placenta, metritis, and laminitis, *Compend Cont Educ Pract Vet* 12:563-569, 1990.

RETAINED FETAL MEMBRANES

MICHAEL S. SPENSLEY
MATS H.T. TROEDSSON

Retained fetal membranes represent the failure of the entire or partial placenta to be expelled within physiologic time limits. Although variation exists among species regarding the duration of time that must pass before a placenta is considered retained, the condition is one of the most common complications occurring in animals after parturition.[135]

RETAINED FETAL MEMBRANES IN THE MARE

The anatomic structure of the equine placenta is described as diffuse, epitheliochorial, and microcotyledonary. It is composed of the allantochorion, the allantoamnion, and the umbilical cord.[136] During most normal foalings, the separation of fetal membranes from the endometrium and their subsequent expulsion occurs within ½ hour to 3 hours of the delivery.[135] The incidence of retained fetal membranes is 2% to 10% in the mare, with a higher incidence in draft horses than in lighter horse breeds.[135] The cause of retained fetal membranes remains unclear, but it is believed that allantochorionic microcotyledons near the tip of the nongravid uterine horn have failed to separate as a result of an endocrine unbalance, a disturbance in normal myometrial contractions, or any swelling at the site of microcotyledons[137] (Box 12-18).

BOX 12-18

Causes of Retained Fetal Membranes in the Mare

COMMON CAUSES
Dystocia
Preterm parturition
Abortion
Endometritis, metritis
Twinning
Induced parturition
Stillbirth

LESS COMMON CAUSES
Fetotomy
Cesarean section
Placental edema at uterine horn tip
Placentitis
Drugs
Prolonged gestation
Fescue toxicity
Poor condition, poor environment, fatigue, increasing age, and other debilitating conditions
Hypocalcemia
Dropsy of fetal membranes
Entrapped placenta

Diagnosis of retained fetal membranes in the mare is straightforward when it is based on the observation of membranes hanging from the vulva beyond 3 hours after foaling. However, if the fetal membranes fall cranially over the pelvis, they remain within the uterus without being visible, and the diagnosis must be made using vaginoscopy or ultrasonography or by digital intrauterine examination. If an early diagnosis of complete or partial retention of fetal membranes has been missed, the diagnosis may be made 1 to 2 days after foaling. At this time, clinical signs indicative of metritis are often present (i.e., fever, depression, colic, and/or laminitis).

After their expulsion, the fetal membranes should be stored until they can be scrutinized to determine if they are complete. The clinician should rinse the fetal membranes with water and, on a flat surface, thoroughly examine them for completeness.[138] Evidence that a part of the placenta is retained in the uterus or that an area of microvilli has been sheared off and retained in the endometrial crypts is an indication for digital endometrial examination or ultrasonographic examination, and institution of appropriate therapy (see Chapter 41, Retained Fetal Membranes).

Approach to Diagnosis of Retained Fetal Membranes

HISTORY. Many cases of retained fetal membranes follow episodes of dystocia, cesarean section, and fetotomy. An increased incidence of retained fetal membranes has been reported in mares that abort after the seventh month of gestation.[139] However, no increase in the incidence of retained fetal membranes associated with abortion, stillbirth, twinning, and delivery of a weak or diseased foal was observed if it occurred without dystocia.[140]

PHYSICAL EXAMINATION. Fetal membranes must be examined after their expulsion to determine their entirety and integrity. Tears, missing areas of tissue, and areas of chorionic surface devoid of microvilli should be considered evidence of partly retained fetal membranes, and immediate action should be taken to enhance expulsion of retained tissue and minimize complications.

Vital signs may be normal early in cases of retained fetal membranes. A rectal examination should be performed to determine the degree of uterine involution. Aseptic intrauterine palpation can be performed to determine the area and extent of retention and the integrity of involved tissues and fluid.[138] Systemic signs of dehydration, septicemia, toxemia, and laminitis may accompany fetal membranes retained for 24 to 36 hours.[141] Occasionally mares with retained fetal membranes show signs of colic. Therapeutic approaches for retained fetal membranes in mares are discussed in Chapter 41.

RETAINED FETAL MEMBRANES IN RUMINANTS

The anatomic structure of the ruminant placenta is described as cotyledonary and epitheliochorial.[135] It is composed of the allantochorion, the allantoamnion, and the umbilical cord. Fetal membranes are considered pathologically retained in the cow if they are not expelled by 8 to 12 hours after calving.[135] The incidence of retained fetal membranes in dairy cattle is 3% to 12% after normal parturition.[142] Dairy cows are more commonly affected than beef cows.[142] The incidence of retained fetal membranes may exceed 50% after abnormal parturition or abortion and in brucellosis-infected herds.[142] The retained placenta itself is relatively innocuous, but the condition is important because cows with retained fetal membranes experience an increased incidence of postpartum complications such as metritis, pyometra, ketosis, mastitis, delayed conception, and abortion.[143,144] The principal cause of retained placenta in cattle is a disturbance in the

Causes of Retained Fetal Membranes in Ruminants

COMMON CAUSES
Multiple births
Induced parturition
Placentitis (bacterial, fungal infection)
Hypocalcemia
Abortion
Stillbirth
Dystocia
Abnormal gestation length

LESS COMMON CAUSES
Injury, inflammation, or edema of placentome
Cesarean section
Uterine torsion
Necrotic placentomes secondary to uterine and systemic
    disease
Excessive weight gain during dry period
Uterine atony
Dropsy of fetal membranes
Entrapment of separated placenta
Prostaglandin $F_{2\alpha}$ deficiency
Trace mineral deficiencies (selenium and iodine)
Vitamin deficiencies (carotene, vitamins A and E)
Mineral deficiencies, imbalances (calcium and
    phosphorus)
Heat stress
Increasing age
Nitrate toxicity
High milk production

PHYSICAL EXAMINATION. In cows that have calved spontaneously and without problem after a normal gestation period, little illness tends to be associated with retained fetal membranes, and treatment may be unnecessary. Transient decreases in appetite and milk production may be observed.[142] However, metritis, toxemia, and septicemia may be observed when retention of fetal membranes is associated with gestation of abnormal length, dystocia, nutritional deficiencies, or certain infectious diseases. Metritis affects up to 90% of cows with retained fetal membranes.[149] For considerations for the treatment of retained fetal membranes in cows, see Chapter 41.

REFERENCES
135. Roberts SJ: *Veterinary obstetrics and genital diseases (theriogenology)*, ed 3, North Pomfret, Vt, 1986, SJ Roberts, pp 44-49; 353-396.
136. Asbury AC, LeBlanc MM: The placenta. In McKinnon AO, Voss JL, eds: *Equine reproduction*, Philadelphia, 1993, Lea & Febiger.
137. Threlfall WR: Retained placenta. In McKinnon AO, Voss JL, eds: *Equine reproduction*, Philadelphia, 1993, Lea & Febiger.
138. Blanchard TL, Varner DD: Therapy for retained placenta in the mare, *Vet Med* 88:55-59, 1993.
139. Vandeplaasche M, Spincemaille J, Bouters R: Aetiology, pathogenesis, and treatment of retained placenta in the mare, *Equine Vet J* 3:144-147, 1971.
140. Provencher R et al: Retained fetal membranes in the mare: a retrospective study, *Can Vet J* 29:903-910, 1988.
141. Zent WW: Postpartum complications. In Robinson NE, ed: *Current therapy in equine medicine*, ed 2, Philadelphia, 1987, WB Saunders.
142. Arthur GH: Retention of the afterbirth in cattle: a review and commentary, *Vet Ann* 19:26-36, 1979.
143. Gilbert RO, Schwark WS: Pharmacologic considerations in the management of peripartum conditions in the cow, *Vet Clin North Am* 8:29-57, 1992.
144. Fahning ML: Retained fetal membranes. In Howard JL, ed: *Current veterinary therapy 3: food animal practice*, Philadelphia, 1993, WB Saunders.
145. Eilert H: Retained placenta. In Youngquist RS, ed: *Current therapy in large animal theriogenology*, Philadelphia, 1997, WB Saunders.
146. Bretzlaff K: Physiology and pharmacology of the postpartum cow and retained fetal membranes, *Proceedings of the American Association of Bovine Practitioners*, 1988, pp 71-76.
147. East NE: Pregnancy toxemia, abortions, and periparturient diseases: symposium on sheep and goat medicine, *Vet Clin North Am (Large Anim Pract)* 5:601-618, 1983.
148. Franklin JS: Retained placenta, metritis, and pyometra. In Morrow DA, ed: *Current therapy in theriogenology: diagnosis, treatment, and prevention of reproductive diseases in small and large animals*, ed 2, Philadelphia, 1986, WB Saunders.
149. Olson JD et al: The metritis-pyometra complex. In Morrow DA, ed: *Current therapy in theriogenology: diagnosis, treatment, and prevention of reproductive diseases in small and large animals*, ed 2, Philadelphia, 1986, WB Saunders.
150. Paisley LG, Mickelsen WE, Anderson PB: Mechanisms and therapy for retained fetal membranes and uterine infections of cows: a review, *Theriogenology* 25:353-381, 1986.
151. McClary D: Retained placenta. In Howard JL, ed: *Current veterinary therapy 2: food animal practice*, Philadelphia, 1986, WB Saunders.

loosening process between the fetal cotyledons and the maternal caruncles[145] (Box 12-19). The processes that lead to successful loosening and separation of the placentomes occur during the months preceding parturition. Many infectious and noninfectious factors are believed to disrupt the separation and expulsion processes. An endocrine causal relationship does not appear to exist.[146]

Clinical signs of retained fetal membranes in the doe and ewe are similar to those in the cow. The placenta of the ewe and doe is considered retained if it is not expelled within 24 hours after parturition.[147] The incidence of retained placentas in does is 6.4%.[148] Placental retention for longer than 24 hours may cause metritis in ewes and does. Inadequate dietary selenium and inadequate nutrition and exercise during gestation have been seen as factors predisposing does to retained placentas.[148] There have been several reports on factors that predispose to retained fetal membranes.[135,142-145,149,150] Many infectious and noninfectious factors apparently contribute to the disruption of the process of loosening and separation of the placentome. Accordingly, it has been suggested that a retained placenta should be considered to be a sign of an underlying disease.[151]

Approach to Diagnosis of Retained Fetal Membranes

HISTORY. A review of accurate breeding records correlates retention of fetal membranes with the duration of pregnancy. Gestational periods of abnormal lengths result in a higher incidence of retained placenta than do normal-term parturitions. Induced parturition, twinning, and late-term abortions have been associated with retained fetal membranes in cows. Many periparturient diseases and conditions affect the incidence of retained fetal membranes.[135,142-145,149,150]

ALTERATIONS IN LACTATION

MICHAEL S. SPENSLEY

The mammary glands are modified cutaneous glandular structures considered accessory reproductive organs that function to secrete milk for the nourishment of the young.[152] The mammary glands are located in the prepubic region in the mare, cow, ewe, and doe. The cow's udder is composed of four mammary glands, whereas in the doe, ewe, and mare the udder has two mammary glands. One teat serves each mammary gland, and in the cow, ewe, and doe each teat has one streak canal. The mare has two streak canals per teat.

The mammary glands are ectodermal in origin, and most of their fetal development occurs during the first half of gestation.[153] Except for growth that occurs in association with some of the anomalous conditions of the mammary gland

or as a result of the deposition of fat, there is little growth of mammary tissue between birth and puberty. Further mammary gland development occurs with each estrous cycle after the onset of puberty. Development of the duct system is primarily attributable to estrogen. Progesterone is the principal stimulant to development of secretory tissue. However, neither estrogen nor progesterone alone or in combination can cause optimum mammary gland growth and development.[154] Insulin, cortisol, thyroxine, prolactin, and growth hormone are necessary for full mammary gland development. During pregnancy the mammary gland attains maximum development under the control of pituitary, ovarian, adrenal, and placental hormones.[155] During parturition a process of interrelated neuroendocrine processes initiates lactogenesis, the production of milk. The secretion of milk and its release from the mammary gland after parturition depend on the availability of appropriate amounts of the hormones named above, especially prolactin and oxytocin.

In addition to mastitis, conditions that manifest themselves as alterations in the mammary gland and lactation are fairly common in ruminants and horses. Problems caused by conditions that affect the mammary gland are often multifactorial in that they compromise the well-being of the patient, the nutrition of the offspring, and ultimately the economics, especially in commercial dairies.

ENLARGED MAMMARY GLAND

Many conditions and diseases of the mammary gland cause swelling or enlarging of the gland[156] (Boxes 12-20 and 12-21). Enlargement may involve one or more of the glands of the udder. However, the enlarged mammary gland is not necessarily inflamed. Several anomalies of the mammary gland cause noninflammatory enlargement of the gland (e.g., gynecomastia and precocious udder development).[156-158] It is important to determine whether the enlargement of the gland is attributable to an infectious or a noninfectious etiology. Trauma is probably the most likely cause of noninfectious inflammation of the mammary gland. Mastitis, with which a large number of organisms has been associated, is the most common cause of mammary gland inflammation (see Chapter 34).

Evaluation of a patient with an enlarged mammary gland should include the medical and reproductive histories. The age and sex of the animal may limit the considerations. Gynecomastia is seen in young bucks, rarely in rams and bulls, and never in stallions.[156,158] Congenital anomalies such as stenotic or absent teat canals are not determined until parturition occurs and lactation commences.[156] The animal should be given a complete physical examination, with emphasis on the affected mammary gland. Examination of the gland should include observation, palpation, and expression of its contents. Cytologic and bacteriologic examination of the secretion from the mammary gland may be helpful in determining the cause and establishing the prognosis of enlarged mammary glands. In postpartum cows the most common causes of enlarged mammary glands are periparturient udder edema and mastitis. Mastitis occurs most often in mares after weaning. Trauma to the udder is more likely to be problematic in cows and goats than in ewes and mares because the udder is more pendulous in the former.[156] Undesirable udder traits of genetic origin occur in the goat (i.e., hanging or saclike udder, polythelia, and blocked teat).[159] Lacerations, superficial contusions, and seromas are detected by close examination of the affected gland. Diagnoses of other injuries may rely on examination of the gland's secretion for evidence of increased cellularity and hemorrhage. Mammary gland neoplasia is rare in mares, cows, and small ruminants.[156,160-162]

BOX 12-20

Causes of Enlarged Mammary Glands in the Mare

COMMON CAUSES
Mastitis
Abscessation
Periparturient udder edema (physiologic)
Gland distention associated with weaning

LESS COMMON CAUSES
Trauma (contusion, hematoma, seroma, laceration)
Neoplasia (malignant melanoma, carcinoma)
Cutaneous histoplasmosis (*Histoplasma farciminosus*)

BOX 12-21

Causes of Enlarged Mammary Glands in Ruminants

COMMON CAUSES
Mastitis
Periparturient udder edema
Abscessation
Trauma (contusion, hematoma, seroma, laceration)
Pendulous udder (B, C)
Blind quarters (aplastic duct) (B)

LESS COMMON CAUSES
Eczema
Urticaria (irritants, caustic chemicals; contact dermatitis; insect bites)
Sarcoptic and psoroptic mange
Primordial mammarian tissue swelling (accompanies witch's milk)
Photosensitization
Sunburn
Frostbite
Cowpox (B)
Pseudocowpox (B)
Goat pox
Contagious ecthyma (orf) (C, O)
Furunculosis, abscesses
Staphylococcal folliculitis
Papillomatosis, warts
Caprine arthritis-encephalitis (C, O)
Zearalenone toxicity
Neoplasia (lymphosarcoma, malignant melanoma [C], squamous cell carcinoma [C])
Milk allergy (B)
Tuberculosis (B)
Ovarian neoplasia
Caseous lymphadenitis (O, C)
Cutaneous lipomatosis
Enzootic mycobacterial nodular-ulcerative mammillitis (B)
Bovine herpesvirus mammillitis (BHV-2) (B)
Precocious udder development (B, C)
Udder cysts (C)
Gynecomastia (C)
Pseudopregnancy (C)
Foot and mouth disease (exotic)

B, Bovine; C, caprine; O, ovine.

Causes of Udder Edema

MARES
Periparturient udder edema (physiologic)

RUMINANTS
Periparturient udder edema (physiologic)
Hereditary predisposition
Overfeeding of grain prepartum
Excess dietary protein
Obesity
Excess dietary sodium, potassium
Hypomagnesemia (chronic udder edema)
Disturbances in udder blood and lymph circulations
Excessively long dry period
Anemia

UDDER EDEMA

Udder edema, one of the most common causes of enlarged mammary glands, results from the excessive accumulation of intercellular fluid in the mammary gland (Box 12-22). The disorder is observed during the late gestation and early postpartum periods and is common in both horses and ruminants, but it is probably more frequently seen in dairy cattle. One study reported an udder edema incidence of 18% in dairy cattle, of which less than 1% required veterinary treatment.[163]

Two forms of udder edema are seen in cattle.[164] In the physiologic or acute form, there is edema of the mammary gland during the late gestation and early postpartum periods.[164] The entire udder is usually symmetrically involved, and the edema may involve adjacent abdominal and perineal areas.[164] The condition is usually not obviously painful but may cause the cow some difficulty in lying down and walking because of the mammarian swelling. Chronic bovine udder edema differs from the acute form in that affected cows develop udder edema within 6 weeks after calving, and the edema may persist for several months.[164] The swelling may be localized in the form of plaques on the ventral aspect of the rear of the udder or it may involve the ventral abdominal wall.[164]

Udder edema is a relatively common condition of dairy goats.[165] Two-year-old does kidding for the first time are most commonly affected; however, all ages can be affected. Affected does usually have colostrum at parturition, but within a few hours the udder is warm, hard, and agalactic.

Brood mares affected with udder edema have generalized ventral edema during the last 1 to 2 weeks of gestation and for as long as 2 to 3 days after foaling. The extent of ventral edema varies, ranging from local swelling of the udder and immediately adjacent subcutaneous tissues to a generalized swelling that may extend from posterior to the mammary glands forward, along the ventral abdomen and thorax, to the axillary or pectoral area. In the mare such edematous accumulations are referred to as plaques of edema. Affected brood mares seem to be uncomfortable and reluctant to move. Younger brood mares, especially primiparous mares affected with udder edema, appear to be more painful than older mares, and some of the mares so affected refuse to allow their foals to suckle.

AGALACTIA

Any disease or condition that adversely affects the dam has the potential to compromise lactation. Agalactia, the failure

Causes of Agalactia and Hypogalactia in the Mare

COMMON CAUSES
Mammary aplasia, hypoplasia
Abscessation
Mastitis
Abortion
Premature birth
Postpartum complication

LESS COMMON CAUSES
Endocrine dysfunction
Nutritional deficiencies, malnutrition
Neoplasia
Squamous cell carcinoma
Malignant melanoma
Pituitary adenoma
Lymphosarcoma
Other tumors
Fescue toxicity
Trauma to mammary gland
Periparturient disease
Dystocia
Anemias
Severe toxicity

Causes of Agalactia and Hypogalactia in Ruminants

COMMON CAUSES
Mammary aplasia, hypoplasia
Mastitis
Abscessation
Caseous lymphadenitis (udder involvement) (C, O)
Caprine arthritis-encephalitis (CAE; hard udder) (C, O)

LESS COMMON CAUSES
Endocrine dysfunction
Malnutrition
Water deprivation
Self-sucking (B, C)
Trauma
Chapped teats; teat dip irritation (B, C)
Milk allergy
Neoplasia
Malignant melanoma (C)
Lymphosarcoma
Squamous cell carcinoma
Carcinomas
Fescue toxicity
Papillomatosis
Mycoplasmal agalactia (C, O)
Anemias
Severe toxicity

B, Bovine; *C,* caprine; *O,* ovine.

of lactation after parturition, may be attributable to a primary endocrinologic or mammary gland problem, or it may be secondary to any of a multitude of systemic conditions and diseases (Boxes 12-23 and 12-24). True agalactia may be attributable to mammary gland anomalies or inadequacies among the numerous endocrinologic factors of development and

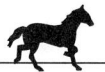

pregnancy. Agalactia may be a complication of many conditions. In some animals the conditions to which agalactia is secondary manifest as alterations in a specific system, whereas other animals with agalactia may demonstrate such signs as fever, weight loss, anorexia, and anemia. Inadequate nutrition is rarely the cause of clinically observed agalactia. Fescue grass toxicity, caused by ingestion of the ergot alkaloid–producing *Acremonium coenophialum*, is an important cause of agalactia and hypogalactia[166,167] (see Fescue toxicity).

Agalactia should not be confused with failure of milk ejection (milk letdown). Administration of oxytocin may enhance milk letdown but does not affect milk production. Oxytocin stimulates a release phenomenon that acts on previously secreted and stored milk. Although somatotropin may increase milk production in a normally lactating cow, its effect on agalactia has not been adequately studied.

Inexperienced or nervous mares with adequate milk are often reluctant to allow their offspring to nurse, in part because of the mare's inexperience. Such nervous mares need not necessarily be primiparous mares. Although not allowing their offspring to nurse is usually a manageable behavior problem, the mare's udder should be examined for evidence of periparturient edema, inflammation, and painful conditions.

Approach to Diagnosis of Agalactia

An accurate reproductive history should be obtained. It should be determined whether the dam is primiparous or multiparous. If primiparous, is she manifesting anxiety in the presence of her offspring? If multiparous, has she been agalactic at previous parturitions? Has she sustained recent trauma, perhaps during parturition, or has there been exposure during gestation to infectious diseases or toxic plants? After a history has been determined and the dam and neonate have been observed, attempts to facilitate the youngster's suckling might be indicated. Is the dam agalactic, or does she simply refuse to let the neonate suckle? Such measures as twitching or tranquilizing the nervous and inexperienced mare may resolve that problem. If assessing the dam's behavior toward her offspring does not resolve the problem, a thorough physical examination should be initiated. The objective now should be to rule out or incriminate infectious and inflammatory conditions contributing to the agalactic state. The dam herself may be systemically affected, or the problem may be localized in the udder or a mammary gland.

In listing causes of agalactia and hypogalactia in Boxes 12-23 and 12-24, only those that have a direct effect on the anatomic integrity of the mammary gland or its function are included. Abnormalities involving any system may compromise lactation.

GALACTORRHEA AND PRECOCIOUS MAMMARY GLAND DEVELOPMENT

Galactorrhea, the abnormal manifestation of lactation (not the secretion of true milk), occurs occasionally from the primordial mammary gland of young foals and ruminants, including neonates.[156] The serous secretion occurs in association with swelling of mammarian tissue in males and females and may be caused by transplacental transmission of maternal steroid hormones[168] (Box 12-25). The secretion is popularly known as witch's milk.

Precocious mammary gland development and galactorrhea occur in pregnant and nonpregnant mares and in some of the ruminant species. Such premature udder development and subsequent lactation has been observed in nonpregnant and nonsuckled doelings and heifers.[156,169] Udder development and subsequent lactation have been observed in young nonpregnant heifers and does being suckled by other young

---

BOX 12-25

Causes of Galactorrhea and Precocious Mammary Gland Development in the Horse and Ruminants

Impending abortion
In utero death of one twin fetus
Spontaneous (inappropriate prolactin secretion)
Placental separation
Zearalenone toxicity
Pregnancy (especially multiple fetuses)
Suckling
Pseudopregnancy (caprine)
Ascending infection during pregnancy, placentitis
Ovarian tumors

---

animals.[156] In addition to the continued stimulation of suckling, other causes of premature mammarian development and lactation may be trauma and diseases of the pituitary, ovarian, and adrenal glands.[156] Zearalenone toxicity has been implicated in precocious mammary gland development and lactation in heifers.[170] Milk production is nonphysiologic in that it is of insufficient quality and quantity and does not justify milking the affected animals. There is no evidence that such abnormal development compromises normal lactation after parturition.[156]

Inappropriate lactation has been observed at various stages of pregnancy in most domestic species.[156] The most common cause of galactorrhea is abortion. Lactation may commence before or even without expulsion of the dead fetus. Lactation during pregnancy has also been observed in association with multiple fetuses, placentitis, and ovarian tumors. Accordingly, premature mammary gland development during gestation should be considered a warning of impending abortion, and the dam should be examined. Occasionally pregnant mares develop mammarian enlargement during middle to late gestation that spontaneously regresses.[167] Some of these mares begin to lactate before parturition. It must be kept in mind that premature lactation and subsequent loss of colostrum is one of the most important causes of failure of passive transfer of immunoglobulins.[171]

Gynecomastia, the abnormal development of the male's mammary glands, has been observed in bucks in which rudimentary mammary glands and associated teats underwent development.[156,169] The aberrant structures, located on both sides of the buck's scrotum, can secrete up to 1 L daily of substance that resembles milk. The cause is presumed to be endocrine imbalance but has not been determined. Lofstedt, Laarveld, and Ihle[172] reported adrenal neoplasia as a cause of lactation in a wether.

REFERENCES

152. Getty R: *Sisson and Grossman's the anatomy of the domestic animals,* ed 5, Philadelphia, 1975, WB Saunders.
153. Schmidt GH: Mammary gland development. In Freeman, WH *Biology of lactation,* San Francisco, 1971, WH Freeman.
154. Speroff L, Glass RH, Kase NG: *Clinical gynecologic endocrinology and infertility,* Baltimore, 1973, Williams & Wilkins.
155. Salazar H, Tobon H: Morphologic changes of the mammary gland during development, pregnancy, and lactation. In Josimovich JP, ed: *Lactogenic hormones, fetal nutrition, and lactation,* New York, 1974, John Wiley & Sons.
156. Heidrich HJ, Renk W: *Diseases of the mammary glands of domestic animals,* translated by Van den Heever LW, Philadelphia, 1967, WB Saunders.
157. McDonald NR: Lactation in a calf, *NZ Vet J* 1:55, 1952.
158. Basrur PK: Congenital abnormalities of the goat, *Vet Clin North Am (Food Anim Pract)* 9:183-202, 1993.
159. Basrur PK, Yadar BR: Genetic diseases of sheep and goats, *Vet Clin North Am (Food Anim Pract)* 6:779-801, 1990.

160. Seahorn TL et al: Mammary adenocarcinoma in four mares, *J Am Vet Med Assoc* 200:1675-1677, 1992.
161. Ford TS et al: Primary teat neoplasia in two yearling heifers, *J Am Vet Med Assoc* 195:238-239, 1989.
162. Andreasen CB, Huber MJ, Mattoon JS: Unilateral fibroepithelial hyperplasia of the mammary gland in a goat, *J Am Vet Med Assoc* 202:1279-1280, 1993.
163. Snider GW, Brightenback GE, Siegmund OH: A new approach to edematous conditions of cattle, *Can Vet J* 3:150-155, 1962.
164. Vestweber JGE, Al-Ani FK: Udder edema in cattle, *Compend Cont Educ Pract Vet* 5(suppl):5-12, 1983.
165. East NE, Birnie EF: Diseases of the udder: symposium on sheep and goat medicine, *Vet Clin North Am (Large Anim Pract)* 5:591-600, 1983.
166. Porter JK, Thompson FN: Effects of fescue toxicosis on reproduction in livestock, *J Anim Sci* 70:1594-1603, 1992.
167. McCue PM: Lactation. In McKinnon AO, Voss JL, eds: *Equine reproduction*, Philadelphia, 1993, Lea & Febiger.
168. Roberts SJ: *Veterinary obstetrics and genital diseases (theriogenology)*, ed 3, North Pomfret, Vt, 1986, SJ Roberts, pp 93-122.
169. Smith MC, Roguinsky M: Mastitis and other diseases of the goat's udder, *J Am Vet Med Assoc* 171:1241-1248, 1977.
170. Bloomquist C, Davidson JN, Pearson EG: Zearalenone toxicosis in prepubertal dairy heifers, *J Am Vet Med Assoc* 180:164-165, 1982.
171. Jeffcott LB: Passive transfer of immunity to foals. In Robinson NE, ed: *Current therapy in equine medicine 2*, Philadelphia, WB Saunders.
172. Lofstedt RM, Laarveld B, Ihle SL: Adrenal neoplasia causing lactation in a castrated male goat, *J Vet Int Med* 8:382-384, 1994.

Musculoskeletal Abnormalities

JOHN MAAS

Consulting Editor

MAJOR CLINICAL SIGN/PROBLEM ENCOUNTERED

LAMENESS AND STIFFNESS

CARTER E. JUDY
JOHN MAAS

Definition

Lameness is the term used to describe a condition in which an animal is incapable of normal locomotion. Generally lameness is characterized by an inability to maintain a normal gait, manifested by asymmetry in movement, apparent incoordination or weakness, and inefficient or ineffective motion of the limbs. Thus lameness usually can be assessed only when the animal is moving under its own power, although lameness severe enough to cause an inability to bear weight can be assumed at a standstill. The onset of lameness can be acute (e.g., fracture), chronic (e.g., degenerative joint disease), or acute on chronic (e.g., catastrophic fracture secondary to stress fractures).

Mechanisms of Lameness and Stiffness

The ultimate effects of any cause of lameness are restricted movement of the limbs or body, reduced performance, and abnormal gait. Causes of lameness are generally associated with conditions of the musculoskeletal system or nervous system. Most causes of lameness have both a musculoskeletal component (e.g., atrophy of the supraspinatus and infraspinatus muscles) and a neurologic component (e.g., suprascapular neurapraxia). Some causes of lameness have only a musculoskeletal component (e.g., upward fixation of the patella) and are not principally associated with either afferent

(i.e., pain) or efferent (i.e., motor dysfunction) nerve signs. Similarly, other causes of lameness are solely related to a motor nerve deficit (e.g., radial neurapraxia).

Unlike the usual definition of lameness, "stiffness" refers to a generalized restriction in freedom of movement in a limb, the neck, or back. Stiffness is manifested by a limited range of motion by a joint, reduced length of stride, or decreased flexibility during bending or turning. For example, cellulitis and soft tissue swelling in the area of the arsocrural joint can cause restricted freedom of movement of the hindlimb and an apparent lameness, yet there may be no specific musculoskeletal or neurologic cause. Therefore stiffness may have either congenital or acquired causes, and the clinical signs may be mild and transient or severe and persistent. Stiffness may or may not be associated with pain.

Approach to Diagnosis of Lameness and Stiffness in the Horse

The lameness examination is the most commonly performed assessment of the musculoskeletal system in the horse. The examination should be well planned, consistent, and thorough. Knowledge of all diseases capable of causing lameness is not required, as long as the examiner maintains an open mind and objectivity during the examination (Box 13-1). The goals of the lameness examination are to: (1) determine which limb(s) is (are) affected, (2) differentiate between supporting leg and swinging leg lameness, and (3) establish the musculoskeletal and/or neurologic components producing the lameness.

BOX 13-1

Causes of Lameness and Stiffness in the Horse

COMMON CAUSES
Infections of the foot
Bruised or punctured sole
Hoof wall defects
Fractures
Septic (infectious) arthritis
Laminitis
Secondary (degenerative) joint disease
Navicular disease
Osteomyelitis
Fibrotic/ossifying myopathy
Rhabdomyopathy (tying-up)
Sprain
Strain
Tenosynovitis
Contracted tendons (flexural deformity)
Ankylosis/arthrogryposis
Osteochondrosis or bone cyst
Cruciate/meniscal rupture
Luxation/subluxation (dislocations)
Upward fixation of the patella (locking patella)
Sesamoiditis
Muscle injury, soreness, bruise, trauma, compartment
   syndrome
Subcutaneous abscess, cellulitis
Angular limb deformities
Disruption of the suspensory apparatus (broken down)
Postanesthetic equine myasthenia
Tendon rupture, damage, tendonitis (bowed tendon)
Osteomalacia, osteodystrophy (rickets)
Bucked shins
Epiphysitis (physeal injuries)
Purpura hemorrhagica

LESS COMMON CAUSES
Shivers (shivering)
Borreliosis (Lyme disease)
Equine monocytic ehrlichiosis (Potomac fever)
Chronic selenium toxicity
Hemangioma, hemangiosarcoma, angiosarcoma
Skeletal neoplasia
Rabies
Spondylitis, diskospondylitis
Spinal/vertebral neoplasia
Vertical column malformation
White muscle disease (nutritional myodegeneration)
Gunshot injury

LESS COMMON CAUSES—cont'd
Corynebacterium pseudotuberculosis
Hypothyroidism (goiter)
Actinobacillosis
Hyperparathyroidism
Ulcerative lymphangitis
Myotonia congenita
Vesicular stomatitis
Fistulous withers (*Brucella abortus* or other organisms)
Sporadic equine lymphangitis
Acute necrotizing equine vasculitis (with or without
   thrombocytopenia)
Peripheral arteriovenous fistula
Hypertrophic osteopathy/osteodystrophy

UNCOMMON CAUSES
Nocardiosis
Cutaneous blastomycosis
Pemphigus foliaceus
Tuberculosis
Multisystemic postexhaustion syndrome
Generalized steatitis
Cutaneous vasculitis
Sterile nodular panniculitis
Multiple clotting defects in ill foals
Salmonellosis
Factor VIII deficiency (hemophilia A)
Idiopathic equine aplastic anemia
Idiopathic equine thrombocytopenia
Hemimelia (radial, tibial, ulnar hypoplasia, agenesis)
Lupus erythematosus (rheumatoid arthritis)
Phycomycosis

POISONS, TOXINS, DEFICIENCIES, AND EXCESSES
Moldy sweet clover poisoning
Strychnine toxicity
Tetrachlorodibenzodioxin (dioxin) toxicity
Warfarin (Dicumarol) toxicity
Vitamin K–induced renal toxicity
Calcinosis resulting from plant poisoning
Zinc toxicity
Phosphorus toxicity
Phosphorus deficiency
Vitamin D toxicity
Locoweed-associated limb deformities or stringhalt-like gait
Chronic fluoride toxicity

1. History. The lameness examination begins with the client interview. A summary of the important historic features of the lameness should include answers to basic questions about the following:
   - Onset
   - Characteristics of the lameness
   - Associated or inciting factors (e.g., injury) that may have contributed to or caused the lameness
   - Changes in the characteristics, intensity, and duration of the lameness
   - Responsiveness to treatment
   - Time since the last hoof trimming and shoeing
     In addition the signalment and the activity that the horse undertakes (e.g., jumping vs. racing) should be ascertained and may be a guide in determining potential etiologies of the lameness (e.g., stress fractures are more common in racing thoroughbreds, and osteochondrosis is more commonly diagnosed in young animals).

2. Observe from a distance—stationary phase. Observing the horse from a distance while it is stationary enables one to assess the horse's position and posture. The horse should be viewed from the front, hind, and both sides. From the front, special note should be made of any abnormality in the following:
   - Position of the head (e.g., tilted, turned)
   - Distribution and equality of muscle mass along the neck and trunk
   - Topographic symmetry of the front limbs, from the dorsal region of each scapula to the hoof. From the rear, the height and mass of the hip musculature and the symmetry between the hindlimbs should be assessed. From each side, abnormalities in stance (e.g., camped out in front) or load-bearing (e.g., dropped elbow) and the position of the head and neck (e.g., hyperflexed poll) should be compared.

3. Observe from a distance—mobile phase. Observations

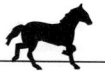

BOX 13-2

Causes of Spontaneous Fractures in the Horse and Ruminants

Pathologic fractures
Subclinical stress fractures
Tumors
Infection
Inflammation
Osteoporosis
Copper deficiency
Molybdenum excess
Phosphorus deficiency
Protein deficiency
Osteomalacia
Osteodystrophy (rickets)
Rapid growth
Lactation
Advanced pregnancy

TABLE 13-1

A Five-Grade Lameness Scheme

Grade	Description
1	An inconsistently observable lameness visible under special circumstances (in a circle, flexion tests, hard surface, etc.).
2	A consistently observable lameness visible only under special circumstances (in a circle, flexion test, hard surface, etc.).
3	A consistently observable lameness at a trot in a straight line.
4	A consistently observable lameness at a walk.
5	A non–weight-bearing lameness. Horse is unable to use the leg.

Modified from *American Association of Equine Practitioners Newsletter*, March 1983, p 12, Lexington, Ky.

made from a distance while the horse is moving can be evaluated critically once clues provided by the history and observations made of any postural deformities direct the practitioner's attention to a specific area of the horse's body. This part of the examination is conducted while the horse is moving in at least two gaits, the walk and the trot. Sometimes it is also helpful diagnostically to observe the horse move at other gaits (e.g., canter) or while under saddle. It may also be beneficial to observe the horse on different surfaces (hard and soft) to amplify different lamenesses. If possible, the horse should be evaluated under similar conditions as that under which it performs.

If a fracture is suspected (e.g., nondisplaced long-bone fracture) or if there is the possibility of exacerbating preexisting trauma, this part of the examination should either be abbreviated or not performed at all to preclude further damage or trauma. In such cases, immediate radiographic or other definitive diagnostic tests should be performed (Box 13-2).

During the examination, the freedom of movement, symmetry, and head carriage at each gait should be evaluated. At a walk, the horse should be observed moving toward and away from the examiner. The breakover of the foot at the toe, the arc of the foot flight, the distance covered by the foot in the swing phase, and the placement of the foot should be evaluated for each limb and should be compared between pairs of limbs. The same observations should be made during the trot, noting especially how the horse tracks and the length of stride. Although many abnormalities often can be observed only during a trot, some conditions may cause a subtle alteration in gait that can be observed only at a walk (e.g., fibrotic myopathy). Trotting in a circle at the end of a lunge line is a useful method for stressing one limb in contrast to the opposite limb (e.g., lameness caused by trauma to the right front hoof may be exacerbated by trotting the animal in a circle to the right). A head nod also may be more noticeable in a circle than on a straightaway. It often helps to listen to the sounds of the feet striking the ground during each stride; the unaffected limb lands more heavily than the lame limb when working the horse on a hard surface.

Characteristic signs of stiffness include reduced range of motion of the fetlock joint, dragging of a toe in the swing phase of the stride, advancing a limb by swinging it forward and to the outside, and general unwillingness to move.

A few general guidelines can help the examiner differentiate a forelimb from a hindlimb lameness. Clues that can help identify the affected limb include shortened stride, dragged toe, and reduced fetlock joint motion at a trot. Abnormal head carriage and asymmetric hip height or movement can be especially useful in localizing the origin of the lameness. When present, a head nod can be very informative but also confusing, especially if the nod is caused by a hindlimb lameness. In contrast to the head nod that occurs on landing of the sound forelimb associated with forelimb lameness during a trot, the head nod appears on the landing of the forelimb *opposite* the affected hindlimb during hindlimb lameness. For example, with lameness of the left hindlimb, the head will nod or "not raise" when the affected left hindlimb and the opposite (unaffected) right forelimb of the diagonal pair land. The hip of the unaffected hindlimb also appears to drop during the trot while the opposite hip (the affected hindlimb) is carried higher. Observing the horse while it is trotting after a stress test (e.g., flexion test) often helps localize lameness to a specific region of a limb, but it cannot selectively distinguish lamenesses originating from between closely related articulations.

Thorough and useful systems for grading the severity of lameness are available. Most systems are designed to enable the practitioner to compare how a lameness changes with time, assess the characteristic of a lameness among horses, and accurately record information and communicate information to other veterinarians. Simple and consistent schemes that are easy to remember and modify can be developed (Table 13-1).

4. Palpation. Palpation enables a closer inspection of the horse and identification of abnormalities that may or may not otherwise be noticed. The examination can be started anywhere on the limb, as long as it is conducted consistently and thoroughly. Abnormal findings should be described as to their location on the limb, their size, and their orientation relative to normal anatomic landmarks. Certain signs indicating trauma (e.g., wounds, swelling, hair loss, pain) may lead to more important findings such as underlying evidence of a fracture (e.g., bony crepitus, warm or cold areas, bony protuberance).

Stressing articulations by flexion and extension enables an assessment of range of motion and pain. Joint distention should be distinguished from distention of tendon sheaths or generalized swelling of the region. Comparing limbs is often useful for distinguishing an abnormality from an unusual or unique conformation. The pelvis, iliac arteries, and sublumbar musculature can be evaluated by rectal palpation while the horse is standing quietly; movement or crepitation can be assessed while swaying the horse from side to side.

The relative size, shape, and condition of the feet (e.g., contracted heel, scuffed toe), length of heel, and pattern of

TABLE 13-2

Structures Desensitized by Commonly Performed Nerve Blocks

Nerve Block	Nerve(s) Affected	Structures Desensitized*
Palmar (plantar) digital	Palmar (plantar) digital	Heel bulbs, frog, bars, navicular bone and bursa, and palmar regions of the third phalanx, distal interphalangeal joint, sole, and soft tissues
Abaxial sesamoid	Palmar (plantar)	Coronary band, interphalangeal joints, lamellar and solar corium
Low palmar (volar)	Palmar, palmar metacarpal†	Skin of medial and lateral pastern, metacarpophalangeal joint, proximal sesamoids, flexor tendons, and tendon sheath
High palmar (volar)	Palmar, palmar metacarpal†	Skin and deep structures of palmar cannon region (flexor tendons, suspensory ligament except origin, interosseous ligaments of splint bones)
High two-point	Lateral palmar, medial palmar	Origin of suspensory ligament

*Includes all structures listed up to and including the particular block; first structure listed in each block—also the area that can be tested with point pressure to evaluate the effectiveness of the block.
†For hindlimbs, additional anesthetic (i.e., ring block) is needed at the level of the particular perineural block to achieve the desired effect.

shoe wear (e.g., thinner branch on the outside of the shoe than on the inside) give clinically significant but often overlooked clues to the site and cause of lameness. Evaluation of the feet with hoof testers is mandatory; most lameness arises from problems in the forefeet.

Except in cases in which catastrophic disruption of a nondisplaced fracture may occur, an attempt should be made to reduce the intensity of the lameness by selective anesthesia of sensory nerves and joints. Nerve blocks help to localize the origin of the lameness and to identify a bilateral lameness. It is essential to know what structures are affected by peripheral nerve blocks (Table 13-2). Intraarticular anesthesia can be used to selectively evaluate a joint that is incriminated as the source of lameness. This technique can be used in association with peripheral nerve anesthesia: a single joint in a group of joints blocked by anesthesia of the regional peripheral nerves can be selectively blocked by intraarticular anesthesia. The risk of introducing contaminants into the joint and iatrogenic induction of infectious arthritis can be reduced by aseptic preparation of the skin, sterile technique, and use of anesthetic from an unopened bottle. The volume of local anesthetic infused into a joint depends on the size of the joint. Lameness may be erroneously associated with a joint if intraarticular anesthesia of several joints is performed within a short period of time; ample time (30 to 60 minutes) must be allowed between joint blocks to allow for adequate articular desensitization. An improvement in gait indicates a favorable response to a nerve or joint block; complete elimination of gait asymmetry is unusual and generally should not be expected following intraarticular or peripheral nerve anesthesia. If necessary, improvement in gait can be confirmed by repeating the successful block the next day. By that time residual effects from multiple blocks performed previously should be absent.

Once the lameness has been described and localized, a radiographic or ultrasonographic examination can be performed as the next step to confirm a clinical diagnosis. Radiography should be performed using proper technique, an ideal film/screen combination, and multiple views to construct a thorough study (Table 13-3). Comparing radiographs of affected and unaffected limbs can help confirm or refute a suspected abnormality, evaluate the severity of the disease, and identify possible bilateral limb involvement.

When radiographic or ultrasonographic techniques are nondiagnostic, other methods such as thermography, nuclear scintigraphy, treadmill evaluation, computerized videographic gait analysis, force plate evaluation, computed axial tomography, or magnetic resonance imaging may be useful. University hospitals and major regional referral centers often are the only locations where adjunctive procedures such as these can be performed because such procedures are expen-

TABLE 13-3

Recommended Radiographic Views of Extremities

Radiographic Series	Minimum Radiographic Views
Distal extremity (navicular)	45 degrees DP, 65 degrees DP (2), LM, Flexor*
Pastern	45 degrees DP, LO, MO, LM
Fetlock	45 degrees DP, LO, MO, LM
Metacarpal/metatarsal	DP, LO, MO, LM
Carpus	DP, LO, MO, LM, flexed skylines (distal radius, proximal and distal rows of carpal bones)
Tarsus	0 degrees DP, 10 degrees DP, LO, MO, LM
Radius-ulna/tibia-fibula	Cr-Cd, LO, MO, LM
Elbow	Cd-Cr, LO, LM, patellar
Shoulder	ML

Cd-Cr, Caudocranial; *Cr-Cd*, craniocaudal; *DP*, dorsopalmar (dorsoplantar); *LM*, lateromedial; *LO*, lateral oblique; *ML*, mediolateral; *MO*, medial oblique.
*View to highlight the flexor cortical margin of the navicular bone (50 degrees proximal palmaropalmaro distal oblique).

sive and technically complex and require specialized equipment and experienced personnel. However, even these techniques have limitations; for example, nuclear scintigraphy may not identify the origin of insidious (e.g., osteochondrosis) or chronic lameness as successfully as an acute lameness.

Approach to Diagnosis of Lameness and Stiffness in Ruminants

1. History. An accurate history is the first step in reaching a correct diagnosis for the cause of lameness in ruminants (Box 13-3). For example, although stiffness can occur at any time in life, it occasionally occurs at birth (e.g., arthrogryposis); therefore acquired and congenital signs can be differentiated on the basis of a complete history. Further, other ruminants on a property may demonstrate similar clinical signs, and the onset and duration of signs may be important diagnostically. It also is useful to examine the environment and determine how the ruminant could have been traumatized or injured. Finally, any evidence of systemic disease manifested by fever, anorexia, or depression should be determined.

2. Observe from a distance—stationary phase. Next, the ruminant should be observed standing to assess posture and stance. For example, a cross-legged stance may indicate an abnormality of the medial claw of the hoof. A dairy cow with painful heels in the hind feet may stand with its heels over the gutter while in a stanchion. Alternatively, a ruminant resting its feet farther forward than usual may have a

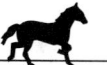

BOX 13-3

Causes of Lameness and Stiffness in Ruminants

COMMON CAUSES
Infections of the foot
Hoof defects
Interdigital dermatitis (infectious footrot)
Underrun heel
Rusterholtz ulcer, granuloma of sole
Laminitis
Corkscrew claw and other growth abnormalities
Interdigital fibroma
Overgrown feet
Bruised or overworn sole
Puncture wound
Septic infectious arthritis
Contracted tendons
Arthrogryposis
Chlamydial arthritis of sheep
Caprine arthritis-encephalitis in goats
Fractures
Blackleg
Muscle abscess
Mycoplasma polyarthritis of sheep and goats
Osteomyelitis
Ruptured anterior cruciate ligament
Ligament rupture (e.g., torn collateral ligament of stifle)
Foot warts (digital dermatitis)

LESS COMMON CAUSES
Erysipelothrix arthritis
Vesicular stomatitis
Secondary (degenerative) joint disease
Luxations and subluxations
Sprain
Strain
Hygroma
Spinal abscess
Spinal lymphosarcoma
Osteomalacia
Bluetongue virus in sheep (coronitis and myopathy)
Dorsal fixation of the patella (bovine)
Septic tenosynovitis
Angular limb deformities
Malignant edema

COMMON CAUSES—cont'd
Malignant catarrhal fever
Muscle injury
Ruptured tendon

UNCOMMON CAUSES
Sporadic bovine encephalomyelitis
Ulcerative lymphangitis
Salmonellosis
Dactylomegaly in shorthorn cattle
Bovine virus diarrhea (coronitis)
Physeal injuries (epiphysitis)
Clotting factor deficits
Hyperparathyroidism
Phycomycosis
Neoplasia
Angioneurotic edema
Hemimelia (radial, tibial, ulnar, hypoplasia, or agenesis)
Meliodosis (exotic)
Ibaraki disease (exotic)
Ephemeral fever (exotic)
African bovine malignant catarrhal fever (exotic)
Akabane disease (exotic)
Foot-and-mouth disease (exotic)
Lumpy skin disease (exotic)

POISONS, TOXINS, DEFICIENCIES, AND EXCESSES
Nutritional myodegeneration (white muscle disease selenium deficiency)
Fescue foot (ergot poisoning)
Polybrominated biphenyl (PPB) toxicity
Acorn calves
Kaley-pea poison in cattle
Calcinosis caused by plant poisoning
Sweet clover poisoning
Copper deficiency
Locoweed toxicity
Lupine alkaloid poisoning
Zinc deficiency
Nicotinic acid toxicity
Hemlock poisoning
Sweet vernal grass poisoning (exotic)

painful toe region. Small ruminants with problems in both front feet may attempt to move around on their carpi.

3. Observe from a distance—mobile phase. In ruminants these observations are usually made while walking rather than trotting the animal. This enables the examiner to identify the affected limb; to determine whether the lameness is a supporting or swinging-leg lameness; and to assess how much of the lameness is solely mechanical, associated with pain, or both.

4. Palpation. The most important part of lameness examination in ruminants is examination of the foot. As with horses, most lameness in ruminants involves the foot. The examiner should look closely between toes, around the coronary band, and at the hoof wall. The sole should be pared with a hoof knife to identify discoloration or draining tracts beneath the sole or into the corium. A black discoloration may indicate infections of deeper structures of the foot. Applying pressure to the sole with a hoof tester or tapping over the wall may elicit pain.

   The limb should also be palpated to detect swelling, heat, or soreness, which may indicate inflammation from infection or soft tissue trauma. Crepitation found by

manipulating the limb may indicate a fracture or dislocation. Stiffness or pain on joint flexion may indicate joint disease, either septic or degenerative.

Flexion tests and nerve blocks are not used for diagnosis as routinely in ruminants as they are in horses, but they may be useful in certain instances. The technique is similar to that described for horses, but the location of the nerves is different. Radiographs are not necessary in most cases, although they can identify bony or articular lesions that may not be readily apparent or palpable. Examination of synovial fluid obtained by arthrocentesis can be used to differentiate septic from traumatic arthritis.

POSTURAL DEFORMITIES

CARTER E. JUDY
JOHN MAAS

Definition

A postural deformity in horses or ruminants is an abnormal stance caused by neurologic deficit, pain, or a musculoskeletal problem. Postural deformities can range from subtle

TABLE 13-4

Examples of Postural Deformities and Possible Origins

Postural Defect	Likely Site of Origin
Contracted heels	Foot; flexor tendons
Bucked knees	Suspensory ligament
Dropped elbow	Motor nerves to forelimb; olecranon
Tiptoe stance	Foot; flexor tendons; interphalangeal joints
Non–weight-bearing	Foot; any long bone; any limb articulation
Broken down (hyperextension) of fetlock; dropped fetlock	Suspensory apparatus
Toe-out hindlimb and elevated hip	Coxofemoral joint; femoral neck
Basewide behind	Coxofemoral joint; femoral neck
Hyperextension of stifle and hock	Patella
Camped out in front	Bilateral forefeet
Carpal valgus	Distal metaphysis, physis, epiphysis, or carpal bones
Stiffly elevated head	Withers; cervical spine
Shifting weight between forefeet	
Recumbency	Any long bone; feet; spinal cord; myopathy

BOX 13-4

Causes of Postural Deformities in the Horse

COMMON CAUSES
Infections of the foot
Hoof wall defects
Fractures
Septic (infectious) arthritis
Secondary (degenerative) joint disease
Laminitis
Angular limb deformities
Osteomyelitis
Sprain
Strain
Tenosynovitis
Contracted tendons (flexural deformity)
Laxity of flexor tendons in foals
Tendon rupture, damage, tendonitis (bowed tendon)
Upward fixation of the patella (locking patella)
Epiphysitis
Septic tenosynovitis
Muscle injury, soreness, bruise, trauma, compartment
 syndrome
Navicular disease
Congenital
Cuboidal bone hypoplasia

LESS COMMON CAUSES
Disruption of the suspensory apparatus (broken down)
Lateral or medial patellar luxation
White muscle disease (nutritional myodegeneration)
Brucellosis
Sesamoiditis
Hypertrophic osteopathy/osteodystrophy
Ankylosis/arthrogryposis
Luxation/subluxation
Snakebite
Equine monocytic ehrlichiosis (Potomac fever)
Spondylitis, diskospondylitis

LESS COMMON CAUSES—cont'd
Spinal/vertebral neoplasia
Tick paralysis
Vertebral column malformation
Nigropallidal encephalomalacia (star thistle poisoning)
Postanesthetic equine myasthenia
Abscess caused by *Clostridium perfringens*
Hyperparathyroidism
Osteomalacia, osteodystrophy (rickets)

UNCOMMON CAUSES
Lupus erythematosus (rheumatoid arthritis)
Osteochondrosis
Cruciate/meniscal rupture
Patellar ligament injury
Malnutrition
Splenic rupture
Neonatal maladjustment
Subcutaneous abscess, cellulitis, foreign body
Vesicular stomatitis
Bucked shins (dorsal metacarpal disease)
Hemimelia (radial, tibial, ulnar hypoplasia, agenesis)
Botulism (Shaker foal)
Myotonia congenita
Skeletal neoplasia
Shivers (shivering)
Borreliosis (Lyme disease)

POISONS, TOXINS, DEFICIENCIES, AND EXCESSES
Vitamin A deficiency
Vitamin D toxicity
Strychnine toxicity
Phosphorus deficiency
Chronic fluoride toxicity
Chronic selenium toxicity

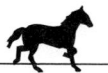

BOX 13-5

Causes of Postural Deformities in Ruminants

COMMON CAUSES
Congenital
Crooked calf syndrome (lupinosis)
Syndactyly
Hemimelia (radial, tibial, ulnar hypoplasia)
Osteogenesis imperfecta
Dactylomegaly in shorthorns
Contracted tendons
Idiopathic deformities
Angular limb deformities
Shortened long bones (acorn calves)
Acquired hoof wall defects
Infections of the foot
Secondary contracted tendons
Muscle atrophy caused by denervation
Fractures
Luxations
Severed or ruptured tendons
Septic arthritis with ankylosis
Arthritides (e.g., mycoplasma, caprine arthritis encephalitis, septic arthritis)
Osteomalacia

COMMON CAUSES—cont'd
Rickets
Epiphysitis
Septic tenosynovitis
Chronic laminitis
Degenerative joint disease
Hypertrophic osteopathy
Hyperparathyroidism
Osteomyelitis
Ruptured gastrocnemius (goats)
Ruptured peroneus tertius
Upward fixation of the patella (locking patella)

POISONS, TOXINS, DEFICIENCIES, AND EXCESSES
Primary copper deficiency or secondary copper deficiency (molybdenosis) (e.g., physitis, spontaneous fractures)
Selenium poisoning
Fluoride poisoning
Phosphorus deficiency
Monensin toxicity
Calcinosis caused by plant poisoning
Locoweed-associated limb deformities

---

conformational faults such as broken forward foot axis to severe and unusual positions, such as when the animal is camped out in front. Inability to bear weight on a limb, asymmetric angles between joints, and lateral or medial deviations in the alignment of limbs are examples of postural deformities. Often the postural deformity itself is specific for certain diseases and conditions (Table 13-4).

Mechanisms of Postural Deformities

Postural deformities can be either congenital or acquired and result from maldevelopment, trauma, or disease (Box 13-4). Congenital deformities may be caused by tendon contracture or laxity, osseous malformation, and hypoplasia or aplasia of osseous structures or soft tissues. Acquired deformities are most often caused by trauma or disease. Disuse atrophy secondary to an unrelated musculoskeletal abnormality can result in abnormal posture. Occasionally diseases affecting proprioception and consciousness may cause an abnormal stance that appears as a postural deformity (e.g., headpressing) but is unrelated to neurologic pain or a musculoskeletal problem.

Approach to Diagnosis of Postural Deformities in the Horse

A history can help the examiner determine if a postural deformity is congenital, as with arthrogryposis, or acquired. Because most postural deformities in horses arise from traumatic injuries or overuse, a complete lameness examination is essential. Occasionally a postural deformity does not cause lameness; in these instances the veterinarian must consider nontraumatic causes associated with abnormal development, improper nutrition, and seemingly unrelated disease such as carpal valgus deformity.

Diagnosis of the cause of a postural deformity begins with a detailed description of the deformity and assessment of the position and asymmetry of the anatomic structures involved. If the nature and severity of the deformity cannot be determined by direct observation, palpation and manipulation of the affected structure are required. Radiography and ultrasonography also can assist in the diagnosis and provide information on which to base treatment recommendations and prognosis.

Approach to Diagnosis of Postural Deformities in Ruminants

Because of the many differences in husbandry and management practices between ruminants and horses, most postural deformities in ruminants are congenital or arise from dietary nutritional imbalances or plant poisonings (Box 13-5). Traumatic injures play a smaller role, except in dairy cattle, which commonly slip on concrete and injure themselves. History, visual inspection, manipulation, and palpation are important in the diagnosis of postural deformities in ruminants. In addition, other ruminants in the herd with similar abnormalities should be identified. Plant, feed, soil, and water samples should be taken to identify toxins that may have been ingested, resulting in the deformity. Often the signalment helps rule out certain breed- or species-specific genetic defects. Because goats jump off heights, they are subject to numerous fractures, sprains, and luxations, including unilateral or bilateral rupture of the gastrocnemius tendon.

SWELLINGS AND ENLARGEMENTS (SOFT AND HARD TISSUE)
CARTER E. JUDY
JOHN MAAS

Definition

Swelling and enlargements consist of soft (e.g., tendon) or hard (e.g., osseous) tissue and can occur anywhere on an animal's body. Generally clinically significant swellings and enlargements associated with the musculoskeletal system occur on the limbs.

Swellings and enlargements can be further divided into two principal groups, depending on whether or not they are associated with a specific anatomic structure. For example, a soft fluctuant swelling in the region of the left carpus may be caused by an abnormality of the antebrachialcarpal joint (e.g., septic synovial effusion) or may not involve the joint at all (e.g., subcutaneous abscess). Although lameness can be associated with such a swelling, clearly it is important to determine the cause of the abnormality because the one involving the joint may require the more immediate treatment.

Mechanisms of Swellings and Enlargements

The mechanism by which swelling or enlargement develops depends on the tissue involved (Box 13-6). Soft tissue swelling often is produced by trauma, inflammation, infection, or neoplasia; and it can consist of interstitial fluid (e.g., edema), fluid within an open space (e.g., synovial hernia), or a localized accumulation of cells or fibrous tissue. Localized edematous swelling commonly is caused by inflammation and/or obstruction of venous blood or lymph flow. Generalized edema is usually the result of increased hydrostatic pressure caused by circulatory failure or an altered capillary-tissue osmotic gradient stemming from hypoalbuminemia. Fluctuant swellings such as hematoma, synovial effusion, a purulent abscess, or a plasma-filled cyst contain free fluid. Granulation tissue, fibrous scar tissue, and tumor cells are the most common constituents of firm soft tissue swellings. Rupture of supporting or confining structures (e.g., prepubic tendon

rupture) can result in unusual forms of soft tissue swelling caused by herniation of internal organs.

Many factors influence new bone formation. Trauma and infections initiate bony enlargement (e.g., callus) by disrupting the periosteum, producing inflammation and eventually ossification. The extent of periosteal new bone formation depends on the etiology of the stimulus and the size of the affected area. Remodeled bone may also arise from nontraumatic events, usually associated with altered metabolism or neoplasia. Bony enlargements associated with the metaphysis and physis in young, growing animals are usually secondary to a combination of nutritional and traumatic factors. For example, dietary calcium, phosphorus, and vitamin D imbalance can lead to abnormal bone growth. A bony swelling develops gradually and may become noticeable only after it enlarges, interferes with normal function, or becomes a source of lameness.

Approach to Diagnosis of Swellings and Enlargements in the Horse

1. History. A history should determine the number of horses involved, the duration of clinical signs, and the possibility that traumatic events or environmental factors are responsible for causing a swelling or enlargement. In addition, changes over time in the appearance and size of the swelling or enlargement can be informative.
2. Inspection and palpation. The location of the swelling and its proximity to anatomic structures often reveal the tissue involved and the probable cause of the condition. For example, swelling around a joint may indicate arthritis, periarthritis, or hygromas. Tendon swelling may indicate tendonitis or ruptured tendons. Swelling over ligaments may indicate rupture, subluxation, or inflammation around a ligament. Muscle swelling results from abscessation or fascial tears. Subcutaneous swelling may indicate hematomas, edema from inflammation around a ligament, or cellulitis. Bony enlargements often can be localized to the shaft of a bone (e.g., periosteal callus) or at the ends of a bone (e.g., metaphyseal flaring). Periarticular new bone may be readily apparent (e.g., ringbone) or may not be found even on deep palpation. New bone formation also can be found associated with the axial skeleton and head.

   Palpation of a swelling can determine its consistency and association with anatomic structures. Osseous swelling indicates calcification, proliferation of bone, or fracture. Firm soft tissue swelling indicates inflammation, abnormal proliferation of soft tissue (e.g., granulation, tumor), or herniation.

   Warmth, redness, and pain associated with swelling indicate active inflammation. While new bone is forming, the swelling may be soft and sensitive to palpation. Cold and insensitivity to palpation suggest inadequate blood supply and possibly ischemia (e.g., gangrene).

   Lameness caused by an injury or condition that results in a hard swelling or enlargement may be accentuated by performing a stress test, such as trotting the horse in hand after direct pressure on the swelling. Intraarticular anesthesia may substantially reduce a lameness caused by joint effusion associated with periarticular new bone.
3. Radiography, ultrasonography and alternative imaging techniques. In addition to identifying definitively the nature of an osseous swelling or enlargement, radiography can gauge the severity and progression of the disease and help establish a therapeutic plan and prognosis. Ultrasound often can determine the position (e.g., depth, area) and volume of a soft tissue swelling and the optimum site for aspiration or biopsy. Thermography may help to identify subtle heat production secondary to inflamma-

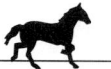

BOX 13-7

Causes of Swellings and Enlargements in Ruminants

SOFT TISSUE
Septic arthritis
Mycoplasma arthritis
Caprine arthritis-encephalitis in goats
Hygroma
Tenosynovitis
Chronic tendonitis
Ruptured tendon
Footrot
Gangrene of the foot
Fescue foot
Neoplasia
Bee stings
Snake bite
Abscess
Hematoma
Capped hock
Interdigital fibroma
Digital dermatitis (foot warts)
Skin neoplasia

SOFT TISSUE—cont'd
Granulomas (such as woody tongue)
Habronemiasis
Phycomycosis

HARD TISSUE
Osteomyelitis (periosteal new bone formation)
Septic arthritis
Secondary (degenerative) joint disease
Epiphysitis
Sequestrum
Lumpy jaw (actinomycosis)
Rickets
Fracture
Tumoral calcinosis
Osteosarcoma
Calcinosis circumscripta
Traumatic stifle injury with fibrosis
Primary or secondary copper deficiency (molybdenosis) (e.g., physitis, spontaneous fractures)

---

tion and increased blood flow, before onset of a swelling, allowing for early treatment. Nuclear scintigraphy may help to localize the etiology of swellings and identify whether they are bony or soft tissue in origin (e.g., tarsal effusion secondary to a sustentaculum tali osteomyelitis). Computed axial tomography (CAT scan) is useful for evaluating bony swellings, especially of the head when swellings of the mandible and maxilla may be related to infected teeth and the determination of which teeth are involved is necessary before surgical intervention. Magnetic resonance imaging (MRI) may prove useful for accurate imaging of soft tissue masses that cannot be accurately characterized with other diagnostic techniques.

4. Cytology, microbiology, and histology. A fine-needle aspiration, using aseptic techniques, should be performed to obtain samples for microbiologic culture (e.g., bacterial and fungal) of soft tissue swellings. If the material is very viscous, a large-gauge needle may be required. Fluid collected for cytology should be placed in tubes containing EDTA to prevent clotting before analysis. Tissue samples obtained by biopsy should be placed in 10% buffered formalin.

Approach to Diagnosis of Swelling and Enlargements in Ruminants

1. History. The history should determine the duration of a swelling and whether it is congenital or acquired (Box 13-7). The rate of growth of a mass may be significant. The signalment of the ruminant sometimes gives a clue to the origin of the swelling; other ruminants in the herd should be examined for similar signs. Systemic manifestations (e.g., fever, anorexia, depression, and elevated pulse and respiratory rates) may indicate such things as blackleg, malignancies, and septic abscesses.

2. Inspection and palpation. The origin of a swelling may be identified by the density and position of the mass on the ruminant. Masses over joints may represent hygromas or distention caused by synovial effusion. Skin masses may be edematous or parasitic nodules or neoplastic tumors. Muscle masses could be abscesses, herniations through torn fascia, or, in rare cases, neoplasia. Lymph nodes are most frequently enlarged because of abscessation, but neoplasia must be considered. Foot masses include interdigital fibromas and granulation tissue from chronic infections. Large osseous masses indicate calcification, bone proliferation, or a foreign body. When drainage is present in the center of a firm mass, a bone sequestrum is very likely. Firm soft tissue masses may be granulomatous tissues, neoplasia, or a connective tissue scar.

3. Radiography and ultrasonography. (See comments for equine section.)

4. Cytology, microbiology, and histology. In some cases the density and location of a mass will be diagnostic and eliminate other possible diagnoses, but in many cases a microscopic examination of the tissue is necessary. Tissue can be obtained by needle aspiration, biopsy, or sometimes complete excision. Abscesses can simply be lanced, drained, and flushed. Unidentified tissue should be sectioned and stained for histopathologic examination and, in some cases, cultured.

PARESIS AND WEAKNESS

RICHARD A. LeCOUTEUR

Definition

Paresis may be defined as a deficit of voluntary movement. It may be monoparesis (paresis of a single limb), paraparesis (paresis of both pelvic limbs), tetraparesis (paresis of all four limbs), or hemiparesis (paresis of a thoracic and pelvic limb on the same side). Paresis results from disruption of the voluntary motor pathways that extend from the cerebral cortex, through the brainstem and spinal cord, to the motor unit (peripheral nerve, neuromuscular junctions, and muscle fibers). Complete loss of voluntary movement is referred to as paralysis (plegia). Voluntary movements must be differentiated from reflex movements on the basis of neurologic examination findings and general observations.

Weakness may be defined as impairment of strength and power. Most authors use the terms *paresis* and *weakness*

---

synonymously; however, this may be confusing in some circumstances. For example, weakness may occur in the absence of paresis in some disorders of the nervous system, and weakness may result from many disease processes that do not primarily involve the nervous system (e.g., heart failure, respiratory insufficiency). The clinical signs of weakness may vary considerably and may include: paresis, gait abnormalities, dysphagia, regurgitation, dyspnea, and dysphonia. Weakness may be present at rest, or may occur after exercise. The distribution of involvement may be local, regional, or generalized. In addition there may be gross deformities of muscle mass (i.e., atrophy, hypertrophy, and skeletal deformities) associated with weakness.

This section focuses on paresis and weakness caused by conditions that affect the motor unit (Box 13-8). Diseases of other systems (e.g., respiratory and cardiovascular diseases or central nervous system disorders) that may result in paresis and weakness are discussed separately in other sections.

Mechanisms of Paresis and Weakness

Voluntary movement is initiated by the cerebral cortex. Muscular activity occurs subconsciously following activation of successively lower levels of the nervous system: basal nuclei, midbrain, pons and medulla, cerebellum, brainstem, spinal cord, and motor unit. The function of these lower levels is vital and without their input voluntary movements become impossible.

Monoparesis (or monoplegia) is a common problem in horses and ruminants. It may be caused by dysfunction of the lower motor neuron, or neuromuscular junction. Monoparesis is commonly caused by trauma to a nerve or plexus, although neoplasia (e.g., lymphoma, neurofibroma) and inflammation or infection (e.g., early stages of rabies) of peripheral nerves have been reported to cause monoparesis.

Bilateral pelvic limb paresis, ataxia, or paralysis may occur as a result of a neurologic disorder localized to the spinal cord caudal to the T2 spinal cord segment. Various congenital vertebral and spinal cord malformations may result in pelvic limb paresis. Equine protozoal myeloencephalitis and equine degenerative myeloencephalopathy may result in lameness, weakness, and ataxia that may progress to tetraparesis. Musculoskeletal disorders resulting only in bilateral pelvic limb weakness and paresis are unusual. Possible causes include trauma (e.g., postcalving/postfoaling paralyses caused by lumbosacral nerve root compression/contusion), vascular disorders (e.g., thrombosis), and early stages of an infectious disorder that may progress to tetraparesis.

The causes of tetraparesis are numerous and include progression of many of the disorders mentioned above. Outbreaks of intoxication with *Clostridium botulinum* occur spo-

radically in horses and ruminants and results in a flaccid paralysis that starts with the pelvic limbs and progresses cranially. Depending on the amount of toxin involved, large numbers of animals may be affected. Polyneuropathies (congenital and acquired), and polymyopathies (congenital, metabolic, infectious, immune-mediated) are causes of tetraparesis.

Muscle weakness may result either from a primary neuromuscular disease or disorders that affect muscle secondarily. In the latter category, problems of horses and ruminants that commonly result in weakness include poor diet, underfeeding, toxicity, and anorexia. Systemic diseases and disorders such as dehydration, low circulating blood volume, anemia, and metabolic abnormalities (e.g., acidosis or alkalosis) also may result in weakness. Disorders of bones (e.g., fractures) and joints (e.g., septic arthritis) affecting one limb also may affect the contralateral limb through overuse or misuse, and weakness of the contralateral limb may result.

Primary neuromuscular diseases usually are classified on the basis of the anatomic component of the motor unit that is involved. Such diseases broadly are subdivided into neuropathies—disorders of the neuron, its cell body, axon, and/or Schwann cells (myelin); junctionopathies—disorders of the neuromuscular junction; myopathies—disorders of muscle fibers; and neuromyopathies—disorders of both the neurons and muscle fibers.

Dysfunction of the motor unit results in lower motor neuron signs, seen clinically as muscle weakness. The expression of this weakness may vary considerably, and the distribution of involvement may be local, regional, or generalized. Atrophy, hypertrophy, and skeletal deformities may accompany the muscle weakness. Any patient presenting with some form of clinical weakness should be viewed as potentially having a motor unit disorder. Conclusions that the patient is "merely weak because it is sick" should not be readily assumed without meticulous evaluation of the motor unit.

Approach to Diagnosis of Paresis and Weakness in the Horse

Establishing a diagnosis requires an informed and coordinated approach to defining a problem list through associations and direct observations (i.e., a diagnostic plan) (Box 13-9).
1. Signalment. Breed, age, sex, and use of the horse.
2. History. Feeding program, vaccination and deworming schedules, course of complaint, response to treatment, and possibility of exposure to toxins or trauma.
3. Physical examination. Presence and distribution of abnormal findings on physical and neurologic examinations should be recorded. Normal functions must be known before abnormal functions may be recognized. Abnormal

BOX 13-9

Causes of Paresis and Weakness in Horses

DEGENERATIVE
Equine degenerative myeloencephalopathy

ANOMALOUS/CONGENITAL
Hydrocephalus
Vertebral and spinal cord malformations

METABOLIC
Exertional rhabdomyolysis
Hyperkalemic periodic paralysis
Hypothyroidism
Hyperthermia
Hypocalcemia
Hypokalemia
Equine hepatic lipidosis
Vitamin A deficiency

NUTRITIONAL
Malnutrition, vitamin E/selenium deficiency

NEOPLASTIC
Brain or spinal cord tumor
Lymphosarcoma
Melanoma
Leukemia

INFECTIOUS/INFLAMMATORY
Encephalitis, myelitis
Equine protozoal myeloencephalitis

INFECTIOUS/INFLAMMATORY—cont'd
Diskospondylitis
Botulism
Rabies
Ehrlichiosis
Tuberculosis
Rhinopneumonitis
Hepatoencephalopathy
Tick paralysis
Cerebrospinal nematodiasis
Equine protozoal myeloencephalitis

TOXIC
Snake bite
Plant poisons (star thistle poisoning, oleander, moldy
    corn poisoning, white snake root, locoweed, larkspur,
    delphinium, onion, moldy sweet clover)
Vitamin D
Phosphorus
Heavy metals (lead, arsenic)

TRAUMATIC
Vertebral fracture/luxation

VASCULAR
Postanesthetic hemorrhagic myelopathy

---

functions must be recognized because neurologic diseases are manifested clinically almost entirely by dysfunction. It is uncommon for the clinical signs to include readily detectable anatomic changes. Therefore a clinician must rely on clinical signs of abnormal function to identify the location of the neurologic dysfunction.

The first step in locating a neurologic lesion is to determine the level of the abnormality along the longitudinal plane of the neuraxis (i.e., brain, spinal cord or motor unit). The second step is to further localize the lesion within an anatomic region (e.g., motor unit should be further localized to either peripheral nerve, neuromuscular junction, or muscle). The third step is to determine the location of the lesion in the transverse plane at the appropriate longitudinal level (e.g., left or right side).

4. Minimum database. Complete blood count, serum biochemistry panel (including electrolyte determinations), fecal analysis, and urinalysis. Measurement of muscle-specific serum enzymes, such as creatine kinase (CK), as well as aspartate aminotransferase (AST), and lactic dehydrogenase (LDH), may be helpful in identifying neuromuscular disorders in which myonecrosis is a principal pathologic feature. Elevated serum enzyme activities may help to differentiate myopathies from other neuromuscular disorders. Immunologic procedures for the detection of myoglobin that are becoming available may provide a sensitive means of detecting myolysis in the future.
5. Specific diagnostic tests
   A. Electrodiagnostic testing. Electromyography (EMG) involves the detection and characterization of electrical activity (potentials) recorded from a patient's muscles.

A systematic study of individual muscles permits an accurate determination of the distribution of muscles affected by a pathologic process.
   B. Nerve and muscle biopsy examination. This procedure evaluates the morphology of portions of the motor unit and may differentiate between neuropathies, junctionopathies, and myopathies. In some instances, results of muscle biopsy analysis may provide a definitive diagnosis (e.g., polysaccharide storage myopathy of horses).

Approach to Diagnosis of Paresis and Weakness in Ruminants

The approach to the diagnosis of disorders causing paresis and weakness in ruminants is essentially the same as that for horses (Box 13-10). Differences may be encountered as a result of the intended use of ruminants. Most ruminants live in a herd setting and the level of human supervision and care of the herd will vary. In some cases, animals will be monitored daily for signs of abnormal behavior, whereas in other cases animals may not be observed for varying periods of time. Infectious diseases, disorders arising from nutritional problems, parasites, or toxicity may progress to affect several individuals before a problem is noticed. Signalment, history, and a physical and neurologic examination are essential to determine first if the paresis and weakness are neurologic in origin and second to make a neuroanatomic diagnosis. These findings should be combined with a knowledge of diseases/disorders that produce this clinical picture in order to arrive at a diagnosis.

MUSCLE SPASMS AND MYOCLONUS

RICHARD A. LeCOUTEUR

Definition

Muscle spasms are sudden, transient, and involuntary contractions of a single muscle or group of muscles, attended by pain and loss of function. Often all the muscles affected by a spasm are supplied by a single nerve. A painful, tonic, spasmodic muscular contraction is often referred to as a cramp.

Myoclonus may be defined as a disturbance of neuromuscular activity characterized by abrupt, brief, rapid, jerky, arrhythmic, asynergic, involuntary contractions involving portions of muscles, entire muscles, or groups of muscles, regardless of their functional association. The movements may be single or repetitive (10 to 50 per minute) and are similar to those that follow stimulation of a muscle. Myoclonus is seen primarily in muscles of the limbs, where involvement is often diffuse or widespread. Myoclonus also may be present in facial or masticatory muscles and muscles of the tongue, larynx, and pharynx. Myoclonus usually disappears during sleep.

This section describes muscle spasm and myoclonus as specific clinical signs associated with dysfunction of the musculoskeletal system.

Mechanisms of Muscle Spasms and Myoclonus

Spasms usually are of reflex origin, and may result from irritation or stimulation at any level of the nervous system from the cerebral cortex to the muscle fibers. In most cases, however, spasms are caused by peripheral irritation affecting either muscles or nerves. Pain may cause either tonic or clonic spasms of muscles, especially should the painful stimulus be focal or discrete. Mechanical irritation may cause a localized spasm. There may be prolonged and characteristic muscle spasm associated with the hyperirritability of nerves and muscles in tetany or tetanus. Spasms may follow injury or irritation of peripheral nerves, particularly during the process of regeneration. Spasms may also result from irritation or diseases affecting cortical centers in the brain, motor nuclei in the brainstem, or descending motor pathways in spinal cord.

There has been much discussion regarding the pathologic process underlying myoclonic movements. Whereas originally it was thought that the neural discharge that excites the muscular contraction of myoclonus was confined to the motor unit, it is now known that myoclonus also may result from dysfunction of the brain (cerebral cortex, brainstem, basal nuclei, thalamus, etc.), spinal cord, peripheral nerve, neuromuscular junction, or the muscle itself, alone or in combination. A variety of processes evidently lead to hyperexcitability of the cerebral cortex, subcortical structures, or even the lower motor neurons alone. Myoclonic movements or muscle spasms may occur in a variety of conditions. They have been observed in association with encephalitis, meningitis, toxic and postanoxic states, metabolic disorders, degenerative diseases, and vascular and neoplastic conditions. Myoclonus has also been reported in association with lesions of peripheral nerves, nerve roots, and spinal cord.

Specifically, disturbances in plasma electrolyte concentrations, certain drugs, toxins, and poisons may elicit involuntary muscle activity. In general, the mechanism that is common to all causes of spasm or myoclonus involves an inappropriate stimulation of a nerve or muscle cell, causing the cell to fire a series of action potentials, resulting in muscle contraction. For example, toxins may act directly on the muscle cell membrane to stimulate the release of calcium into the cell from the sarcoplasmic reticulum, thereby causing involuntary muscle contraction. Alternatively, some toxins may cause efferent neurons to release neurotransmitter across the neuromuscular junctions, thereby stimulating receptors on the muscle cell membrane.

Approach to Diagnosis of Muscle Spasms and Myoclonus in the Horse

A broad spectrum of diseases may be associated with muscle spasms or myoclonus in horses (Box 13-11). A thorough investigation is needed to achieve an accurate diagnosis.

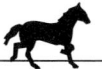

BOX 13-11

Causes of Muscle Spasms and Myoclonus in Horses

ANOMALOUS/CONGENITAL
Myotonia congenita

METABOLIC
Hyperkalemic periodic paralysis
Hypocalcemia
Hypoglycemia
Hypothermia
Exhaustion
Shivering

NEOPLASTIC
Insulinoma

INFECTIOUS/INFLAMMATORY
Tetanus
Rabies
Equine influenza
Tick-borne encephalitis
Meningitis

IDIOPATHIC
Neonatal maladjustment syndrome

TOXIC
Strychnine
Organochlorines
Chlorinated hydrocarbons

BOX 13-12

Causes of Muscle Spasms and Myoclonus in Ruminants

ANOMALOUS/CONGENITAL
Congenital posterior paralysis of Danish red calves
Inherited congenital myoclonus (formerly known as neur-axial edema) of polled Herefords and their crossbreeds
Maple syrup urine disease in polled Herefords and their crossbreeds
Lethal spasms in Jersey and Hereford calves
Congenital brain edema in Herefords

METABOLIC
Hypomagnesemia
Hypocalcemia
Hypoglycemia

INFECTIOUS/INFLAMMATORY
Tetanus
Rabies
Pseudorabies
Meningitis
Coccidiosis

TOXIC
Chlorinated hydrocarbons
Strychnine
Cockelbur
Buckeye

1. History. A comprehensive history including evaluation of the environment, stablemates, description of any traumatic episodes, and any potential drug or toxin exposure.
2. Physical examination. Complete lameness and neurologic examinations should be done as extensions of a thorough physical examination.
3. Minimum database. Complete blood count, serum biochemistry panel (including muscle enzyme determinations), and cerebrospinal fluid analysis should be performed. In the case of muscle spasm and myoclonus, elevation in muscle enzymes may indicate secondary muscle damage rather than a primary muscle disease. A tetany panel, including serum calcium, phosphorus, and magnesium determinations, may be completed. Hypocalcemia may be a cause of muscle spasms in lactating horses, exhausted endurance horses, or horses transported long distances.
4. Specific diagnostic tests.
   A. Electrodiagnostic testing. A systematic study of individual muscles using electromyography permits an accurate determination of the distribution of muscles affected by a pathologic process.
   B. Nerve and muscle biopsy examination. This procedure evaluates the morphology of portions of the motor unit and may differentiate between neuropathies, junctionopathies, and myopathies. In some instances, results of muscle biopsy analysis may provide a definitive diagnosis (e.g., phosphorylase deficiency of Charolais cattle).

Approach to Diagnosis of Muscle Spasms and Myoclonus in Ruminants

The approach to diagnosis of muscle spasms and myoclonus in ruminants is essentially the same as that described for horses (Box 13-12). In ruminants a tetany panel (consisting of serum calcium, phosphorus, and magnesium determinations) should be completed in any animal exhibiting these signs. In lactating cattle on grass pasture, and in sheep transported long distances, hypomagnesemia and hypocalcemia, respectively, are highly suspected initially. Several infectious (e.g., rabies, pseudorabies), toxic, and inherited causes of muscle spasms and myoclonus should be suspected in ruminants. In postparturient animals and animals with wounds or bites, or animals recently castrated or tail docked, tetanus should be considered as a possible cause of muscle spasms and myoclonus.

SUGGESTED READINGS

Auer JA, Stick JA: *Equine surgery,* ed 2, Philadelphia, 1999, WB Saunders.
Greenough PR, Weaver AD: *Lameness in cattle,* ed 3, Philadelphia, 1997, WB Saunders.
McIlwraith CW, Trotter GW: *Joint disease in the horse,* Philadelphia, 1996, WB Saunders.
Nixon AJ: *Equine fracture repair,* Philadelphia, 1996, WB Saunders.
Stashack TS: Diagnosis of lameness. In *Adams' Lameness in horses,* ed 4, Philadelphia, 1987, Lea & Febiger, pp 100-151.
White NA, Moore JN: *Current techniques in equine surgery and lameness,* ed 2, Philadelphia, 1998, WB Saunders.

Collapse/Sudden Death

STAN W. CASTEEL

JAMES R. TURK

MAJOR CLINICAL SIGN/PROBLEM ENCOUNTERED

The ruminant or horse that collapses and dies within 24 hours while being observed or is found dead with no premonitory signs of illness is often a diagnostic challenge. In these situations, clients often are distressed and frequently pressure the veterinarian to declare an immediate diagnosis. Sudden death in the absence of observed clinical illness is usually the most perplexing. Obligation to clients necessitates a systematic approach to derive a specific etiologic diagnosis, to determine the source and extent of the problem, and to recommend corrective measures. These goals are best accomplished by delineating the characteristics of normal animals within the herd and analyzing the distribution of the disease with respect to time, place, and a variety of exposure factors and environmental influences. These factors are then correlated with necropsy results and additional diagnostic testing.

COLLAPSE VERSUS SUDDEN DEATH

Collapse is easily identified as a state of extreme prostration and depression. However, sudden death has a somewhat tenuous meaning, lending itself to subjective impression. The timing parameter used to define sudden death ranges from 1 to 24 hours from the onset of the fatal episode. Some veterinarians restrict the definition to a narrower time span. The 12- to 24-hour interval is sometimes selected to coincide with the frequency of owner observation of the livestock. For our purposes, sudden death means clinically unexplained rapid death (12 to 24 hours) occurring during normal activity in apparently healthy animals. Generally a condition of this nature is associated with fatal dysfunction of the cardiovascular, nervous, respiratory, or gastrointestinal systems. In addition, perturbations in general cellular metabolism (cyanide or hydrogen sulfide) may result in peracute death.

Approach to Diagnosis of Sudden Death

The causes of sudden death are investigated in much the same way as any disease. The accompanying tables of differential diagnoses include infectious, metabolic/nutritional, physical, cardiovascular, toxic, and miscellaneous causes of sudden death. Diagnostic laboratories provide an array of tests and analytic procedures based on the needs of veterinarians in their service areas. Use of these facilities to support a definitive diagnosis is essential in sudden death cases. Diagnosis is rarely based on a single item of evidence and usually requires input from multiple testing procedures. Unless the cause of death is apparent, some important considerations required for effective use of a diagnostic laboratory include the following.

1. History. A detailed history, which consists of the herd incidence, management changes, past medical problems, vaccination records, new additions to the herd, a complete description of the environment, and a recognition of the frequency of animal observation. Owners and managers may not be candid for fear of being considered negligent. Inconsistencies between involved parties should be carefully evaluated. Recent changes in management practices should be scrutinized, including feeding habits and whether there have been any illnesses in commingled animals. Animals trailed or transported for long distances or introduced onto unfamiliar ranges often are poisoned by plant species normally avoided by indigenous livestock. The chance of foul play should be considered without creating undue alarm. Assigning blame should be left to the discretion of owners. Consideration of disgruntled former employees and equine insurance claims are particularly critical situations that may have legal implications. The precise cause of death is crucial for insured livestock

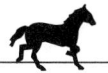

(mostly horses) because of exclusion clauses in many insurance policies. Heavily insured horses should be subjected to a detailed documented and witnessed diagnostic evaluation; toxicologic testing is especially critical in these cases. Evaluation of the environment before the animal is moved is necessary to eliminate questionable procedures in insurance claim cases. Evidence of struggling in the immediate area indicates a more protracted illness in contrast to collapse and death without a struggle. Suspicions should be aroused when evidence suggests the animal may have been dragged or carried to the current location.

2. Specimen. The appropriate specimen is required by the diagnostic laboratory to perform the requested examination. Many cases of sudden death are attributed to central nervous system dysfunction, so it is necessary to remove the brain. Busy practitioners frequently do not take the time to remove this organ. There is a higher-than-normal probability of a poison being involved in sudden death cases, especially in equine insurance claims. For toxicologic examination, toxicants remaining in the gastrointestinal tract, major excretory organs, liver, and kidneys must be considered.

3. Sample. The correct *amount and preservation of the sample* depends on the specific test. Medicolegal cases demand that stringent photographic and written documentation, witnessing, and chain of custody protocol be followed during necropsy and sample collection. The amount of the sample is particularly important for chemical analysis. Sending insufficient quantities of sample may preclude multiple testing procedures. In general, 100 to 200 g of tissue or ingesta, 50 ml of urine, all fluid from both eyes, and 5 to 10 ml of blood or serum suffice for most analytical procedures. A midsagittal cut through the brain is performed to allow freezing of one half for chemical analysis and formalin preservation of the other. When poisoning is suspected, samples from possible sources such as feed, water, baits, poisonous plants, and suspect materials should be submitted. Usually 1 kg of each is adequate. Samples submitted for chemical analysis should be frozen in individual containers and labeled with date, location, and identity of the specimen. Specimens for bacteriology and virology are to be packaged separately and chilled. Dry ice should be avoided because gaseous carbon dioxide may kill some infectious agents. Tissues for histopathologic examination require fixing in 10% formalin with tissue slices 4 to 5 mm thick. Suspected poisonous plants are properly preserved by placing them in a plastic bag with wet paper towels or by drying them between sheets of paper.

CAUSES OF COLLAPSE/SUDDEN DEATH

Infectious Causes of Sudden Death in the Horse (Box 14-1)

Foal actinobacillus is an acute fulminant septicemia caused by *Actinobacillus equuli*, a gram-negative bacterium found in the upper respiratory tract, feces, and genital tract of normal adult horses. Predisposing factors to foal septicemia with any agent include prematurity, failure of passive transfer, dam malnourishment during gestation, and environmental stress. A characteristic histologic finding is multiple bacterial emboli in renal glomerular capillaries without inflammatory infiltrate in neonatal foals. Acute anthrax may be rapidly fatal to horses after a period of excitement, depression, convulsions, and coma. Isolating the etiologic agent from blood confirms the diagnosis. Babesiosis is an erythrocytic parasite that may cause death within 24 hours. Identification of the organism in blood smears or complement fixation test for parasite antibodies confirm the diagnosis.

BOX 14-1

Infectious Causes of Collapse/Sudden Death in the Horse

Acute colitis
Babesiosis
Botulism*
Clostridial myopathy
Clostridium difficile diarrhea
Clostridium perfringens enterotoxemia
Clostridium sordellii dysentery
Equine monocytic ehrlichiosis (Potomac fever)
Guttural pouch mycosis (hemorrhage from)
Hemorrhagic enterotoxemia in foals
Neonatal septicemia
Neonatal diarrhea
Salmonellosis*
Tyzzer's disease

*Likely to involve several animals.

Acute clostridial disease involving the clostridial species *septicum, chauvoei, novyi,* and *perfringens* has been associated with intramuscular injections of various parenterals such as ivermectin, vitamin B complex, prostaglandin, antihistamines, and flunixin meglumine when asepsis has been ignored. Clostridial myopathies also are associated with deep stab or puncture wounds. Botulism in foals (Shaker foal syndrome) is caused by *Clostridium botulinum* (usually type B). Toxin may sometimes be demonstrated in feed and gut contents. The organism may be cultured from tissues or gut contents in toxicoinfectious cases. *Clostridium sordellii* should be suspected in cases of foals having a history of colic, bloody diarrhea, and death within a few hours.[1] *C. perfringens* type C may induce a hemorrhagic enterotoxemia and death in foals as young as 4 days.[2] Severe intestinal lesions are caused by the beta toxin produced by this species. Organisms may be demonstrated in smears of intestinal contents. *C. perfringens* type D also induces sudden death in the most aggressive foals in group feeding situations. Similar enterotoxemia also has been associated with toxin-producing *Clostridium difficile*[3] and *Bacteroides fragilis.*[4]

Equine monocytic ehrlichiosis (Potomac fever), caused by *Ehrlichia risticii*, is a severe colitis with diarrhea and dehydration, followed by ileus, endotoxemia, and death in adult horses. Diagnosis is based on clinical findings and antibody and antigen detection using immunofluorescent antibody (IFA) and enzyme-linked immunosorbent assay (ELISA) methods, respectively. Guttural pouch mycosis often results in nonfatal intermittent unilateral epistaxis. Occasionally a single episode of severe epistaxis from rupture of an aneurysm in the internal carotid artery may result in sudden death. Necropsy reveals blood in the nasal passages and guttural pouch with a diphtheritic plaque in the dorsocaudal aspect of the medial compartment. Salmonellosis is responsible for many cases of acute enterocolitis, especially when several animals are involved. The peracute syndrome may resemble colitis-X in mature horses with a course of 6 to 12 hours. Horses may die before diarrhea develops. Postmortem diagnosis is based on isolation of *Salmonella* spp. from bowel contents, bowel wall, or associated lymph nodes. Tyzzer's disease is a rapidly developing fatal hepatitis of foals. The incidence is sporadic, and, because of the peracute development, clinical signs may not be observed before death. Diagnosis is based on histologic demonstration of the bacilli in bundles within hepatocytes surrounding necrotic areas.

Infectious and Parasitic Causes of Sudden Death in Ruminants

Sudden death caused by infectious agents ranges from acute septicemias and toxemias to rupture and release of abscess contents into the systemic circulation (Box 14-2). A liver abscess rupturing into the caudal vena cava or endocarditis, especially of the right atrioventricular valve, with subsequent pulmonary thromboembolism, or the rupture of a pituitary abscess are occasional causes of sudden death in individual animals. Acute anthrax and the clostridial infections, as well as ingestion of their preformed toxins, are more common causes of sudden death in ruminants. Anaplasmosis may cause sudden death in mature cattle under stress, without apparent icterus. In these cases, anthrax may be mistaken for anaplasmosis because of the gross enlargement of the spleen. Anaplasma organisms may be demonstrated in blood smears whereas newer diagnostic methods involve immunofluorescence assay (IFA) and deoxyribonucleic acid (DNA) probes. Of all domestic animals, cattle are the most susceptible to clostridial infections in which tissue invasion is present (e.g., blackleg). Because of this, vaccination status is important to ascertain. In addition, a fluorescent antibody test and isolation of the bacterium confirm the diagnosis. *C. perfringens* of various types is responsible for heavy losses caused by enterotoxemia in calves, lambs, kids, and feedlot cattle in apparent good health and on full feed. *C. perfringens* type D has been associated with focal symmetric encephalomalacia in lambs.[5] Coliform mastitis may result in peracute systemic disease and rapid death if not treated early. Diagnosis is based on culture of the organism from the affected gland. *Leptospira* may cause an acute septicemia with hemolytic anemia and rapid death in young ruminants. Demonstration of leptospires in fresh urine or by immunohistochemical staining of tissues may assist in making the diagnosis. The course of listeriosis in sheep and goats is rapid, and death may occur in 4 to 48 hours following the appearance of clinical signs.[6]

Bacteriologic culture (isolation) or immunohistochemical staining of the organism in tissues is diagnostic. Acute fascioliasis *(Fasciola hepatica)* occurs seasonally in sheep and may cause sudden death within 6 weeks of initial infection. Anaerobic conditions induced by flukes in hepatic parenchyma predispose ruminants to the highly fatal clostridial hepatopathies such as *Clostridium hemolyticum* infection. Evidence of fluke infection is visible grossly. Peracute malignant catarrhal fever (MCF) is a sporadic cause of sudden death in cattle that is usually associated with contacting ovine carriers, but most cases of MCF have diarrhea, keratitis, and other obvious clinical signs for days before death occurs. A septicemic form of mycoplasmosis has induced rapid death in kids.[7] Isolation of the causative organism is diagnostic. Sudden death is the usual manifestation of septicemic pasteurellosis in lambs. Pseudorabies is a consideration in sudden death cases of ruminants having contact with infected swineherds in the midwestern United States. Brain for microscopic examination and virus isolation should be submitted to confirm the diagnosis. Acute septicemic salmonellosis mainly affects young ruminants and may result in death within 24 hours. Acute septic metritis usually occurs secondary to complications of parturition. Endotoxic shock and rapid death may occur in severe cases. Thromboembolic meningoencephalomyelitis caused by *Haemophilus somnus* is a peracute septicemic disease of young calves. Many cattle die without showing clinical signs. It may be associated with prior respiratory problems in the herd or feedlot. Typical lesions or isolation of the causative organism is diagnostic. Adult lymphosarcoma associated with bovine leukemia virus can be a cause of sudden cardiac death when neoplastic cells infiltrate the cardiac conduction system.

Metabolic and Nutritional Causes of Sudden Death in the Horse

Hypocalcemia in horses is most common in lactating mares, but it also occurs after transit. Animals may develop tetany, synchronous diaphragmatic flutter (thumps), muscle tremors, and sweating. Low serum calcium is diagnostic. White muscle disease (nutritional myodegeneration) is associated with selenium and vitamin E deficiency. Sudden death in adult horses following severe exercise is attributed to degenerative lesions in cardiac and skeletal musculature. Death in foals may occur within hours from pulmonary edema and heart failure. Diagnosis is based on measuring whole blood and/or liver selenium and vitamin E concentrations.

Metabolic and Nutritional Causes of Sudden Death in Ruminants

Metabolic and nutritional diseases often are not considered in cases of sudden death. The primary lesion in a disorder of cattle known as "falling disease" is progressive fibrosis of the myocardium. Sudden deaths characteristic of the disease are attributed to exercise-induced heart failure.[8] Rapid development of hypocalcemia usually is associated with the onset of lactation in cattle, with stressful circumstances in older lactating ewes, or with transport associated with fasting and weather stress. Hypomagnesemia also may develop under similar conditions, especially in ewes and cows in heavy lactation and on lush grass pastures. Polioencephalomalacia occurs most commonly in animals raised under intensive production techniques and can sometimes be traced to excessive sulfates in the diet and/or water. The clinical course tends to be most rapid in sheep. Severe cases of ruminal lactic acidosis, especially in animals unaccustomed to high levels of soluble carbohydrate in the diet, may induce death within 24 hours. Nutritional myodegeneration of the heart is a frequent

---

BOX 14-2

Infectious and Parasitic Causes of Collapse/Sudden Death in Ruminants

Abscesss rupture at liver hilus or pituitary
Anaplasmosis* (B)
Anthrax*
Black disease, infectious necrotic hepatitis
Blackleg
Botulism*
Bovine lymphosarcoma
Clostridium hemolyticum, bacillary hemoglobinuria, redwater*
Clostridium perfringens, enterotoxemia
Coliform mastitis
Endocarditis
Leptospirosis
Listeriosis (C, O)
Liver flukes (O)
MCF (B)
Mycoplasmosis (C)
Neonatal septicemia
Neonatal diarrhea
Pasteurellosis, septicemic* (O)
Pseudorabies
Salmonellosis*
Septic metritis
Thromboembolic meningoencephalomyelitis* (B)

B, Bovine; *C,* caprine; *O,* ovine.
*Likely to involve several animals.

cause of sudden death in young ruminants born to dams fed selenium-deficient diets during gestation. Diagnosis is based on histopathology and measurement of liver selenium concentration. Some cases of sudden death associated with myocardial necrosis are idiopathic.[9]

Cardiovascular Causes of Sudden Death in the Horse

Diagnosis of sudden death caused by cardiovascular failure depends on a careful and methodic technique (Box 14-3). Usually a single animal is affected. Necropsy is necessary to identify the location and characteristics of the lesion, and further analysis may be necessary to establish the exact cause of death. Aortic ring (root) rupture in stallions usually is seen early in the breeding season, occurring immediately after servicing a mare. Rupture of the aorta may occur just distal to the aortic valve, resulting in cardiac tamponade and rapid death. Acute central nervous system embolism results from detached thrombi originating from endocarditic lesions or accidental intracarotid injection. Cerebral hematoma also can result from intracarotid injection. Endocarditis, especially of the aortic valve, may result in coronary thromboembolism and myocardial infarction. Coronary occlusion as a result of damage induced by *Strongylus vulgaris* larvae can be diagnosed by the presence of the larvae in the coronary thrombus. Massive abdominal or thoracic hemorrhage is found at necropsy, and the cause may be difficult to ascertain.[10] Racehorses mostly die from severe hemorrhage in the thorax. Myocarditis in horses up to 4 years of age resulting from recent respiratory infection may be diagnosed with histopathologic examination. Pericardial rupture and the associated heart damage is a result of violent trauma. Splenic rupture and fatal hemorrhage rarely occur because of the protection afforded by the thoracic wall. Massive thrombi of verminous origin have been observed in young horses that die suddenly while exercising. Uterine arterial rupture involving ovarian, uteroovarian, uterine, or external iliac arteries is observed in older mares, with death ensuing in 30 minutes to 20 hours postpartum.

Physical Causes of Sudden Death in the Horse

Fatal air embolism can result from any open vein above the heart. Open needles or catheters and severe head wounds involving teeth and sinuses have resulted in sudden death from air emboli. Air is aspirated into the vein by the Venturi effect from blood surging past a portal and creating the necessary negative pressure to aspirate air into the vein. Between 700 and 6000 ml of air may produce a fatal air embolus in the right cardiac ventricle where it obstructs the pulmonary

artery. Cecal or colonic rupture in parturient mares results in sudden death within 8 hours.[11]

Physical Causes of Sudden Death in Ruminants

Physical causes of sudden death often display gross evidence indicative of the diagnosis. Abomasal bloat occurs in calves and lambs drinking excessive quantities of warm milk replacer at infrequent intervals. Abomasal ulcers occasionally may perforate and cause rapid death in calves or adult cattle. Ruminal bloat is one of the more common physical causes of sudden death in intensively raised ruminants. When differentiating postmortem from antemortem bloat, note that bloat is the primary cause of death when there is congestion and hemorrhage in the anterior parts of the carcass and edema in the scrotal and ventral perineal areas. Bloat and hypersalivation are the most consistent clinical signs seen in cases of choke. Firm fruits, tubers, or green ears of corn may occlude the esophagus and result in rapid rumenal tympany and death.

Sudden death is a major concern in feedlots because most occur in cattle near market weight. Gastrointestinal disturbances are seen with a high frequency in cattle in these late stages of the feeding program. Sudden death is the result of interactions between factors such as rumen acidosis, bloat, and endotoxemia.

Exposure to high-voltage currents in the form of lightning or electrical transmission wires may cause instantaneous death. The diagnosis of lightning strike is based on a history of an electrical storm, linear singe marks, food in the mouth, several animals dead in the same vicinity, and evidence of lightning damage in the immediate environment. Gunshot wounds may be deliberate or accidental, but in any case involving sudden death the head or heart is the usual site of injury. Bullets may pass through or lodge in obscure locations, making retrieval difficult. Radiography can assist in locating a bullet. Heatstroke is a sporadic condition characterized by hyperthermia and collapse. High humidity, dehydration, obesity, and poor heat tolerance associated with young or old age are all factors that predispose animals to overheating. Summer slump induced by consumption of endophyte-infected fescue potentiates the heat intolerance. Internal bleeding may cause sudden death when a uterine artery is ruptured during parturition. This is readily apparent on necropsy. Tracheal edema, or "honker" syndrome, of feeder cattle is seen sporadically in feedlot cattle of the southern plains during hot weather. The pathoanatomic basis of this syndrome is extensive edema of the mucosa and submucosa of the lower trachea, with attendant dyspnea and obstructive asphyxiation. Increased respiratory movements stimulated by hot weather or exercise trigger the clinical illness, especially in heavy cattle during the latter part of the feeding period.[12] Traumatic reticuloperitonitis/reticulopericarditis is associated with lack of oral discrimination in cattle. Sudden death occurs because of acute hemorrhage or dysrhythmia when the heart is punctured.

Toxic Causes of Sudden Death in the Horse

Toxic causes of sudden death are frequently related to management practices. An increase in specific disease syndromes or sudden death in a population of livestock with common potential exposures suggests involvement of a toxic agent. Investigation of the premises and a familiarity with poisonous plants and pesticides used in the practice area should help narrow the list of possible etiologic agents (Box 14-4).

Horses ingesting a lethal dose of the avicide 4-aminopyridine have died within 2 hours of the onset of clinical signs. Diagnosis is based on chemical analysis of stomach contents.

BOX 14-3

Cardiovascular Causes of Collapse/Sudden Death in the Horse

Aortic ring (root) rupture
Central nervous system embolism
Coronary occlusion
Endocarditis
Massive abdominal or thoracic hemorrhage
Myocarditis
Pericardial rupture
Splenic rupture
Thrombi of verminous origin
Uterine arterial rupture

BOX 14-4

Toxic Causes of Collapse/Sudden Death in the Horse

4-Aminopyridine
Arsenic
Black flies
Cantharidin*
Ferrous fumarate
Fusarium monoliforme–associated mycotoxicosis
Insulin and potassium
Monensin*
Nitrogen dioxide
Organophosphate and carbamate insecticides

TOXIC PLANTS
Acer rubrum (red maple)
Blue-green algae*
Cicuta spp. (water hemlock)
Conium maculatum (poison hemlock)
Cyanogenic plants
Meliotus spp. (sweet clover)
Nerium spp. (oleander)
Nicotiana spp. (tobacco)
Ricinus communis (castor bean)
Taxus spp. (Japanese yew)

*Likely to involve several animals.

Fatal doses of arsenic-containing pesticides may induce cardiovascular collapse and death in horses within hours of ingestion. The presence of edema and fluid in the GI tract suggests the diagnosis, and chemical analysis of contents, liver, or kidney confirms it. Black flies swarm where swiftly flowing water provides the aeration necessary for the development of larvae. Massive attacks of these blood-sucking insects can rapidly kill livestock because a toxin present in the saliva of the flies increases capillary permeability.[13] Cantharidin poisoning can occur after ingestion of 4 to 5 g of blister beetles. Lesions suggestive of cantharidin toxicosis include blistering and ulceration of mucous membranes of the GI and urinary tracts and myocardial degeneration and necrosis. Sustained hypocalcemia and hypomagnesemia are features of the clinical pathology consistent with blister beetle poisoning. Identification of blister beetles in the hay and chemical analysis of urine and GI contents are suitable for diagnostic confirmation. In the past, ferrous fumarate, present in digestive inoculate and administered to foals immediately after birth, has resulted in death in some cases in 12 to 96 hours. This illustrates the acute toxicity of iron to young animals in particular. Lesions induced were those of gross liver damage. *Fusarium monoliforme*–contaminated corn causes rapid death in horses after the sudden onset of bizarre neurologic deficits and behavioral effects. The lesion of this mycotoxin-induced leukoencephalomalacia is liquefactive necrosis in the subcortical white matter.

High intravenous doses of insulin[14] and potassium[15] induce sudden death without significant lesions. Chemical detection is often overlooked and very difficult to perform and interpret in cases of deliberate poisoning. Immediate analysis of blood and circumstantial evidence of needle punctures in the jugular furrow are of diagnostic value. Monensin is quite toxic to horses, and fatal poisoning can occur within 12 hours of ingestion of poultry feed containing 100 g/ton or cattle premixes containing 300 g/ton. Lesions related to heart failure are seen on postmortem examination. Tissues collected for microscopic examination should include heart and diaphragm. Chemical analysis of feed samples and stomach contents will confirm

exposure. Toxic gases such as nitrogen dioxide, hydrogen sulfide, and carbon monoxide may be responsible for sudden death in horses housed in poorly ventilated buildings with associated gas sources nearby. Organophosphate and carbamate insecticides may induce acute intoxication and death within hours. Diagnosis is based on a history of exposure, determination of acetylcholinesterase activity in the caudate nucleus of the brain, and chemical detection of specific compounds in gut contents.

Circumstances surrounding toxic plant ingestion and diagnosis of intoxication are described in the ruminant section of this chapter. Ingestion of wilted *Acer rubrum* (red maple) leaves may induce massive methemoglobinemia, causing marked tissue anoxia and death.[16] Red maple poisoning usually occurs during the late summer and early fall when trees are in full leaf. Ready access to wilted leaves follows windstorms. *Ricinus communis,* or castor bean, is also unique to this section. Seeds of this plant contain a phytotoxin called ricin, which causes severe enteritis and rapid death in horses. About 150 beans (50 g) are sufficient to kill a 450-kg horse. Diagnosis can be verified by finding a toxic amount of ingested seeds in the gut contents.

Toxic Causes of Sudden Death in Ruminants

Intoxication of livestock is frequently suggested as a simple explanation for very complex situations involving sudden death. Suspicions are warranted when a large number of animals die suddenly within a short time. Toxicants should be considered when the appearance of a disease or sudden death is temporally associated with a change in the environment (Box 14-5). An accurate diagnosis in many of these cases requires qualitative and quantitative analyses for suspect poisons. Selecting toxicants for which to analyze requires reasoned judgment supported by an extensive investigation of the environment and postmortem findings.

The avicide 4-aminopyridine usually is formulated with corn, making it a palatable poison for nontarget herbivorous livestock. Diagnosis is confirmed by chemical analysis of rumen contents or urine. Anticoagulant intoxication may induce sudden death when hemorrhage occurs in the cranial vault, abdominal cavity, pericardial sac, mediastinum, or thorax. The antemortem or postmortem sample for chemical analysis is whole blood or liver. Failure to detect an anticoagulant is not unusual because of the time lag between consumption and presence of the clotting defects, as well as the metabolism of the compound. Arsenic derivatives are a significant hazard to ruminants, especially in areas where such chemicals are widely used as cotton desiccants. Postmortem findings are consistent with microvascular injury to the gastrointestinal tract. Diagnosis is confirmed by chemical analysis of rumen contents, liver, or kidney. In rare cases large doses of botulinum toxin may cause sudden death in ruminants. Sources of the toxin include the bones of dead animals eaten by osteophagic livestock, poultry carcasses in manure fed to cattle, stagnant pond water, animal tissues in silage or baled hay, and improperly ensiled silage or haylage.

Acetylcholinesterase-inhibiting agents such as the carbamate and organophosphate pesticides can kill livestock within hours. Agricultural practices result in the use of these pesticides in close proximity to livestock. This situation may lead to disaster. Acetylcholinesterase activity in the caudate nucleus of the brain is readily determined and interpreted, and specific compounds may be identified in rumen contents. Toxic gases such as carbon monoxide, hydrogen sulfide, and nitrogen dioxide become important differentials for sudden death in ruminants housed in poorly ventilated buildings, particularly over waste pits. Chlorinated hydrocarbon pesticides do not enjoy the widespread use they once did; however, old containers remain in obscure locations on

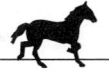

Toxic Causes of Collapse/Sudden Death in Ruminants

4-Aminopyridine (Avitrol), an avicide
Anticoagulants
Arsenic
Botulism*
Carbamates
Carbon monoxide
Chlorinated hydrocarbons
Copper (B, O)
Crude oil
Gossypol*
Hydrogen sulfide gas*
Ionophores*
Lead*
Metaldehyde
4-Methyl-imidazole, bovine bonker's syndrome (B, O)
Nicotine sulfate
Nitrogen dioxide gas*
Organophosphates
Selenium, parenteral overdose
Strychnine
Urea, nonprotein nitrogen*
Water deprivation, sodium ion toxicity

TOXIC PLANTS
Aconium spp. (monkshood)
Asclepias spp. (milkweed)
Blue-green algae*
Calycanthus fertilis (bubby bush) (B)
Cicuta spp. (water hemlock)
Conium maculatum (poison hemlock)
Cyanogenic plants
Delphinium spp. (larkspur) (B)
Drymaria pachyphylla (inkweed)
Halogeton glomeratus (halogeton) (B, O)
Kalmia spp. (laurel)
Kochia scoparia (summer cypress)
Laburnum anagyroides (golden chain tree)
Lupinus spp. (lupine) (O)
Meliotus spp. (sweet clover)
Nerium spp. (oleander)
Nicotiana spp. (nightshades)
Nitrate-accumulating plants
Perilla frutescens (perilla mint)
Phalaris spp. (canary grass) (O)
Sarcobatus vermiculata (greasewood) (B, O)
Solanum spp. (nightshades)
Taxus spp. (yew)
Xanthium spp. (cocklebur) (B, O)
Zygadenus spp. (death camas) (O)

B, Bovine; O, ovine.
*Likely to involve several animals.

Close proximity of livestock to petroleum exploration and production activities in the major oil-producing states results in a variety of clinical problems, including sudden death.[18] Consumption of the more volatile petroleum constituents may induce rapid bloating and coating of the respiratory membrane when aspirated into the lungs. Gossypol toxicosis reportedly causes death without premonitory signs in calves (occasionally cows) and lambs fed cottonseed products containing this toxic pigment.[19,20] Poisoning appears abruptly after livestock have been fed the gossypol-containing ration for a period of weeks to months. Sudden death is attributed to heart failure. Postmortem examination reveals edema, centrilobular hepatic necrosis, and an enlarged heart. Ionophores may induce sudden death in species exposed to large overdoses, but delayed death is the usual course. Conditions conducive to lethal overdose include insufficient mixing or top dressing with monensin- or lasalocid-supplemented mineral. Degenerative-to-necrotic lesions in the heart are compatible with a diagnosis of ionophore poisoning.

Acute lead intoxication is another differential from the list of possibilities in sudden death cases. Lead poisoning is the most common toxicosis in cattle. Blood, liver, and kidneys are suitable specimens for lead analysis. Metaldehyde is an uncommon poison for ruminants; however, intoxication in cattle has occurred in low wetland areas where the chemical is used as a molluscicide. The palatability of metaldehyde baits promotes ingestion. Ammoniation of high-quality forage such as forage sorghum and Sudan grass, cereal grain, brome, and fescue hays is responsible for bovine bonker's syndrome, reportedly caused by the formation of 4-methyl-imidazole.[21] This sporadic intoxication causes central nervous system derangement and rapid death in cows and nursing calves. Ruminants may be poisoned by nicotine sulfate from ingestion of solution, treated foliage, and food or water from contaminated containers. The onset and progression of the syndrome are rapid, and death may occur within hours. Detection of nicotine in urine is easily performed by most toxicology laboratories. Iatrogenic selenium toxicosis and death in young ruminants can result from parenteral administration of excess doses. Rapid onset of violent tetanic seizures ending in death characterizes strychnine toxicosis. Samples suitable for chemical analysis include rumen contents, liver, and urine.

Urea toxicosis is a frequent cause of sudden death in feedlot livestock. In one particular case, 48 feedlot steers died within 2 days of delivery of a new lot of feed supplemented with urea.[22] Unusually high rumen pH, excess ammonia in serum, rumen contents, and eyeball fluid support the diagnosis. Water deprivation, with attendant sodium ion intoxication, is a known cause of sudden death in ruminants.[23] Some cases occur in hot weather, but frozen water supplies in cold weather can be equally devastating.

Poisonous plant problems frequently present a unique set of circumstances associated with their ingestion. Overgrazing of pastures is probably the most significant factor affecting the ingestion of toxic plants. Other situations conducive to poisonous plant ingestion include lack of suitable forage in periods of drought and the incorporation of toxic forbs in hay or greenchop. Plants normally avoided because of poor palatability may become acceptable when frosted or sprayed with herbicide. Toxic plants also may be the first green plant available early in the spring, when livestock are hungry for anything green and succulent. Livestock trailed or transported for long distances without food or water and then suddenly introduced to new pasture may fail to avoid toxic plants and often will eat anything within immediate reach. In general, diagnosis of plant poisoning is based on availability, grazing evidence or presence in the hay, and the existence of plant parts in the rumen contents. Diagnostic lesions are usually lacking, and analytic methods for toxic components are severely limited.

many farms. When acute intoxication with these compounds is suspected, samples for analysis should include liver, brain, and rumen contents. In subacute cases, fat and milk are appropriate samples. Copper toxicosis is a frequent cause of sudden death in sheep and has been reported in cattle fed chicken litter.[17] Cattle feeds normally contain twice as much copper as sheep feeds and may cause copper toxicosis in sheep. Copper from treated fence posts also may poison sheep, either when they chew the posts or ingest contaminated forage in the vicinity. Samples required for chemical confirmation consist of whole blood or serum and liver.

Aconitum spp. (monkshood) rarely are a cause of sudden death because of their limited availability. *Delphinium* spp. (larkspur), however, are closely related to monkshood and are responsible for more cattle losses in the western United States than any other poisonous plant. Larkspur grows densely in the mountainous west and is readily consumed especially during an early stage of growth. Mature stands are less palatable and not as toxic. Cattle poisoned by larkspur often are found close to a stand, collapsed and bloated. Death from the cardiotoxic- and neuromuscular-blocking effects may occur within a few hours of ingestion. Sheep are less susceptible to larkspur and are seldom poisoned by it, partly because of their different grazing habits.[24] *Asclepias* spp. (milkweed) contain either cardioactive glycosides or neurotoxic compounds.[25] The most toxic species reside in the west and southwest United States. These plants are not very palatable but are somewhat less objectionable when dried. Livestock will graze them in a drought, but the biggest problem is contamination of hay or greenchop. Blue-green algae may cause sudden death in all classes of livestock within minutes of ingestion of toxins from certain neurotoxic species. Toxins from other hepatotoxic species may require 24 hours to induce death. Toxic blooms occur sporadically during certain environmental conditions of late summer and fall. Diagnosis is usually based on a history of exposure to a concentrated bloom, but some laboratories perform chemical and bioassays.

Calycanthus spp. (bubby bush) contain an alkaloid similar to strychnine in structure and mechanism of action. These species are of minor importance to the livestock industry in the southeast and west but have induced death in cattle. Seeds and other plant parts may be identified in rumen contents. *Cicuta* spp. (water hemlock) may induce violent convulsions and death within an hour. Intoxication is most common in early spring, when plants growing along waterways are easily uprooted and the tuberous parts are eaten. A single root system from a large plant can kill a cow. This is one of the most toxic plants in North America, and it has been responsible for the deaths of numerous livestock and humans. *Conium maculatum* (poison hemlock) grows throughout the United States. Cattle are most sensitive and sheep are relatively resistant. Poisoning is usually associated with heavily grazed pastures.

Cyanogenic glycosides are present at toxic concentrations in more than 250 plant genera, including *Sorghum*, *Prunus*, *Triglochin*, and *Linum*. Ruminants are especially susceptible to these glycosides, because they possess the microorganism enzyme systems necessary for rapid liberation of hydrocyanic acid. Death may occur within 15 to 30 minutes of ingestion. Hyperoxygenated venous blood will be cherry red and slow to clot, and rumen contents may have the odor of almond extract. Samples of forage, blood, and rumen contents should be collected immediately, placed in airtight containers, and frozen for analysis. Negative results are often questionable because of the highly volatile nature of hydrogen cyanide. *Drymaria pachyphylla* (inkweed) has caused sudden death in cattle in the southwestern United States. The differential diagnosis in this part of the country includes anthrax; diagnosis is based on examination of rumen contents for plant parts.

Halogeton glomeratus is a soluble oxalate-containing plant that grows best in disturbed soil along roadsides in the western intermountain states. *Sarcobatus vermiculata* (greasewood) grows in semiarid regions of the west; it also contains toxic levels of soluble oxalate. Unadapted sheep are most frequently intoxicated with these plants, and death may occur within 9 to 11 hours of onset of intoxication. Sudden death results from hypocalcemia and inhibition of cellular respiration. Postmortem findings include hemorrhagic rumenitis, hydrothorax, ascites, and the presence of oxalate crystals in the kidney and rumen wall. *Kalmia* spp. (laurel) are an occasional problem in winter or early spring, when they are the only conspicuously green plant available. Laurel grows in the wild in the eastern and western regions of the United States. Death may occur in 12 to 14 hours. Fragments of glossy, leathery leaves may be visible in rumen contents. *Kochia scoparia* (summer cypress or burning bush) sporadically causes a thiamine-responsive polioencephalomalacia in cattle. *Laburnum anagyroides* (golden chain tree) is a large ornamental shrub considered to be the second most poisonous plant in the United Kingdom; it also grows in much of the United States. The shrub contains quinolizidine alkaloids that may induce rapid death from respiratory failure. *Lupinus* is a genus with about 200 species in North America. There is considerable seasonal variation in toxicity, with the toxic species presenting a problem when plants are very immature or when they have reached the seedpod stage. Acute intoxication and rapid death are likely only when large quantities of seeds are ingested within a short time. Toxic species cause more deaths in sheep than any other plant in Montana, Idaho, and Utah. Improperly cured hay and silage derived from *Melilotus* spp. (white and yellow sweet clover) may cause sudden death in cattle when hemorrhage occurs in the cranial vault, pericardial sac, mediastinum, or thorax. Induction of the disease requires consumption of the moldy forage for several weeks to allow sufficient depletion of vitamin K–dependent clotting factors. *Nerium* spp. (oleander) are widely cultivated in the Southern and Western United States. Toxic in the green or dry state, these plants may border hay fields, and significant mortality of livestock may occur when dropped leaves or trimmings are incorporated into forage. Livestock often are poisoned when prunings are mixed with grass clippings and the bitter taste is disguised. Diagnosis is based on evidence of consumption and identification of plant parts in rumen contents.

The genus *Nicotiana* contains toxic species of wild and cultivated tobacco. Poor palatability usually hinders consumption; however, opportunities for intoxication and death sometimes occur in areas of the west where forage is scarce and in parts of the country where tobacco is cultivated. Nitrate-accumulating plants include certain annuals, weeds, and cool-season crops and grasses. Notable examples include pigweed, lamb's-quarter, Sudan grass, and oat hay. Under the right environmental conditions most plants can accumulate toxic concentrations of nitrate. Plant-associated nitrate poisoning is a serious problem only in ruminants because of the nitrate-reducing ability of rumen microbes. Onset of nitrate intoxication is rapid, and death may result within 6 to 24 hours of rapid ingestion of a toxic dose. Diagnosis is based on a brownish cast to the viscera and blood, together with chemical analysis of serum, aqueous humor, and forage for nitrate concentration.

Acute bovine pulmonary emphysema is associated with an abrupt change from dry range forage to lush green pasture high in L-tryptophan concentration. Less commonly, the pulmonary toxins of *Perilla frutescens* (perilla mint) can induce dyspnea and death in a few hours. Necropsy reveals incomplete collapse of lungs that are heavy and firm, with froth-filled airways. Histologic examination shows a proliferation of type II pneumocytes. *Phalaris* spp. (canary grass) recently were reported to have caused sudden collapse and death of sheep in California.[26] Sheep that had been grazing a field containing canary grass were herded a short distance when six ewes collapsed and died. Bilaterally symmetric, greenish-gray discoloration was seen in the midbrain. The same gross discoloration also was seen in the renal cortex. Microscopic examination confirmed the presence of intracytoplasmic accumulation of this granular pigment. *Solanum* spp. (nightshades) grow throughout the United States, especially in waste areas and overgrazed pastures. Rapid ingestion of large quantities of highly toxic fruit can result in coma and rapid death. *Taxus* spp. (yew) poisoning in ruminants commonly results in sudden death. Poisoning is most likely to occur when ruminants are pastured adjacent to residential areas where yew is a common ornamental shrub. Diagnosis is based on evidence of exposure and identification of yew leaves in rumen contents. *Xanthium* spp. (cocklebur) are most toxic at the cotyledonary stage of growth. These species may induce death in calves within 12 hours of onset of clinical intoxication. Hypoglycemia and centrilobular hepatic necrosis are consistent findings. *Zygadenus* spp. (death camas) are of major importance to sheep grazing on western ranges. These plants begin growth in early spring, presenting a significant hazard at this time.[27]

Miscellaneous Causes of Sudden Death in the Horse

Allergic reactions capable of causing sudden death include rupture of warble fly larvae. Warble fly larvae are seldom able to penetrate equine skin, and the fully matured larvae either die or are killed when the horse is saddled or harnessed. Anaphylactic shock results, and pulmonary edema and foam in the airways are found on necropsy. Penicillin or other antibiotics may cause an anaphylactic reaction with a similar outcome.

Perinatal sudden death may occur in foals as a result of meningeal hemorrhage caused by birth trauma. The sudden onset of profuse, watery diarrhea and rapid development of hypovolemic shock characterize colitis-X. A severe necrotic typhlitis is seen at necropsy, with destruction of colonic and cecal mucosa. Diaphragmatic rupture and hernia are associated with violent exercise or trauma, with or without bowel herniation. Electrocution occurs when a horse chews through or contacts an uninsulated hot-wire while well grounded. Death is instantaneous, usually with negative necropsy findings. Lightning strike may reveal burning or singeing of skin, hair, or underlying tissue. Gastrointestinal maladies that may cause sudden death include volvulus, intussusception, torsion, incarceration, gastric rupture from grain overload, tympanites, and small intestine rupture from ascarid impaction.

Gunshot wounds may be another cause of sudden death that is surprisingly difficult to verify, because bullet retrieval is necessary to establish the diagnosis. Finding the bullet lodged in tissue is a time-consuming task at best. Heat or work stress is seen in horses in hot, poorly ventilated quarters or in poorly conditioned horses overworked in hot, humid weather. Collapse and coma are followed by death in a few hours. Necropsy reveals skeletal and cardiac muscle damage, gastrointestinal ulceration, and renal necrosis. In pregnancy, unrecognized and untreated torsion of the gravid uterus may result in sudden death.

Exercise-induced respiratory tract injury may cause sudden death in well-conditioned horses.[28] Epistaxis and pulmonary hemorrhage occur at the peak of training, with most cases being of little concern. However, in fatal cases, horses that die immediately after exercise often have subpleural hemorrhages in the caudal lung lobes, and rupture of these hematomas has resulted in extensive intrathoracic hemorrhage and sudden death. Rupture of lung tissue while exercising also may result in fatal hemorrhage.

Serum sickness (acute hepatitis) can be traced to administration of biologic agents of equine origin 50 to 90 days before the onset of clinical signs. Death may occur within 12 to 48 hours. The main lesion seen is liver necrosis, with discoloration and accentuation of the lobular pattern on the cut surface. Fracture of the junction between the basisphenoid and basioccipital bone usually results from rearing over backward and striking the poll on the ground.

Miscellaneous Causes of Sudden Death in Ruminants

Fatal anaphylaxis occurs in sensitized animals after parenteral use of drugs or vaccines. This is most common with the peni-cillins and vaccines containing gram-negative bacteria or cell walls. Anaphylactic shock also may be an outcome of blood transfusion reactions. Immune-mediated hemolytic anemia (neonatal isoerythrolysis) from ingestion of colostrum-containing antibodies against a neonate's erythrocytes may induce sudden death if the specific antibody concentration is sufficiently high. A sudden death syndrome occurs in feeder cattle on high-concentrate diets. It usually occurs in warmer months and is limited to cattle fed high-concentrate rations for several weeks.[29] A malignant tumor that has been associated with sudden death is thymoma, or thymic lymphosarcoma, which is seen most commonly in old goats. It appears as a large, pale, fleshy mass in the cranial mediastinum.[30]

REFERENCES

1. Hibbs CM et al: *Clostridium sordellii* isolated from foals, *Vet Med (Small Anim Clin)* 72:256-258, 1977.
2. Dickie CW et al: Enterotoxemia in two foals, *J Am Vet Med Assoc* 173:306-307, 1978.
3. Jones RL et al: Hemorrhagic necrotizing enterocolitis associated with *Clostridium difficile* infection in four foals, *J Am Vet Med Assoc* 193:76-79, 1988.
4. Myers LL, Shoop DS, Byars TD: Diarrhea associated with enterotoxigenic *Bacteroides fragilis* in foals, *Am J Vet Res* 48:1565-1568, 1987.
5. Gay C, Blood DC, Wilkinson JS: Clinical observations of sheep with focal symmetrical encephalomalacia, *Aust Vet J* 51:266-269, 1975.
6. King JM: Sudden death in sheep and goats, *Vet Clin North Am (Large Anim Pract)* 5:703, 1983.
7. DaMassa AJ et al: Mycoplasmosis in goats, *Am J Vet Res* 44:322-325, 1983.
8. Osweiler GD et al: *Clinical and diagnostic veterinary toxicology*, ed 3, Dubuque, Iowa, 1985, Kendall Hunt.
9. Bradley R, Markson LM, Bailey J: Sudden death and myocardial necrosis in cattle, *J Pathol* 135:19-38, 1981.
10. Gelberg HB et al: Sudden death in training and racing thoroughbred horses, *J Am Vet Med Assoc* 187:1354-1356, 1985.
11. Platt H: Caecal rupture in parturient mares, *J Comp Pathol* 93:343-346, 1983.
12. Williams DE, Pier AC: The "honker" syndrome in feedlot cattle: a possible etiology, *Bovine Pract* 8:60, 1973.
13. Mote DC: Outbreak of black flies causing death in livestock, *Can Insect Pest Rev* 22:139-170, 1944.
14. Given BD et al: Severe hypoglycemia attributable to surreptitious injection of insulin in a mare, *J Am Vet Med Assoc* 193:224-226, 1988.
15. Casteel SW, Thomas BR, South PJ: Postmortem diagnosis of potassium poisoning, *J Equine Vet Sci* 9:247-249, 1989.
16. McConnico RS, Brownie CF: The use of ascorbic acid in the treatment of 2 cases of red maple (*Acer rubrum*)-poisoned horses, *Cornell Vet* 82:293-300, 1992.
17. Banton MI et al: Copper toxicosis in cattle fed chicken litter, *J Am Vet Med Assoc* 191:827-828, 1987.
18. Edwards WC: Toxicology of oil field wastes, *Vet Clin North Am (Food Anim Pract) (Clin Toxicol)* 5:363-374, 1989.
19. Hudson LM, Kerr LA, Maslin WR: Gossypol toxicosis in a herd of beef calves, *J Am Vet Med Assoc* 192:1303-1305, 1988.
20. Morgan et al: Clinical, clinicopathologic, pathologic, and toxicologic alterations associated with gossypol toxicosis in feeder lambs, *Am J Vet Res* 49:493-499, 1988.
21. Morgan SE, Edwards WC: Bovine bonkers: new terminology for an old problem—a review of toxicity problems associated with ammoniated feeds, *Vet Hum Toxicol* 28:16-18, 1986.
22. Casteel SW, Cook WO: Urea toxicosis in cattle: a dangerous and avoidable dietary problem, *Vet Med* 79:1523-1524, 1984.
23. Scarratt WK, Collins TJ, Sponenberg DP: Water deprivation: sodium chloride intoxication in a group of feeder lambs, *J Am Vet Med Assoc* 186:977-978, 1985.
24. Cheeke PR, Shull LR: *Natural toxicants in feeds and poisonous plants*, Westport, Conn, 1985, AVI.
25. Burrows GE, Tyrl RJ: Plants causing sudden death in livestock, *Vet Clin North Am (Food Anim Pract) (Clin Toxicol)* 5:263-290, 1989.
26. East NE, Higgins RJ: Canary grass (*Phalaris* spp) toxicosis in sheep in California, *J Am Vet Med Assoc* 192:667-669, 1988.
27. Fuller TC, McClintock E: *Poisonous plants of California*, Berkeley, 1986, University of California Press.
28. Gunson DE, Sweeney CR, Soma LR: Sudden death attributable to exercise-induced pulmonary hemorrhage in racehorses: nine cases (1981-1983), *J Am Vet Med Assoc* 193:102-106, 1988.
29. Cecil Reedy Workshop on Sudden Death. In Proceedings of the Academy of Veterinary Consultants, March 11, 1977.
30. King JM: Sudden death in sheep and goats, *Vet Clin North Am (Large Anim Pract)* 5:710, 1983.

DISORDERS AND MANAGEMENT OF THE NEONATE

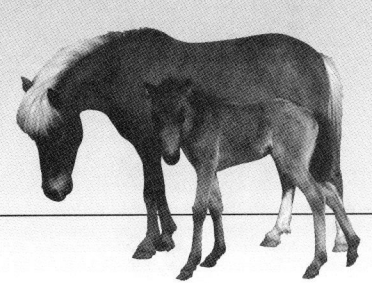

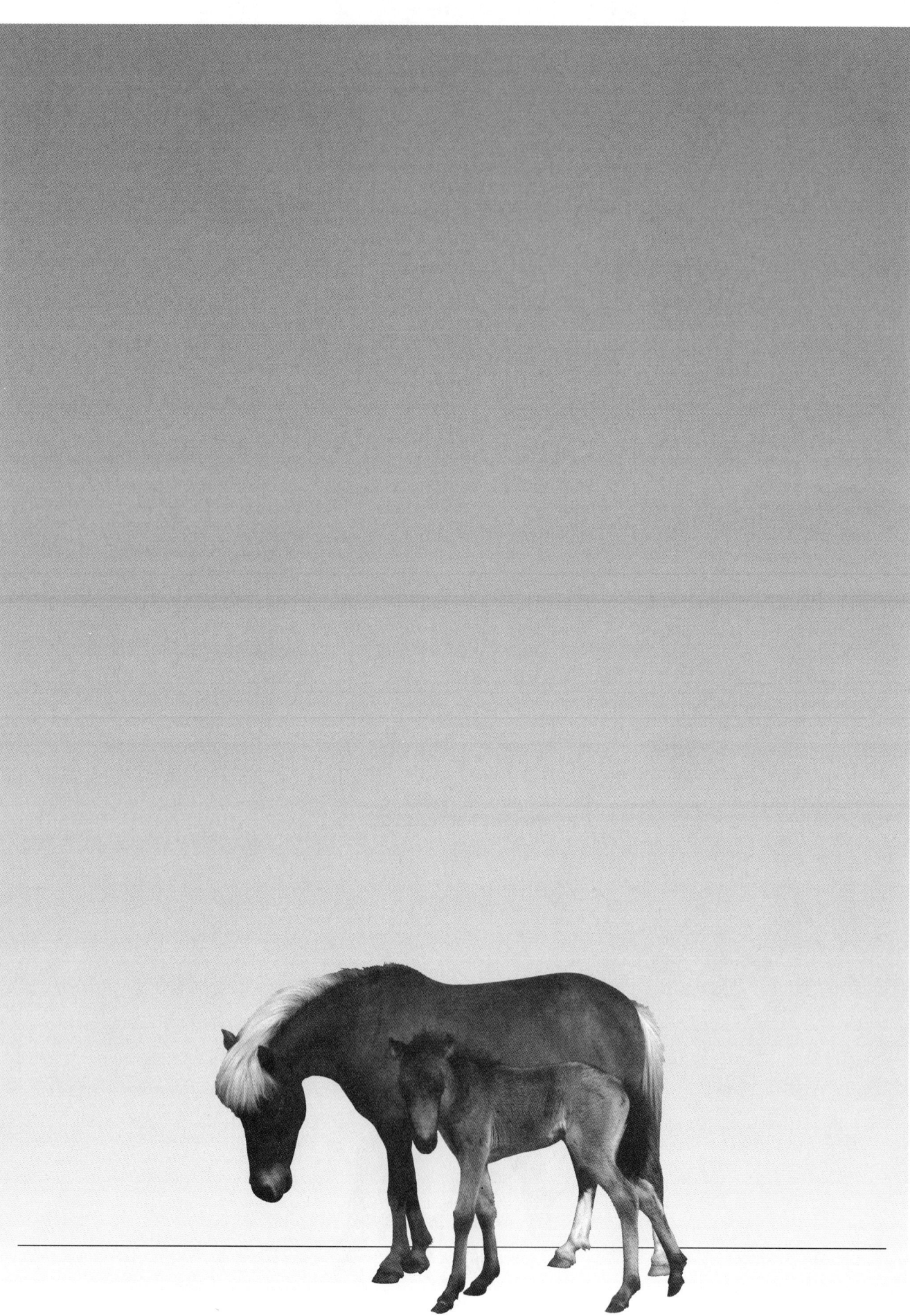

The Peripartum Period

WENDY E. VAALA

JOHN K. HOUSE

ASSESSMENT OF THE MARE DURING LATE GESTATION

WENDY E. VAALA

It has been estimated that between 25% and 40% of mares that are bred do not produce a live foal.[1-4] Many factors contribute to this poor outcome, including infertility, early fetal loss, abortion, stillbirth, and perinatal death.[2] During late gestation, two of the most important causes of reproductive loss are fetoplacental infection and complications of delivery including dystocia and perinatal asphyxia.[2,5] As mares age, their pregnancy and foaling rates decline and their foals experience higher morbidity and mortality rates and decreased athletic ability.[1,3]

Septicemia, asphyxia, and dysmaturity, including prematurity and postmaturity syndromes, are the leading causes of neonatal foal mortality during the first 2 weeks of life. Despite dramatic advances in neonatal intensive care, many foals still die, not because their primary problem is untreatable, but because veterinary intervention was delayed, delivery was unattended, neonatal compromise was not recognized in a timely fashion, or critical care was unavailable or not economically feasible. Foals surviving severe peripartum illness often experience increased morbidity associated with chronic infections, suboptimal growth, or developmental orthopedic disease. Therefore the focus of equine neonatology has shifted from a strictly therapeutic approach to a preventive one. This new direction emphasizes assessment of fetoplacental well-being during late pregnancy. The three periparturient events that have the most devastating effect on neonatal survival are hypoxia, infection, and derangement of in utero development. These events can result in behavioral abnormalities, multiorgan system failure, neonatal death, abnormal fetal development, or premature delivery.

Many of the periparturient events associated with increased fetal/neonatal morbidity and mortality have been identified in the mare (Box 15-1). In human obstetrics, prepartum detection of placental dysfunction and fetal distress has become an important factor influencing the management of the last stages of pregnancy and the newborn infant. Following the lead in human perinatology, biochemical and biophysical techniques for monitoring fetoplacental well-being are being developed for use in the pregnant mare.[6-9] Mares with high-risk pregnancies should be identified early, treated appropriately, and monitored carefully through the birth process. Accurate assessment of fetal well-being is complicated and difficult in humans. Fetal monitoring in the equine species is less developed and is handicapped by the size of the dam and fetus.

Vaala has suggested that mares experiencing problem pregnancies be assigned to one of three categories: (1) mares with histories of abnormal pregnancies, deliveries, or newborn foals, (2) mares at risk for a problem with the current pregnancy because of systemic illness or reproductive tract abnormality, and (3) mares with no apparent risk factor that experience an abnormal periparturient event.[9] A list of important perinatal risk factors is presented in Box 15-2. Ideally, mares with high-risk pregnancies should receive some type of late-gestation fetal monitoring or at least be carefully watched during late gestation and attended at the delivery. Personnel attending the delivery of a high-risk foal should be trained in resuscitation techniques.

A variety of biochemical and biophysical parameters can be measured in the late-term mare or fetus, but the ideal combination of tests is not yet known. Maternal progestagen concentration may be increased in mares with placental pathology[9-12] and may decrease to very low levels (<2 ng/ml) in pregnant mares subjected to stressful circumstances, such as colic and uterine torsion, that go on to abort their fetuses.[13] Measurement of progestagens may therefore be indicated to determine the need for progestin supplementation.[9] An enzyme-linked immunosorbent assay (ELISA) has been developed to measure equine fetal protein, and elevated concentrations have been associated with twinning, placentitis, premature placental separation, uterine trauma, and fetal death.[9,14] Additional studies are required before this test can be applied accurately in a clinical setting. Another reproductive hormone that holds promise as a marker of fetoplacental well-being and periparturient complications in the mare is relaxin. The placenta is the primary source of relaxin in horses.[15] In healthy pregnant mares, relaxin concentrations increase from about day 80 to a peak of 80 to 100 ng/ml at day 175, which persists until birth.[16,17] In mares with problematic pregnancies, low relaxin levels during late pregnancy have been indicative of placental insufficiency associated

257

with a variety of causes including fescue toxicosis,[18] oligohydramnios, placentitis, and pituitary neoplasia.[19]

Several studies have demonstrated that ultrasound-guided transabdominal amniocentesis and allantocentesis can be performed relatively safely in the late-gestation mare as long as the procedure is performed aseptically and multiple attempts are not made.[9,20] However, the clinical usefulness of fetal fluid analysis in the horse remains to be determined. Studies attempting to relate the phospholipid profile in amniotic fluid with equine fetal lung maturation have been inconclusive to date.[9,20,21] Transabdominal-guided ultrasound amniocentesis has been used to detect experimentally induced equine herpes virus (EHV-1) fetal infection in utero.[22] This technique holds promise as a diagnostic aid to detect specific fetal diseases and as a potential therapeutic avenue to deliver medication in utero.

Electrolyte concentrations in prepartum mammary secretions may be monitored to predict impending parturition in the mare. As parturition nears, calcium and sodium concentrations increase and potassium decreases. An increase in calcium concentration to over 40 mg/dl is considered the most reliable indicator of readiness for birth and may be used to help determine whether elective induction or cesarean section should be performed. Test strips are commercially available to measure calcium and magnesium concentrations in a field setting.*

A scoring system using calcium, sodium, and potassium concentration in the mammary secretions to assess fetal maturity has also been described.[23] Both false-negative and false-positive results may occur with both types of tests. False-positive results have been associated with vaginal discharge, placentitis, and premature lactation. On the other hand, in many mares the changes in the electrolytes occur only within hours of delivery, so if monitoring is not performed fre-

---

*Predict-a-foal test, Animal Health Care Products, Vernon, CA 90054; Foalwatch Kit, Chemetrics, Calverton, CA.

---

quently, the changes will be missed.[9,24] Therefore the decision on whether or not to induce parturition in a mare should not be based on the results of this type of testing alone.

Fetal heart rate (FHR) monitoring is routinely used in the human fetus to detect fetal distress, particularly hypoxia, during late-gestation labor and delivery. Doppler ultrasound is the most common technique used for FHR monitoring; this technology has been adapted for use in the mare.[25] First, the fetal heart is located using an ultrasound transducer, then the Doppler transducer is placed on the mare's abdominal wall directly over the fetal heart. Fetal movement is detected by a pressure transducer or by a hand placed on the mare's abdomen. Continuous FHR monitoring for at least 10 minutes is preferred to better detect abnormalities in heart rate and rhythm. Use of M-mode echocardiography makes it easier to obtain an FHR measurement because of the rapid motion of the normal equine fetus. Heart rate is normally regular and decreases from greater than 120 beats/min before day 160 of gestation to between 60 and 90 beats/min in late gestation.[7,25-27] An average of 10 heart rate accelerations (25 to 40 beats/min) was observed in a 10-minute period; 95% of these were associated with fetal movement.[25] Cardiac accelerations in response to fetal movement are an indicator of fetal well-being. Cardiac rhythm should be regular. Persistent bradycardia is associated with fetal distress and is mediated by a vagal response to hypoxemia. Severe tachycardia and arrhythmias have been associated with impending fetal demise. Although persistent fetal tachycardia and bradycardia suggest fetal compromise, normal heart rate alone does not guarantee that the fetus is healthy. Prolonged periods of fetal inactivity, in the absence of maternal sedation, are also suggestive of fetal compromise.

Fetal electrocardiogram (ECG) may also be used to assess FHR and rhythm after day 150 of gestation.[26,27] The procedure is relatively easy to perform. The left arm electrode is placed on the dorsal midline of the mare at the lumbar region, and the left leg electrode is placed 15 to 20 cm cranial to the mare's udder on the ventral midline. The hair should be clipped and ample gel or alcohol should be placed to ensure good contact of the electrodes. Poor fetal signals may result from poor electrode contact or placement, fetal movement, or electrical interference.[9]

Transabdominal ultrasonography allows noninvasive evaluation of the intrauterine environment and fetal well-being. A biophysical profile (BPP) using five parameters is used in women to evaluate fetal distress late in pregnancy.[28,29] The BPP evaluates the following: fetal tone, fetal movement, fetal breathing, FHR reactivity (i.e., increased FHR during fetal activity), and amniotic fluid volume. The BPP was predicated on the theory that during asphyxia the most complex activity, FHR reactivity, disappears first, followed sequentially by fetal breathing, fetal movements, and fetal tone. Decreases in fetal fluids are associated with chronic intrauterine stress/hypoxia, dysmaturity, and placental insufficiency.[30]

In the mare, transabdominal ultrasonography can be used to evaluate the equine fetus after day 90 when the gravid uterus contacts the ventral abdominal wall. This technique is used more commonly during the second and third trimesters. Recent studies have focused on the development of a modified BPP using FHR reactivity, fetal activity, fetal breathing movements, qualitative and quantitative fetal fluid assessment, evaluation of placental integrity, and measurement of fetal size. Transducers with lower frequencies (2 to 4 MHz) are required because of the deep tissue penetration needed. The mare's ventral midline must be cleaned and clipped from the level of the umbilicus caudally to the mammary gland and a viscus coupling gel applied. Minimal maternal restraint is usually required. Chemical sedation should be avoided because drugs such as xylazine and detomidine induce fetal bradycardia and retard fetal movement.

In the pregnant mare, transabdominal ultrasonography has been used to detect twins, document fetal position, estimate fetal size using fetal aortic diameter, evaluate fetal activity, evaluate placental integrity, determine fetal fluid clarity and volume, and monitor FHR and fetal breathing. After 9 months of gestation most fetuses are in an anterior presentation and are unlikely to change that presentation before delivery.[31] The mean fetal thoracic aortic diameter averages between 2.2 and 2.5 cm in horse fetuses.[7] Fetal activity increases with advancing gestational age and FHR decreases. During late gestation the equine fetus should demonstrate good tone and moderate activity, with only brief episodes of inactivity (<20 minutes). During the last month of gestation the FHR averages between 60 to 90 beats/min with transient bouts of tachycardia (25 to 40 beats/min above baseline) observed during or immediately after fetal activity. Cardiac rhythm should be regular. Persistent bradycardia is associated with fetal distress and is mediated by a vagal response to hypoxemia. Severe tachycardia and arrhythmias have been associated with impending fetal demise. Fetal breathing is characterized by excursion of the diaphragm between the thorax and the abdomen, with accompanying rib cage expansion. Regular breathing movements are observed intermittently in most late-term fetuses. It is difficult to differentiate fetal from maternal breathing movements. The maximum ventral fetal fluid pocket depths average 8 cm for amniotic fluid and 13 cm for allantoic fluid.[7] Excessive fetal fluid accumulation is observed in cases of hydrops. Markedly decreased amounts of fetal fluids have been associated with placental dysfunction and the birth of a dysmature, hypoxic foal. As gestation advances, fetal fluids increase in turbidity. Sudden increases in turbidity may be associated with meconium passage, hemorrhage, or inflammatory debris. Average uteroplacental thickness viewed transabdominally ranges between 8 and 15 mm.[7] Thicker uteroplacental units may indicate placental edema, placental separation, or placentitis. Areas of separation between the uterus and chorion appear as black anechoic areas.

Transabdominal real-time ultrasonography can provide both structural and functional information about the health and environment of the fetus. Because of the depth of penetration required, 2- to 4-MHz transducers should be used. As in other procedures involving ultrasonography, familiarity with the normal appearance of the placenta and fetus is essential to detect abnormalities. Details on how to perform the evaluation can be found in other texts.[25,32-34] In the mare, this procedure has been used in late gestation to determine fetal position, estimate fetal size, evaluate the placenta and fetal fluids, detect premature placental separation, and to assess fetal movement and viability.[9,33] Overall, fetal activity tends to increase with advancing gestational age; periods of inactivity longer than 15 minutes may indicate the need for further evaluation. A BPP has been developed that uses several parameters to establish an idea of the size and overall health of the equine fetus.[8,25,35] The parameters include fetal weight, as estimated by the fetal aortic diameter (mean 2.1 cm at 300 days' gestation to 2.7 cm at term), heart rate, movement, uteroplacental thickness (mean 1.26 ± 0.33 cm), qualitative allantoic fluid appearance, and allantoic volume estimation. Additional studies are needed to establish the validity of this profile in predicting fetal health or compromise in a larger group of mares.

EFFECTS OF PLACENTAL INSUFFICIENCY

The effects of uteroplacental vascular insufficiency on the newborn depend on the severity of placental compromise and the severity and duration of prenatal and perinatal asphyxia. Conditions associated with chronic asphyxia in the large animal fetus include chronic placentitis, villous atrophy, twin and postterm pregnancies, ingestion of endophyte-infected fescue grass by the pregnant mare,[36] and ingestion of ponderosa pine by pregnant cattle.[37]

If decreased uteroplacental blood flow is long-standing, growth is concomitantly inhibited in the fetus. The pattern of growth restriction associated with chronic placental insufficiency is usually asymmetric. This type of growth restriction is characterized by visceral wasting with relative preservation of fetal length and head circumference. Affected human infants are expected to be long and thin, with loss of subcutaneous fat and a large head relative to the body size. The same is probably true in the large animal neonate. It has long been recognized that twin equine neonates and other abnormally small foals tend to have heads that are disproportionately large for their small, wasted bodies.[38]

In placental vascular insufficiency, the fetus has the ability to avoid overgrowing its nutrient supply and to maximize organ growth. Under metabolic stress, there is a fetal antiinsulin response with loss of fat and glycogen stores and muscle mass. Associated with the decrease in uteroplacental blood flow is an increase in uterine and fetal vascular resistance, and redistribution of cardiac output, with a greater percentage of blood flow going to organs such as the brain and heart. Unless uteroplacental insufficiency is very severe, brain growth continues at a relatively normal rate. In the human fetus, the redistribution of cardiac output also results in decreased blood flow to the lung and kidney and decreased production of fetal urine and lung liquid, two major components of amniotic fluid. A decrease in amniotic fluid volume is therefore associated with chronic fetal asphyxia. The regulation of these adaptations is not completely understood, but corticosteroids, catecholamines, and vasopressin, among others, play a role.[39,40]

It is thought that repeated episodes of hypoxemia during gestation slowly deplete cardiac glycogen stores and impair the ability of the heart to pump blood effectively during subsequent hypoxemic episodes, such as during labor. The newborn with depleted glycogen stores may also be at increased risk of developing hypoglycemia and hypothermia. Meconium aspiration and persistent arterial hypertension in the newborn period are secondary to chronic fetal hypoxia. Immature skeletal ossification, particularly of the carpal and tarsal bones, has also been associated with growth restriction in the foal.[38]

There are certain advantages associated with fetal adaptation to chronic placental insufficiency. Growth-restricted premature human infants have a lower incidence of hyaline membrane disease than infants of the same gestational age that are appropriately sized.[41] Presumably, fetal hormones, such as the corticosteroids and catecholamines that are released in response to nutrient deprivation, stimulate the early maturation of the lung and surfactant system. Accelerated neurologic maturity has also been documented along with accelerated pulmonary maturity.[42] Therefore the fetus that has been chronically exposed to an adverse in utero environment may be in some ways more tolerant of premature delivery and independent life outside the uterus than the "normal" fetus that is abruptly displaced through induction of labor or cesarean section. The low-birth-weight fetus therefore represents a successful adaptation to a nutrient-deprived environment. Its smaller size, decreased metabolic needs, and early organ maturation actually place it at lower risk of hypoxic injury at birth and aid its transition to independent life after delivery.[40] Further discussion of the characteristics, treatment, and prognosis of growth-restricted premature foals may be found in Chapter 20.

Premature lactation, purulent vaginal discharge, previous history of growth-restricted foals, advanced maternal age, and prolonged gestation are problems that should raise the suspicion of chronic uteroplacental insufficiency. The labor and delivery should be attended to minimize the chances of acute asphyxia. The newborn animal should be examined for evidence of growth restriction; infection, particularly pneumonia acquired in utero secondary to placentitis; and metabolic and acid-base derangements. Ample colostrum should be administered, and body temperature and blood glucose should be monitored closely.

One author has suggested that intrauterine growth restriction is unlikely to pose any substantial additional threat to the neurodevelopment of premature human infants unless it is accompanied by chromosome abnormalities or severe perinatal asphyxia or hypoglycemia or unless growth restriction is very severe.[43] Human infants who display characteristics of asymmetric growth restriction commonly "catch up" by late infancy or early childhood. Similar observations have been made in the foal. Many mildly to moderately growth-restricted newborn foals have also done well after discharge from the hospital and have grown to a normal size. Problems secondary to an immature musculoskeletal system, such as angular limb deformities, have been the most common complications noted in these individuals, but careful orthopedic management can result in a successful outcome.

MANAGEMENT OF THE HIGH-RISK LATE-GESTATION MARE

Each mare should receive a complete physical examination and a complete foaling history should be obtained. She should be evaluated regularly for clinical signs of impending parturition (sacroiliac ligament and perineal relaxation, mammary development, and mammary secretion electrolyte concentration). The reproductive tract may be evaluated by rectal palpation, and transabdominal ultrasonography may be performed at regular intervals to detect changes in the fetus, fetal fluids, or placenta. Prolonged periods of starvation are best avoided to prevent maternal hypoglycemia.[9] For current recommendations concerning management recommendations for specific maternal or fetal conditions, the reader is referred to a recent text.[9]

When treating the pregnant mare for any medical or surgical condition there are two patients to consider: the dam and the fetus. Any illness or disease that affects the mare's cardiovascular system has the potential to affect placental perfusion and the integrity of the fetoplacental unit. Hypotension, endotoxemia, and hypoxemia are examples of conditions that can alter uteroplacental blood flow and jeopardize the pregnancy. Diseases that stimulate prostaglandin production have the potential to initiate labor and delivery. Illnesses that produce prolonged periods of anorexia in the late-term mare can also contribute to premature delivery. The effect of various drugs on the placenta and fetus should be considered when treating the pregnant mare. If delivery is not imminent, many drugs will pass through the placental and fetal circulation and be cleared by the maternal liver and kidneys. Because of the epitheliochorial nature of the mare's placenta, some drugs will not cross the placental barrier at all. If drugs are administered to the mare and the fetus is delivered shortly thereafter, then the neonate must rely on its renal and hepatic function to process, degrade, and excrete those drugs. In most instances, as long as fetal well-being and placental integrity are closely monitored, the goal of most therapies is to treat the maternal condition and maintain the pregnancy as long as possible to achieve an acceptable degree of fetal maturation. If premature delivery appears unavoidable, then one or two doses of maternal steroids can be used with the hope of stimulating and accelerating fetal lung maturation through enhanced surfactant production.

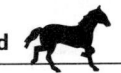

It is very important that the delivery of the high-risk mare be attended by knowledgeable personnel, and that all supplies, drugs, and equipment required for diagnosing and correcting a dystocia and stabilizing the mare and foal be organized and close at hand. A spontaneous vaginal delivery is generally preferred in the high-risk mare, because of both the profound problems associated with the untimely delivery of a premature foal and the complications sometimes associated with induced labor or cesarean section.[44,45] (See Chapter 20, Prematurity). There are instances, however, when an induced birth or cesarean section is indicated or preferred. Induction of parturition should be considered with the following:

- Severe fetal distress noted on prenatal assessment
- Evidence of premature placental separation or a history of premature placental separation associated with dead or asphyxiated foals
- Hydrops allantois and/or amnion
- Unproductive stage I labor
- Uterine inertia
- Impending prepubic tendon rupture
- Life-threatening maternal illness
  Indications for cesarean section may include the following:
- Pelvic injury or abnormality resulting in obstruction of the birth canal
- Gastrointestinal crisis requiring surgery
- Severe dystocia
- Insufficient, thickened placenta associated with fescue toxicity in the mare
- Catastrophic and terminal illness or injury in the mare, such as gut rupture or fractured limbs

If induction of parturition or cesarean section is elected, every effort should be made to ensure that the fetus is mature and is ready to be born; the usual result of induction at an inappropriate time is a nonviable newborn. Three essential criteria are a gestation of longer than 330 days, good-quality colostrum in the udder, and softening of the cervix.[44] The scheduling needs of the veterinarian or owner should never be the only criterion used for determining the timing of delivery! A slow, continuous oxytocin infusion administered at a rate of 1.0 U/min usually results in delivery within 20 to 40 minutes.[9] Alternatively, multiple intravenous or intramuscular injections of 10 to 20 U of oxytocin every 10 minutes have been recommended.[44,46] Other investigators have shown that smaller intravenous doses of oxytocin (2.5 IU administered every 15 to 20 minutes until rupture of the chorioallantois or a total of 20 IU of oxytocin has been administered) is an effective and perhaps more physiologic method of induction.[47]

Induction of parturition in the mare has been associated with more violent, painful contractions than spontaneous labor and a higher incidence of premature placental separation and neonatal asphyxiation. Cesarean section also predisposes to neonatal peripartum asphyxia. Maternal hypotension secondary to general anesthesia and the weight of the maternal abdominal contents on the aorta and vena cava may both compromise uteroplacental circulation. For further details concerning anesthesia of the late-term mare, the reader is referred to other texts.[48,49]

THE PERIPARTUM RUMINANT

JOHN K. HOUSE

The peripartum period is a high-risk period for the fetus and dam. Approximately 5% to 10% of the annual calf crop and 15% to 20% of the annual lamb crop in the United States dies before weaning.[50,51] Between 50% and 70% of neonatal

mortality occurs in the first 3 days of life, with dystocia, starvation, and hypothermia responsible for 50% to 60% of these losses.[51,52]

Reduced fetal viability often reflects mismanagement of maternal nutrition and or the maternal environment during the last trimester of pregnancy and or during the prepartum and peripartum period. Investigation of perinatal morbidity and mortality should begin with assessment of maternal management. Some of the more common causes of stillbirth and perinatal mortality are listed in Box 15-3.

Forty percent to 60% of stillbirths are associated with dystocia. Maternal variables correlated with dystocia and consequently calf mortality at birth include parity and conformation. Dystocia and stillbirths in heifers are most commonly secondary to fetopelvic incompatibility. Fetopelvic incompatibility accounts for a lower proportion of dystocias in multiparous cows but weak labor secondary to hypocalcemia, uterine torsion, and incomplete cervical dilation are more common in older cows.[53] In a large study of Holstein calving records, 8.3% of calves born to heifers were stillborn compared with 3.6% of calves born to multiparous cows.[54] Dam pelvic diameter is an important determinant of dystocia for heifers.[55] Pelvic measurements can be used to identify abnormally small or abnormally shaped pelvises. Large frame size of the dam correlates with a reduced risk of dystocia; however, continued selection for large frame size tends to select for larger birth weight and dimensions of calves.[56] Age at first calving for heifers is not correlated with risk of dystocia as long as heifers are fed and managed to achieve appropriate growth and stature before calving.[57-59] Appropriate nutrition and management of replacement heifers to achieve appropriate size and stature at parturition reduces maternal and neonatal losses by reducing the incidence of dystocias. Maternal consequences associated with calving difficulty and delivery of a stillborn calf include decreased milk production and reduced reproductive efficiency. Reductions in milk production ranging from 100 to 400 kg have been reported to be associated with the birth of a stillborn calf. If the stillborn calf is delivered by cesarean section the reduction in milk yield is in the order of 300 to 500 kg.[54] Delivery of a stillborn calf is also associated with depressed conception rates, increased services per conception, and delayed conception.

Use of calving ease bulls over primiparous cows helps to reduce the incidence of dystocia and subsequently mortality during parturition. The heritability of calving ease is relatively low; estimates of maternal calving ease range from 0.03 to 0.24[53,60,61] and paternal heritability is approximately 0.147. Despite the relatively low heritability of calving ease, selection for calving ease should not adversely affect other production parameters in dairy cattle because the genetic correlation between calving ease and other dairy production traits are generally close to zero.[53] Calving ease evaluations are intended to increase the use of artificial insemination for heifers. To facilitate sire selection, most breed associations provide guidelines regarding calving ease or expected progeny difference for calf birth weights. An example of such a scheme is the calving ease and reliability values assigned to AI Holstein bulls. In this system the calving ease score is the expected percentage of difficult births predicted for calves delivered by primiparous cows.[62] The reliability score provides an indication as to the number of births that were considered in deriving the calving ease score. The higher the reliability score, the larger is the number of observations the calving ease score is based on and the more likely it is that the calving ease prediction will accurately reflect the outcome.

Management variables that influence the risk of dystocia and perinatal mortality include stocking density of preparturient

---

BOX 15-3

Common Causes of Stillbirth and Perinatal Death in Ruminants[50,51,105,106]

Dystocia
Cold stress
Pneumonia (lambs)
Nutrition
    Energy deficiency
    Protein deficiency
    Pregnancy toxemia
    Mineral
        Copper excess/deficiency
    Iron excess
    Iodine excess/deficiency
    Selenium deficiency
    Vitamin A deficiency

INFECTIOUS
Viruses
    Infectious bovine rhinotracheitis virus
    Bovine virus diarrhea
    Border disease
    Bluetongue
    Akabane
    Cache Valley
Bacteria
    Hemophilus somnus
    Brucella abortus
    Leptospira spp.
    Clostridium perfringens types C and D
    Streptococci spp.
    Campylobacter spp.
    Campylobacter fetus var fetus
    Listeria monocytogenes
    Yersinia pseudotuberculosis
    Histophilus ovis
    Brucella ovis
Protozoa
    Neospora

INFECTIOUS—cont'd
    Toxoplasma gondii
    Tritrichomonas foetus
Fungus
    Aspergillus spp.
Rickettsia
    Chlamydia spp.
    Coxiella burnetti

TRAUMA
Obstetric
Castration, tail docking

TOXINS
Plant toxins
    Monterey pine *(Pinus radiata)*
    Perennial broomweed *(Gutierrezia* spp.)
    Locoweed *(Astragalus lentiginosis)*
    Lupines *(Lupinus sericeus* and *Lupinus caudatus)*
    Poison hemlock *(Conium maculatum)*
Chemical toxins
    Nitrate

GENETIC
Epitheliogenesis imperfecta
Cardiac abnormalities (ventricular septal defects, tetralogy of Fallot)
Internal hydrocephalus
Cerebellar hypoplasia
Arthrogryposis/cleft palate
α-Mannosidosis
Spider lamb syndrome
β-Mannosidosis
Bovine citrullinemia
Bovine maple syrup urine disease

---

cows, timing of calving, and cow grouping. In a study of 123 beef herds the dystocia rate was highest for cows housed in a barn and decreased progressively through barn/yard, barn/pasture, and pasture-only calving location categories.[63] The most common cause of dystocia in penned heifers was vulval constriction, whereas dystocias in paddocked heifers were most commonly associated with malpresentations.[64] Calving beef heifers 6 weeks before cows has been recommended to allow the heifers longer to recover and conceive after calving than cows.[65] In a herd level comparative study this practice was associated with a higher incidence of dystocia and stillborn calves.[63] Presumably because of better nutritional management, heifer dystocia rate is reduced the longer heifers are maintained as a separate group from cows before calving.[63]

Fetal variables that influence the risk of mortality include gender, size, and number. Calves born to primiparous cows, twins, and bull calves are more likely to die at birth than calves born from multiparous cows, single calves, and heifer calves.[66,67] Low- and high-birth-weight calves are at greater risk of mortality than average-birth-weight calves.[66] Small calves experience greatest mortality at parities greater than one and large calves at first parity.[57] Fetal viability may be compromised in utero by a number of infectious agents. Common infectious agents associated with abortion or birth of weak calves are listed in Box 15-3. Manifestations of disease in the newborn are dependent on the time of exposure to the infectious agent.

Environmental stress before or around the time of parturition can compromise the fetus or neonate. Heat stress affects fetal viability by impeding calf growth in the last trimester of pregnancy[68] and by depressing colostral quality[69] and immunoglobulin transfer.[70] Uterine blood flow and placental mass are reduced and endocrine profiles altered when cattle are heat stressed during the last trimester of pregnancy. Heat stress during the last 3 weeks of pregnancy lowers dry matter intake, contributing to a negative energy balance at this time, which promotes mobilization of body fat and ketogenesis. Transfer of immunoglobulins to colostrum is impaired, and the concentration of protein, casein, lactalbumin, fat, and lactose in colostrum is reduced.[69] Cold, windy, and wet conditions also adversely affect calf survival. The magnitude of the effect of climate on neonatal survival depends on the age of the dam, gender and size of the calf, and on the incidence of dystocia in the herd.[66] Cold stress sufficient to cause hypothermia in calves leads to subcutaneous hemorrhages and delayed absorption of colostral immunoglobulins.[71]

Maintenance of adequate nutrition throughout pregnancy is essential to provide for the growing fetus and to maintain a healthy dam capable of delivering and nursing the fetus.

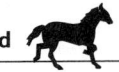

Pregnancy toxemia, hypocalcemia, protein energy malnutrition, micronutrient deficiencies, and obesity may all impair the health of the fetus directly or indirectly by affecting the health or capacity of the dam to deliver the fetus. Protein energy malnutrition and copper deficiency have been associated with impaired fertility, weak calves, and high calf mortality.[72]

ASSESSMENT OF FETAL VIABILITY

Fetal viability is rarely evaluated during the prepartum period in production animals but is a serious consideration when the prepartum dam is diseased or debilitated. Assessment of fetal viability is diagnostically challenging, but several methods are available to evaluate the fetus and fetal environment. During the physical examination of cattle, uterine blood flow, uterine tone, and presence of a vaginal discharge may be evaluated via rectal palpation and a vaginal speculum examination. Reduced fremitus in the uterine arteries and increased uterine tone may be appreciated by rectal palpation following fetal death. Abdominal ultrasound is useful for examining the uterus, placenta, and fetuses of small ruminants. The uterus and placenta of cattle can be examined by transrectal ultrasound, but examination of the fetal calf via transrectal or transabdominal ultrasound is often compromised by limited access. After fetal death, some of the following may be observed: thickening of the uterine wall, increased echogenicity of chorioallantoic and amniotic fluid, altered fetal posture, altered contour of the amnion, and reduced definition and ultimately reduced size of the caruncles. Examination of the fetus may detect gross congenital abnormalities and ultrasound of the fetal chest allows visualization of a beating heart and determination of fetal heart rate. The normal heart rate of full-term lambs is 108 to 126 beats/min.[73] Measuring the heart rate of fetal calves is more difficult than measuring that of small ruminants but can be done via transabdominal Doppler using a 1.5-MHz probe. The normal heart rate of full-term calves is 90 to 125 beats/min.[74] In human medicine, FHR is used as a measure of fetal viability. FHR accelerations associated with fetal movement are considered a sign of fetal well-being, and persistent bradycardia or tachycardia is a sign of fetal stress.[75] Normal fetal heart rate patterns of ruminants need to be characterized in more detail before FHR measurements are used for prenatal clinical assessment of ruminant fetal well-being.[76]

Fetal loss associated with abnormal placentation occurs sporadically and is reflected by alterations in volume and composition of allantoic and amniotic fluid. In a study of 60 cases of bovine hydrops, 88% were hydrallantois, 5% hydramnios, and 7% a combination of both.[77] Hydrallantois is often associated with disease of the uterus and hydramnios with genetic or congenital defects of the fetus (e.g., Dexter cattle with bulldog calves, Angus calves with osteopetrosis, Guernsey calves with pituitary hypoplasia or pituitary aplasia).[78] The concentration of sodium and chloride in allantoic fluid of cattle during the last 12 weeks of gestation is normally low (Na is 52 ± 20 mmol/L and Cl is 17 ± 11 mEq/L) and the concentration of creatinine high (1224 ± 458 μg/ml).[79] With hydrallantois, allantoic fluid sodium and chloride concentrations rise toward extracellular fluid concentrations (Na is 116 ± 13 mEq/L and Cl is 81 ± 12 mEq/L) and allantoic creatinine concentration decreases (193 ± 73 μg/ml).[79] Normal amniotic fluid has electrolyte concentrations similar to plasma (Na is 132 ± 7 mEq/L and Cl is 115 ± 8 mEq/L) and a lower creatinine concentration than allantoic fluid (70 ± 26 μg/ml).[79] Cows with hydrallantois are also often hyponatremic and hyperglycemic.[77,80]

Estrone sulfate is a marker of a viable fetoplacental unit and has been used to assess fetal viability in cattle.[81] Estrogen synthesized by embryonic tissue is converted to estrone sulfate by the endometrium, which contains the enzyme sulfotransferase. Estrone sulfate assays can be used to diagnose pregnancy in small ruminants after 50 days[82] and in cattle after 100 days.[83] Estrone sulfate may be measured in plasma or milk[68,83]; baseline values are low after fetal loss, regardless of the stage of pregnancy. Compromise of the fetoplacental unit reduces estrone sulfate production. In a study of the effects of heat stress on pregnant cattle, plasma estrone sulfate concentrations were significantly lower throughout pregnancy in cows that gave birth to low-birth-weight calves.[68] Plasma concentrations of estrone sulfate rise slowly during the second trimester of pregnancy from 0.74 ng/ml to 3.66 ng/ml from day 90 to day 210 of pregnancy. The last trimester of pregnancy is associated with a rapid rise in the concentration of estrone sulphate to 13.36 ng/ml around 10 days before parturition.[84]

In human medicine, diagnosis of surfactant deficiency is based on the ratio of two phospholipids in amniotic fluid, lecithin (L) and sphingomyelin (S). If the L/S ratio is greater than 2, the surfactant system is mature and respiratory distress syndrome is rare.[85] The L/S ratio in amniotic fluid collected from cattle may also be used to assess surfactant system maturity,[86] providing a measure of readiness for birth, but is rarely employed in clinical veterinary medicine.

INDUCTION OF PARTURITION IN RUMINANTS

Manipulation of parturition may be considered for maternal, fetal, or management reasons. Fetal viability following induced parturition is variable between species. The viability of calves induced within 14 days of anticipated calving date is good.[87] Viability of lambs and kids induced greater than 5 days before anticipated parturition date is poor.[78] Absorption of colostral immunoglobulins by premature calves is reduced so colostral transfer should be monitored closely in induced neonates.[88] Induction of parturition or cesarean section is often necessary to prevent mortality of small ruminants with pregnancy toxemia.[89] Fetal viability is often improved by induction of parturition with dexamethasone; however, delivery of the fetuses via cesarean section is often necessary because of the debilitated state of the dam. Steroids stimulate production of surfactant phospholipids by alveolar type II cells, enhance the expression of surfactant-associated proteins, reduce microvascular permeability, and accelerate overall structural maturation of the lungs.[90] Administration of flumethasone (10 mg) or dinoprost (25 mg) to pregnant cows 30 hours before elective cesarean section increases the lecithin/sphingomyelin ratio, thereby improving lung function and reducing complications associated with respiratory acidosis in the calf.[91] Induction of parturition has been used to reduce the incidence of dystocia in herds or breeds experiencing a high incidence of dystocia associated with fetomaternal disproportion.[92] Large birth weights are strongly correlated with fetomaternal disproportion.[93,94] Induction of parturition within 14 days of anticipated calving date is associated with good calf viability and a 3.2-kg reduction in birth weight of beef calves.[87]

Exogenous glucocorticoids, prostaglandin $F_{2\alpha}$ ($PGF_{2\alpha}$) or a combination may be used to induce parturition in cattle (dexamethasone 20 to 30 mg alone or in combination with 25 mg of $PGF_{2\alpha}$) and sheep and goats (10 to 20 mg dexamethasone and/or 15 mg $PGF_{2\alpha}$).[78] Glucocorticoids are more effective than prostaglandin for inducing parturition in sheep.[95] A lower incidence of dystocia and higher viability of calves has been reported in cattle induced with glucocorticoids compared with cows induced with prostaglandin.[96] Cows treated with dexamethasone or prostaglandin within 14 days of anticipated calving date usually calve within 72 hours of treatment.[87]

Combination of dexamethasone with prostaglandin increases the efficacy and reduces the interval to parturition (36 hours).[97,98] Retention of fetal membranes is a common complication of induced parturition in cattle.[99] Retention of fetal membranes may be associated with reduced first service conception and subsequent pregnancy rates.[100] Treatment of cows with prostaglandin at calving was reported to reduce the incidence of retained fetal membranes,[101] but subsequent studies have failed to support this.[97,102] Induction of cattle by administration of 25 mg of triamcinolone (Opticortinol) at day 270 followed by treatment with dexamethasone and prostaglandin 6 days later appears to reduce the incidence of retained fetal membranes associated with induction.[99,103] Coliform mastitis is an uncommon complication observed after induced parturition.[104]

REFERENCES

1. Bruck I, Anderson GA, Hyland JH: Reproductive performance of thoroughbred mares on six commercial stud farms, *Aust Vet J* 70:299-303, 1993.
2. Giles RC et al: Causes of abortion, stillbirth, and perinatal death in horses: 3,527 cases (1986-1991), *J Am Vet Med Assoc* 203:1170-1175, 1993.
3. Morley PS, Townsend HGG: A survey of reproductive performance in thoroughbred mares and morbidity, mortality and athletic potential of their foals, *Equine Vet J* 29:290-297,1997.
4. Roberts SJ: *Veterinary obstetrics and genital diseases*, ed 2, Ann Arbor, Mich, 1971, Edwards Brothers, p 512.
5. Hong CB et al: Equine abortion and stillbirth in central Kentucky during 1988 and 1989 foaling seasons, *J Vet Diagn Invest* 5:560-566, 1993.
6. Adams-Brendemuehl C, Pipers FS: Antepartum evaluations of the equine fetus, *J Reprod Fertil Suppl* 35:565-573, 1987.
7. Reef VB et al: Transabdominal ultrasonographic evaluation of the fetus and intrauterine environment in healthy mares during late gestation, *Vet Radiol Ultrasound* 36:533-541, 1995.
8. Reef VB et al: Ultrasonographic assessment of fetal well-being during late gestation: development of an equine biophysical profile, *Equine Vet J* 28:200-208,1996.
9. Vaala WE, Sertich PL: Management strategies for mares at risk for periparturient complications, *Vet Clin North Am (Equine Pract)* 10:237-265, 1994.
10. Cottrill CM et al: The placenta as a determinant of fetal well-being in normal and abnormal equine pregnancies, *J Reprod Fertil Suppl* 44:591-601, 1991.
11. Holtan DW et al: Plasma progestagens in the mare, fetus and newborn foal, *J Reprod Fertil Suppl* 44:517-528, 1991.
12. Rossdale PD et al: Effects of placental pathology on maternal plasma progestagen and mammary secretion calcium concentrations and on neonatal adrenocortical function in the horse, *J Reprod Fertil Suppl* 44:579-584, 1991.
13. Santschi EM, LeBlanc MM, Weston PG: Progestagen, oestrone sulphate and cortisol concentrations in pregnant mares during medical and surgical disease, *J Reprod Fertil Suppl* 44:627-634, 1991.
14. Vaala WE: Equine fetal protein and high risk pregnancy in the mare, *Proceedings of the 9th Annual Veterinary Medicine Forum*, 1991, p 483.
15. Klonisch et al: Partial complementary deoxyribonucleic acid cloning of equine relaxin messenger ribonucleic acid, and its localization within the equine placenta, *Biol Reprod* 52:1307-1315, 1995.
16. Stewart DR, Stabenfeldt G: Relaxin activity in the pregnant mare, *Biol Reprod* 25:281-289, 1981.
17. Stewart DR: Development of a homologous equine relaxin radioimmunoassay, *Endocrinology* 119:1100-1104, 1986.
18. Ryan PL et al: Effects of fescue toxicosis and fluphenazine on relaxin concentrations in pregnant pony mares, *Proc 44th Annu Conv Am Assoc Equine Pract* 44:60-61, 1998.
19. Ryan PL, Vaala WE, Bagnell C: Evidence that equine relaxin is a good indicator of placental insufficiency in the mare, *Proc 44th Annu Conv Am Assoc Equine Pract* 44:62-63, 1998.
20. Williams MA, Goyert NA, Goyer GL: Preliminary report of transabdominal amniocentesis for the determination of pulmonary maturity in an equine population, *Equine Vet J* 20:457, 1988.
21. Williams MA et al: Amniotic fluid analysis for evaluation of equine foetal development (abstract), *Proceedings of the Second International Conference on Veterinary Perinatololgy*, St John's College, Cambridge 38:1990.
22. Smith KC et al: Use of transabdominal ultrasound-guided amniocentesis for detection of equid herpesvirus 1-induced fetal infection in utero, *Am J Vet Res* 58:997-1002, 1997.
23. Ousey JC, Dudan F, Rossdale PD: Preliminary studies of mammary secretions in the mare to assess foetal readiness for birth, *Equine Vet J* 16:259, 1984.
24. Ley WB et al: Daytime management of the mare. I, Pre-foaling mammary secretions testing, *Equine Vet Sci* 9:88, 1989.
25. Adams-Brendemuehl C: Fetal assessment. In Koterba AM, Drummond WH, Kosch, PC, editors: *Equine clinical neonatology*, Philadelphia, 1990, Lea and Febiger, p 16.
26. Colles CM, Parkes RD, May CJ: Foetal electrocardiography in the mare, *Equine Vet J* 10:32, 1978.
27. Holmes JR, Darke PGG: Foetal electrocardiography in the mare, *Vet Rec* 82:651, 1968.
28. Manning FA, Platt LD, Sipos L: Antepartum fetal evaluation: development of a fetal biophysical profile, *Am J Obstet Gynecol* 136:787-795, 1980.
29. Schifrin SS, Clement D: Why fetal monitoring remains a good idea, *Contemp Obstet Gynecol* 35:70, 1990.
30. Manning FA, Hill LM, Platt LD: Qualitative amniotic fluid volume determination by ultrasound: antepartum detection of intrauterine growth retardation, *Am J Obstet Gynecol* 139:254-258, 1981.
31. Ginther OJ: Entry and retention of fetal hindlimbs in a uterine horn, *Theriogenology* 41:795-807, 1994.
32. Reef VB et al: Transabdominal ultrasonographic evaluation of the fetus and intrauterine environment in healthy mares during late gestation (abstract), *Proceedings of the Fortieth Annual Convention of the American Association of Equine Practitioners*, 1994, p 35.
33. Pipers FS, Adams-Brendemuehl CS: Techniques and applications of transabdominal ultrasonography in the pregnant mare, *J Am Vet Med Assoc* 185:766-771,1984.
34. Reef VB: Fetal ultrasonography. In Reef VB, editor: *Equine diagnostic ultrasound*, Philadelphia, 1998, WB Saunders, pp 425-445.
35. Adams-Brendemuehl C, Pipers FS: Antepartum evaluations of the equine fetus, *J Reprod Fertil Suppl* 35:565-573, 1987.
36. Green EM, Loch WE, Messer NT: Maternal and fetal effects of endophyte fungus infected fescue, *Proceedings of the Thirty-seventh Annual Convention of the American Association of Equine Practitioners*, 1991, p 29.
37. Ford SP et al: Effects of Ponderosa pine needle ingestion on uterine vascular function in late-gestation beef cows, *J Anim Sci* 70:1609-1614, 1992.
38. Koterba AM: Prematurity. In Koterba AM, Drummond WH, Kosch PC, editors: *Equine clinical neonatology*, Philadelphia, 1990, Lea and Febiger, p 66.
39. Lockwood CJ, Weiner S: Assessment of fetal growth, *Clin Perinatol* 13:3, 1986.
40. Warshaw JB: Intrauterine growth retardation: adaptation or pathology? *Pediatrics* 76:998, 1985.
41. Gluck L, Kulvich MV: Lecithin-sphingomyelin ratios in amniotic fluid in normal and abnormal pregnancy, *Am J Obstet Gynecol* 115:539, 1973.
42. Gould JB, Gluck L, Kulovich MV: The relationship between accelerated pulmonary maturity and accelerated neurological maturity in certain chronically stressed pregnancies, *Am J Obstet Gynecol* 127:181, 1977.
43. Chiswick ML: Intrauterine growth retardation, *Br Med J* 291:845, 1985.
44. LeBlanc MM: Induction of parturition in the mare: assessment of readiness for birth. In Koterba AM, Drummond WH, Kosch PC, editors: *Equine clinical neonatology*, Philadelphia, 1990, Lea and Febiger, p 34.
45. Freeman DE et al: Caesarean section and other methods for assisted delivery: comparison of effects on mare mortality and complications, *Equine Vet J* 31:203-207, 1999.
46. Macpherson ML, Chaffin KM, Carroll GL: Three methods for oxytocin-induced parturition: effects on the neonatal foal, *Proceedings of the Forty-second Annual Convention of the American Association of Equine Practitioners*, 1996, pp 150-151.
47. Ley WB, Nikola AP, Bowen JM: How we induce the normal mare to foal, *Proceedings of the Forty-fourth Annual Convention of the American Association of Equine Practitioners*, 1998, pp 194-197.
48. Brock KA: Anesthesia of the late-term mare. In Koterba AM, Drummond WH, Kosch PC, editors: *Equine clinical neonatology*, Philadelphia, 1990, Lea and Febiger, p 87.
49. Wilson DV: Anesthesia and sedation for late-term mares, *Vet Clin North Am* 10:219-236, 1994.
50. Wikse SE, Kinsel ML, Field RW, et al: Investigating perinatal calf mortality in beef herds, *Vet Clin North Am (Food Animal Pract)* 10:147-166, 1994.
51. Rook JS et al: Diagnosis and control of neonatal losses in sheep, *Vet Clin North Am (Food Anim Pract)* 6:531-562, 1990.
52. Patterson D et al: Occurrence of neonatal and postnatal mortality in range beef cattle. I, Calf loss incidence from birth to weaning, backward and breech presentation and effects of calf loss on subsequent pregnancy rates of dams, *Theriogenology* 28:557, 1987.
53. Meijering A: Dystocia and stillbirth in cattle: a review of causes, relations and implications, *Livestock Prod Sci* 11:143-177, 1984.
54. Mangurkar BR, Hayes JF, Moxley JE: Effects of calving ease: calf survival on production and reproduction in Holsteins, *J Dairy Sci* 67:1496-1509, 1984.
55. Price TD, Wiltbank JN: Predicting dystocia in heifers, *Theriogenology* 9:221-249, 1978.
56. Ali TE, Burnside EB, Schaeffer LR: Relationship between external body measurements and calving difficulties in Canadian Holstein-Friesian cattle, *J Dairy Sci* 67:3034-3044, 1984.

57. Thompson JR, Pollak EJ, Pelissier CL: Interrelationships of parturition problems, production of subsequent lactation, reproduction, and age at first calving, *J Dairy Sci* 66:1119-1127, 1983.
58. Simerl NA et al: Prepartum and peripartum reproductive performance of dairy heifers freshening at young ages, *J Dairy Sci* 74:1724-1729, 1991.
59. Radcliff RP et al: Effects of diet and injection of bovine somatotropin on prepubertal growth and first-lactation milk yields of Holstein cows, *J Dairy Sci* 83:23-29, 2000.
60. Cue RI, Hayes JF: Correlations of various direct and maternal effects for calving ease, *J Dairy Sci* 68:374-381, 1985.
61. Thompson JR, Rege JE: Influences of dam on calving difficulty and early calf mortality, *J Dairy Sci* 67:847-853, 1984.
62. Berger PJ: Genetic prediction for calving ease in the United States: data, models, and use by the dairy industry, *J Dairy Sci* 77:1146-1153,1994.
63. McDermott JJ et al: Patterns of stillbirth and dystocia in Ontario cow-calf herds, *Can J Vet Res* 56:47-55, 1992.
64. Dufty JH: The influence of various degrees of confinement and supervision on the incidence of dystocia and stillbirths in Hereford heifers, *N Z Vet J* 29:44-48, 1981.
65. Wiltbank JN: Maintenance of a high level of reproductive reproductive performance in the beef cow-calf herd, *Vet Clin North Am (Large Animal Pract)* 5:41-52, 1983.
66. Azzam SM et al: Environmental effects on neonatal mortality of beef calves, *J Animal Sci* 71:282, 1993.
67. Gregory KE, Echternkamp SE, Cundiff LV: Effects of twinning on dystocia, calf survival, calf growth, carcass traits, and cow productivity, *J Animal Sci* 74:1223-1233, 1996.
68. Collier RJ et al: Effects of heat stress during pregnancy on maternal hormone concentrations, calf birth weight and postpartum milk yield of Holstein cows, *J Anim Sci* 54:309-319, 1982.
69. Nardone A et al: Composition of colostrum from dairy heifers exposed to high air temperatures during late pregnancy and the early postpartum period, *J Dairy Sci* 80:838-844, 1997.
70. Stott GH et al: Influence of environment on passive immunity in calves, *J Dairy Sci* 59:1306-1311, 1976.
71. Olson DP et al: Effects of maternal nutritional restriction and cold stress on young calves: clinical condition, behavioral reactions, and lesions, *Am J Vet Res* 42:758-763, 1981.
72. Wikse SE et al: Impaired fertility and weak calf syndrome due to inadequate nutrition, *Comp Cont Educ Pract Vet* 1309-1316, 1997.
73. Aiumlamai S, Fredriksson G, Nilsfors L: Real-time ultrasonography for determining the gestational age of ewes, *Vet Rec* 131:560-562, 1992.
74. Jonker FH et al: Feasibility of continuous recording of fetal heart rate in the near-term bovine fetus by means of transabdominal Doppler, *Vet Q* 16:165-168, 1994.
75. Wood C, Renou P: Fetal heart rate monitoring. In Beard RW, Nathanielsz PW, editors: *Fetal physiology and medicine*, London, 1976, WB Saunders.
76. Jonker FH et al: Fetal heart rate patterns and the influence of myometrial activity during the last month of gestation in cows, *Am J Vet Res* 54:158-163, 1993.
77. Vanderplassche M et al: Wien Tierarztl Monatsschr 52:461, 1965.
78. Roberts SJ: *Veterinary obstetrics and genital diseases (theriogenology)*, ed 3, Ann Arbor, Mich, 1986, Edwards Brothers.
79. Skydsgaard JM: The pathogenesis of hydrallantois bovis. I, The concentrations of sodium, potassium, chloride and creatinine in the foetal fluids in cases of hydrallantois and during normal pregnancy, *Acta Vet Scand*, 6:193-207, 1965.
80. Wintour EM, Laurence BM, Lingwood BE: Anatomy, physiology and pathology of the amniotic and allantoic compartments in the sheep and cow, *Aust Vet J* 63:216-221, 1986.
81. Heap RB, Hamon M: Oestrone sulphate in milk as an indicator of a viable conceptus in cows, *Br Vet J* 135:355-363, 1979.
82. Chaplin VM, Holdsworth RJ: Oestrone sulphate in goats' milk, *Vet Rec* 111:224, 1982.
83. Hatzidakis G, Katrakili K, Krambovitis E: Development of a direct and specific enzyme immunoassay for the measurement of oestrone sulfate in bovine milk, *J Reprod Fertil* 98:235-240, 1993.
84. Zhang WC et al: The relationship between plasma oestrone sulphate concentrations in pregnant dairy cattle and calf birth weight, calf viability, placental weight and placental expulsion, *Anim Reprod Sci* 54:169-178, 1999.
85. Farrell PM, Avery ME: Hyaline membrane disease, *Am Rev Respir Dis* 111:657-688, 1975.
86. Eigenmann UJ et al: Neonatal respiratory distress syndrome in the calf, *Vet Rec* 114:141-144, 1984.
87. Peters AR, Poole DA: Induction of parturition in dairy cows with dexamethasone, *Vet Rec* 131:576-578, 1992.
88. Johnston NE, Stewart JA: The effect of glucocorticoids and prematurity on absorption of colostral immunoglobulin in the calf, *Aust Vet J* 63:191-192, 1986.
89. Hunt ER: Treatment of pregnancy toxemia in ewes by induction of parturition, *Aust Vet J* 52:338-339, 1976.
90. Robertson B: Corticosteroids and surfactant for prevention of neonatal RDS, *Ann Med* 25:285-288, 1993.
91. Zaremba W, Grunert E, Aurich JE: Prophylaxis of respiratory distress syndrome in premature calves by administration of dexamethasone or a prostaglandin F2 alpha analogue to their dams before parturition, *Am J Vet Res* 58:404-407, 1997.
92. Baker AA et al: The induction of parturition as an aid in the management of dystocia in beef herds, *Aust Vet J* 65:32-33, 1988.
93. Rice LE, Wiltbank JN: Factors affecting dystocia in beef heifers, *J Am Vet Med Assoc* 161:1348-1358, 1972.
94. Rice LE: Dystocia-related risk factors, *Vet Clin North Am (Food Anim Pract)* 10:53-68, 1994.
95. Harman EL, Slyter AL: Induction of parturition in the ewe, *J Animal Sci* 50:391-393, 1980.
96. Kordts E, Jochle W: Induced parturition in dairy cattle: A comparison of a corticoid (flumethasone) and a prostaglandin (PGF$_{2\alpha}$) in different age groups, *Theriogenology* 3:171-178, 1975.
97. Garcia A, Barth AD, Mapletoft RJ: The effects of treatment with cloprostenol or dinoprost within one hour of induced parturition on the incidence of retained placenta in cattle, *Can Vet J* 33:178-183, 1992.
98. Lewing FJ, Proulx J, Mapletoft RJ: Induction of parturition in the cow using cloprostenol and dexamethasone in combination, *Can Vet J* 26:317, 1985.
99. Bo GA et al: Reduced incidence of retained placenta with induction of parturition in the cow, *Theriogenology* 38:45-61, 1992.
100. Browning JW et al: A collapse syndrome associated with gram-negative infection in cows treated with dexamethasone to induce parturition, *Aust Vet J* 67:28-29, 1990.
101. Gross TS, Williams WF, Moreland TW: Prevention of the retained fetal membranes syndrome (retained placenta) during induced calving in dairy cattle, *Theriogenology* 26:365-370, 1986.
102. Mapletoft RJ et al: Controlling the incidence of retained placenta with induction of parturition in the cow, *Rev Brasil Reprod Anim* 3:140-148, 1991.
103. Nasser LF et al: Induction of parturition in cattle: effect of triamcinolone pretreatment on the incidence of retained placenta, *Can Vet J* 35:491-496, 1994.
104. Bellows RA, Short RE, Staigmiller RB: Exercise and induced-parturition effects on dystocia and rebreeding in beef cattle, *J Anim Sci* 72:1667-1674, 1994.
105. Mickelsen WD, Evermann JF: In utero infections responsible for abortion, stillbirth, and birth of weak calves in beef cows, *Vet Clin North Am (Food Anim Pract)* 10:1-14, 1994.
106. Haughey KG: Perinatal lamb mortality: its investigation, causes and control, *J S Afr Vet Assoc* 62:78-91, 1991.

Perinatal Adaptation, Asphyxia, and Resuscitation

WENDY E. VAALA

JOHN K. HOUSE

PERINATAL ADAPTATION

JOHN K. HOUSE

At birth the fetus must successfully make a series of structural and physiologic changes to survive. Perinatal mortality is often attributable to cardiovascular, pulmonary, thermoregulatory, or metabolic physiologic abnormalities. Dystocia and severe birth asphyxia compromise physiologic transitions, thereby increasing the risk of neonatal mortality. Compromised neonates that survive the birth process are less likely to consume adequate colostrum and are subsequently more likely to die of hypothermia and infectious diseases. A good review of physiologic mechanisms of adaptation at birth is presented by Kasari.[1]

The placenta functions as the respiratory organ of the developing fetus and efficiency of oxygen transfer to the fetus is increased by the high oxygen affinity of fetal versus adult hemoglobin.[2] In utero the potential spaces of alveoli and the tracheobronchial tree are distended with fluid secreted by pulmonary tissue.[3] Oxygenated blood is delivered to the fetus via the umbilical vein, which anastomoses with the portal vein near the liver, and approximately two thirds of the blood flow is shunted via the ductus venosus directly into the caudal vena cava.[1] The caudal vena cava drains into the right atrium, where over 50% of the volume shunts directly into the left atrium via the foramen ovale.[1] The relatively hypoxic in utero environment causes constriction of pulmonary vessels and dilation of the ductus arteriosus.[1] Because pulmonary arterial resistance is higher than systemic arterial resistance, nearly 70% of pulmonary artery flow is shunted via the ductus arteriosus into the aorta, with the remainder per-

fusing the lung.[4] Left ventricular output is distributed to the systemic circulation via the aorta. The two umbilical arteries arise from the aorta in the region of the last lumbar vertebra to carry predominantly venous blood back to the placenta via the umbilicus.

At birth some of the lung fluid is evacuated through the trachea during spontaneous delivery.[5] When the umbilicus ruptures, asphyxia triggers reflex gasping, respiratory movements, and increased peripheral vascular resistance.[4] The majority of lung fluid is absorbed through alveolar walls in the initial stages of ventilation.[5] This mechanism is prompted by activation of adrenaline-mediated β-adrenergic receptors in the pulmonary epithelium.[6] The rapidity of lung fluid absorption by the body is optimized at thoracic pressures between 35 and 40 cm H_2O.[5] Pulmonary ventilation reduces pulmonary vascular resistance, promoting perfusion of the ventilated alveolar tissue.[1] The increased O_2 saturation of blood stimulates closure of the ductus arteriosus within 4 to 5 minutes of birth.[4] The foramen ovale functionally closes within 5 to 20 minutes of birth when increased pulmonary venous return raises blood pressure in the left atrium, reversing the right to left shunt.[4] The septum secundum, a thin fold of tissue that lies in close apposition to the foramen, acts as a valve closing the opening. Healthy calves have mean pulmonary arterial pressures ranging from 40 to 82 mm Hg immediately after birth, declining to 22 to 25 mm Hg by 2 weeks of age.[7] Systemic arterial pressure is approximately 100 mm Hg and arterial saturation is greater than 90%.[1] Transient mild metabolic and respiratory acidosis are observed following rupture of the umbilical cord because of anaerobic glycolysis

TABLE 16-1

Arterial and Venous Blood Gas Values for Newborn Calves

	Calf Age (hr)	pH	po_2	pco_2	HCO_3^-	Base Excess
			Parameters			
Venous*	1	7.219 (0.05)	N/A	41.0 (5.9)	24.2 (2.7)	−2.9 (3.2)
Arterial†	1	7.3 (0.05)	58.43 (11.61)	50.40 (5.27)	23.52 (2.78)	N/A

N/A, Not available.
Values represent mean with standard deviation in parentheses. N/A = not available.
*Blood taken from the jugular vein immediately postpartum.[8]
†Blood was taken from the brachial artery while the calf was in lateral recumbency (*N* = 30).[63]

in poorly perfused tissues during the transition from placental oxygen delivery to the establishment of respiratory function. The mild acidosis is normally corrected within 1 to 4 hours of birth.[8] Anatomic closure of the foramen ovale and ductus arteriosus may take several weeks.[4] Normal blood gas values for the calf during the immediate postpartum period are presented in Table 16-1.

Dystocia is commonly associated with prolonged hypoxia and acidosis. Hypoxia and acidosis maintain constriction of pulmonary arterioles, and the subsequent maintenance of high pulmonary vascular resistance favors continuation of in utero right to left vascular shunts, which contributes to systemic hypoxia. Following dystocia, neonates are less active, slow to stand, slow to nurse, and prone to hypothermia and hypogammaglobulinemia. The normal duration of stage 2 labor (from appearance of fetal membranes at the vulva to delivery of the fetus) in ruminants is generally shorter in multiparous animals (~30 min) than primiparous animals (~60 min).[9] Fetal viability is improved with early intervention; multiparous animals should be assisted after 30 to 60 minutes of stage 2 labor and primiparous animals after 60 to 90 minutes.[10]

The range in ambient temperatures over which newborn animals are able to maintain homeothermy is much narrower than in growing or adult animals. Neonates are more susceptible to fluctuations in environmental temperature because of their large surface area to mass ratio, evaporation of amniotic fluid, and limited caloric reserves. Starvation and hypothermia is the second leading cause of death of neonatal lambs.[11] Neonatal mortality increases with decreasing ambient temperature and with increasing precipitation on the day of birth.[12] Thermoneutrality is maintained by shivering and metabolism of brown adipose tissue. Normally at birth, blood glucose concentration in calves ranges between 50 and 60 g/dl, rising to 100 mg/dl within the first 24 hours of life.[1] Lambs born in warm weather can survive for up to 4 days without supplemental nutrition. Severe weather stress may increase energy requirements by 500% and deplete the energy reserves of newborn lambs in 6 to 16 hours.[13] Starvation exacerbates the effects of environmental stress by reducing the available substrates for heat production, and energy depletion leads to hypoglycemia. Administration of glucose to hypothermic neonates before and during warming is important to avoid deaths from cerebral hypoglycemia induced by increased utilization of glucose by peripheral tissues.[14] Warming hypothermic lambs by immersion in 38° C (100.4° F) water is more efficient than infrared lamps or wrapping the lamb in a cotton cloth.[15]

No intrauterine transfer of immunoglobulin occurs in ruminants, so at birth neonatal ruminants are agammaglobulinemic and immunologically naive. Infectious disease is the leading cause of morbidity and mortality in calves greater

than 3 days of age.[16] Failure of passive transfer increases the risk of neonatal mortality.[17] Colostrum provides a concentrated source of energy and immunoglobulins. Immunoglobulins are concentrated in colostrum by an active, receptor-mediated transfer of IgG_1 from the blood of the dam across the mammary gland secretory epithelium beginning several weeks before parturition.[18] Colostral IgG_1 concentrations may be 5 to 10 times the maternal serum concentrations. IgM, IgA, and IgG_2 concentrations in colostrum are much lower.[19] The large numbers of leukocytes also contribute to providing passive immunity to the newborn.[20] Methods of assessing passive transfer and management of failure of passive transfer are discussed in detail in Chapter 49.

ACUTE ASPHYXIA IN THE NEONATE
WENDY E. VAALA

Peripartum asphyxia produces hypoxic ischemic encephalopathy (HIE), ischemic renal failure, and varying degrees of necrotizing enterocolitis (NEC). Diagnosis relies on prepartum transabdominal ultrasonography of the fetoplacental unit, postpartum placental and neonatal foal examination, and immediate assessment of creatinine and presuckle glucose in the foal after delivery. Patient survival depends on management of CNS, gastrointestinal, and renal dysfunction.

Asphyxia is a multifactorial disease process that develops when tissue oxygenation is disrupted. It is most commonly encountered when pregnancy and labor are complicated by problems resulting in impaired oxygen delivery to fetal tissues, on either a short-term or long-term basis. Peripartum asphyxia has been associated with rapid, seemingly uncomplicated deliveries, dystocia, induced delivery, cesarean section, premature placental separation and other placental abnormalities, umbilical cord abnormalities, twinning, meconium staining, postdate pregnancy, and severe maternal illness.[21] Asphyxia may also occur in the neonatal period; causes include severe hemorrhage, resulting in hypovolemia and shock, and severe cardiorespiratory dysfunction, as in severe pneumonia, cardiac malformations, pulmonary hypertension, and airway obstruction.

The overall incidence of the condition in the foal is not known, because of the high incidence of unmonitored and unobserved deliveries, and the diagnostic confusion of asphyxial problems with other perinatal problems.[22] In a recent study of causes of equine perinatal death, complications of birth, including asphyxia, dystocia, and trauma, were listed as the second most common cause of death after infection (19% of 3527 cases). This figure does not include acute placental or umbilical cord abnormalities, problems that could have also caused acute fetal asphyxiation.[23]

Pathophysiologic Considerations

Asphyxia is the result of impaired oxygen delivery to cells and usually results from a combination of hypoxemia (decreased oxygen concentration in the blood) and ischemia (decreased tissue perfusion). Pure hypoxemia implies a decrease in oxygen concentration in the blood with preservation of blood flow, which allows organs to respond by increasing their efficiency in extracting oxygen from the circulation. The effects of hypoxemia and ischemia are not identical, but they are difficult to distinguish clinically. Ischemia is far more devastating and results in anaerobic metabolism, increased lactate concentrations, intracellular acidosis, and is a preamble for reperfusion injury. Metabolites of anaerobic metabolism, such as lactic acid, cannot be removed from the tissues until blood supply is restored. As a result, severe acidosis may develop locally, which interferes with cellular function and may cause irreversible cell damage.

In utero the mammalian fetus adapts to a relatively hypoxic environment by increased oxygen affinity of fetal hemoglobin, increased ability to extract oxygen from the blood, and a greater tissue resistance to acidosis. Fetal compensatory mechanisms against increasing asphyxia include bradycardia, decreased oxygen consumption, anaerobic glycolysis, reflex redistribution of blood flow with preferential perfusion of the brain, heart, and adrenal glands at the expense of circulation to kidneys, gut, liver, lungs, and muscle.[24] The extent of tissue injury depends on whether the asphyxial insult is acute or chronic, or partial or complete, and whether the neonate is premature or full term. During severe in utero hypoxia there is sequential loss of fetal reflexes with the most oxygen-demanding fetal activities disappearing first. Fetal reflexes are lost in the following order: (1) fetal heart rate reactivity (the ability to increase heart rate in response to fetal activity), (2) fetal breathing, (3) generalized fetal movements, and (4) fetal tone.

In mild hypoxia there is decreased heart rate, slight increase in blood pressure, and little change in cardiac output, but as asphyxia progresses there is a further decrease in heart rate, decreased cardiac output, and finally, falling blood pressure, as oxidative phosphorylation fails and energy reserves are depleted.[25] Without sufficient energy, cellular ion pumps eventually fail, with accumulation of sodium, chloride, water, and calcium intracellularly, and excitatory amino acid neurotransmitters in the brain, such as glutamate, extracellularly.

Several lines of investigation suggest that the fast excitatory neurotransmitters glutamate and aspartate play an important role in hypoxic-ischemic brain injury. Glutamate injection into specific regions of the brain results in neuronal injury identical to that seen after hypoxia-ischemia. Specific glutamate antagonists can also prevent cell death from anoxia. Therefore research is focusing on pharmacologic agents that would either inhibit glutamate release or block its actions. At high extracellular concentrations, glutamate acts as a neurotoxin and mediates opening of ion channels that permit sodium to enter cells followed by an influx of chloride ions and water resulting in osmotic lysis and immediate neuronal death.[26,27] Glutamate also mediates delayed cell death by provoking calcium influx through depolarization-induced opening of calcium channels and by direct stimulation of N-methyl-D-aspartate (NMDA) receptors that open additional calcium channels.[26,27] High intracellular levels of free calcium result in activation of lytic enzyme systems that attack the structural integrity of the cell, generation of free radicals, and impairment of mitochondrial function resulting in delayed neuronal death. Because of the important role of calcium in regulation of cellular function, drugs such as NMDA and calcium antagonists that prevent calcium influx into damaged cells are being investigated to help reduce delayed ischemic brain injury. It is likely that as the pathophysiology of hypoxic-ischemic injury is better understood, better and more specific drugs will be identified to decrease the severity of cellular injury.[25,28]

Oxygen-free radicals are generated during the reperfusion phase of hypoxic-ischemic injury. It is thought that these radicals contribute to brain injury by their ability to attack the fatty acid moiety of cellular membranes and cause membrane fragmentation.[28] The physical integrity of the circula-

Table 16-2

Clinicopathologic Conditions Associated With Peripartum Asphyxia[64]

Clinical Signs	Laboratory Findings	Pathology Lesions
CENTRAL NERVOUS SYSTEM		
Hypotonia	Increased ICP	CNS hemorrhage
Hypertonia	Increased BBB permeability and albumin	Edema
Seizures	quotient	Ischemic necrosis
Coma		
Loss of suckle		
Proprioceptive deficits		
Apnea		
RENAL SYSTEM		
Oliguira	Azotemia	Tubular necrosis
Anuria	Hyponatremia	
Generalized edema	Hypochloremia	
	Abnormal urinalysis	
GASTROINTESTINAL SYSTEM		
Colic	Occult blood (+) feces and reflux	Ischemic mucosal necrosis
Ileus	Pneumatosis intestinalis	Enterocolitis
Abdominal distention		Ulceration
Bloody diarrhea		
Gastric reflux		

BBB, Blood-brain barrier; *CNS,* central nervous system; *ICP,* intracranial pressure; *PFC,* persistent fetal circulation.

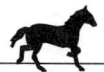

tion is often severely compromised after a period of ischemia. It is suspected that oxygen-derived free radicals are at least partially responsible for the increased capillary permeability, edema formation, and tissue damage that commonly follows the restoration of blood flow to ischemic tissues.[29]

Potential Postnatal Sequelae of Birth Asphyxia

The consequences of an episode of asphyxia can be far-reaching and profound. Many organ systems can be adversely affected and contribute to the commonly observed clinical signs of weakness and depression in the neonate. Management can be difficult and complex, but with good supportive care, dramatic recoveries can be made in even severely affected individuals. Unfortunately, it is virtually impossible at the onset of treatment to predict either the severity of injury or the prognosis. Chronic asphyxia in premature individuals or those who develop sepsis carries the poorest prognosis for intact neurologic survival.

Clinical signs related to the asphyxial injury may not appear until hours or days after the insult. Blood volume abnormalities, such as severe hypovolemia, occurring at delivery, may not be obvious until several hours later. Blood pressure may actually be normal at first because capillary capacitance beds are constricted by substances such as catecholamines and angiotensin II. Then as the peripartum stresses decrease over time, circulating hormone levels fall and progressive hypotension and acidosis often develop.[22]

Table 16-2 lists specific clinical conditions and organ system derangements that have been associated with asphyxial injury. Table 16-3 presents therapies for specific organ system dysfunction.

CENTRAL NERVOUS SYSTEM. Asphyxia produces hypoxic ischemic encephalopathy (HIE) associated with hemorrhage, edema, and necrosis. Mild asphyxia produces transient tissue ischemia with potentially reversible damage. Prolonged ischemia results in disruption of tight junctions in the capillary endothelium and leakage of osmotic agents and fluid into surrounding brain interstitium causing vasogenic edema.[30] Brain necrosis occurs and is accompanied by increased intracranial pressure, progressive brain swelling, reduced cerebral blood flow, and exacerbation of existing ischemia. In critically ill foals, cerebral edema has been associated with cerebellar herniation.[31]

An important mediator of CNS damage is the fast excitatory neurotransmitter glutamate. At high extracellular concentrations, glutamate acts as a neurotoxin and mediates both immediate and delayed neuronal death. Additional brain injury occurs as a result of repeated seizures, which are common during severe encephalopathy. Repeated seizures cause brain injury through (1) hypoventilation and apnea resulting in hypoxemia and hypercapnea, (2) elevation in arterial blood pressure and cerebral blood flow, (3) progressive neuronal injury because of excessive release of excitatory amino acids such as glutamate, and (4) depletion of the brain's limited energy stores to support seizure activity.

Neonatal foals suffering from HIE display a wide spectrum of neurologic signs that include jitteriness, hyperalertness, stupor, somnolence, obtundation, lethargy, hypotonia, clonic seizures, extensor rigidity, hypertonia, subtle seizures, tonic posturing, coma, death, aimless wandering, head pressing, loss of affinity for the dam, inability to find the udder, abnormal vocalization (barking, high-pitched cry), loss of suckle, dysphagia, decreased tongue tone, odontoprisis, central blindness, anisocoria, mydriasis, nystagmus, eye deviation, head tilt, head and neck turn, irregular respiration, apnea, abnormally slow respiratory rate, proprioceptive deficits, and spastic dysmetric gait.

Foals with HIE exhibit a variety of seizurelike activities. Seizures can vary in clinical severity from subtle, which may not be recognized as seizure activity, to generalized and severe (see Seizures, Chapter 20). Jitteriness is associated with mild hypoxia and is not a true seizure but a movement disorder consisting of tremors that can be stopped by gentle restraint. Subtle seizures are called motor automatisms and are characterized by paroxysmal events including eye blinking, eye deviation, nystagmus, pedaling movements, a variety of oral-buccal-lingual movements such as intermittent tongue

---

Table 16-2

Clinicopathologic Conditions Associated With Peripartum Asphyxia[64]—cont'd

Clinical Signs	Laboratory Findings	Pathology Lesions
RESPIRATORY SYSTEM		
Respiratory distress, tachypnea	Hypoxemia	Hyaline membrane disease
Dyspnea	Hypercapnia	Atelectasis
Rib retractions	Respiratory acidosis	Meconium aspiration
		Pulmonary hypertension
CARDIAC SYSTEM		
Arrhythmia	Hypoxemia	Myocardial infarcts
Weak pulses	Elevated myocardial enzymes	Valvular insufficiency
Tachycardia		Persistent fetal circulation
Edema		
Hypotension		
HEPATIC SYSTEM		
Icterus	Hyperbilirubinemia	Hepatocellular necrosis
Abnormal mentation	Elevated liver enzymes	Biliary stasis
ENDOCRINE SYSTEM—ADRENALS, PARATHYROIDS		
Weakness	Hypocortisolemia	Necrosis
Apnea	Hypocalcemia	Hemorrhage
Seizures		

TABLE 16-3

Drugs Used to Treat Foals With Peripartum Asphyxia[64]

Organ System	Clinical Signs	Drug Therapy
Central nervous system (CNS)	Seizures	**Diazepam:** 0.11-0.44 mg/kg IV
		Phenobarbital: 2-10 mg/kg IV q12hr; give slowly, monitor serum levels
		Pentobarbital: 2-10 mg/kg IV
	CNS edema	**Dimethyl sulfoxide:** 0.5-1g/kg IV as 20% solution over 1 hr; can repeat q12hr
		Mannitol: 0.25-1 g/kg IV as 20% solution over 15-20 min; q12-24hr
Renal	Oliguria, anuria	**Dopamine infusion:** 2-10 μg/kg/min; monitor blood pressure and pulse
		Furosemide infusion: 0.25-2 μg/kg/hr or 0.25-0.5 mg/kg IV q1-6hr; monitor serum electrolytes and hydration status
		Mannitol: 0.5-1 g/kg IV as 20% solution over 15-20 min
		Dobutamine infusion: 2-15 μg/kg/min; use if cardiac dysfunction is contributing to hypotension and poor renal perfusion
Gastrointestinal	Ileus, GI distention	**Erythromycin:** 1-2 mg/kg PO q6hr; 1-2 mg/kg/hr as IV infusion q6hr
		Cisapride: 10 mg PO q6-8hr
		Metoclopramide: 0.25-0.5 mg/kg/hr infusion q6-8hr
	Ulcers	**Sucralfate:** 20-40 mg/kg PO q6hr
		Ranitidine: 8-10 mg/kg PO q6-8hr, 1-2 mg/kg IV q8hr
		Cimetidine: 15-20 mg/kg PO q6hr; 6.6 mg/kg IV q6hr
		Omeprazole: 2 mg/kg PO q24hr
Cardiac	Hypotension	**Dopamine infusion:** 2-10 μg/kg/min
		Dobutamine infusion: 2-15 μg/kg/min
		Digoxin: 0.02-0.035 mg/kg PO q24hr if cardiac failure is suspected
Respiratory	Hypoxemia	**Intranasal, humidified oxygen:** 2-10 L/min
	Apnea	**Caffeine:**
		Loading dose: 10 mg/kg PO
		Maintenance dose: 2.5-3 mg/kg PO q24hr
Endocrine	Hypocortisolemia	**ACTH (depot):** 0.26 mg IM q8-12hr
Immune	FPT, leukopenia	**Hyperimmune plasma:** 10-20 ml/kg IV; monitor serum IgG and WBC

ACTH, Adrenocorticotropic hormone; *FPT,* failure of passive transfer; *GI,* gastrointestinal; *IgG,* immunoglobulin G; *IV,* intravenously; *PO,* orally; *WBC,* white blood cells.

protrusion, sucking behavior, purposeless thrashing, and other vasomotor changes such as apnea, abnormal breathing patterns, and changes in heart rate. Tonic posturing is another subtle seizure activity characterized by symmetric limb hyperextension or flexion and may be accompanied by abnormal eye movements and apnea. Clonic seizures are true epileptiform seizures with a distinct EEG signature and are characterized by rigid jerky motions that cannot be suppressed by restraint.

Not all neurologic abnormalities in large animal neonates are the result of peripartum asphyxia. Other causes of neonatal neurologic disease include the following:

- Metabolic disorders: hypocalcemia, hypomagnesemia, hyponatremia, hypernatremia, hyperosmolality (e.g., hyperlipidemia, hyperglycemia), severe azotemia, hepatoencephalopathy
- Infectious conditions: septic meningitis, septicemia/endotoxemia, EHV1 infection
- Malformation: hydrocephalus, agenesis of the corpus callosum, vertebral and spinal cord malformations, cerebellar abiotrophy, occipitoatlantoaxial malformation
- Cranial or vertebral trauma
- Toxins

If severe metabolic derangements, infections, and congenital defects are ruled out, then asphyxia is the most likely cause of the neonate's neurologic deficits. Normal serum chemistries help rule out metabolic disturbances. A normal leukogram or the absence of severe leukopenia, neutropenia, and toxic neutrophil changes help rule out septic conditions. Cerebrospinal fluid analysis is indicated if septic meningitis is a possible differential. Septic meningitis produces an increased nucleated cell count, protein concentration, and IgG index in the CSF. Hypoxic brain damage may result in an increased albumin quotient in the CSF compatible with increased blood-brain barrier permeability.

Other diagnostic aids that have enjoyed limited use in large animals include cranial ultrasonography, computed tomography (CT), magnetic resonance imaging (MRI), EEGs, and auditory evoked brainstem potentials. The increased availability of CT or MRI scans may in the future help to document the location, severity, and progression of brain injury in asphyxiated large animal neonates.

Currently, suggested treatment of CNS dysfunction in asphyxiated large animal neonates includes seizure control, nursing care to prevent self-trauma, and careful fluid therapy to avoid overhydration and hypoglycemia or hyperglycemia. Diazepam is used initially to control seizures because of its rapid onset of action. Phenobarbital is used to control severe or repeated seizures. Foals receiving high doses of anticonvulsants should have their vital signs monitored closely because the combination of diazepam and phenobarbital can produce profound respiratory depression, loss of thermoregulatory control, and hypotension. Cerebral edema may occur in some hypoxic neonates. Intravenous dimethyl sulfoxide (DMSO 0.5 to 1 g/kg of a 10% to 20% solution, slowly over 1 to 2 hours) therapy may be useful in some patients for several reasons, including its ability to reduce brain swelling, intracranial pressure, and inflammation and to act as a diuretic.[21] The osmotic agent mannitol has also been used to reduce cerebral edema. To prevent exacerbation of cerebral edema, fluid therapy should be conservative and sudden changes in osmolality should be avoided. Controversy surrounds the benefits of glucose administration. Hyperglycemia immediately after prolonged hypoxic ischemic injury has been associated with severe neonatal brain injury.[32] Other studies suggest glucose administration after global

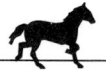

hypoxic injury may offer neuroprotection by stimulating insulin release and by reducing glycolysis, free radical formation, and glutamine-mediated injury.[33] Therefore the safest recommendation is to maintain serum glucose concentration within a normal range.

CARDIOPULMONARY EFFECTS. The response of pulmonary vasculature to hypoxia and acidemia includes (1) increased pulmonary vascular resistance, (2) pulmonary hypertension, (3) increased atrial pressure, and (4) persistent right-to-left flow of blood across fetal pathways (e.g., patent ductus arteriosus, foramen ovale). The neonatal pulmonary circulation reflexly constricts in response to hypoxemia and acidosis.[34] This pulmonary vasoconstriction results in increased pulmonary vascular resistance, pulmonary hypertension, and increased right atrial pressure. If pulmonary arterial pressure exceeds systemic pressure, right to left blood flow may result in the reestablishment of fetal circulation (right to left flow through the ductus arteriosus and foramen ovale). Persistent fetal circulation (PFC) is associated with severe hypoxemia unresponsive to oxygen therapy caused by severe right to left shunting of unoxygenated blood away from the lungs.

When PFC patterns exist, hypoxemia is exacerbated. During asphyxia-induced pulmonary vasoconstriction, substrate delivery to the pneumocytes is impaired and surfactant production decreases, with secondary pulmonary atelectasis. Perinatal asphyxia may adversely affect the respiratory control centers of the brain and result in hypoventilation (increased CO_2) secondary to periods of apnea or abnormal breathing patterns.

Adequate surfactant production is dependent on adequate function of the type II pneumocytes and the ongoing delivery of lipid precursors by the blood. If pulmonary blood flow is compromised, surfactant production may stop, and a secondary surfactant deficiency may result.[22,25] The altered permeability characteristics of the lung that have been associated with asphyxial injury also interfere with the function of surfactant, predisposing to atelectasis.[35]

If asphyxia induces in utero passage of meconium, then the fetus may aspirate meconium. Meconium can caused mechanical obstruction of airways resulting in suffocation or regional lung atelectasis. Partial obstruction produces a ball-valve phenomenon with distal air trapping, ventilation-perfusion mismatching, alveolar overdistention and possible rupture, interstitial emphysema, and pneumothorax.[36] Meconium also induces chemical pneumonitis accompanied by alveolar collapse and edema.[37] The free fatty acids in meconium displace surfactant, resulting in additional atelectasis and decreased lung compliance.[38] See Respiratory Distress, Chapter 20, for further information. Adverse effects of asphyxia on myocardial function include (1) reduced myocardial contractility, (2) left ventricular dysfunction, (3) tricuspid valve insufficiency, and (4) cardiac failure. As a result of cardiac insufficiency the foal may develop systemic hypotension, further impairment of renal blood flow, and decreased pulmonary perfusion. In the human infant, perinatal asphyxia has been associated with myocardial and papillary muscle ischemia and infarction, with decreased myocardial contractility, tricuspid valve insufficiency, and congestive heart failure often resulting. Cardiac isoenzymes may be increased. Treatment is directed at correcting hypoxemia, acidosis, and hypoglycemia, and maintaining cardiac output and blood pressure. Inotropic drugs, such as dopamine and dobutamine, are commonly used.

If pulmonary hypertension develops, thoracic radiographs show diminished vascular markings caused by pulmonary hypoperfusion. Surfactant dysfunction produces diffuse lung atelectasis and a diffuse reticulogranular parenchymal pattern with air bronchograms. Meconium aspiration may produce perihilar infiltrated and focal atelectasis. Echocardiography helps identify arrhythmias.

Support of the respiratory system involves maintenance of oxygenation and ventilation of the patient. Mild to moderate hypoxemia can be treated by increasing the amount of time the foal spends in sternal recumbency or standing and by administering modest flows of humidified intranasal oxygen (2 to 8 L/min). Foals suffering severe hypoxemia and hypercapnea (PaO_2 <40 mm Hg; $PaCO_2$ >65 mm Hg) require positive-pressure ventilation. Respiratory stimulants are used to treat periodic apnea and abnormally slow breathing patterns associated with central depression of the respiratory center. Caffeine is used most frequently to stimulate the respiratory neuronal activity and increase receptor responsiveness to elevated CO_2 concentrations. Overdosing with respiratory stimulants leads to excessive CNS, myocardial, and gastrointestinal stimulation resulting in agitation, seizures, tachycardia, hypertension, colic, and diarrhea. Caffeine is the safest methylxanthine to use.

RENAL EFFECTS. During asphyxia, redistribution of blood flow away from the kidneys frequently results in decreased renal perfusion and acute tubular necrosis. In human infants, oliguria (<1 ml urine/kg/hr) is the most common clinical sign of acute renal failure; it has also been observed in asphyxiated foals.[21,22] Other signs of renal ischemic damage include peripheral edema, elevated concentrations of serum creatinine and urine γ-glutamyltransferase, and electrolyte disturbances such as hypocalcemia, hyponatremia, and hypochloremia caused by renal tubular damage. The oliguric animal should be identified by careful monitoring of fluid intake and output to avoid fluid overload and edema formation. Based on studies in other neonates, renal blood flow and urine output may be increased by the use of low to moderate doses of dopamine (2 to 10 µg/kg/min infusion) or dobutamine (2 to 10 µg/kg/min infusion). Higher doses of dopamine are contraindicated to avoid peripheral vasoconstriction and a decrease in renal blood flow.[21] Therefore blood pressure and urine output should be carefully monitored during infusion of these substances. Diuretics, such as furosemide (0.5 to 2.5 mg/kg/hr) as an infusion, or 1 mg/kg IM or IV every 12 hours) or mannitol (0.25 to 1 g/kg as 20% solution, infused slowly intravenously over 1 to 2 hours) have also been successfully used to improve urine output in asphyxiated foals.[21]

GASTROINTESTINAL EFFECTS. Hypoxia results in reduced mesenteric and splanchnic blood flow and varying degrees of intestinal ischemia. The most severe form of intestinal dysfunction is necrotizing enterocolitis (NEC) (see Abdominal Distention, Chapter 20). During gastrointestinal ischemia, mucosal cell metabolism diminishes and production of the protective mucus layer ceases, allowing proteolytic enzymes to begin autodigestion of the mucosal barrier. Bacteria within the lumen can then colonize, multiply, and invade the bowel wall. Intramural gas is produced by certain species of bacteria and pneumatosis intestinalis develops. Possible complications include intestinal rupture, pneumoperitoneum, severe bacterial peritonitis, and septicemia.[39] Reflux and feces may be positive for blood. Generalized sepsis often accompanies NEC. As a result of varying degrees of intestinal dysmotility, some foals develop intussusceptions that can be visualized with ultrasound.

Many asphyxiated foals demonstrate mild signs of gastrointestinal malfunction, including meconium impactions and intolerance to enteral feeding (delayed gastric emptying, abdominal distention, diarrhea, and colic). Colic, bloody diarrhea, and sudden death have been observed secondary to extensive intestinal mucosal sloughing in severe cases. Ileus associated with hypoxic gut damage can result in bowel distention and colic. Nasogastric decompression relieves proximal gut distention. Enema administration stimulates distal colonic function and encourages passage of gas. Metoclopramide and erythromycin may improve gastric emptying and upper gastrointestinal function. Metoclopramide infusion (0.25 to 0.3 mg/kg infusion every 6 hours) has been suggested to improve gastric emptying and improve small intestinal motility.[21] Cisapride and erythromycin have been used to stimulate small and large intestinal motility. Be certain to allow adequate time for healing of damaged bowel before using prokinetics in a compromised foal. Sonographic examination of the abdomen helps rule out the presence of intussusceptions and other obstructive lesions before administering motility modifiers. Severe large bowel distention may require percutaneous trocarization. Alternatively, exploratory celiotomy may be performed, but the multisytemic derangements often make these animals poor surgical risks.

To reduce the risk of NEC, asphyxiated foals should have enteral feeding withheld until intestinal motility has returned. Reassuring signs include manure passage, normal borborygmi, and stable vital signs (temperature, blood pressure). Enteral feeding should be started cautiously with fresh mare's milk or colostrum. Foals with severe gastrointestinal dysfunction should have enteral feeds withheld and should be started on parenteral nutrition. Because intestinal ischemia may predispose to ulceration, histamine-2 blockers (cimetidine, ranitidine), proton pump inhibitors (omeprazole), or cytoprotective agents (sucralfate) are recommended.

HEPATIC AND ENDOCRINE FUNCTION. Hypoxic liver damage produces an increase in hepatocellular and biliary enzymes. Affected neonates are usually icteric. Impaired hepatic function renders the neonate more susceptible to alteration in glucose homeostasis and can result in decreased hepatic defense mechanisms and increased susceptibility to sepsis. Endocrine organ damage associated with hypoxia includes adrenal gland hemorrhage and necrosis with hypocortisolemia. Parathyroid damage may result in hypocalcemia; pancreatic injury and abnormal insulin activity can occur.

IMMUNE DYSFUNCTION. Maladjusted foals are at increased risk for failure of passive transfer (FPT) because of their abnormal nursing behavior. Serum IgG levels should be evaluated and colostrum and/or plasma administered to treat FPT.

Supportive Care and Prognosis of the Acutely Asphyxiated Foal

A summary of therapies for specific organ dysfunction associated with peripartum asphyxia is presented in Table 16-3. Blood glucose, blood gases, and fluid and acid-base balance should be monitored closely. In severely affected animals, both arterial and central venous pressure are monitored. Nursing care must be carefully performed to avoid secondary infection.

Prognosis varies with the severity and duration of clinical signs. In one intensive care unit, 70% of asphyxiated foals recovered, with most making a complete recovery. A poor prognosis was associated with foals that failed to show any signs of improving neurologic function in the first 5 days after delivery; foals that remained comatose or experienced severe, recurrent seizures; and foals that developed septicemia.[21]

RESUSCITATION OF THE NEONATE

JOHN K. HOUSE

Assisted deliveries are usually associated with moderate to severe fetal stress. Survival of the compromised fetus is facilitated by prompt initiation of supportive care. Prior preparation of a "crash box" or "crash cart" (Fig. 16-1) expedites location of the necessary supplies and equipment. Passage and subsequently aspiration of meconium often accompany fetal stress. Suction is useful for clearing the airway if available, but should be used judiciously as prolonged pharyngeal and tracheal aspiration induces vagally mediated bradycardia.[40] Vigorously rubbing the skin over the legs stimulates a somatic-respiratory reflex and may help initiate respiratory effort.[41] Thermoregulation is important because recovery from acidosis is delayed by hypothermia.[42] Cold stress leads to increased metabolic needs and produces hypoxia, hypercarbia, metabolic acidosis, and potentially hypoglycemia-metabolic sequelae that resuscitation is aimed at correcting.[43] Weak fetuses are often born with strongly beating hearts but have difficulty initiating adequate inspiratory efforts to expand their lungs. Positive-pressure ventilation is required to overcome surface tension in alveoli and the elastic recoil of lung tissue. Fluid within alveolar spaces and the lumen of the tracheobronchial tree is absorbed into the pulmonary interstitium most efficiently at thoracic pressures between 35 and 40 cm H_2O.[5] Less pressure is usually needed for succeeding breaths. Intrathoracic pressure that exceeds 40 cm H_2O increases the risk of damaging the alveolar epithelium. Observation of chest wall movement is a more reliable sign of appropriate inflation pressures than pressure readings from a manometer. Nasal insufflation with oxygen does not facilitate resorption of lung fluid and is largely ineffective.

If an endotracheal tube and laryngoscope are available, the fetus should be intubated. Placing a rigid stylet in the endotracheal tube and positioning the neonate in sternal recumbency with head and neck extended makes intubation easier. Calves may also be intubated blindly via palpation of the larynx. Ventilation of asphyxiated newborn neonates with 100% oxygen is usually recommended, but experimental work with newborn pigs and a study in humans suggests that room air may be as effective.[44,45] Ventilation using a pulmonary resuscitation bag (Ambu bag) with a pressure relief valve set at 42 cm H_2O avoids inadvertent overinflation.[46] If a laryngoscope and endotracheal tube are not available, positive-pressure ventilation can be achieved using an esophageal feeding tube. The tube is passed into the esophagus with the fetus in right lateral recumbency. The distal end of the tube is located approximately one third of the distance "down" the neck. The esophagus is compressed distal to the end of the tube with one hand, taking care not to trap the trachea, and the muzzle is gripped with the other hand to seal the nares. The operator then blows into the tube and, if the esophageal and muzzle seals are good, air is delivered into the lungs.[47] Direct mouth-to-mouth resuscitation is unhygienic and delivers air mainly into the abomasum. Respiratory stimulant (analeptic) drugs, such as doxapram hydrochloride, may be used to stimulate respiration in neonates but should be used judiciously because the stimulatory action of the drug is nonselective. Convulsions may be observed with repeated dosing, increasing the demand for O_2 in an already hypoxic neonate.[48] Analeptics should not be used as a substitute for ventilatory support.

Progressive hypoxia and tissue acidosis lead to bradycardia, decreased cardiac contractility, and eventually cardiac arrest. If apnea progresses to cardiopulmonary arrest, artificial circulation in the form of cardiac massage needs to be provided along with positive pressure ventilation. Cardiac massage in lambs and kids is performed by compressing the ventral thorax behind the elbows between the thumb and two fore fingers. Cardiac compression in calves is achieved by placing the patient in lateral recumbency and compressing the ventral thorax behind the elbows against a sandbag placed under the calf in a position opposite the resuscitator's hands. Effectiveness of cardiac compression may be monitored by

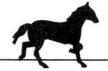

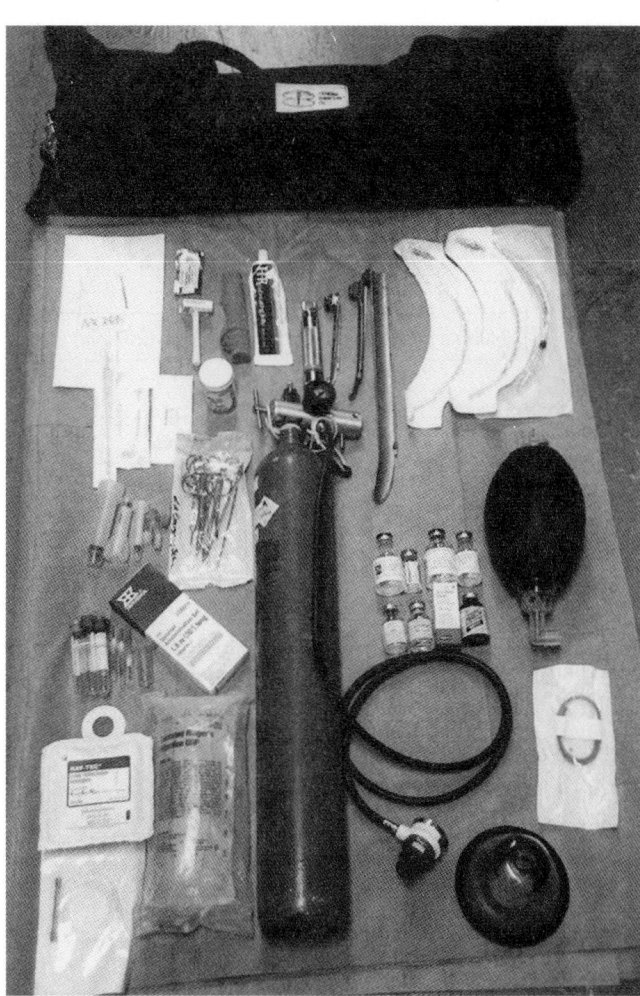

Ambu bag
Oxygen mask
Oxygen cylinder, regulator, and pressure relief valve
Nasal insufflation tubing
Endotracheal tubes
Laryngoscope
KY jelly
Brown gauze, umbilical tape, and adhesive tape
Razor
IV catheters, T-ports, PRNs, and suture
J wire
Needles and syringes
Emergency surgery pack, scalpel blades and surgical gauze
Fluids (saline, lactated Ringer's, and dextrose), administration and
    extension sets
Blood collection tubes and needles
Drugs (epinephrine, lidocaine, prednisolone, doxapram, sodium
    bicarbonate, calcium chloride, and dopamine) (observe neces-
    sary storage requirements)

FIG. 16-1 ▌▌ Supplies for a "crash box."

checking for a palpable pulse and by observing changes in mucous membrane color. When available, an electrocardiogram is useful to monitor the electrical activity of the heart. Abdominal wrapping is used in human and small animal medicine during cardiopulmonary resuscitation to improve myocardial perfusion by returning pooled venous blood from the abdomen and limbs to the central compartment and by reducing the runoff of arterial blood to the caudal periphery.[49] Treatment with epinephrine is recommended for asystole or if the heart rate stays below 60 beats/min. Epinephrine increases systemic vascular resistance, redistributing circulation away from the periphery to the cerebral and myocardial circulation, and increases myocardial contractility, heart rate, and cardiac output. Epinephrine is initially administered at a dose of 0.02 mg/kg either intravenously or intratracheally (via the endotracheal tube). There are reports of cases in the human literature in which there was no response to this dose, but responses were observed to doses as high as 0.2 mg/kg.[50] High-dose epinephrine therapy may increase the risk of acute renal failure and intracranial hemorrhage and is not recommended as a primary treatment.[43] Peak plasma concentrations of epinephrine are achieved 60 seconds after endotracheal administration. Plasma concentrations of epinephrine after endotracheal administration are approximately 10 times lower than those achieved with intravenous administration so intravenous access should be established as soon as possible.[51] Administration of large doses of epinephrine endotracheally

to compensate for the reduced absorption is associated with prolonged hypertension and is not recommended.[52] In an emergency the endotracheal route of drug administration may be used for other lipid-soluble drugs such as lidocaine or atropine, but should not be used for drugs that are not lipid soluble.[53] When drugs are administered by the endotracheal route they should be instilled as deeply as possible into the tracheobronchial tree using a catheter inserted beyond the tip of the endotracheal tube.[54] Dilution of the drug in 1 to 2 ml of saline may aid drug delivery. Rapid intravenous infusion of warm isotonic fluid (lactated Ringer's solution 20 to 40 ml/kg) increases the circulating fluid volume and may help to compensate for the increased vascular volume. The use of sodium bicarbonate, atropine, and calcium chloride in cardiopulmonary resuscitation of neonates is controversial. A basic protocol for resuscitation of the newborn neonate is presented in Figure 16-2.

The rationale for sodium bicarbonate administration in the presence of lactic acidosis is to increase extracellular pH and thereby improve cardiac function, perfusion, and oxygenation of peripheral tissues; intracellular pH; and lactate metabolism.[55] Sodium bicarbonate administration is associated with production of CO_2; correction of the acidosis requires removal of the CO_2, which is dependent on adequate ventilation and pulmonary blood flow. If pulmonary ventilation or pulmonary blood flow is inadequate, administration of sodium bicarbonate will result in hypercarbia. Excessive

1. Clear airway (postural drainage, nasopharyngeal suction).
2. Stimulate respiration by rubbing thorax and limbs.
3. Provide an external heat source (infared lamps, blankets, avoid drafts).

Assessment (Note the time)

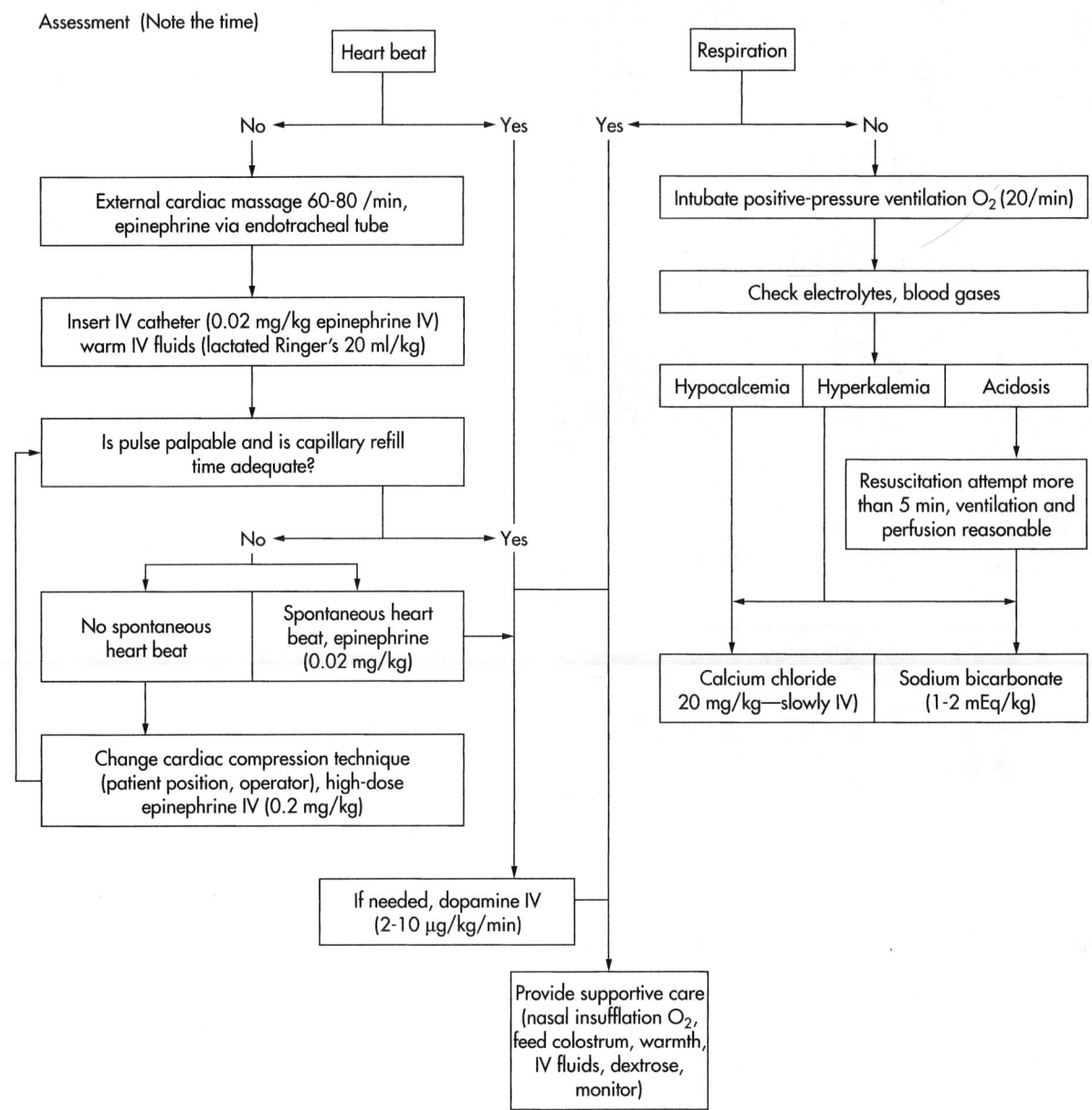

FIG. 16-2 ▓ Resuscitation of the newborn neonate.

administration of sodium bicarbonate causes alkalemia and a right shift in the oxygen/hemoglobin dissociation curve, reducing oxygen availability to tissues. Paradoxic central nervous system acidosis has been documented in association with bicarbonate administration during cardiopulmonary resuscitation,[56] and acute intracellular potassium shifts secondary to sodium bicarbonate therapy may be associated with an increased incidence of cardiac arrhythmias.[57] Administration of sodium bicarbonate is only recommended if adequate ventilation has been established and when all other measures are not successful.[58] The dose is 1 to 2 mEq/kg administered by slow intravenous injection. Because catecholamines are inactivated by bicarbonate and calcium will precipitate when mixed with bicarbonate, intravenous catheters should be flushed between infusions of drugs.[54]

Use of atropine in resuscitation is based on its peripheral effects as a competitive antagonist of acetylcholine, reducing vagal tone and increasing conduction through the atrioventricular node. The effect of atropine is dependent on the degree of vagal stimulation that is causing the bradycardia. Vagal stimulation is not the cause of bradycardia in hypoxic newborns; therefore a response is unlikely. Possible deleterious effects of atropine administered at therapeutic doses are increased myocardial oxygen consumption and precipitation of atrial and ventricular tachyarrhythmias.[59] In low doses atropine stimulates the medullary vagal nuclei, causing paradoxic bradycardia with slowing of atrioventricular conduction.[60]

The belief that increasing the availability of calcium during cardiac arrest might improve myocardial function led to inclusion of calcium chloride in cardiopulmonary resuscitation protocols. Calcium has been implicated as a cause of postresuscitation cerebral ischemia because high levels of calcium promote prolonged vasoconstriction, exacerbating cerebral and myocardial hypoperfusion.[61] Currently, administration of calcium chloride is only recommended in cases of known hypocalcemia and hyperkalemia.

Postresuscitation Care

After resuscitation it is important to monitor cardiopulmonary function closely. Steroids have been recommended to reduce postischemic cerebral edema via preservation of membrane integrity, inhibition of prostaglandin and free radical formation, lysosomal membrane stabilization, and preservation of vascular membrane permeability, but there is no documented evidence demonstrating their effectiveness.[62] The β_1 agonist dopamine may be administered via a continuous slow intravenous infusion (2 to 10 µg/kg/min) if peripheral perfusion is poor, as indicated by decreased capillary refill, absent or decreased pulses, cool extremities, tachycardia, and oliguria. Infiltration of dopamine into tissues can produce local tissue necrosis. Dopamine, like epinephrine, is inactivated in alkaline solutions and should not be administered in sodium bicarbonate.[54] Serum electrolytes, blood gases, and blood glucose should be periodically monitored if laboratory support is available, and appropriate fluid therapy administered to correct deficits. Positioning the newborn in sternal recumbency and provision of oxygen via nasal insufflation helps the compromised neonate maintain blood oxygen saturation. Body temperature should be monitored closely and heating lights and pads provided. During the course of the first 24 hours of life the newborn should receive approximately 15% of its body weight in colostrum. If the coordination of the newborn is questionable, colostrum should be tube fed to avoid aspiration. Immunoglobulins are often absorbed poorly by the compromised neonate, so passive transfer should be evaluated at 18 hours of age and plasma administered if the plasma immunoglobulin concentration is less than 400 mg/dl.

REFERENCES

1. Kasari TR: Physiologic mechanisms of adaptation in the fetal calf at birth, *Vet Clin North Am (Food Anim Pract)* 10:122-136, 1994.
2. Harvey JW: Hemoglobin oxygen affinity. In Kaneko JJ, editor: *Clinical biochemistry of domestic animals*, ed 8, San Diego, 1989, Academic Press.
3. Adams FH et al: The expanded lung of the term fetus, *J Pediatr* 75:59, 1969.
4. Detweiler DK, Riedesel DH: Regional and fetal circulations. In Swenson MJ, Reece WO, eds: *Dukes' physiology of domestic animals*, ed 11, Ithaca, NY, 1993, Cornell University Press.
5. Egan EA, Olver RE, Strang LB: Changes in non-electrolyte permeability of alveoli and the absorption of lung liquid at the start of breathing in the lamb, *J Physiol* 244:161, 1975.
6. Brown MJ et al: Effects of adrenaline and of spontaneous labour on the secretion and absorption of lung liquid in the fetal lamb, *J Physiol* 344:137-52, 1983.
7. Reeves JT, Leathers JE: Circulatory changes following birth of the calf and the effect of hypoxia, *Circ Res* 15:343, 1964.
8. Szenci O: Role of acid-base disturbances in perinatal mortality of calves, *Acta Vet Hung* 33:205, 1985.
9. Doornbos D, Bellows R, Burgening P: Effects of obstetrical assistance on post-partum reproduction in beef females, *J Anim Sci* 59:1-10, 1984.
10. Rice LE: Dystocia-related risk factors, *Vet Clin North Am (Food Anim Pract)* 10:53-68, 1994.
11. Rook JS et al: Diagnosis and control of neonatal losses in sheep, *Vet Clin North Am (Food Anim Pract)* 6:531-562, 1990.
12. Azzam SM et al: Environmental effects on neonatal mortality of beef calves, *J Anim Sci* 71:282, 1993.
13. Alexander G: Temperature regulation in the newborn lamb, *Aust J Agri Res* 12:1152-1174, 1961.
14. Eales FA: Detection and treatment of hypothermia in newborn lambs, *In Pract* 4:20-22, 1982.
15. Robinson JB, Young BA: Recovery of neonatal lambs from hypothermia with thermal assistance, *Can J Anim Sci* 68:183-190, 1988.

16. Garry FB: Focal and generalized bacterial infection in neonatal calves, *Proceedings of the Third International Conference on Veterinary Perinatology*, University of California, Davis, Calif, 1993, pp 63-65.
17. Gay CC: The role of colostrum in managing calf health, *Proc Am Assoc Bovine Pract* 16:79-84, 1984.
18. Butler JE: Bovine immunoglobulins: an augmented review, *Vet Immunol Immunopathol* 4:43-152, 1983.
19. Besser TE, Gay CC: The importance of colostrum to the health of the neonatal calf, *Vet Clin North Am (Food Anim Pract)* 10:107-117, 1994.
20. Riedel-Caspari G: The influence of colostral leukocytes on the course of an experimental *Escherichia coli* infection and serum antibodies in neonatal calves, *Vet Immunol Immunopathol* 35:275-288, 1993.
21. Vaala WE: Peripartum asphyxia, *Vet Clin North Am (Equine Pract)* 10:187-218, 1994.
22. Drummond WH, Koterba AM: Neonatal asphyxia. In Koterba AM, Drummond WH, Kosch PC, editors: *Equine clinical neonatology*, Philadelphia, 1990, Lea and Febiger.
23. Giles RC et al: Causes of abortion, stillbirth, and perinatal death in horses: 3527 cases (1986-1991), *J Am Vet Med Assoc* 203:1170-1175, 1993.
24. Behrman RE et al: Distribution of the circulation in the normal and asphyxiated fetal primate, *Am J Obstet Gynecol* 108:956-969, 1970.
25. Snyder EY, Cloherty JP: Perinatal asphyxia. In Cloherty JP, Stark AR, editors: *Manual of neonatal care*, ed 3, Boston, 1991, Little, Brown.
26. Clark GD: Role of excitatory amino acids in brain injury caused by hypoxia-ischemia, status epilepticus, and hypoglycemia, *Clin Perinatol* 16:459-474, 1989.
27. Rothman SM, Olney JW: Glutamate and the pathophysiology of hypoxic-ischemic brain damage, *Ann Neurol* 19:105-111, 1986.
28. Vannucci RC: Current and potentially new management strategies for perinatal hypoxic-ischemic encephalopathy, *Pediatrics* 85:961-968, 1990 (comments).
29. McCord JM: Oxygen-derived free radicals in postischemic tissue injury, *N Engl J Med* 312:159-163, 1985.
30. Goldstein GW: Pathogenesis of brain edema and hemorrhage: role of the brain capillary, *Pediatrics* 64:357-360, 1979.
31. Kortz GD et al: Cerebral edema and cerebellar herniation in four equine neonates, *Equine Vet J* 24:63, 1992.
32. Sheldon RA, Partridge JC, Ferriero DM: Postischemic hyperglycemia is not protective to the neonatal rat brain, *Pediatr Res* 32:489-493, 1992.
33. Hattori H, Wasterlain CG: Posthypoxic glucose supplement reduces hypoxic-ischemic brain damage in the neonatal rat, *Ann Neurol* 28:122-128, 1990.
34. Rudolph AM, Yuan S: Response of the pulmonary vasculature to hypoxia and H ion concentration changes, *J Clin Invest* 45:399, 1966.
35. Jobe A: Respiratory distress syndrome: new therapeutic approaches to a complex pathophysiology, *Adv Pediatr* 30:93-130, 1983.
36. Tyler DC, Murphy J, Cheney FW: Mechanical and chemical damage to lung tissue caused by meconium aspiration, *Pediatrics* 62:454-459, 1978.
37. Lopez A, Bildfell R: Pulmonary inflammation associated with aspirated meconium and epithelial cells in calves, *Vet Pathol* 29:104-111, 1992.
38. Clark DA et al: Surfactant displacement by meconium free fatty acids: an alternative explanation for atelectasis in meconium aspiration syndrome, *J Pediatrics* 110:765-770, 1987.
39. Santulli TV: Acute necrotizing enterocolitis: recognition and management, *Hosp Pract* 9:174, 1974.
40. Apgar V: Infant resuscitation, *Postgrad Med* 19:447-450, 1956.
41. Scarpelli EM, Condorelli S, Cosmi EV: Cutaneous stimulation and generation of breathing in the fetus, *Pediatr Res* 11:24, 1977.
42. Adamsons K, Gandy GM, James LS: The influence of thermal factors upon oxygen consumption of the newborn human infant, *J Pediatr* 66:45, 1965.
43. Leuthner SR, Jansen RD, Hageman JR: Cardiopulmonary resuscitation of the newborn: an update, *Pediatr Clin North Am* 41:893-907, 1994.
44. Rootwelt T et al: Hypoxemia and reoxygenation with 21% or 100% oxygen in newborn pigs: changes in blood pressure, base deficit, and hypoxanthine and brain morphology, *Pediatr Res* 32:107-113, 1992.
45. Ramji S et al: Resuscitation of asphyxic newborn infants with room air or 100% oxygen, *Pediatr Res* 34:809-812, 1993.
46. Kasari TR: Weakness in the newborn calf, *Vet Clin North Am (Food Anim Pract)* 10:167-180, 1994.
47. Lester WA, Benson R, Froehlich P: Lamb resuscitation. *Vet Record* 126:296-297, 1990.
48. Martens RJ: Neonatal respiratory distress: a review with emphasis on the horse, *Compend Cont Educ Pract Vet* 4:S23-S34, 1982.
49. Young LE: Current developments in cardiopulmonary resuscitation, *J Small Anim Pract* 33:138-145, 1992.
50. Goetting MG, Paradis NA: High-dose epinephrine improves outcome from pediatric cardiac arrest, *Ann Emerg Med* 20:22-26, 1991.
51. Burchfield DJ: Medication use in neonatal resuscitation: epinephrine, sodium, bicarbonate, *Neonat Pharmacol Q* 2:2, 1993.
52. Ralston SH: Endotracheal versus intravenous epinephrine during electromechanical disassociation with CPR in dogs, *Ann Emerg Med* 14:1044-1048, 1985.
53. Johnston C: Endotracheal drug delivery, *Pediatr Emerg Care* 8:94-97, 1992.
54. Association AH: Pediatric advanced life support, *J Am Med Assoc* 268:2262-2275, 1992.

55. Staepoole PW: Lactic acidosis: the case against bicarbonate therapy, *Ann Intern Med* 105:276-278, 1986.

56. Van Pelt DR, Wheeler SL, Wingfield WE: The use of bicarbonate in cardiopulmonary resuscitation, *Compend Cont Ed Pract Vet* 12:1393-1399, 1990.

57. Association AH: Standards and guidelines for cardiopulmonary resuscitation (CPR) and emergency cardiac care (ECC), *JAMA* 255:2905-2952, 1986.

58. Pediatrics: *AHAAA textbook of neonatal resuscitation*, Elk Grove Village, IL, 1990, AAP.

59. Massumi RA et al: Ventricular fibrillation and tachycardia after intravenous atropine for treatment of bradycardias, *N Engl J Med* 287:336-338, 1972.

60. Kottmeier CA, Graverstevi JS: The parasympathomimetic activity of atropine and atropine methylbromide, *Anesthesiology* 29:1125, 1986.

61. Hughes WG, Ruedy JR: Should calcium be used in cardiac arrest? *Am J Med* 81:285-296, 1986.

62. Muir WW: Brain hypoperfusion post resuscitation, *Vet Clin North Am* 19:1151-1166, 1989.

63. Adams R et al: Arterial blood gas values in newborn beef calves, *Proceedings of the International Society of Veterinary Perinatology*, Cambridge, England, 1990, p 33.

64. Vaala WE: Peripartum asphyxia syndrome in foals, *Proceedings of the 45th Annual Convention of American Association of Equine Practitioners*, 1999, 247-253.

Initial Management and Physical Examination of the Neonate

WENDY E. VAALA

JOHN K. HOUSE

JOHN E. MADIGAN

APPROACH TO THE HIGH-RISK OR COMPROMISED NEONATAL FOAL

WENDY E. VAALA

The abnormal large animal neonate often presents diagnostic and management challenges to the veterinarian. Familiarity with neonatal characteristics and behavior, as well as with neonatal disease processes, is crucial for a successful outcome. Despite dramatic advances in neonatal intensive care, many foals die, not because their primary problem is untreatable but because veterinary intervention was delayed, delivery was unattended, neonatal compromise was not recognized in a timely fashion, or critical care was unavailable or not economically feasible. It is absolutely essential to recognize abnormalities early in the course of the disease process. Large animal neonates are born with few nutritional, physiologic, or immunologic reserves. Any condition that prevents them from standing and nursing soon after birth represents a potentially fatal condition. Unfortunately, signs of illness in the neonate are frequently vague and nonlocalizing. Many high-risk newborn animals look relatively good during the first hours following birth. This grace period is often followed in 12 to 24 hours by a worsening of condition because of the specific disease process itself and disruption of normal adaptive processes. The presence of one localizing sign, such as diarrhea, may obscure the fact that other organ systems are involved as well. Multiple problems in the same individual seem to be the rule rather than the exception. Many weak foals begin to fade as a result of a series of problems that need to be systematically addressed. Therefore diagnosis on the basis of physical examination alone is extremely difficult. Prompt collection of a complete database (history, hematology, clinical chemistries, immunoglobulin status, radiographs, and ultrasonography) is often necessary to form a realistic idea of the neonate's problems and prognosis. The veterinarian must initiate treatment for the specific disease process while addressing the unique metabolic demands and physiologic instability of the newborn.

Another neonatal tendency that is extremely important in dictating the time course of clinical diagnosis, monitoring, and intervention is the rapidity with which changes in condition can occur, either for better or worse. Even a short delay in institution of therapy can make the difference between success and failure. The placentation of the large animal fetus does not allow transfer of immunoglobulins from mother to fetus in utero, and the newborn is dependent on the ingestion of colostrum shortly after birth for the majority of its immunoglobulins. Even with a normal level of circulating immunoglobulin, the immune system of the neonate is not as effective as that of the adult, and if failure of passive transfer of immunoglobulins occurs (see Chapter 49), the neonate is at higher risk of acquiring severe, generalized infections.

ROUTINE POSTPARTUM CARE OF THE NEWBORN FOAL

The newborn foal's behavioral patterns should be observed closely following parturition. Healthy full-term foals are precocious neonates that have an effective suckle reflex within 20 minutes of birth, can stand within 1 hour, and nurse from the udder within 2 hours of delivery. A veterinarian should examine all foals within the first day of life, but a foal that deviates from this simple time line should receive prompt attention. Any foal that fails to stand and nurse within 2 to 3 hours of delivery may be suffering from a variety of problems, including peripartum asphyxia, septicemia, prematurity, and musculoskeletal abnormalities.

Immediately postpartum, the modified Apgar score (Table 17-1) can be used to detect early signs of peripartum asphyxia. Each parameter in the score is assigned a value from 0 to 2. The optimal score is 10. The Apgar is best performed within 10 to 15 minutes of delivery.

Mucous membrane color is used to determine appearance. Pulse is self-explanatory and should be 60 beats/min soon after delivery and then increase above 100 beats/min within the first hour. Reflexes represent grimace. The thoracolumbar stimulus is performed by briskly running the thumb and forefingers down either side of the foal's spine. Attitude is translated into muscle tone and the ability to sit sternal. Respirations are shallow and should be greater than 30 breaths/min immediately after birth. Healthy foals have a score between 9 and 10. Scores between 6 and 8 indicate mild asphyxia. Such foals respond to brisk rubbing and limb manipulation to stimulate breathing. Foals with scores between 3 and 5 require intranasal oxygen and cardiovascular support. Foals with scores below 3 require more aggressive resuscitation (see Chapter 16).

The behavior of the mare toward her foal should be assessed, and care should be taken to minimize activities that disrupt the bonding process. Maternal behavior is an instinctual behavior that occurs during the immediate postpartum period. In some mares it is absent or replaced by direct aggression toward the foal or fear of the foal. The incidence of foal rejection is highest among primiparous mares and Arabians.[2] Mare rejection is probably multifactorial and may involve breed, familial, and hormonal factors, as well as environmental and physical stresses and past experience. It is important to distinguish fearful behavior from truly aggressive behavior. Many maiden mares are afraid of their foals. These mares may have nuzzled, nickered to, and licked their foals initially, but then become uneasy around the stag-gering, unpredictable newborn once it stands and begins searching for the udder.

Possible causes of foal rejection include pain associated with udder edema, uterine trauma following a difficult delivery, uterine contractions associated with stage III labor or gastrointestinal discomfort, interference with normal bonding by too much stall traffic during the peripartum period, and lack of maternal experience. A thorough examination of the dam and review of the foaling events may help uncover contributing factors. If maternal discomfort seems to be the problem, banamine administration may help. If a tender udder and poor milk letdown are contributing to pain associated with nursing, then application of warm compresses, udder massage, and the administration of oxytocin (10 to 20 U IM) may be effective. Acepromazine administration calms nervous mares and stimulates lactation through prolactin release without making the mare ataxic. When working with a fearful mare, introduce her to the foal's hindquarters rather than the foal's face. The hindquarters and tail are far less threatening and are the parts of the foal's anatomy that all mares see and sniff during normal nursing. Giving continuous physical and verbal reprimands whenever the mare tries to bite or kick her foal frustrates the mare and handler and intensifies the stress associated with nursing. If the mare is cow kicking, attach soft rope or leather hobbles to her hindlegs. If the mare is biting the foal, attach a grazing muzzle to her halter. Using sedation and mechanical restraints reduces the number of people who must be present when the foal tries to nurse and creates a calmer atmosphere while protecting the foal from a potentially fatal bite or kick. Frightened, hurting, or nervous mares should be given a reasonable length of time to bond with their foals. However, if the mare is demonstrating unprovoked aggression toward the foal or if a sick foal is failing to maintain homeostasis, then protection and stabilization of the foal should be considered a higher priority and the mare and foal should be separated.

In most cases the umbilicus breaks spontaneously about 2 inches (5 cm) from the body wall, when the mare or foal attempts to rise. If for some reason the cord does not break, it is best to break it manually by placing one hand on the abdominal wall and one hand distal to where the cord would naturally break and exerting a sharp, pulling force. Clamping a hemostat on the proximal end of the umbilicus helps crush the umbilical vessels to improve hemostasis and provides a more secure grip when bluntly tearing the cord. The umbilicus may also be clamped and cut, but this method does not promote the natural retraction of the umbilical structures and is associated with a higher incidence of hem-

TABLE 17-1

Apgar Score: Assessment of Neonatal Asphyxia*[1]

Parameter	0 Points	1 Point	2 Points
APPEARANCE	Gray/blue mucous membranes	Pale pink mucous membranes	Pink mucous membranes
PULSE (beats/min)	Absent	<60, irregular	>60, regular
GRIMACE			
Nasal stimulation	No response	Grimace	Strong grimace, sneeze
Ear tickle	No response	Head/neck motion	Ear tickle, head shake
Thoracolumbar stimulus	No response	Head/neck motion	Attempt to stand with head, neck, limb motion
ATTITUDE: (MUSCLE TONE)	Limp, lateral recumbency	Semisternal, some limb flexion	Sternal
RESPIRATION (breaths/min)	Absent	<30, irregular	>30, regular, can whinny

*Performed 1 min after delivery. A total score of 7 to 8 indicates a normal foal, 4 to 6 indicates moderate depression, and 0 to 3 indicates marked depression. Repeat evaluation in 4 min.

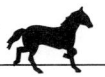

orrhage and patent urachus. It is routine practice to apply a disinfectant solution to the umbilical stump shortly after delivery. The results of a recent study suggest that a 0.5% chlorhexidine solution is preferable to the traditional 1% povidone or 2% or 7% iodine as an umbilical disinfectant in the foal. The chlorhexidine was more effective than the povidone or the 2% iodine solution in suppressing the number of organisms that colonize the umbilicus and did not have the caustic effects of the 7% iodine solution.[3] The umbilicus should be disinfected several times during the first 48 hours or until the umbilical stump is dry.

The nursing behavior of the newborn animal should be observed closely. If it has not nursed effectively by 2 to 3 hours of age, at least 20 ml/kg good-quality colostrum should be provided by bottle or gavage feeding to a foal and 40 ml/kg to the calf, ideally within the first 6 hours of age. Opinion varies regarding the need for routine measurement of immunoglobulin G (IgG) levels in apparently healthy, low-risk foals that are nursing well from the mare. Healthy foals that have consumed adequate amounts of good-quality colostrum should have a serum IgG concentration greater than 800 mg/dl by 18 to 24 hours of age. Failure of passive transfer (FPT) of colostral immunoglobulins, defined as serum IgG values below 400 mg/dl, is one of the common predisposing causes of infection in foals younger than 2 weeks of age.[4,5] In the high-risk foal, however, serum IgG determination should be performed within 18 hours of delivery. A foal should be considered high risk if any of the abnormal periparturient events listed in Box 17-1 have been observed.

Tetanus immunization (1500 U of tetanus antitoxin) should be administered to the newborn foal only if the neonate is suffering from FPT and does not receive timely immunoglobulin supplementation in the form of colostrum or

---

BOX 17-1

Periparturient Events Associated With High-Risk Neonates

PREPARTUM EVENTS
Premature udder development or precocious lactation in the dam
Severe maternal illness
Severe maternal malnutrition
Exposure to endophyte-infected fescue within 2 months of delivery
Inadequate prenatal maternal immunization
Advanced maternal age

PARTURIENT EVENTS
Premature delivery
Prolonged gestation
Premature placental separation
Meconium staining of fetus, placenta, or fluids
Agalactia
Severe dystocia
Cesarean section
Induced delivery
Grossly abnormal or heavy placenta (>11% foal's body weight)

POSTPARTUM EVENTS
Failure of neonate to stand and nurse within 3 hours of delivery
Low Apgar score
Abnormal physical examination findings, including generalized weakness, poor suckle, severe angular limb deformities, enlarged or bleeding umbilicus, patent urachus, respiratory distress, diarrhea, colic, or other signs of localized infection

---

intravenous plasma administration. Foals born in regions of the country known to have selenium-deficient soils should receive selenium supplementation soon after birth if their mares have not received additional selenium supplementation during pregnancy.

In an effort to prevent the discomfort and straining often accompanying the passage of meconium, enemas are often administered routinely to the newborn foal. The most commonly used enemas are the commercially available phosphate-based type (e.g., Fleet). Proper restraint and careful passage of the applicator tip are important to avoid traumatizing the rectal mucosa. Alternatively, a gravity enema may be given using a soft stallion urinary catheter to infuse warm, dilute soapy water into the rectum.

Although I highly recommend that all high-risk newborn foals receive hematologic evaluation early in life, the cost effectiveness of routine hematology in apparently normal foals has not been established. The routine administration of one injection of penicillin or penicillin-streptomycin to low-risk newborn foals is not recommended. If the newborn foal is a high-risk individual or if there is reasonable suspicion of infection, appropriate diagnostic tests and cultures should be taken and broad-spectrum bactericidal antibiotic therapy should be started as soon as possible.

POSTPARTUM ASSESSMENT AND CARE OF NEWBORN RUMINANTS

JOHN K. HOUSE

Calves and lambs normally have a head-righting reflex almost immediately after birth. Sternal recumbency usually is attained within 2 to 3 minutes, followed rapidly by attempts to stand at 10 to 20 minutes for lambs and 15 to 30 minutes for calves.[6,7] Hypoxic neonates may struggle and appear bright initially but have difficulty maintaining sternal recumbency, have depressed or absent suck reflex, are slow to stand or remain recumbent, and develop a depressed mentation within hours. After experimentally induced hypoxia, nonviable hypoxic calves had similar heart rates (118 ± 36 beats/min) and body temperatures (39.6° ± 0.2° C) as viable calves but lower respiratory rates (14 and 18 vs. normal 49 ± 12).[6] The normal time taken to stand and nurse varies between species and breeds. In cattle the average time from birth to standing and nursing varies according to breed. The average time from birth to standing and nursing for beef calves is 35 and 81 minutes respectively. Dairy calves take approximately twice as long.[8] Small ruminants are generally quicker to stand and nurse than calves, with most lambs standing within 30 minutes[7] and nursing within 90 minutes of birth. Failure of the newborn to nurse may result from reduced neonatal vigor, poor mothering, poor maternal conformation, or adverse conditions such as slippery flooring. Calves have difficulty locating teats on low-slung udders (less than 45 cm from the ground)[9] and difficulty nursing teats greater than 35 mm in diameter.[10] Observation of interaction between the newborn and dam in the immediate postnatal period allows early recognition of the compromised neonate and facilitates timely intervention if maternal conformation or behavior threatens to impede the neonate's efforts to nurse.

Failure of maternal bonding is more common with primiparous dams, multiple offspring, and after delivery via cesarean section. Maternal bonding in sheep is mediated by an olfactory mechanism.[11] Parturition alters the release of monoamines, amino acids, and oxytocin within the olfactory bulb, stimulating an attraction to amniotic fluid and acceptance of the lamb.[12] Artificial vaginocervical stimulation with a gloved hand induces similar alterations in the release of

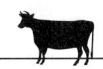
monoamines, amino acids, and oxytocin within the olfactory bulb and is useful for triggering formation of maternal bonds to foster lambs for at least 27 hours postpartum.[12]

Abnormal neonatal behavior in the immediate postnatal period is commonly secondary to perinatal hypoxia. Resuscitation of the newborn is discussed in Chapter 16. In utero infections and congenital neurologic abnormalities should also be considered as possible causes of abnormal neonatal behavior. Collection of sera before feeding colostrum is useful for diagnosing in utero infections. Precolostral serum immunoglobulin concentrations in calves are very low (IgM, 0.126 ± 0.015 mg/ml, IgG, 0.044 ± 0.003 mg/ml).[13] Elevated serum concentrations of immunoglobulins before ingestion of colostrum may be observed with in utero infections.[13] Specific serologic tests are available for Cache Valley virus, Akabane virus, bovine virus, diarrhea virus, *Neospora* spp., toxoplasma, and bluetongue virus.[14] Teratogens and inherited diseases that may cause the birth of weak neonates are listed in Table 15-3.

Tube feeding colostrum during the first 12 hours of life is appropriate if free choice consumption is questionable. Drying, warming, and tube feeding colostrum may revive weak newborn lambs and kids. Tube feeding dairy calves 3 L of colostrum at birth is recommended because failure of passive transfer is high (61%) in dairy calves left to nurse their dams.[15]

Literature on the efficacy of navel treatment at reducing calf mortality is divided. In a study of 104 dairy farms a farm policy of navel treating newborn calves had no significant effect on calf mortality rates. A significant beneficial effect was observed when the navels of calves that had assisted deliveries were dipped with chlorhexidine; other navel treatments such as iodine tended to be associated with an increased odds of dying.[16] Navel treatment with iodine was associated with significantly higher mortality in another study of 48 farms; however, the association of navel treatment with mortality on these farms may have reflected the response of producers to high neonatal mortality rather than indicating that navel treatment is a risk factor for high calf mortality.[17] Prophylactic administration of antibi-

otics to young calves has been associated with an increased incidence of diarrhea[18] and increased calf mortality.[19]

In regions deficient in selenium nutritional myodegeneration can be a major cause of death in neonates if the dam has not been supplemented with selenium during pregnancy. Nutritional myodegeneration has also been observed when selenium levels are adequate but α-tocopherol levels are low.[20,21] The concentration of vitamin E in sheep colostrum is 5 to 11 times higher than milk and appears to be an important source of vitamin E for lambs because vitamin E is transferred poorly across the placenta. Nutritional myodegeneration secondary to vitamin E deficiency is observed when pregnant ewes are maintained on forage low in vitamin E. Vitamin E–associated nutritional myodegeneration may be prevented by supplementing lambs and kids at birth with α-tocopherol (500 IU orally) or by supplementing ewes during pregnancy either via a single dose of 500 mg IM 2 weeks before lambing or via dietary supplementation, delivering 150 mg daily for 3 to 4 weeks before lambing.[21] Neonatal nutritional myodegeneration associated with selenium deficiency may similarly be prevented by supplementing neonates at birth (2.5 to 3 mg selenium/ 45 kg) or via supplementing the dam during pregnancy, and is discussed further in Chapter 40.

PHYSICAL EXAMINATION OF THE NEONATE

WENDY E. VAALA

JOHN K. HOUSE

JOHN E. MADIGAN

GENERAL EXAMINATION

A complete physical examination is an important component of the workup of the large animal neonate. Although many parameters are similar in the adult and neonatal animal,

---

TABLE 17-2

Normal Physical Examination Parameters of the Neonatal Foal and Calf

Parameter	Foal	Calf
Gestational age	241 days (327-365) < 320 days = premature	278-282 (Holstein) 281-282 (Shorthorn) 292 (271-310) (Brahma)
Time to suckling reflex (stimulated by placing a finger in the mouth)	2-20 min	2-20 min
Time to stand	57 min (15-165 min) > 2 hr abnormal	60-158 min 60-228 min without dam
Time to nurse from mother	111 min (35-420 min) > 3-4 hr abnormal	1-4 hr
Body temperature	37°-38° C (99°-102° F) AM nonstressed value	37°-38° C (100°-102° F)
Heart rate	1-5 min postfoaling > 60 beats/min 6-60 min postfoaling 80-130 beats/min Day 1-5 80-120 beats/min	90-110 beats/min
Respiratory rate	Postfoaling for 30 min 60-80 breaths/min 1-12 hours in sternal recumbency 30-40 breaths/min	

there are important differences, which are outlined in this section. An initial assessment of the sick neonate should be made to determine if there is a need for immediate intervention and stabilization (e.g., if respiratory distress, cyanosis, hypothermia, hypotension, or shock are present). Particular attention should also be paid to identification of any congenital malformations. Normal parameters for the foal and calf are listed in Tables 17-2 to 17-5.[22-33] A newborn foal should be considered potentially abnormal if it takes longer than 2 hours to stand or longer than 3 hours to suckle from the mare.

Physical examination begins with a quick assessment of the foal's body language. Healthy foals are bright, alert, and inquisitive. The first sign of neonatal weakness is a drooping head carriage and ears at half-mast. Sick foals spend increasing amounts of time recumbent and less time nursing, resulting in udder distention in the dam and a milk-stained face on the foal. Sick foals are often more difficult to arouse from sleep.

Cardiovascular System

Peripheral pulses, such as at the great metatarsal and brachial arteries, should be strong and regular, and the limbs should be warm. Hypotension is common in foals that are seriously ill or very premature. Indirect blood pressure measurement can provide important information regarding the cardiovascular status of the patient. Commercially available units

TABLE 17-3

Normal Hematology Reference Values (for Neonatal Foals)

Parameter	Gestational Age (Premature Foals)			Postnatal Age (Term Foals)	
	300-309 Days Mean	310-319 Days Mean	320-334 Days Mean	1 Day Mean ± SD	2-7 Days Mean ± SD
RBC ($\times 10^6/\mu l$)	9.6	10.1	11.3	10.5 ± 1	9.26 ± 0.8
Hb (g/dl)	13.1	14.1	13.2	14.4 ± 1.1	13.2 ± 1.2
PCV (%)	41	42	43	42.0 ± 3.6	36.5 ± 3.1
MCV (fl)	42.7	42.2	38.6	40.2 ± 3.6	39.4 ± 2.3
MCH (pg)	14	14.4	11.8	13.6 ± 1.1	14.5 ± 1.1
MCHC (%)	32.4	33.8	30.5	33.8 ± 2	36.2 ± 1.1
Icterus index (u)				40.0 ± 15	30.0 ± 15
Total plasma protein (g/dl)				6.1 ± 0.8	6.4 ± 0.6
Fibrinogen (mg/dl)				243 ± 74	310 ± 90
Total WBC/μl	5000	6800	4900	8632 ± 2570	9075 ± 2200
Neutrophils/μl	1230	1540	1940	6381 ± 2225	6528 ± 2000
Bands/μl				< 50	> 50
Lymphocytes/μl	3720	5090	2960	2021 ± 2225	2203 ± 575
Monocytes/μl				222 ± 160	305 ± 145
Eosinophils/μl				0	22
Basophils/μl				8	17
Neutrophil:lymph ratio	0.33	0.3	0.66	3.16	2.96

Hb, Hemoglobin; *MCH,* mean corpuscular hemoglobin; *MCHC,* mean corpuscular hemoglobin concentration; *MCV,* mean corpuscular volume; *PCV,* packed cell volume; *RBC,* red blood cell; *WBC,* white blood cell.

TABLE 17-4

Normal Serum Biochemical Reference Values for Normal-Term Postnursing Foals

Parameter	Age		Parameter	Age	
	1 Day Mean ± SD	4-7 Days Mean ± SD		1 Day Mean ± SD	4-7 Days Mean ± SD
Sodium (mEq/L)	139.7 ± 6	139.5 ± 4.2	Total bilirubin (mg/dl)	4.3 ± 2.2	4.4 ± 1.1
Potassium (mEq/L)	4.4 ± 0.9	4.5 ± 0.4	Direct bilirubin (mg/dl)	0.5 ± 0.2	0.8 ± 0.4
Chloride (mEq/L)	103.5 ± 3	101.3 ± 4	Indirect bilirubin (mg/dl)	3.8 ± 1.5	3.5 ± 1.1
Bicarbonate (mEq/L)	22.9 ± 3.4	24.3 ± 2.1	Alkaline phosphatase (IU/L)	2282 ± 1100	1949 ± 1100
Calcium (mg/dl)	11.7 ± 1.1	11.4 ± 0.8	GGT (IU/L)	29.6 ± 15	18.3 ± 7.3
Inoganic phosphorus (mg/dl)	5 ± 0.85	6.4 ± 0.8	SDH (IU/L)	2 ± 0.9	2 ± 0.9
Magnesium (mg/dl)	2.2 ± 0.35	2.7 ± 0.15	AST (SGOT) (IU/L)	154 ± 55	225 ± 60
Glucose (mg/dl)	136 ± 40	150 ± 30	LDH (IU/L)	487 ± 100	490 ± 100
BUN (mg/dl)	18.9 ± 4.3	13.6 ± 5.6			
Creatinine (mg/dl)	2.3 ± 0.6	1.3 ± 0.3			

AST, Aspartate aminotransferase (SGOT); *BUN,* blood urea nitrogen; *GGT,* γ-glutamyltransferase; *LDH,* lactate dehydrogenase; *SDH,* sorbitol dehydrogenase.

TABLE 17-5

Normal Hematology Reference Values (for Neonatal Calves)

Parameter	Age			
	Birth	24 hours	48 hours	3 weeks
Red blood cells ($\times 10^6/\mu l$)	9.35 ± 1.02	8.17 ± 1.34	7.72 ± 1.09	8.86 ± 0.68
Hemoglobin (g/dl)	12.86 ± 1.85	10.93 ± 2.05	10.49 ± 1.8	11.32 ± 1.02
Packed cell volume (%)	41 ± 6	34 ± 6	32 ± 6	35 ± 3
Mean corpuscular volume (fl)	43.2 ± 2.4	41 ± 2.8	41.1 ± 2.3	39.1 ± 1.9
Mean corpuscular hemoglobin concentration (g/dl)	31.3 ± 1.1	32.1 ± 0.8	32.6 ± 1.0	32.8 ± 1.6
Total WBC/μl	13.99 ± 5.73	9.81 ± 2.8	7.76 ± 1.95	8.65 ± 1.69
Neutrophils/μl	10,940 ± 5,700	6,480 ± 2,660	4,110 ± 2,040	2,920 ± 1,140
Bands/μl	100 ± 150	310 ± 460	210 ± 450	10 ± 30
Lymphocytes/μl	2,980 ± 2,730	2,730 ± 820	2,850 ± 880	5,050 ± 800
Monocytes/μl	590 ± 660	230 ± 210	350 ± 280	620 ± 330
Eosinophils/μl	0	20 ± 40	20 ± 30	20 ± 40
Basophils/μl	0	0.02 ± 0.05	0.02 ± 0.05	0.02 ± 0.04
Total plasma protein (g/dl)	4.8 ± 0.3	6.4 ± 0.7	6.4 ± 0.7	6.4 ± 0.3
Fibrinogen (mg/dl)	258 ± 138	288 ± 105	335 ± 116	283 ± 147
Urea nitrogen (mg/dl)	6.36 ± 2.36	7.52 ± 2.13	6.93 ± 3.13	
Creatinine (mg/dl)	4.14 ± 1.27	1.69 ± 0.35	1.27 ± 0.24	
Total bilirubin	0.34 ± 0.66	1.28 ± 0.5	0.89 ± 0.41	
Sodium (mEq/L)	141 ± 3.77	135 ± 2.86	135 ± 3.68	
Potassium (mEq/L)	6.1 ± 1.86	5.46 ± 0.56	5.63 ± 0.96	
Chloride (mEq/L)	97.39	95.76	95.28	
Calcium (mg/dl)	12.24 ± 1.64	10.22 ± 1.2	10.65 ± 0.56	
Phosphorus (mg/dl)	8.16 ± 1.39	7.22 ± 0.87	7.46 ± 0.87	
Creatinine phosphokinase (IU/L)	83 ± 42	531 ± 532	256 ± 364	
Aspartate aminotransferase (IU/L)	18 ± 19	99 ± 18	72 ± 25	
γ-Glutamyl transferase (IU/L)	8 ± 3	1761 ± 1058	846 ± 517	

Data from Adams R et al: *Am J Vet Res* 53:944-950, 1992; and Adams R et al: *Cornell Vet* 83:13-29, 1993.

provide reasonably accurate results if the procedure is performed carefully.[34]

Mucous membranes should be moist and pale pink, with a capillary refill time of less than 2 seconds. Hyperemic membranes accompanied by scleral injection and red coronary bands are the hallmark of early sepsis. Icteric mucous membranes in a newborn foal that has not nursed suggest sepsis or possible EHV-1 infection. Jaundice in an older foal that has had several meals of colostrum raises the possibility of neonatal isoerythrolysis as a cause of icterus. Petechiae on the oral or nasal mucous membranes or inside the pinna are indicative of early sepsis. Petechiae may be the result of sepsis-induced vasculitis and thrombocytopenia. Gray or cyanotic mucous membranes are associated with severe hypoxia (i.e., Pao_2 <35-40 mm Hg) or circulatory collapse as seen with hypotensive, endotoxic, or hypovolemic shock. Cardiac and pulmonary causes of cyanosis must be distinguished.

Cardiac murmurs usually mean less during the newborn period than at any other time in an animal's life. Very serious heart anomalies may not be accompanied by any murmur, whereas a closing ductus arteriosus may cause a murmur that is very loud and therefore quite worrisome and misleading. This normal ductal murmur is best auscultated on the left side of the chest at the third intercostal space at the level of the shoulder. In most foals this murmur disappears by 48 to 96 hours of age. In some instances, however, it is described as a continuous machinery type of murmur, but far more commonly a grade II to V/VI holosystolic murmur is auscultated. Although the holosystolic murmur has usually disappeared by the time the foal is 1 week of age, in some foals it can be auscultated for the first 2 to 3 months of age in the absence of any detectable cardiac abnormalities.[35] In the majority of foals the patent ductus arteriosus (PDA) is benign because birth-induced changes in intracardiac and pulmonary pressures result in a reversal of blood flow: vena cava to right atrium to right ventricle to pulmonary artery to lungs to pulmonary vein to left atrium to left ventricle to aorta to PDA and back through the pulmonary artery into the lungs or into the descending and ascending aorta into the systemic circulation. In this scenario the PDA shunts a small volume of already oxygenated blood back through the lungs. Such foals may have hypervascularity of the lungs on radiographs but otherwise suffer no untoward effects. Pathologic causes of a persistent murmur include PDA, ventricular septal defect (VSD), and other valvular defects. Bacterial endocarditis should be considered if a cardiac murmur is associated with recurrent fevers and repeated pyogenic infections. Myocardial dysfunction has been documented in septicemic foals.[36]

Dyspnea and coughing are often the predominant clinical signs of congestive heart failure in calves. Close examination may reveal distention of the jugular veins and brisket edema, but if heart failure is predominantly left sided these may be absent. Cardiomyopathy secondary to selenium deficiency, gossypol, monensin, or lasalocid toxicity may present as a syndrome of sudden death during periods of excitement precipitated by feeding or moving calves out of hutches into group pens.[37]

Cardiac arrhythmias are observed sporadically in neonates, often associated with diarrhea. Metabolic acidosis secondary to losses of electrolytes and water causes a transcellular shift of potassium ions into the extracellular fluid in exchange for hydrogen ions.[38] As serum potassium increases (>5.5 mEq/L), aberrations in cardiac excitability occur and are manifested as progressive atrial standstill, progressing to ventricular fibrilla-

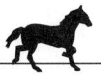

tion and asystole.[39] Foals with hyperkalemia, hyponatremia, and hypochloremia associated with uroperitoneum may experience a variety of cardiac arrhythmias including ventricular premature contractions, ventricular tachycardia, ventricular fibrillation, and third-degree atrioventricular block. Tachyarrhythmias may be observed in calves with cardiomyopathies, ionophore toxicosis,[40] or hypomagnesemia.

The most common cardiac defect in the large animal neonate is a ventricular septal defect, but a variety of other malformations have been described and are discussed in Chapters 6, 28, and 47. Ancillary tests for evaluating the cardiovascular system are discussed in Chapter 28.

Respiratory System

The respiratory rate and work of breathing are best observed from some distance away before the neonate is handled, so that the excitement of being restrained does not influence the assessment. The breathing pattern in the awake, standing foal should be regular. During rapid eye movement sleep, the pattern of breathing may become markedly irregular, with alternating periods of apnea and tachypnea. The visible effort of breathing should be minimal, with no excessive rib retraction or grunting. Conditions causing partial occlusion of the upper airway, such as stenotic nares, choanal atresia, collapsing trachea, guttural pouch tympany, and subepiglottic cyst, often induce pronounced inspiratory stridor. Expiratory stridor and increased and prolonged expiratory effort are usually associated with lower airway disease.[41] A malodorous breath may be present with necrotic pharyngeal injuries, necrotic laryngitis, or aspiration pneumonia. Age is an important signalment for respiratory disease in calves. Enzootic pneumonia is common in calves between 4 weeks and 6 months of age but uncommon in calves less than 4 weeks of age. Outbreaks of pneumonia in calves less than 4 weeks of age are occasionally observed in calves fed milk contaminated with *Mycoplasma* spp.[42,43] This scenario is one of the risks associated with feeding calves unpasteurized "hospital milk." *Mycoplasma* pneumonia in calves may be associated with arthritis, tenosynovitis, otitis media,[43] and decubital abscesses.[44] Clinical signs associated with mycoplasma otitis include cranial nerve 7 and 8 deficits and unilateral or bilateral ear droop, ptosis, epiphora, head tilt, and recumbency in severely affected calves. Aspiration pneumonia is common in calves less than a week of age, often reflecting inappropriate feeding practices (large holes in teat nipples) or pharyngeal dysfunction.

Lung sounds of neonates are typically much easier to hear than those of adults, but the loudness of the large airway sounds may obscure subtle abnormalities in the smaller airways. *Frequently, lung sounds do not correlate well with the severity of pulmonary pathology present.* Animals with few or no audible thoracic abnormalities may have severe respiratory disease, particularly interstitial pulmonary involvement and atelectasis. On the other hand, increasingly obvious adventitial lung sounds may be associated with resolution rather than with deterioration of the disease process. Fine inspiratory rales are often heard immediately postpartum and are associated with inflation of fluid-filled alveoli. Because of the difficulty in accurately assessing the respiratory system through physical examination alone, chest radiology, thoracic ultrasonography, and arterial blood gas analysis have become integral components of the workup of the abnormal neonate. Ultrasound evaluation can be particularly useful in the diagnosis of diaphragmatic hernias; pleural effusions, such as hemothorax; and pulmonary abscessation.[45,46]

Lung disease in the newborn is usually diffuse and is the result of infection acquired in utero or postpartum or lung atelectasis associated with immaturity, recumbency, or surfactant dysfunction. Signs of lung disease include increased work of breathing characterized by nostril flare, rib retractions, and increased abdominal effort. A cough and nasal discharge, salient features of respiratory disease in older neonates, are infrequent findings in newborn foals with lung disease. Work of breathing is a more accurate way to assess the severity of lung pathology in the newborn during a physical examination. Foals on the brink of respiratory failure begin to grunt at the end of expiration as a form of physiologic positive end-expiratory expiration (PEEP) in an attempt to keep alveoli inflated. Affected foals also demonstrate paradoxical respiration associated with collapse of the chest wall during inspiration because of respiratory muscle fatigue and increasing lung stiffness. Periodic apnea and abnormally slow respirations are often the result of metabolic disturbances (e.g., hypoglycemia, hypocalcemia), hypothermia, advanced prematurity, or hypoxia-induced suppression of the respiratory center. Tachypnea is often a response to pain or stress. If birth was difficult, check carefully for fractured ribs. In addition to palpating crepitus over the broken ribs, a faint clicking sound can be heard during inspiration on the side of the chest with the rib fracture(s).

Congenital defects of the upper airways of the neonate include various malformations of the larynx, nares, and trachea, including collapsed trachea, stenotic nares, choanal atresia, subepiglottal cyst, and guttural pouch tympany (foal). Congenital malformations of the lower respiratory system are quite rare but include diaphragmatic hernias and agenesis of a lung lobe.

Gastrointestinal Tract and Abdomen

In contrast to the adult, rectal palpation of the abdominal structures of the large animal neonate is of very limited value. External palpation of the abdomen can be more rewarding, depending on the cooperation of the individual and how tense the abdominal musculature is. The inguinal rings and umbilical area should be palpated for hernias. In the foal with a relaxed abdominal wall, palpation can sometimes detect impactions of the large and small colon and other masses, and the urinary bladder may be palpated and expressed. Hairballs (trichobezoars) may be palpated in the rumen of calves.

Abdominal auscultation should reveal borborygmi in all quadrants in the normal large animal neonate. Colostrum ingestion and the act of suckling enhance gastrointestinal motility and manure passage. Simultaneous auscultation and percussion identify areas of tympany.

The first manure passed is meconium and is dark black or brown and pelleted or pasty in consistency. Meconium consists of glandular secretions of the intestinal tract, swallowed amniotic fluid, and other cell debris. Before birth it is moved along the gastrointestinal tract by peristalsis and stored in the colon and rectum. Meconium is generally dark brown to black in color and may be found in hard pellets or in a paste-like mass. A change in the color and consistency of the feces to a lighter brown, less tenacious material indicates that the meconium has been passed. Meconium is expelled before delivery only if the fetus is subjected to stressful conditions, particularly asphyxia. If meconium contaminates the amniotic fluid, when the newly born animal takes its first breath, aspiration of the meconium-contaminated fluid can result in severe respiratory distress (see Chapter 20). Within a few hours after birth many newborn animals display some degree of straining and pass most of the meconium within the first 48 hours of life. The ingestion of colostrum seems to stimulate gastrointestinal motility and aids the passage of meconium.

Meconium impaction is the most common cause of colic in the otherwise healthy newborn foal (particularly colts) and in most instances resolves uneventfully with medical therapy, which includes enema(s) and oral stool softeners. However, any medical condition interfering with gastrointestinal motility, such as asphyxia and enteritis, can impede the passage of meconium and result in a severe impaction. Any newborn large animal that fails to pass any meconium within the first 12 to 24 hours of life and on digital examination has only mucus in the distal rectum should be considered at high risk of having an incomplete gastrointestinal tract such as atresia coli or recti. Further discussion on the causes of abdominal distention in the neonate can be found in Chapter 20.

Distention of the small or large bowel results in generalized abdominal enlargement that is readily apparent because of the neonate's thin body wall. Abdominal distention and colic may be associated with ileus, peritonitis, enteritis, hypoxic gut damage, meconium impaction, or other intestinal obstruction (e.g., intussusception, volvulus).

Abdominal radiographs and/or ultrasound examination can be very helpful in diagnosing abdominal problems in the neonate and in distinguishing causes of abdominal distention.[47-49] Transabdominal ultrasonography can be used to locate a suitable site for abdominocentesis. Normal peritoneal fluid values for equine neonates include a nucleated cell count of less than 1500 cells/µl and total protein of 2 g/dl or less.[50] Normal peritoneal fluid from calves has a higher nucleated cell count than that of adult cattle (3350 cells/µl vs. 1371 cells/µl). Total protein concentration in peritoneal fluid of calves is similar to that of adults (2.5 g/dl vs. 3.1 g/dl).[51]

Common congenital defects of the gastrointestinal tract include cleft palate, poor jaw conformation (brachygnathism, inferior and superior), atresia coli, atresia recti, and atresia ani. The spiral loop of the ascending colon (spiral colon) is the most commonly affected segment of intestine in calves.[52] Matings between two Overo paint horses may result in a lethal white foal, which is characterized by terminal ileocolonic aganglionosis.[53] Affected foals retain meconium and demonstrate progressive colic beginning on day 1. There is no cure for the disease. Coat color and aganglionosis are probably related because both melanocytes and intestinal ganglia cells originate from the neural crest. Inheritance is most likely autosomal recessive.

Passage of melena may be associated with infectious enteritis (e.g., clostridiosis, salmonellosis) and necrotizing enterocolitis caused by hypoxic-ischemic bowel injury. Infectious diarrhea is the leading cause of mortality in calves between 3 and 21 days of age. Typically more than one pathogen is involved and the physical examination provides no indication of the etiologic agent. Fecal pH may be used as an indicator to distinguish secretory diarrhea (enterotoxigenic *Escherichia coli*) from diarrhea associated with malabsorption and maldigestion. Secretory diarrhea produces an alkaline pH, whereas malabsorption and maldigestion is associated with an acidic fecal pH.[54] Infectious agents causing diarrhea, and ancillary tests available to establish an etiologic diagnosis are discussed in Chapter 20.

Abnormal forestomach function in neonatal ruminants, like adults, is often reflected by altered abdominal contour as described in Chapter 30. Left and right abomasal displacement and abomasal torsion are observed sporadically in calves. Succussion (simultaneous auscultation and percussion) is useful for delimiting the boundaries of distended visci. Passage of a stomach tube helps distinguish rumen and abomasal distention and facilitates collection of a rumen fluid sample. A putrid odor to neonatal rumen fluid is common with putrefactive indigestion when milk is delivered to the rumen in greater quantities than normal by escaping the esophageal groove or via excessive backflow from the abomasum. Reflux of abomasal contents into the reticulum and rumen, independent of feeding, occurs in connection with abomasal inflammation and obstructions.[55] Evaluation of rumen fluid pH and renin activity are useful for distinguishing abomasal reflux from esophageal groove overflow. Rumen fluid pH is usually 7 or greater with rumen putrefaction, and low to normal with abomasal reflux.[55] Chymosin (renin) is normally present in abomasal juice, and renin activity in rumen fluid suggests abomasal reflux.[56] Renin activity is measured by adding 2 ml of rumen juice to 2 ml of whole milk on a California Mastitis Test (CMT) plate. Presence of renin in the ruminal fluid causes coagulation of the casein in the milk. Chloride ion concentration in rumen fluid from calves is higher than adults (55 to 102 mmol/L in calves[57]; 25 mmol/L in adults[55]), possibly reflecting the high chloride content of milk 45 mmol/L; therefore the chloride concentration of rumen fluid is not useful for identifying abomasal reflux in calves.

Urogenital System

The mean time to first urination in pony foals was found to be 8.5 hours, with fillies first urinating at 10.8 hours and colts at 6 hours of age.[58] Because of the large volume of milk normal nursing foals drink each day, the volume of urine voided is large (148 ml/kg/day), the urine osmolarity is low (102 ± 24 mOsm/L), and urination occurs at frequent intervals.[59] Normal urine osmolarity in the 2- to 3-day-old calf has been reported to be 286 to 391 mOsm/L, and urine volume voided per day has been reported to be 34 ml/kg/day.[60] Because of a persistent frenulum, some colts may not extend their penis to urinate during the first week of life.

Congenital abnormalities of the urinary system include ruptured urinary bladder, ruptured ureter, ectopic ureter, blocked urethra, renal agenesis, fused kidney, and polycystic kidneys. Rupture of the urinary bladder at parturition is common in male foals but uncommon in ruminants. Clinical signs of a ruptured bladder include dysuria, stranguria, progressive abdominal distention, and depression. Some foals with ruptured bladders are able to urinate small volumes of urine. A percussion wave may be felt with ballotment of the distended abdomen. Ancillary tests including abdominal ultrasound, abdominocentesis, and assessment of serum and peritoneal electrolytes are useful to verify the diagnosis. In the filly, increasing protrusion of the vulva has been associated with a ruptured ureter and retroperitoneal accumulation of urine.[61] The mucous membranes of the vulva should be examined for the presence of jaundice, petechial hemorrhages, and edema.

The testicles may be in the scrotum at birth or should descend by 6 months of age. In horses the definitive diagnosis of cryptorchidism is usually reserved until a colt is 1 year of age. Abdominal cryptorchidism is a dominantly inherited trait. The external genitalia of both sexes should be examined for congenital malformations. In the calf, congenital defects described include ovarian aplasia, duplication of the cervix in Hereford cattle, persistence of the hymen (white heifer disease), and rectovaginal constriction in Jersey cattle. Congenital urolithiasis has been described in calves and lambs. Calcium oxalate is the most commonly reported congenital form of urolithiasis and may be associated with other congenital abnormalities.[62] A report of renal oxalosis in a number of beefmaster calves suggests a possible recessively inherited metabolic defect resulting in primary hyperoxaluria in this breed.[63] Freemartins (XX/XY chimeras) occur in over 90% of bovine[64] and 1% of ovine[65] female heterosexual twins. Typically freemartins are sterile and have hypoplastic ovaries and internal tubal genitalia; the external genitalia normally are not affected. Males should be examined for cryptorchidism and male pseudohermaphroditism and both sexes for evidence of hermaphroditism (gonads of both sexes).

Hemodynamically mediated renal disease is observed sporadically in calves after chronic enteritis.[66] Prolonged reduced renal perfusion secondary to hypovolemia may lead to ischemia and acute tubular necrosis. Failure to thrive following apparent recovery from diarrhea may reflect compromised renal function. Renal failure has also been observed after drug-induced acute tubular necrosis in foals.[67]

Examination of the Umbilicus

Umbilical cord remnant infections represent an important problem in neonates.[46] The infection generally develops during the first 2 weeks of life. Complications associated with umbilical infections include umbilical abscess, acquired patent urachus, omphalitis, omphalophlebitis, and omphaloarteritis and can progress to septicemia, septic arthritis, and osteomyelitis.[68,69] Early detection of umbilical abnormalities can be a decisive step in the success of neonatal management. An umbilical infection may be present when alternative sites of sepsis exist or when an inflammatory profile of unknown origin is present.[46,68]

The umbilicus should be examined closely for patency, increased size, moistness or discharge, and tenderness. Abdominal palpation, using both hands pressing together, is useful for evaluating the umbilicus of ruminants. Enlargement of the umbilical arteries can be palpated coursing caudally toward the bladder, and enlargement of the umbilical vein can be palpated coursing cranially to the liver. Application of pressure caudal to the xiphoid often elicits a soft grunt from calves with a septic umbilicus and associated peritonitis. Extensive adhesion of bowel to inflamed umbilical structures produces a large, easily palpable intraabdominal mass. Common abnormalities of the calf umbilicus include umbilical hernias, omphalophlebitis, external umbilical abscess, urachal abscess, and omphaloarteritis. Patent urachus is uncommon in calves. Only a small portion of the umbilical structures of foals can be evaluated on physical examination, however, and many umbilical abnormalities are missed on the basis of physical examination alone. Therefore ultrasound examination of the intraabdominal umbilical structures has become an important diagnostic tool.

A common abnormality of the umbilicus in the foal is the patent urachus. A patent urachus may be congenital but is more commonly acquired. Usually the urachus closes normally following delivery; however, with illness, debilitation, or improper umbilical treatment at birth, it spontaneously reopens a few days later. A high incidence of patent urachus has been observed in foals in which the umbilicus has been cut, clamped, or tied after delivery rather than being allowed to break and retract spontaneously. Closure of the patent urachus usually occurs in a few days to 2 weeks; silver nitrate sticks are frequently used with the hope of speeding healing, but their efficacy has not been proven. In a few cases, surgery is required to ligate the urachus. The ultrasonographic appearance of a patent urachus is shown in Fig. 17-1.

Bleeding from the umbilicus may occur intermittently after birth, particularly if the umbilicus was cut or tied. Occasionally, hemoperitoneum results from substantial hemorrhage from an umbilical vessel within the abdominal cavity, and shock and death may occur.

Although traditionally it has been noted that a patent urachus predisposes to ascending infection, cystitis, and joint illness, these complications have been infrequently encountered in the young foal undergoing intensive care, perhaps because of concurrent antibiotic administration. The vast majority of patent urachus cases in foals that occurred as a complication during hospitalization often resolve uneventfully

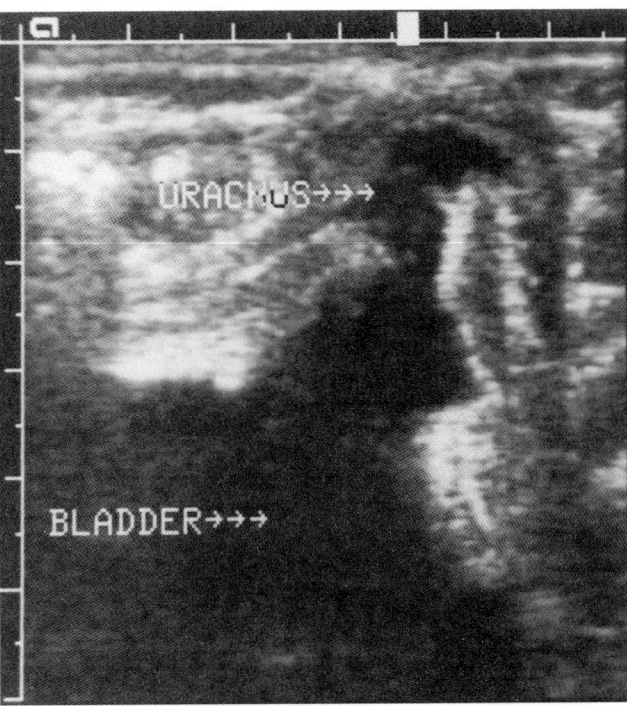

FIG. 17-1 ■ Ultrasound longitudinal section of the urinary bladder of a foal with a patent urachus *(arrows)* leading from the apex of the bladder toward the body wall.

with medical therapy. Once recumbent foals are ambulatory, improved body wall tone and more regular micturition facilitates closure of the patent urachus. On the other hand, particularly in the slightly older foal (1 week to 1 month), umbilical infections are relatively common. In foals this age, the spontaneous development of a patent urachus is more likely to indicate umbilical infection. If there is reason to suspect that the urachus or remnants of the umbilical vessels are infected (pain on palpation, unexplained inflammatory hemogram, fever of unknown origin, purulent discharge), ultrasound examination is often very useful in identifying the infected or abscessed structures.[70]

DIAGNOSIS OF UMBILICAL DISORDERS USING ULTRASOUND

JOHN E. MADIGAN
JOHN K. HOUSE

Ultrasonography has been used to quantitatively correlate umbilical structural changes with age in foals. Mean diameters for selected umbilical structures derived from 13 foals ranging from 6 hours to 4 weeks of age have been reported.[71] Foals may be examined in a stall adjacent to their dams and near the stall door. Foals are made to lie down without sedation, using the method depicted in Fig. 17-2. Foals will usually become quiet and still within a few minutes of recumbency. All ultrasound examinations are performed with the foal in left lateral recumbency with the ultrasound machine behind the examiner (Fig. 17-3.)

Fig. 17-3 depicts a diagram of the anatomic locations of the structures examined during the ultrasound evaluation. A 5- to 8-cm-wide strip of hair can be clipped along the ventral midline, extending from the umbilical stump cranial to the xiphoid to facilitate examination of the umbilical vein. In

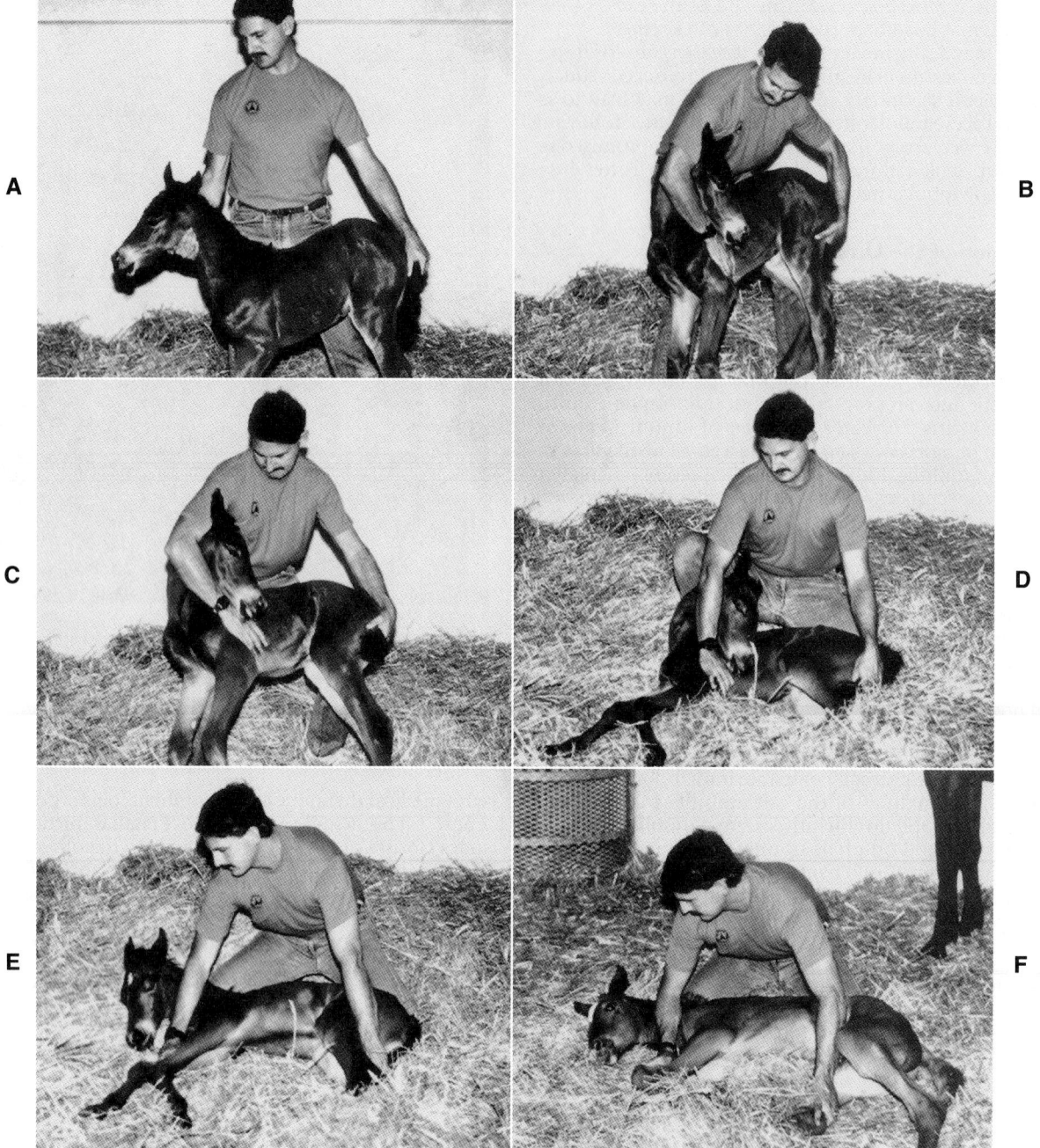

FIG. 17-2 ▪ Procedure for placing neonatal foals in lateral recumbency for umbilical ultrasound. **A,** The foal is restrained by placing the arms around the neck area and rump and holding the tail. **B,** The left forearm of the handler is placed against the head of the foal and the head folded back toward the rump area while pressure is applied to the rear quarters with the other arm. **C,** The foal leans backward and sags toward the handler, becoming recumbent. **D,** The foal is allowed to sag to the ground and is kept in the folded position until completely recumbent and relaxed. **E,** The front legs are then grasped with left hand and the forearm is placed on the neck area. The rear legs are held with the right hand. **F,** The foal is held steady in this position until blindfolded and struggling stops. The foal is in left lateral recumbency.

addition, an area 5 cm by 5 cm caudal to the umbilical stump is clipped to visualize the umbilical arteries and urachus. The ultrasound examination is performed with a 7.5-MHz sector scanning transducer; a built-in standoff is preferred. Eight views of the umbilical vessels and linear measurements of the vertical and horizontal dimension of each vessel can be taken. This allows examination of the umbilical vein (three views) and umbilical stump (one view) (Fig. 17-4), and urachus/umbilical arteries (four views) (Fig. 17-5). The umbilical vein is visualized at a site approximately 1 cm cranial to the umbili-

cal stump (view 1); another view taken approximately halfway between the umbilicus and the liver (view 2) and at a point where the vein curves away from the body wall and angles toward the liver (view 3). A single cross-sectional view of the external umbilical stump is made at the body wall. The combined urachus/left and right umbilical artery is visualized in a single cross-sectional view just caudal of the umbilical stump. The comparative mean umbilical vessel diameter normal data is summarized in Table 17-6. All but one of the ultrasound views demonstrated a significant reduction in mean

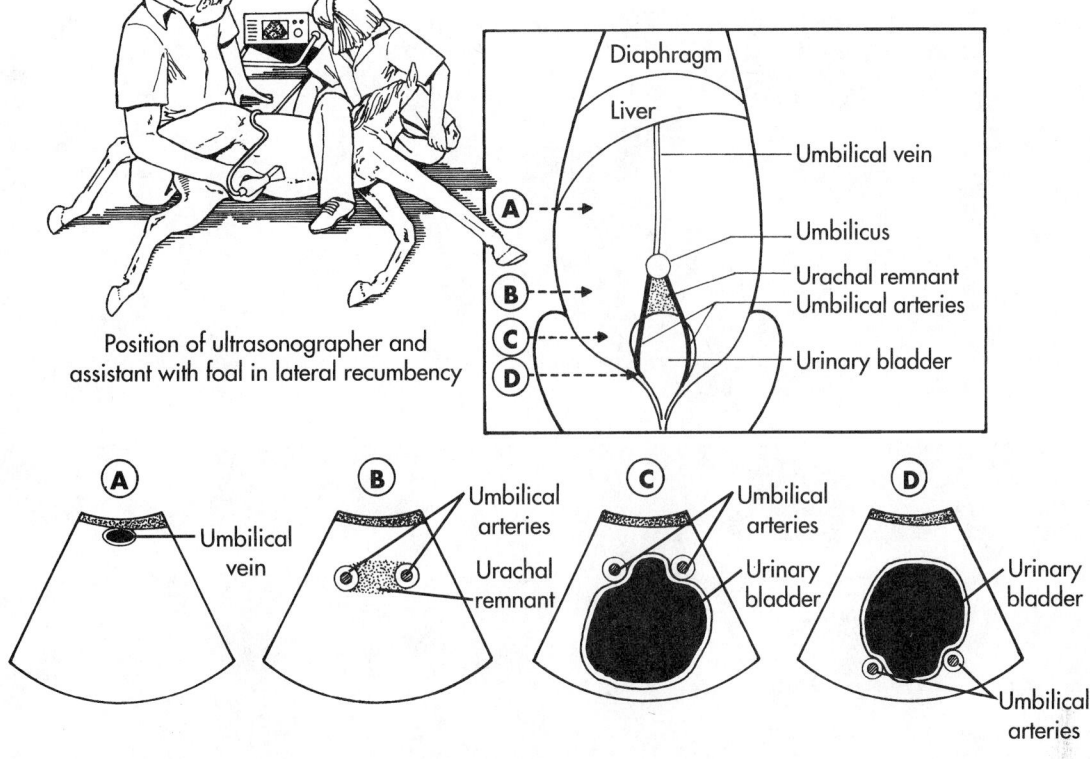

Position of ultrasonographer and
assistant with foal in lateral recumbency

Diaphragm

Liver

Umbilical vein

Umbilicus

Urachal remnant

Umbilical arteries

Urinary bladder

(A) Umbilical vein

(B) Umbilical arteries — Urachal remnant

(C) Umbilical arteries — Urinary bladder

(D) Urinary bladder — Umbilical arteries

FIG. 17-3 ▦ Ultrasound evaluation of equine umbilical structures. Diagram depicts the positioning of the ultrasonographer and the assistant and illustrates the selected anatomic locations recommended for ultrasound examination.

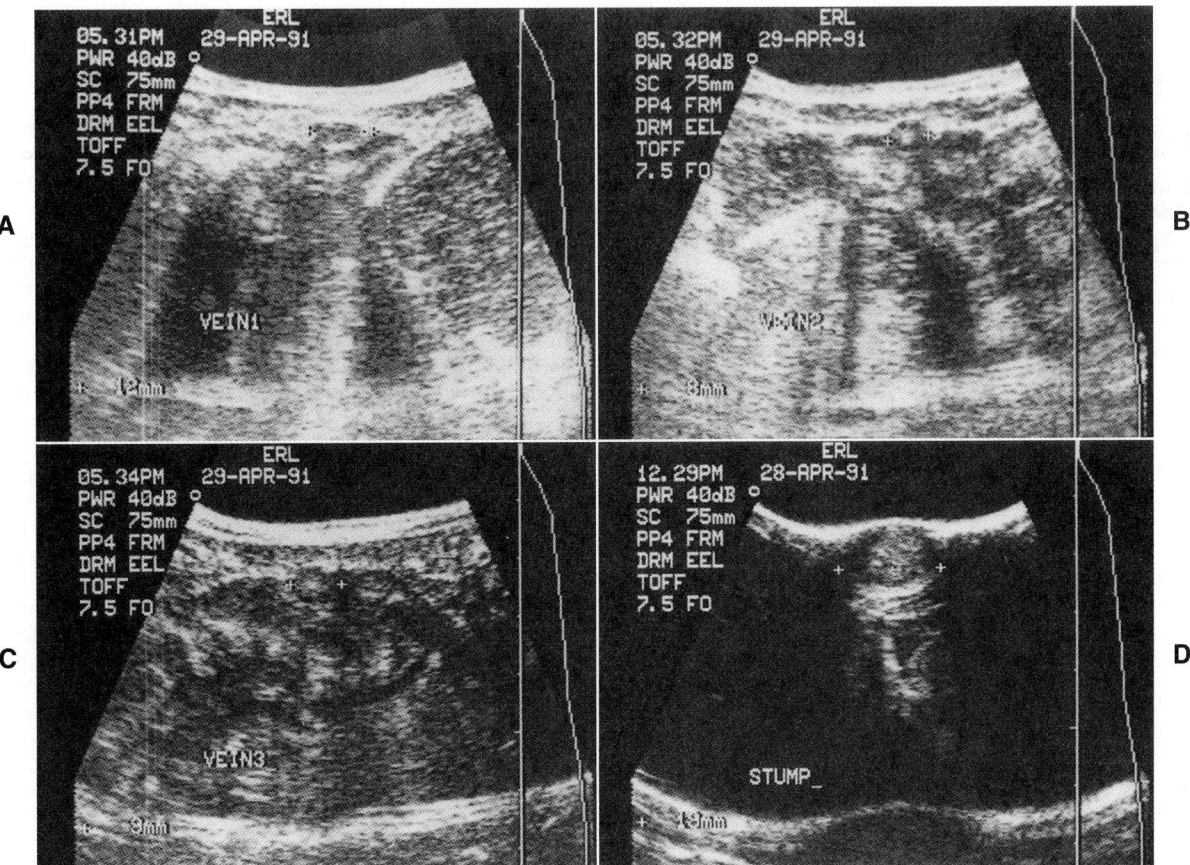

FIG. 17-4 ▦ Ultrasonographic images of four views of umbilical structures. **A,** Urachus. **B** through **D,** Umbilical arteries. Refer to the text for the definition of the views.

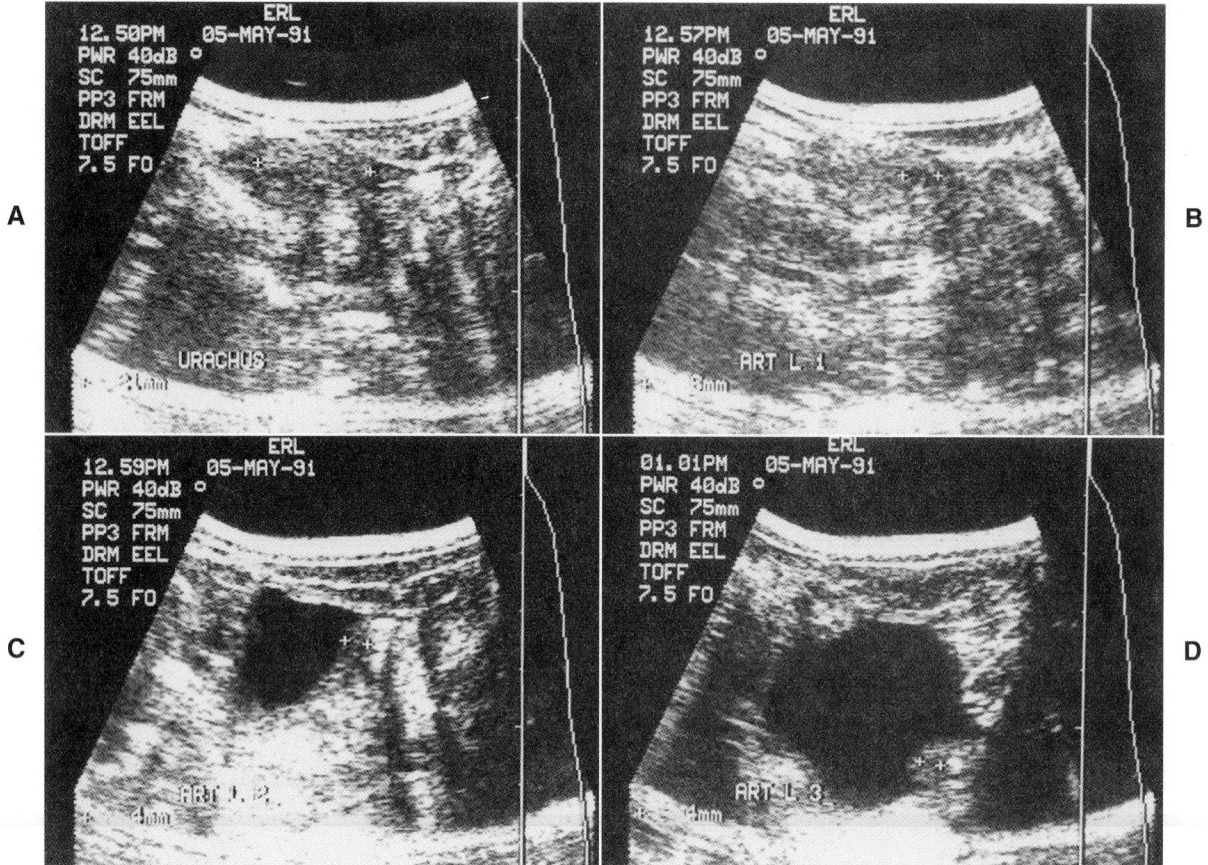

FIG. 17-5 ■ Ultrasonographic images of four views of umbilical structures. A through C, Umbilical vein. D, Umbilical stump. Refer to the text for the definition of the views.

TABLE 17-6

Comparative Mean Umbilical Vessel Diameters (mm) for 31 Clinically Normal Foals on the First and Seventh Days of Age (Mean ± SD)

Postnatal Age	2-24 Hours	7 Days	p Value
UMBILICAL VEIN			
View 1	8.3 ± 3.0	5.8 ± 1.5	$p < .0001$
(range)	(5.0-18.5)	(4.0-11.5)	
View 2	7.5 ± 1.4	5.4 ± 0.8	$p < .0001$
(range)	(5.0-11.0)	(4.0-7.0)	
View 3	8.3 ± 1.4	5.4 ± 1.3	$p < .0001$
(range)	(6.0-11.0)	(3.5-10.5)	
Overall	8.0 ± 2.1	5.6 ± 1.3	$p < .0001$
(range)	(5.0-18.5)	(3.5-11.5)	
Umbilical stump	15.5 ± 2.7	12.5 ± 2.3	$p < .0001$
(range)	(10.5-20.5)	(7.5-18.0)	
Urachus + arteries	17.7 ± 2.7	17.8 ± 2.6	$p = .4781$
(range)	(13.5-24.0)	(13.0-25.0)	
UMBILICAL ARTERIES			
View 1	7.8 ± 1.7	6.4 ± 1.5	$p < .0001$
(range)	(4.5-13.0)	(4.0-10.0)	
View 2	7.4 ± 1.6	6.7 ± 1.3	$p < .002$
(range)	(4.0-13.5)	(4.0-10.5)	
View 3	7.1 ± 1.6	6.5 ± 1.4	$p < .01$
(range)	(4.0-12.5)	(3.5-9.5)	
Overall	7.4 ± 1.6	6.5 ± 1.4	$p < .0001$
(range)	(4.0-13.5)	(3.5-10.5)	

Refer to text for definition of Views 1, 2, 3.

vessel diameter over the first 7 days of life in normal foals; only the urachus and umbilical arteries in a single structure remain static during the first week of life. Enlargements in these structures are suggestive of inflammation, infection, or hematoma and should be correlated with clinical signs and laboratory findings for choosing an optimal treatment plan.

Ultrasonography of the umbilical structures of calves has been described by Watson and colleagues.[72] Ultrasound examination of the calf is performed with the calf standing; occasionally the umbilical vein is easier to identify with the patient in left lateral recumbency. The anatomy of the umbilicus of calves differs slightly from foals requiring alterations in ultrasound technique. In both species the umbilical vein courses from the umbilicus to the liver, which in the calf is located on the right side as opposed to a midline location in the foal. Also in cattle the umbilical arteries and urachus retract into the abdominal cavity when the cord ruptures and thus cannot be identified in the external umbilical stalk in normal calves.[72] The umbilical vein of calves is scanned from the umbilical stalk to the liver along the right abdominal wall. The umbilical vein enters the liver caudoventral to the gallbladder. The umbilical arteries are most easily located adjacent to the urinary bladder and cannot normally be identified much beyond the apex of the urinary bladder, unless enlarged and abnormal. Identification of a urachal remnant in calves is abnormal.[72]

Musculoskeletal System

The musculoskeletal system should be examined for evidence of birth trauma including fractured ribs, long bones, and mandibles; brachial plexus injuries; and soft tissue trauma

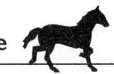

including an edematous head and tongue from excessive traction or compression in the pelvic canal. Occasionally, marked swelling of one hindlimb may be observed because of an expanding hematoma that is the result of blunt trauma or vessel injury associated with a femoral fracture. If birth was difficult, check carefully for fractured ribs. In addition to palpating crepitus over the broken ribs, a faint clicking sound can be heard during inspiration on the side of the chest with the rib fracture(s). Strenuous manipulation during a dystocia can also result in Salter-Harris type 1 fractures characterized by disruption of the distal physis in one or more limbs. Femoral nerve paralysis occurs as a sporadic complication of dystocias associated with "hip lock" in calves.[73]

The limbs should be examined carefully. The passive range of motion of the joints should be assessed for evaluation of prematurity or dysmaturity. In the immature-appearing or growth-restricted newborn foal, radiographs of at least one carpus and one tarsus are recommended to assess the degree of ossification present.[74] Ultrasonography has also been used to assess the degree of cuboidal bone ossification.[75]

All four legs should be examined for both flexural and angular limb deformities. The most commonly seen congenital abnormality is the contracted foal syndrome that is characterized by bilateral contracture of the joints of the forelimbs or hindlimbs or both. The joints most frequently involved are the metacarpophalangeal and metatarsophalangeal joints. In addition to limb contractions, scoliosis, torticollis, and cranial asymmetry have been observed. Although most mild to moderate limb deformities correct themselves in a few days, others may need splinting, casting, or surgery for a successful result. A single, large dose of intravenous oxytetracycline (2 to 3 g diluted in 500 ml saline) may be an effective treatment of mild to moderate contraction in ambulatory foals.[76,77] Complications of this treatment are apparently few, but include teeth staining, phlebitis, and nephrotoxicity.[67] In severe cases of congenital contracture, which are often associated with dystocia, even heroic measures such as surgical resection of flexor tendons may provide little or no benefit.

If the limb deformities have impaired the ability of the newborn foal to stand and nurse, it is of paramount importance to supply the foal with ample colostrum in the first 6 hours of life, to minimize the chance of postnatal infection. The foal may also require assistance to suckle ample quantities of milk. Details concerning the orthopedic management of limb deformities in neonatal foals may be found elsewhere.[78,79]

Any heat, swelling, edema, pain around the joints or physes, or lameness, should be noted. A swollen joint should be considered infected until proven otherwise. All too frequently, lameness or joint swelling in an otherwise bright and active neonate is incorrectly assumed to be a result of trauma by the mother, and the resulting delay in therapy can be devastating. In older neonates, metabolic bone disease should be considered as a differential diagnosis for lameness associated with flaring of the physis. Diets high in energy and protein that have low calcium and high phosphorus promote rapid weight gain, increasing the physical load on metabolically compromised growing bones. Damage to the growing physis may result in the subsequent development of angular limb deformities. Calcium deficiency in calves leads to reduced mineralization of bone. The transverse processes of the lumbar vertebrae become soft and bend when palpated. Copper deficiency causes metabolic bone disease that is manifested by physitis and brittle bones, reflected by a propensity to spontaneous fractures.

Skeletal muscle myopathy is an important differential for lame neonatal ruminants. Lambs and kids with selenium and/or vitamin E deficiency are often mentally bright and reluctant to stand and walk with a stiff gait and cry when forced to move. Evaluation of serum creatinine phosphokinase, blood

selenium, and plasma vitamin E concentrations is useful to confirm the diagnosis.

The skull should be examined for excessive doming of the forehead and symmetry. A moderately domed forehead is most commonly the result of intrauterine growth restriction rather than hydrocephalus. The entire vertebral column should be examined for scoliosis, kyphosis, lordosis, and other malformations. Arthrogryposis is characterized by multiple skeletal malformations, including severely contracted limbs and malformations of the vertebrae, and has been associated with the ingestion of toxins, such as locoweed and sudan grass, by the pregnant mare.[80,81]

Umbilical and scrotal hernias are the most common congenital malformations. The greatest danger associated with a hernia is strangulation of a portion of the gastrointestinal tract outside the body wall, with compromise of its vasculature. Many umbilical and scrotal hernias in foals close spontaneously but should be monitored closely and reduced periodically. Umbilical hernias in cattle do not tend to close spontaneously and are believed to be hereditary.[82] Dwarfism is a relatively common inherited problem in most cattle breeds. Osteopetrosis has been reported in Angus, Hereford, and Simmental breeds of cattle and in Peruvian Paso foals.[83] Syndactyly is considered an inherited disorder in Holstein-Friesan cattle, and affected animals are also predisposed to hyperthermia.

NEUROLOGIC EXAMINATION OF THE NEONATAL FOAL

A more complete description of the neurologic examination of the adult large animal is provided in Chapter 8 and of the neonatal foal elsewhere in this text.[84,85] In this section the emphasis is on differences in the neurologic examination of the neonatal foal and the adult horse.

General Behavior

The foal generally stands and nurses within 2 hours of birth. During the first few weeks of age the foal spends much time recumbent but is easily aroused and should run to the mare. During the first week of life the foal nurses an average of seven times an hour, with the frequency of nursing decreasing and length of nursing periods increasing as the foal matures.[86] When a foal is restrained tightly, after an initial struggle it often sinks limply into the restrainer's arms and becomes very relaxed. Head movements are jerky and exaggerated. Seizure activity, as in newborn human infants, may be subtle and difficult to recognize (see Chapter 20).

Hypotonia, seizures, and hyperesthesia are often associated with hypoxic-ischemic encephalopathy. Jitteriness is a sign of mild hypoxia. More severe hypoxia results in progressive hypotonia. Such foals are more difficult to arouse from sleep. With more global central nervous system hypoxic-ischemic damage, foals exhibit signs of grand mal seizures followed by periods of postictal stupor. Respiratory center depression may occur and is accompanied by irregular breathing patterns, prolonged bouts of apnea, or episodes of unprovoked tachypnea. Many normal foals will exhibit rapid eye movement sleep (REM) accompanied by random twitching and occasional vocalizing. These events should not be mistaken for seizures.

Septic meningitis is a less common cause of seizures. Affected foals display concurrent signs of sepsis including mucous membrane and scleral injection, depression, and tachycardia. Most foals with septic meningitis exhibit head and neck pain and severe scleral injection. Diagnosis is confirmed with a spinal tap. Other causes of seizures include hypocalcemia, hypoglycemia, azotemia, and hepatoencephalopathy.

Congenital defects of the brain and spinal cord include cerebellar abiotrophy of Arabian foals. It is an inherited disorder with an 8% incidence in some Arabian lines. It is also reported in Oldenburgs and Gotland ponies. The condition occurs in both sexes. Signs include intention head tremor, base-wide stance, dysmetria, ataxia, spasticity, swaying while standing, preservation of strength, absent menace reflex (disruption of neuronal tracts form the occipital cortex through the cerebellum in the facial nucleus), and a tendency to fall over backward with the head raised. There is degeneration of Purkinje cells and thinning of the granular and molecular layer of the cerebellar cortex. There is no treatment. Occipitoatlanto-axial malformation is more common in Arabian foals and results in progressive ataxia, tetraparesis, restricted neck movement, and an audible clicking noise associated with luxation of the dens during head/neck movement. Cervical radiographs demonstrate fusion of occiput and atlas and hypoplasia of the dens. There is limited success with surgical stabilization. Other developmental abnormalities associated with abnormal CNS behavior and possible seizures include hydrocephalus, hydrencephaly, and hypomyelinogenesis.

Cranial Nerve Examination

Because the menace reflex is usually absent in the neonatal foal until about 2 weeks of age, evaluation of sight must be done by observation of the foal's activities or movement of the head away from threatening gestures. Foals should blink in response to a bright light, but this reaction does not guarantee that they are visual. Pupils should be responsive to light and of equal size. Anisocoria may occur secondary to primary ophthalmologic abnormalities, retrobulbar problems, or a variety of neurologic disorders (brainstem, oculomotor, cervical sympathetic trunk, guttural pouch, and cervical spinal cord). Foals that are excited may have dilated pupils that do not readily constrict in response to light. Pupil dilation is associated with retinal, optic nerve, or tract abnormalities; botulism; and severe neurologic dysfunction. In foals up to about 1 month of age, the pupil forms a slight ventromedial angle with the horizontal axis of the palpebral fissure, in contrast to the slight dorsomedial angle formed by the pupil of the adult.

Foals are normally hypersensitive to stimuli applied over the face and nose. In testing the facial nerve, local reflexes are the same as in the adult but are accompanied by exaggerated and jerky head movements. Foals respond to noise with the same jerky movements that they show to tactile stimulation. The ability to swallow can be tested by laryngeal palpation or by passage of a stomach tube. Nursing is a complicated activity involving a swallowing reflex (cranial nerves IX, X, and XI), a movement of the lips (cranial nerve VII), jaw (motor nerve V), and tongue (cranial nerve XII), as well as recognition of the mare's udder (cerebrum). Presence of milk at the nostrils can indicate a cleft palate, pharyngeal paresis, inflammation or malformation, dysphagia associated with white muscle disease, gastric distention or gastrointestinal stasis, or merely a depressed, weak foal. Some foals may have no other obvious abnormalities except some milk at the nostril; these foals usually return to normal by 3 to 4 days of age. In very depressed foals the tongue may hang out of the mouths even though there is no specific neurologic disorder.

Gait and Posture

A righting reflex should be present after birth. During its first days of life the foal assumes a base-wide stance and has a choppy, dysmetric gait, gradually acquiring agility as it matures. The neck and forelimbs should be palpated for symmetry and muscle tone. The foal is very sensitive to tactile stimuli. In lateral recumbency, newborn foals exhibit hyperreflexic spinal reflexes compared with the adult and have substantial resting extensor tone. The limbs of the normal foal relax with repeated passive flexion, in contrast to the abnormal individual with upper motor neuron disease and extensor rigidity. In the normal foal, a prominent crossed extensor reflex of the contralateral limb may accompany the flexor or withdrawal reflex until around 3 weeks of age. The trunk and hindlimbs should also be palpated for symmetry, muscle tone, passive range of motion, and musculoskeletal deformities. A panniculus response is elicited as in the adult. The patellar and other spinal reflexes of the hind limbs are also hyperreflexive compared to the adult response.

NEUROLOGIC EXAMINATION OF NEONATAL RUMINANTS

Neurologic disease in neonates during the perinatal period often results from birth asphyxia, congenital disease, or sepsis. Congenital central nervous system abnormalities in the large animal neonate may be inherited or result from in utero infections, toxins, and other environmental factors (see Chapters 47 and 48 for complete tables of congenital problems in foals, calves, kids, and lambs). In both the calf and foal, hydrocephalus, hydranencephaly, and anencephaly may occur. In the calf both Akabane and bluetongue virus may cause hydranencephaly and other problems, including arthrogryposis and premature births. Hydrocephalus is fairly common and appears to be inherited as a simple autosomal-recessive trait in many breeds. Internal hydrocephalus may result from a simple recessive gene or congenital bovine virus diarrhea (BVD) infection. Fetal infection with BVD virus may result in a number of other problems, including cerebellar dysplasia, ocular defects, hypomyelinogenesis, and intrauterine growth restriction. Cerebellar hypoplasia may also result from an autosomal-recessive gene and is seen in some cattle breeds.

Disorders of amino acid metabolism that result in primarily neurologic signs include maple syrup urine disease[87,88] and citrullinemia.[88] Maple syrup urine disease is analogous to branched-chain keto acid decarboxylase deficiency and results in clinical signs of extensor spasms, weakness, dullness, recumbency, and opisthotonos shortly after birth. The most striking lesion of the central nervous system histologically is widespread spongy vacuolation in the white and gray matter of the brain. Citrullinemia, an inborn error of metabolism of the urea cycle, was reported in five neonatal Friesian calves.[89] The calves appeared normal for a short period after birth, but at 24 hours to 5 days of age they developed progressive neurologic signs of depression, tremors, seizures, and opisthotonos, which were followed by death.

Congenital myoclonus (neuraxial edema) is an autosomal-recessive inherited disorder of polled Herefords.[90] Clinical signs included premature delivery, inability to stand after birth (with the majority remaining in lateral recumbency), normal mentation, and prominent, sensory stimuli–induced myoclonic jerking of the whole body with extension of the head and limbs. The majority of cases also display traumatic hip lesions, presumably as a result of the severe myoclonic contractions. Severe alterations in spinal cord glycine-mediated neurotransmission result from a marked decrease or defect in glycine receptors and an increase in neuronal (synaptosomal) glycine uptake. Alterations are also present in the major inhibitory system (GABA receptors) in the cerebral cortex.[91] Storage diseases in cattle, usually inherited as an autosomal recessive gene, include α-mannosidosis in purebred Angus, β-mannosidosis in Salers, GM-1 gangliosidosis in inbred Friesians, neuronal lipodystrophy in beefmasters, and Shaker calf syndrome in horned Hereford calves. The latter condition was recently recognized as an inheritable neurodegenerative disorder characterized by excessive accumulation of neurofilaments within neurons of the central, peripheral, and autonomic nervous systems. Clinical signs included a normal birth but inability to stand unassisted after delivery. Several hours later the calves developed fine gener-

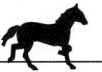

alized tremors, hyperesthesia to tactile stimulation, weakness, ataxia, and aphonia.[92]

Most acquired neurologic disease in neonates is associated with disease in other organ systems. Sepsis and diarrhea are both commonly associated with depressed mentation secondary to toxemia and or metabolic derangements. Bacterial meningitis is common in neonates following bacteremia; diarrhea, septic arthritis, omphalophlebitis, and uveitis are frequent concurrent clinical problems. The clinical signs of meningitis in neonates, lethargy, anorexia, and recumbency are nonspecific. Concurrent metabolic derangements may appear to provide an adequate explanation for the observed depressed mentation. In a retrospective study of 32 cases of bacterial meningitis in calves, concurrent metabolic derangements included hyperkalemia (15/25, 60%), respiratory acidosis (11/24, 46%), hypernatremia (3/20, 15%), and hypoglycemia (3/7, 43%).[92] The more classical clinical signs described for bacterial meningitis in older animals (fever, opisthotonos, extension of the head, convulsions, hyperesthesia, and signs of neck pain) may not be evident or perceived in neonates. Seizures in calves are often subtle, manifested as facial twitches or jaw champing. Common causes of cerebral disease in lambs and kids include polioencephalomalacia and focal symmetric encephalomalacia. Affected animals are typically depressed and blind but have normal pupillary light reflexes.

Posterior paresis is common in neonates; causes include border disease, enzootic ataxia, vertebral body abscesses, caprine arthritis, encephalomyelitis virus, and vertebral body fractures associated with dietary copper deficiency or calcium phosphorus imbalance. These neurologic problems are discussed in Chapter 33.

EXAMINATION OF THE EYE

Eyes should be examined for the presence of entropion, ectropion, corneal abrasions or ulcers, uveitis and hyphema, congenital cataracts, microphthalmia, corneal dermoids, scleral injection, and scleral hemorrhage. Retinal hemorrhages may be observed in hypoxic foals. Scleral hemorrhage is usually the result of birth trauma and can take several weeks to resolve. A list of other congenital eye problems can be found in Chapters 47 and 48.

A common cause of corneal edema and ulceration, conjunctivitis, and lacrimation is acquired or congenital entropion. Acquired entropion is associated with self-trauma, dehydration or prematurity, and the lack of periorbital fat. Entropion should be corrected promptly before serious corneal ulceration and keratitis develops. Mild cases may respond to subcutaneous injections of procaine penicillin G into the lower eyelid. Most foals with entropion will require placement of vertical or horizontal mattress sutures (e.g., 4-0 absorbable on a curved cutting needle) in the lower eyelid to correct the problem. The affected eye should be stained to detect concurrent corneal ulceration. Varying degrees of miosis secondary to pain and ciliary body spasm is common. Treatment after correction of entropion includes topical administration of 1% atropine to dilate the pupil and relieve ciliary body spasm and topical antibiotics to prevent bacterial infection.

Uveitis may be observed in the newborn animal exposed to an infected uterine environment or may be a result of generalized infection acquired after birth. Scleral injection suggests sepsis. Observation of fibrin in the anterior chamber of the eye of a neonate is highly indicative of sepsis.

EXAMINATION OF POSTPARTUM MARE AND PLACENTA

When accompanying a sick newborn foal, the mare should be evaluated thoroughly, and a complete foaling history should be acquired (Chapter 15).

If available, the fetal membranes should be weighed and examined for integrity, abnormal thickening, discharges, villous atrophy, and other abnormalities. The placenta should be scrutinized systematically for valuable information about the in utero environment.[94,95] Fetoplacental infection, associated with bacterial, viral, and fungal agents, is one of the most important causes of abortion, stillbirth, and perinatal mortality in the equine species.[96] Normal placental weight for thoroughbreds ranges from 4.5 to 6.4 kg (10 to 14 lb) or about 11% of the foal's body weight[97]; placentas that weigh over 6.4 kg should be considered potentially abnormal (edema or placentitis), and those that weigh less than 4.5 kg may be incomplete or have severe villous atrophy.

Cases of chronic placentitis are usually recognized by thickening and discoloration of the chorion. Because most intrauterine infections begin as an ascending placentitis of the chorioallantois, the area of discoloration and thickening originates at the cervical star and extends up the body of the placenta. Acute cases of placentitis may require histopathologic examination for a diagnosis.[98] If placentitis is suspected, fetal fluids or membranes should be cultured, and sections of amnion and chorioallantois should be saved in formalin for histopathologic examination. Organisms most commonly associated with endometritis may also be associated with placentitis. Pathogens include *Streptococcus zooepidemicus*, *Leptospira* sp., *E. coli*, *Nocardioform actinomycetes*, fungi, *Pseudomonas aeruginosa*, *Streptococcus equisimilis*, *Enterobacter agglomerans*, *Klebsiella pneumoniae*, and α-hemolytic *Streptococcus* spp.[99,100] Diffuse placentitis is associated with hematogenous spread of infection such as seen with *Leptospira* infection. *Nocardioform placentitis* is characterized by focally extensive placentitis at the base of the placental horns at the junction of the horns and the body of the uterus.[100] The affected placenta is usually covered with thick, tenacious brown exudate. Fungal placentitis often presents with a sticky brown mucoid exudate covering parts of the chorion and is often associated with the birth of a small, emaciated foal.[98] Sabouraud's agar should be used to isolate suspected fungal pathogens. A direct smear of the exudate can be examined with Gomori's methenamine silver stain.[99] *Aspergillus* and *Mucor* spp. are the most fungal pathogens isolated.[101] Systemic fungal infection of the foal is relatively rare.

Pending culture results, the foals from grossly abnormal placentas should be considered at high risk of being infected. Such foals should have a blood culture submitted and their leukogram and creatinine concentration evaluated. Prophylactic treatment with broad-spectrum antibiotics is indicated.

If the chorioallantois is unusually heavy it may fail to rupture at the cervical star, resulting in premature or abnormal placental separation with the rupture of membranes occurring near the base of one horn. Foals may experience bouts of hypoxia associated with such deliveries. Early postpartum treatment with drugs, such as dimethyl sulfoxide (DMSO) or mannitol, to decrease cerebral edema are indicated at the first signs of neonatal hypoxic ischemic encephalopathy (i.e., dummy foal syndrome).

Adenomatous hyperplasia of the allantois may appear as hyperplasia and hypertrophy of the epithelial cells of the allantois with the formation of intraepithelial glands. More severely affected membranes may have raised firm tan nodules on the allantoic surface of the chorioallantois.[101] These lesions consist of dilated, anastomosing glands surrounded by loose, collagenous stroma. Inflammatory changes are thought to be secondary to the adenomatous dysplasia. The cause of this lesion is not known, but it is seen with chronic placentitis, placental edema, and fetal diarrhea.[99,102] Umbilical cord abnormalities may also affect the fetus.[103] Granular debris and golden meconium particles on the amniotic portion of the cord suggest local inflammation. An excessively long umbilical cord (normal range is 36 to 83 cm) may result in strangulation of the fetus with evidence of edema and vascular occlusion around the head and neck. If there is excessive twisting of the cord, compromised fetal circulation or obstruction of the urachus may occur. Urachal obstruction may contribute to urachal patency or bladder rupture. An unusually short cord is prone to premature rupture and hemorrhage and may predispose the foal to hypoxic injury.

The mare's udder, milk, and reproductive tract should be carefully examined. After birth, the quality of colostrum may be assessed by visual inspection (thick, sticky) or by colostrometer (specific gravity >1.060 is normal). A full, distended udder usually indicates that the foal is not nursing adequately, but in rare instances it may accompany mastitis. In mares with mastitis the milk may appear normal on visual inspection. A flaccid, empty udder may indicate either an aggressively nursing foal or a mare that is not lactating sufficiently. One way to distinguish the two is to muzzle the foal for 1 to 2 hours and then check the amount of milk in the udder.

The mare's reproductive tract should be evaluated if there is a history of vaginal discharge, retained placenta, or traumatic birth or if the mare appears sick or febrile. The mare's appetite and manure production should be monitored. Postpartum mares are at increased risk for developing gastrointestinal disease. Causes of colic in the postpartum mare include impaction of the large colon or cecum; cecal rupture; large colon displacement; large colon torsion; rectal prolapse with rupture of the mesocolon; ischemic necrosis of the descending colon; diaphragmatic herniation of abdominal viscera into the thorax; rupture of the uterine artery, hematoma formation within the broad ligament or uterine wall; peritonitis secondary to uterine trauma, rupture, or prolapse; and metritis.

Diagnostic aids include a careful history of events surrounding delivery. Prepartum maternal problems such as hydrops or prepubic tendon rupture or ventral abdominal hernia formation predispose to specific problems. Hydrops, if severe, can result in uterine rupture, leading to postpartum peritonitis. Prepubic tendon rupture and rectus abdominis damage can produce intraperitoneal inflammation, leading to intraabdominal adhesions, bowel trauma, and peritonitis. A history of dystocia increases suspicions of intrauterine trauma, uterine rupture, metritis, and peritonitis.

Dystocias have also been associated with bowel damage including cecal rupture. If the mare experienced rectal prolapse, she is at increased risk for rupture of the mesocolon and secondary disruption of blood supply to the descending colon, resulting in intestinal ischemic necrosis and peritonitis. Retained fetal membranes increase the risk of metritis and secondary peritonitis. It is common practice to feed mares a laxative diet following parturition to reduce the risk of impaction. The mare should be dewormed within 24 hours of delivery to reduce the foal's parasite exposure.

RESTRAINT OF THE FOAL

The uncooperative nature of many neonatal foals can seriously limit the quality of care provided, and identification of effective restraint techniques often becomes a concern equal in importance to medical therapy. In general, procedures should be performed as quickly and quietly as possible. For minor procedures such as venipuncture, most foals can be successfully restrained in the standing position, with the foal held against a wall or in a corner of the stall. One of the restrainer's arms is placed around the foal's chest and the opposite hand grasps the tail base and holds the tail up over the rump. If foals are held too tightly, they tend to collapse, then leap forward. Alternatively, most foals stand well when both ears are held tightly at the base; this technique also provides excellent access to the jugular vein.

To perform procedures that are more involved and time consuming, it is highly recommended that foals less than 2 weeks of age be placed in lateral recumbency. The use of local anesthetic placed with a small needle facilitates catheter placement and arterial blood gas collection. Additional details concerning foal restraint can be found in other texts.[104]

REFERENCES

1. Vaala WE: Assessment of the critically ill foal. *Proceedings of the Postgraduate Foundation in Veterinary Science,* Sydney, NSW, Australia, 1996, p 267.
2. Juarbe-Díaz SV, Houpt KA, Kusunose R: Prevalence and characteristics of foal rejection in Arabian mares, *Eq Vet J* 30:424-428, 1998.
3. Lavan RP et al: Effect of disinfectant treatments on bacterial flora of the umbilicus of neonatal foals, *Proceedings of the Fortieth Annual Convention of the American Association of Equine Practitioners,* 1994, p 37.
4. McGuire TC, Poppie MJ, Banks KL: Hypogammaglobulinemia predisposing to infection in foals, *J Am Vet Med Assoc* 166:71-75, 1975.
5. McGuire TC et al: Failure of colostral immunoglobulin transfer as an explanation for most infections and deaths of neonatal foals, *J Am Vet Med Assoc* 170:1302-1304, 1977.
6. Dufty JH, Sloss V: Anoxia in the bovine foetus, *Aust Vet J* 53:262-267, 1977.
7. Smith FV: Instinct and learning in the attachment of lamb and ewe, *Anim Behav* 13:84-86, 1965.
8. Selman IE, McEwan AD, Fisher EW: Studies on natural suckling in cattle during the first eight hours postpartum. II, Behavioural studies (calves), *Anim Behav* 18:284-289, 1970.
9. Ventorp M, Michanek P: The importance of udder and teat conformation for teat seeking by the newborn calf, *J Dairy Sci* 75:262-268, 1992.
10. Frisch JE: The use of teat-size measurements or calf weaning weight as an aid to selection against teat defects in cattle, *Anim Prod* 32:127, 1982.
11. Balwin BA, Shillito E: The effects of ablation of the olfactory bulbs on parturition and maternal behaviour in Soay sheep, *Anim Behav* 22:220-223, 1974.
12. Kendrick KM, Levy F, Keverne EB: Importance of vaginocervical stimulation for the formation of maternal bonding in primiparous and multiparous parturient ewes, *Physiol Behav* 50:595-600, 1991.
13. Ivanoff MR, Renshaw HW: Weak calf syndrome: serum immunoglobulin concentrations in precolostral calves, *Am J Vet Res* 36:1129-1131, 1975.
14. Oberst RD: Viruses as teratogens, *Vet Clin North Am (Food Anim Pract)* 9:23-31, 1993.
15. Besser TE, Gay CC, Pritchett L: Comparison of three methods of feeding colostrum to dairy calves, *J Am Vet Med Assoc* 198:419-422, 1991.
16. Walter-Toews D, Martin SW, Meek AH: Dairy calf management, morbidity and mortality in Ontario Holstein herds. IV, Association of management with mortality, *Prev Vet Med* 4:159-171, 1986.
17. Lance SE et al: Effects of environment and management on mortality in preweaned dairy calves, *J Am Vet Med Assoc* 201:1197-1202, 1992.
18. Walter-Toews D, Martin SW, Meek AH: Dairy calf management, morbidity and mortality in Ontario Holstein herds. III, Association of management with morbidity, *Prev Vet Med* 4:137-158, 1986.
19. Thurmond MC: Epidemiologic approaches used in a herd health practice to investigate neonatal calf mortality, *Prev Vet Med* 4:317-328, 1986.
20. Rammell CG et al: Selenium, vitamin E and polyunsaturated fatty acid concentrations in goat kids with and without nutritional myodegeneration, *N Z Vet J* 37:4-6, 1989.
21. Pehrson B, Hakkarainen J, Blomgren L: Vitamin E status in newborn lambs with special reference to dl-alpha-tocopheryl acetate supplementation in late gestation, *Acta Vet Scand* 31:359-367, 1990.
22. Harvey JW et al: Haematology of foals up to one year old, *Equine Vet J* 16:347-353, 1984.
23. Jeffcott LB, Rossdale PD, Leadon DP: Haematological changes in the neonatal period of normal premature foals, *J Reprod Fertil Suppl* 32:537-544, 1982.
24. Medeiros LO et al: Haematological standards for healthy newborn foals, *Biol Neonate* 17:351-360, 1971.
25. Sata T, Oda K, Kubo M: Haematological and biochemical values of thoroughbred foals in the first 6 months of life, *Cornell Vet* 69:3-19, 1978.
26. Schalm OW, Carlson GP: The blood and blood-forming organs. In Mansmann RA McAllister ES, eds: *Equine medicine and surgery,* ed 3, Santa Barbara, Calif, 1982, American Veterinary Publications, pp 377-414.
27. Wilson WD: Hematology reference values. In JE Madigan, ed: *Manual of equine neonatal medicine,* Woodland, Calif, 1987, Live Oak Publishing.
28. Bauer JE et al: Clinical chemistry reference values for foals during the first year of life, *Equine Vet J* 16:361-363, 1984.
29. Gossett KA, French DD: Effect of age on liver enzyme activities in serum of healthy quarter horses, *Am J Vet Res* 45:354-356, 1984.
30. Rumbaugh GE, Adamson PJW: Automated serum chemical analysis in the foal, *J Am Vet Med Assoc* 183:769-772, 1983.
31. Schmitz DG, Joyce JR, Reagor JC: Serum biochemical values in quarter horse foals in the first 6 months of life, *Equine Pract* 4:24-30, 1982.

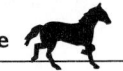

32. Varner DD, Vaala WE: Equine perinatal care. II, Routine management of the neonatal foal, *Compend Cont Educ Pract Vet* 8:581-594, 1986.

33. Wilson WD: Blood chemistry values. In Madigan JE: *Manual of equine neonatal medicine*, Woodland, Calif, 1987, Live Oak Publishing.

34. Vaala WE, Webb AI: Cardiovascular monitoring of the critically ill foal. In Koterba, AM, Drummond, WH, Kosch, PC, eds: *Equine clinical neonatology*, Philadelphia, 1990, Lea & Febiger, p 262.

35. Lombard CW et al: Blood pressure, electrocardiogram, and echocardiogram measurements in the growing pony foal, *Equine Vet J* 16:342, 1984.

36. Marr CM et al: Myocardial dysfunction in neonatal septicemia, *Proceedings of the British Equine Veterinary Association*, 1993.

37. Cawley GD, Bradley R: Sudden death in calves associated with acute myocardial degeneration and selenium deficiency, *Vet Rec* 103:239-240, 1978.

38. Fisher EW: Hydrogen ion and electrolyte disturbances in neonatal calves, *Ann NY Acad Sci* 176:223-230, 1971.

39. Weldon AD, Moise NS, Rebhun WC: Hyperkalemic atrial standstill in neonatal calf diarrhea, *J Vet Intern Med* 6:294-297, 1992.

40. Benson JE et al: Lasalocid toxicosis in neonatal calves, *J Vet Diagn Invest* 10:210-214, 1998.

41. Kosch PC et al: Developments in management of the newborn foal in respiratory distress. I, Evaluation, *Equine Vet J* 16:312, 1984.

42. Stalheim OH: Failure of antibiotic therapy in calves with mycoplasmal arthritis and pneumonia, *J Am Vet Med Assoc* 169:1096-1097, 1976.

43. Walz PH et al: Otitis media in preweaned Holstein dairy calves in Michigan due to *Mycoplasma bovis*, *J Vet Diag Invest* 9:250-254, 1997.

44. Kinde H et al: Mycoplasma bovis associated with decubital abscesses in Holstein calves, *J Vet Diagn Invest* 5:194-197, 1993.

45. Reef VB: Equine pediatric ultrasonography, *Comp Cont Educ Pract Vet* 13:1277-1285, 1991.

46. Bernard WV, Reimer JM: Examination of the foal, *Vet Clin North Am (Equine Pract)* 10:37-66, 1994.

47. Campbell ML, Ackerman N, Peyton LC: Radiographic gastrointestinal anatomy of the foal, *Vet Radiol* 25:194-204, 1984.

48. Cudd TA, Toal RL, Embertson RM: The use of clinical findings, abdominocentesis, and abdominal radiographs to assess surgical vs. nonsurgical abdominal disease in the foal, *Proc 33rd Annu Conv Am Assoc Equine Pract* 33:41-53, 1988.

49. Reimer JM: Sonographic evaluation of gastrointestinal diseases in foals, *Proceedings of the Thirty-ninth Annual Convention of the American Association of Equine Practitioners*, 1993, pp 245-246.

50. Grindem CB et al: Peritoneal fluid values from healthy foals, *Equine Vet J* 22:359, 1990.

51. Anderson DE et al: Comparative analyses of peritoneal fluid from calves and adult cattle, *Am J Vet Res* 56:973-976, 1995.

52. Smith DF et al: Clinical management and surgical repair of atresia coli in calves: 66 cases (1977-1988), *J Am Vet Med Assoc* 199:1185-90, 1991.

53. Hultgren BD: Ileocolonic aganglionosis in white progeny of overo spotted horses, *J Am Vet Med Assoc* 180:289-292, 1982.

54. Bergeland ME, Henry SC: Infectious diarrheas of young pigs, *Vet Clin North Am (Large Animal Pract)* 4:389-399, 1982.

55. Dirksen GU, Garry FB: Diseases of the forestomachs in calves. I, *Comp Cont Educ Pract Vet* 9:F140-F147, 1987.

56. Jorgensen RJ et al: A simple test for the demonstration of abomasal juice in rumen samples of young calves, *Acta Vet Scand* 33:105-107, 1992.

57. Dirksen G, Dirr L: Oesophageal groove dysfunction as a complication of neonatal diarrhea in the calf, *Bovine Pract* 24:53-60, 1989.

58. Jeffcott LB: Observations on parturition in crossbred pony mares, *Equine Vet J* 4:209, 1972.

59. Brewer BD et al: Renal clearance, urinary excretion of endogenous substances and urinary diagnostic indices in healthy neonatal foals, *J Vet Int Med* 5:28, 1989.

60. Dalton RG: The effect of starvation on the fluid and electrolyte metabolism of neonatal calves, *Br Vet J* 123:237, 1967.

61. Divers TJ, Byars TD, Spirito M: Correction of bilateral ureteral defects in a foal, *J Am Vet Med Assoc* 192:384-386, 1988.

62. Gopal T, Leipold HW, Cook JE: Renal oxalosis in neonatal calves, *Vet Pathol* 15:519-524, 1978.

63. Rhyan JC et al: Severe renal oxalosis in five young beefmaster calves, *J Am Vet Med Assoc* 201:1907-1910, 1992.

64. David JSE, Long SE, Eddy R: The incidence of freemartins in heifer calves purchased from markets, *Vet Rec* 98:417-418, 1976.

65. Kennedy PC: The female genital system. In Jubb KVF, Kennedy PC, Palmer N, eds: *Pathology of the domestic animals*, vol 3, ed 3, New York, 1985, Academic Press, pp 305-408.

66. Mechor GD, Cebra C, Blue J: Renal failure in a calf secondary to chronic enteritis, *Cornell Vet J* 83:325-331, 1993.

67. Vivrette S et al: Hemodialysis for treatment of oxytetracycline-induced acute renal failure in a neonatal foal, *J Am Vet Med Assoc* 203:105-107, 1993.

68. Madigan JE: Umbilical problems. In Madigan JE, ed: *Manual of equine neonatal medicine*, Woodland, Calif, 1991, Live Oak Publishing, pp 179-183.

69. Adams SB, Fessler JF: Umbilical cord remnant infections in foals: 16 cases (1975-1985), *J Am Vet Med Assoc* 190:316-318, 1987.

70. Reef VB et al: Clinical, ultrasonographic, and surgical findings in foals with umbilical remnant infections, *J Am Vet Med Assoc* 195:69-72, 1989.

71. Reef VB, Collatos C: Ultrasonography of umbilical structures in clinically normal foals, *Am J Vet Res* 49:2143-2146, 1988.

72. Watson E et al: Ultrasonography of the umbilical structures in clinically normal calves, *Am J Vet Res* 55:773-780, 1994.

73. Tryphonas L, Hamilton GF, Rhodes CS: Perinatal femoral nerve degeneration and neurogenic atrophy of quadriceps muscles in calves, *J Am Vet Med Assoc* 164:801-807, 1974.

74. Adams R, Poulos PW: A skeletal ossification index for neonatal foals, *Vet Radiol* 29:217, 1988.

75. Ruohoniemi M: Use of ultrasonography to evaluate the degree of ossification of the small tarsal bones in 10 foals, *Equine Vet J* 25:539-543, 1993.

76. Lokai MD, Meyer RJ: Preliminary observations on oxytetracycline treatment of congenital flexural deformities in foals, *Mod Vet Pract* April, 1985, p 237.

77. Madison JB et al: Effect of oxytetracycline on metacarpophalangeal and distal interphalangeal joint angles in newborn foals, *J Am Vet Med Assoc* 204:246-249, 1994.

78. Orsini JA, Kreuder C: Musculoskeletal disorders of the neonate, *Vet Clin North Am (Equine Pract)* 10:137-166, 1994.

79. Adams R: Noninfectious orthopedic problems. In Koterba AM, Drummond WH, Kosch PC, eds: *Equine clinical neonatology*, Philadelphia, 1990, Lea & Febiger, p 333.

80. McIlwraith CW, James LF: Limb deformities in foals associated with ingestion of locoweed by mares, *J Am Vet Med Assoc* 181:255-258, 1982.

81. Prichard JT, Voss JL: Fetal ankylosis in horses associated with hybrid Sudan pasture, *J Am Vet Med Assoc* 150:871-873, 1967.

82. Angus K, Young GB: A note of the genetics of umbilical hernia, *Vet Rec* 40:245-247, 1972.

83. Berry CR, House JK, Poulos PP: Radiographic and pathologic features of osteopetrosis in two Peruvian Paso foals, *Vet Radiol Ultrasound* 35:355-361, 1994.

84. Adams R, Mayhew IG: Neurological examination of newborn foals, *Equine Vet J* 16:306, 1984.

85. Adams R, Mayhew IG: Neurologic diseases, *Vet Clin North Am (Equine Pract)* 1:209-234, 1985.

86. Carson K, Wood-Gush DGM: Behaviour of thoroughbred foals during nursing, *Equine Vet J* 15:257, 1983.

87. Baird JD et al: Maple syrup urine disease in five Hereford calves in Ontario, *Can Vet J* 28:505, 1987.

88. Harper PA, Healy PJ, Dennis JA: Maple syrup urine disease as a cause of spongiform encephalopathy in calves, *Vet Rec* 119:62-65, 1986.

89. Harper PA et al: Citrullinaemia as a cause of neurological disease in neonatal Friesian calves, *Aust Vet J* 63:378-379, 1986.

90. Harper PA, Healy PJ, Dennis JA: Inherited congenital myoclonus of polled Hereford calves (so-called neuraxial oedema): a clinical, pathological and biochemical study, *Vet Rec* 119:59-62, 1986.

91. Lummis SCR et al: Increased gamma-aminobutyric acid receptor function in the cerebral cortex of myoclonic calves with an hereditary deficit in glycine/strychnine receptors, *J Neurochem* 55:421-426, 1990.

92. Rousseaux CG, Ribble CS: Developmental anomalies in farm animals. II, Defining etiology, *Canadian Vet J* 29:30, 1988.

93. Green SL, Smith LL: Meningitis in neonatal calves: 32 cases (1983-1990), *J Am Vet Med Assoc* 201:125-128, 1992.

94. Sertich PL: Clinical anatomy and evaluation of equine fetal membranes, *Proceedings of the Annual Meeting of the Society for Theriogenology*, Jacksonville, Fla, 1993, pp 178-184.

95. Sertich PL: Diagnostic value of fetal membrane evaluation in the management of neonates *Proceedings of the Annual Meeting of the Society for Theriogenology*, Kansas City, Mo, 1996, pp 249-252, 1996.

96. Giles RC et al: Causes of abortion, stillbirth, and perinatal death in horses: 3527 cases (1986-1991), *J Am Vet Med Assoc* 203:1170-1175, 1993.

97. Roberts SJ: *Veterinary obstetrics and genital disease*, Ann Arbor, 1971, Edwards Brothers, p 46.

98. Whitwell KE: Infective placentitis in the mare, *Proceedings of the Fifth International Conference on Equine Infectious Diseases*, 1988, pp 172-180.

99. Hong CB et al: Etiology and pathology of equine placentitis, *J Vet Diagn Invest* 5:56-63, 1993.

100. Williams NM, Donahue JM: Placentitis in mares in Kentucky, *Proceedings of the Havemeyer Foundation Workshop on Equine Placentitis*, 1998.

101. Prickett ME: Abortion and placental lesions in the mare, *J Am Vet Med Assoc* 157:1465-1470, 1970.

102. McEntee M, Brown T, McEntee K: Adenomatous dysplasia of the equine allantois, *Vet Pathol* 25:387-389, 1988.

103. Whitwell KE: Morphology and pathology of the equine umbilical cord, *J Reprod Fertil*, 1975, pp 599-603.

104. McDonald PG et al: Nursing care of the neonatal foal. I, Nursing techniques. In Koterba AM, Drummond WH, Kosch PC, eds: *Equine clinical neonatology*, Philadelphia, 1990, Lea & Febiger, p 625.

Supportive Care of the Abnormal Newborn

WENDY E. VAALA

JOHN K. HOUSE

The vulnerability of neonates to contagious and opportunistic pathogens is amplified by adverse environmental conditions. Maintenance of a "friendly" environment is a crucial component of neonatal medicine. Any condition that prevents neonates from standing and nursing within 3 hours of delivery represents a potentially fatal condition. Forced recumbency alone interferes with pulmonary function, contributes to dependent lung atelectasis and increases the risk of pneumonia, compromises gastrointestinal function and predisposes to constipation, increases the risk of aspiration after milk meals, exacerbates preexisting musculoskeletal weakness and favors tendon contracture, delays absorption of colostral antibodies and calories (which increases the risk of infection and hypoglycemia), predisposes to decubital sores, and contributes to poor hygiene, urachal patency, and omphalitis. Supportive care is aimed at protecting the patient from self-inflicted injury; maintaining fluid, electrolyte, and metabolic homeostasis; providing adequate caloric intake; and preventing nosocomial infections.

If recumbent, foals should be kept on soft, absorbent bedding (mattress covered in synthetic fleece, straw on top of a deep bed of shavings or rubber mats) and turned and assisted to stand every 2 hours. If the foal is thrashing, it should be manually restrained to prevent self-trauma. Padded walls and strategic placement of pillows helps protect the recumbent patient. Using a temporary barrier between the mare and recumbent foal facilitates treatment of the foal, yet keeps the dam within sight, sound, touch, and smell of her foal, thereby fostering bonding. The foal's eyes are prone to injury with the development of entropion, corneal edema, and ulceration. To prevent these injuries, artificial tears or other sterile ocular lubricant should be applied topically every few hours. If entropion develops, it should be corrected promptly using one or two vertical mattress sutures. A small bleb of procaine penicillin injected into the lower eyelid provides temporary improvement for mild cases of entropion.

If the animal's body temperature is less than 37° C (100° C), efforts should be made to warm it by raising the environmental temperature, using radiant heat lamps, applying blankets, and using heating pads judiciously. An effective heat pack can be made by placing a wet towel inside two rectal sleeves and microwaving them to the desired temperature. The hot pack remains dry and can be nestled alongside the foal's abdomen. If the animal is wet, it should be dried off to reduce convective heat loss. Volume expansion to restore normal cardiovascular function, peripheral circulation, and systemic blood pressure is an essential part of the warming process. Rewarming the periphery only with external heat without simultaneously warming the core can produce peripheral vasodilation with cardiovascular collapse. The thermoneutral zone for a term foal is 23° to 25° C (73° to 77° F).[1]

Generalized seizure activity should be controlled as soon as possible. Diazepam at 5 to 20 mg IV, given slowly to effect to a 45-kg foal, is an appropriate first choice (see Chapter 20, Seizures). If seizures are severe or recurrent, phenobarbital should be administered (3 to 10 mg/kg IV slowly over 5 to 10 minutes). Multiple doses of diazepam can cause respiratory depression and should be avoided.

Respiratory rate, effort of breathing, mucous membrane color, heart rate, and fluid balance are quickly assessed to establish the need for immediate intervention and stabiliza-

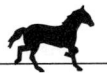

TABLE 18-1

Physical Examination: Normal and Abnormal Parameters

Parameter	Normal Finding	Abnormal Observation
Attitude	Bright, alert	Depression: sepsis, hypoxia, pain, metabolic disturbances (acidosis, hypoglycemia); seizures: hypoxic brain damage or meningitis
Body tone	Erect head and neck posture	Hypotonia: sepsis, immaturity, hypoxia; extensor rigidity: hypoxia, meningitis
Suckle reflex	Present <20 min after birth	Absent or weak with sepsis, immaturity, or hypoxia
Body temperature	37.2°-38.6° C (99°-102° F)	Fever with well-established infection, hypothermia with acute sepsis; temperature instability with prematurity
Mucous membranes	Pink, moist	Pale membranes: anemia from excessive umbilical cord hemorrhage, blood loss into body cavities associated with birth trauma, hemolysis caused by NI or DIC Icteric: liver disease, EHV-1 infection, sepsis, NI Cyanotic: shock, hypoxia Hyperemic: sepsis
Capillary refill time	<2 sec	>2 sec with dehydration, shock
Petechiation	Absent	Present with DIC, sepsis
Pulse	70-100 beats/min, regular	Tachycardia: fever, pain, shock, sepsis, hypocalcemia Bradycardia: severe septic shock, hypothermia, hypoglycemia, hyperkalemia
Pulse quality	Strong peripheral pulses	Hypotension: hypovolemic and septic shock; hyperkinetic pulses during early sepsis
Respiration	30-40 breaths/min, regular	Tachypnea: stress, pain, fever, lung disease, acidosis; slow, irregular rate with apnea caused by hypoxia, prematurity
Nostril flare, rib retractions	Absent	Increased with impending respiratory failure, pneumonia
Lung sounds	Easily heard over all of chest	Rales, rhonchi, ventral dullness with pneumonia, consolidation, atelectasis
Eyes, eyelids	Clear cornea, no entropion	Blepharospasm, miosis, lacrimation, corneal edema and ulceration with self-trauma during recumbency, and entropion
Abdominal distention; borborygmi	Distention absent; borborygmi heard on both sides of abdomen	Distention with ileus, hypoxic gut damage, meconium impaction, uroperitoneum, enteritis; borborygmi decreased with ileus and increased with enteritis
Fecal volume, consistency; color	4-6 oz two to four times/day; pasty; yellow or tan	Constipation with meconium impaction, dehydration Diarrhea: sepsis, hypoxic gut damage, diet changes
Urine volume, concentration	4-6 ml/kg/hr; dilute with specific gravity usually <1.02	Decreased volume with renal failure, hypoxic kidney damage, dehydration, ruptured bladder
Umbilicus	Dry, small	Moist and inflamed because of infection, urachal patency
Joints	No distention or lameness	Warm, distended joints, lameness with septic synovitis
Limbs	Straight with mild carpal valgus common	Tendon laxity with immaturity; carpal and fetlock contracture associated with fetal malpositioning, hypothyroidism, plant toxins

DIC, Disseminated intravascular coagulation; *EHV-1,* equine herpesvirus type 1; *NI,* neonatal isoerythrolysis.

tion. Depending on the type and severity of the animal's condition, postural drainage, suction, oxygen therapy, or positive-pressure ventilation may be indicated. If shock, severe dehydration, or metabolic derangements, such as hypoglycemia, are present, fluid therapy should be initiated as soon as an intravenous catheter is placed and secured. Table 18-1 highlights the significance of abnormal findings on the physical examination.

NEONATAL CHARACTERISTICS INFLUENCING FLUID AND DRUG THERAPY

It is often observed that neonatal animals are more "sensitive" to the actions of drugs administered at normal adult dosage levels and less tolerant of inappropriate fluid administration than the adult animal. Differences between neonatal and adult animals in drug effects generally can be attributed to differences in drug distribution, metabolism, or excretion.[2] Some general characteristics of the neonatal period include better absorption of drugs from the gastrointestinal tract, less drug binding to plasma proteins, increased apparent volume of distribution of drugs that are distributed in the extracellular fluid volume, increased permeability of

the blood-brain barrier, and slower elimination (i.e., longer half-life) of many drugs. It is important to remember, however, that the foal and the calf are relatively precocious newborns, and much of the data on neonatal differences were generated in considerably less mature species. For instance, glomerular filtration rate (GFR) reaches adult values at 2 days of age in calves versus at 14 days of age or more in puppies. Studies of the development of renal function in foals,[3] as well as indirect evidence provided by pharmacokinetic studies of antibiotic agents eliminated primarily by renal excretion,[4] suggest that full-term, 2- to 4-day-old foals also have relatively mature renal function. For a more detailed discussion of neonatal drug disposition, the reader is referred to other texts.[2,5,6]

In the neonate the relative volumes of fluid differ from the adult. Total body water in the equine neonate constitutes 70% to 75% of the total body weight versus about 60% in the adult horse. During growth, the intracellular fluid compartment remains relatively consistent relative to size, whereas the extracellular fluid compartment decreases as a percentage of body weight, with an increasing body fat percentage. In the 2-day-old foal, ECF volume was 394 ± 29 ml/kg, blood volume was 151 ± 32.8 ml/kg, and plasma volume was 94.5 ± 8.9 ml/kg; however, at 4 weeks at age, ECF volume was 348 ml ± 45 ml/kg and plasma volume was 61.9 ± 5.9 ml/kg.[7] In another study, in the 1-week-old term foal, extracellular fluid (ECF) volume was 44 ± 1.3% of body weight and plasma volume was 6.5 ± 1% of body weight. The ECF volume at 3 weeks of age had decreased to 28 ± 2% of body weight.[8]

Although the neonate has a higher percentage of total body water than the adult, it is more vulnerable to water loss than the adult for several reasons, including: (1) increased basal metabolic rate; (2) relatively greater surface area, predisposing to increased heat and water losses; and (3) reduced urine-concentrating ability.

BASIC FLUID THERAPY IN THE NEONATE

The goal of fluid therapy is to expand vascular volume in an attempt to restore and maintain cardiovascular function; improve organ perfusion and blood pressure; and correct dehydration, acid-base balance, osmolality, and electrolyte disturbances. Fluid therapy is a crucial part of the supportive care of the abnormal neonate. In assessment of the need for fluid therapy, both the state of hydration (sunken eyeballs, decreased skin turgor, dry mucous membranes, generalized weakness, decreased urine output) and the state of circulating volume (heart rate, pulse quality, capillary refill time, temperature of limbs, blood pressure) should be assessed. If the losses are very acute, gross abnormalities in effective circulating volume may not yet be reflected in decreased skin turgor or sunken eyeballs, but heart rate or pulse quality may be abnormal. On the other hand, pulse quality and perfusion may be relatively normal in a neonate with severely sunken eyes and reduced skin turgor. Neonates that appear very thin and malnourished may actually be very dehydrated; with fluid therapy alone, their appearance can dramatically change in a short period. In sick foals fluid therapy should replace existing deficits while supplying maintenance requirements. A foal or calf with moderately to severely sunken eyes is estimated to be 8% to 10% (of body weight) dehydrated. The estimated fluid deficit in a 40-kg animal that is 10% dehydrated would be approximately 4 L.

Laboratory parameters are useful for formulating a fluid therapy plan. Serum electrolyte concentrations may be life-threateningly deranged in foals with conditions such as uroperitoneum or enteritis, and knowledge of specific values can be of great benefit in selection of an appropriate fluid. The affordability of portable blood chemistry analyzers* makes determination of electrolyte values feasible even in field situations. A neonate that is nursing poorly can be detected by measurement of urine specific gravity. The normal nursing foal produces large quantities of dilute urine (specific gravity 1.000 to 1.012). In some cases, laboratory values can be misleading. For example, packed cell volume or total plasma protein is often within the normal range in clinically dehydrated neonates.

The fluid therapy plan is calculated to supply maintenance needs and to replace deficits and current losses. Calculation of fluid deficits is based on the equation:

Replacement fluid deficits (L) = % Dehydration × Body weight (kg)

Table 18-2 lists fluid replacement volumes for foals based on clinical assessment of dehydration.

Foals experiencing septic or hypovolemic shock may require fluid administration rates of 40 to 80 ml/kg/hr initially

TABLE 18-2

Calculation of Fluid Deficits

Severity of Dehydration	Percentage of Dehydration	Fluid Deficits for 50-kg Foal (Liters)
Mild	5-6	2.5-3.0
Moderate	7-8	3.5-4.0
Severe	>10	>5.0

BOX 18-1

Blood Pressure Ranges and Maintenance Fluid Requirements for Newborn Foals

BLOOD PRESSURE (BP)
Systolic BP = 80 to 120 mm Hg
Diastolic BP = 65 to 90 mm Hg
Mean BP = 70 to 100 mm Hg

MAINTENANCE FLUID REQUIREMENT
Approximately 4 to 6 ml/kg/hr = 200 to 300 ml/hr for a 50-kg foal

until their blood pressure is stable. Normal blood pressure ranges are shown in Box 18-1. Blood pressure can be easily measured indirectly using the coccygeal artery and the noninvasive Doppler or oscillometric methods.[9] The maintenance fluid requirement for a newborn foal is shown in Box 18-1. Maintenance fluid administration in large animal neonates at the rate of approximately 100 ml/kg/day usually results in adequate fluid balance and good urine output, in the absence of fluid deficits or increased fluid losses. If severe diarrhea is present, the daily fluid requirements can reach 15 to 20 L (500 ml/kg/day) or more.

If an animal is mildly to moderately dehydrated and the gastrointestinal tract is not seriously compromised, fluid requirements can be provided by the enteral route, using milk or commercially available dextrose and electrolyte mixtures. However, if the gut is abnormal or if moderate-to-severe dehydration is present, the intravenous route is the preferred method of fluid administration.

Many types of intravenous catheters are suitable for use in the large animal neonate. Teflon catheters tend to be more thrombogenic than silastic or polyurethane catheters and therefore should be replaced at more frequent intervals. A 5-inch-long, 16-gauge Teflon catheter* placed in the jugular vein and a 2-inch, 16-gauge Teflon catheter† placed in the cephalic vein have both worked well to deliver intravenous fluids to the neonatal calf and foal. Short catheters placed in peripheral veins can be difficult to maintain and are not suitable for large-volume, rapid fluid replacement. We prefer to use a long-term 8-inch, 16-gauge polyurethane catheter‡ inserted in the jugular vein. This catheter is inserted over a flexible J-wire and can be left in place for 2 to 3 weeks. The use of polyurethane catheters reduces the incidence of thrombophlebitis and eliminates the need for frequent catheter replacement. Smaller-diameter catheters may be more suitable

---

*For example, IRMA Blood Analysis System, Diametrics Medical, St. Paul, Minnesota.

---

*Abbocath, Abbott Hospitals, North Chicago, Illinois.
†Quik-cath, Baxter Healthcare Corporation, Deerfield, Illinois.
‡Arrow Catheter, Arrow International, Reading, Pennsylvania.

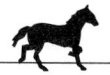

for lambs and kids. Regardless of the type used, it is essential to use aseptic techniques for catheter placement and to secure the catheter firmly to the skin. A combination of superglue and sutures is effective in keeping the catheters in place. Catheter sites are kept as clean as possible, and the site of venipuncture and the vein are watched closely for signs of infection. Specific information on catheter placement and maintenance can be found in other texts.[10,11]

The intraosseous infusion technique is an alternative method for rapid delivery of fluids in the critically ill neonate when intravenous access is not possible. This procedure uses the intramedullary vessels in the bone marrow to gain access to the central circulation. A description of this technique is described in other texts.[12] In calves, intraosseous fluids may be administered via placement of a 14- or 16-gauge needle in the head of the femur or humerus. A 16- or 14-gauge needle is inserted in a longitudinal plane. Neonatal bones are soft, so the needle can be drilled into the bone using finger pressure. Commonly a core of bone will plug the needle, requiring the drilling needle to be discarded and replaced with a new needle placed in the same hole. After placement of the needle, attach a 60-cc syringe and inject sterile saline under slight pressure to start the flow. As the fluid is administered, check for subcutaneous leakage to ensure that the needle is correctly placed within the bone marrow. One to 2 L of saline or isotonic bicarbonate administered to the severely dehydrated calf is often enough to restore blood pressure sufficiently for placement of an intravenous catheter. The optimum type of intravenous fluid administered depends on the electrolyte and acid-base status of the patient. Fluids are available as either crystalloids (e.g., polyionic fluids such as Plasmalyte, Normosol, lactated Ringer's solution, saline) or colloids (e.g., Plasma, Hetastarch). Polyionic fluids are usually used for rapid rehydration and maintenance fluid therapy. These fluids should be isotonic (osmolality = 270 to 300 mOsm/L). In most circumstances, in the absence of appropriate laboratory services, the use of a balanced electrolyte solution such as lactated Ringer's or Plasmalyte is satisfactory to replace fluid deficits. Saline solutions may be a more appropriate choice in certain situations: foals with diarrhea are often hyponatremic and hypochloremic; premature foals with immature renal and endocrine function conserve electrolytes poorly and have a tendency to become hyponatremic and hypochloremic; foals receiving diuretics often require additional sodium chloride. Other exceptions to this rule include animals with hyperkalemia, when potassium-containing fluids are best avoided, and animals with hypernatremia, when controlled slow reduction of body sodium content is required.

Fresh or frozen plasma is often more effective than crystalloid fluids for volume expansion in seriously ill neonates. Endotoxemia and sepsis produce inflammatory changes in vessel walls. Capillary endothelial permeability is increased, resulting in increased extravasation of fluid and albumin from the capillaries into the interstitium. Rapid infusion of large volumes of crystalloids reduces colloidal oncotic pressure while transiently increasing intravascular hydrostatic pressure. These forces favor movement of fluid out of vessels. Colloidal solutions contain large-molecular-weight molecules that do not freely pass though the capillary membrane. Therefore colloid administration results in increased plasma oncotic pressure, increased plasma volume, and more effective improvement in circulating blood volume. Both synthetic colloids (e.g., dextran, hetastarch) and natural colloids (e.g., plasma, whole blood) are available. Plasma has several advantages over synthetic colloids. It is a good source of protein, opsonins, complement, clotting factors, and immunoglobulins. The disadvantages of plasma include the possibility of an anaphylactic reaction and the need to thaw frozen plasma, which makes it less suitable when rapid fluid

resuscitation is necessary. An effective commercially available synthetic colloid is hetastarch.* Hetastarch has been used successfully for rapid fluid resuscitation in equine patients and has had few adverse reactions.[13]

If a neonate remains hypotensive in spite of volume expansion and fluid replacement, pressor agents such as dopamine and dobutamine may be indicated. Dopamine with its combined α- and β-adrenergic and dopaminergic activity is preferred. Higher doses will be required for patients in severe septic shock. If the foal fails to respond to high doses (>10 to 15 μg/kg/min), norepinephrine, which is a more potent α-adrenergic agent, can be tried. Safe and effective infusion of these agents requires continuous monitoring and some type of infusion pump. Recently, nitric oxide (NO) has been shown to play a role in sepsis-induced hypotension.[14] Intravenously administered new methylene blue, an NO antagonist, has been used to try and reverse severe life-threatening hypotension.

The rate of fluid administration is determined by the degree of dehydration, severity of cardiovascular compromise, and maintenance requirements. Most normal foals can tolerate rapid fluid infusion, but asphyxiated, septic, or premature foals may be oliguric and therefore far less tolerant of overzealous fluid administration. In these cases, generalized edema may result. A general rule of thumb is to replace one half of the calculated deficit in the first 6 hours of fluid therapy and the rest over 12 to 24 hours. A flow rate of 20 ml/kg/hr or higher (40 to 80 ml/kg/hr) may be needed to treat hypovolemic or septic shock.

In any depressed, weak, or seizing animal, blood glucose levels should be checked because hypoglycemia is one of the most frequently observed metabolic derangements accompanying many neonatal diseases. The rapid blood glucose reagent strips and hand-held glucometers are very useful in making this determination in a field setting. For treatment of hypoglycemia, a continuous infusion of 5% to 10% dextrose is sufficient to reach and maintain adequate blood glucose levels in most neonates. Hypertonic glucose boluses (25% to 50%) may aggravate preexisting central nervous system insults and frequently result in rebound hypoglycemia 30 to 40 minutes after infusion; thus they should be avoided. One regimen for treating hypoglycemia is 10% dextrose infusion at 5 to 10 ml/kg fairly rapidly, followed by a continuous infusion to supply 4 to 8 mg/kg/min (approximately 5 ml/min of 5% dextrose for a 40-kg neonate). The appropriateness of the therapy should be judged by frequent blood and urine glucose determinations. If hyperglycemia results, the rate of infusion or concentration of solution is decreased (to deliver perhaps 2 mg/kg/min) but not stopped.

Another metabolic derangement commonly observed in the large animal neonate is metabolic acidosis. This disorder may be caused by accumulation of acid, by loss of buffers from the body, or by a combination of the two. Whenever possible, treatment should be directed at correcting the underlying cause of the acidosis. Acidosis caused by low cardiac output or decreased peripheral oxygen delivery should be treated by measures to increase tissue perfusion (e.g., plasma volume expansion, cardiac inotropes, nasal oxygen insufflation). In this type of acidosis there is no actual loss of bicarbonate from the body, and bicarbonate therapy often produces disappointing results and adverse reactions. If respiratory dysfunction is present, considerable caution should be exercised in the use of sodium bicarbonate. Bicarbonate functions as a buffer only in an "open" system in which carbon dioxide can be transported to the lungs and eliminated.[15] Profound fluctuations in blood pressure and

---

*Hespan, DuPont Pharmaceuticals Co., Wilmington, Delaware.

cerebral blood flow, intracranial hemorrhage, and decreased oxygen delivery to tissues are possible adverse effects of sodium bicarbonate infusion in humans.[16] In many mildly to moderately acidotic neonates, simple volume expansion with isotonic fluids alone is very effective in correcting the base deficit by improving perfusion. Other more compromised individuals need more aggressive support of the cardiovascular system. Mild acidosis (HCO_3^- deficit 5 to 10 mEq/L) associated with dehydration can be corrected by simple rehydration. Bicarbonate supplementation is recommended when HCO_3^- deficits are greater than 10 mEq/L (serum HCO_3^- <15 mEq/L) or whenever the pH is less than 7.2. Bicarbonate deficits can be calculated using the following equation:

Bicarbonate deficit (mEq) =
$$0.6 \times \text{Body weight (kg)} \times \text{Base deficit (mEq)}$$

An isotonic bicarbonate solution is preferred because excessive bicarbonate administration results in increased CO_2 production leading to respiratory embarrassment and increased risk of CNS acidosis and hemorrhage. Isotonic bicarbonate can be made by adding 150 ml 8.4% bicarbonate solution to 850 ml sterile water or by adding 200 ml 5% bicarbonate solution to 800 ml of sterile water. Bicarbonate solutions should be given slowly. Hyperkalemia is often observed with metabolic acidosis because of the transcellular shift of potassium ions into the extracellular fluid in exchange for hydrogen ions.[17] As the metabolic acidosis is corrected, the hyperkalemia resolves. Bicarbonate solution should not be combined with any calcium-containing solution or precipitation will occur.

The effect of the bicarbonate replacement therapy should be monitored closely and the dose adjusted accordingly. Neonates with severe diarrhea because of ongoing losses of bicarbonate through the feces may need considerably more than the calculated deficit to maintain an adequate blood pH until the diarrhea subsides. As in any type of fluid therapy, a plan is devised, the animal's response to the plan is monitored, and changes are made accordingly.

Hypokalemia can occur in anorexic foals, foals with diarrhea, and those receiving diuretic therapy. Potassium supplementation can be estimated using the following equation:

Replacement K (mEq) = 0.4 × Body weight (kg) × K deficit (mEq)

Potassium can safely be added to fluids at a rate of 20 to 30 mEq/L. The rate of potassium administration should not exceed 1 mEq/kg/hr. If acidosis is present, hydrogen ions are exchanged for intracellular potassium ions, resulting in a relative increase in serum K. As the acidosis is corrected there will be an influx of K ions back into cells, resulting in potential hypokalemia; hypokalemia must always be anticipated during fluid therapy.

Hypernatremia is observed sporadically in calves and is associated with errors in mixing milk replacer and oral electrolyte preparations. Hypernatremia produces cerebral depression similar to metabolic acidosis and will not be recognized if serum electrolyte concentrations are not measured. Correction of hypernatremia with hypotonic solutions has been described but was associated with 100% mortality.[18] Experimentally, during rapid restoration of plasma osmolality in chronically hypernatremic animals, the development of brain edema correlates with the onset of seizures.[19] Correction of hypernatremia via controlled, gradual reduction of serum sodium over 2 to 3 days has been successful in calves[20] and pigs.[21] Strict regulation of sodium fluid load (intravenous and oral) and repetitive monitoring of serum electrolytes is required. Fluid therapy of diarrheic calves is discussed more specifically in Chapter 20.

NUTRITIONAL SUPPORT OF THE ABNORMAL NEONATAL FOAL

Provision of adequate nutritional support to the compromised neonate is an essential part of critical care but often becomes a major management problem. Reasons for the common failure to provide adequate nutrition to the neonate include underestimating the needs of the ill, stressed animal; a disinterest in nursing on the part of the sick neonate; the need to use alternative methods and routes of delivery for continued oral feeding; and a gastrointestinal tract that is compromised and intolerant of nutrient intake.

Nutrition of the premature or sick neonate is a science in the early stages of development; this is true in human neonatology, and much less is known in veterinary medicine. The exact nutritional requirements for optimum growth of the normal-term foal have not even been defined, let alone for the premature, growth-restricted, or debilitated animal whose caloric, protein, mineral, and vitamin requirements might be very different.

Measurements of milk production of mares combined with data concerning the free-choice milk intake of normal orphan foals and premature and sick foals recovering from various illness suggest that about 125 to 150 kcal/kg/day or even higher is close to the normal caloric intake.[22] Healthy full-term foals nurse an average of 2 minutes, seven times an hour,[23] consume between 20% and 30% of their body weight in mare's milk daily, and gain 0.5 to 1.4 kg/day. On this diet a 50-kg foal would consume 10 to 12.5 L of milk a day to provide 120 to 150 kcal/kg/day. Nutritional requirements may be even higher in disease states such as generalized septicemia, pulmonary disease, thermal stress, or after surgery.

If there is no medical contraindication for oral feeding, and the gastrointestinal tract is functional, then enteral nutrition is the preferred and most effective route of nutritional supplementation. Enteral feeding is more physiologic, stimulates normal gut maturation, growth of intestinal villi, production of crypt cells, hepatic and biliary secretions, and brush border disaccharidase enzyme activity. Enterocytes rely on absorption of volatile fatty acids (VFA) such as glutamine and β-hydroxybutyrate from the gut lumen as their primary energy source. Therefore, even in foals that must be fed parenterally, small volumes of enteral feeds are given to "feed the gut" to prevent gut atrophy.

Foals that are not nursing from the mare can be fed by bottle, bucket, or nasogastric tube. If an effective swallow reflex is present, bottle-feeding can be used. Udder bumping and teat-seeking behavior can be stimulated by allowing the foal to approach the bottle from behind and under the handler's armpit. This technique also reduces the risk of aspiration by preventing overextention of the head and neck. Bucket feeding allows the foal to drink with its head and neck in a flexed position and is helpful for foals with a weak swallow reflex or foals who will be hand raised. Milk should be introduced in a shallow hand-held bowl and the foal encouraged to suckle the finger or nipple as its head is lowered into the milk. "On demand" feeding is ideal but often impractical and labor intensive. Foals less than 7 days of age should be fed every 2 hours.

Nasogastric intubation is required if ineffectual swallowing and suckling are present. A small-bore flexible silicone tube (5 to 7 mm internal diameter) with a weighted tungsten end is preferred. Individual choice dictates whether the tube is passed for each feeding or left in-dwelling. In-dwelling tubes can be sutured to the nares or taped to half a tongue depressor, which is then taped to the foal's muzzle and/or fleece halter. Tubes should be sealed between feedings to prevent aerophagia. Recumbent foals should be maintained in sternal recumbency immediately after tube feeding to reduce the risk of gastroesophageal reflux and aspiration.

If the foal's mother is available and milk production is adequate, free-choice nursing is optimal. A nurse mare is probably the next best substitute. Popular enteral formulas include mare's milk, goat's milk, and artificial milk replacers. Mare's milk is preferred. Goat's milk is acceptable and is higher in fat, total solids, and gross energy than mare's milk. Foals raised on goat's milk occasionally become constipated. Cow's milk is not as digestible, but can be used if additional sugar is added and some of the fat is removed. This can be accomplished by using 2% skim milk and adding 20 g of dextrose per liter of milk. A variety of artificial milk replacers are available. The ideal replacer should have 22% crude protein, 15% fat, and less than 0.5% fiber on a dry matter basis. Complications associated with enteral feeding include colic, abdominal distention, diarrhea, constipation, flatulence, misplacement of the nasogastric tube, aerophagia, nasal and pharyngeal irritation from the tube, and aspiration pneumonia.

Delayed gastric emptying and gastroduodenal dysmotility can be improved in some foals with metoclopramide given intravenously as a slow infusion (0.25 mg/kg/hr) or orally (0.3 to 0.6 mg/kg every 4 to 6 hours). Overdosage is associated with excitement. Other prokinetic agents are erythromycin (2 mg/kg PO every 6 hours or given as hourly infusions every 6 hours), which works throughout the gastrointestinal tract, and cisapride (0.1 to 0.2 mg/kg PO or per rectum every 6 hours), which also affects the entire gut. All prokinetic agents are contraindicated if gastrointestinal obstruction is suspected. Diarrhea is treated symptomatically with oral bismuth subsalicylate (1 to 2 ml/kg PO every 4 to 6 hours) and/or loperamide (0.1 to 0.2 mg/kg PO every 6 hours). Diarrhea may also respond to administration of active-culture yogurt or an intestinal inoculant containing lactobacillus organisms. Nasopharyngeal irritation from repetitive tubing can be treated with insufflation of a nasopharyngeal spray containing prednisone, furacin, glycerin, and dimethyl sulfoxide (DMSO).

More details on the feeding of both orphan and sick neonatal foals are contained in review papers[22,24-27] and in Chapter 46.

NUTRITIONAL SUPPORT OF THE SICK CALF

Although the neonatal calf has a stomach with four parts, it functions very differently from that of the adult. At birth the abomasum is the only truly functional part and has a capacity twice that of the other compartments. Liquid is shunted past the reticulorumen into the abomasum through a tube that is formed by the esophageal groove. The groove is closed by a reflex that is stimulated by the intake of liquids (milk is the best, electrolyte and glucose water are usually effective, but straight water becomes ineffective in closing the groove fairly early in life).

The first enzyme to start the process of milk digestion is salivary lipase. Shortly after the milk reaches the abomasum, it begins to clot as a result of the enzyme renin. Shortly after feeding, whey is released from the abomasal milk clot to the duodenum, and partially digested casein follows. The age at which ruminal digestion begins is very dependent on the calf's diet. Transition to ruminal digestion begins at 3 to 4 weeks of age; the earlier dry feed with a fiber source is provided, the earlier ruminal development starts. If liquid diet is limited, the calf will start to consume dry food at a few days of age.

The energy requirements of the calf may be divided into maintenance and growth requirements. Blaxter and Wood[28]

found the maintenance requirement for the neonatal calf to be 52.4 kcal/kg of body weight per day, whereas Brisson, Cunningham, and Haskell[29] estimated 44.7 kcal/kg per day. Energy requirements for growth have been estimated at 307[26] and 268[29] kcal/100 g of body weight gain. Because whole milk contains about 70 kcal/100 ml, a neonatal calf would need about 3 L of whole milk for maintenance and 4 to 5 additional L to gain 1 kg of weight. The requirements for the sick, stressed calf are not as well established. Digestible protein requirement for maintenance is 0.5 g/kg of body weight, and the amount required for growth is about 22 g/100 g gain in body weight. Digestibility of the protein is an important concern in the evaluation of milk replacers. Many milk replacers substitute legume proteins for milk-derived proteins. Legume-derived proteins contain antinutritional factors (ANF) that include antigenic proteins, lectins, and trypsin inhibitors.[30] Trypsin provides a protective mechanism against clostridial disease by cleaving the clostridial β toxin.[31] Soybean flour has been used to experimentally induce *Clostridium perfringens* type C enterotoxemia in lambs.[32]

After provision of ample colostrum, dairy calves are routinely fed milk replacer at the rate of 5% to 6% of body weight twice a day (see Chapter 21 for discussion of milk replacers). To avoid abomasal bloat, no more than 2 L is provided per feeding, and solid feed is introduced at an early age. Although the normal neonatal calf tolerates this feeding regimen well, the amount of milk supplied is probably insufficient for optimum growth. In addition, the nutritional requirements of the infected or premature calf probably far exceed this. In the compromised individual a smaller volume of milk should be provided more frequently.

PARENTERAL NUTRITION

In the past, parenteral nutrition was more frequently used to supply at least a portion of the daily nutritional requirements to critically ill foals and calves. Parenteral nutrition is indicated whenever feeding via the gut is inadequate or contraindicated. Candidates for partial or total parenteral nutrition include those individuals with chronic diarrhea, gastroduodenal ulcer disease (foal), a variety of postsurgical patients, foals with botulism, premature and infected animals, and other individuals with gastrointestinal tracts poorly tolerant of enteral feedings.

Parenteral nutrition involves administration of hypertonic solutions containing dextrose, amino acids, lipids, vitamins, electrolytes, and trace minerals. These parenteral nutrition solutions must be administered continuously through a jugular catheter. Complications include metabolic disturbances such as hyperglycemia/hypoglycemia, glucosuria/osmotic diuresis, hyperlipemia, azotemia, and imbalances of trace minerals, vitamins, and electrolytes. Catheter-related problems include thrombosis, phlebitis, and sepsis. Commonly used stock solution for parenteral nutrition include 50% dextrose, 8.5% or 10% amino acids, and 10% or 20% lipid emulsion. Sample calculations are shown in Box 18-2.

Foals receiving parenteral nutrition should have their blood and urine glucose monitored. Serum glucose concentration should remain greater than 80 mg/dl and less than 180 mg/dl. Serum should be checked for gross lipemia. Heparin can be administered at 10 units/kg as an IV bolus to treat lipemia. The amount of glucose, lipid, and amino acids can be varied for each individual foal. Foals must be weaned onto and off parenteral nutrition slowly. All intravenous lines must be checked routinely for signs of infection. Additional information regarding the use of parenteral nutrition in foals is presented in other articles.[27]

Currently the applications of parenteral nutrition are on a fairly short-term basis compared with human medicine, usually 2 to 3 weeks at the most. Most commonly, parenteral and enteral nutrition has been used in combination; parenteral nutrient delivery is used to supplement, not totally replace, oral intake. Enteral nutrition helps to maintain the intestinal mucosa. Prolonged total parenteral nutrition is associated with reduced intestinal epithelial cell renewal, villous atrophy, and decreased enzymatic activity.[33]

Although parenteral nutrition can be expensive and difficult to manage, the benefits, such as prevention of a catabolic state or starvation, improved body condition at discharge, and better healing, can far outweigh the drawbacks. Details concerning the use of parenteral nutrition compounds can be found in other references[34] and in Chapter 46.

NOSOCOMIAL AND ZOONOTIC INFECTIONS

Immunologically naive neonates are particularly susceptible to opportunistic and contagious pathogens. Nosocomial infections increase mortality and amplify environmental contamination, perpetuating further dissemination of the infecting organism. Prevention of nosocomial infection requires attention to detail. Patients may be exposed to pathogens via environmental contamination, biologic vectors, equipment, and personnel. Provision of a pathogen-free environment requires disinfection between patients and verification of disinfection via culture. Control of vermin is important as birds, rodents, and insects have all been implicated in dissemination of infectious pathogens. Equipment (shovels, brushes, nasogastric tubes, etc.) function as vectors if not disinfected between stalls and or animals. Most importantly, personnel have to appreciate their potential role in nosocomial infections. Personnel schedules need to consider the workload demands and implications these may have on infectious disease control over the whole 24-hour

period of each day. Separate personnel for management of infected and high-risk patients is desirable. Attention to detail, basic hygiene, and common sense should prevail. Washable foot-wear, disinfectant footbaths, patient-specific protective clothing, and hand washing between patients are infectious disease control protocols that have been successfully applied in controlling infectious disease outbreaks in veterinary hospitals. Many of the pathogens that affect neonates are potentially zoonotic (salmonella, cryptosporidia, *Giardia*, and clostridia); personal hygiene is in the interest of health care providers and their patients.

IMMUNE SYSTEM SUPPORT: PLASMA AND COLOSTRUM

Controversy persists as to what serum immunoglobulin G (IgG) concentration is protective for newborn foals. There is little argument, however, that healthy foals have postsuckle IgG exceeding 1000 to 2000 mg/dl within 24 hours of birth. There is also agreement that there a correlation between very low IgG concentrations (IgG <200 mg/dl) and increased foal morbidity and mortality. By definition, a serum IgG level less than 200 mg/dl is complete failure of passive transfer (FPT), and a serum IgG level between 200 and 800 mg/dl is partial failure of passive transfer. Causes of FPT include poor-quality colostrum, failure to ingest adequate colostrum, and inability to absorb adequate amounts of colostral immunoglobulins. Mares produce an average of 1.5 to 2.0 L of colostrum. Ideally, foals should receive a minimum of 1 L of good-quality colostrum within the first 8 hours of life. In addition to IgG, colostrum contains IgA for local gut immunity, IgM, high caloric density, growth factors, lactoferrin, laxative properties, and leukocytes. If fresh or frozen colostrum is not available, there are some sources of lyophilized IgG products for oral administration that have a longer shelf life and do not require freezing. These products are expensive and may have variable absorption. Regardless of the product, a rule of thumb is to administer a minimum of 40 g of IgG (or 1 g/kg body weight) to colostrum-deprived foals. Always measure serum IgG concentrations to determine if the supplementation was adequate.

Plasma administration becomes necessary if the foal's IgG is low, it is too old to absorb colostrum, or gut function is abnormal. I recommend IgG supplementation for any foal with a serum IgG level less than 200 mg/dl regardless of its health status or environment. If the foal's IgG is between 200 and 800 mg/dl, I recommend IgG supplementation if one or more of the following conditions exist:

- Gestation length less than 320 days or signs of prematurity/dysmaturity
- Difficult delivery (e.g., dystocia, premature placental separation, meconium staining)
- Grossly abnormal or heavy placenta (>11% of foal's body weight)
- 5- and 10-minute Apgar scores lower than 6.
- High environmental stresses including overcrowding and poor farm hygiene
- Anticipated transportation off the farm within 7 to 10 days of foaling
- Failure to stand and nurse within 3 hours of delivery
- Abnormal physical examination within 24 hours of birth; significant abnormalities include generalized weakness, infected mucous membranes, poor suckle, severe angular limb deformities, enlarged umbilicus, patent urachus, colic, meconium retention, increased respiratory effort, other signs of localized infection.
- Poor postpartum surveillance

Plasma is administered through an aseptically placed catheter using a blood administration set with an in-line filter. The volume of plasma to give depends on the foal's IgG

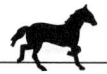

TABLE 18-3

Transfusion Reactions: Signs, Causes, Therapy

Signs of Reaction	Cause	Treatment
Hemolysis, hemoglobinuria, hemoglobinemia	Incompatibility between donor RBCs/recipient's plasma	Stop transfusion; give IV fluids; cross match for suitable donor
Fever, chills	Allergic or nonspecific reaction to donor protein	Give antipyretics
Allergic reaction, urticaria	Recipient reacts to soluble antigens in donor's plasma	Slow transfusion, give antihistamine
Anaphylactic reaction, respiratory distress, hypotension, shock	Anaphylaxis	Stop transfusion, give epinephrine (5-10 ml of 1:10,000 epinephrine IV/SC)
Circulatory overload, hypertension, pulmonary edema, cardiac dysfunction	Excessive volume expansion	Stop or slow transfusion; give diuretic
Endotoxemia, fever, tachycardia, tachypnea, leukopenia	Contaminated transfusion	Stop transfusion, give banamine, and antibiotics

IV, Intravenous; *SC*, subcutaneously; *RBCs*, red blood cells.

level, the desired IgG level, the foal's body weight, and the IgG level in the plasma and the general health of the foal. The old rule of thumb for plasma administration for FPT is 20 ml/kg or approximately 1 L for a 45-kg foal. In healthy foals, 1 L of plasma with IgG of 1200 mg/dl raises the serum IgG 200 to 250 mg/dl. The same amount of plasma has less effect in septic foals. Ill foals require relatively more plasma because the serum half-life of IgG is less, IgG may be sequestered in intravascular spaces or at sites of inflammation, and IgG may be catabolize more readily. A complete discussion of FPT and its treatment is presented in Chapter 49.

Plasma should be administered at an average rate of 10 ml/kg/hr. Give the first 100 ml slowly and monitor the foal's pulse, respiratory rate, and temperature. Possible transfusion reactions and treatment are listed in Table 18-3.

RESPIRATORY SUPPORT

Thoracic radiographs and arterial blood gas analysis help determine the severity of lung disease. Lateral radiographs with the foal standing or recumbent help characterize the nature and extent of pulmonary pathology. Diffuse pulmonary infiltrates occur with bacterial or viral pneumonia and atelectasis. Cranioventral and caudoventral pulmonary infiltrates are seen with aspiration pneumonia and bacterial bronchopneumonia. Nodular infiltrates suggest discrete abscessation.

Arterial blood gas analysis determines the degree of pulmonary dysfunction. Portable blood gas machines now make blood gas analysis easy and affordable. The preferred site for arterial puncture is the great metatarsal artery. A small 25-gauge needle attached to a heparinized 1- or 3-ml Luer slip syringe is used. Hypoxemia (Pao_2 <60 mm Hg) with a normal $Paco_2$ is caused by ventilation/perfusion mismatching, right to left shunting, low inspired O_2, and impaired gas exchange. Hypoxemia accompanied by elevated concentrations of CO_2 is usually the result of hypoventilation caused by respiratory muscle fatigue, central depression of the respiratory center, or neuromuscular weakness as with botulism. Mild hypoxemia can be improved by positioning the laterally recumbent foal into a sternal position. Oxygen supplementation is best administered through a soft nasal cannula inserted into the nasal passage to the level of the medial canthus. The cannula can be sutured or taped to the external nares. Humidified oxygen is administered using a tank or wall oxygen source and humidifier filled with distilled water. Oxygen flows between 2 and 10 L/min are regulated using a flowmeter. Flow rates are adjusted to keep the Pao_2 between 70 to 100 mm Hg. Long oxygen lines attached to a surcingle allow even ambulatory foals to benefit from continuous oxygen therapy.

Mechanical ventilation is necessary for persistent hypoxemia that is refractory to nasal insufflation or is accompanied by $Paco_2$ greater than 70 to 75 mm Hg. A long, cuffed nasotracheal tube is required and a ventilator capable of delivering tidal volumes of 10 to 15 ml/kg, respiratory rate of 15 to 25 breaths/min, proximal airway pressure between 18 and 25 cm H_2O, end-expiratory pressure (PEEP) of 0 to 10 cm H_2O, and an inspired oxygen concentration between 0.21 to 1.0. Ventilators that allow the foal to breathe spontaneously between preset ventilator-delivered breaths are tolerated the best by the foal. Guidelines regarding ventilatory support for foals are presented in other review articles.[35] More recently investigations have been conducted using noninvasive mechanical ventilation in neonatal foals.[36]

Foals have a poorly developed cough reflex. Tracheobronchial secretion removal may be enhanced using chest coupage and nebulization with mucolytic agents such as acetylcysteine or dilute bicarbonate solution. Ultrasonic nebulizers using solutions or an Equine Aero Mask using metered-dose aerosol inhalers can be used.

Chemical respiratory stimulants can be used to stimulate the central respiratory center. Theophylline, caffeine, and aminophylline are xanthine derivatives commonly used as bronchodilators, but they can also be used to improve diaphragmatic contractility and to treat periodic apnea associated with hypoxia and prematurity. The safest stimulant is caffeine: loading dose of 10 mg/kg PO once daily followed by 2.5 mg/kg PO once daily as a maintenance dose.

ANTIBIOTIC THERAPY

Foals that become ill or compromised during the first few days of life are at increased risk for infection. Because of the neonate's immature immune system, localized infections tend to become systemic and may lead to septicemia. This explains how foals that present with diarrhea can develop uveitis and septic joints. Antibiotics are administered to foals for two reasons: (1) prophylactically to prevent infection, and (2) therapeutically to treat existing infection. The most serious infections are those caused by gram-negative bacteria (e.g., *Escherichia coli*, *Klebsiella*, *Salmonella*, *Pasteurella*, and *Actinobacillus* spp.). The most common gram-positive pathogen is *Streptococcus* sp., which is often encountered as part of a mixed infection involving the respiratory tract and umbilicus. Occasionally, anaerobic infections (e.g., *Clostridia* and

Bacteroides spp.) are encountered as causes of umbilical infections, diarrhea, or aspiration pneumonia.

When used prophylactically, the oral and intramuscular routes of administration can be considered. Penicillin or ampicillin and an aminoglycoside administered intramuscularly or intravenously are good choices if the risk of infection is great. Ceftiofur (intramuscularly) or trimethoprim-sulfamethoxazole (orally) are reasonable choices. Prophylactic antibiotics should be given for 3 to 5 days or until the risk factors for sepsis are gone. Once sepsis is confirmed, intravenous therapy is the preferred route because gut absorption is too variable. Antibiotic therapy should be continued for a minimum of 7 to 10 days. If localized infections develop, then antibiotics may need to be given for 2 to 3 weeks. In cases of abscess formation and bone infections, therapy is often extended for 1 to 2 months.

TRANSPORT AND REFERRAL

A decision should be made early in the clinical course as to whether the neonate can be taken care of at the farm or whether it should be referred to a neonatal intensive care facility for treatment. If the support staff on a farm is experienced and committed to provision of good nursing care and if appropriate diagnostic facilities are available, many mildly to moderately ill individuals can be successfully treated on the farm and recover within 2 to 4 days. When the neonate is more compromised and in need of considerable supportive care, including continuous intravenous fluid therapy and oxygen supplementation, a more rational decision is to make a referral if the animal's value warrants the expense. The sicker or more immature the neonate, the more complications it is likely to develop during the course of treatment. It is much better to refer a sick neonate early in the course of disease rather than as a last resort before death.

If a decision is made to refer the animal, the method of transportation is extremely important to the outcome of the case. If the foal is recumbent and is showing signs of hypothermia or respiratory distress, consider shipping the foal ahead of the mare in a heated vehicle. The mare can be stripped of colostrum and then sedated. Colostrum can be sent with the foal. The mare can be sent later, once the foal's condition has been evaluated and stabilized at the referral clinic. Save and send the placenta with all compromised foals. Recumbent foals can be restrained in a car by wrapping them in a sleeping bag or blanket. Ideally, an attendant should travel with any weak, recumbent, or potentially recumbent foal.

Cold foals can be warmed during transport by increasing the inside temperature of the vehicle and by placing water bottles or heat packs beside the foal. Body temperature, blood glucose, and oxygenation must be maintained during the trip. In the hypoglycemic patient, a continuous glucose infusion during the trip is far better than a glucose bolus given before departure.

If the foal is dyspneic, administer intranasal oxygen at 3 to 6 L/min using an indwelling intranasal cannula. Portable oxygen tanks can be rented from home care pharmacies with a veterinarian's prescription. A recumbent foal should be kept sternal and turned every 2 hours to minimize dependent lung atelectasis. If the foal is apneic or demonstrating an unusually slow respiratory rate consider a loading dose of caffeine (10 mg/kg) given orally or per rectum before transport.

REFERENCES

1. Ousey J, Murgatroyd P, Rossdale PD: Thermoregulation in the neonatal foal, *Equine Vet J Suppl* 5:50, 1988.
2. Baggot JD: Drug therapy in the neonatal foal, *Vet Clin North Am (Equine Pract)* 10:87-107, 1994.
3. Brewer BD et al: A comparison of inulin, para-aminohippuric acid, and endogenous creatinine clearances as measures of renal function in neonatal foals, *J Vet Intern Med* 4:301-305, 1990.
4. Cummings LE, Guthrie AJ, Harkins JD: Pharmacokinetics of gentamicin in newborn to 30-day-old foals, *Am J Vet Res* 51:1988-1992, 1990.
5. Brock KA: Sedation and anesthesia. In Koterba AM, Drummond WH, Kosch PC, eds: *Equine clinical neonatology,* Philadelphia, 1990, Lea & Febiger, p 653.
6. Caprile KA, Short CR: Pharmacologic considerations in drug therapy in foals, *Vet Clin North Am (Equine Pract)* 3:123-144, 1987.
7. Spensley MS, Carlson GP, Harrold D: Plasma, red blood cell, total blood, and extracellular fluid volumes in healthy horse foals during growth, *Am J Vet Res* 48:1703-1707, 1987.
8. Kami G, Merritt AM, Duelly P: Preliminary studies of plasma and extracellular fluid volume in neonatal ponies, *Equine Vet J* 16:356, 1984.
9. Vaala WE, Webb AI: Cardiovascular monitoring of the critically ill foal. In Koterba AM, Drummond WH, Kosch PC, eds: *Equine clinical neonatology,* Philadelphia, 1990, Lea & Febiger.
10. Spurlock SL, Furr M: Fluid therapy. In Koterba AM, Drummond WH, Kosch PC, eds: *Equine clinical neonatology,* Philadelphia, 1990, Lea & Febiger, p 671.
11. Orsini JA, Kreuder C: Intravenous catheter placement. In Orsini JA, eds: *Manual of equine emergencies,* Philadelphia, 1998, WB Saunders, pp 15-16.
12. Orsini JA, Kreuder C: Intraosseous infusion technique. In Orsini JA, eds: *Manual of equine emergencies,* Philadelphia, 1998, WB Saunders, pp 15-16.
13. McFarlane D: Hetastarch: a synthetic colloid with potential in equine patients, *Compend Contin Educ* 21:867-871, 1999.
14. Symeonides S, Balk RA: Nitric oxide in the pathogenesis of sepsis, *Infect Dis Clin North Am* 13:449-463, 1999.
15. Ostea EM, Odell GB: The influence of bicarbonate administration on blood in a "closed system": clinical implications, *J Pediatr* 80:671, 1972.
16. Howell JH: Sodium bicarbonate in the perinatal setting: revisited, *Clin Perinatol* 14:807-816, 1987.
17. Fisher EW: Hydrogen ion and electrolyte disturbances in neonatal calves, *Ann NY Acad Sci* 176:223-230, 1971.
18. Pringle JK, Berthiaume LMM: Hypernatremia in calves, *J Intern Vet Med* 2:66-70, 1988.
19. Hogan GR et al: Pathogenesis of seizures occurring during restoration of plasma tonicity in animals previously chronically hypernatremic, *Pediatrics* 43:54-64, 1969.
20. Angelos SM et al: Treatment of hypernatremia in an acidotic neonatal calf, *J Am Vet Med Assoc* 214:1364-1367, 1335, 1999.
21. Holbrook TC, Barton MH: Neurologic dysfunction associated with hypernatremia and dietary indiscretion in Vietnamese pot-bellied pigs, *Cornell Vet J* 84:67-76, 1994.
22. Koterba AM, Drummond WH: Nutritional support of the foal during intensive care, *Vet Clin North Am (Equine Pract)* 1:35-40, 1985.
23. Carson K, Wood-Gush DGM: Behaviour of thoroughbred foals during nursing, *Equine Vet J* 15:257, 1983.
24. Koterba AM: Nutritional support: enteral feeding. In Koterba AM, Drummond WH, Kosch PC, eds: *Equine clinical neonatology,* Philadelphia, 1990, Lea & Febiger, p 728.
25. Naylor JM, Bell R: Raising the orphan foal, *Vet Clin North Am (Equine Pract)* 1:169-78, 1985.
26. Pugh DG, Williams MA: Feeding foals from birth to weaning, *Comp Cont Educ Pract Vet* 14:526, 1992.
27. Vaala WE: Nutritional management of the critically ill neonate. In Robinson NE, ed: *Current therapy in equine medicine,* ed 3, Philadelphia, 1992, WB Saunders, pp 741-751.
28. Blaxter KL, Wood WA: The nutrition of the young Ayrshire calf, *Br J Nutr* 5:55, 1951.
29. Brisson GJ, Cunningham HM, Haskell SR: The protein and energy requirements of young dairy calves, *Can J Anim Sci* 37:157, 1957.
30. Lalles JP: Nutritional and antinutritional aspects of soybean and field pea proteins used in veal calf production: a review, *Livestock Prod Sci* 34:181-202, 1993.
31. Niilo L: *Clostridium perfringens* type C enterotoxemia, *Can Vet J* 29:658-664, 1988.
32. Niilo L: Experimental production of hemorrhagic enterotoxemia by *Clostridium perfringens* type C in maturing lambs, *Can J Vet Res* 50:32-35, 1986.
33. Levine GM et al: Role of oral intake in maintenance of gut mass and disaccharide activity, *Gastroenterology* 67:975-982, 1974.
34. Hansen T: Nutritional support: parenteral feeding. In Koterba AM, Drummond WH, Kosch PC, eds: *Equine clinical neonatology,* Philadelphia, 1990, Lea & Febiger, p 747.
35. Palmer JE: Ventilatory support of the neonatal foal, *Vet Clin North Am (Equine Pract)* 10:167-185, 1994.
36. Hoffman AM, Kupcinskas RL, Paradis MR: Comparison of alveolar ventilation, oxygenation, pressure support, and respiratory system resistance in response to noninvasive versus conventional mechanical ventilation in foals, *Am J Vet Res* 58:1463-1467, 1997.

Neonatal Infection

WENDY E. VAALA

JOHN K. HOUSE

Infection, general and localized, is an important cause of morbidity and mortality in the large animal neonate. In both calves and foals, bacteria cause most infections. The prognosis of neonatal infection varies considerably depending on the type and severity of infection. During septicemia, the release of bacterial endotoxins results in overactivation of the host immune system and uncontrolled release of endogenous mediators. This response precipitates a cascade of metabolic and hemodynamic changes that often culminate in multiple organ system failure.[1,2] Circulatory failure, perfusion deficits, and an inability of the body to use existing metabolic substrate effectively characterize septic shock, the end point of that continuum. If the neonate survives acute sepsis, localized areas of infection may then appear, such as pneumonia, uveitis, synovitis, physitis, meningitis, hepatitis, and enteritis.

In the past decade the survival rates of septicemic foals have improved considerably because of advances in early detection and critical care management,[3-8] but it is far preferable to prevent septicemia through good management techniques and by ensuring that the newborn acquires good colostrally derived immunity. The prognosis for septicemic neonates admitted for treatment in the late stages of the disease remains dismal, because bacteria usually are already well established in many organs, particularly the bones and joints. In these cases, even if the neonate survives in the short term, some chronic complications result in an unfavorable long-term outcome. Devastating, rapidly developing multiorgan infections refractory to treatment are common in neonates with failure of passive transfer (FPT) of immunoglobulins.[9] (Chapter 49 presents detailed information on the detection, prevention, and treatment of failure of passive transfer.)

ETIOLOGY AND NEONATAL IMMUNITY

Most neonatal infections are caused by opportunistic bacteria that normally live in the genital tract, on the skin, or in the environment of normal horses, cows, sheep, and goats. Infection may be acquired prenatally, through the placenta, from the birth canal, or from the environment after birth. Portals of entry include the respiratory and gastrointestinal tracts, the placenta, and the umbilicus. Several abnormalities in the late-gestation mare make infection more likely in the

neonate (see Chapter 15). Bacterial placentitis is a common cause of premature delivery and infection in the newborn foal; most cases are caused by an infection that ascends through the cervix. Perinatal stress, including chronic in utero hypoxia, prematurity, dystocia, and birth asphyxia, renders the neonate more susceptible to infection. Unsanitary environmental conditions, overcrowding, poor ventilation, contamination of the environment with pathogenic bacteria such as *Salmonella* organisms, and other poor management techniques also predispose to infection.[6]

The propensity for contagious and opportunistic infections in neonates reflects the immature status of their immune system. At birth foals, calves, lambs, and kids are hypogammaglobulinemic or agammaglobulinemic and immunologically naive. Bovine colostrum contains approximately 45 mg/ml[10] of immunoglobulin and 10[6] leukocytes per milliliter.[11] Passively derived immunoglobulins enhance neonatal immunity by functioning as neutralizers and opsonins. The association between failure of passive transfer of immunoglobulins and neonatal infection has been well established in the calf[12,13] and suggested by several studies in the foal.[9,14-16] Colostral leukocytes participate in regulation of the neonate's immune response. Comparison of the immune response of calves fed leukocyte-replete or leukocyte-depleted colostrum indicates that colostral leukocytes enhance humoral immunity and phagocytic function.[17-21] After experimental *Escherichia coli* infection, calves fed leukocyte-replete colostrum recovered more quickly and shed fewer bacteria than calves fed leukocyte-depleted colostrum.[11] Transfer of cellular immunity via colostral leukocytes has also been demonstrated in sheep.[22] Colostral leukocytes are destroyed when colostrum is frozen, pasteurized, or fermented.

The phagocytic and bacterial killing function of neutrophils (polymorphonuclear neutrophils [PMNs]) is a crucial component of the primary immune response against invading pathogens. Even though normal calves at birth have a larger number of neutrophils in the circulation than adults, the neutrophils from neonatal calves are functionally less effective than adult cells. Reduced Fc-receptor expression in neonatal PMNs may contribute to impaired phagocytosis and antibody-dependent cellular cytotoxicity.[23-25] Depressed PMN bacterial killing[26] may be related to reduced superoxide anion[27] and myeloperoxidase-hydrogen peroxide-halide antibacterial activity.[25] Adult-level superoxide activity in fetal PMNs suggests that some of the deficits in neonatal PMN function may be a manifestation of perinatal PMN suppression.[28] Calves have elevated cortisol levels for the first 10 days of life, which may contribute to depression of neutrophil function.[29] Dexamethasone depresses neutrophil phagocytosis, antibody-dependent cellular cytotoxicity, and bacterial killing.[30,31]

Undefined serum factors also appear to be important for PMN function, because phagocytosis and bacterial killing by neonatal PMNs are similar to those of adult PMNs when bacteria are opsonized with adult serum, but they are reduced when bacteria are opsonized with neonatal serum.[26] T-helper (CD 4+) cells play a central role in humoral and cell-mediated immunologic memory. Lymphokines produced by CD 4+ cells, specifically interleukin-2 (IL-2), interleukin-4 (IL-4), and interferon-γ (IFN-γ), are essential components of antigen-specific immunity. Virtually all IL-4 and most IFN-γ produced by polyclonally activated adult human CD4+ cells are mediated by a subset of "functional memory cells."[32] Leukocyte production of IL-4 and IFN-γ is reduced in human neonates,[32] and IFN-γ is reduced in bovine neonates,* possibly reflecting their antigenically naive status. Depressed lymphocyte proliferation and IL-2 activity in the perinatal period correlates with elevated cortisol levels.[29]

Acquisition of humoral immune competence is age and antigen dependent.[33] Neonates are capable of producing humoral immune responses to good immunogens (protein antigens) but may fail to respond to lesser immunogens (sugars and lipids). Calves under 3 months of age vaccinated with modified live or killed salmonella vaccines produce an adult type of humoral immune response to salmonella protein antigens but do not respond to salmonella lipopolysaccharide.[34] Ingestion of colostrum suppresses the humoral response to some antigens but not others.[33]

Adverse management and environmental conditions further compromise neonatal immunity. Cold stress depresses neutrophil chemotaxis, and vasoconstriction reduces delivery of leukocytes to peripheral tissues.[35] Protein-energy malnutrition in calves is associated with depressed lymphocyte IL-2 activity, lymphocyte proliferation, and humoral immune responses.[29] Micronutrient deficiencies also depress immunity. Selenium, zinc, copper, and vitamin E deficiencies depress lymphocyte and phagocyte function.[36,37]

Inherited defects in immune function are sporadically observed in neonates and should be considered when recurrent or atypical infections are observed, such as *Pneumocystis carinii* pneumonia in foals. Inherited immune deficiencies are discussed in Chapter 49.

PATHOGENESIS OF SEPSIS

One of the most potent mediators of gram-negative sepsis is endotoxin, the lipopolysaccharide (LPS) component in the outer cell membrane of gram-negative bacteria. Endotoxin is released whenever the bacterial cell membrane is disrupted, such as occurs during rapid growth or cell death. More specifically, endotoxin is composed of hydrophilic heteropolysaccharide and hydrophobic lipid. The surface portion of lipopolysaccharide is the O-antigenic determinant, consisting of sugar chains that are highly variable between species. Deeper in the LPS molecule is the lipid moiety, which is responsible for most of the endotoxin's biologic activities. The reticuloendothelial system is responsible for detoxification of endotoxin.

The initiating event in the sepsis cascade is the release of endotoxin into the circulation. Endotoxin's interaction with neutrophils, mononuclear cells, lymphocytes, and vascular endothelial cells results in the release of a second wave of endogenous mediators that include tumor necrosis factor, interleukins, kinins, myocardial depressant factor, β-endorphins, free radical oxygen species, lysosomal enzymes, prostaglandins, interferons, and eicosanoids.[1,2,38] Most of these mediators have direct effects on the vascular endothelium, resulting in increased endothelial permeability. The endothelium releases two additional substances: endothelium-derived relaxing factor (EDRF) and endothelin-1. EDRF has been identified as nitric oxide and is responsible for relaxing smooth muscle, depressing myocardial function, decreasing vasopressor responsiveness, and inhibiting platelet aggregation.[39,40] Endothelin-1 is a potent vasoconstrictor. After the increase in vascular permeability, interstitial and pulmonary edema, hypovolemia, and decreased cardiac output develop, as do pulmonary and systemic hypotension. Splanchnic perfusion decreases, and coagulation pathways are activated, resulting in varying degrees of disseminated intravascular coagulation (DIC). Most patients that die of septic shock suffer multiple organ failure.[2]

Respiratory failure is a common complication of septic shock. As pulmonary capillary permeability increases, leukocytes accumulate and degranulate in the pulmonary microvascualture, resulting in endothelial damage and increased capillary leakiness and alveolar flooding. Lung collapse (atelectasis), intrapulmonary shunting, and ventilation/perfusion mismatch develop. Terminally, hypoxemia, pulmonary hypertension, progressive lung collapse, pulmonary edema, and respiratory failure develop.[2]

Myocardial depression occurs during sepsis. Endotoxin and nitric oxide exert a direct inotropic depressant effect on the heart. During early sepsis, stimulation of the sympathetic nervous system results in tachycardia, increased cardiac output, improved myocardial contractility, and increased oxygen consumption. As sepsis progresses, vascular tone and oxygen extraction by peripheral tissues decrease, and metabolic acidosis and anaerobic metabolism develop. During late sepsis, myocardial failure develops, accompanied by decreased cardiac output and severe hypotension.

Sepsis is best characterized nutritionally by hypermetabolism, catabolism, and protein wasting.[41] During sepsis, intermediary metabolism is disrupted and the foal loses sequentially the ability to utilize glucose, then fat, and finally protein as an energy source. Elevated concentrations of catecholamines and glucagon contribute to insulin resistance and increased lipolysis. These changes explain the hyperglycemia and lipemic serum occasionally observed in septic foals.

INFECTIOUS AGENTS ASSOCIATED WITH NEONATAL DISEASE

In all studies conducted in the United States, Europe, and Australia in the past 15 years, gram-negative bacteria have been the predominant cause of infection in large animal neonates, and *E. coli* has been by far the most common bacterium isolated.[3,4,6,7,42-47] Other common bacterial organisms include *Actinobacillus* spp. (foals), *Pasteurella* spp. (calf and foal[48] [rare]), *Klebsiella* spp., *Salmonella* spp. (calf and foal), and less commonly, *Pseudomonas* spp., *Listeria monocytogenes*,[49] *Clostridium perfringens* and *Clostridium septicum*,[50] *Staphylococcus aureus*, and *Streptococcus* spp. Although *Streptococcus* organisms are most commonly isolated in mixed infections with gram-negative bacteria,[3,4] both α-hemolytic and β-hemolytic *Streptococcus* organisms have been isolated in pure culture in foals with large subcutaneous abscesses and physitis and septic arthritis. *Streptococcus pneumoniae* type 3,

---

*Dr. David Van Metre, University of California-Davis, Unpublished data.

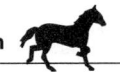

typically a human pathogen, was identified as the cause of severe respiratory distress in a neonatal foal.[51] Polymicrobial infections are common in septicemic calves (28%).[44]

More recent surveys examining blood culture results of foals admitted to neonatal intensive care units reflect a trend in the type of bacterial organisms contributing to septicemia. The number of gram-positive bacterial isolates has increased, including *Streptococcus* (α and β), *Staphylococcus, Enterococcus,* and *Clostridium* organisms.[52] These statistics serve to remind clinicians not to ignore the pathologic significance of gram-positive organisms when selecting an antibiotic regimen for the septic neonate. Although newer antibiotics, including some of the cephalosporins, β-lactam antibiotics, and fluoroquinolones, have an extended gram-negative spectrum, their gram-positive spectrum may be inadequate for pathogens such as *Streptococcus* spp.

Most organisms known to cause placental and fetal disease may cause disease of the newborn. Infectious agents associated with stillbirths and birth of weak ruminant neonates are listed in Box 15-3. Infections of neonates contracted in utero are uncommon compared with postnatally acquired infections. Clinical signs of in utero infections depend on the age of the fetus at the time of infection and the tissue tropism and virulence of the infecting organism. Abortion storms and outbreaks of perinatal weakness, congenital defects, and mortality are often manifestations of widespread herd or flock infections. Subclinically infected neonates may remain chronically infected, providing a continuing reservoir of infection in the population. Transplacental infection is important in the epidemiology of some diseases, including Johne's disease (*Mycobacterium paratuberculosis*), bovine virus diarrhea, and bovine leukosis.[53-55]

Although viral agents are most commonly associated with abortion in the mare, viral infections may also occasionally cause disease in the newborn foal. Equine herpesvirus infection may result in a weak newborn foal that responds very poorly to conventional supportive care; antemortem diagnosis is very difficult.[56,57] Equine viral arteritis has been reported in a full-term neonatal foal.[58] Equine influenza may be associated with interstitial pneumonia in foals.[59]

Fungal infections have been only rarely observed in the foal. The development of severe, generalized candidiasis has been observed in debilitated or immunocompromised foals undergoing intensive care. The diagnosis has been made using blood cultures or cultures of joint aspirates.

CLINICAL SIGNS

The spectrum of clinical signs associated with septicemia depends on the integrity of the host immune system, the duration of illness, the severity and route of infection, and the target organs. Early in the clinical course, clinical signs usually are nonexistent or vague, nonspecific, and easily attributed to other diseases. During the early hyperdynamic phase of sepsis, clinical signs include lethargy, hypotonia, more time spent sleeping, decreased nursing frequency followed by complete loss of suckle reflex, hyperemic mucous membranes with rapid capillary refill time associated with peripheral vasodilation and increased cardiac output, tachycardia, bounding peripheral pulses, extremities that are still warm, tachypnea, and variable body temperature. Capillary leakiness contributes to the early appearance of petechiae on the gums and sclera, inside the ears, and on the coronary bands. As soon as the foal's nursing vigor decreases, the mare's udder becomes warm and distended and may stream milk spontaneously. When the foal does nurse from the overdistended udder, the weak foal often comes away with a milk-stained face because of the spontaneous milk letdown that it is too weak too swallow. Dehydration develops rapidly,

resulting in decreased urine output and constipation. Obviously, the earlier the infection is diagnosed, the better chance the treatment has of being successful. Localizing signs may or may not be present. Prompt and aggressive intervention at this stage of the disease process frequently results in a successful outcome.

During late sepsis, when infection overwhelms the host's immune system, septic shock develops. Affected foals are usually recumbent, dehydrated, and almost moribund. Clinical signs include severe hypotension associated with hypovolemia and decreased cardiac output, tachycardia, altered mentation, cold extremities, weak peripheral pulses, and dry, injected mucous membranes with a toxic ring and prolonged capillary refill time. Hypothermia is common. Gut motility usually is decreased and is accompanied by gastric reflux, abdominal distention, and constipation or diarrhea. Colic may be present if the ileus and abdominal distention are severe. Liver dysfunction is associated with cholestasis and increasing clinical jaundice. Decreased pulmonary perfusion and increased vascular permeability contribute to progressive respiratory compromise. Signs of respiratory distress include tachypnea, dyspnea with nostril flare, rib retractions, and expiratory grunting. Salvage of the patient in late septic shock usually is not successful. Although an encouraging response to intensive therapy may be noted initially, most neonates presented in late septic shock do not survive.

Fever is inconsistently present in infected foals; the possibility of infection should *never* be ruled out because of the absence of fever.[3] In one study, diarrhea was the most common early localizing sign in a group of septicemic foals.[3] Other signs include seizures (with or without the presence of meningitis or encephalitis), colic, respiratory distress, uveitis, subcutaneous abscesses, joint distention, or periarticular edema (or both), and umbilical abscessation. The signs of osteomyelitis or physeal infection may be extremely subtle, with no obvious areas of inflammation detectable on the limbs. The only clues may be a reluctance to move or a choppy, stilted gait or an inflammatory hemogram (increased fibrinogen, in particular).

The time of onset of clinical signs of infection in the neonate depends on whether the infection was acquired in utero or postnatally. Animals infected in utero generally begin to show signs sometime during the first 24 hours of life, whereas postnatally infected animals often appear relatively normal for the first 2 days of life or longer. *Actinobacillus* infections in foals may become apparent at a somewhat earlier age (24 to 48 hours of age) and are commonly characterized by an acute onset of depression, diarrhea, or rapidly distending, painful joints. Bone and joint infections in neonates may not be obvious for several days to weeks, and their appearance may either follow an improvement in systemic signs of illness or not be accompanied by any signs of systemic illness.

Similar to the condition in foals, septicemia in ruminant neonates commonly involves multiple organs, with the respiratory and gastrointestinal systems most commonly affected.[44] Clinical signs are often nonspecific and may include lethargy, poor suckle reflex, weakness, dehydration, tachycardia, tachypnea, and recumbency. Findings suggestive of involvement of a particular organ system include diarrhea, lameness, omphalophlebitis, neurologic and ocular signs, and cardiac murmurs. Depressed mentation, diarrhea, and dehydration are the most common clinical signs of sepsis in neonatal ruminants, but the clinical presentation varies.[46] The rectal temperature, heart rate, and respiratory rate are poor predictors of sepsis in calves.[46,47] Fecteau and others[47] have developed a clinical score for predicting sepsis in calves to promote better use of antimicrobial drugs by producers. Criteria included in the model were fecal consistency, hydration status, attitude (mental awareness), and umbilical and scleral vessel assessment. The sensitivity and specificity of the model were 76% and 75%, respectively. In the calves examined, the presence of severe diarrhea or a localized infection (e.g., infected navel) was associated with an increased probability of bacteremia as determined by blood culture.

DIAGNOSIS OF BACTERIAL INFECTION IN THE NEONATAL FOAL

It is not difficult to diagnose an infected neonate when overwhelming sepsis is present and every body fluid is swarming with bacteria. Unfortunately, if treatment is instituted at this time, it is unlikely to be successful. Because of the necessity of early diagnosis and treatment of infection for a favorable outcome, a reliable, rapidly available field test to establish the presence of infection would be highly desirable; however, such a test is not currently available. Positive blood culture results are the only definitive antemortem proof of bacteremia, but a minimum of 24 hours usually is required for preliminary results.

Because of the difficulty in identifying early sepsis at a treatable stage, a scoring system has been developed for the neonatal foal that incorporates a group of historic parameters, physical examination findings, and laboratory values, which together have been found to be considerably more accurate than any single parameter in establishing the likelihood of infection (Fig. 19-1).[60] The sepsis score is intended for use as a diagnostic aid only and is not 100% accurate. If the score is low for an individual foal but clinical suspicion of infection is high, antibiotic therapy should be instituted, and further assessment should then be performed.

White Blood Cell Count and Differential

The white blood cell (WBC) count and differential are an important part of the sepsis score. Some foals in the early stages of septicemia have a normal total WBC count, but most have either an increased number of band neutrophils (more than 50 cells/μl) or toxic changes in the neutrophils (Döhle bodies, toxic granulation, vacuolization). Foals dying of septicemia generally have very low WBC counts with considerable toxicity, but a low WBC count in a septic patient does not necessarily predict death. The WBC count may make dramatic changes in a short period, often preceding changes in the clinical condition.

Fibrinogen Level

The fibrinogen level is of particular value in detecting newborn foals that have been infected or exposed to inflammatory placental disease in utero. Fibrinogen values in these cases may be 1000 mg/dl or higher at birth (normal is 300 mg/dl or less). In the early stages of postnatally acquired infections, fibrinogen values may only be mildly increased (400 to 500 mg/dl), but with increasing chronicity resulting from pneumonia or bone and joint infections, plasma fibrinogen levels may increase dramatically.

The total plasma protein concentration varies considerably and may be influenced by dehydration, catabolism, and ingestion of colostral immunoglobulins. The range of presuckle protein concentration varies so much between foals that it is not a reliable indicator of FPT.

Hypoglycemia

Hypoglycemia (a glucose level below 60 mg/dl) commonly accompanies generalized infection and is associated with bacterial consumption and reduced glycogen reserves. Serum glucose values can be very low, with the animal showing few signs other than depression and weakness. See p. 297 for details on the treatment of hypoglycemia.

IgG Determination

IgG determination has been shown to be an important component of the sepsis evaluation, because low IgG levels have strongly correlated with the presence of sepsis. Severe, overwhelming infections are seen far less commonly in foals with normal IgG levels (over 800 mg/dl), but they can occur, particularly in individuals with in utero–acquired infections and severe enteric infections caused by pathogenic bacteria such as *Salmonella* spp. and in clostridial intestinal infections. Because serum IgG levels can change dramatically as a result of the protein catabolism associated with sepsis, it often is difficult to determine whether hypogammaglobulinemia in a sick foal is the cause or result of sepsis.

The possibility of using hematologic evaluation of neonates for early detection of sepsis is illustrated in a study reported by Adams and colleagues.[61] Hematologic values in 35 newborn beef calves were evaluated; five calves subsequently developed clinical signs of sepsis at 3 weeks of age. Comparison of the hematologic values from the five diseased calves with values for healthy calves revealed significant differences at each sample collection time (birth, 24 hours, 48 hours, and 3 weeks), although disease was not clinically evident at the three early sample times. Compared with the clinically normal calves, the five septic calves had more band neutrophils and a higher neutrophil to lymphocyte ratio at birth. At 24 hours, the monocyte count was higher, and at 48 hours, the total leukocyte, mature neutrophil, and monocyte counts and the neutrophil to lymphocyte ratio were higher in the five calves. At 3 weeks, when clinical signs of disease were detectable in the five calves, the total leukocyte, band neutrophil, and mature neutrophil counts, neutrophil to lymphocyte ratio, and plasma total protein and fibrinogen concentrations were higher.[61]

Hematologic abnormalities observed in septic calves with clinical signs of disease are not consistent. In a retrospective study of 25 septic calves, a noticeable feature of the pattern of laboratory abnormalities was the contrast of severe clinical signs with minor complete blood count (CBC) and serum biochemical alterations in numerous calves.[44] Abnormal laboratory findings included neutrophilia or neutropenia, immature neutrophils, toxic neutrophils, and hyperfibrinogenemia.[44] Low serum immunoglobulin concentrations are also commonly observed in septic calves.[44,47]

Other abnormal serum chemistries associated with sepsis include metabolic acidosis (bicarbonate level below 19 mEq/L), caused by the increased anaerobic metabolism and azotemia (creatinine greater than 2 mg/dl) that occur secondary to dehydration, and also because of the primary renal damage. During the terminal stages of septicemia, foals frequently display a mixed respiratory and metabolic acidosis accompanied by hypoxemia. Lipemia and hyperbilirubinemia reflect altered endocrine and hepatic function. Thrombocytopenia, hypofibrinogenemia, a prolonged prothrombin time (PT) and partial thromboplastin time (PTT), and an increase in fibrin degradation products characterize DIC.

Positive Blood Culture Results

Positive blood culture results are essential to make the diagnosis of septicemia. However, it is clear that treatment cannot be delayed until the results of blood cultures are obtained. Although it does not help to make the initial decision about therapy, a positive blood culture result allows a more accurate prognosis to be given to the owner, provides

COLLEGE OF VETERINARY MEDICINE

J. Hillis Miller Health Center

University of Florida
Gainesville, FL 32610

Large Animal Hospital

Sepsis Score

Foal's Name _____   Date _____   Total Score _____

Case Number _____   Check One:

Age _____   ____ At admission?

____ Day subsequent to admission?
Indicate day

❋: _____

Number of points to assign:

Information collected:	Record exact ❋	4	3	2	1	0	This case
I. CBC							
1. Neutrophil count (NOT TOTAL WBC!)			<2000/mm³	2000-4000 or >12,000	8000-12,000	Normal	
2. Band neutrophil count			>200/mm³	50-200		<50	
3. Doehle bodies, toxic, granulation, or vacuolization in neutrophilis		Marked	Moderate	Slight		None	
4. Fibrinogen mg/dl				>600	401-600	≤400	
II. Other Laboratory Data 1. Blood glucose mg/dl				<50	50-80	>80	
2. IgG quick test mg/dl		<200	200-400	401-800		>800	
III. Clinical Examination 1. Petechiation or scleral injection not secondary to eye disease or trauma			Marked	Moderate	Mild	None	
2. Fever				>102°F	<100°F	Normal	
3. Hypotonia, coma, depression, convulsions				Marked	Mild	Normal	
4. Anterior uveitis, diarrhea, respiratory distress, swollen joints, open wounds			Yes			No	
IV. Historical data 1. Placentitis, vulvar discharge prior to delivery, dystocia, long transport of mare, mare sick, foal induced, GA >365d			Yes			No	
2. Prematurity			<300 days	300-310	311-330	>330	

Total Points _____

1. IF a foal is older than 12 h, compute the score using the ZST value you get back from the lab.
2. IF it is less than 12 h, give it a +2 for ZST if it has a history of nursing what appeared to be good colostrum. Give the foal a +4 if it has not nursed or if in doubt.
3. A score of 11 or higher correctly predicts sepsis 93% of the time. A score of 10 or less predicts non-sepsis correctly 88% of the time.

FIG. 19-1 ▦ Sepsis scoring system in use at the Equine Neonatal Intensive Care Unit of the University of Florida (College of Veterinary Medicine. From Brewer BD, Koterba AM: *Equine Vet J* 10:18, 1988.)

information on the type of bacteria and its susceptibility pattern, and helps guide the decision as to length of antibiotic treatment.

Blood cultures are easy to perform but must be done carefully for accurate results. The hair should be shaved and the site of venipuncture surgically scrubbed. Depending on the type of culture bottle or tube, a set amount of blood is withdrawn from the vein aseptically and deposited into both the anaerobic and aerobic blood culture bottles. A liquid or solid blood culture media can be used. One popular culture media is Columbia Broth Medium with sodium polyanetholesulfonate as anticoagulant for aerobic cultures (Septi-Chek, Roche Laboratories, Nutley, NJ) and a brain-heart infusion media for anaerobic cultures. If the media is not readily available, the sample can be transferred in a yellow-top tube containing the anticoagulant acid citrate dextrose. Serial cultures are preferred. A clean needle is used to transfer the blood into each bottle, and the bottles are then incubated. A positive culture is characterized by marked turbidity, usually within 12 to 48 hours of incubation. The media with bacterial growth is then Gram stained and plated for identification and susceptibility testing. Working with a local human hospital may provide the ideal resource when trying to identify bacteria and establish antibiotic susceptibility patterns.

Other samples that can be used for culture in addition to urine and blood are synovial fluid, cerebrospinal fluid (CSF), peritoneal fluid, feces, and transtracheal aspirate. In cases of physeal osteomyelitis, a physeal aspirate may be beneficial.

In our opinion, all abnormal neonatal foals should have a blood culture performed once on admission to the hospital, regardless of whether they had received antibiotics previously, and they should then be given antibiotic therapy if infection is suspected. Specimens for bacterial cultures are also taken from specific areas (CSF, joint, feces, trachea) if local infections are suspected. With only one blood culture routinely taken per foal, some false-negative results have been obtained, but the number of positive results has been surprising.[3,43] However, foals with in utero–acquired pneumonia have rarely shown a positive result on a blood culture, and additional cultures (e.g., with tracheal aspirate) should also be done. If a fever spike occurs during the hospital stay, if the WBC count changes dramatically, or if the clinical condition of an infected foal deteriorates, the blood is recultured. The development of resistant infections has been observed in both community- and hospital-acquired infections, and prompt detection is important.

TREATMENT OF BACTERIAL INFECTION

Antibiotic therapy currently is the cornerstone of treatment of neonatal infection. Because sepsis can progress with devastating speed in the neonate, antibiotic therapy should be started as soon as sepsis is suspected. Broad-spectrum coverage should be initiated pending culture results, keeping in mind the preponderance of gram-negative bacteremia, the reemergence of gram-positive pathogens, and the possibility of polymicrobial infections. Bactericidal drugs are favored for the treatment of sepsis in neonates because of the immaturity of the neonatal immune system. The immaturity of mechanisms involved in drug absorption, distribution, biotransformation, and excretion contributes to the altered pharmacokinetics of antimicrobials in neonates. Implications of altered pharmacokinetics in neonates include the potential for suboptimal therapeutic concentrations, toxic effects and, an effect important in food animals, violative residues if adult dosing regimens are used. In general, antimicrobials have longer elimination times in neonates (under 2 weeks of age) than in adults, and therefore larger doses are administered with a longer dosage interval to achieve similar peak and trough antimicrobial concentrations. More complete discussions of antibiotic therapy in neonatal foals[7,62,63] and food animals can be found in other texts.[64-67]

The duration of antibiotic therapy in infected neonates depends on the clinical status of the patient and the type of infection documented. One week to 10 days of therapy may be adequate for suspected but undocumented cases of sepsis if the CBC results, the fibrinogen level, and the patient's condition are normal at the end of that interval. A minimum of 2 weeks of treatment is suggested when the blood culture result is positive but there is no evidence of localized infections. Three to 4 weeks of antibiotic treatment (or longer) often are required when the infection has localized, particularly in the joints or lungs. Therapy usually is discontinued when the WBC count, fibrinogen level, and radiographs have returned to normal. Although there was concern in the past about the use of aminoglycoside antibiotics in the neonatal foal, 10 years of extensive use of amikacin sulfate in a clinical setting without routine serum monitoring suggests that a well-hydrated neonatal foal tolerates the drug very well, even after extended periods of treatment (2 to 4 weeks).

Treatment of established sepsis in the neonate has a poor prognosis, with a survival rate of less than 12% of septic calves in a referral hospital.[44] Client education to facilitate early recognition and treatment of septic neonates improves outcome and reduces cost.

Antibiotic Therapy in Foals

The combination of a penicillin and an aminoglycoside, such as gentamicin (3 mg/kg given IV or IM every 8 to 12 hours) or amikacin (7 to 10 mg/kg IV or IM twice every 8 to 12 hours), usually provides good antimicrobial coverage. Many clinicians working in referral intensive care units prefer amikacin to gentamicin because it seems to be less nephrotoxic and less likely to be associated with the development of resistant bacterial infections.[7,63,68] Ideally, peak and trough serum aminoglycoside concentrations are monitored to ensure that the proper dose and dosing interval are used, but this is not often possible in a field setting. Unfortunately, no studies have been conducted in the foal to determine the specific peak and trough serum concentrations that result in optimal survival rates in septic individuals.[69] Based on work involving in other species, a target peak concentration of 15 to 30 µg/ml and a trough concentration of 1 to 3 µg/ml have been suggested.[70] Daily monitoring of amikacin serum levels in studies of critically ill foals revealed a need to change the intravenous dosing rate from 7 mg/kg twice a day to 9 to 12 mg/kg at 10- to 12-hour intervals in 40% of full-term hypoxic patients.[70] The amikacin dose was changed to 8.5 to 10.5 mg/kg at 12- to 24-hour intervals in six of seven premature hypoxic foals, based on serum monitoring results.[71] Studies conducted more recently have demonstrated the efficacy of high-dose, once-daily dosing of amikacin (21 mg/kg IV every 24 hours).[72] Gentamicin dosages for neonatal foals have also been altered from 3.5 mg/kg IV twice a day to 6.6 mg/kg every 24 hours.[73] During long-term aminoglycoside therapy, efforts are made to prevent dehydration, and the patient's urinalysis results and serum creatinine level are monitored at least weekly.

Other antibiotics that may be useful in the empiric treatment of the infected neonate include certain third-generation cephalosporins, such as cefotaxime (20 to 30 mg/kg IV or IM every 8 hours), ceftriaxone, and ceftazidime. In studies of susceptibility patterns of bacteria cultured from foals undergoing treatment in intensive care units, antibiotics such as ampicillin, kanamycin, and tetracycline were of very little value for treatment of gram-negative infections. Twenty percent to 40% of isolates were resistant to trimethoprim-sulfonamide combinations (15 mg/kg IV or PO every 12 hours), ceftiofur (2.2 to 6.6 mg/kg IM every 12 hours), chloramphenicol (25 to 50 mg/kg IV or PO every 6 hours), and ticarcillin-clavulanate (50 mg/kg IV every 6 to 8 hours).[4,6,43,74] A susceptibility pattern should document that the organism is indeed susceptible before these antibiotics are selected for use. Fluconazole may be effective in the treatment of localized and generalized candidiasis. One recommended dosage for foals is a loading dose of 400 mg followed by 200 mg at 24-hour dosing intervals.[7]

Antibiotic Therapy in Neonatal Ruminants

Common medical conditions in neonatal calves that require antimicrobial therapy include diarrhea, pneumonia, bacteremia, omphalophlebitis, osteomyelitis, meningitis, and septic arthritis.

Bacteremia is a common problem in debilitated neonatal ruminants. Quick recognition and treatment of sepsis improves the likelihood of a successful outcome. Blood culture studies of debilitated calves indicate that gram-negative bacteria account for approximately 80% of bacterial isolates, E. coli being the bacteria most often isolated.[44,46,75] In a study of 190 recumbent calves on a large calf-raising facility, 31% were determined to be bacteremic as follows: E. coli accounted for 51% of the isolates; other gram-negative organisms, 25%; gram-negative anaerobes, 6%; gram-positive cocci, 12%; and gram-positive rods, 6%.[75] Empiric antimicrobial therapy

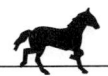

should include a gram-negative and gram-positive spectrum. Other considerations pertinent to antimicrobial selection include the pharmacokinetics and pharmacodynamics of the drug in neonates, the likelihood of antimicrobial resistance, and the potential for violative antimicrobial tissue residues. Determination of antimicrobial susceptibility (minimal inhibitory concentration [MIC]) before therapy is desirable but often not possible. As an alternative, a drug may be selected and given at a dosage that has been shown to be effective for 90% or more of similar isolates tested (MIC 90%). The objective of measuring antimicrobial MICs is to facilitate antimicrobial selection that is likely to achieve a therapeutic concentration of drug for the target pathogen. The MIC data are of limited value without information on the serum and tissue concentrations attainable using the intended drug dose. Data on microbial susceptibility to antimicrobial drugs are

provided in Table 19-1, and pharmacologic data on the volume of distribution, half-life, and breakpoint MICs of common antimicrobial drugs are presented in Table 19-2. The data are intended as a guide. The data obtained from different studies reflects the magnitude of differences that may be observed over time and between sources.

Antimicrobial drugs with a gram-negative spectrum of activity include third-generation cephalosporins (ceftiofur), trimethoprim-sulfonamides (TMS), fluoroquinolones (enrofloxacin), aminoglycosides, sulfonamides, and tetracyclines. In Herd Health Memo No. 9 for 1993-1994, the National Cattlemen's Association (NCA) recommended that "until further scientific information becomes available alleviating safety and efficacy concerns, aminoglycoside antibiotics should not be used in cattle except as specifically approved by the FDA." The bacteriostatic action and frequency

TABLE 19-1

Antimicrobial Susceptibility Data for Bacterial Pathogens from Bovine Sources

Organism (Number of Isolates)	Drug	Percentage Susceptible	Minimal Inhibitory Concentration (μg/ml) 50%	90%	Range
PASTEURELLA HAEMOLYTICA*					
(n = 461)[82]	Ampicillin	60.5	0.25	32	≤0.03->64
(n = 89)[83]	Ampicillin		4	>16	0.25->16
(n = 421)[84]	Ampicillin		128	128	
(n = 461)[82]	Ceftiofur	100	≤0.03	0.06	≤0.03-0.13
(n = 50)[85]	Ceftiofur		0.0078	0.015	≤0.003-0.03
(n = 121)[86]	Enrofloxacin		0.06	0.06	0.03-0.12
(n = 461)[82]	Erythromycin	5.4	4	4	≤0.03->64
(n = 89)[83]	Erythromycin		2	16	0.5->16
(n = 421)[84]	Erythromycin		4	4	
(n = 243)[87]	Florfenicol			1	
(n = 89)[83]	Gentamicin		1	2	0.25-8
(n = 421)[84]	Gentamicin		2	4	
(n = 89)[83]	Kanamycin		4	>16	2->6
(n = 89)[83]	Penicillin G		8	>16	4->6
(n = 461)[82]	Spectinomycin	83.5	32	64	0.5->128
(n = 89)[83]	Spectinomycin		12	>32	8->32
(n = 421)[84]	Spectinomycin		8	16	
(n = 89)[83]	Sulfadimethoxine		200	>400	12.5->400
(n = 421)[84]	Sulfadimethoxine		>256	>256	
(n = 461)[82]	Sulfamethazine	46.2	128	>512	0.5->512
(n = 461)[82]	Tetracycline	57	1	32	≤0.06-64
(n = 89)[83]	Tetracycline		>16	>16	0.5->6
(n = 421)[84]	Tetracycline		32	64	
(n = 461)[82]	Tilmicosin	69.1	4	8	0.06-16
(n = 89)[83]	Tylosin		>16	>16	8->16
(n = 421)[84]	Tylosin		64	128	
PASTEURELLA MULTOCIDA					
(n = 318)[82]	Ampicillin	88.1	0.25	8	≤0.03->64
(n = 32)[83]	Ampicillin		1	>16	0.25->16
(n = 158)[84]	Ampicillin		2	4	
(n = 318)[82]	Ceftiofur	100	≤0.03	0.06	≤0.03-0.25
(n = 50)[85]	Ceftiofur		0.0078	0.0078	≤0.003-0.0078
(n = 108)[86]	Enrofloxacin		0.015	0.03	≤0.008-0.06
(n = 318)[82]	Erythromycin	16	2	8	≤0.03->64
(n = 32)[83]	Erythromycin		4	>6	1->16
(n = 158)[84]	Erythromycin		4	4	
(n = 183)[87]	Florfenicol			0.5	
(n = 32)[83]	Gentamicin		1	4	0.25->8
(n = 158)[84]	Gentamicin		4	8	
(n = 32)[83]	Kanamycin		4	16	1->6

*New name is *Mannheimia haemolytica*.

Continued

TABLE 19-1

Antimicrobial Susceptibility Data for Bacterial Pathogens from Bovine Sources—cont'd

Organism (Number of Isolates)	Drug	Percentage Susceptible	Minimal Inhibitory Concentration (µg/ml)		
			50%	90%	Range
PASTEURELLA MULTOCIDA—cont'd					
(n = 32)[83]	Penicillin		4	>16	0.12->16
(n = 158)[84]	Penicillin		2	4	
(n = 318)[82]	Spectinomycin	76.4	32	>128	0.13->128
(n = 32)[83]	Spectinomycin		12	>32	4->32
(n = 158)[84]	Spectinomycin		8	16	
(n = 32)[83]	Sulfadimethoxine		>400	>400	100->400
(n = 158[84]	Sulfadimethoxine		>256	>256	
(n = 318)[82]	Sulfamethazine	27.4	128	>512	0.5->512
(n = 318)[82]	Tetracycline	71.1	0.5	16	≤0.06->32
(n = 32)[83]	Tetracycline		>16	>16	1->16
(n = 158)[84]	Tetracycline		2	16	
(n = 318)[82]	Tilmicosin	58.9	4	8	0.25-32
(n = 32)[83]	Tylosin		>16	>16	16->16
(n = 158)[84]	Tylosin		32	64	
HAEMOPHILUS SOMNUS					
(n = 109)[82]	Ampicillin	90.1	0.06	1	≤0.03->64
(n = 109)[82]	Ceftiofur	100	≤0.03	0.06	≤0.03-0.13
(n = 59)[85]	Ceftiofur		≤0.0019	≤0.0019	≤0.0019
(n = 104)[86]	Enrofloxacin		0.015	0.03	≤0.008-0.5
(n = 109)[82]	Erythromycin	88.9	0.25	2	≤0.03->32
(n = 34)[87]	Florfenicol			0.5	
(n = 109)[82]	Spectinomycin	87.1	8	32	≤0.13->128
(n = 109)[82]	Sulfamethazine	35.8	256	>512	≤0.5->512
(n = 109)[82]	Tetracycline	98.2	0.5	1	≤0.03-32
(n = 109)[82]	Tilmicosin	90.4	2	4	≤0.03-32
MYCOPLASMA BOVIS					
(n = 20)[88]	Enrofloxacin		0.1	0.25	0.05-1
(n = 100)[87]	Florfenicol			0.5	
(n = 20)[88]	Oxytetracycline		1	2.5	0.1-10
(n = 20)[88]	Tylosin		1	5	0.025->100
MYCOPLASMA MYCOIDES SSP. MYCOIDES SMALL COLONY TYPE					
(n = 20)[89]	Florfenicol		1	2	0.25-8
(n = 20)[89]	Oxytetracycline		0.5	1	0.125-4
(n = 20)[89]	Spectinomycin		8	16	4->128
(n = 20)[89]	Tilmicosin		0.015	0.03	<0.008-0.25
FUSOBACTERIUM NECROPHORUM					
(n = 21)[90]	Ampicillin		1.6	2.3	
(n = 68)[91]	Ampicillin	100			
(n = 17)[92]	Ceftiofur	100	≤0.062	≤0.062	≤0.062
(n = 68)[91]	Chloramphenicol	100			
(n = 21)[90]	Erythromycin		3.1	6.3	
(n = 12)[87]	Florfenicol			0.25	
(n = 21)[90]	Oxytetracycline		0.08	0.2	
(n = 365)[93]	Penicillin	96			
(n = 68)[91]	Penicillin	100			
(n = 21)[90]	Penicillin G		0.1	1.9	
(n = 365)[93]	Tetracycline	99			
(n = 68)[91]	Tetracycline	100			
(n = 21)[90]	Tylosin		3.1	6.3	
CLOSTRIDIUM PERFRINGENS					
(n = 67)[93]	Chloramphenicol	99			
(n = 67)[93]	Penicillin G	93			
(n = 67)[93]	Tetracycline	70			
OTHER CLOSTRIDIA					
(n = 109)[93]	Chloramphenicol	99			
(n = 109)[93]	Penicillin	90			
(n = 109)[93]	Tetracycline	77			

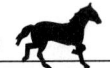

TABLE 19-1

Antimicrobial Susceptibility Data for Bacterial Pathogens from Bovine Sources—cont'd

Organism (Number of Isolates)	Drug	Percentage Susceptible	Minimal Inhibitory Concentration (μg/ml)		
			50%	90%	Range
FUSOBACTERIUM NECROPHORUM SPP. FUNDILIFORME					
$(n = 16)^{90}$	Ampicillin		1.3	2.7	
$(n = 16)^{90}$	Erythromycin		3.1	6.3	
$(n = 16)^{90}$	Oxytetracycline		0.2	4.1	
$(n = 16)^{90}$	Penicillin G		0.2	0.8	
$(n = 16)^{90}$	Tylosin		4.7	21.3	
BACTEROIDES MELANINOGENICUS					
$(n = 11)^{87}$	Florfenicol			0.25	
BACTEROIDES FRAGILIS					
$(n = 29)^{92}$	Ceftiofur	69	1	16	≤0.0625-≥16
$(n = 192)^{93}$	Chloramphenicol	99			
$(n = 192)^{93}$	Penicillin G	15.9			
$(n = 192)^{93}$	Tetracycline	77.3			
NON-BACTEROIDES FRAGILIS ORGANISMS					
$(n = 12)^{92}$	Ceftiofur	58	2	16	0.125-≥16
$(n = 114)^{93}$	Chloramphenicol	100			
$(n = 114)^{93}$	Penicillin G	89			
$(n = 114)^{93}$	Tetracycline	96			
PEPTOSTREPTOCOCCUS ANAEROBIUS					
$(n = 57)^{91}$	Ampicillin	100			
$(n = 12)^{92}$	Ceftiofur	100	0.25	2	0.125-2
$(n = 57)^{91}$	Chloramphenicol	100			
$(n = 193)^{93}$	Chloramphenicol	100			
$(n = 57)^{91}$	Penicillin	97			
$(n = 193)^{93}$	Penicillin	96			
$(n = 57)^{91}$	Tetracycline	100			
$(n = 193)^{93}$	Tetracycline	100			
ESCHERICHIA COLI					
$(n = 24)^{83}$	Ampicillin		4	>16	1->16
$(n = 40)^{85}$	Ceftiofur		0.25	0.5	0.13-1
$(n = 24)^{83}$	Gentamicin		1	2	0.5->8
$(n = 24)^{83}$	Oxytetracycline		16	>16	1->16
$(n = 24)^{83}$	Spectinomycin		16	>32	8->32
$(n = 24)^{83}$	Sulfachlorpyridazine		200	>400	12.5->400
ARCANOBACTERIUM PYOGENES*					
$(n = 42)^{94}$	Ampicillin		0.025	0.05	≤0.0125-0.05
$(n = 42)^{94}$	Benzylpenicillin		≤0.0125	0.25	≤0.0125-0.05
$(n = 42)^{94}$	Ceftiofur		0.78	1.56	0.39-1.56
$(n = 42)^{94}$	Chloramphenicol		1.56	1.56	0.39-1.56
$(n = 42)^{94}$	Erythromycin		0.025	0.025	≤0.0125-0.025
$(n = 42)^{94}$	Florfenicol		1.56	1.56	0.78-1.56
$(n = 42)^{94}$	Gentamicin		1.56	1.56	0.2->100
$(n = 42)^{94}$	Oxytetracycline		6.25	25	0.2-25
$(n = 42)^{94}$	Tilmicosin		0.05	0.05	≤0.0125-0.05
SALMONELLA SPP.					
$(n = 9)^{83}$	Ampicillin		>16	N/A	2->6
$(n = 48)^{83}$	Ampicillin		16	>16	0.5->16
$(n = 28)^{85}$	Ceftiofur		1	1	0.6-2
$(n = 9)^{83}$	Gentamicin		0.5	N/A	0.5-4
$(n = 48)^{83}$	Gentamicin		0.5	2	0.25-8
$(n = 9)^{83}$	Oxytetracycline		2	N/A	1->16
$(n = 48)^{83}$	Oxytetracycline		>16	>16	1->16
$(n = 9)^{83}$	Spectinomycin		12	N/A	8->32
$(n = 48)^{83}$	Spectinomycin		32	>32	12-32
$(n = 9)^{83}$	Sulfachlorpyridazine		150	N/A	50->400
$(n = 48)^{83}$	Sulfachlorpyridazine		400	>400	12.5->400
$(n = 48)^{83}$	Sulfamethoxine		>400	>400	12.5->400

*Formerly known as *Actinomyces pyogenes*.
N/A, Not available.

TABLE 19-2

Pharmacokinetics of Antimicrobial Drugs in Calves and Adult Cattle

Drug	Neonate Volume of Distribution (L/kg)	Adult Volume of Distribution (L/kg)	Drug Half-Life in Neonates (hr)	Drug Half-Life in Adults (hours)	Breakpoint Minimal Inhibitory Concentration (μg/ml)
Ampicillin	0.5[95]		3.8	0.95[67]	≤2
Ceftiofur	0.385[96]	0.3[96]	16.1[96]	7[96]	≤2[84]
Enrofloxacin		1.46		6.4[67]	≤0.25
Erythromycin		1.7[97]		3.2[67]	≤2[84]
Florfenicol	0.907[98]	0.35[99]	3.8[98]	2.9[99]	≤0.5
Gentamicin	0.42[100]	0.21[100]	2.9[100]	1.7[100]	≤4[84]
Oxytetracycline	2.48[101]	0.8[101]	13.5[101]	10.3[101]	≤4
Penicillin G	0.77[102]		0.98[102]	0.7[67]	≤1[84]
Spectinomycin					≤32[82]
Sulfadimethoxine		0.31[103]		12.5[103]	≤100[84]
Sulfamethazine		0.44		8.2	≤32
Sulfadiazine	0.72[104]	0.75	4.4[104]	2.5[105]	
Tilmicosin		>2		4.18	≤4[82]
Trimethoprim			1 day old = 8.4 7 days old = 2.1 42 days old = 0.9[104]		
Tylosin	4.4[106]	4.4[106]	2.31[106]	1.26[106]	≤5[84]

The data presented reflects intravenous administration. The half-life of drugs is often longer with intramuscular injection, reflecting absorption rate–dependent elimination.[99]

of antimicrobial resistance to tetracyclines and nonpotentiated sulfonamides limits their effectiveness in septic neonates. TMS may be used to treat sepsis in neonatal calves, but its half-life rapidly declines as rumen function develops. In ruminating calves (6 to 8 weeks old), subcutaneous or oral administration of trimethoprim-sulfa leads to high serum levels of sulfadiazine but little or no serum trimethoprim.[76] Bacterial resistance to trimethoprim-sulfa is less common than resistance to sulfa drugs alone but still may be high.[46,77]

Fluoroquinolones such as enrofloxacin are bactericidal and have an appropriate gram-negative spectrum of activity suitable for treatment of gram-negative sepsis. *However, in the United States enrofloxacin is conditionally licensed for treatment of respiratory disease in beef cattle.* In countries where it is legal to use enrofloxacin for treatment of neonatal sepsis, a dosage rate of 2.5 to 5 mg/kg every 24 hours has been suggested as appropriate for calves.[78] Enrofloxacin has demonstrated good efficacy in the treatment of *E. coli* septicemia, *Salmonella* enteritis, and *Mycoplasma* and *Pasteurella* pneumonia in calves.[79-81] Prolonged administration of enrofloxacin (weeks) is not recommended because it causes articular erosions in immature animals of other species. Ceftiofur has an appropriate antimicrobial spectrum, is bactericidal, and has been used to treat septic calves with good clinical results at a dosage of 5 mg/kg twice a day.* The label dosage of 1 mg/kg once a day may not achieve minimal inhibitory tissue drug concentrations for some bacteria commonly isolated from neonates. Deviation from the labeled dose requires implementation of a withholding period. Information about drug withholding times for extralabel use of antimicrobials is available from the Food Animal Residue Avoidance Databank (FARAD), and a database of U.S. Food and Drug Administration (FDA)-approved drugs is accessible via the Internet (http://www.cvm.fda.gov/index/iHN ADA.html).

The use of antimicrobial therapy in the management of

calf diarrhea is controversial. Many of the agents responsible for causing diarrhea in neonatal ruminants are not susceptible to antibiotics. A number of studies have reported no benefit associated with antimicrobial treatment of diarrhea in neonatal calves.[107-109] Conversely, attenuation of disease and reduced mortality has been demonstrated in other studies.[110-113] Antimicrobial therapy is likely to be beneficial in severely debilitated calves and specifically for treatment of bacterial enteric pathogens (*Salmonella* spp., enterotoxigenic *E. coli*, and *Clostridium perfringens*).

Several respiratory disease syndromes may be observed in neonatal calves. Pneumonia in calves under 3 days of age typically reflects aspiration of milk subsequent to inappropriate feeding practices or pharyngeal dysfunction (white muscle disease). A mixture of gram-positive, gram-negative, and anaerobic bacteria may be introduced into the lungs, inciting a severe inflammatory response that requires broad-spectrum antimicrobial and antiinflammatory therapy. *Pasteurella haemolytica* and *Pasteurella multocida* infrequently cause pneumonia in calves under 2 weeks of age. However, outbreaks of respiratory disease may be associated with mixed infections with *Mycoplasma bovis* in this age-group or may occur secondary to bovine virus diarrhea infection. Outbreaks of *Mycoplasma* pneumonia are often associated with the feeding of mastitic milk contaminated with *Mycoplasma bovis*. *Mycoplasma* spp. are susceptible to antimicrobial agents that affect DNA, RNA, protein synthesis, or the integrity of the cell membrane; they are not susceptible to agents that interfere with synthesis of folic acid or that act on the cell wall. Tylosin, tetracyclines, erythromycin, tilmicosin, florfenicol, aminoglycosides, and fluoroquinolones have been shown to be active against one or more *Mycoplasma* species.[114]

Septic arthritis in neonatal calves usually occurs by hematogenous spread. Common primary sources of infection include enteritis, pneumonia, and inflamed umbilical structures. FPT increases the risk of sepsis. The pathogens most commonly isolated from septic joints of neonatal calves are enteric organisms, including *E. coli* and *Salmonella* spp., *Strepto-*

*Dr. Lisle George, University of California-Davis, personal communication.

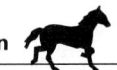

coccus spp., *Staphylococcus* spp., and *Arcanobacterium pyogenes* are less common isolates. In older calves *A. pyogenes* is isolated more frequently. Treatment options include joint lavage or arthrotomy to remove destructive inflammatory products and long-term antimicrobial therapy. Accumulation of fibrin in the joint space in cattle often makes it difficult to lavage septic joints effectively using needles. Joint lavage may be facilitated by using a rigid arthroscope or, in the case of simple joints (elbow and stifle), arthrotomy. Empiric antimicrobial therapy should include a gram-negative and gram-positive spectrum. Culture of synovial fluid facilitates antimicrobial selection.

Therapeutic synovial concentrations of penicillin, oxytetracycline, ampicillin, and cephapirin can be attained in inflamed and normal joints of calves with systemic administration.[102,115-117] The distribution of trimethoprim-sulfadiazine, penicillin, oxytetracycline, and cephapirin in joints is neither enhanced nor reduced by inflammation.[102,115,116] Penicillin, trimethoprim, and sulfadiazine equilibrate in $1/2$ to 1 hour, oxytetracycline in $4^{1}/2$ to 6 hours.[102] The subsequent decline in antibacterial drug concentration in synovial fluid parallels that in serum.[115] Synovial inflammation accelerates the distribution of antimicrobial drugs into joints[102] but has little effect on the peak drug concentration achieved in synovial fluid.[102,115] The peak concentration of ampicillin in synovial fluid after a single intramuscular injection of ampicillin trihydrate at a dosage of 10 mg/kg is higher in normal and inflamed synovial fluid than in sera.[117] Little bovine-derived data are available about the distribution of the newer generation antimicrobials into synovial fluid with systemic administration. Studies in other species suggest that most classes of antibacterial drugs are capable of crossing the synovial membrane. Synovial tissue is very vascular and does not have a basement membrane. In humans, synovial fluid concentrations of most antibacterials generally average at least 60% to 70% of serum drug concentrations at the time of peak serum concentrations and frequently exceed those in serum immediately before the subsequent systemic dose in patients with septic arthritis.[118] Antimicrobial dosing is targeted to achieve a peak antibacterial concentration that exceeds the MIC of the infecting organism by fivefold to tenfold.[118] The duration of therapy depends on the antimicrobial sensitivity of the pathogen and the patient's immune status; prolonged antimicrobial therapy (4 to 8 weeks) commonly is required.

Meningitis in neonatal calves is most commonly caused by gram-negative enterics. In a review of 32 cases, mortality was reported to be 100%.[119] In our experience treating calves in a hospital environment, the mortality rate is high, but aggressive early treatment can be successful. Empiric antimicrobial therapy for meningitis in neonatal calves should include a gram-negative and gram-positive spectrum. Antibiotics enter the CSF predominantly by means of passive diffusion down a concentration gradient. The major determinant of CSF penetration is lipid solubility. Lipophilic agents diffuse via transcellular pathways; peak concentrations in the CSF occur relatively rapidly, and entry into the CSF is affected minimally by the presence of inflammation. In contrast, hydrophilic agents enter the CSF through paracellular pathways; their transport depends on the opening of tight junctions, and peak concentrations are relatively delayed.[120] Only one report documents the pharmacokinetics of an antimicrobial agent in the CSF of calves. Table 19-3 shows the CSF to blood concentration ratios (penetration) derived from multiple species for some antimicrobial drugs available for use in cattle.

In a CSF pharmacokinetic study of florfenicol in calves, the maximum concentration of florfenicol attained in the CSF was 4.67 ± 1.51 μg/ml after a single IV dose of 20 mg/kg. The levels remained above the MIC for *Haemophilus somnus* over a 20-hour period.[121] Bactericidal antibiotics are thought to be more effective for treatment of meningitis in humans. Generally in animals it is recommended that the

TABLE 19-3

Penetration* of Antibiotics for Treatment of Meningitis in Calves[120,121]

Antimicrobial Drug	Concentration CSF/Concentration Serum (%)	
	Humans	Animals
Ampicillin	13-14	8-12
Florfenicol	N/A	46 (calves)
Gentamicin	0-30	21-25
Penicillin	5-10	5-6
Trimethoprim-sulfamethoxazole	<41	35-39

Modified from Lutsar I, McCracken GH Jr, Friedland IR: *Clin Infect Dis* 17:1117-1129, 1998; and de Craene BA et al: *Antimicrob Agents Chemother* 41:1991-1995, 1997.
CSF, Cerebrospinal fluid; *N/A*, not available.
*Cerebrospinal fluid to blood concentration ratios; the list is based on the little data that is available.

concentration of antibiotic in the CSF should be maintained at 10 times the MIC of the target pathogen.[120] Ceftiofur may be used to treat meningitis in calves. In one calf the author measured the concentration of ceftiofur in the CSF 28 hours after initiation of treatment with 10 mg/kg IM twice a day. The concentration of ceftiofur in the CSF at this time was 1.27 μg/ml, which happened to be five times the MIC of the *E. coli* isolated from the CSF of the calf. Unfortunately the lack of CSF pharmacokinetic data in cattle makes antimicrobial treatment of meningitis an inexact science.

Circulatory Support

Maintenance or restoration of effective circulating volume is a top priority in cases of sepsis. Aggressive IV fluid therapy is the mainstay of cardiovascular support and should be administered at the maximal rate tolerated by the foal. Severe septic shock may require fluid rates of 40 to 80 ml/kg/hr. Volume expansion should be achieved using a balanced electrolyte solution (crystalloid) or plasma (colloid). Colloid solutions are preferred and may reduce the incidence of pulmonary and systemic edema during fluid resuscitation. Infusion of crystalloid solutions equivalent to one half to one and one half times the estimated blood volume of the patient have been used, but hemodilution is a common consequence.[122] If hemodilution is severe or if hypotension or vasoconstriction continue or recur, additional fluid administration in the form of colloid, such as plasma, or hypertonic crystalloid fluid should be considered. Additional discussion of hypertonic saline administration may be found in other references.[123,124]

When fluid resuscitation alone is inadequate to improve cardiovascular function and restore acceptable blood pressure, pharmacologic intervention with sympathomimetic agents is necessary. Peripheral and cardiac adrenergic receptor downregulation necessitates the use of larger doses of pressor agents than usual. In patients that are hypotensive, dopamine, with its combined α- and β-adrenergic and dopaminergic activity, is preferred. Higher doses are required for patients in severe septic shock. If the foal fails to respond to high doses (over 10 to 15 μg/kg/min), then norepinephrine, a more potent α-adrenergic agent, can be tried. Recently NO has been shown to play a role in sepsis-induced hypotension. If oliguria continues despite restoration of circulating volume, diuretics such as furosemide or mannitol are used to promote renal vasodilation and urine flow.[122]

Because most septic foals are hypoglycemic, a slower, continuous infusion of solutions containing dextrose should be run simultaneously with the rehydration fluids. Too rapid infusion of dextrose should be avoided, because it could cause hyperglycemia that can induce an osmotic diuresis that further exacerbates the dehydration.

Endotoxemia probably is responsible for many of the clinical signs that accompany gram-negative infection.[125] Endotoxin, a component of lipopolysaccharide in the outer membrane of gram-negative bacteria, is considered the most potent initiating mediator of septic shock. Endotoxins are released during periods of rapid bacterial growth or with lysis of the bacteria and are removed from the circulation by the mononuclear phagocyte system. Macrophages are activated by LPS to secrete various cytokines, including tumor necrosis factor (TNF), IL-1, IL-6, and procoagulant activity (PCA), which begin the cascade activation of the membrane-bound enzyme phospholipase A_2; the end result of this pathway causes septic shock. The interaction of the LPS and macrophages also results in the production of prostaglandins and leukotrienes. The cytokines, leukotrienes, and prostaglandins mediate many of the behavioral, hematologic, and hemodynamic alterations observed in endotoxemia. A number of studies have investigated the specific effects of endotoxemia in the foal,[125,126] and calf,[127] cytokine production in natural occurring cases of neonatal sepsis,[128] and the effects of selected drugs in the treatment of endotoxemia in the large animal neonate.[129]

Treatment with antiprostaglandin drugs has been found to counteract several of the clinical and hemodynamic changes associated with endotoxemia and septic shock, including the decrease in cardiac output and systemic hypotension. However, these drugs have little effect on the leukopenia, thrombocytopenia, or coagulopathies that develop in septic shock.[122] Based on the effect of these drugs in models of endotoxemia in the adult horse[130,131] and neonatal calf[129] and in models of septic shock in other species,[122] they would be expected to be of some benefit in the treatment of the septic large animal neonate. Pharmacokinetic studies of flunixin meglumine in neonatal foals suggest that despite prolonged elimination of flunixin in healthy newborn foals, the physiologic activity appears similar to that in the adult, and the adult dose of 1.1 mg/kg body weight would be appropriate in at least some patients.[132] Lower doses of flunixin meglumine (Banamine) (0.25 mg/kg IV every 8 hours) may be effective in ameliorating some of the signs of endotoxemia. Other treatments include plasma administration from hyperimmunized donors to treat not only failure of passive transfer but to provide opsonins and improve foal neutrophil function. Plasma also represents an ideal colloid for rapid volume expansion.

Other, newer therapies for endotoxemia and sepsis include naloxone, an opiate antagonist, that has been used experimentally to counteract the detrimental vasodilatory effects of endorphins released during sepsis. NO inhibitors, such as new methylene blue, have been used to treat refractory hypotension in septic patients.[39,40] Pentoxifylline, a methylxanthine derivative, has been used for treatment of conditions characterized by inadequate regional blood flow.[133,134] The drug increases red cell deformability, reduces blood viscosity, decreases platelet aggregation, and decreases thrombus formation. Pentoxifylline administration also results in decreased plasma fibrinogen, increased action of plasminogen activators and antithrombin III, decreased platelet thromboxane synthesis, and increased synthesis of prostaglandins 1 and 2. The net effect of the drug is to increase regional blood flow and inhibit coagulation. When the drug was used in animal models of endotoxic shock, it increased overall survival rates and prevented endotoxin-induced renal failure, synthesis of TNF, and coagulopathies. Horses receiv-

ing the drug showed a decrease in packed cell volume and red blood cell (RBC) sedimentation rate and beneficial effects on RBC deformability. Intravenous doses used experimentally in horses include a single bolus of 7.5 mg/kg body weight followed by a continuous infusion of 1.5 mg/kg/hr.[133]

Polymyxin B, administered at low, nontoxic doses, is an investigational treatment being used to neutralize systemic endotoxin. Low doses of the drug result in decreased concentrations of circulating endotoxin, improved immune function, and decreased mortality rates among shock patients. Polymyxin B binds and neutralizes endotoxin in vitro and has been shown to remove endotoxin from the circulation in vivo. Use of this drug in the horse is investigational. A suggested dose is 6000 IU/kg diluted in 300 to 500 ml of 5% dextrose and given as a slow intravenous infusion.

Immunologic Support

When failure of passive transfer of antibodies accompanies neonatal infection, plasma is routinely used to increase immunoglobulin levels. Between 1 and 4 L of plasma have been infused intravenously to raise immunoglobulin G (IgG) levels, but the optimum amount is not known. Important factors influencing the amount of plasma indicated include the total IgG content of the plasma and the specific antibody concentration against foal pathogens, as well as the degree of circulatory impairment of the neonate. The efficacy of plasma in preventing or treating septicemia in foals has not been established as of this writing.

Several immunologic products are currently under investigation as potential treatments of foal septicemia; their efficacy has not yet been proven. These include serum or plasma containing high levels of antibodies to the common core structures of lipopolysaccharide[131,135] and granulocyte colony-stimulating factor, which markedly increases white blood cell counts in foals.[136] Monoclonal antibodies to TNF and other inflammatory mediators may also be of use in the future.[137]

Several bovine colostrum supplements are available. The immunoglobulin content varies among products and should be considered when comparing prices. Colostrum supplements generally fail as colostrum substitutes because of the relatively low mass of immunoglobulin delivered per dose.[138] In two separate clinical trials, peak serum immunoglobulin concentrations were not significantly different in calves fed 3 or 4 L of maternal colostrum with or without colostrum supplement.[138,139] Administration of a colostrum supplement before 18 hours of age is indicated when an adequate supply of colostrum is not available. If a colostrum supplement is to be used as a colostral substitute, multiple doses are required to deliver a minimum of 100 g of immunoglobulin.

Supportive Therapy

Nutritional support of septic foals is critical. Gram-negative bacterial sepsis, a leading cause of death in neonatal foals, disrupts intermediary metabolism, increases the metabolic rate, and sequentially hinders utilization of carbohydrates, lipids, and finally protein for energy. The release of endotoxin precipitates a neurohormonal cascade of events mediated by TNF and increased levels of catecholamines, glucocorticoids, and glucagon. Elevated concentrations of antidiuretic hormone (ADH), aldosterone, and thyroxin and low levels of insulin accompany low perfusion states associated with septic shock. Sepsis results in glycolysis, lipolysis, and proteolysis, increased urinary excretion of potassium and nitrogen, and water and sodium retention. Suppressed insulin production and peripheral insulin resistance result in glucose intolerance and hyperglycemia. During sepsis the transport, oxidation, and clearance of free fatty acids (FFAs) is impaired because

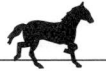

of a deficiency of the carrier peptide carnitine and decreased lipoprotein lipase activity. Lipemia develops. The final fuel source becomes protein degradation. Uremia, production of false neurotransmitters, hepatoencephalopathy, and neurologic signs occur when excessive amino acid degradation overwhelms hepatic metabolic capacity.

Provision of adequate nutrition is vital for a successful outcome in the treatment of infected neonates. Poor nutritional support leads to debilitation, a poorly functioning immune system, poor healing, persistent infection, and other complications, such as decubital ulcers. A healthy newborn foal requires 15% to 25% of its body weight in milk per day. Foals too weak to nurse from the mare or a bottle should be tube fed a minimum of 10% of their body weight per day in milk, administered in small feedings every 2 to 3 hours. Because many sick foals have poor gut function, enteral nutrition is not a viable option initially. If a foal is not consuming at least 10% of its body weight in milk within the first 36 to 48 hours, it should be started on parenteral nutrition using a formula containing dextrose, lipids, amino acids, vitamins, and trace minerals. Solutions of 5% to 10% glucose can be administered to help maintain a normal blood glucose level. These solutions provide temporary nutritional support but do not contain nearly enough calories for long-term nutritional support. It would require 35 L of a 5% dextrose solution per day to provide a 50-kg foal with adequate calories (120 kcal/kg/day). Use of a combination of oral and parenteral nutritional support has considerable merit in treating the infected neonate.

Septic foals are susceptible to pulmonary dysfunction because of a variety of factors, including dependent lung atelectasis, pneumonia, pulmonary edema, and surfactant dysfunction. The focus of respiratory support is to minimize ventilation and perfusion mismatching. Fluid therapy helps increase left ventricular, left atrial, and diastolic pressures to create more uniform lung perfusion. Recumbent foals should be turned and repositioned frequently to minimize dependent lung atelectasis and the formation of pulmonary edema. Mild to moderate hypoxemia can be treated with humidified intranasal oxygen (2 to 10 L/min). Severe hypoxemia (a partial pressure of oxygen [PO_2] below 50 mm Hg) despite oxygen supplementation and persistent hypercapnea (a partial pressure of carbon dioxide [PCO_2] above 65 to 70 mm Hg) require positive-pressure ventilation with positive end expiratory pressure (PEEP) to prevent further lung collapse, reduce interstitial edema, and prevent respiratory muscle fatigue. Debilitated septic foals that require mechanical ventilation and nasotracheal intubation are at increased risk for nosocomial infections. Nebulization using bronchodilators, wetting agents, and mucolytic agents, accompanied by coupage therapy, help relieve foals with respiratory distress and facilitate removal of tracheal secretions.

The nursing care of the septic neonate is very important. Maintenance of body temperature and fluid, blood gas, and acid-base balance, as well as a clean environment, are all critical to a successful outcome. Every neonate undergoing intensive care, regardless of its primary problem, should be monitored closely for fever spikes, neutropenia, increasing lethargy, or localizing signs of infection that could indicate early sepsis or a different bacterial infection resistant to the antibiotics being used.

Management of Suspected Placentitis

Placentitis is a common cause of reproductive losses in horses in the United States. During the 1998-1999 foaling season in Kentucky, 24.7% of cases of aborted, stillborn, and premature foals were associated with placentitis.[140] The most common cause of placentitis is infection that ascends from the lower urogenital tract via a relaxing cervix. A far less com-

mon route of infection is the hematogenous avenue, resulting in a diffuse or multifocal placentitis. Most cases of placentitis are the result of bacterial infection caused by typical equine pathogens, including *Streptococcus zooepidemicus, Enterobacter agglomerans, Klebsiella pneumoniae,* and *Pseudomonas aeruginosa.* In Kentucky a slightly different form of placentitis has been recognized that is characterized by focally extensive placentitis located predominantly at the base of the placental horns at the junction of the horns and the body of the placenta. The affected area is covered with thick, tenacious, brown mucoid exudate, and the underlying chorionic villi are necrotic and absent or reduced in size. This form is associated with infection by a group of gram-positive, branching, filamentous nocardioform organisms.[140]

Clinical signs of placentitis include vaginal discharge that may be evident on the mare's vulva, tail, or inner thighs, premature udder development, and precocious lactation. Premature udder development is the result of placental compromise, fetal stress, a precocious increase in maternal progestogen concentration, and enhanced fetal adrenocortical activity. Despite even voluminous vaginal discharge, most mares with placentitis do not become febrile and do maintain a normal appetite. The dam's hemogram and fibrinogen concentration usually remain within normal limits. A transrectal ultrasound examination can be done to detect early areas of placental separation and increased uteroplacental thickness in the pericervical area. The combined thickness for the uterus and placenta should be less than 10 mm between days 271 and 300 of gestation, less than 10 mm between days 301 and 330, and less than 12 mm after day 330.[141] A transabdominal ultrasound examination can be done to evaluate other areas of the placenta to detect loss of placental integrity or increased uteroplacental thickening. Using transabdominal ultrasound, the uteroplacental unit should be less than 16 mm thick during late gestation. Other signs suggestive of placentitis include increased fetal fluid echogenicity, which may be the result of hemorrhage, and purulent exudate of the brown mucoid material associated with nocardioform placentitis.[142] If the placentitis is severe enough to alter placental function, reduced fetal movement, loss of heart rate variability, and absolute fetal bradycardia indicate fetal compromise.

Samples of vaginal discharge should be cultured, and Gram staining should be done. The goal of maternal therapy is to treat the placental infection and maintain the pregnancy, provided there is no evidence of severe fetal distress or demise. In many cases, because the infection is of long duration, the fetus has been chronically stressed and therefore is relatively mature for its gestational age and better prepared to tolerate premature birth. Often medical treatment of the placental infection and prolongation of pregnancy is associated with a good outcome. Maternal treatment involves administration of systemic antibiotics, flunixin meglumine (Banamine), and progesterone.[143] Because of the usual presence of mixed gram-positive and gram-negative placental and fetal infections, a broad-spectrum antibiotic that reaches therapeutic levels in the fetus and fetal fluids should be selected. In normal pregnant mares, penicillin and gentamicin levels were undetectable in the fetus and fetal fluids after maternal drug administration, and trimethoprim-sulfonamide concentrations achieved reasonable levels.[144] However, if placental inflammation is present, higher fetal antibiotic levels may be achieved.[143] Other antibiotic choices include potassium penicillin and gentocin, or ceftiofur. Low doses of flunixin meglumine can be administered to reduce inflammation and prevent prostaglandin-mediated induction of delivery. Regumate (Altrenogest, 10 to 20 ml PO once daily) is given to help maintain the pregnancy. If large areas of placental thickening are found, dimethyl sulfoxide (DMSO) (0.5 to 1 g/kg IV) can be administered to reduce placental

6. Brewer BD: Neonatal infection. In Koterba AM, Drummond WH, Kosch PC, eds: *Equine clinical neonatology,* Philadelphia, 1990, Lea & Febiger.
7. Baggot JD: Drug therapy in the neonatal foal, *Vet Clin North Am (Equine Pract)* 10:87-107, 1994.
8. Axon J: Short- and long-term athletic outcome of neonatal intensive care unit survivors, *Proceedings of the Forty-first Annual Convention of the American Association of Equine Practitioners,* 1995, pp 224-225.
9. Robinson JA et al: A prospective study of septicemia in colostrum-deprived foals, *Equine Vet J* 25:214, 1993.
10. Besser TE, Gay CC, Pritchett L: Comparison of three methods of feeding colostrum to dairy calves, *J Am Vet Med Assoc* 198:419-422, 1991.
11. Riedel-Caspari G: The influence of colostral leukocytes on the course of an experimental *Escherichia coli* infection and serum antibodies in neonatal calves, *Vet Immunol Immunopathol* 35:275-288, 1993.
12. Tyler JW et al: Partitioning the mortality risk associated with inadequate passive transfer of colostral immunoglobulins in dairy calves, *J Vet Intern Med* 13:335-337, 1999.
13. Selim SA et al: Serum immunoglobulins in calves: their effects and two easy reliable means of measurement, *Vet Med* 90:387-404, 1995.
14. McGuire TC et al: Failure of colostral immunoglobulin transfer as an explanation for most infections and deaths of neonatal foals, *J Am Vet Med Assoc* 170:1302-1304, 1977.
15. Stoneham SJ, Digby NJ, Ricketts SW: Failure of passive transfer of colostral immunity in the foal: incidence and the effect of stud management and plasma transfusions, *Vet Rec* 128:416-419, 1991.
16. Clabough DL et al: Factors associated with failure of passive transfer of colostral antibodies in standardbred foals, *J Vet Intern Med* 5:335-340, 1991.
17. Riedel-Caspari G, Schmidt FW: Colostral leukocytes and their significance for the immune system of newborns, *Dtw Dtsch Tierarztl Wochenschr* 97:180-186, 1990.
18. Riedel-Caspari G, Schmidt FW, Marquardt J: The influence of colostral leukocytes on the immune system of the neonatal calf. IV, Effects on bactericidity, complement and interferon: synopsis, *Dtw Dtsch Tierarztl Wochenschr* 98:395-398, 1991.
19. Riedel-Caspari G, Schmidt FW: The influence of colostral leukocytes on the immune system of the neonatal calf. III, Effects on phagocytosis, *Dtw Dtsch Tierarztl Wochenschr* 98:330-334, 1991.
20. Riedel-Caspari G, Schmidt FW: The influence of colostral leukocytes on the immune system of the neonatal calf. II, Effects on passive and active immunization, *Dtw Dtsch Tierarztl Wochenschr* 98:190-194, 1991.
21. Riedel-Caspari G, Schmidt FW: The influence of colostral leukocytes on the immune system of the neonatal calf. I. Effects on lymphocyte responses, *Dtw Dtsch Tierarztl Wochenschr* 98:102-107, 1991.
22. Schnorr KL: Cell tracing with fluorescein isothiocyanate and maternal transfer of cellular immunity in sheep, doctoral dissertation, Fort Collins, Colo, 1983, Colorado State University.
23. Zwahlen RD, Wyder-Walther M, Roth DR: Fc receptor expression, concanavalin A capping, and enzyme content of bovine neonatal neutrophils: a comparative study with adult cattle, *J Leukoc Biol* 51:264-269, 1992.
24. Toman M, Psikal I, Mensik J: Phagocytic activity of blood leukocytes in calves from birth to 3 months of age, *Vet Med* 30:401-408, 1985.
25. Hauser MA, Koob MD, Roth JA: Variation of neutrophil function with age in calves, *Am J Vet Res* 47:152-1153, 1986.
26. Moiola F et al: Comparative in vitro phagocytosis and F-actin polymerization of bovine neonatal neutrophils, *Zentralbl Veterinarmed [a]* 41:202-214, 1994.
27. Dore M, Slauson DO, Neilsen NR: Decreased respiratory burst activity in neonatal bovine neutrophils stimulated by protein kinase C agonists, *Am J Vet Res* 52:375-380, 1991.
28. Clifford CB et al: Ontogeny of inflammatory cell responsiveness: superoxide anion generation by phorbol ester–stimulated fetal, neonatal, and adult bovine neutrophils, *Inflammation* 13:221-231, 1989.
29. Griebel PJ, Schoonderwoerd M, Babiuk LA: Ontogeny of the immune response: effect of protein-energy malnutrition in neonatal calves, *Can J Vet Res* 51:428-435, 1987.
30. Reddy PG et al: Bovine recombinant granulocyte-macrophage colony-stimulating factor enhancement of bovine neutrophil functions in vitro, *Am J Vet Res* 51:1395-1399, 1990.
31. Blecha F, Baker PE: Effect of cortisol in vitro and in vivo on production of bovine interleukin 2, *Am J Vet Res* 47:841-845, 1986.
32. Lewis DB et al: Cellular and molecular mechanisms for reduced interleukin 4 and interferon-γ production by neonatal T cells, *J Clin Invest* 87:194-202, 1991.
33. Smith AN, Ingram DG: Immunological responses of young animals. II, Antibody production in calves, *Can Vet J* 6:226-232, 1965.
34. Roden LD et al: Effect of calf age and *Salmonella* bacterin type on ability to produce immunoglobulins directed against *Salmonella* whole cells or lipopolysaccharide, *Am J Vet Res* 53:1895-1899, 1992.
35. Olson DP: In vitro migration responses of neutrophils from cows and calves, *Am J Vet Res* 51:973-977, 1990.
36. Pollock JM et al: Effects of dietary vitamin E and selenium on in vitro cellular immune responses in cattle, *Res Vet Sci* 56:100-107, 1994.
37. Graham TW: Trace element deficiencies in cattle, *Vet Clin North Am (Food Anim Pract)* 7:153-215, 1991.
38. Polin RA, St Geme JWD: Neonatal sepsis, *Adv Pediatr Infect Dis* 7:25-61, 1992.

BOX 19-1

Complications Associated With Septicemia and Its Therapy in the Neonate

Pneumonia (common); pleuritis (less common)
Osteomyelitis, septic arthritis, septic physitis
Enteritis
Peritonitis
Gastrointestinal ulceration (often asymptomatic)
Meningitis
Brain or spinal cord hemorrhage
Corneal ulceration (often secondary to entropion)
Patent urachus
Omphalophlebitis
Resistant bacterial infections
Anemia
Progressive debilitation, starvation
Uroperitoneum (secondary to umbilical infection, cystitis)

---

edema. Pentoxifylline has also been administered in attempts to improve placental perfusion.

If placentitis is suspected, after delivery the foal should be considered a high-risk individual. Commonly encountered problems in the newborn foal exposed to placentitis are pneumonia, uveitis, growth restriction, incompletely ossified bones, and sometimes septicemia.

PROGNOSIS AND COMPLICATIONS OF SEPTICEMIA AND RELATED INFECTIONS

If a large animal neonate has FPT and is septicemic with several organ systems involved, its long-term outcome must be considered guarded even with intensive nursing care.[5] A recent study reported a short-term survival rate of 81% for neonatal intensive care unit survivors.[8] Secondary complications that often accompany multifocal bone and joint infections may have an adverse effect on the final outcome (Box 19-1). A retrospective study that examined the factors associated with the prognosis for survival and athletic use in foals with septic arthritis showed that with treatment, the prognosis for survival was favorable, but the prognosis for ability to race was unfavorable. Approximately 78% of treated foals survived, and a third of those foals raced. Multisystem disease, isolation of *Salmonella* organisms from synovial fluid, involvement of multiple joints, and a synovial fluid neutrophil count over 95% were associated with a poor prognosis.[145] Some possible complications of septicemia are listed in the Box 19-1. If blood culture results are negative and localized infection (enteritis, pneumonia) is present, the outcome can be much more positive with aggressive therapy. If in utero–acquired infections in the foal are treated appropriately early in the clinical course and good IgG levels are attained by the newborn, the outcome can be quite favorable (survival rate exceeding 75%).

REFERENCES

1. Bone RC: The pathogenesis of sepsis, *Ann Intern Med* 115:457-469, 1991.
2. Rackow EC, Astiz ME: Pathophysiology and treatment of septic shock, *JAMA* 266:548-554, 1991.
3. Koterba AM, Brewer BD, Tarplee FA: Clinical and clinicopathological characteristics of the septicaemic neonatal foal: review of 38 cases, *Equine Vet J* 16:376-382, 1984.
4. Paradis MR: Update on neonatal septicemia, *Vet Clin North Am (Equine Pract)* 10:109-135, 1994.
5. Koterba AM: Equine neonatal intensive care at the University of Florida 1982-1987: an update, *Proceedings of the Thirty-third Annual Convention of the American Association of Equine Practitioners,* 1987, p 805.

39. Symeonides S, Balk RA: Nitric oxide in the pathogenesis of sepsis, *Infect Dis Clin North Am* 13:449-463, 1999.
40. Lowenstein CJ, Dinerman JL, Snyder SH: Nitric oxide: a physiologic messenger, *Ann Intern Med* 120:227-237, 1994.
41. Cerra FB et al: Septic autocannibalism: a failure of exogenous nutritional support, *Ann Surg* 192:570-580, 1980.
42. Platt H: Septicaemia in the foal: a review of 61 cases, *Br Vet J* 129:221-229, 1973.
43. Wilson WD, Madigan JE: Comparison of bacteriologic culture of blood and necropsy specimens for determining the cause of foal septicemia: 47 cases (1978-1987), *J Am Vet Med Assoc* 195:1759, 1989.
44. Aldridge BM, Garry FB, Adams R: Neonatal septicemia in calves: 25 cases (1985-1990), *J Am Vet Med Assoc* 203:1324-1329, 1993.
45. Joshi DV, Kaul PL, Shan NM: Bacterial agents associated with lamb mortality, *Indian J Anim Sci* 62:120-121, 1992.
46. Hariharan H et al: Blood cultures from calves and foals, *Can Vet J* 33:56-57, 1992.
47. Fecteau G et al: Predicting bacteremia in the bovine neonate, *Proceedings of the Twelfth ACVIM Annual Convention*, San Francisco, 1994, pp 626-628.
48. Bourgault A, Bada R, Messier S: Isolation of *Pasteurella canis* from a foal with polyarthritis, *Can Vet J* 35:244-245, 1994.
49. Wallace SS, Hathcock TL: *Listeria monocytogenes* septicemia in a foal, *J Am Vet Med Assoc* 207:1325-1326, 1995.
50. Jones SL, Wilson WD: *Clostridium septicum* septicemia in a neonatal foal with hemorrhagic enteritis, *Cornell Vet* 83:143-151, 1993.
51. Meyer JC et al: Bacteremia and pneumonia in a neonatal foal caused by *Streptococcus pneumoniae* type 3, *Equine Vet J* 24:407, 1992.
52. Marsh PS, Palmer JE, Fitzsimmons M: A survey of results of bacteriologic culture of blood from critically ill neonatal foals: 56 cases (1996-1998), *Proceedings of the Second Dorothy Havemeyer Foundation Neonatal Septicemia Workshop*, Boston, 1998.
53. Agresti A et al: Use of polymerase chain reaction to diagnose bovine leukemia virus infection in calves at birth, *Am J Vet Res* 54:373-378, 1993.
54. Moerman A et al: A long-term epidemiological study of bovine viral diarrhea infections in a large herd of dairy cattle, *Vet Rec* 132:622-626, 1993.
55. Sweeney RW, Whitlock RH, Rosenberger AE: *Mycobacterium paratuberculosis* isolated from fetuses of infected cows not manifesting signs of the disease, *Am J Vet Res* 53:477-480, 1992.
56. Bryan LA et al: Fatal, generalized bovine herpesvirus type 1 infection associated with a modified live infectious bovine rhinotracheitis and parainfluenza-3 vaccine administered to neonatal calves, *Can Vet J* 35:223-228, 1994.
57. Whitwell KE: Investigations into fetal and neonatal losses in the horse, *Vet Clin North Am (Large Anim Pract)* 2:313-331, 1980.
58. Vaala WE et al: Fatal, congenitally acquired infection with equine arteritis virus in a neonatal thoroughbred, *Equine Vet J* 24:155, 1992.
59. Buergelt CD et al: A retrospective study of proliferative interstitial lung disease of horses in Florida, *Vet Pathol* 23:750-756, 1986.
60. Brewer BD, Koterba AM: The development of a scoring system for the early diagnosis of equine neonatal sepsis, *Equine Vet J* 20:18, 1988.
61. Adams R et al: Hematologic values in newborn beef calves, *Am J Vet Res* 53:944-950, 1992.
62. Brumbaugh GW: Clinical pharmacology and the pediatric patient, *Proc Am Assoc Equine Pract* 45:226-234, 1999.
63. Koterba AM: Antibiotic therapy. In Koterba AM, Drummond WH, Kosch PC, eds: *Equine clinical neonatology*, Philadelphia, 1990, Lea & Febiger.
64. Prescott JF, Baggot JD, eds: *Antimicrobial therapy in veterinary medicine*, ed 2, Ames, Iowa, 1993, Iowa State University Press.
65. Wilcke JR: Clinical pharmacology of antimicrobial drugs for the treatment of septic neonatal calves, *Vet Clin North Am (Food Animal Practice)* 7:695-711, 1991.
66. Schwark WS: Factors that affect drug disposition in food-producing animals during maturation, *J Anim Sci* 70:3635-3645, 1992.
67. Prescott JF, Baggot JD: Principles of antimicrobial drug disposition. In Prescott JF, Baggot JD, eds: *Antimicrobial therapy in veterinary medicine*, ed 2, Ames, Iowa, 1993, Iowa State University Press.
68. Orsini JA et al: Resistance to gentamicin and amikacin of gram negative organisms isolated from horses, *Am J Vet Res* 50:923-925, 1989.
69. Golenz MR et al: Effect of route of administration and age on the pharmacokinetics of amikacin administered by the intravenous and intraosseous routes to 3- and 5-day-old foals, *Equine Vet J* 26:367, 1994.
70. Green SL et al: Effects of hypoxia and azotemia on the pharmacokinetics of amikacin in neonatal foals, *Equine Vet J* 24:475, 1992.
71. Green SL, Conlon PD: Clinical pharmacokinetics of amikacin in hypoxic premature foals, *Equine Vet J* 25:276, 1993.
72. Magdesian KG, Wilson WD, Mihalyi J: Pharmacokinetics and nephrotoxicity of high dose, once daily administered amikacin in neonatal foals, *Proceedings of the Forty-third Annual Convention of the American Association of Equine Practitioners*, 1997, pp 396-397.
73. Magdesian KG et al: Pharmacokinetics of gentamicin administration once daily by the intravenous and intramuscular routes in horses, *Proceedings of the Fortieth Annual Convention of the American Association of Equine Practitioners*, 1994, pp 115-116.
74. Brewer BD, Koterba AM: Bacterial isolates and susceptibility patterns in foals in a neonatal intensive care unit, *Compend Cont Educ Pract Vet* 12:1773-1781, 1990.
75. Fecteau G et al: Bacteriological culture of blood from critically ill neonatal calves, *Can Vet J* 38:95-100, 1997.
76. Guard CL et al: Age-related alterations in trimethoprim-sulfadiazine disposition following oral or parenteral administration in calves, *Can J Vet Res* 50:342-346, 1986.
77. Hariharan H et al: Resistance to trimethoprim-sulfamethoxole of *Escherichia coli* isolated from pigs and calves with diarrhea, *Can Vet J* 30:348-349, 1989.
78. Berg JN: *Clinical indications for enrofloxacin in domestic animals and poultry*, Lawrenceville, NJ, 1988, Veterinary Learning Systems, pp 25-33.
79. Bauditz R: Results of clinical studies with Baytril in calves and pigs, *Vet Med Rev* 2:122, 1987.
80. Giles CJ et al: Efficacy of danofloxacin in the therapy of acute bacterial pneumonia in housed beef cattle, *Vet Rec* 128:296-300, 1991.
81. Lekeux P, Art T: Effect of enrofloxacin therapy on shipping fever pneumonia in feedlot cattle, *Vet Rec* 123:205-207, 1988.
82. Watts JL et al: A 4-year survey of antimicrobial susceptibility trends for isolates from cattle with bovine respiratory disease in North America, *J Clin Microbiol* 32:725-731, 1994.
83. Burrows GE, Morton RJ, Fales WH: Microdilution antimicrobial susceptibilities of selected gram negative veterinary bacterial isolates, *J Vet Diagn Invest* 5:541-547, 1993.
84. Post KW, Cole NA, Raleigh RH: In vitro antimicrobial susceptibility of *Pasteurella haemolytica* and *Pasteurella multocida* recovered from cattle with bovine respiratory disease complex, *J Vet Diagn Invest* 3:124-126, 1991.
85. Salmon SA, Watts JL, Yancey RJ Jr: In vitro activity of ceftiofur and its primary metabolite, desfuroylceftiofur, against organisms of veterinary importance, *J Vet Diagn Invest* 8:332-336, 1996.
86. Ewert KM: Food animal pharmacology. III. Baytril, *Proceedings of the Seventeenth ACVIM Annual Convention*, Chicago, 1999, pp 259-261.
87. Simmons RD, Varma KJ, Johnson JC: Food animal pharmacology. II. Nuflor, *Proceedings of the Seventeenth ACVIM Annual Convention*, Chicago, 1999, pp 256-258.
88. Hannan PC et al: Comparative susceptibilities of various animal-pathogenic mycoplasmas to fluoroquinolones, *Antimicrob Agents Chemother* 41:2037-2040, 1997.
89. Ayling RD et al: Comparison of in vitro activity of danofloxacin, florfenicol, oxytetracycline, spectinomycin and tilmicosin against *Mycoplasma mycoides* subspecies *mycoides* small colony type, *Vet Rec* 146:243-246, 2000.
90. Lechtenberg KF, Nagaraja TG, Chengappa MM: Antimicrobial susceptibility of *Fusobacterium necrophorum* isolated from bovine hepatic abscesses, *Am J Vet Res* 59:44-47, 1998.
91. Hirsh DC et al: Changes in prevalence and susceptibility of obligate anaerobes in clinical veterinary practice, *J Am Vet Med Assoc* 186:1086-1089, 1985.
92. Samitz EM, Jang SS, Hirsh DC: In vitro susceptibilities of selected obligate anaerobic bacteria obtained from bovine and equine sources to ceftiofur, *J Vet Diagn Invest* 8:121-123, 1996.
93. Jang SS, Hirsh DC: Broth-disk elution determination of antimicrobial susceptibility of selected anaerobes isolated from animals, *J Vet Diagn Invest* 3:82-84, 1991.
94. Yoshimura H, Kojima A, Ishimaru M: Antimicrobial susceptibility of *Arcanobacterium pyogenes* isolated from cattle and pigs, *Zentralblatt fur Veterinarmedizin Reihe B* 47:139-143, 2000.
95. Nouws JF et al: Comparative plasma ampicillin levels and bioavailability of five parenteral ampicillin formulations in ruminant calves, *Vet Q* 4:62-71, 1982.
96. Brown SA, Chester ST, Robb EJ: Effects of age on the pharmacokinetics of single dose ceftiofur sodium administered intramuscularly or intravenously to cattle, *J Vet Pharmacol Ther* 19:32-38, 1996.
97. Burrows GE et al: A comparison of the various routes of administration of erythromycin in cattle, *J Vet Pharmacol Ther* 12:289-295, 1989.
98. Adams PE et al: Tissue concentrations and pharmacokinetics of florfenicol in male veal calves given repeated doses, *Am J Vet Res* 48:1725-1732, 1987.
99. Soback S et al: Florfenicol pharmacokinetics in lactating cows after intravenous, intramuscular and intramammary administration, *J Vet Pharmacol Ther* 18:413-417, 1995.
100. Burrows GE, Barto PB, Martin B: Comparative pharmacokinetics of gentamicin, neomycin and oxytetracycline in newborn calves, *J Vet Pharmacol Ther* 10:54-63, 1987.
101. Nouws JF, van Ginneken CA, Ziv G: Age-dependent pharmacokinetics of oxytetracycline in ruminants, *J Vet Pharmacol Ther* 6:59-66, 1983.
102. Guard CL, Byman KW, Schwark WS: Effect of experimental synovitis on disposition of penicillin and oxytetracycline in neonatal calves, *Cornell Vet* 79:161-171, 1989.
103. Boxenbaum HG et al: Pharmacokinetics of sulphadimethoxine in cattle, *Res Vet Sci* 23:24-28, 1977.
104. Shoaf SE, Schwark WS, Guard CL: Pharmacokinetics of sulfadiazine-trimethoprim in neonatal male calves: effect of age and penetration into cerebrospinal fluid, *Am J Vet Res* 50:396-403, 1989.

105. Nielsen P, Rasmussen F: Half-life, apparent volume of distribution and protein binding for some sulfonamides in cows, *Res Vet Sci* 22:205-208, 1977.

106. Burrows GE et al: Comparative pharmacokinetics of antibiotics in newborn calves: chloramphenicol, lincomycin, and tylosin, *Am J Vet Res* 44:1053-1057, 1983.

107. Fisher EW, De la Fuente GH: Antibiotics and calf diarrhoea: the effect of serum immune globulin concentrations, *Vet Rec* 89:579-582, 1971.

108. Radostits OM et al: A clinical evaluation of antimicrobial agents and temporary starvation in the treatment of acute undifferentiated diarrhea in newborn calves, *Can Vet J* 16:219-227, 1975.

109. Buntain BJ, Selman IE: Controlled studies of various treatments for neonatal calf diarrhoea in calves of known immunoglobulin levels, *Vet Rec* 107:245-248, 1980.

110. Lister EE, McKay RR: Effect of medication with antibiotics and mature bovine plasma on mortality, morbidity, rate of growth and serum immunoglobulins of Holstein calves, *Can J Anim Sci* 50:645-650, 1970.

111. Palmer GH, Bywater RJ, Francis ME: Amoxicillin: distribution and clinical efficacy in calves, *Vet Rec* 100:487-491, 1977.

112. Bywater RJ, Palmer GH, Wanstall SA. Discrepancy between antibiotic (amoxicillin) resistance in vitro and efficacy in calf diarrhoea, *Vet Rec* 102:150-151, 1978.

113. Grimshaw W, Colman PJ, Petrie L: Efficacy of sulbactam-ampicillin in the treatment of neonatal calf diarrhoea, *Vet Rec* 121:162-166, 1987.

114. McCormack WM: Susceptibility of mycoplasmas to antimicrobial agents: clinical implications, *Clin Infect Dis* 17(suppl 1):S200-S201, 1993.

115. Shoaf SE et al: Pharmacokinetics of trimethoprim-sulfadiazine in neonatal calves: influence of synovitis, *J Vet Pharmacol Ther* 9:446-454, 1986.

116. Brown MP et al: Pharmacokinetics and synovial fluid concentrations of cephapirin in calves with suppurative arthritis, *Am J Vet Res* 52:1438-1440, 1991.

117. Brown MP, Mayo MB, Gronwall RR: Serum and synovial fluid concentrations of ampicillin trihydrate in calves with suppurative arthritis, *Cornell Vet* 81:137-143, 1991.

118. Hamed KA, Tam JY, Prober CG: Pharmacokinetic optimization of the treatment of septic arthritis, *Clin Pharmacokinet* 31:156-163, 1996.

119. Green SL, Smith LL: Meningitis in neonatal calves: 32 cases (1983-1990), *J Am Vet Med Assoc* 201:125-128, 1992.

120. Lutsar I, McCracken GH Jr, Friedland IR: Antibiotic pharmacodynamics in cerebrospinal fluid, *Clin Infect Dis* 27:1117-1127, 1128-1129, 1998.

121. de Craene BA et al: Pharmacokinetics of florfenicol in cerebrospinal fluid and plasma of calves, *Antimicrob Agents Chemother* 41:1991-1995, 1997.

122. Haskins SC: Management of septic shock, *J Am Vet Med Assoc* 200:1915-1924, 1992.

123. Constable PD et al: Respiratory, renal, hematologic, and serum biochemical effects of hypertonic saline solution in endotoxemic calves, *Am J Vet Res* 52:990-998, 1991.

124. Bertone JJ, Shoemaker KE: Effect of hypertonic and isotonic saline solutions on plasma constituents of conscious horses, *Am J Vet Res* 53:1844-1849, 1992.

125. Lavoie JP et al: Hemodynamic, clinical pathologic, haematologic and behavioural changes during endotoxin infusion in equine neonates, *Equine Vet J* 22:23, 1990.

126. Allen GK et al: Serum tumor necrosis factor-α concentrations and clinical abnormalities in colostrum-fed and colostrum-deprived neonatal foals given endotoxin, *Am J Vet Res* 54:1404-1410, 1993.

127. Cullor JS: Shock attributable to bacteremia and endotoxemia in cattle: clinical and experimental findings, *J Am Vet Med Assoc* 200:1894-1902, 1992.

128. Morris DD, Moore JN: Tumor necrosis factor activity in serum from neonatal foals with presumed septicemia, *J Am Vet Med Assoc* 199:1584-1589, 1991.

129. Semrad SD: Comparative efficacy of flunixin, ketoprofen, and ketorolac for treating endotoxemic neonatal calves, *Am J Vet Res* 54:1511-1516, 1993.

130. Bottoms GD et al: Endotoxin-induced hemodynamic changes in ponies: effects of flunixin meglumine, *Am J Vet Res* 42:1514-1518, 1981.

131. Moore JN et al: Prevention of endotoxin-induced arterial hypoxemia and lactic acidosis with flunixin meglumine, *Equine Vet J* 13:95, 1981.

132. Semrad SD, Sams RA, Ashcraft SM: Pharmacokinetics of and serum thromboxane suppression by flunixin meglumine in healthy foals during the first month of life, *Am J Vet Res* 54:2083-2087, 1993.

133. Barton MH: Use of pentoxifylline for the treatment of equine endotoxemia, *Proceedings of the Twelfth ACVIM Forum*, San Francisco, 740-742, 1994.

134. Geor RJ: Effects of pentoxifylline on blood flow properties in the horse, *Proceedings of the Tenth ACVIM Forum*, San Diego, 818-820, 1992.

135. Morris DD, Whitlock RH: Therapy of suspected septicemia in neonatal foals using plasma-containing antibodies to core lipopolysaccharide (LPS), *J Vet Intern Med* 1:175-182, 1987.

136. Zinkl JG et al: Haematological, bone marrow and clinical chemical changes in neonatal foals given canine recombinant granulocyte colony-stimulating factor, *Equine Vet J* 26:313, 1994.

137. Moore JN, Morris DD: Endotoxemia and septicemia in horses: experimental and clinical correlates, *J Am Vet Med Assoc* 200:1903-1914, 1992.

138. Zaremba W, Guterbock WM, Holmberg CA: Efficacy of a dried colostrum powder in the prevention of disease in neonatal Holstein calves, *J Dairy Sci* 76:831-836, 1993.

139. Abel Francisco SF, Quigley JD: Serum immunoglobulin concentrations after feeding maternal colostrum or maternal colostrum plus colostral supplement to dairy calves, *Am J Vet Res* 54:1051-1054, 1993.

140. Williams NM, Donahue JM: Placentitis in mares in Kentucky, *Proceedings of the Havemeyer Foundation Workshop on Equine Placentitis*, Lexington, Ky, 1998.

141. Troedsson MHT et al: Transrectal ultrasound evaluation of the placenta in normal mares and mares with impending abortion, *Proceedings of the Havemeyer Foundation Workshop on Equine Placentitis*, Lexington, Ky, 1998, p 136.

142. Reimer JM: Transabdominal ultrasound evaluation of placentitis, *Proceedings of the Havemeyer Foundation Workshop on Placentitis*, Lexington, Ky, 1998, p 38.

143. Vaala WE, Sertich PL: Management strategies for mares at risk for periparturient complications, *Vet Clin North Am (Equine Pract)* 10:237-265, 1994.

144. Sertich PL, Vaala WE: Concentrations of antibiotics in mares, foals, and fetal fluids after antibiotic administration during late pregnancy, *Proceedings of the Thirty-eighth Annual Convention of the American Association of Equine Practitioners*, 1992, pp 727-733.

145. Steel CM et al: Factors associated with prognosis for survival and athletic use in foals with septic arthritis: 93 cases (1987-1994), *J Am Vet Med Assoc* 215:973-977, 1999.

Manifestations of Disease in the Neonate

WENDY E. VAALA

JOHN K. HOUSE

Consulting Editors

MAJOR CLINICAL SIGNS/PROBLEMS ENCOUNTERED

PREMATURITY

WENDY E. VAALA
JOHN K. HOUSE

TERMINOLOGY AND CLINICAL SIGNS. During the past 20 years, several terms have been used to describe small or immature appearing foals; these include *premature, immature, dysmature, intrauterine growth retarded or restricted, small for dates, unready for birth,* and *viable or nonviable.* One commonly used definition of prematurity is a foal that is the product of a curtailed gestation of 320 days or less.[1] This definition was derived from the following three sources:

1. A study of birthweight of Thoroughbred foals with gestational ages ranging from 300 to 371 days in which those born between 300 and 320 days were significantly lighter.[2]
2. Optimal survival of foals delivered in the gestational age range of 320 to 360 days.[3]
3. The lower limit of the norm around the distribution of 340 days (the mean gestational length of Thoroughbreds) is 320 days.[4]

However, the normal gestational length of an individual mare varies considerably, and it has been recommended that gestational age be only one of several criteria used to assess the viability of the fetus.[1] For example, a 335-day-old fetus may be totally unprepared for birth if its normal gestational length is really 365 days. Dysmaturity implies delayed or inappropriate fetal growth and development resulting from an abnormal intrauterine environment associated with conditions such as placentitis, twinning, hydrops, and placental insufficiency. Dysmature foals can have shortened, normal, or prolonged gestation lengths.

A small body size, short and silky haircoat, increased range of motion of joints, and immature skeletal ossification are seen in most foals that are born before 320 days' gestation. Severely lax flexor tendons in the front and rear, marked periarticular ligamentous laxity, general weakness or "floppiness," including floppy ears, and progressive deterioration in neurologic function and ability to maintain homeostasis (e.g., body temperature, blood pressure, serum glucose concentration) are clinical signs more commonly associated with a specific group of premature foals. That group includes those

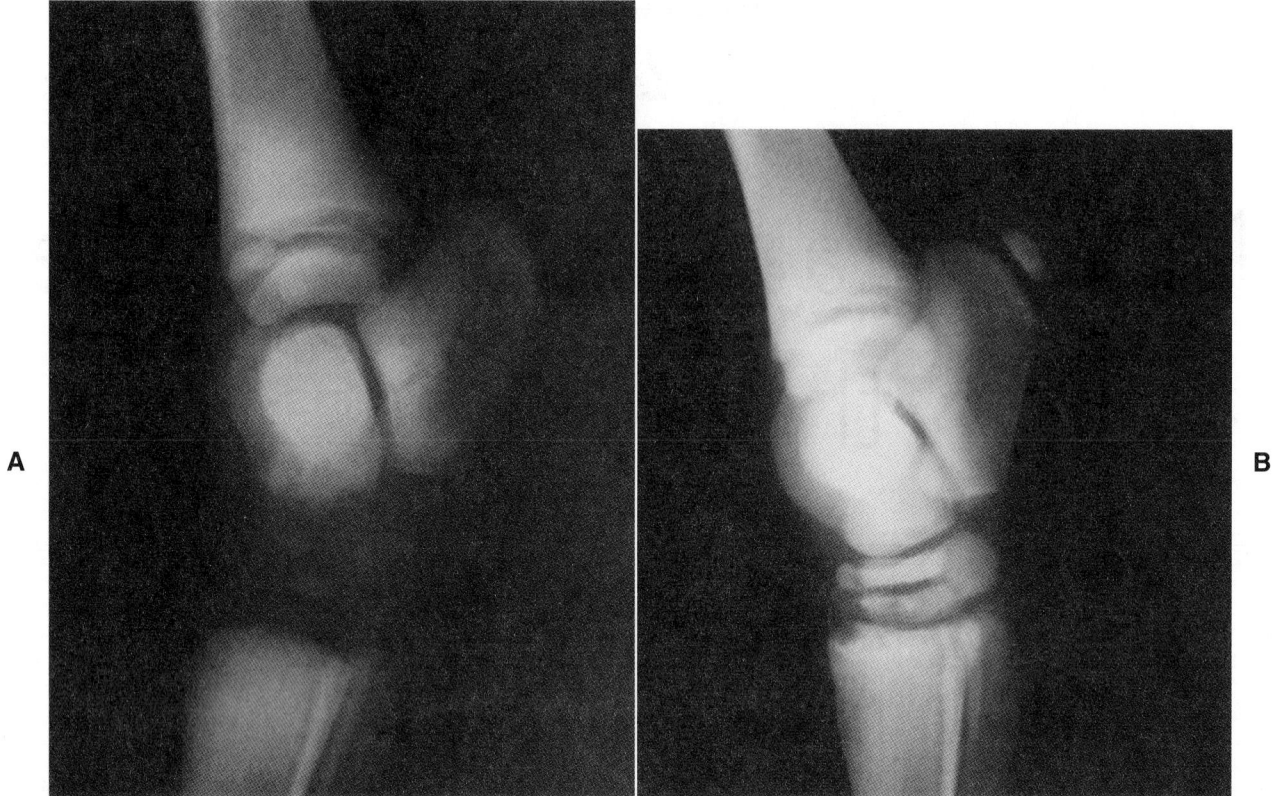

FIG. 20-1 ▓ **A,** Lateral tarsus of a 1-day-old, 305-day gestational age colt. Note the lack of ossification of the small tarsal bones. **B,** Lateral tarsus of the same foal as in **A,** at 3 weeks of age, showing irregular ossification. Without the initial radiograph, increasing ossification could have been confused with bone lysis and osteomyelitis. The foal is reported to be sound at 6 months of age.

fetuses that were normal in other ways, but were delivered early and abruptly by induction of parturition, cesarian section, or acute placentitis or because of severe systemic maternal illness. Rossdale and colleagues[5] coined the term "unready for birth" to describe the clinical syndrome associated with this type of premature foal. Rossdale and colleagues studied various aspects of the physiology of the "unready for birth" foal by using a model involving early induction of parturition.[5] Abnormal hematologic and endocrinologic findings in the first 24 hours postpartum include abnormally low plasma cortisol concentrations and peripheral blood neutrophil to lymphocyte ratios, along with a lack of responsiveness of plasma cortisol to endogenous adrenocorticotrophic hormone (ACTH) or ACTH administration.[6] These findings led the investigators to suggest that the low level of cortisol was secondary to a lack of responsiveness of the adrenal gland. Whether this is the only endocrinologic abnormality present, or merely one of many, has not yet been determined.

It is common practice in human medicine to compare gestational age with body weight and appearance to assess whether the infant is small for its gestational age (SGA). Thus a neonate can be classified as both premature and SGA. This term implies that some type of chronic derangement during gestation interrupted normal growth processes. Intrauterine growth restriction (IUGR) has replaced SGA as the term used to describe unusually small birth weight neonates. IUGR is pathologic and is due to genetic causes or epigenetic causes that disrupt normal placental function. In humans, IUGR is defined as an infant whose birth weight is below the 10th percentile for a given gestational age.[7] Detailed fetal weights throughout gestation are not available for the horse. Despite

some variation between breeds, the average relative weight of the term foal to its dam is approximately 10%.[8,9] Using these definitions, a 45-lb twin Thoroughbred foal would be an example of SGA and IUGR.

Fetal growth rate and size at birth are affected by various factors including genetics,[8] gestation length, placental surface area,[10] uterine blood flow,[10] maternal age, and fetal chromosomal abnormalities.[8] Genetic factors, predominantly maternal genes, play a significant role in the size of the foal at birth with size of the dam correlating directly with the relative size of the foal. Curtailed gestation length is associated with reduced neonatal birth weights. Abnormally long gestation lengths have also been associated with small birth weight neonates because of derangements in the intrauterine environment. Fungal infection resulting in reduced placental surface area has been associated with small birth weight foals.[11] Advancing maternal age of the dam has been correlated with decreasing birth weight in the foal.

Poor fetal growth is associated with decreased growth potential (type 1 IUGR) or restriction of growth secondary to diminished oxygen and nutrient supplies (type 2 IUGR).[7] In humans, type 2 IUGR is the most common form of IUGR and results in a newborn that has a relatively large head and small body. In humans, most cases of type 2 IUGR are suspected to occur during the third trimester and are associated with placental vascular lesions, maternal starvation, twinning, intrauterine infections caused by bacterial or fungal pathogens, and chronic hypoxia. Most available evidence suggests that a decrease in placental function resulting in chronic hypoxia is a critical element in the development of IUGR. Fetal adaptations to hypoxia include a redistribution of blood flow with preferential perfusion of the heart, brain,

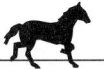

and adrenal glands at the expense of blood flow to kidneys, gut, lungs, liver, and muscle.[12-14] The dysproportionately large head size in infants with IUGR is due to relative brain sparing compared with other organs.

Other characteristics of severe growth restriction in the foal include a head that is disproportionately large for the body and a forehead that seems excessively domed. However, accurate identification of the less severely growth restricted fetus is seriously limited by a lack of breed-specific fetal and postnatal growth curves, by lack of information on normal body proportions of foals, and on the normal rate and pattern of fetal skeletal ossification.

IUGR may reflect fetal infection as observed with bovine virus diarrhea virus infection in bovine fetuses.[15] Growth restriction is indicated when the developmental age is less than the chronological age. Crown to anus length is useful for determining the developmental age of ovine fetuses from 50 to 100 days and bovine fetuses up to 210 days of gestation. In late gestation, significant variation in measurements of gestational age (crown to anus length, long bone length, body weight, and skeletal ossification) is observed between breeds. Near term, the rate of increase in crown-anus length, body weight, and diaphyseal length of bones decreases. The length of long bone diaphyses provides the best measure of gestational age for bovine fetuses greater than 260 days gestational age.[16-18]

With reference to foals the term *premature* is used to describe a foal that is 320 days or less gestational age. Regardless of the cause of the premature birth, most foals less than 320 days' gestation display some characteristics of prematurity. Even if certain organ systems, such as the brain and lungs, have matured secondary to chronic prenatal stress, and the foal is ready for birth, it usually still has specific problems related to prematurity that require special consideration, such as an immature musculoskeletal system. It is also important to identify the newborn that has grown poorly in response to chronic in utero stress, regardless of its gestational age. The term used in human medicine, *intrauterine growth restriction*, seems adequate at this time, until specific studies are performed in the horse. The physiologic stability of the newborn should also be assessed, particularly in terms of endocrinologic function (Fig. 20-1). The term "readiness for birth" has been used relative to adrenocortical function. Until we more completely understand the defects predisposing to the clinical appearance of the unready for birth foal, a more specific description is not really possible. Assessment of the degree of skeletal maturity, the presence of peripartuient asphyxia and the likelihood of generalized or localized infection are also important considerations when formulating a rational treatment plan.

FORMATION OF PROGNOSIS FOR THE PREMATURELY DELIVERED FOAL

The prognosis for life for a prematurely delivered foal depends greatly on the cause of the premature delivery, the events of the perinatal period, the degree of immaturity the animal displays, the level of support available to care for it, and the financial commitment of the owner. For example, a severe asphyxial episode at birth can greatly complicate the clinical course of the premature foal. Premature foals that experienced a normal, spontaneous delivery and were treated appropriately during the first 24 hours of life had a considerably better survival rate (>70%) than all other premature foals that resulted from early cesarian section or induction of parturition or that were born spontaneously from a systemically ill mare (20% to 25% survival rate).[19,20] In general, the lower the gestational age and birth weight, the greater the number of complications observed. Rossdale[2] has suggested that most foals younger than 300 days' gestation are nonvi-

able; this statement probably is correct for induced and cesarian section premature foals. However, some foals born at 285 to 300 days' gestation have survived and done well, although most required long and expensive stays in an intensive care facility. Virtually all of these foals were born spontaneously because of chronic placental insufficiency, and their organ systems were probably maturationally advanced secondary to chronic prenatal stress (see Chapter 15).

For a successful outcome in the premature animal, extremely careful management of the cardiopulmonary system, generalized and localized (e.g., pneumonia) infection, unstable metabolism (e.g., hypoglycemia), and an immature musculoskeletal system is crucial. Complications observed after discharge of premature foals from the hospital have included chronic pneumonia; musculoskeletal problems, often as a result of bone and ligament immaturity; and small size.

Favorable and unfavorable short-term prognostic signs in premature foals are listed in Table 20-1. As stated earlier, the clinical appearance of a spontaneously born premature foal exposed in chronic uteroplacental disease is typically different from that of the premature foal that is "unready for birth" (see below). Physical examination of the former type often revealed a small newborn with a head relatively large in proportion to its thin body. Initially, most were weak and depressed and experienced difficulties maintaining blood glucose and body temperature. Respiratory distress has been the most common localizing clinical sign; the radiographic pattern of pulmonary infiltration was usually suggestive of a pneumonic process (presumed secondary to placentitis) rather than hyaline membrane disease (see Respiratory Distress). With intensive management, including antibiotics, fluid therapy, enteral and parenteral nutrition, and respiratory support, including oxygen therapy in most patients and short-term positive-pressure ventilation in several, these foals usually improved rapidly in strength and awareness after the first 24 hours postpartum. Physically, they tended to have a short, silky haircoat, but erect ears. Although many had fairly lax rear flexor tendons, most had had relatively normal front limb conformation once weight bearing began; a few even had contracted front flexor tendons. Mentation generally improved rapidly, with some foals appearing almost hyperalert. In most cases, their appetite was excellent after the initial postnatal period, and some appeared almost ravenous. Typical hematologic values and trends in surviving premature foals are listed in Table 20-1. In particular, a high plasma fibrinogen concentration and increasing white blood cell count on day 2 were associated with a favorable outcome. Rossdale and colleagures[21] have reported on certain endocrinologic characteristics of a group of premature foals with evidence of chronic placental pathology. They found premature increases of maternal progestagen concentrations, elevated circulating progestagens, and some degree of enhanced adrenocortical activity in the newborn foal. This suggests that chronic stress in late gestation may also cause early maturation of the adrenal gland in the horse, enhancing the likelihood of survival in the prematurely delivered foal.[21]

In our clinical experience, nonsurviving premature foals have usually been victims of early cesarian section delivery, poorly timed induction of parturition, in utero sepsis or severe hypoxia or they have been "aborted" from very ill mares. They have shown a relatively consistent pattern of deterioration. After initial resuscitation, the first 12 to 18 hours are often deceptively uneventful, with slight improvement in condition often noted. This period is usually followed by a marked decline in awareness, seizure activity, and worsening acidosis, usually both respiratory and metabolic in nature. The WBC count is usually low (<5000 cells/μl), and plasma fibrinogen is usually normal (100 to 300 mg/dl). Chest radiographs usually show a diffuse interstitial infiltrate.

TABLE 20-1

Prognostic Signs* for the Prematurely Delivered Foal

Parameter	Favorable	Unfavorable
Placenta	Chronic placental changes, such as villous atrophy, placentitis	Normal placenta, or edematous, without evidence of infection
Delivery process	Spontaneous, no dystocia	Induction of parturition, dystocia
Systemic disease in dam	None	Severe colic, especially surgery, endotoxemia
Neurologic status at 24 hours	No seizures, aware of environment, suckling reflex present	Deteriorating, some seizure activity noted; poor or no suckle reflex
Total WBC count	>5000 cell/μl on day 1, or low on day 1 and increases on day 2 to 3	<5000 cells/μl persistently
N:L ratio	>2, or if low on day 1, increases on day 2-3	<2 persistently
Plasma fibrinogen (mg/dl)	>400 mg/dl at birth	100-300 mg/dl at birth
Metabolic acidosis	Not present, pH >7.3	Present, with pH persistently <7.3
Plasma cortisol within 2 hours of birth	Increasing levels (120-140 ng/ml) at 30-60 min postpartum	Low levels (<30 ng/ml)
Plasma ACTH over first 2 hours of life	Declining values from peak (300 pg/ml at birth)	Peak values (about 650 pg/ml) at 30 min postpartum and then decline
Response to synthetic ACTH (short-acting synacthen, dose of 0.125 mg IM)	Good response shown by doubling of plasma cortisol and widening of N:L ratio	Poor response shown by little increase in plasma cortisol and no change in N:L ratio
Glucose tolerance test (0.5 mg/kg glucose IV)	Clear response demonstrated by a 250% increase in plasma insulin at 5 min after administration	Slight response demonstrated by a 100% increase in plasma insulin 15 min after administration
Renin angiotensin aldosterone system, plasma renin substrate	Low (>0.6 μg/ml) and declining levels during 15-30 min postpartum	Higher and/or increasing levels during 15-60 min after foaling

ACTH, Adrenocorticotrophic hormone; *N:L ratio,* neutrophil/lymphocyte ratio; *WBC,* white blood cell.
*Caution: No single parameter should be used to formulate a prognosis. The presence of several unfavorable parameters, however, usually indicates a very compromised individual in need of intensive monitoring and support.

Intolerance to enteral feeding is usually noted, with abdominal distention and gastric reflux. Pulse quality often declines, coinciding with the development of generalized edema, oliguria, and deteriorating neurologic function. At this stage, these patients are frustratingly refractory to treatment. Severe shock and coma result in death or euthanasia at 48 to 72 hours postpartum in most cases. Postmortem examination is usually unremarkable, the most consistent finding being pulmonary atelectasis, with or without neutrophil infiltration. Bacterial cultures may be negative.

With the present state of neonatal equine critical care, many foals that are described above and display several of the poor prognostic signs listed in Table 20-1 are lost. Whether the poor survival rates are the result of an inherent, irreversible problem, or simply a matter of ignorance of the most appropriate treatment approach, is not known. Presumably, with more knowledge of the physiology of these patients, a greater percentage of these patients will be salvagable, although it remains to be determined if the necessary treatment will be cost-effective. Therefore a newborn foal with poor prognostic signs should not be automatically considered a lost cause, but rather an animal in need of extremely careful monitoring and aggressive treatment for impending or existing shock.

APPROACH TO DIAGNOSIS IN THE PREMATURE FOAL

Prematurity in animals is associated with immaturity of many organ systems, placing the preterm individual at higher risk than the term foal of developing respiratory, metabolic, and infectious problems. In particular, glycogen stores may not be completely formed or may be depleted by in utero stress (Chapter 15). Glucose homeostasis may be precarious because of inadequate insulin production or peripheral insulin resistance. Normal blood pressure may be difficult to maintain because of an immature neuroendocrine system

that predisposes to hypotension. An immature immune system increases the neonate's susceptibility to generalized and localized infections caused by bacteria, viruses, and fungi, and immaturity of the lung surfactant system may predispose to hypoxemia and atelectasis. The musculoskeletal system is often incompletely developed, the gastrointestinal tract may be unready to handle an oral diet, the kidneys and liver may be less efficient in their ability to eliminate drugs, and the immature brain may be less tolerant to the effects of asphyxia. Additionally, the actual cause of the premature delivery may also be detrimental to the neonate's well-being. Sepsis resulting from acute baterial placentitis or acute hypoxia caused by placental insufficiency or separation may overwhelm the premature foal during the critical period of postpartum adaptation. Therefore the clinician may be faced with treatment of several abnormalities.

The reason for the premature delivery should be established, if possible. Any maternal problems during late gestation should be identified, and the foal should be evaluated for IUGR. The placenta should be thoroughly examined grossly and histologically, and appropriate cultures should be taken. A useful guideline is to submit sections obtained from the following areas of the chorioallantois: fetal and nonfetal horns, the body, and the cervical star region. The most common causes of prematurity in the foal are probably placentitis and/or chronic placental insufficiency.[20] Therefore it is important to establish the likelihood of infection as early as possible (see Chapter 18). The most common locations of in utero acquired infections appear to be the lungs and the eyes (anterior uveitis), but pulmonary disease may not be obvious on physical examination until the condition is well advanced. Therefore, in any case in which the suspicion of in utero acquired infection is high, chest radiographs and arterial blood gases are indicated to detect early disease.

The animal should be closely examined for any obvious congenital malformations that will limit its viability. After delivery, the ability of the neonate to maintain homeostasis (e.g.,

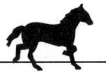

body temperature, respiratory rate and effort, blood pressure, blood glucose concentration) should be carefully monitored on a regular basis for a minimum of 48 hours. Arterial blood gases should be closely monitored. The premature or growth-restricted fetus may be dependent on a constant infusion of dextrose to maintain blood glucose levels because of low glycogen stores. Conversely, some premature neonates suffering from concurrent sepsis or asphyxia may exhibit a rebound hyperglycemia associated with inadequate production and release of insulin or peripheral insulin resistance.

Finally, assessment of whether the foal is ready for birth includes a white blood cell (WBC) count and differential, measurement of blood gases or plasma bicarbonate concentration to identify metabolic acidosis, and possibly, an ACTH stimulation test. This is performed by giving 0.125 mg synthetic $ACTH_{1-24}$ IM during the first 24 hours postpartum. The neutrophil to lymphocyte ratio (N:L) in the peripheral blood (and plasma cortisol, if testing is available) is measured before and 1 to 2 hours after injection. A good response is indicated by a substantial increase in plasma cortisol and a widening of the N:L ratio.[22]

The degree of skeletal ossification should be determined by radiography[23] or possibly ultrasonography[24] of the tarsus and carpus. The musculoskeletal system should also be evaluated for angular limb and flexural deformities.

TREATMENT CONSIDERATIONS IN THE PREMATURE FOAL[20]

Several factors may predispose the premature foal to failure of passive transfer. Chronic placental pathology is frequently accompanied by premature lactation, and as a result after delivery the colostrum is often of poor quality. If early delivery has occurred because of acute serious illness in the mare or early induction of labor, the mammary gland is often poorly developed and has insufficient colostral antibody levels. It is also possible that the immature gastrointestinal tract of the compromised premature foal is not capable of absorbing colostral antibodies as efficiently as is the mature tract, but no such studies have been published to date. Prematurity in a variety of animal species is associated with an increased susceptibility to infection; therefore it is crucial to ensure that the premature neonate receive ample amounts of high-quality colostrum (at least 20 ml/kg) in the first 6 hours after delivery, provided its condition is stable. A cold, hypotensive, hypoxic foal is likely to have secondary gastrointestinal compromise that includes ileus, delayed gastric emptying, and impaired digestive capabilities. These foals should not be fed until their vital signs are stable. Such foals should receive intravenous hyperimmune plasma as soon as possible to provide immunoglobulins and other opsonins useful in disease prevention. As soon as gut function seems adequate, small aliquots of colostrum should be administered. A serum immunoglobulin (IgG) level should be measured at 18 to 24 hours of age to ensure successful passive transfer of immunity (>800 mg/dl).

Many premature foals are born early because of in utero infection, and antibiotic therapy is an important part of treatment. Although some cases of congenital pneumonia resolve quickly, it is not unusual for pulmonary disease to persist for 2 to 4 weeks or longer, even with appropriate therapy. Treatment should be continued until chest radiographs and hematologic parameters are normal (Chapter 17). The suspicion of nosocomial infection should be high in the premature foal, particularly if failure of passive transfer was diagnosed or if the nutritional status of the patient is poor. In such patients, multiresistant bacterial[25] and generalized *Candida* spp. infections are not uncommonly associated with long-term antibiotic therapy. Fever spikes, changes in the WBC count, or

deterioration in the clinical appearance of the animal suggests the need for additional cultures, and possibly a change in antimicrobial therapy.

The first 12 to 24 hours after delivery can be deceptive with many premature foals showing varying degrees of improvement which often delays timely referral. The surge of hormones accompanying delivery is probably responsible for the initial improvement in awareness, strength, heart rate, and pulse quality. During the next 24 hours, many immature foals begin to fade. Body temperature may decrease, and breathing effort increases with an unpredictable change in rate. If the respiratory center is intact, the foal's respiratory rate should increase after birth. Foals experiencing hypoxic-ischemic damage to the respiratory center may demonstrate a gradually decreasing respiratory rate, which may be mistaken as an encouraging sign. Newborn foals should have ventilatory rates above 25 to 35 breaths/min. Premature foals may fail to respond normally to rising carbon dioxide concentrations and decreasing oxygen levels in arterial blood. Other premature foals that were breathing rapidly and with increased effort become fatigued and cannot maintain adequate work of breathing resulting in progressive lung atelectasis and respiratory distress. Hypoxia, hypercapnea, and acidosis may also stimulate a reversion to fetal circulation with the development of pulmonary hypertension. Pulmonary hypertension is characterized by is characterized by a significant elevation of the pulmonary artery pressure and cyanosis caused by right-to-left shunting through the ductus arteriosus and foramen ovale. Monitoring arterial blood gases becomes critical in the successful management of pulmonary function in premature foals suffering from advanced prematurity and hypoxia or sepsis.

Because the majority of premature foals develop some degree of pulmonary dysfunction, appropriate respiratory support is often a critical part of their therapy. The tendency for atelectasis is increased in premature foals, presumably as a result of both lung and chest wall immaturity. Maintenance in sternal recumbency, frequent turning from side to side, and encouragement of lung expansion (deep breathing, coughing, etc.) may all minimize the tendency for lung collapse. Intranasal humidified oxygen therapy is frequently necessary to maintain adequate oxygenation, and positive-pressure ventilation may be required if respiratory distress is severe and hypoventilation is progressive. The usefulness of surfactant replacement products in premature foals has not been determined to date (see Respiratory Distress). Administration of caffeine, a methylxanthine, as a respiratory stimulant helps reduce lung atelectasis associated with hypoventilation and prolong apnea caused by depression of the central respiratory center. Methylxanthines have a stimulatory effect on the central respiratory center and peripheral effects on the neuromuscular junction.[26] The central effect results from nonspecific inhibition of cerebral adenosine receptors. Caffeine may also alter the sleep-wake cycle, with an increased amount of time spent awake or in active sleep, which results in a decreased frequency of apnea. Methylxanthines increase minute ventilation and chemoreceptor CO_2 sensitivity. These drugs also work on the neuromuscular junction to increase skeletal muscle tone and decrease diaphragmatic fatigue while increasing metabolic rate and oxygen consumption. One of the most common causes of apnea and respiratory center depression is hypoxic-ischemic encephalopathy. Other causes of respiratory depression, including hypothermia, hypoglycemia, and hypocalcemia should be addressed.

Little is known about the special nutritional requirements of the premature, growth restricted or skeletally immature foal, so no specific recommendations regarding nutritional support can be made. The immature gastrointestinal tract is often intolerant of enteral feeding, yet the caloric requirements of these foals is probably great. Therefore a combination of parenteral and enteral nutrition is often helpful in supplying at least part of the daily nutritional needs. Premature and growth-restricted foals have poorly defined nutrient requirements. Some foals suffering from prematurity, sepsis, or peripartum asphyxia may have blunted insulin responses and lower glucose concentrations at birth than full-term neonates. In the absence of species-specific information, the nutritional needs of the premature infant can be considered when designing a feeding regimen for premature foals. Premature infants have higher energy (114 to 181 kcal/kg/day) and protein (4 to 6 g/kg/day) requirements. Fat absorption is reduced because of decreased bile salt synthesis and hepatic immaturity, resulting in inefficient lipid solubilization by micelle formation. Dysmature foals with incomplete skeletal ossification have increased calcium and phosphorus requirements that may not be met by mare's milk alone and must be considered when feeding such foals parenterally for prolonged periods.

The best way to support the immature musculoskeletal system is currently not known. There is often a conflict between the needs of the whole individual and the needs of the musculoskeletal system. Weight bearing on an incompletely ossified cartilage matrix may cause collapse or permanent malformation. On the other hand, forced prolonged restraint in lateral recumbency of a foal strong enough to ambulate is not practical and predisposes to secondary complications, such as pneumonia and decubital sores. Treatment of incomplete ossification of tarsal bones should be aimed at maintaining the longitudinal axis of the limb so ossification proceeds without distortion of the cartilaginous precursors. Depending on the degree of skeletal immaturity, exercise is usually restricted to the stall or a small area until tarsal and carpal ossification is near normal. If lax flexor tendons are present, heel extensions are usually helpful. If angular limb deformities are present or develop, bandages, light splints or braces are often used to reduce the compressive forces acting on the dorsal aspects of the tarsal bones. Care should be taken to avoid devices that are too heavy for the small, weak individual and interfere with its ability to stand and walk.[27] Severe tarsus valgus that persists despite external support may require hemicircumferential periosteal transection or growth restriction.

One study examined the outcome of foals with varying degrees of incomplete ossification of their tarsal bones. Foals with incomplete ossification and greater than 30% collapse of the central or third tarsal bone or both with pinching or fragmentation of the dorsal aspects of affected bones were classified as having type II lesions. Foals with less than 30% collapse of the central and third tarsal bones were classified as having type I lesions. Foals with type II lesions all developed degenerative joint disease and had a guarded prognosis for future athletic performance.[28]

The use of corticosteroids in treatment of the premature foal is controversial. Many premature foals with the favorable prognostic signs listed in Table 20-1 have been managed successfully without steroid administration. It is probable that their adrenal function is relatively mature and that exogenous steroids are unnecessary and possibly detrimental. On the other hand, the apparent immaturity of the adrenal gland and low plasma cortisol levels in the nonviable group of premature foals suggest that corticosteroid administration could be of benefit. It would seem appropriate to provide a daily dose that would result in physiologic rather than immunosuppressive levels until adrenal function improves, but an effective dosing regimen cannot be recommended at this time. The effect of steroid administration on the development of the neonatal adrenal gland or on the susceptibility of the foal to infection is not known at the time of this writing.

In human obstetrics, premature deliveries are prevented, if possible, using tocolytic agents. β-Sympathomimetics, such as isoxsuprine, are being investigated to produce tocolysis in pregnant mares.[29] If delivery is inevitable, corticosteroids may be given to the mother to accelerate fetal lung maturation and to decrease the incidence of hyaline membrane disease. Human mothers are treated with corticosteroids when delivery is not expected for at least 24 hours and when fetal membranes are not infected. In the horse, these criteria are seldom met. However, if circumstances are appropriate, maternal steroid administration might be attempted, but the best drug and dose is not known. Transabdominal ultrasonography allows evaluation of fetal well-being and placental integrity. If bacterial placentitis is suspected, the pregnancy often can be maintained using broad-spectrum antibiotics to treat bacterial infection, flunixin meglumine to reduce inflammation and prevent prostaglandin induced abortion, pentoxyfylline to improve microcirculation, and tocolytic agents to delay delivery.[29]

WEAKNESS AND/OR DEPRESSION

WENDY E. VAALA
JOHN K. HOUSE

When confronted with a neonate with the primary complaint of weakness with or without accompanying depression, several differential diagnoses must be ruled out (Box 20-1). The gestational and postnatal age of the neonate should be established. If weakness has been present since birth, in utero acquired bacterial or viral infections, birth asphyxia and trauma, chronic placental problems, and congenital anomalies should be placed higher on the list of differential diagnoses. Neonatal calves with storage diseases primarily affecting the nervous system may appear reasonably normal for a short period after birth and then show progressive signs of neurologic dysfunction, including tremors, spasms, depression, recumbency, and coma. Lethargy and loss of suckle are often the first signs of neonatal illness. A full udder on the dam accompanies poor nursing behavior in the neonate. If the neonate is depressed and has injected mucous membranes and hyperemic coronary bands, then septicemia is the primary differential and the most life threatening. If the neonate is relatively bright but is becoming a "dishrag," consider peripartum hypoxia and early signs of hypoxic-ischemic encephalopathy. If the newborn shows signs of immaturity such as tendon laxity and silky hair coat, weakness may be the result of progressive fatigue, hypothermia, hypoxia, or hypoglycemia. Unfortunately, many weak foals and calves begin to fade as a result of multiple problems.

If weakness is present without accompanying depression, several other differentials for primary neuromuscular or musculoskeletal disease should be considered. Neuromuscular diseases include botulism, white muscle disease, and congenital myopathies. Botulism is an infection acquired via the gastrointestinal tract. Consequently, signs appear in neonates that are usually 10 days or older. Although most cases of nutritional myodegeneration (NMD) occur during the first year of life among rapidly growing, large animal neonates, an in utero form of NMD may occur, resulting in clinical signs in affected neonates soon after birth. If weakness is detected in one or more limbs immediately after birth, peripheral nerve and muscle damage associated with birth trauma should be ruled out. Femoral nerve paralysis may be observed in calves following a "hip lock" dystocia.[30] A condition resembling congenital myasthenia gravis has also been described in Brahman calves.[31]

It should be determined whether any drugs or anesthetics were administered to the mother before or at the time of de-

BOX 20-1

Differential Diagnoses for the Weak or Depressed Large-Animal Neonate

BACTERIAL INFECTION: IN UTERO OR POSTNATALLY ACQUIRED
Septicemia
Joint and bone
Enteritis
Pneumonia
Meningitis
Peritonitis (primary or secondary)

CONGENITAL VIRAL INFECTION
Equine herpesvirus (E)
Equine viral arteritis (E)
Bovine virus diarrhea virus (B)
Bluetongue virus (B, O)
Infectious bovine rhinotracheitis virus (B)
Akabane virus (B)
Parainfluenza (B)
Caprine herpes (C)
Border disease virus (O)

PREMATURITY/POSTMATURITY
Placentitis, prolonged gestation associated with fescue toxicosis
Intrauterine growth restriction
Weak calf syndrome
Insufficient fetoplacental matching (twin foals)
Bacterial or fungal placentitis

BIRTH ASPHYXIA
Placentitis
Dystocia
Cesarean section
Premature placental separation
Induced parturition

BIRTH TRAUMA
Brachial plexus injuries
Fractured rib, pneumothorax, hemothorax
Ruptured bladder

CONGENITAL MALFORMATIONS
Cardiac malformations
Central nervous system malformations (e.g., hydrocephalus, hydranencephaly)
Angular limb deformities
Arthrogryposis

METABOLIC DERANGEMENTS
Hypoglycemia
Hyponatremia
Hypokalemia/hyperkalemia
Hypocalcemia
Acidosis (respiratory or metabolic)
Uroperitoneum (with electrolyte abnormalities)
Renal failure

SEVERE ANEMIA
Neonatal isoerythrolysis
Blood loss

BRAIN DISEASE
Hemorrhage
Ischemia/edema/necrosis
Traumatic injury
Meningitis
Malformations
Narcolepsy-cataplexy syndrome (intermittent weakness)

SPINAL CORD DISEASE
Spinal cord hemorrhage
Vertebral malformation (e.g., atlantooccipital)
Vertebral abscessation or osteomyelitis
Vertebral fracture or other trauma to spinal cord

PERIPHERAL NERVE AND MUSCLE DISEASE
Botulism (foal)
White muscle disease
Tetanus
Congenital myopathy, polymyositis
Neuropathy of spinal roots or peripheral nerves
Aminoglycoside-induced neuromuscular blockade
Collagen disorder

LIVER DISEASE
Tyzzer's disease (2 weeks and older foal)
Toxin ingestion (iron fumarate, in foals)
Hepatitis
Severe hypoxic insult

ENDOCRINE ABNORMALITIES
Hypoadrenocorticism
Hypothyroidism

STORAGE DISORDERS
Maple syrup urine disease
Citrullinemia
Shaker calf syndrome (neurofilament accumulation)
GM-1 gangliosidosis

INGESTION OF DRUGS OR TOXINS
Transplacental transfer of anesthetics and sedatives
Inadvertent oversedation of neonate

GASTROINTESTINAL DISEASE
Gastrointestinal ulceration
Necrotizing enterocolitis

B, Bovine; *C,* caprine; *E,* equine; *O,* ovine.

livery, because many agents cross the placenta and can exert depressive and other adverse effects on the fetus. For example, one study reported that phenylbutazone administered to normal pregnant mares crossed the placenta and resulted in substantial concentrations of phenylbutazone and its active metabolite oxyphenbutazone. Although clinical signs of phenylbutazone toxicity were not noted in the foals post-

natally,[32] adverse effects are possible, particularly if other problems are present. Drug-induced neonatal depression is particularly important after cesarean section deliveries. Maternally administered anesthetics and analgesics can suppress respiration and heart rate in the newborn. In horses, both xylazine and detomidine cause maternal and fetal bradycardia and reduced cardiac output.[33,34] These effects will cause a reduction in placental perfusion and fetal oxygenation. If the newborn shows depression associated with maternal administration of these drugs, yohimbine can be given as an antagonist. Weakly basic drugs, when given to the mare, tend to concentrate in the fetus. Diazepam is an example of such a drug that crosses the placenta rapidly and accumulates in the fetal circulation resulting in lethargy, hypotonia, and hypothermia in the neonate after delivery. Flumazenil has been used to reverse the sedative effects of benzodiazepines. Maternal systemic illness of various types may also result in a weak newborn.

Starvation and hypothermia resulting from mismothering is a common cause of weakness in neonatal lambs. Similarly, weakness, poor body condition, and increased susceptibility to infectious diseases are observed with protein-calorie malnutrition induced by feeding poor quality or incorrectly mixed milk replacers.[35] Weakness associated with micronutrient deficiencies results from myodegeneration (white muscle disease, selenium, and vitamin E) or demyelination (copper, enzootic ataxia).

Many neonatal disorders are associated with severe electrolyte and metabolic derrangements. Weakness is a common clinical manifestation of hypoglycemia, metabolic acidosis, hyponatremia, hypernatremia, and hyperkalemia. Such abnormalities may occur before or at the time of birth, and laboratory assessment of the weak newborn is essential for accurate diagnosis. Profound weakness associated with metabolic acidosis is commonly observed in foals and calves with diarrhea and sporadically in kids ("floppy kid syndrome") and calves without other clinical signs of disease.[36,37] Correction of the acidosis by intravenous administration of bicarbonate produces a rapid recovery.

Several congenital bacterial, fungal, and viral infections that cause abortions and stillbirths may also result in the birth of a live, weak neonate. In cattle brucellosis, salmonellosis, leptospirosis, listeriosis, *Escherichia coli*, *Corynebacterium* spp., and *Aspergillus* spp. may cause placentitis and disease in the newborn. In sheep, in utero infection with chlamydia, campylobacter, coxiella, bluetongue virus, and border disease may cause disease in the newborn. Congenital viral infections of ruminants are listed in Box 15-3. Clinical manifestations of fetal infections depend on the age of the fetus and virulence and trophism of the infecting agent (see individual diseases).

Generally weakness secondary to uroperitoneum, renal, and liver failure, postnatally acquired infections, and neonatal isoerythrolysis is not expected to first appear during the first 24 hours of age. Rather, foals with neonatal isoerythrolysis usually present between 24 and 72 hours of age, foals with uroperitoneum at 2 to 5 days or older, and neonates with postnatally acquired infections most commonly at 2 to 5 days of age or older.

Nutritional myodegeneration associated with selenium and or vitamin E deficiencies may produce localized (dysphagia) or generalized paresis. Neonatal small ruminants appear to be particularly susceptible. Affected lambs may be unable to rise. Others can stand but may be unable to nurse because they are unable to raise their heads. Diagnosis is based on clinical signs, increased serum creatinine kinase concentration, and reduced whole blood glutathione peroxidase and or selenium concentrations (see Chapter 40). Vitamin E deficiency is observed when pregnant ewes are fed stored forage low in vitamin E. The clinical signs in affected lambs are identical to selenium deficiency but selenium status is adequate. Because vitamin E is labile, serum should be harvested quickly after blood collection, frozen, wrapped in aluminum foil, and sent via express courier on ice.

Paraplegia and tetraplegia are commonly associated with spinal cord compression. Compression of the spinal cord in neonates most commonly results from vertebral body malformations, osteomyelitis, or fractures. Generally, vertebral body malformations occur sporadically; genetic, nutritional, and environmental factors have been implicated.[38,39] In older calves, underlying metabolic bone disease (copper, vitamin D, or phosphorus deficiency) may increase the propensity for fractures to occurr. Osteomyelitis and vertebral body abscess may be a sequela to bacteremia after neonatal septicemia or pneumonia.[40] The frequent isolation of *Arcanobacterium pyogenes* from vertebral body abscesses in ruminants suggests that chronic respiratory infections is more frequently the source in these species.[41,42] Vertebral body abscesses in lambs are occasionally a sequela to infected docking wounds. *Rhodoccus equi* vertebral osteomyelitis with or without associated pulmonary infection has been reported in foals.[43,44] Leukocytosis and hyperfibringogenemia are commonly observed in neonates with vertebral body abscesses. In most instances, vertebral abscesses do not infiltrate the pachymeninges, so the cerebrospinal fluid (CSF) either is normal or has a mild elevation of protein and or a mild pleocytosis.[40,41]

Differential diagnoses for paresis in goat kids include caprine arthritis encephalitis virus (CAEV) and enzootic ataxia. Enzootic ataxia is also common in lambs. Progressive ataxia and paresis or paralysis is a feature of both diseases. There are two forms of enzootic ataxia (swayback): the neonatal type and the delayed type. In the neonatal condition, animals are affected at birth; in the delayed type signs of incoordination appear at 14 to 30 days of age.[45] Most affected kids are afebrile, bright and alert, and will continue to eat if it is physically possible. Enzootic ataxia is associated with low liver copper content and, occasionally, low serum copper concentration.[46] It has been proposed that reduction in the activity of the copper-dependent enzyme cytochrome oxidase impairs phospholipid synthesis and subsequently myelin production. Microcytic anemia and increased fragility of bones may be observed in more chronic cases.[47] The copper, molybdenum, and sulfur content of the maternal diet should be evaluated and adjustments made for copper deficiency or molybdenum or sulfur excess (see Chapter 30).

Goat kids with the neurologic form of CAEV will have mild to moderate fevers and evidence of cerebral involvement. Cerebral signs commonly identified include depression, head tilt, torticollis, and circling.[48] Evidence for CAEV would include CSF pleocytosis and increased CSF protein and a positive CAEV (AGID) or enzyme linked immunosorbent assay (ELISA) test. Both the neurologic form of CAEV and enzootic ataxia carry a poor prognosis.

A complete neurologic examination is an important component of the work-up of the weak neonate. In particular, it should be noted if the weakness is accompanied by signs of depression and diffuse cerebral disease. It should be remembered that strength is preserved if ataxia is caused by cerebellar disease. Limb reflexes should be tested to establish whether components of the spinal reflex pathways are involved in the disease process (sensory nerve, lower motor neuron, neuromuscular junction, muscle). For example, foals with severe spinal cord hemorrhage may have relatively normal mentation, but spinal reflexes may be greatly diminished and profound weakness may be present. Animals with other types of spinal cord disease (e.g., trauma, vertebral malformations, enzootic ataxia) may also show weakness and ataxia yet appear clinically to have normal cerebral function. Virtually any severe systemic disease such as generalized infection can cause both profound depression and weakness in a neonate without the presence of actual brain pathology. Intermittent signs of severe weakness and depression may be caused by the narcolepsy-cataplexy syndrome.

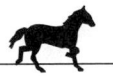

RESPIRATORY DISTRESS

WENDY E. VAALA
JOHN K. HOUSE

Diseases involving the respiratory system are common in the neonatal period, both as primary conditions and as conditions that occur secondary to other disease processes (Box 20-2). In many instances, abnormalities result from failure of the lungs to make a complete transition from a collapsed, fluid-filled organ to an air-filled structure responsible for sufficient gas exchange for the entire body. Even if the lungs are reasonably normal at birth, lung pathology often develops during the course of treatment for other neonatal diseases, most notably prematurity, birth asphyxia, neonatal maladjustment syndrome (foals), and septicemia. The onset of the pulmonary component of the disease, however, may be extremely insidious and therefore difficult to diagnose by physical examination alone. Signs of respiratory distress and hypoxemia are frequently vague, with some severely hypoxemic individuals showing only restlessness and considerable resistance and struggling when handled. Failure to make an early identification of pulmonary disease often results in an unfavorable outcome, with chronic, severe pneumonia resulting. Malformations, inflammation, or other abnormalities of the upper respiratory tract can cause clinical signs of respiratory distress, stridor, and dysphagia and result in lower respiratory tract problems as well. Several nonrespiratory conditions also cause clinical signs that mimic respiratory disease.

BOX 20-2

Causes of Respiratory Distress

AIRWAY OBSTRUCTION
Choanal atresia (nasopharyngeal atresia)
Laryngeal edema
Tracheal malformation: stenosis, collapse

DEVELOPMENTAL DISORDERS
Pulmonary hypoplasia
Diaphragmatic hernia

LUNG PARENCHYMAL DISEASES
Pneumonia (bacterial or viral)
Atelectasis
Hyaline membrane disease
Pulmonary edema, congestion
Aspiration syndromes
Air leaks (e.g., pneumothorax)
Pulmonary hemorrhage
Transient tachypnea syndromes

NONPULMONARY CAUSES
Congestive heart failure
Central nervous system lesions
Metabolic derangements (e.g., acidosis, hypoglycemia)
Severe anemia
Hypovolemia
Persistent pulmonary hypertension
Birth asphyxia
Pain, abdominal crisis
Fever, high environmental temperatures
Excitement
Pleural effusion (e.g., pleuritis)
Endotoxemia/gram-negative sepsis

APPROACH TO DIAGNOSIS OF RESPIRATORY DYSFUNCTION

Physical Examination of the Respiratory System

Assessment of the pattern and effort of breathing is an important part of the examination of the respiratory system. Any obvious abnormal noises associated with respiration should be noted. Absence of cyanosis is not a reliable indicator of adequacy of oxygenation in the neonate, because the partial pressure of oxygen may reach very low levels (<35 to 40 mm Hg) before cyanosis is observed. Fever, cough, and nasal discharge are usually absent in the early stages of pneumonia in the neonate. Pulmonary complications are common with prematurity, sepsis, and asphyxial injury. Careful assessment of the respiratory system should take place early in the disease course, and the animal should be monitored closely for worsening respiratory function.

Thoracic Radiology

Thoracic radiographs are often helpful in diagnosing the presence of respiratory disease and in determining the type and extent of pulmonary involvement. In human neonatology, thoracic radiographs have been useful in identifying certain diseases with characteristic radiographic appearances, including hyaline membrane disease and meconium aspiration. In large animal neonatology, interpretation has not yet advanced to that point. Unfortunately there are large voids in our knowledge of normal thoracic radiographic appearance at different gestational and postnatal ages, and it is difficult to distinguish lung "immaturity" from disease.

Shortly after birth the smaller vessels posterior to the heart and in the caudodorsal lung fields should be clear. The heart, posterior vena cava, and aorta should be clearly defined. When the radiographic appearance of the lung fields is evaluated, the type of infiltrate (interstitial, nodular, alveolar, mixed), severity, and location (diffuse, cranioventral, caudodorsal) should be noted. Other soft tissue structures (including the heart, vessels, and diaphragm) and bones (ribs, vertebrae, long bones) should also be evaluated. Thoracic radiographs are routinely taken only in the standing or recumbent lateral position in foals, with dorsoventral positioning reserved for the anesthetized or very depressed foal. Thus interpretation can be limited because of positioning limitations. If the neonate has been in lateral recumbency for extended periods, atelectasis may result in diffuse or localized interstitial infiltrates that usually resolve once lung reexpansion occurs. It can be difficult to accurately distinguish bacterial pneumonia from atelectasis and pulmonary edema on the basis of radiographic appearance alone. In these cases, additional diagnostic aids (cultures, hematology, necropsy) should be used in conjunction with radiology to reach an accurate diagnosis.

Serial chest radiographs are useful in monitoring the progress of a respiratory condition. Radiographic changes may either follow or precede changes in clinical condition, and sometimes major changes can occur surprisingly rapidly (Fig. 20-2). Clinical signs of pneumonia frequently resolve much earlier than chest radiographs and hemograms return to normal.

With the use of rare earth screens, thoracic radiology of the foal and calf is feasible using a portable x-ray machine in the field. The major disadvantage of the use of portable x-ray equipment is that motion is often present, particularly when the respiratory rate is high, and there is a tendency to overread such films. Alternatively, most small animal x-ray units are capable of taking good-quality chest films if the patient can be transported to such a facility.

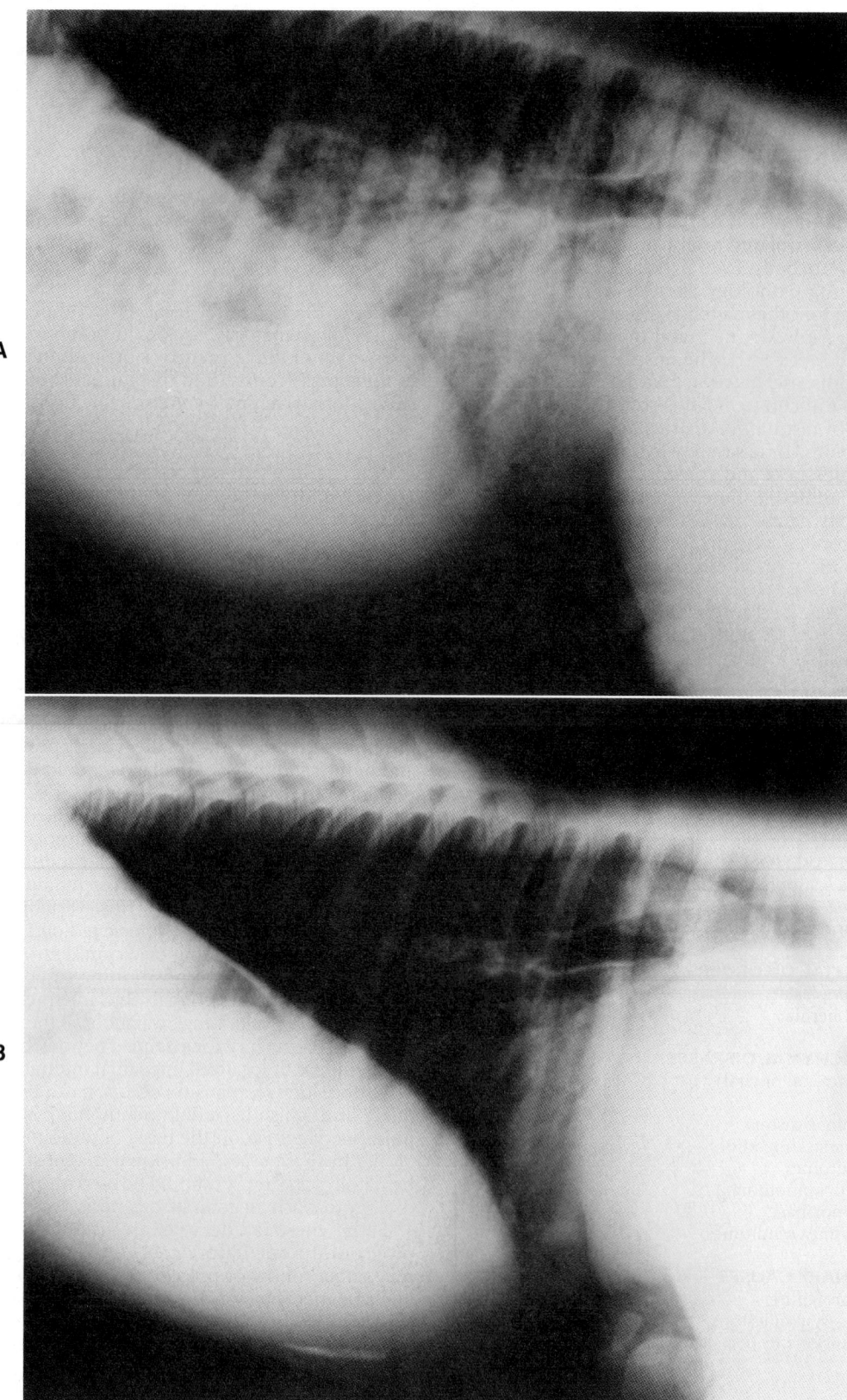

FIG. 20-2 ▓ **A,** Standing lateral chest radiograph of a 7-day-old Thoroughbred filly with severe angular limb deformities that experienced an acute onset of severe respiratory distress and cyanosis after a walk outside the stall. Entubation and 100% oxygen administration only raised the Pao₂ to 48 mm Hg. Severe pulmonary interstitial disease is present in the caudoventral lung fields, and the tentative diagnosis was bacterial pneumonia. Modifications were not made in the treatment regimen (the same antibiotics being given for a wound were continued), and over the next 24 hours the filly clinically improved. **B,** Repeat radiographs taken 3 days after the first ones revealed marked resolution of the infiltrates. The diagnosis remains open, but pulmonary edema was suspected.

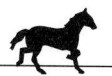

Thoracic Ultrasonography

Ultrasonographic evaluation of the foal's thorax can yield useful information in a variety of disease processes, including pleural effusion, such as hemothorax or pleuritis, bronchopneumonia, or abscessation. It is also the preferred method for diagnosing congenital heart disease, and thus is often a useful technique to differentiate cardiac and pulmonary causes of hypoxemia.[49]

Arterial Blood Gas Analysis

Arterial blood gases can be obtained by direct puncture from several different sites from foals, including the great metatarsal, brachial, femoral, facial, and carotid arteries (listed in order of preference). If pulse quality is reasonable, the great metatarsal is preferred for repeated sampling because of its location and the lack of a major vein in close proximity. The sample is usually collected while the patient is restrained in sternal or lateral recumbency. A small bleb of local anesthetic (2% lidocaine, without epinephrine) can greatly facilitate proper collection and minimize needless struggling and subsequent hyperventilation. A small-gauge needle (No. 25, $5/8$ inch) attached to a 1- or 3-ml syringe with the hub filled with heparin is used for arterial sampling. Any air bubbles are removed promptly, and the syringe is sealed with a cork and placed in ice slush until analysis is performed. After removal of the needle, direct pressure is placed on the artery for 1 to 2 minutes to minimize hematoma formation and preserve the artery for future sampling. A sealed blood gas sample may be stored on ice for 6 hours without major changes in PaO_2. The optimal site for collection of arterial blood samples from neonatal calves is the brachial artery.[50] The calf is placed in lateral recumbency, with one hand on the neck and the other pulling the upper leg caudally. The brachial artery is located on the proximomedial aspect of the elbow of the lower limb. The area over the artery is thoroughly scrubbed and the artery stabilized by placing the index and second finger of one hand above and below the proposed site of puncture. The arterial blood sample is collected using a 25- or 27-gauge, $3/4$-inch needle and a 3-ml syringe.[50]

Problems caused by poor patient compliance and vessel trauma after multiple punctures can be serious limitations to adequate blood gas monitoring. If proper technique is used, however, most arteries can be maintained for many days of frequent sampling. Alternatively, percutaneous placement of an indwelling arterial catheter is not difficult, but maintenance of catheter position and patency can be frustrating. An umbilical arterial catheter may also be placed in known high-risk cases if the birth is attended; the advantages of continuous access to arterial blood must be weighed against the possible disadvantages, including infection and hemorrhage.

Normal arterial blood gas values for neonates of different postnatal and gestational ages are presented in Table 20-2. Several factors can interfere with accurate interpretation of blood gases in the neonate. First, significant inaccuracies can occur if the blood sample is collected, handled, or measured improperly. The most common artifact is the introduction of room air into the sample, with an artificially increased PaO_2, decreased $PaCO_2$, and more alkaline pH resulting. Excessive struggling during sampling may cause transient changes in all blood gas values. The position of the foal when the sample is taken influences interpretation. In both premature and term foals, repositioning from upright (standing or sternal) to lateral recumbency quickly results in a significant decrease in PaO_2.[51-53] The mean decrease in PaO_2 when normal, term neonatal foals were placed in lateral recumbency was 14 mm Hg (95 mm Hg while standing to 80.5 mm Hg in lateral position). In premature foals or foals with significant pulmonary disease, the difference may be much greater.[51] This finding obviously also has important treatment ramifications as well (see Treatment, below). The inspired oxygen concentration must also be considered when analyzing arterial blood gas values. With supplemental oxygen, PaO_2 is increased variably, depending on the inspired oxygen concentration (FIO_2), the amount of pathology present, particularly the extent of right-to-left shunting, and the respiratory rate and tidal volume of the foal, if the oxygen is delivered by nasal insufflation. A flow rate of 10 L/min, delivered by nasal insufflation, increased the PaO_2 to 298 ± 69 mm Hg in the normal, term newborn foal[54]; this flow rate was thought to approximate an FIO_2 of 1.0.[55] In the induced premature foal,

TABLE 20-2

Blood Gas Normals

Age-group	Arterial					Venous			
	O_2 (mm Hg)	CO_2 (mm Hg)	pH	Base Excess	HCO_3^- (mEq/L)	O_2 (mm Hg)	CO_2 (mm Hg)	pH	HCO_3^- (mEq/L)
EQUINE NEONATES (LATERAL RECUMBENCY)									
Immediate post-foaling[39]	40-50	52-60	7.2-7.3	+2	24-26	—	—	—	—
2 hours[40]	68±10	49±2	7.37±0.01	+4	26±2	42±2	56±2	7.33±0.01	28±2
4-12 hours[40]	75±5	47±2	7.39±0.01	+6	28±2	42±2	52±2	7.38±0.01	30±2
24 hours[40]	81±6	48±2	7.4±0.01	+6	28±2	42±2	52±2	7.38±0.01	30±3
1-3 days[40]	90±6	48±2	7.4±0.01	+6	28±2	43±2	52±2	7.38±0.01	29±2
4-14 days[40]	86±5	45±2	7.41±0.01	+6	28±1	38±2	53±2	7.38±0.01	31±2
Premature[39] birth	39±5	55±4	7.27	−3	24±1	—	—	—	—
(320-330 days' gestation)—1 hour	52±4	48±3	7.33	−1.3	25±1	—	—	—	—
CALVES									
1 hour	58.43±11.61	50.40±5.27	7.30±0.05		23.52±2.78				
4 hours	62.3±9.27	47.92±3.97	7.34±0.03		24.49±2.35				
12 hours	67.23±9.32	45.36±3.97	7.38±0.03		25.74±2.37				
24 hours	70.53±11.47	44.04±3.45	7.40±0.03		26.44±1.87				
48 hours	63.85±10.82	45.25±3.69	7.42±0.01		27.98±1.91				

the PaO_2 increased only to 111 ± 35 mm Hg.[54] If the respiratory rate of a foal is rapid and shallow, the supplemental oxygen will be "diluted" by room air because of the large quantity of room air entering the upper respiratory tract, and the concentration of alveolar oxygen will probably be much less than 100%.

If an abnormality is detected on blood gas analysis, one of two patterns of derangement is usually encountered: hypoxemia (PaO_2 <70 mm Hg) with low or normal $PaCO_2$ and hypoxemia with hypercapnia ($PaCO_2$ >50 mm Hg). If there is hypercapnia and resulting respiratory acidosis, hypoventilation is diagnosed. In the neonate, hypoventilation may occur for several reasons. One of the most common is the inability of the animal's respiratory muscles to work hard enough to adequately ventilate the abnormal lung. In animals with neurologic dysfunction, chemosensitivity also may be altered, resulting in inappropriate ventilatory responses to changes in blood gas values. In foals with botulism and other neuromuscular diseases, hypoventilation occurs primarily because the respiratory muscles become too weak to adequately ventilate relatively normal lungs. Clinical signs must be evaluated along with blood gas analysis, in order to choose the most appropriate therapy. Certain hypoxic or hypercapnic neonates do not display signs of respiratory distress, whereas others with similar or worse blood gas pictures are markedly distressed. The reasons for these discrepancies may include the rapidity of the development of the problem, developmental or pathologic variation in chemoreceptor function, and the type of lung pathology present.

Venous Blood Gas Analysis

Interpretation of blood gas values of venous blood (see Table 20-2) can be deceptive and should be restricted to evaluation of metabolic conditions (e.g., metabolic acidosis) and not pulmonary gas exchange. To avoid problems associated with regional blood sampling, peripheral venous blood should be taken from a free-flowing jugular vein, because the metabolic status of the head is usually stable. To obtain a sample representative of the whole body, mixed venous blood is drawn from the right atrium. Determination of mixed venous blood oxygen saturation is a good test for assessing the overall adequacy of oxygen delivery to tissues because it reflects the balance between oxygen delivery and oxygen use.

SPECIFIC RESPIRATORY CONDITIONS

Upper Respiratory Tract Disorders

Upper respiratory tract disorders are relatively uncommon in neonates. Conditions affecting pharyngeal and laryngeal function are important because they predispose to aspiration pneumonia. Dyspneic neonates also have difficulty nursing and are subsequently likely to become malnourished. Congenital defects of the upper respiratory tract include collapsed trachea, stenotic nares, choanal atresia, epiglottal cyst, and guttural pouch tympany (foal). There have also been recent reports of dorsal displacement of the soft palate as a cause of acute dyspnea, stridor, and dysphagia in neonatal foals.[56,57] Endoscopic examination of the upper airways of these foals revealed that the dorsally displaced soft palate was edematous, flaccid, and redundant. To varying degrees, flaccidity and swelling of other pharyngeal and laryngeal structures (e.g., arytenoid cartilages, epiglottis, or palatopharyngeal arch) were also noted.[57] Both medical[57] and surgical[56] treatment of the condition have been suggested. In one study, medical management with antiinflammatory drugs, enteral feeding via nasogastric tube, and broad-spectrum antibiotics (for the coexisting aspiration pneumonia) resulted in dramatic and permanent resolution of the problems within 2 to 4 days. The cause of these abnormalities remains unknown at this time, but may involve primary pharyngeal and palatal muscular laxity.[57]

Impaired pharyngeal and laryngeal function may result from physical deformation or neuromuscular disorders. Sporadic outbreaks of pharyngeal and laryngeal injuries are often associated with improper application or use of damaged feeding tubes and oral medication equipment. Compression of the larynx by a retropharyngeal abscess or mass tends to cause inspiratory dyspnea. Edema and necrosis of the larynx may be observed with infectious bovine rhinotracheitis virus infections in neonatal calves; aspiration pneumonia is a common sequela.[58,59] *Fusobacterium necophorum* typically causes necrotic laryngitis in weaned calves but sporadically infects neonates following pharyngeal trauma.[60] Partial occlusion of the upper airway induces turbulent airflow and subsequently mucosal edema. Placement of a tracheostomy tube provides an alternative, sometimes lifesaving, airway and rests the inflamed mucosa.

Nutritional myodegeneration, hyperkalemic periodic paralysis, and botulism may induce laryngeal paresis. Dysphagia and subsequent aspiration pneumonia is a common sequelae of pharyngeal and laryngeal dysfunction associated with nutritional myodegeneration and botulism. Exercise- and excitement-induced respiratory stridor has been described in foals with hyperkalemic periodic paralysis.[61]

Collapsed trachea is a rare congenital or acquired condition. Clinical signs include an intermittent honking cough, stridor, and dyspnea with mild exercise. There is no stenosis of the trachea; rather there is a dynamic dorsoventral collapse during inspiration. The caudal cervical and cranial thoracic sections of the trachea in the area of the thoracic inlet are most frequently affected. Acquired tracheal collapse is commonly associated with fractured ribs and compression of the trachea at the thoracic inlet by the subsequent bony callus. Treatment of collapsed trachea in the calf by surgical reconstruction has been attempted but the prognosis is poor.[62-65]

Diagnosis of most upper airway disorders can usually be made with a combination of radiography and endoscopy. A 7-mm outside diameter (OD) endoscope is usually small enough to pass through the ventral meatus of horse and pony foals weighing over 30 lb. An integral part of the diagnostic approach to the neonate with suspected upper airway obstruction is assessment of the lungs for aspiration pneumonia. If the primary upper respiratory problem is not corrected and normal nursing is allowed, the pneumonic process will likely persist and become chronic.

Respiratory Infection

Neonatal respiratory infection in large animals most commonly takes the form of pneumonia. In most cases, pneumonia is part of a generalized septicemia caused by opportunistic pathogens infecting an immunologically compromised host. Contagious respiratory pathogens commonly affect young stock greater than 4 weeks of age, but neonates may be affected in disease outbreaks. Bovine respiratory syncytial virus, infectious bovine rhinotracheitis virus, bovine virus diarrhea virus, *Mycoplasma* spp., and bovine coronavirus may all produce respiratory disease in neonatal calves. In the horse, fetal equine herpesvirus 1 infection may cause bronchopneumonia and result in an aborted fetus or in a live, but weak, foal. Viral infections increase the risk of opportunistic bacterial infections by their immunosuppressive effects and damage to the respiratory epithelium and pulmonary clearance mechanisms. Pleuritis is an uncommon feature of most neonatal respiratory infections but may be a manifestation of a generalized polyserositis with specific pathogens such as my-

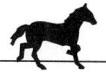

coplasma infections of ruminant neonates[66] and occassionaly pasteurella infections in lambs.[67]

FACTORS PREDISPOSING TO NEONATAL PNEUMONIA. Immaturity of the immune system, environmental stress, and exposure to pathogens predispose the neonate to respiratory infections. Little has been reported on the developmental anatomy of the foal and calf lung. In human infants an immature ciliary apparatus leads to inefficient removal of bacteria and inflammatory debris. Many neonatal mammalian species have a much lower number of alveolar macrophages than the adult,[68] and bacterial clearance is probably considerably reduced. Several studies have shown that complement values in newborn calves are less than 50% of the values in adult cows, with levels decreasing to even lower values the day after birth, possibly as a result of an increase in plasma volume.[69] Complement plays an important role in primary host defense against invading organisms. If colostrum intake is insufficient and IgG levels are low, not only is the neonate deprived of specific antibody protection, but neutrophil function, as measured by the chemiluminescence assay, is also seriously impaired.[70]

Environmental risk factors include extremes of temperature, poor ventilation, dust, ammonia, and overcrowding. Poor cleaning practices that promote aerosolization may effectively disperse pathogens in the environment.

Neonatal respiratory pathogens may be acquired in utero, during the birth process, or from contaminated milk, the environment, or other affected animals. In utero acquired bacterial infections are not uncommon in the foal, and pneumonia is the most common manifestation of the disease process. In human infants, pneumonia may result from aspiration of pharyngeal secretions and seems to occur more commonly in infants born after difficult deliveries.[71] Although the fetus may be infected by hematogenous transmission of bacteria across the placenta, it appears that ascending infection of the placenta occurs more frequently, with aspiration of infected amniotic fluid being the most common route of infection. During delivery the fetus becomes colonized by bacteria living in the vagina, and after delivery is exposed to a variety of bacteria living on and around the dam. Initial bacterial colonization of the neonate probably occurs on the skin and mucosal surfaces, including the nasopharynx. Although bacteria may proliferate at these sites, they rarely cause disease unless other predisposing factors are present. The respiratory system may serve as the primary portal of entry of bacteria into the body, or it may be infected secondarily as a resulted of septicemia and hematogenous spread of bacteria. Bacteria that cause pneumonia are essentially the same as those listed in the section on generalized infections (see Chapter 19). Early in life, localizing clinical signs of respiratory infection may be absent, even in the presence of extensive disease, with weakness and depression the only abnormal physical examination findings.

Pathogens shed in milk that have a trophism for the respiratory system include *Mycoplasma* spp.,[66,72,73] caprine arthritis encephalitis virus,[74,75] and *Salmonella dublin*. The practice of feeding mastitic milk (hospital milk) to neonates increases the risk of disease transmission. Rapid growth of salmonella in warm milk quickly produces a lethal challenge. *S. dublin* is an invasive salmonella serotype host adapted to cattle. Calves commonly become septicemic; however, respiratory disease may be the predominant clinical manifestation. *Mycoplasma* spp. infection typically produces an acute polyserositis; goat kids infected with *Mycoplasma mycoides* subspecies *mycoides* (large colony type) are often in pain, febrile, and reluctant to stand and have multiple hot swollen joints. Approximately 50% of kids develop pneumonia or pleuropneumonia manifested by an increase in respiratory rate and auscultable lung sounds.[66] Pasteurizing goat's milk at 56° C for 1 hour kills

Mycoplasma spp. and caprine arthritis encephalitis virus. Mycoplasma arthritis and pneumonia has also been reported in neonatal calves infected with *Mycoplasma* spp.[72] Caprine arthritis encephalitis virus produces several disease syndromes including mastitis, arthritis, encephalitis, and pneumonia. Encephalitis and subclinical respiratory disease typically occurrs in kids 2 to 4 months of age and occassionally in kids as young as 1 month of age.[74,76]

Environmental contamination increases exponentially during the course of infectious disease outbreaks because of the large number of organisms shed during clinical disease. Isolation of affected animals, disinfection of the environment and equipment, segregation of age-groups, and separate management of neonates helps to reduce the potential for disease transmission. In the hospital setting, nosocomial infections may be introduced by exposure to contaminated equipment such as endotracheal tubes and humidifiers.

CLINICAL ASSESSMENT AND LABORATORY EVALUATION. Microbiologic cultures are important in confirming the diagnosis of pneumonia. With in utero–acquired infections in foals, blood cultures are frequently negative. In these individuals, cultures and cytology (including Gram stain) of tracheal secretions (obtained through placement of a nasotracheal tube or transtracheal aspiration), gastric aspirate, pharynx (if newborn), or urine should be performed, in addition to blood cultures. If pneumonia is acquired postnatally, blood cultures have been helpful in identifying the pathogen. Transtracheal aspiration provides a sample for both cytologic and microbiologic analysis (see Chapter 29 for specific details on technique and interpretation). If the neonate is in respiratory distress, this technique can be a difficult and dangerous procedure. Alternatively, a guarded brush catheter can be passed into the trachea through a nasotracheal tube and a sample of tracheal secretions can be obtained. Most studies in humans have employed quantitative methods to identify bacterial pathogens, usually using a finding of $>10^3$ colony-forming units (CFU)/ml to distinguish infection from colonization.[77] An advantage of this method is that an airway is available for resuscitation if the animal is compromised by the stress of the procedure. When mycoplasma or chlamydia infection is suspected the laboratory must be notified because specific media and growth conditions are required to isolate these pathogens.

Viral infections are diagnosed directly by viral isolation (cell culture) or indirectly by demonstrating the presence of a virus (polymerase chain reaction and fluorescent antibody techniques) or an immunologic response to a virus (seroconversion). Specific tests available for specific respiratory viral pathogens are discussed in Chapter 29.

TREATMENT. Antibiotic therapy is an important part of the medical treatment of pneumonia. Pending culture results, broad-spectrum antibiotic therapy should be instituted. Ampicillin or penicillin and gentamicin is a reasonable initial empiric treatment for foals and ceftiofur for calves. In a hospital setting, with the documentation of a resident population of resistant bacteria, a combination of ampicillin and amikacin or cefotaxime may be a better choice. The third-generation cephalosporins present certain advantages over aminoglycosides in the treatment of neonatal pneumonia. They have been found to have good penetration into lung tissue; the concentrations achieved greatly exceed the concentrations needed to kill susceptible bacteria.[77] Aminoglycosides penetrate lung tissue in amounts equal to 10% to 45% of serum levels,[78] but in the acidic environment of infected airways the activity of these drugs is markedly reduced, and levels attained may not be sufficient to kill the offending bacteria.[79] One major disadvantage of the routine use of the third-generation cephalosporins seems to be the rapid induction of resistance in a hospital setting.[80]

Because premature discontinuation of antibiotic therapy resulted in relapse in some cases, repeat radiographs and hematology (complete blood cell count and plasma fibrinogen) are highly recommended before discontinuation of antibiotic therapy. A course of therapy of 3 to 4 weeks' duration is not unusual in cases of severe pneumonia. Premature foals with pneumonia should be monitored particularly closely for the development of bacterial pneumonia resistant to the antibiotics being used or for noninfectious chronic respiratory disease such as has been described in humans and foals as bronchopulmonary dysplasia (BPD).[81]

If failure of passive transfer is present, the patient is routinely treated with plasma (see Chapter 49). Respiratory supportive care is an extremely important part of the treatment of pneumonia. Maintenance in a sternal position or at least frequent turning from side to side, routine coupage, and good airway hygiene, including suction if indicated, are important routine procedures. Physical examination findings combined with blood gas results determine the need for oxygen or other more aggressive ventilatory support.

Lung Maturity and the Surfactant System

PATHOPHYSIOLOGY. Surfactant, a mixture of phospholipids (primarily dipalmitoyl phosphatidylcholine and phosphatidylglcerol and proteins), is produced and stored in the type II alveolar pneumocytes of the mammalian lung. It is an extremely effective surfactant mixture and under dynamic compression is capable of lowering surface tension dramatically. In 1959, Avery and Mead[82] reported that saline extracts of lung removed from premature babies dying of respiratory distress syndrome (RDS) lacked the capacity to effectively reduce surface tension. They suggested that RDS was caused by either the absence or the delayed appearance of pulmonary surfactant caused by an immaturity of the type II alveolar epithelial cells. Since that time a great deal has been published regarding the biochemical and physiologic aspects of the fetal and newborn surfactant systems.

Maturation of the lung involves not only maturation of the surfactant system but also thinning of the alveolar capillary barrier, a decrease in alveolar epithelial permeability, and maturation of the chest wall. Although lack of surfactant is an important factor in the initiation of RDS, a highly compliant chest wall, altered permeability characteristics of the lung, and the type of perinatal treatment also play important roles in its expression. The structural immaturity of the lung and chest wall of the premature neonate decreases lung compliance and allows a low end-expiratory lung volume. This predisposes to airway collapse and necessitates high pressures to reopen closed airways, thus increasing the work of breathing. Permeability characteristics of the lung may be directly influenced by the fluid balance of the patient, cardiovascular function, presence of a patent ductus arteriosus, degree of pulmonary hypertension, and extent of ischemic injury present. An increase in permeability of the alveoli allows protein exudation into air-spaces. Hyaline membranes, aggregates of proteinaceous material and cellular debris, disrupt alveolar architecture and the gas-exchange surfaces.[83]

Surfactant system dysfunction may occur as a result of primary deficiency (as in RDS of premature infants) or secondary deficiency. Several other conditions are known to interfere with the activity of surfactant, including asphyxia, acidosis, hypercarbia, pulmonary edema with protein leak into the alveoli, sepsis, shock, hypoperfusion, prolonged atelectasis, and overinflation.[84]

Hyaline membrane formation and atelectasis are not pathognomonic for primary surfactant deficiency; they have been observed in human neonates in which the presence of surfactant is documented.[85] In human infants, pulmonary infection with group B *Streptococcus* in term infants can cause a syndrome clinically, radiographically, and pathologically similar to hyaline membrane disease.[86] A similar syndrome has been described in a foal with *Streptococcus pneumoniae* type 3.[87]

Clinical Syndromes of Hyaline Membrane Disease: An Overview

Hyaline membrane disease (HMD) or RDS has been reported in the premature human infant and in the premature lamb, pig, calf, and foal. RDS has been defined as progressive respiratory failure in a premature infant caused by inadequate surfactant function superimposed on a structurally immature lung.[83] It should not be confused with the generic term *respiratory distress*, which simply describes the clinical signs of increased respiratory effort or rate.

TYPICAL CLINICAL COURSE (HUMAN). After birth the infant may have little or mild evidence of respiratory distress, but over the next 24 to 48 hours increasingly severe respiratory distress is noted, followed by a plateauing of clinical signs. This period is then followed by rapid improvement over the next few days.

DIAGNOSIS. Diagnosis is based on a characteristic clinical course, negative blood cultures, and a typical diffuse, ground-glass radiographic appearance, with air bronchograms.

PREVENTION. One of the best ways to prevent RDS is to prevent premature births, but this can be difficult to do, particularly in the veterinary patient. Birth asphyxia can markedly worsen the clinical course of RDS in the premature individual, so conditions of labor and delivery should be optimized. While investigating corticosteroid induction of parturition in the sheep, Liggins[88] found that lambs that had been infused with steroids or ACTH in utero were viable and showed alveolar stability at 118 to 123 days' gestation, whereas previous studies had indicated that RDS normally developed in lambs less than 125 days' gestation at delivery. Because of these studies and further work in sheep, which showed that the appearance of surfactant was accelerated in lungs of cortisol-treated fetal lambs,[88] maternally administered steroids were administered to human pregnancies to enhance fetal lung maturation. Since these discoveries, the use of steroids for this purpose is widespread in human medicine. Better results have been observed in female infants than in male infants whose mothers received steroids. The use of steroids is usually avoided if amnionitis is present and if birth is likely to take place in less than 24 hours.

TREATMENT. Treatment of RDS has traditionally been directed at trying to prevent lung atelectasis and to maintain an adequate end-expiratory lung volume and gas exchange. This usually involves some combination of oxygen therapy, continuous positive airway pressure, and mechanical ventilation, depending on the severity of the condition. Common complications associated with therapy of RDS in the human infant include air leaks resulting in pneumothorax and chronic pulmonary disease (e.g., bronchopulmonary dsyplasia).

In the past 5 years, surfactant replacement therapy using both natural and surfactant products has become an integral part of the therapy of RDS in premature human infants. In large multicenter, double-blind studies, both commercially available products* have been clearly shown to improve survival, decrease the requirements for ventilatory support, and reduce the incidence of pneumothorax.[89,90]

RDS IN THE FOAL. The results from one study of surfactant in the foal[91] based on limited numbers (at 300 days, n = 1) suggest that maturation of surfactant occurs quite late in ges-

---

*Survanta, Abbott Laboratories, and Exosurf, Burroughs-Wellcome.

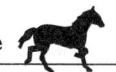

tation, at or after 300 days (88% of gestation). This compares with full development in the sheep at around 90% of gestation and 75% to 80% in human infants. The information concerning the foal should be considered preliminary pending further investigations.

Primary surfactant deficiency as a cause of respiratory distress has not been well documented in the foal. The only report of respiratory disease accompanied by low surfactant levels concerned a full-term foal that was normal at birth but showed signs of central nervous system derangement at 32 hours of age. Pathologic findings included atelectasis and edema, with no true hyaline membrane formation, but with a decrease in lung lining film.[92] Respiratory distress in foals has been associated with neonatal asphyxia, hypovolemia, prematurity, dysmaturity, and bronchial obstructions,[93] but little effort has been made to correlate these conditions with surfactant quantity or function. Analysis of L/S ratios and phosphatidylglycerol levels in equine amniotic fluid of normal term and premature foals that showed subsequent signs of respiratory distress have yielded conflicting results.[94] Some premature and term foals undergoing intensive care, many of which were victims of complicated deliveries (e.g., cesarean section, early induction of labor), have displayed signs, such as progression of respiratory distress over the first 24 to 48 hours, diffuse interstitial infiltrate on radiographs, and diffuse atelectasis on postmortem examination, that were suggestive of RDS. However, air bronchograms were rarely observed radiographically (rather, interstitial pattern only), hyaline membrane formation was rarely observed on postmortem examination (rather, atelectasis with or without inflammatory cell infiltrate), and the outcome was usually poor, with progressive neurologic and cardiovascular deterioration, in spite of mechanical ventilation and intensive care. Unfortunately, surfactant measurements were not made in any of these cases. Additional studies are clearly indicated to clarify the importance of surfactant deficiency in syndromes of respiratory distress in both premature and term foals.

RDS IN THE CALF. Several reports have documented RDS in the calf. In one study 35 calves were delivered by cesarean section near term (range of 247 to 284 days), lecithin/sphingomyelin (L/S) ratios were measured in calves with and without evidence of respiratory distress, and the lungs of calves that died were examined histologically.[95] Of the 35 calves, 20 developed signs of respiratory dysfunction within the first hours after birth. In the normal calves, there were no deaths, and the L/S ratio was 2.6; whereas, in the calves showing signs of respiratory disease, 11 died, and the L/S ratio was 1.5, statistically lower than in the normal individuals. Only 2 calves with an L/S ratio greater than 2 developed respiratory distress, whereas 18 of 19 calves with a ratio less than 2 developed respiratory disorders during the first hour of life. However, there was a fairly poor correlation between gestational age and L/S ratio. The most striking findings on postmortem examination were pulmonary lesions (hyaline membranes, interstitial and alveolar edema) and intracranial hemorrhages. Thus RDS in the calf seems to be similar to that in the human infant.

RDS IN THE PIG. All piglets affected by "barker" syndrome or HMD were sired by the same boar, and analysis of the breeding data suggests that the condition was inherited. The three major features of these "barker" piglets were abnormally immature lungs with hyaline membranes, a deficiency of surfactant in lung washings, and abnormally small thyroid glands accompanied by clinical signs of hypothyroidism. The relationship between the abnormalities in the thyroid glands and pulmonary immaturity in these piglets remains unknown.[96-97]

Meconium Aspiration Syndrome

In utero asphyxia or umbilical cord occlusion can result in fetal passage of meconium into amniotic fluid. Hypoxia induces a redistribution of blood flow away from less vital organs including the gastrointestinal tract resulting in mesenteric vasoconstriction and secondary intestinal ischemia. Transient hyperperistalsis and anal sphincter relaxation occur, thereby allowing passage of meconium. Meconium aspiration may occur before, during, or immediately after delivery as a result of fetal gasping. Meconium can produce a variety of clinical signs including mechanical airway obstruction (ball-valve effect) and regional air trapping, chemical pneumonitis and alveolitis, alveolar edema, and displacement of surfactant by free fatty acids in meconium leading to decreased lung compliance, small airway obstruction and focal atelectasis.[98-101] These events lead to increased pulmonary vascular and airway resistance and ventilation/perfusion mismatching. Meconium may also enhance the growth of bacterial species within the respiratory tract, resulting in secondary bacterial pneumonia. It may be difficult to differentiate meconium aspiration from bacterial pneumonia, especially if the birth was unattended. Occasionally, chronic placentitis is associated with both bacterial pneumonia and meconium aspiration.

If meconium has been aspirated into the pharynx, gentle suctioning of the nasal and oral cavities is recommended. The ideal time to suction the airways is while the animal is still in the birth canal, before it has taken its first breath. If the foal shows signs of meconium aspiration below the vocal cords, nasotracheal intubation and careful, aseptic suctioning are recommended. Intranasal oxygen should be administered during suctioning. Arterial blood gas analysis dictates what long-term respiratory and metabolic support is necessary. Mild to moderate hypoxemia van be treated with humidified intranasal oxygen (2 to 10 L/min). Severe hypoxemia with accompanying hypercapnea requires positive pressure ventilation (PPV) and is associated with increased mortality. If surfactant displacement and secondary atelectasis is contributing to hypoxemia, continuous positive-airway pressure (CPAP) alone may improve oxygenation while avoiding any unnecessary increase in peak airway pressure. Exogenous surfactant administration has been advocated to treat the surfactant dysfunction. Intravenous dimethyl sulfoxide (DMSO) (0.5 to 1.0 g/kg) administered as a 10% solution may help reduce alveolar and interstitial edema. Systemic antibiotic therapy is recommended to prevent secondary bacterial pneumonia. Good airway hygiene and coupage are crucial.

A diagnosis of meconium aspiration is based on a history of meconium-contaminated amniotic fluid and a meconium-stained newborn. Radiographs typically show a ventrocranial distribution of pulmonary infiltrate characteristic of aspiration. Clear, brownish fluid may drip from the nose.

Pneumothorax and Hemothorax

Pneumothorax[102] is usually an iatrogenic sequela of positive-pressure ventilation of diseased lungs, but it may occur spontaneously or as a result of birth trauma. During mechanical ventilation, uneven alveolar ventilation leads to alveolar rupture and dissection of air into the interstitium. The air moves along bronchioles and other lung structures to pleural surfaces, forming blebs. This air may rupture into the pleural space.

Pneumothorax should be suspected if the respiratory condition suddenly worsens while an animal is being ventilated (decreased PaO_2, increased peak inspiratory airway pressure).

Clinical signs may include respiratory distress, shift of cardiac point of maximum intensity, cyanosis, and hypotension. Although auscultation may reveal decreased breath sounds, it may be misleading because of the wide referral of breath sounds. Percussion is usually fairly unremarkable, unless the condition is severe. Radiographs are indicated to confirm the diagnosis, but, if radiology is unavailable or the animal is distressed, a direct needle aspirate is diagnostic and therapeutic.

Pneumothorax may be treated conservatively if no distress is associated with the air leak and the condition appears stable. Stress should be minimized. Chest tube insertion is indicated in human infants with continuing air leak, if underlying pulmonary disease is causing respiratory distress, and in those patients receiving mechanical ventilation. A trocar catheter is sterilely introduced into the chest cavity, and the catheter is secured, with the suture material crisscrossed tightly around the catheter. Suction is applied at -15 cm H_2O after confirmation of chest tube position by chest radiograph. Suction is discontinued when the tube has drained no air for 24 to 48 hours and when extrapulmonary air has been resolved radiographically for 24 to 48 hours. The tube may then be placed under water seal for an additional 24 hours, and, if no air accumulates, the tube may be removed.

Hemothorax is occasionally noted in the large animal neonate. It has occurred secondary to unstable fractured ribs, with puncture of the lung parenchyma resulting in hemorrhage into the pleural space. Occasionally hemothorax may remain undiagnosed until clinical signs of anemia, hypovolemia, or shock appear in the young animal.

Disorders of Breathing Pattern

IDIOPATHIC TACHYPNEA IN THE NEONATE. A syndrome observed in Clydesdale, Thoroughbred, and Arabian neonatal foals has been the combination of fever and tachypnea. It has also been observed in calves of several breeds. The condition appears to be more frequent during hot, humid weather conditions. The pathogenesis of the condition is unknown, but it is speculated that it results from a transient problem in central or peripheral control of thermoregulation or respiratory rate and pattern. Unfortunately little is known about these normal control mechanisms in the foal and calf.

Affected foals are usually of normal gestation and experience a normal birth. Most display normal activity for a variable period after birth, with a sudden onset of clinical signs. Occasionally, a foal may show mild signs of central nervous system derangement (e.g., lack of affinity for the mare, wandering). In human infants, transient tachypnea syndromes have been attributed to a delay in resorption of lung liquid, but in foals there is usually no sign of pulmonary abnormalities on chest radiographs or blood gas analysis. Body temperature is variable among foals, ranging from 102° to 108° F (39° to 42.2° C). A generally poor response to antipyretics has been noted. The respiratory rate and breathing pattern often resemble panting (respiratory rate >80 beats/min). The condition usually resolves spontaneously within a few days to weeks.

Before idiopathic tachypnea is diagnosed, it is extremely important to rule out a pneumonic process or other pulmonary abnormality, other forms of infection, metabolic acidosis, and other causes of an increased respiratory rate. Hematology, chest radiographs, and arterial blood gases should be within normal limits, and bacterial cultures should be negative.

Treatment is directed at controlling the body temperature; body clipping, alcohol baths, and maintaining in a cool environment are the most effective methods. If infection cannot be entirely ruled out, antibiotic therapy should be considered.

NEONATAL APNEA AND IRREGULAR BREATHING PATTERNS. Periods of apnea in the neonate are commonly associated with nonrespiratory factors, including infection, central nervous system disorders, hypothermia, and metabolic causes such as hypoglycemia. Seizure activity may be expressed by changes in breathing rate and pattern, and neonatal asphyxia may induce respiratory depression, whether or not cerebral lesions are present.[26] Neonatal respiratory distress may also cause apnea resulting from respiratory center depression or diaphragmatic fatigue. There are two mechanisms of apnea: central apnea, resulting from cessation of diaphragmatic activity; and obstructive apnea, resulting from obstruction of the airway, usually at the pharyngeal level. Both types have been observed in the foal.

Foals with irregular breathing patterns characterized by frequent pauses in breathing activity often show evidence of hypoventilation (increased P_{CO_2}) and hypoxemia on blood gas analysis. Oxygen therapy usually corrects the mild hypoxemia but does not affect the hypercapnia. Treatment of the condition in human infants includes increasing the amount of external stimulation, continuous positive airway pressure, pharmacologic treatment with methylxanthines such as theophylline and doxapram, and intermittent positive-pressure ventilation if prolonged apnea persists in spite of other treatments. In my experience, some hypoventilating foals have responded well to short-term doxapram infusion in the range of 0.02 to 0.05 mg/kg/min diluted IV (or 1.0 to 2.5 mg/kg/hr) for a few hours. Signs of toxicity in the human infant include hyperactivity, seizures, hypertension, and hyperglycemia.[103] In most foals with the condition, if the neurologic problem is resolved, the abnormalities in breathing pattern will be resolved.

TREATMENT OF RESPIRATORY DISTRESS

It is beyond the scope of this book to provide detailed information on the respiratory support of the large animal neonate, and the reader is referred to other articles and text for additional information on mechanical ventilation and other topics.[104-106]

Oxygen therapy is extremely useful in the treatment of the large animal neonate with respiratory disease. The decision as to when to institute oxygen therapy is somewhat subjective and is based both on clinical signs and on blood gas analysis. Increased respiratory rate, labored respiration, increased intercostal and abdominal muscle activity, and restlessness are considered indications for a trial of oxygen therapy. A Pa_{O_2} <55 to 60 mm Hg in lateral recumbency is considered an objective indication for oxygen therapy, although many foals with a Pa_{O_2} of 50 to 55 mm Hg on room air that were recovering from pneumonia apparently did well and displayed no signs of hypoxia. If blood gas analysis is not available, clinical signs indicating a favorable response to oxygen therapy include a decrease in effort of breathing, decrease in respiratory rate, and a more comfortable appearing animal. An absence of response may indicate a nonrespiratory origin of the clinical signs, severe lung pathology, cardiac malformation resulting in right-to-left shunting of blood, or inadequate inspired oxygen concentration.

The inspired oxygen concentration is most easily increased by nasal insufflation using a bias flow of humidified oxygen. Although an oxygen-delivery mask can be used, its presence interferes with nursing or feeding, and it may be poorly tolerated by the alert foal. Depending on the severity of disease and size of the individual, oxygen is initially delivered at a flow rate of about 5 L/min, and the response is noted. The catheter's tip should be advanced into the nasopharynx, and the opposite end should be secured to the nostril using tape or sutures in active foals. The actual oxygen concentration de-

livered to the alveoli depends on several factors, including the position of the tube and the depth and rate of breathing. Oxygen therapy should be directed at maintaining a PaO_2 of 80 to 100 mm Hg, and the flow rate should be adjusted according to blood gas results. Oxygen therapy should be on a continuous basis, and weaning from support should be done gradually. Transtracheal oxygen delivery may beneficial in larger foals, hypoxemic neonatal foals that have a rapid, shallow breathing pattern, or foals with severe pulmonary disease that are unresponsive to nasal insufflation.[107] A percutaneous catheter system is placed using local anesthetic and secured to the skin. The distal location of the catheter bypasses a substantial volume of dead space and probably results in a higher alveolar oxygen concentration. One advantage of this method of oxygen delivery was the ability to provide long-term oxygen therapy to unrestrained foals.[107]

Unfortunately, oxygen therapy is not effective in correcting hypoventilation, and, if hypercapnia is progressive and accompanied by signs of increasing respiratory distress, some type of mechanical ventilatory support is usually indicated. This decision to provide mechanical ventilation must take into account several considerations, including the worth of the individual, commitment of the owners, facility and manpower availability, and type of disease process present.

Regardless of the level of respiratory support provided, the importance of meticulous respiratory supportive technique cannot be overemphasized. Maintenance in sternal position, frequent turning from side to side, regular coupage, and use of proper suction technique are all important components of respiratory support.

LONG-TERM OUTCOME IN FOALS WITH RESPIRATORY DISEASE

A few studies have attempted to describe the long-term outcome of foals that had pneumonia or other respiratory disease early in life. Studies that followed somewhat older foals successfully treated for *Rhodococcus equi* pneumonia concluded that even severely affected individuals did not have detectable evidence of residual lung damage after recovery.[108,109] Follow-up studies of neonatal foals receiving treatment in intensive care facilities did not detect a higher incidence of poor performance, exercise intolerance, or other respiratory abnormalities in horses treated for pneumonia or other respiratory disease as neonates.[110,111] However, poor growth, malnutrition, and chronic multiresistant pneumonia have been observed in premature foals in which respiratory disease was overlooked or treated inappropriately.

DISTENDED AND/OR PAINFUL ABDOMEN

WENDY E. VAALA
JOHN K. HOUSE

APPROACH TO DIAGNOSIS OF DISTENDED AND/OR PAINFUL ABDOMEN

The large animal neonate with a painful or distended abdomen can present a diagnostic challenge to the clinician. Medical and surgical causes of colic and gastrointestinal disease in the foal include ileus and bowel distention associated with peritonitis, hypoxic gut damage and metabolic disturbances, enteritis resulting from dietary changes, viral infections and bacterial pathogens, gastroduodenal ulcer disease, impaction associated with ascarid infections, intussusception, thromboembolic disease, small intestinal volvulus, colon tor-

sion, uroperitoneum, strangulating abdominal hernias, and congenital gastrointestinal lesions. The clinical challenge is to distinguish medical from surgical lesions to permit rapid and appropriate therapy. Abdominal surgery in young foals, particularly neonates, is associated with increased morbidity and mortality and a higher incidence of intraabdominal adhesion formation compared with mature horses.[112] Medical causes of gastrointestinal disease such as enteritis and peritonitis carry an increased risk of generalized sepsis and death if the patient's cardiovascular status and metabolic parameters are not monitored and stabilized in a timely manner.

Box 20-3 lists some of the more common conditions associated with the acute abdomen in large animal neonates. Physical examination findings can be similar between neonates requiring surgical intervention and those with only an infectious problem, such as enteritis. If abdominal distention is present, every effort should be made to identify its cause. Because the neonatal foal or calf is considerably smaller than the adult, some of the diagnostic techniques routinely used in the adult (rectal palpation, assessment of shape of abdomen) are of limited value in assessing the acute abdomen in the neonate. Bilateral, tympanitic distention of the paralumbar fossae is suggestive of generalized ileus or large bowel obstruction (e.g., meconium impaction). Other diagnostic aids including abdominal radiographs, transabdominal ultrasonography,

---

BOX 20-3

Causes of Distended or Painful Abdomen (Acute Abdomen)

MECONIUM IMPACTION
Primary (mainly foal)
Secondary to other causes: sepsis, asphyxia

OBSTRUCTION
Foreign body (hairballs in calf)
Malformation (atresia coli, recti, ani)
Intussusception
Volvulus, torsion/strangulation

UROPERITONEUM
Ruptured bladder (mainly foal)
Torn or necrotic urachus, ureter

PERITONITIS
Generalized infection
Devitalized bowel
Perforated gastric or intestinal ulcer
Severe umbilical infection

GAS/FLUID ACCUMULATION IN STOMACH, ABOMASUM, INTESTINAL TRACT
Aerophagia
Intolerance to diet
Ileus
Gastric, abomasal, duodenal ulceration
Necrotizing enterocolitis
Ruminal bloat

MISCELLANEOUS
Hemoperitoneum
Ruptured umbilical vessels
Ruptured spleen or liver
Congenital tumor

ASCITES
Severe liver or renal failure
Severe hypoproteinemia

abdominal ballottment, and transcutaneous abdominal palpation are not practical in the adult but may be helpful in the large animal neonate.

The approach to the neonate with a painful or distended abdomen should include a complete history, including any abnormalities noted during the perinatal period, the type and dose of any analgesics previously administered, and whether there is history of diarrhea in other foals or horses on the farm. The age of the foal helps determine the risk of certain conditions. Young foals less than 2 weeks of age are more likely to experience colic as a result of meconium retention, peritonitis associated with generalized sepsis, hypoxic gut damage, uroperitoneum, and congenital deformities, including lethal white syndrome (e.g., mesenteric aganglionosis), inguinal and scrotal hernias and atresia of the anus or colon.[113-115] We have also seen increasing numbers of young foals with clostridial enteritis that present for colic. Older foals are more likely to suffer from intussusceptions, enteritis, gastroduodenal ulceration, and thromboembolic disease.[113,114]

The neonate's age at the onset of abdominal distress also may provide diagnostic clues. For example, foals with meconium impaction or congenital gastrointestinal malformations, such as atresia coli, tend to be presented for treatment during the first 12 to 36 hours of age, whereas foals with uncomplicated ruptured urinary tracts are usually presented at about 3 days of age, when the abdomen is visibly distended. The character, quantity, and frequency of defecation and urination should be determined. Surgical gastrointestinal tract lesions such as intussusception and large colon displacement have occurred secondary to enteritis. On the other hand, in the early stages, enteritis alone can cause severe abdominal distention or severe pain in the absence of diarrhea. Necrotizing enterocolitis and clostridial enteritis can be particularly painful conditions. Most foals with ruptured urinary bladders display abnormalities in urination, but, in some cases, normal micturition has been noted. Reduction in urine output from a neonate with a distended abdomen is not pathognomonic for uroperitoneum. Urine volume is typically reduced as a result of dehydration secondary to a variety of abnormalities, including gastrointestinal disease.[116] The colic associated with uroperitoneum is not usually severe.

Assessment of the degree of pain being exhibited is an important part of the examination of the neonate with a distended abdomen. Foals more commonly show signs of abdominal discomfort than do calves. In a retrospective study of foals undergoing exploratory celiotomy, uncontrollable pain and severe abdominal distention were the primary reasons the animals were taken to surgery. Unfortunately severe abdominal pain is not pathognomonic for a surgical lesion, because several foals with severe enteritis alone were taken to surgery for this reason.[117] However, persistent tachycardia in a neonate with a heart rate in excess of 150 beats/min despite administration of analgesics and in the absence of fever is suggestive of a surgical gastrointestinal lesion.

The degree of compromise to the cardiovascular and pulmonary systems should be assessed. A neonate with an abdominal crisis is often in need of immediate stabilization because of shock secondary to endotoxemia or hypovolemia. Exploratory celiotomy in neonates that receive inadequate presurgical supportive therapy is associated with a number of complications, including poor tolerance to anesthesia. The degree of respiratory compromise secondary to the abdominal problem should also be considered, particularly if the animal is a surgical candidate. For example, foals with long-standing uroperitoneum may have pleural effusion and pulmonary abnormalities as well as serum electrolyte abnormalities, all of which may predispose to anesthetic problems (hypoxemia, hypercapnia, cardiac arrhythmias)

It is important to establish the likelihood of generalized or localized infection such as enteritis. Generalized sepsis can interfere with the function of many organ systems, including the gastrointestinal tract. The first signs of enteritis are often severe abdominal distention and colic, with diarrhea becoming apparent a few hours to days later (Fig. 20-3); the severity of these signs may warrant surgical exploration of the abdomen. Leukopenia may be observed in foals with septicemia, enteritis, peritonitis, and surgical gastrointestinal lesions. An unexplained metabolic acidosis may also indicate impending enteritis.

Additional information on the physical examination of the abdomen and gastrointestinal tract can be found in Chapter 17. It is difficult to distinguish fluid accumulation in the large colon from accumulation in the peritoneal cavity using physical examination alone, and additional diagnostic procedures are usually required to distinguish the two (see below). In general, nasogastric intubation in the neonatal foal does not seem to be as useful a diagnostic technique as it is in the adult horse. Gastric reflux can be difficult to obtain, even if the stomach appears markedly distended on radiographs, and a moderate amount may be obtained in cases of ileus. If large volumes of reflux are obtained, however, obstructive disease (e.g., of the pylorus and small intestine) is considered more likely.[117]

Neonates with enteritis, uroperitoneum, and other abdominal problems can have markedly deranged serum electrolyte concentrations (hyperkalemia, hyponatremia, and metabolic acidosis are typical). Failure to recognize the severity of these abnormalities or adequately treat them can result in the death of the patient.

Abdominal radiographs can be helpful in identifying segments of the intestinal tract that are distended, fluid in the peritoneal cavity, and the composition of ingesta in the gastrointestinal tract (e.g., sand, meconium) (Figs. 20-4 and 20-5). A good knowledge of normal radiographic anatomy of the intestinal tract is important for accurate interpretation (Fig. 20-6). Adequate radiographs are obtained in foals up to 250 kg if available radiograph equipment includes a grid, rare earth screens and sufficient mAs (5 to 28) and kVp (75 to 95). With experience in viewing normal and abnormal abdominal radiographs the likelihood of an obstructive lesion versus simple ileus can be established in some but not all cases. The presence of erectile, distended loops of small intestine is most consistent with a diagnosis of obstructive disease. Intramural gas is suggestive of necrotizing enterocolitis. It can be difficult to differentiate large colon torsion or displacement from simple gas and fluid distention secondary to ileus. Contrast radiography can help to define the location and nature of gastrointestinal problems such as duodenal stricture and abnormalities of the small colon or rectum.[118,119]

Abdominal ultrasonography can be of value in diagnosing certain conditions that may be contributing to a distended or painful abdomen, including fluid-distended small and large intestine, ascarid impaction, intussusception, colonic impaction, uroperitoneum, and abnormalities of the umbilical vessels and urachus. Ultrasonography also permits characterization of small intestinal motility, distention, and bowel wall thickness. Healthy foals have flaccid, fluid-filled loops of small intestine. The presence of rounded, distended loops of small intestine is suggestive of an ileus, enteritis, or possible small bowel obstructive disease. The location, amount, character, and echogenicity of free peritoneal fluid can also be determined[49,114,120] (Fig 20-7). A large accumulation of peritoneal fluid with increased echogenicity (or fibrin) is suggestive of peritonitis, whereas an excessive volume of hypoechogenic peritoneal fluid is suggestive of uroperitoneum.

In my opinion, except in a couple of specific conditions, peritoneal taps are of limited value in diagnosis of the acute

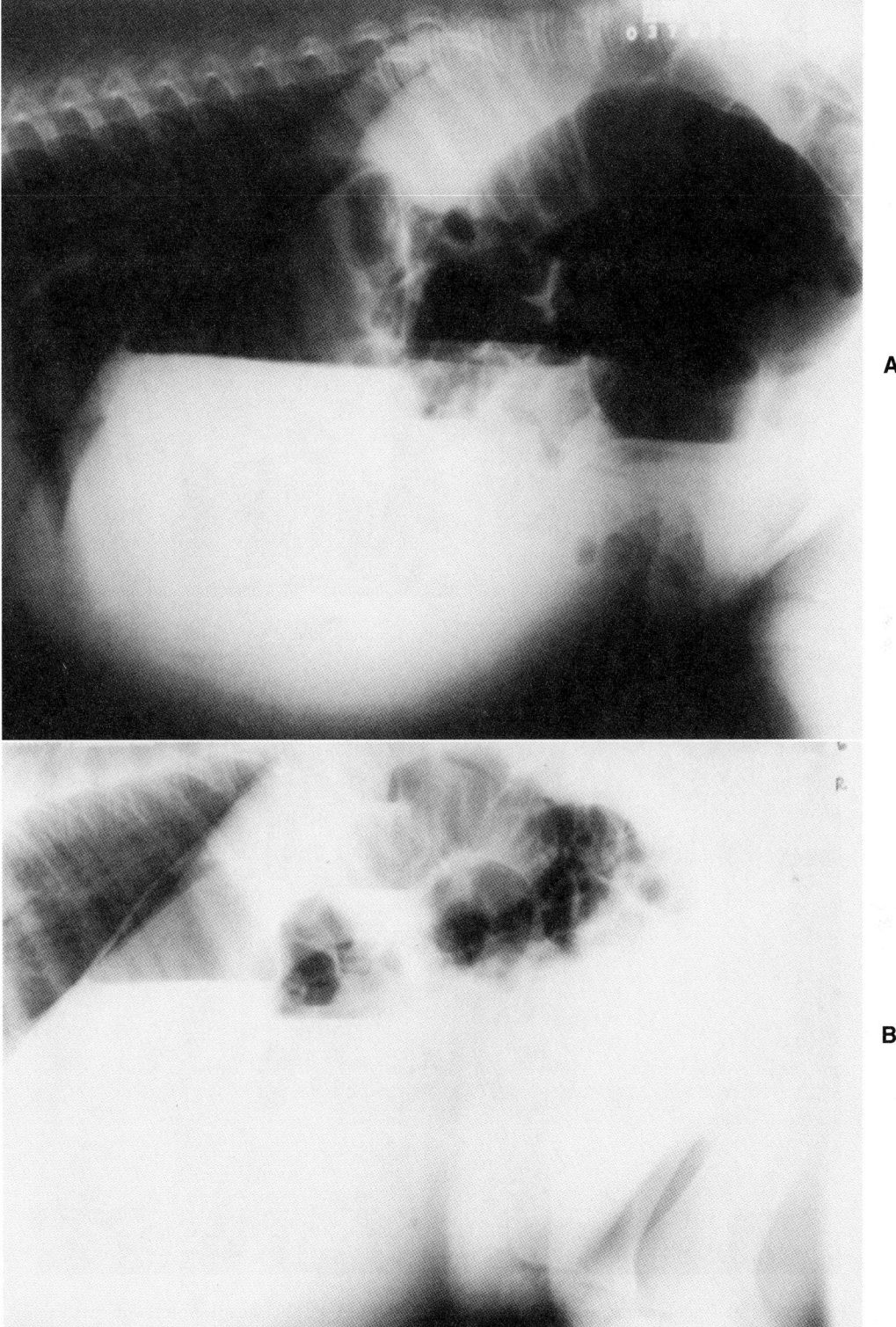

FIG. 20-3 ▓ **A,** Abdominal radiograph (standing) of a 48-hour-old foal that presented with meconium impaction and a distended abdomen. The foal also had a metabolic acidosis, hypoglycemia, and leukopenia. Note the gaseous distention of the large intestines, which was suggestive of ileus and possibly obstruction. **B,** Standing abdominal radiograph of the same foal 24 hours later after passage of diarrhea. After removal of the meconium, profuse bloody diarrhea was observed, suggesting enteritis. With passage of the diarrhea, gas distention resolved.

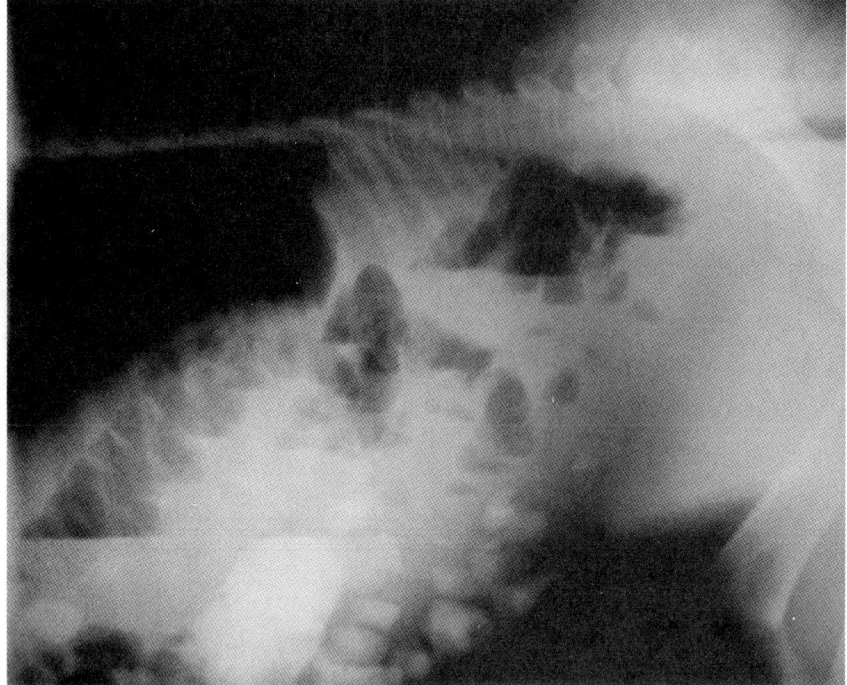

FIG. 20-4 ▉ Sand accumulation in the ventral colon of a 1-month-old foal with chronic diarrhea and intermittent colic.

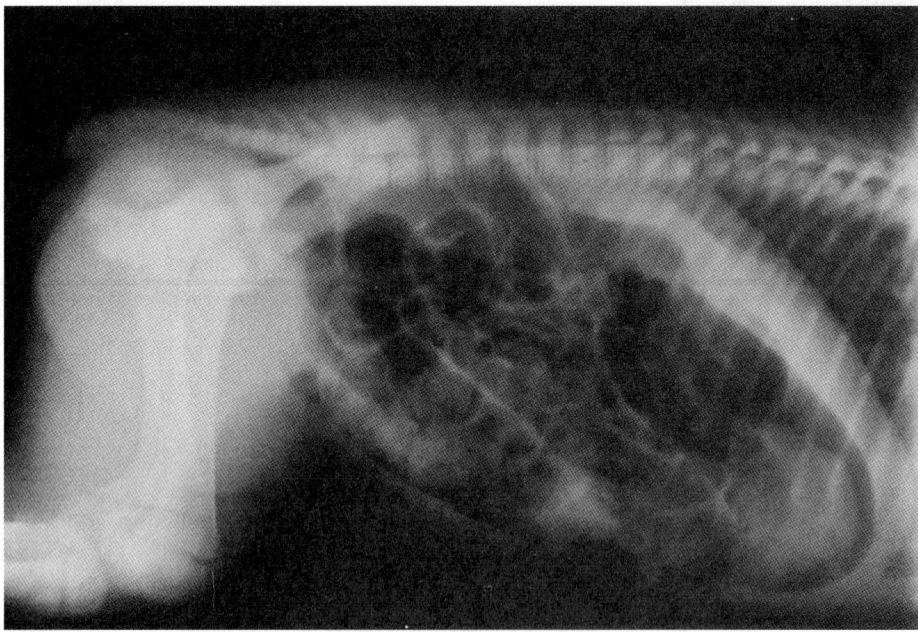

FIG. 20-5 ▉ Abdominal radiograph (lateral recumbency) of a 7-hour-old Miniature Horse foal with atresia ani, showing meconium packed into a gas-distended large colon. The extent of the atresia proximally from the anus is not visible.

abdomen in the neonate. Extreme caution should be exercised to avoid perforating the bowel while attempting to acquire a sample of peritoneal fluid, particularly if intestinal distention is present. The intestine of the neonate is easily ripped by inadvertent perforation with a needle or teat cannula, even if the neonate is well restrained. It is probably safest to perform the procedure using ultrasonography to image the fluid pocket and the needle position. Foals with

uroperitoneum are the ideal candidates for abdominocentesis. Clear yellow, urinelike peritoneal fluid is easily and safely obtained in these patients because the excessive volume of peritoneal fluid allows the abdominal viscera to float well above the ventral floor of the abdomen.

Normal peritoneal fluid is similar to that of the adult, except that the normal WBC count is lower (1500 cells/μL or less).[121] Cytologic examination should also be performed to

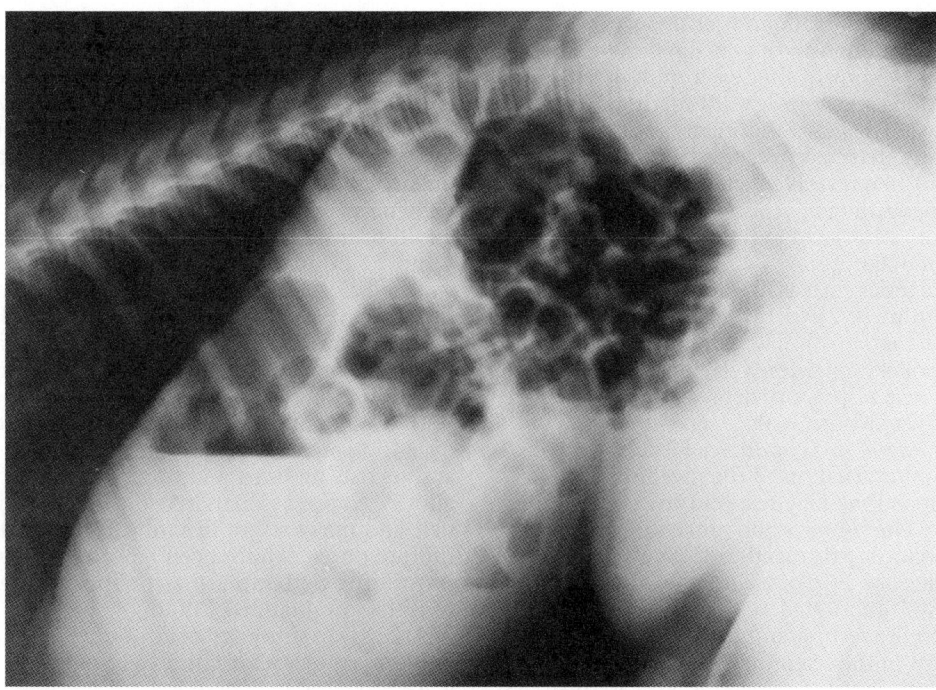

FIG. 20-6 ▓ Normal standing abdominal radiograph in a neonatal foal. Note the prominent fluid line in the stomach and the presence of gas in various portions of the tract.

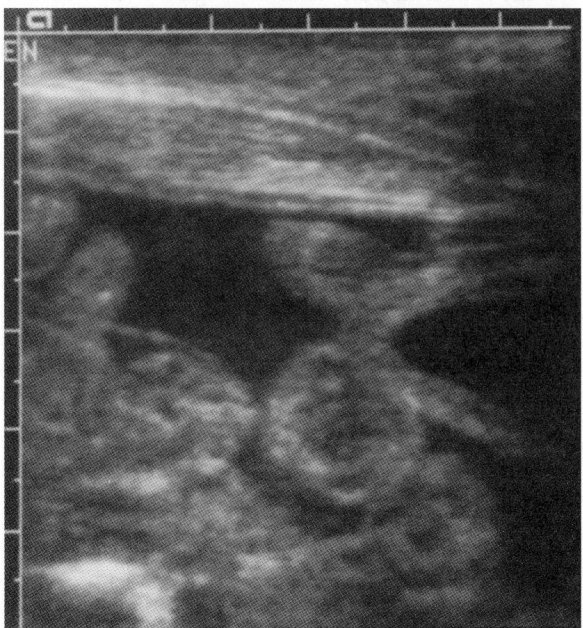

FIG. 20-7 ▓ Ultrasound view of the caudal abdomen of a 24-hour-old premature foal with a torn urachus, showing *(from top to bottom)* the ventral abdominal wall, free abdominal fluid *(black)*, the urinary bladder *(oval structure to the right)*, and small intestinal loops *(cross-sectional view)*.

determine the cell types present and to detect the presence of bacteria and toxic neutrophils (suggesting peritonitis), and fecal material (suggesting either inadvertent gut tap or bowel rupture). The total protein and WBC count may be elevated in a variety of conditions. These include severe enteritis; urachal, umbilical, or severe bladder infection; and primary peritonitis, in addition to conditions in which there is ischemic bowel requiring surgical resection. On the other hand, as in the adult,

normal peritoneal fluid has accompanied a number of surgical intestinal lesions, such as large colon displacement. Therefore peritoneal fluid analysis is of limited value in distinguishing the surgical patient, but can be useful in the diagnosis of peritonitis. In addition, peritoneal fluid analysis usually results in a straightforward diagnosis of uroperitoneum. In virtually all cases of uroperitoneum observed to date, peritoneal creatinine level was greater than the serum level (usually >2:1). Also, the acquisition of free-flowing blood from the abdominal tap usually allows a diagnosis of hemoperitoneum.

Endoscopy of the upper and lower gastrointestinal tract of the foal can be performed if appropriately sized equipment is available (8 to 10 mm OD, 180 to 250 cm long).[116] The esophagus and stomach can be examined for erosion, ulceration, perforation, and other abnormalities. Suspected impactions or malformations of the rectum and small colon can also be examined.[114]

In summary, accurate identification of foals with acute abdominal problems requiring surgery can be difficult even with the use of ancillary diagnostic procedures, and mistakes are commonly made because there are no clear-cut and consistent differences between medical and surgical cases. Findings suggestive of the need for surgical exploration include severe and unrelenting pain and persistent tachycardia.[117-118,122]

SPECIFIC CONDITIONS

Meconium Impaction

Meconium impaction is the most common cause of colic in the newborn foal. This condition is more common in colts because of the narrow pelvic canal. Many foals show some degree of straining and discomfort while passing meconium, but in most instances it is passed uneventfully by 24 to 48 hours of age. The meconium most commonly becomes impacted in the rectum or small colon. The clinical signs associated with meconium impaction in the otherwise normal foal include repeated attempts to defecate, straining with the back arched, swishing of the tail, and restlessness. Nursing stimulates defecation through an oral-anal reflex, so signs of discomfort may appear shortly after each milk meal. If left untreated, meconium impactions lead to varying degrees of abdominal distention. The foal's abdomen becomes gas distended with tympany detected over the paralumbar fossa. Digital examination often reveals a rectum packed with hard fecal balls. Occasionally, the impaction is located more proximally (large or small colon) and radiography or ultrasonography is required for diagnosis.

Low doses of analgesics such as dipyrone (10 to 22 mg/kg IV), flunixin meglumine (0.25 to 1.0 mg/kg IV), and butorphenol (0.01 to 0.1 mg/kg IV) may be required to prevent self-trauma during colicky episodes. Xylazine may exacerbate gut stasis and can cause respiratory depression; it should be used with caution in newborn foals. A gravity enema with mild soap and warm water or a commercial Fleet enema usually results in prompt evacuation of the meconium. Refractory meconium impactions may respond to acetylcysteine retention enemas.[123] The supplies and procedure for a retention enema are as follows: Mix together 150 ml water, 6 g of acetylcysteine powder, and 20 g of sodium bicarbonate (baking soda). Insert a well-lubricated 12- or 14-Fr, cuffed Foley urinary catheter into the rectum and inflate the cuff. Slowly infuse 120 to 180 ml of the retention enema solution. Plug the end of the catheter. Tape the catheter loosely to the foal's tail. Leave in place a minimum of 15 minutes, then deflate the cuff and remove the catheter. This procedure can be repeated several times. Care must be taken to avoid traumatizing the rectal mucosa by stiff tubing or multiple enemas with harsh detergents. Clinical signs associated with meconium impaction in the compromised foal may be absent. In asphyxiated or premature individuals that are receiving little or no enteral feeding, meconium may remain in the large colon for days, gradually forming into hard concretions that are diagnosed by palpation or radiographs or at postmortem examination. In these cases the routine administration of an enema is often ineffective in mobilizing the impaction because it is high in the large colon. Additional therapy includes intravenous fluids, oral fluids, and laxatives (60 to 120 ml of mineral oil with ½ to 1 oz of psyllium, 60 to 120 ml of milk of magnesia). If the gas distention becomes severe, transcutaneous bowel trocarization can be pursued. We avoid the use of dioctyl sodium sulfosuccinate (DSS) as an oral cathartic because it can cause excessive irritation resulting in diarrhea and colic. Analgesics may also be helpful in controlling the neonate's discomfort and reducing the risk of self-trauma. Although most meconium impactions can be successfully treated with aggressive medical therapy, those few foals that are refractory to treatment or display uncontrollable pain are candidates for surgical intervention. Meconium impaction is rare in neonatal ruminants.

Uroperitoneum

Uroperitoneum is a relatively common cause of abdominal distention and depression in the neonatal foal. The condition predominates in males, but may occur in females as well. Uroperitoneum may be congenital or acquired. The congenital form occurs as a result of failure of the dorsal wall of the bladder to close during development.[124] The most common cause of uroperitoneum is a ruptured urinary bladder, but other sites in the urinary tract may also leak, including the ureters, urachus, and urethra. Most cases of ruptured bladders are presumed to occur during parturition because of external pressure on a distended bladder. This form occurs most commonly in colts. With the recent development of neonatal critical care, there have also been an increasing number of reports of uroperitoneum secondary to the necrotic or infected urinary bladder or urachus in the compromised foal.[117] Critically ill, recumbent foals may rupture their bladders while being lifted and turned with a full bladder or from chronic overdistention associated with their generalized disease state. Foals with botulism may also rupture their bladder secondary to bladder atony and chronic overdistention. Older foals of either sex may experience bladder rupture secondary to focal infection of the umbilical arteries or urachus or ischemic necrosis of the apex of the bladder.

Clinical signs of uroperitoneum are rarely noticed before 48 to 72 hours of age, particularly if the foal is not being watched closely. The first signs may be urinary incontinence or frequent attempts to urinate, with only small amounts voided. Sometimes, particularly in those animals that rupture sometime after birth, there is a history of a period of normal urination, which at some point stopped or became abnormal. Loss of suckle, mild colic, and increasing abdominal distention are usually accompanied by worsening depression and increasing heart and respiratory rate. If the condition is allowed to persist, foals become increasingly weak and dyspneic and may present in cardiovascular collapse. Fillies with ruptured ureters have been reported to have a characteristic protruding perineum, presumably as a result of retroperitoneal accumulation of fluid.[125]

Laboratory findings commonly associated with uroperitoneum are elevated serum creatinine and blood urea nitrogen (BUN), hyperkalemia, hyponatremia, hypochloremia, and metabolic acidosis. These changes are probably a result of the normal diet of the foal (milk being relatively high in potassium [25 mEq/L] and low in sodium [12 mEq/L]) and the third spacing of urine in the peritoneal cavity. With urine potassium concentration relatively higher than serum and urine sodium concentration lower than serum levels, the net effect of partial equilibration of serum with peritoneal fluid across a semipermeable membrane is hyponatremia and hyperkalemia, along with an inability to excrete the waste products of metabolism. Hyperkalemia may be severe enough to induce potentially fatal bradyarrhythmias. In hospitalized foals that developed uroperitoneum as a secondary complication, these typical electrolyte abnormalities were not consistently observed. Because most of those foals were receiving replacement intravenous fluids (high in sodium, low in potassium) and little milk, it was theorized that intake has a great influence on the electrolyte abnormalities associated with uroperitoneum.[117] On the other hand, the electrolyte abnormalities typically associated with uroperitoneum are not pathognomonic for that disorder. Foals with renal failure, blocked urethra, white muscle disease, and enteritis have shown the same electrolyte changes.

A diagnosis of uroperitoneum often can be made quickly using transabdominal ultrasound and a 5- or 7.5-MHz transducer to visualize large volumes of free, nonechogenic fluid within the abdomen, and a small, irregularly shaped, collapsed bladder. Abdominocentesis usually produces a free flow of peritoneal fluid that contains a low cell count, low specific gravity, and at least twice the creatinine concentration of peripheral blood. If the creatinine is the same in both serum and peritoneal fluid, other explanations for the clinical signs should be investigated. The WBC count, total protein, and cytology of the fluid should also be determined. Most uncomplicated cases of ruptured bladders have fairly normal values for peritoneal fluid. In some cases, however, an increased WBC count and total protein and the presence of bacteria may suggest peritonitis. This may be a result of the urine in the abdomen, but more commonly there is a primary ongoing infectious problem (necrotic urachus or bladder, enteritis), and the prognosis becomes worse. If laboratory facilities are not available, new methylene blue can be injected into the bladder using a urinary catheter, and a few minutes later a sample of peritoneal fluid should have a blue

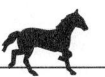

discoloration if a ruptured bladder is present. However, this technique may not detect other causes of uroperitoneum such as a ruptured ureter or distal urachus. Positive contrast cystography using a 10% solution of water-soluble media may be helpful in detecting the location of the urinary tract leakage. The ability to obtain urine on catheterization of the urinary bladder does *not* rule out uroperitoneum. Hematology and blood cultures should be performed to detect primary or secondary sepsis.

Treatment of uroperitoneum is surgical repair. However, the foal with uroperitoneum should not be rushed to surgery without first carefully stabilizing it. Serum electrolytes and blood gases should be run to determine the extent of hyperkalemia, hyponatremia, and acidosis present. Although the total amount of water in the body is usually grossly increased by the peritoneal accumulation of urine, effective circulating volume may be drastically reduced. If the eyeballs are sunken and pulse quality and capillary refill time are poor, aggressive fluid therapy is indicated to support the circulation. This is best performed by concurrently removing as much fluid as possible from the abdomen with a teat cannula, 14-gauge catheter, or peritoneal dialysis catheter to avoid worsening fluid overload and respiratory distress. The fluids of choice to treat the typical electrolyte alterations associated with uroperitoneum are saline, dextrose, and possibly sodium bicarbonate solutions, depending on the degree of acidosis present. In most instances, continuous dextrose infusion is effective in decreasing the serum potassium level to an acceptable level, but values should be rechecked before anesthesia is induced. Insulin and dextrose may also be used to treat hyperkalemia, but the patient must be monitored for hypoglycemia. One suggested regimen is regular insulin at 0.1 to 0.2 U/kg SC or IV accompanied by a continuous intravenous dextrose infusion (4 to 8 mg/kg/min). Some individuals also have pleural fluid accumulation and atelectasis secondary to the abdominal distention, so oxygenation and ventilation during and after surgery should be closely monitored. Broad-spectrum antibiotics should be started immediately after samples are taken for culture if infection is suspected.

The prognosis for uncomplicated ruptured urinary bladders is usually good (>80% survival), provided the animal is stabilized before anesthesia. The presence of concurrent septicemia carries with it a considerably poorer prognosis.[126] In one retrospective study among foals with uroperitoneum, 100% of those foals with a negative sepsis score lived and only 57% of foals with a positive septic score survived.[126]

Gas or Fluid Accumulation in the Gastrointestinal Tract: Ileus

Abdominal distention and colic secondary to excessive gas or fluid accumulation in all or a portion of the gastrointestinal tract are common complications in the compromised neonate undergoing intensive care. The exact mechanisms responsible for the presumably altered gastrointestinal motility are not well defined. Ileus is associated with the absence of intestinal sounds, abdominal distention, and intolerance of oral feeds characterized by gastric reflux. Auscultation of reduced gastrointestinal borborymi does not always correlate with the degree of intestinal compromise and decreased motility. Transabdominal ultrasonography helps identify absence of intestinal motility and the location and degree of intestinal distention. Ileus and the attending abdominal distention can cause severe colic and can induce respiratory distress in a weak or premature foal with preexisting pulmonary compromise.

Metabolic and infectious causes of ileus in the foal include hypokalemia, hypocalcemia, hypoxic-ischemic bowel injury, bowel obstruction, peritonitis, enterocolitis, and endotoxemia.

Hypokalemia is associated with anorexia, diarrhea, and renal loss. Hypocalcemia is associated with prematurity, decreased dietary intake, excessive bicarbonate administration, diuretic therapy and those conditions such as asphyxia, toxemia, and sepsis that stimulate release of cortisol and catecholamines. Peripartum hypoxia results in a preferential decrease in blood-flow to the gut and kidneys. Poor perfusion of the intestines leads to varying degrees of mucosal damage and decreased motility. Severely damaged bowel requires a period of gut rest to allow healing to occur before restarting oral feeds. Premature resumption of enteral feeding is associated with colic, maldigestion, diarrhea (often bloody), and translocation of intraluminal bacteria across damaged bowel wall into the bloodstream. Some of the more common causes of bowel distention in the neonate include meconium retention, intussusception, ascarid impaction, and small intestinal volvulus. Peritonitis may be associated with intraabdominal abscessation, severe enteritis or gastroduodenal ulcer disease, and generalized septicemia. The most common causes of enteritis in foals include rotavirus, *Clostridium* spp., *Salmonella* spp., and dietary changes. Endotoxemia is usually part of generalized septicemia. Chronic bowel distention, regardless of the cause, further impedes return of normal gut motility. In the foal, aerophagia, particularly in the struggling or hypoxic neonate, often results in gas distention that is not easily removed through a nasogastric tube, because gas tends to move quickly through the gastrointestinal tract (Fig. 20-8). Abdominal distention is also commonly observed during mechanical ventilation in the foal and as a result of overfeeding in the calf. Foals with botulism are often intolerant of enteral feeding, probably because of altered gastrointestinal motility. Use of certain milk replacers can result in bloat, colic, and diarrhea, even in the apparently healthy orphan neonate (see Evaluation of Milk Replacers, Chapter 21). Discontinuation of or a decrease in the amount of enteral feeding and, if possible, increased activity of the patient usually results in resolution of the problem.

Abdominal radiographs reveal gas-distended loops of small or large intestine and may identify bowel obstruction. Sonographic examination permits evaluation of bowel wall thickness, peritoneal fluid volume and echogenicity, gut patency, intramural gas accumulation, location and degree of intestinal distention, and presence or absence of motility. An abdominal sonogram should be performed to rule out the presence of an intussusception or other obstructive lesion before initiating any prokinetic therapy.

Management of ileus includes nasogastric decompression, cessation or reduced volume and frequency of enteral feeds if gastric reflux is present, parenteral alimentation if enteral feeding cannot be maintained at a rate of at least 10 % of body weight/day, enema administration to relieve distal meconium or fecal retention, correction of any underlying electrolyte abnormalities, exercise for ambulatory foals, judicious use of prokinetic agents, and, occasionally, percutaneous trocarization and decompression of severely distended large bowel. The gut atrophies without enteral feeding. Glutamine and butyrate are essential fuels for the small and large bowel, respectively, and have been added to enteral formulas for humans and some oral fluid replacement formulations for animals to help maintain and restore enterocyte health.[127] The procedure for percutaneous bowel trocarization is described in detail elsewhere.[128] Prokinetic drugs should not be used when bowel obstruction or compromised bowel integrity is suspected. Prokinetic agents that have been used include cisapride, metaclopramide, bethanechol, and erythromycin.

Surgical Gastrointestinal Lesions

Most types of displacement, torsion, volvulus, and entrapments that occur in the adult horse may also occur in the

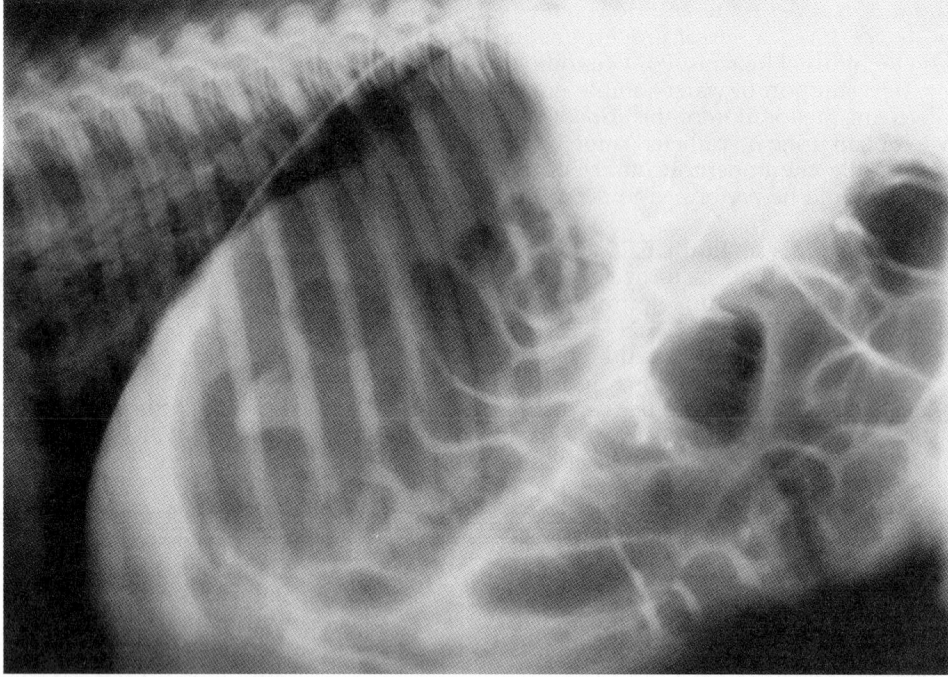

FIG. 20-8 ▮▮ Marked gastric and generalized small intestinal gas distention in a septic, collapsed, 3-day-old Thoroughbred colt. There is no evidence of obstruction. The patient was treated with supportive therapy and recovered.

neonatal foal, though probably at a lower frequency (Fig. 20-9). Large colon displacement, intussusception, and small intestinal volvulus have also been observed secondary to enteritis and colitis.

Surgical correction of congenital gastrointestinal defects may be attempted. Atresia ani, atresia recti, and atresia coli have been well documented in the foal and calf, and intestinal aganglionosis has been observed in association with recessive lethal white foals, which are usually the products of mating between two overo paint horses.[115] Acute colic, progressive abdominal distention, and lack of meconium staining after repeated enemas have been the most common findings in newborn foals with atresia coli. Barium enemas may be of use in identifying foals with a short small colon, but may also be misleading.[129] Surgical exploration of the abdomen offers definitive diagnosis of the severity of the malformation and the possibility of correction, but the owner should be informed before surgery of the high frequency of inoperable lesions and the high failure rate after reattachment.[129] Before any surgery is contemplated, a thorough physical examination should be performed to identify any other congenital malformations. Surgical correction of atresia ani is often successful, particularly if the atresia is limited only to a persistent membrane blocking the anus and the anal sphincter is normal. The prognosis for atresia coli is guarded. Poor intestinal motility, technical difficulties of attaching bowel segments that are so different in size, anastomosis breakdown, and peritonitis after surgery are common complications.[129]

An inguinal hernia is another congenital lesion occasionally requiring surgical intervention. These hernias occur in colts and may be caused by compression during parturition. Most congenital inguinal hernias are handled conservatively because the condition is often self-limiting by the time the foal is 3 to 6 months old. Treatment includes daily manual reduction of the hernia and frequent observation to detect possible bowel strangulation. Indications for surgical intervention in foals with congenital hernias include rupture of the common vaginal tunic, persistent colic, severe edema of the prepuce and scrotum, and trauma to the skin overlying the hernial sac. Surgical hernias are difficult to reduce manually, and loops of intestines are often palpable in the subcutaneous tissues of the scrotum and medial thigh.[130] Unilateral castration is usually performed on the affected side.

Other gastrointestinal lesions in foals that may require an exploratory laparotomy include intussusception, small or large intestinal volvulus, and mechanical obstruction (e.g., food or ascarid impaction, phytobezoar, fecalith). Intussusceptions are reported in horses younger than 3 years of age. An intussusception is formed when one segment of intestine and its mesentery invaginates into the lumen of the adjacent bowel immediately aboral to it. The invaginated segment is referred to as the intussusceptum and the enveloping segment is referred to as the intussuscipiens. Small intestinal intussusceptions can involve the jejunum, ileum, or ileocecal junction. Other sites of obstruction include cecocecal and cecocolic junctions. Intussusceptions are most common in foals less than 6 weeks old.[131]

Causes of intussusception include segmental motility differences (e.g., a hypermotile section of bowel adjacent to an atonic segment of bowel) and local changes in the bowel wall (e.g., abscessation). Causes of altered peristalsis include enteritis, heavy ascarid infestation, mesenteric arteritis, and sudden dietary changes.[132] Changes in the bowel wall have included granulomas, papillomas, and intramural leiomyoma. Anoplocephala perfoliata has been associated with ileocecal intussusceptions. Clinical signs include varying degrees of discomfort, depending on the site of obstruction and its duration. Abdominal pain can be severe but is often low-grade and intermittent and accompanied by decreased manure production. Ultrasonography is a useful diagnostic aid. Sonographically the cross-sectional view of the intussusception reveals a targetlike pattern with a thick hypoechoic rim. The outer rim is created by severe edema of the entering and returning bowel walls of the intussusceptum.

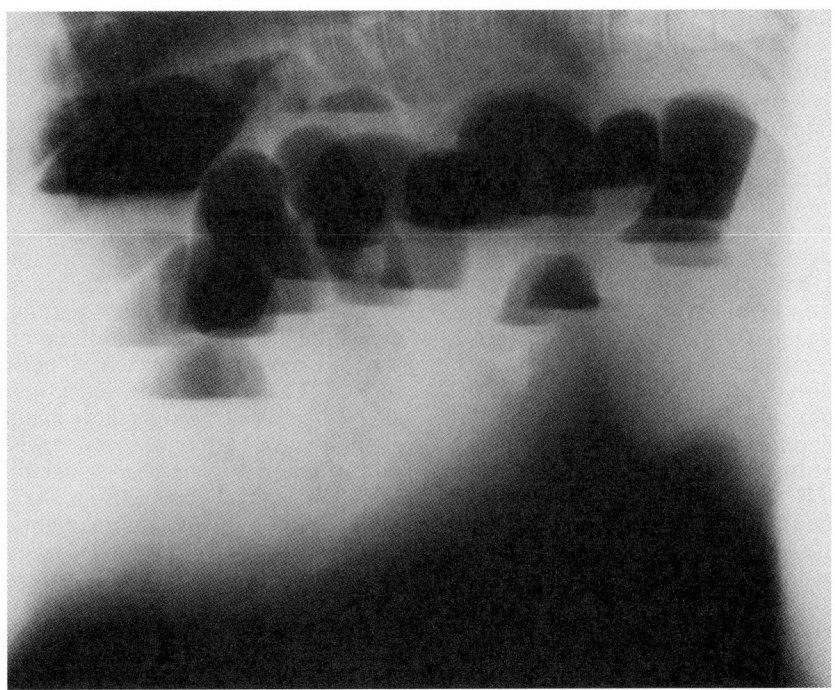

FIG. 20-9 ▓ Standing abdominal radiograph of a 3-week-old foal that presented with signs of severe pain. Note the multiple, erectile loops of distended small intestine with fluid lines. Obstructive disease was suspected. On surgical exploration of the abdomen, obstructing adhesions secondary to a previous surgery were found.

Treatment involves a surgical exploratory. Early cases can be manually reduced followed by surgical resection. Because of the ileum's tenuous blood supply and the inaccessibility of the ileocecal junction, intussusceptions involving the ileum are usually treated with a side-to-side jejunostomy or ileocecostomy. Ileoileal intussusceptions have been reported to have a better prognosis than jejunal or ileocecal intussusception. Foals that have multiple sites of intussusception have a poor prognosis.

Volvulus may involve the small or large intestines. Small intestinal volvulus is the most common, especially among foals between 2 and 4 months of age. Signs include abdominal distention, gastric reflux, persistent tachycardia, severe pain, and sonographic evidence of uniform, severe bowel distention with bowel wall edema (>3 to 4 mm), and absence of motility. As expected, survival is poorer after correction of strangulating versus nonstrangulating lesions. Strangulating lesions of the small intestines have a poor survival compared with large intestinal lesions and a higher incidence of fatal complications. Parasitic migration and abrupt dietary changes are among conditions thought to predispose to volvulus development.

Surgical colic in foals carries a poorer long-term prognosis than in adult horses. One study[133] examined the survival rate among 67 foals younger than 150 days of age undergoing colic surgery. The most common lesions requiring a celiotomy were small colon impaction, large colon impaction, jejunal volvulus, and ascarid impaction. A poor prognosis was associated with strangulating lesions. Foals younger than 14 days of age experienced more early postoperative complications and suffered poor long-term survival because of adhesion formation. Only 25% of foals younger than 14 days of age survived in the short term compared with 71% of foals older than 15 days of age.

Another study[134] examined the outcome among 119 young horses less than 1 year of age that underwent exploratory celiotomy. Among all foals the most common cause for surgery was small intestinal strangulation. Uroperitoneum and meconium impaction were the most common conditions in neonatal foals, and intussusception and enteritis were more common among older foals. Significant elevations in packed cell volume (PCV) (37% to 54%), heart rate (80 to 134 beats/min), nucleated cell counts, and total protein concentration in peritoneal fluid (3.1 to 32.8 × 10³/μl, 2.9 to 4.9 g/L), and rectal temperature (38.2 to 39.2° C) were observed in nonsurvivors compared with survivors. Nonsurvivors had significantly decreased serum bicarbonate, chloride, sodium, and venous pH values. Thirty-three percent of foals surviving surgery had evidence of intraabdominal adhesions.

Surgical gastrointestinal lesions in neonatal ruminants include intestinal atresia, intussusception, torsion of the mesentery, intestinal strangulation/incarceration/volvulus, torsion of the cecum, and abomasal displacement.

Intestinal atresia is the most common cause of abdominal distention of calves in the first week of life.[135] Typically calves are born normally but develop progressive abdominal distention shortly after birth. Signs of mild colic are occasionally observed. The spiral loop of the ascending colon is the most common site of atresia.[136] Other congenital abnormalities may be present (18% of cases).[136] Pregnancy diagnosis by palpating the amniotic sac before 40 days' gestation may cause colonic atresia in cattle[137]; however, an autosomal-recessive inheritance in Holstein cattle has recently been proposed.[138] Surgical repair by resection of the distended proximal blind end, and anastomosis of the proximal segment of intestine to the descending colon has been described, but breeding affected animals is not recommended.[136] Long-term survivors are likely to have loose feces and do not tend to grow well.[136]

Intussusception occurs most commonly in the jejunum, but the frequency of ileocecal and colon intussusceptions appears higher in calves than adults.[139] Commonly there is a history of diarrhea. Clinical signs may include intermittant colic, abscence of feces, and melena; however, these are inconsistent. The inconsistency of clinical signs and inability to perform a rectal examination makes the diagnosis more difficult in calves than adults.[139] Abdominal ultrasound may be useful. The prognosis after surgical correction is strongly influenced by the duration of the condition before correction.

Twisting of the intestinal mass around the cranial root of the mesentery is a rare event but occurs more frequently in calves than adults.[139] Clinically the condition is characterized by a sudden onset of severe colic (kicking at the abdomen, dropping to the ground) that rapidly progresses (abdominal enlargement, tachycardia, tachypnea, reduced or absent fecal passage) to signs of shock and recumbency.

Abomasal displacement is rare in neonatal ruminants. Clinical signs include reduced appetite, poor weight gain, recurrent tympany (left side), and diarrhea. An association of left-sided abomasal displacement with pneumonia in calves suggests altered vagal function may be involved in the pathogenesis of the condition.[140,141] Typically left-sided abomasal displacement in calves occurs between 6 and 14 weeks of age, but younger calves may be affected. Displacement of the abomasum is diagnosed by auscultation and percussion; affected animals may have a hypochloremia metabolic alkalosis. Correction can be attempted by rolling the calf on its back or via surgery.

Necrotizing Enterocolitis

Necrotizing enterocolitis (NEC) is one of the most common serious surgical disorders of human infants undergoing intensive care, and has been described in two equine neonates.[142] It is a syndrome of acute intestinal necrosis.[143] In human infants, prematurity is the single greatest risk factor. The causes of NEC are not well defined, but predisposing factors include ischemic hypoxic gut injury, presence of intraluminal bacteria, and enteral feeding. After gastrointestinal ischemia, mucosal cell metabolism diminishes and the protective mucous layer is lost. This allows enzymes to break down the mucosal barrier, and intraluminal bacteria can then invade and multiply within the bowel wall. Enteral feeding provides substrate for the bacteria. Pneumatosis intestinalis develops, and the bowel frequently ruptures. Abdominal signs include abdominal distention, tenderness, ileus, and ascites. The condition may appear as a fulminant, rapidly progressive disease or progress at a much slower pace.[143,144] One of the affected equine neonates was premature and was undergoing treatment for respiratory distress when the abdominal crisis occurred. The other was a term foal that had experienced a prolonged delivery and was presented at 24 hours of age for weakness and abdominal pain. Abdominal distention and abdominal pain, followed by ventral colon rupture, were noted in both foals.[142]

Clinical signs associated with varying degrees of hypoxic, ischemic gut injury include ileus, gastric reflux, colic, lethargy, abdominal distention, and diarrhea. Reflux and feces may be positive for blood. Generalized sepsis often accompanies NEC. NEC should be distinguished from intestinal ileus secondary to other neonatal diseases, other surgical gastrointestinal tract lesions, bacterial or viral enterocolitis, and intolerance to a milk diet. Although no single laboratory test is specific for NEC, the abdominal radiograph often reveals pneumatosis cystoides intestinalis, bowel wall edema, and an abnormal gas pattern consistent with ileus. Ultrasonography may reveal intramural gas accumulation. If intestinal perforation has occurred, pneumoperitoneum and septic peritonitis may also be noted.[142,143] Intestinal perforation is associated with a poor prognosis.

Abomasal Tympany

Acute abdominal distention, colic, depression, and sudden death have been reported in neonatal calves with abomasal ulcers, abomasitis, and abomasal tympany. Possible sequelae to abomasal dilation include abomasal torsion, perforation, or rupture. Numerous causes have been postulated including dietary changes, in particular, the addition of coarse roughage feeds, abomasal bezoars, copper deficiency, and various microorganisms. Roeder and colleagues[145] isolated *Clostridium perfringens* type A from a group of 8 calves affected by this syndrome and subsequently experimentally reproduced the disease by intraruminal inoculation of the organism.[146] *Campylobacter* spp. have been incriminated in other studies. Histopathologic evaluation of abomasums from 38 affected calves at necropsy revealed 31 contained abundant gram-positive bacteria associated with the damaged abomasal mucosa.[147] *Campylobacter*-like organisms were demonstrated in 9 and *C. perfringens* in 14 of the 38 cases.[147] Studies of range cattle in west central Nebraska and Wyoming suggest subclinical trace mineral deficiencies of copper or selenium may be involved in the pathogenesis of the condition in this region.[148]

Onset of clinical signs is rapid, and afflicted animals become anorexic, depressed, or occasionally restless. Signs of abdominal discomfort manifesting as treading on the spot and kicking at the abdomen are observed in approximately half of the cases. On physical examination, splashing and metallic sounds are heard on succussion of the distended abdomen; passage of a stomach tube fails to releave the distension. Fecal output is reduced and occasionally melena is observed. Early in the clinical course, calves are likely to have a marked metabolic alkalosis; however, rapid deterioration and onset of shock is common and accompanied by metabolic acidosis. Observation of metabolic acidosis carries a poor prognosis.

Management of abomasal tympany requires rapid relief of the abomasal distention. Paracentesis through the right flank often fails to completely drain the abomasum and carries a high risk of inducing peritonitis.[149] Kumper[150] describes good results with paracentesis using a 1.4- by 50-mm needle when the calf is turned upside down and the abomasum is deflated by inserting a needle in the highest point of the distended abdominal wall between the umbilicus and xiphoid. Of 21 calves suffering from abomasal tympany, 20 were successfully managed without complications using this technique. Repeated paracentesis carries a high risk of inducing peritonitis. If after paracentesis the calf's condition deteriorates or tympany recurs, a right flank laparotomy is performed in order to correct a possibly torsed abomasum.[150] Intravenous fluids are administered to correct dehydration, electrolyte, and metabolic derangements.

A decreased prevalence of abomasal tympany and ulceration were reported in neonatal calves from herds having a history of these problems after implementation of a *C. perfringens* vaccination program.[148,151]

Abomasal bloat is a significant problem in artificially raised lambs. Feeding systems that allow lambs to drink large quantities of milk replacer at infrequent intervals and housing lambs on litter are predisposing factors.[152,153] Proliferation of lactobacilli, *Escherichia coli*, and *C. perfringens* have been implicated in the disease process.[153,154] Fermentation of sugars contained in milk replacer produces carbon dioxide, distending the abomasum.[155] Lambs may die within hours as a result of acute abdominal tympany compromising vascular return and respiration. Early treatment of bloated lambs with oral doses of antibiotics is sometimes an effective treatment. Addition of 0.1% formalin (37% formaldehyde) to milk replacer reduces the incidence of the condition.[154]

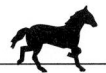

Ruminal Bloat

Ruminal bloat is uncommon in calves younger than 5 weeks of age because of the relatively undeveloped state of the neonatal rumen. Causes of rumen bloat in calves include rumen putrefaction, obstruction of the cardia or esophagus, and vagal indigestion.

If milk arrives in the rumen in greater quantities than normal by escaping the esophageal groove, it can be subjected to putrefative decomposition by proteolytic bacteria. Normally the rumen of neonatal calves has a stable aerobic bacterial population. Anaerobic conditions are rapidly established when appreciable amounts of fermentable substances enter the rumen.[156] Clinical signs include diarrhea, poor development, rough haircoat, and recurrent bloat. Reducing the volume of milk fed per feeding, feeding from nipples rather than buckets, and introduction of calf starter to promote rumen development helps prevent the condition. A course of oral antibiotics (500 mg oxytetracycline) once daily for 3 to 4 days may help affected calves by killing the putrefactive gut flora.

Bloat is occasionally observed as a complication of severe bronchopneumonia in calves as a consequence of swollen mediastinal lymph nodes compressing the esophagus or compression or inflamation of the vagus.[157] Relief of rumen distention is important for return of rumen function. Chronic rumen bloat may be relieved by placement of a rumen fistula (Buff's screw trocar). Correct placement of the screw, as described by Dirksen and Garry,[158] reduces the risk of inducing peritonitis. The rumen must be bloated so that it lies firmly against the body wall as the trocar is screwed into place. The site for the trocar is shaved and scrubbed, a small skin incision is made, and the trocar is quickly and forcefully screwed into the belly wall and rumen. After removal of the stylet, the outer rim of the trocar is kept under constant outward tension so that the ruminal wall is held tightly against the parietal peritoneum by the last ridge of the screw. To fix the trocar in this position, gauze soaked in antibiotic should be wrapped around the stem of the trocar between the outer rim and the body wall.[158]

Gastrointestinal Ulceration

Gastroduodenal disease in the slightly older foal is covered in greater detail in Chapter 30. Gastrointestinal ulceration has also been associated with several neonatal diseases, including neonatal maladjustment syndrome, asphyxiation, enteritis, and septicemia.[159] It is also observed in a many clinically normal neonates. In endoscopic surveys of neonatal foals in the United States, England, and Ireland, approximately one half of foals younger than 3 months of age had evidence of gastric ulceration.[160,161] The prevalence of lesions was greatest in 2- to 9-day-old foals and 30- to 59-day-old foals. In the young foals, typical lesions were golden-colored crusts in the squamous mucosa next to the margo plicatus along the greater curvature in association with diffuse ulceration/erosion and, commonly, squamous epithelial desquamation.[161] In one of these studies, foals that had a previous disorder (e.g., diarrhea, illness, transport) were more likely to have a glandular mucosal lesion than those that had not (9% vs. 4%).[161]

The clinical signs of bruxism, excessive salivation, and colic that are commonly associated with gastroduodenal ulcer disease in the 1- to 4-month-old foal are rarely observed in the neonatal foal. Frequently, gastric perforation is the first indication of the problem. Perforated and bleeding gastric ulcers have been diagnosed as early as 24 hours of age. There is also a high incidence of abomasal ulceration in calves, but rarely do they become symptomatic unless perforation occurs. Currently the etiology and pathophysiology of the condition in the neonatal period is not known. Because of the difficulty of diagnosing the condition without specialized endoscopic equipment and the often catastrophic consequences of subsequent perforation or pyloric or duodenal stricture formation, antiulcer medications are often used prophylactically in the compromised neonatal foal. Foals at highest risk for ulcers are sick neonates that are not recumbent and foals suffering from hypoxic gut damage, enterocolitis, and painful orthopedic conditions. Foals that are chronically recumbent frequently maintain a high pH that may be due to ileus and enterogastric reflux.[162] In normal foals the mean hourly baseline gastric pH ranged from 3.2 to 3.7. Milk intake had a dramatic but transient alkalinizing effect on pH. H_2 blockers, including ranitidine and omeprazole, significantly raised gastric pH. Ranitidine administered intravenously at 2.0 mg/kg or orally at 6.6 mg/kg significantly raised gastric pH. Initial therapy includes the use of H_2 blockers (cimetidine 15 to 20 mg/kg PO every 6 hours, ranitidine 6 to 8 mg/kg PO every 8 hours), cytoprotective agents (sucralfate 20 mg/kg PO every 6 hours), and a new class of drugs, proton pump inhibitors (omeprazole [Gastrogard] 4 mg/kg PO once daily). Omeprazole is highly effective and has the advantage of once-daily administration. Treatment regimens should continue for a minimum of 21 to 28 days. In acute stages, some foals receive additional pain relief from Digel* (simethicone calcium carbonate, and magnesium hydroxide) administration (10 to 20 ml every 3 to 4 hours). Some foals are in too much pain to nurse, and they benefit from withholding enteral feeds temporarily and maintaining them on a brief course of parenteral alimentation using a mixture of amino acids, lipids, dextrose, electrolytes, and vitamins. Currently recommended dosages for antiulcer medications are listed in Chapter 30.

Abomasal ulcers are usually asymptomatic in young calves, but, if perforation occurs, peritonitis and shock rapidly develop. Clinical signs include abdominal distention, pain on abdominal palpation, expiratory grunt, drooling saliva, bruxism, and melena. Less commonly a syndrome of chronic abdominal pain is observed after abomasal perforation.[135] Absence of inflammatory changes suggest the gut is unlikely to be perforated or necrotic. Severe hypoproteinemia is common with diffuse peritonitis presumably because of the combination of poor colostral uptake and loss of protein into the abdominal exudate. Obtaining peritoneal fluid from normal calves is difficult; if peritonitis is suspected, collection of abdominal fluid is facilitated by locating pockets of peritoneal fluid via abdominal ultrasound.

Clinically, more abomasal ulcers seem to appear during or shortly after a period of weather-induced stress.[163] This may be associated with higher endogenous cortisol secretion.[148] Perforating abomasal ulcers in calves have also been associated with *C. perfringens* abomasitis,[145] copper deficiency, dietary changes, mycotic infections, and abomasal bezoars.

Perforated abomasal ulcers are repaired surgically by a right paracostal approach. The ulcers are commonly located on the midpart of the fundus, on the greater curvature of the abomasum. Prognosis is guarded (40%).[163]

Hemoperitoneum

Hemoperitoneum is a relatively uncommon cause of abdominal distention in the large animal neonate. The structures usually responsible for the hemorrhage are the umbilical vessels and rupture of the liver or spleen secondary to trauma. Other structures such as a ruptured granulosa cell tumor may bleed.[164] Depending on the cause, time course, and

---

*Digel, Schering Plough Health Care, Memphis, TN 38151.

severity of the hemorrhage, clinical signs relating to hypovolemia and anemia may be mild or severe. Diagnosis of hemoperitoneum is based on the retrieval of free-flowing blood on peritoneal tap and the detection of free fluid in the abdomen. Ultrasound examination may be of benefit in detecting the source of the bleeding. Prevention of hypovolemic shock is critical, regardless of the source of the hemorrhage, and intensive patient monitoring and intervention are often indicated. Whole blood transfusion may be necessary (see Chapter 35). If an internally bleeding animal with an unstable cardiovascular system is rushed to surgery without prior stabilization, profound shock may occur, and a poor outcome usually results.

SEIZURES

JOHN K. HOUSE

IDENTIFICATION OF NEONATAL SEIZURE ACTIVITY

Seizures may be generalized or partial, depending on the part of the cerebral cortex affected by abnormal electrical activity. Involuntary muscle activity, opisthotonos, paddling, and extensor rigidity are signs associated with a generalized convulsion. In the neonate, more subtle neurologic signs also may be associated with seizure activity. In the human infant, particularly the premature infant, the neuromuscular system is not fully developed at birth and is therefore unable to fully express the abnormal electrical activity in cerebral neurons. Abnormal breathing patterns, lip smacking, chomping, rapid eye movements, small limb movements, and tremor may be the only signs indicating seizure activity in the human infant. Similar signs in the abnormal neonatal foal also have been attributed to seizure activity.[165]

In the large animal neonate, several conditions should be distinguished from seizure activity. Bizarre movements associated with rapid eye movement (REM) sleep, particularly prominent in the premature foal, are frequently confused with seizure activity by the inexperienced observer. Signs can be similar and include rapid eye movement, rhythmic paddling of the limbs, and chomping. The two conditions can be distinguished by attempting to arouse the animal; if activity is associated with REM sleep, the animal should be easily aroused to full consciousness. A foal that is simply resisting restraint in lateral recumbency also may appear to be seizing, and violent paddling of the limbs and occasionally opisthotonos are noted. If confusion exists as to the cause of the activity, the animal is encouraged to stand, and its behavior is then evaluated. Finally, in the foal the cataplexy-narcolepsy syndrome may be confused with convulsions. This "fainting foal syndrome" was first described in 1924 in three Suffolk foals that showed signs within a few hours after birth,[166] and a familial occurrence was recently reported in Miniature Horse foals.[167] Any exciting stimulus, including petting and restraint, can trigger the attacks, during which affected foals suddenly appear to be asleep, with flaccid limbs yet open eyes.

DIAGNOSIS OF THE ETIOLOGY OF SEIZURE ACTIVITY

Once seizure activity is identified, its cause should be investigated (Box 20-4). A complete history is obtained, including a detailed description of the delivery process, and complete physical and neurologic examinations are performed. Any signs of trauma, infection, or congenital malformations

---

BOX 20-4

Causes of Neonatal Seizures

PERINATAL COMPLICATIONS
Hypoxic-ischemic brain injury
Intracranial hemorrhage
Cerebral contusion, secondary to birth trauma

METABOLIC DERANGEMENTS
Hyponatremia
Hypernatremia
Hypocalcemia
Hypoglycemia
Hypomagnesemia
Metabolic acidosis

INFECTION
Generalized sepsis without evidence of meningitis
Bacterial meningitis or encephalitis
Botulism
Central nervous system parasite migration
Tyzzer's disease
Viral encephalitis

TRAUMA (DRUG-ASSOCIATED)
Premature withdrawal from anticonvulsant medication
Theophylline at toxic blood levels
Ingestion or administration of toxins
Intracarotid injection of oil or water-soluble drugs

DEVELOPMENTAL MALFORMATIONS AND ABNORMALITIES
Hydrocephalus
Hydranencephaly
Hypomyelinogenesis
Defects in amino acid metabolism (maple syrup urine disease, citrullinemia in calves)
Storage diseases (GM-1 gangliosidosis [B], "shaker" calf)
Congenital myoclonus (extensor spasms) (B)

LIVER FAILURE

IDIOPATHIC EPILEPSY

RABIES

HEAT STROKE

B, Bovine.

---

should be noted. Evaluation of hematologic data and IgG status, combined with historic and physical examination parameters, results in an assessment of the likelihood of sepsis (see Diagnosis of Bacterial Infection, Chapter 19). Blood glucose and serum electrolyte concentrations should be determined promptly. A chemistry panel, blood gas analysis, and bacterial cultures of blood and other body fluids and possibly cerebrospinal fluid (CSF) analysis and skull radiographs complete the database in most cases.

Before attempting to collect CSF (see Chapter 33), the benefit of the information likely to be obtained must be weighed against the small risk to the patient and the inconvenience of having to analyze the sample within 30 minutes of collection. In the large animal neonate, as in the adult, either the atlantooccipital or lumbosacral site may be used. Depending on the state of consciousness of the neonate, local anesthesia with manual restraint or light sedation, or general anesthesia may be required to obtain the fluid. For collection of fluid from the atlantooccipital site, a 20-gauge, 1- to 2-inch

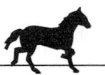

needle with a clear hub may be used. A change in resistance is felt when the needle penetrates the dural membranes, and CSF appears in the plastic hub as soon as the subarachnoid space is entered. Approximately 5 to 10 ml of fluid may be removed safely from foals.[165]

Urinary reagent strips can be used to rapidly obtain general information on the fluid. If blood is detected, the sample should be spun down after the cytologic examination. Red blood cells contaminating the sample will settle, and the supernatant should be colorless. If hemorrhage occurred before the procedure, the sample remains xanthochromic (yellow). Glucose should be present in "trace" or "+" amounts in the normal sample. Negative values in the adult suggest severe meningitis, but in the neonate may also be caused by profound hypoglycemia. The total protein level is increased in neonatal foal CSF compared with the level in the CSF of the adult horse, averaging 1.38 ± 0.5 g/L (138 ± 50 mg/dl) during the first 40 hours after delivery,[168] and slight xanthochromia is often present. Immaturity of the blood-brain barrier is postulated as one reason for the difference in CSF protein between adult and neonatal animals.

Vascular accidents in the neonate are tentatively diagnosed on the basis of a xanthochromic sample, elevated total protein levels, increased numbers of erythrocytes, and microscopic identification of erythrophagocytosis (best). CSF analysis is most useful in determining the presence of septic meningitis. Elevation of the total protein level (>150 mg/dl) and neutrophil count in addition to a positive Gram stain and bacterial culture results in a straightforward diagnosis of bacterial meningitis, and the prognosis is considered poor for the animal.[169] Infection in the central nervous system (CNS), however, can be difficult to detect until the process becomes generalized; the lack of positive cultures and Gram stain does not rule out CNS infection. An elevated albumin quotient suggests increased blood-brain permeability and can be seen in both hypoxic-ischemic brain injury and meningitis, but an elevated IgG index indicates increased intrathecal IgG production and is more compatible with a diagnosis of meningitis.[170]

Ultrasonography and computerized tomography (CT) are important procedures for evaluating anatomic causes of seizures (hemorrhage, infarct, malformations) in the human infant. Because the fontanelles are usually closed in the large animal neonate, ultrasound imaging is of limited or no use. Although CT or magnetic resonance imaging (MRI) are potentially useful techniques for diagnosis of brain abnormalities in large animal neonates, historically, facilities with CT scans have not often been available to the veterinary neonate. Currently, more referral veterinary hospitals are obtaining this type of imaging capacity, and several human and research facilities are available for veterinary patients. Antemortem diagnosis of agenesis of the corpus callosum and associated malformations was made using CT scanning in a foal that had an abnormally shaped head and seizures refractory to anticonvulsant therapy.[171] Identification of the specific abnormalities early in the clinical course allowed the owners to make a more informed decision regarding the treatment of the foal, and the clinicians to acquire valuable information regarding the prognosis of a specific malformation in the horse.

TREATMENT OF NEONATAL SEIZURES

Generalized seizures should be controlled immediately. Diazepam* is often the initial drug chosen for seizure control because of its rapid effect. A dose of 5 to 20 mg for a 45-kg neonate is slowly administered and its effect monitored. In some individuals, one dose controls the seizure, and repeat seizures are not observed; in others, multiple doses at frequent intervals may become necessary. In these animals, other longer-acting anticonvulsants are often required.

Phenobarbital* acts by raising the seizure threshold, and its peak effect is seen at approximately 30 minutes. An initial dose of 10 to 20 mg/kg diluted in saline and given intravenously over 15 minutes has been used successfully to control seizures in clinical patients. This initial dose is followed by a maintenance dosage of 10 mg/kg IV every 12 hours. Oral tablets also may be used. The major side effect of phenobarbital in foals has been mild sedation and ataxia. Interactions between phenobarbital and other drugs usually involve induction of the hepatic microsomal enzyme system. Weaning from anticonvulsant therapy should be gradual to avoid recurrence of seizure activity.

Phenytoin† also has been used for seizure control in the newborn foal. The initial dose is 5 to 10 mg/kg IV followed by 1 to 5 mg/kg every 2 to 4 hours. This dosage has resulted in effective seizure control in several foals unresponsive to both diazepam and phenobarbital, but it also appeared to cause marked depression in some patients. Little is known about the pharmacokinetics of the drug in the large animal neonate.

Pentobarbital anesthesia also has been used to control seizures, but its use has been associated with marked respiratory depression, hypotension, hypothermia, and prolonged anesthesia. Xylazine is also a potent sedative in the foal, but its side effects also have included markedly depressed cardiovascular and respiratory function and prolonged recovery in abnormal foals. Neither pentobarbital nor xylazine is recommended for seizure control in the foal, unless other agents are not available.

SPECIFIC DISORDERS CAUSING SEIZURES

Neonatal Maladjustment Syndrome in the Foal

The term *neonatal maladjustment syndrome* (NMS) has been used to describe a noninfectious central nervous system (CNS) disorder of newborn foals of normal gestational length associated with gross behavioral abnormalities. Synonyms for the condition include "barkers," "wanderers," and "dummies." The time of onset of signs varies from immediately after birth to about 24 hours of age. A variety of neurologic disorders have been lumped together and placed in this category, and the etiology is probably not the same for all of them. More specific terminology is needed to describe abnormalities of neurologic function and behavior in the neonatal foal, but at the current time, the foal's brain largely remains a "black box." Until we have a better understanding of the etiology of the condition(s) causing neurologic dysfunction, a better classification system is probably impossible. It is important, however, to avoid the tendency to apply the term *NMS* to any individual showing neurologic signs, without making the effort to rule out other conditions, particularly infection, that frequently cause similar clinical signs.

HISTORY. The history may include a description of a fast, uncomplicated delivery of a term foal or, alternatively, a known dystocia and period of asphyxia. In one study, 20% of foals with the clinical diagnosis of NMS experienced dystocia.[171]

CLINICAL SIGNS. Affected foals may primarily show deranged cerebral function, signs primarily of spinal cord

---

*Valium, Hoffman-LaRoche, Inc, Nutley, NJ 07110.

*Eli Lilley, Indianapolis, IN 46285.
†Dilantin, Parke-Davis, Detroit, MI 48063.

damage, or both. Commonly observed head signs include loss of suckle reflex, aimless wandering and apparent central blindness, hyperexcitability or depression, extensor spasms or clonic convulsions, excessive chewing and salivation, abnormal vocalization, and abnormal respiratory patterns. Spinal cord signs include weakness in front, hind, or all limbs, depending on the location of the lesion; ataxia; and depressed spinal reflexes. Foals may show normal behavior for a variable period after birth, which may be suddenly followed by a period of worsening neurologic function.

PATHOLOGY. CNS lesions could not be identified grossly or histologically in approximately 60% of foals with the clinical diagnosis of NMS that received necropsies. In the remaining 40% the most common findings included necrosis of the brainstem, diencephalon, and cerebral cortex; hemorrhage in the white and gray matter of the cerebral cortex and cerebellum; subarachnoid hemorrhage in the brain and spinal cord; and edema surrounding the areas of hemorrhage.[172]

ETIOLOGY. The etiology of the condition is not well defined. The necrotic CNS lesions are similar to lesions resulting from experimentally induced asphyxia in neonates of other species. In many cases of NMS, however, a clear-cut episode of hypoxia is not observed. Johnson and Rossdale[173] suggested that an increase in intracranial vascular pressure during delivery could be responsible for the observed pathology. They also presented evidence that substantial CNS vascular pressure increases can occur in response to partial asphyxia and airway obstruction. Premature human infants have a high incidence of intraventricular hemorrhage which, unlike as in foals, originates primarily from the germinal matrix of the subependymal region. The vessels in this area are thought to lack structural maturity and autoregulatory ability and therefore are predisposed to damage by hypoxic events and increased arterial pressures. Unfortunately, the regulation of the vasculature in the CNS of the foal is not well understood.

DIAGNOSIS. To make a diagnosis of NMS, other disease processes causing similar signs must be ruled out. In particular, septicemia, meningitis, and metabolic disturbances can closely mimic NMS. Thus collection of a complete database as outlined previously is essential to differentiate the possibilities. It is important to obtain a complete history and in particular to establish the peripartum events and time of birth. NMS would be unlikely in a previously normal foal with onset of seizure activity at 3 days of life; septicemia or electrolyte abnormalities would be more probable diagnoses. Foals with NMS should have a relatively normal WBC count and fibrinogen and normal electrolytes. CSF analysis may reveal increased xanthochromia, protein, and red blood cells (RBCs), but in many cases is normal. Thoracic radiographs and arterial blood gas analysis commonly indicate some degree of respiratory dysfunction. Moderate hypoxemia and hypercapnia and interstitial infiltrates suggestive of pneumonia or atelectasis are common. Blood and other bacterial cultures should be negative, at least at the time of onset of clinical signs. IgG determination at 18 to 24 hours of age commonly reveals failure of passive transfer (FPT) of immunity, usually resulting from insufficient colostral intake during the first hours of life as a result of the onset of behavioral abnormalities. This FPT predisposes the individual to secondary bacterial infection, which, if treated improperly, frequently results in the demise of the animal.

TREATMENT. Therapy is directed at control of seizures and aimless thrashing. Diazepam and phenobarbital are the most commonly used anticonvulsants, but careful manual restraint on a well-padded surface is also important to avoid self-inflicted trauma if the foal is down. In particular, entropion and corneal ulceration must be identified and treated promptly to avoid needless prolongation of hospital stay. Appropriate nursing care is crucial for a favorable outcome.

Body temperature, hydration, caloric intake, electrolyte, blood-gas and acid-base balance, and cleanliness must be maintained during the period of convalescence. Once the foal is coherent, it often must relearn how to walk, nurse, and follow its mother; and the process is usually extremely labor intensive. FPT is best prevented by ensuring that the foal ingests at least 1 L of good-quality (specific gravity >1.06) colostrum in the first 6 hours of life. If FPT occurs, plasma and antibiotic therapy is indicated, and the foal should be monitored closely for signs of infection. Gastric ulceration is also common in foals with NMS, and antiulcer medication (see Chapter 30) is usually administered empirically, particularly if a nasogastric tube is being used for nutritional support.

Dimethyl sulfoxide (DMSO) has been used intravenously in foals showing neurologic abnormalities suggestive of NMS. It is used to reduce cerebral edema, as well as to scavenge oxygen free radicals that may result from asphyxial damage. Adverse effects have not been noted at a dosage of 1 g/kg diluted to a 10% to 20% solution and given intravenously once or twice a day, nor is there clear-cut evidence of efficacy.

Multisystem dysfunction often accompanies neurologic signs in asphyxiated foals, and failure to recognize and address these problems until late in the clinical course often results in a poor outcome (see Chapter 16).

CLINICAL COURSE AND PROGNOSIS. Despite often severe signs of neurologic dysfunction, many foals diagnosed as having NMS make a complete recovery with intensive nursing care and become normal, athletic performance horses as adults; usually no residual neurologic deficits are present on neurologic examination. The best prognosis is associated with a normal IgG level at 18 hours of age and an apparently normal, spontaneous delivery with the term foal standing and making efforts to nurse before showing signs of maladjustment. In one multicenter study, foals with these characteristics had a 91% discharge rate from the hospital.[174] In the same study, if term foals showed neurologic signs immediately after a known difficult delivery or period of asphyxia, the discharge rate fell to 50%. If failure of passive transfer results in secondary infection or if the foal never stood or demonstrated a suckling response, the prognosis also decreased.

Despite these overall statistics, it is still difficult, if not impossible, to predict early in the clinical course which individual neonates are going to fully recover from neurologic disease and which will not, either because of congenital brain abnormalities or permanent damage secondary to asphyxia or other injury. Most foals that recover from NMS show some plateauing of severity of clinical signs at 24 to 48 hours and gradual improvement after 48 to 72 hours. If more than 4 days pass without any signs of improvement, the prognosis becomes considerably more guarded. If the head is malformed, or if the foal shows little improvement after 4 to 5 days, additional diagnostic procedures, such as MRI, are probably indicated to rule out anatomic malformations or severe brain injury. As more data are collected and analyzed, it is hoped that improvement will be made in the understanding of brain injury in the large animal neonate.

Meningitis

Although bacterial meningitis may occur as a primary entity, it more commonly is a result of generalized septicemia in neonates with FPT. Agents causing meningitis are the same that cause septicemia, most commonly the gram-negative enteric bacteria such as *E. coli*, *Enterobacter* spp., and *Salmonella* spp. Because clinical signs of meningitis are easily confused with NMS and septicemia without localization in the CNS, diagnosis depends on CSF analysis (see Chapter 33). Treatment recommendations for treating bacterial CNS infections may be found in Chapter 33. Although there is one report on

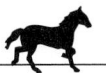

the successful treatment of two neonatal foals with suspected meningitis using third-generation cephalosporins,[175] in many cases, once the diagnosis is made the infectious process is often well advanced both in the brain and other tissues, resulting in a poor outcome.

In a recent review of 32 cases of meningitis in calves by Green and Smith,[176] the clinical signs of CNS disturbance observed were lethargy, recumbency, anorexia, loss of suckle reflex, coma, opisthotonos, convulsions, tremor, and hyperesthesia. Leukocytosis and a left shift were evident in 11 of 15 (73%) calves. Concurrent metabolic problems were common and included hyperkalemia, respiratory acidosis, hypernatremia, hyponatremia, hypomagnesemia, and hypoglycemia. Analysis of CSF revealed pleocytosis, xanthochromia, turbidity, and high total protein concentration. Cytologically, neutrophils predominated in the CSF in calves with acute disease. Mononuclear cells dominated in calves with chronic disease. Microscopically, bacteria were evident in 10 of 22 (45%) of the antemortem CSF samples, and bacteria were isolated from slightly more than half (11/19). The prognosis for recovery, even with appropriate antimicrobial therapy, is poor.[176]

DIARRHEA IN NEONATAL FOALS

JOHN E. MADIGAN

Diarrhea in the neonatal foal is a common disorder that carries the potential for more rapid development of systemic manifestations of illness than in the adult. Great variation in causes for diarrhea in this age-group and the varying degree of illnesses produced make careful evaluation important (Box 20-5). Evaluation of the neonate with diarrhea requires careful observation for signs of depression, dehydration, colic, or abdominal distention. A history should be obtained for age-related causes of diarrhea (foal heat) and use of antimicrobials or other agents capable of producing alterations in gastrointestinal function. Neonates with colic symptoms present difficult diagnostic dilemmas because they may have enteritis that results in diarrhea or mechanical intestinal problems such as volvulus, intussusception, foreign bodies, or colon torsion. In contrast to adult horses with diarrhea, the neonate is especially prone to developing septicemia concurrent with diarrhea. Endotoxemia and bacteremia may produce rapid development of adverse signs and death. Diarrhea may accompany bacteremia, especially in foals less than 7 days of age, and may be associated with signs of depression or loss of suck reflex and should be rapidly and more completely assessed. Causes of diarrhea include bacteria, viruses, nutrition, parasites, foal heat, gastric ulcers, mechanical displacements or blockages, and antimicrobial usage.

DIFFERENTIAL DIAGNOSES

Bacteria

Clostridial species have gained increased recognition as causes of diarrhea in the equine neonate. *C. perfringens* types A, B, and C and *Clostridium septicum* can cause signs of colic, bloody diarrhea, and rapid progression to death within the first 48 hours of life.[177-181] Age-related susceptibilities may be related to a lack of intestinal proteases or trypsin inhibitors in colostrum. Diagnosis is based on demonstration of large numbers of gram-positive rods within the small intestine, toxin neutralization tests in mice, or blood culture.[181,182] Hematologic findings often reveal a severe neutropenia and lymphopenia and hyperfibrinogenemia with hypoalbuminemia and metabolic acidosis. Blood culture may reveal other gram-negative bacteria, presumably from breakdown of the gut barrier. Exotoxins produced cause hemorrhagic necrosis in the gut wall. *Clostridium difficile* and its toxins have been identified from foals with watery diarrhea from 2 to 5 days of age.[183] *C. difficile* was detected in non–antibiotic-treated foals from an outbreak involving several cases, resulting in several fatalities. Clinical signs varied from mild to severe diarrhea with abdominal cramping and hemorrhagic necrotizing enteritis.[183] Diagnosis requires culture on selective media for *C. difficile* (*C. difficile* agar plates) or demonstration of cytotoxin in feces. The presence of other pathogenic agents must be ruled out because *C. difficile* has been isolated from normal foals. Foals that recover from severe enterocolitis may later develop colic as a result of adhesions.[183] Treatment provided in cases identified early include oral metronidazole to lower numbers of clostridial species and systemic antimicrobials for concurrent gram-negative septicemia; intensive care is usually required and mortality is high.

Salmonellosis in foals younger than 14 days of age often presents with acute septicemia and bacteremia that initially may be without signs of diarrhea. Other less virulent strains or factors of stress and immunity may allow signs of enteritis with only mild diarrhea. Depression, mild colic, dehydration, and toxic mucous membranes may be noted initially. In cases with bacteremia, lung, joint, vertebral body, renal, ocular (uveitis), or nervous system involvement may be noted. Hematologic signs include neutropenia, left shift, and toxic granulation of neutrophils (these are not pathognomonic for *Salmonella* infection). Many serotypes produce disease in foals, including *Salmonella typhimurium* and *Salmonella saintpaul*. Newborn foals may acquire infection from asymptomatic shedding of *Salmonella* strains by the mare that are not virulent in adult horses.

Diagnosis is made by culture of the organism from feces, rectal biopsy, or blood.[184] Because the organism is not shed

---

BOX 20-5

Causes of Diarrhea in Foals

FOAL HEAT
Cause unknown, possibly diet changes

NUTRITION
Milk (lactase deficiency)
Milk replacers
Concentrates

PARASITES
Strongyloides westeri
Strongylus vulgaris
Cryptosporidia

VIRUSES
Rota
Corona

BACTERIA
Salmonellosis
Clostridium perfringens types A, B, and C, necrotizing enterocolitis
Clostridium difficile
Campylobacter spp.
Bacteriodes fragilis
Rhodococcus equi

MECHANICAL OBSTRUCTIONS

FOREIGN BODIES

ANTIBIOTICS

in a constant manner, five or more fecal cultures may be required to identify the organism. Ten to 15 g of feces placed in enrichment media is recommended at a ratio of 1:10.[184]

Foals less than 2 months of age appear to be more susceptible to bacteremia than adults exposed to the same enteric bacterial pathogens. Consequently, in addition to the fluid and electrolyte considerations, blood cultures, and determination of a sepsis score (see Fig. 19-1), the use of antimicrobials with a gram-negative spectrum is appropriate in some cases of suspected bacterial diarrheas.

Several different bacteria have been implicated but not proven to be causes of foal diarrhea. Enterotoxigenic *Bacteroides fragilis* has been isolated from foals less than 7 days old with diarrhea.[185] *Campylobacter* spp. can be found in feces of foals with or without diarrhea and in foals with intestinal perforations, but the overall significance is not known.[186-188] Although *E. coli* is a well-documented cause of diarrhea in other species, it has not proved to be a primary cause of diarrhea in foals, except from one report of effacing *E. coli* in a foal.[189-192] However, *E. coli* is the most frequent blood culture isolate from septicemic foals.[190,193] *Rhodococcus equi* may cause abscesses and enteric disease, leading to diarrhea in foals 2 to 6 months of age.[191,194]

Viruses

Rotavirus is an established cause of diarrhea in foals (either alone or in conjunction with other bacterial agents).[190,191,195-206] Rotavirus affects the small intestine and invades the villus epithelial cells, causing loss of absorptive cells.[207] Villus atrophy and compensatory crypt cell proliferation combine to cause decreased fluid absorption and increased secretion. Initial signs may be depression and anorexia, which progress to watery diarrhea. Disease occurs in foals less than 2 months of age. Severely affected foals may show severe dehydration, weight loss, poor growth rate, and unthriftiness for some time after cessation of severe diarrhea. Lactase deficiency has been suggested to play a role after epithelial cell damage. Because epithelial cells that normally produce lactase are lost, lactose moves undigested into the colon where it is fermented, releasing osmotically active particles in the colon. Rotavirus is prevalent; most adult horses have evidence of exposure (by demonstration of serum antibody). Infections can occur as outbreaks of diarrhea in susceptible foals following periods of crowding and stress, which may allow amplification of rotavirus numbers. Initial sources of infection may be adult horses or recovered foals that, under some circumstances, may intermittently shed the virus for up to 8 months.[195] In recent studies 10 days was the longest shedding time detected in foals after recovery from clinical rotavirus diarrhea.[198] Rotavirus persists in the environment for up to 9 months.[196] Rotavirus disinfection requires the use of phenolic disinfectants because bleach is not effective.

Diagnosis of rotavirus requires detection of virus in feces and tests to rule out pathogens causing concurrent infection. Tests include electron microscopy, enzyme-linked immunosorbent assay (ELISA), and latex agglutination Virogen Rotatest.*

Both of the rotavirus serotypes identified in the equine are detected by these tests, and the latter two commercial tests have good correlation with electron microscopy.[186,195] Virus is shed in large concentration early on during infection.[208] Prevention involves good hygiene and reduction in crowding. The use of bovine rotavirus vaccines is not uniformly pre-

ventive in the foal.[206] There is limited cross protection in calves and pigs among human, calf, pig, and foal rotaviruses.[199] Colostrum containing high levels of antirotaviral antibodies prevents infection on a short-term basis.[208] Coronavirus and adenovirus have been isolated from foals with diarrhea, but the causative relationship with overt clinical signs requires further investigation.[209-213]

Parasites

Strongyloides westeri is a common parasite of foals, with early infection of the foal occurring through mare's milk. Experimental studies have indicated that higher numbers of infective larvae than are found in milk are needed to produce diarrhea.[214] In addition, foals with high egg counts (prepatent period 8 to 14 days) are often asymptomatic. *S. westeri* is susceptible to a variety of anthelmintics, including ivermectin (200 µg/kg),[215] thiabendazole (50 mg/kg),[190,215] cambendazole (20 mg/kg),[190,215] and oxibendazole (10 mg/kg).[190,215] *Strongylus vulgaris* can migrate into arteries by 14 to 20 days after infection and therefore may be a potential cause of gastrointestinal disturbances during this phase. Fever, abdominal pain, and diarrhea have been observed in experimental cases[190,216,217] and may occur naturally in the foal. The long prepatent period of *S. vulgaris* precludes use of fecal egg counts for diagnosis. *Eimeria leukarti* is commonly found in feces of foals from approximately 30 to 125 days of age.[218] It is unlikely to be a cause of diarrhea in foals, although definitive proof is lacking.[219]

Cryptosporidium spp. have been isolated from feces of foals with diarrhea and may play a role as a causative agent.[220] A recent study using a direct immunofluorescence staining method detected *Cryptosporidium* spp. in 15% to 31% of normal foals in Ohio and Kentucky. Foals start excreting *Cryptosporidium* spp. between 4 and 19 weeks of age. Infection is much lower in weanlings and not detectable in yearlings and mares.[221] Foals with *Cryptosporidium* spp. detected in those studies did not have diarrhea. *Giardia* spp. may be found in normal foals, with infection rates reported from 17% to 35%. *Giardia* spp. are present in all age-groups, and it is believed foals acquire infection from nursing mares. Concurrent infection with *Cryptosporidium* and *Giardia* spp. may be observed.[221]

Nutrition

Nutritional causes of diarrhea include overingestion of milk (as might occur when the mare and foal are separated and rejoined) or overfeeding orphaned or sick foals. Overwhelming the ability of the small intestine to digest and absorb results in presentation of milk to the colon, where it is fermented and produces osmotically active sugars and acids.[222] In a controlled study of foals less than 5 days of age,[223] an elemental isotonic diet (Osmolyte) produced diarrhea in healthy foals when fed as the sole source of nutrition. Older foals fed a similar diet apparently did not develop diarrhea.[224] Caution should be exercised in using elemental diets designed for humans in the foal without adequate prior testing of tolerance to the diet. Orphan foals and foals fed commercial milk replacer may experience diarrhea associated with these diets.

Transient lactase deficiency has been proposed in foals.[225-227] An oral lactose tolerance test is conducted by a 4-hour fast and administration of 1 g/kg of body weight in a 20% solution of α-lactose powder and observing an increase of plasma glucose of 35 mg/dl by 90 minutes.[227] It has been postulated that agents such as rotavirus that damage epithelial cells may cause prolongation of the diarrhea because of temporary lactase deficiency (lactase is produced in mucosal cells). Lactase and cellulobiase are present at birth and decline after 4 months

---

*Rotazyme, Abbott Laboratories, North Chicago, IL 60064; Wampole Laboratories, Cranbarry, NJ 08512.

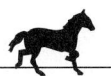

of age.[228] Yogurt has been used successfully in humans as a source of lactase.[229]

Foal Heat Diarrhea

Diarrhea developing during days 7 to 14 of life has been termed foal heat diarrhea because of the time relationship to the occurrence of postfoaling estrous in the mare. Diarrhea has developed in foals in this age-group that have been raised separated from the dam on a consistent diet and isolated from pathogens, so it does not appear to be causally related to estrus. Clinical and experimental investigations have not determined the etiology of this condition.[230-232] There is no demonstrable change in the composition of mare's milk during this time period.[232] *S. westeri* has been investigated and is not believed to be the etiologic agent of foal heat diarrhea.[214] Because foals eat hay and grain and practice coprophagia by 5 to 7 days of age, new bacterial flora and more fiber may be introduced into the gut and changes in fecal consistency may be produced.[233]

Most foal heat diarrheas are mild and require no specific therapy. Continued diarrhea, fever, or depression with signs of reduced sucking activity on the mare should be evaluated carefully, and a complete blood count (CBC) and electrolyte and acid-base determinations performed. Appropriate fluids should be administered orally or intravenously. In some persistent cases of foal heat diarrhea, intestinal protectants may be beneficial. Younger foals with profuse diarrhea require more aggressive evaluation and treatment because of the risk of septicemia associated with diarrhea.

Miscellaneous Causes

Gastric ulceration has been associated with diarrhea in foals. Ingestion of sand and irritants such as mare's tail hairs and ropes may produce diarrhea. Digital examination of the rectum may reveal sandy, gritty material in some foals.

CLINICAL PATHOLOGY AND RADIOLOGY

In addition to the fecal tests described under specific etiologies, tests for signs of systemic involvement are indicated in foals with frequency and amounts of diarrhea that may produce dehydration or in foals with fever and depression or loss of suck reflex. CBCs may indicate an enteritis or septicemia with low neutrophil count and left shift. Computation of a sepsis score (see Fig. 19-1) is indicated in foals with diarrhea that are less than 7 days of age. Assessment of renal function through serum urea nitrogen (SUN), creatinine, and urinalysis may reveal renal azotemia of prerenal or renal origin and warrant prolonged fluid therapy. Assessment of electrolyte and acid-base balance are warranted in neonatal diarrheas because hyponatremia caused by losses in the gastrointestinal tract and renal compromise can be significant. Prolonged diarrhea can lead to significant metabolic acidosis requiring fluid and bicarbonate replacement (see Chapter 19). Fecal culture and determination of fecal leukocytes and occult blood are additional diagnostic tests that may indicate a more severe disease condition.

A special problem in the foal with enteritis and pain is the differentiation of nonobstructive ileus from obstructive disease, which requires surgery. Enteritis in the foal may cause mild to severe pain. Abdominal radiography may indicate large and small bowel distention with multiple gas-filled interfaces within the small bowel that mimic obstruction.[234] However, long, erectile, inverted loops seen in cases of obstructive disease were not observed (see Figs. 20-8 and 20-9). In addition, peritoneal fluid examination is usually normal in cases of nonobstructive enteritis. However, serial evalua-

tion at 2- to 3-hour intervals for clinical signs, peritoneal fluid, and ultrasonographic and radiographic changes may be required to differentiate surgical from nonsurgical cases.[226] Abdominal ultrasonography can detect loops of small intestine. Normal findings include flaccid fluid-filled loops.[235] The bowel distends and the loops become larger and rounded with enteritis, ileus, and small intestinal obstructive disease. Intussusception is demonstrated by target or donut-shaped patterns.[235] Abdominal fluid, uroperitoneum, and peritonitis can be visualized with abdominal ultrasonography.

TREATMENT AND PROGNOSIS

The three main components of therapy of diarrhea in the neonatal foal are (1) fluid therapy (either oral or intravenous), (2) intestinal protectants/adsorbents, and (3) systemic antibiotics if indicated to treat bacteremia and/or oral antibiotics for suspected clostridial agents. Sodium-containing isotonic intravenous fluids (see Tables 20-5 and 20-6) are an important component of diarrhea therapy in the compromised neonate. Potassium is lost in severe diarrhea and, if hyperkalemia is not present, should be supplemented by adding 15 to 20 mEq/L of potassium chloride to fluids. Foals that are not nursing normally may have hypoglycemia and may need glucose-containing fluids. Acid-base correction by volume expansion and replacement of bicarbonate as needed can be lifesaving and should be monitored frequently when significant intestinal fluid losses occur.

Withholding milk has been advocated in human neonates with diarrhea, but this is more difficult to accomplish in the horse. It can be an important part of therapy, however, especially with the clostridial diarrheas. The foal can be muzzled for 8 to 12 hours while the mare is milked out, and the foal provided with oral fluids through a stomach tube or a bottle if a suck reflex is present. Although labels of electrolyte replacers do not always specify for use in foals, many preparations used in calves (see Table 20-7) have been used successfully in foals. Most of these preparations provide insufficient energy and should be used for short intervals of no more than 24 to 36 hours unless parenteral nutrition of some type is provided to maintain blood glucose levels.

Intestinal protectants may be all that are required in uncomplicated cases or may be used in conjunction with other therapies. Bismuth subsalicylate, kaolin or pectin, and activated charcoal have been used for this purpose. Suggested advantages of bismuth subsalicylate[220] are its neutralization of bacterial toxins and antisecretory effect through its local antiprostaglandin activity.[236,237] Preventive antiulcer therapy in ill foals may be beneficial in foals requiring more than basic symptomatic therapy because gastric and duodenal ulcers (see Chapter 30) may be a sequela of gastroenteritis in the foal.

Systemic antibiotics should be used in the neonate with diarrhea that may be septicemic or have compromised immunity. Blood cultures (see Chapter 19) should be obtained before initiating antimicrobial therapy. Antibiotics with a spectrum against gram-negative and gram-positive organisms should be used. Because foals with diarrhea may be dehydrated, monitoring of renal function is indicated when using potentially nephrotoxic drugs such as aminoglycosides. Plasma therapy for hypoproteinemia associated with failure of passive transfer or protein-losing enteropathy is useful to maintain plasma oncotic pressure and expected protein binding of medications. Foals with albumin levels below 2 g/dl may benefit from plasma therapy.

PREVENTION AND CONTROL

Prevention is best accomplished by minimizing density of populations of horses, separating of age-groups, providing

TABLE 20-3

Evaluation of the Pathogenicity of Various Infectious Agents as Gauged by Their Ability to Experimentally Produce Diarrhea in Calves, Field Surveys of the Incidence of Infection in Diarrheic and Healthy Calves, and Similarity in the Distribution of Intestinal Pathology and the Infectious Agent

Group	Agent Name	Experimental Production of Diarrhea		Isolated With Higher Frequency From Diarrheic Calves	Organism Associated With Intestinal Pathology
		Gnotobiotic Calves	Conventional Calves		
BACTERIAL					
	Enterotoxigenic *E. coli*		+	++/−	+
	Enterohemorrhagic *E. coli*	+	+/−		++++s
	Salmonella sp.	++	+	+	
	Campylobacter				
	fecalis		+		
	coli		++	−−	
	jejuni		++	+/−	
	Clostridium perfringens				
	type A	+	−		+
	type C	+			++
	Clostridium sordelli	+			
VIRAL					
	Rotavirus	++	++	+++	+++
	Coronavirus	+++	+	+	+++
	Bovine virus diarrhea	+	+++		+
	Breda virus	+++		+	+
	Calici virus	+	−		+
	Parvo virus		+/−		+
	Astro virus		−		
PARASITIC					
	Cryptosporidium sp.		++++	++	+
	Eimeria sp.		++		+

−, Negative finding, +, Postive finding.

appropriate sanitation and hygiene, and obtaining adequate colostrum of good quality (see Chapter 49).

NEONATAL RUMINANT DIARRHEA

JONATHAN M. NAYLOR

In approaching a problem of neonatal death losses in housed calves, the veterinarian should evaluate calf immunoglobulin status, calf feeding, calf housing, disinfection of the environment, calving area sanitation, and cow vaccination status and health. Successful calf raising is based on good management. A goal of less than 5% death loss from diarrhea is achievable.

In approaching a problem of neonatal death losses in pasture or range animals, the nutritional status of the cow, cleanliness of the calving and nursing areas, and the provision of shelter from wind should be evaluated.

Traditionally, rotavirus, cryptosporidia, coronavirus, and enterotoxigenic *E. coli* were recognized as the major causes of diarrhea in beef calves (Fig. 20-10).[238-240] However, recent surveys suggest that the incidence of infection with enterotoxigenic *E. coli* bearing the F5 (K99) antigen has fallen considerably.[241] However, other *E. coli* are probably of considerable importance. *Salmonella* spp. are particularly important in dairy calves.[239,240,242] Bovine virus diarrhea can infect calves and cause severe illness. A variety of other agents have been implicated as causes of neonatal diarrhea, but their importance in the field situation is unknown (Table 20-3). The incidence of the various etiologic agents varies with the age of the calf and this is useful in establishing the likelihood that a particular agent is involved

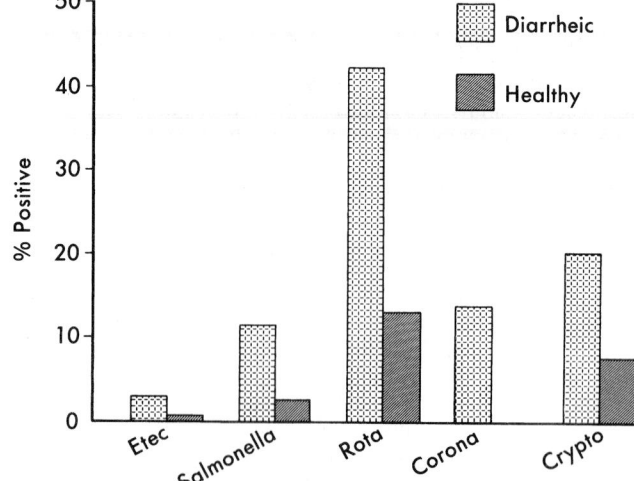

FIG. 20-10 ▓ Common enteropathogens in dairy calves. The comparative incidence of isolation from diarrheic and normal calves is shown. (From Snodgrass DR et al: *Vet Rec* 119:31-34, 1986.)

(Fig. 20-11). It is usually impossible to make a definitive etiologic diagnosis on clinical grounds. It is possible to detect signs of straining or passage of frank blood and mucus that suggest the presence of a colitis, implicating possible *Salmonella* spp., *Campylobacter* spp., bovine virus diarrhea or attaching and effacing *E. coli* infections.

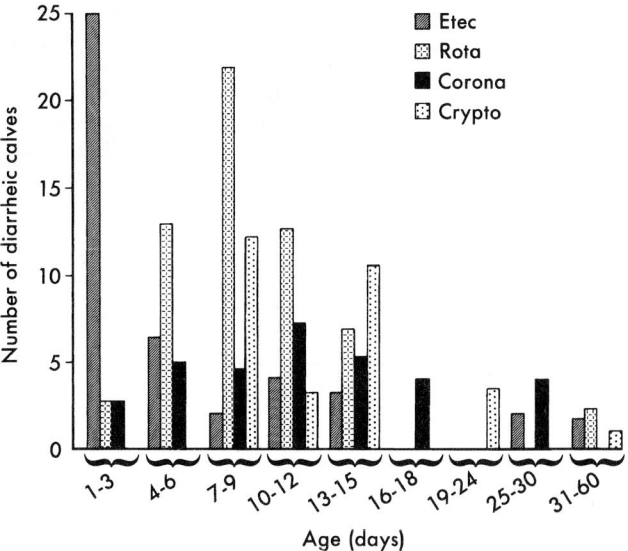

FIG. 20-11 ▦ Age incidence of isolation of different enteropathogens from diarrheic beef calves. The data are based on a retrospective records survey of 245 diarrheic calves admitted to the Western College of Veterinary Medicine over a 2-year period.

PATHOGENESIS

Diarrhea can be the result of either increased secretion or decreased absorption. Bacteria such as enterotoxigenic *E. coli* and to some extent *Salmonella* spp. and possibly *Campylobacter* spp. and rotavirus cause neonatal diarrhea by secreting enterotoxins which stimulate increased intestinal secretions.[243-245] These changes are thought to be mediated by cyclic AMP or cyclic GMP, calmodulin, and changes in protein kinase activity.[246,247] The cell's structure is not affected, but the activity of the membrane pumps is altered, and there is increased secretion of chloride, sodium, and potassium.[248] Sodium absorption linked to glucose and amino acid transport across the mucosal epithelium is not affected.[243,244] Bovine enterotoxigenic *E. coli* do not stimulate intestinal bicarbonate secretion.[248]

Protozoa and enteric viruses cause neonatal diarrhea as a result of the destruction of the absorptive villous epithelial cells.[249-252] In rotavirus and coronavirus infections there is compensatory hyperplasia of the crypt cells. Diarrhea results because intestinal digestive secretions continue and absorption is impaired.[253,254] The crypt cells have secretory functions and their multiplication adds to the secretory load.[253] In addition, continued feeding may result in more nutrients being presented to the small intestine than the damaged villi can absorb.[255,256] Excess nutrients ferment in the large intestine and promote bacterial overgrowth,[246,257] which can generate organic acids and other deleterious compounds. The osmotic effect of the unabsorbed nutrients drags water into the gut and contributes to the diarrhea.[253] Marked inflammation is a feature of salmonellosis and clostridiosis. This contributes to diarrhea by increasing mucosal pore size and hydraulic pressures within the intestinal wall, by destroying absorptive cells, and by increasing prostaglandin production, which in turn stimulates secretory mechanisms within the enterocytes.[246,253]

On an individual animal basis, diarrhea is significant because of fluid and electrolyte losses. As long as the neonate can compensate for these losses it will remain fairly bright and continue to suck. If the losses exceed intake, systemic ef-

fects of dehydration (salt and water loss) or acidosis are seen. Fluid is lost preferentially from the vascular compartment,[258,259] and cardiovascular collapse results. Acidosis has several causes including fecal loss of bicarbonate, generation of acids within the gastrointestinal tract, and endogenous synthesis of L-lactic acid in response to dehydration and poor tissue perfusion.[260,261] Emerging evidence suggests that production of novel acids, such as D-lactic acid, by bacterial fermentation of undigested or malabsorbed milk within the gastrointestinal tract plays an important role in the development of acidosis.[262,263] D-Lactic acid is only slowly metabolized by the calf and is more likely to accumulate than L-lactic acid, which can be rapidly removed by healthy tissue.[259] Acidosis contributes to the calf's malaise by increasing vascular resistance, and impairing cardiac function by direct effects, and inhibiting the action of catecholamines. The neonate becomes depressed, loses its suck reflex, and becomes weak; if the disease progresses, recumbency and coma may develop. One cause of death is believed to be heart failure as a result of myocardial potassium imbalance caused by the combined effects of potassium losses into the diarrhea and the redistribution of potassium from the cells to extracellular fluid as a result of acidosis.[264-266] Hypothermia will also contribute to cardiac failure. In cases of enterotoxigenic *E. coli*, cryptosporidia, and rotavirus and coronavirus infections, correcting the fluid, electrolyte, and acid-base imbalances restores the neonate's ability to walk and suck. A residual degree of malaise may persist, which can be attributed to inflammation within the gut wall and damage to the integrity of the mucosal barriers allowing invasion of enteric microbes or their toxins. If malabsorption persists, cachexia can develop—particularly if milk is withheld as part of therapy— and death from malnutrition or hypoglycemia may occur.

Salmonella are invasive and release endotoxins in the systemic circulation. Clostridia produce exotoxins. Both endotoxins and exotoxins have profound systemic effects that are often directly responsible for malaise, microcirculatory failure, and cardiovascular collapse. Correcting fluid and electrolyte disturbances in these infections will aid the neonate but will not overcome the effects of toxemia or bacteremia.

On a herd basis the diarrheic neonate is a major source of contamination of the environment. Once a herd begins to experience problems with diarrhea the level of infectious agents in the environment can rise rapidly, leading to a marked increase in morbidity.

ETIOLOGY

Bacteria

E. coli cause diarrhea in calves as a result of septicemia or enteric infection. Enteric *E. coli* infection has been divided into enterotoxigenic, enteropathogenic, enterohemorrhagic, enteroadherent, and enteroinvasive forms.[267] Each form is associated with the production of specific pathologies by different toxins. In calves, enterotoxigenic colibacillosis is the most common form, but enterohemorrhagic disease has also been described.

Septicemic invasion can produce shock with a low-grade diarrhea in young calves; most commonly they are under 4 days of age. Differentiation of this disease from simple enteropathies depends on demonstration of signs of bacteremia such as hypopyon, arthritis, or hyperesthesia and neck rigidity associated with meningitis. Fever is not a consistent feature of septicemia in neonates and cannot be used to rule out septicemia. Diarrhea is not profuse and is presumably secondary to endotoxemia. In bacteremic neonates the degree of collapse cannot be adequately explained by the severity of dehydration. Low-grade bacteremia does not produce obvious signs, but the organisms can localize in joints and lead to the development of septic arthritis in older calves.

Enterotoxigenic *E. coli* produce a profuse watery diarrhea. They are mainly a problem in calves up to 4 days old,[238] although they can occasionally produce diarrhea in older calves (Fig. 20-12). The incidence of this cause of diarrhea may be decreasing in recent years, perhaps because of the introduction of effective vaccines. Enterotoxigenic *E. coli* are often hemolytic and usually belong to O serogroups 8, 9, 20, 26, 101, or 141.[268] In susceptible calves, enterotoxigenic *E. coli* multiply in large numbers in the small intestine. They are pathogenic because of fimbria or pili that allow them to bind to enterocytes.[268] Fimbrial antigens that bind to calf en-

Bicarbonate requirements for diarrheic calves		Base deficit (mmol/L)	Therapy							≤8 days of age
Clinical assessment										
Visual	**Descriptive**	30 kg	35 kg	40 kg	45 kg	50 kg	55 kg	60 kg		
	Standing, strong suck reflex	0				Oral*				
	Standing, weak suck reflex	5				Intravenous+				
	Sternal recumbency	10	150	175	200	225	250	275	300	
	Lateral recumbency	10	150	175	200	225	250	275	300	

* Should contain at least 60 mmol/L of acetate or bicarbonate.
\+ Total bicarbonate requirement for intravenous fluid therapy, mmol.

Bicarbonate requirements for diarrheic calves		Base deficit (mmol/L)	Therapy							>8 days of age
Clinical assessment										
Visual	**Descriptive**	30 kg	35 kg	40 kg	45 kg	50 kg	55 kg	60 kg		
	Standing, strong suck reflex	5				Oral*				
	Standing, weak suck reflex	10				Intravenous+				
	Sternal recumbency	15	225	262.5	300	337.5	375	412.5	450	
	Lateral recumbency	20	300	350	400	450	500	550	600	

* Should contain at least 60 mmol/L of acetate or bicarbonate.
\+ Total bicarbonate requirement for intravenous fluid therapy, mmol.

FIG. 20-12 ▇ Prediction of severity of metabolic acidosis from body position, strength of suck reflex, and age.

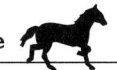

terocytes were initially given K designates, but are more correctly named using the F designation; important antigens include F5 (K99) and F41.[269] Enterotoxigenic *E. coli* also secrete an enterotoxin that stimulates secretion of water, sodium, and chloride. Heat-labile (LT) and heat-stable (ST) varieties of toxin exist. Many bovine enterotoxigenic *E. coli* were F5 positive and secreted ST$_a$.[268,270,271] Today, however, the association between enterotoxin production and the F5 adhesion factor is weaker, possibly because of the widespread use of vaccines against the F5 (K99) adhesion factor.[272] The affinity of F5 antigen for enterocytes declines rapidly with age.[273] Evidence indicates that viral enteritis can modify the type of enterocytes present and increase susceptibility to *E. coli* binding[274]; thus enterotoxigenic *E. coli* infections may complicate enteropathies produced by other infectious agents in older calves. Enterotoxigenic F5 *E. coli* also attack lambs under a week of age.[275]

Calves infected with enterotoxigenic *E. coli* have a mild inflammatory reaction in the small intestinal wall and some villous atrophy. In fresh specimens, sheets of gram-negative bacilli can be seen adhering to the small intestinal mucosa.[276]

Enterotoxigenic F5 *E. coli* can produce a discrete clinical syndrome characterized by diarrhea, dehydration, and weakness in calves 1 to 4 days of age. The course is rapid, and the calf may progress from health to recumbency and death within 6 to 12 hours. Weakness may be noted before diarrhea is observed. When the diarrhea breaks, it is profuse and watery and is passed without straining. The progression of the disease can be halted by appropriate antibiotic therapy, but fluids and electrolytes are needed to restore hydration and vigor. Milder forms of the disease exist that cannot be clinically differentiated from other forms of diarrhea.

Other types of pathogenic *E. coli* exist. Some attach to the enterocytes of the colon and sometimes of the distal small intestine and are described as attaching and effacing *E. coli* because they distort and destroy the microvilli of the brush border. They are subdivided into enterhemorrhagic and enteropathogenic groups depending on whether or not they produce shigalike toxin; both have been associated with calf diarrhea.[272,277-282] Enterohemorrhagic shigalike toxin (Vero and HeLa cytotoxic factors) producing *E. coli* produce a mucohemorrhagic colitis, with petechial or ecchymotic hemorrhages in the wall of the colon and rectum.[272,277-279] *E. coli* that carry this toxin are F5 (K99) negative and may belong to O serogroups 5, 26, and 111.[278,283] There are reports of outbreaks of bloody diarrhea in calves 2 days to 4 weeks old associated with enterohemorrhagic *E. coli*[284] In some of these outbreaks, other agents were also involved. The most common clinical sign is diarrhea, but dysentery and dehydration are seen in some cases.[272,283-286] Occasionally there were signs of abdominal pain manifested by bruxism and pain on abdominal palpation. The disease has been reproduced by inoculation with enterohemorrhagic *E. coli*.

Salmonella spp. are an important cause of diarrhea and septicemia in dairy and veal calves, particularly in situations where calves are brought together from a variety of sources and raised intensively on milk replacer diets. *Salmonella typhimurium*, *Salmonella dublin*, and *Salmonella newport* are commonly isolated serotypes. Infections are not common in single suckle beef calves.[274,287] Signs of septicemia often predominate.[288] Affected calves are dull and often have fever and a profuse diarrhea; dysentery is an inconsistent feature.[289] Bacteremia is common in calves under a month of age and may result in clinically swollen joints. In older calves, joint involvement is less common. In sheep, abortions in pregnant ewes may be seen, as well as diarrhea and septicemia in lambs.[275,290] The depression in salmonellosis cannot be completely explained by dehydration and acidosis and is probably due in part to endotoxemia.

Campylobacter jejuni and *Campylobacter fecalis* are thought to be of minor importance in calves and lambs.[275] Experimental infections in calves are characterized by mild diarrhea with blood and mucus. In the early stages of infection a mild ileitis is present and progresses to a colitis.[264,291]

C. perfringens type C mainly causes disease in calves under 10 days of age. Typical signs include sudden death or weakness and prostration. Signs of colic, nervous derangement, and a terminal diarrhea are less common.[292,293] At necropsy hemorrhagic enteritis with necrosis of the small intestine are observed. The mesenteric lymph nodes may be swollen and hemorrhagic and petechial or ecchymotic hemorrhages may be observed, especially on the pericardium and thymus.[294] *C. perfringens* type A may be responsible for a mucoid diarrhea in calves.[295] *C. perfringens* type B causes lamb dysentery. This is characterized by a severe ileitis with profuse blood-stained diarrhea, colic, and sudden death in lambs under 10 days of age.[275] *Clostridium sordelli* can cause mild inflammatory changes in the intestinal tract of calves resulting in loose feces that contain blood and mucus.

Viruses

Intestinal viruses multiply within enterocytes. As the epithelial cells are destroyed, villous atrophy develops. The various agents cannot be readily separated on clinical grounds. Diarrhea can vary in severity from soft to watery feces.

Rotaviruses are the most common cause of neonatal diarrhea in calves.[296,297] Typically they belong to serogroup A and cause diarrhea in calves 4 to 14 days old, but they can also be a problem in younger and older calves (see Fig. 20-11). This age predilection is thought to be because many cows secrete antirotavirus antibody in their colostrum, which confers local protection against rotavirus attack until antibody levels in milk decline 48 to 72 hours postpartum.[298,299] Rotaviruses also cause diarrhea in lambs, but atypical (serogroup B) viruses may be more common than in calves.[300] Different strains are associated with disease in different species, and there are also strain differences in virulence. However, calves are fully susceptible to disease when challenged with rotaviruses isolated from monkeys, pigs, and rabbits.[301] The virus invades small intestinal villus epithelial cells; the attack is usually self limiting because once susceptible epithelial cells have been destroyed there are no further target cells.[252] Although infection is short lived, it takes time for the villi to repair. The shrunken villi are initially covered by squamous and cuboidal cells from the crypts; the villi gradually regenerate as these differentiate into absorptive columnar epithelium.[252,302]

One method by which rotaviruses persist is through the infection of adult cattle. Clinical signs are not seen in adults, but viral excretion is a potential source of infection for their calves.[303]

Coronaviruses cause problems in calves of most ages, although they are particularly common in 4- to 30-day-old calves. Pathology involves both the small and large intestine. In the small intestine, they destroy the absorptive epithelial cells of the intestinal villi, where they can cause a more severe villous atrophy than that produced by rotavirus. In the spiral colon, they cause widespread destruction of the cells of the colonic ridges.[249,251] Because coronaviruses produce more widespread pathology than rotaviruses, they are more likely to be associated with signs of colitis. such as straining and passage of mucus, or occasionally blood, in the feces. Experimentally, coronavirus can also invade the upper respiratory tract and lung and produce a mild interstitial pneumonia.[304] In some studies the incidence of respiratory and enteric disease are linked. Aerosol transmission is possible.[305]

Coronavirus particles are also excreted by adult cattle. Excretion tends to increase around the time of parturition, and calves born to dams excreting virus are at higher risk of developing diarrhea.[306] Adults are usually asymptomatic excreters, but coronavirus has been implicated as a cause of winter dysentery.[307,308] Once infected, calves initially excrete high levels of virus and are potent sources of contamination. Infection persists for weeks in apparently recovered calves, and these excrete low levels of virus for weeks.[309]

Parvoviruses are proven pathogens in neonatal calves.[310] They have been associated with postweaning diarrhea, but their exact importance in neonatal diarrhea is unknown. *Caliciviruses*[311,312] and *Breda* virus[311,312] are pathogenic in calves; the extent of their contribution to field outbreaks is uncertain.[313-315]

Bovine viral diarrhea (BVD) sometimes produces diarrhea in neonatal calves.[316-320] The virus attacks the bone marrow, lymphoid tissue (Peyer's patches), and platelets and the epithelium of the digestive system. Affected calves usually show oral ulcerations, particularly on the hard and soft palate. The buccal papillae are often blunted and the tips may be ulcerated.[320] Some variants of the virus produce intestinal bleeding, petechiation, ecchymosis, or prolonged bleeding from venipuncture sites secondary to thrombocytopenia.[318,319,321,322] Hematologic findings often include leukopenia and thrombocytopenia. The disease must be differentiated from other causes of enteritis that are complicated by bovine papular stomatitis infection. Bovine papular stomatitis is common in neonatal calves. It produces oral lesions that are hyperemic and red, with a central white area of necrosis and often a raised rim of proliferating epithelial cells. These lesions often involve the mucosa around the molars. They are usually of little consequence, and their importance lies in the fact that they may be confused with BVD. One feature that helps identify BVD ulcers is that they lack the zones of epithelial proliferation seen in bovine papular stomatitis.

Protozoa

Cryptosporidium is a major cause of calf diarrhea.[323] The cryptosporidia that infect mammals are divided into several species.[323-326] *Crytosporidium parvum* is probably the most important pathogenic species in calves, although the slightly larger *Crytosporidium muris* has also been isolated from cattle.[328-331] In birds, respiratory and gastrointestinal involvement occurs, whereas the intestine is the predilection site in ruminants. Cryptosporidia are capable of infecting most domestic mammals and humans. Cross infection between mice, lambs, calves, and pigs is possible.[332,333] An outbreak of cryptosporidiosis has been described in caregivers in a veterinary hospital treating diarrheic calves. Affected humans suffered from watery diarrhea, cramping, flatulence, and headache.[334] One person became infected as a result of handling soiled clothing.

The parasite invades the enterocytes of the distal small intestine and large intestine.[335] It lives in the space just under the cell membrane, not in the cytoplasm. Pathology is usually most severe in the distal small intestine and is characterized by villous atrophy and villous fusion. Late in the disease, inflammatory changes are also seen. Diarrhea is the result of villous atrophy leading to malabsorption and secondary milk fermentation. The disease is common in 1- to 4-week-old calves. The feces vary in consistency from loose to watery and may contain undigested milk, blood, mucus, and bile. Tenesmus may be seen.[335] Although the disease is usually characterized by a high morbidity and low mortality,[336,337] autoinfection (without the protozoa leaving the host) occurs, so relapses and protracted infections leading to chronic diarrhea and cachexia may be seen. Oocyst secretion starts at the same time as diarrhea and usually persists for a few days after the end of the diarrheic phase. Cryptosporidia cause diarrhea and

sometimes death in 3- to 30-day-old lambs. Protracted infections and mortality is most common in lambs infected in the first few days of life, because age resistance is seen after about 3 weeks of age.[260,275,329,338] Cryptosporidiosis has also been described in goats, affecting 5- to 20-day-old kids; signs lasted from 3 to 7 days, relapses were not uncommon, and there was a moderate mortality.[339] Cryptosporidia are resistant to all commonly available antimicrobial/anticoccidial agents and most disinfectants and can survive for long periods in the environment.

Eimeria spp. produce clinical signs of coccidiosis in calves and lambs over 3 to 4 weeks of age.[275,340,341] The diarrhea is usually characterized by the presence of fresh blood and tenesmus. Signs are particularly common when calves or lambs are kept in crowded conditions that promote fecal-oral contamination and when the weather is warm and wet.

Giardia has been implicated in some cases of calf diarrhea, sometimes in concert with other pathogens.[342]

Nutrition

At one time, nutritional diarrhea was thought to be common in calves. With the identification of viral and parasitic causes of diarrhea, the use of this diagnosis has declined. It is still recognised, however, that there is a relationship between diet and scours. For example, rotavirus does not produce diarrhea in weaned calves, even though infection can be successfully established.[343] Villous atrophy as a result of attack by an enteropathogen reduces the ability of the calf to digest nutrients,[254,256] and this predisposes to gastrointestinal overload with fermentation of milk in the large intestine. Healthy calves can handle large quantities (16% to 20% of body weight/day) of whole cow's milk without getting diarrhea.[344] However, experiments with calves infected with multiple enteric pathogens indicate that feeding normal amounts of whole cow's milk (10% of body weight) exacerbates diarrhea and depression during the initial stages of diarrhea. The composition of milk replacers can also be a problem. Calves seem to experience more problems with diarrhea on certain milk replacers. One study showed that calves performed well on soy protein–containing milk replacers when healthy but that during an outbreak of salmonellosis there was better weight gain and less mortality in calves fed whole milk.[345]

Although restricting intake of milk and milk replacers may be beneficial in calves with diarrhea, deliberate underfeeding in healthy calves predisposes to diarrhea.

Septicemia and Bacteremia

Recent work shows that calves with severe systemic signs and diarrhea may be bacteremic or septicemic. *E. coli* organisms are most commonly isolated along with other gram-negative enteric bacteria. *Campylobacter fetalis* has also been identified in a small but important percentage of diarrheic calves.[346,347] These infections likely result from fecal flora entering the systemic circulation across damaged or devitalized intestinal mucosa. Direct damage by many enteric pathogens results in shortening of villi rather than exposure of the submucosa. However, it is likely that the effects of direct viral attack and damage from poor perfusion of villi as a result of circulatory disturbances combine to disrupt the mucosal barrier. In one study, experimentally infected calves were unlikely to become septicemic if maintained in normal fluid and acid-base balance, whereas calves infected with the same agents and allowed to become severely acidotic had a higher rate of septicemia.[348] Septicemia is more likely to be present in calves that are recumbent, under a week of age, and have no suck reflex.[346]

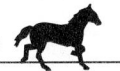

ESTABLISHING AN ETIOLOGIC DIAGNOSIS

An etiologic diagnosis is useful in selecting specific diagnostic and preventative regimens for bacterial infections. Establishing an etiologic diagnosis for viral infections may be more important now that there is some indication that effective vaccines are being developed. Diagnosis of salmonellosis, cryptosporidiosis, and giardiasis can have public health implications. Once an agent has been identified, one of the major problems is in interpretation of whether or not that agent is responsible for diarrhea in the individual or herd, because most agents can also be found in a percentage of normal calves (see Fig 20-10).

Necropsy diagnosis usually rests on the demonstration of the agent associated with damaged intestinal tissue together with the presence of widespread pathology typical of that produced experimentally by the agent. It is important to examine several calves so that a representative sample is obtained. Best results are obtained when the calves are early in the course of disease and are examined fresh (euthanitized immediately before autopsy), because autolysis and bacterial invasion of gut mucosa occur within 5 minutes after death. Samples should be fixed by laying a square of gut on paper, serosal side down, and dropping into fixative, or by tying off sections of gut, injecting fixative into the segment, then dropping the segment into fixative. These techniques help minimize distortion of the mucosal architecture. Tissues are then examined by high-power light or electron microscopy for the presence of bacteria adhering to the mucosa and cryptosporidia associated with the brush border of epithelial cells. Fluorescent antibodies techniques can be used for F5 (K99) *E. coli* and virus identification. Identification of one agent in pathologic material does not preclude the possibility that other agents are also contributing to the condition.

Clinical diagnosis is based on the isolation of proven enteropathogens from diarrheic calves. This approach is valid when the agent is known to be enteropathogenic, is only released on lysis of the enterocyte and the calf has diarrhea. However, it does not mean that this is the only enteropathogenic agent or even that it is the major cause of diarrhea. Multiple infections are common, and evidence indicates that several agents may be required to produce severe disease.[349] The quantitative role of an infectious agent can be partially characterized by excluding the presence of other known enteropathogens and by the response to specific therapy. This approach can be complemented by collecting multiple fecal samples from diarrheic and healthy calves on the same farm and looking for an increased incidence of the agent in diarrheic calves. Infectious agents can be isolated from the feces of healthy calves that show no signs of diarrhea; this is because pathology is sufficiently mild that other parts of the gut compensate for localized loss of function. Variations in virulence occur and this also influences the likelihood of seeing clinical signs.[350] *E. coli*, *Campylobacter* spp., and *C. perfringens* are normal inhabitants of the gastrointestinal tract, and isolation of these agents by themselves is commonplace and of no significance[291,351,352] unless one can identify virulent strains.

The biotype of a particular *E. coli* as determined by its ability to ferment sugars, decarboxylate amino acids, or produce hemolysins is of no significance in determining whether or not it is enterotoxigenic.[353,354] Definitive diagnosis of enterotoxigenicity rests on demonstration of the ability of the *E. coli* to dilate intestinal loops. Enterotoxigenic *E. coli* can also be identified by the presence of the F5 (K99) antigen, which allows them to attach to the mucosa. Slide agglutination tests are available for the F5 antigen, but the immunoflorescent antibody test is thought to be the most reliable. Newer strains

of enterotoxigenic *E. coli* may use other attachment factors that are not detected by these tests. At present, identification of enterohemorrhagic *E. coli* is difficult in most diagnostic laboratories,[278] although the histologic demonstration of gram-negative bacilli adherent to the colonic mucosa in necropsy specimens should suggest this diagnosis.

C. perfringens that belong to pathogenic strains produce exotoxins. These can only be readily identified by collecting intestinal fluid at necropsy. Bacterial free filtrates can be made and injected into groups of mice that have also received various antitoxins. The demonstration of *C. perfringens* toxin together with hemorrhagic and necrotizing enteritis is evidence for disease caused by *C. perfringens*. Finding many large positive bacilli in the mucosa of fresh specimens is suggestive of the diagnosis of clostridial enterotoxemia when lesions are compatible.

It is difficult to determine when the isolation of *Campylobacter* spp. is of significance. Only *Campylobacter jejuni* can be regarded as a pathogen of calves at the present time, but it is unclear whether toxin production or the numbers of organisms present determine pathogenicity in calves. The organism may become bacteremic and detection of *Campylobacter* spp. in blood cultures is significant.

Salmonellae can be excreted by healthy animals. Ruminants suffering from salmonellosis can be presumptively identified by the presence of Salmonellae in the feces together with typical necropsy findings. The organism often causes bacteremia and positive blood or postmortem tissue cultures are diagnostic.

Viruses are usually identified by direct examination of the feces or fluorescent antibody examination of gut tissues. Viral isolation is not commonly used because enteric viruses are difficult to grow. Feces can be examined for the presence of viral antigens by a variety of immunologic methods. Tests such as enzyme-linked immunosorbent assay (ELISA) are sensitive but will fail to detect virus if it is already complexed to host antibody (i.e., late in the infectious process) or if the ELISA antibody does not recognize the virus.[355] For example, atypical rotaviruses, called pararotaviruses or group B rotaviruses, carry a different group antigen to the more common group A rotaviruses. These atypical rotaviruses are not picked up by standard immunologic tests[356]; this is likely to be a particular problem in lambs, in which group B infections are common.[300] Direct immunofluorescence utilizes antibodies that are conjugated to a fluorescein label to identify virus infected cells in fecal smears.[287] This test works best in the acute stages (first 48 hours) of infection when infected epithelial cells detach from the villi. It is also useful for demonstrating the presence of virus infected epithelial cells in pathologic samples of intestinal wall. Electron microscopic examination has the advantage that many different types of viruses can be detected, including those such as parvovirus that are not recognized as common causes of diarrhea. However, there can be problems in identifying coronaviruses, because they may not exhibit typical morphology. The sensitivity of electron microscopic examination can be increased using techniques that concentrate viral particles before examination. Some comparative studies with feces have shown that ELISA and electron microscopy give similar results when searching for specific pathogens; the agreement between these two methods varies from 65% to 100%.[355,357] Direct immunoflorescence testing of fecal samples gives good agreement (90%) with electron microscopic examination for rotaviruses when samples are collected during the first 24 hours of diarrhea.[358] Examination of intestinal fragments obtained at necropsy using immunofluorescence has a low false-positive rate and gives good agreement with electron microscopy and ELISA tests on intestinal contents in some studies.[359]

TABLE 20-4

Guidelines for Assessing Dehydration in Neonatal Calves

% Dehydration	Eyeball Sunkenness	Neck Skin Tent (seconds)	Mucous Membranes
0	None	<1	Moist
1-5	None/slight	1-4	Moist
6-8	Slight separation of eyeball and globe	5-10	Tacky
9-10	Gap, <0.5 cm, between eyeball and orbit	11-15	Tacky to dry
11-12	Gap, 0.5 to 1 cm, between eyeball and orbit	16-45	Dry

Others report poor agreement between these tests, probably because epithelial cells slough rapidly after death and are not present in fragments taken from calves that had experienced a long course of disease or had been dead for a few hours.[357]

Protozoa are detected by fecal flotation. *Eimeria* oocysts are readily detectable and diagnosis is facilitated by the fact that oocyst counts parallel signs of disease.[360] Cryptosporidia present a diagnostic challenge because they are small (3 to 5 μ) and easily missed. Diagnosis of cryptosporidiosis is usually based on fecal flotation with Schearer's solution (sucrose) followed by staining for the oocysts, which are acid fast, with modified Ziehl-Neelsen stains.[361] The sensitivity of detection can be increased by using 36% salt solutions or Ritchie's ether extraction to separate the oocysts and auramine/carbol fuschin stain.[362] The organisms are stable in feces for many days at room temperature.[363] Fecal excretion begins with the onset of clinical signs and persists past the diarrheic period, so detection of this infection should be easy if appropriate techniques are used.

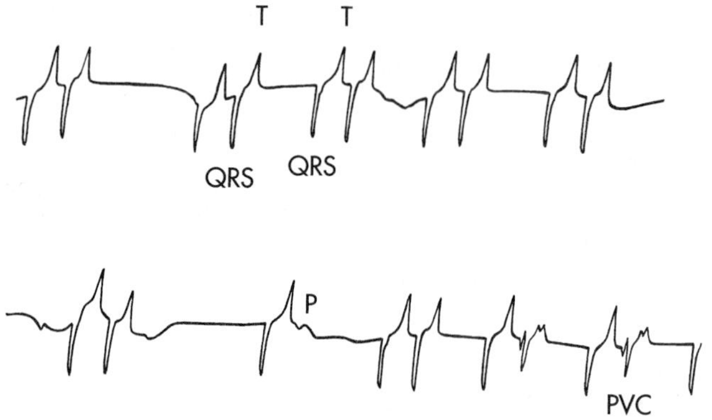

TREATMENT OF INDIVIDUAL CALVES

Examination

Physical examination of the diarrheic calf is the first step in establishing therapeutic needs. It is important to determine the presence of any intercurrent disease. Treatment of uncomplicated cases of diarrhea depends on the estimation of dehydration, severity of acidosis, likelihood of intercurrent infection, presence or absence of hypothermia, and hypoglycemia. The severity of dehydration is gauged from the eyeball position and skin tent (Table 20-4). Skin tent can be measured over the eyelids and neck. Best results are obtained when the neck is held straight and the skin of the mid-neck is tented in the direction of the long axis of the neck to avoid the natural skin folds that run across the neck. Some have claimed a relationship exists between severity of dehydration and acidosis. However, this has not been borne out in studies of diarrheic calves.[364] Instead, acidosis can be gauged from the calf's sucking/drinking drive and the degree of weakness and the age of the calf (see Fig. 20-12).[364,365] Estimation of severity of acidosis either from laboratory or physical findings is important to the successful therapy of severely depressed calves. Rectal temperature measurement will determine whether or not the calf is hypothermic.

Heart rate is variable in diarrheic calves. Bradycardia (<90 beats/min) is clinically important and may indicate the presence of hypothermia, hypoglycemia or hyperkalemia. Cardiac arrhythmias occur[365] and are usually due to severe hyperkalemia (K$^+$ above 8 mEq/L) (Fig. 20-13). Hyperkalemic arrhythmia can usually be differentiated from arrhythmia resulting from cardiomyopathy (selenium deficiency) because the heart rate is not elevated. The presence of bradycardia or arrhythmia indicates the need for immediate fluid therapy with bicarbonate containing solutions to prevent death.

FIG. 20-13 ■ Bradycardia and atrial standstill in a severely hyperkalemic diarrheic calf. Heart rate is 84 beats/min. There is bigeminy and the T waves are abnormally large. There is only one P wave, and it is not conducted. Serum potassium was 8.9 mmol/L and sodium 116 mmol/L.

Body condition is usually good at the start of an attack of diarrhea. Poor condition often indicates chronic infection, mismothering, or poor feeding programs, which may be exacerbated by milk withdrawal for therapeutic purposes.

It is important to check for intercurrent infections; these are easily missed even with careful examination. The lungs should be examined for signs of pneumonia; the navel palpated for pain, swelling, and wetness; and the joints checked for signs of distention and lameness. The boundary between calves in which the primary insult is septicemia with a secondary diarrhea and those in which primary diarrhea is complicated by septicemia is blurred. Calves that are recumbent, under a week of age, have lost their suck reflex, or have evidence of intercurrent infection are more likely to be septicemic and require concurrent antibiotic therapy.[346] Calves in which septicemia has progressed to produce signs of meningitis (e.g., extended neck with reluctance to flex neck), joint involvement, or ophthalmic signs (congested scleral vessels with hypopyon or iridospasm) carry a poor to very poor prognosis. It is best to identify these cases before instigating therapy so that the owner can decide whether treatment is economically feasible.

The laboratory is useful in quantitating metabolic disturbances in diarrheic calves. Blood gas analysis will accurately determine the degree of metabolic acidosis. This is not routinely available to most practitioners. However, it may be worthwhile to make special efforts to get measurements when setting up a fluid therapy protocol for your area or when dealing with cases that fail to respond to treatment. Blood can be collected into a heparinized syringe, capped, placed in a styrofoam cup surrounded by ice, and transported 4 hours or more to a laboratory. Alternatively the practice laboratory may have a total CO_2 (Harleco) analyzer or access to serum bicarbonate estimation as part of serum chemistry

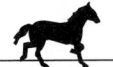

profile. Total CO_2 or bicarbonate is a useful index of the severity of metabolic acidosis. Blood glucose can be readily determined using a handheld glucometer.

Fluid Therapy

The most common causes of death in diarrheic calves are dehydration and acidosis.[366] The immediate objective in treating depressed diarrheic calves is to restore them to a normal systemic state. In some calves it may also be necessary to correct hypoglycemia or hypothermia, restrict milk intake, or give antibiotics.

The estimated severity of dehydration can be combined with estimates of losses through diarrhea and for the maintenance of essential functions to give the total daily fluid requirement (Box 20-6). Bicarbonate requirements can be calculated from base deficit values (based on blood gas measurements or estimated from physical findings) as follows:

mmol bicarbonate = Body weight,
Kilograms × Base deficit, mmol/L × 0.5

A chart of bicarbonate requirements for various body weights and base deficit values is available (Table 20-5).

Measurements of serum total carbon dioxide content or bicarbonate are also reliable estimates of bicarbonate requirements.[367] Bicarbonate requirements are as follows:

mmol bicarbonate = Body weight,
Kilograms × (30 − TCO₂) × 0.5

For example, a 40-kg calf has a serum bicarbonate or TCO_2 of 10 mmol/L. The calf has a bicarbonate deficit of 30 mmol/L − 10 mmol/L = 20 mmol/L, so 40 kg × 20 mmol/L × 0.5 = 400 mmol bicarbonate is required to replace existing deficits. Ongoing diarrhea may require additional bicarbonate.

Calves that are unwilling to suck and are severely depressed are best treated with intravenous fluids. Calves that are only moderately depressed may also be treated with intravenous fluids if the condition is worsening rapidly. Catheterization is easier if a No. 15 scalpel blade is used to nick the skin, which is about a centimeter thick and tough in dehydrated calves. If it proves difficult to catheterize the calf, it can be suspended upside down so that blood will pool and distend the jugular veins. The calf's neck should be clipped and prepared before inversion and the calf laid flat as soon as the catheter is placed. It should be possible to place a catheter in less than a minute, even in severely dehydrated calves using this technique. Once the catheter is placed, fluids can be administered. If the calf is hypothermic, fluids should be warmed before administration because cold fluids can decrease cardiac output and may kill a critically ill calf. Fluids can be warmed by several methods; one convenient technique is to run the fluids through a coil of tubing immersed in a bucket of hot water (check the temperature regularly) on the way to the calf.

Saline-based fluids are suitable for rehydration (Table 20-6) but most severely depressed calves are acidotic and more consistent recovery is obtained if an alkalizing agent is also used. A wide variety of alkalizing agents are available (lactate, acetate, gluconate), but clinical trials show that only bicarbonate is consistently effective in severely acidotic calves[261,368] (Fig. 20-14). Many diarrheic calves require large amounts of bicarbonate to correct their acidosis,[259] and these are best given as isotonic solutions to avoid problems with hypertonicity and salt overload. An isotonic solution (156 mmol/L) of bicarbonate can be readily made by dissolving 13 g of sodium bicarbonate (baking soda) in 1 L of water.[369] Sodium bicarbonate solutions can be mixed with saline; there is a possibility that precipitates may form if bicarbonate is mixed with calcium containing solutions such as Ringer's lactate.

BOX 20-6

Calculation of Daily Fluid Requirements for Diarrheic Calf

Replacement = % Dehydration × Body weight in kilograms
Maintenance = 50 ml/kg/day
Ongoing losses in diarrhea, 1 to 4 L/day

TOTAL, L/DAY
The total requirement can either be given intravenously or orally. If the oral route is chosen, an allowance must be made for partial absorption of the fluid (60% to 80%). The success of therapy is monitored based on the calf's clinical signs and restoration of urination.

TABLE 20-5

Calculation of Bicarbonate Requirement From Calf Body Weight and Severity of Acidosis

Calf Weight kg (lb)	Base Deficit (mmol/L)	Bicarbonate Requirements (mmol)	Volume in Liters 1.3% NaHCO₃⁻ (L)
30 (66)	5	75	0.5
	10	150	1.0
	15	225	1.5
	20	300	1.9
35 (77)	5	88	0.5
	10	175	1.1
	15	263	1.6
	20	350	2.3
40 (88)	5	100	0.6
	10	200	1.3
	15	300	1.9
	20	400	2.6
45 (99)	5	113	0.7
	10	225	1.4
	15	338	2.1
	20	450	2.9
50 (110)	5	125	0.8
	10	250	1.6
	15	375	2.4
	20	500	3.2
55 (121)	5	138	0.9
	10	275	1.8
	15	413	2.7
	20	550	3.6
60 (132)	5	150	1.0
	10	300	1.9
	15	450	2.9
	20	600	3.8

NOTE: Isotonic 1.3% sodium bicarbonate solution is prepared by adding 13 g of sodium bicarbonate to 1 L distilled water (155 mmol bicarbonate/L).

Some may prefer to rehydrate the neonate first and then reconsider the need for bicarbonate if it is not up and sucking within 12 hours of therapy. However, this is time consuming. It is not always necessary to completely correct acidosis; blood pH from 7.25 to 7.45 has little adverse affect (normal calves have a venous blood pH of 7.34, bicarbonate of 30 mmol/L, and a base excess of 5 mmol/L).

Ideally, dehydration and acidosis should be corrected over a 24-hour period. However, it is unusual to see problems when the fluid and acid-base deficits are corrected over

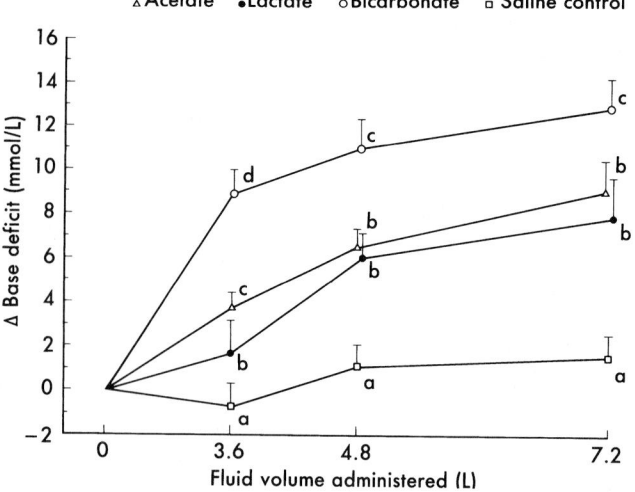

FIG. 20-14 ▓ Comparison of the alkalizing effect of various bases in diarrheic calves suffering from severe dehydration and acidosis. At the start of the trial, all calves were at least 8% dehydrated and had a mean blood pH of 7.032 and a base deficit of 18 mmol/L. All calves received a total of 7.2 L of fluid containing 102 mmol/L of saline plus 50 mmol/L of the sodium salt of the respective alkalizing agent. Letters (a, b, c, d) are statistically different ($p < 0.5$) from each other at that point. (From Kasari TR, Naylor JM: *J Am Vet Med Assoc* 187:392-397, 1985.)

TABLE 20-6

Fluids Commonly Used in Intravenous Therapy

Item	Concentration (mmol/L)									
	Na^+	K^+	Ca^{++}	Mg^{++}	Cl^{1-}	HCO_3^-	$Lactate^-$	$Acetate^-$	$Gluconate^-$	Glucose
0.9% saline	155				155					
1.3% sodium bicarbonate*	156					156				
Ringer's	147	4	5		156					
Lactated Ringer's†	130	4	3		107		30			
Ionalyte (diluted)†	139	10		3	101			55		167
Normosol R†	140	5		3	98			25	25	
Plasma-lyte 148†	140	5		3	98			27	23	
5% Dextrose (D_5W)‡										278

*Do not mix sodium bicarbonate with calcium-containing solutions; precipitates may form. Mixtures of 1.3% sodium bicarbonate and saline are usually used for treating recumbent diarrheic calves.

†Multiple electrolyte solutions are equivalent, with the exception that one should be careful of using Ionalyte in severely hyperkalemic neonates. All are suitable for rehydrating neonates that can stand.

‡Intravenous fluids are often spiked with 50% dextrose to give a final concentration of 5% dextrose in the drip when hypoglycemia is suspected.

4 hours, although the calf may continue to improve after this period. After 24 hours of appropriate therapy, one would expect the calf to be standing and show a good suck reflex. Persistent depression is usually a sign of uncorrected acidosis or toxemia.

Most diarrheic calves are not markedly hypoglycemic, but glucose supplementation is needed to treat severe hypoglycemia (glucose concentrations <2 mmol/L or <36 mg/dl). Severe hypoglycemia is treated by adding glucose to the intravenous fluids to a final concentration of 2.5% to 5%. Severe hyperkalemia is seen in some dehydrated diarrheic calves but this responds to rehydration (restores renal perfusion and dilutes out potassium) and correction of acidosis (redistributes potassium into the cells). Nutritional support is not needed if the calf is in good body condition but should be given if the calf is emaciated or if the calf has been deprived of milk for more than 3 days.

There are increased losses of potassium in diarrhea; the significance of this is uncertain, although potassium depletion can result in weakness. Usually there is no need to add potassium to intravenous fluids—the majority of calves respond to infusion of saline and 1.3% sodium bicarbonate. After 12 to 24 hours of intravenous fluid therapy most calves start on oral electrolyte solutions—these usually contain 10 to 30 mmol of potassium/L. Clinical trials comparing the efficacy of low- and high-potassium solutions have not been reported.

Once the calf is able to nurse or drink, therapy is usually switched to oral electrolytes. This is also the route of choice for treatment of mildly affected calves on the farm. Calves with weak suck reflexes and calves that are unused to hand feeding can be tubed. There are a wide variety of oral electrolyte preparations on the market, and different products are suited to different situations. Almost all the products contain water and electrolytes and are suitable for rehydration (Table 20-7). Beware of products that are designed for medicating hundreds of liters of water—the final solution is often dilute (<10 g electrolytes/L) and will not rehydrate sick calves. These products are often marketed as "boosters" and "stress relievers." Glucose and glycine are usually added to oral electrolyte solutions to facilitate sodium absorption. Research in humans has shown that adding glycine to solutions containing 110 mmol/L of glucose aids rehydration. It is probable, however, that there is little additional benefit to supplementing solutions that contain more than 200 mmol/L of glucose with glycine. This glucose/glycine–sodium cotransport mechanism remains intact in calves with enterotoxigenic *E. coli* diarrhea,[243] but is likely to be less functional in viral diarrhea that results in destruction of the absorptive cells. Solutions that contain large amounts of glucose are hyperos-

TABLE 20-7

Composition of Oral Electrolyte Solution in Water and Use in Calves

Product	Company	Other*	Na (mmol/L)	K (mmol/L)	Cl (mmol/L)	HCO₃⁻ (mmol/L)	Acetate (mmol/L)	Citrate (mmol/L)	Alkalinizing Ability (mEq/L)	Glucose (mmol/L)	Glycine (mmol/L)
Biolyte, 110-g package	Pharmacia & Upjohn	Indications mention nutrition	195	33	110	118	0	0		549	0
Biolyte, bottle or pail	Pharmacia & Upjohn	Indications mention nutrition	142	24	80	86	0	0		400	0
Calf Quencher	Vedco	Indications mention diarrhea	142	24	80	86	0	0		399	0
Calf Rehydrate	Durvet		120	10	70	40	0	10	70	56	40
Elpak-G†	Vedco	Contains gelling agent, alginate	180	10	70	40	0	?	?	55	50
Elpak-360	Vedco	Isotonic	120	10	70	40	0	?	?	56	40
Entrolyte	Pfizer	Indications mention nutritional supplement	105	25	51	80	0	0	80	166	36‡
Entrolyte HE	Pfizer	Indications mention energy	106	25	51	80	0	0	80	422	54
Fluid Formula-360	Bio-Ceutic	Isotonic	120	10	70	40	0	0		58	40
Hydra-Lyte	Vet-A-Mix		126	30	45	0	99	0	99	405	15
Hy-sorb	Rhone Merieux	Isotonic	120	10	70	40	0	0	40	56	40
Oral rehydration	Anchor	Source of nutrients	120	10	70	40	0	0	40	58	40
Renew	AgriLabs	Insufficient information									
Replenish	Aspen	Insufficient information									
Re-sorb	Pfizer	Indications mention diarrhea	80	25	80	0	0	1	3	129	45
RESTART	Biostar	Indications mentions diarrhea; not available in United States	120	20	50	0	80	0	72	120	40
RESTART HE	Biostar	Indications mention diarrhea; not available in United States	120	20	50	0	80	0	72		40
Respond	AgriLabs	Contains gelling agents—pectin and alginate	69	28	37	0	60	0	60	435	50

Modified from Naylor JM: Oral electrolyte therapy, *Vet Clin North Am (Food Anim Pract)* 15:487-504, 1999.
NOTE: Concentrations of calcium, magnesium, phosphate, and sulfate not included.
?, Compendium provides insufficient information to provide reasonable estimate.
*Consult formulary for details.
†Also contains other amino acid.

molar and are absorbed more slowly than isotonic solutions, but the differences are too small to be clinically important.[370] The ionic composition also affects absorption; mixtures of sodium chloride and citrate, bicarbonate or acetate have improved absorption over chloride salts alone. Oral electrolyte solutions are almost completely absorbed in healthy calves, but absorption can be as low as 60% in severe *E. coli* diarrhea.[371]

The ability to counteract acidosis varies greatly among oral electrolytes. Some have a net acidifying effect and others alkalinize blood (Fig. 20-15). These differences are therapeutically important and are responsible for differences in survival rates between products. Highly alkalinizing solutions give the best results—one study showed that it was more important that an electrolyte solution contain bicarbonate than chloride.[372] This is particularly important in older calves. Acetate, lactate, citrate, gluconate, and bicarbonate are all used as alkalizing agents in oral electrolyte solutions. Bicarbonate combines with hydrogen ions directly, whereas the other agents remove hydrogen ions during their metabolism within the body. A body of research is available concerning the use of different amounts and types of alkalinizing agents in oral electrolyte solutions.[218,348,372-374] Basically this shows that acetate is the best choice for treating calves that are still receiving milk—it has excellent alkalinizing ability and does not interfere with milk clotting in the abomasum. Bicarbonate is also an excellent alkalinizing agent, but it interferes with milk clotting. Breakdown of abomasal milk clots results in gradual release of some nutrients into the small intestine. Some studies with diarrheic calves show that bicarbonate can greatly reduce milk digestibility. Citrate is an effective alkalinizing agent but it is a strong inhibitor of milk clotting. Thus any of the commonly used alkalinizing agent are likely acceptable if the calf is held off milk. Acetate-based solutions are the best choice for calves that are also receiving milk.[373] We recommend that oral electrolyte solutions contain 50 to 80 mmol/L of alkalinizing agent.

Recently there has been interest in adding glutamine to oral electrolyte solutions because it is an important fuel for the gastrointestinal tract and can promote mucosal repair.[375-377] However, studies show that oral electrolytes containing glutamine as the sole amino acid are no more effective in diarrheic calves than other well-designed solutions that use glycine as the amino acid.[378] Psyllium has been added to some oral electrolyte solutions for several perceived benefits, but controlled studies show no clinical advantages, although there may be some moderation of bacterial fermentation within the gastrointestinal tract.[379,380]

The other problem to be considered in the chronically scouring calf is the need for nutritional support. Maintenance metabolizable energy requirements for a 50-kg calf are about 2000 kcal, and 3500 kcal are required to support a weight gain of 0.5 kg/day. These requirements can be met by 3.3 and 5.7 L of whole cow's milk, respectively. Comparative studies indicate that weight loss in calves fed oral electrolytes are inversely proportional to the energy content of the solutions.[381] Assuming a 4-L daily intake and 100% digestibility of oral electrolyte nutrients, regular electrolyte solutions supply between approximately 15% and 25% of energy needs. As a result, diarrheic calves that are held off milk for prolonged periods lose weight[382] and can become emaciated. When maintaining body condition is a concern, and little milk or solid food is being ingested, then a high-energy oral electrolyte should be fed. Products such as Biolyte, Lifeguard/Enterolyte HE* provide about 50% of energy requirements if fed twice a day (total intake 4 L) and about 75% if fed 3 times a day (total intake approximately 6L) (Fig 20-16).

Milk withdrawal can reduce the severity of diarrhea and depression in severe scours. This is because malabsorption exacerbates diarrhea through the osmotic effect of unabsorbed milk nutrients and also promotes bacterial overgrowth and

---

*Biolyte, Pharmacia and Upjohn Co, Kalamazoo, MI 49001; Lifeguard/Enterolyte HE, Rochester Midland, Rochester, NY 14603-1515.

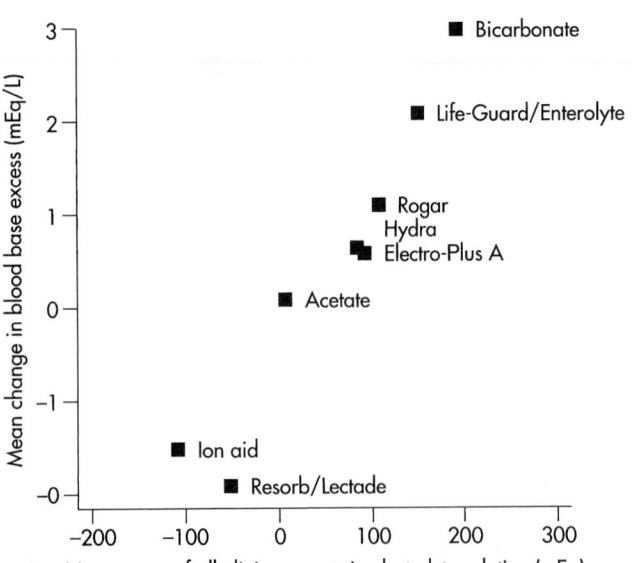

FIG. 20-15 ■ Comparison of the alkalizing abilities of various oral electrolyte solutions. The Y axis shows the mean alkalizing effect following administration of 1 treatment (1.9 to 2.25 L) of the fluid to healthy calves, the X axis shows the net amount of alkalizing agents in the solution. Bicarbonate and acetate are experimental solutions. (Life-Guard/Enterolyte is manufactured by SmithKline Beecham Labs, Rogar is Rogar STB's electrolyte powder, Hydra is manufactured by Vetrepharm, Electro-Plus A by Pitman-Moore, Ion Aid by Syntex and Resorb by Beecham.) (Modified from *Proc 14th World Congr Dis Cattle* 1:362-367, 1986.)

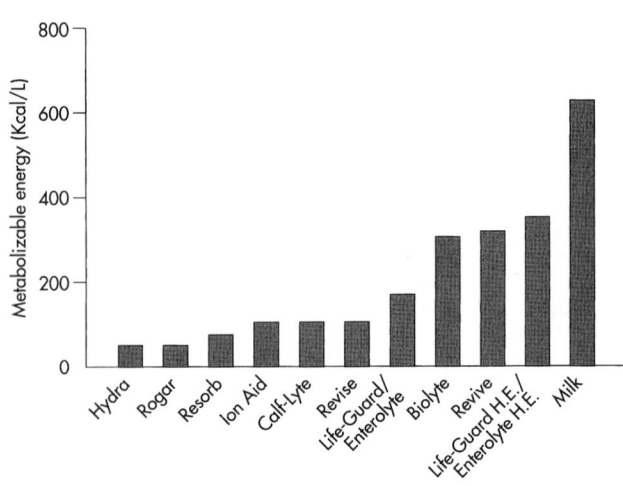

FIG. 20-16 ■ Comparison of the energy contents of various oral electrolyte solutions. Milk is also shown for comparative purposes. (See text for manufacturers.)

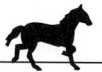

possibly malfermentation with production of organic acids. However, milk withdrawal reduces weight gain in diarrheic calves[374] and can result in severe cachexia and other signs of malnutrition. In many calves, particularly the less severely affected, there is often a considerable degree of residual absorptive capacity—enough to support body weight gain if limited amounts of milk are fed. I recommend milk withdrawal while the calf is depressed and not interested in sucking. In most cases, electrolyte therapy will restore a calf's vigor and sucking drive within 1 to 2 days. Milk can then be reintroduced in small amounts, for example, 1 L given 2 to 4 times daily. If the calf is not interested in drinking or becomes depressed when reintroduced to milk, a high-energy oral electrolyte preparation can be tried instead. Studies indicate that diarrheic calves have a generalized malabsorption rather than specific lactose intolerance.[256] Thus it may be more important to manage calves with milk intolerance by giving smaller amounts of milk in each feed rather than by changing carbohydrate source. There is little point in withdrawing milk from calves that remain alert and interested in nursing; it is unlikely to result in clinical improvement. This is particularly likely to be the case when the calf receives whole cow's milk in frequent small quantities, that is, by natural sucking of the dam.

Antibiotic Therapy

Antibiotics are frequently used in the treatment of the diarrheic calf, even though enterotoxigenic *E. coli* and *Salmonella* sp. are the only common agents that respond to antimicrobials.[383] Controlled studies show that oral antibiotics shorten the diarrheic period by about 1 day in enterotoxigenic *E. coli* diarrhea. Our experience indicates that there is a marked improvement in fecal quality (e.g., from watery to loose feces) within 24 hours of the instigation of appropriate oral or systemic therapy in calves with *E. coli* diarrhea. Calves with *Salmonella* infections are frequently bacteremic and appropriate antibiotic therapy reduces mortality and shortens the diarrheic period in infected calves. Antibiotic resistance is high in *E. coli*[384,385] and *Salmonella* sp., and culture and sensitivity is useful in selecting an appropriate antibiotic. Indiscriminate use of antibiotics leads to selection for resistant strains and complicates future therapeutic efforts.

Giardiasis has been reported to cause calf diarrhea but is thought to be a relatively unimportant cause. The condition responds to nitrofurazone, metronidazole, or fenbendazole. The use of nitrofurazone or metronidazole in food animals is illegal in the United States.

Most other causes of diarrhea in calves are viral or parasitic and are not directly sensitive to antibiotics. Several studies document that cryptosporidia are resistant to all therapeutic agents routinely available to veterinarians, including ionophores, the potentiated sulfonamides, and a variety of anticoccidials.[351,386,387] Despite this, there may be benefit to systemic antimicrobial therapy in diarrheic calves, particularly those with severe systemic signs. Intercurrent disease is not uncommon, and evidence has been shown for leakage of microbes across damaged intestine, leading to bacteremia or septicemia.[347] This is particularly likely in diarrheic calves under a week of age that are recumbent or have a poor suck reflex.[346] Survival is enhanced in calves treated with systemic antibiotics, partly because of the benefits in controlling intercurrent infections.[388] Diarrheic calves that are known to have secondary pneumonia can have a high mortality rate and individuals should be treated with systemic antibiotics for at least 5 days. Omphalophlebitis can respond to systemic antimicrobial therapy but sometimes requires surgical excision to effect a complete cure. Calves that have obvious joint infections are difficult to treat; the success rate is poor and the attempt is not usually economically justifiable.

Prolonged use of oral antibiotics has led to diarrhea in

some studies, and this mode of therapy should be discouraged in calves over 5 days of age unless there is specific evidence of giardiasis. Oral antibiotics are effective in calves with *E. coli* diarrhea, and 3 days of therapy is usually sufficient. Systemic antibiotics are also effective.

Other treatments are occasionally used in treating diarrheic calves. Flunixin meglumine and bismuth subsalicylate (Pepto Bismol) may help reduce the severity of secretory *E. coli* diarrhea.[389,390] Kaopectate may help decrease diarrhea. Mucopolysaccharides have been advocated as agents to improve electrolyte absorption, but one controlled study was unable to demonstrate any benefit on fecal consistency or glucose absorption. Pregelatinized starch is also used as an antidiarrheic agent. On an experimental basis, weak acids such as nicotinic acid have been shown to reduce the secretory effects of enterotoxigenic *E. coli*, but these are not currently used commercially.[391,392]

Prognosis for recovery decreases with the severity of depression. Severe hypothermia and the presence of intercurrent disease are grounds for a guarded prognosis.[393-395]

In summary, an initial examination should be performed. Calves with a primary problem of septicemia usually are not worth treating because of the poor prognosis. The severity of dehydration, hypothermia, and acidosis should be estimated. Recumbent calves are usually treated intravenously with a saline-based rehydrating fluid (0.9% saline, Ringer's, lactated Ringer's, etc.) and isotonic sodium bicarbonate (especially for older and comatose calves). Calves that can suck are treated with oral electrolytes that contain 50 to 80 mmol/L of alkalinizing agent. Products that use mainly acetate as the alkalinizing agent are best for calves that are still drinking cow's milk (small quantities, frequently). Any alkalinizing agent is likely effective in calves held off milk.

PREVENTION

The principles of prevention are to:
1. Ensure adequate colostral intake
2. Boost specific and nonspecific immunity
3. Reduce the possibility of introduction/spread of infectious agents

Adequate Colostral Intake

Numerous surveys indicate that colostrum is important in preventing morbidity and mortality from calf scours.[396-401] It is clearly established that local (enteric) immunity is important in this protection; the major benefits appear to last for about 3 to 4 days after birth.[402-404] After this period, milk contains little immunoglobulin and most colostral antibody has been cleared from the intestine. Colostral antibody is responsible for the low incidence of rotaviral infections in calves under 4 days of age[298,299]; in contrast, anti-F5 (K99) (*E. coli*) antibody is present in low amounts in unvaccinated cows,[405] and enteric *E. coli* infections are usually seen in very young calves. After 4 days the protective effects of colostrum primarily are due to systemic antibodies, and evidence indicates that these can leak back into the gut and probably give limited long-term protection against diarrhea.[398]

The principles of colostrum feeding and evaluation are discussed in detail elsewhere. In general, colostrum deprivation is seen in 25% to 50% of dairy calves,[399,400,406] but is much less common in single suckle beef operations.[407] Colostrum deprivation, poor mothering, and early separation of dam and calf are the major causes of failure of transfer in dairy calves. Beef calves are usually mothered well,[408-410] and volume of colostrum production, which is strongly influenced by nutrition, is one limiting factor.[411-413] Thus adequate colostrum intake is best ensured in dairy calves by assisted sucking of the dam or hand feeding 2 to 3 L of colostrum within 2 to 4 hours of birth. If colostrum is given by stomach tube, 4 L should be administered, because the efficiency of absorption is reduced. In beef cattle, adequate nutrition during late pregnancy is important. The calving area should be carefully monitored, and any calves that fail to suck soon after birth should be caught and tubed with colostrum.

Boosting Immunity

Vaccination against enterotoxigenic *E. coli* is effective because most enteropathogens share a common antigen F5 (K99), colostral antibody titers against F5 (K99) are often low in unvaccinated cows, and the disease strikes in the first few days of life. Experimental studies have confirmed the feasibility of boosting colostral antibody titers by vaccinating the dam with bacterins containing F5 (K99) positive *E. coli*.[414] This preparation was superior to a multivalent vaccine in protecting the dam's calves against experimental *E. coli* diarrhea.[405] The vaccine was also shown to be effective in field trials.[415] In general, it is recommended that the vaccines are given 6 and 3 weeks before calving. Studies with some vaccines have shown that the vaccine is still effective if the priming dose is given 18 months before calving, and boosting is carried out in the second half of gestation.[416] Clinical experience in beef farms suffering severe outbreaks of *E. coli* F5 (K99) diarrhea indicates that vaccinating cows that are more than 10 days from parturition can give considerable protection against death from enterotoxigenic *E. coli* infection.

Products containing monoclonal antibodies against F5 (K99) antigen have been shown to reduce the severity of diarrhea when calves are experimentally challenged a few hours after receiving the product.[417] In field situations, however, monoclonal products can have a low efficacy, presumably because a single dose only provides a short period of enteric protection. Antibody supplements are expensive, and vaccination of the dam to boost colostral immunity will usually be more cost effective. On farms experiencing an outbreak of neonatal diarrhea caused by F5 (K99) *E. coli*, there may be a place for the use of these products until vaccinated cows begin to calve. However, short-term administration (once a day for first 3 days of life) of an antibiotic to which the *E. coli* is susceptible is also highly effective in preventing diarrhea in herds experiencing outbreaks of enterotoxigenic *E. coli*.

The relatively low incidence of diarrhea associated with *E. coli* F5 in recent years may be due to widespread use of vaccine. However, *E. coli* with other attachment factors may still be important.

Vaccination against rotavirus and coronavirus diarrhea has had a checkered history. Early work indicated that vaccinating calves orally with a tissue-culture adapted rotavirus vaccine would protect against rotavirus diarrhea. However, it appears that the vaccine is inactivated in many calves by antirotaviral antibody from colostrum. Field studies with beef herds failed to show any benefit from this vaccine.[418] Vaccines can also be given to the dam to boost colostral immunity to higher levels. Studies with some early vaccines demonstrated that these did not cause significant seroconversion in the cows and did not boost colostral antirotavirus antibody titers.[419,420] Field studies failed to show any protection against viral scours in calves born to vaccinated dams[420] or any protection against diarrhea in calves vaccinated against scours.[349] Vaccines developed in Europe have produced seroconversion, boosted colostral antibody titers,[419,420] and reduced the incidence of rotavirus diarrhea in field trials.[422-424] In the United States, Norden* modified its calf diarrhea vaccine, and Scourguard 3(K)* boosts colostral antirotavirus antibody titers.[425] Titers

decline fairly rapidly, and at the present time it is not clear whether the vaccine provides protection. In hand-rearing operations it is possible to provide extended periods of protection by storing immune colostrum and feeding small amounts (200 ml) daily throughout the first few weeks of the calf's life.[419,426] One problem with vaccines is that even within serogroup A rotaviruses there are sufficient strain differences that vaccination with one strain does not necessarily protect against challenge with other strains.[427,428]

Some producers routinely administer vitamin A to neonatal calves. Many, but not all, studies in children indicate that supplementation can reduce the incidence of diarrhea in areas where clinical and subclinical vitamin A deficiency is endemic.[429] In cattle, vitamin A deficiency is most likely when a diet of unsupplemented straw and grain is fed. Calves born to cows fed good-quality, green forage or cattle receiving a vitamin A supplement should not require supplementation—particularly if they received adequate colostrum. Enteric absorption of vitamin A is diminished in calves with cyptosporidiosis, so the systemic route should be used in calves with this type of infection.[430]

Reducing Entry and Spread of Infectious Agents

Most enteropathogens can survive for long periods in the environment. Salmonellae and *E. coli* can survive in a damp environment for months. In one instance, salmonella organisms persisted in a calf-rearing unit despite the fact that the unit was depopulated, cleaned, disinfected, and kept free of calves for 6 months.[431] Rotaviruses survive for about 2 weeks in fresh water, but survival is enhanced by cool temperatures. Dirt also stabilizes viral particles. Under favorable conditions, rotaviruses can persist for months.[432] Cryptosporidia are also resistant and can survive for 2 to 6 months at 4° C. They die off more rapidly in airy locations and are killed by freezing.[328]

In dairy systems, where calves are reared by hand, the number of young stock on the farm and the incidence of respiratory disease are positive predictors for calf diarrhea.[421] In addition, cleanliness of the calving area appears to be important; bedding should be changed between each calving, and large numbers of cows should not be cycled through a few stalls.[421] There should be sufficient stalls to allow thorough cleaning before each calving and disinfection on a regular basis. Before calving, the udder and the perineum of the cow should be cleaned. The calf should receive adequate colostrum.[433] In recent years the use of calf hutches has gained widespread acceptance for managing calves after they have been separated from their dam. This system provides individual isolated housing for each calf. Cleaning is facilitated because the hutches can be moved to new sites between calves. Keeping preweaned calves in groups larger than six puts them at increased risk of diarrhea.[434]

Cleaning and disinfection after each batch of calves plays an important role in reducing contamination in housed calves. The key to decontamination is cleaning. All movable equipment should be removed and scrubbed down. After the electricity has been turned off, the building can be wetted down to trap dust and then thoroughly cleaned; this removes about 90% of bacteria. High-pressure hosing is an effective cleaning method and can remove 99.98% of contamination, even when no disinfectants are used.[435] The most easily cleanable surfaces are made of smooth, impervious materials such as plastic and varnished wood (Table 20-8). Usually buildings are cleaned and then either disinfected or fumigated.[436] Many disinfectants are inactivated by organic matter; viruses, coccidia, and particularly cryptosporidia, may be resistant to their action (Table 20-9). They may also be toxic and are best applied by personnel wearing rubber gloves and respirators (if indoors). Generally, potent phenolics such as cresol (cresylic acid) are useful for disinfecting dirty surfaces because they are

---

*Pfizer Animal Health, Exter, PA 19341.

not inactivated by organic matter and are effective against gram-negative organisms and viruses. The phenolics are highly toxic and leave lingering odors. Hypochlorite solutions (5 g available chlorine/L) have a broad spectrum of action but are rapidly inactivated by organic matter. They would be useful as a final disinfectant on previously cleaned surfaces. Because hypochlorite is unstable, it is unlikely to leave toxic residues. Iodophors are not effective against rotavirus, particularly if organic matter is present. Formaldehyde is one of the few agents that is effective against cryptosporidia. It requires a long contact time and is highly toxic. It is usually used for terminal fumigation in buildings that can be tightly sealed. Formaldehyde gas is best generated by heating paraformaldehyde (5 g/m³ of building) in an electrically heated pan at 204° C. Some manufacturers of paraformaldehyde provide

pans specially designed for this purpose. The pans should be placed no more than 30 m apart. The set up should be arranged so that electricity to the pan can be controlled from outside the building, and there must be some mechanism for ensuring that the pan does not overheat and cause a fire. The building must be sealed for at least 24 hours and cannot be entered until it has been thoroughly ventilated. Formaldehyde gas can also be generated by boiling formalin or by adding potassium permanganate to formalin. The latter method generates a violent chemical reaction and carries risks of explosion. Formalin aerosol generators are ineffective.[437] After cleaning and disinfection, one should allow a rest period for the building to ventilate before reintroducing calves. It is important that cleaning and disinfection be thorough. Attention should also be given to rodent control because these can be a reservoir for *Salmonella*.[438]

In addition to cleaning between batches it is important to clean nipple buckets and other feeding utensils between each feed. Adequate ventilation may also be important because some enteric pathogens also infect the respiratory tract, and the incidence of respiratory and enteric disease in calf units is related. In some surveys a factor that made a systematic difference to calf survival was the sex and age of the caregiver. Women and children did a better job than men.[434,439]

Operations that buy in calves for rearing purposes should be encouraged to buy from as few sources as possible. Direct purchase from one farm is best; assembling collections of calves through auction markets should be avoided if possible. In some cases, calves may be infected with *Salmonella* on the farm of origin from carrier cows. Culturing calves and cows can help detect this problem.

Diet is an important factor in preventing diarrhea. Calves that are fed milk from mastitic quarters or antibiotic-containing milk are at increased risk of diarrhea.[434] After fresh colostrum feeding, young calves have less diarrhea if placed on whole cow's milk rather than other diets. Feeding surplus colostrum and waste cow's milk is thought to be intermediate, whereas milk replacers, particularly those containing vegetable protein, can give a higher incidence of diarrhea. Pasteurizing surplus colostrum and waste milk reduces the

TABLE 20-8

Ability of Bacteria to Persist on Various Types of Surfaces Found in Farm Buildings

Material	Total Bacterial Count per 100 cm²	
	Uncleaned	Cleaned
Brick	76,000	
Painted wood	34,000	
Block board	116,000	
Ply board	77,000	23,000
Fiber board	57,000	
Chip board	35,000	
Formica	29,000	
Polystyrene	29,000	
Metal		14,000
Concrete		13,000
Plastic	16,000	100
Varnished wood	5,000	

Modified from Morgan-Jones SC: In Collins E et al: *Disinfectants: their use and evaluation of effectiveness*, London, 1981, Academic Press, pp 199-212.

TABLE 20-9

Efficacy of Disinfectants Against Enteropathogens

Group	Compound	Efficacy		
		Gram-negative Bacteria	Rotavirus	Cryptosporidia
Phenolics				
	Hexachlorophene	+	++	
	Tricloson	+	++	
	Cresol (coal tar derivation)	++	++	−
	Phenol	±	−	
Halogens				
	Povidone-iodine	+	−	−
	Hypochlorite	+	+	
Biguamides				
	Chlorhexidine	++	−	
Aldehydes				
	Formaldehyde*	+	+	+
	Glutaraldehyde	+		
Quaternary ammonium				
	Benzalkonium chloride	+	+	
	Cetrimide	+		
Ammonia				
	Ammonia			+

Based on information in references 408, 446-451.
++, Highly effective, not inactivated by organic matter; +, moderately effective/inactivated by organic matter; ±, some effect; −, little effect.
*Requires long contact time—18 hours to kill cryptosporidia.

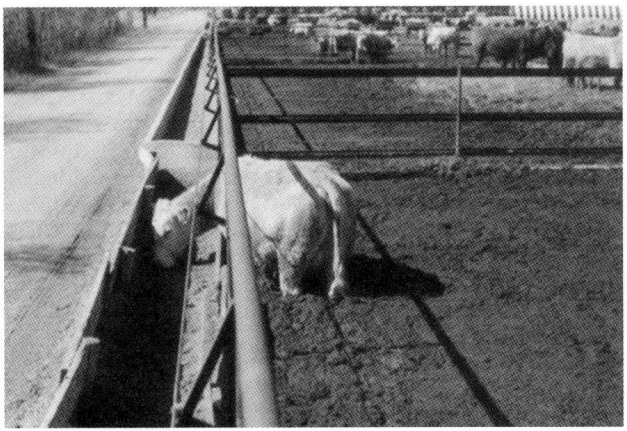

FIG. 20-17 ▌ Cow on a farm with a high incidence of neonatal diarrhea. Note that the mud is so deep around the feeders that it covers the cow's hocks. As a result the teats will be contaminated by manure and enteric pathogens.

incidence of diarrhea on these diets.[440] It is also important to offer good-quality hay from about 2 days of age; at first, little will be ingested, so offer small amounts and keep it fresh.[440]

Studies of beef herds indicate that diarrhea is more likely to be a problem in large herds.[441] Viral agents are known to be excreted in low numbers by adult cows,[442,443] so this may be one method by which infection is introduced into the calf population. Bacterial agents such as *Salmonella* and *E. coli*, and protozoa are also often brought into or maintained in a herd by asymptomatic carrier cows. The organisms multiply in calves, and the infection is magnified until it reaches epidemic proportions in neonates.

Epidemiologic studies show that a high percentage of heifers in the herd, intensive stocking, poor drainage, and dirty or wet calving and rearing areas are major risk factors. Cattle should also be moved from the wintering area to a clean calving area.[444] Beef cattle are best overwintered in separate groups from cows and heifers, and it is important that heifers are calved in a separate area and their calves managed separately.[445] This gives the opportunity to provide better feed to the heifers and to slow the transmission of disease from susceptible calves born to heifers to the rest of the herd. Large herds are best split into groups of 50 to 75 head. Just before calving the cows or heifers should be moved to a clean, well-drained calving area. The group size should be small, and there should be a minimum of 100 m² (1000 ft²) per cow and ideally 200 m². The area should provide plenty of clean bedding and good wind breaks.[433] During this period the cow can be carefully observed for dystocia. Once the calf is born, it should be checked frequently to make sure it is up and sucking. Calves that are not sucking within 4 hours of birth can be tube fed colostrum for a colostrum bank. When cow and calf are successfully bonded, they can be moved to a separate nursing area. Again, the area should be clean, well-drained, and spacious. If more than 5% of the area is poorly drained (prone to standing water) or if the cows have mud above their hocks (and thus likely on their udders), the risk of diarrhea is increased (Fig. 20-17). Early cases of diarrhea are best isolated from the main group to reduce contamination. Buying in replacements for calves lost at birth should be discouraged—it is easy to buy in diseased calves.

SUMMARY

Calf scours is caused by a variety of infectious agents. At the present time the need to make a definitive diagnosis of en-

terotoxigenic *E. coli* and salmonella infections has been established; these diseases can be controlled by antibiotics and prevented by vaccination.[446] There are public health implications to the diagnosis of cryptosporidiosis and salmonellosis. New vaccines may help control rotavirus and coronavirus infections. Treatment of neonate diarrhea is primarily based on correcting dehydration and acidosis through the use of oral and intravenous electrolytes. Only in the case of bacterial infections can direct action be taken against the invading organism, but antibiotics may still be useful in preventing secondary bacteremias. Colostrum feeding will help reduce diarrhea in the first days of life. Management is thought to be important in the control of diarrhea, and because infectious agents are almost always present at some exposure level, the underlying theme must be reduction of stress on the calf.

To approach a problem of neonatal death losses, the areas to be examined should include calf immunoglobulin status, calf feeding, calf housing, cleanliness of environment, calving area, cow vaccinations, diagnosis of specific infectious agents, and the treatment protocol.

LAMENESS AND RELUCTANCE TO WALK

JOHN E. MADIGAN
JOHN K. HOUSE

INFECTIOUS LAMENESS

ETIOLOGY. Septic arthritis, septic physitis, and osteomyelitis as a complication of or sequel to bacteremia (septicemia) produce lameness and reluctance to move. Terminology to describe this condition has included "joint-ill," "navel-ill," septic physitis, septic polyarthritis, and septic epiphysitis.[452] Blood-borne bacteria from a previous illness or concurrent with an active nidus of infection produces infection in synovial membranes, growth plates, or periarticular bone. Sources of infection include primary bacteremia (septicemia) associated with failure of passive transfer[453] (FPT) (see Chapter 49), pneumonia, umbilical infection, enteritis, and extension of local infection from penetrating wounds. A recent study demonstrated that only 38 of 140 foals had abnormal umbilicus with confirmed septic arthritis. In foals, bacteria that produce septic arthritis include the etiologic agents of septicemia: *Escherichia coli, Klebsiella* spp., *Actinobacillus equuli, Salmonella* spp., *Rhodococcus equi*, and *Streptococcus* spp.[453] A recent review of 78 foals with septic arthritis ranked the frequency of isolation of bacterial agents. Gram-negative bacteria were cultured from 51 of 78 foals. In addition, the probability of susceptibility of these isolates to various antibiotics was determined. Blood culture produced more bacterial isolates, although joint aspiration yielded bacteria in 69% of foals sampled.[454] Bacterial species cultured from blood and synovial fluid were identical in 16 of 88 foals. Negative cultures occurred in 31% of foals with later confirmed septic arthritis.[454] Gram-negative bacteria were more common with younger foals and gram-positive infections became increasingly more common with advancing age of the foal.[454]

Bacteria commonly isolated from septic joints in lambs include *Streptococcus* spp., coliforms, *Arcanobacterium pyogenes, Erysipelothrix rhusiopathiae*, and *Fusobacterium necrophorum*.[455] Predisposing factors include poor docking hygiene and contaminated sheep dip. In neonatal calves, streptococci and coliforms (*E. coli, Salmonella* spp.) are the most commonly isolated organisms from septic joints; *A. pyogenes* is the most frequently isolated organism from joints of older calves.[456-458] Sporadic outbreaks of polyarthritis in lambs,

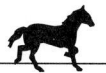

kids,[459,460] and calves[461] are associated with *Chlamydia* and *Mycoplasma* spp. infections. *Chlamydia* infections may occur in utero or postnatally, *Mycoplasma* infections often result from ingestion of mycoplasma-contaminated milk.

CLINICAL SIGNS AND DIFFERENTIAL DIAGNOSES. Signs may be extremely variable. Sudden onset of lameness in one leg in an apparently healthy neonate with or without joint distention, pain, or edema may be noted. Other presentations may be observed, consisting of sudden onset of lameness with systemic signs of illness or evidence of multiple joint distention, pain, and edema in a neonate with obvious illness and a diagnosis of septicemia. Prematurity or failure of passive transfer should raise the index of suspicion. The chief differential is trauma; lameness is often blamed by the owner on the dam's stepping on the newborn. Any neonate less than 45 days of age with sudden onset of lameness should be considered infected until proven otherwise. Lambs and kids with septic arthritis often fail to nurse and may present with significant weight loss. Typically polyarthritis caused by *Mycoplasma* spp. and *Chlamydia* is associated with high fevers and respiratory and occasionally neurologic disease. High morbidity and mortality are common. Conjunctivitis is commonly observed with chlamydial infections.[462]

CLINICAL PATHOLOGY AND RADIOLOGY. Diagnosis may be obvious, with signs of septicemia; a positive sepsis score (see Chapter 19); and a swollen, hot, and painful joint. Peripheral leukocyte counts, temperature, alertness, and appetite may be normal with localized infections. Joint aspiration may reveal normal synovial fluid if the infection is in the early stages of synovial membrane inflammation or physeal or bone involvement.[452] Synovial fluid with greater than 10,000 white blood cells (WBC)/μl and greater than 70% neutrophils indicates that infection is likely.[453] Gram stain of the synovial fluid smear for intracellular and extracellular bacteria may aid diagnosis. Thin, turbid, or brown synovial fluid with increased leukocytes is considered evidence of infection.[452] Culture of synovial fluid is often negative, even when infection is present. Improved recovery of bacteria may be obtained with thioglycolate broth or brain heart broth with an agar slant and sodium polyanethole sulfonate (SPS) to prevent clotting and inhibit aminoglycoside and trimethoprim antibiotics.[463] Chlamydial inclusions may be found in Giemsa-stained smears of synovial cells and the organism isolated from joint fluid or plasma in early cases.[462] Isolation of *Mycoplasma* spp. requires specific media (Hayflick's media) and microaerophilic conditions. Normal synovial fluid does not rule out septic physitis or osteomyelitis, because the infection may be in the physis or small tarsal bones.[452]

Careful examination of high-quality radiographs is important for the detection of bone lysis indicating infection. Initial radiographs may be normal because the degree of damage is often not detectable for 10 to 14 days after initial infection occurs.[452] Radiographic features of septic arthritis include soft tissue swelling, widening or collapse of the joint space, osteoporosis, and osteosclerosis. Repeat radiographs taken at 7-day intervals are valuable for assessing the degree of damage.[452] Ultrasound may be used to confirm involvement of the joint and rule out periarticular or tenosynovial infection to avoid iatrogenic contamination of the joint during arthrocentesis. Joint distention and hyperechogenic fragments in the synovial fluid are suggestive of septic arthritis.[464] Normal synovial fluid is anechoic. Bone scans or computerized tomography (CT) may facilitate early detection.[465]

PATHOPHYSIOLOGY. Hematogenous bacteremia resulting in bone infection may follow a variety of pathways.[452] A nidus of infection may develop in a junction of cartilage and subchondral bone. The low pressure/slow flow and reduced oxygen pressure of the blood supply at cartilage-bone junctions may predispose to establishment of infection in these

---

---

areas. Level of immunity and degree of maturation of bone of the foal may be additional predisposing factors.[452] Destruction of the epiphysis and extension of infection into the joint may be primary in some cases, rather than starting as a primary synovial membrane infection that spreads to the epiphysis/physis. A classification has been proposed to reflect the various pathogeneses of infection (Box 20-7). Infection of the small bones of the tarsus has been reported to be more common than that of the carpus,[466] and the metaphysis of ribs and vertebral bodies may be involved.[453] Synovitis produces severe inflammation and depletion of the cartilage matrix and collagen framework, which can cause irreversible damage.[452,453] Eburnation of cartilage leads to exposure of subchondral bone and extension of infection in bone.[452]

TREATMENT. Aims of treatment are to (1) remove the infectious agent, (2) protect and minimize cartilage damage, and (3) minimize secondary osteoarthrosis. If FPT has occurred, an additional aim is to provide immunoglobulins through plasma transfusion (2 or more liters intravenously).[452] Treatment described for bacteremia (septicemia) should be used promptly. Umbilical ultrasound should be considered if another nidus of infection is not found. Systemic antibiotics provide adequate levels of antibiotic in normal and inflamed joints.[452,467] Antibiotics with gram-negative spectrum should be used initially, and selection modified by culture results from synovial fluid, blood, or tracheal wash. A recent review found the administration of ampicillin or a first-generation cephalosporin in conjunction with amikacin had a good probability of antimicrobial sensitivity.[454] Antimicrobials (antibiotics) should be continued for at least 3 weeks. Joint lavage with 1 to 3 L of balanced polyionic buffered (pH-adjusted) fluids helps to remove bacteria and inflammatory mediators that damage cartilage and improves outcome.[454] An infected joint is a medical emergency, and treatment should be carried out immediately after clinical diagnosis of probable sepsis, even before all cultures and clinical pathology tests are back. Arthrotomy for joints with fibrin and debris has been advocated and appears effective.[463,468] Delivery of antibiotics to chronically infected tissues via regional limb perfusion has been described.[469] Confinement and limb immobilization may decrease pain, inflammation, and cartilage damage. Short-term use (24 to 48 hours) of nonsteroidal antiinflammatory drugs (NSAIDs) such as flunixin or phenylbutazone at prescribed dosages may be indicated, although the risk of these agents inducing gastric ulceration in foals is well described.

Acute septic arthritis in neonatal ruminants may be treated effectively via joint lavage combined with systemic and local antimicrobial treatment. Typically, however, neonatal ruminants are presented with a chronic disease process. Joint lavage is rarely efficacious in the treatment of chronic septic arthritis in calves as accumulation of fibrin and pocketing of purulent material often make adequate joint drainage impossible.[470]

Systemic antibacterial treatment is often insufficient to eliminate joint infections, particularly in the subacute or chronic stages. Bacteria trapped in fibrin clots are partially protected from the effects of systemically administered antibiotics.[471] Joint drainage and arthrotomy improve the success rate, but the recovery may be protracted and complications from the procedure are not uncommon. Arthroscopy may be used to explore and debride infected joints. Advantages include excellent exposure, thorough lavage under pressure, decreased postoperative management, and fewer complications.[464] Carpal arthrodesis is the most effective way to treat calves with chronic septic carpitis with secondary flexor tendon contraction and extensor sheath infection.[470]

Antimicrobial selection is guided by bacterial isolation and determination of drug sensitivities. Broad-spectrum antimicrobial treatment should be initiated pending culture results anticipating the high probability of a coliform, streptococcal, or *Arcanobacterium* infection. An extensive review of antimicrobial treatment of infectious arthritis and osteomyelitis in ruminants is presented by Trent and Plumb.[472] In calves the concentration of trimethoprim-sulfadiazine, oxytetracycline, cephapirin, or penicillin in synovial fluid following chemically induced synovitis were no different than the drug concentrations in normal joints.[473-475] Suppurative inflammation reduces the concentration of ampicillin in synovial fluid compared with normal joints; however, the synovial drug concentration reached is still greater than the mean inhibited concentration for *Arcanobacterium pyogenes*.[470,476]

PROGNOSIS. Duration, extent of bone involvement, and degree of damage affect the prognosis. A recent study determined 79% of foals with septic arthritis had IgG levels less than 8 g/L (800 mg/dl). Infection of multiple joints, delay in onset of treatment, and presence of concurrent bony lesions on radiographs were associated with a poorer prognosis.[454] In one study, 67% of foals with septic arthritis were discharged when treatment was initiated within 24 hours of the onset of clinical signs.[454] Better outcomes were observed when treatment included joint lavage. Of foals treated for septic arthritis, 26% went on to perform their intended function.

If FPT has occurred and multiple joints are involved, the prognosis is poor because, in foals with FPT and lameness, multiorgan involvement is common.[453] Initial detection should warrant a guarded prognosis. The long duration of treatment and sometimes costly multiple therapeutic modalities should be discussed with the owner at the outset. Reevaluation of the patient at regular intervals is indicated. Recurrence after cessation of therapy sometimes occurs.

In a review of 81 cases of septic arthritis in cattle, a 72% recovery was achieved with a combination of surgical treatment (opening of the joint capsule; debridement; and excision of the synovium, infected cartilage, and bone), joint immobilization, and systemic antibiotic therapy. Of cattle treated conservatively with systemic and intraarticular antimicrobials, 43% recovered.[477]

NONINFECTIOUS LAMENESS

Rhabdomyolysis in foals deficient in vitamin E and selenium may be precipitated by stress such as septicemia. Affected foals are reluctant to move, paretic, and occasionally dysphagic. Pelvic limb muscles are often palpably firm. Elevated serum creatinine kinase and electrolyte disturbances of hyponatremia and hyperkalemia may be observed.[478] Neonatal ruminants with nutritional myodegeneration often have a stiff, stilted gait. Lambs and kids may have difficulty nursing if they are unable to lift their head and may cry with pain when assisted to stand (see Chapter 40).

In foals, rupture of the common digital extensor tendon may be present at birth or develop within a few days of life.

Rupture occurs within the carpal synovial sheath and produces swelling over the dorsolateral surface of the carpus at the level of the intercarpal and carpometacarpal joints. Palpation of the fibers reveals tearing of the tendon. Splinting of the limb for 3 to 4 weeks usually results in healing.[479]

Contracture of joints or tendons of the limbs produces difficulty in movement and predisposes to failure of passive transfer by impeding the ability to adequately nurse. Degree of contracture varies from mild to severe and may be associated with scoliosis and/or torticollis.[480] Foals with congenital contracture of tendons of the front limbs may spontaneously rupture the common digital extensor tendon. Conservative therapy consisting of splinting the front limbs to induce tendon laxity may be helpful. Calves with severe digital flexor tendon contractures often require surgical resection of one or both digital flexor tendons, followed by bandaging or casting and stall rest for 3 to 4 weeks.

Developmental Causes

Incomplete ossification of the cuboidal bones (see Fig. 20-1) of the carpus and tarsus of newborn foals is considered to be related to the development of flexural and angular deformities of the foal.[481] Twins, premature foals, foals that are small for gestational age, and foals with in utero–acquired infection are likely to have incomplete ossification of cuboidal bones at birth.[481,482] Radiographic analysis and grading of the degree of ossification have been suggested for these foals.[482] Foals with substantially reduced ossification may damage bone with limb loading. Limited exercise may be prudent until ossification begins to increase radiographically, which can be within 7 days. Hypothyroidism (see Chapter 39) has been identified in foals with angular limb deformities, contracted tendons, and tarsal bone collapse.[483,484]

PATENT URACHUS, OMPHALITIS, AND OTHER UMBILICAL ABNORMALITIES

JOHN E. MADIGAN
JOHN K. HOUSE

PATENT URACHUS

DEFINITION. Patent urachus is a persistence after birth of the tubular connection between the bladder and umbilicus. The urachus drains the bladder into the allantoic sac during gestation. Urine flow should gradually change, with some urine entering the amniotic sac through the urethra in later gestation. At birth, with umbilical cord rupture the urachus should be closed, and urine should be voided through the urethra. Foals with a patent urachus may dribble urine from the urachus during or after urination or may simply present with a constantly wet umbilical stump.

ETIOLOGY. A variety of causes have been suggested for failure of the urachus to close and completely involute. Early severance or ligation of the umbilical cord, inflammation, infection, and excessive physical handling of the neonate have been implicated.[485] Rather than being the original cause for hospital admission, patent urachus develops as a complication of hospitalization in a significant percentage of foals in neonatal intensive care.

CLINICAL SIGNS AND DIFFERENTIAL DIAGNOSIS. Differentials include concurrent infection of the navel (omphalophlebitis). Ultrasound may assist the diagnosis and determine the involvement of umbilical arteries or vein.[486]

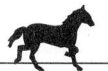

Moist hairs around the umbilicus and visualization of fluid coming from the navel are diagnostic.

CLINICAL PATHOLOGY. Identification of concurrent infection is essential. A complete physical examination should be performed. If abnormalities are noted, serum IgG, complete blood count, and urinalysis are helpful for detecting susceptibility to infection and presence of systemic or urinary tract infection.

PATHOPHYSIOLOGY. Congenital patent urachus caused by excessive torsion on the umbilical cord in utero occurs in 6% of normal foals.[487] The obstruction of the urachus caused by the torsion causes retention of urine in the bladder and overdistends the proximal urachus, which interferes with normal involution.[487] Infection of umbilical structures or the urachus itself may result in inflammation and failure to completely involute. In a review of 16 cases of umbilical cord infections in foals, 13 had patent urachus.[488] The majority of these foals had acquired patent urachus after birth, with the youngest age of onset 3 days and the mean age of onset 12 days. Excessive manipulation and improper lifting of the foal's abdomen in the presence of high urethral sphincter tone may force urine within the bladder out into the involuting urachus. In our experience, farms have experienced outbreaks of patent urachus when procedures (such as tests for failure of passive transfer) have been implemented that require handling of foals in the first 12 to 24 hours of life. A similar cause may be responsible for the increased incidence of patent urachus in hand-reared calves.

TREATMENT AND PROGNOSIS. Therapy consists of either conservative management through monitoring or medical treatment for infection and cauterization of the urachus with iodine, phenol, or silver nitrate sticks applied into the urachus. Persistence of urine dribbling after 2 to 3 days of cauterization, the detection of involvement of other umbilical structures through ultrasound, and a rent in the urachus that produces subcutaneous swelling are indications for surgery. Not all foals that have persistent patent urachus have an infected umbilicus.[416] Use of general anesthesia and removal of the entire urachus to the tip of the bladder are performed in foals or ruminants with an infected or enlarged urachus. Associated arteries and veins should be ligated and removed if they are infected or necrotic. Merely ligating the exterior stump can trap organisms and cause infection. In our neonatal unit the majority of patients with acquired patent urachus respond to conservative therapy. Late-onset patent urachus (5 days of age) may be more refractory to conservative therapy.[488] Complications of delaying surgery relate to development of bladder necrosis and uroperitoneum caused by extension of infection and inflammation of the urachus.

PREVENTION. Allowing the umbilical cord to rupture without ligation or the careful use of specific umbilical clamps after birth has been suggested to decrease the incidence of patent urachus. Minimum handling of neonates and careful restraint may prevent pressure build-up in the bladder and subsequent patent urachus.

OMPHALITIS/OMPHALOPHLEBITIS

DEFINITION AND ETIOLOGY. Omphalitis is inflammation of umbilical structures that may include the umbilical arteries, umbilical vein, urachus, or tissues immediately surrounding the umbilicus. The umbilicus consists of three types of structures and undergoes functional and anatomic changes at birth. Two umbilical arteries connect internal iliac arteries to the placenta. These later regress and become the round ligaments of the bladder. One umbilical vein connecting the placenta to the liver and porta cava regresses to become the round ligament of the liver within the falciform ligament. The urachus connects the fetal bladder to the allantoic cavity.

Umbilical abscess or infection of any of the three components of the umbilicus may produce local infection or be a source of septicemia. The source of infection is most commonly the external environment, coupled with failure of passive transfer. Organisms isolated in foals include *E. coli* and *Proteus* and *Streptococcus* spp. Bacteria isolated from calf umbilical cord remnant infection include *A. pyogenes*, *E. coli*, and *Proteus* and *Enterococcus* spp. The urachus is the most commonly affected structure in calves and the umbilical arteries the least.[489] Omphalophlebitis may extend the length of the umbilical vein into the liver and result in liver abscessation.

CLINICAL SIGNS AND DIFFERENTIAL DIAGNOSIS. When the umbilicus is enlarged and draining purulent material, infection is easily noted. In other cases the umbilicus may be dry and larger in diameter than expected. In addition, neonates may have a completely normal-appearing, dry external navel and be severely ill from infection of the urachus, umbilical arteries, or vein.[416] In a septic neonate without external signs of infection, involvement of the umbilicus can be difficult to determine. The presence of pain on palpation of the umbilicus indicates inflammation. Ultrasound has recently been shown to aid the detection of involvement of urachus or arteries and vein by detection of size abnormalities.[486] The umbilical area of neonates less than 20 days of age with fever of unknown origin should be scanned. Hematoma developing after umbilical rupture may produce distention of the umbilical stump shortly after birth.

Overt signs of infection are heat, swelling, purulent discharge, or pain. Concurrent signs of systemic infection such as joint infection, pneumonia, diarrhea, meningitis, or uveitis may be noted. Calves with urachal abscesses may show signs of dysuria or pollakiuria.[490,491] Infection in more than one umbilical vessel in the neonate is common, and urachal involvement is frequent.[418] Umbilical abscessation that is walled off and does not involve deeper structures is a less severe problem and may be treated with drainage without surgical removal of the entire umbilicus. The depth of involvement may be determined by standing behind the neonate and pressing the hands together above the umbilicus to detect internal masses and painful areas.

DIAGNOSTIC METHODS. In addition to detection of overt umbilical inflammation as described, ultrasonography may aid in evaluating a normal-appearing navel.[486] The umbilical vein, arteries, and urachus may be imaged in the newborn (see Chapter 17). The umbilical arteries leave the umbilical stalk and course on the outer edges of the urachus in a parallel fashion.[486] In the foal the urachus connects the apex of the bladder with the umbilicus and is located along the midline immediately adjacent to the body wall. Persistent dilation of the umbilical vein or arteries with a hypoechoic-to-echogenic fluid is seen with infection. In calves the urachus normally retracts up into the abdomen at birth, and ultrasonographic identification of a urachal remnant is abnormal.[492] In the hands of a skilled ultrasonographer familiar with normal ultrasonographic findings of the umbilicus, there is an excellent correlation between surgical and ultrasound findings.[486]

TREATMENT AND PROGNOSIS. Early treatment with antibiotics and supportive care as described for the septicemic foal (see Chapter 19) may allow resolution before development of abscessation and distention of the urachus or the umbilical arteries and vein. Established infection, which may occur within 24 hours, usually requires surgical removal of involved structures in addition to medical therapy.[488,489] When omphalophlebitis extends into the liver, the umbilical vein may be marsupialized to facilitate drainage and flushing.[493] Surgical removal of urachal abscesses in calves often requires resection of the apex of the bladder. Prognosis is improved when adequate passive transfer of colostral immunoglobulins has occurred and when joints or other structures are not involved. Sequelae such as renal abscessation, joint or bone infection, peritonitis, and other complications described for septicemia may develop if therapy is started too late or discontinued prematurely.

ANEMIA

JOHN E. MADIGAN

DEFINITION AND ETIOLOGY. Anemia in the neonate should be interpreted in the context of the realization that normal hematologic values of the neonate may vary from the adult. In foals, values of hemoglobin and packed cell volume (PCV) are similar to those of adult horses but decrease during the first weeks and months of life to below that of adults.[494] Foals have low iron stores during the first 5 months of life; this is reflected in decreased serum ferritin concentration, increased serum total iron binding capacity, and decreasing mean corpuscular hemoglobin concentration.[495] Microcyte production is observed rapidly after birth.[495] Absolute red blood cell (RBC) and total blood volume decrease between 2 days and 2 weeks of age and then progressively increase.[496] In calves the incidence of anemia (hemoglobin <10 g/dl) is quite high, ranging from 15% to 30% in many herds[497,498] and is normocytic, normochromic, and poikilocytic. Previous reports had indicated an iron deficiency as a cause of the anemia.[497,498] Potential causes are reduced amounts of iron in milk, poor placental transfer of iron, or decreased intestinal absorption. Recent work[499] revealed that anemic calves with poikilocytosis have similar levels of serum iron, total iron binding capacity, and marrow iron and plasma copper levels compared with normal calves. Anemic calves do not appear to have an increased incidence of disease or decreased growth rates.[500] An overall higher plane of nutrition versus iron supplementation alone produces higher PCVs and hemoglobin levels.[499] Calves less than 6 weeks of age have three types of hemoglobin in various amounts (adult 28%, fetal 40%, and neonatal 25%). The poikilocytosis may be a function of erythrocyte membrane defects or maturation transitions.[499]

In addition to frank blood loss from an injury, diseases causing anemia in the neonate include neonatal isoerythrolysis (NI), non–NI immune-mediated hemolytic anemia, blood loss caused by gastric ulcer or ovarian cyst rupture producing hemoperitoneum, anemia of chronic disease associated with localized infections, piroplasmosis, and equine infectious anemia.

CLINICAL SIGNS AND DIFFERENTIAL DIAGNOSIS. Rapidly developing anemias such as those associated with neonatal isoerythrolysis in the foal and hemolytic disease of the newborn in ruminants produce signs of weakness, pale or jaundiced mucous membranes, fever, and depression. Hemoperitoneum produces weakness and pale mucous membranes. Suspected drug-induced, immune-mediated hemolytic anemia and thrombocytopenia have been reported in the foal.[501] Intestinal parasitism does not normally lead to anemia during the neonatal period. Chronic localized infection may produce anemia of chronic disease.

CLINICAL PATHOLOGY. Intravascular hemolysis may produce hemoglobinuria and hemoglobinemia. Icterus develops when the ability of the liver to conjugate bilirubin is exceeded. Mainly, indirect bilirubin is elevated. Anisocytosis is observed in responsive anemias. Nonspecific stimulation of bone marrow may produce a leukocytosis.

PATHOPHYSIOLOGY. Hemolytic disease of newborn calves is uncommon but has occurred after vaccination of pregnant cows against anaplasmosis or babesiosis. The presence of red cell antigens in the vaccine causes the production of antierythrocyte antibody, primarily against the A and F systems.[502] Cows mated to bulls carrying these red cell antigens may have hemolytic disease develop in their A- and F-positive calves after ingestion of colostrum-containing alloantibodies.

THERAPY. Determination of the nature of the anemia may allow specific treatment. NI is discussed in Chapter 49. Drug-induced or autoimmune anemias may be treated with corticosteroids (0.05 to 0.1 mg/kg dexamethasone twice a day intramuscularly or intravenously). Blood transfusion following crossmatch may be indicated when anemia develops rapidly or PCV drops below 14%. Massive red cell destruction may trigger disseminated intravascular coagulation, and the actual cause of death may be a result of activation of the clotting system by RBC destruction and reticuloendothelial system removal.[502] Associated conditions such as metabolic acidosis and hypoglycemia should be corrected. Anemia of chronic disease requires correction of the primary disease condition.

FEVER

JOHN E. MADIGAN

DEFINITION AND ETIOLOGY. Fever (rectal temperature >38.9° C [102° F]) as a clinical sign must be interpreted differently in neonates than in the adult because of the variations of anticipated response to systemic illness, temperature regulation control differences, and susceptibility to environmental changes in temperature. In septicemic foals, fever greater 38.9° C [102° F]) was present in fewer than 30% of cases, and hypothermia was noted in approximately 20%.[169] This finding is similar in neonatal ruminants. Consequently fever is considered an unreliable clinical sign for determination of sepsis in neonates. Older ruminants and foals with localized infection such as in joints or bone are more likely to have fever.

DIFFERENTIAL DIAGNOSIS. The chief differentials for fever in neonates are fever caused by infections with viral or bacterial pathogens, seizures with subsequent generation of heat by muscular overactivity, pyrogens generated from massive hemolysis in NI, and environmentally induced hyperthermia. The condition of transient tachypnea of the newborn may produce significantly elevated temperatures in warm environments.[503] Neonatal foals have a rapid respiratory rate that appears to be an attempt at heat loss through a panting type of mechanism. Extreme care must be used in attributing the pyrexia and fever to transient tachypnea syndrome alone by ruling out the presence of infection through physical examination, chest radiographs, blood gases, and computation of a sepsis score.

Pathophysiology is similar to that in the adult and is discussed thoroughly in Chapter 4.

TREATMENT AND PROGNOSIS. Although a conservative approach to fever in older animals may be appropriate, the presence of a fever in a neonate warrants rigorous diagnostic evaluation and aggressive therapeutic intervention. The immaturity of the neonatal immune system, the high fatality rate, and the frequency of devastating sequelae to bacterial infection warrant a complete examination of the neonate.

Because fever may be beneficial to the animal, the need to administer antipyretics to the febrile neonate is controversial. Body temperatures lower than 40.8° C (105.4° F) are not considered detrimental unless they are associated with heat stroke or seizures,[504] in which case cooling and antipyretics are indicated. Because many antipyretics are antiprostaglandins that can cause deleterious gastrointestinal and renal effects, these agents should be used judiciously. Dipyrone is often used in neonates in our clinic for antipyretic response because it lacks most of the adverse gastrointestinal side effects found with most nonsteroidal antiinflammatory drugs. Correction of the initiating cause and maintaining fluid balance are also important. Prognosis depends on

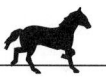

immunoglobulin status and stage of disease when treatment is initiated. Significant fatality rates occur in neonates with bacterial infections. Transient tachypnea has an excellent prognosis, with neonates becoming normothermic within 2 to 3 weeks of age. Clipping a long and thick haircoat, use of fans in stalls, and removal from direct sunlight may reduce heat stress to the neonate.

CYANOSIS
JOHN E. MADIGAN

DEFINITION AND ETIOLOGY. Cyanosis is the purple-blue coloration observed on mucous membranes or skin caused by reduced or poorly oxygenated hemoglobin in blood.[505] Causes for this condition include congenital heart disease, respiratory impairment, or any circulatory condition producing a right-to-left shunt. The degree of cyanosis depends on the arterial oxygen saturation, hemoglobin concentration, pH, peripheral circulation, and temperature of the neonate.[505] Shock and hypothermia are important causes of peripheral cyanosis (Box 20-8).

PATHOPHYSIOLOGY. The affinity of hemoglobin for oxygen is reflected in the standard oxyhemoglobin dissociation curve. This curve is similar for neonates but is affected by the amount of 2,3-diphosphoglycerate (DPG) in the erythrocyte. The foal does not have a fetal hemoglobin but has decreased amounts of 2,3-DPG, which causes oxygen to bind more tightly to hemoglobin and thus to be released in lesser amounts to the tissues.[506] Calves' erythrocytes have higher levels of 2,3-DPG, but the higher levels do not affect the affinity of hemoglobin for oxygen. A separate fetal hemoglobin exists in calves to increase affinity for oxygen.[507] Severe hypothermia and acidosis cause the oxygen dissociation curve to shift to the right and therefore contribute to tissue hypoxia. Cyanosis can be either central or peripheral.[505] Peripheral cyanosis results from increased peripheral extraction of oxygen from normally saturated blood or a significant decrease in the perfusion to an extremity.[505] In the neonate, causes include septic shock and severe hypothermia. Central cyanosis is more common in neonates and is related to congenital heart disease that causes right-to-left shunting or severe respiratory conditions that result in hypoxia. Paroxysmal atrial fibrillation in three foals with cyanosis shortly after birth is described.[508]

TREATMENT. Examination and clinical pathologic evaluation for metabolic causes of cyanosis, hypothermia, and cardiac abnormalities should be conducted. History, medication use, auscultation, thoracic radiographs, and arterial blood gases are useful in determining the degree of respiratory component to cyanosis. Therapy for respiratory causes are discussed under Respiratory Distress. Electrocardiogram (ECG) and echocardiography may be required for identification of cardiac anomalies. Circulatory compromise caused by hypothermia, hypoglycemia, and shock requires aggressive fluid therapy, respiratory support, and environmental temperature correction.

OLIGURIA AND STRANGUIRA
JOHN E. MADIGAN

DEFINITION AND ETIOLOGY. In the neonate, urination is usually observed within 6 to 10 hours after birth. Frequency of voiding is every few hours. Urine volume produced in the foal is approximately 148 ml/kg/day.[509] Urine specific gravity is low (1.001 to 1.0012) because of the high water content of milk. Specific gravity readings of 1.018 to 1.025 are approaching maximum in concentrated urine.[510,511]

The major causes of slow or painful discharge of urine (stranguria) in neonatal foals are ruptured bladder, bacterial cystitis, and reduced urine production (oliguria) resulting from reduced renal perfusion. In neonatal ruminants, hypovolemia following diarrhea is a common cause of reduced renal perfusion. Pollakiuria, dysuria, and cystitis are complications occasionally observed with urachal abscesses.[510,511]

PATHOPHYSIOLOGY. Ruptured bladder (see also Chapter 32) occurs most frequently in male foals and is believed to be caused by occlusion of the male urethra during birth, a full bladder, and great pressures during birth when the mare pushes to expel the fetus. Inadequate pressure flow to the kidney producing oliguria may be caused by congenital cardiac anomalies, asphyxia, sepsis, diarrhea, or endotoxemia. Straining from cystitis can be severe and mimic meconium impaction. Infection of the bladder may be associated with urachal infection. Inappropriate antidiuretic hormone (ADH) secretion occurs in stressed human infants, resulting in decreased urine production and electrolyte abnormalities. Ovine neonatal kidneys are responsive to ADH at birth but, unlike the adult kidneys, excrete sodium and potassium in response to ADH.[510] In the calf, glomerular filtration rate (GFR) increases to adult values by 2 days of age.[512] During periods of reduced GFR, drugs excreted by the kidney may accumulate, resulting in toxicity. Inability to excrete a water load associated with excessive fluid therapy may result in fluid accumulation and pulmonary or generalized edema. Uroperitoneum may result in stranguria or oliguria. Postrenal obstruction syndromes are rare in the neonate. Ectopic ulcers have been reported in foals[513] and ruminants as a cause of incontinence and hydronephrosis. A syndrome of apparent pain on attempting the first urination is observed in some male foals; urinary bladder catheterization for 1 to 3 days may resolve the problem.

CLINICAL SIGNS. A carefully obtained history of events of the birth and neonatal period is important. Observation of

---

BOX 20-8

Causes of Cyanosis

CARDIOVASCULAR ORIGIN
Tetralogy of Fallot
Tricuspid atresia
Truncus arteriosus
Pentalogy of Fallot
Double outlet right ventricle
Single ventricle
Eisenmenger complex
Ventricular septal defect
Patent ductus arteriosus

RESPIRATORY CAUSES
Alveolar hypoventilation
Drug-induced central nervous system (CNS) depression
CNS trauma or hemorrhage
Hypoglycemia or hypocalcemia
Altered neurologic function of spinal nerves (of respiratory muscles)
Thoracic cage abnormalities: pneumothorax, fractured ribs
Diaphragmatic hernia
Upper airway obstruction
Restrictive pleural space disorders: hemothorax, pleuritis
Hypoplastic lung

IMPAIRED DIFFUSION
Pulmonary: pneumonia, edema, atelectasis
Shunting
Anatomic (congenital heart defects)
Pathologic: pulmonary hypertension
Ventilation/perfusion mismatch

defecation, posture during urination, frequency, and estimated amounts of urination should be noted. Excessive stretching of the front legs, dorsoventral flexion of the back, and colic may be observed with uroperitoneum. Detection of oliguria requires careful observation or catheterization of the bladder to determine presence of urine and amount of urine production. Free catch of urine and examination for white blood cells aid in diagnosis of cystitis.

Azotemic neonates with oliguria have signs of depression, dehydration, poor pulse quality, prolonged capillary refill, reduced jugular distensibility, and retracted eyeballs. Elevated levels of serum urea and creatinine may be observed with uroperitoneum, often with concurrent electrolyte abnormalities of hyponatremia, hyperkalemia, and hypochloremia. If the presence of uroperitoneum is suspected, abdominocentesis should be performed. The fluid can be analyzed for potassium and creatinine and compared with serum values. Urea rapidly equilibrates between abdominal fluid and serum. Peritoneal fluid creatinine levels will be 1.8 to 2 times that of serum with uroperitoneum. A syndrome of high creatinine in newborn foals associated with maternal conditions or events of birth and without renal disease has been reported.[440] Serial creatinine determinations reveal a gradual decline toward normal values over several days. Consequently a single serum creatinine determination should not be used to determine prerenal, renal, or postrenal uremia in the foal.

TREATMENT. Administration of balanced electrolyte solutions such as lactated Ringer's solution or saline and determination of urine production are important. Specific electrolyte and acid-base disturbances should be corrected slowly. Prolonged ischemia of the kidneys may result in permanent renal parenchymal damage. Lack of urine production after restoration of fluid balance should be an indication for diuretic therapy with furosemide (0.5 to 2 mg/kg IV) or osmotic diuresis with mannitol (0.25 to 0.5 mg/kg IV over 20 minutes and repeated in 4 hours if no response occurs). If adequate urine production has not developed, administration of dobutamine (2 to 10 g/kg/min) or dopamine (2 to 5 μg/kg/min) may be attempted. Treatment of concurrent sepsis, endotoxemia, hypoproteinemia, respiratory distress, or other abnormality should be attempted. If adequate urine flow is not produced, maintenance levels of fluids should be administered to prevent fluid overload. Body weight determinations three to four times a day help to prevent overhydration by detecting fluid accumulation. Urinalysis and clearance calculations may add further insight to the origin and degree of primary renal involvement. Progressive development of uremia and generalized edema is associated with a poor prognosis. When oliguria is present, serial blood urea nitrogen (BUN) and creatinine determinations should be performed and urine production monitored. Recumbent neonates may be catheterized and urine production quantitated.

SHOCK
JOHN E. MADIGAN

DEFINITION AND ETIOLOGY. A variety of definitions have been applied to describe shock. In the neonate, if pulse quality is poor, capillary refill time is prolonged, and appendages are cold, the neonate is likely in shock, possibly from hypothermia, hypovolemia, cardiac insufficiency, or sepsis.[514]

DIFFERENTIAL DIAGNOSIS. Weak or recumbent neonates should be approached in a systematic manner that will allow detection of the cardinal signs of shock. Hypoglycemia, hypothermia, and septicemia are important to rule out. Because sepsis is common in neonates and the mortality rate is high, blood cultures followed by early use of broad-spectrum antibiotics with coverage against gram-negative infections is appropriate.

TREATMENT. Assessment of blood pressure is helpful in determining therapy. In all forms of shock, arterial pressure is low. Venous pressure is low, except in cardiogenic shock. Pressor agents, including dopamine and dobutamine infusions (2 to 5 μg/kg/min IV), have been attempted with severe hypotension and shock in addition to fluid therapy. If blood glucose is normal, fluid therapy should consist of lactated Ringer's solution (40 to 100 ml/kg) given rapidly intravenously if central venous pressure is low. In the absence of a venous pressure monitoring system, fluid therapy should probably not exceed 2 L/50 kg/hr. The neonate is more susceptible to pulmonary edema than the adult. Determination of acid-base status should be performed, and bicarbonate should be administered if base deficit is greater than 8 mEq/L and ventilation is adequate to remove generated carbon dioxide. If hypoglycemia is present, fluids containing 5% to 10% dextrose are indicated to raise blood sugar to 160 to 180 mg/dl. Urination should be observed or the bladder catheterized to determine urine production rate. The use of corticosteroids is controversial, and because of the high incidence of septic shock in the neonate, the decision for use should be made carefully. When thought to be absolutely essential, a short-acting soluble corticosteroid such as prednisolone sodium succinate should be used at a dose of 5 to 10 mg/kg. Recent studies have indicated no advantage to corticosteroid use in septic shock in humans.[515] A minimum database of serum IgG, complete blood count, and determination of initiating factors for sepsis should be ascertained.

Neonates that are collapsed and hypothermic and in shock may need resuscitation in addition to the therapy previously described. Oxygen or ventilation therapy may be indicated to raise arterial oxygen levels and reduce carbon dioxide to appropriate levels (see Respiratory Distress).

HEART MURMUR
JOHN E. MADIGAN

DEFINITION AND ETIOLOGY. Heart murmurs in the neonate may be heard normally before physiologic closing of the ductus arteriosus during the first 1 to 5 days of life. Other causes for murmurs include congenital anomalies, severe anemia, or infectious valvular disease.

CLINICAL SIGNS AND DIFFERENTIAL DIAGNOSIS. Physical examination for other signs of heart disease helps determine the severity of the murmur. Jugular pulse, weak or irregular arterial pulse, and palpable thrill indicate a serious condition. Signs of weakness, cyanosis, and tachypnea are indications of poor cardiac performance. Timing and location of the heart murmur should be determined. The electrocardiogram (ECG) may detect atrial or ventricular enlargement. Thoracic radiography may aid in determining heart size and in detecting pulmonary edema or distended pulmonary vessels. Echocardiography may reveal atrial or ventricular enlargement, thickened ventricular walls, anomalous orientations of outflow tracts, or ventricular septal defects.[516]

Patent ductus arteriosus (PDA) produces a continuous murmur localized over the left heart base.[517] The diastolic component may not be heard with auscultation over other parts of the heart. As pulmonary hypertension develops, the murmur is shortened to a holosystolic type with normal arterial pulse. Large shunting of blood produces a bounding arterial pulse caused by wide fluctuations of systolic and diastolic pressures.[517] The ECG is normal unless atrial enlargement is present and increasing QRS amplitudes are observed.[516] Radiographs may reveal an enlarged heart with increased vascularity due to left-to-right shunting of blood. Echocardiography may reveal an increased left atrial and left ventricular diastolic dimension/volume and hyperdynamic septal and left ventricular wall systolic motion (depending on the degree of right-to-left shunt).[516] Catheterization and

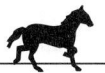

angiography may further delineate the degree of shunting.[518] Recent studies have indicated the ductus architecture changes days before birth, which prepares the ductus for closure. Triggering factors for closure include increased blood oxygenation and lower pressures resulting from vasodilation of pulmonary vasculature at birth.

Ventricular septal defect (VSD) produces a large, harsh, holosystolic murmur that is heard loudest on the right cranial region of the thorax and is softer over the left heart base.[519] Electrocardiography may be normal or show increased amplitude of the QRS, with larger shunts and alterations in chamber size. Radiography may reveal heart size increase, left atrial enlargement, and dilated pulmonary vasculature.[516] Two-dimensional echocardiography may show aortic and septal discontinuity.[516] Injection of saline bubbles into the left ventricle and observation of bubbles in the right atrium or ventricle document a left-to-right shunting of blood.[516] Tetralogy of Fallot or other types of complex malformations often produce loud murmurs and are associated with cyanosis, weakness, fatigue, and stunted growth.[520] Tetralogy of Fallot produces a systolic ejection murmur heard at the left heart base.[516] Electrocardiography may reveal negative QRS complexes in leads I, II, and aVF, suggesting right ventricular hypertrophy.[516] Echocardiography may reveal a thickened right ventricular wall, septal echo dropout in the area of the VSD, rightward displacement of the aortic root, and an abnormal pulmonary outflow region.[516] Saline injection into the jugular vein demonstrates right-to-left flow from the right ventricle to the left ventricle or the aorta.

TREATMENT. PDA has been treated by chemical closure using indomethacin in human neonates, but it has not been used in veterinary medicine.[521] Other global antiprostaglandins, including flunixine meglumine, have been used in attempts to assist with chemical closure of the ductus arteriosus in foals. The efficacy of this procedure has not been determined. Minimal fluid administration is also suggested to be of assistance. Ventricular septal defects may pose few problems if the degree of shunting is small. Other complex cardiac anomalies producing murmurs may be treated symptomatically for a short time, but the long-term prognosis is extremely poor.

ICTERUS

JOHN E. MADIGAN

DEFINITION AND ETIOLOGY. Jaundice producing a yellow discoloration of mucous membranes and sclera is a nonspecific sign in the equine neonate, as it is in the adult horse. Icterus may be observed with sepsis, anorexia, liver disease (Tyzzer's disease), equine herpesvirus I, and hemolytic anemia.

CLINICAL SIGNS AND DIFFERENTIAL DIAGNOSIS. Liver disease in the neonate may be caused by toxic hepatic failure or systemic involvement from sepsis producing bacterial hepatitis, or it may be secondary to hypoxia. Toxic hepatic failure was described in foals less than 7 days of age that had all received a digestive tract inoculum* shortly after birth (see Chapter 31). Mild jaundice was observed in septic foals but was considered nonspecific and likely related to hypoxia and hypoperfusion of tissues during shock.[522] Hemolytic anemia seen with neonatal isoerythrolysis produces significant elevation in bilirubin, principally unconjugated bilirubin (see Chapter 49). Tyzzer's disease is an acute multifocal hepatitis seen in foals 5 to 42 days of age. The causative agent is *Clostridium piliformis*, formerly termed *Bacillus piliformis*, a filamentous gram-negative pleomorphic rod bacteria (see Chapter 31). *Clostridium perfringens* type A has been impli-

cated in an enterotoxemic condition in nursing lambs, kids, and calves characterized by icterus, hemoglobinuria, anemia, and intravascular hemolysis.[523] Equine herpesvirus 1 (EHV-1) may produce weak newborn foals in addition to commonly causing abortion. Foals are weak and may show icterus with central nervous system signs that may be confused with primary liver disease. Severe leukopenia and bone marrow necrosis are associated with foal EHV-1.

FAILURE TO THRIVE: CACHEXIA AND WEAK CALF SYNDROME

JOHN MAAS

DEFINITION AND ETIOLOGY. Neonates that are born weak or fail to grow as anticipated pose important problems. In the foal, twins, prematurity, hypothyroidism, and congenital heart or other organ defects may produce failure to thrive. Infections acquired shortly after birth that produce chronic pneumonia, nephritis, endocarditis, arthritis, or gastric ulcers are a cause of morbidity in the neonatal period. Nutritional problems in sick and convalescing foals have been identified as being previously unrecognized factors in stunting. Daily consumption of 25% to 30% of their body weight as milk in convalescing foals has been reported. This is not surprising, as normal foals gaining 1 kg/day consume 20% of their body weight in milk.

In calves the weak calf syndrome has been reproduced by feeding low-protein diets to prepartum cows that subsequently calved in environments in which the temperature was well below the thermoneutral zone for calves.[524] The dietary recommendation for crude protein intake for third-trimester pregnant cows and heifers is 0.9 kg (2 lb) of total crude protein/day. This is particularly important for heifers and cows calving early in the spring calving season when temperatures well below freezing can occur. Cold rains, however, also can produce the hypothermic conditions that aid in precipitating this syndrome.

Cows weighing 450 kg (1000 lb) therefore need to consume 9.9 kg (20 lb) dry matter of good to excellent quality hay that is 10% crude protein or more. A quadratic equation has been developed to predict crude protein (CP) intake of the dams if their serum total proteins, urea nitrogen, and creatinine are known.[525] This equation predicts the daily crude protein intake on a continuing basis.

$$\text{Daily CP consumption (kg)} = 0.1806 + 0.04327\,(BUN) - 0.33497\,(creat) + 0.06963\,(TP) - 0.00025\,(BUN)^2 + 0.06049\,(creat)^2 - 0.00666\,(BUN \times creat)$$

where *BUN* is serum urea nitrogen (mg/dl), *creat* is serum creatinine (mg/dl), and *TP* is serum total protein (g/dl).

Also, the use of this formula could predict CP intake for pregnant heifers and pregnant cows. This relationship may prove to have important clinical applications when weak calf syndrome or protein-calorie malnutrition is suspected and the gestation diet of the dams is not available for analysis (as under some range conditions). Supplements such as molasses licks that contain urea may tend to overestimate CP intake.[526]

REFERENCES

1. Rossdale PD, Silver M: The concept of readiness for birth, *J Reprod Fertil* 32:507-510, 1982.
2. Rossdale PD: Perinatal development: a clinician's view of prematurity and dysmaturity in Thoroughbred foals, *Proc Royal Soc Med* 69:631-632, 1976.
3. Laing JA, Leech FB: The frequency of infertility in Thoroughbred mares, *J Reprod Ferti* 307-310, 1975.
4. Rossdale PD: Clinical studies on the newborn Thoroughbred, *Perinal Behav* 123:470, 1967.
5. Rossdale PD et al: Studies on equine prematurity. I, Methodology *Equine Vet J* 16:275-278, 1984.

---

*Primapaste, Ethco Lab., St. Joseph, MO. (No longer on market.)

6. Silver M et al: Studies on equine prematurity. II, Postnatal adrenocortical activity in relation to plasma adrenocorticotrophic hormone and catecholamine levels in term and premature foals, *Equine Vet J* 16:278-286, 1984.

7. Johnson MP, Evans MI: Intrauterine growth retardation: pathophysiology and possibilities for intrauterine treatment, *Fetal Ther* 2:109-122, 1987.

8. Platt H: Growth of the equine foetus, *Equine Vet J* 16:247-252, 1984.

9. Willoughby DP: The physique of the horse in various of its breeds. In Willoughby DP, ed: *Growth and nutrition in the horse*, New York, 1975, Barnes, pp 33-48.

10. Harding JE, Jones CT, Robinson JS: Studies on experimental growth retardation in sheep: the effects of a small placenta in restricting transport to and growth of the fetus, *J Dev Physiol* 7:427-442, 1985.

11. Platt H: Infection of the horse fetus, *J Reprod Fertil Suppl* 101:605-610, 1975.

12. Behrman RE et al: Distribution of the circulation in the normal and asphyxiated fetal primate, *Am J Obstet Gynecol* 108:956-969, 1970.

13. Peeters LL et al: Blood flow to fetal organs as a function of arterial oxygen content, *Am J Obstet Gynecol* 135:637-646, 1979.

14. Perlman JM: Systemic abnormalities in term infants following perinatal asphyxia: relevance to long-term neurologic outcome, *Clin Perinatol* 16:475-484, 1989.

15. Done JT et al: Bovine virus diarrhoea-mucosal disease virus: pathogenicity for the fetal calf following maternal infection, *Vet Rec* 106:473-479, 1980.

16. Richardson C, Hebert CN, Terlecki S: Estimation of the developmental age of the ovine fetus and lamb, *Vet Rec* 99:22-26, 1976.

17. Richardson C et al: Estimation of the developmental age of the bovine fetus and newborn calf, *Vet Rec* 126:279-284, 1990.

18. Richardson C et al: Growth rates and patterns of organs and tissues in the bovine fetus, *Br Vet J* 147:197-206, 1991.

19. Koterba AM: Equine neonatal intensive care at the University of Florida 1982-1987: an update. In *Proceedings of the Thirty-third Annual Convention of the American Association of Equine Practitioners*, 1987, p 805.

20. Koterba AM: Prematurity. In Koterba AM, Drummond WH, Kosch PC, eds: *Equine clinical neonatology*, Philadelphia, 1990, Lea & Febiger, p 66.

21. Rossdale PD et al: Effects of placental pathology on maternal plasma progestagen and mammary secretion calcium concentrations and on neonatal adrenocortical function in the horse, *J Reprod Fertil Suppl* 44:579-584, 1991.

22. Rossdale PD et al: Studies on equine prematurity. VI, Guidelines for assessment of foal maturity, *Equine Vet J* 16:300-302, 1984.

23. Adams R, Poulos PW: A skeletal ossification index for neonatal foals, *Vet Radiol* 29:217, 1988.

24. Ruohoniemi M: Use of ultrasonography to evaluate the degree of ossification of the small tarsal bones in 10 foals, *Equine Vet J* 25:539-543, 1993.

25. Vaala WE: Neonatal sepsis in clinical practice. Dorothy Havemeyer Foundation Workshop on Neonatal Septicemia, Tufts University, School of Veterinary Medicine, Boston, Nov 19-22, 1998.

26. Marchal F, Bairam A, Vert P: Neonatal apnea and apneic syndromes, *Clin Perinatol* 14:509-529, 1987.

27. Adams R: Noninfectious orthopedic problems. In Koterba AM, ed: *Equine clinical neonatology*, Philadelphia, 1990, Lea & Febiger, p 66.

28. Dutton DM et al: Incomplete ossification of the tarsal bones in foals: 22 cases (1988-1996), *J Am Vet Med Assoc* 213:1590-1594, 1998.

29. Vaala WE, Sertich PL: Management strategies for mares at risk for periparturient complications, *Vet Clin North Am (Equine Pract)* 10:237-265, 1994.

30. Tryphonas L, Hamilton GF, Rhodes CS: Perinatal femoral nerve degeneration and neurogenic atrophy of quadriceps femoris muscle in calves, *J Am Vet Med Assoc* 164:801-807, 1974.

31. Thompson PN: Suspected congenital myasthenia gravis in Brahman calves, *Vet Rec* 143:526-529, 1998.

32. Crisman MV et al: Concentrations of phenylbutazone and oxyphenbutazone in post-parturient mares and their neonatal foals, *J Vet Pharmacol Therapeut* 14:330-334, 1991.

33. Smith LJ, Schott H: Xylazine-induced bradycardia bradycardia. In *Proceedings of the Second International Conference on Veterinary Perinatology*, Cambridge, England, 1990, p 36.

34. McGladdery AL, Cottril CM, Rossdale PD: Effects upon the fetus of sedative drugs administered to the mare. *Proceedings of the Second International Conference on Veterinary Perinatology*, Cambridge, England, 1990, p 14.

35. Erskine RJ, Ridell MG, Wolfe DF: Protein-calorie malnutrition in dairy calves fed a poor-quality milk replacer, *Agri Pract* 14:38-42, 1993.

36. Tremblay RRM et al: Metabolic acidosis without dehydration in seven goat kids, *Can Vet J* 32:308-310, 1991.

37. Kasari TR, Naylor JM: Metabolic acidosis without clinical signs of dehydration in young calves, *Can Vet J* 25:394-399, 1984.

38. Doige CE et al: Congenital spinal stenosis in beef calves in western Canada, *Vet Pathol* 27:16-25, 1990.

39. Leipold HW, Hiraga T, Dennis SM: Congenital defects of the bovine musculoskeletal system and joints, *Vet Clin North Am (Food Anim Pract)* 9:93-104, 1993.

40. Scott PR, Penny CD, Murray LD: A field study of eight ovine vertebral body abscess cases, *N Z Vet J*, 39:105-107, 1991.

41. Sherman DM, Ames TR: Vertebral body abscesses in cattle: a review of five cases, *J Am Vet Med Assoc* 188:608-611, 1986.

42. Finley GG: A survey of vertebral abscesses in domestic animals in Ontario, *Can Vet J* 16:114-117, 1975.

43. Giguere S, Lavoie JP: Rhodococcus equi vertebral osteomyelitis in 3 quarter horse colts, *Equine Vet J*, 26:74-7, 1994 [see comments].

44. Desjardins MR, Vachon AM: Surgical management of *Rhodococcusequi* metaphysitis in a foal, *J Am Vet Med Assoc* 197:608-12, 1990.

45. Watt A: Neonatal losses in lambs, *In Pract*, March 1980, pp 5-9.

46. Lofstedt J et al: Ataxia, arthritis, and encephalitis in a goat herd, *J Am Vet Med Assoc* 193:1295-1298, 1988.

47. Chalmers GA: Swayback (enzootic ataxia) in Alberta lambs, *Can J Comp Med* 38:111-117, 1974.

48. Norman S, Smith MC: Caprine arthritis-encephalitis: review of the neurologic form in 30 cases, *J Am Vet Med Assoc* 182:1342-1345, 1983.

49. Reef VB: Equine pediatric ultrasonography, *Compend Cont Educ Pract Vet* 13:1277-1285, 1991.

50. Adams R et al: Arterial blood sample collection from the newborn calf, *Vet Res Commun* 15:387-394, 1991.

51. Kosch PC et al: Developments in management of the newborn foal in respiratory distress. I, Evaluation, *Equine Vet J* 16:312, 1984.

52. Stewart JH, Rose RJ, Barko AM: Respiratory studies in foals from birth to seven days old, *Equine Vet J* 16:323-328, 1984.

53. Madigan J, Thomas WP: Cardiopulmonary function in normal newborn foals from 1-14 days of age, *Proc ACVIM* 10:101, 1986.

54. Rose RJ, Rossdale PD, Leadon DP: Blood gas and acid-base status in spontaneously delivered, term-induced and induced premature foals, *J Reprod Fertil* 1982, pp 521-528.

55. Stewart JH, Rose RJ, Barko AM: Response to oxygen administration in foals: effect of age, duration and method of administration on arterial blood gas values, *Equine Vet J* 16:329-331, 1984.

56. Shappell KK et al: Staphylectomy for treatment of dorsal displacement of the soft palate in two foals, *J Am Vet Med Assoc* 195:1395-1398, 1989.

57. Altmaier K, Morris EA: Dorsal displacement of the soft palate in neonatal foals, *Equine Vet J* 25:329-332, 1993.

58. Ross HM et al: Fatal infection of neonatal calves by infectious bovine rhinotracheitis virus, *Vet Rec* 113:217-218, 1983.

59. Baker JA, McEntee K, Gillespie JH: Effects of infectious bovine rhinotracheitis-infectious pustular vulvovaginitis (IBR-IPV) virus on newborn calves, *Cornell Vet* 50:156-170, 1960.

60. Gasthuys F et al: Laryngotomy as a treatment for chronic laryngeal obstruction in cattle: a review of 130 cases, *Vet Rec* 130:220-223, 1992.

61. Traub-Dargatz JL et al: Respiratory stridor associated with polymyopathy suspected to be hyperkalemic periodic paralysis in four quarter horse foals, *J Am Vet Med Assoc* 201:85-89, 1992.

62. Scarratt WK, Bliss E: Collapsed trachea in two calves, *Compend Cont Educ Pract Vet* 7:S45-S49, 1985.

63. Vestweber JG, Leipold HW: Tracheal collapse in three calves, *J Am Vet Med Assoc* 184:735-736, 1984.

64. Watt BR: Collapse of the trachea in two calves, *Aust Vet J* 60:309-310, 1983.

65. Kasari TR: Weakness in neonatal calves associated with dystocia, *Agri Pract* 10:19-25, 1989.

66. East NE et al: Milkborne outbreak of *Mycoplasma mycoides* subspecies mycoides infection in a commercial goat dairy, *J Am Vet Med Assoc* 182:1338-1341, 1983.

67. Haughey KG: Perinatal mortality: its investigation, causes and control, *J S Afr Vet Assoc* 62:78-91, 1991.

68. Liu IK et al: Bronchoalveolar lavage in the newborn foal, *J Reprod Fertil Suppl* 35:587-592, 1987.

69. Mueller R et al: Changes of complement values in calves during the first month of life, *Am J Vet Res* 44:747-750, 1983.

70. LeBlanc MM: Responses to plasma transfusion in clinically healthy and clinically ill foals, *Proceedings of the Thirty-fourth Annual Convention of the American Association of EquinePractitioners*, 1988, p 755.

71. Dennehy PH: Respiratory infections in the newborn, *Clin Perinatol* 14:667-682, 1987.

72. Hughes KL et al: Polyarthritis in calves caused by *Mycoplasma* spp, *Vet Rec* 78:276-280, 1966.

73. Villalba EJ et al: An outbreak caused by *Mycoplasma mycoides* species in goats in the Canary Islands, *Vet Rec* 130:330-331, 1992.

74. Crawford TB, Adams DS: Caprine arthritis-encephalitis: clinical features and presence of antibody in selected goat populations, *J Am Vet Med Assoc* 178:713-719, 1981.

75. Cork LC, Hadlow WJ, Gorham JR: Pathology of viral leukoencephalomyelitis of goats, *Acta Neuropathol* 29:281-292, 1974.

76. Cork LC et al: Infectious leukoencephalomyelitis of young goats, *J Infect Dis* 129:134-141, 1974.

77. Koterba AM: Respiratory disease: approach to diagnosis. In Koterba AM, Drummond WH, Kosch PC, eds: *Equine clinical neonatology*, 1990 Lea & Febiger, pp 153-176.

78. Pennington JE: Penetration of antibiotics into respiratory secretions, *Rev Infect Dis* 3:67-73, 1981.

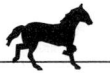

79. Bodem CR et al: Endobronchial pH: relevance of aminoglycoside activity in gram-negative bacillary pneumonia, *Am Rev Respir Dis* 127:39-41, 1983.

80. Bryan CS et al: Gentamicin vs cefotaxime for therapy of neonatal sepsis: relationship to drug resistance, *Am J Dis Child* 139:1086-1089, 1985.

81. Freeman KP et al: Recognition of bronchopulmonary dysplasia in a newborn foal, *Equine Vet J* 21:292-296, 1989.

82. Avery ME, Mead J: Surface properties in relation to atelectasis and hyaline membrane disease, *J Dis Child* 97:517, 1959.

83. Jobe A: Respiratory distress syndrome: new therapeutic approaches to a complex pathophysiology, *Adv Pediatr* 30:93-130, 1983.

84. Kotas RV: Surface tension forces and liquid balance in the lung. In Thibeault PW, Gregory GA, eds: *Neonatal pulmonary care*, Menlo Park, Calif, 1979, Addison-Wesley, p 125.

85. Reynolds EOF, Roberton NRC, Wigglesworth JS: Hyaline membrane disease, respiratory distress and surfactant deficiency, *J Pediatr* 1968, p 768.

86. Katzenstein AL, Davis C, Braude A: Pulmonary changes in neonatal sepsis to group B beta-hemolytic streptococcus: relation of hyaline membrane disease, *J Infect Dis* 133:430-435, 1976.

87. Meyer JC et al: Bacteraemia and pneumonia in a neonatal foal caused by *Streptococcus pneumoniae* type 3, *Equine Vet J* 24:407-410, 1992.

88. Liggins GC: Premature delivery of foetal lambs infused with glucocorticoids, *J Endocrinol* 45:515-523, 1969.

89. Pramanik AK, Holtzman RB, Merritt TA: Surfactant replacement therapy for pulmonary diseases, *Pediatr Clin North Am* 40:913-936, 1993.

90. Long W et al: A controlled trial of synthetic surfactant in infants weighing 1250 g or more with respiratory distress syndrome. The American Exosurf Neonatal Study Group I and the Canadian Exosurf Neonatal Study Group, *N Engl J Med* 325:1696-1703, 1991.

91. Pattle RE et al: The development of the lung and its surfactant in the foal and in other species, *J Reprod Fertil* 1975, pp 651-657.

92. Rossdale PD, Pattle RE, Mahaffey LW: Respiratory distress in newborn foals with failure to form lung lining film, *Nature (Lond)* 215:1498, 1967.

93. Sonea I: Respiratory distress syndrome in neonatal foals, *Compend Cont Educ Pract Vet* 7:S462-S469, 1985.

94. Paradis MK: Lecithin/sphingomyelin ratios and phosphatidylglycerol in term and premature equine amniotic fluid, *Proc 5th Annu ACVIM Vet Med Forum* 5:789, 1987.

95. Eigenmann UJ et al: Neonatal respiratory distress syndrome in the calf, *Vet Rec* 114:141-144, 1984.

96. Slauson DO: Naturally occurring hyaline membrane disease syndromes in foals and piglets, *J Pediatr* 95:889-891, 1979.

97. Gibson EA et al: The "barker" (neonatal respiratory distress) syndrome in the pig: its occurrence in the field, *Vet Rec* 98:476-479, 1976.

98. Lopez A, Bildfell R: Pulmonary inflammation associated with aspirated meconium and epithelial cells in calves, *Vet Pathol* 29:104-111, 1992.

99. Clark DA et al: Surfactant displacement by meconium free fatty acids: an alternative explanation for atelectasis in meconium aspiration syndrome, *J Pediatr* 110:765-770, 1987.

100. Tran N et al: Sequential effects of acute meconium obstruction on pulmonary function, *Pediatr Res* 14:34-38, 1980.

101. Tyler DC, Murphy J, Cheney FW: Mechanical and chemical damage to lung tissue caused by meconium aspiration, *J Pediatr* 62:454-459, 1978.

102. Stiles AD: Airleak: pneumothorax, pneumomediastinum, pulmonary interstitial emphysema, pneumopericardium. In Cloherty JP, Stark AR, eds: *Manual of neonatal care*, Boston, 1985, Little, Brown, p 185.

103. Stark AR: Apnea. In Cloherty JP, Stark AR, eds: *Manual of neonatal care*, Boston, 1991, Little, Brown, p 225.

104. Webb AI et al: Developments in management of the newborn foal in respiratory distress. II, Treatment, *Equine Vet J*, 16:319-323, 1984.

105. Coons TJ, Kosch PC, Cudd TA: Respiratory care. In Koterba AM, Drummond WH, Kosch PC, eds: *Equine clinical neonatology*, Philadelphia, 1990, Lea & Febiger, pp 200-239.

106. Palmer JE: Ventilatory support of the neonatal foal, *Vet Clin North Am (Equine Pract)* 10:167-185, 1994.

107. Hoffman AM, Viel L: A percutaneous transtracheal catheter system for improved oxygenation in foals with respiratory distress, *Equine Vet J* 24:239-241, 1992.

108. Bernard B et al: The influence of foal pneumonia on future racing performance, *Proceedings of the Thirty-eighth Annual Convention of the American Association of Equine Practitioners*, San Francisco, Dec 1992.

109. Ainsworth DM et al: Lack of residual lung damage in horses in which *Rhodococcus equi*-induced pneumonia had been diagnosed: evaluation the effectiveness of equine neonatal care, *Am J Vet Res* 54:2115-2120, 1993.

110. Freeman L, Paradis MR: Evaluating the effectiveness of equine neonatal care, *Vet Med*, Sept 1992, p 921.

111. Baker SM et al: Follow-up evaluation of horses after neonatal intensive care, *J Am Vet Med Assoc* 189:1454-1457, 1986.

112. Santschi E et al: Racing performance after colic surgery in 209 juvenile thoroughbreds, *Proceedings of the Forty-fifth Annual Convention of the American Association of Equine Practitioners*, 1999, pp 245-246.

113. Cohen ND, Chaffin MK: Intestinal obstruction and other causes of abdominal pain in foals, *Compend Cont Educ Pract Vet* 16:780-790, 1994.

114. Cohen ND, Chaffin MK: Assessment and initial management of colic in foals, *Compend Cont Educ Pract Vet* 17:93, 1995.

115. Hultgren BD: Ileocolonic aganglionosis in white progeny of overo spotted horses, *J Am Vet Med Assoc* 180:289-292, 1982.

116. Cudd TA: Gastrointestinal system dysfunction. In Koterba AM, Drummond WH, Kosch PC, eds: *Equine clinical neonatology*, Philadelphia, 1990, Lea & Febiger, pp 367-369.

117. Adams R et al: Exploratory celiotomy for gastrointestinal disease in neonatal foals: a review of 20 cases, *Equine Vet J*, 20:9-12, 1988.

118. Bernard WV: Differentiating enteritis and conditions that require surgery in foals, *Compend Cont Educ Pract Vet* 14:535, 1992.

119. Cudd TA, Wilson JH: Diagnostic techniques for abdominal problems. In Koterba AM, Drummond WH, Kosch PC, eds: *Equine clinical neonatology*, Philadelphia, 1990, Lea & Febiger, pp 279-412.

120. Reef V: Abnormalities of the neonatal umbilicus detected by diagnostic ultrasound, *Proceedings of the Thirty-third Annual Convention of the American Association of Equine Practitioners*, 1987, p 157.

121. Grindem CB et al: Peritoneal fluid values from healthy foals, *Equine Vet J* 22:359, 1990.

122. Embertson RE: Gastrointestinal tract disorders, small intestinal and colonic obstruction in foals. In White NA, Moore JM, eds: *Current practice of equine surgery*, Philadelphia, JB Lippincott, 1990, pp 311-318.

123. Madigan JE, Goetzman BW: Use of an acetylcysteine solution enema for meconium retention in the neonatal foal, *Proceedings of the Thirty-seventh Annual Convention of the American Association of Equine Practitioners*, Lexington, Ky, Dec 1991.

124. Hodgson DR: Rupture of the urinary bladder. In Robinson NE, ed: *Current therapy in equine medicine*, ed 2, Philadelphia, 1987, WB Saunders, pp 717-718.

125. Divers TJ, Byars TD, Spirito M: Correction of bilateral ureteral defects in a foal, *J Am Vet Med Assoc* 192:384-386, 1988.

126. Kablack KA: Uroperitoneum in the septic equine neonate: retrospective study of 331 cases, 1988-1997. In *Proceedings of the Dorothy Havemeyer Neonatal Septicemia Workshop 2*, Boston, Nov 1998, pp 27-28.

127. Argenzio RA: Short chain fatty acids and glutamine: Influence on mucosal transport and repair, *Proc 12th Annu ACVIM Forum*, 1994, p 539-540.

128. Vaala WE, Webb AI: Cardiovascular monitoring of the critically ill foal. In Koterba AM, Drummond WH, Kosch PC, eds: *Equine clinical neonatology*, Philadelphia, 1990, Lea & Febiger, p 262.

129. Young RL, Linford RL, Olander HJ: Atresia coli in the foal: a review of six cases, *Equine Vet J* 24:60-62, 1992.

130. Spurlock GH, Robertson JT: Congenital inguinal hernias associated with a rent in the common vaginal tunic in five foals, *J Am Vet Med Assoc* 193:1087-1088, 1988.

131. Platt H: Etiologic aspects of perinatal mortality in Thoroughbreds, *Equine Vet J* 5:116-170, 1973.

132. Becht JL, Semrad SD: Gastrointestinal disease of foals, *Compend Cont Educ Pract Vet* 8:S367-S373, 1986.

133. Vatistas NJ: Surgical treatment for colic in the foal, *Proceedings of the Forty-second Annual Convention of the American Association of Equine Practitioners*, 1996, pp 256-257.

134. Cable SC: Abdominal surgery in foals: a review of 119 cases (1977-1994), *Equine Vet J* 29:257-261, 1997.

135. Naylor JM, Bailey JV: A retrospective study of 51 cases of abdominal problems in the calf: etiology; diagnosis and prognosis, *Can Vet J* 28:657-662, 1987.

136. Smith DF et al: Clinical management and surgical repair of atresia coli in calves: 66 cases (1977-1988), *J Am Vet Med Assoc* 199:1185-1190, 1991.

137. Ness H, Leopold G, Muller W: Zur Genese des angeborenen Darmverschlusses (atresia coli und jejuni) des kalbes, *Monatsh Veterinaermed* 37:89, 1982.

138. Syed M, Shanks RD: Atresia coli inherited in Holstein cattle, *J Dairy Sci* 75:1105-1111, 1992.

139. Dirksen G, Doll K: Ileus and subileus in the young bovine animal, *Bovine Pract* 21:33-40, 1986.

140. Dennis R: Abomasal displacement and tympany in a nine-week-old calf, *Vet Rec* 114:218-219, 1984.

141. Medina-Cruz M et al: Description of abomasal displacements in dairy calves, *Bovine Pract* 25:95-98, 1990.

142. Cudd TA, Pauley TH: Necrotizing enterocolitis in two equine neonates, *Compend Cont Educ Pract Vet* 9:88, 1987.

143. Vaala WE: Peripartum asphyxia, *Vet Clin North Am (Equine Pract)* 10:187-218, 1994.

144. McAlmon KR: Necrotizing enterocolitis. In Cloherty JP, Stark AR, eds: *Manual of neonatal care*, Boston, 1991, Little, Brown.

145. Roeder BL et al: Isolation of *Clostridium perfringens* from neonatal calves with ruminal and abomasal tympany, abomasitis, and abomasal ulceration, *J Am Vet Med Assoc* 190:1550-1555, 1987.

146. Roeder BL et al: Experimental induction of abdominal tympany, abomasitis, and abomasal ulceration by intraruminal inoculation of *Clostridium perfringens* type A in neonatal calves, *Am J Vet Res* 49:201-207, 1988.

147. Mills KW et al: Laboratory findings associated with abomasal ulcers/tympany in range calves, *J Vet Diagn Invest*, 2:208-212, 1990.

148. Lilly CW et al: Linking copper and bacteria with abomasal ulcers in beef calves, *Vet Med* 80:85-88, 1985.
149. Doll K: Tympany and torsion of the abomasum in calves, *Bovine Pract,* 1991, pp 96-99.
150. Kumper H: New therapy for acute abomasal tympany in calves, *Tierarztl Prax,* 22:25-27, 1994.
151. Johnson JL et al: Diagnostic observations of abomasal tympany in range calves, *Proc Int Symp World Assoc Vet Lab Diagn* 2:485-491, 1983.
152. Gorrill ADL et al: Growth, mortality and meat quality of lambs fed milk replacers containing full-fat soybean flour, *Can J Anim Sci* 55:731-740, 1975.
153. Lutnaes B, Simensen E: An epidemiological study of abomasal bloat in young lambs, *Preventive Vet Med* 1:335-345, 1983.
154. Gorrill A, Nicholson J, MacIntyre TM: Effects of formalin added to milk replacers on growth, feed intake, digestion and incidence of abomasal bloat in lambs, *Can J Anim Sci* 55:557-563, 1975.
155. Large RV: The artificial rearing of lambs, *J Agri Sci,* 65:101-108, 1965.
156. Jayne-Williams DJ: The bacterial flora of the rumen of healthy and bloating calves, *J Appl Bacteriol* 47:271-284, 1979.
157. Dirksen GU, Garry FB: Diseases of the forestomachs in calves. I, *Compend Cont Educ Pract Vet* 9:F140-F147, 1987.
158. Dirksen GU, Garry FB: Diseases of the forestomachs in calves. II, *Compend Cont Educ Pract Vet* 9:F173-F179, 1987.
159. Andrews FM, Nadeau JA: Clinical syndromes of gastric ulceration in foals and mature horses, *Equine Vet J Suppl* 12:30-33, 1999.
160. Murray MJ, Hart J, Parker GA: Equine gastric ulcer syndrome: Endoscopic survey of asymptomatic foals, *Proceedings of the Thirty-third Annual Convention American Association Equine Practitioners,* 1987, p 769.
161. Murray MJ et al: Prevalence of gastric lesions in foals without signs of gastric disease: an endoscopic survey, *Equine Vet J* 22:6-8, 1990.
162. Sanchez LC, Lester GD, Merritt AM: Gastric acid in the newborn foal: Profiles and responses to H2-receptor antagonism in health and disease, *Proceedings of the Forty-fifth Annual Convention of the American Association of Equine Practitioners,* 1999, pp 243-244.
163. Tulleners EP, Hamilton GF: Surgical resection of perforated abomasal ulcers in calves, *Can Vet J* 21:262-264, 1980.
164. Green SL et al: Hemoperitoneum caused by rupture of a juvenile granulosa cell tumor in an equine neonate, *J Am Vet Med Assoc* 193:1417-1419, 1988.
165. Adams R, Mayhew IG: Neurologic diseases, *Vet Clin North Am (Equine Pract)* 1:209-234, 1985.
166. Sheather AL: Fainting in foals, *J Comp Pathol Ther* 37:106, 1924.
167. Lunn DP et al: Familial occurrence of narcolepsy in Miniature Horses, *Equine Vet J* 25:483-487, 1993.
168. Rossdale PD et al: Biochemical constituents of cerebrospinal fluid in premature and full term foals, *Equine Vet J* 14:134-138, 1982.
169. Koterba AM, Brewer BD, Tarplee FA: Clinical and clinicopathological characteristics of the septicaemic neonatal foal: review of 38 cases, *Equine Vet J* 16:376-383, 1984.
170. Andrews FM et al: Albumin quotients, IgG, and IgG index determinations in CSF of neonatal foals, *Proceedings of the Third International Conference on Veterinary Perinatology,* Davis, Calif, 1993, p 19.
171. Cudd TA, Mayhew IC, Cottrill CM: Agenesis of the corpus callosum with cerebellar vermian hypoplasia in a foal resembling the Dandy-Walker syndrome: premortem diagnosis by clinical examination and CT scanning, *Equine Vet J* 21:378, 1989.
172. Clement SF: Behavioral alterations and neonatal maladjustment syndrome in the foal, *Proceedings of the Thirty-second Annual Convention of the American Association of Equine Practitioners,* 1986, pp 145-148.
173. Johnson P, Rossdale PD: Preliminary observations on cranial cardiovascular changes during asphyxia in the newborn foal, *J Reprod Fertil* 23:695-699, 1976.
174. Cudd TA, Koterba AM: Results of the 1988 member survey of equine neonatal disease, *Int Soc Vet Perinatol News* 3:1, 1990.
175. Morris DD, Rutkowski J, Lloyd K: Therapy in two cases of neonatal foal septicaemia and meningitis with cefotaxime sodium, *Equine Vet J* 19:151-154, 1987.
176. Green SL, Smith LL: Meningitis in neonatal calves: 32 cases (1983-1990), *J Am Vet Med Assoc* 201:125-128, 1992.
177. Dickie CW, Klinkerman DL, Petrie RJ: Enterotoxemia in two foals, *J Am Vet Med Assoc* 173:306-307, 1978.
178. Niilo L, Chalmers GA: Hemorrhagic enterotoxemia caused by *Clostridium perfringens* type C in a foal, *Can Vet J* 23:299-301, 1982.
179. Sims LD et al: Haemorrhagic necrotising enteritis in foals associated with *Clostridium perfringens,* *Aust Vet J* 62:194-196, 1985.
180. Dart AJ et al: Enterotoxaemia in a foal due to *Clostridium perfringens* type A, *Aust Vet J* 65:330-331, 1988.
181. Jones SL, Wilson WD: *Clostridium septicum* septicemia in a neonatal foal with hemorrhagic enteritis, *Cornell Vet* 83:143-151, 1993.
182. Howard-Martin M et al: *Clostridium perfringens* type C enterotoxemia in a newborn foal, *J Am Vet Med Assoc* 189:564-565, 1986.
183. Jones RL, Adney WS, Shideler RK: Isolation of *Clostridium difficile* and detection of cytotoxin in the feces of diarrheic foals in the absence of antimicrobial treatment, *J Clin Microbiol* 25:1225-1227, 1987.
184. Smith BP: Salmonella infection in horses, *Compend Cont Educ Pract Vet* 3(suppl):1-9, 1981.
185. Myers LL, Shoop DS, Byars TD: Diarrhea associated with enterotoxigenic *Bacteroides fragilis* in foals, *Am J Vet Res* 48:1565-1567, 1987.
186. Powell DG: The first report of the Lloyd's foal enteric disease project, Lexington, 1987, Department of Veterinary Science, College of Agriculture, University of Kentucky.
187. Prescott JF, Bruin-Mosch CW: Carriage of *Campylobacter jejuni* in healthy and diarrheic animals, *Am J Vet Res* 42:164-165, 1981.
188. Atherton JG, Ricketts SW: *Campylobacter* infection from foals, *Vet Rec* 107:264-265, 1980.
189. Cimprich RE: Differential diagnosis of neonatal diarrhea in domestic animals, *Compend Cont Educ Pract Vet* 3:S26, 1981.
190. Martens RJ, Scrutchfield WL: Foal diarrhea: pathogenesis, etiology, and therapy, *Compend Cont Educ Pract Vet* 4:S175, 1982.
191. Urquhart K: Diarrhea in foals, *Equine Pract* 3:22, 1981.
192. Whitlock RH: Acute diarrheal disease in the horse *Proceedings of the Twenty-second Annual Convention of the American Association of Equine Practitioners,* Dallas, 1976 [review].
193. Carter GK, Martens RJ: Septicemia in the neonatal foal, *Compend Cont Educ Pract Vet* 8:S256-S271, 1986.
194. Cimprich, RE, Rooney JR: *Corynebacterium equi* enteritis in foals, *Vet Pathol* 14:95-102, 1977.
195. Conner ME et al: Detection of rotavirus in horses with and without diarrhea by electron microscopy and rotazyme test, *Cornell Vet* 73:280-287, 1983.
196. Conner ME, Darlington RW: Rotavirus infection in foals, *Am J Vet Res* 41:1699-1703, 1980.
197. Eugster AK, Whitford HW, Mehr LE: Concurrent rotavirus and salmonella infections in foals, *J Am Vet Med Assoc* 173:857-858, 1978.
198. Dwyer RM, Powell DG: The third report of the Lloyd's Foal Disease Project, Department of Veterinary Science, Gluck Equine Research Center, College of Agriculture, University of Kentucky, 1989.
199. Flewett TH, Woode GN: The rotaviruses: brief review, *Arch Virol* 57:1, 1978.
200. Kanitz CL: Identification of an equine rotavirus as a cause of neonatal foal diarrhoea, *Proceedings of the Twenty-third Annual Convention of the American Association of Equine Practitioners,* Vancouver, 1977.
201. Mitchell WC: Rotaviral diarrhea in foals, *Mod Vet Pract* 63:896, 1982.
202. Scrutchfield WL et al: Rotavirus infections in foals, *Proceedings of the Twenty-sixth Annual Convention of the American Association of Equine Practitioners,* 1980, pp 217-223.
203. Strickland KL et al: Diarrhoea in foals associated with rotavirus, *Vet Rec* 111:421, 1982.
204. Traver DS, Trimmell BJ, Armstrong C: Salmonellosis in foals, *Proceedings of the Twenty-sixth Annual Convention of the American Association of Equine Practitioners,* 1980, 225-233.
205. Tzipori S, Walker M: Isolation of rotavirus from foals with diarrhoea, *Aust J Exp Biol Med Sci* 56:453-457, 1978.
206. Woode GN et al: Morphological and antigenic relationships between viruses (rotaviruses) from acute gastroenteritis of children, calves, piglets, mice, and foals, *Infect Immun* 14:804-810, 1976.
207. Whipp SC: Physiology of diarrhea: small intestines, *J Am Vet Med Assoc* 173:662-666, 1978.
208. Snodgrass DR, Wells PW: Passive immunity in rotaviral infections, *J Am Vet Med Assoc* 173:565-568, 1978.
209. Bass EP, Sharpee RL: Coronavirus and gastroenteritis in foals, *Lancet* 2:822, 1975.
210. Ward A, Evermann JF, Reed SM: Presence of coronavirus in diarrheic foals, *Vet Med Small Anim Clin* 78:563-564, 1983.
211. Corrier DE, Montgomery D, Scrutchfield WL: Adenovirus in the intestinal epithelium of a foal with prolonged diarrhea, *Vet Pathol* 19:564-567, 1982.
212. Gleeson LJ, Studdert MJ, Sullivan ND: Pathogenicity and immunologic studies of equine adenovirus in specific-pathogen-free foals, *Am J Vet Res* 39:1636-1642, 1978.
213. Studdert MJ, Blackney MH: Isolation of an adenovirus antigenically distinct from equine adenovirus type 1 from diarrheic foal feces, *Am J Vet Res* 43:543-544, 1982.
214. Lyons ET, Drudge JH, Tolliver SC: On the life cycle of *Strongyloides westeri* in the equine, *J Parasitol,* 1973, pp 780-787.
215. Ludwig KG et al: Efficacy of ivermectin in controlling *Strongyloides westeri* infections in foals, *Am J Vet Res* 44:314-316, 1983.
216. Martens RJ: Non-infectious diarrhea in the foal, *Proceedings of the Thirty-fifth Annual Convention of the American Association of Equine Practitioners,* 1989, 205-216.
217. Duncan JL, Pirie HM: The pathogenesis of single experimental infections with *Strongylus vulgaris* in foals, *Res Vet Sci* 18:82-93, 1975.
218. Barker IK, Remmler OI: The endogenous development of *Eimeria leukarti* in ponies, *J Parasitol,* 58:112-122, 1972.
219. Lyons ET, Drudge JH, Tolliver SC: Natural infection with *Eimeria leuckarti:* prevalence of oocysts in feces of horse foals on several farms in Kentucky during 1986, *Am J Vet Res* 49:96-98, 1988.
220. Becht JL, Semrad SD: Gastrointestinal disease of foals, *Compend Cont Educ Pract Vet* 8:S367-S373, 1986.
221. Xiao L, Herd RP: Epidemiology of equine *Cryptosporidium* and *Giardia* infections, *Equine Vet J* 26:14-17, 1994.

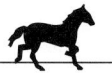

222. Merritt AM: Pathophysiology of diarrhea in the foal, *Proceedings of the Twenty-sixth Annual Convention of the American Association of Equine Practitioners,* 1980, pp 197-203.
223. Madigan J: Unpublished information.
224. Kohn CA: Personal communication.
225. Roberts MC: Carbohydrate digestion and absorption studies in the horse, *Res Vet Sci* 18:64-69, 1975.
226. Breukink HJ: Oral mono- and disaccharide tolerance tests in ponies, *Am J Vet Res* 35:1523-1527, 1974.
227. Martens RJ, Malone PS, Brust DM: Oral lactose tolerance test in foals: technique and normal values, *Am J Vet Res* 46:2163-2165, 1985.
228. Roberts MC: The development and distribution of mucosal enzymes in the small intestine of the fetus and young foal, *J Reprod Fertil* 23:(suppl):717-723, 1975.
229. Kolan JC et al: An auto digesting source of lactose, *N Engl J Med* 310:1-3, 1984.
230. Udall DH: *The practice of veterinary medicine,* ed 4, New York, 1943, Udall Publishing.
231. Doll ER: *Disease of foals: yearbook of agriculture,* Washington, DC, 1956, US Government Printing Office.
232. Johnston RH et al: Mare's milk composition as related to "foal heat" scours, *J Anim Sci* 31:549, 1970.
233. Francis-Smith K, Wood-Gush D: Coprophagia as seen in thoroughbred foals, *Equine Vet J* 9:155-157, 1977.
234. Cudd TA, Toal RL, Embertson RM: The use of clinical findings, abdominocentesis, and abdominal radiographs to assess surgical vs. nonsurgical abdominal disease in the foal, *Proceedings of the Thirty-fourth Annual Convention of the American Association of Equine Practitioners,* 1988, pp 41-53.
235. Bernard WV et al: Ultrasonographic diagnosis of small-intestinal intussusception in three foals, *J Am Vet Med Assoc,* 194:395-397, 1989.
236. Goldenburg MM et al: The antidiarrhael action missing of bismuth subsalicylate in the mouse and rat, *Am J Dig Dis* 20:955-959, 1975.
237. Ericsson CD et al: Bismuth subsalicylate inhibits activity of crude toxins of *Escherichia coli* and *Vibrio cholerae, J Infect Dis* 136:693-696, 1977.
238. Acres SD, Saunders JR, Radostits OM: Acute undifferentiated neonatal diarrhea of beef calves: the prevalence of enterotoxigenic *E. coli,* reo-like (rota) virus and other enteropathogens in cow-calf herds, *Can Vet J* 18:113-121, 1977.
239. Reynolds DJ et al: Microbiology of calf diarrhoea in southern Britain, *Vet Rec* 119:34-39, 1986.
240. Snodgrass DR et al: Aetiology of diarrhoea in young calves, *Vet Rec* 119:31-34, 1986.
241. Ganaba R et al: Importance of *Escherichia coli* in young beef calves from northwestern Quebec, *Can J Vet Res* 59:20-25, 1995.
242. Waltner-Toews D, Martin SW, Meek AH: An epidemiological study of selected calf pathogens on Holstein dairy farms in southwestern Ontario, *Can J Vet Res* 50:307-313, 1986.
243. Bywater RJ: Evaluation of an oral glucose-glycine-electrolyte formulation and amoxicillin for treatment of diarrhea in calves, *Am J Vet Res* 38:1983-1987, 1977.
244. Fromm D et al: Ion transport across isolated ileal mucosa invaded by *Salmonella, Gastroenterology,* 66:215-225, 1974.
245. Ball JM et al: Age-dependent diarrhea induced by a rotaviral nonstructural glycoprotein, *Science* 272:101-104, 1996 [see comments].
246. Argenzio RA: Pathophysiology of neonatal calf diarrhea, *Vet Clin North Am (Food Anim Pract)* 1:461-469, 1985.
247. Argenzio RA et al: Effect of heat-stable enterotoxin of *Escherichia coli* and theophylline on ion transport in porcine small intestine, *Can J Comp Med* 48:14-22, 1984.
248. Bywater RJ, Logan EF: The site and characteristics of intestinal water and electrolyte loss in *Escherichia coli*-induced diarrhoea in calves, *J Comp Pathol,* 1974, pp 599-610.
249. Mebus CA, Newman LE, Stair E, Jr: Scanning electron, light, and immunofluorescent microscopy of intestine of gnotobiotic calf infection with calf diarrheal coronavirus, *Am J Vet Res* 36:1719-1725, 1975.
250. Mebus CA et al: Neonatal calf diarrhea: propagation, attenuation, and characteristics of a coronavirus-like agent, *Am J Vet Res,* 34:145-150, 1973.
251. Mebus CA et al: Pathology of neonatal calf diarrhea induced by a coronavirus-like agent, *Vet Pathol,* 1973, pp 45-64.
252. Stair EL et al: Neonatal calf diarrhea: electron microscopy of intestines infected with a reovirus-like agent, *Vet Pathol,* 1973, pp 155-170.
253. Moon HW: Mechanisms in the pathogenesis of diarrhea: a review, *J Am Vet Med Assoc* 172:443-448, 1978.
254. Woode GN, Smith C, Dennis MJ: Intestinal damage in rotavirus infected calves assessed by D-xylose malabsorption, *Vet Rec* 102:340-341, 1978.
255. Halpin CG, Caple IW: Changes in intestinal structure and function of neonatal calves infected with reovirus-like agent and *Escherichia coli, Aust Vet J* 52:438-441, 1976.
256. Nappert G et al: Determination of lactose and xylose malabsorption in preruminant diarrheic calves, *Can J Vet Res* 57:152-158, 1993.
257. Blaxter KL, Wood WA: Some observations on the biochemical and physiological events associated with diarrhea in calves, *Vet Rec* 65:889-892, 1953.
258. Phillips RW, Lewis LD, Knox KL: Alterations in body water turnover and distribution in neonatal calves with acute diarrhea, *Ann N Y Acad Sci* 176:231-243, 1971.
259. Naylor JM: Severity and nature of acidosis in diarrheic calves over and under one week of age, *Can Vet J* 28:168-173, 1987.
260. Tzipori S et al: Diarrhea in lambs experimentally infected with cryptosporidium isolated from calves, *Am J Vet Res* 42:1400-1404, 1981.
261. Naylor JM, Forsyth GW: The alkalinizing effects of metabolizable bases in the healthy calf, *Can J Vet Res* 50:509-516, 1986.
262. Omole OO et al: High-performance liquid chromatographic assay of (±)-lactic acid and its enantiomers in calf serum, *J Chromatogr Biomed Sci Appl* 727:23-29, 1999.
263. Schelcher F et al: Metabolic acidosis without dehydration and no or minimal diarrhoea in suckler calves is caused by hyper D-lactatemia, *Proc World Buiatrics,* Sydney, 1998.
264. Al-Mashat RR, Taylor DJ: Production of enteritis in calves by the oral inoculation of pure cultures of *Campylobacter fecalis, Vet Rec* 109:97-101, 1981.
265. Fisher EW: Death in neonatal calf diarrhoea, *Br Vet J* 121:132-138, 1965.
266. Fisher EW, McEwan AD: Death in neonatal calf diarrhoea. II, The role of oxygen and potassium, *Br Vet J* 123:4-6, 1967.
267. Levine MM: *Escherichia coli* that cause diarrhea: Enterotoxigenic, enteropathogenic, enteroinvasive, enterohemorrhagic, and enteroadherent, *J Infect Dis* 155:377-389, 1987.
268. Acres SD: Enterotoxigenic *Escherichia coli* infection in newborn calves, *J Dairy Sci* 68:229-256, 1985.
269. Morris JA, Chanter N, Sherwood D: Occurrence and properties of FY (Att25)+ *Escherichia coli* associated with diarrhoea in calves, *Vet Rec* 121:189-191, 1987.
270. Harnett NM, Gyles CL: Enterotoxin plasmids in bovine and porcine enterotoxigenic *Escherichia coli* of O groups 9, 20, 64 and 101, *Can J Comp Med* 49:79-87, 1985.
271. Sherwood D, Snodgrass DR, Lawson G: Prevalence of enterotoxigenic *Escherichia coli* in calves in Scotland and northern England, *Vet Rec* 113:208-212, 1983.
272. Mahdi-Saeed A et al: The role of pathogenic *Escherichia coli* in the etiology of veal calf hemorrhagic enteritis, *Prev Vet Med* 17:65-75, 1993.
273. Runnels PL, Moon HW, Schneider RA: Development of resistance with host age to adhesion of K99+ *Escherichia coli* to isolated intestinal epithelial cells, *Infect Immun* 28:298-300, 1980.
274. Runnels PL et al: Effects of microbial and host variables on the interaction of rotavirus and *Escherichia coli* infections in gnotobiotic calves, *Am J Vet Res* 47:1542-1550, 1986.
275. Mitchell G, Linklater K: Differential diagnosis of scouring in lambs, *In Practice* 5:6-10, 1983.
276. Bellamy J, Acres SD: A comparison of histopathological changes in calves associated with K99- and K99+ strains of enterotoxigenic *Escherichia coli, Can J Comp Med,* 47:143-149, 1983.
277. Mainil JG et al: Shiga-like toxin production and attaching effacing activity of *Escherichia coli* associated with calf diarrhea, *Am J Vet Res* 48:743-748, 1987.
278. Sherwood D, Snodgrass DR, O'Brien AD: Shiga-like toxin production from *Escherichia coli* associated with calf diarrhea, *Vet Rec* 116:217-218, 1985.
279. Pearson GR et al: Natural infection with an attaching and effacing *Escherichia coli* in the small and large intestines of a calf with diarrhea, *Vet Rec* 124:297-299, 1989.
280. Fischer J et al: Pathogenicity of a bovine attaching effacing *Escherichia coli* isolate lacking Shiga-like toxins, *Am J Vet Res* 55:991-999, 1994.
281. Wieler LH, Bauerfeind R, Baljer G: Characterization of Shiga-like toxin producing *Escherichia coli* (SLTEC) isolated from calves with and without diarrhoea, *Zentralb Bakteriol* 276:243-53, 1992.
282. Aidar L et al: Subtypes of intimin among non-toxigenic *Escherichia coli* from diarrheic calves in Brazil, *Can J Vet Res* 64:15-20, 2000.
283. Chanter N et al: Dysentery in gnotobiotic calves caused by atypical *Escherichia coli, Vet Rec,* 1984, p 114.
284. Janke BH et al: Attaching and effacing *Escherichia coli* infection as a cause of diarrhea in young calves, *J Am Vet Med Assoc* 196:897-901, 1990.
285. Chanter N et al: Dysentery in calves caused by an atypical strain of *Escherichia coli* (S102-9), *Vet Microbiol* 12:241-253, 1986.
286. Hall GA et al: Dysentery caused by *Escherichia coli* (S102-9) in calves: natural and experimental disease, *Vet Pathol* 22:156-163, 1985.
287. Acres SD et al: Acute undifferentiated neonatal diarrhea in beef calves. I. Occurrence and distribution of infectious agents, *Can J Comp Med* 39:116-132, 1975.
288. Forbes D, Oakley GA, Mackenzie JA: Experimental *Salmonella dublin* infection in calves, *Vet Rec* 101:220-224, 1977.
289. Petrie L et al: Salmonellosis in young calves due to *Salmonella enteritidis, Vet Rec* 101:398-402, 1977.
290. Hunter AG et al: An outbreak of *S. typhimurium* in sheep and its consequences, *Vet Rec* 98:126-130, 1976.
291. Morgan JH, Hall GA, Reynolds DJ: The association of *Campylobacter* species with calf diarrhoea, *Proc World Congr Dis Cattle,* 1:325-330, 1986.

292. Fleming S: Enterotoxemia in neonatal calves, *Vet Clin North Am (Food Anim Pract)* 1:509-514, 1985.

293. Griner LA, Braken FK: *Clostridium perfringens* (type C) in acute hemorrhagic enteritis of calves, *J Am Vet Med Assoc* 122:99-102, 1953.

294. Niilo L, Harries WN, Jones GA: *Clostridium perfringens* type C in hemorrhagic enterotoxemia of neonatal calves in Alberta, *Can Vet J*, 1974, pp 224-226.

295. Wood AM, Al-Mashat RR, Taylor DJ: *Clostridium perfringens* type A in the calf intestine. *Proceedings of the Fourth International Symposium on Neonatal Diarrhea, Veterinary Infectious Disease Organization*, University of Saskatchewan, 4:666-673, 1983.

296. Ganaba R et al: A seroepidemiological study of the importance in cow-calf pairs of respiratory and enteric viruses in beef operations from northwestern Quebec, *Can J Vet Res* 59:26-33, 1995.

297. Athanassious R et al: Detection of bovine coronavirus and type A rotavirus in neonatal calf diarrhea and winter dysentery of cattle in Quebec: evaluation of three diagnostic methods, *Can Vet J* 35:163-169, 1994.

298. Burki F, Schusser G, Szekely H: Clinical, virological and serological evaluation of the efficacy of peroral live rotavirus vaccination in calves kept under normal husbandry conditions, *Zentrabl Vet Med B* 30:237-250, 1983.

299. Lecce JG, King MW: Rotaviral antibodies in cow's milk, *Can J Comparative Med* 46:434-436, 1982.

300. Chasey D, Banks J: The commonest rotaviruses from neonatal lamb diarrhoea in England and Wales have atypical electropherotypes, *Vet Rec* 115:326-327, 1984.

301. Castrucci G et al: A study on neonatal calf diarrhea induced by rotavirus, *Comp Immunol Microbiol Infect Dis* 17:321-331, 1994.

302. Mebus CA et al: Pathology of neonatal calf diarrhea induced by a reo-like virus, *Vet Pathol* 8:490-505, 1971.

303. Kodituwakku SN, Harbour DA: Persistent excretion of rotavirus by pregnant cows, *Vet Rec* 126:547-549, 1990.

304. Saif LJ et al: Experimentally induced coronavirus infections in calves: viral replication in the respiratory and intestinal tracts, *Am J Vet Res* 47:1426-1432, 1986.

305. Heckert RA et al: Epidemiologic factors and isotype-specific antibody responses in serum and mucosal secretions of dairy calves with bovine coronavirus respiratory tract and enteric tract infections, *Am J Vet Res* 52:845-851, 1991.

306. Bulgin MS et al: Detection of rotavirus and coronavirus shedding in two beef cow herds in Idaho, *Can Vet J* 30:235-239, 1989.

307. Tsunemitsu H, Saif LJ: Antigenic and biological comparisons of bovine coronaviruses derived from neonatal calf diarrhea and winter dysentery of adult cattle, *Arch Virol* 140:1303-1311, 1995.

308. Durham PJK et al: Coronavirus-associated diarrhea (winter dysentery) in adult cattle, *Can Vet J* 30:825-827, 1989.

309. Kapil S, Trent AM, Goyal SM: Excretion and persistence of bovine coronavirus in neonatal calves, *Arch Virol* 115:1-2, 1990.

310. Storz J, Bates RC: Parvovirus infections in calves, *J Am Vet Med Assoc*, 163:884-886, 1973.

311. Bridger JC, Hall GA, Brown JF: Characterization of a calici-like virus (Newbury agent) found in association with astrovirus in bovine diarrhea, *Infect Immun* 43:133-138, 1984.

312. Hall GA et al: Lesions of gnotobiotic calves experimentally infected with a calicivirus-like (Newbury) agent, *Vet Pathol* 21:208-215, 1984.

313. Bridger JC et al: Calici-like viruses in calf diarrhoea, *Proceedings of the Fourth International Symposium on Neonatal Diarrhea, Veterinary Infectious Disease Organization University of Saskatchewan*, 1983, pp 154-161.

314. Brown D, Morgan JH, Bridger JC: Survey of Breda virus in neonatal calf diarrhoea, *Vet Rec* 126:337, 1990.

315. Koopmans M et al: Breda virus (Toroviridae) infection and systemic antibody response in sentinel calves, *Am J Vet Res* 51:1443-1448, 1990.

316. Lambert G, McClurkin AW, Fernelius AL: Bovine viral diarrhea in the neonatal calf, *J Am Vet Med Assoc* 164:287-289, 1974.

317. Holland RE: Investigation of an epizootic of bovine viral diarrhea virus infection in calves, *J Am Vet Med Assoc* 202:1849-1854, 1993.

318. Corapi WV, French TW, Dubovi EJ: Severe thrombocytopenia in young calves experimentally infected with noncytopathic bovine viral diarrhea virus, *J Virol* 63:3934-3943, 1989.

319. Castrucci G et al: A study of some pathogenetic aspects of bovine viral diarrhea virus infection, *Arch Virol Suppl* 3:101-108, 1991.

320. Nuttall PA, Stott EJ, Thomas LH: Experimental infection of calves with two strains of bovine viral diarrhoea virus: virus recovery and clinical reactions, *Res Vet Sci* 28:91-95, 1980.

321. Corapi WV et al: Thrombocytopenia and hemorrhages in veal calves infected with bovine viral diarrhea virus, *J Am Vet Med Assoc* 196:590-596, 1990.

322. Bolin SR, Ridpath JF: Differences in virulence between two noncytopathic bovine viral diarrhea viruses in calves, *Am J Vet Res* 53:2157-2163, 1992.

323. Wilson JB et al: A case-control study of selected pathogens including verocytotoxigenic *Escherichia coli* in calf diarrhea on an Ontario veal farm, *Can J Vet Res* 56:184-188, 1992.

324. Awad-el-Kariem FM, Warhurst DC, McDonald V: Detection and species identification of *Cryptosporidium* oocysts using a system based on PCR and endonuclease restriction, *Parasitology* 109:19-22, 1994.

325. Leng X, Mosier DA, Oberst RD: Differentiation of *Cryptosporidium parvum, C. muris,* and *C. baileyi* by PCR-RFLP analysis of the 18S rRNA gene, *Vet Parasitol* 62:1-7, 1996.

326. Xiao L et al: Species and strain-specific typing of *Cryptosporidium* parasites in clinical and environmental samples, *Memoriasdo Instituto Oswaldo Cruz*, 93:687-691, 1998.

327. Nichols GL, McLauchlin J, Samuel D: A technique for typing *Cryptosporidium* isolates, *J Protozool* 38:237S-240S, 1991.

328. Tzipori S: Cryptosporidiosis in animals and humans, *Microbiol Rev* 47:84-96, 1983.

329. Tzipori S: *Cryptosporidium:* notes on epidemiology and pathogenesis, *Parasitol Today* 1:159-165, 1985.

330. de Souza JCP, Lopes CWG: Criptosporidiose em bezerros de rebanhos da bacia leiteira sul-fluminense, Estado do Rio de Janeiro, *Rev Brasil Parasitol Vet* 4:33-36, 1995.

331. Bukhari Z, Smith HV: Detection of Cryptosporidium muris oocysts in the faeces of adult dairy cattle in Scotland, *Vet Rec* 138:207-208, 1996.

332. Klessius PH, Haynes TB, Malo LK: Infectivity of *Cryptosporidium* sp isolated from wild mice for calves and mice, *J Am Vet Med Assoc* 189:192-193, 1986.

333. Tzipori S et al: Cryptosporidium: evidence for a single species genus, *Infect Immun* 30:884-886, 1980.

334. Reif JS et al: Human cryptosporidiosis associated with an epizootic in calves, *Am J Public Health* 79:1528-1530, 1989.

335. Tzipori S et al: Experimental cryptosporidiosis in calves: clinical manifestations and pathological findings, *Vet Rec* 112:116-120, 1983.

336. Anderson BC, Bulgin MS: Enteritis caused by *Cryptosporidium* in calves, *Vet Med Small Anim Clin* 76:865-868, 1981.

337. Current WL: Cryptosporidiosis, *J Am Vet Med Assoc* 187:1334-1338, 1985.

338. Anderson BC: Cryptosporidiosis in Idaho lambs: natural and experimental infections, *J Am Vet Med Assoc* 181:151-152, 1982.

339. Tzipori S et al: Diarrhoea in goat kids attributed to cryptosporidiosis infection, *Vet Rec* 111:35-36, 1982.

340. Fitzgerald PR, Mansfield PE: Effects of bovine coccidiosis on certain blood components, feed consumption and bodyweight changes of calves, *Am J Vet Res* 33:1391-1397, 1972.

341. Stockdale P: The pathogenesis of the lesions produced by *Eimeria zuernii* in calves, *Can J Comp Med* 41:338-344, 1977.

342. Xiao LH, Herd RP, Rings DM: Concurrent infections of Giardia and Cryptosporidium on two Ohio farms with calf diarrhea, *Vet Parasitol* 51:41-48, 1993.

343. Bridger JC, Morgan JH: Variation in bovine rotaviruses: The influence of calf age, virus strain, calf type and diet on the outcome of infection, *Proceedings of the Association of Veterinary Teachers and Research Workers*, 1990, p 4.

344. Mylrea PJ: Digestion in young calves fed whole milk ad lib and its relationship to calf scours, *Res Vet Sci* 7:407-416.

345. Kertz AF: Calf health, performance and experimental results under a commercial-research facility and program, *J Dairy Sci* 60:1006-1015, 1977.

346. Lofstedt J, Dohoo JR: A model for the prediction of sepsis in diarrheic neonatal calves, *Proc ACVIM*, San Antonio, Tex, 1996, p 14.

347. Fecteau G et al: Bacteriological culture of blood from critically ill neonatal calves, *Can Vet J* 38:95-100, 1997.

348. Naylor JM et al: A comparison of three oral electrolyte solutions in the treatment of diarrheic calves, *Can Vet J* 31:753-760, 1990.

349. Hall GA et al: Pathogenesis of diarrhoea in rotavirus-infected calves, *Proc 14th World Vet Congr Dis Cattle World Assoc Buiatrics* 1:331-335, 1986.

350. Bridger JC, Oldham G, Pocock DH: Variation in virulence of bovine rotaviruses: relevance to diagnosis and vaccination in bovine enteritis, *Proc14th World Congr Dis Cattle Dublin* 1:336-341, 1986.

351. Mylrea PJ: Passage of antibiotics through the digestive tract of normal and scouring calves and their effect upon the bacterial flora, *Res Vet Sci* 9:5-13, 1968.

352. Wray C, Thomlinson JR: Factors influencing occurrence of colibacillosis in calves, *Vet Rec* 96:52-56, 1975.

353. Godbout-DeLasalle F, Higgins R: Biotyping of clinical isolates of *Escherichia coli* of animal origin, using the Analytab API 20E system, *Can J Vet Res* 50:418-421, 1986.

354. Braaten BA, Myers LL: Biochemical characteristics of enterotoxigenic and nonenterotoxigenic *Escherichia coli* isolated from calves with diarrhea, *Am J Vet Res* 38:1989-1991, 1977.

355. Reynolds DJ et al: Evaluation of ELISA and electron microscopy for the detection of coronavirus and rotavirus in bovine faeces, *Vet Rec* 114:397-401, 1984.

356. Chasey D, Davies P: Atypical rotaviruses in pigs and cattle, *Vet Rec* 114:16-17, 1984.

357. Benfield DA et al: Comparison of a commercial enzyme-linked immunosorbent assay with electron microscopy, fluorescent antibody, and virus isolation for the detection of bovine and porcine rotavirus, *Am J Vet Res* 45:1998-2002, 1984.

358. McNulty MS et al: Comparison of methods for diagnosis of rotavirus infection of calves, *Vet Rec* 98:463-464, 1976.

359. Opdenbosch Ev et al: A simple ELISA test for the detection of bovine coronavirus antigen in fecal and intestinal homogenates: a comparative study, *Vlaams Diergen Tijdschrift* 54:385-391, 1985.

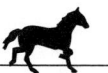

360. Stockdale P et al: Some pathophysiological changes associated with infection of *Eimeria zuernii* in calves, *Can J Comp Med* 45:34-37, 1981.

361. Pohjola S, Jokipii L, Jokipii A: Dimethylsulphoxide-Ziehl-Neelsen staining technique for detection of cryptosporidial oocysts, *Vet Rec* 116:442-443, 1985.

362. Casemore DP, Armstrong M, Sands RL: Laboratory diagnosis of cryptosporidiosis, *J Clin Pathol* 38:1337-41, 1985.

363. Anderson BC: Patterns of shedding of cryptosporidial oocysts in Idaho calves, *J Am Vet Med Assoc* 178:982-984, 1981.

364. Naylor JM: A retrospective study of the relationship between clinical signs and severity of acidosis in diarrheic calves, *Can Vet J* 30:577-580, 1989.

365. Naylor JM: Oral fluid therapy in neonatal ruminants and swine, *Vet Clin North Am (Food Anim Pract)* 6:51-67, 1990.

366. Phillips RW, Knox KL: Diarrheic acidosis in calves, *J Comp Lab Med* 3:1-3, 1969.

367. Naylor JM: Evaluation of the total carbon dioxide apparatus and pH meter for the determination of acid-base status in diarrheic and healthy calves, *Can Vet J* 28:1-2, 1987.

368. Kasari TR, Naylor JM: Clinical evaluation of sodium bicarbonate, sodium L-lactate, and sodium acetate for the treatment of acidosis in diarrheic calves, *J Am Vet Med Assoc* 187:392-397, 1985.

369. Radostits OM: Treatment and control of neonatal diarrhea in calves, *J Dairy Sci* 58:464-470, 1975.

370. Bywater RJ, Dupe RJ, Groddard M: Osmolality of solutions for oral rehydration in calves, *13th World Vet Congr Abstr* 10:1-5, 1987.

371. Guard CL, Tennant BC: Rehydration of neonatal calves with experimental colibacillosis: oral v. intravenous fluids, *Proc14th World Congr Dis Cattle Dublin* 1:356-361, 1986.

372. Booth AJ, Naylor JM: Correction of metabolic acidosis in diarrheal calves by oral administration of electrolyte solutions with or without bicarbonate, *J Am Vet Med Assoc* 191:62-68, 1987.

373. Naylor JM: Effects of electrolyte solutions for oral administration on clotting of milk, *J Am Vet Med Assoc* 201:1026-1029, 1992.

374. Heath SE et al: The effects of feeding milk to diarrheic calves supplemented with oral electrolytes, *Can J Vet Res* 53:477-485, 1989.

375. Nappert G, Zello GA, Naylor JM: Oral rehydration therapy for diarrheic calves, *Compend Cont Educ Pract Vet (Food Anim Pract)* 19:S181-S190, 1997.

376. Nappert G, Zello GA, Naylor JM: Intestinal metabolism of glutamine and potential use of glutamine as a therapeutic agent in diarrheic calves, *J Am Vet Med Assoc* 211:547-553, 1997.

377. Nappert G et al: Nutrient uptake by viscera drained by the portal vein in neonatal calves during intravenous infusion of glutamine, *Am J Vet Res* 60:446-451, 1999.

378. Naylor JM, Leibel T, Middleton DM: Effect of glutamine or glycine containing oral electrolyte solutions on mucosal morphology, clinical and biochemical findings, in calves with viral induced diarrhea, *Can J Vet Res* 61:43-48, 1997.

379. Cebra ML et al: Treatment of neonatal calf diarrhea with an oral electrolyte solution supplemented with psyllium mucilloid, *J Vet Intern Med* 12:449-455, 1998.

380. Naylor JM, Liebel T: Effect of psyllium on plasma concentration of glucose, breath hydrogen concentration, and fecal composition in calves with diarrhea treated orally with electrolyte solutions, *Am J Vet Res* 56:56-59, 1995.

381. Fettman MJ et al: Evaluation of commercial oral replacement formulas in healthy neonatal calves, *J Am Vet Med Assoc* 188:397-401, 1986.

382. McLean DM, Bailey LF: The effectiveness of three treatments for scouring in calves, *Aust Vet J* 48:336-338, 1972.

383. Osborne AD, Nazer AH, Shimeld C: Treatment of experimental calf salmonellosis with amoxicillin, *Vet Rec* 103:233-237, 1978.

384. Chaslus-Dancla E, Lafont JP: Resistance to gentamicin and apramycin in *Escherichia coli* from calves in France, *Vet Rec* 117:90-91, 1985.

385. Hinton M, Linton AH: Antibacterial drug resistance among *Escherichia coli* isolated from calves fed on a milk substitute diet, *Vet Rec* 112:567-568, 1983.

386. Angus KW et al: Prophylactic effects of anticoccidial drugs in experimental murine cryptosporidiosis, *Vet Rec* 114:166-168, 1984.

387. Moon HW, Woode GN, Ahrens FA: Attempted chemoprophylaxis of cryptosporidiosis in calves, *Vet Rec* 110:181, 1982.

388. Grimshaw W, Colman PJ, Petrie L: Efficacy of sulbactam-ampicillin in the treatment of neonatal calf diarrhoea, *Vet Rec* 121:162-166, 1987.

389. Bywater RJ: Pathophysiology and treatment of calf diarrhoea, *Proc 12th World Congr Dis Cattle The Netherlands*, 1982, pp 291-297.

390. Ericsson CD et al: Bismuth subsalicylate inhibits activity of crude toxins of *Escherichia coli* and *Vibrio cholerae*, *J Infect Dis* 136:693-696, 1977.

391. Forsyth GW, Kapitany RA, Hamilton DL: Organic acid proton donors decrease intestinal secretion caused by enterotoxins, *Am J Physiol* 241:G227-G234, 1981.

392. Forsyth GW, Kapitany RA, Scoot A: Nicotinic acid inhibits enterotoxin-induced jejunal secretion in the pig, *Can J Comp Med* 45:167-172, 1981.

393. Dickson J: Saline injections in the treatment of severe cases of scour in young suckled calves, *Vet Rec* 83:428-433, 1968.

394. Larouche Y, Black WD: A survey of calves treated for calf diarrhea at the Ontario Veterinary College 1966-1971, *Can Vet J*, 1973, pp 307-310.

395. Peters AR: Some husbandry factors affecting mortality and morbidity on a calf-rearing unit, *Vet Rec* 119:355-357, 1986.

396. Boyd JW, Baker JR, Leyland A: Neonatal diarrhoea in calves, *Vet Rec*, 1974, pp 310-313.

397. Dardillat J, Trillat G, Larvor P: Colostrum immunoglobulin concentration in cows: relationship with their calf mortality and with the colostrum quality of their female offspring, *Ann Rech Vet* 9:375-384, 1978.

398. Fisher EW et al: Studies of neonatal calf diarrhoea. II, Serum and faecal immune globulins in enteric colibacillosis, *Br Vet J* 402-415, 1975.

399. Gay CC et al: Gamma globulin levels and neonatal mortality in market calves, *Vet Rec* 77:148-149, 1965.

400. McEwan AD, Fisher EW, Selman IE: Observations on the immune globulin levels of neonatal calves and their relationship to disease, *J Comp Pathol* 80:259-265, 1970.

401. Penhale WJ et al: Observations on the absorption of colostral immunoglobulin by the neonatal calf and their significance in colibacillosis, *Ann Rech Vet* 4:223-233, 1973.

402. Leeuw Pd et al: Rotavirus infections in calves in dairy herds, *Res Vet Sci* 29:135-141, 1980.

403. Snodgrass DR, Wells PW: The influence of colostrum on neonatal rotaviral infections, *Ann Rech Vet* 9:335-338, 1978.

404. Woode GN, Jones J, Bridger J: Levels of colostral antibodies against neonatal calf diarrhoea virus, *Vet Rec* 97:148-149, 1975.

405. Acres SD et al: Immunization of calves against enterotoxigenic colibacillosis by vaccinating dams with purified K99 antigen and whole cell bacterins, *Infect Immun* 25:121-126, 1979.

406. Irwin VC: Disease incidence in colostrum deprived calves under commercial conditions and the economic consequences, *Vet Rec* 94:406, 1974.

407. McBeath DG, Penhale WJ, Logan EF: An examination of the influence of husbandry on the plasma immunoglobulin level of the newborn calf, using a rapid refractometer test for assessing immunoglobulin content, *Vet Rec* 88:266-270, 1971.

408. Bradley JA, Niilo L: A re-evaluation of routine force feeding of dam's colostrum to normal newborn beef calves, *Can Vet J* 25:121-125, 1984.

409. Selman IE, McEwan AD, Fisher EW: Studies on natural suckling in cattle during the first eight hours post partum. II, Behavioural studies (calves), *Anim Behav* 18:284-289, 1970.

410. Selman IE, McEwan AD, Fisher EW: Studies on natural suckling in cattle during the first eight hours post partum. I, Behavioural studies (dams), *Anim Behav* 18:276-283, 1970.

411. Fishwick G, Clifford D: The effects of a low protein intake by beef cows during pregnancy on the voluntary intake of roughage, the composition of the colostrum and the serum immune globulin concentration of their calves, *Nutr Soc* 34:74a-75a, 1975.

412. Logan EF: The influence of husbandry on colostrum yield and immunoglobulin concentration in beef cows, *Br Vet J* 133:120-125, 1977.

413. Petrie L, Acres SD, McCartney DH: The yield of colostrum and colostral gamma globulins in beef cows and the absorption of colostral gamma globulins by beef calves, *Can Vet J* 25:273-279, 1984.

414. Acres SD, Forman AJ, Kapitany RA: Antigen-extinction profile in pregnant cows, using a K99-containing whole-cell bacterin to induce passive protection against enterotoxigenic colibacillosis of calves, *Am J Vet Res* 43:569-575, 1982.

415. Myers LL: Vaccination of cows with an *Escherichia coli* bacterin for the prevention of naturally occurring diarrheal disease in their calves, *Am J Vet Res* 37:831-834, 1976.

416. Nagy LK, MacKenzie T, Painter KR: Re-vaccination of cows with *E. coli* K99/rotavirus vaccine in early gestation. *Proceedings of the Fourth International Symposium on Neonatal Diarrhea*, Veterinary Infectious Disease Organization, University of Saskatchewan, 1983, pp 448-455.

417. Sherman DM: Protection of calves against fatal enteric colibacillosis by orally administered *Escherichia coli* K99 specific monoclonal antibody, *Infect Immun* 42:653-658, 1983.

418. Acres SD, Radostits OM: The efficacy of a modified live reo-like virus vaccine and an *E. coli* bacterin for prevention of acute undifferentiated neonatal diarrhea of beef calves, *Can Vet J* 17:197-212, 1976.

419. Saif LJ et al: Passive immunity to bovine rotavirus in newborn calves fed colostrum supplements from immunized or nonimmunized cows, *Infect Immun* 141:1118-1131, 1983.

420. Waltner-Toews D: A field trial to evaluate the efficacy of a combined rotavirus-coronavirus/*Escherichia coli* vaccine in dairy cattle, *Can J Comp Med* 49:1-9, 1985.

421. Frank NA et al. Management risk factors associated with calf diarrhea in Michigan dairy herds: risk factors for mortality from diarrhea in beef calves in Alberta, *J Dairy Sci* 76:1313-1323, 1993.

422. McNulty MS, Logan EF: Effect of vaccination of the dam on rotavirus infection in young calves, *Vet Rec* 120:250-252, 1987.

423. Dauvergne M et al: Vaccination of dams with a combined rotavirus-coronavirus vaccine to protect newborn calves against diarrhea, *Proceedings of the Fourth International Symposium on Neonatal Diarrhea*, Veterinary Infectious Disease Organization, University of Saskatchewan, 1983, pp 424-434.

424. Snodgrass DR: Evaluation of a combined rotavirus and enterotoxigenic *Escherichia coli* vaccine in cattle, *Vet Rec* 119:39-42, 1986.

425. Sharpee RL et al: Enhancement of lactogenic immunity in cattle against rotavirus, coronavirus and *Escherichia coli* K99 by vaccination with an inactivated and adjuvanted combination vaccine, *Proc 14th World Congr Dis Cattle Dublin* 1:398-401, 1986.

426. Snodgrass DR et al: Diarrhoea in dairy calves reduced by feeding colostrum from cows vaccinated with rotavirus, *Res Vet Sci* 32:70-73, 1982.

427. Woode GN et al: Antigenic relationships among some bovine rotaviruses: serum neutralization and cross-protection in gnotobiotic calves, *J Clin Microbiol* 18:358-364, 1983.

428. Parwani AV et al: Characterization of field strains of group A bovine rotaviruses by using polymerase chain reaction-generated G and P type-specific cDNA probes, *J Clin Microbiol* 31:2010-2015, 1993.

429. Glasziou PP, Mackerras DEM: Vitamin A supplementation in infectious diseases: a meta-analysis, *Br Med J* 306:366-370, 1993.

430. Holland RE et al: Malabsorption of vitamin A in preruminating calves infected with *Cryptosporidium parvum*, *Am J Vet Res* 53:1947-1952, 1992.

431. McLaren IM, Wray C: Epidemiology of *Salmonella typhimurium* infection in calves: persistence of salmonellae on calf units, *Vet Rec* 29:461-462, 1991.

432. Smith EM, Gerba CP: Survival and detection of rotaviruses in the environment, *Proceedings of the Third International Symposium on Neonatal Diarrhea*, University of Saskatchewan, 1980, pp 67-81.

433. Radostits OM: The role of management and the use of vaccines in the control of acute undifferentiated diarrhea of newborn calves, *Can Vet J* 32:155-159, 1991.

434. Losinger WC, Heinrichs AJ: Management practices associated with high mortality among preweaned dairy heifers, *J Dairy Res* 64:1-11, 1997.

435. Morgan-Jones SC: Cleansing and disinfection of farm buildings. In Collins CH et al, eds: *Disinfectants: their use and evaluation of effectiveness*, London, 1981, Academic Press, pp 199-212.

436. Anonymous: *The cleansing and disinfection of calf houses*, no 645, Ministry of Agriculture Fisheries and Food, UK, 1981, pp 1-8.

437. Scarlett CM, Matheson GK: Terminal disinfection of calf houses by formaldehyde fumigation, *Vet Rec* 101:7-10, 1977.

438. Tablante N, Jr, Lane VM: Wild mice as potential reservoirs of *Salmonella dublin* in a closed dairy herd, *Can Vet J* 30:590-592, 1989.

439. James RE, McGilliard ML, Hartman DA: Calf mortality of Virginia dairy herd improvement herds, *J Dairy Sci* 67:908-911, 1984.

440. Jamaluddin AA et al: Economics of feeding pasteurized colostrum and pasteurized waste milk to dairy calves, *J Am Vet Med Assoc* 209:751-756, 1996.

441. Church TL: An analysis of production, disease, and veterinary usage in selected beef cow herds in Saskatchewan, Medical Science Thesis, 1978.

442. Collins JK et al: Shedding of enteric coronavirus in adult cattle, *Am J Vet Res* 48:361-365, 1987.

443. Crouch CF, Acres SD: Prevalence of rotavirus and coronavirus antigens in the feces of normal cows, *Can J Comp Med* 48:340-342, 1984.

444. Schumann FJ, Townsend HG, Naylor JN: Risk factors for mortality from diarrhea in beef calves in Alberta, *Can J Vet Res* 54:366-372, 1990.

445. Clement JC et al: Use of epidemiologic principles to identify risk factors associated with the development of diarrhea in calves in five beef herds, *J Am Vet Med Assoc* 207:1334-1338, 1995.

446. Smith BP, Spier S: How to approach control of *S. dublin* on a dairy, *Proc ACVIM* 6:561-563, 1988.

447. Angus KW et al: Evaluation of the effect of two aldehyde-based disinfectants on the infectivity of faecal cryptosporidia for mice, *Res Vet Sci* 33:379-381, 1982.

448. Campbell I et al: Effect of disinfectants on survival of *Cryptosporidium* oocysts, *Vet Rec* 111:414-415, 1982.

449. Ferrari M, Gualandi GL, Minelli MF: A study on the sensitivity of bovine rotavirus to some chemical agents, *Microbiologica* 9147-150, 1986.

450. Harvey SC: Antiseptics and disinfectants; fungicides; ectoparasiticides, In.Gilman AG et al, eds: *Goodman and Gilman's the pharmacological basis of therapeutics*, ed 7, New York, 1985, Macmillan, pp 959-979.

451. Snodgrass DR, Herring JA: The action of disinfectants on lamb rotavirus, *Vet Rec*, 101:81, 1977.

452. Firth EC: Hematogenous osteomyelitis in the foal, *Proceedings of the Thirty-third Annual Convention of the American Association of Equine Practitioners*, 1987, pp 795-804.

453. Martens RJ, Auer JA, Carter GK: Equine pediatrics: septic arthritis and osteomyelitis, *J Am Vet Med Assoc* 188:582-585, 1986.

454. Wilson WD et al: Septic arthritis in foals: bacterial isolates and antimicrobial susceptibility. In *Proceedings of the Seventh International Conference on Equine Infectious Disease*, 1994, p 163.

455. Angus K: Arthritis in lambs and sheep, *In Practice* 13:204-207, 1991.

456. Firth EC et al: Haematogenous osteomyelitis in cattle, *Vet Rec* 120:148-152, 1987.

457. Van Pelt RW: Infectious arthritis in cattle caused by *Corynebacterium pyogenes*, *J Am Vet Med Assoc* 156:457-465, 1970.

458. Van Pelt RW, Langham RF, Sleight SD: Lesions of infectious arthritis in calves, *J Am Vet Med Assoc* 149:303-311, 1966.

459. East NE et al: Milkborne outbreak of *Mycoplasma mycoides* subspecies mycoides infection in a commercial goat dairy, *J Am Vet Med Assoc* 182:1338-1341, 1983.

460. Rodriquez JL et al: Polyarthritis in kids associated with *Mycoplasma putrefaciens*, *Vet Rec* 135:406-407, 1994.

461. Stipkovits L, Rady M, Glavits R: Mycoplasmal arthritis and meningitis in calves, *Acta Vet Hung* 41:1-2, 1993.

462. Shewen PE: Chlamydial infection in animals: a review, *Can Vet J* 21:2-11, 1980.

463. Bertone AL, McIlwraith CW: A review of current concepts in the therapy of infectious arthritis in the horse, *Proceedings of the Thirty-third Annual Convention of the American Association of Equine Practitioners*, 1987, pp 323-339.

464. Munroe GA, Cauvin ER: The use of arthroscopy in the treatment of septic arthritis in two highland calves, *Br Vet J* 150:439-449, 1994.

465. Markel MD, Ryan AM, Madigan JE: Vertebral and costal osteomyelitis in a foal, *Compend Cont Educ Pract Vet* 10:856-861, 1988.

466. Firth EC et al: Tarsal osteomyelitis in foals, *Vet Rec* 116:261-266, 1985.

467. McIlwraith CW: Treatment of infectious arthritis, *Vet Clin North Am (Large Anim Pract)* 5:363-379, 1983.

468. Martens RJ, Auer JA: Hematogenous septic arthritis and osteomyelitis in the foal, *Proceedings of the Twenty-sixth Annual Convention of the American Association of Equine Practitioners*, 1980, 47-63.

469. Whitehair KJ et al: Regional limb perfusion with antibiotics in three horses, *Vet Surg* 21:286-292, 1992.

470. Huffel X et al: Carpal joint arthrodesis as a treatment for chronic septic carpitis in calves and cattle, *Vet Surg* 18:304-311, 1989.

471. Hau T, Nishikawa RA, Phuangsab A: The effect of bacterial trapping by fibrin on the efficacy of systemic antibiotics in experimental peritonitis, *Surg Gynecol Obstet* 157:252-256, 1983.

472. Trent AM, Plumb D: Treatment of infectious arthritis and osteomyelitis, *Vet Clin North Am (Food Anim Pract)* 7:747-778, 1991.

473. Brown MP et al: Pharmacokinetics and synovial fluid concentrations of cephapirin in calves with suppurative arthritis, *Am J Vet Res* 52:1438-1440, 1991.

474. Shoaf SE et al: Pharmacokinetics of trimethoprim/sulfadiazine in neonatal calves: influence of synovitis, *J Vet Pharmacol Ther* 9:446-454, 1986.

475. Guard CL, Byman KW, Schwark WS: Effect of experimental synovitis on disposition of penicillin and oxytetracycline in neonatal calves, *Cornell Vet* 79:161-171, 1989.

476. Brown MP, Mayo MB, Gronwall RR: Serum and synovial fluid concentrations of ampicillin trihydrate in calves with suppurative arthritis, *Cornell Vet* 81:137-143, 1991.

477. Verschooten F et al: Surgical and conservative treatment of infectious arthritis in cattle, *J Am Vet Med Assoc* 165:271-275, 1974.

478. Moore RM, Kohn CW: Nutritional muscular dystrophy in foals, *Compend Cont Educ Pract Vet* 13:476-486, 1991.

479. Yovich JV, Staska TS, McIlwarith CW: Rupture of the common digital extensor tendon in foals, *Compend Cont Educ Pract Vet* 6:S373-S378, 1984.

480. Crowe MW, Swerczek TW, Ward-Crowe M: Equine congenital defects, *Am J Vet Res* 46:353-358, 1985.

481. Auer JA, Martens RJ, Morris EL: Angular limb deformities in foals. I, Congenital factors, *Compend Cont Educ Pract Vet* 4:330-339, 1982.

482. Adams R, Poulos P: Radiographic evaluation of the tarsal and carpal regions of neonatal foals, *Proceedings of the Thirty-third Annual Convention of the American Association of Equine Practitioners*, 1987, pp 677-682.

483. McLaughlin BG, Doige CE: A study of ossification of carpal and tarsal bones in normal and hypothyroid foals, *Can Vet J* 23:164-168, 1982.

484. McLaughlin BG, Doige CE: Congenital musculoskeletal lesions and hyperplastic goitre in foals, *Can Vet J* 22:130-133, 1981.

485. Turner TA, Fessler JF, Ewert KM: Patent urachus in foals, *Equine Pract* 4:24-31, 1982.

486. Reef VB: Abnormalities of the neonatal umbilicus detected by diagnostic ultrasound, *Proceedings of the Thirty-third Annual Convention of the American Association of Equine Practitioners*, 1987, pp 157-162.

487. Whitwell KE: Morphology and pathology of the equine umbilical cord, *J Reprod Fertil* 23(suppl):599-603, 1975.

488. Adams SB, Fessler JF: Umbilical cord remnant infections in foals: 16 cases (1975-1985), *J Am Vet Med Assoc* 190:316-318, 1987.

489. Trent AM, Smith DF: Surgical management of umbilical masses with associated umbilical cord remnant infections in calves, *J Am Vet Med Assoc* 185:1531-1534, 1984.

490. Diefenderfer DL, Brightling P: Dysuria due to urachal abscessation in calves diagnosed by contrast urography, *Can Vet J* 24:218-221, 1983.

491. Trent AM: Pollakiuria due to urachal abscesses in two heifers, *J Am Vet Med Assoc* 184:984-986, 1984.

492. Watson E et al: Ultrasonography of the umbilical structures in clinically normal calves, *Am J Vet Res* 55:773-780, 1994.

493. Steiner A, Lischer CJ, Oertle C: Marsupialization of umbilical vein abscesses with involvement of the liver in 13 calves, *Vet Surg* 22:184-189, 1993.

494. Harvey JW et al: Haematology of foals up to one year old, *Equine Vet J* 16:347-353, 1984.

495. Harvey JW et al: Serum ferritin, serum iron, and erythrocyte values in foals, *Am J Vet Res* 48:1348-1352, 1987.

496. Spensley MS, Carlson GP, Harrold D: Plasma, red blood cell, total blood, and extracellular fluid volumes in healthy horse foals during growth, *Am J Vet Res* 48:1703-1707, 1987.

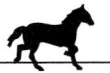

497. Raleigh RJ, Wallace JP: The influence of iron and copper on hematologic values and on body weight of range calves, *Am J Vet Res* 23:276-299, 1962.

498. Tennant B et al: Hematology of the neonatal calf. III, Frequency of congenital iron deficiency anemia, *Cornell Vet* 65:543-556, 1975.

499. McGillivray SR, Searcy GP, Hirsch VM: Serum iron, total iron binding capacity, plasma copper and hemoglobin types in anemic and poikilocytic calves, *Can J Comp Med* 49:286-290, 1985.

500. Katunguka-Rwakishaya E, Larkin H, Kelly WR: Blood values of neonatal calves, and blood values and live weight gains of calves fed on different levels of milk replacer, *Br Vet J* 143:184-190, 1987.

501. Sockett DC, Traub-Dargatz J, Weiser MG: Immune-mediated hemolytic anemia and thrombocytopenia in a foal, *J Am Vet Med Assoc* 190:308-310, 1987.

502. Tizard I: *Veterinary immunology*, ed 3, Philadelphia, 1987, WB Saunders, p 299.

503. Madigan JE: *Manual of equine neonatal medicine*, Woodland, Calif, 1987, Live Oak Publishing, p 208.

504. Van der Jagt E: Fever. In Hackelman RA, ed: *Primary pediatric care*, St Louis, 1987, Mosby, p 956.

505. Krotje LJ: Cyanosis: physiology and pathogenesis, *Compend Cont Educ Pract Vet* 9:271-278, 1987.

506. Comline RS, Silver M: A comparative study of blood gas tensions, oxygen affinity, and red cell 2,3 DPG concentrations in fetal and maternal blood in the mare, cow, and sow, *J Physiol* 242:805-826, 1977.

507. Bunn HF, Kitchen H: Hemoglobin function in the horse: the role of 2,3-diphosphoglycerate in modifying the oxygen affinity of maternal and fetal blood, *Blood* 42:471-479, 1973.

508. Machida N, Yasuda J, Too K: Three cases of paroxysmal atrial fibrillation in the thoroughbred newborn foal, *Equine Vet J* 21:66-68, 1989.

509. Brewer BD et al: Renal clearance, urinary excretion of endogenous substances and urinary diagnostic indices in healthy neonatal foals, *J Vet Intern* 5:28, 1989.

510. Koterba AM et al: Renal and urinary tract function and dysfunction in the neonatal foal, *Proceedings of the Thirty-second Annual Convention of the American Association of Equine Practitioners*, 1986, pp 659-671.

511. Parker HR, Murphy JA: Kidney development in newborn lambs: response to water load and antidiuretic hormone (ADH), *Theriogenology* 6:273-292, 1976.

512. Short CR: Drug disposition in neonatal animals, *J Am Vet Med Assoc* 184:1161-1162, 1984.

513. Houlton J et al: Urinary incontinence in a Shire foal due to ureteral ectopia, *Equine Vet J* 19:244-247, 1987.

514. Haskins SC: Shock. In Madigan JE, ed: *Manual of equine neonatal medicine*, Woodland, Calif, 1987, Live Oak Publishing, pp 77-78.

515. Bone RC et al: A controlled clinical trial of high-dose methylprednisolone in the treatment of severe sepsis and septic shock, *N Engl J Med* 317:653-658, 1987.

516. Thomas WP: Congenital cardiac anomalies. In Madigan JE, ed: *Manual of equine neonatal medicine*, ed 2, Woodland, Calif, 1993, Live Oak Publishing, pp 186-191.

517. Amorosao EC, Dawes GS, Mott JC: Patency of the ductus arteriosus in the newborn foal, *Br Heart J* 20:92-96, 1958.

518. Scott EA, Kneller SK, Witherspoon DM: Closure of ductus arteriosus determined by cardiac catheterization and angiography in newborn foals, *Am J Vet Res* 36:1021-1023, 1975.

519. Lombard CW, Scarratt WK, Buergelt CD: Ventricular septal defects in the horse, *J Am Vet Med Assoc* 183:562-565, 1983.

520. Bayly WM et al: Multiple congenital heart anomalies in five Arabian foals, *J Am Vet Med Assoc* 181:684-689, 1982.

521. Harper RG, Yoon JJ: Respiratory distress. In Harper RG, ed: *Handbook of neonatology*, ed 2, St Louis, 1987, Mosby, p 256.

522. Koterba AM, Brewer BD, Tarplee FA: Clinical and clinicopathological characteristics of the septicaemic neonatal foal: review of 38 cases, *Equine Vet J* 16:376-382, 1984.

523. Roeder BL et al: Isolation of *Clostridium perfringens* from neonatal calves with ruminal and abomasal tympany, abomasitis, and abomasal ulceration, *J Am Vet Med Assoc* 190:1550-1555, 1987.

524. Olson DP et al: Effects of maternal nutritional restriction and cold stress on young calves: clinical condition, behavioral reactions, and lesions, *Am J Vet Res* 42:758-763, 1981.

525. Bull RC et al: Evaluation of blood metabolite profiles to predict crude protein consumption in pregnant beef cattle, *J Anim Sci* 66(suppl 1):509-510, 1988.

526. Bull RC: Personal communication, 1988, University of Idaho, Moscow, Idaho.

Milk Replacers

A. JUDSON HEINRICHS

LORRAINE DOEPEL

RICK CORBETT

In recent years research in the area of milk replacers has burgeoned. It has focused on improving the quality of milk replacers to enhance calf performance, while minimizing the cost of calf rearing. The goals of the milk-replacer feeding program are to (1) achieve optimum growth rates, (2) develop a strong immune system, (3) minimize health disorders, (4) stimulate and optimize rumen development, and (5) minimize the cost of feeding the preweaning calf.

CALVES

Digestive Physiology of the Preruminant Calf

The gastrointestinal physiology of the newborn calf is poorly developed, and the calf is unable to digest a variety of feedstuffs normally provided for ruminant animals. The gastrointestinal tract of newborn calves undergoes maturation during the first 3 or more weeks of life and continues to grow and mature for an extended period. The calf is technically a monogastric at this time, and its diet must be easily digestible and consist of predominantly high-quality, human-grade feedstuffs.

The size and proportion of the compartments of the calf's stomach change dramatically during the first few weeks of life and are affected by diet.[1] At birth the reticulorumen makes up approximately 30% of the stomach compartments, although it is nonfunctional, the omasum makes up 10%, and the true stomach, or abomasum, makes up 60%. The abomasum is the only truly functional part of the four stomach compartments in the newborn. By 4 weeks of age the reticulorumen makes up slightly more than half the total, the omasum remains about the same at 12%, and the true stomach makes up about 36%. By 16 weeks of age the reticulorumen accounts for more than two thirds of the total stomach weight. The omasum makes up about the same proportion (18%), but the abomasum now constitutes only 15%. It is still functional, as it was at birth, and has even grown, but the increase in size and functionality of the reticulorumen makes it the major part of the stomach system.

As mentioned previously, the rumen at birth is nonfunctional, with little tissue development and no microbial population. The enzymes produced by the microorganisms in ruminants are largely responsible for breaking down complex carbohydrates and fiber. Having no ruminal microbial population, the calf depends on digestive enzymes released primarily from the abomasum, pancreas, and small intestine to digest fats, carbohydrates, and protein. After colostrum, milk, or casein-containing milk replacer is swallowed, the ingested liquid bypasses the rumen through the esophageal groove and enters the abomasal canal for digestion. The esophageal groove consists of muscular folds from the reticulorumen that come together with the stimulus of suckling. This fold works well with the calf's head in any position, but only when colostrum or milk is fed. Interestingly, it does not function when the calf drinks water; therefore water enters the rumen rather than the abomasum.

During the first feeding of colostrum, the esophageal groove closes and the colostrum passes directly into the abomasum.[2] The liquid forms a clot as a result of the action of chymosin, pepsin, and hydrochloric acid. Chymosin, also known as rennin, is the enzyme that specifically binds with the casein protein of colostrum or milk. The clotting action causes the casein and fat in colostrum to form a hard lump, or curd. The lump of fat and protein is digested and emptied into the small intestine over the next 12 to 18 hours. The enzymes of the stomach and small intestine are produced in small amounts in the first 48 hours of life. Curd formation allows the digestive tract, which has limited digestive capacity, to slowly yet efficiently break down the nutrients and assimilate them completely, thereby preventing digestive scours caused by the delivery of undigested nutrients to the large intestine. The second feeding of colostrum or transition milk adds to the already formed curd in the stomach. This system allows the calf to receive a steady supply of nutrients over the first 24 to 48 hours of life as long as it is fed casein-containing liquids.[3]

The fraction of the colostrum that does not form a curd is whey. Whey is passed to the small intestine for digestion or absorption or both. Whey is composed of water, minerals, lactose, and a variety of proteins. Immunoglobulins are one of the important protein groups in whey. Immunoglobulins pass out of the abomasum to the small intestine within 10 minutes after feeding, which allows them to be quickly absorbed into the calf's bloodstream. The rapid absorption of these essential immunoglobulins is critical because no placental transfer of immunoglobulins from the dam occurs.

Digestion of carbohydrates by the newborn calf is relatively poor; the exception is lactose, or milk sugar. Calves younger than 1 month of age are limited in their ability to use starch, maltose, sucrose, or dextrin because they lack sufficient amounts of the necessary digestive enzymes. By 3 weeks of age, the calf shows a marked improvement in the ability to digest starch. Over 3 weeks of age, the ability to digest vegetable proteins also improves.

Within a few days of birth, the rumen begins to develop a microbial population. The number and types of bacteria that develop are a function of the type of feeds the calf eats. When the calf eats dry feed, the esophageal groove does not function and the feed enters the rumen. Inoculation of the rumen with microorganisms occurs by way of the environment, hair coat, bedding, and feeds eaten. The types of ruminal microbes that proliferate are those that best digest and use the feedstuffs being consumed. In addition to feed, ruminal microbes require water to grow properly and digest feedstuffs. If the calf is not provided with water in early life, ruminal microbial growth will be limited. The neural stimulus that forms the esophageal groove does not generally function when water is fed separate from milk or milk replacer. Much of the water a calf drinks does not bypass the rumen and thus is available to support the growth of ruminal microbes.

Milk Replacer Quality and Formulation for the Dairy Calf

The first few weeks of life are critical to the growth and long-term performance of a dairy calf. After birth the calf normally receives colostrum for a first feeding and, under many farm situations, for several feedings up to 3 days of age. The length of time before other feeds are offered to the calf depends primarily on the management of the particular dairy farm. Often the calf consumes only a liquid diet for the first 2 weeks of life. Even when dry feed (grain) is offered, very little if any is consumed for the first 7 to 10 days. Therefore the liquid feeding portion of the rearing program is important to the calf's health and initial growth.

More than 60% of the dairy calves in the United States are fed milk replacers for most or all of their liquid feeding period.[4] A dairy calf typically is fed a milk replacer for 6 to 8 weeks and then weaned. Farmers wean calves at anywhere from 3 weeks of age to, in extreme cases, 6 months of age. It is recommended that calves be weaned by 6 weeks of age, with a goal for most of the calves, most of the year, being 4 to 5 weeks of age at weaning. The national average in 1992 was 8.1 weeks[5]; however, this average is declining, with the more progressive farms leading the way toward a 4-week weaning age.

Convenience and economics are the two major factors driving the increase in the use of milk replacers. Feeding milk replacer often is more convenient than feeding whole milk or waste milk because calves generally are housed in different areas on the farm than the milking cows, and the transport of saleable or waste milk is difficult. This issue becomes more pronounced as the size of the farm increases. Often, supplying the transition milk from the dam to the calf up to the time the milk is saleable is all that is possible from a labor and management standpoint.

Milk replacers can be manufactured with a variety of ingredients and levels of nutrients to match the management requirements of a wide variety of farms. Various additives that cannot be easily used in whole milk or waste milk feeding systems can be supplied in milk replacers to improve the nutrition and health of the calf.

PROTEIN. One major reason for the use of milk replacers is the cost savings over the alternative of using whole milk. Savings are realized because milk replacers are composed primarily of by-products of the cheese industry. Casein removed for dried skim milk production and casein and fat removed for cheese production carry much of the original value of the whole milk. The whey that remains is less valuable and, although its demand on a world market is growing, it still commands a much lower price than skim milk. The trend for increased use of milk replacers likely will continue as long as the price differential between milk and milk replacers remains.

The composition and quality of a milk replacer will influence the calf's growth, health, and overall performance. Composition and nutrient levels vary greatly among the various products. Milk replacers used in the United States typically are composed of whey and whey protein concentrate compounds. Dried whey contains 12% crude protein, mainly lactalbumin, and 74% lactose. Whey protein concentrate, which is produced by ultrafiltration of liquid whey to remove lactose and other soluble components, contains about 34% crude protein. Skim milk is rarely used in appreciable amounts in the United States because of its high cost.

The protein in skim milk differs from that in whey, varying in several amino acids, as shown in Table 21-1 (the amino acid composition of common ingredients used in manufacturing milk replacers also is shown). The table lists the average amounts of the various amino acids, but it does not show the availability of each amino acid to the calf. Availability depends on the method and conditions of processing and can vary greatly between feeds and processors. In general, for a very young calf the milk proteins are highly digestible (92% to 98%) and the plant proteins somewhat less digestible (85% to 94%). In some milk replacers the essential amino acids lysine and methionine are supplemented from synthetic sources to compensate for low content or reduced availability in a particular ingredient. This most often occurs when soy or other plant proteins are used in the product. Manufacturers use available data to best fortify the product in an economical manner. Some evidence suggests that the amino acid composition of whey is actually more correct for meeting the calf's requirements for optimum growth than the amino acid composition of skim milk. In any case, research trials using skim milk or whey proteins have proved both to be completely satisfactory in meeting the newborn calf's needs for growth.[6]

Some milk replacers contain vegetable proteins, primarily of soy origin, but wheat and potato proteins may also be used. The soy proteins include soy protein isolates, soy protein concentrates, and chemically treated soy flours. Soy flour is obtained by grinding defatted soy flakes that have been heated to remove trypsin inhibitor or washed in aqueous ethanol to remove glycinin and β-conglycinin. Soy protein concentrate is produced by washing defatted soy flakes with aqueous alcohol to remove the soluble carbohydrates. Isolated soy protein is produced by washing defatted soy flakes in alkali followed by acid precipitation and alkali resolubilization of extracted protein. Wheat gluten is derived from wheat flour by wet processing or milling. Milk replacers that include wheat gluten (33% of total protein) and those without it have resulted in comparable calf gains.[7] Animal proteins, including animal plasma, or hydrolyzed red blood cells, are also used to replace some of the whey protein concentrate. Many of the amino acids in these ingredients are present at very high levels compared with milk proteins. Dairy calf research on these proteins is limited, but they appear promising. Hydrolyzed red blood cells can replace up to 43% of protein from whey protein concentrate without adversely affecting the calf's health or performance.[8] Bovine or porcine plasma products also can be

TABLE 21-1

Composition of Ingredients Used in Milk Replacers

	Whey	Whey Protein Concentrate	Delactosed Whey	Skim Milk	Whole Dried Milk	Isolated Soy Protein	Soy Protein Concentrate	Soy Flour	Modified Wheat Protein	Spray-Dried Blood Meal	Spray-Dried Animal Plasma
	Expressed on an "as is" basis (%)					Expressed on an "as is" basis (%)					
Dry matter	98	98	98	98	97	94	95	95	94	92	92
Protein	12	34	23	34	26	66	67	53	82	80	78
Fat	0.2	3.5	1.5	0.1	28.5	0.5	0.3	0.2	2	1.3	1.1
Lactose	74	52	55	54	34	—	—	—	—	—	—
Ash	8.5	8	16	7.9	6	4.5	7	6.3	3	5.3	8.9
Calcium	0.9	0.54	1.95	1.25	0.95	0.1	0.35	0.35	0.04	0.32	0.15
Phosphorus	0.81	0.67	1	1.05	0.75	0.76	0.18	0.73	0.4	0.24	1.7
	Essential amino acids (g/100 g protein)					Essential amino acids (g/100 g protein)					
Lysine	8.92	9.09	8.91	8.24	8.23	6.07	6.32	6.15	1.6	8.19	6.9
Methionine	1.92	1.94	1.91	2.65	2.62	1.11	1.32	1.26	1.85	1.01	0.7
Cysteine	2.25	2.47	2.09	1.51	1.5	1.41	1.47	1.42	2.47	0.9	1.8
Arginine	2.92	2.53	2.91	3.65	3.85	7.79	8.1	7.17	3.95	3.87	4.5
Tryptophan	2.09	2.15	2.09	1.41	1.41	1.01	1.32	1.28	0.99	1.16	1.3
Histidine	1.75	1.91	1.74	2.74	2.73	2.73	2.65	2.6	2.22	5.87	2.5
Isoleucine	6.08	5.97	8.09	6.99	7	4.85	4.65	4.62	4.44	4	2
Leucine	10.33	10.47	10.35	10.01	10	8.09	7.94	7.62	7.78	2.34	7.4
Phenylalanine	3.5	3.24	3.48	4.71	4.69	4.95	5	4.91	5.93	6.2	4.8
Threonine	7	7.29	7	4.25	4.23	3.84	4.12	4.06	2.59	3.78	4.3
Valine	5.92	5.82	5.91	5.58	6.65	5.06	5.15	4.89	4.44	7.81	5.2

used successfully in milk replacers as a partial replacement (23% of total protein) for milk proteins.[9] In addition to being highly digestible protein, plasma proteins supply a source of immunoglobulins that may have a beneficial effect in the calf's intestinal lumen. In performance and cost, these products rank between all-milk protein replacers and soy-based replacers.

Historically, the rennet coagulation test was used to evaluate the quality of milk replacers. This technique checks for the presence of undamaged casein, the predominant protein in skim milk. When the price of this ingredient was low enough to allow it to be included in milk replacers, it was sometimes heat damaged or altered during manufacture and therefore was indigestible to the calf, resulting in scouring and poor growth. The rennet coagulation test was an easy means of checking for this problem during the 1950s and 1960s. Today, there is no reason to use this test because we can be quite certain that the world market price and product competition in the United States will minimize the use of skim milk powder in dairy calf milk replacers. Those that do have skim milk have been dried in a manner that does not denature the casein protein. Milk replacers containing plant proteins are often higher in protein content to counteract their lower digestibility relative to milk proteins. Most of the soy protein isolates or concentrates used today are highly digestible for the young calf.

Wheat flour, soy flour, meat solubles, and fish proteins are among the least recommended ingredients in a dairy calf milk replacer. Some of the soy protein compounds are patented, and the label may bear the registered name and not the generic soy protein name (isolate or concentrate).

The ingredients on the milk replacer tag should be listed in descending order of predominance, as specified by the U.S. Food and Drug Administration. Many states use a Uniform State Feed Bill that does not specify the need to list ingredients in order of predominance; however, in these states most companies list ingredients in order of predominance to facilitate comparison of products. It is important to read and understand the ingredients in a milk replacer to compare and evaluate products.

ENERGY. Energy (calories) in milk replacers is derived primarily from lactose and fat. The effects of the energy content of milk replacers are not always clear in practical applications because of interactions with environmental temperature, energy derived from dry calf starter, the stage of rumen development, and differences in the metabolic efficiency of fat- and carbohydrate-derived energy.[10] During periods of extreme stress, which include cold temperatures with outside-housed calves, the calf's energy intake should be increased. This can be done by increasing by 30% to 50% the amount of replacer fed daily or by increasing the fat content of the replacer. Fats added to calf milk replacers are mainly edible animal fats, with some use of vegetable fats such as palm oil or refined coconut oil (digestibility 94% to 95%). The animal fats used can be bleached tallow, lard, and white grease (digestibility 87% to 92%).[10] It is important to note that when dry matter intake from milk replacer is increased, it will substitute for some dry matter intake from grain. The long-term effects of this are reduced grain intake and delayed rumen development.

ADDITIVES. An obvious reason to use milk replacers is that nutrient fortification and additives for promoting growth and health can be incorporated without extra steps. Such fortification includes extra vitamins and minerals, along with various other additives. The most common additives found in milk replacers are lasalocid and decoquinate, which prevent coccidiosis, and oxytetracycline and neomycin, which help prevent bacterial scours.

Summary

It is noteworthy that much of the current research related to milk replacers is done by individual manufacturers, with less done in the public domain. This means that much of the peer-reviewed journal research is dated and often does not account for modern feed-manufacturing technology. It is likely that recommended levels of nutrients based on older research are overestimated or underestimated. The recommended ranges of nutrients (Table 21-2) are broad in many cases, to account for some of these differences and for the variety of protein sources and energy content in milk replacers. Many farms want high growth rates in their young calves, and these farms therefore need milk replacers with marginally increased nutrient density; other farms want only economy. The milk-replacer industry has a variety of products to meet the needs of these different customers. As with most purchased items, quality is related to price.

Although milk replacers are important in the dairy feed industry today, many studies show that only 24% of growth before weaning can be accounted for by the energy provided in milk replacers. Calf starter makes up the remaining 76% of the energy for body weight gain in the first 2 months of life. It is important to note that overfeeding milk replacer, either the amount or concentration, primarily replaces dry matter intake that normally would come from grain. This slows rumen development and is less economical for the producer.

FOALS

Milk replacer must be used for foals if the mare has an inadequate milk supply or the foal is orphaned at an early age. Milk replacers for foals should contain 18% to 22% crude protein, 12% to 16% crude fat, and 10% to 11% total solids. The replacer should be highly digestible, easily reconstituted, and palatable.

Orphan foals should be fed milk replacer from 1 day of age (after receiving colostrum within 24 hours of birth) to at least 1 month of age.[11] General guidelines for feeding milk

TABLE 21-2

General Nutrient Recommendations for Dairy Calf Milk Replacers*

Nutrient	Recommended Concentration
Crude protein	18-24s
Fat	10-22
Calcium	0.7
Phosphorus	0.6
Potassium	0.8
Magnesium	0.07
Sodium	0.09
Chlorine	0.18
Sulfur	0.26
Iron (ppm)	90
Cobalt (ppm)	0.09
Copper (ppm)	9
Manganese (ppm)	36
Zinc (ppm)	36
Iodine (ppm)	0.23
Selenium (ppm)	0.27
Vitamin A (IU/lb)	25,000-35,000
Vitamin D (IU/lb)	5000-7500
Vitamin E (IU/lb)	50-125

*Percentage of dry matter unless otherwise indicated.

TABLE 21-3

Typical Feeding Recommendations for Foal Milk Replacers

Age (Days)	Number of Daily Feedings	Approximate Amount (ml/Meal)	Amount of Water (ml/Day)	Total Amount of Powder (g/Day)
0-3	12	300	3000	480
4-5	8	500	3500	560
6-7	8	770	5300	860
8-10	8	1000	7000	1100
11-14	6	1660	8625	1335
15-21	4	3225	11,130	1750
over 21	3-4	?	>15%-20% body weight	>2.5% body weight

Cymbaluk N: Managing orphan foals and early weaned foals, *Proceedings of the Alberta Horse Breeders and Owners Conference*, Red Deer, Alberta, Canada, 1994.

replacers can be found in Table 21-3. Feeding less often than recommended may reduce the growth rate as a consequence of inadequate intake of milk replacer. It is important that the foal receive the recommended amount of milk-replacer powder daily to avoid starvation from underfeeding or diarrhea from overfeeding.

LAMBS AND KIDS

Milk replacers generally are used to raise extra lambs from multiple births and orphaned lambs and also can be used for kids. Most of the principles discussed previously for calves apply to lambs and kids. Milk replacers for lambs usually contain 21% to 24% crude protein and 24% to 30% crude fat. The lactose level in lamb milk replacers should not exceed 25%, because higher levels may result in abomasal bloat and diarrhea. Milk replacers for lambs generally are fed cold ad libitum from automatic nipple feeders. Lambs that are fed warm milk replacer a few times during the day drink too much at each feeding and may develop abomasal bloat.

Creep feed can be offered to lambs after 1 week of age. It should contain 17% to 20% crude protein, should be highly digestible, and should be fed fresh daily. Introduction of creep feed at an early age helps the lamb develop a fully functional rumen by 35 to 40 days of age.

REFERENCES

1. Church DC: *Digestive physiology and nutrition of ruminants,* Corvallis, Ore, 1969, DC Church.
2. Cruywagen CW, Brisson GJ, Meissner HH: Casein curd-forming ability and abomasal retention of milk replacer components in young calves, *J Dairy Sci* 73:1578-1585, 1990.
3. Longenbach JI, Heinrichs AJ: A review of the importance and physiological role of curd formation in the abomasums of young calves, *Animal Feed Science and Technology* 73:85-97, 1998.
4. Heinrichs AJ, Wells SJ, Losinger WC: A study of the use of milk replacers for dairy calves in the United States, *J Dairy Sci* 78:2831-2837, 1995.
5. Heinrichs AJ et al: The National Dairy Heifer Evaluation Project: a profile of heifer management in the United States, *J Dairy Sci* 77:1548-1555, 1994.
6. Lammers BP, Heinrichs AJ, Aydin A: The effect of whey protein concentrate or dried skim milk in milk replacer on calf performance and blood metabolites, *J Dairy Sci* 81:1940-1945, 1996.
7. Terui H, Morrill JL, Higgens JJ: Evaluation of wheat gluten in milk replacers and calf starters, *J Dairy Sci* 79:1261-1266, 1996.
8. Quigley JD III et al: Effects of hydrolyzed spray-dried red blood cells in milk replacer on calf intake, body weight gain, and efficiency, *J Dairy Sci* 83:788-794, 2000.
9. Morrill JL et al: Plasma proteins and a probiotic as ingredients in milk replacer, *J Dairy Sci* 78:902-907, 1995.
10. Tomkins T, Sowinski J, Drackley JK: New developments in milk replacers for preruminants, Minnesota Nutrition Conference, Sept 1994.
11. Cymbaluk N: Managing orphan foals and early weaned foals, *Proceedings of the Alberta Horse Breeders and Owners Conference*, Red Deer, Alberta, Canada, 1994.

COLLECTION OF SAMPLES AND INTERPRETATION OF LABORATORY TESTS

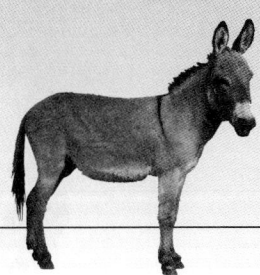

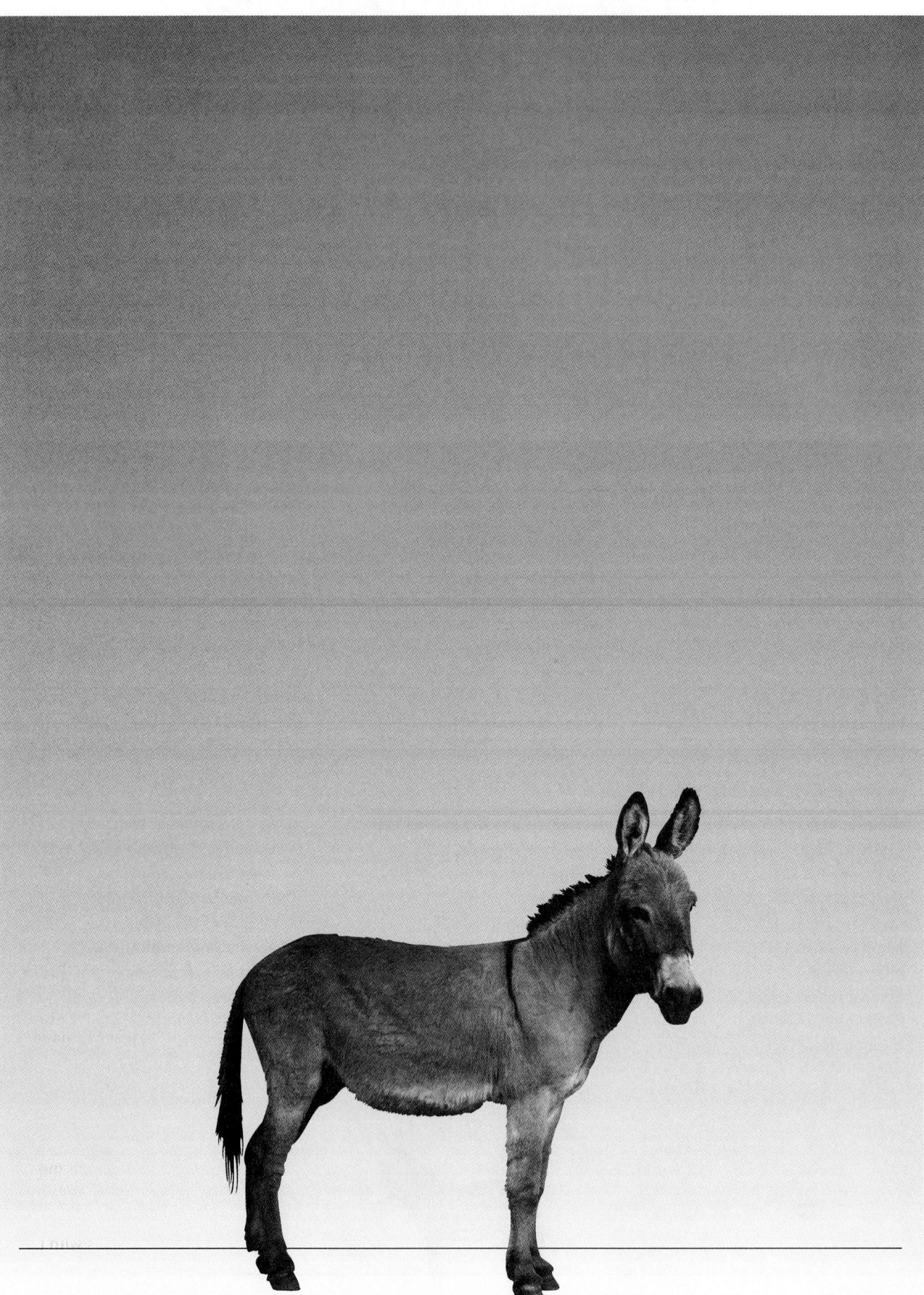

Clinical Chemistry Tests

GARY P. CARLSON

MAJOR BIOCHEMICAL ABNORMALITIES/PROBLEMS ENCOUNTERED

This chapter deals with interpretation of clinical laboratory data in relation to case management. The discussion focuses on interpretation of an abnormality in the typical clinical situation; detailed pathophysiologic explanations of these changes are beyond the scope of this section. If additional information is required, a textbook on veterinary clinical pathology should be consulted.[1,2]

All laboratory samples should be submitted with specific objectives in mind. In general, these objectives fall into one of the following categories:

1. Evaluating organ system involvement or functional impairment
2. Confirming a diagnosis or ruling out a disease condition
3. Assessing response to therapy
4. Formulating a more accurate prognosis

SUBMISSION OF LABORATORY SAMPLES

Veterinary Diagnostic Services

Laboratory diagnostic services must provide accurate results promptly to be of benefit in clinical case management. However, the clinician also must be aware of the inherent limita-

tions of laboratory evaluation in certain clinical settings. In general, veterinary diagnostic laboratories are preferred to general medical laboratories, because human medical laboratories may be less familiar with animal diseases and the responses of animals to disease. Test methodologies and interpretation may also be different. These species differences can cause confusion when results are evaluated on the basis of human criteria that often don't apply to animals.

Several desktop or portable, hand-held, point-of-care devices are available to veterinarians for determination of serum chemistry, electrolytes, and acid-base balance. Many of these devices use self-contained strips, cartridges, or rotors, thereby reducing errors associated with maintaining, measuring, and mixing reagents. A number of these devices can use whole blood, which eliminates the need to wait for clot formation and centrifugation to obtain clear serum samples. The results may be available in minutes, although most devices recommend that refrigerated cartridges be warmed to room temperature for the most accurate results. Relatively little independently published data are available comparing the results obtained with these point-of-care devices with the results of standard laboratory procedures for large animal species in a typical range of clinical settings. One of the most widely used hand-held devices (iSTAT)* has been shown to yield comparable results for blood electrolyte concentrations and acid-base balance in dogs and horses.[3] However, it was noted that the correlation between results from this device and standard laboratory techniques was poor for sodium in the dog and for hematocrit in the horse.

Point-of-care devices that can provide rapid, accurate, and relatively inexpensive results have obvious advantages. As the technology improves, wider application of this equipment in many large animal practices can be expected. For each of these devices, however, it will be important to have well-established normal values for all large animal species and a clear delineation of their limitations and possible idiosyncratic reactions in certain species or clinical settings.

Selection of Procedures

Careful selection of specifically indicated laboratory procedures has its advantages. This approach fosters logically integrated thinking and concentrates on evaluation of the primary medical problems while avoiding submission of samples for unnecessary diagnostic procedures. However, the sophisticated autoanalyzers used by large commercial laboratories can perform a wide battery of tests quickly and efficiently with little additional cost. These panels may be broadly defined (e.g., a general large animal health panel) or may offer a more focused evaluation of a specific organ system (e.g., liver, kidney, or muscle). The clinician must ensure that the panel selected contains all the appropriate tests for a thorough evaluation of the individual patient's medical problems.

The following recommendations should be used as guidelines for selecting laboratory procedures. They are presented as diagnostic panels that should provide a clear, comprehensive indication of organ damage or dysfunction. The most directly applicable diagnostic procedures are listed under "Recommended," and additional procedures that may be beneficial in certain circumstances are listed under "Optional."

General Panel

The broadly based general chemistry panel should provide a balanced evaluation of the most likely medical problems.

RECOMMENDED
Glucose
Blood urea nitrogen (BUN)
Creatinine
Creatine kinase (CK)
Aspartate aminotransferase (AST)
Sorbitol dehydrogenase (SDH)
γ-Glutamyltransferase (GGT)
Alkaline phosphatase (ALP)
Bilirubin (direct, indirect, and total)
Total protein
Albumin
Globulin
Albumin/globulin ratio (A/G ratio)
Bicarbonate or total carbon dioxide (total CO_2)
Sodium
Potassium
Chloride
Calcium
Phosphate

*i-STAT Corporation, Holliston, MA.

OPTIONAL
Venous blood gases
Ionized calcium

Muscle Panel

The muscle panel should detect active skeletal and cardiac muscle destruction (rhabdomyolysis) and the degree of secondary renal damage. The possible causal factors are evaluated as optional procedures, depending on the history, clinical findings, or special circumstances.

RECOMMENDED
CK
AST
Muscle biopsy
Urinalysis
BUN or creatinine
OPTIONAL
Blood selenium
Venous blood gases
Thyroid hormones
Calcium (ionized and total)
Magnesium
Fractional excretion of:
  Sodium
  Potassium
  Chloride

Liver Disease Panel

The liver panel should detect active damage to the hepatic parenchyma, involvement of the biliary system, or alteration in hepatic function.

RECOMMENDED
SDH
AST
GGT
ALP
BUN
Blood glucose
Fibrinogen
Total protein
Albumin
Globulin
Bilirubin (direct, indirect, and total)
Complete urinalysis
OPTIONAL
Liver ultrasound
Liver biopsy
Bile acids
Blood ammonia
Bromsulphalein clearance halftime (BSP $t_{1/2}$)
Clotting panel

Renal Disease Panel

The kidney panel should provide a rough quantitative estimation of compromised renal function and indicate the location and nature of the damage to the urinary tract.

RECOMMENDED
BUN
Creatinine
Calcium
Phosphate
Protein or albumin
Complete urinalysis
OPTIONAL
Renal ultrasound
Renal biopsy

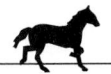

Urine culture
Urine/plasma osmolality ratio
Urinary CK/creatinine ratio
Fractional excretion of:
Sodium
Potassium
Chloride
Endogenous creatinine clearance
Sulfanilate clearance

Gastrointestinal Disease Panel

The gastrointestinal disease panel should include evaluation of acid-base status, fluid and electrolyte balance, and renal function, which are common complicating features of gastrointestinal diseases. Additional optional or special diagnostic procedures may be necessary in calves or foals with neonatal diarrhea, in horses with colic, and in ruminants with gastrointestinal stasis or displacement.

RECOMMENDED
Packed cell volume (PCV)
Total plasma protein (TPP)
Sodium
Potassium
Chloride
Calcium (ionized and total)
Venous blood gases, pH, bicarbonate
Anion gap
BUN
Creatinine
Glucose
Peritoneal fluid cytology
Fecal occult blood
Fecal parasites
Ruminal fluid pH
OPTIONAL
Peritoneal fluid (glucose and pH)
Serum immunoglobulin
Plasma lactate
Fecal protozoa
Fecal culture
Fecal *Clostridium difficile* toxin
Fecal cytology
Rectal biopsy
Absorption test:
Glucose
Xylose

Metabolic Profiling

The health status and productivity of dairy cattle, swine, and other food animals maintained in large, confined groups are the result of a fragile balance involving metabolic events, nutrition, agents of disease, management, and environmental factors. In these production units the health status of the herd as a whole is of paramount importance. Subclinical disease or nutritional imbalance may be contributing to suboptimal productivity. Most productivity problems in these settings are caused by several factors, and defining and resolving these problems before they become too costly is a difficult, complicated task. Sequential assessment of weight gains, body condition scores, milk quality, and milk production are useful for recognizing subclinical production disorders.

Another tool that has been used in some situations is metabolic profiling. Blood samples are drawn from a number of individual animals as representative of the group as a whole. Some experts have recommended the submission of pooled serum samples from representative individuals, much like the use of bulk tank tests, as a reflection of the general level of mastitis in the herd. Sampling may be done routinely and sequentially. In dairy cattle this may be done during gestation or lactation but frequently focuses on the periparturient period, when a combination of nutritional and metabolic events often contribute to costly production disorders.

Metabolic profiles might include most of the recommended parameters listed previously under the general panel, with the addition of magnesium, total cholesterol, nonesterified fatty acids (NEFA), and β-hydroxybutyrate (BHB). The BHB, NEFA, and cholesterol values may provide an indication of energy balance, and the BUN, creatinine, total protein, albumin, and CK levels may be helpful in assessing protein status. In certain settings trace minerals or fat-soluble vitamins may be important indicators of underlying nutritional problems. Metabolic profiling is not a substitute for careful clinical examination, sound animal husbandry, or ration analysis, but it may play a useful role in some modern, large-scale operations, in which a variety of subclinical problems can quickly translate into financial disaster.

SOURCES OF VARIATION IN NORMAL VALUES

Laboratory

One of the most commonly overlooked sources of variation in clinicopathologic data is the difference in results obtained by different laboratories. This can result in fivefold to tenfold differences in the normal range of certain enzyme activities between laboratories using similar but not identical methodologies. In the past the units of measure used to express the activities of different serum enzymes varied markedly. The standard method of representing serum enzyme activity is in international units per liter (IU/L), which is used in this text. Correction factors for converting the commonly used but older units of measure to international units are shown in Table 22-1. The normal values given in Tables 22-2 and 22-3 are those used at the University of California Veterinary Medical Teaching Hospital or are from the literature.[2,3] It is always best to use the normal values and reference intervals determined by the clinical pathology laboratory service chosen for the tests.

Species

Relatively modest variation exists between species for most clinicopathologic parameters. Notable exceptions are the plasma electrolyte concentration, the erythrocyte potassium concentration in some breeds of sheep, and the serum bilirubin concentration, which is higher in horses than in other species. The BUN is a less reliable indicator of renal function in ruminants and horses because urea nitrogen is metabolized by the intestinal microflora. Donkeys and burros have a much higher GGT level than horses and cattle.

Breed

Significant differences in hematologic parameters exist between hot-blooded and cold-blooded horses. Hot-blooded horses include most of the athletic breeds (thoroughbred, quarter horse, standardbred, and Arabians). Cold-blooded horses include the pony and draft breeds. Cold-blooded horses have lower red cell values both at rest and after exercise and maintain a slightly lower leukocyte count; they also have lower resting and fasting indirect bilirubin concentrations.

Age

There are several important differences in hematologic and clinical chemistry between neonatal and adult animals. The

TABLE 22-1

Conversion of Conventional Units to International Units

Component	Conventional Unit	Multiply By	International Unit (IU)
CHEMISTRY			
Ammonia	μg/dl	0.5872	μmol/L
Bilirubin	mg/dl	17.1	μmol/L
Cholesterol	mg/dl	0.02586	mmol/L
Creatinine	mg/dl	88.4	μmol/L
Glucose	mg/dl	0.05551	mmol/L
Lactate	mg/dl	0.111	mmol/L
Urea nitrogen	mg/dl	0.357	mmol/L
ELECTROLYTE			
Sodium	mEq/L	1	mmol/L
Potassium	mEq/L	1	mmol/L
Chloride	mEq/L	1	mmol/L
Calcium	mg/dl	0.2495	mmol/L
Magnesium	mg/dl	0.4114	mmol/L
Phosphorus	mg/dl	0.3229	mmol/L
BLOOD GAS			
P_{O_2}	mm Hg	0.1333	kPa
P_{CO_2}	mm Hg	0.1333	kPa
Bicarbonate	mEq/L	1	mmol/L
T_{CO_2}	mEq/L	1	mmol/L
PROTEIN AND HEMATOLOGY			
Protein	g/dl	10	g/L
Albumin	g/dl	10	g/L
Fibrinogen	mg/dl	0.01	g/L
Hemoglobin	g/dl	10	g/L
Iron	μg/dl	0.1791	μmol/L
Transferrin	mg/dl	0.01	g/L
Haptoglobin	mg/dl	0.01	g/L
HORMONE			
Cortisol	μ/dl	27.59	nmol/L
Triiodothyronine (T_3)	ng/dl	0.01536	nmol/L
Thyroxine (T_4)	μg/dl	12.87	nmol/L

From Kaneko JJ, Harvey JW, Bruss ML, eds: *Clinical biochemistry of domestic animals*, ed 5, New York, 1997, Academic Press.
kPa, Kilopascal; *P_{O_2},* partial pressure of oxygen; *P_{CO_2},* partial pressure of carbon dioxide; *T_{CO_2},* total carbon dioxide.

effects of age have been studied most carefully in horses and cattle. Suckling neonatal animals tend to have a lower BUN, slightly lower total protein and globulin, moderately higher GGT and phosphate, and markedly greater alkaline phosphatase than do adult animals.

Sex

With the obvious exception of sex hormone concentrations, few recognized differences in clinical chemistry values are seen between sexes. In most domestic animals the intact male tends to have a slightly higher erythrocyte count, hemoglobin concentration, and PCV than the female or neutered male. This sex-related difference has been demonstrated most clearly in the horse.

Factors Influencing Results or Their Interpretation

Many factors influence the results obtained in laboratory analysis. Two important factors are sample collection and handling. The sample collection site (e.g., jugular vein, mammary vein, or carotid artery) can have an important effect on the results of tests such as blood gas evaluation, glucose, or ketones. The choice of anticoagulants depends on whether the samples are to be submitted for serum, plasma, or whole blood determinations. The specific sample requirements for the most commonly ordered clinical chemistry determinations are listed in Table 22-4. Serum is required for most chemistry determinations, and serum separator tubes work very well in most settings. There have been some indications that the results of some serum hormone assays may be influenced by collection of blood in serum separator tubes. Heparin is the anticoagulant of choice for most chemical determinations requiring plasma. Formerly, fluoride-oxalate was the anticoagulant of choice for blood glucose determination because it halts glycolysis by the red cells. However, fluoride may interfere with certain chemical procedures (i.e., the glucose oxidase method of blood glucose determination) and should be used only for blood lactate determination or selected circumstances when glucose determinations are required and samples must be held for a time without refrigeration. Citrate is the anticoagulant of choice for clotting tests and blood typing. Ethylenediamine tetraacetic acid (EDTA) is the anticoagulant most often used for hematologic evaluation, but both citrate and EDTA are chelating agents, which interfere with a variety of chemical determinations.

Samples should be submitted as soon after collection as possible, but circumstances may require storage of some samples for 12 to 24 hours. With serum samples, blood should be allowed to clot before refrigeration. Serum should be separated from the red cells immediately after clot formation and then kept refrigerated. Samples should be stored in clean containers and kept free of exposure to sunlight, medications, or chemicals. If whole blood is left at room temperature for longer than 60 minutes, the blood glucose reading will be falsely low as the result of red cell glycolysis. Storage of whole blood may result in in vitro hemolysis, with the potential for misleading increases in the serum or plasma enzymes AST and LDH as a result of hemolysis of red cells. Failure to separate serum or plasma from the red cells within an hour of collection may lead to leakage of erythrocyte potassium and a falsely elevated serum or plasma potassium concentration.

Stress, transport, excitement, and handling produce physiologic responses in animals that affect a variety of hematologic and biochemical parameters. This is most evident in the horse, which shows marked increases in red cell mass and, to a lesser extent, the plasma protein concentration in response to excitement, exercise, or catecholamine administration. The red cell count and hemoglobin concentration can increase by as much as 50%; the plasma protein concentration may increase by 1 to 2 g/dl. Leukocytosis is induced as the marginating leukocyte pool is mobilized into the general circulation. Prolonged stress results in the release of endogenous corticosteroids, which produce the typical "stress response" in the leukogram. The combination of catecholamine and glucocorticoid release associated with stress, transport, and excitement, as well as with many gastrointestinal catastrophes, may result in markedly elevated blood glucose concentrations (up to 400 mg/dl). Modest elevations (two to four times normal) in muscle-derived enzymes occur in association with prolonged transport or vigorous exercise.

Dehydration and decreases in the effective circulating fluid volume commonly are associated with certain disease processes in large animals. Large losses or compartmentalization of sodium-containing fluid accompanies many systemic disorders, particularly digestive disorders such as diarrhea, colic, displacement of viscera, excessive sweat losses, and some urinary tract diseases. These forms of dehydration lead to decreases in plasma volume, which are indicated by

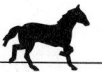

TABLE 22-2

Clinical Chemistry: Normal Range for Large Animals

Component	Unit	Equine	Bovine	Ovine	Caprine
CHEMISTRY					
Total bilirubin	mg/dl	0.5-2.3	0-0.1	0.1-0.2	0-0.1
Direct	mg/dl	0-0.6	0	0	0
Indirect	mg/dl	0.2-2	0-0.1	0-0.12	0-0.1
Cholesterol	mg/dl	75-150	80-120	52-76	80-130
Creatinine	mg/dl	0.9-2	0.9-1.3	0.8-1.3	0.7-1
Glucose	mg/dl	89-112	33-66	56-92	53-81
Fibrinogen	mg/dl	100-400	100-600	100-500	100-400
Protein (total serum)	g/dl	5.8-7.7	6.8-8.6	6.6-8.6	6.8-8.3
Albumin	g/dl	2.3-3.6	3-4.3	2.7-3.7	3.2-3.8
Globulin	g/dl	1.7-4.7	3-4.9	2.8-5.4	3.1-4.8
Urea nitrogen	mg/dl	12-27	8-23	14-37	19-31
ENZYME					
ALP	IU/L	86-285	27-107	50-300	27-210
AST	IU/L	138-409	43-127	60-280	46-161
CK	IU/L	119-287	105-409	100-547	104-219
GGT	IU/L	8-22	15-39	40-94	34-65
LDH	IU/L	162-412	697-1445	238-440	123-392
LDH-1	%	6.3-18.5	39.8-63.5	45.7-63.6	29.3-51.8
LDH-2	%	8.4-20.5	19.7-34.8	0-3	0-5.4
LDH-3	%	41-65.9	11.7-18.1	16.4-29.9	24.2-39.9
LDH-4	%	9.5-20.9	0-8.8	4.3-7.3	0-5.5
LDH-5	%	1.7-16.5	0-12.4	10.5-29.1	14.1-36.8
SDH	IU/L	0-8	12-53	18-77	2-57
ELECTROLYTE					
Sodium	mEq/L	132-146	132-152	139-152	142-155
Potassium	mEq/L	2.4-4.7	3.9-5.8	3.9-5.4	3.5-6.7
Chloride	mEq/L	99-109	97-111	95-103	99-110
Calcium	mg/dl	11.2-13.6	9.7-12.4	11.5-12.8	8.9-11.7
Phosphorus	mg/dl	3.1-5.6	5.6-6.5	5-7.3	6.5
Magnesium	mg/dl	2.2-2.8	1.8-2.3	2.2-2.8	2.8-3.6
Osmolality	mOsm/kg	270-300	270-300	N/A	N/A
Anion gap	mEq/L	6-15	14-20	N/A	N/A
ACID-BASE (VENOUS BLOOD)					
pH		7.32-7.44	7.31-7.53	7.32-7.54	N/A
P_{CO_2}	mm Hg	38-46	35-44	37-46	N/A
Bicarbonate	mEq/L	20-28	17-29	20-25	N/A
TCO_2	mEq/L	24-32	21-32	21-28	26-30
SPECIAL					
Acetylcholinesterase					
Red cell	IU/L	450-790	1270-2430	640	270
Ammonia	µg/dl	13-108	N/A	N/A	N/A
BSP ($t_{1/2}$)	min	2-3.7	2.5-4	1.6-2.7	2.1
Serum iron	µg/dl	73-140	57-162	166-222	N/A
TIBC	µg/dl	200-262	63-186	N/A	N/A
Lactic acid	mmol/L	1.11-1.78	0.56-2.22	1.00-1.33	N/A
Ketones					
Acetone	mg/dl	N/A	0-10	0-10	N/A
Acetoacetate	mg/dl	N/A	0-1.1	N/A	N/A
BHB	mg/dl	N/A	0-10	N/A	N/A

Data from Kaneko JJ, Harvey JW, Bruss ML, eds: *Clinical biochemistry of domestic animals*, ed 5, New York, 1997, Academic Press; Duncan JR, Prasse KW: *Veterinary laboratory medicine*, ed 3, Ames, Iowa, 1994, Iowa State University Press; and the Normal Values Clinical Pathology Laboratory, Veterinary Medical Teaching Hospital, University of California at Davis, 2000.
ALP, Alkaline phosphatase; *AST,* aspartate aminotransferase; *BHB,* β-hydroxybutyrate; *BSP (t₁/₂),* bromsulphalein clearance halftime; *CK,* creatine kinase; *GGT,* γ-glutamyl transferase; *LDH,* lactate dehydrogenase; *N/A,* not applicable; *P_{CO_2},* partial pressure of carbon dioxide; *SDH,* sorbitol dehydrogenase; *TIBC,* total iron-binding capacity; *TCO_2,* total carbon dioxide.

TABLE 22-3

Serum Protein Electrophoresis: Normal Range for Large Animals

Component	Unit	Equine	Bovine	Ovine	Caprine
Total protein	g/dl	5.2-7.9	6.74-7.46	6-7.9	6.4-7
Albumin	g/dl	2.6-3.7	3.03-3.55	2.4-3	2.7-3.9
Globulin	g/dl	2.62-4.04	3-3.48	3.5-5.7	2.7-4.1
α_1	g/dl	0.06-0.7	N/A	N/A	N/A
α_2	g/dl	0.31-1.31	N/A	N/A	N/A
α	g/dl	N/A	0.75-0.88	0.3-0.6	0.5-0.7
β_1	g/dl	0.4-1.58	N/A	0.7-1.2	0.7-1.2
β_2	g/dl	0.29-0.89	N/A	0.4-1.4	0.3-0.6
β	g/dl	N/A	0.8-1.12	N/A	N/A
γ_1	g/dl	N/A	N/A	0.7-2.2	N/A
γ_2	g/dl	N/A	N/A	0.2-1.1	N/A
γ	g/dl	0.55-1.9	1.69-2.25	N/A	0.9-3
Albumin/globulin (A/G) ratio		0.62-1.46	0.84-0.94	0.42-0.76	0.63-1.26

Data from Kaneko JJ, Harvey JW, Bruss ML, eds: *Clinical biochemistry of domestic animals,* ed 5, New York, 1997, Academic Press; and Duncan JR, Prasse KW: *Veterinary laboratory medicine,* ed 3, Ames, Iowa, 1994, Iowa State University Press.
N/A, Not applicable.

TABLE 22-4

Recommended Anticoagulant for Hematologic or Clinical Chemistry Evaluation

Anticoagulant	Specimen	Test or Procedure
Ethylenediamine tetraacetic acid (EDTA)	Whole blood	Complete blood count, cross-match, platelet count
	Whole blood	Blood selenium
	Plasma	Refractometric protein and fibrinogen
	Peritoneal fluid	Fluid analysis
	Bone marrow	Hematologic evaluation
	Synovial fluid	Fluid analysis
Heparin	Whole blood	Blood pH, blood gases
	Plasma	Electrolytes, osmolality
	Synovial fluid	Mucin clot test
Fluoride/oxalate	Plasma	Lactate
Citrate	Whole blood	Blood typing
	Plasma	Coagulation tests (PT, PTT, factor analysis)
None, serum separator tubes	Serum	Most chemistries, electrolytes, osmolality
		Protein electrophoresis
		Hormones (cortisol, T_3, T_4)
		Immunoglobulins (IgG, IgM, IgA)

Modified from Brobst DF, Parry BW: Normal clinical pathology data. In Robinson NE, ed: *Current therapy in equine medicine,* ed 2, Philadelphia, 1987, WB Saunders.
PT, Prothrombin time; *PTT,* partial thromboplastin time; T_3, triiodothyronine; T_4, thyroxine.

moderate to marked increases in the PCV and the TPP concentration. The concentrations of other compounds dissolved in the plasma may also increase as a result of decreases in the plasma volume. The concentrations of compounds that are largely protein bound, such as calcium, are generally closely related to the protein concentration. Over 50% of the serum calcium is bound to albumin. Increases or decreases in the plasma protein concentration normally result in proportional changes in the total serum calcium concentration, although the physiologically active ionized calcium may remain unchanged.

Diseases that cause a reduction of effective circulating fluid volume often also cause alterations in renal function. This may result in prerenal azotemia with moderate to marked elevation of BUN and creatinine. Although this is generally considered primarily a prerenal azotemia, real pathologic changes in the kidneys often are associated with the systemic processes initiated by these disorders. Reevaluation of renal function (urinalysis, BUN, creatinine) during the course of the disease is important, because renal function affects the prognosis, response to fluid administration, and potential for nephrotoxicity and systemic toxicity of a variety of chemotherapeutic agents.

Fasting laboratory data are important for evaluation of many disease conditions in human and small animal patients. True fasting conditions are rather difficult given the large and complex gastrointestinal tract of most herbivores and are thus seldom used. However, the feeding of animals in relation to sample collection can affect the data obtained. Hay feeding in horses is reported to affect sodium, potassium, and protein concentrations within the first few hours after feeding. Animals feeding on lush green pasture or large amounts of silage may have slightly different parameters from those fed high-concentrate rations. The anion-cation balance of the ration has an impact on the relative serum electrolyte concentration, acid-base balance, urine pH, and urinary electrolyte excretion. Lactescent (cloudy) plasma may be observed in samples from nursing foals or calves. The fluid intake of the normal nursing neonate may range from 100 ml/kg/day to more than 250 ml/kg/day, and this high fluid intake is reflected by a commensurately high urine output of low specific gravity and low osmolar content.

Certain medications also may have an impact on some laboratory parameters. Tranquilization may be necessary for animal restraint and sample collection, but the practitioner should be aware that tranquilizers often decrease the red cell mass and plasma protein concentration. This is particularly true of the phenothiazine-derivative tranquilizers when used in the horse. Xylazine administered to large animals produces a modest catecholamine release, which may be evidenced by the slight sweating response seen in many horses sedated with this drug. The glucose concentration increases modestly in response to the xylazine-induced catecholamine release. Repeated intramuscular injections with certain antibiotics (especially erythromycin and tetracycline) or other preparations that are locally irritating may produce slight to moderate elevations in muscle-derived serum enzyme activities. Intravenous administration of certain drugs and compounds can produce intravascular hemolysis and hematuria. The amount of hemolysis in these circumstances is relatively small and of little consequence, except that it can cause confusion as to why hemoglobinuria occurred.

FLUID AND ELECTROLYTE BALANCE

Packed Cell Volume and Total Plasma Protein

Changes in the plasma volume generally are reflected by changes in the PCV and the TPP concentration. In dehydrated humans, changes in the PCV are believed to be the more reliable guide to changes in plasma volume because substantial protein fluxes occur into and out of the circulation. However, in most animal species the range of normal for the PCV is much wider than for the TPP concentration. This is particularly true of horses, in which excitement, pain, or catecholamine release can produce variable mobilization of splenic erythrocytes, making it difficult to obtain a truly resting PCV. For these reasons, precise quantitative estimation of a change in plasma volume using these parameters is more complex and less reliable in large animal species. As plasma volume increases or decreases, the change in the PCV is always less than the change in the TPP concentration. However, a large disparity in the changes in the PCV and the TPP concentration in a patient with a history of loss of sodium-containing fluid and clinical evidence of reduced effective circulating fluid volume suggests blood or protein loss. Marked increases in the PCV with a normal to low TPP concentration frequently are encountered in animals with acute protein-losing enteropathy such as salmonellosis or equine toxic enteritis. In horses being treated for diarrhea, excessive administration and retention of sodium-containing fluids are common factors that contribute to edema and hypoproteinemia. Blood loss generally results in a decrease in the PCV and the TPP concentration.

Serum Sodium

The serum sodium concentration is a function of the exchangeable cation content (i.e., the exchangeable sodium [Na] in the extracellular fluid volume plus the exchangeable potassium [K] in the intracellular fluid volume relative to total body water), as indicated in the following formula:

$$\text{Serum Na (mEq/L)} = \frac{\text{Exchangeable (Na + K)}}{\text{Total body water}}$$

Changes in the sodium concentration reflect the net changes in this relationship and often do not represent accurately the changes in sodium balance. Changes in water balance are thus primarily responsible for changes in the serum sodium concentration. Hyponatremia is an indication of a relative water excess, whereas hypernatremia is an indication of a relative water deficit.

Dehydration is defined as a loss of body water (fluid volume contraction). It occurs in a variety of clinical circumstances. The serum sodium concentration provides a means of categorizing dehydration in a physiologically meaningful way. Hypertonic dehydration, which occurs when water losses exceed the losses of sodium and potassium, is indicated by hypernatremia. The response of horses to feed and water deprivation is an example of this form of dehydration. Isotonic dehydration occurs with a balanced loss of water and electrolytes; that is, about 140 to 150 mEq of sodium plus potassium (Na + K) for each liter of water lost. Because the relative water balance has not changed, the serum sodium concentration remains unchanged despite the accumulation of what may have been a substantial sodium deficit. The early stages of acute diarrhea and the dehydration of heavily sweating endurance horses are examples of isotonic dehydration. Hypotonic dehydration occurs when the losses of exchangeable cations (Na + K) exceed the net change in water balance; this condition is indicated by hyponatremia. Hypotonic dehydration often is seen in animals with subacute or chronic diarrhea that develop substantial water and electrolyte deficits but then replace part of the water deficit by water consumption. Fig. 22-1 shows the compartmental distribution of fluid between the extracellular fluid (ECF) volume and the intracellular fluid (ICF) volume in four situations.

Hyponatremia

Hyponatremia is often but not invariably associated with conditions that cause sodium depletion such as vomiting, diarrhea, excessive sweat losses, and adrenal insufficiency. The fluid losses in these conditions are most often hypotonic or isotonic, and initial fluid and electrolyte deficits do not result in hyponatremia until water intake or renal water retention (or both) disturb the balance between the remaining exchangeable cations and the total body water.

The accumulations of sodium-containing fluid in body cavities or the gut lumen caused by ascites, peritonitis, or rupture of the bladder or by displacement, torsion, or volvulus of the gut are referred to as third space problems. When these accumulations develop rapidly, the plasma volume is reduced, and the serum sodium concentration subsequently may decrease as compensating renal responses cause water retention. Rupture of the bladder in neonatal foals is associated with a marked hyponatremia and hypochloremia. As fluid intake continues and dilute urine accumulates in the abdomen, sodium, chloride, and other ions are drawn from the rest of the ECF into this accumulating fluid. No sodium or chloride has been lost from the body, and the observed decreases in the electrolyte concentration are caused by changes in the relative water balance. The neurologic signs seen in these foals are largely caused by the effects on the central nervous system of the rapidly developing and marked hypotonic hyponatremia. Progressively severe neurologic disturbances may be seen as the serum sodium concentration falls below 115 mEq/L and then below 100 mEq/L. The severity of the neurologic abnormalities is a function both of the rate at which hyponatremia develops and the absolute degree of hyponatremia. Neurologic disturbances can occur iatrogenically if excessive amounts of free water (usually given as 5% dextrose) are administered to patients with altered renal function.

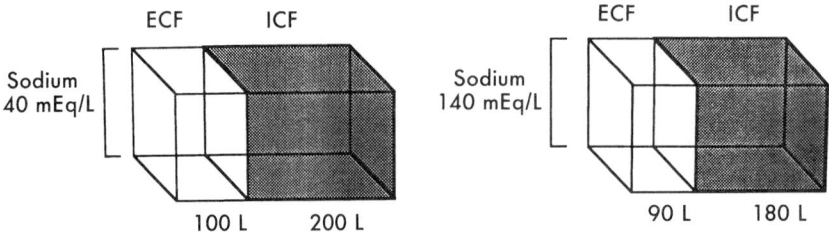

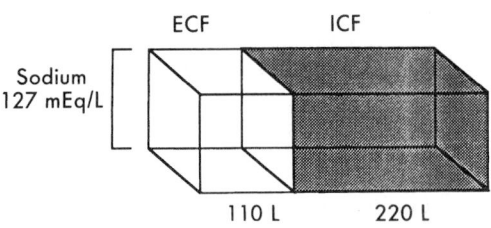

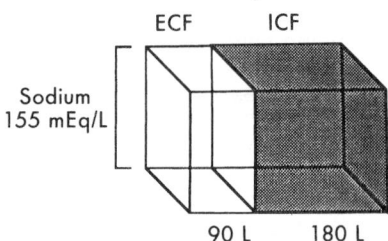

FIG. 22-1 ▉ Compartmental distribution of fluid between the extracellular fluid (ECF) volume and the intracellular fluid (ICF) volume in a 450-kg horse with normal fluid balance; with isotonic fluid volume contraction; with hypotonic fluid volume expansion; and with hypertonic fluid volume contraction. (Modified from Kaneko JJ, Harvey JW, Bruss ML, eds: *Clinical biochemistry of domestic animals*, ed 5, New York, 1977, Academic Press.)

BOX 22-1

Causes of Hyponatremia

COMMON CAUSES
Relative water excess
  Loss of sodium-containing fluid (decreased effective
    circulating volume)
    Diarrhea
    Excessive sweating
    Blood loss
    Fluid drainage
      High-volume gastric reflux
      High-volume pleural drainage
  Adrenal insufficiency
  Sequestration of fluid (third space problems)
    Peritonitis
    Ascites
    Ruptured bladder

COMMON CAUSES—cont'd
  Torsion or volvulus of the gut
  Excessive administration of 5% dextrose to patient
    with renal disease
  False hyponatremia
    Hyperlipidemia
    Hyperproteinemia
    Hyperglycemia

UNCOMMON CAUSES
Water retention with normal effective circulating volume
  Psychogenic polydipsia
  Renal disease
  Inappropriate antidiuretic hormone secretion

Mastitis results in an increased loss of sodium in the milk, and a low-grade mastitis problem in a dairy herd on a marginal dietary salt intake may result in sodium depletion and medullary washout. Decreased milk production, polyuria, hyposthenuria, and a low urine sodium level may be noted, although the serum sodium concentration may remain within the lower range of normal.

The most common causes of hyponatremia are listed in Box 22-1. Marked hyperlipidemia or hyperproteinemia produces a falsely low sodium concentration value, because lipid or protein occupies a significant volume in the serum or plasma sample, and sodium is present only in the aqueous phase. This potential cause of hyponatremia is indicated by an increase in the osmolar gap between measured and calculated osmolality. The use of direct ion-specific electrodes for electrolyte determinations avoids this potential cause of a falsely low sodium concentration value.

Marked hyperglycemia causes a reduction in the measured serum sodium concentration of approximately 1.6 mEq/L for every 100 mg/dl increase in the glucose concentration. Increases in the plasma glucose concentration generate osmotic forces that result in the movement of cellular water into the ECF, diluting the plasma sodium concentration.

Hypernatremia

Hypernatremia can occur in the initial stages of diarrhea, vomiting, or renal disease if water loss exceeds electrolyte loss

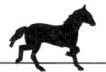

BOX 22-2

Causes of Hypernatremia

COMMON CAUSES
Pure water losses
   Panting
   Water deprivation
Sodium excess (water restriction)
   Salt poisoning
   Feeding only electrolytes, no free water

UNCOMMON CAUSES
Water loss exceeds electrolyte loss
   Vomiting
   Diarrhea
   Burns
   Intrinsic renal disease
   Diuretics
   Diabetes insipidus
      Central
      Nephrogenic
   Hypertonic saline or sodium bicarbonate
      administration
   Mineralocorticoid excess

BOX 22-3

Causes of Hypokalemia

COMMON CAUSES
Altered External Balance*
Vomiting
Vagal indigestion with internal vomiting
Diarrhea
Third space problems (gut or abomasal torsion or
   volvulus; peritonitis)
Excessive sweat losses
Dietary deficiency
Prolonged anorexia

Altered Internal Balance
Metabolic alkalosis

UNCOMMON CAUSES

Altered External Balance
Mineralocorticoid excess
Diuretics
Renal tubular acidosis
Postobstruction diuresis

Altered Internal Balance
Excessively rapid bicarbonate administration
Insulin and/or glucose administration
Catecholamine administration or endogenous release

*External balance refers to the relative changes in potassium intake and output; internal balance refers to the distribution of potassium between the extracellular and the intracellular fluid compartments.

(Box 22-2). When water losses are replaced by increased water consumption, enhanced renal water retention, or both, the serum sodium concentration decreases. Food and water deprivation in normal horses and cattle is associated with substantial reduction of renal and fecal output, but continued cutaneous and respiratory insensible water loss may result in hypernatremia. In this case the hypernatremia is the result of a primary water loss. Hypernatremia may occur transiently as a result of sodium excess after administration of hypertonic saline or sodium bicarbonate if water intake is restricted or impaired. Hypernatremia has been reported in calves fed an inappropriately mixed oral electrolyte replacement solution as their only fluid intake.[4] The hypernatremia observed with salt poisoning in cattle and swine is the result of water restriction in animals that have been maintained on a high-salt intake.

Serum Potassium

The serum potassium concentration is influenced by factors that alter internal balance (the distribution of potassium between the ECF and the ICF) and those that change external balance (potassium intake and output). Changes in the serum potassium concentration occur in a wide variety of clinical circumstances and have profound neuromuscular effects that are largely the result of changes in cell membrane potential. The responses to dehydration and acid-base imbalance often complicate the evaluation of the potassium concentration. For example, calves with acute diarrhea often develop potassium depletion because of excessive losses and inadequate intake, but the serum potassium concentration of these animals usually is normal to increased as the result of renal shutdown and the metabolic acidosis induced by dehydration, sodium depletion, and hypovolemia. Hypokalemia may become evident only as other fluid and electrolyte losses are replaced.

Measuring the erythrocyte potassium concentration is relatively easy and has been suggested as an aid in assessing the need for potassium supplementation for racehorses with recurrent muscle disease. However, experimental studies in horses indicate that the erythrocyte potassium concentration does not always accurately reflect potassium deficits.

Hypokalemia

Hypokalemia may result from depletion of the body's potassium stores or from a redistribution of potassium from the ECF into the ICF space (Box 22-3). Hypokalemia is most commonly seen with altered intake and absorption and with excessive potassium losses from the gastrointestinal tract caused by vagal indigestion, torsion of the abomasum, ileus, or diarrhea. Excessive renal loss may result from mineralocorticoid excess, certain diuretics, or altered renal function, as reported in horses with renal tubular acidosis. Marked hypokalemia develops when reduced dietary intake caused by anorexia is associated with excessive potassium losses.

Hypokalemia without potassium depletion results from the movement of extracellular potassium to the intracellular space. This form of hypokalemia occurs in response to an acute alkalosis and to the administration of insulin or glucose. Overzealous and rapid administration of sodium bicarbonate can produce an alkalosis with a profound and rapidly developing hypokalemia. Animals with moderate potassium deficits that are vigorously treated with sodium bicarbonate to correct a coexisting mild metabolic acidosis may be particularly prone to this problem. The initial response to catecholamine administration is a modest, transient increase in potassium caused by α-adrenergic stimulation, which often is followed by hypokalemia caused by β-adrenergic receptor responses.

Hyperkalemia

Hyperkalemia may develop in vitro as a result of hemolysis or leakage of erythrocyte potassium after storage of whole blood (Box 22-4). The release of potassium from leukocytes or platelets into the serum after clot formation is a potential

---

BOX 22-4

Causes of Hyperkalemia

COMMON CAUSES
False hyperkalemia
    In vitro hemolysis
    Prolonged storage of blood (over 6 hours) without
        separation of serum or plasma
Altered external balance
    Hypovolemia with renal shutdown
Altered internal balance
    Metabolic acidosis
    Vigorous exercise

UNCOMMON CAUSES
False hyperkalemia
    Markedly elevated leukocyte or platelet count
Altered internal balance
    Hyperkalemic periodic paralysis in quarter horses
    Diabetes mellitus
    Tissue necrosis
    Renal disease
    Addison's disease

BOX 22-5

Causes of Hyperchloremia

WITH PROPORTIONAL INCREASE IN SODIUM
Common Causes
Relative water deficit
    Panting
    Water deprivation
    Salt poisoning

Uncommon Causes
Vomiting
Diarrhea
Burns
Intrinsic renal disease
Diuretics
Diabetes insipidus
    Central
    Nephrogenic
Hypertonic saline administration
Mineralocorticoid excess

WITHOUT PROPORTIONAL INCREASE IN SODIUM
Common Causes
Hyperchloremic metabolic acidosis
Renal tubular acidosis

Uncommon Cause
Compensation for respiratory alkalosis

---

cause of hyperkalemia if marked leukocytosis or thrombocytosis is present. Hyperkalemia also results from renal potassium retention in Addison's disease, acute renal failure, and renal shutdown. A number of factors contribute to the movement of intracellular potassium into the ECF, resulting in hyperkalemia. Hyperkalemia often is associated with a metabolic acidosis, particularly when the acidosis results from volume depletion and is complicated by renal shutdown. Hyperkalemia has been reported in animals with massive muscle necrosis, but neither hyperkalemia nor a metabolic acidosis is a common feature in horses with exertional rhabdomyolysis. Vigorous short-term exercise of horses at high intensity results in a marked but transient hyperkalemia (9 to 10 mEq/L) that may be associated with the profound lactic acidosis seen with anaerobic workloads.[5] Potassium returns to normal within minutes, and often a modest hypokalemia occurs later in the recovery period. Episodic hyperkalemia and muscular weakness are associated with the condition known as hyperkalemic periodic paralysis (HYPP).[6] HYPP is inherited as an autosomal-dominant trait in horses, with a specific quarter horse lineage[7] (see Chapter 40 for a more complete discussion of this disorder). The disease is the result of a single DNA base pair substitution that leads to the production of an abnormal voltage-regulated sodium channel at the cell membrane.[8] Sudden marked increases in the serum potassium concentration, up to 8 to 9 mEq/L, are the result of transcellular movement of potassium and are associated with profound electrocardiographic abnormalities and fluid shifts.

Serum Chloride

Alterations in the chloride concentration usually are associated with nearly proportional changes in the sodium concentration as the result of changes in relative water balance. In addition, the chloride concentration tends to vary inversely with the bicarbonate concentration; thus when disproportionate changes in the chloride concentration relative to sodium occur, significant acid-base imbalances should be anticipated. Disproportionate increases in chloride are associated with a normal to low anion gap hyperchloremic metabolic acidosis, but they also are seen as a result of the compensating responses for a primary respiratory alkalosis (Box 22-5). A striking hyperchloremic metabolic acidosis has been reported in horses with renal tubular acidosis.[9,10] Disproportionate decreases in chloride relative to sodium characteristically are seen in a metabolic alkalosis but also may be seen as part of the compensating response for a chronic primary respiratory acidosis (Box 22-6). Hypochloremic metabolic alkalosis is a common feature in many digestive disorders of ruminants and is caused by loss of chloride-rich fluids or sequestration of such fluids in the abomasum and forestomachs.

Osmolality

Measurement of the serum osmolality provides an indication of relative water balance in much the same way as the serum sodium concentration does. In most circumstances these parameters are closely correlated. Comparing the measured osmolality with the calculated osmolality, as determined from the measured concentrations of the major solutes in serum (sodium, glucose, and urea), provides a means of determining if the serum water content deviates widely from normal or if foreign, low-molecular-weight substances are present in the blood. The difference between the measured osmolality and the calculated osmolality is called the osmolar gap. Decreases or increases in the osmolar gap could indicate laboratory error, but increases of more than 10 mOsm/kg generally are the result either of a decrease in the serum water content (caused by hyperlipidemia or hyperproteinemia) or of the presence of abnormally high concentrations of low-molecular-weight substances in the serum. These substances can include a variety of exogenous and potentially toxic compounds such as mannitol, ethanol, methanol, propylene glycol, ethylene glycol, isopropanol, ethyl ether, acetone, trichloroethane, and paraldehyde.

BOX 22-6

Causes of Hypochloremia

WITH PROPORTIONAL DECREASE IN SODIUM
Common Causes
Relative water excess
 Diarrhea
 Excessive sweating
 Blood loss
 Fluid drainage
 High-volume gastric reflux
 High-volume pleural drainage
 Sequestration of fluid (third space problems)
  Peritonitis
  Ascites
  Ruptured bladder
 Renal disease
False hypochloremia
 Hyperlipidemia
 Hyperproteinemia
 Hyperglycemia

Uncommon Causes
Psychogenic polydipsia
Inappropriate antidiuretic hormone secretion
Adrenal insufficiency

WITHOUT PROPORTIONAL DECREASE IN SODIUM
Common Causes
Metabolic alkalosis
 Exhaustive disease syndrome
 Abomasal torsion
 Vagal indigestion with internal vomiting
Response to furosemide in horses

Uncommon Cause
Compensation for respiratory acidosis

BOX 22-7

Causes of Hypocalcemia

COMMON CAUSES
Parturient paresis (milk fever)
Grass tetany
Hypoalbuminemia (decreased total calcium; ionized calcium may remain unchanged)
Fat necrosis
Lactation tetany
Transport tetany
Synchronous diaphragmatic flutter
Blister beetle toxicosis (cantharidin)
Acute renal failure
Anorexia in lactating cows

UNCOMMON CAUSES
Acute toxemia and associated anorexia in lactating dairy cows
Hypoparathyroidism
Exertional rhabdomyolysis
Malignant hyperthermia
Pancreatic disease
Oxalate toxicity
Tetracycline administration
Furosemide administration
Alkalosis induced by excessive bicarbonate administration

Serum Calcium

Calcium plays a vital role in many of life's processes, including maintenance of neuromuscular excitability, permeability of cell membranes, conduction of nerve impulses, muscle contraction, and blood clotting. For these reasons the serum calcium concentration or, more correctly, the ionized calcium concentration normally is maintained within a relatively narrow range, despite wide variation in intake and output. Calcium metabolism is regulated by dietary factors, vitamin D and its active metabolites, and the hormones parathormone and calcitonin. The serum calcium concentration is maintained by adjusting intestinal absorption, renal excretion, and mobilization of available calcium from the large stores in bone. Calcium exists in the serum in three forms: ionized calcium, complexed calcium, and protein-bound calcium. Ionized calcium, which normally constitutes 40% to 60% of the total calcium, is the physiologically active form of calcium. Protein binding, which normally constitutes 40% to 50% of the total calcium, can cause confusion. Hyperalbuminemia may result in a modest hypercalcemia, whereas hypoproteinemia, especially hypoalbuminemia, regularly results in a moderate hypocalcemia. The ionized calcium concentration generally remains within normal limits, despite increases or decreases in total calcium associated with the change in protein concentration. The acid-base balance has additional influence on the amount of ionized and protein-bound calcium. Alkalosis reduces ionized calcium and increases protein binding, whereas acidosis produces the opposite effect. Ion-specific electrodes are available for determining the ionized calcium level, which can be very useful if blood samples are handled appropriately. Most diagnostic laboratories provide the total serum calcium value, which comprises ionized, complexed, and protein-bound calcium.

Hypocalcemia

Large increases or decreases in the serum calcium concentration generally are the result of a failure in the normal mechanisms of calcium homeostasis rather than a reflection of absolute calcium deficits or calcium-phosphorus imbalances. Hypocalcemia occurs with some frequency in domestic animals, particularly in high-producing dairy cattle near the onset of lactation. In cattle the serum calcium concentration normally decreases to less than 8 mg/dl with the stress of parturition and the onset of lactation (Box 22-7). Failure to mobilize sufficient calcium to maintain serum calcium results in the clinical syndrome of parturient paresis (see Chapter 39 for a more detailed discussion of this syndrome). Most animals are recumbent with a calcium level of 6 mg/dl or less, and fatalities may occur if the level drops below 4 mg/dl. Parturient paresis is associated with a normal to increased serum magnesium level, hypophosphatemia, and hypocalcemia. Change in the cation-anion balance in the diet of dairy cattle during the periparturient period has modest effects on the acid-base balance and enhances calcium mobilization from storage sites, thus reducing the incidence of milk fever in cows at high risk. Grass tetany is associated with marked hypomagnesemia and modest hypocalcemia, whereas the inorganic phosphorus level remains within the normal range.

Systemic diseases resulting in anorexia (e.g., ketosis, traumatic reticuloperitonitis, and displaced abomasum) or acute toxemic conditions (e.g., coliform mastitis, septicemia, or aspiration pneumonia) that produce anorexia in lactating cattle frequently result in hypocalcemia. Hypocalcemia also is

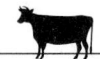

seen in sheep on marginal rations if stressed by inclement weather or when being moved. Hypocalcemia is seen in cattle with fat necrosis, presumably as the result of incorporation of calcium with the fat as a form of soap. Horses with exhaustive disease syndrome or transit tetany often develop decreases in ionized calcium with resultant muscle cramps and synchronous diaphragmatic flutter, which generally respond to intravenous calcium administration. Horses, cattle, and sheep usually respond initially to acute renal tubular damage with mild hypocalcemia and hyperphosphatemia.

Hypercalcemia

Marked hypercalcemia, with a serum calcium level ranging from 14 to 20 mg/dl, and modest hypophosphatemia frequently are observed in horses with chronic renal failure that are fed a high-calcium diet such as alfalfa hay (Box 22-8). In these horses blood samples collected in standard EDTA tubes may actually clot. This occurs because the serum calcium concentration is so high that there is insufficient EDTA to bind all the calcium, and some free calcium is available to complete the clotting process. Vitamin D intoxication can develop as a result of excessive dietary supplementation or the ingestion of certain plants such as *Cestrum diurnum* (day blooming jasmine) and *Solanum malacoxylon*, which contain toxic quantities of vitamin D analogs. Primary hyperparathyroidism is exceedingly rare in large animals, but pseudohyperparathyroidism with hypercalcemia occasionally can develop in animals with tumors that produce protein substances with parathormone-like biologic activity. This has been reported in a few animals with lymphosarcoma or gastric squamous cell carcinoma.

Serum Phosphorus

Phosphorus is found primarily in the skeleton and teeth in close association with calcium in the intricate and dynamic crystalline structure of bone. Intracellularly, phosphate plays an essential role in the degradation and synthesis of many compounds. Also, as adenosine triphosphate (ATP), adenosine diphosphate (ADP), and adenosine monophosphate (AMP), it is the primary form of energy storage and transfer required for almost all of life's processes. Phosphorus in the ECF exists primarily as the buffer pair H_2PO^{-3} and HPO^{-4} and plays a role in acid-base balance. Like calcium, phosphorus is regulated by dietary factors, the active metabolites of vitamin D, and the hormones parathormone and calcitonin. Imbalances of calcium and phosphorus or the presence of compounds that bind these substances in the gut can produce serious imbalances that are not always evident on analysis of serum samples. Measurement of urinary output or creatinine clearance ratios for calcium and phosphate are simple and helpful procedures. They provide an indication of an imbalance while more definitive procedures such as ration analysis are contemplated.

Hypophosphatemia

Serum phosphorus concentrations are not always an accurate guide to phosphate balance, but dietary deficiencies of phosphorus are frequently manifested by hypophosphatemia. Hypophosphatemia is a common feature in cattle with parturient paresis (see also Chapter 39) and horses with chronic renal failure (Box 22-9). It has been reported with experimental oxalate toxicity, in animals in chronic wasting states, or with starvation. Postparturient hemoglobinuria is a disorder of cattle, primarily lactating dairy cattle, that often is associated with diets low in phosphorus. Although marked hypophosphatemia is often reported, it is not an invariable feature of this disorder.

BOX 22-8

Causes of Hypercalcemia

COMMON CAUSES
Chronic renal failure in horses
Hypervitaminosis D
  Excessive dietary supplements
  Plant intoxication
    Cestrum diurnum (day blooming jasmine)
    Solanum malacoxylon
Excessive or too rapid intravenous administration
  of calcium

UNCOMMON CAUSES
Neoplasia (pseudohyperparathyroidism)
  Lymphosarcoma
  Gastric squamous cell carcinoma
Hyperparathyroidism

BOX 22-9

Causes of Hypophosphatemia

COMMON CAUSES
Chronic renal failure in horses
Parturient paresis in cattle
Postparturient hemoglobinuria

UNCOMMON CAUSES
Brassica toxicity
Inadequate dietary intake
Starvation or chronic wasting diseases
Hyperparathyroidism, pseudohyperparathyroidism

Hyperphosphatemia

Age-related differences exist in the normal range of serum phosphorus concentration. Young animals have much higher values than adults, with values for neonates commonly up to 7 to 9 mg/dl. The serum phosphate concentration declines progressively with age. Hyperphosphatemia is seen in animals with vitamin D toxicity, transiently in horses after long-distance endurance rides, and initially in horses with acute renal failure (Box 22-10).

Serum Magnesium

Disturbances of magnesium metabolism occur principally in cattle and sheep. Complex nutritional and environmental interactions contribute to a variety of clinical syndromes attributed to magnesium deficiency and the onset of tetany in grazing animals.

Hypomagnesemia

Hypomagnesemia is reported in cattle with grass tetany and in sheep with grass staggers (Box 22-11) (see also Chapter 39). A serum magnesium level below 1.8 mg/dl is considered low; values below 1 mg/dl are considered severe and are likely to be associated with clinical signs. Hypomagnesemia caused by dietary magnesium deficiency has been reported in calves reared in confinement and fed a milk diet exclusively.

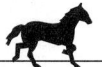

BOX 22-10

Causes of Hyperphosphatemia

COMMON CAUSES
Acute renal failure
Nutritional secondary hyperparathyroidism (excess phosphate intake)
Endurance exercise in horses
Higher normal range in neonates

UNCOMMON CAUSES
Acute rhabdomyolysis
Vitamin D toxicity

BOX 22-11

Causes of Hypomagnesemia

COMMON CAUSES
Grass tetany
Winter tetany
Grass staggers
Calves on a milk-only, magnesium-deficient diet
Endurance exercise

UNCOMMON CAUSE
Undernutrition (B)

BOX 22-12

Causes of Hypermagnesemia*

Epsom salt (MgSO$_4$) overdose given orally or as an enema
Intravenous administration of magnesium in excessive amounts

*Hypermagnesemia is an uncommon condition in large animals.

Hypermagnesemia

Hypermagnesemia occurs infrequently but may be seen with overzealous administration of Epsom salts (MgSO$_4$), either orally as a drench by means of nasogastric intubation or as an enema for the treatment of digestive disorders (Box 22-12). Intravenous administration of magnesium produces muscle relaxation but does not alter consciousness, and hypertonic MgSO$_4$ solutions are not considered a humane means of euthanasia.

ACID-BASE IMBALANCE

Using the traditional approach to acid-base balance, the four primary acid-base imbalances and their compensating responses are presented in Table 22-5. Acidosis is associated with an increase in the hydrogen ion concentration (decreasing pH), whereas alkalosis is caused by a decrease in the hydrogen ion concentration (increasing pH). When the primary imbalance is associated with a change in the bicarbonate concentration, the acid-base imbalance is called a meta-

TABLE 22-5

Acid-Base Imbalances and Compensatory Responses

Disorder	ph	[H$^+$]	Primary Imbalance	Compensatory Response
Metabolic acidosis	↓	↑	↓ [HCO$_3^-$]	↓ PCO_2
Metabolic alkalosis	↑	↓	↑ [HCO$_3^-$]	↑ PCO_2
Respiratory acidosis	↓	↑	↑ PCO_2	↑ [HCO$_3^-$]
Respiratory alkalosis	↑	↓	↓ PCO_2	↓ [HCO$_3^-$]

[HCO$_3^-$], Bicarbonate concentration; PCO_2, partial pressure of carbon dioxide.

bolic disorder. The compensating response for a metabolic acid-base imbalance is mediated by the respiratory tract, which alters the partial pressure of carbon dioxide (PCO_2) to counterbalance the primary imbalance and to partly restore the pH toward normal. Primary respiratory imbalances are related to changes in alveolar ventilation, which result in an increased PCO_2 in a respiratory acidosis and a decreased PCO_2 with respiratory alkalosis. The compensating response for these primary respiratory acid-base imbalances is mediated by the kidneys through alterations in the excretion or retention of hydrogen ions and bicarbonate. Heparinized blood samples for acid-base evaluation must be drawn anaerobically and sealed immediately. Arterial blood samples should be submitted for evaluation of primary respiratory disorders and for evaluation of ventilation in patients under general anesthesia. Venous blood samples are easier to obtain and provide reliable data for most primary metabolic acid-base abnormalities.

Blood gas analysis should be done as soon after collection as possible. However, appropriately collected blood samples yield reliable results for as long as 4 hours if held in ice water. The patient's rectal temperature should be provided to the laboratory so that corrections can be made for variation in body temperature. Changes in body temperature have a major impact on the partial pressure of oxygen (PO_2) as well as the PCO_2 but relatively little effect on estimations of bicarbonate or base balance. During brief exercise at maximal intensity, the temperature of the central venous blood may exceed the rectal temperature by as much as 3° C. In these circumstances, the central blood temperature is more appropriate than the rectal temperature for correcting blood gas determinations. The blood sampling site (arterial, venous, or capillary blood) has a significant impact on the blood gas values obtained.[11] Arterial blood samples yield higher values for pH and lower values for PCO_2 than venous blood, but the bicarbonate is higher in venous blood. The use of blood gas data for evaluation of acid-base imbalances in animals has been reviewed.[12,13] In addition, an excellent review of the traditional and nontraditional approaches to evaluation of acid-base balance as related to fluid therapy in small animals has application to many large animal situations and is well worth reading.[14]

Metabolic Acidosis

Metabolic acidosis is characterized by a decrease in pH and bicarbonate concentration. Metabolic acidosis is traditionally thought to be produced by the addition of hydrogen ions or the loss of bicarbonate ions. The most common causes include the lactic acidosis of rumen overload, hypovolemia associated with loss or compartmentalization of sodium-containing fluid, ketoacidosis in ketosis and pregnancy toxemia, loss of bicarbonate-rich saliva with oral diseases or esophagostomy in cattle, gastrointestinal loss of bicarbonate as a result of diarrhea, and renal failure, which may result in decreased ability to excrete hydrogen and thus to retain bicarbonate (Box 22-13). Other causes include ingestion of certain drugs or toxic compounds such as salicylate, methanol, ethylene glycol, or paraldehyde. Increased ventilation provides the compensating respiratory response for a metabolic acidosis, and a decline in the P_{CO_2} generally begins within minutes. This temporarily minimizes the fall in blood pH, but long-term correction of a metabolic acidosis requires renal bicarbonate retention and enhanced acid excretion. Complete correction of a metabolic acidosis may be difficult in patients with intrinsic renal disease or those with diseases such as renal tubular acidosis that impair the ability of the kidneys to excrete acid or retain bicarbonate, or both.

Metabolic Alkalosis

Metabolic alkalosis is characterized by an increase in pH and bicarbonate. It occurs fairly commonly in domestic animals, particularly in association with digestive disturbances in ruminants. An initiating process capable of generating alkalosis is necessary and must be coupled with additional factors to maintain metabolic alkalosis. Generation of metabolic alkalosis is traditionally thought to be caused by excessive hydrogen loss, bicarbonate retention, or contraction alkalosis (Box 22-14). Contraction alkalosis occurs when the ECF volume is reduced because of loss or sequestration of fluids high in sodium and chloride but without proportionate loss of bicarbonate. This is a contributing mechanism for generation of the metabolic alkalosis reported in heavily sweating endurance horses and in response to the diuretic furosemide in the horse. The most common causes of increased hydrogen ion loss are the gastrointestinal losses caused by salivary secretions in ponies after surgical esophagostomy[15]; massive gastric reflux associated with anterior enteritis, ileus, or small bowel obstruction in horses; or sequestration of fluid in the abomasum and forestomach associated with a variety of gastrointestinal displacements or functional disturbances (vagal indigestion) of ruminants. Continuous salivary losses in horses after surgical esophagostomy result in transient metabolic acidosis followed by progressive metabolic alkalosis. Most of these disorders cause significant dehydration and sodium, chloride, and potassium deficits.

The factors responsible for maintaining metabolic alkalosis involve impaired renal bicarbonate excretion. These factors are associated with the renal response to decreases in the effective circulating fluid volume, chloride depletion, or potassium depletion. Renal tubular sodium resorption is enhanced in response to hypovolemia. Maintenance of electroneutrality requires that sodium resorption in the proximal tubule be accompanied by a resorbable anion, whereas in the distal tubule sodium resorption is associated with the secretion of another cation, usually hydrogen or, to a lesser extent, potassium. Chloride is the only resorbable anion normally present in appreciable quantities in the proximal tubular fluid. In metabolic alkalosis, plasma bicarbonate is increased and the chloride concentration is generally decreased as the result of disproportionate chloride losses. The relative lack of the resorbable anion, chloride, in the proximal tubule thus allows a larger amount of sodium to reach the distal tubule, where aldosterone and other factors enhance hydrogen or potassium loss into the tubular lumen in exchange for sodium. Potassium depletion reduces or eliminates potassium exchange as a means of sodium retention, thus placing greater emphasis on hydrogen ion exchange. Because renal hydrogen excretion is linked with bicarbonate resorption, the

---

BOX 22-13

Causes of Metabolic Acidosis

COMMON CAUSES
Rumen overload (lactic acidosis)
Ketosis
Pregnancy toxemia
Hypovolemic shock
Acute diarrhea
Colic with strangulated bowel
Strangulating abomasal torsion
Peritonitis
Uroperitoneum (ruptured bladder)
Exercise above anaerobic threshold (normal response in horses)

UNCOMMON CAUSES
Renal failure
Renal tubular acidosis
Urea toxicity
Salicylate toxicity
Methanol toxicity
Paraldehyde toxicity
Ethylene glycol toxicity

BOX 22-14

Causes of Metabolic Alkalosis

COMMON CAUSES
Sequestration of fluid in the abomasum and forestomach in ruminants
Gastric reflux in horses with ileus
Massive sweat loss in horses (endurance horses)
Chloride depletion
Potassium depletion
Contraction alkalosis (extracellular fluid volume contraction without bicarbonate loss)
Salivary loss of chloride in horses with esophagostomy
Use of diuretics (especially furosemide)

UNCOMMON CAUSES
Excessive bicarbonate supplementation or therapy
Mineralocorticoid excess
Vomiting

---

excess bicarbonate cannot be eliminated, and metabolic alkalosis is maintained. This is the reason for the *paradoxical aciduria* seen in some patients with metabolic alkalosis, and it is the reason these patients respond when given intravenous fluids containing chloride and potassium. The compensating respiratory response to a metabolic alkalosis is hypoventilation, resulting in an increase in the P_{CO_2}. Excessive bicarbonate administration is an additional potential cause of metabolic alkalosis. Most normal animals can tolerate large doses of bicarbonate, and excesses are rapidly eliminated by renal excretion.[16] However, patients with decreases in effective circulating fluid volume, particularly when coupled with potassium or chloride deficits, may not tolerate a bicarbonate load because renal clearance of excess bicarbonate is likely to be impaired. Attempts to alter the acid-base balance, and thereby affect the athletic performance of rac-

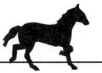

ing horses, by prerace administration of high doses of sodium bicarbonate–containing "milk shakes" has become a major concern around the world. This has stimulated substantial research on the acid-base balance of horses before and after racing. In many racing jurisdictions stringent prerace or postrace standards for blood pH or bicarbonate levels (or both) have been enacted to control this practice.

Respiratory Acidosis

Respiratory acidosis is characterized by a decrease in pH and an increase in PCO_2, which develop because of decreased effective alveolar ventilation. Carbon dioxide diffuses through the lungs much more readily than oxygen; thus diseases that compromise ventilation normally result in decreases in PO_2 before significant increases in PCO_2 develop. The most common causes are acute upper respiratory obstruction and primary pulmonary diseases, including pneumonia, pneumothorax, and chronic obstructive lung disease (Box 22-15). Diseases or drugs that affect the respiratory center of the central nervous system also may produce a respiratory acidosis, as can general anesthesia. The compensating response for a respiratory acidosis is renal retention of bicarbonate. This response requires days to develop and is seen only in chronic respiratory acidosis. Exogenous bicarbonate does not correct a respiratory acidosis and should not be administered to these patients.

Respiratory Alkalosis

Respiratory alkalosis is caused by hyperventilation, which may be stimulated by hypoxemia associated with pulmonary disease, congestive heart failure, severe anemia, or neurologic disorders (Box 22-16). The initial compensating response to acute respiratory alkalosis is a modest decline in the ECF bicarbonate concentration, the result of cellular buffering. Subsequent renal responses result in a decrease in the ECF bicarbonate concentration through reduced renal bicarbonate resorption. The decline in bicarbonate may be offset by chloride retention; thus hyperchloremia and decreased PCO_2 may be associated with compensated respiratory alkalosis, as well as with compensated metabolic acidosis. Compensating responses for chronic respiratory alkalosis that lasts several weeks actually may be sufficient to return pH to normal.

Mixed Acid-Base Imbalances

Mixed acid-base disorders occur when several primary acid-base imbalances coexist.[17] Metabolic acidosis and alkalosis can coexist, and either or sometimes both may occur with either respiratory acidosis or alkalosis. The following factors should be considered when evaluating possible mixed acid-base disorders:

1. Compensating responses to primary acid-base disturbances do not result in overcompensation.
2. Compensating responses rarely correct pH to normal. A normal pH in a patient with an acid-base imbalance is an indicator of a mixed acid-base disturbance.
3. A change in pH in the opposite direction to that predicted for a known primary disorder indicates a mixed disturbance.
4. Bicarbonate and PCO_2 always deviate in the same direction with primary acid-base disturbances. If these parameters deviate in opposite directions, a mixed abnormality exists.
5. If the change in the anion gap does not approximate the change in bicarbonate, a mixed acid-base imbalance should be suspected.

Mixed acid-base abnormalities occur with some frequency in domestic animals and often are overlooked. The practi-

---

BOX 22-15

Causes of Respiratory Acidosis

COMMON CAUSES
Primary pulmonary disease
  Obstruction of the upper airway
  Laryngeal edema
  Aspiration pneumonia
  Pneumonia
  Pneumonia/pleuritis complex
  Pneumothorax
  Chronic obstructive pulmonary disease
Depression of the respiratory center of the central nervous system
  General anesthesia with inappropriately assisted ventilation
  Drugs
    Opiates
    Anesthetics
    Tranquilizers
Central nervous system diseases

UNCOMMON CAUSES
Cardiac arrest
Muscle weakness or dysfunction
  Tetanus
  Botulism
  Myasthenia
  Severe hypokalemia
Neonatal respiratory distress syndrome

BOX 22-16

Causes of Respiratory Alkalosis

COMMON CAUSES
Hypoxemia
  Pulmonary diseases
  Congestive heart failure
  Severe anemia
Stimulation of the respiratory center of the central nervous system
  Psychogenic hyperventilation
  Excitement, fear, transport, pain
  Gram-negative septicemia
  Neurologic disorders

UNCOMMON CAUSES
After correction of metabolic acidosis
Inappropriate mechanical ventilation
Salicylate toxicity

---

tioner must be aware of the potential for mixed acid-base imbalances to correctly interpret blood gas data in complex clinical situations.

Anion Gap

The anion gap can be an extremely helpful tool for categorizing causal factors in acid-base imbalances and may prove a useful prognostic guide in animals with serious digestive disorders. The anion gap can be calculated as the difference between the major cations (sodium plus potassium) and the measured anions (chloride plus bicarbonate). The anion gap normally is 12 to 16 and provides an approximation of the so-called unmeasured anions. These are anions that are not measured routinely in the clinical laboratory; they include the anionic equivalents of plasma proteins (particularly albumin), sulfate, phosphate, lactate, ketones, and a variety of inorganic anions. Significant differences exist in the normal range of the anion gap between species, and there also may be age-related differences. Foals are reported to have a larger anion gap than adult horses.

Hypoalbuminemia and hyperchloremic metabolic acidosis are the most common causes of a decrease in the anion gap resulting from decreases in unmeasured anions. The cause of normal to low anion gap hyperchloremic metabolic acidosis often can be differentiated on the basis of the serum potassium concentration. Animals with hyperchloremic metabolic acidosis associated with gastrointestinal fluid losses or renal tubular acidosis most often manifest hypokalemia, whereas hyperkalemia generally is seen in patients with decreased mineralocorticoid secretion (Addison's disease) or renal failure with renal shutdown. Decreases in the anion gap can be seen with increases in cationic proteins associated with polyclonal gammopathy or multiple myeloma. Decreases in the anion gap also result from overhydration caused by decreases in the protein concentration and changes in the relative concentration of plasma sodium and chloride.

Most commonly, high anion gap acidosis is associated with accumulation of a metabolizable acid such as lactic acid associated with anaerobic exercise, grain overload, or hypovolemic shock. Ketoacidosis, uremic acidosis, and poisoning with a variety of anionic poisons result in increases in nonmetabolizable acids that are also causes of an increased anion gap. When a high anion gap metabolic acidosis is found, a thorough search for the potential causes of the accumulated unmeasured anions is indicated. The anion gap also is useful for identifying mixed acid-base imbalances. A mixed metabolic acid-base imbalance should be suspected when the change in the anion gap does not approximate the change in bicarbonate. Increases in the anion gap can be associated with dehydration and contraction alkalosis caused by changes in the protein concentration and the relative concentration of plasma sodium and chloride.

Bicarbonate and Total Carbon Dioxide

Bicarbonate accounts for approximately 95% of the measured CO_2; thus the total CO_2 (TCO_2) or "CO_2 content" of serum or plasma provides a measure of metabolic changes in the acid-base balance. Most automated chemistry profiles now provide the bicarbonate level directly, whereas some may still provide the TCO_2. Bicarbonate or TCO_2 is decreased in metabolic acidosis and increased in metabolic alkalosis. However, the bicarbonate or TCO_2 values provide only a crude indication of acid-base status. When acid-base abnormalities are suspected, appropriate samples should be submitted for blood gas determination.

Buffer Base, Standard Bicarbonate, and Base Excess or Base Deficit

The terms *buffer base*, *standard bicarbonate*, and *base excess* (or *base deficit*) represent derived calculated estimates of the metabolic component of acid-base balance. The buffer base indicates the sum of all the buffer anions in blood under standardized conditions. The standard bicarbonate is the plasma bicarbonate concentration that would be found under specific conditions that eliminate respiratory influences

on the values obtained. The base excess or base deficit often is supplied in routine assessment of acid-base balance; it indicates the deviation of bicarbonate from normal. The calculated base deficit provides a means of estimating the amount of bicarbonate required to correct a metabolic acidosis. The bicarbonate estimate is calculated by multiplying the base deficit by the probable bicarbonate space (about 40% to 60% of body weight), as in the following equation:

$$mEq\ HCO_3\ needed = mEq\ base\ deficit \times kg\ body\ weight \times 0.5$$

Nontraditional Approach to Acid-Base Balance

The current edition of this book would not be complete without a brief introduction to the new, nontraditional approach to acid-base balance. Some years ago Dr. Peter Stewart[18,19] undertook a careful study of factors that determine hydrogen ion concentration in aqueous solutions and extended the concept to the acid-base balance of body fluids.

According to Stewart, acid-base balance is solely determined by three independent variables:

Strong ion difference (SID)
Partial pressure of carbon dioxide (Pco_2)
Total weak acids in solution (A_{tot})

In this approach, the hydrogen ion concentration or pH and the bicarbonate concentration are considered *dependent variables* and do not determine acid-base balance directly. The SID generally is taken as the concentration difference between plasma (sodium + potassium) minus (chloride + lactate). This is somewhat analogous to the base balance of the traditional approach. When the SID is increased, bicarbonate is elevated and the animal probably has a metabolic alkalosis. When the SID is decreased, bicarbonate is decreased and the animal probably has a metabolic acidosis. The change in Pco_2 is essentially the same as the respiratory component of the traditional approach. Increases in Pco_2 are associated with respiratory acidosis and decreases in Pco_2 with respiratory alkalosis. The term A_{tot} represents the sum of the activity of all weak acids in solution. In plasma this largely consists of the plasma proteins, particularly albumin. Increases in albumin tend to promote a decrease in bicarbonate and an increase in the hydrogen ion concentration (decrease in pH), whereas decreases in albumin have the opposite effects. The contribution of proteins to acid-base balance is generally overlooked in the traditional approach to acid-base balance.

The Henderson-Hasselbalch equation has been the central component of the traditional approach to acid-base balance. Although this equation is correct, Stewart noted that a variety of other interrelationships must also be solved simultaneously.[18] He defined these interrelationships with a series of seven equations that use the three independent variables (SID, Pco_2, and A_{tot}). All of these relationships can be combined as a single third-order quadratic equation that can be solved to yield the hydrogen ion concentration.

A number of attempts have been made to introduce these concepts into human medicine,[20] veterinary medicine,[21-23] and exercise physiology.[24,25] Stewart's approach is appealing because it relates more closely to the causal events that affect acid-base balance. However, it has not gained general acceptance for practical application. Nonetheless, this approach can be helpful when trying to conceptualize the interrelationships between electrolyte and acid-base balance. For example, using the traditional approach, it is not clear why heavy sweat losses by endurance horses should result in a hypochloremic metabolic alkalosis. As viewed by the Stewart approach, the disproportionately large losses of chloride in horse sweat result in a decrease in plasma chloride with relatively little change in plasma sodium or potassium. The net effect is to

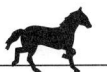

increase the plasma SID, with a resultant increase in bicarbonate and thus a mild metabolic alkalosis. In due time many aspects of the nontraditional approach to acid-base balance likely will find practical application. The selected references provide the interested reader with a fuller understanding of the Stewart approach to acid-base balance.[18-25]

SERUM ENZYMES

Some of the common and less common causes of elevated serum enzyme activity are listed in Box 22-17.

Sorbitol Dehydrogenase

Sorbitol dehydrogenase is a liver-specific enzyme in all large animal species, and increases in this enzyme indicate hepatocellular damage and leakage of enzymes. Increases in SDH also are seen with obstructive or strangulating gastrointestinal lesions and with acute toxic enteritis as the result of liver damage associated with absorption of bacteria or their toxins (or both) from the damaged bowel into the portal circulation. This enzyme is a sensitive indicator of liver damage, and modest increases may be seen with anoxia, acute anemia, or general anesthesia. The half-life of SDH in the circulation is short (a matter of hours), and elevations indicate active and ongoing liver damage. This enzyme is not stable when stored at room temperature, but refrigerated samples may yield useful results after several days of storage.

Creatine Kinase

Creatine kinase is a highly sensitive and specific indicator of muscle damage in domestic animals. Although CK is found in both cardiac and skeletal muscle, elevations of this enzyme most commonly are associated with exertional myopathies (rhabdomyolysis) and also are seen as musculoskeletal manifestations of systemic disease. Intramuscular injections, vigorous exercise, or prolonged shipping may result in modest releases (up to a fourfold increase over resting values) of CK into the circulation without producing histologic evidence of muscle damage. The half-life of this enzyme in the circulation is very short (2 hours in horses and 4 hours in cattle), and even marked elevations in CK may return to normal within 12 to 24 hours after a single muscle insult. Although marked elevation of CK can be a guide to the extent of muscle damage, the short half-life and the potential for continuing myonecrosis have marked influence on the enzyme activity observed at any point in time. A persistent elevation of CK suggests a process resulting in active and continuing muscle damage and provides grounds for resting athletic horses. Elevated CK provides no information on the factors responsible for the rhabdomyolysis. Hemolysis may produce falsely high values for CK.

Aspartate Aminotransferase

Aspartate aminotransferase is found in high concentration in a variety of tissues, including skeletal and cardiac muscles, the erythrocytes and kidneys, and the liver. This enzyme is a nonspecific indicator of tissue damage and tends to be less sensitive to mild insults than the tissue-specific enzymes SDH or CK. The half-life of AST in the circulation is relatively long, and elevations may persist for as long as 10 days after an episode of myonecrosis or liver damage. As a general rule, extensive muscle necrosis tends to produce much higher elevations of AST than severe liver necrosis. This enzyme is most useful when compared with the tissue-specific enzymes as determined sequentially over the time course of a disease process. Elevations of CK and AST indicate muscle damage, whereas elevations of SDH and AST indicate liver damage. Marked but transient elevations of CK and SDH are associated with a single insult to the muscles and liver, respectively, whereas AST increases gradually and remains elevated for a much longer time. Thus a moderate to marked increase in AST in an animal with progressively declining SDH or CK indicates that some tissue damage occurred within the past 7 to 10 days but also that the process may no longer be active. This often is a favorable prognostic indicator. Persistent elevation of or a progressive increase in CK or SDH and AST over time indicates an active, continuing process of tissue damage, and the prognosis is more guarded. AST is relatively stable at room temperature, but hemolysis or lipemia may interfere with the assay.

γ-Glutamyltransferase

γ-Glutamyltransferase is an important marker of hepatobiliary disorders and cholestasis in large animals. GGT is quite stable, and reliable results can be obtained from samples submitted several days after blood samples have been drawn, provided the serum is refrigerated. The activity of this enzyme is highest in the cells of the periportal region of the liver, in the pancreas, and in the renal tubular cells. Pancreatic diseases resulting in inflammation and necrosis are relatively rare in large animal species. Damage to the renal tubular cells leads to a release of GGT into the tubular lumen and the urine. Because this enzyme is a relatively large molecule, it is not resorbed into the systemic circulation, and renal tubular damage does not result in elevated serum GGT activity. Increases in GGT relative to creatinine in the urine have been used as an index of acute renal tubular damage. However, the validity of the normal range for this ratio in horses has been questioned.

In large animal species an elevation in serum GGT is one of the more reliable indicators of damage to the liver and biliary obstruction. Disease processes such as pyrrolizidine alkaloid intoxication, chronic active hepatitis, cholangiohepatitis, and cholelithiasis produce liver damage, primarily in the periportal region, leading to marked and persistent elevation of GGT activity in the serum. In these instances elevations in serum alkaline phosphatase activity generally are associated with the increase in GGT. Two syndromes, fatty liver syndrome in dairy cows and hyperlipemia syndrome of periparturient mares of pony and miniature horse breeds, are associated with liver damage, which is often reflected by elevation of GGT.

Most suckling neonatal large animals have high levels of GGT activity in their serum. This is the result of absorption of maternal GGT, which is present in relatively high levels in the colostrum. Elevation of GGT in neonates should be regarded as a normal finding unless it is associated with other evidence of liver disease. The normal range of serum GGT activity for burros, donkeys, and asses may be substantially higher (two to three times) than the normal range of serum GGT activity for horses. Caution should thus be used when evaluating this enzyme in these species. Elevation in serum GGT activity has been reported in thoroughbred racehorses that are performing below expectations. The reasons for the increase in GGT are not known, but horses often respond to a period of rest or reduction in workload. These horses show little histologic evidence of liver damage, and other indices of liver damage and dysfunction usually are within normal limits. The stress of training may be associated with an elevated GGT. Certain trainers, often highly successful trainers, appear to have a disproportionately large number of horses with elevations in this enzyme. The normal range for GGT of thoroughbreds in race training may be slightly higher than that of normal sedentary horses.

BOX 22-17

Causes of Elevated Serum Enzymes

ELEVATION OF SORBITOL DEHYDROGENASE (SDH)
Common Causes
Severe anoxia
Acute liver failure
Liver abscess
Secondary to damaged bowel
　Strangulating intestinal lesion
　Acute toxic enteritis
Chronic liver failure

Less Common Causes
Acute and severe anemia
General anesthesia
Anoxia

ELEVATION OF γ-GLUTAMYLTRANSFERASE (GGT)
Common Causes
Acute liver failure
Chronic liver failure
Pyrrolizidine alkaloid toxicity
Aflatoxicosis
Cholangiohepatitis
Cholelithiasis
Liver flukes

Uncommon Causes
Higher normal range in young animals
Fatty liver

ELEVATION OF ALKALINE PHOSPHATASE (ALP)
Common Causes
Acute liver failure
Chronic liver failure
Pyrrolizidine alkaloid toxicity
Cholangiohepatitis
Cholelithiasis
Liver flukes

Uncommon Causes
Higher normal range in young animals
Fatty liver

ELEVATION OF CREATINE KINASE (CK)
Common Causes
Exertional rhabdomyolysis (azoturia, myositis,
　tying-up)
Polysaccharide storage myopathy
Streptococcus equi–associated myopathy
Nutritional myodegeneration (selenium, vitamin E
　deficiency)
Postendurance ride multisystemic disorder
Alert downer cow syndrome (muscle crush syndrome)
Malignant hyperthermia
Malignant edema
Prolonged recumbency with inability to rise

Uncommon Causes
Normal postexercise modest increase
Acute cardiomyopathy
Purpura hemorrhagica
Equine influenza

ELEVATION OF CREATINE KINASE (CK)—cont'd
Uncommon Causes—cont'd
Sarcosporidiosis
Local irritation from intramuscular injections

ELEVATION OF LACTATE DEHYDROGENASE (LDH)
Common Causes
Muscle disease
　Exertional rhabdomyolysis (azoturia, myositis, tying-up)
　Polysaccharide storage myopathy
Streptococcus equi–associated myopathy
　Nutritional myodegeneration (selenium, vitamin E
　deficiency)
　Postendurance ride multisystemic disorder
　Alert downer cow syndrome (muscle crush syndrome)
　Malignant hyperthermia
　Malignant edema
Liver disease
　Acute liver failure
　Chronic liver failure
　Cholangiohepatitis
　Cholelithiasis
In vitro hemolysis

Uncommon Causes
Hemolytic anemia
Acute cardiomyopathy
Purpura hemorrhagica
Equine influenza
Sarcosporidiosis
Local irritation from intramuscular injections
Fatty liver

ELEVATION OF ASPARTATE AMINOTRANSFERASE (AST)
Common Causes
Muscle disease
　Exertional rhabdomyolysis (azoturia, myositis, tying-up)
　Polysaccharide storage myopathy
Streptococcus equi–associated myopathy
　Nutritional myodegeneration (selenium, vitamin E
　deficiency)
　Postendurance ride multisystemic disorder
　Alert downer cow syndrome (muscle crush syndrome)
　Malignant hyperthermia
　Malignant edema
Liver disease
　Acute liver failure
　Chronic liver failure
　Cholangiohepatitis
　Cholelithiasis
　Liver flukes
In vitro hemolysis

Uncommon Causes
Hemolytic anemia
Acute cardiomyopathy
Purpura hemorrhagica
Equine influenza
Sarcosporidiosis
Local irritation from intramuscular injections
Fatty liver

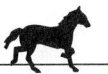

Alkaline Phosphatase

Alkaline phosphatase is used in most species as a marker for intrahepatic or extrahepatic obstruction of the biliary system. The enzyme is also released by osteoblasts from metabolically active bone. This may be the reason that young, rapidly growing animals normally have high levels of serum ALP. Elevations in ALP are also reported in cases of rickets and healing fractures. The intestinal isoenzyme of ALP is very similar to the ALP isoenzyme found in neutrophils. Elevations in the ALP activity of abdominal fluid in horses with intraabdominal disease may reflect the release of this enzyme from the neutrophils rather than be a specific marker of damage to the bowel.

ALP has been useful for evaluating liver disease in large animals, particularly in horses with pyrrolizidine alkaloid intoxication, chronic active hepatitis, and cholangiohepatitis, and in some patients with cholelithiasis. A profound elevation in ALP activity is thought to reflect periportal liver damage and biliary obstruction in these patients. A moderate to marked elevation in ALP may be observed with a wide range of disorders resulting in hepatic necrosis and intrahepatic cholestasis. Because this enzyme is not organ specific in large animals, elevations in ALP activity must be interpreted in relation to more organ-specific enzymes such as SDH and GGT.

Other Enzymes

Lactate dehydrogenase is found in relatively high concentrations in a variety of organs and tissues of the body from the heart, liver, muscle, and kidney to the erythrocytes and leukocytes. An elevation in serum LDH enzyme activity must be evaluated in relation to other, more organ-specific enzymes. LDH isoenzyme analysis can be helpful in differentiating organ system damage, but the analysis is time-consuming and not always available. An elevation in LDH activity is expected in hepatic necrosis and serves as an indicator of an active disease process. Extensive muscle damage and rhabdomyolysis tend to result in a more massive release of enzyme and much higher serum enzyme activity. A modest elevation in LDH may be seen in some hemolytic disorders and some cases of leukemia. Blood samples must be handled with care, because hemolysis results in falsely elevated serum LDH activity.

Glutamic dehydrogenase and ornithine carbamoyltransferase are two enzymes that are reported to be sensitive indicators of hepatic necrosis in ruminants. Alanine aminotransferase (ALT) is an important liver-specific enzyme that has wide application in small animals and is often included in automated chemistry profiles. This enzyme has not been useful for evaluation of liver disease in large animal species, and occasionally horses with marked rhabdomyolysis and no other evidence of liver disease show an elevation in serum ALT activity.

BILIRUBIN

Bilirubin is a breakdown product of the heme component of the hemoglobin molecule. Bilirubin exists in the serum in two forms and is responsible for the yellow color known as icterus, or jaundice, of the mucous membranes. Unconjugated, prehepatic, albumin-bound bilirubin is also known as "indirect-reacting" bilirubin, as determined by the van den Bergh reaction. Indirect-reacting bilirubin must be taken up by the liver cells, where it is conjugated and then excreted in the bile. Conjugated bilirubin is known as "direct-reacting" bilirubin, as determined by the van den Bergh reaction. The horse normally has a much higher serum bilirubin level than ruminants, and hot-blooded horses have a higher bilirubin level than cold-blooded horses of the pony and draft breeds.

The horse also differs from ruminants in that horses often develop moderate icterus in response to fasting or anorexia associated with many systemic diseases. The increase in the bilirubin concentration in these horses is caused almost entirely by an increase in unconjugated (indirect-reacting) bilirubin, and within a few days the bilirubin can increase from the normal range up to 6 to 8 mg/dl. Therefore the total serum bilirubin concentration is of little diagnostic value in the horse unless both the direct- and indirect-reacting bilirubin values are determined.

Total serum bilirubin is elevated in animals with a hemolytic anemia, and this increase is caused largely by an increase in indirect-reacting bilirubin (Box 22-18). The degree to which bilirubin is elevated in hemolytic anemia is a function of the rate of red cell destruction and the capacity of the liver to excrete the newly formed bilirubin. The total bilirubin rarely exceeds 10 mg/dl in hemolytic anemia. An exception is the hemolytic anemia of neonatal isoerythrolysis in newborn foals, which often is associated with marked clinical icterus. In these foals the serum bilirubin may exceed 25 mg/dl, a variable but substantial proportion of which (40% to 60%) is likely to be direct-reacting bilirubin.

The second major cause of clinical icterus and increased serum bilirubin is liver failure. Liver failure results in impaired uptake and excretion of bilirubin. Acute liver failure caused by hepatic necrosis results in marked to moderate increases in both direct- and indirect-reacting bilirubin. In horses, bilirubin often exceeds 10 mg/dl, and this increase is caused primarily by increases in indirect-reacting bilirubin. Direct-reacting bilirubin rarely exceeds 25% of the total bilirubin in the horse, and increases of this magnitude suggest an intrahepatic or extrahepatic biliary obstruction. With chronic liver failure, icterus is more variable, and total bilirubin rarely

---

BOX 22-18

Causes of Elevated Serum Bilirubin

ELEVATION OF TOTAL SERUM BILIRUBIN
Common Causes
Hemolytic anemia
Liver failure
Condition occurs secondary to systemic disease or
  anorexia in horses

Uncommon Cause
Chronic liver failure in cattle

ELEVATION OF INDIRECT-REACTING BILIRUBIN
Common Causes
Condition occurs secondary to systemic disease or
  anorexia in horses
Liver failure
Hemolytic anemia

Uncommon Cause
Chronic liver failure in cattle

ELEVATION OF DIRECT-REACTING BILIRUBIN
Common Causes
Liver failure
Cholelithiasis
Cholangiohepatitis
Neonatal isoerythrolysis

Uncommon Cause
Hemolytic anemia

---

exceeds 10 mg/dl. Liver failure in ruminants, particularly chronic liver failure, is associated with a much less striking elevation in serum bilirubin than occurs in the horse. In the absence of hemolytic anemia, a bilirubin above 2 mg/dl indicates impaired hepatic function in ruminants.

GLUCOSE

The concentration of glucose in the blood normally is regulated by the hormones insulin and glucagon, but it is influenced by several other factors as well.

Hypoglycemia

Fasting usually does not result in hypoglycemia except in neonatal animals (Box 22-19). Newborns have limited energy reserves, and any disease, injury, congenital defect, maternal rejection, agalactia, or management error that limits energy intake can result in marked hypoglycemia associated with profound depression, even coma. Rapid, semiquantitive field tests for blood glucose (Dextrostix,* Chemstrip BG†) provide a practical means of early recognition of this problem. Hypoglycemia may be seen in animals with acute toxic enteritis, coliform mastitis, septicemia, and colic associated with strangulated bowel, as well as in the later stages of endotoxemia and in some horses with exhaustion after prolonged exercise. Hypoglycemia is a reasonably consistent feature with primary ketosis and fat cow syndrome in cattle, with pregnancy toxemia in sheep and goats, and in hyperlipemia syndrome, which is seen primarily in pregnant or lactating ponies.

Hyperglycemia

Hyperglycemia may be seen with excitement, transportation, or stress and probably is mediated by increases in catecholamine and glucocorticoid hormones (Box 22-20). The stress and pain of acute severe colic in horses frequently results in hyperglycemia, and elevations of blood glucose above 250 mg/dl are associated with a poor prognosis in such cases. Endotoxemia initially results in a transient hyperglycemia that may be followed by marked hypoglycemia in the terminal stages of the toxemia. The later stages of Cushing's syndrome in horses generally are associated with a noninsulin-responsive hyperglycemia and glycosuria. Similar changes can be induced transiently when exogenous glucocorticoid hormones are administered at a high dose rate.

Insulin-responsive diabetes mellitus rarely occurs in large animals but has been reported in association with destructive pancreatic lesions.[23]

CREATININE

Creatinine is derived from the cyclic use of phosphocreatine, the muscle energy store, resulting in the production of inorganic phosphate and creatinine. In the resting animal this process occurs at a relatively constant rate. The absolute muscle mass and level of physical activity may influence the rate of creatinine production and thus the serum concentration. Starvation, with loss of muscle mass, may result in a slightly reduced serum creatinine level, whereas serum creatinine may be slightly higher in muscular, athletic individuals than in sedentary animals. Creatinine is distributed throughout the body water and is not reused. Creatinine is normally excreted by the kidneys, primarily by glomerular filtration. In azotemic patients a substantial part of creatinine is metabolized and excreted by nonrenal routes. Serum or urine creatinine concentrations determined by the standard alkaline picrate reaction may be falsely elevated by the presence of noncreatinine chromogenic compounds in the serum. These chromogens include glucose, fructose, ascorbic acid, hippuric acid, urea, ketones, and several other compounds. The contribution of these compounds can be reduced or eliminated, and most automated chemical laboratories use such methodology. However, if inappropriately high creatinine is reported in patients without other evidence of renal failure, the method of creatinine measurement should be ascertained.

Alterations in renal blood flow caused by decreases in effective circulating fluid volume (hypovolemia) produce an elevation in serum creatinine and BUN; this can be considered a prerenal azotemia (Box 22-21). It occurs with some frequency in animals with acute enteritis, peritonitis, acute heart failure, massive blood loss, and some forms of colic and in horses with exhaustive disease syndrome. An important point is that many of these disorders initiate the release of vasoactive mediators, which may cause renal damage and impaired renal function above and beyond that associated with impaired renal blood flow and hypovolemia. Prerenal azotemia usually is seen in animals that are dehydrated and volume depleted and that have a history of loss or compartmentalization of sodium-containing fluid. The azotemia often can be marked (creatinine level above 6 mg/dl), but if uncomplicated, it generally responds rapidly to fluid replacement therapy. Urine production, the urine sodium concentration, and the fractional excretion of sodium usually are low, and the urine specific gravity usually is elevated. The ratio of urine to plasma urea or creatinine, as well as the urine to plasma ratio of osmolality, are reported to be higher in horses with prerenal azotemia compared with renal azotemia.[16]

---

*Ames Division, Miles Laboratories, Inc., Elkhart, Ind.
†Boehringer Mannheim Diagnostics, Inc., Indianapolis, Ind.

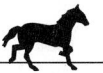

BOX 22-21

Causes of Elevated Creatinine

COMMON CAUSES
Prerenal azotemia
    Reduced renal perfusion
    Hypovolemia
    Congestive heart failure
    Dehydration after endurance exercise
Renal azotemia
    Acute renal failure
    Chronic renal failure
Postrenal azotemia
    Urolithiasis
        Renal calculi
        Ureteral calculi
        Urethral calculi
    Ruptured bladder

UNCOMMON CAUSES
False azotemia
    Noncreatinine chromogens in serum or plasma
Perirenal abscess
Renal carcinoma
Renal dysgenesis
Carcinoma of the bladder
Postexhaustion multisystemic syndrome in horses
Severe exertional rhabdomyolysis with myoglobinuria
Severe intravascular hemolysis with hemoglobinuria
Intoxication or poisoning
    Heavy metal poisoning
    Nonsteroidal antiinflammatory drug intoxication
    Aminoglycoside intoxication

BOX 22-22

Causes of Decreased Blood Urea Nitrogen

COMMON CAUSES
Liver failure
Neonatal animals (BUN is normally lower than in adults)

UNCOMMON CAUSES
Low-protein diet
Anabolic steroid administration

BOX 22-23

Causes of Increased Blood Urea Nitrogen

COMMON CAUSES
Prerenal azotemia
Reduced renal perfusion
    Hypovolemia
    Congestive heart failure
    Dehydration after endurance exercise
Renal azotemia
    Acute renal failure
    Chronic renal failure
Postrenal azotemia
    Urolithiasis
        Renal calculi
        Ureteral calculi
        Urethral calculi
    Ruptured bladder

UNCOMMON CAUSES
Gastrointestinal bleeding
Perirenal abscess
Renal carcinoma
Renal dysgenesis
Carcinoma of the bladder
Postexhaustion multisystemic syndrome in horses
Severe exertional rhabdomyolysis with myoglobinuria
Severe intravascular hemolysis with hemoglobinuria
Intoxication or poisoning
    Heavy metal poisoning
    Nonsteroidal antiinflammatory drug intoxication
Aminoglycoside intoxication

The serum creatinine concentration provides a crude measure of the glomerular filtration rate. However, serum creatinine, like the BUN, is not a very sensitive or early indicator of changes in renal function. In ruminants, creatinine is a more reliable indicator of renal failure than the BUN. Urea nitrogen can be secreted in saliva and metabolized by the ruminal microflora; this frequently results in a disparity between the BUN and creatinine levels in ruminants with renal failure. Although small increases in creatinine may be seen with progressively compromised renal function, nearly two thirds to three fourths of the nephrons must be nonfunctional before the serum creatinine level clearly exceeds the normal range. Both acute and chronic renal failure usually are associated with elevated creatinine. Acute renal failure, especially in animals with anuria or oliguria, is usually associated with progressive daily changes in blood parameters. In contrast, blood parameters of animals with chronic renal failure tend to remain relatively constant. A transient but markedly elevated serum creatinine has been observed in some newborn foals that have no other evidence of compromised renal function. Many of these foals are born to mares that had medical problems before parturition. Alterations in placental function may allow the accumulation of creatinine in the foal's circulation. In most of these otherwise normal foals this marked elevation in serum creatinine resolves within the first few days of life.

BLOOD UREA NITROGEN

The term blood urea nitrogen is ingrained in the veterinary literature, despite the fact that urea nitrogen determinations usually are performed on serum or plasma samples. This is of little consequence, because the actual difference in urea concentrations of whole blood and serum or plasma is relatively

small. Urea provides a nontoxic means of excreting ammonia generated by amino acid catabolism and the intestinal microflora. It is distributed throughout the body water. In the intestine urea is broken down by urease, which is produced by the intestinal microflora, and the nitrogen, as ammonium ion, is recycled to the liver. Urea is excreted by the kidneys, primarily by glomerular filtration.

Urea production occurs almost exclusively in the liver, and liver failure is frequently associated with a decrease in the BUN (Box 22-22). Urea nitrogen tends to be low in nursing animals because of their high fluid intake and urine output and their anabolic state of rapid growth. Urea nitrogen may be reduced slightly in animals given anabolic steroids or fed diets low in protein but of adequate calorie content.

Starvation or other processes that result in rapid tissue catabolism such as fever, burns, or corticosteroid administration may result in modest increases in the BUN (Box 22-23). The BUN, along with creatinine, provides a crude index of altered renal function in most animal species. The BUN is influenced more directly by dietary factors than is creatinine, and creatinine is generally a better guide to renal failure. This is particularly true in ruminants, in which the BUN may remain within normal limits in animals with marked impairment of renal function. With these considerations in mind, the discussion of prerenal, renal, and obstructive causes of azotemia in the section on creatinine apply to the BUN.

SERUM PROTEIN

The serum or plasma proteins consist of albumin and globulin fractions. These are discussed in Chapter 26.

URINALYSIS

Urinalysis can be an extremely useful diagnostic tool, providing information on many systemic disorders. It is essential in the evaluation of primary renal disease. Urine normally is collected as a voided sample or after catheterization. Voided urine samples are safe and easy to collect but are easily contaminated. Catheterization is preferred for bacteriologic evaluation, but the resultant mild trauma may result in a slight increase in urine red cells and protein. Because of the urethral diverticulum at the level of the pelvis, it is difficult to successfully catheterize male ruminants. Urethral obstruction is common in male small ruminants, and percutaneous aspiration may be the only way to obtain a urine sample in affected animals. Urinalysis should be performed as soon after collection as possible (within 30 minutes) to avoid degeneration of cellular elements, changes in pH, or bacterial overgrowth. If this is not possible, samples should be refrigerated. Urine volume and composition are influenced by feed and water intake, salt supplementation, environmental factors, exercise, stress, systemic disease, and drug administration. Urine samples collected after administration of a diuretic are dilute and unsuitable for routine urinalysis. The tranquilizer xylazine, which is often used to assist in the catheterization of male horses, may alter the results of the urinalysis because it produces a diuresis as the result of glycosuria.

Specific Gravity

Specific gravity is defined as the weight of urine relative to the weight of distilled water. The specific gravity of serum is approximately 1.008-1.012. The urine specific gravity is an indicator of renal function, because it reflects the action of the renal tubules and collecting ducts on the glomerular filtrate by providing an estimation of the number of particles dissolved in the urine. It is usually measured by refractometry. Urine dipsticks with reagent pads for estimating the urine specific gravity in humans should not be used for this purpose in domestic animals, because a poor correlation has been reported compared with refractometry in large animals.[26] Normal animals have the capacity to dilute their urine specific gravity to less than 1.010 and to concentrate to greater than 1.050. The normal range reported for most adult large animals is 1.020 to 1.050. Suckling neonatal animals normally produce a very dilute urine with a specific gravity below 1.010. Although this could represent immature renal function, it more likely reflects their high-volume fluid intake, because normal neonates can concentrate their urine if fluids are withheld.

Failure to produce a concentrated urine, as reflected by a specific gravity below 1.020, in the face of dehydration is an indication of altered renal function, which may be caused by primary renal disease, diabetes insipidus, medullary washout, or nephrogenic diabetes insipidus. With severe and chronic sodium depletion, tubular sodium may be insufficient to sustain normal countercurrent mechanisms for water resorption. This process is called medullary washout and has been reported as a cause of polyuria in lactating dairy cattle on a salt-deficient diet. At least 50% of renal function must remain to produce a highly concentrated urine. Isosthenuria, a urine specific gravity that remains around 1.010 despite variation in hydration, occurs when renal disease progresses to the point where renal function is reduced to less than a third of normal. Altered renal function in these animals is usually reflected by a moderate to marked elevation in the BUN and creatinine levels and by other changes in the urinalysis. Hyposthenuria occurs when the specific gravity remains below 1.010; this indicates altered release of or response to antidiuretic hormone, as occurs with diabetes insipidus, medullary washout with chronic sodium depletion, nephrogenic diabetes insipidus, psychogenic polydipsia, and chronic liver failure in some horses.

pH

The normal range of urine pH for adult herbivores is alkaline, with values ranging from 7 to 9. Neonatal foals tend to have a slightly acid urine with a pH below 7. Aciduria in adults may be seen in postrace samples collected from racehorses, after prolonged fasting, with ketosis in ruminants, or in response to metabolic acidosis. A paradoxical aciduria frequently is seen in ruminants with hypochloremic, hypokalemic metabolic alkalosis, as was explained earlier.

Protein

Protein normally is not detected in urine, although a false positive protein reaction may be noted on urine dipsticks if the sample is strongly alkaline. Urine with a positive reaction for protein on dipsticks should be checked for protein by a chemical method. Proteinuria should be evaluated in relation to the other findings in the urinalysis. Persistent and strongly positive reactions for protein in the absence of leukocytes, red cells, bacteria, or casts suggest glomerular protein loss, as in glomerulonephritis or amyloidosis. The presence of bacteria and leukocytes with proteinuria suggests sepsis in the urinary tract, whereas hemorrhage or inflammation in the urogenital tract often is associated with proteinuria.

Glucose

Glucose is not found in the urine of normal large domestic animals unless the blood glucose level increases above the renal threshold, which is thought to be around 100 to 140 mg/dl in ruminants and approximately 160 to 180 mg/dl in horses. The causes of hyperglycemia and glycosuria have been described in a previous section; they include Cushing's syndrome, stress, and catecholamine or glucocorticoid hormone release. Hyperglycemia and glycosuria can be created iatrogenically when glucose-containing fluids are administered at an excessive rate. Glycosuria is a fairly consistent finding in sheep with enterotoxemia type D (pulpy kidney). The presence of glycosuria without hyperglycemia strongly suggests renal tubular damage resulting from a toxic or ischemic insult.

Occult Blood

Both myoglobin and hemoglobin give a positive reaction on urine occult blood dipsticks. In most instances proteinuria shows a positive result as well. A tentative clinical impression sometimes can be formed to differentiate myoglobin from hemoglobin in dark urine if the sample is shaken vigorously in a closed, transparent container. Myoglobin tends to produce a brown foam, whereas hemoglobin produces a reddish

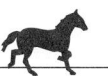

foam. Hemoglobinuria caused by intravascular hemolysis is generally associated with clinical and hematologic evidence of a hemolytic anemia. Hematuria may result in a positive occult blood reaction if lysis of some of the intact red blood cells has occurred. This is likely to happen if the urine is very dilute or if it is held at room temperature for an extended period before analysis. False positive reactions can occur if microbial peroxidase or oxidizing contaminants are present.

Myoglobin

Myoglobinuria should be associated with clear clinical and clinicopathologic evidence of extensive muscle damage. The ammonium sulfate precipitation method of differentiating hemoglobin from myoglobin is imprecise and frequently fails to detect myoglobin in the dark, coffee-colored urine of horses with severe rhabdomyolysis. Accurate differentiation of these compounds in urine requires more sophisticated procedures.

Cells

The normal range for cells generally is considered to be up to five red cells or leukocytes per high-power field. An increased number of erythrocytes indicates hematuria, which may be caused by neoplasia, trauma, inflammation, or coagulopathy. Pyuria, an increase in urine leukocytes, indicates an inflammatory process, and when associated with bacteriuria, it indicates a septic process in the urinary tract. The presence of sheets or rafts of transitional cells suggests neoplasia.

Casts

Casts are accumulations of protein and cellular material that form in the renal tubules, and when present in the urine, they indicate renal damage or tubular disease. Casts can consist of erythrocytes, leukocytes, or renal tubular cells. As cellular degeneration proceeds, the cell type is more difficult to determine, and the casts become granular and then waxy. Hyaline casts are noncellular and are formed from mucoprotein. They may be seen with glomerulonephritis, fever with passive congestion, or severe dehydration with altered renal blood flow.

Crystals

The crystalline structures in the urine of large animals are those usually associated with an alkaline urine. Calcium carbonate crystals normally are found in abundance in horse urine, particularly if the horse has been fed alfalfa hay. Triple phosphate and calcium oxalate crystals frequently are observed in relatively small numbers. The major crystals involved in urolithiasis of feedlot cattle is struvite ($Mg\,NH_4PO_4 \cdot 6H_2$). In the western United States silicate stones are most common in livestock under range conditions. Carbonate and oxalate stones are common causes of urolithiasis in small flocks of backyard sheep and goats fed alfalfa hay.

Bacteria

Bacteria sometimes are seen in small numbers in voided urine samples and may represent surface contaminants. Bacterial infections of the urinary tract usually are associated with significant pyuria. When this is noted, a catheterized sample (horse) or clean midstream catch (ruminant) should be obtained for Gram stain, culture, and sensitivity testing. Results from ruminant samples must be carefully interpreted, because male ruminants routinely urinate within the prepuce, thus heavily contaminating samples. Fortunately urinary tract infections in male ruminants and horses are rare.

Urine Creatinine Clearance Ratio

Urinary electrolyte excretion is affected by a variety of factors, including dietary intake, alterations in renal function, and specific hormones that regulate renal electrolyte excretion. Determination of electrolyte concentrations from randomly collected urine samples is easily done and can be clinically useful when these concentrations are compared with serum concentrations. The presence of substantial amounts of sodium in the urine of an animal with hyponatremia suggests excessive renal sodium loss caused by altered renal function or hormonal control. However, marked variation in the rate of urine production can lead to serious problems in the interpretation of urine electrolyte concentrations. The standard physiologic methods of determining renal electrolyte clearance are complicated by the need for quantitative urine collection and are not well suited to most practical clinical situations. One means of overcoming these difficulties is expression of the renal electrolyte clearance relative to the endogenous creatinine clearance. Expression of the renal clearance as a ratio eliminates the need for quantitative urine collection. This derived value is known as the creatinine clearance ratio or the fractional excretion (FE), and is calculated by the following formula:

$$FE = \frac{Urine\ (X)}{Serum\ (X)} \times \frac{Serum\ (C)}{Urine\ (C)} \times 100$$

where X represents the electrolyte concentration and C represents the creatinine concentration.

The FE fluctuates somewhat during the day in relation to physical activity and feed and water intake. However, under standardized conditions, there is close agreement between the FE determined from single random samples of blood and urine and that based on samples quantitatively collected during a 12- to 24-hour period.[16] The FE of electrolytes has a very wide range of normal values. The principal sources of this variation are differences in dietary intake and environmental or experimental conditions. The FE of electrolytes has been useful for detecting specific dietary deficiencies or imbalances. Dietary salt deficiency is associated with an extremely low FE of sodium and chloride, whereas the plasma concentration of these ions generally remains within normal limits. In a similar fashion, dietary calcium and phosphorus imbalances seldom are reflected by the serum concentrations of these ions. Calcium deficiency and phosphorus excess are relatively common dietary problems in large animals and result in a low FE for calcium and a high FE for phosphorus. There are technical problems with the determination of the urine calcium concentration in horses because of their normally alkaline urine and the resultant precipitation of calcium carbonate in the urine. Mixed urine samples from horses must be acidified (hydrochloric acid can be used) to solubilize the calcium.

Increases in the FE of sodium are noted with renal tubular damage and impaired sodium resorption. The sodium FE increase has been a useful indicator for the differential diagnosis of prerenal azotemia, which almost invariably results in a low sodium FE, from the azotemia caused by primary renal disease in which the FE for sodium often is markedly increased.

REFERENCES

1. Duncan JR, Prasse KW: *Veterinary laboratory medicine*, ed 3, Ames, Iowa, 1994, Iowa State University Press.
2. Kaneko JJ, Harvey JW, Bruss ML: *Clinical biochemistry of domestic animals*, ed 5, New York, 1997, Academic Press.
3. Looney AL et al: Use of a hand-held device for analysis of blood electrolyte concentrations and blood gas partial pressures in dogs and horses, *J Am Vet Med Assoc* 213:526-530, 1998.

4. Pringle JK, Berthiaume LMM: Hypernatremia in calves, *J Vet Intern Med* 2:66-70, 1988.
5. Harris P, Snow DH: Alterations in plasma potassium concentrations during and following short-term strenuous exercise in the horse, *J Physiol* 376:46P, 1986.
6. Cox JH: An episodic weakness in four horses associated with intermittent serum hyperkalemia and the similarity of the disease to hyperkalemic periodic paralysis in man, *Proc Ann Meet Am Assoc Equine Pract* 31:383-391, 1985.
7. Spier SJ et al: Genetic study of hyperkalemic periodic paralysis in horses, *J Am Vet Med Assoc* 202:933-937, 1993.
8. Rudolph JA et al: Periodic paralysis in quarter horses: a sodium channel mutation disseminated by selective breeding, *Nat Genet* 2:144-147, 1992.
9. Ziemer EL et al: Clinical features and treatment of renal tubular acidosis in two horses, *J Am Vet Med Assoc* 190:289-293, 1987.
10. Ziemer EL et al: Renal tubular acidosis in two horses: diagnostic studies, *J Am Vet Med Assoc* 190:294-296, 1987.
11. Speirs VC: Arteriovenous and arteriocentral venous relationships for pH, P_{CO_2}, and actual bicarbonate in equine blood samples, *Am J Vet Res* 41:199-203, 1980.
12. Carlson GP: Fluid-electrolyte and acid-base balance. In Kaneko JJ, Harvey JW, Bruss ML, eds: *Clinical biochemistry of domestic animals*, ed 5, New York, 1997, Academic Press.
13. DiBartola SP: Introduction to acid-base disorders. In DiBartola SP, ed: *Fluid therapy in small animal practice*, Philadelphia, 2000, WB Saunders.
14. deMorais HAS: A nontraditional approach to acid-base disorders. In DiBartola SP, ed: *Fluid therapy in small animal practice*, Philadelphia, 1992, WB Saunders.
15. Stick JA, Robinson NE, Krehbiel JD: Acid-base and electrolyte alterations associated with salivary loss in the pony, *Am J Vet Res* 42:733-737, 1981.
16. Rumbaugh GE, Carlson GP, Harrold DR: Clinicopathologic effects of rapid infusion of 5% sodium bicarbonate in 5% dextrose in the horse, *J Am Vet Med Assoc* 178:267-271, 1981.
17. Wilson EA, Green RA: Clinical analysis of mixed acid-base disturbances, *Compend Cont Educ Pract Vet* 7:S364-S371, 1985.
18. Stewart PA: *How to understand acid-base: a quantitative acid-base primer for biology and medicine*, New York, 1981, Elsevier.
19. Stewart PA: Modern quantitative acid-base chemistry, *Can J Physiol Pharmacol* 61:1444-1461, 1983.
20. Fencl V, Rossing TH: Acid-base disorders in critical care medicine, *Annu Rev Med* 40:17-29, 1989.
21. Leith DE: The new acid-base: power and simplicity, *Proc Am Coll Vet Intern Med* 8:449-455, 1990.
22. Constable PD: A simplified strong ion model for acid-base equilibria: application to horse plasma, *J Appl Physiol* 83(1):297-311, 1997.
23. Stampfli HR et al: Weak acid concentration Atot and dissociation constant Ka of plasma proteins in racehorses, *Equine Vet J* (suppl 30):438-442, 1999.
24. Heigenhauser GJF et al: The role of the physiochemical systems in plasma in acid-base control in exercise. In Taylor AW, Gollnick PD, Green HJ et al, eds: *International series on sports sciences*, Champaign, Ill, 1990, Human Kinetics Books.
25. Carlson GP: The interrelationships between fluid, electrolyte, and acid-base balance during maximal exercise, *Equine Vet J* (suppl 18):261-269, 1995.
26. Kohn CW, Chew DJ: Laboratory diagnosis and characterization of renal disease in horses, *Vet Clin North Am (Equine Pract)* 3:585-615, 1987.

Collection and Submission of Samples for Cytologic and Hematologic Studies

DEBRA DEEM MORRIS

BLOOD

Accurate assessment of hematologic data depends heavily on the proper collection, preparation, and transportation of blood samples. Factors that must be considered are (1) the most appropriate venipuncture site, (2) proper restraint, (3) the correct technique, (4) the type of anticoagulant, (5) the necessary volume of blood, and (6) handling of the samples before laboratory analysis. Many of these factors are determined by the test or tests to be performed.

Venipuncture Site and Technique

Because they are large and easily accessible, the jugular veins most often are used in horses and small ruminants. In adult cattle the subcutaneous abdominal (milk) vein and coccygeal (tail) vein also are easily accessible. The disadvantages of using a milk vein are the danger to the operator and the relatively common occurrence of hematomas. In horses alternate sites for collection are the cephalic, lateral thoracic, and saphenous veins.

Blood should be drawn from animals at rest under conditions of least excitement to minimize physiologic variations in cell counts. Evacuated tubes (Vacutainer)* containing the appropriate anticoagulant and their needles are most convenient for collecting blood. These tubes must be filled to capacity to ensure the proper blood to anticoagulant ratio. The chosen vein is raised by digital occlusion proximally; an 18- to 20-gauge, $1^1/_2$- to 2-inch needle is then plunged through the skin into the vein at approximately a 30-degree angle. A clean venipuncture is important to avoid contamination of the blood by tissue thromboplastin, which en-

courages clot formation and invalidates hemostatic function tests.

The coccygeal vein in cattle is punctured between the sixth and seventh coccygeal vertebrae, where the caudal folds end[1] with the tail directly over the animal's back. The needle is inserted at a right angle to the skin to bone and then is withdrawn gradually while vacuum is applied to the syringe, until sufficient blood has been obtained. This technique should not be used to collect blood for hemostatic testing.

Blood for hemostatic tests should be carefully transferred to the anticoagulated vial to prevent hemolysis. Because goat erythrocytes are very sensitive to hemolysis, a Vacutainer is not recommended for blood collection in goats.[2]

Anticoagulants

An anticoagulant must be added to all blood samples collected for hematologic examination, because cell counts and morphology cannot be evaluated in clotted blood. Commonly used anticoagulants include ethylenediamine tetraacetic acid (EDTA), heparin, and sodium citrate. The minimum amount of blood needed for most routine blood studies is 2 ml. Regardless of the volume withdrawn, the proper blood to anticoagulant ratio must always be maintained.

The preferred anticoagulant for the complete blood count (CBC) is EDTA at a concentration of 1 to 2 mg/ml. An excessive EDTA concentration causes erythrocyte shrinkage and may invalidate the packed cell volume, mean corpuscular volume, and mean corpuscular hemoglobin concentration.[2] Vac-

---

*Becton Dickinson, Inc., Rutherford, NJ.

413

utainers contain the appropriate amount of EDTA for the full volume of blood; therefore these tubes should be allowed to fill until the vacuum stops. In addition to the CBC, EDTA-anticoagulated blood is suitable for platelet counts, total plasma protein levels, and plasma fibrinogen determinations.

Trisodium citrate (3.8% aqueous solution) is used to anticoagulate blood to be used for hemostatic function tests.[3] It should be used in a 1:9 proportion with blood.

Handling and Transportation of Samples

The vial containing blood and anticoagulant should be inverted several times to ensure adequate mixing. Blood samples for hematologic studies (CBC) are best processed as soon as possible after collection. If delay is expected, the samples should be refrigerated at 4° C (39.2° F). Air-dried blood smears for the differential count should be prepared immediately if samples must be held longer than 2 hours. If refrigerated, the remainder of the blood sample produces an acceptable CBC for 24 hours. Cold packs and an insulated container should be used to transport blood samples to a laboratory. Blood smears can be held several days before staining with Wright stain or any modified Romanovsky stain.

Blood samples for laboratory examination of the hemostatic system must be collected and handled with special care to prevent platelet clumping and activation of coagulation. If blood is collected into a Vacutainer, discarding the first tube ensures that the sample does not contain tissue fluids.[3] Optimally, the samples are placed on ice and delivered to the laboratory within 1 hour of collection. If the sample must be stored for several hours, plasma should be collected immediately by centrifugation (800 to 1000 g for 15 minutes), harvested with a plastic pipette, and frozen, preferably at −70° C (−94° F). Platelet counts must be performed immediately. The platelet count may be estimated by examining a peripheral blood smear and comparing the number of platelets per oil immersion field to the number of red or white cells.

BONE MARROW

Air-dried smears can be made directly from a bone marrow aspirate or after the sample has been anticoagulated with EDTA. Because the volume of most aspirates is less than 0.5 ml, it is better to collect the sample in a syringe containing 1 to 2 drops of EDTA solution than to place it in a tube containing proportionately too much anticoagulant. Anticoagulant may not be required if smears can be made immediately after collection. These aspirates and smears should be handled as outlined for blood samples to be used for hematologic studies.

A bone marrow core must be preserved by placing it in a 10% neutral buffered formalin solution. Impression smears may be made from these samples by gently rolling them on a clean glass slide before placing them in the formalin solution.

LYMPH NODE ASPIRATES

Air-dried smears of lymph node aspirates are handled in the same way as blood smears for the differential count.

REFERENCES

1. Rosenberger G: *Clinical examination of cattle,* Philadelphia, 1979, WB Saunders.
2. Jain NC: *Schalm's veterinary hematology,* ed 4, Philadelphia, 1986, Lea & Febiger.
3. Dodds WJ: Hemostasis. In Kaneko JJ, ed: *Clinical biochemistry of domestic animals,* ed 4, San Diego, 1989, Academic Press.

Alterations in the Erythron

DEBRA DEEM MORRIS

MAJOR ALTERATIONS

Anemia, 415

Erythrocytosis (polycythemia), 419

The erythron is composed of all data pertaining to erythrocytes in the peripheral blood. In most instances the routine complete blood count (CBC), which includes microscopic evaluation of a blood smear, provides the data discussed in this chapter. After evaluation of the CBC, additional data on the erythroid compartment may be necessary, such as can be obtained from staining for Heinz bodies, the Coombs' test, or the erythrocyte fragility test. All pertinent tests associated with erythroid diseases are discussed in this chapter except bone marrow analysis.

Any description of hematologic alterations in large animals would be incomplete without a brief discussion of the unique features of the equine erythron. To correctly interpret hematologic data, the practitioner must appreciate the characteristics that distinguish the horse from other domestic animals.

1. *Unstable packed cell volume (PCV).* The horse has a highly innervated muscular spleen that normally contains up to one third of the potentially circulating red cell mass. On adrenergic stimulation (which normally accompanies exercise, excitement, or blood loss), the spleen contracts and releases its reservoir of erythrocytes into the peripheral circulation, causing the PCV to increase by as much as 50%. For this reason the resting PCV of horses is highly unstable and must be evaluated serially under different levels of excitement. Also, the response of the spleen to massive hemorrhage precludes using the PCV to estimate the magnitude of blood loss for at least 24 hours.

2. *Rouleau formation.* Equine erythrocytes show a tendency for marked rouleaux formation (aligning like stacked coins), which causes cells to separate rapidly from plasma (high erythrocyte sedimentation rate). This characteristic necessitates thorough mixing of blood in the sample vial before analysis and must be differentiated from autoagglutination (see p. 417).

3. *Icteric plasma.* Although hyperbilirubinemia causes plasma to become more intensely yellow or orange, equine plasma is normally yellow (icteric).

4. *Lack of peripheral signs of regeneration.* Equine erythrocytes are retained in the bone marrow until hemoglobin synthesis is complete; thus polychromasia (reticulocytosis), macrocytosis, and other peripheral blood signs of bone marrow regeneration are extremely rare in horses. The erythron of anemic horses cannot be assessed by peripheral blood alone.

5. *Howell-Jolly bodies.* Small numbers of these eccentric erythrocytic inclusions normally are found in equine blood. Their presence does not indicate a responsive anemia, as in other species.

ANEMIA

Anemia is functionally defined as decreased oxygen-carrying capacity of the blood. The most accurate laboratory indication of anemia is a drop in the PCV or hematocrit below the normal range. The PCV must always be interpreted in light of the animal's hydration status and level of excitement, especially in horses. Because goats have very small erythrocytes (Table 24-1), the PCV for these animals must be determined by microhematocrit centrifugation (12,000 g for 5 minutes) to prevent plasma trapping in the erythrocyte column.[1] This is the most accurate method of PCV determination in all species.

The three pathophysiologic mechanisms for the development of anemia are blood loss, increased erythrocyte destruction (hemolysis), and inadequate erythrocyte production. In the first two instances the bone marrow is normal and responds by increased erythropoiesis (regenerative or responsive anemias). In ruminants, regenerative anemias are attended by the appearance of immature erythrocytes in the

TABLE 24-1

Normal Values for Erythron Data in Ruminants and the Horse

	Cattle	Sheep	Goats	Horses
PCV (%)	24-46	27-45	22-38	32-53
Erythrocytes ($\times 10^6$/L)	5-10	9-15	8-18	6.7-12.9
Hemoglobin (g/dl)	8-15	9-15	8-12	11-19
MCV (fl)	40-60	28-40	16-25	37-58.5
MCH (pg)	11-17	8-12	5.2-8	12.3-19.7
MCHC (g/dl)	30-36	31-34	30-36	31-38.6
Reticulocytes	0	<0.5%	0	0
Erythrocyte diameter (m)	4-8	3.2-6	2.5-3.9	5-6
Erythrocyte fragility (percent NaCl)				
Minimum (beginning hemolysis)	0.52-0.66	0.58-0.76	0.74	0.54
Maximum (complete hemolysis)	0.44-0.52	0.40-0.55	0.44	0.34
Erythrocyte sedimentation rate (mm/1 hour)	0	1-2.5	0	50-60
Erythrocyte life span (days)	160	140-150	125	140-150

PCV, Packed cell volume; *MCV,* mean corpuscular volume; *MCH,* mean corpuscular hemoglobin; *MCHC,* mean corpuscular hemoglobin concentration; *NaCl,* sodium chloride.

peripheral blood. Inadequate erythrocyte production is caused by a bone marrow abnormality, and by definition the anemia is nonregenerative. Often anemia in large animals is caused by a combination of pathophysiologic mechanisms (Boxes 24-1 and 24-2).

Alteration in Mean Corpuscular Volume

The mean corpuscular volume (MCV) is a reflection of mean erythrocyte size, as expressed in the equation below:

$$\text{MCV (fl)} = \frac{\text{Hematocrit} \times 10}{\text{Erythrocyte count (millions/}\mu\text{l)}}$$

An *increased* MCV (macrocytosis) indicates a regenerative anemia, because immature erythrocytes are larger than mature ones. Iron deficiency results in a *decreased* MCV (microcytosis), because cells undergo an extra division as a result of inadequate hemoglobin concentration. Inadequate spinning of blood causes a spurious elevation of the MCV by trapped plasma. This is most commonly a problem in goats.

Alteration in Mean Corpuscular Hemoglobin

The mean corpuscular hemoglobin (MCH) is an estimation of the amount of hemoglobin (Hb) in the blood per erythrocyte. It is calculated according to the following equation:

$$\text{MCH (pg)} = \frac{\text{Hb (g/dl)} \times 10}{\text{RBC count (millions/}\mu\text{l)}}$$

An *increased* MCH may indicate (1) the presence of reticulocytes (immature erythrocytes) in the peripheral blood or (2) hemolysis, either in vivo *or* in vitro. Iron deficiency results in a *decreased* MCH.

Alteration in Mean Corpuscular Hemoglobin Concentration

The mean corpuscular hemoglobin concentration (MCHC) is the most accurate of erythrocytic indices. It can be expressed as a percentage or as grams per deciliter:

$$\text{MCHC (\%)} = \frac{\text{Hb (g/dl)} \times 100}{\text{Hematocrit (\%)}}$$

Reticulocytosis (erythroid regeneration) or iron deficiency results in a *decreased* MCHC; hemolysis (in vivo or in vitro) causes an *increased* MCHC. Inadequate spinning of blood produces a spurious reduction in the MCHC.

Anisocytosis

Variation in the size of erythrocytes is caused by the presence of macrocytes or microcytes (or both) among normal cells. Slight to moderate anisocytosis is normal in cattle, but marked anisocytosis in ruminants is a sign of regenerative anemia. Macrocytic erythrocytes may be seen at the peak of erythrocyte release during equine regenerative anemia, but in most horses effective regeneration occurs without macrocytosis.[2]

Polychromasia

Variation in color among the cells (using Romanovsky stains) is caused by the presence of reticulocytes that stain bluish because of residual DNA. In ruminants polychromasia is a sign of regenerative anemia. Reticulocytosis can be quantitated most accurately by using new methylene blue stain, which causes cytoplasmic DNA to appear as blue granules. Insufficient cellular hemoglobin caused by iron deficiency results in decreased staining intensity and increased central pallor of erythrocytes (hypochromia). Hypochromia is difficult to recognize in large animals because their erythrocytes are small.

Poikilocytosis

The presence of abnormally shaped erythrocytes indicates increased erythrocyte fragility or diseases characterized by erythrocyte fragmentation. In rare cases, poikilocytosis may accompany iron deficiency or disseminated coagulopathy in large animals.

Basophilic Stippling

Tiny blue granules occasionally are observed in Romanovsky-stained erythrocytes containing residual DNA. This is a normal feature of regenerative anemia in cattle and sheep. In cattle basophilic stippling also may indicate chronic lead poisoning.

BOX 24-1

Causes of Anemia in the Horse

COMMON CAUSES
Through Blood Loss
Intestinal parasitism (strongylosis)
Ectoparasites (lice, ticks)
Gastric ulcers
Immune-mediated thrombocytopenia
Gastric squamous cell carcinoma
Equine purpura hemorrhagica

Through Hemolysis
Neonatal isoerythrolysis
Equine infectious anemia
Red maple leaf toxicosis
Equine ehrlichiosis

Through Inadequate Erythrocyte Production
Abdominal abscess or other chronic abscess
Chronic pneumonia or pleuritis
Equine purpura hemorrhagica
Equine ehrlichiosis
Lymphosarcoma

LESS COMMON CAUSES
Through Blood Loss
Disseminated intravascular coagulation
Moldy sweet clover toxicosis
Warfarin toxicosis
Hemophilia A or other congenital factor deficiencies
Guttural pouch mycosis

Through Hemolysis
Onion toxicosis
Autoimmune hemolytic anemia
Babesiosis (piroplasmosis)
Clostridial infections
Incompatible blood transfusion

Through Inadequate Erythrocyte Production
Myelogenous leukemia
Equine viral arteritis
Chronic renal failure (glomerulonephritis)
Radiation toxicosis
Idiopathic aplastic anemia

BOX 24-2

Causes of Anemia in Ruminants

COMMON CAUSES
Through Blood Loss
Intestinal parasitism
Ectoparasites (lice, ticks)
Abomasal ulcer (B)

Through Hemolysis
Anaplasmosis
Brassica toxicosis
Onion toxicosis
Bacillary hemoglobinuria
Leptospirosis
Chronic copper toxicosis (O)

Through Inadequate Erythrocyte Production
Lymphosarcoma
Liver abscess
Chronic bovine virus diarrhea
Johne's disease
Chronic pneumonia
Chronic abscessation

LESS COMMON CAUSES
Through Blood Loss
Moldy sweet clover toxicosis
Disseminated intravascular coagulation
Pulmonary abscess with hemorrhage associated with thrombosis of the posterior vena cava
Severe acute pyelonephritis

Through Hemolysis
Postparturient hemoglobinuria
Immune-mediated hemolytic anemia

Through Inadequate Erythrocyte Production
Chronic renal failure (amyloidosis, pyelonephritis)
Bracken fern toxicosis (also hemorrhage in enzootic hematuria)
Radiation toxicosis
Myelofibrosis (pygmy goats)

B, Bovine; *O*, ovine.

Howell-Jolly Bodies

Basophilic nuclear remnants commonly are seen in immature erythrocytes during responsive anemia in ruminants. In healthy horses a few Howell-Jolly bodies occur normally.

Nucleated Erythrocytes

Nucleated erythrocytes and metarubricytes occasionally appear in the peripheral blood during the responsive phase of severe anemia in ruminants.

Heinz Bodies

Oxidative stress to erythrocytes causes denaturation of hemoglobin, which precipitates as aggregates, called Heinz bodies. Heinz bodies appear as round structures projecting from one edge of the red cell and are most easily visible on new methylene blue preparations. Erythrocytes containing Heinz bodies are susceptible to intravascular hemolysis and removal in the mononuclear phagocyte system (MPS). Heinz body hemolytic anemia is seen in cattle that have ingested toxic amounts of onions or plants of the *Brassica* genus. Horses develop Heinz body anemia in association with toxicoses caused by phenothiazine, red maple leaves and, in rare cases, onions.

Autoagglutination

Aggregation of erythrocytes may be observed grossly or microscopically during immune-mediated anemia in horses or cattle. Marked rouleaux formation, which occurs normally in horses, may be differentiated from agglutination by diluting the blood sample 1:4 with 0.9% saline. Both rouleaux formation and autoagglutination, rarely induced by severe inflammation, are dispersed by saline dilution.

Increased Erythrocyte Fragility

The erythrocyte fragility test is a measure of the susceptibility of erythrocytes to hemolysis in a range of hypotonic saline concentrations (see Table 24-1). An increase in osmotic fragility is *indirectly* suggestive of immune-mediated anemia; the Coombs' test is more specific.

Positive Direct Antiglobulin (Coombs') Test Result

A positive Coombs' test result indicates the presence of antibodies on the surface of erythrocytes. A positive test result may be found in idiopathic autoimmune hemolytic anemia in any species and in horses with neonatal isoerythrolysis or equine infectious anemia. The Coombs' reagent is a mixture of antibodies directed against immunoglobulins and complement of a certain species. Because the end point of this test is agglutination, it cannot be performed on blood that is autoagglutinating. There are many false negative results.

Erythrocytic Parasites

During the acute stages of bovine anaplasmosis and babesiosis in horses, cattle, sheep, and goats, intraerythrocytic parasites can be found. *Anaplasma marginale* is seen as a round, basophilic inclusion at the edge of cells, present in highest numbers before a hemolytic crisis. *Babesia* trophozoites occur in erythrocytes as round, bizarre, rod-shaped, or typical piriform (teardrop-shaped) structures. Absence of intraerythrocytic parasites does not rule out anaplasmosis or babesiosis.

Clinical Signs of Anemia

The major clinical signs of anemia (e.g., tachycardia, tachypnea, reduced exercise tolerance, and depression) reflect physiologic adjustments to inadequate oxygen transport to body tissues. The PCV level at which clinical signs occur depends on the rate of development, the severity of the anemia, and the physical demands placed on the animal. Other clinical signs depend on the cause and mechanism of anemia development. Anemia is accompanied by mucosal pallor except when it is caused by hemolysis, which results in icterus. Red urine (hemoglobinuria) indicates intravascular hemolysis, which may be accompanied by fever. Melena, hematuria, and petechial hemorrhages may indicate chronic blood loss.

Although diagnosing anemia is easy, determining the cause, which dictates proper treatment, may be complex. The practitioner first must determine the pathophysiologic classification of the anemia and then consider possible causes.

Approach to Diagnosis of Anemia in the Horse

1. Take the history. Important factors are the diet, housing, pasture conditions, drug history, date of the most recent Coggins' test, travel history, time course of current signs, and any past illnesses. In considering neonatal isoerythrolysis, the number of the dam's previous foals and their sires must be ascertained.
2. Perform a physical examination. Take note of the mucous membranes. Icterus in horses may be associated with fasting or cholestatic liver disease, as well as hemolysis. Hemoglobinuria, which is uncommon in horses, indicates intravascular hemolysis (this is difficult to distinguish from myoglobinuria; therefore the plasma should be examined). Epistaxis or other signs of bleeding diathesis suggest a source of chronic blood loss. A thorough search should be made for evidence of chronic disease affecting the respiratory and gastrointestinal tracts. Take note of any weight loss and the character of feces. Any chronic inflammatory disease such as abdominal abscess, pneumonia, or lymphosarcoma causes a mild to moderate non-

regenerative anemia. Immune-mediated hemolytic anemia often is associated with equine lymphosarcoma.
3. Perform a CBC.
   a. PCV is reduced.
   b.
   $$\frac{\text{PCV (\%)}}{\text{Hb (g/dl)}}$$
   Result below 3 suggests intravascula hemolysis.
   c. Pink plasma suggests intravascular hemolysis.
   d. MCV above 60 fl (rare) suggests regenerative anemia.
   e. Heinz bodies (substantiate by new methylene blue staining) suggest toxicosis caused by phenothiazine, red maple leaves, or wild onions.
   f. Agglutination (substantiate by diluting blood 1:4 with 0.9% saline) suggests immune-mediated anemia. Perform Coggins' test in adult. In newborn foal perform hemolytic cross-match with dam.
4. Evaluate leukogram and plasma proteins.
   a. Neutrophilia, hyperglobulinemia, and/or hyperfibrinogenemia suggests chronic infection.
   b. Hypoproteinemia may indicate blood loss anemia or an underlying disease causing protein loss (e.g., granulomatous bowel disease or intestinal lymphosarcoma). In horses gastric squamous cell carcinoma causes chronic blood loss anemia associated with iron deficiency.
5. Perform bone marrow analysis. This is necessary to adequately characterize anemia in horses as regenerative or nonregenerative.
6. Analyze urine. A positive result for occult blood without microscopic hematuria indicates hemoglobinuria (intravascular hemolysis) or myoglobinuria (myopathy). Hemoglobinuria is associated with pink plasma. Saturated ammonium sulfate usually precipitates and removes color caused by hemoglobin; however, spectrophotometric tests are best for differentiating from myoglobin.[3]
7. Test feces for occult blood. A positive result may indicate gastrointestinal blood loss as a cause of chronic anemia. Gastric ulcers (foals) and gastric squamous cell carcinoma should be considered.
8. Test serum iron and total iron-binding capacity (TIBC). Low serum iron and a high TIBC are consistent with iron deficiency (chronic blood loss). Low serum iron with normal TIBC suggests the anemia of chronic disease.
9. Perform a Coggins' test. A positive result indicates equine infectious anemia.
10. Perform a Coombs' test. A positive result indicates immune-mediated anemia.

Approach to Diagnosis of Anemia in Ruminants

1. Take the history. Note the type of diet, access to pasture, other herd or flock members with clinical signs of systemic disease, immunization status, and exposure to new animals.
2. Perform a physical examination. Icterus in ruminants is rare except in association with hemolysis. Pallor indicates blood loss or inadequate erythrocyte production. Fever may be a sign of hemolysis or of an underlying systemic disease. Most hemolytic anemias in ruminants, *except anaplasmosis,* cause hemoglobinuria. Check the breath for onion odor.
3. Perform a CBC.
   a. PCV is reduced.
   b. Pink plasma suggests intravascular hemolysis.
   c. Regenerative changes indicate blood loss or hemolysis with normal marrow.
   d. If no signs of regeneration are present, abnormal bone

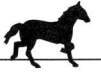

BOX 24-3

Causes of Erythrocytosis in Large Animals

RELATIVE ERYTHROCYTOSIS
Dehydration
Endotoxic shock
Strangulating intestinal obstruction
Salmonellosis
Colitis X (E)
Septic metritis
Septic mastitis (B)

ABSOLUTE ERYTHROCYTOSIS
Common Causes
Congenital cardiovascular disease
Residence at high altitudes
Chronic obstructive pulmonary disease

Less Common Causes
Familial (B)
Chronic hepatic disease
Hepatoma
Leiomyoma
Hemangioblastoma
Pheochromocytoma
Nephroma
Hydronephrosis
Polycystic kidneys
Nephrocalcinosis

B, Bovine; *E*, equine.

marrow, acute blood loss (less than 4 days), or acute hemolysis is indicated.

    e. Increased Hb, MCH, and/or MCHC with a low PCV indicates intravascular hemolysis.

    f. Basophilic stippling without other signs of regeneration may indicate chronic lead poisoning.

    g. Heinz bodies suggest ingestion of onions or *Brassica* plants. May need to do new methylene blue stain to observe.

    h. Autoagglutination suggests immune-mediated anemia. Perform dilution tests.

4. Evaluate plasma proteins.

    a. Hypoproteinemia suggests blood loss.

    b. Hyperproteinemia, hyperglobulinemia, and/or hyperfibrinogenemia suggests chronic inflammatory disease.

4. Analyze urine. See discussion under Approach to Diagnosis of Anemia in the Horse. Myoglobinuria is associated with clear plasma.

5. Test feces for occult blood. Bleeding abomasal ulcers cause acute or chronic anemia in cattle.

6. Perform bone marrow analysis. This test is necessary in the absence of peripheral blood signs of regeneration.

ERYTHROCYTOSIS (POLYCYTHEMIA)

Erythrocytosis is defined as an increase in the PCV, erythrocyte count, and hemoglobin concentration above the normal range. Erythrocytosis may be absolute or relative (apparent), caused by hemoconcentration (dehydration, shock) or splenic contraction (Box 24-3). Absolute erythrocytosis (primary or secondary) is caused by increased erythropoiesis that creates a greater total circulating erythrocyte mass.

Primary absolute erythrocytosis (polycythemia vera) is an idiopathic, myeloproliferative disorder associated with a normal partial pressure of oxygen (Po_2) and reduced erythropoietin levels. Secondary absolute erythrocytosis is caused by an increase in erythropoietin. Chronic tissue hypoxia, which may accompany residence at high altitudes, chronic pulmonary disease, and heart defects that produce arteriovenous shunting, induce a physiologic or compensatory increase in serum erythropoietin that results in absolute secondary erythrocytosis. Inappropriate elaboration of erythropoietin (normal Po_2) and secondary erythrocytosis rarely occur in chronic renal, hepatic, or endocrine disorders, especially those caused by neoplasia.

In domestic animals, absolute erythrocytosis usually occurs secondary to chronic diseases that produce tissue hypoxia. Primary absolute erythrocytosis and inappropriate secondary erythrocytosis caused by hepatocellular carcinoma have been described in horses.[4] Familial erythrocytosis has been described in cattle, and the source of the increase in erythropoietin has not been identified.[5] Clinical signs of erythrocytosis are vague; they include lethargy, weight loss, mucosal hyperemia, and signs of underlying disease.

Diagnosis of erythrocytosis is based on persistent elevation of the PCV, hemoglobin, and erythrocyte count in the absence of clinical evidence of shock or dehydration and without response to intravenous fluid therapy. Chronic hypoxia can be ruled out by determining the arterial oxygen concentration. Thoracic radiographs and echocardiography can delineate cardiorespiratory function more thoroughly. Examination of the bone marrow is indicated, although erythroid hyperplasia is not specific for primary or secondary erythrocytosis. In the absence of hypoxemia and a demonstrable disease that could lead to appropriate secondary erythrocytosis, polycythemia vera and inappropriate secondary erythrocytosis must be considered. Renal and hepatic disease should be excluded by determining the serum creatinine, hepatic enzyme, and bile acid levels. The only way clearly to differentiate primary from secondary absolute erythrocytosis is to determine the serum erythropoietin. This is a bioassay, which is not routinely available, and it is relatively insensitive to minor changes in erythropoietin concentrations.

REFERENCES

1. Jain NC: *Schalm's veterinary hematology*, ed 4, Philadelphia, 1986, Lea & Febiger.
2. Radin MJ, Eubank MC, Weiser MG: Electronic measurement of erythrocyte volume and volume heterogeneity in horses during erythrocyte regeneration associated with experimental anemias, *Vet Pathol* 23:656-660, 1986.
3. Duncan JR, Prasse KW, Mahaffey EA: *Veterinary laboratory medicine: clinical pathology*, ed 3, Ames, Iowa, 1994, Iowa State University Press.
4. Beech J, Bloom JC, Hodge TG: Erythrocytosis in a horse, *J Am Vet Med Assoc* 184:986-989, 1984.
5. Tennant B et al: Familial erythrocytosis in cattle, *J Am Vet Med Assoc* 150:1493-1509, 1967.

Alterations in the Leukogram

DEBRA DEEM MORRIS

MAJOR ALTERATIONS

The leukogram (white blood cell count, differential analysis, and white blood cell morphology) provides extremely useful laboratory data when considered with the history, clinical signs, and physical findings. To fully use the leukogram, the practitioner must know the types of white blood cells (WBCs), their kinetics and functions, and the pathologic and physiologic conditions that can cause deviations from normal. Normal values for leukogram data are given in Table 25-1.

Mature WBCs include neutrophils, lymphocytes, monocytes, eosinophils, and basophils. Immature leukocytes that may or may not be present in the peripheral blood include band or nonsegmented neutrophils, metamyelocytes, myelocytes, and progranulocytes. These immature forms usually are found only in the bone marrow, but they may be released in response to disease.

LEUKOCYTES

Leukocytes, or WBCs, are divided into two main categories: polymorphonuclear (PMN) leukocytes (granulocytes) and mononuclear leukocytes. PMN leukocytes include neutrophils, eosinophils, and basophils, which are produced in the bone marrow. The mononuclear leukocytes are the lymphocytes and monocytes. Lymphocytes are produced in the bone marrow (the primary source), lymphoid organs (thymus, spleen, and lymph nodes), and gut-associated lym-

phoid tissues (Peyer's patches, tonsils). Monocytes, the largest of the WBCs, originate in the bone marrow.

Neutrophils

Neutrophils develop in the bone marrow as myeloblasts, progranulocytes or promyelocytes, myelocytes, metamyelocytes, band cells, and segmented neutrophils. Myeloblasts arise from bipotential committed stem cells (colony-forming unit–granulocyte, macrophage) that are derived from pluripotent hematopoietic stem cells.[1]

Myeloblasts, promyelocytes, and myelocytes are capable of cell division, but metamyelocytes, bands, and segmented neutrophils (about 80% of the bone marrow granulocytes) do not divide.[2] The normal interval for progression from myeloblast to mature blood neutrophil is 4 to 9 days, depending on the species. A functional storage compartment of neutrophils exists in the marrow to prevent marrow depletion by the sudden imposition of a greatly increased peripheral use. The storage pool, which is limited to segmented neutrophils and some bands, varies in size among species and is relatively small in adult cattle.[1] A marginal pool of neutrophils adheres to endothelium throughout the microvasculature. Neutrophils in the circulating pool are the only part of the total neutrophil population enumerated by the peripheral blood neutrophil count. In large animals the

TABLE 25-1

Normal Values for Leukogram Data (Adult Animals)

	Cattle	Sheep	Goats	Horses
White blood cells ($\times 10^3/\mu l$)	4-12	4-12	4-13	5.4-14.3
Neutrophils ($\times 10^3/\mu l$)	0.6-4	0.7-6	1.2-7.2	2.3-8.6
Bands ($\times 10^3/\mu l$)	0-0.12	Rare	Rare	0-1
Lymphocytes ($\times 10^3/\mu l$)	2.5-7.5	2-9	2-9	1.5-7.7
Monocytes ($\times 10^3/\mu l$)	0.025-0.84	0-0.75	0-0.55	0-1
Eosinophils ($\times 10^3/\mu l$)	0-2.4	0-1	0.05-0.65	0-1
Basophils ($\times 10^3/\mu l$)	0-0.2	0-0.3	0-0.12	0-0.29
Neutrophil/lymphocyte (N/L) ratio	0.3-0.6	0.3-0.7	0.6-3.6	0.8-2.8

marginal neutrophil pool is approximately equal in size to the circulating pool.[1]

After entering the bloodstream, neutrophils have a half-life of 6 to 14 hours, depending on the species. The entire blood pool of neutrophils is replaced two to two and one half times per day. Neutrophils move randomly into the tissues by diapedesis through vascular endothelium and do not return to the blood. Neutrophils migrate into tissues within 2 hours of injury, infection, or inflammation. In the absence of such lesions, the neutrophils are destroyed by macrophages of the bone marrow, liver, and spleen or are lost into body secretions and excretions within 96 hours of exiting the marrow.[2]

The major function of neutrophils is to phagocytize and destroy foreign material, especially pathogenic bacteria. Bacterial products and substances released from activated lymphocytes (lymphokines), macrophages, and cellular damage are responsible for attracting the neutrophils, which move by chemotaxis and bind to the foreign particle.[3] Opsonins are protein components of serum that adhere to foreign particles and make them more liable to phagocytosis.[4] Opsonization by specific antibodies increases the rate and magnitude of ingestion for most bacterial organisms. Once drawn into the cell, the bacteria are enclosed in a phagocytic vacuole, which fuses with lysosomes in the neutrophil cytoplasm that release hydrolytic enzymes to destroy the contents. Degranulation, which occurs within 5 seconds of a phagocytic event, can lead to release of lysosomal enzymes into the surrounding milieu and cause tissue destruction.

Gram-negative bacteria are more resistant to digestion in the neutrophil than gram-positive bacteria because of the structure of their outer wall. *Brucella abortus, Mycobacterium paratuberculosis, Listeria monocytogenes,* and some *Salmonella* serotypes are extremely resistant to lysosomal destruction and may survive and multiply within the neutrophil.

EOSINOPHILS

Eosinophils are produced in the bone marrow and follow the same maturation sequence and kinetics as neutrophils, except that eosinophils arise from the colony-forming unit–eosinophil.[1] There is a large marrow reserve of eosinophils, and their circulatory half-life varies from 30 minutes to 10 hours, depending on the species. Eosinophils also are found in many body tissues, particularly the gut, subcutis, uterus, and respiratory tract, where they have a half-life of 12 days.

Eosinophils are most important in controlling parasitic infections and in regulating inflammatory and allergic reactions. Eosinophils are less efficient phagocytes than neutrophils and provide little host resistance to bacterial infection but are important in protective parasitic immunity.[2] Eosinophils are believed to regulate immediate (type I) hypersensitivity and inflammatory responses by inactivating

histamine, leukotrienes, platelet-activating factor, and other chemical mediators involved in these processes. Other, less characterized effects of eosinophils include tissue damage, augmentation of coagulation and fibrinolysis, and inhibition of granulopoiesis.

BASOPHILS

Basophils are relatively scarce in the blood of large animal species. The blood basophil resembles the tissue mast cell and is believed to perform similar functions. Basophils are produced in the bone marrow by mitosis of basophilic promonocytes through the same sequential stages of maturation as neutrophils. Basophils have a mean circulatory half-life of about 6 hours. They then enter tissues, where they survive for about 10 to 12 days.[1] Mast cells, found in many body tissues, originate from undifferentiated connective tissue mesenchymal cells, especially near blood vessels. There is evidence in some species that mast cells also originate from a precursor in the bone marrow.[1]

Basophils and mast cells contain stored intragranular substances that mediate their function in allergic and inflammatory processes. The most important function of basophils and mast cells is to elicit an immediate hypersensitivity reaction through secretion of vasoactive mediators, including histamine, leukotrienes, platelet-activating factor, and others. Vasodilation, pooling of fluid in tissue spaces, and systemic reactions may occur, with signs of dyspnea, urticaria, coughing, and even severe anaphylactic shock. Eosinophils are attracted to these areas to neutralize the histamine and attenuate the inflammatory response.

Lymphocytes

Lymphocytes are produced in the bone marrow, lymph nodes, thymus, spleen, and Peyer's patches. They are classically divided into two groups: T cells, or thymus-derived lymphocytes, and B cells, or bone marrow–derived lymphocytes. Null cells have been identified in humans and in some animals that lack specific markers for T or B cells.[1] Both T and B cell populations are present in the peripheral blood of large animal species, with T cells making up the majority. B cells are few during fetal life but steadily increase to make up about 20% of circulating lymphocytes in most adult domestic animals.[1] Observations in cattle indicate that various inflammatory states are associated with an increase in B cells and a decrease in T cells. Leukemic cows infected with bovine leukosis virus (BLV) and those with persistent lymphocytosis have a higher number of B cells, which constitute up to 97% of lymphocytes.[1] Lymphocytes can recirculate and continue to undergo mitosis. Information is unavailable on domestic animals, but most blood lymphocytes in humans have an average life span of 4.3 years.[1]

B lymphocytes transform into plasma cells that produce antibodies under the regulation of T lymphocytes. T lymphocytes are primarily responsible for delayed-type hypersensitivity (DTH), graft and tumor rejection, autoimmunity, and resistance to certain intracellular pathogens. Some types of T cells have a direct cytotoxic function to destroy foreign cells, and null cells express natural killer activity. Lymphocytes produce important immunologic mediators called lymphokines, which include macrophage-activating factor, interferons, and interleukins.

The number of lymphocytes in the peripheral blood reflects a balance between cells leaving and entering the circulation; thus changes do not necessarily mean altered lymphopoiesis. Besides considering the total number in the leukogram, lymphocytes can be evaluated by measuring the ratio of T cells to B cells (normal range is 1:1 to 3:1), antibody levels and response to vaccination, in vitro lymphocyte stimulation tests, and skin tests of DTH.

Monocytes

Monocytes are produced in the bone marrow from the colony-forming unit–granulocyte, macrophage, which differentiates into either myeloblasts or monoblasts (precursors of monocytes).[1] Monoblasts undergo mitosis to promonocytes and then divide one to two more times to produce monocytes. Once released into the blood, monocytes circulate for 1 to 3 days and then enter body cavities and tissues and transform into macrophages. Tissue macrophages survive in tissues for weeks to years. Once in tissue, these macrophages are described as "fixed" or "free." Free macrophages are found in the peritoneal and pleural cavities, in joints, in alveolar spaces, and at areas of inflammation. Fixed macrophages include Kupffer's cells of the liver, osteoclasts, microglial cells, and macrophages found in the spleen, bone marrow, and lymph nodes.

The blood monocytes and tissue macrophages constitute the mononuclear phagocyte (reticuloendothelial) system.[1,2] The functions of tissue macrophages include sustained phagocytic activity to remove dead and damaged tissue; microbicidal action against some bacteria, viruses, fungi, and protozoa; regulation of the immune response in both afferent and efferent limbs; tumor defense; regulation of hematopoiesis; tissue repair and remodeling; and secretion of monokines, lysosomal enzymes, and other substances, such as coagulation factors, that have wide-ranging biologic importance. The tissue macrophages are better equipped than neutrophils to combat intracellular organisms and those that cause granulomatous inflammation such as fungal infections, listeriosis, brucellosis, Johne's disease, tuberculosis, and salmonellosis.

Interleukin-1 and tumor necrosis factor are important macrophage-derived mediators of the inflammatory response.[5] These and other cytokines are released when macrophages are exposed to bacterial products (especially endotoxin), antigens, and injured tissue. Interleukin-1 stimulates bone marrow release of neutrophils and attracts them to areas of bacterial infection or inflammation. Tumor necrosis factor is responsible for many of the physiologic derangements associated with endotoxemia that end in shock, tissue injury, and death.

GENERAL PRINCIPLES OF LEUKOGRAM INTERPRETATION

When interpreting the leukogram, the practitioner must consider (1) the established normal values for the species, (2) the animal's age and condition, and (3) the species-specific WBC

BOX 25-1

Causes of Neutrophilia in the Horse

COMMON CAUSES
Excitement, exercise
Stress, exogenous corticosteroid administration
Chronic pneumonia, pleuritis
Strangles (*Streptococcus equi* infection)
Chronic peritonitis, abdominal abscess
Other internal abscessation
Chronic salmonellosis or colitis
Thrombophlebitis
Purpura hemorrhagica (vasculitis)

LESS COMMON CAUSES
Bacterial endocarditis
Cellulitis
Pyelonephritis
Chronic hepatitis, cholangiohepatitis
Cholelithiasis
Lymphosarcoma
Other internal neoplasia
Pituitary adenoma (equine Cushing's syndrome)
Autoimmune hemolytic anemia
Granulocytic leukemia
Systemic fungal infections

---

responses. Leukocytosis may be attributed to physiologic or pathologic causes, whereas leukopenia always is considered pathologic.[1,6]

Physiologic Leukocytosis

Physiologic leukocytosis occurs when epinephrine is released, as with stress, excitation, anxiety, or exercise. The elevated WBC count is transient and caused by both neutrophilia and lymphocytosis, although it is primarily the result of temporary mobilization of the marginal neutrophil pool.[2] Corticosteroids, either exogenous or endogenous, cause neutrophilia and lymphopenia. Younger animals may have higher lymphocyte and total WBC counts than those considered normal for adults.[1]

Neutrophilia

Bacterial infection is the most common cause of pathologic neutrophilia (Boxes 25-1 and 25-2). In the acute stage of the infection, a left shift (presence of increased immature neutrophil granulocytes in the peripheral blood) may appear.[1,6] Left shift with concomitant mature neutrophilia is called a regenerative left shift. Rebound neutrophilia often follows neutropenia associated with endotoxemia, and it is usually a good prognostic indicator. Neutrophilia is most pronounced while bacterial infections are being localized, especially with abscess formation. Chronic localized infections rarely are attended by a left shift, and in cattle the neutrophil count may increase only minimally or not at all. Horses with chronic bacterial infections often show only a mild mature neutrophilia attended by lymphopenia and a normal total WBC count.

Neutrophilia may also accompany inflammation caused by neoplasia or severe injury or may arise during the postoperative period. Less common causes of neutrophilia include parasitic and mycotic infections, tumors that cause secretion of endogenous corticosteroids, toxins, and some metabolic diseases such as pregnancy toxemia.

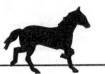

BOX 25-2

Causes of Neutrophilia in Ruminants

COMMON CAUSES
Stress, exogenous corticosteroid administration
Chronic pneumonia
Chronic traumatic reticuloperitonitis
Peritonitis
Internal abscessation
Caseous lymphadenitis (O, C)
Mycoplasmal or chlamydial polyarthritis (O, C)
Chronic pyelonephritis
Chronic metritis
Liver abscesses
Enteritis
Umbilical abscessation
Chronic salmonellosis
Septic arthritis

UNCOMMON CAUSES
Autoimmune hemolytic anemia
Toxins
Pregnancy toxemia (O, C)
Bovine granulocytopathy syndrome

C, Caprine; *O,* ovine.

BOX 25-3

Causes of Neutropenia in the Horse

COMMON CAUSES
Acute salmonellosis
Acute toxic colitis
Acute peritonitis (ruptured viscus)
Gram-negative septicemia, endotoxemia
Neonatal septicemia
Acute pleuritis
Acute metritis
Proximal enteritis (duodenitis, proximal jejunitis)
Equine influenza
Equine herpesvirus type 1 infection

LESS COMMON CAUSES
Equine ehrlichial colitis (Potomac fever, *Ehrlichia risticii* infection)
Equine ehrlichiosis (*Ehrlichia equi* infection)
Idiopathic aplastic anemia
Equine viral arteritis
Radiation toxicosis
Myelophthisic disease (e.g., eosinophilic leukemia)

BOX 25-4

Causes of Neutropenia in Ruminants

COMMON CAUSES
Gram-negative septicemia, endotoxemia
Septic metritis
Septic (coliform) mastitis
Diffuse peritonitis
Ruptured uterus with peritonitis
Ruptured abomasal ulcer
Acute salmonellosis
Acute pneumonia
Toxemia- or toxin-induced bone marrow suppression
Fat cow syndrome (fatty liver)
Clostridial infection

UNCOMMON CAUSES
Bovine virus diarrhea
Bracken fern toxicosis
Trichloroethylene toxicosis
Radiation toxicosis
Idiopathic aplastic anemia

In large animals the total WBC or neutrophil count may not reflect chronic inflammation; for this reason, examination of neutrophil morphology is paramount in interpreting the leukogram. Bacterial infections, especially those caused by gram-negative organisms, often result in neutrophil cytoplasmic and nuclear alterations, which are referred to as "toxic changes." These changes occur in the bone marrow and include cytoplasmic foaminess, vacuolation, and/or basophilia; reddish purple "toxic" granules; bluish cytoplasmic inclusions called Döhle bodies; and bizarre giant forms with or without polyploidy. The changes do not accompany other causes for neutrophilia.

Neutropenia

The usual causes of neutropenia in the large animal species are bacterial septicemia and endotoxemia caused by gastrointestinal disease, metritis, or coliform mastitis (Boxes 25-3 and 25-4). Some viral diseases and anaphylaxis also cause neutropenia.

A degenerative left shift, generally associated with neutropenia, occurs when immature neutrophils appear in the peripheral blood in greater numbers than mature neutrophils. In species other than cattle, degenerative left shift is an extremely poor prognostic sign. Because cattle have a small bone marrow reserve of neutrophils, immature neutrophils appear quickly in the blood during acute inflammatory diseases and often exceed the mature neutrophils. A marked fall in the WBC count commonly is seen in cattle during the developmental stage of an acute localizing inflammatory process such as mastitis or metritis. Once neutrophil production has intensified, the left shift disappears and mature neutrophilia intervenes. Neutropenia that persists longer than 4 days is a sign of inadequate granulopoiesis, which sometimes occurs subsequent to severe toxemia. Neutropenia apparently is rare in goats.

The severity of toxemia is reflected by the number of "toxic" neutrophils and the degree of toxic changes. In diseases causing severe toxemia, precursor cells in the bone marrow become vacuolated and fail to divide, thereby contributing to the existing neutropenia. This bone marrow hypoplasia subsequent to severe infection and inflammation is seen most often in cattle.

In rare cases, neutropenia may develop subsequent to myelophthisic disease, idiopathic aplastic anemia, myelofibrosis, or bone marrow suppression by drugs, chemicals, or ionizing radiation. Lymphosarcoma may involve the bone marrow in rare cases.

Lymphocytosis

Pathologic lymphocytosis is uncommon, occurring occasionally with chronic viral infections and autoimmune

---

BOX 25-5

Causes of Lymphocytosis in the Horse

COMMON CAUSE
Excitement, exercise

UNCOMMON CAUSES
Lymphocytic leukemia
Equine infectious anemia

BOX 25-6

Causes of Lymphocytosis in Ruminants

Persistent lymphocytosis (bovine leukosis virus infection)
Lymphocytic leukemia
Chronic infections (pneumonia, peritonitis, pericarditis, liver abscess)

BOX 25-7

Causes of Lymphopenia in the Horse

COMMON CAUSES
Stress, exogenous corticosteroid administration
Equine influenza
Equine herpesvirus type 1 infection
Endotoxemia, septicemia
Acute peritonitis (gastrointestinal rupture)

LESS COMMON CAUSES
Malnutrition, starvation
Equine viral arteritis
Combined immunodeficiency disease

BOX 25-8

Causes of Lymphopenia in Ruminants

COMMON CAUSES
Stress, exogenous corticosteroid administration
Gram-negative septicemia, endotoxemia
Septic mastitis
Diffuse peritonitis
Ruptured abomasal ulcer
Acute pneumonia
Infectious bovine rhinotracheitis

UNCOMMON CAUSES
Bovine virus diarrhea
Immunodeficiency

BOX 25-9

Causes of Monocytosis in Large Animals

UNCOMMON CAUSES
Granulomatous disease
Chronic bacterial infections

BOX 25-10

Causes of Eosinophilia in the Horse

UNCOMMON CAUSES
Internal parasitism
Cutaneous habronemiasis
Systemic hypersensitivity reaction
Lymphosarcoma
Eosinophilic leukemia

---

disease processes (Boxes 25-5 and 25-6). Lymphocytic leukemia is rare in large animals. Thirty percent of cattle infected with BLV are leukemic (see Chapter 35), and lymphocytosis may persist in the absence of lymphoma or leukemia. Physiologic lymphocytosis associated with epinephrine release caused by excitement or exercise is common in horses under 2 years of age.

Lymphopenia

Causes of lymphopenia include acute viral diseases, endotoxin release, severe bacterial infection, septicemia, rickettsial diseases, malnutrition, tumors that cause increased release of corticosteroids, and immunodeficiency (Boxes 25-7 and 25-8). Persistent lymphopenia is a poor prognostic indicator. Increasing lymphocyte counts represent recovery.

Monocytosis

Monocytosis occurs with chronic inflammation (Box 25-9). Because the monocyte count is not highly responsive to inflammatory disease in large animals, it is not an especially useful part of the leukogram.[6]

Monocytopenia

Endotoxin release and viremia may cause monocytopenia. Monocytopenia occurs initially during stress periods associated with corticosteroid release and may be followed by monocytosis.

Eosinophilia

Eosinophilia is uncommon in large animals but may occur with diseases that involve an interaction between antigen, IgE antibody, and mast cells or basophils, such as parasitic infections, allergic respiratory diseases, and dermatoses (Boxes 25-10 and 25-11). In contrast to humans and small animals, visceral larval migrans rarely induce peripheral eosinophilia. Tissue protein breakdown (malignancies, chronic suppurative processes) may cause eosinophilia in rare cases through the release of histamine or eosinophilic chemotactic factor of anaphylaxis from mast cells. Histamine in the blood attracts bone marrow eosinophils to the circulation. For eosinophilia to occur in response to parasitism, a parasite protein must be released and processed by cells infiltrating the tissue site of parasitic lodgement.[1] Thus eosinophilia is unlikely to

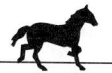

accompany intestinal parasitism when the parasite is free-living in the lumen.

Eosinophilic granulocytic leukemia is rare in large animal species but has been reported in horses.[7] The circulation of bizarre, immature eosinophils differentiates this from other causes of eosinophilia.

Eosinopenia

Eosinopenia is difficult to evaluate, because the leukograms of clinically normal animals may contain very few eosinophils. Eosinopenia may occur secondary to an increase in endogenous or exogenous corticosteroids. Eosinopenia also may be seen with active inflammatory processes.

Basophilia and Basopenia

Basophils are rarely seen in the peripheral blood of the large animal species, although they are more frequently encountered than in dogs and cats.[1] Changes in the number of basophils are difficult to interpret. Stress causes a reduction in their number, whereas basophilia may be seen with allergic dermatitis and delayed hypersensitivity reactions.

APPROACH TO INTERPRETATION OF THE LEUKOGRAM IN THE HORSE

The equine neutrophil to leukocyte (N/L) ratio declines from approximately 2.8 at birth to 1.1 between 1 and 2 months of age and to 0.9 between 6 and 8 months. An N/L ratio near 1 persists through 2 years and increases with age to approximately 2 as lymphocyte numbers are reduced. The total WBC count increases from birth through 3 months of age, is slightly above adult values between 3 months and 2 years of age, and then starts to decline. Physiologic leukocytosis is quite common in horses under 2 years of age.[1]

During chronic and established inflammatory diseases, horses generally have a mature neutrophilia and lymphopenia that may or may not result in leukocytosis.[6] The degree of leukocytosis in chronic suppurative diseases rarely exceeds 20,000/µl. Peracute diseases of the gastrointestinal tract and septicemia (especially in neonates), usually attended by endotoxemia, are characterized by leukopenia and a degenerative left shift, the severity of which is correlated with the prognosis. In the most severe cases, the left shift includes myelocytes and neutrophils that show marked "toxic" changes. Survival and recovery are attended by a rebound

neutrophilia (with or without left shift) and monocytosis. Neonates have a small neutrophil reserve and have more sluggish granulopoiesis in response to disease.

Lymphopenia and eosinopenia often occur readily in response to stress or corticosteroid administration. Chronic diseases commonly result in a reduction of the lymphocyte count, which may be under 1000/µl during severe systemic stress. The monocyte is not particularly responsive to disease in horses,[1] but the blood monocyte generally decreases acutely and may increase above normal during chronic inflammatory diseases, especially those associated with tissue necrosis.

APPROACH TO INTERPRETATION OF THE LEUKOGRAM IN RUMINANTS

The general trend is for the WBC count to be higher in calves through 2 years of age and then decline with advancing age. Sheep and goat leukocyte counts increase through 2 to 3 months of age and then decline in adulthood to levels seen at birth. In cattle and sheep, neutrophils exceed lymphocytes at birth, but the ratio is reversed within the first week of life, and this ratio persists as a species characteristic. A reduction in the number of lymphocytes without similar changes in neutrophils produces an N/L ratio near unity in goats over 3 years of age.

Acute inflammatory disease and infection in cattle (e.g., neonatal septicemia, salmonellosis, enteritis, metritis, and coliform mastitis) cause a rapid drop in the WBC count because of migration of mature neutrophils to the site of inflammation, margination of neutrophils, and stress-induced loss of lymphocytes. The bone marrow has a small reserve of mature neutrophils, and immature forms (bands, metamyelocytes) are released into the circulation, creating a degenerative left shift during the first 2 to 3 days of acute inflammation. By the fourth day bone marrow granulopoiesis usually has increased sufficiently to meet the tissue demand for neutrophils, causing a normal leukocyte count with a left shift. If the inflammatory stimulus persists, a mature neutrophilia may develop. Generally, the N/L ratio increases without leukocytosis. Severe systemic toxemia or chronic infections (or both) may cause granulopoietic depression and neutropenia.

Approximately 30% of cattle infected with BLV develop a benign persistent lymphocytosis, defined as an absolute blood lymphocyte count over 3 standard deviations above the normal mean for at least 3 months. Although these cells are BLV infected, cattle with lymphocytosis are clinically normal, and most do not develop enzootic bovine lymphosarcoma (EBL).[8] Approximately 50% of cattle with EBL have a mild to moderate lymphocytosis, and leukemia is present in 10% to 30% of cases.[1] Lymphocytosis, usually attended by neutrophilia, occurs sometimes as a result of chronic pyogenic conditions such as liver abscess, pericarditis, pulmonary abscess, and traumatic reticuloperitonitis.

The leukogram changes in sheep generally are similar to those of cattle. Parturition and adverse weather conditions induce typical corticosteroid-induced neutrophilia, lymphopenia, and eosinopenia.

Goats differ from cattle and sheep in that the leukogram typically has an equal or slightly greater number of neutrophils than lymphocytes.[1] The total WBC count during inflammatory diseases may attain levels higher than 25,000/µl because of neutrophilia. A regenerative left shift is a common response to subacute or chronic inflammation. Leukopenia is rare.

An inherited syndrome characterized by marked neutrophilia and an increased susceptibility to bacterial infections has been recognized in Holstein-Friesian cattle under 2 years of age.[9] Affected calves have a history of anorexia, weight loss, and failure to thrive, with signs of chronic, intermittent pneumonia and diarrhea. Lymphadenopathy, periodontitis, and generalized dermatitis are also features of the syndrome. The neutrophils of these animals are dysfunctional because of a single mutation in CD 18 that causes a lack of surface glycoproteins, called β_2-integrins, that are important in cell adhesion processes.[10] Calves that are heterozygous for the defect do not have dysfunctional leukocytes compared with those of clinically normal calves.[11]

REFERENCES

1. Jain NC: *Schalm's veterinary hematology*, ed 4, Philadelphia, 1986, Lea & Febiger.
2. Duncan JR, Prasse KW, Mahaffey EA: *Veterinary laboratory medicine: clinical pathology*, ed 3, Ames, Iowa, 1994, Iowa State University Press.
3. Becker EL: Chemotaxis, *J Allergy Clin Immunol* 66:97-105, 1980.
4. Roitt I, Brostoff J, Male D: *Immunoloyg*, St Louis, 1998, Mosby.
5. Morris DD, Moore JN, Crowe N: Serum tumor necrosis factor activity in horses with colic attributable to gastrointestinal disease, *Am J Vet Res* 52:1565-1595, 1991.
6. Morris DD: The haemolymphatic system. In Higgins AJ, Wright IM, eds: *The equine manual*, London, 1995, WB Saunders.
7. Morris DD et al: Eosinophilic myeloproliferative disorder in a horse, *J Am Vet Med Assoc* 185:993-996, 1984.
8. Ferrer JR: Bovine lymphosarcoma, *Adv Vet Med* 24:1-68, 1980.
9. Gerardi AS: Bovine leukocyte adhesion deficiency: a review of a modern disease and its implications, *Res Vet Sci* 61:183-186, 1996.
10. Nagahata H et al: Expression and rate of adhesion of molecule CD 18 on bovine neutrophils, *Can J Vet Res* 59:1-7, 1999.
11. Syses KM et al: Analysis of surface antigen expression and host defense functions in leukocyte from calves heterozygous or homozygous for bovine leukocyte adhesion deficiency, *Am J Vet Res* 60:1255-1216, 1999.

Alterations in Blood Proteins

DEBRA DEEM MORRIS

JANET K. JOHNSTON
Consulting Editors

MAJOR ALTERATIONS

Proteins play an integral role in numerous physiologic processes. Not only are they important to the basic structural integrity of most body tissues, but as enzymes and hormones, they also regulate many of the body's biochemical reactions. Hemostasis, resistance to infection, and acid-base balance depend on protein metabolism. Plasma proteins also act as carriers for other plasma constituents, and albumin provides osmotic pressure to help maintain proper intravascular volume and prevent edema. Because of the central role proteins play in the body's homeostasis and the close relationship between plasma proteins and tissue proteins, much information about the body's response to disease can be obtained by measuring the total plasma protein and its fractions—albumin, the globulins, and fibrinogen.

Filtration between intravascular and extravascular space, metabolic demands, hormonal balance, nutritional status, and water balance determine the plasma protein concentration of an individual at any given time. Through colostrum absorption, passive transfer of immunoglobulins causes a rise in the total protein concentration of the newborn (see Chapter 49). With time, however, the passively absorbed immunoglobulin concentration declines through natural catabolic degradation. The rate of decline varies among species and classes of immunoglobulins. The time required to reach levels that are no longer protective depends on the initial concentration of the immunoglobulin. The total protein concentration also declines over the next several weeks, even though immunoglobulins are actively produced (Fig. 26-1). In adults the protein concentration remains relatively stable. Pregnancy alters plasma proteins because fetal development imposes additional stress on the dam's protein reserve,[1] and the concentration and response of each protein fraction to different stressors varies among the species.[2,3] In general, however, albumin decreases and globulin (especially α_2-globulin) increases in response to stress.

Several methods are available for determining the concentration of serum or plasma protein. The biuret test is a simple colorimetric technique that has been widely adapted for use in

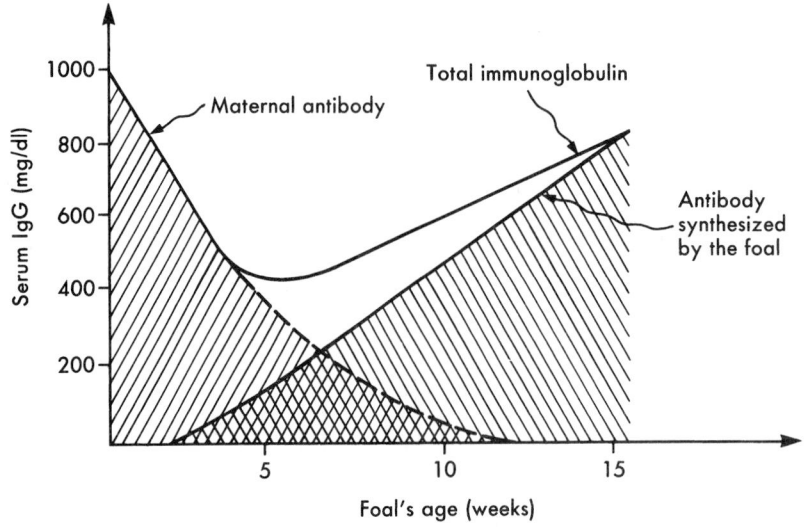

FIG. 26-1 ■ Immunoglobulin in foal serum during the first 15 weeks of life. (From Tizard I: *Veterinary immunology*, ed 3, Philadelphia, 1987, WB Saunders.)

TABLE 26-1

Normal Serum Protein Values for Horse, Cow, Sheep, and Goat

	Value	Horse	Cow	Sheep	Goat
Total	g/dl	5.2-7.9	6.74-7.46	6-7.9	6.4-7
Albumin	g/dl	2.6-3.7	3.03-3.55	2.4-3	2.7-3.9
Globulin	g/dl	2.62-4.04	3-3.48	3.5-5.7	2.7-4.1
α_1	g/dl	0.06-0.7			
α	g/dl		0.75-0.88	0.3-0.6	0.5-0.7
α_2	g/dl	0.31-1.31			
β_1	g/dl	0.4-1.58	0.7-1.2		0.7-1.2
β	g/dl		0.8-1.12		
β_2	g/dl	0.29-0.89		0.4-1.4	
γ_1	g/dl		0.7-2.2		
γ	g/dl	0.55-1.9	1.69-2.23		0.9-3
γ_2	g/dl		0.2-1.1		
A/G ratio		0.62-1.46	0.84-0.94		0.63-1.26
Fibrinogen	mg/dl	200-400	200-700	200-500	200-300

Kaneko JJ: In Kaneko JJ, ed: *Clinical biochemistry of domestic animals*, ed 4, San Diego, Calif, 1989, Academic Press.
A/G, Albumin to globulin ratio.

automated chemical analyzers. It is highly specific for protein, especially in the range of 1 to 10 g/dl. Unfortunately the biuret technique is not precise enough for evaluation of very low levels, such as those found in cerebrospinal fluid. Refractometry is a useful method for rapidly determining the protein level in serum, plasma, or other body fluids because the refractive index of a solution is proportional to its protein concentration. Mild hemolysis or icterus of a solution does not interfere with its accuracy; however, turbid or lipemic solutions may alter the transmission of light and provide inaccurate results.

The concentration of the total plasma protein and of the individual fractions varies between species (Table 26-1). When a dysproteinemia is suspected, the total plasma (or serum) protein concentration, albumin to globulin (A/G) ratio, serum protein electrophoresis results, and plasma fibrinogen concentration should be evaluated. The A/G ratio can easily be calculated from most automated serum chem-

istry profiles. Changes in the A/G ratio often are the first indication of a dysproteinemia. Because this method of albumin measurement can be inaccurate when values are markedly low,[4] the A/G ratio is most accurately obtained from serum protein electrophoresis.

When the practitioner is confronted with a dysproteinemia, serum protein electrophoresis (SPE) is necessary to quantitate the individual protein fractions that make up the total. Fig. 26-2 shows normal equine and bovine SPE results. Albumin is identified as a discrete molecular compound by a sharp, narrow-based peak nearest the anode. The sharpness of the albumin peak is a measure of the quality of the SPE procedure and is used to differentiate polyclonal globulin peaks. The α-, β-, and γ-globulins form broad-based peaks during their migration in the electrical field, and depending on the species, one or two types of the individual fraction normally are present.

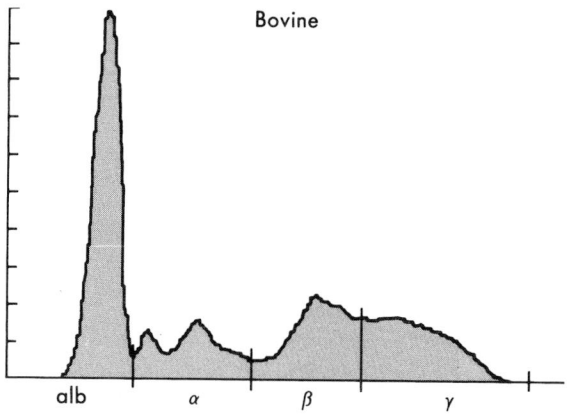

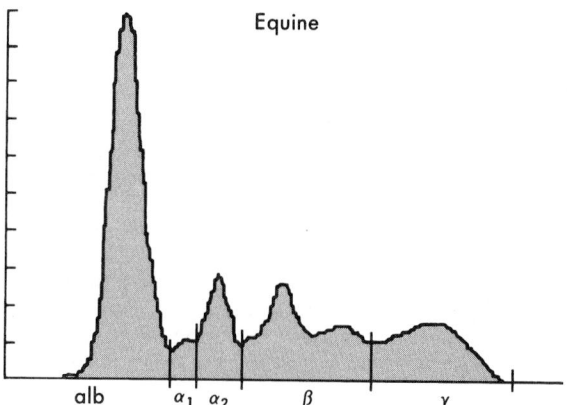

FIG. 2-2 ▍▍ Normal bovine and equine serum protein electrophoresis. *alb*, Albumin. (Courtesy Dr. Dennis DiNicola, Purdue University, West Lafayette, Ind.)

BOX 26-1

Causes of Hyperproteinemia in the Horse

PANHYPERPROTEINEMIA-DEHYDRATION
Common Causes
Acute toxic colitis of unknown etiology
Acute salmonellosis
Potomac horse fever
Intestinal clostridiosis
Intestinal strangulating obstruction
Proximal enteritis
Gram-negative sepsis, endotoxemia
Botulism
Choking (esophageal obstruction)

Less Common Causes
Chronic renal failure
Chronic hepatic disease
Guttural pouch mycosis with dysphagia
Equine protozoal myelitis
Salt toxicity
Toxins, poisonous plants
Lead toxicity
Yellow star thistle poisoning (dysphagia)
Dysphagia of unknown etiology

HYPERGLOBULINEMIA
Common Causes
Abdominal (mesenteric) abscess (including "bastard" strangles)
Pulmonary abscess
Chronic pleuritis
Purpura hemorrhagica
Equine infectious anemia

Less Common Causes
Chronic hepatic disease
Strongylosis
Lymphosarcoma
Immune-mediated cytopenia

HYPERPROTEINEMIA

Hyperproteinemia can result from an elevation in the concentration of all plasma proteins (panhyperproteinemia) or an absolute increase in globulins (hyperglobulinemia) (Boxes 26-1 and 26-2).

Panhyperproteinemia

An increase in the concentration of all blood proteins most commonly results from loss of the fluid component of the blood. Dehydration (decreased fluid intake or excessive fluid loss or both) causes hyperproteinemia with an associated increase in packed cell volume (PCV); however, a dehydrated, anemic animal will have hyperproteinemia with a normal or subnormal PCV. The A/G ratio will be normal. In large animals a total plasma protein concentration above 8 g/dl can be expected with severe dehydration. Initially dehydration causes withdrawal of tissue fluid into the intravascular space as the body attempts to maintain adequate blood volume. As dehydration proceeds, intravascular fluid is lost; hemoconcentration results with a relative increase in total protein and progressive peripheral circulatory failure. If renal function is adequate, urine concentration increases and output decreases in an attempt to compensate for the fluid loss; water is ab-

sorbed from the gastrointestinal (GI) tract, assuming that GI function is normal.

A decrease in fluid intake can result from unavailability of water, lack of thirst caused by depression or toxemia, or dysphagia.

In rare cases polyuria with renal failure, exudation from extensive skin wounds, and excessive sweating can cause dehydration. Dehydration most commonly occurs after excessive fluid loss, especially from diarrhea. Other causes of increased fluid loss from the blood include fluid sequestration with an intestinal obstruction, vagal indigestion with internal vomiting, and grain engorgement.

Clinical signs of dehydration include tachycardia, an increase in the capillary refill time, and a decrease in pulse pressure, skin elasticity, and urine output. Improvement with appropriate fluid therapy is evidenced by improvement in clinical signs and a decrease in the PCV and the plasma protein concentrations. A decline in the plasma proteins while the PCV remains elevated often indicates protein loss into a third space (this occurs most commonly in horses with severe colitis) and is a poor prognostic sign. Massive plasma transfusions are indicated in such patients.

BOX 26-2

Causes of Hyperproteinemia in Ruminants

PANHYPERPROTEINEMIA-DEHYDRATION
Common Causes
Ruminal acidosis (grain overload)
Abomasal torsion
Acute salmonellosis
Peritonitis
Sepsis, toxemia (mastitis, metritis)
Intussusception
Vagal indigestion
Oral or pharyngeal foreign body with dysphagia
Coccidiosis
Diarrhea, undifferentiated
Salt toxicity
Toxins, poisonous plants

Less Common Causes
Renal amyloidosis
Lymphosarcoma
Johne's disease
Pregnancy toxemia
Rabies

HYPERGLOBULINEMIA
Common Causes
Abdominal abscess (traumatic reticuloperitonitis, uterine
    tear, other)
Chronic pneumonia
Umbilical abscess
Lymphosarcoma
Caseous lymphadenitis (sheep and goats)
Other abscess

Less Common Causes
Parasitism
Pregnancy

Hyperglobulinemia

Hyperproteinemia in a patient with apparently normal hydration usually is due to hyperglobulinemia, because hyperalbuminemia is due to dehydration. The most common cause of hyperglobulinemia is a generalized increase in γ-globulins (polyclonal gammopathy). This represents the activity of plasma cells in response to chronic antigenic stimulation. Chronic infection, abscess, amyloidosis, and neoplasia typically result in a generalized increase in γ-globulins. Some immunoglobulins (particularly IgM) migrate in the β-globulin region, and polyclonal increases in β-globulins usually are associated with an increase in γ-globulins. A concomitant decrease in albumin synthesis commonly occurs. Chronic hepatitis, hepatic abscess, and suppurative diseases are usually accompanied by an increase in the γ-globulin concentration. Immune-mediated disease processes (e.g., autoimmune hemolytic anemia and autoimmune thrombocytopenia), lymphosarcoma, and other tumors of the reticuloendothelial system typically demonstrate polyclonal increases in γ-globulin.

An abnormal increase in a single immunoglobulin class is known as monoclonal gammopathy. On SPE, the monoclonal peak is as sharp or sharper than the albumin peak and is the result of a single clone of plasma cells producing an increased amount of immunoglobulin. Monoclonal gammopathies can be caused by multiple myeloma, lymphocytic leukemia, and other tumors of the reticuloendothelial system

(e.g., lymphosarcoma). The clinical signs depend on the degree of organ involvement, plasma cell proliferation, and protein production. Increased susceptibility to infection can be expected as a result of decreased production of normal immunoglobulins, leukopenia, and/or impaired granulocyte function. Internal parasitism, especially strongylosis, may cause an associated β-globulin spike that does not usually cause hyperglobulinemia. An increase in both β- and γ-globulin fractions (β-bridging) can occur with intense antigenic stimulation, chronic active hepatitis, or lymphosarcoma.

The α-globulins are divided into α_1 and α_2 fractions in most species except ruminants. α-Globulins are known as acute-phase reactants because their concentration rapidly increases after tissue injury or inflammation. α_2-Antiplasmin rapidly increases,[5] whereas ceruloplasmin[6] increases several days after the onset of inflammation.[7] An increase in C-reactive protein has been associated with pneumonitis, enteritis, and arthritis in horses.[8] The increase does not generally cause hyperglobulinemia.

HYPOPROTEINEMIA

Hypoalbuminemia

Hypoalbuminemia often exists despite normal total plasma protein levels. The three most common causes of hypoalbuminemia are a decrease in production, an increase in loss by the gut, and renal loss (Boxes 26-3 and 26-4).

Albumin is produced by the liver, has the lowest molecular weight, and is the most abundant of the plasma proteins, accounting for 75% of plasma osmotic activity. In addition to maintaining osmotic pressure, a major function of albumin is to bind and transport plasma components that do not have a specific transport protein. Hypoalbuminemia causes a decrease in the A/G ratio.

Starvation, malnutrition, and chronic GI disorders that interfere with digestion and absorption may lead to inadequate provision of amino acid substrate for general protein production. Hypoalbuminemia often precedes the development of panhypoproteinemia with dietary protein deficiencies. In certain cases diets that appear to be well balanced and to provide adequate protein nutrition may actually be inadequate in demanding conditions.

Although albumin is produced by the liver, synthesis does not usually decrease in acute liver disease. Chronic, diffuse liver diseases such as chronic hepatitis, fibrosis, and hepatic neoplasia may cause hypoalbuminemia. Because the half-life of albumin is prolonged in horses and cattle compared with that of dogs and human beings,[9] hypoalbuminemia rarely occurs with large animal hepatic disease.[10] If it does, it often is accompanied by increases in β- and γ-globulins. Because these changes occur late in the course of the disease, they may be of more prognostic than diagnostic value.

Increased metabolic demands such as occur with fever, trauma, surgery, and neoplasia can lead to a state of negative nitrogen balance with excessive albumin breakdown. Chronic antigenic stimulation can also result in increased albumin catabolism to provide necessary amino acids for immunoglobulin production; however, this increased albumin catabolism typically does not result in a change in the total plasma protein concentration.

Excessive protein loss usually occurs through the urinary and GI tracts. Normally urine contains little or no protein, but transient physiologic proteinuria occurs with exercise, stress, convulsions, and excessive protein intake, as well as in neonates; however, none of these factors cause hypoproteinemia.

Clinically significant proteinuria consists primarily of albumin, resulting in subsequent hypoalbuminemia. Because of its small size and low molecular weight, albumin is readily filtered through defects in the glomerular basement

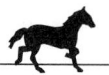

BOX 26-3

Causes of Hypoproteinemia in the Horse

HYPOALBUMINEMIA
Common Causes
Parasitism
Glomerulonephritis
Pyelonephritis
Idiopathic granulomatous enteritis
Intestinal lymphosarcoma
Parasitism
Salmonellosis
Equine ehrlichial enterocolitis (Potomac horse fever)
Colitis X
Clostridiosis
Nonsteroidal antiinflammatory drug toxicosis

Less Common Causes
Chronic hepatic fibrosis (pyrrolizidine alkaloid toxicity
    and other causes)
Hepatic neoplasia
Chronic hepatitis
Amyloidosis
Tuberculosis
Histoplasmosis
Chronic eosinophilic gastroenteritis
Starvation

PANHYPOPROTEINEMIA
Common Causes
Excessive fluid therapy or water intake
Acute blood loss
Gastrointestinal ulceration
Strangulating gastrointestinal obstruction, infarction
Protein-losing enteropathy (chronic granulomatous bowel
    disease)
Acute severe peritonitis
Nonsteroidal antiinflammatory drug toxicity
Glomerulonephritis

Less Common Causes
Blood-sucking gastrointestinal or external parasites
Intestinal lymphosarcoma
Urinary blood loss
Congenital vascular disorders:
    Renal trauma
    Renal calculi
    Pyelonephritis
    Neoplasia
    Cystic calculi
Disseminated intravascular coagulation
Immune-mediated thrombocytopenia
Congestive heart failure

BOX 26-4

Causes of Hypoproteinemia in Ruminants

HYPOALBUMINEMIA
Common Causes
Protein malnutrition, starvation
Amyloidosis
Pyelonephritis
Glomerulonephritis
Salmonellosis
Johne's disease
Trichostrongylus infection

Less Common Causes
Chronic liver failure
Intestinal lymphangiectasia
Intestinal lymphosarcoma

PANHYPOPROTEINEMIA
Common Causes
Excessive intravenous fluid therapy or water intake
Acute blood loss
Abomasal ulceration
Blood-sucking gastrointestinal or external parasites
Gastrointestinal ulceration

Less Common Causes
Ingestion of caustic chemicals
Strangulation, infarction of intestine
Congestive heart failure
Pyelonephritis
Urinary tract blood loss

membrane. Glomerulonephritis, amyloidosis, and less commonly pyelonephritis cause albuminuria, which may lead to hypoproteinemia.[7]

Protein-losing enteropathy refers to the excessive loss of plasma proteins into the GI tract, with resultant hypoproteinemia. The diagnosis of protein-losing enteropathy usually is made after ruling out protein loss through other routes (urine), increased protein catabolism, and inability to produce protein (liver disease). The clinically important mechanisms of GI protein loss are defective lymphatic drainage, increased mucosal permeability, exudation as a result of inflammation, and ulceration. In a study of horses with diarrhea, albumin was lower in horses that died than in those

that survived.[11] Panhypoproteinemia eventually develops, especially when inflammation is a cause.

The most common cause of protein-losing enteropathy in the horse is idiopathic granulomatous enteritis.[12] Tuberculosis and histoplasmosis also cause "granulomatous changes." Lesions are most commonly located in the small intestine, and weight loss results. Other causes of chronic protein-losing enteropathy in the horse include eosinophilic gastroenteritis, intestinal lymphosarcoma, and strongyle larval migrans. Salmonellosis, nonsteroidal antiinflammatory drug (NSAID) toxicity, and other causes of acute colitis and enteritis may result in hypoalbuminemia and a general loss of all plasma proteins. A decreasing plasma protein level that occurs with an elevated PCV indicates acute protein loss from the gut.

The most common cause of chronic protein-losing enteropathy in ruminants is Johne's disease. Hypoalbuminemia causes hypoproteinemia. *Trichostrongylus* infection, intestinal lymphangiectasia, and intestinal lymphosarcoma can cause a primary hypoalbuminemic hypoproteinemia.

Clinical signs of hypoalbuminemia include edema of the distal extremities, ventral body wall, and face. The albumin level generally must be below 1.5 g/dl in the horse and below 1 g/dl in ruminants before these clinical signs occur. Pharyngeal and laryngeal edema may result in upper airway obstruction, necessitating a tracheostomy.

Panhypoproteinemia

Vigorous fluid therapy or excess water intake can cause dilution of the plasma proteins, with subsequent panhypoproteinemia. Panhypoproteinemia occurs most often in animals that have acute protein-losing colitis or enteritis and that are receiving intravenous fluid therapy. Similarly, animals that lose large amounts of sodium through diarrhea and then drink fresh water may become hyponatremic as a result of a relative water excess.

Acute blood loss results in loss of plasma proteins and a dilution of the remaining protein by rapid movement of interstitial fluid into the intravascular space to help maintain intravascular volume. This dilutional effect is intensified by the excess water intake that commonly occurs after acute blood loss. Acute hemorrhage resulting from trauma, severe epistaxis, or internal vascular rupture should be ruled out in a hypoproteinemic, anemic animal.

GI blood loss can result from abomasal or gastric ulcers, blood-sucking parasites (particularly *Haemonchus contortus* in ruminants), viral or bacterial infection, azotemia, neoplastic invasion, or exposure to caustic chemicals. NSAID toxicosis and strangulating GI obstructions and infarctions can result in mucosal necrosis and leakage of plasma proteins into the gut lumen. Although protein-losing enteropathy initially results in hypoalbuminemia, it eventually results in panhypoproteinemia.

Blood loss from the urinary tract can result from congenital vascular disorders, renal trauma, renal calculi, pyelonephritis, neoplasia, or cystic calculi. Coagulation dysfunction, such as disseminated intravascular coagulation (DIC) or immune-mediated thrombocytopenia, may cause blood loss by way of the GI or urinary tract.

Congestive heart failure may cause hypoproteinemia by a number of mechanisms. Extracellular fluid is diluted by the retained sodium and water, and plasma protein is lost into interstitial spaces, ascitic fluid, and the GI tract. Hypoproteinemia also can occur as a result of acute severe peritonitis with massive protein exudation, as is seen with a ruptured GI viscus.

ALTERATIONS IN PLASMA FIBRINOGEN

Fibrinogen is a large molecular weight protein produced by the liver. Its primary function is to serve as substrate for thrombin in the formation of fibrin during hemostasis. Fibrinogen, as an acute-phase reactant protein, increases its concentration during active inflammatory disease and is a useful marker in assessment of the inflammatory response.

Hyperfibrinogenemia

Plasma fibrinogen is nearly always increased during severe inflammatory conditions and may increase with milder inflammation that is not associated with a leukocytosis or neutrophilia (Boxes 26-5 and 26-6). After surgical treatment for subchondral bone cysts and osteochondrosis dessicans, horses still had hyperfibrinogenemia 15 days after surgery.[13] Hyperfibrinogenemia generally occurs with infectious, suppurative, traumatic, and neoplastic diseases and subsides as the condition improves. Chronic inflammation is associated with hyperfibrinogenemia, but the degree of hyperfibrinogenemia is not always directly correlated with the severity of the disease. Fibrinogen is an especially useful indicator of inflammation in cattle because of their greater capacity to produce fibrinogen,[14] which is a more sensitive indicator of inflammation than the leukocyte count (see Table 26-1).

Hypofibrinogenemia

A decrease in the fibrinogen concentration may result from increased consumption of fibrinogen or decreased synthesis. Severe, diffuse liver damage, such as occurs with severe pyrrolizidine alkaloid toxicity, causes a decrease in the fibrinogen concentration, whereas mild to moderate inflammatory liver disease can result in an increase in plasma fi-

---

BOX 26-5

Causes of Hyperfibrinogenemia in the Horse

Abscess (abdominal or other)
Chronic peritonitis
Pleuritis
Pneumonia
Osteomyelitis
Septic arthritis
Cholelithiasis
Neoplasia with inflammatory response
Vasculitis (equine purpura hemorrhagica)
Cellulitis
Gastrointestinal inflammation
Salmonellosis

BOX 26-6

Causes of Hyperfibrinogenemia in Ruminants

Acute mastitis, especially coliform
Abscess
Traumatic reticuloperitonitis, pericarditis
Salmonellosis
Gastrointestinal inflammation
Pyelonephritis
Endocarditis
Pleuritis
Pneumonia
Chronic peritonitis
Necrotic rumenitis
Lymphosarcoma
Septic arthritis
Cellulitis
Omphalophlebitis
Osteomyelitis

---

brinogen. With DIC and fibrinolysis a decrease in the fibrinogen concentration would be expected; however, hypofibrinogenemia is not common in horses with DIC. Inflammatory disorders often are the cause of DIC, and a compensatory increase in production masks the increased consumption. In rare cases rapid removal of fibrinogen from the circulation may occur as a result of primary hyperfibrinolysis. An erroneous finding of hypofibrinogenemia may result if the fibrinogen concentration is quantitated from samples containing clotted blood.

REFERENCES

1. Larson BL, Kendall KA: Changes in specific blood serum protein levels associated with parturition in the bovine, *J Dairy Sci* 40:659, 1957.
2. Kaneko JJ: Serum proteins and the dysproteinemias. In Kaneko JJ, ed: *Clinical biochemistry of domestic animals*, ed 4, San Diego, 1989, Academic Press.
3. Cornelius CE et al: Distribution and turnover of iodine-131-tagged bovine albumin in normal and parasitized cattle, *Am J Vet Rec* 23:837, 1962.
4. Mattheeuws DRG et al: Compartmentalization and turnover of I-labeled albumin and globulin in horses, *Am J Vet Res* 27:699, 1966.
5. Topper MJ, Prasse KW: Analysis of coagulation proteins as acute phase reactants in horses with colic, *Am J Vet Rec* 59(5):542-545, 1998.
6. Okumura M et al: Isolation, characterization, and quantitative analysis of ceruloplasmin, *Am J Vet Rec* 52:1979, 1991.
7. Morris DD, Lee JW: Renal insufficiency due to chronic glomerulonephritis in two horses, *Equine Pract* 4(8):21-32, 1982.

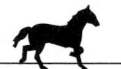
8. Takiguchi M et al: Isolation, characterization, and quantitative analysis of C-reactive protein from horses, *Am J Vet Rec* 51:1215, 1990.
9. Dixon FJ: Half-lives of homologous serum albumins in several species, *Proc Soc Exp Biol Med* 83:287, 1953.
10. Farrago ME et al: Serum protein concentrations in horses with severe liver disease: a retrospective study and review of the literature, *J Vet Intern Med* 9:154-161, 1995.
11. Mair TS, Cripps PJ, Ricketts SW: Diagnostic and prognostic value of serum protein electrophoresis in horses with chronic diarrhea, *Equine Vet J* 25:324, 1993.
12. Eades SC: Diseases affecting plasma proteins. In Colahan PT et al, eds: *Equine medicine and surgery,* ed 5, St Louis, 1999, Mosby.
13. Allen BV, Kold SE: Fibrinogen response to surgical tissue trauma in the horse, *Equine Vet J* 20:441, 1988.
14. McSherry BJ et al: Plasma fibrinogen levels in normal and sick cows, *Can J Comp Med* 34:191, 1970.

Alterations in the Clotting Profile

DEBRA DEEM MORRIS

MAJOR ALTERATIONS

Thrombocytopenia, 434
Prolonged prothrombin time, 435
Prolonged activated partial thromboplastin time, 436
Elevated fibrin/fibrinogen degradation products, 437

Reduced plasma antithrombin III, 437
Hypofibrinogenemia, 438
Abnormalities in other tests, 438

The minimum laboratory data needed to evaluate hemostasis in large animals are a platelet count, plasma fibrinogen, the prothrombin time (PT), activated partial thromboplastin time (APTT), and serum fibrin/fibrinogen degradation products (FDPs). Proper collection and preparation of blood samples is paramount in obtaining accurate results (see Chapter 23). If the laboratory does not have normal values for the species in question, plasma from two or more healthy animals should be collected and assayed in a similar manner for comparison. Table 27-1 shows some normal values that have been published.

THROMBOCYTOPENIA

Thrombocytopenia (a platelet count below 100,000/µl) is caused by one of three basic mechanisms: a decrease in the production of platelets, platelet sequestration, or a shortened platelet life span (Boxes 27-1 and 27-2). *Reduced production* of platelets is the result of a bone marrow abnormality such as infiltration by neoplastic tissue (myelophthisic disease) or aplastic anemia. Occasionally immune-mediated destruction of megakaryocytes causes selectively reduced platelet production. Familial myelofibrosis occurs in some lines of pygmy goats.

Splenomegaly that may occur in acute and chronic infections and in noninfectious inflammatory disorders causes platelet *sequestration,* although this does not generally predispose the animal to hemorrhage. Congestive splenomegaly occurs when venous outflow is occluded by intestinal displacements or congestive heart failure.

Shortened platelet life span is the most common cause of thrombocytopenia in large animals. Excessive consumption of platelets occurs with disseminated intravascular coagulation (DIC), overwhelming septicemia or endotoxemia, and in rare cases in systemic vasculitides. Platelet destruction by immune-mediated mechanisms is a common cause of thrombocytopenia in horses. Viral and rickettsial diseases may cause consumption or immune-mediated thrombocytopenia (IMTP).

Platelets form the initial hemostatic plug, provide phospholipid and a surface for clot formation, and maintain vascular integrity. Thrombocytopenia is characterized by petechial hemorrhages on the oral, nasal, and/or vaginal mucous membranes and the nictitans, sclerae, and pinnae. Epistaxis, melena, hyphema, or hematuria may occur, although spontaneous hemorrhage is rare unless the platelet count drops below 10,000/µl. Prolonged bleeding from injections or wounds and a propensity to form hematomas with minor trauma are quite common when the platelet count drops below 40,000/µl.

Anemia and mild hypoproteinemia accompany significant, chronic blood loss. Other components of the hemostatic system also should be evaluated (e.g., PT, APTT, and FDPs), because thrombocytopenia may be only part of a disseminated coagulopathy. Evaluation of a bone marrow specimen (aspirate, core) is necessary to document adequate

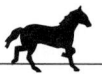

TABLE 27-1

Normal Values for Hemostatic Data in Ruminants and the Horse

	Cattle	Sheep	Goats	Horses
Platelet count ($\times 10^{-3}$/L)	100-800	250-750	300-600	100-600
Fibrinogen (mg/dl)	200-500	100-500	100-400	200-400
Prothrombin time(s)	22-55	—*	9.5-12.5	7-9
Activated partial thromboplastin time(s)	44-64	—	28-52	37-54
Fibrin/fibrinogen degradation products (μg/ml)	<8	<8	—	<32

Modified from Duncan JR et al: *Veterinary laboratory medicine*, ed 3, Ames, 1994, Iowa State University Press; and Kaneko JJ: *Clinical biochemistry of domestic animals*, ed 4, San Diego, Calif, 1989, Academic Press.
*Inadequate data available.

BOX 27-1

Causes of Thrombocytopenia in the Horse

COMMON CAUSES
Disseminated intravascular coagulation (DIC)
Immune-mediated thrombocytopenia (IMTP)
Endotoxemia, septicemia (e.g., acute toxic colitis, intestinal strangulating obstruction, neonatal septicemia)
Equine infectious anemia
Equine ehrlichiosis (*Ehrlichia equi*)
Lymphosarcoma

LESS COMMON CAUSES
Salmonellosis
Equine viral arteritis
Equine influenza
Myeloproliferative disease (myelogenous leukemia)
Plasma cell myeloma
Aplastic anemia
Stachybotryotoxicosis

BOX 27-2

Causes of Thrombocytopenia in Ruminants

COMMON CAUSES
Disseminated intravascular coagulation (DIC)
Bracken fern (*Pteridium aquilinum*) toxicosis
Septic mastitis or metritis (endotoxemia)

LESS COMMON CAUSES
Salmonellosis
Gram-negative sepsis

LESS COMMON CAUSES—cont'd
Trichloroethylene-extracted soybean meal
Lymphosarcoma
Plasma cell myeloma
Immune-mediated thrombocytopenia (IMTP)
Stachybotryotoxicosis
Myelofibrosis (pygmy goats)

---

megakaryocyte numbers if thrombocytopenia is the only laboratory abnormality *or* if pancytopenia is present.

PROLONGED PROTHROMBIN TIME

The prothrombin time is a measure of the extrinsic and common pathways of coagulation (Fig. 27-1). It becomes prolonged when the fibrinogen level drops below 100 mg/dl or with a marked deficiency (less than 50% of normal concentration) of prothrombin and/or clotting factors V, VII, and X. Besides deficiencies of these factors, functional abnormalities or factor inhibitors may be reflected by changes in the PT. The most common mechanisms for prolonging the PT are increased consumption of the relevant clotting factors or failure of the liver to produce these factors. Congenital afibrinogenemia in goats may prolong the PT.[1]

Increased factor consumption usually is caused by DIC, which also causes prolonged APTT and thrombocytopenia (Boxes 27-3 and 27-4). Reduced production occurs as a result of hepatocellular disease or vitamin K deficiency. Vitamin K is necessary for hepatic production of factors II, VII, IX, and X. The action of vitamin K is inhibited by coumarin compounds, which may be found in moldy sweet clover hay or rodenticides. Coumarin derivatives (warfarin) sometimes are used therapeutically in horses.

Clinical signs of clotting factor deficiencies relate to the tendency for spontaneous hemorrhage (e.g., epistaxis, melena, hematuria) or prolonged bleeding after trauma, diagnostic procedures, or surgery. Hematomas or hemarthroses are common after minor trauma or normal exercise. The clotting times are designed primarily for screening purposes and are very insensitive to minor abnormalities of one or more

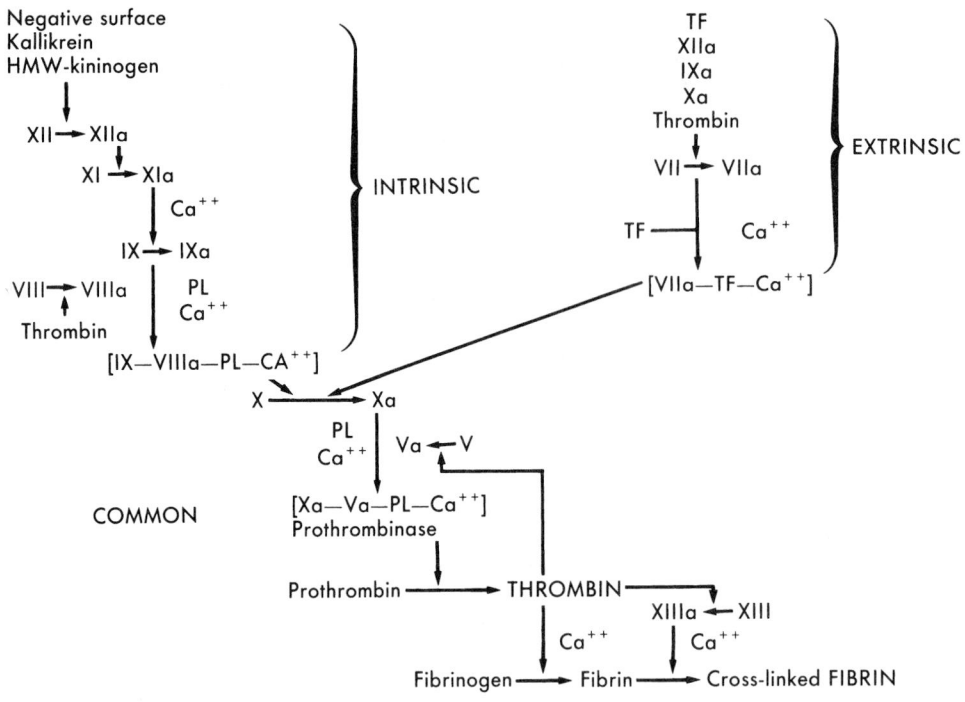

FIG. 27-1 ▓ Coagulation pathways.

BOX 27-3

Causes of Prolonged Prothrombin Time (PT) in the Horse

COMMON CAUSES
Disseminated intravascular coagulation (DIC)
Rodenticide (warfarin) toxicosis
Acute hepatic necrosis
Pyrrolizidine alkaloid toxicosis
Aflatoxicosis
Chronic hepatic fibrosis

LESS COMMON CAUSES
Moldy sweet clover toxicosis

BOX 27-4

Causes of Prolonged Prothrombin Time (PT) in Ruminants

COMMON CAUSES
Moldy sweet clover (*Melilotus* spp.) toxicosis
Disseminated intravascular coagulation (DIC)

LESS COMMON CAUSES
Rodenticide (warfarin) toxicosis
Pyrrolizidine alkaloid toxicosis
Rubratoxicosis
Aflatoxicosis
Bitterweed (*Hymenoxys odorata*) toxicosis
Chronic hepatic fibrosis

factors. Patients with mild bleeding tendencies may require more specialized diagnostic procedures.

PROLONGED ACTIVATED PARTIAL THROMBOPLASTIN TIME

The activated partial thromboplastin time screens the function of the intrinsic coagulation pathway (see Fig. 27-1) and is sensitive to deficiencies or abnormal activity of factors VIII:coagulant (VIII:C), IX, XI, and XII. Insufficiencies of prekallikrein and high molecular weight kininogen may prolong the APTT, depending on the thromboplastin reagent used in the assay. Thromboplastin in which ellagic acid is used as the activator will not demonstrate a prekallikrein deficiency because ellagic acid activates factor XII directly. Kaolin activates factor XII by means of prekallikrein. Of course, the APTT is abnormal if deficiencies of factors in the common pathway exist. The activated coagulation time (ACT) is a simplified variation of the APTT that can be tested by mixing whole blood with activator and calcium.

The most common cause of a prolonged APTT is the increased consumption of clotting factors induced by DIC (Boxes 27-5 and 27-6). Liver failure and vitamin K deficiency prolong both the APTT and PT, because factors II, IX, and X are tested by both. Inherited deficiencies of factors VIII,[2] IX, XI,[3] and prekallikrein[4] have been described in horses, and these are associated with prolonging the APTT without affecting the PT. Congenital factor VIII deficiency is sex linked, occurring only in males.[2,5] A mixed deficiency of intrinsic coagulation was reported in an aged horse with lymphosarcoma.[6] Inherited factor XI deficiency is transmitted in Holstein cattle by an autosomal recessive trait.[7]

Clinical signs of clotting factor deficiencies are those of hemorrhagic diathesis, as described in the previous section. Cattle deficient for factor XI seem to have complete in vivo coagulation competency. The level of factor VIII:C or factor IX

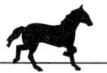

BOX 27-5

Causes of Prolonged Activated Partial Thromboplastin Time (APTT) in the Horse

COMMON CAUSES
Disseminated intravascular coagulation (DIC)
Warfarin toxicosis
Acute hepatic necrosis

LESS COMMON CAUSES
Moldy sweet clover toxicosis
Hemophilia A (deficient factor VIII:C)
Congenital deficiencies of factors IX, XI, prekallikrein, or high molecular weight kininogen
Hepatotoxins (pyrrolizidine alkaloids, rubratoxins, aflatoxins, bitterweed)

BOX 27-6

Causes of Prolonged Activated Partial Thromboplastin Time (APTT) in Ruminants

COMMON CAUSES
Moldy sweet clover toxicosis
Disseminated intravascular coagulation (DIC)

LESS COMMON CAUSES
Congenital deficiency of factor XI
Rodenticide (warfarin) toxicosis
Hepatotoxins (pyrrolizidine alkaloids, rubratoxins, aflatoxins, bitterweed)

BOX 27-7

Causes of Elevated Fibrin/Fibrinogen Degradation Products (FDPs) in Large Animals

COMMON CAUSES
Disseminated intravascular coagulation (DIC)
Thrombophlebitis
Postoperative state
Severe inflammation
Immune-mediated thrombocytopenia (IMTP)

UNCOMMON CAUSES
Massive internal hemorrhage
Primary hyperfibrinolysis

must drop below 5% of normal before spontaneous bleeding occurs. Hemophilia A is a deficiency in factor VIII:C.

A disseminated coagulopathy should be manifested by several abnormalities in the coagulation profile, although variable use, synthetic rates, and the half-lives of clotting factors may result in abnormality of only one clotting time (PT *or* APTT). Serial analyses should reveal a trend toward prolonged PT and APTT, with dropping platelet numbers. When a persistently prolonged APTT is the only laboratory abnormality, hereditary deficiency of one or more clotting factors should be suspected. Specific quantitative assays of intrinsic clotting factors usually are reserved for experienced coagulation laboratories.

ELEVATED FIBRIN/FIBRINOGEN DEGRADATION PRODUCTS

Measurable levels of fibrin/fibrinogen degradation products in the serum generally indicate increased fibrinolysis in response to excessive activation of coagulation (i.e., DIC) (Box 27-7). Severe inflammatory processes, hemorrhagic disorders, or postoperative states that cause extensive intravascular fibrin deposition may exceed the clearance capacity of the mononuclear phagocyte system (MPS) and elevate serum FDPs. Primary (spontaneous) hyperfibrinolysis has not been described in large animals.

Elevated serum FDPs contribute to the hemorrhagic manifestations of DIC by interfering with thrombin activity, fibrin monomer polymerization, and platelet function. Interpretation of this test depends on evaluation of the other components of the clotting profile (platelet count, PT, APTT) in concert with the patient's clinical signs. A serum FDP level above 40 µg/ml most often occurs secondary to DIC; however, values below 40 µg/ml do not exclude the diagnosis of DIC, because there may be considerable compensation by the MPS, degradation of FDPs, or both.

REDUCED PLASMA ANTITHROMBIN III

The physiologically most important inhibitor of coagulation is the α-globulin called antithrombin III (AT-III). This low-molecular-weight glycoprotein contributes up to 70% of the total procoagulant-inhibiting activity in plasma and can neutralize thrombin-activated factors IX, X, XI, and XII, kallikrein, and plasmin. Heparin is a necessary cofactor for the action of AT-III, causing a 200-fold acceleration of the interaction between the inhibitor and its substrates. Plasma AT-III may be reduced by failure of production in the liver, excessive use, loss from the intravascular compartment, or increased catabolism.

Chronic liver disease may result in failure to produce AT-III and a number of other important plasma proteins; however, horses with chronic liver disease were shown to have a higher than normal plasma AT-III level in addition to hyperfibrinogenemia.[8] These findings suggest that AT-III may behave as an acute-phase protein in horses, as has been shown in cats.[9]

In conditions such as DIC, AT-III is consumed as a result of irreversible binding to activated clotting factors. Any pathologic generation of thrombin and other activated clotting factors, such as can occur with trauma, neoplasia, or endotoxemia (all known initiators of DIC), would be expected to cause some reduction in plasma AT-III (Boxes 27-8 and 27-9).

Diseases that cause massive proteinuria or protein-losing enteropathy result in reduced plasma AT-III, in addition to loss of other plasma proteins. Because of the small size of AT-III (molecular weight ≈65,000), it is lost in approximately the same proportion as albumin. Starvation or sepsis resulting in massive protein catabolism may cause a reduction in plasma AT-III.

The major clinical sequela of AT-III deficiency is a tendency to develop venous thrombosis. A hypercoagulable state with nephrotic syndrome has been recognized in humans,[10] dogs,[11] and cattle.[12] Venous thrombosis is commonly recognized in horses with severe toxic colitis or endotoxemia; whether this involves AT-III is not known. The contribution of AT-III consumption in DIC to the clinical manifestations

---

of this syndrome is difficult to evaluate; however, use of AT-III concentrates in human patients with acute DIC has improved survival in some circumstances.[8] As with all components of the hemostatic system, plasma AT-III must be evaluated in the light of other clotting data.

HYPOFIBRINOGENEMIA

Hypofibrinogenemia may result from impaired hepatic synthesis, increased consumption with DIC, degradation during primary hyperfibrinolysis, or uncompensated loss during massive hemorrhage (Boxes 27-10 and 27-11). A reduction in plasma fibrinogen is rare under any circumstances in large animals. This protein is produced exclusively by the liver, and it functions as an acute-phase reactant, being rapidly released in response to a variety of inflammatory and procoagulant stimuli. The equine liver seems to have a remarkable reserve capacity to produce fibrinogen, because hypofibrinogenemia is a feature only of acute fulminant hepatic necrosis, which is attended by DIC.

Hereditary afibrinogenemia has been recognized in a family of Saanen dairy goats.[1] This incompletely dominant trait causes a hemorrhagic diathesis in newborn kids that is characterized by umbilical bleeding, recurrent hemarthroses, and bleeding into the skin and mucous membranes. Heterozygotes have hypofibrinogenemia.

OTHER TESTS OF HEMOSTATIC FUNCTION

Other tests of hemostasis are performed less routinely in large animals because of lack of specificity or sensitivity, technical difficulty, or expense. Some of these tests may be useful in a particular disease situation.

Thrombin Time

The time required for a standard thrombin solution to clot plasma is a measure of the rate of fibrinogen to fibrin conversion. In large animals a prolonged thrombin time usually indicates the presence of FDPs that interfere with fibrin polymerization.

Factor Assays

(See previous discussion of prolonged APTT.) For consumptive states such as DIC, factor analyses rarely provide significantly more information than the PT and APTT. Factor VIII:C functions as an acute-phase reactant and may be increased by inflammatory disease. Specific factor analyses are indicated for the diagnosis of hereditary factor deficiencies.

Platelet Factor 3

The platelet factor 3 (PF_3) test is an indirect assay for the presence of serum antibodies directed against platelets. Because of its low sensitivity for the diagnosis of IMTP, it is no longer routinely available.

Plasminogen

The zymogen precursor of plasmin is reduced in the plasma during states that cause pathologic increased fibrinolysis such as DIC. Plasminogen levels have been explored in horses with colic.[13]

α_2-Antiplasmin

α_2-Antiplasmin, a plasma glycoprotein, is the main physiologic inhibitor of fibrinolysis. In humans, α_2-antiplasmin (α_2-AP) is decreased by severe liver disease (reduced production) and with DIC (consumption). Limited experimental studies in ponies suggest that α_2-AP may be reduced significantly with chronic DIC.[14]

Fibronectin

The soluble form of fibronectin is a large glycoprotein that promotes clearance of plasma particulates by the MPS. Fibronectin initially is consumed by binding to fibrin breakdown products and platelet microaggregates; however, it is replenished rapidly in the acute-phase response. A persis-

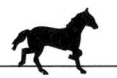

tently low fibronectin level is associated with a high mortality rate in humans with DIC.

Eicosanoids

During activation of coagulation, thromboxane A_2 (TxA$_2$) and prostacyclin are produced and released by platelets and endothelial cells, respectively. TxA$_2$ is a potent vasoconstrictor and aggregates platelets, whereas prostacyclin has the opposite effect. Plasma concentrations of thromboxane B_2 (TxB$_2$), the stable hydrolysis product of TxA$_2$, are elevated during acute, severe DIC in humans. Although not actually evaluated in DIC, both eicosanoids are increased in horses and cattle with endotoxemia.

Protein C

The protein C pathway provides the second major anticoagulant mechanism that regulates hemostasis. Protein C is activated by thrombin and then proteolytically destroys factors V and VIII. In humans, plasma protein C may be reduced by liver failure or by disseminated coagulopathy, inducing a tendency for thrombotic disease. The same may be true in horses.[13]

REFERENCES

1. Dodds WJ: Hemostasis. In Kaneko JJ, ed: *Clinical biochemistry of domestic animals,* ed 4, San Diego, 1989, Academic Press.
2. Archer RK, Allen BG: True hemophilia in horses, *Vet Rec* 91:655-656, 1972.
3. Hinton M et al: A clotting defect in an Arab colt foal, *Equine Vet J* 9(1):1-3, 1977.
4. Turrentine MA et al: Prekallikrein deficiency in a family of miniature horses, *Am J Vet Res* 47:2464-2467, 1986.
5. Feldman BF, Giacopuzzi RL: Hemophilia A (factor VIII deficiency) in a colt, *Equine Pract* 4:24-30, 1982.
6. Ainsworth DM, Dodds WJ, Brown CM: Deficiency of the contact phase of intrinsic coagulation in a horse, *J Am Vet Med Assoc* 187:71-72, 1985.
7. Gentry PA, Ross ML: Failure of routine coagulation screening tests to detect heterozygous state of bovine factor XI deficiency, *Vet Clin Pathol* 15:12-16, 1986.
8. Johnstone IB, Peterson D, Crane S: Antithrombin III (AT III) activity in plasmas from normal and diseased horses and in normal canine, bovine, and human plasmas, *Vet Clin Pathol* 16:14-18, 1987.
9. Welles EG et al: Platelet function and antithrombin, plasminogen, and fibrinolytic activities in cats with heart disease, *Am J Vet Res* 55:619-627, 1994.
10. Bick RL, ed: *Disorders of thrombosis and hemostasis: clinical and laboratory practice,* Chicago, 1992, American Society of Clinical Pathology Press.
11. LaRue MJ, Murtaugh RJ: Pulmonary thromboembolism in dogs: 47 cases (1986-1987), *J Am Vet Med Assoc* 197:1368-1372, 1990.
12. Murray M, Rushton A: Bovine renal amyloidosis: a clinicopathologic study, *Vet Rec* 90:210-216, 1972.
13. Prasse KW et al: Analysis of hemostasis in horses with colic, *J Am Vet Med Assoc* 203:685-693, 1993.
14. Morris DD et al: Effects of equine ehrlichial colitis on the hemostatic system of ponies, *Am J Vet Res* 49:1030-1036, 1988.

DISORDERS
OF THE ORGAN SYSTEM

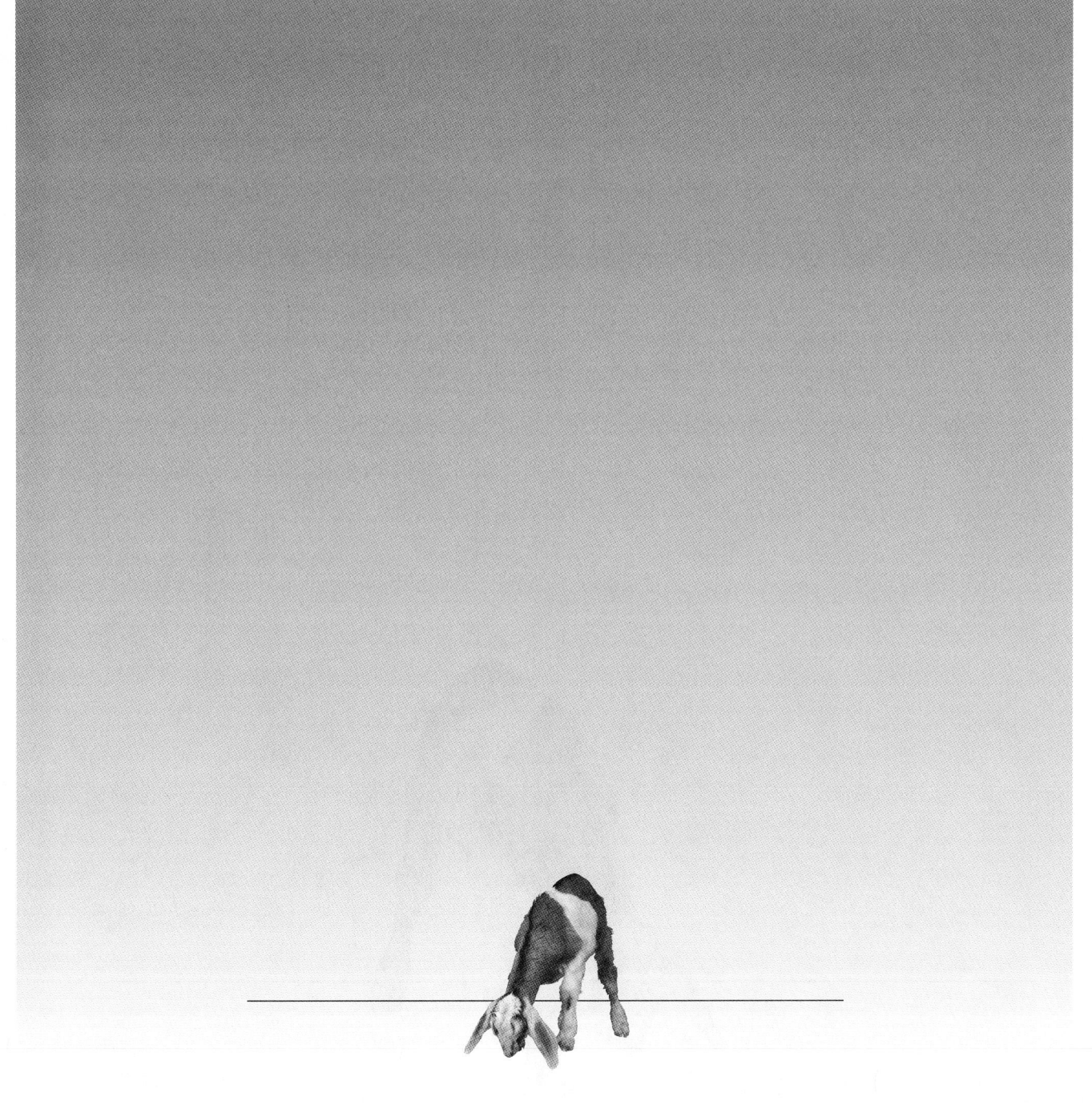

Diseases of the Cardiovascular System

VIRGINIA B. REEF

SHEILA M. McGUIRK

PERFORMING THE ELECTROCARDIOGRAM

No single electrocardiographic lead system has been universally accepted for use in large animals. Bipolar leads (I, II, III, base-apex, X, Y, and Z of the orthogonal lead system) and unipolar leads (aV_F, aV_R, aV_L, thoracic) have been described, but the amplitude, duration, and configuration of the different wave forms vary widely, depending on an animal's breed, size, body type, and sex. In addition, there is lability of certain wave forms within each animal depending on the level of exercise, excitement, or organic heart disease. Large animals have a deeply penetrating Purkinje system, and depolarization from ventricular endocardium to epicardium occurs explosively and in many directions at once. This period of ventricular activation is responsible for the electrocardiographic criteria indicative of ventricular enlargement in small animals but contributes little to the generation of the QRS complex of large animals. Thus establishing specific diagnostic criteria for chamber enlargement in large animal species has been difficult because changes in the QRS complex are not sensitive or specific for ventricular enlargement.

Therefore the electrocardiogram (ECG) is used primarily to detect cardiac arrhythmias. For this purpose a single-channel machine can be used, and the lead system chosen can be any that generates distinctive P, QRS, and T complexes. The lead system should be easy to apply and the tracing free of artifacts created by muscle tremors, skin movement, shifting of weight, and changes in limb position. Two such leads commonly used for the diagnosis of cardiac arrhythmias are the Y lead of the orthogonal lead system[1] and the base-apex lead.[2]

Lead Y is attached by placing the positive electrode over the xiphoid and the negative electrode cranially to the front of the chest. The base-apex lead is attached by placing the positive electrode on the left thorax in the fifth intercostal space at the level of the elbow or at the location where the apex beat is most readily palpable. The negative electrode is attached to the skin of the right jugular furrow two thirds of the way from the ramus of the mandible to the thoracic inlet or at the top of the right scapular spine. The ground electrode can be attached to any site remote from the heart. Electrical contact is improved by clipping hair or wetting the skin with alcohol. The base-apex lead ECG is recorded by attaching a positive, a negative, and a ground electrode in the designated locations and dialing the ECG machine to one of three standard bipolar leads designed for use in humans (Table 28-1). A suitable bipolar lead is created by switching the machine to one of these leads and using the appropriate limb leads. The attachment sites are positioned to suit the operator and are not limited to the limbs.

Continuous electrocardiographic recording over a 24-hour period (Holter monitoring) or with radiotelemetry is also useful for evaluating horses with arrhythmias. Continuous recording of the electrocardiogram can be performed with contact electrodes, electrode patches that are held against the skin with a surcingle, or electrode patches attached to shaved skin with a cyanoacrylate adhesive and protected underneath a surcingle.[3,4] The contact electrodes or electrode patches held against the skin with a tight surcingle appear to work the best for obtaining a continuous ECG recording. With bipolar contact electrodes the positive electrode is placed over the left cardiac silhouette or over the sternum while the negative electrode is placed over the dorsum to the left of the withers where the electrode will lie flat and remain in contact with the skin.[3] The electrodes are kept moist with alcohol. The electrodes are then covered with moist sponges to maintain contact and are held in position with a tight surcingle. The electrodes are connected to a recorder (reel-to-reel, cassette, or digital) that records the animal's heart rhythm for the entire monitoring period (Holter monitor) or a telemetry device that sends the ECG signal back to the receiver to be displayed on a monitor. The continuous 24-hour Holter monitor is useful for diagnosing arrhythmias that occur intermittently or for monitoring cardiac rhythm during exercise. Radiotelemetry electrocardiography is useful for monitoring cardiac rhythm during treatment or during exercise.

In the base-apex lead the P wave is positive in most horses and ruminants. The P wave is most frequently bifid in horses. In many horses a T_a wave, indicative of atrial repolarization, occurs as a negative deflection after the P wave (Fig. 28-1). The QRS complex begins with a small positive deflection (*rS*)

and is followed by a large negative deflection, which terminates in the ST segment. The T wave is variable and can be positive, negative, or biphasic in horses and ruminants. Frequently the appearance of the T wave is variable within one recording. Fig. 28-2 illustrates a typical base-apex ECG recorded from a cow and a horse at 25 mm/second paper speed with the gain set at 10 mm/mV.

When a systematic approach is used to analyze the ECG, diagnosing arrhythmias is not difficult. The following step-by-step approach can be used:

1. Identify all the QRS complexes. Each QRS complex should be followed by a T wave and the QT interval should be similar for all QRS configurations, unless there is a marked change in heart rate. Identify the remaining complexes. Are P waves, "F" (flutter) waves or "f" (fibrillation) waves present? Are there any artifacts?

2. Determine the atrial and ventricular rates. Are they identical? This determines whether there is a tachycardia or bradycardia.

3. Are the P-P and R-R intervals regular? Determine whether an irregular rhythm has underlying regularity that is interrupted by irregular intervals or whether the rhythm is consistently irregular. Second-degree AV block and atrial and ventricular premature beats are arrhythmias with underlying regularity, whereas atrial fibrillation, sinus arrhythmia, and sinus arrest are truly irregular rhythms.

4. Are P waves present? If so, is there a P wave preceding every QRS complex? If not, there are premature depolarizations, escape beats, or atrial fibrillation. Are all P waves followed by QRS complexes? If not, second-degree AV block may be present. Is the resultant P-R interval constant? If not, there may be a wandering pacemaker or first-degree AV block.

TABLE 28-1

Standard Bipolar ECG Leads

Lead	Positive Electrode	Negative Electrode
I	Left arm	Right arm
II	Left leg	Right arm
III	Left leg	Left arm

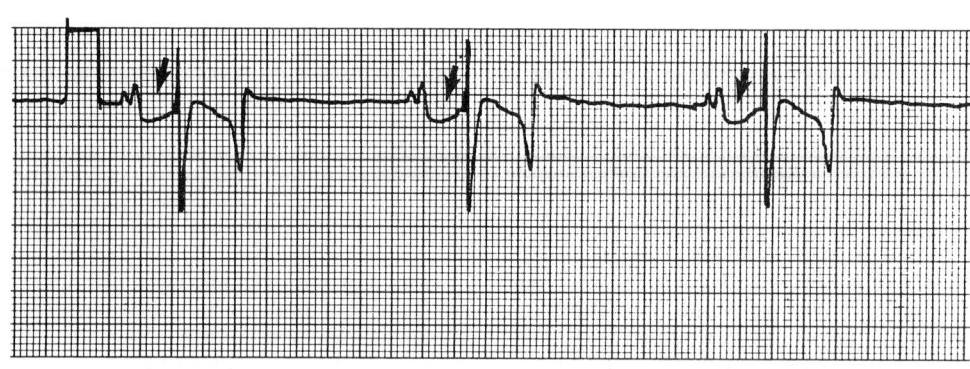

FIG. 28-1 ▓ Base-apex lead ECG recorded from a horse. *Arrows* point to the atrial repolarization wave (Ta) frequently seen in normal horses. It follows the notched P wave and precedes the QRS complex. Paper speed 25 mm/sec, calibration 1 cm/mV.

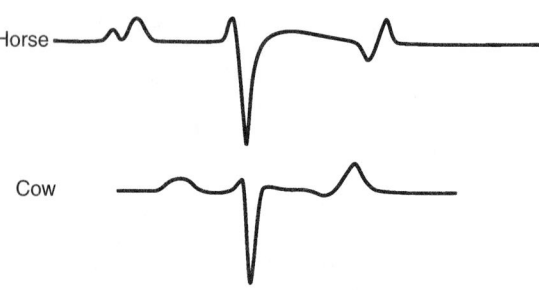

FIG. 28-2 ▓ Schematic representation of a typical base-apex lead ECG recorded from a cow and horse. In horses the P and T waves may be variable in appearance.

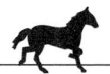

5. Are all P waves and QRS complexes identical or normal in contour? If not, this signifies more than one pacemaker, premature depolarizations, or escape beats.

REFERENCES

1. Holmes JR: Equine electrocardiography: some practical hints on technique, *Equine Vet J* 16:477-479, 1984.
2. Hilwig RW: Cardiac arrhythmias in the horse, *J Am Vet Med Assoc* 170:153-163, 1977.
3. Reef VB: Cardiovascular. In Orsini JA, Divers TJ, eds: *Manual of equine emergencies*, vol 1, Philadelphia, 1998, WB Saunders, pp 94-156.
4. Bussadori C et al: Applicazioni cliniche dell'electrocardiographia Holter in cardiologia equina, *Ippoloogia* 8:5-11, 1997.

USE OF ECHOCARDIOGRAPHY IN LARGE ANIMALS

Echocardiography is a noninvasive diagnostic tool that uses sound waves in the range of 2.25 to 10 MHz to visualize the heart in motion, using either a single ice-pick (M-mode) or a two-dimensional (B-mode) image. Noninvasive evaluation of blood flow in the heart and great vessels is performed with pulsed wave, color flow, and continuous wave Doppler echocardiography. Precise localization of abnormal flow within the heart and great vessels is performed with pulsed wave and color flow Doppler echocardiography, whereas continuous wave Doppler echocardiography is used to determine the peak velocity of blood flow and to noninvasively estimate pressure gradients. In contrast with M-mode and two-dimensional echocardiography, in which the best image is obtained with the ultrasound beam perpendicular to the structures being imaged, optimal Doppler signals are obtained with the ultrasound beam parallel to the blood flow being evaluated. For accurate peak blood flow velocities to be recorded with continuous wave Doppler echocardiography, the ultrasound beam should be as close to parallel as possible (less than a 20-degree angle) to the direction of blood flow being measured. This alignment is difficult or impossible to achieve in most large animals with valvular heart disease but is possible with a ventricular septal defect. Therefore accurate peak blood flow velocities often cannot be obtained from large animals with valvular heart disease. Noninvasive estimations of pressure gradients are inaccurate in these instances. A more extensive review of the theory and application of echocardiography in horses has been published.[5-8] Echocardiography is particularly useful in evaluating large animals with cardiovascular disease because the examination is noninvasive and can be performed in most standing, unsedated animals in a timely fashion. Diagnostic criteria for valvular, myocardial, pericardial, and congenital lesions of the heart are well established, and the information obtained assists the practitioner in confirming a diagnosis, assessing the extent of the disease, determining the severity of cardiac dysfunction, monitoring treatment response, and providing an accurate prognosis. Large animal echocardiographic equipment should provide satisfactory resolution of images at depths of 24 to 30 cm. Portable ultrasound machines that can be used in large animals are available with pulsed, continuous wave, and color flow Doppler. However, Doppler echocardiography is used mainly in specialty practices and referral institutions because performing and interpreting a complete echocardiogram, including Doppler, requires a significant amount of training and expertise and state-of-the-art color flow Doppler equipment remains fairly expensive.

Echocardiographic examination is performed in a systematic way, using standardized images to obtain information about chamber size, wall thickness, myocardial function, valve appearance, valve function, great vessels, blood flow, and presence of abnormal structures or echodensities. The standard equine or bovine echocardiogram is performed from the right parasternal window (the right fourth intercostal space in horses and third intercostal space in ruminants) with a 2.5-MHz transducer. Higher-frequency transducers should be used to examine younger animals and small ruminants. Both long- and short-axis views of all cardiac structures should be evaluated. The cardiac valves should be carefully examined for any abnormalities of structure or function (thickening, prolapse, ruptured chordae tendineae, fenestrations, flail valve leaflet, vegetative lesion, or high-frequency vibrations). The relative size, shape, and relationship of the cardiac chambers and great vessels should be assessed and an evaluation of myocardial function and blood flow performed. Standard measurements of left ventricular internal diameter, left ventricular free wall thickness, interventricular septal thickness, and right ventricular internal diameter should all be obtained at end diastole and peak systole from the M-mode echocardiogram, and also the diameter of the aortic root and left atrial appendage, the distance between the interventricular septum and the peak opening of the septal leaflet of the mitral valve (septal to E point separation) and the ejection time. End diastolic measurements are obtained at the Q wave of the ECG, whereas peak systolic measurements are made from the peak downward deflection of the interventricular septum. Calculations of fractional shortening and ejection fraction can then be performed to assess left ventricular function using the following formulas:

$$FS = \frac{LVIDd - LVIDs}{LVIDd} \times 100$$

$$EF = \frac{LVIDd - LVIDs}{LVIDd} \times ET \times 100$$

in which *LVIDd* is the left ventricular internal diameter at end diastole (cm), *LVIDs* is the left ventricular internal diameter in systole (cm), and *ET* is the ejection time (sec).

Echocardiograms should also be performed from the left cardiac window when the entire heart cannot be successfully imaged from the right side; a pericardiocentesis is planned; atrial fibrillation is present; abnormalities of the mitral valve, aortic valve, pulmonic valve, aorta, pulmonary artery, left atrium, left ventricle, or outflow portion of the interventricular septum are detected; or murmurs originating from the mitral, aortic, or pulmonic valves are detected. The maximal diameter of the left atrium should be obtained from the left cardiac window. The diameters of the aorta and pulmonary artery should be measured from comparable areas in the vessel on the two-dimensional echocardiogram and compared. Echocardiography should be considered a useful diagnostic test to evaluate patients with the following complaints, physical examination findings, or tentative diagnoses:

1. Cardiac murmur, to determine whether the murmur is functional or pathologic
2. Congenital heart defects, especially atrial and ventricular septal defects
3. Acquired valvular heart disease
4. Cardiac enlargement
5. Cardiac arrhythmias not associated with high resting vagal tone
6. Unexplained exercise intolerance or that attributed to cardiac causes
7. Muffled heart sounds, pericardial friction rubs, or pericardial effusion
8. Myocarditis or myocardial dysfunction
9. Cardiovascular neoplasia
10. Prominent third heart sound
11. Congestive heart failure
12. Pulmonary hypertension

13. Aortic rupture or other abnormalities of the great vessels
14. Ionophore toxicity

Pulsed wave or color flow Doppler echocardiography should be used to map the size and location of a turbulent jet associated with an intracardiac or extracardiac shunt, valvular regurgitation, or stenosis (rare), and thus to semiquantitate its severity. Continuous wave Doppler echocardiography can then be used to estimate the peak velocity of blood flow in the jet, estimating (noninvasively) the pressure difference between cardiac chambers and assessing the hemodynamic significance of the lesion. This can be accurately performed in most patients with a ventricular septal defect, but is difficult to impossible to accurately perform in many patients with valvular insufficiencies because of the limited windows available for interrogating blood flow in large animals and the inability to align the ultrasound beam to within 20 degrees of the abnormal blood flow. Contrast echocardiography, a technique involving microbubble-laden injections of saline, carbon dioxide, or indocyanine green, can be used to demonstrate valve dysfunction and the direction of intracardiac shunts (ventricular and atrial septal defects) and extracardiac shunts (patent ductus arteriosus, truncus arteriosus).

REFERENCES

5. Bonagura JD, Herring DS, Welker F: Echocardiography, *Vet Clin North Am (Equine Pract)* 1:311-333, 1985.
6. Reef VB: Echocardiographic examination in the horse: the basics, *Compend Cont Educ Pract Vet* 12:1312-1320, 1990.
7. Reef VB: Advances in echocardiography, *Vet Clin North Am (Equine Pract)* 7:435-450, 1991.
8. Long KJ: Two-dimensional and M-mode echocardiography, *Equine Vet Educ* 4:303-310, 1992.

CARDIAC CATHETERIZATION IN LARGE ANIMALS

Cardiac and great vessel catheterization can be performed in standing, unsedated large animals to determine the following:
1. Pressure and wave forms (shape of the pressure curve)
2. Oxygen tension, oxygen saturation, oxygen content
3. Cardiac output and other indicators of ventricular size and function

Cardiac catheterization is also used for special diagnostic studies such as angiocardiography, nuclear angiocardiography, and indicator dilution studies. These data are used to determine the direction and size of intracardiac and extracardiac shunts, chamber size and contractility, and valvular and myocardial function. Much of this same information can now be obtained noninvasively with echocardiography and can help the practitioner establish a diagnosis, more accurately assess the prognosis, and can provide a direction for therapy.

Cardiac catheterization is usually reserved for specialty practices and referral institutions because of the equipment needed and the skills required for acquiring and interpreting accurate data. Results are not always specific, but catheterization can add quantitative measurements that increase the accuracy of the diagnosis and prognosis of certain cardiac conditions.

Blood Pressure Measurements

The normal pressures for cattle and horses are listed in Table 28-2.[9-12] The values for horses represent a summary of data from numerous authors as cited in the references given. The accuracy of pressure recordings is greatly influenced by the choice of catheter and the recording equipment used. The pulmonary arterial wedge pressure is an indicator of the left atrial mean pressure, as long as balloon inflation of the catheter occludes flow in the segment of the pulmonary artery that is catheterized. Pulmonary arterial wedge pressure is superior to

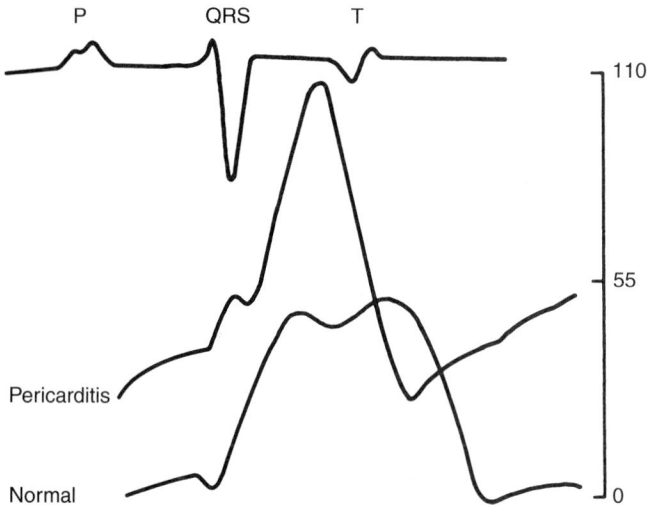

FIG. 28-3 ▮ Schematic representation of ventricular pressure curves recorded from a normal horse and a horse with pericarditis, showing the relationship between pressure changes and the ECG. With pericarditis, the ventricular end-diastolic and systolic pressures are elevated, and pressure declines sharply in early diastole.

TABLE 28-2

Cardiac Pressure Measurements in Normal Horses and Cattle*

	Horses[9]	Cattle[10]
RA	12 to 28/22 to 5 (4 to 10)	(5)
RV	30 to 59/24 to 14 (9 to 25)	42 to 56/0 to 1 (19 to 28)
PA	34 to 48/14 to 22 (16 to 30)	33 to 46/19 to 21 (24 to 31)
PAW	13/3 (8)	(5 to 21)[11]
LV	140 to 148/15 to 17	(120 to 144)[12]
AO	131 to 144/86 to 100 (110 to 115)	
CA	142 to 157/98 to 119 (113 to 124)	160 to 208/110 to 147 (135 to 175)

*Pressure ranges are reported as systolic/diastolic (mean) in mm Hg unless otherwise designated. *AO*, Aorta; *CA*, carotid artery; *LV*, left ventricle; *PA*, pulmonary artery; *PAW*, pulmonary arterial wedge; *RA*, Right atrium; *RV*, right ventricle.

central venous pressure as a monitor of left ventricular function and fluid therapy.

The shape of the pressure curve in the ventricles, aorta, or pulmonary artery may have diagnostic significance in conditions such as constrictive pericardial disease (Fig. 28-3), pulmonic stenosis (giant A wave), or tricuspid or mitral valve regurgitation (large V wave). These conditions are more commonly assessed by echocardiography. An abnormal rise in pressure going from one chamber to the next indicates a stenotic lesion (uncommon in large animals) at the level of the pressure gradient. The size of the pressure gradient can be used to determine the severity of the lesion.

Blood Oxygen Measurements

Blood oxygen measurements are taken from the chambers on the right side of the heart to detect abnormal elevations indicative of a left-to-right shunt (atrial septal defect, ven-

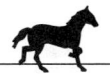

tricular septal defect, patent ductus arteriosus). Criteria for oxygen step-ups have not been established for large animals, but human guidelines have been accepted for qualitative assessment of shunts.[13,14] In humans, oxygen content step-ups of the following magnitude are considered abnormal and indicative of a left to right shunt[15]:

1. ≥1.9 volume percent from the superior vena cava to right atrium
2. ≥0.9 volume percent from the right atrium to right ventricle
3. ≥0.5 volume percent from the right ventricle to pulmonary artery

Oxygen content depends on the hemoglobin concentration; therefore oxygen saturation, which is independent of hemoglobin concentration, may be a more accurate indicator of shunts in anemic or polycythemic patients. Changes in the animals' physiologic status during sampling (cardiac output, ventilation, oxygen consumption), incomplete mixing of shunted blood, and variable time intervals between sampling can be potential sources of error. Several samples within a single chamber improve the reliability of results. Small shunts and shunts in animals with low systemic arterial oxygen tension may not be detected by this technique.

Shunt calculations can be made once oxygen saturation or content has been measured in each of the right heart chambers, pulmonary artery, and a systemic artery. For a left-to-right shunt, the pulmonary flow/systemic flow ratio (QP/QS) is determined as follows:

$$QP/QS = \frac{(SAO_2 - MVO_2)}{(SAO_2 - PAO_2)}$$

in which SAO_2 is the arterial blood oxygen content, MVO_2 is the mixed venous blood oxygen content, and PAO_2 is the pulmonary artery oxygen content. A 2:1 QP/QS represents a 50% left-to-right shunt, indicating that 50% of the pulmonary flow is from the left heart. For a right-to-left shunt, the QP/QS is determined as follows:

$$QP/QS = \frac{(SAO_2 - MVO_2)}{(PVO_2 - MVO_2)}$$

in which PVO_2 is the pulmonary venous oxygen content (assumed to be 98% of oxygen capacity plus 0.3 ml of dissolved oxygen).[16]

Cardiac Output and Ventricular Function Assessment

Cardiac output is determined by indicator dilution methods (usually by dye dilution or thermodilution) or by the Fick method. The Fick method requires the use of a face mask and simultaneous determination of mixed venous and arterial blood samples. Dye dilution and thermodilution results are comparable when 30 to 40 ml of 5% dextrose are injected rapidly at 32° F (0° C).[17] Representative cardiac output values in the horse have been summarized, with most reported values being approximately 73 ml/kg/min.[17] In cattle, cardiac output values of approximately 110 ml/kg/min have been reported.[12] Cardiac output measurements in clinical patients vary with heart rate, excitement, hydration, and many other factors and are best determined in the pulmonary artery. Electronic integration and computation of area under curve by means of battery-powered units that can display results instantly provide the most reliable results.[18]

Cardiac output results or indicator dilution curves can provide quantitative and qualitative assessment of cardiac shunts. Characteristic changes in the temperature-time curve (thermodilution methods) or dye concentration–time curve

indicate the presence of a left-to-right, right-to-left, or bidirectional shunt. Calculation of the cardiac output in the chamber just proximal to the shunt and distal to it can give a quantitative estimate of the size of the shunt.[14]

Angiocardiography

Angiocardiography is used in neonates or animals small enough to have the entire cardiac silhouette visualized on a single radiograph cassette. The contrast medium must be injected rapidly, and in most cases this is done with a pressure injector. Specialized radiographic requirements include rapid film change capabilities or cineradiography. Angiocardiography is used to confirm the presence of an intracardiac shunt (atrial septal defect, ventricular septal defect) or extracardiac shunt (patent ductus arteriosus, truncus arteriosus), or valve dysfunction, to visualize chamber size, or to estimate contractility. Angiocardiography is performed in anesthetized animals.

Nuclear Angiocardiography

In nuclear angiocardiography, specialized equipment captures sequential digitized images of the right side of the heart, lung, and left side of the heart after rapid injection of radiographic tracer into peripheral circulation. A more extensive review of this subject has been published.[19] Nuclear angiocardiography can be used to confirm valvular dysfunction, which is manifested by chamber enlargement or prolonged washout of affected vessels or cardiac chambers and is quantitated by the regurgitant fraction. It also can reveal enlargement of chambers and prolonged washout resulting from cardiac failure. The presence of intracardiac or extracardiac shunts can be demonstrated by the simultaneous visualization of left- and right-side cardiac chambers or slow washout downstream of the shunt. In addition, nuclear angiocardiography can be used to calculate cardiac output and ejection fraction and other indices of cardiac function.

REFERENCES

9. Fregin GF: The cardiovascular system. In Mansmann RA, McAllister ES, eds: *Equine medicine and surgery*, ed 3, vol 1, Santa Barbara, Calif, 1982, American Veterinary Publications, pp 645-704.
10. Doyle JT et al: Observations on the circulation of domestic cattle, *Circ Res* 8:4-15, 1960.
11. Reeves JT et al: Hemodynamics in normal cattle, *Circ Res* 10:166-171, 1962.
12. Sodhi SPS: Cardiovascular hemodynamic changes in the crossbred calves during the early postnatal life, *Indian J Anim Sci* 56:1030-1035, 1986.
13. Lombard CW, Scarratt WK, Buergelt CD: Ventricular septal defects in the horse, *J Am Vet Med Assoc* 183:562-565, 1983.
14. McGuirk SM et al: Thermodilution curves for diagnosis of ventricular septal defect in cattle, *J Am Vet Med Assoc* 184:1141-1145, 1984.
15. Franch RH, King SB, Douglas JS: Techniques of cardiac catheterization including coronary arteriography. In Hurst JW, editor: *The heart*, ed 6, vol 2, New York, 1986, McGraw-Hill, pp 1768-1809.
16. Gore JM, Sloan K: Use of continuous monitoring of mixed venous saturation in the coronary care unit, *Chest* 86:757-761, 1984.
17. Muir WW, Skarda RT, Milne DW: Estimation of cardiac output in the horse by thermodilution techniques, *Am J Vet Res* 37:697-700, 1976.
18. Miller RJ, Holmes JR: Computer processing of transaortic valve blood pressures in the horse using the first derivative of the left ventricular pressure trace, *Equine Vet J* 16:210-214, 1984.
19. Koblik PD, Hornof WJ: Diagnostic radiology and nuclear cardiology, *Vet Clin North Am (Equine Pract)* 1:289-309, 1985.

CONGENITAL CARDIOVASCULAR DISEASE

The cause of congenital cardiac defects has not been established, although hereditary factors may be responsible for some defects. In humans, additional factors such as maternal infection, age, and nutritional status have been identified. Fetal anoxia from placental insufficiency, fetal infection or metabolic dysfunction, or other causes may contribute to the

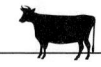

development of congenital cardiac defects. These same factors may apply in animals. Congenital cardiac defects in large animals can occur alone or in combination. The most commonly reported is a ventricular septal defect.[20-25] Multiple cardiac anomalies including patent ductus arteriosus,[26] tetralogy of Fallot,[27,28] truncus arteriosus in Arabian foals,[30] and Eisenmenger's complex in calves[29] have been reported. Single congenital anomalies of the tricuspid,[30-33] mitral,[34] and pulmonic valves[30,35,36] are uncommon. Disorders of the aorta are reported in calves and foals but are also uncommon.[25,37,38] Atrial septal defect occurs more commonly in calves than in foals and is frequently accompanied by other defects.[25,39] Hypoplasia of the left and right ventricles has been infrequently reported in calves and foals.[25,40,41]

Congenital cardiovascular disease should be suspected in a young patient if examination reveals a holosystolic (pansystolic), holodiastolic, or continuous murmur or a murmur with a palpable thrill or wide radiation over the thorax. Cyanosis at rest or with exercise in a patient with a cardiac murmur warrants consideration of a right-to-left cardiac shunt, obstructive pulmonary disease, or severe stenosis of the structures of the right side of the heart. Any of the above findings in a young animal with a history of lethargy, weakness, or failure to thrive are grounds to suspect congenital cardiovascular disease.

Ventricular Septal Defect

DEFINITION AND ETIOLOGY. A ventricular septal defect (VSD) is an opening in the interventricular septum, creating a communication between the left and right ventricles. In large animals, most defects occur in the membranous septum and are imaged ventral to the septal leaflet of the tricuspid valve and the right and/or noncoronary leaflet of the aortic valve.[21-25] VSD can occur as a single defect or as part of a complex anomaly. Many cardiac malformations such as tetralogy and pentalogy of Fallot, truncus or pseudotruncus arteriosus, common atrioventricular canal defect, tricuspid atresia, and double outlet right ventricle include a VSD. The cause of VSD is unknown, although it has been documented to be a heritable defect in Limousine[25] and possibly Hereford[42] cattle. The defect is thought to result either from failure of fusion of a part of the endocardial cushion and the muscular ventricular septum or failure of fusion of the truncal and conal septa.[43]

CLINICAL SIGNS AND DIFFERENTIAL DIAGNOSIS. The clinical signs of an isolated VSD vary and depend on the size of the defect, the direction of the shunted blood, and the presence of concurrent valvular or myocardial disease. In isolated VSD, the blood flow is shunted from the left ventricle to the right ventricle through the defect in the interventricular septum. The size of the shunt depends on the size of the defect and the pressures in the left ventricle, right ventricle, and pulmonary artery.

VSD is suspected when a harsh, plateau-shaped pansystolic murmur is heard on both sides of the thorax. The point of maximum intensity of the murmur is usually on the right side in the tricuspid valve area, but the intensity may be equal on the left side. The murmur on the left side has its point of maximal intensity (PMI) in the pulmonic valve area, associated with a relative pulmonic stenosis (increased blood flow across a normal pulmonic valve). If the murmur is loudest on the left side of the thorax, a subpulmonic VSD or a complex anomaly with pulmonic stenosis (or some form of right ventricular outflow tract obstruction) should be suspected.[23,24,44] A palpable cardiac thrill usually is present and occasionally there is splitting of the second heart sound. The murmur may be the only clinical sign identified

if the defect is small. On the other hand, poor growth, lethargy, dyspnea, exercise intolerance, and signs of congestive heart failure can be exhibited by animals with a moderate to large VSD. This usually develops by the time the animal is 5 years old. Occasionally there is a diastolic murmur of aortic insufficiency associated with a large VSD, the location of which compromises the support of one of the aortic valve cusps.[23,24] Cardiac arrhythmias, particularly atrial fibrillation, may be associated with VSD when there is cardiac enlargement or failure.

Diagnosis of VSD is frequently based on the finding of the loud pansystolic murmur in the tricuspid valve area and a slightly softer, more crescendo-decrescendo holosystolic murmur loudest in the pulmonic valve area. If the murmurs in the tricuspid and pulmonic valve areas are of equal intensity or the pulmonic murmur is louder, a complex cardiac abnormality that includes a VSD should be considered. The murmurs associated with tetralogy of Fallot are usually of equal intensity in the tricuspid and pulmonic valve areas or the pulmonic murmur is louder. A systolic murmur that is loudest in the pulmonic valve area is common in any large animal with complex congenital cardiac disease that includes right ventricular outflow tract obstruction. Large animals with tetralogy of Fallot may have cyanosis at rest or with exercise or exertion. Cyanosis is also a distinguishing feature of Eisenmenger's complex, a defect in which right heart resistance to blood flow causes the shunt associated with VSD to become right to left. Congenital abnormalities of the mitral and tricuspid valves cause a loud systolic murmur audible on both sides of the thorax. The PMI of the left-sided systolic murmur is more caudally located (in the mitral to aortic valve area) than the relative pulmonic stenosis murmur. However, congenital mitral or tricuspid valve dysplasia is rare in large animals. An innocent flow murmur of neonates can usually be distinguished from VSD by its crescendo-decrescendo shape, point of maximum intensity at the left heart base, lack of radiation, and low to moderate intensity.

CLINICAL PATHOLOGY. Echocardiography is the diagnostic technique of choice for identifying a VSD. With two-dimensional echocardiography the VSD can be imaged directly (Fig. 28-4) and the shunt size, location, and direction demonstrated with pulsed wave Doppler, continuous wave Doppler, color flow echocardiography, or the injection of microbubbles. Careful scanning of the interventricular septum should be performed with two-dimensional echocardiography to directly image the VSD and measure its maximal diameter in two mutually perpendicular planes.[23,24] The typical membranous VSD (≤ 2.5 cm in both planes) is missed if the long-axis view of the left ventricular outflow tract is not examined. The membranous VSD is located underneath the septal leaflet of the tricuspid valve and the right or noncoronary leaflet of the aortic valve. If a membranous defect is not found, the entire septum should be carefully scanned in all image planes to detect the VSD. The subpulmonic location, more common in calves, is easy to miss. This defect is usually best imaged in the short-axis view scanning the interventricular septum between the left and right ventricular outflow tracts. With a right-to-left shunt a reddish orange jet is depicted originating in the left ventricle, traversing through the hole in the interventricular septum into the right ventricle with color flow Doppler echocardiography (blood flow towards the transducer in the right cardiac window), whereas a negative contrast jet is imaged in the right ventricle with a right-sided injection of microbubbles.[23,24] A left ventricular injection of microbubbles is necessary to visualize echo-laden blood in the right ventricle with a typical VSD. M-mode echocardiography may show septal discontinuity when traversing the ventricular septum from the apex of the heart to

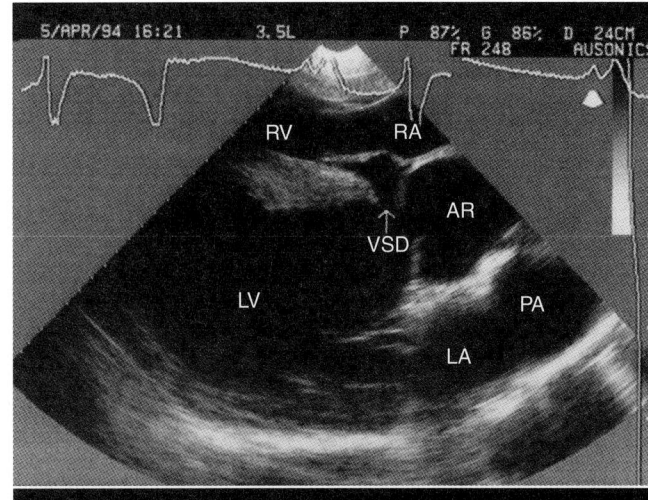

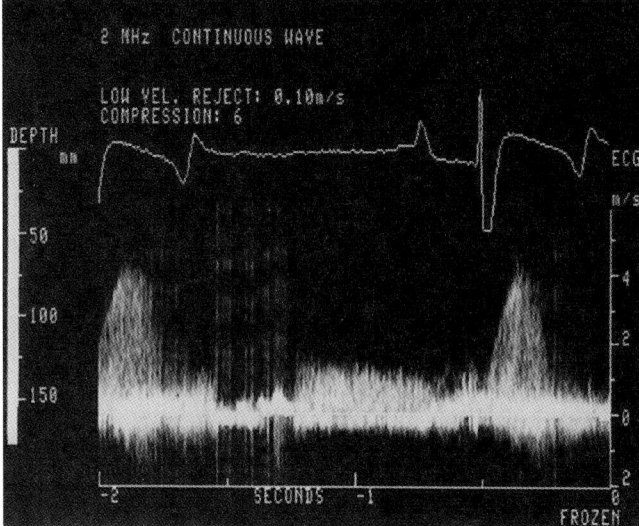

FIG. 28-4 ▓ Two-dimensional echocardiographic image **(A)** and continuous wave Doppler spectral tracing **(B)** of a ventricular septal defect *(arrow)* in a weanling colt. The ventricular septal defect *(VSD)* is located just underneath the septal leaflet of the tricuspid valve and right coronary cusp of the aortic valve. The VSD is best imaged in this left ventricular outflow tract view. There is significant left ventricular enlargement in this colt. The right atrium *(RA)*, right ventricle *(RV)*, left ventricle *(LV)*, left atrium *(LA)*, aortic root *(AR)*, and pulmonary artery *(PA)* are all visible in this view. The spectral tracing shows a peak shunt velocity of slightly under 4 m/sec in systole, with some turbulent flow (spectral broadening) also detected in diastole with a peak flow velocity of approximately 1.3 m/sec.

the aortic root (septal dropout). Moderate to large VSDs show left atrial (see Fig. 28-4) and left ventricular enlargement, right ventricular enlargement, and pulmonary artery dilation. The left atrial to aortic root ratio is increased. Aortic valve prolapse and aortic regurgitation may also be detected because of loss of support of the aortic root from the VSD. Myocardial dysfunction and subsequent congestive heart failure may occur with a large VSD. Continuous wave Doppler echocardiography can be used to noninvasively assess the hemodynamic significance of the shunt. A peak shunt flow velocity of greater than or equal to 4 m/sec indicates a restrictive VSD with normal or near normal right ventricular pressures. Nuclear angiocardiography can also be used to demonstrate simultaneous opacification of the left and right ventricles. The radiographic presence of cardiomegaly and increased vascularization of the lungs provides only nonspecific evidence of

VSD. If polycythemia is found, a complicated VSD should be suspected.

Cardiac catheterization can be used for qualitative and quantitative assessment of the VSD but has largely been supplanted by echocardiographic diagnosis. Elevated cardiac pressures provide qualitative evidence of a VSD. Right ventricular systolic pressure elevation is most common and may equal left ventricular pressure with a large VSD. Pulmonary artery pressure can be increased as a result of increased blood flow from the left-to-right shunt or increased pulmonary vascular resistance and decreased flow (restrictive pulmonary hypertension). Elevation of left or right ventricular diastolic pressure provides evidence of cardiac failure in the patient with VSD. Oximetric data (oxygen content or oxygen saturation) can be used to locate the shunt and provide some evidence of the size of the defect. A step-up in oxygen content or saturation between the right atrium and the pulmonary artery suggests a moderate or large VSD. Because most VSDs are located high in the right ventricular outflow tract, there may be inadequate mixing of shunted blood in the right ventricle to detect the shunt in this chamber unless the catheter is directed to the outflow tract for sampling. When the oxygen step-up is detected first in the pulmonary artery, a patent ductus arteriosus cannot be ruled out. A small shunt may be missed by oximetry as described above under oxygen sampling.

Using indicator dilution methods described previously, the shape of the concentration-time or temperature-time curve can be used to demonstrate the left-to-right shunt of a VSD. A comparison of the cardiac output measured in the right ventricle with the cardiac output measured in the pulmonary artery can give an estimation of the percent of pulmonary blood flow coming from shunted blood and therefore an estimation of the size of the defect.[45]

Angiocardiography can be performed in the anesthetized neonate and definitively demonstrate VSD if there is simultaneous opacification of the left and right ventricles when dye is injected into the left ventricle.

PATHOPHYSIOLOGY. A small VSD may provide enough resistance to flow that the left-to-right shunt is minimal and the patient remains asymptomatic. Horses can race successfully with small VSDs (≤2.5 cm in diameter with peak shunt velocities ≥4 m/sec), although are not usually successful as elite racehorses.[24] Ventricular septal defects produce a left-to-right shunt because the pressure in the left ventricle exceeds the pressure in the right ventricle. A peak shunt velocity of 3 to 4 m/sec indicates an increased right ventricular pressure and a less restrictive VSD; however, the defect is usually compatible with a normal life expectancy. A peak shunt velocity of less than 3 m/sec is indicative of a large shunt that is hemodynamically significant. These animals usually develop congestive heart failure by 5 years of age. Occasionally the VSD is so large that the pressure between the two chambers is equalized. The right ventricle, pulmonary circulation, left atrium, and left ventricle must compensate for this volume overload, which generally results in dilation of cardiac chambers and the development of pulmonary hypertension.

Pulmonary vascular resistance can increase because of simultaneous pulmonary disease or left heart failure from chronic volume overload. In addition to volume overload, the right ventricle is subjected to a chronic pressure overload, which may be sufficient to reverse the direction of the shunt (Eisenmenger's complex—more common in cattle than horses). Because of the pressure and volume overload with moderate to large VSDs, patients with this condition run a greater risk of developing congestive heart failure.

Considerable turbulence associated with the left-to-right shunts and endocardial damage increase the risk of endocarditis in patients with VSD. Because the VSD usually is located high in the left ventricular outflow tract, structural support of the aortic valve cusps may be lost, and aortic insufficiency may develop. Significant aortic regurgitation adds to the left ventricular volume overload caused by the VSD.

EPIDEMIOLOGY. The true incidence of VSD in large animals is unknown, although it is recognized as the most common congenital cardiac defect. In one study, 36 calves had 78 congenital cardiac defects, of which 11 were VSD.[25]

NECROPSY FINDINGS. VSD is usually located high in the interventricular septum just ventral to the aortic valve in the left ventricle and underneath the septal leaflet of the tricuspid valve or caudal or ventral to the crista terminalis in the right ventricle. It can be an isolated defect or accompanied by other cardiac or organ anomalies. If the defect is moderate or large, there is right ventricular, left atrial, and left ventricular enlargement, and pulmonary artery dilation. The lungs may be congested because of increased pulmonary blood flow, and secondary pneumonia is not uncommon. If pulmonary vascular resistance was increased, right ventricular hypertrophy may be present. There may be secondary endocarditis (infrequent in large animals) or endocardial lesions as a result of turbulent blood flow across the defect.

TREATMENT AND PROGNOSIS. There is no practical treatment for VSD in large animals. A complete echocardiographic examination is indicated to identify the presence and significance of a VSD. It is important to identify those animals with moderate to large defects, because the prognosis for normal production or function is poor. Animals with small defects may remain asymptomatic throughout life. It is important to recognize that small defects, which provide a large resistance to flow, can produce loud murmurs. Because of this, the intensity of the murmur is not a good predictor of the size of the defect.

Currently there is limited evidence that VSD is inherited in cattle or horses. However, breeding animals with VSD is not advised because of the increased risk of heart failure and other cardiac complications. As a general rule, bull studs do not accept animals with this defect into a breeding program.

Patent Ductus Arteriosus

DEFINITION AND ETIOLOGY. A patent ductus arteriosus (PDA) is the persistent patency of a vessel (normally present in the fetus) that connects the pulmonary arterial system to the aorta. The ductus arteriosus fails to close at birth when breathing begins and placental circulation is removed. Closure of the ductus arteriosus occurs in response to decreasing pulmonary vascular resistance and increased systemic vascular resistance.

A PDA can occur as a single defect (rare in large animals) or with other cardiac anomalies. In large animals the most common other defects reported with PDA are tetralogy and pentalogy of Fallot and pseudotruncus arteriosus.

CLINICAL SIGNS AND DIFFERENTIAL DIAGNOSIS. The clinical signs of PDA depend on the length and diameter of the ductus arteriosus, the direction of the shunted blood, and the presence of other cardiac defects. A PDA should be suspected when a continuous, high-pitched murmur, frequently referred to as a "machinery murmur" because of its alternating intensity, is auscultated. The murmur may be heard on the left and right sides of the thorax but is usually loudest in the left third or fourth intercostal space at the level of the shoulder. The intensity of the murmur increases with increased heart rate, exercise, or excitement. The arterial pulses are usually bounding because of the run off of blood from the systemic to the pulmonary circulation. Occasionally the PDA is manifested by a holosystolic murmur[46] because the diastolic component is barely audible except at the left heart base. Large PDAs can exist without producing a murmur. In

the animal with increased pulmonary vascular resistance and reversal of the shunt, there may be cyanosis of the caudal parts of the body if the PDA enters the aorta caudal to the brachiocephalic trunk.

Other causes of a continuous murmur in large animals are extremely rare; however, the detection of a continuous machinery murmur should lead the veterinary clinician to suspect a complex congenital cardiac defect that includes a PDA, rather than an isolated defect. A systolic and diastolic murmur can be present in young animals with a large VSD causing aortic insufficiency. A similar murmur is possible with vegetative endocarditis of one of the atrioventricular or semilunar valves, producing insufficiency and stenosis of the affected valve. These conditions should not have the machinery murmur characteristics of the PDA. A loud systolic ejection murmur, which is confused with a PDA, frequently can be heard at the left heart base of foals shortly after closure of the PDA. This murmur may persist for 2 to 3 months.[26]

CLINICAL PATHOLOGY. No characteristic clinicopathologic changes are associated with a PDA. Radiography may show enlargement of the cardiac silhouette and pulmonary overcirculation in an uncomplicated PDA. Pulmonary venous congestion, interstitial pulmonary edema, and alveolar edema are evidence of a large PDA with left heart failure. These signs are not specific for PDA and can be present with any congenital heart defect that results in a left-to-right shunt. No consistent electrocardiographic pattern has been identified with PDA. Echocardiographic evidence of a PDA is provided by the detection of an enlarged left atrium and left ventricle with a pattern of left ventricular volume overload and increased values for the ratio of the left atrial to aortic root dimension.[23,46-48] Direct visualization of the ductus arteriosus is difficult with echocardiography but is most successful when performed from the left cardiac window. High-velocity turbulent flow throughout the cardiac cycle in the pulmonary artery and ductus arteriosus is detected with pulsed wave, continuous wave, or color flow Doppler echocardiography.[47]

Cardiac angiocardiography and nuclear angiocardiography using a selective aortic angiogram provide definitive evidence of a PDA. Oximetric data show a step-up in oxygen content or saturation in the pulmonary artery that is proportional to the size of the shunt. Indicator dilution methods also provide evidence of a left-to-right shunt occurring in the pulmonary artery in cases of an uncomplicated PDA. Pulmonary arterial and right ventricular pressures may be increased with a large PDA.

PATHOPHYSIOLOGY. Normally the ductus arteriosus narrows near term and constricts rapidly after birth in response to lowered pulmonary vascular resistance, increased systemic vascular resistance, increased blood volume, and increased left ventricular pressure when breathing begins and the placental circulation is removed. If the ductus arteriosus is large or the resistance to flow across the ductus is minimal, there is a significant left-to-right shunt, which produces a large left ventricular volume overload. The left ventricular response may be failure or, with time, dilation (primarily) and hypertrophy. Pulmonary hypertension and congestion result. The right ventricle can be affected by the pulmonary pressure load, and right ventricular hypertrophy can also develop. If the pulmonary resistance equals or exceeds the systemic vascular resistance, a right-to-left shunt occurs.

EPIDEMIOLOGY. Normal foals may have a PDA for a few days after birth, but closure of the ductus arteriosus is expected by 96 hours of age.[46] Normal ruminants rarely have a PDA after birth, and if one is present, it is considered abnormal. Functional closure may precede anatomic closure of the PDA. This defect is uncommon in older animals. Currently

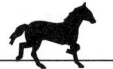

there is no evidence to suggest that this is an inherited defect in horses or cattle.

NECROPSY FINDINGS. The ductus arteriosus can be of variable length and diameter but is patent between the aorta and the pulmonary artery. Frequently the PDA enters the aorta caudal to the origin of the brachiocephalic trunk. Changes in the left and right ventricles and lung and pulmonary vasculature are variable and depend on the size of the shunt. When the PDA is large, there may be cardiomegaly with left atrial and left ventricular dilation, right ventricular hypertrophy, pulmonary congestion, and edema.

TREATMENT AND PROGNOSIS. There is insufficient evidence on which to base a prognosis for animals with PDA. The condition can be corrected surgically in neonates, but future performance has not been documented. Animals with small defects may remain asymptomatic throughout life. The prognosis is poor if the defect is large, because the risk for left (primarily) and right ventricular failure is increased. Pharmacologic closure of the PDA using inhibitors of prostaglandin synthesis has been successful in humans but is not without risk of complications and recurrence. The efficacy of prostaglandin inhibitors has not been evaluated in large animals.

Tetralogy and Pentalogy of Fallot

DEFINITION AND ETIOLOGY. Tetralogy and pentalogy of Fallot are characterized by biventricular origin (overriding) of the aorta, ventricular septal defect, right ventricular hypertrophy, and obstruction of pulmonary arterial flow. When there is an associated atrial septal defect, the anomaly is referred to as pentalogy of Fallot. The defect is caused by abnormal development of the conal septum in the embryonic heart, which leads to narrowing of the right ventricular infundibulum (pulmonic stenosis), an inability of the conal septum to participate in closure of the interventricular foramen (ventricular septal defect), and overriding of the aorta. Right ventricular hypertrophy develops as a result of the pulmonary outflow obstruction.

CLINICAL SIGNS AND DIFFERENTIAL DIAGNOSIS. Tetralogy of Fallot is one of the more common congenital cardiac defects that cause cyanosis in large animals. Resting cyanosis is rare in horses, although may be detectable after exercise. Cyanosis of the oral and nasal mucosa, the tongue, the vaginal mucous membranes, and occasionally the nose and skin of light-colored animals is noticed when more than 5 g/dl of hemoglobin is reduced (unoxygenated). Exercise intolerance is often marked and is characterized by dyspnea or collapse in most cases and frequently the owner complains of slow growth or small size. A loud pansystolic murmur, which is associated with a palpable thrill, is loudest in the left third to fourth intercostal space. The murmur may be a crescendo-decrescendo murmur of pulmonic stenosis or the harsh, plateau-shaped murmur of a VSD; one of these usually predominates. A harsh band-shaped pansystolic murmur is also auscultated in the tricuspid valve area but is usually one or two grades softer than the pulmonic stenosis murmur. Excitement of the animal may result in auscultation of a gallop rhythm or an early systolic ejection click. A continuous machinery murmur can be auscultated in some patients, associated with continuous shunting through the patent ductus arteriosus.

Tetralogy and pentalogy of Fallot must be distinguished from other causes of cyanosis in young animals. Respiratory distress syndrome of neonates can be distinguished by the presence of tachypnea, dyspnea, and abnormal lung sounds in the absence of a cardiac murmur. Cyanosis caused by central nervous system disease has other neurologic manifestations. Cyanosis from congenital cardiac disease may be caused by a right-to-left shunt or by heart failure with pulmonary edema. Cyanosis resulting from heart failure or respiratory disease improves with oxygen administration, whereas the patient with a right-to-left cardiac shunt fails to improve. Right-to-left cardiac shunting does or can occur with tetralogy and pentalogy of Fallot, reverse PDA or VSD, tricuspid valve or right ventricular atresia, left ventricular hypoplasia, persistent truncus arteriosus, pseudotruncus arteriosus, and other complex congenital cardiac disease, all of which may occur with cyanosis and a cardiac murmur. A complete echocardiographic examination using a segmental approach to cardiac anatomy is needed to accurately diagnose the correct congenital cardiac malformation and has widely supplanted other methods of diagnosing complex congenital cardiac disease in large animals. Radiography and cardiac catheterization provide supplemental information that may be helpful in distinguishing between the causes of right-to-left cardiac shunting.

CLINICAL PATHOLOGY. Increased packed cell volume (PCV), red blood cell count, and hemoglobin concentration (polycythemia) may be present in some animals with tetralogy and pentalogy of Fallot.[28] However, polycythemia is uncommon in foals with cyanotic congenital cardiac disease and is usually less than 45% in most calves. Electrocardiographic changes are usually nonspecific, but a right-axis deviation may be detected.[28] Radiographs of the lungs may show decreased vascularity. The four components of tetralogy of Fallot are easily visualized echocardiographically. The ventricular septal defect and overriding aorta usually are clearly visible with two-dimensional echocardiography. The malalignment VSD is usually large and located just below the right cusp of the aortic valve, separated from the pulmonic valve by the crista supraventricularis. The aortic root is usually large and overrides the septal defect. Echocardiography shows increased thickness of the right ventricular wall, ventricular septal hypertrophy, paradoxic septal motion, and similar left and right ventricular internal dimensions. Narrowing of the right ventricular outflow tract, pulmonic stenosis, or a hypoplastic pulmonary artery (most common) may be imaged as the cause of the right ventricular outflow tract obstruction. Pulsed wave and color flow Doppler echocardiography can be used to further characterize the abnormalities of blood flow associated with tetralogy of Fallot, in particular the severity of the right ventricular outflow tract obstruction. Contrast echocardiography also nicely demonstrates the path of blood flow with a peripheral venous injection. Contrast echoes are imaged entering the right ventricle from the right atrium and then simultaneous opacification of the pulmonary artery, left ventricle, and aorta occur.

Cardiac catheterization can be used to demonstrate equalization of ventricular pressures and a pressure gradient between the right ventricle and pulmonary artery. Oximetry should demonstrate decreased oxygen content in the left ventricle compared to the pulmonary vein. Angiocardiography demonstrates simultaneous filling of the right ventricle, left ventricle, and overriding aorta with decreased pulmonary artery filling and increased right ventricular trabeculation (hypertrophy).

PATHOPHYSIOLOGY. VSD is usually large, resulting in equalization of pressures in the two ventricles and aorta. The degree of shunting is controlled by the resistance across the stenotic right ventricular outflow tract compared to the resistance across the aortic valve. If the right ventricular outflow tract is severely obstructed, the clinical signs of cyanosis are more marked. Excitement, drugs, or increased myocardial contractility from any cause decreases right ventricular volume and worsens clinical signs. Right ventricular failure usually is not a consequence of the pressure overload because of equalization of the ventricular pressures.

EPIDEMIOLOGY. The prevalence of tetralogy and pentalogy of Fallot in large animals has not been documented, but these defects seem to be more common in calves than in foals. There is no evidence that these disorders are inherited.

NECROPSY FINDINGS. Examination of the heart reveals a rounded apex caused by right ventricular enlargement. There is a high, usually large VSD, an overriding aorta that straddles the VSD and the left and right ventricle, right ventricular hypertrophy, and septal hypertrophy. There is usually right ventricular infundibular narrowing and a hypoplastic pulmonary artery although there may be valvular pulmonic stenosis with a poststenotic dilation. The right and left atria may be enlarged.

TREATMENT AND PROGNOSIS. There is no practical treatment for tetralogy and pentalogy of Fallot in large animals. When cyanosis or exercise intolerance is present or growth is stunted (the latter two are common findings in affected animals), the prognosis for long-term survival, production, or performance is poor. Affected foals should not be used for performance or broken to ride if they live long enough. As with many congenital cardiac diseases, the intensity of the murmur is not a good predictor of the severity of the condition and further diagnostic tests are suggested.

Other Congenital Cardiac Defects

ATRIAL SEPTAL DEFECT. Atrial septal defect (ASD) is a connection between the left and right atria at the septal level. The most common type of defect is the ostium secundum defect, of which patent foramen ovale is seen most frequently. Patent foramen ovale is relatively common in calves and is caused by the failure of the septum primum, the valve of the foramen ovale, to become adherent to the crista dividens after birth, when changes in left and right atrial pressures produce functional closure of the foramen ovale. Patent foramen ovale is frequently associated with PDA in calves.[25]

Animals frequently are asymptomatic with an ASD, but a holosystolic, crescendo-decrescendo murmur may be heard at the left heart base. The shunt is usually left to right, and the murmur is the result of increased volume being ejected across the pulmonic valve. If the defect is large, right atrial, right ventricular, and left atrial dilation may be present. Differential diagnostic considerations are a functional murmur, pulmonic stenosis, VSD, or PDA. A definitive diagnosis can be made by two-dimensional echocardiography in which an enlarged right atrium, right ventricle, and left atrium are imaged. Pulsed wave Doppler, color flow, or contrast echocardiography can be used to demonstrate the shunt through the ASD.

PULMONIC VALVE STENOSIS. Pulmonic valve stenosis is uncommon as a single defect but has been reported in a foal with VSD and as one of multiple defects in calves and foals.[25,35,36] Clinical signs of cardiac murmur, cyanosis, and polycythemia are variable and depend largely on the other cardiac defects present. Characterization of the severity of the pulmonic stenosis and other associated cardiac defects can be performed with a complete echocardiographic examination.

TRICUSPID VALVE ATRESIA. This defect has been reported in foals[30-33] in conjunction with other cardiac defects. The abnormalities associated with tricuspid atresia include patent foramen ovale, VSD, small right ventricle, large left ventricle, and large mitral valve orifice. The foals showed cyanosis and a crescendo-decrescendo or band-shaped holosystolic or pansystolic murmur audible over the left and right heart base. Tachycardia, tachypnea, and weak peripheral pulses also were present. Polycythemia was commonly reported. Echocardiographic diagnosis of tricuspid atresia in foals has been reported.[30,32] A thick echo in the region of the tricuspid valve that does not separate in diastole (absent tricuspid valve), an ASD (usually patent foramen ovale), a VSD,

a small right ventricle, a large left ventricle, and a large mitral valve orifice are the echocardiographic findings in tricuspid atresia. Blood flow (right to left) through the patent foramen ovale into the left atrium and left ventricle followed by simultaneous opacification of the aorta and right ventricle is detected with contrast echocardiography. Necropsy showed tricuspid atresia, along with ASD, VSD, small right ventricle, and large left ventricle. Pulmonic valve stenosis and dextropositioning of the aorta have also been reported.

MITRAL VALVE CHORDAE RUPTURE. This defect was reported in three foals between 3 and 8 months old.[34] The defects most likely were acquired because of sepsis and degenerative valvular changes, but congenital abnormalities of the mitral valve or papillary muscle could not be ruled out. The foals showed signs of congestive heart failure and loud, coarse, plateau-shaped, pansystolic murmurs heard over a wide area. Supraventricular arrhythmias were not uncommon. Diagnosis was made echocardiographically and confirmed at necropsy (see section on Valvular Heart Disease). Myocardial necrosis of a papillary muscle was associated with chordal rupture in one of the foals and bacterial endocarditis probably predisposed another foal to chordal rupture.

VENTRICULAR HYPOPLASIA. Ventricular hypoplasia has been reported in foals and calves.[25,40] The defect may be present with other cardiac defects and is usually associated with early death. The defect was present in three closely related Holstein calves, suggesting possible genetic factors.[25]

TRUNCUS OR PSEUDOTRUNCUS ARTERIOSUS. Persistent truncus arteriosus refers to the condition in which one arterial vessel leaves the heart above a VSD. The coronary and pulmonary arteries and aorta arise from this vessel. Subclassifications of this condition have been applied to humans, depending on the origin of the pulmonary trunk or arteries. Pseudotruncus arteriosus has also been described in foals and a calf and is characterized by the presence of a remnant of an atretic pulmonary trunk.[30,49] With pseudotruncus arteriosus, the pulmonary blood supply comes from bronchial arteries or a PDA. Clinical manifestations of these conditions include tachycardia, exercise intolerance, and a cardiac murmur. The murmur may be a continuous machinery murmur if a PDA is also present, holosystolic and crescendo-decrescendo, loudest at the left heart base, or the coarse murmur of the VSD may be auscultated, although the relative pulmonic stenosis component is absent. Cyanosis, dyspnea, or syncope may be seen with exercise or excitement. Congestive heart failure and stunted growth may be noticed. Polycythemia was detected in a calf with a pseudotruncus arteriosus.[49] The presence of cyanosis with the cardiac murmur helps differentiate this condition from a simple VSD or PDA. Definitive diagnosis may be made by echocardiography, angiocardiography, or nuclear angiocardiography.

AORTIC ANOMALIES. Dextropositioning or transposition of the aorta are the most common aortic anomalies of foals and calves and are seen most frequently with other defects. Other aortic anomalies of foals and calves are persistence of the right aortic arch and double aortic arch, which may cause esophageal compression. The clinical presentation is one of esophageal obstruction. Interruption of the aortic arch in two foals with VSD, ASD, and PDA has been reported.[38] The foals showed weakness, lethargy, cyanosis, and tachycardia. The murmur was pansystolic and plateau-shaped with the point of maximum intensity on the right side of the thorax. Radiology showed cardiomegaly and increased vascularization of the lungs. Cardiac catheterization showed left ventricular failure. Bicuspid and quadricuspid cusps of the aortic and pulmonic valve occur in large animals and usually result in both stenosis and valvular insufficiency.

EISENMENGER'S COMPLEX. Eisenmenger's complex has been described in a stunted, 24-month-old Holstein heifer that had a loud, crescendo-decrescendo, pansystolic murmur heard best over the pulmonic valve.[29] The heifer had a prominent gallop rhythm from a loud fourth heart sound and exercise intolerance without cyanosis. Polycythemia was present, however. Cardiac catheterization showed increased pressures in the right atria, right ventricle, and pulmonary artery, with normal left-sided pressures. The echocardiogram was characterized by a VSD, overriding aorta, and dilation of the pulmonary trunk, a feature that distinguished this from tetralogy of Fallot. Left ventricular function was decreased, and at necropsy the heart was enlarged and rounded with a dilated pulmonary trunk and small aorta. The right ventricle was dilated and hypertrophied, whereas the left atria and ventricle were only mildly dilated.

ECTOPIA CORDIS CERVICALIS. Ectopia cordis cervicalis is a relatively common defect of cattle.[25,37] Although this defect usually results in the heart being in the cervical region, a few animals may have the heart in the pectoral region (14%) or the abdomen (3%).[37] Various defects are associated with ectopia cordis cervicalis, including defects of the heart, great vessels, neck (torticollis), ribs, and sternebrae. The heart is usually contained within the pericardium under the muscles of the skin in the ventral cervical area, with the double apex of the heart pointing craniodorsally. The ligaments of the pericardium are most frequently attached to the mandibles and the parotid fascia cranially, the cervical fascia laterally, and the first rib or manubrium caudally. The lung may lack the cardiac notch and often protrudes to the base of the heart. Although the prognosis for a productive life is poor, some calves lived until approximately 1 year of age.

MISCELLANEOUS CARDIAC DEFECTS. Other cardiac defects can occur, but the significance of the lesion is questioned or the defect has been recorded infrequently. Anomalous coronary artery development has been reported at postmortem examination, but the lesion was not necessarily the cause of death in a calf.[50] Anomalous origin of the coronary artery has been thought to be the cause of death in horses.[51] Congenital hematomas of the atrioventricular valves also have been noted, but the significance is unknown.[25] Endocardial fibroelastosis, an anomalous development of the endocardium associated with left ventricular hypertrophy, is usually a severe defect resulting in death of the animal. The frequency of this defect in large animals is not established.

REFERENCES

20. Huston R, Saperstein G, Leipold HW: Congenital defects in foals, *J Equine Med Surg* 1:146-161, 1977.
21. Lombard CW, Scarratt WK, Buergelt CD: Ventricular septal defects in the horse, *J Am Vet Med Assoc* 183:562-565, 1983.
22. Pipers FS, Reef V, Wilson J: Echocardiographic detection of ventricular septal defects in large animals, *J Am Vet Med Assoc* 187:810-816, 1985.
23. Reef VB: Echocardiographic findings in horses with congenital cardiac disease, *Compend Cont Educ Pract Vet* 13:109-117, 1991.
24. Reef VB: Echocardiographic evaluation of ventricular septal defects in horses, *Equine Vet J Suppl* 19:86-95, 1995.
25. Gopal T, Leipold HW, Dennis SM: Congenital cardiac defects in calves, *Am J Vet Res* 47:1120-1121, 1986.
26. Machida N, Yasuda J, Too K: Auscultatory and phonocardiographic studies on the cardiovascular system of the newborn thoroughbred foal, *Jpn J Vet Res* 35:235-250, 1987.
27. Prickett ME, Reeves JT, Zent WW: Tetralogy of Fallot in a thoroughbred foal, *J Am Vet Med Assoc* 162:552-555, 1973.
28. Lacuata AQ et al: Tetralogy of Fallot in a heifer, *J Am Vet Med Assoc* 178:830-836, 1981.
29. Machida N et al: Eisenmenger's complex in a Holstein heifer, *Jpn J Vet Sci* 48:1031-1035, 1986.
30. Bayly WM et al: Multiple congenital heart anomalies in five Arabian foals, *J Am Vet Med Assoc* 181:684-689, 1982.
31. Button C et al: Tricuspid atresia in a foal, *J Am Vet Med Assoc* 172:825-830, 1978.
32. Reef VB, Mann PC, Orsini PG: Echocardiographic detection of tricuspid atresia in two foals, *J Am Vet Med Assoc* 191:225-228, 1987.
33. Wilson RB, Haffner JC: Right atrioventricular atresia and ventricular septal defect in a foal, *Cornell Vet* 77:187-191, 1987.
34. Reef VB: Mitral valve insufficiency associated with ruptured chordae tendineae in three foals, *J Am Vet Med Assoc* 191:329-331, 1987.
35. Critchley KL: An interventricular septal defect, pulmonary stenosis and bicuspid pulmonary valve in a Welsh pony foal, *Equine Vet J* 8:176-178, 1976.
36. Hinchcliff KW, Adams WM: Critical pulmonary stenosis in a newborn foal, *Equine Vet J* 23:318-320, 1991.
37. Hiraga T, Abe M: Eight calves of cervical ectopia cordis and their sternums, *Jpn J Vet Sci* 48:1199-1206, 1986.
38. Scott EA et al: Interruption of aortic arch in two foals, *J Am Vet Med Assoc* 172:347-350, 1978.
39. Ecke P, Malik R, Kannegieter NJ: Common atrioventricular canal in a foal, *NZ Vet J* 39:97-98, 1991.
40. Musselman EE, LoGuidice RJ: Hypoplastic left ventricular syndrome in a foal, *J Am Vet Med Assoc* 185:542-543, 1984.
41. Rooney JR, Franks WC: Congenital cardiac anomalies in horses, *Pathol Vet* 1:454-464, 1964.
42. Blood DC, Radostits OM, Henderson JA: *Veterinary medicine*, ed 6, London, 1983, Baillière Tindall.
43. van Mierop LHS, Kutsche LM: Embryology of the heart. In Hurst JW, editor: *The heart*, ed 6, vol 1, New York, 1986, McGraw-Hill, pp 3-16.
44. Glazier DB, Farrelly BT, O'Connor J: Ventricular septal defect in a 7-year-old gelding, *J Am Vet Med Assoc* 167:49-50, 1975.
45. McGuirk SM et al: Thermodilution curves for diagnosis of ventricular septal defect in cattle, *J Am Vet Med Assoc* 184:1141-1145, 1984.
46. Reef VB: Cardiovascular disease in the equine neonate, *Vet Clin North Am (Equine Pract)* 1:117-129, 1985.
47. Reef VB: Cardiovascular ultrasonography. In Reef VB, editor: *Equine diagnostic ultrasound*, Philadelphia, 1998, Saunders, pp 215-272.
48. Stewart JH, Rose RJ, Barko AM: Echocardiography in foals from birth to three months old, *Equine Vet J* 16:332-341, 1984.
49. Lane VM, Anderson BC, Bulgin MS: Polycythemia and cyanosis associated with hypoplastic main pulmonary segment in the bovine heart, *J Am Vet Med Assoc* 183:460-461, 1983.
50. Sandusky GE, Smith CW: Anomalous left coronary artery in calf, *J Am Vet Med Assoc* 173:475-477, 1978.
51. Karlstam E et al: Anomalous origin of the left coronary artery in a horse, *Equine Vet J* 31:350-352, 1999.

VALVULAR HEART DISEASE

DEFINITION AND ETIOLOGY. In adult animals, disorders of the tricuspid, pulmonic, mitral, or aortic valves usually are acquired and most commonly result in insufficiency of the affected valve. These disorders may be the result of degenerative changes, infection (bacterial or viral endocarditis or myocarditis), inflammation (valvulitis), trauma, or unknown causes (cardiomyopathy). They are usually manifested by a cardiac murmur, most frequently of valvular regurgitation, with the PMI at the location of the affected valve or in the direction of the regurgitant blood flow. Predisposing causes such as microembolism or infarction have not been identified in large animals. Chronic active infection such as foot abscesses, rumenitis, reticular abscess, or other septic process may lead to sustained or recurrent bacteremia, predisposing the animal to the development of bacterial endocarditis, particularly in cattle, or a nonvegetative valvulitis, probably more common in horses. Experimentally, valvular vegetative endocarditis can be induced by intravenous administration of bacteria without preliminary damage to a valve.[52] Rupture of a valve leaflet or chordae tendineae can cause valvular heart disease, as can dilation of a cardiac chamber from any cause or rupture of the aortic root or of a sinus of Valsalva aneurysm.[53-55] In rare cases, neoplasia, primarily lymphosarcoma of cattle, can cause valvular heart disease. Congenital valvular heart disease in adult animals is rare. The most common bacterial isolates from equine and bovine endocarditis cases are streptococci and *Arcanobacterium pyogenes* (formerly *Actinomyces pyogenes*) in horses and cattle, respectively, although a wide variety of organisms have been isolated from large animals with endocarditis.[56-59]

CLINICAL SIGNS AND DIFFERENTIAL DIAGNOSIS. Most animals with valvular heart disease have no clinical signs but have a cardiac murmur that is detected during a routine examination. The clinical signs vary depending on

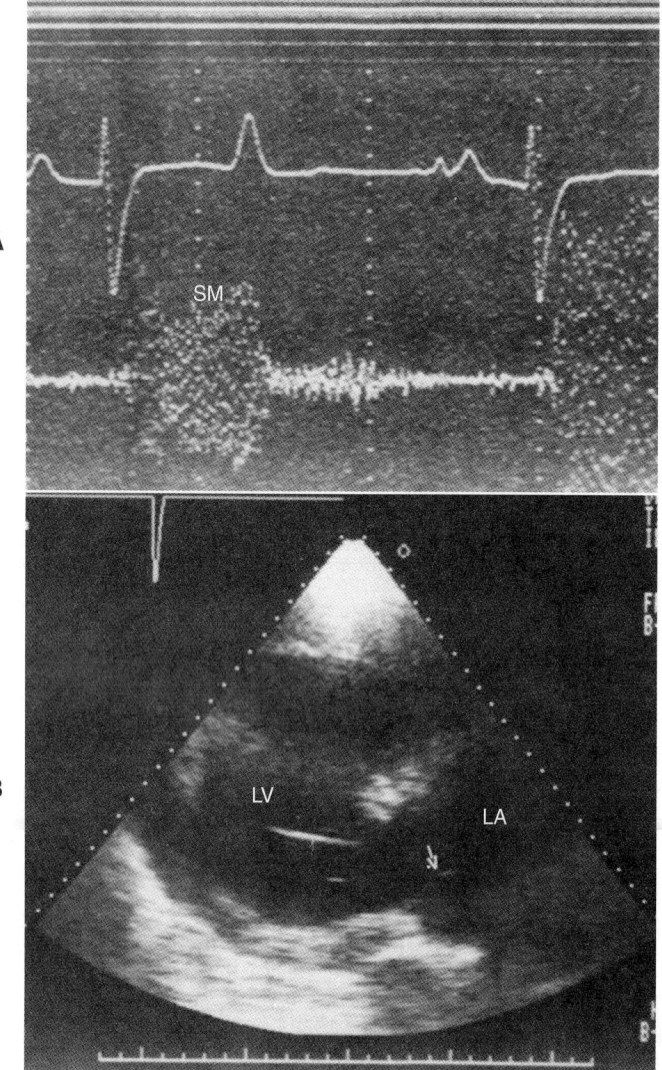

FIG. 28-5 ▊ Phonocardiogram **(A)** and two-dimensional echocardiogram **(B)** obtained from a horse with a ruptured mitral valve chordae tendineae. A loud, plateau-shaped holosystolic murmur *(SM)*, which is variable in intensity, occurs when the free wall leaflet of the mitral valve is prolapsing into the left atrium *(arrow)*. The left atrium *(LA)* is enlarged (13.7 cm). *LV,* Left ventricle.

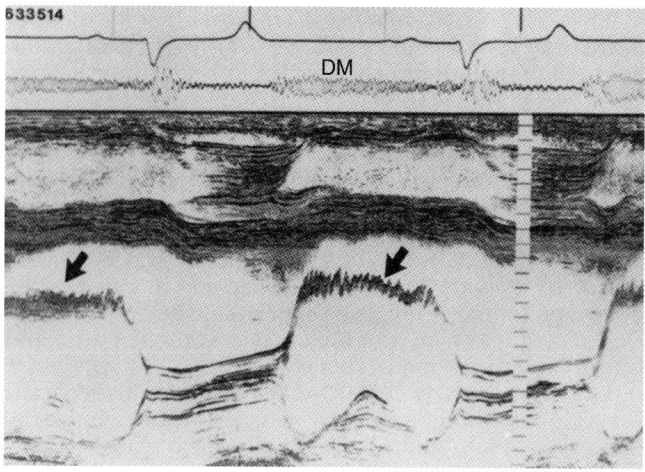

FIG. 28-6 ▊ Phonocardiogram and M-mode echocardiogram obtained from a horse with a holodiastolic murmur *(DM)* caused by aortic valve regurgitation. The M-mode echocardiogram shows diastolic flutter *(arrows)* of the septal mitral valve leaflet, characteristic of aortic valve insufficiency.

the severity of the lesion and its rate of development. Murmurs of valvular heart disease are frequently holosystolic (Fig. 28-5), pansystolic, or holodiastolic (Fig. 28-6). They radiate from the point of maximum intensity (PMI) in the direction of the abnormal blood flow, are coarse and band-shaped, crescendo or honking (if systolic), and decrescendo and/or musical (if diastolic), and are moderate to loud in intensity (≥ grade 3/6). All of these characteristics help distinguish these murmurs from functional or innocent murmurs, which generally occur early or late in systole or diastole, are soft and blowing or crescendo-decrescendo in quality, are localized to a small area, don't radiate, and are soft to moderate in intensity (≤3/6). The intensity of the murmur is not a reliable indicator of the severity of the lesion, except in horses with tricuspid regurgitation in which the longer, louder murmurs are associated with a larger jet of tricuspid regurgitation.[60] In cattle, in particular, severely involved valves (usually

in cattle with endocarditis) commonly have faint or no audible murmurs.

The location of the PMI of the murmur is helpful in distinguishing which valve is involved, although more than one valve can be affected in the same animal. The PMI for lesions of the mitral valve frequently is at the left apex of the heart, although murmurs of mitral regurgitation usually radiate dorsally and toward the left heart base and aortic valve area. Therefore loud systolic murmurs with the PMI in the aortic or mitral valve area in horses are usually mitral regurgitation murmurs. Disorders of the tricuspid valve commonly have the PMI on the right side of the thorax (third to fourth intercostal spaces [horses] or second to third intercostal spaces [cattle]). Infrequently, the murmur may also be heard on the left thorax cranial to the pulmonic valve location in the second intercostal space. Aortic and pulmonic valve lesions produce murmurs with the PMI at the left heart base in the third or fourth intercostal space. Acquired valvular lesions of the mitral and tricuspid valves produce primarily systolic murmurs.[56,57,59-63] Diastolic tricuspid flow murmurs have been reported, however, and may be associated with right-sided mural or valvular masses in horses or may be physiologic, associated with normal blood flow across the atrioventricular valves.[64,65] Lesions of the aortic and pulmonic valves may produce diastolic murmurs, systolic murmurs, or both.[56,63,66-68] However, diastolic murmurs of regurgitation are most common in large animals. Aortic regurgitation associated with degenerative valve disease is most common in horses whereas pulmonic regurgitation associated with bacterial endocarditis is more common in cattle. Aortic valve lesions in horses have primarily holodiastolic, decrescendo, musical murmurs (see Fig. 28-6) and are accompanied by a water-hammer or bounding arterial pulse if the aortic regurgitation is associated with a significant left ventricular volume overload.[56,69] The musical quality of the murmur (harmonic) indicates that some part of the aortic valve is vibrating during diastole. The arterial pulse quality becomes more bounding as the aortic regurgitation becomes more severe, and is a good clinical indicator of the degree of left ventricular volume overload. Ventricular premature beats and atrial fibrillation may also be detected in horses with significant aortic regurgitation.

Besides the cardiac murmur, animals with valvular heart disease may have exercise intolerance, weight loss or signs of congestive heart failure evidenced by tachycardia, coughing, respiratory distress, jugular venous distention, subcutaneous edema, and ascites (uncommon in large animals). In adult cattle, mammary vein distention is another sign of congestive heart failure.[57] Cardiac enlargement may be noticed as an increased area of auscultation and/or percussion or caudal dislocation of the apical impulse of the heart. Atrial fibrillation may be present. This development is usually an indicator of atrial enlargement in animals with valvular heart disease. If tricuspid valve regurgitation is present, there may be abnormal systolic jugular venous pulsations. If mitral regurgitation is present there may be tachycardia, tachypnea, poor recovery to resting respiratory rate after exercise, coughing, and frothy pulmonary edema. Lung sounds may be harsh at rest and on deep inspiration with rare crackles or moist bubbly sounds. Most horses with pulmonary edema have only harsh breath sounds that are detected at rest and on deep inspiration.

One of the clinical signs of bacterial endocarditis is a cardiac murmur, the PMI and timing of which depend on the valve or valves affected. Other signs may include tachycardia, arrhythmias, auscultation of prominent heart sounds, tachypnea, coughing, recurring fever, anorexia, weight loss, or signs of congestive heart failure. Evidence of disseminated sepsis such as pneumonia, hematuria, or pyuria is usually present. Shifting leg lameness and swollen joints or tendon sheaths are common but are usually immune-mediated in etiology. Mastitis and decreased milk production are common in cattle. The presence of weight loss, fever, and signs of recurring sepsis help distinguish bacterial endocarditis from other forms of acquired valvular disease.

The clinical signs of mitral valve chordal rupture (major chorda tendineae) or its characteristic murmur distinguish this disease from other mitral valve diseases. The murmur is usually a widely radiating murmur of mitral valve regurgitation (see Fig. 28-5) with a distinctive honking quality (again the honking quality is consistent with vibration of the mitral valve chorda tendineae or leaflet with blood flow in systole). There may be evidence of acute hemodynamic collapse. Acute onset of respiratory distress with coughing and expectorating foamy pulmonary edema fluid (this fluid is also detected at the external nares) is a relatively consistent feature with rupture of a major chorda tendineae. Signs of right heart failure (jugular venous distention, subcutaneous edema, and ascites) may develop rapidly. Atrial arrhythmias, most frequently atrial fibrillation, often develop secondary to atrial enlargement. The acute onset of respiratory distress, along with a honking systolic murmur, distinguishes mitral valve chordae rupture from other causes of mitral valve regurgitation. The murmur of mitral valve prolapse is also a distinctive murmur and should be suspected in horses whenever a mid to late crescendo systolic murmur is auscultated with the PMI over the mitral valve area.[70] A similar murmur is frequently auscultated in horses with tricuspid valve prolapse. Murmurs of mitral or tricuspid valve prolapse can be detected in horses with all degrees of valvular insufficiency. Most frequently, however, there is little or no valvular regurgitation associated with valvular prolapse. An increased prevalence of mitral and tricuspid regurgitation has been reported in young horses in training.[71]

CLINICAL PATHOLOGY. Diagnosis of valvular disease is best performed with a complete echocardiographic examination including M-mode, two-dimensional, and Doppler echocardiography. Two-dimensional echocardiography is superior to M-mode for detection of valvular abnormalities, measurement of valvular masses (Fig. 28-7), and the global assessment of ventricular function, but chamber enlargement, high-frequency vibrations of the valve leaflets, and

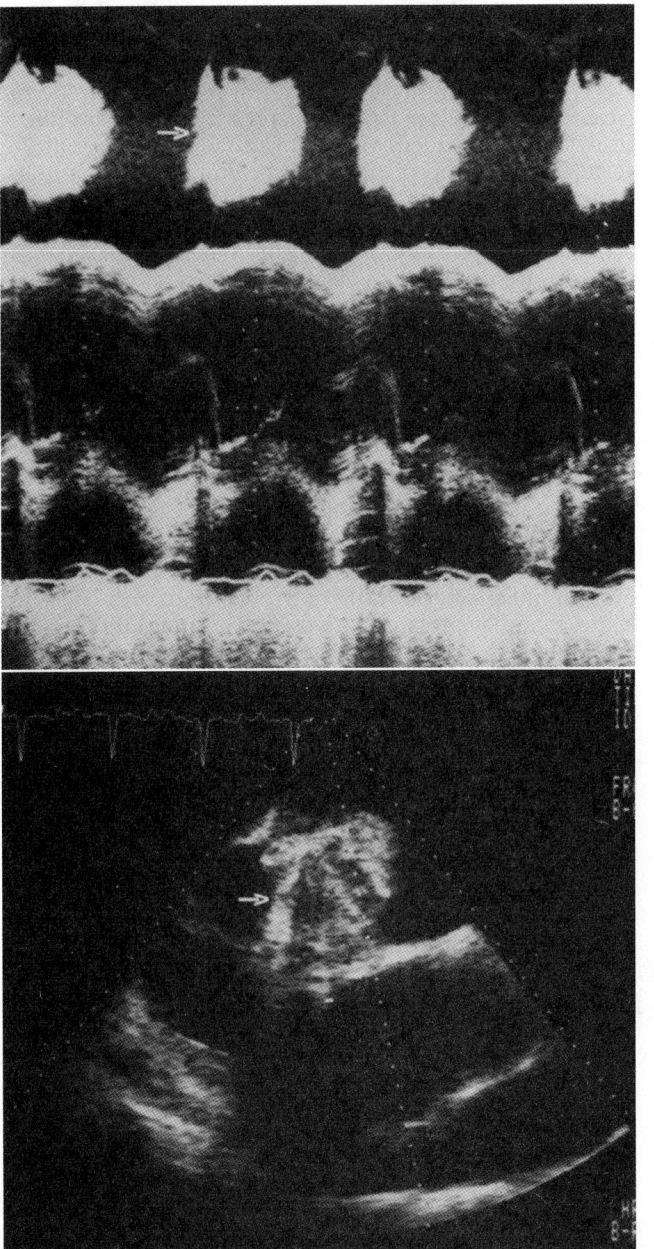

FIG. 28-7 ■ M-mode (**A**) and two-dimensional (**B**) echocardiograms obtained from a cow with tricuspid valve vegetative bacterial endocarditis. The valvular mass (*arrows*) can be seen in the right ventricle in both echocardiograms, but the two-dimensional image is superior to M-mode in demonstrating the size and shape of the vegetation.

shortening fraction (an indication of ventricular systolic function) can be determined by both. Pulsed wave, continuous wave, and color flow Doppler echocardiography can be used to semiquantitate the severity of valvular regurgitation.[70-75] The size of the regurgitant jet detected with pulsed wave or color flow echocardiography is an indicator of the severity of the valvular insufficiency.[76] Clinically insignificant jets of regurgitation are detected only just behind the valve when it is closed. Mild valvular insufficiency is when the jet occupies one third or less of the receiving chamber, moderate is a jet that occupies greater than one third but less than two thirds of the receiving chamber, and severe valvular insufficiency is when the jet occupies greater than two thirds of the receiving chamber.

Echocardiographic signs of mitral regurgitation are increased left atrial (see Fig. 28-5) and left ventricular dimensions and a left-sided volume overload. The cause of the valvular regurgitation can often be determined. Endocarditis, ruptured mitral valve chordae, a flail valve leaflet, valvular prolapse, or thickening of the valve leaflet are readily imaged echocardiographically.[77] The regurgitant jet detected with pulsed wave or color flow Doppler echocardiography usually originates from the site of the valvular abnormalities detected with two-dimensional echocardiography. In some animals the regurgitant lesion is not visualized with two-dimensional echocardiography but the regurgitant orifice is detected with pulsed wave or color flow Doppler echocardiography.[73-75,78] Left ventricular function may be normal (if the mitral regurgitation is mild) or the fractional shortening may be increased (if there is a significant left ventricular volume overload associated with moderate to severe mitral regurgitation), unless there is concomitant myocardial disease. A ruptured mitral valve chordae is diagnosed by finding a mobile linear echo everting into the left atrium or a flail leaflet that may prolapse into the left atrium during systole (see Fig. 28-5), systolic and chaotic diastolic mitral valve flutter, rapid mitral valve opening with increased excursion of the affected leaflet, and lack of coaptation of the mitral valve in systole. The asynchronous movement of any portion of the valve leaflet during any phase of the cardiac cycle indicates the presence of a flail valve leaflet.[77,79] A larger than normal pulmonary artery (larger than the aortic root) is compatible with severe pulmonary hypertension and left-sided heart failure. A smaller than normal aortic root is detected echocardiographically in horses in low-output left-sided heart failure.[76,77,79]

Tricuspid regurgitation may produce echocardiographic evidence of right atrial and right ventricular enlargement with paradoxical septal motion. Frequently the cause of tricuspid valve regurgitation in cattle is bacterial endocarditis, and the incompetent valve can be visualized (see Fig. 28-7). In cattle, neoplasia of the right atrium, tricuspid valve, or right ventricle can usually be visualized when present.[80] Tricuspid regurgitation is common in horses with no obvious valvular lesion.[65,71,81]

Aortic valve regurgitation is diagnosed echocardiographically by observing left ventricular dilation, increased aortic root diameter, increased left ventricular fractional shortening (if the aortic regurgitation is moderate to severe and left ventricular function is normal), diastolic fluttering of the septal mitral valve leaflet, or less frequently, the interventricular septum or aortic valve (see Fig. 28-6).[67,69,74,76] Rarely, premature closure of the mitral valve is detected. Thickening of the left cusp of the aortic valve is frequently detected echocardiographically, but prolapse, fenestration, and tears of the aortic cusps also occur.

Acquired pulmonic valve lesions are uncommon in large animals and when present are usually associated with bacterial endocarditis.[63,68,82] Diagnosis is established by finding the mass associated with the pulmonic valve. Severe pulmonic regurgitation associated with pulmonic valve rupture has been reported in one horse.[83] Pulmonic regurgitation is most common in horses with pulmonary hypertension and congestive heart failure but is rarely detected clinically.

Lesions of bacterial endocarditis may have a shaggy, ragged, or cystic appearance with two-dimensional echocardiography.[59,63,67,68] Occasionally the only abnormality noticed is valve thickening with ventricular hyperkinesis and enlargement of the chambers on the side of the affected valve. Acoustic reverberation and production of microbubbles have

also been associated with valvular bacterial endocarditis.[63,64] Other laboratory evidence of bacterial endocarditis includes anemia, neutrophilia (a left shift may be present), an increased serum globulin concentration, and hyperfibrinogenemia. Liver enzymes are frequently mildly elevated, and a urinalysis sometimes shows hematuria or pyuria. Positive blood cultures taken during febrile episodes confirm the diagnosis when associated with the above findings. However, many times the culture results are negative in large animals with bacterial endocarditis. Other laboratory evidence of disseminated sepsis includes neutrophilic response in peritoneal, tracheal wash, or joint fluid. Ventricular arrhythmias are frequently detected electrocardiographically in individuals with mitral or aortic valve endocarditis. Radiographic or sonographic evidence of disseminated pneumonia also may be found with bacterial endocarditis, usually in large animals with a right-sided lesion.

Other laboratory evidence of valvular heart disease is nonspecific. The ECG is not reliable for detecting chamber enlargement associated with valvular incompetence. The ECG is valuable for documentation of cardiac arrhythmias occurring secondary to chamber enlargement or the underlying myocardial disease. Radiographic findings of cardiac enlargement, increased pulmonary vascular pattern, or pulmonary edema are also nonspecific. Cardiac catheterization can be performed, and pressure measurements help determine the degree of cardiac dysfunction. Nuclear angiocardiography shows cardiac enlargement or prolonged washout of contrast material. Time-activity curves can be helpful in accurately documenting ventricular dysfunction and the valvular regurgitant fraction.[84]

PATHOPHYSIOLOGY. Acquired valvular heart disease that is slow in onset or gradually progressive may be asymptomatic at first, but cardiac changes occur that eventually may lead to congestive heart failure. Valvular incompetence from endocarditis, degenerative changes, chordal rupture, or other causes results in volume overload of the recipient chamber. Initially the output of the chamber is increased to maintain forward output, but the increased end-diastolic volume of the recipient chamber leads to compensatory dilation and a mild elevation in end-diastolic pressure. Compensatory hypertrophy may also result. In the later stages of valvular regurgitation contractile function of the volume-overloaded chamber may diminish, leading to further elevation of end-diastolic pressure and decreased compliance. In the case of severe aortic and mitral regurgitation, this causes elevation of left atrial pressure and eventually pulmonary venous hypertension. With severe tricuspid regurgitation, right atrial or central venous pressure increases. Increased myocardial oxygen consumption is a natural sequela, and biventricular failure can ensue.

If valvular heart disease is acute in onset, as with mitral valve chordae rupture, the regurgitation and volume overload is imposed on the left atrium, which cannot dilate and adapt acutely to the increased diastolic filling. The sudden hemodynamic change leads to pulmonary venous hypertension and acute pulmonary edema. However, most horses with mitral regurgitation do not have acute pulmonary edema. Instead, chronic pulmonary hypertension leading to subtle respiratory signs and the subsequent development of right-sided congestive heart failure are common in horses with severe mitral regurgitation.

In addition to the hemodynamic load placed on the heart from an incompetent valve, bacterial endocarditis also results in disseminated sepsis. The vegetations are made up of layers of fibrin, blood cells, necrotic tissue, and bacteria and are relatively resistant to short-term antimicrobial therapy. The disseminated sepsis may be the cause of death or the reason for culling of the animal.

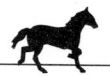

EPIDEMIOLOGY. Acquired valvular heart disease is common in large animals, involving 356 of 1557 horses (22.9%) in one abattoir survey.[85] Endocarditis, one form of valvular heart disease, was reported in 4% of cattle in another study.[86] Bacterial endocarditis most commonly affects the tricuspid valve in cattle but has been reported on the pulmonic, mitral, or the aortic valve as well.[57,67,68,80] Most cases of tricuspid valve bacterial endocarditis have been reported in horses with septic jugular vein thrombophlebitis.[56,59,87] Aortic and mitral valve endocarditis are most common in horses, occurring with nearly equal frequency.[58,59] In the largest survey of acquired valvular heart disease in horses, the aortic valve was affected most commonly with degenerative valve changes, followed by the mitral valve, tricuspid valve, and, uncommonly, the pulmonic valve.[85] Not all valvular lesions are associated with incompetency of the valve. Degenerative valvular changes are seen more commonly in older horses, particularly changes involving the aortic valve.

NECROPSY FINDINGS. Acquired valvular disease is associated with finding nodular thickening, fibrous bands, valve fenestrations, rupture of mitral valve chordae, fibrinous masses typical of endocarditis, and combinations of these lesions on postmortem examination. There may be associated or secondary changes varying from enlargement of a chamber or vessel to hematomas, degeneration, inflammation, and fibrosis. Enlargement (primarily dilation) of the chamber receiving the regurgitant flow, in addition to enlargement (primarily dilation) of the chamber or vessel from which the regurgitant flow arises, is commonly detected. Jet lesions are usually found in the receiving chamber associated with the high-velocity turbulent regurgitant blood flow.

Subcutaneous edema, increased pericardial, pleural, or peritoneal fluid, and congestion and mottling of the liver may be present and indicate congestive heart failure. Ascites associated with congestive heart failure is uncommon in large animals, particularly in horses. A primary source of chronic or active infection, along with evidence of bacterial embolization, may be seen in cases of endocarditis, primarily in cattle.

TREATMENT AND PROGNOSIS. The treatment and prognosis of acquired valvular heart disease depend on the etiology, onset, duration, and severity of the lesion. In general, the prognosis is guarded to poor when evidence of valvular incompetence includes tachycardia, exercise intolerance, signs of congestive heart failure, or echocardiographic evidence of severe chamber enlargement. Degenerative valve disease may be asymptomatic except for a cardiac murmur, or it may be mild; but it generally is slowly progressive and therefore historically has been given a guarded prognosis. A more accurate prognosis for horses with murmurs can now be obtained from a complete echocardiographic examination, including Doppler. The valve affected, the lesions detected on the valve leaflets, the degree of chamber enlargement and volume overload detected, the echocardiographic assessment of myocardial function, and the severity of the regurgitation determined with Doppler echocardiography, coupled with the animal's age and intended use, can be used to formulate a prognosis.[74,76] Valvular regurgitation associated with no detectable abnormalities, valvular prolapse, and mild valvular thickening usually has a fair to good prognosis if the amount of valvular regurgitation is small. Individuals with ruptured chordae tendineae, flail valve leaflets, and marked valvular thickening usually have moderate to severe regurgitation, which is likely to progress more rapidly and usually warrants a guarded to poor prognosis. Mitral regurgitation is the most likely valvular insufficiency to be associated with clinical signs of cardiovascular disease, whereas primary aortic regurgitation and tricuspid regurgitation infrequently result in the development of congestive heart failure or result in

the death of the animal, except in horses with severe aortic regurgitation. Bacterial endocarditis has a guarded to grave prognosis even with long-term antibiotic therapy and frequently results in sudden death of the animal, although bacteriologic cures have been reported.

Despite the guarded long-term prognosis, palliative therapy can be applied for most forms of acquired valvular heart disease. Bacterial endocarditis is treated with long-term use of bacteriocidal antimicrobials, ideally intravenously, the choice of which is based on blood culture and sensitivity results. In cattle and horses, initial therapy is directed at the likelihood of a gram-positive infection. Combination antibiotic therapy of a penicillin and aminoglycoside can be used for gram-negative organisms. Recently, using rifampin at a dose of 5 mg/kg twice daily orally in combination with another antibiotic with appropriate spectrum has improved the short-term outlook for large animals with bacterial endocarditis. Aspirin (100 mg/kg/day, ruminants; 17 mg/kg every other day, horses) and low-dose heparin (30 U/kg subcutaneously twice daily, ruminants and horses) may be used in patients with valvular endocarditis in an attempt to prevent platelet adhesion and increased size of the valvular mass. Early diagnosis and aggressive treatment with the appropriate antimicrobials for a prolonged period are important for successful treatment of bacterial endocarditis. The long-term outcome for successfully treated cases is still poor because the scarring that results as the endocarditis lesion heals may lead to severe valvular regurgitation and the death of the animal, particularly with left-sided bacterial endocarditis lesions.[76,88] Compliance and economics are also major drawbacks in treating endocarditis.

The hemodynamic consequences of valvular heart disease (volume overload or congestive heart failure) may be improved by using diuretics. Furosemide has been used most commonly at a dose of 0.5 to 1 mg/kg as needed. Digoxin can be used to improve contractility when congestive heart failure has occurred. Conditions such as aortic valve or mitral valve regurgitation may show little or no long-term improvement, although many individuals improve for 2 to 6 months before the congestive heart failure becomes refractory to treatment. In horses the intravenous loading dose of 12 to 14 μg/kg is followed by a maintenance dose of 6 to 7 μg/kg daily.[89] Digoxin can also be administered orally to horses at a dose of 34 to 70 μg/kg for loading and 17 to 35 μg/kg for maintenance.[89] The administration of a maintenance dose of digoxin at 2.2 μg/kg IV twice daily or 11 μg/kg orally twice daily has resulted in therapeutic plasma digoxin concentrations and clinical improvement in horses in congestive heart failure with no significant adverse effects.[90] Digoxin is administered intravenously to cattle at a loading dose of 22 μg/kg followed by a maintenance dosage of 11 μg/kg three times daily or, preferably, at an infusion rate of 0.86 μg/kg/hr.[91] The efficacy of vasodilators for reducing the regurgitant fraction in acquired valvular heart disease in large animals has not been established with a controlled study. However, clinical impression is that horses, like other species, benefit from the use of vasodilators. Clinical and echocardiographic improvement has been seen in horses in congestive heart failure. Clinical and echocardiographic improvement has been seen in several horses with moderate mitral or aortic regurgitation treated with angiotensin converting enzyme (ACE) inhibitors. Clinical improvement has been seen with hydralazine at 0.05 to 1.5 mg/kg orally twice daily. The ACE inhibitor enalapril has also been effective in horses with moderate to severe mitral or aortic regurgitation and in horses with congestive heart failure, at a dose of 0.5 mg/kg orally once or twice daily. Until recently the expense of these drugs limited the usefulness of enalapril and the other ACE inhibitors. However, a generic form of enalapril maleate has just become available, making this treatment more affordable for most owners. Although the short-term outlook may be improved with use of cardiovascular drugs, the prognosis is guarded for long-term survival or production.

PREVENTION AND CONTROL. Many causes of acquired valvular heart disease cannot be controlled. Appropriate therapy of chronic active infections and careful attention to asepsis with intravenous medication and other invasive procedures may help prevent endocarditis. Effective parasite control measures may eliminate some predisposing causes of valvular heart disease such as trauma to heart valves, microembolism, or infarction in horses.

REFERENCES

52. Dewar HA et al: A study of experimental endocarditis in pigs, *J Comp Pathol* 97:567-574, 1987.
53. Roby KA et al: Rupture of an aortic sinus aneurysm in a 15-year-old broodmare, *J Am Vet Med Assoc* 189:305-308, 1986.
54. Lester GD, Lombard CW, Ackerman N: Echocardiographic detection of a dissecting aortic root aneurysm in a thoroughbred stallion, *Vet Radiol Ultrasound* 33:202-205, 1992.
55. Marr CM et al: Clinical and echocardiographic findings in horses with aortic root rupture, *Vet Radiol Ultrasound* 39:22-31, 1998.
56. Brown CM: Acquired cardiovascular disease, *Vet Clin North Am (Equine Pract)* 1:371-382, 1985.
57. Power HT, Rebhun WC: Bacterial endocarditis in adult dairy cattle, *J Am Vet Med Assoc* 182:806-808, 1983.
58. Buergelt CD et al: Endocarditis in 6 horses, *Vet Pathol* 22:333-337, 1985.
59. Maxson AD, Reef VB: Bacterial endocarditis in horses: ten cases (1984-1995), *Equine Vet J* 29:394-399, 1997.
60. Blissitt KJ, Bonagura JD: Colour flow Doppler echocardiography in horses with cardiac murmurs, *Equine Vet J Suppl* 19:82-85, 1995.
61. Holmes JR, Miller RJ: Three cases of ruptured mitral valve chordae in the horse, *Equine Vet J* 16:125-135, 1984.
62. Brown CM et al: Rupture of mitral chordae tendineae in two horses, *J Am Vet Med Assoc* 182:281-283, 1983.
63. Yamaga Y, Too K: Diagnostic ultrasound imaging of vegetative valvular endocarditis in cattle, *Jpn J Vet Res* 35:49-63, 1987.
64. Rantanen NW et al: Spontaneous contrast and mass lesions in the hearts of race horses: ultrasound diagnosis—preliminary data, *Equine Vet Sci* 4:220-223, 1985.
65. Kriz NG, Hodgson DR, Rose RJ: Prevalence and clinical importance of heart murmurs in racehorses, *J Am Vet Med Assoc* 216:1441-1445, 2000.
66. Bonagura JD: Equine heart disease: an overview, *Vet Clin North Am (Equine Pract)* 1:267-274, 1985.
67. Bonagura JD, Pipers FS: Echocardiographic features of aortic valve endocarditis in a dog, a cow, and a horse, *J Am Vet Med Assoc* 182:595-599, 1983.
68. Ware WA, Bonagura JD, Rings DM: Echocardiographic diagnosis of pulmonic valve vegetative endocarditis in a cow, *J Am Vet Med Assoc* 188:185-187, 1986.
69. Reef VB, Spencer P: Echocardiographic evaluation of equine aortic insufficiency, *Am J Vet Res* 48:904-909, 1987.
70. Bonagura JD: Clinical evaluation and management of heart disease, *Equine Vet Educ* 2:31-37, 1990.
71. Young LE, Wood JLN: Effect of age and training on murmurs of atrioventricular valvular regurgitation in young thoroughbreds, *Equine Vet J* 32:195-199, 2000.
72. Hagio M, Otsuka H: Pulsed Doppler echocardiography in normal dogs and calves and three cases of valvular regurgitation, *Jpn J Vet Sci* 49:1113-1125, 1987.
73. Long KJ: Doppler echocardiography: clinical applications, *Equine Vet Educ* 5:161-166, 1993.
74. Reef VB: The use of diagnostic ultrasound in the horse, *Ultrasound Q* 9:1-34, 1991.
75. Reef VB: Advances in echocardiography, *Vet Clin North Am (Equine Pract)* 7:435-450, 1991.
76. Reef VB: Heart murmurs in horses: determining their significance with echocardiography, *Equine Vet J Suppl* 19:71-80, 1995.
77. Reef VB, Bain FT, Spencer PA: Severe mitral insufficiency in horses: clinical, echocardiographic, and pathologic findings, *Equine Vet J* 30:18-27, 1998.
78. Bonagura JD: Echocardiography, *Vet Clin North Am (Equine Pract)* 1:311-333, 1985.
79. Reef VB: Mitral valve insufficiency associated with ruptured chordae tendineae in three foals, *J Am Vet Med Assoc* 191:329-331, 1987.
80. Yamaga Y, Too K: Echocardiographic detection of bovine cardiac diseases, *Jpn J Vet Res* 34:251-267, 1986.
81. Patteson MW, Cripps PJ: A survey of cardiac auscultatory findings in horses, *Equine Vet J* 25:409-415, 1993.
82. Nilsfors L, Lombard CW: Diagnosis of pulmonic valve endocarditis in a horse, *Equine Vet J* 23:479-482, 1991.
83. Reimer JM, Reef VB: Echocardiographic detection of pulmonic valve rupture in a horse with right-sided failure, *J Am Vet Med Assoc* 198:880-882, 1991.
84. Koblik PD, Hornof WJ: Diagnostic radiology and nuclear cardiology, *Vet Clin North Am (Equine Pract)* 1:289-301, 1985.
85. Else RW, Holmes JR: Cardiac pathology in the horse. I. Gross pathology, *Equine Vet J* 4:1-8, 1972.
86. Evans ET: Bacterial endocarditis in cattle, *Vet Rec* 69:1190-1206, 1957.
87. Pipers FS, Hamlin RL, Reef V: Echocardiographic detection of cardiovascular lesions in the horse, *J Equine Med Surg* 3:68-77, 1979.
88. Dedrick P et al: Treatment of bacterial endocarditis in a horse, *J Am Vet Med Assoc* 193:339-342, 1988.
89. Muir WW, McGuirk SM: Drugs to treat cardiovascular disease in horses, *Vet Clin North Am (Equine Pract)* 1:335-352, 1985.
90. Sweeney RW, Reef VB, Reimer JM: Pharmacokinetics of digoxin administered to horses with congestive heart failure, *Am J Vet Res* 54:1108-1111, 1993.
91. Koritz GD et al: Pharmacokinetics of digoxin in cattle, *J Vet Pharmacol Ther* 6:141-148, 1983.

BRISKET DISEASE: COR PULMONALE/ PULMONARY HYPERTENSION

DEFINITION AND ETIOLOGY. Cor pulmonale is a term used to refer to the effect of lung dysfunction on the heart and is therefore a secondary form of heart disease. Regardless of the cause, the underlying feature is pulmonary hypertension that leads to right ventricular hypertrophy, dilation, or failure. The primary cause of the disease (also called high mountain disease or high altitude disease in cattle) is hypoxic vasoconstriction from high-altitude dwelling. The disease is worsened by the ingestion of locoweed (*Oxytropis* and *Astragalus* spp.).[92] Chronic pulmonary disease such as bronchopneumonia or lungworm infection also can result in cor pulmonale. In the horse, right heart dysfunction (i.e., decreased cardiac output, increased right ventricular end-diastolic pressure, increased right atrial or central venous pressure, jugular venous distention, or subcutaneous edema) associated with chronic pulmonary disease is rare. However, right heart dysfunction associated with pulmonary hypertension and left heart dysfunction is a common cause of congestive heart failure.

CLINICAL SIGNS AND DIFFERENTIAL DIAGNOSIS. Frequently the primary presenting clinical sign of brisket disease is subcutaneous edema of the brisket, ventral thorax, submandibular area, and occasionally the limbs. Jugular venous distention or pulsations may be present. Dyspnea and tachypnea frequently are exhibited. Tachycardia is present, and a gallop rhythm may be auscultated. Splitting of the second heart sound (S_2) is a variable finding. Pulmonary hypertension may accentuate the separation of the aortic and pulmonic valve closures, producing audible splitting of S_2 that is most noticeable during inspiration. In some horses with moderate or severe chronic obstructive pulmonary disease and increased vascular impedance; however, pulmonic valve closure occurs early, and only a single S_2 is audible.[93]

A cardiac murmur may be auscultated, caused either by tricuspid insufficiency or a pulmonic valve ejection murmur. The murmur of tricuspid insufficiency, which is secondary to right ventricular dilation, is regurgitant or plateau-shaped with the PMI over the right thorax or, less frequently, the left second intercostal space. The pulmonic valve ejection murmur, found less commonly, is audible as a crescendo-decrescendo murmur at the left heart base.[94] Pleural or pericardial effusion is not common with cor pulmonale.[95]

These clinical signs are not specific for brisket disease (cor pulmonale) and largely reflect right-sided heart failure. Other considerations when signs of right-sided heart failure are present should be bacterial endocarditis or tricuspid insufficiency from any cause, cardiomyopathy, cardiac lymphosarcoma or other thoracic neoplasms, pericarditis, left-sided

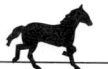

heart failure, pleuritis or pleural effusion, and congenital pulmonic valve stenosis (rare). With pericarditis, heart sounds may be muffled, or the characteristic "washing machine murmur" may be audible. Left-sided heart failure is frequently accompanied by pleural effusion, pulmonary edema, and weak peripheral pulses. In horses, however, expectoration of pulmonary edema fluid only occurs with sudden onset of severe left-sided heart failure. In horses with chronic left-sided heart failure, tachypnea, coughing, poor recovery after exercise, and harsh lung sounds may be all that is detected.

CLINICAL PATHOLOGY. A complete blood count may reveal a neutrophilia in cases of cor pulmonale caused by primary lung disease. Radiography of the thorax reveals primary pulmonary disease such as bronchopneumonia, bronchiectasis, or chronic bronchitis in cattle that have developed this disease at low altitudes. Arterial blood gases demonstrate the presence of hypoxia and may also show hypercapnea. Transtracheal wash fluid cytology and bacterial culture may provide evidence of the cause of the primary lung disease. Fecal sedimentation helps rule out parasitic bronchitis or pneumonia. Electrocardiographic findings are not specific. An echocardiogram may provide further evidence of pulmonary hypertension and right-sided heart dysfunction by showing right ventricular hypertrophy and dilation, increased septal thickness, and abnormal septal motion (Fig. 28-8).[96] Dilation of the pulmonary artery is also detected with two-dimensional echocardiography and is a sensitive indicator of pulmonary hypertension or increased flow through the pulmonary artery. Cardiac catheterization reveals elevated pressure in the pulmonary artery (see Fig. 28-8), right ventricle, and right atrium.

Elevation of right ventricular end-diastolic pressure is a sign of right ventricular failure.

PATHOPHYSIOLOGY. Pulmonary arteriolar constriction is the response to hypoxia from high-altitude dwelling or pulmonary disease. The response to hypoxia varies, depending on the amount of smooth muscle in the pulmonary arteries. In cattle, increased pulmonary vascular resistance and pulmonary hypertension frequently develop. Chronic pulmonary artery hypertension causes a pressure overload on the right ventricle, which responds to the increased work load with hypertrophy, dilation, or failure, depending on the speed with which the condition develops. The disease is progressive, and at some stage the right ventricular myocardium is unable to compensate, dilates, and fails. With failure come the typical signs of jugular venous distention and development of subcutaneous edema. Chronic right-sided heart failure may result in diastolic dysfunction of the left ventricle.

EPIDEMIOLOGY. The disease is more common in cattle than in other animal species, especially when cattle are kept at altitudes over 6000 feet, in which cases the incidence has been estimated at 0.5% to 2%.[97] Mainly calves are affected, and some herds with a higher prevalence are thought to have a genetic predisposition to develop pulmonary arterial constriction when subjected to hypoxia at high altitude. Ingestion of locoweed (*Oxytropis* and *Astragalus* spp.) also predisposes cattle to right-sided heart failure at high altitudes by causing toxic myocardial damage.[92]

NECROPSY FINDINGS. There is evidence of right-sided heart failure such as subcutaneous edema in the submandibular area, brisket, and ventral abdomen. There is dilation and hypertrophy of the right ventricle, congestion of the liver, and ascites. The lung may have changes of pneumonia, bronchitis, bronchiectasis, or emphysema. Lesions of locoweed toxicity may be found in other organs.[92]

TREATMENT AND PROGNOSIS. Removing the animal from high altitude, treating the primary lung disease, and administering oxygen may help eliminate the hypoxia and thus the pulmonary artery hypertension. Cor pulmonale from high altitude is potentially reversible when the animal is returned to a lower altitude. The heart failure can be treated with digoxin and diuretics. Beneficial effects of vasodilator therapy have not been documented. Once heart failure signs have developed, the prognosis is guarded even with appropriate treatment.

PREVENTION AND CONTROL. Selection of breeding stock with low or normal pulmonary arterial pressures at altitudes above 5000 feet (mean pulmonary artery pressure less than 35 mm Hg) helps to eliminate the predisposing genetic susceptibility to the effects of hypoxia of high altitude.[97] The disease can also be controlled by removing susceptible animals from high altitude and preventing locoweed ingestion. Herd health practices such as avoiding crowding and poor ventilation and using appropriate vaccinations to reduce the incidence of pulmonary disease help to reduce the incidence of other causes of cor pulmonale.

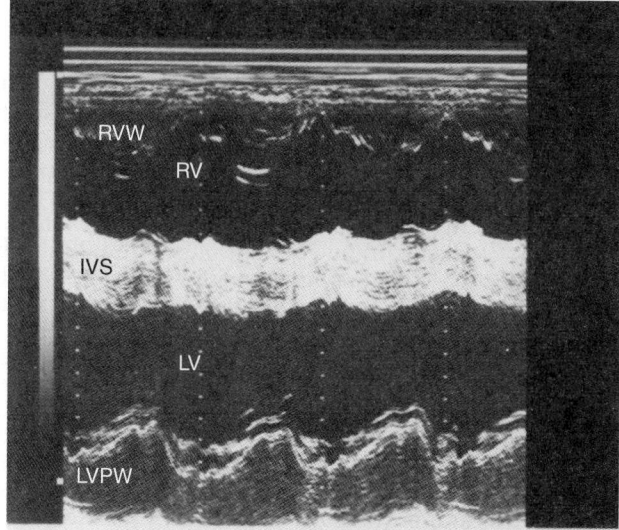
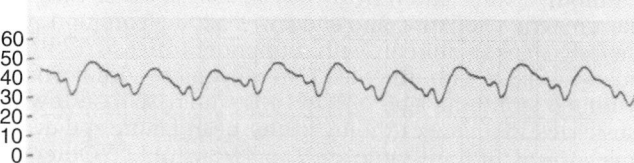

FIG. 28-8 ▓ M-mode echocardiogram and pulmonary artery pressure curve obtained from a cow with pulmonary hypertension and cor pulmonale. The echocardiogram shows mild thickening of the right ventricular wall *(RVW)* and interventricular septum *(IVS)*, dilation of the right ventricle *(RV)*, and abnormal septal motion. *LV,* Left ventricle, *LVPW,* left ventricular free wall. The pulmonary artery pressure curve demonstrates elevated systolic and diastolic pressures. (Pulmonary artery pressure curve in mm Hg.)

REFERENCES

92. James LF et al: Locoweed *Oxytropis sericea* poisoning and congestive heart failure in cattle, *J Am Vet Med Assoc* 189:1549-1556, 1986.
93. Welker FH: Investigation of the second heart sound in the horse, master's thesis, Columbus, Ohio, 1984, Ohio State University College of Veterinary Medicine.
94. Brown CM: Acquired heart disease, *Vet Clin North Am (Equine Pract)* 1:371-382, 1985.
95. Fellers G, Ardington P, Cimprich R: Clinico-pathologic conference, *J Am Vet Med Assoc* 166:700-706, 1975.
96. Bertoli L et al: Echocardiographic and hemodynamic assessment of right heart impairment in chronic obstructive lung disease, *Respiration* 44:282-288, 1983.
97. Knight AP: Clinical forum: brisket disease, *Agri-Pract* 7:21-22, 1986.

MYOCARDIAL DISEASE: MYOCARDITIS AND CARDIOMYOPATHY

DEFINITION AND ETIOLOGY. Myocarditis is an inflammation in the myocardium caused by bacterial, viral, or parasitic organisms or thromboembolic disease caused by these organisms. In large animals, recognized bacterial causes include *Staphyloccus aureus, Streptococcus equi, Clostridium chauvoei,* and *Mycobacterium* spp. Myocarditis also can occur after bacteremia, septicemia, pericarditis, or endocarditis, regardless of the etiologic agent. Known viral causes of myocarditis include foot-and-mouth disease, equine infectious anemia, equine viral arteritis, equine influenza, and African horse sickness. Parasitic causes of myocarditis may include strongylosis[98] or onchocerciasis in horses, toxoplasmosis, cysticercosis, or sarcocystis infection in ruminants.[99,100] Currently it is thought that infection with the spirochete *Borrelia burgdorferi* may be a cause of myocarditis in domestic animals, as it is in human beings.[101] Cardiomyopathy is a subacute or chronic disease of the ventricular myocardium that occurs without anatomic valvular disease, congenital malformations of the heart or vessels, or pulmonary disease. In large animals, dilated cardiomyopathy is the only cardiomyopathy of known significance. Dilated cardiomyopathy is associated with ventricular dilation, increased ventricular mass, and decreased systolic function. Although the cause is frequently undetermined,[102-104] several conditions have been related to or identified with cardiomyopathy. The most common cause of cardiomyopathy in horses is probably myocarditis, although the inciting insult is usually difficult to identify. An inherited cardiomyopathy, which is thought to be linked to the red Holstein gene, has been found in Holstein-Friesian cattle in Canada, Japan, Australia, the Netherlands, and Switzerland.[105-107] There is also a cardiomyopathy associated with a curly hair coat in polled Herefords.[108] Cardiomyopathy has been associated with ingestion of monensin, lasalocid, salinomycin, gossypol, *Cassia occidentalis,* and *Phalaris* spp. Vitamin E and selenium deficiency, copper deficiency, excessive molybdenum, or high sulfates (secondary copper deficiency) may cause cardiomyopathy.[109-117] Myocardial infiltration by neoplasia such as lymphosarcoma or fibrosarcoma also may cause cardiomyopathy.

CLINICAL SIGNS AND DIFFERENTIAL DIAGNOSIS. The manifestations of myocarditis are highly variable, depending on the extent of the disease, location of the inflammation within the myocardium, and associated systemic illness. Myocarditis can easily be missed because of the lack of specific cardiac signs or the predominance of signs related to the organ system with primary involvement (e.g., strangles in horses or mastitis in cattle). Animals with myocarditis are often febrile or have a recent history of fever and may have tachycardia. The elevated heart rate may be caused by sinus tachycardia or other paroxysmal or sustained supraventricular or ventricular arrhythmias, because cardiac arrhythmias are common. Premature beats are also commonly detected in large animals with myocarditis and may be present in animals with a normal or increased heart rate. Occasionally acute myocarditis is associated with auscultation of a pronounced gallop rhythm or a cardiac murmur of either tricuspid or mitral valve insufficiency. Jugular venous distention, other signs of congestive heart failure such as peripheral edema, and signs of circulatory collapse may be present. Horses may show evidence of myalgia, reluctance to move, or exercise intolerance. With these signs it may be difficult to distinguish myocarditis from colic, respiratory disease, lameness, or septicemia. If signs are more clearly cardiac (e.g., murmur, arrhythmia, jugular venous pulsations), the practitioner should rule out endocarditis, cardiomyopathy, cardiac neoplasia, or congestive heart failure from another cause.

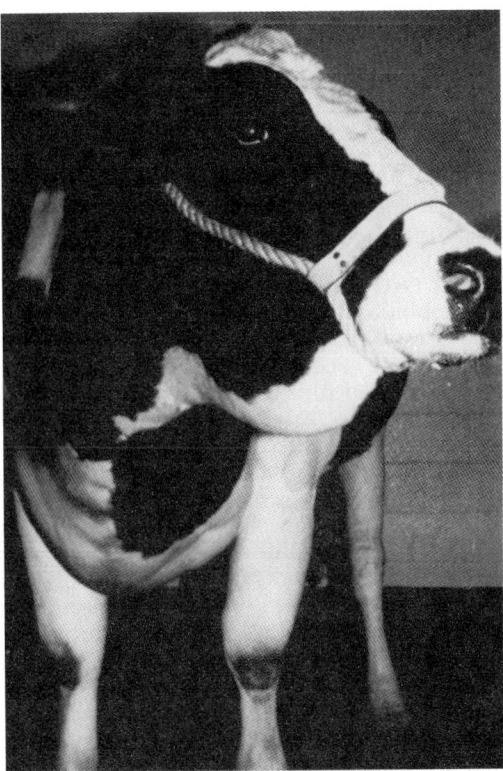

FIG. 28-9 ▓ Holstein cow with cardiomyopathy showing signs of congestive heart failure (submandibular and brisket edema, jugular venous distention, and pulsations).

The clinical signs associated with dilated cardiomyopathy can also be variable but are usually more clearly associated with heart disease. Most animals have signs of cardiac failure such as peripheral edema and jugular venous distention or pulsations (Fig. 28-9). Auscultation frequently reveals tachycardia, gallop rhythm, muffled heart sounds, or a cardiac arrhythmia. Cardiac murmurs of tricuspid or mitral valve insufficiency are usually present secondary to the ventricular dilation. The breath sounds are increased, tachypnea is present, and, frequently, percussion of the thorax reveals sign of pleural or pericardial fluid. Occasionally respiratory distress is evident with hyperpnea, dyspnea, coughing, and the presence of a bloody froth at the nostril. Nonspecific signs of cardiomyopathy such as exercise intolerance, syncope, diarrhea, or anorexia may also be present. In cattle, decreased milk production and abomasal displacement have been associated with dilated cardiomyopathy.[105]

Sudden death can be a feature of myocarditis or dilated cardiomyopathy, and it frequently follows stress or exercise. Recumbency, collapse, and sudden death are common presenting signs in animals with ionophore toxicosis.[109-117] In many animals with inherited cardiomyopathy, death occurs within 6 months of age.[106,108] In Holstein-Friesian cattle with suspected inherited cardiomyopathy, heart failure and death may not occur until cattle are 2 to 4 years old.[105] Other acquired causes of cardiomyopathy can occur at any age.

When animals show clinical signs of dilated cardiomyopathy, many differential diagnoses should be considered. If the animal is young, other congenital heart defects, cor pulmonale, and nutritional myodegeneration should be considered. In adults, bacterial endocarditis, cardiac neoplasia, thoracic abscess, pericarditis, pleuritis, and diaphragmatic hernia may also have similar clinical manifestations. Although the

cause of dilated cardiomyopathy may be difficult to determine, nutritional (vitamin E, selenium, or copper deficiency), toxic (monensin, gossypol, salinomycin, lasalocid, *Cassia* spp., or *Phalaris*), infectious (viral, bacterial, or parasitic) or drug-induced causes should be investigated.

CLINICAL PATHOLOGY. Depending on the cause of the myocardial disease, the clinicopathologic findings may vary. Routine complete blood count may be normal, or a neutrophilic leukocytosis may be present. No consistent changes are expected in the serum chemistry profile, but serum albumin concentration may be slightly decreased and serum urea nitrogen, creatinine, γ-glutamyltranspeptidase (GGT), sorbitol dehydrogenase (SDH), and bilirubin concentrations may be increased because of congestive liver disease when signs of congestive heart failure are present. Serum concentrations of creatine kinase (CK) and lactic dehydrogenase (LDH) may be elevated but hepatic and skeletal muscle contribution to these elevations cannot be ruled out. A better indication of myocardial disease may be the elevation of cardiac troponin I or the myocardial isoenzymes of CK (myocardial bound [MB]) and LDH (LDH_1), but the sensitivity and specificity of these tests have not been documented in large animals. Large elevations of the myocardial isoenzymes of CK and LDH were detected in one recent outbreak of monensin toxicosis[112] and have been detected in other horses with myocardial necrosis of unknown etiology. Marked elevations of cardiac troponin I have also been reported in a horse with ventricular tachycardia and aortic septal rupture.[118] Analysis of pericardial or pleural fluid reveals a transudate with low protein concentration (less than 2.5 g/dl) and cellularity (WBC less than 2500/μl), with the predominant cell type being mononuclear cells, unless the myocarditis is an extension of pericarditis. Serum should be tested for serologic evidence of bovine leukosis (BLV) infection in adult cattle, α-tocopherol, glutathione peroxidase, and copper concentrations. Whole blood selenium levels should be determined. In infectious myocarditis or inherited cardiomyopathy, these tests are most likely normal. A negative BLV test essentially eliminates lymphosarcoma as a cause of the myocardial disease; a positive test does not confirm a causal relationship. In horses, serum should be tested for serologic evidence of a variety of equine viruses, particularly influenza, equine viral arteritis, and herpes virus. Hemoglobinuria, if present, suggests consideration of monensin, gossypol, or nutritional myodegeneration as the cause of myocardial disease. Arterial blood oxygen tension may be reduced below 80 mm Hg in animals with myocardial disease.

An ECG may demonstrate sinus tachycardia or other cardiac arrhythmias; the frequency and severity of these arrhythmias are best demonstrated with continuous electrocardiographic monitoring. There may be some evidence of conduction abnormalities in the base-apex lead, but these findings are not specific for myocardial disease. Echocardiography may be normal in animals with myocarditis or the abnormalities detected may be caused by the arrhythmias present. More frequently, however, there is increased ventricular chamber size, decreased thickness of the interventricular septum and left ventricular free wall, and decreased myocardial function (decreased fractional shortening, decreased ejection fraction, and myocardial dyskinesis), especially in more severe cases of myocarditis and in animals with dilated cardiomyopathy. In humans with myocarditis there may be evidence of abnormal left ventricular wall motion, paradoxical motion of the interventricular septum, or an echo-free pericardial space.[119] Additional echocardiographic features of dilated cardiomyopathy are increased end-systolic and end-diastolic dimensions of the left and right ventricles (Fig. 28-10), increased left atrial size, and an increased left atrial to aortic root dimension ratio. There may be abnormal mitral

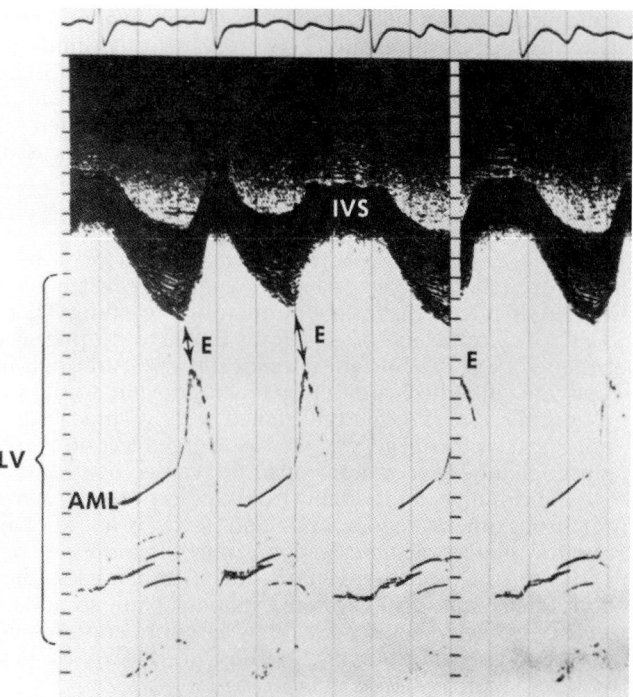

FIG. 28-10 ▓ M-mode echocardiogram obtained from a horse with dilated cardiomyopathy, showing a markedly dilated left ventricle (21 cm in diastole), increased septal mitral valve EF slope, and E point to interventricular septal separation *(arrows)*. *SML,* Septal mitral valve leaflet; *IVS,* interventricular septum.

valve closure (increased EF slope) and increased separation of the septal mitral valve leaflet and the interventricular septum (see Fig. 28-10). A decreased aortic root diameter may be imaged in animals with low-output left-sided heart failure and an enlarged pulmonary artery indicative of pulmonary hypertension.

Cardiac catheterization may reveal elevated intracardiac pressures (right atrial, right ventricular, pulmonary artery, pulmonary capillary wedge, and left ventricular end-diastolic) in animals with dilated cardiomyopathy. Humans with acute infectious myocarditis may show hypotension and a narrow pulse pressure. Nuclear angiocardiography may be used to show decreased ejection fraction[120] in animals with myocardial disease.

PATHOPHYSIOLOGY. The pathophysiologic changes associated with myocardial disease depend on the specific nature and extent of the disease. Acute myocarditis or angiopathic myocardial lesions[98] may go on to develop idiopathic dilated cardiomyopathy. It is speculated that changes in cellular metabolism occur with either acute myocarditis or dilated cardiomyopathy, resulting in ECG abnormalities and reduced myocardial performance (reduced cardiac output). In an attempt to compensate for reduced cardiac output, circulating fluid volume is increased by activation of the renin-angiotensin-aldosterone system, and arterial resistance is increased. These compensatory mechanisms frequently lead to only minor improvement in the cardiac output of the failing heart, and the increase in ventricular preload (venous return) and afterload (arterial resistance) may cause pulmonary edema and a further reduction in cardiac contractility. Ventricular dilation, further reduction in cardiac output, and signs of heart failure occur.

EPIDEMIOLOGY. The prevalence of acute myocarditis is difficult to estimate, because frequently the disease goes undiagnosed or is mild, is masked by disease in another organ system, or the animal recovers spontaneously. Similarly, it is difficult to assess the clinical significance of postmortem findings of myocardial inflammation and fibrosis. The morbidity of myocarditis in large animals probably is underestimated because it is rarely the cause of mortality and is associated with viral, bacterial, and parasitic infections that manifest themselves without specific signs of cardiovascular disease.

Inherited cardiomyopathy has been reported in cattle in Japan, Australia, the Netherlands, Canada, and Switzerland, with the incidence in inbred populations reaching 3% to 5%.[106] These cattle may be genetically linked by the presence of the red gene in Holstein-Friesian cattle.[105] Although in some cattle inherited cardiomyopathy resulted in death by 6 months of age,[106,108] other cattle failed to show clinical signs until 2 to 4 years of age.[103-105,107] No sex predilection is recognized in inherited cardiomyopathy of cattle.

The morbidity and mortality from cardiomyopathy stemming from other causes in cattle and horses is not known. From the number of clinical reports, inherited cardiomyopathy seems to be more prevalent in cattle than in horses. Idiopathic dilated cardiomyopathy or cardiomyopathy secondary to viral or bacterial infections may be more common in horses and is a common cause for the acute onset of congestive heart failure in horses of racing age.

NECROPSY FINDINGS. There may be no gross lesions associated with myocarditis. Depending on the relationship between death and the occurrence of myocarditis, microscopic examination of the myocardium may show no inflammatory cells but increased fibrous tissue in the interstitium or there may be foci of inflammatory cells (typically mononuclear cells), degeneration of adjacent myocardial fibers, myocardial necrosis, and fibrosis. Samples of gastric or rumenal contents should be obtained and submitted for analysis of ionophores if ionophore toxicosis is suspected. Similarly, feed samples should also be obtained and submitted for ionophore analysis in these cases.

The lesions of cardiomyopathy are recognized more easily grossly as enlargement of the heart, which may be rounded to globose. Biatrial, biventricular, and pulmonary artery dilation are usually present. Patchy or uniform streaks of myocardial pallor may be detected. In rare cases, one of the chambers or major vessels (usually pulmonary artery) may rupture. Generalized edema is frequently found as ascites (uncommon in horses), pericardial or pleural effusion, and edema of the mesentery and subcutaneous tissues. There may be evidence of vascular congestion of the liver, lungs, and spleen. The kidneys may be pale and swollen, and have an irregular, granular, pitted surface.

Microscopically the lesions of cardiomyopathy are characterized as myocardial vacuolation and degeneration with necrosis and fibrosis. Calcification may be associated with these lesions. Occasionally there is increased vascularization with proliferative regeneration of myofibers. In some cases, no histopathologic abnormalities are found.

TREATMENT AND PROGNOSIS. The treatment of myocarditis includes treatment of the underlying etiologic agent if it is recognized and control of the complications such as arrhythmias, congestive heart failure, or shock. Thromboembolism is rarely a complication recognized in animals. Performance animals should be rested. Corticosteroids may be beneficial in animals with severe toxemia, complicated arrhythmias, or intractable heart failure but their use in early cases of myocarditis or in infections suspected of having a viral etiology is controversial because viral recrudescence may occur. However, in many cases the corticosteroids appear to have a beneficial effect. Prognosis is good if there are no signs

of heart failure and if cardiac arrhythmias are managed successfully. Prognosis is guarded to poor if signs of congestive heart failure are present.

Therapeutic strategies currently used for treatment of dilated cardiomyopathy include positive inotropic agents (digoxin), diuretics, vasodilators, rest, and in some cases removal of pleural or abdominal fluid. The advantages of vasodilators (venodilators to relieve pulmonary edema and arterial dilators to reduce preload and afterload and improve contractility) in the treatment of cardiomyopathy are recognized in humans and small animals[121] but these drugs have not been widely used in large animals because of the lack of pharmacokinetic studies and clinical trials.

Digoxin is the positive inotropic agent used almost exclusively in large animals but is contraindicated in animals with acute monensin toxicosis. A priming or loading dose can be used in horses with acute severe congestive heart failure followed with a maintenance dose or the horse can be started on a maintenance dose from the onset of therapy. In horses the drug can be administered orally or parenterally. In cattle, low bioavailability limits its use to the intravenous route of administration.[122] The following dosage schedules serve as guidelines for the use of digoxin[123-125]:

Horses:	Priming dose IV:	12 to 14 µg/kg
	Priming dose PO:	34 (Elixir) to 70 (powdered tablets in suspension) µg/kg
	Maintenance dosage IV:	6 to 7 µg/kg/24 hr
	Maintenance dosage PO:	17 (Elixir) to 35 (powdered tablets in suspension) µg/kg/24 hr
Cattle:	Priming dose IV:	22 µg/kg
	Maintenance dosage IV:	Infusion of 0.86 µg/kg/hr or give 11 µg/kg three times daily

Dehydration, acid-base imbalance, and electrolyte abnormalities should be corrected before digoxin therapy. The dose of digoxin should be decreased in animals with elevated creatinine or BUN, until these values return to normal. In horses the intravenous loading dose of digoxin should be administered slowly or divided and given at a rate of one third of the loading dose hourly until completion.[123] Alternatively, therapy can be initiated with the maintenance dose. Close monitoring of body weight, appetite, electrolyte concentrations, creatinine or BUN concentrations, and cardiac rhythm are essential during therapy. Therapeutic drug monitoring with digoxin plasma concentrations can be helpful during initial therapy, when the volume of distribution of the drug and the patient's body weight may be in a state of flux. Samples for determination of peak serum digoxin concentrations should be obtained 1 to 2 hours after digoxin administration and should not exceed 2.5 ng/ml.[125,126]

The diuretic used most commonly in large animals is furosemide. It is administered parenterally at the rate of 0.5 to 1 mg/kg twice daily or as needed to control edema. The half-life and diuretic effect of bumetanide, a sulfonamide diuretic, are shorter than that of furosemide in horses.[127] Electrolyte concentrations and water consumption should be monitored closely in patients receiving diuretics.

The vasodilators used most frequently in horses include hydralazine and enalapril, an ACE inhibitor. Both have resulted in clinical improvement in animals treated for congestive heart failure. Hydralazine is administered orally at a dose of 0.5-1.5 mg/kg twice daily. Enalapril has been used at a dose of 0.5 mg/kg orally once or twice daily. Enalapril has also been beneficial in the management of horses with moderate to severe mitral or aortic regurgitation.

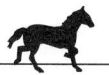

Control of cardiac arrhythmias should be attempted in animals that are hemodynamically unstable or threatened with the development of worsening arrhythmias. Quinidine is usually the drug of choice for control of atrial and ventricular arrhythmias in cattle and is one of the drugs of choice in horses. Procainamide, lidocaine and propafenone have also been successful in the treatment of ventricular arrhythmias in horses (see Table 28-3). Although administration is limited to the intravenous route in cattle, oral or intravenous administration in horses results in adequate plasma concentrations to control arrhythmias. Quinidine is administered intravenously by infusion or by divided bolus injections as follows:

Cattle:	IV:	48 mg/kg infused intravenously over a 4-hr period
Horses:	IV:	1.5 to 2 mg/kg every 20 min until conversion or desired effect but not to exceed a total dosage of 12 mg/kg
	PO:	22 mg/kg (1 g/100 lb of body weight) q2h until conversion or desired effect; not to exceed a total dosage of 132 mg/kg q2h

When quinidine is used intravenously, concurrent IV administration of a balanced electrolyte solution at the rate of 3 to 4 ml/kg/hr is desirable to maintain blood pressure in animals with a severely compromised cardiovascular status.

Prognosis for animals with dilated cardiomyopathy is poor. Echocardiography is useful in determining the severity of the myocardial dysfunction and in formulating a prognosis. The results of the initial echocardiographic examination were the best prognostic indicator of survival in a recent outbreak of monensin toxicosis.[112] Recovery of animals with cardiomyopathy is unusual, constant therapy is required for maintenance of animals in congestive heart failure, and sudden death can occur at any time. Some animals may have significant myocardial dysfunction without congestive heart failure and are "cardiac cripples," comfortable at pasture but not safe to use for performance. These animals may later develop congestive heart failure.

PREVENTION AND CONTROL. Maintenance of a good vaccination program may limit the bacterial and viral causes of myocarditis. Parasite control may also reduce myocardial injury that predisposes to myocarditis or cardiomyopathy in horses. Toxic myocardial diseases are prevented by proper mixing of feeds containing monensin, salinomycin, or lasalocid and by preventing horses from ingesting these medicated feeds. Gossypol toxicity can be prevented by feeding no cottonseed meal or cottonseed meal with low gossypol content, especially when feeding preruminants.[128] Feeding of cottonseed meal can be limited by providing more forage or additional protein sources in the diet of ruminants so that ingestion of gossypol is limited to concentrations of 1 to 2 g/kg or less of feed for adult cattle and 0.5 to 1 g/kg or less of feed for immature cattle.[129] Nutritional myocardial disease can be prevented by adequate feeding of vitamin E, selenium, and copper with supplementation as required. Inherited cardiomyopathy is controlled by avoiding breeding of known or suspected carriers of the polled Hereford and Holstein-Friesian breeds.

REFERENCES

98. Cranley JJ, McCullagh KG: Ischaemic myocardial fibrosis and aortic strongylosis in the horse, *Equine Vet J* 13:35-42, 1981.
99. Dubey JP et al: Caprine toxoplasmosis: abortion, clinical signs, and distribution of *Toxoplasma* in tissues of goats fed *Toxoplasma gondii* oocysts, *Am J Vet Res* 41:1072-1076, 1980.
100. Dubey JP: A review of sarcocystis of domestic animals and other coccidia of cats and dogs, *J Am Vet Med Assoc* 169:1061-1078, 1976.
101. Madigan JE, Teitler J: *Borrelia burgdorferi* borreliosis, *J Am Vet Med Assoc* 192:892-896, 1988.
102. Dudan F, Rossi GL, Luginbihl H: Ètude cardiovasculaire chez le cheval: relation entre les alterations vasculaires et tissulaires du myocarde. III, Suite et fin, *Schweiz Archiv Tierheikld* 127:369-378, 1985.
103. Lacuata AQ, Yamada H, Hirose T: Atrial fibrillation in a cow with postpartum cardiomyopathy: case report, *J Vet Med* 19:97-99, 1980.
104. Yamaga Y, Too K: Echocardiographic detection of bovine cardiac diseases, *Jpn J Vet Res* 34:251-267, 1986.
105. Baird JD: Dilated cardiomyopathy in Holstein cattle: clinical and genetic aspects, *Proceedings of the sixth annual Veterinary Medicine Forum*, Washington, DC, 1988, pp 175-177.
106. Watanabe S et al: Evidence for a new lethal gene causing cardiomyopathy in Japanese black calves, *J Hered* 70:255-258, 1979.
107. Martig J et al: Gehnufte fnlle von herzinsuffizienz beim rind vorlnufige mitteilung, *Schweiz Archiv Tierheikld* 124:69-82, 1982.
108. Morrow CJ, McOrist S: Cardiomyopathy associated with a curly hair coat in poll Hereford calves in Australia, *Vet Rec* 117:312-313, 1985.
109. Muyelle E et al: Delayed monensin sodium toxicity in horses, *Equine Vet J* 13:107-108, 1981.
110. Doonan GR et al: Monensin poisoning in horses: an international incident, *Can Vet J* 30:165-169, 1989.
111. Boemo CM et al: Monensin toxicosis in horses: an outbreak resulting in the death of ten horses, *Aust Vet J* 9:103-107, 1991.
112. Reef VB: A monensin outbreak in horses in the eastern United States: pathogenesis, clinical signs and epidemiology, *Proceedings of the Eighth annual Veterinary Medicine Forum*, 1990, pp 619-622.
113. Rollinson J, Taylor FGR, Chesney J: Salinomycin poisoning in horses, *Vet Rec* 121:126-128, 1987.
114. Newsholme SJ et al: Fatal cardiomyopathy in feedlot sheep attributed to monensin toxicosis, *J South Afr Vet Assoc* 54:29-32, 1983.
115. Geor RJ, Robinson WF: Suspected monensin toxicosis in feedlot cattle, *Aust Vet J* 62:130-131, 1985.
116. van Amstel SR, Guthrie AJ: Salinomycin poisoning in horses: case report, *Proc Am Assoc Equine Pract* 31:373-382, 1985.
117. Whitlock RH et al: Monensin toxicosis in horses: clinical manifestations, *Proc Am Assoc Equine Pract* 24:473-486, 1978.
118. Cornelisse CJ et al: Concentration of cardiac troponin I in a horse with a ruptured aortic regurgitation jet lesion and ventricular tachycardia. *J Am Vet Med Assoc* 217:231-235, 2000.
119. Iknheimo MJ, Takkunen JT: Echocardiography in acute infectious myocarditis, *Chest* 89:100-102, 1986.
120. Koblik PD et al: Left ventricular ejection fraction in the normal horse determined by first-pass nuclear angiocardiography, *Vet Radiol* 26:53-62, 1985.
121. Miller MS, O'Grady MR, Smith FWK: Current concepts in vasodilator therapy for advanced or refractory congestive heart failure, *Can Vet J* 29:354-361, 1988.
122. Koritz GD et al: Pharmacokinetics of digoxin in cattle, *J Vet Pharmacol Ther* 6:141-148, 1983.
123. Button C et al: Digoxin pharmacokinetics, bioavailability, efficacy, and dosage regimens in the horse, *Am J Vet Res* 41:1388-1395, 1980.
124. Pedersoli WM et al: Pharmacokinetics of a single, orally administered dose of digoxin in horses, *Am J Vet Res* 42:1412-1414, 1981.
125. Sweeney RW, Reef VB, Reimer JM: Pharmacokinetics of digoxin administered to horses with congestive heart failure, *Am J Vet Res* 54:1108-1111, 1993.
126. Davis LE, Neff-Davis CA, Wilcke JR: Monitoring drug concentrations in animal patients, *J Am Vet Med Assoc* 176:1156-1158, 1980.
127. Delbeke FT, Desmet M, Stevens M: Pharmacokinetics and diuretic effect of bumetanide after intravenous and intramuscular administration to horses, *J Vet Pharmacol Ther* 9:310-317, 1986.
128. Morgan S et al: Clinical, clinicopathologic, pathologic, and toxicologic alterations associated with gossypol toxicosis in feeder lambs, *Am J Vet Res* 49:493-499, 1988.
129. Hudson LM, Kerr LA, Maslin WR: Gossypol toxicosis in a herd of beef calves, *J Am Vet Med Assoc* 192:1303-1305, 1988.

PERICARDITIS

DEFINITION AND ETIOLOGY. Pericarditis is inflammation of the pericardium that results in the accumulation of fluid or exudate between the visceral and parietal pericardium. Pericarditis in large animals can be caused by trauma from penetration of ingested foreign objects or external wounds, hematogenous spread (septicemia) of infection, extension of infection from the lung or pleura, viral infections such as equine viral arteritis or equine influenza, and neoplasia. Idiopathic pericarditis, characterized by an aseptic inflammatory exudate, is not uncommon in horses.[130-134] Autoimmune, hereditary, and metabolic causes of pericarditis have not been documented in large animals.

CLINICAL SIGNS AND DIFFERENTIAL DIAGNOSIS.
The clinical presentation of pericarditis can vary, depending on the volume and rate of development of the pericardial effusion and the cause. The nonspecific clinical signs of fever, anorexia, depression, or weight loss may be the chief complaints; but more frequently peripheral edema, jugular venous distention and pulsations, tachypnea, or dyspnea are the presenting clinical signs. Cattle may exhibit pain by an abnormal stance characterized by abducted elbows, a spontaneous or induced expiratory grunt, reluctance to move, or preference to stand with the forequarters elevated. Horses may show signs of colic or syncopal episodes.

The most consistent findings on auscultation are tachycardia, muffling of heart sounds, and absence of lung sounds in the ventral thorax. Dorsally the lung sounds are louder than normal. These findings are in contrast to pleuritis, an important diagnostic ruleout for pericarditis, in which the lung sounds are muffled ventrally but the heart sounds are not and radiation of the heart sounds occurs over a wider area than normal.[135] In cattle, splashing sounds frequently are audible in the cardiac auscultation area, a sound some refer to as a "washing machine murmur." This is attributed to the accumulation of gas and fluid in the pericardium and is indicative of the presence of gas-forming (anaerobic) organisms and a grave prognosis. In cattle, this murmur distinguishes pericarditis from cardiac neoplasia or other causes of congestive heart failure. The splashing sounds are absent in horses and muffled heart sounds are the rule, but pericardial friction rubs may be auscultated, especially after pericardial fluid accumulation has been relieved.[132] A gallop rhythm may be auscultated in either horses or cattle.

Mucous membranes may be congested and have a prolonged capillary refill time. Jugular venous distention and pulsations usually are present. Arterial pulses are weak. The latter findings may help distinguish pericarditis from primary pleuritis. Percussion of the thorax reveals ventral dullness, and pleural effusion is frequently present in horses with pericarditis. Ascites is infrequently detected in horses with pericarditis, but concurrent peritonitis has been reported.[136]

CLINICAL PATHOLOGY. The changes shown in a complete blood count are not specific and depend on the cause of the pericarditis. There may be hemoconcentration if the animal is dehydrated or toxemic, or there may be a mild ane-

mia associated with chronic infectious pericarditis. The white blood cell (WBC) count may be normal or increased. There may be an absolute neutrophilia or a lymphopenia. Frequently the fibrinogen concentration is elevated. The serum chemistries are usually normal except for albumin concentration, which may be low[131,132] and accompanied by an elevation in globulin concentration. Liver enzyme, bilirubin, serum urea nitrogen, and creatinine concentrations are frequently mildly elevated, consistent with the development of congestive heart failure. Laboratory evidence of dehydration (increased packed cell volume, total protein, serum urea nitrogen, and creatinine concentrations) may be exaggerated when diuretics have been administered previously. Although total serum LDH concentration may be elevated, more specific information may come from finding an increase in the cardiac troponin I or the myocardial isoenzymes of CK and LDH. Electrolyte concentrations are frequently normal, but serum calcium and potassium concentrations may be low because of anorexia. Decreased sodium and chloride concentrations have been reported in horses with pericarditis.[132] No consistent abnormalities in arterial or venous blood gas concentrations have been reported in large animals with pericarditis.

Radiography is not a sensitive diagnostic test for pericarditis in horses. In cattle, traumatic pericarditis frequently results in fluid and gas accumulation in the pericardium that is detectable radiographically and is relatively specific for this disease. A metallic foreign body is usually detected radiographically in the cranial reticulum or caudal thorax in cattle with traumatic pericarditis. Radiographic changes may not be detected in early or uncomplicated pericarditis and, if fluid accumulation is large and there is concurrent pleural effusion, are indistinguishable from pleuritis. An enlarged, rounded cardiac silhouette can be seen with pericarditis or other causes of generalized cardiomegaly. An obscured cardiac silhouette, vena cava, and diaphragm with dorsal displacement of the trachea may be seen with pericarditis or pleuritis. The lungs, which may be aerated only dorsally, frequently have interstitial infiltrates.

The ECG changes most commonly associated with pericarditis in large animals are decreased amplitude of the QRS complexes (less than 1.5 mV in the base-apex lead)[132,133,136] (Fig. 28-11), electrical alternans (altered configuration of the P, QRS, or T complexes on a regular basis), and ST segment

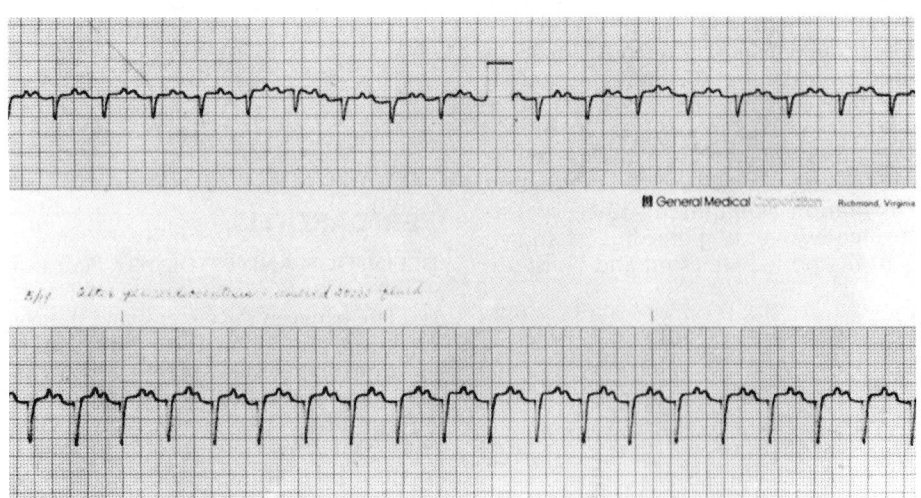

FIG. 28-11 ▓ Base-apex lead ECG taken from a cow before (upper strip) and after (lower strip) removal of 2 L of pericardial fluid. The markedly decreased amplitude (0.6 mV) of the QRS complexes is improved (1.2 mV) after pericardiocentesis.

elevation or slurring.[131,132,136-138] A right-axis deviation in the standard limb leads may be apparent.[131,137] In some animals, no ECG changes are evident.[139]

Echocardiography reveals findings specific for pericarditis and is used to confirm the diagnosis noninvasively. An echo-free space between the visceral and parietal pericardium is evident and apparent even with a minimum amount of fluid accumulation.[135,138] Frequently, hypoechoic to echoic strands that correspond to fibrin are imaged in the pericardial space with a hypoechoic to echoic layer covering the epicardial surface of the heart in large animals with pericarditis (Fig. 28-12). The pericardial effusion is often anechoic to hypoechoic but more echoic pericardial fluid is occasionally seen consistent with a more exudative fluid. Bright hyperechoic pinpoint echoes representing free gas are often imaged in cattle with pericarditis. Gas in the pericardial sac of cattle with splashy heart sounds may limit the ability to obtain an echocardiographic evaluation of all cardiac structures. The visualization of intrapericardial gas is a sensitive indicator of anaerobic pericarditis. Pericardial effusion is differentiated from pleural effusion by finding the echo-free space surrounding the right ventricle and left ventricular free wall, but pericardial effusion is rarely imaged behind the left atrium.[140] Unlike pleural effusion, pericardial effusion produces an echo-free space between the descending aorta and the left ventricular free wall.[140] Right ventricular diastolic collapse and right atrial collapse are common findings with large pericardial effusions and are an indication of the development of cardiac tamponade and hemodynamically significant pericardial effusion.[133] Other echocardiographic findings consistent with pericarditis are decreased left ventricular chamber dimension, decreased left ventricular free wall motion, and decreased parietal pericardial motion.[133,134,138,141] Increased or paradoxical motion (cranial motion beginning before the QRS complex) of the interventricular septum may be apparent (see Fig. 28-12).[140,141]

The site for pericardiocentesis should be selected echocardiographically. Pericardial fluid is obtained most commonly from the left fifth intercostal space 2.5 to 10 cm dorsal to the olecranon, above the level of the lateral thoracic vein, the safest site to perform a pericardiocentesis. When there is a large volume of pericardial effusion, pericardiocentesis can be productive from the right at approximately this same location. If at all possible, a pericardial catheter (large-bore Argyle tube) should be inserted into the pericardial space at the time the initial pericardiocentesis is performed to enable repeated drainage and lavage of the pericardial sac. Fluid analysis and bacterial and viral culture results depend on the etiology. In cattle with traumatic pericarditis, fluid analysis usually reveals elevated protein concentration (>3.5 g/dl) and an elevated WBC count (>2500/μl), composed primarily of neutrophils. The fluid is urine colored to slightly blood tinged and foamy, and it has a foul odor. A mixed population of gram-positive and gram-negative aerobic and anaerobic (gastrointestinal flora) bacteria usually are present. Protozoa may be found in unusual circumstances. In horses, protein concentration of the pericardial fluid is elevated ($\geq$2.5 g/dl) and the WBC count is normal or elevated with a population predominantly of neutrophils, although red blood cells, lymphocytes, eosinophils, mesothelial cells, and histiocytes have been observed.[131-133,136,138] Bacterial (aerobic and anaerobic) cultures and viral cultures may be negative. Paired serum may support a viral etiology. Analysis of pleural and peritoneal fluid (when present) usually reveals fluid characterized as a modified transudate or that is mildly inflammatory.

Cardiac catheterization demonstrates an elevation in central venous or right atrial pressure, and the atrial and ventricular pressure curve may be abnormal in appearance. Right atrial, right ventricular, and pulmonary artery end-diastolic pressures may equilibrate.[137] In combination these findings are relatively specific for pericarditis.

PATHOPHYSIOLOGY. The accumulation of fluid in the pericardium occurs as a result of inflammation. The rate of fluid accumulation and the degree to which the pericardial pressure increases determine the pathophysiologic consequences. Generally pericarditis results in decreased distensibility (increased ventricular end-diastolic pressure) of the heart, which impairs the ability of the heart to fill during diastole. The elevation in end-diastolic pressure and impairment of ventricular filling elevate atrial pressure and reduce venous flow or venous return to the heart and diastolic perfusion of the myocardium. The result is a depression of ventricular contractility, stroke volume, and consequently cardiac output. In addition, arterial pressure and renal blood flow are decreased. Initially compensatory mechanisms consisting of vasoconstriction, increased heart rate, and sodium retention (increased vascular volume) may maintain cardiac output. Failure to maintain cardiac output results in circulatory collapse.

Pericarditis can be classified as primarily effusive, constrictive, or a combination of both.[137] The hemodynamic consequences of effusive pericarditis are primarily caused by the physical presence of pericardial fluid, whereas constrictive pericarditis is classified as such because the reduction in ventricular compliance is caused by fibrinous or fibrotic involvement of the pericardium and epicardium. Removal of pericardial fluid results in improved cardiac performance in effusive pericarditis but is of limited usefulness in constrictive pericarditis.

EPIDEMIOLOGY. Pericarditis is uncommon in horses; when it does occur, it is most frequently idiopathic and can occur in a horse of any age. History of a recent respiratory tract infection is not uncommon. Traumatic pericarditis has been reported in horses but is rare.[142] Traumatic pericarditis is not uncommon in cattle, but it occurs in less than 10% of cattle with traumatic reticuloperitonitis.[143] Most cattle are affected in late gestation or at parturition. Idiopathic pericarditis is rare in cattle.

NECROPSY FINDINGS. Gross postmortem examination shows distention of the pericardial sac with serosanguineous or urine-colored fluid that is foamy and may be malodorous (cattle). There may be organization of fibrinous exudate and

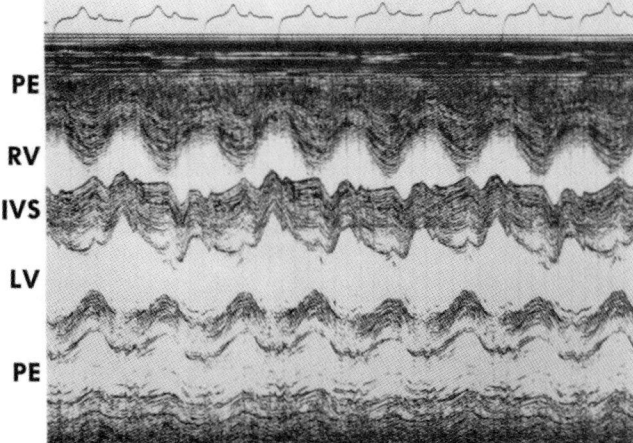

FIG. 28-12 ▓ M-mode echocardiogram obtained from a cow with traumatic pericarditis. There is a separation between the visceral and parietal pericardium cranial to the right ventricle (RV) and caudal to the left ventricle. The cranial pericardial effusion (PE) is echogenic, suggesting that fibrin or debris is present. The left ventricular (LV) dimension is reduced, and there is marked cranial motion of the interventricular septum (IVS) just before the QRS complex.

fibrosis that is also evident on the epicardium (Fig. 28-13) and may infiltrate the myocardium. Pleural effusion may be present. Other signs of congestive heart failure such as pulmonary congestion, pulmonary edema, and chronic passive congestion of the liver may be present. If the cause is traumatic, the offending object may be well contained in a fibrous tract located between the reticulum and the pericardium.

Histopathologic examination reveals pericardial, epicardial, and occasionally myocardial fibrosis and inflammation with neutrophilic, lymphocytic, eosinophilic, or plasma cell infiltrates. Bacteria may be visualized. The liver may show diffuse, centrilobular necrosis, fatty change, dilation and congestion of sinusoids, and perivenous fibrosis.

TREATMENT AND PROGNOSIS. Treatment of traumatic pericarditis in cattle is unrewarding and usually is addressed toward salvage or short-term survival to calving. Repeated pericardial drainage by means of pericardiocentesis or a fifth rib resection, lavage, or pericardiectomy may be useful for short-term survival, but the prognosis for return to normal function is poor, because congestive heart failure results from involvement not only of the pericardium but also of the epicardium and myocardium (see Fig. 28-13). Thoracotomy by a split-rib technique followed by pericardiectomy has been effective in treating some cattle with traumatic, restrictive pericarditis.[144]

Treatment of pericarditis not caused by trauma has been successful in horses, but the initial prognosis should be guarded. Aggressive treatment of horses with moderate to large pericardial effusions should include the placement of a large-bore indwelling chest tube into the pericardial sac under echocardiographic guidance and drainage and lavage of the pericardial sac, with local infusion of antibiotics. Obtaining a sample for cytology and culture and sensitivity testing via a pericardiocentesis should be postponed until an indwelling catheter can be safely inserted because it is difficult to insert the catheter once the pericardiocentesis has been performed. The pericardial drainage and lavage, performed once or twice daily as needed, has been very effective in treat-ing idiopathic or septic pericarditis in horses.[133,134,136,138] The indwelling tube should remain in situ until the fluid recovered at the time of drainage is consistently less than or equal to that instilled in the pericardial sac with antimicrobials 12 to 24 hours earlier. The electrocardiogram should be monitored, because occasionally cardiac arrhythmias occur during the therapeutic procedure or during a routine pericardiocentesis. All horses with pericarditis should initially be treated for septic pericarditis with systemic broad-spectrum bacteriocidal antimicrobial drugs. The antimicrobial choice should be based on the most likely etiologic agents and modified as needed by the results of culture and sensitivity testing. Fibrinous pericarditis has been successfully treated in horses with broad-spectrum bacteriocidal antimicrobials when the amount of pericardial fluid detected echocardiographically was too small to safely obtain a sample for cytology and culture and sensitivity testing. Treatment of idiopathic pericarditis with corticosteroids should only be initiated once the results of the cytology, culture, and sensitivity testing demonstrate no evidence of sepsis. Pericardiotomy or preferably pericardiectomy is the treatment of choice if signs of restrictive (constrictive) pericarditis are present. The surgical procedure is prolonged, expensive, and of considerable risk. A partial pericardiectomy was performed in one horse with constrictive pericarditis but was only transiently successful.[145]

In traumatic pericarditis the antibiotic selected must be capable of covering gram-positive and gram-negative aerobic and anaerobic bacteria. Nonsteroidal antiinflammatory drugs have been deemed useful as adjunctive therapy, as have corticosteroids if bacterial culture of the fluid is negative and there is no evidence of sepsis detected cytologically.

Although diuretics are effective in eliminating the severity of peripheral edema, they further reduce venous return and preload in animals with pericarditis. The result is further compromise of cardiac output and worsening of heart failure.

PREVENTION AND CONTROL. Traumatic pericarditis in cattle can be prevented by routine administration of magnets to heifers at the time of pregnancy diagnosis. At each subse-

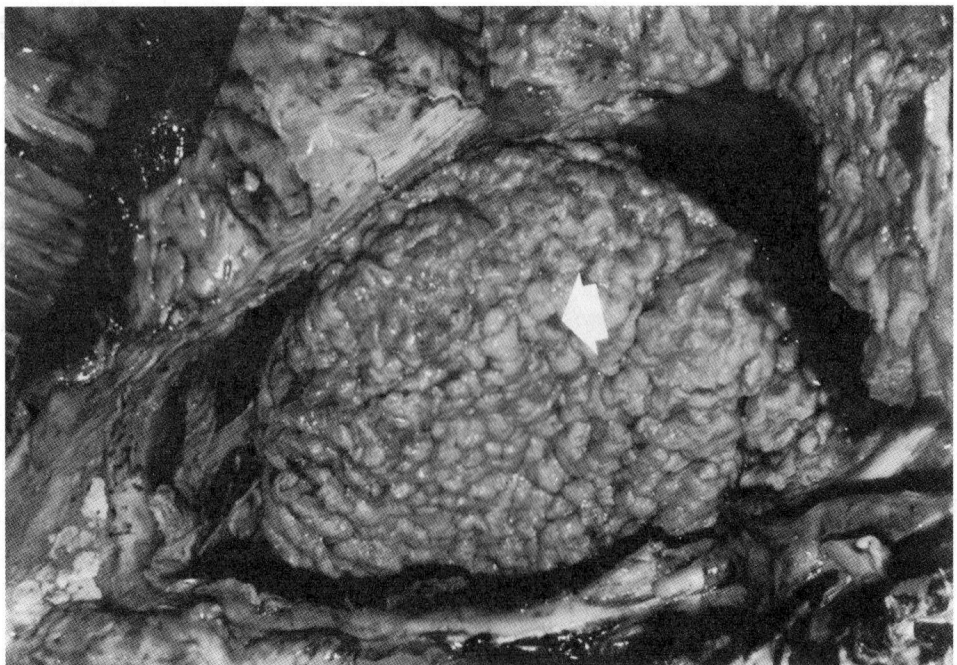

FIG. 28-13 ▒ Postmortem photograph of a cow with constrictive pericarditis. The pericardium is opened and reflected, revealing the epicardium (*arrow*) covered in fibrinopurulent exudate.

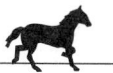

quent pregnancy diagnosis, the cattle should be checked for the presence of the magnet in the reticulum. It is not beneficial to have more than one magnet present at one time.

Some types of infectious pericarditis in horses may be controlled by routine vaccination for the common respiratory pathogens.

REFERENCES

130. Wagner PC et al: Constrictive pericarditis in the horse, *J Equine Med Surg* 1:242-247, 1977.
131. Dill SG et al: Fibrinous pericarditis in the horse, *J Am Vet Med Assoc* 180:266-271, 1982.
132. Freestone JF et al: Idiopathic effusive pericarditis with tamponade in the horse, *Equine Vet J* 19:38-42, 1987.
133. Robinson JA et al: Idiopathic, aseptic, effusive, fibrinous, nonconstrictive pericarditis with tamponade in a standardbred filly, *J Am Vet Med Assoc* 201:1593-1598, 1992.
134. Worth LT, Reef VB: Pericarditis in horses: 18 cases (1986-1995), *J Am Vet Med Assoc* 212:248-253, 1998.
135. Smith BP: Pleuritis and pleural effusion in the horse: a study of 37 cases, *J Am Vet Med Assoc* 170:208-211, 1977.
136. Reef VB, Gentile DG, Freeam DE: Successful treatment of pericarditis in the horse, *J Am Vet Med Assoc* 185:94-98, 1984.
137. Foss RR: Effusive-constrictive pericarditis: diagnosis and pathology, *Vet Med* 80:89-97, 1985.
138. Bernard W et al: Pericarditis in horses: six cases (1982-1986), *J Am Vet Med Assoc* 196:468-471, 1990.
139. Wingfield WE, Rawlings CR, Steinkamp SJ: Physiologic changes in awake goats after experimentally induced pericardial effusion, *Am J Vet Res* 41:1130-1133, 1980.
140. Salcedo E: *Atlas of echocardiography,* ed 2, Philadelphia, 1985, WB Saunders, pp 294-295.
141. Bonagura JD, Pipers FS: Echocardiographic features of pericardial effusion in dogs, *J Am Vet Med Assoc* 179:49-56, 1981.
142. Voros K et al: Two-dimensional echocardiographically guided pericardiocentesis in a horse with traumatic pericarditis, *J Am Vet Med Assoc* 198:1953-1956, 1991.
143. Blood DC, Radostits OM, Henderson JA: *Veterinary medicine: a textbook of the diseases of cattle, sheep, pigs, goats, and horses,* ed 6, Philadelphia, 1983, Baillière Tindall, pp 237-238.
144. Krishnamurthy D et al: Thoracopericardiotomy and pericardiectomy in cattle, *J Am Vet Med Assoc* 175:714-718, 1979.
145. Hardy J, Robertson JT, Reed SM: Constrictive pericarditis in a mare: attempted treatment by partial pericardiectomy, *Equine Vet J* 24:151-154, 1992.

CARDIAC TUMORS

DEFINITION AND ETIOLOGY. The heart may be the primary site of neoplastic disease, or it may be involved secondarily by tumors from adjacent structures such as the lungs, pleura, lymph nodes, or diaphragm. Cardiac neoplasia is uncommon in large animals. The most common primary cardiac tumor is lymphosarcoma. Mesotheliomas, fibrosarcoma, adenocarcinomas, and other carcinomas, especially squamous cell carcinomas in horses, may involve structures adjacent to the heart and extend to the heart or heart base, producing signs of heart disease.[146,147] An infiltrative cardiac lipoma has been reported in a horse, but no signs of cardiac disease were attributed to it.[148] A metastatic anaplastic pulmonary carcinoma has been reported in a horse that did cause signs of congestive heart failure.[147]

CLINICAL SIGNS AND DIFFERENTIAL DIAGNOSIS. The clinical signs of cardiac neoplasia are not specific and depend on the cardiac site involved, and on the other sites of tumor manifestation. Nonspecific signs of neoplasia are common and include anorexia, depression, weight loss, and fever. These signs can be produced by any site of chronic disease; and in large animals pneumonia, peritonitis, enteritis, and liver and kidney disease are considered differential diagnoses, among others. If the tumor involves the pericardium, signs of pericarditis or pericardial effusion such as tachycardia, pain, jugular venous distention, peripheral edema, and weak arterial pulses may be seen. Myocardial involvement of the neoplasia, as is most common with lymphosarcoma, may result in cardiac signs that include tachycardia, cardiac ar-

rhythmias, and cardiac murmur (atrioventricular valve insufficiency) or signs of congestive heart failure such as peripheral edema, ascites, and diarrhea. Clinical signs attributable to tumor involvement of the endocardium (i.e., obliteration of a cardiac chamber, valvular obstruction or damage, embolic showering) are rare in large animals.

Tumor involvement of other organ systems and tissues can be manifested by lymphadenopathy, peripheral edema, diarrhea, melena, rectal palpation of abdominal masses, dysphagia, tachypnea, or pleural effusion.

CLINICAL PATHOLOGY. Cardiac tumors present no consistent clinicopathologic feature. The complete blood count from horses or cattle with lymphosarcoma may reveal neoplastic lymphocytes. The absence of leukemic changes does not rule out lymphosarcoma. Cattle with lymphosarcoma may be positive for fecal occult blood. A serum chemistry profile may reveal nonspecific changes such as hypoalbuminemia, hyperglobulinemia, or elevated liver enzyme concentrations, depending on the other organ systems affected by the tumor or the animal's debilitation. Diagnosis of the cardiac tumor is based on histopathology of tumor tissue. Tumor cells may be found in pericardial or pleural fluid or adjacent lymph nodes. Serologic evidence (agar gel immunodiffusion or radioimmunoassay) for BLV infection does not confirm a diagnosis of lymphosarcoma, but a negative test virtually rules out the adult or enzootic form of lymphosarcoma in cattle. No evidence of BLV infection will be found in cattle or horses with the thymic form of lymphosarcoma.

If electrocardiographic evidence of cardiac tumors is present, it is nonspecific. Cardiac tumors may produce cardiac arrhythmias; reduce amplitude of the QRS complexes; or alter the normal appearance of the P, QRS, and T complexes. Two-dimensional echocardiography or ultrasound of the lungs or pleura may show evidence of the cardiac tumor by providing direct evidence of abnormal echogenic masses involving the heart or surrounding tissue, abnormal fluid accumulation, or myocardial functional changes. The ultrasound findings can direct the practitioner to the best site for biopsy to confirm the diagnosis of cardiac tumor.

Radiographs may provide evidence of cardiac tumors by showing abnormal soft-tissue densities in the thorax that obscure the cardiac silhouette or the ventral lung borders.

PATHOPHYSIOLOGY. The most common cause of cardiac tumors in cattle, lymphosarcoma, has a predilection for the right atrial myocardium. Right ventricular myocardial involvement is not uncommon; left atrial or left ventricular involvement is rarer. Involvement of the right heart may result in little or no evidence of heart disease. More commonly the myocardial involvement results in dilation of the chamber involved. As a consequence, the tricuspid valve ring may be dilated, and tricuspid valve insufficiency occurs. Either because of chamber enlargement or infiltration of the myocardial conduction system, cardiac arrhythmias may develop. Myocardial function may be impaired, so that signs of right heart failure become apparent, including tachycardia, peripheral edema, jugular venous distention or pulsations, pericardial or pleural effusion, hepatic congestion, and ascites.

EPIDEMIOLOGY. Cardiac tumors are rare in large animals. The most common cause in cattle is lymphosarcoma. Although more than 50% of cattle in some parts of the United States are infected with BLV, less than 1% develop lymphosarcoma.[149,150] In herds with more than 50% of cattle infected with BLV, the incidence of lymphosarcoma may be higher. Cardiac involvement is common in cattle with the adult or enzootic form of bovine leukosis, a disease that occurs most commonly in cattle over 4 years old. Thymic lymphosarcoma, which is not associated with BLV infection, also involves the heart but is much less common, occurring in cattle under 30 months of age.

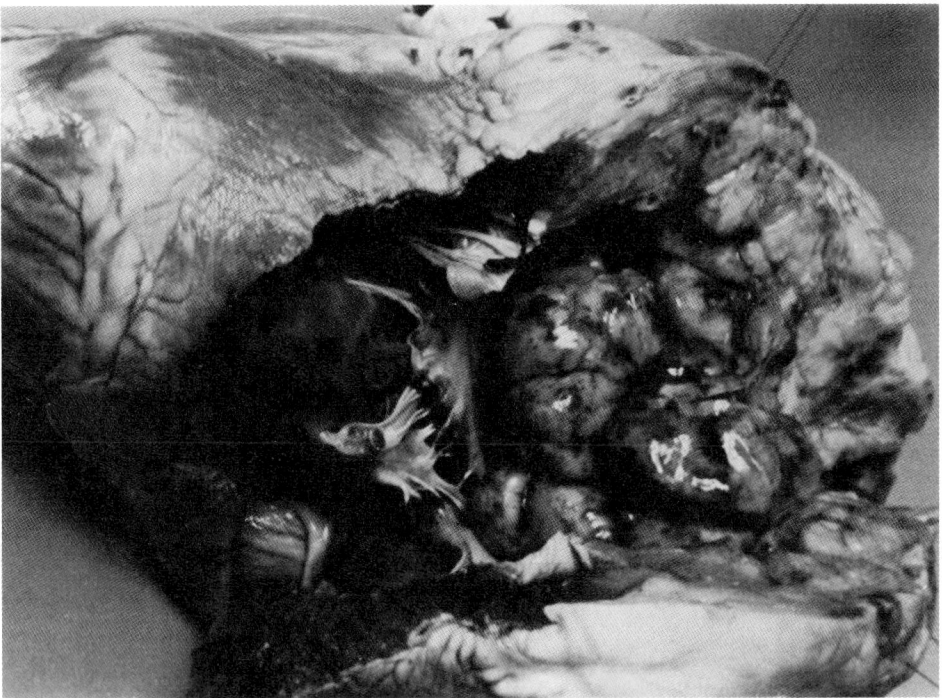

FIG. 28-14 ▮ Postmortem photograph of a cow with lymphosarcoma demonstrating right atrial myocardial infiltration by a tumor and extension of the tumor into the atrial lumen.

Lymphosarcoma, mesothelioma, and squamous cell carcinoma probably are the most common causes of neoplastic involvement of the equine heart, but the prevalence is not documented.

NECROPSY FINDINGS. Necropsy findings depend on the type of cardiac tumor. Direct involvement of the myocardium by lymphosarcoma is associated with finding diffuse infiltration by a pale, tan, homogenous tissue that frequently causes enlargement of the cardiac chamber. Involvement of the right atrium (Fig. 28-14) is the most common manifestation of adult enzootic BLV, but any area of the myocardium and pericardium may be involved. Intracavitary extension of the tumor may be evident (see Fig. 28-14). Histologic evaluation of the tumor shows diffuse infiltrates of lymphoblastic cells that obliterate the normal architecture of the myocardium.

Other tumors such as fibrosarcoma, squamous cell carcinoma, pulmonary carcinoma, and thymic lymphosarcoma may involve the heart by extension or metastasis from other sites in the thorax.

TREATMENT AND PROGNOSIS. No definitive treatment exists for neoplasias involving the heart, and the prognosis for survival is poor. Death can be expected within 6 months with most cardiac tumors. Lymphosarcoma of the heart in cattle has a grave prognosis and is usually associated with death within a few months. Short-term improvement has been achieved in cattle with lymphosarcoma treated with a combination of corticosteriods, L-asparaginase, and cytotoxin, but no published treatment regimens exist.

PREVENTION AND CONTROL. The prevention and control of BLV can be accomplished by isolation of BLV-positive and BLV-negative animals; use of individual or sterilized supplies such as needles, rectal examination sleeves, tattooing, dehorning, and ear-tagging equipment on each animal; rigorous attention to a vector control program; and feeding colostrum from serologically negative cows only.[150,151] Frequent testing (at least every 6 months) and isolation of serologically positive animals over 6 months of age should be performed.

Prevention and control of other cardiac tumors is not possible.

REFERENCES

146. Wallace SS et al: Mesothelioma in a horse, *Compend Cont Educ Pract Vet* 9:210-216, 1987.
147. Dill SG, Moise NS, Meschter CL: Cardiac failure in a stallion secondary to metastasis of an anaplastic pulmonary carcinoma, *Equine Vet J* 18:414-417, 1986.
148. Baker D, Kreefer J: Infiltrative lipoma in the heart of a horse, *Cornell Vet* 77:258-262, 1987.
149. House C, House JA, Glover FL: Antibodies to the glycoprotein antigen of bovine leukemia virus in the cattle population of five states, *Cornell Vet* 67:510-522, 1977.
150. Miller JM: A review of bovine leukosis, *Proc Am Assoc Bovine Pract* 15:30-32, 1983.
151. Johnson R, Gibson CD, Kaneene JB: Bovine leukemia virus: a herd-based control strategy, *Prev Vet Med* 3:339-349, 1985.

VASCULAR DISEASE: ANEURYSMS/THROMBOSIS/EMBOLISM

DEFINITION AND ETIOLOGY. Aneurysms, which are vascular dilations, develop from weakening of the medial elastic coat of blood vessels. The medial weakness may be primary or caused by a progression of an intimal atherosclerotic lesion that has enlarged from hemorrhage, calcification, ulceration, and thrombus formation. The specific causes of aneurysms in large animals are unknown, but trauma (internal or external), sepsis, parasite migration, degenerative vascular disease, atherosclerosis, or aging changes (dilation, elongation, and loss of elasticity of blood vessels) may play a role.[152-154] Hypertension can accelerate the degeneration of the wall.

Thrombosis is the formation of a clot that obstructs blood flow in the circulatory system. The causes of thrombosis are numerous and include trauma, venous stasis, and catheterization for administering medication or fluids. Needle penetration, indwelling catheters themselves, thrombogenic solutions, or bacterial contamination can cause thrombosis associated with catheterization. Secondary thrombosis can result from perivascular inflammation caused by cellulitis, lymphangitis, or other sources of bacterial invasion around the blood vessel. Mural thrombi, which occur in cardiac chambers dilated from valvular regurgitation or chronic atrial fibrillation in humans and which are associated with low flow states, also may occur in large animals, although they have been rarely diagnosed antemortem. Thrombosis usually occurs when intimal disease is present, but it may occur in arteries with no intimal disease when a hypercoagulable state exists such as with dehydration, endotoxemia, anemia, hypotension, stress, or stasis.[155] This type of thrombosis is frequently a complication of acute infectious disease (particularly acute toxic enteritis/colitis), neoplasia, or any chronic debilitating disease.

An embolism is foreign material carried in the bloodstream. Emboli frequently arise from an arterial or venous thrombus, but unusual emboli include catheters and other foreign bodies inadvertently introduced into the circulatory system. In large animals, emboli occur most commonly in bacterial endocarditis, thrombophlebitis, omphalophlebitis, and parasitic arteritis. Emboli may also originate from detachment of mural thrombi in other forms of cardiac disease such as chronic atrial fibrillation and valvular heart disease.

CLINICAL SIGNS AND DIFFERENTIAL DIAGNOSIS. Sites of thrombosis associated with thrombophlebitis are likely to have pain, swelling, redness, and palpable thickening of the involved vein. These signs frequently occur within 12 to 24 hours after catheter removal when the thrombus is associated with catheterization. If there is bilateral jugular venous thrombosis, sudden, marked swelling of the head may occur. If the thrombosis involves the terminal aorta and iliac arteries in horses, the signs are frequently a vague hindlimb lameness, exercise intolerance, or poor performance. These nonspecific signs make it necessary to rule out lameness from other causes, cardiac disease, or respiratory problems. Aortoiliac thrombosis in horses also is characterized by heavy sweating after exercise, except over the hindlimbs, which are cool. Saphenous vein filling is slow or nonexistent in affected horses, and the metatarsal and other peripheral arterial pulses of the hindlimbs are weak. Rectal examination may be normal; or weak, absent, or asymmetric iliac pulses may be palpated. Fremitus of the iliac arteries or terminal part of the aorta may be palpated. The terminal part of the aorta may feel larger or firmer than normal, or an aneurysmal dilation may be detected. Similarly with verminous arteritis of the cranial mesenteric artery, a thickened, dilated cranial mesenteric artery or aorta may be palpated that may be firmer than normal and have a weak pulse, or fremitus may be palpated.

The signs attributable to embolism and thrombosis may be identical. Embolism usually is manifested by an acute episode of pain or fever, abnormal pulsation in a peripheral vessel, or a change in skin temperature. If there is peripheral vessel showering, superficial veins may be collapsed, and muscular weakness may be present. Embolic showering usually occurs in animals suspected of having or known to have thrombus formation.

Clinical signs associated with an aneurysm depend on the location of the aneurysm and may vary from being asymptomatic to being a noticeable enlargement or mass associated with a blood vessel, to causing colic, syncope, seizures, or sudden death on rupture. In a peripheral artery a pulsatile, expansile mass may be visualized or palpated. Other considerations for this finding are a false aneurysm and an arteriovenous fistula. A false aneurysm is clinically indistin-

guishable from a true aneurysm but can be distinguished ultrasonographically. A false aneurysm is caused by a break in the continuity of all three coats of the arterial wall rather than in the tunica media alone. This results in extravascular accumulation of blood in adjacent tissues. Signs attributed to low blood flow such as lameness, colic, or edema may be present with arterial aneurysms. Aneurysms of the cranial mesenteric artery frequently are manifested as chronic episodes of colic. With involvement of major cardiac vessels, there may be pain, an auscultable heart murmur, rapid tachycardia, signs of congestive heart failure, acute onset of pulmonary edema, or sudden death when the aneurysm ruptures. The latter signs make aneurysms difficult to distinguish from valvular heart disease or cardiomyopathy.

CLINICAL PATHOLOGY. Aneurysms or pseudoaneurysms may be visualized radiographically as soft-tissue density masses continuous with (true aneurysm) or extending outward from a vessel wall (false aneurysm).[153,154] However, the majority of the aneurysms involving the aorta and aortic root are not visible radiographically. Angiography can be used in the diagnosis of peripheral vessel swelling or suspected thrombosis but is of little use in diagnosis of aneurysms of major vessels in adult animals. Ultrasonography may be used for the diagnosis of aneurysms or thrombosis of major arteries and peripheral vessels. In aortoiliac thrombosis of horses, ultrasound has been used to determine the origin of the thrombus and the extent of occlusion of the involved arteries.[156] Similarly, diagnostic ultrasound has been used to image the cranial mesenteric artery, its branches, and the aorta in horses with verminous arteritis.[157] Aneurysms appear as dilated vascular structures or vascular outpouchings continuous with the vessel wall,[158] whereas a thrombus is apparent as a hypoechoic to echogenic mass within a blood vessel.[159] Cavitation of an occlusive thrombus is suggestive of septic thrombophlebitis whereas a nonseptic thrombus usually has a homogeneously hypoechoic to echoic appearance.[159] Complete occlusion of the vessel can be determined ultrasonographically, or flow within an aneurysm or alongside a thrombus determined. Doppler ultrasound provides a more sophisticated method for determining blood flow and vessel patency. Computer-assisted radiographic techniques such as computerized tomography and digital subtraction angiography may also be useful but have not yet been widely used in large animals. The latter methods may be limited in usefulness by the size of large animals and the cost of the equipment and procedures.

In the case of catheter-associated thrombosis, a positive catheter tip culture ($>10^3$ colony-forming units), along with a positive blood culture, provides evidence of septic thrombophlebitis.[160] An aseptic ultrasound-guided aspirate of the cavitary lesion within a heterogeneous thrombus can be performed and submitted for culture and sensitivity testing. Septic thrombophlebitis from any cause or embolic showering of septic thrombi may be accompanied by neutrophilic leukocytosis and elevation in fibrinogen concentration.

PATHOPHYSIOLOGY. Irritation of the intimal lining of a blood vessel, stasis of blood flow, or the existence of a hypercoagulable state triggers the clotting cascade and sets the stage for the development of thrombosis. Further injury causes hemorrhage, more thrombosis, ulceration, and calcification. These in turn can compromise the media of the vessel, predisposing to aneurysm formation, and impinge on the lumen of the vessel, causing obstruction to blood flow. Either aneurysm or thrombosis can occlude blood flow to vital structures or organs, resulting in ischemia.

Thrombosis in any sizable vein causes venous hypertension, passive congestion, and subsequent edema and pain of the structure. As the thrombus matures, it adheres to the wall more, but with clot retraction and lysis, recanalization may occur. However, parts of the thrombus may protrude into the

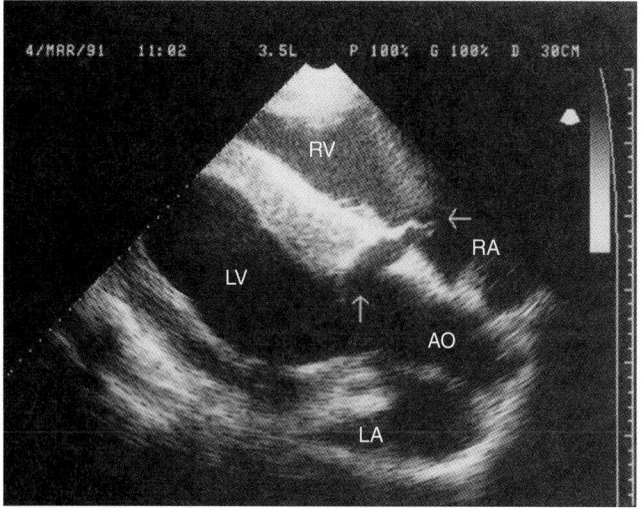

FIG. 28-15 ▓ Two-dimensional echocardiogram of a horse with a ruptured sinus of Valsalva aneurysm. Notice the defect in the right side of the aorta at the sinus of Valsalva (*vertical arrow*) extending into the right atrium (*horizontal arrow*). The right atrium *(RA)*, right ventricle *(RV)*, left ventricle *(LV)*, left atrium *(LA)*, and aorta *(AO)* can be seen in this left ventricular outflow tract view.

moving bloodstream and serve as the source of embolic showering, even during thrombus organization. The most common site for an embolus to lodge has not been established in large animals; the femoral and iliac arteries are common locations in humans. Emboli usually lodge at bifurcations, where the caliber of the artery is suddenly reduced.

The most common outcome of aneurysm of a major vessel is thought to be rupture. Rupture of sinus of Valsalva aneurysms into the right atrium, right ventricle, and interventricular septum has been reported in the horse (Fig. 28-15).[161-163] Ventricular tachycardia often occurs with rupture of an aortic sinus of Valsalva aneurysm and dissection into the interventricular septum.[162,163] Unruptured aneurysms may have other complications such as thrombosis or embolization of the thrombus. The frequency of rupture or embolic showering from thrombosis is unknown in animals.

EPIDEMIOLOGY. The significance of thromboembolism in large animals is poorly defined. Spontaneous thromboembolism is most commonly associated with parasitism in horses, and the aorta and cranial mesenteric arteries are the sites most frequently involved.[164] Aortoiliac thrombosis is also a recognized syndrome diagnosed most frequently in heavily exercised horses. Although parasitism has been associated with aortoiliac thrombosis in horses, other causes of this syndrome are probable but have not been elucidated. Thrombotic disease can occur in any animal having repeated intravenous injections or being catheterized for administration of medication or fluids, but is particularly common in horses with acute toxic enteritis/colitis.

Arteriosclerosis is recognized in horses and in cattle. In cattle the lesion is most frequently caused by excessive vitamin D_3 supplementation or with ingestion of calcinogenic plants such as *Solanum malacozylon*, *Cestrum diurnum*, or *Trisetum flavescens*.[165] In horses the arteriosclerotic lesions were caused by lesions induced by *Strongylus vulgaris*.[166]

Aneurysms are uncommon in large animals but have been documented as the cause of sudden death in breeding stallions and racing Thoroughbred and Standardbred horses.[163,166] Aneurysms of the sinus of Valsalva are probably a common cause of aortic rupture in older horses and are probably congenital in horses as they are in human beings.[158,161-163] Aortic root rupture

also occurs with the presence of a preexisting aneurysm and has been associated with medial necrosis of the aorta.

NECROPSY FINDINGS. Aneurysms are detected grossly as dilations of the involved blood vessel. Aneurysms of the sinus of Valsalva are characterized by an absent tunica media in the wall of the aorta, causing the aneurysmal dilation.[158,163] Rupture of a sinus of Valsalva aneurysm may occur into the right atrium, right ventricle, or interventricular septum, resulting in an aortic cardiac fistula and volume overload.[158,161-163] Rupture through the tricuspid valve or chordae tendineae may also occur. Subendocardial dissection of blood down the interventricular septum may occur with rupture into the left ventricle and of the mitral chorda tendineae also reported. Aneurysms of the major vessels leaving the heart may involve more than one vessel by dissection and hemorrhage. Aneurysms may contain thrombi or parasites, and there may be evidence of embolic showering of thrombi into peripheral vessels or other organ systems, especially the lungs. Histologically there may be necrosis and inflammation at the site of the aneurysm with foci of mineralization.

Thrombosis and arteriosclerotic lesions are recognized as rounded, well-demarcated fibrous plaques frequently located in the thoracic and cranial abdominal aorta. The plaques may contain a central calcified core or parasitic larvae. Microscopically there is a thin layer of fibrin, platelets, and inflammatory cells in early lesions, whereas older lesions have a greater fibrous component. Thrombotic lesions may be associated with proliferation of the underlying aortic intima. In horses, parasitic larvae may be found.

TREATMENT AND PROGNOSIS. Aneurysms of major vessels carry a guarded to grave prognosis because surgical correction is rarely attempted and spontaneous rupture is thought to be relatively common. Intact aneurysms of the sinus of Valsalva can be detected echocardiographically and, once detected, the horse should be removed from all athletic competition because of the risk of rupture.[158]

Treatment of thrombosis consists of removal of the catheter, if present, and resting the affected vessel. Warm compresses or hydrotherapy may be helpful in some animals. Support wraps may be useful to control swelling. The effectiveness of anticoagulant therapy (aspirin at 100 mg/kg once daily PO or heparin at 30 U/kg subcutaneously twice daily) or antiinflammatory drugs for dissolving a thrombus is questionable. Anticoagulant therapy may be useful in preventing additional thrombus formation or propagation of the existing thrombus. Ultrasonographic guidance can be used to obtain a sterile aspirate of the cavitated area of the thrombus for culture and sensitivity testing when septic thrombophlebitis is suspected.[159] Broad-spectrum bacteriocidal antimicrobial therapy should be instituted for suspected septic thrombophlebitis or when a cavitated thrombus is detected ultrasonographically and modified, if necessary, based on the results of culture and sensitivity testing.[159] Bacterial endocarditis, particularly involving the tricuspid valve, is a potential complication of septic jugular vein thrombophlebitis. With the exception of a jugular venous thrombus, surgical removal of an embolism or thrombus is rarely attempted in large animals. Surgical resection of a jugular vein with septic thrombophlebitis has been performed successfully when the surgeon could ligate the affected vein above and below the thrombus. Although the prognosis is guarded for complete resolution of the thrombophlebitis, especially if the thrombus is infected, many veins do recannulate with complete resolution of the thrombus and without vascular stricture. However, the time course is slow, and persistent local induration and obstruction to blood flow may persist.

PREVENTION AND CONTROL. Thrombosis and embolization from intravenous catheters can be prevented by aseptic insertion, stabilization of the catheter, use of topical

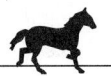

antiseptics, application of a sterile dressing, daily inspection of the catheter and vein, and replacement of the catheter at another site (preferably in another vein) if phlebitis occurs. Attempts should be made to place long-term catheters in large peripheral or central veins where contact between the endothelium and catheter is minimized and medications administered are diluted by the large volume of blood flow. Catheters left in place for prolonged periods should be of silicone rubber or polyurethane.[160] Aspirin (100 mg/kg PO once daily, ruminants; 17 mg/kg every other day, horses) and low-dose heparin (30 U/kg subcutaneously twice daily, ruminants and horses) therapy should be considered in maintaining a catheter without thrombus formation in septic or endotoxic patients. Horses are much more prone to jugular thrombosis than are ruminants.

Parasite control is important in the control of thromboembolic disease and aneurysm in horses. Aneurysms of the sinus of Valsalva may be detected by routine echocardiographic screening of horses. In cattle, arteriosclerotic lesions are prevented by proper calcium and vitamin D supplementation.

REFERENCES

152. Derksen FJ, Reed SM, Hall CC: Aneurysm of the aortic arch and bicarotid trunk in a horse, *J Am Vet Med Assoc* 179:692-694, 1981.
153. Watrous BJ et al: Spontaneous resolution of pseudoaneurysm in a horse following angiographic diagnosis, *Vet Radiol* 28:49-52, 1987.
154. Wagner PC et al: Treatment of a dorsal metatarsal arterial aneurysm in a horse, *Compend Cont Educ Pract Vet* 9:580-582, 1987.
155. Lindsay JL, DeBakey ME, Beall AC: Diseases of the aorta. In Hurst JW, editor: *The heart*, ed 6, vol 2, New York, 1986, McGraw-Hill, pp 1321-1372.
156. Reef VB et al: Use of ultrasonography for the detection of aortic-iliac thrombosis in horses, *J Am Vet Med Assoc* 190:286-288, 1987.
157. Wallace KC et al: In vitro ultrasonographic appearance of the normal and verminous equine aorta, cranial mesenteric artery, and its branches, *Am J Vet Res* 50:1774-1778, 1989.
158. Reef VB et al: Echocardiographic detection of an intact aneurysm in a horse, *J Am Vet Med Assoc* 197:752-755, 1990.
159. Gardner SY, Reef VB, Spencer PA: Ultrasonographic evaluation of 46 horses with jugular vein thrombophlebitis: 1985-1988: a retrospective study, *J Am Vet Med Assoc* 199:370-373, 1991.
160. Spurlock SL et al: Long-term jugular vein catheterization in horses, *J Am Vet Med Assoc* 196:425-430, 1990.
161. Roby KA et al: Rupture of an aortic sinus aneurysm in a 15-year-old broodmare, *J Am Vet Med Assoc* 189:305-308, 1986.
162. Lester GD, Lombard CW, Ackerman N: Echocardiographic detection of a dissecting aortic root aneurysm in a thoroughbred stallion, *Vet Radiol Ultrasound* 33:202-205, 1992.
163. Marr CM et al: Clinical and echocardiographic findings in horses with aortic root rupture, *Vet Radiol Ultrasound* 39:22-31, 1998.
164. Cranley JJ, McCullagh KG: Ischemic myocardial fibrosis and aortic strongylosis in the horse, *Equine Vet J* 13:35-42, 1981.
165. Bundza A, Stevenson DA: Arteriosclerosis in seven cattle, *Can Vet J* 28:49-51, 1987.
166. Brown CN: Acquired cardiovascular disease, *Vet Clin North Am (Equine Pract)* 1:371-382, 1985.

ATRIAL FIBRILLATION

DEFINITION AND ETIOLOGY. Atrial fibrillation is a cardiac arrhythmia characterized by a lack of coordinated atrial electrical activity. It is caused by an abnormality of impulse conduction that results from unidirectional conduction block and random reentrant activation of the atria. High resting vagal tone, commonly found in horses, shortens the action potential duration in atrial myocardial cells, making atrial fibrillation more likely to occur. Atrial fibrillation can occur when there is atrial enlargement from atrial myocardial disease, atrioventricular valvular regurgitation, ventricular failure (organic atrial fibrillation), myocarditis, autonomic nervous system imbalance, electrolyte or acid-base disturbances, anesthetic drugs or tranquilizer administration, or unknown causes (functional or benign atrial fibrillation).

CLINICAL SIGNS AND DIFFERENTIAL DIAGNOSIS. Large animals with atrial fibrillation may be asymptomatic at rest, and atrial fibrillation may be detected as an incidental finding in an otherwise normal horse. Horses usually have a history of exercise intolerance or poor performance. Other complaints may be exercise-induced epistaxis, respiratory disease, weakness, syncope, myopathy, colic, or congestive heart failure. Cattle with atrial fibrillation usually have gastrointestinal disease. Footrot and pneumonia also have been associated with atrial fibrillation in cattle. Anorexia and decreased milk production are common in cattle with atrial fibrillation. Atrial fibrillation and the clinical signs associated with it in horses and in cattle can be paroxysmal. Paroxysmal atrial fibrillation usually lasts no more than 24 to 48 hours before spontaneous conversion to sinus rhythm occurs.[167] Spontaneous conversion usually only occurs in horses with small atria or in cattle with correction of the underlying problem. Transient potassium depletion associated with the administration of furosemide is a common cause of paroxysmal atrial fibrillation in horses. The administration of bicarbonate "milkshakes" has also been implicated in horses with paroxysmal atrial fibrillation.

Animals with atrial fibrillation have an irregular cardiac rhythm with no underlying regularity. The heart sounds vary in intensity, and no fourth heart sound is audible. The heart rate may be slow, normal, or elevated. In cattle with severe abdominal disease, the heart rate usually reflects the severity of the underlying disease. In horses the resting heart rate is usually normal to slightly elevated and is rarely above 50 beats/min, unless there is underlying myocardial or valvular disease. During exercise, horses with atrial fibrillation develop abnormally high heart rates that are usually 40 to 60 beats/min higher than expected for each level of exercise, far exceeding the peak heart rate of 240 beats/min at maximal exercise.[168,169] The arterial pulse varies in intensity. A pulse deficit occurs when two beats occur in rapid succession and is infrequent unless the heart rate is elevated. Cardiac murmurs of grade 3/6 or louder are present in less than 50% of the horses and in even fewer cattle with atrial fibrillation.[170-172] Signs of congestive heart failure (peripheral edema, jugular venous distention) may be present in some animals, but they are not caused by the arrhythmia. In these cases the atrial fibrillation occurs secondary to the atrial enlargement that occurs with the underlying valvular or myocardial disease.

The lack of an auscultable fourth heart sound in the presence of an irregular cardiac rhythm with no underlying regularity distinguishes atrial fibrillation from other cardiac arrhythmias. Sinus arrhythmia, which is also an irregular rhythm, has an audible fourth heart sound. Ventricular and atrial ectopic beats usually occur with a relatively regular underlying rhythm. A complicated ventricular rhythm with more than one focus of activation may have characteristics similar to those of atrial fibrillation and must be distinguished from it by an ECG. Atrial tachycardia with varying degrees of atrioventricular block has similar characteristics, and the underlying fourth heart sounds may be missed if the animal is auscultated in a noisy environment.

CLINICAL PATHOLOGY. In cattle with atrial fibrillation, acid-base and electrolyte disturbances occur frequently and are most likely attributable to the underlying primary disease. Most cattle with atrial fibrillation have gastrointestinal disease, and the most consistent acid-base disturbance is metabolic alkalosis.[172] Hypocalcemia, hypokalemia, and hypochloremia may also be seen in cattle with atrial fibrillation. Experimental induction of metabolic alkalosis with hypokalemia in cattle has been associated with the development of atrial fibrillation.[173] Most horse with atrial fibrillation have normal electrolytes although the fractional excretion of potassium may be low, particularly in horses that sweat excessively or are routinely receiving furosemide for exercise-induced pulmonary hemorrhage.

The diagnosis of atrial fibrillation is made by ECG. The arrhythmia is characterized by an irregular R-R interval. The ventricular response rate is low, normal, or high, depending on the presence of heart disease or the severity of the primary disease. The ventricular complexes have normal polarity and amplitude but vary slightly in appearance from beat to beat. Similarly, the Q-T interval and the appearance of the T wave vary. P waves are absent, replaced by fine undulations of the baseline called fibrillation or f waves. In some leads the "f" waves are barely visible, particularly in cattle (Fig. 28-16).

The echocardiogram is used to determine whether cardiac disease is present. The most significant change associated with the arrhythmia is a mild reduction in shortening fraction (24% to 32%) that occurs, in part, secondary to the loss of the atrial contribution to ventricular filling.[174] Absence of the cranial motion of the mitral valve, corresponding to atrial contractions, is also detected with atrial fibrillation.[175] Conversion to sinus rhythm results in these echocardiographic findings returning to normal within several days, if there is no underlying myocardial disease. In many large animals with atrial fibrillation, no evidence of heart disease can be detected echocardiographically. Abnormal echocardiographic dimensions suggest that heart disease is present. Measurement of the maximal left atrial dimension in the two-chambered view of the left atrium and left ventricle from the left cardiac window should be performed to determine whether there is left atrial enlargement, because this measurement is a more sensitive indicator of left atrial enlargement than the left atrium to aortic root ratio. In normal horses the left atrial diameter in this view should be less than or equal to 13.5 cm.

Cardiac catheterization reveals normal cardiac output and blood pressure measurements in most conscious horses with atrial fibrillation, but conversion to normal sinus rhythm may induce a reduction in mean right atrial, pulmonary arterial, and aortic pressures.[176] Similar studies have not been reported in cattle.

PATHOPHYSIOLOGY. Experimentally rapid stimulation of the atrium can initiate atrial fibrillation, which can be sustained if there is a large heart and sufficient vagal tone.[177,178] In horses and cattle the normal atria may be large enough to support atrial fibrillation once it is established. In addition, both species have high vagal tone at rest. This combination of factors may be responsible for the large number of benign or functional cases of atrial fibrillation in large animals. Cardiac diseases such as endocarditis, atrioventricular valvular regurgitation, and congestive heart failure that result in atrial enlargement and rapid stimulation of the atria provide a setting in which atrial fibrillation can develop and be sustained naturally. Microscopic cardiac pathology might also create the proper setting for the development of conduction block and reentry.

During atrial fibrillation there is no coordinated contraction of the atria; thus ventricular filling is passive. Although this might be expected to reduce cardiac output, there is no evidence that this occurs in resting horses, unless there is concomitant congestive heart failure.[176] During exercise, however, the heart rate of horses with atrial fibrillation exceeds normal limits, and atrial fibrillation probably is responsible for a fall in cardiac output and resulting exercise intolerance.[168] Blood flow to other organs and viscera, though not studied, may be altered in large animals with atrial fibrillation, resulting in reduced gastrointestinal motility, colic, reduced muscle blood flow, and poor milk production.

Atrial pressures are elevated in horses with atrial fibrillation.[176,179] Sustained high pressure is likely to produce dilation of the atria. With progressive dilation, secondary atrioventricular valve regurgitation may occur. During atrial fibrillation blood flow to the atrial myocardium is reduced, and progressive fibrosis can also be a consequence of chronic atrial fibrillation. Sustained atrial fibrillation most likely results in progressive cardiac disease.

EPIDEMIOLOGY. Standardbred, Thoroughbred, and draft horses have been reported to have the highest incidence of atrial fibrillation.[169-171] Racehorses have been diagnosed most frequently, but atrial fibrillation has been found in all types of horses.[170,171] Geldings have been more frequently reported with atrial fibrillation than intact male or female horses.[171] Horses of all ages are susceptible to atrial fibrillation; however, atrial fibrillation occurs infrequently in ponies, foals, weanlings, and yearlings. Older horses, ponies, foals, weanlings, and yearlings with atrial fibrillation more frequently have underlying heart disease associated with the arrhythmia, rather than being benign fibrillators.

In cattle, atrial fibrillation is diagnosed more frequently in dairy cattle than beef cattle, but there is no apparent breed predilection.[172,180] It is commonly associated with gastrointestinal disease or abdominal pain in cattle.[172,180] Footrot and pneumonia can also be associated with the development of atrial fibrillation in cattle.

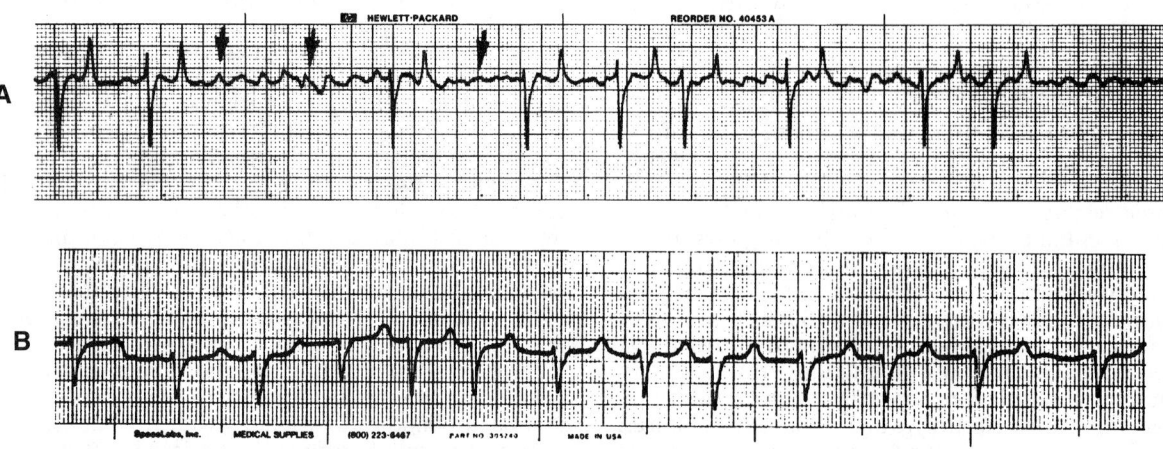

FIG. 28-16 ECGs showing atrial fibrillation in a horse (**A**) and cow (**B**). The irregular Q-T intervals and absence of P waves are apparent. Arrows point to fibrillation waves, which are apparent only in **A**.

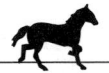

NECROPSY FINDINGS. Many cattle and horses are benign fibrillators without apparent underlying heart disease, so the necropsy findings reflect the primary disease. Microscopic cardiac pathology has been found in horses with atrial fibrillation that consists of focal atrial myocardial fibrosis, microvascular alterations, and cardiac nerve abnormalities.[181-183] Whether these changes predisposed to the development of atrial fibrillation, were a consequence of atrial fibrillation, or are aging changes has not been established. A minority of horses and cattle have endocarditis, congestive heart failure, or valvular lesions; and the necropsy findings reflect these conditions. In horses with atrial fibrillation, mitral valve disease was the most common valvular lesion.[171]

TREATMENT AND PROGNOSIS. Quinidine is the drug of choice to convert atrial fibrillation to normal sinus rhythm in horses and cattle. The drug is a negative inotrope at high dosages, causes systemic hypotension, increases the ventricular response rate, and can produce undesirable side effects and toxicity; thus it must be used with caution. In animals with congestive heart failure, quinidine therapy has considerable risk.[171] Because most large animals are benign fibrillators without underlying cardiac pathology, treatment with quinidine is successful in restoring normal sinus rhythm. Treated animals should be monitored frequently by physical examination, with careful auscultation and ECG recording. Continuous ECG recording should be performed throughout treatment, if possible.[184] Animals should have normal acid-base balance and electrolyte concentrations before treatment. They should be adequately hydrated, allowed to drink and eat, or given additional oral fluids (horses) or intravenous fluids (cattle) during therapy. The intravenous administration of quinidine gluconate is successful in converting horses with recent onset atrial fibrillation to sinus rhythm.[185] Quinidine gluconate is most successful when administered to horses with a not more than 2 week duration of atrial fibrillation but has been successful in converting horses with atrial fibrillation of 2 to 4 weeks duration. Horses with longer durations of atrial fibrillation should be treated orally with quinidine sulfate. Quinidine is poorly absorbed after oral administration to cattle and so must be given by intravenous infusion to obtain therapeutic concentrations. Cattle should be given intravenous fluids during quinidine infusion. Quinidine therapy should always be discontinued when conversion to normal sinus rhythm occurs.

Quinidine sulfate is the preparation most economically used in large animals. Before therapy, a baseline ECG is recorded. Horses are given a dose of 22 mg/kg (1 g/100 lb body weight) in a suspension of water via nasogastric tube. At 2 hours (time of peak blood concentration), horses are evaluated closely for idiosyncratic or toxic reactions such as nasal edema, cutaneous reactions, laminitis, colic, diarrhea, or ataxia. If no abnormalities are noticed, an ECG is recorded. If conversion to normal sinus rhythm has not occurred and the QRS duration is not greater than 25% of the pretreatment QRS duration, an additional dose is administered. Two hours after each oral dose, an ECG is recorded. If there has been no conversion to normal sinus rhythm, another dose is administered, up to a maximum of four to six doses. If the QRS complex is prolonged by more than 25% of the pretreatment value or if a fast (more than 100 beats/min) supraventricular arrhythmia, ventricular rhythm, colic, diarrhea, ataxia, nasal edema or laminitis develops, therapy should be discontinued or the treatment intervals prolonged to every 6 hours (half-life of quinidine). Although laminitis is a frequently reported complication of quinidine sulfate therapy, the actual incidence of laminitis associated with the administration of quinidine is rare and much less frequent than the development of colic, diarrhea, ataxia, nasal edema, QRS prolonga-

tion greater than 25% of the pretreatment value, rapid supraventricular tachycardia greater than 100 beats/min, or ventricular arrhythmias.[184] Nasal mucosal edema, colic, neurologic signs and prolongation of the QRS duration to greater than 25% of the pretreatment value are all signs of quinidine toxicity that, if detected, should prompt discontinuation of every 2 hour administration of the drug and, if the signs do not resolve within the next 4 hours, discontinuation of quinidine treatment altogether (at least for this attempt at conversion). If conversion has not occurred after a total of four to six doses (one every 2 hours) or a cumulative dosage of 88 to 132 mg/kg of quinidine sulfate has been administered or toxic or adverse side effects occur, treatment intervals should be prolonged to every 6 hours.[184] The every-6-hour treatment can be continued until the horse converts, shows toxic or adverse side effects, or the owner elects to discontinue treatment. The advantage of this treatment regimen is that steady state plasma and myocardial concentrations of the drug are achieved, there is less quinidine toxicity, a lower total dose of quinidine sulfate is used and horses that did not convert after the standard every 2-hour dosing may convert with this treatment regimen. Digoxin at 0.011 mg/kg orally twice daily can then be added to the therapeutic regimen if conversion has not occurred in 24 to 48 hours and appears to be helpful in some horses.

Quinidine sulfate at a dosage of 48 mg/kg is suspended in 4 L of saline or lactated Ringer's solution when cattle are treated for atrial fibrillation. This dosage is administered at a rate of 1 L/hr. Intravenous fluids are administered simultaneously in the opposite jugular vein. Cattle should be monitored continuously during infusion. Cattle frequently become depressed and develop diarrhea during infusion of quinidine. These signs are side effects, and therapy can be continued. The infusion rate should be slowed if the ventricular response rate exceeds 100 beats/min. If the QRS complex is visibly prolonged or a fast (more than 120 beats/min) supraventricular arrhythmia or ventricular rhythm develops, therapy is temporarily discontinued. Just before conversion, some cattle have blepharospasm and are ataxic. The infusion should be discontinued as soon as conversion occurs. Therapy should be discontinued after the 4 L infusion, even if conversion to normal sinus rhythm has not occurred.

During quinidine therapy the ECG shows predictable changes. The fibrillation waves become more coarse and less frequent. The R-R interval becomes more regular as the heart rate increases. Before conversion there may be an occasional P wave or two or three P waves for each QRS complex (atrial tachycardia with atrioventricular block). At the time of conversion, a single P wave is present for each QRS complex. Frequently a large T_a wave is present, and the ST segment is elevated. The ECG should be normal within 12 hours of conversion. A continuous 24-hour electrocardiogram is recommended in horses with atrial fibrillation after conversion to determine if frequent atrial premature depolarizations are present. If the continuous ECG is normal during the 24 hours after conversion and myocardial function has returned to normal, the horse can be returned to training. If frequent supraventricular premature extrasystoles are detected, the horse should be rested and treatment with corticosteroids may be considered for a possible myocarditis. The horse should not be returned to work until the atrial premature depolarizations have resolved.

Digoxin is used before quinidine therapy in horses and cattle with fast heart rates. The ventricular response rate should be less than 60 beats/min in horses and 100 beats/min in cattle before quinidine therapy. Digoxin is administered for one to two doses in horses with only mild tachycardia to up to 5 to 7 days before initiation of quinidine therapy in horses with very labile heart rates or problems with supraventricular tachycardia during a previous conversion. Digoxin should be administered at the dose of 11 μg/kg twice daily orally to horses. Cattle are given digoxin intravenously by infusion of 0.86 μg/kg/hr or 11 μg/kg three times daily. The side effects of quinidine treatment such as rapid supraventricular tachycardia may be decreased in animals pretreated with digoxin. Digoxin is also indicated as a pretreatment in horses with atrial fibrillation and very low fractional shortening (<24%) indicative of underlying myocardial disease before the administration of quinidine sulfate.

Cattle with primary gastrointestinal disease that is treated successfully frequently convert to normal sinus rhythm spontaneously. Spontaneous conversion usually occurs within 5 days of resolution of the primary problem; therefore treatment is delayed for this period.[172] Cattle that do not convert spontaneously in 5 days, have chronic gastrointestinal problems, or have atrial fibrillation with adverse hemodynamic effects (poor peripheral perfusion, weak arterial pulses, pulse deficit) are selected for quinidine therapy. The prognosis for cattle with atrial fibrillation is good if the primary problem has been resolved and conversion to normal sinus rhythm occurs. Prognosis for cattle with chronic gastrointestinal disease is guarded, but many show improved appetite and milk production when atrial fibrillation is resolved. Unless heart disease is present, few cattle revert to atrial fibrillation. A small percentage of cattle fail to respond to quinidine therapy, and their prognosis is guarded to poor, because milk production and appetite are intermittently poor, and heart disease can be progressive.

Horses with paroxysmal atrial fibrillation have a good prognosis for return to performance, and few have a recurrence of the arrhythmia. Predisposing factors such as transient potassium depletion should be removed, if possible, by discontinuing the furosemide administration or adding oral KCl to the diet. Oral bicarbonate milkshakes should be avoided. Horses with benign atrial fibrillation have a good prognosis for conversion to normal sinus rhythm and a return to previous performance level.[170,171] Horses with heart rates greater than 60 beats/min or with signs of congestive heart failure have a guarded to grave prognosis, and conversion to sinus rhythm is rarely warranted. Treatment of the underlying cardiac disease, if possible, is warranted, and the horse should be treated for congestive heart failure with digoxin, diuretics, and vasodilators as needed. Recurrence of atrial fibrillation and side effects of quinidine therapy are more frequent in horses that have had atrial fibrillation longer than 4 months before treatment.[171] The recurrence rate for horses with atrial fibrillation of greater than 4 months duration increases to 60% from 25%. This may be the result of microscopic cardiac lesions that developed with chronic atrial fibrillation.

REFERENCES

167. Holmes JR et al: Paroxysmal atrial fibrillation in racehorses, *Equine Vet J* 18:37-42, 1986.
168. Amada A et al: Atrial fibrillation in the horse: clinical and histopathological studies of two cases. I, Clinical study, *Exp Rep Equine Health Lab* 11:51-69, 1974.
169. Holmes JR, Drake PGG, Else RW: Atrial fibrillation in the horse, *Equine Vet J* 1:212-222, 1969.
170. Deem DA, Fregin GF: Atrial fibrillation in horses: a review of 106 clinical cases, with consideration of prevalence, clinical signs, and prognosis, *J Am Vet Med Assoc* 180:261-265, 1982.
171. Reef VB, Levitan CW, Spencer PA: Factors affecting prognosis and conversion in equine atrial fibrillation, *J Vet Intern Med* 2:1-6, 1988.
172. McGuirk SM et al: Atrial fibrillation in cows: clinical findings and therapeutic considerations, *J Am Vet Med Assoc* 182:1380-1386, 1983.
173. Goetze VL et al: Atemmechanik-and EKG-befunde bei experimenteller metabolischer alkalose des rindes, *DTW* 91:307-313, 1984.
174. Marr CM et al: An echocardiographic study of atrial fibrillation in horses before and after conversion to sinus rhythm, *J Vet Intern Med* 9:336-340, 1995.
175. Wingfield WE et al: Echocardiography in assessing mitral valve motion in 3 horses with atrial fibrillation, *Equine Vet J* 12:181-184, 1980.
176. Muir WW, McGuirk SM: Hemodynamics before and after conversion of atrial fibrillation to normal sinus rhythm in horses, *J Am Vet Med Assoc* 184:965-970, 1984.
177. Detweiler DK: Experimental and clinical observations on auricular fibrillation in horses, *J Am Vet Med Assoc* 1:119-129, 1952.
178. Kubo K, Senta T, Sugimoto O: Changes in cardiac output with experimentally induced atrial fibrillation in the horse, *Exp Rep Equine Health Lab* 12:101-108, 1975.
179. Miller PJ, Holmes JR: Effect of cardiac arrhythmia on left ventricular and aortic blood pressure parameters in the horse, *Res Vet Sci* 35:190-199, 1983.
180. Brightling P, Townsend HGG: Atrial fibrillation in ten cows, *Can Vet J* 24:331-334, 1983.
181. Kiryu K et al: Atrial fibrillation in the horse: clinical and histopathological studies of two cases. II, Formal pathogenesis, *Exp Rep Equine Health Lab* 2:70-86, 1974.
182. Kiryu K: Histopathogenesis of atrial fibrillation in the horse: cardiopathology of an additional case, *Exp Rep Equine Health Lab* 14:54-63, 1977.
183. Else RW, Holmes JR: Pathological changes in atrial fibrillation in the horse, *Equine Vet J* 3:56-64, 1971.
184. Reef VB, Reimer JM, Spencer PA: Treatment of equine atrial fibrillation: new perspectives, *J Vet Intern Med* 9:57-67, 1995.
185. Muir WW, Reed SM, McGuirk SM: Treatment of atrial fibrillation in horses by intravenous administration of quinidine, *J Am Vet Med Assoc* 197:1607-1610, 1990.

VENTRICULAR TACHYCARDIA

DEFINITION AND ETIOLOGY. Ventricular tachycardia is a cardiac arrhythmia characterized by a rapid rhythm originating in the ventricle. This rhythm originates below the bundle of His in the specialized conduction system, the surrounding ventricular myocardium, or both.[186] Ventricular tachycardia may be caused by disorders in impulse formation or impulse conduction or a combination of these two mechanisms.[186] Ventricular reentry is an important mechanism in the genesis of sustained ventricular tachycardia, whereas abnormal automaticity is probably responsible for idioventricular rhythms and parasystole. Changes in autonomic tone may also be important in the genesis of ventricular tachycardia. Early afterdepolarizations are thought to be the mechanism responsible for ventricular tachyarrhythmias associated with sympathetic stimulation. Late coupled ventricular complexes or a very premature ventricular depolarization are usually required to initiate ventricular tachycardia. Ventricular tachycardia can occur when there is myocarditis, myocardial necrosis or fibrosis, bacterial endocarditis (especially involving the aortic or mitral valve), autonomic nervous system imbalance, hypoxia, ischemia, electrolyte or metabolic disturbances, anesthesia, drug administration, sepsis, endotoxemia, toxic myocardial injury, or aortic root rupture; or it may be associated with other unknown causes.[187-189]

CLINICAL SIGNS AND DIFFERENTIAL DIAGNOSIS. The clinical signs detected depend on the ventricular rate, the type of ventricular tachycardia (uniform or multiform), the duration of ventricular tachycardia, and the severity of the underlying cardiac disease.[188] Large animals with ventricular tachycardia may be asymptomatic at rest, if the rhythm is relatively slow and uniform, or present with severe congestive heart failure with rapid uniform or multiform ventricular tachycardia.[188] Exercise intolerance is common and may be so severe that the animal has frequent syncope. Other complaints include depression, weakness, colic, respiratory distress, coughing, ventral edema, and pulmonary edema. Acute viral or bacterial respiratory disease with high fever may precede the development of ventricular tachycardia in horses or occur concurrently with it.[190] Gastrointestinal disease and primary myocardial disease are common in horses with ventricular tachycardia.[187] In cattle, ventricular tachycardia occurs most frequently secondary to sepsis and toxemia. Anorexia and decreased milk production are common in affected cows.

Animals with sustained ventricular tachycardia have a rapid heart rate with a regular (uniform) or irregular (multiform) rhythm.[191-194] Heart rates as high as 300 beats/min have been detected in horses with ventricular tachycardia. Heart sounds vary in intensity with some very loud booming sounds (bruit de cannon). Arterial pulse may be variable or uniform, with normal (slower rate) or weak (rapid rate) intensity pulses. Pulse deficits frequently occur, particularly with rapid or multiform ventricular tachycardia. Jugular pulses are frequently detected in large animals with ventricular tachycardia. The large pulse waves seen in the jugular vein are cannon "a" waves that occur when the atria and ventricle contract simultaneously. Cardiac murmurs are not commonly detected. Signs of congestive heart failure are usually present when ventricular tachycardia is rapid and sustained but are uncommon in animals with slower or paroxysmal ventricular tachycardia.[191-193] Signs of right-sided congestive heart failure (ventral edema, venous distention) usually predominate with sustained uniform ventricular tachycardia and increase in severity the longer the duration and more rapid the rate of the arrhythmia. Signs of left-sided congestive heart failure (coughing, expectoration of foamy fluid, respiratory distress) usually predominate with multiform ventricular tachycardia.[190]

The presence of jugular pulses and bruit de cannon in an animal with a rapid regular rhythm helps distinguish ventricular tachycardia from sinus or supraventricular tachycardia. Multiform ventricular tachycardia can be difficult to distinguish from atrial fibrillation, because both arrhythmias have an irregular rhythm with heart sounds that vary in intensity. Jugular pulses may also be detected in large animals with atrial fibrillation but are usually less prominent than in animals with ventricular tachycardia. Although large animals with multiform ventricular arrhythmias usually have more severe clinical signs, an ECG is necessary to distinguish these arrhythmias.

CLINICAL PATHOLOGY. Electrolyte, metabolic, or toxic causes of ventricular tachycardia may be present in large animals with primary gastrointestinal disease. Hypomagnesemia and hypokalemia has also been associated with the development of ventricular tachycardia.[194] Serum creatinine and blood urea nitrogen may be elevated in horses and cattle in congestive heart failure associated with prerenal azotemia. Serum osmolality, blood urea nitrogen, and creatinine increases; and urine osmolality decreases acutely in horses with experimental monensin toxicosis.[190,195] Initial decreases in serum potassium and serum calcium have also been reported in these animals. Marked elevations of cardiac troponin I have been seen in horses with ventricular tachycardia.[196] Cardiac troponin I is a more sensitive indicator of myocardial injury in human beings and appears to have a similar sensitivity in the horse. Cardiac isoenzymes of CK and LDH are often elevated if there is recent myocardial injury associated with the ventricular tachycardia. Elevation of the myocardial fraction of CK (CK-MB) in excess of 5% of the total CK is compatible with myocardial injury in horses.[190,195] A neutrophilic leukocytosis and hyperfibrinogenemia may be detected in animals with an infectious myocarditis or bacterial endocarditis or may be elevated associated with the primary underlying disease. In most large animals with ventricular tachycardia, however, the hematology is normal.

The diagnosis of ventricular tachycardia is made from the ECG. A series of four or more ventricular premature depolarizations is diagnostic of ventricular tachycardia.[187,197] The electrocardiographic appearance of the ventricular premature depolarizations may be widened and bizarre, or the QRS duration and appearance of the QRS and T may be near normal, especially in horses (Fig. 28-17).[187,188] Although the duration of QRS complexes that are ventricular in origin is usually within the normal range reported for horses, it is usually longer than the QRS duration of the horse's normal sinus beats.[187] The major direction of the QRS complex is usually oriented opposite to that of the T wave. The R-R intervals may be regular or irregular. The morphology of the QRS complexes may be similar (uniform) or vary widely (multiform). Atrioventricular dissociation is usually present with a slower atrial than ventricular rate. Fusion beats and capture beats may be detected (Fig. 28-18). Ventricular tachycardia can be sustained or paroxysmal.

The echocardiogram is used to determine whether cardiac disease is present. The echocardiogram is usually abnormal in large animals with primary myocardial disease and normal in large animals with secondary ventricular tachycardia, except for the changes associated with the ventricular tachycardia itself. Abnormal echocardiographic findings that may be detected in large animals with primary myocardial disease include myocardial dyskinesis, hypokinesis, and akinesis; abnormal myocardial echogenicity; decreased fractional shortening, ejection time, and ejection fraction; loss of the normal

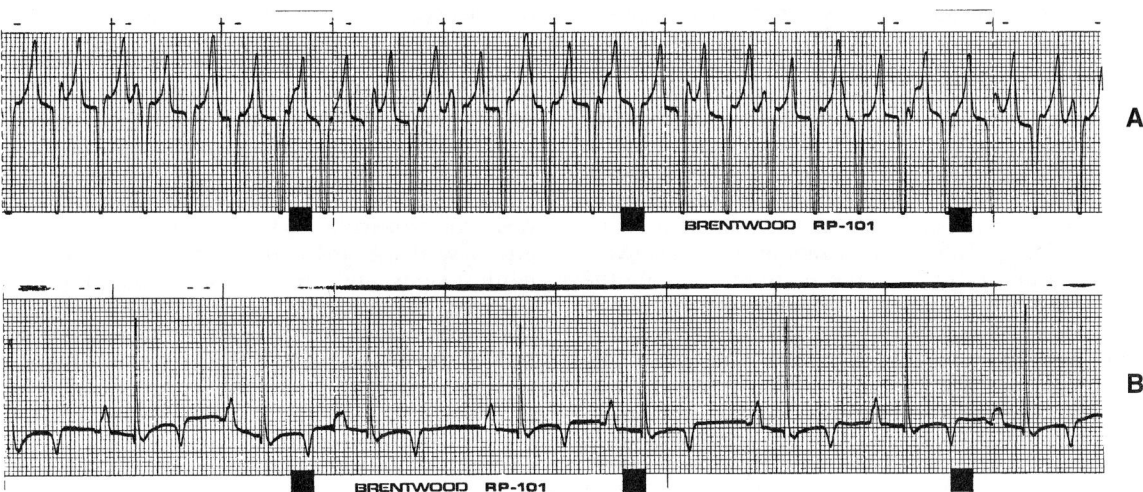

FIG. 28-17 ▓ Lead II ECG obtained from a horse with sustained uniform ventricular tachycardia and congestive heart failure before (**A**) and after (**B**) conversion to sinus rhythm. Notice the abnormal QRS and T configuration and slower atrial rate during the sustained ventricular tachycardia.

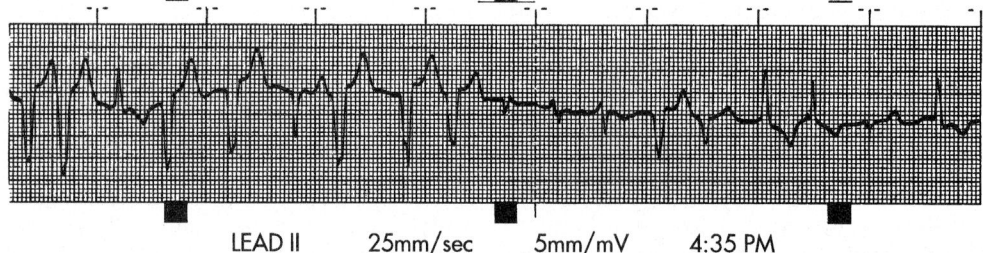

FIG. 28-18 ▌▌ Lead II ECG obtained from a horse with multiform ventricular tachycardia and acute onset of pulmonary edema. Notice the multiple different QRS and T configurations and the elevated ventricular rate.

systolic and diastolic undulations of the aortic root; the detection of spontaneous contrast, small aortic root, and large pulmonary artery. Occasionally the echocardiographic abnormalities created by ventricular tachycardia may be difficult to distinguish from those of primary myocardial disease. Rupture of the aortic root in the right sinus of Valsalva may be detected in horses with acute onset of uniform ventricular tachycardia and colic.

Cardiac catheterization may reveal severe hypotension and low cardiac output. In healthy ponies with pacing-induced ventricular tachycardia, stroke volume decreased significantly when the ventricle was paced at 150, 200, and 250 beats/min.[198] Mean left atrial pressure, mean pulmonary arterial pressure, and right ventricular systolic pressure increased significantly when the ventricle was paced at 220 and 250 beats/min. Aortic pressure and cardiac output decreased in these ponies at 250 beats/min, but the decrease from resting values was not statistically significant. Myocardial perfusion in the papillary muscles and subendocardium decreased significantly with pacing-induced ventricular tachycardia at a rate of 250 beats/min. Decreases in cardiac output, arterial blood pressure, and myocardial perfusion are even more marked in animals with underlying myocardial disease or multiform ventricular tachycardia, as are the changes in left atrial, pulmonary arterial, and right ventricular pressure.

PATHOPHYSIOLOGY. Ventricular tachycardia is probably initiated spontaneously by late coupled ventricular complexes, whereas one very early ventricular premature depolarization can often initiate ventricular tachycardia electrically.[186] Sympathetic stimulation may also provoke ventricular tachycardia by increasing the amplitude of the early afterdepolarizations, culminating in a run of ventricular tachycardia.[186] This may be the mechanism of some of the exercise-induced ventricular tachycardia in horses. Reentry in the ventricle is an important cause of sustained ventricular tachycardia, particularly in human patients with dilated cardiomyopathy and ischemic heart disease. The area of reentry is reportedly small, less than 1.4 cm^2.[186] Reentry is also thought to be an important mechanism in horses with sustained ventricular tachycardia.[193,199,200] Delayed afterdepolarizations may trigger ventricular tachycardia in humans and dogs and may be the mechanism for digitalis-induced ventricular tachycardia.[186] Abnormal action potentials have also been demonstrated in ventricular myocardium resected from human beings with recurrent ventricular tachycardia.[186] Depressed automaticity and afterdepolarizations have been associated with acute myocardial ischemia, whereas automaticity and afterdepolarizations are enhanced in Purkinje fibers surviving myocardial infarction. Idioventricular rhythms and parasystole may be caused by abnormal automaticity.

Cardiac diseases such as endocarditis may result in septic myocardial emboli and myocardial ischemia. Aortic root rupture and the dissection of blood into the interventricular septum disrupts conduction and usually results in a uniform ventricular tachycardia. Myocarditis, myocardial necrosis, and fibrosis also may result in abnormalities of impulse formation and conduction leading to ventricular tachycardia.[201] The excitement of the high-performance situation and the decreased myocardial perfusion that may occur at peak exercise may make exercise-induced ventricular tachycardia more common in racehorses and other types of high-performance horses.

EPIDEMIOLOGY. Ventricular tachycardia has been reported in all large animals, although horses may have the highest incidence. Ventricular tachycardia leading to ventricular fibrillation is thought to be one of the leading causes of sudden death in horses when other causes of death cannot be found on postmortem examination.[200] Male horses are at increased risk for aortic root and sinus of Valsalva rupture and are usually at least 10 years old at the time of rupture. Ventricular tachycardia is also more likely in large animals of any age with primary gastrointestinal disease.

NECROPSY FINDINGS. If the ventricular tachycardia is not associated with primary myocardial disease, the necropsy findings reflect the underlying disease. Gross and microscopic cardiac pathology has been found in horses with ventricular tachycardia, although in some horses no cardiac pathology is found. Areas of myocardial necrosis, inflammatory cell infiltrate, fibrosis, infarction, microvascular alterations, and cardiac nerve abnormalities have been reported in horses with ventricular tachycardia.[193,199-201] Congestive heart failure is most likely in large animal patients with multiform ventricular tachycardia and heart rates in excess of 180 beats/min. A minority of large animal patients have bacterial endocarditis with septic emboli disseminated through the coronary arteries associated with ventricular tachycardia. Aortic root rupture and rupture of a sinus of Valsalva aneurysm with dissection of blood into the interventricular septum are infrequently detected in horses.

TREATMENT AND PROGNOSIS. The treatment and prognosis for ventricular tachycardia depends on the suspected etiology of the arrhythmia, the severity of the animal's clinical signs, and the electrocardiographic abnormalities detected.[187,188] Relatively slow uniform ventricular tachycardia often resolves or improves significantly with the correction of the underlying electrolyte or metabolic imbalances, without requiring antiarrhythmic therapy. These animals usually have an excellent prognosis for conversion with correction of the underlying problem. Similarly, in large animals with sepsis or toxemia, hemodynamically and electrically stable ventricular tachycardia often resolves with treatment of the underlying disease. Uniform, hemodynamically stable ventricular tachycardia in animals with myocarditis may re-

TABLE 28-3

Drug Therapy for Ventricular Tachycardia

Drug	Usual Dose
Bretylium tosylate	0.5 mg/kg IV for life-threatening ventricular tachycardia or ventricular fibrillation
Dexamethasone	0.05-0.22 mg/kg, IV or IM
Furosemide	1-2 mg/kg as needed for pulmonary edema
Lidocaine	Equine: 0.1-0.25 mg/kg as a bolus; repeat up to total of 0.5 mg/kg in 10-15 min
	Bovine: 0.5 mg/kg, slowly IV; can repeat in 15 min
Magnesium SO_4	IV infusion at 1 g/min, to effect, up to a maximum of 25 g
Procainamide	1 mg/kg/min, IV to a maximum of 20 mg/kg
Propafenone	2 mg/kg PO tid
	0.5-1 mg/kg in 5% dextrose slowly IV over 5-8 min for refractory sustained ventricular tachycardia (not available in United States)
Propranolol	0.03 mg/kg, IV
Quinidine gluconate (IV)	1-10 mg/kg, IV, total dose in 0.25-0.5 mg/kg boluses 5-10 min apart

solve with rest and/or corticosteroid therapy. A minimum of 4 to 8 weeks of rest is indicated in these patients before returning to work, once the ventricular tachycardia has resolved.

Treatment with antiarrhythmics is indicated in any animal with hemodynamically unstable or life-threatening ventricular tachycardia. Treatment with antiarrhythmics is indicated if clinical signs of congestive heart failure or cardiovascular collapse are present or if the rate of sustained ventricular tachycardia is extremely high. In horses with sustained uniform ventricular tachycardia, a heart rate in excess of 120 beats/min usually warrants antiarrhythmic therapy, whereas in cattle, antiarrhythmic therapy may not be indicated until the heart rate exceeds 140 beats/min or greater. Horses with rapid sustained uniform ventricular tachycardia (120 beats/min or faster) need antiarrhythmic therapy because signs of congestive heart failure will develop after several days or weeks with this arrhythmia, if not already present. The rapidity of onset of congestive heart failure is related to the heart rate and type of primary myocardial disease, if present. These horses usually have a good prognosis for conversion and return to their previous performance level, with appropriate antiarrhythmic therapy (many times three or more antiarrhythmic drugs must be tried before conversion occurs) and rest before returning the horse to work.

The electrocardiographic findings associated with life-threatening ventricular tachycardia include a multifocal origin for the ventricular premature depolarizations, torsades de pointes (wide ventricular tachycardia) and the presence of an R wave superimposed on the preceding T wave ("R on T"). Large animal patients with clinical signs of congestive heart failure and hemodynamic collapse with rapid (heart rate >120 beats/min) multiform ventricular tachycardia (±R on T) should be treated as a cardiovascular emergency, because sudden death from ventricular fibrillation is likely without antiarrhythmic therapy. Large animals with multiform ventricular tachycardia (±R on T) must be given a guarded to grave prognosis for survival, because most have severe underlying myocardial disease. Often conversion to sinus rhythm may not be successful before the animal develops ventricular fibrillation and dies. If successfully converted to sinus rhythm, many of these animals die or are euthanized because of the severity of the underlying cardiac disease.

Several antiarrhythmic choices are available to the large animal practitioner for the correction of life-threatening ventricular tachycardia (Table 28-3). Lidocaine hydrochloride is the most readily available drug for most large animal practi-

tioners, is rapidly acting, is administered intravenously, and has a short duration of action and minimal hemodynamic effects. Lidocaine hydrochloride does, however, have central nervous system side effects in horses (hyperexcitability and seizures) and must be used at a lower dosage than in cattle. Quinidine gluconate (or quinidine sulfate in cattle) is very effective in large animals but is less rapidly acting, has negative inotropic effects at large doses or if primary myocardial disease is present, causes hypotension, and can produce undesirable adverse or toxic reactions. Magnesium sulfate has no recognized adverse cardiovascular effects, is less rapidly acting than lidocaine, but may be effective when other antiarrhythmics fail, in both normomagnesemic and hypomagnesemic patients. Intravenous procainamide and oral propafenone have also been used successfully in horses with ventricular tachycardia. Intravenous propafenone has been used successfully in one horse with refractory sustained uniform ventricular tachycardia that did not respond to lidocaine, quinidine, procainamide, or magnesium sulfate; but it is not available at this time in the United States. Other antiarrhythmics such as propranolol have been used with less success but have converted large animals with sustained ventricular tachycardia.

REFERENCES

186. Zipes DP: Genesis of cardiac arrhythmias: electrophysiological considerations. In Braunwald E: *A textbook of cardiovascular medicine*, ed 4, Philadelphia, 1992, Saunders, pp 603-614.
187. Reimer JM, Reef VB, Sweeney RW: Ventricular arrhythmias in the horse: twenty-one cases (1984-1989), *J Am Vet Med Assoc* 201:1237-1243, 1992.
188. Bonagura JD, Miller MS: Junctional and ventricular arrhythmias, *J Equine Vet Sci* 5:347-350, 1985.
189. Lester GD, Lombard CW, Ackerman N: Echocardiographic detection of a dissecting aortic root aneurysm in a thoroughbred stallion, *Vet Radiol Ultrasound* 33:202-205, 1992.
190. Reef VB: Pericardial and myocardial diseases. In Koblick CN et al: *The horse: diseases and clinical management*, New York, 1993, Churchill Livingstone, pp 185-197.
191. Nielsen IL: Ventricular tachycardia in a thoroughbred racehorse, *Aust Vet J* 67:140-142, 1990.
192. Senta T et al: A case report on ventricular paroxsysmal tachycardia (permanent type) in a thoroughbred colt, *Exp Rep Equine Health Lab* 8:61-71, 1971.
193. Machida N et al: Cardiopathological observation on a case of persistent ventricular tachycardia in a pony mare, *J Vet Med Sci* 54:1213-1216, 1992.
194. Marr CM, Reef VB: ECG of the month, *J Am Vet Med Assoc* 198:1533-1534, 1991.
195. Reef VB: A monensin outbreak in horses in the eastern United States: pathogenesis, clinical signs and epidemiology, *Proceedings of the Eighth Annual Veterinary Medicine Forum*, 1990, pp 619-622.

196. Cornelisse CJ et al: Concentration of cardiac troponin I in a horse with a ruptured aortic regurgitation jet lesion and ventricular tachycardia, *J Am Vet Med Assoc* 217:231-235, 2000.

197. McGuirk SM, Muir WW: Diagnosis and treatment of cardiac arrhythmias, *Vet Clin North Am (Equine Pract)* 1:353-370, 1985.

198. Parks C, Manohar M, Lundeen G: Regional myocardial blood flow and coronary vascular reserve in unanesthetized ponies during pacing-induced ventricular tachycardia, *J Surg Res* 35:119, 1983.

199. Kiryu K et al: Cardiopathological observation on a case of paroxysmal ventricular tachycardia in a thoroughbred colt: formal pathogenesis, *Exp Rep Equine Health Lab* 12:74-88, 1975.

200. Kiryu I et al: Cardiopathology of sudden death in the race horse, *Heart Vessels Suppl* 2:40, 1987.

201. Traub-Dargatz JL et al: Ventricular tachycardia and myocardial dysfunction in a horse, *J Am Vet Med Assoc* 205:1569-1573, 1994.

Diseases of the Respiratory System

PAMELA A. WILKINS

JOHN C. BAKER

TREVOR R. AMES

Consulting Editors

◼ DIAGNOSTIC PROCEDURES FOR THE RESPIRATORY SYSTEM ◼

ANGELINE E. WARNER

GENERAL EVALUATION OF THE PATIENT WITH RESPIRATORY DISEASE

History

A well-taken history should include several questions with direct bearing on respiratory disease. It is important to establish exercise levels, because the pastured animal may not manifest signs of respiratory function limitation and exercise intolerance that would be immediately apparent in an athletic counterpart. Immediate environment has direct bearing on potential allergen, parasite, and infectious disease exposure. Accurate knowledge of current immunization status and medications, especially analgesics or antipyretics, is essential.

Presenting Signs

Several physical findings or presenting complaints (see also Chapter 5) call attention to the respiratory system and should suggest implementation of more specialized procedures discussed in the next section. The upper respiratory system is suspect when sneezing or stertorous breathing is found. Findings that require follow-up evaluation with consideration of possible abnormality in either the upper or lower respiratory tract include coughing, tachypnea, dyspnea, cyanosis, hemoptysis, nasal discharge, and epistaxis.

Coughing is a nonspecific sign that indicates stimulation of irritant receptors, impaired mucociliary clearance, or ex-cessive production of secretions. Coughing that produces thick yellow or green exudate indicates the presence of numerous leukocytes (neutrophils or eosinophils) in respiratory secretions, confirming presence of an inflammatory process, but not always bacterial infection.

Dyspnea is the sensation of "shortness of breath" that is inferred from the attitude or behavior in veterinary patients. Dyspnea is distinct from tachypnea, or increased rate, and the latter may be present without dyspnea. The sensation of dyspnea can arise from obstruction to airflow, parenchymal disease (especially restrictive disease), and cardiovascular or pulmonary vascular disease. Either pleural effusion or pneumothorax can cause profound dyspnea. Regardless of the cause, inadequate gas transport stimulates deeper ventilatory efforts, manifest by abduction of the elbows, open-mouthed breathing, signs of apprehension in ruminants (Fig. 29-1), and increased abdominal muscle activity and flaring of the nostrils in horses.

Cyanosis is bluish discoloration of the oral, nasal, or vulvar mucous membranes. It is not apparent until 5 mg/100 ml of deoxygenated hemoglobin is present (normal hemoglobin content is 15 mg/100 ml blood), and thus it reflects a profound decrease in the oxygen being transported to the tissues. In the anemic patient the total quantity of desaturated hemoglobin may be less than the amount required to produce a blue color. Thus severe anemia can make appreciation of cyanosis impossible.

Hemoptysis is the coughing up of blood from the airways or lungs. It is important to determine conclusively that the

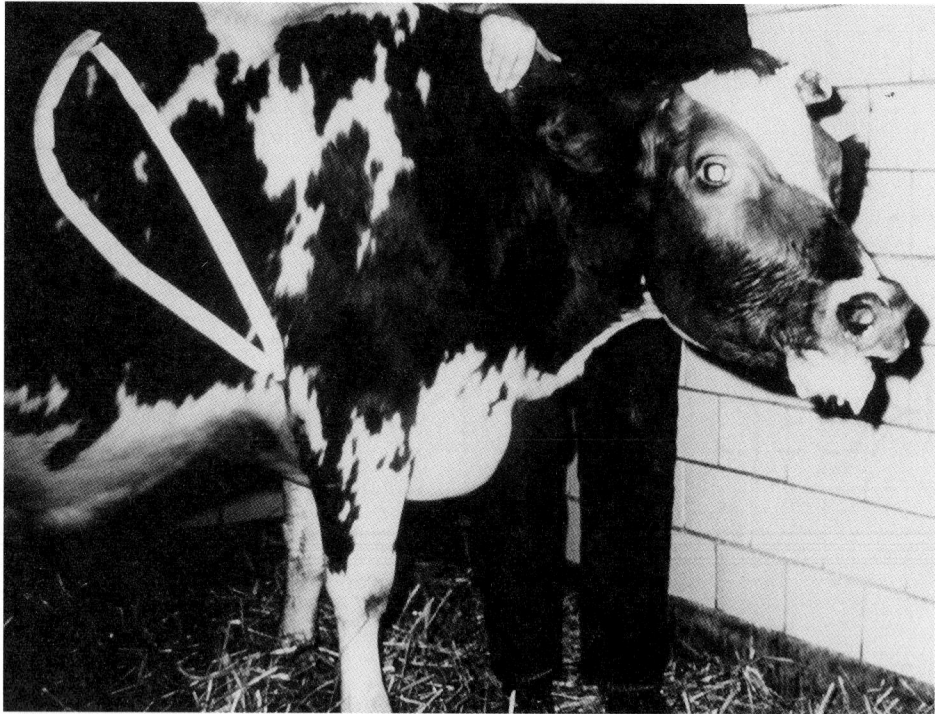

FIG. 29-1 ▊ Dyspnea in the cow. The cow appears apprehensive and shows open-mouthed breathing. (Courtesy Dr. T. Divers, Cornell University.)

blood has come from the respiratory system and not the upper gastrointestinal tract. Epistaxis is defined as blood produced at the nares and often signifies origin in the nasal passages, sinuses, turbinates, nasopharynx, or equine guttural pouches. Bilateral epistaxis indicates a source caudal to the choanae (nasal septum). Intrathoracic airways and lung parenchyma can also be the source of blood visualized at the nostrils (as in equine exercise-induced pulmonary hemorrhage), yet the presentation may be unilateral. Because animals tend to swallow excessive respiratory secretions, bleeding can be occult and is often witnessed only when the animal drops its head toward the ground. Skin depigmentation of the ventral nares or presence of mucoid material in feed or water containers is a clue to presence of a nasal discharge. A unilateral discharge is characteristic of sinus inflammation, whereas bilateral discharge suggests a more caudal source.

Physical Examination

When possible, resting respiration should be observed to allow accurate determination of rate without excitement or fear caused by handling. Normal adult resting rates are as follows: horses, 12 to 20 breaths/min; cattle, 15 to 35 breaths/min; and sheep and goats, 12 to 20 breaths/min. Heavily wooled sheep with normal respiratory function frequently pant in warm weather. Tachypnea can be a valuable early sign of respiratory disease in calves and foals. The normal rate for foals is 30 to 40 breaths/min at birth, and fewer than 30 breaths/min by 1 month of age; it decreases toward the adult rate with age. The normal rate for neonatal ruminants is 20 to 50 breaths/min. The general pattern of respiration should be noted, including prolonged inspiration, expiratory abdominal lift, and grunting or other signs of associated pain.

A thorough physical examination includes attention to both upper and lower respiratory systems. The nasal alar folds and passages should be palpated, followed by examination using an external light source. Symmetry of airflow and any facial swelling or asymmetry over the sinuses should be noted. The hair over inflamed sinuses may stand erect. Further evaluation of the sinuses includes oral examination and tapping of the teeth to elicit a pain response. Ventral deviation of the hard palate suggestive of sinus distortion should be looked for. Percussion of the sinuses can indicate presence of fluid or abnormal soft-tissue density. Holding the mouth open with the examiner's thumb in the interdental space during the procedure increases the normal resonance of the sinuses. The larynx should be palpated especially for asymmetry or abnormal prominence of the muscular process in the horse. The strength required to elicit a cough on laryngeal palpation should be noted. At the same time, any induced coughing may elicit exudate for cytologic examination. The lymph nodes and trachea should be palpated and the jugular veins checked for patency.

Auscultation

The lower respiratory tract is assessed by means of auscultation, and it is essential to have a quiet environment in which to listen, which is often a limiting factor in examination of large animals in a barn setting. It is important to obtain deep inspirations from the patient by raising the inspired carbon dioxide levels either through holding the nostrils to prevent ventilation for several seconds or by making the patient take several breaths into a plastic rebreathing bag. The first deep breaths taken after this procedure can reveal abnormal sounds not heard during resting respiration. Auscultatory changes can be subtle and allow early detection of disease, facilitating additional diagnostic procedures or timely therapy. In general, early auscultatory changes are more frequently heard in horses than in ruminants with bronchopneumonia. Thus, in many ruminants, significant pulmonary disease may not be detected by auscultation.

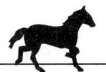

TABLE 29-1

Normal Lung Boundaries for Horses and Ruminants

Equine		Bovine		Ovine	
Landmark	Intercostal Space	Landmark	Intercostal Space	Landmark	Intercostal Space
Tuber coxae	17	Tuber coxae	11	Tuber coxae	11
Tuber ischii	16	Midthorax	9	Midthorax	8
Midthorax	13	Olecranon	5	Olecranon	5
Pt. shoulder	11				
Olecranon	6				

Lung sounds heard by auscultation are generated by changes in airflow, and sound intensity is related to airstream velocity. Turbulence in the large airways is the predominant mechanism of sound generation, because turbulent flow of adequate velocity cannot occur in small airways. Only airways from the larynx to segmental bronchi contribute to sound generation, and normally generated "bronchial" and "vesicular" sounds both represent larger airway flow events. Vesicular sounds correlate best with regional ventilation and mainly represent segmental bronchial sounds; they do not represent gentle flow in terminal airways, which is actually silent.

Once generated, airway sounds are attenuated to a variable degree by transmission through lung parenchyma. An inflated lung strongly attenuates airway sounds, but a consolidated lung is a good acoustic-conducting medium. Further modification on the way to the stethoscope bell depends on presence of pleural inflammation or effusion, pneumothorax, body fat thickness, and hair coat characteristics. Bronchial sounds are heard over the site of production: trachea, hilar area, and mainstream bronchi. Vesicular sounds are heard over the lung periphery after filtration through lung tissue. Increased intensity of these normal sounds indicates greater air velocity caused by deeper or more rapid ventilation, which can be initiated by exercise, anxiety, hyperthermia, acidosis, and cardiac or pulmonary disease. Normal sounds are also heard with increased intensity when transmitted through consolidated parenchyma. Thus ventral consolidation, which frequently occurs with bronchopneumonia in ruminants, causes harsh, loud, auscultable inspiratory and expiratory airway sounds rather than absence of airway sounds ventrally. Sounds are less well transmitted to the listener when emphysematous bullae, pneumothorax, or pleural effusion is present. Absence of lung sounds ventrally usually indicates pleural effusion, whereas absence of lung sounds dorsally suggests pneumothorax.

Until recently the terminology for adventitious, or abnormal, lung sounds has been plagued by considerable ambiguity, but a simplified uniform terminology that has greatly improved communication among clinicians in human and veterinary medicine has been agreed upon.[1] Adventitious lung sounds are divided into discontinuous sounds (<20 ms, intermittent or explosive) called crackles and continuous sounds (>250 ms, often musical) called wheezes. These replace the older terms rales and rhonchi, respectively, although the latter is currently accepted as equivalent to wheezes.

Crackles suggest bubbling of air through secretions, but most commonly are generated by explosive equalization of upstream and downstream pressures when collapsed segments reopen. Although an air/fluid interface is required, crackles do not necessarily imply excessive secretions or pulmonary edema. They are often end-inspiratory, as peak transpulmonary pressure is achieved, correlating with reinflation of atelectatic lung. Disease processes that generate crackles include pneumonia, interstitial fibrosis, chronic obstructive lung disease, congestive heart failure, and atelectasis.[2]

Continuous adventitious sounds (wheezes) commonly represent oscillation of airway walls before complete closing (expiratory wheezes) or opening (inspiratory wheezes). Extrathoracic airways may be involved, usually generating inspiratory or stridorous sounds. Intrathoracic airways are generally involved in expiratory wheezes and include the lower trachea, main, lobar, and segmental bronchi. The airflow rate in small airways is too slow to initiate these sounds. Disappearance of a wheeze after coughing indicates that a secretory rather than a tissue component is involved in oscillation. Disease processes responsible for wheezes include airway stenosis or external compression; airway lumen compromise by foreign body, purulent material, cyst or neoplasm, and airway wall thickening as in chronic bronchitis; and bronchoconstriction.[3] Expiratory wheezes are a hallmark of obstructive lung disease. These sounds are modulated by the degree of aeration of the adjacent lung tissue. A final category of adventitious sounds are the "rubbing" or "creaking" sounds generated by sliding or stretching of inflamed pleural surfaces.

Percussion

Percussion of the lungs depends on the resonant sounds obtained by tapping the chest wall over inflated lungs versus the dull sound obtained over fluid (pleural effusion) or consolidated lung tissue devoid of air. The procedure is performed by tapping the extended fingers of one hand with the fingertips of the opposite hand, with a specially designed plexor and pleximeter, or with a rubber neurologic reflex hammer and large spoon. The latter are readily obtainable and produce excellent results. The spoon is moved from dorsal to ventral along each individual rib space while tapping continuously. The point at which a change occurs from resonant to dull can be marked with adhesive tape. Thus the outline of aerated lung immediately beneath the chest wall is delineated (Fig. 29-2). Over the cranial aspect of the lungs, some difficulty is usually encountered because of body fat and triceps musculature. There is a distinct region of cardiac dullness for all species on the left side. Normal lung boundaries for horses and ruminants are indicated in Table 29-1.

Percussion allows delineation of pleural effusion (see Fig. 29-2) and intrathoracic masses or consolidated lung up to 7 cm beneath the pleural surface, but cannot distinguish among these. The procedure is noninvasive, inexpensive, and should be performed whenever pleural effusion is suspected on the basis of auscultatory findings (absence of ventral airway sounds) and in all ruminants as part of the physical examination to uncover occult pneumonia.[4] Because the parietal pleura is well innervated and often becomes painful with inflammation, the patient's response to the procedure may also be clinically important.

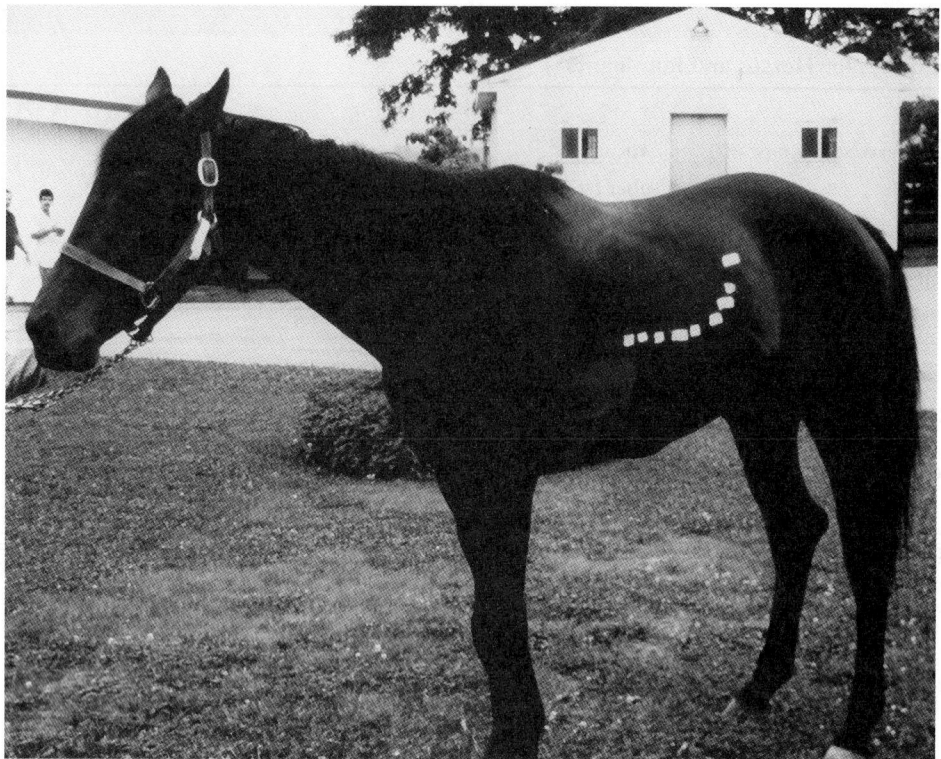

FIG. 29-2 ▌▐ Abnormal aerated lung boundaries demonstrated by thoracic percussion. The horizontal line shown here is consistent with a pleural effusion, and several liters of pleural fluid were subsequently drained from this horse.

SPECIALIZED DIAGNOSTIC PROCEDURES FOR EVALUATING THE RESPIRATORY SYSTEM

The respiratory system is evaluated on a macroscopic level by several procedures, including radiology, ultrasonography, endoscopy, intradermal allergic skin testing, and nuclear medicine. Microscopic evaluation includes those techniques that yield specimens for culture or cytologic study: tracheobronchial aspirate or bronchoalveolar lavage, thoracocentesis, sinus tap, and guttural pouch catheterization. Evaluation on a functional level is limited to pulmonary function tests and arterial blood gas evaluation. Additional general clinical pathologic data are often needed, including total peripheral white blood cell (WBC) count and differential, plasma fibrinogen, serologic evaluation for viral respiratory diseases, and the use of fluorescent antibody or viral isolation. If lungworms are suspected, a fecal sample for Baermann examination for larvae should be submitted, with the recognition that patent infections do not develop in many horses.

Thoracic Radiographs

Thoracic radiographs offer an excellent opportunity for visualization of fluid-dense structures, both normal and abnormal, within the lungs, contrasted naturally by pulmonary air. In addition to the spine, ribs, heart, and mediastinum, the lungs can be evaluated for presence of opacities falling within four major categories: vascular (Fig. 29-3), bronchial, interstitial, or alveolar.

Thoracic radiographs in adult horses and cattle require equipment usually only available at larger referral centers and veterinary teaching hospitals, and at least four films are required to image equine lungs adequately. It is possible, however, for ambulatory practitioners to produce diagnostic films of young animals with a portable radiograph capable of 80 to 100 kVp and 20 mA using only one 14- × 17-inch film.[5] Because of its configuration, the thorax in adult horses and cattle is filmed as a standing lateral; thus the benefit of the ventrodorsal view in which the two lungs may be compared is lost. Neonates and small ruminants can be handled as large dogs, and multiple recumbent views can be obtained. Ventrodorsal views are somewhat limited in very deep-chested animals, except for demonstration of consolidation in the dorsocaudal region.

Radiographs are indicated when the clinician suspects a congenital anomaly involving any thoracic structure; infectious disease of the pleura, pulmonary parenchyma (Fig. 29-4), tracheobronchial tree, or mediastinum; pneumothorax (Fig. 29-5) or pneumomediastinum; thoracic neoplasia of any origin; or trauma. They are also valuable in assessing the degree of ventilation, and thus aeration, in neonatal lungs. Unfortunately, numerous pulmonary diseases, including tracheitis, bronchitis, bronchiolitis, alveolitis, alveolar emphysema, and hypersensitivity pneumonia,[5] exhibit few if any radiographic signs.

Although lateral projection radiographic analysis of the lungs allows visualization of the entire lungs (unfortunately superimposed), it is limited in resolution. Solitary uncalcified lesions of less than 6 mm may not be detected, although presence of multiple nodular densities enhances the probability of detection. Radiographs are an appropriate initial imaging method in cases of pulmonary disease, but they often must be used with clinical parameters, other imaging methods, and diagnostic techniques, for example, in patients with pleural disease or peripheral lung lesions.

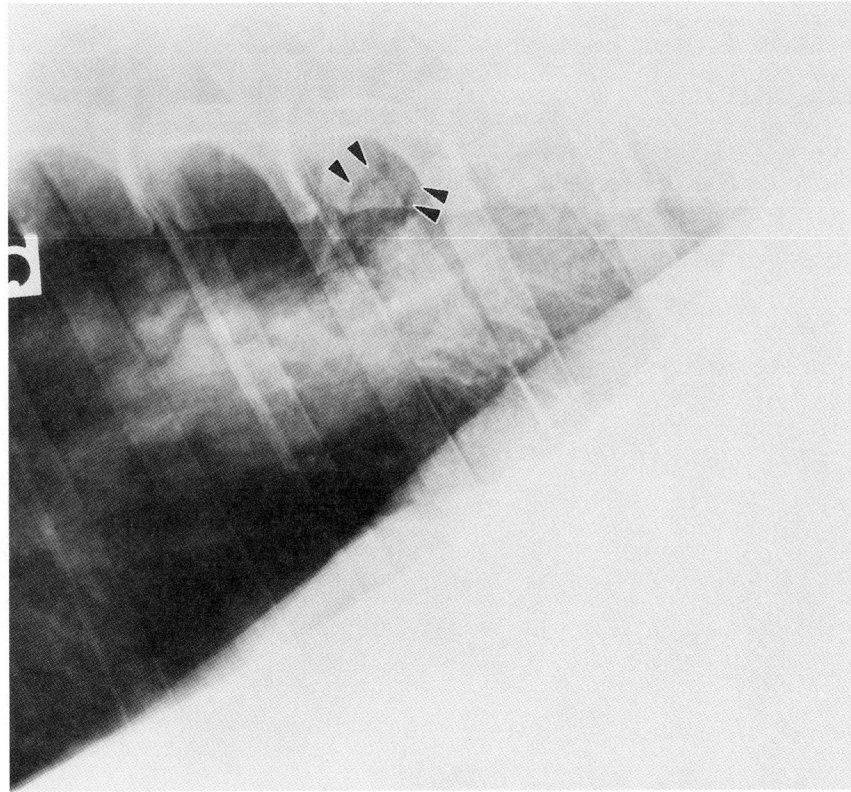

FIG. 29-3 ▓ Left lateral radiograph of the dorsocaudal lung fields in an adult Thoroughbred racehorse with a history of exercise-induced pulmonary hemorrhage (EIPH). The dorsocaudal angle of the lung demonstrates a localized dense area of mixed bronchointerstitial marking that almost obscures the vascular pattern. Along the caudal and dorsal margins of this opacity *(arrowheads)*, air bronchogram formation indicates an air-space ("alveolar") pattern more suggestive of recent involvement than the interstitial marking seen in the remainder of the lesion. This radiographic appearance is seen in a small proportion of EIPH cases. (Courtesy Dr. M. O'Callaghan, Tufts University School of Veterinary Medicine.)

In addition to thoracic radiographs, skull and cervical radiograph films offer diagnostic information for the upper respiratory tract. For large animal species, standing lateral skull films are easily obtained, but ventrodorsal and oblique projections require general anesthesia. Skull films offer visualization of the sinuses, pharynx, and larynx. Sinuses affected by neoplasia or inflammation may show abnormal tissue density, a horizontal fluid line on a standing lateral film, bone lysis around the affected sinus, or alveolar periostitis.

The equine guttural pouches are evident on lateral skull projection, and abnormal fluid accumulation, distortion by enlarged retropharyngeal lymph nodes, or emphysema are radiographically apparent. Structural distortion of the larynx or upper trachea and presence of foreign bodies can also be assessed radiographically.

Ultrasonography

Ultrasonography is performed with the patient standing, and sound waves are generated by piezoelectric crystals and transmitted to the area of interest through a skin coupling gel. Reflected echoes are detected by the same crystal. The image is made by displaying echo signals from all tissue interfaces contained in a plane defined by the scanning beam. The screen image can be photographed for a permanent record.

Aerated lung parenchyma is not penetrated by the ultrasound beam, rendering only the pleura and superficial lung surface available for study. It is in the study of the pleural surfaces and space, however, that ultrasound offers a great advantage over diagnostic radiology. Small amounts of pleural fluid that would be missed on auscultation, percussion, or thoracic radiographs can be detected.[6] The amount of pleural effusion in each hemithorax can be separately evaluated. Often compression atelectasis of the ventral lung is also visible (Fig. 29-6). The character of pleural exudate can also be noninvasively assessed. Clear fluid is anechoic, but accumulation of inflammatory cells and fibrin is echogenic, causing opacities that can be seen floating in pleural fluid. Ultrasound is the technique of choice for monitoring pleural disease; the efficacy of fluid removal, its recurrence, the development of loculation, and the position of indwelling catheters are easily assessed. Ultrasonography can be used to guide catheter placement, especially to drain isolated fluid pockets.[6] Gas echoes in pleural fluid are significantly correlated with positive culture results for anaerobic bacteria in tracheobronchial aspirate or pleural fluid.[7] In patients with pneumothorax, dorsal accumulation of air is best visualized radiographically, but ultrasound can be used to determine the ventral margin of free air for needle introduction and aspiration.

The pleural surfaces themselves are well visualized by ultrasound, and thickened or roughened areas easily detected. Adhesions are characterized by lack of normal independent movement of the visceral and parietal pleural surfaces during the respiratory cycle.

Consolidated lung is a better acoustic medium than aerated parenchyma and can be well visualized. If there is pleu-

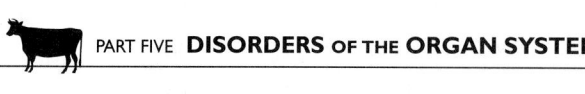

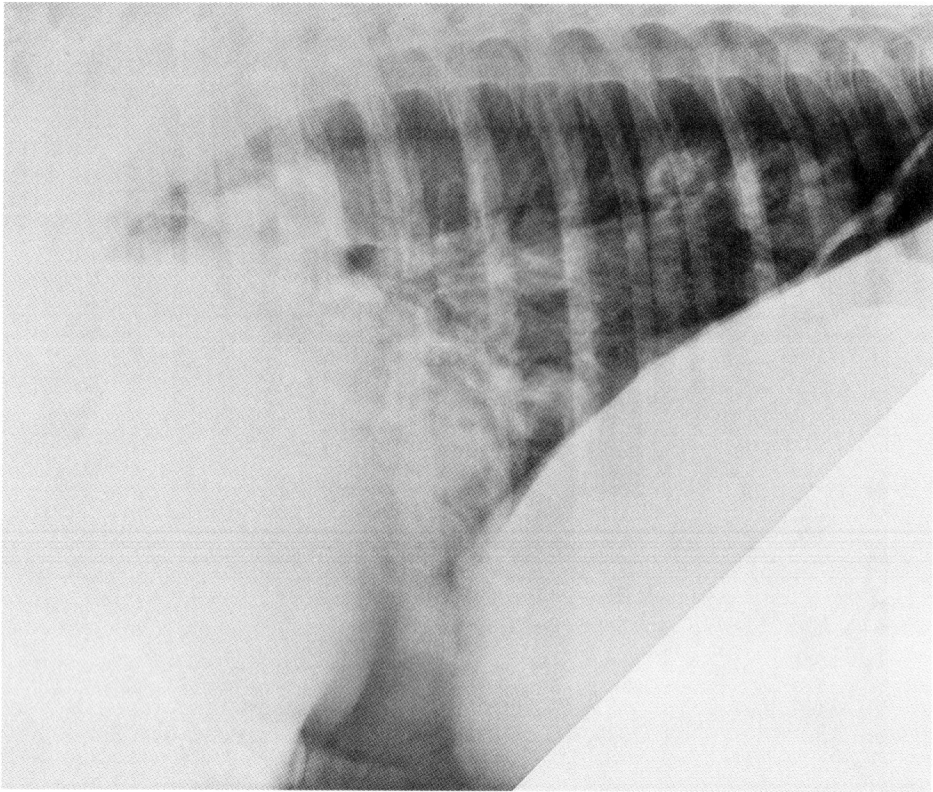

FIG. 29-4 ▓ Lateral standing thoracic radiograph in a young foal. The midventral lung area shows a mixed pattern of air-space ("alveolar") bronchial and interstitial patterns, almost completely obscuring the cardiac silhouette. In the dorsocaudal lung fields and cranially overlying the heart, multiple spherical opacities containing gas/fluid interfaces indicate abscess formation. This appearance is typical of resolving but still active *Rhodococcus* bronchopneumonia. (Courtesy Dr. M. O'Callaghan, Tufts University School of Veterinary Medicine.)

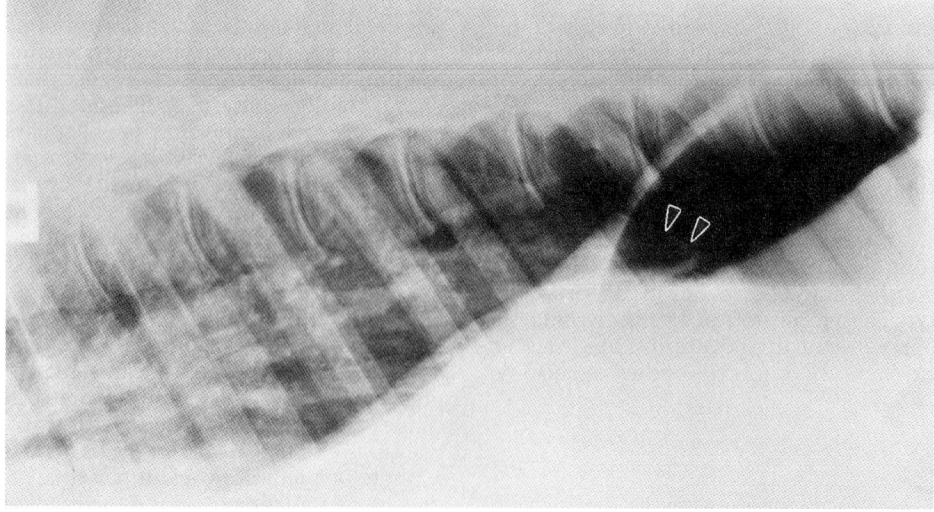

FIG. 29-5 ▓ Lateral standing radiograph of the dorsocaudal lung field in an adult horse with a thoracic laceration. A moderage degree of pneumothorax is demonstrated by the retracted apex of one lung *(arrowheads)* silhouetted against surrounding air. The remainder of the visible lung field demonstrates a moderate bronchointerstitial pattern overlying a horizontal gas-fluid interface, indicative of pleural effusion. The ventral lung is totally obscured by this fluid opacity. (Courtesy Dr. M. O'Callaghan, Tufts University School of Veterinary Medicine.)

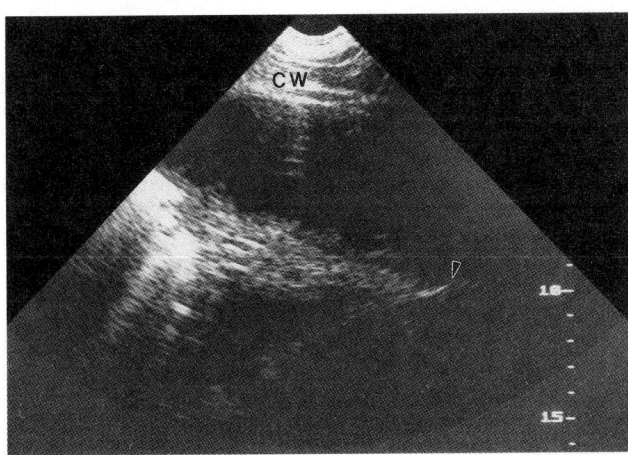

FIG. 29-6 ▮ Sector scan ultrasound image of the ventral pleural space in a horse with severe pleuritis and effusion. Collapsed lung at the costophrenic angle *(arrow)* is identified as a moderately echoic structure floating in a large volume of relatively anechoic fluid *(black)*. On the surface of the lung, irregular echoicity suggests the presence of fibrinous tags adhered to the visceral pleura. Air-filled lung *(intense white area in the middle left of the image)* has reflected most of the sound beam, obscuring underlying detail. The chest wall *(CW)* is identified at the top of the image. Depth marks (in centimeters) are shown on the right of the image. (Courtesy Dr. M. O'Callaghan, Tufts University School of Veterinary Medicine.)

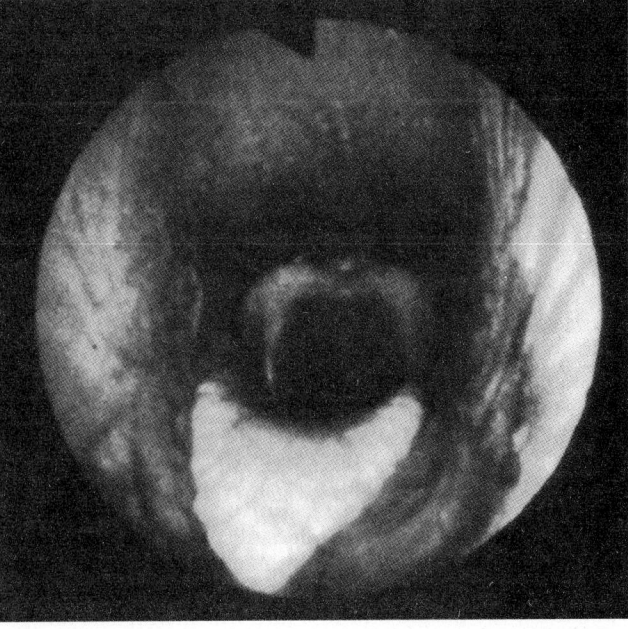

FIG. 29-7 ▮ Normal equine larynx. The larynx is directly visualized by endoscopy. Both structure and symmetry of movement can be evaluated. (Courtesy Dr. C. Sweeney, New Bolton Center, University of Pennsylvania.)

ropneumonia with consolidation or atelectasis caused by compression of the ventral lung by pleural effusion, it will be evident. A pulmonary abscess or neoplastic mass extending to the surface can also be delineated, and a needle guided to it under ultrasound surveillance for diagnostic aspiration and drainage if necessary. Radiographs are superior to ultrasound in diagnosis of pulmonary parenchymal disease, because the air-filled parenchyma can be visualized.

Endoscopy

The upper airway is amenable to direct visual study with the endoscope. The size of the airways and the distance from the nares that can be examined are limited by the technology that is available. The standard flexible fiberoptic endoscope allows direct examination of the nasal passages, ethmoid turbinates, nasal maxillary opening of the sinuses, pharynx, guttural pouch openings, larynx, and cranial trachea (Fig. 29-7). An 8- to 10-mm-diameter endoscope can be introduced into the equine guttural pouches with minimum difficulty. Endoscopes longer than 150 cm and greater than 10 mm in diameter are now available and allow examination of the mainstem bronchi and their initial branches in large animals. Accessory equipment includes a small brush for collecting exfoliated cells for cytologic study and a biopsy instrument. The latter is designed for obtaining small samples from airway walls but is most useful in equine patients for guiding the instrument into the guttural pouches.

Endoscopy allows confirmation of pharyngeal lymphoid hyperplasia, laryngeal hemiplegia, epiglottic entrapment by arytenoepiglottic folds, dorsal displacement of the soft palate, pharyngeal cysts, retropharyngeal masses, and epiglottic deformities. Dynamic upper respiratory tract function can be assessed in equine athletes during treadmill exercise, and freeze-frame images produced with video-endoscopy during exercise can be used to make objective measurements.[8] In cases of guttural pouch emphysema, exudate may be seen at the guttural pouch orifice without the

necessity of introducing the endoscope into the pouch. Direct endoscopic visualization of blood in the trachea is far more sensitive in the diagnosis of exercise-induced pulmonary hemorrhage in the horse than is appearance of blood at the nostrils.

Tranquilization should be avoided for evaluation of equine laryngeal and pharyngeal function, but any other examination is facilitated by sedation. Equine airways are well innervated, and introduction of the endoscope into the trachea usually incites coughing. Bronchoscopic examination is usually limited by severe coughing unless local anesthesia is used. Polyethylene tubing can be advanced though the biopsy port to allow small amounts of 2% lidocaine to be directly applied just before advancing the endoscope. With this method the mainstem bronchi and their branches can be viewed with minimal patient discomfort.[9]

Cattle have less irritable airways, and examination usually requires only adequate restraint to prevent damage to the equipment. Sheep and goats have irritable airways, and local anesthetic must be used. Lidocaine should be diluted to prevent administration of a toxic dose (20 mg/kg). Instrument size determines whether the endoscope can be passed though the nares or through the mouth using a bite block in small ruminants. If the endoscope is passed through the mouth, great care must be taken to prevent crush damage by cheek teeth; patient sedation is strongly advised.

Tracheobronchial Aspirate/Bronchoalveolar Lavage

Various spaces in the respiratory system can be aspirated or lavaged for diagnostic or therapeutic purposes. The most commonly performed procedure is the tracheobronchial aspirate. By aspirating from the airways caudal to the larynx, a sample without pharyngeal contamination is obtained.

In both the horse and the ruminant the procedure is performed with the animal standing. Sedation or restraint may be needed. A 10-cm area over the trachea in the middle to lower third of the neck is clipped and sterilely prepared. The skin is anesthetized, and a small stab incision made. A trocar or angiocatheter needle is introduced on the midline between muscle bundles, and the ventral tracheal wall is punctured between cartilaginous rings. Sterile polyethylene tubing or the catheter from the angiocatheter is introduced about 30 cm, using the cannula or needle to direct the tubing downward. A needle or sharp trocar should be withdrawn to prevent severing the tubing or catheter, but a cannula with rounded edges may be left in place. Approximately 30 ml of sterile saline solution is introduced quickly. Commercial saline solution containing bacteriostatic preservatives must be avoided. Intermittent aspiration is performed as the tubing is gradually withdrawn. The tubing can be advanced again if a guarding cannula has been left in place to prevent introduction of skin contamination. Additional saline solution aliquots can be introduced. Once an adequate sample has been obtained, the tubing is completely withdrawn. Injectable antibiotic can be infiltrated at the skin incision site if a septic sample is suspected. In horses and small ruminants a sterile dressing is applied for 24 hours.

Possible complications include subcutaneous emphysema (which is usually peritracheal but may extend into the mediastinum), local cellulitis at the incision site, or cutting of the catheter at the needle and loss into the airway. The latter is usually resolved because the catheter is rapidly coughed up, but good technique should prevent this complication. Airway aspiration can also be performed during routine endoscopy of the trachea using an aspiration catheter advanced through the endoscope biopsy channel, but there is potential for pharyngeal contamination. Results comparing culture from a protected aspiration catheter passed through an endoscope compared favorably with traditional percutaneous tracheobronchial aspirate.[10] The sample should be cultured for aerobic bacteria. Anaerobic colonization is possible, and appropriate cultures should be made if these organisms are suspected (evidence of pleural effusion, consolidation, abscessation, fetid breath, history of aspiration). For patients with prior antimicrobial therapy, it is advised to discontinue antibiotics for 72 to 96 hours before culture, although a recent study has shown reliable recovery of bacteria using bronchoalveolar lavage fluid from foals receiving therapy.[11] A direct smear and Gram stain can be used to suggest antimicrobial therapy pending culture results. Cytologic evaluation can be extremely valuable in differentiating among infectious, allergic, parasitic, and neoplastic processes. A differential cell count is performed, but a total cell count is not useful because the sample is obtained by a saline lavage, and variable amounts are retrieved. Normally, columnar ciliated epithelial cells, a few neutrophils, and multiple mononuclear cells are present. Increased percentages of neutrophils and presence of mast cells, eosinophils, giant cells, and hemosiderophages have been demonstrated in aspirates from normally performing Thoroughbred racehorses, indicating some airway inflammation in "normal" equine atheletes.[12] Mucus, large spores, and fungal hyphae may be found in the absence of airway disease. Allergic bronchiolitis is characterized by increased numbers of nondegenerate neutrophils and occasional eosinophils. A recent study suggests that aspirates obtained after strenuous exercise are more likely to reveal airway disease.[13] In cases of pneumonia, neutrophils may constitute 40% to 90% of the cellular sample. Bacterial pneumonia causes a more degenerate appearance of neutrophils, and intracellular bacteria may be found. Equine lungworm is characterized by finding large numbers of eosinophils and occasionally a larva. In ruminants the most important information gathered in patients with bronchopneumonia is usually the result of culture and antimicrobial sensitivity testing.

Bronchoalveolar lavage involves obtaining a sample from the terminal airways and alveolar region. It is performed using a long endoscope or double-lumen tube introduced through the nares. The outer tube or the endoscope is wedged in a bronchus, and the smaller tube advanced. Saline solution aliquots of 60 to 300 ml are introduced, followed by continuous aspiration. The procedure has the advantage of sampling the airways nearest the parenchymal region, but only a limited area of the lung is sampled instead of the pooled secretions from a tracheobronchial aspirate. Thus bronchoalveolar lavage may be superior to tracheobronchial aspirate in evaluation of horses with chronic lung diseases,[14] but false-negative results can be obtained from horses with pneumonia or pleuropneumonia.[15] Bronchoalveolar lavage cytology is valuable in evaluation of inflammatory airway disease[16] and assessment of therapeutic response.[17]

Skin Testing

Sensitivity to allergens that may elicit an airway hypersensitivity response in horses can be determined by intradermal skin testing. The procedure is aimed at diagnosis of allergic bronchiolitis or chronic obstructive pulmonary disease (COPD) rather than dermatologic disease. A collection of allergens, including numerous mold species isolated from barns, an extract of hay and straw dust, and common feed components, has been developed at the George Widener Hospital, University of Pennsylvania, for such testing.[18] Intradermal responses to histamine, saline, or 0.1 ml of antigen are read at 30 minutes, 4 hours, or 24 hours. Positive responses can be used to plan environmental modification for avoidance and often are of greatest value in convincing owners of the need to minimize stabling and thus exposure.

Thoracocentesis

Aspiration from the pleural space is a simple, inexpensive procedure that can be both diagnostic and therapeutic. In the horse with septic or neoplastic effusion, sedation is often unnecessary, because the procedure causes only minimum discomfort. The thorax should be widely clipped from the olecranon caudally to the tenth intercostal space and from the point of the shoulder to well below the olecranon. The area should be surgically prepared. A site is chosen in the sixth or seventh intercostal space 10 cm dorsal to the olecranon and above the lateral thoracic vein. A sonogram may be valuable in determining the site in horses with loculated pockets of fluid in the pleural cavity. The skin and intercostal tissue down to the pleura are anesthetized with lidocaine and a stab incision made. A sterile 2- to 3-inch teat cannula or bitch catheter is introduced immediately cranial to the rib border to avoid the intercostal nerve and vessel along the caudal aspect of the ribs. The cannula should be attached to sterile intravenous extension tubing and a three-way stopcock. While the cannula is advanced bluntly through the parietal pleura, a sudden loss of the force required to advance is felt. Aspiration should be attempted at this point. The orientation of the cannula can be varied to reach as much fluid as possible. Normally only a few milliliters of straw-colored fluid is obtained. In cases of pleural effusion, as much as 30 L may be removed from each side of the chest. If fluid is excessive, the tubing can be extended over a bucket for gravity drainage (Fig. 29-8), or a vacuum pump with fluid trap attached. Once the procedure is complete, a purse string suture is placed around the stab incision, and the cannula withdrawn while the suture is tightened.

Increasing opacity, presence of fibrin clumps, and malodor of pleural fluid all suggest relative progression from transudate to septic exudate containing inflammatory cells and debris. A putrid odor suggests the presence of anaerobic bacteria. Samples should be cultured for aerobic and anaer-

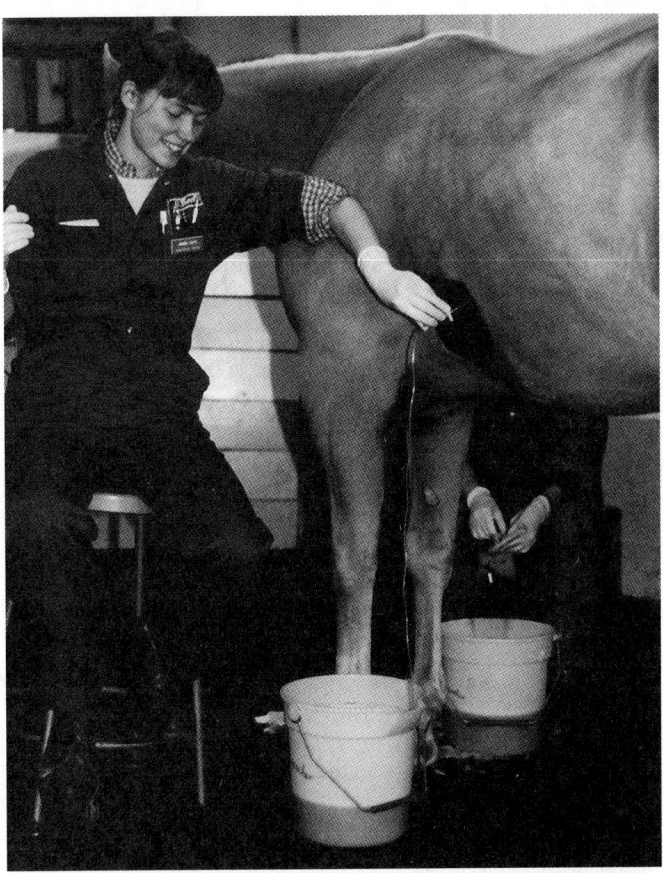

FIG. 29-8 ▓ Thoracocentesis and therapeutic drainage in the horse. Pleural effusion can be excessive and bilateral. Samples should be obtained for culture and cytologic examination, and free fluid removed by gravity drainage or a vacuum pump. (Courtesy Dr. C. Sweeney, University of Pennsylvania, New Bolton Center.)

obic organisms. Because no lavage fluid is introduced, the total cell number and total protein are valuable numbers. A WBC count of 10,000/μl or less is considered normal; fewer than 60% are normally neutrophils, the remainder being lymphocytes and macrophages. The proportion and total number of neutrophils increase with pleuritis. Erythrocytes are normally not present in the absence of a traumatic tap. The protein concentration is normally less than 3.5 g/dl, and pH should be approximately 7.4. Additional metabolic values that give early indication of sepsis can be obtained on pleural fluid samples collected after filtration through a blood administration set to remove fibrin and debris potentially detrimental to analytical equipment. Pleural fluid pH, P_{CO_2}, and concentration of glucose, lactate, and bicarbonate can be directly compared with similar analysis of venous blood from the patient. A septic pleural exudate is acidic, with decreased glucose and bicarbonate but elevated lactate and P_{CO_2} compared with venous blood levels, apparently reflecting metabolic activity of phagocytic cells and bacteria and development of an anaerobic environment.[19] Of these values, low pleural fluid glucose concentration (<40 mg/dl) has the best correlation with sepsis.[20]

Neoplastic cells may be found in cases of lymphosarcoma or adenocarcinoma. Equine gastric squamous cell carcinoma occasionally presents with a neoplastic pleural effusion. If a neoplastic effusion is suspected, but diagnostic cells do not exfoliate into the pleural fluid, pleuroscopy under sedation and local anesthesia can be used directly to visualize and obtain biopsy samples of intrathoracic lesions.

When a septic process is suspected, results of the thoracocentesis should be evaluated in the light of other diagnostic findings, including hematology, radiology, and ultrasonog-

raphy. Because any mediastinal fenestrations may be occluded by fibrin and cell debris, each side of the thorax should be evaluated separately. In the horse a transtracheal aspirate for culture should also be performed because of the common association of pleuritis with bacterial pneumonia and pulmonary abscessation. Often the airway aspirate yields the causative organism on culture, whereas the pleural fluid does not.

Sinus Trephination

Sinusitis is not uncommon in horses or ruminants. Clinical signs include foul-smelling purulent nasal discharge (the most consistent sign with dental disease or invasive tumors), facial malformation, exophthalmos, stertorous breathing, and epistaxis. Roots of the three molars are within the floor of the maxillary sinus, and dental disease can initiate sinus inflammation and infection. Sinus cysts, neoplasms, or hematomas occasionally occur and result in serosanguineous discharge. When the physical examination, especially percussion, and radiographic findings indicate, the sinus should be trephined for diagnostic aspiration, drainage, and flushing, if necessary.

In the horse the frontal, sphenopalatine, and ethmoidal sinuses all communicate with the posterior chamber of the maxillary sinus and drain through the nasal maxillary opening into the middle meatus. The anterior chamber of the maxillary sinus is separated by an osseous septum that often breaks down with infection, making the posterior chamber of the maxillary sinus the most productive site for diagnostic aspiration. A line is drawn from the medial canthus of the eye perpendicularly to the facial crest. After tranquilization and local anesthesia, the sinus is approached with a Steinmann pin midway on this line. Once the sinus has been entered, it should be aspirated by using a sterile 16-gauge needle or a canine urinary catheter. One skin suture will suffice for closure. If purulent material or fluid within the sinus is under pressure, some leakage into the subcutaneous space may occur, with resulting cellulitis. The sample should be cultured for aerobic and anaerobic bacteria and examined cytologically for signs of septic inflammation or neoplastic cells.

The frontal sinus is trephined more often for flushing in chronic cases than for diagnostic purposes. The approach is 2.5 cm lateral to the midline of the face and 2.5 cm caudal to the point where the nasal bones begin to diverge.

In cattle the frontal sinus is most often affected with septic inflammation as a consequence of dehorning. Purulent material frequently accumulates in the postorbital diverticulum of the sinus. This site is approached for trephination 4 cm from the edge of the orbital cavity just dorsal to the temporal (lateral) canthus of the eye.

Postdehorning sinusitis in goats can be a severe condition, especially in animals dehorned when mature. The frontal sinus contains numerous septae, creating poor drainage; the bony plate protecting the brain is thin, so that septic necrosis of bone leading to meningitis may occur. Therefore, in mature goats with sinusitis, appropriate systemic antimicrobial therapy and vigorous curettage of the affected areas should be used. A bone flap similar to the technique used in chronic maxillary sinusitis may be required to expose the frontal sinuses to curettage adequately.

Guttural Pouch Catheterization

When indicated by radiography and/or endoscopy, the equine guttural pouches are easily catheterized for diagnostic sampling and flushing. The patient should be tranquilized so that the head drops, facilitating drainage of the secretions by gravity. A Chambers mare catheter can be passed through the ventral meatus into the pharynx. The curved end is directed beneath the flap of the medial lamina of the pouch ipsilateral to the nostril used for passage. Successful passage is indicated by lack of resistance while the catheter is inserted deeper than if it were in the pharynx. The position of the catheter tip in the pharynx can be observed through the endoscope placed up the opposite nasal passage. Once the catheter is within the pouch, it can be used to obtain a sample, to drain excessive secretions, or to act as a conduit for flushing. A self-retaining uterine catheter can be left in place for repeated flushing, but the Chambers catheter can be passed repeatedly with no complications.

Lung Biopsy

Lung biopsies are indicated to obtain a histologic diagnosis or prognostic information primarily in cases of diffuse lung disease, because the sample obtained is very small. A more useful parenchymal sample is obtained by means of percutaneous rather than endobronchial biopsy; complications of percutaneous biopsy are uncommon. Lung biopsy is most often done in the horse and should be used in conjunction with other, less invasive diagnostic techniques such as ultrasonography, radiography, and transtracheal aspiration. A 14-gauge, 15-cm TruCut biopsy needle* provides an excellent sample. Discomfort is minimal, and sedation may or

may not be needed. The preferred site is on the right side, in the seventh or eighth intercostal space, approximately 8 cm above a horizontal line through the olecranon. The specimen is obtained from the right middle lung lobe. The site should be widely clipped, surgically prepared, and infiltrated with local anesthetic down to the pleura. The biopsy needle is inserted through a stab incision just cranial to the rib and directed medially and cranially through the intercostal muscles and parietal pleura. The needle should be advanced 2 cm into the lung parenchyma, and the biopsy taken. If no specimen is obtained, the procedure can be repeated. After the needle is withdrawn, a single skin suture can be placed at the incision site, but no additional aftercare is needed. The specimen should be placed directly in 10% formalin or glutaraldehyde for fixation. Complications of lung biopsy have been restricted to transient hemoptysis, and no long-term complications have been reported.[21]

Pulmonary Function Testing

The techniques described thus far provide cytologic or histopathologic information, but they provide no information as to the degree of impairment in pulmonary function caused by the disease process. The major functions of the lungs are to transport gas from the periphery to the site of gas exchange (i.e., the "bellows" function) and to provide gas exchange with the blood, facilitating gas transport to the tissues. The first of these is assessed by means of pulmonary function tests, and the second by arterial blood gas evaluation.

Pulmonary function tests have thus far mainly been used in horses and in most cases as a research tool in veterinary teaching hospitals. They involve measurement of pressure, flow, and volume during breathing to allow computation of ventilatory functional values. These techniques have become increasingly automated and available to equine practitioners. They are valuable in assessment of equine athletes, especially those suspected of inflammatory obstructive airway disease. Baseline measurements can be compared, and airway hyperreactivity can be evaluated using histamine or methacholine bronchoprovocation protocols.[22] Responses to environmental changes[23] or therapy[24,25] can be noninvasively evaluated.

To perform pulmonary function tests, flow is measured using a tight-fitting face mask sealed above the nostrils and attached to a pneumotachograph. Transpulmonary pressure is measured using an esophageal balloon attached to a catheter and pressure transducer. Flow and pressure are measured directly and used to calculate tidal volume (V_T) and maximal pleural pressure change (ΔPPL_{max}). Pulmonary resistance (R_L) and dynamic compliance (C_{dyn}) are computed, the latter by $V_T/\Delta PPL$. Flow-volume loops can also be generated and used to evaluate obstructive disease. The most valuable measurements for comparison among horses or assessment of responses have been ΔPPL_{max}, R_L (both increased in cases of obstructive airway disease), and C_{dyn} (decreased in cases of obstructive airway disease).

Arterial Blood Gas Evaluation

Unlike pulmonary function tests, arterial blood gas determination is a routine procedure in most veterinary hospitals. The procedure is simple and provides valuable information concerning pulmonary gas exchange and ventilation. In horses the carotid in the lower third of the neck is the preferred site for arterial puncture, although peripheral limb arteries or the femoral artery may be used in foals or neonatal ruminants. Pulsations should be palpated with two fingers

---

*Travenol Laboratories, Inc, Deerfield, IL 60015.

on one hand; puncture using an 18- or 20-gauge needle (25-gauge in neonates) is performed with the other. Pulsation of blood from the needle, spontaneous filling of the syringe, and bright color of the blood all confirm a successful arterial puncture. If the practitioner is uncertain whether the sample is arterial, a jugular vein sample can be compared. Once the sample has been drawn, the vessel should be manually compressed for 2 to 5 minutes to prevent hematoma formation. If the carotid attempt is unsuccessful, the facial, submandibular, radial, or great metatarsal may be used, especially in the anesthetized horse. In cattle the coccygeal artery on the ventral aspect of the tail head is easily accessible. If an arterial sample cannot be obtained, venous blood from a well-perfused area may be used to give a reasonable estimate of acid-base status and P_{CO_2}, but not of oxygen available to the tissues.

The sample may be obtained in a glass or plastic syringe; the latter is safer to use around large animals. Heparin is the only acceptable anticoagulant for blood gas samples, and all gas bubbles must be removed and the syringe capped to prevent equilibration of the sample with room air. If the sample will not be analyzed within 10 minutes, it should be placed on ice to slow metabolism of blood cells. The iced sample will be valid if analyzed within $1^{1}/_{2}$ hours. Arterial blood gases can now be analyzed using a handheld device, eliminating any delay necessitated by transport to a specialized laboratory.[26] The patient's body temperature at the time of sampling should also be recorded because the results of the analysis will be corrected for temperature.

Pa_{O_2} reflects pulmonary gas exchange and oxygen available to the tissues. Hypoxia is defined as Pa_{O_2} less than 85 mm Hg with the patient inspiring room air. Causes of hypoxia include decreased inspired P_{O_2}, hypoventilation, right-to-left shunting of blood, diffusion impairment, and ventilation/perfusion mismatching, with the last the most common cause. Alveolar gas exchange is most effectively evaluated by using the alveolar-arterial (A-a) gradient for oxygen, computed by subtracting the Pa_{O_2} measured by the arterial blood gas from the calculated alveolar oxygen partial pressure (PA_{O_2}). The PA_{O_2} is effectively estimated using the partial pressure of inspired oxygen (PI_{O_2}) as follows[27]:

$$PA_{O_2} = \frac{PI_{O_2} - Pa_{CO_2}}{0.8}$$

The PI_{O_2} equals the total barometric pressure (760 mm Hg) minus the partial pressure of water vapor (42 mm Hg) multiplied by the fraction of room air that is oxygen (0.21), and thus equals 150 mm Hg for room air. For patients on supplemental inspired oxygen, the practitioner must remember to recalculate the PI_{O_2} with the new oxygen fraction in the inspired gas. The Pa_{CO_2} is obtained from the arterial blood gas measurement. The A-a gradient is normally only 4 to 10 mm Hg; an increase beyond this indicates impaired gas exchange within the lungs, most often the result of ventilation/perfusion mismatching.

Pa_{CO_2} is the most accurate measure of pulmonary ventilation, because increased Pa_{CO_2} is the major stimulus for increasing ventilation. An elevated Pa_{CO_2} indicates the patient cannot increase ventilation in response to this stimulus. Thus in many cases hypoxemia alone suggests ventilation/perfusion mismatch, but hypercapnia suggests impaired ventilation. *Hypoxia with a markedly elevated Pa_{CO_2} defines respiratory failure and indicates the need for ventilatory support in addition to supplemental oxygen.*

Increased or decreased ventilation also changes the acid-base status of the patient. Primary respiratory acidosis is characterized by decreased pH and an elevated Pa_{CO_2}, in-

dicating inadequate CO_2 elimination. Causes include pulmonary disease, impaired chest wall function, pneumothorax, central nervous system depression, and inadequate assisted ventilation. Primary respiratory alkalosis is characterized by increased pH and depressed Pa_{CO_2}, indicating hyperventilation. Causes include hypoxia, fear, pain, strenuous exercise, hyperthermia, gram-negative sepsis, and overzealous assisted ventilation. Metabolic compensation for primary respiratory acid-base disorders acts to maintain the pH within the physiologic range but requires 1 to 2 days for maximum effect. Acute, severe respiratory disorders can result in marked pH abnormalities. The ranges of normal values for various species are listed in Table 29-2.[28]

Nuclear Imaging

Gamma-emitting radioisotopes can be used with an external detector in the assessment of regional pulmonary ventilation and perfusion, thus giving functional and topographic information that augments structural information obtained by radiographs and ultrasound. Lung scans have been an important diagnostic tool in human medicine for a number of years and now are available for large domestic species at a few veterinary teaching hospitals. The procedure is safe and painless. Anesthesia is not needed, and the only requirement for sedation is that the patient stand quietly in front of the gamma camera. After the study the patient must be kept in an isolated area to allow decay and excretion of the radiopharmaceutical (normally no more than 48 hr).

The principle behind perfusion scanning is use of a radioisotope, usually technetium-99m (^{99m}Tc), bound to albumin aggregates of 10 to 15 micrometer diameter. When injected into a peripheral vein, these aggregates become physically trapped in the pulmonary vasculature. Provided the radioisotope is evenly mixed in the right ventricle, the resulting gamma camera image demonstrates the perfusion distribution of the pulmonary arterial system. The technique is valuable in diagnosis of pulmonary emboli (more common in humans than veterinary patients) and areas of poor pulmonary arterial perfusion or hemorrhage.

Ventilation scans are made by allowing the patient to inspire either a radioactive gas such as krypton-81m or an aerosol containing a short-lived radioisotope (^{99m}Tc).[29] Again, the gamma camera image demonstrates the regional ventilation pattern (of both lungs superimposed in lateral view). Valuable information can be obtained, especially in equine obstructive airway disease (Fig. 29-9, *A* and *B*) and response to therapy can be assessed. [30] Advanced computer technology now allows superimposition of ventilation and perfusion images from the same patient to obtain objective regional ventilation/perfusion ($\dot{V}/\dot{Q}$) ratio data and highlight areas of poor $\dot{V}/\dot{Q}$ matching. This technology is specialized and expensive. It has greatest application in the equine athlete or the valuable equine patient.

TABLE 29-2

Normal Respiratory Values for Various Species

Species	Blood pH	P_{CO_2} (mm Hg)	HCO_3^- (mEq/L)
Bovine	7.32-7.45	35-53	21-27
Ovine	7.32-7.54	37-46	20-25
Equine	7.32-7.44	38-46	24-34
Caprine	7.42-7.46	33-38	24-27

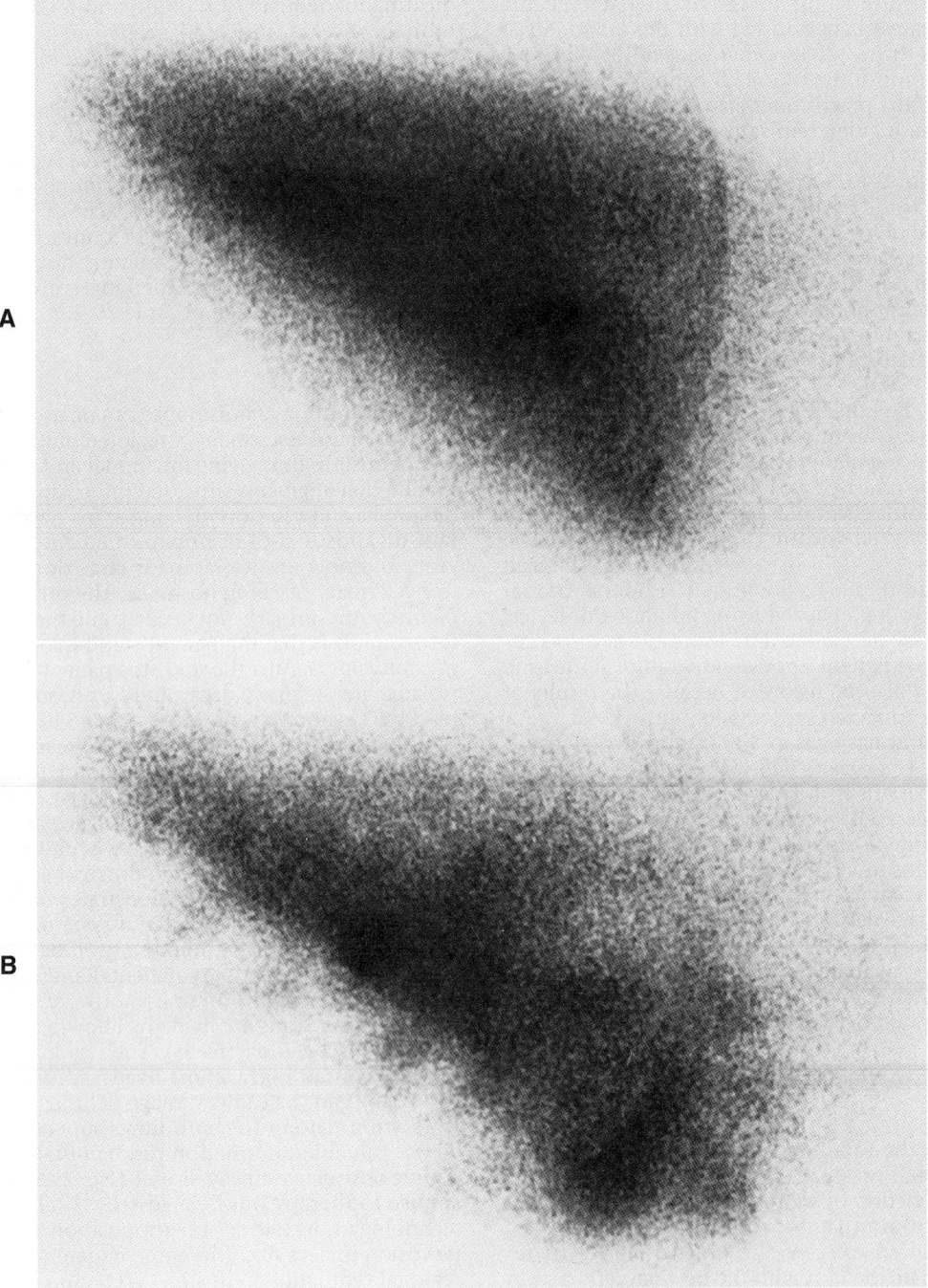

FIG. 29-9 ▌ Composite scintigraphic images of ventilatory distribution of ^{99m}Tc-DTPA aerosol in the right lungs of a normal horse **(A)** and a horse with moderate chronic obstructive pulmonary disease (COPD) **(B)**. Note the even distribution of radioaerosol in the normal horse compared with the patchy, irregular distribution in the affected animal. The small zone of intense activity in the center of the lungs fields is a radioactive marker placed on the skin to allow accurate computerized merging of the composite images. (Courtesy Dr. M. O'Callaghan, Tufts University School of Veterinary Medicine.)

REFERENCES

1. Roudebush P, Ryan J: Breath sound terminology in the veterinary literature, *J Am Vet Med Assoc* 194:1415-1417, 1989.
2. Murphy RL: Discontinuous adventitious lung sounds, *Semin Respir Med* 6:210-219, 1985.
3. Waring WW, Beckerman RC, Hopkins RL: Continuous adventitious lung sounds: site and method of production and significance, *Semin Respir Med* 6:201-209, 1985.
4. Tyler JW et al: Something old, something new: thoracic acoustic percussion in cattle, *J Am Vet Med Assoc* 197:52-57, 1990.
5. Lamb CR, O'Callaghan MW: Diagnostic imaging of equine pulmonary disease, *Compend Cont Educ Vet Pract* 11:1110-1118, 1989.
6. Reef VB et al: Comparison between diagnostic ultrasonography and radiography in the evaluation of horses and cattle with thoracic disease: 56 cases (1984-1985), *J Am Vet Med Assoc* 198:2112-2118, 1991.
7. Reimer JM, Reef VB, Spencer PA: Ultrasonography as a diagnostic aid in horses with anaerobic bacterial pleuropneumonia and/or pulmonary abscessation: 27 cases (1984-1986), *J Am Vet Med Assoc* 194:278-282, 1989.
8. Hammer EJ et al: Videoendoscopic assessment of dynamic laryngeal function during exercise in horses with grade-III left laryngeal hemiparesis at rest: 26 cases (1992-1995), *J Am Vet Med Assoc* 212:399-403, 1998.
9. Sweeney CR et al: Bronchoscopy of the horse, *Am J Vet Res* 10:1953-1956, 1992.

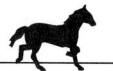

10. Darien BJ et al: A tracheoscopic technique for obtaining uncontaminated lower airway secretions for bacterial culture in the horse, *Equine Vet J* 22:170-173, 1990.

11. Hoffman AM et al: Sensitivity and specificity of bronchoalveolar lavage and protected catheter brush methods for isolating bacteria from foals with experimentally induced pneumonia caused by *Klebsiella pneumoniae*, *Am J Vet Res* 54:1803-1807, 1993.

12. Sweeney CR, Humber KA, Roby KAW: Cytologic findings of tracheobronchial aspirates from 66 thoroughbred racehorses, *Am J Vet Res* 53:1172-1175, 1992.

13. Martin BB, Beech J, Parente EJ: Cytologic examination of specimens obtained by means of tracheal washes performed before and after high-speed treadmill exercise in horses with a history of poor performance, *J Am Vet Med Assoc* 214:673-677, 1999.

14. Derksen FJ et al: Comparison of transtracheal aspirate and bronchoalveolar lavage cytology in 50 horses with chronic lung disease, *Equine Vet J* 21:23-26, 1989.

15. Rossier Y, Sweeney CR, Ziemer EL: Bronchoalveolar lavage fluid cytologic findings in horses with pneumonia or pleuropneumonia, *J Am Vet Met Assoc* 198:1001-1004, 1991.

16. Moore BR et al: Cytologic evaluation of bronchoalveolar lavage fluid obtained from Standardbred racehorses with inflammatory airway disease, *Am J Vet Res* 56:562-567, 1995.

17. Rush BR et al: Cytologic evaluation of bronchoalveolar lavage fluid from horses with recurrent airway obstruction after aerosol and parenteral administration of beclomethasone dipropionate and dexamethasone, respectively, *Am J Vet Res* 59:1033-1038, 1998.

18. Halliwell RE et al: The role of allergy in chronic pulmonary disease of horses, *J Am Vet Med Assoc* 174:277-281, 1979.

19. Brumbaugh GW, Benson PA: Partial pressures of oxygen and carbon dioxide, pH, and concentrations of bicarbonate, lactate, and glucose in pleural fluid from horses, *Am J Vet Res* 51:1032-1037, 1990.

20. Schott HC, Mansmann RA: Thoracic drainage in horses, *Compend Cont Educ Pract Vet* 12:251-261, 1990.

21. Raphel CF, Gunson DE: Percutaneous lung biopsy in the horse, *Cornell Vet* 71:439-448, 1981.

22. Hoffman AM, Couetil LL, Miller CJ: Airway responses to histamine aerosol in clinically normal foals, *Am J Vet Res*, 60:965-968, 1999.

23. Jean DJ, Vrins A, Lavoie J: Monthly, daily, and circadian variations of measurements of pulmonary mechanics in horses with chronic obstructive pulmonary disease, *Am J Vet Res* 60:1341-1346, 1999.

24. Rush BR et al: Pulmonary function in horses with recurrent airway obstruction after aerosol and parenteral administration of beclomethasone dipropionate and dexamethasone, respectively, *Am J Vet Res* 59:1039-1043, 1998.

25. Derksen FJ et al: Aerosolized albuterol sulfate used as a bronchodilator in horses with recurrent airway obstruction, *Am J Vet Res* 60:689-693, 1999.

26. Looney AL et al: Use of a handheld device for analysis of blood electrolyte concentrations and blood gas partial pressures in dogs and horses, *J Am Vet Med Assoc* 213:526-530, 1998.

27. West JB: *Pulmonary pathophysiology: the essentials*, ed 2, Baltimore, 1982, Williams & Wilkins, p 22.

28. Coles EH: *Veterinary clinical pathology*, ed 4, Philadelphia, 1986, WB Saunders, p 210.

29. O'Callaghan MW et al: Ventilation imaging in the horse with ^{99m}technetium-DTPA radioaerosol, *Equine Vet J* 19:19-24, 1987.

30. Rush BR et al: Pulmonary distribution of aerosolized technetium Tc99m pentetate after administration of a single dose of aerosolized albuterol sulfate in horses with recurrent airway obstruction, *Am J Vet Res* 60:764-769, 1999.

EQUINE RESPIRATORY SYSTEM

PAMELA A. WILKINS, Consulting Editor

DISEASES OF THE LUNGS

BACTERIAL PNEUMONIA IN ADULT HORSES

ANGELINE E. WARNER

ETIOLOGY AND PATHOGENESIS. Bacterial pneumonia is colonization of the pulmonary parenchyma by pathogenic microorganisms. It is characterized by influx of inflammatory cells, especially neutrophils; tissue destruction; and loss of normal function. The lower airways and alveolar spaces are normally sterile and are protected by defense mechanisms that effectively remove or destroy bacterial contaminants under normal circumstances. Infection of lung tissue occurs when these defense mechanisms are overwhelmed.

Bacterial pneumonia in adult horses is most often caused by *Streptococcus zooepidemicus*, a β-hemolytic Streptococcus sp. that is found in mucous membranes, skin, and tonsillary tissue of normal horses. It rapidly invades mucous membranes damaged by viral infection and can be responsible for abscess formation.[31] *Streptococcus equi*, the organism responsible for "strangles," is far less often a cause of pneumonia than of lymph node abscessation. *Streptococcus pneumoniae* (an important pathogen that causes lobar pneumonia in humans) has been isolated from horses with clinical signs of respiratory disease and from asymptomatic carriers.[32] Gram-negative organisms can complicate streptococcal pneumonia, with *Pasteurella* spp. the most common offender, followed by *Escherichia coli*, *Enterobacter* spp., *Klebsiella* spp., and *Pseudomonas* spp.[33] Over half the pneumonia cases at a referral hospital had more than one species of microorganism isolated from the tracheobronchial aspirate.[33] Table 29-3 shows the prevalence of tracheobronchial aspirate isolates in that study.

More and more commonly, anaerobes, especially *Bacteroides* spp. and *Clostridium* spp., are being recognized as complicating organisms in equine pleuropneumonia.[33] These organisms gain access to the respiratory tract most often by aspiration of oropharyngeal bacteria. They are not isolated from tracheobronchial aspirates of normal horses and should be considered significant when cultured.[34] Anaerobic bacteria are not usually primary isolates in pneumonia; rather, they often complicate aerobic infection, especially with *E. coli*, enhancing aerobic bacterial growth and often causing a necrotizing process.[35]

CLINICAL SIGNS AND DIFFERENTIAL DIAGNOSIS. Horses with bacterial pneumonia most often clinically manifest fever, increased respiratory rate, nasal discharge, coughing, and exercise intolerance. Fever may be intermittent, necessitating several daily determinations to demonstrate a fever spike. Cough may or may not be spontaneous but generally can be easily induced on tracheal palpation and may be productive. The respiratory rate is usually elevated, and the resting rate is a very sensitive indicator. In chronic cases, weight loss usually occurs with or without a decreased appetite. Physical examination may reveal enlarged submandibular lymph nodes.

When physical signs indicate pulmonary dysfunction in horses, the major clinical task is differentiating infectious from noninfectious causes. Among infectious causes, bacterial pneumonia is most common. Viral infections are usually confined to the upper respiratory tract. Pulmonary aspergillosis most often follows gastrointestinal (GI) disease that results in mucosal compromise, and respiratory disease unresponsive to antimicrobial therapy should arouse suspicion of fungal pneumonia.[36] Parasitic pneumonitis in horses involves larval migration and is not common, but may pre-

TABLE 29-3

Organisms Isolated From Cultures of Equine Tracheobronchial Aspirates (TBAs) and Pleural Fluid (PF) in Horses With Pneumonia or Pleuropneumonia[33]

Organisms	No. of Horses With Organism Isolated From TBA Only (%)	No. of Horses With Organism Isolated From TBA and PF (%)	Total
AEROBES			
β-Hemolytic *Streptococcus* spp.	28 (35)	48 (60)	80
Pasteurella spp.	21 (57)	15 (40)	37
Escherichia coli	12 (48)	9 (36)	25
Enterobacter spp.	13 (69)	5 (26)	19
Pseudomonas spp.	5 (72)	1 (14)	7
Klebsiella pneumoniae	8 (73)	2 (18)	11
ANAEROBES			
Bacteroides spp.	9 (35)	11 (42)	26
Clostridium spp.	8 (44)	5 (28)	18
Eubacterium spp.	4 (45)	1 (10)	9
Fusobacterium spp.	4 (80)	1 (20)	5
Peptostreptococcus spp.	5 (42)	6 (50)	12

dispose to secondary bacterial pneumonia. The list of noninfectious causes of respiratory embarrassment in the horse is headed by allergic obstructive bronchiolitis (chronic obstructive pulmonary disease). In severe cases, obstructive disease can cause profound dyspnea and, over time, be responsible for weight loss. Primary neoplastic lung disease is rare in the horse, but thoracic lymphosarcoma and metastatic lesions (from renal or gastric carcinoma or melanoma) can occur.

DIAGNOSTIC APPROACH. Diagnosis of equine pneumonia should begin with a thorough physical examination, auscultation of the lungs, and percussion of the thorax. The earliest auscultatory changes heard include increased harshness and intensity of expiratory sounds. When expiratory sounds are as loud as inspiratory sounds, significant airway disease is present. In cases of more advanced pneumonia, auscultation usually demonstrates end-inspiratory crackles, signifying transient atelectasis or increased secretions. Expiratory wheezes may be present if airways are inflamed or narrowed by thick secretions. In these cases, elevated resting respiratory rate and presence of fever are very useful indicators. Extension of inflammation to the pleura causes audible rubbing sounds on auscultation. The ventral thorax may be quiet, suggesting subpleural abscessation or pleural effusion. If a pleural effusion has developed, a horizontal line can be demonstrated on percussion.

The clinical pathology database for infectious respiratory disease should begin with a complete blood count, including fibrinogen. In cases of pneumonia, an elevated peripheral WBC count with an absolute neutrophilia is often found. Band forms may or may not be present. Bacterial pneumonia is an inflammatory process that stimulates hepatocytes to synthesize fibrinogen, and elevations in the range of 500 to 1000 mg/dl are often seen. Especially high levels are characteristic of chronic pneumonia or pulmonary abscessation. Total plasma protein, specifically the immunoglobulin fraction, is usually elevated in pneumonia that lasts for weeks or months as a result of chronic antigenic stimulation.

Thoracic radiographs are extremely valuable for the diagnosis, prognosis, and progressive evaluation of equine pneumonia. The most common finding is opacity in the anteroventral thorax consistent with loss of normal aeration in the cranial lung lobes (Fig. 29-10). Often the entire radiolucent space ventral to the caudal vena cava and caudal to the heart is lost because of increased tissue density. Multiple opacities suggesting abscesses (see Fig. 29-10, dorsal) may be

seen in some cases. Large cavitary lesions with a horizontal line suggest involvement of gas-forming organisms in abscesses (Fig. 29-11).

A horizontal line across the ventral thorax suggests free fluid in the pleural space on one or both sides. However, the pleural space is most sensitively evaluated by ultrasonography. Each side can be separately examined for presence of abnormal fluid accumulation. The presence of fibrin within pleural fluid or of consolidated ventral lung can be detected.

When bacterial pneumonia is suspected, a tracheobronchial aspirate should be performed to obtain a sample for culture, Gram stain, and cytologic examination. Techniques are described in the diagnostic procedures section. Once fluid is obtained, an aliquot should be placed in an ethylenediamine tetraacetic acid (EDTA) anticoagulant tube for cytologic examination, and a sample submitted in a closed syringe for aerobic and anaerobic culture. In cases unresponsive to prior therapy, antimicrobial agents should be withheld for at least 24 hours before a sample is taken for culture and sensitivity.

Degenerated neutrophils, often containing engulfed bacteria, are found in aspirates from horses with pneumonia. Precipitated protein and necrotic material may be present, along with damaged epithelial cells. These findings differentiate a bacterial infection from (1) allergic bronchiolitis, which is characterized by nondegenerated neutrophils, possibly eosinophils, and absence of bacteria, or (2) neoplasia, which often yields neoplastic cells on aspiration. Gram stain results from the cytologic sample can be very helpful in guiding therapy until culture results are final. At that time, antibiotic therapy should be reevaluated in light of culture and sensitivity results.

If a pleural effusion is detected by percussion, thoracic radiography, or ultrasonography, the pleural space should be aspirated and therapeutically drained. Drainage can be of great value when effusion volume is large enough to restrict ventilation. Thoracocentesis technique is described in the diagnostic procedures section. Cytologic examination, culture, and sensitivity determination should be performed on the sample. As with the tracheobronchial aspirate, anaerobic culture is warranted. When a septic pleural effusion is found, a transtracheal aspirate often yields pathogenic organisms, whereas the pleural aspirate may not.

Clinical suspicion of anaerobic infection should be aroused whenever a foul odor, necrotic tissue, or gas forma-

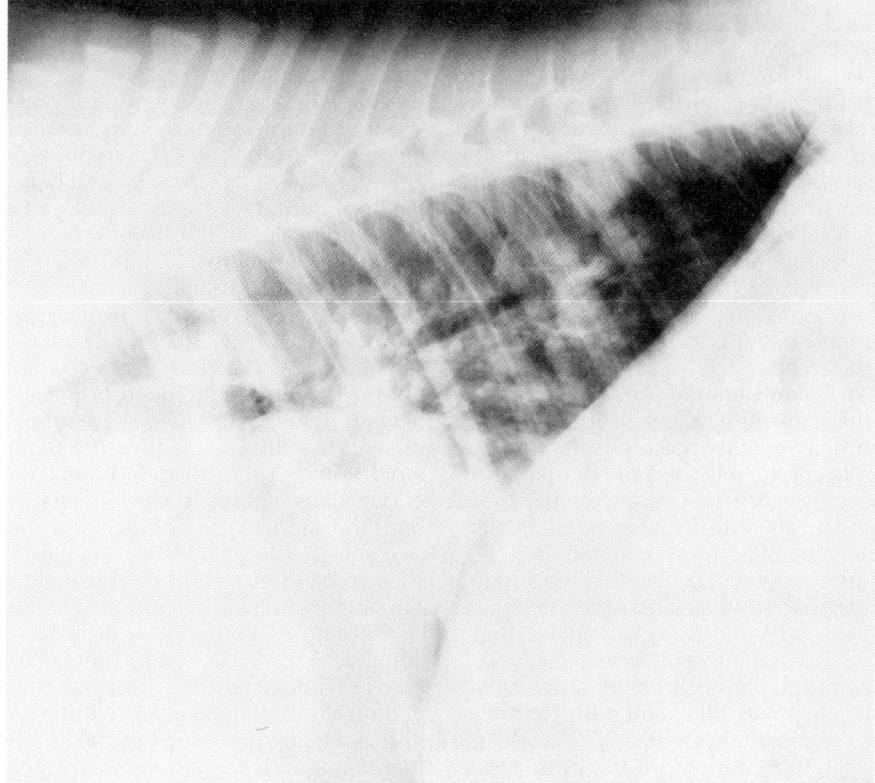

FIG. 29-10 ▋▋ Lateral standing thoracic radiograph in a young foal. A diffuse interstitial and air-space pattern obscures most of the cardiac silhouette, giving way to a predominant bronchointerstitial pattern in the caudodorsal lung field. Dorsally numerous large nodular opacities, some of which contain gas/fluid interfaces, are evident. These represent multiple lung abscesses accompanying ventral bronchopneumonia. The latter changes are often associated with *Rhodococcus* lung infections. (Courtesy Dr. M. O'Callaghan, Tufts University School of Veterinary Medicine.)

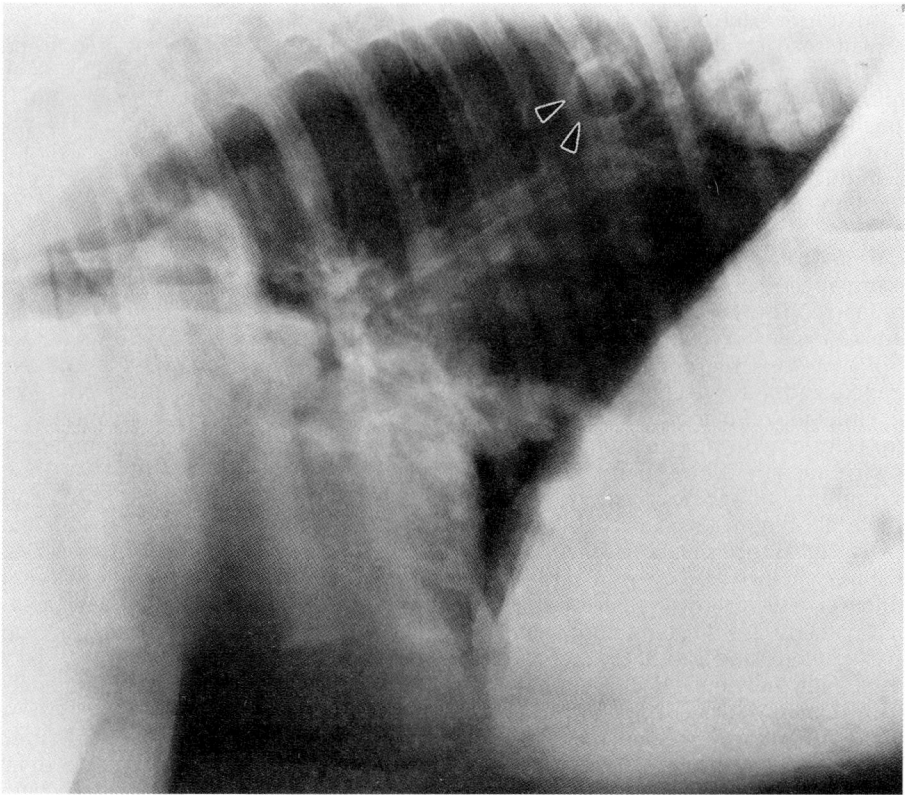

FIG. 29-11 ▋▋ Lateral standing radiograph of a foal's thorax demonstrates multiple abscesses containing gas/fluid interfaces *(arrowheads).* In the area caudal and ventral to the hilus there is patchy bronchointerstitial opacity that partially obscures the cardiac silhouette and is indicative of bronchopneumonia. A broad zone of lung in the middorsal lung field is normally aerated and free of obvious nodular opacities. (Courtesy Dr. M. O'Callaghan, Tufts University School of Veterinary Medicine.)

tion develops and in cases of foreign body penetration. Purulent exudate that fails to yield aerobic bacteria on culture and organisms seen on Gram stain that subsequently fail to grow point to the presence of anaerobes.[37] The foul odor is caused by volatile fatty acids produced during anaerobic metabolism. Foul odor is not uniformly found in cases of anaerobic infection, but it is a sensitive indicator when present. Anaerobic culture requires appropriate medium to minimize exposure to atmospheric oxygen. Aspirated fluid can be transported in a syringe from which air has been expressed. Isolation of obligate anaerobes is less affected by prior antibiotic treatment than is that of aerobes.[37]

PATHOPHYSIOLOGY. Colonization of lung tissue occurs when normal defense mechanisms have been compromised or overwhelmed. Pulmonary defense mechanisms include mucociliary clearance, phagocytic cells, and the cellular and humoral immune systems. Mucociliary clearance consists of waves of beating cilia on tracheobronchial epithelial cells that move a blanket of mucus and trapped material progressively away from the pulmonary parenchyma. The primary line of phagocyte cell defense is the alveolar macrophage, which engulfs foreign material and microorganisms that reach the alveolar spaces. Bacterial infection results in an outpouring of neutrophils into the alveolar space. These cells then play an important role in engulfing and killing pathogenic bacteria. Immune defense of the respiratory tract is centered in the major hilar lymph nodes and the bronchus-associated lymphoid tissue (BALT), where antigens processed by airway and alveolar macrophages induce proliferation of lymphocytes and immunoglobulin synthesis. The upper airways are protected predominantly by secretory IgA, and the lower respiratory tract by IgG.[38] Cellular immune defense, provided by T lymphocytes, affords protection, especially against intracellular organisms.

Infectious organisms reach the lower respiratory tract by means of inhalation, aspiration, or hematogenous spread. Infection occurs when the normal defense mechanisms are compromised or overwhelmed by sheer numbers of the inoculum. Mucociliary clearance is most often impaired by viral infection with epitheliotropic strains. Temporary structural damage to the tracheobronchial mucosa retards transport of bacteria out of the respiratory tract. Equine herpesvirus 1 and equine influenza virus A1 have been shown to cause loss of cilia or entire epithelial cells.[39] Ciliary function is also inhibited by toxic gases. In a poorly ventilated barn, ammonia from urine-soaked bedding can reach noxious levels. Causes of impaired phagocytic cell function include viral infection of macrophages, which reduces their capacity to kill ingested bacteria; endotoxemia, which reduces alveolar macrophage phagocytosis and microbicidal capacity[40]; and severe neutropenia. Immune defenses can be compromised by defects in either the cellular or humoral system; causes include protein-calorie malnutrition, hypoproteinemia, immunosuppressive therapy, and primary immunologic disease (such as combined immunodeficiency).

Stress plays a major role in pathogenesis of infectious equine respiratory disease. Stress includes such situations as cold temperature (stimulating shivering, increased oxygen consumption, and deeper ventilation, which carries inhaled bacteria deeper into the respiratory tract), crowding and poor ventilation (allowing buildup of ammonia and aerosolized pathogens and rapid transmission among individuals), and transportation (often involving dehydration, which changes the properties of mucus and mucociliary transport). There is an anecdotal association between long-distance transport of horses and development of pneumonia or pleuropneumonia. Experimental studies have suggested transportation stress adversely affects the number and function of alveolar macrophages and inflammatory cells.[41,42] Increased endogenous corticosteroid levels that occur as a physiologic response to stress are known to impair function of phagocytic and immune cells.

Stress, endotoxemia, or strenuous exercise with pulmonary hypertension can result in pulmonary endothelial damage that triggers vascular thrombosis and hemorrhagic infarction. Pulmonary infarcts and tissue necrosis can lead to sanguinous pleural effusion. A recent study of such cases of pulmonary infarction demonstrated that most involve bacterial infection and septic pleuropneumonia.[43]

Once pulmonary colonization has occurred, bacterial growth is greatly facilitated in a mixed infection. Microbial synergy occurs between *Bacteroides* spp. and facultative aerobes, with enhanced growth of the aerobic species. Synergy may result in the protection of aerobes from engulfment and phagocyte killing in the presence of anaerobic capsular material.[35] Encapsulated strains of anaerobes develop from unencapsulated strains in chronic mixed infection, enhancing both the pathogenicity of the anaerobes and the growth rate of associated aerobes.[44] The synergistic response means that early recognition of and specific therapy for anaerobic infection are essential.

Once normal pulmonary defense mechanisms have been compromised, bacteria can colonize the parenchyma. In the case of pathogenic strains such as *Streptococcus* spp. and the gram-negative organisms listed previously, bacterial growth is associated with tissue destruction and recruitment of inflammatory cells, especially neutrophils. The influx of neutrophils, accumulation of cellular debris, exudation of serum from capillaries, and deposition of fibrin in the alveolar space locally impair gas exchange. As the inflammatory process spreads by means of the airways, ventilation to the region decreases, and mismatching of ventilation and perfusion develops. Such ventilation/perfusion mismatching is a major cause of hypoxemia but results in hypercapnia only in extreme cases. Thus arterial blood gases taken from horses with severe pneumonia most often show an oxygen deficit without carbon dioxide retention.

EPIDEMIOLOGY. Bacterial pneumonia in adult horses is associated most often with antecedent viral infection, stress, general anesthesia, endotoxemia, immunosuppression, or aspiration. Both viral infection and stress serve to compromise normal lung defense mechanisms.[38,45] Because *S. zooepidemicus* is part of normal equine pharyngeal flora, potential for aspiration into the lungs is frequent, and colonization vs. clearance of infection depends on degree of function of the pulmonary defense mechanisms. Stress factors are associated with competitive athletic performance, especially racing, and with long-distance transportation. Because of competitive pressure, horses recovering from viral respiratory infections may not be adequately rested before returning to strenuous athletic activity. Thus the racing population is often at greatest risk for development of pneumonia. Management factors and vaccination status of the population are very important in reducing individual risk.

NECROPSY FINDINGS. Necropsy in cases of bacterial pneumonia shows extensive consolidation of affected areas, especially the anterior and ventral regions. In early stages the lungs may be merely edematous, reflecting inflammation and early exudation; in chronic, severe cases the airways may be filled with purulent material and necrotic debris. If inflammation has extended to the pleural space, adhesions can be found between the visceral and parietal pleura, and a fibrinous exudate may be present. Extension into the mediastinal space also occasionally occurs. Histologic samples should be taken from areas in various stages of involvement, because chronically infected tissue is often characterized mainly by necrotic debris. Multiple cultures, including cultures for anaerobes, should be taken, especially in cases of necrotizing pneumonias that have been resistant to therapy.

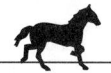

THERAPY AND PROGNOSIS. Therapy for equine bacterial pneumonia should be based on culture and sensitivity results from a tracheobronchial aspirate. These determinations are crucial in cases that have proved resistant to initial treatment. In early cases of pneumonia, the practitioner is justified in suspecting *S. zooepidemicus* as the causative organism and treating accordingly. The possibility of a mixed infection, especially involving gram-negative organisms, must be kept in mind when such empiric therapy is unsuccessful. *S. zooepidemicus* is generally sensitive to potassium or sodium penicillin at a dose of 22,000 U/kg IV four times daily or procaine penicillin at 22,000 U/kg IM twice daily. Therapy should be continued at least 7 days or until clinical signs resolve; the duration needed may preclude continuous intramuscular therapy because of muscle soreness. In mixed infections, ampicillin (11 mg/kg IM or IV four times daily) can be used to broaden the spectrum of sensitive organisms. Trimethoprim-sulfadiazine (30 mg/kg twice daily) offers a broad-spectrum alternative that can be administered orally or intravenously. The oral form is convenient for owners to administer.

Complicated infections with multiple or resistant organisms necessitate choice of antimicrobial agents specifically directed against the pathogens isolated. Aminoglycosides, including kanamycin, gentamicin, and amikacin, are effective alternatives for gram-negative pathogens; the second- and third-generation cephalosporins are effective for gram-positive and selected gram-negative pathogens. The antimicrobial sensitivity of aerobic tracheobronchial isolates listed in Tables 29-4 and 29-5 can be used to guide therapy.

Early and vigorous antimicrobial therapy directed at both the aerobic and anaerobic components of a mixed infection is essential for resolution. Aminoglycosides are uniformly ineffective against anaerobes because these bacteria lack the oxidative transport system for intracellular drug accumulation. Penicillin has been a mainstay of anaerobe therapy, but some isolates (especially *Bacteroides* spp.) produce β-lactamase that renders penicillin and some cephalosporins inactive.[46] Widespread resistance to tetracycline among anaerobes has also developed. Chloramphenicol (20 to 50 mg/kg PO) is effective, but concerns regarding human exposure during administration of the drug preclude its use in most cases. Metronidazole (15 to 25 mg/kg PO or IV four times daily) is effective against nearly all anaerobic species and has resulted in marked clinical improvement in many cases. It may, however, contribute to anorexia in patients already prone to loss of weight and body condition. Metronidazole should be used in conjunction with appropriate therapy against the aerobic isolates, however, because it has no activity against them. Rifampin is bactericidal and is effective against most species of *Bacteroides* and *Clostridium*. It penetrates well into abscesses and may be helpful in anaerobic infections with walled-off abscesses.[47] A relatively new class, the fluoroquinolones are bactericidal and broad spectrum with high potency against aerobic gram-negative organisms, but have poor activity against anaerobes. They penetrate tissues and abscesses well,

TABLE 29-4

Susceptibility of Bacteria of Equine Neonatal Origin to Selected Antibiotics

Bacterial Species	Antibiotic								
	CEF	CEPH	AK	GM	CHL	T/C	TMS	AMP	PEN
E. coli	100	81	95	94	90	89	70	8	0
A. suis	95	95	76	97	99	79	90	75	72
A. equuli	100	100	72	100	100	100	97	87	87
K. pneumoniae	100	81	100	73	65	50	63	0	0
P. aeruginosa	0	1	71	28	4	33	3	0	0
β-Hemolytic *Streptococcus*	100	100	16	26	100	96	96	98	99
Enterobacter spp.	91	10	100	82	65	30	48	9	0
Citrobacter spp.	100	56	100	85	53	50	67	6	5
Salmonella spp.	100	74	100	94	49	30	80	22	0

From Wilson WD, Spensley MS, Adamson PJW: Considerations for the selection of antibiotics in equine neonates, Proceedings of the sixth annual medical forum, ACVIM, Washington, DC, 1988, pp 628-634.
CEF, Ceftizoxime; *CEPH,* cephalothin; *AK,* amikacin; *GM,* gentamicin; *CHL,* chloramphenicol; *T/C,* ticarcillin/clavulanic acid; *TMS,* trimethoprim-sulfonamide; *AMP,* ampicillin; *PEN,* penicillin G.

TABLE 29-5

Probability of Susceptibility to Selected Antibiotics of Isolates From Neonatal Foals With Bacterial Infections

Probability of Susceptibility (%)	Septicemia	Pneumonia	Septic Arthritis
>90			CEF
85-90	CEF	CEF	
80-84	AK, GM, CHL	AMP, CHL	CHL, CEPH, T/C
75-79	T/C	T/C, CEPH, GM	TMS, GM
70-74			AK
60-69	TMS, KAN	TMS, KAN	KAN, TIC
<60	TIC, OTC, AMP, PEN	TIC, OTC, AMP, PEN	OTC, AMP, PEN

From Wilson WD, Spensley MS, Adamson PJW: Considerations for the selection of antibiotics in equine neonates, Proceedings of the sixth annual medical forum, ACVIM, Washington, DC, 1988, pp 628-634.
CEF, Ceftizoxime; *CEPH,* cephalothin; *AK,* amikacin; *GM,* gentamicin; *CHL,* chloramphenicol; *T/C,* ticarcillin/clavulanic acid; *TMS,* trimethoprim-sulfonamide; *AMP,* ampicillin; *PEN,* penicillin G; *TIC,* ticarcillin; *KAN,* kanamycin; *OTC,* oxytetracycline.

resulting in excellent activity within cells and in pus. They are well tolerated in adult animals, even when given for prolonged periods, and thus have potential for therapy in equine pneumonia.

In bacterial pneumonia of any cause, inadequate duration of therapy frequently results in relapse or treatment failure. The response should be monitored by using clinical signs, especially respiratory rate and temperature. The temperature should be monitored carefully at the cessation of antibiotic therapy, and use of nonsteroidal antiinflammatory agents that mask fever should be avoided at that time. Stall rest must be enforced during therapy of pneumonia, and return to exercise should be gradual and permitted only after the horse is clinically normal and antibiotic therapy has been completed. Progress should be monitored radiographically, especially in infections with nodular or cavitary lesions.

In uncomplicated pneumonia with adequate duration of antibiotic therapy and adequate rest, the prognosis is excellent. Many equine patients have returned to competitive athletic activity even after severe pulmonary infection. The most common intrathoracic complications are development of pulmonary abscesses and extension of inflammation and sepsis into the pleural space. If febrile episodes continue despite appropriate antibiotic therapy, clinical suspicion of either complication should be aroused, and further evaluation using thoracic radiography or ultrasonography is warranted. Pulmonary abscesses are amenable to prolonged antimicrobial therapy (i.e., several months), and progress should be evaluated radiographically. Pleural effusion should be drained, and samples cultured to reassess antimicrobial therapy. The prognosis depends on the organism responsible and response to initial therapy. Pleuropneumonia involving anaerobic organisms has a more guarded prognosis with expectation of prolonged therapy and expense.[33,41]

PREVENTION AND CONTROL. Prevention of equine bacterial pneumonia depends on management of factors that affect the normal defense mechanisms of the respiratory tract. Thus adequate ventilation to provide fresh air and prevent buildup of pathogenic aerosols is important, especially in winter months when horses are stabled. Damp, warm barns with moisture condensation on windows provide poor air quality and prolong the life of aerosolized pathogens. Such conditions also maximize the probability of exposure to potentially allergenic aerosols, contributing to symptoms of allergic bronchiolitis. Every effort should be made to use the least dusty bedding possible and to avoid moldy or dusty hay. Stress minimization, especially in competitive athletes, is important because pathogen exposure is impossible to control when horses are gathered for competitive events.

Because viral infections compromise the integrity of the respiratory epithelium, immunization programs may be helpful in reducing predisposition to bacterial pneumonia. Adults should be immunized against equine herpesvirus 1 (rhinopneumonitis) and equine influenza at 3- to 4-month intervals.

REFERENCES

31. Beech J: Diseases of the lung, *Vet Clin North Am (Large Anim Pract)* 1:149-169, 1979.
32. Burrell MH, Mackintosh ME, Taylor CED: Isolation of *Streptococcus pneumoniae* from the respiratory tract of horses, *Equine Vet J* 18:183-186, 1986.
33. Sweeney CR et al: Aerobic and anaerobic bacterial isolates from horses with pneumonia or pleuropneumonia and antimicrobial susceptibility patterns of the aerobes, *J Am Vet Med Assoc* 198:839-842, 1991.
34. Sweeney CR, Beach J, Roby KA: Bacterial isolates from tracheobronchial aspirates of healthy horses, *Am J Vet Res* 46:2562-2565, 1985.
35. Brook I: Enhancement of growth of aerobic and facultative bacteria in mixed infections with *Bacteroides* species, *Infect Immun* 50:929-931, 1985.
36. Sweeney CR, Habecker PL: Pulmonary aspergillosis in horses: 29 cases (1974-1997), *J Am Vet Med Assoc* 214:808-811, 1999.
37. Dow SW, Jones RL: Anaerobic infections. II, Diagnosis and treatment, *Compend Cont Educ Pract Vet* 9:827-839, 1987.
38. Mair RS, Stockes CR, Bourne FJ: Quantification of immunoglobulins in respiratory tract secretions of the horse, *Vet Immunol Immunopathol* 14:197-203, 1987.
39. O'Neill FD, Issel CJ, Henk WG: Electron microscopy of equine respiratory viruses in organ cultures of equine fetal respiratory tract epithelium, *Am J Vet Res* 45:1953-1960, 1984.
40. Jacobs RF, Kiel DP, Balk RA: Alveolar macrophage function in a canine model of endotoxin-induced lung injury, *Am Rev Respir Dis* 134:745-751, 1986.
41. Chaffin MK, Carter GK: Equine bacterial pleuropneumonia. I, Epidemiology, pathophysiology, and bacterial isolates, *Compend Cont Educ Pract Vet* 15:1642-1650, 1993.
42. Traub-Dargatz JL et al: Effect of transportation stress on bronchoalveolar lavage fluid analysis in female horses, *Am J Vet Res* 49:1026-1029, 1988.
43. Carr EA et al: Acute hemorrhagic pulmonary infarction and necrotizing pneumonia in horses: 21 cases (1967-1993), *J Am Vet Med Assoc* 210: 1774-1778, 1997.
44. Brook I: Role of encapsulated anaerobic bacteria in synergistic infections, *CRC Crit Rev Microbiol* 14:171-193, 1987.
45. Overson P et al: The effect of experimental stress on pulmonary alveolar macrophage function, *Clin Res* 20:879, 1972.
46. Tally FP, Cuchural GJ, Malamy MH: Mechanisms of resistance and resistance transfer in anaerobic bacteria: factors influencing antimicrobial therapy, *Rev Infect Dis* 6:S260-S269, 1984.
47. Moore RM: Diagnosis and treatment of obligate anaerobic bacterial infections in horses, *Compend Cont Educ Pract Vet* 15:989-994, 1993.

PNEUMONIA IN FOALS

MARY ROSE PARADIS

Pneumonia is a concern in both the neonatal and the older foal.[48-50] Though the etiologic agents and the mode of infection are different for each age-group, there is a common thread in the underlying cause. This thread is a compromise in the immunologic protection of the foal.

In the neonate, septicemia has been stated as the primary cause of illness and death in foals less than 8 days of age.[49] Bacterial pneumonia is a frequent manifestation of neonatal septicemia.[50,51] Lack of adequate transfer of maternal antibodies from the dam to the foal results in an immunocompromised foal that is susceptible to environmental bacteria. Bacteria, such as *E. coli*, *Klebsiella*, *Streptococcus* spp., and *Staphylococcus* spp., gain entry to the foal by inhalation, ingestion, or through the umbilicus and spread hematogenously to the lungs.[51]

Pneumonia is also the greatest cause of morbidity and mortality in foals greater than 1 month of age.[49] It is thought that affected foals are predisposed to developing bacterial pneumonia because of a low immunoglobulin status created by a lag between the waning of maternal antibodies and the production of the foal's own antibodies. It has been shown that a subgroup of foals with undifferentiated respiratory disease had significantly lower serum IgA and IgM levels.[52]

Young foals have a decreased number of cells in their bronchoalveolar lavage fluid when compared to bronchoalveolar samples from adult horses, the predominant cell being the macrophage, with low levels of lymphocytes.[53] The number and distribution of the cell types approach adult levels around 3 to 6 weeks of age.[53] It has recently been suggested that perhaps a natural cellular immunodeficiency may occur in foals between 2 and 4 months of age.[54] A CD4+ and CD8+ T lymphocytopenia was found in one filly with a concurrent *Pneumocystis carinii* pneumonia.[55] More work needs to be done on determining the role of these cells in immunity against intracellular pathogens such as *P. carinii* and *Rhodococcus equi* of foals.[54]

The clinical signs and diagnostic procedures needed to make a diagnosis of pneumonia in the neonate and the older foal are often different. With the exception of tachypnea and increased respiratory effort, neonatal foals with pneumonia may not exhibit signs that lead the practitioner to suspect lower respiratory involvement. Thoracic radiographs and arterial blood gas analysis are important in confirming the presence of pneumonia. Attempts to isolate the causative

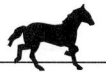

agent are usually made through the use of blood cultures, because transtracheal aspirates and bronchoalveolar lavage can be dangerous in the compromised septic foal.[50,51]

The older foal, on the other hand, will generally exhibit signs that focus on the respiratory tract, such as abnormal auscultation of the lungs, nasal discharge, cough, fever, tachypnea, and increased respiratory effort. Thoracic radiographs are important in determining the degree of involvement and the presence or absence of abscesses. Transtracheal aspirate or bronchoalveolar lavage is important in the determination of the etiologic agent.[56]

The treatment goals in dealing with bacterial pneumonia in either age group are the same—appropriate antibiotic administration and supportive care. Supportive care involves the provision of oxygen in hypoxic situations, fluid therapy when septic shock is evident, inhaled bronchodilators when obstructive airways are suspected, and ventilatory assistance in cases of hypercapnia.

Because neonatal septicemia and pneumonia are discussed more fully in Chapter 19, the remainder of this section will address pneumonia in the older foal. Lower respiratory disease in this age-group can be separated into etiologic categories—undifferentiated respiratory tract disease, pneumonia caused by *R. equi*, *P. carinii* infection, and acute respiratory distress syndrome (atypical bronchointerstitial pneumonia).

Undifferentiated Respiratory Tract Disease

Foals between the ages of 4 and 5 months appear to be highly susceptible to respiratory tract disease. Morbidity of up to 80% and 90% has been reported on some farms.[57] The clinical presentation of the affected foals includes auscultable abnormalities in the lung fields, including crackles and wheezes; mucopurulent nasal discharge; a spontaneous and inducible cough; and tachypnea. High fevers are not a prominent sign. Mucopurulent bronchial exudate, and bronchial erythema and edema are found on endoscopic examination of affected foals.[57] Mild to moderate bronchointerstitial pattern without consolidation may be seen on thoracic radiographs. Hematology is generally within normal limits, though a mild neutrophilia may be present. Bronchial lavage fluid contains a high number of neutrophils as compared to normal, unaffected foals.[10] Intracellular cocci are often seen.

Though viral disease has been cited as a possible predisposing factor in this disease, attempts to isolate equine influenza, equine herpes virus 1 and 2, equine rhinovirus, and equine adenovirus in acute cases have failed. Acute and convalescent serologic examinations have shown no significant change with the exception of an occasional conversion for equine herpes 1.[58]

Gram-positive cocci with a prominent capsule can usually be seen on Gram-stained smears of bronchial lavage. In one study gram-negative organisms were seen on a Gram stain in 40% of the cases. Bacterial culture of bronchial lavage fluid has yielded *S. zooepidemicus* as the most prominent isolate. Other gram-positive organisms cultured that may be considered pathogenic include *R. equi* and *Staphylococcus epidermidis*. Other gram-positive isolates, such as *Bordetella bronchiseptica*, *Mycoplasma equirhinis*, and α-hemolytic streptococci, are not associated with specific disease outcome.[58] Despite the incidence of gram-negative organisms seen on the Gram stain in the above study, they could not be isolated through normal procedures. When cultures were enriched, a *Pasteurella ureae*–like organism could occasionally be isolated; however, there was no correlation between the presence of the organism in the culture and the Gram-stained slides.[58]

The microbiologic susceptibility of *S. zooepidemicus* in a field study of undifferentiated respiratory disease in foals included

β-lactams antibiotics and trimethoprim-sulfamethoxazole. It appears that a combination of both drugs may provide better coverage than either one alone. β-Lactam antibiotics include penicillin (22,000 U/kg IM twice daily) and ampicillin (10 to 20 mg/kg IM twice daily). Potentiated sulfa drugs can be dosed orally at 20 to 30 mg/kg twice daily. The clinical response to this treatment should include a significant reduction in nasal discharge, cough, and adventitious lung sounds.[59] Reculturing of the broncholavage fluid posttreatment should demonstrate a decrease of *S. zooepidemicus* numbers.

One of the most frustrating features of this disease process is a 30% relapse rate. The relapse usually occurs between 7 and 35 days after treatment withdrawal.[59] It is suggested that the relapse is due to the continued predisposing immunodeficiency.[59]

The long-term prognosis of foals that have experienced this type of pneumonia is hard to assess. One study suggested that affected foals that reached the racetrack did not perform as well as horses that had not had respiratory problems as foals.[60] This may be hard to judge because the high morbidity of the problem may make it difficult to find control animals.

Rhodococcus equi Pneumonia

Foals infected with *R. equi* have a slightly different clinical picture. The morbidity of the disease is more sporadic except on endemic farms. Affected foals tend to be younger, with a mean age of 2 months.[61,62] Infection can be seen as early as 1 month of age and as late as 6 months. The most common clinical signs are related to the respiratory system and include auscultable wheezes and crackles over both lung fields, fever (38.5° to 41° C), mucopurulent nasal discharge, and tachypnea. Generally the signs appear to develop acutely and the foals may be in respiratory distress. The mean duration of illness is 12 days.[61,62] Radiographically these foals have pulmonary consolidation and abscessation.

R. equi infection can manifest in other body systems as well. It can present as diarrhea, peritonitis, subcutaneous abscessation, joint effusion or "reactive" arthritis, and osteomyelitis with subcutaneous abscessation or septic arthritis.[63] If the osteomyelitis is located in a vertebral body, then ataxia and recumbency may be the presenting sign.[64-67]

The diagnosis of *R. equi* pneumonia is made by a combination of the clinical signs, evidence of pulmonary abscessation on radiographs, and a positive culture of a transtracheal aspirate, abdominal fluid, or synovial fluid. *R. equi* appears as a gram-positive pleomorphic rod.[61] A recent polymerase chain reaction test was developed and tested to analyze its effectiveness in diagnosing the disease compared to culture. Bacterial isolation proved to be more effective.[68,69]

Hematologically, affected foals have a leukocytosis with a neutrophilia. They characteristically have a high fibrinogen level. Several serologic tests have been developed to aid in the diagnosis of *R. equi*. It was hoped that they would be useful in the early diagnosis of this disease, before severe clinical signs, but they are probably more useful in herd monitoring[61,62] One enzyme-linked immunosorbent assay (ELISA) test measured maternally derived antibodies against the virulence-associated proteins of *R. equi* and found that they were lowest at 4 to 8 weeks of age.[70]

Pyogranulomatous pulmonary lesions are found on postmortem of foals that do not respond to treatment. Abscessation of the bronchial and mediastinal lymph nodes is common.[61,71]

The antibiotic combination of choice for the treatment of *R. equi* is erythromycin estolate (25 mg/kg PO four times daily) and rifampin (10 mg/kg PO twice daily). This combination is particularly effective because of its lipophilic nature, which enables the drugs to penetrate the abscesses and also cells. This is important because *R. equi* lives and multiplies inside of the macrophage. Although other antibiotics, such as gentamycin, may have an in vitro sensitivity to *R. equi*, they do not reach high levels in the phagocytes where the organism resides. Prolonged treatment of affected animals is needed. Treatment should continue until there is no longer radiographic evidence of pneumonia, approximately 6 to 8 weeks.[61,62]

Several side effects of erythromycin therapy have been noted. These include a mild diarrhea in the foals, clostridial colitis in the dams of affected foals (reportedly from ingesting the active metabolites of the drug from the foal's feces), and hyperthermia in treated foals.[56,61]

R. equi tends to be sporadic except on some farms where it is endemic. The organism is a normal inhabitant of soil and can be cultured from horse feces. Affected foals pass higher numbers of bacteria in their feces and can be a source of continued contamination of the premises. A dry, dusty environment tends to promote aerosolization of the bacteria. Manure removal and the elimination of dusty areas may decrease the spread of the bacteria.[61]

Hyperimmune plasma has been administered to foals on endemic farms during the first few weeks postpartum in an attempt to provide immunologic protection against infection. Harris and colleagues showed a significant reduction in the number of foals affected using this method. It has been suggested that the serum from foals less than 2 to 3 weeks of age is deficient in factors that enhance opsonization of *R. equi*.[72]

The long-term athletic prognosis for foals with *R. equi* pneumonia is guarded. Foals that make it to the racetrack do as well as foals that did not experience pneumonia as foals, but the number of foals that actually get to the racetrack is significantly reduced.[60,73]

Pneumocystis carinii Infection

P. carinii (PC) is a unicellular eukaryote that has been classified as a fungus by DNA studies.[74] It is most commonly seen in humans and animals that have a concurrent immunodeficiency. It was first recovered in Arabian foals with combined immunodeficiency syndrome.[75] It has since been recovered from foals of other breeds with no specific history of immunodeficiency, though for the most part, no direct testing for immunocompetence was performed in the reported cases. However, one recently reported case demonstrated a low number of circulating CD4+ and CD8+ lymphocytes in a filly with PC.[55]

The onset of clinical signs in affected foals ranged from a 3-week history of weakness, weight loss, and nasal discharge to acute dyspnea. Half of the reported non-Arabian cases had concurrent infections with *R. equi*, *Enterobacter cloaca*, *E. coli*, or *S. zooepidemicus*.

A severe interstitial, sometimes miliary and alveolar pattern was seen on radiographs of the lungs. The majority of the reported foals died and the diagnoses of PC were made on necropsy.[55,75-80] On postmortem examination the lungs were uniformly heavy and consolidated. A diffuse interstitial pneumonia was found. Trophozoites and cysts were found in the alveolar epithelial cells and macrophages in the alveoli. Silver staining and streptavidin-biotin immunolabeling of histologic sections provide a better visualization of the organisms in the pulmonary tissue.[79] A few foals were diagnosed by visualization of the organism on a bronchoalveolar lavage sample. Two surviving foals responded to trimethoprim-sulfamethoxazole therapy.

Bronchointerstitial Pneumonia (Acute Respiratory Distress Syndrome)

There is a subset of foals with severe respiratory distress that shares some of the clinical characteristics of the foals with *R. equi* and PC but for which a consistent causative organism,

either bacterial or viral, cannot be found. In a report of 23 cases, bacteria were not grown in culture attempts in nine foals. Cultures from six foals grew an *E. coli*, five grew *S. zooepidemicus*, four grew *R. equi*, and single cultures grew *K. pneumoniae*, *Bordetella bronchiseptica*, *Enterobacter* spp., *Pseudomonas mirabilis*, *Fusobacterium* spp., *Actinobacillus suis*, and *Flavobacterium*. One foal was positive for equine herpesvirus type 2.[81] Buergelt in Florida and Prescott in Canada reported similar inconsistent etiologic findings.[82,83]

The reported cases have been between 1 and 7 months of age. They were either found dead or they presented with acute onset of respiratory distress. Some foals were normal before the onset of the respiratory distress or they were being treated for a respiratory problem that escalated into the respiratory distress. The general signs include tachypnea, increased respiratory effort, cyanosis, hypoxemia, and hypercapnia resulting in respiratory acidosis. A severe diffuse interstitial to bronchointerstitial pulmonary pattern is generally found on thoracic radiographs. In some instances this pattern coalesced into an alveolar pattern.[81-83]

Affected foals do not respond well to antibiotic treatment. The use of oxygen insufflation, bronchodilators, antiinflammatory medication, and corticosteroids appears to improve recovery rate. Environmental control, such as air-conditioned stalls and alcohol baths, is important in decreasing the core body heat.[81]

On postmortem examination, lungs from these foals are generally heavy and fail to collapse. They may be edematous and exude fluid when cut or bulge on cut surfaces. Histopathologic lesions include bronchiolitis, foci of alveolar septal necrosis with infiltration of neutrophils, congestion, hyaline membrane formation, interstitial fibrosis, and type II pneumocyte hyperplasia.[81-83]

Etiologies that have been proposed include endotoxemia with severe inflammatory response syndrome, an inhaled or ingested toxin, viral infection, such as equine herpesvirus type 2, and heat shock.[81-84] In one study, all foals were hyperthermic and presented on days with high ambient temperatures. It was felt that the stress of transport on hot days could be responsible for some of the clinical signs.[81]

Prognosis for foals presenting with signs of respiratory distress is guarded for both life and for future athletic ability. Survivors may have persistent pulmonary pathology.[81]

REFERENCES

48. Zent WW: Foal pneumonia, *Proceedings of the Thirty-second Annual Convention of the American Association of Equine Practitioners*, 1986, pp 269-275.
49. Cohen ND: Causes of and farm management factors associated with disease and death in foals, *J Am Vet Med Assoc* 204:1644, 1994.
50. Lester GD: Respiratory disease in the neonatal foal, *Equine Vet Educ* 11:208-217, 1999.
51. Paradis MR: Update on neonatal septicemia, *Vet Clin North Am (Equine Pract)* 10:109-135, 1994.
52. Hoffman AM, Viel L, Prescott JF: Clinical endoscopic study of lower respiratory-tract infections in foals on Ontario breeding farms, *Proceedings of the Thirty-seventh Annual Convention of the American Association of Equine Practitioners*, 1992, pp 191-192.
53. Hines MT: Development of pulmonary immunity in foals, *Proceedings of the Seventeenth ACVIM Forum*, Chicago, 1999, pp 604-605.
54. Prescott JF: Immunodeficiency and serious pneumonia in foals: the plot thickens, *Equine Vet J* 25:88-89, 1993.
55. Flaminio MJBF et al: CD4+ and CD8+ T-lymphocytopenia in a filly with *Pneumocystis carinii* pneumonia, *Aust Vet J* 76:399-402, 1998.
56. Wilson WD: Foal pneumonia: an overview, *Proceedings of the Thirty-seventh Annual Convention of the American Association of Equine Practitioners*, 1992, pp 203-229.
57. Hoffman AM et al: Clinical and endoscopic study to estimate the incidence of distal respiratory tract infection in thoroughbred foals on Ontario breeding farms, *Am J Vet Res* 54:1602-1607, 1993.
58. Hoffman AM et al: Association of microbiologic flora with clinical, endoscopic, and pulmonary cytologic findings in foals with distal respiratory tract infection, *Am J Vet Res* 54:1615-1622, 1993.
59. Hoffman AM, Viel L, Prescott JF: Microbiologic changes during antimicrobial treatment and rate of relapse of distal respiratory tract infections in foals, *Am J Vet Res* 54:1608-1614, 1993.

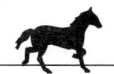

60. Bernard B et al: The influence of foal pneumonia on future racing performance, *Proceedings of the Thirty-sixth Annual Convention of the American Association of Equine Practitioners*, 1991, pp 17-18.
61. Ainsworth DM: Rhodococcal infections in foals, *Equine Vet Educ* 11:191-198, 1999.
62. Giguère S, Prescott JF: Clinical manifestations, diagnosis, treatment, and prevention of *Rhodococcus equi* infections in foals, *Vet Microbiol* 56:313-334, 1997.
63. Paradis MR: Cutaneous and musculoskeletal manifestations of *Rhodococcus equi* infection in foals, *Equine Vet Educ* 9:266-270, 1997.
64. Olchowy TWJ: Vertebral body osteomyelitis due to *Rhodococcus equi* in two Arabian foals, *Equine Vet J* 26:79-82, 1994.
65. Giguère S, Lavoie JP: *Rhodococcus equi* vertebral osteomyelitis in 3 quarter horse colts, *Equine Vet J* 26:74-77, 1994.
66. Prymak-Oldick KE, Edens LM, Hawkins DL: Challenging cases in internal medicine: what's your diagnosis? *Vet Med* 14-20, 1995.
67. Chaffin MK et al: Cauda equina syndrome, diskospondylitis, and a paravertebral abscess caused by *Rhodococcus equi* in a foal, *J Am Vet Med Assoc* 206:215-220, 1995.
68. Takai S et al: Identification of virulent *Rhodococcus equi* by amplification of gene coding for 15- to 17-kilodalton antigens, *J Clin Micro* 33:1622-1627, 1995.
69. Anzai T et al: Comparison of tracheal aspiration with other tests for diagnosis of *Rhodococcus equi* pneumonia in foals, *Vet Microbiol* 56:335-345, 1997.
70. Prescott JF et al: Use of a virulence-associated protein based enzyme-linked immunosorbent assay for *Rhodococcus equi* serology in horses, *Equine Vet J* 28:344-349, 1996.
71. Wada R et al: Pathogenicity and virulence of *Rhodococcus equi* in foals following intratracheal challenge, *Vet Microbiol* 56:301-312, 1997.
72. Harris JA et al: Effects of anti-*Rhodococcus equi* hyperimmune serum on equine neonatal alveolar macrophage function, *Proceedings of the Seventh International Conference on Equine Infectious Diseases*, Tokyo, 1994, p 94.
73. Ainsworth DM et al: Associations between physical examination, laboratory, and radiographic findings and outcome and subsequent racing performance of foals with *Rhodococcus equi* infection: 115 cases (1984-1992), *J Am Vet Med Assoc* 213:510-515, 1998.
74. Edman JC et al: Ribosomal RNA sequence shows *Pneumocystis carinii* to be a member of the Fungi, *Nature* 334:519-522, 1988.
75. Shively JN et al: *Pneumocystis carinii* pneumonia in two foals, *J Am Vet Med Assoc* 162:648-652, 1973.
76. Shively JN, Moe KK, Dellers RW: Fine structure of spontaneous *Pneumocystis carinii* pulmonary infection in foals, *Cornell Vet* 64(suppl 4):72-88, 1974.
77. Ainsworth DM et al: Recognition of *Pneumocystis carinii* in foals with respiratory distress, *Equine Vet J* 25:103-108, 1993.
78. Ewing PJ et al: *Pneumocystis carinii* pneumonia in foals, *J Am Vet Med Assoc* 204:929-933, 1994.
79. Whitwell KE: *Pneumocystis carinii* pneumonia in thoroughbred foals, *Seventh International Conference on Equine Infectious Diseases*, Tokyo, Japan, 1994, p 98.
80. Lepage MFP, Gerber V, Suter MM: A case of interstitial pneumonia associated with *Pneumocystis carinii* in a foal, *Vet Pathol* 36:621-624, 1999.
81. Lakritz J et al: Bronchointerstitial pneumonia and respiratory distress in young horses: clinical, clinicopathologic, radiographic, and pathological findings in 23 cases (1984-1989), *J Vet Intern Med* 7:277-288, 1993.
82. Buergelt CD et al: A retrospective study of proliferative interstitial lung disease in horses in Florida, *Vet Pathol* 23:750-756, 1986.
83. Prescott JF et al: Sporadic, severe bronchointerstitial pneumonia of foals, *Can Vet J* 32:421-425, 1991.
84. Ames TR, O'Leary TP, Johnston GR: Isolation of equine herpesvirus type 2 from foals with respiratory disease, *Comp Equine* 8:664-670, 1986.

FUNGAL PNEUMONIAS

CORINNE R. SWEENEY

DEFINITION AND ETIOLOGY. Fungi are ubiquitous, and their constant aerosol exposure to respiratory tissue is inevitable. In most samples of stable air, more than 90% of particles visible under a light microscope were spores of fungi or actinomycetes.[85] When a horse stood quietly in its stable without access to hay, the mean concentration of dust was very low (approximately 12 particles per cubic centimeter [of particles less than 5 mm in diameter]). When the bedding was disturbed during normal "bedding down" operation, the concentration of respirable dust increased sixfold.[86]

Pulmonary disease caused by fungi is acquired by the inhalation route; sporular diameter is small enough to allow penetration into the distal airways and alveoli. Tissue invasion usually occurs in the immunocompromised host, although on occasion the normal individual may be affected. Important predisposing factors include (1) qualitative and

especially quantitative granulocyte abnormalities and (2) the presence of devitalized tissue. In vitro studies support the critical role of phagocytic cells in host defense against opportunistic fungi.

Pathogenic fungi such as *Coccidioides immitis, Histoplasma capsulatum*, and *Cryptococcus neoformans* usually infect immunologically normal horses. However, in a recent report of cryptococcosis in seven horses, five had a history of illness that may have predisposed them to cryptococcosis.[87] The relatively high frequency of cryptococcosis in Western Australia suggests that a regional factor may contribute to its occurrence.[89] A separate group of fungal pathogens infect only those equine patients with abnormal host defenses. These so-called opportunistic fungi include *Aspergillus* spp., the *Phycomycetes, Mucor, Rhizopus*, and *Candida* spp. For example, in the immunocompromised patient *Aspergillus* spp. may produce a fulminant invasive pulmonary infection.

In a survey of horses with fungal pneumonias examined at the George Widener Hospital, University of Pennsylvania, the majority of those with fungal pneumonia had a serious primary problem such as enterocolitis, peritonitis, nephritis, endotoxemia, or septicemia. Many of the horses showed no respiratory signs, and the diagnosis of fungal pneumonia was made at the time of postmortem examination. Most had been on antimicrobial therapy for a varying period for their primary problem. Immunosuppression in combination with severe enteritis has resulted in pulmonary aspergillosis, suggesting invasion of *Aspergillus* spp. from damaged intestine.[88,89]

DIAGNOSIS. Clinicians must be careful in attributing significance to presence of fungal elements in a transtracheal aspirate or the isolation of fungus from these samples. Fungal hyphae are often present either free or in large mononuclear cells in tracheal aspirates from healthy horses.[90] Sixteen percent of healthy horses are reported to have fungal growth on the tracheal aspirate bacterial culture plates.[91] A study of healthy Thoroughbred racehorses showed 70% had fungal elements detected in their tracheal aspirates.[92] None of the horses from either of the studies had other evidence of fungal pneumonia. To be significant, cytologically large numbers of fungi should be involved in the inflammatory process within the lung. If fungal pneumonia is suspected, a percutaneous lung biopsy can confirm the diagnosis. However, the lesions, though multiple, are usually small and not detectable by ultrasound examination. Therefore biopsy is done blindly and may or may not sample an affected site.

In patients with suspected *Aspergillus* spp. infection, careful examination of the nose and paranasal sinuses may be rewarding. Biopsy of a nasal erosion or ulcer that reveals organisms histologically is highly predictive of concomitant or future invasive pulmonary aspergillosis. Serologic analysis is not helpful, because many horses have titers to *Aspergillus* spp. Clinical signs suggestive of pulmonary aspergillosis include coughing and hemoptysis. Radiographs of affected patients may reveal virtually any infiltrative pattern. Although miliary patterns are occasionally seen, the most common initial finding is a patchy bronchopneumonia. Multiple focal sites are common, and lesions tend to be peripheral in distribution.

TREATMENT. Treatment of fungal pneumonia is usually frustrating. Most equine cases occur secondary to a severe primary disease (e.g., enterocolitis, liver failure), which often is responsible for the death of the horse. The drug of choice depends on the opportunistic fungus involved. Specific antifungal agents include amphotericin B, ketoconazole, miconazole, 5-fluorocytosine, and iodides. Often therapy is not attempted because of the severity of the primary disease, expense, or the poor prognosis.

Prevention of invasive fungal pneumonia is difficult. It is impossible for the horse to avoid large inhaled inocula, given its environmental conditions. Improving ventilation and minimizing exposure to inspired spores are most beneficial in immunocompromised patients. At present the most important methods of disease prevention are treating predisposing illnesses promptly and effectively and judiciously avoiding overuse of corticosteroids and broad-spectrum antibiotics.

REFERENCES

85. Clark AF: Air hygiene and equine respiratory disease, *Vet Res In Practice* 9:196-204, 1987.
86. Webster AJF et al: Air hygiene in stables. I. Effects of stable design, ventilation and management on the concentration of respirable dust, *Equine Vet J* 19:448-453, 1987.
87. Riley CB, Bolton JN, Thomas JB: Cryptococcosis in seven horses, *Aust Vet J* 69:135-139, 1992.
88. Slocombe RF, Slauson DO: Invasive pulmonary aspergillosis of horses: an association with acute enteritis, *Vet Pathol* 25:277-281, 1988.
89. Hattel AL et al: Pulmonary aspergillosis associated with acute enteritis in a horse, *J Am Vet Med Assoc* 199:589-590, 1991.
90. Beech J: Cytology of tracheal bronchial aspirate in horses, *Vet Pathol* 12:157-164, 1975.
91. Sweeney CR, Beech J, Roby KAW: Bacterial isolates from tracheal bronchial aspirates from healthy horses, *Am J Vet Res* 46:2562-2565, 1985.
92. Sweeney CR, Humber KA, Roby KAW: Cytologic findings of tracheobronchial aspirates from 66 thoroughbred racehorses, *Am J Vet Res* 53:1172-1175, 1992.

PLEUROPNEUMONIA

CORINNE R. SWEENEY

Bacterial pleuropneumonia, frequently referred to as pleuritis, is a common and often severe disorder of horses.[93-97] The condition involves bacterial colonization of the pulmonary parenchyma, development of pneumonia or pulmonary abscesses, and subsequent extension to the visceral pleura and pleural space. In humans it is noted that up to 40% of patients with bacterial pneumonia have accompanying pleural effusions. Although similar data are not available for the horse, the increased use of thoracic ultrasound has documented that pleural effusion is not uncommon in any horse with pneumonia and is not restricted to those horses with severe pleuropneumonia.

PATHOGENESIS. The first stage of bacterial pleuropneumonia is an exudative stage characterized by rapid outpouring of sterile pleural fluid into the pleural space in response to inflammation of the pleura. The associated pneumonic process is usually contiguous with the visceral pleura and results in increased permeability of the capillaries in the visceral pleura. If appropriate antimicrobial therapy is initiated at this stage, the pleural effusion may progress no further.

With progression the bacteria invade the pleural fluid from the contiguous pneumonic process and the second, fibropurulent, stage evolves. This stage is characterized by the accumulation of large amounts of pleural fluid with many neutrophils, bacteria, and cellular debris. Fibrin is deposited in a continuous sheet covering both the visceral and parietal pleural in the involved area (Fig. 29-12). As this stage progresses, the tendency is to loculation and the formation of limiting membranes. These loculations prevent extension of the empyema, but make drainage of the pleural space with chest tubes increasingly difficult.

The last stage is the organization stage, in which fibroblasts grow into the exudate from both the visceral and parietal pleura surfaces and produce an inelastic membrane called the pleural peel. This inelastic pleural peel encases the lung and renders it virtually functionless. At this stage the exudate is thick.

Although pleuropneumonia can occur spontaneously, it is often associated with a stressful event such as transportation over an extended distance or recent illness from acute viral disease. It is most commonly seen in Thoroughbred and Standardbred racehorses. Aspiration of pharyngeal secretions may play a significant role in the etiology of pleuropneumonia, as suggested by the bacterial populations responsible for pleuropneumonia. Transportation of horses usually involves

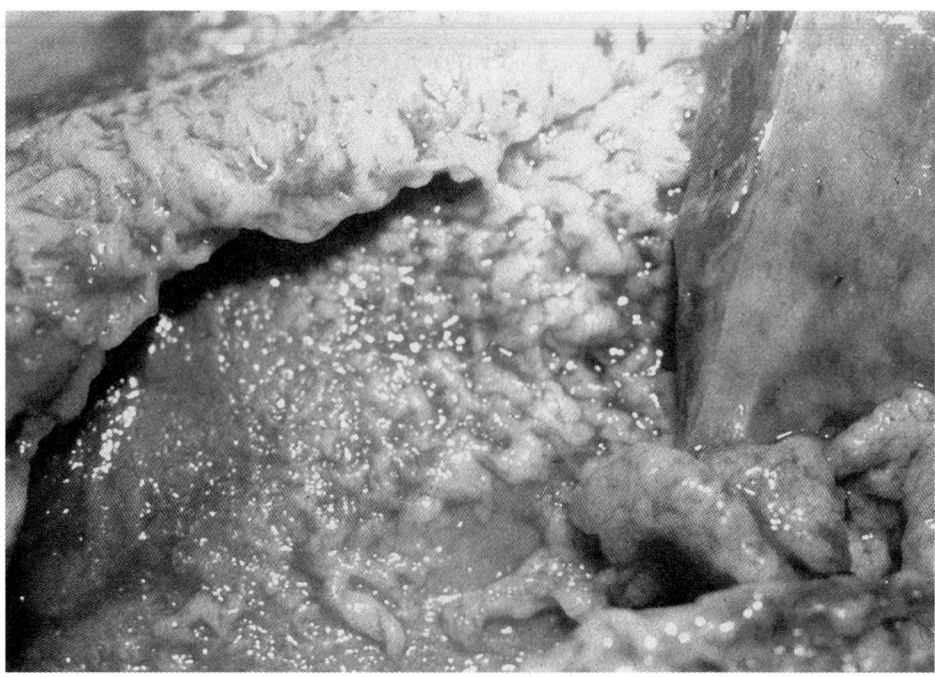

FIG. 29-12 ▮▮ Postmortem view of lungs with severe pleuropneumonia with thick fibrin layer covering the pleura soon to develop into a pleural peel.

an elevation in environmental temperature and relative humidity and increase in the number of bacterial organisms within the air. These changes, combined with the stress of transportation, may predispose the animal to development of lower respiratory disease. The aerobic bacteria most commonly involved in equine pleuropneumonia include β-hemolytic *Streptococcus* spp., *Pasteurella* spp., *Actinobacillus* spp., *E. coli*, and *Klebsiella pneumoniae*. The majority of the horses have a mixed infection, with both aerobic and anaerobic bacteria. Commonly isolated anaerobes include *Bacteroides* spp. and *Clostridium* spp. A wide variety of other anaerobes are commonly found in these horses.

CLINICAL SIGNS. Clinical signs include fever, anorexia, depression, cough, respiratory distress, stiff gait, weight loss, sternal or limb edema, and colic. In the acute stage of pleuritis, pain in the thorax may be elicited by palpation over the thoracic wall. Pain is demonstrated by grunts, intercostal muscle spasm, or even escape maneuvers by the patient. Horses may abduct their elbows and have a "catch" to inspiration. As more fluid accumulates in the pleural space and the disease becomes chronic, pain is less evident. Auscultation of a horse with pleuropneumonia reveals a normal lung sound in the dorsal lung field with no sounds or only bronchial tracheal sounds heard ventrally. Pleural friction rubs are often not heard because they are present only in the acute stage of the disease. If they are heard, friction rubs are present predominantly at the end of inspiration and the early part of expiration. They disappear as inflammation decreases or as pleural fluids accumulate. Cardiac sounds are often heard over a wider area of the chest than normal, probably as a result of enhanced conduction of sound through the pleural fluid. Thoracic percussion frequently confirms the impression gained from auscultation. Pleural effusion causes a dullness of the ventral aspects of the lung field and is often delineated by a horizontal line (Fig. 29-13).

DIAGNOSTIC PROCEDURES

Cytology and Culture Specimens. Airway and pleural fluid specimens should be submitted for cytology and aerobic and anaerobic culture. Percutaneous transtracheal aspiration is preferred to avoid contamination from the upper airway. Bronchoalveolar lavage can be used, but because only a limited segment of the lung is sampled, the diseased region(s) may be missed. Thoracocentesis is performed to collect pleural fluid samples for analysis.

Thoracic Ultrasonography. Because air is a near-perfect reflector of ultrasound waves, the practitioner might expect ultrasound to have limited value in examination of the lung, "an air-filled structure." With close to 25 years of experience, thoracic ultrasonography is currently regarded as the preferred method to diagnose pleuropneumonia in the horse. Although the value of the art of thoracic auscultation and percussion should not be unestimated, clinicians managing horses with thoracic disease recognize the limitations of these tools. With the widespread use of thoracic ultrasound, the equine practitioner currently has the ability to determine not only the presence of pleuropneumonia, but also the location and the extent of the disease.

Thoracic ultrasonography in horses with pleuropneumonia allows the clinician to characterize the fluid and to evaluate the severity of the underlying pulmonary disease.[98,99] The presence of adhesions, pleural thickening, pulmonary necrosis, and compression atelectasis can also be detected (Fig. 29-14). The detection and further characterization of the above abnormalities improve the clinician's ability to form a more accurate prognosis. Notation of free gas echoes often associated with anaerobic infection, severe fibrinous pleuritis, or loculation all suggest a guarded prognosis. Adhesions can be detected that ultimately may affect the horse's return to its previous performance level. Horses with compression atelectasis and a nonfibrinous pleuritis have an

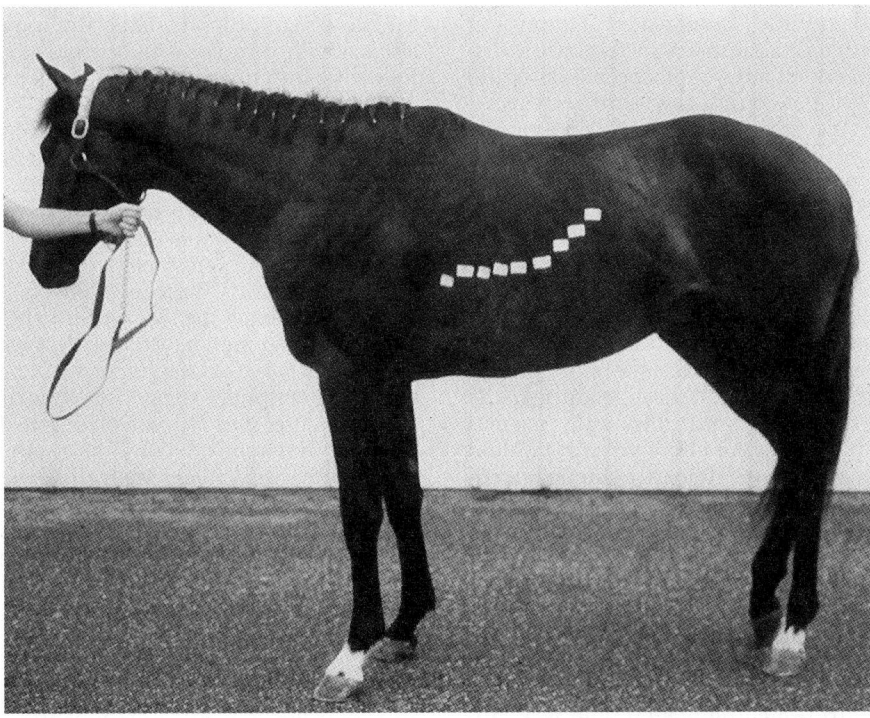

FIG. 29-13 ▮ Horse with pleural effusion secondary to pleuropneumonia. Horizontal line marked by tape indicates fluid level in thorax detected by auscultation and percussion.

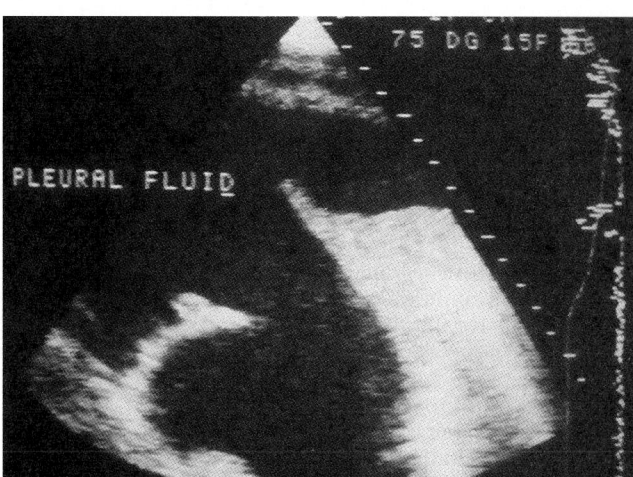

FIG. 29-14 ▓ Anechoic pleural fluid and compression atelectasis of a horse with pleuropneumonia.

excellent prognosis for survival and return to performance. The detection of areas of consolidation, pulmonary necrosis, or abscesses all increase the probable treatment and recovery time and the prognosis for survival decreases as these become more extensive. Ultrasonography can be used as a guide to sample or drain the area with a large fluid accumulation or the least loculation. These patients often benefit from progressive scanning to assess response to treatment and the need for drainage. Ultrasonography is a valuable diagnostic aid in the evaluation of the pleura, lung, and mediastinum of horses with pleuropneumonia.

Thoracocentesis. If pleural effusion is suspected, thoracocentesis should be considered. In the acute stages of pleuropneumonia with small volumes of pleural effusion, thoracocentesis is not necessary if the horse is improving or is not showing signs of respiratory distress. Moderate amounts of pleural effusion may be resorbed quite readily. However, if fluid accumulates rapidly, if the horse is in respiratory distress, or if its condition deteriorates, thoracocentesis should be performed. The procedure is quick, easy, and inexpensive, and is considered safe. The preferred site is the sixth or seventh intercostal space just dorsal to the palpable costochondral junction. Choosing a site farther caudal may provide a sample but does not allow adequate drainage of the chest. When attempting to aspirate pleural fluid from a horse with a minimum amount of effusion, the practitioner should choose a space no farther back than the sixth or seventh intercostal space. Thoracic ultrasound aids the site selection. If the procedure has caused some trauma, the first fluid obtained may be blood tinged, but this clears as more fluid is withdrawn. If the pleural fluid is blood tinged because of the underlying disease process, the red coloration persists throughout the entire procedure. An aliquot of pleural fluid is transferred from the syringe into tubes containing anticoagulant solution (EDTA) so that appropriate laboratory evaluation may be performed. Part of the fluid should be saved in sterile containers with transport media for subsequent Gram stain and culture. Fluid should be removed as long as it flows freely. Both sides of the thorax should be tapped.

Examination of Pleural Fluid. The color, turbidity, viscosity, and odor should be noted. Normal pleural fluid is clear and yellow; cloudiness reflects an increased number of white blood cells (WBCs). Putrid-smelling pleural fluid is a hallmark of anaerobic infection; however, the absence of odor does not exclude anaerobic infection. In addition to the odor

of the pleural fluid, the odor of the horse's breath should be noted, particularly after coughing. The majority of horses with anaerobic infections have a putrid odor associated with the pleural fluid or breath. These horses have a low survival rate.

The WBC count of normal pleural fluid is generally less than 10,000/µl. WBC count of pleural fluid in pleuropneumonia can range from 1600 to 300,000 cells/µl varying in the same pleural fluid sample between the beginning and the end of the thoracocentesis. There is no association between the WBC count in pleural fluid and survival. Pleural fluid protein is greater than 3 g/dl in horses with pleuropneumonia, but this is also not a prognostic indicator.

Pleural fluid should be Gram stained and cultured for bacteria. The Gram stain may provide tentative identification until the culture results are obtained. Both aerobic and anaerobic cultures should be performed. Anaerobes occur in 46% of horses with pleuropneumonia. The pleural fluid used for anaerobic cultures should be transferred to the laboratory immediately after collection in a manner that prevents or minimizes exposure to air. Anaerobic transport media are commercially available and should be routinely used. Specimens submitted for isolation of anaerobes should not be refrigerated, because many anaerobes are intolerant to cold. Isolation of anaerobic bacteria from either the pleural fluid or tracheobronchial aspirate provides a poor prognosis.

TREATMENT

Antimicrobial Therapy. The most important treatment in bacterial pleuropneumonia is the use of systemic antimicrobial agents. Ideally an etiologic agent is identified from either the tracheobronchial aspirate or pleural fluid, and antimicrobial sensitivity determined. Without bacterial culture results, broad-spectrum antibiotics should be used because many horses have mixed infections of both gram-positive and gram-negative and aerobic and anaerobic organisms. Commonly used therapy is penicillin combined with an aminoglycoside such as gentamicin, trimethoprim and sulfamethoxazole, or chloramphenicol. Because of the need for long-term therapy, initial intravenous or intramuscular antimicrobials may need to be followed by oral antimicrobials. Preferably the oral antimicrobials are not administered until the horse's condition is stable and improving because blood levels obtained by this route are not as high as those achieved following intramuscular or intravenous administration.

Treatment of anaerobic pleuropneumonia is usually empiric, because antimicrobial susceptibility testing of anaerobes is difficult because of their fastidious nutritive and atmospheric requirements. Thus familiarity with antimicrobial susceptibility patterns is helpful in formulating the treatment regimen when an anaerobe is suspected. The majority of anaerobic isolates are sensitive to relatively low concentrations of penicillin. *Bacteroides fragilis* is the only frequently encountered anaerobe that is routinely resistant to penicillin, although other members of the *Bacteroides* family are known to produce β-lactamases and are potentially penicillin resistant. Chloramphenicol is effective against most aerobes and anaerobes that cause equine pleuropneumonia. However, because of human health concerns, the availability of chloramphenicol may decrease. Metronidazole has in vitro activity against a variety of obligate anaerobes including *B. fragilis.* Pharmacokinetic studies indicate a dose of 15 mg/kg intravenously or orally four times a day is necessary to maintain adequate serum levels. Oral administration rapidly results in adequate serum levels and thus is an acceptable route of administration for horses with pleuropneumonia. Metronidazole is not effective against aerobes and therefore should always be used in combination therapy. The aminoglycosides are ineffective in the treatment of anaerobic pleuropneumonia because the amount of the aminoglycosides needed to inhibit the growth of the anaerobic bacteria far exceeds the levels that are safely achieved in the blood and tissue. Thus aminoglycosides should not be considered for the treatment of pleuropneumonia caused by an anaerobe unless used in combination therapy (i.e., with penicillin).

Pleural Drainage. Following selection of an appropriate antimicrobial agent, the next decision to be made is whether to drain the pleural space. Ideally the decision is based on an examination of the pleural fluid. If the pleural fluid is thick pus, drainage using a chest tube should be initiated. If the pleural fluid is not thick pus but the Gram stain is positive and WBC counts are elevated, pleural drainage is recommended. Another indication for therapeutic thoracocentesis is the relief of respiratory distress secondary to a pleural effusion.

There are many options for thoracic drainage including the following: intermittent chest drainage, indwelling chest tube, pleural lavage, pleuroscopy and debridement, open chest drainage/debridement with no rib resection (standing), open chest drainage/debridement with rib resection (standing), open chest drainage and debridement (general anesthesia), and lung resection (general anesthesia). Drainage of a pleural effusion can be accomplished by (1) using a cannula, (2) indwelling chest tubes, or (3) thoracostomy. Thoracostomy is reserved for severe abscessation of the pleural space. Thoracocentesis is easily accomplished in the field and may not need to be repeated unless considerable pleural effusion reaccumulates. Indwelling chest tubes are indicated when continued pleural fluid accumulation makes intermittent thoracocentesis impractical. If properly placed and managed, they provide a method for frequent fluid removal and do not exacerbate the underlying pleuropneumonia or increase the production of pleural effusion. A one-way flutter valve may be attached to allow for continuous drainage without leakage of air into the thorax. The chest entry site and end of the drainage tube must be maintained aseptically. If a chest tube is placed aseptically and managed correctly, it can be maintained for several weeks. It should be removed as soon as it is no longer functional. Heparinization of tubing after drainage helps maintain patency. Local cellulitis may occur at the site of entry into the chest, but is considered a minor complication. Bilateral pleural fluid accumulation requires bilateral drainage in most horses.

Open drainage or thoracostomy may be considered when tube drainage is inadequate. It is important not to begin open drainage too early in the disease. An incision is made in the intercostal space, exposing the pleural cavity and causing a pneumothorax, unless the visceral and parietal pleura adjacent to the drainage site have not been fused by the inflammatory process. The wound is kept open for several weeks while the pleural space is flushed and treated as an open draining abscess.

Pleural Lavage. Pleural lavage may be helpful to dilute fluid and remove fibrin, debris, and necrotic tissue. Lavage appears to be most effective in subacute stages before loculae develop; however, pleural lavage may help break down fibrous adhesions and establish communication between loculae. Care must be exercised that infused fluid is communicating with the drainage tube. Lavage can be performed by infusing fluid through a dorsally positioned tube and draining it through a ventrally positioned tube (Fig. 29-15). Ten liters of sterile, warm lactated Ringer's solution is infused into each affected hemithorax by gravity flow. After infusion, the ventrally placed chest tube is opened and the lavage fluid is allowed to drain. Pleural lavage is probably contraindicated in horses with bronchopleural communications because it may result in spread of septic debris up the airways. Coughing and drainage of lavage fluid from the nares during infusion suggest the presence of a bronchopleural communication.

Other Therapy. Antiinflammatory agents help reduce pain and may decrease the production of pleural fluid. This in turn may encourage the horse to eat and maintain body weight.

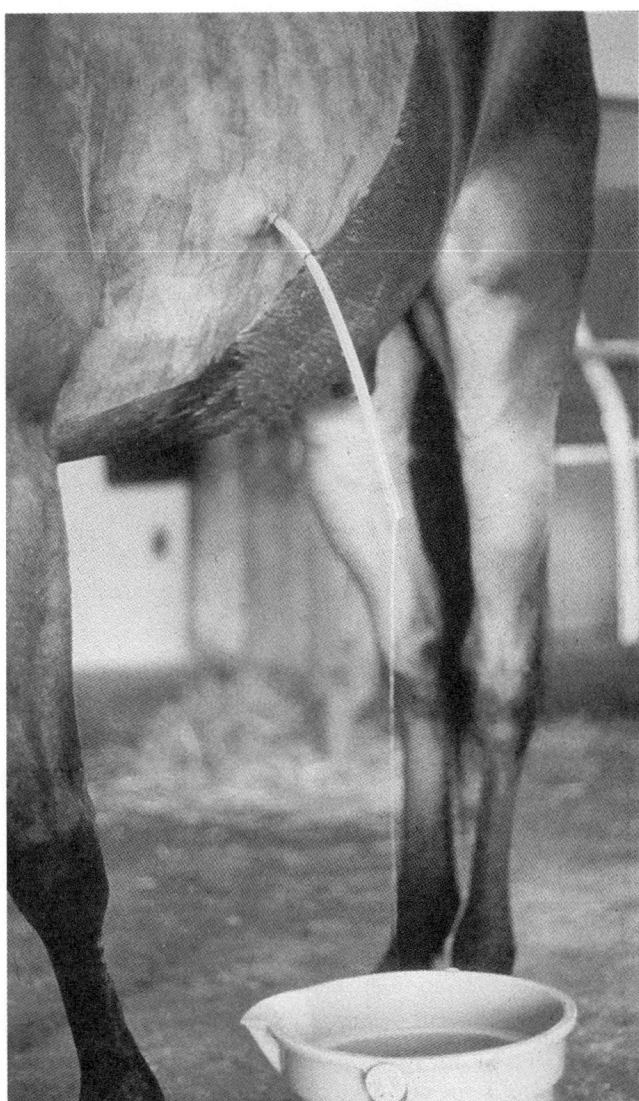

FIG. 29-15 ▨ Chest tube drainage of pleural fluid in horse with severe pleuropneumonia after pleural lavage.

Phenylbutazone (1 to 2 g twice a day) or flunixin meglumine (500 mg once or twice daily) is commonly used for this purpose. The author believes that corticosteroids are *contraindicated* in bacterial pleuropneumonia.

Rest and the provision of an adequate diet are important components of the treatment of pleuropneumonia. Because the disease course and period of treatment are usually prolonged, attempts should be made to encourage eating.

PROGNOSIS AND SEQUELAE. A guarded prognosis must always be given in cases of equine pleuropneumonia. Prognosis for survival and return to normal athletic function is determined by the severity and duration of the disease process and the development of complications. In general, when an early diagnosis is made and aggressive therapy is provided, the prognosis for survival is good for many horses with pleuropneumonia.

Earlier studies reported that approximately 40% to 45% of horses recover from pleuropneumonia and 50% of the recovered group return to normal function. Others are well enough to use as breeding or pleasure horses. With the improved ability to diagnosis and treat the disease, survival rates are increasing to approximately 75%.

Serial examinations to monitor response to therapy are critical to dictate alterations in treatment and to detect complications. Frequent sonographic exams are critical for assessing changes in location, character, and amount of pleural fluid, fibrin, debris, and abscessation.

REFERENCES

93. Chaffin MK, Carter GK: Equine bacterial pleuropneumonia. I, Epidemiology, pathophysiology, and bacterial isolates, *Compend Cont Educ Pract Vet* 15:1642-1650, 1993.
94. Chaffin MK, Carter GK, Redford RL: Equine bacterial pleuropneumonia. II, Clinical signs and diagnostic evaluation, *Compend Cont Educ Pract Vet* 16:362-378, 1994.
95. Chaffin MK, Carter GK, Byers TD: Equine bacterial pleuropneumonia. III, Treatment, sequelae, and prognosis, *Compend Cont Educ Pract Vet* 16:1585-1589, 1994.
96. Chaffin MK, Carter GK: Bacterial pleuropneumonia. In Robinson NE, ed: *Current therapy in equine medicine*, ed 4, Philadelphia, 1997, WB Saunders, pp 449-452.
97. Sweeney CR, Divers TJ, Benson CE: Anaerobic bacteria in 21 horses with pleuropneumonia, *J Am Vet Med Assoc* 187:721-724, 1985.
98. Sweeney CR, Maxson AD: Equine pleuropneumonia: the value of thoracic ultrasonography in diagnosis and management, *Equine Vet Educ* 7:330-333, 1995.
99. Reimer JM: Diagnostic ultrasonography of the equine thorax, *Compend Cont Educ Pract Vet* 12:S1321-1327, 1990.

STREPTOCOCCUS EQUI INFECTION (STRANGLES)

CORINNE R. SWEENEY

ETIOLOGY. Strangles, or *Streptococcus equi* subspecies *equi* infection, was one of the first equine diseases described in the early veterinary science publications. In 1664, Solleysel, concerned for strangles's contagious nature, recommended isolation of the affected animals and pointed out that the most common source of infection for horses was water buckets that had been used for infected animals. This advice remains valid today because strangles is probably the perfect example of contagious infection as manifested in the horse. The organism may vary in strength from strain to strain and situation to situation, but the severity of infection is much more related to the health and inherent resistance of the horse than to variations in the organism itself.

PATHOGENESIS. Following entry into a new host, *S. equi* attaches primarily to cells on the tonsillar crypts and the ventral surface of the soft palate and is detectable in the mandibular or retropharyngeal lymph nodes a few hours after infection. The organism slowly multiplies extracellularly in the lymph node, forming long chains and attracting large numbers of neutrophils. Pus in the resulting abscesses contains large numbers of *S. equi* that remain viable in the face of antibody responses. Resistance to phagocytosis mediated by a combination of the hyaluronic acid capsule and antiphagocytic SeM protein is the key feature of *S. equi* virulence. The guttural pouch is commonly infected during the early stages of strangles. In a small percentage of animals the infection may persist for many months, with intermittent nasal shedding.[100]

CLINICAL SIGNS AND DIAGNOSIS. Strangles is characterized by sudden onset of fever and upper respiratory tract catarrh (Fig. 29-16), followed by acute swelling and subsequent abscess formation in submaxillary, submandibular, and retropharyngeal lymph nodes (Fig. 29-17). The name strangles was coined because affected horses that were not treated often suffocated because the lymph nodes became enlarged and obstructed the pharynx.

The first clinical signs are seen 7 to 12 days after exposure to an infected horse. The horse is depressed, anorectic, and febrile. Submandibular lymph node enlargement can be observed and palpated. The horse may stand with its neck stretched and may be reluctant to swallow. These signs are ac-

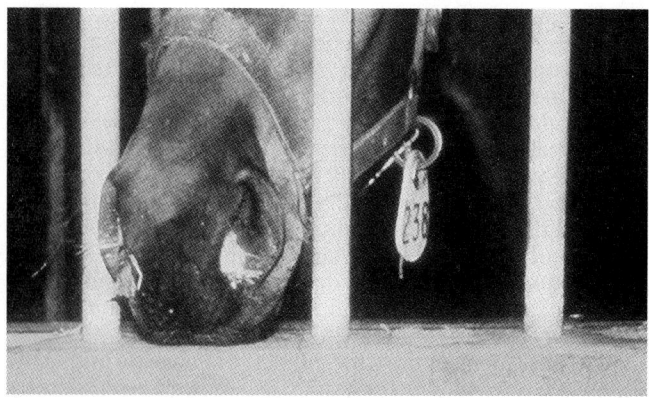

FIG. 29-16 Horse with bilateral thick purulent nasal discharge typical of strangles.

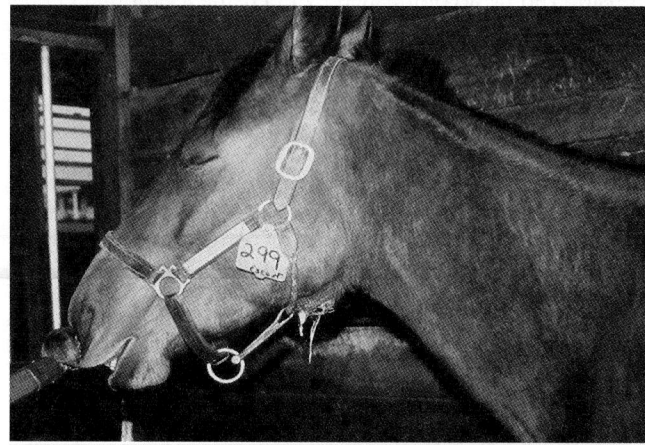

FIG. 29-17 Submandibular lymphadenopathy in a Standardbred yearling with strangles.

companied by a serous nasal discharge that rapidly becomes mucopurulent. The onset of fever is 2 to 9 days before nasal shedding is detectable.

Acute inflammatory swelling of the lymph nodes is firm, but the nodes begin to fluctuate as liquefaction and suppuration develop. The typical and favorable outcome of the lymphadenitis is for the abscess to rupture onto the skin. Rupture is preceded by epilation and oozing of serum. In most horses, abscess of one, some, or all of the submandibular, submaxillary, or retropharyngeal lymph nodes develops 7 to 14 days after the initial onset of signs. With extensive abscessation, there may be respiratory obstruction and dyspnea. Lymph nodes may drain and cause empyema of the guttural pouches. Reported morbidity rates range from 30% to 100%, whereas mortality rates range from 0% to 10% of affected horses. Horses usually recover completely after rupture of the lymph nodes, though complications may develop.[101]

In older animals with residual immunity to *S. equi*, strangles may present as an atypical or catarrhal form of the disease. Atypical strangles is clinically milder in character, with a slight nasal discharge, cough, slight fever in some animals, and abscessation of lymph nodes in only a small proportion of cases.[100]

Diagnosis of strangles is usually based on the presence of classic clinical signs of lymphadenopathy with subsequent abscessation and rupture. A diagnosis of *S. equi* infection can

only be confirmed by isolation of the *S. equi* from either a nasal or a lymph node discharge. Nasal washes are more sensitive in detection of small numbers of organisms because a greater surface area within the internal nares is sampled. The only reliable means of identifying guttural pouch carriers is endoscopic examination to confirm empyema and/or chondroids and to sample pouch content. Polymerase chain reaction (PCR) testing combined with culture greatly increases the carrier detection rate, but long-term carriers may remain PCR positive for months after viable organisms are cultured, suggesting that DNA persists for some time following death of *S. equi*. In contrast, nasal swabs and washes become PCR negative shortly after viable organisms are no longer detectable. This is explained by rapid mucociliary clearance from the nasopharynx. PCR is at least three times as sensitive as culture in detection of *S. equi* in nasal swabs and cultures and can be completed in 4 to 6 hours.[100]

Because in both natural and experimental outbreaks of strangles nasal swab cultures are not consistently positive for *S. equi*, the author's rule of thumb is "if it looks like strangles, treat it like strangles."

EPIDEMIOLOGY. Strangles can occur in horses of any age, but the 1-to-5-year-old group is predisposed, most likely because they are immunologically naive. Although the majority of animals with strangles are subsequently immune, some may contract the disease a second or even a third time. Strangles is highly contagious, with transmission occurring by the oral and nasal routes. An obligate parasite of equids, *S. equi* relies on its host for survival and interepizootic maintenance.

S. equi is transmitted through direct contact with the mucopurulent discharges from infected horses or from such fomites as feeding utensils, buckets, and other equipment. Transfer from horse to horse usually involves direct face to face contact or exposure of horses to contaminated feed, water, hands, veterinary instruments, grooming tools, or twitches. There is enormous potential for environmental contamination with *S. equi*. *S. equi* may survive for several weeks in water troughs but dies quickly in soil and on pasture. Communal drinking sources play an important role in the rapid dissemination of infection because of contamination by nasal discharges. The organism will remain viable in frozen discharges. Otherwise, survival requires moisture and protection from sunlight and environmental microbial contaminants. With the exception of drinking water, the environment is probably not a significant source of *S. equi* except during an epizootic and for a few days thereafter.

Because the organism is not known to persist in the environment, the usual source of infection is an infected horse. Interepizootic maintenance of the organism has not been well explained other than by survival in herds experiencing cases of strangles or rarely in carrier animals. Introduction of infection into a herd or stable is usually by means of an animal that is either incubating the disease or is asymptomatic. Occasionally, however, the disease breaks out in stables that have had no recent arrival and no known contact with infected horses. In this situation, the organism has apparently persisted in the tissues of the nasopharynx of recovered or carrier animals for long periods and is subsequently transmitted to susceptible in-contact animals.[101]

TREATMENT. Treatment of horses with strangles depends on the stage of the disease in the individual. This section distinguishes the following four phases:

1. Horses with the early clinical signs of strangles, including pyrexia and depression
2. Horses with lymph node abscessation associated with strangles
3. Horses exposed to strangles but not currently showing any clinical signs
4. Horses with strangles-associated complications

Horses with Early Clinical Signs. Often the first clinical signs of strangles are fever, anorexia, depression, and purulent nasal discharge. If these signs are suggestive of *S. equi*, efforts should be directed at isolation of the affected horse. Further development of clinical signs of strangles, including submaxillary, submandibular, and retropharyngeal lymph node abscessation, can be arrested at this time with the appropriate antimicrobial treatment. However, there is a high probability of relapse following cessation of therapy if the horse remains exposed to infected horses. Protective immune responses are poor in antibiotic-treated horses, and thus these horses are susceptible to *S. equi* infection upon future exposure. Immediate treatment of horses that show early clinical signs should be an effective way of controlling strangles outbreaks in racing stables or riding barns, although the disadvantages of treatment just discussed should be weighed.

Horses with Lymph Node Abscessation. The second category of therapeutic consideration is treating strangles-affected horses that have already developed lymph node abscessation. Therapy should be direct toward enhancing maturation and drainage of the abscesses. Recommended procedures include: isolation of the sick horse, local application of hot packs and poultices to the abscess, and possible lancing of the ventral surface of the abscess. After an abscess is draining, it should be flushed regularly with 3% to 5% povidone-iodine. Most authors agree that using antibiotics in not beneficial after an abscess has formed. Parenteral antibiotics given after abscess formation tend to prolong rather than arrest the disease.

Some horses with advanced signs of strangles require antimicrobial treatment. If a horse shows signs of prolonged fever, anorexia, depression, lethargy, or dyspnea resulting from severe swelling of retropharyngeal lymph nodes, systemic treatment with penicillin is recommended. Rarely, affected horses may require intensive supportive therapy, including intravenous fluids, feeding by nasogastric tube, and tracheostomy. Any animal requiring a tracheostomy should be given systemic antimicrobial drugs to prevent secondary bacterial infections of the lower respiratory tract.

Horses Exposed to Strangles. Antimicrobial therapy at the time of exposure may prevent the "seeding" of the pharyngeal lymph nodes by *S. equi*. Ideally, a horse that is exposed to other horses with strangles could be treated with penicillin until the affected horses are isolated and no longer serve as sources of infection for the susceptible horse. I believe penicillin therapy can prevent an exposed horse or foal from contracting strangles during the period of therapy. If the animal is still exposed when the antibiotics are discontinued, infections may then develop.

Horses with Complications. Horses that develop complications from strangles must receive therapy directed at treatment of the specific problems. Antimicrobial therapy with penicillin is appropriate for metastatic abscessation to either the thoracic or peritoneal cavity. Horses with purpura hemorrhagica require systemic antibiotics (penicillin) and corticosteroids. Guttural pouch empyema must be treated locally either by flushing of the pouches through the pharyngeal openings or by surgical incision into the pouches through Viborg's triangle.

SEQUELAE AND COMPLICATIONS. In the majority of horses with strangles, after the lymph node abscesses rupture and drain naturally or are surgically lanced and flushed, the disease runs its course and the horse recovers uneventfully. A number of complications have been reported to occur and complication rates of 20% have been reported.[102] Mortality rates for horses with complications have been reported to be as high as 40% with the most common complication resulting in death being the development of lower respiratory tract disease.

Metastasis of *S. equi* to lymph nodes other than submaxillary, submandibular, or retropharyngeal lymph nodes or to

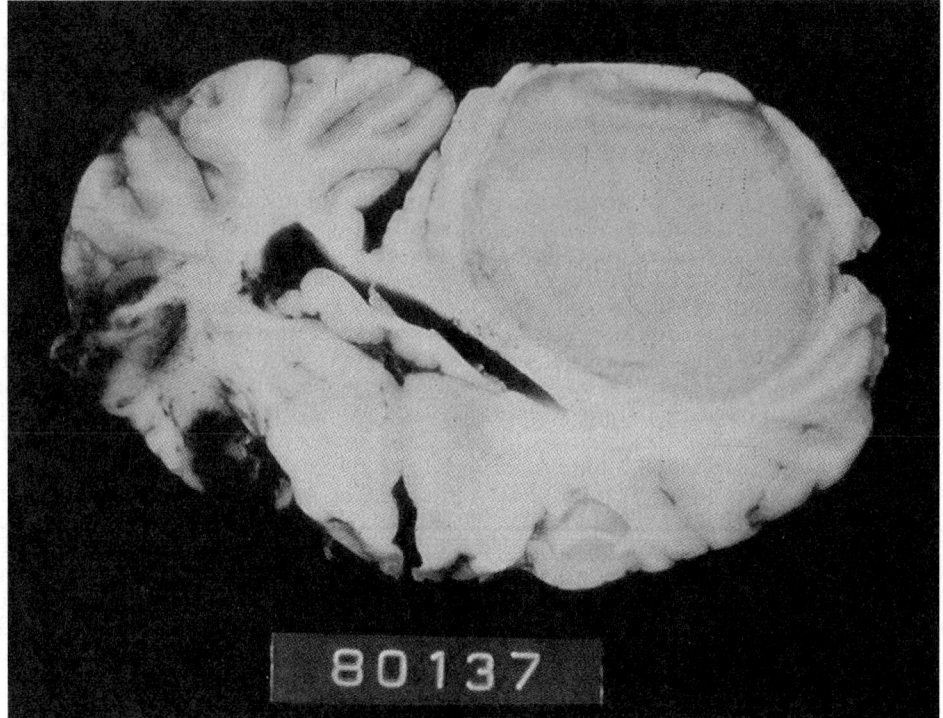

FIG. 29-18 ▮▮ "Bastard strangles," a brain abscess caused by *Streptococcus equi* in a yearling Arab colt.

other body areas is referred to as "bastard strangles." Although metastatic abscesses can occur anywhere in the body, more common locations include the lungs, mesentery, liver, spleen, kidneys, and brain (Fig. 29-18). Although the prevalence of bastard strangles is reported to be low, when the disease does occur it is difficult to treat successfully and often results in death of the infected animal. If abscesses form in the retropharyngeal lymph nodes, a horse may present for acute upper respiratory tract obstruction. The enlarged lymph nodes compress the larynx or trachea, and an emergency tracheotomy may be necessary to relieve the signs of respiratory dyspnea.

Suppurative necrotic bronchopneumonia has been reported as a sequela of strangles. Either aspiration of pus from the upper respiratory tract or metastatic spread of the organism to the lungs could be the cause. Laryngeal hemiplegia is reported as the result of damage to the recurrent laryngeal nerve from the abscessation of the anterior cervical lymph nodes or the retropharyngeal lymph nodes.

Another common complication of *S. equi* infection is guttural pouch empyema (Fig. 29-19). Myocarditis and endocarditis associated with *S. equi* infection have been reported. Purpura hemorrhagica is a serious and potentially fatal sequela to streptococcal infection.

VACCINATION AND CONTROL. Strangles continues to be a serious and common disease of horses throughout the world despite the availability of various vaccines.[103] The efficacy of these vaccines has been questioned and naturally occurring outbreaks of severe disease have been described in vaccinated populations. Vaccines consisting of bacterins or M-protein rich extracts, although immunologically potent, do not stimulate a satisfactory level of resistance. The level of immunity stimulated by vaccines is lower than that produced during recovery from strangles because of failure to produce mucosal antibodies. Vaccination during an outbreak is of no value to horses already infected. In the case of noninfected

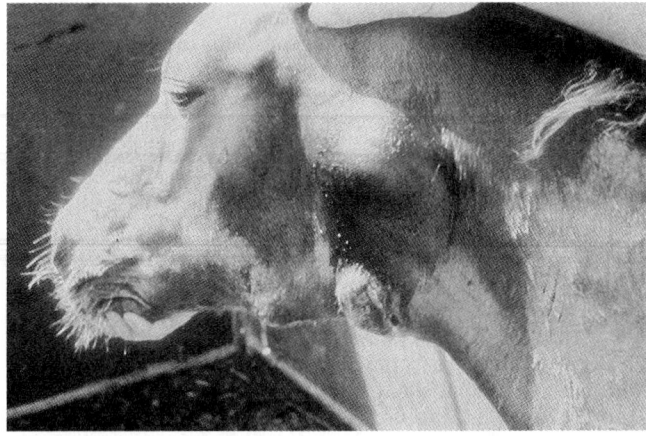

FIG. 29-19 ▮▮ Guttural pouch empyema with marked distention of the guttural pouch in a foal with strangles infection.

animals the results of one study of weanlings foals have shown the clinical attack rate was reduced by 50% during the weeks immediately after the last vaccination.

A live, attenuated, nonencapsulated mutant of *S. equi* was developed that stimulated mucosal and systemic antibody responses similar to those produced during convalescence. This mutant became the progenitor of intranasal strangles vaccine, marketed in the United States since 1998. Rapid progress is being made in development of alternative methods of intranasal immunization of horses with other antigens of *S. equi*.[100]

The lack of 100% efficacy of vaccines has placed a premium on nonimmunologic strategies of control.[104] Any plan to control strangles on a farm is designed to minimize mor-

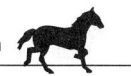

bidity, severity, and reduce the numbers and virulence of *S. equi.* If used, the duration of an outbreak is shortened. Recommendations for a control plan include the following:

- Newly introduced animals should be isolated for 2 to 3 weeks and observed for signs of strangles or other diseases.
- Rectal temperatures of new arrivals should be checked twice daily, and horses observed closely for signs of nasal discharge, cough, and so on.
- Horses suspected of being affected should be immediately quarantined.
- All tools and equipment used in the area of the infected horses, including feeding utensils, bits, bridles, bedding, tractors, wagons, and other vehicles, should be isolated from healthy horse.
- Fly control should be attempted.
- People who care for the infected horses should avoid any contact with healthy horses. This is one of the most difficult quarantine provisions.
- Rectal temperature of in-contact horses should be measured twice daily and recorded for 2 or 3 weeks.
- Horses showing temperature elevations should be cultured on three occasions at 4- to 7-day intervals after abscess drainage to determine cessation of nasal shedding and clearance of infection.
- Only severely affected animals should be treated with an antibiotic such as penicillin G administered intramuscularly. Most cases recover uneventfully without antibiotics and develop strong protective immune responses.
- An appropriate disinfectant should be used to destroy the *S. equi* organisms on the surfaces where they are located, such as stalls, feed tubs, water buckets, and vans. Because of their effectiveness in the presence of organic matter, phenolics are recommended for use in horse facilities. Bleach and quaternary ammonium compounds become inactivated by organic matter. Iodophores and chlorhexidine are most appropriately used for handwashing; formaldehyde, although highly germicidal, is too dangerous for routine use.

REFERENCES

100. Timoney JF: Equine strangles, *Proceedings of the Forty-fifth Annual Convention of the American Association of Equine Practitioners*, 1999, pp 31-37.
101. Sweeney CR: Strangles: *Streptococcus equi* infections in horses, *Equine Vet Educ* 8:317-322, 1996.
102. Sweeney CR et al: Complications associated with *Streptococcus equi* on a horse farm, *J Am Vet Med Assoc* 191:1446-1448, 1987.
103. Timoney JF: Protecting against "strangles": a contemporary view, *Equine Vet J* 20:392-396, 1988.
104. Timoney JF: Controlling strangles, *Equine Dis Q* 4:3-4, 1996.

EQUINE THORACIC NEOPLASIA

FABIO DEL PIERO
PAMELA A. WILKINS

Surveys of equine neoplasms indicate a low incidence of thoracic neoplasia in the horse (Fig. 29-20, *A* and *B*). In an abattoir survey in London of 1308 horses, 2 horses had pulmonary tumors, one granular cell tumor and one bronchiolar adenoma.[105] Two other necropsy surveys of 155 and 687 equines reported no thoracic neoplasms.[106,107] A report on chronic pulmonary disease in the horse states that the practical importance of lung tumors is negligible.[108] University of Pennsylvania researchers examined 5629 horses between 1968 and 1987. Thirty-five horses had neoplasia involving the thoracic cavity, for an incidence of 0.62%.[109]

Primary pulmonary tumors are rare in the horse. The incidence of primary lung tumors of any type is reported to be less than 1% of all reported tumors in domestic animals.[110] The lungs are susceptible to tumor emboli because of the fil-

ter action of the capillary bed associated with small capillary diameter and, perhaps, specific adhesion factors. It can sometimes be difficult or impossible to distinguish gross and microscopic patterns of metastatic disease from those of primary lung neoplasia; thus an important part of the diagnosis is exclusion of possible primary sites elsewhere in the body. Primary pulmonary tumors reported in the horse include granular cell tumor, bronchial myxoma, adenoma, adenocarcinoma, anaplastic bronchogenic carcinoma, and pulmonary carcinoma and perhaps undifferentiated sarcoma. Other primary thoracic tumors reported in the horse include pulmonary chondrosarcoma, plural mesothelioma, thymoma, and malignant lymphoma. All these neoplasms generally occur in the mature or aged horse. The exception is malignant lymphoma, which may also be observed in young animals.

Antemortem diagnosis of thoracic neoplasia depends first on recognition of thoracic disease. Most of the reported cases of thoracic neoplasia involve metastatic disease. The horses' clinical signs are generally related to the primary site of the neoplasm; thus the clinician often has no reason to suspect thoracic involvement. When respiratory signs such as dyspnea, tachypnea, hemoptysis, cough, cyanosis, nasal discharge, or epistaxis are present, relevant diagnostic tests are more likely to be performed. Ultrasonography and bronchoscopy increase the frequency of antemortem diagnosis of thoracic neoplasia.

Granular cell tumor is the most frequently reported primary pulmonary tumor of the horse with at least 15 communications in the literature. Granular cell tumors in horses are usually confined to the lungs. The neoplasia usually has consisted of single to multiple well-defined whitish compact nodules associated with a major bronchus, often protruding into the bronchial lumen or more distally within the parenchyma. Most granular cell tumors have been diagnosed only at postmortem examination, often as incidental findings. On a population of 350 mature and elderly horses examined in an abattoir by the one of the authors (FDP), two pulmonary granular cell tumors were observed. These homogeneous growths of granular eosinophilic cells expressed S-100 and occasionally neuron specific enolase, as previously observed.[111] The ultrastructural morphology of this tumor may suggest a neural origin, leading to the definition of granular cell schwannoma.

Primary pulmonary chondrosarcoma has been reported in the horse.[112] In this horse, cytologic examination of pleural fluid and an antemortem needle aspirate of the pulmonary mass revealed neoplastic chondrocytes. Another report describes metastatic chondrosarcoma in the lungs of a horse with a primary tumor in a rib.[113] A primary bronchial myxoma, characterized by loose spindloid mesenchymal cells, was reported in a 25-year-old Arabian mare with a history of intermittent coughing, hyperpnea, and respiratory disease of 2 years' duration.[114]

Primary pleural tumors are also rare. The specific type reported in the horse is pleural mesothelioma. The tumor frequently is associated with a large volume of pleural effusion. Cytologic examination of the pleural effusion revealing numerous pleomorphic mesothelial cells may aid in the antemortem diagnosis.

Thymomas are neoplasms of thymic epithelial cells, regardless of the presence or absence of lymphocytes. They are infrequently reported in the horse.[115-117] Equine malignant lymphoma occurs in mediastinal, alimentary, multicentric, cutaneous, and generalized forms; combinations of one or more of these are not infrequent. In a 1973 review of 54 cases of equine malignant lymphoma,[118] the lung was involved in 16.6% of the cases, whereas the thoracic lymph nodes were involved in 35.2%.[120] In the University of Pennsylvania sur-

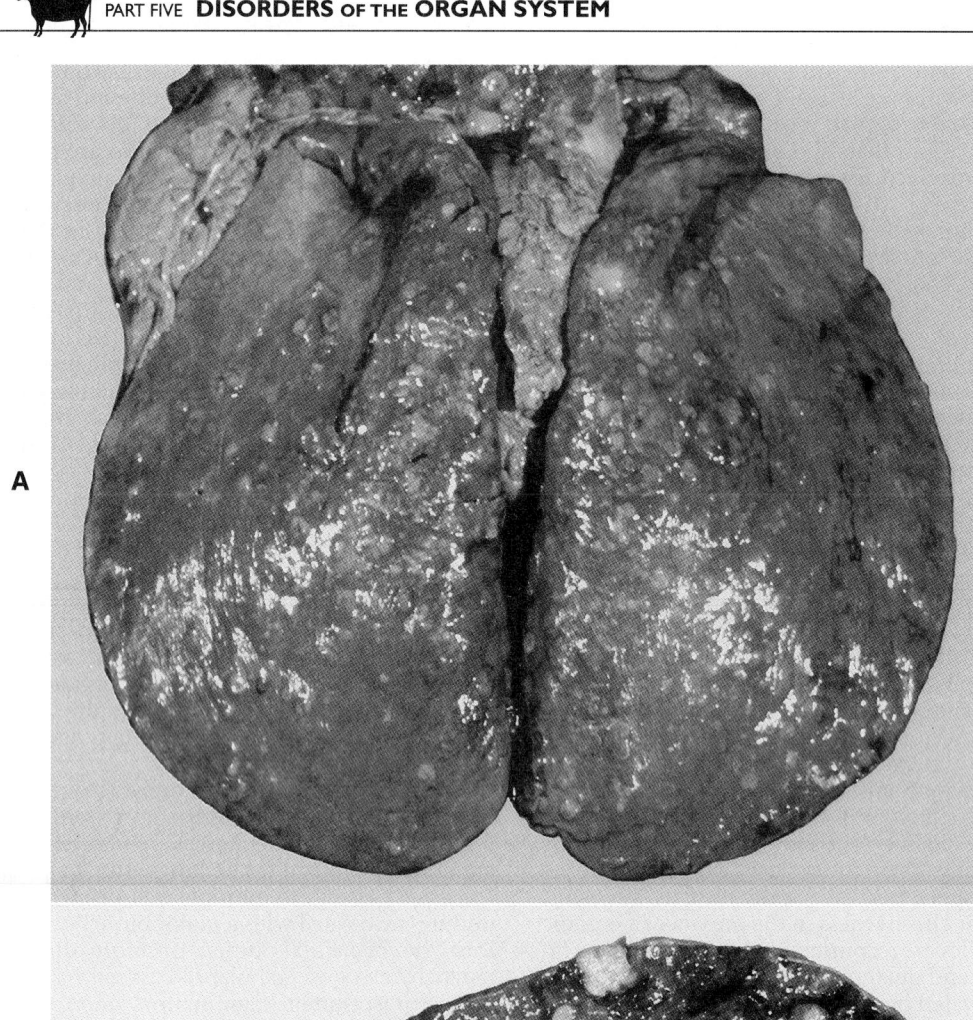

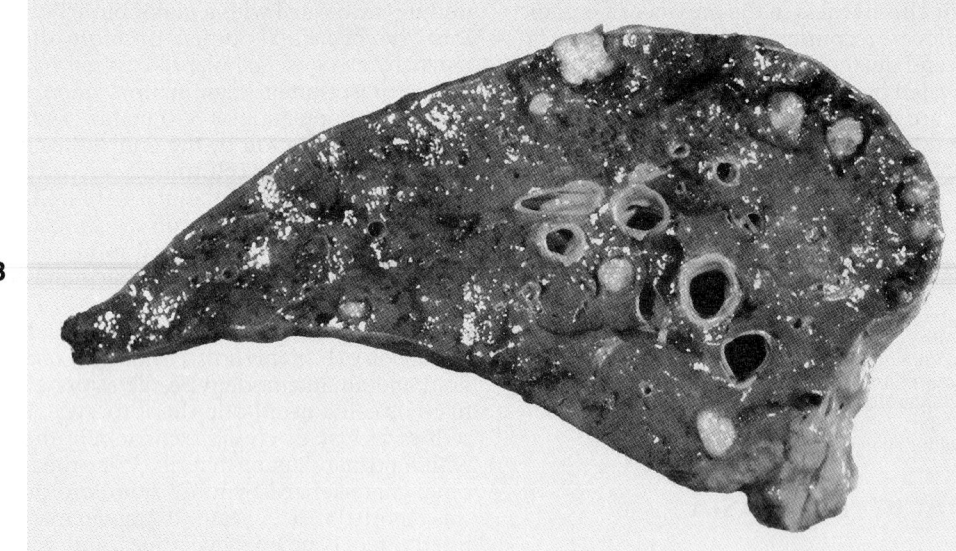

FIG. 29-20 ▍ **A,** Lung with undifferentiated sarcoma. Multiple variably sized nodules are contained within the pulmonary parenchyma and can be seen at the pleural surface. **B,** Cross section of the above lung shown in **A.**

vey, thoracic malignant lymphoma was the single most common neoplasia of the thorax and was present in 19 (54%) of the cases.[109] Pleural fluid cytologic evaluation was diagnostic in six (75%) of the eight horses. Diagnosis was made by biopsy of a peripheral lymph node in several cases. In a report from the University of Bristol, thoracic malignant lymphoma accounted for 74% of the cases of thoracic neoplasia.[120] Metastatic adenocarcinoma accounted for 20% of the cases in the University of Pennsylvania study[109] and 11% of the cases in the University of Bristol study.[120] The primary

sites of the tumor were thought to be kidney, uterus, thyroid, and ovary.

Gastric squamous cell carcinomas commonly metastasize to the thoracic cavity. Cytology of pleural fluid with identification of neoplastic epithelial pleomorphic and squamous cells has allowed for antemortem diagnosis of the carcinoma in several cases. Metastatic squamous cell carcinoma (SCC) of the thorax was found in 14% and 5% of the cases in the University of Pennsylvania[109] and University of Bristol[120] surveys, respectively. Neoplastic epithelial cells may also be iden-

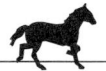

tified in biopsy specimens using "cocktails" of primary antisera containing antibodies recognizing cytokeratins of various molecular weights.

Hemangiosarcoma with pulmonary involvement has been previously reported and was found in 9% of the horses in the University of Pennsylvania survey.[109] Hemothorax, anemia, and dyspnea were commonly seen with pulmonary hemangiosarcoma. Tentative antemortem diagnosis of the hemangiosarcoma has been made by transcutaneous direct thoracoscopy and observation of the hemorrhages distributed over the visceral and parietal pleural surfaces and biopsy of these sites. Identification of neoplastic endothelial cells demarcating variously irregular sometimes blood-filled cavities allows diagnosis on the biopsy specimen. Neoplastic endothelium still expresses a variable amount of immunohistochemically identifiable factor VIII.

Malignant melanoma in a 20-year-old gelding had widespread infiltration of many organs including the lungs and pleura.[120] This pattern of distribution is not uncommon in malignant, less pigmented melanomas. Amelanotic melanomas are very rare in the horse and microscopic identification of melanin simplifies the diagnosis of these tumors. Melanocytes express S-100 protein and may present cross-reactivity to melanoma cell markers of other species.

Other pulmonary metastatic tumors reported are mammary carcinoma,[121] seminoma,[122] and malignant pheochromocytoma.[123] Metastatic pulmonary tumors have been so far examined only morphologically. The use of immunohistochemistry for the detection of specific cell markers and other sophisticated molecular studies may lead to different diagnoses.

Occasionally, a myxomatous multifocal to coalescing infiltrative neoplastic-like growth can be observed within the lung of mature and aged horses generally as an incidental finding. This infiltration is composed of loosely arranged mesenchymal cells with moderate collagen deposition.

Pulmonary hamartomas are occasionally observed in the newborn foal. Although they are nonneoplastic growths, they appear as tumorlike masses that can compress the surrounding parenchyma and cause systemic passive congestion and hydrops of the amnion in the fetus. Histologically they may be characterized by an organized proliferation of bronchiolar-like structure lined by cuboidal epithelium with lack of alveolar development or by normal alveoli, bronchi, and blood vessels but with alveolus:artery ratio greater than normal. Generally they are not compatible with a long period of extrauterine life.

An unusual progressive idiopathic multifocal granulomatous pneumonia of adult horses may resemble behaviorally and morphologically neoplasia during clinical examination.[124] Pulmonary biopsy may allow the identification of diagnostic histiocytic infiltrate with multinucleated giant cells.

Clinical signs of thoracic neoplasia are often inapparent or nonspecific, for example, depression, inappetence, weight loss, and pyrexia. More specific signs include cough, epistaxis, or dyspnea. Cytologic examination of a tracheobronchial aspirate, bronchoalveolar lavage fluid, or pleural fluid, or histologic examination of a thoracic mass biopsy with ancillary histochemistry and immunohistochemistry may allow for antemortem diagnosis of the tumor. Occasionally, electron microscopy may provide additional information. In equine patients with respiratory signs, all causes of infectious or allergic lung disease should be eliminated before considering neoplasia in the differential diagnosis.

REFERENCES

105. Cotchin E, Baker-Smith J: Tumours in horses encountered in an abattoir survey, *Vet Rec* 97:339, 1975.
106. Baker JR, Leyland A: Histological survey of tumours of the horse with particular reference to those of the skin, *Vet Rec* 96:419-422,1975.
107. Sundberg JP et al: Neoplasms of equidae, *J Am Vet Med Assoc* 170:150-152, 1977.
108. Gerber H: Chronic pulmonary disease in the horse, *Equine Vet J* 5:26-33, 1973.
109. Sweeney CR, Gillette DM: Thoracic neoplasia in equids: 35 cases (1967-1987), *J Am Vet Med Assoc* 195:374-377, 1989.
110. Priester WA, McKay FW: The occurrence of tumours in domestic animals (monograph 54), vol 56, Washington, DC, 1980, National Cancer Institute, pp 56-57.
111. Bouchard PR et al: An immunohistochemical study of three equine pulmonary granular cell tumors, *Vet Pathol* 32:730-734, 1995.
112. Clem MF et al: Pulmonary chondrosarcoma in a horse, *Compend Cont Educ* 8:964-969, 1986.
113. Sullivan DJ: Cartilaginous tumors (chondroma and chondrosarcoma) in animals, *Am J Vet Res* 21:531-535, 1960.
114. Murphy JR, Breeze RG, McPherson EA: Myxoma of the equine respiratory tract, *Mod Vet Pract* 59:529-532, 1978.
115. Whiteley LO, Leininger JR, Wolf CB: Malignant squamous cell thymoma in a horse, *Vet Pathol* 23:627-629, 1986.
116. Blanchard L, Poisson J, Drieux H: Pathologic compare des tumeurs du thymus: con interet pour l'histogenese, *Rec Med Vet* 115:129, 1939.
117. Moulton JE, Dungsworth DL: Tumors of the lymphoid and hemopoietic tissues. In Moulton JE: *Tumors of domestic animals*, ed 2, Los Angeles, 1978, University of California Press, p 177.
118. Parker GA, Casey HW: Thymomas in domestic animals, *Vet Pathol* 15:353, 1976.
119. Theilen GH, Fowler ME: Lymphosarcoma (lymphocytic leukemia) in the horse, *J Am Vet Met Assoc* 140:923-930, 1962.
120. Mair TS, Brown PJ: Clinical and pathological features of thoracic neoplasia in the horse, *Equine Vet J* 25:220-223, 1993.
121. Kato M et al: Lactalbumin-positive mammary carcinoma in a mare, *Equine Vet J*, 30: 358-360, 1998.
122. Trigo FG, Miller RA, Torbeck RL: Metastatic equine seminoma: report of two cases, *Vet Pathol* 21:259-260, 1984.
123. Froscher BG, Power HT: Malignant pheochromocytoma in a foal, *J Am Vet Med Assoc* 181: 494-496, 1982.
124. Del Piero F et al: Granulomatous pneumonia in five adult horses, *Vet Pathol* 36:498, 1999.

EQUINE RESPIRATORY VIRUSES

MARY ROSE PARADIS

Equine respiratory viruses are a major economic concern in the horse industry. Losses caused by recuperation time in the equine athlete, abortions in reproductive animals, and veterinary costs for all affected animals can be formidable to the large and small breeder and owner alike.

Most of the viruses discussed in this chapter appear clinically as upper respiratory tract problems, although the abnormality may extend to the lungs and distal airways.[125] One exception is the Hendra virus, which primarily affects the lung.[126] On presentation it may be very difficult to distinguish one viral disease from another. The major clinical signs seen on physical examination of an affected animal are elevated temperature, cough, and nasal discharge. The severity of the signs depends on two factors: the specific immunologic experience of the horse to the infecting agent and the type of virus to which the animal is exposed.[125]

Both the humoral and cellular immunities of the host appear to play a role in protecting the horse in viral disease. In most species immunoglobulin A (IgA), a secretory immunoglobulin, is the dominant antibody produced in the nasal passage in response to viral infection. It acts to neutralize and immobilize the infecting agent and aids in blocking viral penetration of the mucosa but is not effective in killing the organism. In contrast, IgM and IgG are located in higher concentrations in the lungs and are capable of enhancing phagocytosis of the virus by neutrophils and macrophages. Previous infection or vaccination stimulates production of these antibodies. Reexposure to the antigen produces an anamnestic response. This response can provide full or partial protection from the disease.[127] An important epidemiologic principle to consider in viral respiratory disease in horses is the contact rate. This will determine the likelihood of an epidemic and the speed of its propagation. The more common respiratory viruses are spread by aerosolization and inhalation of the viral particles, and by contact with infected buckets or other equipment. This makes the potential contact rate very high, especially in the racetrack and show barn environments. Combine the high contact rate with a short incubation period and an unvaccinated population and an explosive epidemic can occur. This is in contrast to the Australian Hendra virus, which does not appear to be spread via aerosol and has a lower infection rate.[128]

DIAGNOSIS OF VIRAL DISEASE. The diagnosis of viral respiratory disease in the horse is largely a presumptive diagnosis made solely from the clinical signs seen on the physical examination. In depth viral testing is not usually performed for the following reasons:

- Currently there is no therapeutic benefit derived from knowing the specific viral agent that is causing the disease.
- Diagnostic techniques available to the field veterinarian are limited, and several weeks may be required for a conclusive answer. By the time an answer is obtained the affected animal has recovered. It is hard to justify the cost of the tests to the individual client whose animal does not receive any benefit from the answer. The development of new polymerase chain reaction (PCR) testing for the different viruses with the possibility of stall-side testing would increase the usefulness of viral testing in the horse.[129-131]

Justification for viral testing can certainly be made when multiple animals are at risk of infection. Specific recommendations can be made about the vaccination program of a horse population if the prevalence of the local viral pathogens is known. A sufficiently rapid diagnosis can allow the use of specific vaccines in an outbreak. Indiscriminate use of antibiotics can be avoided if a viral origin is documented.

The three most common methods available for the diagnosis of equine viral disease are virus isolation, serologic evaluation, and direct detection of the viral particle. Nasopharyngeal swabs (with guarded culturettes) and transtracheal aspirates are the best specimens to send for isolation of the respiratory viruses. It is crucial to communicate with the laboratory to obtain a suitable viral transport medium. The inherent problems with virus isolation are that it is expensive, time consuming (2 to 4 weeks) to grow the virus, and frequently unsuccessful.[132]

The least expensive and most used method of viral diagnosis in the horse is the serologic demonstration of an antibody response in an animal. This is accomplished by comparing antibody titers during the acute phase of the disease with those of the convalescent phase 10 to 14 days later.[132] A 10-ml sample of blood is drawn from the horse and placed into a tube with no anticoagulant. The serum should be separated from the clot and frozen. The acute- and convalescent-phase serums should be submitted to the laboratory together, to ensure a valid comparison. Titers requested should include equine influenza, equine herpesvirus (EHV-1 and EHV-4), and equine viral arteritis.

A fourfold or greater increase in antibody titer is considered significant. A falling titer may also be informative. If the acute phase serum was taken 7 to 10 days after the clinical signs were first seen, the titers may be declining by the time the second serum sample is taken. The vaccination history is important when interpreting antibody levels.[132]

A single antibody titer is usually not diagnostic. However, another method of obtaining acute and convalescent titers in a herd of infected animals is to collect blood from animals that are just beginning to show signs of illness and from animals that appear to be recovering. A significant difference in the titers of these two groups of animals suggests a recent infection.[132]

Direct detection of the viral particle with fluorescent antibodies or viral RNA/DNA with PCR is available. PCR has been used in the diagnosis of equine viral arteritis, influenza, and herpes 1 and 4.[129-131] An advantage of the PCR technique is the speed at which the virus can be identified.[133]

TREATMENT. Isolation of horses that exhibit clinical signs of upper respiratory disease is important in decreasing the spread of the virus. Specific antiviral drug therapy is limited by the lack of a rapid diagnostic test for viral infection. The drugs that are currently under investigation (adamantanamine, acyclovir) may be of little therapeutic value after a horse has become infected with the virus.[132,134]

General supportive care should include a well-ventilated stall or shed with protection from foul weather. Nonsteroidal antiinflammatory drugs help to lower the high fevers, encourage the animals to eat, and provide some analgesia for possible myalgia. Rest should be enforced for a minimum of 1 week after the clinical signs have resolved. If coughing occurs when exercise is resumed, rest should continue. A convalescent period of 3 to 4 weeks is generally needed for complete resolution of an uncomplicated viral respiratory problem.[125,134-136]

In cases in which the fever persists for more than 5 days and the nasal discharge changes from serous to mucopurulent, a secondary bacterial infection should be suspected. A transtracheal aspiration should be performed, and the exudate should be submitted for culture and sensitivity testing. Antibiotic therapy can then be initiated.[136] The most common secondary bacterial infectious agent is *Streptococcus equi* var. *zooepidemicus*.

EQUINE INFLUENZA

Equine influenza has a worldwide distribution and is frequently seen in mobile populations of horses. In a surveillance study preformed in Colorado, influenza was the most common cause of upper respiratory infection in horses.[137] It has a sudden onset and a short incubation period (1 to 3 days). Disease outbreaks usually occur in horses 1 to 3 years of age. This time corresponds with the general mixing of susceptible animals at the racetrack or showgrounds. Influenza also infects older horses, but signs are usually milder and may be subclinical despite rises in titers. Although infections can occur at any time of the year, they appear more frequent in the winter and spring.[125,134,135,138] Low ambient temperatures and humidity enhance viral survival.[139]

CLINICAL SIGNS. The first clinical sign that may be evident in an infected horse is the sudden onset of a high fever. This temperature elevation may reach 41° C (106° F) and it often is biphasic. A cough and a serous nasal discharge accompany the fever, or they may appear several days later. The cough may persist up to 3 weeks and is easily induced with tracheal palpation. Pharyngitis and tracheitis may be diagnosed on endoscopic examination of the upper airways. A reluctance to move about is often interpreted as myalgia. In an outbreak in California, in several yearlings with influenza and very high fevers, severe myopathies developed with creatine phosphokinase values as high as 60,000 IU. Slightly enlarged intermandibular lymph nodes may be felt on palpation.

Early in the clinical disease transient changes can be seen in the differential leukocyte numbers. Circulating lymphocytes and eosinophils decrease.[140] This can be followed by an increase in monocytes a few days later. Because of the transient nature of the complete blood count (CBC) changes, the timing of the test is important if it is to be of diagnostic value. A fourfold rise in antibody titer for the influenza virus during a 2-week course of the disease is highly suggestive of a recent infection.[138]

PATHOGENESIS. The influenza virus belongs to the orthomyxovirus group. It has a lipid envelope that can be destroyed by common disinfectants. Chlorine bleaches are

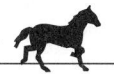

among the most inexpensive and highly effective virus disinfectants. Hemagglutinin and neuraminidase glycoproteins are surface antigens on the virus envelope that are important in the antigenic variability seen between the two equine influenza subtypes, A/equine/1 (H7N7) and A/equine/2 (H3N8).[128] An antigenic "drift" occurs when there is a minor difference in these glycoproteins. Major differences constitute an antigenic "shift." There has been minimal change in the A/equine/1 subtype since its isolation in Prague in 1956. However, the isolation of A/equine/2/Miami/63 (H3N8) represented a major shift from A/equine/1 (H7N7). A/equine/2 has undergone antigenic drifts, creating several subgroups of the H3N8 that cause epizootics around the world.[128] The Chinese strain A/equine/Gansu/1/94 infected more than a million horses and was associated with 30,000 equine deaths.[141]

Infection in a susceptible horse begins with the inhalation of the virus. Incubation time is 1 to 3 days. The virus then attaches to and propagates in the epithelial cells of the entire equine respiratory tract. In in vitro studies, equine influenza virus was associated with a scattered loss and clumping of ciliated epithelium in equine fetal tracheal and nasal turbinate organ cultures.[142] Studies show that tracheal mucociliary clearance rates, measured by nuclear scintigraphy, are reduced in horses infected with equine influenza for up to 32 days, despite clinical improvement.[143] Presumably this damage impairs mucociliary transport in affected animals, predisposing them to secondary bacterial infection. A horse with influenza may be unfit for competition for 50 to 100 days.[144]

The differential diagnosis that should be considered when an acutely febrile horse has a nasal discharge and a cough are equine influenza, EHV-1, EHV-4, equine viral arteritis, and *Streptococcus equi* infection. A commercially available enzyme immunoassay that detects influenza A nucleoprotein in humans* has been tested in the horse. Because influenza nucleoprotein is highly conserved across species, it will react with many influenza viruses despite the subtype. The test requires a nasopharyngeal swab and gives a positive or negative result in 15 minutes.[145,146]

PREVENTION. Vaccination is the key to disease prevention. It has been suggested that over 70% of the population should be vaccinated to prevent occurrence of epidemics.[144] If the vaccinated animal does become infected while its immunity is waning, the partial protection may not prevent infection, but it may decrease the duration and intensity of the illness. On the other hand, some surveillance studies suggest that vaccination doesn't make any difference in the expression of disease, the recovery of specific infectious agents, or subsequent antibody response.[147,148] Failure of a vaccination program may occur for several reasons. These reasons include noncompliance by owners because of the inconvenience of local vaccine reactions, the short-lived nature of the protection afforded by the vaccine, and the presence of antigenic variants that may not be present in the vaccine.[148] Failure of the vaccine to produce an adequate immune response in susceptible horses has also been cited.[148]

The vaccines that are presently available in the United States contain bivalent (A/1,A/2) or trivalent chemically inactivated influenza viruses. Manufacturers recommend an initial vaccination followed by a booster in 3 to 4 weeks. The animal is then revaccinated on a yearly basis. Unfortunately, in the young horse this is not sufficient for maintaining protective levels of antibody. Young horses (2 years old) appear to be less responsive to vaccination than older horses (older than 5 years).[148] It is more beneficial to revaccinate young horses and horses that may be heavily exposed at a 4- to

6-month interval. A less frequent schedule (i.e., every 9 to 12 months) may be adequate for the older regularly vaccinated animal.[136]

Antibodies against equine influenza can be found in the colostrum of foaling mares. The half-life of these maternally derived antibodies in the newborn foal is approximately 38 days.[149] Vaccination trials were conducted on foals born to mares that were vaccinated approximately 30 days before foaling. It was concluded that maternal antibodies to equine influenza interfered with the foal's response to the vaccine even up to 8 months of age. Foals from mares that had not been vaccinated against influenza were able to mount an immune response at 2 to 3 months of age, thus proving that young foals can respond to inactivated vaccines and that maternal antibodies do interfere with a foal's response to influenza vaccine.[150,151]

EQUINE HERPESVIRUS (RHINOPNEUMONITIS)

Equine herpesvirus 1 (EHV-1) and equine herpesvirus 4 (EHV-4) are the most clinically important α-herpesviruses affecting the equine respiratory tract. Formerly thought to be subtypes of the same virus (EHV-1), they were reclassified as EHV-1 and EHV-4 in the early 1990s on the basis of their different responses to monoclonal antibodies.[152] They can also be differentiated through the use of PCR.[133]

The mode of transmission of EHV-1 and EVH-4 in susceptible horses is through the respiratory system. The incubation period is 3 to 7 days. After inhalation the virus attaches to and replicates in the mucosal epithelial cells of the nasal passages, pharynx, and tonsillar tissue. The virus is then transported to other organs by mononuclear cells; the T lymphocyte is the predominant cell that harbors the infective particle.[152,153] It has been established that both EHV-1 and EHV-4 have a latent state. In one abattoir study with the use of PCR, both viruses were demonstrated to be present in leukocytes and 70% of the bronchial lymph nodes. EHV-1 was frequently found in other lymph nodes, whereas EHV-4 was only occasionally seen outside the bronchial lymph nodes.[154] Equine herpesvirus (EHV-2) has also been found to be present in 90% of the equine population.[154] Current work suggests that it may play a role in transactivating EHV-1. Viral inoculation of tracheal and nasal turbinate organ cultures with EHV can produce extensive damage to the epithelial layer.[142] In vivo, these lesions represent edema, hyperemia, and petechial hemorrhages of the upper respiratory tract of the horse. The demonstration of viral inclusion bodies in these animals is inconsistent.[155] The differential diagnosis for a horse with the respiratory signs of EHV is the same as that considered in equine influenza.

CLINICAL SIGNS. The respiratory signs of EHV-1 and EHV-4 infection are clinically indistinguishable. The respiratory form is commonly seen in the horse's first year of life or soon after entry into a training situation. The distribution of the virus appears to be worldwide. The acute respiratory disease has a sudden onset of pyrexia, which is often biphasic, reaching spikes of 41° C (106° F). A serous nasal discharge progresses to mucopurulence. Coughing is not a dependable sign.[152] It has been stated that one third of the upper respiratory diseases seen at the racetrack can be attributed to EHV.[136,137] EHV-1 infection in the horse can also present as neonatal deaths, abortions, and myeloencephalopathy.[134,135,152,155]

Neonatal foals infected with EHV-1 may be normal at birth but within the first week of life become weak and lethargic. The illness progresses to respiratory distress, tachycardia, hyperemic mucous membranes, and intractable diarrhea. Prognosis is poor. Postmortem interstitial pneumonia accompanied by hypoplasia of the thymus and spleen is

---

*Directigen Flu A, Becton-Dickinson Microbiological Systems, Cockeysville, Md; Directigen Kit, Centaur Inc, Overland Park, Kan.

found.[155] The abortion and myeloencephalopathy forms of EHV-1 are discussed elsewhere under the appropriate system.

The clinical pathologic findings in respiratory EHV infection include a leukopenia and a fourfold rise in antibody titer from the acute to the convalescent sera. Care must be taken to obtain the two sera samples at the appropriate times because the EHV-1 antibodies are short-lived and will be decreasing if the second sample is taken late. Diagnostic serologic testing is not as helpful in the confirmation of the abortigenic form of EHV-1 because the initial infection may occur several months before the abortion takes place.[132] PCR has been useful in detecting EHV-1 DNA in an aborted fetal sample in which a pathologic diagnosis of infection was made but virus isolation was negative.[130]

PREVENTION. Vaccines for EHV-1 and EHV-4 are currently available as a monovalent modified live vaccine or a divalent killed vaccine. They can be combined with equine influenza virus vaccine. Though adequate antibody response occurs after vaccination, this titer is short-lived. Vaccinated animals may actually become infected and shed virus in nasal secretions, but the severity and length of illness are usually attenuated. High levels of circulating antibody to EHV-1 provide some cross-reactivity to EHV-4 but type-specific vaccination offers more specific antibody protection.[152] The monovalent modified live vaccine may offer an enhanced cell-mediated immunity.[156,157] Vaccination does not offer protection against the neurologic form of EHV-1. Because of a short-lived immune response, revaccination every 2 to 3 months is recommended. Maternal antibodies against EHV are present in colostrum. The half-life of these colostral antibodies is approximately 1 month. Foals from vaccinated dams become susceptible to the disease at 3 months of age.[156] Foals appear to be less responsive to vaccination than adults.[156]

Equine herpesvirus 2 (EHV-2) is a slow-growing virus, sometimes referred to as equine cytomegalovirus. It is highly cell-associated and establishes a persistent infection in the horse. Most adult horses have antibody titers to EHV-2, and virus can be isolated from their leukocytes.[158] Viral antigens have been isolated from macrophages harvested from bronchoalveolar lavage of horses with chronic pulmonary disease.[159]

Clinically EHV-2 has been linked to respiratory disease in foals. One author[160] has suggested that EHV-2 played an initiating role in a chronic nonresponsive pneumonia in four Arabian foals. Nasal scrapings from the foals and frozen sections from the lungs of a foal that died of the pneumonia all gave positive results for EHV-2 using fluorescent antibody techniques. Bacterial culture findings were also positive but were thought to be secondary to the viral disease. Firm, rubbery, enlarged lungs that failed to collapse were found at necropsy. Microscopically there was thickening of the septal walls by increased numbers of mononuclear cells. No exudate was seen in the airways or alveoli. These foals had none of the signs of immunodeficiency.[160]

Because of the widespread distribution of EHV-2 in the equine population and the relative lack of clinical disease associated with the virus, its significance as a respiratory pathogen is questioned. There is no vaccine available for prevention of EHV-2.

EQUINE VIRAL ARTERITIS

Equine viral arteritis (EVA) was first identified in 1953, when an outbreak of a respiratory/abortion syndrome occurred on a Standardbred breeding farm in Ohio. Concern over the virus declined over the years until 1984, when it was isolated from an outbreak in Kentucky.[161-163] The most recent outbreak in the United States occurred in the summer of 1993 at Arlington International Race Course in Illinois. Equine viral arteritis has been isolated from horses in the United States,

Austria, Australia, and Switzerland. A serosurvey for EVA antibodies adds France, South Africa, Poland, Morocco, Germany, Tunisia, Sicily, Spain, United Kingdom,[164-171] and Canada to the list of countries that have evidence of EVA infection.[164-175] Some authors have shown that the virus tends to spread slowly, with the incidence of seropositive animals increasing with age. Outbreaks in the United States have occurred in areas where there is a high concentration of horses and where these animals are very transient (i.e., at racetracks and on breeding farms). For some undetermined reason there appears to be a breed predilection. Seroprevalence in the Standardbred population can be as high as 80%.[161]

CLINICAL SIGNS. The clinical signs of EVA infection can vary from subclinical to severe disease and death. Each individual may not show all the following signs. Typically the affected animals are pyrexic, with temperatures reaching 40.5° C (105° F) for 1 to 5 days. Anorexia, depression, serous nasal discharge, lacrimation, and coughing may also occur. Edema of the limbs, palpebra, and scrotum has been reported.[161,162,176,177] In a study on the abortigenic effect of EVA, it was found that 71% of seronegative pregnant mares aborted after they were exposed to the virus by natural transmission.[178] In the 1984 Kentucky outbreak, some of the cases were so mild that only the heightened awareness of the disease made it possible to identify these animals and subsequently to isolate virus from them.[162]

Neonatal foals infected with EVA show severe respiratory signs and a high mortality. In foals that survive more than 24 hours, a fever and leukopenia or thrombocytopenia are present. Interstitial pneumonia, lymphocytic arteritis/periarteritis, renal tubular necrosis, and fibrinoid necrosis of the tunic media are seen on pathologic examination.[179]

A fourfold increase in the EVA titer is highly suggestive of a recent infection with the virus. A leukopenia is the only clinical pathologic finding seen on the CBC.[176]

PATHOGENESIS. EVA is classified in the *Arterivirus* genus and family Arterivirdae.[180] Only one serotype has been identified.[177] Both venereal and inhalation transmission of the virus occurs in EVA. It has been shown that chronic carrier stallions can continue to shed virus in the semen for months to years.[161,163] The carrier state in the stallion is testosterone dependent and serves as the natural reservoir for EVA.[181,182] EVA can be transmitted through artificial insemination of chilled semen.[177] Of seronegative mares 85% to 100% become infected when bred to a carrier stallion. Infected mares can spread the virus laterally through aerosolization.[161] EVA virus can also be isolated from the urine.[183]

EVA is a panvasculitis, with all areas of the cardiovascular system involved. The virus is picked up by macrophages in the lung and transported to the bronchial lymph nodes, from which it is spread to the circulatory system. Replication occurs in the macrophages and the mesothelium and endothelium of various organs. A necrotizing arteritis of the small arteries of the muscle is seen on histopathologic examination of the tissues from affected animals.[161,166] This accounts for the edema that is seen clinically.

PREVENTION. Both a modified live and a killed vaccine against EVA have been developed in recent years. The modified live vaccine provides complete or partial protection against the clinical signs of EVA, but viral replication still occurs after challenge. This has been shown with the secondary humoral response in serum antibody titers.[184,185] The duration of vaccinal protection appears to be as long as 2 years. No significant secondary rise in antibody titer was noted after challenge of horses previously vaccinated with the killed vaccine, indicating that this vaccine provides protection from EVA infection.[186] Foals gain some protection against EVA through the absorption of colostral antibodies from the mare. These passively derived antibodies can no longer be found after 2 to 6 months.

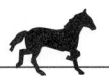

Timoney and McCollum[177] report that an important step in EVA control is the identification of carrier stallions. Mares being bred to carrier stallions should either be positive themselves or be vaccinated against EVA. Negative stallions should be on an annual vaccination program. Consideration should be given to vaccinating young colts before they reach sexual maturity to minimize the risk of infection. Fresh and frozen semen from carrier stallions is also infective and negative mares receiving this semen should be vaccinated.[177]

EQUINE RHINOVIRUS

Equine rhinovirus (ERV), a picornavirus, is another virus of questionable clinical significance. Two subtypes have been identified, ERV-1 and ERV-2. It is thought that their genetic structure is related to foot and mouth disease virus.[187] Antibodies can be found in 60% to 80% of horses over the age of 5 years. In contrast to the extensive damage produced by EHV-1, very little abnormality is found in organ cultures of equine respiratory tract epithelia inoculated with ERV.[142] In a study of 2-year-old racehorses, horses that seroconverted for ERV-1 exhibited minor, transient temperature elevations and minimal, but significant changes, in their polymorphonuclear cells during the presumed time of infection.[188] In a Canadian study, 28 of 92 horses exhibiting mild respiratory disease cultured positive for ERV-2.[147]

The reported clinical signs in ERV range from fever, anorexia, nasal discharge, and pharyngitis to a transient fever with no other signs. No vaccine is available for prevention of infection.

EQUINE ADENOVIRUS

Equine adenovirus (EAV) infection results in severe respiratory disease in Arabian foals that have the inherited condition of combined immunodeficiency (CID) (see Chapter 49). Newborn non-CID foals that were experimentally inoculated with EAV generally had a mild, transient lymphopenia followed by a lymphocytosis. In these foals, cough, fever, tachypnea, and nasal and ocular discharges developed. The clinical signs disappeared by day 10 after infection. In colostrum-deprived foals the lesions seen on postmortem examination were more severe than in those foals that received colostrum.[189]

Equine adenovirus is widespread in the equine population. It persists in the upper respiratory tract of adult horses, which acts as a carrier or reservoir host for the virus. Infection can be confirmed by serum titers. This virus is of little consequence except in the immunocompromised animal.[190]

HENDRA VIRUS

Hendra virus (HeV, equine morbillivirus, EMV), a member of a new genus within the Paramyxoviridae family, was first isolated in Hendra, a suburb of Brisbane, Queensland, Australia in 1994 from an acute outbreak of respiratory disease in which 21 horses and 2 humans were affected. The affected horses exhibited signs of respiratory difficulty and high fevers (up to 41° C). Fourteen of the horses died or were euthanized.[191] One of the affected humans also died.[126] Necropsy findings in the naturally affected horses included pulmonary edema, interstitial pneumonia with hemorrhage, dilated lymphatics, alveolar thrombosis and necrosis, and necrosis of the walls of small blood vessels. Endothelial syncytial giant cells were found in the capillaries and arterioles of the lungs.[126]

A second focus of infection involving two horses and one human was discovered retrospectively. This incidence occurred about a month before the reported outbreak, on a farm approximately 1100 km away. One horse exhibited signs of severe respiratory distress, ataxia, and swelling of the head. The second horse was reported to wander aimlessly and to have muscle fasciculation and a hemorrhagic nasal discharge. There was an 11-day interval between the deaths of the horses, which was consistent with a proposed 8 to 14 day incubation suggested by the Hendra outbreak. Histopathology of the lungs was only available in one of these animals, but it was similar to the findings of the Hendra outbreak with vasculitis and multinucleate giant cells or syncytial cells in the vascular endothelia. These cells were positive on indirect immunofluorescence test for HeV.[192,193]

Extensive serologic studies of HeV in the Queensland horse population were negative for the virus.[193] Serologic studies of other animal species were also negative except for the fruit bat (flying foxes, *Pteropus* spp.). There was a high prevalence of antibody to HeV in the fruit bat, indicating that it may be a wildlife reservoir for the virus. Clinical signs of the disease can be reproduced experimentally in the horse and cat but although the fruit bat seroconverts postinfection, it does not appear to develop clinical signs.[128] Transmission studies between inoculated bats, cats, and horses indicate that it is not a highly infectious disease under experimental circumstances. Virus has been isolated from the kidney and the urine and not from the nasal cavity or trachea of experimentally infected horses. This suggests a possible oral inoculation from infected urine contamination of the environment.[128]

REFERENCES

125. Kohn CW: Recognition and management of equine viral respiratory diseases, *Compend Cont Educ* 3:S101, 1981.
126. Murray K et al: A morbillivirus that caused fatal disease in horses and humans, *Science* 268:94-97, 1995.
127. Wilkie BN: Respiratory resistance to microbial pathogens, *Proceedings of the Twenty-eighth Annual Convention of the American Association of Equine Practitioners,* 1982, p 317.
128. Williamson MM et al: Transmission studies of Hendra virus (equine morbillivirus) in fruit bats, horses and cats, *Aust Vet J* 76:813-818, 1998.
129. Belak S et al: Evaluation of a nested PCR assay for the detection of equine arteritis virus infection, *Proceedings of the Seventh International Conference on Equine Infectious Diseases,* Newmarket, 1994, R&W Publications, pp 33-38.
130. Mackie JT et al: Diagnosis of equine herpesvirus 1 abortion using polymerase chain reaction, *Aust Vet J* 74:390-391, 1996.
131. Oxburgh L, Hagstrom A: A PCR based method for the identification of equine influenza virus from clinical samples, *Vet Microbiol* 67:161-174, 1999.
132. Crawford TB: Diagnostic virology in equine practice, *Proceedings of the Twenty-fourth Annual Convention of the American Association of Equine Practitioners,* St Louis, 1978, p 49.
133. Kirisawa R et al: Detection and identification of equine herpesvirus-1 and -4 by polymerase chain reaction, *Vet Microbiol* 36:57-67, 1993.
134. Scott JC, Dutta SK, Myrup AC: In vivo harboring of equine herpesvirus-1 in leukocyte populations and subpopulations and their quantitation from experimentally infected ponies, *Am J Vet Res* 44:1344, 1983.
135. Allen GP, Bryans JT: Molecular epizootiology, pathogenesis, and prophylaxis of equine herpesvirus 1 infections, *Prog Vet Microbiol Immunol* 2:78, 1986.
136. Bryans JT: Control of equine influenza, *Proceedings of the Twenty-sixth Annual Convention of the American Association of Equine Practitioners,* 1980, p 279.
137. Mumford EL et al: Monitoring and detection of acute viral respiratory tract disease in horses, *J Am Vet Med Assoc* 213:385-390, 1998.
138. Wilson WD: Equine influenza, *Vet Clin North Am (Equine Pract)* 9:257-282, 1993.
139. Beech J: *Equine respiratory disorders,* Philadelphia, 1991, Lea & Febiger, pp 153, 170.
140. Allen BV, Frank CJ: Haematological changes in two ponies before and during an infection with equine influenza, *Equine Vet J* 14:171, 1982.
141. Webster RG: China's "flu," *Equine Dis Q* 2:1, 1994.
142. O'Niell FD, Issel CJ, Henk WG: Electron microscopy of equine respiratory viruses in organ cultures of equine fetal respiratory tract epithelium, *Am J Vet Res* 45:1953, 1984.
143. Willoughby R et al: The effects of equine rhinovirus, influenza virus and herpesvirus infection on tracheal clearance rate in horses, *Can J Vet Res* 56:155-221, 1992.
144. Baker DJ: Rationale for the use of influenza vaccines in horses and the importance of antigenic drift, *Equine Vet J* 18:93, 1986.

145. Chambers TM et al: Rapid diagnosis of equine influenza by the Directigen FLU-A enzyme immunoassay, *Vet Rec* 135:275-279, 1994.
146. Morley PS et al: Evaluation of Directigen Flu A assay for detection of influenza antigen in nasal secretions of horses, *Equine Vet J* 27:131-134, 1995.
147. Carman S et al: Infectious agents in acute respiratory disease in horses in Ontario, *J Vet Diagn Invest* 9:17-23, 1997.
148. Morley PS et al: Efficacy of a commercial vaccine for preventing disease caused by influenza virus infection in horses, *J Am Vet Med Assoc* 215:61-66, 1999.
149. Van Oirschot JT et al: Maternal antibodies against equine influenza virus in foals and their interference with vaccination *Zentralblatt Fur Veterin-Reihe B* 38:391-396, 1991.
150. Van Maanen C et al: Interference of maternal antibodies with the immune response of foals after vaccination against equine influenza, *Vet Q* 14:13-17, 1992.
151. Conboy HS et al: Failure of foal seroconversion following equine influenza vaccination, *Proceedings of the Forty-third Annual Convention of the American Association of Equine Practitioners*, 1997, pp 22-23.
152. Ostlund EN: The equine herpesviruses, *Vet Clin North Am (Equine Pract)* 9:283-294, 1993.
153. Edington N: Latency of equine herpesviruses. In Plowright W, Rossdale PD, Wade JF, editors: *Proceedings of the Sixth International Conference on Equine Infectious Diseases VI*, Cambridge, England 1991, pp 195-200.
154. Welch HM et al: Prevalence of latent equid herpesviruses among a thoroughbred population. In Plowright W, Rossdale PD, Wade JF, editors: *Proceedings of the Sixth International Conference on Equine Infectious Diseases VI*, Cambridge, England 1991, pp 338-339.
155. Bryans JT et al: Neonatal foal disease associated with perinatal infection by equine herpesvirus, *J Equine Med Surg* 1:20, 1977.
156. Burrows R, Goodridge D: Equid herpesvirus 1 (EHV-1): some observations on the epizootiology of infection and on the innocuity testing of live virus vaccines, *Proc Am Assoc Equine Pract*, 1978, p 17.
157. Ellis JA, Kanara EW: Rhino-Flu EHV-1 vaccine induces specific immune response to EHV-4, *Top Vet Med* 6:8-11, 1995.
158. Gleeson LJ, Coggins L: Equine herpesvirus type 2: cell-virus relationship during persistent cell-associated viremia, *Am J Vet Res* 46:19, 1985.
159. Schlocker N, Gerber-Bretscher R, von Fellenberg R: Equine herpesvirus 2 in pulmonary macrophages of horses, *Am J Vet Res* 56:749-754, 1995.
160. Ames TR, O'Leary TP, Johnston GR: Isolation of equine herpesvirus type 2 from foals with respiratory disease, *Compend Cont Educ Pract Vet* 8:664, 1986.
161. Timoney PJ, McCollum WH: Equine viral arteritis, *Vet Clin North Am (Equine Pract)* 9:295-309, 1993.
162. Timoney PJ: Clinical, virological, and epidemiological features of the 1984 outbreak of equine viral arteritis in the thoroughbred population in Kentucky, USA, *Proceedings of the Grayson Foundation International Conference of Thoroughbred Breeders Organizations*, 1984, p 24.
163. Timoney PJ, McCollum WH: The epidemiology of equine viral arteritis, *Proceedings of the Thirty-first Annual Convention of the American Association of Equine Practitioners*, 1985, p 545
164. Bryans JT: Equine viral arteritis prior to 1984, *Proceedings of the Grayson Foundation International Equine Viral Arteritis Seminar*, Ireland, 1984, p 11.
165. Lang G, Mitchell WR: A serosurvey by ELISA for antibodies to equine arteritis virus in Ontario racehorses, *J Equine Vet Sci* 4:153, 1984.
166. Mumford JA: Preparing for equine arteritis, *Equine Vet J* 17:6, 1985.
167. Huntington PJ, Forman AJ, Ellis PM: The occurrence of equine arteritis virus in Australia (published erratum appears in *Aust Vet J* 68:49, 1991), *Aust Vet J* 67:432-435, 1990.
168. Paweska JT, Barnard BJ: Serological evidence of equine arteritis virus in donkeys in South Africa, *Onderstepoort J Vet Res* 60:155-158, 1993.
169. Golnik W, Paweska J: Prevalence of equine viral arteritis infection in foals before weaning, *Med Wet* 53:654-656, 1997.
170. El Harrak M et al: Epidemiology of equine viral arteritis in Morocco, *Pract Vet Equine* 28:285-292, 1996.
171. Eichhorn W, Heilmann M, Kaaden OR: Equine viral arteritis with abortions: serological and virological evidence in Germany, *J Vet Med Series B* 42:573-576, 1995.
172. Ghram A et al: The seroprevalence of equine viral rhinopneumonitis and viral arteritis in the northeast of Tunisia, *Arch L'Institut Pasteur Tunis* 71:5-12, 1994.
173. Guercio A, Orlandella BM: Equine viral arteritis: serological survey in Sicily, *Acta Med Vet* 40:325-329, 1994.
174. Monreal L et al: Clinical features of the 1992 outbreak of equine viral arteritis in Spain, *Equine Vet J* 27:301-304, 1995.
175. Wood JLN et al: First recorded outbreak of equine viral arteritis in the United Kingdom, *Vet Rec* 136:381-385, 1995.
176. Traub-Dargatz JL, Collins JK, Bennett DG: Equine viral arteritis, *Compend Cont Educ* 7:S490, 1985.
177. Timoney PJ, McCollum WH: Equine viral arteritis, *Equine Vet Educ* 8:97-100, 1996.
178. Cole JR et al: Transmissibility and abortigenic effect of equine viral arteritis in mares, *J Am Vet Med Assoc* 189:769, 1986.
179. Del Piero F et al: Equine viral arteritis in newborn foals: clinical, pathological, serological, microbiological and immuno-histochemical observations, *Equine Vet J* 29:178-185, 1997.
180. Cavanagh D et al: Revision of the taxonomy of the coronavirus, torovirus and arterivirus genera, *Arch Virol* 135:27, 1994.
181. Holyoak GR et al: Pathological changes associated with equine arteritis virus infection of the reproductive tract in prepubertal and peripubertal colts, *J Comp Path* 109:281-293, 1993.
182. McCollum WH et al: Resistance of castrated male horses to attempted establishment of the carrier state with equine arteritis virus, *J Comp Path* 111:383-388, 1994.
183. McCollum WH, Timoney PJ: The pathogenic qualities of the 1984 strain of equine arteritis virus, *Proceedings of the Grayson Foundation International Conference of Thoroughbred Breeders Organizations*, 1984, p 34.
184. Harry TO, McCollum WH: Stability of viability and immunizing potency of lyophilized, modified equine arteritis live-virus vaccine, *Am J Vet Res* 42:1501, 1981.
185. McCollum WH: Responses of horses vaccinated with a virulent modified-live equine arteritis virus propagated in the E. Derm (NBL-6) cell line to nasal inoculation with virulent virus, *Am J Vet Res* 47:1931, 1986.
186. Fukunaga Y et al: Immune potency of lyophilized, killed vaccine for equine viral arteritis and its protection against abortion in pregnant mares, *J Equine Vet Sci* 16:217-221, 1996.
187. Wutz G et al: Equine rhinovirus serotypes 1 and 2: relationship to each other and to aphthoviruses and cardioviruses, *J Gen Virol* 77:1719-1730, 1996.
188. Klaey M et al: Field case study of equine rhinovirus 1 infection: clinical signs and clinicopathology, *Equine Vet J* 30:267-269, 1998.
189. McChesney AE et al: Experimental transmission of equine adenovirus in Arabian and non-Arabian foals, *Am J Vet Res* 35:1015, 1974.
190. Baratt RM, England JJ, McChesney AE: Serologic comparison of seventeen equine adenoviruses isolated in the United States, *J Equine Med Surg* 1:410, 1977.
191. Rogers RJ et al: Investigation of a second focus of equine morbillivirus infection in coastal Queensland, *Aust Vet J* 74:243-244, 1996.
192. Hooper PT et al: The retrospective diagnosis of a second outbreak of equine morbillivirus infection, *Aust Vet J* 74:244-245, 1996.
193. Ward MP et al: Negative findings from serological studies of equine morbillivirus in the Queensland horse population, *Aust Vet J* 74:241-242, 1996.

EQUINE LUNGWORMS

BRETT DOLENTE

Dictyocaulus arnfieldi, the equine lungworm, may cause chronic coughing in an individual horse or pony or affect several animals simultaneously. Donkeys, mules, and asses appear to be inapparent carrier natural hosts that contaminate pastures. Up to 70% of donkeys in certain parts of the world may be affected.

In a patent infection the larvae are ingested, migrate through the gut wall, travel to the lungs, and mature in peripheral bronchi. The parasite may grow up to 16 cm long and has been seen during endoscopic examination of the airways. After a prepatent period of 2 to 3 months, the eggs are laid in the bronchi and then transported through mucociliary clearance to the pharynx, swallowed, and passed out in the manure. Egg laying is not seasonal, but because winter kills larvae on pastures, infections occur only in warm months in temperate geographic areas.

Infections are usually nonpatent in adult ponies and horses but, in foals, a patent infection may develop in the absence of clinical signs.[194] Clinical signs are those of obstructive pulmonary disease: chronic coughing, increased expiratory effort, exudate in the airways, and often audible wheezes and rales in the lungs.

The Baermann flotation technique, which can be used on feces, soil, and tissues, identifies only patent infections and is not useful in diagnosing the more common, and more important, nonpatent infections. Multiple fecal examinations may be needed to make diagnosis in patent infections. When fecal examination results are negative, presumptive diagnosis must be based on the clinical signs plus exposure to donkeys and the elimination of other causes of chronic coughing. Tracheobronchial aspirates can be very helpful; there may be an eosinophilia without neutrophilia and larvae may be visible.[195] Eosinophilia in the tracheobronchial aspirate is not pathognomonic for lungworm infection. It has been suggested that direct examination of smears of tracheobronchial

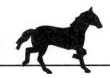

aspirates should be performed in addition to routine staining. Larvae may be seen with the former technique yet be absent after stain processing.[196] Blood eosinophilia is variable and not diagnostic. Ivermectin is effective against both mature and immature stages of the parasite and horses being dewormed every 4 to 6 weeks with ivermectin are unlikely to have clinical disease.

Necropsy of infected horses, even those with no clinical signs, reveals circumscribed, pale, raised, hyperinflated areas in the lungs that are most numerous in the caudal lobes. The small airways to the hyperinflated foci are often obstructed with mucus and parasites. The adult worm incites minimal mucus exudation, unlike the first-stage larvae.[197] On histologic examination, goblet cell hyperplasia of the airway epithelium and mucopurulent reaction with eosinophils and neutrophils surrounding the hatched first-stage larvae, are present.[197] Application of the Baermann flotation technique to diced lung tissue may be helpful in finding the larvae.

Pasturing nontreated donkeys, mules, or asses with horses should be avoided. Pastures around fairgrounds or other areas that have had a concentrated population of mules and donkeys may be especially contaminated with parasites. Frequent collection of manure from pastures is helpful and decreases the general parasite burden. Controlled studies on donkeys showed that mebendazole, 15 to 20 mg/kg/day for 5 days, was effective in decreasing worm burdens and larval counts.[194] Although fenbendazole (15 mg/kg) has been reported to be effective in causing remission of coughing, even higher doses were found to cause only a 3- to 4-week suppression of fecal larval counts in donkeys. Ivermectin (200 μg/kg PO) is effective against mature and immature stages of *D. arnfieldi* in donkeys and horses.[198,199]

REFERENCES

194. Clayton HM, Trawford AF: Anthelminthic control of lungworm in donkeys, *Equine Vet J* 13:192-194, 1981.
195. Mair TS: Value of tracheal aspirates in the diagnosis of chronic pulmonary disease in the horse, *Equine Vet J* 19:463-465, 1987.
196. George LW et al: Chronic respiratory disease in a horse infected with *Dictyocaulus arnfieldi*, *J Am Vet Med Assoc* 179:820-822, 1981.
197. Clayton HM: Lung parasites. In Robinson NE, ed: *Current therapy in equine medicine*, Philadelphia, 1983, WB Saunders, pp 520-522.
198. Britt DP, Preston JM: Efficacy of ivermectin against *Dictyocaulus arnfieldi* in ponies, *Vet Rec* 116:343-345, 1985.
199. Lyons ET, Drudge JH, Tolliver SC: Ivermectin: treating for naturally occurring infections of lungworms and stomach worms in equids, *Vet Med* 80:58-64, 1985.

HEMOTHORAX

JANE AXON

Hemothorax may result from trauma that causes lacerations to pleural or pulmonary vessels, or rupture of the large thoracic vessels. Traumatic hemothorax is often accompanied by pneumothorax. Other causes of hemothorax include rupture of lung parenchymal bullae, vessel erosion by severe lung abscessation or neoplasia, hemangiosarcoma involving the pleural surfaces, and coagulopathy. Iatrogenic causes include tube thoracostomy and lung biopsy. Hemothorax can be unilateral or bilateral depending on etiology and whether the mediastinum is intact.

Diagnosis is based on clinical examination and thoracocentesis. The horse may be dyspneic and tachycardic, depending on the volume of blood loss into the pleural cavity and underlying disease condition. Auscultation reveals a decrease in lung sounds ventrally. Heart sounds are often muffled and radiate over a wider range. Percussion, which may be painful, reveals a change from the normal resonance of aerated lung to dullness over the hemothorax. Thoracic radiographs show a loss of the diaphragmatic and cardiac silhouettes and opacity of the ventral lung fields with a horizontal fluid line. Ultra-

sonography demonstrates fluid within the pleural cavity. Thoracocentesis is necessary for assessment of the pleural fluid. Fluid should be collected for cytologic evaluation, cell count, packed cell volume, and total protein. It should be cultured if there is a possible infectious etiology. When a respiratory tract infection is suspected, a transtracheal aspirate should be obtained for culture, sensitivity and cytology. Cytologic evaluation should always be performed to determine whether there is evidence of neoplasia or infection. Absence of neoplastic cells does not eliminate neoplasia as a diagnosis. If there is bleeding elsewhere, or if a coagulopathy is suspected, a clotting profile and platelet count should be performed. The horse may develop anemia and hypoproteinemia associated with the blood loss. The thorax should be palpated to detect any palpable rib fracture or change in thoracic excursion. If there is a rib fracture, pain and shallow respiration may be exhibited.

The underlying cause should be identified and treated. Medical therapy such as intranasal oxygen administration, analgesics, intravenous fluids or whole blood if the blood loss is severe, may be required to stabilize cardiopulmonary function. Blood may be removed via a tube thoracostomy; however, a recent report documents the successful treatment of two cases of hemothorax without blood drainage.[200] When blood is injected into a normal pleural cavity it coagulates rapidly and then defibrinates, because of agitation caused by the movement of thoracic viscera. There is minimal pleural reaction and the erythrocytes are reabsorbed via the pleural lymphatics. Thus nontraumatic or noninfectious hemothorax may resolve spontaneously. However, in cases of lung or pleural trauma and infection, drainage may be necessary because there is a suggested increased chance of an organized hemothorax, and subsequent fibrothorax, forming. In cases of hemothorax resulting from coagulopathy, drainage is not recommended unless respiratory distress occurs. Fractured ribs should be stabilized. Broad-spectrum antimicrobials are recommended, because blood is an excellent culture medium.

Prognosis depends on the underlying disease. Horses with uncomplicated trauma should respond well. If trauma is the result of a penetrating wound, the prognosis is very poor because of ensuing pleuritis. Clotting disorders associated with hepatic disease have a very poor prognosis. Those secondary to drugs or chemicals may respond well to appropriate therapy and removal of the offending agent. Neoplasia has an extremely poor prognosis.

REFERENCES

200. Perkins G, Ainsworth DM, Yeager A: Hemothorax in 2 horses, *J Vet Intern Med* 13:375-378, 1999.

PNEUMOTHORAX

JANE AXON

Pneumothorax is uncommon in horses and usually associated with trauma. Puncture or laceration of the trachea, ruptured esophagus, penetration of foreign objects into the thoracic cavity, external wounds resulting in subcutaneous emphysema and pneumomediastinum, and rib fractures with subsequent damage of the lung can be causes. Horses with pleuropneumonia can develop bronchopleural fistulas and develop pneumothorax, although the air is usually contained by fibrinous adhesions. Additional causes of pneumothorax are ruptured emphysematous lung bullae and iatrogenic causes such as tube thoracostomy, mechanical ventilation, and transtracheal aspiration. The latter is usually asymptomatic and detected incidentally if thoracic radiographs are taken after the procedure.

Pneumothorax can be closed, in which air is trapped in the pleural space, or open, in which there is free communication between the pleural space and external environment.

A tension pneumothorax occurs when there is a greater influx of air into the thorax than escapes, so intrapleural pressure exceeds atmospheric pressure. A tension pneumothorax may lead to vena cava compression and decreased venous return to the heart. Pneumothorax is usually bilateral because of the incomplete mediastinum of horses. The normal fenestrations in the mediastinum may be blocked as a result of inflammatory thoracic disease or a collapsed lung.

Clinical signs seen with pneumothorax are dyspnea, tachypnea, cyanosis, and evidence of trauma. Auscultation reveals absence of normal breath sounds in the dorsal thorax. The area of abnormality will depend on the extent of the pneumothorax and volume of collapsed lung. Percussion reveals hyperresonance over the area of pneumothorax. Concurrent subcutaneous emphysema complicates interpretation. If a horse with subcutaneous emphysema is unduly dyspneic or distressed, pneumothorax should be suspected, because the former does not usually cause dyspnea unless it involves the neck and face, causing airway compression. Radiographs show the presence of pleural surfaces and lack of pulmonary vasculature in the dorsal aspect of the caudal lung fields. Ultrasonography reveals an absence of lung excursions and presence of comet tail artifacts during respiration; however, subcutaneous emphysema in tissue and fascial planes may prevent accurate sonographic imaging. Aspiration of air from the thorax is also diagnostic.

Treatment consists of relieving the pneumothorax if the horse is showing signs of respiratory distress, and treating the underlying cause. Treatment of simple pneumothorax may simply require rest and close observation while gradual reabsorption of air occurs. If hypoxemia (PaO_2 <80 mm Hg) or dyspnea is present, nasal insufflation of oxygen (15 L/min) should be administered. An open sucking wound should be occluded. Pneumothorax is treated by inserting a teat cannula or thoracostomy tube, with a suction device attached, into the dorsal thoracic cavity to facilitate the removal of air. If the pneumothorax reoccurs or continues, tubes should be left in place to allow constant air removal. A Heimlich chest drainage valve* provides continual drainage and if correctly placed is effective for long periods. Gradual reexpansion of the lungs is recommended to avoid reexpansion pulmonary edema and parenchymal trauma. Broad-spectrum antimicrobial therapy is recommended as long as the tube is in place. The wound should be explored for any residual foreign material and the extent of the wound determined to eliminate the possibility of involvement of the abdominal cavity. If the cause of the pneumothorax requires correction under general anesthesia, the horse must first be stabilized and chest tubes should be inserted for decompression, to correct atelectasis and improve ventilation. Fractured ribs should be stabilized. Tracheal defects should be sutured when possible.

The prognosis for pneumothorax is good, provided that air is removed and leaks are sealed, and infections are treated successfully. Major parenchymal lesions resulting in air leakage and esophageal ruptures have a very poor prognosis.

PULMONARY EDEMA

PAMELA A. WILKINS

Pulmonary edema rarely occurs as a primary event in the horse and, when present, is usually secondary to some other pathologic process. Extravascular fluid accumulates within the lung following events that alter hydrostatic and colloid osmotic interstitial and vascular forces, change the surface area and pore size of the blood gas barrier, or diminish lymphatics drainage.[201] Pulmonary edema can be classified as cardiogenic or noncardiogenic. Pulmonary capillary pressure can be increased by any increase in left atrial or pulmonary artery pressure. In the horse, this can occur secondary to acute renal failure, left ventricular failure, or very high cardiac output conditions, such as extreme exercise. Increases in microvascular permeability may occur with sepsis, disseminated intravascular coagulation, hypoxic acidosis, or primary pulmonary pathology resulting in the release of mediators of inflammation that increase vascular endothelial permeability. Pulmonary edema associated with airway obstruction has been termed negative-pressure pulmonary edema (NPPE) and has been reported in horses.[202,203] Negative pressure pulmonary edema occurs secondary to inspiratory efforts against a closed glottis that result in a precipitous fall in intrathoracic pressure. The large decrease in intrathoracic pressure increases the transmural pressure gradient for all intrathoracic vascular structures, favoring movement of water into the extravascular space.

Diagnosis is based on clinical examination, a history of predisposing causes, and radiographs. Horses have a shallow rapid respiratory pattern and may be dyspneic. Arterial blood gas analysis may reveal hypoxemia and hypercapnia. Fine crackles or wheezes may be audible on auscultation. Cases with volume overload (associated with renal failure or too rapid fluid administration) or primary cardiac problems may have an increased central venous pressure with pronounced venous distention. Fluid (clear or slightly yellow or pink-tinged) may drip from the nostrils and can increase in volume without necessarily becoming frothy. Progression to this stage warrants a very grave prognosis. Radiographic findings are nonspecific but include peribronchial and perivascular cuffing, increased prominence of vessels, and a hazy reticular interstitial pattern. Underlying pulmonary disease may obscure signs of edema and radiographs of sufficiently high quality to show relatively subtle changes may not be obtainable in mature horses.

TREATMENT. Treatment consists of correcting the cause, reversing hypoxemia, decreasing plasma volume and left atrial pressure, and increasing plasma colloid osmotic pressure. Intranasal oxygen and even ventilation may be needed in severe cases. Improvement in oxygenation can be monitored by sequential arterial blood gas analysis or by using transcutaneous oxygen saturation monitoring equipment applied to the nasal mucosa. In cases of NPPE, maintaining an adequate, low-resistance airway is very important to prevent further damage and tracheostomy may be necessary. Intravenous fluid therapy should be guided by the patient's needs and monitored by serial measurement of central venous pressure if necessary. Furosemide may be given intravenously or intramuscularly at a dose of 1 to 2 mg/kg and repeated in 1 hour. If helpful, the dosage can be titrated for each patient. At a dose of 1 mg/kg, approximately 8 L of urine is produced in about 1 hour.[204] Few studies have been conducted on the effects of furosemide on pulmonary hemodynamics in the horse.[205-208] The effects in horses with pulmonary edema have not been reported. Colloid solutions should be administered cautiously or in conjunction with use of diuretics because they can initially increase vascular pressure. Plasma may be safer than other colloid preparations such as dextrans or hetastarch. Colloid solutions are of little benefit in raising intravascular osmotic pressure in patients with increased microvascular permeability.

Antiprostaglandin drugs (flunixin meglumine, phenylbutazone) and antihistamines may help. Bronchodilators may be of benefit. The use of corticosteroids remains controversial; if used, antimicrobial coverage is advisable, because pulmonary edema has been shown to impair pulmonary bacterial defense mechanisms.

---

*Heimlich chest drainage valve, Band-Parker, Division of Becton-Dickson Co., Rutherford, NJ, 07070.

REFERENCES

201. Mellins RB, Stalcup SA: Pulmonary edema. In Kendig EL, Chernick, eds: *Disorders of the respiratory tract in children*, ed 4, Philadelphia, 1983, WB Saunders, pp 458-475.
202. Kollias-Baker CA et al: Pulmonary edema associated with transient airway obstruction in three horses, *J Am Vet Med Assoc* 202:116-118, 1993.
203. Tute A et al: Negative pressure pulmonary edema (NPE) as a postanesthetic complication associated with upper airway obstruction in a horse, *Vet Surg* 25:519-523, 1996.
204. Tobin T et al: The pharmacology of furosemide in the horse. III, Dose and time response relationships, effects of repeated dosing, and performance effects, *J Equine Med Surg* 2:216-226, 1978.
205. Muir WW, Milne DW, Sharda RT: Acute haemodynamic effects of furosemide administered intravenously in the horse, *Am J Vet Res* 37:1177-1180, 1976.
206. Dixon PM: Effects of furosemide on pulmonary arterial pressures of normal horses and horses affected with chronic obstructive pulmonary disease (COPD), *Equine Vet J* 12:28-29, 1980.
207. Hinchcliff KW, Muir WW: Pharmacology of furosemide: a review, *J Vet Intern Med* 5:211-218, 1991.
208. Milne DW et al: Effects of furosemide on cardiovascular function and performance when given prior to simulated races: a double blind study, *Am J Vet Res* 41:1183-1189, 1980.

SMOKE INHALATION

PEGGY MARSH

Smoke inhalation injury is typically associated with exposure to fires and there are often concurrent problems in other body systems, in particular burns. Extensive or severe burns can magnify the severity of the injuries. Extensive burns can lead to hypoproteinemia, which can worsen edema. Also, the risk of infection increases with burn-induced immunosuppression. Multiple systems are generally affected and cases can be a challenge to manage.

Insult to the respiratory system by smoke inhalation is initiated by three mechanisms. The first is direct thermal injury, which can be limited to the upper respiratory tract (URT) by laryngeal reflexes and efficient heat exchange within the nasal passages. Toxic chemicals in the smoke can cause damage, both directly and indirectly, through inflammatory mediators.[209] Finally, with combustion there is consumption of oxygen and the resulting low PA_{O_2} can lead to pulmonary vasoconstriction.

Three phases of pulmonary dysfunction have been described.[209,210] The first stage is acute pulmonary insufficiency caused by three mechanisms. Carbon monoxide (CO) may be present in sufficiently high concentration to cause toxicity within a short time after exposure. Carbon monoxide combines with hemoglobin to form carboxyhemoglobin, resulting in hypoxia. CO also shifts the oxyhemoglobin dissociation curve to the left, thereby decreasing oxygen release at the tissue level, exacerbating the tissue hypoxia. During this acute phase, progressive edema and necrosis in the URT can lead to airway obstruction. In the lower respiratory tract the irritating effects of noxious products can cause bronchoconstriction.

These insults produce the second stage; formation of pulmonary edema. Within 48 to 72 hours after exposure, driven by pulmonary macrophages, neutrophils are called into the area of insult. They release cytokines, proteolytic enzymes, and oxygen-derived free radicals. Expression of the inflammatory cascade in excess of balance causes microvascular damage, leading to increased extravascular lung water. Debris from the inflammatory cascade, along with material directly deposited from smoke inhalation, can create pseudomembranous casts, which can obstruct the small airways.

Bronchopneumonia is the last stage and occurs as a result of the impaired host immune system, both locally and systemically. This phase can occur up to 1 to 2 weeks after the initial injury.

Signs vary depending on the duration and type of exposure, and the length of time from the insult. Acutely, within the first 6 hours, signs of CO toxicity and shock may occur.

The patient shows signs of severe hypoxemia and may be depressed, disoriented, irritable, ataxic, or even moribund and comatose. As edema and necrosis progress in the URT, dyspnea and stridor may develop. Auscultation may reveal decreased air movement, crackles, or wheezes, but these may not become apparent for 12 to 24 hours. If edema of the airways is sufficiently severe, airflow may be severely restricted. Edema fluid may be visible at the nostrils and, later, may be replaced by inflammatory exudate. Signs of infection may be difficult to ascertain from other signs. All that may be noticed is a fever and a worsening of respiratory signs after initial improvement.

Diagnosis is typically based on history and physical examination. A normal initial examination does not rule out exposure because the onset of clinical signs may be delayed several days. Within a short time after exposure, carboxyhemoglobin concentration in venous blood can be measured. A level above 10% is consistent with carbon monoxide toxicity.[209] Various diagnostic tests are useful in determining the extent of injury. These include endoscopy of the URT and tracheobronchial tree, thoracic radiographs, blood gas analysis, hematology, and cytologic evaluation of tracheal aspirates. Any or all of these tests can be performed on a serial basis as prognostic aids. Serum chemistry analysis uncovers problems in other body systems.

Treatment depends on stage of injury. Initially, oxygen support is of benefit. It is a treatment for CO toxicity and helps reduce hypoxemia.[211] Humidified oxygen can be supplied by nasal insufflation or via transtracheal catheter. URT obstruction may require a tracheostomy. Attention should be paid to keeping the airways clear, and nebulization may be useful, especially when pseudomembranous casts are suspected. Bronchodilators may be useful in counteracting reflex bronchoconstriction. Decreasing inflammation and pulmonary edema may require the use of diuretics and nonsteroidal antiinflammatory drugs. Use of corticosteroids is controversial because of potential for immunosuppression and laminitis.[209] Agents with mineralocorticoid effects should be avoided because edema formation may be increased by retention of sodium. Analgesia may be needed. Secondary complications require attention. Burns and signs of shock often require the judicious use of intravenous fluids. To prevent infection, strict hygiene, meticulous nursing care, and optimal nutritional support should be provided. Prophylactic antimicrobial use is not recommended in human patients. Documented infection should be treated with appropriate antimicrobial agents based on results of culture and sensitivity patterns.

REFERENCES

209. Geor RJ, Ames TR: Smoke inhalation injury in horses, *Compend Contin Educ Pract Vet* 13:1162-1168, 1991.
210. Kirkland KD et al: Smoke inhalation injury in a pony, *Vet Emerg Crit Care* 3:83-89, 1992.
211. Kemper T et al: Treatment of smoke inhalation in five horses, *J Am Vet Med Assoc* 202:91-94, 1993.

CHRONIC OBSTRUCTIVE PULMONARY DISEASE (CHRONIC RECURRENT AIRWAY OBSTRUCTION)

JILL BEECH

Chronic obstructive pulmonary disease ("heaves" in its severe form) has been a major equine affliction for years. In most cases, chronic obstructive pulmonary disease (COPD) is associated with stabling and exposure to hay, straw, and molds, although in some areas it may be associated with summer pastures.[212-214] Both conditions are believed to be hypersensitivity diseases, but the role of IgE is still debated.

Although allergens appear to be most important, it is possible that viruses and bacteria also contribute to lower airway inflammation. In several studies of tracheal aspirates from young Thoroughbred racehorses, an association was found between lower airway inflammation and bacteria, especially *Streptococcus equi* var. *zooepidemicus*.[215,216] However, decreased mucociliary clearance and airway inflammation itself may promote secondary colonization by bacteria, and horses with COPD were reported to have more bacteria colonizing their airways compared with normal horses.[217] The role of viruses still remains undefined. In humans with asthma, especially children, viral infections are recognized triggers of bronchospasm. The incidence of COPD increases with age but it is unknown whether lower airway inflammation in young horses, if untreated or unmanaged, will progress to COPD with age. A hereditary basis has been reported, although no genetic markers have yet been identified. If one parent is affected, the risk of offspring developing chronic bronchitis was reported to be increased approximately threefold; the risk increased approximately fivefold when both parents were affected with chronic bronchitis.[218]

When horses susceptible to, or affected by, COPD are exposed to antigens an inflammatory response occurs in the airways with airway hyperresponsiveness and bronchospasm. Numerous inflammatory mediators are secreted that directly contract small airway smooth muscle and augment bronchospasm caused by other factors (such as cholinergic responses), attract neutrophils, and increase mucus production.[219-223] In addition to the above causing airflow obstruction, in vitro studies have demonstrated an absence of the inhibitory nonadrenergic, noncholinergic (NANC) system in airways from horses with COPD.[224,225] If this primary inhibitory system to airway smooth muscle is also absent in vivo in horses with COPD, susceptibility to bronchospasm would be enhanced.

CLINICAL SIGNS. Diagnosis of chronic lower airway inflammation and chronic airway disease, or COPD, may be difficult in horses that show signs intermittently or only when challenged. If horses are examined during asymptomatic periods, the diagnosis may be missed because auscultation of the thorax may be normal. Horses with mild COPD may breathe normally or have only slightly accentuated end-expiratory effort. Lung sounds may be normal or only slightly increased in loudness, but with deep breaths occasional wheezes may occur and the horse may cough. Coughing may be the major complaint of the owner. Use of a rebreathing bag to force deep breathing helps in evaluation of the lung fields. Percussion of the lung fields is normal in these cases and physical condition of the horse is unaffected. Exposure of mildly affected horses to dust or molds can increase the expiratory effort and precipitate unequivocal signs of airway obstruction. A hot, humid environment, or very cold air, may also accentuate signs, and these horses usually show exercise intolerance. In the horse that is symptomatic at the time of examination the diagnostic tests that are most helpful are a combination of clinical signs, history, response to bronchodilators such as atropine or β-adrenergic drugs, or response to changing the environment. Horses with more severe COPD have a frequent deep cough that may be explosive, paroxysmal, and sometimes accompanied by flatulence. Nasal discharge may be copious, thick, and mucopurulent or may be absent even when there is significant exudate in the lower airways, presumably because the horse swallows most of the material. Inspiration is shorter than expiration and the latter is increased in effort, which may lead to a "heave line" caused by hypertrophy of the external abdominal oblique muscles. Pumping of the anus with breathing may be seen in severe cases. Nostrils are frequently flared and the horse may appear anxious. Wheezing or mucus clicking may be audible at the nostrils. Membrane color is usually normal but may

be pale; even in very severe cases membranes are rarely cyanotic. These horses may lose considerable amounts of weight and become emaciated. Auscultatory findings vary with the severity of the disease. There may be low- to high-pitched inspiratory and expiratory wheezes. These may be diffuse or loudest ventrally or in the hilar area bilaterally. Fine crackles may be most audible in the peripheral lung fields and rales may be heard when airways contain significant exudate. A combination of wheezes and crackles, or a predominance of one sound, may be heard. Percussion of the thorax reveals normal or expanded lung fields. If right ventricular failure has developed, jugular distention and pulsation may be evident. However, despite right ventricular hypertrophy and increased weight in very severe cases, signs of heart disease are very rare.[226,227] Fever is rare, although occasionally a severe allergic reaction can elicit a fever spike. A persistent fever should make the practitioner suspect an infection.

OTHER DIAGNOSTIC TESTS. Even horses fairly severely affected, intermittently, with COPD can have normal pulmonary function test results during unchallenged times. Tidal breathing flow volume loops can differentiate between affected and normal horses even when the former are in remission, but this testing is not readily available.[228] Reportedly, lung function can vary over the day; however, results in horses with COPD have been inconsistent. One study found that horses with severe COPD had worse lung function at night with significantly different night and day values,[229] whereas another found no significant daily variations.[230] A transportable esophageal instrument for measuring intrapleural pressure is marketed for use by practitioners and has been used in horses[231] but, in my opinion, would not be very useful in most clinical situations. Raised intrapleural pressures are not consistently found in horses with COPD and are not pathognomic for COPD. Direct intrapleural pressure measurements are invasive and placement of an esophageal balloon can be problematic. Raised intrapleural pressure was reported to correlate well with clinical dyspnea regardless of the cause.[232] Radiographs are not helpful in the diagnosis of COPD per se, except for detection of other pulmonary conditions possibly contributing to, or causing, a horse's respiratory distress. In older horses, interpretation of radiographs may be difficult because with age there may be an increased interstitial pattern and some peribronchial thickening. Also, the size of the horse can confound interpretation of radiographs because size and fat affect the quality of the films. In most cases, practitioners do not have access to the type of equipment necessary to obtain adequate radiographs of large mature horses' thoraces. Ultrasonography is helpful in determining whether there is pleural disease or superficial lung pathology, and may be helpful in ruling out other diseases, but it is not diagnostic for airway inflammation or COPD. Scintigraphic demonstration of altered alveolar clearance has been reported to be a sensitive indicator of lung damage in horses with COPD, even when clinical signs and pulmonary function tests were not abnormal.[233,234] Cost effectiveness may be a factor in the use of this diagnostic tool and it is not presently readily available.

Tracheobronchial aspirates and bronchoalveolar lavage (BAL) are used to diagnose airway disease. Even when physical examination findings are relatively normal, cytologic evaluation of a tracheobronchial aspirate may reveal increased mucus, Curschmann's spirals, increased numbers of neutrophils, and sometimes eosinophils and damaged epithelial cells. Presence of eosinophils is inconsistent and eosinophilia is not characteristic of COPD. The absence of eosinophils does not rule out allergic COPD. A Gram stain usually does not demonstrate a large number of bacteria, and neutrophils do not show evidence of sepsis unless there is a superimposed bacterial infection. Culture may yield a light growth of secondary invaders, but if there is a pure heavy growth of a pathogen with cellular evidence of sepsis, significant bacterial infection may be superimposed on underlying inflammatory airway disease. Culture results should always be interpreted in conjunction with the cellular characteristics of the aspirate and the horse's clinical signs. If the aspirate is adequate in volume and quality, and is retrieved from the lower airways, but lacks excessive numbers of neutrophils, diffuse bronchiolitis can be excluded as a diagnosis, although functional broncho-constriction could still be present. The accuracy of tracheo-bronchial aspirates has been questioned and many clinicians believe BAL is more useful in diagnosing diffuse lung diseases. Tracheobronchial aspirates retrieve material from both large and small airways, whereas BAL lavage collects material from the smaller peripheral airways. (The term BAL is somewhat of a misnomer; because most of the fluid retrieved from a BAL is from the small airways, a more correct term for the procedure would be bronchial lavage.) A wide variation in the number of neutrophils in tracheal aspirates from ponies without COPD and a lack of significant correlation in cytologic findings between tracheal aspirates and BALs have been reported, suggesting the tracheal cell population differs from that in the lower airways.[235] BAL from horses with COPD show an increase in neutrophils and occasionally eosinophils or mast cells. Because of the sample collection method, BALs generally are not suitable for culture. Cell counts can vary with volumes used. BAL is not likely to be useful in an asymptomatic horse, because studies in ponies with COPD have shown the lavage cytology is not abnormal except during disease exacerbation.[236] Percentage of neutrophils in the airways varies somewhat with the environment. Exposing normal and COPD horses to a barn results in an increase in neutrophils in both groups, although the increase is significantly higher in ponies with COPD.[236] One study reported that neutrophils increased from 9% to 28% in BAL from control horses when they were stabled and fed hay.[237] However, this finding may demonstrate the difficulty of classifying horses as normal in the absence of clinical symptomatology. When deciding which method to use, the practitioner should always consider the patient's status, because the BAL procedure has been associated with distress in horses with severe COPD.[238] Partial lack of association between severity of airway obstruction and inflammatory changes in airway secretions, including BAL, has been reported in horses.[238-240] It is my opinion that tracheal aspirates can still be very useful. Obviously, if only a small sample is retrieved or the sample is contaminated with upper airway secretions, the sample will not be representative of the lower respiratory tract. Also, if many inflammatory cells are seen in the tracheal aspirate, the practitioner cannot tell if there is a focal highly exudative lesion or more diffuse inflammation. Interpretation of both BAL and tracheal aspirates must be combined with results from other tests and clinical evaluation of the animal. Blood gases indicate whether a horse is hypoxemic; however, single test results are unlikely to be helpful in prognosticating whether the horse will be responsive to treatment or the ease of management. Large variations in PaO_2 values have been reported for horses with respiratory disease, and only 72% of horses with COPD were reported to have PaO_2 values less than 85 mm Hg.[232] Blood gases have been used to help monitor response to treatment, but on a practical basis, clinical signs plus the horse's exercise tolerance are usually more important. A CBC and fibrinogen measurement may help when trying to decide if there is an infection versus bronchiolitis solely caused by allergies. However, occasionally horses with focal lung infections have a normal CBC and fibrinogen. Endoscopic examination should be a routine part of the evaluation of horses with respiratory disease. Excess secretions may be visible even when there is no nasal discharge.

Attempts to diagnose whether a horse has an allergic etiology for its respiratory disease remain problematic. Allergen skin testing has been used in horses but there is controversy over its validity. Selection of pertinent antigens for testing may be a problem, especially if the practitioner cannot identify all potential offending allergens. Interpretation must always be based on the patient's history and responses in the normal population. A positive skin test reaction does not mean that particular antigen is causing a clinical problem. Skin test reactivity to certain molds was reported not to correlate with the reactivity of the lung to inhalation challenge with those molds.[241,242] However, inhalation challenges in themselves can be problematic. Challenge with *Faenia rectivirgula (Micropolyspora faeni)*, the mold most frequently implicated in COPD, does not totally reproduce COPD.[240] A good agreement between inhalation and skin test responses was reported for *M. faeni*.[243] Individual overlap between normal horses and those with COPD has been demonstrated for numbers of reactions to many antigens.[243-245] Serologic testing to determine levels of IgE against certain antigens is commercially available but, to my knowledge, there are no published data supporting its use or comparing responses in normal horses versus abnormal horses. Disparate results can be expected amongst different laboratories because of lack of standardization of the test protocols. Studies comparing antibody levels to certain molds in the serum and BAL fluid from horses have not found a correlation.[246,247] Local production of IgE can increase without an increase in serum concentrations. Studies on pulmonary and systemic *Aspergillus fumigatus*–specific IgE and IgG antibodies in horses with COPD showed no differences in serum levels compared with control horses, although antibody levels were higher in BAL.[246,247]

TREATMENT AND MANAGEMENT. Treatment and management of horses with COPD can be difficult. Environmental changes are of utmost importance, but it may be almost impossible to eliminate the offending antigens if a horse with barn-induced COPD has to be stabled inside. One study showed that both peat and newspapers had fewer fungi and actinomycetes than shavings or straw, and hay had the most, suggesting that in many cases elimination of hay is more important than changes in bedding.[248] Some horses can tolerate hay as long as it is dampened, whereas others require its complete removal from their diet. An attempt should be made to determine whether one hay in particular is important in the pathogenesis. Hay cubes, if not dusty, may be used, or alfalfa pellets may be fed. Whenever possible the horse should be kept outside, and hay, which is usually the major source of inhaled molds, eliminated from the diet. Complete feeds can be used, but horses usually want roughage. Dust levels close to the horse's nostrils when it is eating hay can be many times higher than levels a few feet away. When hay was replaced by a pelleted diet, dust concentrations decreased to 3% of the former levels.[248] If horses cannot be housed outside, bedding should be changed to shavings or shredded paper in both their own and neighboring horses' stalls. The importance of removing hay for most of these horses cannot be overemphasized. Dampening hay may decrease respirable particles, but is not as effective as elimination of hay, and in established COPD cases it was ineffective in preventing disease.[249]

When horses are transported their heads should not be tied close to a hay net. This practice superimposes close proximity to a concentrated source of molds upon decreased mucociliary clearance caused by head position.[250] Although horses may show a rapid improvement following environmental changes, in some cases weeks may be necessary before a response is seen. When hot, humid weather or certain pastures exacerbate the condition, these further complicate management. If summer pasture–associated obstructive pulmonary disease occurs, horses must then be maintained inside. Frequently, ideal management is not possible or may be inadequate and medication is necessary.

Antiinflammatory drugs, usually steroids, are usually effective. However, side effects of chronic steroid usage can be serious and steroids may not be allowed because of drug testing of competitive horses. Intramuscular triamcinolone (0.09 mg/kg IM) significantly decreased airway obstruction in five horses with COPD for several weeks in the absence of improved air hygiene; however, in most horses improvement was incomplete, probably because of irreversible airway obstruction.[239] This dosage is more than double the manufacturer's recommended dose, and I do not recommend it. Dexamethasone has long been used to treat COPD, but clinically effective dosage appears to vary amongst individual horses. The major potential side effect accompanying systemic use of corticosteroids is laminitis, which appears to be idiosyncratic, with some horses tolerant of relatively high doses and others not. Although prednisolone has been used, in my opinion it is less effective than dexamethasone and one study evaluating response of COPD horses to 10 days of treatment with prednisone (400 mg PO once daily) showed no significant clinical response, although there was a decrease in mast cells in the BAL.[238] Beneficial effects of both inhaled beclomethasone (1320 μg twice daily) and intravenous dexamethasone (0.1 mg/kg once daily) have been reported; these drugs resulted in a decrease in pulmonary resistance, increase in dynamic compliance, decrease in maximum pleural pressure changes, and a decrease in numbers of neutrophils in the BAL.[251] Although inhaled steroids should circumvent some of the adverse effects of systemic steroids, absorption does occur and adrenal gland suppression has been documented following inhaled beclomethasone.[251] Inhaled fluticasone (2 mg) appeared effective in preliminary trials in horses with COPD.[252]

Bronchodilators have been administered orally, as well as by inhalation. The latter appears to be increasing in usage. Some studies showed an effect of inhaled pirbuterol (600 μg), albuterol (360 μg), and fenoterol.[253-255] Albuterol and pirbuterol have the same duration of action (less than 1 to 2 hours). Doubling the dosage of albuterol from 360 μg to 720 μg neither increased nor prolonged bronchodilation.[254] Most inhaled β-adrenergic drugs have a short duration of action. Salmeterol lasts 12 hours in humans, but duration of effect in horses has not yet been reported. A handheld metered-dose inhaler and a tight-fitting mask have been used for delivering pressurized inhalant drugs. When drugs are nebulized, drug deposition beyond the larynx is usually low, even with appropriately sized aerosol particles. Some horses, however, may not initially tolerate a pressurized aerosol. Intramuscular or intravenous use of β-adrenergic drugs can be complicated by side effects such as excitement, tremors, and sweating and these routes are usually not advisable. Although different β-adrenergic drugs have been administered orally to horses, to my knowledge only one field study in a large number of horses has been reported. Varying doses of clenbuterol were evaluated.[256] Incremental dosing (0.8 to 3.2 μg/kg twice daily) resulted in clinical improvement in 75% of the horses with 25% not responding to any of the dosages. However, only 24% of the horses responded to the recommended dose of 0.8 μg/kg twice daily.[256] The incidence of side effects (sweating, muscle tremor, and nervousness) was less than 7%; the low incidence of side effects was attributed to incremental dosing. Administration of large dosages of β-agonists to naïve patients is likely to cause more severe or a greater incidence of side effects.[256] Another study failed to show a significant clinical response to a 10-day course of 0.8 μg/kg clenbuterol orally twice daily.[238]

Aminophylline, a phosphodiesterase inhibitor, has been used in both horses and humans, although it has not had widespread use in the former. It can be administered orally and is effective in some horses. However, the dosage must be carefully calculated to avoid toxicity. I usually initiate treatment with 6 mg/kg orally twice daily and increase it as needed. Signs of toxicity similar to those of β-adrenergic drugs (excitement, tremors, sweating, tachycardia, etc.) can be seen, although they are unlikely at low doses and when serum theophylline levels are less than 80 μmol/L (15 μg/L). Some animals are more responsive than others to aminophylline, with bronchodilation measurable at a low serum level, but, below 59 μmol/L bronchodilator activity has been inconsistent.[257] If other drugs are concurrently administered with aminophylline, the practitioner should check for possible interactions and effect on pharmacokinetics of aminophylline because certain drugs can potentiate toxicity of aminophylline. Pharmacokinetics of theophylline in the horse has been reported.[258-260] The slow-release preparation of aminophylline does not appear to afford any advantage.[261]

Antimuscarinic drugs such as atropine and ipratropium are effective bronchodilators in horses with COPD. Intravenous administration of even a low dose of atropine (e.g., 5 to 7 mg/450 kg horse) usually evokes a rapid improvement in clinical signs of COPD. A rapid increase in dynamic compliance and decrease in lung resistance has been documented after administration of intravenous atropine.[262] However, the systemic effects (ileus, tachycardia, etc.) and potential for drying mucous secretions, deter its clinical use. Intravenous or inhaled atropine delays tracheal mucus transport rate in normal horses, although the duration of effect was not evaluated.[263,264] The inhaled anticholinergic drug ipratropium has been shown to have a bronchodilatory effect in horses with COPD without undesirable side effects.[265-267] Bronchodilation is dose dependent; 1 to 3 μg/kg has been used, with maximal effect on dynamic compliance and pulmonary resistance occurring at 2.5 μg/kg.[268] A dosage of 2400 μg was used in one study, but doses as low as 180 to 360 μg through a metered-dose inhaler reportedly have been effective.[268] Ipratropium has a short duration of action (4 to 6 hours). Although ipratropium had a bronchodilating effect in horses with COPD at rest, no effect was measured on the horses' pulmonary function after exercise.[269] Whether tiotropium, a drug with greater than 12 hours duration of action in other species, will be available or beneficial for use in horses remains to be determined. Although glycopyrrolate was reported to be clinically effective when given by inhalation or injection in a single horse with COPD,[270] it is not widely used in treating horses with COPD. Furosemide (Lasix) has been shown to decrease work of breathing but is usually not used on a routine basis in horses with COPD. Single dose studies with furosemide (1.0 mg/kg IV or by aerosol) relieved airway obstruction for several hours in ponies with COPD,[224] but effects of repeated dosing have not been reported. The drug reverses bronchospasm partially by the release of prostanoids, and pretreatment with flunixin therefore prevents its beneficial effect.[224] Dehydration of a horse with excessive secretions would be ill advised because an increase in stickiness could make expectoration more difficult and increase bronchial obstruction. No effect of furosemide itself on tracheal mucus transport rate was seen after single intravenous dose studies in normal horses.[263] Mast cell stabilizers such as cromolyn (disodium cromoglycate) have been administered by inhalation, but results have been rather inconsistent. An early study showed that cromolyn was prophylactic in horses with COPD but another failed to show any marked beneficial prophylactic effect in horses with severe COPD.[271,272] It is possible that use of the new delivery devices, which should aid delivery to the lower airways, will enhance efficacy. In humans, leukotriene synthesis inhibitors and leukotriene receptor antagonists have been used for treating allergic airway disease. To my knowledge, their usefulness in equine COPD remains to be determined. Because leukotrienes are potent chemoattractants for neutrophils and cause bronchospasm and mucosecretion in horses,[219,222,273,274] their inhibition should be beneficial.

Antihistamines have been used in horses with COPD but have limited efficacy, not unexpected because of the numerous mediators and neurologic pathways involved in COPD. Serotonin may be involved in bronchospasm but, to my knowledge, serotonin antagonists have not been used to treat COPD. Whether cyproheptadine, a drug with anticholinergic, antiserotonin, and antihistamine activity has any beneficial effect has not, to my knowledge, been reported. Calcium ascorbate was reported to have a beneficial clinical effect within 45 days in six horses with COPD[275]; but I am unaware of any subsequent blinded trials on ascorbic acid. Methyl sulfonyl methane, a purported antiinflammatory drug and a metabolite of DMSO, has been used, but, I have seen only one report evaluating its use. At a dosage of 10 g/horse ($n = 6$) PO twice daily for 10 days, no significant effect on clinical signs, arterial blood gases, or cytology of tracheal washes or BAL was seen.[238]

Acupuncture has been used to treat horses with COPD. A study on 12 COPD horses evaluated pulmonary function tests, clinical signs, radiographs, and cytology of BAL.[276] There was approximately 50% improvement in clinical scores, a worsening of pulmonary function, and a decrease in percent neutrophils in the BAL.[276] The clinical improvement and decrease in BAL neutrophils was similar to the effect of prednisone treatment but, unlike acupuncture, the latter improved pulmonary mechanics. More studies are needed to critically evaluate acupuncture as a treatment for COPD. Immunotherapy, or desensitization, has been used for many years in treating allergic respiratory disease in humans; although most studies have shown a beneficial effect, reports have not been consistent. Several different hyposensitization regimens have been used for treating equine respiratory disease. A positive effect was reported in a study of 121 horses treated with hyposensitization.[277] Similarly, another study reported amelioration of clinical signs in 31 of 36 horses within 6 months of starting hyposensitization treatment.[278] However, in neither study was there a placebo group for comparison. Miscellaneous other treatments have also been used and over-the-counter herbal remedies are also available to horse owners. Despite introduction of new treatments, most important and beneficial for affected horses is appropriate environmental management.

REFERENCES

212. Seahorn TL, Beadle RE: Summer pasture–associated obstructive pulmonary disease in horses: 21 cases (1983-1991), *J Am Vet Med Assoc* 202:779-782, 1993.
213. Seahorn TL et al: Chronic obstructive pulmonary disease in horses in Louisiana, *J Am Vet Med Assoc* 208:248-251, 1996.
214. Dixon PM, McGorum B: Pasture-associated seasonal respiratory disease in two horses, *Vet Rec* 126:9-12, 1990.
215. Wood JLN et al: Streptococci and *Pasteurella* spp. associated with disease of the equine respiratory tract, *Equine Vet J* 25:314-318, 1993.
216. Burrell MH et al: Respiratory disease in thoroughbred horses in training: the relationship between disease and viruses, bacteria and environment, *Vet Rec* 139:308-313, 1996.
217. Traub-Dargatz JL et al: Effect of transportation stress on bronchoalveolar lavage fluid analysis in female horses, *Am J Vet Res* 49:1026-1029, 1988.
218. Marti E et al: The genetic basis of equine allergic diseases. I, Chronic hypersensitivity bronchitis, *Equine Vet J* 23:457-460, 1991.
219. Olszewski MA et al: Mediators of anaphylaxis but not activated neutrophils augment cholinergic responses of equine small airways, *Am J Physiol* 276 (Lung Cell Mol Physiol 20): L522-L529, 1999.
220. Fairbairn SM et al: Early neutrophil but not eosinophil or platelet recruitment to the lungs of allergic horses following antigen exposure, *Clin Exp Allergy* 23:821-828, 1993.
221. Gray PR et al: The role of cyclooxygenase products in the acute airway obstruction and airway hyperreactivity of ponies with heaves, *Am Rev Respir Dis* 140:154-160, 1989.
222. Marr KA et al: Inhaled leukotrienes cause bronchoconstriction and neutrophil accumulation in horses, *Res Vet Sci* 64:219-224, 1998.
223. McGorum BC, Dixon PM, Halliwell REW: Quantification of histamine in plasma and pulmonary fluids from horses with chronic obstructive pulmonary disease before and after "natural (hay and straw) challenges," *Vet Immunol and Immunopathol* 36:227-236, 1993.
224. Broadstone RV et al: *In vitro* responses of airway smooth muscle from horses with recurrent airway obstruction, *Pulm Pharmacol* 4:191-202, 1991.
225. Yu M et al: Inhibitory nerve distribution and mediation of NANC relaxation by nitric oxide in horse airways, *J Appl Physiol* 76:339-344, 1994.
226. Dixon PM et al: Chronic obstructive pulmonary disease anatomical cardiac studies, *Equine Vet J* 14:80-82, 1982.
227. Littlejohn A, Bowles F: Studies on the physiopathology of chronic obstructive pulmonary disease in the horse. II, Right heart haemodynamics, *Onderstepoort J Vet Res* 47:187-192, 1980.
228. Petsche VM, Derkson FJ, Robinson NE: Tidal breathing flow volume loops in horses with recurrent airway obstruction (heaves), *Am J Vet Res* 55:885-891, 1994.
229. Stadler P, Deegen E, Reinhard H-J: Circadian rhythm of lung function parameters in horses with chronic airway disease. *Pherdeheilkunde* 1:47-54, 1985.
230. Jean D, Vrins A, Lavoie JP: Monthly, daily and circadian variations of pulmonary function tests in COPD and healthy horses, *Proceedings of the Fifteenth Annual ACVIM Forum*, Lake Buena Vista, Fla, 1997, p. 655.
231. Deegan EH, Klein K: Interpleural pressure measurement and bronchial spasmolysis tests in the horse performed with a transportable oesophageal pressure measuring instrument, *Pferdeheilkunde* 3:213-221, 1987.
232. Dixon PM, Railton DI, McGorum BC: Equine pulmonary disease: a case control study of 300 referred cases. III. Ancillary diagnostic findings, *Equine Vet J* 27:428-435, 1995.
233. Votion DM et al: Alveolar clearance in horses with chronic obstructive pulmonary disease, *Am J Vet Res* 60:495-600, 1999.
234. Votion D et al: Analysis of scintigraphical lung images before and after treatment of horses suffering from chronic pulmonary disease, *Vet Rec* 144:232-236, 1999.
235. Derksen FJ et al: Comparison of transtracheal aspirate and bronchoalveolar lavage cytology in 50 horses with chronic lung disease, *Equine Vet J* 21:23-26, 1989.
236. Derkson FJ et al: Bronchoalveolar lavage in ponies with recurrent airway obstruction (heaves), *Am Rev Respir Dis* 132:1066-1070, 1985.
237. Tremblay GM et al: Effect of stabling on bronchoalveolar cells obtained from normal and COPD horses, *Equine Vet J* 25:194-197, 1993.
238. Traub-Dargatz JL et al: Evaluation of clinical signs of disease, bronchoalveolar and tracheal wash analysis, and arterial blood gas tensions in 13 horses with chronic obstructive pulmonary disease treated with prednisone, methyl sulfonmethane, and clenbuterol hydrochloride, *Am J Vet Res* 53:1908-1916, 1992.
239. Lapointe JM, Lavoie JP, Urins AA: Effects of triamcinolone acetonide on pulmonary function and bronchoalveolar lavage cytologic features in horses with chronic obstructive pulmonary disease, *Am J Vet Res* 54:1310-1316, 1993.
240. Grünig G et al: Partial divergence between airway inflammation and clinical signs in equine chronic pulmonary disease, *Equine Vet J* 21: 145-148, 1989.
241. McGorum BC, Dixon PM, Halliwell REW: Responses of horses affected with chronic obstructive pulmonary disease to inhalation challenges with mould antigens, *Equine Vet J* 25:261-267, 1993.
242. McGorum BC, Dixon PM, Halliwell REW: Evaluation of intradermal mould antigen testing in the diagnosis of equine chronic obstructive pulmonary disease, *Equine Vet J* 25:273-275, 1993.
243. McPherson EA et al: COPD in horses: etiological studies, responses to intradermal and inhalation antigen challenge, *Equine Vet J* 11:159-166, 1979.
244. Halliwell REW et al: The role of allergy in chronic pulmonary disease of horses, *J Am Vet Med Assoc* 174:227-281, 1979.
245. Evans AG, Paradis MR, O'Callaghan M: Intradermal skin testing of horses with chronic obstructive pulmonary disease and recurrent urticaria, *Am J Vet Res* 53: 203-208, 1992.
246. Halliwell REW et al: Local and systemic antibody production in horses affected with chronic obstructive pulmonary disease, *Vet Immunol Immunopathol* 38:201-215, 1993.
247. Schmallenbach KH et al: Studies on pulmonary and systemic *Aspergillus fumigatus* specific IgE and IgG antibodies in horses affected with chronic obstructive pulmonary disease (COPD), *Vet Immunol and Immunopathol* 16:245-256, 1998.
248. Woods PSA et al: Airborne dust and aeroallergen concentration in a horse stable under two different management systems, *Equine Vet J* 25:208-213, 1993.
249. Dixon PM et al: Equine pulmonary disease: a case control study and 300 referred cases. IV, Treatments and re-examination findings, *Equine Vet J* 17:436-439, 1995.
250. Raidal SL, Love DN, Bailey GD: Inflammation and increased numbers of bacteria in the lower respiratory tract of horses within 6-12 hours of confinement with the head elevated, *Aust Vet J* 72:45-50, 1995.
251. Rush BR et al: Inhaled beclomethasone dipropionate for treatment of heaves, *Proceedings of the Fifteenth Veterinary Respiratory Symposium*, Liege, Belgium, 1997, The Comparative Respiratory Society, p S18.
252. Viel L, Celly C: Preliminary efficacy results of fluticasone propionate in heavy horses, *Proceedings of the Fifteenth Veterinary Respiratory Symposium*, Liege, 1997, The Comp. Respiratory Society, p S19.

253. Derkson FJ et al.: Use of a hand-held metered dose delivery device to administer pirbuterol acetate to horses with "heaves," *Equine Vet J* 28: 306-310, 1996.

254. Derksen FJ et al: Aerosolized albuterol sulfate used as a bronchodilator in horses with recurrent airway obstruction, *Am J Vet Res* 60:689-693, 1999.

255. Tesarowski DB et al: The rapid and effective administration of a β_2 agonist to horses with heaves using a compact inhalation device and metered dose inhalers, *Can Vet J* 35:170-173, 1994.

256. Erichsen DF et al: Clinical efficacy and safety of clenbuterol HCl when administered to effect in horses with chronic obstructive pulmonary disease (COPD), *Equine Vet J* 26:331-336, 1994.

257. McKiernan BC et al: Plasma theophylline concentration and lung function in ponies with recurrent obstructive lung disease, *Equine Vet J* 22: 194-197, 1990.

258. Ayres JW, Pearson EG, Riebold TW: Theophylline and dyphylline pharmacokinetics in the horse, *Am J Vet Res* 46:2500-2506, 1985.

259. Kowalczyk DF, Beech J, Littlejohn D: Pharmacokinetic disposition of theophylline in horses, *Am J Vet Res* 45:2272-2275, 1984.

260. Errecalde JO et al: Pharmacokinetics bioavailability of theophylline in horses, *J Vet Pharmacol Ther* 7:255-264, 1984.

261. Errecalde JO, Landoni MF: The pharmacokinetics of a slow-release theophylline preparation in horses after intravenous and oral administration, *Vet Res Commun* 16:131-138, 1992.

262. Broadstone RV et al: Effects of atropine in ponies with recurrent airway obstruction, *J Appl Physiol* 65:2720-2725, 1988.

263. Maxson AD et al: Effects of furosemide, exercise and atropine on tracheal mucus transport rate in horses, *Am J Vet Res* 56:908-912, 1995.

264. Kiely RG, Jenins WL, Martens RJ: Mucociliary transport rate in the horse and its modification with various pharmacologic agents, *Proceedings of the Fourth Veterinary Respiratory Symposium*, 1985, The Comparative Respiratory Society, p 7.

265. Robinson NE et al: The airway response of horses with recurrent airway obstruction (heaves) to aerosol administration of ipratropium bromide, *Equine Vet J* 25:299-303, 1993.

266. Duvivier DH et al: Airway response of horses with COPD to dry powder inhalation of ipratropium bromide, *Vet J* 154:149-153, 1997.

267. Duvivier DH et al: Effects of inhaled dry powder ipratropium bromide on recovery from exercise of horses with COPD, *Equine Vet J* 31:20-24, 1999.

268. Robinson NE: Structure and function of the tracheobronchial system (p 87-94), Pharmacology of the equine tracheobronchial tree (p 95-105), Pathogenesis and management of airway disease (p 106-115), *Proceedings of the Forty-third Annual Convention of the American Association of Equine Practitioners*, 1997.

269. Bayly WM et al: Effects of inhaled ipratropium bromide on pulmonary mechanics and gas exchange during exercise in horses with COPD, *Proceedings of the Fifteenth Veterinary Respiratory Symposium*, Liege, Belgium, 1997, The Comp. Respiratory Society, S17.

270. Goetz TE: Successful management of equine chronic obstructive pulmonary disease, *Vet Med* 79:1073-1078, 1984.

271. Thomson JR, McPherson EA: Prophylactic effects of sodium cromoglycate on chronic obstructive pulmonary disease in the horse, *Equine Vet J* 13:243-246,1981.

272. Soma LR, Beech J, Gerber NH: Effects of cromolyn in horses with chronic obstructive pulmonary disease, *Vet Res Commun* 11:339-351, 1987.

273. Doucet MY, Jones TR, Ford-Hutchinson AW: Responses of equine trachealis and lung parenchyma to methacholine, histamine serotonin, prostanoids and leukotrienes *in vitro*, *Can J Physiol Pharmacol* 68: 279-283, 1990.

274. Marr KA, Less P, Page CP: Effects of inhaled LTD_4 and LTB_4 on bronchoconstriction and radiolabeled neutrophil accumulation in the horse, *Am J Respir Crit Care Med* 151:A825, 1995.

275. Newman NL: Use of a calcium ascorbate supplement in therapy of obstructive pulmonary disease, *Proceedings of the Forty-third Annual Convention of the American Association of Equine Practitioners*, 1997, p 401-402.

276. Paradis MR et al: The efficacy of acupuncture as compared to prednisone treatment for chronic obstructive pulmonary disease (COPD) in horses, *Proceedings of the Fifteenth ACVIM Forum*, Lake Buena Vista, Fla, 1997, p 655.

277. Beech J, Merryman LS: Immunotherapy for equine respiratory disease, *Equine Vet Sci* 6:6-10, 1986.

278. Tallarico NJ, Tallarico CM: Results of intradermal allergy testing and treatment by hyposensitization of 64 horses with chronic obstructive pulmonary disease, urticaria, headshaking and/or reactive airway disease, *Vet Allergy and Clin Immunol* 6:25-35, 1998.

TUBERCULOSIS

JILL BEECH

Tuberculosis is extremely rare in horses, especially in the United States. The organism is usually ingested, although primary respiratory infection may occur. Spread is hematogenous, and the organism frequently settles in lymph nodes and the spleen. The lungs may be most severely affected when the spread is miliary and multiple diffuse small nodules occur. Miliary lesions are reported to cause more rapid progression of disease because organ function is more rapidly compromised.

The most frequent presenting complaint is chronic weight loss with ensuing weakness and lethargy. Terminally ill horses with the pulmonary form are febrile and dyspneic and have a cough. Osteomyelitis of the cervical vertebrae and associated signs have been reported.

Diagnosis is based on isolation of the organism or demonstration of its presence cytologically or histologically. Radiographs of the thorax are helpful in defining the pattern and distribution of lesions. Biopsy of the lesion(s) is necessary for a definitive diagnosis. Culture of a transtracheal wash with cytologic evaluation is advisable; when tuberculosis is suspected, an acid-fast stain should be used. If the sample submitted for culture is not sterile, it should be placed in special transport medium such as 10% cetyl pyridinium chloride (CPC). The intradermal skin test is not reliable and should not be used as a diagnostic tool. Diagnosis is probably most frequently made after the horse's death.

Treatment is not usually attempted, because of the associated risk of transmission to humans. If the horse is to be treated, rifampin and isoniazid should be used. Isoniazid has been used in horses for other conditions at an oral dosage of 5 to 15 mg/kg orally twice daily.[279] Although a study on rifampin pharmacokinetics in horses recommended using 10 to 25 mg/kg orally twice daily,[280] clinical results in foals with *Rhodococcus equi* pneumonia suggest that 5 to 10 mg/kg orally twice daily is adequate.

Streptomycin may also be used; a dosage regimen of 15 mg/kg/day for 1 month, followed by 15 mg/kg twice weekly for 3 months, has been suggested in humans.[281] However, in humans streptomycin is routinely used only in conjunction with other drugs, and never alone, because of the development of resistance.[282] I know of no published reports on treating horses with tuberculosis. If treatment is undertaken, the horse should be isolated, with precautions taken to prevent spread of disease. In humans, treatment periods frequently exceed 1 year. Periodic cultures and sensitivity testing should be performed. If radiographic lesions are present, periodic radiographs may be helpful in revealing any change. Prognosis is very poor. Bacillus Calmette-Guerin (BCG) vaccine has been used in humans with potential exposure, but its benefit in increasing resistance of exposed horses to tuberculosis infection is unknown. If a horse is to be treated, consultation with the handler's physician or public health officials is advisable, because tuberculosis is a reportable disease in other species.

REFERENCES

279. Roberts WD: Isoniazid in equine therapy, *Proceedings of the Seventeenth Annual Convention of the American Association of Equine Practitioners*, 1971, pp 33-34.

280. Burrows GE et al: Rifampin in the horse: comparison of IV, IM, and oral administration, *Am J Vet Res* 46:442-446, 1985.

281. Peel JE: Tuberculosis. In Robinson NE, ed: *Current therapy in equine medicine*, Philadelphia, 1983, WB Saunders, pp 29-31.

282. Kendig EL: Tuberculosis disorders of children. In Kendig EL, Chernick V, eds: *Disorders of the respiratory tract in children*, ed 4, Philadelphia, 1983, WB Saunders, pp 662-702.

PNEUMOCONIOSIS (SILICOSIS)

BRETT DOLENTE

The most complete case series of pneumoconiosis in horses originates from the Monterey-Carmel Peninsula in California.[283] In humans, onset of clinical signs of silicosis usually

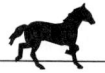

occurs decades after exposure. Severity of clinical signs depends on genetic factors, presence of coexisting diseases, amount and type of silica, and duration of exposure.[284] The small (0.5 to 5 mm) particles that are deposited in small airways and alveoli, and subsequently phagocytosed, initiate the disease process. In decreasing order of frequency, fibrosis and cytotoxicity are most likely to be caused by the tridymite, cristobalite, quartz, and ceosite forms of silica. In the reported horses, cristobalite was the major silica species identified.[283] Usually this form of silica, associated with volcanic igneous rocks, is a minor component of soils; it is found in an unusually high concentration in the Monterey region. Whether other geographic areas have a similarly high content is not known. A more recent report of 12 cases of silicate and aluminum pneumoconiosis arose from one county in China.[284] The reported age range is 5 to 18 years.[283-285] Although most cases are symptomatic, two asymptomatic cases have been diagnosed on the basis of histopathologic evaluation within the Monterey region.

Clinical signs are similar to chronic obstructive pulmonary disease, and include weight loss, cough, exercise intolerance and, sometimes, exercise-induced respiratory distress (sweating, nostril flaring, abducted elbows, reluctance to move, and shaking). Resting respiratory rates are often increased.

Physical examination reveals a restrictive pattern of breathing. Auscultation reveals harsh breath sounds and some wheezing, which is exacerbated by exercise. Hematologic analysis is nondiagnostic. Transtracheal aspirates obtained in six horses contained primarily alveolar macrophages, some of which had cytoplasmic inclusions.[283] Small numbers of bacteria and/or fungi may be isolated. Radiographs of the thorax may reveal a variety of patterns including interstitial patterns (miliary, reticulonodular, and linear) most severe in the caudodorsal lung fields. Other radiographic abnormalities noted were lymphadenopathy, pleural effusion or thickening, hyperinflation, and pulmonary consolidation.[286]

Gross pathologic analysis revealed interstitial granulomatous pneumonia and fibrosis. Histologic examination with both light and electron microscopy may reveal peribronchitis, perivasculitis, and cellular infiltrates consisting of mostly macrophages and giant cells, with refractile inorganic dust particles noted both intracellular and extracellularly.[285,286]

One horse was reported to be treated with corticosteroids and bronchodilators with no change in clinical signs noted.[283]

REFERENCES

283. Schwartz LW et al: Silicate pneumoconiosis and pulmonary fibrosis in horses from the Monterey-Carmel Peninsula, *Chest* 80:82S-85S, 1981.
284. Davis GS: The pathogenesis of silicosis: state of the art, *Chest* 89:166S-170S, 1986.
285. Chen HT et al: Pathological study of heaves in horses in Gansu province, *Acta Vet Zoot Sinica* 20:55-59, 1989.
286. Berry CR et al: Thoracic radiographic features of silicosis in 19 horses, *J Vet Intern Med* 5:248-256, 1991.

MYCOPLASMA

BRETT DOLENTE

Mycoplasma species are a group of bacteria that differ from other bacteria because they lack a cell wall, are much smaller than most bacteria, and need cholesterol to survive. These organisms are proven to cause respiratory disease in humans, cattle, and pigs. The relative importance of *Mycoplasma* species as a pathogen in equine lower respiratory disease is still controversial. Several reports that exist in the literature suggest *Mycoplasma felis* is a pathogen that causes pleuritis and pericarditis in the horse.[287-289] Experimental infection in ponies with *M. felis* induced pleuritis.[290] Although multiple

other species have been isolated from the equine respiratory tract, evidence only exists confirming *M. felis* as a pathogen.

Clinical signs of mycoplasma infection, including fever, depression, and pleurodynia, mimic other bacterial pleuritis cases. Auscultation of the thorax may reveal pleural friction rubs and dull lung sounds over the cranioventral thorax. Sonographic examination of the thorax reveals pleural effusion, often bilateral. Thoracocentesis should be performed for both diagnostic and, if necessary, therapeutic purposes. The fluid is most often an exudate, lacking any odor. Cytologic examination reveals large numbers of neutrophils within the pleural fluid.

Crucial to diagnosis of mycoplasma infection is the elimination of more common pathogens, such as streptococcal infections. Thus routine cultures for aerobic and anaerobic bacteria should be performed in any case of pleuritis. Culture for the presence of mycoplasma is difficult. Immediate centrifugation of pleural fluid is ideal, because supernatants are the preferred culture samples.[291] These samples should then be placed in Hayflick's media.[291] Seroconversion can also be an aid in diagnosis, with seroconversion occurring in a large number of the reported cases of *M. felis* infection.[287-289] Experimental infection revealed that once seroconversion occurs, the organism can no longer be isolated from culture samples.[290] Seroprevalance in this country is not known.

Experimentally infected ponies recovered without treatment in one study, so the requirements of treatment are unclear.[290] Although sensitivity testing should be performed on any isolate, *Mycoplasma* species have been found to be sensitive to gentamicin, tetracyclines, and erythromycin.[292] The role these organisms play in equine respiratory disease is still unclear and more investigation is needed.

REFERENCES

287. Wood JL et al: An outbreak of respiratory disease in horses associated with *Mycoplasma felis* infection, *Vet Rec* 140:388-391, 1997.
288. Morley PS et al: Pericarditis and pleuritis caused by *Mycoplasma felis* in a horse, *Equine Vet J* 28:237-240, 1996.
289. Hoffman AM et al: *Mycoplasma felis* pleuritis in two show-jumper horses, *Cornell Vet* 82:155-162, 1992.
290. Ogilvie TH et al: *Mycoplasma felis* as a cause of pleuritis in horses, *J Am Vet Med Assoc* 182:1374-1376, 1983.
291. Rosendal S et al: Detection of antibodies to *Mycoplasma felis* in horses, *J Am Vet Med Assoc* 188:292-294, 1986.
292. Carter GR, Chengappa MM: *Essentials of veterinary bacteriology and mycology*, ed 4, Philadelphia, 1991, Lea & Febiger, pp 242-243.

DISEASES OF LYMPH NODES, VASCULATURE, AND PHARYNX

RETROPHARYNGEAL LYMPH NODE ABSCESSATION

CLIFFORD M. HONNAS

JOHN R. PASCOE

DEFINITION AND ETIOLOGY. In horses the retropharyngeal lymph nodes consist of medial and lateral lymphoid chains. The lateral chain (8 to 15 nodes) is located ventral to the atlas and along the lateral sides of the guttural pouches. These lymph nodes are covered by the parotid gland and are not clearly distinguishable from the medial retropharyngeal lymph nodes (20 to 30 nodes). The medial retropharyngeal lymph nodes are located ventral to the lateral chain on the dorsolateral aspect of the pharynx and the caudoventral aspect of the guttural pouches.[293]

Retropharyngeal lymph node abscesses in horses are generally caused by *Streptococcus equi* ssp. *equi* infection (see Strangles, p. 504) or are secondary to trauma.[294,295] Other bacterial isolates have included *Streptococcus equi* ssp., *Streptococcus zooepidemicus*, *Corynebacterium pseudotuberculosis*, and *Actinobacillus* spp. An unusual case of granulomatous infection of the guttural pouch caused by *Mycobacterium avium* complex was believed to have originated from the retropharyngeal lymph nodes.[296] Extension of guttural pouch infections into the retropharyngeal space has been suggested as another source of infection.[297] Lymphadenopathy of the retropharyngeal nodes may also occur during viral respiratory infections, including equine herpesvirus, influenza, and viral arteritis.[298] Retropharyngeal abscesses not associated with regional lymph nodes can result from perforation of the oropharynx or nasopharynx by ingested foreign bodies,[299] or by passage of a nasogastric tube,[300] or use of a balling gun.

In ruminants the medial retropharyngeal lymph nodes are located on the dorsolateral aspect of the pharynx, one on each side of the midline. One to three lymph nodes may be present in cattle. The lateral retropharyngeal lymph nodes are located caudal to the medial retropharyngeal lymph nodes in the cranial neck region and are caudal to the retropharyngeal space.[293]

Abscessation of the medial retropharyngeal lymph nodes in cattle may result from pharyngeal actinobacillosis, foreign body penetration, or traumatic perforations by balling guns or dose syringes.[301,302] Frequently *Actinomyces (Corynebacterium) pyogenes* or *Actinobacillus* spp. can be isolated.[303] Cattle with abscessed pharyngeal lymph nodes often have a small ulcer in the mouth, most frequently at the junction of the base and shaft of the tongue. This is more likely to occur when cattle are eating dry scabrous roughage. In addition to traumatic perforations and foreign bodies, caseous lymphadenitis caused by *C. pseudotuberculosis* frequently results in abscessation of these lymph nodes in sheep and goats.[298]

CLINICAL SIGNS AND DIFFERENTIAL DIAGNOSIS. The clinical signs associated with retropharyngeal lymph node infection or abscessation in horses include dysphagia, odynophagia (painful swallowing), nasal or oral regurgitation, excess salivation, difficult and often noisy breathing, painful throatlatch swelling, mucoid to mucopurulent nasal discharge, extension of the head and neck, and weight loss.[293] In a retrospective study of 46 horses referred for retropharyngeal lymph node abscessation, the frequency of abnormal clinical signs was fever and increased heart and respiratory rates (80%), unilateral or bilateral throatlatch swelling (65%), respiratory stertor or distress (35%), purulent nasal discharge (20%), inappetence and signs of depression (15%), and dysphagia (9%).[304] Other clinical signs observed endoscopically include reduction in size or collapse of the pharyngeal lumen, asymmetry of the dorsal pharyngeal wall, and deviation of the laryngeal aperture away from the retropharyngeal mass.[294,304] The differential diagnosis for a retropharyngeal mass should include abscess, cellulitis, guttural pouch empyema or tympany, parotiditis, lymphadenopathy, neoplasia, and hematoma.

Clinical signs observed in cattle with infection or abscessation of the medial retropharyngeal lymph nodes include difficult breathing, excessive salivation, extension of the head and neck, anorexia, enlarged submandibular lymph nodes, nasal discharge, and swelling in the retropharyngeal space.[301] Other disease conditions that affect the oropharynx and surrounding lymph nodes should be considered in the differential diagnosis. These include actinobacillosis, lymphosarcoma, sialolithiasis, and necrotic laryngitis, laryngeal edema, or severe tracheitis caused by infectious bovine rhinotracheitis virus.[298,301]

Affected sheep and goats may exhibit excessive salivation, increased respiratory rate, stertorous breathing, mucopurulent nasal discharge, regurgitation, gagging, depression, sub-

cutaneous crepitation, weakness, and fetid breath. A false carotid aneurysm in the retropharyngeal space has been reported; on external examination it may be confused with abscessation of the medial retropharyngeal lymph nodes.[305] Enlarged retropharyngeal lymph nodes are usually easily palpated and identified in sheep and goats. Caseous lymphadenitis (see Chapter 35) is the most frequent cause of enlarged retropharyngeal lymph nodes in these species.

CLINICAL PATHOLOGY. Collection of purulent material from abscessed lymph nodes may assist in identification of the causal agent. Leukocytosis may be evident on the hemogram, with neutrophilia peaking as the lymph nodes abscess.

LABORATORY AIDS AND DEFINITIVE DIAGNOSTIC TESTS. Lateral radiographs of the pharynx, diagnostic ultrasound, and endoscopy aid in the diagnosis of retropharyngeal infections or abscesses. In horses, radiography may reveal a large soft-tissue mass impinging on the guttural pouch from a caudoventral direction (Fig. 29-21, *A*), as well as thickening of the pharyngeal roof. The soft-tissue swelling may contain gas (Fig. 29-21, *B*). Compression of the larynx and trachea with ventral displacement may also be evident (Fig. 29-21, *C*).[294] Observation of a gas/fluid interface on radiographs of the pharynx generally indicates abscessation, but care should be taken to distinguish a retropharyngeal abscess from guttural pouch empyema.[296] Foreign bodies associated with pharyngeal trauma are not usually radiopaque and therefore not visible radiographically unless outlined by contrast medium. Exceptions include small wire foreign bodies likely ingested from baled hay that can perforate the tongue or oropharynx causing cellulitis and dysphagia,[299] or in cattle, magnets that have been inadvertently placed retropharyngeally.

On endoscopy, asymmetry or collapse of the pharyngeal lumen or both signs suggest a retropharyngeal space-occupying mass. Recognition of drainage from the guttural pouch openings or examination of the guttural pouches may be necessary to differentiate between guttural pouch empyema and retropharyngeal lymphadenopathy or pharyngeal neoplasia. Occasionally the pharyngeal wall ruptures, allowing endoscopic observation of retropharyngeal drainage into the pharynx, usually near the esophageal entrance.[294] Percutaneous needle aspiration may yield a definitive diagnosis if purulent material is obtained. Ultrasonography improves diagnostic precision by permitting more accurate identification of the abscess and highlighting its anatomic relationships as an aid to surgical drainage.

Clinical examination, radiography, ultrasonography, endoscopy, and percutaneous centesis may all prove helpful in making a diagnosis of medial retropharyngeal lymph node infection or abscessation in ruminants. In cattle, localized swelling cranial to the larynx may be detected by digital palpation of the oropharynx.[301] Oropharyngeal examination must be performed carefully in animals with respiratory distress, to prevent further airway compromise.

PATHOPHYSIOLOGY. Upper respiratory disease, trauma, and foreign body penetration with resulting infection and drainage to local lymph nodes result in clinically apparent infection and abscessation of the retropharyngeal lymph nodes. In horses the retropharyngeal space is occupied primarily by the guttural pouches. Because the vagus, glossopharyngeal, hypoglossal, spinal accessory, and sympathetic nerves traverse this area, their function can be affected by infectious or inflammatory processes involving the retropharyngeal space.[294] If such infections are contained within the lymph nodes or are confined within the fibrous capsule of the abscess, cranial nerve dysfunction is not usually evident.[294] Clinical evidence of dysphagia or odynophagia such as the presence of feed and saliva at the external nares may result from inflammation or injury of the glossopharyngeal nerve or pharyngeal branch of the vagus nerve,[294] compression, or obstruction of pharynx or esophagus,

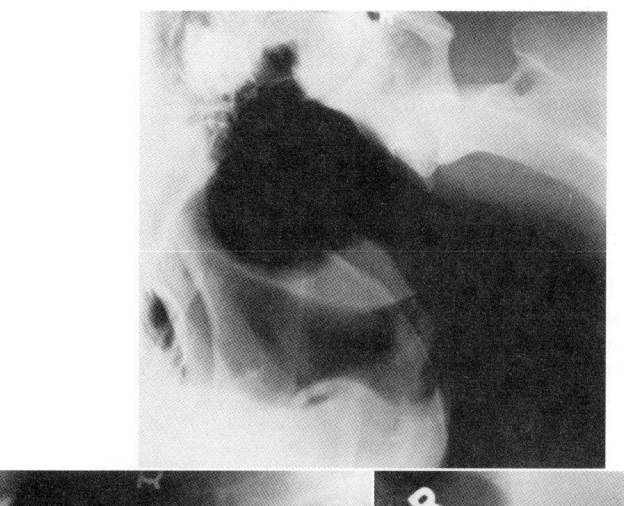

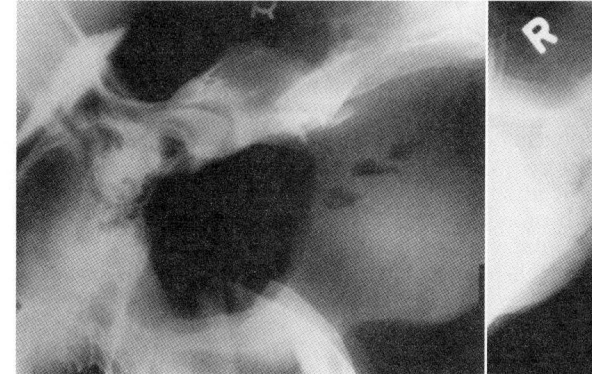

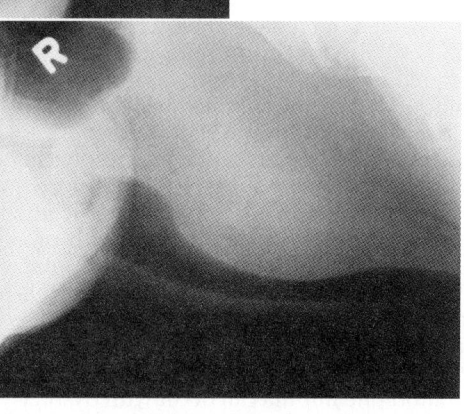

FIG. 29-21 ▓ **A,** Lateral radiograph. A soft-tissue density (retropharyngeal abscess) is distorting the floor of the guttural pouch. **B,** Lateral radiograph. There is increased soft-tissue density with gas shadows ventral to the cervical vertebrae. These changes are consistent with abscessation of the retropharyngeal lymph nodes. **C,** Lateral radiograph. There is increased soft-tissue density ventral to the cervical vertebrae, with compression of the dorsal border of the trachea. These changes were caused by cellulitis and abscessation of the retropharyngeal lymph nodes.

and from angina. It has been suggested that retropharyngeal lymphadenitis may result in neuritis of the pharyngeal branch of the vagus nerve in young horses and contribute to the pathogenesis of dorsal displacement of the soft palate.[306]

Respiratory distress may result when enlargement of the retropharyngeal lymph nodes compresses or obstructs the nasopharyngeal, laryngeal, or tracheal lumen,[294,301] and the disease caused by *S. equi* ssp. *equi* in horses is appropriately named strangles.

The most common cause of pharyngeal inflammation and infection in cattle is pharyngeal trauma associated with balling guns, dose syringes, paste wormer guns, esophageal feeders, or stomach tubes. A careful history to determine whether any of these devices were used is important in ascertaining the source of pharyngeal abscessation. Such infections usually involve a mixed bacterial flora, because they are directly connected with the oral pharynx.

EPIDEMIOLOGY. Infection with *S. equi* usually results from contact (inhalation or ingestion) with pasture, feed, or water contaminated with nasal discharge from infected horses. Asymptomatic carrier horses have also been implicated as source of infection.[309] The likely bacterial reservoir in carrier horses is the guttural pouch, particularly if chondroids are present in one or both pouches.[307] Infection of the pharyngeal and nasal mucosa results in an acute pharyngitis and rhinitis, and drainage to regional lymph nodes results in lymphadenopathy and, possibly, abscessation.[298]

Caseous lymphadenitis is spread through the discharges from ruptured lymph nodes. The causal agent *C. pseudotuber-*

culosis may persist in the environment for long periods, and infection results from contact of shearing, docking, or castration wounds with contaminated soil, equipment, or freshly ruptured abscesses. Sheep dips have been reported as another important source of infection.[298] Spread of infection from skin wounds often leads to involvement of local nodes and abscess formation. The mode of spread in goats is still not well understood, but the disease usually spreads in a low-grade contagious manner, often involving most of the herd over a period of years.

NECROPSY FINDINGS. Fatalities are rare and most likely result from respiratory compromise or septicemia. Postmortem lesions include cellulitis with compression and ventral displacement of the larynx and cranial cervical trachea. Abscesses are variable in size and may contain either caseous (*C. pseudotuberculosis*) or liquid material (*S. equi* ssp. *equi*). A thick, fibrous capsule may occur in response to the infectious process and account for the surrounding tissue compression. Occasionally, draining tracts may connect the abscess to the pharynx, guttural pouch, or skin.[300,308]

TREATMENT AND PROGNOSIS. Treatment goals are relief of respiratory distress and control of infection. Temporary tracheotomy may be needed for relief of respiratory distress. After surgical drainage appropriate systemic antibiotics are administered and supportive therapy to further reduce swelling may be beneficial.

Surgical approaches include percutaneous drainage, intraoral drainage, and marsupialization.[294,301] In horses an intraoral approach is very difficult because of the long narrow oral cavity, and for this reason percutaneous drainage is commonly used. For abscesses visible through the mucosal lining of the guttural pouch, endoscopically assisted drainage into the pouch can also be considered. Surgical access to the retropharyngeal space has been described including a dorsal and ventral approaches, an approach through Viborg's triangle, and a lateral approach.[304,309] A ventral surgical approach is recommended because of the relative lack of vital structures encountered and the excellent ventral drainage achieved. A less invasive drainage technique can be accomplished in standing sedated horses, by ultrasound-guided percutaneous needle placement into abscessed lymph nodes. Respecting regional anatomy, incision directly along the needle shaft provides exterior drainage and access for cavity lavage with antiseptic solutions or use of a seton or gauze packing. If the abscess is endoscopically visible beneath the guttural pouch mucosa, drainage into the guttural pouch and subsequent lavage of the purulent material can be accomplished. Before or at the time of abscess drainage or excision, the horse should be started on broad-spectrum antimicrobials, followed by the appropriate specific antimicrobial drug when results of the culture and susceptibility test are known.

Occasionally, medical management alone may resolve infection; however, this is less likely if abscessation has occurred. Because the most common bacterial isolate in the horse is *S. equi*, parenteral antimicrobial therapy with procaine penicillin G (22,000 IU/kg IM twice daily) or potassium penicillin (20,000 IU/kg IV four times daily) is recommended. Systemic nonsteroidal antiinflammatory agents are useful to reduce inflammation and swelling and fluid and electrolyte therapy may be necessary if there is odynophagia or dysphagia. Aspiration pneumonia can occur with dysphagia or if there is oral or nasal regurgitation associated with painful swallowing.

In cattle with pharyngeal trauma, an existing wound is often draining from the retropharyngeal area to the oropharynx, making surgical drainage unnecessary. Such animals tend to respond well to parenteral broad-spectrum antimicrobial therapy.[310] Parenteral antimicrobial therapy alone has been ineffective in treating retropharyngeal abscesses when there is no draining tract.[301,302] Intraoral or percutaneous drainage has been used successfully in conjunction with broad-spectrum, parenteral antimicrobial therapy.[302] After drainage, the abscess cavity is flushed daily with an antiseptic or antibiotic solution.[301] Surgical drainage into the oral cavity must be handled with caution. The patient's head should be lowered so that exudate or flush solution is not aspirated; inspection of the granulating abscess cavity is necessary if feed impaction is suspected.[294,301] Aspiration pneumonia may be a serious complication when dysphagia is present.

In sheep and goats, walled-off *C. pseudotuberculosis* abscesses may often be most safely drained by suturing the skin to the heavy abscess capsule (a procedure known as marsupialization) before opening the capsule. Marsupialization prevents contamination of other retropharyngeal structures with infected material and markedly reduces postsurgical cellulitis. Although *C. pseudotuberculosis* is susceptible in vitro to a number of antimicrobial agents, abscesses associated with the condition have not been well controlled by antimicrobial therapy. Walled-off *C. pseudotuberculosis* abscesses are difficult to eliminate solely with antimicrobial therapy, and drainage or removal of the entire lymph node gives the best results.

PREVENTION AND CONTROL. Preventive measures to limit infection and abscessation of retropharyngeal lymph nodes include proper administration of therapeutic agents with balling guns and dose syringes, isolation of horses affected with viral or bacterial upper respiratory disease, vaccination against strangles, and vigorous treatment in the early stages of streptococcal infection. Preventing contamination

of shearing equipment and dipping vats with *C. pseudotuberculosis* is important in limiting the spread of this organism in sheep. Culling affected sheep and goats may also help to reduce the incidence of caseous lymphadenitis.

REFERENCES

293. Getty R, ed: *Sisson and Grossman's the anatomy of the domestic animals*, ed 5, Philadelphia, 1975, WB Saunders, pp 619-620, 1024-1027, 1043, 1050.
294. Todhunter RJ, Brown CM, Stickle R: Retropharyngeal infections in five horses, *J Am Vet Med Assoc* 187:600-604, 1985.
295. Raker CW: The nasopharynx. In Mansmann RA, McAllister ES, eds: *Equine medicine and surgery*, ed 3, Santa Barbara, Calif, 1982, American Veterinary Publications, pp 747-748.
296. Sills RC et al: Bilateral guttural pouch infection due to *Mycobacterium avium* complex in a horse, *Vet Pathol* 27:133-135, 1990.
297. Peyton LC, Delahanty DD: What is your diagnosis? *J Am Vet Med Assoc* 168:67-68, 1976.
298. Blood DC, Radostits OM, Henderson JA: *Veterinary medicine: a textbook of the diseases of cattle, sheep, pigs, goats, and horses*, ed 6, London, 1983, Baillière Tindall, pp 148-149, 502-518.
299. Kiper ML et al: Metallic foreign bodies in the mouth or pharynx of horses: seven cases (1983-1989), *J Am Vet Med Assoc* 200:91-93, 1992.
300. Rashmir-Raven AM et al: What is your diagnosis? *J Am Vet Med Assoc* 198:1991-1992, 1991.
301. Vestweber JG, Roeder B: Medial retropharyngeal lymph node abscess as a cause of respiratory dyspnea in cattle, *Compend Cont Educ Pract Vet* 8:F71-F74, 1986.
302. Horney FD, Wallace CE: Surgery of the bovine digestive tract. In Jennings PB, ed: *The practice of large animal surgery*, Philadelphia, 1984, WB Saunders, p 502.
303. Mackey DR: The respiratory system. In Gibbons WJ, Catcott EJ, Smithcors JF, eds: *Bovine medicine and surgery*, Wheaton, Ill, 1970, American Veterinary Publications, pp 467-468.
304. Golland LC et al: Retropharyngeal lymph node infection in horses: 46 cases (1977-1992), *Aust Vet J* 72:161-164,1995.
305. Rings DM, Constable P, Biller DS: False carotid aneurysm in a sheep, *J Am Vet Med Assoc* 189:799-801, 1986.
306. Holcombe SJ et al: Effect of bilateral blockade of the pharyngeal branch of the vagus nerve on soft palate function in horses, *Am J Vet Res* 59:504-508, 1998.
307. Newton JR et al: Naturally occurring persistent and asymptomatic infection of the guttural pouches of horses with *Streptococcus equi*, *Vet Rec* 140: 84-90, 1997.
308. Knight AP et al: Experimentally induced *Streptococcus equi* infection in horses with resultant guttural pouch empyema, *Vet Med Small Anim Clin* 70:1194-1199, 1975.
309. Haynes PF: Surgery of the equine respiratory tract. In Jennings PB, ed: *The practice of large animal surgery*, Philadelphia, 1984, WB Saunders, pp 465-470.
310. Davidson HP, Rebhun WC, Habel RE: Pharyngeal trauma in cattle, *Cornell Vet* 71:15-25, 1981.

EXERCISE-INDUCED PULMONARY HEMORRHAGE (EIPH)

JOHN R. PASCOE

DEFINITION AND ETIOLOGY. Exercise-induced pulmonary hemorrhage (EIPH) is bleeding from the lung as a consequence of exercise.[311] Synonymous terms include epistaxis and "bleeders." Although they are still common in clinical practice and in racing vernacular, continued use of these descriptive terms serves to confuse those less familiar with EIPH by suggesting that the problem results from a nosebleed or is somehow related to a defect in hemostasis.

CLINICAL SIGNS AND DIFFERENTIAL DIAGNOSIS. The predominant clinical sign is blood within the airways,[311] which can be observed by careful endoscopic examination. Less commonly, epistaxis is the most readily observable clinical sign, but fewer than 10% of horses experiencing EIPH exhibit epistaxis.[312] Because EIPH occurs as a consequence of strenuous exercise, other likely signs include those indicative of impaired performance, such as slowing or stopping toward the end of a race and difficult, labored, or abnormal breathing. Riders and trainers use a variety of other colorful terms to describe what they perceive the horse is experiencing. Examples include "bobbling," "choking," and "gurgling." Because

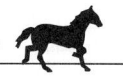

of their lack of specificity, these terms convey different meanings to different individuals; thus horses with one of these signs as a primary complaint must be evaluated carefully for other conditions that might contribute to these signs.

Astute trainers may observe excessive swallowing after racing.[311] This is usually associated with clearance of blood from the respiratory tract. Coughing after exercise may accompany clearance of airway blood but usually is associated with hypersensitivity of upper airway irritant receptors or clearance of inhaled material such as dirt or grass.[313] The specificity of the differential diagnosis is determined largely by the precision of the presenting sign(s) and the results of the clinical examination. For example, if the clinical sign is blood in the lower respiratory tract after exercise, its most probable source is the lung vasculature. Although EIPH is the most likely diagnosis, consideration should also be given to bleeding from a lung abscess, neoplastic mass, or foreign body. When epistaxis is the presenting sign, other diagnostic considerations include nostril lacerations, nasal trauma, nasal turbinate necrosis, ethmoid hematoma, guttural pouch mycosis, airway foreign bodies, and neoplasia. Epistaxis has been reported in association with acute esophageal obstruction and sinusitis in horses, but is a fairly uncommon finding in these diseases.

When the presenting complaint or sign(s) is exercise intolerance (see Chapter 5) the differential diagnosis must include the entire spectrum of conditions that can cause reduced performance. It is important to evaluate each organ system for abnormalities that might influence performance. Conversely, it cannot be overemphasized that recognition of EIPH in a horse with a history of performance problems does not preclude a complete examination for other possible causes of poor performance.

Excessive swallowing may be caused by clearance of blood, respiratory secretions, or inhaled material from the upper airway. Similarly, coughing can indicate attempts to clear material from the respiratory tract or increased hypersensitivity of airway irritant receptors. Although horses with EIPH swallow often after the completion of exercise, most do not appear to cough in response to the presence of blood in their airways. The cause of both signs can be elucidated by careful endoscopic examination.

Inappropriate breathing efforts after exercise may be associated with a variety of clinical conditions. Careful evaluation of the respiratory, cardiovascular, and thermoregulatory systems is essential to determine the cause. In horses with EIPH this finding suggests extensive lung injury such as diffuse pulmonary hemorrhage, subpleural or parenchymal hematoma, or concurrent focal or diffuse pulmonary disease such as pneumonia, pleural effusion, diffuse interstitial or granulomatous lung disease, or neoplasia. Many horses that experience EIPH often "cool out" slowly after exercise; this is manifested by an increased respiratory rate and prolonged peripheral vasodilation and sweating.

CLINICAL PATHOLOGY. In the absence of other systemic disease, horses with EIPH do not usually have abnormalities in their hemogram or in their biochemical or hemostatic profiles.[313-315] Recognition of variations from normal demands careful reexamination of the horse for evidence of other systemic disease. If pneumonia or pleural effusion is concurrent, hematologic or biochemical changes typically seen with these conditions may be present. There are no apparent abnormalities in the intrinsic and extrinsic pathways of coagulation, and there is no evidence of enhanced fibrinolysis.[315] Platelets from horses known to experience EIPH were reported to be less responsive to platelet agonists (adenosine diphosphate, collagen, and platelet activating factor) in vitro than platelets from normal horses[315]; however, both hematocrit and choice of anticoagulant have an effect on measured platelet aggregation.[317] Platelets from blood collected in low-molecular-weight heparin during supramaximal treadmill exercise had enhanced aggregability compared with platelets collected in sodium citrate.[316] An increase in circulating platelet-neutrophil aggregates has been reported in near maximally exercised horses.[317]

LABORATORY AIDS AND DEFINITIVE DIAGNOSTIC TESTS. Cytologic examination of respiratory secretions can help differentiate horses with EIPH from normal horses. Observation of macrophages containing erythrocytes (erythrophages) or hemosiderin (hemosiderophages) is considered supportive evidence that a horse has previously experienced EIPH.[312,317-320] Identification of hemosiderophages can be enhanced by use of special stains (Sano's trichrome stain or Perls' stain) selective for iron-containing pigment.[318,321] One study reported that most (>90%) horses in full training had hemosiderophages in their respiratory secretions and that neutrophils and eosinophils were more common in respiratory secretions of horses known to have experienced EIPH than in normal horses.[318] Microscopic examination of lungs from horses with a known history of EIPH has confirmed the presence of large numbers of alveolar hemosiderophages, and, although eosinophils were seen in some horses, these were usually in lung areas with few hemosiderophages.[322] The interrelationship between these two cell types in EIPH is unknown. In the same study hemosiderophages were recovered from the respiratory secretions at least 150 days after the last known observation of EIPH.[314]

In the absence of a visible source of hemorrhage rostral to the larynx, endoscopic observation of blood in the tracheobronchial airways after exercise is considered definitive evidence of EIPH. Because individual variation in the temporal relationship between onset of hemorrhage and endoscopic observation may exist, it is generally recommended that horses be examined within 90 minutes of the completion of exercise.[312] If EIPH is strongly suspected but not observed during the initial examination, reexamination within 30 to 60 minutes is advised. Horses with epistaxis should be examined as soon as possible to determine the origin of the hemorrhage.

When endoscopy is not possible, cytologic examination of tracheobronchial secretions or bronchoalveolar lavage (BAL) samples for hemosiderophages is recommended. In some racing jurisdictions in North America a signed affidavit from a veterinarian attesting to identification of hemosiderophages on a smear of a transtracheal aspirate or BAL is diagnostic evidence of EIPH for the purpose of legally administering permitted prerace medication. Experimentally increased numbers of hemosiderophages are observed in BAL 1 week after strenuous exercise and remain elevated for at least 3 weeks after exercise.[319] Similar observations have been made after inoculation of autologous blood into equine lungs; erythrocytes are initially removed by mucociliary clearance, but free erythrocytes and erythrophages were recovered by BAL 3 weeks after blood instillation.[320] Hemosiderophages have been recovered up to 150 days after exercise.[314]

Thoracic radiography and ultrasonography should only be considered adjunctive diagnostic aids.[323] Although radiographic and ultrasound changes have been recognized in the lungs of some horses that have experienced EIPH, a definitive diagnosis of EIPH cannot be made solely on the basis of either radiographic or ultrasonographic findings, although horses with EIPH may have abnormal radiographic or ultrasonographic signs in the dorsal caudal lungfields. Spontaneous echocardiographic contrast, thought to be associated primarily with aggregated platelets and some aggregated leukocytes, has been identified more frequently in horses known to have experienced EIPH and reportedly is reduced after daily oral aspirin administration with a concurrent reduction in EIPH and improvement in performance.[324]

PATHOPHYSIOLOGY. The etiopathogenesis of EIPH is unknown. Many causes have been suggested[325] but three possible mechanisms are currently popular: capillary stress failure,[326] locomotry impact–induced pulmonary trauma,[327] and hemorheologic alterations.[328] A unifying concept that links known physiologic and pathologic evidence suggests that disruption of pulmonary capillaries as a consequence of the high cardiac outputs necessary to sustain metabolic function during strenuous exercise may be the initiating event.[325] Pathologic studies have highlighted several consistent features in lungs from horses with a confirmed history of EIPH: bilaterally symmetric distribution of hemosiderin within the dorsal regions of the caudal lung lobes in association with increased small airway disease, interstitial fibrosis, and development of an extensive collateral circulation.[329] Instillation of autologous blood in the airways of horses elicits a profound inflammatory response similar to early lesions observed in horses with EIPH.[330] Likewise, acute exposure of horses to ozone during exercise induces injury of terminal bronchioles and pulmonary hemorrhage.[331] If stress failure of pulmonary capillaries is accepted as the initiating event in EIPH, it is likely that hemorrhage into interstitium and air-spaces elicits an inflammatory reaction that with time causes small airway disease, which is exacerbated by exposure to inhaled particulate matter and environmental pollutants. Bronchial arterial neovascularization occurs in response to the marked inflammatory changes, and leakage from these developing vessels likely also contributes to EIPH. Interpretation of the sequence of events is further complicated by the complex vascular architecture of the distal air spaces where bronchopulmonary anastomoses are believed to occur.[332,333] Because systemic arterial pressures during exercise are higher than pulmonary arterial pressures, capillaries perfused by blood of bronchial vessels are even more likely to be subjected to transmural pressures of sufficient magnitude to result in vascular disruption. Some profound hemorheologic alterations also occur with strenuous exercise, notably increased blood viscosity and decreased erythrocyte deformability. It is likely that these changes increase microvascular shear stress and may contribute to overall increases in vascular pressure but are unlikely to be the sole initiating event in EIPH.[327]

Locomotry induced impact trauma to the lung has been modeled experimentally[334] and postulated as a cause of EIPH.[326] Whereas there is some evidence that footfall affects pleural pressure and that pressure waves move from cranial to caudal along the dorsum of the lung,[335] it is uncertain if the magnitude of these changes is sufficient to induce pulmonary barotrauma and thus EIPH. Despite this, substantial evidence implicates capillary stress failure as the likely initiating event for EIPH[326,336] with other events contributing to continued development of the parenchymal lesions.

EPIDEMIOLOGY. EIPH occurs in horses used for many athletic activities. Racing horses, particularly thoroughbreds, have been most widely studied. On the basis of endoscopic observation of Thoroughbreds, quarter horses, and Appaloosas used for flat racing, the reported frequency of EIPH has varied between 43% and 75%.[313] Considering the results of cytologic studies, it is likely that most, if not all, thoroughbred horses in race training experience EIPH after moderately strenuous exercise.[318,319]

Endoscopic surveys after a race in Thoroughbred horses used for steeplechase, timber races, and jumping indicate similar frequencies of EIPH for these events.[328] The reported frequency of EIPH in racing Standardbreds (pacers and trotters) varies between 25% and 87%[313,337,338]; 11% of polo ponies have endoscopic evidence of EIPH.[339] Although I am aware of anecdotal reports of epistaxis in horses used for endurance events, two endoscopic surveys of endurance horses (primarily Arabian and Anglo-Arabian horses) at the end of 50- and 100-mile rides have failed to detect EIPH.[312] Collation of published data suggests that there is little geographic variation, either within a country or between countries, in the incidence of EIPH.[312,314] There is no apparent gender difference in the frequency of EIPH, but the relationship between a horse's age and EIPH is less clear. On the basis of available survey data, it is generally accepted that EIPH probably occurs soon after training begins, especially after fast galloping (>14 m/sec), and continues to occur in association with moderately strenuous exercise throughout the rest of the horse's racing career. Most studies have reported that older horses bleed more frequently; this might be expected in view of the chronic nature of the lung lesions reported in horses with EIPH.

NECROPSY FINDINGS. Symmetric, bilateral subpleural blue to blue-brown staining distributed in the dorsal part of the caudal lung lobe is noted when the lungs are collapsed.[340] These stained areas of lung are slightly raised and firm in comparison with the surrounding normal lung. An apparent increase in the size and number of subpleural vessels is noted in association with these stained areas of lung. With lung inflation the subpleural parenchymal staining becomes light brown or bronze and has a fine reticular pattern. The prominent subpleural vessels originate from the bronchoesophageal arteries in the pulmonary ligament.[331]

Transverse (dorsoventral) slices through fixed lung show the rust-colored staining extending ventrally from the dorsum of the caudal lobe toward and slightly beyond the level of the principal bronchus.[333] The area of stained lung progressively diminishes toward the hilar region. Examination of slices from lungs with colored latex injected into the pulmonary and bronchial arterial circulations shows increased bronchial arterial vessels in the rust-stained areas of lung.

Microscopic findings include bronchiolitis and increased fibrous connective tissue in interlobular septa around abnormal airways and some vessels.[321] Large numbers of hemosiderophages are observed within alveolar and bronchiolar lumens and in connective tissue septa, both interlobular and interalveolar septa. Although small airway disease is observed in areas without hemosiderophages, the converse is not true. Blood vessels appear more numerous around affected airways, and in some of these vessels the elastic membranes are duplicated and fragmented.[340] Ultrastructural changes in lungs of treadmill-exercised horses and ponies include capillary disruption and leakage of erythrocytes and proteinaceous material into airspaces and interstitial spaces.[336,341]

TREATMENT AND PROGNOSIS. The relatively chronic nature of the pulmonary lesions combined with our poor understanding of their development make it difficult to recommend specific guidelines for management or therapy. This is complicated further by the large number of "treatments" currently in use. Few of these therapies have been critically evaluated for their efficacy in treating or preventing EIPH, and reported studies have been limited in their scope by racing regulations.

If EIPH is caused by high transmural vascular pressures as a consequence of high cardiac outputs during strenuous exercise it seems unlikely that a suitable treatment that will prevent EIPH and not impair cardiovascular function or performance will be accepted as a permitted prerace medication. It may be that different training programs that achieve fitness and stimulate a stronger blood/gas barrier without impairing gas exchange function could be developed to prevent or reduce the prevalence of EIPH. If attention is focused on small airway disease as an important contributory factor, the spectrum of management considerations must include providing an environment relatively free of dust and infectious respiratory disease. Given the methods used to raise, train, and house horses, this would seem to be an impossible task. Nevertheless, efforts must be made to improve our understanding of stable ventilation and design. Also, improved predictors of adequate convalescence after infectious respiratory disease are needed so that the lung has a chance to heal completely before training resumes. If inhaled materials are a major contributory factor, different racing surfaces or nasal filters could be considered as methods to reduce this source of lung insult. Once small airway disease is established, therapeutic measures are largely limited to palliation of adverse effects such as bronchoconstriction, which may occur during exercise. Unfortunately, drugs that might be useful such as bronchodilators often stimulate the cardiovascular system; this poses regulatory problems with respect to their potential influence on performance. Administration of bronchodilators, broad-spectrum antibiotics, and low-dose corticosteroids can be used to improve airway health during convalescent periods in horses with recurrent, performance limiting EIPH. This efficacy of this therapeutic strategy has not been critically evaluated although anecdotally, affected horses often have less tracheal mucopus after strenuous exercise, however, EIPH usually still occurs.

Furosemide (0.3 to 0.6 mg/kg IV) is probably the most commonly used medication for prevention of EIPH[342,343] and is used with higher frequency in Thoroughbreds (up to 75%) than in quarter horses and standardbreds.[344] When approved for use as a prerace medication, furosemide usually cannot be administered less than 3 hours before racing. It is generally believed that furosemide was initially used on the assumption that EIPH occurred as a consequence of pulmonary edema. At least 50% of furosemide-treated horses still experience EIPH, and, although furosemide may reduce the amount of hemorrhage, it is not effective in preventing EIPH in most horses.[312,345,346] Furosemide's effect on performance remains controversial, but accumulating evidence suggests a performance enhancing effect in Thoroughbred[344,346-348] but not Standardbred racehorses.[349] Despite improvements in study design and sample size for Thoroughbred horses, disagreement about methodologic approaches for controlling potential performance influencing variables that improve confidence in longitudinal comparison of performance data and lack of discrete knowledge about individual horse EIPH and medication status continue to confound interpretation of the data.

Administration of furosemide increases urine production, reduces blood and plasma volume and body weight, causes hypochloremia and metabolic alkalosis, and decreases cardiac output and vascular pressures, changes that persist during exercise provided the fluid loss is not replaced.[344] Available evidence implicates the reduction in body weight associated with diuresis as the most likely factor enhancing performance, whereas changes in cardiovascular function are the most likely factors to be of benefit in reducing EIPH.[344] In treadmill-exercised horses, furosemide causes significant decreases in vascular pressures, particularly in right atrial, pulmonary arterial, and pulmonary capillary wedge pressure, for at least 4 hours after administration.[350] A reduction in pulmonary capillary pressure has also been reported after furosemide administration in treadmill-exercised Standardbreds.[351] These extrarenal effects of furosemide do not appear to be mediated through prostaglandin production.[352] If EIPH occurs because of high transmural vascular pressures, furosemide may attenuate these increases in vascular pressures sufficiently to reduce the likelihood of EIPH in some horses for at least 4 hours after administration. Occasionally, a second administration of furosemide either intramuscularly or closer to race time is practiced for horses with chronic severe

EIPH (so-called problem bleeders). In treadmill-exercised horses, administration of furosemide 4 hours and again 2 hours before exercise provided no further attenuation of vascular pressures observed after a single administration 4 hours before exercise.[353]

In ponies with recurrent airway obstruction, furosemide administration decreased pulmonary resistance and increased dynamic compliance without improvement in blood gases.[354] If horses with EIPH experience exercise-induced bronchoconstriction, prerace administration of furosemide may also benefit pulmonary function. Clinical experience suggests that higher doses of furosemide (1 mg/kg) intravenously or intramuscularly have an adverse effect on the horse's attitude and performance. Other therapies include prerace administration of conjugated estrogens and feed supplementation with various substances, including hesperidin-citrus bioflavonoids, vitamins C and K, and bee pollen.[353] With the exception of the bioflavonoids, which were shown not to be effective, none of the other commonly used products has been critically evaluated for efficacy in the treatment of EIPH.[352] The continued introduction of new treatments and cures reflects the general level of frustration experienced by both trainers and veterinarians dealing with EIPH.

Although most horses in race training apparently experience EIPH, few seem to be adversely affected in terms of performance. Unfortunately, preventing EIPH and improving performance in these horses remain a major challenge. Although enforced rest (3 to 6 months) will help some horses, most continue to experience EIPH when training resumes. Thus, in those horses in which EIPH is the major cause of impaired or poor performance, the prognosis for continued competitive racing is poor.

PREVENTION AND CONTROL. As outlined in the preceding section, our understanding of the etiopathogenesis and therapy of EIPH is still rudimentary. Consequently, recommendations for control and prevention can only be speculative. The economic dictates of racing and other competitive equine events are such that major changes in management and preventive medicine will need to induce substantial reductions in the magnitude of this problem if they are to gain industry acceptance.

REFERENCES

311. Pascoe JR et al: Exercise-induced pulmonary hemorrhage in racing thoroughbreds: a preliminary study, *Am J Vet Res* 42:703-707, 1981.
312. Pascoe JR, Raphel CF: Pulmonary hemorrhage in exercising horses, *Compend Cont Educ* 4:S411-S416, 1982.
313. Clarke AF: Review of exercise induced pulmonary haemorrhage and its possible relationship with mechanical stress, *Equine Vet J* 17:166-172, 1985.
314. O'Callaghan MW et al: Exercise-induced pulmonary haemorrhage in the horse: results of a detailed clinical, postmortem, and imaging study. I, Clinical profile of horses, *Equine Vet J* 19:384-388, 1987.
315. Johnstone IB et al: Hemostatic studies in racing Standardbred horses with exercise-induced pulmonary hemorrhage: hemostatic parameters at rest and after moderate exercise, *Can J Vet Res* 55:101-106, 1991.
316. Kingston JK et al: The effect of supramaximal exercise on equine platelet function, *Equine Vet J Suppl* 30:181-183, 1999.
317. Weiss DJ et al: Evaluation of platelet activation and platelet neutrophil aggregates in thoroughbreds undergoing near-maximal treadmill exercise, *Am J Vet Res* 59:393-396, 1998.
318. Whitwell KE, Greet TRC: Collection and evaluation of tracheobronchial washes in the horse, *Equine Vet J* 16:499-508, 1984.
319. Meyer TS et al: Quantification of exercise-induced pulmonary haemorrhage with bronchoalveolar lavage, *Equine Vet J* 30:284-288, 1998.
320. McKane SA, Slocombe RF: Sequential changes in bronchoalveolar lavage cytology after autologous blood inoculation, *Equine Vet J Suppl* 30:126-130, 1999.
321. Beech J: Cytology of tracheobronchial aspirates in horses, *Vet Pathol* 12:157-164, 1975.
322. O'Callaghan MW et al: Exercise-induced pulmonary haemorrhage in the horse: results of a detailed clinical, postmortem and imaging study. V, Microscopic observations, *Equine Vet J* 19:411-418, 1987.

323. O'Callaghan MW et al: Exercise-induced pulmonary haemorrhage in the horse: results of a detailed clinical, postmortem and imaging study. VI, Radiological/pathological correlations, *Equine Vet J* 19:419-422, 1987.

324. Rantanen NW: Evaluation of the respiratory system. In Rantanen NW, McKinnon AD, eds: *Equine diagnostic ultrasonography,* Baltimore, Williams & Wilkins, 1998, p 593.

325. Pascoe JR: Exercise-induced pulmonary hemorrhage: a unifying concept, *Proceedings of the Forty-second Annual Convention of the American Association of Equine Practitioners,* 1996, pp 220-226.

326. West JB, Mathieu-Costello O: Stress failure of pulmonary capillaries as a mechanism for exercise-induced pulmonary haemorrhage in the horse, *Equine Vet J* 26:441-447, 1994.

327. Schroter RC, Marlin DJ, Denny E: Exercise-induced pulmonary haemorrhage (EIPH) in horses results from locomotry impact induced trauma: a novel, unifying concept, *Equine Vet J* 30:186-192.

328. Weiss DJ, Smith II CM: Haemorrheological alterations associated with competitive racing activities in horses: implications for exercise-induced pulmonary haemorrhage (EIPH), *Equine Vet J* 30:7-12, 1998.

329. O'Callaghan MW et al: Exercise-induced pulmonary haemorrhage in the horse: results of a detailed clinical, postmortem and imaging study. VIII, Conclusions and implications, *Equine Vet J* 19:428-434, 1987.

330. Tyler WS et al: Morphologic effects of autologous blood in airspaces of equine lungs, *Proceedings of the Tenth Veterinary Respiratory Symposium,* Michigan State University, Lansing, Mich, September 22, 1991, p S-7.

331. Tyler WS et al: Effects of ozone on exercising horses: a preliminary report, *Equine Exer Physiol* 3:490-502, 1991.

332. McLaughlin RF, Tyler WS, Canada RO: A study of the subgross pulmonary anatomy in various mammals, *Am J Anat* 108:149-165, 1961.

333. O'Callaghan MW et al: Exercise-induced pulmonary haemorrhage in the horse: results of a detailed clinical, postmortem, and imaging study. III, Subgross findings in lungs subjected to latex perfusion of the bronchial and pulmonary arteries, *Equine Vet J* 19:394-404, 1987.

334. Schroter RC et al: Modelling impact-initiated wave transmission through lung parenchyma in relation to the aetiology of exercise-induced pulmonary haemorrhage, *Equine Vet J Suppl* 30:34-38, 1999.

335. Roberts CA, Erickson HH: Exercise-induced pulmonary haemorrhage workshop, *Equine Vet J Suppl* 30: 642-644,1999.

336. Erickson HH, McAvoy JL, Westfall JA: Exercise-induced changes in the lung of Shetland ponies: ultrastructure and morphometry, *J Submicrosc Cytol Pathol* 29: 65-72, 1997.

337. LaPointe JM, Vrins A, McCarvill E: A survey of exercise-induced pulmonary haemorrhage in Quebec Standardbred racehorses, *Equine Vet J* 26:482-485, 1994.

338. Sweeney CR, Soma LR: Exercise-induced pulmonary haemorrhage in horses after different competitive exercises. In Snow DH, Rose RJ, Persson SGB, eds: *Equine exercise physiology,* Cambridge, 1982, Granta, pp 51-56.

339. Voynick BT, Sweeney CR: Exercise-induced pulmonary hemorrhage in polo and racing horses, *J Am Vet Med Assoc* 188:301-302, 1986.

340. O'Callaghan MW et al: Exercise-induced pulmonary haemorrhage in the horse: results of a detailed clinical, postmortem and imaging study. II, Gross pathology, *Equine Vet J* 19:389-393, 1987.

341. West JB et al: Stress failure of pulmonary capillaries in racehorses with exercise-induced pulmonary hemorrhage, *J Appl Physiol* 75:1097-1109, 1993.

342. Sweeney CR: Exercise-induced pulmonary hemorrhage. In Robinson NE, ed: *Current therapy in equine medicine,* ed 2, Philadelphia, 1986, WB Saunders, pp 603-605.

343. Pascoe JR: Exercise-induced pulmonary hemorrhage. In Robinson NE, ed: *Current therapy in equine medicine,* ed 4, Philadelphia, 1997, WB Saunders, pp 441-443.

344. Hinchcliff KW: Effects of furosemide on athletic performance and exercise-induced pulmonary hemorrhage in horses, *J Am Vet Med Assoc* 215:630-635,1999.

345. Pascoe JR, McCabe AE, Franti CE: Efficacy of furosemide in the treatment of exercise-induced pulmonary hemorrhage in thoroughbred racehorses, *Am J Vet Res* 46:2000-2003, 1985.

346. Sweeney CR et al: Effects of furosemide on racing times of thoroughbreds, *Am J Vet Res* 51:772-778, 1990.

347. Soma LR et al: Effects of furosemide on the racing time of horses with exercise induced pulmonary hemorrhage, *Am J Vet Res* 46:763-768, 1985.

348. Gross DK et al: Effect of furosemide on performance of thoroughbreds racing in the United States and Canada, *J Am Vet Med Assoc* 215:670-675, 1999.

349. Tobin T et al: The pharmacology of furosemide in the horse. III, Dose and time relationships, effects of repeated dosing and performance effects, *J Equine Med Surg* 2:216-226, 1978.

350. Manohar M: Furosemide attenuates the exercise-induced increase in pulmonary artery wedge pressure in horses, *Am J Vet Res* 54:952-958, 1993.

351. Gleed RD et al: Effects of furosemide on pulmonary capillary pressure in horses exercising on a treadmill, *Equine Vet J Suppl* 30:102-106, 1999.

352. Manohar M: Pulmonary vascular pressures of strenuously exercising thoroughbreds after administration of flunixin meglumine and furosemide, *Am J Vet Res* 55:1308-1312, 1994.

353. Goetz T, Manohar M, Magid JH: Repeated administration of furosemide does not offer an advantage over single dosing in attenuating exercise-induced pulmonary hypertension in thoroughbred horses, *Equine Vet J Suppl* 30:539-545, 1999.

354. Broadstone RV et al: Effects of furosemide on ponies with recurrent airway obstruction, *Pulm Pharmacol* 4:203-208, 1991.

PHARYNGITIS

JOHN R. PASCOE

DEFINITION AND ETIOLOGY. Pharyngitis is inflammation of the pharyngeal tissues. It is not generally considered to be a specific disease entity but rather a response to other diseases, particularly viral and bacterial respiratory disease, and to a lesser extent to local physical, chemical, or allergic causes. Acute and chronic forms of pharyngitis are recognized.

Although physical and chemical causes of pharyngitis may be identified with certainty, the role and specificity of microbial pathogens as causative agents remain controversial. In horses, *Streptococcus* spp., picornavirus, rhinovirus 1 and 2, herpesvirus (equine herpesvirus [EHV-1, EHV-2]), myxovirus (influenza A/equi 1, A/equi 2), and paramyxovirus (parainfluenza 3) have been incriminated as specific causes of pharyngitis.[355-359] In cattle, *Corynebacterium pyogenes, Actinobacillus* spp., and *Fusiformis necrophorus* are frequently isolated.[360]

In horses, synonyms for chronic pharyngitis include pharyngeal lymphoid hyperplasia (also PLH), chronic pharyngitis, chronic lymphoid follicular hyperplasia, follicular pharyngitis, and follikelkatarrh.[361-363]

CLINICAL SIGNS AND DIFFERENTIAL DIAGNOSIS. In acute pharyngitis, signs are associated with pharyngeal pain (odynophagia, dysphagia), nasal discharge (serous, seromucous, mucopurulent, purulent, feed-contaminated), regional lymphadenopathy (submandibular, retropharyngeal nodes), ptyalism (especially in cattle), respiratory noise (often inspiratory), pharyngeal swelling, and cough. Mouth breathing may occur in cattle when there is increased resistance to breathing associated with excessive exudate, diphtherous membranes, and lymphadenopathy or lymph node abscess. When pharyngitis results from local pharyngeal trauma or incarcerated foreign bodies, there may also be odor associated with either the breath or the nasal discharge. Calves with necrotic laryngitis, pharyngitis, and stomatitis also have a characteristic malodorous breath. Acute laryngeal inflammation and edema of unknown cause can occur in horses and ruminants and is characterized by marked inspiratory dyspnea and stertor without malodorous breath. Treatment of acute edema with dexamethasone (0.05 mg/kg IM) and broad-spectrum antimicrobials or penicillin has produced rapid clinical improvement.

Signs observed on endoscopic or oropharyngeal examination in cattle include hyperemia and edema of the pharynx, lymphonodular swelling, and either a moist appearance of the pharyngeal surface or the presence of exudate or a diphtherous membrane adhering to the pharyngeal surface. Focal necrosis or ulceration of the mucous membrane and tonsillar tissue may occur; signs associated with rhinitis and laryngitis may also be evident. Signs of chronic pharyngitis are similar. In horses, there may be endoscopic evidence of more marked hyperplasia of the lymphonodular follicles within the pharyngeal mucosa and single or multiple lymphonodular masses may be within, or protrude from, the pharyngeal mucosa. Biopsy and cytologic evaluation are recommended to rule out neoplasia, particularly squamous cell carcinoma, lymphoma, and lymphosarcoma. Differential diagnostic possibilities include rhinitis and laryngitis, and in cattle, rabies should be strongly considered before oropharyngeal examination. If the predominant sign is dysphagia (see Chapter 7), other diagnostic ruleouts include tongue foreign bodies, fractures of the hyoid apparatus or jaws, and in the horse, dis-

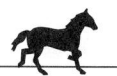

eases of the guttural pouches. If exercise intolerance is the primary complaint in a horse, pharyngitis should only be considered after all other possible causes of impaired performance have been eliminated (see Chapter 5).[364-368]

Upper airway inspiratory pressures recorded during strenuous exercise in horses with grade IV lymphoid hyperplasia do not appear to be different from those recorded in normal horses under the same exercise conditions.[367] If the assumption is made that airflow in both groups of horses is comparable, then severe lymphoid hyperplasia does not appear to cause functional upper airway obstruction. It is conceivable that pharyngeal pain associated with lymphoid hyperplasia may contribute to bronchoconstriction and impaired performance; however, this effect remains to be proved.

CLINICAL PATHOLOGY. Changes in the hemogram and biochemical profiles are likely to result from concurrent respiratory disease (increases or decreases in absolute or differential leukocyte counts, hyperfibrinogenemia, anemia) or reflect abscess formation (neutrophilia, hyperfibrinogenemia) or dehydration and fasting associated with dysphagia.

LABORATORY AIDS AND DEFINITIVE DIAGNOSTIC TESTS. Although a presumptive diagnosis can be made from the clinical signs, definitive diagnosis requires observation of the pharynx (Fig. 29-22) and, more important, exclusion of other conditions that might have similar signs. Radiography of the pharynx can provide information on pharyngeal anatomy, radiodense foreign bodies, soft-tissue masses, fractures, and in horses, guttural pouch disorders. Ultrasonography of the pharyngeal region and, if indicated from the clinical examination, both radiographic and ultrasound examination of the thorax may help define the extent of concurrent pulmonary disease.

Microbial culture of pharyngeal secretions can be considered, but interpretation of results is difficult because (1) the pharynx normally has a resident microflora that has considerable individual variation, and (2) many of the microorganisms isolated are capable of opportunistic infection. In horses with grades III and IV pharyngeal lymphoid hyper-

plasia, the number of bacteria recovered per gram of pharyngeal secretion was almost 100-fold greater than in normal horses.[368] The pattern of microbial isolation was not consistent among horses, suggesting that these organisms were not the source of the pharyngitis but rather other factors had made conditions for colonization more favorable.

Biopsy and cytologic examination are indicated in refractory cases and when abnormal masses are present to rule out neoplasia.

PATHOPHYSIOLOGY. Acute pharyngitis occurs as a sequela to inflammation of regional lymphoid tissue. In horses the pharyngeal tonsil consists of discrete lymphoid follicles diffusely distributed in the dorsal and lateral walls of the pharynx. In ruminants the pharyngeal tonsil is located caudal to the pharyngeal septum in the caudodorsal wall of the pharynx and is bounded by long ridges and grooves into which mucous glands open. In response to local or lymphogenous spread of infection, the tonsillar tissue becomes inflamed and the tonsillar crypts become filled with desquamated epithelium, leukocytes, and bacteria. Clinically this is seen as hyperemia and edema of the pharyngeal tonsil with diffuse white or yellow tips to the lymph nodules. The edematous appearance is associated with hyperplasia of the lymph nodules and sequestration of perinodular inflammatory fluid.

If extensive destruction of the lymphoid cells or subsequent invasion of the nodules or supporting soft tissue is evident, the result is focal or diffuse necrosis, which may be seen as pinpoint areas of follicular necrosis or diffuse necrosis with associated purulent or fibrinonecrotic exudate. With resolution, atrophy of some follicles and increased fibrosis are present. Follicular atrophy also occurs with aging.

EPIDEMIOLOGY. No specific epidemiologic data are available on pharyngitis. When pharyngitis occurs as a sequela to respiratory tract infection, the population demographics should be similar to those known for the specific respiratory disease. For example, grade II pharyngeal lymphoid hyperplasia was identified in 60% of foals with distal respiratory tract infection and in only 13% of control foals.[369] Because physical and chemical injury to the pharynx occur sporadically, no universal epidemiologic characteristics would be anticipated.

Pharyngeal lymphoid hyperplasia has been reported to be particularly prevalent in horses younger than 5 or 6 years of age.[361,365,370-372] In an endoscopic survey of 479 horses, primarily Thoroughbreds in race training, 141 (29%) had pharyngeal lymphoid hyperplasia. Of the 2-year-olds, 63% were affected, and the prevalence decreased with age; less than 20% of horses older than 5 years were affected.[365] In a subsequent survey of 678 Thoroughbred horses in training, the prevalence of pharyngeal lymphoid hyperplasia was 34%: the prevalence was again age-related and severe grades of pharyngeal lymphoid hyperplasia were observed more often in younger horses.[370] Grade II pharyngeal lymphoid hyperplasia was observed in 45% of 2-year-old horses, whereas only 16%, 15%, and 12% of 3-, 4-, and 5-year-old horses were classified as grade II. Similar results were reported from Japan for racing Thoroughbreds with a history of cough or abnormal respiratory noise.[371]

TREATMENT AND PROGNOSIS. The approach to treatment is largely symptomatic and directed to palliation of pharyngeal pain and maintenance of unobstructed breathing until the initiating disease process has abated. In many instances the signs are sufficiently mild that treatment is unnecessary. When pharyngeal angina is causing inappetence or dysphagia, administration of nonsteroidal antiinflammatory drugs should be considered. Dehydration should be corrected by either parenteral or enteral fluid administration. Enteral fluid therapy may be difficult because passage of a

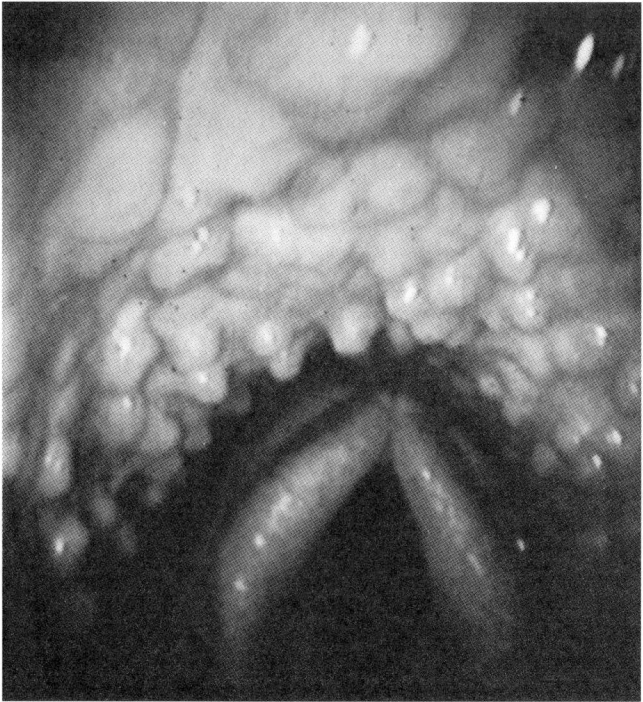

FIG. 29-22 ■ Endoscopic view showing the nodular appearance of pharyngeal lymphoid hyperplasia.

nasogastric tube may elicit too much pain. If the animal has been inappetent for several days, nutritional support may be necessary until pharyngeal pain subsides sufficiently to allow normal eating to resume. Soft feeds, especially green grass, should be offered when available to encourage animals with pharyngeal discomfort to eat.

Although routine antimicrobial therapy is probably not indicated, it is often given to limit development of secondary bacterial infection. Infections caused by foreign body injuries should be treated with antibiotics that have broad aerobic and anaerobic sensitivity. Daily lavage of any cavitary wounds, debridement, and removal of feed material may be necessary to prevent additional abscess formation and hasten healing.

Custom topical preparations, usually containing an antibiotic, an antiinflammatory drug, and a hygroscopic agent (glycerine) or dimethyl sulfoxide, are often used for palliation of clinical signs, especially in horses with pharyngeal lymphoid hyperplasia.[372,373] These preparations are usually administered two or three times daily through a transnasal catheter and sprayed onto the pharyngeal surface. Despite their frequent use, it is not known whether this form of therapy is effective or whether the response merely reflects natural resolution of the predisposing cause.

Treatment of pharyngeal lymphoid hyperplasia is also empiric and generally palliative. Rest from training for 4 to 8 weeks is commonly advocated, and, although some horses experience recurrence when training resumes, this enforced rest is beneficial as a convalescent period for any concurrent subclinical respiratory disease. Horses that are kept in training are often initially treated empirically with sulfa compounds and topical throat preparations. With continued clinical signs, penicillin or broad-spectrum antibiotics are often given. If the pharyngeal lymphoid hyperplasia does not improve or resolve after this therapy, pharyngeal cautery is often used. Techniques for pharyngeal cautery include topical application of trichloroacetic acid, electrocautery, freezing with liquid nitrogen or freon, or photoablation by Nd:YAG laser in either contact or noncontact technique.[372-375] Cauterization techniques have received considerable testimonial support, but it should be realized that cautery does not really effect a cure but rather obliterates the reactive tissue so that it is no longer clinically evident.

Routine immunization at frequent intervals for known viral respiratory pathogens is also advocated for both treatment and prevention of pharyngeal lymphoid hyperplasia.[372,376]

PREVENTION AND CONTROL. Methods used to control and prevent most of the common viral and bacterial respiratory diseases (see Chapter 44) should limit herd problems with acute pharyngitis. Nonrespiratory disease–related causes such as trauma from balling guns, nasogastric tubes and dose syringes, foreign objects, and chemical burns—can be minimized by improvement of husbandry practices.

Although preventing pharyngeal lymphoid hyperplasia in horses by prophylactic immunization for common equine viral respiratory agents at regular intervals has been discussed at length, there are no substantive data to support this practice. Nevertheless, racetrack veterinarians maintain that frequent immunization (60-day intervals) against influenza and rhinopneumonitis markedly reduces the severity of pharyngeal lymphoid hyperplasia and improves exercise tolerance.[376] Considering the mobility of racing and show horse populations, this approach should at least be beneficial for limiting outbreaks of viral respiratory disease and consequently perhaps limiting chronic pharyngeal lymphoid hyperplasia. Until more is understood about the clinical appearance of the pharyngeal tonsil in horses, along with normal variations that occur with aging in exercised and nonexercised horses, and these findings can be correlated with immunopathologic events and indexes of performance, it will remain difficult to treat, control, and prevent pharyngitis in a systematic manner.[377]

REFERENCES

355. Fallon EH: The clinical aspects of streptococcic infections of horses, *J Am Vet Med Assoc* 155:413-415, 1969.
356. Platt H: The role of respiratory viruses in equine disease, *Vet Rec* 91:33-36, 1972.
357. Lewis PF: Epidemiology of major respiratory diseases of the horse, *Aust Vet J* 45:231-236, 1969.
358. Blakeslee JR et al: Evidence of respiratory tract infection induced by equine herpesvirus, type 2, in the horse, *Can J Microbiol* 21:1940-1946, 1975.
359. Follicular pharyngitis, *American Association of Equine Practitioners Newsletter*, No 2, 1980, pp 92-94.
360. Mackey DR: Pharyngitis. In Amstutz HE, ed: *Bovine medicine and surgery*, vol 2, Santa Barbara, 1980, American Veterinary Publications, pp 711-712.
361. McAllister ES, Blakeslee JR: Clinical observations of pharyngitis in the horse, *J Am Vet Med Assoc* 170:739-741, 1977.
362. Raker CW, Boles CL: Pharyngeal lymphoid hyperplasia in the horse, *J Equine Med Surg* 2:202-207, 1978.
363. Boening KH: Klinische und endoskopische Beobachtungen beim "Follikelkatarrh" der Pferde, *Tierarztl Prax* 4:300-302, 1978.
364. Ferraro GL: Equine follicular pharyngitis, *Proceedings of the Twenty-seventh Annual Convention of the American Association of Equine Practitioners*, 1981, pp 55-56.
365. Raphel CF: Endoscopic findings in the upper respiratory tract of 479 horses, *J Am Vet Med Assoc* 181:470-473, 1982.
366. Burrell MH: Endoscopic and virological observations on respiratory disease in a group of young thoroughbred horses in training, *Equine Vet J* 17:99-103, 1985.
367. Williams JW et al: Upper airway function during maximal exercise in horses with obstructive upper airway lesions: effect of surgical treatment, *Vet Surg* 19:142-147, 1990.
368. Hoquet F et al: Comparison of the bacterial and fungal flora in the pharynx of normal horses and horses affected with pharyngitis, *Can Vet J* 26:342-346, 1985.
369. Hoffman AM et al: Clinical and endoscopic study to estimate the incidence of distal respiratory tract infection in thoroughbred foals on Ontario breeding farms, *Am J Vet Res* 54:1602-1607, 1993.
370. Sweeney CR, Maxson AD, Soma LR: Endoscopic findings in the upper respiratory tract of 678 thoroughbred racehorses, *J Am Vet Med Assoc* 198:1037-1038, 1991.
371. Hobo S, Matsuda Y, Yoshida K: Prevalence of upper respiratory tract disorders detected with a flexible videoendoscope in thoroughbred horses, *J Vet Med Sci* 57:409-413, 1995.
372. Bayly WM: Pharyngitis. In Robinson NE, ed: *Current therapy in equine medicine*, Philadelphia, 1983, WB Saunders, pp 490-493.
373. Haynes PF: Pharyngeal lymphoid hyperplasia. In Jennings PB, ed: *The practice of large animal surgery*, Philadelphia, 1984, WB Saunders, pp 418-423.
374. Dean PW: Upper airway obstruction in performance horses: differential diagnosis and treatment, *Vet Clin North Am (Equine Pract)* 7:123-148, 1991.
375. Palmer SE: Neodymium:YAG laser treatment of pharyngeal lymphoid hyperplasia, pharyngeal polyps, subepiglottic cysts and granulation tissue in the upper airway of the horse. In Rantanen NW, Hauser ML, editors: *Proceedings of Dubai International Equine Symposium: The Diagnosis and Treatment of Respiratory Disease*, 1997, pp 425-436.
376. Montgomery T: A clinical consideration of the causes of chronic equine pharyngitis in the equine, *Equine Pract* 3:26-36, 1981.
377. Kester WO: Equine pharyngitis report, *American Association of Equine Practitioners Newsletter*, No 3, 1976, pp 19-25.

GUTTURAL POUCH DISEASES

CLIFFORD M. HONNAS
JOHN R. PASCOE

DEFINITION AND ETIOLOGY. The guttural pouches are paired air-filled diverticula of the eustachian tubes that communicate between the middle ear and the pharynx. They are located ventral to the atlas, dorsocaudal to the pharynx, and rostrodorsal to the retropharyngeal lymph nodes and occupy a large part of the retropharyngeal space. Each pouch is divided into medial and lateral compartments by a stylohyoid bone that courses through the caudolateral aspect of each pouch. The medial compartments appose each other on the midline. The lateral walls of each guttural pouch contain cranial nerves VII (facial), IX (glossopharyngeal), X (vagus), XI (spinal accessory), and XII (hypoglossal); the cranial sympathetic trunk; the internal carotid artery; and branches of the external carotid artery.[378] The intimate relationship of these vessels and nerves with the mucous membrane lining the guttural pouches explains why epistaxis and nerve dysfunction frequently accompany guttural pouch disease. Each pouch has a capacity of approximately 300 ml, with the medial compartment accounting for approximately two thirds of this volume. Communication with the pharynx occurs through a slitlike opening situated rostral and ventral to the pharyngeal recess. The pharyngeal opening of the guttural pouch is funnel-shaped and wider rostrally than caudally. The plica salpingopharyngea is a fold of mucous membrane that contributes to the caudal narrowing of the pharyngeal opening and makes catheterization of the guttural pouch difficult. Redundancy of this fold of tissue may contribute to guttural pouch tympany.[378]

The guttural pouch is not a sterile environment; as an extension of the pharynx, it normally contains bacteria. In one report of 30 normal horses, 59% of percutaneous guttural pouch lavage aspirates had bacterial growth, although only 7% were considered to have bacteria considered to be pathogenic; no fungi were isolated.[379] Inflammatory cell counts and distribution were correlated with recovery of bacteria. Aspirates were considered normal if there were less than 5% neutrophils; typical cell distribution was primarily ciliated columnar epithelial cells, a few nonciliated cuboidal epithelial cells, and less than 1% monocytes, lymphocytes, and macrophages.[379] Horses exercised strenuously on a regular basis had lower total cell counts, lower neutrophil counts, and fewer bacteria isolated.[379]

Three disease conditions commonly affect the guttural pouches: tympanitis, empyema, and mycosis.[37] Less common conditions include neoplasia,[380] fractures of the hyoid bone, foreign bodies,[378,381] and cystic structures.[382]

GUTTURAL POUCH TYMPANY

Tympany of the guttural pouch occurs infrequently and is recognized in foals after birth up to $1\frac{1}{2}$ years of age.[378,383,384] It is characterized by unilateral or bilateral distention of the guttural pouch with air. The exact cause is unknown, but numerous reports have implicated a congenital redundancy of the plica salpingopharyngea, which acts as a one-way valve that apparently permits airflow into but not out of the pouch.[383] It has also been postulated that upper airway infections and inflammation may result in enlargement of this fold of tissue, with subsequent air trapping in the pouch.[385]

CLINICAL SIGNS AND DIFFERENTIAL DIAGNOSIS. Affected foals usually have a nonpainful, soft, fluctuant swelling in the retropharyngeal space (Fig. 29-23, *A*) with variable respiratory distress, extension of the head and neck, and signs of dysphagia.[383,384] Mild tympany may not result in signs other than swelling of the throatlatch region.[385] Respiratory distress occurs when continued distention of the pouch compresses the pharyngeal area. The differential diagnosis should include guttural pouch empyema and retropharyngeal abscesses or cellulitis.

CLINICAL PATHOLOGY. Stress leukocytosis may occur if there is marked respiratory distress.

DIAGNOSTIC AIDS. Diagnosis of guttural pouch tympany is based on recognition of characteristic swelling in the retropharyngeal space and confirmation by physical examination. Although the distention is most often unilateral, extreme distortion of a single pouch may give the impression of bilateral involvement.[386] Differentiation between unilateral

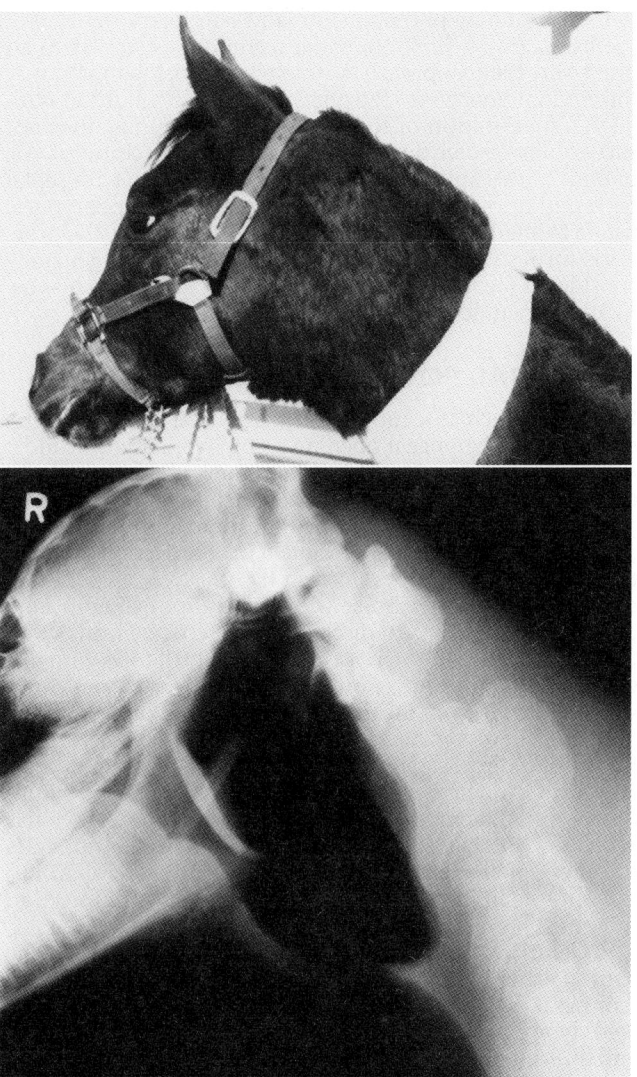

FIG. 29-23 ■ **A,** Foal with guttural pouch tympanitis. Note the protrusion of the soft tissues over the lateral and ventral aspects of the throatlatch. **B,** Lateral radiograph of a foal with tympanites of both guttural pouches.

and bilateral involvement can be difficult and may require deflation of the affected guttural pouch by catheterization or percutaneous needle aspiration combined with external compression. Other adjunctive diagnostic procedures include radiographic demonstration of gas distention of one or both pouches (Fig. 29-23, *B*) and endoscopic observation of pouch distention and pharyngeal distortion.

TREATMENT AND PROGNOSIS. Guttural pouch tympany and respiratory distress can be alleviated temporarily by aspiration of air from the affected pouch by means of either percutaneous decompression at the point of greatest distention through Viborg's triangle or introduction of a catheter through the pharyngeal opening of the guttural pouch.[378] These measures are palliative, and the pouch rapidly refills when decompression is discontinued. Treatment methods of choice include surgical excision or photoablation of the redundant plica salpingopharyngea; fenestration of the medium septum between the two pouches by excision, electrosurgery, or photoablation; or creation of a salpingopharyngeal fistula by photoablation and temporary stenting of the fistula.[383,384,387-389] The latter technique is similar to an older, successful approach that involved incising the floor of the guttural pouch into the pharynx.[390] If the condition is bilateral, fenestration of the median septum alone does not successfully resolve the condition and either excision of one or both plica salpingopharyngea in combination with septal fenestration or septal fenestration and salpingopharyngeal fistula formation must be performed. After surgery, the prognosis for resolution of guttural pouch tympany is generally considered favorable unless complicating factors such as aspiration pneumonia exist.[384]

GUTTURAL POUCH EMPYEMA

Guttural pouch infections are introduced either directly through the pharyngeal opening or by lymphatic spread.[391] Accumulation of purulent material (empyema) is considered to be a secondary, chronic, localized manifestation of a more generalized ascending respiratory infection. Empyema is usually unilateral and is often a sequela to an infectious respiratory disease, especially infection by *Streptococcus equi* ssp. *equi*.[392-394] Typically a horse with guttural pouch empyema displays continued nasal discharge after recovery from streptococcal infection.[386] In a case control study of foals with distal respiratory tract infection, 21% had concurrent mucopurulent drainage from the pharyngeal openings of the guttural pouches.[395] *Streptococcus equi* ssp. *zooepidemicus* was isolated from respiratory secretions of the majority of infected foals and from exudate collected from guttural pouches.[396] Rupture of retropharyngeal abscesses into the guttural pouch has also been associated with empyema, suggesting that strangles or other upper respiratory tract infections may have an important role in the development of guttural pouch infection in horses.[393,397]

CLINICAL SIGNS AND DIFFERENTIAL DIAGNOSIS. The clinical signs of guttural pouch empyema include intermittent nasal discharge that may worsen when the head is lowered, lymphadenitis, parotid swelling and pain, dysphagia, and difficult breathing. The nasal discharge can be unilateral or bilateral, even if only one pouch is affected, because the pharyngeal openings of the guttural pouches are located caudal to the nasal septum. The nasal discharge is generally nonodorous, white, and opaque. Signs of dysphagia may be observed secondary to pharyngeal compression or paresis. Labored breathing may result from gradual collapse of the pharynx as the guttural pouch distends. Inspissation of the purulent material results in chondroids, which are hard concretions of inspissated pus.[398] The differential diagnosis of guttural pouch empyema should include those diseases with chronic mucopurulent nasal discharge such as pneumonia, sinusitis, upper respiratory tract infections, and guttural pouch tympany.

CLINICAL PATHOLOGY. Leukocytosis is often present. Plasma fibrinogen levels are often increased, and these changes generally parallel the development of leukocytosis, pyrexia, and clinical signs of strangles or primary guttural pouch empyema. Analysis of fluid obtained by catheterization of the guttural pouch often reveals a β-hemolytic *Streptococcus* sp.[393,398]

DIAGNOSTIC AIDS. Guttural pouch empyema should be considered in any patient with a chronic, nonresponsive nasal discharge.[386] Diagnostic aids include radiography, endoscopy, percutaneous centesis, and aspiration of material from the pouch through the pharyngeal opening.[378] Recognition of fluid (Fig. 29-24) or radiodense masses (chondroids) within the pouch on standing lateral radiographs supports a diagnosis of empyema. Physical and endoscopic examination or oblique radiographic projections may be nec-

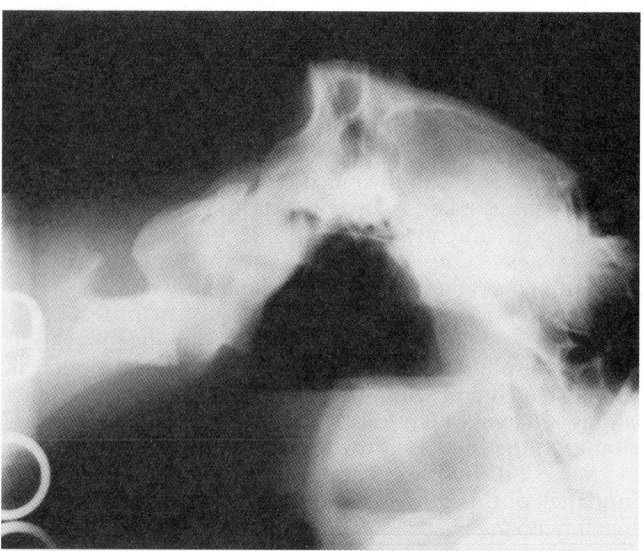

FIG. 29-24 ▓ Lateral radiograph demonstrating distinct fluid lines in both guttural pouches.

essary to identify which pouch is involved. Endoscopic examination permits identification of the affected pouch and evaluation of the character of the fluid. The absence of fluid at the pharyngeal ostium does not preclude the possibility of guttural pouch empyema, especially if the fluid has become inspissated.[386] Fluid identified on radiographs should be characterized by endoscopic examination of the pouches or aspiration of the fluid with appropriate cytologic and microbial analysis. Fluid samples can be aspirated through the pharyngeal ostium with a sterile artificial insemination pipette, a Chambers catheter, or tubing advanced through the biopsy channel of an endoscope. Alternately, fluid can be aspirated percutaneously, but this may lead to cellulitis along the needle tract if pathogenic bacteria are tracked through tissues on needle withdrawal.

PATHOPHYSIOLOGY. Strangles is a common upper respiratory disease affecting young horses. Primary clinical signs of strangles usually develop after a short incubation period of 2 to 6 days and include depression, pyrexia, coughing, and ocular and nasal discharges that become mucopurulent as the disease progresses. Lymph nodes of the head and neck become enlarged and painful, often forming abscesses. Guttural pouch empyema may result from extension of the upper respiratory infection with *S. equi* (strangles) to the guttural pouches or from rupture of retropharyngeal lymph node abscesses into the guttural pouch.[392,393] Many patients with empyema do not have a history of strangles, and empyema appears to occur by many of the same mechanisms as middle ear infection: that is, fluid accumulates in the area and uncontrolled growth of bacteria normally present results in inflammation and exudation.

TREATMENT AND PROGNOSIS. Treatment of guttural pouch empyema is complicated by poor drainage from the affected pouch.[378] In the normal horse the pharyngeal opening of the guttural pouch is located rostrodorsal to the floor of the guttural pouch, and drainage can only be achieved by lowering the horse's head.[378,387,391] However, in horses with empyema, lowering the head may not achieve adequate drainage if there is ventral distortion of the pouch.[378] Inflammation of the lining mucosa may result in swelling of the tissue surrounding the pharyngeal opening, further compromising normal drainage.[378]

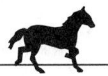

Choice of medical or surgical treatment depends on the duration and nature of the empyema. Parenteral antimicrobial therapy may reduce the quantity of the nasal discharge, but relapse often follows cessation of treatment.[386] The early stages of empyema may respond to daily lavage of the affected guttural pouch with saline antibiotic solutions injected through a catheter. A volume of 500 ml should be flushed into the involved pouch under moderate pressure to create contact with as much of the interior of the guttural pouch as possible.[399] During lavage the head should be lowered to prevent aspiration of fluid. Purulent fluid from the affected guttural pouch should be aspirated on initial catheterization and submitted for bacterial culture and antimicrobial susceptibility testing. This can be accomplished with most flexible uterine culturettes under direct endoscopic observation. Parenteral antimicrobial drugs should be administered on the basis of susceptibility testing results; although they may be of benefit in treating empyema, adequate drainage and local therapy are of primary therapeutic importance.

Irrigating the guttural pouch with an indwelling catheter may result in the development of severe inflammatory changes in the guttural pouch.[400] Indwelling catheters placed in horses with normal guttural pouches have caused increasing purulent discharge with time; nasal discharge diminished after catheter removal and was absent after 3 days. Povidone iodine (1% available iodine) diluted to a 10% solution (0.1% available iodine) for lavage of the guttural pouch caused considerable reaction, including inflammatory infiltrates, hemorrhage, necrosis, and lymphoid reaction. Therefore, if possible, other means should be used to achieve antiseptic or antimicrobial therapeutic goals.[400] Consideration should be given to using nonirritating solutions to prevent initiating cranial nerve neuritis. Although indwelling catheters are convenient, it may be well to suggest daily catheterization and irrigation with an artificial insemination (AI) pipette or Chambers catheter to diminish the inflammatory response associated with indwelling catheters in an already inflamed guttural pouch. Consideration of daily catheterization must be weighed against stress, possible tissue trauma, and time requirements for intermittent catheterization.[400]

Treatment with parenteral antimicrobials and local lavage is successful, but the course of treatment may be protracted. If response to treatment is poor or if secretions reaccumulate and empyema returns, surgical drainage of the guttural pouch should be considered.[378] Surgery is generally indicated when purulent material becomes inspissated or chondroids have formed,[378,401] although resolution has been reported in one horse after prolonged lavage (14 days) through an indwelling catheter.[402]

The prognosis for guttural pouch empyema is generally favorable if it is recognized promptly and treated appropriately.

GUTTURAL POUCH MYCOSIS

Guttural pouch mycosis is a fungal disease of the guttural pouch that typically affects the dorsocaudal region of the medial compartment, although lesions have been seen affecting larger areas, including the lateral compartment.[386,403-406] Fungal invasion of neurovascular structures coursing through the walls of the guttural pouches results in clinically apparent disease. Although the exact cause of guttural pouch mycosis is not known, a number of fungi, especially *Aspergillus (Emericella) nidulans,* have been isolated from the lesions.[378,406-411]

CLINICAL SIGNS AND DIFFERENTIAL DIAGNOSIS. Lesions are usually unilateral, occasionally bilateral. The wide spectrum of clinical signs that can occur in association with guttural pouch mycosis reflects the degree of fungal invasion and subsequent inflammation of vascular structures or nerves beneath the mucous membrane lining the guttural pouch.

Common clinical signs include intermittent spontaneous epistaxis and dysphagia.[378,403] Epistaxis generally results from fungal erosion of the wall of the internal carotid artery in the roof of the medial compartment and, less commonly, from erosion of the external carotid artery and maxillary artery in the lateral compartment.[378,403] Epistaxis is usually unilateral, occurring from the ipsilateral nostril, but can also be bilateral because the pharyngeal openings of the guttural pouches are located caudal to the caudal border of the nasal septum.[405] Episodes of epistaxis generally occur while the horse is at rest and can vary from mild to severe, with several premonitory bleeds that generally culminate in a fatal episode of epistaxis.[404,405] Occasionally a horse dies of a single episode of epistaxis without previous clinical signs. Epistaxis may recur at intervals varying from 24 hours to 3 weeks.[405]

Dysphagia, the second most common clinical sign, likely results from damage to the pharyngeal branches of the vagus and glossopharyngeal nerves and generally occurs later than epistaxis in the course of the disease.[405] Horses with dysphagia cough during attempts to eat solid food, and, in addition to nasal discharge containing food material, a considerable quantity of food is coughed out the mouth. Recovery from dysphagia may occur,[405] but in general the prognosis for full recovery is poor.

Other clinical signs include parotid pain, abnormal head posture, unilateral or bilateral nasal discharge, head shyness, abnormal respiratory noise, sweating and shivering, Horner's syndrome, visual disturbances, colic, and facial paralysis.[404,405,410-412] These symptoms are the result of angina and dysfunction of cranial nerves and the sympathetic nervous system.

The differential diagnosis for the horse with epistaxis should include exercise-induced pulmonary hemorrhage, ethmoid hematoma, guttural pouch or pharyngeal neoplasia, tracheobronchial foreign bodies, and guttural pouch mycosis.[405] Differentiation of these diseases is aided by a thorough history and endoscopic examination. Differential diagnosis for dysphagia should include fractures of the hyoid apparatus; pharyngeal/guttural pouch fistula; cleft palate; esophagitis; pharyngeal paralysis; foreign body entrapment in the mouth or esophagus; pharyngeal neoplasia; lead poisoning; bacterial, viral, and mycotic central nervous system infections; and guttural pouch mycosis.[405,411]

CLINICAL PATHOLOGY. If epistaxis is the presenting complaint, there may be a moderate to severe anemia with an accompanying hypoproteinemia. Differential white cell distributions may be normal or indicate a stress response. If dysphagia becomes a dominant clinical sign, other hematologic changes indicative of infection secondary to aspiration pneumonia may be evident.

DIAGNOSTIC AIDS. Clinical signs of epistaxis or cranial nerve dysfunction are suggestive of a diagnosis of guttural pouch mycosis. A thorough physical examination may reveal abnormal sensitivity on digital palpation of the parotid area on the affected side.[404] A definitive diagnosis of guttural pouch mycosis requires endoscopic observation of the characteristic diphtheritic lesion in the dorsocaudal aspect of the medial compartment or elsewhere within the guttural pouch.[405] A healed lesion may be identified by the presence of scar tissue within the mucous membrane.[405] Lesions may vary in color (brown, yellow, black, or white) and in size, from discrete nodules to diffuse irregular patches covering the roof of both the medial and lateral compartments[406,412]; erosion with fistula formation can occur into the opposite guttural pouch or pharynx. Occasionally the characteristic lesion is obscured by clotted blood, so that the diagnosis is based on the clinical signs of epistaxis correlated with blood present in the guttural pouch. Because hemorrhage may originate from the internal carotid, external carotid, or maxillary

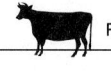

arteries, it is important to identify the source of bleeding before therapy, particularly if surgical intervention is being considered.[403] Care should be taken not to dislodge a thrombus and produce further hemorrhage. If dysphagia is apparent, food and saliva may be identified during endoscopy of the pharynx and nasal passages.[378]

In guttural pouch mycotic infections, radiographs are of limited value because only minimum suppuration is associated with mycotic infections[411]; however, the lateral view may allow assessment of the degree of fibrous reaction and loss of normal air space.[411] Radiography may also aid in diagnosing some of the long-term sequelae such as fibrous deposits in the pouch and associated bony changes.[413]

Serum titers to *Aspergillus fumigatus* are not diagnostic; however, reactivity to 22-kd and 26-kd serum antigens measured by immunoblot analysis may be diagnostic for guttural pouch mycosis.[414]

PATHOPHYSIOLOGY. The pathogenesis and predisposing factors leading to guttural pouch mycosis and arterial erosion are unknown, but it is believed that the disease is initiated by some stress to the soft tissues where the mycotic plaques are generally found.[406] Potential stresses include inflammation, trauma, or vascular insult.[397] Aneurysm formation is not well correlated with the severity of the plaque formation. Although the nature of the initiating lesion remains unclear, it is generally agreed that the later stages are associated with deep fungal infections.[406] *A. nidulans* and other *Aspergillus* spp. have been isolated in several of the reported cases and may be the causal agents.[406-413] *A. nidulans* is rarely pathogenic, but in the warm humid environment of the guttural pouch it may grow as an opportunist under certain circumstances.[406] The mycotic lesions show no predilection for either the right or left guttural pouch.[405] Fungal infection of the pouch and erosion of major blood vessels and involvement of nerves (IX, X, XI, XII, cranial cervical ganglion and postganglionic sympathetic fibers) that traverse the area explain the epistaxis, local pain, and neurologic signs associated with guttural pouch mycosis.[405,406]

EPIDEMIOLOGY. No apparent age, sex, breed, or geographic predispositions have been observed. Guttural pouch mycosis is a sporadic disease that tends to arise during the warmer months of the year and rarely affects more than one horse in a particular stable.[405] Affected horses are afebrile; infection is diagnosed when clinical signs such as epistaxis and dysphagia occur.[405]

NECROPSY FINDINGS. At postmortem examination, lesions are confined to the pharyngeal muscles, guttural pouch, and bones of the skull.[404] Gross findings may include large blood clots in the nasal passages and at the pharyngeal opening of the guttural pouch.[413] Unilateral denervation atrophy of the ipsilateral pharyngeal or laryngeal muscles may occur if there is involvement of the pharyngeal and recurrent laryngeal branches of the vagus.[404] Examination of the guttural pouch generally reveals clotted blood and a diphtheritic plaque in the dorsocaudal aspect of the medial compartment that is firmly adherent to the underlying tissue and is clearly demarcated from surrounding tissue.[406,413] The lesion may be localized or affect the entire roof of the pouch. If hemorrhage has occurred, the lesion may be obscured by clotted blood, pus, or mucus.[406] An intense inflammatory reaction may be evident in response to acute fungal infection, whereas the inflammation may subside with chronic healing lesions so that scar tissue is evident.[406,411] Active inflammation may also predispose to osseous lesions of the petrous temporal and stylohyoid bones.[404,406,410] Some cases of guttural pouch mycosis may remain asymptomatic and only be diagnosed at routine postmortem examination.[405]

TREATMENT AND PROGNOSIS. Without treatment a poor prognosis is warranted, because horses affected with guttural pouch mycosis are at risk from a fatal episode of epistaxis. Both medical and surgical treatments have been advocated for horses affected with guttural pouch mycosis with variable results.[415,416] Spontaneous regression of guttural pouch mycosis may occur, and this must be considered when evaluating the various medical or surgical treatments for this disease.[378,405]

Medical treatment is generally aimed at topical therapy of the mycotic lesion through the pharyngeal opening of the guttural pouch by means of a catheter.[378] Bathing of the lesion may be facilitated by anesthetizing the horse and placing it in dorsal recumbency.[404] Instilling fungicidal and fungistatic drugs, topical enzymes, and organic iodine compounds into the guttural pouch has been attempted with variable success.[417,418] The necessity and efficacy of these treatments are unknown, and systematic treatment is hampered by a lack of knowledge of the pathogenesis of guttural pouch mycosis.[419] Parenteral administration of antibiotics, corticosteroids, thiabendazole, ketoconazole, and iodine compounds also has questionable efficacy.[413,415,419] The response of guttural pouch mycosis to local and parenteral treatment is protracted; thus the risk of fatal hemorrhage exists long after treatment has commenced.[421]

Surgical treatment of guttural pouch mycosis appears to offer the best prognosis for eventual cure. The internal carotid artery is not an end artery, and blood may enter this vessel from the bifurcation of the common carotid or may return from the cerebral arterial circle. Although various surgical techniques have been described, it appears that insertion of a balloon-tipped catheter into the distal internal carotid artery, combined with proximal ligation of the internal carotid artery, induces thrombus formation and prevents hemorrhage from normal and retrograde blood flow.[413,420-422] It has been observed that thrombosis sufficient to prevent hemorrhage may develop in the distal internal carotid artery within 10 days of catheter placement.[422] Mucosal healing and complete regression of the fungal plaque have been reported to occur as early as 5 weeks after arterial catheterization.[420] In a series of 13 cases the insertion of the balloon-tipped catheter successfully prevented fatal epistaxis in all horses.[420] Topical or systemic treatment of the mycotic plaque is believed to be unnecessary after arterial catheterization.[420] Intraarterial insertion of latex balloons or embolization coils also results in lesion resolution.[423-425]

REFERENCES

378. Freeman DE: Diagnosis and treatment of diseases of the guttural pouch. I, *Compend Cont Educ Pract Vet* 2:S3-S11, 1980.
379. Chiesa OA et al: Cytological and bacteriological findings in guttural pouch lavages of clinically normal horses, *Vet Rec* 144:346-349, 1999.
380. Baptiste KE, Moll HD, Robertson JL: Three horses with neoplasia including growth in the guttural pouch, *Can Vet J* 37:499-501, 1996.
381. Freeman DE: Diagnosis and treatment of diseases of the guttural pouch. II, *Compend Cont Educ Pract Vet* 2:S25-S31, 1980.
382. Hance SR, Robertson JT, Bukowiecki CF: Cystic structures in the guttural pouch (auditory tube diverticulum) of two horses, *J Am Vet Med Assoc* 200:1981-1983, 1992.
383. Wheat JD: Tympanites of the guttural pouch of the horse, *J Am Vet Med Assoc* 140:453-454, 1962.
384. McCue PM, Freeman DE, Donawick WJ: Guttural pouch tympany: 15 cases (1977-1986), *J Am Vet Med Assoc* 184:1761-1763, 1989.
385. Holmes RA: The guttural pouches of the horse, *Mod Vet Pract* 43:45-49, 1962.
386. Haynes PF: Surgery of the equine respiratory tract. In Jennings PB, ed: *The practice of large animal surgery*, Philadelphia, 1984, WB Saunders, pp 456-470.
387. Cook WR: Clinical observations on the anatomy and physiology of the equine upper respiratory tract, *Vet Rec* 79:440-446, 1966.
388. Sullins KE: Standing endoscopic electrosurgery, *Vet Clin North Am (Equine Pract)* 7:571-581, 1991.
389. Tate LP, Blikslager AT, Little EDE: Transendoscopic laser treatment of guttural pouch tympanites in eight foals, *Vet Surg* 24:367-372, 1995.
390. Kinsley AT: Tympanites of the guttural pouch, *Am Vet Rev* 32:599-600, 1907.

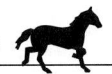

391. Johnson JH: The relationship of the guttural pouch to upper respiratory conditions, *Proceedings of the Sixteenth Annual Convention of the American Association of Equine Practitioners,* 1970, pp 247-250.

392. Mansmann RA, Wheat JD: The diagnosis and treatment of equine upper respiratory diseases, *Proceedings of the Eighteenth Annual Convention of the American Association of Equine Practitioners,* 1972, pp 375-379.

393. Knight AP et al: Experimentally induced *Streptococcus equi* infection in horses with resultant guttural pouch empyema, *Vet Med Small Anim Clin* 70:1194-1199, 1975.

394. Sweeney CR et al: Complications associated with *Streptococcus equi* infection on a horse farm, *J Am Vet Med Assoc* 191:1446-1448, 1987.

395. Hoffman AM et al: Clinical and endoscopic study to estimate the incidence of distal respiratory tract infection in thoroughbred foals on Ontario breeding farms, *Am J Vet Res* 54:1602-1607.

396. Hoffman AM et al: Association of microbiologic flora with clinical, endoscopic, and pulmonary cytologic findings in foals with distal respiratory tract infection, *Am J Vet Res* 54:1615-1622, 1993.

397. Baker GJ: Diseases of the auditory tube diverticula (guttural pouches). In Rose RJ: *Proceedings of Symposium of Surgery and Diseases of the Oral Cavity and Respiratory Tract,* Artarmon, Australia, 1981, Australian Equine Veterinary Association, pp 62-63.

398. Riggs WR: Guttural pouch mycosis and chondroids in a mare, *Southwest Vet* 25:61-65, 1971.

399. Boles C: Treatment of upper airway abnormalities, *Vet Clin North Am (Large Anim Pract)* 1:127-147, 1979.

400. Wilson J: Effects of indwelling catheters and povidone iodine flushes on the guttural pouches of the horse, *Equine Vet J* 17:242-244, 1985.

401. Seahorn TL, Schumacher J: Nonsurgical removal of chondroid masses from the guttural pouches of two horses, *J Am Vet Med Assoc* 199:368-369, 1991.

402. Adkins AR, Yovich JV, Colbourne CM: Nonsurgical treatment of chondroids of the guttural pouch in a horse, *Aust Vet J* 75:332-333, 1997.

403. Smith KM, Barber SM: Guttural pouch hemorrhage associated with lesions of the maxillary artery in two horses, *Can Vet J* 25:239-242, 1984.

404. Cook WR: Observations on the aetiology of epistaxis and cranial nerve paralysis in the horse, *Vet Rec* 78:396-406, 1966.

405. Cook WR: The clinical features of guttural pouch mycosis in the horse, *Vet Rec* 83:336-345, 1968.

406. Cook WR, Campbell RSF, Dawson C: The pathology and aetiology of guttural pouch mycosis in the horse, *Vet Rec* 83:422-428, 1968.

407. Kosuge J, Takatori K, Anzai T: [Biological characteristics of *Emericella nidulans* isolated from horse guttural pouch mycosis], *Nippon Ishinkin Gakkai Zasshi* 40:169-173, 1999.

408. Guillot J et al: Detection of antibodies to *Aspergillus fumigatus* in serum of horses with mycosis of the auditory tube diverticulum (guttural pouch), *Am J Vet Res* 58:1364-1366, 1997.

409. Guillot J et al: *Emericella nidulans* as an agent of guttural pouch mycosis in a horse, *J Med Vet Mycol* 35: 433-435, 1997.

410. Hatziolos BC et al: Ocular changes in a horse with gutturomycosis, *J Am Vet Med Assoc* 167:51-54, 1975.

411. Wagner PC et al: Mycotic encephalitis associated with a guttural pouch mycosis, *J Equine Med Surg* 2:355-359, 1978.

412. Johnson JH, Merriam JG, Attleberger M: A case of guttural pouch mycosis caused by *Aspergillus nidulans, Vet Med Small Anim Clin* 68:771-774, 1973.

413. Grant BD, Miller RA, Fadok VA: Fatal epistaxis and guttural pouch mycosis, *Western Vet* 15:23-26, 1977.

414. Owen RR, McKelvey WAC: Ligation of the internal carotid artery to prevent epistaxis due to guttural pouch mycosis, *Vet Rec* 104:100-101, 1979.

415. Church S et al: Treatment of guttural pouch mycosis, *Equine Vet J* 18:362-365, 1986.

416. Greet TR: Outcome of treatment in 35 cases of guttural pouch mycosis, *Equine Vet J* 19:483-487, 1987.

417. Davis EW, Legendre AM: Successful treatment of guttural pouch mycosis with intraconazole and topical enilconazole in a horse, *J Vet Intern Med* 8:304-305, 1994.

418. Van Nieuwstadt RA, Kalsbeek HC: Air sac mycosis: topical treatment using enilconazole administered via indwelling catheter, *Tijdschr Diergeneesk* 119:3-5, 1994.

419. Speirs VC et al: Is specific antifungal therapy necessary for the treatment of guttural pouch mycosis in horses? *Equine Vet J* 27:151-152, 1995.

420. Caron JP et al: Balloon-tipped catheter arterial occlusion for prevention of hemorrhage caused by guttural pouch mycosis: 13 cases (1982-1985), *J Am Vet Med Assoc* 191:345-349, 1987.

421. Freeman DE, Donawick WJ: Occlusion of internal carotid artery in the horse by means of a balloon-tipped catheter: clinical use of a method to prevent epistaxis caused by guttural pouch mycosis, *J Am Vet Med Assoc* 176:236-240, 1980.

422. Freeman DE, Donawick WJ: Occlusion of internal carotid artery in the horse by means of a balloon-tipped catheter: evaluation of a method designed to prevent epistaxis caused by guttural pouch mycosis, *J Am Vet Med Assoc* 176:232-235, 1980.

423. Cheramie HS et al: Evaluation of a technique to occlude the internal carotid artery of horses, *Vet Surg* 28:83-90, 1999.

424. Matsuda Y, Nakanishi Y, Mizuno Y: Occlusion of the internal carotid artery by means of microcoils for preventing epistaxis caused by guttural pouch mycosis in horses, *J Vet Med Sci* 61:221-225, 1999.

425. Leveille R et al: Transarterial coil embolization for prevention of hemorrhage from guttural pouch mycosis in horses, *Proceedings of the Forty-fifth Annual Convention of th American Association of Equine Practitioners,* 1999, pp 94-95.

DISEASES OF THE PARANASAL SINUSES

SINUSITIS

CLIFFORD M. HONNAS
JOHN R. PASCOE

DEFINITION AND ETIOLOGY. Sinusitis refers to inflammation of the paranasal sinuses, generally as a result of either primary or secondary bacterial infection. The paranasal sinuses are lined by respiratory mucosa and are therefore at risk of developing diseases that affect the respiratory tract.[426,427] Sinus empyema, accumulation of pus within a sinus cavity, may result from bacterial or viral infection.

In the horse, sinusitis occurs primarily in the frontal or maxillary sinus and corresponding conchal sinuses. The incidence of sinus empyema appears highest between 4 and 10 years of age.[428] Maxillary sinusitis occurs most often secondary to dental disease as a result of the close association between the maxillary sinus and the tooth roots. Alveolar periostitis, patent infundibula, and fractured or split teeth are the most common dental causes of maxillary sinus empyema.[427] These dental defects permit access of food material or bacteria to the tooth root and sinus cavity. Extension of maxillary sinusitis to the frontal sinus may occur through the frontomaxillary opening. Primary sinusitis as a result of bacterial or viral upper respiratory tract infections occurs less frequently. Primary sinusitis is usually caused by *Streptococcus* spp. and may be an acute or chronic manifestation of the associated upper respiratory disease.[426] Additional causes of sinusitis in the horse include trauma, developmental disorders (maxillary follicular cysts), neoplasia, and fungal granulomas.[429-431] Reported neoplasms include osteoma, osteosarcoma, adenocarcinoma, lymphosarcoma, squamous cell carcinoma, and fibroma.[429,431-433]

CLINICAL SIGNS AND DIFFERENTIAL DIAGNOSIS. Signs of sinusitis vary, depending on the cause, location, and extent of sinus involvement. Physical examination of a horse with sinusitis should include observation for facial asymmetry that may indicate distention from infection, neoplasia, or fracture. The most common presenting complaint is chronic unilateral nasal discharge that varies from serous to mucopurulent.[428,434] Nasal discharge only occurs on the involved side because the nasomaxillary opening is located rostral to the caudal edge of the nasal septum. The discharge may be intermittent or continuous and need not be related to a previous upper respiratory infection. Submandibular lymphadenopathy may occur with acute and chronic sinusitis. Primary sinusitis is usually accompanied by mucopurulent or purulent nasal discharge without an unpleasant odor whereas fetid-smelling breath generally accompanies sinusitis caused by dental disease or tissue necrosis within the sinus.

Paranasal sinus or nasal neoplasia or turbinate necrosis should also be considered when fetid nasal odors are noted in the absence of dental disease.[435] Facial distortion occurs as a result of space-occupying lesions or fluid accumulation in a closed sinus compartment. Occasionally exophthalmos can occur with marked sinus distortion. Patency of the nasomaxillary opening usually precludes facial distortion. Loss of patency occurs when inspissated exudate accumulates or tissue reaction obstructs the opening.[426] Expansion of the sinus may result in reduced nasal airflow, particularly ipsilaterally, caused by distortion of the architecture of the nasal passages, and in such instances abnormal respiratory noise rather than nasal discharge may be the primary presenting sign.[428,432] Percussion of the affected sinus may reveal dullness or pain, although normal resonance does not preclude the possibility of sinusitis.[428,435] If there is bone thinning over gas above a fluid line (as can occur with some maxillary sinus cysts), percussion may elicit increased resonance. Additional signs include ipsilateral ocular discharge as a result of compromise of the lacrimal canal and fistula formation.[428,431] Careful examination of the oral cavity for signs of dental or periodontal disease should be performed when any of these signs are present. Particular attention should be paid to examination of the occlusal surface of the teeth with a very fine dental pick (e.g., 22-gauge needle); however, it should be recognized that periapical abscess formation can occur without defects in the occlusal surface.

In horses, nasal discharge is suggestive of diseases involving the upper respiratory tract. Other differential diagnoses should include guttural pouch empyema or mycosis; acute pharyngitis (strangles, rhinopneumonitis, and influenza); neoplasia or necrosis of the turbinates; and ethmoidal hematoma. One report of 28 horses considered chronic unilateral nasal discharge to be almost pathognomonic for paranasal sinus empyema.[428] Nasal discharge characterized by hemorrhage suggests ethmoid hematoma, guttural pouch mycosis, pulmonary hemorrhage, nasal turbinate necrosis, and neoplastic or granulomatous lesions.[426]

CLINICAL PATHOLOGY. The hemogram in animals with sinusitis generally remains within the normal range, although acute sinusitis of infectious origin may be associated with neutrophilia. With chronic sinusitis concurrent hyperfibrinogenemia may be present. Sinus fluid obtained by percutaneous centesis should be examined cytologically (including a Gram stain) and submitted for microbial culture and susceptibility testing.[426] This allows differentiation between bacterial and fungal diseases and may aid in the identification of neoplasia. Flecks of feed material indicate sinusitis secondary to dental abnormalities.

LABORATORY AIDS AND DEFINITIVE DIAGNOSTIC TESTS. A presumptive diagnosis of sinusitis can be made from the physical examination and associated clinical signs.[436] Procedures most helpful in establishing a diagnosis of sinus disease in 85 horses were radiography (92%), endoscopy (38%), percutaneous centesis (21%), and examination of the oral cavity (20%).[431] Examination of the paranasal sinuses can also be accomplished by sinoscopy using an arthroscope[437] or flexible endoscope[438] inserted through small trephine holes in either the maxillary or the frontal sinus. Diagnostic accuracy, especially determination of the extent of involvement of structures within the skull, can be enhanced by computed tomography.[439] Radiographic findings include fluid lines within the sinus, space-occupying soft-tissue densities, areas of decreased bone density, fractures, or dental abnormalities. Dental root disease is identified radiographically by a loss of continuity of the lamina dura and lysis of the tooth root or surrounding bone, combined with new bone formation and cement deposition.[440] Standard radiographic projections include the standing lateral, dorsoventral, and right and left oblique views.[440,441] Scintigraphic examination may improve specificity in identification of dental involvement in sinusitis.[442] Endoscopic examination of the nasal cavity may permit identification of exudate draining from the nasomaxillary opening or, in advanced cases, may reveal distortion of the nasal cavity secondary to sinus enlargement.

Percutaneous sinus centesis may provide a definitive diagnosis and allow an avenue for subsequent therapy.[426] Cytologic evaluation, with concurrent microbial culture and antibiotic susceptibility testing, may elucidate the cause of the sinusitis.[431] Isolation of a single organism such as *Streptococcus* spp. generally indicates a primary sinusitis, whereas polymicrobial infection is more compatible with sinusitis of dental origin. Visual examination of the oral cavity and careful probing of the occlusal surfaces with a dental pick may identify dental abnormalities.

NECROPSY FINDINGS. Affected sinuses contain fluid or tissue of variable color and consistency. Fluid character ranges from clear and odorless with cystic sinus disease to white, yellow, or green purulent fluid with a variable, but often putrid, odor in sinusitis resulting from other causes. Sinusitis of dental origin has a characteristically pungent and unpleasant odor. Granulomatous lesions have been reported to appear as large lobular gelatinous masses, filling the involved sinus cavity.[430] The gross appearance of neoplastic lesions within the sinus cavity depends on the type of neoplasm. Malignant neoplasms may cause surrounding soft-tissue and bony destruction, whereas large, benign space-occupying lesions may result in distortion of the nasal turbinates and nasal septum, as well as external facial bone distortion.

TREATMENT AND PROGNOSIS. Not infrequently, horses with a chronic mucopurulent nasal discharge from sinusitis have a history of response to antimicrobial therapy, followed by recurrence of the discharge after antibiotic therapy was stopped. A definitive diagnosis of sinusitis can be reached using the techniques described earlier. Sinoscopy is a technique that permits examination of the paranasal sinuses and in some instances facilitates treatment.[438,443]

Suggested treatment for primary sinusitis or empyema involves daily lavage of the sinus through a percutaneous centesis site with 1 L of saline, to which a broad-spectrum antibiotic or antiseptic has been added. Once the results of culture and susceptibility testing are available, the appropriate antibiotic should be administered locally in the flush solution, as well as systemically, for 14 days. Resolution or reduction in the volume of nasal discharge is an indication of successful therapy. If little progress is made after 10 to 14 days or if drainage recurs, sinusotomy (trephination or bone flap technique) may be required to resolve the condition.[435,444] The prognosis is generally favorable in cases of primary sinusitis if the condition is not chronic and if the mucous membrane is not markedly thickened.[426] Chronic sinus disease (longer than 6 months) has a poor prognosis, and, for resolution to occur, surgical removal of the thickened, infected mucous membrane is required. Isolation of *Pseudomonas* spp. from a sinus aspirate generally indicates an unfavorable prognosis.[434]

Sinusitis that results from secondary factors is generally not responsive to medical management. Such conditions include diseased teeth, granulomas, or neoplasia; surgical removal of the inciting cause is required. The prognosis for sinusitis associated with dental abnormalities is usually favorable once the diseased tooth has been removed.[445] If the periodontal ligament is intact, endodontic therapy can be used to save the tooth.[446] This is accomplished by surgical apicoectomy and retrograde occlusion of the root canal after debridement of the pulp. In geriatric horses with dental-associated sinusitis, when economic constraints limit surgical options, sinusotomy and periodic sinus lavage and antibiotic therapy have been used successfully to manage nasal discharge.[435] The prognosis for resolution of granulomatous lesions is generally guarded and depends on surgical access and extent of the lesion. Neoplastic lesions are often well established and have metastasized, either locally or regionally, by the time they become clinically apparent; they generally have a guarded to poor prognosis for resolution.[426,429] In a series of 16 horses with sinus neoplasia, 11 were euthanized because of the extent of the lesion, four lesions recurred after surgical removal, and 1 horse with squamous cell carcinoma was suc-

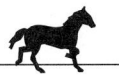

cessfully treated and had no recurrence at a 2-year follow-up evaluation.[431]

PREVENTION AND CONTROL. Prevention of sinusitis in horses is difficult because of the variety of etiologic agents that can precipitate disease. Isolation of horses from those affected with upper respiratory bacterial or viral diseases may be of benefit in preventing primary sinusitis. Regular dental care and a proper diet may help circumvent sinusitis caused by dental abnormalities, although many cases most likely result from a variety of causes not yet defined or over which the owner or veterinarian has no control.

REFERENCES

426. Haynes PF: Surgery of the equine respiratory tract. In Jennings PB, ed: *The practice of large animal surgery*, Philadelphia, 1984, WB Saunders, pp 405-411.
427. Trotter GW: Paranasal sinuses, *Vet Clin North Am (Equine Pract)* 9:153-169, 1993.
428. Mason JE: Empyema of the equine paranasal sinuses, *J Am Vet Med Assoc* 167:727-731, 1975.
429. Dixon PM, Head KW: Equine nasal and paranasal sinus tumors. II, A contribution of 28 case reports, *Vet J* 157: 279-294, 1999.
430. Scott EA, Duncan JR, McCormack JE: Cryptococcosis involving the postorbital area and frontal sinus in a horse, *J Am Vet Med Assoc* 165:626-627, 1974.
431. Boulton CH: Equine nasal cavity and paranasal cavity disease: a review of 85 cases, *J Equine Vet Sci* 5:268-275, 1985.
432. Leyland A, Baker JR: Lesions of the nasal and paranasal sinuses of the horse causing dyspnoea, *Br Vet J* 131:339-346, 1975.
433. Head KW, Dixon PM: Equine nasal and paranasal sinus tumors. I, Review of the literature and tumour classification, *Vet J* 157: 261-278, 1999.
434. Cannon JH, Grant BD, Sande RD: Diagnosis and surgical treatment of cyst-like lesions of the equine paranasal sinuses, *J Am Vet Med Assoc* 169:610-613, 1976.
435. Merriam JG: Field sinusotomy in the management of chronic sinusitis and alveolitis, *Proceedings of the Thirty-ninth Annual Convention of the American Association of Equine Practitioners*, 1993, pp 235-237.
436. Bertone JJ, Biller DS, Ruggles A: Diagnostic techniques for evaluation of the paranasal sinuses, *Vet Clin North Am (Equine Pract)* 9:75-91, 1993.
437. Ruggles AJ, Ross MW, Freeman DE: Endoscopic examination of normal paranasal sinuses in horses, *Vet Surg* 20:418-423, 1991.
438. Worster AA, Hackett RP: Equine sinus endoscopy using a flexible endoscope: diagnosis and treatment of sinus disease in the standing sedated horse, *Proceedings of the Forty-fifth Annual Convention of the American Association of Equine Practitioners*, 1999, pp 128-130.
439. Tietje S, Becker M, Bockenhoff G: Computed tomographic evaluation of head diseases in the horse: 15 cases, *Equine Vet J* 28:98-105, 1996.
440. Pascoe JR: Dental radiography/radiology, *Proceedings of the Thirty-seventh Annual Convention of the American Association of Equine Practitioners*, 1991, pp 99-111.
441. Gibbs C: Dental imaging. In Baker GJ, Easley J, eds: *Equine dentistry*, Philadelphia, 1999, WB Saunders, pp 139-169.
442. Semevolos SA, Hackett RP, Scrivani PV: Nuclear scintigraphy as a diagnostic aid in the evaluation of tooth root abscessation, *Proceedings of the Forty-fifth Annual Convention of the American Association of Equine Practitioners*, 1999, pp 103-104, 1999.
443. Ruggles AJ, Ross MW, Freeman DE: Endoscopic examination and treatment of paranasal sinus disease in 16 horses, *Vet Surg* 22:508-514, 1993.
444. Schumacher J, Honnas C, Smith B: Paranasal sinusitis complicated by inspissated exudate in the ventral conchal sinus, *Vet Surg* 16:373-377, 1987.
445. Prichard MA, Hackett RP, Erb HN: Long-term outcome of tooth repulsion in horses: a retrospective study of 61 cases, *Vet Surg* 21:145-149, 1992.
446. Schumacher J, Honnas CM: Dental surgery, *Vet Clin North Am (Equine Pract)* 9:133-152, 1993.

ETHMOID HEMATOMA

JOHN R. PASCOE

DEFINITION AND ETIOLOGY. Also termed progressive ethmoidal hematoma[447] and hemorrhagic nasal polyps,[448] ethmoid hematomas are slowly expanding angiomatous masses that appear to originate principally from the mucosal lining of the ethmoid conchae. Although smaller hemangiomas arising from the mucosal lining of the frontal, maxillary, and sphenopalatine sinuses have been recognized, the relationship between these benign endothelial tumors and ethmoid

hematoma is uncertain. The cause of ethmoid hematoma is unknown and it remains a relatively uncommon condition.[449-453] Although reported in a 4-week-old foal and in 3-year-old horses, most affected horses are older than 8 years; generally Thoroughbred, Arabian, or warmblood horses.[449-455]

CLINICAL SIGNS. A nasal discharge with intermittent epistaxis from one or both nostrils is the most common clinical sign. Epistaxis can be unilateral or bilateral and vary from blood-tinged mucoid or mucopurulent discharge to blood spots or a trickle of blood. Fulminant or fatal epistaxis as can occur with guttural pouch mycosis is uncommon. If the hematoma occupies the choana(e) or nasal cavity, a mucopurulent, often malodorous nasal discharge with some blood discoloration is more commonly seen. Typically these horses have a history of abnormal respiratory noise, both inspiratory and expiratory, especially during exercise. Facial distortion or asymmetry is uncommon and is more likely to occur when the hematoma occupies the frontal and maxillary sinuses. Less commonly there may be an associated history of coughing, choking, ptyalism, increased respiratory effort during resting breathing, and either head shyness or head shaking.[447] If the hematoma has expanded into the paranasal sinuses, percussion yields a dull sound. Airflow is usually reduced or may be absent on the affected side.

LABORATORY AIDS AND DEFINITIVE DIAGNOSTIC TESTS. Confirmation of ethmoid hematoma requires endoscopy of the ethmoid conchae and skull radiography (Figs. 29-25 and 29-26). The origin and extent of the mass can be determined more accurately by computed tomographic examination of the skull. Because ethmoid hematoma occurs bilaterally in approximately 30% of affected horses, it is prudent to examine both the left and right ethmoidal conchae. The ethmoidal labyrinth is visible approximately 25 cm from the nares with the endoscope positioned in the ventral nasal meatus and the viewing tip deflected dorsally. The rostral surface of the ethmoidal concha does not protrude beyond the caudal nasal cavity and has a bulbous shape and a moist pink to pale red mucosal covering.

Beyond the rostral surface the numerous pillars that form the ethmoidal conchae and separate the ethmoidal spaces (cellulae ethmoidales) are visible. Ethmoidal hematomas that project into the ventral meatus or through the choana into the nasopharynx often obscure the ethmoidal concha. In some instances of unilateral ethmoid hematoma, if the expanding mass has entered the nasopharynx, it may also protrude into the contralateral ventral meatus, obscuring view of the ethmoidal labyrinth on that side also. The origin of hematomas that expand dorsally into the frontal sinus may not be visible on endoscopy, but hemorrhage that originates deep to the visible portion of the ethmoidal conchae may be evident or may be noticed from the region of the nasomaxillary opening in the middle meatus. Visible ethmoid hematomas can vary in color from deep red to red-purple or may have a yellow-brown, yellow-green-brown-to-bronze color. The hematoma usually has an irregular rounded surface, with small punctate hemorrhages or erosions and may be partially covered in yellow-white mucopurulent material that may be admixed with fresh blood. Often the floor of the ventral meatus and the regions of contact with the nasal cavity have pooled exudate of blood and mucopurulent matter. Manipulation of the visible surface of the hematoma with the tip of the endoscope may elicit bleeding or oozing.

Recognition of a discrete, often smooth-surfaced homogeneous radiodensity originating from the ethmoidal conchae and extending into the frontal, maxillary, or sphenopalatine sinuses or into the pharynx or nasal cavity is suggestive of an ethmoid hematoma. Radiography is beneficial in determining the extent of expansion of the hematoma and also in identifying suspected ethmoid hematomas that

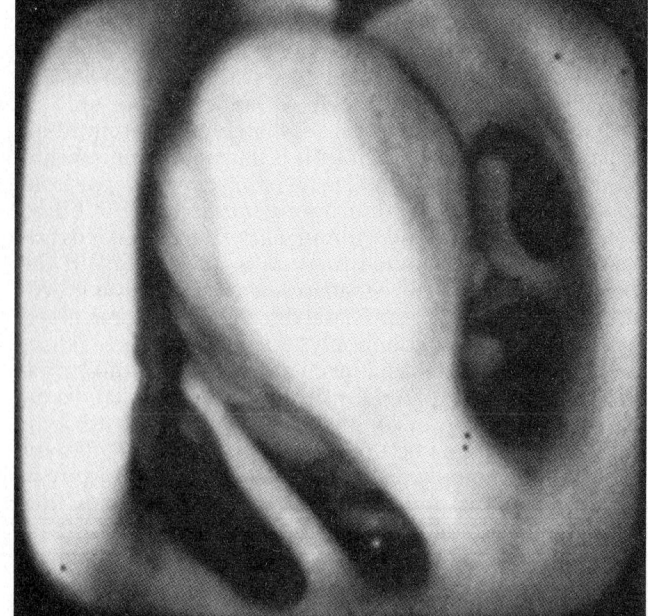

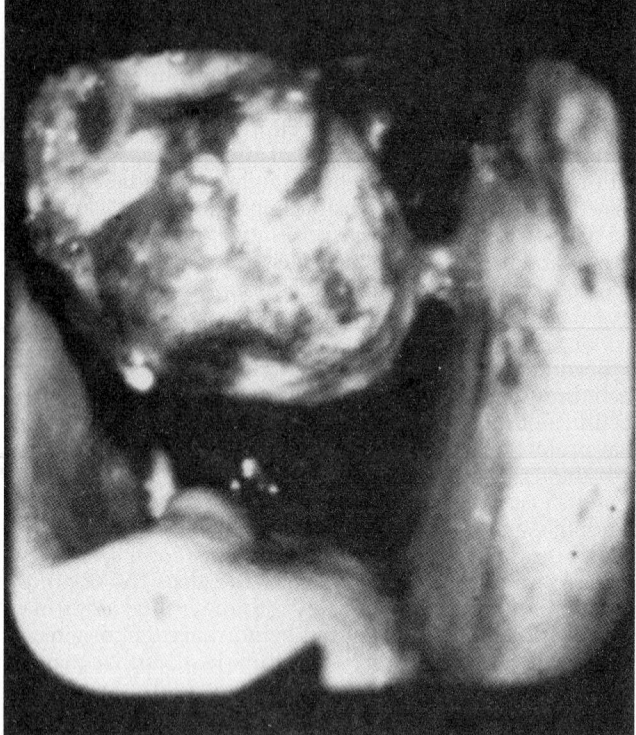

FIG. 29-25 Endoscopic view of left ethmoturbinate. **A,** Normal appearance. **B,** Ethmoturbinate obscured by an ethmoid hematoma.

FIG. 29-26 Lateral radiograph demonstrating an ethmoid hematoma.

regions with necrosis or secondary infection associated with contact with the sinus or nasal cavity walls, the hematoma is a smooth-surfaced saclike structure containing blood in various stages of organization. The sac lining is generally healthy respiratory mucosa originating from a pedunculated region of the mucosal covering of the ethmoturbinal or sinus wall. On section the contents are amorphous red-black to chocolate brown, and in larger masses some evidence of irregular compartmentalization by fibrous tissue exists, especially on the inner surface of the sac.

Morphologic features include an outer covering of respiratory epithelium overlying an irregular zone of submucosal fibrous tissue, containing hemosiderophages and occasional plasma cells, that forms a pseudocapsule around hemorrhage in varying states of organization. Endothelial cells do not show evidence of neoplasia. Thin endothelium-lined sinuses are often present within the myxomatous stroma. The respiratory epithelium is sometimes ulcerated and infiltrated with neutrophils, and occasionally there are squamous metaplastic changes.

TREATMENT AND PROGNOSIS. Because these masses slowly and progressively increase in size and can result in distortion of skull architecture, hematoma removal is recommended. The method of treatment depends on the location and size of the hematoma. Surgical ablation has been the preferred method; however, destruction of the hematoma by intralesional injection of formaldehyde solution is associated with less morbidity, although recurrence rates are similar to other methods.[452-457] Surgical access is usually achieved by sinusotomy and then hematoma ablation by curettage, cryosurgery, or use of an Nd:YAG laser[458,459]; photoablation can also be accomplished through the biopsy channel of an endoscope. After sinusotomy, the pedunculated origin of the hematoma is identified by digital palpation and then dissected, frozen, or photoablated and the hematoma removed. If the hematoma is friable, intact removal may not be possible and hemorrhage from the disrupted hematoma may make observation of the origin of the mass difficult. After removal, the paranasal sinuses and nasal cavity are packed with gauze to control postoperative hemorrhage.

Although commonly used as the initial treatment, surgical curettage can have the disadvantage of being associated with marked intraoperative blood loss typically from the turbinates or sinus mucosa rather than the hematoma. Temporary occlusion of both carotid arteries[460] during extirpation of the hematoma can substantially decrease blood loss until the sinus cavity is packed with gauze. Blood loss is minimized by cryosurgical extirpation, but this technique is not always practical when initially dealing with large hematomas. Likewise blood loss is minimized by photoablation techniques, especially when the origin of the hematoma can be

are not visible by endoscopy. Small hematomas contained within the ethmoid labyrinth may not be visible on radiographs. Computed tomographic examination of the skull allows more accurate assessment of the origin of the ethmoid hematoma,[455] allows determination of the extent of involvement of the paranasal sinuses and conchae, and facilitates surgical planning.

NECROPSY FINDINGS. Most of the morphologic features have been described from surgical specimens; few skulls with intact ethmoid hematomas have been examined.[448] Except in

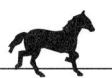

identified. There is also minimum blood loss with transnasal photoablation; however, this technique requires multiple procedures to destroy large masses but can be performed in the standing sedated horse.[459] Recent experience with destruction of ethmoid hematomas by endoscopically guided intralesional injection of formalin in standing sedated horses indicates that this technique may reduce the need for surgical ablation in many horses.[457,461] A catheter passed through the biopsy channel of an endoscope is advanced through the rostral surface of the mass toward its origin, then 10 ml of 10% formalin (4% formaldehyde solution) is injected intralesionally. Tissue necrosis and slough occur in 5 to 10 days and the technique can be repeated at 10- to 14-day intervals until the mass has been destroyed. Removal of necrotic tissue can be facilitated by use of long grasping forceps and hydropulsion. Irrespective of treatment method, recurrence of the hematoma occurs in 30% to 50% of cases from several months to years after the initial surgery.[448,451-454,456,457]

REFERENCES

447. Cook WR, Littlewort MCG: Progressive haematoma of the ethmoid region in the horse, *Equine Vet J* 6:101-108, 1974.
448. Platt H: Haemorrhagic nasal polyps of the horse, *J Pathol* 115:51-55, 1975.
449. Leyland A, Baker JR: Lesions of the nasal and paranasal sinuses of the horse causing dyspnoea, *Br Vet J* 131:339-347, 1975.
450. Bonfig H: Diagnose and therapie des progressiven hämatoms der siebbeinregion—dargestellt an 13 klinischen fallen, *Pferdheilkunde* 2:71-79, 1989.
451. Specht TE et al: Ethmoidal hematoma in nine horses, *J Am Vet Med Assoc* 197:613-616, 1990.
452. Greet TRC: Outcome of treatment in 23 horses with progressive ethmoidal haematoma, *Equine Vet J* 24:468-471, 1992.
453. Laing JA, Hutchins DR: Progressive ethmoidal hematoma in horses, *Aust Vet J* 69:57-58, 1992.
454. Colbourne CM, Rosenstein DS, Steficek BA: Surgical treatment of progressive ethmoidal hematoma aided by computed tomograph in a foal, *J Am Vet Med Assoc* 211: 335-338, 1997.
455. Meagher DM: Ethmoid hematoma. In White NA, Moore JN, eds: *Current practice of equine surgery*, Philadelphia, 1990, Lippincott, p 227.
456. Schumacher J et al: Transendoscopic chemical ablation of progressive ethmoidal hematoma in standing horses, *Vet Surg* 27:175-181, 1998.
457. Tate LP: Application of lasers in equine upper respiratory surgery, *Vet Clin North Am (Equine Pract)* 7:165-195, 1991.
458. Rothaug PG, Tulleners EP: Neodymium:yttrium-aluminum-garnet laser assisted excision of progressive ethmoid hematomas in horses: 20 cases (1986-1996), *J Am Vet Med Assoc* 214:1037-1041.
459. Wyn-Jones G, Jones RS, Church S: Temporary bilateral carotid artery occlusion as an aid to nasal surgery in the horse, *Equine Vet J* 18:125-128, 1986.
460. Marriot MR, Dart AJ, Hodgson DR: Treatment of progressive ethmoidal hematoma using intralesional injections of formalin in three horses, *Aust Vet J* 77:371-373, 1999.

RUMINANT RESPIRATORY SYSTEM

JOHN C. BAKER AND TREVOR R. AMES, Consulting Editors

UPPER RESPIRATORY TRACT DISEASES

JOHN C. BAKER
JOHN A. SMITH

DISEASES OF THE NASAL CAVITY

JOHN C. BAKER
JOHN A. SMITH

Mycotic Nasal Granuloma (Mycetoma)

Fungal-induced granulomas in the nasal cavity of ruminants are not common. Documented causes include *Rhinosporidium seeberi* and other *Rhinosporidium* spp. (which cause "rhinosporidiosis"), *Helminthosporium* spp. (which cause "maduromycosis"), *Drechslera rostrata*, *Aspergillus* spp., *Phycomycetes* spp., *Stachybotrys* spp., and *Bipolaris* spp. Phycomycosis is discussed in the dermatology section in Chapter 38. There is no apparent age, breed, or seasonal predilection, and cases are sporadic. The major clinical signs are upper respiratory noise (stridor), dyspnea, and mucopurulent nasal discharge, sometimes with epistaxis.[461,462] Nasal airflow may be reduced, and open-mouth breathing may occur in advanced cases. Hot or dusty weather may accentuate the signs, giving the appearance of seasonal exacerbation, but the lesions are progressive. The granulomas may be single or multiple, unilateral or bilateral, and located anywhere in the nasal cavity. They consist of 0.5- to 5-cm yellow to yellow-green or red nodules or polyps, which may be sessile or pedunculated. Rhinosporidiosis tends to be a single unilateral polyp in the posterior nasal cavity, and maduromycosis tends to occur in the anterior cavity, but these distinctions are not consistent. Red and black spots (spores) may occur on the masses, and some may become secondarily infected with bacteria and ulcerate. Differential diagnoses include allergic rhinitis, foreign bodies, tumors, nasal actinobacillosis, and actinomycosis.

Endoscopy, biopsy, and culture of the lesions aid in the diagnosis. Histopathologic analysis reveals granulation tissue containing eosinophils, mononuclear cells, round sporangia, and sometimes hyphae.[461] The pathogenesis of the disease involves inoculation of eroded nasal mucosa with fungal spores from the environment. The fungus causes a chronic delayed (type IV) hypersensitivity reaction, which eventually leads to the formation of a granuloma. Because of the fungal cause, the condition is more common in warm, wet climates. The granulomas can be difficult to treat, and, although rarely fatal, the disease is chronically debilitating, with salvage often being the most practical solution.

Recommended treatments include surgical removal of the granulomas when possible and long-term sodium iodide (NaI) therapy. NaI can be administered at a dose of 66 mg/kg IV as a 20% solution, repeated at 10- to 14-day intervals until remission or until iodism occurs. Iodism is characterized by lacrimation, cough, and scaling of the skin. The use of antifungal drugs for this condition, either topically or systemically, has not been investigated in cattle.

REFERENCES

461. McKenzie RA, Connole MD: Mycotic nasal granuloma in cattle, *Aust Vet J* 53:268-270, 1977.
462. Patton CS: *Helminthosporium speciferum* as the cause of dermal and nasal maduromycosis in a cow, *Cornell Vet* 67:236-244, 1977.

Allergic Rhinitis and Enzootic Nasal Granuloma

Allergic rhinitis occurs in cattle and in its chronic stages may lead to the formation of granulomas. A similar condition may occur in sheep.[463] The inciting antigen is frequently a plant pollen or more likely a fungal spore.[464] Once homocytotropic antibody (immunoglobulin E or possibly other classes in cattle) to the allergen has developed, subsequent exposure results in a localized, ongoing, immediate (type I) hypersensitivity reaction.[464,465] If recurrent exposure to the allergen occurs, repeated tissue damage by mast cell factors results in chronic epithelial, duct, and goblet cell hyperplasia and metaplasia, as well as mucus hypersecretion and granulomatous inflammation.[465] Allergic rhinitis in cattle has recently been reviewed.[466]

Any breed may be affected, but Channel Island breeds and Friesians seem most susceptible.[464] The disease occurs sporadically in the United States. A familial predisposition has been reported.[467] Most affected animals are between 6 months and 2 years of age. The signs are initially seasonal, usually occurring in warm, moist conditions; they include rhinorrhea, sneezing, nasal pruritus, a sudden onset of dyspnea, and stertorous inspiration.[467,468] There is a profuse bilateral nasal discharge. Intense pruritus is characteristic and associated with sneezing, head shaking, and nose rubbing.[468] In severe cases, facial swelling, tachypnea, hyperpnea, and ulceration of the nasal mucosa may occur.[465,468] Nasal foreign objects may result from the animal's attempts to scratch the nasal mucosa. Lacrimation, chemosis, and blepharitis may also be present. In the chronic stages (the "enzootic nasal granuloma"), the signs are more constant, with seasonal exacerbations.[465,468] The granulomas tend to be multiple, firm, white, raised nodules 1 to 2 mm in diameter with an intact mucosa, or pale pink flat plaques scattered throughout the nasal cavity. Differential diagnoses include fungal granulomas, foreign bodies, respiratory viruses, nasal actinomycosis or actinobacillosis, tumors, and inhalation of hot or irritant gases.

Endoscopy, biopsies, cultures (viral, bacterial, fungal), antigen detection tests, and serologic analysis can be used to rule out these differentials. Eosinophil counts in nasal secretions correlate with the susceptibility of the animal and activity of the disease, but no absolute level is diagnostic.[464] Intradermal allergen testing has been suggested to aid in diagnosis, but interpretation of results needs to be done in conjunction with historical and clinical findings.[466] This condition should be differentiated from fungal granuloma because the therapy is different.

Treatment and control entail removal of the allergen, or removal of the animal from the allergen, and therapy to block the hypersensitivity reaction. Recommended drugs include various antihistamines, meclofenamic acid, and corticosteroids at standard antiinflammatory doses (0.04 to 0.22 mg/kg dexamethasone IM or IV or 1.0 to 2.2 mg/kg prednisolone IM or IV daily). Topical corticosteroids are a consideration in severe, acute occurrences of the disease. The adverse effects of corticosteroids on milk production and their potential to induce abortion or parturition should be considered before their use. Antihistamine therapy has had equivocal results.[466]

REFERENCES

463. Wilke BN: Allergic respiratory disease, *Adv Vet Sci Comp Med* 26:233-266, 1982.
464. Carbonell PL, Muller HK: Bovine nasal granuloma: nasal eosinophilia, *Aust Vet J* 59:97-101, 1982.
465. Allan EM, Gibbs HA, Wiseman A: Pathologic features of bovine nasal granuloma (atopic rhinitis), *Vet Rec* 112:222-223, 1983.
466. Van Metre DC: Allergic respiratory disease, *Vet Clin North Am (Food Anim Pract)* 13:495-514, 1997.
467. Krahwinkel DJ et al: Familial allergic rhinitis in cattle, *J Am Vet Med Assoc* 192:1593-1596, 1988.
468. Wiseman A, Gibbs HA, McGregor AB: Bovine nasal granuloma (atopic rhinitis) in Britain, *Vet Rec* 110:420-421, 1982.

Nasal Foreign Bodies

Cattle are more prone than small ruminants to the acquisition of nasal foreign bodies. Foreign objects may be acquired as a result of attempts to scratch the nose in cases of allergic rhinitis or of the cow's aggressive eating habits. Depending on the size and duration of residence of the object, signs may include head shaking, stridor, sneezing, snorting, frequent nose licking, unilateral decreases in airflow, foul odors, and serous, mucopurulent, or hemorrhagic discharges. Differential diagnoses include fungal granulomas, allergic rhinitis, tumors, nasal actinomycosis or actinobacillosis, and bots. Many objects can be visualized on careful examination of the nasal cavity with an adequate light source, whereas some may require endoscopy for diagnosis and removal.

Nasal Trauma and Fractures

Trauma to the facial bones, sinuses, and turbinates may result from fighting, accidents caused by improper restraint, farm machinery accidents, human maliciousness, and passage of excessively large nasogastric tubes. Severe fractures can lead to facial swelling, subcutaneous emphysema, obstruction of airflow, stertor, and epistaxis. Secondary infection causes foul odors and mucopurulent nasal discharge. Differential diagnoses for the acute external swelling and stertor include snakebite, actinobacillosis, actinomycosis, and phlegmon (*Fusobacterium, Clostridium* spp.). Unless severe depression fractures, formation of sequestra, or severe obstruction of airflow occurs, surgery is usually not indicated. Radiographs confirm the diagnosis and help determine the need for surgical removal of potential sequestra or elevation and fixation of large displaced segments. Prophylactic antibiotics (typically penicillin, 22,000 U/kg IM or SC twice daily) are recommended to prevent fracture infection and sinusitis; and nonsteroidal antiinflammatory drugs (aspirin, 100 mg/kg PO twice; phenylbutazone, 6 mg/kg PO daily; flunixin meglumine, 0.5 to 1.1 mg/kg IV or IM daily to three times daily) may help relieve pain, swelling, and stridor. The prognosis is usually good.

Nasal Tumors and Polyps

Tumors and polyps of the nasal cavity and sinuses are rare in ruminants. Nasal tumors reported in cattle are osteomas and osteosarcomas of the sinuses, squamous cell carcinomas,[469] neuroblastomas, and adenocarcinomas of the ethmoid mucosa. Ethmoid adenocarcinomas are speculated to be caused by viruses on the basis of an endemic pattern in some cases.[470] They tend to occur in cattle 6 to 9 years of age and are frequently unilateral. Metastasis occurs to the lymph nodes and lungs. There is a report of a hemangiosarcoma involving the external naris of a cow.[471] Signs common to all nasal tumors include mixed or inspiratory dyspnea, stridor, nasal discharge, epistaxis, foul breath odors, unilateral decreases in airflow, open-mouth breathing, and distortion of the facial bones. Differential diagnoses include fungal granulomas, atopic granulomas, foreign bodies, sinusitis, fractures, and nasal actinobacillosis/actinomycosis. Treatment has not been investigated.

The majority of nasal neoplasms in sheep are adenopapillomas, adenomas, or adenocarcinomas.[472] Squamous cell carcinoma has also been reported.[473] Although nasal adenocarcinoma in sheep was initially thought to have a hereditary basis, there is increasing evidence that this neoplasm is contagious and caused by a retrovirus.[472,474,475] Nasal adenocarcinomas have also been described in goats.[476] There is no breed or sex predisposition; most adenocarcinomas occur in yearling to adult sheep, but the tumor has been seen as early as 4 months of age.[474] Signs in sheep are progressive inspiratory dyspnea;

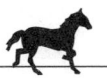

stridor; exercise intolerance; mouth breathing; serous, mucoid, or mucopurulent nasal discharge; tachypnea; decreased airflow; head shaking; sneezing; exophthalmos; and facial asymmetry.[472,474] Differential diagnoses in sheep are nasal actinobacillosis, actinomycosis, bots, and sinusitis. The lesions may be unilateral or bilateral, occur in the olfactory region of the ethmoid turbinates, and are probably derived from Bowman's glands.[474] They begin as small nodules and grow into soft, gray to grayish pink, mucoid, nodular, cystic masses. The tumor is benign but locally expansive, and death usually occurs within 90 days of recognition of signs as a result of inanition, asphyxia, or aspiration pneumonia. The tumors grossly resemble mucoid polyps, which also occur with chronic rhinitis in sheep. Endoscopy and, to a lesser extent, radiology are helpful in establishing an initial diagnosis of a nasal mass. Preoperative or antemortem pinch biopsies and exfoliative cytologic analysis frequently are nondiagnostic and findings may be misleading.[472,473] Surgical management has been described.[477]

REFERENCES

469. Pycock JF, Pead MJ, Longstaffe JA: Squamous cell carcinoma in the nasal cavity of a cow, *Vet Rec* 114:542-543, 1984.
470. Popischil A, Haenichen T, Schaeffler H: Histological and electron microscopic studies of endemic ethmoidal carcinomas in cattle, *Vet Pathol* 16:180-190, 1979.
471. Queen WG, Masterson MA, Weisbrode SE: Hemangiosarcoma of the external naris in a cow, *J Am Vet Med Assoc* 201:1411-1412, 1992.
472. Rings DM, Rojko J: Naturally occurring nasal obstructions in 11 sheep, *Cornell Vet* 75:269-276, 1985.
473. Johnson R et al: Nasal squamous-cell carcinoma in a sheep, *Mod Vet Pract* 63:897-900, 1982.
474. McKinnon AO et al: Enzootic nasal adenocarcinoma of sheep in Canada, *Can Vet J* 23:88-94, 1982.
475. DeMartini JC, York DF: Retrovirus-associated neoplasms of the respiratory system of sheep and goats, *Vet Clin North Am (Food Anim Pract)* 13:55-70, 1997.
476. De las Heras M, Garcia de Jalon JA, Sharp JM: Pathology of enzootic intranasal tumor in thirty-eight goats, *Vet Pathol* 28:474-481, 1991.
477. Trent AM, Smart ME, Fretz PB: Surgical management of nasal adenocarcinoma in sheep, *J Am Vet Med Assoc* 193:227-229, 1988.

Congenital Cystic Nasal Turbinates in Cattle

An apparently developmental anomaly that results in signs of nasal obstruction has been reported in cattle.[478] The nasal conchae lack the normal communication with the nasal cavity and become filled with a thick white fluid, which may account for the enlargement. Signs are evident at or near birth and include progressive stridor, tachypnea, decreased airflow, exercise intolerance, mouth breathing, and short, convex nasal bones. Digital, radiographic, and endoscopic examinations of the nasal cavity reveal large, smooth, bilateral cystic ventral nasal conchae, often bilobate. Differential diagnoses include foreign bodies, trauma, and tumors. Surgical removal of the conchae with bilateral dorsolateral nasal bone flaps relieves the obstruction. Transnasal removal using obstetric wire has been described.[479]

REFERENCES

478. Ross MW et al: Nasal obstruction caused by cystic nasal conchae in cattle, *J Am Vet Med Assoc* 188:857-860, 1986.
479. Cohen ND et al: Cystic nasal concha in a calf, *J Am Vet Med Assoc* 198:1035-1036, 1991.

DISEASES OF THE SINUSES

CLIFFORD M. HONNAS
JOHN R. PASCOE
NANCY E. EAST

Sinusitis

DEFINITION AND ETIOLOGY. Inflammation of the paranasal sinuses is most common in cattle and occurs infrequently in sheep and goats. Typically the frontal or maxillary sinuses are involved and a variety of bacteria may be isolated. The proximate cause for infection is usually dehorning (frontal sinusitis) or infected teeth (maxillary sinusitis). Other causes include extension of actinomycosis or nasal neoplasia into the sinus, injuries to the horn, facial fractures, respiratory viruses (including malignant catarrhal fever, infectious bovine rhinotracheitis, and parainfluenza viruses), sinus cysts,[480,481] lymphosarcoma,[482] and bots (in sheep).[483-486]

CLINICAL SIGNS AND DIFFERENTIAL DIAGNOSIS. Sinusitis associated with dehorning may be acute or occur weeks to months later; typically only one sinus is affected. Nonspecific clinical signs include anorexia, lethargy, reluctance to move, and fever. When sinusitis occurs acutely after dehorning, the portal of entry is frequently open and discharging pus, and the animal is often febrile (39.5° to 40.5° C). In chronic sinusitis, signs may include unilateral or bilateral nasal discharge, mild stridor, changes in airflow, and foul breath odors that are frequently unilateral; fever is not common. The animal may hold its head at an odd angle (extended up or down, tilted) and may squint the eyelids as if in pain.[485,487] With chronicity, frontal bone distortion, exophthalmos, and neurologic signs may occur.[487,488] In one report of 12 cattle with frontal sinusitis, 4 cattle had abnormal posture, with an extended head and neck, partially closed eyes, and a tendency to head-press or to rest the head on a stationary object; the other 8 cattle were apprehensive and intolerant of head manipulation.[487] Extension of infection may involve the central nervous system.

Occasionally sinusitis irritates the animal sufficiently that it may rub its head on the ground, driving more debris into the sinus.[486] Maxillary sinus cysts have been observed in cattle.[480] Typical signs included unilateral facial swelling over the affected sinus, mucopurulent, nonfetid nasal discharge, and radiographic evidence of septal deviation. One cow had stertorous respiration with diminished airflow. Differential diagnoses for sinusitis include facial fractures, nasal tumors, actinomycosis, actinobacillosis, and retrobulbar abscess, or lymphosarcoma.

CLINICAL PATHOLOGY. Diagnosis can usually be made on clinical signs. Diagnostic aids may be useful in selected cases, particularly when there is no recent history of dehorning, or in cases of maxillary sinusitis. The hemogram is quite variable and is of little assistance in diagnosis. Percussion of the sinus may reveal a dull, full sound, and elicit pain. If the bone has been greatly thinned and has gas underlying it, percussion may produce a hyperresonant sound. Fractures, soft-tissue masses, dental disease, fluid in the frontal sinus, or lysis of bony septa may be evident on radiographs.[487] Sinus centesis may yield purulent material, which should be cultured and examined cytologically. A small area over the affected sinus is clipped and surgically prepared, and local anesthetic is infiltrated subcutaneously. Then a small stab incision is made through the skin and periosteum, and a Steinmann pin is used to drill a small hole. Polyethylene tubing is inserted, and attempts are made to aspirate material. A small amount of sterile isotonic fluid can be injected and aspirated to obtain a washing. The stab incision is closed unless sinusitis is confirmed.

TREATMENT AND PROGNOSIS. Trephine sites for sinusotomy (Fig. 29-27) are:

1. Dorsal frontal sinus
2. Postorbital diverticulum
3. Rostral frontal sinus
4. Turbinate portion of the frontal sinus
5. Maxillary sinus

Cattle with frontal sinusitis after dehorning should be treated by sinusotomy and drainage of the sinus.[489] Sinusotomy sites should be based on anatomic landmarks[487] and modified as needed to accommodate any frontal bone distortion or wounds related to dehorning.[487] Sinusotomy

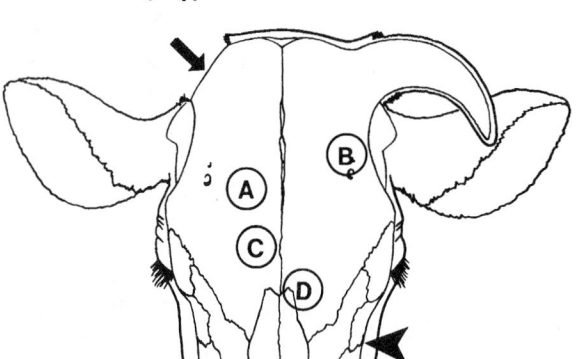

FIG. 29-27 ▉ Trephine sites for sinusotomy. *A,* Dorsal frontal sinus. *B,* Post-orbital diverticulum. *C,* Rostral frontal sinus. *D,* Turbinate portion of frontal sinus. The maxillary sinus is trephined ventral to a line from the infraorbital foramen to the medial canthus *(arrowhead).* If draining tracts are present at the poll, an additional sinusotomy can be made in the cornual portion of the frontal sinus *(arrowhead).*

should be performed 3 to 4 cm from midline, intersecting a line drawn between the caudal aspect of the orbits. If draining tracts are present at the poll, an additional sinusotomy can be made in the cornual portion of the frontal sinus.[487] Sinusotomy is performed after sedation and local anesthetic infiltration of the centesis site(s). A 2-cm-diameter circular piece of skin is excised, and a 19-mm (3/4-inch) trephine used to create an opening into the sinus, through which purulent fluid should be evacuated and the sinus lavaged.

Additional trephine sites that permit access to other regions of the frontal sinus include the postorbital diverticulum, which is trephined approximately 4 cm caudal to the dorsal rim of the orbit, just above the temporal crest of the frontal bone; the rostral frontal sinus, which is trephined just caudal to a line between the centers of the orbits and to either side of the midline; and the turbinate portion of the frontal sinus, which is trephined just rostral to the line described and to either side of the midline.

Access to the maxillary sinus is achieved by trephining ventral to a line from the infraorbital foramen to the medial canthus. If an infected tooth is the cause of maxillary sinusitis, a sinusotomy is created with a trephine over the affected tooth to repel it; otherwise, the hole is usually made just dorsal and caudal to the facial tuberosity. The trephine site should be higher in the sinus of younger animals because the tooth roots are longer.

If the frontomaxillary and nasomaxillary openings are still patent, one trephine site may be sufficient, with the natural opening providing ventral drainage. In more chronic cases, two trephine sites (for ingress and egress) are needed. Another alternative in chronic sinusitis is the use of a curved steel sinus probe (1 cm diameter × 55 cm long), which is forcefully driven through the septal plates of the frontal sinus into the nasal meatus for ventral drainage.[490] The frontal sinus is very compartmentalized in mature sheep and goats, and effective drainage is difficult. Therapy should therefore

be aggressive in these species, even in early cases, and double trephination or bone flaps for exposure and curettage should be considered.

If a tooth has been repelled, a roll of gauze or dental impression material should be used to occlude the alveolar socket to prevent feed material from entering the sinus. A strip of umbilical tape tied around the gauze roll or a wire in the dental material is passed through socket, sinus, and trephine hole and secured to the face by tying around another roll of gauze as a stent. These gauze packs are replaced each time the sinus is flushed. The sinus is lavaged daily with dilute antiseptic solutions such as 0.1% povidone iodine or chlorhexidine in saline, or 1:1000 potassium permanganate. Lavage is continued until infection is resolved. Enzymes (papain or 200,000 U of streptokinase and 50,000 U of streptodornase in at least 10 ml of normal saline solution) may help remove thick exudate.

Parenteral antibiotics and nonsteroidal antiinflammatory drugs (aspirin, 100 mg/kg PO twice daily; phenylbutazone, 17.6 mg/kg PO loading dose for the first 48 hours followed by 4.4 mg/kg PO once daily[491]; or flunixin meglumine, 0.5 to 1.1 mg/kg IM or IV daily to three times daily) are indicated if systemic signs are present. In the absence of microbial culture and susceptibility results, penicillin (22,000 U/kg IM twice daily) is recommended as the antibiotic of choice because *Arcanobacterium (Actinomyces) pyogenes* is the most common organism isolated from cattle with chronic frontal sinusitis resulting from dehorning. *Pasteurella multocida* is the most common organism isolated from infections of the frontal sinus not associated with dehorning.[487] Antimicrobial therapy should be modified according to bacteriologic susceptibility test results. Early cases often resolve in 10 to 14 days, with a good prognosis. Long-term therapy (weeks) is frequently needed in chronic cases; the prognosis is more guarded and salvage is often the best option.

PREVENTION AND CONTROL. Dehorning ruminants as neonates, particularly if a "closed" method such as a dehorning iron is used, is the most effective way to prevent frontal sinusitis. In larger cattle, surgical dehorning with primary skin closure achieved under aseptic conditions minimizes the likelihood of sinusitis.[492] When this is not practical, dehorning should be avoided in rainy, windy, or dusty conditions and fly control must be used. The dehorning of mature sheep or goats leaves massive wounds that typically take 4 to 6 weeks to close by second intention and so are susceptible to infection, and special care such as bandaging for the initial 7 to 10 days, must be taken.[493] Sinusitis did not occur in goats aged 2 to 24 months dehorned with a technique in which primary skin closure was achieved.[494]

REFERENCES

480. McPike Mundell LD, Smith BP, Hoffman RL: Maxillary sinus cysts in two cattle, *J Am Vet Med Assoc* 209:127-129, 1996.
481. Miller M et al: What is your diagnosis? Right maxillary sinusitis or sinus cyst in a cow, *J Am Vet Med Assoc* 208:829-830, 1996.
482. Crocker CB, Rings DM: Lymphosarcoma of the frontal sinus and nasal passage in a cow, *J Am Vet Med Assoc* 213:1472-1474, 1998.
483. Mackey DR: The respiratory system. In Gibbons WJ, Catcott EJ, Smithcors JF, eds: *Bovine medicine and surgery,* Wheaton, Ill, 1970, American Veterinary Publications, pp 466-467.
484. Gibbons WJ: *Diseases of cattle,* Santa Barbara, Calif, 1963, American Veterinary Publications, pp 157-158.
485. Nyack B, Padmore CL, Bernard N: Conservative therapy for right frontal sinusitis in a Brahma bull, *Vet Med Small Anim Clin* 77:107-109, 1982.
486. Greenough PR, Johnson L: The integumentary system. In Oehme FW, Prier JE, eds: *Textbook of large animal surgery,* Baltimore, 1974, Williams & Wilkins, p 205.
487. Ward JL, Rebhun WC: Chronic frontal sinusitis in dairy cattle: 12 cases (1978-1989), *J Am Vet Med Assoc* 201:326-328, 1992.
488. Schneider JE: The respiratory system. In Oehme FW, Prier JE, eds: *Textbook of large animal surgery,* Baltimore, 1974, Williams & Wilkins, pp 350-352.

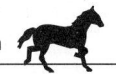

489. Schneider JE: The respiratory system. In Oehme FW, ed: *Textbook of large animal surgery*, ed 2, Baltimore, 1988, Williams & Wilkins, pp 356-357.
490. Misra SS, Angelo SJ: Sinus-probe in the clinical management of frontal sinusitis in zebu cattle, *Indian Vet J* 60:154-156, 1983.
491. Roussel AJ: Personal communication, 1994.
492. Hoffsis G: Surgical (cosmetic) dehorning in cattle, *Vet Clin North Am (Food Anim Pract)* 11:159-169, 1995.
493. Hull BL: Dehorning the adult goat, *Vet Clin North Am (Food Anim Pract)* 11:183-185, 1995.
494. Hague BA, Hooper RN: Cosmetic dehorning in goats, *Vet Surg* 26:332-334, 1997.

Oestrus ovis Infestation

Infestation of the nasal cavity with the bots of *Oestrus ovis* occurs most commonly in sheep and occasionally in goats. Zoonotic infection is rare but has been reported as an ocular myiasis occurring in shepherds working closely with infested flocks. *O. ovis* has a worldwide distribution and is endemic in some regions.[495] The adult is a fly about the size of a honeybee and dark gray to brown with small black spots. It is active only in warm months (spring through autumn in most regions). The mature bot is fat and yellow-white and has a dark stripe on the dorsum and a row of spines on the ventrum of each segment. Adult flies deposit larvae in or around the nostrils. Larvae migrate to the dorsal turbinates and sinuses, develop through three instars over several weeks to months, migrate back to the nostrils where they are expelled by sneezing, and pupate in the ground. Overwintering occurs as first instar larvae in the nasal passages or as pupae in the soil; in warm areas, adults emerge in 3 to 6 weeks. In endemic regions, larvae are present in untreated sheep throughout the year. Third-stage larvae are often found in water troughs and feeders in endemically infested flocks.

Adult female flies annoy sheep as they approach to deposit larvae at the nares and elicit avoidance behaviors like head shaking, sneezing, blowing, nasal rubbing on the ground, feet stamping, and loss of grazing time. Sheep stop grazing when bot flies are active and flock together in tight groups standing nose to nose with heads held close to the ground. Sheep on the outside of the group stamp their feet and run into the center of the flock shaking their heads, snorting, and rubbing their noses as the bot flies attempt to deposit larvae. The bots cause a rhinitis with sneezing, snorting, mucopurulent (intermittently blood tinged) nasal discharge, stridor, and reduced airflow. In regions with hot dry climates, the nasal discharge can become encrusted and may interfere with breathing. Chronic sinusitis is common as instar development occurs. Secondary bacterial infections occur,[496,497] and interstitial pneumonia from aspiration of respiratory secretions contaminated with bacteria, activated inflammatory cells, and cytokines.[500] Rarely, L3 larvae will enter the brain from an infected sinus.

Goats, even when run together with sheep, are not usually infested with *O. ovis*, although occasionally bots will be found in the sinus or brain at necropsy. Most goats with *O. ovis* infestation are debilitated from chronic illness such as caprine arthritis and encephalitis virus (CAEV), Johne's disease, or parasites. Variations in response to experimental infestation of goat kids with L1 instars from naturally infected sheep or goats have led to speculation that there may be ovine and caprine strains of *O. ovis*, although this remains unproven.[498] The clinical signs in goats are generally milder than those seen in sheep and may reflect differences in relative larval load or sensitivity to infestation.[498]

Differential diagnoses for oestrosis should include foreign bodies, nasal adenocarcinoma, pneumonia, trauma, actinobacillosis, actinomycosis, sinusitis, bluetongue, and nonspecific central nervous system signs as might occur with brain abscess or gid. Diagnosis is typically inferred from clinical signs and can be confirmed by necropsy examination of the nasal passages or, if practical, by endoscopy. Serodiagnosis of

O. ovis infections has also been reported.[499] Opinion differs as to the importance of treatment solely for nasal bots, and control is often accomplished coincidentally by other gastrointestinal parasite control programs.[500] Ivermectin, 200 μg/kg PO, is an effective treatment and apparently kills all instars[501]; the dead larvae are sneezed out. Strategically timed treatments should reduce infestations and administration of controlled-release capsules of ivermectin may offer a means of parasite control. Orally administered controlled-release capsules of ivermectin (20 μg/kg/day for 100 days) treat existing infection and prevent new infestation.[500,502]

REFERENCES
495. Dorchies P: Comparative physiopathology of *Oestrus ovis* (Linne 1761) myiasis in animals and man, *Bull Acad Nat Med* 181:673-683, 1997.
496. Jensen R, Swift BL: *Diseases of sheep*, ed 2, Philadelphia, 1982, Lea & Febiger, pp 219-221.
497. Marsh H: *Newsom's sheep diseases*, ed 3, Baltimore, 1965, Williams & Wilkins, pp 195-198.
498. Dorchies P, Duranton, C, Jacquiet P: Pathophysiology of *Oestrus ovis* infection in sheep and goats: a review, *Vet Rec* 142:487-489, 1998.
499. Goddard P, Bates P, Webster KA: Evaluation of a direct ELISA for the serodiagnosis of *Oestrus ovis* infections in sheep, *Vet Rec* 144:497-501, 1999.
500. Rugg D et al: Efficacy of ivermectin controlled-release capsules for the control and prevention of nasal bot infestations in sheep, *Aus Vet J* 75:36-38, 1997.
501. Roncalli RA: Efficacy of ivermectin against *Oestrus ovis* in sheep, *Vet Med* 79:1095-1097, 1984.
502. Rehbein S et al: Efficacy of an ivermectin controlled-release capsule against nematode and arthropod endoparasites of sheep, *Vet Rec* 142:331-334, 1998.

DISEASES OF THE PHARYNX, LARYNX, AND TRACHEA

JOHN C. BAKER
JOHN A. SMITH

Pharyngeal Trauma and Abscesses

DEFINITION AND ETIOLOGY. Pharyngeal trauma may result in hematomas, foreign body granulomas, cellulitis, or abscesses. Trauma usually results from careless use of balling guns, dose syringes, paste-type anthelmintics or calcium preparations, specula, and stomach tubes. Rough, stemmy feeds (especially when chopped), grass awns, briars, and foreign objects (e.g., nails, baling wire) may also cause punctures. Migrating foreign objects or medications (e.g., mineral oil, anthelmintics) may cause pharyngeal granulomas. Hematomas and puncture wounds often result in abscess formation. Diffuse cellulitis may also result. Common bacteria involved include *Arcanobacterium (Actinomyces) pyogenes, Actinobacillus* spp., *Pasteurella* spp., *Bordetella* spp., *Fusobacterium necrophorum,* and *Streptococcus* spp. In cases of particularly virulent bacterial invasion, the condition can become rapidly fatal. *Corynebacterium pseudotuberculosis* (caseous lymphadenitis) may localize in the pharyngeal nodes of sheep and especially goats. Caseous lymphadenitis is discussed further on p. 583 and also in relation to the hemolymphatic system in Chapter 38.

CLINICAL SIGNS AND DIFFERENTIAL DIAGNOSIS. Signs of pharyngeal trauma vary with the severity of the resulting reaction (e.g., cellulitis, abscess). Prominent signs include inspiratory dyspnea with stertorous inspiratory sounds and a prolonged inspiratory phase; extended head and neck; ptyalism, which is often profuse; quidding; evident pain on swallowing or reluctance to swallow solid feed but willingness to drink liquids; prolonged chewing of boluses; regurgitation of food or saliva through the nostrils caused by pharyngeal paresis; mucopurulent to bloody nasal discharge and fetid odors, usually bilateral; cough; bloat; and visible or palpable swelling in the pharyngeal area.[503,504] Megaesophagus has been reported subsequent to pharyngeal trauma.[505]

Palpation of the pharynx may increase the stertor and cause pain. In severe cases, systemic signs of fever, anorexia, depression, dehydration, and forestomach stasis may be present. Aspiration pneumonia may be a secondary complication. A thorough manual examination of the oral pharynx or a visual examination with an adequate speculum and light source usually confirms the diagnosis of a pharyngeal swelling and often reveals a puncture that is discharging pus. Cases in which the infection is diffuse can be more difficult to recognize, and endoscopy or radiography can be particularly helpful.[503] Restraining the jaws with a McAllum speculum allows a guarded needle attached to a length of tubing and a syringe to be inserted into the swelling. This helps to differentiate localized abscesses from granulomas, hematomas, cellulitis, and tumors; allows culture and sensitivity determinations on abscesses; and may aid in cytologic diagnosis of granulomas or tumors. Radiographs may reveal foreign bodies (Fig. 29-28) or air densities (Fig. 29-29) in the pharyngeal tissues. Differential diagnoses include pharyngeal tumors; lymphosarcoma; sialoliths; rabies; botulism; actinobacillosis; necrotic laryngitis; laryngeal abscesses, trauma, edema, or paralysis; and laryngeal tumors.

CLINICAL PATHOLOGY. The complete blood count (CBC) usually reflects a chronic inflammatory process, with a neutrophilic leukocytosis and a left shift, or a neutrophil-lymphocyte reversal. Dehydration is frequently evident. If the animal is unable to swallow, large amounts of bicarbonate may be lost through the saliva, which may be reflected in blood gas and electrolyte values.

TREATMENT AND PROGNOSIS. Discrete pharyngeal abscesses are usually best drained into the pharynx. Whenever possible, the procedure should be done on the standing animal without sedation to preserve the cough reflex and prevent aspiration. A good oral speculum and excellent restraint are needed. The head should be kept lowered. A guarded blade such as a hook blade from a fetotomy set is introduced into the pharynx, and the abscess is lanced. The cavity is flushed with a mild antiseptic such as 0.2% povidone iodine in saline solution, again taking care to prevent aspiration. Other options include drainage to the exterior, drainage and flushing with a large-gauge needle and tubing, and extirpation.[504] Systemic antibiotics are administered in accordance with culture and sensitivity results, or, in their absence, procaine penicillin G (22,000 U/kg IM or SC twice daily), tetracyclines (11 mg/kg IM, IV, or SC daily or twice daily), or sulfonamides (a 140-mg/kg IV loading dose followed by 70 mg/kg IV daily) are used. Nonsteroidal antiinflammatory drugs (aspirin, 100 mg/kg PO twice daily; phenylbutazone, 6 mg/kg PO daily; or flunixin, 0.5 to 1.1 mg/kg IM or IV daily to 3 times daily) help relieve pain, swelling, and stertor. In severe cases, tracheostomy may be necessary. Granulomas and diffuse cellulitis are treated medically. Supportive therapy such as intravenous fluids or feeding through a rumenostomy site may be necessary if the animal refuses to eat or drink. The prognosis for most pharyngeal abscesses, hematomas, cellulitis, and granulomas is usually good with appropriate therapy.

REFERENCES

503. Davidson HP, Rebhun WC, Habel RE: Pharyngeal trauma in cattle, *Cornell Vet* 71:15-25, 1981.
504. Vestweber JG, Roeder B: Medial retropharyngeal lymph node abscess as a cause of respiratory dyspnea in cattle, *Compend Cont Educ Pract Vet* 8:F71-F74, 1986.
505. Ross CE, Rebhun WC: Megaesophagus in a cow, *J Am Vet Med Assoc* 188:623-624, 1986.

Dorsal Displacement of the Soft Palate

Although rare, dorsal displacement of the soft palate has been reported in cattle.[506] Respiratory noise is apparent on inspiration and expiration, but is loudest on inspiration. Diagnosis can be made by endoscopic examination. Treatment is similar to that used in horses and can include conservative therapy, which consists of antiinflammatory drug therapy and rest, or the condition can be surgically corrected.

REFERENCE

506. Anderson DE et al: Persistent dorsal displacement of the soft palate in two young bulls, *J Am Vet Med Assoc* 204:1071-1074, 1994.

Subepiglottic Cyst

Although rare, a subepiglottic pharyngeal cyst causing upper airway obstruction has been reported in cattle.[507] Surgical removal by a peroral approach has been described.[507]

REFERENCE

507. Mattoon JS et al: Subepiglottic cyst causing upper airway obstruction in a neonatal calf, *J Am Vet Med Assoc* 199:747-749, 1991.

Necrotic Laryngitis (Calf Diphtheria, Laryngeal Necrobacillosis)

DEFINITION AND ETIOLOGY. Acute to chronic infection of the laryngeal mucosa and cartilage of young cattle is very common, particularly in feedlots. Laryngeal contact ulcers[508] probably provide a damaged mucosal surface, which then allows invasion of the cartilage by *Fusobacterium necrophorum*, which is the proximate cause of the lesions. It has also been suggested that *Haemophilus somnus* is the primary agent inducing a perilaryngeal vasculitis and that *F. necrophorum* represents a secondary bacterial invader.

CLINICAL SIGNS AND DIFFERENTIAL DIAGNOSIS. The problem occurs most commonly in calves from 3 to 18 months of age, up to about 24 months. It is characterized by an acute onset of a moist, painful cough, which the animal may attempt to suppress because of pain. Frequently a severe inspiratory dyspnea with a loud guttural stertor and open-mouth breathing with the head and neck extended are observed. The animal may salivate, make frequent painful swallowing movements, and stand and sip water continually. Severe systemic signs of anorexia, depression, fever (as high as 106° F [41.1° C]), and hyperemic mucous membranes are present. There is often a bilateral nasal discharge and a fetid odor to the breath. The larynx may be visibly or palpably swollen, and palpation may elicit a cough, cause pain, and markedly increase the dyspnea and stertor. The diagnosis can usually be made on clinical signs alone. A laryngoscopic or endoscopic examination can help confirm the diagnosis, but care must be taken to prevent further stress and respiratory embarrassment. If untreated, many calves will die in 2 to 7 days as a result of toxemia and upper airway obstruction. Recovered cases may have a chronic roaring respiration and a harsh, dry cough because of the misshapen larynx. Aspiration pneumonia and chronic "poor doers" are common sequelae. Differential diagnoses include pharyngeal trauma (abscess, cellulitis), severe viral laryngitis (e.g., infectious bovine rhinotracheitis), actinobacillosis, and laryngeal edema, abscesses, trauma, paralysis, and tumors.

CLINICAL PATHOLOGY. Acute cases show changes in the CBC consistent with any acute septic condition: a leukopenia caused by a neutropenia with a left shift.

PATHOPHYSIOLOGY. *F. necrophorum* normally does not penetrate intact mucous membranes. Laryngeal contact ulcers are thought to provide the portal of entry for *F. necrophorum*, which is ubiquitous, especially in feedlots. Laryngeal contact ulcers are also very common in slaughter cattle, and they in turn are speculated to be caused by the following combination of factors: (1) an acute mucositis from mixed upper respiratory infections (viruses such as infectious bovine

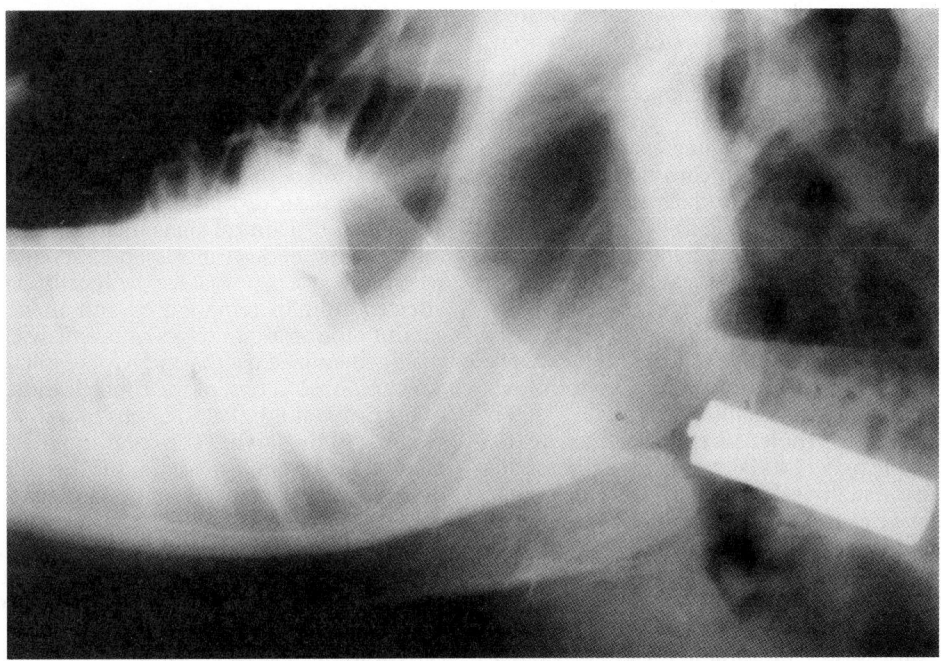

FIG. 29-28 ▦ Radiograph of the pharyngeal area of a cow. Note magnet located in the retropharyngeal tissue.

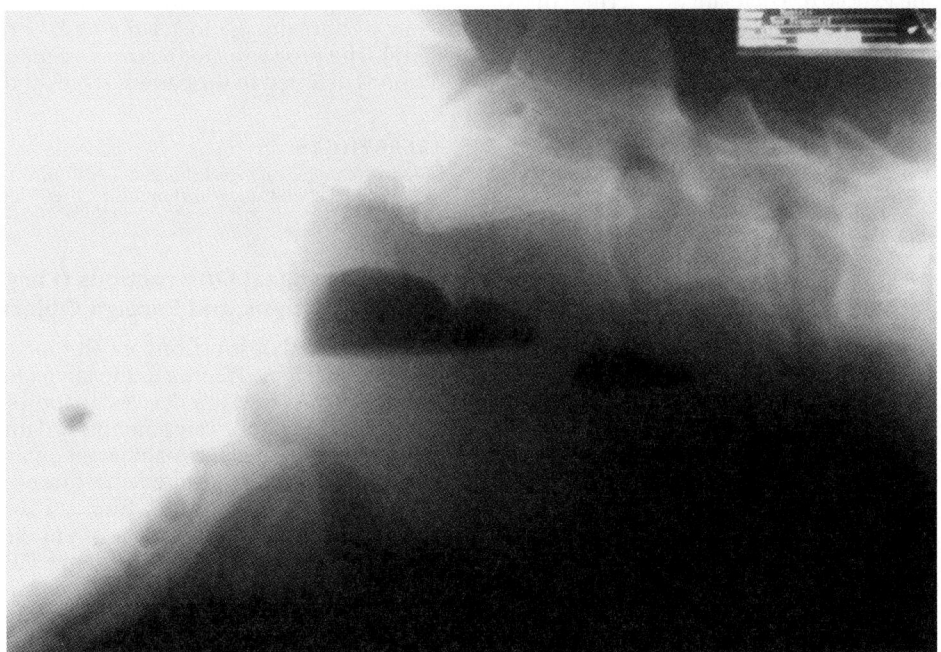

FIG. 29-29 ▦ Radiograph of the pharyngeal area of a cow. Note air densities in the tissue suggestive of abscess formation.

rhinotracheitis [IBR], bovine respiratory syncytial virus [BRSV], and parainfluenza virus 3 [PI3], mycoplasma, and bacteria, including *Pasteurella* and *Hemophilus* spp.); (2) reflex coughing and swallowing, which accelerate the rate of laryngeal closure; and (3) resulting erosion of the swollen membranes over the vocal processes and medial angles of the arytenoid cartilages.[509] It has also been proposed that necrotic laryngitis results from a perilaryngeal vasculitis initiated by *H. somnus* with secondary invasion by *F. necropho-*

rum.[510] Necrotic laryngitis can alter pulmonary function such that the growth rate is impeded and also predisposes to secondary bacterial pneumonia.[511]

EPIDEMIOLOGY. The disease is most common where cattle are housed in dirty or crowded conditions and in feedlots. Most feedlot cases occur in animals on feed for longer than 30 days. The incidence is sporadic. Cases occur year round, but there appears to be a higher incidence in fall and winter. The disease has a worldwide distribution.

NECROPSY LESIONS. The lesions are typically located over the vocal processes and medial angles of the arytenoid cartilages. Acute lesions consist of marked edema, hyperemia, and swelling of the mucous membrane around a necrotic ulcer, with accumulated exudate. The lesions spread along the vocal processes and vocal folds and may extend into the cricoarytenoideus dorsalis muscles. In chronic cases the lesions consist of a focus of necrotic cartilage surrounded by purulent exudate, with a tract extending to the mucosal surface. The tract opening is surrounded by granulation tissue and may drain pus. The arytenoid cartilage may be rotated into the lumen or may contain mucosal cavities lined with thin, hyperemic epithelium.[509]

TREATMENT, PROGNOSIS, PREVENTION, AND CONTROL. Sulfonamides (a 140-mg/kg IV loading dose followed by 70 mg/kg daily) or procaine penicillin G (22,000 U/kg IM or SC twice) are the drugs of choice; streptomycin, oxytetracycline, and tylosin (11 mg/kg IM daily or twice daily for all three drugs) are also usually effective. Nonsteroidal antiinflammatory drugs (aspirin, 100 mg/kg PO twice daily; phenylbutazone, 6 mg/kg PO daily; or flunixin, 0.5 to 1.1 mg/kg IM or IV daily to 3 times daily) reduce swelling, inflammation, and fever. A tracheostomy may be necessary in severe cases to relieve dyspnea and rest the larynx. Good nursing and supportive care are also important, including shelter, adequate ventilation, easy access to feed and water, and oral or intravenous fluids if needed. The prognosis is good when the condition is detected very early and treated vigorously; when extensive cartilage necrosis occurs, a fatal outcome or a chronic roarer can be expected. There are no specific control measures. The proposed pathogenesis would suggest that measures to control other respiratory diseases may reduce the incidence of necrotic laryngitis.

REFERENCES

508. Jensen R et al: Laryngeal contact ulcers in feedlot cattle, *Vet Pathol* 17:667-671, 1980.
509. Jensen R et al: Laryngeal diphtheria and papillomatosis in feedlot cattle, *Vet Pathol* 18:143-150, 1981.
510. Beeman KB: *Haemophilus somnus* of cattle: an overview, *Compend Cont Educ Pract Vet* 7:S259-S263, 1985.
511. Lekeux P, Art T: Functional changes induced by necrotic laryngitis in double muscled calves, *Vet Rec* 121:353-355, 1987.

Laryngeal Granulomas

Laryngeal granulomas have been described in cattle.[512] These may originate from laryngeal contact ulcers that have been described in feedlot cattle at slaughter.[508]

REFERENCE

512. Gamboa JC et al: Laryngeal granuloma in a bull, *J Am Vet Med Assoc* 201:460-462, 1992.

Laryngeal Papillomatosis

Papillomas of the larynx are common in feedlot cattle. They are caused by a papovavirus, which is thought to enter laryngeal contact ulcers (see Necrotic Laryngitis, p. 546).[513] Characteristic signs of laryngeal papillomatosis are stertorous respiration and cough. Differential diagnoses include chronic necrotic laryngitis, pharyngeal trauma, actinobacillosis, and laryngeal abscesses, trauma, edema, paralysis, and tumors. The lesions are sessile to pedunculated, yellow, frondlike, 1- to 10-mm growths over the vocal processes of the arytenoid cartilages.[513] Treatment usually is not indicated, but involves surgical removal. Measures to decrease other respiratory infections and thereby decrease contact ulcers may lower the incidence of papillomas.

REFERENCE

513. Jensen R et al: Laryngeal diphtheria and papillomatosis in feedlot cattle, *Vet Pathol* 18:143-150, 1981.

Laryngeal Abscesses

Abscessation of the arytenoid cartilages caused by *Arcanobacterium (Actinomyces) pyogenes* has been reported in calves[514] and sheep.[515] Clinical signs include tachypnea, extension of the head and neck, cyanosis, and a severe progressive dyspnea with marked stertor that can be localized to the larynx. Many affected animals remain alert and afebrile and continue to eat until the terminal stages of severe dyspnea. Endoscopy reveals generalized edema and hyperemia of the laryngeal mucosa and obstruction of the rima glottidis by swelling of one or both arytenoids. Radiographs may demonstrate soft-tissue swelling of the larynx. The condition has been speculated to be initiated by grass awns, trauma, hereditary predisposition, or congenital cavitations in the cartilages. In sheep, rams appear to be more commonly affected than ewes, and two reports found a breed predisposition in Texels and Southdowns, although other reports have indicated that various breeds are affected.[515] The necropsy lesions consist of encapsulated abscesses containing pus and necrotic debris in the arytenoid cartilage, usually in the vicinity of the vocal cord. A tract from the abscess typically opens in an area of granulation tissue in the laryngeal mucosa. Treatment consists of tracheostomy, antibiotics (usually penicillin at 22,000 U/kg IM or SC twice daily), and antiinflammatory drugs (aspirin, 100 mg/kg PO twice daily; phenylbutazone, 6 mg/kg PO daily; or flunixin, 0.5 to 1.1 mg/kg IM or IV daily to 3 times daily). The prognosis for recovery is guarded unless the condition is detected in the earliest stages and treated vigorously.

REFERENCES

514. Lawrence JA: Laryngeal abscesses in calves, *Vet Rec* 81:540-541, 1967.
515. Lane JG et al: Laryngeal chondritis in Texel sheep, *Vet Rec* 121:81-84, 1987.

Other Laryngeal Obstructions (Laryngeal Trauma, Edema, Paralysis, and Foreign Objects)

Other laryngeal obstructions are all sporadic and may present with similar signs. Trauma to the larynx may result from roping or injury in restraint devices. Inappropriate placement of an endotracheal tube can potentially damage the larynx. The respiratory system is the main target organ for anaphylaxis in ruminants, and laryngeal edema can be a prominent component of this syndrome, which is discussed fully in this chapter on p. 576. Inhalation of smoke or other noxious gases also may cause laryngeal edema. Paralysis of the larynx was reported in a sheep with a false carotid aneurysm[516]; presumably other lesions of the neck or anterior mediastinum could cause laryngeal paralysis through involvement of the recurrent laryngeal nerves. Foreign objects more commonly lodge in the pharynx, but sharp objects and food materials may be aspirated and lodge in the larynx. Signs common to these laryngeal obstructions include inspiratory dyspnea, prolongation of the inspiratory phase, mouth breathing, stertor, cyanosis, salivation, and extension of the head and neck. Palpation of the larynx may reveal swelling and may exaggerate the dyspnea and stertor. Differential diagnoses include necrotic laryngitis, laryngeal abscesses, severe viral laryngitis, actinobacillosis, and tumors. Endoscopy and radiology are required in most cases to differentiate these conditions. Hematologic analysis may give some indication of the presence of bacterial infection; a stress leukogram is expected otherwise. Tracheostomy is indicated in all severe cases. Surgical correction of laryngeal obstruction by tracheolaryngostomy has been described in cattle.[517]

Laryngeal trauma and paralysis may resolve spontaneously or may require reconstructive surgery. The therapy of anaphylaxis is discussed on p. 576. Foreign objects should be removed surgically or endoscopically. Nonsteroidal antiinflammatory drugs (aspirin, 100 mg/kg PO twice daily; phenylbutazone, 6 mg/kg PO daily; or flunixin, 0.5 to 1.1 mg/kg IM or IV daily to 3 times daily) may help reduce swelling, edema, and respiratory embarrassment in all forms of obstruction.

REFERENCES

516. Rings DM, Constable P, Biller DS: False carotid aneurysm in a sheep, *J Am Vet Med Assoc* 189:799-801, 1986.
517. West HJ: Tracheolaryngostomy as a treatment for laryngeal obstruction in cattle, *Vet J* 153:81-86, 1997.

Tracheal Stenosis, Collapse, and Stricture

DEFINITION AND ETIOLOGY. Tracheal collapse is infrequently reported in cattle. The cause is usually unknown, but the problem may result from cranial thoracic trauma, roping, tracheostomies, or possibly congenital defects. All cases recently reported have been in calves in which signs were usually first evident at several weeks of age.[518-521] The majority of these cases also involved the thoracic trachea (Fig. 29-30), suggesting a congenital lesion. However, most calves with tracheal collapse have been cases of dystocia at birth, especially breech presentations; thus suggesting a traumatic etiology.[522]

CLINICAL SIGNS AND DIFFERENTIAL DIAGNOSIS. A variety of beef and dairy breeds and both sexes have been represented.[521] Tracheal collapse has been reported in a young goat also.[523] Clinical signs may include fever, tachycardia, tachypnea, cyanosis, and mucosal hyperemia with vessel engorgement, but many of the animals have normal vital signs and are otherwise alert and in good condition. Dyspnea is usually induced or exacerbated by excitement or exercise or may be severe at rest. Stertorous respiration is usually evident, is frequently worse on inspiration, and can often be localized to the trachea on auscultation. The inspiratory phase is prolonged, and a "honking" cough is characteristic, especially with intrathoracic collapse. Palpation may reveal or induce the collapse when the cervical trachea is involved. Tracheal palpation or elevation of the head may increase the stertor or induce the honking cough. In some cases there may be other evidence of trauma (fractured ribs, sternebrae), and in some, pneumonia may be present. There is no response to antibiotics, steroids, or tracheostomy. Other possible disorders with similar signs are tracheal foreign bodies, tracheal actinobacillosis, neoplasms, bronchopneumonia, necrotic laryngitis, and extratracheal compressive lesions (e.g., abscesses, tuberculosis, hematomas).

CLINICAL PATHOLOGY. Any deviation of the hemogram from normal is probably a reflection of associated pneumonia or stress. Endoscopy and radiography are the most helpful ancillary aids. Care must be taken when restraining, sedating, and passing the endoscope in these animals; oxygen should be available. Radiography (see Fig. 29-30) and endoscopy usually reveal a dorsoventral flattening, most typically in the caudal cervical and cranial thoracic trachea, although lateral collapse and collapse in other locations (cranial cervical, intrathoracic) are occasionally encountered.

PATHOPHYSIOLOGY. Proposed causes of tracheal collapse in other species include congenital malformations, genetic or nutritionally induced weakness of cartilage, deficient innervation of the trachealis muscles, trauma, ischemic lesions from endotracheal tube cuffs, and primary pulmonary disease. No histologic differences were noted in tracheal rings from collapsed and normal segments in calves in one report.[518]

As previously mentioned, most calves with tracheal collapse have a history of being a case of dystocia at birth. During delivery, compression of the chest wall with fracture of the first pair of ribs may cause injury at the thoracic inlet.[524] However, signs of tracheal collapse are not immediately evident at birth, but develop over time.

TREATMENT AND PROGNOSIS. Mild cases may respond to confinement sufficiently to be fed out for slaughter. A number of surgical treatments have been proposed in other species, including anastomosis, bisection of tracheal rings, internal and external prostheses, and plication of the dorsal membrane.[518] External prostheses have been used success-

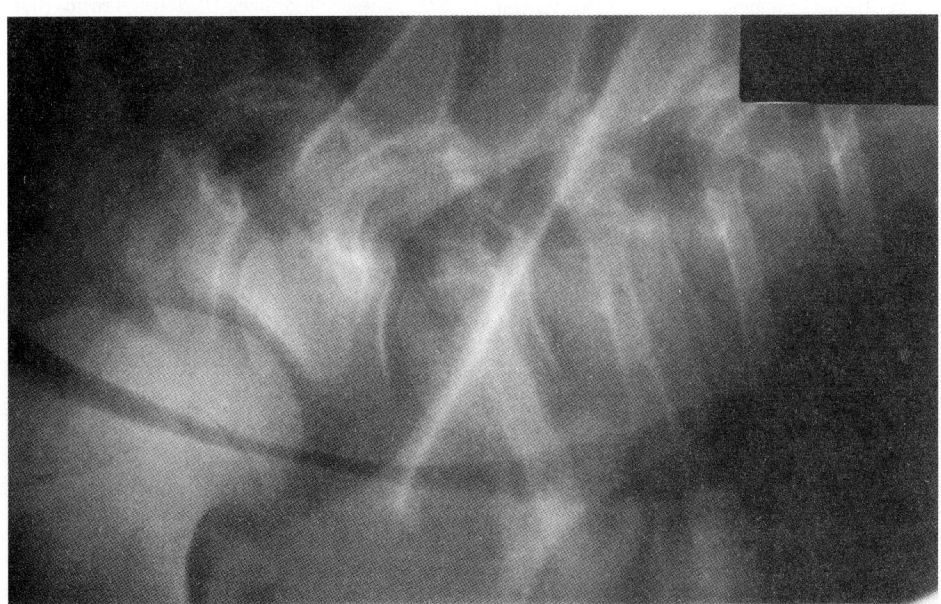

FIG. 29-30 ▦ Radiograph demonstrating collapse of the thoracic trachea in a calf.

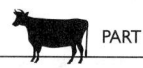

fully in calves[518,522,524] and a goat.[523] A favorable prognosis for surgical correction is estimated at approximately 30%.[522] A detailed description of surgical repair in calves by external prostheses has been published.[522]

REFERENCES
518. Horney FD: Tracheal prosthesis in a calf, *J Am Vet Med Assoc* 167:463-464, 1975.
519. Vestweber JG, Leipold HW: Tracheal collapse in three calves, *J Am Vet Med Assoc* 184:735-736, 1984.
520. Watt BR: Collapse of the trachea in two calves, *Aust Vet J* 60:309-310, 1983.
521. Scarratt WK et al: Collapsed trachea in two calves, *Compend Cont Educ Pract Vet* 7:S45-S49, 1985.
522. Rings DM: Tracheal collapse, *Vet Clin North Am (Food Anim Pract)* 11:171-175, 1995.
523. Jackson PGG et al: Tracheal collapse in a goat, *Vet Rec* 119:160, 1986.
524. Fingland RB, Rings DM, Vestweber JG: The etiology and surgical management of tracheal collapse in calves, *Vet Surg* 19:371-379, 1990.

Tracheal Foreign Bodies and Masses

Ruminants may occasionally inhale foreign objects that lodge in the trachea. There are also two reports of tracheal actinomycosis that resulted in signs of tracheal obstruction.[525] Signs include a chronic cough, inspiratory dyspnea, audible stridor that can be localized to the trachea, extension of the head and neck, open-mouth breathing, and salivation. Differential diagnoses should include pharyngeal trauma; necrotic laryngitis; laryngeal abscesses, trauma, edema, or paralysis; tracheal collapse; and extratracheal compressive lesions. Endoscopy and radiology are important aids to diagnosis. Care must be exercised in restraint and in passage of the endoscope. Some small objects may be retrieved by a snare passed through an endoscope; others may require tracheostomy. When possible, the tracheostomy should be performed below the object. The actinomycotic masses are soft, pedunculated lesions with a granular surface containing small yellow foci. Of the two reported cases of tracheal actinomycosis, one died of asphyxiation, and the other responded initially to partial surgical removal of the masses, tracheostomy, and therapy with sodium iodide, penicillin, and streptomycin but relapsed some months later.[525]

REFERENCE
525. Bertone AL, Rebhun WC: Tracheal actinomycosis in a cow, *J Am Vet Med Assoc* 185:221-222, 1984.

Tracheal Edema Syndrome of Feedlot Cattle

Tracheal edema syndrome has also been referred to as tracheal stenosis in feedlot cattle. In this condition, extensive edema and hemorrhage in the dorsal wall of the trachea result in coughing, dyspnea, and stertor, which has given rise to the term "honker cattle."[526] The tracheal edema syndrome occurs in two forms, an acute dyspnea or a chronic cough. It is not known whether the two forms are related. The cause is also unknown, but theories include infections with upper respiratory viruses and bacteria such as *Pasteurella multocida* or *Haemophilus somnus*, trauma to the trachea from feedbunks, passive congestion and edema from excessive fat accumulation in the thoracic inlet, hypersensitivity reactions, and mycotoxins.[527]

The acute dyspnea syndrome occurs mainly in heavy feedlot cattle in the latter two thirds of the feeding period and is most common in southern plains feedlots. It is sporadic and more common in summer, possibly because of exacerbation by hot weather. At one extreme, sudden deaths without the onset of noticeable clinical signs have been reported, and at the other extreme subclinical disease was evidenced by lesions in animals at slaughter that did not have clinical signs. Other factors that increase respirations also may cause signs to appear. Signs include an acute onset of dyspnea and loud guttural inspiratory sounds that can be localized to the lower trachea. Open-mouth breathing, extension of the head and neck, and cyanosis, leading to recumbency and death by asphyxiation, are present. Differentials for this form include pharyngeal trauma; necrotic laryngitis; infectious bovine rhinotracheitis (IBR); laryngeal abscess, tumor, foreign object, edema, or paralysis; tracheal foreign object, mass, or collapse; and atypical interstitial pneumonia.

The chronic form occurs in lighter cattle (135 to 400 kg [300 to 900 lb]) and is more common in western plains feedlots. It is also sporadic but less seasonal. Affected animals may have a history of IBR or pneumonia. The main sign is a continuous, frequent, deep, hacking, nonproductive cough. The animal may be unthrifty but is otherwise normal in appearance. The main differential diagnosis is mild, chronic suppurative pneumonia. Endoscopy and visualization of the lesions described in the following paragraph aid in the diagnosis. Necropsy of the acute form reveals an edematous thickening of the submucosa and mucosa of the dorsal trachea, as much as 5 cm thick and extending 20 to 30 cm from the midcervical area to the thoracic inlet or tracheal bifurcation. There is also extensive mucosal, submucosal, and peritracheal hemorrhage, probably related to agonal breathing. There are no other lesions of the airway or lungs.[527] Lesions in the chronic form consist of hyperemia of the mucosa of the caudal third of the trachea, with a thin layer of mucopurulent exudate. The mucosa may have a cobblestone appearance or even large, fiberlike projections and polyps. No effective treatment exists for the chronic form. Broad-spectrum antibiotics and corticosteroids (dexamethasone, 0.04 to 0.22 mg/kg IM or IV; prednisolone, 1 to 2.2 mg/kg IM or IV daily) are recommended for the acute form, as well as such practices as preventing stress, providing shade, and cooling with water sprays and fans. Tracheostomy, insertion of an endotracheal tube to the tracheal bifurcation, and administration of oxygen may be needed in severe cases. Recovered patients tend to relapse and should be salvaged.

REFERENCES
526. Erickson ED, Doster AR: Tracheal stenosis in feedlot cattle, *J Vet Diagn Invest* 5:449- 451, 1993.
527. Panciera RJ, Williams DE: Tracheal edema (honker) syndrome of feeder cattle. In Howard JL, editor: *Current veterinary therapy 2: food animal practice*, Philadelphia, 1986, WB Saunders, p 800.

LOWER RESPIRATORY TRACT DISEASES

TREVOR R. AMES
JOHN C. BAKER
STEVEN E. WIKSE

CLINICAL CLASSIFICATION OF PNEUMONIA

TREVOR R. AMES
JOHN C. BAKER
STEVEN E. WIKSE

In an effort to simplify the differential diagnosis of the bewildering array of lower respiratory diseases of cattle, a classification system based on pathophysiology and clinical signs has been suggested.[528] Three classifications were proposed:

1. Bronchial pneumonia is characterized pathophysiologically by invasion of pathogenic organisms that gain

access to the lung through the pulmonary tree. It is characterized clinically by depression, fever, and other signs of sepsis such as hyperemic mucous membranes or scleral injection, and an anterior-ventral distribution of abnormal lung sounds and lesions (see the following section). Bronchial pneumonia is the final outcome of the respiratory disease complex of ruminants and because viruses play an important role in this disease complex, viral causes of respiratory tract disease in ruminants are placed in this category.

2. The interstitial pneumonias are a very diverse group of (usually) noninfectious diseases. Although it is difficult to make generalizations, these diseases are characterized pathophysiologically by an interstitial reaction that results from ingestion or inhalation of toxins or allergens. Clinically they are "atypical" (compared with the more common infectious diseases) because affected animals tend not to be as depressed and septic, the abnormal lung sounds and lesions are diffusely distributed, and there is no response to routine therapy such as antibiotics.

3. Metastatic pneumonia is characterized pathophysiologically by septic embolization of the lungs from other foci in the body, classically liver abscesses and postcaval thrombi. Clinically, cases of metastatic pneumonia exhibit signs of sepsis as with bronchopneumonia, but with widespread pulmonary lesions and abnormal lung sounds, and the eventual development of hemoptysis (see Vena Caval Thrombosis and Metastatic Pneumonia in this chapter).

THE BRONCHOPNEUMONIAS (RESPIRATORY DISEASE COMPLEX OF CATTLE, SHEEP, AND GOATS)

TREVOR R. AMES
JOHN C. BAKER
STEVEN E. WIKSE

DEFINITION. The respiratory disease complex of ruminants consists of the single clinical entity of bronchopneumonia, but is caused by numerous combinations of infectious agents, compromised host defenses, and environmental conditions. Bronchopneumonia causes greater economic losses than any other disease of feedlot calves or lambs and is one of the most common causes of dairy calf mortality.

In dairy calves, bronchopneumonia, often called enzootic pneumonia, is most common in housed calves. It is called "shipping fever" in beef calves because the greatest incidence of bronchopneumonia occurs after shipment to stocker operations or feedlots. The infectious agents and risk factors of bronchopneumonia of sheep and goats are very similar to those of calves.

Bronchopneumonia of ruminants is a disease of multifactorial causation that only occurs when a certain combination of host, environment, and infectious agent characteristics (risk factors) is active. The numerous infectious agents (Boxes 29-1 and 29-2) that are associated with bronchopneumonia are ubiquitous in the cattle population, and the bacteria most often associated with pneumonic lesions are part of the normal resident flora of the nasopharynx of cattle. An understanding of the epidemiologic characteristics of bronchopneumonia of ruminants is the basis for developing successful programs of prevention.

EPIDEMIOLOGY

Enzootic Calf Pneumonia. Enzootic calf pneumonia (ECP) has traditionally been described as affecting calves from 2 to 6 months of age. Recent prospective studies examining cohorts

---

BOX 29-1

Bacteria, *Mycoplasma*, *Ureaplasma*, and *Chlamydia* spp. Associated With Bronchopneumonia of Cattle, Sheep, and Goats

BACTERIA
Facultative Anaerobes
*Mannheimia (Pasteurella) haemolytica**
*Pasteurella multocida**
*Haemophilus somnus**
Arcanobacter pyogenes
Pseudomonas aeruginosa
Escherichia coli
Streptococcus spp.
Staphylococcus spp.
Moraxella spp.
Salmonella spp.

Anaerobes
Bacteroides spp.
Peptococcus indolicus
Fusobacterium spp.

OTHER AGENTS
Mycoplasma bovis
Mycoplasma dispar
Ureaplasma spp.
Chlamydia spp.
Mycoplasma mycoides
Mycoplasma ovipneumonia†

*Principal primary invaders.
†Can be primary cause of pneumonia in young goats.

BOX 29-2

Viral Agents Associated With Respiratory Tract Diseases in Ruminants

BOVINE
Bovine herpesvirus type 1 (IBR)*
Alcelaphine herpesvirus 1 & 2/ovine herpesvirus 2 (malignant catarrhal fever)*
Bovine herpesvirus type 4 (DN-599, Movar 33/63, FTC-2)
Bovine parainfluenza virus type 3
Bovine viral diarrhea virus
Bovine respiratory syncytial virus*
Bovine adenovirus
Bovine rhinovirus
Bovine reovirus
Bovine enterovirus
Bovine coronavirus
Calicivirus
Influenza virus

OVINE AND CAPRINE
Parainfluenza virus type 3
Adenovirus
Respiratory syncytial virus
Bluetongue virus*
Ovine progressive pneumonia (maedi-visna) virus of sheep†
Pulmonary carcinoma of sheep

*Capable of causing severe acute respiratory disease.
†Progressive pneumonias, capable of causing severe chronic respiratory disease.

of calves have found calves may be affected with ECP as early as 2 weeks of age.[529] Slaughter surveys of dairy calves 4 to 14 days of age have found ECP to be the second most common cause of slaughter condemnation.[530] Virtala and colleagues[529] found that veterinarian-diagnosed ECP occurred at a younger age than did caretaker-diagnosed ECP. As a whole, these studies suggest that ECP may start much earlier than previously recognized.

Pneumonia of dairy calves occurs both as endemic disease and as outbreaks of respiratory disease. Chronic endemic disease is the most common manifestation of this disease and as a result pneumonia of dairy calves is commonly called enzootic calf pneumonia. The distinction between enzootic and epizootic calf pneumonia is important in reference to etiology because different causes are more important in each form of the disease.

Waltner-Toews, Martin, and Meek[531] determined from producer diagnosis that 15% of Ontario Holstein dairy calves were treated for pneumonia before weaning. Curtis, Erb, and White[532] reported that Holstein calves in New York had a crude incidence risk of 7.4% for respiratory tract illness, as diagnosed by the farmer. Sivula and colleagues[533] found that 7.6% of 845 Minnesota dairy calves were diagnosed by producers as having pneumonia. Van Donkersgoed and colleagues[534] found that the risk of pneumonia in Saskatchewan dairy calves was 39%, as diagnosed by the farmer, and 29% when the pneumonia was veterinarian diagnosed. Virtala and colleagues[529] found that the risk of pneumonia was 11% in New York dairy calves when diagnosed by producers and 25.6% when diagnosed by a veterinarian.

Mortality rates reported for ECP vary from 1.8%[533,534] to 4.2%.[529] Case fatality rates reported for calves with ECP range from 2.2% to 9.4% and will vary with the sensitivity of the initial detection method (veterinarian versus producer).[529]

Pneumonia accounts for a significant proportion of the mortality (proportionate mortality) in dairy calves raised on dairy farms. Pneumonia accounted for 24% of deaths in New York calves[529] and 30% in Minnesota calves.[533] In one study examining Ontario veal calves raised in veal barns, pneumonia accounted for 52% of mortality in 4863 calves on six farms.[535] Producer accuracy in diagnosing causes of mortality was examined by Sivula and colleagues.[533] Producers were found to be moderately accurate, but often listed the cause of death as unknown. This emphasizes the importance of laboratory confirmation of mortality over producer diagnosis.

Shipping Fever. Despite the undisputed economic importance of the disease, surprisingly little has been established regarding the behavior of pneumonic pasteurellosis or shipping fever at the population level, and even the question of whether the disease is truly contagious has yet to be answered from the epidemiologic perspective. Reviews of the literature from North American feedlot studies before 1985 found that published measures of morbidity in calves ranged from 0% to 69%, whereas measures of population mortality ranged from 0% to 15%. Incidence of disease was found to peak within 3 weeks of calves arriving at the feedlot. In view of the lack of uniformity in methods used to define cases of respiratory disease and calculate disease incidence, however, these data may not be reliable. In most of the studies, the crude measures of total morbidity and total mortality were used as outcomes, and case definitions for these were often highly variable or absent. This lack of uniformity with respect to case definition and nomenclature, along with the inherently subjective nature of morbidity assessment, makes it difficult to draw legitimate comparisons between reports. Recently one observational study specifically addressing epidemiology of fibrinous pneumonia (the classic lesion of shipping fever caused by *Mannheimia [Pasteurella] haemolytica*) was conducted by Ribble and colleagues.[536] Because of the difficulty and expense inherent in making definitive diagnoses of the causes of illness and death among feedlot

cattle, most epidemiologic studies have used crude mortality as an estimate of death losses caused by shipping fever, and treatment rate as a measure of respiratory morbidity. The results of several necropsy surveys and the previously cited epidemiologic study, however, indicate that crude mortality is unreliable as a surrogate measure of fibrinous pneumonia mortality and may lead to erroneous conclusions regarding risk factors contributing to this important disease.

In the observational study of fatal fibrinous pneumonia conducted by Ribble and colleagues in 1995,[536] risk factors specifically associated with shipping fever mortality in western Canadian feedlot calves were investigated. Data were collected on all 58,885 spring-born calves entering a single feedlot in southwestern Alberta between September 1 and December 31 over a 4-year period (1985-1988). The vast majority of calves were purchased from auction marts throughout western Canada and transported to the feedlot by truck. A complete necropsy was performed on all dead cattle within 24 hours of death, and a gross diagnosis recorded. Cases were assigned a diagnosis of fatal fibrinous pneumonia on the basis of pathologic evidence of acute fulminating lobar bronchopneumonia with fibrinous exudate, and data from each year were analyzed separately. Crude mortality ranged from 2.44% to 4.78%, whereas the mortality caused specifically by fibrinous pneumonia varied more than tenfold (0.25% to 2.73%) between years. Proportionate mortality caused by fibrinous pneumonia ranged from 10% to 57%, and this large annual variation was interpreted as evidence that crude mortality should not be used as a measure of fibrinous pneumonia mortality in epidemiologic studies. Epidemic curves constructed for each of the 4 years showed that peak mortality occurred approximately 16 days after arrival at the feedlot, and that at least 50% of fibrinous pneumonia mortalities occurred within 3 weeks of arrival. Epidemic curves using the time of first treatment for all cases that eventually died of fibrinous pneumonia revealed that peak fatal disease onset occurred within 8 days of arrival, and that 75% of fibrinous pneumonia mortalities were already sick within 2 weeks of arrival. The consistent onset of fatal disease in calves within days of their arrival at the feedlot indicates that the disease process may have been well underway in affected calves before their installation in a home pen, and that preventive measures should be implemented at the time of arrival, or possibly even before. In one of the study's most important findings Ribble and colleagues[536] demonstrated that, when the incidence of fatal shipping fever was high (greater than 2%), the disease clustered within truckload groups of calves and also, in 1 year, within pens. This was contrary to the conclusions of other studies, and lends credence to anecdotal reports from feedlot owners that shipping fever mortality is not randomly distributed in calves throughout the feedlot, but may often be abnormally high in individual truckloads or pens, indicating a contagious nature to the disease.

It may be argued that *Haemophilus somnus* should not be discussed under the epidemiology of fatal fibrinous pneumonia or shipping fever. This argument is based on the fact that *H. somnus* is not commonly isolated from pneumonic lungs with fibrinous pneumonia. In addition, epidemic curves evaluating the day of first treatment of calves ultimately dying of disease caused by *H. somnus* are distinct from epidemic curves of cattle dying of fibrinous pneumonia caused by *M. haemolytica*. The median days after arrival for the onset of fatal disease caused by *H. somnus* is 28 days as opposed to 8 days after arrival for fatal fibrinous pneumonia.[536-538]

Host and Environmental Risk Factors of Enzootic Pneumonia of Dairy and Veal Calves

The documented host and environmental risk factors of dairy and veal calf bronchopneumonia involve inadequate passive transfer of immunoglobulins, nutritional deficiencies, and adverse environmental conditions (Fig. 29-31). Calves are generally affected at less than 2 months of age. Successful passive transfer is the foundation of protection against pneumonia at this age and older and is effective except in situations where the other risk factors are so severe that even calves with high concentrations of passively acquired immunoglobulins are at high risk. Successful passive transfer requires good-quality colostrum (first milk or tested by colostrometer) and adequate volume (4 L in the first 12 hours for 45-kg calves). In addition, regular herd vaccination, especially in dry cows, should increase the levels of specific antibody in calves provided passive transfer is accomplished. Vaccination of calves after colostral immunity has declined or with intranasal vaccines in the face of passive immunity may produce a protective immune response in calves that prevents or limits the severity of ECP from certain infectious agents.

Nutritional problems that predispose to calf pneumonia include deficiencies of energy, protein, vitamins, or the minerals necessary for the immune response. Deficiencies of copper, selenium, zinc, manganese, iron, and vitamins A and E are of special concern. Dairy managers sometimes create energy and protein deficiencies by feeding calves a low volume of milk during the first few weeks of life to minimize the incidence of neonatal diarrhea.

The calf's immediate environment affects the calf in a number of ways. Ambient temperature is an important factor affecting dairy calf health.[539] Cold weather is especially detrimental to young calves, which have little body insulation. Increased humidity or precipitation in the calf's environment worsens the calf's ability to maintain thermal neutrality. Warm weather can also be undesirable, because young calves are capable of greater perspiration per pound of body weight than adults, and warm weather may predispose young calves to dehydration.[539]

The bacterial content of air in cattle barns can be as high as 10^6 organisms per cubic meter.[540] Disease incidence can be affected by length of pathogen survival time as an aerosol and the concentration of the pathogen in the air space. Humidity is an important limiting factor affecting pathogen survival. The optimum zone for limiting survival time of bovine pathogens is 55% to 75% relative humidity. Adequate fresh airflow into the calf's environment is important in limiting humidity and reducing the concentration of noxious gases and pathogens. The flow of air should be from younger, more susceptible cattle to older, less susceptible cattle to limit moving pathogens from older cattle to younger cattle. Adequate fresh airflow and proper directional movement of air are important goals of ventilation.

Calf housing with overcrowding of calves or excessive stocking densities results in increased transmission of pathogens, especially if there is mixing of age-groups. Overcrowding also puts additional stress on the building ventilation through build-up of noxious gases and pathogens. Cleaning of calf crates with high-pressure water sprayers is associated with new cases of pneumonia several days later. Bates and Anderson[541] have recommended standards for ventilation, including building location, fan capacity and location, intake location and design, temperature regulation, air space needed and airflow directions, and acceptable humidity levels. Individual calf hutches that are properly located provide the calf with adequate fresh air free of pathogens and noxious gases and overcome many of the problems found with calf barns. Calves moved out of hutches can then be put into small

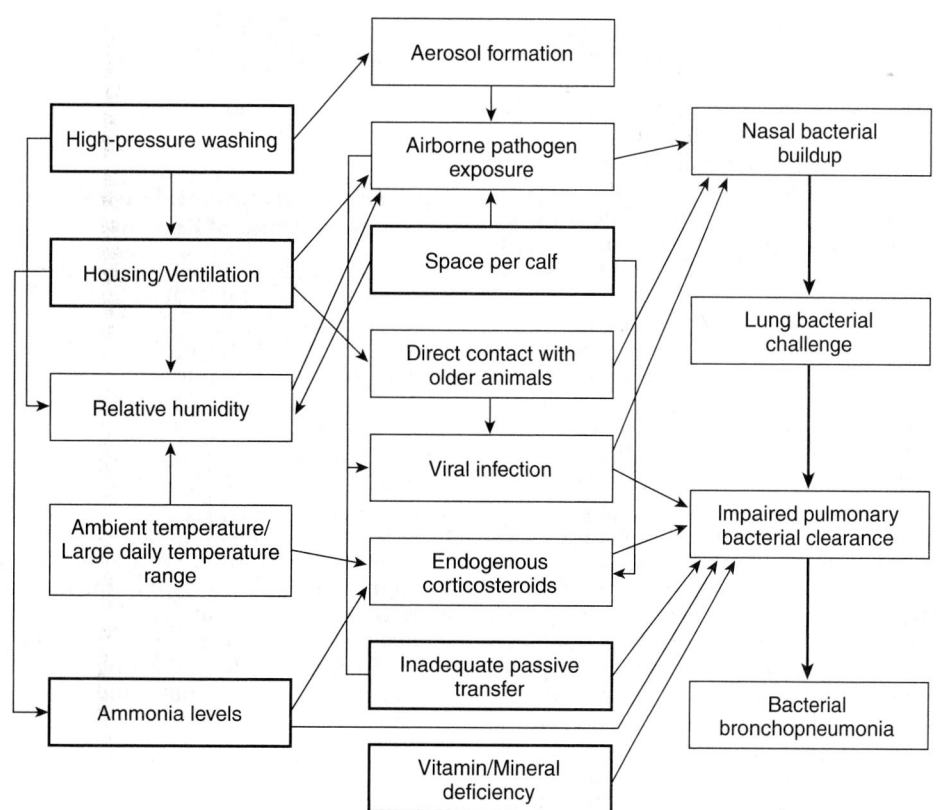

FIG. 29-31 ▮▮ Path model for risk factors for enzootic calf pneumonia. NOTE: Risk factors in bold-faced rectangles indicate those that may be altered by management.

TABLE 29-6

Standards for Adequacy of Ventilation of Calf Housing[533,541]

Housing Type	Ventilation Standards
Calf hutch	■ One calf per hutch ■ Minimum of 4 ft between hutches ■ Hutches further than 50 ft from exhaust outlets of other buildings ■ Hutches 10 ft from fenced enclosure with older cattle
Mechanically ventilated calf barn	■ 200 ft³ of air space per calf ■ Barrier walls to separate age-groups of cattle housed in building ■ Fan capacity to achieve 4 air changes per hour in winter, 15 air changes per hour in spring and fall, and 40 air changes per hour in summer ■ Humidity levels between 50% and 80% ■ Ammonia levels less than 10 ppm ■ Intake velocity for fresh air intakes of 200 to 800 feet/sec
Naturally ventilated calf housing	■ Adjustable opening on sidewalls ■ Open ridge for dual slope (2 inches/10 feet of building width) ■ Eve opening for monoslope buildings (2 inches/10 feet of width) ■ Barrier walls between age-groups (especially first postweaning age-group and older animals) ■ Separate waterer for first postweaning age-group

groups (7 or 8 calves) separated from older cattle using super hutches. Like the calf hutch the super hutch also serves to limit pathogen transmission and build-up of noxious gases in this susceptible group of calves. Alternatively, calves can be moved out of hutches and placed in pens in pole sheds provided groups are small (7 to 10 calves), air quality is good, and proper segregation from older age-groups is maintained. Standards of housing for calves are shown in Table 29-6.

Sivula and colleagues[533] found that 80% of calf barns provided housing that failed to meet adequate standards of ventilation and housing[541] regardless of whether calves were housed individually or in groups. In addition, calf housing where calves shared the same air space as adults never met the adequate standards of ventilation and housing.[533] A much higher percentage of calf housing that used calf hutches met these adequate standards of ventilation and housing, and virtually 100% would have been adequate housing if the hutches had been positioned correctly.[533] Calves raised in inadequate housing have significantly poorer growth rates than do calves raised in housing that is considered adequate,[533] which emphasizes the importance of adequate housing. The percentage of producers who use calf hutches continues to increase, as the benefits of their use are documented and published.

Veal calves are at greatest risk because they are reared in rooms that are filled to high stocking density with calves from multiple dairies that put minimal effort into ensuring that the calves are fed adequate amounts of high-quality colostrum.

The respiratory defenses of the calf lung include aerodynamic filtration, particle removal, adhesion resistance, secretory defenses, and cellular defenses. The physical respiratory defenses (filtration, removal, adhesion resistance) can be compromised by inhaled noxious gases, temperature extremes, dehydration, and viral infections causing impairment through damage to the mucosal lining of the upper respiratory tract, or by increased viscosity of respiratory secretions. Noxious gases, such as ammonia, methane, hydrogen sulfide, or carbon dioxide, which become increased from inadequate manure handling or poor ventilation, can also impair secretory defenses via damage to the mucosal lining and impair cellular defenses by direct effect on alveolar macrophages. Viral infection may also damage the mucosal lining and impair production of secretory defenses, such as lysozymes, lactoferrin, complement, or secretory immunoglobulin. Viral infections can also have a direct effect on cellular defenses, including alveolar macrophages, and for some viruses, the neutrophils. Stress caused by overcrowding, temperature ex-

tremes, commingling, surgical procedures, or vaccination may impair cellular defenses and immunoglobulin production and enhance bacterial adherence.

Calves that have neonatal diarrhea are at greater risk of pneumonia.[542] Thus risk factors that are unique to neonatal diarrhea, such as poor sanitation in the calving area, must be added to those outlined in Fig. 29-31 as possible risk factors of dairy calf bronchopneumonia. Calves born in loose housing have a higher risk of illness than those that are born in individual maternity pens. Treatments at birth can affect subsequent calf health. All dairy calves must have the navel treated with strong iodine. Injections of vitamin A and iron at birth may increase the disease resistance of dairy calves, which can be deficient in these nutrients at birth.

Other risk factors associated with enzootic calf pneumonia include large herd size, weather extremes (hot and cold), birth to a heifer, and low antibody titers to certain respiratory pathogens.[529,534]

Host and Environmental Risk Factors of Shipping Fever Pneumonia of Feedlot Calves

Risk factors of feedlot calf bronchopneumonia are active in three areas: (1) at the farm of origin, (2) during transit, and (3) in the feedlot[543-545] (Fig. 29-32).

Several on-farm management practices have a large impact on feedlot cattle pneumonia. Weaning, creep feeding, and performance of routine surgeries at least 3 weeks before shipment have been shown to reduce morbidity rate 20% to 25%.[546] Vaccination on the farm against respiratory pathogens would be expected to reduce the incidence of feedlot cattle pneumonia but has not always been beneficial. Other farm factors are deficiencies of nutrients necessary for normal immune responses. Pneumonia has a higher incidence in young calves, and severe outbreaks sometimes occur in early-weaned calves that enter feedlots.

Risk factors that are active during transport from the farm to the feedlot include sale through auctions, feeding of low-energy diets before shipping, and prolonged time in market channels (sales barns, transport vehicles). Excessive dehydration or "shrink" from transport has been shown to account for significant morbidity and mortality in the feedlot. Movement through multiple auctions greatly increases the risk of pneumonia.

Feedlot risk factors that influence morbidity and mortality rates include processing procedures, numbers of calves and number of different origins of calves per pen, diet, on-arrival

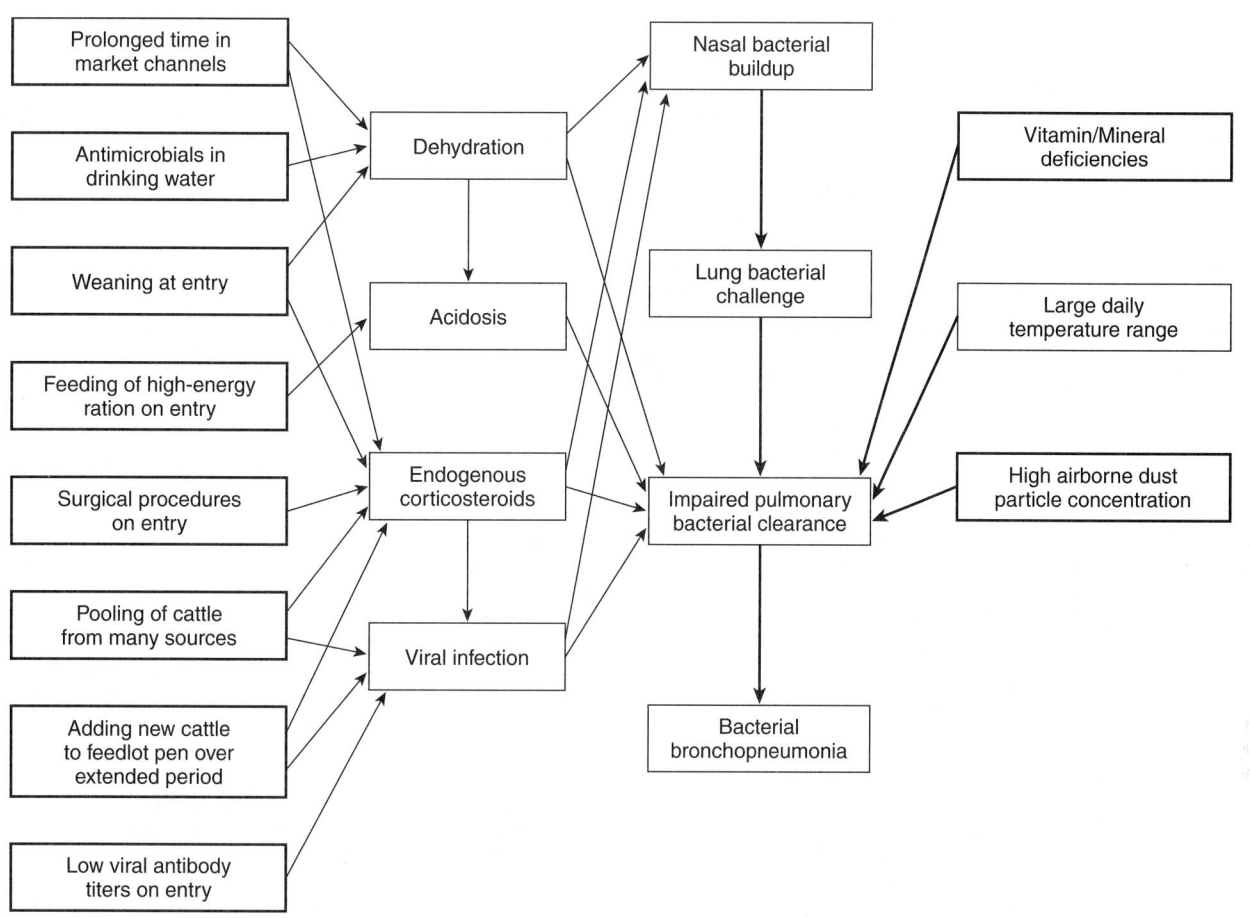

FIG. 29-32 ▨ Path model for risk factors of feedlot cattle pneumonia. NOTE: Risk factors in bold-faced rectangles indicate those that may be altered by management.

surgeries (i.e., dehorning), and environmental conditions. Calves that arrive in the feedlot with moderate levels of antibodies against the respiratory viruses have been shown to have a decreased incidence of pneumonia, indicating that natural exposure or vaccination at the ranch, rather than the feedlot, is protective. Mixing of calves from different origins and filling of feedlot pens with calves over a prolonged period increase mortality and morbidity rates because infectious agents spread more readily in large populations. Starting calves on diets containing 75% concentrate or greater or feeding corn silage as a major dietary component during the first month is associated with higher mortality and morbidity rates, probably because of an inhibition of alveolar macrophage function caused by acidosis. Nonprotein nitrogen, such as urea, fed to stocker calves at any time or to feedlot calves on arrival is associated with increased levels of pneumonia. The addition of antibiotics to the drinking water of newly arrived feedlot cattle has been shown to be detrimental to their health, possibly because of decreased water consumption.

Environmental conditions that tend to result in an increased incidence of pneumonia in feedlot cattle include fluctuations in daily temperature and increased concentrations of dust particles small enough to be inhaled into the alveoli.[544]

Pneumonia of beef calves on the farm has the greatest incidence after weaning. The occasional outbreaks of pneumonia in suckling beef calves are likely to be associated with adverse weather, parasitism, or nutritional deficiencies.

As mentioned in the previous discussion regarding respiratory defenses of dairy calves, endogenous corticosteroid release caused by physical stressors (overcrowding, mixing of calves, surgical procedures, starvation, dehydration), environmental

stressors (weather extremes), and damage to respiratory defenses (vehicle exhaust, environmental dust, noxious fumes, acidosis, dehydration, and viral infections) may also weaken or overwhelm the respiratory defenses of feedlot calves.

Host and Environmental Risk Factors of Bronchopneumonia of Sheep and Gaots

Many of the risk factors that have been found to predispose to bronchopneumonias of sheep and goats are similar to those affecting cattle.[547] Pneumonia is more common in younger animals, after shipping or storms, and under crowded conditions. In addition, cold stress is an important risk factor of pneumonia in young lambs and recently shorn adult sheep and goats. In contrast, heat stress may predispose to pneumonia in unshorn sheep that do not have access to shade. Pneumonia also is associated with semiconfinement or total confinement of sheep in poorly ventilated barns.

Infectious Agents Associated With the Respiratory Complex of Cattle, Sheep, and Goats

Numerous infectious agents, usually in combination, have been isolated from cases of bronchopneumonia (see Boxes 29-1 and 29-2) and are necessary components of its multifactorial causation.

Viral Agents

Respiratory viruses usually act in combination with other infectious agents, in particular bacteria, in the production of respiratory disease. The viruses associated with respiratory diseases of ruminants are listed in Box 29-2. They are not of equal importance to agents of respiratory disease and the importance of some is not well known. Currently, commercially produced vaccines are available only for bovine herpesvirus 1 (BHV-1), bovine virus diarrhea virus (BVDV), parainfluenza virus type 3 (PI-3), and bovine respiratory syncytial virus (BRSV). These viruses are generally thought to be the most important causes of viral respiratory disease in cattle. Although this may be true, it does not exclude the possibility that other viruses are of equal or greater importance in this disease complex. For example, there is an increasing accumulation of evidence that bovine coronavirus may have a more important role in bovine respiratory disease than previously recognized.

In addition, several retroviruses can cause progressive pneumonia in sheep and goats. These viral-caused progressive pneumonias include ovine progressive pneumonia (maedi-visna) and ovine pulmonary carcinoma (adenomatosis, jaagziekte) in sheep. Progressive pneumonia may be associated with caprine arthritis encephalitis (CAE) virus infections in adult goats. This section deals only with acute viral respiratory disease in sheep and goats; the progressive pneumonias are discussed later in this chapter.

Bovine Herpesvirus Type 1 (Infectious Bovine Rhinotracheitis Virus)

DEFINITION AND ETIOLOGY. Bovine herpesvirus 1 (BHV-1) is a deoxyribonucleic acid (DNA) virus that is classified as an α-herpesvirus. It is associated with multiple, distinct disease syndromes of cattle that include infectious bovine rhinotracheitis (IBR), conjunctivitis (see Chapter 37), infectious pustular vulvovaginitis (IPV), balanoposthitis, abortion (see Chapter 41), encephalomyelitis (see Chapter 33), and mastitis.[548,549] Although only a single serotype of BHV-1 is recognized, three types have been identified on the basis of restriction endonuclease cleavage patterns. These three types are referred to as BHV-1.1 (respiratory infections), BHV-1.2 (respiratory and genital infections), and BHV-1.3 (neurologic infections). BHV-1.3 has been reclassified as a distinct herpesvirus and is designated as bovine herpesvirus type 5.[550] Only the respiratory manifestations of infection with BHV-1 are discussed here. The respiratory form is characterized by rhinitis, tracheitis, and pyrexia, and is referred to as IBR.

CLINICAL SIGNS. Clinical signs vary and range from mild to severe, depending on the presence of secondary bacterial pneumonia. Genetic factors also appear to be an important determinant of the severity of BHV-1 infection, specifically the type-I interferon genotype.[551] Clinical signs include pyrexia, anorexia, dramatic drop in milk production in dairy cattle, increased respiratory rate, a slight degree of hyperexcitability, ptyalism, coughing, and nasal discharge that progresses from serous to mucopurulent. BHV-1 infection can predispose to the development of secondary bacterial pneumonia. Dyspnea characterized by open-mouth breathing may appear if the larynx or trachea becomes partially blocked with mucopurulent material. Auscultation of the lungs reveals increased breath sounds and referred tracheal sounds. Severe hyperemia and reddening of the muzzle led to the common name of "red nose." Pustules may develop on the nasal mucosa and later form diphtheritic plaques. Conjunctivitis with excessive ocular discharge may be present. Conjunctivitis with corneal opacity can also occur as the principal manifestation of BHV-1 infection and may be misdiagnosed as infectious bovine keratoconjunctivitis (pinkeye). Abortions may occur concurrently with respiratory disease, but they can also occur as late as 100 days after infection.[548,549] Abortions may also occur in cattle that escape serious respiratory disease.

On rare occasions, neonatal calves may suffer from both an acute respiratory and a systemic form of BHV-1 infection. The infection is characterized by rhinitis, marked lacrimation, inflammation and necrosis of the soft palate, laryngotracheitis, and ulceration of the gastrointestinal tract.[549]

EPIDEMIOLOGY. Studies of antibody prevalence to BHV-1 indicate that infection is widely distributed in the cattle population.[548,549] Infections of the respiratory tract by BHV-1 are prevalent when large concentrations of beef or dairy cattle are assembled, although BHV-1 does not appear to have an important role in enzootic pneumonia of dairy calves. Feedlot cattle appear to have higher attack rates, more severe disease, and higher case fatality rates than do range or dairy cattle. This is likely because of the stressful conditions experienced by feeder calves at the time of entry into feedlots. Entry into feedlots may also coincide with decline of passive immunity. The case fatality rate is generally low unless complicated with secondary bacterial pneumonia. The route of infection is aerosol and adult cattle are thought to be the principal reservoirs of infection.[548,549] The fact that BHV-1 is capable of establishing latent infections in neural tissue is undoubtedly important in its epidemiologic characteristics. Under periods of stress, latent infections can become reactivated, resulting in viral shedding. Modified-live BHV-1 vaccines are also capable of causing latent infections.[548,549]

NECROPSY FINDINGS. Infectious bovine rhinotracheitis is rarely fatal in mature cattle unless it occurs during periods of severe stress or is complicated by secondary bacterial infection of the lung. Postmortem examination may reveal congestion of the tracheal mucosa with petechial and ecchymotic hemorrhages and severe bronchopneumonia. Usually the inflammatory lesions induced by BHV-1 do not extend into airways contained within the lung. Pustular lesions (sometimes referred to as plaques) may be observed. Although they are not pathognomonic, observation of these pustular lesions that coalesce to form adherent necrotic lesions on respiratory, ocular, and reproductive mucosa may be helpful in diagnosis. Conjunctivitis may be present. Although intranuclear inclusion bodies are a feature of herpesvirus infections, they are not a common histologic feature of BHV-1.

Herpesviruses in Sheep and Goats

Herpesviruses have been isolated from sheep and goats. It remains undetermined whether herpesviruses have a role, and if so, to what extent, in respiratory disease of small ruminants.

Bovine Virus Diarrhea Virus

BVDV is a ribonucleic acid (RNA) virus and is a member of the genus *Pestivirus* in the family Flaviviridae.[552] A wide spectrum of disease has been associated with BVDV infection, including subclinical infection, bovine viral diarrhea/mucosal disease (see Chapter 30), immunosuppression, repeat breeding problems, abortion, and fetal mummification (see Chapter 41), congenital defects, immunotolerance, and persistent infections. Only the contribution of this virus to respiratory disease is discussed here.

The role of BVDV in the bovine respiratory disease complex is controversial and this topic has recently been reviewed.[553,554] Because of the immunosuppressive effects of BVDV infection, it is likely that this virus is an important respiratory pathogen in cattle. It is a frequent isolate in cattle affected with shipping fever pneumonia, most often in association with *Mannheimia (Pasteurella) haemolytica*. Synergistic interactions between BVDV and *M. haemolytica*,[555] BHV-1,[556] and BRSV[557] have been demonstrated. Epidemiologic studies that investigated the role of BVDV in respiratory disease outbreaks have had equivocal results, with some studies implicating and other studies show-

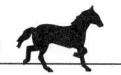

ing no role for BVDV.[554] It was reported to be the virus most frequently associated with multiple viral infection of the respiratory tract of calves.[558] Thus the suggested role of BVDV in respiratory tract disease of cattle appears to be that of a viral agent capable of inducing immunosuppression, which allows secondary infections by opportunistic microorganisms.

Respiratory Syncytial Viruses of Cattle, Sheep, and Goats

DEFINITION AND ETIOLOGY. Bovine respiratory syncytial virus (BRSV) has been recognized as an important pathogen involved in bovine respiratory disease. It is classified as a nonhemagglutinating pneumovirus of the paramyxovirus family. This virus was named for the characteristic cytopathic effect it produces in vitro and in vivo, which is the formation of syncytial cells. BRSV shares many similarities in its biology and epidemiology with the human respiratory syncytial virus (HRSV). HRSV is considered to be the most important respiratory tract pathogen of infancy and early childhood. Although BRSV and HRSV are closely related, they appear to be distinct viruses.[559] An ovine and a caprine respiratory syncytial virus have been described. Studies using RNAse mismatch cleavage analysis indicate that ovine RSV may be distinct from HRSV and BRSV, whereas caprine RSV may be more closely related to BRSV.[560,561] Recently the existence of antigenic subtypes has been demonstrated for the HRSV. It is not known whether antigenic subtypes exist for BRSV, but there are preliminary findings that suggest this possibility.[562,563] Definition of antigenic variation in BRSV will be important to future vaccine development. The topic of BRSV has recently been reviewed.[559]

CLINICAL SIGNS. In feeder-age calves, respiratory signs predominate in BRSV infections, including elevated body temperature of 40° C to 42.2° C (104° F to 108° F), depression, decreased feed intake, elevated respiratory rates, ptyalism, cough, and nasal and lacrimal discharges. Signs of disease may progress rapidly and early signs may be missed. There are increased bronchial and bronchovesicular sounds, and fine crackles may be heard that are consistent with the presence of emphysema in the lung. In later stages of the disease, dyspnea becomes pronounced and is characterized by mouth breathing. Subcutaneous emphysema and intermandibular edema are sometimes noted. Secondary bacterial pneumonia has been reported, but may not always be present. Dramatic reduction in milk production has been reported in dairy cattle. Duration of disease is variable, lasting 1 to 2 weeks. A biphasic clinical course has been described but does not appear to be a consistent finding. In dairy calves, signs similar to those described may be present at the onset, followed by rapid progression of the disease.

EPIDEMIOLOGY. Prevalence of antibodies to BRSV in the cattle population of the United States ranges from approximately 60% to 80%.[564] The virus has been recognized in association with respiratory tract disease in nursing beef calves, in feeder-age calves on introduction to feedlots, and in dairy calves. Bovine respiratory syncytial virus was demonstrated to be involved in 14.4% of respiratory infections on a large farm in England, 32.2% of the outbreaks of calf pneumonia in Northern Ireland, 71.4% of the outbreaks of calf pneumonia in Minnesota, and 53% of fall respiratory outbreaks in Belgium.[565] Seroconversion to BRSV has been reported to be significantly associated with treatment for respiratory disease. Bovine respiratory syncytial virus represents a very important virus in the bovine respiratory disease complex on the basis of its frequency of occurrence and predilection for causing infection of the lower respiratory tract. Bovine respiratory syncytial virus infections associated with respiratory disease predominantly occur in young animals but are capable of causing disease in adult cattle, although the occurrence is

sporadic. Subclinical infections with BRSV have been documented. In general, morbidity rate tends to be high in outbreaks of BRSV, whereas case fatality rate is variable, ranging from none to as high as 20%. Observations from experimental infection studies and natural outbreaks indicate that passively derived antibody does not prevent BRSV infections in calves but does modify the severity of the disease.[566,567]

The means of transmission appears to be contact with infected cattle and aerosols. The incubation period is 3 to 5 days. Cattle are most likely the principal reservoirs of infection, although the mechanism by which the virus persists in the cattle population is not known. Possibly a similar epidemiologic pattern to the one that has been described for human respiratory syncytial virus (HRSV) also exists for BRSV. HRSV is capable of reinfecting the host throughout his or her life; however, severe lower respiratory tract disease only occurs in association with the initial exposure. Subsequent exposure results in mild upper respiratory tract disease. Similarly, adult cattle may periodically undergo subclinical to mild infections and serve as a source of infection for susceptible young stock. However, a recent study concluded that transmission among seropositive cattle was not a plausible mechanism of BRSV persistence in a dairy herd.[568] It has been proposed that a persistent BRSV infection in individuals is a more plausible explanation of population persistence of BRSV, although a persistent or chronic infection with BRSV has never been demonstrated.

NECROPSY FINDINGS. Bovine respiratory syncytial virus infections have been demonstrated to be significantly associated with pulmonary lesions described as atypical interstitial pneumonia.[569] Gross examination of the respiratory tract reveals a diffuse interstitial pneumonia with the presence of subpleural and interstitial emphysema and interstitial edema. Emphysematous bullae may be present between lung lobules. At necropsy, pulmonary emphysema often prevents the lungs from collapsing when the thoracic cavity is opened. The gross lesions are similar to and must be differentiated from other causes of atypical interstitial pneumonia (see later discussion). Histopathologic findings depend on the stage of disease at the time of death but may reveal syncytial cells in bronchiolar epithelium and throughout the lung parenchyma. Intracytoplasmic inclusion bodies, proliferation or degeneration of bronchiolar epithelium, alveolar epithelialization, edema, and hyaline membrane formation are commonly observed.

RESPIRATORY SYNCYTIAL VIRUSES IN SMALL RUMINANTS. Respiratory syncytial virus (RSV) has been isolated from sheep and goats with respiratory disease. The possibility of interspecies transmission has not been defined. Experimental infections of lambs with ovine RSV caused a mild primary pneumonia and were also capable of causing lower respiratory tract lesions in calves and deer.[570] Experimentally a synergistic relationship between RSV and *Mannheimia (Pasteurella) haemolytica* has been demonstrated in lambs.[547] It is difficult to draw firm conclusions on the importance of this agent in small ruminants because further epidemiologic studies need to be conducted.

Parainfluenza Virus Type 3 of Cattle, Sheep, and Goats

DEFINITION AND ETIOLOGY. Parainfluenza virus type 3 (PI-3) is a ribonucleic acid (RNA) virus classified in the paramyxovirus family. It hemagglutinates and hemadsorbs red blood cells of certain species. Variation in virulence between strains of PI-3 has been reported. This topic has recently been reviewed.[571]

CLINICAL SIGNS. Uncomplicated PI-3 infections result in subclinical to mild signs. Clinical signs include fever, cough, nasal and ocular discharge, increased respiratory rate, and increased breath sounds. The most important role of PI-3 is in predisposing the respiratory tract to subsequent infection by other viruses and bacteria such as *Mannheimia (Pasteurella) haemolytica.*[549] Severity of signs increases with the development of secondary bacterial pneumonia, and, if death occurs, it is usually the result of secondary bacterial infection. PI-3 infection is widespread in sheep and probably in goats.[547] Only one serotype of ovine PI-3 has been identified, and it is related to, but distinct from, the bovine strain. Most infections are inapparent to mild.

EPIDEMIOLOGY. The widespread prevalence of antibodies to this virus indicates that it is ubiquitous in the cattle population. This finding suggests the possibility of repeat infections or at least the persistence of antibodies after infection. In calves, passively derived immunity wanes at approximately 2 months of age. Inapparent or subclinical infections with PI-3 are common; however, if environmental and managerial practices are suboptimal, PI-3 may become an important initiator of respiratory tract disease. PI-3 infection appears to have its greatest impact on weaned beef calves after introduction to feedlots and on housed dairy calves. Infection appears to spread rapidly in susceptible cattle housed at high population densities and in close contact. Although PI-3 is capable of damaging the epithelial mucosa of the respiratory tract, uncomplicated infection results in subclinical or mild signs of respiratory tract disease.

NECROPSY FINDINGS. Lesions of PI-3 infection alone are rarely seen during postmortem examination. Experimental PI-3 infection results in congestion of the respiratory mucosa, swelling of lymph nodes associated with the respiratory tract, and mild pneumonitis.[549] Bronchiolitis and peribronchiolitis are seen histologically with both proliferative and degenerative changes in the epithelial cells of the bronchioles and alveoli. Intranuclear and intracytoplasmic inclusion bodies may be seen. In many respects, pathologic features of PI-3 infection are similar to those caused by BRSV, although the lesions produced by the latter are generally more extensive.

Malignant Catarrhal Fever Virus

The African (wildebeest-associated) form of malignant catarrhal fever (MCF) is caused by alcelaphine herpesvirus types 1 and 2. A causative agent for the American (sheep-associated) form is believed to be ovine herpesvirus type 2. The occurrence of MCF in the cattle population is sporadic. There is multisystemic involvement, including involvement of the respiratory tract. MCF is discussed in detail in Chapter 30.

Bovine Herpesvirus Type 4

The bovine type 4 herpesviruses are serologically distinct from other herpes viruses such as BHV-1 and BHV-2 (bovine mammillitis).[549] Although the level of antibody prevalence to bovine herpesvirus type 4 (BHV-4) is high in the cattle population of the United States, the pathogenic role of this virus remains unclear. It has been implicated in several disease conditions of cattle, including respiratory tract disease, reproductive disorders (abortions and metritis), mammillitis, and enteric disease.[572] It has also been isolated from apparently healthy cattle. Several of these viruses (DN-599, Movar 33/36, FTC-2) have been isolated from cattle with respiratory tract disease. Intranasal inoculation of DN-599 into calves produced respiratory disease, but the importance of this group of viruses in the bovine respiratory disease complex is poorly defined. Currently they are not thought to be important enough to warrant vaccine development.

Adenoviruses of Cattle, Sheep, and Goats

Adenoviruses are DNA viruses; 10 serotypes of bovine adenovirus (BAV) are currently recognized.[573] BAV infection is widespread and is frequently subclinical. BAV is often isolated in association with other viruses and bacteria. It appears to be associated with a wide spectrum of diseases, including pneumonia, enteritis, pneumoenteritis, conjunctivitis, keratoconjunctivitis, weak calf syndrome, and abortion.[549] BAV serotype 3 is most often associated with respiratory infection. Although most infections are subclinical, signs of both upper and lower respiratory tract disease and concurrent enteritis may be present.

Six antigenic types of ovine adenovirus and two types of caprine adenovirus have been identified.[574] Little information concerning the incidence and distribution of adenovirus infection in the sheep and goat population is available; however, it appears likely that this virus causes widespread infection. A study in Iowa reported that adenovirus infections were widespread in the sheep population and that the prevalence of active infection based on seroconversion rates was approximately 45%.[575] The majority of isolations of this virus have been from young lambs, and it has been isolated in association with respiratory and enteric disease. Experimental infections result in mild disease with anorexia, pyrexia, increased respiratory rates, coughing, and diarrhea. Gross lesions observed include atelectasis, edema, and consolidation of the lungs.[576] Ovine adenovirus serotype 6 has been shown under experimental conditions to act synergistically with *Mannheimia (Pasteurella) haemolytica* in the production of pneumonia in lambs.[577]

Bovine Coronavirus

Bovine coronavirus is a major cause of calf diarrhea and has also been implicated as a cause of winter dysentery in cattle. Although it has been known for some time that bovine coronavirus can infect the respiratory tract of calves,[578] there is evidence accumulating that bovine coronavirus may have a more important role in the bovine respiratory disease complex than previously thought. One reason for the lack of awareness is that standard cell lines used for virus isolation may not be permissive to all isolates of bovine respiratory coronavirus. The bovine respiratory coronavirus can readily be recovered by using human rectal tumor-18G cell lines.[579] A high rate of coronavirus recovery by virus isolation has been reported from feeder calves with signs of respiratory disease on arrival at feedlots. A Canadian-based study in feeder calves did not clearly define a role for bovine coronavirus in respiratory disease.[580] The importance of respiratory coronaviruses in the bovine respiratory disease complex still requires further definition.

Bovine Rhinovirus

Bovine rhinovirus is a RNA virus classified in the picornavirus family. Two serotypes of bovine rhinovirus are officially recognized.[549] Infection with this virus appears to be widespread in the cattle population. By 10 to 12 months of age virtually 100% of beef and dairy cattle in Missouri are seropositive to rhinovirus.[581] Clinical signs of rhinovirus infections range from inapparent signs to fever, depression, decreased appetite, increased respiratory rate, lacrimation, conjunctivitis, salivation, coughing, and nasal discharge.

Bovine Reovirus

Bovine reovirus is an RNA virus classified in the reovirus family. Three mammalian serotypes are recognized. Reoviruses have been isolated from the respiratory and digestive tracts of apparently healthy cattle. Infections appear to be common in cattle, and bovine isolates are antigenically identical to human serotypes. The importance of reovirus infections in bovine respiratory tract disease is unclear. Subclinical infections appear to predominate under field conditions.

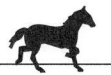

Bovine Enterovirus

Enteroviruses are small RNA viruses belonging to the picornavirus family. Over 60 strains of bovine enterovirus have been isolated from the respiratory, reproductive, and digestive tracts of cattle. The majority of these isolates have been obtained from healthy animals, although isolations have been made from cattle in association with abortions, enteritis, and respiratory disease. In general, infections with enteroviruses are common and transient and usually not considered to be pathogenic.

Calicivirus

A calicivirus has been isolated from dairy calves from a herd with a persistent respiratory disease problem.[582] This virus caused only minimum disease in experimentally infected calves, but a persistent infection was produced.

Bacterial, Mycoplasmal, Ureaplasmal, and Chlamydial Agents

Mannheimia (Pasteurella) haemolytica serotype A1, one of 16 typeable serotypes in addition to a number of untypeable strains of *M. haemolytica* that have been identified in cattle, is the most common bacterium isolated of pneumonic lungs in cattle.[583] Although *M. haemolytica* is more commonly isolated from fibrinous necrotizing lobar pleuropneumonia of feedlot animals, *Pasteurella multocida* is more frequently isolated from the lungs of calves experiencing enzootic calf pneumonia (ECP) and is associated with a purulent bronchopneumonia. *M. haemolytica* and *Haemophilus somnus* are also isolated from lungs of calves with ECP. *H. somnus* is being isolated with increasing frequency from feedlot animals experiencing not only pneumonia but also pleuritis. Pulmonary abscesses often yield *Arcanobacterium (Actinomyces) pyogenes* and *Bacteroides melaninogenicus* and are considered opportunistic of existing lesions. Anaerobic bacteria are isolated from approximately one third of the lungs of cattle that die of bronchopneumonia.[584] They are opportunists that are inhaled with eructated rumen gases. Other bacteria are less frequently isolated from pneumonic bovine lungs (see Box 29-1).

Mycoplasmas are isolated, usually in combination with other pathogens, from 50% to 90% of beef and dairy cattle pneumonias.[585,586] The species of mycoplasmas (see Box 29-1) prevalent in North America are generally considered to be mild respiratory pathogens, mainly causing subclinical infections unless coupled with environmental stresses or infections by other pathogens.[587] Tracheal bronchial aspirates performed on dairy calves at random found that calves with both *Mycoplasma* spp. and *Pasteurella* spp. present in the aspirate were at significantly greater risk of developing ECP than calves with only one organism or no organisms. Mycoplasma known effects of immunosuppression[588] and inhibition of the mucociliary transport mechanism[589] suggest that they may play an important contributory role in the pathogenesis of bovine pneumonia.

Chlamydial agents are occasionally isolated from pneumonic ruminant lungs. These organisms are thought to produce only mild respiratory infections by themselves but may enhance the pathogenicity of concurrent infections. Experimental challenge of calves to a combination of chlamydia and *M. haemolytica* results in clinical disease more severe than either agent produces alone.[590]

Many of the bacterial agents that are associated with bovine bronchopneumonia have also been isolated from pneumonic lungs of sheep and goats. Twelve serotypes of *M. haemolytica* have been identified in sheep in the United States. Other bacteria, including *P. multocida*, *Haemophilus* spp., and *Salmonella* spp., have been associated with bronchopneumonia in sheep and goats. Experimental infections of lambs with PI-3 or adenovirus followed in several days by *M. haemolytica* cause severe pneumonia.[547,591] *Mycoplasma ovipneumonia* is often isolated from pneumonic lungs of sheep and goats, usually accompanied by *M. haemolytica*. On its own, *M. ovipneumonia* is capable of causing mild, subacute to chronic bronchiolitis or bronchopneumonia that probably predisposes to *M. haemolytica* infections.

PATHOPHYSIOLOGY. *M. haemolytica*, *P. multocida*, and *H. somnus* are normal inhabitants of the nasal pharyngeal mucosa,[592,593] but not the lung, and are considered "opportunistic pathogens." Calves and lambs become infected at an early age and carry pasteurella as a minor part of the upper respiratory tract flora. Only a small percentage of nasal swabs yields positive results for *M. haemolytica* serotype A1 in healthy, unstressed calves, but if several areas of the nasal mucosa are cultured at necropsy, it is often possible to isolate *M. haemolytica* from animals that previously had negative findings on nasal swabs.[594] The stress of transportation causes a breakdown of the defense mechanisms that hold the nasal mucosa infections in check, resulting in a rapid proliferation of virulent *M. haemolytica* serotype A1. A greater number of calves will yield positive nasal mucosa swab *M. haemolytica* results during and after transport, and there is a large increase in the numbers of *M. haemolytica* in positive samples. BHV-1 and PI-3 viruses have been shown to have the same effect as transportation on pasteurella populations of the nasal mucosa. *M. haemolytica* has been demonstrated in the tracheal air of stressed, healthy calves harboring the organism on their nasal mucosa. Some of these inhaled organisms are deposited deep within the lung and normally are cleared within hours. But under conditions of impaired pulmonary defenses caused by stress, nutritional deficiencies, or preexisting viral infection, *M. haemolytica* is able to proliferate rapidly within the lung and with the aid of its virulence factors and toxins produce a severe lobar necrotizing fibrinous pleuropneumonia.

Calves infected with respiratory viruses, including BHV-1, PI-3, BVDV, and BRSV, or *Mycoplasma* spp., have increased susceptibility to severe bronchopneumonia when exposed to *M. haemolytica*.[592] Once bacterial pathogens become established in the lungs, interactions between the bacteria and the host defenses result in tissue damage and elimination of the invaders. The capsules of *M. haemolytica*, *P. multocida*, and *H. somnus* contain a lipopolysaccharide (LPS) endotoxin that initiates the complement and coagulation cascades, recruits neutrophils, and activates neutrophils and alveolar macrophages. *M. haemolytica* also produces an exotoxin, called leukotoxin, that causes cytolysis of platelets, macrophages, and neutrophils.[595] This leukotoxin is also capable of activating macrophages to produce inflammatory cytokines, resulting in a massive influx of neutrophils, which is a key factor in lung tissue destruction.

Calves experimentally depleted of neutrophils are completely protected from gross and microscopic lesions of the severe fibrinonecrotic bronchopneumonia that is induced by intratracheal inoculation of *M. haemolytica* in calves with normal neutrophil levels.[596] Lysis of neutrophils results in the release of lysosomal products, including elastase, collagenase, and reactive oxygen intermediates. These chemicals are bactericidal, but also capable of destroying the neutrophils themselves and surrounding tissues. Neutrophil-mediated damage to the endothelial cells results in exudation and thrombosis, which produce the classic lesions of necrosis and fibrinous exudation.[597]

Little is known regarding the pathogenesis of *P. multocida*. Its prominent role in ECP and rather minor role in shipping fever would suggest that prolonged impairment of the respiratory defense mechanisms is necessary to establish this organism in the lungs in sufficient numbers to create bronchopneumonia. It is likely that the organism is chronically inhaled in small numbers into the lung of calves with persistent damage to the respiratory defenses from infectious agents such as mycoplasma, and environmental damage from inadequate housing and ventilation, allowing it to colonize and produce an expanding lesion. In addition to LPS, the organism also has a capsule that allows it to resist phagocytosis. This proposed pathogenesis agrees with the insidious onset that is commonly observed with ECP. It should be noted that culture of *P. multocida* from pneumonic lung does not exclude the possibility of other bacteria such as *M. haemolytica* being the primary pathogen, because *P. multocida* has been shown to overgrow *M. haemolytica* in challenge studies using large doses of pure cultures of *M. haemolytica*.[598]

H. somnus produces a complex of disease syndromes often called hemophilosis, which include reproductive, respiratory, and septicemic (meningoencephalitis polyarthritis, myocarditis, pleuritis, pericarditis) forms. The septicemic forms result from hematogenous spread from the respiratory tract, whereas respiratory infections occur from mechanisms similar to that already discussed with *M. haemolytica* and *P. multocida*. The organism is inhaled from the upper respiratory tract into the lungs and is able to replicate in part based on compromised respiratory defenses. This organism has been reported to produce a number of virulence factors in addition to LPS. These include soluble factors that resist phagocytic killing and toxic factors that produce cytotoxic changes in endothelial cells.[599,600] This latter toxic principle may be important in producing the thrombotic changes characteristic of this organism in certain disease states such as thrombotic meningoencephalitis.

CLINICAL SIGNS AND DIFFERENTIAL DIAGNOSIS. Clinical signs associated with specific viral infections of the respiratory tract have previously been presented. In general the clinical signs observed are dependent on the stage of the disease and particularly on whether secondary bacterial pneumonia has been superimposed. In the early stages of viral pneumonia common clinical features include mild depression and anorexia, often marked elevation in body temperature, serous to mucopurulent lacrimal and nasal discharges, cough, and elevated respiratory rates. On auscultation of the lungs there may be an increase in breath sounds. In the presence of secondary bacterial pneumonia, the severity of clinical signs becomes more pronounced. Ruminants affected by bronchopneumonia exhibit signs of respiratory tract inflammation and toxemia. In early stages, animals stand off by themselves and do not approach feed. They hold their heads and ears low, appear depressed, and move slowly. Respirations become rapid and shallow, there is frequent licking of the muzzle, and a moist cough is often present. In later stages, animals have a fever of 40° C to 41° C (104° F to 105.8° F) and they appear gaunt, have deep labored respirations, and may hold the head extended. Dyspnea is both inspiratory and expiratory. Ocular and nasal discharges progress from serous to mucopurulent. Normal lung sounds are difficult to hear except in calves, goats, and sheep. Sheep normally have harsh inspiratory sounds. The heavy chest wall of larger cattle makes it difficult to hear normal airway sounds. The first auscultable lung changes are increased harshness of inspiratory sounds while purulent material accumulates in the airways. By the time expiratory sounds are as loud as or louder than inspiratory sounds, severe bronchopneumonia exists. In the most severe cases, auscultation of the anterior ventral lung fields reveals crackles and wheezes and an increase in bronchial sounds, especially on inspiration. When ventral consolidation occurs, harsh tracheal breathing is still audible ventrally, but percussion reveals ventral dullness. Percussion is best accomplished on young calves and goats of any age. Recently shorn sheep can be readily percussed, but heavy wool makes percussion difficult. Animals in which a fibrinous pleuritis develops are reluctant to move because of pain, have shallow respirations, and sometimes have pleural friction rubs detectable by auscultation.

Nasal discharge, dyspnea, abnormal lung sounds, cough, and high fevers are cardinal signs of bronchopneumonia. Other respiratory tract conditions that must be considered as differential diagnoses include acute bovine pulmonary emphysema, interstitial pneumonia, pulmonary edema, pleuritis, laryngitis, tracheitis, and lungworms. Rare conditions include thoracic neoplasia and diaphragmatic hernia. Systemic conditions that result in respiratory signs include septicemia, heart failure, acid-base imbalances, and poisonings such as nitrate toxicity. An important feature that separates systemic conditions from bronchopneumonia is that, in addition to signs of pulmonary dysfunction, systemic conditions often are manifested by clinical signs of damage to other organ systems. In sheep and goats, ovine progressive pneumonia, caprine arthritis encephalitis, and lung or mediastinal abscesses caused by *Corynebacterium pseudotuberculosis* or other bacterial invaders are additional differentials.

CLINICAL PATHOLOGY. Complete blood counts or serum biochemical analyses are rarely of value in diagnosis of viral respiratory disease. Some viruses, such as BVDV, may cause leukopenia, but when bacterial pneumonia is superimposed the white blood cell count is most often in the high normal range to mildly elevated with a left shift. Specimens for cytologic evaluation can be obtained by transtracheal aspiration or bronchoalveolar lavage and with most bacterial and viral infections a high percentage of neutrophils is found. Thoracocentesis can be a useful diagnostic procedure with fluid accumulation in the thorax and shows elevated neutrophilia and high total protein if bacterial pleuropneumonia is the cause of fluid accumulation.

NECROPSY FINDINGS. Shipping fever pneumonia of calves is characterized pathologically as a fibrinopurulent bronchopneumonia. The infection is aerogenous; it begins in the bronchioles and extends through their walls into the surrounding parenchyma. The cranial ventral areas of affected lungs are swollen, red, firm, and heavy. The inflamed areas are sometimes covered with variable amounts of yellow fibrin and the pleural cavity may contain straw-colored fluid. The dorsal regions of the caudal lobes often are mottled by patches of inflammation and normal parenchyma. In up to one third of bronchopneumonia cases, forced respirations result in vesicular to bullous pockets of emphysema in the dorsal areas of the caudal lobe. These changes are common with BRSV infections, but can also occur with other viral infections. Some 60% to 80% of the lung tissue is usually involved in fatal cases of uncomplicated bacterial pneumonia. However, when other diseases such as BHV-1, BVD, salmonellosis, mycotic rumenitis, or traumatic pharyngitis occur concurrently, only 30% to 50% of the lung may be affected. Abscesses may appear by 3 weeks but are not encapsulated until at least 4 weeks. Bronchial lymph nodes are swollen, wet, and dark red.

Information concerning cause can be obtained by careful gross examination of pneumonic lungs. Large amounts of yellow fibrin may overlie affected areas, accompanied by a straw-colored effusion in cases caused by *M. haemolytica*, with red-black dry areas of coagulation necrosis resembling infarcts seen in cut sections of lungs. As previously mentioned, the lesions of fibrinous necrotizing lobar pleuropneumonia are classically associated with shipping fever of feedlot cattle.

P. multocida produces a purulent bronchopneumonia with plum-colored cranioventral consolidation and purulent exudate on cut section within the airways. This lesion is considered classic for ECP of housed dairy calves. *H. somnus* produces lesions similar to that of *P. multocida* and rarely may produce lesions that resemble *M. haemolytica*, creating a fibrinous pneumonia. Interestingly, *M. haemolytica* may also

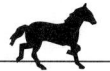

produce lesions in dairy calves that are not typical fibrinous pneumonia. In all cases of bacterial pneumonia and especially ECP, lung culture is essential to definitively determine the etiology.

A massive fibrinous pleuritis with pleural effusion sometimes results from septicemic spread of *H. somnus*. This condition can be differentiated from the fibrinous necrotizing lobar pleuropneumonia of shipping fever caused by *M. haemolytica*, because the *H. somnus* lesion involves only the pleural surface, not the lung.

Mycoplasmas have been associated with peribronchial and peribronchiolar lymphoid hyperplasia, which is sometimes referred to as a "cuffing pneumonia." Mycoplasmas have also been recovered from lesions of acute and chronic bronchopneumonia in which a cuffing pneumonia was not apparent. Recently, *Mycoplasma bovis* has been associated with a bronchopneumonia in cattle with the formation of abscesses.[601] The abscesses appear very similar to those associated with *Arcanobacterium (Actinomyces) pyogenes*, as seen in chronic bronchopneumonia. There is also a recent report of *M. bovis* causing otitis media in preweaned dairy calves.[602]

Animals that die after chronic persistent coughing and weight loss exhibit lesions of chronic suppurative pneumonia. Bronchi and bronchioles are filled with purulent exudate, there are multiple mature lung abscesses, and greatly dilated bronchioles contain malodorous exudate. When bronchiectasis is severe, the lung lobes have a nodular appearance. Pulmonary abscesses and bronchiectasis are common findings in cases of chronic pneumonia and explain poor weight gains.

Lambs that die of bronchopneumonia caused by *M. haemolytica* have swollen lungs with reddish purple anterior ventral consolidation. An extensive fibrinous pleuritis with large amounts of straw-colored exudate is often present. Chronic cases have multiple abscesses and pleural adhesions.

Identification of Infectious Agents

VIRUSES. A specific viral diagnosis requires laboratory confirmation. Most laboratories direct their diagnostic efforts toward the viruses for which vaccines are available. Diagnosis of other respiratory viruses may require the assistance of specialized laboratories. Because of the time and expense that specific viral diagnosis entails, care must be taken in the collection, storage, and transport of appropriate specimens to a diagnostic facility.

Virus Isolation. Virus isolation is time-consuming and expensive, but it is a sensitive method for identifying viruses. Virus isolation is performed in cell culture; a variety of specimens can be used, including nasopharyngeal, conjunctival, and tracheal swabs; transtracheal aspirates or bronchoalveolar lavage fluids; and a variety of respiratory tract tissues that can be obtained at postmortem examination. Fluids, tissues, and swabs may be frozen; alternatively, swabs and tissue specimens may be placed in viral transport medium and kept refrigerated until arrival at the diagnostic laboratory, preferably within 24 hours. BRSV does not appear to survive freezing or transport well, and it is important that specimens be inoculated onto cell cultures as soon as possible. In general, better success at virus isolation is obtained when specimens are collected in the acute phase of disease. Chances of successful isolation may be improved by sampling asymptomatic animals that are in close contact with affected animals. These animals may be in an incubation phase of infection. Some viruses appear to be more difficult to isolate than others. For example, BRSV is very difficult to isolate by routine procedures, and other diagnostic procedures (discussed later) should be performed in conjunction with attempts at virus isolation. During isolation procedures, viruses are detected by production of cytopathic changes in cell monolayers. Viral identification

is accomplished by a variety of procedures such as neutralization with specific antiserum, fluorescent antibody staining, immunoperoxidase staining, and examination by electron microscopy and immunoelectron microscopy. An immunoperoxidase monolayer assay has been developed for detection of BVDV and is in routine use for screening serum samples for detection of cattle persistently infected with BVDV.

Detection of Viral Antigens. Immunofluorescence is a rapid method for identification of specific respiratory viruses. Antemortem identification can be made from conjunctival or nasal smears, and from cells obtained by tracheal or bronchoalveolar lavage. Postmortem identification can be made from frozen tissue sections prepared from a variety of respiratory tract tissues.

Another technique that is being used to detect viral antigen in tissues is immunoperoxidase staining. This is a very useful procedure that allows histologic examination of tissues in conjunction with immunologic identification of the causative agent.

Antigen capture enzyme immunoassay (EIA) provides a rapid means for detection of respiratory viruses. These tests can be performed on fluids obtained from the respiratory tract. There are commercially available antigen capture EIAs for diagnosis of HRSV infections in infants and young children that are also capable of detecting BRSV,[603] and these are in use in some veterinary diagnostic laboratories. This same technique has been developed for the detection of BVDV and is in use for screening serum samples to detect cattle persistently infected with BVDV.

Detection of Viral Nucleic Acids. The nucleotide sequence has been determined for the genome or partial genome for many of the ruminant respiratory viruses. Although they are not currently in routine use, the possibility exists of using nucleotide probes for the detection of these viruses. Recently a polymerase chain reaction has been developed for the detection of nucleic acid sequences of BRSV.[604] Similar approaches can potentially be used for diagnosis of other ruminant respiratory viruses.

Serologic Diagnosis. Retrospective diagnosis of viral infections can be made by determination of antibody titers in paired sera from individual animals. The first sample is collected in the acute phase of the disease, and the second is collected 2 to 4 weeks later. In a respiratory disease outbreak multiple animals should be tested to achieve a serologic diagnosis. Serologic diagnosis is made by demonstrating a rising antibody level to a specific virus. Because BRSV and PI-3 infections can occur in the presence of passively derived antibodies, serologic diagnosis of infections by these viruses may not be possible in outbreaks of ECP involving young calves. This problem may be overcome by inclusion of older calves in the population sampled, which are likely to have lost passively derived antibody to these viruses. Also, BRSV antibody levels appear in some instances to peak at the onset of severe disease, and a decreasing antibody level is seen on paired serologic analysis rather than a rising level. Serologic testing of normal appearing, in-contact cattle that may be in early stages of infection may be helpful in demonstrating seroconversion to BRSV. A wide variety of serologic procedures are available for antibody determinations, but most laboratories use a microtiter serum-virus neutralization test for IBRV, BVDV, PI-3, and BRSV. A hemagglutination-inhibition test can also be used for PI-3. Some laboratories are beginning to use more rapid procedures such as EIA for determination of serum antibody titers. By using an isotype specific EIA, diagnosis of BRSV can be achieved on a single serum sample by measurement of IgM levels.[605]

BACTERIA. A wide variety of bacteria have been isolated from the respiratory tract of ruminants in association with respiratory disease. However, the most frequent and most important isolates are *M. (Pasteurella) haemolytica*, *P. multocida*, and

H. somnus. The isolation of *A. pyogenes,* coliforms, or anaerobic bacteria often is indicative of chronic pneumonia or aspiration pneumonia and may be associated with lung abscessation.

Before attempting bacterial culture the status of any recent antibacterial therapy should be determined and if possible specimens from untreated cattle should be collected. It is important to remember that *M. haemolytica, P. multocida,* and *H. somnus* are normal inhabitants of the nasal passages of cattle and may be cultured in the absence of respiratory disease. Although isolates obtained from nasal swabs may reflect the organisms causing pneumonia on a group level, specificity can be increased by obtaining specimens from the lower respiratory tract.[606] Specimens appropriate for bacterial culture are similar to those discussed for viruses, such as nasopharyngeal and tracheal swabs, transtracheal aspirates, and bronchoalveolar lavage or lung aspirates. Swabs are acceptable for transferring samples directly to culture medium, but if transport is necessary, the swab must be placed in a transport chamber such as a Culturette* to ensure adequate moisture for the sample during transport. Specimens of respiratory tract tissues such as lung and bronchial lymph nodes can be placed in sterile containers such as Petri dishes or self-sealing plastic bags, and transported to the laboratory on ice. If preferred, swab specimens of lung can be obtained by first searing the lung surface, then making an incision with a sterile scalpel, followed by sampling with a swab through the incision.

Generally, neither serologic tests nor direct means of detection of bacteria are performed (such as polymerase chain reaction [PCR] procedures or immunofluorescence testing) and diagnosis relies upon bacterial culture. Recently, diagnostic laboratories have begun using immunohistochemical staining for certain antigens of *M. haemolytica, M. bovis,* and *H. somnus.* This technique offers many advantages, including correlation of the pathogenic organism with the lesion and detection of pathogens not found on bacterial culture because of overgrowth of other organisms such as *A. pyogenes* or *P. multocida.* Specimens are routinely streaked onto MacConkey and blood agar plates. Blood agar plates are incubated at 37° C in the presence of 5% CO_2 and MacConkey agar plates should be incubated at 37° C under atmospheric conditions.

MYCOPLASMAS. Collection of samples is similar to those procedures previously described for bacteria. Specimens can be placed in Amies transport medium for shipment to a diagnostic laboratory. Special media are required for the isolation of mycoplasmas and ureaplasmas, such as Friis and Hayflicks T-mycoplasma media. Plates are incubated in 3% to 10% CO_2 at 37° C. Plates are examined by low-power microscopy, and colonies are identified by their characteristic "fried egg" appearance. Isolates can be speciated by growth inhibition by specific antiserum or by immunofluorescent examination.

CHLAMYDIA. Chlamydial organisms may be demonstrated by staining smears and sections of lesions with a Gimenez stain or by immunofluorescence techniques. Isolation attempts are done by inoculation of yolk sacs of embryonated chicks. Serologic tests such as complement fixation are also available.

Treatment

Successful intervention with a pneumonia outbreak is based on identification and alteration of the risk factors associated with the outbreak. An investigation begins with a thorough history and is followed by examinations of the animals and the environment. The history questions are directed to management practices that predispose to pneumonia. It is important to observe personally as many management practices as possible to ensure that what is planned is actually implemented.

Animal examinations may include collection of blood or serum samples for measurement of the concentrations of trace minerals that are necessary for proper function of the immune system. The success of passive transfer in dairy or veal calves should be determined by measurement of immunoglobulins in the serum of calves 1 to 7 days of age. The zinc sulfate turbidity test, sodium sulfite test, and measurement of total serum protein with a refractometer are practical, satisfactory procedures for estimation of serum immunoglobulin concentrations.

Examination of the environment includes evaluation of the nutrition program to determine whether any of the dietary factors that predispose to pneumonia are present. Evaluation of the microclimate of housed calves is of critical importance in the control and prevention of pneumonia. Equipment useful for evaluating mechanically ventilated buildings includes a smoke generator to visualize airflow patterns, an anemometer to measure air velocity, a psychrometer to determine air temperature and relative humidity, and a gas detector kit to measure ammonia concentrations in the air. Naturally ventilated buildings should also be evaluated for adequate sidewall and ridge openings, adequate segregation of age-groups, and stocking densities. Hutches should be evaluated for proper placement in relation to other hutches, other buildings, prevailing winds, exposure to sun, bedding and draining, and ventilation of the hutch.

Management practices surrounding the purchase, transport, processing, and placement of background and feedlot calves must be carefully reviewed. The feeding practices used to bring weaned calves on to high-energy rations should also be carefully reviewed, as should pen management (i.e., does feedlot observe "all-in-all-out" management?).

Antimicrobial Therapy. The basic foundations of antimicrobial therapy for bacterial bronchopneumonia are treat early enough, treat long enough, and treat with the appropriate antimicrobial agent. Treating early enough is far more important than what is used for therapy. It should be remembered that a major reason for treatment failure is the presence of a lesion that is too far advanced for successful therapy. The role of antimicrobial therapy in treating bacterial bronchopneumonia is to control or stop bacterial replication. This will limit or prevent release of virulence factors from organisms like *M. (Pasteurella) haemolytica* A1 such as the leukotoxin and endotoxin that are responsible for thrombosis, exudative edema, and necrosis. If this lesion becomes too far advanced, the antimicrobial agents will have difficulty reaching areas of necrosis and suppuration, and the regenerative response will not be able to return this tissue to normal lung parenchyma.

Although antibacterial agents for the treatment of bacterial bronchopneumonia may reduce losses caused by fatality and retarded growth, they do not serve as a substitute for preventive management practices. Cattle requiring treatment do not perform as well as those that have not needed treatment. Calves receiving treatment that respond to initial therapy without relapse will, however, often have the same average daily gain as cattle not requiring therapy, unlike calves that experience treatment failure (relapse and not responding.) This further emphasizes the need for effective antimicrobial therapy for bacterial bronchopneumonia, because animals with treatment failure will have decreased growth rate.

Early detection relies on a systemic approach by trained personnel to identify cattle in pens that are subjectively different from pen mates. Animals identified by this means should be removed from the pen and placed in a chute or restrained in some manner so that body temperature can be determined. It is important that while the animal is being taken to the restraint facility it be monitored closely for clinical signs referable to the respiratory system such as coughing, labored breathing, and nasal discharge, versus those that are referable to some other system, such as ataxia, lameness, or

---

*Marion Scientific, Kansas City, MO.

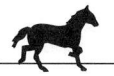

diarrhea. This, in effect, is the physical examination that will be used, along with the temperature, by the animal caretakers to make a decision as to whether to treat and for what condition. In general, cattle that are febrile without obvious symptomatology of other organ systems and with or without signs of respiratory system dysfunction are considered to have bacterial bronchopneumonia (case definition). Early detection is especially critical with ECP, in which disease onset and lesion progression may be insidious and chronic.

The precise temperature used to determine whether animals need treatment depends on the balance between the costs of overtreatment (drugs and labor) and undertreatment (treatment failures and mortality.) This temperature may vary depending on the animal type. The cut-off commonly used for feedlot cattle is 104° to 104.5° F (40 to 40.3° C) but may be 103.5° F (39.7° C) for dairy calves. This recommendation is based on the long-term effects that ECP has been shown to have on growth rate, age at first calving, culling before calving, and culling after calving, indicating that ECP can have long-lasting effects if not properly treated with early antibiotic therapy. When outbreaks of respiratory disease occur, surveillance of the affected group must be increased to ensure early detection of diseased animals.

Treatment of sufficient duration can be achieved only if the response to therapy is monitored. Therapy should be continued for at least 48 hours after clinical signs of fever, dyspnea, and toxemia have abated. Frequently, antibiotics are evaluated over a standard 3-day treatment period, with cases failing to provide a reduction in temperature being classified

as non-responders. With ECP, treatment for more than 3 days may be indicated. This is in part based on an attempt to prevent the long-term effects of ECP previously discussed. A longer course of antibiotic therapy may also be indicated with ECP because of the insidious nature of the disease, in which a lesion may already be well established when first detected. Animals classified as non-responders to the first-line antibiotics may then be placed on an alternate antibiotic (second-line antibiotic) for a set period (4 days.) It is important that the criteria used to define a favorable therapeutic response be closely adhered to. Determination of therapeutic response by evaluation of general appearance without regard to restoration of normal body temperature has been shown to result in high relapse rates. A typical decision tree for treating feedlot cattle with antibiotics is shown in Figure 29-33.

Selection of the appropriate antibiotic tends to be what most veterinarians focus on when treating respiratory disease because this is the aspect of therapy over which they have the greatest control. Factors such as cost, route of administration, treatment interval, drug licensure, necessity of extra label doses, and withholding times quickly cull a number of antibiotics, leaving a short list of suitable alternatives for use as first-line antimicrobial agents. Antibiotics that are associated with severe injection site reactions such as erythromycin or those associated with complications of administration such as balling gun injuries with oral boluses are often avoided. Only antibiotics that are licensed and effective at label doses should be considered for routine use in food animals. Table 29-7 lists the approved antimicrobials for treating respiratory

TABLE 29-7

Antimicrobials Approved by the FDA for Treatment of Bronchopneumonia of Beef Cattle

Antimicrobial	Label Dosage	Route of Administration	Treatment Interval (hr)	Withdrawal for Slaughter
STANDARD PREPARATIONS				
Amoxicillin	11 mg/kg	IM, SC	12	25 days
Ampicillin	2-5 mg/kg (22 mg/kg)*	SC	12	6 days
Ceftiofur (sodium)	1.1 mg/kg	IM, SC	24	None
Ceftiofur (HCl)	1.1 mg/kg	IM, SC	24	48 hr
Enrofloxacin	2.5-5.5 mg/kg	SC	24	28 days
Erythromycin	2.2-4.4 mg/kg (11-22 mg/kg)*	IM	24	14 days
Oxytetracycline	11 mg/kg	IV, IM, SC	24	15-22 days†
Procaine penicillin G	6600 U/kg (22,000 U/kg)*	IM, SC	24	7 days
Spectinomycin	10-15 mg/kg	SC	24	11 days
Sulfachloropyridazine	33-50 mg/kg	IV (injectable)	12	7 days
Sulfadimethoxine	200 mg/kg, initial treatment 130 mg/kg daily thereafter	IV (injectable) Oral (bolus)	24	10 days
Tylosin	17 mg/kg	IM	24	21 days
LONG-ACTING PREPARATIONS				
Ceftiofur HCl	2.2 mg/kg	IM, SC	48	48 hr
Enrofloxacin	7.5-12.5 mg/kg	SC	Licensed for one treatment only	28 days
Florfenicol	20 mg/kg	IM	48	28 days
	40 mg/kg	SC	Licensed for one treatment only	38 days
Oxytetracycline	20 mg/kg	IM, SC	48	28 days
Penicillin G benzathine/ penicillin G procaine	8800 U/kg	IM, SC	48	30 days
Sulfadimethoxine (sustained release bolus)	137.5 mg/kg	PO	96	21 days
Tilmicosin	10 mg/kg	SC	72	28 days

*Author-suggested dose that would be required to achieve adequate treatment response. Higher dose can be given by the same route of administration and with the same treatment interval, but use of extralabel dosages must comply with the Animal Medicinal Drug Use Clarification Act (AMDUCA), and withdrawal times must be significantly extended.
†Varies with preparation.

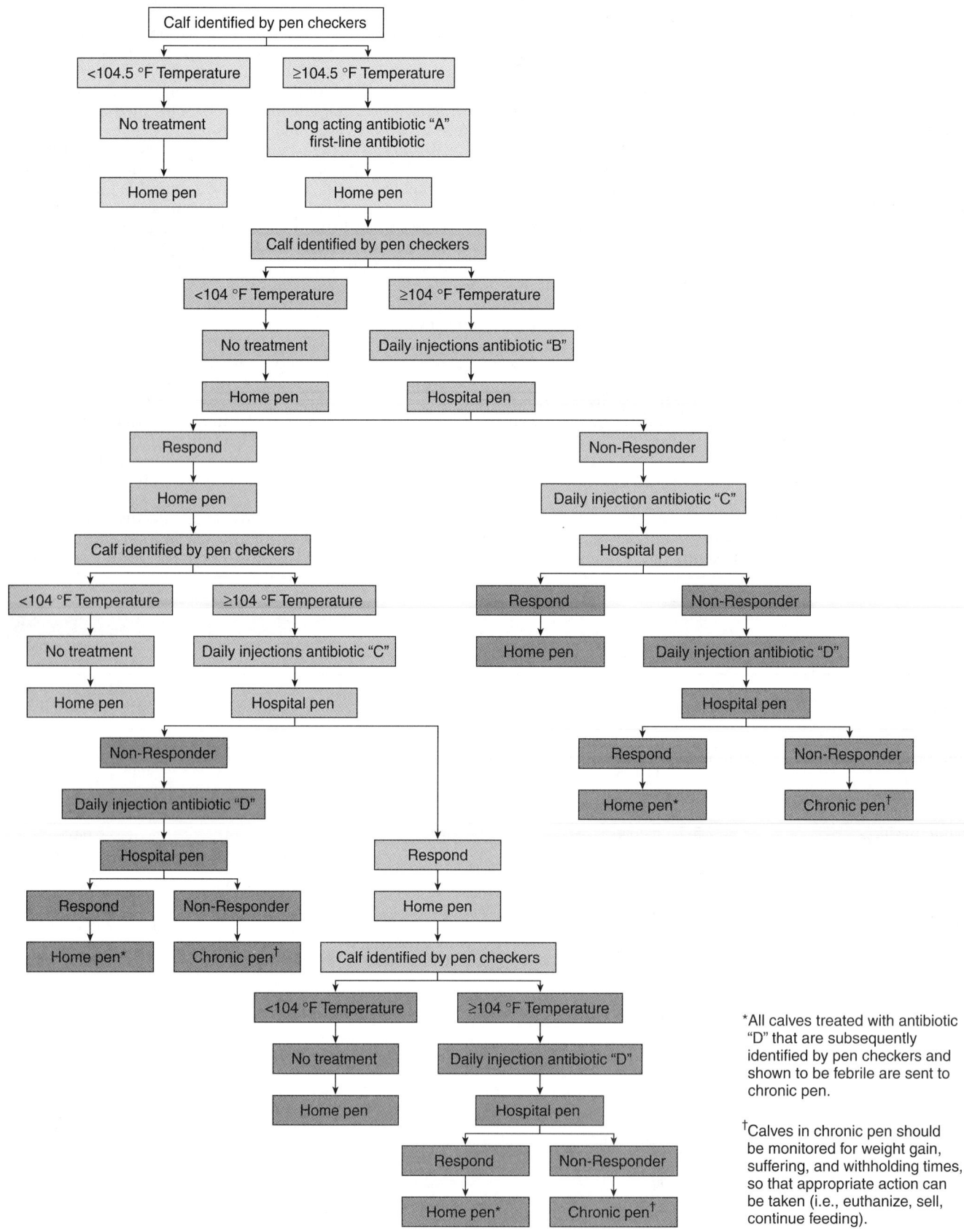

FIG. 29-33 ▌▌ Decision tree for antibiotic treatment of feedlot cattle.

*All calves treated with antibiotic "D" that are subsequently identified by pen checkers and shown to be febrile are sent to chronic pen.

†Calves in chronic pen should be monitored for weight gain, suffering, and withholding times, so that appropriate action can be taken (i.e., euthanize, sell, continue feeding).

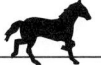

disease in cattle. This list is then modified based on pharmacokinetic behavior and the minimum inhibitory concentration (MIC) of the organism being treated. More simply stated, the clinician will have to have the confidence that the antimicrobial agent can achieve tissue levels above the MIC of the organism being treated in the pneumonic lungs.

Determining the MIC or sensitivity of the causative agents such as *M. haemolytica* A1 in the case of bacterial bronchopneumonia can be difficult. In reviewing any MIC or sensitivity results it should be kept in mind that *M. haemolytica* can develop plasmid-mediated multiple antimicrobial resistance by bacterial conjugation so that, for example, exposure to oxytetracycline may induce resistance to oxytetracycline and penicillin. Therefore, *M. haemolytica* A1 recovered from cattle treated with antibiotics will have a different sensitivity pattern than *M. haemolytica* A1 cultured from untreated cattle. This is especially important when reviewing publications of antimicrobial susceptibility of *M. haemolytica* isolates cultured at diagnostic laboratories, because these results will have a bias toward cases that have been treated with antimicrobial agents. The findings of these studies may be looked at as a worst case scenario demonstrating antimicrobial agents for which acquired resistance is rarely or never a problem versus those for which acquired antimicrobial resistance occurs commonly. In general, few drugs, with the possible exception of ceftiofur, and enrofloxacin, and, to a lesser extent, florfenicol and spectinomycin, are found to have limited resistance in *M. haemolytica* lung isolates.

Feedlot operators and calf raisers who keep accurate records of drugs used, treatment responses, relapses, and chronic cases may also select first-line antibiotics based on historical performance of a drug. This may be the best approach to antimicrobial selection. A final method of choosing a first-line antimicrobial drug is reliance on published treatment trials. Published trials give comparisons between treatment response for various antibiotics in cattle with naturally occurring bacterial bronchopneumonia. The outcomes for these trials are often expressed as both health and production values. When evaluating published treatment trials that use cases of naturally occurring bacterial bronchopneumonia, it is useful to realize that the results may not be applicable to the cattle and pathogens in a given geographic area, but if the trial is well designed, it should provide useful comparisons. To determine if the trial is well designed, it should be controlled and random, use multiple experimental groups, and be statistically analyzed.

Sensitivity testing using isolates from clinic cases raises concerns over where to sample and from which cattle. Antibacterial sensitivities of isolates cultured from nasal swabs may not represent sensitivities of organisms causing pneumonia. This is unusual, because pneumonia usually is preceded by multiplication of *M. haemolytica* in the upper respiratory tract, and the nasopharynx serves as the source of bacteria colonizing the lungs. Nevertheless, there are discrepancies between sensitivities of bacteria isolated from nasal swabs and clinical outcome. Ideally specimens for sensitivity testing should be collected from pneumonic lung, tracheal swabs, or tracheobronchial aspirates from cattle before treatment. Unfortunately this may not always be a practical alternative.

Recently, long-acting antibiotics have replaced antibiotics given daily as first-line drugs in feedlots. The perceived benefit of higher blood and tissue levels achieved with daily injections of cattle kept in hospital pens is more than outweighed by the improved performance observed when cattle are returned to the home pens after an injection of long-acting antibiotic. This avoids constant use of hospital pens and transfer of pathogens among hospitalized animals and increased labor costs of daily injections.

Mass medication with antibiotics at full therapeutic doses during an outbreak of feedlot cattle pneumonia dramatically curtails the daily number of new cases and improves feed consumption. Ceftiofur HCl, enrofloxacin, florfenicol, tilmicosin, long-acting oxytetracycline, or sustained-release sulfonamides (or a combination of oxytetracycline and sulfonamides) can be given to every calf, or sulfonamides can be administered in the drinking water for 5 days. Pneumonia cases that follow administration of mass medication have an increased high possibility of being resistant to therapy with the antimicrobial used in mass treatment and have a greater than usual resistance to other antimicrobials. Thus mass medication should not be a standard practice but is warranted to control severe outbreaks of pneumonia. It is important to base a decision to mass medicate on measurable criteria. Some feedlot veterinarians implement mass medication when the pull rate of sick animals is 10% on any 1 day or is 25% over a 3- to 5-day period. A sudden drop in feed consumption, especially in high-risk cattle, is another situation in which mass antibiotic medication should be cost-effective. Long-acting antibiotics have extended withdrawal times to slaughter. It is of critical importance that animals that receive them are properly identified and that the withdrawal times are observed.

The same principles of therapy of pneumonia apply to sheep and goats.[547] Tetracycline given intramuscularly at 5 mg/kg twice a day for 5 to 6 days is usually effective. Long-acting tetracycline at 10 mg/kg is very effective against experimental *M. haemolytica* infections. Administration of tetracycline subcutaneously to goats is effective and less painful than intramuscular injection. Other antimicrobials used to treat pneumonia of sheep and goats include sulfonamides, penicillin, and erythromycin. Drugs without established withholding times should be avoided when treating feeder lambs or lactating goats.

Antiinflammatory Therapy. Favorable responses to treatment with corticosteroids and antihistamines have been reported from field outbreaks of BRSV infection. However, corticosteroids should not be used indiscriminately in the treatment of respiratory disease because of the potential for immunosuppression. Corticosteroids may have a place in treatment of respiratory diseases such as necrotic laryngitis or tracheal edema syndrome of feedlot cattle.[607] It is unlikely that a single administration of a glucocorticoid will have a detrimental effect on the immune system of cattle. The dose for dexamethasone in cattle is 5 to 25 mg given IM or IV, and the dose for isoflupredone acetate is 10 to 20 mg IM. Treatment with corticosteroids may cause recrudescence of BHV-1 infections.

Nonsteroidal antiinflammatory drugs (NSAIDs) such as acetylsalicylic acid (aspirin), flunixin meglumine, phenylbutazone, and ibuprofen have been reported to be beneficial in the treatment of respiratory disease in ruminants. Aspirin (100 mg/kg every 12 hours) is approved for use in cattle and flunixen meglumine (1.1 to 2.2 mg/kg either as a single dose or divided into two doses at 12-hour intervals) has recently been approved for use in cattle. Flunixin meglumine administered intravenously at 2.2 mg/kg to calves with pneumonia induced by PI-3 virus results in a marked improvement in clinical signs and reduction in lung consolidation.[607] Unlike corticosteroids, NSAIDs do not impair immune function and they are analgesic and antipyretic. The clinical responses of calves with either experimental or naturally occurring pneumonic pasteurellosis are markedly improved by adding intramuscularly administered flunixin meglumine to tetracycline therapy. In contrast, supplementation of antibiotic therapy with corticosteroids usually results in poorer responses, more relapses, and prolonged illness, although there is still some controversy over the use of corticosteroids for treatment of pneumonia. Because of the potential for renal toxicity with NSAIDs, dehydrated animals should be rehydrated before administration of these drugs. Care should also be taken not to overdose with NSAIDs or use them for prolonged periods, because they may also result in abomasal ulceration.

There has been little work done to evaluate the use of antihistamines as an ancillary treatment for bovine respiratory disease. Tripelenamine HCl is labeled for cattle at a dose of 1.1 mg/kg, which can be repeated in 6 to 12 hours if needed.

Tilmicosin, a macrolide antibiotic approved in the United States for use in cattle, has been shown to also have antiinflammatory effects in cattle with pneumonic pasteurellosis.[608] This antibiotic induces apoptosis in leukocytes. Following the induction of programmed cell death, LTB$_4$ synthesis is impaired in the lungs of tilmicosin-treated cattle, thus further preventing amplification of the inflammatory process.[608]

Antiviral and Immunomodulating Therapy. Because respiratory viral infections predispose to development of secondary bacterial infections, antibiotic therapy (discussed previously) is indicated to prevent or limit bacterial pneumonia. There are few antiviral drugs available in human medicine, and none of these is in routine use in veterinary medicine for the treatment of viral respiratory disease in ruminants. Ribavirin is an antiviral drug that also has immunomodulating effects and is used for treatment of HRSV infections in infants. The drug is administered to infants by continuous pulmonary aerosolization over a 12- to 18-hour period per day. No studies have been done on the use of this drug for BRSV infections in cattle. Ribavirin is expensive and difficult to administer, thus precluding its use in routine veterinary practice. Interferon has potential as an immunomodulating and antiviral drug in the prevention and treatment of viral respiratory disease. Human leukocyte interferon is currently approved in Texas for the prophylactic treatment of "shipping fever" associated with BHV-1 infections. Levamisole and Isoprinosine have been used in attempts to stimulate the bovine immune system with equivocal success and cannot yet be recommended as supportive treatments.[607] It is important to recognize that the immunostimulatory benefits of levamisole occur at doses in the 2- to 3-mg/kg range, compared with the anthelmintic dose of 6 mg/kg. A decreased immune response has been observed after an 8-mg/kg dose of levamisole. High doses of vitamin C (1 g/45 kg; 1 g/100 lb) have been shown to enhance the activity of bovine neutrophils and reverse dexamethasone-induced suppression of neutrophil activity.[609] Isoprinosine has been evaluated as an immunomodulating drug for treatment of bovine respiratory disease and has shown some potential on the cellular level.[607]

Supportive Therapy. Supportive treatment of any kind will relieve stress, thus fostering the resistance of the patient, a very important component of the successful therapy of pneumonia cases. Ill animals should be provided shelter that protects them from rain, cold, wind, or hot sun. They should not be crowded, and the best-quality feed should be provided. Mineral and vitamin deficiencies should be corrected with the use of injections or oral preparations. An intramuscular vitamin A injection should be a standard part of the first day's treatment. In the future, immunopotentiation may be part of supportive therapy.

PREVENTION AND CONTROL

Management (Enzootic Calf Pneumonia). Bronchopneumonia of dairy and veal calves is prevented by eliminating or altering as many predisposing risk factors as possible. Control is based on healthy, well-vaccinated dams giving birth in maternity facilities that limit pathogen exposure. Good colostral management is needed to ensure adequate passive transfer. The calves must have their navels disinfected and be moved to calf housing that limits pathogen exposure by overcrowd-

ing and direct contact, provides good-quality air, and protects the calf from environmental extremes. Calf hutches that are managed properly provide most, if not all, of the housing requirements previously mentioned. Calves need to move to postweaning housing that allows small groups to be segregated from older age-groups. Super hutches or pens in pole sheds separated by barrier walls can effectively provide this postweaning housing. Calves should be fed proper nutrition for protein, energy, minerals, and vitamins and should be vaccinated appropriately with effective vaccines. Vaccination programs are often used in dairy calves beginning at 1 to 2 months of age in situations where housing or mixing of calves results in a high incidence of ECP.

Management (Feedlot Pneumonia). Preconditioning of calves is an attempt to eliminate certain risk factors that influence the occurrence of feedlot cattle pneumonia. Preconditioned calves are weaned at least 3 weeks before shipment and are trained to eat in feed bunks. They are castrated and dehorned, treated for internal and external parasites, and vaccinated against respiratory pathogens. A summary of eight studies comparing the health of preconditioned calves to control calves indicated that, on average, preconditioning reduced morbidity rate by 23% and mortality rate by 50% in the feedlot.[546] It is not surprising that preconditioning does not consistently influence feedlot pneumonias, because it has no effect on many risk factors active during transit and in the feedlot. Thus optimal control of feedlot pneumonia should begin with preconditioning and continue with avoidance of auction yards, minimization of transport time to the feedlot, limited mixing of calves from different sources, limited number of calves per pen, control of dust, and careful diet management in the feedlot. Correction of vitamin and/or mineral deficiencies if known or detected, using vitamin injections in entering calves, may be a very important aspect of prevention of feedlot pneumonias that are associated with immunodeficiencies of nutritional origin.

Processing procedures on arrival at the feedlot affect the incidence of pneumonia. General recommendations for handling incoming cattle can be made that are appropriate for any category of animals. In a receiving program, rest, rehydration, and rumen restoration need to be addressed because cattle are physically and psychologically stressed by the marketing and transportation processes. It is useful for these cattle to be rested for 12 to 24 hours before processing to allow the immune system to overcome the effects of stress. Prolonged holding before processing is associated with increased illness and holding times over 48 hours should be avoided. Holding pens should be clean and dry or have dry bedding (if pens are wet from excessive precipitation) because this allows all cattle to lie down and rest. Shelter from wind, sun, rain, and dust should also be present in the receiving pen.

Holding pens should have 150 to 200 square feet of pen space per animal, 12 to 16 inches of bunk space per animal, and be located close to the processing facility. Excess mixing of cattle in the receiving pens should also be avoided.

It is important that incoming cattle have access to clean, fresh water. Raised spigots have been suggested as a way to teach incoming cattle to drink out of automatic watering devices because cattle will be attracted to the sound of splashing water. Incoming cattle should also be offered good-quality, long grass hay on arrival. This is the most similar to what cattle are used to on range. Hay is the best foodstuff for restoring or refilling the rumen. Hay can be put in the feed bunks as well as in feeders in the pen as a way of teaching cattle to eat out of bunks. Hay feeders may also be put along the pen perimeter to decrease walking the fence line and encourage eating. The starter ration is an important source of energy and should be highly palatable. The proportion of the starter ration dry matter that is forage is not usually less than 50% to prevent problems of acidosis. Starter rations often contain a coccidiostat, because coccidiosis can occur in calves after commingling.

Processing protocols may be tailored to the category of the incoming cattle. Pharmaceutical processing options include vaccination (respiratory and nonrespiratory), vitamin injections, implanting, deworming for internal parasites and acaricides for external parasites (may be the same product for both), long-acting antibiotic therapy, drugs for aborting pregnant heifers, and probiotic administration. Management procedures for processing include ear tagging, branding, tail trimming, castration, tip dehorning, and temperature sorting. Some management procedures such as castration and dehorning could be left for a later time such as at reimplanting at 70 to 90 days on feed (if cattle are expected on feed for more than 150 days). "Temping" on arrival can be very useful, because even cattle that look bright can have very high temperatures and thus can be identified as "sick" by this procedure. Variation in processing protocols for high- and low-risk cattle are shown in Box 29-3.

Management (Sheep and Goat Pneumonia). Prevention of pneumonia in sheep and goats is also based on altering the risk factors that predispose to pneumonia. Minimizing cold and heat stress, providing properly ventilated housing, avoiding overcrowding, and avoiding long transports in adverse weather aid in prevention. Mass medication can be used to control outbreaks of pneumonia in flocks. Sulfonamides are administered in the drinking water or orally at 200 mg/kg on the first day and 66 mg/kg each subsequent day of treatment, or long-acting tetracycline is given subcutaneously at 10 mg/kg.

Antibiotics for Metaphylaxis of Bacterial Bronchopneumonia. Use of antibiotics for on-arrival mass medication of feedlot cattle to prevent bacterial bronchopneumonia has been advocated in various forms for many years. It is useful to examine the theoretical mechanisms of how metaphylactic antibiotics may work to evaluate or choose a particular antimicrobial agent and the most suitable route of administration.

As part of its pathogenic mechanisms, *M. (Pasteurella) haemolytica* A1 can proliferate in large numbers in the upper respiratory tract of cattle. The exact site of replication is thought to be the tonsillar crypt; this replication is a crucial phase in lesion development because large numbers of bacteria can be inhaled into the lung allowing colonization, proliferation, and production of virulence factors. There appears to be a short time after arrival in the feedlot when cattle that will subsequently develop bacterial bronchopneumonia have large numbers of *M. haemolytica* A1 present in their upper respiratory tract. Antimicrobial therapy timed to coincide with this pathologic event and designed to provide therapeutic levels can have a profound effect on bacterial bronchopneumonia morbidity and mortality. Metaphylactic antimicrobial therapy is aimed at reducing the number of *M. haemolytica* A1 present in the upper respiratory tract of calves, which could also limit colonization of the lung and prevent horizontal transmission of *M. haemolytica* from calf to calf. Long-acting antibiotics have been reported to significantly alter the number of calves from which *M. haemolytica* can be cultured.[610] An additional rationale for mass medication of feedlot cattle on arrival with antimicrobial agents is based on the epidemic curve of fatal disease onset for bacterial bronchopneumonia, which shows that feedlot calves dying from fatal fibrinous pneumonia are sick on arrival or become ill within days of arrival. Although mass medication through feed and water has been used for many years, the focus in recent years has shifted to mass medication using injectable antimicrobial agents. The ability of these drugs to reach therapeutic levels quickly in all animals gives them a clear advantage given the previously discussed rationale for bacterial bronchopneumonia metaphylaxis.

A number of trials have been published that examine various antimicrobial agents and their effectiveness for bacterial bronchopneumonia metaphylaxis. Most of these studies have examined both health and production values. Tilmicosin given to calves on arrival at the feedlot was shown to reduce the treatment rate, extend the time from arrival to the onset of therapy, and increase the average daily gain and feed efficiency over the trial period compared to nonmedicated control animals.[611] When long-acting oxytetracycline was compared to trimethoprim-sulfadoxine for prophylaxis of bacterial bronchopneumonia, the long-acting oxytetracycline reduced bovine respiratory disease morbidity and fatal fibrinous pneumonia mortality compared with controls and trimethoprim-sulfadoxine–treated animals.[612] This indicates that there is an advantage to using long-acting or sustained-release formulations rather than products designed for daily injection. In a separate bacterial bronchopneumonia metaphylaxis study, tilmicosin-treated calves, when compared with long-acting oxytetracycline–treated calves, showed lower morbidity and mortality attributable to pneumonia, lower morbidity and mortality attributable to all causes, and decreased case fatality.[613] The tilmicosin-treated calves had significantly greater weight gains than the calves that received long-acting oxytetracycline.[613]

Similar use of long-acting antimicrobials in dairy calves may also be of value. The disease process does not have the same narrow windows of therapeutic intervention that occur in calves entering the feedlot. Dairy calves properly managed in maternity facilities and raised in hutches rarely experience any respiratory disease until they are moved to the postweaning housing. Injectable mass medication is often used at the time calves are moved and then again at some time later (7 to 10 days after entering the postweaning housing) as a means of controlling postweaning ECP. The use of injectable mass medication for small ruminants is limited by cost constraints. Some feedlots inject lambs on arrival with long-acting oxytetracycline.

Vaccination. Vaccination for prevention of respiratory disease has been controversial and does not appear to be totally effective under all circumstances. Vaccines are not available

---

BOX 29-3

Various Processing Protocols for High- and Low-Risk Cattle Entering a Feedlot

PROCESSING PROTOCOL FOR HIGH-RISK, FALL-WEANED, AUCTION MARKET CALVES
1. Modified live IBR, BVD, BRSV, and PI-3 vaccine
2. Eight-way clostridial bacterin
3. Ivermectin type "pour-on"
4. *Pasteurella* and *Haemophilus* vaccine
5. Implant
6. Ear tag identification
7. Bulls castrated with bander (if needed)
8. Tip dehorning (if needed)
9. "Temp" all incoming cattle and sort by temperature, (i.e., >105 °F (40.5 °C)—treat with tilmicosin; all others treat with long-acting oxytetracycline)

PROCESSING PROTOCOL FOR HEALTHY YEARLINGS PREVIOUSLY FED IN BACKGROUND OPERATIONS
1. Modified live IBR, BVD, BRSV, and PI-3 vaccines
2. Eight-way clostridial vaccine
3. Ear tag identification
4. Implant
5. Ivermectin type or organophosphate type "pour-on" if days on feed will allow for withholding times needed

for all of the infectious agents implicated in the respiratory disease complex of ruminants. The effectiveness of vaccines and bacterins is often hard to determine under field conditions. Although the efficacy of some viral vaccines to prevent their specific viral disease has been established, questions remain about their effectiveness in preventing undifferentiated respiratory disease.[614] Under some circumstances viral vaccines have been associated with an increase in mortality rates for respiratory disease.[615] In the past, *Pasteurella* bacterins have been ineffective and potentially dangerous.[616] The multifactorial nature of the ruminant respiratory disease complex contributes to the difficulty of conducting field trials. Also, the tremendous environmental variation that can affect the occurrence of respiratory disease makes controlled studies essential. Because of the lack of control over environmental factors, more replicates are required under a variety of circumstances. With multivalent products, it is often difficult to determine which components are responsible for the outcomes observed.

Because respiratory disease in feeder calves most often occurs shortly after their introduction into feedlots, it is preferable to establish immunity to respiratory pathogen infection before arrival. This can be accomplished through preconditioning programs, but these programs have not gained total acceptance. More often than not, vaccination is performed on arrival at feedlots. Vaccination at this time coincides with severe periods of stress, which may cause a poor immune response. ECP generally occurs at an age when passive immunity is a calf's main defense against infectious disease. Thus the successful use of vaccination to prevent enzootic pneumonia involves vaccination of the dam in the periparturient period to boost concentrations of immunoglobulins against respiratory pathogens in the colostrum and secondarily in the calf's serum. This has been successful with a commercially available pasteurella vaccine in herds with proper colostral management but has failed in herds with poor colostral management.[617] There is also evidence accumulating that neonatal calves can be immunologically primed against respiratory virus infections by vaccination with modified live virus vaccines.[618]

No single, simple recommendation for vaccination of cattle for control of respiratory disease can be made. The veterinarian must individualize each vaccination program to the situation at hand. Many factors need to be considered in formulating recommendations for vaccination, including type of production unit, age of animals, system of management, housing facilities, amount of stress imposed on animals, open or closed herd, type of ration, and level of sanitation. In addition, some infectious agents such as BHV-1, BVDV, and *H. somnus* can cause other disease problems not associated with the respiratory tract. Thus the complete spectrum of disease caused by these agents must be considered in formulating a vaccination program.

Viruses. PI-3 vaccines are available and are generally found in combination with BHV-1. In general, their use has centered around the BHV-1 component rather than PI-3. Both inactivated and attenuated forms have been produced. The modified live virus vaccines are available in intramuscular and intranasal forms. Inactivated and attenuated BHV-1 vaccines are available. Temperature-sensitive, modified live BHV-1 vaccines are available for intranasal vaccination. Because some of the BHV-1 vaccines can induce abortion, the manufacturer's recommendations should be closely followed. Intranasally administered BHV-1/PI-3 vaccines have the advantage of inducing a local immune response and may have an advantage when vaccinating calves in the presence of passive immunity.[619] Modified live BHV-1 vaccines are capable of causing latent infections.[549] Recently BHV-1 vaccines that have gene deletions have been developed.[620] These vaccines allow serologic differentiation of vaccinated from naturally

infected animals and have application for control or eradication programs for BHV-1. For complete discussion of the topic of BVDV vaccination, the reader is referred to Chapters 30 and 44 and a recent review article.[621] Both live and killed vaccines are available, but there are no intranasal BVDV vaccines. Previously, BVDV vaccines contained only the type 1 BVDV genotype, but currently both live and inactivated BVDV vaccines containing the type 1 and 2 genotypes are commercially available in the United States. The advantage of live BVDV vaccines is that they achieve high levels of immunity without booster vaccination. Additionally, modified live BVDV vaccines provide broader protection with respect to the antigenic variation that occurs among BVDV isolates. The disadvantage is that they can cross the placenta and induce all of the known consequences of fetal BVDV infection. Also, modified live BVDV virus vaccines have been shown to be immunosuppressive, although this may be of concern only when used in cattle subjected to severe stress. Inactivated BVDV vaccines are safe for pregnant animals but require booster vaccination, do not achieve as high a level of immunity, and may not protect as long as the modified live vaccines.

The topic of BRSV vaccination has been reviewed.[622] Currently, modified live and inactivated BRSV vaccines for intramuscular administration are available in the United States. The modified live BRSV vaccines are not thought to replicate after administration. Because of this, booster vaccination is necessary. This vaccine appears to be safe and can be adapted into a preconditioning program or given to calves at time of arrival at feedlots. Dairy calves can be vaccinated when passive immunity has declined. However, there is also evidence that vaccination of calves with modified live BRSV vaccine in the presence of passively derived immunity can result in systemic and local memory responses.[623] Furthermore, it has been demonstrated that T cell responses can be stimulated in young calves by modified live BRSV vaccines in the presence of maternal antibodies.[618] A single report originating from Europe indicated that vaccination of cattle that were incubating a BRSV with a modified live BRSV vaccine enhanced the severity of the infection.[624] Inactivated BRSV vaccines are commercially available. There has been little published with respect to their development, methods of virus inactivation, means of adjuvanting, and outcomes of field trials. There have been no published reports of inactivated vaccines causing immunopotentiation of disease in BRSV-infected cattle. There have been reports that some of the commercially available BRSV vaccines stimulate predominantly nonneutralizing antibodies, but how this relates to protection or immunoenhancement of disease is not known.[622] In Europe there is a unique commercially inactivated vaccine available under the trade name of Torvac.* This vaccine is reported to be more immunogenic than modified live vaccine or natural infection and can immunize in the presence of passively derived maternal antibodies.[622]

The following basic principles must be applied in decisions on the use of inactivated versus modified live viral vaccines[625]:

- Noninfectious vaccines generally require multiple doses (2 to 6 weeks apart) to immunize and one dose has no benefit at all.
- The immunity generated by noninfectious vaccines is short-lived, requiring boosters every few months to 1 year for maintenance.
- Noninfectious vaccines do not stimulate local immunity at all and either do not stimulate or poorly stimulate cellular immunity.
- Noninfectious vaccines are very effective in stimulating humoral immunity and are more effective than modified live

---

*C-Vet Veterinary Products, Leyland, United Kingdom.

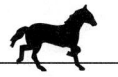

vaccines in stimulating a secondary immune response, because of the increased amount of antigen in the noninfectious vaccine.

- Modified live vaccines provide cellular and humoral immunity that persists for years to life and are the first choice for successful immunization of young animals.
- Modified live vaccines can cause abortion in unprotected pregnant animals or disease in immunologically compromised animals.

There are no approved respiratory vaccines for sheep and goats in the United States. Modified live bovine PI-3 vaccines may be of benefit, but if these vaccines contain modified live BHV-1, their use cannot be recommended. No information is available on the use of BRSV vaccines in sheep and goats. It is important to remember that administration of these bovine vaccines to sheep and goats constitutes "extralabel" usage of these products.

Bacteria. Vaccination for pneumonic pasteurellosis has been controversial. *Mannheimia* whole-cell bacterins were the first products developed, but are now considered to be ineffective. The use of *M. haemolytica* bacterins has been associated with increased incidence and severity of bovine respiratory disease.[626] Live attenuated *M. haemolytica* vaccines have been developed, but the results from use of these products have been variable.[626] Complaints against this type of vaccine have included localized skin swelling with the intradermal vaccine and transient lameness and pyrexia with the intramuscular vaccine. In contrast to the bacterins, the attenuated vaccines have not been associated with enhanced morbidity or mortality rate and were shown to provide protection against disease caused by this organism.[627] Although the original live attenuated *Pasteurella (Mannheimia)* vaccines are no longer commercially available in the United States, a new modified live streptomycin-dependent mutant is now available. Recent advances have been made in the development of biologics that contain concentrated leukotoxin and soluble cell surface antigens of *M. haemolytica*. Immunity against the leukotoxin is critical to protection against this organism.[628] Bacterin-toxoids are currently available in the United States and Canada and have a proven beneficial effect.[629,630] *P. multocida* modified live vaccines have been developed with the technologies used in the *M. haemolytica* streptomycin-dependent mutants and are available in combination with that organism. *P. multocida* subunit vaccines containing antigen extracts are also available in combination with *M. haemolytica* subunit vaccines. Protective immunity for *P. multocida* is not as well understood as with *M. haemolytica*. *Pasteurella* bacterins are the only products licensed for use in small ruminants.

H. somnus–killed whole-cell bacterins are commercially available. *H. somnus* is involved in several disease syndromes of cattle, including thrombotic meningoencephalitis, septicemia, arthritis, respiratory infections, and reproductive failure.[631] The ability of the bacterins to control all the different manifestations of *H. somnus* infections is not well defined, although feedlot-based studies in Canada have indicated that the *H. somnus* bacterin does provide a sparing effect against bovine respiratory disease.[632]

REFERENCES

528. Pierson RE, Kainer RA: Clinical classification of pneumonias in cattle, *Bovine Pract* 15:73-79, 1980.
529. Virtala AK et al: Epidemiologic and pathologic characteristics of respiratory tract disease in dairy heifers during the first three months of life, *J Am Vet Med Assoc* 208:2035, 1996.
530. Biss ME et al: Lesions in the carcasses and viscera of very young slaughter calves condemned at post mortem meat inspection, *N Z Vet J* 42:121, 1994.
531. Waltner-Toews D, Martin SW, Meek AH: Dairy calf management, morbidity and mortality in Ontario Holstein herds. II: Age and seasonal patterns, *Prev Vet Med* 4:125, 1986.
532. Curtis CE, Erb HN, White ME: Descriptive epidemiology of calfhood morbidity and mortality in New York Holstein herds, *Prev Vet Med* 5:293, 1988.
533. Sivula NJ et al: Descriptive epidemiology of morbidity and mortality in Minnesota dairy heifer calves, *Prev Vet Med* 27:155, 1996.
534. Van Donkersgoed J et al: Epidemiologic study of enzootic pneumonia in dairy calves in Saskatchewan, *Can J Vet Res* 57:247, 1993.
535. Sargeant JM et al: Production practices, calf health and mortality on six white veal farms in Ontario, *Can J Vet Res* 58:189, 1994.
536. Ribble CS et al: The pattern of fatal fibrinous pneumonia (shipping fever) affecting a large feedlot in Alberta (1985-1988), *Can Vet J* 36:753-757, 1995.
537. Ribble CS et al: Using epidemiology as an aid in feedlot diseases, *Proceedings of the Twenty-fourth Annual Convention of the American Association of Bovine Practitioners,* 1992, pp 122-127.
538. Van Donkersgoed J, Janzen ED, Harland RJ: Epidemiologic features of calf mortality due to haemophilosis in a large feedlot, *Can J Vet* 31:821-825, 1990.
539. Thompson GE: Climactic physiology of cattle: review of the progress of dairy science, *J Dairy Res* 40:441, 1973.
540. Fisher A: Microbial air contamination on large farms, *Acta Veterinaria (BRNO) (Brünn)* 45:235, 1976.
541. Bates DW, Anderson JF: Environmental design for a total animal health care system, *Bovine Pract* 19:4, 1984.
542. Van Donkersgoed J et al: Epidemiological study of enzootic pneumonia in dairy calves in Saskatchewan, *Can J Vet Res* 57:247-254, 1993.
543. Lofgreen GP: Nutrition and management of stressed beef calves, *Vet Clin North Am (Large Anim Pract)* 5:87-101, 1983.
544. MacVean DW et al: Airborne particle concentration and meteorologic conditions associated with pneumonia incidence in feedlot cattle, *Am J Vet Res* 47:2676-2682, 1986.
545. Martin SW et al: Factors associated with mortality and treatment costs in feedlot calves: the Bruce County beef project, 1978, 1979, 1980, *Can J Comp Med* 46:341-349, 1982.
546. Cole NA: Preconditioning calves for the feedlot, *Vet Clin North Am (Food Anim Pract)* 1:401-411, 1985.
547. Robinson RA: Respiratory disease of sheep and goats, *Vet Clin North Am (Large Animal Pract)* 5:539-555, 1983.
548. Kahrs RF: Infectious bovine rhinotracheitis: a review and update, *J Am Vet Med Assoc* 171:1055-1064, 1977.
549. Kahrs RF: *Viral diseases of cattle,* Ames, Iowa, 1981, Iowa State University Press.
550. Roizmann B et al: The family Herpesviridae: an update, *Arch Virol* 123:425-449, 1992.
551. Ryan AM, Hutcheson DP, Womack JE: Type-I interferon genotypes and severity of clinical disease in cattle inoculated with bovine herpesvirus 1, *Am J Vet Res* 54:73-79, 1993.
552. Collett MS, Moenning V, Horzinek MC: Recent advances in pestivirus research, *J Gen Virol* 70:253-266, 1989.
553. Potgieter LND: Bovine respiratory tract disease caused by bovine viral diarrhea virus, *Vet Clin North Am (Food Anim Pract)* 13:471-481, 1997.
554. Grooms DL: Role of bovine viral diarrhea virus in the bovine respiratory disease complex, *Bovine Pract* 32:712, 1999.
555. Potgieter LND et al: Experimental production of bovine respiratory tract disease with bovine viral diarrhea virus, *Am J Vet Res* 45:1582-1585, 1984.
556. Potgieter LND et al: Effect of bovine viral diarrhea virus infection on distribution of infectious bovine rhinotracheitis in calves, *Am J Vet Res* 45:687-690, 1984.
557. Broderson BW, Kelling C: Effects of concurrent experimentally induced bovine respiratory syncytial virus and bovine viral diarrhea virus infection on respiratory tract and enteric diseases in calves, *Am J Vet Res* 59:1423-1430, 1998.
558. Richer L, Marois P, Lamontagne L: Association of bovine viral diarrhea virus with multiple infections in bovine respiratory disease outbreaks, *Can Vet J* 29:713-717, 1988.
559. Baker JC, Ellis JA, Clark EG: Bovine respiratory syncytial virus, *Vet Clin North Am (Food Anim Pract)* 13:425-454, 1997.
560. Duncan RB, Potgieter LND: Antigenic diversity of respiratory syncytial viruses and its implication for immunoprophylaxis of ruminants, *Vet Microbiol* 37:319-341,1993.
561. Alansari H et al: Analysis of ruminant respiratory syncytial virus isolates by RNAse protection of the G glycoprotein transcripts, *J Vet Diagn Invest* 11:215-220, 1999.
562. Baker JC et al: Identification of subgroups of bovine respiratory syncytial virus, *J Clin Microbiol* 30:1120-1126, 1992.
563. Furze J et al: Antigenic heterogeneity of the attachment protein of bovine respiratory syncytial virus, *J Gen Virol* 75:363-370, 1994.
564. Baker JC: Bovine respiratory syncytial virus: pathogenesis, clinical signs, diagnosis, treatment and prevention, *Compend Cont Educ Pract Vet* 8:F31-F38, 1986.
565. Ames TR: The epidemiology of BRSV infection, *Vet Med* 88:881-885, 1993.
566. Kimman TG et al: Epidemiological study of bovine respiratory syncytial virus infections in calves: influence of maternal antibodies on the outcome of disease, *Vet Rec* 123:104-109, 1988.

567. Belknap EB et al: The role of passive immunity in bovine respiratory syncytial virus infected calves, *J Infect Dis* 163:470-476, 1991.

568. De Jong MCM et al: Quantitative investigation of population persistence and recurrent outbreaks of bovine respiratory syncytial virus on dairy farms, *Am J Vet Res* 57:628-633, 1996.

569. Collins JK et al: Association of bovine respiratory syncytial virus with atypical interstitial pneumonia in feedlot cattle, *Am J Vet Res* 49:1045-1049, 1988.

570. Bryson DG et al: Studies on the pathogenesis and interspecies transmission of respiratory syncytial virus isolated from sheep, *Am J Vet Res* 49:1424-1430, 1988.

571. Kapil S, Basaraba RJ: Infectious bovine rhinotracheitis, parainfluenza-3, and respiratory coronavirus, *Vet Clin North Am (Food Anim Pract)* 13:455-469,1997.

572. Evermann JF, Henry BE: Herpetic infections of cattle: a comparison of bovine cytomegalovirus and infectious bovine rhinotracheitis, *Compend Cont Educ Pract Vet* 2:205-213, 1989.

573. Russell WC: Adenoviridae. In Francki FIB et al, editors: Classification and nomenclature of viruses. Fifth report of the international committee on taxonomy of viruses, *Arch Virol Suppl* 2:140-144, 1991.

574. Mattson D: Ovine and caprine adenoviruses. In Howard JL, ed: *Current veterinary therapy 3*, Philadelphia, 1993, WB Saunders, p 461.

575. Lehmkuhl HD, Cutlip RC, Brogden KA: Seroepidemiologic survey of adenovirus infection in lambs, *Am J Vet Res* 54:1277-1279, 1993.

576. Davies DH, Herceg M, Thurley DC: Experimental infection of lambs with an adenovirus followed by *Pasteurella haemolytica*, *Vet Microbiol* 7:369-381, 1982.

577. Cutlip RC et al: Lesions in lambs experimentally infected with ovine adenovirus serotype 6 and *Pasteurella haemolytica*, *J Vet Diagn Invest* 3:296-303, 1996.

578. McNulty MS et al: Coronavirus infection of the bovine respiratory tract, *Vet Microbiol* 9:425-434, 1984.

579. Storz J, Stine L, Liem A: Coronavirus isolations from nasal swabs samples in cattle with signs of respiratory tract disease after shipping, *J Am Vet Med Assoc* 208:1452-1455, 1996.

580. Martin SW et al: The association of titers to bovine coronavirus with treatment for bovine respiratory disease and weight gain in feedlot calves, *Can J Vet Res* 62:257-261, 1998.

581. Rosenquist BD: Bovine rhinoviruses. In Howard JL, ed: *Current veterinary therapy 3*, Philadelphia, 1993, WB Saunders, p 437.

582. Smith AW et al: Isolation and partial characterization of a calicivirus from calves, *Am J Vet Res* 44:851-855, 1983.

583. Al-Ghamdi G et al: Serotyping *Pasteurella haemolytica* isolates from the upper midwest, *J Vet Diagn Invest* 12:576-578, 2000.

584. Chirino-Trejo JM, Prescott JF: The identification and antimicrobial susceptibility of anaerobic bacteria from pneumonic cattle lungs, *Can J Comp Med* 47:270-276, 1983.

585. Hjerpe CA: The role of mycoplasma in bovine respiratory disease, *Vet Med* 75:297-298, 1980.

586. Jensen R et al: Shipping fever pneumonia in yearling feedlot cattle, *J Am Vet Med Assoc* 169:500-506, 1976.

587. Stalheim OHV: Mycoplasmal respiratory diseases of ruminants: a review and update, *J Am Vet Med Assoc* 182:403-406, 1983.

588. Bennett RH, Jasper DE: Immunosuppression of humoral and cell-mediated responses in calves associated with inoculation of *Mycoplasma bovis*, *Am J Vet Res* 38:1731-1738, 1977.

589. Jarstrand C, Camner P, Philipson K: *Mycoplasma pneumoniae* tracheobronchial clearance, *Am Rev Resp Dis* 110:41-44, 1975.

590. Palotaz JL, Christensen NR: Bovine respiratory infections. I, Psittacosis-lymphogranuloma venereum group of viruses as etiologic agents, *J Am Vet Med Assoc* 134:222-230, 1959.

591. Davies DH, Hercez M, Thurley DC: Experimental infection of lambs with an adenovirus followed by *Pasteurella haemolytica*, *Vet Microbiol* 7:369-381, 1982.

592. Yates WDG: A review of infectious bovine rhinotracheitis, shipping fever pneumonia and viral-bacterial synergism in respiratory disease of cattle, *Can J Comp Med* 46:225-263, 1982.

593. Brown LN, Dillman RC, Dierks RE: The *Hemophilus somnus* complex, Proceedings of the meeting of the U.S. Animal Health Association, 1970.

594. Pass DA, Thomson RG, Ashton GC: Regional histological variations of the nasal mucosa in cattle, *Can J Comp Med* 35:212-217, 1971.

595. Clinkenbeard KD et al: Role of *Pasteurella haemolytica* leukotoxin in virulence and immunity in shipping fever pneumonia, *Compend Cont Educ* 14:1249-1262, 1992.

596. Slocombe RF et al: Importance of neutrophils in the pathogenesis of acute pneumonic pasteurellosis in calves, *Am J Vet Res* 46:2253-2258, 1985.

597. Whitely LE et al: *Pasteurella haemolytica* AI and bovine respiratory disease: a review of its pathogenesis, *J Vet Int Med* 6:11-22, 1992.

598. Ames TR et al: Pulmonary response to intratracheal challenge with pasteurella, *Can J Comp Med* 49:395-400, 1985.

599. Czuprynski CJ, Hamilton HL: Bovine neutrophils ingest but do not kill *Haemophilus somnus*, *Infect Immun* 50:431-436, 1985.

600. Thompson KG, Little PB: Effect of *Haemophilus somnus* on bovine endothelial cells in organ culture, *Am J Vet Res* 42:748-754, 1981.

601. Adegboye DS et al: *Mycoplasma bovis*-associated pneumonia and arthritis complicated with pyogranulomatous tenosynovitis in calves, *J Am Vet Med Assoc* 209:647-649, 1996.

602. Walz PH et al: Otitis media in preweaned Holstein dairy calves in Michigan due to *Mycoplasma bovis*, *J Vet Diagn Invest* 9:250-254, 1997.

603. Osorio FA et al: Detection of bovine respiratory syncytial virus using a heterologous antigen capture enzyme immunoassay, *J Vet Diagn Invest* 1:210-214, 1989.

604. Oberst RD et al: Identifying bovine respiratory syncytial virus by reverse transcription-polymerase chain reaction with oligonucleotide hybridizations, *J Clin Microbiol* 31:1237-1240, 1993.

605. Westenbrink F, Kimman TG: Immunoglobulin M-specific enzyme-linked immunoabsorbent assay for serodiagnosis of bovine respiratory syncytial virus infections, *Am J Vet Res* 48:1132-1137, 1987.

606. Allen JW et al: The microbial flora of the respiratory tract in feedlot calves: associations between the nasopharyngeal and bronchoalveolar lavage cultures, *Can J Vet Res* 55:341-346, 1991.

607. Apley M: Ancillary therapy of bovine respiratory disease, *Vet Clin North Am (Food Anim Pract)* 13:575-592, 1997.

608. Chin AC et al: Anti-inflammatory benefits of tilmicosin in calves with *Pasteurella haemolytica*-infected lungs, *Am J Vet Res* 6:765-771, 1998.

609. Roth JA, Kaeberle ML: In vivo effect of ascorbic acid on neutrophil function in healthy and dexamethasone-treated cattle, *Am J Vet Res* 46:2434-2436, 1985.

610. Frank GH et al: Effects of tilmicosin treatment of *Pasteurella haemolytica* organisms in nasal secretion specimens of calves with respiratory tract disease, *Am J Vet Res* 61:525-529, 2000.

611. Schujmann FJ, Janzen ED, McKinnon JJ: Prophylactic tilmicosin medication of feedlot calves at arrival, *Can Vet J* 31:285-288, 1990.

612. Harland RJ et al: Efficacy of parenteral antibiotics for disease prophylaxis in feedlot calves, *Can Vet J* 32:163-168, 1991.

613. Morck DW et al: Prophylactic efficacy of tilmicosin for bovine respiratory tract disease, *J Am Vet Med Assoc* 202:273-277, 1993.

614. Martin SW: Vaccination: is it effective in preventing respiratory disease and influencing weight gain in feedlot calves? *Can Vet J* 24:10-19, 1983.

615. Martin SW et al: Factors associated with morbidity and mortality in feedlot calves: the Bruce County beef project, year two, *Can J Comp Med* 45:103-112, 1981.

616. Janzen ED: Clinical management of bovine respiratory disease, *Can Vet J* 32:215-218, 1991.

617. Hodgins DG, Shewen PE: Passive immunity to *Pasteurella haemolytica* A1 in dairy calves: effects of preparturient vaccination of the dams, *Can J Vet Res* 58:31-35, 1994.

618. Ellis JA et al: Effects of perinatal vaccination on humoral and cellular immune response in cows and young calves, *J Am Vet Med Assoc* 208:393-400, 1996.

619. Todd JD: Intranasal vaccination of cattle against IBR and PI-3: field and laboratory observations in dairy, beef, and neonatal calf populations, *Dev Biol Stand* 33:391-395, 1976.

620. Flores EF et al: Efficacy of a deletion mutant herpesvirus-1 (BHV-1) vaccine that allows serologic differentiation of vaccinated from naturally infected animals, *J Vet Diagn Invest* 5:534-540, 1993.

621. Bolin SR: Control of bovine viral diarrhea infection by use of vaccination, *Vet Clin North Am (Food Anim Pract)* 11:615-625, 1995.

622. Baker JC, Velicer LF: Bovine respiratory syncytial virus vaccination: current status and future vaccine development, *Compend Cont Educ Pract Vet* 13:1323, 1991.

623. Kimman TG et al: Priming for local and systemic antibody responses to bovine respiratory syncytial virus: effect of amount of virus, virus replication, route of administration and maternal antibodies, *Vet Immunol Immunopathol* 22:145-160, 1989.

624. Kimman TG et al: A severe outbreak of respiratory tract disease associated with bovine respiratory syncytial virus probably enhanced by vaccination with a modified live vaccine, *Vet Q* 11:250-253, 1989.

625. Schultz RD: Certain factors to consider when designing a bovine vaccination program, *Proceedings of the Twenty-sixth Annual convention of the American Association of Bovine Practitioners*, Albuquerque, 1993, pp 19-26.

626. Confer AW, Panciera RJ, Mosier DA: Bovine pneumonic pasteurellosis: immunity to *Pasteurella haemolytica*, *J Am Vet Med Assoc* 10:1308-1316, 1988.

627. Srinand S et al: Efficacy of various vaccines against pneumonia pasteurellosis in cattle: a meta-analysis, *Prev Vet Med* 25:7-18, 1996.

628. Srinand S et al: Evaluation of three experimental subunit vaccines against pneumonia pasteurellosis, *Vaccine* 14:147-154, 1996.

629. Srinand S et al: Evaluation of efficacy of three commercial vaccines against experimental bovine pneumonia pasteurellosis, *Vet Micro* 52:81-90, 1996.

630. Jim K, Guichon T, Shaw G: Protecting feedlot calves from pneumonic pasteurellosis, *Vet Med* 83:1084-1087, 1988.

631. Beeman KB: *Haemophilus somnus* of cattle: an overview, *Compend Cont Educ Pract Vet* 7:S259-S263, 1985.

632. Ribble CS, Jim GK, Janzen ED: Efficacy of immunization of feedlot calves with a commercial *Haemophilus* bacterin, *Can J Vet Res* 52:191-198, 1988.

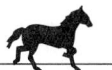

THE INTERSTITIAL PNEUMONIAS

JOHN A. SMITH

DAN GROOMS

Understanding of the "atypical" interstitial pneumonias has undergone considerable evolution in the past 15 to 20 years. Unfortunately, confusion still exists, particularly in regard to terminology. Terms such as acute bovine pulmonary emphysema (ABPE), atypical interstitial pneumonia (AIP), fog fever, pulmonary adenomatosis, farmer's lung, and acute respiratory distress syndrome (ARDS) have been used interchangeably for all of the conditions that follow. This text uses a classification presented by Breeze,[633] which places the interstitial pneumonias in four groups: (1) the acute respiratory distress syndromes (ARDS), (2) hypersensitivity diseases, (3) chronic conditions that may be sequelae of ARDS or hypersensitivity diseases, and (4) parasitic diseases. The bovine respiratory syncytial virus also has been associated with an "atypical interstitial pneumonia" of feedlot cattle; this disease is discussed in relation to the respiratory disease complex of cattle, sheep, and goats earlier in this chapter.

REFERENCE

633. Breeze RG: Respiratory disease in adult cattle, *Vet Clin North Am (Food Anim Pract)* 1:311-346, 1985.

▣ *Acute Respiratory Distress Syndromes*

An acute respiratory distress syndrome (ARDS) is any respiratory condition characterized clinically by a sudden onset of (usually severe) dyspnea and pathologically by any combination of the following pulmonary lesions: (1) congestion and edema, (2) hyaline membranes, (3) alveolar epithelial hyperplasia, and (4) interstitial emphysema.

Acute Bovine Pulmonary Edema and Emphysema

DEFINITION AND ETIOLOGY. Acute bovine pulmonary edema and emphysema (ABPEE), classically known as "fog fever," is an ARDS of adult (over 2 years old) cattle that are changed from dry, sparse forages to lush green pastures. It is caused by the conversion of L-tryptophan ingested in the lush forages to a pneumotoxic compound (3-methylindole), which leads to the development of pulmonary edema, alveolar epithelial hyperplasia, hyaline membranes, and emphysema.[634]

CLINICAL SIGNS AND DIFFERENTIAL DIAGNOSIS. Adult brood cows are most commonly affected because this is the type of animal most likely to be subjected to the abrupt pasture change required to produce the condition. No breed is resistant.[634] The type of pasture appears to be unimportant, as long as it is lush; ABPEE has been reported on a wide variety of grasses, alfalfa, rape, kale, and turnip tops.[635] Signs usually occur within 2 weeks of the pasture change.[634] In severe cases there is an acute onset of very severe dyspnea with a loud expiratory grunt, frothing at the mouth, mouth breathing, and tachypnea (35 to 75 breaths/min).[635] The animals are obviously distressed (as opposed to exhibiting the typical depression that occurs with infectious diseases) and stand with the head and neck extended and elevated and the nostrils dilated.[636] Temperature and heart rate may be elevated secondary to the severe dyspnea and hypoxia.[636] On auscultation, the breath sounds are usually surprisingly soft in view of the gross dyspnea and tachypnea; a few crackles may be heard.[635] Even mild exercise increases the dyspnea and may precipitate collapse and death. As many as 30% of severely affected patients may die, usually within 2 days.[635] Those that survive typically show a dramatic improvement after 3 days.[635] Recovering patients and those that are less severely affected exhibit tachypnea (50 to 80 breaths/min), hyperpnea, harsh breath sounds, and crackles and wheezes, particularly in the caudal lung fields.[635] Subcutaneous emphysema may develop. The demeanor of the entire group tends to become more tranquil.[635] In cattle that have repeated episodes of nonfatal ABPEE, a chronic respiratory condition characterized by diffuse pulmonary fibrosis and alveolitis may develop.[637] For purposes of differential diagnosis, it is important to note that coughing is not prominent in the individual or the group.[635] The main differential diagnoses are those diseases that cause ARDS in pastured adult cattle, usually in outbreak form. The association of ABPEE with the typical management conditions (i.e., changes of pasture) and the absence of coughing, signs of sepsis, and adventitious lung sounds in early cases are also very important features. Primary considerations should include the other plant toxicities (moldy sweet potatoes, perilla mint, and possibly others) that can be differentiated only by identifying the source. Parasitic bronchitis may also be considered, but it is characterized by more coughing, signs of depression, and more prominent adventitious sounds.

CLINICAL PATHOLOGY. There are no significant hematologic or biochemical changes.[636] A stress leukogram is often seen.

PATHOPHYSIOLOGY. L-Tryptophan in lush forages is converted by ruminal microorganisms to indole acetic acid and eventually to 3-methylindole (3-MI), which is rapidly absorbed from the rumen into the blood. Metabolism of 3-MI by the cytochrome P-450 mixed function oxidase system in the nonciliated bronchiolar epithelial (Clara) cells and type 1 pneumocytes results in one or more highly reactive intermediates that bind to intracellular proteins or other macromolecules. It is thought that these intermediates produce the damage to these cells. These intermediates are detoxified by conjugation with glutathione.[638] Cellular damage results in degeneration, necrosis, exfoliation of type 1 pneumocytes and Clara cells, and edema. These lesions in turn cause hyaline membrane formation, proliferation of type 2 pneumocytes, and, to a lesser extent, proliferation of Clara cells.[638] The proliferation of type 2 cells is also known as adenomatosis. Emphysema is probably secondary to the severe dyspnea.[638]

EPIDEMIOLOGY. As indicated, ABPEE is consistently related to management practices in which hungry adult cattle are suddenly moved from sparse, dry grazing to lush green pastures. The British name "fog fever" arose from the association of the disease with "fog" pastures, which are the lush green regrowth pastures after hay or silage has been cut. The problem usually occurs in the fall. In the typical pattern in the western United States, cattle are moved from dry summer range onto irrigated or fertilized aftermath pastures.[634] The disease usually appears as a herd outbreak, but individuals may be affected to widely varying degrees; morbidity rate commonly approaches 50%, with a case fatality rate as high as 30%. Nursing calves are apparently not at risk, and yearlings are less susceptible than adults.[641]

NECROPSY FINDINGS. In animals that die of ABPEE, ecchymotic to petechial hemorrhages occur in the larynx, trachea, and bronchi, and frothy fluid is present in the airways. Congestion, edema, and hyaline membranes cause deep red-to-purple coloration of the cranial lung lobes and a smooth, glistening appearance to the cut surface. Interstitial emphysema with large bullae and gelatinous yellow interlobular edema is common. Histologically eosinophilic hyaline membranes line alveoli and alveolar ducts, and there are edema and proliferation of epithelial cells.[634] In animals that are killed after 3 to 4 days, emphysema and edema are less obvious, and the lungs tend to be light brown, firm, heavy, and rubbery. There is severe diffuse alveolar epithelial hyperplasia ("adenomatosis"), and large mononuclear cells, multinucleated giant cells, and hyaline membranes are present in alveolar spaces. Edema, eosinophils, and interstitial cells occupy the septae.[634]

TREATMENT AND PROGNOSIS. The stress of handling cattle can precipitate further losses. Some authors maintain that most cases in an outbreak occur within 4 days, that removing the herd from the pasture does not prevent additional cases, and that leaving the herd on the pasture does not result in additional cases; consequently the recommendation has been to handle severely affected cattle only if necessary to remove them to shade or to slaughter.[640] Others[634,641] recommend careful removal from the offending pasture. Antihistamines, corticosteroids, epinephrine, atropine, diethylcarbamazine, and diuretics are alleged to be of palliative value,[634,643] but none of these has been properly tested.[634] Pretreatment with antagonists to postulated mediators of inflammation, including acetylsalicylic acid, mepyramine, sodium meclofenamate, diethylcarbamazine citrate, and betamethasone, did not influence the clinical course or lesions of experimental 3-MI toxicity.[642] Likewise, pretreatment with chloramphenicol or disodium cromoglycate failed to alter signs or lesions.[642] However, in one small trial, flunixin meglumine at 1.1 mg/kg IV daily given after the onset of 3-MI–induced disease in calves was effective in lessening signs and lesions.[643] Recovery often occurs without therapy in the less severe cases. In view of the dangers of handling affected cattle, the questionable efficacy of medical treatment, the probable irreversible nature of severe lesions, and the probability of spontaneous recovery in less severe cases, the best treatment may be no treatment. If treatment must be attempted, affected cattle should be handled very cautiously, and furosemide (0.4 to 1 mg/kg IM or IV twice daily)[636] and flunixin meglumine (0.5 to 1.1 mg/kg IM or IV daily to twice daily) may be given. Most fatalities occur in the first 2 days. Severely affected animals that survive may develop chronic emphysema or heart failure secondary to cor pulmonale.[640] Moderate to mild cases often show marked improvement after day three, with recovery over about 10 days; relapses do not occur.

PREVENTION. Prevention is based on management and prophylactic drugs. Management strategies that prevent the exposure of susceptible cattle to potentially toxic pastures include the following:

1. Place the cattle in a drylot, feed palatable hay for several days, and turn them onto the lush pasture for 2 hours the first day. Gradually decrease the amount of hay fed and increase the time on pasture over a period of 10 to 12 days.[640]
2. Delay use of lush pastures until after a hard frost.[641]
3. Cut and windrow the pasture before turning cattle out.[642]
4. Use the pasture for young stock (less than 15 months old) or sheep or other livestock[641]; turn adult cattle out only after the pasture has been thoroughly grazed over.
5. Use the pasture before it becomes particularly lush.[638]
6. Use continuous strip-grazing.[640]

Because such management changes are frequently not feasible, prophylactic medication is a promising alternative. Monensin or lasalocid at 200 mg/head/day PO reduces the conversion of tryptophan to 3-MI.[635] Treatment with monensin should be started at least 1 day before pasture change and should be continued an additional 10 days, whereas lasalocid requires a longer pretreatment period of 6 days.[644] For example, 1 kg/head/day of a protein or energy supplement containing 0.15% Rumensin 60 supplies 200 mg of monensin.[634] Monensin or lasalocid are not expected to be beneficial after the onset of signs.[634] Future possibilities include blockers of the mixed function oxidase system and enhancers of intracellular glutathione levels.

REFERENCES

634. Breeze RG: Respiratory disease in adult cattle, *Vet Clin North Am (Food Anim Pract)* 1:311-346, 1985.
635. Selman IE et al: Differential diagnosis of pulmonary disease in adult cattle in Britain, *Bovine Pract* 12:63-74, 1977.
636. Dickinson EO, Spencer GR, Gorham JR: Experimental induction of an acute respiratory syndrome in cattle resembling bovine pulmonary emphysema, *Vet Rec* 80:487-489, 1967.
637. Ciszewski DK, Baker JC, Slocombe RF: Acute bovine pulmonary emphysema and edema, *Compend Cont Educ Pract Vet* 10:767-774, 1988.
638. Breeze RG, Carlson JR: Chemical-induced lung injury in domestic animals, *Adv Vet Sci Comp Educ* 26:201-231, 1982.
639. Heron BR, Suther DE: A retrospective investigation and random sample survey of acute bovine pulmonary emphysema in Northern California, *Bovine Pract* 14:2-8, 1979.
640. Blood DC, Radostits OM, Henderson JA: *Veterinary medicine*, ed 6, London, 1983, Baillière Tindall, pp 1255-1261.
641. Blake JT, Thomas DW: Acute bovine pulmonary emphysema in Utah, *J Am Vet Med Assoc* 158:2047-2052, 1971.
642. Breeze RG: Fog fever and heaves: studies on respiratory diseases of adult cattle and horses, *Proceedings of the Annual Scientific Meeting of the American College of Veterinary Internal Medicine*, Dallas, 1978, pp 87-119.
643. Gibbs HA: The use of antiprostaglandins in respiratory disease in cattle, *Proceedings of the Tenth Annual Food Animal Medicine Conference*, Ohio State University, Columbus, 1984, pp 62-79.
644. Wikse SE, Craig TM, Hutcheson DP: Nutritional and dietary interrelationships with diseases of grazing beef cattle, *Vet Clin North Am (Food Anim Pract)* 7:143-152, 1991.

Acute Respiratory Distress Syndrome of Feedlot Cattle

DEFINITION AND ETIOLOGY. In feedlot cattle, an acute respiratory distress syndrome occurs sporadically and is commonly referred to as atypical interstitial pneumonia (AIP). The exact cause of this syndrome in feedlot cattle is often undetermined. Feedlot management practices typically do not include exposure of cattle to forages high in L-tryptophan. The sporadic nature of the disease usually rules out exposure to toxic causes of ARDS such as moldy sweet potatoes.[645] A higher incidence of ARDS in feedlots has been reported in summer and fall months, suggesting that dust may be involved.[646] Using immunohistochemistry for detection, evidence of BRSV has been found in some cases of feedlot ARDS and may be a factor in AIP.[647] Similar to fog fever, abnormal production of or metabolism of 3-methylindole may also be involved.[648]

EPIDEMIOLOGY. Occurrence of ARDS in feedlot cattle is sporadic and can occur at all stages of the feeding period.[646] In one study, mortality from ARDS in feedlot calves and yearlings was reported to be 0.498% and 0.107%, respectively. In Colorado a higher incidence of ARDS was reported in the summer and fall, possibly related to increased amounts of dust.[646]

CLINICAL SIGNS AND DIFFERENTIAL DIAGNOSIS. Feedlot cattle affected by ARDS are often found dead in the pen. Clinical presentation includes rapid onset of tachypnea and expiratory dyspnea. Calves typically stand with their heads extended and exhibit open-mouth breathing. Frothing from the mouth may also be observed. Rectal temperatures are variable, ranging from normal to elevated. Physical examination may reveal cyanosis, tachycardia, and subcutaneous emphysema that extends from the cervical to dorsal thoracic area.[649] Auscultation of lungs reveals dull areas throughout the lungs along with some crackles. Differential diagnoses of bronchopneumonia, tracheal edema, tracheal obstruction, and hypersensitivity pneumonitis should be considered.

NECROPSY FINDING. When examined grossly, lungs fail to collapse when the thoracic cavity is entered.[650] They are typically dark pink to red, rubbery to firm feeling, and heavy when removed from the thorax. Foam often fills the airways and prominent interlobular edema and emphysema are present. This is especially noticeable in the diaphragmatic lobes.[650]

TREATMENT AND PREVENTION. Because of the similar pathophysiologic mechanisms to those of ABPEE, similar treatments are recommended. High case fatality rates may warrant immediate slaughter salvage if proper drug withdrawals are observed.[651] No control measures for this syndrome, because it occurs in feedlot cattle, have been suggested. Management strategies to reduce dust, abrupt dietary changes, and infection with BRSV may be of some value.

REFERENCES

645. Johnson B: Nutritional and dietary interrelationships with diseases of cattle, *Vet Clin North Am (Food Anim Pract)* 7:133-142,1991.
646. Jensen R et al: Atypical interstitial pneumonia in yearling feedlot cattle, *J Am Vet Med Assoc* 169:507-510, 1976.
647. Collins JK et al: Association of bovine respiratory syncytial virus with atypical interstitial pneumonia in feedlot cattle, *Am J Vet Res* 49:1045-1049, 1988.
648. Glock RD, DeGroot BD: Sudden death of feedlot cattle, *J Anim Sci* 76:315-319, 1998.
649. Kerr LA, Linnabary RD: A review of interstitial pneumonia in cattle, *Vet Hum Toxicol* 31:247-254, 1989.
650. Wiske SE: Feedlot cattle pneumonias, *Vet Clin North Am (Food Anim Pract)* 1:289-310, 1985.
651. Griffin D: Feedlot diseases, *Vet Clin North Am (Food Anim Pract)* 14:199-231,1998.

4-Ipomeanol (Moldy Sweet Potato) Toxicity

DEFINITION AND ETIOLOGY. This ARDS is caused by the ingestion of a furanoterpenoid toxin produced by sweet potatoes (*Ipomoea batatas*) in response to infestation with the fungus *Fusarium solani (javanicum)*. It should be emphasized that this disease is an intoxication and not an allergic response to the fungus.[652]

CLINICAL SIGNS AND DIFFERENTIAL DIAGNOSIS. There is an acute onset of tachypnea, tachycardia, hyperpnea, and dyspnea, with loud expiratory grunting, frothing at the mouth, extension of the head and neck, flaring of the nostrils, and frequent deep coughing. Crackles and harsh bronchial sounds are heard on auscultation.[653] Signs usually occur within 1 day of exposure, and deaths may occur 2 to 5 days later.[652] Differential diagnoses are as for acute bovine pulmonary emphysema (see earlier discussion), which this condition closely resembles, except for the history of exposure and the more prominent cough and adventitious lung sounds.

PATHOPHYSIOLOGY. When *F. solani* (or closely related species) grows on sweet potatoes, the potato produces several 3-substituted furans, including 4-hydroxymyoporone, which is hepatotoxic. This is converted by the fungus to a series of pneumotoxins, the most abundant of which is 4-ipomeanol. When ingested by cattle in sufficient amounts, this toxin is absorbed, carried to the lungs in the blood, and converted to a highly reactive metabolite by a cytochrome P-450–dependent mixed function oxidase system.[652] From this point the pathogenesis is similar to that of ABPEE; that is, the toxin binds to intracellular macromolecules in the cell, causing cellular damage, particularly in Clara cells, type I pneumocytes, and endothelium; edema, hemorrhage, cellular necrosis, hyaline membrane formation, and proliferation of cuboidal epithelium result, with secondary emphysema.

EPIDEMIOLOGY. The disease usually occurs in outbreak form when groups of cattle are fed damaged sweet potatoes. Morbidity and case fatality rates are high. Calves nursing affected cows are unaffected.[654]

NECROPSY FINDINGS. The lungs are wet, firm, and large and fail to collapse. Hemorrhages, yellow gelatinous edema fluid, and emphysema with bullae occur throughout. Lobules are dark red and firm.[653,654] Microscopic lesions include edema, emphysema, hyaline membranes, hemorrhage, mixed interstitial infiltrates, alveolar epithelial hyperplasia, peribronchiolar fibrosis, and bronchiolitis obliterans.[654]

TREATMENT AND CONTROL. Treatment has not been investigated. Because the pathophysiologic mechanisms are similar to those of ABPEE, similar recommendations are offered here: handle affected animals with extreme care; if treatment is attempted, furosemide (0.4 to 1.0 mg/kg IM or IV twice daily) and flunixin meglumine (0.5 to 1.1 mg/kg IM or IV daily to twice daily) may be given. The prognosis for moderate to severe cases is grave, regardless of management. Because toxicity is difficult to predict and is usually severe and irreversible when it occurs, the feeding of mold-damaged sweet potatoes should be strictly prevented.

REFERENCES

652. Breeze RG: Respiratory disease in adult cattle, *Vet Clin North Am (Food Anim Pract)* 1:311-346, 1985.
653. Doster AR et al: Effects of 4-ipomeanol, a product from mold-damaged sweet potatoes, on the bovine lung, *Vet Pathol* 15:367-375, 1978.
654. Peckham JC et al: Atypical interstitial pneumonia in cattle fed moldy sweet potatoes, *J Am Vet Med Assoc* 160:169-172, 1972.

Perilla (*Perilla frutescens*) Ketone Toxicity

DEFINITION AND ETIOLOGY. Perilla ketone toxicity is an ARDS caused by ingestion of a pneumotoxin found in the leaves and seeds of *Perilla frutescens*, a common weed in the southeastern United States. This plant is also known as purple mint, perilla mint, wild coleus, and beefsteak plant.[655] It is an erect herbaceous annual about 2 m high, with characteristic square stems, an aromatic odor, and opposite, coarsely serrated ovate leaves 5 to 10 cm long and 4 to 8 cm wide, with a purplish tint at maturity. The seed/flower stage, which occurs in August to October, appears to be most toxic.[655] The flowers are small, white to purple blooms on a long raceme.[655] The plant prefers semishade, such as damp, open wooded areas.

CLINICAL SIGNS AND DIFFERENTIAL DIAGNOSIS. Animals are often found dead.[655] Signs observed include a sudden onset of moderate to severe dyspnea, wheezing, frothing at the mouth, and an expiratory heave or grunt.[655,656] In less severe cases the cow may pant.[656] Exertion worsens the signs and may precipitate death. Mature cows are most often affected, but deaths have been reported in yearlings and calves.[655] Death occurs in 3 to 7 days in experimental toxicity.[655] Differential diagnoses are as for acute bovine pulmonary emphysema (see earlier discussion), which this condition closely resembles and from which it can be differentiated only by history of exposure.

PATHOPHYSIOLOGY. The volatile oils of *P. frutescens* contain a number of 3-substituted furans that are chemically similar to 4-ipomeanol, the moldy sweet potato toxin. One of these, perilla ketone, predominates in the later growing season (when most toxicities occur) and has been shown to be pneumotoxic when given parenterally to mice, hamsters, goats, calves, and sheep.[655] The toxin is absorbed from the rumen, carried to the lungs through the blood, and probably metabolized to the toxic form by the mixed function oxidase system, as for 4-ipomeanol and 3-MI.[657] The pathogenesis from this point parallels that of ABPEE or moldy sweet potato toxicity.

EPIDEMIOLOGY. *P. frutescens* seems to thrive in late summer, when pastures in the southeastern United States are frequently dry and dormant.[656] This also corresponds with the more toxic stage of the plant.[655] Cattle normally avoid the plant when other pasture is available but may be forced to consume it during this critical period.[656] However, under experimental conditions, calves were noted to prefer the mint.[655] The preseed stage appears to be of relatively low toxicity; the green seed-stage plant is most toxic, especially the seed parts; dried hay from seed-stage plants is less toxic than green plants but is still potentially lethal; and frosted plants appear to have relatively low toxicity.[655] The exact toxic dose is unknown, but 2.3 kg of green seed-stage plant and 11.2 kg of hay were lethal for cattle in one trial.[655]

NECROPSY FINDINGS. The lungs are distended (often bearing the impressions of the ribs), fail to collapse, and are moist, heavy, edematous, and emphysematous. There are often bullae, pleural effusions, and froth in the airways. Histologic characteristics are edema, extensive alveolar epithelial hyperplasia, emphysema, and congestion.

TREATMENT AND CONTROL. Treatment has not been investigated. On the basis of the similar pathophysiologic mechanisms, the recommendations for acute bovine pulmonary emphysema should be followed (see earlier discussion). The prognosis for severe cases is grave, regardless of management. Cattle should be provided sufficient forage so that they do not seek out perilla mint; once they have begun to eat it, they should be fenced away from stands of the plant, and other forage should be provided.

REFERENCES

655. Kerr LA, Johnson BJ, Burrows GE: Intoxication of cattle by *Perilla frutescens* (purple mint), *Vet Human Toxicol* 28:412-416, 1986.
656. Linnabary RD et al: Acute bovine pulmonary emphysema (ABPE): perilla ketone, another cause, *Proceedings of the Twentieth Annual Meeting of the American Association of Veterinary Laboratory Diagnosticians,* Minneapolis, 1977, pp 323-326.
657. Breeze RG: Respiratory disease in adult cattle, *Vet Clin North Am (Food Anim Pract)* 1:311-346, 1985.

Other Toxic Plants

Zieria arborescens (stinkwood) leaves cause a fatal acute respiratory distress syndrome (ARDS) in Tasmanian and Eastern Australian cattle after ingestion of 15 to 30 kg over 2 to 4 weeks. An oil isolated from the leaves has produced the same lung lesion in rabbits. The signs are as for the other ARDS: acute tachypnea, grunting, extension of the head, mouth breathing, abdominal respiration, tachycardia, and fever secondary to the respiratory effort. Death occurs in 1 to 21 days; some animals survive. Lesions include massive pulmonary edema and emphysema.[658] Treatment has not been investigated, and recommendations as for acute bovine pulmonary emphysema (see earlier discussion) are suggested. As mentioned in relation to ABPEE, *Brassica* spp. (rape, kale, turnip tops) are currently regarded as one of the types of pasture that can precipitate the 3-MI–associated disease. The possibility that other specific toxins may be identified in these species has not been excluded. Morbidity and mortality rates appear to be much higher on *Brassica* spp. pastures than on other lush forages.[659] The hepatotoxic effects of pyrrolizine alkaloids are well known, but they also cause lung lesions. Lung lesions develop only in animals with chronic liver lesions, and the minimum dose necessary to produce lung lesions is never less than that which is hepatotoxic; therefore signs of liver disease usually predominate. *Crotalaria* and *Trichoderma* spp. are the most common offenders; to a lesser extent, *Senecio* spp. are a cause. Horses, sheep, cattle, and pigs have been affected. Pulmonary lesions include edema, congestion, hemorrhage, proliferation of bronchiolar and alveolar epithelial cells with megalocytosis, and interstitial fibrosis and cellular infiltration. As with 3-MI, 4-ipomeanol, and perilla ketone, the toxicity of the pyrrolizine alkaloids depends on activation by the mixed function oxidase system; in this case, however, the toxin is probably formed in the liver and spills over into the blood to reach the lungs. Vascular endothelium is probably the primary target for injury (vs. the Clara cells and type 1 pneumocytes in the other ARDS).[660]

REFERENCES

658. Blood DC, Radostits OM, Henderson JA: *Veterinary medicine,* ed 6, London, 1983, Baillière Tindall, p 1188.
659. Breeze RG: Respiratory disease in adult cattle, *Vet Clin North Am (Food Anim Pract)* 1:311-346, 1985.
660. Breeze RG, Carlson JR: Chemical-induced lung injury in domestic animals, *Adv Vet Sci Comp Med* 26:201-231, 1982.

Toxic Gases

Food animals may be exposed to a variety of toxic gases in the environment. The most important are ammonia, hydrogen sulfide, carbon dioxide, and methane from excreta and respiration; these can be especially important when excreta is collected in pits or tanks. Other gases include nitrogen dioxide from silos; carbon monoxide from machinery exhausts and heaters; zinc oxide from welding of galvanized metal in barns; chlorine, formaldehyde, insecticides, and other fumes from agricultural chemicals and cleaners; and smoke from fires. In most cases, concentrations usually remain below overtly toxic levels, and effects are very subtle. Such chronic low-level exposure may result in decreased disease resistance and depression of growth rates.[661] Slightly higher levels of chronic exposure may cause clinically vague syndromes of lethargy, mild dyspnea, anorexia, depressed growth, excessive lacrimation and salivation, low incidence of sudden deaths over weeks or months, and stillbirths.[661] Acute, severe outbreaks usually occur in tightly enclosed facilities and are related to accidents, power outages, agitation or pumping of manure pits, or other combinations of unusual circumstances. Such outbreaks are characterized by an ARDS of variable morbidity and frequently a high case fatality rate.

NITROGEN DIOXIDE. Nitrogen dioxide (NO_2) is a yellow-orange to brown gas with an acrid odor that is produced by anaerobic fermentation of green plant material. It is a major component of "silo gas." Acute exposure of farm workers to high concentrations of NO_2 causes a respiratory condition known as "silo-filler's disease," characterized by severe acute edema and congestion and followed by bronchiolitis obliterans and progressive interstitial pulmonary fibrosis. A similar condition has been induced experimentally in cattle,[662] and apparent (although unproved) spontaneous field cases have been reported.[663,664] Clinical signs in experimental and apparent field cases include cough, tachycardia, tachypnea, respiratory grunting, depression, anorexia, hypogalactia, extension of the head, open-mouth breathing, fever, salivation, lacrimation, and subcutaneous emphysema. Auscultation reveals decreased breath sounds and crackles.[663,664] The primary differential diagnoses should include other ARDS of housed cattle that occur in outbreak form, especially other toxic gases (manure pit gases, zinc oxide, chlorine, carbon monoxide), and hypersensitivity pneumonitis from moldy hay. Nitrate toxicity should also be considered. Clinical pathologic evaluation is of limited benefit. Leukocyte counts remained normal in experimental cases; methemoglobin levels increased to a peak at 30 minutes after exposure and returned to normal in 12 to 24 hours.[662] The pathophysiologic mechanism probably involves the dissolution of the NO_2 in the water of the respiratory tract to form nitric acid. Nitrates and nitrites are also formed; these are irritating, and the nitrites cause methemoglobinemia.[664] Nitrogen dioxide is also an oxidant itself and may contribute directly to the injury. The disease occurs as an outbreak, usually in housed cattle in proximity to a silo chute in a tight or poorly ventilated barn.[663,664] Nitrogen dioxide is heavier than air and layers on the top of silage or spills out around the bottom of the silo. Corn silage produces more gas than hay, and a high nitrate content increases the danger. The levels are highest in the first 48 hours after filling the silo but may remain dangerous for 2 to 3 weeks.

Necropsy findings in experimental disease include hyperemia of the upper airways; hemorrhages, fibrinous membranes, and froth in the trachea; distended, noncollapsing

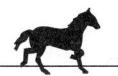

lungs with rib imprints; a mottled appearance caused by consolidated lobules alternating with emphysematous lobules; and bullae. Microscopic lesions include alveolar epithelial hyperplasia, large foamy alveolar macrophages, hyaline membranes, hyperemia, hemorrhage, and edema.

Treatment involves the establishment of adequate ventilation; cows should be completely removed from closed buildings if necessary. Corticosteroids have apparently been beneficial in field cases,[663,664] but no controlled studies have been performed. Because of the obvious differences in pathophysiologic characteristics, it would be unwise to extrapolate treatment regimens from those of ABPEE. Suggested empiric therapy might include corticosteroids (dexamethasone at 0.04 mg/kg or more IM or IV daily), furosemide (0.5 to 1.1 mg/kg IM or IV daily to 3 times daily), and appropriate antibiotics to prevent secondary bacterial infections.

ZINC OXIDE. Zinc oxide fumes have been associated with an ARDS in cattle.[665] Oxyacetylene cutting or arc welding of galvanized pipe results in production of white fumes of zinc oxide containing colloidal particles of 0.3 to 0.4 mm in diameter, which can reach the terminal alveoli when inhaled.[665] Construction activities in closed barns containing animals may result in toxicity in animals in close proximity or in the path of ventilation. All ages may be affected.

Clinical signs in severe cases include acute onset of anorexia, frothing at the mouth, anxiety, extension of the head and neck, mouth breathing, expiratory grunting, tachypnea, tachycardia, mild fever, subcutaneous emphysema, and crackles on auscultation of the lungs. Death may occur within 12 hours. Less severe cases exhibit depression, mild fever, and tachypnea.[665] Differential diagnoses include other ARDS of housed cattle that occur in outbreak form such as other toxic gases (nitrogen dioxide, manure pit gases) or hypersensitivity pneumonitis. The pathophysiologic process presumably involves direct damage to cells by the ZnO and its products dissolved in the fluid lining the respiratory tract. Necropsy findings include purulent conjunctivitis; subcutaneous emphysema; congestion of the airways; tracheal hemorrhages; stiff, noncollapsing lungs; and pulmonary congestion, edema, and emphysema with bullae.[665] Histologic lesions include pulmonary congestion, emphysema, edema, and mixed cellular infiltrates with a prominent eosinophil component. Treatment of severe cases with epinephrine, antihistamine, atropine, and corticosteroids had no effect in one outbreak,[665] whereas mild cases recover spontaneously. Suggested empiric therapy could include ventilation of the area, dexamethasone (0.04 mg/kg or more IM or IV daily), furosemide (0.5 to 1.1 mg/kg IM or IV daily to 3 times daily), and appropriate antibiotics to control secondary bacterial invaders.

CHLORINE. Chlorine is a greenish yellow gas widely used in manufacturing. Animal exposure is usually the result of industrial accidents. Exposed animals may be found dead. Signs include depression, profuse nasal discharge, lacrimation, and dyspnea; crackles may be heard on auscultation.[666] The toxic effects are the result of the formation of hydrochloric and hypochlorous acids; the latter breaks down to hydrochloric acid and oxygen, both of which are toxic to tissues. Necropsy findings include congestion of the nasal mucosa, tracheitis, and pulmonary edema, hemorrhage, and emphysema. Histologic lung lesions include edema, emphysema, hemorrhage, atelectasis, hyaline membrane formation, and lymphocytic bronchitis.[666] Treatment is empiric; suggestions include corticosteroids (dexamethasone at 0.04 mg/kg or more IM or IV daily), furosemide (0.5 to 1.1 mg/kg IM or IV daily to 3 times daily), and appropriate antibiotics to prevent secondary bacterial infection.

MANURE GASES. Manure gases include mixtures of hydrogen sulfide, ammonia, carbon dioxide, methane, and carbon monoxide.[667] Accumulation of these gases can result in asphyxiation of animals in enclosed barns over manure pits.

SMOKE INHALATION. Smoke inhalation injury may occur in animals that survive barn fires. Many clinical changes may not become evident for 24 to 48 hours after the fire. It is important to assess the degree of damage as early as possible and to attempt to anticipate sequelae so that early aggressive therapy can be instituted.[668] Common problems for which to check include oral burns, conjunctivitis, and laryngospasm. Hoarseness, expiratory wheezes, and carbonaceous sputum indicate potentially serious sequelae. Crackles and wheezes on auscultation may occur very early or may be delayed for hours. Cough, stridor, and tachypnea may also occur. Bright red mucous membranes may indicate CO poisoning or burns and may mask cyanosis.[668] Carboxyhemoglobin determinations on iced venous blood (often available at human hospitals), serial arterial blood gas determinations, transtracheal wash, and bronchoscopy are useful in delineating the extent of damage and prognosis.[668]

The pathophysiology of smoke inhalation is complex and involves two main mechanisms: CO toxicity and smoke toxicity. CO toxicity results in tissue hypoxia in all organs, especially the brain; O_2 consumption in the fire and the pulmonary effects of smoke may aggravate this hypoxia. Heat damage in animals is usually limited to the upper airways. Smoke toxicity is related to the inhalation of soot, superheated particles, and a variety of noxious gases (e.g., aldehydes, oxides of sulfur and nitrogen, benzene from plastics), which results in the formation of dissolved acids, alkaloids, and other direct irritants in pulmonary fluids. These mechanisms eventually (usually 2 to 24 hours after inhalation) result in alveolar damage, interstitial edema, hypoxia, and secondary bronchopneumonia.[668]

Treatment involves establishing a patent airway with intubation or tracheostomy if necessary. Oxygen, up to 100% for short periods, is indicated[668]; care must be exercised because 100% oxygen can also cause pulmonary damage. Intravenous fluids should be given, with careful monitoring for pulmonary edema. The use of corticosteroids is controversial and appears to be losing favor in human and small animal medicine.[668] Antibiotics are indicated to prevent secondary bronchopneumonia. Bronchodilators such as aminophylline at 6 to 10 mg/kg IV or PO 3 times daily may help relieve soot-induced bronchospasm.

REFERENCES

661. Curtis SE: Toxic gases. In Howard JL, ed: *Current veterinary therapy 2: food animal practice,* Philadelphia, 1986, WB Saunders, pp 456-457.
662. Cutlip RC: Experimental nitrogen dioxide poisoning in cattle, *Pathol Vet* 3:474-485, 1966.
663. Brightwell AH: "Silo gas" poisoning in cattle, *Can Vet J* 13:224-225, 1972.
664. Haynes NB: "Silo filler's disease" in dairy cattle, *J Am Vet Med Assoc* 143:593-594, 1963.
665. Hilderman E, Taylor PA: Acute pulmonary emphysema in cattle exposed to zinc oxide fumes, *Can Vet J* 15:173-175, 1974.
666. MacDonald DW et al: Chloride gas poisoning in farm livestock: case report and review, *Can Vet J* 13:33-40, 1971.
667. Breeze RG: Respiratory disease in adult cattle, *Vet Clin North Am (Food Anim Pract)* 1:311-346, 1985.
668. Tams TR: Aspiration pneumonia and complications of inhalation of smoke and toxic gases, *Vet Clin North Am (Small Anim Pract)* 15:971-989, 1985.

Hypersensitivity Pneumonitis

DEFINITION AND ETIOLOGY. Hypersensitivity pneumonitis, also known as extrinsic allergic alveolitis (EAA), is an allergic respiratory disease caused by inhalation of organic dusts. Several such conditions are recognized in humans, differing only in the nature of the antigen and the circumstances under which exposure occurs. The classic example, of which the bovine disease is probably the counterpart, is "farmer's lung." EAA is caused by exposure to the dust from moldy hay, grain, or other plant matter containing spores and products of thermophilic actinomycetes such as *Micropolyspora faeni* and *Thermoactinomyces vulgaris*.[669] Other unidentified forms of hypersensitivity pneumonitis probably occur in cattle.

CLINICAL SIGNS AND DIFFERENTIAL DIAGNOSIS. EAA is a disease of confined adult cattle; consequently it is more common in dairy than beef breeds. Typically a succession of acute cases occurs during the winter housing period, so that the clinician is presented with a group problem in which animals are in varying stages of the disease. The acute form is indicative of recent exposure and is characterized by a sudden onset of dullness, decreased appetite, hypogalactia, coughing, expiratory tachypnea, dyspnea, and cranial-ventral crackles on auscultation of the lungs.[669,670] There is a moderate transient fever, which is frequently missed.[669] The chronic form is insidious at onset and may not be detected until there is considerable fibrosis. Animals with the chronic disease may have acute exacerbations as a result of heavy antigen exposure; some may not be detected until turned out in the spring, when increased exercise causes an acute crisis. There is a history of weight loss and coughing for several winters, with remission in the grazing season. Chronic signs include hypogalactia, weight loss, productive coughing, tachypnea, obvious hyperpnea, and widespread crackles and wheezes on auscultation of the lungs, especially in the rostral-ventral areas.[669] Differential diagnoses should include respiratory diseases affecting groups of housed adult cattle in winter. Infectious diseases (viral and bacterial pneumonias) can usually be differentiated from farmer's lung by careful evaluation of factors such as clinical signs of fever and consolidation. Therefore the main differentials are the toxic gases. It should be emphasized that hypersensitivity pneumonitis is not considered an ARDS and that no evidence exists for the involvement of hypersensitivity in the pathogenesis of the ARDS described previously. However, severe cases of EAA with prominent dyspnea and moderate, nonfatal cases of gas intoxication may appear clinically similar. If the group outbreak aspect of EAA is ignored, the clinician who examines one individual may be unable to distinguish this condition from fibrosing alveolitis.

CLINICAL PATHOLOGY. Precipitating antibodies to *M. faeni* are found in the serum in most cases.[669] However, two precautions are necessary. First, the presence of precipitating antibodies only indicates exposure to the antigen; many normal animals also have antibodies. Second, it is possible that other as yet unidentified antigens may cause allergic respiratory disease in cattle. The presence or absence of titers is therefore not necessarily diagnostic of the clinical status of the animal, and the magnitude of the titer does not reflect the extent of disease.[669]

PATHOPHYSIOLOGY. The spores of the thermophilic actinomycetes are 0.7 to 1.3 mm in diameter and can easily reach the alveoli, where they induce both humoral (precipitating) and cellular immune responses. It is thought that repeated exposure results in the activation of a number of immunologically specific and nonspecific cellular and humoral effector mechanisms at the alveolar level, which results in tissue damage.[669]

EPIDEMIOLOGY. EAA is a problem in areas with wet summers and severe winters, a situation characterized by the combination of moldy hay and housing of cattle in winter. In North America, EAA occurs primarily in the Great Lakes region of the United States and the eastern provinces of Canada.[669] Baling and stacking of hay with a high moisture content (over 30%) results in overheating of the stacks. Thermophilic molds become dominant and produce billions of spores, which are released when the hay is distributed for feeding. A similar situation can occur in stored grains. Affected hay is usually dry, friable, discolored, and dusty; however, it is not necessary for hay to be grossly dusty and poor in quality to release large numbers of spores.[669]

NECROPSY FINDINGS. In acute cases the lungs are superficially grossly normal. Closer inspection reveals small gray spots in many lobules, which represent interstitial and peribronchiolar accumulations of lymphocytes. Other lobules exhibit dark red centers of atelectasis surrounded by pale pink raised edges of trapped air that are caused by narrowing of airways with lymphocytic infiltrates. Histologic evaluation confirms the presence of these lymphocytic infiltrates and aggregations, as well as epithelial granulomas, bronchiolitis, and bronchiolitis obliterans. The gross appearance in chronic cases is similar, with the addition of focal areas of interalveolar fibrosis and epithelial hyperplasia; epithelioid granulomas are absent unless a recent acute exposure has occurred.[669]

TREATMENT AND PROGNOSIS. Treatment and control center around removal of the offending antigen, which is frequently difficult from an economic and management standpoint. Corticosteroids (dexamethasone at 0.04 mg/kg IV daily) may be beneficial in acute cases. Suggestions to decrease the molding of hay or degree of exposure include making silage instead of hay, ensuring proper drying before baling, and feeding hay outside. If the condition can be arrested before significant fibrosis occurs, the prognosis is good.

REFERENCES

669. Breeze RG: Respiratory disease in adult cattle, *Vet Clin North Am (Food Anim Pract)* 1:311-346, 1985.
670. Wilkie BN: Allergic respiratory disease, *Adv Vet Sci Comp Med* 26:233-266, 1982.

Anaphylaxis

In ruminants the lung is the major target organ in immediate (type I) hypersensitivity reactions. Precipitating antigens include vaccines, drugs, blood, *Hypoderma bovis* or *Hypoderma lineatum* larvae, insect bites, and bee stings. Signs of anaphylaxis usually develop in 10 to 20 minutes and include severe acute dyspnea, with flaring of the nostrils, extension of the head and neck, open-mouth breathing, frothing of the mouth, hyperpnea, and abduction of the elbows. Pharyngeal and laryngeal edema cause stertor and inspiratory dyspnea. Urticaria may occur in some cases, such as milk allergy in Jersey cows. Shivering, salivation, lacrimation, pruritus, diarrhea, fever, edema (eyes, muzzle, anus, and vulva), collapse, nystagmus, cyanosis, and discharge of froth from the nostrils also may occur. On auscultation there are harsh breath sounds, large airway sounds, and crackles. The primary differential is peracute pneumonia. The pathogenesis involves an initial exposure to the antigen, which results in a genetically determined production of homocytotropic antibodies. In humans and dogs, this is immunoglobulin E (IgE); in ruminants various classes may be involved.[671] This antibody attaches to receptors on mast cells and basophils. On subsequent exposure to the antigen, bridging of the Fab parts of the antibody on these cells results in degranulation, with release of a variety of mediators such as histamine, bradykinin, 5-hydroxytryptamine, serotonin, slow-reacting substance-anaphylaxis (SRS-A), eosinophil chemotactic factor A, platelet activating factor, kinins, and prostaglandins.[671-673] These mediators result in a cascade of vascular events, notably increased vascular permeability, which in turn results in acute severe edema. Pulmonary venous constriction, pulmonary artery hypertension, splanchnic pooling, increased mucus secretion, and bronchospasm also occur. Ruminants that die of anaphylaxis have severe pulmonary congestion and edema, laryngeal edema, and froth in the airways. Lung lesions of ARDS may be present.

The treatment of choice is epinephrine, 4 to 8 mg (4 to 8 ml of 1:1000 solution) IV or SC or 1 to 5 mg IV for an average 500-kg cow and 1 to 3 mg IV or SC for an average adult sheep or goat. Epinephrine has a short half-life, and animals should be observed closely for relapse. Ancillary therapy includes corticosteroids (dexamethasone, 0.22 mg/kg IM or IV; prednisolone, 2.2 mg/kg IM or IV daily), nonsteroidal anti-inflammatory drugs (aspirin, 100 mg/kg PO twice daily; phenylbutazone, 6 mg/kg PO daily; or flunixin meglumine, 0.5 to 1.1 mg/kg IM or IV daily to 3 times daily), and diethylcarbamazine. Other supportive therapies include shock doses of intravenous fluids (40 ml/kg/hr) with added sodium bicarbonate; aminophylline; diuretics such as furosemide; oxygen therapy; and tracheostomy if necessary.

REFERENCES
671. Black L: Hypersensitivity in cattle. I, Mechanism of causation, *Vet Bull* 49:1-9, 1979.
672. Black L: Hypersensitivity in cattle. II, Clinical reactions, *Vet Bull* 49:77-88, 1979.
673. Black L: Hypersensitivity in cattle. III, Mediators of anaphylaxis, *Vet Bull* 49:303-308, 1979.

▓ *Chronic Interstitial Pneumonias*

At least two chronic interstitial pneumonias of uncertain cause have been identified in cattle: fibrosing alveolitis and bronchiolitis obliterans. These are typically chronic diseases of individual animals.

Fibrosing Alveolitis

Fibrosing alveolitis (FA) is, by definition, a chronic disease of unknown and possibly multiple causes, characterized by diffuse inflammation of the lung beyond the terminal bronchiole. Approximately 50% of cases produce positive results for precipitating antibody to *Micropolyspora faeni*, and it is possible that these cases represent chronic farmer's lung, whereas others (that have negative *M. faeni* results) may be the chronic stage of hypersensitivity to other unidentified antigens.[674] Field investigations have failed to substantiate any connection between FA and repeated episodes of ARDS such as acute bovine pulmonary edema (ABPE). Furthermore, recovery from a single dose of 3-methylindole does not result in lesions typical of FA. However, repeated doses of 3-methylindole at weekly intervals experimentally cause FA-like lesions.[674] FA occurs in individual adult cattle (usually over 6 years of age) in both housing and pasture conditions. The history is usually that of a chronic progressive respiratory disease several weeks to 2 years in duration. Affected cattle remain bright and alert and continue to eat until the terminal stages of cor pulmonale and heart failure intervene. Signs include marked weight loss; consistent coughing; tachypnea (40 to 70 breaths/min); very marked hyperpnea, even at rest; and dyspnea after mild exertion. Auscultation may reveal crackles in the rostral-ventral lung field and widespread wheezes. Fever is not apparent.[674] The primary differential diagnoses to consider are other chronic respiratory conditions of individual adult cattle. Chronic suppurative pneumonia and metastatic pneumonia can usually be differentiated from FA by careful physical examination and detection of depression, anorexia, shallow respiration, thoracic pain, and hemoptysis. ARDS and lungworms are typically group problems, with at least some severe cases in the group. Differentiation from EAA may be impossible if the group outbreak nature of farmer's lung is not appreciated; in fact, at least some cases of fibrosing alveolitis may represent chronic farmer's lung. At necropsy the lungs are very pale, firm, and heavy throughout. Scattered lobules are gray-red, slightly collapsed, and edematous. Thick mucus may be found in the airways, and there is frequently right ventricular hypertrophy as a result of cor pulmonale. Histologic changes are diffuse and include interalveolar fibrosis and infiltration with plasma cells, lymphocytes, mast cells, and interstitial cells; obliteration of alveolar spaces; mononuclear exudates in alveoli; alveolar epithelial hyperplasia; bronchitis; and bronchiolitis. The epithelioid granulomas characteristic of acute farmer's lung are absent.[674] No treatment exists, and the lesions are obviously irreversible.

Bronchiolitis Obliterans

Bronchiolitis obliterans is a chronic respiratory condition of yearling or young adult cattle characterized by a deep infrequent cough, tachypnea, hyperpnea, and an exaggerated expiratory effort. There is no fever. The cause is unknown; the condition is speculated to be a sequela to viruses (respiratory syncytial virus, parainfluenza virus type 3, infectious bovine rhinotracheitis), parasites such as *Dictyocaulus viviparus*, or hypersensitivity pneumonitis. The lungs appear grossly normal at necropsy, except that they do not collapse. Histologic examination reveals extensive bronchiolitis and bronchiolitis obliterans, with epithelium-covered polyps with a connective tissue core projecting into and obstructing the lumen.[674]

REFERENCE
674. Breeze RG: Respiratory disease in adult cattle, *Vet Clin North Am (Food Anim Pract)* 1:311-346, 1985.

▓ *Parasitic Bronchitis and Pneumonia*
ANNE M. ZAJAC

Two parasites in cattle (*Dictyocaulus viviparus* and aberrant migration of *Ascaris suum* larvae) and three in sheep and goats (*Dictyocaulus filaria*, *Protostrongylus rufescens*, and *Muellerius capillaris*) may cause respiratory disease characterized by alveolar and interstitial pneumonia. Other species of lungworms also parasitize small ruminants, but are less widely distributed throughout the world.

Dictyocaulus viviparus

DEFINITION AND ETIOLOGY. *D. viviparus* is a trichostrongylid nematode parasitizing the bovine trachea and bronchi. Adult worms may reach 8 cm in length. The life cycle of *D. viviparus* is direct. Adult female worms in the trachea and bronchi lay eggs that hatch almost immediately. First-stage larvae are coughed up, swallowed, and passed in the feces. Larvae develop in a minimum of 5 days (usually longer under normal environmental conditions) to the infective third stage, migrate onto grass, are ingested, penetrate the intestine, and move to the mesenteric lymph nodes, where they molt. Fourth-stage larvae travel through lymph and blood to the lungs and tend to lodge in the pulmonary capillaries of the ventral parts of the caudal lobes. Approximately 7 days after ingestion, they enter the alveoli and molt to the fifth (final) stage in the bronchioles several days later. Egg-laying adults are present in the bronchi 21 to 28 days after ingestion of larvae. Clinically evident infection with *D. viviparus* typically occurs in two forms: (1) a primary infection, in which young stock (less than 12 months old) or previously unexposed yearling or adult cattle are exposed for the first time, and (2) a reinfection syndrome in which previously infected (and therefore immune) adults are subjected to massive challenge with infective larvae. The primary infection can be further broken down clinically into a prepatent phase, a patent phase, and a postpatent phase.[675,676]

CLINICAL SIGNS AND DIFFERENTIAL DIAGNOSIS. No signs are associated with the initial penetration of larvae until they reach the alveoli, where they provoke an eosinophilic exudate that blocks small airways. During the prepatent phase (approximately 7 to 25 days after ingestion), there is a gradual onset of coughing and tachypnea (35 to 60 breaths/min), which becomes increasingly apparent from day 14 to day 25. The severity of signs in this stage is proportional to the number of larvae ingested, the rate of ingestion, and the proportion reaching the lungs.[675] Severe illness and death can occur in cases of heavy infection. In the patent phase (approximately 25 to 55 days after ingestion), a parasitic pneumonia with consolidation develops in the ventral areas of the caudal lung lobes as a result of aspiration of eggs and larvae into these areas. Tracheitis and bronchitis associated with the adult worms also develop. Clinical signs vary in severity and range from intermittent to marked coughing, tachypnea (respiratory rate may increase to more than 70 breaths/min), dyspnea, anorexia, and weight loss. Fever may develop with secondary bacterial infection. Auscultation reveals harsh breath sounds and widespread crackles and wheezes. Severe cases may exhibit open-mouth breathing, extended head and neck, protrusion of the tongue, and an expiratory grunt. Death is common in untreated, heavily infected animals.[675,676]

Recovery begins in the late patent phase, and the signs gradually resolve, sometimes over several months. During the postpatent phase (about days 55 to 90), adult parasites are expelled by a self-cure phenomenon. In approximately 25% of severe cases the postpatent phase is characterized by a sudden exacerbation of dyspnea at days 45 to 60 that is often fatal, after secondary bacterial infection or alveolar epithelialization.[675,676] The reinfection syndrome occurs 14 to 16 days after adult cattle are placed on heavily contaminated pastures. Signs include acute hypogalactia; severe, frequent coughing; marked tachypnea; and depression. Auscultation reveals only harsh breath sounds with no crackles or wheezes.[675,676]

Differential diagnosis should be straightforward if both the clinical signs and epidemiologic characteristics of the disease are taken into account, especially in endemic areas. This is a disease of groups of cattle at pasture, typically in late summer or fall in northern temperate climates; the situation thus resembles acute bovine pulmonary edema and emphysema, which differs in clinical signs (i.e., less coughing and fewer adventitious lung sounds). The signs associated with lungworm infection are reminiscent of those of farmer's lung, which occurs in quite different circumstances. In typically nonendemic areas, outbreaks associated with climatic changes are frequently mistaken for acute bacterial bronchopneumonia.[675]

CLINICAL PATHOLOGY. Larvae of *D. viviparus* are large, slow-moving, and contain dark food granules. They are detected by the Baermann examination[677] and may also be seen on a transtracheal wash. It is best to check several animals in the herd. Rectal fecal samples are preferred for parasite examination because samples picked up off the ground may contain free-living nematodes that can be difficult to differentiate from lungworm larvae. Recovery of larvae from fecal samples is substantially diminished if the sample is stored at room temperature for more than a few hours. If the Baermann test cannot be set up soon after fecal collection, the sample can be safely refrigerated for 24 to 48 hours without serious larval loss.[678] No larvae are detected in the reinfection syndrome. In some European countries an ELISA technique is also available that indicates whether infection has occurred in the current grazing season.[679] An increase in eosinophils in the peripheral blood may also occur about 2 weeks after infection and peak at 4 to 7 weeks after infection.[680]

PATHOPHYSIOLOGY. Once the fourth-stage larvae enter the alveoli, they incite an eosinophilic exudate that blocks small bronchi and bronchioles, resulting in atelectasis and

causing the cough and tachypnea of the prepatent phase. As these larvae mature and migrate up the airways, these lesions may resolve. However, the adult worms produce an inflammatory response in the larger airways, and aspirated eggs and larvae cause a marked macrophage and giant cell response, with consolidation of the ventral caudal lobes; these lesions are the cause of the signs in the patent phase. At any point in the pathogenesis (prepatent, patent, or postpatent stage), complications may occur that account for acute exacerbation and death. These complications are as follows:

- Development of pulmonary edema, caused either by heart failure or by extensive alveolar epithelial damage and hyaline membrane formation
- Severe interstitial emphysema from the severe dyspnea
- Alveolar epithelial hyperplasia
- Secondary bacterial infection, which is actually relatively uncommon

In the reinfection syndrome the immune response cannot completely overcome a massive challenge, and a small number of larvae reach the lungs. The signs are caused by the immune reaction to the migrating larvae. Lymphoid nodules develop around dead larvae in the bronchioles.[675]

EPIDEMIOLOGY. Parasitic bronchitis and pneumonia occur most often in areas of mild climate and high rainfall or intense irrigation. Primary infections are usually seen in dairy calves when they are first turned out onto infected pastures. Older animals exhibit this syndrome when circumstances result in the exposure of previously unexposed adult animals, such as purchase and transport of animals from a nonendemic to an endemic area. Beef animals are less often affected because management practices are more extensive and levels of infective larvae on pastures are generally lower. The reinfection syndrome occurs in such circumstances as placing immune adults on a pasture previously contaminated very heavily by calves with patent disease. Both forms of the disease should be recognized as a group problem.[675,676] Recently, variation from the typical pattern of primary infection has been observed in Great Britain. Outbreaks of primary parasitic bronchitis have become an important cause of respiratory disease in adult dairy cows. The increased prevalence of disease in this older age-group may be the result of decreased levels of immunity in adult cattle following a decline in the rate of vaccination and increased use of powerful suppressive anthelmintic regimens in first and second season grazing animals. Other management factors, such as isolation of calves from adult carrier animals and increased movement of livestock, may also contribute to a decline in levels of immunity.[679]

In northern temperate climates, the infection is carried from year to year by overwintering of larvae on pasture in some areas, by spreading of manure from infected housed calves in the spring, and by carrier cattle. Lungworm larvae also may be inhibited in the lungs of calves in winter (as with *Ostertagia* spp. in the abomasum) and mature in the spring.[675,676] Usually there is a gradual build-up of pasture contamination over the spring and early summer, and infections become severe enough that clinical signs begin to appear in July through September. Evidence from Louisiana, however, indicates that in the southern United States maximum transmission of *D. viviparus* to calves occurs between December and March.[681]

NECROPSY FINDINGS. In the prepatent phase the lungs are largely normal, with a few atelectatic lobules in the ventral caudal lobes; adult worms are not present until late in this phase, but larvae may be detectable by microscopic examination of smears of bronchial exudate. In the patent phase there is usually bilaterally symmetric red consolidation of the ventral caudal lobes. Adult worms can be recognized on necropsy by their relatively large size and location in the trachea and bronchi. The lesions of the postpatent phase are similar, but no adult worms or larvae are present. In those patients that die of an acute exacerbation, there is extensive pulmonary edema and emphysema, with hyaline membranes and alveolar epithelial hyperplasia.

In the reinfection syndrome the pulmonary lymphoid nodules may be 3 to 4 mm in diameter and thus grossly visible as raised, gray-red to greenish yellow nodules under the pleura. Initially these are composed of a core of eosinophilic parasitic debris surrounded by macrophages, multinucleated giant cells, hyperplastic bronchiolar epithelium, eosinophils, and plasma cells. The lesions eventually mature to lymphoreticular nodules with a germinal center. There is also greenish mucus in the airways and a greenish discoloration to the tissues, both caused by eosinophil infiltration. There is no edema or emphysema, and the rare lungworms that may be found are small and stunted.[675]

TREATMENT, PROGNOSIS, PREVENTION, AND CONTROL. *D. viviparus* infection can be treated with a number of bovine anthelmintics available in the United States and other countries (Table 29-8). Animals with only cough and tachypnea respond well, whereas those with dyspnea, fever, anorexia, and depression have a more guarded prognosis; some of these can be expected to die or remain chronically unthrifty.[675] Control (see also Chapter 45) involves the strategic use of these anthelmintics to prevent build-up of infection in the herd and on pastures. Several strategic deworming programs have been developed in Europe, which effectively suppress lungworm infection throughout the grazing season. These programs include use of ivermectin at 3, 8, and 13 weeks after turnout and use of doramectin or eprinomectin at 0 and 8 weeks. Use of an oxfendazole pulse release bolus (not available in the United States) also provides strategic treatments. Alternatively, use of a continuous release ivermectin or fenbendazole bolus (fenbendazole bolus not available in the United States) will prevent development of lungworm infection during its period of efficacy.[679] Anthelmintic treatment with moxidectin or fenbendazole followed by movement of calves to safe pasture 9 weeks after turnout was also effective in controlling lungworm.[682] None of these control programs have been extensively tested under the variety of grazing conditions in the United States. Despite concern that suppressive programs may limit exposure to larvae and interfere with the development of immunity to lungworm, several studies conducted in Europe have shown that stimulation of the immune response still occurs, although relative levels of immunity may vary.[682-684] In Europe, methods of control also include a highly effective irradiated larval vaccine. Delay of spring turnout is an adjunct to control but should not be relied on as the sole means of control.[685]

Ascaris suum

Cattle exposed to large numbers of *A. suum* eggs in areas contaminated by swine may have an interstitial pneumonia. Animals are typically affected about 10 days after exposure. Signs include depression, anorexia, fever, tachycardia, tachypnea, dyspnea with an expiratory grunt, variable coughing, rumen stasis, and bloat. Auscultation of the lungs reveals increased breath sounds without adventitious sounds. Some deaths may occur. Differential diagnosis is difficult. Differentiation from the other interstitial pneumonias depends more on history of exposure to the causative agents (i.e., lush pastures, moldy sweet potatoes, *Perilla frutescens*, toxic gases, and moldy hay). Differentiation from viral pneumonia (such as that caused by respiratory syncytial virus) and *D. viviparus* reinfection syndrome requires necropsy and demonstration of larvae. Ascarid larvae have characteristic lateral alae in histologic sections. Patent *D. viviparus* infection can be differentiated by Baermann examination of the feces. In fatal cases the lung lobes are firm and mottled blue, red, and gray. The cut surface oozes thin yellow exudate. There is emphysema in the dorsal diaphragmatic lobes and subpleural hemorrhage with neutrophil infiltration and necrosis of bronchiolar and alveolar epithelium. In chronic cases the cellular infiltrate is lymphocytic, and there are proliferation of bronchiolar epithelium and peribronchial fibrosis. Recommended treatments include corticosteroids (dexamethasone, 0.04 mg/kg IM or IV, or prednisolone 1 mg/kg IM or IV daily) and antibiotics to control secondary bacterial infection.[686] Clinical signs resolved after treatment with oxfendazole in one outbreak of suspected *A. suum* migration.[687] Cattle should not be exposed to areas heavily contaminated by swine.

Lungworms of Sheep and Goats

Three species of lungworms are of primary importance in sheep and goats: *Dictyocaulus filaria*, and the two metastrongylid nematodes, *Muellerius capillaris* and *Protostrongylus rufescens*. Other genera of metastrongylid lungworms of minor pathogenic importance in sheep and goats include *Cystocaulus*, *Spiculocaulus*, and *Neostrongylus*. These parasites are rare or absent from North America.[688]

DICTYOCAULUS FILARIA. *D. filaria* has a life cycle essentially identical to that of *D. viviparus*; the time from ingestion to the appearance of larvae in the feces is about 4 weeks. Mainly young animals are affected but disease can also occur in adults. Dyspnea, tachypnea and coughing, and loss of condition occur in clinical cases.[688,689] Differential diagnosis in-

---

TABLE 29-8

Anthelmintics Approved for Treatment of *D. viviparus* in the United States

Anthelmintic	Formulation	Residual Efficacy of a Single Treatment	Approved for Dairy Cattle of Breeding Age
Levamisole	Drench, bolus, pour-on, injectable, feed additive		
Fenbendazole	Paste; suspension; mineral, molasses and protein blocks		(Paste and suspension only)
Oxfendazole	Suspension, intraruminal injection		
Albendazole	Paste, suspension		
Ivermectin	Injection, pour-on, sustained release bolus	Injection, 28 days (Bolus active 135 days)	
Eprinomectin	Pour-on	21 days	—
Doramectin	Injection, pour-on	Injection, 28 days Pour-on, 21 days	
Moxidectin	Pour-on	42 days	

cludes the progressive viral pneumonias. Diagnosis is made by finding larvae in fresh feces by the Baermann technique. Samples should be tested soon after collection because larval recovery is significantly reduced in stored samples.[678] Larvae of *D. filaria* are similar in size and appearance to those of *D. viviparus* but also have a distinctive knob on the anterior end. The pathogenesis is similar to that of *D. viviparus* (see earlier discussion). The adults are found largely in the dorsal-caudal regions of the diaphragmatic lobes. Bronchitis and peribronchitis, along with cone-shaped areas of pneumonia and atelectasis, and emphysema are present. Secondary bacterial infections may also occur.[688,689] Levamisole (8 mg/kg), fenbendazole (5 to 10 mg/kg), ivermectin (0.2 mg/kg PO),[689] and moxidectin (0.2 mg/kg, PO or SC)[690,691] can be used for treatment. When outbreaks occur, all animals should be treated and moved to fresh pasture when possible. Clinical *D. filaria* infections seem to occur most frequently in areas with warm climates. In temperate areas the parasite overwinters either as arrested larvae in ewes or as larvae on pasture.[688]

MUELLERIUS CAPILLARIS. *M. capillaris* is probably the most common of the lungworms of sheep and goats. Infection is more pathogenic in goats than in sheep. Recent surveys in Maryland and Georgia detected the parasite in 64% and 68% of goats, respectively.[692,693] The life cycle is indirect. First-stage larvae are coughed up, swallowed, and passed in the feces. These larvae are relatively resistant and may survive for several months in the environment. Following penetration of an appropriate molluscan intermediate host, the infective third stage develops in a minimum of about 12 days, is ingested with the snail, and passes to the mesenteric lymph nodes. The fourth stage larva proceeds to the lungs where adults develop in the alveoli. The prepatent period of *M. capillaris* infection is about 6 weeks.[694] Although many infections are subclinical, clinical disease may develop. Goats appear to be more likely than sheep to develop unthriftiness, coughing, and dyspnea. Infection may also predispose to secondary bacterial infection.[689,694] The difference in clinical signs between sheep and goats is probably due to a difference in the pathogenesis of infection. The adult worms live in the pulmonary parenchyma, particularly the subpleural tissue. In sheep they produce grayish nodules typically 2 to 3 mm in diameter. On palpation at necropsy, these nodules have been described as feeling like "lead shot."[694] Each nodule contains a worm and necrotic leukocytes and pulmonary tissue surrounded by a connective tissue wall and giant cells.[688] They may calcify or become secondarily infected with bacteria. There are few reports of the lesions in goats, and these indicate that *M. capillaris* causes an interstitial pneumonia. The lungs are resilient and firm, fail to collapse, and have tan, yellow, or gray patches located especially in the dorsal diaphragmatic lobes. The histologic lesion in goats is a diffuse thickening of alveolar septae, with a mononuclear cell infiltrate and alveolar epithelial hyperplasia that extends far beyond the area immediately around the parasite. The local reaction around the worm is quite variable and does not appear to produce the nodules seen in sheep.[695] Diagnosis is made by Baermann examination of the feces. The larvae are smaller than those of *D. filaria* and have a kink at the end of the tail with a characteristic subterminal accessory spine.

Control of *M. capillaris* infections can be difficult. Although larvae may initially disappear in the feces following treatment, they often reappear in fecal samples again after 1 to 2 months, either because anthelmintics are ineffective against immature worms and/or because of resumption of development by inhibited larvae.[696] Treatments that appear to eliminate adult parasites in goats include fenbendazole (15 to 30 mg/kg),[694-698] albendazole (10 mg/kg),[698] oxfendazole (7.5 to 10 mg/kg),[699] and ivermectin (0.3 mg/kg).[696,700] *M. capillaris* is largely resistant to levamisole.[689] One strategy

that appears to provide better control of immature or inhibited larvae is the administration of fenbendazole (1.25 to 5 mg/kg) for 7 to 14 days, although a regimen of 1 week on/ 1 week off/1 week on appeared to provide the most effective treatment. Albendazole (1 mg/kg) orally daily for 7 to 14 days was also effective.[698] Possible teratogenic effects of extended benzimidazole treatment in goats have not been thoroughly investigated and benzimidazole should be used cautiously in the first 35 days of pregnancy.[689] Administration of ivermectin (0.3 mg/kg) or fenbendazole (15 mg/kg) two or three times at 35-day intervals has also been suggested for treatment.[696] Control methods include avoiding wet pastures and treatment of animals before the start of the grazing season to reduce infection levels in the intermediate host.[689]

PROTOSTRONGYLUS RUFESCENS. *P. rufescens* also uses molluscan intermediate hosts and adults develop in the small bronchioles of sheep and goats.[694] Most infections are probably subclinical or produce only mild signs of chronic bronchitis or bronchopneumonia with nasal discharge and cough. Occasionally *P. rufescens* may produce severe or even fatal disease.[701] The diagnosis of *Protostrongylus* spp. infection is made by finding larvae in the feces with the Baermann technique. The larvae are similar to those of *Muellerius* except *Protostrongylus* larvae lack the subterminal accessory spine on the tail. Fenbendazole and levamisole can be used for treatment at the dosages used for *Dictyocaulus*. Other modern anthelmintics may also be effective but have not been thoroughly tested. Control strategies are identical to those for *M. capillaris*. Few cases of infection have been reported in the United States, but nonspecific clinical signs, presence of subclinical carriers, and need for a special diagnostic technique may produce an underestimation of the prevalence of *P. rufescens* infection in sheep and goats.[701]

REFERENCES

675. Breeze RG: Parasitic bronchitis and pneumonia, *Vet Clin North Am (Food Anim Pract)* 1:277-287, 1985.
676. Eysker M: Dictyocaulosis in cattle, *Compend Cont Ed Pract Vet* 16:669-675, 1994.
677. Sloss MW, Kemp RL, Zajac AM: *Veterinary clinical parasitology*, ed 6, Ames, Iowa, 1994, Iowa State University Press, pp 11-12.
678. Rode B, Jorgensen RJ: Baermannization of *Dictyocaulus* spp from faeces of cattle, sheep and donkeys, *Vet Parasitol* 30:205-211, 1989.
679. David G: Strategies for the control of parasitic bronchitis in cattle, *In Pract* 21:62-68, 1999.
680. Lekeux P, Hajer R, Breuking HJ: Longitudinal study of the effects of lungworm infection on bovine pulmonary function, *Am J Vet Res* 46:1392-1395, 1985.
681. Eddi CS, Williams JC, Swalley RA: Epidemiology of *Dictyocaulus viviparus* in Louisiana (USA), *Vet Parasitol* 31:37-48, 1989.
682. Eysker M et al: Comparison between fenbendazole and moxidectin applied in a dose and move system for the control of *Dictyocaulus viviparus* infections in calves, *Vet Parasitol* 64:187-196, 1996.
683. Schneider T et al: The development of protective immunity against gastrointestinal nematode and lungworm infections after use of an ivermectin bolus in first-year grazing calves, *Vet Parasitol* 64:239-250, 1996.
684. Taylor SM et al: Protection against *Dictyocaulus viviparus* in second year cattle after first year treatment with doramectin or an ivermectin bolus, *Vet Rec* 141:593-597, 1997.
685. Jacobs DE, Fox MT: Relationship between date of spring turnout and lungworm infection in calves, *Vet Rec* 116:75-76, 1985.
686. Morrow DA: Pneumonia in cattle due to migrating *Ascaris lumbricoides* larvae, *J Am Vet Med Assoc* 153:184-189, 1968.
687. Borgsteede FHM et al: Illness in two dairy herds suspected of being due to *Ascaris suum* infection, *Tijdschr Diergeneesk* 117:296-298, 1992.
688. Urquhart GM et al: *Veterinary parasitology*, London, 1996, Blackwell Scientific, pp 41-42.
689. Smith MC, Sherman DM: *Goat medicine*, Baltimore, 1994, Lea & Febiger, pp 261-263.
690. Oosthuizen WTJ et al: Efficacy of moxidectin against internal parasites of sheep, *J S Afr Vet Assoc* 64:28-30, 1993.
691. Dorchies P, Cardinaud B, Fournier R: Efficacy of moxidectin as a 1% injectable solution and a 0.1% drench against nasal bots, pulmonary and gastrointestinal nematodes in sheep, *Vet Parasitol* 65:163-168, 1996.
692. Ashraf M, Nepote KH: Prevalence of gastrointestinal nematodes, coccidia and lungworms in Maryland dairy goats, *Small Rum Res* 3:291-298, 1990.

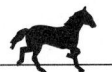

693. Anderson DL, Roberson EL: Gastrointestinal and respiratory parasitism in Georgia goats, *Agri-Prac* 17:20-24, 1996.

694. Levine ND: *Nematode parasites of domestic animals and man,* ed 2, Minneapolis, 1980, Burgess, pp 241-245.

695. Nimmo JS: Six cases of verminous pneumonia (*Muellerius* spp) in goats, *Can Vet J* 20:49-52, 1979.

696. McCraw BM, Menzies PI: Treatment of goats infected with the lungworm, *Muellerius capillaris, Can Vet J* 27:287-290, 1986.

697. Bliss EL, Greiner EC: Efficacy of fenbendazole and cambendazole against *Muellerius capillaris* in dairy goats, *Am J Vet Res* 46:1923-1925, 1985.

698. Helle O: The efficacy of fenbendazole and albendazole against the lungworm *Muellerius capillaris* in goats, *Vet Parasitol* 22:293-301, 1986.

699. Cabarnet J et al: Le traitement de la muelleriose caprine: efficacité comparée de l'oxfendazole, Les maladies de la Chevre, *Les Colloques de l'INRA*, number 28, pp 358-366, 1984.

700. Gregory E, Foreyt WJ, Breeze R: Efficacy of ivermectin and fenbendazole against lungworms, *Vet Med* 80:114-117, 1985.

701. Mansfield LS et al: Lungworm infection in a sheep flock in Maryland, *J Am Vet Med Assoc* 202:601-606, 1993.

PROGRESSIVE BACTERIAL AND VIRAL PNEUMONIAS OF SHEEP AND GOATS

JEANNE LOFSTEDT

Chronic progressive pneumonias are diagnosed with some frequency in mature small ruminants. In sheep, ovine progressive pneumonia (OPP) and caseous lymphadenitis (CLA) are the chief causes of chronic respiratory disease. Chronic respiratory disease in goats is commonly associated with the pneumonic form of CLA and less frequently with caprine arthritis encephalitis virus (CAEV)-induced lung lesions. Differential diagnoses that should be entertained in sheep and goats exhibiting signs of chronic respiratory disease include ovine pulmonary carcinoma (OPC), chronic suppurative pneumonia, verminous pneumonia, mycotic pneumonia, tuberculosis, and pulmonary neoplasia.

Ovine Progressive Pneumonia (Maedi-Visna)

DEFINITION AND ETIOLOGY. Ovine progressive pneumonia (OPP) and maedi-visna (MV) are North American and European names for slow virus diseases of sheep characterized by chronic, progressive, debilitating pneumonia, wasting, and indurative mastitis.[702,703] Synonyms are Marsh's progressive pneumonia, zwoegerziekte, la bouhite, and Graaff-Reinet disease.[702] The ovine progressive pneumonia virus (OPPV) and maedi-visna virus (MVV) are nononcogenic exogenous retroviruses that belong to the subfamily Lentiviridae.[704] These enveloped, single-stranded RNA viruses contain the enzyme RNA-dependent DNA polymerase (reverse transcriptase). With this enzyme they use cellular machinery to transcribe a segment of DNA from a template of single-stranded viral RNA; the DNA strand or provirus is then incorporated into the host genome. Close similarity of causal viruses, clinical signs, and lesions produced in tissues permits discussion of OPP and MV as a single disease entity.[702] The ovine lentiviruses (OvLVs) are also related to the CAEV of goats, but differences have been demonstrated through nucleic acid hybridization studies.[705]

CLINICAL SIGNS AND DIFFERENTIAL DIAGNOSIS. Conditions in sheep attributed to infection with OvLV include progressive emaciation ("thin ewe syndrome"), progressive respiratory failure, indurative lymphocytic mastitis ("hard bag"), posterior paresis, chronic nonsuppurative arthritis, and vasculitis.[702-706] In North America progressive pneumonia and aseptic mastitis are the most common clinical manifestations.[702] Natural disease is usually observed in 2- to 3-year-old sheep, but adult sheep of any age can be affected.[702,703,705] Emaciation despite a good appetite is one of the earliest symptoms. Clinical signs of progressive pneumonia include exercise intolerance, tachypnea, expiratory dyspnea, open-mouth breathing, and occasionally a nonproductive cough. Thoracic auscultation reveals increased breath sounds, but crackles and wheezes are inapparent. Pyrexia and purulent nasal discharge suggest the presence of secondary bacterial pneumonia. Affected ewes give birth to small, weak lambs. Death from anoxia or secondary bacterial infection results within 6 to 12 months of first appearance of signs.

Chronic pneumonias of sheep that have to be differentiated from OPP include chronic bronchopneumonia caused by *M. (Pasteurella) haemolytica*, OPC, verminous pneumonia, and pulmonary and lymph node abscesses caused by *Corynebacterium pseudotuberculosis*.[704] Thoracic radiographs, culture of tracheal wash material, and fecal examination by the Baermann technique are useful for antemortem differentiation. Gross and histopathologic evaluations of pulmonary tissues obtained at necropsy are useful for diagnosis of a flock problem.

CLINICAL PATHOLOGY. Hematologic changes in sheep with OPP are nonspecific and may include lymphocytosis early in the course of disease, and mild hypochromic anemia and hypergammaglobulinemia in advanced disease.[705] A presumptive diagnosis of OPP can be made on the basis of clinical signs, lack of response to treatment, and serologic test results. The serologic tests commonly used to detect antibodies to OvLV in serum are the agar gel immunodiffusion test (AGID), enzyme-linked immunosorbent assay (ELISA), and indirect immunofluorescent test (IIFT).[702,703] The simplicity and low cost of the AGID makes it the test of choice for most eradication programs.[707] However, the ELISA is more sensitive and is able to detect infected sheep earlier than the AGID test.[708] Antibodies detected by the AGID are usually present 6 months after infection, but it may take years before seroconversion can be documented.[702] Passively acquired antibodies in noninfected offspring decrease to undetectable levels by 6 months of age.[702,705] A negative AGID result indicates freedom from infection or presence of antibody at a level that is not measurable. A positive AGID result indicates infection but does not correlate with disease expression or prove that clinical signs are attributable to OvLV infection. Currently, virus isolation is the only definitive way to identify OvLV-infected animals.[704] Virus isolation, which is time-consuming and expensive, is accomplished by coculture of infected fresh or frozen tissue with indicator cell lines. In culture, retroviruses form characteristic multinucleated syncytia.[705] Viral antigens can be detected in these syncytia by use of immunofluorescent staining.[705] In the future the polymerase chain reaction (PCR) may be used to detect viral antigen in tissues.[703,710]

PATHOPHYSIOLOGY. OvLV are thought to gain access to the body via the oral or respiratory route. Infection is then established in the monocyte/macrophage cell line and spreads via these infected cells to the lungs, lymph nodes, choroid plexus, spleen, bone marrow, mammary glands, and kidneys.[705] The virus is able to persist in the face of humoral and cellular immunity through (1) latent infection of host cells by DNA provirus, (2) long-term nonproductive infection of blood monocytes (virus replicates only upon differentiation of monocytes into macrophages), and (3) virus mutation with emergence of new antigenic variants that are not neutralized by preexisting antibody.[705] Persistent low-grade viral replication results in continuous antigenic stimulation and development of immunologically mediated inflammatory lesions in various target tissues. B-cell hyperplasia, not accompanied by significant plasmacytosis, predominates in lymph nodes of sheep with OPP, suggesting aberrant immunoregulation in affected sheep.[710]

EPIDEMIOLOGY. The seroprevalence of OPP in cull ewes in the United States ranges from 1% to 70% and increases with advancing age.[711] With the exception of Texas with an infection rate of 1%, serologic surveys in cull ewes in other states have revealed infection rates of 30% to 67%. Low seroprevalence in Texas has been attributed to the hot dry climate and extensive grazing practices.[705] Certain breeds of sheep (Rambouillets) appear to be more resistant to infection, whereas other breeds are highly susceptible (Finnish Landrace and Texel).[705] Disease expression and severity have been shown to be greater in Border Leicester than Columbia sheep regardless of infection method or virus strain used.[702] Although the ewe-lamb relationship has been shown to be an important factor in transmission of MVV, and OPPV is readily isolated from ewe colostrum, colostral transmission of OvLV has not been definitively shown.[705] Nose-to-nose or droplet transmission in confinement is considered the major route of MVV transmission. However, because OvLV are associated with cells (macrophages, monocytes, lymphocytes), fomite (saliva, nasal discharge, urine, feces) contamination of feed and water is the most likely mechanism for spread of disease.[705] Transmission through the uterine wall, or via germ cells, can occur but is rare.[712] Prolonged heavy exposure to OvLV in sheep reared in close confinement appears to accelerate seroconversion and lesion development; lambs reared in confinement can be seropositive and exhibit clinical signs at 1 year of age.[712]

NECROPSY FINDINGS. Lesions may develop in any or all of the following tissues of OPPV-infected sheep: lungs and regional lymph nodes, brain, joints, mammary glands, and blood vessels.[702] Changes are most obvious in the lungs, which do not collapse on opening the thorax.[704,705] Vertical rib impressions may be seen on the exterior lung surface. Affected lungs are heavy and have a mottled to uniform pink-brown to gray-blue discoloration. Secondary bacterial pneumonia may cause anterior-ventral pulmonary consolidation. Tracheobronchial and mediastinal lymph nodes are markedly enlarged, bulge on cut surface, and are homogeneous, gray-white throughout. Histologic examination reveals a diffuse lymphoproliferative pneumonia characterized by prominent lymphoid follicle formation adjacent to bronchioles and small vessels; discrete nodules of lymphocytes, unrelated to vessels or airways, are also found in the lung parenchyma.[702-705] Lymphocytes, plasma cells, and macrophages infiltrate into interalveolar septae, and hyperplasia of alveolar epithelium and terminal bronchial smooth muscle may be seen.

TREATMENT AND PROGNOSIS. OPP is not treatable. Antibiotics can be used to control secondary bacterial pneumonia, but most sheep die within a year of first exhibiting clinical signs.[702,703]

PREVENTION AND CONTROL. OPPV is difficult to eradicate from a flock once infection is established.[705] Control methods include (1) a "test and cull" practice and (2) isolation of infected adults and artificial rearing of their offspring.[702] With the first method, all sheep are tested annually for antibody and seropositive animals and their progeny younger than 1 year of age are culled or isolated from the negative flock; culling is preferred because of the danger of cross-contamination. New additions should be seronegative and originate from seronegative flocks. Annual testing should be performed until two consecutive negative herd test results are obtained to be reasonably confident that the flock is virus free. With the second method, progeny are removed from their dams before they nurse and are fed cow's colostrum and raised in isolation. The clean herd should be kept isolated from infected sheep and goats and from humans and equipment in contact with infected sheep. Herd additions and annual testing should be handled as described for method one.

REFERENCES

702. Cutlip RC et al: Ovine progressive pneumonia (maedi-visna) in sheep, *Vet Microbiol* 17:237-250, 1988.

703. Concha-Bermejillo A de la: Maedi-visna and ovine progressive pneumonia, *Vet Clin North Am (Food Anim Pract)* 13:13-32, 1997.

704. Ellis J, DeMartini JC: Retroviral diseases in small ruminants: ovine progressive pneumonia and caprine arthritis encephalitis, *Compend Cont Educ Pract Vet* 5:S173-S183, 1983.

705. Bulgin MS: Ovine progressive pneumonia, caprine arthritis-encephalitis, and related lentiviral diseases of sheep and goats, *Vet Clin North Am (Food Anim Pract)* 6:691-704, 1990.

706. Narayan O, Cork LC: Lentiviral diseases of sheep and goats: chronic pneumonia, leukoencephalomyelitis and arthritis, *Rev Infect Dis* 7:89-98, 1985.

707. Dawson M: Comparison of serological tests used in three state veterinary laboratories to identify maedi-visna virus infection, *Vet Rec* 111:432-434, 1982.

708. Houwers DJ, Gielkens ALJ, Schaake J: An indirect enzyme-linked immunosorbent assay (ELISA) for detection of antibodies to maedi-visna virus, *Vet Microbiol* 7:209-219, 1982.

709. Smith C: Research roundup: ovine lentivirus: a real or imagined threat? *J Am Vet Med Assoc* 200:139-143, 1992.

710. Ellis JA, DeMartini JC: Immunomorphologic and morphometric changes in pulmonary lymph nodes of sheep with progressive pneumonia, *Vet Pathol* 22:32-41, 1985.

711. Gates NL, Everson DO, Hulet CV: Serologic survey of prevalence of ovine progressive pneumonia in Idaho range sheep, *J Am Vet Med Assoc* 173:1575-1577, 1978.

712. Houwers DJ: Importance of ewe lamb relationship and breed in the epidemiology of maedi-visna infections, *Res Vet Sci* 46:5-8, 1989.

Ovine Pulmonary Carcinoma

DEFINITION AND ETIOLOGY. Ovine pulmonary carcinoma (OPC) (sheep pulmonary adenomatosis or jaagsiekte) is a transmissible bronchiolo-alveolar carcinoma of sheep that has been associated etiologically with a type B/D retrovirus (jaagsiekte sheep retrovirus [JSRV]).[713] Ovine lentiviruses (OVLV) and herpesviruses have been isolated from OPC tumors; however, they are not consistently present[714] and do not induce OPC when inoculated experimentally.[715,716] One theory is that these viruses act as cofactors in tumor induction. Defining the role of JSRV in OPC has been complicated by the presence of JSRV-related endogenous sequences in the genomes of sheep and goats.[717] Recent research has indicated that exogenous JSRV-like viruses are likely not of endogenous origin. There has been speculation that the endogenous viruses may modify the genome of exogenous JSRV, either by inducing the expression of an oncogene, or by inactivating a tumor suppressor gene.[713]

CLINICAL SIGNS AND DIFFERENTIAL DIAGNOSIS. OPC usually affects mature sheep between 2 and 4 years of age although lambs as young as 3 months of age have been diagnosed with the disease.[713] Clinical manifestations include progressive weight loss, exercise intolerance, tachypnea, dyspnea, occasional cough, and crackles and wheezes on thoracic auscultation. In many cases, presence of abundant watery nasal discharge can be demonstrated by raising the rear limbs and lowering the head of the affected sheep ("wheelbarrow test").[713] Appetite and rectal temperature are usually normal unless secondary infection and intercurrent disease are present. Sheep with OPC die within a few weeks to months after first exhibiting clinical signs.

CLINICAL PATHOLOGY. The only reported laboratory abnormality in sheep with OPC is hypergammaglobulinemia. Some researchers have demonstrated the utility of serologic assays to identify OPC infected sheep, but other investigators have been unable to demonstrate antibodies to JSRV in the sera of affected sheep.[713] Modern molecular diagnostic tests, for example, PCR to demonstrate viral nucleic acids in OPC infected tissue, are being developed. In order to be useful, such tests must be able to differentiate between exogenous and endogenous JSRV.[713]

EPIDEMIOLOGY. OPC has been reported in many countries in Europe, Africa, and Asia, but surprisingly has never been documented in Australia.[713] OPC has an average annual morbidity of 2% and mortality of 100%. In some countries,

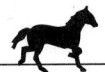

notably South Africa, Peru, and Scotland, disease prevalence is very high, approaching 20% in some flocks. OPC is rarely diagnosed in the United States and Canada, and has been eradicated from Iceland.[713]

OPC has been reproduced experimentally by intratracheal inoculation of lung homogenates or pulmonary lavage fluids obtained from infected animals.[718] Lambs between birth and 5 weeks of age have been shown to be more susceptible to experimental infection than 10-week-old lambs.[718] This age-related susceptibility to OPC suggests that natural virus transmission occurs in the neonatal period. Aerosol transmission and contamination of feed and water by respiratory secretions are likely methods of disease spread, particularly in confined sheep.

NECROPSY FINDINGS. Lungs of OPC sheep are heavy (two to three times normal weight) and exude clear fluid from the cut surface. The trachea and bronchi often contain clear, foamy fluid. Large, firm, gray masses are commonly encountered in the cranioventral regions of one or both lungs. Smaller (1- to 2-cm) nodules are occasionally visualized in the caudodorsal lung regions.[713] Regional pulmonary lymph nodes may be enlarged. Some cases are complicated by secondary acute or chronic bacterial pneumonia.

OPC is classified by the WHO as a brochiolo-alveolar carcinoma arising from alveolar type II pneumocytes or nonciliated bronchiolar cells.[719] Neoplastic masses consist of columnar or cuboidal cells arranged in an acinar or papillary pattern. Some tumors are surrounded by areas of fibroplasia. Metastases to regional lymph nodes occur in approximately 10% of cases; metastases to cardiac and skeletal muscles are infrequently reported.

TREATMENT AND PROGNOSIS. There are no known treatments for this disease. Antibiotics may prolong the life of OPC-affected sheep through control of secondary bacterial pneumonia.[713]

PREVENTION AND CONTROL. Because antemortem tests cannot identify infected sheep, control is difficult. The disease was eradicated from Iceland by slaughtering all sheep in endemic areas.

REFERENCES

713. DeMartini JC, York DF: Retrovirus-associated neoplasms of the respiratory system of sheep and goats, *Vet Clin North Am (Food Anim Pract)* 13:55-70, 1997.
714. Perk K, Yaniv A: Lack of maedi viral related RNA in pulmonary carcinoma of sheep (jaagsiekte), *Res Vet Sci* 24:46-48, 1978.
715. DeMartini JC, Rosadio RH, Lairmore MD: The etiology and pathogenesis of ovine pulmonary carcinoma (sheep pulmonary adenomatosis), *Vet Microbiol* 17:219-236, 1988.
716. Sharp JM: Sheep pulmonary adenomatosis: a contagious tumor and its cause, *Cancer Surv* 6:73-83, 1987.
717. Hecht SJ, Carlson JO, DeMartini JC: Analysis of type D retroviral capsid gene expressed in ovine pulmonary carcinoma and present in both affected and unaffected sheep genomes, *Virology* 202:480-484, 1994.
718. Rosadio RH et al: Retrovirus-associated ovine pulmonary carcinoma (sheep pulmonary adenomatosis) and lymphoid interstitial pneumonia. I. Lesion development and age susceptibility, *Vet Pathol* 25:475-483, 1988.
719. Stunzi H, Head KW, Nielson SW: Tumors of the lung (International Histological Classification of Tumors of Domestic Animals), *Bull World Health Organ* 50:9-19, 1974.

Caprine Arthritis Encephalitis

Caprine arthritis encephalitis (CAE) is a naturally occurring retroviral disease of goats with two major clinical presentations: leukoencephalomyelitis in kids 2 to 6 months of age, and chronic, hyperplastic polysynovitis in mature goats.[720,721] Mild interstitial pneumonia, which is silent clinically, is a common postmortem finding in goat kids with leukoencephalomyelitis.[721] In one study 60% of goats serologically positive for CAEV had lesions of severe chronic interstitial pneumonia at slaughter.[721] Similarly, chronic interstitial pneumonia, accompanied by exercise intolerance and dyspnea, was described in dairy goats originating from herds that had clinical cases of arthritis and leukoencephalomyelitis.[722] The lung lesions in these goats resembled those of ovine progressive pneumonia[722,723] and were positive for CAEV. However, CAEV has been recovered from the lungs of goats with advanced arthritis, but without pneumonia. In addition, goats inoculated intratracheally with purified CAEV did not develop pulmonary lesions.[722] This may indicate that there is no causal relationship between CAEV and interstitial pneumonia in goats, or that the lesions have a multifactorial etiology. Caprine arthritis encephalitis is discussed in detail in Chapter 36.

REFERENCES

720. Phelps SL, Smith MC: Caprine arthritis-encephalitis virus infection, *J Am Vet Med Assoc* 203:1663-1666, 1993.
721. Cork LC, Naraya O: The pathogenesis of viral leukoencephalomyelitis-arthritis of goats. I, Persistent viral infection with progressive pathologic changes, *Lab Invest* 42:596-602, 1980.
722. Ellis TM, Robinson WF, Wilcox GE: The pathology and aetiology of lung lesions in goats infected with caprine arthritis-encephalitis virus, *Aust Vet J* 65:69-73, 1988.
723. Sims LD, Hale CJ, McCormick BM: Progressive interstitial pneumonia in goats, *Aust Vet J* 60:368-371, 1983.

Caseous Lymphadenitis

Caseous lymphadenitis (CLA), caused by *Corynebacterium pseudotuberculosis* (previously known as *C. ovis*), is a worldwide disease of sheep and goats characterized by the development of pyogranulomatous abscesses in the lymph nodes and lungs.[724] CLA usually manifests as subcutaneous abscesses involving superficial lymph nodes. The visceral form of CLA is characterized by development of internal abscesses in the mediastinal and mesenteric lymph nodes, and internal organs, including the lungs. Clinical signs associated with abscesses in the lung parenchyma and mediastinal lymph nodes include exercise intolerance, tachypnea, dyspnea, and chronic cough.[725] Visceral CLA with lung involvement is a common cause of severe weight loss in sheep and goats.[726,727] Because of the encapsulated nature of pulmonary abscesses and lack of exudate in airways, pulmonary crackles are not routinely ausculted.[725] Nonspecific laboratory findings in sheep and goats with CLA include leukocytosis, hyperfibrinogenemia, hyperproteinemia, and hypergammaglobulinemia; however, laboratory findings are frequently normal in animals with chronic abscesses.[725] A definitive diagnosis can be reached by demonstrating abscesses in the lungs and mediastinal lymph nodes of affected small ruminants, and by isolating *C. pseudotuberculosis* from a transtracheal aspirate.[725] Failure to isolate the organism from tracheal wash fluid does not rule out CLA as the cause of pulmonary disease. Characteristic postmortem findings of the respiratory form of CLA are one to multiple thick-walled, laminated, encapsulated, caseopurulent abscesses in the bronchial lymph nodes, mediastinal lymph nodes, and lung parenchyma. The synergistic hemolysis inhibition (SHI) test, which measures antibodies to *C. pseudotuberculosis* toxin, was developed to diagnose early infections before the development of subcutaneous abscesses, and to assist in the diagnosis of internal abscesses.[728] False-negative results with this test are rare, but false-positive results have been reported in 10% of sheep, and 20% of goats. The SHI test is not specific enough to justify its use in culling practices. A double-antibody sandwich ELISA directed at *C. pseudotuberculosis* is being employed in Europe to detect subclinically affected sheep and goats and has contributed to successful disease eradication from some flocks.[729] CLA is discussed in more detail in relation to the hemolymphatic system (see Chapter 35).

REFERENCES

724. Ellis JA: Ovine caseous lymphadenitis, *Compend Cont Educ Pract Vet* 5:S504-S509, 1983.
725. Smith MC, Sherman DM: Respiratory system. In Smith MC, Sherman DM, eds: *Goat medicine*, Philadelphia, 1994, Lea & Febiger, pp 247-273.
726. Smith MC, Sherman DM: Wasting diseases. In Smith MC, Sherman DM, eds: *Goat medicine*, Philadelphia, 1994, Lea & Febiger, pp 495-502.
727. Gates NL, Everson DO, Hulet CV: Effects of the thin ewe syndrome on reproductive efficiency, *J Am Vet Med Assoc* 171:1266-1267, 1984.
728. Brown CC et al: Serodiagnosis of inapparent caseous lymphadenitis in goats and sheep, using the synergistic hemolysis-inhibition test, *Am J Vet Res* 47:1461-1463, 1986.
729. Schreuder BEC, ter Laak EA, Dercksen DP: Eradication of caseous lymphadenitis in sheep with the help of a newly developed ELISA technique, *Vet Record* 135:174-176, 1994.

OTHER PNEUMONIAS

STEVEN E. WIKSE

Aspiration Pneumonia

Aspiration pneumonia is caused by inhalation of large amounts of foreign material, often liquids. It is also called gangrenous pneumonia, foreign-body pneumonia, medication pneumonia, or lipid pneumonia. The most common cause is careless drenching or passage of stomach tubes during administration of milk or liquid medication. It also occurs occasionally in pail-fed calves, animals with pharyngeal paresis, animals with necrobacillary laryngitis, lambs with nutritional myodegeneration, anesthetized animals, sheep that are dipped, cattle that have parturient paresis, and cattle that ingest crude oils or fuel oils.[730,731] Meconium aspiration secondary to fetal distress has been recognized as a possible risk factor of neonatal calf mortality.[732] The condition is characterized by a mild diffuse alveolitis that results in hypoxia and acidosis, which lead to impaired absorption of colostral antibodies and inadequate passive transfer.

If large quantities of fluid are aspirated, death may be almost instantaneous, but generally a gangrenous bronchopneumonia develops as a result of infection and the irritating properties of the inhaled material. Affected animals exhibit depression, polypnea, dyspnea, coughing, and fever, and may have putrid breath. Crackles, wheezes, and occasionally pleural friction rubs can be heard on auscultation.

Diagnosis is based on the history, sudden onset, and severe signs. Differential diagnoses include acute bronchopneumonia and septicemia. Necropsy reveals consolidation of the anterior ventral areas of the lungs. Affected areas are severely hemorrhagic in acute cases and contain suppuration and liquefactive necrosis in subacute cases.

The prognosis is guarded in all cases of aspiration pneumonia, but some animals can be saved. Antibiotics combined with antiinflammatory agents should be promptly administered intravenously. Both nonsteroidal antiinflammatory drugs (NSAIDs) and corticosteroids should be administered immediately, and long-term antimicrobial therapy is required. Prevention of aspiration pneumonia centers on careful administration of medication and avoidance of other risk factors that may promote inhalation of foreign materials.

REFERENCES

730. Radostits OM et al: *Veterinary medicine*, ed 9, London, 1999, Baillière Tindall, p 450.
731. Rowe LD, Edwards WC: Crude oils, fuel oils, and kerosene. In Howard JL, ed: *Current veterinary therapy 2*, Philadelphia, 1986, WB Saunders, pp 451-454.
732. Lopez A, Bildfell R: Pulmonary inflammation associated with aspirated meconium and epithelial cells in calves, *Vet Path* 29:104-111, 1992.

MYCOTIC PNEUMONIAS

Ruminants may occasionally have pulmonary infections with *Coccidioides immitis*, *Aspergillus* spp., *Histoplasma capsulatum*, *Candida albicans*, and fungi of the order Mucorales.[733] Coccidioidomycosis occurs in cattle and much less commonly in sheep and goats in the southwestern United States. It causes very few clinical signs in ruminants, but the occasional animal may exhibit a chronic cough and weight loss. Differential diagnoses include tuberculosis and caseous lymphadenitis. Radiologic evaluation is helpful in establishing the presence of pulmonary masses. The diagnosis may be confirmed by culture, histologic identification of the characteristic spherules, and intradermal and complement-fixation tests. The organism is obtained from the soil and is not easily transmitted from animal to animal or to human, but nevertheless it represents a serious zoonotic disease concern. The major lesion is a granuloma with creamy pus in the bronchial and mediastinal lymph nodes. There is no treatment. Control of dust may lessen the incidence.[733]

Aspergillosis is a rare condition that usually occurs in housed calves, particularly in those that have had chronic antibiotic or steroid therapy or that are otherwise immunosuppressed or chronically ill. There are three forms. The acute form is characterized by a fibrinous pneumonia with fever, dyspnea, tachypnea, cough, nasal discharge, groaning, and a short course to death. The subacute and chronic forms are less severe and exhibit mainly anorexia, weight loss, and mild respiratory signs. Differential diagnoses include enzootic pneumonia, tuberculosis, and lungworms. Radiographs, transtracheal washings, histopathologic evaluation (with demonstration of branching septate hyphae), and culture of lesions help establish the diagnosis. The subacute and chronic lesions consist of multiple small, white, discrete granulomas with necrotic centers. The acute lesions are those of a severe fibrinous pleuropneumonia.[733] Treatment is frequently ineffective; antifungal agents such as nystatin, amphotericin B, and ketoconazole may be tried in individual cases. Doses for these drugs are not established for ruminants.

Histoplasmosis is rare in ruminants. It is a polysystemic disease with chronic emaciation, dyspnea, diarrhea, and anasarca. An intradermal delayed hypersensitivity test, culture, or histopathologic identification of the yeastlike organism helps to confirm the diagnosis. Lesions include ascites, liver enlargement, gut edema, pulmonary emphysema, and pulmonary edema with abscesses. There is no treatment.[733]

Pulmonary candidiasis has been reported as an outbreak in a feedlot. It was characterized by a chronic pneumonia with severe dyspnea but only moderate fever; a mucopurulent, brown-streaked nasal discharge; diarrhea; a crusted muzzle; and lacrimation without conjunctivitis. Differential diagnoses should include the various upper respiratory viruses, particularly infectious bovine rhinotracheitis (IBR) and bovine viral diarrhea virus (BVDV), and bacterial bronchopneumonia. The diagnosis is made by the presence of the budding yeastlike organism in smears and cultures. Lesions include lung consolidation and abscesses.[733] Treatment has not been investigated.

Zygomycosis, phycomycosis, and mucormycosis are synonyms for a very rare opportunistic disease in ruminants. This is a systemic fungal infection that may affect the lung, stomach, liver, brain, and lymphatic system. Cattle with *Mucorales* spp. pneumonia exhibit tachypnea, dyspnea, nasal discharge, fever, and anorexia. The pulmonary lesions are a fibrinous pleuritis with firm, heavy, wet, mottled lungs. Histopathologic demonstration of broad aseptate hyphae in affected tissue and culture are the best means of diagnosis.[733] Treatment has not been investigated.

REFERENCE

733. Armstrong CH, Carlton WW: Systemic mycoses. In Amstutz HE, editor: *Bovine medicine and surgery*, ed 2, vol 1, Santa Barbara, Calif, 1980, American Veterinary Publications, pp 387-401.

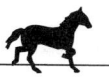

Contagious Bovine Pleuropneumonia

DEFINITION AND ETIOLOGY. Contagious bovine pleuropneumonia (CBPP) is a highly fatal bronchopneumonia caused by *Mycoplasma mycoides* ssp. *mycoides* (small-colony type). The disease originated in Central Europe and in the 1800s spread to many other countries, including the United States. In 1887, Congress established the Bureau of Animal Industry to control CBPP. It was eradicated from the United States through intensive slaughter and quarantine by 1892, 6 years before isolation of its causative organism. The agent of CBPP was the first mycoplasma to be identified and grown on artificial media. Contagious bovine pleuropneumonia now occurs mainly in portions of Asia, Central Africa, Spain, and Portugal.[734]

CLINICAL SIGNS AND DIFFERENTIAL DIAGNOSIS. There is a sudden onset of severe illness after an incubation period that is usually 3 to 6 weeks but can be up to 6 months. Respirations are shallow and rapid with an expiratory grunt. Affected animals cough and exhibit pain by being reluctant to move and standing with their backs arched and elbows out. Auscultation reveals pleural friction sounds in the early stages and fluid sounds with moist wheezes in the later stages. Percussion of the lung fields elicits pain and may identify dull areas. In the later stages there may be a mucopurulent nasal discharge and edematous swellings of the throat and brisket. Pregnant cows may abort, and in young calves a polyarthritis sometimes develops. Approximately 50% of affected animals die after an illness of several days to 3 weeks. Another 25% become recovered carriers with or without clinical signs. Morbidity rate ranges from 50% to 90% and mortality rate from 10% to 50%.

CLINICAL PATHOLOGY. Carrier animals can be detected by the complement-fixation (CF) test, the agglutination test, or an intradermal test similar to the tuberculin test. The strength of the CF test at various serum dilutions is correlated to the duration of illness.[735] All the tests sometimes fail to identify early cases and animals that have recovered for some time. This is a serious problem, particularly in Europe where CBPP infections are often subclinical. More sensitive tests such as polymerase chain reaction (PCR) are under evaluation as solutions to this problem.[736]

PATHOPHYSIOLOGY. Disease probably follows deposition of the organisms in the bronchioles. Mycoplasmas are capable of attaching to the surface of epithelial cells lining the trachea and bronchioles. The events that lead to severe tissue damage have not been completely elucidated. An important aspect of the pathogenesis is a prominent vasculitis that may be caused by exotoxins of the mycoplasma or may be immune mediated. *M. mycoides* ssp. *mycoides* shares common antigens with lung tissue.

EPIDEMIOLOGY. Contagious bovine pleuropneumonia is spread by inhalation of infected droplets disseminated by coughing. Active cases also shed numerous organisms in urine, potentially causing transmission when urine droplets are inhaled. Close contact between animals that are housed or transported fosters transmission. Recovered carrier animals commonly harbor sequestra of infection in their lungs that can serve as potential sources of organisms for years. These animals may not be obviously dangerous to unexposed herd mates because they are often in good flesh.

NECROPSY FINDINGS. Contagious bovine pleuropneumonia is manifested as a fibrinonecrotic bronchopneumonia with abundant serofibrinous pleuritis.[737] The gross lesions are similar to the bronchopneumonia of pasteurellosis, but CBPP differs as follows: (1) often only one lung is affected, (2) the lesions are never symmetric when both lungs are involved, (3) lesions are more common in caudal lung lobes, (4) the marbled appearance on cut sections is more pronounced, and (5) sequestra are more common.

TREATMENT AND PROGNOSIS. Tylosin, tetracycline, and erythromycin had identical very low minimum inhibitory concentrations, and chloramphenicol was the next most active of nine antibiotics tested against *M. mycoides* ssp. *mycoides*.[738] Tylosin is commonly used at a dosage of 10 mg/kg IM every 12 hours for six injections.

PREVENTION AND CONTROL. In countries free of the disease, the obvious method of control is eradication by test and slaughter of reactors. In endemic areas, prevention is accomplished by annual vaccination of the highest percentage of susceptible animals possible.

REFERENCES

734. Radostits OM et al: *Veterinary medicine*, ed 9, London, 1999, Baillière Tindall, pp 999-1004.
735. Dannacher G et al: Report on evaluation of the European comparative trial concerning complement fixation test for diagnosis of contagious bovine pleuropneumonia, *Ann Rech Vet* 17:107-114, 1986.
736. Bashiruddin JB, Taylor TK, Gould AR: A PCR-based test for the identification of *Mycoplasma mycoides* subspecies *mycoides* SC, *J Vet Diag Invest* 6:428-434, 1994.
737. Jubb JVF, Kennedy PC, Palmer N: *Pathology of domestic animals*, ed 4, vol 2, New York, 1993, Academic Press, pp 656-658.
738. Lee DH, Miles RJ, Inal JRM: Antibiotic sensitivity and mutation rates to antibiotic resistance in *Mycoplasma mycoides* spp. *mycoides*, *Epidemiol Infect* 98:361-368, 1987.

Contagious Caprine Pleuropneumonia

Contagious caprine pleuropneumonia (CCPP) is a highly fatal disease of goats in Africa, the Middle East, and Western Asia. Several mycoplasmas have been incriminated as its etiologic agent, but only *Mycoplasma* F38 is currently considered the cause of classic CCPP.[739,740] The disease is highly contagious for goats but not for sheep or cattle.

The infection is introduced into susceptible herds by an asymptomatic carrier or a goat that is in the incubation stage.[740] Rapid spread by inhalation results in a 100% morbidity and 60% to 100% case mortality rate. After an incubation period of 6 to 10 days, affected animals have a fever (40.5° C to 41.5° C [104.9° F to 106.7° F]) and cough, have labored breathing, and become recumbent. In the terminal stages they stand with open-mouth breathing and tongues extended and dribble frothy saliva. Death usually occurs in several days, but it can occur within 2 days.

Diagnosis of clinical or subclinical cases can be accomplished by several serologic tests, including a complement-fixation test, passive hemagglutination, and an ELISA. Recently a latex slide agglutination test has been developed that can easily be performed on serum or whole blood in the field.[741] It is much more sensitive than the complement-fixation test in detecting subclinical infection in goats.

Necropsy of goats dying in the acute stages reveals an excessive amount of clear, straw-colored fluid with small pieces of fibrin in the pleural cavity.[742] The lungs are enlarged and covered with plaques of thick, yellow fibrin. Cut sections of the lung have a mosaic pattern of red, brown, yellow, and gray lobules as a result of different stages of inflammation. Large necrotic areas are also present. Chronic cases have fibrous adhesions between the lungs and thoracic wall, and the lung contains areas of dry white or yellow friable material surrounded by fibrous capsules.

Treatment of cases of CCPP with tylosin tartrate (10 mg/kg) or oxytetracycline (15 mg/kg daily) is highly successful.[743] Tiamulin, a semisynthetic antibiotic, has a very low minimum inhibitory concentration range for the *M. mycoides* group and has been shown to reverse the clinical signs of experimental CCPP rapidly.[744]

Prevention of CCPP can be accomplished by prevention of the introduction of carrier goats into the herd and vaccination. All purchased goats should be held in quarantine for 2 weeks and not mixed with the herd until they are shown

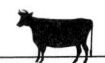

to have negative serologic results for *Mycoplasma* F38. In the past, infective fluids from tissues of field cases have been inoculated subcutaneously to provide immunity.[740] Short-term protection results, and there is no local inflammation or clinical effect of the vaccination. A safer approach is to use inactivated vaccine. An inactivated saponized vaccine has been shown to produce excellent protection for at least 12 months.[745] Control of outbreaks of CCPP is based on slaughter of goats with clinical cases and asymptomatic infections and vaccination of the remaining animals.

REFERENCES

739. MacOwan KJ, Minette JE: The role of mycoplasma strain F38 in contagious caprine pleuropneumonia (CCPP) in Kenya, *Vet Rec* 101:380-381, 1977.
740. McMartin DA, MacOwan KJ, Swift LL: A century of classical contagious caprine pleuropneumonia: from original description of aetiology, *Br Vet J* 136:507-515, 1980.
741. Rurangirwa FR et al: A latex agglutination test for field diagnosis of contagious caprine pleuropneumonia, *Vet Rec* 121:191-193, 1987.
742. Kaliner G, MacOwan KJ: The pathology of experimental and natural contagious caprine pleuropneumonia in Kenya, *Zentralbl Veterinarmed* 23:652-661, 1976.
743. Radostits OM et al: *Veterinary medicine*, ed 9, London, 1999, Baillière Tindall, pp 1004-1005.
744. Ojo MO, Kasali OB, Bamgboye DA: In vitro and in vivo activities of tiamulin against caprine mycoplasmas, Paris, 1984, *International Colloquium on Goat Diseases*, Institut National de la Recherche Agronomique (France), pp 287-293.
745. Rurangirwa FR et al: An inactivated vaccine for contagious caprine pleuropneumonia, *Vet Rec* 121:397-402, 1987.

Mycoplasma Pneumonia of Goats

DEFINITION AND ETIOLOGY. Caprine pneumonias that are not contagious among adults are caused by several species of *Mycoplasma*. *Mycoplasma capricolum* has not been associated with disease in the United States since 1955, and *Mycoplasma mycoides* ssp. *capri* has not been identified in the United States.[746] In recent years the large colony type *M. mycoides* ssp. *mycoides* (Mmm) has emerged as a very serious cause of mortality among goat kids and does throughout the United States.[747,748]

CLINICAL SIGNS AND DIFFERENTIAL DIAGNOSIS. In herds with Mmm infections, goat kids usually appear clinically normal until 2 to 8 weeks of age, when the following three clinical syndromes occur[747,748]:

1. A peracute illness characterized by high fevers (41.1° C to 42.2° C [105.8° F to 107.9° F]) and death within 12 to 24 hours
2. A central nervous system (CNS) syndrome with opisthotonos and death within 24 to 72 hours
3. An acute to subacute syndrome with high fevers, multiple hot swollen joints, and pneumonia

The most common manifestations are swollen joints, lameness, and recumbency. About one half of affected kids have increased lung sounds on expiration and elevated respiratory rates. During an outbreak, 80% to 90% of kids die or are euthanized because of permanent recumbency. Mmm infection in adult does is also life-threatening. Forty-six does died in 1 week on a 600-goat dairy during an acute outbreak of arthritis/polyarthritis, mastitis, and interstitial pneumonia caused by Mmm infection.[749]

In the United States the main differential diagnosis of Mmm infection in goats is caprine arthritis encephalitis (CAE), which is a chronic, sporadic disease. Animals with CAE are generally alert and nonfebrile and continue to eat well. Affected kids exhibit a CNS syndrome at 8 to 16 weeks of age characterized by ataxia and posterior paresis progressing to tetraparesis in 2 weeks to 2 months. They also have a progressive interstitial pneumonia that is usually inapparent. The arthritic form of CAE usually occurs in goats 1 to 2 years of age. In addition, the joints of animals with acute Mmm contain fibrinopurulent exudate, whereas mononuclear cells are present in the joint fluid of CAE cases.

CLINICAL PATHOLOGY. The definitive diagnosis of Mmm infection in individuals requires isolation of the agent from milk, joint fluid, blood, urine, or tissue. Infected goat herds can be readily identified by culturing bulk tank milk because infected does shed up to 10^{10} Mmm per milliliter of milk.[747] Inapparent carriers can be identified by milk culturing, but false-negative results are a risk because organisms are shed intermittently. An enzyme-linked immunosorbent assay to detect specific antibodies against Mmm has been developed but has not been evaluated for detection of carrier animals.[750]

PATHOPHYSIOLOGY. Field cases of Mmm infection show evidence of widespread thrombosis, suggesting disseminated intravascular coagulation. A coagulopathy, indicated by increases in prothrombin and partial thromboplastin times and a decrease in number of platelets, has been demonstrated in experimental infections.[751] Mmm has been shown to cause direct damage to cultured endothelial cells and to activate complement.[752]

EPIDEMIOLOGY. Localization of Mmm in the udder with no overt signs of mastitis is a key feature of transmission of the disease. In other does udder infections develop through contact with the organisms during milking, and their kids become infected by ingestion of colostrum.[753] The localization of Mmm, often associated with mites in the external ear canal of asymptomatic goats, may also play a role in the epidemiologic process of Mmm infections.[754]

NECROPSY FINDINGS. The most common necropsy finding in goat kids that die of Mmm infections is a fibrinopurulent polyarthritis.[747,748] Approximately one half of field cases have pneumonia. One or more lung lobes have areas of patchy to diffuse red consolidation that is sometimes covered with a fibrinous exudate. Clear, golden yellow to serosanguineous fluid is found in the thorax in half of the cases. In some patients there are fibrinous adhesions between the lungs and thoracic wall. Affected lungs have microscopic evidence of bronchopneumonia or interstitial pneumonia. Other common lesions include pericarditis, peritonitis, and enlargement of the kidneys, liver, and spleen.

TREATMENT AND PROGNOSIS. Conventional antibiotic therapy for goats with Mmm infections is almost always unsuccessful.[747,748] Tylosin or tetracyclines are commonly used. A low percentage of kids make a clinical recovery from the septicemic illness but often have arthritis by the time they freshen. Does that recover from mastitis become chronic carriers.

PREVENTION AND CONTROL. Prevention is based on maintaining herds free of Mmm infection. Purchased does should originate only from herds that have no history of mortality in kids from arthritis and pneumonia and that have negative bulk tank cultures for Mmm. Purchased individuals should be held separate from the milking herd until they have an Mmm-negative milk culture result and are treated for ear mites.[755] A vaccine is not commercially available; however, an experimental formalin-killed vaccine has been shown to be protective.[756]

Control of Mmm outbreaks is centered on prevention of the systemic infection in kids and mastitis in milking does. Rapid prevention of new cases in kids can be expected from a program of feeding heat-treated goat colostrum (56° C [132.4° F] for 1 hour) or cow colostrum at birth, pasteurized milk up to 1 month of age, and pasteurized milk or a high-quality milk replacer from 1 month to weaning.[747,755] All kids with swollen joints should be culled. Milking hygiene should be improved to prevent transmission of infection during milking. Udders should be dried with individual cloths or paper towels, teats should be dipped with an organic iodine base preparation, and

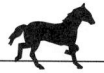

teat cups should be backflushed. Milk samples from all does in the milking herd should be cultured to identify carrier does. Infected does should be kept in a separate string and milked last or culled, depending on production. Colostrum of dry does should be cultured as they freshen, and the does should be hand-milked separately until their milk is found to be free of Mmm. Monthly cultures of the bulk tank milk from the non-infected string should be performed to ensure that it is free of Mmm infection. The goal of control procedures is eradication of Mmm from the herd.

REFERENCES

746. DaMassa AJ et al: Brief account of caprine mycoplasmosis in the United States with special reference to *Mycoplasma mycoides* subsp *mycoides*, *US Anim Health Assoc* 88:291-302, 1984.
747. DaMassa AJ, Brooks DL, Adler HE: Caprine mycoplasmosis: widespread infection in goats with *Mycoplasma mycoides* subsp *mycoides* (large colony type), *Am J Vet Res* 44:322-325, 1983.
748. East NE et al: Milkborne outbreak of *Mycoplasma mycoides* subspecies *mycoides* infection in a commercial goat dairy, *J Am Vet Med Assoc* 182:1338-1341, 1983.
749. Kinde H et al: Mycoplasma infection in a commercial goat dairy caused by *Mycoplasma agalactia* and *Mycoplasma mycoides* subsp. *mycoides* (caprine biotype), *J Vet Diagn Invest* 6:423-427, 1994.
750. Lebel E et al: Vaccination trials against caprine *Mycoplasma mycoides* subsp *mycoides* (large colony) infection in young goats. II, Detection of antibodies by an enzyme-linked immunosorbent assay, *Refuah Vet* 39:85-90, 1982.
751. Rosendal S: Experimental infection of goats, sheep and calves with the large colony type of *Mycoplasma mycoides* subsp *mycoides*, *Vet Pathol* 18:71-81, 1981.
752. Rosendal S: Pathogenic mechanisms of *Mycoplasma mycoides* subsp *mycoides* septicemia in goats, *Israel J Med Sci* 20:970-971, 1984.
753. DaMassa AJ, Brooks DL, Holmberg CA: Induction of mycoplasmosis in goat kids by oral inoculation with *Mycoplasma mycoides* subsp *mycoides*, *Am J Vet Res* 47:2084-2089, 1986.
754. DaMassa AJ: Prevalence of mycoplasmas and mites in the external auditory meatus of goats, *Calif Vet* 37:10-13, 17, 1983.
755. East NE: Personal communication, 1988.
756. Bar-Moshe B et al: Vaccination trials against caprine *Mycoplasma mycoides* subsp *mycoides* (large colony) infection in young goats. I. Infectivity trials, vaccination and challenge, *Refuah Vet* 39:77-85, 1982.

VENA CAVAL THROMBOSIS AND METASTATIC PNEUMONIA

DEFINITION AND ETIOLOGY. Metastatic or embolic pneumonia in cattle, also called caudal vena caval thrombosis, pulmonary thromboembolism, and embolic pulmonary aneurysm, is a distinct syndrome associated with multifocal abscessation of the lungs caused by septic thromboembolism of the pulmonary arterial system. The septic emboli arise from septic thrombi of the caudal vena cava, or, less commonly, the cranial vena cava. Vena caval thrombi are in turn a sequela to various septic conditions such as jugular phlebitis, mastitis, metritis, foot rot, or, most often, liver abscesses secondary to rumenitis.[757] A variety of bacteria may be involved; those most frequently encountered include *Fusobacterium necrophorum*, *Arcanobacterium pyogenes*, staphylococci, streptococci, and *Escherichia coli*.

CLINICAL SIGNS AND DIFFERENTIAL DIAGNOSIS. Because of its association with rumenitis, this condition is most commonly seen in feedlot cattle, but any age, breed, sex, and class of cattle may be affected. The problem is unusual in cattle less than 1 year of age. Cattle with metastatic pneumonia usually exhibit respiratory disturbance or weight loss or occasionally thoracic pain. The duration of signs is quite variable, ranging from acute respiratory distress to a chronic history of weight loss and coughing for weeks to months.[758,759] The classic presentation includes tachycardia, tachypnea (respiratory rate over 30 breaths/min), expiratory dyspnea and groaning, hyperpnea, coughing, hemic murmurs and pale mucous membranes (caused by anemia), widespread wheezes, epistaxis, and hemoptysis.[757,758] Other signs, which are more variable, include fever, thoracic pain on deep palpation of the sternum and intercostal spaces, hepatomegaly (indicated by the ability to palpate the caudal edge of the liver in the right paralumbar fossa), subcutaneous emphysema, froth at the muzzle, and melena caused by coughing up and swallowing blood.[757,758] Nonspecific accompanying signs include depression, anorexia, rumen stasis, scant feces, and decreased milk production. In chronic cases, cor pulmonale may lead to signs of right ventricular failure such as jugular distention and brisket edema.[758] The combination of respiratory signs with anemia, widespread wheezes, and especially hemoptysis is generally regarded as pathognomonic for this syndrome.[758] Animals usually deteriorate rapidly once hemoptysis becomes evident, and the condition is essentially 100% fatal. Many patients die suddenly with an acute episode of severe intrapulmonary hemorrhage or hemoptysis after a variable course of respiratory disease. Some of these cases in which the respiratory signs were overlooked may account for the reports of sudden death attributed to vena caval thrombosis.[758] Caudal vena caval thrombosis can also lead to hepatomegaly and extensive ascites, but most of these animals also have respiratory signs.[759] Sudden erosion of a large hepatic abscess into the caudal vena cava may also result in a massive embolic shower, with acute respiratory distress and death.[759]

In patients with the pathognomonic signs (the majority of cases), no differential diagnoses need be considered. However, many patients are examined before the onset of hemoptysis, and a few may die without exhibiting these signs.[759] Differential considerations in such cases, which usually manifest as acute dyspnea, should include anaphylaxis, the various acute respiratory distress syndromes, hypersensitivity pneumonitis, lungworms, and acute bronchopneumonia. Patients with right ventricular failure should be differentiated from those with pericarditis, lymphosarcoma, cardiomyopathy, and endocarditis.

CLINICAL PATHOLOGY. The complete blood count may reveal anemia and a neutrophilic leukocytosis with a regenerative left shift. Hyperglobulinemia is frequently present. Serum chemical analysis may reflect chronic passive congestion of the liver, with elevation of bilirubin and liver-derived enzymes. Radiographs often reveal only an irregular increase in lung density. Small discrete densities (areas of embolic infarction and collapse); large, discrete, spheric opacities (hematomas); cavitating nodules, sometimes with gas/fluid interfaces (abscesses); bullae; and areas of consolidation may be observed in some cases.[758,759]

PATHOPHYSIOLOGY. The classic pathogenesis of this disease begins with the development of rumenitis secondary to lactic acidosis caused by highly fermentable diets such as those used in feedlots, some dairies, and some growing rations. Bacteria such as *F. necrophorum* and *A. pyogenes* are then able to penetrate the damaged rumen epithelium and are transported to the liver in the portal drainage system, where they are filtered out and result in abscesses. If an abscess is located next to the caudal vena cava (where the vessel is closely applied to the left border of the liver), a septic thrombus may form in the vena cava as a result of infiltration of its wall by the abscess. Septic emboli detach from the thrombus and reach the lungs through the pulmonary arterial system. Alternatives to this classic pathway are rare; they include the following: thrombosis of the cranial vena cava from primary lesions such as jugular phlebitis, thrombosis of the caudal vena cava from other subdiaphragmatic abscesses, right-sided endocarditis, and emboli arising from other septic foci such as mastitis, metritis, and foot rot. Large emboli may block lobar or larger arteries, causing an acute crisis and death. More typically, smaller emboli lodge in arterioles, where they cause arterial thromboembolism, arteritis, endarteritis, and pulmonary abscesses. The widespread arterial embolism also results in pulmonary arterial hypertension. Arteritis and endarteritis weaken the vessel walls and, in combination with pulmonary hypertension, lead to the formation of aneurysms. In some cases a perivascular abscess not only erodes an arterial wall to produce an aneurysm, but simultaneously erodes a bronchial wall; when the aneurysm ruptures, the abscess cavity channels the blood into the bronchus, resulting in massive hemoptysis. In other cases, rupture of aneurysms results in large interstitial hematomas. Both processes result in anemia; when coughed-up blood is swallowed, melena may result. Coughing and wheezes are probably caused by blood clots in airways, peribronchial aneurysms and abscesses, and suppurative pneumonia. Pain results from dissecting aneurysms and hematomas.[758]

EPIDEMIOLOGY. Metastatic pneumonia accounted for 1.3% of necropsy diagnoses in one large feedlot survey, with a rate varying between 1.6 and 7.3 cases per 100,000 head on feed. Cases occurred year round and during all stages of fattening, although 68% of cases occurred during the first 90 days on feed.[760] The case fatality rate is usually 100%.

NECROPSY FINDINGS. Almost all patients with significant hemoptysis have a thrombus in the posterior vena cava between the liver and the right atrium. There is usually an adjacent hepatic abscess, varying degrees of venous congestion of the liver, and hepatomegaly. The lungs are large, uncollapsed, and firm. Aneurysms may occur in either lung or both. Hematomas associated with ruptured aneurysms are frequently 3 to 10 cm in diameter.[760] Large blood clots may be found in the airways, aspirated blood in the alveoli, and swallowed clots in the rumen. Areas of suppurative pneumonia and multiple abscesses are present.

TREATMENT AND PROGNOSIS. The prognosis is grave, so treatment is rarely indicated, and salvage is the most feasible recommendation. In valuable individuals, antibiotics and supportive therapy may be attempted. Penicillin is the drug of choice for the most common organisms involved; large doses (22,000 U/kg IM or SC twice daily as a minimum) for extended periods (weeks to months) are recommended. Supportive therapy for cases with acute severe dyspnea includes furosemide (0.4 to 1.1 mg/kg IV or IM twice daily), flunixin meglumine (0.5 to 1.1 mg/kg IM or IV daily to 3 times daily), and atropine (0.04 mg/kg SC daily).

PREVENTION AND CONTROL. On the basis of the assumption that rumenitis and liver abscesses are the first steps in the pathogenesis of most cases, measures to reduce the incidence of these problems may be beneficial. Recommendations include slow adaptation of animals to high-energy rations and feeding of antibiotics to reduce the incidence of liver abscesses (see Chapter 31).

REFERENCES

757. Gudmundson J, Radostits OM, Doige CE: Pulmonary thromboembolism in cattle due to thrombosis of the posterior vena cava associated with hepatic abscessation, *Can Vet J* 19:304-309, 1978.
758. Breeze RG et al: Hemoptysis in cattle, *Bovine Pract* 11:64-72, 1976.
759. Rebhun WC et al: Caudal vena caval thrombosis in four cattle with acute dyspnea, *J Am Vet Med Assoc* 176:1366-1369, 1980.
760. Jensen R et al: Embolic pulmonary aneurysms in yearling feedlot cattle, *J Am Vet Med Assoc* 169:518-520, 1976.

TUBERCULOSIS

H. MICHAEL CHADDOCK

DEFINITION AND ETIOLOGY. Mycobacterium bovis is the most common cause of tuberculosis in cattle and goats, which are quite susceptible.[761] Sheep have been regarded as relatively resistant, but reports from New Zealand indicate that large numbers can be affected.[762,763] Other *Mycobacterium*

spp., particularly *M. avium* and *M. tuberculosis*, occasionally cause clinical disease, but their main importance lies in the problems that they create in eradication programs through cross-sensitization to mammalian tuberculin.

CLINICAL SIGNS AND DIFFERENTIAL DIAGNOSIS. Unfortunately the signs of *M. bovis* infection are very nonspecific. Most infected animals do not show clinical abnormalities, yet they pose health risks to other livestock and to humans. Patients may have chronic weight loss, variable appetite, and fluctuating fevers, which may be accentuated after calving. Other signs depend on the organs involved. The route of invasion in ruminants is usually respiratory; however, recent research has demonstrated the capability of contaminated feed to transmit the disease.[764] Signs related to the respiratory system are relatively common although usually mild. Respiratory signs in ruminants include a soft, moist, chronic cough. Obvious dyspnea, tachypnea, hyperpnea, and adventitious lung sounds occur only in the terminal stages. Lung sounds include crackles, wheezes, and silent spots occupied by granulomas; pleural friction rubs may occur rarely. Enlarged mediastinal nodes may cause bloat. Intestinal ulceration and diarrhea may occur, and enlarged mesenteric nodes may cause transport failure or obstructions. Involvement of retropharyngeal nodes may cause dysphagia, stridor, and salivation. Lesions occur rarely in the peripheral nodes, the reproductive tract (causing infertility, abortion, metritis, and vaginitis), and the mammary gland. Other chronic pulmonary infections should be considered (e.g., chronic suppurative pneumonia, *Arcanobacterium pyogenes* abscesses, *Corynebacterium pseudotuberculosis* caseous lymphadenitis in sheep and goats, and mycotic pneumonias). Pharyngeal lesions should be differentiated from pharyngeal trauma, abscesses, lymphosarcoma, other tumors, rabies, botulism, actinobacillosis, necrotic laryngitis, and laryngeal abscesses, trauma, edema, paralysis, and tumors.

CLINICAL PATHOLOGY. The intradermal tuberculin test is the only clinicopathologic test routinely used. In the United States, accredited veterinarians are authorized to administer 0.1 ml of mammalian tuberculin purified protein derivative intradermally in the caudal tail fold. The test result is read in 72 ± 6 hours as negative or suspect. State or federal veterinarians use the comparative cervical test to determine the disposition of suspect cattle; biologically balanced mammalian and avian tuberculin are injected simultaneously in two sites on the same side of the neck, 12 cm apart and one above the other. The results are read with calipers in 72 hours and applied to a nomogram to determine status. State or federal veterinarians may also use a 0.2-ml cervical test in known infected herds. Other tests no longer in use include the subcutaneous and intravenous thermal tests, in which a temperature spike to over 40° C (104° F) in 4 to 8 hours is the positive response; and the Stormont test, in which the intradermal test is performed twice in the same area 7 days apart. The response is determined 24 hours after the second test and an increase in skin thickness of 5 mm or greater is the positive result. A tuberculin test may result in locally increased sensitivity for about 12 days; thereafter there is a temporary generalized hyposensitization that may last for up to 6 months. Repeat tests must therefore be performed within the 12-day window (before 10 days or after 60 days in the United States). A relative hyposensitization also may occur just before and for 4 to 6 weeks after calving. Finally, animals with advanced pulmonary lesions may be anergic, and early cases less than 6 weeks after infection may not react. False-positive reactions may occur as a result of human or avian tuberculosis, Johne's disease, saprophytic *Mycobacterium* spp., or other agents such as *Nocardia* spp.[761] Radiographs may be helpful in establishing the presence of pulmonary masses in

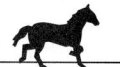

individual cases. Cultures of nasal exudate, tracheal sputum, and lesions, and histopathologic evaluation of lesions, are used by researchers to determine shedding and to make a positive diagnosis. Slaughter examination at slaughter facilities inspected by the Food Safety Inspection Service and necropsy are used by control officials to determine the presence of lesions. Histopathologic examination, polymerase chain reaction (PCR) testing, and bacterial culture are all used to determine the positive diagnosis in animals with lesions, suspect, or reactor animals.

PATHOPHYSIOLOGY. The organism usually enters ruminants through the respiratory route, occasionally by ingestion. A small necrotic granulomatous lesion usually occurs in the lungs but is less common when the gut is involved. From this site of entry the organism invades the local lymph nodes (bronchial, mediastinal, pharyngeal, mesenteric), where it causes necrosis surrounded by a granuloma containing mononuclear cells. This combination of lesions at the site of entry and the local lymph nodes is called the primary complex. From there a postprimary dissemination occurs to various organs and can result in diffuse miliary tuberculosis, discrete nodular lesions in various organs, or chronic organ tuberculosis. In ruminants the disease is progressive.

EPIDEMIOLOGY. Infected animals are the usual source, and the organism occurs in exhaled droplets, sputum, feces, milk, urine, vaginal discharge, semen, and draining nodes. Tuberculous lesions occur in the respiratory lymph nodes in about 90% of reactors with confirmed infections. However, lung lesions are found in only 1% to 2% of these animals at slaughter examinations. Such animals have been regarded as nonexcreters and thus unimportant in transmission of the disease. Recent studies have shown that, if careful laboratory examinations are made, over 70% of cattle with lesions in respiratory lymph nodes have small lung lesions, and in 19% of confirmed cases, *M. bovis* is present in the tracheal mucus. All cattle with tuberculous lesions are therefore potential shedders.[765] Feces can remain infective for 6 to 8 weeks, and stagnant water for 18 days. Milk historically was a common route of infection in young animals. Housing and crowding increase spread. Brahman-type cattle are thought to be more resistant than European breeds. Bovine tuberculosis is an important zoonotic disease because of its potential for spread in nonpasteurized milk from infected animals. Wild ruminants, white-tailed deer, and other species such as badgers in Europe and opossums in New Zealand may serve as reservoirs. Recently, bovine tuberculosis has been recognized to be endemic in the white-tailed deer population in Michigan. Transmission is thought to have occurred from white-tailed deer to cattle in Michigan. The incidence of tuberculosis has been greatly reduced by control programs in many countries, including the United States. However, the residual cases are the most difficult and expensive to detect and remove, and consequently outbreaks still occur. Fairly large-scale outbreaks have been reported recently in dairies that were previously free of the disease,[766] and the proportion of feeder animals that account for slaughter cases has increased in recent years.[767] In the southwestern United States importation of feeder cattle from Mexico is a major source of the disease.[766]

NECROPSY LESIONS. Tuberculous granulomas are typically encapsulated, with thick, yellow to orange, creamy to caseous pus and may be calcified. They occur in any lymph node, but especially the bronchial, mediastinal, and mesenteric nodes, and in a variety of organs, particularly the lungs and liver. The organs may be riddled with small miliary tubercles, and in the lungs these may coalesce into a suppurative bronchopneumonia. They must be differentiated from caseous lymphadenitis lesions in sheep and goats.

TREATMENT, PROGNOSIS, PREVENTION, AND CONTROL. In most countries the disease is not treated, and affected animals are slaughtered. In the United States, animals may be required to test for interstate movement; and examinations are made at slaughter facilities inspected by the Food Safety Inspection Service. Reactors are quarantined and identified and must be sent to an approved slaughter plant or destroyed under regulatory supervision. Reactors are also traced back to the herd of origin, and this herd and any herds in contact are tested for tuberculosis. Affected herds are depopulated if possible or must pass two herd tests at 60-day intervals, followed by another negative test result in 6 months.[768] Suspect animals are either retested or slaughtered. Herds are accredited as free of tuberculosis when all animals over 24 months of age (12 months for goats) and any animal other than natural additions under 24 months of age pass two consecutive annual tests. States are certified as free when no evidence of tuberculosis is disclosed for 5 years.[768]

REFERENCES

761. Blood DC, Radostits OM, Henderson JA: *Veterinary medicine*, ed 6, London, 1983, Baillière Tindall, pp 631-642.
762. Davidson RM, Alley MR, Beatson NS: Tuberculosis in a flock of sheep, *NZ Vet J* 29:1-2, 1981.
763. Cordes DO et al: Observations on tuberculosis caused by *Mycobacterium bovis* in sheep, *NZ Vet J* 29:60-62, 1981.
764. Palmer MV et al: Deer to deer transmission of *Mycobacterium bovis*, *Proceedings of the International Workshop on Tuberculosis in Animals*, Ames, Iowa, Sept 1999.
765. McIlroy SG, Neill SD, McCracken RM: Pulmonary lesions and *Mycobacterium bovis* excretion from the respiratory tract of tuberculin-reacting cattle, *Vet Rec* 118:718-721, 1986.
766. Mathis BM, Langley J: Bovine tuberculosis in an Arizona dairy herd, *J Am Vet Med Assoc* 178:141-142, 1981.
767. Essey MA, Searles WL: Tuberculosis in feedlot animals, *Proceedings of the eighty-sixth annual meeting of the United States Animal Health Association*, Nashville, Nov 7-12, 1982, pp 542-545.
768. Anonymous: Bovine tuberculosis eradication: uniform methods and rules effective March 13, 1985, United States Department of Agriculture, Animal and Plant Health Inspection Service, Veterinary Services.

DISEASES OF THE THORACIC WALL AND CAVITY

JOHN A. SMITH

Pleuritis and Pleural Effusions

DEFINITION AND ETIOLOGY. Acute, primary pleuritis is rare in ruminants. It is almost always a secondary condition. Probably the most common primary cause is bronchopneumonia. Other possible causes of pleuritis and pleural effusions include traumatic reticulopericarditis, extension from other causes of peritonitis, tuberculosis, liver abscesses, tumors (especially lymphosarcoma), external trauma, fractured ribs, gunshot, perforating injuries, sporadic bovine encephalomyelitis (SBE), contagious bovine and caprine pleuropneumonia, various septicemic conditions, acorn toxicity and other causes of uremia, uroperitoneum, right ventricular failure, hypoproteinemia, ruptured thoracic duct, and hemothorax from trauma or hemangiosarcoma.

CLINICAL SIGNS AND DIFFERENTIAL DIAGNOSIS. The signs depend upon, and may be overshadowed by, the primary disease process. Pleuritis is a painful, septic process, whereas the signs associated with nonseptic effusions depend largely on the cause. Signs referable to pleuritis itself include anorexia, depression, fever, weight loss, decreased milk production, progressive dyspnea, and a characteristic stance and respiratory pattern, with the head and neck extended, elbows abducted, restricted excursion of the thorax, abdominal breathing, tachypnea, and a grunting or groaning with respiration. The animal may be reluctant to move. If a cough is

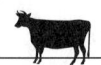

present, it is often soft and suppressed because of pain. Jugular distention and pulsation may result from interference with venous return.[769] Auscultation may reveal creaking or rubbing noises in dry pleuritis or a cranial-ventral masking of sounds caused by effusion. Percussion may reveal dullness ventral to the fluid line and elicit pain. Differential diagnoses for dyspnea with abnormally quiet lung fields may include the atypical pneumonias, pneumothorax, and space-occupying lesions such as large abscesses, tumors, and diaphragmatic hernia. Once pleuritis or pleural effusion has been identified, the main differential diagnostic consideration is the determination of the underlying cause, as listed previously.

CLINICAL PATHOLOGY. A complete blood count helps to separate infectious from noninfectious causes and distinguish relatively acute conditions (with significant left shifts) from those of a more chronic nature (with mature neutrophilia, hyperglobulinemia, and nonregenerative anemia of chronic disease). Serum chemical determinations and urinalysis identify hypoproteinemia and azotemia. A thoracocentesis should be performed and submitted to cytologic and cultural examination for bacteria, mycoplasma, and chlamydia. Nonseptic transudates indicate conditions such as neoplasia, heart failure, hypoproteinemia, and uremia. Effusions of sporadic bovine encephalomyelitis are relatively acellular with high protein and fibrinogen levels, whereas septic exudates high in both cells and protein occur with pneumonia, hardware, peritonitis, abscesses, penetrating trauma, and septicemias. A transtracheal wash is usually indicated because of the common association with pneumonia. Pericardiocentesis, abdominocentesis, and radiographs may indicate the primary source of an infection. Tuberculosis tests, leukemia virus titers, chlamydial titers for SBE, ECG, echocardiographic examinations, ultrasonographic examination of the liver, and exploratory laparotomy may also help to detect other primary processes.

TREATMENT AND PROGNOSIS. The primary problem should be treated. Effusions should be drained, either periodically or continuously through a Heimlich valve or a suction device fashioned from a syringe with the plunger transfixed with a pin. Effective drainage can be difficult in ruminants because of their propensity for fibrin formation and loculation of the fluid. Intermittent drainage is as effective as continuous drainage and simpler to maintain. Attempts at lavage have rarely been successful because of adhesions. Appropriate antibiotics are indicated in the presence of sepsis. Nonsteroidal antiinflammatory drugs (aspirin, 100 mg/kg PO twice daily; phenylbutazone, 6 mg/kg PO daily; flunixin meglumine, 0.5 to 1.1 mg/kg IM or IV daily to 3 times daily) or narcotic analgesics (Demerol, morphine, or butorphanol) are useful to relieve pain, ease respiration, and improve appetite. Rest and good nursing care are essential. The prognosis obviously depends on the extent and duration of the disease. Although many animals that have severe cases survive, such animals often remain chronically underweight.

REFERENCE
769. Nigam JM, Singh AP, Mirakhur KK: Radiographic diagnosis of bovine thoracic disorders, *Mod Vet Pract* 61:1021-1025, 1980.

Pneumothorax

Pneumothorax is not common in ruminants. Most cases result from the rupture of an emphysematous bulla associated with straining, coughing, or pneumonia or from puncture of the lung by a fractured rib. A case has been described in a postparturient cow with no other underlying cause found.[770] The bullae that occur in bovine respiratory syncytial virus–induced pneumonia are a common source. Penetration from the exterior is possible but less common. Ruminants have a complete mediastinum; thus collapse is usually unilateral, and the animal survives on one lung. An inspiratory dyspnea, sometimes severe, with open-mouth breathing is present,[770] and one side of the thorax may be relatively collapsed and immobile, with a compensatory increase in the size and excursion of the other side. However, this latter finding is often subtle and difficult to appreciate. Unless an infectious disease is responsible, affected animals are often alert and anxious. They may attempt to stand with the forefeet elevated. There is a pronounced abdominal component to the respirations. Cyanosis may occur, and airflow may be markedly reduced in severe cases. On auscultation there is an obvious disparity between the two sides; the collapsed side is almost silent. Those lung sounds that are audible have a harsh, high-pitched, large airway character similar to those of a consolidated lung, especially over the carina; these sounds seem to be distant, as if the animal were breathing in a barrel. The point of maximum intensity of the heart may be displaced, and tachycardia is often present. Percussion may reveal an abnormal resonance when compared with that of the normal side, and simultaneous auscultation and percussion may produce a "ping." Subcutaneous emphysema is a fairly common feature, and pleuritis is often a sequela. Differential diagnoses of the inciting cause should include the atypical pneumonias, bronchopneumonia, viral pneumonias (especially bovine respiratory syncytial virus), pleural effusions, diaphragmatic hernia, other space-occupying lesions (large abscesses, tumors), and clostridial infections.[770] Radiographs are the best means of confirming the diagnosis. If a wound is present, it should be closed, and the air aspirated. In cases of internal pneumothorax, dorsal aspiration should be attempted, using a three-way stopcock on a teat cannula and a large syringe or a vacuum pump. This may fail because the lesion reopens and admits more air; the air is gradually resorbed once the lesion heals. Appropriate antibiotics are indicated if a bacterial infection underlies the pneumothorax.

REFERENCE
770. Guard C: Pneumothorax after parturition in a cow, *Compend Cont Educ Pract Vet* 7:S191-S194, 1985.

Diaphragmatic Hernia

DEFINITION AND ETIOLOGY. Diaphragmatic hernias are uncommon in ruminants but have been reported in calves, cattle, sheep,[771] and domestic buffalo.[772,773] The condition appears to be much more prevalent in the buffalo but otherwise is analogous to that in cattle.[774] Hernias may be congenital, but most appear to be acquired, including those occurring in neonates. A congenital weakness in the diaphragm may predispose to some cases. Causes include difficult parturition, external trauma, and, by far the most common cause, traumatic reticuloperitonitis (TRP).

CLINICAL SIGNS AND DIFFERENTIAL DIAGNOSIS. Affected animals can be asymptomatic for a prolonged period.[774] Most affected cattle are in late gestation or have calved recently. The history may include decreased milk production, weight loss, capricious appetite, difficulty in swallowing or regurgitation, previous signs of abdominal pain (possibly associated with acute TRP), vomiting, and abnormal posturing of the head and neck on swallowing or regurgitation. Respiratory signs are actually fairly uncommon, with the exception of large congenital hernias, in which there is obvious severe dyspnea and abdominal respiration from birth. An occasional cough and dyspnea have been reported, and auscultation may reveal asymmetric sounds, with lack of lung or heart sounds in the affected area, or splashing sounds

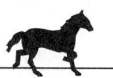

similar to those heard with pericarditis. Gastrointestinal signs are actually more common and include bloat, signs consistent with TRP, difficulty or pain on passage of a stomach tube, diarrhea, constipation, and rumen hypomotility. Some cows may retch or vomit on regurgitation. Pain is evidenced by odontoprisis or grunting on regurgitation. The primary differentials are TRP, pericarditis, esophageal stricture, esophageal foreign body (choke), neoplasia, and abscessation.[774]

CLINICAL PATHOLOGY. Radiographs are the best means of confirming the diagnosis. The normal outline of the diaphragm and heart may be obscured,[772,773] and the honeycombs or foreign objects in the reticulum may be seen in the thorax,[773] because this organ is most commonly involved. Oral barium may also aid in the radiographic interpretation, particularly in early small hernias that will be missed on plain films. Pleuritis and other masses such as tumors and abscesses can also mimic hernias on plain films.[773] Because TRP is frequently involved, the complete blood count (CBC), pleural effusions, and abdominocentesis may reflect the septic process. In cases not associated with TRP, the pleural effusion may be hemorrhagic in acute cases and normal in chronic cases.[774]

NECROPSY LESIONS. The hernial ring is usually located at the junction of the musculotendinous portion of the diaphragm, about 12 cm ventral to the vena cava and slightly lateral to the midline. The ring is usually round to oval, with a diameter of 7 to 20 cm. The reticulum is usually herniated, most frequently to the right side of the chest. The liver, spleen, rumen, omasum, abomasum, intestine, and omentum may also be involved. Extensive adhesions usually develop between the herniated organs and the thoracic organs, and evidence of hardware can often be found.[776]

TREATMENT AND PROGNOSIS. Treatment is surgical. A two-stage approach is usually used. First, a standing left flank laparotomy and rumenotomy are performed; the defect is identified, foreign bodies are removed, and the ruminoreticulum is emptied. Because of the complete mediastinum, ventilatory assistance is rarely needed during this stage. Next, the animal is placed under general anesthesia with positive pressure ventilation. A variety of approaches have been used for this portion, including ventral midline, paramedian, semilunar postxiphoid, paracostal, and transthoracic with rib resection. The hernia is reduced, and the rent repaired with sutures or mesh grafts. Mesh grafts are contraindicated if infection is present.[774]

REFERENCES

771. Ahmed SS, El-Hamamsy H: Diaphragmatic hernia in a sheep, *Vet Rec* 115: 441, 1984.
772. Nigam JM, Singh AP, Mirakhur KK: Radiographic diagnosis of bovine thoracic disorders, *Mod Vet Pract* 61:1021-1025, 1980.
773. Kumar R et al: Radiographic diagnosis of diaphragmatic hernia in cattle, *Vet Med Small Anim Clin* 75:305-309, 1980.
774. Bristol DG: Diaphragmatic hernias in horses and cattle, *Compend Cont Educ Pract Vet* 8:S407-S412, 1986.
775. Deshpande KS et al: Pathoanatomy of herniation of the reticulum through the diaphragm in the bovine, *Can Vet J* 22:234-236, 1981.

Pleural Mesothelioma

Mesotheliomas have been reported in cattle and goats,[776] including a congenital form in calves.[777] Most are peritoneal, but pleural mesotheliomas also occur.[778] Mesotheliomas result in the accumulation of large amounts of fluid in the involved body cavity; signs of pleural mesothelioma are therefore related to pleural effusion. They include dyspnea, tachypnea, decreased lung and heart sounds (sometimes unilateral, with a concomitant increase in sounds on the normal side), dullness on percussion, exercise intolerance, cyanosis, tachycardia, anorexia, weight loss, decreased production,

cough, and weak pulses. If peritoneal lesions are also present, as is common but not universal, ascites is also present. Radiographs confirm the pleural effusion, and thoracocentesis yields a serous, sometimes blood-tinged or gelatinous fluid. Cytologic examination may reveal reactive mesothelial cells. At necropsy the pleura is thickened and contains multiple nodules of gray to yellowish white tissue measuring several millimeters to several centimeters in diameter. Metastasis is uncommon. The tumor can be difficult to diagnose histologically and may resemble inflammation, pleural tuberculosis ("pearl disease"), or metastasis of another tumor.[777] There is no treatment.

REFERENCES

776. McCullagh KA, Mews AR, Pinsent PJN: Diffuse pleural mesothelioma in a goat, *Vet Pathol* 16:119-121, 1979.
777. Baskerville A: Mesothelioma in the calf, *Pathol Vet* 4:149-156, 1967.
778. Wolfe DF, Carson RL, Hudson RS: Mesothelioma in cattle: eight cases (1970-1988), *J Am Vet Med Assoc* 199:486-491, 1991.
779. Klopfer U et al: Mesothelioma in cattle: a rare or an unidentified tumor? *Zentralbl Veterinarmed (B)* 30:785-788, 1983.

MISCELLANEOUS CONDITIONS

JOHN C. BAKER
JOHN A. SMITH

Lung Tumors

Lung tumors are uncommon in large animals, with slaughterhouse surveys reporting an incidence of 19 per million cattle.[780] Those reported include pulmonary alveolar carcinomas, pulmonary adenomas, pulmonary adenocarcinomas, bronchogenic carcinoma, and pulmonary blastoma.[781-783] Malignant forms metastasize to regional lymph nodes and occasionally to other organs. Lymphosarcoma is the most frequent neoplasm to become metastatic to the lung, and uterine and ovarian adenocarcinoma may undergo metastasis to the lung.[783] Because many lung neoplasms in cattle are incidental findings at slaughter or necropsy, clinical signs are therefore not well documented. The lesions are typically discrete, round, yellow to gray masses distributed throughout the lung tissue. Tumors are most likely to be detected antemortem by radiographic examination. Differential diagnoses in such cases include pulmonary abscesses, mycotic pneumonias, and tuberculosis.

REFERENCES

780. Anderson LJ, Sandison AT: Pulmonary tumours found in a British abattoir survey: primary carcinomas in cattle and secondary neoplasms in cattle, sheep and pigs, *Br J Cancer* 22:47-57, 1968.
781. Migaki G, Helmboldt CF, Robinson FR: Primary pulmonary tumors of epithelial origin in cattle, *Am J Vet Res* 35:1397-1400, 1974.
782. Sanford SE, Bundza A: Multicentric bronchiolo-alveolar neoplasm in a steer, *Vet Pathol* 19:95-97, 1982.
783. Andrews GA, Kennedy GA: Respiratory diagnostic pathology, *Vet Clin North Am (Food Anim Pract)* 13:515-547, 1997.

Bronchobiliary Fistula

A communication between the bile duct and a cavitating lesion in the lung has been described in a 3-year-old Charolais cow.[784] The cow had weight loss of 8 months' duration, before which she had been normal. Clinical signs were tachypnea, an expiratory press, bilateral crackles and friction rubs in the ventral lung fields, and a greenish yellow nasal discharge. The adventitious sounds were slightly more prominent on the right, and a silent area was detected in the caudodorsal right lung field. Radiographs revealed a cavitation with a fluid line in this area, and thoracocentesis yielded a sterile green fluid. At surgery, pleural-diaphragmatic adhesions and a mass in the right diaphragmatic lobe were found. A drain was installed, and fluid similar to bile, with a bilirubin of 3.1 mg/dl and alkaline phosphatase concentration of 2694 IU/L, was drained. At necropsy the lesion was a smooth-lined cyst communicating by way of tracts through the adhesions with the biliary system and the bronchioles. Greenish fluid was found in the airways of both lungs.

REFERENCE

784. Welker FH et al: Bronchobiliary fistula in a cow, *J Am Vet Med Assoc* 185:440-441, 1984.

Diseases of the Alimentary Tract

MICHAEL J. MURRAY

BRADFORD P. SMITH

Consulting Editors

▮ EQUINE ALIMENTARY SYSTEM

MICHAEL J. MURRAY, Consulting Editor

DIAGNOSTIC PROCEDURES IN THE EXAMINATION OF THE EQUINE ALIMENTARY SYSTEM (for Ruminants, See p. 694)

MICHAEL J. MURRAY
ANDREW T. FISCHER, JR.

After a thorough physical examination has been performed and a minimum database (complete blood count, serum chemistries, and urinalysis) collected, a clinician may choose to use several diagnostic procedures in the evaluation of a horse with a known or suspected disorder involving the alimentary system. Each procedure is limited in the type and extent of information that can be obtained, and thus the clinician should select the complement of procedures that is most likely to provide the information required to make a proper diagnosis and determine the appropriate therapy.

RECTAL EXAMINATION

A systematic approach to examining the abdominal and retroperitoneal viscera should be established and applied during each examination to ensure that all pertinent regions and structures are examined. When feasible and if required,

the patient should be sedated to allow a more thorough examination.

In the pelvic region of the normal horse, the urethra and accessory sex glands (male) or the vaginal vault and cervix (female) can be palpated. The urethra is usually not discernible in the female, but abnormalities such as uroliths may be felt. In the caudal abdominal cavity the bladder, the uterus in females, and the pelvic flexure and small colon typically should be felt. The pelvic flexure and left ventral and left dorsal colons are normally located ventrally, on midline or toward the left side of the abdomen. The small colon, with formed fecal balls palpable, courses throughout the caudal abdomen, mostly on the left side. In females the left ovary can be felt in the left dorsal, caudal region of the abdomen. Both ovaries should be palpated in conjunction with palpation of the uterus. The peritoneal surface should be felt along the surface of the abdominal wall and the surfaces of the viscera. It should feel smooth, with no crepitus or irregularities. Advancing along the left side of the abdomen, the spleen can be felt as a smooth structure, with the caudal border having a well-delineated, tapered border. The size and location of the spleen are variable, because it can extend from the left body wall to the right ventral region of the abdomen. Advancing cranially and dorsally, the left kidney can be palpated. The kidney should feel smooth with the renal pelvic fissure discernible, although in the overweight horse extensive perirenal fat may obscure this detail.

From the left kidney, moving toward midline and extending from the abdominal aorta, the cranial mesenteric and ileocecocolic arteries may be felt. Palpation of fremitus in these arteries may be associated with arteritis and thrombus formation, secondary to *Strongylus vulgaris* larval migration, although this association has been very inconsistent. Fremitus is frequently absent when severe arteritis exists, or the arteries may be entirely normal and fremitus felt. Fremitus can often be elicited by compressing the wall of the normal artery, thus accelerating flow through the compressed lumen. The mesenteric root of the colon can be felt ventral to the cranial mesenteric artery. This should palpate as a mildly taut band of tissue, extending from the dorsal midline ventrally. Excessive tension, displacement, thickening, or masses within the mesentery should be considered abnormalities. It may be possible to palpate an enterolith, fecalith, or gravel impaction in the transverse colon, although this may be beyond the reach of the examiner, because the transverse colon is located cranial and medial to the left kidney.

Sweeping to the right side of the abdomen, the base and cupola of the cecum can be felt. The body of the cecum can be followed, partially, by sweeping along the medial aspect of the cecum, cranially toward midline. The cecum has a prominent ventral band and sacculations. Gas, together with ingesta that is soft and mainly of a fluid consistency, can be felt within the cecum. Firm ingesta, or excessive ingesta, suggests an abnormality.

Findings that are different from normal often must be differentiated as being variations of normal or truly abnormal. Some common abnormal findings include abnormalities of the peritoneal surface. Crepitus, or a "plastic wrap" texture is indicative of gas secondary to trauma or infection. An irregular or rough surface may be indicative of fibrin on a visceral surface or neoplasia, or with a perforated intestine there may be ingesta adhered to a visceral surface. There are many abnormal presentations of the large colon, most of which are associated with signs of colic. Thickening of the wall of the colon may be appreciated on rectal palpation and is indicative of edema or cellular infiltration of the colon. Palpation of abnormal masses in the wall of the colon or associated with the colonic mesentery is indicative of infection, infarction, granulomatous colitis, or neoplasia.

Normally the small intestine is not discerned by palpation. Occasionally, though, peristaltic contractions may be felt in the small intestine as it courses across midline toward the base of the cecum. In some cases, this will cause the small bowel to palpate as a firm, tubular structure. Relaxation of the peristaltic contraction should be discerned in such cases. Distention of small intestine is abnormal. In some cases the bowel may feel thickened, which can occur with ileal muscular hypertrophy, edema, or inflammatory disorders of the small bowel.

Other abnormal findings that may accompany disorders of the abdominal alimentary system include masses, adhesions, enlarged and thickened mesenteric arteries, and caudal displacement of the spleen (secondary to gastric distention, neoplasia).

PARACENTESIS

Abdominal paracentesis is performed routinely in patients with suspected disorders of the abdominal viscera. The technique is described on p. 670.

ENDOSCOPY

There are two basic types of endoscopic equipment available: equipment based entirely on a fiberoptic system and equipment based on a video chip system. A typical endoscope found in many private practices is a fiberoptic endoscope that has an insertion tube that is 100 to 110 cm in length and 10 to 14.5 mm in outer diameter. The larger-diameter tube can only be inserted through the nasal passages of older yearlings and adults and is not suitable for alimentary endoscopy, whereas a diameter of 10 mm allows passage through the turbinates of young foals. An insertion tube of 100 cm is sufficient for esophagoscopy in foals up to approximately 3 months of age. For older animals, an insertion tube length of 150 to 180 cm is required for esophagoscopy.

An insertion tube length of 110 cm is sufficient to reach the stomach of foals up to 30 to 40 days of age only. A length of 150 to 180 cm is required for weanlings, and 200 cm is usually required for yearlings and adults. An insertion tube length of 200 cm is sufficient to reach the stomach of all adults of warm-blooded breeds, although 280 to 300 cm is required to examine the pylorus in adult horses. A 280- to 300-cm-long insertion tube permits duodenoscopy in adult horses.

Before a gastroscopic examination, suckling foals up to 20 days of age are not routinely withheld from nursing for more than 1 hour. Older foals and mature horses should not have solid feed for 6 to 10 hours so that ingesta from the stomach may be adequately emptied. Longer duration of feed deprivation (18 hours) is desirable to view the antrum and pylorus of horses. Many foals less than 30 days old do not require sedation for gastroscopy, although sedation with 0.5 mg/kg xylazine may facilitate the procedure. Sedation is required if the foal is to be placed in a recumbent position so that the entire glandular portion of the stomach can be examined. Sedation of older foals and horses is required. Xylazine (0.5 mg/kg, IV) usually provides adequate sedation. For greater sedation, combinations of xylazine and butorphanol (0.01 mg/kg) or xylazine and acepromazine (0.02 mg/kg) are effective.

After insertion of the endoscope, the stomach is distended with air until the nonglandular and glandular regions of the gastric surface can be observed. Distention with air is tolerated by foals and horses and has been associated only rarely with adverse effects. Occasionally, sick neonates with poor intestinal motility developed small intestinal distention and experienced discomfort after gastroscopy.

More complete descriptions of techniques of gastroduodenal endoscopy can be found elsewhere.[1,2]

Endoscopy of the rectum and distal small colon can be performed with most flexible endoscopes in use in equine practice and should be preceded, as much as possible, by evacuation and saline lavage of the rectum and distal small colon. The mucosal surface should appear pink to pale red and should have a smooth, "velvety" appearance. Mucosal edema or thickening, hyperemia, irregularities, defects, tears, and intraluminal masses are abnormal findings. Because of the concern for trauma to the rectum and small colon, the horse should be adequately sedated and restrained before preparation and examination of the distal alimentary tract.

LAPAROSCOPY

Laparoscopy can offer valuable diagnostic information regarding the abdominal cavity while being only minimally invasive.[3,4] It should always be preceded by a thorough physical examination, including abdominal palpation per rectum, paying particular attention to the sites for trocar insertion to ascertain that there are no adherent masses or viscera in the area. If abdominocentesis is to be part of the diagnostic workup, it should be performed before laparoscopy because of the effect of laparoscopy on abdominal fluid values. In experimental animals undergoing diagnostic laparoscopy with carbon dioxide insufflation, both the abdominal white blood cell count and the abdominal total protein increased.[5]

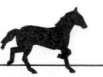

The indications for laparoscopy include palpable abdominal masses, enlarged viscera, adhesions, acute or chronic colic, weight loss, or the desire to obtain visceral biopsy specimens. Contraindications include adherent viscera or masses at the site of laparoscopic trocar insertion, diaphragmatic hernias, or extreme bloating. Horses with acute colic can be safely examined laparoscopically, if one is careful when inserting the trocars and telescopes.

The basic instruments for laparoscopic examinations include a laparoscopic telescope, laparoscopic cannula and trocar assembly, fiberoptic light source and cable, insufflator, and biopsy and manipulation instruments. The 30-degree laparoscope allows better visualization of the less accessible areas compared to the 0-degree telescopes. Video cameras make visualization easier with less eyestrain but require more powerful light sources (250-watt). The cost of laparoscopic instrumentation has decreased recently as a result of the explosion of popularity of laparoscopy in humans, increasing the supply and availability of used instruments.

Horses should be fasted for 18 to 24 hours before most laparoscopic procedures; water is allowed ad lib. Fasting increases intraabdominal visualization and decreases the possibility of penetrating a gas-distended viscus. The animal is restrained in standing stocks if the procedure is to be done while it is standing. Preoperative antibiotics, antiinflammatory drugs, tetanus prophylaxis, and a sedative analgesic combination are administered. It is important to administer the analgesics before abdominal insufflation. The flank areas are prepared for aseptic surgery. Local anesthetic agents are infiltrated subcutaneously and intramuscularly in the middle of the paralumbar fossa slightly above the crus of the internal abdominal oblique muscle for the insertion of the laparoscopic telescope. If additional instruments are to be used, their insertion sites are similarly anesthetized.

It is preferable to begin the laparoscopic procedure on the left side of the abdomen to minimize the chance of penetrating the cecal base. The horse is then draped and a stab incision is made. The laparoscopic cannula and trocar assembly are inserted through the musculature and into the abdominal cavity. It is useful to orient the trocar toward the opposite coxofemoral joint when inserting it. The trocar is exchanged for the telescope, and confirmation of entry into the abdominal cavity is made before commencing insufflation. If the abdominal cavity has not been penetrated, quick thrust with the telescope will usually penetrate the peritoneum. Insufflation of the abdomen with CO_2 to 8 to 10 mm Hg will usually be sufficient for most examinations.

Systematic examination of the abdominal cavity is then carried out. On the left side of the abdomen the spleen, left kidney, nephrosplenic ligament (Fig. 30-1), stomach, left side of liver, diaphragm, and ventral colon may be visualized cranially. Looking caudally, the root of the mesentery, the isolated small intestinal and small and large colon sections, the urogenital tract, the bladder, and the terminal rectum will be seen. The procedure is repeated on the right side of the abdomen. Looking cranially, the liver, epiploic foramen, right kidney, descending duodenum, cecal base, and large colon are visible. Looking caudally, the urogenital tract, root of mesentery, and isolated pieces of intestine are seen. Liver biopsies and right kidney biopsies are taken from the right side. Left kidney and spleen biopsies are taken from the left side of the abdomen. Mesenteric lymph nodes are usually obtained from the left flank. Other masses are biopsied from the more accessible side. At the end of the procedure, the abdomen is deflated, and the skin is closed with skin sutures only. Closure of the skin incision should wait until examination of both sides is completed in order to minimize subcutaneous emphysema.

In some horses with ventral or cranial abdominal masses as determined with ultrasound, it is useful to anesthetize the

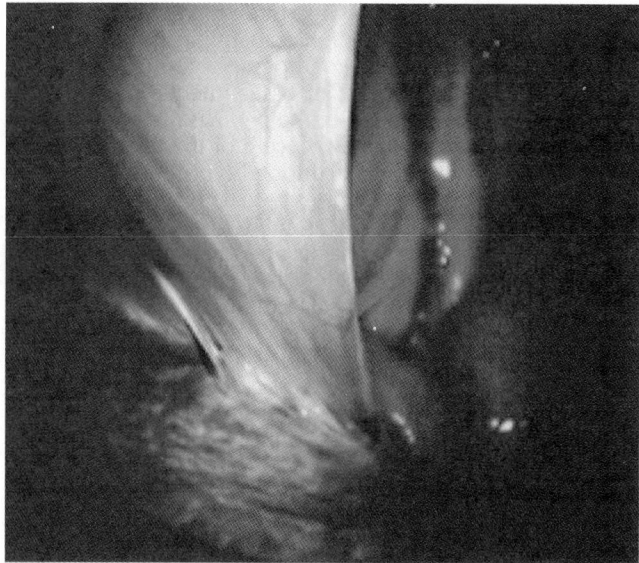

FIG. 30-1 ■ Laparoscopic view of nephrosplenic ligament in a horse.

animal in dorsal recumbency for better characterization of the mass. Biopsies may be readily obtained. In horses with acute colic but without obvious signs indicating the necessity for surgery, laparoscopy can help in making the decision to continue medical therapy or proceed to surgery. Strangulated sections of small intestine can be seen, proximal enteritis can be diagnosed, and edema and vascular compromise to the large colon can be seen. No abnormalities may be detected in some animals with very localized lesions, or lesions may be inaccessible, depending on location.

Laparoscopic complications are similar to those of any other abdominal exploratory procedure. Inadvertent penetration of a viscus may occur. The left kidney may be perforated if the laparoscope is inserted too far dorsally. The spleen may be penetrated if the laparoscope is inserted too far ventrally or is not aimed toward the opposite coxofemoral joint. The cecum may be perforated when entering from the right side. Fasting the horses and carefully inserting the laparoscopic trocars will minimize the occurrence of these problems. Subcutaneous emphysema occurs commonly but has not caused any clinical problems. The peripheral white blood cell count increased but stayed within normal limits in experimental animals undergoing laparoscopy.[5]

IMAGING OF THE ALIMENTARY TRACT

Radiography

Radiography of the alimentary tract can be a useful diagnostic tool in the evaluation of alimentary disorders in horses. The oral, esophageal, and abdominal portions of the alimentary system can be examined with radiography. The size of the patient and the capabilities of radiographic equipment available determine which procedures can be used. Radiography of the abdomen of weanlings, yearlings, and adult horses requires a high-exposure technique and may be accompanied by significant scatter radiation. But it often provides the most valuable information in the evaluation of certain cases.

Many portable units, with settings ranging from 60 kV and 30 mA to 90 kV and 15 mA, are suitable to take good-quality radiographs of the teeth, pharynx, and esophagus in adults and the entire alimentary tract in young foals. The use of rare earth screens with high-latitude film, in conjunction with a focused grid, enhances the capabilities and quality of films taken with a portable radiography unit. Also, techniques that take advantage of air/tissue interfaces, such as an oblique view of the teeth with the paranasal sinuses superimposed on the dorsal arcade of teeth or the use of positive contrast media, allow the practitioner to produce diagnostic films at lower exposure times.

Radiography is particularly useful in the evaluation of disorders of the thoracic esophagus and abdominal viscera in foals. In young foals obstructions caused by meconium impactions, fecal impactions, displacements, volvulus, stricture, and congenital malformations can be deduced from the appearance of visceral distention and accumulation of gas. The presence of peritonitis and abscessation also can be determined in some cases. Barium contrast medium is useful in evaluating the esophagus, the stomach, the proximal small intestine, and the intestinal transit. With a barium contrast enema, the distal colon and rectum can be outlined. To evaluate the esophagus, use Intropaste® 70% Barium sulfate paste (Lafayette Pharmaceuticals, Lafayette IN 47904) at a dose of $^3/_4$ to 1 tube (a tube is 454 gms) for adult horses, half as much for foals. To evaluate the stomach use 60% barium suspension at a dose of 400 to 800 ml. for adult horses, 150 ml. for foals. Disorders such as megaesophagus, cardia stricture, severe gastric ulceration, pyloric stricture, duodenal stricture, colon impaction, meconium impaction, and atresia coli may be diagnosed with contrast radiography. Radiography is indispensable in many cases of colic in young foals in determining whether surgery is indicated. In a retrospective report on the use of radiography in abdominal disorders in foals, a positive radiographic diagnosis of abdominal disease was confirmed at surgery or necropsy in 25 of 26 patients.[6] The films were all reviewed by radiologists, emphasizing that the accuracy of the diagnosis is related to the experience and skill of the individual interpreting the film.

The average exposure for a 100-lb foal is 30 mA and 80 to 100 kvp. Accumulations of gas in the stomach and cecal base are normal. Isolated segments of the small and large intestine will also have small amounts of gas (Fig. 30-2). Marked distention of the small intestine is recognized as multiple hairpin loops with gas-fluid interfaces. The hairpin loops can be seen in cases of small intestinal obstruction or enteritis. Frequently in cases of small intestinal disease, gastric dilation will be evident. The gas pattern tends to be more diffuse in enteritis cases. Obstructions of the large colon are evidenced by long gas-fluid interfaces occurring in the middle to ventral abdomen. Sand accumulations are common in young foals but do not necessarily cause an obstruction.

In young foals with large colon gas distention, retrograde administration of barium sulfate is performed to demonstrate patency of the small colon and the absence of meconium obstructions.[7] Thirty percent barium sulfate (weight/volume) solution is administered to the sedated foal by gravity administration through a Foley catheter placed rectally. If the foal has an obstruction, it will be difficult to administer more than 100 to 200 ml of contrast. Adequate filling of the small colon and transverse colon verifies patency of the distal gastrointestinal tract and is usually noted when 500 to 750 ml of contrast medium enters the foal. If the obstruction is higher in the large colon, more barium should be administered (up to 20 ml/kg). Both ventrodorsal and lateral radiographs should be obtained. In cases of meconium obstruction, the ventrodorsal radiograph may be of greater diagnostic value. Obstructions are noted by a sudden stop of the dye column. If the dye tapers off, insufficient administration of contrast media has occurred. The most common cause of obstruction in the neonate in our practice is meco-

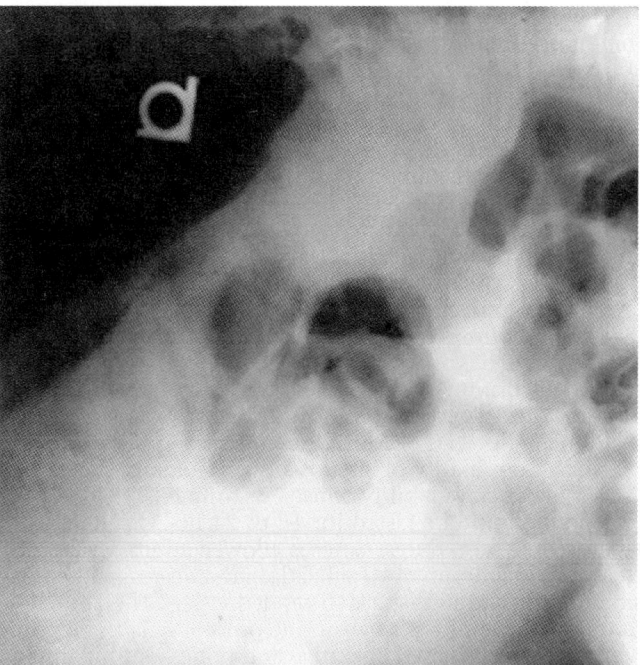

FIG. 30-2 ▮▮ Lateral radiograph of abdomen of a normal neonatal foal.

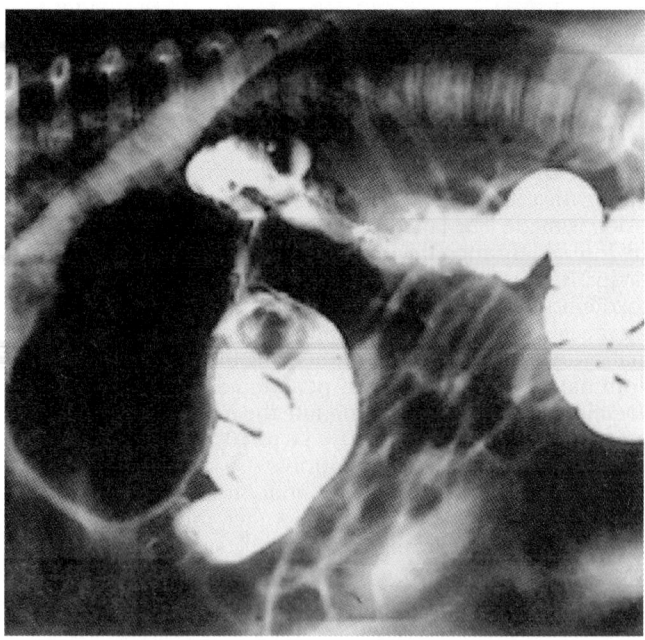

FIG. 30-3 ▮▮ Lateral retrograde contrast radiograph of abdomen of a foal with meconium impaction in proximal small colon.

nium retention, and this is readily identified on retrograde contrast radiography (Fig. 30-3).

The adult horse has a large body mass, which makes it difficult to radiograph unless high mA and high kvp settings can be obtained. Effective exposures may be obtained using a 300-mA head, and good-quality abdominal radiographs can be obtained on most 500- to 600-mA machines capable of 140 kvp. A high-speed, rare earth film screen combination and an 8:1, 80-line-per-inch grid should be used to minimize exposure times. A cassette holder is attached to the tube column perpendicular to the primary beam at a film-focal distance of 122 cm. A 1-mm sheet of lead is placed behind the cassette to reduce scatter.

The abdomen is divided into multiple regions and radiographed. Techniques will vary from 300 mA to 600 mA and 80 to 140 kvp. A typical technique for a 500-kg horse is 450 mA and 100 kvp. Less radiation is required for exposures of the diaphragmatic area and the small colon. In some cases, it is helpful to radiograph the animal from both sides. An average 500-kg horse will require at least three to four radiographs to cover the abdominal cavity. Enteroliths are most commonly seen in the middle of the abdomen viewed laterally[8] (Fig. 30-4). The area examined by this image is the right dorsal and transverse colons. Small colon enteroliths are usually visualized lower along the ventral aspect of the abdomen unless the enterolith is in the very beginning of the small colon.

If the horse has an obstruction or a very large impaction, enteroliths in the small colon can be difficult to image because of their smaller size. Fortunately this is not usually a clinical problem because the animals are obstructed and painful, indicating the need for surgical intervention. If diagnostic radiographs cannot be obtained because of size or large quantities of ingesta, the animal is fasted, and radiographs are repeated in 24 hours.

Sand accumulations are also commonly seen and can be difficult to distinguish from enteroliths if the shape is spherical, such as occurs in the transverse colon. Sand accumulations may obscure enteroliths. If a large accumulation of sand is present, radiographs are repeated when the sand obstruction has broken up and been passed.

Ultrasonography

Ultrasonography can be very useful in evaluating soft tissue structures associated with the alimentary system. Ultrasonography and radiography are often complementary, and in many cases (particularly in adult horses) ultrasonography provides more useful information than radiography. Abdominal ultrasonography is limited by the size of the patient, the quality of the equipment used, and the skill of the examiner. The most limiting features of ultrasonography in its application to the abdominal viscera are the depth of penetration available, 25 to 30 cm, loss of resolution as depth of penetration increases, and interference by gas within the intestine. Use of transrectal probes can increase the area of the abdominal cavity that can be examined.

When examining abdominal viscera, it is preferable to clip the site to be examined, although in young foals and horses with a short hair coat this may not be necessary. Application of mineral oil to the skin often yields satisfactory results without clipping. When hair is clipped, ultrasound couplant gel should be applied to the site before the examination. Often, abdominal ultrasonography can be performed without clipping by wetting the animal's hair coat with alcohol. Caution must be advised because some ultrasound heads are sensitive to alcohol and will be damaged.

With adults, a 2.5- to 3.5-MHz scanhead is used initially for transcutaneous ultrasonography. A 5.0- to 7.5-MHz scanhead can be used for transrectal ultrasonography in horses. In foals a 5.0- to 7.5-MHz scanhead can be used for transcutaneous ultrasonography. Increasing the scanhead frequency improves the resolution but decreases the depth of penetration. An ultrasonic examination of the abdomen should be performed in a standard manner, so that pertinent structures are examined each time. A protocol for examining the abdomen has been described.[9]

Gas within the bowel stops the penetration of the sound waves, and often structures deep to the gas/bowel wall inter-

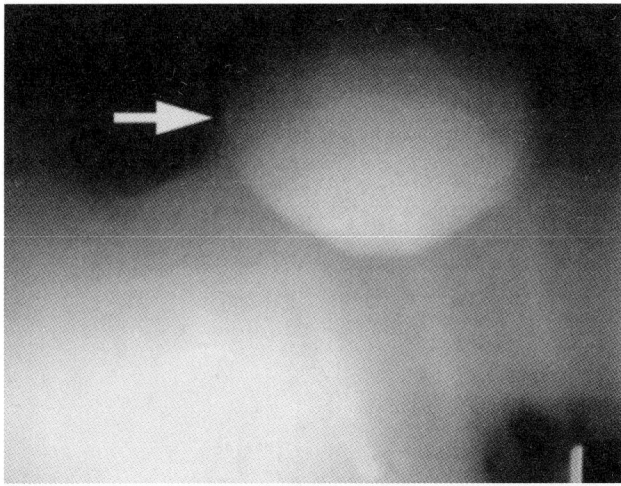

FIG. 30-4 Lateral radiograph of abdomen of a horse demonstrating an enterolith in the right dorsal colon *(arrow)*. The film was produced using rare earth screens and a technique of 450 mA and 106 kvp.

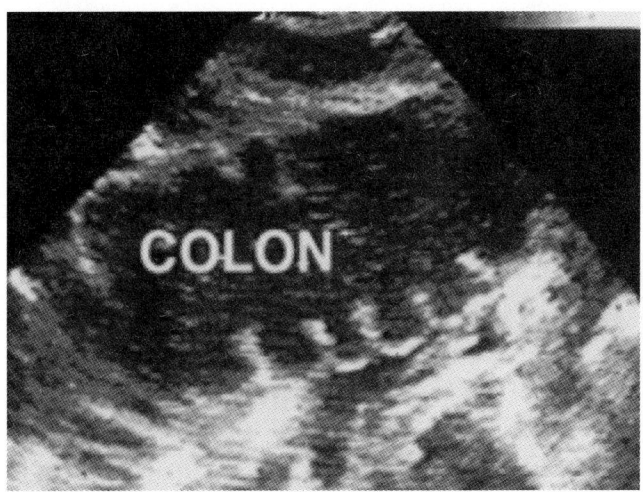

FIG. 30-5 Ultrasonography of abdomen of a 2-day-old-foal with necrotizing enterocolitis. The colon was filled with bloody fluid, noted as a composite hypoechoic appearance on ultrasonography.

face cannot be examined. This fact can be used to the practitioner's advantage, because clear visualization of proximal and distal bowel walls suggests that fluid, not gas, is present within the bowel lumen (Fig. 30-5).

In horses that present with colic, ultrasonography may reveal small intestinal distention (Fig. 30-6), adynamic ileus, or increased bowel wall thickness (Figs. 30-7 and 30-8). Increased bowel wall thickness can result from edema, congestion, or inflammatory cell infiltration. The presence of distended, thickened loops of small intestine without visible motility is strongly suggestive of the presence of a small intestinal strangulation obstruction, whereas if motility is present, peritonitis may be suspected. In one report, transabdominal ultrasound was more accurate in the detection of small intestinal strangulation obstructions than palpation by rectal examination.[10]

In foals with colic, ultrasonography may aid in determining whether there is ileus, fluid accumulation/distention in

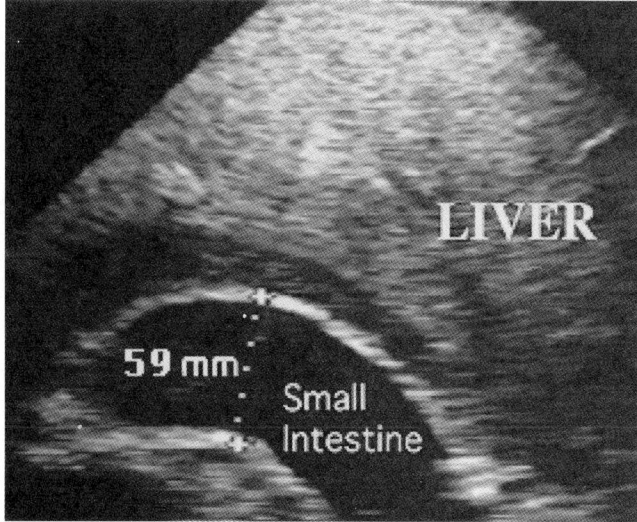

FIG. 30-6 ▦ Ultrasonography of right cranial abdomen in a 14-year-old mare that presented with signs of colic. There is distention of small intestine that was secondary to ileus. There also are hyperechoic foci within the liver (*bright areas toward the top of the illustration*) that represent neoplastic masses.

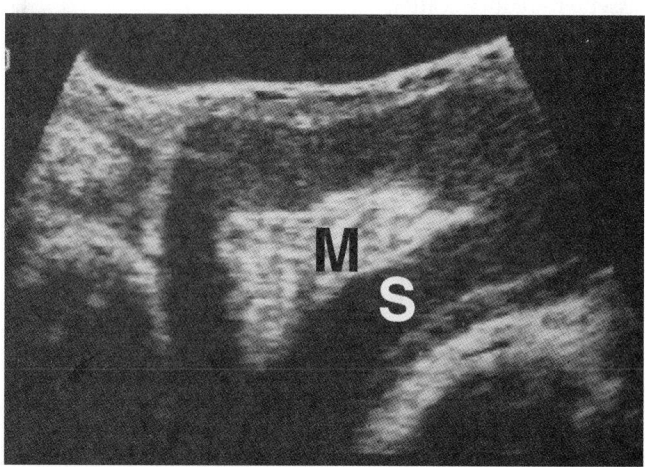

FIG. 30-8 ▦ Ultrasonographic view of a segment of large intestine obtained during a transrectal examination using a 5.0-MHz frequency scanhead. This segment is grossly thickened, including the hyperechoic mucosa (*M*) and the darker-appearing submucosa (*S*). Postmortem examination revealed pronounced edema of the colon submucosa.

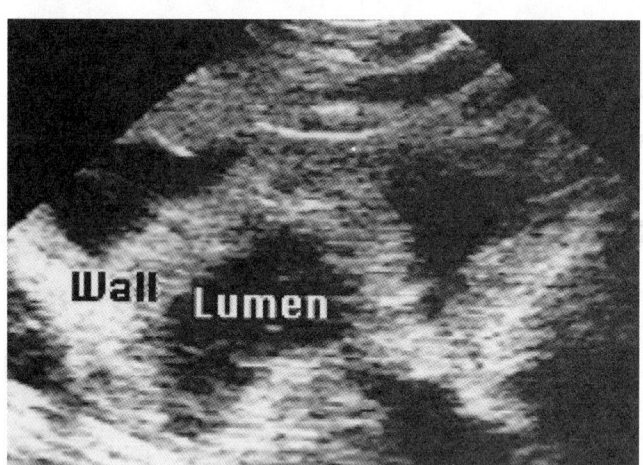

FIG. 30-7 ▦ Ultrasonography of cranial ventral abdomen of a 14-year-old gelding that presented with colic. Distended small intestine could not be felt on rectal examination, but ultrasonography revealed distended small intestine with walls that appeared thickened. At surgery incarceration of the jejunum through the epiploic foramen was found. The wall of the incarcerated jejunem appeared to be edematous and congested.

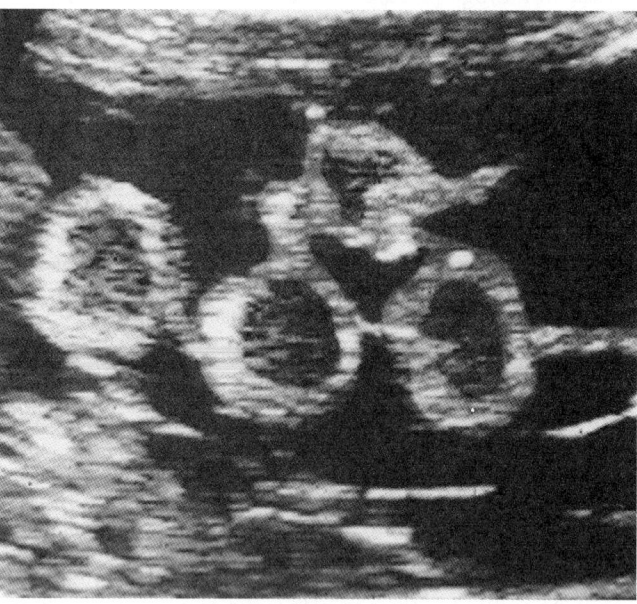

FIG. 30-9 ▦ Ultrasonography of abdomen of a 3-day-old foal with a ruptured bladder. Note that there is increased fluid in the peritoneal cavity and that segments of small intestine with their mesenteric attachments are clearly visible. The diameter and wall thickness of the small intestine are normal.

bowel (see Fig. 30-5), bowel wall thickening, or bowel wall necrosis (presence of hyperechoic gas within the bowel wall). Other abnormalities that may be detected by ultrasonography include peritoneal effusion, hemoperitoneum, ruptured bladder (Fig. 30-9), adhesions, masses, intussusception, and dorsal displacement of the colon over the nephrosplenic ligament. Ultrasonography of the liver may detect areas of heterogenous echo reflection in the hepatic parenchyma (neo-plasms, abscesses, severe fibrosis), bile duct distention or choledocolithiasis.

Scintigraphy

Nuclear imaging can be used selectively in gastrointestinal diagnostics,[11] and it is particularly useful for evaluation of gastrointestinal transit time.[12,13] One useful clinical application

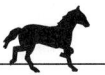

is the determination of the rate of gastric emptying.[12] The isotope technetium-99m–labeled sulfur colloid (^{99}Tc) is added to cooked egg white, which is placed into the stomach via nasogastric tube. Serial measurements of gamma emissions are recorded and the half life ($t_{1/2}$) is calculated. Normal is considered to be 90 minutes or less. Injection of autologous isotope-labeled white blood cells may be useful to diagnose abdominal abscesses and inflammatory conditions of the bowel, although these procedures have been done infrequently with variable success.

BIOPSY

The decision of whether to obtain a biopsy is often based on the ease of obtaining a sample and the relative value of the evaluation that can be made. Very small samples, such as those obtained with an endoscope biopsy instrument, are relatively easy to obtain, but they provide limited information. Full-thickness bowel specimens, obtained by means of ventral midline or flank laparotomy, are more difficult to obtain, but they provide much more information.

Taking a biopsy by endoscopy allows the practitioner to choose the biopsy site on the basis of the appearance of the mucosal surface, which most frequently reflects an inflammatory disorder. Conversely, when a biopsy is obtained through laparotomy, the serosal surface of the bowel may not reflect a disorder within the bowel wall. In such instances, it may be useful to obtain several biopsy specimens. Rectal mucosal biopsies are easily obtained. Many instruments can be used to obtain the biopsy, and a uterine biopsy forceps works well. A fold of mucosa can readily be pinched between two fingers, and a biopsy of this tissue is obtained. The size of the sample is adequate for histologic or bacteriologic examination.

FECAL EXAMINATION

Cytologic, biochemical, bacteriologic, immunologic, and electron microscopic evaluations can be performed on fecal samples. In addition, observation of the consistency and color, the presence of foreign material such as sand or gravel, and the presence of parasites should be included in the examination of the alimentary system. In addition to fecal consistency, fecal particle size can be used to evaluate the efficiency of mastication or the colonic transit time. Increased particle size, with loose or watery stool, is suggestive of decreased colonic transit time.

Cytologic examinations are primarily used to evaluate the parasite burden of the animal. Ova of large and small strongyles, tapeworms, round worms, and *Strongyloides westeri* are most common. Coccidia are occasionally observed, but are clinically unimportant. Examination of fecal white blood cells has been advocated in the evaluation of horses and foals with enterocolitis. Because these cells are very labile, their presence in large numbers indicates that an inflammatory process is present and that the inflammation is in the distal colon or associated with decreased transit time.

Determination of fecal occult blood has been recommended to diagnose gastric ulcers, duodenal ulcers, and other potentially hemorrhagic disorders of the alimentary tract. However, the usefulness of this test has been shown to be quite limited, because negative results can be obtained when blood is present in the proximal portion of the gastrointestinal tract.[14] The sensitivity of most commercially available tests is poor, giving negative results in the face of severe gastric bleeding (see Melena, Chapter 7).

Fecal culture is an essential component in the evaluation of many patients. In bacteriologic culture techniques for fecal samples, selective media that are designed to isolate *Salmonella* are routinely used. These media include selenite broth, tetrathionate broth, brilliant green agar, XLD agar, and *Salmonella-Shigella* agar. Less selective media, McConkey's and eosin methylene blue agars, are desirable to culture other potential gram-negative bacterial pathogens such as *Escherichia coli*, but the mere presence of *E. coli* in the feces does not determine its pathogenicity. Enterotoxigenic *E. coli* have been isolated from foals with diarrhea, but special tests, such as polymerase chain reaction (PCR), must be performed to determine whether an isolate produces enterotoxin.

Tests for detection of enterotoxins of *Clostridium difficile**and *Clostridium perfringens*† in fecal specimens are available at diagnostic laboratories or can be performed using ELISA kits.

The presence of rotavirus in a fecal sample can be determined by use of an enzyme-linked immunosorbent assay (ELISA) or an agglutination test. Both assays test for the presence of viral antigen in the feces. The ELISA test is reported to be more sensitive than the agglutination test, but is less specific. Thus the agglutination test is likely to give more false-negative results, and the ELISA test is likely to give more false-positive results. The ELISA test is more time consuming and inconvenient to perform than the agglutination test. When rotavirus is a concern, particularly as a farm problem, a reasonable approach is to screen fecal samples with the agglutination test and repeat samples that yield negative findings with the ELISA test (see Foal Diarrhea, Chapter 20).

ABSORPTION/DIGESTION TESTS

Tests that evaluate the ability of the equine intestinal tract to digest and absorb nutrients have a more limited clinical application than in human or small animal medicine, but they can be useful in the evaluation of horses with chronic weight loss, suspected small intestinal inflammation or neoplasia, gastric and small intestinal partial obstruction, and postoperative small intestinal malabsorptive disorders. For absorption tests to be diagnostic, the intestinal disorder must either be diffuse or affect the delivery to and transit through the small intestine.

Maldigestion tests are performed to evaluate exocrine pancreatic function and small intestinal mucosal brush border disaccharidase activity. Pancreatic exocrine deficiencies have not been described in the horse, probably because equine pancreatic secretions consist primarily of water and bicarbonate and have less enzymatic activity than in monogastric omnivorous species. Mucosal brush border disaccharidase-related maldigestion is relevant in viral and bacterial enteridites of foals, particularly rotavirus and coronavirus enteridites. As a result of these viral infections, there is loss of the superficial villous epithelial cells of the small intestine, in which the disaccharidases lactase, cellobiase, maltase, sucrase, and trehalase are located.[15] Lactase levels are greatest in young suckling foals, and loss of this enzyme activity, secondary to loss of the mucosal villous cells, leads to lactose maldigestion. Lactose tolerance can be tested by administering a 20% solution of D-lactose at a dosage of 0.5 to 1 g/kg. This dosage should result in an approximate doubling of the serum glucose level within 60 min of administration.[16]

Clinically applicable absorption tests include the D-glucose and D-xylose absorption tests. The glucose absorption test has the advantage of being relatively easy and inexpensive to perform. However, cellular uptake and metabolism of glucose, as well as intestinal absorption, influence the results and thus are undesirable variables. The xylose absorption test is thus advantageous because it more directly measures intestinal absorptive capacity. The results of both tests, though, are affected

---

C. difficile Tox A/B Test, TechLab, Blacksburg, Va.

†*Clostridium perfringens* enterotoxin test, TechLab, Inc., Blacksburg, Va.

by gastric emptying rate and small intestinal transit time. In the United States, D-xylose is available only through chemical suppliers and only for research purposes; its availability for clinical diagnostic use is restricted.

The D-glucose and D-xylose tests are performed similarly. Following an 18- to 24-hour fast, a 10% solution of D-glucose or D-xylose, 0.5 to 1 g/kg, is administered through a nasogastric tube. For the measurement of glucose, blood is collected in sodium fluoride tubes; and for the measurement of D-xylose, blood is collected in heparinized tubes. Samples are taken at 0, 30, 60, 90, 120, 150, 180, 210, and 240 min after administration. Peak levels, which normally range from 20 to 25 mg/dl, occur 60 to 120 min after administration, and levels thereafter should decrease. The normal curve resembles an inverted V. Variability in absorption curves occur as a function of age and type of feed the horse is given.[17] Delay or flattening of the absorption curve may reflect delayed gastric emptying, increased intestinal transit time, or impaired intestinal absorption.[18] Accurate interpretation of the results of these tests depends on the results of other diagnostic evaluations. In addition, different types of diet have been shown to affect the height, although not the shape, of the absorption curves significantly. In general, diets that have a higher digestible energy content result in a lower peak in the curve.

BREATH TESTS

In humans, dogs, and cats, breath tests are used to assess a variety of intestinal disorders. The urea breath test is used as part of an assessment of *Helicobacter* status of the patient,[19] but this is not an issue for horses. The hydrogen breath test is used in assessments of intestinal bacterial overgrowth and in determination of carbohydrate digestion and absorption in the intestine. In patients with an abnormal intestinal bacterial population or carbohydrate malabsorption, there will be excessive bacterial fermentation of carbohydrate, with one by-product being hydrogen. Because hydrogen is freely diffusible from the bowel into the blood, and from the blood into the alveoli, measurement of exhaled hydrogen gas can be used to assess the status of intestinal bacterial fermentation of carbohydrates. In horses, the hydrogen breath test is most applicable to conditions in which there is carbohydrate malabsorption and thus increased delivery of soluble carbohydrate to the large intestine for bacterial fermentation to occur. There are two reports of this technique in horses, one in which different carbohydrate substrates were evaluated in ponies,[20] and another in which the hydrogen breath test was used in conjunction with D-xylose absorption in nine horses with a variety of clinical disorders.[21] In the study with ponies (*n* = 7), fasting resulted in negligible levels of breath hydrogen excretion. Sustained increases in breath hydrogen concentration greater than 10 ppm were observed for all ponies following the ingestion of oats or the administration of wheat flour, for three ponies following the administration of glucose and xylose and for two ponies following the administration of lactulose and lactose. The pattern of breath hydrogen excretion was subject to variation between animals after the ingestion of identical test meals. In the clinical study the diseased horses showed higher fasting breath hydrogen (H$_2$) levels (range 7.5 to 61.5 ppm) than normal horses (range 0 to 5 ppm). After xylose administration, none of the healthy animals showed an increase in breath H$_2$ production and five of diseased animals showed increases in breath hydrogen. In this group of patients, abnormalities in hydrogen breath measurement were more apparent than abnormalities in D-xylose absorption.

REFERENCES

1. Murray MJ, Pipers FS: *Manual of equine alimentary endoscopy* (In press.)
2. Murray MJ: Gastric endoscopy in foals. In Brown CM, Traub-Dargatz JL, eds: *Equine endoscopy*, St Louis, 1997, Mosby.
3. Galuppo LD, Snyder JR, Pascoe JR: Laparoscopic anatomy of the equine abdomen, *Am J Vet Res* 56:518-531, 1995.
4. Fischer AT: Standing laparoscopic surgery. In Freeman DE, ed: *Veterinary clinics of North America: equine practice, surgical management of colic*, Philadelphia, 1997, WB Saunders.
5. Fischer AT et al: Diagnostic laparoscopy in the horse, *J Am Vet Med Assoc* 189:289, 1986.
6. Fischer AT, Kerr LY, O'Brien TR: Radiographic diagnosis of gastrointestinal disorders in the foal, *Vet Radiol* 28:42-48, 1987.
7. Fischer AT, Yarbrough TY: Retrograde contrast radiography of the distal portions of the intestinal tract in foals, *J Am Vet Med Assoc* 207:734-737, 1995.
8. Yarbrough TB et al: Abdominal radiography for diagnosis of enterolithiasis in horses: 141 cases (1990-1992), *J Am Vet Med Assoc* 205:592-595, 1994.
9. Rantanen NW: Diseases of the abdomen. In Rantanen NW, ed: *Veterinary clinics of North America: equine practice, diagnostic ultrasound*, Philadelphia, 1986, WB Saunders.
10. Klohnen A, Vachon AM, Fisher AT: Use of diagnostic ultrasonography in horses with signs of acute abdominal pain, *J Am Vet Med Assoc* 209:1597-1601, 1996.
11. Hightower D, Amoss MS: Gastrointestinal veterinary nuclear medicine. In Anderson NV, ed: *Veterinary gastroenterology*, Philadelphia, 1992, Lea & Febiger.
12. Ringger NC et al: Effect of bethanechol or erythromycin on gastric emptying in horses, *Am J Vet Res* 57:1771-1775, 1996.
13. Lester GD et al: Effect of erythromycin lactobionate on myoelectric activity of ileum, cecum, and right ventral colon, and cecal emptying of radiolabeled markers in clinically normal ponies, *Am J Vet Res* 59:328-334, 1998.
14. Pearson EG, Smith BB, McKim JM: Fecal blood determinations and interpretations, *Proc Am Assoc Equine Pract* 33:77-83, 1987.
15. Roberts MC: Carbohydrate digestion and absorption studies in the horse, *Res Vet Sci* 18:64, 1975.
16. Martens RJ, Malone PS, Brust DM: Oral lactose tolerance test in foals: technique and normal values, *Am J Vet Res* 46:2163-2165, 1985.
17. Murphy D, Reid SW: The effect of age and diet on the oral glucose tolerance test in ponies, *Equine Vet J* 29:467-470, 1997.
18. Mair TS et al: Small intestinal malabsorption in the horse: an assessment of the specificity of the oral glucose tolerance test. *Equine Vet J* 23:344-346, 1991.
19. Savarino V, Vigneri S, Celle G: The 13C urea breath test in the diagnosis of *Helicobacter pylori* infection, *Gut* 45:118-122, 1999.
20. Murphy D, Reid SW, Love S: Breath hydrogen measurement in ponies: a preliminary study, *Res Vet Sci* 65:47-51, 1998.
21. Bracher V, Steiger R, Huser S: Preliminary results using a combined xylose absorption/hydrogen exhalation test in horses, *Schweiz Archiv Tierheilkd* 137:297-305, 1995.

DENTISTRY AND ORAL DISEASE

JACK EASLEY

The equine species has evolved as a continuously grazing animal, developing its own dental form and function along the way. Its dental structure is designed to provide the animal with an ability to detect, prehend, masticate, and begin the digestion of forage. As humans have domesticated and confined the horse, they have, at the same time, altered its diet to consist of less continual grazing and more interval feeding of dry hay, grain, processed forages, and concentrates.

ANATOMY AND FUNCTION

Structures that the horse uses for eating include the hypsodont incisors, premolars and molars, facial bone and sinus construction, tactile and prehensile lips, muscles of mastication, tongue, hard palate, olfactory organs, taste buds, salivary glands and ducts, and the blood, lymph vessels and nerves that support them.

The mature mouth of a horse contains six incisors each in both the upper and lower jaws and six upper and six lower cheek teeth on each side of the mouth (Fig. 30-10). Three cheek teeth are premolars (PMs) and three are molars (Ms). Premolars have deciduous and permanent sets. Molars come in at an older age and only one set is present. The premolars and molars of the upper jaw are broad and square, to facilitate their function of grinding feed. The lower premolars and

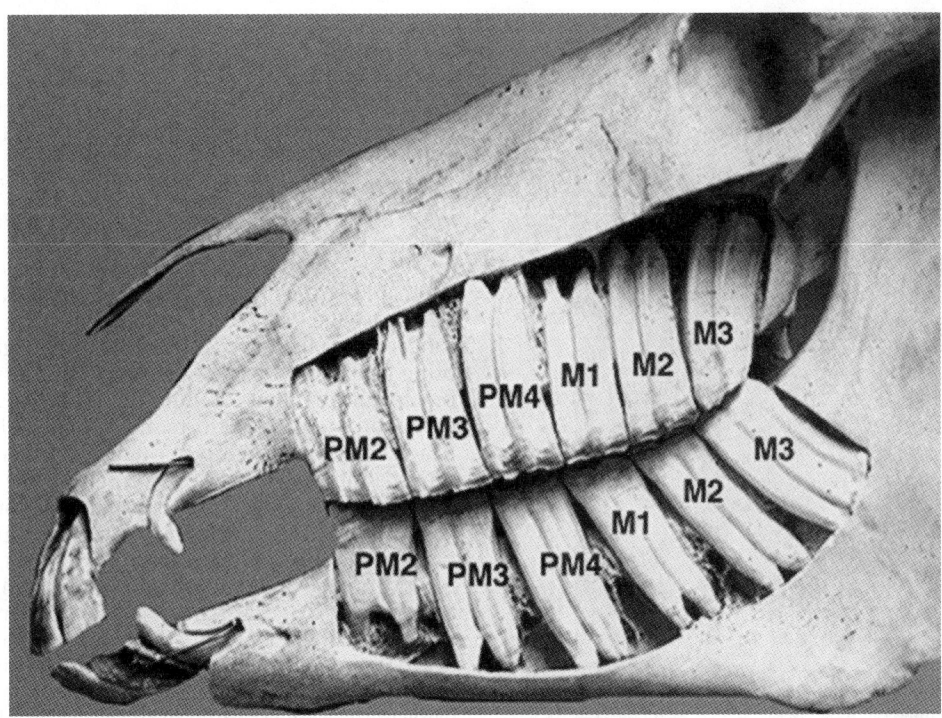

FIG. 30-10 ▓ Lateral view of cadaver equine skull. *M*, Molar; *PM*, premolar.

molars retain a narrower, rectangular shape. The cheek teeth are commonly referred to by number, from rostral to caudal 1 to 6. The coniform vestigial wolf tooth is the first premolar (PM1) and is not included in the 1 to 6 nomenclature. Thus the *first* cheek tooth is the *second* premolar. The following relationships apply: first cheek tooth, PM2; second cheek tooth, PM3; third cheek tooth, PM4; fourth cheek tooth, M1; fifth cheek tooth, M2; and sixth cheek tooth, M3.

To help avoid confusion, the American Veterinary Dental College nomenclature and classification committee has endorsed the use of a modified triadan tooth numbering system. Numbering is based on a fully phenotypic dentition made up of 44 teeth. This three-digit system uses the first digit to designate the quadrant and arch location and whether the dentition is deciduous or permanent. The numbering sequence is upper right, upper left, lower left, and lower right. The permanent dentition uses the numbers 1 to 4 and the deciduous uses numbers 5 to 8. In each quadrant, the first or central incisor is always 01, with incisors numbered 01 to 03. The canines, whether present or not, take up the 04 position in the formula. The premolars are numbered 05 to 08, and the molars are numbered 09 to 11.[22]

The equine incisor, premolar, and molar teeth are hypsodont teeth; these have a long anatomic crown, much of which is held in reserve subgingivally in the alveolar bone, and their roots are relatively short.[23] The root apices complete their development and progressive constriction of the apical foramina continues into early middle age (normally 6 to 9 years). Once fully formed, the tooth no longer grows in length, but continues to erupt throughout life as occlusal wear takes place. As occlusal wear occurs, at the rate of 2 to 3 mm per year, eruption of the tooth into persistent occlusion and function causes the reserve crown length (80- to 90-mm tooth crown in the young horse) in the alveolus and maxillary sinus to decrease. By having this reserve crown in the alveolar bone that erupts continuously as the exposed crown is worn away, horses are able to maintain a functional dental apparatus well into old age.[24]

The cranial position of the premolars and molars is such that the paths of the dental roots of each tooth follow an enlarging circle with the center being just below the temporomandibular joint. There is a consistent relationship between the last cheek tooth and the rostral border of the orbit. The maxillary sinuses store the roots of the upper last premolar (PM4) and three molar teeth in the young horse. The roots of the first two maxillary cheek teeth (PM2, PM3) lie rostral to the sinuses. The caudal root of the third upper cheek tooth (PM4) usually lies in the rostral maxillary sinus. The roots of the first upper molar lie entirely within the rostral maxillary sinus, and the roots of the second molar are beneath the septum separating the maxillary sinuses. The curved roots of upper M2 and M3 are within the caudal maxillary sinus. The cheek teeth of the lower jaw are embedded in the dental alveoli of the mandible.

The horse is anisognathic, which means the bottom jaw is narrower than the upper and the lateral excursion of the jaw during mastication favors occlusal wear of the buccal aspect of the lower and the lingual aspect of the upper molar arcades.

At approximately 6 months of age, the foal will have 24 teeth. Expansion of the cranial and facial bones during the first 2 to 3 years of life allows room for the expansion of the dental formula from 24 to 36 to 44 teeth in the adult horse.

The molar tables are sloped at a 10- to 15-degree angle from dorsal lingual to buccal ventral (Fig. 30-11). As the horse chews, the jaw moves in a rotating motion from side to side with limited rostral-caudal excursion. The construction of the molars with interdigitations of enamel, cementum, and dentin allows for uneven, continuous wear with a sharp, serrating surface when the horse is grazing. The extent of lateral excursion of the mandible during normal mastication is affected by the length of stem or roughage in the horse's ration. A horse on pasture or hay has a full or wide area of mandibular excursion. However, horses eating pellets or concentrates have a limited range of lateral jaw excursion.[25] Horses fed predominantly pellets or limited long-stemmed roughage diets will tend to have incomplete wear of the molar surface, predisposing the arcades to sharp,

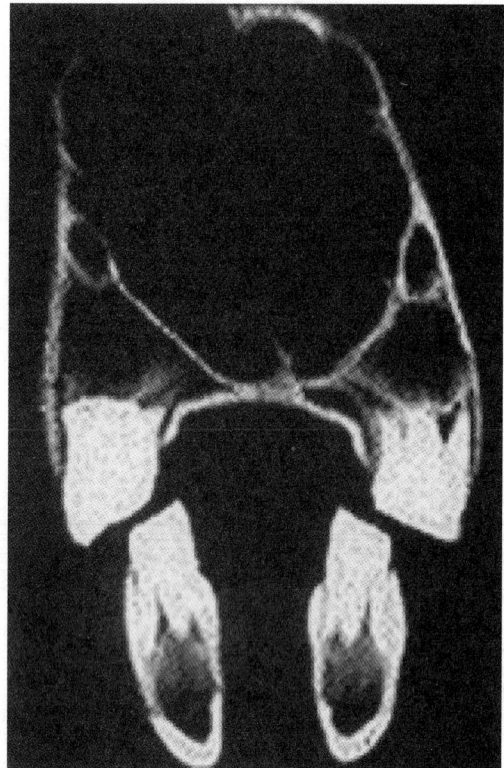

FIG. 30-11 ▮▮ Computed tomography scan of equine skull at the level of the first molars. Dorsal is at top of the illustation. Note that because the upper molars are offset laterally from the lower molars, the molar tables are sloped at a 10- to 15-degree angle from dorsal lingual to buccal ventral.

enamel edges; vaulted ceiling of occlusion; or the equally serious problem of shear mouth. Malocclusion of the incisor or molar arcades perpetuates abnormal wear patterns that eventually lead to severe dental disorders.

Rostral or caudal molar malocclusion or eruption problems (displaced, deformed, delayed eruption, missing or supernumerary teeth) lead to uneven dental wear. Horses with asymmetry between the upper and lower molar arcades (mandibular fracture, facial injury, congenital deformities such as brachygnathism [parrot mouth] and prognathism [sawmouth]) or an abnormally narrow mandible in relation to the maxilla often have abnormal tooth wear in the form of dental hooks, dental overgrowth, vaulted ceiling of occlusion, shear mouth, step mouth, or wave mouth.

Equine males normally have two upper and two lower canine, or bridle, teeth. Lower canines are forward, producing a long lower diastema or interdental space. The upper canine erupts at the suture between the incisive and maxillary bones. Canines are absent or rudimentary in mares.

Rudimentary first premolars (wolf teeth) are constant in fetal life in both the upper and lower jaws. Many never develop to the point of eruption, but instead degenerate and become incorporated in the maxilla or mandible. The uppers erupt in 20% to 50% of horses; the lowers rarely erupt.

The dynamic change that takes place in the horse's head continues at a slower rate throughout life, with continual eruption of the hypsodont premolar, molar, and incisor teeth with their large reserve crowns and slowly forming short root structures.

DENTAL EXAMINATION

Biannual dental examination of the horse should be performed as a routine part of a health maintenance program.

Improved eating efficiency is the first and foremost consideration from a medical standpoint, but often owners are more enthusiastic about dental care because of its positive effects on the horse' athletic performance. Written documentation of dental examination findings is necessary to formulate a problem-oriented treatment plan and to follow a horse's progress after treatment. A consistent routine on the part of the examiner increases the efficacy and quality of the examination (Box 30-1).

Several signs may be obtained from history or observed in a horse suffering from dental problems. A history of abnormal head carriage or head tossing when being ridden or eating, longer time taken to eat, halitosis, dysphagia, drooling, dribbling feed (quidding), or eating hay before grain should lead one to consider that a dental problem is present. Indicators of dental problems in performance horses include tail wringing, head shaking, lugging in or out on the track, and fighting the bit. In addition, dorsal displacement of the soft palate in performance horses may be a sign of dental abnormalities.

Good dental health is highly important to a horse's digestive system. Chronic colic or choke can result from improper mastication of feed, and reluctance to drink cold water may be a result of dental pain. Proper mechanical digestion of feed allows better carbohydrate absorption in the small intestine and improved fiber fermentation in the cecum and large colon. Improperly masticated roughage and concentrate leads to poor digestibility in the small and large intestine because of large feed particles with decreased surface area per mass. This decreased surface area does not allow proper enzyme degradation or bacterial fermentation.[26] Examination of the manure normally should not reveal whole grain or stem particles more than 0.25 inch long.

A horse's overall condition should be evaluated in light of the horse's use and dietary intake as a routine aspect of dental examination. A body score should be assigned because this is a more accurate way to subjectively record body condition.[27] Objective assessment of body condition using a scale, weight tape, or photographs is also beneficial and provides good data to assist in proper management.

The horse's body and head conformation should be considered in evaluating the masticatory system. Horses with small heads have more of an angle in the curve of the mandibular ramus and are predisposed to dental crowding and ramps on the lower dental arcades.

The age of the horse should be taken into consideration, because different conditions need to be addressed for each stage of the horse's growth, development, and maturity. The use of the horse can play a part in whether wearing a bit must be considered in the horse's dental care. Stable surroundings should also be carefully observed for evidence of vices, such as cribbing, or poor eating habits, such as dribbled hay or grain (quidding).

The physical examination itself begins with observing the horse's body condition, attitude, and temperament (Box 30-2). A loose-fitting halter is necessary to properly evaluate the mouth. If the horse is fractious or resists examination, sedation should be administered.

The horse should be approached from the left side of the shoulder. The head should be observed from both sides and the front for symmetry, protuberances, or swelling. Lacrimation should be noted, as well as any nasal discharge. Neurologic evaluation should be considered if any cranial nerve deficit is detected. External palpation of the head should be performed, feeling the mandibular rami, masseter muscles, and temporomandibular joints for enlargements or asymmetry.

The frontal and maxillary sinuses should be percussed with the horse's mouth open. The width between the mandibular ramus should be noted because this correlates with the room in the mouth for the bit. The sides of the head lateral to the upper dental arcade should be compressed from

---

BOX 30-1

Timetable and Checklist for Routine Dental Examinations

IMMEDIATE POSTNATAL PERIOD
Check congenital defects of lips or palate.
Check tongue motion and strength.
Check dental malocclusions.
Evaluate all body systems.

6 TO 8 MONTHS
Check that all incisors are erupted.
Check incisor and premolar occlusion.
Check for sharp enamel points or hooks.
Examine tongue and buccal mucosa for ulcers.
Float teeth if necessary.

16 TO 24 MONTHS
Check for expanded lower wolf teeth eruption.
Check points and hooks on premolars.
Investigate for bit lesions.
Float teeth and round off rostral corner of premolar 2.
Extract wolf teeth.

2 TO 3 YEARS
Check for upper and lower wolf teeth.
Check corners of mouth and interdental space for bite injuries.
Evaluate molars and premolars for points and retained caps (first cheek tooth).
Float outside of upper and inside of lower cheek teeth.
Remove caps if present and ready, and extract wolf teeth.

3 TO 4 YEARS
Check corners of mouth and interdental space for bit injuries.
Evaluate incisors for retained deciduous teeth or supernumerary teeth.

3 TO 4 YEARS—cont'd
Evaluate molars and premolars for points and retained caps (second cheek tooth).
Evaluate size and shape of lower jaw and percuss sinuses.
Check for blind wolf teeth.
Remove caps if present; float teeth, and remove wolf teeth.

4 TO 5 YEARS
Check all incisors for eruption.
Check canine teeth for sharp edges or eruption delays.
Evaluate entire molar arcade for proper eruption and alignment.
Visually check upper rostral and lower caudal cheek teeth for hooks from malocclusion.
Digitally check for points on sharp edges of cheek teeth.
Percuss sinuses.
Float teeth.
Remove deciduous teeth if ready.
Cut or rasp hooks if present.
Remove mucosa over canines if gingival cysts are present.

5 YEARS AND OLDER
Examine mouth visually and digitally, especially noting hooks and uneven wear.
Evaluate canines for sharp edges and tartar.
Percuss sinuses.
Use olfactory senses to detect evidence of oral decay, gingivitis.
Observe incisors for even wear.
Evaluate lateral jaw excursion.
Float teeth; remove hooks with chisel or rasp and level or shorten incisors if indicated.

BOX 30-2

Examination of the Oral Cavity

1. Rinse mouth, noting volume, consistency and smell of material flushed.
2. Evaluate incisors from front and side for evenness of wear.
3. Observe and palpate diastema or interdental space for canine teeth, blind wolf teeth, and unerupted canines.
4. Observe tongue for lesions.
5. Palpate upper rostral premolars for detection of hooks and sharp buccal cusps.
6. Evaluate lateral excursion of the mandible.
7. Palpate oral cavity.
8. Use full-mouth speculum and, with aid of flashlight or headlamp, examine mouth digitally and visually.
9. If necessary, use an endoscope for detailed evaluation of interproximal spaces, gingival pocketing, or defects in the occlusal surfaces of the cheek teeth.

the orbit, moving forward to the first cheek tooth at the level of the nasal notch, noticing any protuberances, depressions, asymmetry, or evidence of pain.

The commissures of the lips should be observed and palpated for evidence of trauma from sharp teeth or improperly fitting bits. Next, a detailed examination of the oral cavity should be performed, as shown in Box 30-2. Because rabies is

a potential cause of dysphagia, the examiner should have an adequate titer for rabies antibodies.

If areas of impacted or trapped feed are present, they should be removed with a digit or dental pick and the mouth rinsed completely. Horses with sharp buccal points on the upper dental arcade resist the full-mouth speculum, and floating the upper arcades may be beneficial before the oral examination is completed.

Dental Radiology

Diagnostic radiology is a valuable aid in management of equine dental disease. The excellent contrast between air, bone, soft tissue, and tooth substance makes the head an excellent area for radiologic evaluation.[28] Good-quality films can be obtained with portable x-ray machines and rare earth intensifying screens without a grid.

Indications for head radiology are any suspicion of dental infection, maleruption, or oral pain of unknown origin. Radiographs should be obtained before and after dental extraction. Any facial swelling, deformity, neoplasm, trauma, or fracture may warrant a radiograph to aid in diagnosis and management.

Radiographs can be taken in the standing animal with the animal under sedation. The head and radiographic cassette can be placed on a stand to decrease motion by the patient. A lateral view centered over the rostral edge of the facial crest will demonstrate fluid lines in the sinuses. Open mouth films are beneficial in evaluating the dental arcades. The lateral view superimposes the dental arcades and should not be relied on to diagnose diseases involving the dental reserve crown and roots. Lesion-oriented oblique films (30 degrees in young horses, 45 degrees in older) taken to demonstrate the roots of the upper or lower cheek teeth are helpful in diagnosis of dental disease. Dorsal ventral views centered over the suspected tooth can demonstrate periodontal disease on the buccal aspect of the upper cheek teeth or infundibular decay. Intraoral occlusal films are useful in demonstrating incisor lesions or fractures from the diastema rostral.

TREATMENT

A plan for treatment based on the results of history, clinical findings, and oral examination should be outlined before proceeding with any dental work. This problem-oriented approach is important because the owner or trainer should be informed of any abnormalities and given a plan for treatment and an estimate of the cost before any corrective procedure is carried out.

It is very important to plan the therapy, making sure all equipment is present to complete the job. The horse should be properly restrained and adequate help present to assist in performing the procedures to completion. A dental record form is an aid in documenting examination results and summarizing the treatment plan (Fig. 30-12).

Routine Dental Maintenance

FLOATING. Dental floating is an age-old and routine method to correct the abnormal wear patterns associated with dental eruption. It also is a procedure that allows the sculpting of the teeth to accommodate the bit. The main purpose of molar floating, or leveling, is to remove points or sharp edges from the buccal aspect of the upper and lingual aspect of the lower molar arcades. Floating may also entail removing minor hooks or ramps from the rostral or caudal aspect of the arcades or leveling minor elevations in the occlusal surface of the arcades.

Proper equipment is required to reach all aspects of the molar surfaces completely, regardless of size of horse.[29] Float blades made of carbide chips or tungsten carbide planing blades make the work of floating more efficient. The outward curve of the upper arcade makes the central buccal area involving PM3 through M2 the easiest to reach with the float. The area around PM2 and M3 requires an offset or angle head on the rasps to reach all extremities. The lower arcade can be floated to remove the lingual enamel points with a flat, long-handled rasp in most cases. To correct rostral and caudal hooks, special equipment, such as carbide planing blades, power burrs, sliding chisel, or simple joint molar cutters, may be needed.

The mouth speculum or a dental wedge may help to make this job easier if the horse closes its mouth, trapping the instrument. In horses with slightly ramped back teeth caused by a greater curvature of spee, a mouth speculum and a slightly curved or swivel head float may be needed to reach the table of the last molar.

In bitted horses the rounding of the first upper and lower cheek teeth and lowering of the buccal cusps from upper PM2 to PM3 usually require an offset head float or an S-

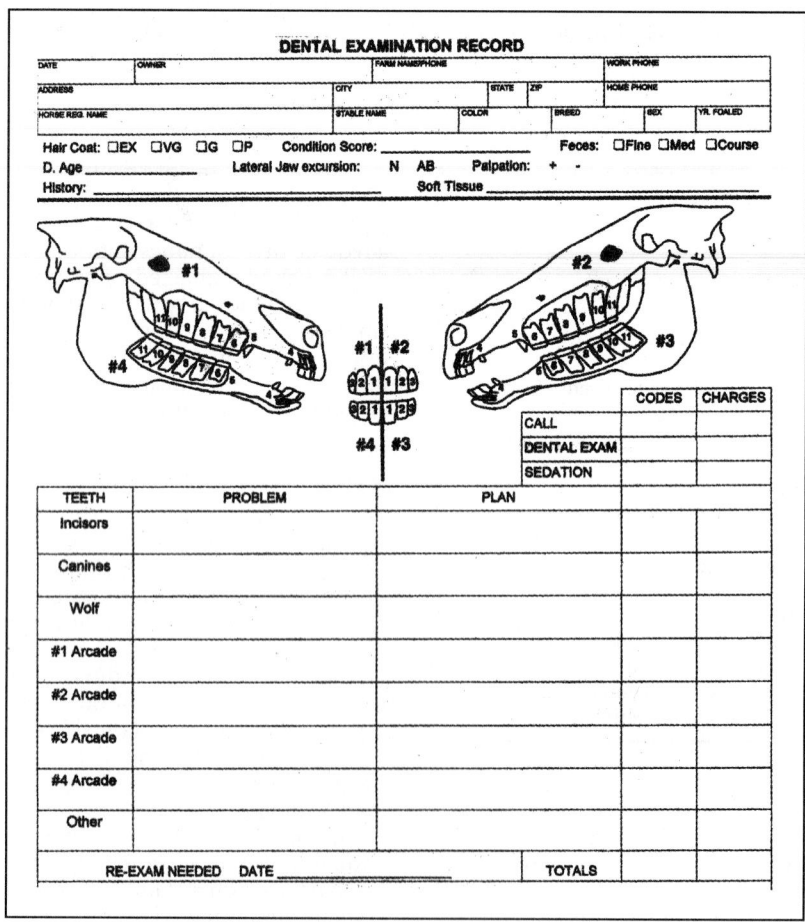

FIG. 30-12 ■ Dental form used to record examination findings.

shaped rasp. The routine floating and other corrective measures in the mouth may require the added physical restraint of a dental halter or mild chemical sedation.

WOLF TEETH. The wolf teeth are caniform first premolars and are present in 20% to 60% of horses in the upper arcade, but rarely are present in the lower arcade. Most animals that are worked with a bit in their mouth benefit from having these teeth removed. Although not all wolf teeth cause problems, a loose or sharp wolf tooth can be a distraction or even cause pain of such severity as to lead to bad bitting habits. In some instances, diagnosis of wolf tooth problems is difficult and confusing. Sometimes they do not erupt in a normal downward path, penetrating the gum, but migrate rostrally under the gum and cause a subgingival enlargement that, in turn, is irritating to the horse. These unerupted first premolars have been referred to as "blind" wolf teeth and should be surgically removed when found.

CANINE TEETH. Canine teeth are present in most male horses over 4 years of age. Because of the unopposed position in the diastema, they cause few problems. Some mares have small or rudimentary canines that do not seem to cause a problem, but can become loose or accumulate tartar, which may indicate removal.

Long or sharp canines in a stallion or gelding can interfere with bitting, be a nuisance or danger to the groomer, or become an area for tartar accumulation. They can be cut or ground down and polished to remedy this problem. Erupting canine teeth in the 4- to 6-year-old horse may cause subgingival pain and bit irritation, which may manifest itself as head shaking or other bad habits. The mucosa should be removed over canines if gingival eruption cysts are present. The canine roots are long and curved, making this tooth extremely difficult to extract in the male. If the canine becomes injured and the root infected, surgical removal through a bone flap is indicated.

DENTAL CAPS. As the developing permanent tooth pushes to the surface, it presses on the roots of the worn down deciduous tooth and gradually cuts off its nutrition. The deciduous tooth becomes loose, loses its blood supply and dies, and is displaced. The osseous alveolar walls adjust to these changes by bone production and resorption, thereby providing a new socket for the embedded portion of the newly formed permanent tooth. The remaining cap portion of the deciduous premolar tooth has up to four legs, or root slivers, that cover the crown of the permanent tooth. If these slivers are broken off and remain subgingival after the cap is shed, gingivitis and periodontal disease can result.

The eruption pattern of permanent molarized dentition follows a sequence that predisposes to entrapment of deciduous PM3 and PM4. Delayed shedding of deciduous premolars can predispose to gingivitis, periodontal irritation, or infection. Retained, split, or displaced deciduous premolars can be distracting to the training process of a young horse and have been an incriminating factor in dorsal displacement of the soft palate.

Impacted caps, manifested as a bony enlargement on the ventral mandibular ramus or maxilla rostral to the facial crest, can cause lingual displacement or delay eruption of permanent teeth. In most cases, these swellings are benign, but they can become diseased if eruption is severely inhibited or bloodborne bacteria inhabit the inflamed dental pulp leading to anachorectic pulpitis and facial swelling with a draining tract on the mandible. Caps should be evaluated by palpation. A crease or neck can be felt at the line separating the deciduous and permanent tooth just above the gum line. Radiographs may be necessary to diagnose retained deciduous premolars in difficult cases.

If one cap has shed and time is past, all others in that corresponding quadruplet should be removed. A molar forceps is placed on the tooth and rotated lingually. The cap is extracted in this manner to ensure that the buccal root slivers are elevated. This will reduce the incidence of retained cap slivers that can be irritating and even predispose to periodontal disease.

INCISORS. After the back teeth have been evaluated and treated as necessary, the horse's mouth should be completely examined, both visually and digitally, to ensure that all sharp or uneven edges have been smoothed and no teeth have been broken or loosened. The speculum is then removed and the mouth closed and the jaw excursion evaluation test repeated to confirm full excursion is present and the mouth is balanced. The incisors should meet evenly and begin to open as the jaw is moved from side to side and the molar arcades make contact. If the incisors are uneven or excessively long, they may need to be aligned or shortened at this time. Minor incisor leveling can be performed with a flat carbide rasp, but any major work should be performed with a motorized burr or cutters.

When the dental examination and floating procedures have been completed, the horse should have full, comfortable range of motion of the jaw with contact between the upper and lower molar arcades.

The Diseased Equine Tooth

Clinical signs referable to dental diseases include the following:

- Abnormal behavior while eating (quidding or head tilting)
- Reluctance to eat
- Loss of condition
- Objectionable odor or halitosis
- Blood or excessive saliva in the mouth
- Abnormal head shaking or shyness
- Abnormal head carriage or signs of pain associated with position or use of the bit
- Oral or facial trauma
- Bumps or swelling in the facial area
- Drainage from the mandible or maxilla
- Chronic fetid nasal discharge

In one survey of 150 horses with no history or clinical signs of dental disease, 8% had broken, missing, or overtly infected teeth.[30]

In addition to the examination, ancillary aids, such as plain and contrast radiography; endoscopy of the oral cavity, nasal turbinates, and paranasal sinuses; cytology; culture; and histopathology may be useful in confirming the clinical diagnosis.

Because no tooth acts independently, but rather as part of the total masticatory apparatus, the management of a diseased tooth must be designed to treat illness that involves the masticatory system as a whole. This approach to dental care has been referred to as "dental treatment planning," which is defined as the development of a series of procedures that are necessary to restore a diseased dentition to a state of health.

Dental disease is related to the age and dental development of the horse. Although dental disease is not easily divided because developmental problems of malocclusion and tooth formation often predispose to many traumatic and infectious problems, diseases can be divided into four categories: developmental, traumatic, infectious, and neoplastic.

Dental disease involving the molars and premolars can be divided into three categories: periradicular disease, dental decay, and periodontal disease. These categories overlap and do not specifically address the etiology of pathogenesis and management of the conditions.

PERIRADICULAR DISEASE. Delayed or abnormal eruption of the permanent teeth is usually caused by retained deciduous teeth (caps). Caps can become trapped, preventing normal eruption of the permanent teeth. The fourth premolar is the last permanent tooth to erupt (average time of eruption is 3 years, 8 months). This tooth must emerge between the permanent third premolar, which usually erupts at 2 years, 8 months, and the first molar, which erupts at 1 year.

A rostral hook may develop on the unopposed second upper or lower deciduous premolar at 1 year of age or less. These hooks occur in 5% to 20% of horses and can cause caudal pressure on the opposite dental arcade.[30] This pressure causes crowding of the permanent teeth and wedging of caps. The erupting permanent teeth beneath the wedged cap may become displaced medially or impacted. The pressure created by the enlarging tooth in the bony mandible or maxilla leads to progressive vascular lysis of the mandible or maxilla surrounding roots of the tooth. Vascular lysis leads to facial or mandibular swelling of the periradicular area of the affected tooth. Osteolysis surrounding the roots can be seen radiographically. It has been referred to as an eruption pseudocyst. The enlargement normally regresses when the tooth completes eruption.

If overcrowding is severe, eruption pseudocysts are accompanied by apical osteitis, pain, and swelling. The involved permanent tooth is in a state of transient hyperemia and opportunistic hematogenous pathogens may infect the area (anachoretic pulpitis). Therapy consists of correcting the predisposing cause. The offending cap, if still present, should be removed. Radiographic evaluation of the position of the tooth roots rostral and caudal to the impacted tooth is indicated. If inadequate space is present for normal tooth eruption, the adjacent surfaces of the offending teeth may have to be ground down.

If heat and soft tissue swelling are present, but there is no fistula, antimicrobial therapy should be instituted. Gram-negative pathogens or anaerobic bacteria are most often involved and can be eliminated with ceftiofur (2 to 4 mg/kg, IM or IV, two to three times daily) or chloramphenicol (30 to 50 mg/kg, PO, four times daily for 30 days) in combination with penicillin. If *Bacteroides fragilis* is suspected, one can combine metronidazole (15 mg/kg, PO, three to four times daily) with penicillin (20,000 U/kg IM, twice daily, or IV, four times daily).

A draining tract in the area of the tooth root indicates advanced changes in the periradicular area. This phenomenon has been referred to as chronic ossifying alveolar periostitis. Good-quality radiographs, with or without insertion of a probe or contrast medium into the tract, can usually pinpoint the area of involvement. The paranasal sinuses may be involved with disease of the fourth upper premolar. Mixed bacterial populations are usually cultured from draining tracts or paranasal sinuses even though the discharge may appear mucoid and sterile. The draining tract usually leads to the apex of the involved tooth root. A draining tract can first be seen up to 2 years after the time the deciduous tooth is shed.

The later in life a draining tract condition develops, the more mature the dental root. The rostral five equine mandibular cheek teeth have two distinct roots and the sixth cheek tooth has three roots. They do not have a pulp chamber that continues as the root canal to the apex, such as occurs in carnivores. The pulp cavity of upper cheek teeth has five main divisions within the folds of enamel and has three roots (one lingual and two buccal). The infundibula and cement lakes add to the complexity of these teeth and may allow for communication between the pulp and crown.

Removal of the apically infected tooth has been the standard method of therapy. Many stable and periodontally sound teeth have been removed, but not without numerous complications and long-term adverse effects.[31] Another approach to the treatment of apically infected teeth has been

periradicular surgery to evaluate the apex of the tooth and to alleviate the infection by root-end resection and apical seal (root canal). If the tooth cannot be saved because it has lost its alveolar attachment, because the surgeon is inexperienced, or because the owner does not comply with this treatment, it can be repelled by the same approach.

DENTAL DECAY. Dental pulp can become infected secondary to imperfect formation of the upper cheek teeth. The enamel folds enclose a lake of cementum (infundibulum). If these lakes of cementum are excessively deep or irregularly formed, they are predisposed to decay from bacterial enzymes. Decay of cementum can allow bacterial toxins to reach the pulp or can simply weaken the architectural structure of the tooth, making it vulnerable to splitting or cracking under the load placed on it during mastication. Decay of the infundibular cementum has been referred to as infundibular necrosis or patent infundibulum.

When oral examination reveals a black spot in the upper cheek tooth (Fig. 30-13), a dental pick or probe can be introduced into the defect for removal of fetid feed and debris. Deep probing and irrigation with a needle and syringe allows determination of the depth of the defect. The defect may progress the entire length of the tooth. Even if the eroded infundibulum does not communicate with the pulp, bacteria or toxins from dental decay may cross into the pulp through small channels in the dentin.

Contrast radiographs may confirm the presence of a channel between the infundibulum and the pulp chamber. The tooth structure should be closely evaluated orally to determine whether the exposed crown is complete. The upper PM4 and M1 can fracture longitudinally along the edge of the cementum and lateral enamel or through the infundibulum. These fractured teeth may have infected pulp, or the pulp may be healthy, with only the unstable portion displaced and periodontally affected. Removal by extraction of the unstable part of the tooth may relieve the clinical signs of dental disease. If the entire tooth is unstable, it should be removed.

Infection of the pulp secondary to infundibular decay can be managed by endodontic therapy or by removal. Periradicular therapy of upper PM2, PM3, M1 with a retrograde filling

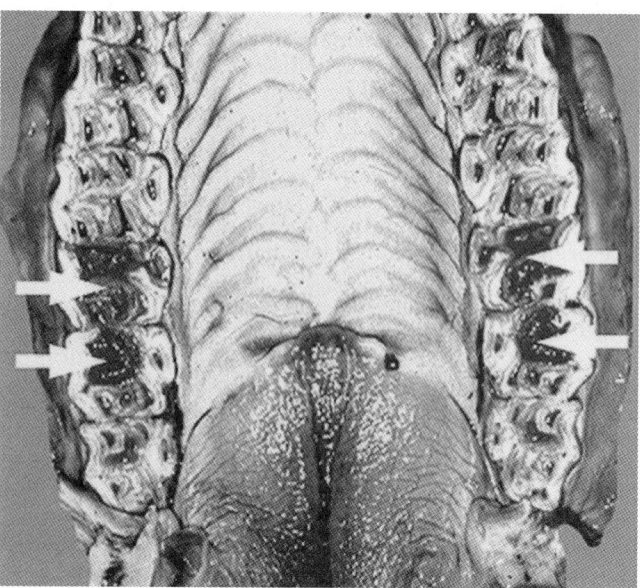

FIG. 30-13 ■ Cadaver specimen of the maxillary dental arcade. Note the black areas of dental decay on the occlusal surfaces of M1 and M2 *(arrows)*.

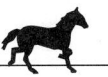

has been done with good results. Infection of the paranasal sinuses can be treated by lavaging the sinuses. If the tooth must be removed, it can be extracted with forceps or repelled through a dorsal bone flap or trephine hole. The tooth can be approached through a lateral buccotomy and can be elevated intact or divided and elevated in several sections.[32,33]

PERIODONTAL DISEASE. Periodontal disease is progressive inflammation of the gingivae, resorption of alveolar bone, degeneration of the periodontal membrane, apical migration of the epithelial attachment, formation of periodontal pockets, and mobility of the tooth.

Shearing forces that are produced by normal mastication are essential for maintenance of a healthy periodontium. Gingivitis can be initiated in any situation in which there is abnormal dental occlusion and alteration in shearing forces. The most severe form of periodontal disease is associated with extreme abnormalities of wear, such as wave mouth, shear mouth, hooks, loss of teeth with corresponding overgrowth of the opposing teeth, and misplaced or split teeth.

Shear mouth can occur when there is a profound difference in width between the upper and lower jaw. This results in excessive angulation of the table surfaces of the cheek teeth and development of long extremely sharp edges. A shear mouth can also develop secondary to chewing on only one side of the mouth, causing the molar table on the opposite side not to wear on the buccal upper table and lingual lower table.

Wave mouth (Fig. 30-14) is brought on by changes in the shape and position of the normal transverse ridges across the occlusal surfaces, resulting in arcades attaining a wave form. In severe cases the teeth in one arcade may be worn to the gum margin, permitting the opposing molar to lacerate the gingivum. Wave mouth also occurs secondary to decay in the upper molars, most frequently PM3 through M2, allowing overgrowth of the opposing lower cheek teeth. Treatment of shear mouth and wave mouth, usually involving cutting and rasping, is helpful but not totally satisfactory. These conditions are best prevented by floating as part of biannual dental maintenance.

Mandibular fracture can lead to acute periodontal disease by exposing the periodontal space to feed. Infection of the tooth root and osteomyelitis can occur subsequently. Malocclusion that often follows mandibular fracture can predispose to a more chronic form of periodontal disease. Fracture to the mandible, premaxilla, or maxilla in a young horse can damage dental buds and cause displaced or malformed permanent teeth.

Periodontal disease has been described as the dental scourge of horses, and its importance must be understood and appreciated. Regular dental examinations and floating to maintain normal occlusion help to prevent periodontal disease. Once the disease is present, a program of oral hygiene can correct, or at least slow, the progression of the disease. I have found that daily cleaning of gingival pockets with an elongated water pick is helpful.

Once the disease has progressed to a point of destroying the bony attachment to the tooth, it loosens the tooth in its socket and the tooth must be removed. The tooth must become quite loose to palpate because of its tight fit between adjacent teeth. Removal can be performed by extraction, elevation through a lateral buccotomy, or repulsion.

EQUINE ORAL TUMORS

Equine oral tumors are rare, making up a very small percentage of the facial or mandibular swellings. These tumors can be divided into three basic types: odontogenic, osteogenic, and secondary.[34]

Odontogenic tumors are derived from remnants of dental epithelium. Five types have been recorded in the maxillae and mandibles of horses. They are ameloblastomas, ameloblastic odontomas, complex odontomas, compound odontomas, and cementomas.[35] Because of their rarity, ill-defined biologic behavior, and poorly defined radiographic features, diagnosis can be difficult. Histopathology can be confusing because of variation in appearance at different sampling sites and age-related changes in tumor appearance.

Primary bone tumors are rare in the horse and are usually benign. More than 80% of equine osteosarcomas occur in the head region.[35] As is the case with odontogenic tumors, disagreement remains on histologic classification, terminology, and nature of bone tumors. In addition to gross and histologic examination, correlation of history, clinical, radiologic, and some biochemical findings by clinicians and pathologists is often essential to establish a diagnosis.

Secondary tumors of the head include extensions of oropharyngeal squamous cell carcinomas, lymphosarcomas, papillomas, and melanomas. Squamous cell carcinoma is the

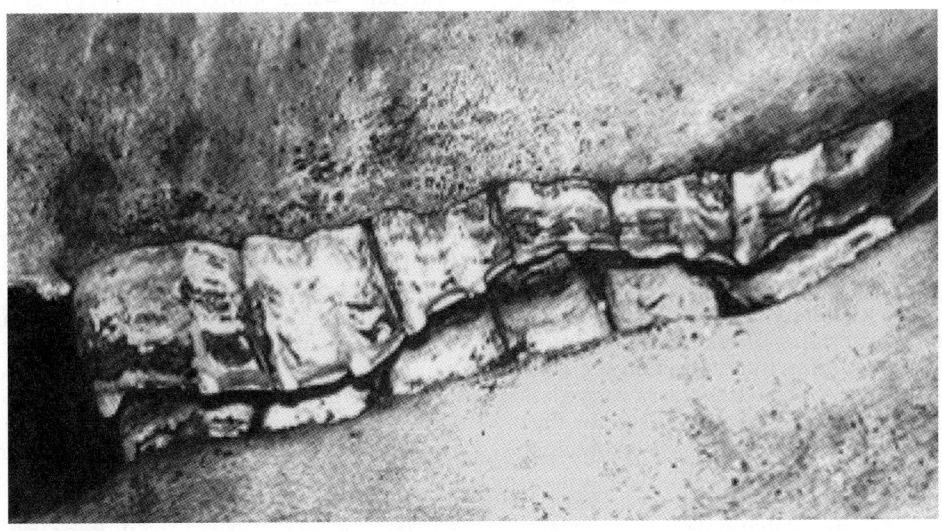

FIG. 30-14 ▒ Lateral view of cadaver equine skull illustrating "wave-mouth."

most frequently reported oral tumor in the horse. Generally, these tumors are seen in older horses, and there is no gender or breed predilection. There are many treatment options and methods to control progression of oral tumors. Radiotherapy, hyperthermia, chemotherapy, cryosurgery, immunotherapy, autogenous vaccines, photodynamic therapy, laser therapy, and surgical resection have been tried with variable results.[36]

SALIVARY GLANDS AND DUCTS

Diseases of the salivary glands, including sialoadenitis, salivary calculi, salivary mucocele, trauma, and neoplasia are uncommon in the horse. During oral examinations, the openings of the salivary ducts should be noted. The parotid salivary ducts enter the mouth at its papilla opposite the last upper premolar. The mandibular salivary duct opens into the oral cavity on the lateral aspect of the sublingual caruncle. The sublingual salivary ducts, approximately 30 in number, are seen as small pores in the sublingual recess.

Salivation may indicate excessive accumulation of saliva in the mouth (sialism, ptyalism, or dysphagia). Heavy-metal toxicity, parasympathomimetic poisoning, neurologic disease, and stomatitis may cause ptyalism. Dysphagia can be caused by esophageal obstruction (choke), oral foreign body, rabies, or other neurologic diseases. Legume grass or hay contaminated with *Rhizoctonia lequminicola* produces a mycotoxin slaframine, which causes sialism.

The salivary glands rarely become involved in any inflammatory process, including infection caused by *Streptococcus equi*. Trauma to one gland may cause an open wound or infection. Sialoadenitis may result from salivary duct obstruction from accumulation of exudate and mucus or an ingested foreign body or sialolith.[37]

Sialoliths occur infrequently in the parotid duct. An organic or vegetable nidus lodges in the duct and the disposition of calcium salt, mainly carbonate, begins to occur around it. The organic nidi are usually cellular debris, resulting from desquamation or inflammatory reaction and bacteria. The vegetable nidus may consist of any small foreign body that enters the duct from the salivary papilla, such as grain husks and spicules or awns of grass, barley, or wheat. Large stones may cause duct obstruction and salivary retention, which may bring about glandular atrophy or acute sialoadenitis with acinar swelling and rupture.

On palpation, sialoliths are usually hard, smooth, movable, and painless enlargements over the cheek at the level of the upper dental arcade. Abscess formation with pain, excessive salivation, and fistula formation can occur. Radiography will reveal a dense oral smooth mass at the level of the upper third and fourth cheek tooth. Surgical removal and primary wound closure yield good results. The diagnosis of sialolith is straightforward but should differ from that of tooth abscess or buccal tumor.

Salivary mucocele is an accumulation of salivary secretions in a single or multiloculated cavity adjacent to a ruptured duct. A ranula is a special type of mucocele that occurs secondary to obstruction of the sublingual salivary duct. Treatment consists of creating a salivary fistula into the oral cavity or excising the mucocele and associated salivary gland.

Lacerations or iatrogenic injury to the salivary ducts can lead to salivary cutaneous fistulas. These injuries should be surgically repaired by reapposing the severed duct, creating an oral opening for the duct, or resecting the salivary gland. Ablation and sclerosis of the gland can be achieved by flushing 1% formalin solution up the duct. Wounds involving the salivary glands can usually be handled by cleansing, debridement, and primary skin closure with good results.

Benign mixed tumors, adenocarcinomas, and acinar cell tumors of the salivary glands have been reported in horses. Local invasion of a salivary gland by tumors originating in adjacent tissue or metastasis of melanomas to the parotid salivary gland in older gray horses is more common. This type of melanoma has been seen to reduce in size after treatment with cimetidine at 6.6 mg/kg, PO, twice daily.

REFERENCES

22. Easley J: Dental and oral examination. In Baker GJ, Easley J, eds: *Equine dentistry*, London, 1999, WB Saunders.
23. Getty R, Sisson, Grossman: *The anatomy of the domestic animals*, ed 5, Philadelphia, 1975, WB Saunders.
24. Kirkland KD et al: Effect of aging on the endodontic system, reserve crown and roots of equine mandibular cheek teeth, *Am J Vet Res* 57:31-38, 1996.
25. Scrutchfield WL, Schumacher J: Examination of the oral cavity and routine dental care, *Vet Clin North Am (Equine Pract)* 9;123-131, 1993.
26. Meyer H et al: Investigations on preileal digestion of oats, corn and barley starch in relation to grain processing, *Proceedings of the Thirteenth Equine Nutrition and Physiology Symposium*, Univ of Florida, 1993.
27. Hennecke DR: A condition score system for horses, *Equine Pract* 7:13-15, 1985.
28. Dik KJ, Gunsser I: *Atlas of diagnostic radiology of the horse part 3: diseases of the head, neck and thorax*, Philadelphia, 1990, WB Saunders.
29. Easley J: *Dental care and instrumentation in veterinary clinics of North America: equine practice*, Philadelphia, 1998, WB Saunders.
30. Uhlinger CA; Survey of selected dental abnormalities in 233 horses aged 6-11, *Proc Am Assoc Equine Pract* 33:577-583, 1987.
31. Prichard MA, Hacket EP, Erb HN: Tooth repulsion in horses: complications and long-term outcome, *Proceedings of the Thirty-fifth Annual Convention of the American Association of Equine Practitioners*, 1989, p 331.
32. Evans LH, Tate LP, LaDow CS: Extraction of the equine 4th upper premolar and 1st and 2nd upper molars through a lateral buccotomy, *Proceedings of the Twenty-seventh Annual Convention of the American Association of Equine Practitioners*, 1981, pp 249-252.
33. Easley J: Equine tooth removal (exodontia). In Baker GJ, Easley J, eds: *Equine dentistry*, London, 1999, WB Saunders.
34. Gorlin RJ, Mesken LH, Brodey R: Odontogenic tumors in man and animals: pathological classification and clinical behavior—a review, *Ann NY Acad Sci* 108:722-771, 1963.
35. Pirie RS, Dixon PM: Mandibular tumors in the horse: a review of the literature and 7 case reports, *Equine Vet Ed* 5:287-294, 1993.
36. Knottenbelt DC; Oral and dental tumors. In Baker GJ, Easley J eds: *Equine dentistry*, London, 1999, WB Saunders.
37. Bouayad H et al: Sialoliths in the horse, *Equine Pract* 13:25-27, 1991.

DISORDERS OF THE ESOPHAGUS

ANTHONY T. BLIKSLAGER
SAMUEL L. JONES

ANATOMIC AND PHYSIOLOGIC CONSIDERATIONS

The cranial-most aspect of the esophagus is located on the median plane immediately dorsal to the trachea. However, at approximately the mid-cervical region (C_4-C_5), the esophagus typically shifts to the left of the trachea and lies just deep to the external jugular vein.[38,39] It is here that intraluminal obstructions or the tip of a stomach tube may be visualized; trauma in this region can readily result in esophageal perforation. When passing a stomach tube, it is critical that the tube be palpated to ensure the tube is in the esophagus, because jugular pulses can be confused with the appearance of the tip of the tube. In addition to its proximity to the external jugular vein, the esophagus is also located adjacent to the vagosympathetic trunk and the common carotid artery.[38] The esophagus is innervated by branches of the vagosympathetic trunk, and blood is supplied to the cervical esophagus by branches of the carotid arteries. The thoracic esophagus, which lies ventral to the trachea until the tracheal bifurcation, where it resumes a dorsal position, receives its blood supply from the bronchoesophageal artery. Venous drainage is via the external jugular veins in the cervical esophagus and via the esophageal vein in the thoracic esophagus.

The muscular wall of the esophagus increases in thickness as the esophagus courses distally, whereas the lumen gets smaller.[38] The esophagus is not covered by a serosa except for a very short segment that traverses the abdominal cavity between the diaphragm and the stomach.[39] Instead, the outer wall of the esophagus is composed of adventitia that is loosely attached to surrounding tissues. This loose connection allows movement of the esophagus during swallowing and during movement of the neck. The cranial two thirds of the esophageal wall consists of skeletal muscle, whereas the distal third of the esophagus is composed of smooth muscle. Although the muscular layers are composed of an outer and inner layer, similar to the remainder of the gastrointestinal tract, the skeletal muscle layers are oriented obliquely to one another.[38] This, and an abundant submucosa, enables extensive dilation of the esophagus as a bolus of food moves toward the stomach. In addition, the velocity of esophageal contraction is faster in the skeletal muscle segment of the esophagus compared with the distal smooth muscle segment.[40] The muscle layers become oriented in more of an outer longitudinal and inner circular configuration in the caudal esophagus.[38] In the resting collapsed state, redundant esophageal mucosa and submucosa becomes oriented in longitudinal folds. The mucosa is composed of stratified squamous epithelium that is continuous with the stratified epithelium of the cardiac portion of the stomach.[38]

The cranial esophageal sphincter is formed by the cricopharyngeus muscle. It maintains a resting intraesophageal pressure of approximately 85 mm Hg and a postdeglutition pressure as high as 200 mm Hg. Although the caudal esophageal sphincter is anatomically indistinct, resting intraesophageal pressure in this region is maintained at approximately 13 mm Hg, and postdeglutition pressure in the caudal esophagus may be as high as 100 mm Hg. The pressure in the caudal esophagus is maintained at approximately 10 mm Hg higher than the intraluminal pressure of the stomach.[40,41] Although the higher pressure in the distal esophagus has been implicated as the cause for the inability of most horses to vomit and for gastric rupture, other factors such as a poorly developed vomiting reflex may be more important.[42]

DIAGNOSTIC CONSIDERATIONS

Esophageal disease should be a differential in any horse that demonstrates excessive salivation. Such signs also indicate the need to assess hydration, electrolyte levels, and acid-base status. In a study in which horses had continual loss of saliva via an experimentally placed esophagotomy, abnormalities included hypochloremia, hyponatremia, and hypokalemia.[43] This results from the relatively high levels of these electrolytes in saliva. Furthermore, because horses depend on dietary intake of potassium, hypokalemia would be exacerbated in a horse that was also unable to eat because of esophageal obstruction. Loss of salivary fluid and bicarbonate also results in dehydration and metabolic acidosis. However, metabolic alkalosis subsequently occurs presumably as a result of renal compensation for electrolyte loss, particularly chloride.[43]

Further examination of horses with esophageal disease may reveal evidence of swelling or emphysema in the region of the cranial or cervical esophagus that should prompt a thorough oral examination, and further diagnostics such as radiography and endoscopy to define the nature of any esophageal abnormalities. If the esophagus has been perforated or ruptured, subcutaneous emphysema is usually evident. The lungs should be carefully auscultated for evidence of aspiration pneumonia. Radiographs of the chest are required for a full pulmonary assessment.

Radiographs of the esophagus should initially include plain films that may reveal evidence of an obstruction or areas of gas opacity within facial planes indicative of esophageal perforation.[44] However, facial and subcutaneous emphysema must be differentiated from other causes, including tracheal perforation.[42] The esophagus is often gas-distended cranial to an obstruction up to the cranial esophageal sphincter. Plain films may be diagnostic, but contrast radiographs are frequently required to fully define the nature of esophageal abnormalities.[44] Administration of barium paste or liquid will reveal linear opacifications as a result of the linear mucosal folds and may help outline intraluminal obstructions or strictures (Fig. 30-15).[44] A double-contrast study

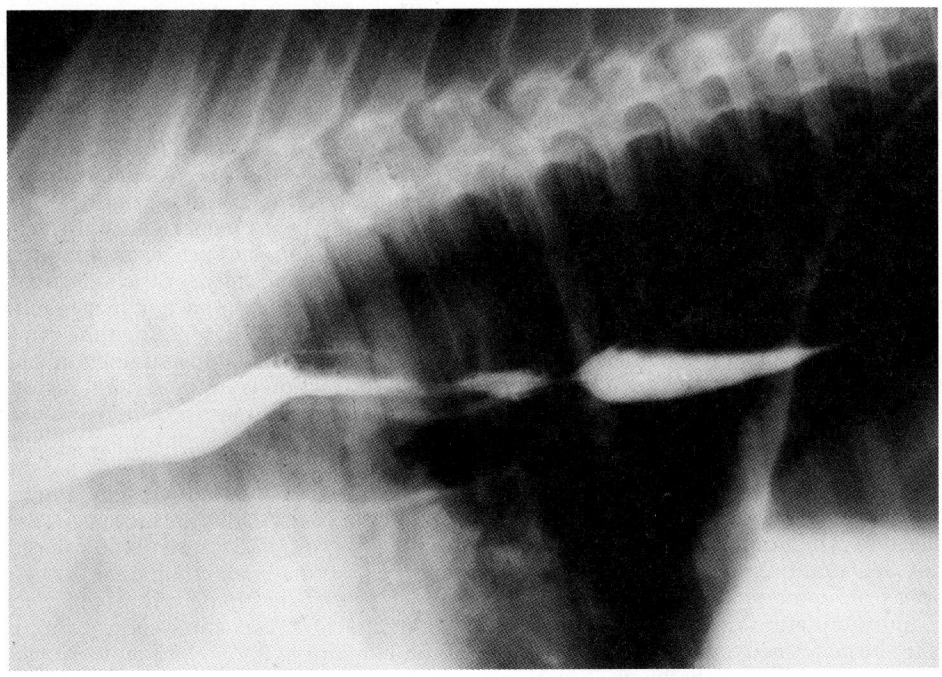

FIG. 30-15 ▌ Barium contrast esophogram, outlining esophageal lumen stricture. (Courtesy Dr. KE Sullins.)

is a useful radiographic technique for defining esophageal wall abnormalities, particularly postobstruction mucosal ulceration. It is performed by placing a cuffed nasogastric tube in the cranial esophagus and injecting 300 to 500 ml of liquid barium followed by a similar volume of air. Care should be taken when evaluating such radiographs, because swallowing can create the false impression that there is a stricture.[45] The incidence of swallowing can be decreased by administration of xylazine. Liquid barium is preferable if swallowing function is compromised, because it is less harmful to pulmonary tissues than paste, and water-soluble iodinated contrast material is particularly damaging to the lung because of its hypertonicity.[42] However, if an esophageal perforation is suspected, water-soluble contrast material is preferable.[42]

Endoscopic evaluation of the esophagus should be performed as part of a complete evaluation of esophageal injuries and abnormalities. Following sedation of the patient, the endoscope should be passed all the way into the stomach before examining the esophagus, which will be more readily viewed as the endoscope is withdrawn.[44] Inflation of the esophagus must also be performed intermittently because the wall of the esophagus collapses around the end of the endoscope. The longitudinal folds of the esophageal mucosa will be readily appreciated, and they can be flattened out as the esophagus is distended to more clearly view the entire circumference of the esophagus. Swallowing may create artifacts such as the appearance of strictures, so the esophagus should be carefully reinflated after each swallow to carefully evaluate such findings.[45]

ESOPHAGEAL OBSTRUCTION

Esophageal obstruction, either primary (simple choke) or secondary to other disease processes, is the most common esophageal disorder seen in horses. Although primary obstructions may be caused by foreign bodies, including corncobs, potatoes, apples, carrots, medicinal boluses, stones, riding crops, or wood fragments, primary obstructions are most often caused by roughage, particularly leafy alfalfa hay, coarse grass hay, bedding, and even grass.[46-56] Prior esophageal trauma or poor mastication caused by dental abnormalities may predispose horses to esophageal impaction.[53] Obstructions from roughage may be precipitated by wolfing or gulping food, particularly if the horse is exhausted or mildly dehydrated, such as after a long ride, or weakened from chronic debilitation. Secondary impactions are caused by intramural or extramural abnormalities that mechanically impede food passage. Examples of intramural obstructions include tumors (squamous cell carcinomas), strictures, diverticula, cysts, and vascular ring anomalies.[52,53,57-63] Mediastinal or cervical masses (tumors or abscesses) may cause extramural obstructions.

The clinical signs associated with esophageal obstructions are similar whether they are classified as primary or secondary and are rarely specific. Horses with esophageal obstruction are often anxious and stand with their neck extended. Gagging or retching may be noted, particularly with acute proximal obstructions. Bilateral frothy nasal discharge containing saliva and food material, coughing, odynophagia, ptyalism, and dysphagia are usually the primary clinical signs, the severity of which varies with the degree and location of the obstruction. Distention of the cervical esophagus may be evident at the site of obstruction. Other clinical signs may be observed related to complications stemming from the obstruction, such as dehydration, weight loss, aspiration pneumonia, or esophageal rupture.

Thorough physical examination, including a complete oral examination, must be performed to rule out other causes of hypersalivation, dysphagia, and nasal discharge. Palpation of the jugular furrow may reveal a mass associated with the impaction. In most horses, the esophagus is located in the left jugular furrow, but may be found in the right furrow in some animals. Crepitus or cellulitis may be evident, suggesting rupture of the esophagus. Auscultation of the lungs is important to determine whether pneumonia or pleural fluid is present as a result of aspiration or intrathoracic esophageal rupture. Passage of a nasogastric tube is a good way to determine whether and where an obstruction is present, but provides little information about the nature of the obstruction or the condition of the esophagus.

Ultrasonography of the cervical region is extremely useful to not only confirm the presence of a cervical esophageal impaction, but also to provide critical information about the location and extent of the impaction and esophageal wall thickness and integrity. Ultrasonography may also provide information about the etiology of the obstruction. Radiography, particularly air or barium contrast studies, may be useful to assess an esophageal impaction, but may be more useful for evaluating the esophagus following rather than before relief of the impaction to demonstrate stricture, dilation, diverticula, esophageal rupture, or masses.[44,64,65] Care should be taken when interpreting radiographic studies in sedated horses, particularly after passage of a nasogastric tube or other esophageal manipulations that may contribute to esophageal dilation.[66] Impacted food material can be detected in the esophagus by a typical granular pattern and gas is often observed to accumulate proximal to the obstruction. Foreign bodies may be identified by contrast radiographic studies.

Definitive evaluation of esophageal obstructions often requires endoscopic examination. Most cases of esophageal obstruction occur at sites of natural narrowing of the esophageal lumen, such as the cervical esophagus, thoracic inlet, base of the heart, or terminal esophagus. Therefore an endoscope longer than 1 meter may be required for complete evaluation. Endoscopic evaluation is useful before relief of an impaction to localize the impaction and to investigate the nature of the impaction if a foreign body is suspected. Foreign bodies may be retrievable via transendoscopic tethering.[54] Critical diagnostic and prognostic information is obtained following resolution of the impaction to determine whether mucosal ulceration, esophageal rupture, masses, or strictures are present.

The primary goal of treatment for esophageal impaction is to relieve the obstruction. Parenteral administration of acepromazine (0.05 mg/kg IV), xylazine (0.25 to 0.5 mg/kg IV) or detomidine (0.01 to 0.02 mg/kg IV), oxytocin (0.11 to 0.22 IU/kg IM) and/or esophageal instillation of lidocaine (30 to 60 ml of 1% lidocaine) may help reduce esophageal spasms due to pain or increased esophageal tone.[51,66-68] Some clinicians advocate parasympatholytic drugs such as atropine (0.02 mg/kg IV) to reduce salivary secretions and lessen the risk of aspiration, but such agents may excessively dry the impaction and inhibit distal gastrointestinal motility.

Resolution of an impaction may require physical dispersal of the material.[51] A nasogastric tube can be used to displace the impacted material in conjunction with external massage if the obstruction is in the cervical region. Often it is necessary to carefully lavage the esophagus with water via an uncuffed or a cuffed nasogastric tube while the head is lowered to aid in breaking up the impaction. Some clinicians advocate a dual tube method whereby a tube is placed through each nasal passage into the esophagus for ingress and egress of the lavage fluid. Because of the risk of aspiration of water and/or food material, esophageal lavage is sometimes done under general anesthesia with a cuffed nasotracheal tube.

In refractory cases, intravenous administration of isotonic fluid containing 0.9% NaCl and KCl (10 to 20 mEq/L) for 24 hr at a rate of 50 to 100 ml/kg/day in conjunction with

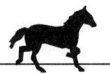

esophageal relaxants such as oxytocin may promote hydration and softening of the impaction and will help prevent or alleviate any electrolyte or acid-base imbalances resulting from salivary losses of chloride, sodium, and potassium.[43] It is important to note that the effects of oxytocin on esophageal tone occur in the proximal two thirds of the esophagus and may not be effective for distal obstructions.[67,68] Refractory cases may require esophagotomy to relieve the impaction. Strict restriction of access to food and water, including access to bedding material, must be enforced until the obstruction is resolved and the esophagus has regained function.

Dilation proximal to the site of obstruction, mucosal injury from trauma, and esophagitis are sequelae to esophageal impaction that predispose patients to reobstruction.[44,53] The rate of reobstruction may be as high as 37%.[53] Depending on the duration of the obstruction and the degree of trauma or dilation, the risk of reobstruction is high for 24 to 48 hours or longer; thus food should be withheld for at least 24 to 48 hours after resolution of the obstruction. After 48 to 72 hours or when the esophageal mucosa has recovered as assessed by endoscopy, soft food (moistened pellets and bran mashes) can be fed. The patient can be gradually returned to a high-quality roughage diet over a period of 7 to 21 days depending on the degree of esophageal damage induced by the impaction and the nature of any underlying disease. The prognosis for survival is good (78%), but some horses may require permanent dietary modification if persistent chronic obstruction is a problem.[53]

Complications of esophageal impaction include metabolic alkalosis from prolonged loss of salivary chloride and sodium,[43] esophageal ulceration, stricture, perforation, aspiration pneumonia, and megaesophagus.[46-53] Esophageal endoscopy or ultrasonography should be performed immediately after the impaction is relieved to determine whether any complications of the impaction have developed or if an inciting cause of the obstruction is present. Endoscopic evaluation is critical to determine the postobstruction treatment and follow-up. Reevaluation should be performed intermittently every 2 to 4 weeks following resolution of the impaction if esophageal dilation or mucosal injury is noted. Additional evaluation via radiography may be warranted to assess motility and transit times.

If the obstruction was present for 48 hours or longer, dehydration, hyponatremia, hypochloremia, and hypokalemia may occur and should be corrected via oral electrolyte solutions or intravenous administration of 0.9% NaCl and KCl (10 to 20 mEq/L). If aspiration is suspected, administration of broad-spectrum antibiotics that are effective against gram-positive and gram-negative organisms, including metronidazole for anaerobes, is advisable. Sucralfate (20 mg/kg PO every 6 hours) may hasten healing if esophageal ulceration is evident, but this is controversial. Some clinicians suggest that administration of a nonsteroidal antiinflammatory drug such as flunixin meglumine (1 mg/kg PO or IV every 12 hours) or phenylbutazone (1.1 mg/kg PO or IV every 12 hours) for 2 to 4 weeks after resolution of the impaction may reduce the development of strictures.

ESOPHAGITIS

Inflammation occurs during many conditions of the esophagus. Esophagitis refers to a clinical syndrome of esophageal inflammation, which may or may not be ulcerative.[47] Causes of esophagitis in horses include trauma (e.g., foreign bodies, nasogastric tube), infection (e.g., mural abscesses), or chemical injury (e.g., medicines, cantharidin).[46,49,52,69,70] An important category of esophagitis is reflux esophagitis, caused by reflux or delayed clearing of gastric contents into the distal esophagus and subsequent chemical injury to the mucosa (Fig. 30-16).[47] Similar to ulceration of the squamous portion of the stomach in horses, a major cause of ulcerative esophagitis is epithelial damage resulting from exposure to acid, which is synergistically exacerbated by bile salts.[47,71] The major protective mechanisms of the esophageal mucosa include salivary and food material buffers, normal peristaltic motility, and the barrier formed by the gastroesophageal sphincter. Thus esophagitis may be seen in conjunction with gastric ulcer disease, motility disorders, increased gastric volume from gastric outflow obstructions, gastric paresis, intestinal ileus, or impaired lower esophageal sphincter function.[47]

The clinical signs of esophagitis are nonspecific and similar to esophageal obstruction and gastric ulcer disease. In fact, esophagitis may occur concurrently with esophageal obstruction or gastric ulcer disease, so that clinical signs may

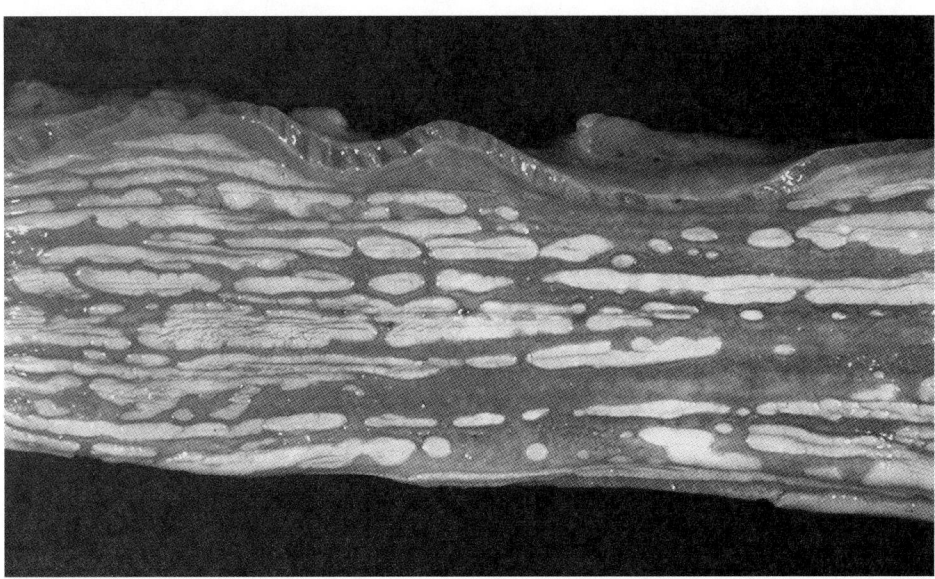

FIG. 30-16 ■ Severe ulceration of the esophagus from a weanling foal that had severe duodenitis and gastric outflow obstruction. (Courtesy Dr. MJ Murray.)

overlap extensively with these diseases. Gagging or discomfort when swallowing may be evident, and hypersalivation and bruxism are signs of esophageal pain. Partial or complete anorexia may be noted such that horses with chronic esophagitis may have significant weight loss. Motility dysfunction secondary to esophagitis may cause recurrent esophageal impaction. Clinical signs of underlying disease that predispose to esophagitis may predominate or mask the signs of esophagitis. Horses with gastrointestinal motility disorders such as anterior enteritis are at high risk of developing reflux esophagitis because of the presence of both gastric acid and bile salts in the fluid reflux. However, signs attributable to esophagitis secondary to ileus may not be noted because of the profound signs caused by the intestinal disorder. Foals with gastric outflow obstructions commonly have reflux esophagitis.

Diagnosis requires endoscopic examination of the esophagus. Diffuse, patchy, linear, or coalescing erosion or ulcerations may be noted. Significant edema or hyperemia may also be observed. It is important to determine whether underlying disease, such as infection, neoplasia, diverticula, or esophageal stricture is present. In addition, the stomach must be examined because reflux esophagitis is commonly accompanied by gastritis or gastric ulcer disease. Contrast radiography may be helpful if endoscopy is not available to detect esophageal ulceration and can be used to assess esophageal motility and transit time.[44]

The principles of therapy for reflux esophagitis include control of gastric acidity and correction of any underlying disorder that is contributing to gastroesophageal reflux. Thus treatment with H_2 histamine receptor antagonists such as ranitidine or proton pump antagonists such as omeprazole* is important for resolution of the disease. Some clinicians advocate sucralfate administration to aid healing of esophageal ulcers. However, the efficiency of sucralfate binding to ulcerated mucosa in the squamous epithelium of the gastrointestinal tract has recently been brought into question.

Foals with reflux esophagitis secondary to delayed gastric

outflow caused by gastroduodenal ulcer disease or gastric paresis may benefit from prokinetic drugs that act on the proximal gastrointestinal tract. Metoclopramide (0.02 to 0.1 mg/kg SQ every 4 to 12 hours) reduces gastroesophageal reflux by increasing lower esophageal sphincter tone, gastric emptying, and gastroduodenal coordination. Caution should be exercised when giving metoclopramide to horses because they are prone to extrapyramidal neurologic side effects. Cholinergic drugs such as bethanecol* (0.025 to 0.035 mg/kg SQ every 4 to 24 hours or 0.035 to 0.045 mg/kg PO every 6 to 8 hours) may improve gastric emptying and are effective for treating reflux esophagitis. For esophagitis from trauma or pressure injury after esophageal impaction, judicious use of nonsteroidal antiinflammatory drugs may be warranted to reduce esophageal inflammation and pain.

Dietary modification may be necessary in patients with esophagitis, depending on the degree of ulceration or if motility is impaired. Horses with less severe esophagitis should be fed frequent small meals of moistened pellets and fresh grass. Severe esophagitis may necessitate withholding food and complete esophageal rest for several days. Although prognosis for esophagitis is good in the absence of underlying disease, the risk of stricture formation is high if severe circumferential or coalescing ulcerations are present. Esophagitis from severe trauma or infection may also be prone to stricture formation.

MOTILITY DISORDERS OF THE ESOPHAGUS

Esophageal hypomotility is the most common motility dysfunction of the equine esophagus, and results in esophageal dilation or megaesophagus. Although megaesophagus in horses is most commonly acquired, there are reports of idiopathic megaesophagus in young horses that is likely congenital.[72-75] Acquired megaesophagus in foals is usually secondary to gastric outlet or duodenal obstruction (Fig. 30-17, Color Plate 1), and in adult horses acquired megaesophagus is usually caused by either primary or secondary esophageal ob-

*Gastrogard, Merial Ltd., Iselin, NJ.

*Urecholine, Merck and Co., Inc., West Point, Pa.

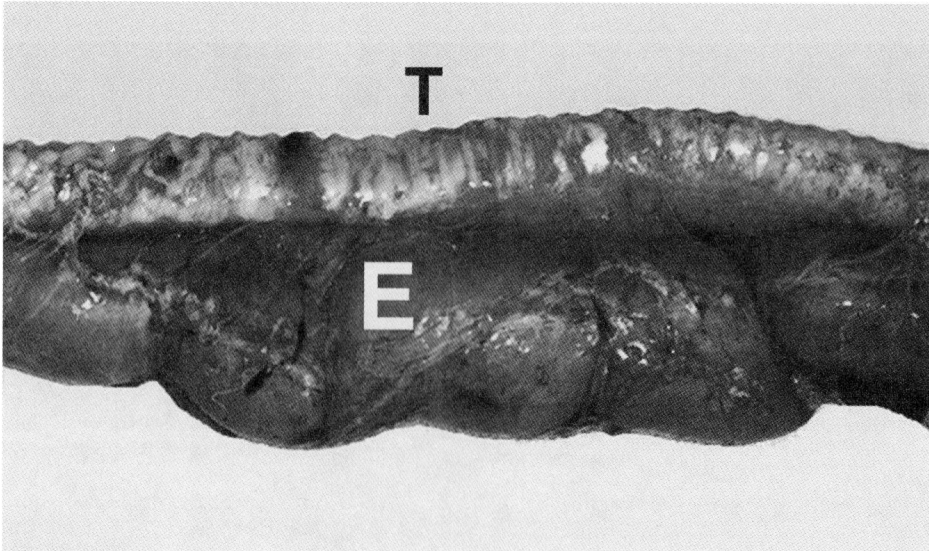

FIG. 30-17 ▦ Megaesophagus in a 10-month-old Paint Horse foal that had two duodenal strictures that appeared to have been present for several months. The trachea *(T)* lies dorsal to the dilated esophagus *(E)*. (Courtesy Dr. MJ Murray.)

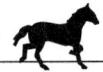

struction.[44,52,53] Esophageal impactions of relatively short duration cause proximal dilation of the esophagus that is generally reversible.[44] However, if the duration of the obstruction is long, the motility of the esophagus may be permanently impaired. Other causes of acquired megaesophagus include extraesophageal obstruction by tumors or abscesses, pleuropneumonia, and vascular ring anomalies.[53,60] In addition, acquired megaesophagus may result from neurologic, neuromuscular, or muscular disorders. Neurologic diseases that cause vagal neuropathy, such as equine protozoal myeloencephalitis, equine herpesvirus myeloencephalitis, and idiopathic vagal neuropathy, have been associated with megaesophagus in horses. Pleuropneumonia may be associated with vagal neuropathy, resulting in megaesophagus. Megaesophagus is also an early sign of equine dysautonomia[76] and may be noted in patients with botulism. Myasthenia gravis is a well-known cause of megaesophagus in other species, but has not been reported in horses. Also in other species, electrolyte disorders, cachexia, primary myopathies, myositis, and Addison's disease may affect esophageal motility, but have not been associated with megaesophagus in horses.

Esophageal inflammation, particularly reflux esophagitis, may affect motility and cause megaesophagus. However, because esophageal hypomotility may predispose to reflux esophagitis, it may be difficult to determine whether the esophagitis or the megaesophagus is the causative disorder. Iatrogenic megaesophagus can be induced by the α_2-adrenergic agonist detomidine, but this is transient and reversible.[66,77] However, the use of this drug may complicate clinical evaluation of esophageal motility. Because esophageal hypomotility is a functional obstruction, the clinical signs of esophageal hypomotility or megaesophagus are similar to esophageal obstruction. Thus the clinical signs include ptyalism, dysphagia, and nasal discharge of saliva and food material.[52,60,72-75] The cervical esophagus may be sufficiently dilated to be evident externally. Weight loss is a common sign, and clinical signs attributable to an underlying disease may be evident.

Diagnosis of esophageal hypomotility requires transit studies. Transit time of a bolus from the cervical esophagus to the stomach can be measured by fluoroscopy or contrast radiography.[44,76] Other signs of esophageal hypomotility and megaesophagus include pooling of contrast material and an absence of peristaltic constrictions.[44,52,72,76] Endoscopy may reveal a dilated esophagus and an absence of peristaltic waves.[52,72] Evidence of underlying disease causing obstruction or esophageal dilation may be observed.[52,53] The esophagus should be evaluated for evidence of esophagitis that is either causing esophageal motility dysfunction or is a result of impaired esophageal clearance of gastric fluid. Esophageal manometry may be useful to document abnormal postdeglutition contraction pressures, contraction time, and propagation times.[41,72] Other diagnostic tests such as a complete blood count and chemistry to help identify an underlying cause should be performed. A careful neurologic evaluation should be performed. Signs of neurologic disease and abnormal cerebrospinal fluid analysis suggest an underlying neurologic disorder. Myopathy may be detected by electromyography.

Treatment of esophageal hypomotility or megaesophagus should be aimed at treating the underlying cause. Dietary modification should be aimed at improving esophageal transit of food. Slurries of pellets should be fed. In addition, it may be beneficial to feed from an elevated position to promote transit. In patients with reflux esophagitis associated with megaesophagus, metoclopramide or bethanecol may be beneficial to increase lower esophageal tone and gastric emptying and reduce gastroesophageal reflux. The prognosis depends on the underlying cause and the degree of dilation. Al-

though many cases of megaesophagus associated with reflux esophagitis respond well to treatment, many other forms of megaesophagus, including congenital megaesophagus, have a poor prognosis.

CONGENITAL DISORDERS

Congenital disorders of the esophagus are rare. Reported congenital abnormalities include congenital stenosis,[78] persistent right aortic arch, congenital strictures,[42] esophageal duplication cysts,[61,63,79,80] and idiopathic megaesophagus.[81] In the one report on congenital stenosis, double-contrast radiography revealed concentric narrowing of the thoracic esophagus in the absence of any vascular abnormalities at the base of the heart. Successful treatment included having the foal stand with the forelimbs elevated off the ground after each feeding.[78]

Persistent right aortic arch is a congenital anomaly in which the right fourth aortic arch becomes the definitive aorta instead of the left aortic arch, which results in constriction of the esophagus by the ligamentum arteriosum as it extends between the anomalous right aorta and the left pulmonary artery.[60] Clinical signs may include dysphagia, drooling of saliva, and distention of the cervical esophagus as a result of partial obstruction of the thoracic esophagus.[60,82] Endoscopic examination typically reveals dilation of the esophagus cranial to the obstruction with evidence of diffuse esophagitis.[82] In addition, evaluation of the thorax usually reveals the presence of aspiration pneumonia. Successful surgical treatment of persistent right aortic arch has been reported in one foal.[82]

Esophageal duplication cysts cause typical signs of esophageal obstruction, including salivation, dysphagia, and swelling of the cervical esophagus as they enlarge.[80] Such signs can make them difficult to differentiate from simple obstruction (choke). However, an aspirate of the mass may aid in the diagnosis by revealing the presence of keratinized squamous cells.[63,83] Cysts may communicate with the lumen of the esophagus.[80] Surgical treatments have included complete surgical resection, and surgical marsupialization.[63,80,83] The latter appears to be more successful and result in fewer complications.[80,83] Complications of surgical resection have included laryngeal hemiplegia secondary to surgical trauma to the recurrent laryngeal nerve in the region of the esophagus, and esophageal fistula formation.[83]

ESOPHAGEAL PERFORATION

Perforation typically occurs in the cervical region in response to external trauma or rupture of an esophageal lesion such as an impacted diverticulum. The esophagus is particularly vulnerable to external trauma in the distal third of the neck because it is only covered by a thin layer of muscle at this point.[84] Iatrogenic perforation may occur in response to excessive force with a stomach tube against an obstruction or a compromised region of the esophagus.[71] Esophageal perforations may be open or closed. They tend to cause extensive necrosis of tissues surrounding the wound because of drainage of saliva and feed material within fascial planes (Fig. 30-18). This may lead to extensive cellulitis and to endotoxemia. Closed perforations of the esophagus are particularly troublesome because wound discharge may migrate all the way to the mediastinum and pleural space via fascial planes.[69,84] In some cases periesophageal abscesses form (Fig. 30-19). In addition, extensive subcutaneous and fascial emphysema can develop, which is usually evident on cervical radiographs.

Treatment should include converting closed perforations to open perforations if possible,[85] extensive debridement and

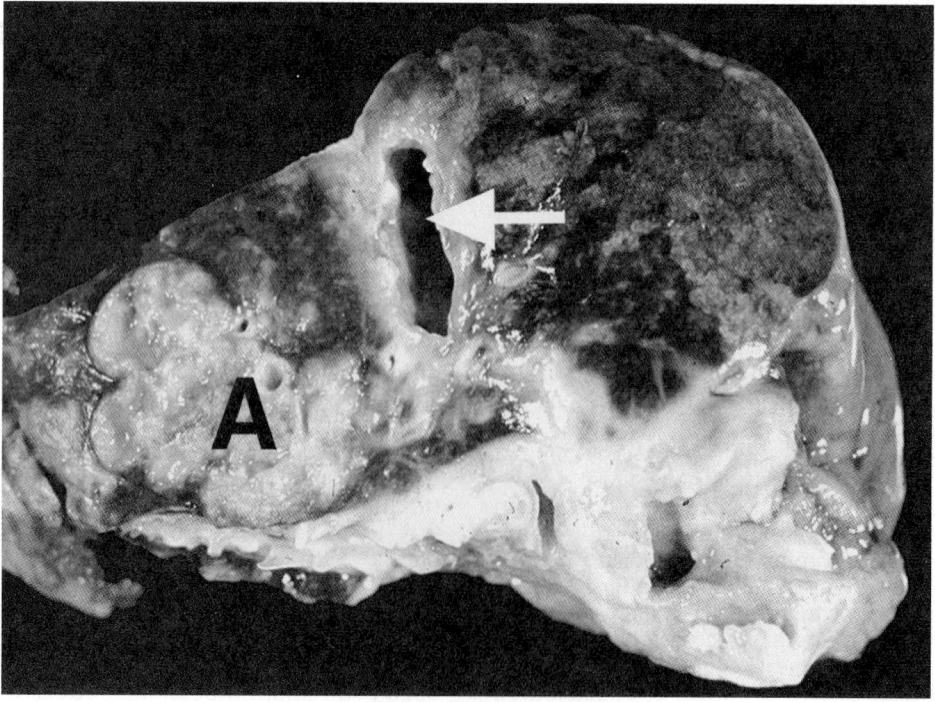

FIG. 30-18 ■ Esophageal perforation in a horse. **A,** An open esophageal laceration was detected on presentation in the mid-cervical region. The wound was treated by lavage and debridement, and the horse was fed via a tube inserted into the esophagus through the wound. **B,** Approximately 14 days later, dissection of esophageal contents within surrounding fascial planes has resulted in extensive sloughing of tissue.

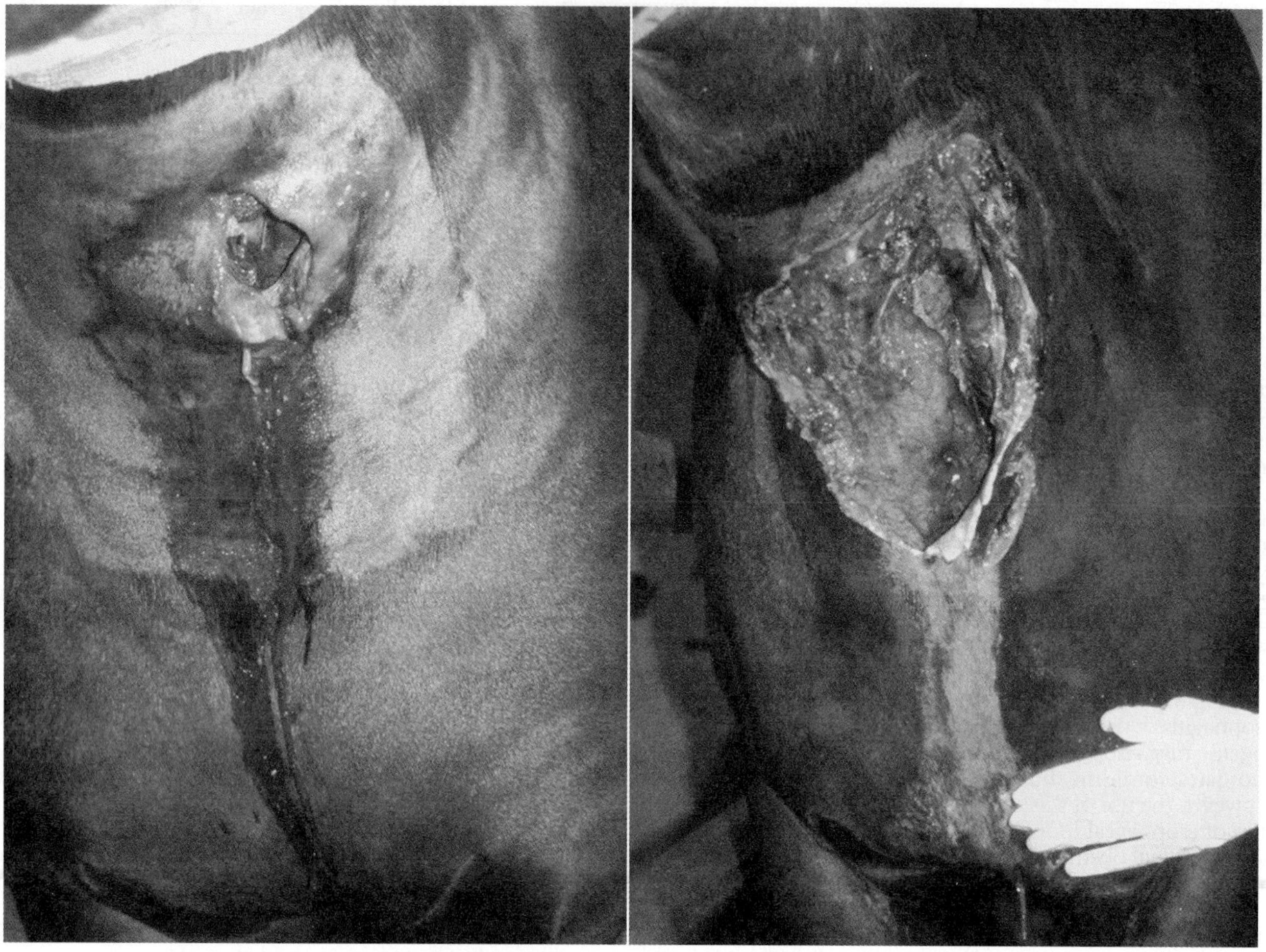

FIG. 30-19 ■ Periesophageal abscess *(A)* and cellulitis that developed secondary to an esophageal obstruction. The esophageal lumen is indicated by the *white arrow.* (Courtesy Dr. MJ Murray.)

lavage of affected tissues, broad-spectrum antibiotics, tetanus prophylaxis, and esophageal rest. The latter may be achieved by placing a feeding tube into the esophagus via the wound. Alternatively, a nasogastric tube should be placed using a small tube (12-Fr diameter).[69] For open perforations, once the wound has granulated and contracted to a small size, oral feeding may be attempted.[84] Extensive loss of saliva via esophageal wounds may lead to hyponatremia and hypochloremia. In addition, transient metabolic acidosis occurs because of salivary bicarbonate loss, followed by progressive metabolic alkalosis.[43] Although there are reports of esophageal wounds healing well by second intention, it takes a prolonged period.[86] In addition, some perforations never completely heal and form permanent esophagocutaneous fistulas that may require surgical correction. The development of esophageal strictures is not common because wounds are usually linear and not circumferential. However, traction diverticula may develop. Other complications of esophageal wounds include Horner's syndrome and left laryngeal hemiplegia.[84]

In a retrospective study on esophageal disorders, only 2 of 11 horses with esophageal perforations survived long term,[53] whereas in a report on esophageal trauma secondary to nasogastric intubation, 4 of 5 horses were euthanized.[69] The prognosis is therefore poor in horses with esophageal perforations, largely because of the extent of cellulitis, tissue necrosis, shock, and local wound complications.

ESOPHAGEAL STRICTURE

Strictures most commonly occur as sequelae to esophageal obstructions that result in circumferential erosion or ulceration of the esophageal mucosa (Color Plates 2 and 3), although strictures may result from oral administration of corrosive medicinal agents and trauma to the neck.[87] Congenital strictures have also been reported.[42] Strictures that result from mucosal and submucosal trauma are termed esophageal webs or rings. Strictures may also originate in the muscular layers and adventitia of the esophagus (mural strictures) or in all of the layers of the esophagus (annular stenosis).[42,88] Horses with these lesions have a similar presentation to those with simple obstructions, because strictures result in partial obstruction and accumulation of feed material in the lumen. Esophageal webs or rings can be observed endoscopically, whereas mural strictures or annular stenosis may require double-contrast esophagrams to confirm their presence.

In one study on esophageal stricture following simple obstruction, maximal reduction in esophageal lumen occurred within 30 days of esophageal obstruction.[87] Surgery has been employed to reduce such strictures; however, initial medical management is warranted because strictures may resolve with conservative therapy and the esophagus continues to remodel for up to 60 days after ulceration. In one report, 7 horses with esophageal obstruction-induced stricture were treated conservatively by feeding a slurry diet and administering antiinflammatory and antimicrobial medications, and 5 of 7 were clinically normal within 60 days.[87] One of the 5 successfully treated horses had a 10-cm area of circumferential ulceration, suggesting that horses with extensive mucosal injury may resolve without permanent stricture formation. If there is insufficient resolution of strictures within 60 days, other methods to increase esophageal diameter should be investigated. Bougienage has been used successfully in small animal patients and humans. The technique involves passage of a tubular dilatable instrument down the esophagus and stretching of the stricture (Fig. 30-20). Some authors have suggested that this may be accomplished by passing a nasogastric tube with an inflatable cuff.[89] However, to be successful the procedure must be performed frequently, and it is not

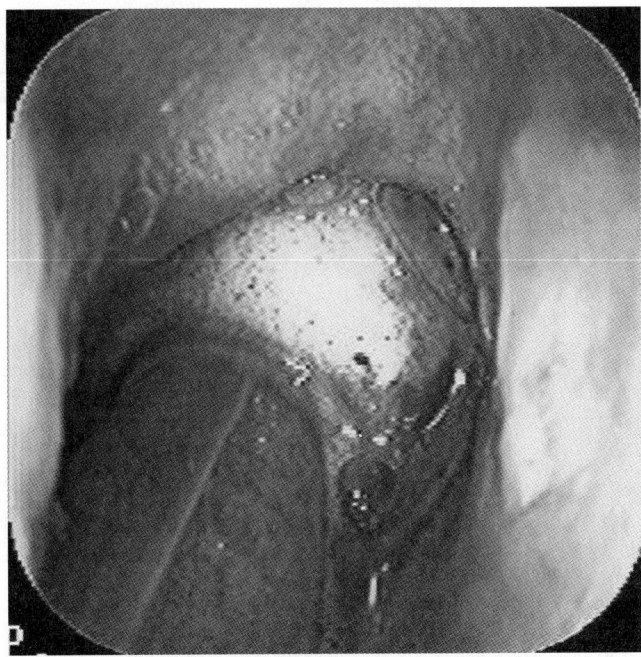

FIG. 30-20 ▇ Attempted dilation of esophageal stricture using bouginage. In this case, a cuffed Silastic tube was passed to the site of stricture aided by endoscopy, and the cuff was then inflated to distend the site of stricture. (Courtesy Dr. MJ Murray.)

well tolerated in the horse.[42] Alternatively, several surgical techniques have been used to resolve strictures, including resection and anastomosis,[90,91] temporary esophagostomy with fenestration of the stricture,[88] esophagomyotomy for strictures of the muscularis and adventitia[90,92] or patch grafting with local musculature.[94] However, such surgeries are fraught with complications, largely because of the propensity of the traumatized esophagus to re-stricture.[53,87] The esophagus lacks a serosal layer and does not rapidly form a fibrin seal as does the remainder of the intestinal tract, so anastomoses tend to leak.[90] In addition, tension on the esophagus during swallowing and movement of the neck impairs healing of anastomoses.[88,91]

ESOPHAGEAL DIVERTICULA

There are two types of diverticula: traction (true) diverticula and pulsion (false) diverticula. Traction diverticula result from wounding and subsequent contraction of periesophageal tissues, with resultant tenting of the wall of the esophagus. Pulsion diverticula arise from protrusion of esophageal mucosa through defects in the muscular wall of the esophagus, and usually result from trauma or acute changes in intraluminal pressure (Fig. 30-21).[42] Traction diverticula appear as a dilation with a broad neck on contrast esophagography, whereas pulsion diverticula typically have a flask shape with a small neck on an esophagram.[62,95] Whereas traction diverticula are usually asymptomatic and of little clinical significance, pulsion diverticula may fill with feed material, ultimately leading to esophageal obstruction.[50,95,96] However, a movable mass in the midcervical region may be noticed before onset of complete obstruction.[42] Pulsion diverticula may be surgically corrected by inverting or resecting prolapsed mucosa and closing the defect in the wall of the esophagus.[62,95,96] Inversion of excessive mucosa may predispose horses to esophageal obstruction and should therefore be reserved for small diverticula.[62]

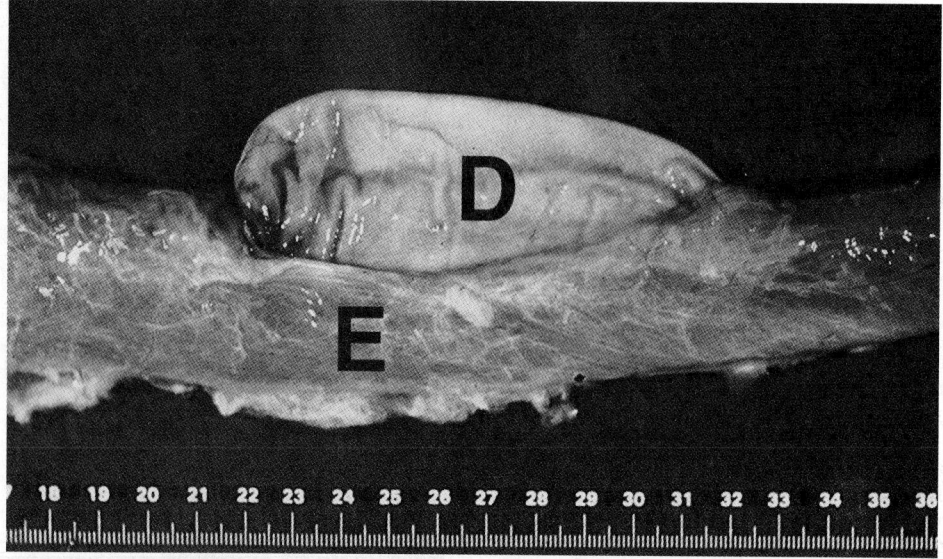

FIG. 30-21 ▓ Pulsion diverticulum *(D)* of the esophagus *(E)* from a horse that had intermittent episodes of esophageal obstruction. (Courtesy Dr. MJ Murray.)

NEOPLASIA

Neoplasia of the esophagus is rare, but squamous cell carcinoma[58,97,98] and leiomyosarcoma[99] have reportedly affected the esophagus either as the primary site[58,97,98] or in association with a lesion in the squamous portion of the stomach.[99] The predominant clinical signs are weight loss, colic, and recurrent esophageal obstruction. The tumor is typically detected antemortem on esophagoscopy and radiography,[97,98] but a definitive diagnosis may require a biopsy during laparotomy.[57,99] When neoplasia affects the lower esophageal sphincter, gastroesophageal reflux may contribute to ulceration of esophageal mucosa. The prognosis for malignant neoplasia of the esophagus is grave.

REFERENCE

38. Schummer A, Nickel R, Sack WO: The alimentary canal. In: *The viscera of the domestic mammals,* New York, 1979, Springer-Verlag, pp 99-202.
39. Sisson S: Equine digestive system. In Getty R, ed: *Sisson and Grossman's anatomy of the domestic animals,* Philadelphia, 1999, WB Saunders, pp 454-475.
40. Stick JA et al: Equine esophageal pressure profile, *Am J Vet Res* 44:272-275, 1983.
41. Clark ES, Morris DD, Whitlock RH: Esophageal manometry in horses, cows, and sheep during deglutition, *Am J Vet Res* 48:547-551, 1987.
42. Fubini SL, Starrack GS, Freeman DE: Esophagus. In Auer JA, Stick JA, eds: *Equine surgery,* Philadelphia, 1999, WB Saunders, pp 199-209.
43. Stick JA, Robinson NE, Krehbiel JD: Acid-base and electrolyte alterations associated with salivary loss in the pony, *Am J Vet Res* 42:733-737, 1981.
44. Greet TR: Observations on the potential role of oesophageal radiography in the horse, *Equine Vet J* 14:73-79, 1982.
45. Stick JA: Surgery of the esophagus, *Vet Clin North Am (Large Anim Pract)* 4:33-59, 1982.
46. Meagher DM, Spier SJ: Foreign body obstruction in the cervical esophagus of the horse: A case report, *J Equine Vet Sci* 9:137-140, 1989.
47. Grubb TL, von Mathiessen W, Scott EA: A stone in the esophagus of a horse: surgical removal without esophagomyotomy, *Equine Pract* 15-18, 1991.
48. Lundvall RL, Kingrey BW: Choke in shetland ponies caused by boluses, *J Am Vet Med Assoc* 132:75-76, 1958.
49. Appt SA et al: Esophageal foreign body obstruction in a mustang, *Equine Pract* 18:8-11, 1996.
50. MacDonald MH, Richardson DW, Morse CC: Esophageal phytobezoar in a horse, *J Am Vet Med Assoc* 191:1455-1456, 1987.
51. Hillyer M: Management of oesophageal obstruction (choke) in horses, *In Pract* 17:450-457, 1995.
52. Murray MJ, Ball MM, Parker GA: Megaesophagus and aspiration pneumonia secondary to gastric ulcation in a foal, *J Am Vet Med Assoc* 192:381-383, 1988.
53. Craig DR et al: Esophageal disorders in 61 horses. Results of nonsurgical and surgical management, *Vet Surg* 18:432-438, 1989.
54. Traver DS, Egger E, Moore JN: Retrieval of an esophageal foreign body in a horse, *Vet Med Small Anim Clin* 73:783-785, 1978.
55. Baird AN, True CK: Fragments of nasogastric tubes as esophageal foreign bodies in two horses, *J Am Vet Med Assoc* 194:1068-1070, 1989.
56. Harris JM: Esophageal obstruction by a wood bolus, *Mod Vet Pract* 62:302-304, 1981.
57. Moore JN, Kintner LD: Recurrent esophageal obstruction due to squamous cell carcinoma in a horse, *Cornell Vet* 66:590-597, 1976.
58. Roberts MC, Kelly WR: Squamous cell carcinoma of the lower cervical oesophagus in a pony, *Equine Vet J* 11:199-201, 1979.
59. Green S, Green EM, Aronson E: Squamous cell carcinoma: an unusual cause of choke in a horse, *Mod Vet Pract* 67:870-875, 1986.
60. Butt TD et al: Persistent right aortic arch in a yearling horse, *Can Vet J* 39:714-715, 1998.
61. Scott EA et al: Intramural esophageal cyst in a horse, *J Am Vet Med Assoc* 171:652-654, 1977.
62. Hackett RP, Dyer RM, Hoffer RE: Surgical correction of esophageal diverticulum in a horse, *J Am Vet Med Assoc* 173:998-1000, 1978.
63. Orsini JA et al: Esophageal duplication cyst as a cause of choke in the horse, *J Am Vet Med Assoc* 193:474-476, 1988.
64. Alexander JE: Radiologic findings in equine choke, *J Am Vet Med Assoc* 151:47-53, 1967.
65. Quick CB, Randano VT: Equine radiology: the esophagus, *Mod Vet Pract* 59:625-631, 1978.
66. King JN, Davis JV, Gerring EL: Contrast radiography of the equine oesophagus: effect of spasmolytic agents and passage of a nasogastric tube, *Equine Vet J* 22:133-135, 1990.
67. Meyer GA et al: Effect of oxytocin on contractility of the equine esophagus: treatment for esophageal obstruction? *Proceedings of the Forty-third Annual Convention of the American Association of Equine Practitioners,* 1997, p 337.
68. Hance SR et al: Treating choke with oxytocin, *Proceedings of the Forty-third Annual Convention of the American Association of Equine Practitioners,* 1997, pp 338-339.
69. Hardy J et al: Complications of nasogastric intubation in horses: nine cases (1987-1989). *J Am Vet Med Assoc* 201:483-486, 1992.
70. Schoeb TR, Panciera RJ: Pathology of blister beetle (*Epicauta*) poisoning in horses, *Vet Pathol* 16:18-31, 1979.
71. Lang J et al: Synergistic effect of hydrochloric acid and bile acids on the pars eosophageal mucosa of the porcine stomach, *Am J Vet Res* 59:1170-1176, 1998.
72. Clark ES, Morris DD, Whitlock RH: Esophageal dysfunction in a weanling thoroughbred, *Cornell Vet* 77:151-160, 1987.
73. Barber SM, McLaughlin BG, Fretz PB: Esophageal ectasia in a quarterhorse colt, *Can Vet J* 24:46-48, 1983.
74. Rohrbach BW: Congenital esophageal ectasia in a thoroughbred foal, *J Am Vet Med Assoc* 177:65-67, 1980.
75. Bowman KF et al: Megaesophagus in a colt, *J Am Vet Med Assoc* 172:334-337, 1978.
76. Greet TR, Whitwell KE: Barium swallow as an aid to the diagnosis of grass sickness, *Equine Vet J* 18:294-297, 1986.

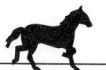

77. Watson TD, Sullivan M: Effects of detomidine on equine oesophageal function as studied by contrast radiology, *Vet Rec* 129:67-69, 1991.
78. Clabough DL, Roberts MC, Robertson I: Probable congenital esophageal stenosis in a thoroughbred foal, *J Am Vet Med Assoc* 199:483-485, 1991.
79. Peek SF, De Lahunta A, Hackett RP: Combined oesophageal and tracheal duplication cyst in an Arabian filly, *Equine Vet J* 27:475-478, 1995.
80. Gaughan EM, Gift LJ, Frank RK: Tubular duplication of the cervical portion of the esophagus in a foal, *J Am Vet Med Assoc* 201:748-750, 1992.
81. Rohrbach BW: Congenital esophageal ectasia in a thoroughbred foal, *J Am Vet Med Assoc* 177:65-67, 1980.
82. Mackey VS et al: Surgical correction of a persistent right aortic arch in a foal, *Vet Surg* 15:325-328, 1986.
83. Sams AE, Weldon AD, Rakestraw P: Surgical treatment of intramural esophageal inclusion cysts in three horses, *Vet Surg* 22:135-139, 1993.
84. Freeman DE: Wounds of the esophagus and trachea, *Vet Clin North Am (Equine Pract)* 5:683-693, 1989.
85. Digby NJ, Burguez PN: Traumatic oesophageal rupture in the horse, *Equine Vet J* 14:169-179, 1982.
86. Lunn DP, Peel JE: Successful treatment of traumatic oesophageal rupture with severe cellulitis in a mare, *Vet Rec* 116:544-545, 1985.
87. Todhunter RJ et al: Medical management of esophageal stricture in seven horses, *J Am Vet Med Assoc* 185:784-787, 1984.
88. Craig D, Todhunter R: Surgical repair of an esophageal stricture in a horse, *Vet Surg* 16:251-254, 1987.
89. Green EM, MacFadden KE: Esophageal disorders of the horse. In Smith BP, ed: *Large animal internal medicine*, St Louis, 1996, Mosby, pp 698-710.
90. Gideon L: Esophageal anastomosis in two foals, *J Am Vet Med Assoc* 184:1146-1148, 1984.
91. Suann CJ: Oesophageal resection and anastomosis as a treatment for oesophageal stricture in the horse, *Equine Vet J* 14:163-164, 1982.
92. Nixon AJ et al: Esophagomyotomy for relief of an intrathoracic esophageal stricture in a horse, *J Am Vet Med Assoc* 183:794-796, 1983.
93. Wagner PC, Rantanen NW: Myotomy as a treatment for esophageal stricture in a horse, *Equine Pract* 2:40-45, 1980.
94. Hoffer RE et al: Esophageal patch grafting as a treatment for esophageal stricture in a horse, *J Am Vet Med Assoc* 171:350-354, 1977.
95. Ford TS et al: Surgical repair of an intrathoracic esophageal pulsion diverticulum in a horse, *Vet Surg* 20:316-319, 1991.
96. Frauenfelder HC, Adams SB: Esophageal diverticulectomy in a horse, *J Am Vet Med Assoc* 180:771-772, 1982.
97. Campbell-Beggs CL et al: Use of esophagoscopy in the diagnosis of esophageal squamous cell carcinoma in a horse, *J Am Vet Med Assoc* 202:617-618, 1993.
98. Ford TS et al: Pleuroscopic diagnosis of gastroesophageal squamous cell carcinoma in a horse, *J Am Vet Med Assoc* 190:1556-1558, 1987.
99. Boy MG et al: Gastric leiomyosarcoma in a horse, *J Am Vet Med Assoc* 200:1363-1364, 1992.

DISORDERS OF THE STOMACH

MICHAEL J. MURRAY

GASTRIC ULCERATION

Just as the term colic describes a clinical presentation and encompasses a large number of disorders, the term equine gastric ulcer syndrome (EGUS) describes a clinical finding, the cause of which is likely to be multifactorial and different from case to case. The umbrella of EGUS includes lesions in the squamous or glandular mucosal linings of the stomach, focal or multifocal ulceration, generalized gastritis, gastric emptying disorders, gastroesophageal reflux disorders, and obstructive disorders. Endoscopic photographs of normal and ulcerated gastric mucosa are presented in Color Plates 4 through 9.

PREVALENCE. Gastric ulceration is a widespread phenomenon, affecting a large number of foals and horses. The overall prevalence of gastric ulceration in foals up to 60 days old has been reported to range from 25% to 50%, and most lesions were observed in the squamous mucosa.[100,101] In the majority of foals with lesions, clinical signs of ulcers were not apparent, and in one study,[102] most lesions observed in foals less than 60 days old healed without treatment.

More than one-half of apparently normal horses had gastric lesions in one endoscopic study,[103] and lesions were more prevalent and severe in horses exhibiting clinical signs

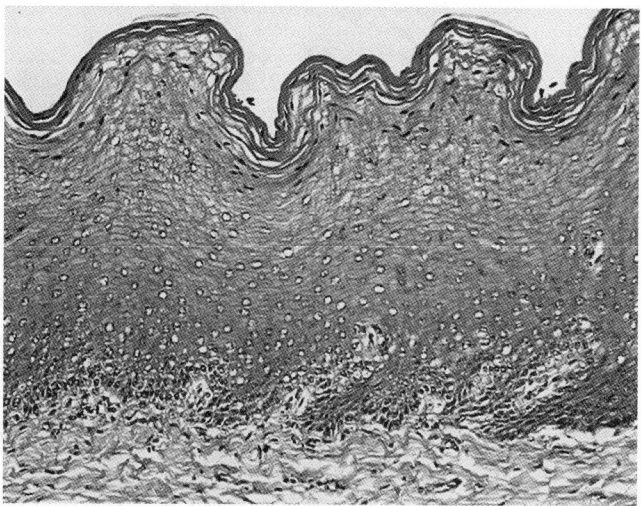

FIG. 30-22 ■ Photomicrograph of equine gastric squamous epithelial mucosa. There are multiple layers of epithelium arranged in parallel with the luminal surface. The most superficial layers of cells are cornified, and superficial to these cells are layers of keratin. (Hematoxylin and eosin stain.)

consistent with gastric ulceration (poor appetite, poor body condition, recurrent abdominal discomfort). Horses in training for racing appear to be at particular risk for developing gastric lesions, 80 to 90% of race horses have had gastric lesions documented endoscopically[103-106] or at necropsy.[107] The majority of gastric lesions in adult horses occurred in the squamous mucosa.

PATHOPHYSIOLOGY. The predominant factor in peptic injury to alimentary mucosa is hydrochloric acid, although the proteolytic enzyme pepsin[108] and bile acids[109] normally refluxed into the stomach may augment hydrochloric acid–induced mucosal injury. The dorsal portion of the equine stomach is lined by a stratified squamous epithelial mucosa, which, like esophageal mucosa, has minimal intrinsic resistance to peptic injury (Fig. 30-22).[110] Studies of esophageal squamous mucosa have revealed that the primary barriers to HCl are intercellular tight junctions and intercellular secretion of bicarbonate ion.[111] These weak barriers to HCl are located in the superficial epithelial layers, and cells deeper in the epithelium actually transport H^+ intracellularly, leading to the death of these cells when exposed to HCl. Studies of porcine gastric squamous mucosa have revealed that short-chain volatile fatty acids (SCFAs) produced in the stomach may increase H^+ permeability,[112] and SCFAs are produced in the equine stomach.[113]

The equine gastric glandular epithelium (Fig. 30-23) is histologically and physiologically similar to the lining of the stomach of other animals and human beings. This tissue is very metabolically active and includes acid-secreting parietal cells, pepsin-secreting chief cells, histamine-secreting enterochromaffin-like cells, gastrin-secreting G cells, and somatostatin-secreting D cells. Histamine and gastrin stimulate acid secretion, whereas somatostatin, as well as prostaglandin E, inhibit acid secretion by parietal cells. This mucosa has developed elaborate mechanisms to protect itself from peptic injury. These include mucus/bicarbonate barrier, prostaglandins, nitric oxide, growth factors, mucosal blood flow, and cellular restitution.[114,115] The mucus/bicarbonate barrier consists of a thin (200 μm) mucus layer that has hydrophobic characteristics and into which bicarbonate ion is secreted.[116] Surface-active phospholipids in the mucus repel aqueous hydrochloric acid, and a pH gradient from the lumen of the stomach to the surface epithelial cells on the order of magni-

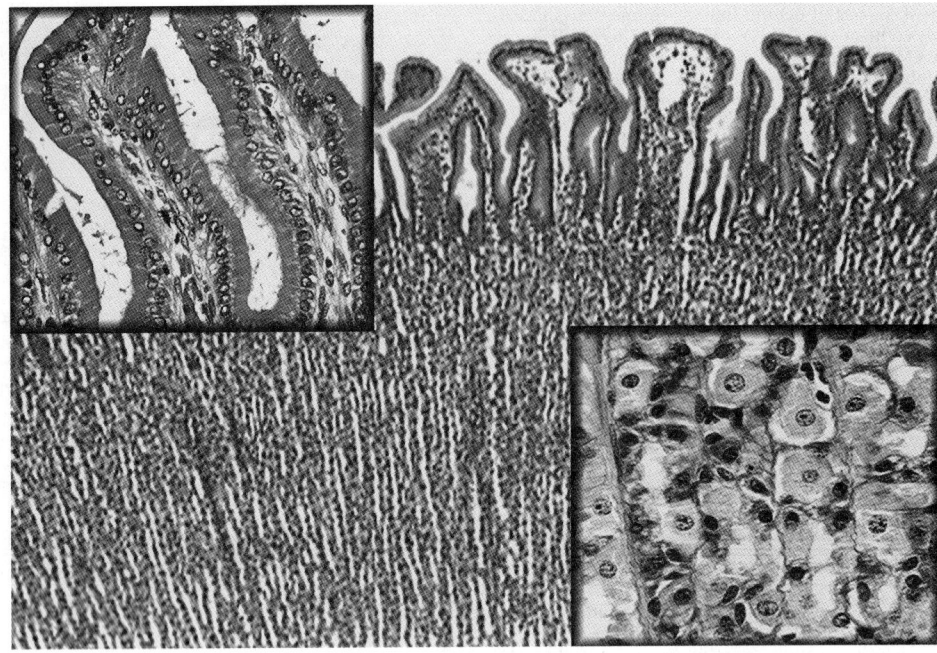

FIG. 30-23 ■ Photomicrograph of equine gastric glandular mucosa. In contrast to the squamous mucosa, the glands are in parallel to each other and perpendicular to the luminal surface. There are multiple cell types within the mucosa, with surface epithelial cells and mucus-secreting cells towards the lumen, and parietal cells, chief cells, enterochromaffin-like cells, G-cells and D-cells deeper in the mucosa. The insert at the top left shows a high-power magnification of cells lining gastric pits on the surface of the epithelium. The insert at the lower right shows a high-power magnification of cells lining the gastric glands deeper in the mucosa. (Hematoxylin and eosin stain.)

tude of 100,000 is created by the bicarbonate that is trapped within the mucus layer. These attributes provide a substantial barrier to back-diffusion of hydrochloric acid.

Mucosal blood flow may be the most important element of [117,118] gastric mucosal protection.[115] Mucosal blood flow is essential in supplying the epithelium with nutrients and oxygen and for disposal of hydrogen ions and noxious agents permeating the mucosa. Nitric oxide (NO) is a key regulator of mucosal blood flow, and inhibition or augmentation of gastric mucosal nitric oxide synthesis has had substantial effects in experimental models. In fact, NO synthesis may be the primary regulator of gastric mucosal blood flow and other mediators related to mucosal blood flow, such as prostaglandins. Prostaglandins E_1 and E_2 have long been recognized as having an important role in gastric mucosal protection, and their primary effects are on mucosal blood flow and gastric mucus.[119]

Although typical, it is not normal for foals and horses to have gastric ulcers. The high prevalence of gastric ulceration, particularly in the squamous mucosa, of young foals may be associated with gastric developmental changes that occur in the first days and weeks of life. At birth the equine gastric squamous epithelium is thin and not highly keratinized.[120] Within days the mucosa becomes hyperplastic and parakeratotic. Desquamation of the squamous epithelium can be observed endoscopically in the first month of life in foals. Histologically, desquamation appears to involve separation of the superficial cornified epithelial layers.

Increasing gastric acidity temporally parallels the proliferation of gastric squamous epithelium, with minimal acidity during the first few days of life, and marked acidity present by 7 to 14 days.[121,122] It is possible that the developing epithelium is less resistant to acid than more mature gastric squamous epithelium, thus predisposing it to peptic injury.

An important, and perhaps the key, factor in whether the gastric squamous mucosa is injured by HCl is the duration of contact of HCl with the mucosa, which is influenced by the eating behavior of the horse or nursing behavior of the foal. Horses and foals secrete HCl continuously,[121,123] and gastric acidity is greatest when foals do not nurse[121] or horses do not eat.[124] Gastric pH can fall to highly acidic levels (<2.0) within minutes of cessation of nursing or eating hay.

Periods of prolonged high gastric acidity (pH <2.0) were created in horses using a protocol of alternating 24-hour periods of feed deprivation with free-choice Timothy hay,[125] which consistently resulted in erosion and ulceration, often severe, in the gastric squamous epithelial mucosa in horses.[124] Erosions, sometimes bleeding, were seen after 48 hours cumulative feed deprivation and ulcers were consistently seen after 96 hours. Concurrent administration of the H_2-receptor antagonist ranitidine during feed deprivation significantly minimized the area of lesions in the gastric squamous epithelial mucosa.

Imposed feed deprivation in the management of cases of colic can result in erosion and ulceration of the gastric squamous mucosa. Similarly, horses that are partly or completely anorectic because of their illness will likely develop erosions or ulcers in their gastric squamous mucosa.

Feeding practices and management of horses can influence gastric acidity and peptic injury to the gastric squamous mucosa. Changing horses from pasture to stall confinement with free choice timothy hay for 7 days resulted in erosion and ulceration of gastric squamous mucosa.[124] Feeding grain and pelleted feed was associated with significantly greater postprandial serum gastrin concentrations compared to feeding only coastal bermuda hay (70 to 80 pg/ml compared with 10 to 20 pg/ml),[126] and whereas gastric acidity was not measured in that study, such high concentrations of serum gastrin should lead to increased HCl secretion in the stomach.

Although eating behavior can affect gastric acidity and the development of gastric squamous epithelial lesions, devel-

Gastric Ulcer Pathophysiology and Healing

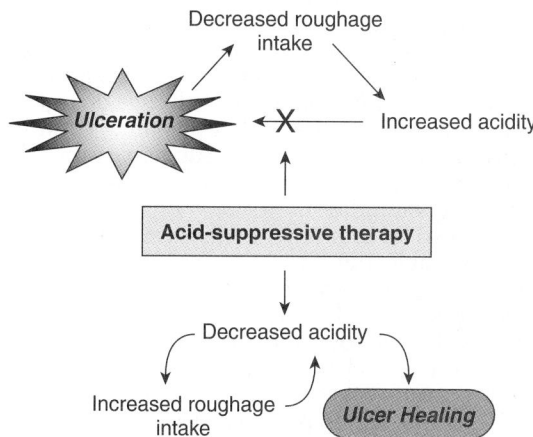

FIG. 30-24 ▓ Diagram representing the pathophysiology of ulceration of the equine gastric squamous mucosal epithelium and the permissive effect acid suppression has on ulcer healing.

opment of lesions can also adversely affect eating behavior. A positive feedback loop can be created in which diminished time consuming roughage may contribute to gastric lesion formation, which in turn can cause discomfort and further reduction in the time the horse spends consuming roughage (Fig. 30-24).

The pathophysiology of lesions in the gastric glandular mucosa of foals and horses is not well understood. Non-steroidal antiinflammatory drugs can induce gastric ulcers, but this is an infrequent cause of ulcers in most horses. Most lesions in the gastric glandular mucosa are observed in the antrum and adjacent to the pylorus. In human beings, *H. pylori* is considered to be the predominant cause of gastric erosions and ulcers,[127] but *Helicobacter* organisms have not been reported to have been identified in equine gastric mucosa.

Illness appears to be a risk factor for foals to develop gastric glandular mucosal lesions, because foals that were sick or had a painful musculoskeletal condition had a greater prevalence of glandular lesions than normal foals.[128] These lesions presumably are associated with stress, and people in intensive care units are known to be at high risk of developing gastric ulcers.[129] The precise mechanism of stress ulceration is not known, but decreased mucosal blood flow is probably an important factor. Stress is frequently cited as the cause of ulcers in horses, by extrapolation from human medicine. But it should be noted that illness is the only stress that has been directly associated with an increased incidence of gastric ulcers in horses[129] or humans.[130] It is possible that other stresses may have an indirect role in the development of ulcers in horses, particularly insofar as it may affect eating behavior.

CLINICAL SYNDROMES. The magnitude of adverse health effects in the majority of foals and horses with gastric lesions remains somewhat speculative, because the disease appears to be occult in most affected animals. In one report, however, the prevalence of gastric ulceration was significantly greater in horses with clinical problems such as colic, poor appetite, and poor bodily condition than in asymptomatic horses.[103]

Foals. The clinical signs that typically are associated with gastric ulcers in foals (e.g., bruxism, dorsal recumbency, salivation, interrupted nursing, diarrhea, and colic) are in fact observed in the minority of foals with endoscopically observed ulcers.[101] Thus, when clinical signs are seen, the clinician

should consider that severe ulceration exists. Diarrhea was the most frequently associated clinical signs in one report.[131] Colic, bruxism, dorsal recumbency, or ptyalism should alert the veterinarian to the probability of severe ulceration. Ptyalism occurs as a result of esophagitis, which often results from gastroesophageal reflux resulting from gastric outlet obstruction or pseudoobstruction. Thus ptyalism in foals often reflects a serious problem in the stomach or duodenum. Weanlings and older foals with chronic gastric ulceration often have intermittent diarrhea and abdominal discomfort, poor growth, rough hair coat, and a pendulous abdomen.

In foals with clinical signs, squamous mucosal lesions often are severe. Most glandular lesions that result in clinical signs are located in the vicinity of the pylorus, although in young foals (<30 days old) with stress ulcers, lesions are often located in the glandular mucosa in the body of the stomach.

Adults. Although most adult horses with gastric lesions do not demonstrate overt clinical signs, low-grade discomfort that results in subtle signs may go unnoticed. Indeed, horses that I have treated solely on the basis of endoscopic findings have frequently demonstrated improved attitude and appetite, yet these were not considered problems as such before treatment began.

In yearlings and horses, gastric lesions have most frequently been associated with colic, poor appetite, and poor bodily condition.[103,132] Other signs associated with ulcers have included attitude changes, stiffness, a tucked-up abdomen, and poor performance.

It should be noted that all the signs attributable to gastric ulcers have also been reported in horses that were referred for gastroscopy but did not have ulcers. Thus, although many signs appear typical for horses with ulcers, none is pathognomonic. Nonetheless, gastric ulcers should be strongly considered in horses with recurrent colic and other vague disorders for which a diagnosis has not been determined.

Hemorrhage (i.e., either active bleeding or darkened, coagulated blood) can occur with deep gastric ulcers in horses. However, bleeding from ulcers in the gastric squamous mucosa does *not* cause anemia or hypoproteinemia in adult horses, and if these abnormalities are present, another cause must be determined.

DIAGNOSIS. Diagnosis of gastric ulceration is based on the presence of age-related characteristic clinical signs, endoscopic findings, and response to treatment. The diagnosis of gastric ulceration in the majority of foals and horses can be definitively determined only by gastroscopic examination. In young foals (<30 days) with an immature colonic flora, the presence of fecal occult blood may be indicative of gastroduodenal ulceration. In older animals, hemoglobin is too extensively degraded by colonic microorganisms for blood originating in the stomach to be detected by fecal occult blood tests.

TREATMENT. Successful treatment (Box 30-3) of gastric ulcers is predicated on addressing the underlying cause and treating with medications that create an environment that is favorable to ulcer healing. Acid-suppressive treatment often is required to break the cycle of inappetence that causes increased gastric acidity, which results in ulceration, which then prolongs and exacerbates the inappetence (see Fig. 30-24).

Decisions concerning whether to treat gastric lesions, what medication to use, and the duration of treatment are best made on the basis of results of a gastroscopic examination. If this is unavailable, some therapeutic guidelines can be used, but the efficacy of the treatment will be determined by clinical signs that are often vague or nonspecific. Usually, clinical conditions such as poor appetite, colic, or diarrhea (foals) that result from gastric ulcers improve in 24 to 48 hours of initiating acid-suppressive therapy. If improvement in clinical signs is not observed, gastric ulceration, if present, should be considered a secondary, not a primary problem.

The primary objective in the treatment of gastric ulcers is to alleviate discomfort, and this is best done by inhibiting or neutralizing acid secretion. Decreasing gastric acidity also creates an environment that is permissive for healing of the gastric mucosal epithelium. Once ulcers form, there are changes in the tissue that promote healing. Suppressing acidity creates an environment within the stomach that permits ulcer healing. Gastric acid secretion can be largely attenuated by use of H_2-receptor antagonists or the proton pump inhibitor omeprazole. Treatment with H_2 antagonists has appeared to be successful in resolving the gastric lesions and in resolving the presenting problem.[132,133] Cimetidine and ranitidine are the most frequently used, and both inhibit gastric acid secretion in the horse.[134-136]

Many dosages of H_2 antagonists have been recommended and used in practice. Before generic forms became available, cimetidine and ranitidine were expensive to use in adult horses and there was pressure to use as little as possible. When deciding on a dose, the clinician must recognize that as the dose of an acid-suppressive agent is lowered, the percentage of patients that will respond poorly or not at all increases.[137] There is tremendous individual variability in the degree and duration of suppression of gastric acidity by H_2 antagonists among horses,[136] presumably as a result of differences in drug absorption. We have found that 6.6 mg ranitidine/kg, given orally every 8 hours provides adequate suppression of acidity in the greatest percentage of horses. This dosage schedule resulted in a median 24-hour gastric pH of 4.6 in horses with free access to hay (compared with a pH of 3.1 in horses fed, but not given ranitidine).[125]

Effective dosages of cimetidine have not been examined as extensively as those of ranitidine, but an effective oral dose may be as high as 50 mg/kg/day. Lower dosages are often given, and sometimes with clinical improvement, but in my experience ulcers have often persisted.

Treatment with cimetidine or ranitidine should continue for at least 21 days to ensure complete healing. The duration of treatment is best determined by the severity of ulcers and the management of the horse. Management changes are as

important as medical treatment, and the two together can lead to complete healing of even severe gastric ulcers within 2 to 3 weeks. When possible, horses should be turned out to graze, grain should be limited, and training should cease.

Other H_2 antagonists, famotidine* and nizatidine† are on the market for use in humans, but effective dosages in the horse have not been established at this time. From limited experience, it would appear that the effect on gastric acidity of oral administration of 3.3 mg/kg famotidine is similar to that with 6.6 mg/kg ranitidine.

Formulations for intravenous administration of H_2 antagonists are available, but are expensive (approximately three times the cost of oral products). Ranitidine should be given intravenously at 1 to 1.5 mg/kg every 8 hours and cimetidine at 6.6 mg/kg three to four times daily.

Omeprazole‡§ is classified as a proton pump inhibitor, which block gastric acid secretion by inhibiting the parietal cell H^+-K^+-ATPase (proton pump) that secretes HCl. Omeprazole is a potent inhibitor of gastric acidity in horses. Because of its potency, once-daily treatment is feasible. Administration of omeprazole granules at a dosage of 1.5 mg/kg, once daily, promoted rapid restoration of normal gastric squamous mucosa in a vehicle-controlled study of Thoroughbred race horses with moderate to severe gastric ulceration.[138] Prilosec is difficult to administer to horses, because it is manufactured in enteric-coated granules, which protect omeprazole from being inactivated in an acidic environment. Daily cost of Prilosec for an adult horse exceeds $100!

A paste formulation of omeprazole was approved in 1999 for use in treating gastric ulcers in foals and horses. In clinical trials, ulcer healing in horses and foals treated once daily with omeprazole was substantially superior to healing in sham-treated horses.[139,140] Of importance, in one set of these trials, ulcer healing occurred in more 77% of omeprazole-treated horses that remained in race training, which has not been noted in horses treated with H_2 antagonists. In fact, we have observed that horses treated with ranitidine at 6.6 mg/kg three times daily for 3 weeks and kept in training did not have endoscopic improvement of gastric lesions. Thus omeprazole brings a new perspective to the treatment of gastric ulcers in horses. Once-daily treatment and a paste formulation should enhance treatment compliance, and the potency of acid suppression permits horses to remain in their activities while being effectively treated for ulcers.

Another important feature of omeprazole paste was the confirmation of its ability to prevent ulcers in horses in race training; the conditions that are most favorable for development of ulcers.[140] The daily dose used for prevention was one-half that used for treatment (2 mg/kg vs. 4 mg/kg, respectively).

The daily cost of omeprazole paste is greater than for cimetidine and ranitidine, which are available in generic form. Also, the label for omeprazole paste indicates that 4 weeks of treatment is required. This label is based on the design of studies submitted for approval of the drug. These studies were conducted for a period of 4 weeks in order to optimize the healing data for omeprazole paste. My experience with H_2 antagonists and omeprazole granules indicate that less time is usually required for healing in horses that are not in intensive training, and healing may occur more rapidly with omeprazole compared with ranitidine or cimetidine. No studies directly comparing these treatments have been reported, however. Also, the use of the animal (racing,

*Pepcid, Merck and Co., Inc., West Point, Pa.
†Axid, Eli Lilly and Co., Indianapolis, Ind.
‡Prilosec, AstraZeneca, Inc., Wayne, Pa.
§Gastrogard, Merial Limited, Iselin, NJ.

show, pleasure, light riding) will probably influence the duration of treatment required for healing to occur. I currently recommend 2 weeks treatment with omeprazole paste at 4 mg/kg, with a follow-up endoscopic examination to determine whether ulcers have healed. *Caution should be exercised when considering using lower doses to reduce treatment costs.* Just as with H_2 antagonists, lowering the dose of omeprazole will increase the percent of poor responders, potentially resulting in treatment failure. The lower the dose, the greater is the individual variability in response.[137] There are no data yet available on the results of using doses less than that recommended on the label for healing gastric ulcers.

Another feature of omeprazole paste that distinguishes it from the H_2 blockers is that at 4 mg/kg, maximum suppression of acidity is achieved between the first and fifth daily doses. It is not known what degree of acid suppression is achieved in the interim period, although it is likely that 90% suppression of acid secretion is accomplished by the third dose. Nonetheless, because the pharmacodynamics of omeprazole differs considerably from that of drugs that have traditionally been used to treat equine gastric ulcers, treatment regimens should not deviate from published recommendations or results of research.

Antacids can effectively reduce gastric acidity, but only briefly. In a study examining administration of 180 ml Maalox,* gastric pH was increased for at most 45 minutes.[136] In another study, 240 ml Maalox TC† increased gastric pH for 2 hours.[141] Thus liquid antacid products must be given both in large volumes (240 ml) and very frequently (6 to 12 times daily!) to be effective in promoting ulcer healing. Some believe that clinical signs are relieved at lower doses given less frequently, but these claims have not been documented. Feed additives that contain antacids are popularly considered to be helpful in controlling gastric ulcers in horses, but there are no supportive data. Also, an acid-neutralizing effect is most desirable when the stomach is empty, not when it is full, because gastric pH naturally is high when horses ingest feed. Antacids containing aluminum may have some effect on healing of gastric glandular lesions, because aluminum hydroxide has been shown to enhance gastric mucosal nitric oxide, which should promote mucosal blood flow.[142]

Sucralfate, the major components of which are sucrose octasulfate (SOS) and aluminum hydroxide, is effective in the treatment of peptic ulcers in humans,[143] although healing rates for sucralfate in treatment of duodenal ulcers were much longer than for H_2 antagonists. Clinical experience suggests that sucralfate can promote healing of lesions in the gastric glandular mucosa of horses. The mechanism of action likely involves adherence to ulcerated mucosa, stimulation of mucus secretion, enhanced mucosal blood flow, and enhanced prostaglandin E synthesis. These are all factors relevant to glandular mucosa, and it is doubtful that sucralfate is effective in treating ulcers in the equine gastric squamous mucosa. In fact, lesions in the squamous mucosa can develop while a horse is being treated with sucralfate.

Sucralfate can be administered concurrently with an H_2 antagonist. Concurrent administration may reduce H_2 antagonist absorption by 10%, but this has not appeared to affect efficacy in humans.[144] Of importance, sucralfate can substantially interfere with the absorption of other drugs, particularly fluoroquinolones, and thus its use with other medications should be determined on a case-by-case basis.

Misoprostol‡ is a prostaglandin E_1 analogue that may promote healing of gastric glandular mucosal lesions by increasing mucosal blood flow. Misoprostol can cause inappetence, diarrhea, and abdominal discomfort, and for these reasons it is not used routinely to treat gastric ulcers. It has been used along with other medications to treat severe gastric glandular mucosal ulcers in a small number of foals and horses, with apparent success. Misoprostol is probably a poor choice for treating gastric ulcers, but it may be effective in treating NSAID-induced colonic ulcers. In humans, misoprostol is used to prevent NSAID-induced gastrointestinal ulceration,[145] but there are no reports of this use in horses.

In some cases, prokinetic drugs may be required to enhance gastric emptying. Use of a prokinetic drug is indicated when there is suspected gastroesophageal reflux, gastric outlet obstruction or peudoobstruction, or duodenal ulceration or inflammation. Drugs available for this purpose include bethanechol* and metoclopramide.

Bethanechol has been used successfully in our clinic to enhance gastric emptying and minimize gastroesophageal reflux with few mild adverse effects. Bethanechol was reported to enhance gastrointestinal motility while not increasing gastric acid output in horses.[146] In cases of acute gastric atony, 0.025 mg/kg SC every 4 to 6 hours has been effective in promoting gastric motility and emptying, followed by oral maintenance dosages of 0.35 to 0.40 mg/kg three to four times daily. Adverse effects can include diarrhea, inappetence, salivation, and colic, but they occur infrequently. Bethanecol can be administered chronically (weeks to months) in horses with pyloric fibrosis and stenosis, although there are no data as to its long-term effectiveness.

Reported experience with metoclopramide in the horse is limited to its use in postoperative ileus. Dosages ranging from 0.10 to 0.25 mg/kg three to four times daily are used by some clinicians to treat suspected delayed gastric emptying, although one report indicated that constant infusion at a rate of 0.04 mg/kg/hr was superior to interval dosing in enhancing postsurgical small intestinal motility.[147] Sudden neurologic excitation is an adverse reaction to metoclopramide, but is more common towards 0.25 mg/kg. In one foal treated in our clinic, administration of metoclopramide over several days resulted in tachycardia, bilateral facial sweating, miosis, and enophthalmos. These signs resolved when the drug was discontinued.

Cisapride can be effective in improving gastric emptying in humans, but investigation into the effect of cisapride on enhancing gastrointestinal motility in horses has yielded inconsistent results. Cisapride in the horse is poorly absorbed orally and per rectum,[148] and it is more expensive than metoclopramide or bethanechol. Cisapride currently is not available in the United States or Europe because of adverse cardiac effects in some patients.

REFLUX GASTRITIS

Reflux gastritis frequently accompanies conditions in which there is small intestinal ileus with large volumes of enterogastric reflux that must be evacuated by nasogastric intubation. This fluid typically has a pH of 5 to 7 and contains substantial biliary and pancreatic secretions. Often, gastroscopy reveals that extensive erosion of the squamous mucosa occurs in association with this reflux. The erosions extend from the margo plicatus dorsally, primarily along the cranial and right sides of the stomach. Presumably, squamous mucosal erosion results from the effect of bile acids on the gastric

---

*Maalox, Novartis Consumer Health, Summit, NJ.
†Maalox TC, Novartis Consumer Health, Summit, NJ.
‡Cytotec, Searle and Co., Chicago, Ill.

*Urecholine, Merck and Co., Inc., West Point, Pa.

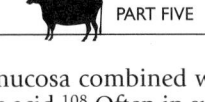

squamous mucosa combined with accumulation of gastric hydrochloric acid.[108] Often in such cases, islands of regenerative squamous epithelium can be observed in the eroded/ulcerated fundus within 2 to 3 days, and in another 2 to 3 days the squamous epithelium can completely regenerate. Intravenous administration of an H_2 antagonist may prevent these lesions from developing or hasten healing, but treatment may not be necessary in all cases.

GASTRIC IMPACTION

True gastric impaction occurs infrequently and may result from ingestion of certain feed stuffs or a horse eating when there is impaired intestinal motility. Potential predisposing feeds include beet pulp, bran, straw, wheat, and barley. Beet pulp and bran can become desiccated within the stomach and may not become rehydrated by water or gastric secretions. Dental disorders may predispose some horses to gastric impaction, if roughage is incompletely masticated. Feeding a horse that has signs of colic may predispose to gastric impaction, because there may be poor gastric emptying associated with generalized decreased gastrointestinal motility.

Definitive diagnosis of gastric impaction is difficult. Gastric impaction is occasionally diagnosed during exploratory laparotomy as the primary cause of colic in horses.[149] Other than at surgery, definitive diagnosis of gastric impaction can be difficult. If the horse has not eaten for several hours, yet poorly macerated or digested feed material is recovered from the nasogastric tube, a gastric impaction may be suspected. On rectal examination, the spleen may be displaced caudally and medially, but this finding is not specific for gastric impaction or dilation. Gastric impactions can be confirmed by gastroscopy, although one cannot differentiate a normally full stomach from an impacted stomach. The key to making this diagnosis is the failure of the stomach to empty appreciably in 12 to 24 hours. Radiography may also reveal a distended stomach that distorts the diaphragm cranially.

Gastric impactions can be effectively treated medically by administering dioctyl sodium succinate (DSS), 5% solution, 4 to 8 ounces, in 4 to 6 L of water. The DSS acts as a surfactant and allows water to penetrate the impacted, desiccated ingesta, facilitating its removal from the stomach. Alternatively, one can lavage the stomach with water repeatedly by pumping 2 to 4 L of water per nasogastric tube and recovering the infused water and ingesta by gravity flow or aspiration through the nasogastric tube. This is particularly effective in treating bran mash impactions, because of the small particle size of the bran. Mineral oil is less effective in treating gastric impactions because the interior of the impacted ingesta is desiccated and compacted. The mineral oil slides around the impaction and does not penetrate it; thus it does not facilitate passage of the impacted ingesta through the pylorus. When diagnosed at surgery, gastric impactions can be effectively treated by the injection of 2 to 4 L of saline transmurally into the stomach, followed by gentle massage of the stomach and the impacted mass. The impaction usually resolves within 12 to 24 hours. Treatment with bethanecol, 0.02 mg/kg SC every 6 to 8 hours to promote gastric emptying may be helpful in conjunction with these therapies. Bethanecol may have reduced effectiveness in a distended stomach, but it should not contribute to stomach rupture and therefore can be used safely.

Gastric impaction can also accompany grass sickness, in which case the prognosis for survival is poor. Grass sickness occurs in the United Kingdom and in areas of South America. The disease does not occur in the United States, but horses recently imported from the United Kingdom have been diagnosed with grass sickness in the United States.

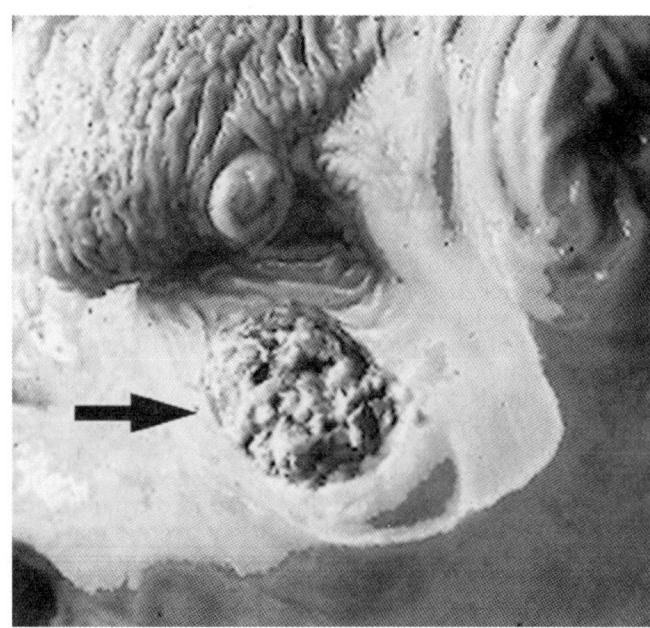

FIG. 30-25 ▓ *Rhodococcus equi* abscess *(arrow)* extending from the abdominal cavity into the stomach of a 4-month-old foal. The abscess has penetrated the stomach along the lesser curvature, between the margo plicatus and the cardia.

GASTRIC RUPTURE

Gastric rupture occurs as a sequel to gastric distention, from ingesta, fluid, or gas. The adult equine stomach can hold 20 to 25 L when maximally distended. Gastric rupture can occur from simple excessive distention, but also the integrity of the wall of the stomach may become compromised because of decreased blood flow. Distention of the small intestine has been demonstrated to significantly reduce mural blood flow, and this likely occurs in the stomach with distention. In some cases, it has appeared that rupture occurred as a result of an infarction of a portion of the stomach wall, without apparent substantial distention. Gastric perforation from ulceration happens rarely in adult horses. Because of extensive contamination of the peritoneal cavity with stomach contents, treatment is not possible and humane destruction of the horse is required.

ABSCESSES

Abscesses in the wall of the stomach are infrequent findings and occur most frequently in foals. Abscesses can form secondary-to-severe gastric ulceration, *R. equi* bacteremia (Fig. 30-25), foreign body penetration, or septic peritonitis. Signs of gastric abscessation are variable and similar to those of abscessation in other organs: fever, neutrophilia, hyperfibrinogenemia, anemia, weight loss, and possibly colic. Diagnosis may be made endoscopically, radiographically, or ultrasonographically. In some cases, use of labelled white blood cell scintigraphy may identify an intrabdominal abscess in the region of the stomach. Usually by the time a diagnosis is made, the abscess is very advanced and often it is adhered to multiple abdominal viscera. Treatment should include long-term antimicrobials, but outcomes are usually poor.

NEOPLASIA

Gastric neoplasia occurs infrequently. Squamous cell carcinoma (Fig. 30-26) is the most common neoplastic disorder stenosis, is permanent, and these horses usually have an active ulcerative process. The treatment objectives are to enhance gastric emptying and promote ulcer healing. Gastric emptying can be promoted by bethanecol (0.02 mg/kg SC every 8 hours or 0.35 mg/kg PO every 8 hours). Ulcer healing can be promoted by a combination of acid suppression and sucralfate. If ulceration is marked, use of omeprazole is recommended for optimal acid suppression.

If medical management is not effective, surgical bypass of the pylorus (gastroenterostomy) is indicated. Whereas pyloromyotomy has been effective in treating cases with primary muscular hypertrophy, the degree of fibrosis that is present in most cases precludes this approach. After surgery, administration of bethanecol is indicated to promote gastric emptying.

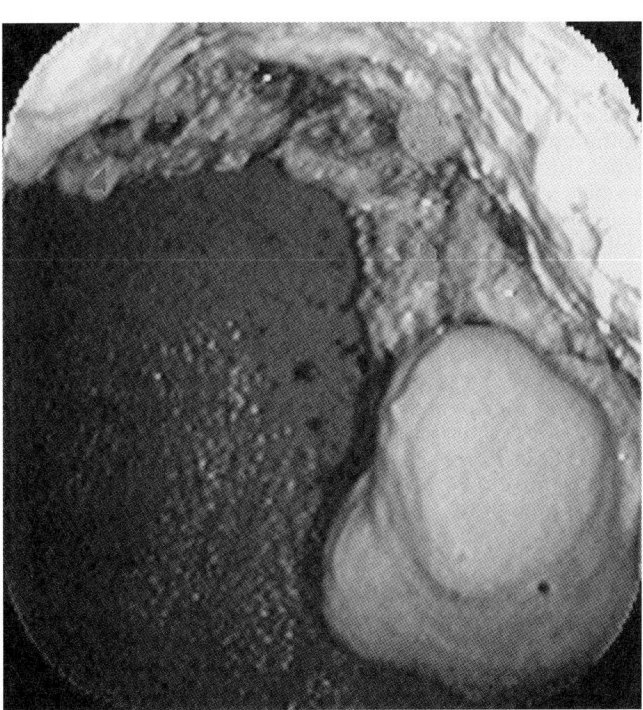

FIG. 30-26 ■ Endoscopic view of a gastric squamous cell carcinoma.

that affects the equine stomach.[150] The tumor originates from the gastric squamous epithelium and can metastasize to the abdominal cavity and viscera or extend into the esophagus. It typically affects horses in their teens or older. Presenting signs include chronic weight loss, anemia, nasal reflux, or colic. Diagnosis can be made by gastroscopy, laparoscopy, barium contrast radiography, or peritoneal fluid analysis when the tumor has metastasized into the abdomen. Metastatic masses may be felt on rectal palpation. When the tumor obstructs the cardia, it is difficult, if not impossible, to pass a nasogastric tube, and saliva and ingesta accumulate within the esophagus. There is no effective therapy.

Primary gastric adenocarcinoma has been described, and metastatic lymphosarcoma, mesothelioma, and bile duct carcinoma have involved the stomach.

PYLORIC STENOSIS

Pyloric stenosis can occur secondary to chronic ulceration and fibrosis or muscular hypertrophy. The majority of cases occur as a result of chronic ulceration at the pylorus. I have diagnosed pyloric stenosis in foals, yearlings, and adult horses up to 20 years old. Pyloric smooth muscle hypertrophy is an unusual finding, but it has been diagnosed in young horses.[151] The clinical presentation was colic with large volumes of acidic reflux obtained on nasogastric intubation.

Diagnosis of pyloric stenosis is best made by endoscopy. Usually there will be active ulceration and inflammation, and the pyloric opening will appear small and fixed. If a biopsy forceps is pushed into the stomach lining at the pylorus, the wall of the stomach will appear to be rigid, because of scar tissue in the stomach wall. With primary muscular hypertrophy, no ulceration of mucosal inflammation should be present. Serum electrolytes and blood gas results are reflective of a hypochloremic metabolic alkalosis, secondary to sequestration of hydrochloric acid in the stomach.

Treatment of pyloric stenosis caused by fibrosis resulting from chronic ulceration is difficult. The fibrosis, and thus the

REFERENCES

100. Wilson JH: Gastric and duodenal ulcers in foals: a retrospective study, *Proceedings of the Equine Colic Research Symposium*, Athens, Ga, Lawrence, NJ, 1986, p 126, Veterinary Learning Systems.
101. Murray MJ, Hart J, Parker GA: Equine gastric ulcer syndrome: endoscopic survey of asymptomatic foals, *Proceedings of the Thirty-third Annual Convention of the American Association of Equine Practitioners*, 1987, pp 769-776.
102. Murray MJ et al: The progression of gastric lesions in young thoroughbred foals: an endoscopic study, *J Am Vet Med Assoc* 196:1623-1627, 1990.
103. Murray MJ et al: Gastric ulcers in horses: a comparison of endoscopic findings in horses with and without clinical signs, *Equine Vet J* 21(suppl 7):68-72, 1989.
104. Vatistas NJ et al: Cross-sectional study of gastric ulcers of the squamous mucosa in Thoroughbred racehorses, *Equine Vet J Suppl* 29:34-39,1999.
105. Murray MJ et al: Factors associated with gastric lesions in Thoroughbred race horses, *Equine Vet J* 28:368-374,1996.
106. Orsini JS, Pipers FS: Endoscopic evaluation of the relationship between training, racing, and gastric ulcers, *Vet Surg* 26:424,1997.
107. Hammond CJ, Mason DK, Watkins KL: Gastric ulceration in mature thoroughbred horses, *Equine Vet J* 18:284, 1986.
108. Lanas A et al: Experimental esophagitis induced by acid and pepsin in rabbits mimicking human reflux esophagitis, *Gastroenterology* 116:97-107,1999.
109. Vaezi MF, Singh S, Richter JE: Role of acid and duodenogastric reflux in esophageal injury: a review of animal and human studies, *Gastroenterology* 108:1897-1907,1995.
110. Orlando RC: Esophageal epithelial defense against acid injury, *J Clin Gastroenterol* 13(suppl 2):S1-S5,1991.
111. Orlando RC et al: Barriers to paracellular permeability in rabbit esophageal epithelium, *Gastroenterology* 102:910-923,1992.
112. Argenzio RA, Eisemann J: Mechanisms of acid injury in procine gastroesophageal mucosa, *Am J Vet Res* 57:564-573, 1996.
113. Argenzio RA, Southworth M, Stevens CE: Sites of organic acid production and absorption in the equine gastrointestinal tract, *Am J Physiol* 226:1043-1050, 1975.
114. Hojgaard L, Mertz NA, Rune SJ: Peptic ulcer pathophysiology: acid, bicarbonate, and mucosal function, *Scand J Gastroenterol Suppl* 216:10-15, 1996.
115. Sorbye H, Svanes K: The role of blood flow in gastric mucosal defense, damage and healing, *Digest Dis* 12:305-317,1994.
116. Ross IN, Bahari HMM, Turneberg LA: The pH gradient across mucus adherent to rat fundic mucosa in vivo and the effect of potential damaging agents, *Gastroenterology* 81:713-718,1981.
117. Brzozowski T et al: Healing of chronic gastric ulcerations by L-arginine: role of nitric oxide, prostaglandins, gastrin and polyamines, *Digestion* 56:463-471,1995.
118. Qiu BS, Cho CH, Pfeiffer CJ: Effects of chronic nitric oxide synthase inhibition in cold-restraint and ethanol-induced gastric mucosal damage in rats, *Digestion* 57:60-66, 1996.
119. Wallace JL, Tigley AW: Review article: new insights into prostaglandins and mucosal defence, *Aliment Pharmacol Ther* 9:227-235,1995.
120. Murray MJ, Mahaffey EA: Age-related characteristics of the equine gastric squamous epithelial mucosa, *Equine Vet J* 25:514-517, 1993.
121. Sanchez LC, Merritt AM, Lester GD: Effect of ranitidine on intragastric pH in clinically normal neonatal foals, *J Am Vet Med Assoc* 212:1407-1412,1998.
122. Baker SJ, Gerring EL: Gastric pH monitoring in healthy, suckling pony foals, *Am J Vet Res* 54:959-964,1993.
123. Campbell-Thompson ML, Merritt AM: Effect of ranitidine on gastric acid secretion in young male horses, *Am J Vet Res* 48:1511-1515, 1987.
124. Murray MJ, Eichorn ES: Effects of intermittent feed deprivation, intermittent feed deprivation with ranitidine, and stall confinement with free access to hay on gastric ulceration in horses, *Am J Vet Res* 57:1599-1603, 1996.

125. Murray MJ, Schusser GF: Application of gastric pH-metry in horses: measurement of 24-hour gastric pH in horses fed, fasted, and treated with ranitidine, *Equine Vet J* 25:417- 421, 1993.
126. Smyth GB, Young DW, Hammond LS: Effects of diet and feeding on post-prandial serum gastrin and insulin concentrations in adult horses, *Equine Vet J* 21(suppl 7):56-59, 1988.
127. Mertz HR, Walsh JH: Peptic ulcer pathophysiology, *Med Clin North Am* 75:799-814,1991.
128. Furr MO, Murray MJ, Ferguson D: The effects of stress on gastric ulceration, T3, T4, rT3, and cortisol in neonatal foals, *Equine Vet J* 24:37-40, 1992.
129. Haglund U: Stress ulcers, *Scand J Gastroenterol* 175:27-33,1990.
130. Schuster DP, Rowley H, Feinstein S: Prospective evaluation of the risk of upper gastrointestinal bleeding after admission to an intensive care unit, *Am J Med* 76:623-630, 1984.
131. Murray MJ: Gastroendoscopic appearance of gastric lesions in foals: 58 cases, *J Am Vet Med Assoc* 195:1135-1142, 1989.
132. Murray MJ: Gastric ulceration in horses: 91 cases (1987-1990), *J Am Vet Med Assoc* 102:117-120, 1993.
133. Furr MO, Murray MJ: Treatment of gastric ulcers in horses with histamine type 2 receptor antagonists, *Equine Vet J* 21(suppl 7):77-79, 1989.
134. Campbell-Thompson ML, Merritt AM: Effect of ranitidine on gastric acid secretion in young male horses, *Am J Vet Res* 48:1511-1515, 1987.
135. Sangiah S, MacAllister CG, Amouzedeh HR: Effects of cimetidine and ranitidine on basal gastric pH, free and total acid contents in horses, *Res Vet Sci* 45:291-295, 1988.
136. Murray MJ, Grodinsky C: The effects of famotidine, ranitidine, and magnesium hydroxide/aluminum hydroxide on gastric fluid pH in adult horses, *Equine Vet J* 24(suppl 11):52-55, 1992.
137. Savarino V et al: Variability in individual response to various doses of omeprazole, *Dig Dis Sci* 39:161-168,1994.
138. Murray MJ et al: The effects of omeprazole on healing of naturally-occurring gastric ulcers in Thoroughbred race horses, *Equine Vet J* 29:425-429,1997.
139. MacAllister CG et al: Effects of omeprazole paste on healing of spontaneous gastric ulcers in horse and foals: a field trial, *Equine Vet J Suppl* 29:77-80, 1999.
140. Andrews FM et al: Efficacy of omeprazole paste in the treatment and prevention of gastric ulcers in horses, *Equine Vet J Suppl* 29:81-86, 1999.
141. Clark CK et al: Effect of an aluminum-magnesium hydroxide antacid and bismuth subsalicylate on gastric pH in horses, *J Am Vet Med Assoc* 208:1687-1691,1996.
142. Lambrecht N et al: Role of eicosanoids, nitric oxide, and afferent neurons in antacid induced protection in the rat stomach, *Gut* 34:329-337,1993.
143. McCarthy DM: Sucralfate, *N Engl J Med* 325:1017-1025, 1991.
144. Mullersman G et al: Lack of clinically significant in vitro and in vivo interactions between ranitidine and sucralfate, *J Pharm Sci* 75:995-998,1986.
145. Scheiman J, Isenberg J: Agents used in the prevention and treatment of nonsteroidal antiinflammatory drug-associated symptoms and ulcers, *Am J Med* 105:32S-38S,1998.
146. Ringger NC et al: Effect of bethanechol or erythromycin on gastric emptying in horses, *Am J Vet Res* 57:1771-1775,1996.
147. Dart AJ et al: Efficacy of metoclopramide for treatment of ileus in horses following small intestinal surgery: 70 cases (1989-1992), *Aust Vet J* 74:280-284,1996.
148. Cook G et al: Pharmacokinetics of cisapride in horses after intravenous and rectal administration, *Am J Vet Res* 58:1427-1430,1997.
149. Barclay WP et al: Primary gastric impaction in the horse, *J Am Vet Med Assoc* 181:682-683, 1982.
150. Olsen SN: Squamous cell carcinoma of the equine stomach: a report of five cases, *Vet Rec* 131:170-173,1992.
151. Allen D: Personal communication, 1988.

THE EQUINE INTESTINE

INTESTINAL INJURY IN THE HORSE

NATHANIEL A. WHITE II

There are numerous causes of intestinal injury during the equine acute abdomen. Classic pathphysiologic explanations use ischemia, ulceration, and inflammation from infection, parasites, trauma, toxins, or immune complexes to categorize and explain intestinal injury. For the clinician, understanding the underlying pathophysiology of injury is important for recognition and treatment. For many of these injuries the signs can be the similar so that clinical differentiation is difficult.

Cellular injury was once characterized by the morphologic change it caused. The new paradigm includes cell injury, which is as much functional as it is structural. The response to a stimulus is mediated by numerous autocrine and paracrine messengers, which include cytokines, prostaglandins, neuropeptides, and proinflammatory substances such as complement, histamine, bradykinin, serotonin, and interferon. In the intestine, inflammatory responses to these messengers can be orchestrated by mucosal cells, fibrocytes, macrophages, mast cells, endothelial cells, neurons, muscle cells, and polymorphonuclear cells.[152] The chain of events is complex with the relationship of all the different cell responses not yet fully understood. It is clear that the inflammatory response from any insult initiates a multitude of chemical and immune reactions that, depending on the severity of the insult, can cause both local and systemic effects.

Several mechanisms can stimulate an inflammatory response including ischemia, reperfusion after ischemia, inflammation from bacterial or viral infection, and inflammation from parasites, trauma (surgical), or toxins. The resulting tissue injuries vary and may be differentiated by their effect on the different layers of the intestine and by the vascular and nervous response. Although the mucosa or serosa is often the cell layer affected first, the inflammatory response frequently involves the remaining layers of the intestine, the submucosa and smooth muscle. The inflammatory response may also vary depending on the specific cause. As an example, ischemia can be caused by strangulation of the blood supply, distention of the intestinal wall, or poor perfusion caused by systemic shock. The response of individual intestinal cells may be similar for each; however, each stimulus appears to evoke different sequences of cell response, thereby resulting in different clinical signs and varying response to treatment. In some instances, injury to the intestine may be secondary to another disease process, but the damage to the intestine can still initiate a systemic response resulting in multiple organ involvement.

INTESTINAL INFLAMMATION: GENERAL CONCEPTS

The cascade of events initiated by infection or ischemia has been extensively studied. Inflammatory mediators increased during bowel inflammation are released from numerous cell types, including mucosal cells, endothelial cells, fibrocytes, myocytes, mesothelial cells, and neurons.[152] There is also evidence that the compounds making up the tissue ground substance can also initiate an inflammatory response and help transmit signals between immunocytes and afferent neurons. Theoretically all cells in the intestine can act as effector cells, both producing cytokines to send messages to other cells, or being activated to respond to the insult.[152] Cytokines, growth factors, and adhesion molecules initiate an inflammatory response.[152] This response also alters cell apoptosis, resulting in delayed removal of mucosal cells and neutrophils or early death of immunocytes.[153] Cytokines such as interleukin-1 (IL-1β) and tumor necrosis factor (TNF-α), platelet activating factor (PAF) complement (C5a), interferon (INF-γ), and histamine, are all reported to be involved in inciting intestinal inflammation.[154] Although describing all the effects and interactions of the inflammatory cytokines and eicosanoids is beyond the scope of this chapter, it is apparent these substances can stimulate and inhibit the inflammatory reaction by directing cell communication and cell response to injury. As a result the disease process should be viewed as a sequence of events altering cell functions that are integrated and designed to protect the intestine from permanent injury.

The cells primarily observed to take part in intestinal injury are mucosal cells, endothelial cells, neurons, fibroblasts, mast cells, eosinophils, neutrophils, and macrophages. Rather than responding independently, these cells likely all respond to the initial insult, each with their inherent cytokine production or cell activation, which stimulates other cells or suppresses cell responses. Envisioned as a group acting simultaneously, the sequence likely proceeds from an initial stimulus to mucosal or serosal cells and subsequent involvement of the vascular endothelium or enteric neurons. Mucosal cells react by releasing cytokines to activate macrophages and lymphocytes in the lamina propria.[155,156] These cells release cytokines and adhesion molecules, which in turn activate other cells while initiating local defenses. Simultaneously, endothelial cells respond to the cytokine message by releasing cytokines to attract neutrophils and eosinophils and subsequently enable them to migrate through the endothelium into the interstium. Afferent neurons detecting cytokine increases initiate neuropeptide, cytokine, or eicosanoid release from the efferent neurons, resulting in activation of numerous cells including those already activated by the initial cell messengers.[157-160] Fibrocytes, responding to the initial cytokine messages and growth factors, subsequently release cytokines and growth factors such as Il-1α, Il-1β, TNF-α, transforming growth factor, and platelet-derived growth factor. Both of these can be proinflammatory or can help to repair the mucosa.[161,162] Metalloproteinases released in response to inflammatory cytokines alter the basement membranes and collagen in the different layers, allowing migration of cells to the extracellular space and stimulating other cells to release chemotactants.[152] Muscle cells, once thought to be neutral in the inflammatory cycle, appear to be able to release cytokines, thereby participating in the inflammatory reaction.[152,163] Bowel dysfunction after surgical manipulation has been linked to neutrophil infiltration as a result of increased adhesion molecule production in the muscle.[164,165]

Although all the cells in the intestine participate in the inflammatory response as effector cells, they can also act a suppressors. Each appears to communicate to other cells locally to cause or suppress the inflammatory response. Production of nitric oxide by endothelial cells can reduce neutrophil adhesion while increased release of growth factor by fibroblasts and the vascular endothelium speeds healing of the mucosa.[161] In response to receptor activation, up-regulation to cytokine production can take only seconds. In some cases the lack of suppression, perhaps the result of chronic or overwhelming stimulation or severe damage to cells that release the inhibitor messengers, allows amplification of inflammation and permanent cell damage.

The role of each cell type as effector and messenger is slowly being unraveled. The role of some cells is better understood than others. Reperfusion, cytokines, and complement initiate endothelial cell changes. Subsequent production of cytokines and prostanoids by endothelial cells attracts neutrophils and macrophages.[166] Endothelial cells also stimulate the inflammatory response by altering capillary permeability, promoting neutrophil adhesion, and physically altering blood flow. The interaction between the endothelial cell and neutrophils or eosinophils is a pivotal response in causing intestinal injury. This response is made possible by PAF, leukotrienes (LTB$_4$), and adhesion molecules produced by endothelial cells and polymorphonuclear neutrophils (PMNs).[166] Neutrophil migration into affected tissues subsequently causes severe damage, including damage to cells and tissue ground substance, which furthers the inflammatory response.

Although all intestinal cells can be involved in the inflammatory process, the nervous system is now known to be integral in the inflammatory response. Release of potassium, ATP, bradykinin, and PGE all stimulate afferent neurons.[157,167] Neuropeptides are released in response to afferent signals from the products of cell injury including cytokines, eicosanoids, and histamine.[157,168] Substance P, neurokinin, calcitonin gene–related protein (CGRP), and vasoactive peptide (VIP) have all been found increased levels in inflamed

tissues, suggesting that they act as messengers to histiocytes or immunocytes that subsequently release cytokines.[154,157] The paracrine response differs in various tissues, but inflammatory responses by mast cells, PMNs, T cells (cytokine release), B cells, macrophages, fibroblasts, and muscle cells are in part due to neuropeptide stimulation. The coordination of this response is not totally understood, but neuropeptides can serve as proinflammatory mediators or suppressors. This system allows for immediate response of cells to a stimulus without humoral involvement and likely can cause persistent inflammatory reactions in response to inflamed tissue.[152]

Local inflammation of the intestine is known to cause change in other organs distant to the intestinal damage, specifically in the lung.[169-171] Circulating cytokines and activated neutrophils rapidly initiate an inflammatory response in the lung after intestine inflammation. This response is well known in experimental models and humans but has not been reported during intestinal disease in the horse. Other organs are likely affected creating signs of multiple organ involvement.

ISCHEMIA AND REPERFUSION

Ischemia is a deficiency of blood flow in tissue or in an organ. The lack of energy production in the cell starts a degenerative process. Within 5 minutes there are alterations in mitochondria, characterized by swelling and disorganization of cristae.[172] Mitochondrial changes precede cytoplasmic and membrane changes, which occurs in the first 30 minutes by activation of phospholipases, cytokine production, and accumulation of arachidonic acid. If ischemia persists, the cell degradation continues with failure of the membrane ion pumps allowing calcium to move into the cytoplasm.[173] This calcium accumulation within the cell activates proteases, which cause cell membrane damage and nuclear clumping. Calcium uptake in the mitochondria is increased, which inhibits oxidative phosphorylation.[173]

In the intestine, microscopic changes become evident at 30 minutes, when the mucosal epithelial cells and serosal mesothelial cells separate from their basement membranes.[174] This appears to be a mechanical separation caused by water movement from the vasculature into the subepithelial space. Metalloproteinases may also be involved in altering the basement membrane. The space, created by the initial separation, named Grunehagan's space, occurs at the tip of the villus in the small intestine (Fig. 30-27).[174] If ischemia continues, the cell damage progresses as the mucosal cells progressively slough off the lamina propria toward the intestinal crypts (Fig. 30-27). The change is similar in the colon, with epithelial cells sloughing off the surface of the mucosa. However, the slough is somewhat slower in the colon as it proceeds into the crypts. The serosa reacts in a similar fashion with mesothelial cells lifting off the basement membrane before there is visible cell membrane or cytoplasmic change. Other than vascular congestion, there is minimal change in the architecture of the supporting tissues in the mucosa or the serosa for the first 60 minutes of total ischemia. After 180 minutes of ischemia the lamina propria and mucosal vascular tuft has lost its architecture. The tissue is necrotic and has become homogeneous with lack of nuclear definition and cell structure.

Estimating the time required to create ischemic lesions depend on the experimental methods used. Different types of anesthesia in the horse and other animals has resulted in different rates of mucosal degeneration during ischemia. For example, animals anesthetized with inhalant anesthetics is different from that required animals breathing air, most likely from higher tissue oxygen concentrations at the beginning of the experiment.[174-176] Also, some cells, such as muscle cells, appear more resistant to ischemia; most likely because of

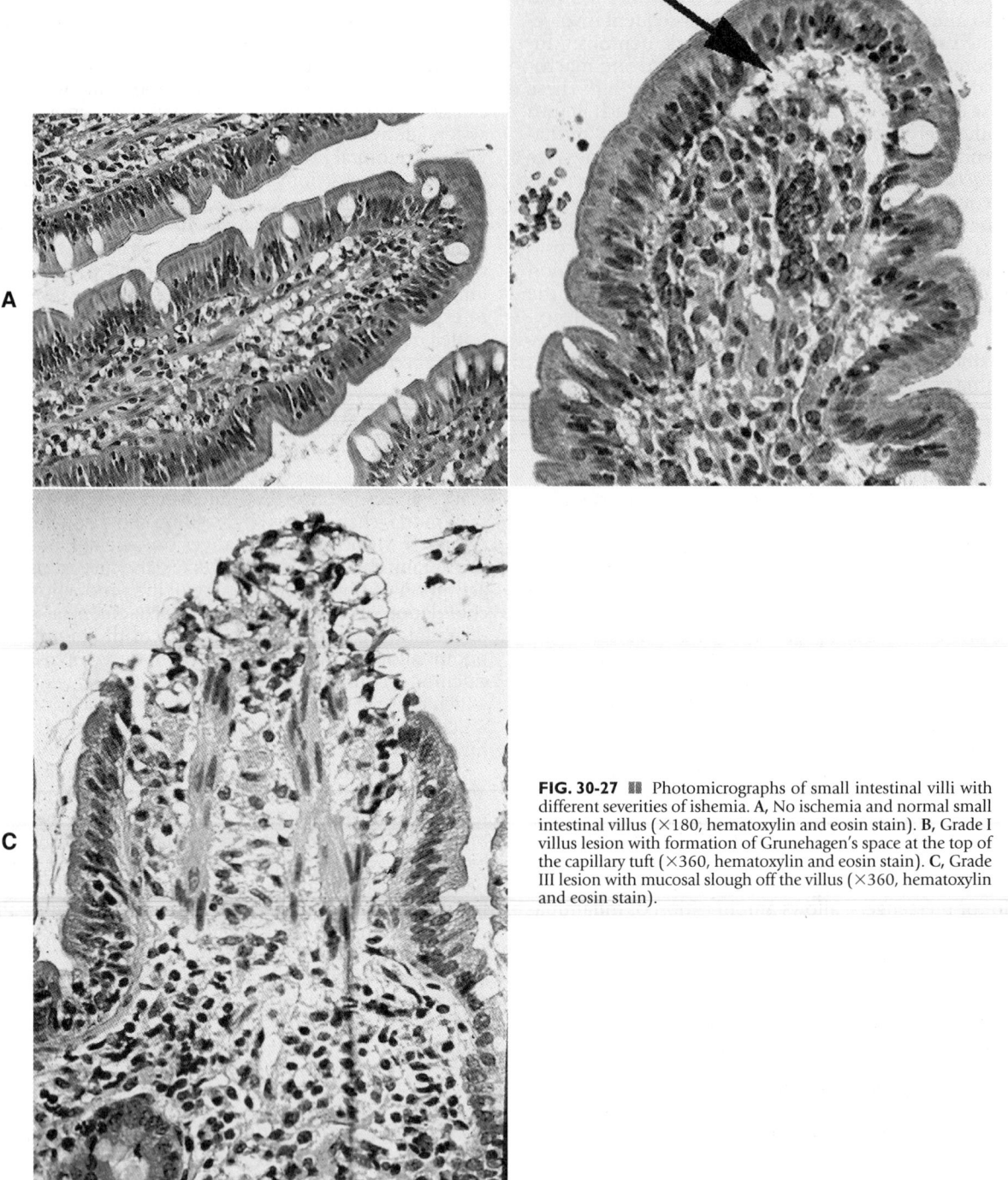

FIG. 30-27 ▦ Photomicrographs of small intestinal villi with different severities of ishemia. **A,** No ischemia and normal small intestinal villus (×180, hematoxylin and eosin stain). **B,** Grade I villus lesion with formation of Grunehagen's space at the top of the capillary tuft (×360, hematoxylin and eosin stain). **C,** Grade III lesion with mucosal slough off the villus (×360, hematoxylin and eosin stain).

the intracellular energy reserves of the cells. There are also differences in the response to low-flow ischemia versus total arteriovenous obstruction. Nevertheless, lesions caused by ischemia progress with reperfusion. If reperfusion, either resumption of blood flow or increased flow after low flow conditions, occurs while cells are still viable, a cascade of events is set in motion by the delivery of oxygen to the previously ischemic tissue.[166,177] The resultant injury is called reperfusion injury and relies on renewed oxygen in the tissue with participation of endothelial cells and afferent receptors to create the subsequent inflammatory response. Although it

makes sense that oxygen is needed to resuscitate the previously ischemic cells, the innate defense system of many cell types is to respond to the ischemic change with an inflammatory response. This response appears to help initiate a defense against bacterial invasion and is aimed at removing the damaged cells from the system. If enough cells have been damaged, the reperfusion effect can cause enough inflammation to prevent cells from surviving, thereby delaying healing.

Reperfusion injury starts as a change in intracellular metabolism in previously ischemic tissue. It does not require exposure to a microbe or toxin, but it does rely on cell production of cytokines and leukotrienes as signals to numerous blood and tissue cells required to complete the process. One primary initiator of reperfusion injury in the intestine is the production of oxygen radicals ($O_2\bullet$). Oxygen has the ability to take on an extra electron during enzymatic processes in the cell. Most cells, including endothelial cells and the small intestinal mucosal cells, contain xanthine dehydrogenase, which, when converted to xanthine oxidase, catalyzes hypoxanthine to xanthine.[177] Hypoxanthine is increased in the cytoplasm of cells during ischemia. Calcium and proteases initiate xanthine dehydrogenase conversion to xanthine oxidase; a process that can be stimulated in endothelial cells by IL-1, TNFα, and C5a, as well as neutrophil adherence. Oxygen is utilized in the reaction and ends up with an extra electron making an $O_2\bullet$ or superoxide.[166]

Once released, $O_2\bullet$ can initiate several chemical reactions that cause cell membrane damage both directly and by stimulating phospholipase activity. During $O_2\bullet$ production, nitric oxide (NO) production is decreased, thereby allowing neutrophil adhesion and migration.[177] Superoxide interaction with iron or catalase causes production of hydroxyl radicals (OH$\bullet$) or hydrogen peroxide (H_2O_2), respectively. Both are cytotoxic. The OH$\bullet$ alter or destroy cell membranes. Affected cells rapidly express cytokines and leukotrienes, which act as chemotactants for neutrophils. After the initial free radical production, cell injury progresses as two main events. Calcium, already increased in the cell, increases further, effectively blocking further energy production in the mitochondria and activating proteases causing further degradation of the cell nucleus and cytoplasm.[173] Secondly, lipoxygenases formed from molecular oxygen can cause cell membrane damage, thereby initiating a similar cellular response. The formation of chemical mediators takes only seconds to minutes after reperfusion and rapidly sets the inflammatory cascade in motion.

Although the mucosal cells and serosal mesothelial cells are damaged early in ischemia and are able to release cytokines to alert other cells locally, endothelial cells appear to be the primary initiators of reperfusion injury. They participate in the cytokine production and are involved with neutrophil adhesion and migration from the vasculature. Endothelial cells are also involved with the changes in blood flow after reperfusion. The platelets and neutrophils accumulate in and obstruct capillaries, altering blood flow. Endothelial cell swelling or contraction causes constriction of the lumens of blood vessels (Fig. 30-28). Changes in endothelial cell shape also increases capillary permeability, allowing fluid and protein to move into the interstium. Even though the metabolic state of the tissue during initial reperfusion initially results in overall increased blood flow, the increased vascular permeability increases interstitial pressure, causing capillary collapse. Combined with endothelial cell change, collapse of the tissue vasculature results in a "no-reflow phenomena" promoting further tissue ischemia.

Endothelial cell membrane changes allow expression of adhesion molecules and receptors, which are necessary for neutrophil adhesion and migration through the capillary and venule endothelium (Fig. 30-29). This migration of neutrophils causes the most prominent inflammation in the tissue, because activated neutrophils release elastase, oxygen radicals, and other serine proteases, which attack collagen, ground substance, and cell membranes.[178] The respiratory burst, a build up of oxygen free radicals in neutrophils during activation, is responsible for most of the inflammation and tissue damage seen during reperfusion. It is also apparent that reperfusion injury can expand the initial injury into the surrounding viable tissue and that it can cause irreversible tissue damage.[179,180] Reperfusion injury can also cause injury

distant to the local damage and has been observed in the lung as a result of cytokine and activated neutrophil circulation.[171] Although not reported in the literature, the resulting lesion can be seen in the lung from horses that succumb to severe intestinal strangulation obstruction and shock.

The importance of oxygen radical generation as a mechanism of injury in strangulating lesions has been questioned in the horse.[181] However, both clinical signs and lesions from clinical cases suggest that intestinal damage progresses after reperfusion. Use of a low-flow to no-flow model of ischemia with subsequent reperfusion responded to treatment to counteract injury from superoxide production and neutrophil accumulation.[182] This suggests that free radical production is part of the cascade of events causing an inflammatory response in the small intestine after bowel strangulation. Lack of malondialdehyde and conjugated diene production in the large intestine suggests less of a role for tissue-generated oxygen radicals and that reperfusion injury is primarily due to the oxygen radical release from migrating neutrophils as seen in xanthine oxidase–deficient rats.[178,183,184]

Recent research suggests that endothelial cells are not the only cells that act as "local effectors" of inflammation during reperfusion. Signs of inflammation are present in all parts of the intestine, including the muscle and myenteric plexus.[163,185-187] Alterations in muscle mitochondrial morphology have been identified in equine jejunum after low-flow ischemia.[188] Similarly, during large colon volvulus the neurons in the myenteric plexus undergo degeneration and decrease in number compared with normal.[186] Evidence of ischemic injury and inflammation occurs in both muscle and myenteric plexuses. This is relevant in horses with colon volvulus, in that survivors had significantly more neurons than nonsurvivors.[186] Perhaps of greater importance is the long-term effect of the inflammation in the myenteric plexus after ischemia and reperfusion. One can speculate that the high rates of repeat colic episodes in horses after colon torsion or large colon impaction are related to damage to the enteric nervous system.[189]

Reperfusion injury occurs after low-flow and no-flow ischemia. These models appear to emulate the clinical event, although the onset of ischemia in strangulation obstruction most likely begins as low-flow progressing to no-flow ischemia. Although the time frame of reperfusion injury is somewhat understood from the experimental models, the functional effects of dynamic events set in motion by reperfusion such as "no-reflow" and persistent inflammation in the serosa and around the intestinal nerve ganglions are not well understood. The relevance of these myenteric plexus lesions is also questioned, because they do not always correlate with severity of clinical signs.[186]

Low Flow Ischemia

The effect of ischemia-reperfusion differs with the type of ischemia. Low-flow ischemia is defined as flow less than 25% of normal blood flow. At this flow rate, vascular and cell damage is minimal, with degeneration occurring over a long time period. When normal flow is returned by increasing vascular volume or release of the arterial obstruction, there is a hyperemic response, doubling the normal blood flow to the affected intestine.[188] Cell damage accelerates during reperfusion, with marked changes in vascular permeability, mucosal damage, serosal damage, and signs of fluid accumulation in the submucosa, muscle, and serosa.[177,188,190,191] Edema in the submucosa and serosa causes vascular collapse leading to decreased blood flow and eventually a "no reflow" phenomena in the serosa and mucosa, with flow to the affected segment decreased below normal.[192,193] The decreased flow is partially due to endothelial cell swelling and neutrophil margination in the vasculature. Neutrophils migrate into all tissues but

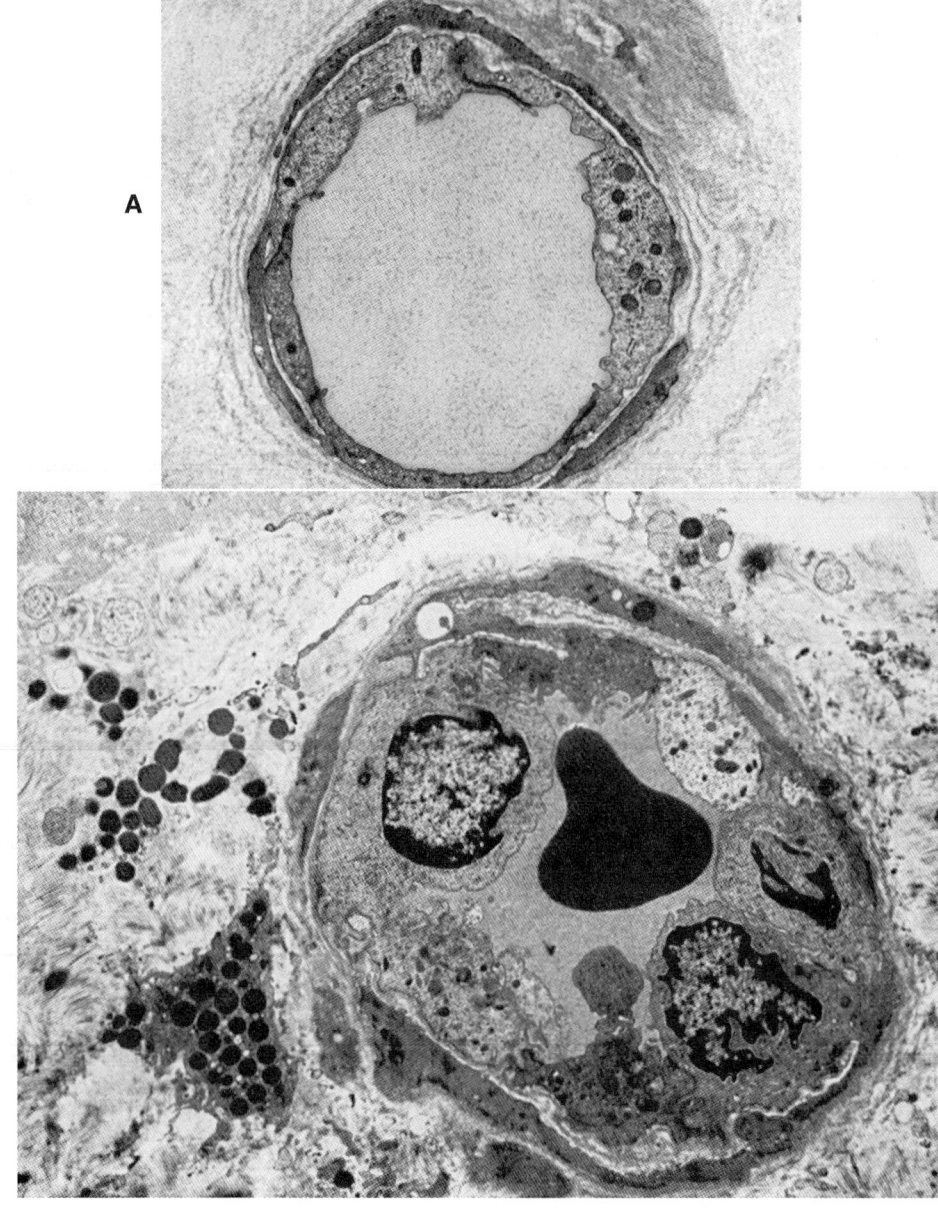

FIG. 30-28 ▮▮ Transmission electron photomicrographs of small vessels in the serosa. **A,** With normal endothelial cells before ischemia ($\times 5800$). **B,** With swollen endothelial cells and accumulation of neutrophils narrowing the vessel lumen during reperfusion ($\times 3600$).

predominately the mucosal and serosal layers. Initially neutrophils accumulate around blood vessels and capillaries. As reperfusion progresses, the greatest injury is observed in the serosa, with marked accumulation of neutrophils beneath the serosal basement membrane. Although neutrophil accumulation is the most marked in the serosa, they can be found in all layers of the intestine. This type of low-flow ischemia is rarely documented in equine abdominal disease, but it likely exists in distended intestine where there is low flow to the affected bowel wall. The flow is directly related to the intraluminal pressure, with pressures common in severe small intestinal distention causing greater than 50% reduction in blood flow.[194]

When examined in experimental models or when observed in clinical cases, most of these changes from acute low-flow ischemia are reversible and the affected intestine survives and heals. The effect varies greatly and depends on the length of ischemia. It is suspected that function is compromised temporarily, resulting in ileus, endotoxin absorption, or enteritis with excess secretion.[164,195] In the small intestine, serosal scarring and adhesions are the most common long-term result and may increase the risk of colic episodes in the future. Even if lesions are not grossly evident and appear minor on microscopic examination, horses with colic, particularly those requiring surgery, likely have intestinal injury, which can result in permanent intestinal dysfunction. Hypothetically this is one possible reason for increased risk of colic after previous colic episodes or previous surgery for colic.[189,196]

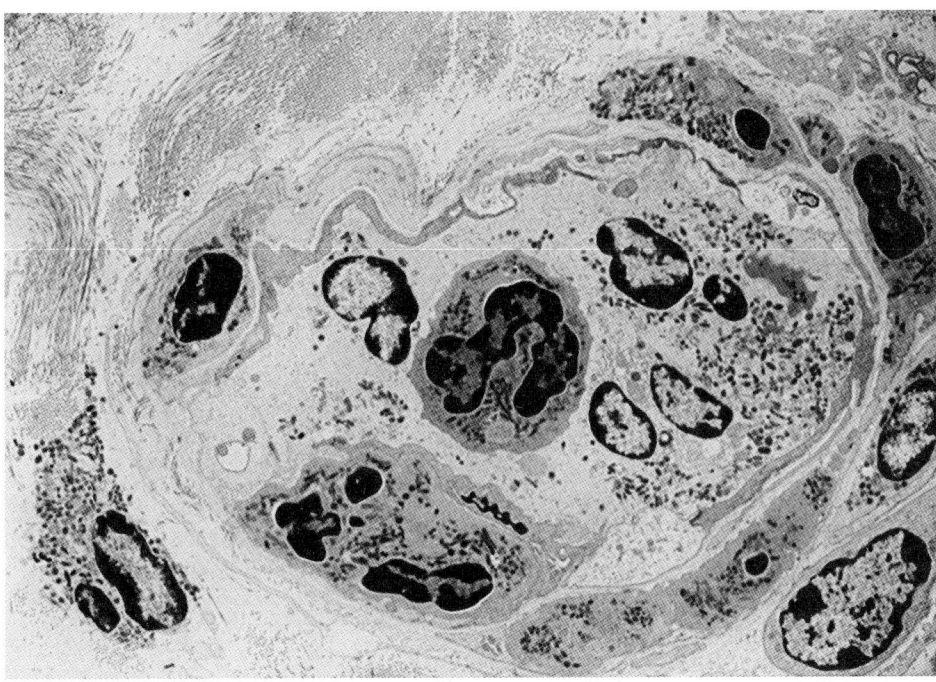

FIG. 30-29 ▓ Transmission electron photomicrograph of neutrophils adhering to the endothelium and perivascular accumulation after migrating through the endothelium (×2900).

Nonstrangulating infarction is the classic example of low-flow ischemia. In the horse, thromboembolic colic is reported to be caused by thrombosis of the mesenteric artery and its branches in horses infected with fourth-stage larva of *Strongylus vulgaris.*[197] The mechanism of infarction is most likely due to reduction of blood flow from a thrombus in the artery or thromboembolism obstructing the peripheral vasculature. In nonstrangulating infarction the intestinal injury most likely results from long-term low-flow ischemia or low-flow ischemia with episodes of reperfusion injury. In clinical cases the injury is severe, often resulting in necrosis in all layers of the bowel, with obvious infarction.

Low-flow ischemia may also occur during shock. Intestinal injury in bowel not directly involved in the primary lesion is suggestive that this injury is frequently present in horses with bowel strangulation obstruction.[198] In horses with obstructing or strangulating lesions, biopsies from nonaffected, grossly normal intestine have evidence of some degree of bowel injury.[179,180] Endotoxin administration also has been reported to cause an inflammatory reaction in the intestines, with loss of mucosa and neutrophil infiltration in the mucosa.[199] This may be relevant to assessing horses in shock.

Total Arteriovenous Occlusion

Total ischemia resulting from arteriovenous occlusion causes total vascular stasis. The most common cause of this form of ischemia is the mesenteric infarction caused by incarceration of bowel in hernias or constricted spaces. Early in the occlusion, capillary congestion is observed in all layers of the intestine. The intestine undergoes degeneration as previously described with ischemia. When total ischemia exceeds 2 hours in the small intestine and 3 hours in the large colon, the tissue changes during blood flow occlusion are extensive and cell necrosis may preclude a response to reperfusion.[174-176,200-203] If the capillary damage is not too extensive during total ischemia, reperfusion causes further degeneration, including mucosal cell loss, increased edema, and neutrophil migration. However, oxygen radical production seen with low-flow ischemia and reperfusion may not be responsible for the continued damage during total arteriovenous occlusion. Furthermore, these events cannot be separated from the systemic shock, which can be cause secondary lesions seen in intestine distant to the lesion.[180] Despite the questions about the validity of reperfusion in the total ischemic event, continued intestinal injury during reperfusion is seen both in the small intestine and large colon after total ischemia.[174,179,180,183,204] The epithelial cell loss after reperfusion is progressive and likely due to either to counter current exchange creating a decreased oxygen concentration in the distant mucosa or from inflammation resulting from oxygen radical-induced inflammation from neutrophil activation.[178,185,205] The response in the serosa includes marked edema with initiation of neutrophil migration.[188] Eventually a massive collection of neutrophils fills the outer limits of the serosa.[206] During this type of ischemia and reperfusion, the damage from the inflammatory reaction can continue for days and, if severe enough, can prevent healing of the mucosa and serosa.

Venous Occlusion

Venous obstruction without arterial obstruction causes increased pressure at the capillary, resulting in decreased blood flow and red blood cell (RBC) and fluid extravasation into the interstium. The result is separation of the tissues with an increased diffusion distance for oxygen and nutrients. The RBC accumulation causes tissue damage and likely a continuation of cell hypoxia, which is irreversible even with reperfusion. Therefore, although reperfusion may be initiated, progressive injury is minimized by the lesion already present.[207] Small intestine can survive 2 hours of venous obstruction, although the resultant degeneration is severe and the intestine permanently scarred after healing.[175] The gross lesion is marked with obvious thickening of the bowel, which at first is red and eventually is purple. With time the color turns black or green with subsequent necrosis and alterations in hemoglobin.

Based on both experimental work and observations in clinical cases, irreversible death of a segment of the intestine occurs after 2 hours in the small intestine and 3 hours in the large colon, although this obviously varies depending on amount of residual blood flow to the affected tissue.[175,201] For the surgeon, venous occlusion is the most difficult type of lesion, because intestinal thickness or amount of hemorrhage may not correlate with the viability. The sequence of mucosal degeneration remains the same in this type of ischemia, making the biopsy the most reliable method to decide if the intestine can survive and heal.[176]

Distention

Although distended intestine may appear to have normal color and motility after decompression, alterations in blood flow in the wall of the distended intestine is a form of low-flow ischemia. During intestinal distention, intraluminal pressure causes collapse of the veins and capillaries, thereby decreasing the vascular capacity. This occurs even when blood pressure is normal. When small intestinal pressure is increased to 18 cm of water, as previously measured in clinical disease,[208] mesenteric blood flow to the intestine is decreased by 50%. Increasing capillary back-pressure while maintaining arterial pressure alters Starling forces in the intestinal wall.[194] The result is secretion of fluid from the vasculature even with an increase in wall tension. Water and some protein escapes into the interstitum causing submucosal and serosal edema. At higher intraluminal pressures there is more secretion than absorption of water, creating a cyclic increase in intraluminal pressure after bowel compliance has reached its limit.[209] Fluid and eventually protein leaks through the serosa into the peritoneal cavity.

If the pressure is maintained, intestinal compliance allows blood flow to gradually increase, acting as a form of reperfusion. Serosal and submucosal edema progresses during the period of distention. The mucosal and serosal lymphatics dilate and RBCs and WBCs migrate into the serosa and submucosa. There is minimal mucosal injury at pressures seen in clinical cases during simple obstruction of the small intestine or colon.

Subsequent decompression of the bowel causes reperfusion with a hyperemic response similar to that seen after low-low or total ischemia. Blood flow to the affected bowel can initially double, but this effect is temporary, with subsequent blood flow decreasing below normal.[194] The mucosa appears relatively resistant to short-term distention, whereas the edema in the serosa causes capillary closure and increased vascular permeability. Serosal edema increases and more neutrophils migrate into the serosa, causing destruction of collagen and ground substance.[179,199,210] Intestinal smooth muscle is also affected, with edema and neutrophil migration evident in the fascial planes around the myenteric plexuses (Fig. 30-30). Though bowel can frequently heal after this type of ischemic insult, the serosa is often thickened by fibrous tissue, with the possibility of adhesion formation and permanent mesenteric constriction.[210]

Although the mucosa appears relatively resistant to the low-flow ischemia experienced with bowel distention, the response is time dependent. Rarely does prolonged distention cause bowel necrosis. Bowel wall necrosis is more common where focal distention is caused by foreign bodies or impactions. Because the response to distention is both time and pressure dependent, the time frame for permanent damage is difficult to determine. The small intestine is more susceptible to distention injury compared with the large colon. Clinical measurement of intraluminal pressure during ob-

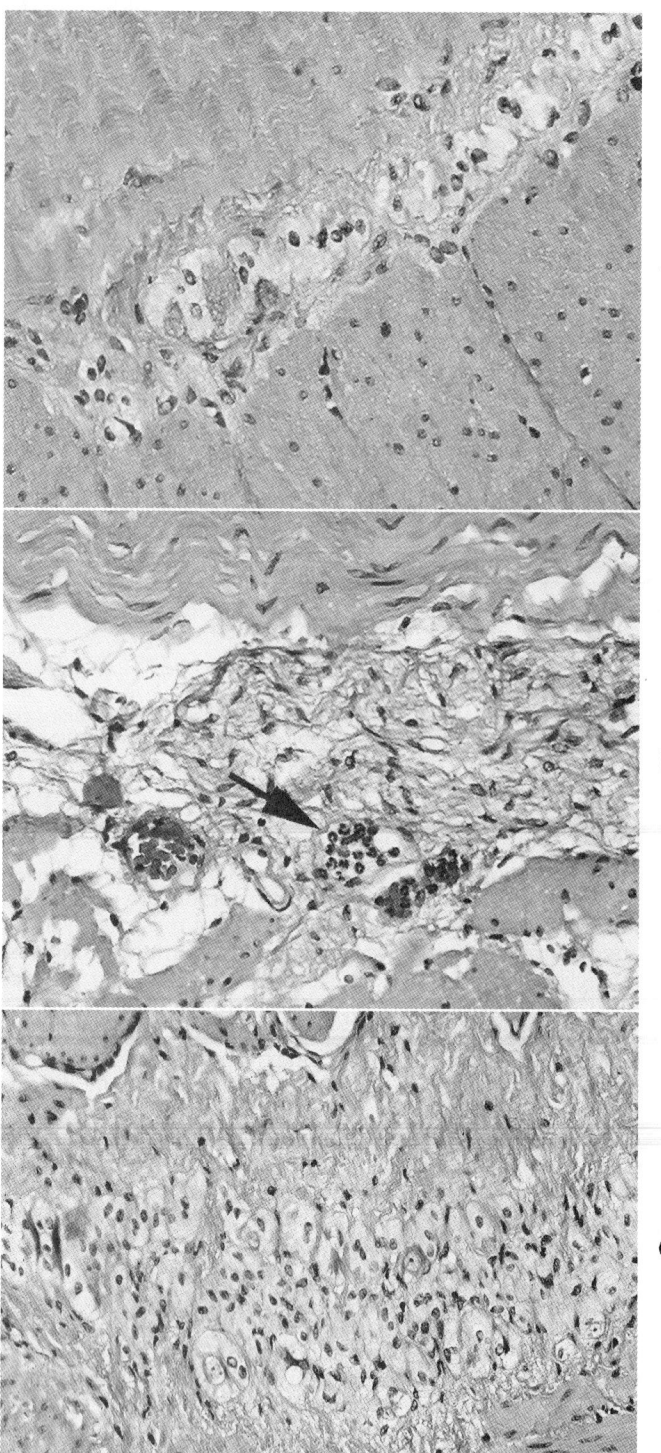

FIG. 30-30 ▪ Photomicrographs of myenteric plexuses from horses. **A,** Normal myenteric plexus with connective tissue surrounding an accumulation of neurons (×360, hematoxylin and eosin stain). **B,** Neutrophil infiltrate in the muscle and around a myenteric plexus after low-flow ischemia and reperfusion (×360, hematoxylin and eosin stain). **C,** Increased glial cells in the myenteric plexus from a horse with chronic obstruction due to large colon displacement (×360, hematoxylin and eosin stain).

struction indicates that the large colon can tolerate at least twice the distention pressure with no adverse affects.[211,212]

Intestinal dysfunction occurs after decompressing bowel that was previously obstructed. Ileus with gastric reflux is common in horses with previously distended small intestine, and the severity can be predicted by the bowel pressure measured

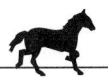

at surgery.[211,212] Although the injury from distention cannot be separated from conditions in the peritoneal cavity or failure of the cardiovascular system, the correlation of increased intraluminal pressures and survival indicates the importance of intestinal distention in causing injury.[193,194,208,210,211]

The enteric nervous system also appears to respond to intestinal distention. Chronic obstruction caused by impaction of the colon or cecum or colon displacement has been associated with a significant decrease in the number of neurons in the myenteric plexuses while the number of myenteric plexuses was similar to that in normal horses.[183,213] This change in neuron number was also associated with increased thickness of the longitudinal muscle in the pelvic flexure or both circular and longitudinal muscle hypertrophy in the cecum.[213] This appears similar to pseudoobstruction in humans and to experimental denervation of intestinal segments in rats. The lack of nervous inhibition is hypothesized to allow constant and uncoordinated muscular contractions with resulting hypertrophy and eventually poor transit of ingesta.

Myenteric plexuses from distended or obstructed large colons also had an increase in the number of glial cells (Fig. 30-30, C). This appears to be an inflammatory response by the enteric nervous system to the conditions involved with bowel distention. Alternatively the inflammation and neuron dropout may have been responsible for colon dysfunction in these horses examined because of colon obstruction.

INFECTION

Enteritis caused by infection is frequently caused by *Salmonella* sp., *Clostridia* sp., *Ehrlichia* sp. or virulent *E. coli*. Viruses such as rotavirus can also cause infection in foals, with subsequent clinical signs. These agents adhere to and attack mucosal cells. When bacteria bind to the mucosal cells the release of endotoxin or exotoxins causes the mucosal cell to release cytokines, which signal immunocytes and neutrophils of impending invasion. The gut has a large number of lymphocytes and macrophages in the lamina propria suggesting the constant stimulus by agents or substances.[154,214] Although the mucosal cell has an innate ability to resist infection, the communication between the immunocytes and the mucosa is likely the chief defense. The infection can change mucosal function without destroying the mucosal barrier, although increased TNF-α concentration has been shown to impair barrier function at the tight junctions.[215] The change can cause lack of absorption or massive secretion of fluid into the bowel causing diarrhea.

Functional secretion is caused by stimulation of adenylcyclase and guanylcyclase, which catalyze formation of cyclic adenosine monophosphate (cAMP) or cyclic guanosine monophosphate (cGMP), respectively. These cyclic nucleotides subsequently activate protein kinases that block the NaCl absorptive process in the absorptive mucosal cell and stimulate Cl secretion in the crypt cell.[216] Inflammation with release of eicosanoids and bradykinin can also initiate the secretory process. The enteric nervous system can also induce inflammation and secretion in the bowel, which can be inhibited by nerve blocking agents or indomethacin.[216,217] Neuropeptides from efferent nerves are hypothesized to initiate this response by affecting mucosal cells, fibroblasts, and endothelial cells.[158,218]

When bacteria cause injury by adhering to the mucosal surface and invading the mucosa, the response of the mucosal cells stimulates both the afferent nervous system and an immediate local immunocytes immune reaction. Cytokines from local macrophages or injured epithelial cells serve as the messengers of recognition that stimulate macrophages and polynucleated cells; both neutrophils and eosinophils to migrate to the region of invasion. Lymphocytes are also activated, releasing cytokines, including interferon-γ.

After an initial delay in mucosal cell apoptosis during bacterial adhesion and invasion, apoptosis is increased, theoretically to increase cell turnover and healing. TNF-α and nitric oxide appear to control mucosal cell apoptosis.

The inflammatory response to invasion often causes massive mucosal necrosis with loss of mucosal cells and a massive infiltrate of neutrophils and lymphoid cells. Fibrin exudate creates a cast on the mucosal surface of the bowel. The vasculature is exposed to the bowel lumen, allowing subsequent invasion of the bacteria, both pathogens and others, as well as bacterial toxins. The remaining mucosal cells are stimulated to secrete water via the stimulation of cAMP within the crypt cells. Water is also retained in the bowel because of the lack of absorptive cells; the result is diarrhea.

The infection can involve the other layers of the intestine, although it rarely involves the serosa. However, some diseases, such as hemorrhagic fibrinonecrotic duodentis-proximal jejunitis, affect all layers of the intestine. A causative organism has never been discovered to explain duodenitis-proximal jejunitis, although the lesion is similar to that seen with clostridial disease in young swine.[219] Similar to reperfusion injury, the inflammatory process creates dysfunction that can last for days. Long-term complications from duodenitis-proximal jejunitis have not been reported, but severe cases have not survived because of the lack of healing and severe residual inflammation in the bowel wall.[219]

PERITONEAL INFLAMMATION

The serosal layer is made of a single-cell mesothelial layer mounted on a layer of connective tissue This layer is important, to maintain a lubricated barrier at the bowel surface necessary for normal intestinal motility. The mesothelial layer attaches to a basement membrane, which is adjacent to an elastic layer. The mesothelial cells vary in type. Some are short and have channels linking the peritoneal surface to the serosa. Others have long microvilli that appear to help trap fluid on the surface of the peritoneum, providing the main mechanism of lubrication on the bowel surface. Mesothelial cells react to circulating or intraperitoneal lipopolysaccide, infection, and surgery by releasing TNF-α, IL-1β, IL-6, and macrophage inflammatory protein.[220] The response in the serosa is attraction and migration of neutrophils into the serosal connective tissue.

The initial response to serosal injury has been studied in laboratory animals predominantly by using scarification of organs or fecal contamination of the peritoneal surface. The response to ischemia or distention of the equine small intestine is similar though often more severe. During ischemia the mesothelium is rapidly lost, with subsequent serosal swelling with edema. During reperfusion the serosal vasculature becomes more permeable and polymorphonuclear cells and mononuclear cells migrate through capillaries or venules and infiltrate into the serosal connective tissue layer. Neutrophils accumulate at the basement membrane around vessels and within lymphatics. Fibrin accumulates within the serosa and on the surface. WBCs release lysozmes, resulting in disruption of collagen, the primary ground substance of the serosa. The denuded serosal surface is covered with a fibrin clot. After 24 to 48 hours there is massive accumulation of cells, predominately neutrophils, within the serosa and at the new surface.

Cytokines are involved in the response to serosal injury and the subsequent healing.[221,222] After intestinal anastomosis in rabbits, macrophages increased in number until about day four. Superoxide levels in these cells is high in the first 24 hours. Prostaglandins, cytokine secretion, and plasminogen activator inhibitor activity are known to increase during the first three days after peritoneal injury. Interleukin-1, and TNF-α are secreted by peritoneal macrophages after injury and appear to modulate peritoneal healing.[222] Peritoneal macrophages also secrete plasminogen activator. The secretion of both plasminogen activator and plasminogen activator inhibitor is stimulated by interleukin-1. After intestinal anastomosis there is a decrease in fibrinolytic activity for the first 5 days. Thereafter, plasminogen activator returns to the normal preoperative level. Normally fibrin will be dissolved by plasmin after plasminogen is activated by tissue plasminogen activator. The severity of the serosal injury is also related to the reduction of tissue plasminogen activator and to the suppression of plasminogen activator normally produced by macrophages. If plasminogen is not activated or is absent, adhesions have a greater likelihood of becoming fibrous and permanent.

As healing progresses, fibroblasts migrate into the fibrin and a layer of granulation tissue forms both beneath and on top of the original basement membrane. Mesothelial cells produce connective tissue growth factor in response to IL-1β, which simulates fibroblast proliferation.[162] During this stage, IL-1 stimulates and PGE_2 inhibits fibroblast activity in the injured serosa. Primordial stem cells migrate to the surface and change to form a new mesothelium, a metaplasia likely under the control of growth factor from fibroblasts. The greater the inflammatory reaction is within the serosa and on the surface, the more fibroplasia occurs, delaying mesothelium resurfacing and increasing the chance for adhesion formation or bowel scarring. Experimentally the severity of adhesions is correlated with increasing concentrations of TNF-α in peritoneal fluid, and antibodies against TNF-α can decrease adhesion formation.[223,224] Healing of the serosa may not result in bowel-to-bowel adhesions but can still cause bowel and mesenteric scarring, which can cause lumen narrowing or kinking. The serosa also becomes thickened, which may result in bowel dysfunction or interrupt the vascular supply.

In the horse the serosal injury is frequently due to bowel distention. The cellular injury is similar to an inflammatory model except for the vascular sequelae. After small intestinal ischemia there is an initial vascular hyperemia in most of the bowel but a reduction of perfusion to the serosa. This same effect occurs during bowel distention and is even greater after alleviating distention. The edema formation in distended bowel takes place immediately and increases serosal tissue pressure, which exerts extravascular pressure and closes capillaries and venules.[193,194] This continues after bowel decompression, resulting in ischemic injury during reperfusion. Reperfusion after decreasing bowel distention also causes serosal endothelial cell swelling and capillary plugging. This helps to explain the adhesions seen in bowel that was only distended proximal to an obstruction or strangulating lesion but was otherwise not involved in an ischemic lesion.

Adhesions resulting from septic peritonitis occur in response to a massive inflammatory response in the serosa. Similar to the response to ischemia there is neutrophil migration and fibrin deposition in and on the serosa.[221] The inflammatory response may be so great that the lysozmes may prevent adhesion between bowel loops by breaking down fibrin. However, in most cases there is massive fibrin production and frequent bowel-to-bowel adhesions.

BOWEL HEALING

After ischemic damage the mucosa heals rapidly.[206,225] Enterocytes migrate along the lamina propria covering the surface within 24 to 38 hours. In the mucosa the crypt cells are responsible for rapid multiplication and physically forcing the older cells to the mucosal surface. Delayed healing is associated with a massive inflammatory response, which can stimulate delayed epithelial apoptosis and lack of cell replacement.[152,226] Connective tissue growth factor stimulates mucosal

growth and may be responsible excessive fibrosis in chronic inflammatory disease.[227]

Similarly the serosal mesothelium also heals rapidly after loss from abrasion, although it takes longer than the mucosa to heal with a functional cell boundary. The mesothelial cells come from multipotent stem cells in the serosal connective tissues. These migrate to the serosal surface and form an initial layer of cuboidal cells before transforming to the more characteristic flattened mesothelial cell. The healing time appears to be dependent on amount of inflammation and subsequent production of fibrous tissue on the serosal surface.

Although healing is thought to be successful when clinical signs of colic, obstruction, or peritonitis are no longer observed, the latent effect of serosal fibrosis, residual mucosal inflammation, and ganglionitis with loss of neurons may increase the risk of future colic episodes. Horses that have had a colic episode or previous abdominal surgery are 3 to 4 times more likely to have a second colic episode than the horse that has never had colic.[196] Whether chronic inflammation is responsible for recurrent colic has not been determined.

REFERENCES

152. Fiocchi C: Intestinal inflammation: a complex interplay of immune and nonimmune cell interactions, *Am J Physiol* 273:g769-g775, 1997.
153. Kim JM et al: Apoptosis of human intestinal epithelial cells after bacterial invasion, *J Clin Invest* 102:1815-1823, 1998.
154. Kunkel SL, Lukacs N, Strieter RM: Cytokines and inflammatory disease. In: Sirica AE, ed: *Cellular and molecular pathogenesis*, Philadelphia, 1996, Lippincott-Raven, pp 23-35.
155. Uguccioni M et al: Increased expression of IP-10, IL-8, MCP-1, and MCP-3 in ulcerative colitis, *Am J Pathol* 155:331-336, 1999.
156. MacDermott RP: Chemokines in the inflammatory bowel diseases, *J Clin Immunol* 19:266-272, 1999.
157. Payan DG: The role of neuropeptides in inflammation. In Gallin JI, Goldstein IM, Synderman R, eds: *Inflammation: basic principles and clinical disorders*, ed 2, New York, 1992, Raven Press, pp 177-192.
158. Raithel M, Schneider HT, Hahn EG: Effect of substance P on histamine secretion from gut mucosa in inflammatory bowel disease, *Scand J Gastroenterol* 34:496-503, 1999.
159. Keates AC et al: CGRP upregulation in dorsal root ganglia and ileal mucosa during *Clostridium difficile* toxin A-induced enteritis, *Am J Physiol* 274(1 Pt 1):G196-202, 1998.
160. Mayer EA, Raybould H, Koelbel C: Neuropeptides, inflammation, and motility, *Dig Dis Sci* 33(suppl 3):71S-77S, 1988.
161. Postlethwaite AE, Kang AH: Fibroblasts and matrix proteins. In Gallin JI, Goldstein IM, Synderman R, eds: *Inflammation: basic principles and clinical correlates*, ed 2, New York, 1992, Raven Press, pp 747-773.
162. Cronauer MV et al: Basic fibroblast growth factor synthesis by human peritoneal mesothelial cells: induction by interleukin-1, *Am J Pathol* 155:1977-1984, 1999.
163. Van Assche G et al: Neurotransmitters modulate cytokine-stimulated interleukin 6 secretion in rat intestinal smooth muscle cells, *Gastroenterology* 116:346-353, 1999.
164. Kalff JC et al: Surgically induced leukocytic infiltrates within the rat intestinal muscularis mediate postoperative ileus [see comments], *Gastroenterology* 117:378-387, 1999.
165. Kalff JC et al: Biphasic response to gut manipulation and temporal correlation of cellular infiltrates and muscle dysfunction in rat, *Surgery* 126:498-509, 1999.
166. Moore RM, Muir WW, Granger DN: Mechanisms of gastrointestinal ischemia-reperfusion injury and potential therapeutic interventions: a review and its implications in the horse, *J Vet Intern Med* 9:115-132, 1995.
167. Bueno L, Fioramonti J: Effects of inflammatory mediators on gut sensitivity, *Can J Gastroenterol* 13(suppl A):42A-46A, 1999.
168. Collins SM et al: Effect of inflammation of enteric nerves: cytokine-induced changes in neurotransmitter content and release, *Ann N Y Acad Sci* 664:415-424, 1992.
169. Mercer-Jones MA et al: Neutrophil sequestration in liver and lung is differentially regulated by C-X-C chemokines during experimental peritonitis, *Inflammation* 23:305-319, 1999.
170. Neumann B et al: Mechanisms of acute inflammatory lung injury induced by abdominal sepsis, *Int Immunol* 11:217-227, 1999.
171. Koike K et al: Gut ischemia/reperfusion produces lung injury independent of endotoxin, *Crit Care Med* 22:1438-1444, 1994.
172. Brown R et al: Ultrastructural changes in the canine ileal mucosal cell after mesenteric arterial occlusion, *Arch Surg* 101:290-297, 1970.
173. Paller MS, Greene EL: Role of calcium in reperfusion injury of the kidney, *Ann NY Acad Sci* 723:59-70, 1994.

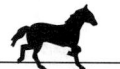
174. White NA, Moore JN, Trim CM: Mucosal alterations in experimentally induced small intestinal strangulation obstruction in ponies, *Am J Vet Res* 41:193-198, 1980.
175. Sullins KE, Stashak TS, Mero KN: Pathologic changes associated with induced small intestinal strangulation obstruction and nonstrangulating infarction in horses, *Am J Vet Res* 46:913-916, 1985.
176. Snyder JR et al: Comparison of histologic findings in naturally occurring colon torsion and experimental colonic ischemia, *Vet Surg* 15:134-135, 1986.
177. Kurose I, Granger DN: Evidence implicating xanthine oxidase and neutrophils in reperfusion-induced microvascular dysfunction, *Ann N Y Acad Sci* 273:158-179, 1994.
178. Nalini S, Mathan MM, Balasubramanian KA: Oxygen free radical induced damage during intestinal ischemia/reperfusion in normal and xanthine oxidase deficient rats, *Mol Cell Biochem* 124:59-66, 1993.
179. Gerard MP et al: The characteristics of intestinal injury peripheral to strangulating obstruction lesions in the equine small intestine, *Equine Vet J* 31:331-335, 1999.
180. Meschter CL et al: Histologic findings in the gastrointestinal tract of horses with colic, *Am J Vet Res* 47:598-606, 1986.
181. Blikslager AT et al: How important is intestinal reperfusion injury in horses? *J Am Vet Med Assoc* 211:1387-1389, 1997 [see comments].
182. White NA, Young BL, Donaldson LL: Unpublished data, Leesburg, Va, 1999, Virginia Polytechnic Institute.
183. Moore RM et al: Histopathologic evidence of reperfusion injury in the large colon of horses after low-flow ischemia, *Am J Vet Res* 55:1434-1443, 1994.
184. Kooreman K, Babbs C, Fessler J: Effect of ischemia and reperfusion on oxidative processes in the large colon and jejunum of horses, *Am J Vet Res* 59:340-346, 1998.
185. Hierholzer C et al: Molecular and functional contractile sequelae of rat intestinal ischemia/reperfusion injury, *Transplantation* 68:1244-1254, 1999.
186. Schusser GE, White NA: Morphologic and quantitative evaluation of the myenteric plexuses and neurons in the large colon of horses, *J Am Vet Med Assoc* 210:928-934, 1997.
187. Burns GA, Karcher LF, Cummings JF: Equine myenteric ganglionitis: a case of chronic intestinal pseudo-obstruction, *Cornell Vet* 80:53-63, 1990.
188. Dabareiner RM et al: Microvascular permeability and endothelial cell morphology associated with low-flow ischemia/reperfusion injury in the equine jejunum, *Am J Vet Res* 56:639-648, 1995.
189. Dabareiner RM, White NA: Large colon impaction in horses: 147 cases (1985-1991) [published erratum appears in *J Am Vet Med Assoc* 206(10):1574, 1995], *J Am Vet Med Assoc* 206:679-685, 1995.
190. Henninger DD et al: Microvascular permeability changes in ischemia/reperfusion injury in the ascending colon of horses, *J Am Vet Med Assoc* 201:1191-1196, 1992.
191. Prichard M et al: Xanthine oxidase formation during experimental ischemia of the equine small intestine, *Can J Vet Res* 55:310-314, 1991.
192. Dabareiner RM et al: Evaluation of the microcirculation of the equine jejunum and ascending colon after ischemia and reperfusion, *Am J Vet Res* 54:1683-1692, 1993.
193. Dabareiner RM et al: Evaluation of the microvasculature in equine large and small intestine following distention or ischemia and reperfusion using scanning electron microscopy, microangiography, and light microscopy, *Vet Surg* 20:333, 1991.
194. Dabareiner RM, White NA, Donaldson LL: Effects of intraluminal distention and decompression on the microvascular permeability and hemodynamics of the equine jejunum, *Am J Vet Res* 62:225-236, 2001.
195. Eskandari MK et al: Lipopolysaccharide activates jejunal muscularis macrophages and suppresses circular muscularis activity, *Transplant Proc* 30:2670, 1998.
196. Cohen ND et al: Case-control study of the association between various management factors and development of colic in horses. Texas Equine Colic Study Group, *J Am Vet Med Assoc* 206: 667-673, 1995.
197. White NA: Intestinal infarction associated with mesenteric vascular thrombotic disease in the horse, *J Am Vet Med Assoc* 178:259-262, 1981.
198. Kalff JC et al: Hemorrhagic shock results in intestinal muscularis intercellular adhesion molecule (ICAM-1) expression, neutrophil infiltration, and smooth muscle dysfunction, *Arch Orthop Trauma Surg* 119:89-93, 1999.
199. Schmall LM, Argenzio RA, Whipp SC: Effects of intravenous *Escherichia coli* endotoxin on gastrointestinal function in the pony, *Proceedings of the Equine Colic Research Symposium*, Athens, Ga, Sept 1982.
200. Snyder JR et al: Angioarchitecture of normal and ischemic equine colon: a correlative study using scanning electron microscopy of vascular replicas, microangiography, and light microscopy, *Vet Surg* 18:67, 1989.
201. Snyder JR et al: Ultrastructural mucosal injury after experimental ischemia of the ascending colon in horses, *Am J Vet Res* 53:1917-1924, 1992.
202. Darien BJ et al: Morphologic changes of the ascending colon during experimental ischemia and reperfusion in ponies, *Vet Pathol* 32:280-288, 1995.
203. Kawcak CE et al: Abnormalities in oxygenation, coagulation, and fibrinolysis in colonic blood of horses with experimentally induced strangulation obstruction, *Am J Vet Res* 56:1642-1650, 1995.
204. Reeves MJ et al: Failure to demonstrate reperfusion injury following ischaemia of the equine large colon using dimethyl sulphoxide, *Equine Vet J* 22:126-132, 1990.
205. Moore RM et al: Neutrophil accumulation in the large colon of horses during low-flow ischemia and reperfusion, *Am J Vet Res* 55:1454-1463, 1994.
206. White NA, Moore JN, Trim CM: Mucosal healing response 48 hours after experimental intestinal strangulation obstruction, *Proceedings of the Equine Colic Research Symposium*, Athens, Ga, Sept 1982.
207. Laws EG, Freeman DE: Significance of reperfusion injury after venous strangulation obstruction of equine jejunum, *J Invest Surg* 8:263-270, 1995.
208. Allen D Jr, White NA II, Tyler DE: Morphologic effects of experimental distention of equine small intestine, *Vet Surg* 17:10-14, 1988.
209. Donawick WJ, Ramberg CF Jr, Topkis GA: Absorption and secretion of water and electrolytes by normal and obstructed ileum of ponies, *Proceedings of the Equine Colic Research Symposium*, Athens, Ga, Sept 1982.
210. Lundin C et al: Induction of peritoneal adhesions with small intestinal ischaemia and distention in the foal, *Equine Vet J* 21:451-458, 1989.
211. Moore RM et al: Colonic luminal pressure in horses with strangulating and nonstrangulating obstruction of the large colon, *Vet Surg* 25:134-141, 1996.
212. Allen D Jr, White NA, Tyler DE: Factors for prognostic use in equine obstructive small intestinal disease, *J Am Vet Med Assoc* 189:777-780, 1986.
213. Schusser GF, Scheidemann W, Huskamp B: Muscle layer thickness and neuron density in the cecum of horses with chronic recurrent cecal impaction, *Proceedings of the Sixth Annual Equine Colic Research Symposium*, Athens, Ga, 1998.
214. Woywodt A et al: Mucosal cytokine expression, cellular markers and adhesion molecules in inflammatory bowel disease, *Eur J Gastroenterol Hepatol* 11:267-276, 1999.
215. Schmitz H et al: Tumor necrosis factor-alpha (TNF-alpha) regulates the epithelial barrier in the human intestinal cell line HT-29/B6, *J Cell Sci* 112(Pt 1):137-146, 1999.
216. Argenzio RA: Pathophysiology of diarrhea. In Anderson NV, ed: *Veterinary gastroenterology*, ed 2, Philadelphia, 1992, Lea and Febiger, pp 163-172.
217. Clarke LL, Argenzio RA: NaCl transport across equine proximal colon and the effect of endogenous prostanoids, *Am J Physiol* 259:g62-g69, 1990.
218. Roberts MC, Clarke LL, Johnson CM: Castor-oil induced diarrhoea in ponies: a model for acute colitis, *Equine Vet J* 7:60-67, 1989.
219. White NA et al: Hemorrhagic fibrinonecrotic duodenitis-proximal jejunitis in horses: 20 cases (1977-1984), *J Am Vet Med Assoc* 190:311-315, 1987.
220. Tsukada K et al: Concentrations of cytokines in peritoneal fluid after abdominal surgery, *Eur J Surg* 159:475-479, 1993.
221. Flessner MF: Changes in the peritoneal interstitium and their effect on peritoneal transport, *Perit Dial Int* 19(suppl 2):S77-S82, 1999.
222. Rogers KE, diZerega GS: Function of peritoneal exudate cells after abdominal surgery, *J Invest Surg* 6:9-23, 1993.
223. Kaidi AA et al: Tumor necrosis factor-alpha: a marker for peritoneal adhesion formation, *J Surg Res* 58:516-518, 1995.
224. Kaidi AA et al: Preoperative administration of antibodies against tumor necrosis factor-alpha (TNF-alpha) and interleukin-1 (IL-1) and their impact on peritoneal adhesion formation, *Am Surg* 61:569-572, 1995.
225. Freeman DE et al: Early mucosal healing and chronic changes in pony jejunum after various types of strangulation obstruction, *Am J Vet Res* 49:810-818, 1988.
226. Papaconstantinou HT et al: Glutamine deprivation induces apoptosis in intestinal epithelial cells, *Surgery* 124:152-159; discussion 159-160, 1998.
227. Dammeier J et al: Connective tissue growth factor: a novel regulator of mucosal repair and fibrosis in inflammatory bowel disease? *Int J Biochem Cell Biol* 30:909-922, 1998.

ENDOTOXEMIA

ROBERT J. MacKAY

The heat-stable endotoxic activity identified by Pfeiffer more than 100 years ago resides in lipopolysaccharide (LPS), the principal component of the outer leaflet of the outer membrane of all gram-negative bacteria. Each LPS molecule has three structural domains: a polar polysaccharide O-region, which projects into the aqueous extracellular environment, a hydrophobic lipid A region, which is largely buried in the bacterial outer membrane, and a core acidic polysaccharide region connecting the two. The O-region is highly variable and contains antigens specific for each bacterial strain, whereas the core glycolipid region is relatively constant among bacteria and mediates most of the toxic effects of endotoxin. On bacterial death or during bacterial proliferation, large (>10^6-dalton molecular mass) aggregates of LPS and membrane protein are released. It is these protein/lipid micelles that constitute native endotoxin and are to be found circulating in naturally acquired cases of endotoxemia.

Endotoxemia is the presence of endotoxin in the blood. When the term is used clinically, it additionally implies the presence of clinical signs caused by circulating endotoxin. This term should not be confused with either *bacteremia*, which refers only to the presence of viable circulating bacteria, or *septicemia*, which is an older term referring to systemic disease caused by circulating microorganisms or their products.

The ability to respond to minute local concentrations of endotoxin by mounting vigorous inflammatory responses is well conserved across species. The gene for the putative LPS receptor of mammals has high sequence homology with the toll gene of fruit flies. Thomas[228] captured nicely the importance of recognition of endotoxin:

> The gram-negative bacteria . . . display lipopolysaccharide . . . in their walls and these macromolecules are read by our tissues as the very worst of bad news. When we sense lipopolysaccharides we are likely to turn on every defense at our disposal; we will bomb, defoliate, blockade, seal off, and destroy all tissues in the area. . . . Cells believe that it signifies the presence of gram-negative bacteria, and they will stop at nothing to avoid this threat.

In the years since this observation was made, a bewildering and biochemically diverse array of endotoxin-induced "bombs" and "defoliants" have been identified. These have included polypeptides, lipids, peptidolipids, molecular radicals, and gases. When properly localized and regulated, these responses serve to protect the host from harmful gram-negative bacterial infections; however, when endotoxin spills into the systemic circulation, global activation of the same inflammatory systems that normally are protective may result in widespread destruction of host tissues and the clinical signs of endotoxic shock. As the yin and yang of inflammation progresses, endogenous *counter-regulatory* systems usually quench inflammation and move to restore homeostasis. If the counter-regulatory response is insufficient, the "auto-cannibalistic" events of the *systemic inflammatory response syndrome* may ensue. Conversely, if the counter-regulatory response is disproportionately large, the endotoxic animal may be tipped into a state of profound and harmful immunosuppression.

Pathophysiology of Endotoxemia

Although the processes initiated by endotoxemia are extremely complex, a sequence of events can be discerned that is critical to the development of associated clinical signs. The following is a description of these events beginning with the initial contact between endotoxin and blood, progressing through humoral and cellular innate inflammatory responses that culminate in death, immunosuppression, or recovery.

STAGE 1: THE PHYSICAL BARRIERS TO ENDOTOXIN ARE BREACHED. Although endotoxin is ubiquitous in the environment, both free and as a component of gram-negative bacteria, it normally is excluded from the body by the skin and mucous membranes. If the protective integument or mucosae are subjected to gram-negative bacterial infection or otherwise damaged, endotoxin may reach the blood in sufficient amount (<1 μg in experimental situations) to cause clinical signs. Gram-negative bacterial enterocolitis (e.g., salmonellosis), metritis, pleuropneumonia, wound infection, and neonatal septicemia are common examples. Because gram amounts of free endotoxin normally are safely sequestered within the intestine of the adult horse, damage to the gut wall as a result of local (e.g., bowel volvulus, infarction, incarceration) or systemic (e.g., hypovolemic shock)

ischemia, inflammation (e.g., duodenitis/proximal jejunitis or clostridial enteritis), mechanical trauma (e.g., rectal perforation, prolonged exercise[?]), or intraluminal acidification (e.g., grain overload) is particularly likely to result in endotoxemia. In highly contaminated environments, potentially harmful amounts of endotoxin can be introduced into the lungs via inhalation.[229] Endotoxin may even be delivered directly into the blood via parenteral solutions (e.g., homemade intravenous fluids).

STAGE 2: ENDOTOXIN INTERACTS WITH CELLS AND PROTEINS OF BLOOD TO PRODUCE INFLAMMATORY MEDIATORS. Most data support the notion that the interaction of endotoxin with mononuclear phagocytes (i.e., monocytes and macrophages) is a pivotal early event in the development of the signs of endotoxemia. When endotoxin contacts blood, some is neutralized by anti-LPS antibodies produced as a result of prior endotoxin exposure; however, most endotoxin binds to LPS-binding protein (LBP), a normal plasma constituent.[230] The endotoxin-LBP complex in turn binds to CD14 on the membranes of intravascular macrophages and, to a lesser extent, monocytes.[231] Pulmonary intravascular macrophages,[232] and Kupffer cells likely are the most important macrophages in this regard. Endotoxin apparently is shuttled from CD14 to toll-like receptor molecules that aggregate with other membrane proteins to initiate intracellular responses.[233]

An important early intracellular event is the activation of nuclear factor β (NF-κB), which induces transcription of a broad array of genes including a small group of extremely potent inflammatory polypeptides known as cytokines.[234] Of particular importance are tumor necrosis factor α (TNF-α) and interleukin 1β (IL-1β).[235] NF-κB activity is affected positively or negatively by many of the mediators found in the inflammatory milieu. Although IL-1 and TNF are unrelated structurally, they share many inflammatory actions of relevance to the pathogenesis of endotoxemia. These cytokines engage specific cell-surface receptors on macrophages and other cells to boost their own secretion and to induce the production of several other cytokines important in the pathogenesis of endotoxemia. In this way, there is tremendous amplification of the original endotoxin signal (note that this amplification can continue in the absence of endotoxin). The second wave of inflammatory cytokines includes granulocyte-monocyte colony stimulating factor (GM-CSF), chemokines, and IL-6.[236] Chemokines are chemoattractant for neutrophils and, with GM-CSF, may accelerate production and release of neutrophils from the bone marrow. IL-6 contributes to endotoxin lethality, as shown by the protective effect of anti–IL-6 in *Escherichia coli* septic shock.[237] TNF, IL-1, and IL-6 not only act locally, but also stimulate "stress" hormone (e.g., cortisol, epinephrine) release and, with macrophage inflammatory peptides, are systemic endogenous pyrogens.

During this period there also is induction, principally in macrophages and endothelial cells, of three important enzymes that, in comparison with constitutive homologues, generate massive amounts of product: (1) cyclooxygenase II (COX-II), which produces prostanoids such as thromboxane, prostacyclin (prostaglandin I_2), and prostaglandin E_2 (PGE$_2$)[238]; (2) inducible nitric oxide synthase (iNOS), which catalyzes formation of nitric oxide (NO) from arginine[239,240]; and (3) heme oxygenase 1, which processes heme to bile pigments and carbon monoxide (CO).[241] These products have potent regulatory effects and are discussed further below.

Simultaneous with cellular activation, endotoxin interacts with normal plasma and tissue proteins to initiate enzymatic reactions that culminate in the production of important mediators of inflammation and hemostasis (Figure 30-31). Thus, via the "contact" system of plasma, endotoxin activates coagulation factor XII (Hageman factor), leading both to lib-

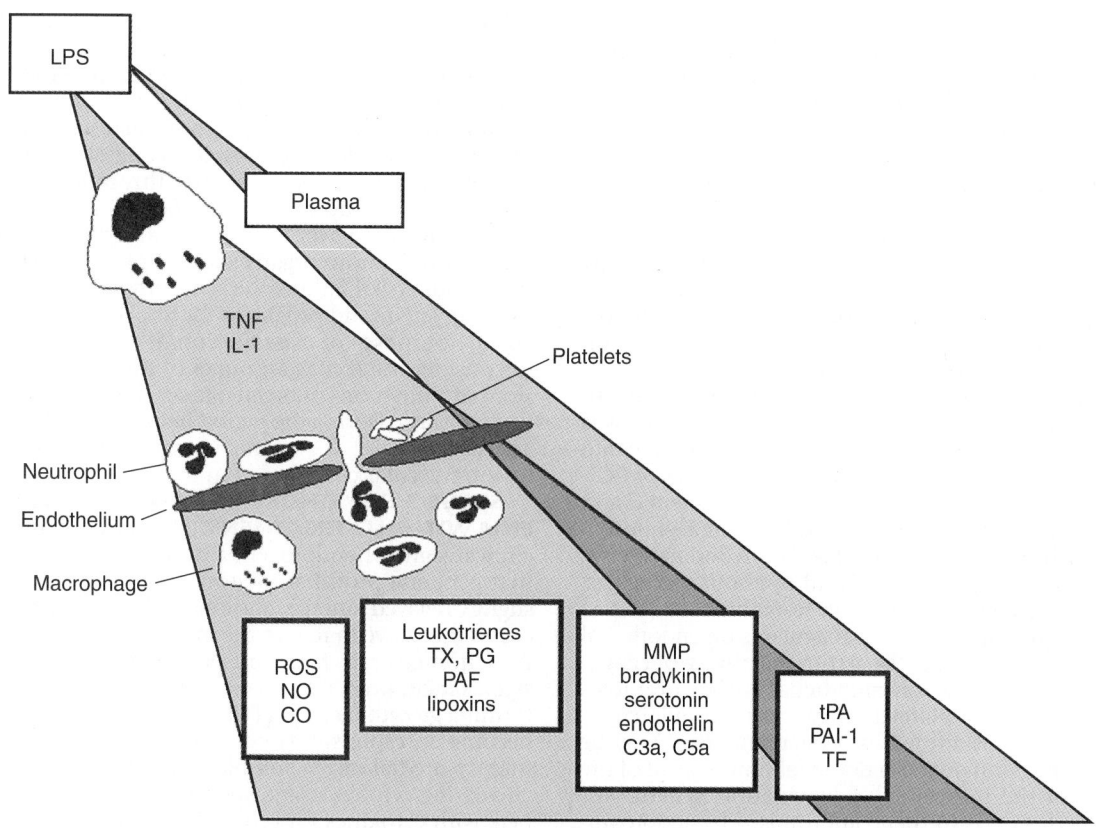

FIG. 30-31 ▓ Endotoxin interacts with cells and plasma to generate inflammatory, vasoactive, and coagulant mediators. The diagram depicts initial contact of endotoxin with plasma and mononuclear phagocytes. Production of inflammatory cytokines by activated mononuclear phagocytes leads to neutrophil-endothelial conjugation and extravasation of neutrophils and other cells. These cells penetrate into tissues producing multiple mediators with overlapping activities. Damage to endothelial surfaces causes aggregation and adhesion of platelets. *CO,* Carbon monoxide; *IL-1,* interleukin 1; *LPS,* lipopolysaccharide; *MMP,* matrix metalloproteinases; *NO,* nitric oxide; *PAF,* platelet-activating factor; *PAI-1,* plasminogen activator inhibitor type 1; *PG,* prostaglandins; *ROS,* reactive oxygen species; *TF,* tissue factor; *TNF,* tumor necrosis factor; *tPA,* tissue plasminogen activator; *TX,* thromboxane.

eration of bradykinin and to initiation of intravascular coagulation. Bradykinin causes venular dilation, increased vascular permeability, and stimulation of neutrophils. Even more importantly, complement is activated by both alternative and classical pathways to yield numerous active peptide products. The anaphylatoxins C3a, C4a, and C5a increase vascular permeability, cause vasodilatation, and have indirect proinflammatory action via induction of mast cell degranulation. C5a also has potent chemotactic and activating activities for neutrophils, monocytes, and macrophages. In rodents, neutralization of C5a has been shown to prevent the lethal effect of endotoxin.[242]

STAGE 3: NEUTROPHILS BIND TO ENDOTHELIAL CELLS AND BECOME ACTIVATED. In response to inflammatory cytokines and complement peptides, endothelial cells express P- and E-selectins and other adhesion molecules.[243] These adhesion molecules "tether" leukocytes via specific cell-membrane ligands (including L-selectin/CD62), and a series of transient interactions between ligands and receptors allows leukocytes to roll along the endothelial surface. Leukocyte capture is most efficient in areas of low shear force, such as the walls of postcapillary venules. During rolling, leukocytes are activated, or "triggered," by selectins, chemokines, and platelet-activating factor (PAF) expressed on endothelial cells. The firm attachment or arrest step of the cascade is mediated by the avid interaction of leukocyte integrins with adhesion molecules of the immunoglobulin superfamily expressed on endothelial cells. During firm attachment, the activated leukocyte spreads out and then squeezes between the intercellular junctions of adjacent endothelial cells. Extravasation of neutrophils accounts for the leukopenia found in most horses with endotoxemia.

As neutrophils become activated and exit the vascular system, "respiratory burst" activity is stimulated and partial degranulation occurs. Such activity is heightened by exposure to inflammatory mediators or phagocytosis of particulate antigen. The NADPH-oxidase–dependent respiratory burst generates toxic but short-lived reactive oxygen species (ROS), including superoxide anion, singlet oxygen, hydrogen peroxide, and hydroxyl radical.[244] In the presence of granule myeloperoxidase,[245] highly toxic hypohalous acids (usually hypochlorous acid) are formed that are corrosive to subendothelial tissues.[246] Other neutrophil granule contents including matrix metalloproteinases (MMP) facilitate the destructive passage of neutrophils across the basement membrane and through tissues.[247] Endothelium is thought also to be an important source of ROS, reflecting the activity of endotoxin-induced xanthine oxidase.[248] During initial passage of neutrophils into inflamed tissues, activation of membrane phospholipase A_2 begins the rapid processing of membrane phospholipids into lipid or peptidolipid mediators such as PAF and leukotriene B_4 (LTB_4). The importance of neutrophil extravasation in the pathogenesis of endotoxemia is evident from the observation that pretreatment of mice with antibodies against CD18, a component of neutrophil integrins, protects against endotoxin-induced mortality.[249]

Once cytokine-initiated activation of neutrophils and endothelial cells occurs, the process may become self-sustaining and malignant. Additional neutrophils are recruited via local secretion of chemokines and LTB$_4$, then activated by these and other locally produced mediators such as PAF (neutrophils) and IL-1 (endothelium). Many of the activities of activated neutrophils are glucose-dependent, and widespread neutrophil activation contributes to hypoglycemia, especially in cases of endotoxemia of neonates.

Global activation of inflammatory systems by mediators derived from plasma and cells is known as the systemic inflammatory response syndrome (SIRS).

STAGE 4: ORGAN PERFUSION IS COMPROMISED. In health the antithrombotic phenotype of endothelial cells is maintained by expression of thrombomodulin and heparan sulfate proteoglycan species, presence of low amounts of PGI$_2$ and NO, and receptor-mediated engagement of protein C and tissue plasminogen activator. During endotoxemia, endothelium supports thrombosis because of leukocyte-induced physical damage, loss of expression of antithrombotic molecules, and up-regulation of plasminogen activator inhibitor 1 (PAI-1) and procoagulant tissue factor. Procoagulants on endothelial cells and phagocytes activate the extrinsic pathway of coagulation; thrombin formation on endothelial surfaces promotes platelet adherence, and platelet activation is stimulated by surface-bound PAF. Additional procoagulant effect may be provided by deposition on the endothelial surface of all of the components of the intravascular coagulation system. Microvascular perfusion is further compromised by endotoxin-induced increase in "stiffness" of both red and white blood cells.[250] Such cells are unable to deform and squeeze through small capillaries.

The effect of endotoxemia on vascular tone depends upon the stage and severity of disease and the particular organ (vascular bed) considered. In the early, pre-TNF phase of experimental endotoxemia, the vasoconstrictive effect of thromboxane is predominant. This effect is especially pronounced in the pulmonary circulation, probably because of the presence of pulmonary intravascular macrophages, and is evident clinically as tachypnea and arterial hypoxemia. It is likely that vasoconstrictors such as arginine vasopressin, angiotensin II, serotonin, norepinephrine, and endothelin are important in the pathogenesis of signs of endotoxemia such as mucous membrane pallor, colic, ileus, and laminitis. In contrast, in the later (post-TNF) stages of high-dosage experimental endotoxemia (and probably also in most naturally acquired cases), there is widespread vasodilation in response to cytokine-induced mediators such as prostacyclin, PGE$_2$ and bradykinin. Nitric oxide and CO are potent endotoxin-induced vasodilators in many species, but their contributions (if any) to the signs of equine endotoxemia have not yet been determined.

Endotoxin-induced mediators such as bradykinin, PAF, C3a, C5a, and LTB$_4$ increase vascular permeability, thereby facilitating the movement of plasma mediators into tissues. Damage to endothelium and basement membranes of all vascular beds by ROS, MMP, local hypoxia, and extravasating neutrophils further permits leakage of plasma into the interstitial spaces. This vascular leak syndrome, if severe, is evident clinically as subcutaneous edema.

The consequences of vasodilatation, vascular leakage, and intravascular cellular plugging and coagulation are systemic arterial hypotension and inadequate tissue perfusion. The effect of tissue hypoperfusion is compounded by an endotoxin-induced defect in oxygen extraction by tissues. Cytokine-induced myocardial depression impairs cardiac function contributing further to hemodynamic failure. Anaerobic glycolysis combined with direct inhibition of pyruvate dehydrogenase by endotoxin generate intense local lactic acidosis.

Impaired organ function (often described as *multiple organ dysfunction syndrome*) may be evident clinically as any combination of stupor and incoordination (central nervous system), weak arterial pulses and congested mucous membranes (cardiovascular system), thrombosis or bleeding diathesis (dyshemostasis), renal failure, ileus and colic (intestine), icterus (liver), laminitis, and respiratory distress. When two or more organs show clinical and clinicopathologic evidence of failure, the syndrome is described as *multiple organ failure* and prognosis for recovery becomes guarded. For the purposes of classification, it probably is reasonable to consider the feet as an organ of the horse. With progression, combinations of organ damage become irreversible and death ensues. During the period before death, blood pressure actually may rise as systemic vascular resistance is increased by intravascular coagulation in multiple capillary beds.

STAGE 5: SOME HORSES RECOVER FROM ENDOTOXEMIA WITHOUT TREATMENT. Obviously, most horses with clinical signs of endotoxemia do not die. The same stimuli that generate proinflammatory responses also evoke, with slightly delayed kinetics, antiinflammatory or regulatory molecules that serve to rein in the inflammatory response and restore homeostasis. Macrophages are exposed to deactivating signals including PGE$_2$, IL-4, IL-10, IL-13, cortisol, and transforming growth factor β (TGF-β). Furthermore, macrophages become unresponsive (tolerant) to the actions of proinflammatory mediators.[251] Soluble cytokine receptors neutralize circulating cytokines, and specific receptor antagonists compete with cytokines for cell-surface receptors. In the yin and yang of inflammation, all of the proinflammatory cascades of plasma proteins induce parallel cascades of regulatory molecules. Reactive oxygen and nitrogen species and degradative enzymes are consumed on host macromolecules. Even intracellularly, proinflammatory pathways are turned off by the actions of inflammation-induced heat-shock proteins. Within hours of extravasation, neutrophils undergo apoptosis in response to signals in the inflammatory milieu such as Fas ligand and TNF. Apoptotic neutrophils undergo cell death in an orderly manner so that lysosomal enzymes are not released extracellularly. Finally, over hours to days, the inflammatory cytokines (especially IL-6), in combination with endogenous corticosteroids, induce the liver to secrete acute-phase proteins (APPs).[252] It is thought that the principal role of APPs, many of which are protease inhibitors, is to suppress or contain inflammatory responses.

STAGE 6: SOME HORSES BECOME DANGEROUSLY IMMUNOSUPPRESSED. As described above, there is a *counter-regulatory* response mounted by the host that is designed to check the inflammatory response.[253] This response may be activated systemically in a way analogous to the proinflammatory phase of endotoxemia. The inflammatory and counter-regulatory systems ideally cancel each other out, allowing repair to begin and homeostasis to be restored. If counter-regulatory systems persist, a state of dangerous generalized immunosuppression may exist—such is the case in human patients with severe burns and is likely in some horses after large intestinal surgery or enterocolitis. In the latter situations, horses likely are particularly susceptible to opportunistic infections of surgical wounds or to bacterial or fungal pneumonia.

Signs of Endotoxemia

CLINICAL SIGNS. The clinical signs of horses given intravenous endotoxin experimentally may range from fever without obvious malaise to multiple organ failure and death. Obviously, signs that are not due exclusively to endotoxin (e.g., severe pain caused by bowel strangulation or diarrhea in horses with *Salmonella* colitis) may greatly influence the overall clinical presentation of horses with naturally acquired endotoxemia.

Typically in an adult horse given a moderate sublethal dose of endotoxin (e.g., 0.1 to 1 μg LPS/kg of body weight), an early period of mild tachypnea peaks within 30 minutes and resolves within 2 hours. During this period, mucous membranes are pale. Beginning within 90 minutes of LPS injection, there is depression, restlessness, and inappetance and rectal temperature begins to rise. Auscultable intestinal sounds usually cease during this period and remain depressed for several hours. Intermittent signs of colic usually are seen, including recumbency (usually without rolling). Small amounts of loose feces usually are passed. Heart rate peaks during the stage of maximal abdominal discomfort (about 2 hours after administration of endotoxin), then temporarily declines. During this time, mucous membranes become congested, the capillary refill time is prolonged, and a dark "toxic" line may become apparent around the gingival margins of the teeth. Beginning at 4 to 6 hours after endotoxin administration, there is a secondary phase of tachycardia and tachypnea that likely is related to development of systemic hypotension and fever. This secondary phase persists for several hours. Horses presented clinically with mild to moderate endotoxemia usually resemble experimental animals during the period 2 to 6 hours after intravenous endotoxin administration.

At higher LPS doses (e.g., 100 μg/kg) in experimental animals or in patients with severe endotoxemia, signs of circulatory failure and disordered hemostasis dominate the clinical picture. Usually these horses are stuporous and totally anorectic. Signs of dehydration such as reduced skin turgor, dry mucous membranes, and sunken eyes are obvious. As systemic blood flow becomes more compromised, rectal temperature may drop into or below the normal range. Urine output is reduced or nonexistent. There are dark, congested mucous membranes, rapid and weak peripheral pulses, cold extremities, and sweating, and the horse may have muscle tremors and become recumbent.

Vascular damage may be seen as petechial and ecchymotic hemorrhages on mucous membranes. A poor prognostic sign is the development of a hypercoagulation syndrome during which routine venipuncture or catheter placement initiates thrombosis along the entire visible length of the jugular veins (or other superficial veins). If both jugular veins are thus occluded, there usually is massive swelling of the soft tissues of the head and associated laryngeal edema may cause signs of upper respiratory tract obstruction. In some horses, thrombosed superficial vessels can easily be palpated through the skin of the legs and abdomen. Infarction of bowel segments or lungs may cause severe clinical signs that are unresponsive to treatment. At the time that hypercoagulation syndrome is recognized clinically, there is often evidence of secondary bleeding tendency (a consequence of platelet and clotting factor depletion and uncontrolled activation of fibrinolysis), seen as prolonged hemorrhage from venipuncture sites and widespread mucosal petechiation. In cases with a severe pulmonary component, there may be hemorrhage into the respiratory tract with progressive tachypnea and dyspnea.

If moderately to severely affected animals survive for more than 24 hours, there usually is visible edema of the ventral abdomen and limbs. Signs of laminitis may first become apparent at this stage and may progress in severity even while the other systemic signs of endotoxemia improve.

CLINICOPATHOLOGIC SIGNS. Although the measured concentration of endotoxin in blood does not correlate well with severity of clinical signs, demonstration of circulating endotoxin obviously is definitive proof of endotoxemia. In one study, 12% of horses with acute gastrointestinal disease had detectable plasma endotoxin.[254] Reported concentrations in these horses were 0 to 30,400 pg/ml with mean of 218 pg/ml. Experimentally, plasma endotoxin usually is assayed by some variant of the *Limulus amebocyte* lysate assay. A simple horse-side test* for endotoxin that was marketed for use in clinical practice is no longer commercially available.

With the exception of early and profound neutropenia (usually accompanied by left shift and a toxic appearance of stained cells) and dose-dependent hypoglycemia, described earlier, the clinicopathologic signs of endotoxemia are nonspecific and reflect altered tissue perfusion, organ dysfunction, or disordered hemostasis. There is lactic acidosis, increased anion gap, and a reduction in Pao_2. Elevations of serum lactate dehydrogenase, creatinine kinase, and alkaline phosphatase activities reflect damage to organs such as the liver, muscle, and intestine. Impaired hepatic function may result in serum bilirubin concentration that is higher than would be expected from anorexia alone. Increased blood urea nitrogen and serum creatinine concentrations occur secondary to reduced blood volume (prerenal azotemia) and, in severe cases, are also associated with renal failure secondary to ischemia. In the latter circumstance, dipstick examination of urine will reveal abnormal amounts of protein and blood.

In moderate and severe cases of endotoxemia, there also may be evidence of dyshemostasis: values affected in blood may include any to all or the following: reduction in the circulating platelet count ($<100,000/\mu l$); reduction in fibrinogen concentration; prolongation of the activated partial thromboplastin, prothrombin, or thrombin times; increased activity of plasminogen activator inhibitor type-1; and increased concentration of fibrin degradation products.[254] In horses with acute gastrointestinal diseases, there also is increased activity in peritoneal fluid of many of the elements of the fibrinolytic system, including tissue plasminogen activator. Depletion of key clotting factors can most simply be detected as prolongation of plasma recalcification time.[255]

Prevention of Clinical Endotoxemia

Solid experimental data from laboratory animal experiments support the concept of protection against effects of all gram-negative bacterial infection by vaccination with endotoxins that lack the O-region and some or all of the core region (R-mutant endotoxins). In food animals, use of J5 vaccine containing an R-mutant *E. coli* endotoxin was associated with significant reduction in mortality in animals with gram-negative infections.[256] An R-mutant *Salmonella typhimurium* bacterin† is marketed for use in horses. When first introduced in the early 1980s, this product caused unacceptable inoculation reactions and was withdrawn from the market; however, it has since been modified to prevent local reactions and reintroduced. A study by the manufacturer indicates that horses vaccinated with this product are partially protected from intravenous endotoxin.[257] Independent evaluation in clinical settings will be required if this product is going to be used routinely. A slightly different approach is the use, in newborn foals, of an oral polyclonal antibody preparation‡ against *E. coli* to prevent death resulting from coliform septicemia.

An interesting experimental approach to dietary manipulation of the response to endotoxin has been developed by researchers at the University of Georgia.[258] They have shown in horses that supplementation of a complete pelleted diet

---

*Etox Dx, Kenland, Ashland, OH 44805.

†Endovac-Equi; Immvac Inc., Columbia, MO 65201.

‡E. colicin-E; EquiLabs, Division of Agri Laboratories, St. Joseph, MO 64503.

with linseed oil (8% by weight) changed the n3/n6 fatty acid ratio in cell membranes of mononuclear cells. Arachidonic acid is an n6 fatty acid that is precursor to many mediators of inflammation such as thromboxane A_2 (TXA_2) and LTB_4, whereas n3-derived mediators are much less potent. When compared with the responses of endotoxin-stimulated mononuclear cells from horses on standard diets, cells from linseed oil–treated animals produced less potent eicosanoids and less TNF. Unfortunately there was no amelioration of clinical signs when supplemented horses were challenged intravenously with endotoxin.[259] More recently, it was shown that IV infusion of horses with n-3-rich lipid emulsion resulted in lower endotoxin-induced thromboxane production than was found in controls.[260]

Treatment of Clinical Endotoxemia

The strategy for management of horses with endotoxemia should include consideration of the following steps: (1) circulatory support, (2) removal of the cause(s) of endotoxemia, (3) neutralization of circulating endotoxin, and (4) inhibition of endotoxin-induced inflammation.

CIRCULATORY SUPPORT. Expansion of blood volume remains the cornerstone of treatment for horses with moderate and severe acute endotoxemia. As detailed earlier, many of the signs of acute endotoxemia relate to leakage of plasma into the interstitial spaces and movement of water into cells. A balanced polyionic solution should be used to restore plasma volume by expanding extracellular fluid. Guidelines for estimating water deficits and administering fluids intravenously are provided on pp. 686-687. Urination should begin during the rapid replacement of estimated losses. Ideally the fine control of fluid replacement should be based on serial measurements of PCV or plasma protein concentration. Some clinicians prefer the early use of compatible plasma (5 L to a 450-kg horse, 1 to 2 L to a neonate) or other colloid solutions such as 6% hydroxyethyl starch solution* to replace the extravasated colloid. Plasma has the advantage of providing immunoglobulin and acute-phase proteins. Unless blood pH at presentation is less than 7.2, HCO_3^- concentration less than 15 mmol/L, or total CO_2 concentration less than 16 mmol/L, sodium bicarbonate probably does not need to be given initially. Improvements in peripheral perfusion and renal function caused by volume expansion likely will improve acid-base balance in these less severe cases. In horses with pH less than 7.2, the estimated deficit should be given during the period in which the initial fluid deficit is being replaced. Acid-base balance should then be reevaluated, and additional bicarbonate provided if the pH is still less than 7.2. Intravenous fluids should be supplemented with potassium (10 to 20 mmol/L) regardless of whether or not there is measured hypokalemia as serum potassium concentration will decline as acidosis is corrected. All fluids given initially to septic neonates or to hypoglycemic adult horses should be supplemented to 5% or 10% glucose and glucose concentration should be closely monitored in the blood and urine.

Hypertonic saline may be given during the initial period of resuscitation of horses with signs of severe fluid-volume contraction. Hypertonic saline is thought to act by shifting water from the intracellular to the extracellular space, by stimulating vagovagal reflexes and myocardial contractility and by reducing vascular leak. Two liters of 7.2% NaCl† can be given rapidly to a 500-kg horse. Use of hypertonic saline should be followed by conventional fluid therapy with isotonic solutions.

Once blood volume has been adequately replaced, if anuria or low blood pressure (mean arterial pressure less than 65 mm Hg as measured by tail cuff manometer) persists, the selective use of vasoactive amines should be considered. Dobutamine (2 to 15 μg/kg/min) is used in an effort to increase systemic blood pressure by improving cardiac myocontractility. Low-dose dopamine (1 to 3 μg/kg/min) may improve renal and brain perfusion by causing selective peripheral vasodilation. A useful protocol that should improve renal perfusion while maintaining or improving systemic blood pressure is as follows: dilute 1 vial each of dobutamine* and dopamine† into 500 ml of saline or 5% dextrose and infuse the mixture at 0.45 ml/kg/hr (200 ml/hr in a 450-kg horse). This will provide 3 μg/kg/min dopamine and 3.6 μg/kg/min of dobutamine. Blood pressure and heart rate should be monitored frequently during the infusion, especially in neonates. If hemodynamic resuscitation is successful, there should be concomitant decline in blood L-lactate concentration.

REMOVAL OF THE CAUSE(S) OF ENDOTOXEMIA. Removal of the cause of endotoxemia usually involves both removal of the source of endotoxin and correction of the abnormality that allows access of endotoxin to blood. In some cases a source of endotoxin can be mechanically removed: for example, gram-negative bacteria and associated inflammatory effusion can be drained from pleural or peritoneal cavities or carefully siphoned from the postpartum uterus. Antimicrobial therapy of gram-negative infection also is essential. In general, bactericidal drugs should be selected because endotoxemic horses may be immunosuppressed. In horses in which endotoxemia is suspected without evidence of extraintestinal gram-negative infection, antimicrobials should only be given in the following situations: (1) the horse is younger than 3 months old, (2) there is suspicion of clostridial enteritis (metronidazole or vancomycin), (3) there is degenerative left shift or total neutrophil count of <1000/μl, or (4) there is clinical evidence of dyshemostasis (e.g., jugular thrombosis or abnormal coagulogram). It should be noted that effective antimicrobial therapy can temporarily worsen clinical signs by causing the release of endotoxin from killed bacteria. This possibility should be anticipated and minimized by the timely use of NSAID or other antiendotoxic therapy (see following paragraphs).

When intestinal strangulation is the cause of endotoxemia, surgical correction obviously is of paramount importance. For the purposes of perioperative management, however, it should be noted that resumption of intestinal blood flow can worsen endotoxemia; sequestered endotoxin may be flushed into the circulation through compromised intestinal walls. At least in the case of small intestinal ischemia, the mucosal barrier to endotoxin may be further compromised by ischemia-reperfusion injury when full blood flow is restored by luminal decompression or other manipulation. Again, prophylactic use of nonsteroidal antiinflammatory drugs (NSAID) and/or ROS scavengers may be warranted.

NEUTRALIZATION OF CIRCULATING ENDOTOXIN

Antiendotoxin Antiserum. An antiserum‡ and a hyperimmune plasma§ produced by immunization of horses against R-mutant endotoxins are used in horses with suspected endotoxemia (in some cases, this is an off-label use). As is the

---

*6% Hetastarch in 0.9% saline; Abbott Laboratories, North Chicago, IL 60064.
†Hyper Saline 8X; The Butler Co., Dublin, OH 43017.

*Dobutrex; EG Lilly & Co., Indianapolis, IN 46285.
†Dopmaine hydrochloride; Abbott Laboratories, North Chicago, IL 60064.
‡Endoserum; Immvac Inc., Columbia, MO 65201.
§Polymune J; Veterinary Dynamics, Templeton, CA 93465.

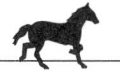

case with studies in humans and small experimental animals, use of cross-reactive endotoxin antibodies in horses with either experimentally or naturally acquired endotoxemia has yielded conflicting results. In several studies there was impressive reduction of mortality rate or improvement in clinical signs when antiendotoxin serum or plasma was given to horses[261,262]; however, in other studies no improvement was demonstrated.[263,264] Pretreatment of foals with antiserum was associated in one report with significant worsening of clinical response to intravenously administered endotoxin compared with that of foals that received no pretreatment.[265] These disparate results probably reflect, at least in part, variation in the quality of antiserums and experimental conditions; thus no blanket recommendation can be made as to the clinical use of such products. Promising results continue to be achieved in experimental animals given monoclonal antibodies against core glycolipid.[266] Hyperimmune plasmas (raised against any antigen[s]) also contain colloid, clotting factors, and increased amounts of substances such as acute-phase proteins that might have nonspecific salutary effect in the setting of endotoxemia. Thus the use of 2 to 10 ml/kg of hyperimmune plasma can be justified in treatment of life-threatening endotoxemia.

Polymyxin B. Polymyxin B is a broad-spectrum cyclic peptide antibiotic with potent endotoxin-binding activity. Potentially lethal side-effects of respiratory paralysis and nephrotoxicity have precluded use of this agent as a systemic antimicrobial drug; however, polymyxin B retains endotoxin-neutralizing capacity at nontoxic dosages. Pretreatment of foals with polymyxin B at a dosage rate of 6000 U (1 mg)/kg significantly suppressed clinical and cytokine responses to intravenous endotoxin without causing toxic side effects.[265] Repeated dosage of ponies with 15,000 U/kg also produced no sign of toxicity.[267] Horses given polymyxin B at 5 mg/kg as a polymyxin B-dextran 70 conjugate were fully protected from the effects of endotoxin but had a transient hypertensive response to treatment infusion.[268] This side effect was prevented by the use of a NSAID. In horses with moderate or severe endotoxemia, consideration should be given to the cautious use of polymyxin B* given intravenously two times daily at a dosage rate of 6000 U/kg. Each treatment should be given over at least 15 minutes.

INHIBITION OF ENDOTOXIN-INDUCED INFLAMMATION

Nonsteroidal Antiinflammatory Drugs. Through inhibition of cyclooxygenase, NSAID reduce the formation of prostanoid metabolites (e.g., thromboxanes and prostaglandins) from arachidonic acid and thereby attenuate much of the adverse effect of endotoxin. Flunixin meglumine, phenylbutazone, ketoprofen, eltenac, and aspirin are examples of this class of drugs used in horses. When flunixin is administered at 0.25 mg/kg every 6 to 8 hours, endotoxin-induced prostanoid production is prevented and maximal antiendotoxic effects are produced in experimental situations without obscuring the signs of colic or risking toxic side effects of the drug.[269] It should be noted that flunixin does not reduce endotoxin-induced leukopenia. Because there is evidence that aspirin does not prevent endotoxin-induced aggregation of platelets,[270] there appears to be no rationale for the common practice of adding aspirin to the NSAID regimen. Because most NSAIDs inhibit constitutive COX-I activity (in addition to endotoxin-induced COX-II activity), there is some morbidity associated with their use. There may be gastric ulceration, right dorsal colitis, renal papillary necrosis and, possibly, impairment of intestinal motility and epithelial restitution.[271,272] It is likely that drugs with specific COX-II activity will increasingly become available for horses in the near fu-

ture and it is presumed that these drugs will have fewer side effects than the drugs currently available.

Methyl Xanthine Derivatives. TNF production by macrophages is inhibited in dose-dependent fashion by methyl xanthine derivatives. This effect appears to be due to phosphodiesterase inhibition and consequent elevation of intracellular cAMP. Pentoxifylline,* a drug that is in widespread use in humans as a hemorheologic agent, has been shown to inhibit TNF production in horse blood and in cultured equine macrophages while increasing secretion of prostacyclin. Studies in other species suggest that pentoxifylline also stimulates production of IL-10, a potent antiinflammatory cytokine. A pharmacokinetic study in horses has indicated that oral dosage at 8.5 mg/kg two times daily provides serum concentration sufficient to increase RBC deformability.[273] In rodents, treatment with pentoxifylline up to 2 hours after endotoxin protected against lethal effect.[274] In addition to TNF suppression, direct stimulation by pentoxifylline of prostacyclin production was thought to contribute to this protective effect; thus there is some concern that concurrent use of flunixin, which is an inhibitor of prostacyclin production, might reduce any useful effect of pentoxifylline in horses. Pentoxifylline has been administered parenterally to horses (7.5 mg/kg IV, followed by 3 mg/kg/hr), beginning 30 minutes after onset of endotoxin infusion, but no clear beneficial clinical effect could be shown when the drug was given alone or with concurrent flunixin meglumine.[275,276] In light of the strong conceptual arguments for its use, however, pentoxifylline therapy (at 10 to 15 mg/kg PO bid) in endotoxemia is reasonable.

Corticosteroids. The coricosteriod class of drugs theoretically has many useful actions in combating the effects of endotoxemia. These include reduced production of cytokines, inhibition of TNF production by macrophages, stabilization of cell membranes, and prevention of neutrophil activation. Surprisingly, however, no beneficial effect of steroid use was found in large, multicenter studies of humans with gram-negative sepsis. Corticosteroids also are widely believed to increase susceptibility to laminitis in endotoxemic horses, perhaps by increasing the sensitivity of digital vessels to the constrictive actions of circulating catecholamines.[277] Use of corticosteroids is contraindicated in the treatment of endotoxemia in adult horses.

Heparin. The use of heparin in horses with endotoxemia is controversial. It prevents microvascular thrombosis principally by promoting the anticoagulant activity of antithrombin III (AT-III). Unfortunately, heparin cannot reverse existing thrombosis, and because AT-III is consumed during severe coagulopathy, it may not prevent additional intravascular coagulation in such cases. Fresh or fresh-frozen plasma are good sources of AT-III, but also provide clotting factors that could potentiate intravascular coagulation. When given at the recommended intravenous or subcutaneous dose of 40 to 150 U/kg bid or tid, unfractionated heparin causes intravascular agglutination of equine red blood cells.[278] Thus it could be argued that the use of heparin might actually exacerbate intravascular cellular plugging. This side effect can be avoided by using low-molecular-weight heparin, which is nonagglutinating but retains anticoagulant activity, principally via inhibition of factor Xa.[279] The use of heparin should be considered in horses that are at high risk for laminitis (e.g., DPJ or grain overload) or hypercoagulation syndrome (early evidence of dyshemostasis such as abnormal coagulogram or spontaneous venous thrombosis). In the latter setting, heparin should be given with plasma at a dose of either 200-300 IU/kg/day for unfractionated heparin (either divided bid subcutaneously or as a continuous intravenous infusion) or

---

*Polymyxin B sulfate: Bedford Laboratories, Bedford OH 44146.

*Trental; Hoescht-Roussel Pharmaceuticals, Somerville, NJ 08876.

50 anti-Xa IU/kg for low-molecular-weight heparin* (subcutaneously sid).

Scavengers of Reactive Oxygen Species. Reactive oxygen species are thought to cause corrosive tissue damage during endotoxemia and may also potentiate the production of inflammatory cytokines. Surgical deflation of distended small intestine is thought to lead to ischemia-reperfusion injury, a process that generates ROS from epithelial xanthine oxidase. The life-saving process of fluid replacement in horses with hypovolemic shock may even lead to whole-body ischemia-reperfusion. Despite these presumed associations between oxidant stress and the signs of endotoxemia, little effort has been made to intervene therapeutically at this level. There is some evidence that allopurinol, a hydroxyl radical scavenger and inhibitor of xanthine oxidase activity, has positive clinical effect during sublethal endotoxin infusion.[248] A recommended dose for allopurinol is 5 mg/kg given intravenously. Because dimethyl sulfoxide (DMSO) has been shown to be a potent scavenger of hydroxyl radicals, it seems reasonable to use this agent in the treatment of equine endotoxemia. Like allopurinol, DMSO may reduce intestinal mucosal injury after ischemia-reperfusion; to date, evidence for efficacy in this setting has been mixed. DMSO can be given by rapid intravenous infusion (or by nasogastric tube) as a 10% to 20% solution in saline at dosage of 0.2 to 1 g/kg every 6 to 12 hours. The 21-aminosteroid (lazaroid) class of drugs, which act in part by suppressing ROS production, have been shown to ameliorate the signs of endotoxemia in calves[280] and may have future use as antiendotoxic agents in horses.

MISCELLANEOUS TREATMENTS. Naloxone, a narcotic antagonist, at dosage of 0.04 mg/kg, blunted some of the cardiovascular effects of high-dose endotoxin[281] but has not been used widely for this purpose. It should be noted that this dose of naloxone likely blocks only the high-affinity μ receptor, which mediates the analgesic effects of endogenous β-endorphins; therefore, use of naloxone at this dose may heighten sensitivity of the horse to pain. The detergent tyloxapol was remarkably effective in preventing the effects of endotoxin in anesthetized horses.[282] The mechanism of antiendotoxic action of tyloxapol is unknown, but the detergent has been shown to have wide-ranging effects on cells and proteins, some of which may preclude its use in clinical cases. For example, the detergent has been shown to inhibit cellular phagocytosis, an important event in innate immunity. Also, this agent induces marked hyperlipidemia (plasma concentration may increase 100-fold) in horses because of interference with lipoprotein metabolism. A recently published report[283] on the use of the suflonyl analog of the alpha-phenyl-N-tert-butyl-nitrone spin trap molecule suggests that this agent was effective in reducing clinical signs in horses given endotoxin. A cautionary note was the observation that some rodents given the same agent at high doses actually suffered enhanced endotoxin-induced mortality.

Future Treatment Considerations

Current research in horses and other experimental animals indicates additional ways in which to inhibit the multiple pathways of endotoxin action. Polyclonal and monoclonal antibodies against TNF, IL-1, IL-6, chemokines, C5a, tissue factor (an important type of procoagulant activity), and leukocyte adhesion molecules have all been shown to protect laboratory animals against the lethal effect of endotoxin.[284] Anti-TNF has also been evaluated in horses given endotoxin and found to minimize adverse clinical effects (not including fever) and leukopenia when given before endotoxin[285] but to have little

effect when given after the onset of endotoxin infusion.[286] Soluble TNF receptor (sTNF-R) has been identified in the supernate of equine leukocyte cultures,[287] and IL-1ra activity has been found in joints of horses with chronic arthritis; the equine gene has been cloned and sequenced.[288] Both sTNF-R and IL-1ra have potent antiendotoxic effect in rodents but have lacked efficacy in clinical trials in humans with sepsis. Nonspecific lipoxygenase inhibitors protect against endotoxin in rodent models; however, specific 5-lipoxygenase inhibitors were ineffective. Lipoxygenase inhibitors have not been evaluated in horses with endotoxemia. Platelet-activating factor inhibitors have been effective antiendotoxic agents in some species but have not yet shown much positive clinical effect in horses or humans.[289] In dogs and other experimental animals, inhibitors of NO production such as N^G-monomethyl arginine reverse endotoxin- or TNF-induced hypotension[290]; however, NOS inhibitors generally have no protective effect in sepsis models. Furthermore, NO production may not be increased in horses with endotoxemia.[291]

As has been mentioned above, it is likely that current but imperfect treatment strategies will be greatly improved in the future. For example, there should soon be truly effective ways of neutralizing circulating endotoxin by "natural" antagonists such as BPI (bactericidal/permeability-increasing protein), an LPS-binding protein produced by neutrophils, or by potent cross-reactive anticore polyclonal antiserums and monoclonal antibodies or nontoxic therapeutic reagents such as analogs of polymyxin B. Also, there should soon be more effective means to suppress or scavenge ROS (with, for example, newer generation lazaroids).

It has to be admitted however, that, almost without exception, potential novel treatments for gram-negative sepsis that have been promising at the experimental level have failed when applied in clinical settings in humans (and, to a limited extent, horses). In a perverse way, this is a relief to equine clinicians whose clients would not be able to afford expensive antimediator therapies. On the horizon are some different approaches that have the potential to be both effective and affordable. One of the most exciting possibilities is that gene therapy might be used to transfect host cells transiently with genes encoding antiinflammatory mediators (e.g., IL-10, TGF-β) or antisense RNA or ribozymes directed against mRNA of proinflammatory mediators. Also at the subcellular level, ways likely will be found to manipulate regulation of NF-κB in order to subvert transcription of genes for cytokines.

REFERENCES

228. Thomas L: *Lives of a cell*, New York, 1974, Viking Press, pp 75-80.
229. McGorum BC, Ellison J, Cullen RT: Total and respirable airborne dust endotoxin concentrations in three equine management systems, *Equine Vet J* 30:430-434, 1998:
230. Tobias PS, Mathison JC, Ulevitch RJ: A family of lipopolysaccharide binding proteins involved in responses to gram-negative sepsis, *J Biol Chem* 263:13479-13481, 1988.
231. Wright R: CD14 and immune response to lipopolysaccharide, *Science* 252:1321-1322, 1991.
232. Longworth KE et al: Pulmonary intravascular macrophages in horses and ponies, *Am J Vet Res* 55:382-388, 1994.
233. Yang RB et al: Signaling events induced by lipopolysaccharide-activated toll-like receptor 2, *J Immunol* 163:639-643, 1999.
234. Zhang FX et al: Bacterial lipopolysaccharide activates nuclear factor-kappa B through interleukin-1 signaling mediators in cultured human dermal endothelial cells and mononuclear phagocytes, *J Biol Chem* 274:7611-7614, 1999.
235. Dinarello C: The proinflammatory cytokines interleukin-1 and tumor necrosis factor and treatment of the septic shock syndrome, *J Infect Dis* 163:1177-1184, 1991.
236. Van Deuren M, Dofferhoff ASM, Van Der Meer, JWM: Cytokines and the response to infection, *J Pathol* 168:349-356, 1992.
237. Starnes HF et al: Anti-IL-6 monoclonal antibodies protect against lethal *Escherichia coli* infection and lethal tumor necrosis factor: a challenge in mice, *J Immunol* 145:4185-4191, 1990.
238. Loll PJ, Garavito RM: The isoforms of cyclooxygenase: structure and function, *Curr Opin Invest Drugs* 3:1171-1180,1994.

*Lovenox: enoxaprin sodium 10,000 IU/ml, Rhone-Poulnec Rorer Pharmaceuticals, Collegeville, PA 19426.

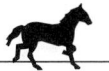
239. Hammond RA et al: Endotoxin induction of nitric oxide synthase and cyclooxygenase-2 in equine alveolar macrophages, *Am J Vet Res* 60:426-431, 1999.

240. Hobbs AJ, Moncada S: Inducible nitric oxide synthesis and inflammation. In Willoughby DA, Tomlinson A, eds: *Inducible enzymes in the inflammatory response,* Basel, 1999, Birkhäuser Verlag, pp 31-54.

241. Willis D: Overview of HO-1 in inflammatory pathologies. In Willoughby DA, Tomlinson A, eds: *Inducible enzymes in the inflammatory response,* Basel, 1999, Birkhäuser Verlag, pp 55-91.

242. Czermak BJ et al: Protective effects of C5a blockade in sepsis, *Nat Med* 5:788-792, 1999.

243. Springer TA: Traffic signals on endothelium for lymphocyte recirculation and leukocyte emigration. In Paul LC, Issekutz TB, eds: *Adhesion molecules in health and disease,* New York, 1999, Marcel Dekker.

244. Rossi F: The O₂-forming NADPH oxidase of the phagocytes: nature, mechanisms of activation and function, *Biochim Biophys Acta* 853:65-89, 1986.

245. Grulke S et al: Plasma myeloperoxidase level and polymorphonuclear leukocyte activation in horses suffering from large intestinal obstruction requiring surgery: preliminary results, *Can J Bet Res* 63:142-147, 1999.

246. Klebanoff SJ: Myeloperoxidase: occurrence and biological function, In Everse J, Everse KE, Grisham MB, eds: *Peroxidases in chemistry and biology,* Boca Raton, 1991, CRC Press, pp 1-35.

247. Elsbach P, Weiss J, Levy O: Oxygen-independent antimicrobial systems of phagocytes, In Gallin JI, Snyderman R, eds: *Inflammation: basic principles and clinical correlates,* ed 3, Philadelphia, 1999, Lippincott Williams & Wilkins, pp 801-817.

248. Lochner F et al: Effects of allopurinol in experimental endotoxin shock in horses, *Res Vet Sci* 47:178-184, 1989.

249. Walsh CJ et al: Anti-CD18 antibody attenuates neutropenia and alveolar capillary-membrane injury during gram-negative sepsis, *Surgery* 110:205-212, 1991.

250. Seahorn TL, Gaunt SD, Berry C: Blood cell deformability in horses with intestinal colic, *Am J Vet Res* 55:321-324, 1994.

251. Allen GK et al: Induction of early-phase endotoxin tolerance in horses, *Equine Vet J* 28:269-274, 1996.

252. Warren HS, Chedid LA: Strategies for the treatment of endotoxemia: significance of the acute-phase response, *Rev Infect Dis* 9(suppl 5):S630-S638, 1987.

253. Bone RC: Immunologic dissonance: a continuing evolution in our understanding of the systemic inflammatory response syndrome (SIRS) and the multiple organ dysfunction syndrome (MODS) [see comments], *Ann Intern Med* 125:680-687, 1996.

254. Barton MH, Collatos C: Tumor necrosis factor and interleukin-6 activity and endotoxin concentration in peritoneal fluid and blood in horses with acute abdominal diseases, *J Vet Intern Med* 13:457-464, 1999.

255. Henry MM, Moore JN: Whole blood re-calcification time in equine colic, *Equine Vet J* 23:303-308, 1991.

256. Fenwick BW et al: Mortality in swine herds endemically infected with *Haemophilus pleuropneumoniae* effect of immunization with cross-reacting lipopolysaccharide core antigens of *Escherichia coli, Am J Vet Res* 47:1888-1891, 1987.

257. Sprouse RF, Garner HE, Lager K: Protection of ponies from heterologous and homologous endotoxin challenges via *Salmonella typhimurium* bacterin-toxoid, *Equine Pract* 11:34-40, 1989.

258. Henry MM et al: Effect of dietary alpha-linolenic acid on equine monocyte procoagulant activity and eicosanoid synthesis, *Circ Shock* 32:173-188, 1990.

259. Henry MM, Moore JN, Fischer JK: Influence of an omega-3 fatty acid-enriched ration on in vivo responses of horses to endotoxin, *Am J Vet Res* 52:523-527, 1991.

260. McCann ME et al: Effect of intravenous infusion of omega-3 and omega-6 lipid emulsions on equine endotoxemia, *Proceedings of the Sixth Equine Colic Research Symposium,* Athens, Ga, Nov 8-11, 1998.

261. Garner HE, Sprouse RF, Lager K: Cross protection of ponies from sublethal *Escherichia coli* endotoxemia by *Salmonella typhimurium* antiserum, *Equine Pract* 10:10-16, 1988.

262. Spier SJ et al: Protection against endotoxemia in horses by using plasma containing antibody to an Rc mutant *E. coli* (J5), *Circ Shock* 28:235-248, 1989.

263. Morris DD, Whitlock RH, Corbeil LB: Endotoxemia in horses: protection provided by antiserum to core lipopolysaccharide, *Am J Vet Res* 47:544-550, 1986.

264. Morris DD, Whitlock RH: Therapy of suspected septicemia in neonatal foals using plasma containing antibodies to core lipopolysaccharide (LPS), *J Vet Intern Med* 1:175-182, 1987.

265. Durando MM, MacKay RJ, Skelley LA: Effects of polymyxin B and *Salmonella typhimurium* antiserum on horses given endotoxin intravenously, *Am J Vet Res* 55:921-927, 1994.

266. Le Roy D et al: Monoclonal antibodies to murine lipopolysaccharide (LPS)-binding protein (LBP) protect mice from lethal endotoxemia by blocking either the biding of LPS to LBP or the presentation of LPS/LBP complexes to CD14, *J Immunol* 162:7454-7460, 1999.

267. Ralsbeck MF, Garner HE, Osweiler GD: Effects of polymyxin B on selected features of equine carbohydrate overload, *Vet Hum Toxicol* 31:422-426, 1989.

268. MacKay RJ et al: Effect of a conjugate of polymyxin B-dextran 70 in horses with experimentally induced endotoxemia, *Am J Vet Res* 60:68-75, 1999.

269. Semrad SD et al: Low dose flunixin meglumine: effects on eicosanoid production and clinical signs induced by experimental endotoxaemia in horses, *Equine Vet J* 19:201-206, 1987.

270. Jarvis GE, Evans RJ: Platelet-activating factor and not thromboxane A₂ is an important mediator or endotoxin-induced aggregation in equine heparinised whole blood in vitro, *Blood Coagul Fibrinolysis* 7:194-198, 1996.

271. Blikslager AT, Roberts MC: Mechanisms of intestinal mucosal repair, *J Am Vet Med Assoc* 211:1437-1441, 1997.

272. Van Hoogmoed L et al: In vitro effects of nonsteroidal anti-inflammatory agents and prostaglandins I₂, E₂, and F₂ alpha on contractility of taenia of the large colon of horses, *Am J Vet Res* 60:1004-1009, 1999.

273. Geor RJ et al: Effects of furosemide and pentoxifylline on blood flow properties in horses, *Am J Vet Res* 53:2043-2049, 1992.

274. Noel P et al: Pentoxifylline inhibits lipopolysaccharide-induced serum tumor necrosis factor and mortality, *Life Sci* 47:1023-1029, 1990.

275. Barton MH, Moore JN, Norton N: Effects of pentoxifylline infusion on response of horses to in vivo challenge exposure with endotoxin, *Am J Vet Res* 58:1300-1307, 1997.

276. Baskett A et al: Effect of pentoxifylline, flunixin meglumine, and their combination of a model of endotoxemia in horses, *Am J Vet Res* 58:1291-1299, 1997.

277. Eyre P, Elmes PJ, Stickland S: Corticosteroid-potentiated vascular responses of the equine digit: a possible pharmacologic basis for laminitis, *Am J Vet Res* 40:135-138, 1979.

278. Mahaffey EA, Moore JN: Erythrocyte agglutination associated with heparin treatment in three horses, *J Am Vet Med Assoc* 189:1478-1480, 1986.

279. Monreal L et al: Comparison of the effects of low-molecular-weight and unfractionated heparin in horses, *Am J Vet Res* 56:1281-1285, 1995.

280. Rose ML, Semrad SD: Clinical efficacy of tirilazad mesylate for treatment of endotoxemia in neonatal calves, *Am J Vet Res* 53:2305-2310, 1992.

281. Weld JM et al: The effects of naloxone on endotoxic and hemorrhagic shock in horses, *Res Commun Chem Pathol Pharmacol* 44:227-238, 1984.

282. Longworth KE et al: Use of detergent to prevent initial responses to endotoxin in horses, *Am J Vet Res* 57:1063-1066, 1996.

283. Harkins JD et al: Effect of alpha-phenyl-tert-butylnitrone on endotoxin toxemia in horses, *Vet Hum Toxicol* 39:268-271, 1999.

284. St John RC, Dorinsky PM: Immunologic therapy for ARDS, septic shock, and multiple-organ failure, *Chest* 103:932-943, 1993.

285. Cargile JL et al: Effect of treatment with a monoclonal antibody against equine tumor necrosis factor (TNF) on clinical, hematologic, and circulating TNF responses of miniature horses given endotoxin, *Am J Vet Res* 56:1451-1459, 1995.

286. Barton MH et al: Effect of tumor necrosis factor antibody given to horses during early experimentally induced endotoxemia, *Am J Vet Res* 59:792-797, 1998.

287. Coyne CP et al: Isolation of an inhibitor of tumor necrosis factor-α–mediated cytotoxicity liberated from chemotaxin-stimulated equine white blood cell populations, *Am J Vet Res* 54:845-855, 1993.

288. Kato H et al: Molecular cloning and functional expression of equine interleukin-1 receptor antagonist, *Vet Immunol Immunopath* 56:221-231, 1997.

289. Carrick JB, Morris DD, Moore JN: Administration of a receptor antagonist for platelet-activating factor during equine endotoxaemia, *Equine Vet J* 25:152-157, 1993.

290. Kilbourn RG et al: Reversal of endotoxin-mediated shock by N^G-methyl-l-arginine, an inhibitor of nitric oxide synthesis, *Biochem Biophys Res Commun* 172:1132-1138, 1990.

291. Bueno AC et al: Plasma and urine nitric oxide concentrations in horses given a low dose of endotoxin, *Am J Vet Res* 60:969-976, 1999.

MEDICAL DISORDERS OF THE SMALL INTESTINE

MICHAEL J. MURRAY

ULCERATIVE DUODENITIS

PATHOPHYSIOLOGY. Duodenal ulceration and ulcerative duodenitis primarily affect foals and to a lesser degree yearling horses. Older horses are rarely affected. Lesions occur primarily in the proximal duodenum and include erosions, focal ulcers, and diffuse inflammation with or without ulceration. The terms duodenal ulceration and ulcerative duodenitis may refer to differing clinical manifestations of the same problem, and the terms are used interchangeably in this section.

The pathophysiology of duodenal ulcer disease in foals is less well understood than gastric ulcer disease. The disorder is classically considered to be a peptic disease, one in which damage to the duodenal mucosa results from excessive exposure to hydrochloric acid and pepsin. This concept may require revision. Equine duodenal ulcer disease has been presumed to be similar to the disorder in humans, but most cases of duodenal ulcer disease in people are associated with *Helicobacter pylori* infection.[292] *Helicobacter pylori* bacteria have not been reported in equine gastrointestinal tissues, however. *Helicobacter pylori* only colonize gastric (glandular) mucosa, and infection of the duodenum must be preceded by metaplasia of areas of duodenal mucosa to gastric mucosa. This is thought to occur from chronic peptic injury. In humans, the incidence of duodenal ulcer disease increases with age,[293] which contrasts with horses, in which duodenal ulcer occurs primarily in animals less than 1 year old.[294]

We have recognized occurrences of duodenal ulceration and inflammation in which cases were clustered geographically (same farm) and temporally. These foals all had moderate to severe gastric ulceration, and they had extensive inflammation with varying degrees of erosion or ulceration in the proximal duodenum (Plates 10, 11). A similar temporal and geographic association was reported in two cases of ulcerative duodenitis in yearlings.[295] These findings seem inconsistent with a purely peptic insult as the cause for the ulcerative duodenitis. In one report of seven foals with ulcerative duodenitis,[296] lesions typically extended into a large area of the proximal duodenum, were characterized by mucosal necrosis, and often had a sharp line of demarcation between affected and more normal-appearing mucosa. In the foals of that report, no common microbial organism, other than *E. coli*, was identified and a cause for the ulcerative duodenitis was not determined. In most foals in which we have diagnosed duodenal disease the lesions were not focal ulcers but rather appeared as more generalized inflammation. An infectious cause seems likely, but has not been identified. In the 1980s, rotavirus infection was thought to be associated with gastroduodenal ulcer disease in foals, but most foals with duodenal ulcer disease do not have rotavirus infection.

Duodenal ulcer disease in foals may have a component of peptic injury. The duodenal mucosa possesses some intrinsic properties that are protective against peptic injury, although these are not as elaborate as in the gastric glandular mucosa. The most important factor that protects the duodenal mucosa from acidic gastric secretions may be the sodium- and bicarbonate-rich secretions that probably originate from the pancreas and that will neutralize acid entering the duodenum from the stomach.[297]

CLINICAL SIGNS. The signs of duodenal ulceration or ulcerative duodenitis have been classically described as being the severe forms of gastric ulcer signs,[298] and in many cases duodenal and gastric ulcers occur simultaneously. However, many foals with ulcerative duodenitis will not have signs similar to gastric ulceration until severe gastric ulceration has occurred. Thus the primary signs of duodenitis can be nonspecific; they include fever, mild to moderate abdominal discomfort, mild obtundation, and diarrhea. A CBC will often reveal peripheral blood leukocytosis and hyperfibrinogenemia.

Gastric ulceration frequently occurs secondary to duodenal ulceration, as a result of physiologic or anatomic obstruction to gastric emptying, and tends to be severe (Plate 12), often leading to gastroesophageal reflux and esophagitis. Foals with esophagitis often exhibit ptyalism. In general the sequelae to duodenal ulceration are more severe than those of primary gastric ulceration. Complications of duodenal ulceration include duodenal perforation with peritonitis or adhesions, duodenal stricture with complete or partial obstruction (Figs. 30-32 and 30-33), ascending cholangitis and hepatitis, and ascending pancreatitis.

DIAGNOSIS. Duodenal ulceration can be difficult to confirm antemortem. Duodenoscopy is the most specific means of diagnosis. It requires an endoscope with at least 200-cm working length in foals up to 6 months of age, and a longer endoscope is required in older foals to examine the duodenal mucosa. Because of the size of the stomach and the anatomic configuration of the duodenum in foals, it is usually not possible to advance the endoscope past the duodenal ampulla. Occasionally the endoscope can be advanced into the descending duodenum.

A diagnosis is most readily made in cases in which lesions are diffuse or located within the ampulla. Excessive enterogastric reflux of bile through the pylorus is consistent with duodenal dysfunction. Ulceration at the pylorus or pyloric antrum may accompany duodenal ulceration and thus provide indication of potential duodenal involvement. Severe gastric ulceration in foals should alert the endoscopist to the potential for duodenal involvement. In such cases, oral histamine type-2 receptor (H_2) antagonist therapy may be less effective in resolving gastric lesions than in cases of primary gastric ulceration, because of delayed gastric emptying secondary to duodenal ulceration. Thus, if a foal has received such treatment before endoscopy and gastric ulceration is severe, suspicion of duodenal ulceration should increase.

Other diagnostic procedures that may be helpful include evaluation of peritoneal fluid; serum liver enzymes, particularly biliary-associated enzymes (γ-glutamyltransferase, alkaline phosphatase); serum bile acids; and radiography. With severe duodenal ulceration, survey radiographs of the cranial abdomen may reveal accumulation of fluid within the stomach and gas ascending the biliary ducts.[299] If barium contrast medium is placed into the stomach, complete emptying is usually delayed (>2 hours) and an irregular mucosal border may be noted in the descending duodenum. It should be recognized that in most cases radiography will not contribute to a diagnosis of duodenal ulcer per se, although duodenal stricture may be noted. If the descending duodenum is to be imaged, the volume of contrast media placed in the stomach should not exceed 0.5 to 1 L in a foal and 1 to 2 L in a weanling/yearling, or the proximal descending duodenum will be obscured by contrast media within the stomach.

TREATMENT. The effectiveness of treatment of duodenal ulceration or ulcerative duodenitis depends on the extent and severity of ulceration and the absence of complications, particularly perforation and stricture of the duodenum. Treatment objectives are to decrease duodenal inflammation, treat secondary gastric and esophageal ulceration, promote gastric emptying, and treat related problems such as peritonitis. If duodenal ulceration is confirmed or even suspected on the basis of clinical signs, treatment should be aggressive.

In acute cases of ulcerative duodenitis, there usually is a pronounced lymphocytic infiltration of the mucosa. In more chronic cases, there is a mixture of neutrophils, macrophages, fibroblasts, and fibrinonecrotic exudate. Definitive antiinflammatory therapy has not been described for these cases, but use of corticosteroids have appeared to be successful in cases in our hospital. In acute cases or those in which delayed gastric emptying is suspected, prednisolone sodium succinate* is given once daily initially at 1 mg/kg IV and then at 0.5 mg/kg IV. When oral medication can be given, prednisone is given at 1 mg/kg PO once daily. Other antiinflammatory therapy can include flunixin meglumine, 1.5 mg/kg/day IV or IM, divided

---

*Solu-Delta-Cortef, Pharmacia and Upjohn, Kalamazoo, Mich.

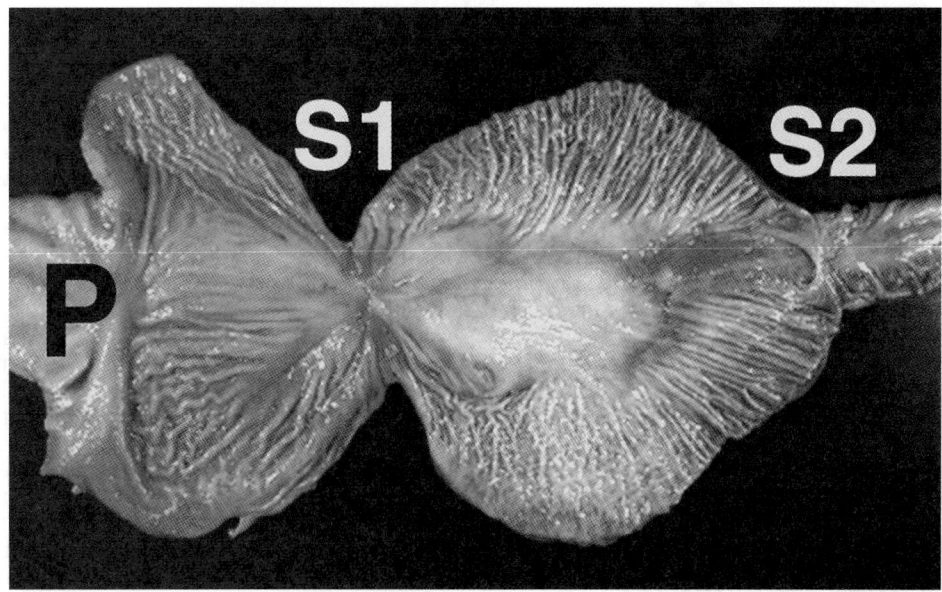

FIG. 30-32 ▮▮ Proximal duodenum of a 10-month-old horse with a history of chronic poor appetite and condition. The pylorus is at the left. There are two strictures in the duodenum: S1 is orad from the major duodenal papilla, and S2 is aborad from the duodenal papilla. The segment of duodenum between the strictures is dilated.

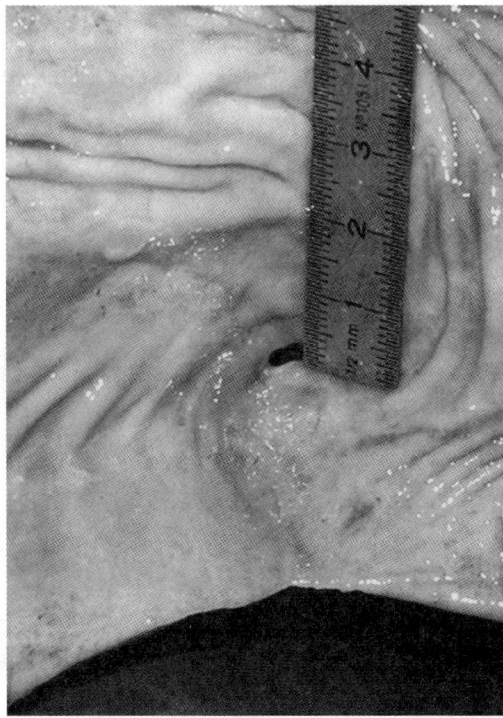

FIG. 30-33 ▮▮ Duodenal stricture *(S1)* of the horse in Fig. 30-32. The diameter of the duodenal lumen at the stricture is only 3 mm.

into 3 to 4 doses and dimethyl sulfoxide diluted to 10% DMSO in a saline solution, 200 mg/kg IV one to two times daily.

Suppression of gastric acid secretion is still an important objective in the treatment of duodenal ulcer/duodenitis in foals, because most of these foals will have gastric ulcers. Initially, acid suppression should be accomplished via par-

enteral administration of H_2 antagonist (cimetidine, 7 mg/kg IV every 6 hours, or ranitidine,* 1.5 mg/kg IV every 8 hours). Oral medications are unlikely to be adequately delivered to and absorbed from the small intestine in the first days of treatment. Gastric emptying can be enhanced with bethanechol† (0.02 mg/kg SC every 6 to 8 hours or 0.35 mg/kg PO every 8 hours when the foal can consume orally). In foals that have severe duodenal disease or that have required surgery, bethanechol has been given for up to 3 months. Once the foal can accept oral medication, it should be treated with the potent acid-suppressive agent omeprazole‡ at a dose of 4 mg/kg once daily for the paste formulation. It should be noted that in the 24 hours after the first dose, acid suppression is incomplete, and maximal suppression of acid secretion is achieved between days 1 and 5.[300] Therefore we usually continue to administer an H_2 antagonist intravenously for the initial 2 days of treatment with omeprazole in foals with duodenitis.

Sucralfate promotes duodenal mucosal healing in humans.[310] The dosage of sucralfate that is effective in humans with duodenal ulceration ranges from 1 to 2 g two to four times daily. Foals treated for duodenal ulceration that do not have impaired gastric emptying should be administered 2 to 4 g of sucralfate three times daily. *Sucralfate should not be used as the sole therapeutic agent for duodenal ulceration.*

Foals with duodenitis must usually be prevented from nursing or eating feed for 1 to 3 days. During this time, parental feeding should be considered. Depending on the age of the foal, administration of parenteral nutrition should provide 40 to 60 kcal/kg/day.

It is impossible to attribute clinical improvement to any one treatment modality. The inclusion of corticosteroid antiinflammatory drugs into the treatment of ulcerative duodenitis is based on the findings of diffuse inflammation,

*Zantac injectable, Glaxo-Wellcome, Research Triangle Park, NC.
†Urecholine, Merck and Co., Inc., West Pointe, Pa.
‡Gastrogard, Merial, Ltd., Iselin, NJ.

sometimes lymphocytic, extending aborally throughout the descending, and occasionally the ascending, duodenum. This type of lesion seems incompatible with a purely peptic insult, but compromise to duodenal defenses can render the duodenum susceptible to peptic injury. Thus combination of antiinflammatory, acid-suppressive, and mucosal protective therapy is warranted.

If medical therapy is ineffective or if sequelae of duodenal ulceration cause complications, surgical intervention may be required. Gastroenterostomy has been reported to be effective in some cases through bypassing the affected portion of duodenum and allowing for an alternative route for gastric emptying.[299] However, short-term survival and long-term quality of life and use are often unsatisfactory. Patients that have a successful surgical outcome require long-term aftercare and usually require long-term maintenance acid suppression and treatment with a prokinetic drug until gastric emptying is normalized. Thus an owner should be prepared to make a significant time and financial commitment before surgery is considered.

DUODENITIS–PROXIMAL JEJUNITIS

Duodenitis–proximal jejunitis (DPJ) (anterior enteritis; proximal enteritis) describes a clinical syndrome that is characterized by inflammation and edema of the duodenum and proximal jejunum, excessive fluid and electrolyte secretion into the small intestine, and, consequently, large volumes of enterogastric reflux. The syndrome of DPJ was first described in 1982[302] and was more fully characterized in 1987.[303] A subsequent report[304] described clinical and clinicopathologic parameters in horses with DPJ that differed somewhat from cases in the 1982 report, suggesting that either the cases were of similar etiopathogenesis but of different severity, or that the cases were of different etiopathogenesis with the only similarity being the segment of bowel affected. A diagnosis of DPJ is often applied to cases in which there is abdominal discomfort, small intestinal distention, and excessive enterogastric reflux without obstruction, yet it is unclear whether all of these cases lie along a spectrum of severity of DPJ or whether there are several disease entities that affect the proximal small intestine and that share clinical features. The latter seems more likely.

PATHOPHYSIOLOGY. In horses with DPJ, lesions are consistently found in the duodenum, but the severity and frequency of lesions in the jejunum are variable. Serositis is a consistent finding, characterized by bright red to dark red petechial and ecchymotic hemorrhages on the serosal surface.[303] Histologic lesions include hyperemia and edema of the mucosa and submucosa, villus epithelial degeneration, epithelial cell sloughing, neutrophilic pleocytosis, hemorrhages in the muscular layers, and fibrinopurulent exudation on the serosa.

With DPJ, there is an increased volume of duodenogastric reflux, typically 50 to 100 ml/min. This reflux has been considered to result from increased intestinal fluid secretion and decreased motility. Mechanisms of intestinal fluid secretion include passive transmucosal exudation, secondary to mucosal and submucosal inflammation and characterized by a protein-rich fluid secretion, and active fluid secretion, caused by increased cyclic nucleotides and characterized by fluid with a high electrolyte and low protein content. The components of fluid in the intestines of horses with DPJ have not been characterized, but it is likely to result from a combination of passive and active secretion. In some horses, the hemorrhagic nature of the gastric reflux implies increased capillary permeability of the duodenal mucosa, whereas in other horses the watery nature of the reflux, the presence of serum

electrolyte disturbances,[305] and the absence of peripheral hypoproteinemia are most consistent with an active secretory process.

Another potential source of the large volume of fluid secreted into the proximal small intestine and refluxed into the stomach is the pancreas. Normally, there is periodic orad movement of duodenal contents into the stomach, which has been observed endoscopically and has been documented by collecting gastric contents with and without pyloric obstruction.[297] The duodenal contents have a large component of water, sodium, and bicarbonate, as well as bile salts from the liver. These secretions are presumed to originate from the pancreas and to a lesser extent the liver, based on one report in the literature, but this has yet to be confirmed. Observation of the major duodenal papilla by endoscopy in normal horses reveals periodic trickles of small volumes of fluid that originate from the pancreas and the liver (Fig. 30-34). In some horses with DPJ, I have observed almost continuous secretion of fluid from the major duodenal papilla into the duodenum, leading to speculation that the pancreas may have an important, even dominant, contribution to the large volume of fluid that must be removed from the stomachs of some horses with DPJ.

CLINICAL SIGNS AND DIFFERENTIAL DIAGNOSIS. Because the primary differential diagnosis is small intestinal obstruction, prompt differentiation of DPJ from obstruction is important, but on a case by case basis this is often very difficult. For this reason, it is not appropriate for a veterinary practitioner in the field to attempt this differentiation. Any case in which small intestinal obstruction is suspected (distended small intestine on rectal examination, greater than 2 L of nasogastric reflux) should be referred to a facility in which abdominal surgery can be performed. Factors that will influence the decision as to whether surgery is indicated are best evaluated in a facility where surgery can be done if needed.

Horses with DPJ present with a history of an acute onset of moderate to severe abdominal pain that often is followed

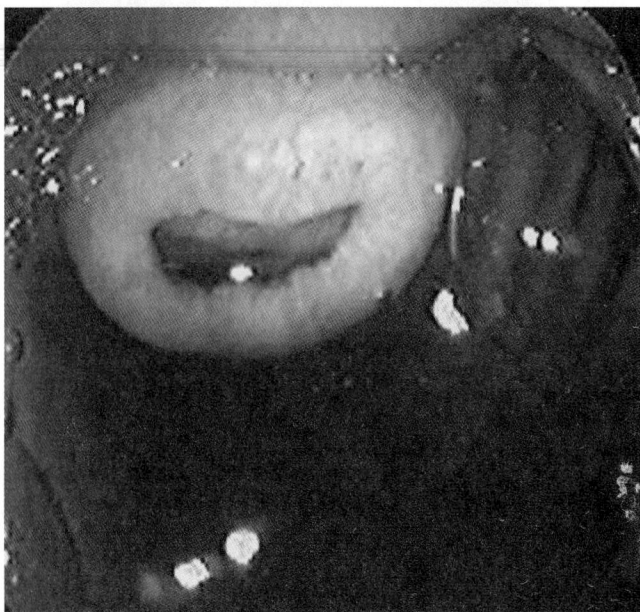

FIG. 30-34 ▓ Endoscopic view of the major duodenal papilla in a horse. Normally, intermittent trickles of green-tinged fluid can be seen to come from the papilla. In some horses with duodenitis-proximal jejunitis, frequent discharge of fluid will be seen.

by varying degrees of obtundation. Nasogastric intubation yields a large volume of enterogastric reflux (frequently orange-brown with a fetid odor), and rectal examination usually reveals moderate small intestinal distention. The initial volume of reflux may be as much as12 L to 16 L. The duration of the reflux may be as short as 24 to 48 hours but usually lasts 3 to 7 days. Horses are often febrile (rectal temperature greater than 38° C [101° F]), dehydrated, and have injected mucous membranes, prolonged capillary refill time, diminished intestinal sounds, tachycardia (>60 beats/min), and tachypnea.[302-304,307,308] Although abdominal pain usually abates after gastric decompression, most horses remain obtunded, which perhaps is the most consistent and characteristic clinical sign of the disease. If the fluid that accumulates in the proximal intestinal tract is not removed periodically, signs of abdominal pain recur.

Assessment of the degree of small intestinal distention and the thickness of the intestinal wall can be useful indicators. Often, horses with DPJ will have generalized distention of small intestine, but when palpated per rectum the intestine does not feel taught. In many cases of small intestinal obstruction, the small bowel will feel tightly distended, but this is not universally true. Ultrasonography can be used, both transrectal and transabdominal, to determine the diameter of the small intestine, evaluate contractions, and to measure the thickness of the wall of the intestine. With acute obstruction one can see several segments of small intestine that are 6 to 10 cm in diameter, have no contraction, and have a wall diameter of 3 to 5 mm. With DPJ small intestinal diameter may be less, and the thickness of the intestinal wall may exceed 6 mm.

CLINICOPATHOLOGIC FINDINGS. Clinical laboratory findings include an increased packed cell volume and total plasma proteins (hemoconcentration), a metabolic acidosis in long-standing or severe cases, an elevated peritoneal fluid protein concentration, and a mild to moderate increase in the peritoneal white blood cell count (>5000 cells/μl).[153,154] The peritoneal fluid is usually yellow and turbid, but in severe cases diapedesis occurs, resulting in a serosanguinous color. The white blood cell count in the peripheral blood may be normal or increased.[303,304] In addition, hyponatremia, hypochloremia, hypokalemia, and acid-base alterations have been reported in horses with DPJ.[305]

TREATMENT. Because the etiologic agent(s) for DPJ are unknown, treatment remains empiric and consists of aggressive supportive therapy. The continuous production of enterogastric reflux requires gastric decompression every 1 to 2 hours to relieve pain and to prevent gastric rupture. Approximately 4 to 8 L of malodorous gastric fluid can be collected during decompression. Horses should receive nothing by mouth until small intestinal function has returned, recognized clinically by cessation or reduction of the nasogastric reflux to 1 to 2 L over a 4-hour period and increased frequency of borborygmi. The time necessary for gastric decompression varies, but 3 to 7 days may be required. Repeated rectal examinations after the first day of therapy will inconsistently reveal distended loops of small intestine, depending on the frequency of removal of the reflux and the severity of the initial lesion. Transrectal ultrasonography may reveal fluid-filled small intestine when such bowel is not discernible by rectal palpation.

Intravenous administration of a balanced electrolyte solution is necessary to maintain intravascular fluid volume and maintain cardiovascular performance. In some horses even rapid administration of fluid fails to adequately restore and maintain intravascular volume because of enteric fluid losses that can be as great as 8 L hour. Additionally, the very large volume of isotonic crystalloid fluid that must be given intravenously to keep pace with enteric fluid losses with DPJ may accelerate the flux of fluid from the vasculature into the intestinal lumen because of a reduced intravascular oncotic pressure, increased capillary perfusion pressure, and increased capillary permeability in the inflamed intestine. Consequently, the balance between adequate hydration and the volume of enterogastric reflux obtained requires careful and frequent monitoring.

Administration of colloid solutions may be of benefit in preserving intravasular volume without promoting enterogastric reflux, but the cost of equine plasma or colloid solutions (dextrans, hetastarch) is exorbitant in the context of the volume of fluid that must be provided. Similarly, it is doubtful whether a relatively small volume (10 L) of colloid solution will have an important impact on DPJ cases. Additionally, some properties of colloid solutions may be undesirable in DPJ patients.[309]

During the initial hours of therapy, even aggressive intravenous fluid administration may result in only moderate clinical improvement. A positive clinical response, as evidenced by improved hydration status, decreased heart rate, decreased nasogastric reflux, improved attitude, and improvement in parameters reflecting kidney function (decreased blood urea nitrogen and serum creatinine), correlates with resolving intestinal inflammation.

Nonsteroidal antiinflammatory agents should be used judiciously to avoid masking the clinical signs of a potential surgical lesion. Flunixin meglumine can be used at dosages of 0.25 to 0.5 mg/kg every 6 hours to reduce the untoward effects of arachidonic acid metabolites.

Antimicrobial agents are typically administered to horses with DPJ, although the necessity for antimicrobial treatment in horses with DPJ is uncertain. Initially, *Clostridium perfringens* was thought to be involved, because gram-positive rods were identified in gastric reflux,[302] but this was an inconsistent finding. Broad-spectrum antimicrobial treatment may be indicated in horses with intestinal inflammation, but care must be taken in selecting an antimicrobial to avoid potential adverse effects, particularly nephrotoxicosis with aminoglycosides in a patient with compromised renal function.

Horses with DPJ may have to be kept from eating for several days and are often in a hypermetabolic state, therefore they rapidly develop a negative energy and nitrogen balance. In these horses, parenteral nutritional support should be considered. Parenterally administered solutions containing glucose, balanced amino acid solutions, lipid emulsions, balanced electrolyte and trace minerals, and vitamins have been administered to adult horses with a variety of intestinal disorders, including DPJ. Providing for part of the horse's nutritional requirements (8000 to 12,000 kCal/day) is possible with glucose/amino acid solutions that are of moderate cost (500 kg horse: $250/day for glucose and amino acids; $500/day for glucose, lipid emulsions, amino acids). The rationale for this treatment is that by providing nutritional support to an anorectic, severely ill horse the healing process will be facilitated, complications will be reduced, and the duration of hospitalization may be shortened. Thus the overall cost of providing nutritional supplementation, enteral or parenteral, to horses with DPJ may well be offset by quicker recoveries and diminished requirements for other costly treatments. This hypothesis has not been proven in horses, but clinical impressions have been favorable.

Medical therapy is sufficient in most cases of DPJ. In patients with prolonged (>7 days) nasogastric reflux, excessive fluid losses that cannot be corrected with conventional fluid therapy, or clinical and laboratory findings strongly suggestive of an intestinal obstruction, surgery should be considered. Surgery is used to make the diagnosis and potentially to alleviate enterogastric reflux by providing an alternative route for fluid that accumulates in the small intestine. This can be done through a standing flank procedure, but it is better accomplished by means of a ventral midline celiotomy. This approach permits a more complete evaluation of the gastrointestinal tract and facilitates development of a more physiologically effective intestinal shunt. On entrance into the abdominal cavity, dilated small intestine is immediately apparent. After the extent of the diseased intestine is determined, a segment of normal distal jejunum is laid side to side to the proximal diseased intestine in an isoperistaltic fashion, as far proximal on the affected bowel as possible without extending to bowel that cannot be removed from the abdominal cavity. A small 1- to 1.5-cm hand-sewn anastomosis can then be made between the two segments of intestine.[310] This provides an adequate stoma for direct intestinal decompression while minimally compromising the digestive and absorptive capacity of the small intestine. Potential complications of this procedure include development of an intestinal incarceration through the loop that is formed and the development of small intestinal adhesions.

COMPLICATIONS. Complications of DPJ include peritonitis, myocardial and renal infarction, aspiration pneumonia, adhesions of the proximal small intestine, and laminitis. Over 90% of horses with DPJ survive the primary intestinal insult with appropriate management.[158] The death/function losses from this disease are more commonly related to the secondary complications such as laminitis and intraabdominal adhesions. In one report, laminitis occurred in 28% of horses with DPJ, and associated factors were high bodyweight and hemorrhagic gastric reflux.[311] Laminitis prophylaxis is routinely incorporated into the medical therapy and can consist of a variety of treatments, none of which is proven to be effective. These include nonsteroidal antiinflammatory drugs, topical glyceryl trinitrate, dimethyl sulfoxide (200 mg/kg given as a 10% solution in normal saline), and heparin at 40 IU/kg SC or in plasma (to activate antithrombin III), among many others.

PROLIFERATIVE ENTEROPATHY

Proliferative enteropathy (PE) is an infrequently diagnosed disorder of the small intestine of young horses. Most horses with PE are weanling foals or yearlings, and in our experience most have been female. The hallmarks of PE are severe hypoproteinemia accompanied by grossly thickened small intestine with mucosal ulceration. Some cases resemble PE in swine, and in a few foals organisms sharing characteristics with *Lawsonia intracelluaris*, the causative agent of porcine proliferative enteropathy, have been identified.[312-314]

CLINICAL SIGNS. Proliferative enteropathy is a chronic, progressive disorder, and, as such, affected animals are typically not presented until the disease is advanced. Horses with PE present with a variety of clinical problems, most notably chronic weight loss, intermittent abdominal discomfort, or diarrhea. Some affected animals are erroneously treated for primary gastric ulceration, and indeed there may appear to be temporary improvement in attitude and appetite. This may reflect successful treatment of gastric ulcers that develop as a secondary problem. Many affected animals are diminished in stature, reflecting retarded growth resulting from a chronic intestinal disorder that probably affects absorption of nutrients. Affected animals typically appear lethargic.

CLINICAL AND LABORATORY FINDINGS. Other than the aforementioned findings, physical examination is usually not remarkable. Ventral edema often is present as a result of hypoproteinemia. Some animals present with tachycardia and tachypnea. Fever is an inconsistent finding. Abdominal

ultrasonography is often useful to identify thickened small intestine. The entire ventral abdomen should be examined, but affected intestine is most often in the distal jejunem and ileum, and this often can be seen along the midline caudally. If transrectal ultrasonography is possible, better detail of the intestinal wall will be appreciated. In affected animals, the intestinal wall diameter will be 6 to 12 mm. More normal surrounding small intestine may be seen, and in contrast the affected segment of bowel will appear more rigid and will have a corrugated appearance to the mucosa, and the diameter of the lumen will be decreased in size because of mucosal proliferation (Fig. 30-35).

Complete blood count findings in horses with PE vary. Leukocystosis is a frequent finding, and this may be characterized by a lymphocytosis. Profound hypoproteinemia (serum protein <3.0 g/dl, albumin <1.5 g/dl) is a consistent finding, although a foal of one report had mildly decreased total serum protein with markedly low albumin (0.6 g/dl) and polyclonal gammopathy (4.6 g/dl). Hyperfibrinogemia occurs in some cases. Other clinicopathologic findings are variable and depend on the chronicity and whether there are excessive fluid and electrolyte losses through diarrhea.

PATHOLOGIC FINDINGS. Gross thickening of the entire small intestine can occur, but in our experience the ileum and distal jejunem are affected the most. All portions of the intestinal wall can be involved, but characteristically there is pronounced mucosal thickening with varying severity of ulceration and transmural edema. The affected bowel appears to be stiff, and the mucosal surface has a corrugated appearance. Mucosal pleocytosis is a common feature, but in different cases the predominating inflammatory cell type will differ. Most of our cases were characterized by a lymphocytic/plasmacytic cellular infiltration, and this histologic appearance was present in two foals in which *L. intracellularis* proliferative enteropathy was diagnosed. Neutrophilic pleocytosis can be seen in areas of intestine in which there is severe mucosal ulceration. In cases with *Lawsonia* infection, there is crypt proliferation, accompanied by crypt elongation and epithelial hyperplasia.

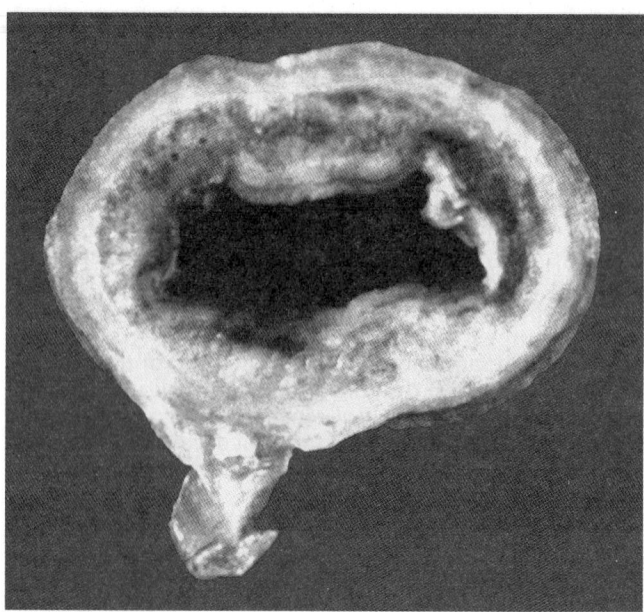

FIG. 30-35 ■ A cross section of ileum from a 6 month-old horse with proliferative enteropathy.

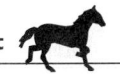

Staining formalin-fixed tissues with Warthin-Starry silver stain will reveal curved bacilli in enterocytes. Confirmation of infection with *L. intracellaris* requires sending tissue specimens to laboratories equipped to diagnose porcine proliferative enteropathy. Identification of *L. intracellularis* is by immunohistochemistry or immunofluorescence using monoclonal antibody to *L. intracellularis* or polymerase chain reaction analysis. Serologic tests for antibody to *L. intracellularis* in equids may be available from some laboratories.

TREATMENT. In many, if not most, cases of proliferative enteropathy, an etiologic agent is not determined. Treatment objectives are to reduce intestinal inflammation and, if pertinent, to eliminate infection. In our experience, corticosteroid administration has been associated with resolution of clinical signs in most cases of PE we have treated. Prednisone, 1 mg/kg per os, once daily for 7 to 10 days, then 0.75 mg/kg per os, once daily for 7 to 10 days, then 0.5 mg/kg per os, once daily for 7 to 10 days has appeared effective, including in severe cases. Antimicrobial therapy is indicated if *Lawsonia* infection is suspected or confirmed. Treatment with erythromycin was associated with clinical improvement in foals in Quebec, Canada that were diagnosed as having PE caused by *L. intracelluaris.* Other supportive treatment can include plasma in cases with severe hypoproteinemia and parenteral nutrition in animals that are anorectic and debilitated. Whereas a diagnosis of PE may be made at exploratory surgery, resection of affected intestine is usually not necessary.

INFLAMMATORY BOWEL DISEASE (IBD)

Several intestinal disorders characterized by inflammatory cell infiltration have been placed under the umbrella of inflammatory bowel disease, including eosinophilic enterocolitis, lymphocytic/plasmacytic enteritis, and basophilic enterocolitis.[316-319] IBD in humans is typically characterized by a neutrophilic inflammation, but neutrophils are just the effector cell in a highly complex disease process.[320] The syndromes described for equine inflammatory intestinal disorders therefore appear to differ from human IBD; given the different types of cellular infiltrates found in affected horses, these disorders presumably reflect different pathophysiologic mechanisms. Thus use of the term inflammatory bowel disease is not intended to imply either a similarity to the condition described in human being or similarity between the various syndromes described in horses.

CLINICAL FINDINGS. Horses with IBD typically have progressive weight loss and may develop a poor appetite and have intermittent abdominal discomfort. If the disease predominates in the small intestine, diarrhea will not be a feature. In some cases, there will be associated dermatitis.[321] Horses often present with peripheral edema secondary to hypoproteinemia from enteric protein losses. Ultrasonography may reveal thickened small intestine (>5 mm wall diameter).

Clinicopathologic abnormalities include anemia, hypoalbuminemia, hypoproteinemia, and malabsorption of glucose and D-xylose. Hypoalbuminemia in the absence of proteinuria or severe liver dysfunction is consistent with protein-losing enteropathy. Some horses may have a relative gammopathy. Serum electrolyte concentrations and total CO_2 are usually normal. Subclinical disseminated intravascular coagulation with thrombocytopenia and increased fibrinogen degradation products have been identified in horses with chronic enteritis.[319,322]

In many horses, inflammatory cells infiltrate throughout the intestinal tract. Thus rectal mucosal biopsy may be useful to identify cases of IBD in horses.[323] A definitive diagnosis often requires biopsy of the small and/or large intestine. With appropriate instruments this can be done by laparoscopy, although an exploration via a ventral midline approach permits a more thorough evaluation of the abdomen. In most horses, cellular infiltration can be found to varying degrees throughout the intestinal tract.

TREATMENT AND PROGNOSIS. Because the specific diseases included in IBD are quite different, a generalized treatment recommendation cannot be made. Most reported cases of IBD in horses have been fatal, even with aggressive treatment with steroidal antiinflammatory drugs. Scott and colleagues[324] reported on 11 cases of IBD that survived long term, but the characterization of these cases as having IBD was not consistent with other reports. None of the reported cases had hypoproteinemia, malabsorption, or evidence of diffuse inflammatory cell infiltration throughout the intestine.

Classically reported cases of eosinophilic, lymphocytic, and basophilic enteritis have failed to respond to treatment. If treatment is attempted, corticosteroids should be used. Clinicians have used immunosuppressive doses of dexamethasone, up to 0.2 mg/kg, once daily.

Granulomatous enterocolitis is a chronic inflammatory disorder that affects the small or large intestine and that can be caused by several factors, including infectious agents, parasites, and exposure to aluminum.[325-329] In some cases the disorder may result from specific defects in the inflammatory cell bacteriocidal capabilities or dysfunctions in the local immune system modulation. The diagnosis of granulomatous enteritis or colitis is based on the histologic appearance of giant cells and epitheloid macrophages in the affected intestinal segments.[316]

The most common clinical sign is weight loss with a good appetite. Hypoalbuminemia may lead to peripheral edema. As the disease progresses to the colon, diarrhea will develop. Dermatitis may accompany the enteric lesions.[330] Diagnosis is made by histologic evaluation of tissue specimens, from rectal mucosal biopsy, surgical biopsy of intestine, or postmortem examination.[316]

Successful remission of granulomatous enteritis was reported in one case that was treated with dexamethasone.[331] However, in the vast majority of cases treatment is unsuccessful.

LYMPANGIECTASIA AND CHYLOABDOMEN

There are few reports of lympangiectasia and chyloabdomen in the literature. Lymphangiectasia is dilation of the lymphatics of the small or large intestine (Fig. 30-36), usually caused by an abscess[332] or neoplasia. There is a report of congenital lymphatic defect in a neonatal foal that resulted in chyloabdomen.[333] Typically, thickening of the intestinal wall and leakage of chyle into the peritoneal cavity result from obstruction of the lymphatics. Animals can present with signs that include abdominal discomfort, diarrhea, and chronic weight loss. Diagnosis is made on the basis of abdominal fluid analysis and ultrasonography. Chylous abdominal fluid will appear milky and may contain a high percentage of lymphocytes. Ultrasonography may reveal segments of thickened small intestine. Diagnosis is confirmed at surgery or postmortem examination, and treatment, if possible, is usually surgical.

NEOPLASIA

Primary and secondary neoplasia involving the alimentary tract of horses is relatively uncommon, although several cases have been reported.[334] Typical signs associated with, but not diagnostic for, small intestinal neoplasia include colic and weight loss. In most horses with focal intestinal neoplasia the problem only becomes apparent when lumen obstruction develops. Lymphosarcoma can be disseminated throughout a

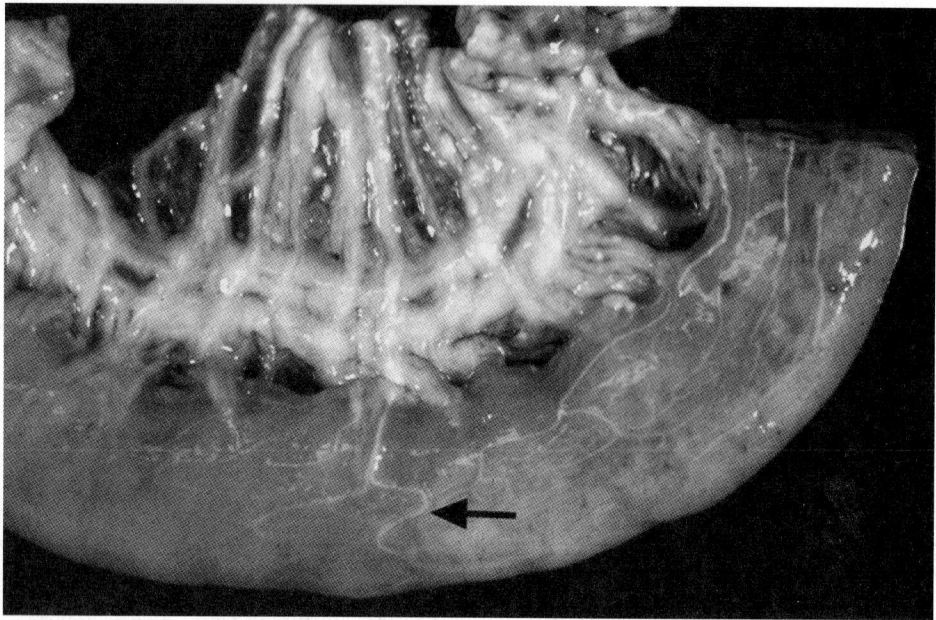

FIG. 30-36 ■ Section of small intestine from a foal with chyloabdomen and a *Rhodococcus equi* abdominal abscess. Mesenteric lymphatics are distended with white chyle, as are serosal lymphatics *(arrow)*.

large portion of intestine, eventually resulting in a malabsorption/weight loss syndrome. Lymphosarcoma affects horses of all ages and can be manifested as an enteric disorder, as well as affecting other systems.[335] The diagnosis of enteric lymphosarcoma can occasionally be made on the basis of cytologic examination of fluid obtained by abdominocentesis. In other cases, intestinal biopsy is required to diagnose the neoplastic disorder. There is no effective treatment, unless the tumor is discrete and can be removed surgically.

Other neoplasms affecting the small intestine are unusual, typically arise from the wall of the bowel, and include adenocarcinoma,[336] leiomyosarcoma,[337] and neurofibroma.[338] These tumors often result in intestinal obstruction and signs of abdominal discomfort. Discrete tumors may be surgically removed.

REFERENCES

292. McColl K, el-Omar EM, Gillen D: The role of *H. pylori* infection in the pathophysiology of duodenal ulcer disease, *J Physiol Pharmacol* 48:287-295, 1997.
293. Miller TA: Bicarbonate secretory breakdown: explanation for increased incidence of duodenal ulcer with age? *Gastroenterology* 100:1471-1472, 1991.
294. Wilson JH: Gastric and duodenal ulcers in foals: a retrospective study. *Proceedings of the Equine Colic Research Symposium*, Athens, Ga, 1986, p 126.
295. Ettlinger JJ, Ford T, Palmer JE: Ulcerative duodenitis with luminal constriction in two horses, *J Am Vet Med Assoc* 196:1628-1630, 1990.
296. Acland HM, Gunson DE, Gillette DM: Ulcerative duodenitis in foals, *Vet Pathol* 20:653-661, 1983.
297. Kitchen DL et al: Source of non-parietal component of pentagastrin-stimulated fasting equine gastric contents, *Proceedings of the Sixth Equine Colic Research Symposium*, Athens, Ga, 1998, p 35.
298. Becht JL, Byars TD: Gastroduodenal ulcers in foals, *Equine Vet J* 18:307-313, 1986.
299. Campbell-Thompson ML et al: Gastroenterostomy for treatment of gastroduodenal ulcer disease in 14 foals, *J Am Vet Med Assoc* 188:840-844, 1986.
300. Jenkins CC et al: Duration of antisecretory effects of oral omeprazole in horses with chronic gastric cannulae, *Equine Vet J* Suppl 13:89-92, 1992.
301. Moshal MG, Spitaels JH, Manion GL: Double-blind placebo-controlled evaluation of one-year therapy with sucralfate in healed duodenal ulcer, *Scand J Gastroenterol* 18(suppl 83):57-59, 1982.
302. Blackwell RB, White NA: Duodenitis proximal jejunitis in the horse, *Proceedings of the First Equine Colic Research Symposium*, Athens, Ga, 1992, p 106.
303. White NA et al: Hemorrhagic fibrinonecrotic duodenitis-proximal jejunitis in horses: 20 cases (1977-1984), *J Am Vet Med Assoc* 190:311-316, 1987.
304. Johnston, JK, Morris, DD: Comparison of duodenitis proximal jejunitis and small intestinal obstruction in horses: 68 cases: (1977-1985), *J Am Vet Med Assoc* 91:849-854,1987.
305. Morris DD: Medical therapy of colic. In Gordon BJ, Allen D, eds: *Colic management in the horse*, Lenexa, Kan, 1988, Veterinary Medicine Publishing, pp 201-212.
306. Alexander F, Hickson JCD: The salivary and pancreatic secretions of the horse. In Phillipson AT, ed: *Physiology of digestion and metabolism in the ruminant*, London, 1970, Oriel, pp 375-389.
307. Seahorn TL, Cornick Il, Cohen ND: Prognostic indication for horses with duodenitis/proximal jejunitis, *J Vet Intern Med* 6:307-311, 1992.
308. Luth B, Robertson J: A retrospective comparison of surgical to medical management of proximal enteritis in the horse, *Proceedings of the Thirty-fourth Annual Convention of the American Association of Equine Practitioners*, 1988, pp 69-79.
309. Roberts JS, Bratton SL: Colloid volume expanders. Problems, pitfalls and possibilities, *Drugs* 55:621-630,1998.
310. Allen D, Clark ES. Duodenitis-proximal jejunitis. In Smith BP, ed: *Large animal internal medicine*, St Louis, 1989, Mosby.
311. Cohen ND et al: Prevalence and factors associated with development of laminitis in horses with duodenitis/proximal jejunitis: 33 cases (1985-1991), *J Am Vet Med Assoc*, 204:250-254, 1994.
312. Brees DJ et al: *Lawsonia intracellularis*-like organism infection in a miniature horse, *J Am Vet Med Assoc* 215:511-514, 1999.
313. Frank N et al: *Lawsonia intracellularis* proliferative enteropathy in a weanling foal, *Equine Vet J* 30:549-552, 1998.
314. Williams NM, Harrison LR, Gebhart CJ: Proliferative enteropathy in a foal caused by *Lawsonia intracellularis*–like bacterium, *J Vet Diagn Invest* 8:254-256, 1996.
315. Lavoie JP: Personal communication, 1999.
316. Platt H: Chronic inflammatory and lymphoproliferative lesions of the equine small intestine, *J Comp Pathol* 96:671-684, 1986.
317. Pass DA, Bolton JR: Chronic eosinophilic gastroenteritis in the horse, *Vet Pathol* 19:486-496, 1983.
318. Pass DA, Bolton JR, Mills JN: Basophilic enterocolitis in a horse, *Vet Pathol* 21:362-364, 1984.
319. MacAllister CG et al: Lymphocytic-plasmacytic enteritis in two horses, *J Am Vet Med Assoc* 196:1995-1998, 1990.
320. Fiocchi C: Intestinal inflammation: a complex interplay of immune and nonimmune cell interactions, *Am J Physiol* 273:G769-775, 1997.
321. Gibson KT: Alders RG Eosinophilic enterocolitis and dermatitis in two horses, *Equine Vet J* 19:247-252,1987.
322. Morris DD, Vaala WE, Sarton E: Protein-losing entropathy in a yearling filly with subclinical DIC and autoimmune hemolytic disease, *Compend Cont Educ* 4:S542-S546, 1982.

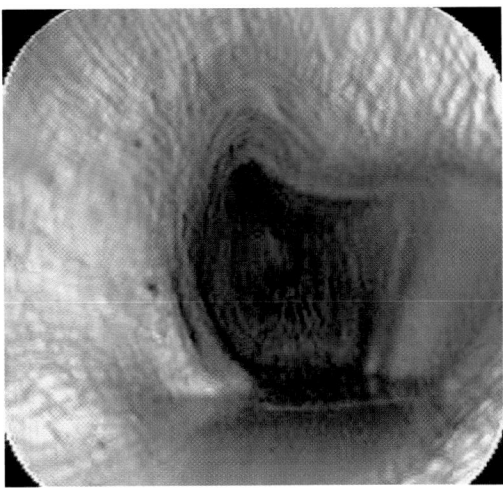

PLATE 1 ▪▪ Endoscopic view of megaesophagus in a 10 month-old foal, also shown in Fig. 30-17. The esophageal lumen is greatly distended, and the mucosa has multifocal erosion. (Courtesy Dr. MJ Murray.)

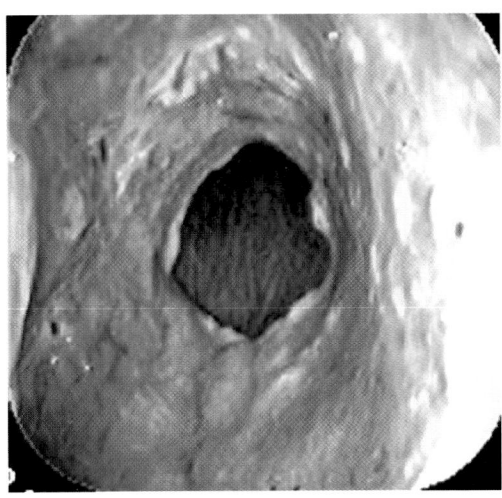

PLATE 2 ▪▪ Endoscopic view of the esophagus of a 20-year-old gelding that presented with a history of 3 days of esophageal obstruction. The horse had recently been "rescued" and its previous history was unknown. After an obstruction consisting of grass was forcefully relieved by flushing water through a nasogastric tube, endoscopy revealed ulceration of the esophageal mucosa just orad to a stricture of the esophageal lumen. (Courtesy Dr. MJ Murray.)

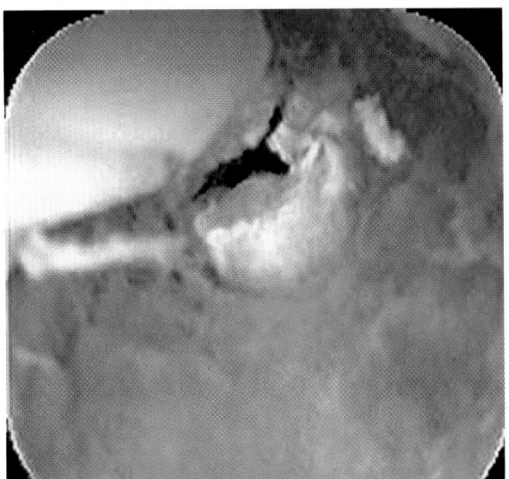

PLATE 3 ▪▪ Same horse as in Plate 2, 14 days later. The mucosa adjacent to the stricture remained ulcerated, and the diameter of the esophageal lumen had progressively diminished. At this point, it was not possible to advance the 10-mm-diameter endoscope through the stricture. (Courtesy Dr. MJ Murray.)

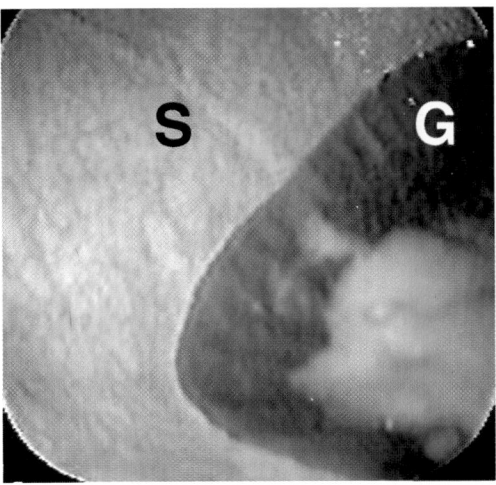

PLATE 4 ▪▪ Endoscopic view of the right side of a normal stomach, showing the pale squamous mucosa (S) and the red glandular mucosa (G).

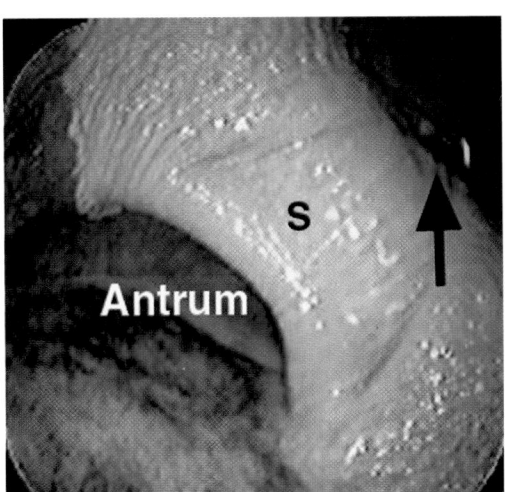

PLATE 5 ▪▪ Endoscopic view of the lesser curvature of a normal stomach, showing the pale squamous mucosa (S). The antrum lies ventral to a fold formed by the squamous mucosa along the lesser curvature, and the pylorus is immediately ventral to the cardia, through which the endoscope (arrow) can be seen entering the stomach.

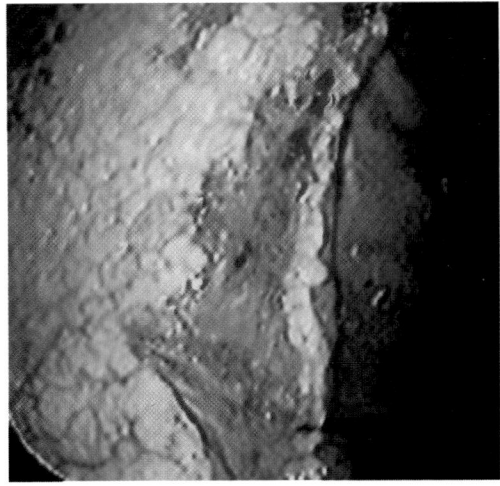

PLATE 6 ▪▪ Endoscopic view of a large area of ulceration of the squamous mucosa adjacent to the margo plicatus along the right side of the stomach.

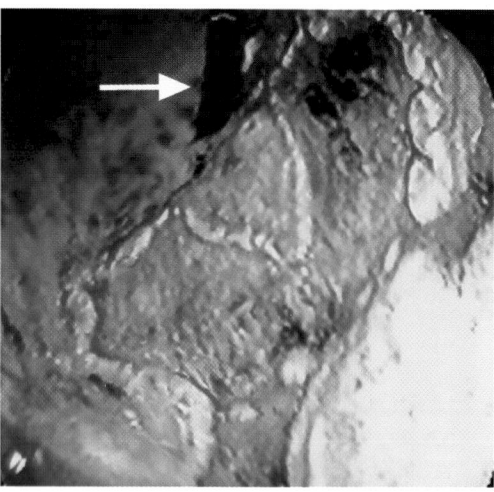

PLATE 7 ■ Endoscopic view of a large area of ulceration of the squamous mucosa along the lesser curvature of the stomach. The ulceration has a "butterfly" pattern, which is typical of ulcers at this site, and this pattern may reflect protection of the mucosa immediately ventral to the cardia by saliva entering the stomach from the esophagus. The *arrow* points at the endoscope entering the stomach through the cardia.

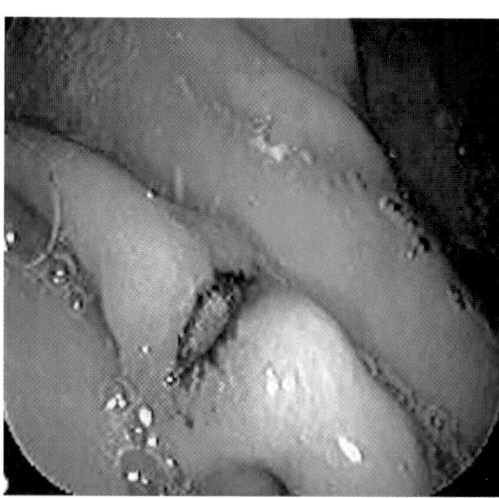

PLATE 8 ■ Endoscopic view of an ulcer in the gastric glandular mucosa. The ulcer is in a rugal fold, which is a typical site of ulcers in the glandular portion of the stomach.

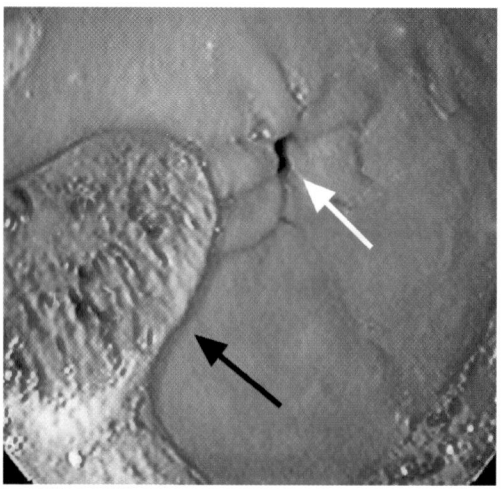

PLATE 9 ■ Endoscopic view of the antrum of the stomach. The *white arrow* points at the pylorus. The *black arrow* points at an area of ulceration and thickening of a rugal fold leading to the pylorus. This is a severe example of a frequent finding in the stomach of adult horses: thickening of a rugal fold in the antrum with associate erosion or ulceration of the mucosa. The cause of these lesions is undetermined.

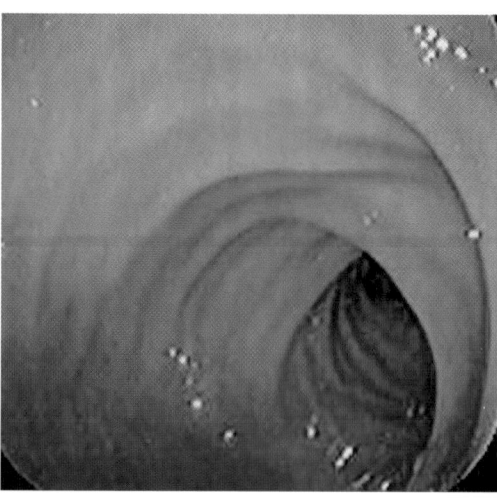

PLATE 10 ■ Endoscopic view of normal duodenal mucosa. In this photograph, the endoscope has advanced aboral to the major duodenal papilla, which in most foals and horses is difficult and unusual to accomplish because of the anatomic configuration of the duodenum with respect to the stomach.

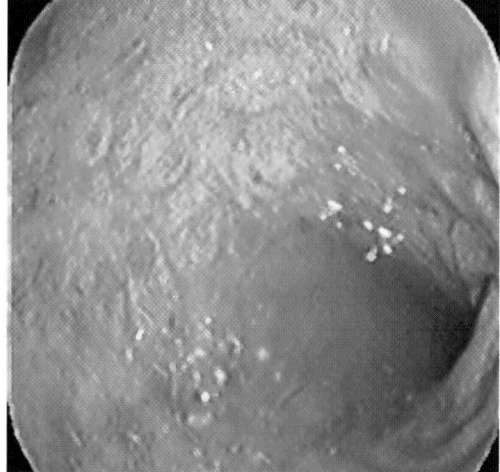

PLATE 11 ■ Duodenum of a foal that presented with fever, depression, leukocytosis, and hyperfibrinogenemia. This endoscopic view is orad to the major duodenal papilla. The mucosa is inflamed and there is yellow-orange fibrinous exudate adherent to the mucosal surface.

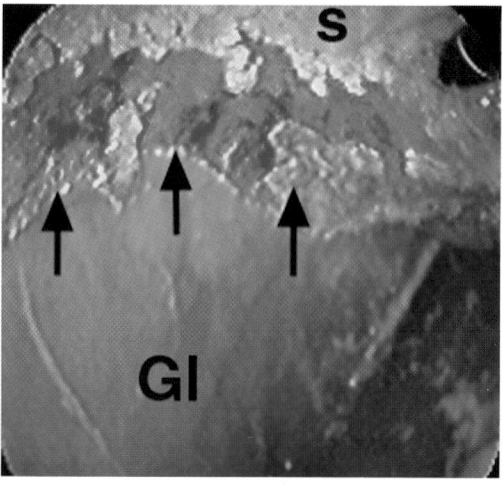

PLATE 12 ■ Endoscopic view of the stomach of the foal in Plate 11. There is severe ulceration of the squamous mucosa *(S)* adjacent to the margo plicatus *(arrows)*, because of delayed gastric emptying secondary to the severe duodenitis. Many foals with duodenitis present with classic gastric ulcer signs, because of delayed stomach emptying, accumulation of acidic peptic secretions in the stomach and often gastroesophageal reflux. *Gl,* Glandular mucosa.

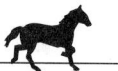

323. Lindberg R, Nygren A, Oersson SGB: Rectal biopsy diagnosis in horses with clinical signs of intestinal disorders: a retrospective study of 116 cases, *Equine Vet J* 28:275-284, 1996.

324. Scott EA et al: Inflammatory bowel disease in horses: 11 cases (1988-1998), *J Am Vet Med Assoc* 214:1527-1530, 1999.

325. Dade AW, Lickfeldt WE, McAllister HA: Granulomatous colitis in a horse with histoplasmosis, *Vet Med Small Anim Clin* 68:279-281, 1973.

326. Larsen AB, Moon HW, Merkal BS: Susceptibility of horses to *Mycobacterium paratuberculosis*, *Am J Vet Res* 33:2185-2189, 1972.

327. Cooley AJ et al: *Molluscum contagiosum* in a horse with granulomatous enteritis, *J Comp Pathol* 97:29-34, 1987.

328. Jasko DJ, Roth L: Granulomatous colitis associated with small strongyle larvae in a horse, *J Am Vet Med Assoc* 185:553-554,1984.

329. Fogarty U et al: A cluster of equine granulomatous enteritis cases: the link with aluminium *Vet Hum Toxicol* 40:297-305, 1998.

330. Woods PR, Helman RG, Schmitz DG: Granulomatous enteritis and cutaneous arteritis in a horse, *J Am Vet Med Assoc* 203:1573-1575, 1993.

331. Duryea JH et al: Clinical remission of granulomatous enteritis in a standardbred gelding long-term dexamethasone administration, *Equine Vet J* 29:164-167, 1997.

332. Hanselaer JR, Nyland TG: Chyloabdomen and ultrasonographic detection of an intra-abdominal abscess in a foal, *J Am Vet Med Assoc* 183:1465-1467, 1983.

333. Campbell-Beggs CL et al: Chyloabdomen in a neonatal foal, *Vet Rec* 137:96-98, 1995.

334. Cotchin C: A general survey of tumours in the horse, *Equine Vet J* 9:16, 1977.

335. Rebhun WC, Bertone A: Equine lymphosarcoma, *J Am Vet Med Assoc* 184:720-721, 1984.

336. Honnas CM et al: Small intestinal adenocarcinoma in a horse, *J Am Vet Med Assoc* 191:845, 1987.

337. Mair, TS, Taylor, FG, Brown, PJ: Leiomyosarcoma of the duodenum in two horses, *J Comp Pathol* 102:119,1990.

338. Kirchhof N, Scheidemann W, Baumgartner W: Multiple peripheral nerve sheath tumors in the small intestine of a horse, *Vet Pathol* 33:727-730,1996.

SURGICAL DISORDERS OF THE SMALL INTESTINE

ANTHONY T. BLIKSLAGER

SIMPLE OBSTRUCTION

Simple intestinal obstruction is a physical obstruction of the lumen without obstruction of vascular flow. Causes include intraluminal masses (e.g., ileal impaction, ascarid impactions) or extraluminal compression (e.g., intestinal adhesions). Because a large volume of fluid enters the small intestinal lumen daily the obstructed intestine becomes distended.[339,340] Therefore, although the blood supply is not directly involved in simple obstructions, progressive distention can result in decreased mural blood flow,[341] and eventual necrosis of tissues.[342]

Ascarid Impaction

Impactions caused by *Parascaris equorum* typically occur in weanling foals (median age, 5 months; range, 4 to 24 months) that have been on a poor deworming program and that are administered an anthelmintic when they have a heavy parasite burden.[343] Products that cause sudden ascarid paralysis or death, including piperazine, organophosphates, and pyrantel pamoate, have been incriminated.[344] Clinical signs include acute onset of colic after administration of an anthelmintic (usually within 1 to 5 days), and signs compatible with small intestinal obstruction, including nasogastric reflux.[343] The onset of the disease varies according to the degree of obstruction.[344] Diagnosis may be tentatively based on a poor deworming history in a foal that appears unthrifty, signs referable to small intestinal obstruction, and presence of dead ascarids in nasogastric reflux.[343] Abdominal radiographs may indicate the presence of multiple loops of distended small intestine, but are not needed if clinical signs indicate the need for surgery. Surgical treatment typically involves an enterotomy made over the in-

traluminal impaction, and removal of ascarids. The mortality rate in these cases is high (up to 92% in one study) as a result of severe intestinal compromise, peritonitis, and development of adhesions.[343]

Ileal Impaction

Ileal impactions occur most commonly in adult horses in the southeastern United States. Although feeding of coastal Bermuda hay has been implicated in the regional distribution of this disease, it has been difficult to separate geographic location from regional hay sources as risk factors.[345] Signs are typical for a horse with small intestinal obstruction, including onset of moderate to severe colic, and palpable loops of distended small intestine per rectum as the condition progresses. The ileum is the distal most aspect of the small intestinal tract; therefore nasogastric reflux may take a considerable time to develop and is found in approximately 50% of horses requiring surgical correction of ileal impaction.[246,347] The diagnosis is usually made at surgery, although an impacted ileum may be palpated per rectum.[348] However, multiple loops of distended small intestine frequently make the impaction difficult to palpate. Ileal impactions may resolve with medical treatment,[348] but frequently require surgical intervention. At surgery, fluids (2 to 3 L) can be directly infused into the mass, allowing the surgeon to break down the impaction. Extensive small intestinal distention and intraoperative manipulation of the ileum may lead to postoperative ileus,[349] but recent studies indicate that this complication is less frequent as the duration of disease before admission has decreased.[346] Although early studies indicated a guarded prognosis,[347] more recent studies indicate that the prognosis is good.[346,348]

Ileal Hypertrophy

Ileal Hypertrophy is a disorder in which the muscular layers (both circular and longitudinal) of the ileum hypertrophy for unknown reasons. In some cases, the jejunum may also be hypertrophied either alone or in combination with the ileum.[350] Clinical signs include chronic intermittent colic as the ileum hypertrophies and gradually occludes the lumen. In one study, partial anorexia and chronic weight loss (1 to 6 months) were documented in 45% of the horses.[350] The diagnosis is usually made at surgery, although in some cases the hypertophied ileum may be palpated per rectum or seen on ultrasonographic evaluation of the abdomen. For treatment, an ileocecal or jejunocecal anastomosis to bypass the hypertrophied ileum is performed. Without surgical bypass, intermittent colic persists, and the thickened ileum may ultimately rupture. According to one recent report of 11 horses with hypertrophy of the ileum, only 1 horse survived, indicating a poor prognosis. The most common reason for euthanasia was spontaneous ileal rupture.[350]

Meckel's Diverticulum

Meckel's diverticulum is an embryonic remnant that may become impacted. The diverticulum arises from the vitelloumbilical duct, which fails to completely atrophy, and becomes a blind pouch projecting from the antimesenteric border of the ileum.[351,352] Occasionally an associated mesodiverticular band may course from the diverticulum to the umbilical remnant and serve as a point around which small intestine may become strangulated. Mesodiverticular bands may also originate from the embryonic ventral mesentery and attach to the antimesenteric surface of the bowel, forming a potential space within which intestine may become entrapped (Fig. 30-37).[353] Clinical signs range from chronic colic, for an impacted Meckel's

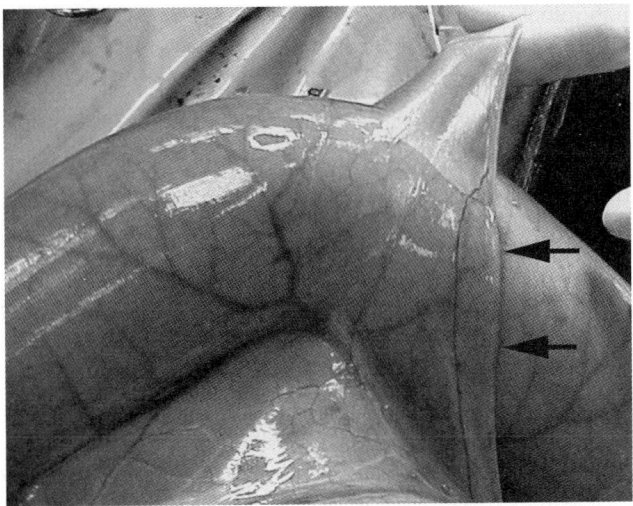

FIG. 30-37 ▓ Jejunal mesodiverticular band. This was an incidental finding during exploration of the abdomen. Intestine may become entrapped within the mesenteric pocket formed by the attachment of the ventral to the dorsal mesentery (arrows).

diverticulum, to acute severe colic if a mesodiverticular band strangulates intestine. The diagnosis is made at surgery, and treatment requires resection of the diverticulum and any associated bands. In one report on strangulation of small intestine by mesodiverticular bands, 2 of 3 horses survived.

STRANGULATING OBSTRUCTION

Strangulation obstruction of the intestine is characterized by simultaneous occlusion of the intestinal lumen and its blood supply. Although strangulation of the intestinal lumen results in clinical signs similar to those of simple obstruction, occlusion of the blood supply results in a more rapid deterioration of the intestinal mucosa and subsequent onset of endotoxemic shock. Therefore clinical signs (including pain, heart rate, mucous membrane color, and capillary refill time) are typically more severe and the prognosis is less favorable.

A great deal of work has been done to characterize mucosal injury that occurs during strangulation[354,355] and, more recently, during reperfusion.[356] In general the lesion that develops during strangulation is severe, leaving little viable bowel for further injury during reperfusion.[357] The severity of the ischemic lesion is partly attributable to the fact that in most cases, initial occlusion of veins and partial occlusion of arterial blood supply during strangulation induces a hemorrhagic lesion. This results in extensive congestion and mucosal degeneration.[354,355] Bowel peripheral to the strangulating lesion may also become injured as a result of distention.[341,353,358] In addition, distended small intestine and bowel that remains viable after surgical correction of strangulation may be subject to reperfusion injury after surgical correction of the lesion, although this has not been documented in natural cases of colic.[359] Furthermore, attempts at reducing mucosal injury in the horse with antioxidants, which would be expected to inhibit injury attributable to reactive oxygen metabolites, have been unsuccessful.

The prognosis for survival in horses with small intestinal strangulating lesions is generally lower than with most types of colic. In a large multicenter study, small intestinal strangulating obstruction had a fatality rate of 67% compared with that of small intestinal simple obstruction, which had a fatality rate of 48%.[361] Although recent studies indicate higher survival rates in general, the relative fatality of strangulating obstruction compared with simple obstruction is probably similar. One study indicated that in excess of 70% of horses were discharged from the hospital after surgical correction of small intestinal strangulating obstruction.[362] These figures should be interpreted cautiously because they are based on the number of horses that are recovered from surgery rather than the number of horses initially presented for evaluation of severe colic. In addition, owners should be warned that the long-term survival rate is closer to 50%.[363] The principal reason for reduced long-term survival in patients that have had small intestinal surgery is intraabdominal adhesions. For example, in one study, 22% of horses that had had small intestinal surgery required further surgery or euthanasia because of adhesions and only 25% of horses that had a clinical problem with adhesions survived.[364]

Epiploic Foramen Entrapment

The epiploic foramen is a potential opening (because the walls of the foramen are usually in contact) to the omental bursa located within the right cranial quadrant of the abdomen. It is bounded dorsally by the caudate process of the liver and caudal vena cava and ventrally by the pancreas, the hepatoduodenal ligament, and the portal vein.[365,366] Clinical signs include acute onset of severe colic with examination findings compatible with small intestinal obstruction. The condition tends to be more prevalent in older horses,[365] possibly because of enlargement of the epiploic foramen as the right lobe of the liver undergoes age-associated atrophy.[367] However, the disease has also been recognized in foals as young as 4 months of age.[368] The diagnosis is definitively made at surgery, although ultrasonographic findings of distended loops of edematous small intestine adjacent to the right middle body wall are suggestive of epiploic foramen entrapment.[365] Entrapped small intestine may enter the foramen from the visceral surface of the liver toward the right body wall, or the opposite direction. Reports differ as to which is the most common form.[365,366] Entrapped small intestine may be limited to a portion of the intestinal wall (parietal hernia),[369] and the large colon may become entrapped within the epiploic foramen.[370] In treating epiploic foramen entrapment, the epiploic foramen must not be enlarged either by blunt force or with a sharp instrument, because rupture of the vena cava or portal vein and fatal hemorrhage may occur. Prognosis has substantially improved over the last decade, with current short-term survival rates (discharge from the hospital) ranging from 74%[371] to 79%.[365] Preoperative abdominocentesis was the most predictive test of postoperative survival in one study in which there was a significant increase in abdominal fluid total protein in the nonsurvivor group compared with the survivor group.[365]

Strangulation by Mesenteric Pedunculated Lipoma

Lipomas form between the leaves of the mesentery as horses age, and develop mesenteric stalks as the weight of the lipoma tugs on the mesentery. The stalk of the lipoma and a loop of small intestine or small colon may become intertwined causing strangulation. Strangulating lipomas should be suspected in mature (>10 years old) horses with acute colic referable to the small intestinal tract.[372] In addition, geldings and ponies appear to be at risk of strangulating lipomas,[373] possibly because of differences in fat metabolism. The diagnosis is usually made at surgery, although on rare occasions a lipoma can be palpated per rectum.[374]

Treatment involves surgical resection of the lipoma and strangulated bowel, although strangulated intestine is not always nonviable.[372] Studies indicate that approximately

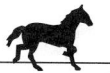

50%[373] to 78%[372] of horses are discharged from the hospital following surgical treatment.

Small Intestinal Volvulus

A volvulus is a twist along the axis of the mesentery, whereas torsion is a twist along the longitudinal axis of the intestine. Small intestinal volvulus is theoretically initiated by a change in local peristalsis or the occurrence of a lesion around which the intestine and its mesentery may twist (such as an ascarid impaction).[375] It is reportedly one of the most commonly diagnosed causes of small intestinal obstruction in foals.[376,377] It has been theorized that young foals may be at risk of small intestinal volvulus because of changing feed habits and adaptation to a bulkier adult diet.[376] Onset of acute, severe colic, a distended abdomen, and radiographic evidence of multiple loops of distended small intestine in a young foal would be suggestive of small intestinal volvulus. However, volvulus is not possible to differentiate from other causes of small intestinal obstruction preoperatively. In adult horses, volvulus frequently occurs in association with another disease process, during which small intestinal obstruction results in distention and subsequent rotation of the small intestinal around the root of the mesentery. Although any segment of the small intestine may be involved, the distal jejunum and ileum are most frequently affected.[375] The diagnosis is made by palpating a twist at the origin of the cranial mesenteric artery during surgical exploration. Treatment includes resection of devitalized bowel, which may not be an option because of the extent of small intestinal involvement. Prognosis is based on the extent of small intestine involved and its appearance after surgical correction of the lesion. In general, horses with greater than 50% of the small intestine devitalized are considered to have a grave prognosis.[378]

Inguinal Hernias

Inguinal hernias are more common in Standardbred and Tennessee Walking horses, which tend to have congenitally large inguinal canals.[375] Inguinal hernias may also occur in neonatal foals, but differ from hernias in mature horses in that they are typically nonstrangulating. Typical historical findings include acute onset of colic in a stallion that recently has been used for breeding. A cardinal sign of inguinal herniation is a cool, enlarged testicle on one side of the scrotum.[379,380] Inguinal hernias can also be detected on rectal palpation. The nature of the hernia (direct versus indirect) is determined based on the integrity of the parietal vaginal tunic. In horses in which the bowel remains within the parietal vaginal tunic, the hernia is referred to as indirect, because strictly speaking the bowel remains within the peritoneal cavity. Direct hernias are those in which strangulated bowel ruptures through the parietal vaginal tunic and occupies a subcutaneous location. These most commonly occur in foals and should be suspected when a congenital inguinal hernia is associated with colic, swelling that extends from the inguinal region of the prepuce, and intestine that may be palpated subcutaneously.[381,382] Although most congenital indirect inguinal hernias resolve with repeated manual reduction or application of a diaper, surgical intervention is recommended for congenial direct hernias.[381]

In stallions with indirect inguinal hernias, manipulation of herniated bowel per rectum can be used to reduce a hernia, but this generally is not recommended because of the risk of rectal tears. In many cases the short segment of herniated intestine will markedly improve in appearance once it has been surgically reduced, and in some cases the affected intestine can be left unresected. The affected testicle will be congested because of vascular compromise within the sper-

matic cord, and although it may remain viable, its is generally recommended that it be resected.[362] The prognosis in adult horses is good, with up to 75% of horses surviving to 6 months of age.[380] Horses that have been treated for inguinal hernias may be used for breeding. In these horses the remaining testicle will have increased sperm production, although an increased number of sperm abnormalities will be noticed after surgery because of edema and increased temperature of the scrotum.

Strangulating Umbilical Hernias

Whereas umbilical hernias are common in foals, strangulation of herniated bowel is rare. In one study, 6 of 147 (4%) horses with umbilical hernias had incarcerated intestine.[383] Clinical signs include a warm, swollen, firm, and painful hernia sac associated with signs of colic. The affected segment of bowel is usually small intestine, but herniation of cecum or large colon has also been reported.[384] In rare cases a hernia that involves only part of the intestinal wall may be found and is referred to as a Richter's hernia. In foals that have a Richter's hernia, an enterocutaneous fistula may develop. In one study, 13 of 13 foals with strangulating umbilical hernias survived to discharge, although at least 3 were lost to long-term complications.[384]

Diaphragmatic Hernias

Herniation of intestine through a rent in the diaphragm is uncommon in the horse, accounting for 0.3% of all cases of colic in a large multicenter study.[361] Any segment of bowel may be involved, although small intestine is most frequently herniated.[385] Diaphragmatic rents may be congenital or acquired, but acquired hernias are more common.[385] Congenital rents may result from incomplete fusion of any of the three embryonic components of the diaphragm: pleuroperitoneal membranes, transverse septum, and esophageal mesentery. In addition, abdominal compression of the foal at parturition may result in a congenital hernia.[385] Acquired hernias are presumed to result from trauma to the chest or a sudden increase in intraabdominal pressure, such as might occur during parturition, distention of the abdomen, a sudden fall, or strenuous exercise.[386] In one study, 19 of 40 (48%) horses diagnosed with diaphragmatic hernia had a history of recent trauma.[387] Hernias have been located in a number of different locations, although large congenital hernias are typically present at the ventral-most aspect of the diaphragm, and most acquired hernias are located at the junction of the muscular and tendonous portions of the diaphragm.[385] In addition, a peritoneopericardial hernia has been documented in at least one horse.[388]

The clinical signs are usually associated with intestinal obstruction rather than respiratory embarrassment.[386] However, careful auscultation may reveal an area of decreased lung sounds associated with obstructed intestine and increased fluid within the chest cavity.[387] Such signs may prompt thoracic radiography or ultrasound, both of which can be used to make a diagnosis. In one review, 7 of 40 (18%) horses reported in the literature with diaphragmatic hernia had dyspnea.[387] Auscultation may also reveal thoracic intestinal sounds, but it is typically not possible to differentiate these from sounds referred from the abdomen. In one report, 2 of 3 horses diagnosed with small intestinal strangulation by diaphragmatic hernia had respiratory acidemia, attributable to decreased ventilation.[389]

Intussusceptions

An intussusception involves a segment of bowel (intussusceptum) that invaginates into an adjacent aboral segment of bowel (intussuscipiens) (Fig. 30-38). The reason for such invagination is not always clear, but may involve a lesion at the leading edge of the intussusception, including small masses, foreign bodies, or parasites. In particular, tapeworms *(Anoplocephala perfoliata)* have been implicated.[390] Ileocecal intussusceptions are the most common intestinal intussusceptions in the horse and typically affect young animals. For example, in one study evaluating 26 cases of ileocecal intussusception, the median age of the horses was 1 year old.[391] Acute ileocecal intussusceptions are those in which the horses has a duration of colic of less than 24 hours and involve variable lengths of intestine that ranged in one study from 6 cm to 457 cm long. In acute cases the involved segment of ileum typically has a compromised blood supply. Chronic ileocecal intussusceptions typically involve short segments of ileum (up to 10 cm long), and the ileal blood supply is frequently intact.[391] Abdominocentesis results are variable because strangulated bowel is contained within the adjacent bowel. There often is evidence of obstruction of the small intestine, including nasogastric reflux and multiple distended loops of small intestine on rectal palpation. Horses with chronic ileocecal intussusceptions have mild, intermittent colic, often without evidence of small intestinal obstruction. A mass may be palpated in the region of the cecal base in approximately 50% of cases.[390] Transabdominal ultrasound may be helpful in discerning the nature of the mass. The intussusception has a characteristic target appearance on cross section.[392]

Other segments of the small intestine may also be intussuscepted, including the jejunum. In one study on 11 jejunojejunal intussusceptions, the length of bowel involved ranged from 0.4 to 9.1 meters.[393] Attempts at reducing intussusceptions at surgery are usually futile because of intramural swelling of affected bowel. Jejunojejunal intussusceptions should be resected. For acute ileocecal intussusceptions, the small intestine should be transected as far distally as possible, and a jejunocecal anastomosis performed. In cases with particularly long intussusceptions (up to 10 meters has been reported), an intracecal resection may be attempted. For horses with chronic ileocecal intussusceptions, a jejunocecal bypass without small intestinal transection should be performed.

In one study that evaluated the survival of horses with ileocecal intussusceptions, 7 of 7 horses with chronic intussusceptions survived long term (>4 months), whereas only 5 of 12 (42%) horses with acute intussusceptions survived long term.[391] In a separate study that evaluated survival in horses with jejunojejunal intussusceptions, 6 of 11 (54%) horses were discharged from the hospital after surgery, and 4 of 11 (36%) horses survived long term (>16 months).[393]

Other Small Intestinal Strangulations

Entrapment of the small intestine may occur through rents in the mesentery; internal ligaments, such as the gastrosplenic ligament[394]; and the broad ligament. Entrapments may also occur through trauma-induced body wall hernias. For all of these conditions, it is often necessary to enlarge the rent or hernia to allow reduction of entrapped small intestine. In the case of body wall hernias, the defect should be closed with suture or patched using mesh.

NONSTRANGULATING INFARCTION

Nonstrangulating infarction occurs secondary to cranial mesenteric arteritis caused by migration of *Strongylus vulgaris*[395] and has become a rare surgical disorder since the advent of broad-spectrum anthelmintics. Although thromboemboli have been implicated in the pathogenesis of this disease, careful dissection of naturally occurring lesions has not revealed the presence of thrombi at the site of intestinal infarctions in most cases.[395] These findings suggest that vasospasm plays an important role in this disease.[396] Clinical signs are highly variable, depending on the extent to which arterial flow is reduced and the segment of intestine affected. Any segment of intestine supplied by the cranial mesenteric artery or one of its major branches may be affected, but the distal small intestine and large colon are more commonly involved.[395] There are no clinical variables that can be used to reliably predict or differentiate this disease from strangulating obstruction. In some cases, massive infarction results in acute, severe colic. Other cases may have intermittent colic as smaller emboli are released into the colonic blood supply.[395] Occasionally an abnormal mass and fremitus may be detected on palpation of the root of the cranial mesenteric artery per rectum. This disease should be considered a differential diagnosis in horses with a history of inadequate anthelmintic treatment and the presence of intermittent colic that is difficult to localize. Although fecal parasite egg counts should be performed, they are neither indicative of the degree nor specific for the type of parasitic infestation.

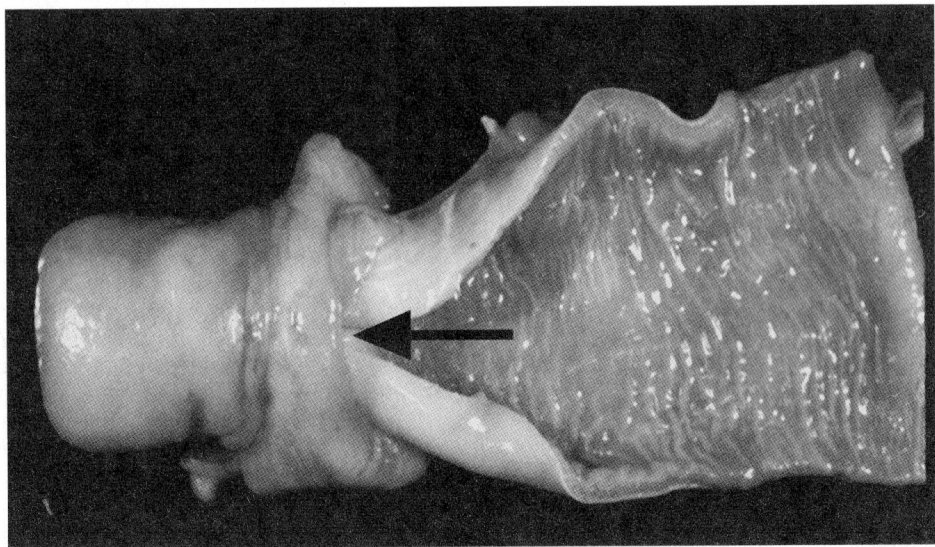

FIG. 30-38 ■ Ileocecal intussusception *(arrow)*. The ileum is at the right, and the cecum at the left. (Courtesy Dr. MJ Murray.)

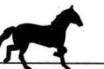

In addition to routine treatment of colic, dehydration, and endotoxemia, medical treatment may include aspirin (20 mg/kg every 24 hours) to decrease thrombosis.[396] Definitive diagnosis requires surgical exploration. Surgical treatment depends on the distribution of infarction. Unfortunately these cases are difficult to treat because of the patchy distribution of the lesions and the possibility of lesions extending beyond the limits of surgical resection. In addition, further infarction may occur following surgery. The prognosis is fair for horses with intermittent mild episodes of colic that may be amenable to medical therapy, but horses that require surgical intervention have a poor prognosis.[395,396]

REFERENCES

339. Clarke LL, Roberts MC, Argenzio RA: Feeding and digestive problems in horses: physiologic responses to a concentrated meal, *Vet Clin North Am (Equine Pract)* 6:433-450, 1990.

340. Clarke LL, Argenzio RA, Roberts MC: Effect of meal feeding on plasma volume and urinary electrolyte clearance in ponies, *Am J Vet Res* 51:571-576, 1990.

341. Dabareiner RM et al: Evaluation of the microcirculation of the equine small intestine after intraluminal distention and subsequent decompression [see comments], *Am J Vet Res* 54:1673-1682, 1993.

342. Allen DJ, White NA, Tyler DE: Morphologic effects of experimental distention of equine small intestine, *Vet Surg* 17:10-14, 1988.

343. Southwood LL et al: Surgical treatment of ascarid impactions in horses and foals, *Proceedings of the Forty-second Annual Convention of the American Association of Equine Practitioners*, 1996, p 258.

344. Clayton HM: Ascarids: recent advances, *Vet Clin North Am (Equine Pract)* 2:313-328, 1986.

345. Parks AH, Allen D: The purported role of coastal Bermuda hay in the etiology of ileal impactions: results of a questionnaire, *Proc Equine Colic Res Symp* 6:37, 1998.

346. Hanson RR et al: Surgical reduction of ileal impactions in the horse: 28 cases, *Vet Surg* 27:555-560, 1998.

347. Parks AH et al: Ileal impaction in the horse: 75 cases, *Cornell Vet* 79:83-91, 1989.

348. Hanson RR et al: Medical treatment of horses with ileal impactions: 10 cases (1990-1994), *J Am Vet Med Assoc* 208:898-900, 1996.

349. Blikslager AT et al: Evaluation of factors associated with postoperative ileus in horses: 31 cases (1990-1992), *J Am Vet Med Assoc* 205:1748-1752, 1994.

350. Chaffin MK et al: Idiopathic muscular hypertrophy of the equine small intestine: 11 cases (1980-1991), *Equine Vet J* 24:372-378, 1992.

351. Hooper RN: Small intestinal strangulation caused by Meckel's diverticulum in a horse, *J Am Vet Med Assoc* 194:943-944, 1989.

352. Grant BD, Tennant B: Volvulus associated with Meckel's diverticulum in the horse, *J Am Vet Med Assoc* 162:550-551, 1973.

353. Freeman DE, Koch DB, Boles CL: Mesodiverticular bands as a cause of small intestinal strangulation and volvulus in the horse, *J Am Vet Med Assoc* 175:1089-1094, 1979.

354. Meschter CL et al: Histologic findings in the gastrointestinal tract of horses with colic, *Am J Vet Res* 47:598-606, 1986.

355. White NA, Moore JN, Trim CM: Mucosal alterations in experimentally induced small intestinal strangulation obstruction in ponies, *Am J Vet Res* 41:193-198, 1980.

356. Laws EG, Freeman DE: Significance of reperfusion injury after venous strangulation obstruction of equine jejunum, *J Invest Surg* 8:263-270, 1995.

357. Blikslager AT et al: How important is intestinal reperfusion injury in horses? *J Am Vet Med Assoc* 211:1387-1389, 1997.

358. Lundin C et al: Induction of peritoneal adhesions with small intestinal ischaemia and distention in the foal, *Equine Vet J* 21:451-458, 1989.

359. Gerard MP et al: The characteristics of intestinal injury peripheral to strangulating obstruction lesions in the equine small intestine, *Equine Vet J* 31:331-335, 1999.

360. Horne MM et al: Attempts to modify reperfusion injury of equine jejunal mucosa using dimethylsulfoxide, allopurinol, and intraluminal oxygen, *Vet Surg* 23:241-249, 1994.

361. White NA, Lessard P: Risk factors and clinical signs associated with cases of equine colic, *Proceedings of the Thirty-second Annual Convention of the American Association of Equine Practitioners*, 1986, pp 637-644.

362. Freeman DE: Surgery of the small intestine. *Vet Clin North Am (Equine Pract)* 13:261-301, 1997.

363. MacDonald MH et al: Survival after small intestine resection and anastomosis in horses. *Vet Surg* 18:415-423, 1989.

364. Baxter GM, Broome TE, Moore JN: Abdominal adhesions after small intestinal surgery in the horse, *Vet Surg* 18:409-414, 1989.

365. Vachon AM, Fischer AT: Small intestinal herniation through the epiploic foramen: 53 cases (1987-1993), *Equine Vet J* 27:373-380, 1995.

366. Turner TA, Adams SB, White NA: Small intestine incarceration through the epiploic foramen of the horse, *J Am Vet Med Assoc* 184:731-734, 1984.

367. Jakowski RM: Right hepatic lobe atrophy in horses: 17 cases (1983-1993), *J Am Vet Med Assoc* 204:1057-1061, 1994.

368. Murray RC et al: Incarceration of the jejunum in the epiploic foramen of a four month old foal, *Cornell Vet* 84:47-51, 1994.

369. Hammock PD et al: Parietal hernia of the small intestine into the epiploic foramen of a horse, *J Am Vet Med Assoc* 214:1354-1355, 1999.

370. Foerner JJ et al: Transection of the pelvic flexure to reduce incarceration of the large colon through the epiploic foramen in a horse, *J Am Vet Med Assoc* 203:1312-1313, 1993.

371. Engelbert TA et al: Incarceration of the small intestine in the epiploic foramen: report of 19 cases (1983-1992), *Vet Surg* 22:57-61, 1993.

372. Blikslager AT et al: Pedunculated lipomas as a cause of intestinal obstruction in horses: 17 cases (1983-1990), *J Am Vet Med Assoc* 201:1249-1252, 1992.

373. Edwards GB, Proudman CJ: An analysis of 75 cases of intestinal obstruction caused by pedunculated lipomas, *Equine Vet J* 26:18-21, 1994.

374. Mason TA: Strangulation of the rectum of a horse by the pedicle of a mesenteric lipoma, *Equine Vet J* 10:269, 1978.

375. Robertson JT: Diseases of the small intestine. In White NA, ed: *The equine acute abdomen*, Philadelphia, 1990, Lea & Febiger, pp 347-368.

376. Orsini JA: Abdominal surgery in foals, *Vet Clin North Am (Equine Pract)* 13:393-413, 1997.

377. Crowhurst RC et al: Intestinal surgery in the foal, *J S Afr Vet Assoc* 46:59-67, 1975.

378. Tate LP et al: Effects of extensive resection of the small intestine in the pony, *Am J Vet Res* 44:1187-1191, 1983.

379. Schneider RK, Milne DW, Kohn CW: Acquired inguinal hernia in the horse: a review of 27 cases, *J Am Vet Med Assoc* 180:317-320, 1982.

380. van der Velden MA: Surgical treatment of acquired inguinal hernia in the horse: a review of 51 cases, *Equine Vet J* 20:173-177, 1988.

381. Spurlock GH, Robertson JT: Congenital inguinal hernias associated with a rent in the common vaginal tunic in five foals, *J Am Vet Med Assoc* 193:1087-1088, 1988.

382. van der Velden MA: Ruptured inguinal hernia in new-born colt foals: a review of 14 cases, *Equine Vet J* 20:178-181, 1988.

383. Freeman DE, Orsini JA, Harrison IA et al: Complications of umbilical hernias in horses: 13 cases (1972-1986), *J Am Vet Med Assoc* 192:804-807, 1988.

384. Markel MD, Pascoe JR, Sams AE: Strangulated umbilical hernias in horses: 13 cases (1974-1985), *J Am Vet Med Assoc* 190:692-694, 1987.

385. Bristol DG: Diaphragmatic hernias in horses and cattle, *Compend Cont Educ Pract Vet* 8:S407-S411, 1986.

386. Wimberly HC, Andrews EJ, Haschek WM: Diaphragmatic hernias in the horse: a review of the literature and an analysis of six additional cases, *J Am Vet Med Assoc* 170:1404-1407, 1977.

387. Everett KA, Chaffin MK, Brinsko SP: Diaphragmatic herniation as a cause of lethargy and exercise intolerance in a mare, *Cornell Vet* 82:217-223, 1992.

388. Orsini JA, Koch C, Stewart B: Peritoneopericardial hernia in a horse, *J Am Vet Med Assoc* 179:907-910, 1981.

389. Santschi EM et al: Diaphragmatic hernia repair in three young horses, *Vet Surg* 26:242-245, 1997.

390. Edwards GB: Surgical management of intussusception in the horse, *Equine Vet J* 18:313-321, 1986.

391. Ford TS et al: Ileocecal intussusception in horses: 26 cases (1981-1988), *J Am Vet Med Assoc* 196:121-126, 1990.

392. Bernard WV et al: Ultrasonographic diagnosis of small-intestinal intussusception in three foals, *J Am Vet Med Assoc* 194:395-397, 1989.

393. Gift LJ et al: Jejunal intussusception in adult horses: 11 cases (1981-1991), *J Am Vet Med Assoc* 202:110-112, 1993.

394. Yovich JV, Stashak TS, Bertone AL: Incarceration of small intestine through rents in the gastrosplenic ligament in the horse, *Vet Surg* 14:303-306, 1985.

395. White NA: Intestinal infarction associated with mesenteric vascular thrombotic disease in the horse, *J Am Vet Med Assoc* 178:259-262, 1981.

396. Sullins KE: Diseases of the large colon. In White NA, ed: *The equine acute abdomen*, Philadelphia, 1990, Lea & Febiger, pp 375-391.

MEDICAL DISORDERS OF THE LARGE INTESTINE

MICHAEL J. MURRAY

ACUTE DIARRHEA

Diarrhea in the horse can be defined as the passage of fecal material that has increased water content. It can vary from soft, formed stools with a mild to moderate increase in water content, to projectile fecal passages that contain little solid matter. The passage of excessive water in the feces reflects dis-

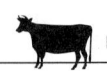

ruption of the normal balance of fluid and electrolyte secretion and absorption in the intestinal tract. In adult horses diarrhea results almost exclusively from disorders of the large intestine, although diarrhea may be a feature of some small colon disorders. Diarrhea can result in significant losses of water, electrolytes, and buffer and is often accompanied by local and systemic inflammatory responses.

Diarrhea disorders in adult horses can be divided into those characterized by inflammation of the cecum and large intestine (typhlitis, colitis) and those in which there typically is not an inflammatory response. Inflammatory disorders can be those characterized by an acute inflammatory response (salmonellosis, clostridiosis), disorders associated with endoparasitism (small and large strongyle larval migration or encystation), and disorders included under the umbrella terms granulomatous enteritis and inflammatory bowel disease (see p. 647). Disorders that can present as diarrhea but that typically do not have colonic inflammation include those in which there is increased intestinal hydrostatic pressure (congestive heart failure, cirrhotic liver disease) and poorly defined disorders in which fluid secretion may be stimulated by the enteric nervous system.

Colitis is active inflammation within the colon that is usually associated with myriad local and systemic pathophysiologic events. Diarrhea is an important problem in horses with colitis, but impaired cardiopulmonary function, coagulopathies, and other sequelae of activation of inflammatory mediator cascades and septicemia can be most life threatening. Complications that occur in colitis patients, regardless of etiology, include overwhelming endotoxemia, laminitis, septicemia and organ colonization by bacteria, immune suppression and susceptibility to superinfection with bacteria or fungi, and cecum or colon infarction.

A variety of inflammatory cells and mediators affect the equine colon. With acute colitis, the neutrophil is the effector cell, and the cascade of activation of inflammatory mediators associated with acute colitis is designed to bring neutrophils to where chemical signals indicative of bacterial infection have been detected. Signs of endotoxemia (see p. 636) frequently accompany, or even precede, diarrhea in horses. Severe tissue inflammation can result in loss of the mucosal epithelium, resulting in chronic malabsorption and protein-losing enteropathy. Malabsorption of volatile fatty acids and metabolic alterations that result from excessive production and release of inflammatory mediators can lead to an energy deficit and catabolism of body tissues.

Specific diseases affecting the equine large colon, such as salmonellosis, Potomac horse fever, and clostridial colitis, may have different activators of local and systemic inflammatory responses, and they can produce unique toxins that further contribute to tissue injury. Regardless of the cause, the clinical problems with which affected horses present are often similar, and the clinician must consider treatments that modify inflammatory changes and replace losses of fluid, electrolytes, and plasma protein. In many cases the cause of the diarrhea is not determined. Descriptions of important causes of diarrhea in horses follow.

Salmonellosis

Salmonella bacteria possess an array of virulence factors that confer attributes of mucosal adhesion and invasion; production of enterotoxins that stimulate intestinal fluid secretion; activation of local immune responses, including recruitment of inflammatory cells and the release of their mediators; local cytotoxic effects; and systemic responses attributable to lipopolysaccharide.

EPIDEMIOLOGY. A large number of *Salmonella* serotypes have been associated with equine colitis, and overall more than 2500 serotypes of *Salmonella* have been described. *Salmonella typhimurium* is the most frequently isolated serotype in horses, with dozens of other serotypes isolated sporadically. There are many reports describing clusters of cases of equine salmonellosis in which specific *Salmonella* serovars predominate. Nosocomial infections associated with *Salmonella krefeld*[397,398] *S. typhimurium*,[397] *Salmonella anatum*,[399] and *Salmonella infantis*[400] have been reported in recent years. Pertinent features of these bacteria are the ability to withstand a wide range of environmental conditions, the ability to rapidly invade and spread within the host (and thus be shed into the environment through the feces), and the range of severity of illness that results from infection.

Other key elements that influence whether clusters of cases will occur given the presence of a particular *Salmonella* serovar in the environment are availability and population density of susceptible hosts and the size of infective dose of the pathogen. It is for these reasons that veterinary hospitals, breeding farms, and other facilities that may have a high density of horses are most vulnerable to the development of *Salmonella* outbreaks. In one study at a veterinary teaching hospital, horses that were at greatest risk for developing salmonellosis were those treated with antimicrobial drugs or admitted for treatment of colic.[401] Such horses will include the majority of patients in any equine referral hospital. Breeding farms are susceptible to *Salmonella* outbreaks (or other enteric infections) because of the concentration of large numbers of immunologically immature animals. In either case the particular *Salmonella* organism involved in disease outbreaks may not have to be especially virulent, because the inherent susceptibility of the host provides the microbe the opportunity to colonize and invade the host. Also of importance is the ability of the organism (inherent or acquired) to persist in the environment, lying in wait, as it were, for both susceptible hosts and environmental conditions that favor its propagation and dissemination.

Serovars or strains of *Salmonella* that have newly acquired virulence plasmids can rapidly become established and spread between farms, sales areas, veterinary clinics, and veterinary teaching hospitals. Often, the origin of these "new" bacteria is undetermined, but in some cases the organism can be traced to contaminated feed,[401a] a specific shedder introduced into the environment, domestic or ferral animals (barn cats), birds, and wildlife.

Salmonellae are ubiquitous in the environment, and the prevalence of fecal shedding varies by the group of horses sampled and the method of detection. Prevalence of fecal shedding, based on fecal culture, in asymptomatic horses admitted to teaching hospitals, varied from 1% to 5%.[402,403] In a nationwide survey of prevalence of *Salmonella* in fecal samples from horses on farms and ranches, *Salmonella* bacteria were cultured from less than 1% of horses.[404] Use of polymerase chain reaction (PCR) to detect *Salmonella* DNA in horse feces resulted in a prevalence rate of 17% in horses admitted to a teaching hospital for lameness examination and greater than 60% in hospitalized horses with gastrointestinal disease.[405] In that report the PCR technique was determined to be specific for *Salmonella* DNA, but the test cannot differentiate between shedding of live bacteria and DNA from dead organisms.

Horses are not considered to be carriers, per se, of *Salmonella*, because no host-adapted *Salmonella* spp. have been identified in horses. *Salmonella abortusequus* has now disappeared in the United States. Horses that shed *Salmonella* spp. in the feces usually do so transiently for several days to weeks; infrequently, horses may shed salmonella bacteria for several months.

In acutely affected horses, large numbers of highly infective salmonellae can be shed in the diarrheic feces. Suscepti-

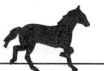

ble animals such as young foals, hospitalized horses receiving antimicrobials, and horses under stress can become ill after becoming infected by numbers of salmonellae 100 to 1000 times less than those required to infect immunocompetent normal horses. Thus particular care should be taken in the management of horses/foals with diarrhea in environments in which there are animals at risk (e.g., hospitals, breeding farms, racetracks). Asymptomatic shedders generally pass relatively small numbers of salmonellae in the feces and do not appear to pose an important threat to healthy horses, although asymptomatic shedders have been responsible for outbreaks of salmonellosis in hospitals and on breeding farms.

CLINICAL FINDINGS. Salmonellosis typically is characterized by an acute colitis that results in profuse diarrhea and, occasionally, abdominal pain. Horses with salmonellosis often have signs compatible with endotoxemia and suffer from cardiovascular shock and coagulopathies. Horses are usually febrile, tachycardic, moderately to severely obtunded, and dehydrated. With other clinical syndromes of salmonella infection, diarrhea is not a feature. These syndromes include fever and leukopenia, colic, and proximal enteritis with gastric reflux.

DIAGNOSIS. Confirmation of salmonellosis requires bacteriologic culture of *Salmonella* bacteria. Multiple fecal cultures for *Salmonella* spp. should be performed on all horses with diarrhea. It is recommended that at least three to five fecal samples be submitted for culture to enhance the chances of isolating *Salmonella*.[406] Samples with little solid matter often yield negative culture results, even when the horse is infected with *Salmonella*. Formed fecal samples are more likely to result in a positive culture from infected horses. A 5- to 10-g amount of feces should be submitted for culture in selective media such as tetrathionate broth or selenite broth and brilliant green agar or XLD agar. Culture of a rectal mucosal biopsy often identifies a positive *Salmonella* finding when fecal cultures are negative.

TREATMENT AND PREVENTION. In most cases of salmonellosis, aggressive treatment facilitates resolution of the severe diarrhea and associated metabolic disorders within 7 to 10 days of the onset of illness. Intravenous administration of polyionic fluids is required to replace fluid and electrolyte losses and to augment preload in horses with poor venous return. Plasma may be required to replace lost plasma proteins. Parenteral nutritional support is often indicated to provide adequate calories and amino acids during the most debilitating period of the illness. Antimicrobial administration to horses with suspected or known salmonellosis is not universally practiced. Antimicrobial administration may decrease the spread of salmonella bacteria to other organs and may have some direct effect on salmonella bacteria in the colon. Traditionally, use of antimicrobials such as chloramphenicol, trimethoprim-sulfa, gentamicin, and cephalosporins has not appeared to accelerate resolution of signs of colitis. Fluoroquinolones, while not approved for horses and potentially arthropathic, particularly in young horses, may be more effective because of high lipid solubility and bacteriocidal activity against salmonella bacteria.

Horses that have severe diarrhea and toxemia for 10 days or longer are unlikely to survive, even with intensive therapy, becausee they often have extensive loss of colonic mucosa and chronic, severe inflammation within the wall of the colon. Complications such as catheter-associated thrombophlebitis, colonic infarction (Fig. 30-39), colonization of other organs by salmonella or other enteric bacteria, and laminitis can occur.

Measures designed to prevent the spread of *Salmonella* in an environment with potentially susceptible hosts need not be excessively laborious nor expensive. The goal is to mini-

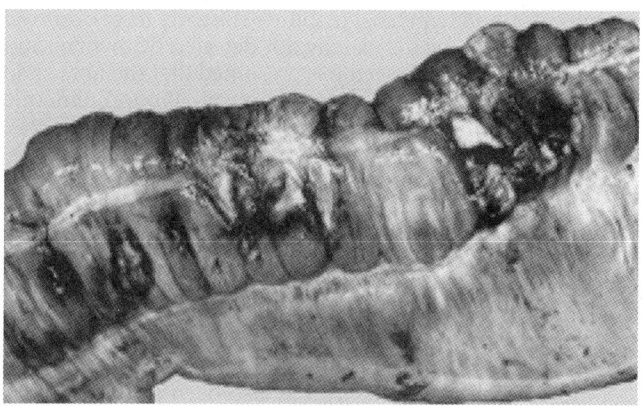

FIG. 30-39 ▦ Colonic infarction in a horse with salmonellosis. Tenesmus and rectal prolapse were early clinical signs associated with the colonic infarction.

mize the size of infective dose of an enteric pathogen to which a susceptible host may be exposed. Thorough cleaning of areas where fecal contamination is likely and preventing mechanical distribution of contaminated material are the most important measures that should be taken. Extensive use of disinfectants may not be necessary if cleaning measures are adequate. Cleaning must include removal of organic debris, which can be accomplished with several products designed for that task. Areas that require particular attention are stalls, including water buckets or automatic watering apparati, drains, and cracks in the floors and wall; stall implements; surgical areas, including drains; and nasogastric tubes and pumps.

If a diarrheic horse is in the environment, it should be isolated to the degree possible. Bedding material should be removed frequently, to minimize accumulation of potential enteropathogens. Personnel entering the stall should be restricted to the professional staff, and they should wear disposable plastic boots. Footbaths with disinfectant often are not effective, because they quickly accumulate organic material that interferes with the disinfectant activity of the footbath. Once a horse vacates a stall, the stall should be thoroughly cleaned, allowed to dry, disinfected (we prefer a 1:30 dilution of chlorine bleach), and determined to be negative for *Salmonella* by culturing selected sites in the stall (floor, drain, waterer). Personnel should use common sense when dealing with diarrheic cases. If bedding is being blown about by wind, or mechanical blowers are used to clean aisles, then potential enteric pathogens may be readily spread to other horses.

Potomac Horse Fever

Potomac horse fever (PHF) is an infectious enterocolonic disorder caused by *Ehrlichia risticii*.[407] The organism is an obligate intracellular parasite, infecting peripheral monocytes and macrophages, colonic and small intestinal epithelial cells, and colon mast cells.[408] The pathophysiology of the disease is incompletely understood, although horses infected with *E. risticii* often have clinical signs and complications similar to those in horses with salmonellosis. After experimental inoculation with *E. risticii* horses had a mild, transient fever 2 to 4 days after infection.[409] By 10 to 14 days after experimental infection horses became febrile, had a poor appetite, and exhibited mild to severe gastrointestinal signs, ranging from mild colic and soft stool to profuse diarrhea.

In clinical cases of PHF, there are signs resembling endotoxemia, including fever, leukopenia, congested mucous membranes, and hypercoagulability. The early fever observed in experimental cases is usually not detected by owners, and when clinical signs are seen it is presumed that the horse had become infected 10 to 14 days previously. Hypoproteinemia is a frequent finding in horses with clinical cases of PHF, which reflects loss of serum protein through inflamed intestinal mucosa. Interestingly, though, the magnitude of intestinal inflammation is typically much less than with salmonellosis, yet the magnitude of hypoproteinemia (toal protein <3.0 g/dl) can be as severe.

Laminitis is a frequent sequela to PHF, and may occur in 30% in horses with PHF. Our clinical impression is that a greater proportion of horses with PHF develop laminitis than horses with salmonellosis, although the latter horses are often more severely ill. E. risticii has also been associated with abortion in mares, although this is an unusual occurrence.[410] In some horses that show significant seroconversion to E. risticii, laminitis is the only clinical sign.

MODE OF TRANSMISSION. Although originally described as a disease of horses living near the Potomac River in Maryland and Virginia, PHF has been confirmed serologically in most states. Because early research on PHF demonstrated that infection was readily transmitted through blood,[409] it was presumed that the natural mode of transmission involved an insect or arthropod vector. However, several studies have failed to demonstrate any such vectors.[411,412]

The association between an affected horse and proximity to a river (within 5 miles) remains strong. Recently, investigators have found a possible link between this association and how the disease may be transmitted. E. risticii and Neorickettsia helmintheca were found to share a high degree of DNA homology,[413] and Neorickettsia helmintheca is transmitted to mammals via a trematode that parasitizes fish. This prompted investigators to search for evidence that E. risticii might reside in trematodes infecting riverine inhabitants. DNA resembling that of E. risticii was identified by nested PCR in operculate snails (Pleuroceridae: Juga spp.) collected from stream water in a northern California pasture in which Potomac horse fever (PHF) is enzootic.[414] The snails released trematode cercariae, and within these cercariae DNA fragments that closely resembled E. risticii were identified.[415] The sequences of these genes were virtually identical to those of the genes of an equine E. risticii strain from a property near the snail collection site. It has been postulated that, in some areas at least, there is a snail-trematode-E. risticii association that either serves as a reservoir for E. risticii or as a source of infection to horses.

Oral transmission of E. risticii with infected cell cultures has been produced experimentally,[416] so ingestion of E. risticii, rather than blood transmission, may prove to be the route of natural infection. Nonetheless, it remains true that horse to horse transmission of E. risticii is highly unlikely, because the organism is an obligate intracellular parasite and will not survive long in feces.

DIAGNOSIS. Accurate confirmation of PHF can be difficult, because clinical signs of disease are nonspecific and available diagnostic tests are not entirely reliable. Conventional recommendation is that paired acute and convalescent blood samples should be submitted for indirect fluorescent antibody (IFA) or enzyme-linked immunosorbent assay (ELISA) testing for antibodies to E. risticii. However, serologic evaluation to confirm the disease is not as straightforward as in many other infectious diseases. A four-fold increase in titer between acute and convalescent sera is considered to confirm infection with E. risticii, but failure to seroconvert does not rule out infection. Because the onset of clinical signs can be delayed as long as 14 days after infection, horses may seroconvert by the time an acute sample is obtained.[416] The magnitude of titer does not always correlate with active infection, because many horses in endemic areas have high titers but no disease. Vaccination also can affect titer, but some vaccinated horses considered to have had PHF on the basis of clinical response to treatment have had no titer. This does not mean that no antibody to E. risticii was produced, but rather may indicate that the test did not detect the antibody.

There is significant inter-laboratory variability in results of IFA and false-positive results occur frequently.[417] Thus it has been suggested that IFA for antibodies to E. risticii not be performed in areas that are not endemic for E. risticii.[417] Some laboratories offer polymerase chain reaction (PCR) testing of blood samples to detect E. risticii DNA. Unfortunately, as with other PCR tests used for identification of pathogenic agents in clinical specimens, there may be excessive false-positive reports with this technique.

TREATMENT AND PREVENTION. Treatment with oxytetracycline, 7 to 11 mg/kg IV twice daily for 4 days, effectively eliminates E. risticii from the horse. Fever should resolve within 48 hours of beginning treatment with oxytetracycline, and diarrhea typically resolves within 24 to 72 hours of beginning treatment. In one horse we treated, clinical signs persisted until the dosage of oxytetracycline was increased to 15 mg/kg twice daily. Orally administered doxycycline (10 mg/kg every 12 hours) may be effective, although in horses with severe GI signs, absorption of doxycycline may be adversely affected. Doxycycline must not be given intravenously, because it will cause the horse to collapse. Some horses have had clinical relapses 2 to 3 weeks after initial resolution of clinical signs that were responsive to tetracycline. Horses do not remain chronic carriers of E. risticii.

In most cases of PHF, intravenous administration of polyionic fluids is required to replace fluid and electrolyte losses and to augment preload in horses with poor venous return. Plasma may be required to replace lost plasma proteins. Because horses improve rather quickly once treatment with oxytetracycline is begun, parenteral nutritional support is usually unnecessary.

Vaccination has appeared to diminish the incidence and severity of disease, but PHF may still develop in vaccinated animals. Experimental results with vaccine were mixed, and the duration of immunoprophylaxis was very limited.[418] Disease severity has appeared to be less in vaccinated animals, although in the summer of 1994 many vaccinated horses developed severe cases of PHF. All of these horses were located in the area where PHF was originally described, and a new strain of E. risticii was identified.[419] In fact, PCR analysis has revealed multiple strains of E. risticii, which may affect vaccination efficacy.[420] Horses in endemic areas should be vaccinated in the early spring and early to midsummer on an annual basis. We recommend vaccinating in April and June.

Clostridial Diarrhea

Enteric clostridiosis was reported as a clinical problem in the 1970s, and clostridial bacteria were implicated as the causative agents of colitis X.[421] Difficulty in substantiating clostridial bacteria as the cause of enterocolitis in horses led to a deemphasis of this potential etiology for diarrhea in adult horses. In the 1990s, improved laboratory techniques for identification of clostridial toxins resulted in increased confirmation of clostridial bacteria as the causative agents of colitis in foals and adult horses.

The two most important clostridial species affecting the equine intestinal tract are Clostridium difficile and Clostridium perfringens. Most reported cases in horses have involved C. difficile, although in a recent report the prevalence of C. difficile toxin A and C. perfringens enterotoxin in fecal samples from horses with diarrhea was similar, and in some horses toxins from both clostridial species were identified.[422]

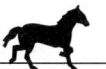

PATHOGENESIS. *C. difficile* is a sporulated obligate anaerobe responsible for most cases of antibiotic-associated colitis, for 15% to 25% of cases of antibiotic-related diarrhea, and for a substantial proportion of nosocomial infections in humans.[423] *C. difficile* produces two important toxins, named toxin A and toxin B. Most isolates of *C. difficile* produce both toxins, but some isolates produce only either toxin A or toxin B. Toxin A can elicit both fluid secretion and a pronounced inflammatory response in the bowel. Toxin A has intestinal secretory and cytotoxic effects,[424,425] increases intestinal permeability,[426] and can activate epithelial cells, neutrophils, mast cells, monocytes, and macrophages to release a multitude of proinflammatory cytokines and vasoactive mediators.[427-429] An interesting feature of toxin A is its induction of the neurotransmitter substance P in both the intestine and dorsal root ganglia, and the apparent dependence on substance P for expression of the full pathologic effects of toxin A in the intestine of rodents.[430] Effects of toxin A appear to be mediated both through direct effects on intestinal cells and via the enteric nervous system.

Toxin B exhibits enterotoxigenic (secretory) activity, but recently also has been demonstrated to have potent cytotoxic effects on human colonic epithelium.[431] Toxin B has little relevance to the pathogenicity of *C. difficile* in animal models, however, and the roles of toxins A and B in the pathogenesis of equine clostridial enterocoltis are not known.

Strains of *C. perfringens* are classified on the basis of the toxins that are produced, with at least a dozen identified to date.[432] *C. perfringens* type A and type C have been recovered from equine specimens,[433] and several *C. perfringens* toxins have been identified in equine specimens.[434,435] *C. perfringens* type A is the most frequently isolated type, and its enterotoxin is released upon sporulation of *C. perfringens* within the intestine. Other exotoxins of *C. perfringens* have phospholipase activity (alpha toxin), necrotizing cytotoxic effects (beta, episilon, iota), and hemolytic effects (theta).

CLINICAL FEATURES. Clostridial enterocolitis affects foals and adult horses. In some reports, toxigenic *C. perfringens* were isolated from more than 50% of foals with diarrhea.[435,436] The clinical presentation in foals can be predominantly gastrointestinal signs (colic, diarrhea); in neonatal foals, clostridiosis may present as septicemia. In some foals, classic necrotizing enterocolitis will be manifested by gas- or fluid-distended intestines and thickened intestinal mucosa. These changes can be appreciated radiographically and ultrasonographically, and intramural gas produced by clostridial bacteria may be detected with ultrasonography as hyperechoic areas within the bowel wall.

Adult horses with clostridial enterocolitis frequently present with diarrhea, but may have abdominal discomfort or fever as the primary presenting problems. There are no clinical features that consistently distinguish clostridiosis from salmonellosis, and a spectrum of clinical signs exists, from moderate illness to severe toxemic colitis. Most horses with clostridial enterocolitis develop diarrhea, but in some cases enteritis manifested by ileus and gas-distention of the small intestine may be the primary problem. *C. perfringens* has been implicated in proximal enteritis,[437] but a cause and effect association has not been proven.

Similar to salmonellosis, clostridial enterocolitis can develop into a widespread problem affecting several animals in a hospital or an equine facility.[438] Risk factors for developing nosocomial clostridial enterocolitis would presumably be similar to nosocomial salmonellosis: antimicrobial administration, concurrent gastrointestinal disease, and age susceptibility (foals). Additionally, *Clostridium* spp. are well suited to persist in the environment because of the production of spores that are resistant to environmental extremes and many disinfectants.

DIAGNOSIS. Diagnosis of clostridial enterocolitis requires identification of toxigenic clostridia from intestinal contents or tissue. There are several direct and indirect methods used to detect toxigenic clostridia and include culture, identification of toxins, and identification of toxin genes. Culture of *C. difficile* or *C. perfringens* requires anaerobic conditions, and the ability to culture these organisms from ingesta or fecal specimens rapidly diminishes with increased time from collection to arrival at a laboratory. It is recommended to transport samples, chilled (not frozen) on ice, immediately or by overnight delivery for best recovery of clostridial organisms. Tissue specimens submitted for culture, toxin identification, or toxin gene identification should be handled similarly. Commercially available tests for clostridial toxins include an ELISA test for *C. difficile* toxin A,* a latex-agglutination test for *C. perfringens* enterotoxin,† and an ELISA test for *C. perfringens* enterotoxin.‡ Tests for other toxins or toxin genes are performed in research laboratories specializing in clostridial bacteria. Identification of toxin is essential to form a putative diagnosis of clostridial enterocolitis, because many isolated *C. difficile* and *C. perfringens* are nontoxigenic.[439]

TREATMENT. Treatment with metronidazole (15 mg/kg every 6 to 8 hours) appears to be effective in eliminating enteric clostridial infection in most cases. In one veterinary teaching hospital, isolates of *C. difficile* were resistant to metronidazole,[440] and vancomycin was used with reported success. Large-scale resistance to metronidazole has not been reported elsewhere, and it should be the first choice in the treatment of suspected clostridial enterocolitis. *Saccharomyces boulardii* is a nonpathogenic yeast used in the treatment of *C. difficile* diarrhea and colitis in humans. The yeast releases a protease that specifically degrades *C. difficile* toxins A and B, and this has been shown to be protective in experimental *C. difficile* colitis in rats and to prevent damage to human colonic epithelium by *C. difficile* toxins A and B in vitro.[441] Use of *S. boulardii* in horses has not been reported. A typical dosage in humans is 1 g PO once daily.[442] The yeast has mild virulence in mice, and its use in immunocompromised patients may not be entirely benign.[443]

Antimicrobial-Associated Diarrhea

The onset of acute diarrhea in the horse has been associated with the use of several antimicrobial drugs. Lincomycin administered orally and tetracycline administered parenterally have been demonstrated to induce severe diarrhea in horses.[444,445] The oral administration of trimethoprim-sulfa, erythromycin, metronidazole, and penicillin and parenteral administration of ceftiofur have been implicated with onset of diarrhea, including fatal colitis, in horses. In one report, there was no association between trimethoprim-sulfa and diarrhea.[446] However, in other reports, prior administration of antimicrobials was positively associated with onset of colitis and negatively associated with prognosis for survival in horses with colitis.[447]

Antimicrobial-associated diarrhea is presumed to be secondary to disruption of normal colonic microflora and the proliferation of an enteropathogen, such as *Salmonella* spp., *C. perfringens*, and *C. difficile*. Of interest, it was reported that mares whose foals were treated with erythromycin for *Rhodococcus* infection developed severe, acute colitis, from which *C. difficile* and its toxins were isolated.[448] The mares had erythromycin detected in their feces, and exposure to the

---

C. difficile Tox A/B test, TechLab, Inc., Blacksburg, Va.
†*Clostridium perfringens* enterotoxin kit, Oxoid Division, Unipath, Ogdensburg, NY.
‡*Clostridium perfringens* enterotoxin test, TechLab, Inc., Blacksburg, Va.

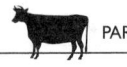

erythromycin was presumed to have occurred by the mares licking erythromycin from the foals' faces.

Other Causes of Acute Diarrhea

The administration of excessive dosages of nonsteroidal antiinflammatory drugs (NSAIDs) (see p. 679) has been associated with the onset of diarrhea secondary to the development of hypoproteinemia and cecal and colonic mucosal edema. The inhibition of prostaglandin synthesis by NSAIDs disrupts mucosal blood flow and other mucosal-protective mechanisms in the bowel. In addition to hypoproteinemia, these horses often have signs of severe endotoxemia. Many horses with diarrhea and toxemia secondary to excessive administration of NSAIDs are slow to respond to therapy and require a long period of intensive care.

Acute diarrhea in the adult horse has also been associated with conditions such as granulomatous enterocolitis, intestinal lymphosarcoma, peritonitis, heavy metal intoxication, anaphylaxis, and stress.

Diagnostic Evaluation

The diagnostic evaluations performed on horses with acute diarrhea are intended to provide the clinician with information to accurately assess the horse's condition and thus direct therapy toward specific requirements. The first part of the evaluation is a thorough physical examination, with particular attention paid to the horse's hydration status (skin turgor, gum moisture, capillary refill time), evidence of toxemia (injected sclera, conjunctiva, oral mucous membranes, mucous membrane color, capillary refill time), cardiovascular system (heart rate and rhythm, character of peripheral pulse, capillary refill time), and signs of laminitis (lameness, digital pulse, palpable temperature of hoof walls). Horses with colitis are often moderately to severely dehydrated, with either purplish or brick-red mucous membranes. Purple mucous membrane color reflects venous congestion and poor venous return, whereas brick-red membrane color reflects venous congestion and poor venous return plus arteriole/venule shunting and poor tissue oxygen exchange.

Blood pressure should be monitored, and whereas direct measurements via an arterial catheter are most accurate, indirect pressure measurements obtained using a Doppler transducer placed over the coccygeal artery are satisfactory. Hypotension and hypertension each occur in horses with colitis, and the blood pressure status of a patient often is unpredictable. Blood pressure can be monitored as frequently as labor permits, and should be done hourly if vasoactive pharmaceutic agents are used.

Laboratory tests that should be performed include complete blood count and plasma protein/total solids. Total hemoglobin and packed cell volume (PCV) are used to assess hydration status. Total protein is used to assess hydration status and degree of protein loss through inflamed intestinal mucosa, and in more chronic cases through protein catabolism. Comparison of clinical hydration, PCV, and total protein is useful in determining the extent of protein loss, and daily evaluations can be used to determine the rate of protein loss.

Total white blood cell (WBC) count, WBC differential, and WBC morphology are used to assess severity of endotoxemia/septicemia; plasma fibrinogen is used to assess the severity of inflammation. Typically the total WBC and neutrophil counts will decrease initially. This is attributable to bacterial endotoxins and the host's mediators of inflammation and occurs in most cases of acute colitis, not just in those caused by *Salmonella* spp. The morphology of the WBCs reflects the severity of the inflammatory response. "Toxic"

changes such as basophilia, granulation, vacuolation of the cytoplasm, and scalloped borders of the cell membrane or adherence of neutrophils to RBCs do not reflect injury to the neutrophils by toxins but reflect the cells' responses to stimulation by pro-inflammatory agents (tumor necrosis factor, interleukin 1) and the production of inflammatory mediators by the neutrophils that are toxic to bacteria. The degree of these changes in circulating neutrophils can be used to assess the severity of disease and also to assess the progress the horse is making. Often the initial sign that the horse is improving is a decrease in the "toxic" appearance to the neutrophils. A horse that continues to have neutrophils with a scalloped cell membrane adhered to red blood cells, together with cytoplasmic vacuolation, granulation, and basophilia for more than 10 days has a severe colitis that is unlikely to resolve.

Serum chemistry tests that should be performed include electrolytes (sodium, chloride, potassium, and calcium), blood urea nitrogen (BUN) and creatinine, and assessment of acid-base status (blood pH and bicarbonate, or total CO_2). Horses with diarrhea often are hyponatremic, hypochloremic, and hypokalemic. With decreased feed intake, hypocalcemia occurs. The severity of these electrolyte disturbances should be monitored, often daily, to allow for appropriate therapy. Parameters that assess renal function, BUN and creatinine, are frequently increased in horses with diarrhea for several reasons. Prerenal azotemia resulting from dehydration and decreased filtration across the glomerulus accounts for some of the increase in these parameters. Hyponatremia and hypochloremia can cause a decrease in glomerular filtration and increase in BUN and creatinine secondary to tubuloglomerular feedback. Horses that are adequately hydrated yet moderately hyponatremic (serum sodium 120 to 128 mEq/L) often remain azotemic until sodium levels increase above 130 mEq/L. Additionally, horses with toxemic colitis often have damage to renal parenchyma, presumably the result of the effects of inflammatory mediators and alterations in renal blood flow.

The acid-base status can be evaluated by estimating serum bicarbonate on the basis of the total CO_2 or directly from a venous or arterial blood gas analysis. Evaluation of a venous blood gas sample is useful in assessing perfusion and oxygen extraction. An increased venous oxygen partial pressure (>60 mm Hg) is indicative of poor capillary perfusion and oxygen delivery to the tissues. Such horses usually have brick-red mucous membranes.

TREATMENT. Because the pathophysiology of equine colitis is complex, treatment often incorporates several medications. Many of these treatments provide well-documented benefit, whereas with others the efficacy is based on empiric judgment only. In addition, in many cases the limiting factor to a successful outcome is a complication of colitis, not a direct effect of colitis.

In cases of acute colitis, fluid administration remains the treatment of primary importance. Most patients require intravenous administration in the early stages. The fluids used must replace fluid, sodium, chloride, and potassium losses. Often, large volumes are required for several days. More specific guidelines for fluid therapy in colitis patients are covered on p. 686.

Most horses with colitis become hypoproteinemic secondary to protein leakage through the inflamed colon and catabolism of albumin secondary to negative energy balance. Hypoproteinemia frequently leads to edema formation in several areas of the body, including the intestinal tract, and can compromise the clinician's ability to keep the patient properly hydrated through fluid administration. Intravenous plasma therapy is often beneficial. Plasma, 3 to 10 L, should be given intravenously. Because the cost of a 900-ml bag of

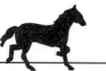

commercial plasma is $100 and $120, the cost of effective plasma therapy in adult horses is often prohibitive.

Plasma contains proteins besides albumin and thus can be of benefit beyond improvement of plasma oncotic pressure. The immunoglobulin present in plasma is of recognized benefit in the treatment of failure of passive transfer in foals. The role of nonspecific immunoglobulin in the treatment of colitis is not known. Fibronectin is essential to the normal function of the monocyte-macrophage system in the processing of a variety of antigens. Other plasma proteins such as elastase and proteinase inhibitors complement inhibitors, anti-thrombin III, and other inhibitors of hypercoagulability may be beneficial to colitis patients.

The nutritional requirements of the colitis patient need to be considered, particularly in a case that may be protracted. Horses with colitis are typically anorectic, and the disruption of normal physiologic processes in the inflamed cecum and colon limits the effectiveness of these organs in the digestion and absorption of nutrients. In addition, several mediators of inflammation and septicemia alter protein/calorie metabolism, resulting in a catabolic state. Thus, even if the horse eats, it is likely to be in a severe caloric deficit for some time. Normally an average horse requires approximately 15 Mcal/day. An endotoxemic horse may require 25 Mcal/day. In a catabolic patient, muscle and fat tissue are mobilized and used in lieu of ingested nutrients. The plasma protein pool, including albumin and immunoglobulins, also is catabolized. In many cases of colitis the decrease in plasma protein may be as much a result of catabolism as of leakage through the inflamed colon. A variety of products can be used for enteral feeding (see Chapter 46).

The use of flunixin meglumine is appropriate in diseases accompanied by production of proinflammatory cytokines. Horses with acute colitis, regardless of the cause, have signs compatible with endotoxemia, as well as local and systemic inflammation. Flunixin doses of 0.25 to 0.5 mg/kg every 6 to 8 hours are used.

Because many of the clinical signs accompanying equine colitis appear attributable to the effects of endotoxin, the development of specific therapy to neutralize endotoxins has been a goal in the past few years. Cross-reactive antibody produced by hyperimmunizing horses to the *Escherichia coli* J5 strain lipopolysaccharide is commercially available.* The efficacy of endotoxin antibody products in treating horses with colitis remains undetermined, although clinical experience suggests that in some cases this treatment is effective in moderating the effects of endotoxemia, particularly when given early in the course of illness. Polymyxin B can neutralize the lipid A moiety of lipopolysaccharide,[451] and its use at a dose of 6000 U/kg early in the course of colitis may moderate the effects of endotoxin.

A medication with potential antiinflammatory benefit in colitis cases is dimethyl sulfoxide (DMSO). DMSO scavenges hydroxyl radicals produced by metabolically activated neutrophils. In the acute stages of equine colitis, there is frequently a pronounced neutrophilic invasion of the cecum and colon, and in this context DMSO may be efficacious. A dosage of 100 to 200 mg/kg/day appears appropriate at this time.

The use of antimicrobials in the treatment of colitis is controversial. In cases of colitis caused by *E. risticii,* the efficacy of tetracycline, 6.6 to 11 mg/kg IV once to twice daily, is documented clinically and experimentally. In other cases of colitis, including *Salmonella* colitis, in which specific antimicrobial sensitivities to the *Salmonella* spp. have been established, the efficacy of antimicrobial administration is less well documented. Many clinicians believe that the use of an antimi-

crobial for which the *Salmonella* spp. have demonstrated sensitivity, such as chloramphenicol, enrofloxacin, gentamicin, amikacin, or a third-generation cephalosporin, does not significantly alter the course of the disease nor hasten the elimination of the organism from the body. In endotoxemic, neutropenic patients the use of broad-spectrum antibiotics is justified to prevent bacteremia or organ colonization by *Salmonella* spp. or other enteric organisms. In clinical practice, the truth probably lies between, with some patients benefitting from the appropriate use of antimicrobials and other patients not requiring such treatment. Deciding prospectively which is the case is the challenge.

Medications that minimize or abolish colonic fluid secretion would be of tremendous benefit in the treatment of equine colitis. Medications such as kaolin, bismuth subsalicylate, and activated charcoal are frequently used in cases of colitis in adult horses, but their efficacy as antisecretory agents in this context has not been established. These medications are more effective in foals with diarrhea, probably as a result of an effect on the small intestine rather than the colon.

CHRONIC DIARRHEA

Chronic diarrhea is one of the most frustrating disorders encountered by equine practitioners, both in determining the cause and in therapeutically managing the diarrhea.[453] Chronic diarrhea may be defined as persistent diarrhea of at least a month's duration. Although there are many causes of chronic diarrhea, these cases can generally be divided into two groups: diarrhea resulting from a chronic inflammatory condition and diarrhea resulting from a disruption in normal physiologic processes. With inflammatory conditions there will be histologic changes in the colon mucosa, including pleocytosis (neutrophils, eosinophils, and lymphocytes), mucosal congestion, and mucosal erosion and ulceration. Submucosal edema, capillary congestion, and lymphatic congestion may be present. With physiologic disorders there are no morphologic changes in the colon, and diarrhea is presumed to result from abnormal volatile fatty acid synthesis or absorption. A small percentage of horses with chronic diarrhea have a primary disorder of a system other than the intestinal tract, such as congestive heart failure or hepatic disease. A thorough physical examination and evaluation of a minimum database (complete blood count, serum chemistry profile, urinalysis) should differentiate horses with primarily nonenteric disorders.

CAUSES. Inflammatory disorders that can cause chronic diarrhea include disorders caused by infectious agents such as chronic salmonellosis; chronic parasitism with *Strongylus vulgaris, Strongylus edentatus,* and larval cyathostomiasis; abdominal abscessation; and, in weanling foals, *Rhodococcus equi* infection of abdominal viscera and rotavirus infection.

Noninfectious inflammatory causes include cellular infiltrative disorders such as granulomatous enteritis and lymphosarcoma, as well as sand enteropathy. Sand causes diarrhea through continued irritation of the mucosal lining of the colon. In weanling foals, gastric ulceration and gastric emptying disorders have been associated with chronic diarrhea that resolved when histamine-2 (H_2) antagonist therapy was started. NSAIDs can cause chronic diarrhea, which is accompanied by varying degress of pathologic change in the large intestine.

Noninflammatory chronic diarrhea of colonic origin is thought to be a result of abnormal fermentation of cellulose by the resident bacteria in the large intestine. In vitro fermentation of feces from normal horses and horses with chronic diarrhea revealed that feces from the diarrheic horses produced more gas, acetate, and propionate than feces from

*Plasma-J, Veterinary Dynamics, San Luis Obispo, CA 93401.

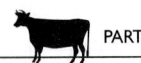

normal horses.[454] Whether this reflects fermentative activity within the colon is not known, but an abnormal increase in acetate could lead to fluid retention within the colonic lumen, because acetate inhibits colonic absorption of sodium and water.

DIAGNOSIS. The diagnostic approach to cases of chronic diarrhea should be based on an attempt to differentiate inflammatory from physiologic causes. The evaluation can be extensive and expensive, and the owner should be prepared for the cause of the diarrhea to remain undetermined. Horses with chronic diarrhea may be adequately hydrated if water consumption has matched water losses. Often, however, such horses are brought to the veterinarian in a condition of mild to moderate dehydration. Moderate weight loss also has often occurred. On physical examination, signs of toxemia (injected mucous membranes, congested or hyperemic mucous membranes) should be noted.

A CBC should be evaluated for signs of chronic inflammation. Such changes include a decrease in the red blood cell count and packed cell volume as a result of decreased erythrogenesis secondary to sequestration of iron by bone marrow macrophages (anemia of chronic inflammation). The WBC count may be normal or moderately increased. The fibrinogen can be normal or increased. Changes in WBC count and fibrinogen levels are influenced by the degree of inflammation and whether the inflammatory response is localized. Thus a normal CBC does not rule out an inflammatory cause of the chronic diarrhea.

Peritoneal fluid analysis may reveal an increase in protein or WBC, which is indicative of an inflammatory process within the peritoneal cavity. Often, however, colon inflammation is not reflected by alterations in the peritoneal fluid.

Serum chemistry values vary in horses with chronic diarrhea. Many cases have evidence of hyponatremia, hypokalemia, hypochloremia, azotemia, and metabolic acidemia. Other horses with less severe chronic diarrhea may have no serum chemistry abnormalities.

The total serum protein is usually decreased with a chronic inflammatory disorder of the colon, reflecting protein leakage from the capillaries and disruption of the colonic mucosal integrity. This is usually reflected by hypoalbuminemia. In some cases, hyperglobulinemia occurs and total protein may be normal to increased.

Increases in hepatic-associated enzymes, including sorbitol dehydrogenase, γ-glutamyltransferase and aspartate amino transferase, and serum bile acids indicate that hepatic disease is present. Hepatic changes and dysfunction such as inflammation, fibrosis or fatty infiltration, or biliary inflammation can be associated with diarrhea.

Feces should be examined for parasite ova; cultured for *Salmonella* spp., *C. difficle,* and *C. perfringens;* and tested for clostridial toxins. In cases of acute diarrhea, it has been recommended that 5 consecutive fecal samples be cultured for *Salmonella* spp., but in cases of chronic diarrhea, many more are often necessary. As many as 15 fecal cultures may be needed to get a positive *Salmonella* spp. culture. In addition, a rectal mucosal biopsy should be cultured. In weanlings the feces should be examined for rotavirus by transmission electron microscopy or ELISA assay. Although it is an unusual cause of diarrhea in weanlings, rotavirus should be considered when dealing with a problem of chronic diarrhea in several foals on the same farm.

An oral glucose absorption test can be done to determine if there is small intestinal malabsorption, which would indicate a widespread small and large intestinal disorder if both diarrhea and glucose malabsorption are present.

A rectal mucosal biopsy may provide evidence of a widespread inflammatory disorder, such as one of the inflammatory bowel diseases (see page 647).[455] Biopsies should be evaluated by a pathologist experienced in examining equine tissue specimens, and some caution should be taken to avoid overinterpretation of the presence of few lymphocytes, plasma cells, and eosinophils.

Frequently the results of the previously mentioned diagnostic procedures do not determine the cause of the chronic diarrhea. In such cases an exploratory laparotomy may be warranted. This is particularly true if episodes of abdominal discomfort accompany the chronic diarrhea. In addition to exploration of the abdomen for the presence of masses or abscesses, the colon and cecum should be thoroughly examined. Biopsies from several sites of the colon, cecum, and mesenteric lymph nodes should be submitted for histopathology and culture for *Salmonella* spp.

TREATMENT. Treatment of horses with chronic diarrhea is often empiric, because either a cause has not been determined or the cause is not amenable to treatment. With inflammatory causes such as lymphosarcoma and granulomatous enteritis, the disease is usually untreatable. Some cases of eosinophilic colitis have been treated successfully with corticosteroids.

Chronic parasitism may be resolved with appropriate anthelmintic therapy, although damage to the mucosa may have become too extensive to allow normal absorption to occur. Administration of larvacidal doses of fenbendazole (15 mg/kg PO daily for 5 days) is usually effective. Concurrent administration of prednisone (1 mg/kg PO once daily for 5 to 7 days) and aspirin (60 grains PO every other day) may minimize inflammation secondary to killing migrating larvae within the vasculature and mucosa of the colon.

Chronic salmonellosis does not lend itself to specific treatment, because antimicrobial therapy is generally unrewarding in resolving *Salmonella* infection in horses.

Administration of products containing bismuth subsalicylate is effective in some cases of chronic diarrhea. The action of bismuth subsalicylate is mediated through inhibition of prostaglandin synthesis and possibly by other undefined mechanisms. In full-size horses a large volume, 1 to 4 L/day, must be administered to be effective.

Iodochlorhydroxyquin* is effective in managing some cases of chronic diarrhea caused by maldigestion of cellulose by colonic microorganisms.[456] The actual mechanism of action of iodochlorhydroxyquin in resolving the diarrhea is not known. The drug was originally administered to horses with chronic diarrhea because an increase in fecal trichomonads was observed. However, this observation likely reflected that trichomonads were washed out of the cecum and colon rather than that they were the cause of the diarrhea. Iodochlorhydroxyquin has minimal effect on colonic protozoal populations. It is not uniformly effective, and in many cases its effectiveness is only transient. Stools may initially become formed, but the diarrhea often recurs within several days. An initial dose of 20 mg/kg/day is recommended. If diarrhea recurs, decreasing the dose to 10 mg/kg/day is sometimes effective. If the medication is effective, it must be continued, because, if it is discontinued, the diarrhea resumes.

Changes in diet occasionally are helpful in horses with noninflammatory chronic diarrhea. Feeding a complete pelleted feed may positively affect the constituent volatile fatty acids produced in the colon and thus facilitate water absorption. Alternatively, trying different types of roughage may result in selecting one that creates a more favorable metabolic environment in the large intestine.

The removal of sand from the colon by nonsurgical means is difficult, and in one report the administration of psyllium was not effective.[457] Other treatments used with anecdotal,

---

*Reaform, Solvay Veterinary, Princeton, NJ 80540.

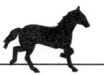

but undocumented, success include fecal transfaunations, probiotics, cultured yogurt, and brewer's yeast.

REFERENCES

396. Sullins KE: Diseases of the large colon. In White NA, ed: *The equine acute abdomen*, Philadelphia, 1990, Lea & Febiger, pp 375-391.
397. House JK et al: Risk factors for nosocomial Salmonella infection among hospitalized horses, *J Am Vet Med Assoc* 214:1511-1516,1999.
398. Par J, Carpenter TE, Thurmond MC: Analysis of spatial and temporal clustering of horses with *Salmonella krefeld* in an intensivecare unit of a veterinary hospital, *J Am Vet Med Assoc* 209:626-628, 1996.
399. Hartmann FA et al: Control of an outbreak of salmonellosis caused by drug-resistant *Salmonella anatum* in horses at a veterinary hospital and measures to prevent future infections, *J Am Vet Med Assoc* 209:629-631, 1996.
400. Tillotson K et al: Outbreak of *Salmonella infantis* infection in a large animal veterinary teaching hospital, *J Am Vet Med Assoc* 211:1554-1557, 1997.
401. Hird DW et al: Risk factors for salmonellosis in hospitalized horses, *J Am Vet Med Assoc* 188:173-177, 1986.
401a. Walker RL et al: Genotypic and phenotypic analysis of *Salmonella* strains associated with an outbreak of equine neonatal salmonellosis, *Vet Microbiol* 43:143-150, 1995.
402. Smith BP, Reina-Guerra M, Hardy AJ: Prevalence and epizootiology of equine salmonellosis, *J Am Vet Med Assoc* 172:353-356, 1978.
403. Roberts MC, O'Boyle DA: Prevalence and epizootiology of salmonellosis among groups of horses in southeast Queensland, *Aust Vet J* 57:27-34, 1981.
404. Traub-Dargatz JL et al: National Animal Health Monitoring System (Nahms) Equine '98 Study: *Salmonella* spp. fecal shedding in the U.S. horse population 1998-1999, *Proc Am Coll Vet Intern Med* 17:153-155, 1999.
405. Cohen ND et al: Comparison of polymerase chain reaction and microbiological culture for detection of salmonellae in equine feces and environmental samples, *Am J Vet Res* 57:780-786, 1996.
406. Palmer JE et al: Comparison of rectal mucosal cultures and fecal cultures in detecting *Salmonella* infection in horses and cattle, *Am J Vet Res* 46:697-698, 1985.
407. Holland CJ, Ristic M, Cole AI: Isolation, experimental transmission, and characterization of causative agent of Potomac horse fever, *Science* 227:522-524, 1985.
408. Rikihisa Y, Perry BD, Cordes DO: Ultrastructural study of ehrlichial organisms in the large colons of ponies infected with Potomac horse fever, *Infect Immun* 49:505, 1985.
409. Ziemer EL et al: Clinical and hematologic variables in ponies with experimentally induced equine ehrlichial colitis (Potomac horse fever), *Am J Vet Res*, 48:63-67, 1987.
410. Long MT et al: Identification of *Ehrlichia risticii* as the causative agent of two equine abortions following natural maternal infection, *J Vet Diagn Invest* 56:201-205, 1995.
411. Burg JG et al: Attempted transmission of *Ehrlichia risticii* (Rickettsiaceae) with *Stomoxys calcitrans* (Diptera: Muscidae), *J Med Entomol* 27:874-877, 1990.
412. Hahn NE et al: Attempted transmission of *Ehrlichia risticii*, causative agent of Potomac horse fever, by the ticks, *Dermacentor variabilis*, *Rhipicephalus sanguineus*, *Ixodes scapularis* and *Amblyomma americanum*, *Exper Appl Acarol* 8:41-50, 1990.
413. Wen B et al: Characterization of the SF agent, an *Ehrlichia* sp. isolated from the fluke *Stellantchasmus falcatus*, by 16S rRNA base sequence, serological, and morphological analyses, *Int J Syst Bacteriol* 46:149-154, 1996.
414. Barlough JE et al:Detection of *Ehrlichia risticii*, the agent of Potomac horse fever, in freshwater stream snails (Pleuroceridae: Juga spp.) from northern California, *Appl Environ Microbiol* 64:2888-2893, 1998.
415. Reubel GH, Barlough JE, Madigan JE: Production and characterization of *Ehrlichia risticii*, the agent of Potomac horse fever, from snails (Pleuroceridae: Juga spp.) in aquarium culture and genetic comparison to equine strains, *J Clin Microbiol* 36:1501-1511, 1998.
416. Palmer JE, Benson CE, Lotz GW: Serological response of experimental ponies orally infected with *Ehrlichia risticii*, *Equine Vet J* 7(suppl):19-20, 1989.
417. Madigan JE et al: Evidence for a high rate of false-positive results with the indirect fluorescent antibody test for *Ehrlichia risticii*, *J Am Vet Med Assoc* 207:1448-1453, 1995.
418. Palmer JE: Prevention of Potomac horse fever, *Cornell Vet* 79:201-205, 1989.
419. Vemulapalli R, Biswas B, Dutta SK: Pathogenic, immunologic, and molecular differences between two *Ehrlichia risticii* strains, *J Clin Microbiol* 33:2987-2993, 1995.
420. Chaichanasiriwithaya W et al: Antigenic, morphologic, and molecular characterization of new *Ehrlichia risticii* isolates, *J Clin Microbiol* 32:3026-3033, 1994.
421. Wierup M: Equine intestinal clostridiosis. An acute disease in horses associated with high intestinal counts of *Clostridium perfringens* type A, *Acta Vet Scand Suppl* 62:1-182, 1977.

422. Donaldson MT, Palmer JE: Prevalence of *Clostridium perfringens* enterotoxin and *Clostridium difficile* toxin A in feces of horses with diarrhea and colic, *J Am Vet Med Assoc* 215:358-361, 1999.
423. Gerding DN et al: *Clostridium difficile*-associated diarrhea and colitis, *Infect Control Hosp Epidemiol* 8:459-477, 1995.
424. Rocha MFG et al: Intestinal secretory factor released by macrophages stimulated with *Clostridium difficile* toxin A: role of interleukin 1 beta, *Infect Immun* 66:4910-4916, 1998.
425. Riegler M et al: Epidermal growth factor attenuates *Clostridium difficile* toxin A- and B-induced damage of human colonic mucosa, *Am J Physiol* 273:G1014-G1022, 1997.
426. Triadafilopoulos G et al: Differential effects of *Clostridium difficile* toxins A and B on rabbit ileum, *Gastroenterology* 93:273-279, 1987.
427. Wershil BK, Castagliuolo I, Pothoulakis C: Direct evidence of mast cell involvement in *Clostridium difficile* toxin A-induced enteritis in mice, *Gastroenterology* 114: 956-964, 1998.
428. Linevsky JK et al: IL-8 release and neutrophil activation by *Clostridium difficile* toxin-exposed human monocytes, *Am J Physiol* 273: G1333-G1340, 1997.
429. Castagliuolo I et al: *Clostridium difficile* toxin A stimulates macrophage-inflammatory protein-2 production in rat intestinal epithelial cells, *J Immunol* 160:6039-6045, 1998.
430. Castagliuolo I et al: Increased substance P responses in dorsal root ganglia and intestinal macrophages during *Clostridium difficile* toxin A enteritis in rats, *Proc Natl Acad Sci USA* 94:4788-4793, 1997.
431. Riegler M et al: *Clostridium difficile* toxin B is more potent than toxin A in damaging human colonic epithelium in vitro, *J Clin Invest* 95:2004-2011, 1995.
432. Shone CC, Hambleton P: Toxigenic clostridia. In Minto NP, Clarke DJ, eds: *Biotechnology handbooks: clostridia*, New York, 1989, Plenum Press, pp 265-292.
433. East LM et al: Enterocolitis associated with *Clostridium perfringens* infection in neonatal foals: 54 cases (1988-1997), *J Am Vet Med Assoc* 212:1751-1756, 1998.
434. Netherwood T et al: Molecular analysis of the virulence determinants of *Clostridium perfringens* associated with foal diarrhoea, *Vet J* 155:289-294, 1998.
435. Herholz C et al: Prevalence of 2-toxigenic *Clostridium perfringens* in horses with intestinal disorders, *J Clin Microbiol* 37:3583-3561, 1999.
436. Netherwood T et al: Foal diarrhoea between 1991 and 1994 in the United Kingdom associated with *Clostridium perfringens*, rotavirus, *Strongyloides westeri* and *Cryptosporidium* spp. *Epidemiol Infect* 117:375-383, 1996.
437. Blackwell RB, White NA: Duodenitis proximal jejunitis in the horse, *Proc First Equine Colic Res Symp* 1982, p 106.
438. Madewell BR et al: Apparent outbreaks of *Clostridium difficile*-associated diarrhea in horses in a veterinary medical teaching hospital, *J Vet Diagn Invest* 7:343-346, 1995.
439. McClane BA: An overview of *Clostridium perfringens* enterotoxin, *Toxicol* 34:1335-1343, 1996.
440. Jang SS et al: Antimicrobial susceptibilities of equine isolates of *Clostridium difficile* and molecular characterization of metronidazole-resistant strains, *Clin Infect Dis* 25(suppl2):S266-S267, 1997.
441. Castagliuolo I et al: *Saccharomyces boulardii* protease inhibits the effects of *Clostridium difficile* toxins A and B in human colonic mucosa, *Infect Immun* 67:302-307, 1999.
442. McFarland LV et al: A randomized placebo-controlled trial of *Saccharomyces boulardii* in combination with standard antibiotics for *Clostridium difficile* disease, *J Am Med Assoc* 271:1913-1918, 1994.
443. McCullough MJ et al: Species identification and virulence attributes of *Saccharomyces boulardii*, *J Clin Microbiol* 36:2613-2617, 1998.
444. Raisbeck MF, Holt GR, Osweiler GD: Lincomycin-associated colitis in horses, *J Am Vet Med Assoc* 179:362-363, 1981.
445. Anderson G et al: Lethal complications following administration of oxytetracycline in the horse, *Nord Vet Med* 23:9-22, 1971.
446. Wilson DA et al: Case control and historical cohort study of diarrhea associated with administration of trimethoprim-potentiated sulphonamides to horses and ponies, *J Vet Intern Med* 10:258-264, 1996.
447. Cohen ND, Woods AM: Characteristics and risk factors for failure of horses with acute diarrhea to survive: 122 cases (1990-1996), *J Am Vet Med Assoc* 214:382-390, 1999.
448. Baverud V et al: A *Clostridium difficile* associated with acute colitis in mares when their foals are treated with erythromycin and rifampicin for *Rhodococcus equi* pneumonia, *Equine Vet J* 30:482-488, 1998.
449. Reference deleted in proof.
450. Scovill WA et al: Opsonic alpha$_2$ surface binding glycoprotein therapy during sepsis, *Ann Surg* 188:521-529, 1978.
451. Durando MM et al: Effects of polymyxin B and Salmonella typhimurium antiserum on horses given endotoxin intravenously, *Am J Vet Res* 55:921-927, 1994.
452. Palmer JE: Update on equine diarrheal diseases: salmonellosis and Potomac fever, *Proceedings of the Am Coll Vet Intern Med Forum* 12:126-132, 1984.
453. Love S, Mair TS, Hillyer MH: Chronic diarrhoea in adult horses: a review of 51 referred cases, *Vet Rec* 130:217-219, 1992.

454. Merritt AM, Smith DA: Osmolality and volatile fatty acid content of feces from horses with chronic diarrhea, *Am J Vet Res* 41:928-931, 1980.
455. Lindberg R, Nygren A, Oersson SGB: Rectal biopsy diagnosis in horses with clinical signs of intestinal disorders: a retrospective study of 116 cases, *Equine Vet J* 28:275-284, 1996.
456. Minder HP, Merritt AM, Chalupa W: In vitro fermentation of feces from normal and chronically diarrheal horses, *Am J Vet Res* 41:564-567, 1980.
457. Hammock PD, Freeman DE, Baker GJ: Failure of psyllium mucilloid to hasten evaluation of sand from the equine large intestine, *Vet Surg* 27:547-554, 1998.

SURGICAL DISORDERS OF THE LARGE INTESTINE

ANTHONY T. BLIKSLAGER

SIMPLE OBSTRUCTION

Simple obstructions of the large intestine tend to have a more gradual onset than those of the small intestine, and in the case of large colon impactions are frequently amenable to medical therapy.[458] Cecal impactions present much more of a dilemma because of the greater propensity of this organ to rupture,[459] and the relative difficulty of surgically manipulating the cecum.[460]

Cecal Impaction

Cecal impaction may develop as a primary condition, or may arise as a complication in hospitalized horses, particularly those that have undergone surgery.[461] Reasons for development of cecal impaction in hospitalized horses are unclear, although motility disturbances arising from postoperative pain or administration of nonsteroidal antiinflammatory drugs may play a role. Cecal impactions may present as one of two types: impaction of the cecum with firm ingesta or gross distention of the cecum with fluid ingesta. The latter has been termed cecal dysfunction; it may be initiated by abnormalities in cecal motility. Evidence in favor of this supposition includes the fact that the right ventral colon is typically empty in horses with cecal dysfunction, suggesting a lack of aboral movement of digesta through the cecocolic orifice.[461] However, clinical differentiation of cecal impaction and cecal dysfunction may be very difficult.[462] In horses with dry ingesta–filled cecal impactions, there is often a gradual onset of abdominal pain over several days.[462] Such impactions have a propensity to rupture before the development of severe abdominal pain or systemic deterioration and therefore must be closely monitored.[459,462] With cecal dysfunction, horses tend to present with elevated heart rates and signs compatible with endotoxemia. In addition, these horses may have evidence of cecal wall degeneration, including a serosanguinous appearance to abdominal fluid with accompanying elevations in total protein.[461] However, analgesic administration and expected degrees of postoperative depression in horses that have recently undergone surgery may mask such clinical signs.

The diagnosis of cecal impaction is based on palpation of a firm, impacted cecum or a grossly distended fluid-filled cecum per rectum. According to one study, such findings were detected in 89% of horses with cecal impaction that underwent per rectal palpation of the abdomen.[462] In some cases, cecal impactions may be difficult to differentiate from large colon impactions. However, careful palpation will reveal the inability to move the hand completely dorsal to the impacted viscus because of the cecum's attachment to the dorsal body wall.[461]

Treatment for horses with dry ingesta–filled cecal impactions may include initial medical therapy, with aggressive administration of intravenous fluids, judicious use of anal-

gesics, and administration of oral laxatives (e.g., 2 to 4 L mineral oil/500 kg).[461,463] Other oral laxatives have also been recommended, including magnesium sulfate (1 mg/kg in 4 L water PO up to twice daily for up to 3 days)[461] and psyllium (1 g/kg every 6 to 8 hours).[463] However, if the cecum is grossly distended, or if medical therapy has had no effect within a reasonable period of time, surgical evacuation of the cecum via a typhlotomy is indicated.[459] In addition, it is advisable to perform an ileocolostomy in order to bypass the cecum, because postoperative cecal motility dysfunction with recurrence of the disease is common.[460,464] However, this aspect of surgical treatment remains controversial, and there are cases of cecal impaction that, if identified early, can be treated via typhlotomy alone.

In horses with cecal dysfunction, immediate surgery is indicated. In addition, cecal bypass is often warranted because it is suspected that motility disturbances initiate the disease, and therefore recurrence in the absence of cecal by-pass may occur. However, this decision can be made based on the appearance of the cecum at surgery.[461]

The prognosis depends on the type of cecal impaction encountered. In a recent report in which dry ingesta–filled cecal impactions were treated by typhlotomy and ileocolostomy or jejunocolostomy, 7 of 9 horses lived long term.[460] Horses in which cecal dysfunction develops have a great propensity to rupture, which is universally fatal.[462] Because these cases can be difficult to identify before surgery, the prognosis for this condition tends to be unfavorable.[462]

Large Colon Impaction

Impactions of the large colon with ingesta occur at sites of anatomic reductions in luminal diameter, particularly the pelvic flexure and the right dorsal colon.[465] Although there are several reported risk factors, most have not been proven. However, a sudden restriction in exercise associated with musculoskeletal injury appears to be frequently associated with onset of impaction.[458] A further consideration is equine feeding regimens, which usually entail twice daily feeding of concentrate. Such regimens are associated with secretion of large volumes of fluid into the small intestine, resulting in transient hypovolemia (15% loss of plasma volume).[466] This leads to activation of the renin-angiotensin-aldosterone system,[466] and because aldosterone stimulates absorption of fluid from the large colon,[467] this may dehydrate colonic contents.[466] Large concentrate meals may decrease small intestinal transit time, resulting in increased presentation of soluble carbohydrate to the cecum and large colon. Large shifts of fluid into the colon occur as concentrates are readily fermented in the large intestine, which would be expected to activate the renin-angiotensin-aldosterone system. This in turn triggers net fluid absorption from the large colon.[467] The effect of these large fluid fluxes on development of large intestinal disorders remains to be fully characterized, but undoubtedly they play some role in the syndrome of colic. From a practical standpoint, intestinal fluid fluxes may be reduced with frequent small feedings in those horses requiring concentrate to maintain condition.[466]

Clinical signs of large colon impaction include slow onset of mild colic that is typically well controlled with administration of analgesics, but becomes increasingly more severe and refractory if the impaction does not resolve. The diagnosis is based on palpation of a firm mass in the large colon per rectum. However, the extent of the impaction may be underestimated by rectal palpation alone because much of the colon will be out of reach.[465] Adjacent colon may be distended if the impaction has resulted in complete obstruction. Initial medical treatment should be attempted. Intermittent abdominal pain is controlled with administration of analgesics (flunixin meglumine 0.25 mg/kg IV every 6 hours to 1.1 mg/kg IV every 12 hours, butorphanol 0.05 mg/kg IV prn, xylazine 0.3 to 0.5 mg/kg IV prn). Detomidine (10 to 20 mg IV prn) can be used with great caution, because this agent readily masks severe pain. In addition to analgesics, mineral oil (2 to 4 L/ 500 kg PO), water with dioctyl sodium sulfosuccinate (180 to 240 ml in 4 L water PO), or magnesium sulfate (1 mg/kg in 4 L water PO) may be administered by stomach tube for their laxative effects. Access to feed should not be permitted. For impactions that persist, aggressive oral and intravenous fluid therapy (2 to 4 times maintenance fluid requirement) should be instituted.[465] If the impaction remains unresolved, the horse develops uncontrollabe pain or extensive gas distention of the colon occurs, surgery is indicated. At surgery the contents of the colon are evacuated via a pelvic flexure enterotomy. The prognosis is good for those horses in which impactions resolve medically (95% long-term survival in one study) and fair in horses that require surgical intervention (58% long-term survival in the same study).[458]

Enteroliths

Enteroliths are mineralized masses that are typically composed of ammonium magnesium phosphate (struvite).[468] One study suggests that an increase in magnesium in the diet may predispose to the formation of enteroliths.[469] Enteroliths almost always form around a nucleus such as a silicon dioxide stone, a nail (Fig. 30-40), or piece of rope that has been ingested,[468] and are most commonly found in the right dorsal and transverse colons.[469] Although enterolithiasis has a wide geographic distribution, horses in California have a high incidence. In one California study, horses with enterolithiasis represented 28% of the surgical colic population. In addition, Arabians, Morgans, American Saddlebreds, and donkeys are at risk for this disease.[470] Initially, clinical signs include intermittent abdominal pain in mature horses (almost always greater than 4 years of age),[471] with few abnormalities on rectal examination. As enteroliths become larger,

they may occlude the lumen of the colon and cause acute pain and large colon distention that necessitates surgical exploration. In some cases, an enterolith is forced into the small colon, where it causes acute small colon obstruction. Enteroliths may be diagnosed by abdominal radiography or at surgery. On rare occasions, an enterolith may be palpated per rectum, particularly if it is present in the distal small colon.

In general, surgery is required for these cases, although there are reports of enteroliths being retrieved per rectum. In fact in one study, 14% of horses that presented for treatment of enterolithiasis had a history of passing an enterolith in the feces.[470] However, enteroliths are typically located in the right dorsal colon, transverse colon, or small colon. At surgery, the enterolith is gently pushed toward a pelvic flexure enterotomy, but removal frequently requires a separate right dorsal colon enterotomy to prevent rupture of the colon. After removal of an enterolith, further exploration must be conducted to determine if other enteroliths are present. Solitary enteroliths are usually round, whereas multiple enteroliths have flat sides. The prognosis is good, (92% 1-year survival of horses recovered from surgery in one study on 900 cases), unless the colon is ruptured during removal of an enterolith. In one recent study, rupture occurred in 15% of cases.[470]

Sand Impactions of the Large Colon

Sand impactions of the large colon are common in horses with access to sandy soils, particularly horses whose feed is placed on the ground. Sand accumulates in the large colon, particularly the right dorsal colon and pelvic flexure.[472,473] In addition, sand may trigger diarrhea, presumably as a result of irritation of the colonic mucosa.[474] In horses with sand impactions, clinical signs are similar to those of horses with large colon impactions.[472] In addition, sand may be found in the feces, and auscultation of the ventral abdomen may reveal sounds of sand moving within the large colon.[475] In addition, sand may be detected on abdominal radiography.[474] The diagnosis is definitively made at surgery, but may be tentatively based on clinical signs compatible with a large colon impaction together with evidence of sand in the feces. To determine the presence of sand, several fecal balls are placed in a rectal palpation sleeve or other container, which is subsequently filled with water. If sand is present, it will accumulate at the bottom of the container. In addition, mineral opacity may be detected within the colon on abdominal radiographs.[473]

Initially, medical therapy is warranted. Administration of *Psyllium hydrophilia* mucciloid in water by stomach tube may facilitate passage of sand, although a recent experimental study has failed to show a benefit of this treatment.[476] If colic becomes intractable, surgical evacuation of the large colon should be performed. The prognosis is good.[472,473]

NONSTRANGULATING OBSTRUCTION OF THE COLON

There are several configurations of displacements, including nephrosplenic entrapment of the colon, that obstruct the colonic lumen, but that do not compromise the colonic blood supply. Therefore technically these are simple obstructions. However, the lumen may not be completely obstructed, and some degree of venous congestion is common.[477] In some cases, nonstrangulating obstructions are difficult to differentiate from large colon volvulus, because a volvulus of less than 270 degrees will not result in strangulation of blood supply but can cause considerable abdominal pain and gas distention of the abdomen. In this regard, nonstrangulating obstructions represent early stages of strangu-

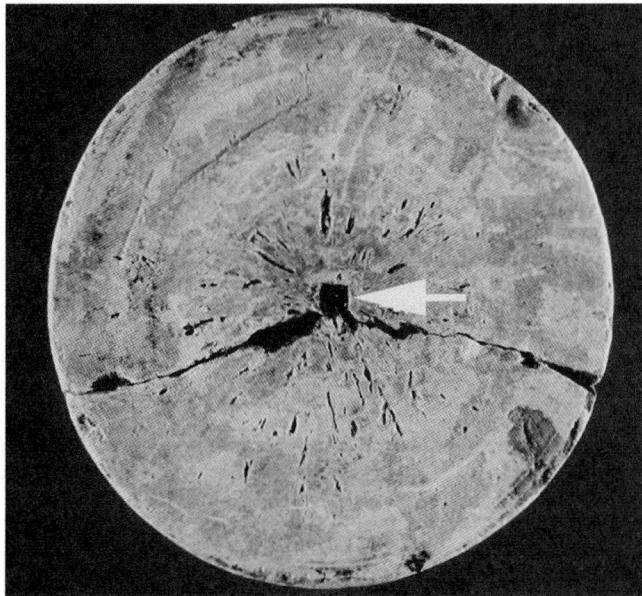

FIG. 30-40 ■ Cut section of an enterolith. The *arrow* points at a nail head that served as a nucleus for the formation of a struvite enterolith. (Photograph courtesy Dr. DG Bristol.)

lating obstructions.[477] Clinical signs include mild to moderate colic, with evidence of large colon distention on palpation of the abdomen per rectum. The diagnosis is confirmed at surgery.[478] If pain is recurrent, particularly if it is of increasing intensity and frequency or if there is evidence of intestinal compromise (particularly progressive changes in abdominal fluid and cardiovascular parameters indicating systemic deterioration), the horse should be taken immediately to surgery. The prognosis is good, with in excess of 80% of horses surviving to hospital discharge in a multicenter study.[479]

Right Dorsal Displacement of the Large Colon

With right dorsal displacement of the colon, the colon displaces to the right of the cecum. Findings on per rectal palpation typically include colonic bands coursing horizontally across the abdomen, with evidence of colon lateral to the cecum.[477] In the most common configuration of the right dorsal displacement, the large colon wraps around the cecum (pivoting counter-clockwise around the cecum looking from above the horse) with the pelvic flexure lying in the left dorsal quadrant. Alternatively, the colon may wrap around the cecum in the opposite direction, with the pelvic flexure lying in the right dorsal quadrant.[480] At surgery a 180-degree volvulus may also be detected at the site of colonic displacement.[477]

Nephrosplenic Entrapment (Left Dorsal Displacement) of the Large Colon

On the left side, colon displacements most commonly involve entrapment of the colon over the nephrosplenic ligament, although left dorsal displacements may be detected before the colon is fully entrapped. Clinical signs include gradual onset of mild to moderate colic as the entrapped colon fills with gas. Palpation per rectum will reveal gas distended ventral colon and displacement of the spleen toward the center of the abdomen. By following colonic bands up to the left dorsal quadrant, careful palpation often reveals the presence of colon between the left kidney and the spleen. Diagnosis may be based on palpation per rectum of the colon traversing the nephrosplenic ligament. Alternatively, a tentative diagnosis can be reached using abdominal ultrasonography.[481] The spleen can be visualized on the left side of the abdomen, but the left kidney will be obscured by gas-distended bowel. Evaluation of this technique indicates that there are no instances of false-positive results, although false-negative results may occasionally occur.[481] Therefore, as with other examination techniques, ultrasonography is not uniformly reliable. A definitive diagnosis may therefore require surgery. Treatment has traditionally been surgical intervention, during which the colon is gently rocked free of the nephrosplenic space. More recently, nonsurgical intervention has been successful in select cases.[481-483] If such manipulations are to be attempted, the clinician must be certain of a diagnosis. The horse is anesthetized and placed in right lateral recumbency. The horse is rotated up to dorsal recumbency, rocked back and forth for 5 to 10 minutes, and then rolled down into left lateral recumbency.[484] The nephrosplenic space should be palpated per rectum to determine whether or not the entrapment has been relieved. Phenylephrine (3 to 6 μg/kg/min over 15 minutes) may be administered to decrease the size of the spleen.[485] If the entrapment remains, further attempts may be tried, but in cases in which the displacement is not corrected the horse should be taken to surgery.[482] More recently, phenylephrine has been used in conjunction with 30 to 45 minutes of light exercise (jogging) to successfully reduce nephrosplenic entrapments in 4 of 6 horses.[477] The authors suggested that the technique be used on horses with

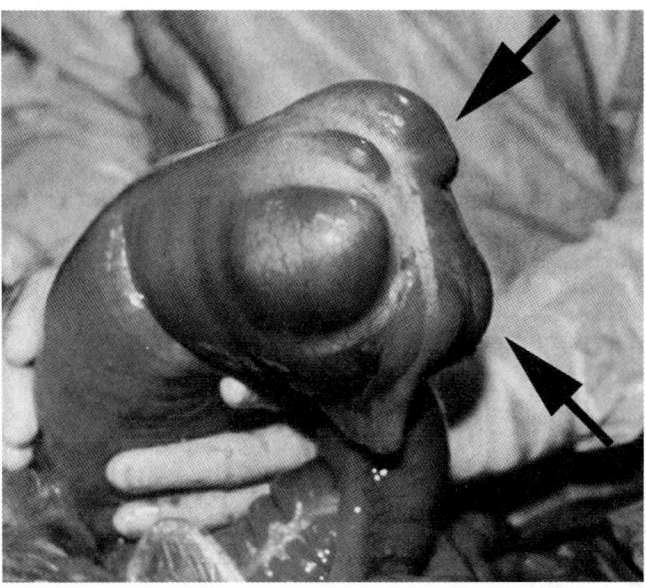

FIG. 30-41 ■ Operative view of atresia coli. Complete atresia of the pelvic flexure resulted in a blind-ended ventral colon *(arrows)* resulting in gas distention of the colon. The ventral colon was subsequently anastomosed to the dorsal colon in this foal.

mild to moderate colonic distention, particularly if signs of colic can be readily controlled.

Regardless of technique, the prognosis is good. In one study, survival was in excess of 90%.[483] There are cases in which nonsurgical interventions do not completely correct the problem and others in which nonsurgical manipulations correct the entrapment but result in large colon volvulus or displacement.[486] Such cases should be taken to surgery promptly.

Atresia Coli

Atresia of any segment of the colon is a rare congenital abnormality in horses (Fig. 30-41).[487] The heritability and causes of the condition is unknown. One potential mechanism for development of the lesion is intestinal ischemia during fetal life, which secondarily results in necrosis of a segment of intestine.[487] Clinical signs include a failure to pass meconium and colic within the first 12 to 24 hours of life. Secondary abdominal distention results from complete intestinal obstruction, and abdominal radiographs may reveal gas-distended colon. The diagnosis is made at surgery. Any portion of the colon may be absent, but the distal segment of the large colon or the proximal small colon is usually most severely affected. If sufficient tissue is present, anastomosis to the proximal blind end of the colon may be attempted.[487] The prognosis depends on which segment of the colon is absent, but is usually poor because of an absence of distal colon.

STRANGULATING OBSTRUCTION

Although simple obstruction of the large colon carries a very favorable prognosis, strangulating obstruction of the large colon is associated with high fatality rates. Two forms of strangulating obstruction are recognized: hemorrhagic strangulating obstruction, in which the arterial blood flow remains patent while veins are collapsed, and ischemic strangulating obstruction, in which both the arteries and veins are collapsed. The differentiating factor between the two is likely

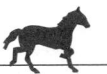

how tightly twisted the volvulus is. It has been suggested that ingesta-filled intestine is more likely to develop a hemorrhagic lesion during volvulus because the intestinal contents prevent the intestine from twisting tightly.[488]

Large Colon Volvulus

Clinical signs include rapid onset of severe, unrelenting abdominal pain.[489] Although postparturient broodmares appear to be at risk,[477] this association has not been conclusively determined. Once the large colon is strangulated ($\geq$270-degree volvulus), gas distention is marked, leading to gross distention of the abdomen, compromised respiration as the distended bowel presses against the diaphragm, and visceral pooling of blood as the caudal vena cava is compressed. Horses with this condition are frequently refractory to even the most potent of analgesics. These horses may prefer to lie in dorsal recumbency, presumably to take weight off the strangulated colon. An abbreviated physical examination is warranted in these cases, because the time elapsed from the onset of strangulation to surgical correction is critical. Experimentally, the colon is irreversibly damaged with 3 to 4 hours of a 360-degree volvulus of the entire colon.[490] Despite severe pain and hypovolemia, horses may present with a paradoxically low heart rate, possibly related to increased vagal tone. In addition, results of abdominocentesis are often not indicative of the degree of colon compromise,[489,491] and in many cases abdominocentesis should not be done because of extreme colonic distention.[477] Palpation will reveal severe gas distention of the large colon, often restricting access to the abdomen beyond the pelvic brim. The diagnosis may be tentatively based on signalment, severity of pain, and degree of distention.

At surgery, the volvulus is typically located at the mesenteric attachment of the colon to the dorsal body wall and the most common direction of the twist is dorsomedial using the right ventral colon as a reference point.[489] However, the colon may twist in the opposite direction, twist greater than 360 degrees (up to 720 degrees has been reported), or twist at the level of the diaphragmatic and sternal flexures.[489] In all cases, the colon should be decompressed as much as possible, and in many cases evacuation of colon contents via a pelvic flexure enterotomy will facilitate correction of the volvulus. A determination must be made after correction of the volvulus as to whether the colon has been irreversibly injured. This is frequently based on mucosal color and bleeding (if an enterotomy has been performed), palpation of a pulse in the colonic arteries, serosal color, and appearance of muscular motility.[488] However, determination of viability based on these parameters is unreliable. Currently, one of the most reliable techniques for determining viability is histologic evaluation of frozen sections of colonic mucosa. Biopsies may be obtained at the pelvic flexure because it has been determined that mucosal changes are uniform throughout strangulated colon. A prediction of viability is based on the degree of crypt epithelial loss and the interstitium to crypt ratio (based on measurements of the crypt width and the width of interstitial space between crypts). In one study, 16 of 18 horses that had greater than 50% loss of crypt epithelium and an interstitium to crypt ratio of greater than 3 typically did not survive, whereas 43 of 46 horses that had less severe mucosal changes survived, suggesting high accuracy.[492] In addition, it has been suggested that accuracy of viability determination can be increased by combining histologic evaluation with surface oximetry or laser Doppler determination of blood flow.[493] Unfortunately, frozen histologic sections are not available at most referral centres on an emergency basis.

If the colon is judged to be irreversibly damaged, the feasibility of a large colon resection can be considered. Although 95% of the colon can be resected (that part of the colon distal to the level of the cecocolic fold), damage from the volvulus usually exceeds that which can be resected. In these cases, surgeons may elect to resect as much damaged bowel as possible or to advise euthanasia.[488]

The prognosis for survival is guarded to poor because of the rapid onset of this disease. In one study, the survival rate was 35%.[491] In a more recent report, the survival rate was 36% for horses with 360-degree volvulus of the large colon compared with 71% for horses with 270-degree volvulus.[489] However, one study in central Kentucky documented a high success rate, most likely because of early recognition of the disease and the proximity of the hospital to the surgical caseload.[494] Postoperative complications include hypovolemic and endotoxemic shock, extensive loss of circulating protein, disseminated intravascular coagulation, and laminitis. In addition, large colon volvulus has a propensity to recur. Although one study documented a recurrence rate of less than 5%,[491] some authors believe recurrence may be as high as 50%.[488] Therefore methods to prevent recurrence should be considered.[495,496]

Intussusception

The most common intussusception of the large intestine is cecocolic intussusception. However, when this is compared to all forms of colic, it is a relatively rare condition of the horse, accounting for 11 of 842 (1.3%) horses taken to surgery for colic at one hospital.[497] The condition tends to occur in young horses (2 to 3 years of age) and may be associated with intestinal parasites, particularly tapeworms. Clinical signs include acute onset of colic that varies in severity according to the degree of intussusception. Initially, the cecal tip inverts, creating a cecocecal intussusception, which does not obstruct flow of ingesta. As the intussusception progresses, the cecum inverts into the right ventral colon (cecocolic intussusception), which obstructs flow of ingesta, and often causes severe colic. In one report on cecocolic intussusception, 10 of 11 horses presented with severe colic.[497] The cause of abdominal pain is often difficult to differentiate in these cases, although it is sometimes possible to detect a mass on the right side of the abdomen and the concurrent absence of a palpable cecum.[497] Treatment involves manual surgical reduction by retracting the intussusceptum directly[497] or via an enterotomy in the right ventral colon.[498] The prognosis is usually regarded as poor because of sever compromise to the cecum and the risk of cecal rupture or severe contamination during surgery.[497] However, a recent report has indicated that 7 of 8 horses that underwent right ventral colon enterotomy and cecal resection survived long term.[498]

Colocolic intussusceptions are rare but have reportedly affected the pelvic flexure and the left colons.[499-502] Although the condition is reportedly more common in young horses,[500-502] older horses may be affected.[499] Clinical findings may include a palpable mass on the left side of the abdomen.[500] Ultrasonography may also be useful. Treatment requires manual reduction of the intussusception at surgery,[500,502] or resection of affected bowel.[499]

REFERENCES

458. Dabareiner RM, White NA: Large colon impaction in horses: 147 cases (1985-1991), *J Am Vet Med Assoc* 206:679-685, 1995.
459. Campbell ML et al: Cecal impaction in the horse, *J Am Vet Med Assoc* 184:950-952, 1984.
460. Gerard MP et al: Jejunocolostomy or ileocolostomy for treatment of cecal impaction in horses: nine cases (1985-1995), *J Am Vet Med Assoc* 209:1287-1290, 1996.
461. Dabareiner RM, White NA: Diseases and surgery of the cecum, *Vet Clin North Am (Equine Pract)* 13:303-315, 1997.
462. Dart AJ, Hodgson DR, Snyder JR: Caecal disease in equids, *Aust Vet J* 75:552-557, 1997.

463. Collatos C, Romano S: Cecal impaction in horses: Causes, diagnosis, and medical treatment, *Compend Cont Educ Pract Vet* 15:976-980, 1993.

464. Craig DR et al: Ileocolostomy. A technique for surgical management of equine cecal impaction, *Vet Surg* 16:451-455, 1987.

465. White NA, Dabareiner RM: Treatment of impaction colics, *Vet Clin North Am (Equine Pract)* 13:243-259, 1997.

466. Clarke LL, Roberts MC, Argenzio RA: Feeding and digestive problems in horses: physiologic responses to a concentrated meal, *Vet Clin North Am (Equine Pract)* 6:433-450, 1990.

467. Clarke LL et al: Short-term effect of aldosterone on Na-Cl transport across equine colon, *Am J Physiol* 262:R939-R946, 1992.

468. Blue MG, Wittkopp RW: Clinical and structural features of equine enteroliths, *J Am Vet Med Assoc* 179:79-82, 1981.

469. Lloyd K et al: Enteroliths in horses, *Cornell Vet* 77:172-186, 1987.

470. Hassel DM et al: Evaluation of enterolithiasis in equids: 900 cases (1973-1996), *J Am Vet Med Assoc* 214:233-237, 1999.

471. Blue MG: Enteroliths in horses: a retrospective study of 30 cases, *Equine Vet J* 11:76-84, 1979.

472. Specht TE, Colahan PT: Surgical treatment of sand colic in equids: 48 cases (1978-1985), *J Am Vet Med Assoc* 193:1560-1564, 1988.

473. Ragle CA et al: Surgical treatment of sand colic: results in 40 horses, *Vet Surg* 18:48-51, 1989.

474. Bertone JJ et al: Diarrhea associated with sand in the gastrointestinal tract of horses, *J Am Vet Med Assoc* 193:1409-1412, 1988.

475. Ragle CA et al: Abdominal auscultation in the detection of experimentally induced gastrointestinal sand accumulation, *J Vet Intern Med* 3:12-14, 1989.

476. Hammock PD, Freeman DE, Baker GJ: Failure of psyllium mucilloid to hasten evaluation of sand from the equine large intestine, *Vet Surg* 27:547-554, 1998.

477. Johnston JK, Freeman DE: Diseases and surgery of the large colon, *Vet Clin North Am (Equine Pract)* 13:317-340, 1997.

478. Hackett RP: Nonstrangulated colonic displacement in horses, *J Am Vet Med Assoc* 182:235-240, 1983.

479. White NA, Lessard P: Risk factors and clinical signs associated with cases of equine colic, *Proceedings of the Thirty-second Annual Convention of the American Association of Equine Practitioners*, 1986, pp 637-644.

480. Huskamp B: Displacement of the large colon. In Robinson NE, ed: *Current therapy in equine medicine*, Philadelphia, 1987, WB Saunders, pp 60-65.

481. Santschi EM, Slone DEJ, Frank WM: Use of ultrasound in horses for diagnosis of left dorsal displacement of the large colon and monitoring its nonsurgical correction, *Vet Surg* 22:281-284, 1993.

482. Sivula NJ: Renosplenic entrapment of the large colon in horses: 33 cases (1984-1989), *J Am Vet Med Assoc* 199:244-246, 1991.

483. Baird AN et al: Renosplenic entrapment of the large colon in horses: 57 cases (1983-1988), *J Am Vet Med Assoc* 198:1423-1426, 1991.

484. Kalsbeek HC: Further experiences with non-surgical correction of nephrosplenic entrapment of the left colon in the horse, *Equine Vet J* 21:442-443, 1989.

485. Hardy J, Bednarski RM, Biller DS: Effect of phenylephrine on hemodynamics and splenic dimensions in horses, *Am J Vet Res* 55:1570-1578, 1994.

486. Sivula NJ, Trent AM, Kobluk CN: Displacement of the large colon associated with nonsurgical correction of large-colon entrapment in the renosplenic space in a horse, *J Am Vet Med Assoc* 197:1190-1192, 1990.

487. Benamou A, Blikslager AT, Sellon D: Intestinal atresia in horses, *Compend Cont Educ Pract Vet* 17:1510-1517, 1995.

488. Hughes FE, Slone DE: Large colon resection, *Vet Clin North Am (Equine Pract)* 13:341-350, 1997.

489. Snyder JR et al: Strangulating volvulus of the ascending colon in horses, *J Am Vet Med Assoc* 195:757-764, 1989.

490. Snyder JR et al: Morphologic alterations observed during experimental ischemia of the equine large colon, *Am J Vet Res* 49:801-809, 1988.

491. Harrison IW: Equine large intestinal volvulus: a review of 124 cases, *Vet Surg* 17:77-81, 1988.

492. Van Hoogmoed L, Snyder JR: Use of pelvic flexure biopsies to predict survivability of horses following large colon torsion, *Proc Equine Colic Res Symp* 6:64, 1998.

493 Van Hoogmoed L, Snyder JR: Adjunctive methods in equine gastrointestinal surgery, *Vet Clin North Am (Equine Pract)* 13:221-242, 1997.

494. Cook G, Embertson RM, Hance SR. Large colon volvulus: surgical treatment of 204 horses (1986-1995), *Proc Equine Colic Res Symp* 5:32, 1994.

495. Hance SR: Colopexy, *Vet Clin North Am (Equine Pract)* 13:351-358, 1997.

496. Hance SR, Embertson RM: Colopexy in broodmares: 44 cases (1986-1990), *J Am Vet Med Assoc* 201:782-787, 1992.

497. Gaughan EM, Hackett RP: Cecocolic intussusception in horses: 11 cases (1979-1989), *J Am Vet Med Assoc* 197:1373-1375, 1990.

498. Hubert J D et al: Cecal amputation via a right ventral colon enterotomy for correction of nonreducible cecocolic intussusception in 8 horses, *Proc Colic Res Symp* 6:62, 1998.

499. Robertson JT, Tate LP: Resection of intussuscepted large colon in a horse, *J Am Vet Med Assoc* 181:927-928, 1982.

500. Dyson S, Orsini J: Intussusception of the large colon in a horse, *J Am Vet Med Assoc* 182:720, 1983.

501. Wilson DG, Wilson WD, Reinertson EL: Intussusception of the left dorsal colon in a horse, *J Am Vet Med Assoc* 183:464-465, 1983.

502. Meagher DM, Stirk AJ: Intussusception of the colon in a filly, *Mod Vet Pract* 55:951-952, 1974.

ABNORMAL CONDITIONS OF THE DESCENDING (SMALL) COLON

VANESSA L. COOK

Abnormal conditions of the small colon are relatively rare. Obstruction of the small colon was identified as the cause of colic in 4.2% of colic surgeries.[503] American Miniature Horses (AMH) appear to be at increased risk for obstruction of the small colon.[504] In a study of colic in AMH, 60% of those admitted had a small colon obstruction.[505] Arabians may also be overrepresented compared with the hospital population.[503,504] Horses over 15 years of age seem to be at an increased risk for small colon conditions.[504] In particular, certain problems such as strangulating lipomas, foaling injuries, and submucosal hematomas have a definite predisposition for older animals.[503] Female horses were found to be at increased risk for small colon disease in one study, possibly because of hormonal fluctuations affecting gastrointestinal motility.[504]

Clinical signs and the rate of physiologic deterioration are less severe than with a higher obstruction, often resulting in later referral.[503,504] Rectal examination and abdominocentesis provide useful information in determining diagnosis and indicating surgical intervention.[503]

Conditions affecting the small colon can be divided into congenital diseases, simple obstructions, vascular lesions, and strangulating lesions.

CONGENITAL DISEASES

Atresia Coli and Aganglionosis

Atresia coli is very rare in foals, with a reported incidence of 0.44%.[506] The pathogenesis of this disease is thought to be an ischemic accident that results in regression of the affected segment.[507] Four types of atresia have been identified,[508] with type 3, blind end atresia, being most commonly reported in foals.[506,509] It is important to differentiate atresia from Overo lethal white syndrome, in which affected foals have myenteric aganglionosis of the distal intestinal tract resulting from a polymorphism in the endothelin receptor type B gene.[510] Loss of neurons in the myenteric plexus of the small colon is also found in equine dysautonomia (grass sickness), although it is less severe than in the ileum.[511]

Foals with atresia are usually normal at birth, but develop progressive abdominal distention, colic, and lack of feces with no meconium staining even after an enema.[506] Digital palpation or proctoscopy can identify a blind ending rectum if a distal segment is affected. Plain radiographs do not usually identify the atresia, but can help to differentiate it from a meconium impaction. Retrograde contrast radiography, as described for meconium impaction (see later discussion of meconium impaction), is a useful diagnostic aid.[512] An increased volume of barium sulfate, up to 20 ml/kg, may be needed if the atresia is proximal to the transverse colon. On radiographs, the contrast agent is seen to end abruptly at the atretic segment.

The only chance for survival is early exploratory celiotomy to assess the affected segment and determine if surgical correction is possible. However, even with resection of the affected segment and anastomosis, the prognosis is grave, with a 100% mortality rate in one study.[506]

SIMPLE OBSTRUCTIONS

Simple Impaction

Impaction of the small colon with firm digesta is the most common abnormal condition of the small colon in adult horses, affecting 1.9 to 2.5% of all horses seen for colic at referral institutes.[513,514] There was a dramatically increased incidence in the fall and winter,[508,509] but the reason for this is unknown.

Rectal palpation is useful for diagnosis of the impaction, with an accuracy of 87% in one study.[513] A solid tube with loss of the normal sacculations is found. Because the rectal mucosa may be edematous, palpation should be performed with care.[515]

Medical therapy should consist of aggressive intravenous and oral fluid therapy, combined with laxatives and lubricants, and flunixin meglumine as necessary.[513,514] The decision for surgical intervention is based on severity of pain and abdominal distention.[513,514] In one study, surgically treated horses had increased mean band neutrophil counts, but other hematologic, biochemical, and abdominocentesis values were within reference ranges.[513] Most impactions can be corrected at surgery by a high enema combined with extra luminal massage by the surgeon. However in severe cases, an enterotomy in the small colon may be necessary to facilitate evacuation.[515] In addition, a pelvic flexure enterotomy is recommended to empty the large colon and reduce the risk of recurrence.[513]

In a recent report, diarrhea developed during hospitalization in 70% of all horses with small colon impaction, and 43% of those treated surgically cultured positive for *Salmonella* sp.[513] This, combined with the results from a similar study,[514] suggest that impaction of the small colon may be a manifestation of *Salmonella* infection.

The prognosis for medical and surgical treatment was similar in one study at 72% and 75% respectively,[513] whereas an earlier study reports a significantly higher long-term success rate in those treated medically.[514]

Fecaliths, Enteroliths, and Foreign Bodies

Simple obstruction of the small colon can also occur as a result of inspissated feces (fecalith), enteroliths, foreign bodies concretions of plant material (phytobezoar), or masses of matted plant material (conglobate).[516]

Fecaliths have been reported in miniature foals.[517] They are larger than normal fecal balls, reaching 15 to 20 cm long by 8 to 12 cm wide in adult horses.[518] Improper fecal ball formation, possibly caused by coarse forage, is the presumed cause.[517,518] Their presence should be suspected in miniature horses with low-grade colic.[517]

Enteroliths are mainly composed of ammonium magnesium phosphate deposited in concentric layers around a nidus.[519] The incidence is increased in the southwestern United States and California, as well as in the Arabian breed. Their formation may be associated with bran and alfalfa in the diet.[519] Abdominal radiographs may be a useful aid in diagnosis, although the sensitivity is reduced when the enterolith is in the small colon.[520] Medical management aimed at reducing colonic pH has been suggested to be useful to prevent recurrence after surgery. However, when an enterolith lodges in the small colon it usually causes complete obstruction and acute colic that require surgical intervention as described below.[519]

Foreign body obstruction of the small colon is usually seen in younger horses and is caused by nondigestible mate-

rial such as twine and rubber.[521] The foreign body usually causes complete obstruction of the small colon, resulting in acute onset of severe colic[522] and abdominal distention.[521] The fibers become covered in crystalline material during their transit through the intestinal tract, and the resulting irregular sharp projections cause mucosal ulceration.[503]

Phytobezoars often contain large quantities of oat hairs, which are found in oat bran and oatmeal fodder.[518] They appear to cause less trauma to the mucosa than foreign bodies because of their smooth surface.[503] Trichobezoars (concretions of hair) are very rare in horses.

The majority of these obstructions require exploratory laparotomy and an enterotomy to allow the mass to be removed.[517,521] If possible, the mass should be manipulated more proximal or distal so that the enterotomy can be performed in unaffected intestine.[503] The enterotomy incision should be made longitudinally through the antimesenteric tenia to preserve lumen diameter and for speed and ease of the procedure.[523,524] Complications include rupture of the small colon at the site of obstruction[521] and adhesion formation, especially in miniature horses.[505]

Meconium Retention

Meconium is composed of glandular secretions and amniotic fluid. It is thick and tarry and is usually passed within 24 hours of birth. Any factors that reduce intestinal motility, such as failure to ingest colostrum and dysmaturity, along with the narrow pelvis in male foals, can result in meconium retention.[525] This results in progressive clinical signs of tenesmus, colic, and tympany.

Diagnosis of meconium retained at the pelvic inlet can be made by careful digital rectal examination. A plain lateral radiograph may reveal more proximal meconium retention. Retrograde contrast radiography provides excellent sensitivity and specificity for evaluation of the small and transverse colon.[512] After obtaining plain radiographs, a Foley catheter is placed into the rectum and up to 20 ml/kg of barium sulfate is carefully allowed to flow in by gravity. Lateral and, more importantly, ventrodorsal radiographs are then obtained. In foals with a meconium impaction, the contrast is seen to stop before it reaches the transverse colon and may outline fecal balls.

Medical therapy should be attempted first, including intravenous fluid therapy, analgesics, and oral laxatives such as mineral oil. However, the most effective therapy is administration of an enema, which can be repeated if necessary. The enema can be a commercial product or simply soap and water. Successful resolution of the impaction has been reported in refractory cases by administration of 4 to 8 oz of 4% acetylcysteine via a Foley catheter in the rectum to allow retention of the solution for 4 to 5 minutes.[526]

If clinical signs persist, combined with abdominal distention and continued pain, an exploratory celiotomy is recommended. Reduction of the impaction is achieved by aboral massage and a concurrent enema, with an enterotomy performed only if this fails. The main postoperative complication in one study was adhesions, resulting in euthanasia in 25% of surgical cases.[527]

VASCULAR LESIONS

Intramural Hematoma

Intramural hematoma of the small colon is relatively rare, although some cases may resolve without being diagnosed if they do not cause complete obstruction.[528] A large clot forms between the mucosa and muscularis layer, which expands to occlude the lumen. The length affected has been reported to range from 24 to 65 cm. The cause is unknown, although chronic mucosal ulceration or iatrogenic rectal trauma have been implicated in some cases.[529] There is an increased incidence in older horses, with those affected having an average age of 11 years in one study.[503]

Exploratory celiotomy with resection of the affected segment and end-to-end anastomosis is necessary. If the entire affected segment can be removed, the prognosis is good, with 75% of horses surviving in one study.[528]

Mesocolic Tears and Rectal Prolapse

Tears in the mesentery of the small colon can occur as a complication of parturition, especially in multiparous mares,[530,531] and result in segmental ischemic necrosis of the small colon. They occur either as a result of direct trauma during parturition[530] or in association with type III or IV rectal prolapse. In a type III rectal prolapse a portion of the small colon intussuscepts into the rectum in addition to prolapse of the rectal ampulla. In type IV rectal prolapse, part of the small colon and the rectum intussuscept through the anus.[532] Palpation and inspection can be used to distinguish the type of prolapse, and abdominocentesis should be performed. Manual reduction alone of the prolapse can be attempted; however, exploratory celiotomy and resection of the devitalized segment is frequently required. Surgical access to viable bowel distally may be impossible, even with caudal extension of the incision, leaving colostomy as the only option.[531,532]

STRANGULATING OBSTRUCTIONS

Strangulating Lipoma

Pedunculated lipomas can cause strangulation of the small colon, but this occurs much less frequently than in the small intestine. Nonstrangulating lipomas resulting in simple obstruction can also occur.[503] The incidence is increased in older horses, with most affected animals being over 15 years of age.[504] There is an increased risk in female Quarter Horses, possibly because these animals are usually inactive, overweight brood mares.[504] Clinical signs typical of a strangulating obstruction are seen, with a significantly elevated heart rate, abnormal abdominocentesis, and distended large colon on rectal examination.[503] Surgery is necessary to free the constricting lipoma, followed by resection and anastomosis if the intestine is nonviable.[503] The prognosis is worse if resection is required, with a 50% survival rate in one study, compared with 100% survival for nonstrangulating lipomas.[503]

Other Causes of Strangulating Obstruction

Several other causes of strangulating obstruction can occur, but each condition is relatively rare. These include volvulus of the small colon[522] and strangulation through internal hernias such as a vaginal tear,[504] a mesenteric tear,[504] or tears in the omentum or uterine broad ligament.[522]

PROGNOSIS. Previous reports have suggested that resection and anastomosis in the small colon may carry a poor prognosis because of a relatively poor blood supply, higher bacterial counts, solid fecal material, and increased collagenase activity.[518] Despite these factors, a good survival rate was found in two large studies reviewing small colon disorders, with 71% and 91% respectively being discharged from the hospital.[503,504] The cases seen at referral institutes had a high rate of surgical intervention, with 85% of cases requiring surgery in one study.[499] Horses with vascular lesions did not have a worse prognosis for survival, if the cases euthanized at surgery were excluded.[504] The main reason for euthanasia at the time of surgery was an inability to completely exteri-

orize the affected segment to allow adequate resection and anastomosis.[503]

REFERENCES

503. Edwards GB: A review of 38 cases of small colon obstruction in the horse, *Equine Vet J Suppl* 13:42-50, 1992.
504. Dart AJ et al: Abnormal conditions of the equine descending (small) colon: 102 cases (1979-1989), *J Am Vet Med Assoc* 200:971-978, 1992.
505. Ragle CA et al: Surgical treatment of colic in American Miniature Horses: 15 cases (1980-1987), *J Am Vet Med Assoc* 201:329-331, 1992.
506. Nappert G et al: Atresia coli in 7 foals (1964-1990), *Equine Vet J Suppl* 13:57-60, 1992.
507. Benamou AE, Blikslager AT, Sellon DC: Intestinal atresia in foals, *Compend Cont Educ Pract Vet* 17:1510-1515, 1995.
508. Van-der-Gaag I, Tibboel D: Intestinal atresia and stenosis in animals: a report of 34 cases, *Vet Path* 17:565-574, 1980.
509. Young RL, Linford RL, Olander HJ: Atresia coli in the foal: a review of six cases, *Equine Vet J* 24:60-62, 1992.
510. Santschi EM et al: Endothelin receptor B polymorphism associated with lethal white foal syndrome in horses, *Mamm Genome* 9:306-309, 1998.
511. Doxey DL et al: Small intestine and small colon neuropathy in equine dysautonomia (grass sickness), *Vet Res Comm* 19:529-543, 1995.
512. Fischer AT, Yarbrough TY: Retrograde contrast radiography of the distal portions of the intestinal tract in foals, *J Am Vet Med Assoc* 207:734-737, 1995.
513. Rhoads WS, Barton MH, Parks AH: Comparison of medical and surgical treatment for impaction of the small colon in horses: 84 cases (1986-1996), *J Am Vet Med Assoc* 214:1042-1046, 1999.
514. Ruggles AJ, Ross MW: Medical and surgical management of small-colon impaction in horses: 28 cases (1984-1989), *J Am Vet Med Assoc* 199:1762-1766, 1991.
515. Rhoads WS: Small colon impactions in adult horses, *Compend Cont Educ Pract Vet* 21:770-775, 1999.
516. Mueller POE: Small colon impaction and foreign bodies (equine), *Proceedings of the American College of Veterinary Surgeons*, San Francisco, 1999.
517. McClure JT et al: Fecalith Impaction in four miniature foals, *J Am Vet Med Assoc* 200:205-207, 1992.
518. Keller SD, Horney FD: Diseases of the equine small colon, *Compend Cont Educ Pract Vet* 7:113-120, 1985.
519. Murray RC: Equine enterolithiasis, *Compend Cont Educ Pract Vet* 14:1104-1111, 1992.
520. Yarbrough TB et al: Abdominal radiography for diagnosis of enterolithiasis in horses: 141 cases (1990-1992), *J Am Vet Med Assoc* 205:592-595, 1994.
521. Gay CC et al: Foreign body obstruction of the small colon in six horses, *Equine Vet J* 11:60-63, 1979.
522. Edwards GB: Diseases and surgery of the small colon, *Vet Clin North Am (Equine Pract)* 13:359-375, 1997.
523. Beard WL, Robertson JT, Getzy DM: Enterotomy technique in the descending colon of the horse: effect of location and suture pattern, *Vet Surg* 18:135-140, 1989.
524. Archer RM et al: A comparison of enterotomies through the antimesenteric band and the sacculation of the small (descending) colon of ponies, *Equine Vet J* 20:406-413, 1988.
525. Wilson JH, Cudd TA: Common gastrointestinal diseases. In Koterba AM, Drummond WH, Kosch PC: *Equine clinical neonatology*, Philadelphia 1990, Lea & Febiger.
526. Madigan JE, Goetzman BW: Use of an acetylcysteine solution enema for meconium retention in the neonatal foal, *Proceedings of the Thirty-sixth Annual Convention of the American Association of Equine Practitioners*, 1990, pp 117-120.
527. Hughes FE, Moll HD, Slone DE: Outcome of surgical correction of meconium impactions in 8 foals, *J Equine Vet Sci* 16:172-175, 1996.
528. Pearson H, Waterman AE: Submucosal haematoma as a cause of obstruction of the small colon in the horse: a review of four cases, *Equine Vet J* 18:340-341, 1986.
529. Speirs VC et al: Obstruction of the small colon by intramural hematoma in three horses, *Aust Vet J* 57:88-90, 1981.
530. Dart AJ, Pascoe JR, Snyder JR: Mesenteric tears of the descending (small) colon as a postpartum complication in two mares, *J Am Vet Med Assoc* 199:1612-1615, 1991.
531. Livesey MA, Keller SD: Segmental ischemic necrosis following mesocolic rupture in postparturient mares, *Compend Cont Educ Pract Vet* 8:763-768, 1986.
532. Freeman DE, Martin BB: Rectum and anus. In Auer JA: *Equine surgery*, ed 1, Philadelphia, 1992, WB Saunders.

PERITONITIS

ROBIN M. DABAREINER

ANATOMY AND PHYSIOLOGY. The peritoneum is the mesothelial lining of the peritoneal cavity and its contained viscera.[533] It forms a closed sac in males but communicates with the external environment in females via the fallopian tubes. The peritoneum consists of a single layer of mesothelial squamous cells resting on a thin basal lamina that is attached to a loose connective tissue layer containing collagen and elastic fibers that allows a variable degree of motion. The peritoneum is coated with a thin serous film that minimizes friction and thus facilitates free movement between abdominal viscera.[534] The peritoneum is divided into the visceral peritoneum, which encloses the intraperitoneal organs and forms the omentum and mesenteries, and the parietal peritoneum, which lines the abdominal walls, pelvis, and diaphragm. The visceral peritoneum, mesentery, and omentum are supplied and drained by the splanchnic vasculature.[535] The parietal peritoneum is supplied by arterial branches of the lower intercostal, lumbar, and iliac vessels and is drained by veins entering into the caudal vena cava. The parietal peritoneum is innervated by branches of the spinal nerves supplying the abdominal wall, and the diaphragmatic peritoneum is supplied by the phrenic nerve. As a result, irritation of the parietal peritoneum gives rise to afferent stimuli that are transmitted by the intercostal and phrenic nerves and perceived as somatic pain.[535] In contrast, there are no pain receptors in the visceral peritoneum, and afferent stimuli are conducted centrally by the visceral autonomic nervous system.

Peritoneal fluid is constantly being produced and absorbed. The movement of fluid and solutes occurs by passive diffusion across the semipermeable peritoneal membrane.[536] Solutions or drugs administered into the peritoneal cavity equilibrate rapidly with plasma. Transperitoneal fluid movement can be increased during peritoneal inflammation, causing a rapid and massive transudation of fluid into the peritoneal cavity that can lead to hypotension and shock.

The peritoneal lymphatics, especially the diaphragmatic lymphatics, play a major role in the removal of fluid and solutes from the peritoneal cavity. The diaphragmatic lymphatic valves provide a unidirectional clearance of peritoneal fluid and debris; these lymphatics empty primarily into the thoracic duct and are probably the first line of defense in peritoneal contamination. The peritoneal lymphatics are aided by movements of breathing, which encourage cranial flow and clearance of peritoneal fluid.[537-539] Cellular defenses are provided by peritoneal macrophages, mast cells, and mesothelial cells. Activated peritoneal T lymphocytes and local antibody production have also been demonstrated experimentally. Peritoneal macrophages have antimicrobial activity resulting from their complement receptors, phagocytic ability, and T cell–mediated immune responses. In addition, peritoneal macrophages are important in neutrophil chemotaxis and fibroblast stimulation, which aid in bacteria localization. Peritoneal mesothelial cells are an abundant source of plasminogen activator, which is responsible for normal fibrinolytic activity on peritoneal surfaces.[537]

PATHOPHYSIOLOGY OF PERITONEAL INJURY. Peritoneal injury can result from any mechanical, chemical, or infectious insult. The initial reaction to inflammatory stimulus is the release of histamine and serotonin from peritoneal mast cells and macrophages, resulting in vasodilation and increased vascular permeability with transudation of fibrinogen-rich plasma into the peritoneal cavity. The concurrent loss of mesothelial cells and release of tissue thromboplastin reduce the fibrinolytic capabilities of the peritoneal surface and activate the extrinsic coagulation pathway, thereby shifting the fibrinolysis-coagulation equilibrium toward fibrin formation.[540,541] This response aids in the fibrin seal of the peritoneal defect and provides the framework for fibroblasts to lay down collagen, which produces fibrous adhesions to localize bacteria.

Peritoneal macrophages stimulate neutrophil chemotaxis both directly and indirectly via the release of tumor necrosis

factor (TNF) and interleukin 1 (IL-1). TNF and IL-1 stimulate neutrophil margination and degranulation and alter the vascular endothelium to promote leukocyte adherence. Metabolism of cell membranes results in phospholipid products such as platelet activating factor (PAF), prostaglandins, and leukotrienes, which contribute to the vasodilatory response; phospholipase A_2 provides the catalyst for activation of these phospholipid products via the arachidonic acid pathway. Within hours, an influx of fluid, protein, and neutrophils enters the peritoneal cavity in response to the inflammatory stimulus.[541]

The combination of enlarged diaphragmatic lymphatics and cellular defenses result in rapid clearance of debris from the contaminated peritoneal cavity. If the inflammatory response resolves, the mesothelial cell lining is restored from either free-floating macrophages or from differentiated subperitoneal connective tissue cells.[541] The normal fibrinolytic activity of the peritoneal mesothelial cells returns, initiating removal of the accumulated fibrin clots. Severe inflammation, foreign bodies, intestinal ischemia, or infection can result in continued fibrin production from proliferating and migrating fibroblasts, causing fibrous scarring and adhesion formation.[540]

Peritonitis in the horse is usually secondary to intestinal leakage or degeneration, resulting in the transmural passage of bacteria into the peritoneal cavity. Any disease process that causes gastrointestinal, hepatic, or urogenital inflammation or compromise can lead to the development of peritonitis (Box 30-4). The adverse effects of intraperitoneal bacteria can be enhanced by the presence of excessive peritoneal fluid accumulation, hemorrhage,[542] fibrin, bile, necrotic tissue, ischemia, anaerobes, and fecal matter. Excessive peritoneal fluid enhances the dissemination of localized bacteria and dilutes opsonic proteins such as complement and immunoglobulins.

BOX 30-4

Gastrointestinal Factors Associated With Peritonitis

IATROGENIC FACTORS
Diagnostic Complications
Enterocentesis during abdominocentesis
Inadvertent rectal tears during palpation
Laceration or leakage of distended bowel during
 percutaneous trocarization
Hemorrhage secondary to splenic abdominal tap

Surgical Complications
Castration
Colpotomy
Surgical trauma to peritoneal surfaces
Enterotomy
Intestinal needle decompression
Intestinal anastomoses
Intraoperative hemorrhage
Break in aseptic surgical procedures
Foreign bodies (sponges, instruments)

FACTORS ASSOCIATED WITH PRIMARY GASTROINTESTINAL DISORDER
Proximal enteritis
Intestinal ischemia or compromise
Gastric, intestinal perforation
Hemorrhage
Uroperitoneum
Parasitic migration
Abscess
Neoplasia

Fibrin formation can be beneficial in confining bacteria; however, excessive amounts can result in abscess formation and prevent phagocytes and antimicrobials from reaching the source of contamination. Fibrinous adhesions may also physically occlude diaphragmatic lymphatics and protect bacteria from opsonins, neutrophils, and antibiotics. Necrotic tissue, fecal matter, and bile all prolong the debridement phase of peritoneal healing and interfere with peritoneal defense mechanisms.

Peritonitis is an inflammation of the peritoneum that can result from many causes, which are classified as primary or secondary, acute or chronic, and localized or diffuse. Primary peritonitis is uncommon in adult horses but may occur by hematogenous spread of bacteria in the septic or immunocompromised neonate or in young horses exposed to *Streptococcus equi* infection.[543] Uroperitoneum and septicemia-induced peritonitis occur predominantly in neonates. Internal abdominal abscesses caused by disseminated *S. equi, Streptococcus zooepidemicus,* or *Rhodococcus equi* infection are usually found in weanlings or young horses.[544]

Peritonitis secondary to another disease process may be caused by perforating abdominal wounds, chemical irritation (bile, urine), neoplasia, breeding and foaling injuries (uterine or vaginal trauma), intestinal parasitism, hepatitis, nephritis, pancreatitis, ruptured bladder or ureter, urinary infection, ruptured or lacerated abdominal viscera (spleen, ovary, liver, diaphragm), castration complications, and factors directly related to gastrointestinal problems, which are divided into preoperative, intraoperative, and postoperative causes (see Box 30-4).

DIAGNOSIS

History and Clinical Signs. The most common presenting clinical signs for horses with peritonitis described in retrospective studies of 21 and 30 horses (age range, 2 months to 16 years) included pyrexia (rectal temperature exceeding 38.5° C), anorexia, mild abdominal pain, reduced or absent borborygmi, diarrhea, increased heart rate, and clinical evidence of dehydration.[545,546] In another retrospective study of 67 horses with peritonitis, clinical signs of abdominal pain, signs of circulatory shock, and diarrhea were significantly less severe in survivors compared with nonsurvivors, regardless of the cause of peritonitis.[547]

Rectal examination often elicits pain, and if adhesions are present and have caused intestinal obstruction, distended bowel may be present. In cases of intestinal rupture, either roughened peritoneal surfaces or an abnormally empty abdomen can be palpated. Occasionally, abdominal masses or abscesses can be palpated and mesenteric lymph nodes may be enlarged; however, in many cases, no abnormalities can be detected. Parietal pain may be characterized by a "guarded" or splinted abdomen with pain on abdominal ballottement and a reluctance to move or defecate.

A urogenital examination should be performed in horses with an undiagnosed etiology of peritonitis to rule out vaginal, cervical, or uterine tears in mares or infected castration sites in males. Gastrointestinal motility is usually decreased secondary to sympathetic stimulation from parietal pain, hemoconcentration, or serosal surface trauma. Ileus frequently results in intestinal stasis with gastric fluid accumulation and intestinal distention, which subsequently intensifies the abdominal pain. The mobilization of fluid into the peritoneal cavity results in an intravascular fluid deficit causing reabsorption of fluid from the large colon and cecum. Findings of intestinal ingesta impactions secondary to these fluid shifts or ileus are found in horses with peritonitis.[541]

Clinicopathology. Abnormal laboratory values are dependent on the etiology and duration of peritonitis. Hematologic abnormalities seen in acute peritonitis include elevated packed cell volume secondary to transudation of fluid into the peritoneal cavity and endotoxemia. Initially a proportional increase in plasma protein levels occurs, reflecting the degree of dehydration; however, in severe cases, protein eventually is sequestered into the abdomen because of increased capillary permeability, resulting in systemic hypoproteinemia. Peripheral blood neutropenia with a degenerative left shift is caused by margination of neutrophils and migration of these cells into the abdomen. Increased plasma fibrinogen levels (up to 1000 mg/dl) can be detected after 48 hours. Peritonitis of longer duration and internal abscesses are associated with greater variability in laboratory values, but these horses often demonstrate a normal or increased systemic neutrophil count, monocytosis, and elevated plasma protein levels as a result of increased immunoglobulin production.[544]

Alterations in blood gas analysis and serum chemistry values often depend on the horse's clinical and hydration status at time of presentation. Increases in blood urea nitrogen and creatinine can occur secondary to dehydration or impaired renal function that may accompany systemic inflammatory response syndrome. Hypokalemia, hypochloremia, and hyponatremia may occur in the anorectic, acidotic patient with gastrointestinal dysfunction. Serum creatinine levels, anion gap, and pH were significantly different between survivors and nonsurvivors at the time of presentation in 67 horses with peritonitis.[547]

Abdominocentesis confirms the diagnosis of peritonitis, although the cause may remain unknown. Normal peritoneal fluid is clear, straw-colored, and serous in consistency. The total nucleated cell count and total protein in peritoneal fluid of normal horses were reported to be less than 5000 cells per microliter and 2.5 g/dl, respectively, with 24% to 60% of the cells being neutrophils.[548] Despite these published values, we have found that normal horses typically have peritoneal fluid protein less than 1.0 g/dl. The cytologic appearance of the leukocytes and mesothelial cells should be normal, although activated mesothelial cells are not an unusual observation.

Colorless fluid is very dilute, and, if it is present in large quantities, the possibility of ascites or uroperitoneum must be considered. Serosanguineous fluid indicates an increase in erythrocytes or free hemoglobin that may be caused by intestinal degeneration and transmural erythrocyte leakage, splenic puncture during abdominocentesis, abdominal viscera laceration, or skin contamination. Green fluid results from enterocentesis or intestinal rupture, and brown fluid is associated with late-stage tissue necrosis. Turbid fluid can reflect an increased cell count or protein concentration, and opalescence suggests chylous effusion. Flocculent fluid with fibrin strands indicates an inflammatory, exudative process in the abdomen. The quantity of fluid varies among horses and can be increased in acute peritonitis (transudate or exudate) or absent in chronic peritonitis with excessive fibrin production.

Peritoneal fluid parameters consistent with peritonitis vary widely, depending on the disease process. High nucleated cell counts ranging from 15,000 to 800,000 cells per microliter, with greater than 90% of neutrophils having toxic or degenerative changes have been reported for horses with peritonitis[545-548] or internal abscesses.[544] Total protein greater than 2.5 g/dl indicates increased capillary permeability of the abdominal viscera or peritoneum resulting in protein exudation and is associated with peritoneal inflammation, intestinal compromise, or blood contamination of the peritoneal fluid. Protein values between 1.5 g/dl and 2.5 g/dl probably reflect mild serosal inflammation. Cytologic evidence of intracellular or extracellular bacteria can result from skin contamination and should be interpreted in combination with clinical signs.

Peritoneal fluid must be interpreted carefully in horses after abdominal surgery, foaling, castration, or multiple abdominocenteses. Nucleated cell counts between 85,000 and 418,000 cells per microliter and protein values from 4.7 to 6.5 g/dl were found on postoperative day 5 in 6 normal horses that had abdominal exploration.[549] Peritoneal fluid 5 days after open castration (*n* = 24) contained 30,000 nucleated white cells per microliter, with more than 85% being neutrophils.[550] By day 7 after castration the cell counts were normal with no toxic or degenerative changes. Parturition can cause increased nucleated and red blood cell counts with elevated total protein values in the peritoneal fluid.[551] In one report, however, postpartum mares having uneventful foaling or uncomplicated dystocias had normal peritoneal fluid except for elevation in percent neutrophils. Mares having complicated dystocia had bloody peritoneal fluid with increased total protein (median 4.0 g/dl) and white blood cell count (median 40,500) one day after foaling.[552] Schumacher, Spano, and Moll found no significant alterations in peritoneal fluid in normal horses that had abdominocentesis every 24 hours for 5 days; however, 48 hours after enterocentesis, nucleated cell counts were 113,333 per microliter in 6 of 9 horses.

Cytologic examination of the peritoneal fluid should include a Wright's and a Gram stain. Macrophages should be examined closely for evidence of cellular engulfment and erythrophagocytosis. The peritoneal fluid cell morphology is an important diagnostic aid and can be evaluated from the Wright's stain. The Gram stain demonstrates the presence of bacteria and can guide initial antimicrobial treatments until culture and sensitivity results become available. Microbiologic culture is performed to identify aerobic and anaerobic bacteria, and antibiotic susceptibility testing is done to identify specific antibiotic therapy. Serial cultures of the peritoneal fluid may be necessary to identify emerging or resistant bacterial strains. Optimal bacteria isolation techniques require the use of an enriching broth, blood culture medium, and, if appropriate, use of an antimicrobial removal device* when culturing peritoneal fluid.

Bacteria were cultured or cytologically identified on 48 of 67 horses (71.6%) with peritonitis and *Escherichia coli* was the most common bacterium isolated from peritoneal fluid samples in one report.[547] Others have reported only a 16% to 25% isolation rate for infective agents.[544,545] Anaerobes have been isolated from approximately 20% of equine peritonitis cases, with *Bacteroides fragilis* most common.[545] Failure to identify or culture bacteria from peritoneal fluid does not rule out septic peritonitis.

Ultrasonography may be helpful in obtaining abdominal fluid, detecting fibrin (Fig. 30-42), finding an abdominal abscess or determining if blood is within the abdomen (Fig. 30-43).

TREATMENT. Horses with peritonitis require early, aggressive therapy. The treatment of peritonitis is based on (1) patient stabilization, (2) correction of the inciting cause, and (3) in most cases, antimicrobials or antihelmintics. Surgical intervention may be required to identify or correct the cause of the peritonitis.

Stabilization includes treatment of systemic hypovolemia and endotoxic shock. Intensive fluid therapy is usually required to replace fluid losses into the peritoneal cavity and combat cardiovascular collapse. Acid-base disorders should be identified and corrected. Electrolytes, especially calcium and potassium, are important for gastrointestinal function and should be supplemented if deficits exist. If intestinal compromise or gram-negative bacterial infections are suspected as the cause of peritonitis, J5 hyperimmune plasma*

(4.4 ml/kg) may moderate the degree of endotoxemia. J5 is a mutant strain of *Escherichia coli* that lacks the variable oligosaccharide side chains and binds to many gram-negative organisms and endotoxin, providing cross protection.[554] If serum hypoproteinemia (total protein less than 4 g/dl) is present, administration of additional plasma should be considered to minimize peripheral edema.

Antimicrobial therapy should be initiated as soon as the diagnosis of peritonitis is made and peritoneal fluid is obtained for culture and sensitivity testing. In a report of 30 horses with peritonitis, 70% were treated successfully with antibiotics and supportive therapy.[546] Cytologic examination of the peritoneal fluid can suggest an antimicrobial regimen until the specific causative organism is identified. Intravenous

---

*Plasma-J, Veterinary Dynamics, Templeton, CA 93456.

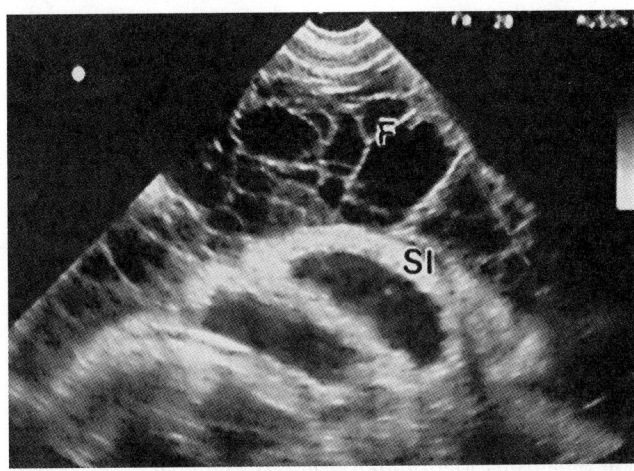

FIG. 30-42 ■ Sonogram of adult horse abdomen showing web of fibrin (*F*) surrounding fluid found in a horse with chronic peritonitis. The wall of the small intestine (*SI*) is thickened. (Courtesy Dr. D Schmitz.)

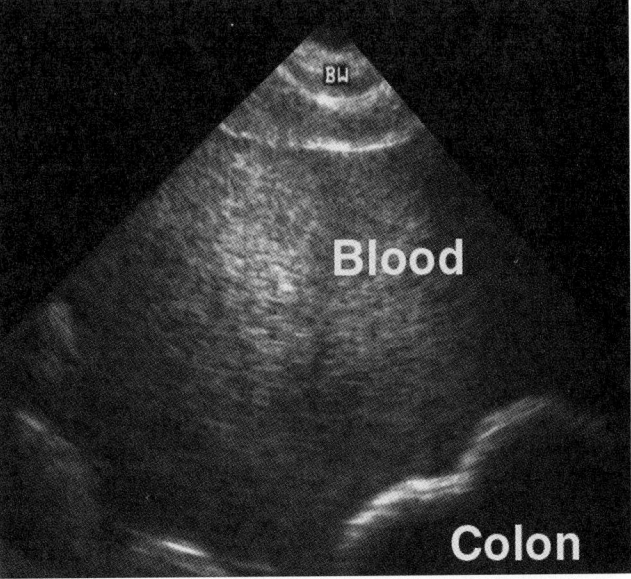

FIG. 30-43 ■ Sonogram of hemoperitoneum. The fluid appears as swirling fluid of heterogenous echogenicity. (Courtesy Dr. D Schmitz.)

*BBL Septi-Chek, Becton Dickinson and Company, Cockeysville, MD 21723.

administration is preferred, especially in the hypovolemic or shocked patient with compromised tissue perfusion. The most common organisms isolated from horses with peritonitis include aerobic bacteria (*E. coli, Staphylcoccus* spp., *Streptococcus* spp., *Rhodococcus equi*) and anaerobic bacteria (*Bacteroides* spp., *Clostridium* spp., *Fusobacterium* spp.).[544-547]

Broad-spectrum antimicrobial therapy is recommended with a combination of an aminoglycoside such as gentamicin (6.6 mg/kg IV every 24 hours) or amikacin sulfate* (20 to 25 mg/kg IV every 24 hours) and potassium penicillin G (22,000 to 44,000 U/kg IV every 6 hours) or ceftiofur (4 mg/kg IV every 8 hours or every 12 hours). After intravenous administration of aminoglycoside antibiotics, antimicrobial activity in the peritoneal fluid reaches 50% to 80% of serum levels; whereas intestinal tissue concentrations are 10% to 25% of serum concentrations.[555]

Aminoglycosides are bacteriocidal and effective against the majority of gram-negative intestinal aerobes, but pharmacologic monitoring is important, especially in the hypovolemic, septic patient. Important considerations during aminoglycoside use include renal toxicoses and potential neuromuscular blocking effects during general anesthesia.[555,556] Most grampositive aerobic bacteria are sensitive to penicillins, but the extended spectrum of antimicrobial activity from sodium ampicillin (11 to 25 mg/kg IV every 6 to 8 hours) or ceftiofur may be beneficial. Trimethoprim-sulfadiazine (30 mg/kg PO every 12 hours), chloramphenicol (25 to 50 mg/kg PO every 6 hours), and enrofloxacin† (5 to 7 mg/kg every 24 hours) are broad-spectrum antimicrobials that have good peritoneal penetration and can be useful if warranted from the culture and sensitivity results. Enrofloxacin has been shown to have adverse effects on cartilage surfaces in young animals and should be reserved for adult horses only.[557]

Anaerobic bacteria, especially penicillin-resistant *Bacteriodes* spp., are reported in 20% to 40% of equine patients with peritonitis.[545,558] Percentages of anaerobic involvement may be artificially low because of difficulty in isolating anaerobic organisms. Metronidazole (15 to 25 mg/kg PO every 6 to 8 hours) is effective against most anaerobic bacteria but should be used in combination with antimicrobials with antibacterial activity against aerobic bacteria.[558] Of 54 horses with positive anaerobic culture results, 95% also had aerobic bacteria isolated from the same specimen.[558] In the face of ileus, an intravenous route of administration can be used, although cost may be prohibitive. Recently the pharmacokinetics of metronidazole (15 mg/kg every 6 to 8 hours) administered to horses per rectum in a suspension of crushed tablets and water (40 ml) was evaluated, and serum minimum inhibitory concentration was reached within 1 hour.[559] Complications attributed to metronidazole administration in horses were reported to be uncommon, with only 4 of 200 horses (2%) undergoing treatment showing appetite suppression. However, peripheral neurologic deficits and CNS dysfunction have been associated with metronidazole treatment in other species.[558]

Antiinflammatory Therapy. Horses with peritonitis often have clinical signs of endotoxemia and tissue trauma eliciting a cascade of inflammatory mediators. Flunixin meglumine, a nonsteroidal antiinflammatory drug, inhibits cyclooxygenase production of prostaglandins and blocks many detrimental effects of endotoxemia.[560] Flunixin also may decrease adhesion formation within the peritoneal cavity. Low doses of flunixin (0.25 mg/kg IV every 6 hours) inhibited prostaglandin production during experimentally induced endotoxemia in horses.[560] Analgesia is also important in the treatment of peritonitis in horses to inhibit sympathetic stimulation secondary to parietal pain; therefore flunixin, at a dosage of 0.5 mg/kg every 6 hours, may be clinically more beneficial.

Anthelmintics. Anthelmintics are required if verminous arteritis secondary to *Strongylus vulgaris* migration is the suspected cause of the peritonitis. A history of mild intermittent colic and a poor or unknown deworming program may be apparent. The abdominal pain arises from ischemia or the initiation of focal infarcts. Often this disease cannot be differentiated from others that cause mild colic. The heart rate is often normal and rectal examination usually has no abnormal findings unless there is concurrent impaction or gas distention. Fremitus to the cranial mesenteric artery is an inconsistent finding. Laboratory findings can also vary greatly. Evidence of peritoneal inflammation is indicated by increased peritoneal protein and white blood cell count. The response to larvacidal therapy may be the best way to diagnose peritonitis secondary to parasitic migration. Horses that respond will usually cease to have colic and become more active and alert several days to weeks after therapy. The larvicidal treatment is fenbendazole* (15 mg/kg PO for 5 days or 50 mg/kg for 3 days) or ivermectin (0.2 mg/kg PO) and aspirin (60 grains PO once daily).[561]

Other Medical Treatment. Gastrointestinal ileus results from peritoneal trauma, intestinal compromise or sympathetic stimulation. Intestinal ileus can cause respiratory compromise from increased abdominal pressure and reduced intestinal perfusion, leading to further compromise. Nasogastric intubation is necessary for relief of gastric fluid accumulation and continued intestinal decompression. Parenteral nutritional support should be considered in the compromised, anorectic patient or in horses with severe, prolonged gastrointestinal dysfunction.

Surgical Treatment. Surgical intervention is often required to identify or correct the inciting cause of peritonitis, which is often secondary to compromised intestine or leakage of the reproductive or urogenital systems. Peritoneal lavage and drainage can be accomplished at the time of surgery to remove any accumulated debris or exudate. Surgical drainage of internal abdominal or perirectal abscesses has been described but is difficult and often results in further contamination of the abdomen.[544] Long-term antimicrobial therapy with marsupialization or aspiration may be the preferred approach in these cases.

A successful technique used in the treatment of peritonitis in small animals and humans is open peritoneal drainage, which allows continuous drainage of the entire abdominal cavity and provides an unfavorable environment for anaerobic bacteria.[562] Open peritoneal drainage was shown to be feasible in horses with experimentally induced peritonitis,[563] but the large size, stall environment, and ambulatory nature of the horse probably restricts its use in the treatment of peritonitis in most clinical cases.

The effectiveness of intermittent peritoneal lavage and drainage in horses with peritonitis is well documented. The benefits of abdominal drainage and lavage include the following:

- Reduction of bacterial numbers, enzymes, and toxins from the large absorptive peritoneal surface area
- Removal of degenerative neutrophils and cellular debris
- Elimination of accumulated blood
- Removal of irritating foreign material such as plant material and urine
- Dilution of adhesion forming substrates such as fibrinogen and fibrin

---

*Amiglyde-V, Ford Dodge Laboratories, Inc., Fort Dodge, IA 50501.
†Baytril, Miles Inc., Shawnee Mission, KS 66201.

*Panacur, Hoechst Roussel Vet, Warren, NJ 07059.

Some claim that only a small part of the equine abdomen is effectively lavaged and that lavage may disseminate a localized infectious focus.[561] In my opinion, peritoneal lavage and drainage is an important and potentially life-saving treatment that should be considered in the treatment of horses with peritonitis. In our hospital, peritoneal drainage and lavage is reserved for acute cases of purulent effusion in the abdomen and in horses not responding to medical therapy as determined by clinical signs and results of abdominocentesis. We also use standing postoperative peritoneal lavage for prevention of abdominal adhesions after surgery for small intestinal obstructions. In an experimental study, horses having abdominal lavage after colic surgery were significantly less likely to develop abdominal adhesions than horses not lavaged.[564]

Stabilization, antimicrobial administration, and hydration of the horse should be performed before abdominal drainage or lavage. Placing an ingress catheter in the paralumbar fossa for fluid infusion and an egress catheter on ventral midline for drainage has been described, but this is probably not effective because the infused fluid usually finds a direct path through the abdomen to the egress catheter, providing inadequate lavage. Retrograde irrigation and drainage through an ingress-egress catheter placed on ventral midline have been used effectively for removal of peritoneal exudate in horses.[565]

The site of drain placement is on ventral midline at the most dependent aspect of the abdomen. Ultrasonography may be useful in locating a site free of abdominal viscera or fetus if the horse is in late gestation. A variety of drains can be used; mushroom drains* and argyle drains are most useful, but a large Foley catheter† is also effective. The horse is properly sedated, and the drain site is prepared aseptically and blocked with local anesthetic. A 1-cm stab incision is made through the skin, subcutaneous tissue, and linea alba. Mushroom and argyle drains should be stretched over a female canine or Chambers mare catheter to aid insertion. If the bowel is inadvertently punctured, the drain should not be removed until the horse is anesthetized to allow removal of the drain and closure of the puncture site.

With the drain acting as an ingress cannula, 10 to 20 L of a warmed balanced polyionic fluid is infused. Abdominal discomfort may be encountered after 10 L of fluid or after rapid infusion. Slowing the infusion rate or further sedation may be required. After fluid infusion, the drain is filled with full strength heparin and clamped closed and the horse is walked for 20 to 30 minutes to promote distribution of the lavaged fluid. The drain is then opened and allowed to drain into a clean calibrated bucket to record the volume of retrieved fluid. The majority of the infused fluid should be collected. This process is repeated two to three times daily for 2 to 3 days until the peritoneal fluid white cell count and total protein values show improvement. Between treatments the abdominal drain should be filled with heparin, closed, and protected from the environment by a sterile bandage.

The addition of povidone-iodine or nitrofurazone to peritoneal lavage solutions has been associated with chemical peritonitis, hypovolemia, hyperosmolarity, and acidosis in normal horses and is not recommended.[565] Adding antimicrobials to the peritoneal lavage solution is probably not necessary; however, plasma concentrations of administered antimicrobials should be measured to assure proper MIC levels in the face of peritoneal lavage and drainage. Horses treated with peritoneal lavage must also be monitored closely for hydration, protein loss (up to 0.5 to 1 g/dl daily), and electrolyte imbalances. Complications of peritoneal drains include visceral puncture during insertion, ascending infection, subcutaneous leakage and edema, and herniation of intestine or omentum through the drain.[566]

Intraperitoneal or systemic administration of heparin has been recommended in the treatment of peritonitis in many species.[567] Heparin is thought to inhibit fibrin deposition, thereby minimizing the localization and entrapment of bacteria, which can decrease the effectiveness of antimicrobials.[541,567] Heparin has also been advocated in the prevention of abdominal adhesions in humans and shown to decrease the formation of adhesions in ponies after experimentally induced intestinal ischemia.[568] There are no controlled studies in horses that describe the outcome of treatment or recommended dosage of heparin therapy in horses with peritonitis, but I use a dose of 20 to 40 IU/kg subcutaneously (SQ) every 8 hours. The horse's hematocrit and platelet count will usually decrease after 4 days of heparin treatment as a result of red blood cell agglutination, but will rebound within 48 hours after the drug is discontinued.

Prognosis. The prognosis depends on the etiology, severity, duration, and complications of the peritonitis. The mortality rate was 59.7% in a recent retrospective study of 67 horses with peritonitis.[547] The prognosis for mortality in that study depended on the inciting cause of peritonitis, with postoperative peritonitis having a high mortality rate (56%).

Laminitis, diarrhea, ileus, and coagulopathies can occur as a part of inflammatory response syndrome, and abdominal adhesions or abscess formation can have a negative affect on long-term prognosis. There are no specific laboratory parameters that can predict prognosis in affected horses; however, a rapid response to therapy is considered a favorable prognostic indicator. With early diagnosis and correction of the inciting cause and a combination of aggressive medical therapy with peritoneal lavage, a fair-to-good prognosis can be given in acute cases of septic peritonitis in the horse.

REFERENCES

533. Barberini S, Correr S, Motta PM: Vascular disease of the gastrointestinal tract. In Marston A, ed: *The peritoneum*, Baltimore, 1985, Williams & Wilkins, pp 243-259.
534. diZerega GS, Rodgers KE: *The peritoneum*, New York, 1992, Springer-Verlag, pp 1-23.
535. Crowe DT, Bjorling DE: Peritoneum and peritoneal cavity. In Slatter DH, ed: *Textbook of small animal surgery*, Philadelphia, 1989, WB Saunders, p 571.
536. Flessner MF, Dedrick RL, Schultz JS: Exchange of macromolecules between peritoneal cavity and plasma, *Am J Physiol* 248:H15-H25, 1985.
537. Hosgood G: Peritonitis part 1: a review of pathophysiology and diagnosis, *Aust Vet Pract* 16:184-189, 1986.
538. Weatherford AL: Role of fenestrated basement membrane in lymphatic absorption from the abdominal cavity, *Am J Physiol* 197:551, 1959.
539. Porter JM, McGregor FH: Fibrinolytic activity of mesothelial surfaces, *Surg Forum* 20:80, 1969.
540. Stangel JJ, Nisbet JD: Formation and prevention of postoperative adhesions, *J Reprod Med* 29:143-155, 1984.
541. Baxter GM: Intraabdominal adhesions in horses, *Compend Cont Educ* 13:1587-1597, 1991.
542. Dunn DL, Nelson RD, Condie RM: Mechanisms of the adjuvant effect of hemoglobin in experimental peritonitis, *Surgery* 93:653-659, 1983.
543. Byars TD: Miscellaneous acute abdominal diseases. In White NA, Moore JN, eds: *The acute abdomen*, Philadelphia, 1990, Lea & Febiger, pp 408-411.
544. Rumbaugh GE, Smith BP, Carlson GP: Internal abdominal abscesses in the horse: a study of 25 cases, *J Am Vet Assoc* 172:304-309, 1978.
545. Mair TS, Hillyer MH, Taylor FG: Peritonitis in adult horses: 21 cases, *Vet Rec* 1990, pp 567-570.
546. Dyson S: Review of 30 cases of peritonitis in the horse, *Equine Vet J* 15:25-30, 1983.
547. Hawkins JF, Bowman KF, Roberts MC: Peritonitis in horses: 67 cases (1985-1990), *J Am Vet Assoc* 203:284-288, 1993.
548. Nelson AW: Analysis of equine peritoneal fluid, Symposium on Gastroenterology, *Vet Clin North Am (Large Anim Pract)* 2:267-274, 1979.
549. Santschi EM et al: Peritoneal fluid analysis in ponies after abdominal surgery, *Vet Surg* 17:6-9, 1988.
550. Schumacher J et al: Effects of castration on peritoneal fluid in the horse, *J Vet Intern Med* 2:22-25, 1988.

---

*Argyle Trochar Catheter, Sherwood Medical, St. Louis, MO 26001.
†Foley Catheter, CR Bard Inc., Murray Hill, NJ, 07974.

551. Wilson J, Gordon BJ: Interpreting the diagnostic tests for colic. In Gordon BJ, Allen D, eds: *Field guide to colic management in the horse,* Lenexa, Kan, 1988, Veterinary Medicine Publishing, pp 157-175.

552. Van Hoogmoed L et al: Peritoneal fluid analysis in peripartum mares, *J Am Vet Med Assoc* 209:1280-1282,1996.

553. Schumacher J, Spano JS, Moll HD: Effects of enterocentesis on peritoneal fluid constituents in the horse, *J Am Vet Med Assoc* 196:1301-1303, 1985.

554. Spier SJ: Use of hyperimmune plasma containing antibody to gram-negative core antigens, *Proceedings of the Thirty-fifth Annual Convention of the American Association of Equine Practitioners,* 1989, pp 91-94.

555. Snyder JR et al: Gentamicin tissue concentrations in equine small intestine and large colon, *Am J Vet Res* 47:1092-1095, 1986.

556. Sojka JE, Brown SA: Pharmacokinetic adjustment of gentamicin dosing in horses with sepsis, *J Am Vet Med Assoc* 189:784-789, 1986.

557. Burkhardt JE et al: Ultrastructural changes in articular cartilages of immature beagle dogs dosed with difloxacin, a fluoroquinolone, *Vet Pathol* 29:230-238, 1992.

558. Sweeney RW, Sweeney CR, Weiher J: Clinical use of metronidazole in horses: 200 cases (1984-1989), *J Am Vet Med Assoc* 198:1045-1048, 1991.

559. Garber JL et al: Pharmacokinetics of metronidazole after rectal administration in horses, *Am J Vet Res* 54:2060-2063, 1993.

560. Semrad SD et al: Low dose flunixin meglumine: effects on eicosanoid production and clinical signs induced by experimental endotoxemia in ponies, *Equine Vet J* 19:201-206, 1987.

561. Semrad SD: Peritonitis in the horse. In Smith B, ed: *Large animal internal medicine,* St Louis, 1990, Mosby, pp 674-679.

562. Greenfield CL, Walshaw R: Open peritoneal drainage for treatment of contaminated peritoneal cavity and septic peritonitis in dogs and cats: 24 cases (1980-1986), *J Am Vet Med Assoc* 191:100-105, 1987.

563. Chase JP et al: Open peritoneal drainage in horses with experimentally induced peritonitis, *Vet Surg* 25:189-194,1996.

564. Hague B et al: Evaluation of standing postoperative peritoneal lavage for prevention of experimentally induced abdominal adhesions in horses, *Proceedings of the Forty-second Annual Convention of the American Association of Equine Practitioners,* 1996, pp 268-269.

565. Valdez H, Scrutchfield WL, Taylor TS: Peritoneal lavage in the horse, *J Am Vet Med Assoc* 175:388-391, 1979.

566. Markel MD: Prevention and management of peritonitis in horses. Management of colic, *Vet Clin North Am (Equine Pract)* 4:145-157, 1988.

567. Hau T, Simmons RL: Heparin in the treatment of experimental peritonitis, *Ann Surg* 1978, pp 294-298.

568. Parker JE et al: Prevention of intraabdominal adhesions in ponies by low-dose heparin therapy, *Vet Surg* 16:459-462, 1987.

GASTROINTESTINAL ILEUS

GUY D. LESTER

Gastrointestinal ileus has been defined as the functional inhibition of propulsive bowel activity, irrespective of its pathophysiologic basis.[569] Ileus of the gastrointestinal tract is most frequently ascribed to the condition that occurs after laparotomy; it is termed simple or uncomplicated postoperative ileus (POI). In humans, gastrointestinal stasis after laparotomy is transient and usually resolves spontaneously within 3 to 5 days. POI of longer duration has been termed complicated or paralytic ileus.[569] Postoperative ileus in horses is most commonly reported after gastrointestinal surgery, particularly after surgical trauma to the small intestine.[570,571] Clinical signs of POI usually develop shortly after the procedure and include abdominal pain, decreased fecal output and borborygmi, and sequestration of fluid within the small intestine resulting in enterogastric reflux. The severity and duration of intestinal stasis is variable lasting from minutes to days.

Ileus is an important clinical feature of other gastrointestinal tract diseases iincluding mechanical obstruction with gas distention, gastroduodenal ulcer disease, duodenitis/proximal jejunitis, enteritis, peritonitis, and a range of neonatal conditions including prematurity, systemic sepsis, and perinatal asphyxia syndromes. It also may occur secondarily to metabolic and electrolyte derangements and endotoxemia.

A specific defect of cecal motility and emptying has been described in horses.[572-574] The condition occurs most commonly after general anesthesia and is best classified as a form of POI, but may also occur spontaneously in animals with or without concurrent diseases. Affected horses demonstrate subtle clinical signs usually 3 to 5 days after anesthesia. Signs include a reduction in feed intake and fecal output, depression, and an auscultable cecal gas cap. An absence of effective cecal motility results in impaction of the organ with moist contents, which is manifested by signs of mild to moderate colic. If recognized late or untreated, the cecum may rupture, resulting in fatal peritonitis.

PATHOPHYSIOLOGY. The control of intestinal motility is complex and involves a combination of central innervation, autonomic innervation, and the enteric nervous system (Fig. 30-44). Intestinal contractions are primarily controlled by the enteric nervous system and do not require extrinsic neural input. Rhythmicity of the intestinal electrical activity is controlled by specialized cells that are electrically coupled to myocytes via gap junctions, the interstitial cells of Cajal (ICC).[575] Cells with immunostaining properties consistent with ICC have been described along the length of horse gastrointestinal tract.[576] These cells are responsible for the generation and propagation of slow wave activity and may be critically involved in a range of motility disorders. Effective coordination and modulation of motility requires both sympathetic and parasympathetic input, along with several hormones. The parasympathetic supply to the gastrointestinal tract is via the vagus and pelvic nerves and the sympathetic supply is through postganglionic fibers of the cranial and caudal mesenteric plexuses. Much of the autonomic input to the enteric nervous system is mediated through cholinergic nicotinic receptors. A complex network of interneurones within each plexus integrates and amplifies neural input; the intensity and frequency of resultant smooth contractions are proportional to the relative amount of sympathetic and parasympathetic input. Additional binding sites for several other endogenous chemicals, including dopamine, motilin, and serotonin, can be found within the enteric nervous system and on smooth muscle cells.[577]

Acetylcholine (ACh) is the dominant excitatory neurotransmitter in the gastrointestinal tract and exerts its action through muscarinic type 2 receptors on smooth muscle cells. Sympathetic nervous system input to the gastrointestinal tract is generally inhibitory. Sympathetic fibers innervating the gastrointestinal tract are adrenergic, postganglionic fibers with cell bodies located in the prevertebral ganglia. Activation of α_2-adrenergic receptors on cholinergic neurons within enteric ganglia inhibits the release of ACh. The inhibitory effects of α_2-agonists, such as xylazine and detomidine, on large colon motility are well described.[578-583] The α_2-antagonist, yohimbine, has a weak, but positive effect on cecal emptying in normal ponies, suggesting that normal motility is under constant α_2-adrenergic tone.[583] β_1, β_2, and β-atypical receptors are directly inhibitory to the intestinal smooth muscle.[584] Inhibitory nonadrenergic, noncholinergic (NANC) neurotransmiters include adenosine triphosphate (ATP), vasoactive intestinal peptide (VIP), and nitric oxide (NO).[585,586] Inhibitory neurotransmitters are critical for mediating descending inhibition during peristalsis and receptive relaxation. Nitric oxide synthase inhibitors have been investigated as potential prokinetics agents. Substance P is a NANC neurotransmitter that may be involved in contraction of the large colon.[587,588] Stimulation of contractile activity by substance P involves neurokinin 1 (NK-1) receptors.[589]

The rate and force of intestinal contractions along the small intestine and large colon of the horse are important determinants of intestinal motility; of even greater importance to the net propulsion of digesta are the cyclic patterns of contractile activity. These patterns have been referred to as the small intestinal and colonic migrating motility (or myoelectric) complexes.[590,591] Recovery of the small intestinal migrating myoelectric complex (MMC) after surgery has been correlated with resolution of the clinical signs of ileus in humans with POI.[569] In humans, POI is considered a primary

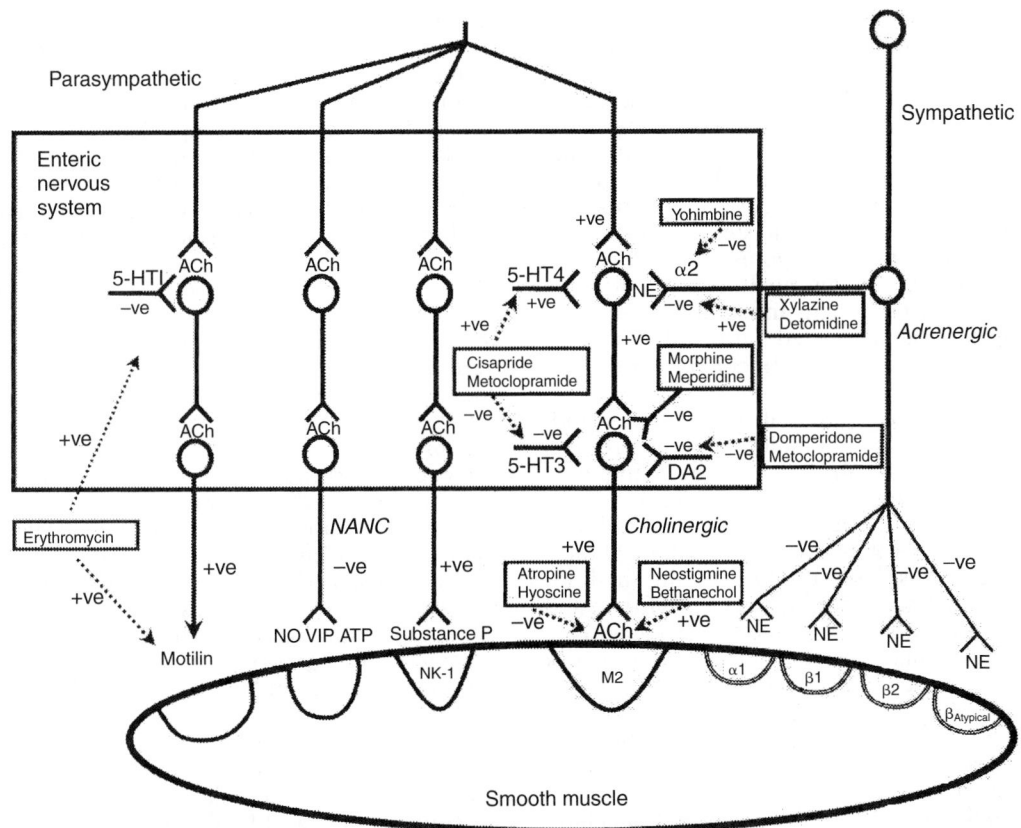

FIG. 30-44 ▓ Schematic representation of some neural and hormonal influences on intestinal motility. *ACh,* Acetylcholine; *ATP,* adenosine triphosphate; *DA2,* dopamine type 2 receptors; *+5-HT1,* 5-hydroxytryptamine type 1 receptors; *M2,* muscurininc type 2 receptors; *NANC,* noncholinergic, nonadrenergic pathway; *NE,* norepinephrine; *NK-1,* neurokinin-1 receptors; *NO,* nitric oxide; *+ve,* excitatory; *−ve,* inhibitory; *VIP,* vasoactive intestinal peptide.

large intestinal disease. Following laparotomy, motor activity resumes initially in the small intestine (5 to 10 hours), then the stomach (24 to 48 hours), and finally the large colon (72 to 120 hours).[569] Similar data is not available in horses, but return of normal myoelectric activity was most delayed in the cecum after surgical implantation of serosal recording electrodes in adult horses.[592]

Peritoneal inflammation or irritation is a well-recognized initiating factor of ileus. Although the exact pathway of this response is yet to be elucidated, it is believed that the inhibition of motility is mediated through neural reflexes.[569,593,594] These reflexes are likely to be important in several diseases in horses, including surgical trauma (POI), nonseptic and septic peritonitis, and inflammatory bowel diseases such as duodenitis/proximal jejunitis. The afferent segment is partly composed of peptidergic fibers that are activated by peritoneal receptors.[595] Afferent fibers terminate in the dorsal horn of the spinal cord, where they can activate inhibitory sympathetic fibers or, alternatively, synapse directly on the sympathetic ganglia. Consequently, the efferent limb of the reflex expresses increased sympathetic outflow, primarily mediated through stimulation of α_2-adrenoreceptors and inhibition of ACh release. This provides the rationale for α_2-blockade in the treatment of ileus.

Hyperactivity of the sympathetic nervous system is the most recognized theory to explain POI, but it is probably only part of a more complex series of events. Recently, attention has been directed to the role of inflammatory cells and their contents as the pivotal event in the development of

POI.[596] Minimal bowel insult, such as that caused through gentle surgical manipulation, increases the expression of P-selectin and intercellular adhesion molecule 1 (ICAM-1) on endothelial cells within the vasculature of the muscularis layer of the intestine. Parallel up-regulation of associated ligands on leukocytes leads to sequential "sticking and rolling," followed by migration into the interstitium, where neutrophil products may interfere with local neurohormonal signaling or smooth muscle responses. There is an associated reduction in intestinal contractility, although the exact mechanism has not been determined. Treatment of rats with antiadhesion molecules prevented leukocyte accumulation in the muscularis and resulted in maintenance of intestinal motility. These data provide the basis for the ileus seen in duodenitis/proximal jejunitis and other acute small intestinal inflammatory diseases, as well as justification for the use of antiinflammatory agents and antioxidants in horses at risk for ileus.

Ileus can also occur in association with intestinal obstruction or displacement. Mild to moderate distention of the bowel, such as that occurring in the early stages of an intraluminal obstruction, evokes an increase in local contractile activity.[597,598] However, excessive distention results in inhibition of motility within the distended segment of bowel. Intestinal stasis is not always detrimental and under certain conditions may be protective. Based on data derived from other species it is likely that intestinointestinal reflexes occur in horses under both normal and diseased conditions.[599] For example, large colon distention may result in delayed gastric emptying and small intestinal transit. Small intestinal distention probably has a similar negative effect on gastric and small intestinal motility.

Endotoxemia is a clinical feature of many diseases of the equine gastrointestinal tract, and endotoxins can independently exert a negative effect on intestinal motility and transit.[600] A variety of mediators are likely involved, but α_2-adrenergic adrenoreceptors appear to be important, through attenuation of blood flow and suppression of contractile activity.[601] In one study, antagonism of endogenous platelet activating factor also partly ameliorated the ileus induced by experimental endotoxin infusion.[602] The same group of investigators demonstrated a protective effect of phenylbutazone or flunixin pretreatment on endotoxin-induced changes in motility.[603]

Certain classes of drugs can induce ileus, the most notorious of which are the anticholinergics such as atropine, hyoscine, and ipratropium. Atropine is a postganglionic blocking agent that binds to muscarinic receptors. When administered intravenously at 0.04 mg/kg, atropine inhibits small intestinal, cecal, and colonic motility for about 2 hours; but, more important, this dose inhibits both the small intestinal and colonic migrating motility complexes for up to 8 hours.[604] The inhibitory effects of α_2-receptor activation are relevant to the medical management of horses either at risk of, or with, ileus. Intravenous xylazine inhibits cecal and large colon motility for 20 to 30 minutes without seriously disrupting small intestinal myoelectric activity.[579-583] The more potent α_2-agonist, detomidine, can reduce large intestinal myoelectric activity for up to 3 hours.[579] Metabolic derangements such as hypokalemia, hypocalcemia, and uremia have been implicated in the pathophysiology of ileus in humans and in other domestic animals. Clinical and experimental data concerning these associations in horses are lacking, but it is important to correct any known abnormalities with appropriate fluid and electrolyte therapy in clinical cases of ileus.

The pathophysiology of cecal motility dysfunction is not known. This syndrome may best mimic POI in humans, which is generally considered a large intestinal disorder.[569] An important difference in horses is that laparotomy is a rare predisposing factor, and most cases occur in horses undergoing routine extra abdominal surgical procedures, such as arthroscopy or laryngeal surgery. General anesthesia itself is a potent inhibitor of gastrointestinal motility in horses, but these effects are short-lived and reversible within hours of anesthetic withdrawal.[590] A link between routine postoperative medications, such as phenylbutazone and aminoglycoside antibiotics, has been suspected but not established. An inhibitory effect of NSAIDs on large colon contractility has been demonstrated using in vitro techniques.[605] Many of the horses with postanesthetic cecal dysfunction are young, intact males that either are currently in work or have recently been in active training. Although this signalment is not common to all cases, it has raised the possibility that sympathetic overstimulation may be an important factor in the pathogenesis of this syndrome.

DIAGNOSIS

It is important to distinguish functional ileus from mechanical obstruction. Collection of routine physical data, including assessment of the pulse rate and character, auscultation and percussion of the abdomen, rectal palpation, and passage of a nasogastric tube, should aid in this assessment. Additional laboratory data, including a complete blood count, fibrinogen estimation, and cytologic analysis of peritoneal fluid, may improve the accuracy of diagnosis. Abdominal pain is a clinical sign in horses with ileus involving the proximal gastrointestinal tract. Signs of colic may be due, in part, to gastric distention and often are relieved by nasogastric intubation and gastric decompression. This procedure

should also result in an almost immediate reduction in pulse rate. Exceptions to this response may include ileus secondary to mechanical obstruction, very severe duodenitis/proximal jejunitis, or peritonitis, in which pain could be expected to persist despite gastric decompression.

Gastric and small intestinal ileus typically results in the sequestration of large volumes of fluid into the intestinal lumen. Consequently, inadequate fluid supplementation can lead to signs of significant dehydration with electrolyte derangements, which can further promote intestinal stasis. Another common clinical sign of ileus is partial or complete anorexia. In horses with some degree of ileus that are not anorectic, consumption of feed or water can induce signs of abdominal pain. Most animals, irrespective of the basis of the ileus, are depressed and have reduced fecal output and intestinal borborygmi. Intestinal sounds should, however, be interpreted with caution because the presence of borborygmi does not always equate to progressive intestinal motility and may merely reflect local, nonpropagated contractions.

Rectal palpation findings in cases of persistent POI or duodenitis/proximal jejunitis are usually nonspecific but may reveal dilated, fluid-filled loops of small intestine. Roughened peritoneal surfaces can occasionally be palpated if there is peritonitis, although cytologic analysis of peritoneal fluid provides a more accurate method of diagnosis. Cecal distention with digesta can be palpated in horses with advanced postanesthetic cecal dysfunction. The signs associated with cecal dysfunction are more insidious than those that occur in small intestinal ileus. Afflicted animals usually develop mild clinical signs 3 to 5 days after general anesthesia; these signs include reduced fecal output, infrequent borborygmi, and palpation of a "doughy" cecum by rectal examination. The horses are usually depressed, but may or may not demonstrate signs of abdominal pain until the cecum becomes impacted. If the animals are not closely monitored, the first signs of cecal dysfunction may be those related to organ rupture and overwhelming septic peritonitis.

TREATMENT

Gastric decompression is an important component of the therapy for ileus involving the proximal gastrointestinal tract. Fluid and electrolyte therapy is critical, particularly with respect to maintaining adequate extracellular potassium, calcium, and magnesium concentrations. Calculation of the volume of fluid to be administered should include maintenance requirements plus an estimate of losses, especially those lost through gastric decompression.

Drugs that may impair normal intestinal motility should be avoided. These include the anticholinergics, such as atropine, and opiate receptor agonists, such as morphine and meperidine. However, butorphanol appears to have little or no adverse effect on either small or large intestinal motility.[582,606,697] α_2-Agonists should be used sparingly because of their inhibitory effects on large intestinal motility.

Antiinflammatory Drugs. Gastrointestinal tract motility is influenced by luminal contents or mucosal inflammation.[608] Inflammatory diseases of the gastrointestinal tract commonly lead to altered motility of both affected and adjacent segments, and, in some conditions, altered intestinal motility may linger long after resolution of the inflammation.[609] Experimental and anecdotal evidence exists to provide a strong rationale for the use of antiinflammatory drugs (NSAIDs) in the prevention and treatment of gastrointestinal ileus, particularly in animals in which endotoxemia may be present.[594,596,603] The analgesic properties of NSAIDs may inhibit the afferent limb of the reflex pathway. Flunixin meglumine* is widely used in equine practice as an analgesic and antiin-

---

*Banamine, Schering-Plough Corp., Kenilworth, NJ 07033.

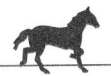

flammatory agent, and it also ameliorates many of the adverse systemic effects of endotoxin, particularly those on the cardiovascular system. A potential negative effect of NSAIDs on large intestinal contractility has been suggested.[605]

Antimicrobials. Broad-spectrum antimicrobials are indicated when sepsis is suspected or if the immune system is compromised, as in cases with moderate to severe endotoxemia. Theoretical concerns have been raised regarding the use of aminoglycoside antibiotics in animals with ileus. Inhibition of intestinal contractions occurred in vitro when sections of intestine were exposed to high concentrations of aminoglycoside antimicrobials,[610] but this inhibitory effect is unlikely to occur at clinically relevant doses.

Prokinetic drugs. Motility-enhancing drugs, or "prokinetics," have been advocated in the treatment of gastrointestinal ileus in humans and domestic animals. Unfortunately information directly pertinent to horses is limited and must be cautiously extrapolated from that of other species. Prokinetic drugs can potentially shorten the length of hospitalization, thereby reducing the cost of treatment and the number of potential complications such as weight loss, thrombophlebitis, and laminitis. In addition, there is experimental evidence that the development of postoperative abdominal adhesions, related to reduced intestinal motility, can be minimized with the use of prokinetic drugs.[611] A potential restriction of their use is the need for normal intestinal integrity; that is, certain drugs require an intact enteric nervous system and smooth muscle layers to be effective at stimulating or enhancing motility. It is unreasonable to assume, therefore, that many of these drugs would be effective in a severe inflammatory insult, such as can occur in the duodenitis/proximal jejunitis syndrome. In addition, some of the agents are associated with significant side effects that could be detrimental to the patient.

Cholinomimetics. Bethanechol* is a true parasympathomimetic agent that can act both at the level of the myenteric plexus and directly on intestinal smooth cells through muscarinic (M2) receptors. The drug is a synthetic ester of ACh and is not degraded by anticholinesterase. Bethanechol has not been used widely in human medicine because of its cholinergic side effects, such as abdominal discomfort, sweating, and salivation. In addition, it has been argued that direct stimulation of the smooth muscle results in contractile activity that is not coordinated. Bethanecol may have efficacy in certain equine diseases, particularly those involving abnormal gastric emptying and delayed small intestinal transit. Side effects appear to be minimal when the drug is administered at 0.025 mg/kg SC or PO. Bethanechol chloride has been shown to increase gastric contractility[612] and hasten the emptying of liquid and solid phase markers from the stomach of normal horses.[613] There are associated increases in small intestinal myoelectric activity.[583] The effects are not restricted to the upper gastrointestinal tract; bethanechol also significantly enhanced the rate of cecal emptying of radiolabeled markers in normal ponies.[583] The latter finding was associated with an increase in relative strength and duration of contractions in the cecum and right ventral colon. Bethanechol, when combined with yohimbine, appeared to have a positive effect on intestinal activity in two Welsh Mountain ponies when contrasted with control animals after experimental ileus.[614] Neostigmine increases receptor levels of ACh by inhibiting the enzyme cholinesterase. The drug (0.022 to 0.025 mg/kg IV) promoted cecal and colonic contractile activity and hastened the emptying of radiolabeled markers from the cecum.[578,582,583] The drug has been used in the management of

small intestinal ileus, but significantly delayed the emptying of 6-mm beads from the stomach of normal adult horses.[615]

Benzamides. Metoclopramide* is a first-generation benzamide. The drug acts principally as a 5-hydroxytryptamine 4-receptor (5HT-4) agonist and 5HT-3 receptor antagonist, but unlike newer-generation benzaimdes, it is also an antagonist at dopamine 1 (DA₁) and 2 (DA₂) receptors.[616] Stimulation of prejunctional DA₂ receptors inhibits the release of ACh; consequently, antagonism of these receptors is expected to facilitate ACh release and smooth muscle contraction. The data surrounding the use of metoclopramide in horses is conflicting. When infused intravenously at 0.25 mg/kg/hr over 60 minutes, metoclopramide was superior to no therapy in restoring motility in experimental ileus in 3 ponies.[614] The drug (2 mg/kg IV) had minimal effects on contractile activity in the ileum, cecum, and colon of small ponies,[617] nor any effect on jejunal or pelvic flexure activity when administered at a bolus intravenous dose (0.03 mg/kg).[606] Metoclopramide crosses the blood-brain barrier, where its antagonist properties on central DA₂ receptors can result in extrapyramidal signs, including seizure. It is these signs that were responsible for poor acceptance of the drug in equine practice. Recently, metoclopramide was examined in a clinical population of 70 horses undergoing small intestinal resection.[618] Constant intravenous infusion of metoclopramide (0.04 mg/kg/hr) significantly decreased the volume and duration of gastric reflux postoperatively over control and intermittent drug infusion groups. Unfortunately, animals were not randomly assigned to groups, and the constant infusion group was smaller in number and underrepresented by horses that had a jejunocecostomy, a procedure associated with a greater risk of postoperative complications. Nevertheless, constant infusion of metoclopramide was well tolerated and appeared superior to intermittent infusion or no treatment at all.

Cisapride† is a second-generation substituted benzamide that is used to treat a variety of conditions in humans, including gastroesophageal reflux disease, peptic ulcer disease, intestinal pseudoobstruction, and constipation.[619] The drug appears to act as a 5HT-4 agonist and 5HT-3–receptor antagonist, but is without antidopaminergic action. Stimulation of 5HT-4 receptors within the enteric nervous system enhances release of ACh from the myenteric plexus.[620] The density and distribution of 5HT-4 receptors varies along the gastrointestinal tract and between species; therefore extrapolation of effects between species should be done with caution. The effects of intravenous cisapride infusion have been investigated in normal ponies, in which increases in gastric, small intestinal, and colonic activity were reported.[621] There are several reports that suggest efficacy of cisapride in the management of intestinal disease in horses, including the resolution of persistent large colon impaction,[622] treatment of equine grass sickness,[623] and as a preventative for POI in horses after small intestinal surgery.[624,625] The latter studies reported significant, albeit modest, effects of the drug after IM administration at 0.1 mg/kg during the postoperative period. The use of cisapride in equine practice in the United States is limited because the drug is available in tablet form only. This formulation is absorbed erratically when administered rectally to horses.[626,627] A method for preparation of a parenteral form of the drug from tablets has been described.[628] Cisapride has adverse cardiac side effects that include lengthening of the QT interval and development of torsades de pointes, a potentially fatal arrhythmia. The cardiac effects are mediated through blockage of the rapid component of the delayed rectifier potassium current, but do not occur commonly.[629]

---

*Urecholine, Merck and Co., Inc., West Point, Pa.

*Metoclopramide, AH Robins Co., Richmond, Va 23220.
†Propulsid, Janssen Pharmaceutica, Titusville, NJ.

Dopamine Antagonist. Domperidone acts as a competitive antagonist at peripheral DA$_2$ receptors.[630] The drug has recently received attention as a therapeutic agent (1.1 mg/kg/day) for mares grazing endophyte-infected tall fescue, principally as a result of drug-enhanced prolactin release.[630,631] The potential prokinetic effects of domperidone have not been extensively studied in horses, but Gerring and King reported modest efficacy of domperidone (0.2 mg/kg IV) in experimental ileus in 2 ponies.[624] The drug is not commercially available in the United States.

Motilides. Erythromycin has prokinetic activity in most species studied, including horses.[613,632] The principal mechanism of action is as a motilin receptor agonist on smooth muscle cells, but it also may act on cholinergic nerves within the enteric nervous system to facilitate the release of ACh and motilin.[633] Erythromycin readily binds to receptors and may displace motilin from receptors. There are regional differences in response to erythromycin within the intestine and differences between species that may correspond to differences in motilin-receptor density. The drug acts preferentially in the stomach and proximal small intestine of humans, dogs, and cats,[633] but the cecum and large colon may be the primary sites of action in horses.[632] Erythromycin does enhance gastric emptying in normal horses,[613] and motilin has been shown to increase small intestinal motility. Motilin (0.6 μg/kg IV) induced premature phase III–like contractile activity in the proximal jejunum of normal adult horses,[634] and synthetic canine motilin (0.06 μg/kg) increased jejunal and ileal myoelectric activity and hastened gastrocecal transit in ponies after experimental ileus.[635] When compared with saline, erythromycin lactobionate,* at doses between 0.1 and 10.0 mg/kg, increased myoelectric activity of the cecum and right ventral colon and hastened the emptying of radiolabled markers from the cecum of normal ponies.[632] The maximal effect on emptying was seen at 1.0 mg/kg and was greater than that induced by neostigmine or bethanechol. Erythromycin also induces colonic MMC-like activity in the colon and is frequently associated with defecation and abdominal discomfort. The drug may be helpful at preventing cecal impaction in horses after anesthesia, although its effectiveness on cecal motility in the immediate postoperative period has been questioned.[592] High doses, constant infusion, or prolonged use of erythromycin induces receptor down-regulation and inhibition of activity.[636] It is therefore recommended to use intermittent, intravenous bolus dosing at 0.5 mg/kg. Erythromycin has been associated with diarrhea in adult horses; consequently dosing over multiple days should be done with caution.

Narcotic Antagonists. Naloxone (0.05 mg/kg IV), has been shown to induce contractile activity in the cecum and left colon.[617,637] The administration of naloxone is commonly followed by defecation within 15 to 20 minutes.

α$_2$-Antagonists. Adrenergic antagonists, specifically α$_2$-antagonists, can act specifically by counteracting the increased sympathetic outflow in response to nociceptive stimulation.[593,601] Endotoxin also exerts its negative effects on propulsive motility partly through stimulation of α$_2$-adrenoreceptors; these effects were attenuated by the slow intravenous infusion of yohimbine† (75 μg/kg).[601] Yohimbine was also useful at restoring intestinal electromechanical activity after ileus was induced experimentally in Shetland ponies.[614]

Lidocaine. Lidocaine has been evaluated in both spontaneous and experimental models of intestinal ileus. Intravenous infusion of lidocaine may suppress primary afferent neurons, thereby limiting reflex efferent inhibition of motility. In addition, local anesthetics have antiinflammatory properties, including inhibition of both granulocyte migration and release of lysosomal enzymes.[638] There is also some evidence that lidocaine may have direct stimulatory properties on smooth muscle.[639] An infusion dose of 15 to 20 mg/min over a period of 5 to 6 hours has been recommended for use in horses.[640] The effects of lidocaine on the incidence and severity of POI were recently evaluated in a multicenter study.[641] Numbers of animals enrolled were limited, but data suggest that lidocaine infusion has a modest positive effect on POI. The systemic analgesic properties of lidocaine infusion may reduce signs of abdominal pain, but could delay detection of laminitis. Lidocaine infusion is associated with reversible side effects that include muscle fasciculations, ataxia, and seizure. Side effects at this infusion rate are uncommon but may include muscle fasciculations.

It is perceived by many that exercise promotes normal intestinal motility. There is little evidence either to support or to discredit this association, with the exception of a study in humans following laparotomy in which early ambulation did not hasten the return to normal intestinal motility.[642]

In summary, after a diagnosis of intestinal ileus has been established it is important to determine the underlying cause. Management of these cases may include gastric decompression, adequate fluid and electrolyte therapy, NSAIDs, and possibly motility-modifying agents. There is experimental evidence to support the use of flunixin and yohimbine in the management of POI. Likewise, several prokinetic agents such as erythromycin, bethanechol, cisapride, and lidocaine may have an important role in the management of certain types of ileus.

REFERENCES

569. Livingston EH, Passaro EP: Postoperative ileus, *Dig Dis Sci* 35:121-132, 1990.
570. Adams S. Recognition and management of ileus, *Vet Clin North Am (Equine Pract)* 4:91-104, 1988.
571. Becht JL, Richardson DW: Ileus in the horse: clinical significance and management, *Proceedings of the Twenty-seventh Annual Convention of the American Association of Equine Practitioners,* 1981, pp 291-297.
572. Campbell ML et al: Cecal impaction in the horse, *J Am Vet Med Assoc* 184:950-952, 1984.
573. Ross MW, Martin BB, Donawick WJ: Cecal perforation in the horse, *J Am Vet Med Assoc* 187:249-253, 1985.
574. Hilbert BJ et al: Caecal overload and rupture in the horse, *Aust Vet J* 64:85-86, 1987.
575. Horowitz B, Ward SM, Sanders KM: Cellular and molecular basis for electrical rhythmicity in gastrointestinal muscles, *Annu Rev Physiol* 61:19-43, 1999.
576. Hudson NPH et al: An immunohistochemical study of interstitial cells of Cajal (ICC) in the equine gastrointestinal tract, *Res Vet Sci* 66:265-271, 1999.
577. Bertaccini G, Coruzzi G: Receptors in the gastrointestinal tract, *Pharmacol Res Comm* 19:87-118, 1987.
578. Adams SB, Lamar CH, Masty J: Motility of the distal portion of the jejunum and pelvic flexure in ponies: effects of six drugs, *Am J Vet Res* 45:795-799, 1984.
579. Roger T, Ruckebusch Y: Colonic alpha-2-adrenoceptor-mediated responses in the pony, *J Vet Pharmacol Ther* 10:310-318, 1987.
580. Clark ES et al: Effects of xylazine on cecal mechanical activity and cecal blood flow in healthy horses, *Am J Vet Res* 49:720-723, 1988.
581. Merritt AM et al: Effect of xylazine treatment on equine proximal gastrointestinal tract myoelectrical activity, *Am J Vet Res* 50:945-949, 1989.
582. Rutkowski JA, Ross MW, Cullen K: Effects of xylazine and/or butorphanol or neostigmine on myoelectric activity of the cecum and right ventral colon in female ponies, *Am J Vet Res* 50:1096-1101, 1989.
583. Lester GD et al: Effect of α2-adrenergic, cholinergic, and nonsteroidal anti-inflammatory drugs on myoelectric activity of ileum, cecum, and right ventral colon and on cecal emptying of radiolabeled markers in clinically normal ponies, *Am J Vet Res* 59:320-327, 1998.
584. Re G et al: Identification of beta-adrenergic receptor subtypes mediating relaxation in isolated equine ileum, *Am J Vet Res* 58:621-625, 1997.
585. Malone ED et al: Adrenergic, cholinergic and nonadrenergic-noncholinergic intrinsic innervation of the equine jejunum, *Am J Vet Res* 60:898-904, 1999.
586. Rakestraw PC et al: Involvement of nitric oxide in inhibitory neuromuscular transmission in equine jejunum, *Am J Vet Res* 57:1206-1212, 1996.
587. Sellers AF, Lowe JE, Cummings JF: Trials of serotonin, substance P and alpha2-adrenergic receptor effects on the large colon, *Cornell Vet* 75:319-323, 1985.

*Erythrocin, Abbott Laboratories, North Chicago, IL 60064.
†Yobine, Lloyd Laboratories, Shenandoah, IA 51601.

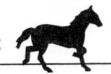

588. Sonea IM et al: Tachykinin receptors in the equine pelvic flexure, *Equine Vet J* 29:306-312, 1997.

589. Sarna SK: Tachykinins and *in vivo* gut motility, *Dig Dis Sci* 44:114S-118S, 1999.

590. Lester GD et al: Effects of general anesthesia on myoelectric activity of the intestine in horses, *Am J Vet Res* 53:1553-1557, 1992.

591. Merritt AM et al: Equine pelvic flexure myoelectric activity during fed and fasted states, *Am J Physiol* 269:G262-G268, 1995.

592. Hooper RN, Roussel AJ, Cohen ND: Erythromycin stimulates myoelectric activity in the ileum and pelvic flexure of horses in the post-operative period. In *Proceedings of the Sixth Equine Colic Research Symposium*, Athens, Ga, 1998, p 42.

593. Sjoqvist A, Hallerback B, Glise H: Reflex adrenergic inhibition of colonic motility in anesthetized rat caused by nociceptive stimuli of peritoneum, *Dig Dis Sci* 30:749-754, 1985.

594. Pairet M, Ruckebusch Y: On the relevance of non-steroidal anti-inflammatory drugs in the prevention of paralytic ileus in rodents, *J Pharm Pharmacol* 41:757-761, 1989.

595. Holzer P, Lippe ITH, Holzer-Petsche U: Inhibition of gastrointestinal transit due to surgical trauma or peritoneal irritation is reduced in capsaicin-treated rats, *Gastroenterology* 91:360-363, 1986.

596. Kalff JC et al: Surgically induced leukocytic infiltrates within the rat intestinal muscularis mediate postoperative ileus, *Gastroenterology* 117:378-387, 1999.

597. Lowe JE, Sellers AF, Brondum J: Equine pelvic flexure impaction: a model used to evaluate motor events and compare drug response, *Cornell Vet* 70:401-412, 1980.

598. MacHarg MA et al: Electromyographic, myomechanical, and intraluminal pressure changes associated with acute extraluminal obstruction of the jejunum in conscious ponies, *Am J Vet Res* 47:7-11, 1986.

599. Bueno L et al: Mediators and pharmacology of visceral sensitivity: from basic to clinical investigations, *Gastroenterology* 112:1714-1743, 1997.

600. King JN, Gerring EL: The action of low dose endotoxin on equine bowel motility, *Equine Vet J* 23:11-17, 1991.

601. Eades SC, Moore JN: Blockade of endotoxin-induced cecal hypoperfusion and ileus with an alpha-2 antagonist in horses, *Am J Vet Res* 54:586-590, 1993.

602. King JN, Gerring EL: Antagonism of endotoxin-induced disruption of equine gastrointestinal motility with the platelet-activating factor antagonist WEB 2086, *J Vet Pharmacol Ther* 13:333-339, 1990.

603. King JN, Gerring EL: Antagonism of endotoxin-induced disruption of equine bowel motility by flunixin and phenylbutazone, *Equine Vet J Suppl* 7:38-42, 1989.

604. Lester GD: The development and application of a computer system for the recording and analysis of intestinal myoelectrical activity in the horse, PhD thesis, Murdoch University, 1990.

605. Van Hoogmoed L et al: In vitro effects of nonsteroidal anti-inflammatory agents and prostaglandins I2, E2, and F2 alpha on contractility of taenia of the large colon of horses, *Am J Vet Res* 60:1004-1009, 1999.

606. Sojka JE et al: Effect of butorphanol, pentazocine, meperidine, or metoclopramide on intestinal motility in female ponies, *Am J Vet Res* 49:527-529, 1988.

607. Merritt AM, Campbell-Thompson ML, Lowrey S: Effect of butorphanol on equine antroduodenal motility, *Equine Vet J Suppl* 7:21-23, 1989.

608. Collins SM: The immunomodulation of enteric neuromuscular function: implications for motility and inflammatory disorders, *Gastroenterology* 111:1683-1699, 1996.

609. MacPherson BR, Shearin NL, Pfeiffer CJ: Experimental diffuse colitis in cats: observations on motor activity, *J Surg Res* 25:42-49, 1978.

610. Paradelis AG: Inhibition of the pendular movements of the intestine by aminoglycoside antibiotics, *Meth Fund Exp Clin Pharmacol* 3:173-177, 1981.

611. Sparnon AL, Spitz L: Pharmacological manipulation of postoperative intestinal adhesions, *Aust N Z J Surg* 59:725-729, 1989.

612. Thompson LP et al: Effect of bethanechol on equine gastric motility and secretion, *Proceedings of the Fifth Equine Colic Research Symposium*, Athens, Ga, 1994, p 12.

613. Ringger NC et al: Effect of bethanechol or erythromycin on gastric emptying in horses, *Am J Vet Res* 57:1771-1775, 1996.

614. Gerring EEL, Hunt JM: Pathophysiology of equine postoperative ileus: effect of adrenergic blockade, parasympathetic stimulation and metoclopramide in an experimental model, *Equine Vet J* 18:249-255, 1986.

615. Adams SB, MacHarg MA: Neostigmine methylsulfate delays gastric emptying of particulate markers in horses, *Am J Vet Res* 46:2498-2499, 1985.

616. MacDonald TM: Metoclopramide, domperidone and dopamine in man: actions and interactions, *Eur J Clin Pharmacol* 40:225-230, 1991.

617. Ruckebusch Y, Roger T: Prokinetic effects of cisapride, naloxone and parasympathetic stimulation at the equine ileo-caeco-colonic junction, *J Vet Pharmacol Therap* 11:322-329, 1988.

618. Dart AJ et al: Efficacy of metoclopramide for treatment of ileus in horses following small intestinal surgery: 70 cases (1989-1992), *Aust Vet J* 74:280-284, 1996.

619. Tollesson PO et al: Treatment of postoperative ileus with cisapride, *Scand J Gastroenterol* 26:477-482, 1991.

620. Briejer MR, Akkermans LMA, Schuurkes JAJ: Gastrointestinal prokinetic benzamides: the pharmacology underlying stimulation of motility, *Pharmacol Rev* 47:631-651, 1995.

621. King JN, Gerring EL: Actions of the novel gastrointestinal prokinetic agent cisapride on equine bowel motility, *J Vet Pharmacol Therap* 11:314-321, 1988.

622. Steinebach MA, Cole D: Use of cisapride in the resolution of pelvic flexure impaction in a horse, *Can Vet J* 36:624-625, 1995.

623. Milne EM et al: An evaluation of the use of cisapride in horses with chronic grass sickness, *Br Vet J* 152:537-549, 1996.

624. Gerring EL, King JN: Cisapride in the prophylaxis of equine post operative ileus, *Equine Vet J Suppl* 7:52-55, 1989.

625. Valden MA, Klein WR: The effects of cisapride on the restoration of gut motility after surgery of the small intestine in horses: a clinical trial, *Vet Q* 15:175-179, 1993.

626. Cook G et al: Pharmacokinetics of cisapride in horses after intravenous and rectal administration, *Am J Vet Res* 58:1427-1430, 1997.

627. Steel CM et al: Unreliable rectal absorption of cisapride in horses, *Equine Vet J* 31:82-84, 1999.

628. Cable CS et al: Preparation of a parenteral formulation of cisapride form Propulsid tablets and pharmacokinetic analysis after its intravenous administration, *J Equine Vet Sci* 18:616-621, 1998.

629. Drolet B et al: Block of the rapid component of the delayed rectifier potassium current by the prokinetic agent cisapride underlies drug-related lengthening of the QT interval, *Circulation* 20:204-210, 1998.

630. Tonini M: Recent advances in the pharmacology of gastrointestinal prokinetics, *Pharmacol Res* 33:217-226, 1996.

631. Redmond LM et al: Efficacy of domperidone and sulpiride as treatments for rescue toxicosis in horses, *Am J Vet Res* 55:722-729, 1994.

632. Lester GD et al: Effect of erythromycin lactobionate on myoelectric activity of ileum, cecum, and right ventral colon, and cecal emptying of radiolabeled markers in clinically normal ponies, *Am J Vet Res* 59:328-34, 1998.

633. Peeters TL: Erythromycin and other macrolides as prokinetic agents, *Gastroenterology* 105:1886-1899, 1993.

634. Sasaki N, Yoshihara T: The effect of motilin on the regulation mechanism of intestinal motility in conscious horses, *J Vet Med Sci* 61:167-170, 1999.

635. Coatney RW, Adams SB: The effect of motilin on equine small intestinal motility during experimental postoperative ileus, *Proceedings of the Third Equine Colic Research Symposium*, Athens, Ga, 1988, p 12.

636. Otterson MF, Sarna SK: Gastrointestinal motor effects of erythromycin, *Am J Physiol* 259:G355-G363, 1990.

637. Roger T, Bardon T, Ruckebusch Y: Colonic motor responses in the pony: relevance of colonic stimulation by opiate antagonists, *Am J Vet Res* 46:31-35, 1985.

638. Rimback G, Cassuto J, Tollesson P: Treatment of postoperative paralytic ileus by intravenous lidocaine infusion, *Anesth Analg* 70:414-419, 1990.

639. Wood J, Marsh D: Effects of atropine, tetrodotoxin and lidocaine on rebound excitation of guinea-pig small intestine, *J Pharmacol Exp Therap* 184:590-598, 1973.

640. Broome TA: The potential use of lidocaine for treatment of ileus in the horse, *Proc North Am Vet Conf* 6:409-411, 1990.

641. Malone ED, Turner TA, Wilson JH: Intravenous lidocaine for the treatment of equine ileus, *Proceedings of the Sixth Equine Colic Research Symposium*, Athens, Ga, 1998, p 42.

642. Waldhausen JH, Schirmer BD: The effect of ambulation on recovery from postoperative ileus, *Ann Surg* 212:671-677, 1990.

NONSTEROIDAL ANTIINFLAMMATORY DRUG TOXICITY

NOAH D. COHEN

Use of nonsteroidal antiinflammatory drugs (NSAIDs) is common in equine practice because of their antipyretic, analgesic, and antiinflammatory properties. These drugs are used to treat horses with colic, endotoxemia, musculoskeletal disorders, and other medical problems. In addition to these therapeutic properties, NSAIDs also exhibit toxic properties. The NSAIDs have a relatively narrow therapeutic range, and when administered at excessive dosages, toxicosis can occur within a few days. Although generally safe when administered at recommended doses,[643] some horses may exhibit signs of toxicosis at these doses within days or weeks.[644,645] Recommended doses for NSAIDs commonly administered to horses include phenylbutazone (2.2 to 4.4 mg/kg every 12 hours), flunixin meglumine (1.1 mg/kg every 12 hours or 0.25 mg/kg every 8 hours), ketoprofen* (2.2 mg/kg every 24 hours), meclofenamic acid† (2.2 mg/kg every 12 to

---

*Ketofen, Fort Dodge Animal Health, Fort Dodge, IA 50501.
†Arquel, Fort Dodge Animal Health, Ford Dodge, IA 50501.

24 hours), naproxen* (5 to 10 mg/kg every 12 to 24 hours), and aspirin (12 to 25 mg/kg every 12 to 48 hours).

PATHOPHYSIOLOGY AND PREDISPOSING FACTORS. The principal mechanism of the therapeutic and toxic effects of NSAIDs is related to their inhibition of prostaglandin synthesis by inhibition of the cyclooxygenase enzyme. Two isoforms of the cyclooxygenase enzyme have been identified: cyclooxygenase-1 (COX-1) and cyclooxygenase-2 (COX-2).[646] COX-1 is largely produced in a constitutive manner and is thought to play an important role in maintaining physiologic homeostasis; it is found in such tissues as the stomach and kidney and in the endothelium and platelets. In contrast, COX-2 is primarily an inducible enzyme thought to be associated with inflammation and is produced by a variety of cells including monocytes, fibroblasts, synoviocytes, and chondrocytes.

It has been postulated that drugs that inhibit COX-1 more than COX-2 have greater toxic potential because they inhibit physiologic functions to a greater extent.[646] In horses, gastric ulcerogenicity of NSAIDs varies (phenylbutazone > flunixin meglumine > ketoprofen).[647] This difference in toxicity among drugs may relate to the extent to which these drugs inhibit the COX-1 isoform. Although the COX-1-versus-COX-2 scheme is currently considered valid, evidence exists that it may be overly simplistic. For example, COX-1 may play an important role in inflammation and is at least partly inducible.[648] In contrast, COX-2 can be induced physiologically in various organs and tissues and by stimuli other than inflammation.[646,649]

The gastrointestinal tract and the kidneys are the most common targets for NSAID toxicity. In the stomach, inhibition of cyclooxygenase can increase acid secretion, decrease output of mucus and bicarbonate, impair vasodilation, and diminish epithelial restitution, cell division, and angiogenesis.[650] Inhibition of cyclooxygenase also impairs the healing of existing ulcers. Although NSAID-induced gastric lesions have been widely studied because of the accessibility of the stomach to endoscopy, NSAID-induced injury can develop anywhere in the gastrointestinal tract (from the mouth to the rectum). Lesions in the large intestine can be particularly troublesome because they can cause chronic debilitation, are difficult to diagnose, and can be refractory to treatment.

In the kidney, PGE_2 and PGI_2 (prostacyclin) produce vasodilation in the autoregulatory response of renal blood flow to hypoperfusion; consequently, hypovolemia, hemorrhage, or renal disease will increase the risk of renal NSAID toxicosis. Damage is greatest at the renal crest (papilla) and papillary crest necrosis may be associated with subsequent nephrolithiasis/uretorolithiasis and chronic renal failure.[651] In humans, the most common side effect of NSAIDS is bleeding, caused in part by reduced function of platelets and in part by gastrointestinal hemorrhage.

Not all of the adverse effects of NSAIDs are attributable to cyclooxygenase inhibition. The NSAIDs also cause injury from a variety of mechanisms, including microvascular damage, increased intracellular concentration of reactive oxygen and other free radicals, direct local injury (particularly with ion trapping in the stomach), inhibition of cell division, and reduced hydrophobicity of the gastric mucus coat.[649,650] Inhibiting cyclooxygenase may shunt arachidonic acid metabolism toward the lipoxygenase pathway, thereby producing other biologically active eicosanoids. The clinical significance of this shunting is unclear, but the potential for deleterious effects exists.

Although the toxicity of NSAIDs is related to the dose and duration of administration, some horses develop toxicosis at recommended doses. Predisposing factors such as dehydra-

tion, renal disease, hepatic disease, or sepsis may contribute to the development of NSAID toxicity. Dehydration, renal disease, and hepatic disease predispose to NSAID toxicosis because of reduced tissue perfusion and reduced drug elimination. Sepsis may predispose to NSAID toxicosis because of secondary hypovolemia, decreased tissue perfusion, and direct and indirect effects of various mediators produced in response to sepsis (e.g., platelet aggregating factor). In humans, risk of NSAID-induced ulceration is increased among those with various gastrointestinal disorders (e.g., inflammatory bowel diseases). Body weight may be a predisposing factor in that NSAIDs are often administered to ponies, miniature horses, and small horses at dosages higher than those recommended for their body weight. Inadvertent overdosing can occur regardless of body weight or size (e.g., administration of a 12-g tube of phenylbutazone paste when administration of an anthelmintic paste was intended).

Some horses may have an idiosyncratic predisposition, particularly for ulceration of the right dorsal colon. Experimentally, arthritic laboratory animals were more susceptible to NSAID-induced gastropathy than healthy animals.[652] This finding may have relevance to horses because NSAIDs are often administered to chronically lame horses. Two or more NSAIDs are used concurrently in some situations. It is important to recognize that the effects of combining NSAIDs are additive, such that administering two NSAIDs at each of their recommended dosages is similar to giving twice the recommended dose of one NSAID. Combination of two NSAIDs will prolong their pharmacologic effect and increase the risk of toxicity.[653]

CLINICAL SIGNS. Clinical signs of NSAID toxicity are usually referable to the gastrointestinal tract. Oral or lingual ulceration may lead to difficulty in prehension and mastication. Esophageal ulceration may result in excessive salivation and apparent signs of pain (stretching of the neck, groaning) during swallowing. Gastric ulceration may result in slow consumption of feed, inappetance (particularly for grain by some horses), or anorexia. Horses that have gastric outflow obstruction associated with gastroduodenal ulceration may exhibit ptyalism, reflux esophagitis, and, in severe cases, spontaneous nasogastric reflux. Horses with ulceration anywhere in their gastrointestinal tract may exhibit signs of colic, which may be intermittent and varying in severity. Horses with colonic ulceration may have soft stool or diarrhea and ventral edema secondary to enteric protein loss. Diarrhea can be severe, even fatal. Endotoxemia may result from intestinal mucosal damage caused by NSAIDs. Clinical signs of endotoxemia (e.g., tachycardia, altered appearance of mucous membranes, fever, and dehydration) may be seen in some horses with NSAID enteropathy. In some horses, hematuria may be seen. Laminitis is often associated with NSAID toxicosis, either preceding or as a sequela to NSAID administration.

Horses may present with clinical signs days to weeks after having been administered NSAIDs. These horses typically present because of recurring colic, weight loss, or loose manure. It is particularly important in these horses to determine whether there was any history of NSAID administration, even if it was several weeks previous to the time of presentation.

DIAGNOSIS. Diagnosis is usually made on the basis of history of NSAID use, clinical signs, and clinicopathologic findings. The most consistent clinicopathologic abnormalities in horses with NSAID toxicosis are hypoproteinemia and hypoalbuminemia, presumably from loss of protein through inflamed intestinal mucosa. These findings are more commonly observed with damage to the distal intestinal tract and are not reliable for diagnosis of NSAID gastropathy. Some horses have decreased serum concentration of calcium, presumably attributable to intestinal loss of protein-bound calcium. In horses with NSAID-induced diarrhea, hyponatremia, hypo-

*Equiproxen, Fort Dodge Animal Health, Fort Dodge, IA 50501.

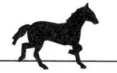

chloremia, hypokalemia, acidemia, and hypovolemia may be observed. In such cases, hypovolemia may make the serum protein concentration appear to be higher than its actual value would be were the horse adequately hydrated.

In chronic cases, horses may be anemic from inflammation, intestinal loss of blood through ulceration, or reduced function of platelets. Occult blood may be found in the feces of horses with lesions in the more distal portions of the intestinal tract. In my experience, tests for occult blood often lack sensitivity and false-positive results may be expected for up to 24 hours after rectal palpation.

The concentration of leukocytes is usually within the reference range, although leukocytosis and hyperfibrinogenemia, associated with inflammation, and leukopenia and neutropenia, presumably caused by endotoxemia, can be seen in some horses with NSAID toxicosis. Generally, results of peritoneal fluid analysis are within reference ranges, but increased concentration of nucleated white blood cells, total protein, and fibrinogen may be seen when there is advanced intestinal damage or intestinal vascular infarction. When findings of cytologic examination of peritoneal fluid are abnormal, results are more consistent with nonseptic than septic inflammation; however, septic inflammation may be observed when severe intestinal ulceration leads to transmural lesions and septic peritonitis.

Several clinicopathologic changes may accompany NSAID-induced renal damage. The most consistent finding is decreased urine specific gravity, from 1.008 to 1.020. Inability to properly dilute urine can be found with acute NSAID toxicosis or years after the original insult. This results from preferential damage to areas of the kidney that contribute most to concentrating urine (medulla, papilla). In chronic cases, urine specific gravity typically ranges from 1.013 to 1.020. Some horses with NSAID toxicosis will be azotemic. In acute cases, azotemia can result from dehydration, NSAID-induced alterations in renal blood flow, and tubuloglomerular feedback mechanisms. Chronic azotemia, with serum creatinine ranging from 2.1 mg/dl to 3.5 mg/dl, results from tubuloglomerular feedback mechnisms that reduce glomerular filtration to compensate for reduced reclamation of solutes in the medullary collecting ducts. In acute NSAID toxicosis, there may be overt hematuria. In other cases, urinalysis may reveal occult blood, increased renal cells, and increased white blood cells. In chronic cases, other than decreased urine specific gravity, urinalysis results are typically normal.

Endoscopy can be useful to visualize the location and extent of esophageal and gastric lesions. NSAID-induced gastric lesions are more common in the glandular epithelium, although nonglandular lesions can be observed. Contrast radiography or scintigraphy may be useful to document delayed gastric emptying in some horses. Lesions of the jejunum, ileum, cecum, and colon can be difficult to identify without celiotomy and enterotomy. Isotope-labeled white blood cell scintigraphic scans may identify colonic ulceration[654]; the sensitivity and availability of the procedure is limited, however. Ultrasonography may reveal thickening of the right dorsal colon or other colonic segments, but the technique appears to lack sensitivity. Ultrasonographically, horses with renal crest necrosis may have increased echogenicity of the renal crest and echogenic debris in the renal pelvis.

MANAGEMENT. Administration of NSAIDs should be discontinued if NSAID toxicosis is suspected. Gastric lavage and administration of 1 gallon per 450 kg of body weight of mineral oil via nasogastric tube may be of benefit in horses with acute NSAID overdose to reduce the absorption of the administered NSAID. Treatment for gastric ulceration with a proton-pump inhibitor (e.g., omeprazole*), an H_2-receptor

blocker (e.g., ranitidine), or sucralfate should be implemented for horses with gastric ulceration.

Regardless of the site of NSAID toxicity, administration of misoprostol* may be of benefit because administration of a synthetic analog of prostaglandin E_2 has been demonstrated to prevent phenylbutazone-induced gastrointestinal lesions in horses.[655] Misoprostol, a synthetic analog of prostaglandin E_1, can be administered orally starting at doses of 5 μg/kg every 12 hours or 2 μg/kg every 6 hours. Some horses will develop signs of abdominal discomfort or diarrhea at these dosages; another protocol is starting at 1.5 μg/kg every 8 hours for 2 to 4 days and increasing at increments of 0.5 μg/kg every 8 hours every 2 to 4 days until a maintenance dose of 2.5 μg/kg every 8 hours to 3 μg/kg every 8 hours is achieved. Because of the paucity of experimental and clinical data for this drug, dosage schedules should be individually tailored for the horse's illness and tolerance to the drug.

For horses with hypovolemia secondary to colitis, administration of crystalloid fluids is indicated. Infusion of plasma may benefit horses with NSAID-induced enteropathies and signs of endotoxemia. The aim of plasma transfusion in a hypoproteinemic horse with colitis need not be to increase the plasma concentration into the reference range because this may be cost-prohibitive and infused protein may be rapidly lost via the intestinal tract. Smaller volumes of plasma (1 to 3 L in an average-size horse) may exert beneficial effects, perhaps by modulating the effects of endotoxemia. Administration of broad-spectrum antimicrobials may be indicated when signs of endotoxemia are observed. Parenterally administered antimicrobials are preferable to orally administered antimicrobials in horses with colitis because of the presumed increased risk of antimicrobial-associated diarrhea with the oral route. Oral administration of metronidazole (10 to 15 mg/kg PO every 8 to 12 hours) might be an exception to this guideline, because evidence exists that metronidazole may exert an antiinflammatory effect and enhance healing in NSAID-induced intestinal ulceration.[656]

For horses with right dorsal colitis (RDC), dietary management directed toward providing a low-bulk diet in the form of a pelleted concentrated and restricting or eliminating ingestion of roughage is recommended. The aims of this approach are to decrease the mechanical and physiologic load of the colon. A complete pelleted diet (i.e., a diet that contains both concentrate and adequate but relatively low dietary roughage) will decrease intestinal fill in the colon. A diet lower in fiber should decrease the physiologic load of the colon because the cecum and large colon are the primary sites in horses of fiber digestion and exchange of fluid and electrolytes. Concentrate should be fed in smaller amounts and frequently (4 to 6 feedings per day). Some horses will not eat complete pellets, and some horses that have roughage withheld will eat bedding or wood as a consequence. These horses should be allowed to eat fresh grass in small amounts on a frequent basis (4 to 6 times daily). The importance of and optimal duration for restriction of roughage is unknown, but it likely requires months for the colon to heal. Horses should be changed from and returned to their usual diet over a period of several days to decrease the risk of inducing other digestive disorders.

Feeding psyllium mucilloid may promote colonic healing in horses with RDC. In other animal species, psyllium mucilloid has been demonstrated to increase the concentration of short-chain fatty acids of the large bowel, and increased short-chain fatty acids can promote colonic mucosal repair.[657] The amount and duration of psyllium mucilloid administered orally that is required to alter the colonic concentration of short-chain fatty acids and the role of short-chain fatty acids

---

*GastroGard, Merial Ltd., Iselin, NJ 08830.

*Cytotec, Searle and Co., Chicago, IL 60680.

in repair of RDC in horses is unknown. Continuous feeding according to manufacturer's recommendations for 3 to 6 months is suggested, or feeding 1 to 2 oz of psyllium mucilloid once or twice daily for the same duration may be considered.

Horses with strictures of the pylorus, duodenum, jejunum, or colon may require surgical management. Bypass or resection of affected intestinal segments may be necessary.

Limiting the extent of predisposing factors, such as dehydration, should decrease the risk of NSAID toxicosis. Avoiding use of NSAIDs or limiting the dose and duration of treatment to the minimum that is required to control the primary problem is recommended to decrease the risk of NSAID toxicosis. Other approaches to analgesia, such as regional (epidural or perineural nerve blocks of distal limbs) anesthesia or administration of butorphanol,* should be considered.

REFERENCES

643. Taylor JB et al: biochemical and hematological effects of a revised dosage schedule of phenylbutazone in horses, *Vet Rec* 112:599, 602, 1983.
644. Lees P et al: Biochemical and hematological effects of phenylbutazone in horses, *Equine Vet J* 15:158-167, 1983.
645. Cohen ND: Medical management of right dorsal colitis in 5 horses: a retrospective study (1987-1993), *J Vet Int Med* 9:272-276, 1995.
646. Griswold DE, Adams JL: Constitutive cyclooxygenase (COX-1) and inducible cyclooxygenase (COX-2): rationale for selective inhibition and progress to date, *Med Res Rev* 16:181-206, 1996.
647. MacAllister CG et al: Comparison of adverse effects of phenylbutazone, flunixin meglumine, and ketoprofen in horses, *J Am Vet Med Assoc* 202:71-77, 1993.
648. Wallace JL et al: Cyclooxygenase 1 contributes to inflammatory responses in rats and mice: implications for gastrointestinal toxicity, *Gastroenterology* 115:101-109, 1998.
649. McCarthy DM. COX-1 and COX-2 in health and disease, *Proc ACVIM* 17:593, 1999.
650. McCarthy DM: Mechanisms of mucosal injury and healing: the role of non-steroidal anti-inflammatory drugs, *Scand J Gastroenterol* 30(suppl 208):24-29, 1995.
651. Ehnen SJ et al: Obstructive nephrolithiasis and ureterolithiasis associated with chronic renal failure in horses: eight cases (1981-1987), *J Am Vet Med Assoc* 197:249-253, 1990.
652. McCafferty DM, Granger DN, Wallace JL: Indomethacin-induced gastric injury and leukocyte adherence in arthritic versus healthy rats, *Gastroenterology* 109:1173-1180, 1995.
653. Semrad SD et al: Effects of concurrent administration of phenylbutazone and flunixin meglumine on pharmacokinetic variables and in vitro generation of thromboxane B2 in mares, *Am J Vet Res* 54:1901-1905, 1993.
654. East LM et al: Nuclear imaging of right dorsal colitis with Tc-99m hexamethylpropyleneamine oxime (99mTc-HMPOA) labeled white blood cells in two horses, *Proc ACVIM* 17:739, 1999.
655. Collins LG, Tyler DE: Experimentally induced phenylbutazone toxicosis in ponies: description of the syndrome and its prevention with synthetic prostaglandin E2, *Am J Vet Res* 46:1605-1615, 1985.
656. Yamada T et al: Mechanisms of acute and chronic intestinal inflammation induced by indomethacin, *Inflammation* 17:641-662, 1993.
657. Fahey GC: Dietary fiber: definition and influence on enteric physiology, colonic proliferation, and inflammatory mediators, *Proc ACVIM*, 1994, pp 536-538.

*Torbugesic, Fort Dodge Animal Health, Fort Dodge, IA 50501.

FLUID THERAPY FOR HORSES WITH GASTROINTESTINAL DISEASES

KEVIN CORLEY

PRINCIPLES OF FLUID THERAPY

The primary goal of fluid therapy is to increase cardiac output by increasing and then maintaining cardiac preload (Starling's Law of the heart). This in turn increases oxygen delivery to the tissues. By varying the electrolyte content of fluids, it is also possible to correct electrolyte and acid-base disturbances.

Formulating a Fluid Therapy Plan

Fluid therapy should be based on an estimation of the horse's percent dehydration, an assessment of the severity of ongoing losses, and any laboratory information available. The plan should consist of a type of fluid, a rate of administration, and an appropriate delivery system. It should also include a schedule of monitoring the effects of the fluid therapy and adjusting as necessary. It is important to consider the practicality of administering fluids in the environmental conditions (e.g., fluids may freeze in cold weather). In horses that are going to be referred from the field, the impact of any delay associated with fluid therapy should be weighed against the perceived benefit, particularly when only small volumes can be administered. The most important part of successful fluid therapy is to frequently adjust the plan according to the patient's response.

Identifying Patients Requiring Fluid Therapy

Gastrointestinal conditions of horses that result in great fluid loss, such as high-volume diarrhea and gastric reflux, obviously require aggressive fluid therapy. However, many other horses with gastrointestinal disease may require fluid therapy because of prolonged mild to moderate fluid losses or prolonged reduced fluid intake. It is the identification of these horses that this section addresses.

CLINICAL SIGNS. The clinical signs of dehydration are listed in Table 30-1. Using these clinical signs it is possible to estimate the fluid deficit of the animal, which is estimated as a percentage of bodyweight (Table 30-1). This percentage is used to estimate the current fluid requirements. For exam-

---

TABLE 30-1

Estimating Percent Dehydration in Adult Horses

Approximate Percentage Dehydration	Skin Tent (Seconds)	Mucous Membranes	Capillary Refill Time	Heart Rate (Pain May Also Increase Heart Rate)	Other Signs
5%	1-3	Moist or slightly tacky	Normal (<2 sec)	Normal	Decreased urine output
8%	3-5	Tacky	Variable Often 2-3 seconds	40-60 beats/min	Decreased arterial blood pressure
10-12%	5 or more	Dry	Variable Often >4 seconds	60 beats/min or greater	Reduced jugular fill Barely detectable peripheral pulse Sunken eyes

Note that not all signs are consistently present in all horses.

ple, a 500-kg horse with 5% dehydration requires 25 L of fluid. The smallest deficit that is detectable clinically is an estimated 5% dehydration, and dehydration of 15% or more is not compatible with life. It is important to assess all of these clinical signs and make a judgement on the fluid status based on the whole patient. For example, tachycardia in horses with colic may be due to pain or hypovolemia. Clinical signs and response to analgesics or fluid loading may help differentiate the two.

LABORATORY INDICATORS OF DEHYDRATION. The most commonly used laboratory tests to assess dehydration are packed cell volume (PCV) and plasma total solids. Unfortunately these tests are neither sensitive nor specific. The PCV may be substantially increased by splenic contraction in the horse, making small increases very hard to interpret. A PCV of greater than 50% usually represents dehydration, and in most cases indicates at least 7% dehydration. Plasma total solids (protein measured by refractometer) or total protein (measured by a chemistry analyzer) concentration also increases with dehydration. However, significant protein loss can occur in gastrointestinal disease (particularly with colitis), resulting in a low or normal protein concentration despite dehydration. Further, hypergammaglobulinemia (e.g., in cyathostomiasis) can increase the plasma total protein concentration without the presence of dehydration. The PCV and plasma total solids are most useful when greatly increased or when used serially to monitor the response to fluid therapy.

Urine specific gravity can easily be measured in the field. High urine specific gravities (>1.040) indicate possible dehydration and normal renal concentration of urine. Isothenuria (1.010) indicates possible renal damage or a recent high fluid load. Urine specific gravity is useful to monitor the response to fluid therapy because rising or continually high specific gravity in the face of fluid therapy may indicate that insufficient fluid is being delivered to the horse.

Plasma or serum creatinine concentrations are useful to assess hydration status in the absence of renal dysfunction. High normal (1.5 to 1.8 mg/dl; 130 to 160 µmol/L) creatinine concentrations can be associated with subclinical dehydration, and should be evaluated in light of the history and clinical signs. Creatinine concentrations up to 3.5 mg/dl (310 µmol/L) are common with moderate to severe dehydration, and concentrations as high as 5.0 mg/dl (450 µmol/L) are possible with prolonged dehydration. Even in severe dehydration, the creatinine concentration will not increase by much more than 2.3 mg/dl (200 µmol/L) per day.[658] If the creatinine concentration is higher than would be suggested by the clinical signs and other laboratory parameters and if the creatinine concentration does not decrease appropriately with fluid therapy, renal dysfunction should be suspected.

Increased blood lactate concentrations in the non-exercising horse are sufficient evidence of a metabolic disturbance to initiate fluid therapy. Blood lactate concentrations are an indicator of tissue perfusion. The most common causes of increased lactate in the horse with gastrointestinal disease are endotoxemia, which can increase tissue lactate production by inappropriate anaerobic metabolism, and dehydration. Increased blood lactate concentration has been associated with worse outcomes in equine colic.[659] Lactate can be measured in the field by handheld blood gas analyzers.* The expected lactate concentration can also be calculated by means of equations (see p. 688) based on electrolyte and acid-base measurements. An increased circulating lactate concentration should be suspected in a metabolic acidosis (de-creased pH, negative base excess) in the absence of hyperchloremia or hyponatremia.[660]

CARDIAC FILLING PRESSURES. Cardiac filling pressures and the changes in these pressures in response to fluids are the most accurate method of determining fluid requirements in the hospitalized animal. It is relatively easy to measure central venous pressure in the horse. A piece of sterile polyethylene tubing (PE 190, outside diameter 1.7 mm, at least 1.5 m long) can be passed through a 12-gauge jugular catheter into the thoracic vena cava or right atrium. The catheter is connected to a pressure transducer or manometer at the level of the sternal manubrium.[661] The normal central venous pressure of the horse is 5 to 14 mmHg.[661] In a horse with normal cardiac function, a high central venous pressure indicates fluid overloading and a low central venous pressure indicates insufficient circulating volume. Perhaps more accurate is the change in central venous pressure in response to a fluid challenge (bolus of fluids),[662] but this has not been evaluated in the horse. The fluid challenge method of monitoring fluid therapy may prove to be particularly useful when factors such as acute renal failure or pulmonary edema complicate the gastrointestinal disease.

TYPES OF FLUIDS

Crystalloids

For most situations in the field, commercial isotonic polyionic crystalloid solutions are the safest fluids to resuscitate dehydrated adult horses. They increase plasma volume without causing profound electrolyte disturbances, because they contain approximately the same electrolyte concentrations as plasma. It also follows that polyionic crystalloid solutions are often not sufficient to correct electrolyte imbalances (see p. 687). Isotonic (0.9%) sodium chloride has a higher ratio of chloride to sodium than plasma and therefore causes a mild hyperchloremic acidosis in normal ponies.[663] Isotonic sodium chloride should not be used for resuscitation unless indicated by measured electrolyte abnormalities. Sodium chloride solution has been advocated in hyperkalemia, in order to avoid the potassium containing polyionic fluids. In adult horses with gastrointestinal disturbances, hyperkalemia is likely to reflect acidosis and polyionic fluids are probably most appropriate.

Two classes of polyionic fluids are available, those for resuscitation and those for maintenance. Maintenance fluids (Normosol-M*, Plasma-lyte M†, etc.) contain higher potassium and lower sodium and chloride concentrations than resuscitation fluids (Normosol-R*, Plasma-lyte 148†, Isolec§, lactated Ringer's solution†, etc.). However, maintenance fluids are not currently commercially available in sizes greater than 1 L. This has led to the practice of adding potassium chloride (at 10 to 20 mEq/L) to resuscitation formulas to use as maintenance fluids in equine medicine.

The different alkalizing agents (or "bicarbonate substitutes") in resuscitation fluids are clinically relevant. The alkalizing agent in plasma is bicarbonate. Bicarbonate-containing fluids are unstable when stored and may result in profound metabolic alkalosis. Therefore Hartmann, an American pediatrician, replaced the bicarbonate with lactate to make lactated Ringer's solution (Hartmann's solution). Lactate is metabolized in the liver, but this process is slow enough to avoid the rapid changes in plasma pH seen with bicarbonate. Sodium bicarbonate and sodium lactate both

*i-STAT, Heska, Fort Collins, Colorado.

*Abbott Laboratories, North Chicago, IL.
†Baxter Healthcare Corporation, Deerfield, IL.
§Ivex Division, Galen Holdings plc, Larne, Northern Ireland.

increase the strong ion difference resulting in a metabolic alkalosis. The cation (sodium) remains in the extracellular fluid while the anion (bicarbonate or lactate) is metabolized.[664] It is the speed of metabolism of the anion and the renal excretion of sodium that determines the ultimate alkalinizing effect. It may seem counter-intuitive to administer lactate-containing fluids to a horse with lactic acidosis resulting from poor tissue perfusion. However, clinical trials in human patients in hemorrhagic shock have shown that lactate-containing fluids do not exacerbate the lactic acidosis of hypoperfusion.[665] It appears that in shock the liver's capacity for metabolizing lactate is not overwhelmed, but the delivery of lactate by the circulation to the liver is impaired. Restoring the circulating volume, even with fluids containing moderate amounts of lactate, is sufficient to allow the liver to clear the circulating lactate. In horses with liver disease, which may have impaired lactate metabolism, lactated Ringer's solution should be used with caution. Alternative alkalizing agents to lactate are found in some commercial polyionic fluids (e.g., acetate and gluconate in Normosol-R). Acetate is metabolized by the muscles and gluconate by a variety of tissues throughout the body. Lactated Ringers' solution contains calcium whereas Normosol-R contains magnesium. Calcium is incompatible with whole blood and sodium bicarbonate and is contraindicated in hypercalcemia; therefore fluids containing magnesium can be used in more clinical situations than those containing calcium.

Five-percent dextrose (D_5W) is used to replace water without accompanying electrolytes, and is effectively hypotonic because the dextrose is rapidly metabolized. It is indicated in cases in which fluid loss exceeds electrolyte loss, which can occur in strangulating intestinal lesions and colitis[666] Horses receiving D_5W should be monitored carefully, because rapid administration can lead to hyperglycemia. If the plasma glucose concentration exceeds the renal threshold (approximately 180mg/dl), an osmotic diuresis will result, which can reduce the benefit of the fluid administration. D_5W should not be considered a form of parenteral nutrition. To provide 11.5 Mcal/day, the maintenance requirement for a 500-kg horse standing in a stall,[667] it would be necessary to administer 67.6 L of D_5W per day, which would result in serious electrolyte abnormalities. Although the glucose in D_5W may be helpful in the initial stages of resuscitation in foals, it is best to use 50% dextrose solution (or total parenteral nutrition solutions) for nutritional support in addition to appropriate crystalloid solutions to meet fluid and electrolyte requirements.

Sodium bicarbonate has been advocated for correction of the acid-base disturbances associated with equine gastrointestinal disease. However, its use in lactic acidosis is controversial, and it should probably be reserved for use in hyponatremia without hypochloremia and for renal tubular acidosis manifested by hyperchloremia without accompanying hypernatremia.[660] Both of these electrolyte disturbances occur occasionally in horses with severe colitis. Sodium bicarbonate should be avoided in horses with respiratory dysfunction, because the bicarbonate is converted to carbon dioxide which, if it is not excreted by the lungs, leads to an increase in plasma carbon dioxide tension and further acidosis.[660]

Homemade or "Carboy" fluids, although considerably cheaper than commercial fluids, have been associated with clinical signs of endotoxemia in normal horses[668] and a sevenfold increase in the risk of thrombophlebitis[669] and thus cannot be recommended.

Hypertonic Saline and Colloids

The large volumes of isotonic fluids required for resuscitation in the horse and the fact that only approximately 30% of the administered fluid remains in the circulation after 30 minutes[670] have prompted the search for alternative fluids. Hypertonic saline and colloid solutions have received the most attention.

Hypertonic saline (2 to 4 ml/kg of 7% to 7.5% NaCl) has been advocated as a method of quickly restoring circulating volume in shock patients. Administration of 7% sodium chloride results in an increase in the extracellular fluid of 2 to 3 times the infused volume for at least 60 minutes after it is infused. This is the result of fluid shifts from the interstitial fluid, principally from the muscle and liver[671] without significant fluid replacement. Hypertonic saline should always be followed by large volumes (at least 10 L for each liter of hypertonic saline) of isotonic polyionic crystalloids within 2.5 hours (the point in experimental studies when cardiac output begins to fall below baseline).[672] As well as restoring plasma volume, hypertonic saline reduces the capillary endothelial swelling that may occur as part of the systemic inflammatory response syndrome and therefore improves tissue microcirculation and oxygen delivery.[673]

Administration of 5 ml/kg hypertonic saline solution immediately after experimental endotoxin infusion in horses was found to attenuate the cardiovascular derangements associated with endotoxemia more effectively than an equivalent volume of isotonic saline.[672] However, the effects of hypertonic saline administration in clinical equine cases have not been published and may be less favorable than in experimental conditions. Hypertonic saline should be used with caution during resuscitation in equine colic and colitis, despite the positive experimental evidence for its use in endotoxemia, because these conditions may be associated with significant dehydration. Resuscitation of dehydrated experimental animals with hypertonic saline resulted in decreased survival and renal dysfunction.[674] Given the beneficial effects of hypertonic saline in experimental endotoxemia and sepsis, it may have a role after initial fluid resuscitation. However, treatment of endotoxic horses with hypertonic saline following fluid resuscitation has not been clinically evaluated.

Combination of dextran 70 (a colloid) with hypertonic saline resulted in acceptable resuscitation in experimental dehydration.[675,676] In the horse, however, hypertonic saline-dextran 70 administration can cause clinically apparent intravascular hemolysis and hemoglobinuria.[677] The combination of hetastarch (10 ml/kg) and hypertonic saline (4 ml/kg) may be an appropriate solution for resuscitation of clinically dehydrated horses, especially in severe colitis, but this has been not been formally evaluated in clinical or experimental cases.

Colloids, particularly hetastarch, have recently been advocated for resuscitation and treatment of severe hypoproteinemia in horses.[678] Colloids contain large branched molecules (450-kD average molecular weight for hetastarch, compared with 69-kD for albumin). These molecules exert a large colloidal oncotic pressure and do not readily leak out of the vasculature and thus hold water in the circulation. Endotoxin[679] and ischemia-reperfusion injury[680] induce capillary damage, which allows plasma albumin to leak out into the interstitium. The large colloid molecules may not leak as readily, allowing their oncotic pressure to draw fluid back into the vasculature. They may also plug the gaps in the capillary endothelium. However, if the capillary damage is severe enough, even the larger colloids may leak into the interstitium and exert their oncotic pressure to draw fluid with them.

In normal ponies, hetastarch was safe but prolonged bleeding times at 20 ml/kg.[681] Although hetastarch has been used clinically in horses,[678] it is still unclear whether its use alters morbidity or mortality. A recent metaanalysis of randomized trials of colloid administration in human critical care patients demonstrated no advantage of colloids compared with crys-

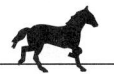

talloids and suggested increased mortality with the use of colloids in some clinical syndromes.[682] The majority of the studies examined in this metaanalysis used albumin rather than hetastarch as the colloid. This research should therefore serve as a note of caution, rather than as a reason to avoid the use of hetastarch in horses. When using colloids, the plasma total solids or total protein concentration is no longer a useful guide to hydration status or plasma oncotic pressure.[678]

Fresh frozen equine plasma has been used extensively in horses with diarrhea. Although classically prescribed for hypoalbuminemia, its utility for replacing protein is unclear. At least 6 to 8 L are required in adult horses to treat clinically significant hypoproteinemia,[683] and the effects may be short-lived. Plasma administration does not have the advantage of the larger colloids of potentially drawing fluid back into the circulation in damaged capillaries, but it may prevent generalized edema arising from low oncotic pressure. Plasma may have a role in replacing antithrombin III and other cofactors that are depleted during the systemic inflammatory response syndrome. This has led to its continued use in diarrhea cases, with apparently favorable results.

Oral Fluid Therapy

It is possible to effectively treat mildly dehydrated horses with oral replacement solutions.[684] Oral fluids do not need to be sterile and are therefore considerably cheaper than intravenous fluids. It is apparently not necessary to add glucose to oral fluids for the horse,[685] but electrolytes should be added if feasible. It is important to administer hypotonic or isotonic fluids.[685] A possible isotonic solution consists of 4.9 g/L table salt and 4.9 g/L Lite salt* to give final concentrations of 123 mmol/L sodium, 34 mmol/L potassium, and 157 mmol/L chloride.[685] If using sodium chloride alone, no more than 9 g should be added per liter. The fluids should be given via a stomach tube to allow measured quantities to be given. The amount given at one time should not exceed 8 to 10 L in a 500-kg horse, with at least 20 minutes between each administration. Before each dose, the stomach should be refluxed and the administration delayed if more than 2 L of fluid are recovered. Some horses will show abdominal pain if large volumes of fluids are given, especially if the fluids are cold. Oral fluids can be a successful adjunct or alternative to intravenous fluids in many mildly dehydrated horses with pelvic flexure impactions. Unfortunately, no protocol has been found to be effective for moderately to severely dehydrated horses. Rapid administration of oral fluids (8 L every 30 minutes) resulted in incomplete fluid absorption and commercially available oral rehydration solutions may not be ideal for fluid replacement in gastrointestinal diseases of horses.[686] In horses with gastrointestinal disease but no apparent dehydration, administration of an electrolyte paste and provision of fresh drinking water may be sufficient to supplement water and electrolytes.[687]

Parenteral Nutrition

Any therapeutic plan in the horse should include a nutritional plan. An enteral diet based on the horse's normal diet is the first choice for nutritional support. However, in adult horses with gastric reflux, ileus, esophageal obstruction and anorexia, parenteral nutrition should be considered if the interruption to enteral feeding is predicted to last at least 3 days.[688] The use of parenteral nutrition may be especially indicated in acute protein-losing enteropathy, in which its use may prolong the oncotic effects of exogenously administered

plasma, possibly by preventing plasma albumin from being metabolized for energy. Total parenteral nutrition solutions commonly consist of dextrose, amino acids, lipids, and a vitamin/mineral mix. The estimated energy requirement of a normal adult horse standing in a stall is calculated by the following equation[667]:

Energy requirement (Mcal/day) =
$$0.975 + (0.021 \times \text{Bodyweight [in kg]})$$

The protein requirements are calculated by the following equation[667]:

Protein requirement (Digestible protein in g/day) =
$$18 \times \text{Energy requirement (in Mcal/day)}$$

Both of these requirements are increased in disease (for example by 25% to 50% in sepsis).[667] The formulation of parenteral nutrition solutions is described elsewhere.[688] Although there is much anecdotal evidence that parenteral nutrition (as opposed to no nutrition) may be beneficial in adult horses with gastrointestinal disorders, it has not been formally studied. The administration of parenteral nutrition increases the risk of thrombophlebitis and sepsis in hospitalized human patients.[689]

FLUID THERAPY DELIVERY SYSTEMS

In the early resuscitation period of moderately to severely dehydrated horses, it is important to use both a large-gauge catheter and a wide-bore sterile delivery system to be able to provide the fast fluid rates required. A 10- to 12-gauge catheter is recommended for severely dehydrated adult horses and a 12- to 14-gauge catheter for moderately dehydrated horses. Moderately dehydrated weanlings and miniature horses can be treated with 14- to 16-gauge catheters. It is necessary to use a large-bore extension set with a large-gauge catheter.

To place a catheter, the hair should be clipped over the vein and the area should be given a surgical scrub, ideally with a chlorhexidine scrub solution.[690] The catheter should be handled and placed with sterile gloves. In young and refractory horses a bleb of local anesthetic placed subcutaneously in the area to be catheterized makes catheterization easier. The sterile scrub should be repeated after the local anesthetic. With 10-gauge and Seldinger ("over the wire") catheters and when local anesthetic is used, a small stab incision through the skin can also be helpful. For fluid therapy the catheter should be directed toward the heart. The catheter should be flushed with heparinized saline (5 U/ml) and fixed with either instant bonding glue (for short-term use) or suture.

The easiest vein to catheterize in the horse is the external jugular vein. The cephalic and the lateral thoracic veins may also be catheterized and carry less serious consequences if they become occluded by thrombophlebitis. However, the maximum fluid rate attainable in these smaller veins (approximately 5 L/hr) is less than with the jugular vein and infectious thrombophlebitis may be serious in any site. If one jugular vein is thrombosed or occluded, it is certainly prudent not to catheterize the contralateral jugular vein because life-threatening head swelling can result from bilateral jugular thrombosis. Both the cephalic and the lateral thoracic vein can be technically difficult to catheterize. Good sedation is required to catheterize the cephalic vein because horses have a tendency to move during catheter placement. The lateral thoracic vein can be difficult to identify and has a flat profile, which can make it difficult to pass the catheter into the lumen. The vein can be identified by ultrasonography and is probably best catheterized using the Seldinger (over the wire) technique. In both of these veins, valves can impede the passing of the catheter stylet or wire.

---

*Morton Salt, Chicago, IL.

TABLE 30-2

Flow Rate Chart: Drops Per 10 Seconds for Various Flow Rates

Bag Size/ Flow Time	Flow Rate (L/hr)	STAT Set* (Drops/10 sec)	Straight Set, Single Spike† (Drops/10 sec)	Coil Set, Single Spike‡ (Drops/10 sec)	Six Spike Set§ (Drops/10 sec)	10 Solution Set‖ (Drops/10 sec)	Mini (60) Set‖ (Drops/10 sec)
5 L/1 hr	5	150				138	—
5 L/1.5 hr	3.33	100				92	—
5 L/2 hr	2.5	75				69	—
5 L/3 hr	1.66	50	32			46	—
5 L/4 hr	1.25	38	23	25		35	—
5 L/5 hr	1	30	21	24	29	28	—
1 L/1 hr	1	30	21	24	29	28	167
1 L/1.5 hr	0.75	—	15	17	21	21	125
1 L/2 hr	0.5	—	11	11	13	14	83
1 L/3 hr	0.33	—	9	8	12	9	55
1 L/4 hr	0.25	—	7	7	11	7	42
1 L/5 hr	0.2	—	6	5	10	—	33
1 L/6 hr	0.16	—	4	4	5	—	28

Part of the data for this table was kindly supplied by William Tan, R&D, Cook Medical Technology.
*Stat Large Animal IV Set, International WIN, Kennett Square, Pennsylvania.
†V-LACT-24-200-S-C-EC1, Cook Veterinary Products, Spencer, Indiana.
‡V-LACT-24-450-S-C-EC2, Cook Veterinary Products, Spencer, Indiana.
§V-LACT-14-60-6S-C-EA3, Cook Veterinary Products, Spencer, Indiana.
‖Baxter Healthcare Corp., Deerfield, Illinois.

Various fluid administration sets are commercially available. Sets that include large-bore tubing and a coil are suitable for most situations in adult horses and are recommended. The flow rate can be estimated by counting the number of drips per 10 seconds in the drip chamber (Table 30-2) or can be set by using an electronic fluid pump. In all situations a record should be kept of the time the infusion was started to ensure that the desired volume is being delivered in the appropriate time.

The frequency of replacement of catheters and administration sets depends on local environmental conditions and the catheter material. Catheters made from polytetrafluoroethylene (Teflon) are associated with an increased incidence of thrombophlebitis and have a tendency to crack and kink.[691] These catheters should not be left in for longer than 72 hours. In contrast, soft catheters made from polyurethane or silicone rubber can often be safely left in place for at least 14 days when properly monitored.[691] These catheters should only be replaced when there is a suspected problem, and in some horses they have been maintained for as long as 6 weeks. It is unclear how frequently administration sets should be replaced when used in a horse barn. The current Centers for Disease Control recommendations for human hospitals is not to replace administration sets more frequently than every 72 hours, except when used to administer blood or lipid-containing parenteral nutrition, in which case they should be changed every 24 hours.[692]

Indwelling cecal catheters have been proposed for fluid therapy in horses, without the expense of sterile fluids. Unfortunately, although it is possible to deliver fluid by this technique, the high rate of serious complications precludes the use of cecal catheters.[693] For repeated administration of oral fluids, an indwelling nasogastric tube may be placed, which should be plugged with a syringe barrel between administrations to prevent excessive air influx. Some horses will not tolerate a large-bore nasogastric tube, and an adult feeding tube* can be sometimes used successfully in its place.

*18-Fr Equine Enteral Feeding Tube, Ross Laboratories, Columbus, Ohio.

RATES OF ADMINISTRATION AND VOLUME TO INFUSE

There are two phases to fluid therapy—initial resuscitation and maintenance therapy. The resuscitation phase aims to rapidly restore current fluid deficits, and the maintenance phase aims to prevent occurrence of further fluid deficits. Correction of electrolyte imbalances usually takes place during the maintenance phase.

Resuscitation

In most adult horses the estimated fluid deficit should be replaced as rapidly as possible, usually within 2 hours. Thus any horse with detectable dehydration should receive at least 5% of its bodyweight as fluid over 2 hours. An exception is with uncontrolled hemorrhage, such as horses with hemoperitoneum presenting for colic, in which more conservative fluid volumes should be used until the hemorrhage is stopped.[694,695] In horses without hemorrhage or with controlled hemorrhage, it is probably advisable not to exceed 60 to 80 ml/kg/hr with crystalloid solutions, based on experimental work in other species.[696] This represents 30 to 40 L/hr for a 500-kg horse, a rate that is difficult to achieve. In adult horses with 10% to 12% dehydration, both jugular veins may be catheterized with large-bore catheters (10 to 12 gauge), which allows approximately 35 L/hr to be administered by gravity if a wide-bore administration set (for example arthroscopy tubing) is used. One of the jugular catheters should be removed immediately after the initial resuscitation phase is over, to reduce the risk of bilateral jugular vein thrombosis. A fluid pump may also be used to achieve high rates of fluid delivery, but the high pressures may cause damage to the intima of the vein and increase the risk of thrombosis. If colloid fluids are being used for initial resuscitation, 1 L should be used to replace each 3 to 4 L of crystalloid. The amount of hetastarch infused should not exceed 10 ml/kg.[681]

Maintenance

The maintenance phase of fluid therapy aims to supply the basal fluid requirement of the horse ("maintenance" rate)

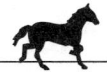

TABLE 30-3

Fluids of Choice for Specific Metabolic Disturbances

Metabolic Disturbance	Recommended Fluid	Dose
Lactic acidosis	Polyionic crystalloids (Normosol-R, lactated Ringer's solution) or	Up to 60 ml/kg/hr
	Hetastarch	Up to 10 ml/kg/hr
Hyponatremia		
with hypochloremia	Sodium chloride	Sodium should be corrected no faster than 1 mEq/L/hr
without hypochloremia	Sodium bicarbonate	
Hypernatremia	5% dextrose or	To lower sodium no faster than 0.5 mEq/L/hr
	2.5% dextrose/0.45% sodium chloride	
Hypochloremia	Sodium chloride	0.9% or 7.5%, to effect
Hyperchloremia		
with hypernatremia	5% dextrose	To lower sodium no faster than 0.5 mEq/L/hr
without hypernatremia	Sodium bicarbonate	5%, slowly, to effect
Hypokalemia	Potassium chloride	0.2 to 0.5 mEq/kg/hr, never to exceed 1 mEq/kg/hr
Hyperkalemia		
with clinical signs	Calcium gluconate	1 ml/kg IV over 10 min
or >7 mEq/L	Sodium bicarbonate	1-2 mEq/L IV over 15 min
	50% dextrose solution	2 ml/kg IV over 5 min
without clinical signs	Polyionic crystalloid fluids	
Hypocalcemia	Calcium gluconate	Typically require 100-300 ml of 23% solution
Hypercalcemia	Non–calcium-containing polyionic fluids	
	Magnesium sulfate IV	4-16 mg/kg as an initial dose
Hypomagnesemia	Magnesium sulfate IV	4-16 mg/kg as an initial dose
	Magnesium oxide PO	8-32 mg/kg as an initial dose
Hypermagnesemia	Calcium gluconate	250-500 ml of 23% solution
Hypoalbuminemia	Fresh or fresh frozen equine plasma	To effect
	Hetastarch	Not to exceed 10 ml/kg

and replace ongoing fluid losses. The mean daily water intake (including water content of feed) of normal resting adult horses is 57 ml/kg/day[697] to 64 ml/kg/day[698] at ambient temperatures of 41 to 77° F (5 to 25° C). Although this may not strictly represent the minimal fluid requirements, it is the usual figure quoted as the "maintenance rate" (2.5 ml/kg/hr) for adult horses. Thus a 500-kg horse requires approximately 30 L of fluid per day for maintenance, in addition to fluids to replace any ongoing losses. Significant ongoing fluid losses occur in horses with diarrhea, continued nasogastric reflux, polyuric renal failure, and profuse sweating. With diarrhea, continued fluid losses may be as high as 200 ml/kg/day (100 L per day for a 500-kg horse).[699] Thus a horse with severe diarrhea might require approximately 260 ml/kg/day (approximately 5.5 L/hr for a 500-kg horse) of crystalloid fluids to provide basal requirements and replace ongoing losses. Horses with less frequent or less watery diarrhea will require less fluid. The rate should be estimated based on the volume and consistency of the diarrhea, and the adequacy of the rate should be frequently reassessed based on clinical and laboratory data. In horses with significant nasogastric reflux, the amount of reflux should be measured and should be directly replaced with intravenous fluids, together with the maintenance requirements. Again the adequacy of the fluid therapy should be frequently monitored. With large urinary fluid losses, as in polyuric renal failure, the amount of urine should be measured or estimated and replaced. In horses with little feed intake or fecal output, serial bodyweight measurements can be useful to monitor fluid losses, replacement, and retention.

A more precise method of ensuring adequate fluid resuscitation and replacement of ongoing losses is to repeatedly measure the response of central venous pressure to fluid therapy as described above, but this is probably only practical in the hospital situation.

FLUID THERAPY, ACID-BASE, AND ELECTROLYTE DISTURBANCES

The rate of delivery and volume infused is only part of developing a fluid therapy plan, albeit the most important one in acute resuscitation. The effect of the fluids on the electrolyte and acid-base status of the horse should also be considered and fluids chosen to help correct physiologic disturbances (Table 30-3). Unfortunately it is not possible to accurately predict electrolyte and acid-base disturbances based on clinical signs because seemingly similar clinical conditions may have quite different physiologic disturbances.[700] This limits the ability of the field veterinarian to monitor and treat these disturbances, although the recent availability of relatively inexpensive, portable blood gas and electrolyte measuring equipment has made determining the acid-base status a possibility in ambulatory equine practice. As stated earlier, in the absence of specific laboratory information, fluid therapy should probably be limited to isotonic polyionic crystalloid fluids, possibly with 10 to 20 mEq/L potassium chloride added in the maintenance phase.

When laboratory information is available within 4 to 6 hours, fluid therapy can be tailored to the individual horse allowing correction of specific physiologic disturbances. Although calculations of whole body electrolyte or base deficits are possible, their relevance to managing the clinical case with ongoing losses and renal responses to changes in plasma electrolyte concentrations is unclear.[701] A safer and more physiologically relevant approach is to frequently monitor clinical and laboratory responses to therapy and adjust treatment accordingly, rather than rely on a calculated electrolyte dose to restore normality.

The most common acid-base disturbance in horses with gastrointestinal disease is metabolic acidosis, which results from lactic acidosis (hypovolemia, endotoxemia), hyponatremia (colitis, peritonitis, intestinal torsion), or hyperchloremia (occasionally seen in colitis cases). Metabolic alkalosis, resulting from hypochloremia (high volume gastric reflux) or hypoalbuminemia (severe enterocolitis, excessive fluid therapy), respiratory alkalosis (hyperventilation resulting from pain), and respiratory acidosis (hypoventilation resulting from extreme abdominal distension, central depression) can also occur.[660]

Although the predominant clinical signs in horses with acid-base disturbances are likely to result from the cause of the disturbance, clinical signs can arise from the physiologic consequences of the derangement. Metabolic acidosis can result in reduced cardiac contractility, constriction of the peripheral vasculature, inhibition of glycolysis, a decrease in oxygen uptake by hemoglobin in the lungs, and CNS depression. Metabolic alkalosis can lead to overexcitability of nervous tissue, blunting of the hypoxic drive, compensatory hypoventilation, susceptibility to cardiac arrhythmias, and inhibition of oxygen release in the tissues.

Treatment of acid-base disturbances should be directed at the underlying cause and the specific plasma constituent imbalance. It is possible to determine the relative contributions of unidentified anions (principally lactate in horses with gastrointestinal disturbances), sodium, chloride, and protein to the measured acid-base status by the use of equations based on the calculated base excess.[660,702] However, decisions for treatment can often be based on the absolute values of these blood constituents, and it is only in complex disturbances with changes in multiple blood constituents that the equations are usually necessary.

Lactate

As discussed above, increased blood or plasma lactate concentrations usually are due to poor tissue perfusion in gastrointestinal diseases, but may also be due to inappropriate anaerobic metabolism in endotoxemia. The clinical signs of lactemia are those of the accompanying metabolic acidosis, but the signs of the cause of the lactic acidosis (those of shock) may predominate.

Although lactate can be directly measured, its plasma concentration can be accurately predicted by the anion gap in horses with normal plasma protein concentrations.[703] The anion gap is calculated from the plasma concentrations of (sodium + potassium) minus the concentrations of (chloride + bicarbonate). The normal range is 7 to 15 mEq/L.[703] At low and high protein concentrations the equations based on base excess,[660,702] or the simplified strong ion gap (= 2.24 × Total protein (g/dl)/$(1 + 10^{6.65\text{-}pH})$ − Anion gap)[703] should be used. Any of these calculations may easily be performed on a pocket calculator.

Lactic acidosis should be treated with large volumes of polyionic crystalloid solutions. The use of sodium bicarbonate in lactic acidosis is highly controversial.[704] It corrects the laboratory value (pH), without addressing the underlying pathophysiology (poor tissue perfusion) by imposing a hypernatremic alkalosis on an already deranged metabolic balance. Although increasing the pH may improve myocardial contractility, this effect may be negated by the myocardial depressant effects of an increased carbon dioxide tension.[705] In

endotoxic ponies, administration of sodium bicarbonate resulted in an increased blood lactate concentration, hypernatremia, hypokalemia, and hyperosmolality.[706]

Sodium

Low plasma sodium concentrations are most commonly seen in acute colitis, such as salmonellosis, Potomac horse fever, and clostridiosis. The hyponatremia is usually accompanied by hypochloremia resulting from an increased loss of electrolytes relative to water.[666] Other gastrointestinal conditions associated with hyponatremia are those that result in third-space loss of sodium (peritonitis, torsion, or volvulus of gut) and sodium-wasting disorders (esophageal obstruction leading to loss of saliva). The clinical signs of hyponatremia are neurologic disturbance, including reduced or absent menace response, intention tremor, and hypermetric gait,[707] but severe clinical signs do not usually occur until the sodium concentration is less than 110 mEq/L.[708] Hyponatremia will also result in a metabolic acidosis.[660]

The fluid choice for hyponatremia depends on whether there is a concurrent hypochloremia. If the plasma chloride concentration is also low, sodium chloride should be used. If the chloride concentration is normal or increased (which is rare in gastrointestinal disease), then sodium bicarbonate should be administered. If the horse is not clinically dehydrated[674] and the hyponatremia is severe, then hypertonic solutions may be administered initially (7 to 7.5% sodium chloride and 5 to 8.4% sodium bicarbonate, respectively). Rapid correction of sodium deficits in other species can cause central pontine myelinosis.[708] It is unclear whether this is a risk in the horse and therefore whether it is necessary to follow the guidelines for sodium restoration in other species. These guidelines state that sodium should be corrected at a rate of 1 mEq/L/hr in acute hyponatremia and at less than 0.5 mEq/L/hr in chronic hyponatremia, in neither case to exceed 8 mEq/L during the first 24 hours.[708]

Hypernatremia is rare in horses with gastrointestinal disease[666,700] and is usually due to water loss in excess of electrolytes and accompanied by hyperchloremia. To correct hypernatremia, low sodium fluids such as 5% dextrose or 2.5% dextrose/0.45% sodium chloride should be administered. Again, in other species, it is recommended not to correct hypernatremia too rapidly: Sodium should be lowered by 0.5 mEq/L/hr, not to exceed 12 mEq/L over the first 24 hours.[708]

Clinical signs associated with hyponatremia and hypernatremia are due to changes in plasma osmolality. Sodium is the major cation in plasma, and sodium and glucose concentrations are the main determinants of plasma osmolality.[666] Changes in plasma osmolality can lead to central nervous system edema or dehydration, resulting in neurologic signs.[709] Rapid changes in plasma sodium concentration may also cause central nervous system edema or dehydration, because the cerebrospinal fluid slowly equilibrates with the plasma but will rapidly change if osmotic gradients are high.

Chloride

Hypochloremia is common in gastrointestinal disease[700] because loss of gastric hydrochloric acid in high-volume reflux (in proximal enteritis and grass sickness) and secretion or lack of absorption of chloride in severe colitis. Hypochloremia in the absence of hyponatremia results in metabolic alkalosis.[660] The alkalosis associated with hypochloremia may also result in increased cellular uptake of potassium, leading to hypokalemia.[708]

Treatment of hypochloremia can usually be achieved with intravenous 0.9% sodium chloride, which contains more

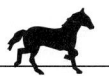

chloride relative to sodium than plasma. In horses with high-volume gastric reflux, administration of intravenous H_2-receptor antagonists (e.g., cimetidine at 6.6 mg/kg IV four times daily) reduces gastric hydrochloric acid secretion and therefore should reduce chloride loss. In humans, intravenous hydrochloric acid has been used to treat severe hypochloremia[710] but carries substantial risks for the patient.[711]

Hyperchloremia is rare in horses with gastrointestinal disease, but may occur in severe colitis as a result of water secretion in excess of electrolytes. It should be treated with 5% dextrose if accompanied by hypernatremia and with sodium bicarbonate if severe and accompanied by a low or normal plasma sodium concentration.[708]

Potassium

Hypokalemia is commonly seen in horses after surgery for colic, because of enhanced mineralocorticoid and glucocorticoid release and infusion of large amounts of sodium-containing fluids that increase distal tubular flow and renal potassium loss.[709] Hypokalemia also occurs in colitis and metabolic alkalosis. The most relevant clinical sign of hypokalemia is reduced intestinal motility.[708,712] However, the association between hypokalemia and ileus remains undetermined in the horse. Other clinical signs include muscle weakness, lethargy, and inability to concentrate urine.[708] Cardiac conduction abnormalities are rare except in severe hypokalemia and in pre-existing cardiac dysfunction.[708] The effect of potassium on acid-base status is small and need not be considered clinically.[660]

Potassium is primarily an intracellular ion and thus decreases in whole body potassium may not be detected by plasma measurements.[713] Although erythrocyte potassium content has been used to estimate whole body potassium,[713] its accuracy is unclear. Moreover, the extracellular potassium concentration (reflected in the plasma) is more relevant to neuromuscular transmission and thus to the important clinical signs than whole body potassium stores.[709] The intervention level for treatment of hypokalemia is unclear. In postoperative colic cases and proximal enteritis, the prevention of ileus is a primary goal and it may be prudent to supplement the plasma potassium concentration below 3.5 mEq/L. In other patients, especially those being fed enterally, it may not be necessary to treat above a plasma potassium concentration of 3.0 mEq/L.

Hypokalemia is treated with intravenous potassium chloride solution. The rate of administration is more important than the amount. The rate should not normally exceed 0.5 mEq/kg/hr and should never exceed 1 mEq/kg/hr.[708] The addition of 40 mEq potassium chloride per liter of crystalloid fluids is safe at rates up to 10ml/kg/hr (5 L/hr for a 500-kg horse). This amount is usually only required in severe hypokalemia (<2.7 mEq/L), and smaller disturbances can often be successfully treated with 20 mEq/L of fluid. If hypokalemia does not respond to potassium chloride administration, magnesium should be supplemented.[714]

Hyperkalemia is not typical in horses with gastrointestinal disease, although it may occur in acidosis, colitis, and secondary renal failure and in horses with hyperkalemic periodic paralysis. Artifactual hyperkalemia may be seen in blood samples stored for longer than 2 hours before plasma separation, as a result of leaching of potassium from the erythrocytes. Clinical signs of hyperkalemia are due to disruption of neuromuscular transmission and are therefore similar to hypokalemia. In the absence of clinical signs, polyionic fluids should be administered. Possible treatments for symptomatic or severe (>7 mEq/L) hyperkalemia include calcium gluconate (1 ml/kg IV over 10 minutes), sodium bicarbonate (1 to 2 mEq/L IV over 15 minutes), and 50% dextrose solution (2 ml/kg IV over 5 minutes).[708]

Calcium

Low plasma ionized calcium concentrations are common in horses with surgical colic[715] and colitis cases. Possible causes of this hypocalcemia include lactic acidosis,[716] endotoxin-induced changes in calcium homeostasis[717] and functional disturbances to the small intestine (the main site of calcium absorption in the horse[718]). Clinical signs of hypocalcemia reported in the horse include synchronous diaphragmatic flutter, tetany, muscle spasm, and seizures.[719] Of these, only diaphragmatic flutter is seen with any regularity in adult horses. Hypocalcemia may be associated with postoperative ileus in the horse,[715] but this has not been formally investigated.

Approximately 50% of the total calcium in plasma is bound to albumin or complexed with small ligands. The remaining ionized fraction is the biologically active form. Where possible the plasma ionized calcium concentration should be measured rather than the total concentration, because the plasma albumin concentration is often decreased in gastrointestinal diseases. If total plasma calcium measurements are used to guide therapy, the calcium concentration should be corrected for changes in albumin concentration. The intervention level for treatment of hypocalcemia is debatable. One report found exacerbation of endotoxemia with calcium administration in a rodent model.[720] While the relevance of this to the horse has not been determined, aggressive supplementation of calcium in endotoxemic horses may be inadvisable. Even in endotoxic horses, calcium should probably be supplemented if the ionized calcium concentration is less than 4.8 mg/dl (1.2 mmol/L).

Hypocalcemia is treated with intravenous 23% calcium gluconate solution. A typical volume required is 100 to 300 ml,[715] but the amount will depend on ongoing losses, and the ionized calcium concentration should be frequently checked during therapy. Calcium solutions are irritating to the veins and should be diluted in crystalloid fluids before administration. They are incompatible with sodium bicarbonate and whole blood. After calcium supplementation the plasma calcium concentration should be checked after 4 to 8 hours because ongoing losses and redistribution into cells may result in further hypocalcemia. Hypocalcemia can be a sequela to magnesium deficiency and therefore magnesium should be supplemented in horses with refractory hypocalcemia.

Hypercalcemia occurs in horses with chronic renal failure, but is rare in gastrointestinal disease. Clinical signs are usually those of the underlying pathophysiology, but soft tissue calcification may occur. Treatment for severe hypercalcemia (ionized calcium greater than 9 mg/dl [2.25mmol/L]) should include non–calcium-containing intravenous fluids (sodium chloride or Normosol-R) and intravenous magnesium sulfate (see discussion of treatment of hypomagnesemia, below).

Magnesium

In a recent study, 44% of horses with gastrointestinal disease had low plasma magnesium concentrations.[721] Causes of hypomagnesemia include decreased intake, gastrointestinal losses (prolonged nasogastric reflux, malabsorption), alterations in distribution (endotoxemia, parenteral nutrition administration), renal losses (prolonged administration of lactated Ringer's solution or other magnesium-free fluids, hypophosphatemia, acidemia, renal tubular acidosis),[722,723] and excessive sweating.[724] Severe hypomagnesemia can result in ventricular arrhythmias and also muscle tremors, ataxia, seizures, and calcification of elastic tissue[725] in the horse. Other clinical manifestations of hypomagnesemia reported in human patients include supraventricular tachycardia, atrial fibrillation, thrombosis, anemia, decreased muscle strength, increased nephrotoxicity of aminoglycoside drugs, increased pulmonary vascular resistance, and sudden death.[722,726-728] Hypomagnesemia can also result in hypokalemia, refractory to potassium supplementation.[714]

Extracellular fluid contains approximately 1% of the total body magnesium, and thus the serum magnesium concentration may not reflect the total body magnesium status,[723] making diagnosis of hypomagnesemia difficult. Fortunately it is safe to administer moderate amounts of magnesium, irrespective of the magnesium status of the horse, providing the horse has normal renal function. Intravenous magnesium sulfate (at 2 mg/kg/min, not to exceed 50 mg/kg) is recommended for ventricular arrhythmias associated with hypomagnesemia.[729] Higher doses should be avoided because they cause significant muscle weakness; 140 mg/kg of intravenous magnesium sulfate can induce recumbency in normal horses.[730] For treatment of hypomagnesemia in the absence of cardiac signs, 4 to 16 mg/kg can be used as an initial dose in horses with normal renal function. Oral supplementation is possible with magnesium oxide, but oral magnesium sulfate should be avoided because of its laxative effects.

In the same study by Costa and colleagues,[721] 11% of horses with gastrointestinal disease were hypermagnesemic, but associated clinical signs were not reported. Severe clinical signs after nasogastric administration of magnesium sulfate were reported in two horses with large colon impactions. The dose given was between 1600 and 2000 mg/kg. Both horses recovered 1 to 6 hours after the onset of clinical signs, which included flaccid paralysis with recumbency, tachycardia, tachypnea, and nondetectable peripheral pulses. The horses were treated with 250 ml of 23% calcium gluconate solution intravenously, repeated after an hour, and polyionic intravenous fluids to promote diuresis.[731]

The phosphorylation of adenosine-diphosphate (ADP) to form adenosine-triphosphate (ATP) depends on the intracellular magnesium concentration,[732] and thus hypomagnesemia can disrupt ATP-dependent cellular processes. The sodium-potassium ATPase pump, the major mechanism for controlling intracellular and extracellular sodium and potassium concentrations, is ATP dependent and thus magnesium dependent. This may explain the relationship of refractory hypokalemia to hypomagnesemia.[714] The relationship between the sodium-potassium ATPase pump and magnesium may also explain the effect of magnesium on calcium flux, because sodium is exchanged down its concentration gradient (controlled by the sodium-potassium ATPase pump) for calcium by the sodium-calcium exchanger.[733] Because of the interaction of the magnesium concentration with these other electrolytes, a main effect of hypomagnesium is to alter depolarization of nerve and muscle cells.[727] Magnesium also directly competes with calcium for some of its binding sites, allowing greater binding of calcium to enzymes in hypomagnesemia. One such enzyme is phospholipase A_2; increased calcium binding results in greater activity of this enzyme, which leads to the increased formation of eicosanoids, particularly thromboxane A_2,[726] which may play a role in thrombophlebitis.[734]

Phosphorus

Hypophosphatemia has been reported in horses with either strangulating intestinal lesions or intestinal ileus[700] and is also a sequela to renal dysfunction.[658] Prolonged administration of lactate-containing fluids,[735] metabolic or respiratory alkalosis, repeated gastric magnesium sulfate administration (because magnesium binds phosphate to form an insoluble complex), and prolonged administration of non–lipid-containing parenteral nutrition solutions[736] may also result in hypophosphatemia. Reduced intestinal phosphate absorption, apparently without hypophosphatemia, is a sequela to large colon resection.[737] Clinical signs reported in small animals and humans with hypophosphatemia include hemolysis, skeletal muscle weakness and rhabdomyolysis, leukocyte dysfunction, ventricular arrhythmias, and reduced cardiac output.[736,738]

Clinical manifestations and treatment of hypophosphatemia have not been reported in the horse, and in humans there is no good evidence for treatment in the absence of clinical signs.[736] Treatment options reported in small animals include intravenous (0.01 to 0.03 mmol/kg/hr) and oral (0.5 to 2 mmol/kg/day) potassium phosphate.[738] The potential effects of potassium phosphate on the plasma potassium concentration must be considered before commencing this treatment. Intravenous glucose-1-phosphate[739] and intravenous sodium phosphate administration has also been reported in humans. The safety of these treatments has not been evaluated in the horse.

Hyperphosphatemia occurs in horses with strangulating intestinal lesions[740] and severe colitis[700] without specifically attributable clinical signs. Clinical findings reported in small animals include diarrhea, hypocalcemia, hypernatremia, and an increased propensity to metastatic soft tissue calcification. Treatment recommended in small animals includes intravenous fluids to correct any acidosis and promote renal phosphorus excretion, and dextrose-containing fluids to promote translocation of phosphorus into cells.[738]

The clinical signs of hypophosphatemia result from the wide range of physiologic functions of phosphate. These include storage of energy as adenosine triphosphate (ATP), which is used for many processes including muscle contraction, neuronal transmission, and electrolyte transport. Because phosphorus and magnesium deficiencies can both result in reduced availability of ATP, the clinical signs can be similar. Phosphate also acts as a buffer in plasma, and is a component of many intracellular compounds, including phospholipids, nucleic acids, enzymatic cofactors, and signaling molecules such as cyclic adenosine phosphate. It appears that increased plasma phosphate concentrations are not directly toxic.[741] Hypocalcemia and metastatic soft tissue calcification caused by hyperphosphatemia result from the calcium/phosphate product exceeding that required for precipitation of calcium phosphate in the tissues.[738,741]

Albumin

Hypoalbuminemia is common in horses with moderate to severe compromise of the colon. It may also occur with over-aggressive fluid therapy and parasitism. Clinical signs of hypoalbuminemia are peripheral edema (caused by reduced plasma oncotic pressure) and tissue and organ edema leading to reduced oxygen uptake by cells (increased perfusion distance) and, in severe cases, organ failure. Albumin is a weak acid, and severe hypoalbuminemia may contribute to a metabolic alkalosis or mask a concurrent metabolic acidosis.[660] A decrease in albumin concentration of 1 g/dl results in an increase in the base excess of +3.7 mEq/L.[702]

Hypoalbuminemia should be treated when acute or if there are clinical signs. Although it is advisable to treat all horses with a plasma total solids concentration of less than 4.0 g/dl, a few horses with chronic hypoproteinemia can have plasma total solids concentrations of 3.5 to 4.0 g/dl with no apparent clinical signs. The treatment options for hypoalbuminemia include fresh or fresh frozen equine plasma, concentrated albumin solutions, and hetastarch. Plasma has the advantage in that it contains other factors, such as antithrombin III, which may be depleted in the disease process. Hetastarch has the advantage of large molecule size and long persistence in the circulation[681] but has questionable efficacy

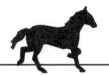

in human patients. Albumin solutions have not been formally tested in horses and are associated with increased mortality in human patients[742] and should therefore not be used outside clinical trials.

COMPLICATIONS OF FLUID THERAPY

Thrombophlebitis

Thrombophlebitis is a common complication of intravenous fluid therapy.[669] It may be a nidus for infection and may cause mechanical blockage of venous drainage resulting in local edema. Fatal edematous occlusion of the upper respiratory tract can result from bilateral jugular vein thrombosis. It is therefore advisable not to catheterize the contralateral jugular vein if one jugular vein shows any signs of thrombosis. Bacterial endocarditis, particularly of the tricuspid valve, can occur as a sequela to infectious thrombosis.

Thrombophlebitis can be identified by heat, swelling, or the presence of exudate around the catheter insertion site or by palpation of a thrombus ("corded" feel) in the catheterized vein. Catheterized veins should be checked at least daily. Ultrasonography of the catheterized vein can help identify thrombus formation. It is prudent to continue to check the vein for 2 to 3 days after catheter removal, because thrombophlebitis may develop or become apparent in this period.

The risk factors for thrombophlebitis include administration of "carboy" fluids,[669] presence of diarrhea[669] or endotoxemia,[734] polytetrafluoroethylene (Teflon) catheter material, and long duration of catheterization.[691] Several other risk factors for thrombophlebitis have been identified in humans but not studied in horses. These include inexperienced personnel placing the catheter,[743] administration of total parenteral nutrition,[689] and larger-bore catheters.[744]

Treatment for thrombophlebitis should include topical nitroglycerin ointment,[745] and probably also hot-packing and topical dimethyl sulfoxide ointment. Catheters from thrombosed veins should be removed aseptically and cultured (preferably by the roll-plate technique[746]) to allow in vitro susceptibility directed antimicrobial therapy, if necessary. A fine-needle aspirate of the thrombus can also be used for bacterial culture. Fluid-filled pockets within the thrombus can often be identified by ultrasound[747] and should be aspirated after a surgical preparation of the skin over them. Empirical antimicrobials should be broad spectrum with activity against *Streptococusi* and *Staphylococcus* species[747] and should have good tissue penetration. These include ceftiofur, gentamicin, enrofloxacin, and chloramphenicol.

Overhydration

Clinical signs of overhydration are rare in adult horses with normal cardiac and renal function. The most important clinical sign is pulmonary edema, manifested by dyspnea and a pink-white foamy nasal discharge. Treatment should include furosemide (0.5 to 1 mg/kg IV) and a reduction in the rate of fluid administration. Intranasal oxygen supplementation is indicated where there is significant hypoxemia (detected by arterial blood gas analysis). Further fluid therapy in these horses should be carefully monitored, ideally by means of central venous pressure measurements.

INOTROPES, PRESSORS, AND VASODILATORS

Some horses with severe cardiovascular compromise will not respond to fluid therapy alone. A proportion of these patients can be successfully managed with inotropes, pressors, or vasodilators. These drugs should be considered in cases with continued tachycardia, lactic acidosis, oliguria, and hypotension or hypertension despite appropriate fluid therapy. In general, horses with a jugular venous oxygen tension of less than 35 mm Hg are most likely to require further cardiovascular support, and those with an oxygen tension over 60 mm Hg are least likely to respond.[748,749] The cause of the cardiovascular insufficiency should be considered before initiating therapy. Horses with necrotic intestine that could not be resected are unlikely to respond to cardiovascular therapy unless the primary problem can be addressed.

The inotropes increase cardiac output by increasing myocardial contractility, resulting in a larger stroke volume. The most commonly used drugs in equine intensive care for this purpose are the β_1-adrenergic agonists. Inotropes that have some β_2-adrenergic activity, such as dobutamine, may also cause mild systemic vasodilation. The pressors cause arterial and venous vasoconstriction, mediated through α-adrenergic receptors, and the vasodilators, such as nitroprusside, cause arterial and venous vasodilation mediated through the nitric oxide pathway.

The decision to use one of these drugs and the choice of drug should be based on as many cardiovascular parameters as can be measured. The minimum information required to select an appropriate drug is heart rate, heart rhythm, indirect (tail cuff) arterial blood pressure, and response to fluid therapy. Direct measurements of central venous pressure, arterial blood pressure, electrocardiogram, and cardiac output, if available, make these treatments safer and easier to titrate. All of these drugs should be carefully titrated to defined endpoints. For inotropes and pressors the goal should be to increase the arterial blood pressure to a set point (mean pressure 65 to 75 mm Hg) sufficient to increase urine output[748] without inducing tachycardia or arrhythmias. For vasodilators the goal should be to reduce the mean arterial pressure to less than 120 mm Hg without inducing hypotension, tachycardia, or acidosis. It is advisable to use an electronic pump to accurately deliver the diluted drug at the correct rate.

It is extremely important to frequently monitor the response to these drugs, because the underlying cardiovascular disturbances may change rapidly. Improvements in arterial blood pressure may not result in improved tissue perfusion. Heart rate and rhythm, the acid-base balance, venous oxygen tension, and urine output should be monitored in addition to arterial blood pressure. If indirect blood pressure is being used to monitor these drugs, it is important to bear in mind the limitations of the technique. All readings should be done in triplicate and the cuff size should be matched to the patient. A small cuff designed for adult humans is appropriate for most adult horse tails.

Endotoxemia is the most common cause of severe cardiovascular disturbances in the adult. The initial cardiovascular response to experimental endotoxin administration is decreased mean arterial pressure, systemic vasodilation, and increased cardiac output.[750] However, this response varies markedly with the dose of endotoxin[751,752] and treatments given,[672,750] and this pattern of disturbance cannot be assumed.

Dobutamine

In the absence of cardiac output measurements, dobutamine should be the first drug used in hypotensive horses (mean arterial pressure less than 65 mm Hg) that have not responded to appropriate fluid therapy. Dobutamine is a β_1-adrenergic agonist and increases cardiac output.[753] Dobutamine also has significant β_2 activity, which can cause vasodilation. This is especially important in neonatal foals, in which increasing the dobutamine dose can lead to a fall in mean arterial pressure resulting from a decrease in systemic vascular resistance.[754] Dobutamine should be diluted in isotonic saline,

5% dextrose or lactated Ringers' solution. The dose should be carefully titrated from a starting dose of 1 to 3 µg/kg/min. The horse should be carefully monitored for tachycardia, which in some cases may indicate inadequate fluid resuscitation, and for dysrhythmias.

In horses with endotoxemia and increased cardiac output,[750] dobutamine is unlikely to improve tissue oxygenation. Despite increasing cardiac output, dobutamine was not found to ameliorate experimental colon ischemia in the pig.[755]

Norepinephrine

In hypotensive horses that either do not respond to dobutamine or have a measured increased cardiac output, norepinephrine (noradrenaline) administration should be considered. Norepinephrine is an α-adrenergic and moderate β1-adrenergic agonist. It is a powerful vasoconstrictor in the horse.[756] Norepinephrine should be diluted in 5% dextrose. A starting dose is 0.1 µg/kg/min, and effects may be seen in some patients at doses as low as 0.01 µg/kg/min. The highest reported dose is 1.5 µg/kg/min in the horse[756] and 3.3 µg/kg/min in human patients.[757] Concurrent infusion of dobutamine (5 µg/kg/min) with norepinephrine has been demonstrated in humans to result in improved tissue perfusion[758] and is especially prudent when cardiac output is not being directly monitored. It is important to carefully monitor urine output when using norepinephrine, because inappropriate doses may reduce renal blood flow.

Dopamine

Dopamine has β-adrenergic (inotropic), α-adrenergic (pressor), and dopaminergic effects. In other species the dopaminergic effects predominate at low doses (1 to 5 µg/kg/min), the β effects at moderate doses (5 to 10 µg/kg/min), and the α effects at high doses (above 10 µg/kg/min),[759] but these distinctions may be blurred in the horse.[760] In anesthetized horses a dopamine infusion started 5 minutes after endotoxin administration improved cardiovascular variables but did not prevent hypoxemia or metabolic acidosis.[761] Dopamine causes significant vasoconstriction of equine colonic arteries at higher doses in vitro[762] and is associated with reduced gastric mucosal perfusion in human septic patients in vivo.[763] Further, dopamine may disrupt normal equine gastrointestinal activity, even after the infusion is stopped.[764] In normal horses, low doses of dopamine (5 µg/kg/min) can cause cardiac arrhythmias.[760]

Dopamine is not recommended for horses with gastrointestinal diseases because of the reported deleterious effects on the gastrointestinal system and because the predominant effects vary with the plasma concentration,[760] which cannot be predicted from the infusion rate.[765] The role of dopamine in preventing or treating acute renal failure has also recently been challenged,[759] and dopamine infusion does not increase creatinine clearance in the normal horse.[760]

Nitroprusside

In severely hypertensive horses, sodium nitroprusside administration should be considered. Hypertension, particularly pulmonary hypertension, has been reported in experimental horses and foals treated with a low dose of endotoxin.[672,766] Nitroprusside liberates nitric oxide by a nonenzymatic one-electron reduction that occurs on exposure to tissues such as vascular smooth muscle membranes.[767] The potential beneficial role of nitroprusside administration in ameliorating laminitis remains to be investigated. Laminitis is associated with hypertension.[768] Nitroprusside induces relaxation of palmar digital arteries and veins isolated from carbohydrate-overloaded horses.[769] Treatment of acute laminitis with glyceryl trinitrate applied topically to the pasterns results in some amelioration of clinical signs.[770] Assuming that this response is due to nitric oxide, parenteral nitroprusside administration would represent a method of delivering a more controlled source of nitric oxide.

Sodium nitroprusside should be diluted in 5% dextrose solution and wrapped in foil to protect the solution from light. The dose should be carefully titrated from a starting dose of 0.1 µg/kg/min to 0.3 µg/kg/min. It is imperative to monitor the blood pressure continuously during the initial titration phase and frequently thereafter. As with all nitric oxide donors, there is a reduced responsiveness with time that may necessitate increasing doses.[767] Hepatic metabolism of nitroprusside produces thiocyanate and cyanide, which may result in altered neurologic status, acidosis, and death at high concentrations.[771] In human patients, cyanide toxicity has not been reported at doses of less than 2 µg/kg/min. Fenoldopam, a selective dopamine-1 receptor agonist, is a possible alternative antihypertensive agent that has been used experimentally in the horse.[772] However, the cost of fenoldopam is likely to prohibit its use in adult horses.

REFERENCES

658. Tennant B, Lowe JE, Tasker JB: Hypercalcemia and hypophosphatemia in ponies following bilateral nephrectomy, *Proc Soc Exp Biol Med* 167:365, 1981.
659. Furr MO, Lessard P, White NA: Development of a colic severity score for predicting the outcome of equine colic, *Vet Surg* 24:97, 1995.
660. Corley KTT, Marr CM: Pathophysiology, assessment and treatment of acid-base disturbances in the horse, *Equine Vet Educ* 10:255, 1998.
661. Hall LW, Nigam JM: Measurement of central venous pressure in horses, *Vet Rec* 97:66, 1975.
662. Webb AR: Fluid management in intensive care: avoiding hypovolaemia, *Br J Intensive Care* 7:59, 1997.
663. Gossett KA et al: Effect of acute acidemia on blood biochemical variables in healthy ponies, *Am J Vet Res* 51:1375, 1990.
664. Kellum JA: Diagnosis and treatment of acid-base disturbances. In Grenvik A et al, eds: *Textbook of critical care*, ed 4, Philadelphia, 1999, WB Saunders, pp 839-853.
665. Lowery BD, Cloutier CT, Carey LC: Electrolyte solutions in resuscitation in human hemorrhagic shock, *Surg Gynecol Obstet* 133:273, 1971.
666. Brownlow MA, Hutchins DR: The concept of osmolality: its use in the evaluation of dehydration in the horse, *Equine Vet J* 14:106, 1982.
667. Ralston SL: Clinical nutrition of adult horses, *Vet Clin North Am (Equine Pract)* 6:339, 1990.
668. Denkhaus H, Van Amstel S: Adverse effects following intravenous fluid therapy in the horse using non-commercial fluids: preliminary findings, *J S Afr Vet Assoc* 57:105, 1986.
669. Traub-Dargatz JL, Dargatz DA: A retrospective study of vein thrombosis in horses treated with intravenous fluids in a veterinary teaching hospital, *J Vet Int Med* 8:264, 1994.
670. Spalding HK, Goodwin SR: Fluid and electrolyte disorders in the critically ill, *Semin Anesth Perioperp Med Pain* 18:15, 1999.
671. Onarheim H: Fluid shifts following 7% hypertonic saline (2400 mosmol/L) infusion, *Shock* 3:350, 1995.
672. Bertone JJ et al: Effect of hypertonic vs isotonic saline solution on responses to sublethal *Escherichia coli* endotoxemia in horses, *Am J Vet Res* 51:999, 1990.
673. Mazzoni MC et al: Capillary narrowing in hemorrhagic shock is rectified by hyperosmotic saline-dextran reinfusion, *Circ Shock* 31:407, 1990.
674. Malcolm DS et al: Hypertonic saline resuscitation detrimentally affects renal function and survival in dehydrated rats, *Circ Shock* 40:69, 1993.
675. Constable PD et al: Use of hypertonic saline-dextran solution to resuscitate hypovolemic calves with diarrhea, *Am J Vet Res* 57:97, 1996.
676. McKirnan MD et al: Hypertonic saline/dextran versus lactated Ringer's treatment for hemorrhage in dehydrated swine, *Circ Shock* 44:238, 1994.
677. Moon PF et al: Effects of a highly concentrated hypertonic saline-dextran volume expander on cardiopulmonary function in anesthetized normovolemic horses, *Am J Vet Res* 52:1611, 1991.
678. McFarlane D: Hetastarch: a synthetic colloid with potential in equine patients, *Compend Cont Educ Pract Vet* 21:867, 1999.
679. Mills PC et al: Kinetics, dose response, tachyphylaxis and cross-tachyphylaxis of vascular leakage induced by endotoxin, zymosan-activated plasma and platelet-activating factor in the horse, *J Vet Pharmacol Therap* 18:204, 1995.
680. Dabareiner RM et al: Microvascular permeability and endothelial cell morphology associated with low-flow ischemia/reperfusion injury in the equine jejunum, *Am J Vet Res* 56:639, 1995.

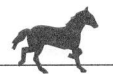

681. Jones PA, Tomasic M, Gentry PA: Oncotic, hemodilutional, and hemostatic effects of isotonic saline and hydroxyethyl starch solutions in clinically normal ponies, *Am J Vet Res* 58:541, 1997.

682. Choi PT et al: Crystalloids vs. colloids in fluid resuscitation: a systematic review, *Crit Care Med* 27:200, 1999.

683. Collatos C: Blood and blood component therapy. In Robinson NE, ed: *Current therapy in equine medicine,* ed 4, Philadelphia, 1997, WB Saunders, pp 290-292.

684. McGinness SG, Mansmann RA, Breuhaus BA: Nasogastric electrolyte replacement in horses, *Compend Cont Educ Pract Vet* 18:942, 1996.

685. Sosa León LA et al: The effects of tonicity, glucose concentration and temperature of an oral rehydration solution on its absorption and elimination, *Equine Vet J Suppl* 20:140, 1995.

686. Ecke P, Hodgson DR, Rose RJ: Induced diarrhoea in horses. II. Response to administration of an oral rehydration solution, *Vet J* 155:161, 1998.

687. Sosa León LA et al: Effects of concentrated electrolytes administered via a paste on fluid, electrolyte, and acid base balance in horses, *Am J Vet Res* 59:898, 1998.

688. Spurlock SL, Ward MV: Parenteral nutrition in equine patients: principles and theory, *Compend Contin Educ Pract Vet* 13:461, 1991.

689. Ioannides-Demos LL et al: A prospective audit of total parenteral nutrition at a major teaching hospital, *Med J Aust* 163:233, 1995.

690. Mimoz O et al: Prospective, randomized trial of two antiseptic solutions for prevention of central venous or arterial catheter colonization and infection in intensive care unit patients, *Crit Care Med* 24:1818, 1996.

691. Spurlock SL et al: Long-term jugular vein catheterization in horses, *J Am Vet Med Assoc* 196:425, 1990.

692. Pearson ML: Guideline for prevention of intravascular device-related infections, *Infect Control Hosp Epidemiol* 17:438, 1996.

693. Mealey RH et al: Indwelling cecal catheters for fluid administration in ponies, *J Vet Intern Med* 9:347, 1995.

694. Burris D et al: Controlled resuscitation for uncontrolled hemorrhagic shock, *J Trauma* 46:216, 1999.

695. Soucy DM et al: The effects of varying fluid volume and rate of resuscitation during uncontrolled hemorrhage, *J Trauma* 46:209, 1999.

696. Kasari TR, Naylor JM: Clinical evaluation of sodium bicarbonate, sodium L-lactate, and sodium acetate for the treatment of acidosis in diarrheic calves, *J Am Vet Med Assoc* 187:392, 1985.

697. Tasker JB: Fluid and electrolyte studies in the horse. III, Intake and output of water, sodium and potassium in normal horses, *Cornell Vet* 57:649, 1967.

698. Groenendyk S, English PB, Abetz I: External balance of water and electrolytes in the horse, *Equine Vet J* 20:189, 1988.

699. Rose RJ: A physiological approach to fluid and electrolyte therapy in the horse, *Equine Vet J* 13:7, 1981.

700. Svendsen CK, Hjortkjaer RK, Hesselholt M: Colic in the horse: a clinical and clinical chemical study of 42 cases, *Nord Vet Med* 31(suppl I):1, 1979.

701. Holliday M: The evolution of therapy for dehydration: should deficit therapy still be taught? *Pediatrics* 98:171, 1996.

702. Whitehair KJ et al: Clinical applications of quantitative acid-base chemistry, *J Vet Int Med* 9:1, 1995.

703. Constable PD, Hinchcliff KW, Muir WW: Comparison of anion gap and strong ion gap as predictors of unmeasured strong ion concentration in plasma and serum from horses, *Am J Vet Res* 59:881, 1998.

704. Sing RF, Branas CA, Sing RF: Bicarbonate therapy in the treatment of lactic acidosis: medicine or toxin? *J Am Osteopath Assoc* 95:52, 1995.

705. Poole-Wilson PA, Langer GA: Effect of pH on ionic exchange and function in rat and rabbit myocardium, *Am J Physiol* 229:570, 1975.

706. Gossett KA et al: Blood biochemical response to sodium bicarbonate infusion during sublethal endotoxemia in ponies, *Am J Vet Res* 51:1370, 1990.

707. Lakritz J, Madigan J, Carlson GP: Hypovolemic hyponatremia and signs of neurological disease associated with diarrhea in a foal, *J Am Vet Med Assoc* 200:1114, 1992.

708. Schaer M: Disorders of serum potassium, sodium, magnesium and chloride, *J Vet Emerg Crit Care* 9:209, 1999.

709. Rose BD: *Clinical physiology of acid-base and electrolyte disorders,* ed 4, New York, 1994, McGraw Hill.

710. Kwun KB et al: Treatment of metabolic alkalosis with intravenous infusion of concentrated hydrochloric acid, *Am J Surg* 146:328, 1983.

711. Rothe KF, Schimek F: Necrotic skin lesion following therapy of severe metabolic alkalosis: a case report, *Acta Anaesth Belg* 37:137, 1986.

712. Gennari FJ: Hypokalemia, *New Engl J Med* 339:451, 1998.

713. Muylle E et al: Determination of red blood cell potassium content in horses with diarrhoea: a practical approach for therapy, *Equine Vet J* 16:450, 1984.

714. Hamill-Ruth RJ, McGory R: Magnesium repletion and its effect on potassium homeostasis in critically ill adults: results of a double-blind, randomized, controlled trial, *Crit Care Med* 24:38, 1996.

715. Dart AJ et al: Ionized calcium concentration in horses with surgically managed gastrointestinal disease: 147 cases (1988-1990), *J Am Vet Med Assoc* 201:1244, 1992.

716. Cooper DJ et al: Plasma ionized calcium and blood lactate concentrations are inversely associated in human lactic acidosis, *Intensive Care Med* 18:286, 1992.

717. Todd JC, Mollitt DL: Effect of sepsis on erythrocyte intracellular calcium homeostasis, *Crit Care Med* 23:459, 1995.

718. Schryver HF et al: The site of calcium absorption in the horse, *J Nutr* 100:1127, 1970.

719. Beyer MJ et al: Idiopathic hypocalcemia in foals, *J Vet Int Med* 11:356, 1997.

720. Malcolm DS, Zaloga GP, Holaday JW: Calcium administration increases the mortality of endotoxic shock in rats, *Crit Care Med* 17:900, 1989.

721. Costa LRR et al: Plasma magnesium concentrations in horses with gastrointestinal tract disease, *J Vet Int Med* 13:274, 1999.

722. Salem M, Munoz R, Chernow B: Hypomagnesemia in critical illness: a common and clinically important problem, *Crit Care Clin* 7:225, 1991.

723. Olerich MA, Rude RK: Should we supplement magnesium in critically ill patients? *New Horiz* 2:186, 1994.

724. Taylor P: Heat stroke, exhaustion and synchronous diaphragmatic flutter (SDF). In Dyson S, ed: *A guide to the management of emergencies at equine competitions,* Newmarket, 1996, Equine Veterinary Journal, Ltd.

725. Harrington DD: Pathological features of magnesium deficiency in young horses fed purified rations, *Am J Vet Res* 35:503, 1974.

726. Gunther T: Biochemical bases of the therapeutic actions of magnesium, *Magnes Bull* 13:46, 1992.

727. Tso EL, Barish RA: Magnesium: clinical considerations, *J Emerg Med* 10:735, 1992.

728. Landon RA, Young EA: Role of magnesium in regulation of lung function, *J Am Diet Assoc* 93:674, 1993.

729. Bonagura JD, Reef VB: Cardiovascular diseases. In Reed SM, Bayly WM, eds: *Equine internal medicine,* Philadelphia, 1998, WB Saunders, 290-370.

730. Bowen JM, Blackmon DM, Heavner JE: Effect of magnesium ions on neuromuscular transmission in the horse, steer, and dog, *J Am Vet Med Assoc* 157:164, 1970.

731. Henninger RW, Horst J: Magnesium toxicosis in two horses, *J Am Vet Med Assoc* 211:82, 1997.

732. Page S, Salem M, Laughlin MR: Intracellular Mg^{2+} regulates ADP phosphorylation and adenine nucleotide synthesis in human erythrocytes, *Am J Physiol* 274:E92, 1998.

733. Zaloga GP: Hypocalcemia in critically ill patients, *Crit Care Med* 20:251, 1992.

734. Morris DD: Thrombophlebitis in horses: the contribution of hemostatic dysfunction to pathogenesis, *Compend Cont Educ Pract Vet* 11:1386, 1989.

735. Walton RJ: Effect of intravenous sodium lactate on renal tubular reabsorption of phosphate in man, *Clin Sci* 57:125, 1979.

736. Bugg NC, Jones JA: Hypophosphataemia: pathophysiology, effects and management on the intensive care unit, *Anaesthesia* 53:895, 1998.

737. Bertone AL, van Soest PJ, Stashak TS: Digestion, fecal, and blood variables associated with extensive large colon resection in the horse, *Am J Vet Res* 50:253, 1989.

738. Macintire DK: Disorders of potassium, phosphorus, and magnesium in critical illness, *Compend Cont Educ Pract Vet* 19:41, 1997.

739. Bollaert PE et al: Hemodynamic and metabolic effects of rapid correction of hypophosphatemia in patients with septic shock, *Chest* 107:1698, 1995.

740. Arden WA, Stick JA: Serum and peritoneal fluid phosphate concentrations as predictors of major intestinal injury associated with equine colic, *J Am Vet Med Assoc* 193:927, 1988.

741. Sutters M, Gaboury CL, Bennett WM: Severe hyperphosphatemia and hypocalcemia: a dilemma in patient management, *J Am Soc Nephrol* 7:2056, 1996.

742. Cochrane Injuries Group Albumin Reviewers: Human albumin administration in critically ill patients: systematic review of randomised controlled trials, *Br Med J* 317:235, 1998.

743. Armstrong CW et al: Prospective study of catheter replacement and other risk factors for infection of hyperalimentation catheters, *J Infect Dis* 154:808, 1986.

744. Swanson JT, Aldrete JA: Thrombophlebitis after intravenous infusion. Factors affecting its incidence, *Rocky Mountain Med J* 66:48, 1969.

745. Berrazueta JR et al: The anti-inflammatory and analgesic action of transdermal glyceryltrinitrate in the treatment of infusion-related thrombophlebitis, *Postgrad Med J* 69:37, 1993.

746. Maki DG, Weise CE, Sarafin HW: A semiquantitative culture method for identifying intravenous-catheter-related infection, *New Engl J Med* 296:1305, 1977.

747. Gardner SY, Reef VB, Spencer PA: Ultrasonographic evaluation of horses with thrombophlebitis of the jugular vein: 46 cases (1985-1988), *J Am Vet Med Assoc* 199:370, 1991.

748. Hollenberg SM et al: Practice parameters for hemodynamic support of sepsis in adult patients in sepsis, *Crit Care Med* 27:639, 1999.

749. Wetmore LA et al: Mixed venous oxygen tension as an estimate of cardiac output in anesthetized horses, *Am J Vet Res* 48:971, 1987.

750. Bottoms GD et al: Endotoxin-induced hemodynamic changes in ponies: effects of flunixin meglumine, *Am J Vet Res* 42:1514, 1981.

751. Burrows GE: Escherichia coli endotoxemia in the conscious pony, *Am J Vet Res* 32:243, 1971.

752. Clark ES, Gantley B, Moore JN: Effects of slow infusion of a low dosage of endotoxin on systemic haemodynamics in conscious horses, *Equine Vet J* 23:18, 1991.

753. Hinchcliff KW, McKeever KH, Muir WW: Hemodynamic effects of atropine, dobutamine, nitroprusside, phenylephrine, and propranolol in conscious horses, *J Vet Int Med* 5:80, 1991.
754. Corley K et al: Unpublished data.
755. Björck M, Bergqvist D, Haglund U: The effect of dobutamine on distal colon ischaemia in the pig, *Intensive Care Med* 24:178, 1998.
756. Corley KTT et al: Initial experience with norepinephrine infusion in hypotensive critically ill foals, *J Vet Emerg Crit Care* 10:267, 2000.
757. Martin C et al: Septic shock: a goal-directed therapy using volume loading, dobutamine and/or norepinephrine, *Acta Anaesth Scand* 34:413, 1990.
758. Duranteau J et al: Effects of epinephrine, norepinephrine, or the combination of norepinephrine and dobutamine on gastric mucosa in septic shock, *Crit Care Med* 27:893, 1999.
759. Denton MD, Chertow GM, Brady HR: "Renal-dose" dopamine for the treatment of acute renal failure: scientific rationale, experimental studies and clinical trials, *Kidney Int* 50:4, 1996.
760. Trim CM, Moore JN, Clark ES: Renal effects of dopamine infusion in conscious horses, *Equine Vet J Suppl* 7:124, 1989.
761. Trim CM, Moore JN, Clark ES: Effects of an infusion of dopamine on the cardiopulmonary effects of *Escherichia coli* endotoxin in anaesthetised horses, *Res Vet Sci* 50:54, 1991.
762. Sedrish SA et al: In vitro response of large colon arterial and venous rings to vasodilating drugs in horses, *Am J Vet Res* 60:204, 1999.
763. Nevière R et al: The contrasting effects of dobutamine and dopamine on gastric mucosal perfusion in septic patients, *Am J Respir Crit Care Med* 154:1684, 1996.
764. King JN, Gerring EL: Biphasic disruption of fasting equine gut motility by dopamine: a preliminary study, *J Vet Pharmacol Therap* 11:354, 1988.
765. Juste RN et al: Dopamine clearance in critically ill patients, *Intensive Care Med* 24:1217, 1998.
766. Lavoie JP et al: Haemodynamic, pathological, haematological and behavioural changes during endotoxin infusion in equine neonates, *Equine Vet J* 22:23, 1990.
767. Harrison DG, Bates JN: The nitrovasodilators: new ideas about old drugs, *Circulation* 87:1461, 1993.
768. Garner HE et al: Equine laminitis and associated hypertension: a review, *J Am Vet Med Assoc* 166:56, 1975.
769. Schneider DA et al: Palmar digital vessel relaxation in healthy horses and in horses given carbohydrate, *Am J Vet Res* 60:233, 1999.
770. Hinckley KA et al: Nitric oxide donors as treatment for grass induced acute laminitis in ponies, *Equine Vet J* 28:17, 1996.
771. Rindone JP, Sloane EP: Cyanide toxicity from sodium nitroprusside: risks and management, *Ann Pharmacother* 26:515, 1992.
772. Clark ES, Moore JN: Effects of fenoldopam on cecal blood flow and mechanical activity in horses, *Am J Vet Res* 50:1926, 1989.

RUMINANT ALIMENTARY DISEASE

BRADFORD P. SMITH, Consulting Editor

DENTAL AND PERIODONTAL DISEASES

GUY ST. JEAN

ERUPTION OF TEETH

Determining an animal's age by examining the teeth is not an exact science, because the appearance of the teeth can be affected by inherited factors, nutrition, and geographic location.[773,774] At birth or within 2 weeks, four deciduous incisors usually are present. The entire eight deciduous incisors erupt within the first month.[775] The fourth incisor (corner) is a modified canine tooth. The incisors meet with the dental pad of the upper jaw for the purpose of gripping and cutting herbage. Usually all three pairs of deciduous premolars have erupted at birth or shortly afterward.[773,774] In cattle the formula of the deciduous teeth is:

$$2 \text{ (incisors } 0/4, \text{ premolars } 3/3) = 20$$

The age at which permanent teeth erupt often is the best criterion for determining the animal's age if a registration certificate is not available. However, systemic illnesses and malnutrition can retard dental development and cause retention of the deciduous teeth.[776] The first molars erupt at 8 months of age and are fully developed at 12 months. At 18 months the second molar is fully developed. The third molar erupts at 24 months and is fully developed at 30 months. The permanent premolar teeth start to replace the deciduous teeth at 24 months, and all three permanent premolars usually are present at 3 years of age.[773,774] The first pair of permanent incisors (centrals) erupts at 18 to 24 months of age, the second pair (medials) appears at 24 to 30 months, the third pair (laterals) erupts at 3 years of age, and the fourth pair (corners) erupts between 3½ and 4 years of age.[775,776] Cattle therefore have a complete set of permanent teeth at age 4 to 4½ years. The formula of the permanent teeth in cattle is:

$$2 \text{ (incisors } 0/4, \text{ premolars } 3/3, \text{ molars } 3/3) = 32$$

The deciduous and permanent dental formulas of the sheep and goat are identical to those of cattle.[775] In sheep and goats the periods of eruption are as follows: The incisors are present at birth or within the first 4 weeks. The premolars erupt 2 to 6 weeks after birth. The first pair of permanent incisors (centrals) replace the deciduous teeth at 12 to 18 months of age. The second pair appears at 18 to 24 months. The third pair (laterals) erupts between 30 and 36 months, and the fourth pair (corners) appears at 3½ to 4 years. The three permanent premolars have erupted by 18 to 24 months of age; the first molar erupts at 3 months, the second molar between 9 and 12 months, and the last molar between 18 and 24 months.[775]

EXAMINATION OF TEETH

Dental disease in ruminants should be considered first on a flock or herd basis.[777,778] Determining dental health is particularly useful when unconventional feeds are incorporated into the herd nutritional program.[779,780] The clinical manifestations of dental diseases include inadequate food intake, inadequate calf development, weight loss, unthriftiness, (low body condition score), quidding, low pregnancy rate in replacement heifers, and mandibular or maxillary swellings or draining tracts.[775,778-781] Examination of the herd should be followed by dental examination of individual animals. To examine the premolars and molars, the tongue should be withdrawn from the mouth and held at the commissure of the mouth opposite the teeth being examined. A small dose of xylazine (0.03 to 0.04 mg/kg IV) and use of a mouth speculum allows for a much more thorough dental examination, including manual palpation in cattle.

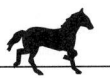

The incisors have a sharp edge in front and are used for gripping and cutting herbage.[775,778] They should be aligned closely, with little space between them.[775,778] In sheep the periodontium of the incisor allows movement of up to 2 mm anteroposteriorly to accommodate rotating or turning forces during grazing.[781] This makes the sheep incisor very prone to loss with periodontal damage. The length of the premolar and molar teeth and their firm placement in the alveolar bone means that they are lost less often than the incisors.[773,774,778]

DENTAL ATTRITION AND EROSION

Rapid wearing of teeth is seen most commonly in grazing sheep 5 years of age or older. Sheep and cattle grazing forage-deficient or sandy pastures and arid ranges in Africa, Australia, New Zealand, and the southwestern United States often show an accelerated rate of tooth wear.[778,782] In Rhodesia the incisors of Hereford cattle showed an increased rate of wear because of the softer enamel of this breed compared with that of indigenous cattle.[783]

Examination of an animal with dental attrition reveals worn incisor or molar teeth (or both); often only short stumps are seen. The teeth also may be loose, fractured, or missing. Dental attrition from excessive wear must be differentiated from periodontal disease that causes tooth loss.[778,784,785] The pathogenesis of excessive tooth wear relates to tooth hardness and diet quality. Ingestion and mastication of soil and sand with forage abrades and wears the incisor and molar teeth. In New Zealand dental attrition in sheep was attributed to the action of the acids and enzymes in the herbage on tooth dentin.[782] A calcium deficiency or calcium-phosphorus imbalance, which results in softness of the tooth enamel and dentin, may accelerate the rate of wear.

In the United States the feeding of fermented sweet potato cannery waste to cattle resulted in substantial increases in incisor erosion.[779,780] Cattle producers who fed the waste noticed a poor growth rate, inadequate calf development, low pregnancy rates in heifers, and worn, mottled, discolored incisors.[779,780] Sweet potato cannery waste is highly acidic (pH 3.2) and causes calcium loss and tooth erosion. Deciduous teeth are etched more rapidly, placing young cattle at higher risk of severe tooth wear and dental infection. In addition the original enamel surface and the pulp chamber are closer together in deciduous teeth than in permanent teeth, which also is more significant in younger cattle.[779,780] Mixing 10% broiler litter with sweet potato cannery waste raised the pH to 4, providing a palatable, high-quality feed and preventing the severe dental problems associated with feeding sweet potato cannery waste alone.[779]

A syndrome involving excessive wear of deciduous incisor teeth, maleruption of permanent incisors, and an increased prevalence of dentigerous cysts in sheep has been reported from New Zealand.[786] Excessive wear of the incisor teeth of cattle was recorded on the same farms. Ingestion of soil during winter because of the inclement weather, overgrazing of pastures, and low blood levels of copper were the main causes of the syndrome.[786] Dental attrition can be prevented by providing supplemental feed to avoid overgrazing of pastures. Adding 1% ground limestone to the feed in calcium-deficient areas is recommended.[787]

PERIODONTAL DISEASE

Periodontal disease is a disease condition of the supporting tissue that surrounds the teeth.[788,789] Periodontal disease of sheep is endemic in parts of New Zealand. A periodontal disease known as cara inchada, or swollen face, has caused losses of cattle in Brazil.[790,781]

Periodontal disease is characterized by protruding, loose incisors.[778,774] With time, incisors, premolars, and molars may be missing. The reason why periodontal disease is prevalent in sheep but less common in cattle is unknown. Periodontal disease causes pain on mastication, leading to poor maceration of food and reduction in food digestibility.

Periodontal disease has been associated with bacterial plaque–induced gingivitis.[788,791-793] The acute gingivitis is replaced progressively by a chronic inflammation in the gingival sulcus. The periodontal ligament is destroyed by plaque-forming oral microorganisms and host enzymes. At this stage, periodontal pockets are formed that lead to loosening of teeth. This process may take months or years. With time the infection extends to the apical area. The gum margin begins to recede over the lesion, food accumulates in the pocket, and the entire alveolus becomes infected. At this point the tooth becomes a sequestrum. The alveolar pyorrhea causes a periostitis of the external surface of the alveolar process, and swelling is observed. Once a tooth has been lost from an affected alveolus, granulation tissue fills the alveolus. Deep to the granulation tissue, alveolar bone is redeposited.

Bacteria such as *Bacteroides* spp., *Actinomyces* spp., and spirochetes, metabolic or immune disorders in the host, and mechanical or chemical agents have been implicated in the pathogenesis of periodontal diseases in sheep.[778,792,794,795] Bacterial invasion in the gingival pockets has been associated with a defect of host immune competence.[796] Hypomagnesemia has been a common finding in sheep with periodontal disease, but this may be a secondary development.[795] Gingival trauma may be important in the etiology.[797] Dissolution of the enamel at the attachment of the gingival epithelium by organic acids from microorganisms of the soil may be a predisposing factor.[798] The serum values for calcium, albumin, and alkaline phosphatase were lower for sheep with periodontal disease than for sheep unaffected by dental disease.[799]

A postmortem examination of Scottish-Hill sheep revealed that 60% of 478 aged sheep had either loose or missing teeth. Gingival pockets were present in 87% of the population and were correlated with tooth looseness.[800] In the United States a 25% mortality rate caused by dental disease in a herd of 300 ewes was reported.[801] The clinical signs were depression, anorexia, ataxia, and emaciation.[801] Necropsy revealed dental disease of the mandibular teeth with plaque, plant fibers in periodontal pockets, and osteomyelitis of the mandibular bone. Initial trauma to the gingivae from cheatgrass awns in the hayfield was implicated.[801]

A particular type of periodontal disease in cattle has been reported from Brazil.[790,791] This condition involves an inflammatory process of the periodontium of calves and older Zebu cattle that results in alveolar periostitis of the maxilla or, less often, the mandible.[790,791] Examination reveals deep periodontal pockets and loss of or loosened teeth. Affected animals suffer from malnutrition, diarrhea, and loss of condition and often die. *Bacteroides* and *Actinomyces* organisms often are found in the lesion and are suspected of causing the disease.[790] This disorder is seen only in certain areas of Brazil, and the cattle improve if moved to unaffected areas. In one trial the development of periodontal disease in calves was avoided by administration of the antimicrobial drug spiramycin.[791]

The assumption that incisor condition is a good indicator of future productivity is not well founded. Little scientific evidence exists on which to base the practice of culling sheep with periodontal disease. Three farms with a high prevalence of periodontal disease were selected, and the body condition and weight of affected sheep were compared to those of sheep with no signs of periodontal disease. On only one farm was a significant association noted between periodontal disease and body condition or weight. It was concluded that periodontal disease in sheep may impair productivity on some farms but not others.[802,803]

Treating periodontal disease on a flock basis often may prove impractical. Dental treatment, drug therapy, and management change have been tried in sheep. One form of dental treatment, tooth grinding, consists of trimming the incisors to the levels of the lower dental pad.[784] Two trials of the productivity effects of tooth grinding have been conducted, and neither showed any benefit from the procedure.[802] An attempt to influence the development of periodontal disease in sheep by long-term treatment with tetracycline and metronidazole has proved ineffective.[793] In commercial sheep surgical treatment could improve conditions such as periapical and gingival abscesses, but such treatment is not economically feasible.

Sheep can live without incisors provided they do not have to graze too closely. Supplementary feeding or improved pasture usage for sheep that have lost incisors should provide a net gain to the owner. However, this approach is unlikely to be effective when premolar and molar teeth are involved because of the inability to chew and ruminate efficiently.

DENTIGEROUS CYSTS

Dentigerous cysts have been described in ruminants, particularly sheep.[786,803] These are odontogenic cysts of unknown etiology that manifest as localized, bony swellings. Radiographs demonstrate the cystic nature of the swelling and reveal one or more teeth in the cyst.[786,803] For valuable individuals, treatment is surgical.

DEVELOPMENTAL ANOMALIES AND RETENTION OF DECIDUOUS TEETH

Developmental anomalies have been reported in cattle.[777] Occasionally tooth buds fail to develop, and the fourth pair of permanent incisors is the set most often absent. The first mandibular premolar on one or both sides also occasionally fails to form. The permanent incisor teeth have been observed to be rotated up to 180 degrees in the alveolus. Rotation of the first permanent mandibular premolar also has been seen; the rotation was 90 degrees, and no cause could be detected. Retention of a deciduous premolar is common in 12- to 18-month-old cattle. This results in difficulty in masticating and excessive salivation. Treatment consists of removing the deciduous premolar with a forceps.

OVERGROWN OR LOOSE MOLAR TEETH

Overgrown molar teeth are found most commonly in old ruminants. The opposite tooth often is missing. Food accumulates between the affected tooth and the cheek, causing obvious swelling of the face. Interference with mastication often is noted. The offending tooth should be rasped regularly or removed. A power tool to grind cheek teeth works well. Premolar or molar teeth can become loose in advanced cases of actinomycosis, affecting the jaw. It may be difficult to determine whether the loose tooth is a cause or result of the bony abnormalities. One cow with maxillary lymphosarcoma and loose teeth has been reported.[804]

BROKEN TEETH

Broken incisors are not common because of the loose alveolar attachment of these teeth. Broken premolars and molars are more common because these teeth are more solidly attached in their alveoli; breakage usually results from attempts to masticate hard objects. Most fractures usually involve only a portion of the tooth, do not involve the root, and are

asymptomatic. A sagittal tooth fracture that includes the root causes pain and may result in reduced feed intake and loss of condition. Treatment is described below in the section Tooth Root Abscess.

DENTAL CARIES

Dental caries, or decay, creates areas of decalcification of the tooth.[775] Dental caries is rare in ruminants,[775] but it sometimes can be found in both temporary and permanent teeth and in both dentin and enamel.[777] Interference with prehension usually is not seen. On oral examination an orange or black pigment is seen in the defective enamel or exposed dentin; these areas should be probed with a fine dental pick or needle. Caries may be filled or the tooth extracted. In rare cases the caries can reach down the pulp cavity to the root apex, causing periodontal abscesses. (See Tooth Root Abscess, below.)

OSTEODYSTROPHIA FIBROSA

Osteodystrophia fibrosa is caused by resorption of calcium from bone and its replacement with connective tissue.[805] It is seen most commonly in the goat. Osteodystrophia fibrosa can result from calcium, phosphorus, or vitamin D deficiencies or from hyperparathyroidism. The affected individual usually is a growing animal with a bilateral, soft, painless swelling of the maxilla or mandible or both.[805] The diagnosis is based on radiographic evidence of poorly mineralized bone and inward rotation of the premolar and molar teeth. Treatment consists of supplementing the ration with adequate mineral levels while maintaining a ratio of calcium to phosphorus of 2:1.

TOOTH ROOT ABSCESS

Dental repulsion is done preferably using general anesthesia with the affected tooth uppermost. A straight incision is made directly over the longitudinal axis of the tooth or a trephine hole over the base of the root can be made. Only the bone lateral to the tooth is removed. If necessary, a chisel is used to free the tooth of bone at its rostral and caudal surface, taking care not to disturb the neighboring teeth. A dental punch is placed on the tooth root, and dental repulsion is performed. The ventral aspect of the incision can be left open for drainage, or the alveolus can be packed with dental wax, gauze, or dental material, such as Optisil. Abscessed maxillary cheek teeth often cause maxillary sinusitis. The sinus must be curetted at the time of surgery and flushed daily for 1 to 2 weeks after surgery. The alveolus must be packed until granulation tissue fills the hole. Antibiotics are administered for 1 week according to culture and antimicrobial sensitivity results. After removal of the affected tooth, the abscess and clinical signs usually resolve, but chronic sinusitis may require a bone flap and extensive curettage.

REFERENCES

773. Andrews AH: First molar eruption in cattle and its use in age determination, *Vet Rec* 107:419-421, 1980.
774. Andrews AH: A comparison of first molar eruption in Friesian steers and heifers, *Br Vet J* 137:31-35, 1981.
775. Hofmeyr CFB: The digestive system. In Oehme FW, ed: *Textbook of large animal surgery,* Baltimore, 1982, Williams & Wilkins.
776. St Clair LE: Teeth. In Getty R, ed: *The anatomy of the domestic animal,* Philadelphia, 1975, WB Saunders.
777. Garlick NL: The teeth of the ox in clinical diagnosis. III, Developmental anomalies and general pathology, *Am J Vet Res* 15:500-508, 1957.
778. Spense J, Aitchison G: Clinical aspects of dental disease in sheep, *In Pract* July, 1986, pp 128-135, 1986.
779. Rogers GM et al: Dental wear and growth performance in steers fed sweet potato cannery waste, *J Am Vet Med Assoc* 214:681-687, 1999.
780. Rogers GM et al: In vitro effects of an acidic by-product feed on bovine teeth, *Am J Vet Res* 58:498-503, 1997.

781. Moxham BJ, Shore RC, Berkovitz BKB: Effects of inflammatory periodontal disease (broken mouth) on the mobility of the sheep incisor, *Res Vet Sci* 48:99-102, 1990.

782. Barnicoat CP, Hall DM: Attritions of incisors of grazing sheep, *Nature* 185:179, 1960.

783. Steenkamp JDG: Effect of the brittle hardness and abrasive hardness of enamel on the degree of attrition of deciduous teeth of representative breeds of *Bos indicus* and *Bos taurus* origin, *Agroanimalia* 1:23-34, 1969.

784. Denholm LJ, Vizard A: Periodontal disease and premature incisor tooth loss (broken mouth) in Australian sheep: is tooth grinding an effective solution? *Wool Tech Sheep Breed* Sept/Oct, 1986, pp 113-120.

785. MacKinnon MM: A pathological study of an enzootic parodontal disease of mature sheep, *N Z Vet J* 7:18-26, 1959.

786. Bruere AN et al: A syndrome of dental abnormalities of sheep. I, Clinical aspects on a commercial sheep farm in the Wairarapa, *N Z Vet J* 27:152-158, 1979.

787. Andrews AH: Acquired diseases of the teeth and mouth in ruminants. In Harvey CE, ed: *Veterinary dentistry,* Philadelphia, 1985, WB Saunders.

788. Cuttress TW, Ludwig TG: Periodontal disease in sheep. I, Review of the literature, *J Periodontal* 40:529, 1969.

789. Cutress TW: Histopathology of periodontal disease in sheep, *Periodontology* 47:643-650, 1976.

790. Blobel VH et al: Bakteriologische Untersuchungen an der "cara inchada," einer periodontalen erkrankung bei Rindern in Brasilien, *Tierärztl Umschau* 42:152-157, 1987.

791. DoBereiner J et al: Efeito de espiramicina na profilaxia DA "cara inchada" dos bovinos, *Pesq Vet Bras* 10:27-29, 1990.

792. McCourtie J: The bacteriology of periodontal disease in sheep, *Rev Med Microbiol* 1:116-123, 1990.

793. Spence JA, Aitchison GH, Fraser J: Development of periodontal disease in a single flock of sheep: clinical signs, morphology of subgingival plaque, and influence of antimicrobial agents, *Res Vet Sci* 45: 324-331, 1988.

794. Spence JA, Aitchison GH: Early tooth loss in sheep: a review, *Vet Ann* 25:125, 1985.

795. Spence JA et al: Skeletal and blood biochemical characteristics of sheep during growth and breeding: a comparison of flocks with and without broken mouth, *J Comp Pathol* 95:505-524, 1985.

796. Van Dyke TE, Levine MJ, Genco RJ: Periodontal diseases and neutrophil abnormalities. In Genco RJ, Mergenhagen SE, eds: *Host-parasite interactions in periodontal diseases,* Washington, 1982, American Society for Microbiology.

797. Healy WB, Ludwig TG: Wear of sheep's teeth, *NZ J Agri Res* 8:737-752, 1965.

798. Mitchum GD, Bruere AN: Solubilization of sheep's teeth: a new look at a widespread New Zealand problem, *Proceedings of the Fourteenth Seminar of the Sheep and Beef Cattle Society of the New Zealand Veterinary Association,* Bulls, NZ, 1984.

799. Cutress TW et al: Periodontal disease in sheep. II, The composition of sera from sheep with periodontosis, *Periodontology* 43:668-676, 1972.

800. Aitchinson GH, Spense JA: Dental disease in hill sheep: an abattoir survey, *J Comp Pathol* 94:285-300, 1984.

801. Anderson BC, Bulgin MS: Starvation associated with dental disease in range ewes, *J Am Vet Med Assoc* 184:737-738, 1984.

802. Orr MB, Mackey D, McNally K: A pilot study of the effects of mechanical shortening of ewes' incisors (bite correction) on body weight and the development of periodontal disease, *Vet J* 39:108-110, 1991.

803. Orr MB et al: A syndrome of dental abnormalities of sheep. II, The pathology and radiology, *NZ Vet J* 27:276-278, 1979.

804. St Jean G et al: Maxillary lymphosarcoma in a cow, *Can Vet J* 35:56, 1994.

805. Andrews AH, Ingram PL, Longstaffe JA: Osteodystrophia fibrosa in young goats, *Vet Rec* 112:404-406, 1983.

SALIVARY GLAND DISEASES

GUY ST. JEAN

The parotid, mandibular, and sublingual glands are the three largest salivary glands in ruminants.[806] In cattle the mandibular gland is larger than the parotid gland. The adult bovine produces 50 L or more of saliva in 24 hours. Saliva is secreted continuously, but the rate of secretion is increased by feeding, rumination, and the presence of coarse feed in the rumen.[806] The saliva provides a fluid medium for transport of ingesta during deglutition and regurgitation. It also maintains adequate phosphate for bacterial digestion of cellulose in the rumen and contains bicarbonate, which acts as a buffer to maintain rumen pH above 5.5. Ruminant saliva contains approximately 80 mEq/L of bicarbonate.

EXCESSIVE SALIVATION

Excessive salivation (ptyalism) is a sign of many pathologic conditions. The volume of saliva may be normal, but if it is not being swallowed, salivation can appear excessive. Gloves should be worn to examine the mouth of any animal that is salivating excessively as a precaution against exposure to rabies. Excessive salivation may be seen with dental disease, stomatitis, foreign objects in the mouth or pharynx, or esophageal obstruction. It also has been seen with ruminal disorders, in cows that have eaten spoiled silage, and with impaction of the abomasum. Ptyalism may be a clinical sign in rabies, pseudorabies, meningoencephalitis, and slaframine toxicity.[806,807] Mercury, iodine, lead, copper, and arsenic also can stimulate secretion by the salivary glands. Treatment depends on the underlying causes.

SIALOCELE

A sialocele develops when saliva escapes from a duct or salivary gland and enters the surrounding tissue. The saliva contains enzymes that irritate the tissue. The accumulation of saliva is surrounded by inflamed tissue, which gives the lesion a cystic appearance. A soft, fluctuant swelling usually is seen. Signs of pain may be observed during mastication. Trauma or foreign body usually is the cause of a sialocele. The diagnosis is based on the history, palpation, paracentesis, and sialography. Needle aspiration may yield mucoid saliva. Two treatments have been described.[808,809] The first involves removal of both the mandibular and sublingual glands and ducts.[808] Surgical extirpation of the mandibular salivary gland in the caudal area of the mandibular spaces has been performed successfully in cows, sheep, goats, and buffaloes.[806] Exposure of the tissue by opening the capsule of the gland facilitates the process of extirpation and prevents trauma of the surrounding nerves and blood vessels.[808] In the second treatment option, the sialocele is opened, drained, and chemically debrided using copper sulfate.[809]

PAROTID GLAND CARCINOMAS

Three cows at slaughter had parotid gland carcinomas.[810] The neoplastic cells appeared to originate from ductal and acinar epithelium.[810] Ocular squamous cell carcinoma may spread locally to the parotid or mandibular lymph nodes.[811]

SIALOADENITIS

Inflammation of the salivary glands usually is caused by nonspecific infections, penetrating wounds, or plant awns. Diffuse swelling of the salivary glands may be observed, and the swelling may be hot and painful on palpation. Abscess formation is a common complication. Treatment consists of systemic antibiotics and antiinflammatory and analgesic drugs. Abscesses should be drained when they localize. Salivary fistulas can be sequelae to salivary abscesses.

REFERENCES

806. Williams EL: The mouth and salivary glands. In Amstutz HE, ed: *Bovine medicine and surgery,* ed 2, Santa Barbara, Calif, 1980, American Veterinary Publication.

807. Hagler WM, Croom WJ Jr: Slaframine: occurrence, chemistry, and physiological activity. In Cheeke PR, ed: *Toxicants of plant origin,* vol 1, Alkaloids, Boca Raton, Fla, 1989, CRC Press.

808. Misk NA, Hifny A, Ahmed IH: Extirpation of the mandibular salivary glands in equine and ruminants, *Vet Med J* 25:169-176, 1991.

809. Mouli SP: Surgical treatment and chemical debridement of parotid salivary cysts in bovines: report of three cases, *Indian Vet J* 65:725-726, 1988.

810. Bundza A: Primary salivary gland neoplasia in three cows, *J Comp Pathol* 93:629-632, 1983.

811. Kainer RA: Current concepts in the treatment of bovine ocular squamous cell tumors. In Moore CP, ed: *Large animal ophthalmology*, Philadelphia, 1984, WB Saunders.

ACTINOBACILLOSIS
(Woody Tongue, Wooden Tongue)

BRADFORD P. SMITH

DEFINITION AND ETIOLOGY. *Actinobacillus lignieresii*, a gram-negative rod, is a normal inhabitant of the rumen and mouth of many cattle and sheep and probably goats. When the organism enters the soft tissues through a lesion, actinobacillosis results in a granulomatous abscessation. Ruminants of all ages can be affected, and the disease appears to have a worldwide distribution. The classic site of infection is the bovine tongue; because the condition causes a very hard, diffuse nodular swelling, it has been given the name "woody tongue" or "wooden tongue." The prevalence of woody tongue in bovines at slaughter is 0.7% to 3.6%.[812] Atypical actinobacillosis lesions of cattle can occur in the lips, nose, or lymph nodes of the head or neck or at other sites.[813-815] Although the lesions normally occur sporadically, herd outbreaks with up to 73% morbidity have been reported.[816,817] Sheep are most commonly affected by hard swellings of the lips, often with fistulous tracts.[818] Actinobacillosis has also been reported to cause tongue lesions in sheep[818,819] and horses.[820] These lesions appear to be rare in goats.

CLINICAL SIGNS AND DIFFERENTIAL DIAGNOSIS. Actinobacillosis lesions usually involve soft tissues. When the tongue is affected, the major clinical signs are inability to prehend food normally, excessive salivation, and sometimes a visibly enlarged tongue that protrudes from the mouth. The submandibular area often is enlarged and firm. On palpation the tongue is firm to very hard, painful, and nodular (Fig. 30-45). Nodular lesions often are slightly ulcerated. The base of the tongue is most frequently affected, but the shaft may also be involved. An ulceration filled with plant awns or stems often is seen in the sulcus lingualis at the junction of the base and shaft of the tongue. Because cattle use the tongue to prehend food, anorexia results when the tongue is painful and inflexible. Actinobacillosis must be differentiated from dental disease, oral foreign bodies, pharyngeal trauma, and other diseases that cause oral pain.

Atypical lesions in cattle involve sites other than the tongue. Lymph nodes of the head and cranial cervical area

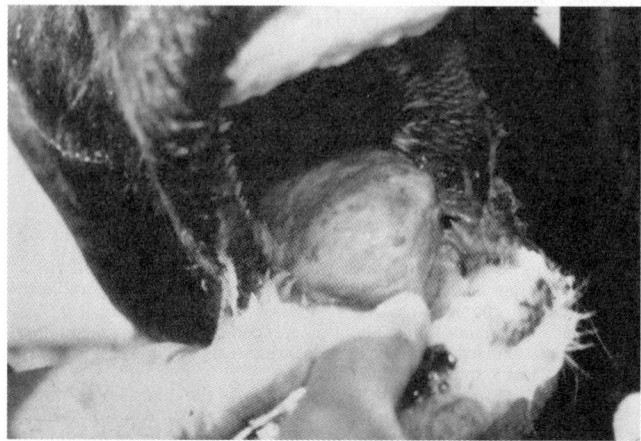

FIG. 30-45 ■ Firm, enlarged bovine tongue typical of woody tongue caused by *Actinobacillus lignieresii*. Partly ulcerated areas of mucosa overlie hard nodules.

are most frequently affected, but where any abrasion is present, granulomas or abscesses may develop, followed by licking or contact with pus draining from a lesion on another animal. Because plant awns and stems create entry sites for the organism in the mouth, most lesions are in the head. Granulomas in the nose and eyelids and needle puncture wounds over the left jugular vein have been reported.[813] These granulomas may be confused with tumors, polyps, or cysts. Granulomas have been reported in the esophagus, pharynx, palate, flank,[814] internal iliac lymph nodes,[815] and testes[815]; multiple subcutaneous lesions with regional lymph node involvement also have been reported.[817] Most granulomatous abscesses in a herd outbreak of actinobacillosis involved the tongue, muzzle, and lips and the submandibular, parotid, and cranial cervical areas.[816] Generalized involvement or granuloma formation in internal organs may also occur.

Lesions in sheep typically involve the lips and face or parotid and submaxillary regions.[819] The nasal cavity and internal organs occasionally may be involved. Soft tissues of the head may be infected through fight wounds.[819] Lesions of the lips must be differentiated from those of contagious ecthyma, and granulomatous abscesses in other sites must be differentiated from caseous lymphadenitis lesions. Lesions of the tongue of sheep, essentially identical to those found in cattle, have been reported as a cause of green staining of the lips and "cud-dropping" in sheep.[818]

CLINICAL PATHOLOGY. Diagnosis of actinobacillosis requires biopsy and culture of the lesion. The pus usually is not malodorous. Pus crushed between two glass slides shows "sulfur granules," "clublike rosettes," or "club colonies." Similar colonies may be found in actinomycosis and some staphylococcal infections.[819] *A. lignieresii* are small, gram-negative rods. Definitive diagnosis relies on culture. No reliable serologic test is available for actinobacillosis, and the hematologic and clinical chemical findings may be normal or typical of a response to chronic infection.

PATHOPHYSIOLOGY. *A. lignieresii* is a normal inhabitant of the mouth of ruminants and can be found in many plant awns. When mucosal lesions occur as a result of plant awns (e.g., foxtails), thistles, or particularly stemmy coarse feed, actinobacillosis may occur. Cattle often have a small ulcer in the sulcus lingualis at the junction of the base and shaft of the tongue. Plant fibers are sometimes found in the granulomatous lesions of actinobacillosis.[816] Once inoculated into tissues the organism may cause a local lesion or lesions in draining lymph nodes, or both. Lesions elsewhere on the body may be contaminated by saliva or by pus from other draining lesions or directly by plant awns on which *A. lignieresii* resides.

EPIDEMIOLOGY. Most cases of actinobacillosis are sporadic. Herd outbreaks may be associated with abrasive feedstuffs and crowded conditions in which the organism is spread rapidly to wounds on other animals by way of saliva. In one herd outbreak, 73% of a group of heifers (4 to 24 months of age) were affected 1 month after feeding of a coarse, stemmy haylage had begun.[816] Atypical lesions often are associated with a previous wound at the site, such as a nose lead wound,[813] multiple needle punctures,[813] or head butting wound.[819] Outbreaks of actinobacillosis in wounds of the head, neck, body, and limbs have been reported.[821]

NECROPSY AND BIOPSY FINDINGS. Actinobacillosis lesions typically are firm, pale, gritty, granulomatous abscesses. Grossly they are similar to exuberant granulation tissue and connective tissue, often appearing to have a yellowish granular (1 to 3 mm) surface. Masses contain multifocal necrotic foci, often filled with nonodorous, thick, yellow-white pus. Histologically the lesion is a granulomatous abscess.[813] An outer capsular region of connective and granulation tissue

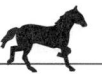

surrounds an area of leukocytes and rosettes ("club colonies"). Mononuclear cells, plasma cells, and eosinophils predominate. Many neutrophils are seen at the center of the lesion. Multinucleated giant cells or plant fibers, or both, may be seen.

TREATMENT AND PROGNOSIS. Treatment usually is successful, and the condition has an excellent prognosis when only the tongue is involved. The prognosis may be only slightly less optimistic when internal organs and atypical sites are involved. Sodium iodide (70 mg/kg given intravenously as a 10% to 20% solution) is the treatment of choice. Intravenous treatment is given once and repeated at least one more time at a 7- to 10-day interval. In refractory cases intravenous therapy may be repeated more often (2- to 3-day intervals). In severe cases daily organic iodides can be administered orally at a rate of 60 mg/kg/day[813] in addition to the intravenous iodide. If signs of iodinism develop (excessive tearing, coughing, inappetence, diarrhea, and/or dandruff), iodine administration should be halted; the adverse signs normally disappear shortly thereafter.

The onset of therapeutic benefit of sodium iodide is remarkably rapid. Within 48 hours after treatment, the tongue is flexible enough to allow the animal to eat. Although the mode by which iodides exert their beneficial therapeutic effect in actinobacillosis is not well understood, it seems most likely that they exert some antiinflammatory effect on the granulomatous inflammation. Iodides have little in vitro bacteriostatic or bactericidal effect at the concentrations given,[822] yet the onset of action is very rapid. They probably act in some way other than by direct antimicrobial effect. The old belief that iodides cause abortion at the recommended dosage has been cast into doubt by my clinical experience and by reports of others,[823] who gave one and one-half to two times the recommended intravenous dose without inducing abortion. Nevertheless, there are anecdotal reports of the association, and when products are labeled with a contraindication for use in pregnant cattle, due caution should be exercised. Iodides should be given slowly and with caution to horses because of the possibility of severe generalized adverse reactions to intravenous sodium iodide.

Most strains of *A. lignieresii* are sensitive in vitro to a number of antimicrobial drugs, including ceftiofur, ampicillin, penicillin, florfenicol, sulfas, aminoglycosides, and tetracyclines. Each isolate should be tested for antimicrobial sensitivity. Therapy with an antimicrobial drug to which the isolate is sensitive is recommended in severe, generalized, or refractory cases of actinobacillosis. Therapy should also include iodides.

Surgical debulking of lesions, particularly if they interfere with airflow, is also possible for atypical cases in which a large granulomatous mass is present and the mass has proved refractory to medical therapy. Hemostasis may be a problem after surgical debulking.

PREVENTION AND CONTROL. Prevention relies mainly on avoidance of coarse, stemmy, scabrous feeds and pastures full of hard, penetrating plant awns (e.g., foxtails) or thistles. If an outbreak occurs, immediate change to a softer feed is advised, and affected animals should be treated individually. Rapid resolution of the outbreak can be expected once these steps have been taken. If atypical lesions occur, a cause of skin wounds in the area should be sought and resolved.

REFERENCES

812. Buttenschon J: The occurrence of lesions in the tongue of adult cattle and their implications for the development of actinobacillosis, *J Vet Med Assoc* 36:393-400, 1989.
813. Rebhun WC, King JM, Hillman RB: Atypical actinobacillosis granulomas in cattle, *Cornell Vet* 78:125-130, 1988.
814. Swarbrick O: Atypical actinobacillosis in three cows, *Br Vet J* 123:70-75, 1970.
815. Palotay JL: Actinobacillosis in cattle, *Vet Med* 2:52-54, 1951.
816. Campbell SG et al: An unusual epizootic of actinobacillosis in dairy heifers, *J Am Vet Med Assoc* 166:604-606, 1975.
817. Hebeler HF, Linton AH, Osborne AD: Atypical actinobacillosis in a dairy herd, *Vet Rec* 73:517-521, 1961.
818. Sproat JB: Cud-dropping in sheep, *Vet Rec* 123:582, 1988.
819. Fubini SL, Campbell SC: External lumps on sheep and goats, *Vet Clin North Am (Large Anim Pract)* 5:457-476, 1983.
820. Baum KH et al: Isolation of *Actinobacillus lignieresii* from enlarged tongue of a horse, *J Am Vet Med Assoc* 185:792-793, 1984.
821. Hofmann VW, Heckert HP, Koberg J: Bestandsweise gehaüfes auftreten von Aktinobazillose bei rindern in Schleswig-Holstein, *Tierärztl Umschau* 46:250-257, 1991.
822. Smith HW: A laboratory consideration of the treatment of *Actinobacillus lignieresii* infection, *Vet Rec* 63:674-675, 1951.
823. Miller HV, Drost M: Failure to cause abortion in cows with intravenous sodium iodide treatment, *J Am Vet Med Assoc* 172:466-467, 1978.

ACTINOMYCOSIS (Lumpy Jaw)

BRADFORD P. SMITH

DEFINITION AND ETIOLOGY. Actinomycosis is caused by *Actinomyces bovis*, a gram-positive, nonencapsulated, branching, filamentous bacterium that is a normal inhabitant of the ruminant mouth. The disease occurs mainly in cattle but on rare occasions may affect sheep or goats. It enters the tissues and bone through oral abrasions, openings, and punctures associated with dental disease, hard plant awns (e.g., foxtails), thorns, stickers, or dry, coarse, stemmy feeds. Lesions are sporadic and occur mainly in the mandible[824-826] and less commonly in the maxilla. The preponderance of mandibular lesions, with the development of periosteal new bone and fibrosis, gives the disease its common name of "lumpy jaw." Lesions occasionally occur in soft tissues of the head, esophagus, forestomachs,[827] and trachea.[828,829] Occasionally *A. bovis* may cause granulomatous abscesses in other soft tissues. Most of the early reports of esophageal groove and forestomach involvement incriminate actinobacillosis rather than actinomycosis.[831]

Osteomyelitis of the mandible in a horse associated with nocardiosis has been reported,[831] but no cases of mandibular actinomycosis in horses have been reported.

CLINICAL SIGNS AND DIFFERENTIAL DIAGNOSIS. Typical bovine actinomycosis causes a hard, immovable, painless, bony mass on the mandible (Fig. 30-46). The lesion is most common on the horizontal ramus. Initially it is nondraining (has no fistulous tracts), but it may develop fistulous tracts and involve tooth roots as the condition progresses. When teeth become involved, evidence of pain when chewing may be seen, and weight loss may result. A careful examination of the mouth is required to detect loose teeth, plant awns, or severe gingivitis and to rule out a pathologic fracture. If a fistula is present, it is useful to flush the tract with organic iodine and perform contrast radiographs to determine if it communicates with the mouth. The differential diagnosis includes tooth root abscess, fracture, tumors, and osteomyelitis caused by other organisms. A mandibular swelling that continues to enlarge despite therapy should be radiographed for evidence of a fracture or sequestrum. Atypical actinomycosis with lesions in soft tissue causes a variety of clinical signs, depending on the location.

CLINICAL PATHOLOGY AND DIAGNOSIS. Hematologic and clinical chemistry findings may be normal or may reflect a chronic infection. Radiographs of the lesion are helpful in determining if there is dental involvement or a pathologic fracture. The radiographic lesion consists of multiple central radiolucent areas of osteomyelitis surrounded by periosteal new bone and fibrous tissue. If a fistulous tract is present, a contrast study done while flushing into the tract may help determine the extent of the fistula. Before flushing, material

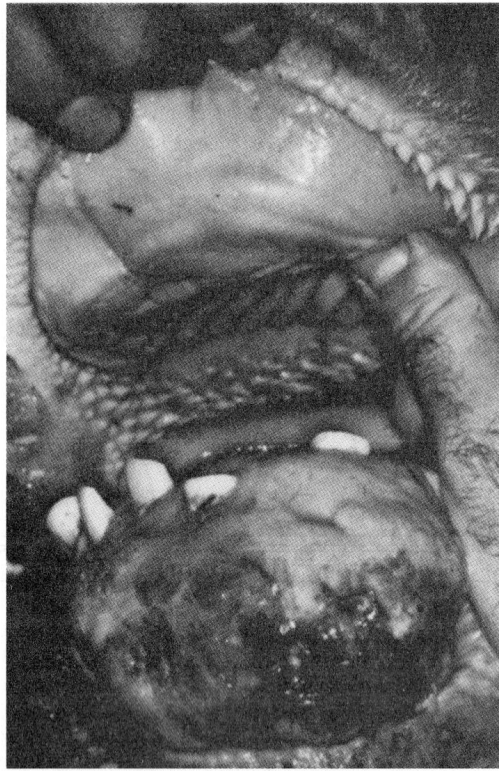

FIG. 30-46 ▓ Hard swelling on the distal mandible of a cow, typical of lumpy jaw caused by *Actinomyces bovis*. Loss of teeth and bone destruction, along with fibrosis and callus formation, are seen in this advanced case. The oral mucosa is secondarily ulcerated by trauma.

from the core of the lesion should be aspirated or biopsied. A Gram stain and culture of pus should be performed. The organism is gram-positive, filamentous, and branching. "Sulfur granules" similar to those described for actinobacillosis may be seen.

PATHOPHYSIOLOGY AND EPIDEMIOLOGY. *A. bovis* appears to enter the bone through mucous membrane punctures caused by foreign bodies, plant awns, or coarse, stemmy feeds or through a diseased tooth or areas of gingivitis that allow oral bacteria access to the bone. Cases usually are sporadic.

NECROPSY AND BIOPSY FINDINGS. Actinomycosis causes a granulomatous abscess.[829] Scattered through the mass of tissue are basophilic clumps of bacteria surrounded by eosinophilic clublike projections. The bacteria are long, filamentous, branching rods. Surrounding them is cellular reaction composed of neutrophils, epithelioid cells, macrophages, and occasional multinucleated giant cells. In the outer fibrous tissue are plasma cells.

TREATMENT AND PROGNOSIS. Treatment of actinomycotic bone lesions usually results in arrest of the lesion, but seldom does the size of the hard mass regress significantly. The prognosis for arrest of the lesion with vigorous treatment is good. If the mass does not have any fistulous tracts and no affected teeth are loose, medical therapy alone may be sufficient. If the mass has fistulous tracts, it should also be vigorously curetted and flushed with povidone-iodine or other organic iodine. The lesion has a rich blood supply, and curettage can result in severe hemorrhage. If the cavity is large, it may be necessary to flush and pack with iodine-soaked gauze daily for several days, then less frequently as healing progresses. If there is an open fistula into the mouth (as judged by vigorous flushing) or if teeth are involved, the affected tooth or teeth should be carefully removed. Care

must be taken to prevent mandibular fracture, and the animal must be sedated or anesthetized to allow for proper intraoral manipulation. The empty alveolus should be carefully packed with gauze or a dental acrylic to which a wire or umbilical tape is attached and pulled through the fistula. The wire is tied externally to a small gauze roll to keep the alveolar packing firmly in place. The wire should be untied daily and the tract flushed thoroughly with povidone-iodine until the wound is completely granulated. Once granulation begins, it may not be necessary to check and flush the lesion more than once a week. The alveolus will take several weeks to close, pushing the gauze or acrylic out as it does so.

Medical treatment of actinomycosis involves the use of sodium iodide, isoniazid, and penicillin or other antimicrobial drug to which the organism is sensitive. Sodium iodide is given intravenously at a dosage of 70 mg/kg as a 10% to 20% solution. It can be given every 7 to 10 days or more often until signs of iodinism occur (i.e., lacrimation, cough, inappetence, diarrhea, and dandruff). If repeated intravenous treatments are difficult, oral organic iodides can be given at the rate of 60 mg/kg/day for 3 weeks. As with actinobacillosis, the beneficial therapeutic effects of iodides appear to lie in their ability to reduce granulomatous inflammation rather than in direct antimicrobial effects.[832] Iodides do *not* appear to cause abortion and can be safely given to pregnant cows,[833] although care should be used because there are anecdotal reports to the contrary, and products are labeled with a contraindication for pregnant cattle.

Isoniazid (10 mg/kg/day given orally for 1 month) is effective at arresting actinomycosis of the mandible in cattle.[824] It is inexpensive and readily consumed in a small amount of grain. A prolonged withdrawal period before slaughter for human consumption is required. The drug appears to be nontoxic at this dosage, but it may cause abortion and should not be used in pregnant cattle.

Penicillin (10,000 U/kg IM twice daily) or another antimicrobial drug such as florfenicol or ampicillin can be added to the treatment regimen in cases involving valuable animals or when twice daily treatment for 7 to 14 days is possible. Streptomycin was found effective in one study,[826] but because of the prolonged persistence of tissue residues, aminoglycosides generally are considered unacceptable in food animals.

PREVENTION AND CONTROL. *A. bovis* is a normal mouth inhabitant of ruminants, therefore the only possible means of prevention is to avoid feeding coarse, stemmy feeds, feeds with hard, penetrating plant awns, or feeds with other sharp materials. The recommendations in this regard are similar to those for actinobacillosis.

REFERENCES

824. Watts TC, Olson SM, Rhodes CS: Treatment of bovine actinomycosis with isoniazid, *Can Vet J* 14:223-224, 1973.
825. Patgiri GP, Bashar SK, Rahman H: Actinomycosis in the bovine: case reports, *Livestock Advis Bangalore* 10:35-36, 1985.
826. Kingman HE, Palen JS: Streptomycin in the treatment of actinomycosis, *J Am Vet Med Assoc* 118:28-30, 1951.
827. Bruere AN: Actinomycosis of the digestive tract in cattle, *NZ Vet J* 3:121-122, 1955.
828. Bertone AL, Rebhun WC: Tracheal actinomycosis in a cow, *J Am Vet Med Assoc* 185:221-222, 1984.
829. Stevenson RG, Taylor RG: Actinomycosis of the trachea in a mature cow, *Can Vet J* 18:278-280, 1977.
830. Begg H: Diseases of the stomach of the adult ruminant, *Vet Rec* 62:797-808, 1950.
831. Tritschler LG, Romach FE: Nocardiosis in equine mandibles associated with bilateral anomalies of the inferior dentition, *Vet Med* 60:605-608, 1965.
832. Smith HW: A laboratory consideration of the treatment of *Actinobacillus lignieresii* infection, *Vet Rec* 63:674-675, 1951.
833. Miller HV, Drost M: Failure to cause abortion in cows with intravenous sodium iodide treatment, *J Am Vet Med Assoc* 172:466-467, 1978.

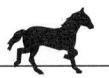

PHARYNGEAL TRAUMA AND ABSCESS

BRADFORD P. SMITH

DEFINITION AND ETIOLOGY. Pharyngeal trauma occurs relatively frequently in cattle, resulting in cellulitis,[834] abscessation,[834] or hematoma formation.[835] One case resulted in megaesophagus.[836] Pharyngeal trauma is almost always associated with use of a balling gun,[834,837] long dose syringe, speculum, paste wormer gun, rigid probe of calf esophageal feeder, or rigid stomach tube.[834] Occasionally a foreign body such as a sharp stick or wire can perforate the pharynx. Hematomas may result from unidentified blunt trauma.[835] The puncture or laceration may be very small and usually is located in the area near the origin of the esophagus. The result is that feed and saliva enter the retropharyngeal area, and eventually inflammation develops (also see Chapter 29, Retropharyngeal Abscess).

CLINICAL SIGNS AND DIFFERENTIAL DIAGNOSIS. The clinical signs include anorexia, drooling of saliva, malodorous breath, extended head and neck, localized or diffuse pharyngeal pain, feed coming from the external nares, and forestomach stasis or bloat.[834] Severe cases may involve obvious pharyngeal swelling, fever, easily elicited cough upon laryngeal palpation, dyspnea, and aspiration pneumonia. Intraluminal submucosal pharyngeal abscesses with similar clinical signs have been reported.[838] Differential diagnosis in cattle must include retropharyngeal abscesses (also see Chapter 29, Retropharyngeal Abscess), pharyngeal foreign body, actinobacillosis, and lymphosarcoma or other tumor involving the pharyngeal lymph nodes.

If megaesophagus occurs, it must be differentiated from diaphragmatic hernia with herniation of the reticulum into the thorax; other outflow obstructions involving the reticulum can result in frequent regurgitation and vomiting, as can a number of other diseases, including esophageal foreign body and esophageal diverticulum. Several toxins also cause vomiting (see Chapter 7). Rabies is easily differentiated, because the only clinical signs common to both are anorexia and salivation. Careful digital palpation of the pharynx often is diagnostic, although restraint is difficult because the area is painful and swollen, causing dyspnea and struggling. A well-lubricated stomach tube should be gently passed to relieve bloat and ascertain that no esophageal obstruction is present. Pharyngeal trauma is rare in sheep and goats, and retropharyngeal abscesses caused by *Corynebacterium pseudotuberculosis* (caseous lymphadenitis) are the most common cause of pharyngeal swelling.

CLINICAL PATHOLOGY AND LABORATORY AIDS. Endoscopy and radiography may be of great help in diagnosing the site of the lesion, the extent of cellulitis, and the presence of a foreign body. Endoscopy reveals a swollen, collapsed pharyngeal air space. The wound may be visible, and it may have exudate at its origin. Endoscopy can help rule out intraluminal masses and foreign bodies. Retropharyngeal cellulitis, abscess, or hematoma often can be visualized radiographically, and radiopaque foreign bodies can be seen (Fig. 30-47). Gas in the soft tissues or a discrete mass can be seen with cellulitis and abscess, respectively. Gas often can be seen in the lumen of the esophagus as well. Radiographs of the lung may be helpful if aspiration pneumonia is suspected. The results of hematologic analysis may reflect an infectious inflammatory process.

PATHOPHYSIOLOGY. Inflammation, swelling, and necrosis in the retropharyngeal tissues interfere with normal swallowing by causing pain when swallowing is attempted, physical interference with passage of a bolus, and neurologic involvement. The resultant dysphagia may predispose the animal to inhalation of feed and saliva.

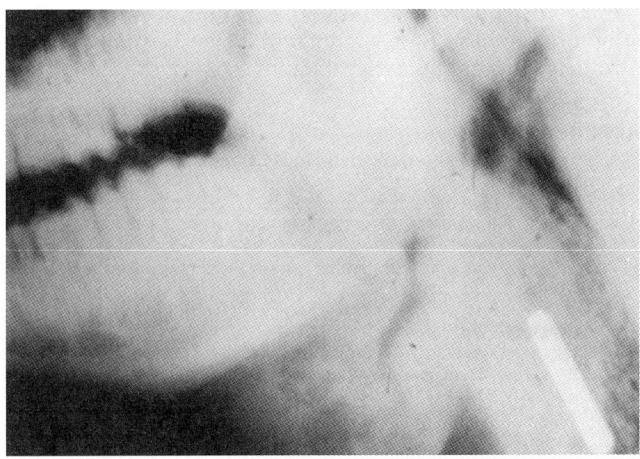

FIG. 30-47 ■ Pharyngeal trauma in a 2-year-old bull caused by a magnet that was given forcefully with a balling gun 24 hours previously. The magnet is visible in the retropharyngeal tissues surrounded by cellulitis, with swelling and gas in the tissues. The area is swollen and painful.

If the retropharyngeal inflammation affects the pharyngeal branch of the vagus nerve on the dorsolateral surface of the pharynx, the esophageal and pharyngeal phases of swallowing and eructation are disturbed.[834,839] The resultant pharyngeal paresis may lead to reflux of feed through the nares. Involvement of the adjacent cranial laryngeal nerve makes the laryngeal mucosa less sensitive to foreign material and thus diminishes the cough reflex.[834] Severe inflammation may involve the vagus nerve itself and cause forestomach stasis with bloat and laryngeal motor dysfunction.[834,840] Eructation also involves pharyngeal muscular activity, and the maneuver is likely to be quite painful when cellulitis is present in the area.

TREATMENT AND PROGNOSIS. In spite of the fact that affected animals often are completely anorectic and febrile and look very ill, most cases of pharyngeal puncture or laceration resolve successfully if the animal can be vigorously treated with broad-spectrum antimicrobial drugs for 7 to 14 days, if aspiration pneumonia can be controlled by limiting access to feed, and if adequate supportive care can be given. Tetracyclines, sulfas, ampicillin, ceftiofur, trimethoprim-sulfa, and florfenicol or penicillin plus an aminoglycoside have been used successfully. Nonsteroidal antiinflammatory drugs should be given for analgesia and for their ability to reduce inflammation. Oral administration of boluses should be avoided.

The animal should have access to water; if it cannot drink, a soft stomach tube should be used several times daily to gently administer a total of 30 to 50 L (8 to 13 gallons) of water plus electrolytes daily. The most important electrolyte to administer is potassium: 60 to 100 g of potassium chloride should be given daily with the water. Once the animal can drink without coughing or nasal reflux, soft green grass or a soft mash should be offered. If this is well tolerated, it should be continued for 2 weeks, after which green pasture or soft, green leafy alfalfa hay or other equally palatable feed should be gradually and carefully introduced into the diet.

If a discrete retropharyngeal abscess forms, it is best first to attempt drainage into the pharynx through the original laceration by pushing a finger into the healing wound until pus escapes. If this fails, a surgical approach to the area may be necessary. Surgery is rarely required in cases of pharyngeal trauma or laceration with cellulitis.

PREVENTION AND CONTROL. Careful use of balling guns, paste wormer guns, and other equipment that can damage the pharynx is the best prevention. Adequate restraint of the head of any animal that is to be orally treated also helps prevent pharyngeal trauma.

REFERENCES

834. Davidson HP, Rebhun WC, Habel RE: Pharyngeal trauma in cattle, *Cornell Vet* 71:15-25, 1981.
835. Farrow CS: Exercise in diagnostic radiology, *Can Vet J* 22:286-287, 1981.
836. Ross CE, Rebhun WC: Megaesophagus in a cow, *J Am Vet Med Assoc* 188:623-624, 1986.
837. Adams GP, Radostits OM: Balling gun–induced trauma of the pharynx in feedlot cattle, *Can Vet J* 29:389-390, 1988.
838. Grymer J, Scott EA: Pharyngeal abscess with lymphoid hyperplasia in a dairy cow, *J Am Vet Med Assoc* 180:942-944, 1982.
839. Dougherty RW, Habel RE, Bond HE: Esophageal innervation and eructation reflex in sheep, *Am J Vet Res* 19:115-118, 1958.
840. Dougherty RW et al: Studies of the pharyngeal and laryngeal activity during eructation of ruminants, *Am J Vet Res* 23:213-219, 1962.

BLUETONGUE

PAUL G. E. MICHELSEN

DEFINITION AND ETIOLOGY. Bluetongue is an arthropod-borne viral disease of domestic and wild ruminants with complex interactions with the host, the host's immune system, the vector or vectors, other similar viruses, and the biopolitical environment. Clinical disease is largely restricted to sheep, but other ruminants may show disease in some circumstances. Epizootics of bluetongue disease such as one on the Iberian peninsula that killed 179,000 sheep in 4 months led to the idea of bluetongue as an emerging exotic disease that threatened livestock industries. Epidemic disease outbreaks, the wide host range, the potential for establishment of endemic disease, and the similarity of some signs of bluetongue to those of vesicular diseases have made bluetongue infection the subject of intense regulatory interest worldwide. Import regulations promulgated in reaction to the disease have been more of a threat than the disease itself to the livestock industries of some countries.[841]

Bluetongue virus (BTV) is the prototypical orbivirus, a genus (or subfamily) within the family Reoviridae. Other viruses in the genus, some of which cross-react serologically with BTV, include Palyam virus, the epizootic hemorrhagic disease of deer virus and the agent of African horse sickness. The virus has a segmented genome of 10 double-stranded (RNA) pieces, each of which codes for one or two polypeptides. The genome of bluetongue virus was recently determined down to atomic resolution using crystallography, the largest molecule known in such detail to date.[842] The serologic classification is based on the protein product of one or two genomic segments, but virulence and other characteristics may not be related to this protein, and genetic reassortment of the pieces occurs in infections of cells with more than one serotype.[843] BTV reproduces in both arthropod and mammalian hosts and must evolve quickly to maintain itself in these imperfectly overlapping realms. Reassortment of the segmented genome contributes to the prodigious genetic diversity and rapid evolution of BTV.[844]

Strains of the virus with the same serotype may have markedly different virulence.[845,846] The discovery of BTV in Australia in 1975 originally was a cause of great concern, because the continent had been thought to be free of the virus. Subsequent investigation showed the presence of antibody in stored sera, and the Australian strains of serotypes that are pathogenic elsewhere proved to have almost no pathogenic capability. Twenty-five serotypes are recognized worldwide, five (2, 10, 11, 13, and 17) in the United States.

CLINICAL SIGNS AND DIFFERENTIAL DIAGNOSIS. Clinical bluetongue disease is manifested in two ways: reproductive syndromes and bluetongue per se, a vasculitic disease of several organ systems. Cattle and goats rarely manifest clinical disease; infected sheep commonly do.

In sheep the first clinical signs appear after an incubation period of 3 to 8 days. These signs include a transient fever (up to 41.1° C [106° F] or higher); edema of the face, lips, muzzle, and ears; excessive salivation; and hyperemia of the oral mucosa. Affected sheep usually produce a profuse serous nasal discharge that becomes mucopurulent after a few days, leaving crusts around the nostrils and muzzle. The tongue may be cyanotic (hence the name), but this is an infrequent sign. The oral lesions progress to petechial hemorrhages, erosions, and ulcers, which are especially prominent on the dental pad and the commissures of the mouth. Pulmonary edema is often marked, and some cases appear to owners to be pneumonia. Secondary bacterial bronchopneumonia frequently complicates bluetongue. Lameness and stiffness caused by coronitis and myopathy are later signs, occurring 7 to 12 days after exposure, and the coronary band shows petechial hemorrhages and hyperemia. Cardiac myopathy may result in sudden death at any time, even in an animal that appears to be recovering. Lameness may progress to "knee walking" or recumbency. The hooves may slough, and breaks in the wool are common. Diarrhea, with or without blood, is frequently seen. Many sheep become depressed, are unable to rise, and die, but some severely affected sheep make a full recovery. The differential diagnosis for sheep showing some of these signs includes sore mouth (contagious ecthyma), foot-and-mouth disease, and sheep-pox.

The reproductive and teratogenic effects of bluetongue virus in sheep and cattle appear to vary greatly depending on the strain, the host, and the ecologic factors. Reproductive effects, including abortions, stillbirths, and weak, live "dummy lamb" births, were prominent when live attenuated vaccine was given to pregnant ewes in California. In South Africa, which has been recognized as bluetongue-endemic since the first descriptions of the disease before 1900, teratogenic effects have not been firmly linked to the virus despite the use of polyvalent attenuated live vaccines and near-continuous exposure to the virus.[845]

The virus has been shown to be both abortigenic and teratogenic in cattle under experimental conditions,[847] but despite evidence of high seroprevalence in cattle, abortion and teratogenesis are very uncommon under field conditions.[848] Early embryonic wastage and decreased reproductive efficiency may be more important in cattle than teratogenesis and abortion; bluetongue-seropositive cows had more services per conception, longer calving to conception intervals, and a greater number of total services compared with age-matched bluetongue-negative cows on the same large California dairy.[849] Experimental early gestation infections in cattle produce severe deformities that preclude live birth; later infections can cause premature delivery of low birth weight, weak, viremic calves.[846]

Clinical disease in cattle is rare, but it can show many of the same signs as in sheep. Excessive salivation may be the first clinical sign. Hyperemia and necrosis of the muzzle ("burnt muzzle") and a patchy dermatitis may also be seen. In cattle, depending on which signs are exhibited, the differential diagnosis should include mucosal disease (BVD), malignant catarrhal fever, vesicular diseases, rinderpest, photosensitization, bovine papular stomatitis, and infectious bovine rhinotracheitis. Clinical disease in cattle can be difficult to distinguish from foot-and-mouth disease and vesicular stomatitis, and appropriate regulatory officials should be notified in such outbreaks.

"White eye calf" syndrome has been described in Harney County, Oregon. The problem has a low incidence on affected ranches (0.5% to 8%). The calves are full-term stillbirths or weak, recumbent animals that rarely survive, even with good nursing care. Most affected calves have congenital cataracts, often bilaterally, which clear between 3 weeks and 3 months in the few that survive. Hydranencephaly and arthrogryposis are seen in a few calves together with the lens opacity. The calves test negative for BTV antibody on agar gel immunodiffusion (AGID) tests, but BTV or epizootic hemorrhagic disease virus, or both, can be isolated from the spleen or bone marrow.[850] Lenticular, other ocular, and brain abnormalities may also be caused by bovine virus diarrhea (BVD) virus, and that etiology should be considered in the differential diagnosis of suspected bluetongue teratogenesis in cattle.

LABORATORY DIAGNOSIS AND IMMUNOLOGY. Two types of viral antigen are involved in bluetongue diagnosis by serologic testing. All bluetongue viruses have one of the type types, the group antigen, which is a protein called P7. The other type of antigen, the P2 protein, determines the serotype (1 through 25) of the virus in question. The serum commonly is tested with complement fixation, agar gel immunodiffusion, or one of several enzyme-linked immunosorbent assays (ELISAs) for P7, which indicates bluetongue infection. Antibodies detected by AGID persist for years in normal animals exposed to BTV. Complement fixation tests detect shorter-lived antibodies and can be difficult to perform but are still used to determine BTV exposure status for export. The AGID test cross-reacts with related orbiviruses and can also produce a rather high number of false negatives. The competitive ELISA (C-ELISA) has proved to be the best serologic test for detecting group antibodies to bluetongue virus.[851,852] Because of the wide pathogenic variability among bluetongue viruses (aided, no doubt, by reassortment of the segmented genome) and the fact that some other nonpathogenic orbiviruses have antigenic similarities to BTV, a positive result on the bluetongue group test does not prove that an animal's clinical disease was caused by BTV.

Virus isolation from blood obtained during the viremic, febrile stage is the most definitive means of bluetongue diagnosis. Splenic tissues or, in the case of aborted fetuses, brain tissues also can be a source of virus for isolation. Virus isolation is done by inoculation of samples into a variety of test animals and culture systems, but it is being at least partly replaced by detection of viral RNA using polymerase chain reaction (PCR) technology. PCR-based tests for bluetongue are extremely sensitive and specific for BTV RNA and currently are being performed on clinical samples at several diagnostic laboratories. A positive PCR result is not synonymous with infection, however, because viral RNA can be detected for some time after viremia (as detected by standard virus isolation methods) has waned.[853]

Other laboratory aids to diagnosis include the presence of leukopenia during the early febrile stage of the disease and an often marked increase in serum creatinine kinase that corresponds to the latter phase of reluctance to move and stiffness.

The development of immune tolerance to BTV (in utero infection producing antibody-negative, virus-positive individuals), as happens in BVD infections, now is regarded by many as rarely if ever occurring under natural conditions,[852,854] but some controversy remains.[855]

PATHOPHYSIOLOGY. BTV is capable of reproducing in a variety of mammalian cells. In clinical cases the disease appears to be a vasculitis caused by infection of vascular endothelial cells. Vasculitis results in edema and necrosis of epithelial and mucosal surfaces. In bulls the virus can cause inflammation and degeneration of the seminiferous tubules.

Teratogenic effects appear to be caused by general disruptions of organogenesis by viral infection of the developing fetus. The development of clinical disease in cattle may require previous sensitization to the virus, operating through an IgE-mediated hypersensitivy reaction.[850] The disease in sheep also appears to be most severe when previous exposure has occurred.[856] Late-term in utero infections produce elevated fetal cortisol in calves, which could be the mechanism for the induction of premature delivery.[847]

EPIDEMIOLOGY. The development of clinical disease is the product of a complex interaction among host, strain, vector, and environmental characteristics. Bluetongue disease provides a model of host-vector-pathogen coevolution; the pathogenicity of endemic virus to endemic livestock breeds usually is low.[857] Epizootics occur when new virus or new animals or new vectors are introduced into the stable prevailing system.

BTV infects both wild and domestic ruminants and camelids, primarily through the bite of the vector midge of the genus *Culicoides*. This midge is most prevalent in midsummer to early fall, and natural bluetongue in animals usually is limited to this time as well. The virus also can be transmitted sexually in infected semen and transplacentally from dam to offspring but apparently not through embryo transfer if the embryo is washed 10 times.[852,855] Vector transmission is by far the most important method of transmission in endemic areas. In the United States, bluetongue prevalence closely mirrors *Culicoides* prevalence, with lower rates in northern climates inhospitable to the midge and higher prevalence in southern regions. *Culicoides sonorensis* (formerly called *C. variipennis*) is the principal vector of BTV in North America, but not all *C. variipennis* populations are competent vectors of the virus.[858,859] In the absence of competent vector populations, animal to animal transmission is incapable of maintaining the endemic state. The overall seroprevalence in cattle in the United States exceeds 18%.[860]

The location of "overwintering" virus or the reservoir for infection in endemic areas is unclear. Cattle have been suspected because of the high seroprevalence in cattle and the longer course of viremia possible in some cattle compared with sheep. In the Iberian epidemic of bluetongue in 1956 that killed 179,000 sheep in 4 months and caused clinical disease in cattle, the disease failed to become established despite the presence of vectors, suggesting that cattle were not an effective reservoir in this instance. White-tailed deer showed a high BTV seroprevalence (81%) in a survey in northeastern Mexico.[861] The virus reproduces in *C. sonorensis*, and the vector may be the overwintering site in some situations. Another intriguing possibility that needs more investigation involves the prolonged presence of viral RNA in blood as detected by PCR; the vector may be able to recover BTV infectivity from PCR-positive but virus isolation–negative blood.[862]

The severity of clinical signs varies by breed. Early in the history of the bluetongue investigation, it was noted that African Landrace breeds showed few if any signs of infection, whereas imported European breeds showed fulminant disease.[863] More recently, breed differences in immunologic response to a bluetongue vaccine have been reported.[864]

NECROPSY FINDINGS. No one gross or histologic lesion points with certainty toward bluetongue. Some animals that die appear surprisingly normal at necropsy. Most show unusual hemorrhage in some organ, particularly the heart. Some experts consider subendocardial hemorrhage at the base of the pulmonary artery to be pathognomonic. Petechial and ecchymotic hemorrhages are also seen under the tongue, on the hard palate, and in the esophagus, forestomachs (especially on the ruminal folds), lymph nodes, bladder, and spleen. Gross hemorrhage may be seen in skeletal muscles (often alternating with linear areas of pallor, indicating Zenker's necrosis) and in the pulmonary artery. Erosions and ulcers are seen on any surface of the oral mucosa, prominently on the dental pad and tongue, and less often in other digestive organs. Gelatinous subcutaneous edema of the head, neck, forelimbs, and trunk is commonly encountered. Pulmonary congestion and edema probably are caused by vasculitis and occur secondary to heart failure.[865] Microscopically, lesions show evidence of inflammatory cell infiltration, cellular vacuolation, blood stasis, hypertrophy of small vessel endothelial cells, and fragmentation of small vessels. Cattle, but not sheep, show eosinophilic infiltrates histologically, suggesting the role of hypersensitivity in the rare clinical cases in cattle.

TREATMENT, PREVENTION, AND CONTROL. Treatment is nonspecific and aimed at supportive and nursing care. Animals with severe oral lesions are reluctant to eat. Valuable animals can be fed gruels of alfalfa pellets by stomach tube and can be encouraged to eat soft feeds or green grass. Muscle and coronary band pain may limit mobility, therefore water and shade must be close at hand. Sulfas or other relatively broad-spectrum antimicrobial drugs should be administered in an attempt to prevent or treat secondary bacterial pneumonia. Nonsteroidal antiinflammatory drugs, including aspirin and flunixin, are commonly used.

Elimination of *C. sonorensis* from the environment usually is not practical, but housing sheep indoors during the peak of activity (dusk, early evening) to avoid the house-shy midge may be beneficial. Grazing wet areas such as irrigated pasture only during the heat of the day also may help. Midges that feed on ivermectin-treated cattle are killed,[850] but the exchange of virus may be made before the insect's demise. *C. sonorensis* larvae develop in fine-grained mud with high organic matter content, such as around farm reservoirs, overflowing watering troughs, and shallow septic systems. Elimination of these breeding grounds combined with larvicidal treatments may help in some situations.

Modified live vaccines are available in some parts of the world and should be based on the local strains and serotypes. Some cross-protection between some serotypes does occur. A modified live virus containing serotypes 10, 11, and 17 is available in California from the California Woolgrowers' Association. The vaccine should be given at least 2 weeks before breeding season to avoid teratogenic effects. In the face of an outbreak lambs and breeding rams should be vaccinated; pregnant ewes in late gestation may be vaccinated, but there is some risk of inducing abortion. Vaccinated breeding rams may have a slight risk of decreased fertility. Pregnant animals cannot be vaccinated with modified live vaccines with impunity, because the teratogenic effects may manifest. Genetic engineering techniques may produce effective killed vaccines, perhaps as subunits, but both cellular and humoral immunity appear necessary for complete protection. The capability of the virus to reassort the genome in mixed infections makes some aspects of modified live vaccines problematic. For example, a host-adapted, low-virulence vaccine strain could gain virulence from wild-type virus and be serologically indistinguishable in its pathogenic form from the mild vaccine virus.

REFERENCES

841. Oveido MT et al: Analysis of evidence of clinical bluetongue disease in Central America and the Caribbean. In Walton TE, Osburn BI, eds: *Proceedings of the Second International Symposium on Blue-tongue, African horse sickness, and related orbiviruses,* Orlando, Fla, 1992, CRC Press.
842. Gouet P et al: The highly ordered double-stranded RNA genome of bluetongue virus revealed by crystallography, *Cell* 97:481-490, 1999.
843. Maia MS, Osburn BI: Differential serological responses to reassortment bluetongue virus recovered from a bull, *Arch Virol* 128:345-346, 1993.
844. de Mattos CC et al: Phylogenetic comparison of the s3 gene of United States prototype strains of bluetongue virus with that of field isolates from California, *J Virol* 70:5735-5739, 1996.
845. Parsonson IM, Della-Porta AJ, Snowden WA: Developmental disorders of the fetus in some arthropod-borne virus infections, *Am J Trop Med Hyg* 30:660-673, 1981.
846. Waldvogel AS et al: Association of virulent and avirulent strains of bluetongue virus serotype 11 with premature births of late-term bovine fetuses, *J Comp Pathol* 106:333-340, 1992.
847. Luedke AJ, Jochim MM, Jones RH: Bluetongue in cattle: effect of *Culicoides variipennis*–transmitted bluetongue virus on pregnant heifers and their calves, *Am J Vet Res* 38:1687-1695, 1977.
848. Oberst RD: Viruses as teratogens, *Vet Clin North Am (Food Anim Pract)* 9:23-31, 1993.
849. Huffman EM et al: An association between bluetongue virus infection and impaired reproductive performance of dairy cattle, *Proceedings of the Annual Meeting of the Society for Theriogenology,* 1985.
850. Odeon AC, Gershwin LJ, Osburn BI: IgE responses to bluetongue virus (BTV) serotype 11 after immunization with inactivated BTV and challenge infection, *Comp Immunol Microbiol Infect Dis* 22:145-162, 1999.
851. Afshar A et al: Comparison of competitive and indirect enzyme-linked immunosorbent assays for detection of bluetongue virus antibodies in serum and whole blood, *J Clin Microbiol* 25:1705-1710, 1987.
852. Osborn BI: Bluetongue virus, *Vet Clin North Am (Food Anim Pract)* 10:547-560, 1994.
853. MacLachlan NJ, Nunamaker RA, Katz JB: Detection of bluetongue virus in the blood of inoculated calves: comparison of virus isolation, PCR assay, and in vitro feeding of *Culicoides variipennis, Arch Virol* 136:1-8, 1994.
854. Osburn BI: The current world status of bluetongue, *Bovine Practitioner* 25:12-14, 1990.
855. Roberts DH, Lucas MH, Bell RA: Animal and animal product importation and the assessment of risk from bluetongue and other ruminant orbiviruses, *Br Vet J* 149:87-89, 1993.
856. Mahrt CR, Osburn BI: Experimental bluetongue virus infection of sheep: effect of previous vaccination—clinical and immunologic studies, *Am J Vet Res* 47:1191-1197, 1986.
857. Gibbs EP, Greiner EC: The epidemiology of bluetongue, *Comp Immunol Microbiol Infect Dis* 17:207-220, 1994.
858. Tabachnick WJ: *Culicoides variipennis* and bluetongue virus epidemiology in the United States, *Annu Rev Entomol* 41:23-43, 1996.
859. Fu H et al: The barriers to bluetongue virus infection, dissemination, and transmission in the vector *Culicoides variipennis* (dipter: Ceratopogonidae), *Arch Virol* 144:747-761, 1999.
860. Metcalf HE, Pearson JE, Klingsporn AL: Bluetongue in cattle: a serologic survey of slaughter cattle in the United States, *Am J Vet Res* 42:1057-1061, 1981.
861. Martinez A et al: Serosurvey for selected disease agents in white-tailed deer from Mexico, *J Wild Dis* 35:799-803, 1999.
862. Katz J et al: Diagnostic analysis of the prolonged bluetongue virus RNA presence found in the blood of naturally infected cattle and experimentally infected sheep, *J Vet Diagn Invest* 6:139-142, 1994.
863. Howell PG: The epidemiology of bluetongue in South Africa: arbovirus research in Australia, *Proceedings of the Second Symposium,* 1979.
864. Berry LJ et al: Inactivated bluetongue virus vaccine in lambs: differential serological responses related to breed, *Vet Res Commun* 5:289-293, 1982.
865. Mahrt CR, Osburn BI: Experimental bluetongue virus infection of sheep: effect of vaccination—pathologic, immunofluorescent, and ultrastructural studies, *Am J Vet Res* 47:1198-1203, 1986.
866. Holbrook FR, Romney SV, Sessions RM: Piggybacking bluetongue vector control and mosquito abatement, *Wingbeats,* Winter, 1993, pp 19-23.

CONTAGIOUS ECTHYMA (Sore Mouth, Orf, Contagious Pustular Dermatitis, Scabby Mouth)

PAUL G.E. MICHELSEN

DEFINITION AND ETIOLOGY. Contagious ecthyma (sore mouth, orf, contagious pustular dermatitis, scabby mouth) is a common disease of sheep and goats that is transmissible to humans and has a worldwide distribution. The colloquial name sore mouth describes the most common presentation of the disease in sheep and goats; the name orf (possibly from the old Norse term *hrufa,* meaning a crust or scab) is more commonly used for the disease in all species in England and for human disease in the United States. The agent is a poxvirus of the parapoxvirus subgroup, which includes the closely related viruses pseudocowpox (the cause of orflike "milker's nodules" in humans) and the agent of bovine papular stomatitis (see p. 706). Biologic differences exist between strains of contagious ecthyma virus, but these differences are not expressed antigenically; only one serotype is recognized.

CLINICAL SIGNS AND DIFFERENTIAL DIAGNOSIS. The most common presentation is of a young animal with crusting, proliferative lesions of the mucocutaneous junctions of the mouth and nose (Fig. 30-48). Proliferative lesions may be seen on the gums (Fig. 30-49). Older immunologically naive animals may be affected, and lesions may occur at the coronary band, on the tongue, interdigitally, on the conjunctiva of the eye, on the external genitalia, or on the udder or teats, the latter site occurring especially in does or ewes nursing affected kids. The disease progresses through papular, vesicular, and pustular stages, which are rarely seen, before the characteristic presentation of proliferative, coalescing, scabbed lesions appears. One recent report described the characteristic proliferative scabs on the margins of healing burn wounds.[867] Affected animals may be reluctant to nurse, eat, walk, or be nursed, depending on the location of lesions. Secondary bacterial infection or myiasis of affected parts may occur. The disease usually runs its course in 3 to 6 weeks, but chronic cases have been reported.[868] Complete healing without scarring is the norm as scabs fall off. Severe infections may result in stunting of growth. Overwhelming infection has been noted on rare occasions, with extension of lesions into the deeper respiratory or gastrointestinal tracts. Does and ewes with severe udder infection may develop mastitis from secondary bacterial infection. Sheeppox and goatpox may occasionally produce lesions similar to those of contagious ecthyma, but they are virulent diseases with systemic signs, including conjunctivitis, pyrexia, anorexia, and rhinitis. Animals afflicted with bluetongue may have a crusted mouth and nose and eye lesions in the convalescent phase, but bluetongue is a disease with more evidence of oral erosive rather than proliferative lesions and systemic signs, including pyrexia, reluctance to move, and conjunctivitis. Bluetongue has a seasonal incidence (late summer, early fall) that coincides with the activity of its insect vector. Contagious ecthyma may be seen at any time but typically occurs in spring in the lamb or kid crop. Ulcerative dermatosis (lip and leg ulcer) is an uncommon disease caused by a virus similar to that of contagious ecthyma, but the lesions are crusted ulcers, to be distinguished from the crusted proliferations of contagious ecthyma. Recently I saw a series of cases of what appeared to be mild contagious ecthyma of long duration (several years in one individual) in a family of Nubian goats. Pseudocowpox virus was diagnosed by immunofluorescence assay.

LABORATORY DIAGNOSIS. The diagnosis usually is made in the field by recognition of the typical lesions in a naive flock or in a naive group (young lambs or kids) in a disease-endemic flock. Definitive diagnosis usually involves identifying the distinctive cross-hatched virus particles in early lesions with electron microscopy or inoculation into known protected or susceptible animals. Vesicular fluid or minced biopsy tissues have been used as a source of virus that is identified by fluorescent antibodies after it has been growing in embryonic ovine kidney cell cultures.[869] Complement fixation tests to detect antibodies (using patient serum) or antigen (using vesicular fluid or a suspension of scabs) have also been used.

PATHOPHYSIOLOGY. The disease follows a similar time course in animals and human beings that lasts about 6 weeks. Six stages have been described,[870] which begin after an incubation period of 3 to 14 days. Each stage lasts about 1 week.

1. *Maculopapular stage:* An erythematous spot becomes elevated. Histologically this stage shows vacuolization of

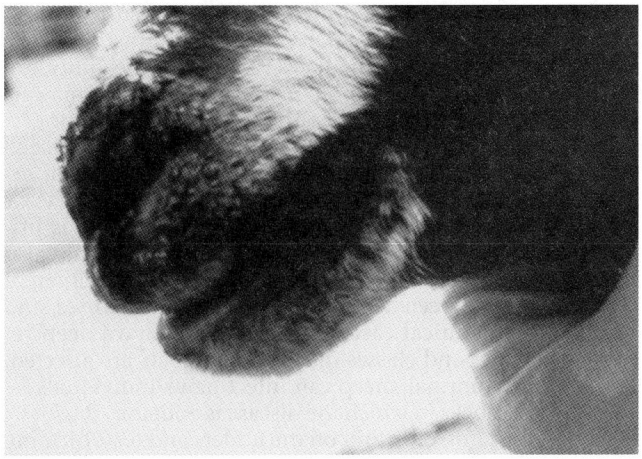

FIG. 30-48 ▨ Typical scabby lesions of contagious ecthyma (sore mouth, orf) on the lips of a young goat. Lesions tend to be proliferative rather than ulcerative.

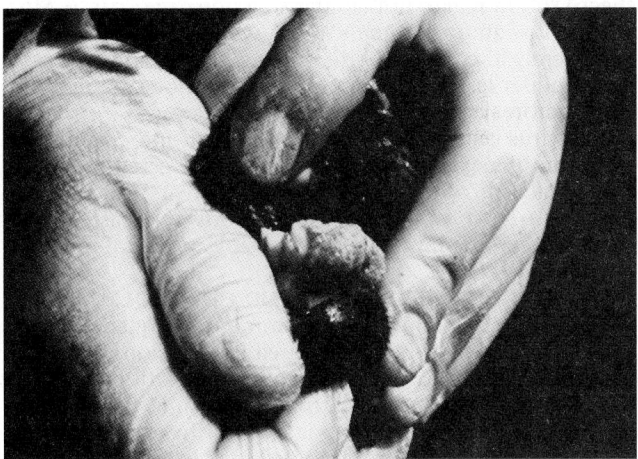

FIG. 30-49 ▨ Typical proliferative lesions of contagious ecthyma (sore mouth, orf) on the gums of a young sheep.

cells in the upper one third of the epidermis with intracytoplasmic eosinophilic inclusions in the affected cells.

2. *Target stage:* A *red halo* of dilated blood vessels and inflammatory cell infiltrates surrounds a *white ring* of vacuolated epidermal cells with intracytoplasmic and intranuclear inclusions, which surrounds a *red center* of pyknotic epidermal cells.

3. *Acute stage:* The lesion is a red, weeping nodule. Microscopically there is reticular degeneration of the epidermis with vesicles. The dermis is infiltrated with macrophages and lymphocytes and is denuded of epidermis in places. The hair follicles are distended with pyknotic epidermal cells.

4. *Regenerative stage:* The nodule is now dry with small black dots (the pyknotic follicle cells, now extruded to the surface) in a thin yellow surface.

5. *Papillomatous stage:* The surface of the nodule is roughened with papillomas, which microscopically prove to be fingerlike, downward projections of epidermis through a full thickness of dermis.

6. *Regressive stage:* The lesion decreases in size and elevation above the surface, the papillomas regress, and several crusts may come off. Microscopically the papillomas and infiltrates regress, leaving normal architecture.

Orf virus encodes for a protein that is apparently homologous to mammalian vascular endothelial growth factors. This family of molecules mediates vascular permeability, angiogenesis, and endothelial cell proliferation, which may account for the swollen, proliferative nature of orf lesions.[871] Transient fever and lymphadenopathy are occasionally seen in humans. Lesions in humans that are not biopsied or excised heal without a scar.

EPIDEMIOLOGY. The naturally occurring disease is primarily one of sheep, goats, and human beings, but it has also been reported in a variety of wild ruminants.[872] Experimental transmission has been achieved in cattle, rabbits, horses, and monkeys. No clinical cases in these species have been reported. All ages and classes of sheep and goats are affected, and clinically normal sheep can infect naive individuals.[873] In herds and flocks in which the disease is endemic, it usually is seen in the lamb crop and on the udders and teats of some of the nursing mothers. Animals that have had a bout of disease are solidly immune for 1 to several years, but morbidity is high (often 80%) among naive individuals. Humans are infected through contact with affected animals or fomites that have contacted affected animals (including one report of transmission by a pickup truck that had been used to haul sheep).[870] Human to human transmission can occur.[872] Mortality is low among animals except when young individuals are severely affected and quit nursing or have mothers with severe udder lesions. Overwhelming infections are rare, but some outbreaks are more severe than others.

The virus is quite resistant to many environmental conditions and persists from year to year on infected premises. Dried scabs allow the virus to persist for years, but wet conditions are less hospitable to it.[874] Reports of persistently infected sheep[875] point to another possible source of infection in wet climates.[874]

TREATMENT, PREVENTION, AND CONTROL. The infection usually is self-limiting and of minor consequence. Young individuals may need to be tube fed if the lesions are severe enough to preclude suckling. Secondary infections, myiasis, or mastitis may be treated with topical disinfectants, antibiotics, or insecticides as appropriate.[875] The hard crusts should not be removed, because doing so may delay healing and promote scarring. Also, humans should limit contact with affected animals and should wear gloves when handling them is necessary. Anecdotal reports, each consisting of one case, have claimed good results for treatment of human orf with intralesional corticosteroids,[876] interferon,[877] idoxuridine in dimethyl sulfoxide (DMSO),[878] or diethyl ether[879] or cryotherapy.[880] Similar good results were obtained in a group of 12 severely affected, bottle-fed lambs with painful intraoral lesions. The proliferative tissues were debrided and cauterized with a portable diathermy unit. The exposed submucosa was then frozen twice with liquid nitrogen spray. Healing occurred by second intention, with rapid recovery of affected lambs.[881]

The infection is prevented by maintaining a virus-free herd or flock by not introducing or contacting infected individuals. Lesions often are not apparent on carriers.[873] Once established, the disease is persistent on the premises because of virus in scabs. Vaccination should be undertaken only if the infection is persistent, because the vaccine consists of virulent live virus. Vaccination can also be achieved with dried scabs from the previous year's outbreak; the scab material is rubbed into scarified skin in an inconspicuous location (inner thigh, under the tail, in the axilla). A localized inflammatory reaction at the site 1 week after vaccination indicates a successful inoculation. Infected or vaccinated animals should not contact unexposed animals (as at shows) until the lesions have healed. Lambs born to immunized ewes may not be protected by colostral antibodies even though their levels of antibody postsuckling are high,[882] pointing to the importance of cell-mediated immunity in protection from the disease. Lambs should be vaccinated at 6 to 8 weeks of age and are immune 3 weeks later.[875] Yearly vaccination of the new lamb crop and new additions to the herd should prevent devastating outbreaks on infected farms. Vaccine failures may be related to virulence of the disease-causing strain rather than to serologic differences between vaccine and field strains.[883]

REFERENCES

867. Hooser SB et al: Atypical contagious ecthyma in a sheep after extensive cutaneous thermal injury, *J Am Vet Med Assoc* 195:1255-1256, 1989.
868. Ndikuwera J et al: Chronic contagious ecthyma and caseous lymphadenitis in two Boer goats, *Vet Rec* 131:584-585, 1992.
869. Lober CW et al: Clinical and histologic features of orf, *Cutis* 32:142-147, 1983.
870. Leavell VW et al: Orf: report of 19 human cases with clinical and pathological observations, *J Am Med Assoc* 204:657-664, 1968.
871. Wise LM et al: Vascular endothelial growth factor (VEGF)–like protein from orf virus NZ2 binds to VEGFR-2 and neuropilin-1, *Proc Natl Acad Sci USA* 96:3071-3076, 1999.
872. Falk ES: Parapoxvirus infections of reindeer and musk ox associated with unusual human infections, *Br J Dermatol* 99:647-654, 1978.
873. Nettleton PF et al: Natural transmission of orf virus from clinically normal ewes to orf-naive sheep, *Vet Rec* 139:364-366, 1996.
874. McKeever DJ, Reid HW: Survival of orf virus under British winter conditions, *Vet Rec* 118:613-614, 1986.
875. Lofstedt J: Dermatologic disease of sheep, *Vet Clin North Am (Large Anim Pract)* 5:427-455, 1983.
876. Reddy J: Intralesional corticosteroids for orf, *Aust Fam Physician* 22:65, 1993.
877. Kacprzak-Bergman I: Orf virus (sheep-pox): a severe infection in an infant-transmitted man to man and treated with interferon, *Abstracts of the Ninth International Congress of Infectious and Parasitic Diseases*, Abstract 819, Munich, 1986.
878. Hunskaar SA: Case of ecthyma contagiosum (human orf) treated with idoxuridine, *Dermatologica* 168:207, 1984.
879. Morgan KL: Orf in man: a treatment? *Vet Rec* 120:539, 1987.
880. Degraeve C et al: Recurrent contagious ecthyma (orf) in an immunocompromised host successfully treated with cryotherapy, *Dermatology* 198:162-163, 1999.
881. Meynink SE, Jackson PGG, Platt D: Treatment of intraoral orf lesions in lambs using diathermy and cryosurgery, *Vet Rec* 121:594, 1987.
882. Buddle BM, Pulford HD: Effect of passively acquired antibodies and vaccination on the immune response to contagious ecthyma virus, *Vet Microbiol* 9:515-522, 1984.
883. Buddle BM, Dellers RW, Schurig GG: Contagious ecthyma virus vaccination failures, *Am J Vet Res* 45:263-266, 1984.

BOVINE PAPULAR STOMATITIS (Proliferative Stomatitis)

BRADFORD P. SMITH

Bovine papular stomatitis (BPS) is a disease principally of young cattle caused by a parapoxvirus closely related to contagious ecthyma (CE) and pseudocowpox. There are many similarities among BPS, CE, and pseudocowpox, and they may indicate a single virus adapted to different species.[884] There are as many antigenic differences between strains of BPS as between BPS, CE, and pseudocowpox.[884] Local strains thus are recommended for vaccination. Infection usually is asymptomatic,[885] but lesions consisting of raised papules may be noted on the muzzle, nose, oral mucosa (particularly the hard palate), or esophagus, where they are important differentials for lesions caused by vesicular stomatitis, foot-and-mouth disease, and bovine virus diarrhea (BVD).[885] In young feedlot cattle, 2- to 10-mm lesions of BPS are common for the first 4 weeks after arrival.[886] Morbidity may approach 100%.[885] BPS may also occur as a chronic disease in young cattle.[887] It may be the same disease as proliferative stomatitis, muzzle disease, mycotic stomatitis, erosive stomatitis, ulcerative stomatitis, and necrotic stomatitis.

Ulcerative esophagitis caused by BPS virus in a 5-month-old, unthrifty calf was associated with a 20% morbidity rate in a group of 25 calves.[888] Outbreaks of severe disease associated with BPS with a mortality rate over 50% have been reported.[888,890] Weight loss and diarrhea accompanied by papular lesions are commonly associated with the severe syndrome. Many lesions are erosions or shallow ulcers with elevated borders,[890] whereas others are obvious raised papules. Lesions are found in the mouth, esophagus, and rumen.[890] There are no lesions on the feet. BPS is commonly seen in calves 1 to 12 months of age and is rare in adult cattle. The disease is spread by animal contact and appears to be worldwide in distribution.[890]

The first evidence of the disease is the appearance of 2- to 4-mm hyperemic foci, most commonly in the ventral margins of the nares. Similar lesions next appear in the mouth. Within 18 hours they become raised papules. Some lesions enlarge to form raised plaques over 1 cm in diameter. Lesions regress in 1 day to 3 weeks, leaving a yellow, red, or brown spot that persists for several weeks more.[885] Secondary lesions come and go, with some calves being visibly infected for 4 months.[885] Most animals have no fever or obvious clinical signs, and they continue to eat normally. Leukopenia was not seen in experimentally infected calves.[885] Secondary lesions appear to be spread through the blood; intravenous inoculation results in similar upper alimentary tract lesions.[891]

Histologic lesions consist of hydropic degeneration of the epithelial cells of the oral mucosa, hyperplasia of the papillae of the lamina propria, and eosinophilic inclusions in the cytoplasm of the degenerating epithelial cells.[890] Lesions reaching the ulcerative stage show secondary necrosis, bacterial invasion, and sloughing of epithelium.

Bovine papular stomatitis has been associated with the "rat tail" syndrome of feedlot cattle.[892] Thirty-six of 84 Texas feedlots reported the problem with a morbidity rate of 1% to 10%. The syndrome consists of diarrhea, salivation, poor weight gain, and loss of hair from the end of the tail.[892] Sarcocystosis has also been mentioned in association with "rat tail" syndrome. Bovine papular stomatitis is capable of causing painful proliferative lesions in human beings.[893] The lesions resemble those caused by contagious ecthyma or pseudocowpox. Most often the affected individual has a recent history of examining the mouths of cattle, often with cuts or abrasions on the hands. Lesions in humans apparently are limited to the primary site of inoculation on the hands.

Although ovine ecthyma vaccines are commercially available, no vaccine is marketed for protection against BPS. Local strains of parapoxviruses would be most likely to be more protective than commercial vaccine strains.

REFERENCES

884. Gonzales GS, Romero RA, Tortora PJ: Antigenic relationships between samples of contagious ecthyma (orf) and bovine parapox by immunodiffusion and counterimmunoelectrophoresis, *Proceedings of the Eighth National Congress of the AZTECA*, 1991, pp 151-157.

885. Griesemer RA, Cole CR: Bovine papular stomatitis. I, Recognition in the US, *J Am Vet Med Assoc* 37:404-410, 1960.

886. Chalmers GA: Papular stomatitis in beef calves, *Can Vet J* 28:108, 1987.

887. Yeruham I, Abraham A, Nyska A: Clinical and pathological description of a chronic form of bovine papular stomatitis, *J Comp Pathol* 111:279-286, 1994.

888. Crandell RA, Gosser HS: Ulcerative esophagitis associated with poxvirus infection in a calf, *J Am Vet Med Assoc* 165:282-283, 1974.

889. Gibbons WJ: USDA report of the preliminary survey on "X disease" (hyperkeratosis) of cattle, February 1949.

890. Gibbons WJ: Bovine papular stomatitis, *Mod Vet Pract* 44:37-39, 1963.

891. Schaaf J, Traub E, Beller K: Untersuchungen uber die stomatitis papulosa des Rindes, *Zeitschrift fur Infektionskr* 56:85-103, 1940.

892. Irwin MR et al: Association of bovine papular stomatitis with the "rat tail" syndrome of feedlot cattle, *Southwest Vet* 29:120-124, 1976.

893. Schnurrenberger PR et al: Bovine papular stomatitis incidence in veterinary students, *Can J Comp Med* 44:239-243, 1980.

DISEASES CAUSED BY BOVINE VIRUS DIARRHEA VIRUS

DAN GROOMS
JOHN C. BAKER
TREVOR R. AMES

DEFINITION AND ETIOLOGY. Disease in cattle resulting from infection with bovine virus diarrhea virus (BVDV) is responsible for economic losses throughout the world. These economic losses are realized through decreased weight gains, loss of milk production, reproductive wastage, and death. More than 50 years ago an enteric disease of cattle was described in North America that was characterized by outbreaks of diarrhea and erosive lesions of the digestive tract.[894,895] The virus was named the bovine virus diarrhea virus. Subsequently the virus was associated with a sporadically occurring, highly fatal disease referred to as mucosal disease (MD). MD occurs only in cattle that are born persistently infected (PI) with BVDV. Persistent infection occurs as a result of in utero exposure of the fetus to BVDV at less than 125 days of gestation.[896]

BVDV is a member of the family Flaviviridae,[897,898] which comprises three genera: *Pestivirus, Flavivirus,* and *Hepacivirus.* BVDV is the prototypic member of the genus *Pestivirus,* which includes two other viruses of veterinary importance, classical swine fever virus (hog cholera virus) and border disease virus. Isolates of BVDV can be classified in vitro as cytopathic (CP) or noncytopathic (NCP); this classification is referred to as the biotype.[899] The NCP biotype predominates in the cattle population and is associated with persistent infection. It has been established that mucosal disease occurs when cattle born immunotolerant to and PI-infected with an NCP-BVDV become superinfected with a CP-BVDV. There also is genetic and antigenic variation between isolates of BVDV.[900] BVDV has been divided into two groups based on genotype, BVDV type I and BVDV type II.[901,902] BVDV type II infections have been associated with a severe acute disease and a hemorrhagic syndrome characterized by thrombocytopenia and death.[902] The significant genotypic and antigenic variations among BVDV isolates may be a factor in achieving complete control of BVDV infections through vaccination.

The virus is unstable at low or high pH and at high temperatures. On the basis of research with the related classical swine fever virus, BVDV probably does not persist in the environment longer than 2 weeks.[903] This same work with the classical swine fever virus also suggests that BVDV is susceptible to common disinfectants such as chlorhexidine, phenols, iodophors, aldehydes, and hypochlorites.[903]

EPIDEMIOLOGY

Prevalence. Evidence of BVDV has been documented in many countries throughout the world. Serologic surveys have demonstrated considerable differences in the prevalence of antibody-positive cattle, ranging from 20% to 90%.[904-906] Cattle density, management practices, and vaccine usage are likely to account for these differences. Several studies have shown the prevalence of PI cattle to be less than 2% of the general cattle population.[907-910] In individual herds the prevalence of PI cattle may be substantially higher. No significant differences have been noted between dairy and beef breeds. The prevalence of herds containing at least one PI animal has been estimated to be 10% to 50%.[909,910] Economic losses attributable to BVDV are difficult to assess. In Europe the annual losses at the population level have been estimated at $10 million to $40 million per million calvings.[911,912]

Transmission. Cattle persistently infected with BVDV shed large amounts of virus their entire life and are the major source of BVDV transmission. Acutely infected cattle are also an important source of BVDV transmission, but the level of virus shed is considerably lower and the length of shedding is limited. Inhalation or ingestion of virus is the most common mode of infection. The most efficient mode of transmission is direct contact with body fluids from PI cattle.[906] Virus has been isolated from nasal swabs, aerosols, saliva, urine, feces, and uterine fluids.[913] Indirect transmission can occur through blood-feeding insects[914] or contaminated mechanical vectors such as common needles, nose tongs, and animal caretakers.[915] Horizontal transmission has also occurred with frozen semen collected from BVDV-infected bulls and inseminated into susceptible cows.[916] Vertical transmission results with transplacental infection of the fetus in cows acutely or persistently infected with BVDV. The role of other species of animals in the transmission of BVDV is unclear. Transmission of BVDV between cattle and sheep has been demonstrated.[917] In addition, BVDV has been isolated from many captive and free-living ruminants as well as pigs.[918]

The rate of transmission of BVDV within a herd varies depending on the source of the virus. Introduction of a PI animal into a herd can result in rapid dissemination of the virus among the majority of susceptible cattle in less than 6 months.[906] Conversely, if acutely infected cattle are the source of the virus, the spread of BVDV may require an extended period.[906]

Spread of BVDV between farms most commonly occurs by the acquisition of new cattle that are PI or pregnant and carrying a PI fetus. Cattle operations that have purchased cattle within the past 5 years are at highest risk for having PI animals.[919] The purchase of new cattle incubating an acute infection is also an important source of virus introduction into a herd. Exposure to other cattle through fence line contact, communal pastures, and animal exhibitions may all be important modes of herd to herd transmission.

CLINICAL DISEASE, DIFFERENTIAL DIAGNOSIS, AND PATHOGENESIS. Infection with BVDV can result in a wide assortment of clinical manifestations ranging from subclinical conditions to death. The clinical outcome after infection is complex and depends on a number of factors. Host factors that influence the clinical outcome include whether the host is immunotolerant or immunocompetent to BVDV, pregnancy status, gestational age of the fetus at the time of infection, immune status (passive or active from exposure or vaccination), and the concurrent level of environmental stress at the time of infection. In addition, genetic diversity, antigenic variation, and differences in virulence among BVDV isolates may account for variations in the clinical response to infection.

Subclinical Bovine Virus Diarrhea Virus Infection

Most animals infected with BVDV have subclinical infections that result in mild fever, leukopenia, and the development of serum-neutralizing antibodies. Subclinical infections explain the positive serum neutralization titers to BVDV found in most unvaccinated cattle. It has been estimated that 70% to 90% of BVDV infections occur without manifestation of clinical signs.[920]

Acute Bovine Virus Diarrhea Virus Infection

Acute BVDV infection often is defined as clinical disease that occurs in immunocompetent cattle that are not PI. This disease syndrome usually occurs in cattle 6 to 24 months of age and traditionally has been thought of as primarily causing disease in cattle that are seronegative (i.e., passive immunity has waned but active immunity has not yet been acquired). The acute BVDV incubation period is 5 to 7 days, with clinical signs of fever, leukopenia, depression, anorexia, oculonasal discharge, oral erosions and ulcerations, diarrhea,

and decreased milk production in lactating cows after infection. A rapid respiratory rate may be observed, which may be interpreted incorrectly as pneumonia. Viremia may last for up to 15 days, with viral shedding in low amounts. This form of the disease, as it was initially described, has been traditionally referred to as bovine virus diarrhea.

Neonatal infection with BVDV may result in enteritis or pneumonia, but this appears to be possible mainly when failure of passive transfer has occurred. Passively derived humoral immunity in calves is thought to be protective unless sufficient antigenic diversity exists between the challenge strain and the strain against which the colostral immunity was developed. Viral infection in young calves without suitable or sufficient passive immunity may result in secondary disease because of the disease's immunosuppressive effects.

The differential diagnosis for acute BVDV infection for the neonatal period includes other causes of diarrhea in young calves such as rotavirus or coronavirus infection, cryptosporidiosis, *Escherichia coli* infection, salmonellosis, and coccidiosis. Other causes of calf pneumonia such as bovine respiratory syncytial virus, salmonellosis, pasteurellosis, hemophilosis, or mycoplasmal infection should also be considered. Diarrheal diseases considered as differential diagnoses for acute BVDV infection in adults include salmonellosis, winter dysentery, Johne's disease, intestinal parasites, malignant catarrhal fever, arsenic poisoning, and copper deficiency. A differential diagnosis for diseases that cause oral lesions in cattle includes malignant catarrhal fever, vesicular stomatitis, papular stomatitis, and bluetongue.

Acute BVDV causes disease in infected cattle by damaging the epithelial tissue of the gastrointestinal, integumentary, and respiratory systems.[922] Viral antigen has been demonstrated in the epithelium of the tongue, esophagus, intestinal crypts and villi, bronchi, and basal layer of the skin of cattle clinically affected with acute BVD or mucosal disease.[922] In infected animals the viral antigens may also be detected in the phagocytic cells of the thymus, lymph nodes, Peyer's patches, tonsils, and spleen. In vitro studies support the theory that phagocytic cells become infected.[923] These phagocytic cells probably represent the antigen-trapping cells of lymphoid structures such as the thymus, lymph nodes, Peyer's patches, tonsils, and spleen. As demonstrated by the presence of viral antigen, the first tissues to be infected are in the respiratory tract and tonsils.[922] From there, BVDV is disseminated to the epithelial surfaces and lymphoid tissue.[922] Mononuclear phagocytic cells in the lymphoid tissue retain the virus.[922]

Severe Acute Bovine Virus Diarrhea Virus Infection

Before 1993 it was believed that most BVDV infections in immunocompetent adult cattle resulted in subclinical or mild disease as described above. Beginning in 1993, however, an atypical form of BVDV infection was recognized in Canada and the United States.[902,924,925] The disease had a peracute course, caused high morbidity, and resulted in a substantial number of deaths in all age-groups. This new form of BVDV infection killed approximately 25% of veal calves in Quebec.[902] Clinical disease in the Ontario outbreaks was characterized by fever, pneumonia, and sudden death in all age-groups of cattle.[924] Abortions in cattle also were a common occurrence. The severity of the disease varied between herds, with some herds experiencing 10% to 20% mortality rates. The gross lesions were similar in appearance to those of MD, which is the primary differential diagnosis (see the section on Acute Mucosal Disease).

Viral isolates obtained from these severe acute outbreaks were obviously of enhanced virulence and have been further

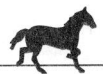

characterized on the molecular level. Nucleotide sequencing of the 5' untranslated end of the RNA of these isolates followed by comparison to classical BVDV isolates revealed a distinct group, designated BVDV type II.[901,902] Classical BVDV isolates are now referred to as BVDV type I.

A further observation from the Ontario outbreaks was that cattle properly vaccinated with BVDV type I vaccines appeared to be protected from clinical disease.[924] It should be emphasized that outbreaks of severe acute BVDV infection should not always be assumed to be caused by BVDV type II. Not all BVDV type II isolates cause severe disease, and it is likely that some type I isolates are capable of causing severe disease.

Hemorrhagic Syndrome

Acute BVDV infections in cattle can cause a hemorrhagic syndrome.[925] These infections are characterized by marked thrombocytopenia, bloody diarrhea, epistaxis, hemorrhages on mucosal surfaces, hyphema, bleeding from injection sites, pyrexia, leukopenia, and death.[925] Hemorrhagic syndrome appears to be associated with noncytopathic isolates of BVDV,[925] and thus far only BVDV type II has been associated with the syndrome.[901,902] Thrombocytopenic BVDV infections have been experimentally reproduced in calves. Diseases that can mimic hemorrhagic syndrome include septicemia with subsequent development of disseminated intravascular coagulation, sweet clover poisoning, and bracken fern poisoning.

The pathogenesis of the hemorrhage relates to the thrombocytopenia induced by the virus. The mechanism by which BVDV infection induces thrombocytopenia has not been clarified. BVDV does appear to be associated with platelets; a recent study demonstrated that in addition to thrombocytopenia, platelet function is altered.[926] Also, BVDV antigen has been demonstrated in megakaryocytes.

Acute Bovine Virus Diarrhea Virus Infections and Bovine Respiratory Disease

Bovine respiratory disease (BRD) is the most common cause of morbidity and mortality in North American feedlots.[927] *Pasteurella haemolytica* is the major contributor to the pneumonic lesions in BRD. (For a more complete description of bovine respiratory disease, see Chapter 29, Ruminant Respiratory Disease.) BVDV has been implicated in bovine respiratory disease complex since its first descriptions. Although this theory has been the subject of controversy, both circumstantial and experimental evidence suggests a role for BVDV in ruminant respiratory disease.[928] The role of BVDV in bovine respiratory disease was recently reviewed.[929] In the United States, BVDV has been reported as the virus most often isolated in outbreaks of BRD. Experimentally it has been difficult to reproduce respiratory disease with BVDV alone, but synergistic effects have been documented between BVDV and *P. haemolytica*,[930] bovine herpesvirus type 1,[931] and bovine respiratory syncytial virus.[932] Differences in pneumopathogenicity have been reported for isolates of BVDV.[933] The results of epidemiologic studies attempting to define the role of BVDV in bovine respiratory disease have been equivocal. Studies have both implicated or shown no evidence of BVDV involvement in outbreaks of respiratory disease.[929] Taken together, the majority of evidence supports the theory that BVDV plays a role in BRD, and the contribution of BVDV to respiratory disease is likely from the immunosuppressive effects of BVDV infection (see below).

Acute BVDV Infections and Immunosuppression

It has been well established that acute BVDV infection can result in immunosuppression, and modified live BVDV vac-

cines have also been demonstrated to induce a degree of immunosuppression.[934] The importance of BVDV-induced immunosuppression is that it increases the host's susceptibility to other pathogens and may enhance the pathogenicity of coinfecting organisms. Stress on the host at the time of BVDV infection undoubtedly adds to the viral-induced immunosuppression. As previously described, synergistic effects of BVDV infection have been demonstrated with *P. haemolytica*, bovine herpesvirus type 1, and bovine respiratory syncytial virus. BVDV infections have also been associated with concurrent salmonellosis, *E. coli* infection, bovine papular stomatitis, and rotavirus and coronavirus infections.[929] The ability of BVDV to cause immunosuppression contributes to the broad range of clinical disease associated with this virus.

The pathogenesis of immunosuppression involves several aspects of the immune system. BVDV targets lymphocytes and macrophages.[935] Acute BVDV infection may result in a transient leukopenia with lymphoid depletion.[936] Also, a decrease in CD 4+ and CD 8+ T lymphocytes, as well as B lymphocytes and neutrophils, has been reported.[937] In vitro studies have suggested different causes of immunosuppression, including decreased responsiveness of infected lymphocytes to mitogen stimulation,[938] decreased production of interferon,[939] monocyte interleukin-1,[940] interleukin-2,[941] and tumor necrosis factor-α,[942] and diminished chemotactic response by monocytes.[923] In addition, neutrophil-mediated, antibody-dependent, cell-mediated cytotoxicity can be impaired by BVDV.[943] Neutrophils from BVDV-infected cattle have reduced bactericidal activity.[944] BVDV-induced immunosuppression also may be the indirect result of prostaglandin production by infected cells.[945]

Reproductive Consequences of Acute Bovine Virus Diarrhea Virus Infections

VENEREAL INFECTIONS. Semen from bulls with acute infection or that are PI with BVDV contains virus and may serve as a source of infection.[916] In acutely infected bulls, shedding of virus in the semen may extend beyond the period of viremia because of local replication in the genital tract. Recently a bull that was immunocompetent with respect to BVDV was found to be persistently shedding virus in his semen.[947] It was hypothesized that the BVDV infection was localized to the testes and was protected from the systemic immune response by the blood-testes barrier. Acceptable and unacceptable semen quality has been reported from acutely infected and PI bulls.

Observations and studies on the consequences of BVDV infection on reproduction in and around the period of insemination of female cattle have resulted in equivocal findings.[946] Taken as a whole, these studies support the theory that BVDV, under certain circumstances, can affect fertility, resulting in decreased conception rates. The adverse effect on conception rates has been attributed to fertilization failure, but the exact cause of infertility after acute BVDV infection is unknown. BVDV has been isolated from the bovine ovary and has been associated with oophoritis. A recent study detected BVDV antigen in ovaries and the development of oophoritis 60 days after experimental infection.[948]

ABORTIONS. Transplacental infection by BVDV virus is a common event and occurs with high efficiency. BVDV has been shown to be detrimental to early embryonic development and a cause of embryonic death.[949] Transplacental infection of the fetus from 50 to 100 days of gestation may result in fetal death.[946] Expulsion of the fetus may occur days to months after infection. In general, late-term fetal infections do not result in abortion, but late-term abortions in association with BVDV have been reported. It should be remembered that BVDV infection can cause abortion during any stage of gestation. Although the incidence of abortion is generally low in immune herds, it can increase dramatically in nonimmune herds. The outbreaks of severe acute infection associated with BVDV type II resulted in a high incidence of abortion.

CONGENITAL DEFECTS. Infection of the fetus at 100 to 150 days' gestation may result in a number of congenital anomalies. This period of fetal development corresponds to the final stages of organogenesis of the nervous system and the development of the fetal immune system, which can result in the generation of an inflammatory response to BVDV infection. At this stage of gestation, BVDV infection may inhibit cell growth or cell differentiation or cause direct cellular lysis. The more common congenital defects induced by BVDV infection include hydrocephalus, cerebellar hypoplasia, hypomyelinogenesis, microphthalmia, cataracts, retinal atrophy or dysplasia, hypotrichosis, brachygnathia and other skeletal abnormalities, growth restriction, and pulmonary hypoplasia.

BVDV INFECTION DURING THE LATER STAGES OF GESTATION. Calves infected with BVDV transplacentally during the later stages of gestation can be normal at birth. These calves are born seropositive to BVDV. To detect this type of infection, serum must be collected for determination of BVDV antibody before the calf ingests colostrum. Late gestational infections can also result in the birth of weak calves.

PERSISTENT INFECTION. Infection of the fetus with NCP-BVDV isolates before the development of fetal immunocompetence may result in the birth of calves that are immunotolerant to and persistently infected with BVDV. The development of immunotolerance to BVDV is rare after 100 days' gestation but has been reported to occur as late as 125 days' gestation.[896] Cattle persistently infected with BVDV are viremic, continuously shed virus, and may appear healthy. PI cattle are immunocompetent with respect to other antigens. The immunotolerance is specific to the infecting NCP-BVDV, therefore PI cattle can respond immunologically to heterologous isolates of BVDV.[950,951] For this reason, PI cattle can be seropositive for BVDV. The prevalence of PI cattle in the population is low, and it has been estimated that a PI calf may occur in every 100 to 1000 births.[905] PI females produce PI offspring,[953] which may result in the production of PI family lines. It appears likely that PI cattle are the main mechanism by which BVDV is maintained in the cattle population.

PI cattle are at risk of developing MD and appear to be at risk for other diseases and have decreased survivorship.[954] PI calves have death rates of 50% in the first 12 months of life,[903] and it is believed that fewer than 10% of PI replacement heifers reach the lactating herd. PI calves may be born undersized and have slower growth rates. Some PI calves appear to be predisposed to infections; this often results in pneumonia and enteritis,[955] which tend to become chronic and unresponsive to treatment. An alteration in immune response, such as suppression of neutrophil and lymphocyte function, also has been reported in PI cattle.[956] Subclinical disease that eventually becomes clinical or immunosuppression that allows secondary bacterial infections may explain unthriftiness and mortality in PI cattle. Postmortem findings such as glomerulitis and encephalitis have been reported in PI animals.[957]

Disease Occurring in Persistently Infected Cattle

MUCOSAL DISEASE. The pathogenesis of MD has been reviewed.[958] MD occurs when cattle that are immunotolerant to and PI with a NCP biotype of BVDV become infected with a CP biotype of BVDV that shares close homology with the persistently infecting noncytopathic virus. Thus not every combination of NCP and CP virus results in MD. The origin of the CP virus can be external, as demonstrated by the documented

occurrence of MD after the use of modified live BVDV vaccines and in experimental studies in which MD was produced by superinfection with CP-BVDV. It is more commonly believed that the CP-BVDV arises de novo from the NCP, persistently infecting BVDV by molecular rearrangement.

MD takes different clinical forms (see below).[946] The differences in the relatedness of the NCP- and CP-BVDV may be responsible for the variations in clinical response. One extreme is acute MD, in which the CP virus shares close homology with the persistently infecting NCP virus. The other extreme is no clinical disease but seroconversion, in which the CP virus is heterologous to the NCP virus. Between these extremes lie other clinical forms of MD (chronic MD and possibly MD with recovery), which are determined by the antigenic relationship of the NCP and CP viruses. A delayed onset form of MD recently was described.[959] As the name implies, delayed onset MD occurs after the expected time frame for acute mucosal disease following exposure of a PI animal to an exogenous CP virus. Although the CP virus is heterologous to the persistently infecting NCP virus, a genetic recombination of the two viruses results in a CP virus that is antigenically identical to the resident NCP, and MD results.

ACUTE MUCOSAL DISEASE. The occurrence of acute MD is sporadic, with less than 5% of the herd being affected. Often the animals affected in a herd are grouped by age and represent calves that were all PI with the same NCP-BVDV. In rare cases, during epizootics, up to 25% of the herd may be involved, but a high number of PI animals would be necessary for this to occur. The case fatality rate for acute MD approaches 100%.

Acute MD is characterized by an incubation period of 10 to 14 days after exposure. Clinical signs of mucosal disease include a biphasic fever, anorexia, tachycardia, polypnea, decreased milk production, and profuse, watery diarrhea (occasionally with frank blood, fibrinous casts, and a foul odor). The oral papillae may be blunted, and the epithelium of the tongue, palate, buccal surfaces, and pharynx may have erosions. Erosive lesions also may be present in the interdigital regions and on the teats and vulva. All erosive lesions may be ulcerative to diphtheric, depending on their duration. Other clinical signs may include nasal and corneal discharge, corneal opacity, excessive salivation, decreased rumination, and bloat. Cattle may have inflammation of the coronary band and, in some cases, laminitis. Acutely infected animals often are neutropenic (without a left shift) and thrombocytopenic. Animals with mucosal disease commonly have secondary bacterial infections, resulting in pneumonia, mastitis, and metritis. Cattle with MD become progressively dehydrated and debilitated and usually die within 3 to 10 days. Some animals survive the acute phase but experience the chronic form of the disease.

The differential diagnosis for bovine diseases with oral lesions and diarrhea includes severe acute BVDV infection, rinderpest, bovine malignant catarrhal fever, and MD. Diseases characterized by oral lesions but no diarrhea include foot-and-mouth disease, vesicular stomatitis, and bovine papular stomatitis. Diseases involving diarrhea but no oral lesions include winter dysentery, salmonellosis, Johne's disease, parasitism, and copper deficiency.

CHRONIC MUCOSAL DISEASE. Some cattle that develop MD do not die in the expected time frame but rather become chronically affected. Cattle with chronic mucosal disease are unthrifty and may have persistently loose feces or intermittent diarrhea, chronic bloat, decreased appetite, weight loss, interdigital erosions, or nonhealing erosive skin lesions. Nasal discharge and persistent ocular discharge are common findings. Areas of alopecia and hyperkeratinization of the skin may develop, typically in the neck area. Long-term lameness problems may develop because of laminitis, interdigital

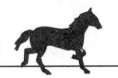

necrosis, or hoof deformities. These animals may be persistently anemic, neutropenic, and thrombocytopenic. Cattle with chronic mucosal disease rarely survive beyond 18 months and ultimately die of severe debilitation. Chronic MD should be distinguished from calves born PI with BVDV that are poor doers from birth.

MUCOSAL DISEASE WITH RECOVERY. A single report exists of several PI calves that showed transient signs of MD and subsequently recovered.[960] These calves remained healthy until slaughtered. The observation is interesting, and MD with recovery is a possibility based on the current understanding of the pathogenesis of MD.

NECROPSY FINDINGS. The postmortem examination findings for animals that died from BVDV vary depending on the form of the disease.

Mucosal Disease. Animals that die of mucosal disease usually have severe, necrotizing erosive or ulcerative lesions involving the mouth, tongue, esophagus, ruminal pillars, omasum, abomasum, intestines, and cecum. Erosive lesions may extend onto the external nares and into the nasal cavity. Ulcers involving the esophagus typically are elongated. The Peyer's patches in the small intestine often are necrotic and hemorrhagic. Bowel contents are watery, hemorrhagic, and foul smelling. Pathologic gastrointestinal conditions may be absent or very mild in cattle with chronic mucosal disease, although histopathologic lesions usually are present. Skin lesions are often found and include patchy hyperkeratosis around the neck, shoulder, and perineal areas. Erosive lesions involving the perineal area, the prepuce, and the interdigital cleft and coronary band of the hoof may be present. Skin lesions are most apparent in cattle suffering from chronic mucosal disease.

Acute Disease. Animals that die of acute BVDV infection have less severe lesions, but some or all of those mentioned for mucosal disease may be present. Often secondary bacterial infections such as pneumonia or mastitis are present and have contributed to the animal's death. Animals that die of hemorrhagic syndrome may have evidence of hemorrhage in many organ systems, including the gastrointestinal, cardiovascular, respiratory, and urinary systems. Petechial or ecchymotic hemorrhages are often apparent on mucosal surfaces, and significant hemorrhage in the gastrointestinal submucosa and Peyer's patches may also be present.

Abortions and Congenital Defects. Fetuses aborted as a result of in utero BVDV infection often are autolytic when expelled. Lesions found in aborted fetuses and the accompanying placenta are nonspecific for BVDV. Under experimental conditions or when aborted fetuses are expelled soon after death, lesions observed include conjunctivitis, peribronchiolar and interalveolar pneumonia, and nonspecific myocarditis. A significant decrease in cerebellar mass may be evident in calves affected by cerebellar hypoplasia as a result of in utero infection with BVDV during the second trimester of gestation. Other common congenital defects associated with BVDV infection that may be noted at necropsy include cataracts and thymic hypoplasia.

DIAGNOSIS. A diagnosis of BVDV infection can be made by serologic evaluation, virus isolation, viral antigen detection, and viral RNA detection using amplification methods such as the polymerase chain reaction technique.

Virus Isolation. Virus isolation is the method most commonly used for identifying cattle infected with BVDV. Serum is most often used to isolate virus from cattle persistently infected with BVDV, whereas buffy coats or nasal swabs are most appropriate for attempting to detect acute infections. Antemortem differentiation of PI cattle from those acutely infected with BVDV requires serial isolation of virus at least 2 weeks apart. At postmortem, BVDV is best isolated from lymphoid tissues such as Peyer's patches, lymph nodes, thymus, and spleen.

BVDV is isolated by inoculating appropriate samples onto bovine cells in culture. Isolates can be characterized as cytopathic or noncytopathic biotypes by the presence or absence of characteristic cytopathic effects in cell culture. Noncytopathic isolates are identified in cell culture using immunoenzymes or immunofluorescence. The immunoperoxidase monolayer assay (IPMA) is a common adaptation of virus isolation and immunoenzymatic antigen detection used for rapid BVDV screening.[961]

Antigen Detection. Virus can be identified in tissue samples using fluorescent antibodies or immunohistochemistry. Immunohistochemistry has been reported to be more accurate than virus isolation and immunofluorescent methods in diagnosing BVDV in cases of abortion and perinatal death.[962] BVDV can also be identified in blood samples using an antigen-capture ELISA. Antigen-capture ELISAs are equal in sensitivity to virus isolation for detection of PI cattle but less sensitive for identification of acute infections with BVDV.[963]

Serologic Evaluation. Serologic detection of BVDV exposure is most commonly done by serum neutralization assays. It is important to realize that serum neutralization titers can vary significantly from laboratory to laboratory.[964] In most situations, evaluation of paired acute and convalescent titers must be used. Single point titers are very difficult to interpret, especially if vaccination programs are used in the herd. Demonstration of a fourfold increase in serum-neutralizing antibodies in association with appropriate clinical signs is considered significant. Use of paired serologic evaluation for diagnosis of abortion may be difficult because seroconversion may already have occurred by the time the event is noticed. PI cattle generally have no or very low serum neutralization titers. However, PI cattle may seroconvert to field virus or vaccination, especially if the vaccine or field virus is antigenically distinct from the virus with which the animal is PI.[965] As a result, the identification of seronegative cattle cannot be used as a sole criterion for determining PI status. Serologic evaluation may be useful in determining the infection status of a herd. High serum neutralization titers in unvaccinated heifers older than 6 months of age indicate that BVDV is currently or has recently been circulating and is highly correlated with the presence of PI cattle in the herd.[910] Table 30-4 summarizes the diagnostic testing that can be used for specific forms of the disease.

TREATMENT AND PROGNOSIS. No specific treatment is available for animals showing clinical signs of BVDV infection. Owners should be informed that severely ill animals may have mucosal disease, which normally is fatal. The goals of therapy for cattle suspected of having acute BVDV infection are supportive care and prevention of secondary bacterial infection. Broad-spectrum antimicrobial agents, fluids, electrolytes, and vitamins may be indicated.

PREVENTION AND CONTROL. Practices aimed at preventing the introduction of BVDV to a farm are applicable only for closed breeding operations (dairy farms or beef cow and calf operations) and cannot be used for feedlot or veal operations. Strict biosecurity systems with isolation and testing of all cattle entering the farm are necessary to ensure that no virus enters the farm; this may be difficult for most dairy and cow and calf operations to achieve. A reasonable compromise is to limit movement of cattle on and off the farm to the essential traffic, to avoid moving pregnant animals, and to purchase replacement animals (including bred heifers) from herds for which accurate records of disease history and vaccination programs are kept. Isolation of new additions for 3 weeks should prevent transmission of virus from acutely infected (non-PI) cattle. Purchased cattle should be tested for BVDV before entering the resident herd. If pregnant cattle are purchased, their offspring should be tested to ensure that they are free of BVDV. Semen used for artificial insemination

TABLE 30-4

Diagnostic Testing for Bovine Virus Diarrhea Virus (BVDV)

Clinical Form	Specimen	Diagnostic Test	Comments
Subclinical disease	1. Paired sera 3-4 weeks apart	1. Serum neutralization	Serology for both types 1 and 2
	2. Buffy coat	2. Virus isolation	BVDV should be performed
	3. Serum	3. PCR	Viremia may be too transient for successful virus isolation
Acute BVD	1. Paired serum	1. Serum neutralization	Serology for both types 1 and 2
	2. Buffy coat	2. Virus isolation	BVDV should be performed
	3. Serum	3. PCR	Type 2 BVDV more commonly associated with mortality
	4. Postmortem tissues (spleen, Peyer's patches, lungs, LN)	4. Fluorescent antibody and immunohistochemical staining Virus isolation PCR	
Repeat breeding	1. Paired serum	1. Serum neutralization	May need to establish serum bank on at-risk animals as seroconversion complete when reproductive problem noticed or compare titers of affected to nonaffected cattle
Abortion/mummification	1. Paired serum	1. Serum neutralization	May need to establish serum bank on at-risk animals as seroconversion complete when reproductive problem noticed or compare titers of affected to nonaffected cattle
	2. Fetal fluid	2. Serum neutralization Virus isolation PCR	Presence of antibodies or BVDV suggestive but not definitive for BVDV-induced abortion
	3. Fetal organs (lymphoid, spleen, thymus)	3. Fluorescent antibody and IHC staining Virus isolation PCR	Presence of BVDV suggestive but not definitive for BVDV-induced abortion
Persistently infected animals	1. Serum or buffy coat	1. Virus isolation	Should be repeated in 3-4 wk to confirm persistent infection
	2. Serum	2. PCR	Buffy coats should be used on calves <4 wk of age
	3. Skin biopsy*	3. IHC staining	Skin biopsy IHC staining. Positive cattle should be confirmed in 3-4 wk with blood sample to confirm persistent infection
Mucosal disease	1. Serum or buffy coat	1. Virus isolation	Isolation of both CP and NCP-BVDV
	2. Serum	2. PCR	
	3. Postmortem tissues	3. Fluorescent antibody or IHC staining Virus isolation PCR	

CP, Cyotpathic; *IHC*, immunohistochemical; *NCP*, noncytopathic biotype; *PI*, persistent Infection; *VI*, virus isolation.
*Ear notch in formalin

should be from bulls that have been tested for BVDV infection. It is important to test embryo transplantation recipients before their use to ensure that they are not PI. Exposure of cattle to small and wild ruminants should be limited through separate housing for sheep and goats and well-maintained fences to reduce contact with deer.

Vaccination programs are routinely used to limit disease from BVDV infection. The goal of a BVDV vaccination program is to induce immunity that will limit viral replication after infection and thus prevent the subsequent effects of viral infection. On dairy farms or in beef cow and calf operations, ensuring adequate immunity in breeding females is aimed at preventing in utero infections and harmful sequelae (infertility, abortion, congenital malformation, birth of weak calves, and persistent infection). An additional benefit of yearly vaccination of breeding stock is enhancement of the level of colostral immunity passed to the offspring.

In stocker/backgrounder and feedlot operations, immunity to BVDV has been shown to be protective against bovine respiratory disease complex.[966] Vaccination against BVDV before the expected occurrence of respiratory disease (as is done in preconditioning programs for beef calves) may minimize the consequences that accompany infection with field strains of BVDV. This, in turn, reduces the severity of infection by other pathogens involved in the respiratory disease complex.

Many practitioners have concerns about commercial BVDV vaccines. Concerns over vaccine safety with modified live BVDV vaccines have traditionally centered around "vaccine breaks," transmission of vaccine strains, and vaccine-induced immunosuppression, abortion, and congenital anomalies. Vaccine breaks, or epizootics of disease after the use of modified live BVDV vaccines, have been reported. Possible explanations for these epizootics include unattenuated BVDV in the vaccine (vaccine contamination), disease caused by a coincidental infection with a field strain of BVDV at the time of vaccination, or vaccination of PI cattle and induction of mucosal disease. Improved testing of vaccine constituents has greatly reduced the occurrence of vaccine contamination. Immunosuppression has been demonstrated experimentally after the use of modified live BVDV vaccines.[967] Vaccinal strains of modified live BVDV are reported to cross the placenta and induce the same detrimental outcomes as seen in fetal infection with field strains of BVD virus except persistent infections. This is of greatest concern during the first and second trimesters. Mod-

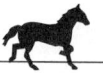

ified live vaccines may or may not induce mucosal disease in PI cattle. The possible induction of mucosal disease in PI cattle should not be a deterrent to using modified live vaccines.

Killed BVDV vaccines are safe for use in pregnant cows and do not result in vaccine breaks or cause immunosuppression unless improperly attenuated. When using a killed virus vaccine in cattle that have never been vaccinated against BVDV, a booster dose must be administered 2 to 4 weeks after the initial vaccination to ensure proper vaccination.

Concerns about the efficacy of BVDV vaccines have centered around the ability of vaccines to stimulate an immune response capable of protecting against the broad antigenic spectrum represented by BVDV types I and II. Current BVDV vaccines appear to be capable of preventing severe disease in cattle infected with heterologous field viruses.[968,969] However, the ability of vaccines to protect against fetal infection is not clear. Research with BVDV has shown that exposure to field virus before breeding can protect fetuses from homologous infection.[970] In another study in which cows were vaccinated with a killed virus vaccine before breeding and then challenged with heterologous strains during pregnancy, protection of the fetuses against the challenge virus was only partial or incomplete.[971] Similar results have been shown using modified live vaccines.[972] The results of these studies suggest that a BVDV vaccine does not produce complete protection against transplacental infections in field situations, especially if the vaccine and field strain are antigenically dissimilar. Despite these concerns, it appears that BVDV vaccines are the best method of controlling the harmful effects of viral replication. BVDV vaccines should be used strategically to optimize immunity during gestation, especially during the first two trimesters when the fetus is most susceptible to the detrimental effects of the virus. This would include vaccination of all breeding stock before they are bred. Replacement heifers should be vaccinated at 5 to 6 months of age when colostral immunity declines and again before breeding. When possible, modified live vaccines should be used to ensure broader and longer protection. In herds in which only killed vaccine is used, cows should be vaccinated before breeding, at midlactation, and at dry off. In calves, vaccination before the decline in colostral antibodies occurs is of questionable value, although some studies indicate that it is beneficial in protecting against calfhood disease associated with BVDV.[968] Vaccination against BVDV should be part of any preconditioning program for beef calves before entry into a commingled environment.

In herds experiencing problems with BVDV infections, screening for PI cattle may be warranted. In breeding herds, PI animals serve as a continuous source of infection to susceptible cattle. In addition, because PI females may produce persistently infected offspring, it is desirable to cull these females before they spread virus to their offspring or before they have disease themselves, resulting in economic loss. Before instituting a herd screening program, several points should be emphasized. First, there should be a definitive diagnosis of BVDV infection in the herd before the expense of testing is undertaken; second, the herd should be experiencing a disease syndrome that is associated with BVDV infection; third, the owner must be willing to implement biosecurity measures aimed at reducing the risk of reintroducing BVDV into the herd. Herd screening involves testing all cattle on the farm for BVDV. This includes in utero calves that are tested after birth. Adaptations of whole herd testing have been advocated, but their usefulness has not been documented.

REFERENCES

894. Childs T: X disease of cattle, *Can J Comp Med* 10:316-319, 1946.
895. Olafson P, MacCallum·AD, Fox FH: An apparently new transmissible disease of cattle, *Cornell Vet* 36:205-213, 1946.
896. Clurkin AW et al: Production of cattle immunotolerant to bovine viral diarrhea virus, *Can J Comp Med* 48:156-161, 1984.
897. Wengler G: Family Flaviviridae. In Fracki RIB et al, eds: *International Committee on Taxonomy of Viruses*, ed 5, Berlin, 1991, Springer-Verlag.
898. Collett MS et al: Recent advances in pestivirus research, *J Gen Virol* 70:253-266, 1989.
899. Donis RO: Molecular biology of bovine viral diarrhea virus and its interaction with the host, *Vet Clin North Am (Food Anim Pract)* 11:393-423, 1995.
900. Dubovi EJ: Genetic diversity and BVD virus, *Comp Immunol Microbiol Infect Dis* 15:155-162, 1992.
901. Ridpath JF, Bolin SR, Dubovi EJ: Segregation of bovine viral diarrhea virus into genotypes, *Virology* 205:66-74, 1994.
902. Pellerin C et al: Identification of a new group of bovine viral diarrhea virus strains associated with severe outbreaks and high mortalities, *Virology* 203:260-268, 1994.
903. Duffell SJ, Harkness JW: Bovine virus diarrhea–mucosal disease infection in cattle, *Vet Rec* 117:240-245, 1985.
904. Loken T, Krogsrud J, Larsen IL: Pestivirus infections in Norway: serological investigation in cattle, sheep, and pigs, *Acta Vet Scand* 32:27-34, 1991.
905. Bolin SR, McClurkin AW, Coria MF: Frequency of persistent bovine viral diarrhea virus infection in selected cattle herds, *Am J Vet Res* 46:2385-2387, 1985.
906. Houe H: Epidemiology of BVDV, *Vet Clin North Am (Food Anim Pract)* 11:521-547, 1995.
907. Harkness JW: The control of bovine virus diarrhea virus infection, *Ann Rech Vet* 18:167-164, 1987.
908. Edwards S, Drew TW, Bushnell SE: Prevalence of bovine virus diarrhoea virus viremia, *Vet Rec* 120:71, 1987.
909. Wittum TE et al: Persistent bovine viral diarrhea infection in beef herds, *Proceedings of the Conference of Research Workers in Animal Diseases*, Chicago, 1998.
910. Houe H, Baker JC, Maes RK: Prevalence of cattle persistently infected with bovine viral diarrhea virus in 20 dairy herds in two counties in central Michigan and comparison of prevalence of antibody-positive cattle among herds with different infection and vaccination status, *J Vet Diagn Invest* 7:321-326, 1995.
911. Bennett RM, Done JT: A case for social cost-benefit analysis? *Proceedings of the Annual Meeting of the Society of Veterinary Epidemiology and Preventive Medicine*, Scotland, 1986, pp 54-56.
912. Houe H, Pedersen KM, Meyling A: A computerized spread sheet model for calculating total annual national losses due to bovine viral diarrhoea virus infection in dairy herds and sensitivity analysis of selected parameters, *Proceedings of the Second Symposium on Pestiviruses*, Annecy, France, 1993.
913. McGowan MR et al: Increased reproductive losses in cattle infected with bovine pestivirus around the time of insemination, *Vet Rec* 133:39-43, 1993.
914. Tarry OW, Tarry L, Edwards S: Transmission of bovine virus diarrhea virus by blood feeding flies, *Vet Rec* 128:82-84, 1991.
915. Gunn HM: Role of fomites and flies in the transmission of bovine viral diarrhoea virus, *Vet Rec* 132:584-585, 1993.
916. Kirkland PD, Mackintosh SG, Moyle A: The outcome of widespread use of semen from a bull persistently infected with pestivirus, *Vet Rec* 135:527-529, 1994.
917. Loken T, Krogsrud J, Bjerkas I: Outbreaks of border disease in goats induced by a pestivirus-contaminated vaccine, with virus transmission to sheep and cattle, *J Comp Pathol* 104:195-209, 1991.
918. Loken T: Ruminant pestivirus infection in animals other than sheep, *Vet Clin North Am (Food Anim Pract)* 11:597-614, 1995.
919. Houe H et al: Comparison of the prevalence and incidence of infection with bovine virus diarrhoea virus (BVDV) in Denmark and Michigan and association with possible risk factors, *Acta Vet Scand* 36:521-531, 1995.
920. Ames TR: The causative agent of BVD: its epidemiology and pathogenesis, *Vet Med* 81:848-869, 1986.
921. Carmen S et al: Severe acute bovine virus diarrhea (BVD) in Ontario in 1993, *Proc Ann Mtg Am Assoc Vet Lab Diagn* 37:19, 1994.
922. Ohmann HB: Distribution and significance of BVD antigen in diseased calves, *Res Vet Sci* 34:5-10, 1983.
923. Ketelsen AT, Johnson DW, Muscoplat CC: Depression of bovine monocyte chemotactic response by bovine viral diarrhea virus, *Infect Immunol* 25:565-568, 1979.
924. Carman S et al: Severe acute bovine viral diarrhea in Ontario, 1993-1995, *J Vet Diagn Invest* 10:27-35, 1998.
925. Corapi WV et al: Thrombocytopenia and hemorrhages in veal calves infected with bovine viral diarrhea virus, *J Am Vet Med Assoc* 196:590-596, 1990.
926. Walz PH, Steficek BA, Baker JC: Effect of type II bovine viral diarrhea virus on platelet function in experimentally infected calves, *Am J Vet Res* 60:1396-1401, 1999.
927. Martin SW et al: Factors associated with mortality and treatment costs in feedlot calves: the Bruce County Beef Project, 1978, 1979, 1980, *Can J Comp Med* 46:341-349, 1982.
928. Yates WDG: Interactions between viruses and bacteria in bovine respiratory disease, *Can Vet J* 25:37-41, 1984.
929. Grooms DL: Role of bovine viral diarrhea virus in the bovine respiratory disease complex, *Bovine Practitioner* 32.2:7-12, 1999.
930. Potgieter LND et al: Experimental production of bovine respiratory tract disease with bovine viral diarrhea virus, *Am J Vet Res* 45:1582-1585, 1984.

931. Potgeiter LND et al: Effects of bovine viral diarrhea virus infection on the distribution of infectious bovine rhinotracheitis virus in calves, *Am J Vet Res* 45:687-689, 1984.

932. Broderson BW, Kelling C: Effects of concurrent experimentally induced bovine respiratory syncytial virus and bovine viral diarrhea virus infection on respiratory tract and enteric diseases in calves, *Am J Vet Res* 59:1423-1430, 1998.

933. Potgeiter LND et al: The comparison of the pneumopathogenicity of two strains of bovine viral diarrhea virus, *Am J Vet Res* 46:151-153, 1985.

934. Potgieter LND: Immunology of bovine viral diarrhea virus, *Vet Clin North Am (Food Anim Pract)* 11:501-520, 1995.

935. Truitt RL, Shechmeister IL: The replication of bovine viral diarrhea–mucosal disease virus in bovine leukocytes in vitro, *Arch Ges Virusf* 42: 78-87, 1973.

936. Bolin SR, McClurkin AW, Coria MF: Effects of bovine viral diarrhea virus on the percentages and absolute numbers of circulating B and T lymphocytes in cattle, *Am J Vet Res* 46:884-886, 1985.

937. Ellis JA et al: Flow cytoflurimetric analysis of lymphocyte subset alteration in cattle infected with bovine viral diarrhea virus, *Vet Pathol* 25:231-236, 1988.

938. Muscoplat CC, Johnson DV, Stevens JB: Abnormalities of in vitro responses during bovine viral diarrhea virus infection, *Am J Vet Res* 34:753-755, 1973.

939. Diderholm H, Dinter Z: Interference between strains of bovine virus diarrhea virus and their capacity to suppress interferon of a heterologous virus, *Proc Soc Exp Biol Med* 121:976-980, 1966.

940. Jensen J, Schultz RD: Effect of infection by bovine viral diarrhea virus (BVDV) in vitro on interleukin-1 activity of bovine monocytes, *Vet Immunol Immunopathol* 29:251-265, 1991.

941. Atluru D et al: In vitro interactions of cytokines and bovine viral diarrhea virus in phytohemagglutinin-stimulated bovine mononuclear cells, *Vet Immunol Immunopathol* 25:47-49, 1990.

942. Alder H et al: Cytokine regulation by virus infection: bovine viral diarrhea virus, a flavivirus, down-regulates production of tumor necrosis factor-α in macrophages in vitro, *J Virol* 70:2650-2653, 1996.

943. Brown GB et al: Defective function of leukocytes from cattle persistently infected with bovine viral diarrhea virus and the influence of recombinant cytokines, *Am J Vet Res* 52:381-387, 1991.

944. Roth JA, Kaekerle ML, Griffith RW: Effects of bovine viral diarrhea virus infection on bovine polymorphonuclear leukocyte function, *Am J Vet Res* 42:244-250, 1981.

945. Markham RJF, Ramnaraine ML: Release of immunosuppressive substances from tissue culture cells infected with bovine viral diarrhea virus, *Am J Vet Res* 46:879-881, 1985.

946. Baker JC: The clinical manifestations of bovine viral diarrhea infection, *Vet Clin North Am (Food Anim Pract)* 11:425-445, 1995.

947. Persistent bovine pestivirus infection localized in the testes of an immunocompetent, nonviremic bull, *Vet Microbiol* 6:165-175, 1998.

948. Grooms DL, Brock KV, Ward LA: Detection of bovine viral diarrhea virus in the ovaries of cattle acutely infected with bovine viral diarrhea virus, *J Vet Diagn Ivest* 10:125-129, 1988.

949. Dubovi EJ: Impact of bovine viral diarrhea virus on reproductive performance in cattle, *Vet Clin North Am (Food Anim Pract)* 10:503-514, 1994.

950. Bolin SR et al: Severe clinical disease induced in cattle persistently infected with noncytopathic bovine viral diarrhea virus by superinfection with cytopathic bovine viral diarrhea virus, *Am J Vet Res* 46:573-576, 1985.

951. Bolin SR et al: Response of cattle persistently infected with noncytopathic bovine viral diarrhea virus to vaccination for bovine viral diarrhea and subsequent challenge exposure with cytopathic bovine viral diarrhea virus, *Am J Vet Res* 46:2467-2470, 1985.

952. Deleted in proof.

953. McClurkin AW, Covia MF, Cutlip RC: Reproductive performance of apparently healthy cattle persistently infected with bovine viral diarrhea virus, *J Am Vet Med Assoc* 174:1116-1119, 1979.

954. Houe H: Survivorship of animals persistently infected with bovine virus diarrhoea virus (BVDV), *Prev Vet Med* 15:275-283, 1993.

955. Werdin RE et al: Diagnostic investigation of bovine viral diarrhea infection in a Minnesota dairy herd, *J Vet Diagn Invest* 1:57-61, 1989.

956. Roth JA, Bolin SR, Frank DE: Lymphocyte blastogenesis and neutrophil function in cattle persistently infected with bovine viral diarrhea virus, *Am J Vet Res* 47:1139-1141, 1986.

957. Cutlip RC, McClurkin AW, Coria MF: Lesions in clinically healthy cattle persistently infected with the virus of bovine viral diarrhea–glomerulonephritis and encephalitis, *Am J Vet Res* 41:1938-1941, 1980.

958. Bolin SR: The pathogenesis of mucosal disease, *Vet Clin North Am (Food Anim Pract)* 11:489-500, 1995.

959. Ridpath JF, Bolin SR: Delayed onset postvaccinal mucosal disease as a result of genetic recombination between genotype 1 and genotype 2 BVDV, *Virology* 212:259-262, 1995.

960. Edwards S et al: Clinical and virological observations of a mucosal disease outbreak with persistently infected seropositive survivors, *Arch Virol* 3(suppl):125-132, 1991.

961. Dubovi EJ: The diagnosis of bovine viral diarrhea infections: a laboratory view, *Vet Med* 85:1133-1139, 1990.

962. Ellis JA et al: Comparison of detection methods for bovine viral diarrhea virus in bovine abortions and neonatal death, *J Vet Diagn Invest* 7:433-436, 1995.

963. Saliki JT et al: Microtiter virus isolation and enzyme immunoassays for detection of bovine viral diarrhea virus in cattle serum, *J Clin Microbiol* 35:803-807, 1997.

964. Vaughn M: SN Titer response comparisons among 14 diagnostic laboratories for antibodies protecting against IBR, BVD, and BRSV virus following the administration of modified live vaccines to weaning age calves, *Bovine Pract* 30:141-143, 1997.

965. Brock KV et al: Changes in levels of viremia in cattle persistently infected with bovine viral diarrhea virus, *J Vet Diagn Invest* 10:22-26, 1998.

966. Martin SW, Bohac JG: The association between serological titers in infectious bovine rhinotracheitis virus, bovine viral diarrhea virus, parainfluenza-3 virus respiratory syncytial virus and treatment for respiratory disease in Ontario feedlot calves, *Can J Vet Res* 50:351-358, 1986.

967. Roth JA, Kaberle ML: Suppression of neutrophil and lymphocyte function induced by a vaccinal strain of bovine viral diarrhea virus with and without the administration of ACTH, *Am J Vet Res* 44:2366-2372, 1983.

968. Cortese VS et al: Clinical and immunologic responses of vaccinated and unvaccinated calves to infection with a virulent type II isolate of bovine viral diarrhea virus, *J Am Vet Med Assoc* 213:1312-1319, 1998.

969. Dean HJ, Leyh R: Cross-protective efficacy of a bovine viral diarrhea virus (BVDV) type I vaccine against BVDV type 2 challenge, *Vaccine* 17:1117-1124, 1983.

970. Meyling A et al: Experimental exposure of vaccinated and nonvaccinated pregnant cattle to isolates of bovine viral diarrhea virus (BVDV). In Harkness JW, ed: *Agriculture: pestivirus infection of ruminants*, Luxembourg, 1987, Office for Official Publications of the EC.

971. Harkness JW et al: The efficacy of an experimental inactivated BVD-MD vaccine. In Harkness JW, ed: *Agriculture: pestivirus infection of ruminants*, Luxembourg, 1987, Office for Official Publications of the EC.

972. Cortese VS et al: Protection of pregnant cattle and their fetuses against infection with bovine viral diarrhea virus type 1 by use of a modified-live virus vaccine, *Am J Vet Res* 59:1409-1413, 1998.

MALIGNANT CATARRHAL FEVER (Bovine Malignant Catarrh; Malignant Head Catarrh)

BRADFORD P. SMITH

DEFINITION AND ETIOLOGY. Acute malignant catarrhal fever (MCF) is a highly fatal disease of cattle, deer, bison, buffalo, and some other ruminants (33 species to date) caused by a herpesvirus. It has been a major problem in zoos. The African strain, identified as alcelaphine herpesvirus type 1 (AHV-1), is a wildebeest-associated γ-herpesvirus.[973] Alcelaphineherpesvirus type 2 is a closely related but apathogenic γ-herpesvirus from other species of African antelope. The name *ovine herpesvirus type 2* (OHV-2) has been proposed for the sheep isolate. Ovine herpesvirus 2, AHV-1, and AHV-2 are closely related antigenically to bovine cytomegalovirus (bovine herpesvirus type 3), which offers some cross-protection.[964] The sheep-associated form of MCF can be acute or chronic, and animals may recover. European, Australian, Asian, and American sheep-associated viruses have been isolated. These herpesviruses appear to represent species-adapted variants of the same virus.[975] The disease usually occurs sporadically, with only one animal affected, but many large outbreaks have been reported. Cattle are considered dead-end hosts and usually do not spread the infection by contact transmission because there is no cell-free virus in secretions.[976] The virus is fragile and unlikely to survive outside a host for more than a day or even hours.

The African and North American forms of the disease are similar except for the reservoir host and the fact that the African herpesvirus appears to be more contagious and is more easily transmitted experimentally. The incubation period for American MCF is more than twice as long as that for African MCF, but the course of clinical disease is one third as long. A higher percentage of cattle develop acute disease with severe diarrhea with the American form.[977]

Some African hoofed ungulates may have clinical signs, and infected animals in wild animal parks may pose a danger to domestic livestock. Both the African and North American viruses can be transmitted to rabbits, in which infection causes an acute, fatal lymphoproliferative disorder.

CLINICAL SIGNS AND DIFFERENTIAL DIAGNOSIS. After an incubation period of 3 to 10 weeks, the disease attacks vascular endothelium (vasculitis), and all epithelial surfaces are affected. In at least one case the incubation period was 200 days. Oral erosions, diarrhea, dysentery, severe keratoconjunctivitis, mucopurulent nasal discharge, thickened, cracking skin, encephalitis, lymphadenopathy with very enlarged nodes, and high fever may be seen (Fig. 30-50). Generalized weakness and dyspnea occur. Ropy saliva may be dropped from the painful mouth, and scabs may develop on the muzzle. The hoof or horns may be shed, and lameness may be pronounced. Hematuria often is present. When particular signs predominate, the condition may be labeled the alimentary form, the encephalitic form, or a skin form. One strain of virus can cause all forms, and animals with most of these signs can be seen in a given outbreak. In California a pygmy goat had vasculitis, sloughing skin, keratitis, neurologic signs, fever, and a positive titer to MCF before dying.

The course of the acute disease usually is 3 to 7 days; some animals survive longer. The mortality rate is very high. In some outbreaks an acute form has predominated, with affected cattle dying in 1 to 3 days after developing a high fever, severe diarrhea, and conjunctivitis.[978,979] Peracute deaths without any visible symptoms also were recorded. A mild form, with transient fever and mild oral and nasal mucosal erosions followed by recovery, has been seen in experimentally infected cattle. In a natural outbreak in the United States, three of the animals survived longer than 3 months with clinical signs, and evidence indicated that some animals seroconverted and remained infected for years. The main lesion in chronic or recovered cases is obliterative arteriopathy.[980] One author recently described chronic MCF cases and animals that have recovered from MCF and concluded that sheep-associated MCF can manifest with a full range of clinical signs.[981] Some animals recovered after treatment with corticosteroids.

Malignant catarrhal fever must be differentiated from bovine virus diarrhea–mucosal disease (BVD-MD), rinderpest, bluetongue, vesicular stomatitis, and foot-and-mouth disease. The last two diseases are not usually associated with diarrhea, and vesicular stomatitis and foot-and-mouth disease tend to have high morbidity and low mortality rates. Clinical bluetongue is rare in cattle and not usually associated with dysentery. Arsenic toxicity and chlorinated naphthalene toxicity have some clinical similarities to MCF.

CLINICAL PATHOLOGY AND SEROLOGY. Some affected animals show a leukopenia caused by neutropenia if sampled early in the course of disease, but this is a very inconsistent finding in natural outbreaks.[978] Joint fluid is cloudy and

may contain increased protein and mononuclear cell numbers. Cerebrospinal fluid has elevated protein concentrations (up to 584 mg/dl) and elevated white blood cell counts (up to 945/mm^3), mainly because of an increase in mononuclear cells.[982] Serologic tests include ELISA, indirect immunofluorescence,[980,983] complement fixation, and virus neutralization. Virus isolation can be attempted. Polymerase chain reaction (PCR)[984,985] tests have been developed for the African MCF herpesvirus and recently for the sheep-associated form of disease. The sheep- and wildebeest-associated viruses appear to be closely related antigenically, cross-react serologically, and offer some cross-protection.[986]

Diagnosis is based on a history of exposure, clinical signs, and gross and histologic lesions. Rabbit inoculations can also be used. Nasal swabs and 500 ml of blood, as well as spleen and lymph node samples, should be collected for viral isolation (these should not be frozen). A cytopathic effect on thyroid cell cultures may be observed 4 to 20 days after inoculation.[987]

PATHOPHYSIOLOGY. Although the incubation period has been described as 3 to 10 weeks, a period of 150 days has been documented between the first and last cases in an outbreak.[978] Persistent asymptomatic infection for 5 months after inoculation with MCF virus followed by 4 weeks of viremia and death was documented in a steer.[988] The MCF virus appears to cause proliferation of cytotoxic T lymphocytes. The evidence suggests that the vasculitis observed with MCF is mediated by lymphoid cell infiltration rather than by virus or immune complexes.[989] Lymphocytes and lymphoblasts are found in all affected tissues, whereas neutrophils and plasma cells are rare. No visible viral particles are involved in the arteritis. Large granular lymphocytes are a subpopulation of T cells that act as natural killer cells and also as T lymphocyte suppressor cells. If these cells are malfunctioning, suppressor dysfunction can result in exuberant T cell proliferation, whereas natural killer cell dysfunction can result in indiscriminant killing of normal cells.[990] Major histocompatibility complex restriction and macrophages also appear to play a role in the pathogenesis. AHV-1 has similarities to other oncogenic lymphotrophic herpesviruses such as the Marek's disease virus and the Epstein-Barr virus.[973] The molecular structure of the MCF virus genome supports this view.

EPIDEMIOLOGY. The African form of MCF is spread to cattle and other susceptible species by wildebeests, especially during the wildebeests' calving season.[991] AHV-1 has been isolated from asymptomatic wildebeests, from the nasal and lacrimal secretions of wildebeest calves,[976] and from a wildebeest fetus.[977] The virus does not survive more than a few hours in the environment. In South Africa, however, MCF occurs in cattle without wildebeest contact (except at a distance) and when wildebeest calves are usually 8 to 10 months old.[992] The exact mode of transmission is thus incompletely understood at present. Hartebeests and topis are also reservoir hosts for the virus. The sheep-associated form of MCF is spread to cattle by contact or housing in nearby fields, even without direct contact between sheep and cattle.[978] The presence of lambs or lambing is associated with many outbreaks. A high proportion of sheep sera yields positive findings for antibody to AHV-1 by indirect immunofluorescence, including some from cesarean-derived lambs, which may indicate transplacental virus transmission.[993]

Although the disease usually occurs sporadically in a single individual, many severe outbreaks involving large numbers of cattle have been reported.[978,986,994] The dairy cow outbreaks[978,986] that occurred in the late 1970s in California and Minnesota were sheep associated, whereas recurrent North American feedlot outbreaks may not be.

Asymptomatic carrier cattle[988] or deer[973] may be sources of the virus, which would explain how outbreaks can occur without apparent contact with wildebeests, hartebeests, topis, or sheep. A steer inoculated with MCF virus was asymptomatic

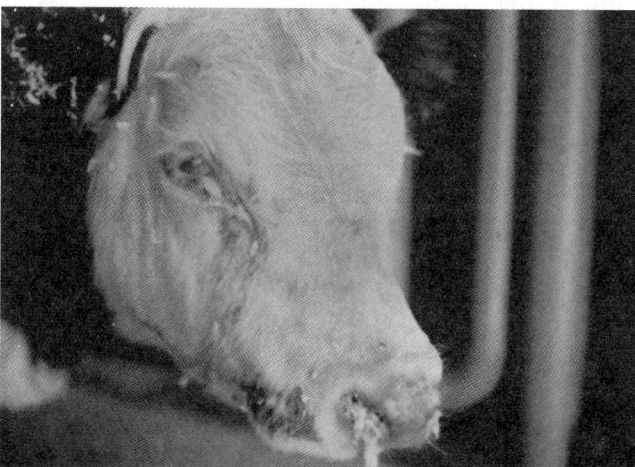

FIG. 30-50 ▪ Yearling steer with malignant catarrhal fever. Note the corneal opacity, lacrimation, and mucopurulent nasal discharge.

for 5 months before becoming viremic for 4 weeks[988] and having clinical MCF. A deer that had previously had MCF as a fawn but had been asymptomatic for 4 months recrudesced (shed virus and had clinical MCF) when given dexamethasone.[973] Cattle traditionally have been considered dead-end hosts for MCF virus because isolated individuals usually are affected, but this may not always be the case if an asymptomatic or symptomatic bovine were to shed cell-free virus in secretions.

NECROPSY FINDINGS. The nasal mucosa is hyperemic to hemorrhagic. The oral mucosa has necrotic papillae and large areas of necrosis and ulceration. Multiple focal ulcerations are seen in the esophagus. Parts of the forestomachs and intestines are thickened, edematous, and occasionally ulcerated and hemorrhagic. The lymph nodes, tonsils, and Peyer's patches are enlarged, moist, and friable. Splenic lymphoid follicles are prominent, and the liver is swollen. The adrenal glands are hemorrhagic. The mucosal surface of the bladder has focal areas of hemorrhage. The eyes are hyperemic and ulcerated and show severe corneal edema. The brain has intersulcal cloudiness and meningeal petechiation. Joints have swollen and reddened synovium with an increased quantity of cloudy fluid.[982]

Microscopic lesions involve blood vessels and epithelial surfaces. There is a marked lymphoid accumulation around vessels, as well as necrosis of the tunica media and intima. There is generalized lymphoid hyperplasia and lymphoid infiltrates in subepithelial and intraepithelial locations, associated with epithelial necrosis and sloughing. Similar changes occur in all epithelial tissues.[982] Chronic cases develop chronic obliterative arteriopathy.[980]

TREATMENT AND PROGNOSIS. Treatment does not appear to be successful. The morbidity rate may be quite high, running to 37% in one outbreak. Although some animals that exhibit mild disease may survive, close to 100% of those with severe clinical signs die.

PREVENTION AND CONTROL. During an epidemic animals that are exposed or that show clinical signs should be separated from unexposed animals, and no across-the-fence contact should be allowed. Exposed or recovered cattle may serve as a reservoir for the virus for months. Sheep should be kept well away from cattle, and cattle should not be exposed to African wildlife, especially wildebeests, hartebeests, and topis which may be infected carriers of the MCF virus. Vaccination with live or killed MCF virus has not proved consistently protective against challenge[995] and generally is not used.

REFERENCES

973. Heuschele WP et al: Dexamethasone-induced recrudescence of malignant catarrhal fever and associated lymphosarcoma and granulomatous disease in a Formosan sika deer (*Cervus nippon taiouanus*), *Am J Vet Res* 46:1578-1583, 1985.
974. Rossiter PB, Gumm ID, Mirangi PK: Immunological relationships between malignant catarrhal fever virus (alcelaphine herpesvirus 1) and bovine cytomegalovirus (bovine herpesvirus 3), *Vet Microbiol* 16:211-218, 1988.
975. Metzler AE: The malignant catarrhal fever complex, *Comp Immunol Microbiol Infect Dis* 14:107-124, 1991.
976. Mushi EZ, Rurangirwa FR: Malignant catarrhal fever virus shedding by infected cattle, *Bull Anim Health Prod Afr* 29:111-112, 1981.
977. Pierson RE et al: Comparison of the African and American forms of malignant catarrhal fever: transmission and clinical signs, *Am J Vet Res* 40:1091-1095, 1979.
978. Weaver LD: Malignant catarrhal fever in two California dairy herds, *Bovine Pract* 14:121-124, 1979.
979. Pierson RE, Liggitt HD, DeMartini JC: Clinical and clinicopathologic observations in induced malignant catarrhal fever of cattle, *J Am Vet Med Assoc* 173:833-837, 1978.
980. O'Toole D et al: Chronic generalized obliterative arteriopathy in cattle: a sequel to sheep-associated malignant catarrhal fever, *J Vet Diagn Invest* 7:108-121, 1995.
981. Penny C: Recovery of cattle from malignant catarrhal fever, *Vet Rec* 142:227, 1998.
982. Liggitt HD et al: Experimental transmission of malignant catarrhal fever in cattle: gross and histopathologic changes, *Am J Vet Res* 39:1249-1257, 1978.
983. Rossiter PB, Jessett DM, Muchi EZ: Antibodies to malignant catarrhal fever virus antigens in the sera of normal and naturally infected cattle in Kenya, *Res Vet Sci* 29:235-239, 1980.
984. Hsu D et al: A diagnostic method to detect alcelaphine herpesvirus 1 of malignant catarrhal fever using the polymerase chain reaction, *Arch Virol* 114:259-263, 1990.
985. Katz JB, Frey ML: New methods for diagnosis of malignant catarrhal fever, *Forgn Anim Dis Rep USDA, APHIS* 20:9-10, 1992.
986. Handy FM et al: Etiology of malignant catarrhal fever outbreak in Minnesota, *Proc US Anim Health Assoc* 82:248-267, 1978.
987. Mebus CA, Kalunda M, Ferris DH: Malignant catarrhal fever, *Bovine Pract* 14:130-132, 1979.
988. Rweyemamu MM et al: Persistent infection of cattle with the herpesvirus of malignant catarrhal fever and observations on the pathogenesis of the disease, *Br Vet J* 132:393-400, 1976.
989. Liggitt HD, DeMartini JC: Lymphoid vasculitis and necrosis in bovine malignant catarrhal fever, *Fed Proc* 38:1463, 1979.
990. Reid HW et al: Malignant catarrhal fever, *Vet Rec* 114:581-583, 1984.
991. Plowright W: Malignant catarrhal fever in East Africa, *Res Vet Sci* 6:56-83, 1965.
992. Barnard BJH, Van De Pypekamp HE: Wildebeest-derived malignant catarrhal fever: unusual epidemiology in South Africa, *Onderstepoort J Vet Res* 55:69-71, 1988.
993. Rossiter PB: Antibodies to malignant catarrhal fever virus in sheep sera, *J Comp Pathol* 91:303-311, 1981.
994. Pierson RE et al: An epizootic of malignant catarrhal fever in feedlot cattle, *J Am Vet Med Assoc* 163:349-350, 1973.
995. Plowright W et al: Immunization of cattle against the herpesvirus of malignant catarrhal fever: failure of inactivated culture vaccines with adjuvant, *Res Vet Sci* 19:159-166, 1975.

VESICULAR STOMATITIS

BRADFORD P. SMITH

DEFINITION AND ETIOLOGY. Vesicular stomatitis (VS) is a rhabdoviral disease of the genus *Vesiculovirus* that causes sporadic (cyclic) outbreaks of disease in cattle, horses, donkeys, mules, and pigs. Cattle under 1 year of age rarely show clinical signs. VS is seen in the United States, Mexico, and Central and South America. Human beings have sometimes been infected with an influenza-like disease. Two distinct antigenic strains have been designated, the New Jersey (NJ) and Indiana (I) serotypes. Vesicles occur in the mouth, on the teats, and in interdigital areas. Lesions may occur only on the teats or only in the mouth.[996,997] The vesicles rapidly turn to painful ulcerations that cause dysphagia and reluctance to eat, frothing at the mouth, drooling, agalactia, weight loss, mastitis, and lameness. Death is rare. Epizootic waves of VS have tended to occur at about 10-year intervals, usually in the summer or fall, but since the major epizootic in 1982 and 1983 in the western United States, the NJ serotype has been identified in the United States each year.[996] An outbreak occurred in 1995 in the western United States, in New Mexico and Colorado.[998] More cases occurred in 1997. Although the NJ serotype has at least 14 distinct genotypes, only a few of these have been found in recent outbreaks in the United States. The NJ serotype should be considered a collection of serologically related but genetically variant viruses.[996] The I serotype has three subtypes; I-1 occurs in the United States. State and federal regulatory veterinarians should be contacted immediately when VS is suspected so that quarantine and disease identification measures can be used quickly to contain an outbreak.

CLINICAL SIGNS AND DIFFERENTIAL DIAGNOSIS. After a mean incubation period of 9 days (the range is 3 to 14 days), there is onset of fever and oral lesions that cause excess salivation and reluctance to eat.[999,1000] From 5% to 60% of cattle on a farm may show clinical signs. Vesicles are only occasionally visible, because the epithelium rapidly necroses and many lesions quickly turn to ulcers. Lesions on the gums and tongue may coalesce to form large eroded areas (Fig. 30-51). Milk yield falls quickly. Teat lesions are common in dairy cattle, and

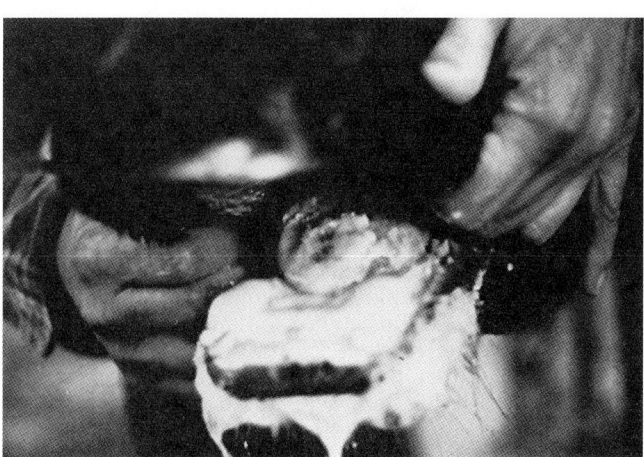

FIG. 30-51 ▦ Severe ulceration of the tongue of a dairy cow caused by vesicular stomatitis. A plaque of dying mucosa covered by fibrin is visible at the tip of the tongue, and excessive salivation is obvious. (Photograph courtesy Dr. Mark Thurmond.)

small ulcers in the interdigital area and on the coronary band are occasionally seen. Recovery varies from 2 to 21 days, depending on the severity of the lesions and management factors such as the type of feed and milking sanitation.[999] Actual healing of the lesions may take 34 to 59 days.[1000]

The major differential diagnostic consideration is foot-and-mouth disease, which causes almost identical clinical signs. Other diseases of cattle that result in oral lesions (bovine virus diarrhea, bovine papular stomatitis, bluetongue) do not usually appear as epidemics but rather in one or a few animals (although bovine papular stomatitis may have a high morbidity). Other causes of oral lesions such as bristle grass irritation and toxins should be ruled out.

CLINICAL PATHOLOGY AND LABORATORY DIAGNOSIS. The VS virus is difficult to isolate from blood, urine, feces, and oral swabs but has been isolated from tongue epithelium.[1000] A complement fixation test and a fluorescent antibody test are available for virus identification. Serum neutralizing (SN) titer rises rapidly after exposure and then gradually falls over the first year. SN titers that follow natural exposure may persist for years. Vaccination with inactivated virus results in a rapid rise in titer followed by a gradual decline for a year.[1001] The presence of an SN antibody titer does not prevent reinfection or development of clinical signs.[1002] ELISAs are also available.[1003] Hematologic and clinical chemistry findings generally reflect an acute to chronic inflammatory disease and are nonspecific in helping to make a diagnosis.

PATHOPHYSIOLOGY. After a short incubation period of 24 hours, fever and viral invasion of oral epithelial cells occur. Oral abrasions or trauma may increase susceptibility.[999] Contact of virus with teats or feet can result in lesions in these areas, especially if the teats are chapped or cracked[999] or the feet are traumatized. The lesions progress rapidly from blanched macules to vesicles and soon rupture, leaving sloughed epithelium and ulcerated areas. Healing occurs quite rapidly if feed is soft and nontraumatic.

EPIDEMIOLOGY. Older, higher-producing dairy cows that have been in milk longer are more susceptible to clinical disease caused by VS than herd mates.[999] Because the virus cannot penetrate intact mucosa, cattle fed coarse feeds or hard pellets that traumatize the oral mucosa are at higher risk.[999] Cows with chapped or cracked teats and those on farms with poor milking hygiene are more likely to get teat lesions.[999] Cow to cow contact is a major mode of transmission in outbreaks, and increased interpen movement of cattle, as well as shared feed and water troughs, unless cleaned frequently, increases the risk

of development of VS.[999] The virus is transmitted by milking machines and human hands during outbreaks. Insect vectors also contribute to the mechanical spread.

Outbreaks are often associated with the movement of animals from another area, but disease epidemics not associated with new animals do occur. The infection tends to be seasonal (occurring in the summer and fall in temperate areas and at the end of the rainy season in the tropics) and behaves like an arthropod-borne virus.[1004] The reservoir and vectors appear to be the sand fly and the black fly. Antibodies have been found in a number of wild species of animals, (deer, raccoon, bobcat, monkey), which may provide a reservoir.[1004] Active cases of VS occur in Mexico between US epidemics, giving rise to the possibility that cattle from Mexico arriving in the United Sates may also act as sources of VS virus.[996] Sheep and goats in contact often seroconvert, although clinical signs in these species are rare. The virus survives several weeks in cool soils and is very resistant to pH changes. Cattle generally show a high morbidity rate and a low mortality rate (1% to 5%). Although many in-contact cattle do not show obvious clinical signs of disease, many more have oral lesions if closely examined, and most animals in the herd seroconvert.[1000]

The economic losses associated with an outbreak of VS can be severe, especially in dairy cattle. In the 1982 epizootic in California, losses on two dairies (principally decreased milk production and culling for mastitis) totaled $225,000 during 2 months.[1005]

NECROPSY FINDINGS. Deaths are rare and usually are attributed to secondary bacterial diseases, including environmental mastitis and pneumonia. Cattle become gaunt and weak as a result of dysphagia and resultant reduced food intake. Erosive and ulcerative lesions are usually confined to the mouth. The teats frequently are involved in lactating cows, and lesions on the coronary band and interdigital area occasionally may be seen.

Histologically, intracellular and extracellular edema, ballooning and degeneration of epithelial cells, and vesicle formation accompanied by neutrophilic infiltration are present. There are no inclusion bodies. The characteristic bullet-shaped structure of the VS virus sometimes can be seen with electron microscope examination of fresh lesions or vesicular fluid.[1004]

TREATMENT AND PROGNOSIS. Mortality can be almost completely prevented if ill cattle are offered shade, fresh water, clean bedding, and soft feed. Offering soft feed hastens recovery and reduces the anorectic period. Debilitated cattle should be given broad-spectrum antibiotics in an effort to control secondary bacterial pneumonia. Cattle with teat lesions are at high risk of developing mastitis and should be carefully milked last and monitored closely for mastitis. The prognosis for survival is very good, but agalactia and mastitis may result in culling of a large number of animals.

PREVENTION AND CONTROL. During an outbreak of VS, quarantine of the premises and isolation of sick animals are required. Regulatory officials will help organize and maintain a quarantine. Feed should be soft and fine, because coarse or hard-pelleted feeds increase the spread of the virus and prolong the recovery time.[999] Leftover feed should be removed from feed bunks twice daily and the bunks disinfected. Water troughs should be cleaned and disinfected daily. Disinfection can be accomplished by using 1% formalin, organic iodines, hexachlorophene, or phenyl-phenolic preparations. Two hours of exposure to lye (2% NaOH) will *not* deactivate the virus.

Vaccination using killed or live virus vaccines[1006] is rarely practiced preventively because the disease occurs as rare epidemics in small areas and because vaccination interferes with serologic testing and monitoring. Vaccination with a killed virus vaccine may be used by regulatory veterinarians in at-risk animals during an epidemic. Owners and managers

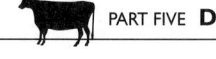
should consult state and federal veterinarians before considering VS vaccination.

REFERENCES

996. USDA: Vesicular stomatitis, *Forgn Anim Dis Rep*, USDA, Animal Plant Health Inspect Service 16:5-11, 1988.
997. Strozzi P, Ramos-Saco T: Teat vesicles as primary and almost exclusive lesions in an extensive outbreak of vesicular stomatitis (New Jersey strain) in milking cows, *J Am Vet Med Assoc* 123:415-418, 1953.
998. Mumford EL et al: Serologic evaluation of vesicular stomatitis virus exposure in horses and cattle in 1996, *J Am Vet Med Assoc* 213:1265-1269, 1998.
999. Hansen DE, Thurmond MC, Thorburn M: Factors associated with the spread of clinical vesicular stomatitis in California dairy cattle, *Am J Vet Res* 46:789-795, 1985.
1000. Thurmond MC et al: Vesicular stomatitis virus (New Jersey strain) infection in two California dairy herds: an epidemiologic study, *J Am Vet Med Assoc* 191:965-970, 1987.
1001. Gearhart MA et al: Serum neutralizing antibody titers in dairy cattle administered an inactivated vesicular stomatitis virus vaccine, *J Am Vet Med Assoc* 191:819-822, 1987.
1002. Rodriguez LL et al: Serological monitoring of vesicular stomatitis New Jersey virus in enzootic regions of Costa Rica, *Am J Trop Med Hyg* 42:272-281, 1990.
1003. DeAnda JH et al: Evaluation of an enzyme-linked immunosorbent assay for detection of antibodies to vesicular stomatitis virus in cattle in an enzootic region of Mexico, *Am J Vet Res* 53:440-443, 1992.
1004. Kahrs RF: *Viral disease of cattle* Ames, Iowa, 1981, Iowa State University Press.
1005. Goodger WJ et al: Economic impact of an epizootic of bovine vesicular stomatitis in California, *J Am Vet Med Assoc* 186:370-373, 1985.
1006. Lauerman LH, Hansen RP: Field trial of live virus vaccination procedure for prevention of vesicular stomatitis in dairy cattle. III. Evaluation of emergency vaccination in Georgia, *Proc US Animal Health Assoc* 67:473-482, 1963.

FOOT-AND-MOUTH DISEASE
(Aftosa; Aphthous Fever)

BRADFORD P. SMITH

DEFINITION AND ETIOLOGY. Foot-and-mouth disease (FMD) is an acute, highly contagious viral disease of cloven-hoofed livestock characterized by vesicular lesions, erosions, and ulcers in the mouth and interdigital areas and on the muzzle, teats, and coronary band.[1007] Natural hosts include cattle, sheep, goats, swine, water buffalo, bison, deer, elk, antelope, bears, llamas, camels, giraffes, elephants, rats, capybaras, and hedgehogs.[1008] Of these, cattle and swine are the most susceptible. Mature sheep and goats usually have mild signs. Livestock of all ages are susceptible, but the mortality rate is higher in young animals because cardiac lesions occur. The horse is resistant to infection. In rare cases, humans have contracted the disease. It is endemic in Asia, Africa, parts of Europe, and most of South America, where losses involve not only those caused by the disease itself but also the monetary losses that result because fewer animal products are available for export due to loss of foreign markets. As this book goes to press (2001), Great Britain is experiencing the first epidemic since 1967, and France is threatened.

The FMD virus is a picornavirus of the genus *Apthovirus*. At least seven immunologically distinct types of FMDV have been identified: A; O; C; SAT 1, 2, and 3; and Asia 1. Within the seven types at least 60 subtypes have been recognized. Vaccination against one subtype may not protect against another.[1009] This fact, together with the fact that immunity is generally short-term, means that effective vaccination programs are difficult. The virus is rapidly inactivated by high or low pH, sunlight, and very high temperatures but is very resistant to normal environmental conditions and drying.[1007] Sodium hydroxide, sodium carbonate, iodophors, chlorine dioxide, and acetic acid are effective disinfectants, but many common disinfectants are ineffective.

CLINICAL SIGNS AND DIFFERENTIAL DIAGNOSIS. FMD is clinically indistinguishable from vesicular stomatitis

except that VS also affects horses. Clinical signs of FMD include fever, depression, anorexia, listlessness, occasional shivering, excess salivation, lip smacking, nasal discharge, and lameness.[1009] Agalactia may occur. In addition to VS the differential diagnosis includes bovine papular stomatitis, bluetongue, rinderpest, malignant catarrhal fever, and severe cases of infectious bovine rhinotracheitis. Teat lesions can be confused with those caused by bovine herpes mammillitis or parapoxviruses.

Vesicular lesions (blisters) 0.5 to 10 cm in diameter rupture within 48 hours, followed by a mucosal slough and large erosion.[1009] These lesions appear to be very painful, and affected animals are reluctant to eat or move. The morbidity rate is high, but the mortality rate is low. The disease is economically devastating because it spreads rapidly and causes weight loss, mastitis, loss of milk production,[1010] and frequent abortion. An outbreak of FMD in a country previously free of the disease can cost billions of dollars in trade losses over ensuing years. Deaths may occur in young calves, mainly from myocardial necrosis, and secondary bacterial pneumonia and foot infections are common.

LABORATORY DIAGNOSIS. Because FMD is clinically indistinguishable from VS and other viral mucosal diseases, laboratory confirmation of the diagnosis is obtained through complement fixation, virus neutralization, agar gel precipitation, ELISA, or fluorescent antibody tests.[1009] ELISA appears to be more sensitive and type specific than complement fixation[1011] and virus neutralization.[1012] When VS or FMD is suspected, state and federal authorities should be contacted immediately. In FMD-free countries, quarantine is practical to control spread. Slaughtered animals are burned. All animals within 3 km may be destroyed during efforts to halt the disease.

PATHOPHYSIOLOGY. The usual primary sites of infection and replication by the FMD virus are the pharyngeal and digestive mucosa[1009] and alveolar epithelium of the udder.[1013] The virus replicates in the cells of the stratum spinosum.[1014] It spreads locally and also enters the circulation and is carried to other susceptible tissues. Within 2 to 21 days a fever begins, and some vesicles occur.[1015] Vesicles develop in the mouth and on the rumen pillars, and myocardial and skeletal muscle degeneration characterized by Zenker's necrosis may occur in young cattle. The mucosal cell disruption results in separation of superficial epithelium from basal epithelium, which fills with tissue fluids. When these epithelial layers slough, erosions are left behind that take days to weeks to heal, depending on their size.[1009]

EPIDEMIOLOGY. Transmission occurs primarily by means of aerosols,[1009,1016,1017] animal contact, and fomites such as shoes, tires, and equipment. The virus may be spread to farms 50 miles in distance. Human beings can carry (and subsequently transmit) the virus on their shoes or clothing or in respiratory tract tissues for longer than 24 hours. Recovered cattle usually stop shedding the virus by 2 weeks, but some harbor it for 6 to 24 months and may act as sources of the virus at the start of an epidemic.[1015] The virus has been isolated from semen,[1018] and the possibility exists of sexual transmission from the African buffalo to cattle.[1019] African Cape buffaloes can be a lifelong carriers.

The virus exists in milk, and it may survive pasteurization. Uncooked or partly cooked meat products or garbage scraps, hides, or other tissues contaminated with the FMD virus from an endemic area of the world may transmit the disease long distances. The virus can persist in frozen meat for years. Besides actively infected animals, sources of infection include bedding, feed, milk, shoes and hands of humans, and equipment.[1009]

NECROPSY FINDINGS. In addition to oral erosions and ulcerations, ulcers may be seen on the rumen pillars. In young cattle myocardial and skeletal muscle degeneration and necrosis may be noted. Histologically, the vesicles are characterized

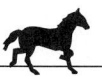

by ballooning, cellular degeneration, intracellular and extracellular edema, and separation of the basal epithelium.[1014] There are no inclusion bodies. Muscle lesions (skeletal and cardiac) are characterized by necrosis (Zenker's degeneration).

TREATMENT AND PROGNOSIS. Where FMD is endemic, quarantine, local eradication, virus typing, and revaccination of contact and at-risk cattle with the appropriate virus subtype should be considered. Good nursing care and administration of systemic antimicrobial drugs to limit secondary bacterial pneumonia and mastitis are recommended. Soft feeds such as chopped green grass are much more palatable than hay to sore-mouthed animals. The prognosis is good for survival, although many animals abort, lose weight, stop lactating, or have severe bacterial mastitis secondary to viral teat lesions and must be culled. The virus destroys mammary alveolar epithelium permanently.[1013]

PREVENTION AND CONTROL. In endemic areas vaccination and quarantine are the basis for prevention and control. In FMD-free areas (Great Britain, the United States, Canada, Japan, New Zealand, and Australia), the method of choice is rapid identification of an outbreak, quarantine, and slaughter of all affected and exposed herds.

Vaccines must be type specific. Most European and South American countries use trivalent inactivated vaccines against types A, O, and C from cell culture virus. Vaccine-induced and naturally occurring immunity is short-lived, and vaccination usually must be repeated two or three times a year.[1009] Newer oil-adjuvanted vaccines can protect for up to 1 year. Because the protection is partial, infection usually results in subclinical or mild disease. Calves nursing immune dams are likewise partly protected by passive antibody for up to 5 months.[1009] In an outbreak the most effective vaccine is autogenous.

REFERENCES

1007. Cottral GE, Callis JJ: Foot-and-mouth disease. In Commission on Foreign Animal Disease, ed: *Foreign animal diseases, their diagnosis and control*, Richmond, Va, 1975, US Animal Health Association.
1008. Fraser CM: Foot-and-mouth disease. In Fraser CM, ed: *The Merck veterinary manual*, ed 6, Rahway, NJ, 1986, Merck.
1009. Kahrs RF: *Viral diseases of cattle*, Ames, Iowa, 1981, Iowa State University Press.
1010. Blackwell JH, Wool SH: Destruction and repair of mammary gland parenchyma of cows infected with foot-and-mouth disease, *J Comp Pathol* 96:227-234, 1986.
1011. Westbury HA et al: A comparison of enzyme-linked immunosorbent assay, complement fixation and virus isolation for foot-and-mouth disease diagnosis, *Vet Microbiol* 17:21-28, 1988.
1012. Hamblin C et al: Enzyme-linked immunosorbent assay (ELISA) for the detection of antibodies against foot-and-mouth disease virus, *Epidemiol Infect* 99:733-744, 1987.
1013. Blackwell JH, Yilma T: Localization of foot-and-mouth disease viral antigens in mammary glands of infected cows, *Am J Vet Res* 42:770-773, 1981.
1014. Yilma T: Morphogenesis of vesiculation in foot-and-mouth disease, *Am J Vet Res* 41:1537-1542, 1980.
1015. Graves JH: Foot-and-mouth disease: a constant threat to US livestock, *J Am Vet Med Assoc* 174:174-176, 1979.
1016. Hurst GH: Foot-and mouth-disease, the possibility of continental sources of the virus in England in epidemics of October, 1967, and several other years, *Vet Rec* 82:610-614, 1968.
1017. Sellers RF, Forman AJ: The Hampshire epidemic of foot-and-mouth disease, *J Hyg (Cambridge)* 71:15-34, 1973.
1018. Cottral GE, Gailuiunas P, Cox BF: Foot-and-mouth disease virus in semen of bulls and its transmission by artificial insemination, *Arch Ges Virus Forsch* 23:362-377, 1968.
1019. Bastos ADS et al: Possibility of sexual transmission of foot-and-mouth disease from African buffalo to cattle, *Vet J* 158:6-13, 1999.

RINDERPEST (Cattle Plague)

BRADFORD P. SMITH

DEFINITION AND ETIOLOGY. Rinderpest (RP) is an acute, highly contagious, and usually fatal disease of ruminants. Cattle and water buffaloes are most frequently affected, but the disease also occurs in sheep, goats, pigs, camels, and other cloven-hoofed animals, in which it is usually less severe. Rinderpest virus (RPV) is in the Paramyxoviridae family, genus *Morbillivirus.* There is only one known strain of RPV. It is closely related serologically to the virus that causes peste des petits ruminants (PPR). The virus can remain viable for at least 1 year in frozen tissue, but it is killed by direct sunlight in 2 hours. The disease currently is active in Africa, the Middle East, and Asia.[1020] Other morbilliviruses pathogenic for animals include canine distemper and the 1995 Australian morbillivirus, which occurred in horses and humans.

CLINICAL SIGNS AND DIFFERENTIAL DIAGNOSIS. The incubation period in cattle is 3 to 15 days, which is followed by sudden onset of fever, depression, and anorexia. The nose is dry, and mucous membranes are congested. Within days oral erosions appear where necrotic foci have sloughed. Purulent lacrimation occurs. Diarrhea is severe and may be bloody. Dehydration and emaciation often lead to death. The disease in sheep and goats usually is mild or subclinical,[1021] but the PPR virus can cause outbreaks with high morbidity and mortality in small ruminants.

In endemic areas RP is suspected when the signs described above occur in groups of animals. In nonendemic areas diseases that appear similar clinically are bovine virus diarrhea, malignant catarrhal fever, arsenic poisoning, severe coccidiosis, and severe fulminating infectious bovine rhinotracheitis. Other causes of severe gastroenteritis and diarrhea (e.g., salmonellosis) must also be considered. Oral lesions of RP are similar to these seen with vesicular stomatitis. In small ruminants, bluetongue, PPR, and Nairobi sheep disease must be ruled out.

LABORATORY DIAGNOSIS. Laboratory confirmation of RP can be accomplished by (1) virus isolation; (2) detection of viral antigen by fluorescent antibody testing, virus neutralization, complement fixation, or agar gel immunodiffusion; (3) detection of rising antibody titer by ELISA or virus neutralization; and (4) histopathologic evaluation.[1022] Virus isolation is most successful in the first days of infection (often before the onset of diarrhea). Blood should be taken in heparin. The lymph nodes and spleen are reliable sources of virus, and in cattle, tears and ocular discharges are also reliable sources.[1023] Lymph node biopsy after day 3 of infection is the most reliable means of diagnosis in a living goat.[1021] Tissues should be shipped on ice to the laboratory for virus isolation or detection of antigen. Detection of a rising antibody titer can help diagnose the disease retrospectively. Leukopenia may be noted in the acute early states of RP.

PATHOPHYSIOLOGY. The virus usually enters through the respiratory mucosa. Lymphoid tissue is the primary target of the rinderpest virus. Lymphocytes are destroyed in the germinal centers of the lymph nodes, Peyer's patches, tonsils, splenic corpuscles, and cecal lymphoid tissue. Immunosuppression occurs as lymphoid tissue is destroyed.[1024] The virus also attacks the alimentary tract mucosa; Peyer's patches are the most severely affected. As alimentary mucosa is lost, diarrhea and emaciation become severe.

EPIDEMIOLOGY. RP is highly contagious; it is spread mainly through airborne droplets, direct contact, feces, and contaminated fomites such as human beings. All secretions and feces of infected animals are contagious throughout the course of the disease. Wild ruminants frequently are a source of infection for livestock. The morbidity rate often approaches 100%, with a 25% to 90% mortality rate, making treatment unrewarding and the prognosis poor. Innate or specific resistance may protect individuals or herds from clinical signs after infection. Recovered animals do not appear to act as carriers. Valuable individuals may be helped by supportive therapy and hydration.

NECROPSY FINDINGS. Lesions are found mainly in the alimentary tract and lymphoid tissues. Subendocardial hemorrhages may also be seen in animals that die of acute illness. Oral erosions, edema, and congestion of the abomasum are typically seen, and ulcers and hemorrhagic to necrotic Peyer's patches occasionally are seen. The cecal and colonic mucosae are hemorrhagic, ulcerated, or necrotic. The lymph nodes have necrotic germinal centers.

PREVENTION AND CONTROL. Because there is only one known strain of RPV and protection after infection usually is lifelong, vaccination of cattle in endemic areas with a live cell culture attenuated virus is an effective means of controlling RP.[1025] Although there is some debate as to whether this vaccine causes immunosuppression,[1026] it has been used safely and effectively in millions of cattle in Africa and Asia.[1025] The vaccine does not produce adverse reactions, has a long shelf life, and produces solid immunity.[1025] Its major disadvantages are that the lyophilized virus has to be kept cold, and once a vial has been reconstituted, it must be used quickly before the virus dies. A vaccinia-vectored gene vaccine currently under field testing is effective and has the advantages of long-term stability in harsh environments and ease of application (scratch on).

Control of epidemics in areas where the disease is not endemic involves quarantine and slaughter of infected and contact animals, as well as other contact ruminants and swine. Disinfection of premises while under government quarantine is essential in controlling the disease. The virus is susceptible to most disinfectants and survives in the environment only for 2 to 3 days.

REFERENCES
1020. Kock RA: Rinderpest epidemic in wild ruminants in Kenya, *Vet Rec* 145:275-283, 1999.
1021. Wafula JS, Wamwayi HM: Development and distribution of rinderpest virus antigen in experimentally infected goats, *Vet Rec* 123:199-200, 1988.
1022. US Department of Agriculture: APHIS Vol. 6: Rinderpest, Peste des Petits Ruminants, Program Aid No. 1581, 1997.
1023. Wafula JS et al: Development and stability of rinderpest virus antigens in cattle tears and lymph nodes, *Trop Anim Health Prod* 18:26-31, 1986.
1024. Scott GR: *Diagnosis of rinderpest*, Rome, 1967, WHO Food and Agriculture Organization.
1025. Rossiter PB, Kariuki DP: Single and combined rinderpest vaccines, *Vet Rec* 121:230-231, 1987.
1026. Jeggo MH, Wardley RC, Cortey N: A reassessment of the dual vaccine against rinderpest and contagious bovine pleuropneumonia, *Vet Rec* 120:131-135, 1987.

CHOKE AND ESOPHAGEAL DISORDERS

CHARLES GUARD

DEFINITION AND ETIOLOGY. Choke is the term used for esophageal obstruction. Of the ruminants, it is most common in cattle because of their eating habits. If the obstruction is complete, the condition is rapidly fatal because of the inability to eliminate the gases of fermentation produced in the rumenoreticulum. Partial obstruction produces dysphagia or anorexia. Obstruction may be caused by the ingestion of foreign objects or large chunks of solid feedstuffs such as apples, potatoes, beet tops, or corn cobs. It also may be the result of space-occupying lesions in or near the esophagus. Choke must be differentiated from diseases that cause dysphagia by means of pharyngeal lesions and resultant neuromuscular dysfunction. Congenital or acquired lesions of the esophagus such as aortic arch anomalies and diverticula may cause signs similar to those of esophageal obstruction.

CLINICAL SIGNS AND DIFFERENTIAL DIAGNOSIS. The earliest signs of complete esophageal obstruction from intraluminal objects are anxiety and ptyalorrhea (i.e., saliva dripping from the mouth because of an inability to swallow). The animal may violently swing the head from side to side and make repeated attempts to swallow. Staggering (which must be differentiated from ataxia caused by neurologic diseases) may be observed. Bloat develops soon after at a rate that depends on the nature of the ruminoreticular contents. Objects such as potatoes, apples, or mangels may be swallowed whole or in chunks too large to pass the entire esophagus, especially in cattle. Dry grain, particularly in pellet form, may be consumed so rapidly that sufficient saliva is not produced to lubricate the passage of the feed boluses. This is more common in sheep than in other ruminants; spontaneous resolution usual occurs within minutes to hours.

Obstruction from intraluminal objects commonly occurs in the cranial part of the cervical esophagus, at the thoracic inlet, or at the base of the heart. External palpation may localize the site of obstruction in the cervical esophagus. With more slowly developing and incomplete obstruction, anorexia and dysphagia may be observed. Bloat may occur repeatedly and resolve spontaneously or after passage of a stomach tube. The underlying cause may cause signs severe enough to mask the esophageal problem. Cellulitis along the cervical esophagus may result in a reluctance to lower the head or bend the neck laterally. Possible causes of cervical cellulitis include perivascular injection of irritating substances, abscesses, and reaction to *Hypoderma lineatum* larvae.

Esophageal stricture may follow a previous episode of esophageal obstruction or inflammation in adjacent tissues.[1027] If no site of obstruction is externally evident, careful attempts to pass a stomach tube usually reveal the site of the problem. Radiography with barium contrast material may help identify the site of strictures, perforations, and diverticula.[1028] Endoscopy of the esophagus may also aid in identifying the specific nature of functional or structural abnormalities. Megaesophagus has been observed after pharyngeal trauma,[1029] as a congenital disorder,[1030] and with hiatal hernia.[1031] An animal with an esophageal stricture or a diverticulum may reflux boluses of feed mixed with saliva or regurgitate liquid rumen contents. Failure to gain weight or progressive weight loss accompanies the failure to swallow feed successfully. Signs may be seen only when forage is consumed, whereas water and grain are swallowed normally.

Systemic diseases may lead to esophageal dysfunction. Rabies must always be considered when dysphagia is present, and appropriate precautions must be taken. Botulism also leads to esophageal transport failure, although dysphagia and a weak tongue are more prominent in the failure of affected animals to eat. Tetanus may be similar in appearance to esophageal obstruction because of the presence of bloat, dysphagia, and drooling. Several poisonous plants, including sneezeweed, larkspur, and milkweed, may cause excessive salivation, drooling, and bloat. Consumption of red clover infected with the fungus *Rhizoctonia leguminicola*, which produces the toxin slaframine, results in copious salivation. Pharyngeal trauma and subsequent cellulitis lead to dysphagia and drooling; severe bloat does not occur unless swelling is sufficient to occlude the esophagus. However, mild bloat frequently accompanies pharyngeal trauma caused by associated vagal nerve inflammation and dysfunction.[1032]

CLINICAL PATHOLOGY. Common features of longstanding choke are dehydration and metabolic acidosis resulting from continued loss of sodium bicarbonate and sodium phosphate in saliva. As sodium depletion develops, the composition of saliva shifts to include more potassium under the influence of aldosterone. Inflammatory diseases lead to predictable changes in the hemogram.

NECROPSY FINDINGS. Animals that die of acute esophageal obstruction are bloated and may have saliva and feedstuffs in the upper airway. Postmortem examination of animals with protracted esophageal dysfunction may reveal focal dilations or stenoses of the esophagus. Esophageal perforation may have occurred because of pressure around an intraluminal foreign body or necrosis caused by extension of an adjacent septic process.

TREATMENT AND PROGNOSIS. In cases of complete esophageal obstruction, relieving bloat is the first concern. Passage of a stomach tube may be attempted if the animal is not in respiratory distress. Trocharization of the rumen or installation of a temporary fistula may be required. Until the esophagus has been cleared, it is important to keep the muzzle level or pointed down to reduce the risk of aspiration of saliva. Sedative drugs such as acepromazine or xylazine may be useful to calm the animal and permit careful examination. Suitable precautions should be taken if rabies is remotely possible. The history and an examination of the environment should enable the clinician to anticipate the nature of the obstructing object. Palpation of the neck along the left jugular furrow may reveal the site of obstruction in lean or thin-necked individuals. A manual oral examination should precede probing attempts with a stomach tube. Gentle pressure on the stomach tube as it passes down the esophagus should allow localization of the obstruction. A small hand can reach into the cranial part of the esophagus and may retrieve some solid objects. If the object is solid (e.g., a potato), it may be possible to massage it into the pharynx by pressing in the jugular furrow on both sides of the neck. Specialized equipment, such as probang, is available with a corkscrewlike or pincerlike end that can be used to grasp or engage a foreign body and expedite its retrieval. If a mass of grain is obstructing the esophagus, external massage, probing with the stomach tube, or pumping fluid against the mass through the tube may break it up.

If the choke is intrathoracic and probing with a stomach tube does not relieve the problem, several courses of action are possible. A small rumen fistula can be inserted to prevent bloat, and the animal can simply be placed in a pen without bedding, feed, or water. Many masses consisting of grain or hay spontaneously pass within 24 hours, whereas solid objects rarely pass spontaneously. If the obstruction does not resolve in 24 hours, the animal can be heavily sedated, a cuffed endotracheal tube passed to prevent aspiration, and vigorous lavage with water through a stomach tube can be attempted. The head should be held lower than the body to minimize the risk of aspiration. If the obstruction still cannot be relieved or it is believed that the obstruction is a solid object, a rumenotomy can be performed. Access to the esophagus through the cardia should allow snaring of the object with a loop of stiff wire or breaking up a mass of grain.

The long-term prognosis after choke is good unless esophageal mucosal damage has occurred. Stricture formation may follow cellulitis or pressure necrosis at the site of the obstruction. Aftercare for the choked animal consists of a soft diet and antiinflammatory drugs to minimize tissue swelling. Well-soaked alfalfa cubes made into a mush may pass partly obstructed areas. Hay and grain should be moistened before feeding, and grain should be offered only in small amounts at each feeding. Broad-spectrum antibiotics should be given if mucosal damage is suspected. Maintenance of an indwelling nasogastric tube for feeding for up to 10 days after severe esophageal trauma may be helpful in preventing strictures during healing.[1028] Thick gruels made from soaked alfalfa cubes or pellets can be pumped into the rumen by a bilge pump designed for boats, or the animal can be fed and watered through a rumen fistula. Surgical exploration may be required for esophageal obstruction from space-occupying lesions or strictures to determine the cause.[1028] Abscesses may be drained, and granulomatous le-

sions resected. Esophageal diverticula, aortic arch anomalies, and intrathoracic surgical problems may not be easily treated.

REFERENCES

1027. Meagher DM, Mayhew IG: The surgical treatment of upper esophageal obstructions in the bovine, *Can Vet J* 19:128-132, 1978.
1028. Verschooten F, Oyaert W: Radiological diagnosis of esophageal disorders in the bovine, *J Am Vet Radiol Soc* 18:85-89, 1977.
1029. Ross CE, Rebhun WC: Megaesophagus in a cow, *J Am Vet Med Assoc* 188:623-624, 1986.
1030. Vestweber JG, Leipold HW, Knighton RG: Idiopathic megaesophagus in a calf: clinical and pathologic features, *J Am Vet Med Assoc* 187:1369-1370, 1985.
1031. Anderson NV et al: Hiatal hernia and segmental megaesophagus in a cow, *J Am Vet Med Assoc* 184:193-195, 1984.
1032. Davidson HP, Rebhun WC, Habel RE: Pharyngeal trauma in cattle, *Cornell Vet* 71:15-25, 1981.

ESOPHAGEAL DILATION (Megaesophagus) AND HIATAL HERNIA

BRADFORD P. SMITH

Megaesophagus rarely occurs in ruminants. It has been reported in association with pharyngeal trauma and resultant inflammatory involvement of the vagus[1033] and with hiatal hernia (diaphragmatic hernia with herniation of the reticulum into the thorax) in which there was a large megaesophagus (10 cm in diameter by 20 cm in length).[1034] Vagotomy and hiatal hernia are recognized as causes of diminished esophageal pressure.[1035] A 4-month-old calf with megaesophagus lacked esophageal muscle cells and ganglion cells, and many fat cells were present.[1036] The esophagus of a 12-month-old ram with megaesophagus was found to be heavily infected with *Sarcocystis arieticanis*, and eosinophilic inflammation and degeneration of muscle fibers were noted.[1037] However, *Sarcocystis* spp. have been found in the esophagus of many sheep without megaesophagus,[1038,1039] making the diagnosis difficult. An 18-month-old heifer with megaesophagus also had eosinophilic submucosal infiltration, but no sarcocysts were seen.[1040]

The principal clinical signs of megaesophagus are regurgitation or vomiting, usually shortly after eating. Mild, recurrent bloat and discomfort when a stomach tube is passed are also observed. In other cattle with a hiatal (diaphragmatic) hernia[1041] or an esophageal diverticulum,[1042] regurgitation or vomiting and bloat have also been reported. Contortion of the neck while eating, apparently caused by pain, was seen in one cow[1034] and is reported in human beings with hiatal hernia.[1043] In some cases of herniation of the reticulum into the thorax, bloat and regurgitation are not seen[1044,1045]; in others diaphragmatic hernia resulted in chronic bloat.[1046] Diaphragmatic hernias may be either congenital or acquired. It appears that acquired diaphragmatic hernias are most common.

A stomach tube should be passed to the rumen to rule out choke or an intraluminal mass obstructing the esophagus as a cause. If a tube can be passed freely to the rumen, plain and contrast radiographs of the esophagus should be taken. If this is not possible, surgical exploration for a diaphragmatic hernia and digital palpation of the cardia and terminal esophagus by means of rumenotomy should be considered.

Megaesophagus associated with pharyngeal trauma has a good prognosis,[1033] whereas megaesophagus associated with hiatal hernia has a more guarded prognosis.[1034,1041] Supportive treatments and stomach tubing with fluids may be required for 1 to 2 weeks until the animal is able to drink unaided. Longer term support can be given to a valuable animal

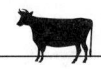

by surgically creating a rumen fistula fitted with a rubber cannula* through which feed and water can be given until normal deglutition is resumed.

REFERENCES

1033. Ross CE, Rebhun WC: Megaesophagus in a cow, *J Am Vet Med Assoc* 188:623-624, 1986.
1034. Anderson NV et al: Hiatal hernia and segmental megaesophagus in a cow, *J Am Vet Med Assoc* 184:193-195, 1984.
1035. O'Brien JA, Harvey CE, Brodey RS: The esophagus. In Anderson NV, ed: *Veterinary gastroenterology*, Philadelphia, 1980, Lea & Febiger.
1036. Vestweber JG, Leipold HW, Knighton RG: Idiopathic megaesophagus in a calf: clinical and clinicopathologic features, *J Am Vet Med Assoc* 187:1369-1370, 1985.
1037. Braun U et al: Regurgitation due to megaesophagus in a ram, *Can Vet J* 31:391-392, 1990.
1038. Duby JP et al: *Sarcocystis arieticanis* and other *Sarcocystis* spp in sheep in the United States, *J Parasitol* 74:1033-1038, 1988.
1039. Bock J et al: *Sarcocystis* und *Toxoplasma* Infektionen bei Schlachtschafen in Bayern, *Berl Munch Tierarztl Wochenschr* 92:137-141, 1979.
1040. Bargai U, Nathan AT, Pearl S: Acquired megaesophagus in a heifer, *Vet Radiol* 32:259-260, 1991.
1041. Kirkbride CA, Noordsy JL: An esophageal hiatus hernia in a bull, *J Am Vet Med Assoc* 152:996-998, 1968.
1042. McGavin MD, Anderson NV: Projectile expectoration associated with an esophageal diverticulum in a cow, *J Am Vet Med Assoc* 166:247-248, 1975.
1043. Kinsbourne M: Hiatus hernia with contortions of the neck, *Lancet* 1:1058-1061, 1964.
1044. Roberts SJ: Diaphragmatic hernia in the bovine, *Cornell Vet* 36:92-97, 1946.
1045. Frost JN, Danks AG: Atypical indigestion in the bovine, *Cornell Vet* 29:70-73, 1939.
1046. Troutt HF et al: Diaphragmatic defects in cattle, *J Am Vet Med Assoc* 151:1421-1429, 1967.

INDIGESTION IN RUMINANTS

FRANKLYN B. GARRY

DEFINITION AND ETIOLOGY. Indigestion is a general term for a group of diseases characterized by dysfunction of the reticulorumen. Some texts have limited the use of the term to a single, poorly defined entity that includes inappetence, decreased reticuloruminal motility, and abnormal feces, with a nonspecific cause that involves intake of abnormal feed.

The more generalized term applied here incorporates a pathophysiologic classification scheme of forestomach disturbances that has been devised by workers in Germany.[1047] An absolute division of the pathologic processes is impossible because the various forestomach functions are interdependent; that is, abnormal motor function affects microbial fermentation by altered mixing or passage of rumen fluid out of the forestomach chambers, whereas abnormal fermentation products secondarily alter motor function. Nevertheless, this classification provides a clinically useful diagnostic framework by emphasizing the underlying pathophysiologic mechanisms of different forestomach disturbances.

The primary indigestions include those diseases in which the reticulorumen is directly affected and responsible for the major disease signs (Box 30-5). These problems can be divided into two categories:

1. Abnormal motor function of the reticulorumen, including disease of the reticuloruminal wall, its innervation, or impedance to the passage of ingesta
2. Abnormal contents of the reticulorumen, with dysfunction of microbial and biochemical fermentation

Secondary indigestions are the sequelae of systemic problems or disease in other organ systems. For example, problems such as endotoxemia, fever, or depression can produce anorexia, secondary rumen hypomotility, and decreased microbial fermentative function. Primary abomasal disease can depress rumen function, inhibit rumen outflow, and reflux abomasal contents back into the rumen.

With the exception of penetrating foreign bodies and sporadic infections of the forestomach wall (e.g., actinomycosis, mucormycosis), indigestions are physiologic abnormalities. In the adult ruminant one or more of the homeostatic processes of the fermentative environment are disturbed (e.g., an excessive carbohydrate intake generates an excessive amount of acid product; abnormal neural regulation of the rumen motility pattern disturbs the mixing or aboral passage of ingesta). In the young ruminant the forestomachs are actively developing, and indigestions can result from disturbances of the developmental mechanisms. The forestomach diseases of young ruminants generally have received little attention, but they can be recognized and appropriately treated within a classification scheme similar to that for adult ruminants.[1048,1049]

PATHOPHYSIOLOGY. Digestion of feedstuffs in the reticulorumen is accomplished by microbial fermentation. The mucosal epithelium absorbs and exchanges products of fermentation but performs essentially no secretory function. Appropriate forestomach fermentation depends on the coordination of processes that provide a fairly constant reticuloruminal environment. The requirements include addition of appropriate amounts and types of feed substrate and water by ingestion; buffering of substances from the saliva to counteract the acid nature of fermentation products; eructation of the gaseous products of fermentation; coordination of reticuloruminal motility to provide mixing; rumination and remastication; aboral passage of ingesta; temperature maintenance; and exchanges of electrolytes and volatile fatty acids (VFAs) across the rumen wall. Because these functions are intimately interrelated, abnormalities of any one of them can lead to digestive disturbances.

---

*Four-inch rumen canula, catalog No 1 C, Bar Diamond, Inc., P.O. Box 60, Parma, ID 83660.

BOX 30-5

Classification of Ruminant Indigestion

PRIMARY INDIGESTIONS
Reticuloruminal Motor Disorders/Diseases of the Rumen Wall
Traumatic reticuloperitonitis (p. 747)
Frothy bloat (p. 754)
Free gas bloat (p. 725)
Reticulitis/rumenitis (p. 725)
Rumenal parakeratosis (p. 726)
Vagal indigestion (failure of omasal transport, failure of pyloric outflow, and free gas bloat) (p. 726)
Obstruction of the cardia (p. 729)
Obstruction of the reticuloomasal orifice (p. 729)
Diaphragmatic hernia (p. 729)

Reticuloruminal Fermentative (Microbial/Biochemical) Disorders
Inactivity of rumen microbial flora (caused by poor quality roughage—rumen impaction) (p. 731)
Simple indigestion (p. 731)
Acute rumen lactic acidosis (p. 731)
Chronic rumen acidosis (p. 733)
Rumen alkalosis (p. 733)
Putrefication of rumen ingesta (p.733)

SECONDARY INDIGESTIONS (SECONDARY TO SYSTEMIC ILLNESS)
Secondary reticuloruminal motor inactivity
Secondary reticuloruminal microflora inactivity
Abomasal reflux

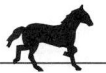

TABLE 30-5

Factors Influencing Vagal Motor Discharge From the Gastric Centers of the Medulla*

Input	Location	Stimulus
EXCITATION OF THE GASTRIC CENTERS (CAUSES INCREASED RUMEN MOTILITY)		
Low-threshold tension receptors	Reticulum, medial wall	Mild distention, and tension generated during contractions
Buccal receptors	Mouth	Feeding (only during chewing)
Acid receptors	Abomasum	Increased acidity as abomasum empties
Tension receptors†	Medial wall of cranial rumen sac	Increased rumen gas pressure
INHIBITION OF THE GASTRIC CENTERS (CAUSES DECREASED RUMEN MOTILITY)		
High-threshold tension receptors	Reticulum and cranial rumen sac	Bloat or other severe ruminal distention
Tension receptors	Abomasum	Abomasal distention
Chemical receptors	Reticulum, rumen	Increased concentration of undissociated volatile fatty acid with rumen acidosis; also locally activated by some toxins
Pain receptors in body increase sympathetic tone and adrenal secretory activity	Anywhere in body; can act directly and through medullary gastric centers	Pain, especially abdominal
Gastric centers	Medulla	Anesthesia, depressant drugs, toxins, endotoxins, fever, acidosis
Hypocalcemia	Reticuloruminal smooth muscle	Hypocalcemia

*There is no inherent reticulorumenal motility such as that found in the intestines.
†Secondary cycle activity; independent of primary cycle activity.

DISORDERS OF RETICULORUMINAL MOTOR FUNCTION

NORMAL MOTOR ACTIVITY. The two reticuloruminal contraction sequences function independently. The primary cycle of contraction occurs approximately once a minute but more often during feeding and rumination. It consists of a biphasic contraction of the reticulum followed by a contraction that runs caudally across first the dorsal and then the ventral rumen sacs. At the height of the second reticular contraction the omasal orifice relaxes and fluid, mostly composed of reticular ingesta, passes into the omasum. This reticuloruminal motility pattern directly influences rumen fermentation by mechanically mixing the ingesta to provide contact with the microbes and to macerate the particulate matter. The mixing function prevents local accumulations of substrate or end products of fermentation, distributes the buffering saliva for neutralization of acids, and provides increased contact of the fluid with the rumen wall to promote VFA absorption. The coordinated sequence of contraction of various parts of the rumen wall maintains a stratification of fluid and particulate matter that selectively sorts the ingesta by particle size. The sorting function serves to retain large particles for further digestive breakdown while promoting passage of small particles (smaller than 6 mm) into the omasum and lower gastrointestinal tract.[1050-1053]

The secondary contraction cycle does not involve the reticulum. It begins in the caudal blind sacs, and a wave of contraction runs cranially across the dorsal rumen, pushing the gas cap into the cardia region. Eructation ensues, eliminating the gases generated by fermentation. Typically one secondary cycle contraction follows two primary cycles, so that three contractions occur every 2 minutes.[1051-1053] Two additional special contractions have been identified in sheep: primary-secondary contractions and prosecondary contractions.[1054,1055] These contractions appear when intraruminal pressure becomes elevated and function as secondary contractions by expelling rumen gas. The primary-secondary and prosecondary contractions appear to help minimize free gas bloat when gas production is high.

Maintenance of the motility patterns requires well-coordinated neural control. The pathophysiologic mechanism of the first group of primary indigestions (i.e., diseases of the reticuloruminal motor function) involves disturbance of the mechanisms of normal rumen motility, which secondarily affects rumen fermentation.

The rumen contraction sequences described rely almost completely on motor nerve activation arising from the medulla oblongata, in contrast to the intrinsic segmental and peristaltic movements of the intestine. Gastric centers in the medulla integrate sensory input and generate motor impulses, both of which are carried in the vagus nerves. The gastric centers have neither spontaneous activity nor an inherent rhythm. Generation of motor impulses relies on a greater excitatory than inhibitory input from the sensory nerves to determine the rate, magnitude, and duration of primary cycle contractions. During the quiescent period between the primary contractions, while the medulla collects the sensory information, there are no tonic vagal motor impulses.[1056-1062]

The splanchnic nerves also affect reticuloruminal motility by direct innervation and by neurohumoral effects of adrenal secretion. These nerves are not required for generation of normal contractions. The effect of splanchnic stimulation is inhibition of reticuloruminal motility. Splanchnic sensory nerves innervate sensory receptors in other areas of the gastrointestinal system, and some abnormalities such as intestinal distention or surgical manipulation produce reticuloruminal inhibition by means of reflex from splanchnic afferent activity.[1052,1060,1063]

PRIMARY CYCLE ACTIVITY. A decrease or absence of normal primary cycle activity (i.e., rumen hypomotility or stasis) implies either a decrease of vagal motor discharges originating from the gastric centers or an ineffective motor response after motor impulse, as in cases of hypocalcemia. Causes of decreased motor discharges can include:

1. Decreased excitatory input to the gastric centers
2. Increased inhibitory input to the gastric centers
3. Depression of the gastric centers
4. Defective vagal transmission of motor impulses
5. Other factors

Decreased Excitatory Input. The three most important excitatory inputs to the gastric centers are from (1) low-threshold tension receptors in the reticulum, (2) buccal receptors in the mouth, and (3) acid receptors in the abomasum (Table 30-5). The tension receptors are located in the musculature of the medial wall of the reticulum. They are stimulated by mild distention during the resting phase and thereby influence contraction frequency. They are further stimulated by the tension generated during contraction and thus increase amplitude and duration of the primary cycle contraction. This mechanism is probably responsible for the increased motility seen after feeding or during incipient bloat. Any cause of anorexia leading to decreased rumen fill decreases this excitatory input, leading to rumen hypomotility. Feeding mechanically stimulates buccal sensory receptors, providing a potent stimulus to both primary and secondary contraction cycles. This reflex can double the rate of primary contractions but is short-lived and declines as soon as chewing activity ceases. Thus anorexia effectively eliminates this potent excitatory input. Abomasal acidity increases as the abomasum empties, and this, too, provides excitatory input to the gastric centers. The resultant increased reticuloruminal motility leads to increased flow of ingesta to the abomasum, diluting the abomasal acid and maintaining normal filling of the abomasum. Certain types of abomasal disease diminish this stimulus to forestomach motility.[1058,1060,1064]

Less well-defined stimuli of reticuloruminal motility include the physical and chemical characteristics of the rumen ingesta. Fiber and water content, as well as the normal chemical products of fermentation, are important for normal rumen contraction. The exact mechanisms through which these factors enhance rumen motility have not yet been clearly defined, but low levels of any of these ingesta characteristics impair normal function, causing decreases of both rumination and primary cycle activity. That these excitatory stimuli are decreased or absent under some feeding regimens and with some of the diseases attributable to abnormal fermentation may account for the impression of hypomotility observed clinically.[1058,1065,1066]

Increased Inhibitory Input. Inhibitory inputs to the gastric center arise from (1) high-threshold tension receptors in the reticulum and cranial rumen sac, (2) tension receptors in the abomasum, (3) epithelial receptors that detect high concentrations of nondissociated VFAs in the rumen, and (4) pain elicited at any site in the body (see Table 30-5). The high-threshold tension receptors are sensory nerve endings below the epithelial basement membrane of the reticulum and cranial rumen sac. They respond to extreme distention of the wall and serve to modify the end stage of reticuloruminal contraction. With severe bloat or gross ruminal distention from other causes, such as overfilling with indigestible fibrous roughage, they can be continuously activated, producing rumen stasis. Abomasal distention can inhibit primary rumen contraction cycles, presumably because of tension receptors in the abomasal wall. In normal circumstances this activity would serve to decrease the flow of ingesta to the abomasum when it is full. With abomasal displacement or impaction, this reflex may partly account for the observed ruminal hypomotility. Epithelial receptors in the reticulum and cranial rumen sac are sensitive to increased concentrations of nondissociated VFAs. Inhibition of forestomach contractions occurs when conditions of excessive fermentation or acidosis increase the concentrations of these substances. Pain can reduce forestomach motility by increasing sympathetic nervous and adrenal secretory activity and by inhibiting the gastric centers. Although painful stimuli in the abdominal viscera are particularly potent, pain from anywhere in the body can inhibit or abolish reticuloruminal motility.[1058,1060,1064]

Depression of the Gastric Centers. Depression of the gastric centers reduces vagal motor activation of forestomach motility and can be induced by central nervous system depressant drugs and anesthetics. Endotoxemia, fever, and possibly blood pH and electrolyte abnormalities can induce rumen hypomotility or stasis through central effects on the

gastric centers. These factors may also inhibit rumen motility by increasing sympathetic nervous activity. In addition, some toxins or other abnormal fermentation products reduce rumen motility. These substances may act locally at the rumen epithelial receptors to generate inhibitory impulses, as do increased VFA concentrations, or they may act centrally after absorption into the blood. For the most part the nature of the substances capable of chemically suppressing rumen function is unknown, but abnormal fermentation end products are the likely cause of rumen stasis in indigestion associated with abnormal rumen contents.[1047,1058,1062,1065-1071]

Defective Vagal Innervation. Failure of vagal nerve transmission of motor impulses has been implicated as the cause of a reticuloruminal contraction abnormality that leads to failure of aborad flow of ingesta (hence the name vagal indigestion). The left and right vagi in the thorax divide into dorsal and ventral branches that unite to form dorsal and ventral vagi as the nerves enter the abdomen. The ventral vagus innervates the cranial and medial parts of the reticulum, the omasum, and the abomasum. The dorsal vagus innervates the rumen and parts of the other segments of the ruminant stomach. Sectioning of more than 50% of the vagal nerve trunks leads to impaired motility function, but most cases of vagal indigestion show much less nerve involvement. The importance of vagal nerve lesions in the pathogenesis of forestomach disease has been a subject of considerable debate and is discussed more fully later in this chapter.[1058,1059,1063]

Other Factors That Affect the Primary Cycles. Other influences on forestomach motility have been identified. Hypocalcemia inhibits motility by preventing contraction of the musculature after motor nerve discharge. This may explain the reduced rumen motility seen in early cases of milk fever.[1071,1072,1073] Low environmental temperatures[1074,1075] and milking[1076] have been shown to increase rumen motility mildly, whereas some drugs,[1062,1063,1077-1079] hyperglycemia,[1080] and gastric hormones[1062,1081] are effective in decreasing reticuloruminal primary cycle contractions. These factors are not discussed further in this text.

SECONDARY CYCLE ACTIVITY. The secondary cycle activity responsible for eructation is elicited independently of the primary cycles. An increase in rumen gas pressure excites tension receptors in the medial wall of the cranial rumen sac. This triggers relaxation of the cardia and eructation of the gas accumulated in the cardia region by the secondary contraction cycle. Receptors that apparently distinguish gas from fluid or solid matter inhibit opening of the cardia if it is covered by material other than gas.[1082] This reflex inhibition of cardia opening is responsible for bloat in cases in which abnormal ingesta cover the area, such as in recumbent animals, in frothy bloat, and when abnormal motility or overfilling of the rumen precludes clearing of the cardia. Under such circumstances and when rumen distention is not yet extreme, both primary and secondary cycle contractions may increase in frequency. In other forms of bloat, hypomotility is a prominent feature, and the gas accumulates as a result of the poor motility function.[1053] This is the most probable cause of bloat in some of the disturbances of fermentative function.

Gross overdistention of the rumen wall may inhibit motility by stretching the musculature beyond its ability to contract forcefully. If the process leading to the distention develops slowly, the high-tension receptor inhibition of motility appears to adapt, and complete inhibition of motor impulses does not seem to occur. Rather, in these cases motility is present but weak and relatively ineffective. This motility disturbance is likely when poorly digestible roughage accumulates in the forestomach. Patients with this condition often have mild to moderate chronic free gas bloat, which may result from poor ability of the weakened rumen to clear the cardia and dispel the gas.[1047]

Free Gas Bloat

Accumulation of free gas in the dorsal rumen should not be considered a primary disease entity but rather a sign of disease (Table 30-6). However, because free gas bloat often is the most prominent sign and because it accompanies several different forms of indigestion, its pathogenesis is reviewed briefly here.

Rumen microbial fermentation and neutralization of salivary bicarbonate continually produce gas as an end product (primarily methane and carbon dioxide) in proportion to the rate of fermentation. Normally the ruminant can eructate volumes of gas that exceed the amount produced even at maximum rates of fermentation.[1054,1055] Thus an excessive production of gas is not the cause of bloat. Bloat develops either because the evacuation of gas is hindered by a physical obstruction or because the mechanisms that expel the gas are inhibited.[1083-1086]

As in choke, physical obstruction of the esophagus by a foreign body can produce dramatic and peracute bloat. Other forms of esophageal occlusion (which may additionally involve inflammation of nerves or rumen muscle malfunction) include muscular spasm (e.g., tetanus), swollen mediastinal lymph nodes (e.g., chronic pneumonia, thymic lymphosarcoma), and tumorous or inflammatory swellings of the cardia region (e.g., papilloma, actinomycosis). These problems tend to show bloat of a slowly progressive or chronic nature, although the degree of bloat may be marked.

Bloat is a common feature of indigestions caused by microbial fermentative disorders. When rumen hypomotility occurs, the fermentative rate may decline, but weak rumen contractions may be inadequate to move the gas layer and to clear the cardia preparatory to eructation. Thus dietary, microbial, or metabolic factors that affect the excitability of the gastric centers or the reticulorumen can result in bloat. Rumen stasis can result in bloat because eructation occurs only with rumen contraction.[1053] Bloat also accompanies indigestions that produce gross distention of the reticulorumen with fluid or solid ingesta (i.e., vagal indigestion, rumen acidosis, and microfloral inactivity caused by indigestible roughage). The cause of bloat in these cases may be a combination of rumen stasis, weakening of the rumen wall caused by the gross distention, and failure to clear the cardia.

Some authors have attributed chronic bloat in calves to a form of vagal nerve damage resulting from mediastinal inflammation.[1087,1088] However, it has not been demonstrated that vagal nerve involvement is the source of the failure to eruc-

tate in these cases. It appears that free gas bloat in calves has numerous causes, as is true in adult cattle, including fermentative indigestions, rumen wall disturbances, and esophageal involvement in an intrathoracic inflammatory process.[1089] Distinguishing between vagal nerve impairment and esophageal compression or inflammation as the cause of free gas bloat requires a thorough assessment of rumen motor function, as described under the section on clinical signs (pp. 736-739).

Reticulitis and Rumenitis

The most important inflammatory problem is reticuloperitonitis caused by sharp foreign body punctures (traumatic reticuloperitonitis, hardware disease). This disease is discussed elsewhere in the text (p. 747). The localized infection established by reticuloruminal perforation causes inflammation of the forestomach wall and adjacent peritoneal cavity and pain in the anterior abdomen, inhibiting forestomach motility, appetite, and aboral flow of ingesta. Other causes of rumen wall inflammation can cause acute or chronic forestomach dysfunction.

Most infections of the rumen wall follow primary mechanical or chemical damage to the mucosa. The secondary invaders colonize the damaged areas and may gain access to the circulation and invade other tissues as well. The rumen wall may be the niche for some of these microorganisms, and isolates from the rumen wall have been matched with those isolated from liver abscesses.[1090] Probably the most common cause of the initial mucosal injury is acute rumen acidosis produced by grain engorgement. Chemical damage resulting in rumen ulcers also occurs in oak or acorn toxicosis and with ingestion of caustic chemicals. Common secondary ulcer invaders include *Actinomyces pyogenes*, *Fusobacterium necrophorum*, and several mycotic species.[1090,1091] Mycotic rumenitis can follow rumen acidosis and septic diseases, especially after the use of oral antibiotics; it also can occur after feeding spoiled and moldy feeds and without apparent predisposing causes.[1092-1096] Diseases that cause anorexia plus abomasal reflux of gastric acids may predispose an animal to mycotic rumenitis and omasitis. Mycotic rumenitis can be severe, with vascular thrombosis and infarction and mural necrosis and gangrene sufficient to cause death. Less frequently occurring specific infections of the rumen wall include actinobacillosis, actinomycosis, and tuberculosis. These infectious inflammatory diseases of the rumen wall may be distributed widely throughout the forestomach, depending on the initial site of mucosal injury, but they tend to localize

TABLE 30-6

Causes of Rumen Tympany (Bloat)

Mechanism	Cause	Disease Examples
Obstruction of eructation	Esophageal obstruction	Choke, tetanus, thoracic inflammation/neoplasia with swollen mediastinal lymph nodes
	Cardia obstruction	Papilloma, fibroma, actinomycosis
	Failure to clear cardia of fluid/ingesta	Lateral recumbency, reticulorumen overfilled with ingesta (as in vagal indigestion, rumen microbial inactivity with poorly digestible roughage, obstruction of the reticuloomasal orifice)
	Gas trapped in stable foam	Frothy bloat
Rumen motor dysfunction	Failure of smooth muscle contraction	Hypocalcemia
	Weakened muscle contraction	Chronic rumen distention with indigestible roughage, outflow obstruction, or vagal indigestion
	Abomasal distention	Displaced abomasum (especially in calves)
	Vagus nerve damage	Thoracic inflammation (especially in calves), neoplasia
Chemical inhibition	Rumen stasis	Rumen acidosis, rumen alkalosis, abnormal fermentation products with simple indigestion

in the ventral regions of the reticulorumen. The granulomatous inflammatory lesions of actinobacillosis and actinomycosis are most commonly found in the cranial forestomach in the area of the esophageal groove.

Neoplastic growths in the rumen have also been identified. These uncommon lesions include papillomas, myxomas, fibromas, carcinomas, and lymphosarcoma.[1047,1097,1098] These lesions are most commonly localized in the reticulum and cranial rumen near the cardia and esophageal groove.

The importance of these inflammatory reticuloruminal lesions depends on their extent and location. Acute and extensive lesions have been associated with signs similar to those of reticuloperitonitis caused by foreign body puncture, including pain, inappetence, impaired forestomach function, and in some cases death. The more chronic cases may cause forestomach motility disturbances and signs of vagal indigestion. Pedunculated masses especially, but not exclusively, may obstruct the cardia or reticuloomasal orifice, leading to bloat or reticuloruminal outflow disturbance.

Reticuloruminal inflammation can also result from certain generalized infections. These include bovine virus diarrhea, foot-and-mouth disease, malignant catarrhal fever, and rinderpest. In these cases the forestomach problems are unlikely to be the most important clinical manifestation.

Ruminal Parakeratosis

In parakeratosis the papillae are darkly colored, enlarged, thickened, and clumped together. Histologic changes of the epithelial cells include a thickened, cornified layer with abnormal retention of nuclei in the cornified cells. These morphologic changes appear to represent a reaction to persistently high concentrations of volatile fatty acids. The changes occur predominantly in animals on pelleted or very finely ground rations, especially when the ration contains a high amount of energy. These rations tend to increase the proportions of propionate and butyrate, reduce the proportion of acetate generated by microbial fermentation, and produce a lowered rumen fluid pH. The growth of the rumen papillae is promoted by contact with the VFAs, especially butyrate, and secondarily propionate.[1050,1085] It appears that a disproportion of the concentrations of these VFAs may be the cause of an excessive change in the epithelium of the papillae. Initial changes in the epithelium under these conditions appear to increase the absorption of the volatile fatty acids, but in severe cases the absorption decreases. This disease of the ruminal wall is not usually diagnosed as a primary problem. Although it may lead to impaired performance of the animal, the disease signs that lead to its discovery are usually those of chronic acidosis, a disease with which it often coexists. Parakeratosis can predispose to other injuries of the rumen wall, however, because the abnormal papillae are more easily traumatized, leading to chronic inflammatory disease of the wall as discussed previously. In calves the problem is also associated with the development of hairballs (trichobezoars) because of the propensity of calves on the rations associated with parakeratosis to lick their hair coat.[1047,1084,1099,1100]

Vagal Indigestion

Vagal indigestion syndrome (vagus indigestion, Hoflund's syndrome) comprises a group of motor disturbances that hinder passage of ingesta from the reticulorumen or abomasum or both. The pathogenesis of the disease has been debated for years and has yet to be completely clarified because many investigations have yielded conflicting information.*

---

*References 1047, 1058, 1059, 1063, 1087, and 1101-1112.

The name vagus indigestion was introduced by Hoflund, who experimentally produced motor defects and disease signs similar to those seen in clinical cases by transecting various branches of the abdominal vagal nerve.[1102] On the basis of his experimental results, he defined four types of functional disturbance, with obstruction of ingesta flow at two sites:

1. *Omasal transport failure* (anterior functional stenosis), which impairs flow of ingesta through the reticuloomasal orifice and occurs with
   a. atony of the reticulorumen, often associated with chronic recurrent bloat or
   b. normal to increased rumen motility
2. *Pyloric outflow failure* (posterior functional stenosis), which impairs flow through the pylorus and occurs
   a. continuously or
   b. in an intermittent, recurrent pattern (incompletely)

Hoflund's description of the syndrome is convenient for explaining the observed functional defects, but its presumed pathogenesis is not supported by the findings of several later investigators.[1062,1101,1104,1109] The use of the term "stenosis" has also led to some confusion, although it was appropriate in its original context. "Functional stenosis" suggested that the defect was a functional one that mimicked a stenosis at the site of outflow. However, vagal denervation does not produce a true stenosis, but rather a paralysis and relaxation of either the reticuloomasal orifice or the pylorus. The paralysis can be appreciated in both experimental and clinical cases.

FAILURE OF OMASAL TRANSPORT. Failure of omasal transport with hypermotility of the rumen is the most common naturally occurring form of the disease. Accumulation of ingesta in the reticulorumen leads to gradually progressive distention of the forestomachs, whereas the omasum and abomasum remain relatively empty. The animal's appetite diminishes as the rumen becomes overfilled, producing one of the most characteristic signs of the disease: inappetence with gross distention of the rumen in the left flank. Continued dilation of the rumen eventually leads to a marked and almost pathognomonic overfilling of the ventral rumen sac. The rumen assumes an L shape because the ventral sac occupies both the right and left ventral quadrants of the abdomen. The resultant characteristic abdominal contour often is called a "papple" shape (Fig. 30-52, *E*) because the left side of the abdomen is distended and assumes the appearance of an apple, whereas the right side assumes the contour of a pear. The diminished passage of ingesta passage results in reduced fecal volume. The normal rumen process of selective retention of fibrous material is disturbed, leading to large particle passage and feces with increased fiber length and a greasy or pasty consistency. Some cases show firm feces with large particle size.[1107,1110] Affected animals often continue to drink water, but absorption from the rumen is poor, and the water accumulates in the forestomach while the animal becomes mildly dehydrated. Vigorous contractions of the rumen can be palpated in the left paralumbar fossa in most affected animals, although some display almost complete atony. The contraction pattern does not produce the typical stratification of material in the forestomach, but rather it churns the rumen contents into a uniform frothy fluid.[1110,1112]

The signs just described, with abnormal flow of ingesta and normal or increased forestomach contractions, can be experimentally reproduced by sectioning the ventral vagal trunk at the cardia and the dorsal trunk just distal to the branching of the ruminal nerves.[1059,1102] The forestomach distention, empty omasum and abomasum, and stasis of the forestomach with resultant free gas bloat can be reproduced by sectioning both abdominal vagal trunks along the esophagus. The paralysis produced by vagal denervation can explain the failure of ingesta flow into the omasum by two

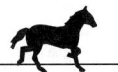

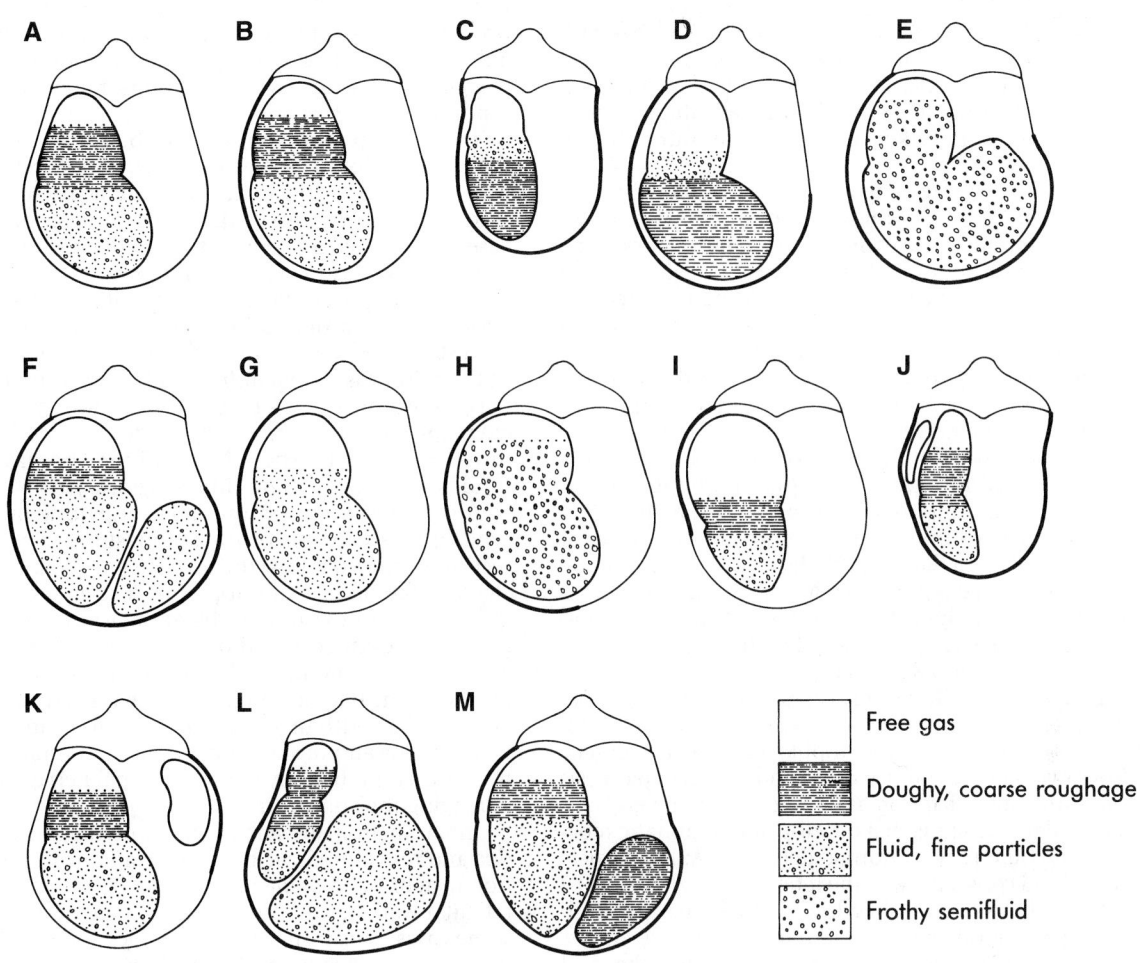

FIG. 30-52 ▓ Abdominal contours (viewed from the rear) and abdominal palpation findings characteristic of cattle with various types of indigestion and other abdominal diseases. A thin line for the abdominal contour indicates the normal configuration. Bold lines indicate areas of the abdominal contour that typically deviate from normal in affected animals. **A,** Normal. **B,** Acute onset of rumen stasis with simple indigestion, traumatic reticuloperitonitis (findings: mild ruminal distention with normal layering of rumen content). **C,** Prolonged rumen stasis, anorexia. The most common result of subacute or chronic disorders such as microbial or fermentative indigestions, traumatic reticuloperitonitis, and secondary indigestions (findings: reduced rumen fill, "tucked-up abdomen," firm, doughy contents that gravitate ventrally). **D,** Rumen inactivity with indigestible roughage (findings: rumen distended with firm, doughy contents that accumulate ventrally; recurrent free gas bloat often present). **E,** Omasal transport failure (findings: L-shaped rumen with gross accumulation of frothy ingesta; rumen hypermotility often present; free gas accumulation varies). **F,** Pyloric outflow failure (findings: fluid accumulation in abomasum; abomasal reflux to rumen common; doughy rumen content that usually accumulates dorsally until rumen stasis or anorexia is prolonged; abdominal contour similar to that for omasal transport failure). **G,** Acute rumen acidosis (findings: rumen distended with fluid; some free gas bloat common). **H,** Frothy bloat. **I,** Free gas bloat or chronic free gas bloat (findings: accumulation of gas in dorsal sac; layering or rumen contents usually normal; with chronicity, rumen fill often decreased; associated with some microbial or fermentative disorders and with esophageal and cardiac disorders). **J,** Left displaced abomasum (findings: gas-filled abomasum that often causes slight bulge of paralumbar fossa; rumen fill usually reduced). **K,** Right displaced abomasum, abomasal volvulus, cecal torsion (findings: distention of right flank with gas-filled viscus; rumen fill and consistency usually normal). **L,** Hydrops (findings: ventral abdomen distended with fluid-filled uterus: rumen fill usually decreased). **M,** Abomasal impaction (findings: abdominal contour similar to E and F; abomasum filled with firm ingesta).

mechanisms. First, the lower end of the esophageal groove is formed by two muscular lips. These overlap in a manner that allows a passive valve effect that blocks flow into the omasum when they are relaxed or paralyzed. Second, it appears that the flow into the omasum is accomplished by an active pumping motion of the omasum that reduces pressure and draws fluid through the reticuloomasal orifice. Paralysis of the omasal musculature after denervation would eliminate this effect. Decreased reticular motility caused by adhesion or paralysis may contribute to the changes in rumen content and the alteration in particle passage.[1110,1112]

The most common predisposing cause of naturally occurring omasal transport failure (anterior functional stenosis) is traumatic reticuloperitonitis. Other causes of anterior functional stenosis include abscesses, adhesions, and peritonitis at the reticulum (especially the right side of the reticulum) or reticuloomasal area without identification of an offending foreign body; hepatic abscesses; diffuse peritonitis; neoplasia of the ruminoreticular fold and esophageal groove; inflammatory disease of the reticular and ruminal walls; papilloma or other mass at the reticuloomasal orifice (see Obstruction of the Cardia or Reticuloomasal Orifice, p. 729); or herniation of the reticulum through a diaphragmatic defect (see Diaphragmatic Hernia, p. 729). Foreign bodies that obstruct the reticuloomasal orifice cause a syndrome indistinguishable from vagal indigestion except by exploratory rumenotomy.[1098] To reconcile the experimental findings with those from clinical cases, the development of omasal transport failure has been explained as involvement of the vagal trunks in the inflammatory process at the reticulum. Several findings make this an unlikely explanation in most clinical cases[1058,1059,1103,1109,1111]:

1. Although sectioning the vagus nerves as described reproduces the syndrome, disturbing only one of the two trunks still allows normal cyclic contractions in most cases. For a clinical lesion to produce disease development, massive involvement of the vagal nerves would be required. By contrast, less than a third of examined cases reported show actual lesions in the nerve branches.

2. The ratio of sensory to motor nerve fibers in the abdominal vagi is approximately 9:1, suggesting the important sensory role of the nerve.

3. Inflammatory lesions of the reticuloruminal wall reported in cases of vagal indigestion are predominantly in the same areas as the important tension receptors that send afferent excitatory impulses to the gastric centers. Induration of the right (medial) wall of the reticulum and in the esophageal groove region may affect intramural nerves and ganglia and reduce the tension receptor activity and therefore the drive for primary cycle activity.

These considerations allow an explanation of some of the inconsistencies found in various cases. Anterior functional stenosis may occur with insufficient vagal sensory excitation, which in turn reduces excitatory input to the gastric centers, diminishes primary cycle motor drive, and results in paralysis of the omasum and reticuloomasal orifice. Alternatively, substantial reticular adhesions that develop after traumatic reticuloperitonitis could prevent normal delivery of small particle ingest, with fluid consistency, to the reticuloomasal orifice.[1112] Because this reduces or abolishes flow into the omasum, both the omasum and abomasum would remain relatively empty, a common finding in these cases. The hypermotility observed in these cases may be the result of secondary rather than primary cycle contractions. Distention of the cranial rumen sac would still be able to induce the secondary contractions if this region is not involved in the induration. Without normal primary cycle activity, the typical stratification of the ingesta would be disturbed, as is usually observed. The existence of hypermotile secondary contractions with absence or severe reduction of primary contractions can be detected clinically (see clinical signs, auscultable findings, p. 738). Damage to the thoracic or abdominal vagi by inflammatory or neoplastic lesions may lead to the occasional cases that show both anterior functional stenosis and atony of the forestomachs, with resultant free gas bloat. This would be similar to the experimental sectioning of both vagal trunks.

Pyloric Outflow Failure. Failure of pyloric outflow (posterior functional stenosis) causes accumulation of ingesta in the abomasum and omasum. Advanced stages of this form of the syndrome also display gross distention of the reticulorumen. Generally the motility of the forestomach is not markedly affected in the early stages, and normal stratification of ingesta is maintained. Overfilling of the forestomach as a result of reflux of ingesta from the abomasum (internal vomiting) may occur, causing the chloride content of the rumen fluid to increase (normal is less than 30 mEq/L). In contrast, the rumen fluid of animals with anterior functional stenosis has a normal chloride content.[1104,1106,1107,1112] With severe distention forestomach motility is reduced, and the rumen contents become more fluid. Failure of ingesta to flow into the intestinal tract, combined with sequestration of chloride-rich fluid in the stomach chambers, can cause both marked dehydration and hypochloremic metabolic alkalosis. In cases with a gradual, prolonged development, however, as in anterior stenosis, any dehydration tends to be mild, and

body fluid electrolyte concentrations do not show remarkable abnormalities. Fecal production in these cases tends to be even less than with the anterior stenosis form of the syndrome.[1101,1112]

Failure of pyloric outflow can be experimentally reproduced by sectioning the ventral vagus trunk at the cardia and the continuation of the dorsal trunk as it crosses the omasum.[1059,1102] This mimics the usual clinical form of the disease, which is characterized by complete inhibition of flow from the abomasum. Combinations of more distal resections of the nerves produce the syndrome of recurrent atony of the abomasum as it occurs in natural clinical cases. Again, the term stenosis is a misnomer, because a true stenosis or spasm of the pylorus is not identified. Rather, the experimental vagal nerve resection and the naturally occurring cases show a flaccid paralysis, and ingesta accumulates as a result of failure of propulsive activity. The dilation of the abomasum is in the fundus and body and not in the pyloric part.[1061,1101,1102]

A common predisposing cause of pyloric outflow failure syndrome is volvulus of the abomasum. After surgical correction of the volvulus, the abomasum remains atonic, and signs of the disease develop within several days. The gross distention and twisting of the abomasum and lesser omentum are presumed to injure the vagal nerves or abomasal wall, or both. The nerve damage may not be irreparable in all cases; return to normal function has been observed. Other abomasal disturbances, including right and left displacements of the abomasum and abomasal ulceration, can cause this disease, perhaps by damaging vagal nerve branches or by damaging the abomasal wall.

Inflammation and adhesions involving the abomasal fundus and reticulum have been associated with posterior functional stenosis in some studies.[1191,1112] Inflammation of the reticular wall may account for the reticular atony reported in some cases. This form of vagal indigestion may be more frequently associated with true vagal nerve impairment than appears to be the case in anterior functional stenosis. Alternatively, reticular adhesions may prevent normal motility, alter the flow of ingesta to the omasum and abomasum, and lead to abnormal filling of the abomasum because of decreased fluidity of abomasal contents.[1112]

Another predisposing cause of pyloric outflow failure is advanced pregnancy with a large fetus. An exact pathogenesis has not been clearly defined. Presumably the large, gravid uterus distorts the positioning of the abomasum or physically compresses and obstructs the anterior small bowel, preventing outflow of ingesta from the abomasum. In these patients the gravid horn typically occupies most of the space in the omental sling. In support of these conclusions, the problem can be resolved by inducing delivery of the calf or performing a cesarean section. Supportive care may be required for severely affected cows, but the gastrointestinal system returns to normal function, suggesting that it was secondarily affected by the pregnancy. This problem is referred to as a form of vagal indigestion because it appears as a pyloric outflow failure. Some patients have such severe obstruction of ingesta passage that they may be diagnosed as having an anterior bowel obstruction. This disease has been called indigestion of late pregnancy.

Animals affected with any form of vagal indigestion for a prolonged time lose body condition because the failure to pass ingesta into the intestinal tract produces a state of starvation. The weight loss may be overlooked because of the impression of full body size produced by the abdominal distention.

CHRONIC RECURRENT BLOAT. Chronic recurrent bloat is commonly identified with vagal indigestion in any of its forms. It is mild to moderate in severity, commonly waxes and wanes, and adds to the visual impression of gross abdominal distention. The pathogenesis of this ruminal tympany varies from case to case. Experimental resection of both abdominal vagal trunks stops eructation by causing complete forestomach stasis. In naturally occurring cases in which lesions of the vagal nerve truly inhibit motor impulse transmission, bloat may arise from this mechanism. When vagal nerve damage does not appear to be involved, other mechanisms may explain the bloat (see Table 30-6). Overfilling of the reticulorumen with frothy ingesta, a common finding, can inhibit the cardia dilation reflex that is a prerequisite of eructation. Gross distention of the forestomach can also weaken the contractile ability of the rumen, so that the contractions are not strong enough to clear the cardia before eructation.

Bradycardia is often identified in association with vagal indigestion but can also occur with other forestomach diseases. The finding that atropine administration can abolish the bradycardia of vagal indigestion suggests increased cardiac vagal tone as the direct cause.[1087,1113] However, the origin of the vagotonia is unclear. When vagal nerve lesions exist distal to the cardiac innervation, reflex excitatory discharges may effect bradycardia. Experimental resection of the vagal nerves causes bradycardia as a striking feature in most cases, although advanced cases show increased heart rates. By contrast, naturally occurring vagal indigestion shows bradycardia as a feature in only a third or fewer of the cases.[1101,1105,1107] These variations may exist because the experimental and natural cases have different causes or because the disease varies in duration. Once the forestomach has become severely distended, the heart rate tends to be elevated, probably as a result of deterioration of hydration and cardiovascular parameters.

Obstruction of the Cardia or Reticuloomasal Orifice

True mechanical obstruction of the forestomach is an uncommon occurrence. The obstruction can be either full or partial and occur at either the cardia or the reticuloomasal orifice. The inflammatory and neoplastic conditions described previously can appear to be obstructive disease when the tissues are sufficiently distorted and lesions involve one of these orifices. Papillomas are most prone to causing an obstruction when they become pedunculated. A variety of foreign bodies create obstruction. In calves, trichobezoars are most commonly the cause, occurring predominantly in animals on a low roughage diet that consequently lick their hair coats vigorously. In adult cows, ingestion of the placenta occasionally results in an obstruction. Curious ruminants, especially goats, sometimes consume plastic bags or discarded rectal palpation sleeves. These and other nondegradable materials can lead to obstruction even after considerable time has passed.

Cardia obstruction leads to the signs typical of esophageal obstruction, with free gas bloat as a prominent, perhaps life-threatening development. Obstruction of the reticuloomasal orifice produces the same consequences as some forms of vagal indigestion. Failure of ingesta flow beyond the rumen results in accumulation of fluid material in the forestomach and diminished or no passage of ingesta through the intestines. The degree and duration of obstruction determine the severity of associated problems such as dehydration, depression, elevated heart rate, forestomach stasis, colic, and muscular weakness. Only rumenotomy can effectively differentiate these obstructive diseases from other problems with similar signs.

Diaphragmatic Hernia

Defects in the diaphragms of cattle are uncommon. Most cases involve a tear through which the reticulum can herniate. Other abdominal organs may also be involved if the rent is large. The diaphragmatic defect may be congenital or an acquired lesion caused by a local inflammatory process (traumatic reticuloperitonitis), sudden external trauma (fighting, hanging up on a fence), or internal pressure (parturition, acute tympany). Entrapment of the reticulum may lead to acute changes in intrathoracic pressure and cause sudden dyspnea, tachycardia, and poor venous return to the heart. Generally, however, this reticular problem causes signs identical to those of vagal indigestion with anterior functional stenosis.[1047,1105] Failure of flow through the reticuloomasal orifice may result from vagal nerve damage, or the anatomic distortion alone may explain the motility defect. Entrapment of the reticulum hinders normal reticular movements and distorts the esophageal groove and reticuloomasal orifice. Reticular ingesta can be heard moving inside the thorax, therefore complete reticular paralysis is unlikely. Motility disturbance is reflected by hypermotility of the rumen, generation of frothy ingesta, persistent or recurrent moderate tympany, and overfilling of the rumen. Signs of pain may also be present, as in cases of traumatic reticuloperitonitis. Rumination usually is impaired, and large volumes of ingesta may be vomited, especially after eating.

DISORDERS OF RETICULORUMINAL FERMENTATIVE FUNCTION (see Box 30-5)

FORESTOMACH MICROBIAL POPULATION. The continuous culture system of the rumen involves an ongoing selection of microorganisms best adapted to grow in a variety of ecologic niches that are in a dynamic state. Numerous control mechanisms govern the environment and the resultant microbial population. Some of these mechanisms are related to the animal itself, such as salivation, mixing and rumination, removal of substances by absorption or diffusion, outflow through the reticuloomasal orifice, and eructation. Others are related to the diet, including nutrient quality of the substrate (feed), balance of required elements, solubility, particle size, presence of inhibitory substances, nutrient quantity, and rate of delivery to the rumen. Control of fermentation also results from microbial interactions such as competition and symbiosis: cross-feeding between species, removal of inhibitory end products, and maintenance of the oxidation-reduction potential. The complexity of the system tends to promote an overall stability. Changes in the controlling factors create selective pressures that lead to population changes in the rumen.[1086,1114,1115]

The rumen bacteria are predominantly anaerobes, with some coexisting facultative anaerobes. Although the facultative organisms are not important in normal rumen function, they may be in some forms of rumen dysfunction. Some microbes ferment the primary nutrients in the feed such as cellulose, hemicellulose, pectin, starch, and simple sugars. Other species ferment the products of the primary group such as pentoses, glucose, lactate, succinate, and formate. Many species are very specialized and have numerous growth requirements that may be supplied by the general fermentation. The second group are important in their role of removing end products and cycling essential factors back to the other organisms.[1086,1114-1116]

EFFECTS OF FEED CHARACTERISTICS. The concentrations and proportions of the microbial species vary with the composition of the diet (Table 30-7). An abundant supply of a certain substrate tends to favor a microbial population with a predilection or high capacity for using that material. The most important factors in the rate of digestion are the properties of the carbohydrates and protein in the feed. High-protein diets favor proteolytic organisms, whereas high-starch, low-fiber diets favor starch users. Cellulolytic bacteria

TABLE 30-7

Effects of Feed Characteristics on Rumen Digestion and Health

Feed	Rumen Content	Effect on Health
Primary forage of high quality, long fiber length, crude fiber >18% of dry matter; with concentrate supplement at 20%-50% of total intake, moderate protein level	pH 6-7, VFA 60-120 mmol/L, acetic > propionic > butyric acid	Normal, healthy, productive
Excessive forage of low nutrient value (late cut) with little concentrate or protein supplementation	pH 6.5-7, VFA decreased, microbial activity decreased	Poor production or growth, microfloral inactivity and rumen impaction, malnutrition caused by protein, energy, mineral, and vitamin deficiency
High level of concentrate feeding (>60%) with decreased forage and/or fiber length	pH 5-6.5, VFA increased, microbial activity increased	High production, rapid growth; possible chronic rumen acidosis, milk fat depression, chronic laminitis, ketosis, rumen parakeratosis, excessively fat condition
Extremely high level of concentrates (especially with sudden exposure to ration), low intake of forage	pH 4-5.5, VFA increased, lactic acid increased	Acute rumen acidosis
Normal levels of forage intake, concentrate with very high protein or NPN supplementation	pH 6.5-7.5, VFA decreased, ammonia increased	Rumen alkalosis, possible urea toxicity

VFA, Volatile fatty acid; *NPN*, nonprotein nitrogen.

are prominent in a high-fiber diet, but their numbers also depend on the fiber size, because this factor determines the rate of passage or retention in the forestomach; thus cellulolytic species can be abundant with a high-concentrate diet if some long-stemmed roughage is included because the retention time of the fiber is prolonged. Diets with readily fermentable carbohydrates and low fiber favor species capable of rapid metabolism and tolerant of low pH. Acid production is rapid and high, and populations of microbes less tolerant of such changes decline.[1114,1116,1117]

The microbial population is also influenced by the limits of supply of certain feed substrates.[1114] High rates of fermentation and microbial growth on the abundant substrates depend on sufficient amounts of the more limited nutrients. Optimum carbohydrate use requires adequate sources of nitrogen, sulfur, and essential mineral nutrients.[1118] When any essential nutrient is deficient, the rate of digestion and thus the digestibility of the feedstuff decrease. Whether the affected animal shows signs of nutrient deficiency or forestomach dysfunction with microbial and forestomach inactivity depends on the limiting nutrient and relative requirement of the host and bacteria for the nutrient. Substances and conditions that inhibit fermentation further reduce digestibility.

The feed material also affects rumen fermentation by influencing the rate of passage from the reticulorumen. Fine grinding and pelleting of feed increase the rate of passage of the particulate matter from the rumen. Very finely ground rations also reduce the stratification of fibrous material in the rumen. This affects the ability to sort material in the rumen selectively by particle size and density, so that larger particles less thoroughly fermented pass more readily into the lower bowel. Microbes associated with the feed particles are passed out of the rumen with the feed. Thus a faster rate of passage influences the bacterial population because it competes with the generation time of the organisms. Populations of slower growing microbes tend to be most influenced by changes in the retention or passage times. Slow-growing cellulolytic bacteria decline in numbers as the passage rate increases (transit time decreases). High passage rates usually produce faster digestion rates. Although these factors are primarily important to the feed efficiency of the animal, they also affect rumen function and the adaptation of microbes to feeding changes.[1119]

Adaptation of the microbial flora to dietary changes requires a week or longer. The abruptness of a dietary change determines the degree of alteration of the rumen microbial population and fermentation pattern and the potential for digestive disturbances. With abrupt and dramatic shifts to higher carbohydrate diets, the facultative species may overwhelm the more normal flora by producing excessive acid and lowering the pH. The importance of microbial adaptation to a particular diet is evidenced by the reduction in forestomach disturbances seen when the rumen is inoculated, before a feeding change, with fluid from animals already adapted to the new ration.[1086,1115]

The end products of microbial fermentation influence not only the microbial population but also rumen function. High concentrations of nondissociated volatile fatty acids (VFAs) excite sensory epithelial receptors that reflexly inhibit rumen motility.[1087,1121,1122] If a sudden increase in concentrate feeding induces a lactic acid fermentation, the rumen pH suddenly declines and a greater proportion of the VFAs shift to the nondissociated state, inducing rumen stasis. A consistently high level of concentrate feeding produces rapid fermentation, high concentration of VFAs, and low pH, and the nondissociated VFA level may reach the threshold for stimulation of the inhibitory epithelial receptors. The rumen stasis reduces the fermentation rate. Mild cases of rumen acidosis may show spontaneous recovery of rumen functions as the absorption of VFAs reduces the concentrations to a noninhibitory level. With more severe rumen acidosis, the generation of acid continues despite the rumen stasis, giving rise to more severe complications of the disease.

In some instances the effects of rumen microbial metabolism and microbial end products extend beyond impacts on nutritional status and digestive system function. Several ruminant diseases represent rumen-generated toxicities. These have extremely variable manifestations and include toxicoses from ammonia, nitrate and nitrite, 3-methylindole, dimethylsulfide (*Brassica* sp., onion toxicity), and sulfur-associated polioencephalomalacia.[1122-1125]

In summary, excesses, deficiencies, or rapid changes of feed substrate can cause imbalance in the microbial population and the fluid milieu. The result can be bacterial overgrowth and overproduction of microbial end products or insufficient microbial growth and fermentation. The effects of

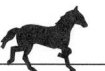

these abnormalities on the animal range from rumen motility dysfunction, to poor growth and performance, to outright toxicity and organic damage.

Inactivity of Rumen Microbial Flora (Caused by Poor-Quality Roughage, Haybelly, or Rumen Impaction)

In rumen microbial flora inactivity, the microbial populations and their metabolic and fermentative processes are diminished as a result of deficiencies of one or more nutrients. This occurs most commonly with poor-quality roughage deficient in protein and readily digestible carbohydrates (late cut, highly lignified hay or straw) (see Chapter 31). Microfloral inactivity can also occur when specific mineral nutrients are deficient or it can be due to inhibitory substances such as antibiotics or some plant products.[1069,1086,1118] Microfloral inactivity also occurs with prolonged anorexia, which abolishes the intake of all nutrients and is the primary pathogenesis of many cases of secondary indigestion.

When microbial digestive processes decline, the breakdown of ingested feedstuffs is prolonged. Failure to reduce the particle size of the ingesta leads to a prolonged retention in the forestomach and gradual accumulation of the undigested feedstuff. Gradual distention of the reticulorumen is commonly observed (haybelly) (see p. 735). In extreme cases this can mimic the signs of vagal indigestion. Forestomach distention can result in weak contractions and moderate recurrent tympany. Rumen hypomotility alters the normal stratification of the rumen contents, and the fibrous components are found mixed in the fluid or compacted ventrally on the rumen floor. Abnormal passage of ingesta from the forestomach results in decreased fecal passage, and the feces usually are dried and contain undigested plant fibers. Other effects on the animal are those of generalized or specific nutrient deficiencies (e.g., decreased growth or production, ketosis, emaciation, and a poor hair coat). When anorexia is the cause of the microbial inactivity, the rumen fill decreases and the lack of normal distention also induces rumen stasis.[1047,1126]

Simple Indigestion

Simple indigestion is the most common sequela of an abrupt change in the ration. Such feed changes present the rumen microflora with nutrient substrates (1) to which they are not metabolically adapted, (2) to which they are adapted but in lesser quantities, or (3) that contain inhibitory substances or produce inhibitory substances upon fermentation. The result is an imbalance in the microflora and its fermentation products. The difference between this problem and some of the other fermentation disorders is mostly a matter of degree. Generally the disease is relatively mild and self-limiting. Most affected animals show anorexia for 1 to 2 days, break with diarrhea in about 24 hours, and return to feed without treatment when the rumen fermentation has stabilized and inhibitory substances have been eliminated. Rumen motility is reduced but usually not absent, the filling of the rumen is not remarkably altered, and if bloat occurs, it is mild. In some cases the rumen fluid pH may change, but usually not dramatically. Mild acidosis or alkalosis of the rumen fluid may develop, depending on the nature of the causative feedstuff and its resultant fermentative degradation. Signs of rumen microfloral inactivity are common. Simple indigestion is an acute problem, in contrast to the microfloral inactivity discussed in the previous paragraphs, in which deficiencies produce microfloral inactivity over time.

Feeds commonly implicated as causes of simple indigestion include moldy or overheated feeds, frosted forages, and partly fermented, spoiled, or sour silages. This form of indigestion also occurs in animals fed high-quality feed, usually after an increase in the rate of feeding or after a change of one of the feed constituents. Thus these mild forms of indigestion can range from a mild acidosis, to an excess of VFAs, to the generation of some bacterial inhibitory products. Because the rumen and its fermentative bacteria are very adaptable, the ways, if any, in which animals given a certain feed experience the problem vary considerably. Often only one or several animals from a group on the ration may have signs.

Acute Rumen Lactic Acidosis (Grain Overload, Toxic Indigestion)

Acute rumen acidosis is the most dramatic of the forms of rumen microbial fermentative disorders and in some cases is lethal in less than 24 hours. It has also received the most research attention, therefore the events in its pathogenesis are more clearly defined than those of the other forestomach disorders. The condition has been named lactic acidosis, acute rumen impaction, rumen overload, acid indigestion, toxic indigestion, grain engorgement, grain overload, and D-lactic acidosis.

This problem is the result of excessive consumption of readily fermentable carbohydrates, which causes a rapid fermentation with production of lactic acid and a decrease in rumen pH to physiologically inappropriate levels. This occurs when animals consume an excess of concentrate feeds (e.g., if animals are suddenly exposed to the feeds without prior adaptation; if animals already on such feeds suddenly consume an excessive quantity because of accidental access; or if animals that have been off feed return to feed and are offered unrestricted access to concentrates). The problem is more common when animals are grouped than when they are separate, probably because the psychology of competition induces them to overconsume. In general the feeds involved include the cereal grains commonly used in high-production rations and fruit and root crops (e.g., feed beets, sugar beets, potatoes) where they are available. Starch and soluble sugars promote an overgrowth of bacteria that produce glucose and organic acids. The acid end products increase rumen acidity and osmolality, inhibit or destroy other rumen microbes, and cause forestomach dysfunction and metabolic disturbances.[1127,1128]

Specific characteristics of the feedstuffs contribute to acidification of the rumen fluid. Cereal grains inherently possess less buffering capacity than the fibrous forages. Low-structured fiber content induces less salivation at the time of ingestion and less rumination subsequently; therefore salivary buffering declines when concentrate feeds are consumed. Some silages contain both high carbohydrate and lactic acid and thus introduce more acid at both ingestion and fermentation.[1127,1129,1130]

Feeding regimens that include significant fibrous roughage limit carbohydrate availability and rates of microbial fermentation and growth. Carbohydrate fermentation efficiency relative to the amount of adenosine triphosphate (ATP) derived from each sugar provides competitive survival value. Slower growing cellulolytic bacteria use substrate most efficiently. When starch or sugar is available in excess, the faster growing species such as *Streptococcus bovis* metabolize carbohydrate faster and produce more ATP per unit time, even though they are less efficient in ATP production per carbohydrate molecule. Under these conditions they can overgrow, producing lactic acid as their end product.[1117,1131]

The severity of rumen acidosis and disease signs vary considerably, depending on the amount and type of carbohydrate-rich feed consumed and the degree of prior rumen microbial adaptation to the carbohydrate substrate. The disease can range from a mild form of indigestion to an overwhelming toxemia that may be difficult to distinguish from other acute toxicities or various diseases with endotoxemia.

If consumption of fermentable carbohydrate is only mildly excessive, *S. bovis* proliferation decreases when the carbohydrate has been fermented, pH rises toward normal, and the efficient fermenters reestablish dominance. If the carbohydrate source is abundant and its supply is not exhausted, the acidosis becomes more severe. Continued production of lactate by *S. bovis* reduces the fluid pH to the range of 5 to 5.5, and the rumen fluid osmolality rises concurrently. Both these factors inhibit or kill the rumen protozoa, which normally use starch and small sugars and help to limit increasing lactic acid levels. There are also numerous species of lactate-using bacteria, of which *Megasphaera elsdenii* and *Selenomonas ruminantium* are the primary examples. These bacteria, which increase in numbers when animals slowly adapt to a high-concentrate diet, are eliminated by abrupt changes and generation of excessive acid, therefore lactate use decreases when the acid is generated too quickly.[1117]

The lactobacilli are the major group of lactic acid producers in the rumen. The increasing acidity of the fluid enhances the growth of these organisms. Because the lactate-using bacteria are killed off before the lactobacilli overgrow, their diverse end products are unavailable as substrate for other bacteria. The lactobacilli are left as the predominant organisms to use the available carbohydrates. Even the *S. bovis* organisms that began the lactic acid production are inhibited below pH 4.5, leaving the lactobacilli, as the most acid-resistant species, to generate more lactic acid.[1129]

The acidification of the fluid milieu enhances the lactic acid production by altering microbial metabolism.[1117,1132] The loss of the fluid bicarbonate buffer and the increase in available hydrogen ions block the conversion of lactate to propionate even before the lactate users die off. Also, when the pH is above 5, as pH declines, rumen fluid amylase activity increases, liberating more free glucose from starch. However, glucose use is reduced, and rumen glucose accumulates. Apparently the lactate-using bacteria such as *S. ruminantium* degrade less lactate to acetate in the presence of increased glucose concentrations. Thus not only does the microbial population change, but the characteristics of the fluid accelerate the lactic acid production when the available carbohydrate is excessive.

The effects on the animal of the rumen fluid changes are numerous and detrimental. In the early stages of the acidic fermentation, the VFAs are produced in abundance. Although VFA production decreases as the microbes are increasingly inhibited, VFA concentrations remain elevated in advanced acidosis. The VFAs are much weaker acids than lactic acid; thus, as pH drops, they accept hydrogen from lactic acid and serve as buffers in the fluid, therefore a greater proportion of the VFAs exist in the nondissociated state. This form is more readily absorbable than free ions through the rumen wall. During absorption some VFAs undergo metabolism by the rumen wall epithelium, resulting in the release of lactate and ketone bodies into the circulation. Excessive absorption of the volatile fatty acids leads to systemic acidosis, and circulating lactate and VFAs may also directly damage the liver.[1132] In addition, the high concentration of nondissociated VFAs at the rumen epithelium provides a strong inhibitory effect on reticuloruminal motility and leads to rumen stasis. This effect tends to protect the animal, because it reduces the absorption of detrimental fermentation products from the rumen.[1120-1129]

The osmotic pressure of the rumen fluid increases as lactic acidosis develops.[1127-1130,1133] In a normal animal, rumen osmolality remains relatively constant at about 280 mOsm/L, but osmolality may double in some cases of acute acidosis. Lactic acid accounts for a major fraction of the increase, but some of the components of this change remain unidentified. The increased osmolality inhibits and kills some of the microflora and draws fluid into the rumen, mostly from the extracellular compartment. This accounts for the increased rumen fluid volume, rumen distention, and severe dehydration observed clinically. The loss of circulating fluid volume leads to circulatory impairment, decreased renal blood flow and glomerular filtration, and in some cases eventual anuria. Poor peripheral circulation results in hypoxic metabolism and contributes to systemic acidosis.

Although it has been assumed that the systemic acidosis that develops with this disease is attributable to rumen lactic acid absorption, such absorption does not appear to occur readily.[1129,1134,1135] Lactate is absorbed from the rumen at a much slower rate than are the volatile fatty acids because it is highly ionized at a pH near physiologic normal, which tends to inhibit absorption. At lower pH the rumen becomes static, thereby also inhibiting absorption. The hypertonicity of the rumen fluid further limits absorption of lactate and other substances. It appears that the peak entry of lactate into the circulation occurs in the early phases of the disease. Some lactate may be absorbed from the intestinal tract from fluid passed before the onset of complete stasis. Many experimental trials do not show the development of severe systemic acidosis in the early phase of the disease. It may be that a large component of the later severe systemic acidosis is attributable to circulatory insufficiency rather than to absorption of lactic acid.

Some absorption of the lactic acid does occur, however, as evidenced by the appearance of D-lactic acid in the circulation.[1084,1129,1134] Microbes produce both the L- and D-form of lactic acid, whereas animal tissues produce only L-lactic acid. The animals' pathways for metabolism of D-lactic acid are not as efficient as those for L-lactic acid, therefore absorption of both forms leads to an accumulation of predominantly D-lactate in the animal's system. The lactate is eliminated by oxidation, gluconeogenesis, and renal excretion. The animal's hydration status, liver and muscle metabolism, and renal function determine how readily it can eliminate excess lactate. Animals that survive rumen acidosis often have metabolic alkalosis after the acidotic phase, as a result of lactate metabolism and production of bicarbonate.

Lactic acid is a strong corrosive agent that can destroy the rumen epithelium, giving rise to the name "toxic rumenitis." The increased rumen fluid osmolality also damages the epithelium as extracellular water influx across the epithelium occurs in response to osmotic pressure imbalance. The effects of epithelial destruction can be far-reaching, because the damage persists after resolution of the acute acidosis.[1130,1136] Some yeast and fungi that are resistant to the high acidity readily colonize the damaged sites, invade the vasculature, and cause thrombosis or spread to the liver and other organs.[1092,1093] Rumen acidosis is considered one of the primary causes of mycotic rumenitis (discussed above under Reticulitis and Rumenitis) and mycotic omasitis, although other predisposing causes have been identified.[1092-1096] Bacterial rumenitis can also result from the chemical damage and may lead to abscess formation, diffuse cellulitis, or perforation and peritonitis. If the animal survives the acute acidosis, it may succumb to secondary rumen damage.[1093,1095] Alternatively, the rumen may heal uneventfully, leaving scars in the rumen wall, but access of bacteria to the circulation through these chemical lesions can result in hepatic abscessation, a common problem of animals fed high-concentrate rations.[1091,1137]

In addition to lactic acid, several toxic factors have been implicated in acute rumen acidosis.[1084,1117,1129] The altered metabolism of the rumen microflora has been shown to generate increased quantities of histamine, ethanol, methanol, tyramine, and tryptamine. These may play a role in the pathogenesis of the disease, but conclusive evidence is lacking. Histamine has been implicated as an agent in the development of laminitis that sometimes accompanies rumen acidosis. However, histamine is poorly absorbed from the rumen, especially at diminished pH levels. The destruction of rumen gram-negative bacteria has been suggested to release large quantities of endotoxin for absorption through damaged mucosal surfaces. Endotoxin would contribute to most of the signs of the disease such as rumen stasis, poor tissue perfusion with cardiovascular deterioration, weakness, and depression. Increased ruminal and blood concentrations of endotoxin and increased blood arachidonic acid metabolites have been found in cattle with experimentally induced rumen acidosis, but their importance in naturally occurring disease is not clear.[1138-1140] With liver impairment or rumen wall damage, toxin absorption and clearance are likely to be altered. Premature delivery and retained placenta may occur in pregnant animals after acute rumen acidosis, possibly resulting from the effects of these circulatory toxins and metabolites.[1141]

Chronic Rumen Acidosis

Like acute rumen acidosis, chronic rumen acidosis is caused by feeding of excessive quantities of concentrate with low levels of well-structured fibrous roughage; however, chronic acidosis results from continued ingestion of these feeds over a prolonged period rather than sudden exposure without adequate adaptation. The rumen microbial population adapts to the high grain ration, and large numbers of lactate-using and lactate-producing organisms are found. The proportion of cellulolytic bacteria decreases, whereas the starch- and glucose-fermenting species proliferate. The overall effect of the adaptation is development of a microbial population that rapidly ferments the ingested feedstuffs. Lactic acid does not accumulate because it is further metabolized by the bacteria. The high rate of fermentation instead produces high concentrations of VFAs, resulting in moderately acidic rumen fluid with pH values usually ranging from 5 to 5.5.[1142] Rumen buffering of the increased acid load is impaired because the fine particle size of the high-energy rations induces less chewing and less saliva production. As the name implies, the effects on the animal are chronic and insidious.

Along with the high concentration of volatile fatty acids and the low pH, a shift occurs in the proportions of the VFAs in the rumen fluid. The proportions of butyric and propionic acids increase, and acetate decreases. Butyric and propionic acids stimulate proliferation of the ruminal papillae epithelium. When this process is exaggerated, it can progress to parakeratosis. The rumen papillae develop an excessively keratinized epithelium and clump together. The parakeratotic changes are associated with decreased absorption of the volatile fatty acids and increased susceptibility to trauma and inflammation. Epithelial damage and the acidic nature of the ingesta appear to be responsible for inflammation of the deeper tissues of the rumen wall in some cases. The ruminal wall lesions allow penetration by bacteria with dissemination to the liver. This commonly results in liver abscessation in a high proportion of affected animals. Liver abscesses usually have no pathognomonic signs. Affected animals tend to show reduced productivity and may have signs of a chronic inflammatory response.*

Cattle with chronic rumen acidosis may have reduced appetite and rumen hypomotility. High rumen VFA concentrations can inhibit rumen motility by stimulating the in-

hibitory receptors in the epithelium. The finely ground ingesta also induces less active rumen motility because it lacks the physical bulk of high-roughage diets that stimulate strong and sustained contractions. Although the bacterial population is metabolically very active, the number of species of bacteria is reduced. Likewise the protozoal population is inhibited when the pH remains in the lower end of this range. The microfloral environment is less stable when fewer species are present and is thus more susceptible to sudden changes in the diet.

A continual high acid load may also reduce metabolic efficiency and overall animal performance. High-concentrate diets have been associated with poor use of dietary protein.[1116,1143] Other pathologic conditions have been attributed to chronic acidosis, including chronic laminitis and cerebrocortical necrosis. These conditions may be induced by some of the toxic by-products of acidic rumen fermentation, such as endotoxins and hydrogen sulfide.[1124,1125,1129,1138-1140]

Rumen Alkalosis

An alkaline rumen fluid pH occurs most commonly when microbial fermentation is reduced while the animal continues to ingest saliva. A rumen fluid pH between 7 and 7.5 is found with prolonged anorexia, microfloral inactivity caused by poorly digestible roughage, and some cases of simple indigestion. The low rate of fermentation does not generate enough acid to neutralize the alkaline pH of the saliva. In addition, the absorption of VFAs through the rumen epithelium proceeds with the generation of bicarbonate in the rumen fluid.[1085,1144] Acetate absorption is associated with greater generation of bicarbonate than is absorption of the other VFAs, and acetate is the predominant VFA produced during fermentation of roughage. Although the fermentation rate is low, the VFA absorption contributes to the rumen alkalinity. Rumen alkalosis occurring with these diseases is not the primary problem, therefore these entities are discussed separately.

Rumen alkalosis can occur with the generation of excessive ammonia. Ammonia concentrations rise when high-protein diets are fermented. The pH usually does not increase above neutral because these diets also contain sufficient readily fermentable carbohydrate to maintain a slightly acidic pH.

More dramatic elevations in the ammonia concentration, with a rumen fluid pH above 7.5, occur with overfeeding of nonprotein nitrogen sources such as urea, biuret, and ammonium phosphate (see Chapter 50). Accidental ingestion of some common fertilizers that contain ammonium salts can produce the same results. For the purpose of this discussion, it is important to realize that some of the signs of urea poisoning involve rumen dysfunction. Severe cases of urea poisoning result in generalized signs such as muscle tremors, incoordination, weakness, tachypnea, and central nervous system excitation, and affected animals die quickly. Signs of forestomach dysfunction such as rumen hypomotility, bloat, vomiting, and abdominal pain are also present. In milder cases, diminished appetite, rumen hypomotility, recurrent tympany, and diarrhea may be the most prominent signs, along with muscular weakness and incoordination. Thus the disease may appear as a form of forestomach disease. The rumen fluid shows an alkaline pH between 7.5 and 8.5 and has a strong odor of ammonia.[1122,1145,1146]

Putrefaction of Rumen Ingesta

Putrefaction of rumen ingesta infrequently results from overgrowth of a microflora that decomposes feed material in a putrefactive manner. The existence of a high rumen fluid pH, such as occurs with high-protein feeds, and repeated inoculation with abnormal bacteria allow the development of the

---

*References 1079, 1085, 1111, 1121, 1124, and 1129-1131.

putrefactive decomposition. Fermented feeds undergoing spoilage, feed and water contaminated with feces, and spoiling, contaminated concentrates supply the offending microflora, which includes the coliform group and *Proteus* spp.[1047] This type of abnormal decomposition is normally inhibited by the existence of an active physiologic microflora. Thus most cattle are remarkably resistant to aberrant digestive patterns even when spoiled feeds are ingested. Cattle affected with this form of indigestion typically follow a chronic course of disease. Rumen motility declines, appetite is poor, and recurrent tympany develops, sometimes with the generation of frothy rumen contents. The rumen fluid characteristically has a blackish green color, a foul, putrefactive odor, poor protozoal and bacterial activity, and a pH in the neutral to alkaline range of 7 to 8.5. The cause of the forestomach hypomotility may be inhibitory products generated by the abnormal fermentation. In cases of prolonged duration, animals lose weight and display a poor hair coat, probably as a result of dietary deficiencies in the abnormal fermentation products.

FORESTOMACH DISEASES OF CALVES

Normal forestomach development and diseases of the forestomachs of calves have recently been reviewed.[1048-1050,1147] The newborn ruminant has the same anatomic division of the stomach into four compartments as the adult ruminant. The abomasum is functional as a secretory digestive organ, like the stomach of monogastrics, and has a capacity approximately twice that of the other compartments. The remaining stomach compartments are small and do not perform digestive functions in the first days of neonatal life. The reticulorumen may not develop an adult-type function until 4 months of age or older and does not completely develop proportional dimensions similar to those of the adult until 9 to 12 months of age.[1047-1050,1147-1149]

The preruminant calf has been viewed as a functionally monogastric animal, and little importance has been assessed to diseases of the forestomachs. Under most management conditions, however, the forestomachs have begun to develop their digestive function within the first week or two after birth. During the development process the calf's forestomach is susceptible to problems different from those of the adult. After the rumen has developed a functional status similar to that of the adult, it is susceptible to the diseases discussed previously. Typically the feeding management of maturing young stock includes pasture or a mainly forage diet and does not predispose to digestive disturbance.

Esophageal (Reticular) Groove Function

Liquid feed bypasses the reticulorumen in the young ruminant, flowing directly into the abomasum through the esophageal groove. The groove consists of two lips that extend from the cardia to the reticuloomasal orifice. These close together, forming a tube to shunt liquid material to the abomasum when the soluble proteins and salts of milk stimulate a reflex through the glossopharyngeal nerve. Other salt solutions and even water can stimulate the reflex in very young animals, but the reflex weakens with age, especially after weaning. The response to stimuli varies among individuals, but generally milk produces the strongest response and plain water the weakest. Both nipple and bucket feeding stimulate closure in very young calves, but beyond 12 weeks of age closure is weak unless stimulated by nipple feeding. In older, weaned animals the reflex can be stimulated weakly for short durations by orally administered strong solutions such as copper sulfate or sodium salts. Intravenous vasopressin can induce more profound closure of the groove and

has been advocated to aid rumen bypass of orally administered treatment.[1150,1151]

Milk replacers that contain nonmilk protein appear to stimulate a weaker closure of the esophageal groove than do whole milk or milk replacers containing real milk protein. Likewise unpalatable fluids and spoiled milk do not seem to induce normal closure of the groove. Even in healthy calves that consume unspoiled whole milk, some overflow into the forestomach may occur.[1152] Failure of esophageal groove closure allows these fluids to pass into the rumen rather than bypassing it. Milk or other fluid administered through stomach tube or esophageal feeder does not contact the pharynx, therefore the reflex closure is not stimulated and the fluid deposits in the forestomachs. Under normal conditions fluid in the forestomach of neonatal calves less than 2 weeks old overflows into the abomasum when more than 400 ml has accumulated.[1153]

Reticuloruminal Milk Accumulation (Ruminal Drinking)

Milk can gain access to the reticulorumen by several means. Failure of esophageal groove closure, just discussed, is one possibility. In addition, if calves are maintained as preruminants for longer than 3 to 4 months, groove closure weakens and may allow greater escape of fluid to the reticulorumen. Fluid can also accumulate in the forestomach from abomasal reflux (Fig. 30-53). Overfeeding fluids beyond the capacity of the abomasum (about 2 L in the newborn, 35-kg calf) promotes backflow into the reticulorumen. Certain fluids affect abomasal motility and emptying times, prolonging their retention in the organ. These include acidic and hypertonic fluids and severely heat-treated skim milk powder. Nonmilk protein does not curd in the abomasum, as does casein, when it contacts the abomasal enzyme renin. Prolonged fluid retention and failure of curd formation in the abomasum may promote backflow into the rumen, especially when more fluid feed is consumed. Abomasal inflammation or ulceration may also inhibit normal emptying and promote abomasal reflux.

Some amount of milk reflux from the abomasum appears to be a physiologically normal occurrence. In fact, this route supplies some of the inoculum for rumen microfloral development and strongly influences the species distribution of the microbial population. But prolonged, repeated, or excessive retention of milk in the forestomach can lead to the development of abnormal fermentation patterns. Although amounts of fluid greater than 400 ml do not normally accu-

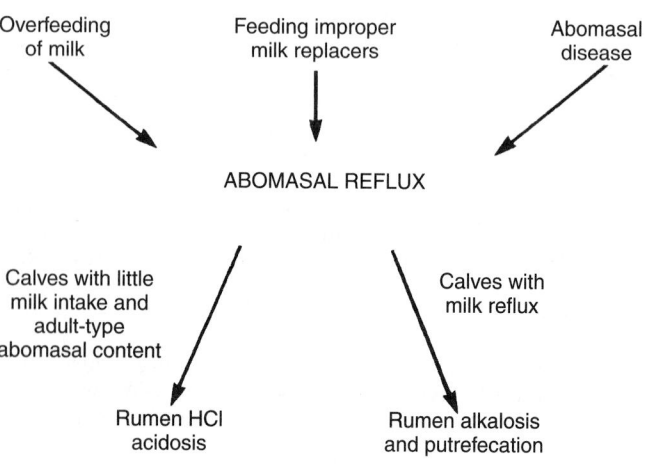

FIG. 30-53 ▮ Abomasal reflux in calves.

mulate in the forestomach of the neonate, more fluid can accumulate when the abomasum is already filled and when rumen size has increased during the development process. In some cases milk flow into the rumen accumulates significantly over prolonged periods.[1152]

The predominant organisms comprising the forestomach microflora of the 1- to 4-week-old ruminant are the coliforms and lactobacilli. These lactose-fermenting, facultative anaerobes tend to maintain the rumen pH in the acidic range before the adult-type, anaerobic, cellulolytic flora becomes established. The high fat and protein content of milk in the rumen can predispose to a flora that decomposes these constituents and produces spoiled and rancid rumen ingesta. Problems associated with rumen milk accumulation are compounded when the milk or other fluid ingested is already contaminated or spoiled. The abnormal microflora established under these circumstances does not supply the young animal with the necessary digestive end products, and signs of dietary insufficiency develop. Affected animals fail to grow normally, show a poor hair coat, and sometimes have a depraved appetite. The stimuli for normal forestomach development are also deficient; affected animals have a potbellied appearance, and the rumen is distended with fluid and clots of milk. Rumen motility is poor, and recurrent bloat is a common sequela. The rumen fluid pH may be alkaline as a result of the proteolytic formation of ammonia, but in most cases the rumen pH is acidic (below 6), and the fluid has a putrid, foul odor. An enteric imbalance also seems to occur, and the feces are commonly pasty or fluid in consistency. Ruminal "drinking" appears to compound problems in calves with infectious enteritis and diarrhea, and affected calves frequently develop systemic acid-base and fluid balance disturbances.[1154-1156]

Problems in Rumen Development

The age at which the calf has reticuloruminal digestion depends largely on its diet. A plentiful supply of milk delays the time until the calf consumes significant quantities of dry feed. Veal calves maintained without access to solid feed do not have forestomach development. The nervous reflexes that drive rumen motility, eructation, and regurgitation are already functional before birth, awaiting only the drive of normal stimuli to begin operating. Dry feeds pass into the rumen, and bacterial inoculation from the environment or from abomasal reflux stimulates fermentation to begin. This process can be initiated as early as 1 week of age when calves are encouraged to consume dry feeds.[1148]

The increase in the size of the forestomach results from the bulk effect of ingestion of bulky, fibrous feeds. Mild distention stimulates rumen motility and the development of the muscular wall. Mucosal development is stimulated by the presence of volatile fatty acids in the rumen fluid, resulting from microbial fermentation. Butyrate and propionate are most effective in this regard, whereas acetate is less stimulatory. The thickness of the mucosa increases with proliferation of the rumen epithelium and elongation of the papillae. These changes serve to increase the ability of the mucosa to absorb the VFAs. Dietary excesses or deficiencies affect the developing rumen by altering the balance of these stimuli.

Calves fed concentrate diets to the exclusion of forages or mixed diets with the hay pelleted or finely ground may experience rumen parakeratosis as a result of the excessive production of the stimulatory VFAs, butyrate, and propionate. These calves can have a form of chronic rumen acidosis that results in a reduced growth rate and poor body condition. Rumen contents are typically fluid with an acidic pH, rumen hypomotility occurs, and recurrent free gas bloat is common. Affected calves often display a craving for fibrous materials. Hair coat licking is common in these individuals, and hairball formation in the reticulorumen is a common sequela. The hairballs may not be deleterious, but occasionally they cause obstructive disease or abrade the parakeratotic papillae or the abomasal mucosa, predisposing to ulcers and inflammatory lesions. Acute rumen acidosis is not typically recognized in the young, developing ruminant, probably because feed consumption is limited and because the predisposing adult-type rumen microflora has not yet developed.

An opposite extreme can occur when the young calf is fed dry forage to the exclusion of more readily digestible carbohydrates. Concentrates and grass contain soluble carbohydrates and are well digested by the developing ruminant. Hays contain much less soluble carbohydrate and an abundance of the structured, slowly digestible forms. These substances are not as well digested by calves because the appropriate cellulolytic microflora is not fully developed. With moderate hay intake and the supply of other sources of nutrition, problems are rarely encountered. When dry roughage is the only available feed, especially when the hay is of poor quality, adequate breakdown of the fiber is prolonged. The low availability of nutrient substrate that results from delayed digestion of the structured carbohydrates decreases microbial proliferation and fermentation. Inadequate fermentation of the feedstuff deprives the animal of required nutrients as well and results in poor performance and growth. When the only available feed source is the hay ration, the calf continues to consume while the long undigested fiber accumulates in the rumen. The rumen continues to expand as a result of the increased filling, eventually becoming grossly distended. Recurrent bloat is common in these animals because of the overfilling and poor rumen contractility. This phenomenon is a frequent occurrence under some management conditions and has commonly been called "haybelly" (see p. 731). Affected animals display a typical abdominal contour, with gross distention of the abdominal wall that is more prominent on the left side. The rumen contents are very firm, the fluid has a pH around neutral and shows little microbial activity or odor, rumen motility is poor and, despite the full abdomen, the animal is thin. This form of microfloral inactivity is more common in calves than in adults because the young ruminant is less able to ferment fibrous roughage.[1047-1049]

Recurrent Bloat (Rumen Tympany)

Moderate gas distention of the rumen is a common sign of disease in calves, usually as a result of free gas accumulation, whereas frothy fermentation is very uncommon in the young ruminant. The pathogenesis of free gas bloat has been discussed, and the same principles hold for the young ruminant. The differences between free gas bloat in the adult and in the young calf are more a matter of chronicity and frequency of occurrence than cause. Digestive disturbances of the adult rumen tend to develop more rapidly and are more readily identified than those of the calf. Because of the involvement of rumen developmental processes in the pathogenesis of calf indigestion, in young ruminants the diseases are more chronic than acute in nature. In most cases the calf continues to consume feed, and the abnormal rumen function and development may be easily overlooked.

Rumen tympany seems to accompany indigestion in calves more often than in adult cattle and also assumes a more prominent appearance in calves than adults. These factors may be reflections of the juvenile anatomy and the incomplete development of adult function. It is worth noting, for instance, that although left-sided abomasal displacement is an uncommon occurrence in young calves, it almost invariably is accompanied by marked rumen tympany.[1157] In contrast, the disease is common in adult cattle, but rumen tympany is an infrequent sign of the disease.

Purulent lung infections appear to be a common cause of bloat in calves, probably as a result of intrathoracic compression or irritation of the esophagus or possibly the vagal nerves. However, other causes of bloat that are associated with abnormal rumen function are also common in calves with indigestion. They include overdistention of the rumen, insufficient clearing of the cardia, and inhibition of motility by abnormal fermentation products. Thus a thorough examination is required to determine the underlying cause of the individual case.

One presumed cause of bloat in calves that is not a cause of adult bloat is sudden filling of the abomasum by milk feeding during weaning. Calves not yet completely converted to a diet of solid feed still consume milk eagerly. In some cases acute free gas bloat occurs immediately after the milk feeding. Because the esophageal groove directs the milk into the abomasum but the abomasum is already partly filled by ingesta from the developing rumen, acute overdistention of the organ can occur and reflexly inhibit forestomach motility. Feeding smaller milk meals or discontinuing the milk feeding resolves the problem in these cases, lending support to the presumed cause.

CLINICAL SIGNS AND DIFFERENTIAL DIAGNOSIS OF INDIGESTION (Table 30-8)

General Signs

A general physical examination allows the practitioner to recognize signs of reticuloruminal problems and to assess whether a disease that could induce reticuloruminal dysfunction as a secondary phenomenon is present. General signs common to all forms of indigestion include a reduction or absence of appetite, dullness or depression, and decreased animal productivity. The most common signs of rumen dys-

function are a decrease, absence, or abnormality of rumen contraction sounds in the left paralumbar fossa or an abnormal left-sided abdominal contour. The left abdominal wall may show gauntness and decreased filling or display gross distention. It is often the failure to detect signs of another primary disease as the cause of ruminal dysfunction that directs attention to the forestomach as the possible primary site of disease. Indigestion in calves effectively produces a state of malnutrition, and additional signs in these growing animals include poor growth rate and long, rough hair coat. The acuteness of onset and the severity of these signs depend on the inciting cause of the indigestion. Specific abnormalities in the rumen motility pattern are discussed in more detail, but most indigestions are marked by decreased or absent ruminations (regurgitation and cud chewing) and depressed rumen contractions. Only early cases of frothy bloat and some cases of vagal indigestion display increased rumen motility.

Body temperature usually is within normal limits because the causes of indigestion are mainly physiologic abnormalities. Exceptions include traumatic reticuloperitonitis and occasional cases of rumenitis with significant inflammation. Disturbances of heart rate, respiratory rate, and body fluid vary tremendously among different forms of indigestion and different cases of any one form of indigestion. For example, an acute onset of severe ruminal bloat can produce severe embarrassment of the cardiovascular and respiratory systems, whereas mild or chronic bloat may produce no remarkable change in these systems. Rapid accumulation of fluid in the forestomach chamber in severe rumen acidosis with grain overload can induce severe dehydration, systemic acidosis, and increased heart and respiratory rates, whereas slow fluid sequestration in some cases of vagal indigestion may not induce marked changes in these parameters.

The anamnesis is important, especially with regard to the animal's feeding. Characteristics of the feed determine the

TABLE 30-8

Clinical Signs Typically Associated With Primary Indigestions

Signs	Associated Problems
Fever	Traumatic reticuloperitonitis, reticuloruminitis
Decreased rumen filling	Fermentative indigestions and secondary indigestions (especially with chronic anorexia) in which passage of material from the rumen is not impeded
Abdominal distention	See Fig. 30-52, p. 727
Excessive fluid (or froth) in the rumen with loss of normal ingesta stratification	Acute rumen acidosis, vagal indigestion, frothy bloat, anterior intestinal obstruction
Excessive firm, fibrous material in rumen	Rumen inactivity caused by poor quality roughage
Firm, doughy ingesta in ventral rumen with decreased rumen filling	Prolonged rumen stasis caused by chronic disease with anorexia
Rumen hypermotility	Early cases of frothy bloat, some cases of vagal indigestion
Abdominal pain present or can be elicited	Traumatic reticuloperitonitis, abomasal ulceration, reticuloruminitis
Abnormal feces	Traumatic reticuloperitonitis, omasal transport failure, rumen inactivity with poor-quality roughage, also dental disease and some abomasal disease
Decreased quantity, firm, dry, with increased fiber length	
Feces with abnormal amounts of whole cereal grains	Acute or chronic rumen acidosis
Greasy consistency with very fine particle size	Pyloric outflow failure, abomasal displacement
Foamy, fluid, yellowish color, acidic odor	Acute rumen acidosis
Pasty to fluid consistency with foul odor	Fermentative indigestions, enteritis
Decreased quantity, dry, otherwise unremarkable	Anorexia (various causes), acute indigestions before later developing abnormalities
Vomiting (rare)	Rumen overdistention with vagal indigestion, inflammation of reticulorumen, reticuloomasal orifice obstruction, diaphragmatic hernia, some intoxications (differentiate from esophageal disease)

type of fermentation pattern to be expected. Knowledge of the nutrient content thus allows an assessment of the biochemistry of microbial digestion. Consumption of a high-concentrate, low-fiber ration or legume pasture may lead to frothy bloat. A ration of poor-quality hay or straw may result in low microbial fermentative activity and accumulation of impacted indigestible roughage. Overeating of carbohydrates or sudden access to concentrate feeds without adequate adaptation time can induce chronic or acute rumen acidosis. The feeding history should agree with the findings from inspection of the rumen contents, or the history should be suspected to be inaccurate. The amount and consistency of the feces should also provide supportive evidence of the type and amount of feed intake.

ABDOMINAL CONTOURS AND ANIMAL STANCE (see Fig. 30-52). Visual inspection of the abdominal contours allows assessment of the degree of abdomen filling. Indigestions can be characterized by decreased, normal, or excessive filling of the reticulorumen. Most primary and secondary indigestions are associated with rumen hypomotility and anorexia. Thus the rumen usually shows no obvious distention and may have less filling than normal, especially when the duration of the disease is prolonged. Forms of indigestion in which abnormal ingesta or abnormal rumen motility prevents effective forward flow of ingesta (overfeeding of poor-quality roughage, vagal indigestion) or in which fluid is actively sequestered in the reticulorumen (acute rumen acidosis) typically cause some degree of forestomach distention (see Fig. 30-52).

A left-sided or bilateral ventral abdominal wall distention indicates ventral ruminal dilation, although advanced pregnancy and hydrops conditions must be considered. Distention of the dorsal left flank results from ruminal tympany with or without distention of the ventral rumen. Abomasal displacement to the left can produce mild distention of the dorsal left flank under the caudal ribs and extending into the paralumbar fossa, but the abdomen usually is gaunt and empty when viewed from the side or the rear. Occasional cases of left displaced abomasum appear to inhibit eructation and produce gross ruminal tympany as the primary sign. Release of free ruminal gas through a stomach tube and reexamination for abdominal pings reveals this cause of secondary rumen dysfunction. Frothy bloat in ruminants is discussed further elsewhere in this text (see p. 754). Free gas accumulation often occurs secondary to the causes of rumen motility inhibition and is important as a sign of indigestion (Table 30-9). Right-sided abdominal distention suggests the various conditions of dilation, displacement, and obstruction or ileus of the intestines and abomasum. The diseases that cause obstruction and reflux of abomasal ingesta into the rumen may result in reticuloruminal distention. Both prolonged cases of gastrointestinal obstruction at any site and generalized peritonitis can produce gross bilateral dorsal and ventral distention of the abdomen.

The animal should be studied for signs of pain. A pain-filled expression, a reluctance to move, an abnormal, stilted gait, an arched back with a tucked up abdomen, and an extended neck are typical signs of anterior abdominal pain. These signs may indicate traumatic reticuloperitonitis, abomasal ulceration, or another source of pain. A similar stilted gait and reluctance to move are typical of laminitis, a common sequela of acute rumen acidosis.

PALPABLE FINDINGS (see Fig. 30-52). Deep palpation of the left side of the abdomen is used to determine the consistency of the rumen contents and thus the nature and volume of the ingesta. In normal animals the organized contraction sequence produces a layering effect.[1050,1113] Ventrally a fluid consistency can be palpated, whereas dorsally the consistency is firm and doughy. The doughy layer consists of the fibrous portion of the feed. Generally an animal fed a high-roughage diet has a more prominent layer of doughy ingesta. The rumen contents of an animal fed concentrate feed are softer. In sheep and goats the normal dorsal rumen is softer than that of cattle no matter what the feed. In the normal condition a small layer of free gas is present in the most dorsal region. Distention with gas or foamy feed produces a taut, elastic tension. With free gas bloat the doughy layer can still be appreciated ventral to the gas accumulation, but in cases of frothy bloat the doughy layer is much less prominent. Most cases of vagal indigestion and some cases of high intestinal obstruction cause a grossly dilated rumen filled with fluid or foamy contents that may fluctuate on ballottement.

Overfeeding of indigestible poor hay or straw with resultant inactivity of rumen microbial fermentation leads to accumulation of more fibrous material than normal that barely yields to deep palpation. With prolonged or severe rumen stasis, as may occur in traumatic reticuloperitonitis, the lack of rumen motility leads to failure to maintain the normal layering of the contents. In these instances the ventral portion of the forestomach is firmer than the area above. During severe rumen acidosis, fluid accumulates in the forestomach. This can lead to some degree of abdominal distention, and on palpation the rumen contents are fluid and may even splash with ballottement.

The rumen should also be palpated per rectum; a comparison of these findings with those obtained externally may

---

TABLE 30-9

Differentiation of Types of Bloat Through Nasogastric Intubation

Results of Intubation	Probable Causes of Bloat
Tube does not pass	Esophageal obstruction
Tube passes with resistance and releases rumen gas	Esophageal compression caused by thoracic inflammatory or neoplastic disease
	Distortion of the cardia caused by inflammation, neoplasia, or abnormal anatomy such as abomasal displacement
Tube passes easily and releases rumen gas	Rumen stasis caused by reticuloruminal fermentative disorder, hypocalcemia
	Obstruction of cardia with ingesta (overfilling of rumen) or pedunculated mass
	Rumenitis (reticulitis)
	Weakened rumen contraction caused by chronic overdistention with ingesta (vagal indigestion, indigestion with poorly digestible forage)
Tube passes easily but does not release gas or releases small amount of foamy ingesta	Frothy bloat
	Frothy rumen contents caused by abnormal motility in some forms of vagal indigestion

be revealing. Moderate degrees of free gas accumulation are often more easily detectable per rectum. Palpation per rectum is also useful in distinguishing the presence of an L-shaped rumen, in which the ventral sac of the rumen is grossly distended in cases of vagal indigestion. It is important to differentiate an L-shaped rumen from either abomasal distention or impaction, which can display a similar external abdominal contour. It is also important to palpate for the size of the lymph nodes in the longitudinal groove of the rumen. These can enlarge to prominent size when rumenitis is present. The organs in the right half of the abdomen should be assessed as sources of abdominal problems.

Rectal examination is impossible in small ruminants and calves. External palpation using both hands can be valuable in these animals. In calves and goats it is the best method for detecting bezoars or clotted clumps of milk in the rumen and for palpating intussusception, umbilical abscesses, or grossly abnormal kidneys.

Palpation of the left paralumbar fossa reveals the presence of rumen contractions. In a normal animal, three contractions should occur over a 2-minute period. One of these contractions should be associated with an eructation of gas, which can be appreciated both visually and audibly. The rate of eructation increases or decreases in proportion to the fermentative production of gas. Most indigestions produce decreased rumen motility or rumen stasis. Early cases of frothy bloat and some forms of vagal indigestion can result in prominent hypermotility. The motility pattern is characterized by changes in both frequency and strength, and weak contractions can also be detected by palpation. Some cases of secondary indigestion, in which the decreased rumen function is a result of inappetence rather than an inhibition of rumen motility, show a normal contraction frequency but decreased contraction strength. The duration and strength of rumen contraction are primarily determined by the nature of the forestomach contents, whereas the frequency relies on medullary gastric center control. Decreased rumen fill, decreased fiber content of the ingesta, or overdistention of the rumen wall musculature results in reduced strength and duration of the contraction sequence. These distinctions can be important in determining the cause of decreased rumen motility.

AUSCULTABLE FINDINGS. Auscultation of abdominal sounds is performed over several sites in the left flank and rib areas. Initial auscultation assesses the nature, frequency, and strength of rumen sounds. This information can be compared with the assessment of rumen motility gathered on palpation. The sounds represent the friction of fibrous ingesta rubbing against the rumen wall as the ruminal sacs contract and mix their contents. In healthy cattle on a roughage diet, the normal rustling sound is prominent and prolonged with each contraction cycle. The rumen contents of animals fed a high-concentrate diet produce less sound because very low fiber rations induce weaker contractions and less fibrous material is in contact with the rumen wall.

As with palpation, both the frequency and the nature of the sounds yield information about reticuloruminal motility. The rumen motility pattern is disrupted in vagal indigestion. Although contractions are present and may be more frequent than normal, their lack of normal coordination can lead to a churning of the ingesta without the usual progression of transport. This disrupts the normal stratification of the contents and produces abnormal sounds that are heard as a rumbling, bubbling, or splashing. When stratification is disrupted because of a hypoactive rumen and more fluid is present in the dorsal area of the rumen, contractions produce splashing sounds. The accumulation of gas under these circumstances may produce ringing tones as the fluid moves, similar to the pings found with a displaced abomasum.

Some circumstances require a distinction between primary and secondary contraction cycles, and they can be differentiated by auscultating for reticular contractions. Holding the stethoscope at the seventh intercostal space at the level of the costochondral junction, the examiner can detect a tinkling fluid sound as the reticulum contracts. A hand held in the paralumbar fossa can detect the tensed bulging of the dorsal sac as it contracts, allowing the examiner to determine if the rumen contraction is associated with a reticular contraction. Reticular contraction and motility can also be assessed by transabdominal ultrasound.[1158] Hyperactivity of primary cycles associated with feeding or the immediate postprandial period is normal. Mechanical stimulation of buccal sensory receptors can lead to an approximate doubling of the primary cycle rate. Hypermotility that results from excessive secondary contractions, without the normal mixing and propulsion of primary contractions, is abnormal and represents ruminal dysfunction.

Combining the auscultation with percussion or ballottement allows assessment of gas or fluid accumulations. The sounds heard in the left flank should be compared with those in the left rib area and right side of the abdomen. High-pitched pings and fluid tinkling sounds suggest a viscus filled with gas and fluid. In the left flank this may represent a displaced abomasum, gas-forming abscess, pneumoperitoneum, or static rumen. Careful comparison of the sounds heard at different sites, combined with the results of rectal palpation, should allow localization of the source. Generally the rumen can be ruled out as the source of pings if palpation reveals normal doughy rumen contents, no rumen tympany is felt per rectum, and sounds of normal rumen contractions are heard in the paralumbar fossa. Prolonged anorexia associated with infectious or inflammatory diseases such as pneumonia or mastitis can result in a static, underfilled rumen, and occasionally a prominent ping can be ausculted in the left flank, where a filled rumen normally would be found. This condition has been called "rumen collapse," and careful evaluation is required to distinguish it from left displaced abomasum.[1159] Ballottement of the rumen may reveal splashing fluid sounds without a high pitch in cases in which the rumen has accumulated significant fluid. This occurs frequently in cases of severe rumen acidosis. It may also occur in cases of marked inactivity of the rumen flora with loss of the normal stratification of rumen contents.

PAIN ELICITATION. Tests of pain sensitivity in the anterior abdomen (percussion, deep palpation, withers pinch, xiphoid pressure) are performed to examine for localized peritonitis caused by traumatic reticuloperitonitis or abomasal ulceration. The same procedures, especially percussion or application of pressure to a localized area in the ventral abdomen, can be used to localize pain associated with rumenitis or rumen abscessation or perforating abosomal ulceration.

FECAL ABNORMALITIES. The rectal examination presents an opportunity to assess the volume and nature of the feces.[1160] The feces are abnormal in most cases of forestomach dysfunction. In adult cattle, passage of ingesta through the digestive tract requires 1½ to 4 days. Changes in the feces caused by acute diseases thus are often delayed by a day or longer beyond the first appearance of other clinical signs. Mature cattle typically pass a total of 30 to 50 kg of feces per day divided into 10 to 24 defecations. The color and consistency of feces are influenced by the feed and should be assessed in light of the feeding history.

Diseases that reduce the flow of ingesta from the rumen to the lower gastrointestinal tract typically result in feces of reduced volume that are firm and dry. These findings are also present with reduced feed or water intake. Assuming that normal intestinal function is present, a decreased flow of ingesta from the forestomach allows longer retention in the bowel with greater resorption of water. In severe instances the feces form into firm disks or balls with a dark, shiny mucus covering. These findings are typical of vagal indigestion and forestomach diseases that produce rumen stasis without a grossly abnormal fermentative pattern. Indigestions with abnormal fermentation may produce decreased quantities of dry feces initially but usually result in other fecal abnormalities as the abnormal ingesta passes into the lower tract. Intestinal obstructions also decrease fecal passage to the point of absence, but usually the material passed also presents other gross abnormalities such as blood, melena, or discolored mucus.

The particle size of fecal material depends on the frequency and duration of rumination, the activity of the rumen flora, and the function of the rumen in appropriately sorting out material for passage through the reticuloomasal orifice. Abnormalities of these digestive functions lead to passage of ingesta of inappropriate particle size. Plant fibers in normal bovine feces measure up to 0.5 cm. Particles with inadequate breakdown may measure 1 to 2 cm or longer. This long particle size may be seen in the feces of cattle with traumatic reticuloperitonitis, some cases of vagal indigestion, and poor-quality roughage with insufficient microfloral activity.[1108,1111,1161] Similar findings occur with tooth disease and some cases of abomasitis or cellulitis at the cardia or esophageal groove, in which rumination or activity of the reticuloomasal orifice is inhibited. Whole cereal grains (especially whole corn) may pass in the feces of normal cattle, but excessive amounts of grain should raise suspicion of excessive intake and acute rumen acidosis. Feces with an abnormally fine particle size and greasy-pasty texture are associated with delayed passage from the forestomach. These are common findings in most cases of vagal indigestion and abomasal displacement.

The odor of bovine feces is relatively inoffensive in healthy individuals. Foul odors are the result of abnormal fermentation or decomposition. Thus abnormal odor typically occurs when the rumen fermentation pattern is altered, as in simple indigestion caused by abnormal feed, rumen acidosis, rumen alkalosis, or rumen content putrefaction. A repugnant odor is also typical of enteritis when blood products, inflammatory products, or tissues decompose in the intestinal tract (e.g., *Salmonella* enteritis). Foamy, fluid feces with a yellow-brown color and acidic smell are typical of rumen lactic acidosis in adult cattle. Abnormal rumen fermentation not only produces feces with abnormal odor but also typically leads to a pasty or fluid consistency as well. Exceptions occur in acute cases, when rumen stasis or the delay in the passage of ingesta from the forestomach can result in normal or firm feces during initial stages of the disease.

ACUTENESS OF SIGNS. The various forms of indigestion may be manifested as acute, subacute, or chronic illness. In general they do not appear as critical emergencies with fulminating systemic signs and life-threatening conditions. The exceptions to this are frothy bloat (discussed elsewhere in the text) and acute rumen lactic acidosis or grain engorgement.

Cattle examined a few hours after engorgement of grain may yet be alert but anorectic with a mildly distended rumen, weak rumen contractions, and mild signs of colic. If the acidosis is mild, affected cattle show the signs of indigestion discussed in previous paragraphs and with or without treatment may show return of appetite within a few days. The severe form of indigestion leads to severe systemic involvement, with depression, severe dehydration, weakness, recumbency, profuse diarrhea, and eventually death. The temperature usually is normal to subnormal. The heart rate elevates with the progression of dehydration and systemic acidosis, with rates above 100 beats/min usually associated with a poor prognosis. Respiration generally is increased (60 to 90 breaths/min)

and shallow. The rumen accumulates fluid. Animals capable of rising may show a staggering gait and appear blind. The pupillary light reflex may be slower than normal. Recumbent animals usually lie quietly and may be stuporous. As the cardiovascular system becomes more severely affected with increasing dehydration and acidosis, the extremities become cool, and mucous membranes dry. Anuria may follow poor renal perfusion. Rapid progression of signs leading to recumbency bespeaks a poor prognosis, and animals may die within 24 to 72 hours. Therefore if the progression of signs is rapid, emergency therapeutic measures are mandatory.

In cattle with intermediate degrees of rumen acidosis, other signs may develop secondarily. Acute or chronic laminitis is a common complication. The damage to the rumen mucosa can lead to mycotic rumenitis or rumen wall abscessation or can disseminate infection through the bloodstream to other organs, most notably the liver, resulting in the formation of hepatic abscesses.

HEART RATE. Bradycardia of 40 to 60 beats/min is frequently associated with certain types of indigestion. This sign suggests reflex vagotonia to the heart and has been considered indicative of vagal indigestion. The bradycardia can be alleviated by subcutaneous administration of 30 mg of atropine, differentiating increased vagal nerve tone from a primary cardiac conduction disturbance. The atropine test is not especially useful because only a minority of vagal indigestion cases show bradycardia.[1102,1106,1108] Advanced cases with severe abdominal distention or fluid imbalances (or both) frequently show elevated heart rates (over 80 beats/min). In most cases the other physical signs are more reliable for establishing the diagnosis. Further, bradycardia may accompany other forms of indigestion when rumen hypomotility is prominent and no significant abnormalities of fluid or electrolyte balance are present. Even in normal cattle, postfasting heart rates may drop below 50 beats/min.[1161] Therefore recognition of bradycardia in association with other signs of rumen dysfunction is probably most useful as evidence that stimuli for an increased heart rate, such as inflammatory, infectious, or fluid balance disturbances, are not prominent factors in the individual disease occurrence.

VOMITING. Vomiting is uncommon in ruminants, but when it does occur, it generally reflects forestomach disease. Regurgitation from the abomasum frequently occurs with abomasal or intestinal disease. Abomasal reflux is not manifested externally and is discussed elsewhere (see pp. 734 and 741) because it relates to forestomach disease. Small volume regurgitation and remastication are routine and normal ruminant functions that do not result in expulsion of material from the mouth. Explosive vomiting of fluid ingesta in large quantity occurs when the reticulorumen is irritated and occasionally when it is overdistended. Vomiting may accompany diaphragmatic herniation of the reticulum, inflammation of the reticulorumen caused by actinobacillosis, vagal indigestion, or obstruction of the reticuloomasal orifice. Animals are more prone than normal to vomiting around an orally passed stomach tube when they have almost any indigestive disturbance. Vomiting also occurs with certain intoxications, most notably azalea, rhododendron, and sneezeweed toxicity and some organophosphate toxicities.

Clinical Pathology

RUMEN FLUID ANALYSIS. Evaluation of rumen fluid characteristics is an essential procedure in establishing the cause of the indigestions of abnormal fermentation.[1113,1127,1162] Several important determinations can be made at cowside in an ambulatory practice. Acquiring an appropriate sample is simplified by using proper equipment. The advantages of various collection techniques and devices have been recently discussed.[1163-1166] Needle puncture of the ventral rumen sac (ruminocentesis) may yield a satisfactory fluid sample, and recent studies demonstrate that rumenocentesis samples provide the most reliable evaluation of rumen fluid pH for field evaluation of subacute rumen acidosis.[1165,1166] Oral or nasal passage of a collection tube produces more fluid volume with no risk of peritoneal contamination but with an increased risk of saliva contamination. An adequate tube for aspiration of a rumen fluid sample should be at least 2.3 m long to reach the ventral rumen sac and should have an internal diameter of 1 cm or larger to reduce the incidence of plugging with ingesta. A plastic stomach tube passed orally or nasally can be adapted for use by cutting multiple holes into the ruminal end of the tube. A digital examination glove can be placed over the end during passage to limit saliva contamination of the sample and then is forcefully blown off before sampling. The sample can then be withdrawn by a dose syringe. This technique is successful when rumen fluid is accessible in the dorsal rumen, but the flexibility of the tube is disadvantageous when a prominent layer of fibrous feed is present. Several instruments with a flexible steel outer tube are commercially available and have the advantage of enough stiffness and weight to penetrate the overlying firm layer of ingesta.

Rumen fluid samples collected in an expeditious manner yield the most useful results. When the animal strongly resists sampling and a prolonged time is required from introduction of the tube until the fluid is obtained, saliva contamination of the sample increases. This contamination alters the pH and consistency of the sample. The specially designed rumen fluid collection tubes reduce this problem. If the sample must be collected with a standard nasogastric tube, passing the tube nasally avoids the presence of a device in the mouth. This reduces the amount of struggling (once the tube has passed the pharynx) and thus reduces excessive salivation.

The sample should be evaluated as soon as possible after collection to minimize the effects of cooling and air exposure on protozoal activity and pH. The more elaborate chemical tests such as chloride, acid, and ammonia concentrations can be delayed up to 9 hours on a room temperature sample and up to 24 hours on a refrigerated sample and still yield reliable results.[1167] Rumen fluid collected for therapeutic transfaunation also retains its beneficial activity for this duration. The rumen fluid parameters important in a clinical examination are listed in Table 30-10.

Color, Consistency, and Odor. The color, consistency, and odor of aspirated fluid are assessed immediately after collec-

tion. Normal color varies, depending on the nature of the feed. Animals fed a hay ration have olive to brownish green rumen fluid, those on grass show a deeper green color, and cattle fed grain or silage, a yellowish-brown color. Fluid from cattle with acidosis tends toward a milky gray. Rumen fluid from animals with prolonged stasis or decomposition of the rumen ingesta (or both) is a darker greenish black, and fluid from calves with milk sequestered in the rumen as a result of abomasal reflux or esophageal groove failure is gray and may contain clots of milk.

Normal rumen fluid has a slightly viscous consistency. The fluid becomes more watery when the microflora is inactive. Saliva contamination causes greater viscosity, therefore the results from a highly viscous sample should be evaluated with care, and it may be best to discard such samples. Rumen fluid has a typical odor that has been called "aromatic." The odor is less prominent when the microflora is inactive. Abnormal odors include the acidic smell of lactic acidosis, the putrid, foul odor of protein decomposition or spoiled milk with putrefaction of rumen ingesta, or the ammonia smell of urea poisoning.

Rumen Fluid pH. The pH of rumen fluid fluctuates within a broad range of normal values. The pH measured in a given fluid sample depends on the type of feed and fermentation pattern and the interval since the last feeding. Physiologic rumen fluid pH typically ranges between 6 and 7 in animals on a mostly forage diet but is lower, at 5.5 to 6.5, in animals fed mostly grain.[1128,1129,1166,1168] The lower pH develops with the faster rate of amylolytic versus cellulolytic fermentation. Immediately after feeding the pH tends toward the high end of normal with the addition of feedstuff and saliva. Over a 2- to 4-hour period the pH decreases to the lower range as the feed undergoes fermentation. With no further feed consumption, fermentation declines and the pH rises with salivary buffering and acid end product absorption.[1145] In animals held off feed the rumen pH rises above 7 within 12 hours after a hay meal and within 24 hours after a high grain meal. Thus consideration of the most recent feed consumption is important to the interpretation of the rumen fluid pH measurement.

Saliva contamination of the sample falsely elevates the measured pH value. Because it is impossible to exclude saliva completely from samples collected by tube, a minor false elevation of the pH likely occurs in all such examinations.[1163,1164,1166] This can be minimized by expedient collection of a large fluid volume (more than 100 to 200 ml). If the collected volume is small and the sample viscosity is high, the pH measurement will be inaccurate. Modest contamination (5% to 10%) raises the measured pH by approximately 0.1 to 0.2 pH units, whereas excessive contamination with approximately 50% saliva may increase pH by 1 pH unit.[1113,1163] Ruminocentesis of the ventral rumen sac below the left paralumbar fossa is preferred by some clinicians for preventing saliva contamination. This is particularly advantageous for samples collected to monitor rumen pH for balancing rations and minimizing chronic rumen acidosis. Recently a sampling strategy that incorporates ruminocentesis and rumen fluid pH measurement in groups of cows in a herd has been developed to optimally identify cow groups with feeding problems that lead to subacute rumen acidosis.[1165,1166]

Rumen pH values of 7 to 7.5 are common in animals with anorexia and in those that have ingested feed that is not suitable for fermentation (e.g., simple indigestion and inactivity of microflora caused by indigestible roughage). Even higher pH values may be measured with rumen alkalosis caused by urea ingestion or putrefaction of rumen ingesta. Low pH values result from engorgement with readily digestible carbohydrates and generation of rumen lactic acidosis. In extreme cases values occasionally decline to 4 to 4.5. It is important

TABLE 30-10

Diagnostic Rumen Fluid Analysis

Parameter	Normal
Color	Olive, brownish-green
Consistency	Slightly viscous
Odor	Aromatic, strong odor
pH	6-7 on roughage
	5.5-6.5 on grain diet
Sedimentation/flotation	4-8 min
Redox potential (methylene blue reduction time)	3-6 min
Protozoal activity	Multiple forms, active motion
Gram stain	Predominant gram-negative bacterial population
Chloride concentration	<30 mEq/L

to remember that prolonged anorexia and continued saliva ingestion result in rising pH values in these cases as well and that the rumen pH of a cow with rumen acidosis can be normal if a sufficient period of anorexia precedes the rumen fluid analysis. Conversely, a rumen pH of 5.5 to 6 is abnormal for a cow fed a roughage diet and may be indicative of unobserved access to grain and resultant lactic acidosis. Subacute or chronic rumen acidosis usually is accompanied by a rumen pH in the range of 5 to 5.5.[1127,1128,1166]Abomasal reflux into the reticulorumen caused by abomasal disease, vagal indigestion, or intestinal obstruction can cause mild decreases in rumen pH because of the acidic nature of abomasal contents. However, rumen pH measurement is a poor means of detecting abomasal reflux because the pH will remain within the wide range of normal values. Abomasal reflux is better assessed by measurement of the rumen chloride concentration.

Sedimentation. The sedimentation activity time, or sedimentation/flotation test, provides a quick evaluation of microfloral activity.[1169] It must be conducted promptly after collection of the sample. The aspirated fluid is allowed to sit in a tube, and the time for completion of sedimentation and flotation of the solid particles is measured. Normally the finer particles settle to the bottom and the coarser particles float, buoyed by the gas bubbles of fermentation. Some of the finer particles sink and then rise again when the fermentation is very active. The normal time for completion of this activity is 4 to 8 min. Grossly inactive fluid shows very rapid sedimentation, and none of the material may float. This occurs with rumen acidosis, prolonged anorexia, and inactive microflora caused by indigestible roughage. When the ingesta is particularly frothy, as in cases of frothy bloat or some cases of vagal indigestion, there may be no appreciable sedimentation or flotation. This test provides a crude evaluation of microfloral activity but does not differentiate well among the different forms of indigestion.

Redox Potential. The redox (reduction-oxidation) potential of rumen fluid is a biochemical characteristic that reflects the anaerobic fermentative metabolism of the bacterial population.[1114] An indirect determination of the redox potential can be achieved by measuring the time required by rumen fluid to decolorize methylene blue dye.[1170] A mixture of 1 ml of 0.03% methylene blue with 20 ml of rumen fluid at normal body temperature is observed in a tube and compared for color with another unaltered tube of the fluid. With a highly active microflora from an animal fed a hay and grain diet, the initial dark blue color of the mixture decolorizes within 3 minutes, leaving a narrow ring of blue color at the top of the decolorized sample. Fluid from a diet of hay alone requires 3 to 6 minutes and from a mostly grain ration requires as little as 1 min for methylene blue reduction. Reduction times up to 15 min and longer occur with diets of indigestible roughage, in anorexia of several days' duration, and after rumen acidosis.[1126,1162] Thus the methylene blue reduction time provides an assessment of the degree of bacterial fermentative activity.

Microscopic Examination. Evaluation of the number and activity of protozoa in the rumen fluid provides a sensitive indicator of the normalcy of the sample.[1113,1114] This is easily accomplished by examining a drop of fresh, warm fluid under a microscope. The examination requires only low magnification (×40 to ×100) and no special stains. In very active fluid samples the largest protozoa can be seen with the naked eye. They are detectable in a tube as small gray specks of material in active motion in the fluid, and they tend to localize above the sedimented particulate matter. Microscopically both ciliate and flagellate forms of varying sizes and shapes can be observed, with ciliates usually outnumbering the flagellates. The protozoa are normal inhabitants of a healthy ruminant's rumen fluid, although their specific function is not completely clear and their presence does not appear to be a prerequisite of normal digestive activity. The importance of the protozoa from a clinical viewpoint is their sensitivity to abnormalities in the fluid milieu. The normal animal should show a wide variety of sizes of protozoa, in large numbers that are easy to see, and with active motility. Reduced numbers occur in inactive fluid samples. The larger species are more susceptible to abnormalities; thus a predominance of only small protozoa would suggest a mild indigestive disturbance. All protozoa are killed off when the rumen pH drops below 5. Thus a recent bout of acidosis results in lack of protozoal activity, even if the pH has subsequently risen back into the normal range. Fluid from such an animal should also show other abnormalities of color and consistency. Very recent disturbances of the fluid may result in the observation of a large number of dead protozoa.

Although elaborate isolation methods for evaluating rumen bacterial growth are not clinically applicable, examination of an air-dried, Gram-stained smear of rumen fluid can be useful in diagnosing rumen acidosis. Normal rumen fluid should contain a variety of morphologically distinguishable bacterial forms, with a predominance of gram-negative organisms. After the overconsumption of readily digestible carbohydrate (grain engorgement), a population of streptococci and lactobacilli proliferates as rumen lactic acidosis develops. This shift in the bacterial population can be distinguished microscopically, and a predominance of gram-positive cocci and rods are seen. The findings are best confirmed by comparing a smear from a herd mate.

Rumen Fluid Chloride. The chloride concentration in rumen fluid can be determined from the supernate from a centrifuged sample using standard chloride titration devices. A delay in measurement does not appreciably affect the value. Saliva contains concentrations of chloride similar to those of normal rumen fluid, so that saliva contamination has minimal effect on the results. The normal rumen fluid chloride concentration is less than 30 mEq/L, with elevated values demonstrating reflux of abomasal ingesta into the rumen or administration of chloride in the feed or as therapy. Accurate assessment of measured values requires information about possible previous administration of electrolytes via the rumen. In the clinical evaluation of forestomach dysfunction, elevated rumen chloride suggests secondary indigestion caused by abomasal disease or obstruction of intestinal flow. This test can be very helpful in differentiating abomasal reflux from rumen lactic acidosis as the cause of low rumen pH and abnormal fluid accumulation in the reticulorumen. With vagal indigestion a high rumen chloride suggests that the failure of aboral flow is posterior at the pylorus rather than anterior at the reticuloomasal orifice.[1106,1112,1113] Generally cattle with elevated rumen chloride also have hypochloremia and metabolic alkalosis as a result of the chloride sequestration in the forestomach, although very slow development of the sequestration may allow the animal to maintain normal plasma levels by altering other excretion rates.

Numerous other tests of the rumen fluid have been described for the evaluation of digestive activity of the rumen microflora. These include cellulose digestion, glucose fermentation, nitrite reduction, and measurements of titratable acidity, volatile fatty acids, lactic acid, and ammonia concentration. These procedures can more clearly define the nature of the rumen fluid but are not generally used in a clinical setting.

HEMATOLOGY. Hematologic abnormalities are not generally a significant feature of the indigestive disorders. The primary exceptions are traumatic reticuloperitonitis or rumenitis, in which neutrophilia and hyperfibrinogenemia are routine findings. This feature of the disease can aid in its differentiation from other forestomach diseases. An inflammatory leukogram can also be observed in some cases of vagal indigestion when inflammatory disease is responsible for dysfunction of vagal innervation and forestomach motility. Chronic bronchopneumonia in calves and traumatic reticuloperitonitis in adult cattle are commonly implicated as causes of vagal dysfunction. A hematologic reflection of an inflammatory response may also be seen after rumen acidosis if the rumen wall and other organs suffer secondary pathogen invasion, and likewise in the occasional cases of primary rumenitis or reticulitis.

The more common hematologic abnormalities associated with indigestion are reflections of fluid disturbance or stress response. Hemoconcentration is routine and may be severe in rumen acidosis. Mild dehydration may also accompany the other forms of indigestion, especially when the disease shows a protracted course. A stress leukogram would be anticipated in cases of indigestion that are acute or distressing, such as acute bloat. The hematologic response in secondary indigestions depends on the primary disease.

When indigestion is chronic, especially in calves, in which the indigestive disturbance may go unrecognized or undiagnosed for a long time, a state of malnutrition may develop. In these instances a mild to moderate anemia may develop that may be attributable to micronutrient or macronutrient deficiencies.

BIOCHEMICAL ABNORMALITIES. Most of the primary forestomach diseases do not induce remarkable changes in the biochemical profile. In lactating or heavily pregnant animals, anorexia may induce a secondary form of acetonemia, which is detected by the presence of urine ketones. The animal must be carefully examined to differentiate ketosis with secondary anorexia and decreased rumen activity from primary indigestion with secondary ketosis. Mild to moderate hypocalcemia and hypokalemia are commonly identified abnormalities in many cases of indigestion, especially when anorexia has been prolonged.

Dramatic alterations of the blood biochemical characteristics may accompany severe rumen acidosis. Usually the laboratory findings correlate with the degree of severity assessed on physical examination. Affected animals have metabolic acidosis with decreased blood pH and plasma bicarbonate. Blood lactate levels rise with the acidosis. The urine pH falls into the acidic range as the kidneys excrete some of the excess acid, but eventually severe dehydration results in renal failure and anuria, eliminating this route of acid excretion. Decreased renal function is reflected by elevated serum creatinine and urea nitrogen concentrations. Other findings commonly include increased serum phosphate concentration, possibly caused by massive cellular destruction, and mildly decreased serum calcium concentration, presumably the result of decreased gut absorption. Other serum electrolyte abnormalities, such as changes in the sodium and chloride concentrations, may reflect fluid balance changes in response to rumen fluid hyperosmolality. Concentrations of serum enzymes of muscle and liver origin rise when acidosis and dehydration produce cardiovascular impairment with poor tissue perfusion, increased recumbency, and cellular destruction. Portal bacteria and toxins from the damaged rumen mucosa contribute significantly to the increased serum liver enzymes: aspartate aminotransferase, sorbitol dehydrogenase, (orthinine carbomyltransferase), and γ-glutamyl transferase.

Vagal indigestion may cause no significant blood biochemical abnormalities or can result in severe disturbances of fluid and electrolyte homeostasis.[1106] Measurement of the serum electrolyte concentrations provides important clues about the site of obstruction of ingesta flow and is useful in adjusting fluid therapy. When the primary problem is failure of flow through the reticuloomasal orifice, the rumen fills and grossly distends with fluid, but significant abomasal reflux does not occur. These patients generally show mild or no serum electrolyte abnormalities. When ingesta fails to pass from the abomasum, reflux of the high-chloride abomasal contents into the rumen results in elevated rumen chloride concentrations and associated hypochloremic, hypokalemic metabolic alkalosis. In some instances these abnormalities can be dramatic. Prolonged or severe hypochloremia and hypokalemia may also result in the paradoxic aciduria associated with avid renal sodium resorption in the face of low concentrations of chloride and potassium. Some slowly developing cases may accumulate significant fluid in the reticulorumen but have minimal blood electrolyte changes.

TREATMENT AND PROGNOSIS

Rumen Wall and Motor Function Disorders

Signs such as rumen tympany, rumen hypomotility or stasis, and forestomach distention can all result from a number of causes. Eliminating the underlying causative problem more effectively resolves the disease than treatment directed at the disease signs. Rumen hypomotility, for example, is commonly a physiologic response to problems such as abnormal rumen contents, a rumen wall lesion, pain, or overdistention. In many cases the rumen motility disturbance serves as a protective role for the animal. Former treatments that were directed at stimulating rumen motility without addressing the causative disturbance included rumenatorics (i.e., nux vomica, ginger, tartar emetic) or parasympathomimetics (i.e., neostigmine, carbamylcholine). Such agents are not indicated under these circumstances.[1062] Likewise the treatment of indigestions with alkalinizing agents such as magnesium hydroxide is indicated only when the pH of rumen contents is low.[1171]

FREE GAS BLOAT. When rumen tympany is a prominent sign, it requires very critical assessment. Frothy bloat and free gas bloat can be differentiated by a thorough physical examination and knowledge of the feeding history. Passage of a stomach tube to help in this differentiation is very important and may alleviate the acute problem if free gas is present (see Table 30-9). Evidence of respiratory or cardiovascular distress indicates that the bloat is an acute, life-threatening problem that requires emergency treatment. With the exception of cardia or esophageal obstruction, the free gas bloat associated with indigestive disturbances is mild to moderate in severity and chronic or recurrent in nature. It does not represent a major threat to the animal and can be handled by treating the primary forestomach disturbance. Chronic free gas bloat does not respond to the antifermentatives or surfactants commonly used for frothy bloat. Only the restoration of physiologically normal reticuloruminal function corrects this type of bloat. Inhibition of eructation caused by lesions of the cardia region can usually be confirmed only by exploratory rumenotomy. This approach also determines whether the lesion is surgically correctable. Inflammatory lesions may respond to long-term administration of broad-spectrum antibiotics. This is also the treatment of choice when purulent lung infections appear to be the cause of the bloat. Failure to respond within about 3 weeks suggests that the treatment is not effective, and slaughter should be recommended after an appropriate withdrawal time. Detection of abnormal forestomach ingesta should direct treatment to the primary fermentative or feeding disorder.

The various causes of chronic or recurrent bloat usually require chronic treatment for correction. It follows that the bloat will also not completely resolve until the underlying disturbance is corrected. Repeated relief of the bloat may be accomplished by passage of a stomach tube during the treatment regimen. In many cases this proves too tedious or too traumatic for the animal, and the most viable alternative of-

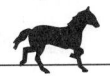

ten is the establishment of a temporary rumen fistula. Several devices are manufactured for this purpose, or the fistula can be created by suturing the rumen to the skin. Release of the fermentative gas in this manner is important for the reestablishment of normal forestomach motility, which is inhibited if distention is extreme. When free gas bloat is the result of an obstruction of eructation or another gastrointestinal tract disease such as abomasal displacement, surgical treatment of the primary problem may be necessary. The tympany responds rapidly in these cases, and rumen fistulation is not required.

LESIONS OF THE RUMEN WALL. Diseases of the rumen wall may be suspected on the basis of the physical examination findings and results of a complete blood count, abdominocentesis, and rumen fluid analysis. In most cases exploratory laparotomy is required to confirm the diagnosis. Rumenitis or reticulitis may respond to antibiotic therapy, but the prognosis in these cases is guarded. Not only is the forestomach inflammation difficult to resolve, but the hematogenous spread of infection to other organs often causes intractable multiple organ system disease. Parakeratosis is best treated by correcting the causal feeding error (reducing the amount of concentrate and increasing the feeding of long-stemmed forage). The rumen papillae can grow or regress in a period as short as 3 weeks when the feed is changed from low- to high-concentrate content or vice versa. Exactly how long it takes for parakeratotic papillae to return to normal is not certain, but it probably depends on the degree of change of the diet. The prognosis of this problem is good if inflammation of the rumen wall is not also involved.

RUMEN DISTENTION. Vagal indigestion is a chronic and insidious problem that generally warrants a guarded to poor prognosis. The syndrome of abdominal distention Λshaped rumen and possibly rumen tympany has several different causes. Exploratory laparotomy and rumenotomy are essential for establishing an accurate assessment (see Fig. 30-52). Diaphragmatic herniation and masses that obstruct the reticuloomasal orifice cause signs indistinguishable from those of vagal indigestion that results from inflammatory lesions of the reticulum. Surgical correction of a diaphragmatic hernia involving the reticulum can be attempted but has usually proved unrewarding, especially if the lesion is chronic, involves a large defect, or is accompanied by inflammatory reaction. Removal of pedunculated masses or foreign bodies at the reticuloomasal orifice can promptly correct such problems.

The two most common causes of vagal indigestion syndrome are inflammatory lesions of the reticuloomasal region and abomasal diseases that involve gross distention, twisting, or vascular impairment of the organ. Vagal indigestion caused by abomasal disease carries a poor prognosis, whereas the prognosis for cases with reticular involvement is more variable. Animals in either category may respond favorably with appropriate therapy[1108,1111,1172] (Box 30-6). Surgical exploration not only allows an assessment of the cause of the problem but may also allow repair. When abscesses are identified at the reticulum or liver, surgical drainage may help resolve the forestomach motor disturbance.[1109,1112] Identification of adhesions and active inflammation indicates that broad-spectrum antibiotic therapy may be beneficial. Gross abomasal distention, indicating pyloric outflow failure, usually warrants a poorer prognosis, as does the presence of granulomatous or neoplastic processes or generalized peritonitis and adhesion formation.[1112] When the presence of a large gravid uterus appears to be the inciting cause of outflow failure, induction of parturition or cesarean section usually resolves the problem completely.

The evaluation of animals with vagal indigestion with a large fluid-filled rumen should include assessment of the fluid and electrolyte status. Abnormalities such as dehydration,

---

BOX 30-6

Principles of Treatment of Vagal Indigestion

1. Determine likely cause, often by means of exploratory laparotomy
2. Administer specific therapy (e.g., antibiotics, antiinflammatory agents, removal of foreign body or relief of obstruction, drainage of abscesses) for causative lesion
3. Relieve forestomach distention; often must be repetitively performed
4. Limit feed and water intake; feed palatable, high-fiber ration
5. Transfaunate
6. Fistulate rumen if chronic bloat is a problem

hypocalcemia, hypochloremia, and hypokalemia should be addressed with supportive fluid therapy. Treatment should be administered parenterally, because oral treatments are ineffective or deleterious. The forestomach should be emptied of the excessive ingesta accumulation either at surgery or with a large-bore stomach tube. This procedure may have to be repeated if the recovery period is prolonged. Relief of persistent forestomach distention is *critical* to the reestablishment of normal motility. Limited feed and water should be offered to prevent repeated accumulations in the reticulorumen, and intravenous fluid therapy should be continued until reticuloruminal motility is reestablished and oral fluid intake can be allowed at normal levels. Once the rumen distention has been alleviated, several liters of rumen fluid transfaunate from a healthy donor should be administered. The limited diet must be palatable and should consist primarily of long-stemmed hay or green feed for maximum stimulation of the normal forestomach motility pattern. A temporary rumen fistula may be indicated if tympany is a prominent sign.

Response to treatment of vagal indigestion usually is a slow process and may require several weeks. Favorable signs include a return of the normal primary and secondary contraction patterns, improvement in appetite, maintenance of normal forestomach dimensions, weight gain, and increased fecal production. Repeated development of forestomach distention, continued scant fecal output, poor rumen motility, and recurrent bloat are indications that the animal is not responding to treatment and the prognosis is grave.

Fermentative Disorders

With the exception of severe acute rumen acidosis, the disturbances of reticuloruminal fermentation generally are not fatal unless the disease is undiagnosed for a prolonged period, leading to extreme debility. Treatment of the fermentation disorders centers around restoring a normal rumen fluid environment that allows normal microbial metabolism. Identification of rumen fluid parameters (see Table 30-10) and the nature of the forestomach ingesta directs the appropriate treatment (Box 30-7).

FEEDING. The first and most important step in treatment of nutritionally related indigestions is correction of the specific causal feeding error. Because the imbalance may have gone on for weeks, especially in cases of calf indigestion, correction of the problem may also take some time. The evolutionary development of the ruminant has adapted it to be a grassland grazer. Economic pressures in the animal industry have caused managers to institute feeding practices that diverge widely from a pasture setting. Fresh green grass, however, remains one of the best means of stimulating normal forestomach digestion and motility. The second best type of diet includes a balance of palatable and digestible sources of energy, protein, fiber, and mineral nutrients. The content of structured roughage should not fall below 10% of the ration dry matter, and a crude fiber component above 17% is desirable for any ration.

ALTERATION OF RUMEN CONTENTS. When the viability or activity of the rumen microflora is in question, as in the primary fermentative disorders and most cases of secondary indigestion, rumen transfaunation is indicated. This should be obtained from a healthy individual that preferably is adapted to a ration similar to the one the patient is expected to consume. The fluid can be obtained from an animal with the rumen fistulated, by removal with a stomach tube, or from a local abattoir. After the large particulate matter has been strained from the fluid (cheesecloth or large stockinette can be used), it can be administered through a stomach tube. The transfer from donor to recipient is best accomplished immediately, but fluid that contains active and healthy microflora remains viable for up to 9 hours at room temperature or 24 hours under refrigeration.[1167] In calves inoculation with 1 L is appropriate, whereas 3 L is minimal in an adult cow, and 8 to 16 L is more desirable.

Many animals with indigestion exhibit decreased rumen fill. As discussed, one of the primary stimuli for active rumen contraction is mild forestomach distention. In addition to the administration of rumen transfaunate, it usually is beneficial in these cases to administer enough oral fluid to produce mild rumen distention. This can be accomplished with water warmed to body temperature, and 20 to 30 L of fluid administered through a tube may be required to achieve the desired effect. The addition of salt (sodium and potassium chloride) in amounts sufficient to produce an isotonic solution (about 2 teaspoons per liter) supplements deficiencies and promotes rapid turnover of the fluid from the rumen to the lower tract. Cathartic agents such as magnesium sulfate have been used and may be beneficial but do not serve to supplement the common electrolyte deficiencies.

Correction of pH abnormalities to the normal range of 6 to 7 is important when rumen acidosis or alkalosis is detected. Alkalinizing agents such as magnesium hydroxide and sodium bicarbonate are indicated for treatment of acidosis at an initial dose of 1 g/kg. Magnesium hydroxide is commonly used by some as a routine treatment for any animals in which rumen hypomotility has been identified. This prac-

tice is not justifiable in most cases of rumen hypomotility because the fluid pH is commonly at or near neutral. The use of magnesium hydroxide in such settings may induce a mild systemic alkalosis, and the agent is better reserved for true cases of acidosis.[1172] Rumen alkalosis can be corrected with the infusion of acetic acid (vinegar, initial dose of 2 ml/kg, up to 12 L). All of these agents are best administered in several liters of warm water to ensure good distribution through the rumen fluid.

Overdistention of the rumen wall may be a primary inhibitor of forestomach motility in some cases of indigestion caused by abnormal fermentation. Treatment of free gas bloat has been discussed. When the distention is caused by accumulation of abnormal ingesta, normal contractions do not return and the rumen tympany is not resolved until the distention is relieved. This situation is best exemplified by cases of microfloral inactivity caused by poor-quality roughage and is the underlying problem in calves with haybelly. One approach to this problem is to restrict the animal to small quantities of readily digestible feed given several times a day. Between meals the animal can be kept in an unbedded stall or muzzled. This process is continued until the accumulated ingesta has passed out of the forestomach. Repeated transfaunations during this time help reestablish a more normal microflora. This approach relies on motility and microbial activity sufficient to break down the ingesta and pass it to the lower tract. An alternative approach is to remove the accumulated ingesta by means of rumenotomy, after which the animal is transfaunated and allowed access to moderate amounts of feed until normal motility is restored. Emptying the rumen surgically is the treatment of choice when spoiled milk, putrefactive rumen ingesta, or severe rumen acidosis is detected. Prolonged cases of microbial inactivity or anorexia (or both) with rumen hypomotility can result in loss of the normal stratification of forestomach ingesta. The fibrous, floating layer sinks to the ventral rumen sac in these cases, forming a dense, firm mass. Return of normal forestomach motility will be delayed unless this accumulation of material can be eliminated. This can be accomplished during the process of microfloral reestablishment by massaging the mass through the lateral and ventral body wall. Dissolution and passage of the material can be enhanced by the administration of mineral oil (4 L), or dioctyl sodium sulfosuccinate (DSS) (4 to 6 ounces in 2 to 3 L of water). Because DSS kills rumen protozoa when given in amounts greater than required to saturate the fibrous matter, at least one rumen transfaunate should be given 1 to 2 days after the last application of this agent.[1173]

Animals with prolonged anorexia caused by a depressant or febrile disease that produced secondary indigestion may not return to feed or have normal rumen motility even after normalcy of the rumen contents has been restored. Chewing activity is one of the strongest stimulants for rumen motility, and these individuals sometimes benefit if palatable hay or grass is placed forcefully into their mouth by hand. An alternative is to give such individuals access to pasture. Both the ruminant and its ruminal microflora have trace mineral requirements that are often not met by the type of diets that may induce microfloral inactivity.[1118] The ruminal microflora is also responsible for supplying the animal with its vitamin B requirements.[1085] The stunted, poor body condition of calves affected by chronic indigestions may reflect these deficiencies, as well as protein energy malnutrition (see Chapter 9). Oral supplementation of minerals and parenteral supplementation of the B vitamins may be helpful until normal rumen digestive function is established. Adult cattle, especially lactating animals with high metabolic demands, may also benefit from B vitamin supplementation when rumen function is impaired.

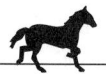

Intraruminal administration of antibiotics has been used to kill undesirable populations of rumen microflora. A 2- to 3-day course of treatment with a broad-spectrum antibiotic that is not readily absorbed is only useful when an overgrowth of undesirable bacterial species is present and should be followed by transfaunation. Drugs used for this effect include neomycin or tetracycline for rumen alkalosis or urea toxicosis, and chlortetracycline or erythromycin for rumen acidosis. Feeding changes and rumen transfaunation are also effective in inhibiting the undesirable population and inoculating the desirable population. When spoiled milk, putrefactive ingesta, or extremely acidic rumen contents are found on rumen fluid analysis, rumenotomy, removal of the contents, and flushing of the rumen seem the more desirable treatment.

ACUTE RUMEN ACIDOSIS. Therapy for cases of mild to moderate or chronic rumen acidosis can follow the guidelines outlined previously. Then prognosis in these cases is usually good, although rumen inflammation and hematogenous dissemination of infection to other organs can produce chronic problems with a poorer prognosis.

Severe grain overload requires prompt and aggressive treatment. Animals showing severe depression, an unresponsive condition, apparent blindness, and gross rumen distention warrant a grave prognosis. Immediate slaughter should be considered for animals with similar signs but still able to stand.

Emergency rumenotomy and removal of the acidic rumen contents may be lifesaving if the procedure can be performed before significant amounts of ingesta have passed into the lower gastrointestinal tract. An alternative treatment in less severe cases is repeating flushing of the rumen with warm water through a large-bore stomach tube. Administration of magnesium hydroxide into the rumen and sodium bicarbonate solution (5%) intravenously is necessary to counter the acidosis. Intravenous fluid therapy should be continued until the animal has recovered to provide support against hypovolemic shock. Other treatments that may be considered include nonsteroidal antiinflammatory drugs and intraruminal antibiotics. The other therapeutic measures discussed such as transfaunation and dietary adjustment should be continued during the recovery phase.

SUPPORTIVE TREATMENTS. Indigestion often is accompanied by varying degrees of dehydration and electrolyte imbalance. When these abnormalities are only mild or moderate, the animal's fluid homeostasis may correct as the normal digestive processes are restored. More rapid recovery is achieved if these problems are addressed during the initial treatment, and animals must be treated if the imbalance is severe. Restoration of normal fluid balance improves attitude and appetite and normal gastrointestinal motility.

When laboratory facilities are available and the specific electrolyte imbalances can be assessed, fluid therapy can be tailored to the individual case. Empiric treatment with a balanced electrolyte solution administered intravenously is sufficient in most cases, because gross disturbances of the body fluid electrolytes are uncommon in most indigestions. The greatest exceptions to this are cases of severe rumen acidosis or vagal indigestion with pyloric outflow failure and sequestration of abomasal chloride. These problems should be identified during the examination.

Hypocalcemia and hypokalemia are routinely present in many cases of indigestion. Low serum concentrations of these elements can produce muscular weakness and impair gastrointestinal motility. Both calcium and potassium should be included in the administered fluids. As an alternative calcium salts should be administered subcutaneously if intravenous fluid administration is not elected. When anorexia has been prolonged, an additional oral dosage of potassium

chloride (120 g/day) may be required even after adequate hydration has been achieved and fluid therapy has been discontinued.

PREVENTION

Some of the sporadically occurring diseases of the forestomach wall such as granulomatous infections, neoplastic invasions, and diaphragmatic herniation cannot be foreseen or prevented. The most common cause of vagal indigestion syndrome is inflammation of the reticular area caused by traumatic reticuloperitonitis. Prevention of this disease by keeping metallic foreign bodies out of the feed or by prophylactic administration of a rumen magnet is the best prevention of vagal indigestion as well.

The microbial-fermentative forestomach disorders are best prevented by proper feeding management. A well-balanced diet of palatable feeds with an adequate amount of well-structured roughage (not finely ground or pelleted) prevents most problems. Dietary changes should be introduced slowly (over 2 to 3 weeks) to allow adaptation of the microbial flora to the new substrate. Calves undergoing rumen development and cattle fed high-production diets or changing between production groups are at risk of oversights in proper feeding management. Some feed additives have proved effective in preventing the overgrowth of the high acid–producing rumen microflora. Feed-grade buffers are widely used in both dairy and beef cattle production, in which high-concentrate diets are fed to maximize production. These buffers stabilize the rumen pH and alter the mechanics of rumen fluid outflow, thus decreasing the chances of overgrowth of the lactate-producing organisms. Commonly used "buffers" include sodium bicarbonate, sodium bentonite, magnesium oxide, and calcium-magnesium carbonate, of which only the bicarbonate is truly a buffering agent in the chemical sense. The other agents do tend to stabilize rumen pH, however, and all of these have shown some benefit in reducing the disease problems associated with heavy grain feeding.[1175] The ionophore antibiotics (e.g., lasalocid, monensin) and some other antibiotics (e.g., the sulfur-containing peptide antibiotic thiopeptin) have also proved effective in reducing lactate production in animals fed high-grain diets. The effect of these agents is to suppress the lactate-producing organisms while not appreciably affecting the lactate users. The ionophores are in common use in feedlot cattle rations because the selective effects on these antibiotics on the rumen microbes alter the rumen metabolism in a manner that promotes increased animal weight gain.[1175,1176]

REFERENCES

1047. Dirksen G: Krankheiten der Haube und des Pansens. In Rosenberger G, ed: *Krankheiten des Rindes*, ed 2, Berlin, 1978, Verlag Paul Parey.
1048. Dirksen GU, Garry FB: Diseases of the forestomachs in calves. I, *Compend Cont Educ* 9:F140-F147, 1987.
1049. Dirksen GU, Garry FB: Diseases of the forestomachs of calves. II, *Compend Cont Educ* 9:F173-F180, 1987.
1050. Van Soerst PJ: *Nutritional ecology of the ruminant*, Corvallis, Ore, 1982, O & B Books.
1051. Wyburn RS: The mixing and propulsion of the stomach contents of ruminants. In Ruckebush Y, Thivend P, eds: *Digestive physiology and metabolism in ruminants*, Lancaster, England, 1980, MTP Press.
1052. Kay R: Rumen function and physiology, *Vet Rec* 113:6-9, 1983.
1053. Sellers AF, Stevens CE: Motor functions of the ruminant forestomach, *Physiol Rev* 46:634-659, 1966.
1054. Peruzzo de Naville LE, Colvin HW, Backus RC: The primary-secondary rumen contraction and gas expulsion in sheep, *Comp Biochem Physiol* 87A:993-1002, 1987.
1055. Mercer SA, Colvin HW, Backus RC: Elevated intrarumen pressure and secondary rumen contractions in sheep, *Comp Biochem Physiol* 90A:481-489, 1988.
1056. Iggo A, Leek BF: An electrophysiological study of some reticuloruminal and abomasal reflexes in sheep, *J Physiol* 193:95-119, 1967.

1057. Iggo A, Leek BF: An electrophysiological study of single vagal efferent units associated with gastric movements in sheep, *J Physiol* 191:177-204, 1967.

1958. Leek BF: Reticuloruminal function and dysfunction, *Vet Rec* 84:238-243, 1969.

1059. Habel RE: A study of the innervation of the ruminant stomach, *Cornell Vet* 46:555-628, 1956.

1060. Titchen DA: Reflex stimulation and inhibition of reticulum contractions in the ruminant stomach, *J Physiol* 141:1-21, 1958.

1061. Harding R, Leek BF: The locations and activities of medullary neurones associated with ruminant forestomach motility, *J Physiol* 219:587-610, 1971.

1062. Ruckebush Y: Pharmacology of reticuloruminal motor function, *J Vet Pharmacol Ther* 6:245-272, 1983.

1063. Dietz O et al: Untersuchungen zur Vagufunktion, zur Vagusbeeinflussung und zu Vagusausfallen am Verdauungsapparat des erwachsenen Rindes, *Arch Exper Vet Med* 24:1385-1439, 1970.

1064. Leek BF, Harding RH: Sensory nervous receptors in the ruminant stomach and the reflex control of reticuloruminal motility. In McDonald IW, Warner ACI, eds: *Digestion and metabolism in the ruminant*, Armidale, NSW, Australia, 1975, New England Publishing Unit.

1065. Ash RW, Kay RNB: Stimulation and inhibition of reticulum contractions, rumination, and parotid secretion from the forestomach of conscious sheep, *J Physiol* 149:43-57, 1959.

1066. Espinasse J, Kuiper R, Schelcher F: Pathophysiology of the bovine stomach, *Bovine Pract* 26:105-110, 1991.

1067. Van Miert AS, van Duin CT, Anika SM: Anorexia during febrile conditions in dwarf goats: the effect of diazepam, flurbiprofen and naloxone, *Vet Q* 8:266-263, 1986.

1068. Van Miert AS: Fever and associated clinical haematologic and blood biochemical changes in the goat and other animal species, *Vet Q* 7:200-216, 1985.

1069. Van Soest PJ: *Nutritional ecology of the ruminant*, Corvallis, Ore, 1982, O & B Books.

1070. Lohuis JA et al: Pathophysiological effects of endotoxins in ruminants. I, Changes in body temperature and reticulorumen motility and the effect of repeated administration, *Vet Q* 10:109-116, 1988.

1071. Froetschel MA et al: Effects of slaframine on ruminal digestive function: ruminal motility in sheep and cattle, *J Anim Sci* 63:1502-1508, 1986.

1072. Jorgensen R et al: Rumen motility during induced hypercalcaemia and hypocalcaemia, *Acta Vet Scand* 39:331-338, 1998.

1073. Daniel R: Motility of the rumen and abomasum during hypocalcaemia, *Can J Comp Med* 47:276-280, 1983.

1074. Westra R, Christopherson RJ: Effects of cold on digestibility, retention time of digesta, reticulum motility and thyroid hormones in sheep, *Can J Anim Sci* 56:699-708, 1976.

1075. Lirette R et al: Effects of psychological stress, acute cold stress and diet on forestomach contractions in cattle, *Can J Anim Sci* 68:399-407, 1988.

1076. Andersson B, Kitchell R, Persson N: A study of rumination induced by milking in the goat, *Acta Physiol Scand* 44:92-102, 1958.

1077. Guard C et al: Effects of metoclopramide, clenbuteronl, and butorphanol on ruminoreticular motility of calves, *Cornell Vet* 78:89-98, 1988.

1078. Sorraing JM, Fioramonti J, Bueno L: Effects of dopamine and serotonin on eructation rate and ruminal motility in sheep, *Am J Vet Res* 45:942-947, 1984.

1079. Brikas P, Tsiamitas C, Wyburn RS: On the effect of xylazine on forestomach motility in sheep, *Zentrabl Vet Med* A 33:174-179, 1986.

1080. Svendson PE: Experimental studies of gastrointestinal atony in ruminants. In McDonald IW, Warner ACI, eds: *Digestion and metabolism in the ruminant*, Armidale, NSW, Australia, 1975, New England Publishing Unit.

1081. Grovum WL: Factors affecting the voluntary intake of food by sheep. III, The effect of intravenous infusions of gastrin, cholecystokinin and secretin on motility of the reticulorumen and intake, *Br J Nutr* 45:183-201, 1981.

1082. Dougherty RW, Habel RE, Bond HE: Esophageal innervation and the eructation reflex in sheep, *Am J Vet Res* 19:115-128, 1958.

1083. Leek BF: Clinical diseases of the rumen: a physiologist's view, *Vet Rec* 113:10-14, 1983.

1084. Dougherty RW: Physiopathology of the ruminant digestive tract. In Swenson MJ, ed: *Dukes' physiology of domestic animals*, ed 10, Ithaca, New York, 1984, Cornell University Press.

1085. Dziuk HE: Digestion in the ruminant stomach. In Swenson MJ, ed: *Dukes' physiology of domestic animals*, ed 10, Ithaca, New York, 1984, Cornell University Press.

1086. Prins RA, Clarke RTJ: Microbial ecology of the rumen. In Ruckebush Y, Thivend P, eds: *Digestive physiology and metabolism in ruminants*, Lancaster, England, 1980, MTP Press.

1087. Whitlock RH: Bovine stomach diseases. In Anderson NV, ed: *Veterinary gastroenterology*, Philadelphia, 1980, Lea & Febiger.

1088. Rebhun WC: Vagus indigestion in cattle, *J Am Vet Med Assoc* 176:506-510, 1980.

1089. Doll K: Bloat in calves: some aspects of differential diagnosis and therapy, *Bovine Pract* 24:49-52, 1989.

1090. Narayanan S et al: Biochemical and ribotypic comparison of *Actinomyces pyogenes* and *A pyogenes*–like organisms from liver abscesses, rumen wall, and ruminal contents of cattle, *Am J Vet Res* 59:271-276, 1998.

1091. Thompson RG: Rumenitis in cattle, *Can Vet J* 8:189-192, 1967.

1092. Taylor RL, Kintner LD: Phycomycosis of feedlot cattle, *J Am Vet Med Assoc* 174:371-372, 1979.

1093. Chihaya Y et al: A pathological study of bovine alimentary mycosis, *J Comp Pathol* 107:195-206, 1992.

1094. Sweeney RW et al: Mycotic omasitis and rumenitis as sequelae to sepsis in dairy cattle: six cases (1979-1986), *J Am Vet Med Assoc* 194:552-553, 1989.

1095. Jensen HE, Basse A, Aalbaek B: Mycosis in the stomach compartments of cattle, *Acta Vet Scand* 30:409-423, 1989.

1096. Jensen HE, Schonheyder H, Basses A: Acute disseminated aspergillosis in a cow with special reference to penetration and spread, *J Comp Pathol* 104:411-417, 1991.

1097. Bertone AL, Roth L, O'Krepky J: Forestomach neoplasia in cattle: report of eight cases, *Compend Cont Educ Pract Vet* 7:S85-S90, 1985.

1098. Gordon PJ: Surgical removal of a fibropapilloma from the reticulum causing apparent vagal indigestion, *Vet Rec* 140:69-70, 1997.

1099. Roy JHB: *The calf*, ed 4, London, 1980, Butterworth.

1100. Herd RM, Cook LG: Hairballs in feedlot-raised calves, *Aust Vet J* 66:372-373, 1989.

1101. Neal PA, Edwards GB: Vagus indigestion in cattle, *Vet Rec* 82:396-402, 1968.

1102. Hoflund S: Investigations of functional defects of the ruminant stomach caused by damage to the vagus nerve, *Svensk Vet Tidskr* 45(suppl), 1940.

1103. Leek BF: Vagus indigestion in cattle, *Vet Rec* 82:498-499, 1968.

1104. Kuiper R, Breukink HJ: Das hoflundsche syndrom nach 47 jahren, *DTW* 94:271-273, 1987.

1105. Dirksen G, Stober M: Beitrag zu den durch Schadigungen des Nervus Vagus bedingten Funktionsstorungen des Rinder-magens: Hoflundsches syndrom, *DTW* 69:213-217, 1962.

1106. Kuiper R, Breukink HJ: Reticuloomasal stenosis in the cow: differential diagnosis with respect to pyloric stenosis, *Vet Rec* 119:169-171, 1986.

1107. Braun U, Hausammann K, Oertle C: Hoflund Syndrome infolge vorderer funktioneller Stenose bei 20 Kuhen, *Berl Munch Tierarztl Wochenschr* 103:192-197, 1990.

1108. Fubini SL et al: Failure of omasal transport attributable to pireticular abscess formation in cattle: 29 cases (1980-1986), *J Am Vet Med Assoc* 194:811-814, 1989.

1109. Stockhofe-Zurwieden N, Rehage J, Yalcin E: Morphological investigations of the forestomach in cows suffering from Hoflund syndrome, *Proc XVII World Buiatrics Congr* 1:127-130, 1992.

1110. Rehage J et al: Hoflund's syndrome: the consequence of failure in the selective retention of particles in the reticulorumen? *Proc XVII World Buiatrics Congr* 1:131-135, 1992.

1111. Fubini SL et al: Vagus indigestion syndrome resulting from a liver abscess in dairy cows, *J Am Vet Med Assoc* 186:1297-1300, 1985.

1112. Rehage J et al: Evaluation of the pathogenesis of vagus indigestion in cows with traumatic reticuloperitonitis, *J Am Vet Med Assoc* 207:1607-1611, 1995.

1113. Dirksen G: Forestomachs. In Rosenberger G, ed: *Clinical examination of cattle*, Berlin, 1977, Verlag Paul Parey.

1114. Van Soest PJ: Rumen microbes. In Van Soest PJ, ed: *Nutritional ecology of the ruminant*, Corvallis, Ore, 1982, O & B Books.

1115. Allison MJ: Microbiology of the rumen and small and large intestines. In Swenson MJ, ed: *Dukes' physiology of domestic animals*, ed 10, Ithaca, New York, 1984, Cornell University Press.

1116. Mackie RI, White BA: Symposium: rumen microbial ecology and nutrition, recent advances in rumen microbial ecology and metabolism—potential impact on nutrient output, *J Dairy Sci* 73:2971-2995, 1990.

1117. Slyter LL: Influence of acidosis on rumen function, *J Anim Sci* 43:910-929, 1976.

1118. Durand M, Kawashima R: Influence of minerals in rumen microbial digestion. In Ruckebush Y, Thivend P, eds: *Digestive physiology and metabolism in ruminants*, Lancaster, England, 1980, MTP Press.

1119. Van Soest PJ, ed: *Nutritional ecology of the ruminant*, Corvallis, Ore, 1982, O & B Books.

1120. Crichlow EC, Chaplin RK: Ruminal lactic acidosis: relationship of forestomach motility to nondissociated volatile fatty acid levels, *Am J Vet Res* 46:1908-1911, 1985.

1121. Crichlow EC, Leek BF: Forestomach epithelial receptor activation by rumen fluids from sheep given intraruminal infusions of volatile fatty acids, *Am J Vet Res* 47:1015-1018, 1986.

1122. Schelcher F, Valarcher JF, Espinasse J: Abnormal ruminal digestion in cattle with dominantly nondigestive disorders, *Dtsch Tierarztl Wschr* 99:175-182, 1992.

1123. Selim HM et al: Rumen bacteria are involved in the onset of onion-induced hemolytic anemia in sheep, *J Vet Med Sci* 61:369-374, 1999.

1124. Gould DH, Cummings BA, Hamar DW: In vivo indicators of pathologic ruminal sulfide production in steers with diet-induced polioencephalomalacia, *J Vet Diagn Invest* 9:72-76, 1997.

1125. Cummings BA et al: Ruminal microbial alterations associated with sulfide generation in steers with dietary sulfate-induced polioencephalomalacia, *Am J Vet Res* 56:1390-1395, 1995.

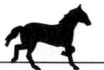

1126. Braun U, Rihs T, Eicher R: Pansensaftuntersuchungen bei Kuhen mit chronischer Inaktivitat der Vormangenflora und fauna vor und nach Therapie und Futterumstellung, *Schweiz Arch Tierheilkd* 130:545-558, 1988.

1127. Owens FN et al: Acidosis in cattle: a review, *J Anim Sci* 76:275-286, 1998.

1128. Leedle JAZ, Coe ML, Frey RA: Evaluation of health and ruminal variables during adaptation to grain-based diets in beef cattle, *Am J Vet Res* 56:885-892, 1995.

1129. Dunlop RH: Pathogenesis of ruminant lactic acidosis, *Adv Vet Sci Comp Med* 16:259-302, 1972.

1130. Gabel G: Pansenazidose: Interaktionen zwischen den Veranderungen im Lumen und in der Wand des Pansens, *Ubers Tierernahrg* 18:1-38, 1990.

1131. Russel JB, Hino T: Regulation of lactate production in *Streptococcus bovis*: a spiraling effect that contributes to rumen acidosis, *J Dairy Sci* 68:1712-1721, 1985.

1132. Bide RW: Excess rumen product anions in cattle. I. Blood clearance rates and reduced liver function from sublethal doses of volatile fatty acids, lactate and succinate, *Can J Comp Med* 47:222-229, 1983.

1133. Huber TL: Effect of acute indigestion on compartmental water volumes and osmolality in sheep, *Am J Vet Res* 32:887-890, 1971.

1134. Giesecke D, Stangassinger M: Lactic acid metabolism. In Ruckebush Y, Thivend P, eds: *Digestive physiology and metabolism in ruminants*, Lancaster, England, 1980, MTP Press.

1135. Dirksen G: Acidosis. In Phillipson AT, ed: *Proceedings of the Third International Symposium on the Physiology of Digestion and Metabolism in the Ruminant*, Newcastle, England, 1970, Oriel Press.

1136. Krehbiel CR et al: The effects of ruminal acidosis on volatile fatty acid absorption and plasma activities of pancreatic enzymes in lambs, *J Anim Sci* 73:3111-3121, 1995.

1137. Nagaraja TG et al: Effects of tylosin on concentrations of *Fusobacterium necrophorum* and fermentation products in the rumen of cattle fed a high-concentrate diet, *Am J Vet Res* 60:1061-1065, 1999.

1138. Andersen PH, Bergeln B, Christensen KA: Effect of feeding regimen on concentration of free endotoxin in ruminal fluid of cattle, *J Anim Sci* 72:487-491, 1994.

1139. Andersen PH, Hesselholt M, Jarlov N: Endotoxin and arachidonic acid metabolites in portal, hepatic and arterial blood of cattle with acute ruminal acidosis, *Acta Vet Scand* 35:223-234, 1994.

1140. Aiumlamai S et al: The role of endotoxins in induced ruminal acidosis in calves, *Acta Vet Scand* 33:117-127, 1992.

1141. Ras A, Janowski T, Zdunczyk S: Einfluss subklinischer und acuter Azidose ante partum bei Kuhen auf den Graviditatsverlauf unter Berucksichtung der Steroidhormonprofile: *Tierarztl Prax* 24:347-352, 1996.

1142. Goad DW, Goad CL, Nagaraja TG: Ruminal microbial and fermentative changes associated with experimentally induced subacute acidosis in steers, *J Anim Sci* 76:234-241, 1998.

1143. Trenkle A: The relationship between acid-base balance and protein metabolism in ruminants. In Hale WH, Meinhadt P, eds: *Regulation of acid-base balance*, Piscataway, NJ, 1979, Church & Dwight.

1144. Aafjes JH: Carbonic anhydrase in the wall of the forestomachs of cows, *Br Vet J* 123:252-255, 1967.

1145. Osweiler GD et al: Urea and nonprotein nitrogen. In *Clinical and diagnostic veterinary toxicology*, ed 3, Dubuque, Iowa, 1985, Kendall/Hunt Publishing, pp 160-166.

1146. air CK: Urea (ammonia) toxicosis in cattle, *Bovine Pract* 24:67-73, 1989.

1147. CL, Drackley JK: *The development, nutrition, and management of the young calf*, Ames, Iowa, 1998, Iowa State University Press.

1148. Giesecke D: Die Funktionelle vormagenentwicklung des Wiederkauers, *Tierarztl Umschau* 22:398-403, 1976.

1149. Franco A et al: Histormorphometric analysis of the rumen of sheep during development, *Am J Vet Res* 53:1209-1217, 1992.

1150. Scholz H: Utilization of the reticular groove contraction in adult cattle: a therapeutic alternative for the practitioner? *Bovine Pract* 23:148-152, 1988.

1151. Schloz H, Mikhail M: Untersuchungen zur Nutzung der Schlundrinnenkontraktion in der Behandlung innerer Erkankungen des erwachsenen Rindes 1. Mittleilung: Auslos-barkeit der Schlundrinnenkontraktion durch intravenose Verabreichung von Vasopressin, *Tierarztl Umschau* 42:280-287, 1987.

1152. Breukink HJ et al: Consequences of failure of the reticular groove reflex in veal calves fed milk replacer, *Vet Q* 10:126-135, 1988.

1153. Chapman HW, Butler DG, Newell M: The route of liquids administered to calves by esophageal feeder, *Can J Vet Res* 50:84-87, 1986.

1154. Dirr L, Dirksen G: Dysfunktion der Schlundrinne ("Pansentrinken") als Komplikation der Neugeborenendiarrho beim Kalb, *Tierarztl Prax* 17:353-358, 1989.

1155. Stocker H, Rusch P: Chronische Indigestion beim Milchkalb, *Schwz Arch Tierheil* 141:407-411, 1999.

1156. Gentile A et al: Systemische Auswirkungen der Panzenazidose im Gefolge von Pansentrinken beim Milchkalb, *Tierarztl Prax* 26:205-209, 1998.

1157. Dirksen G: Linkseitige labmagenverlagerung bei Kalb und Jungrind, *Tierarztl Umschau* 36:674-680, 1981.

1158. Braun U, Gotz M: Ultrasonography of the reticulum in cows, *Am J Vet Res* 55:325-332, 1994.

1159. Rebhun WC: Rumen collapse in cattle, *Cornell Vet* 77:244-250, 1987.

1160. Stober M, Serrano HS: Gross findings in bovine feces, *Vet Med Rev* 4:361-379, 1974.

1161. McGuirk SM, Benarsi RM, Clayton MK: Bradycardia in cattle deprived of food, *J Am Vet Med Assoc* 196:894-896, 1990.

1162. Braun U, Rihs T, Schefer U: Ruminal lactic acidosis in sheep and goats, *Vet Rec* 130:343-349, 1992.

1163. Dirksen G, Smith MC: Acquisition and analysis of bovine rumen fluid, *Bovine Pract* 22:108-116, 1987.

1164. Wagner D, Elmer-Englhard D: Vergleichende Prufung von vier Sonden zur Pansensaftentnahme beim erwachsenen Rind unter Berucksichtigung des Speichelzuflusses in der abgesaugten Probe, *Tierarztl Prax* 16:133-138, 1988.

1165. Nordlund KV, Garrett EF: Rumenocentesis: a technique for collecting rumen fluid for the diagnosis of subacute rumen acidosis in dairy herds, *Bovine Pract* 28:109-112, 1994.

1166. Garrett EF et al: Diagnostic methods for the detection of subacute ruminal acidosis in dairy cows, *J Dairy Sci* 82:1170-1178, 1999.

1167. Dirksen G, Wolf L: Wie lange und bei welcher Auf-bewahrungstemperatur ist pansensaft fur Diagnostische und Therapeutische zwecke brauchbar? *Tierarztl Umschau* 18:282-284, 1963.

1168. Kaufmann W: Uber die regulierung des pH-Wertes im hauben-pansenraum der Wiederkauer, *Tierarztl Umschau* 27:324-328, 1972.

1169. Nichols RE, Penn KE: Simple methods for the detection of unfavorable changes in the ruminal ingesta, *J Am Vet Med Assoc* 133:275-277, 1958.

1170. Dirksen G: Ist die Metylenblauprobe als Schnelltest fur die Klinische Pansensaftuntersuchung geeignet? *DTW* 76:305-309, 1969.

1171. Gartley C, Ogilvie TH, Butler DG: Magnesium oxide contraindicated as a cathartic for cattle in the absence of rumen acidosis, *Proceedings of the Thirteenth Annual Convention of the American Association of Bovine Practitioners* 13:17-19, 1981.

1172. Rebhun WC, Fubini SL, Miller TK: Vagus indigestion in cattle: clinical features, causes, treatments, and long-term follow-up of 112 cases, *Compend Cont Educ* 10:387-391, 1988.

1173. Orpin CG: Studies on the defaunation of the ovine rumen using dioctyl sodium sulfosuccinate, *J Appl Bacteriol* 43:309-318, 1977.

1174. Garry F, Kallfelz FA: Clinical aspects of dietary buffers for dairy cattle, *Compend Cont Educ* 5:S159-S167, 1983.

1175. Nagaraja TG et al: Effect of lasalocid, monensin or thiopeptin in lactic acidosis in cattle, *J Anim Sci* 54:649-658, 1982.

1176. Chalupa W: Chemical control of rumen microbial metabolism. In Ruckebush Y, Thivend P, eds: *Digestive physiology and metabolism in ruminants*, Lancaster, England, 1980, MTP Press.

TRAUMATIC RETICULOPERITONITIS (Hardware Disease; Traumatic Reticulitis; TRP)

CHARLES GUARD

DEFINITION AND ETIOLOGY. Traumatic reticuloperitonitis (TRP), or hardware disease, is a common disease of cattle but rarely seen in small ruminants. The ingestive behavior of cattle predisposes them to the accidental swallowing of metal foreign objects that settle in the reticulum. Subsequently the foreign object may penetrate the reticulum and cause localized or generalized peritonitis. In some cases only the wall of the reticulum is involved; intramural inflammation may result in dysfunction of the rumenoreticulum because of interference with chemoreceptors or mechanoreceptors. The diaphragm, pericardium, and heart muscle are located just cranial to the reticulum and the liver medially and dorsally. These organs may sometimes be penetrated by foreign bodies and become involved in the inflammatory process.

CLINICAL SIGNS AND DIFFERENTIAL DIAGNOSIS. Traumatic reticuloperitonitis in the most severe, acute form is characterized by fever, anorexia, decreased or absent rumen contractions, and evidence of cranial abdominal pain. Pinching of the withers or upward pressure on the xiphoid region may elicit a grunt on expiration. Affected cattle may stand with an arched back and resist ventral flexion of the back when pinched over the withers (normal cattle flex ventrally).

Some cattle grunt spontaneously when forced to move or when defecating or urinating. Lactating cows show a sudden decrease in milk production.[1177,1178] Some cows regurgitate rumen fluid, especially if the oropharynx is mechanically stimulated. Tachycardia, reluctance to move or lie down, mild bloat, constipation, or abducted elbows may also be seen. These typical signs often abate within the first day or two, making diagnosis more difficult. Auscultation may reveal a pounding heart or muffled heart sounds bilaterally if pericarditis has developed by the time of examination. Sudden death has occurred as a result of the laceration of a coronary blood vessel or puncture of the heart by the foreign body.

Less severe or more long-standing cases may have signs that are more subtle and confusing. Cows in early lactation may have ketosis; however, a distinguishing feature of hardware disease is the abrupt onset of anorexia and hypogalactia. Fever may be absent. Weight loss, rough hair coat, diarrhea, or generalized lameness, along with cranial abdominal pain that is difficult to localize, may be the only signs. If the pericardial sac has been seeded with bacteria, pericarditis usually develops. Distended jugular and superficial abdominal veins and other signs of congestive right-sided heart failure are most common after pericarditis. Dyspnea may occur if left-sided failure is also present. The foreign body may penetrate the liver or spleen, leading to abscess formation. These abscesses may be responsible for other signs of gastrointestinal malfunction, particularly ruminoreticular outflow problems. These are further discussed with vagal syndrome and indigestion.

Other diseases to consider in evaluating a potential hardware disease patient are abomasal ulcers, hepatic abscesses from other causes, lymphosarcoma of the abomasum or heart, laminitis, indigestion, cor pulmonale, endoparasitism, intestinal carcinoma, diaphragmatic hernia, and systemic leptospirosis.

CLINICAL PATHOLOGY. The white blood cell count and distribution, plasma proteins, and plasma fibrinogen may be normal in the initial stages of the condition. A standard hemogram may reflect an acute or chronic infectious process, depending on the stage of the disease when examined. Total plasma proteins of 10 g/dl or greater, primarily reflecting globulin levels, were shown to have a predictive positive value of 76% in diagnosing traumatic reticuloperitonitis in a referral population, which reflects a process that has been going on for at least several days.[1179] Abdominocentesis may be rewarding if the peritonitis is not extremely well localized. Abdominal fluid analysis is discussed in the section on peritonitis. Pericardiocentesis may be performed at the level of the point of the elbow in the fifth left intercostal space. Aseptic preparation of the skin and local anesthesia of the region to be punctured are required; pulling the left forelimb forward may be helpful. A 5- to 10-cm spinal needle or intravenous catheter can be used; the length required depends on the size of the animal and the amount of subcutaneous fat. Caution is advised when advancing the needle to prevent laceration of the myocardium. Visual inspection of the fluid obtained is usually adequate to confirm the diagnosis of pericarditis. The fluid may be examined bacteriologically and cytologically. If ileus occurs, the chloride ion concentration in rumen fluid may be elevated as a result of reflux from the abomasum and omasum; hypochloremic metabolic alkalosis may also develop. Radiography can demonstrate the presence of metallic foreign bodies in the reticulum, but surgery may be necessary to confirm their significance. Radiographs may be made with a horizontal beam with the cow standing or cast in dorsal recumbency.[1180]

PATHOPHYSIOLOGY. The indiscriminant eating habits of cattle lead to accidental consumption of foreign bodies. Those that are of high specific gravity initially settle to the bottom of the ventral sac of the rumen. Subsequent contraction cycles of the forestomach dump those objects in the rumen into the reticulum. If the object is large enough and sharp enough, it can be pushed, most often through the cranial wall of the reticulum, by the forceful, normal reticular contractions. Normal forestomach bacteria leak through the hole thus created and may establish infection locally along the foreign body. Infection also may spread as in the pericardium or locally during abscess formation. The pain and inflammation associated with the trauma and infection lead to decreased appetite and rumen hypomotility or stasis. Agalactia is abrupt because of the acute anorexia and subsequent failure to absorb precursors for milk synthesis.

EPIDEMIOLOGY. The ingestive techniques of cattle allow sharp nonfood items to be prehended and swallowed. Ingestion of such items by sheep or goats is extremely rare. The disease affects confined cattle where mechanical processing of forages or construction activities increase the chances that wire or nails will be included in the feed. Most cases are sporadic, but outbreaks have occurred when such things as multistranded cable have been chopped up by a forage harvester and ensiled.

NECROPSY FINDINGS. Cattle that die peracutely may have a lacerated myocardium with resulting hemorrhage or cardiac tamponade. Diffuse peritonitis characterized by copious, foul-smelling peritoneal fluid with an obvious reticular defect may be seen in acute cases. More chronically affected animals may have extensive pericardial effusion with a thick epicardial layer of fibrin. The penetrating foreign body generally is still present in the wall of the reticulum or pericardium.

TREATMENT AND PROGNOSIS. Conservative treatment generally is attempted first and includes the administration of a forestomach magnet, parenteral antibiotic therapy, and confinement. Often the animal is confined to a stanchion or box stall. Many cattle recover after such a course of therapy with resumption of forestomach motility and appetite within 1 to 3 days. Animals that have not significantly improved by the third day may require a rumenotomy to remove the foreign object. Cattle with diffuse peritonitis have a poor prognosis for life. Treatment of peritonitis requires systemic antibiotic therapy, possibly drainage of the affected area, and surgical correction of the inciting cause (see Peritonitis, below). Animals with seemingly uncomplicated short-term recoveries may later experience forestomach outflow problems typical of vagal indigestion syndrome or pericarditis and signs of right-sided heart failure.

PREVENTION AND CONTROL. Eliminating sources of sharp foreign objects in the feed supply prevents traumatic reticuloperitonitis. Installation of large magnets on feed handling equipment and prophylactic administration of forestomach magnets to all animals at 6 to 8 months of age prevent almost all cases caused by magnetizable objects.

REFERENCES

1177. Pinsent PJN: The diagnosis of the surgical disorders of the bovine abdomen, *Bovine Pract* 12:40-47, 1977.
1178. Herringer RW, Mullowney PC: Anterior abdominal pain in cattle, *Compend Cont Educ Pract Vet* 6:S453-S463, 1984.
1179. Dubensky RA, White ME: The sensitivity, specificity and predictive value of total plasma protein in the diagnosis of traumatic reticuloperitonitis, *Can J Comp Med* 47:241-244, 1983.
1180. Ducharme NG, Dill SG, Rendano VT: Reticulography of the cow in dorsal recumbency: an aid in the diagnosis and treatment of traumatic reticuloperitonitis, *J Am Vet Med Assoc* 182:585-588, 1983.

PERITONITIS IN THE RUMINANT

GILLES FECTEAU

Despite the frequency with which peritonitis is included in a list of differential diagnoses, it remains a very frustrating dis-

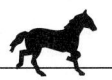

ease for all food animal clinicians. A diagnosis often is based on clinical signs and history and the course often is not confirmed by ancillary tests. If the patient improves with treatment, the clinician often does not learn the cause of peritonitis.

REVIEW OF THE PERITONEAL CAVITY

Histology

The peritoneal cavity is lined by a serous membrane composed of two layers called the peritoneum. The deeper layer (subserosa) is composed of loose connective tissue containing collagen, fat cells, reticulum cells, and macrophages.[1181] Covering that layer is a single-surface layer of mesothelial squamous cells (serosa). On the surface of the diaphragm, special lymphatic collecting vessels are located under the mesothelial basement membrane. Small stomata are found between mesothelial cells. They act as channels for lymphatic drainage from the peritoneal cavity to the thoracic duct.[1182-1184]

Normal Peritoneal Fluid

The peritoneum is a highly permeable membrane. Most of it acts as a bidirectional semipermeable barrier to diffusion of water and low molecular weight solutes between blood and peritoneal fluid.[1182-1186] That is the reason renal failure can be treated effectively by peritoneal dialysis. Normal peritoneal fluid provides lubrication for the movement of abdominal organs and apposed peritoneal surfaces.[1187] It is formed and resorbed constantly. Normal fluid movement is achieved by normal movement of the viscera and contraction of the diaphragm during respiration. A normal animal has no more than 1 ml of peritoneal fluid per kilogram of body weight.[1186] In acute severe peritonitis the inflammatory process may induce a net flow of liters (80 ml/kg/day in humans) of proteinaceous fluid, leading to hypoproteinemia or hypovolemic shock or both.[1182]

Normal bovine peritoneal fluid has a wide range of values.[1184,1188-1191] It should be clear and have a specific density below 1.016 (Table 30-11). The protein content should be less than 3 g/dl, although some authors have reported normal values up to 6.3 g/dl.[1191] Normal bovine peritoneal fluid may contain some fibrinogen and clot when exposed to air.[1192] Normal fluid contains fewer than 10,000 cells, mostly

macrophages. Lymphocytes, eosinophils, and desquamated mesothelial cells may also be present. Normally very few neutrophils are present. Periparturient cattle have significantly more abdominal fluid with a lower protein concentration.[1192] There may even be a complete absence of collectable peritoneal fluid because of dehydration or fibrous adhesions, which are commonly found in bovine peritonitis.

PATHOPHYSIOLOGIC MECHANISMS OF DISEASES IN THE PERITONEAL CAVITY IN RESPONSE TO INJURY

Healing

Peritoneal regeneration is complete within 5 to 7 days, regardless of the defect size. Healing can occur by reperitonealization or creation of an adhesion with an adjacent nearby mesothelial surface. This adherent type of healing occurs more often if the inflammation is severe, with the presence of bacteria or foreign material.[1182,1183,1186]

Host Defenses Against Peritoneal Infection

The first mechanism of defense is physical removal of the bacteria. In normal dogs, for example, it is possible to retrieve bacteria in the bloodstream 12 minutes after an experimental injection into the peritoneum.[1186] The second mechanism of defense relates to the response to noxious stimuli. This is an intense, acute inflammatory response that includes degranulation of peritoneal mast cells with release of vasoactive substances. This creates a net influx of fluid rich in complement and serum opsonins that can bind to the bacteria.[1182,1183,1186] As the third mechanism of defense, the omentum adheres to an infected or damaged area to wall off the problem site. The rapid movement of neutrophils and, later, macrophages is also an important mechanism of control against infection.[1186]

Adhesions

Adhesions are defined as fibrinous or fibrous bands that create an abnormal attachment of two or more surfaces that should be moving freely on each other. Formation of adhesions is part of the healing process and should be interpreted as an effort to control an injury. The omentum is often involved in adhesions and acts as a natural sealing device to control the acute phase of inflammation. Whole blood potentiates adhesion formation by providing more fibrinogen.[1182] Proper ligature and abdominal lavage after a surgical intervention reduce the risk of adhesion formation. The various suture materials are approximately equal in their capacity to induce adhesions, with chromic gut perhaps inducing the most reaction.[1182] Adhesion may or may not be reversible, depending on the amount of organization that takes place in the process. Adhesions that are cut or broken usually reform rapidly As the fibrin deposition process is replaced by capillaries and fibroblasts, the adhesion becomes solid fibrous tissue. The three major elements responsible for dissolution of the fibrinous adhesions are (1) adequate oxygen and nutrient supply for the mesothelium, (2) liberation of plasminogen-activating substance by mesothelial and submesothelial cells, and (3) control of the inflammatory process.[1182,1183] Major undesirable side effects of formation of adhesions are mechanical obstruction to the normal flow of ingesta and subsequent development of bowel obstruction.

PERITONITIS

DEFINITION AND ETIOLOGY. Peritonitis is an inflammatory process that involves the peritoneal cavity and its serosal surface, the peritoneum. This may result from trauma or surgery

TABLE 30-11

Normal Range for Classification of Bovine Peritoneal Fluid According to Different Authors

Parameters	Normal Values	References
Turbidity	Clear	1188,1191,1211
Total protein (g/dl)	0.1-3.1	1211
	<3.0	1188
	2.2-4.0	1212
	1.2-6.3	1191
Specific gravity	1.005-1.015	1211
Total cell count (×1000/μl)	425-2950	1212
	300-5300	1211
	2000-5000	1191
	<10,000	1188
Differential	Ratio 1:1, neutrophils to mononuclear cells	1188, 1211
Neutrophils	45-2183	1212
Lymphocytes	8-168	1212
Mononuclear cells	36-960	1212
Eosinophils	5-545	1212
Comments	Eosinophils may predominate	1188
	Serosa cells may predominate	1191

or from vascular damage associated with an intestinal obstruction or accident or from gastrointestinal ulceration (Box 30-8). Peritonitis is a serious and complex process that often is accompanied by various degrees of abdominal pain, progressive signs of hypovolemia and septicemia, or endotoxemia.

CLASSIFICATION. Peritonitis may be classified according to the clinical presentation or the cause, or both. Clinically relevant classifications include acute or chronic, septic or chemical, localized or generalized, and primary or secondary. Although it is useful to classify types of peritonitis, it is imperative to recognize that it is a dynamic process. An apparently localized, nonseptic peritonitis can evolve into a more diffuse septic process if the primary cause is not resolved.

PATHOPHYSIOLOGY. After peritoneal contamination or injury, mesothelial cells initiate an inflammatory response that modifies the permeability of the peritoneum and its vascular supply. Several blood constituents are then able to move into the peritoneal cavity. Macrophages and polymorphonuclear cells, humoral opsonins, natural antibodies, serum complement, and a protein-rich fluid are the most important. The inflamed peritoneum also becomes more permeable to toxins, allowing them to be absorbed into the bloodstream. Although this initial response is beneficial to the organism, it induces several systemic abnormalities that the clinician must recognize and treat adequately.

Hypovolemia, hypoproteinemia, bacteremia or septicemia, and toxemia are commonly observed in acute diffuse septic peritonitis. The major adverse effects of peritoneal contamination are (1) rapid clearance of bacteria producing endotoxemia and/or bacteremia, (2) rapid influx of fluid rich in protein, leading to hypovolemia and hypoproteinemia, (3) deposition of fibrin, which occludes lymphatic drainage, contributing to abdominal distention and enhancing the chance of abscess formation, (4) ileus, and (5) adhesion formation, which may lead to obstruction (Fig. 30-54).

CLINICAL SIGNS AND DIAGNOSIS. Clinical signs often are nonspecific but suggestive of gastrointestinal dysfunction. The severity of clinical signs ranges from mild, recurrent discomfort caused by a localized abscess to an acute severe onset of toxemia and hypovolemia leading rapidly to death after the sudden rupture of a viscus. Cattle suffering from acute peritonitis tend to show more characteristic signs. As the condition becomes less acute, the ability of the bovine to seal the infection attenuates the clinical signs. Chronic but active peritonitis remains to this day a very difficult diagnosis to make without an exploratory laparotomy. Abdominal rigidity and tenderness, abdominal distention, scleral injection, fever, anorexia, and sudden reduction in milk production are typical but not pathognomonic findings of acute peritonitis. In the acute stage, abdominal pain and the release of catecholamines often lead to a complete gastrointestinal stasis and ileus. The rumen is then completely atonic. Feces are abnormal in quantity and quality. In the acute stage, feces are present in small amounts and often dry. In more chronic cases, feces are present with a tendency to be diarrheic. Pain, decreased plasma volume, and endotoxemia often result in persistent tachycardia. Anterior abdominal pain, evaluated by the "skooch test," or withers pinch, may be difficult to interpret. The skooch test is based on the normal reflex of the bovine to drop its back when the withers and back are pinched (ventroflexion). Cattle with anterior abdominal pain may be reluctant to ventroflex on withers pinch. The sensitivity of this test can be increased by simultaneous auscultation of the trachea during the manipulation. Production of an expiratory grunt is considered a sign of pain during ventroflexion. Cranial ventral pressure with the fist, knee, or some other external force (transverse pole under the abdomen) just behind the xiphoid can help identify the presence of pain (expiratory grunt) and even localize it in some

BOX 30-8

Causes and Examples of Peritonitis in Approximate Order of Frequency

TRAUMATIC PERFORATION
Traumatic reticuloperitonitis
Septic abdominal surgery
Vaginal perforation in heifer during coitus
Penetrating wound

VISCERAL RUPTURE
Perforated abomasal ulcer
Perforated ulcer in other part of gastrointestinal tract (oak toxicity of other cause)
Abomasal rupture after torsion
Small intestinal rupture after volvulus, strangulated hernia, intussusception
Ruptured bladder secondary to urolithiasis
Spontaneous uterine rupture during gestation/dystocia

ABSCESS FORMATION AND POSSIBLE INTRAABOMINAL RUPTURE
Reticuloperitonitis, localized
Liver
Umbilicus
Perimetritis
Pyelonephritis

IATROGENIC
Intraperitoneal injection of irritant solution or contaminated solution
Uterine rupture during dystocia
Perforation of the uterine wall with a pipette
Rectal tear secondary to palpation

MISCELLANEOUS
Hematogenous with systemic infection: tuberculosis, septicemia
Fat necrosis

cases. It is my impression that the most reliable sign of abdominal discomfort in cattle is reluctance to move. Scleral injection, fever, tachycardia, gastrointestinal stasis, and distention are the clinical signs that should be monitored to evaluate peritonitis.

ANCILLARY TESTS. Hematologic findings associated with peritonitis range from a completely normal hemogram, to an increased fibrinogen, to severe leukopenia with degenerative left shift and presence of toxic neutrophils, depending on the severity of the peritoneal contamination. In severe cases variations observed reflect the degree of sepsis and toxemia. Packed cell volume tends to increase as proteins decrease. In less severe cases, a neutrophilic leukocytosis and hyperfibrinogenemia often are present. Hematologic analysis has been a very useful tool for monitoring response to therapy after a diagnosis has been made by other ancillary tests. Immature cells in the peripheral blood or leukocytosis (or both) were better indicators of recurrence than body temperature in one human study.[1193] The plasma fibrinogen concentration also is used to monitor the progress of a particular case.

The blood chemistry profile is rarely altered by peritonitis in a way that is diagnostically useful. Chronic inflammation causes a marked increase in serum proteins, particularly the globulin portion. In acute severe cases, secondary findings may include increased serum urea nitrogen and creatinine, mildly increased liver enzymes, reduction in total carbon

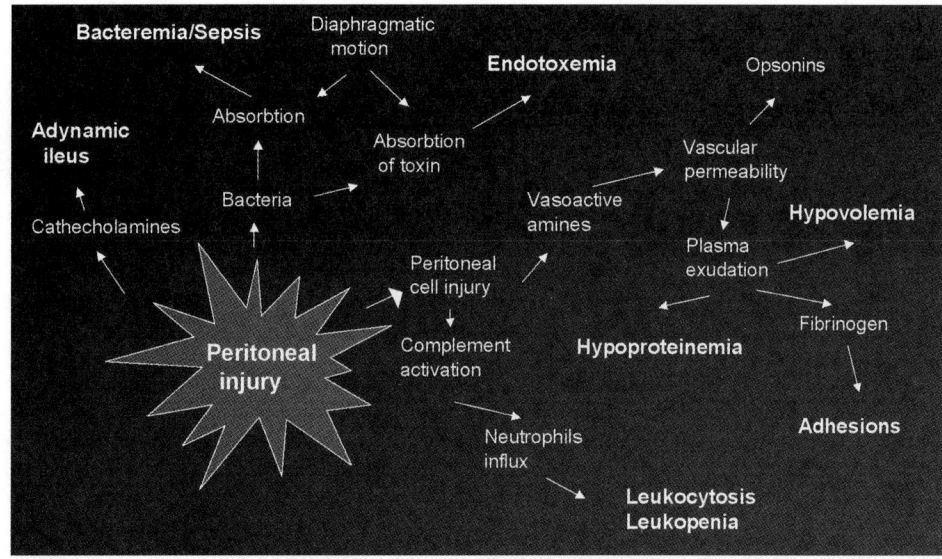

FIG. 30-54 ▌▌ Pathophysiology of peritonitis.

dioxide and strong ion difference and reduction in serum protein (albumin and globulins). Ileus and stasis of the upper gastrointestinal system may result in marked hypochloremia and alkalosis.

Cytologic examination of the peritoneal fluid is a useful aid in making a definitive diagnosis of peritonitis (see Table 30-11).[1194] Abdominocentesis techniques have been described elsewhere.[1182] The right side just cranial to the udder is the preferred site (to avoid the stomach and omentum) (Fig 30-55). Either a needle, a blunt teat cannula, or a bitch catheter may be used with success (Fig. 30-56). The heavy fascia of bulls makes a needle preferable. It is imperative to remember that failure to secure fluid is common and should be interpreted with caution because fibrinous peritonitis with fluid loculation is common. More than one site should be attempted if no fluid is secured on the first attempt. Interpretation and classification of peritoneal fluid analyses have been reviewed by several authors.[1184,1188,1189,1192] The influence of exploratory celiotomy and omentopexy on peritoneal fluid analysis was studied by Anderson et al.[1195] It should be remembered that because of the bovine's ability to deposit fibrin and seal areas of the peritoneal cavity, the interpretation of peritoneal fluid analysis applies only to the immediate area that was sampled. The clinician can be misled and conclude that a nonseptic process is occurring on the basis of a caudal tap, when in fact a septic process has already been sealed by the fibrin deposition in the cranial abdomen.

Abdominal radiographs using a high-power unit are extremely useful when reticuloperitonitis is suspected,[1196] but they are of limited value in other causes of peritonitis. A review of radiography of the bovine cranioventral abdomen is available.[1197]

Ultrasound examination is useful for assessing the size and anatomic relationships of lesions, particularly when drainage, aspiration, or surgical exploration of a mass surrounding vital structures is considered. Knowledge of the underlying anatomy is important to prevent misinterpretation of images. Clarity of the image is affected by the size of the probe and the depth of tissue being evaluated. Higher frequency probes produce finer images but have limited tissue penetration. Images reflect the echogenicity of the tissues viewed; relative echogenicity helps to differentiate structures. Abscesses can have mixed echogenicity, varying from anechoic (absence of internal echoes) to echo-

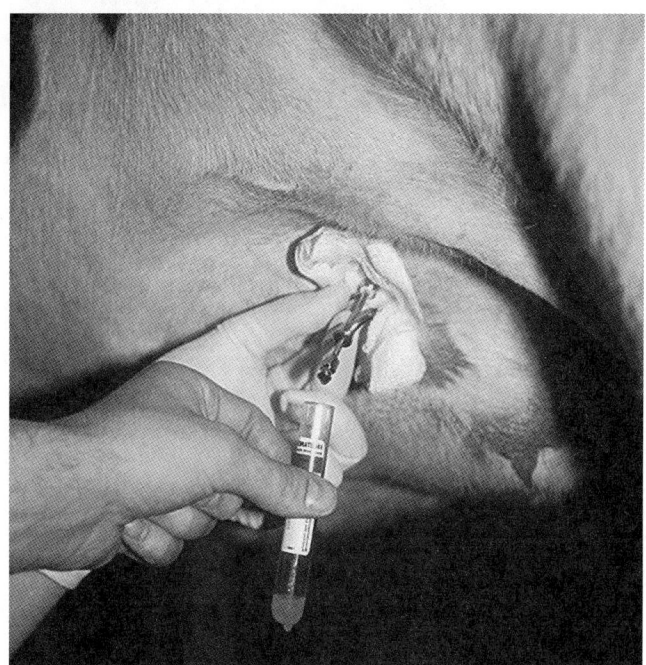

FIG. 30-55 ▌▌ Site of caudal abdominocentesis.

genic, depending on the relative amount of fluid, fibrin, and gas. The fibrous capsule of abscesses may be identified as echogenic bands around the area in question. Ultrasound examination is particularly useful for evaluating the integrity of the body wall for hernias caused by traumatic injuries or that occur secondary to abscessation or incision dehiscence. The umbilical structures' normal and abnormal appearances have been described.[1199,1200] Free abdominal fluid is easily recognized by ultrasound examination, which is also useful to guide a peritoneal tap. Areas that should be scanned include the caudal lower flank area (right and left), right perirenal area, liver, abomasum and pylorus, and right paramedian area. The normal liver and liver abscess formation has been described.[1200,1201]

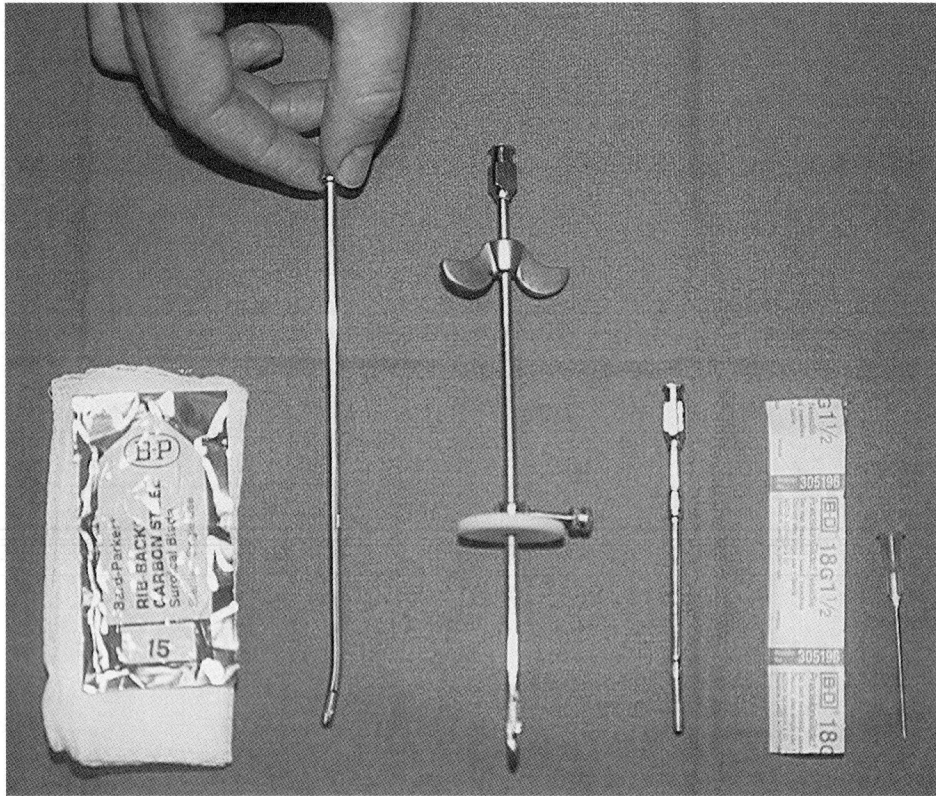

FIG. 30-56 ▌ Material used to perform abdominocentesis in the bovine.

References are available describing the normal appearance of the reticulum and the small intestine in cows.[1202,1203] During an exploratory surgery, ultrasound can be used to image an internal mass or viscera appearing abnormal. Intraoperative ultrasound is performed by placing the probe in a sterile sleeve filled with ultrasound gel.

Surgical exploration often is done to confirm or rule out an intraabdominal problem.[1204] Information obtained from the physical examination and laboratory data often is indicative of a diagnosis of peritonitis but does not provide a specific cause. Cattle are particularly amenable to exploratory surgery, because the procedure is performed while they are standing and is associated with few complications.

TREATMENT. The basic aims of therapy should be as follows[1205]:

1. Stabilize the patient's condition with supportive therapy, including correction of acid-base and electrolyte abnormalities, administration of calcium to promote gastrointestinal motility, and transfaunation
2. Identify and correct the primary cause in a manner that does not compromise the patient's survival
3. Treat the infection by medical procedures and by surgical procedures if indicated

Stabilize: Keep the Patient Alive! Depending on the severity of the process, the patient may appear to be in shock. Large volumes of isotonic intravenous fluids are indicated. Hypertonic saline solution or hypertonic saline-dextran solution has been reported to induce beneficial hemodynamic effects in hypovolemic human beings,[1206] dogs,[1207] horses,[1208] and calves. At this time no studies have been published on these solutions' efficacy in the treatment of acute diffuse peritonitis in cattle. Correction of any acid-base deficit is indicated. Electrolyte abnormalities (hypokalemia and hypocalcemia) should be identified and corrected. If the animal is hypoproteinemic, plasma or whole blood transfusions may be indicated. Nonsteroidal or fast-acting steroidal antiin-

flammatory drugs (or both) are essential to prevent the synthesis of more inflammatory mediators. Control of pain may be beneficial but should be pursued with caution when the exact cause of the problem has not been identified.

Find the Cause, but Above All, Do No Harm! It is useful to identify the primary cause of peritonitis, but not at any price. Successful treatment of gastrointestinal leakage from an ulcer requires surgical repair. However, unnecessary exploratory surgery helps to spread and increase the inflammatory process.

Medically and Surgically Control the Infection; Be Aggressive! Systemic antibiotic therapy should be instituted as soon as a decision to treat is made. Until the results of culture and antimicrobial susceptibility are available, a broad-spectrum antibiotic or a combination of antibiotics should be used. The choice should take into consideration the cost of treatment, the withdrawal period whether the drug is approved for use in food animals, the spectrum of activity, and the treatment regimen (frequency and route). Intravenous (IV) therapy should be recommended when possible, especially early in the course of the disease. A long-term IV catheter* has been used at the farm with good results. Written instructions to the owner should be clear.

When a single antimicrobial drug is to be used, tetracycline or a β-lactam antibiotic (third-generation cephalosporin or synthetic penicillin) probably is the best choice. Diffusion into the peritoneal cavity is not a major limiting factor, because the permeability of the peritoneum is always increased in peritonitis.

Surgical control of peritonitis includes peritoneal debridement, irrigation, and drainage.[1209] Ultrasound guidance can be used to establish drainage from the abdominal cavity. A thoracic chest trocar can be used temporarily until all fluid has been removed. Aseptic preparation is essential, and ul-

---

*Arrow International, Inc., 2400 Bernville Road, Reading, PA 19605.

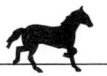

Causes and Examples of Pneumoperitoneum in Approximate Order of Frequency

TRAUMATIC PERFORATION
Traumatic reticuloperitonitis
Septic abdominal surgery
Vaginal perforation in heifer during coitus
Penetrating wound

VISCERAL RUPTURE
Perforated abomasal ulcer
Perforated ulcer in other part of gastrointestinal tract
Abomasal rupture after torsion
Small intestinal rupture after volvulus, strangulated hernia, intussusception
Ruptured bladder secondary to urolithiasis
Spontaneous uterine rupture during gestation
Uterine rupture during dystocia

ABSCESS FORMATION AND POSSIBLE INTRAABDOMINAL RUPTURE
Reticuloperitonitis localized
Liver
Umbilicus
Perimetritis
Pyelonephritis
Iatrogenic
Intraperitoneal injection of irritant solution or contaminated solution
Perforation of the uterine wall with a pipette
Rectal tear secondary to palpation

MISCELLANEOUS
Hematogenous with systemic infection: tuberculosis, septicemia
Fat necrosis

---

trasound guidance makes that procedure safer and more useful. If surgery is performed to identify the cause, the abdomen should be lavaged with an isotonic solution and fluids should be aspirated by gravity or with a suction device. This procedure can be repeated until the fluid comes out clear. In my experience, drainage of the abdomen with Foley catheters or negative pressure drains has been consistently unsuccessful in the bovine species. Because of the bovine's ability to deposit large amounts of fibrin in a short period and because of the presence of the omentum, those drains plug and become inefficient quite rapidly.

PROGNOSIS. The ultimate outcome of an episode of bacterial peritonitis is determined by many factors, some of which are controlled by the clinician. An early decision on treatment (medical and surgical), the correct choice of antimicrobial drugs, and adequate supportive therapy contribute to the success or failure of a therapy. Owner delay in seeking therapy, the primary cause of the peritonitis, and the patient's age are important factors beyond the clinician's control. In animals, when aggressive therapy is economically possible, survival rates are good, but long-term sequelae may compromise a complete recovery.

MISCELLANEOUS CONDITIONS

Ascites

Ascites is a collection of serous fluid in the peritoneal cavity. It must be considered a secondary sign rather than a primary diagnosis.[1210] In that regard the primary cause must be iden-

tified in order to treat the patient adequately. Common causes of ascites in ruminants include severe liver disease and congestive right-sided heart failure. Young cattle with mesothelioma have remarkable ascites. Ascites is an uncommon condition that must be differentiated from septic causes of peritonitis and urine accumulation with a ruptured bladder.

Pneumoperitoneum

Pneumoperitoneum is commonly observed after surgery in the bovine. The presence of air in the abdomen can be recognized by simultaneous percussion and auscultation. A low-pitch resonance can be auscultated in the upper flank on both sides of the abdomen. Air will sometimes accumulate subcutaneously as it escapes. The pneumoperitoneum normally resolves in the week after surgery. No clinical signs seem to be associated with pneumoperitoneum, although some clinicians describe abdominal pain that is associated with no cause other than the presence of air in the peritoneal cavity. Pneumoperitoneum not associated with surgery is indicative of bacterial peritonitis and the presence of gas-producing bacteria (Box 30-9).

REFERENCES

1181. Banks WJ: Digestive system. In *Applied veterinary histology*, Baltimore, 1981, Williams & Wilkins.
1182. Crowe DT, Bjorling DE: Peritoneum and peritoneal cavity. In Slatter DH, ed: *Textbook of small animal surgery*, ed 2, vol 1, Philadelphia, 1993, WB Saunders.
1183. Hosgood GL, Salisbury K: Pathophysiology and pathogenesis of generalized peritonitis, *Probl Vet Med* 1:159-167, 1989.
1184. Kopcha M, Schultze AE: Peritoneal fluid. I. Pathophysiology and classification of nonneoplastic effusions, *Compend Cont Educ Pract Vet* 13:519-524, 1991.
1185. Hosgood G: Peritonitis. I, A review of the pathophysiology and diagnosis, *Aust Vet Pract* 16:184-190, 1986.
1186. Ahrenholz DH, Simmons RL: Peritonitis and other intraabdominal infections. In Simmons RL, Howard RJ, eds: *Surgical infectious diseases*, New York, 1982, Appleton-Century-Crofts.
1187. Bone JF: Digestive system. In *Animal anatomy and physiology*, ed 3, New Jersey, 1988, Prentice-Hall.
1188. Kopcha M, Schultze AE: Peritoneal fluid. II. Abdominocentesis in cattle and interpretation of nonneoplastic samples, *Compend Cont Educ Pract Vet* 13:703-709, 1991.
1189. Oehme FW, Noordsy JL: Examination of peritoneal fluid in differential diagnosis of bovine diseases, *Vet Med Small Anim Clin* 65:54-59, 1970.
1190. Oehme FW: Cytologic examination of the peritoneal fluid in the diagnosis of cattle disease, *J Am Vet Med Assoc* 155:1923-1927, 1969.
1191. Rosenberger G: *Clinical examination of cattle*, Philadelphia, 1979, WB Saunders.
1192. Wilson AD, Hirsch VM, Osborne AD: Abdominocentesis in cattle: technique and criteria for diagnosis of peritonitis, *Can Vet J* 26:74-80, 1985.
1193. Stone HH, Bourneuf AA, Stinson LD: Reliability of criteria for predicting persistence of recurrent sepsis, *Arch Surg* 120:17-20, 1985.
1194. Hirsch VM, Townsend HGG: Peritoneal fluid analysis in the diagnosis of abdominal disorders in cattle: a retrospective study, *Can Vet J* 23:348-354, 1982.
1195. Anderson DA et al: Comparison of peritoneal fluid analysis before and after exploratory celiotomy and omentopexy, *Am J Vet Res* 55: 1633-1637, 1994.
1196. Braun U, Flückiger M, Nägeli F: Radiography as an aid in the diagnosis of traumatic reticuloperitonitis in cattle, *Vet Rec* 132: 103-109, 1993.
1197. Partington BP, Biller DS: Radiography of the bovine cranioventral abdomen, *Vet Radiol* 32:155-168, 1991.
1198. Lischer CJ, Steiner A: Ultrasonography of umbilical structures in calves. I, Ultrasonographic description of umbilical involution in clinically healthy calves, *Schweiz Arch Tierheilk* 135: 221-230, 1993.
1199. Lischer CJ, Steiner A: Ultrasonography of umbilical structures in calves. II, Ultrasonography, diagnosis and treatment of umbilical diseases, *Schweiz Arch Tierheilk* 136: 227-241, 1994.
1200. Braun U: Ultrasonographic examination of the liver in cows, *Am J Vet Res* 51:1522-1526, 1990.
1201. Lechtenberg KF, Nagaraja TG: Hepatic ultrasonography and blood changes in cattle with experimentally induced hepatic abscesses, *Am J Vet Res* 52:803-809, 1991.
1202. Braun U: Ultrasonography of the reticulum in cows, *Am J Vet Res* 55:325-332, 1994.
1203. Braun U, Marmier O: Ultrasonographic examination of the small intestine of cows, *Vet Rec* 136:239-244, 1995.

1204. House JK et al: Ancillary tests for assessment of the ruminant digestive system, *Vet Clin North Am (Food Anim Pract)* 8:221-223, 1992.
1205. Salisbury K, Hosgood GL: Management of the patient with generalized peritonitis, *Probl Vet Med* 1:168-182, 1989.
1206. Holcroft JW et al: 3% NaCl and 7.5% NaCl/dextran 70 in the resuscitation of severely injured patients, *Ann Surg* 206:279-288, 1987.
1207. Lopes OU et al: Hypertonic sodium chloride restores mean circulatory filling pressure in severely hypovolemic dogs, *Proc Inter-Am Soc* 8(suppl): I195-I199, 1986.
1208. Schmall LM, Muir WW, Robertson JT: Haemodynamic effects of small volume hypertonic saline in experimentally induced haemorrhagic shock, *Equine Vet J* 22:273-277, 1990.
1209. McIlwraith CW: Equine digestive system. In Jennings PB, ed: *The practice of large animal surgery,* vol 1, Philadelphia, 1984, WB Saunders.
1210. Kruth SA: Abdominal distension, ascites, and peritonitis. In Ettinger SJ, Feldman EC, ed: *Textbook of veterinary internal medicine,* ed 5, vol 1, Philadelphia, 2000, WB Saunders.
1211. Blood DC, Gay CC, Radostits OM: *Veterinary medicine,* ed 8, London, 1994, Baillère Tindall.
1212. Anderson DA et al: Comparative analyses of peritoneal fluid from calves and adult cattle, *Am J Vet Res* 56:973-976, 1995.

BLOAT (RUMINAL TYMPANY)

CHARLES GUARD

DEFINITION AND ETIOLOGY. Bloat is the abnormal distention of the ruminant forestomach compartments with ingesta or gas. The three causative categories of bloat are (1) frothy bloat caused by diets that lead to the formation of stable froth in the rumen, (2) free gas bloat caused by diets that lead to excessive gas production and concomitant low intraruminal pH, and (3) free gas bloat caused by failure to eructate from extraruminal causes of gas accumulation. Ruminal tympany is synonymous with bloat. The condition may be fatal if the distention is extreme enough to compromise ventilation by compressing the thoracic viscera. Cattle are more susceptible than sheep, but the disease does occur in the same circumstances in small ruminants.

CLINICAL SIGNS AND DIFFERENTIAL DIAGNOSIS. The degree of forestomach enlargement varies from that producing an even filling of the left paralumbar fossa to that causing a uniform, extreme abdominal enlargement when the animal is viewed from the rear. With intermediate degrees of distention, the left paralumbar fossa bulges beyond the contours of the last rib and the tuber coxae. Signs of colic may be seen, including kicking at the abdomen, treading, frequent lying down and rising, and vocalizations. Some animals adopt a stretched stance with the rear feet placed far back. Sheep with heavy fleece may be significantly bloated without the changes in abdominal contour being obvious. As the forestomach enlarges and compresses, the diaphragm breathing becomes more labored. Open-mouth breathing, cyanosis of mucous membranes, and collapse leading to death may occur within a few minutes if the animal becomes frantic from the abdominal pain and dyspnea. Other conditions to consider in the diagnosis of bloat in ruminants are those that cause abdominal enlargement, including advanced pregnancy, hydropic conditions of the uterus, left or right abomasal displacements, vagal indigestion syndrome, cecal dilation of volvulus, intestinal volvulus, omasal bursitis, ascites, diffuse peritonitis, and pneumoperitoneum.

Many systemic conditions influence the motility of the forestomach and thus may produce mild bloat coincidentally. Free gas bloat caused by vagal indigestion and impaired rumen motility is discussed in the section on indigestion in ruminants (see p. 722).

CLINICAL PATHOLOGY. Clinical pathologic measurements are not required for the diagnosis and management of most cases of bloat in ruminants. When no cause for forestomach enlargement is obvious, evaluation of a sample of rumen contents may provide information useful for prescribing treatment and prevention. The presence or absence of froth and the pH are critical features relating to the cause that influence the choice of therapy. The normal pH of the rumen varies with time after feeding but should be between 6 and 6.8. Evaluation of serum calcium and chloride and rumen fluid chloride levels may be useful.

PATHOPHYSIOLOGY. Regardless of the cause of forestomach distention, the process may become self-perpetuating because of reflex inhibition of motility. Low threshold stretch receptors in the rumen wall augment cyclic forestomach contractions when stimulated. However, stimulation of high threshold stretch receptors leads to inhibition of motility. Thus, beyond a certain degree of stretching of the ruminal wall, further contractions that may relieve the distention through eructation are prevented.[1213]

Three classes of bloat may be considered. The first is frothy bloat caused by the retention of gases of fermentation within the mass of ingesta that fail to rise and coalesce into a dorsal gaseous layer. This condition can arise from diets of lush legumes or winter wheat pasture or may be seen with high-concentrate finishing rations in the feedlot. In the case of legume-induced disease, bloat has occurred after grazing or feeding of fresh-cut forages or the feeding of alfalfa hay. The structure of stable froth in the affected rumen contents is not a true foam. The ingesta in the septae between adjacent bubbles forms a complex structure that prevents coalescence. The viscosity of the fluid may prevent gravitational flow through the septae that would lead to the bubbles' rising and coalescing. Frothy ruminal fluid is higher in chloroplast membrane fragments, soluble protein, and very fine particles than nonfrothy ruminal fluid.[1214] The presence of the resulting frothy ingesta at neural receptors believed to be near the cardia prevents the reflex relaxation of the cardia during the secondary contractions of the forestomach that ordinarily lead to eructation.[1215] In addition, the viscosity of the frothy ingesta is such that the cardia may become plugged during attempts to eructate.

Current research[1214] supports both animal and plant characteristics as predisposing to legume bloat. Individual cattle have been classified as having either high or low susceptibility to legume bloat. Thus far, highly susceptible cattle have been shown to have larger rumen volumes and specific salivary proteins in consistently different proportions than bloat-resistant cattle. The actual mechanisms that lead to larger forestomach volume in susceptible cattle have not been determined. There is a relationship between plant factors associated with bloat and the rapidity with which leaf structure is disrupted after ingestion.[1214] Bloat-inducing plants are more readily macerated, thus providing quicker bacterial access to the inner leaf cells. Less bloat-predisposing cultivars of the main bloat-causing species, such as alfalfa (*Medicago sativa*), red clover (*Trifolium pratens*), and white clover (*Trifolium repens*), have a thicker leaf cuticle, smaller stomata, and more fibrous leaf structure. Ionophore antibiotics such as monensin inhibit rumen protozoa that normally ingest chloroplasts, leading to a reduction in the bloat potential of some forages.[1216,1217]

Grain bloat occurs in a manner similar to that caused by legumes; a stable froth is produced from high-concentrate rations. Particle size and the rate of fermentation are thought to be the determining factors in the froth production. A mucoprotein slime composed of bacterial by-products stabilizes the froth.[1216,1218] This material tends to be stable at a lower pH than is found in non–grain-fed ruminants, so that grain feeding promotes slime accumulation by lowering rumen pH. Genetically susceptible cattle lack adequate mucin in their saliva to disrupt the tiny gas bubbles. Animals (such as dairy cattle) that are fed grain and then legumes may be par-

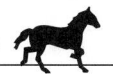

ticularly susceptible to frothy bloat, because all the factors leading to froth production and accumulation are present. Both legume bloat and grain bloat may resolve spontaneously if the animal stops consuming the bloat-producing feed and microbial digestion eliminates the froth-stabilizing factors.

Ruminal tympany *(free gas bloat)* may occur after consumption of an amount of concentrates greater than that to which the animal is adapted. The resulting fermentation leads to the initial production of high concentrations of volatile organic acids, volatile fatty acids (VFAs) and, as the rumen pH drops below 5.3, lactic acid. The rate of VFA and lactic acid production may exceed the capacity for absorption. Compared with VFAs, lactic acid is poorly absorbed from the rumen. Organic acids are absorbed by rumen epithelium mostly in the nondissociated form. Therefore absorption occurs more quickly near the pKA of the respective acids. VFAs have a pKA of 4.9 and lactic acid a pKA of 3.7. FAs can be readily absorbed by the rumen epithelium at low-normal physiologic pH, but at the same pH lactic acid absorption is 92% slower.[1219] The elevated concentrations of nondissociated VFAs and lactic acid and the resulting low intraruminal pH reflexly inhibit cyclic contractions of the forestomach, and gas accumulates.

Causes of the third class of bloat lie outside the forestomach. Obstruction of the esophagus (choke) leads to ruminal distention, with the gases of fermentation produced by the ingesta already in the forestomach before obstruction. Postural bloat occurs if the animal is cast or trapped in a position that keeps the cardia submerged below the ruminal gas cap. Hypocalcemia reduces the strength of or abolishes the cyclic contractions of the forestomach, leading to the accumulation of gas. Severe inflammation, pain, general anesthesia, and some drugs, notably xylazine, reduce or eliminate cyclic forestomach contractions. Most of these causes of bloat lead to mild ruminal distention, with eructation occurring at a reduced frequency. However, drugs or procedures that inhibit forestomach motility should be used with appropriate precautions such as prior withholding of feed or placement of a cannula to allow gas to escape.

Acute distress, often appearing as colic, is caused by overdistention of the forestomach that stimulates pain receptors in the rumen wall. As the abdominal distention increases, the ability to achieve normal respiratory movements of the diaphragm and rib cage is impaired. Death from asphyxia ultimately results as the lungs are compressed by the cranially expanding diaphragm.

EPIDEMIOLOGY. Bloat from causes other than consumption of wet legumes and high-concentrate diets occurs sporadically, whereas frothy bloat often occurs as an epidemic. Pasture bloat occurs wherever alfalfa, red clover, or white clover is grazed. Environmental conditions that produce rapid, early growth lead to a higher incidence of bloat. Frothy bloat also occurs when stocker cattle are grazed on winter wheat pastures in the southern Great Plains of the United States. Death losses at pasture range from 0.5% to 2.5% of cattle at risk on an annual basis. The incidence of feedlot bloat has been estimated at about 1%, with death losses of about 0.1%.[1214]

NECROPSY FINDINGS. Ruminants that die of most causes bloat with free gas after death. The finding of tenacious froth in the rumen along with other evidence of bloat is grounds for a presumptive diagnosis of frothy bloat. The challenge for the diagnostician is to determine if the bloat occurred before death; this may not be possible if the animal has not been observed before death. The increase in intraabdominal pressure prevents venous return from the hindquarters and may lead to obvious edema in the intermuscular areas. Unfortunately this is not a consistent finding; other evidence of impaired circulation or a differential degree of edema between fore and hind parts must be used to make a diagnosis.

TREATMENT AND PROGNOSIS. Passage of a stomach tube generally is sufficient to relieve the discomfort of mild to moderate distention of the rumen with free gas. Manipulation and repositioning of the tube after it enters the stomach are sometimes required to deflate the gas pocket. A sample of the rumen contents for pH measurement should be obtained at this time. Care must be taken to exclude saliva from the tube by blowing into the rumen, flushing water through the tube, or using a rumen sampling device that carries the tip of the stomach tube down into the liquid ingesta. If the pH of the rumen fluid is below 5.5, rumen acidosis is responsible for the bloat. Antacid therapy should be provided in the form of sodium bicarbonate or magnesium hydroxide. For further information on rumen acidosis, see the discussion of indigestion (pp. 743 to 745). If no gas can be released with a stomach tube, the tube should be withdrawn after suction has been applied and examined for the presence of froth. If the animal is not in respiratory distress or extremely colicky, surface-active agents should be administered by means of a stomach tube. Poloxalene (given orally at a dosage of 44 mg/kg) is recommended for forage bloat,[1217] and mineral oil or animal tallow for feedlot bloat.[1220]

Some cattle are in violent pain with bloat but not in respiratory distress. Sedation with xylazine may be necessary for further examination and treatment. Animals with extreme distention of the forestomach and in respiratory distress require immediate surgical intervention. Animals with advanced cases of parturient paresis may be bloated severely enough that deflating the rumen should precede calcium administration. A trocar introduced through the left paralumbar fossa relieves bloat caused by free gas accumulation but may not be adequate for frothy bloat. An emergency rumenotomy may be necessary to evacuate frothy contents.

For animals with free gas bloat of extraruminal cause, a temporary rumen fistula may be required. Either a screw-type trocar that is self-retaining or a small tube, such as a syringe barrel, surgically placed in the left paralumbar fossa provides an avenue for gas escape. On resolution of the primary problem, removal of the trocar usually results in spontaneous closure of the fistula.

PREVENTION AND CONTROL. Prevention of frothy pasture bloat has historically relied on attempts to anticipate when forages were most likely to induce bloat. Cattle were fed other feeds and allowed limited access to the problem forages. Accurately predicting when forages are safe has not been reliable. As an alternative the cattle at risk have been treated with supplemental surface-active agents.

In Australia and New Zealand, oils and tallows have been drenched daily, sprayed on fields, and smeared on the flanks to be later licked off, to prevent pasture bloat. Although poloxalene has proved effective, it is more expensive than oils. It can be fed in molasses blocks or individually administered. More recently ionophore antibiotics have shown promise for controlling bloat. Rumensin (1 mg/kg daily) greatly reduced the incidence of legume bloat, and lasalocid (1.32 mg/kg/daily) effectively reduced the incidence of grain bloat.[1216,1217] In both circumstances, beginning treatment before exposure to the bloat-inducing feed was more effective than waiting until bloat occurred. Agronomists are selecting cultivars of the bloat-producing forages for slower rates of initial fermentation. These are likely to become more widely used in the regions in which bloat is a regular occurrence.

Providing adequate fiber in feedlot rations and slowly introducing higher proportions of concentrates, particularly corn, barley, and soybean meal, permit ruminal adaptation that helps prevent bloat. Preventing ruminal tympany secondary to carbohydrate overload requires provision of balanced diets adequate in fiber and buffers and prevention of accidental consumption of concentrate.

Prevention of sporadic cases of bloat from causes such as milk fever relies on prevention or early treatment of the inciting problem. Cases caused by tumors, allergic reactions, and trauma will continue to provide challenges for the practitioner.

REFERENCES

1213. Reid CSW et al: Physiological and genetical aspects of pasture (legume) bloat. In McDonald IW, Warner ACI, eds: *Digestion and metabolism in the ruminant*, Armidale, NSW, Australia, 1975, University of New England Publishing Unit.
1214. Howarth R et al: Ruminant bloat. In Milligan LP, Grovum WL, Dobson A, eds: *Control of digestion and metabolism in ruminants*, Englewood Cliffs, NJ, 1986, Prentice-Hall.
1215. Grovum WL: The control of motility of the ruminoreticulum. In Milligan LP, Grovum WL, Dobson A, eds: *Control of digestion and metabolism in ruminants*, Englewood Cliffs, NJ, 1986, Prentice-Hall.
1216. Bartley EE et al: Effects of lasalocid or monensin on legume or grain (feedlot) bloat, *J Anim Sci* 56:1400-1406, 1983.
1217. Katz MP, Nagaraja TG, Fina LR: Ruminal changes in monensin- and lasalocid-fed cattle grazing bloat-provocative alfalfa pasture, *J Anim Sci* 63:1246-1257, 1986.
1218. Sakauchi R, Hoshino S: Effects of monensin on ruminal fluid viscosity, pH, volatile fatty acids, and ammonia levels, and microbial activity and population in healthy and bloated feedlot steers, *Tierphysiol Tierernahrg Futtermit-telkde* 46:21-33, 1981.
1219. Williams VJ, Mackenzie DDS: The absorption of lactic acid from the reticulorumen of the sheep, *Aust J Biol Sci* 18:917-934, 1965.
1220. Blood DC, Radostits OM, Henderson JA: *Veterinary medicine*, ed 6, London, 1983, Baillière Tindall.

ABOMASAL DISPLACEMENT AND VOLVULUS

CHARLES GUARD

DEFINITION AND ETIOLOGY. Abomasal displacement occurs either to the right or to the left side of the abdomen when gas accumulates within this viscus. Left displacement of the abomasum is most often encountered. By far the highest incidence is in adult dairy cattle in the early postpartum period, but cases have been seen in all other classes of cattle. Atony of the abomasum caused by an abnormally high volatile fatty acid (VFA) concentration and continued microbial fermentation of ingesta lead to gas accumulation and resultant distention. Hypocalcemia with decreased abomasal smooth muscle tone may also contribute to atony. The abomasum floats up along the lateral abdominal wall on either the left as a left displaced abomasum (LDA) or on the right as a right displaced abomasum (RDA) as a result of the buoyancy of the trapped gas. Unknown mechanical factors sometimes lead to volvulus on right torsion of the abomasum (RTA) during right displacement. The relative frequency of these abomasal problems in dairy cattle can be seen in the following data from my practice in central New York: between January 1988 and April 1989, 301 LDAs, 31 RDAs, and 21 RTAs were diagnosed. Diets high in starch or deficient in roughage are commonly associated with abomasal displacement. Displacement also occurs in association with other common disorders of postpartum dairy cattle.

LEFT DISPLACEMENT OF THE ABOMASUM

CLINICAL SIGNS AND DIFFERENTIAL DIAGNOSIS. Cattle with simple LDA have moderate to total anorexia, decreased fecal output, reduced frequency of rumen contractions, and hypogalactia and do not chew their cud. The last one or two ribs on the left are sprung, but the abdomen is sunken in the paralumbar fossa. The eyes frequently are retracted in the orbit to varying degrees, and mild pain may be evident (treading). The pulse may be slightly elevated to 85 to 90 beats/min.

Ketonuria and acetone on the breath are common. Respirations may be normal or shallow. Gurgling or tinkling rather than normal scratching sounds may be heard on auscultation in the left paralumbar fossa. Simultaneous auscultation and percussion reveal a ping over the gas-filled portion of the abomasum. With LDA the area of ping may be anywhere from the lower third of the abdomen in the eighth intercostal space to the paralumbar fossa. The examiner should percuss along a line from the tuber coxae to the elbow. The area of the ping often is circular and does not generally extend beyond the last rib. With extreme abomasal distention the abomasum may be visible as a bulge in the left paralumbar fossa. In most cases the rumen is not pressed tightly to the abdominal wall when palpated through the left paralumbar fossa. Feces may be drier than normal or scant and watery. During rectal examination the clinician may be able to palpate the abomasum to the left of the caudodorsal blind sac of the rumen or at least perceive that the rumen is displaced medially.

Ruminal tympany, pneumoperitoneum, and collapsed rumen[1221] may all produce pings on the left side of the cow. Physometra (air in the uterus) and dilation and displacement of the cecum to the left of the rumen (which is rare) may also produce left-sided pings. Having an assistant blow on the stomach tube passed into the rumen while auscultating over the left side differentiates the rumen from other structures. Rectal examination permits identification of a displaced cecum or gas-filled uterus. The collapsed rumen creates a void in the upper left quadrant of the abdomen. Percutaneous needle aspiration of fluid or gas from the suspected abomasum aids in correct identification. A pH of less than 4.5 as determined with wide-range pH paper or the odor of abomasal gas (slightly acrid or burnt almonds) confirms the presence of LDA.

CLINICAL PATHOLOGY. The most important abnormalities detected by clinical chemical evaluation usually are the serum electrolyte and acid-base levels.[1222] Sequestration of the hydrochloric acid secreted into the abomasum within the abomasum or by means of reflux in the ruminoreticulum leads to mild metabolic alkalosis. The blood pH and bicarbonate concentration are elevated, with a concomitant decrease in the blood chloride concentration. Cattle examined on the farm usually are hypoglycemic and ketonuric. After transport to a clinic hyperglycemia, often with glycosuria, may be observed. This difference presumably is the result of excitement or stress, which causes endogenous secretion of cortisol. The serum calcium level may be below normal as a result of decreased intake and absorption. Other serum electrolytes may be elevated slightly because of dehydration. The urine pH often is acidic despite the metabolic alkalosis.[1223] Hypokalemia may develop as a consequence of both the metabolic alkalosis and reduced intake and absorption. The hypokalemia and dehydration result in the renal response of sodium retention and hydrogen excretion, leading to an acid urine, the so-called paradoxic aciduria.[1224]

PATHOPHYSIOLOGY. The precise cause of LDA is unknown, but many have observed the association between the occurrence of LDA and stress, adverse weather, high relative proportions of concentrate in the diet, and concurrent disease. Some clinicians have observed that exercise (walking to pasture) reduced the incidence of LDA. Svendson[1225] demonstrated an inhibition of abomasal motility by direct infusions of VFAs or by feeding of high-concentrate diets, but other workers failed to reproduce his results with corn silage diets.[1221] Despite this failure to reproduce abomasal atony with high-concentrate diets, the relationship between feed particle sizes large enough to be considered adequate mechanical stimuli for rumination and the prevention of LDA has been noted by many clinicians. The substitution of citrus pulp for some of the long-stemmed hay in rations (producing equivalent neutral detergent fiber content) led to a high incidence of LDA, which was abated by return to the larger particle size of the hay.[1227] In addition to stimulating rumination (through touch receptors) and salivary buffer production, larger particles may serve to trap smaller ones in the ruminal raft that facilitates microbial digestion in the forestomach. This delay of passage of fermentable substrate associated with long-stemmed fiber provides less opportunity for gas production in the abomasum. Gas can be produced in the abomasum as a by-product of microbial fermentation there and from carbon dioxide released in the reaction of bicarbonate and hydrochloric acid. In the high-producing dairy cow, it is desirable to have high flow rates of ingesta from the ruminoreticulum to increase nutrient intake. Higher intake rates can be achieved with smaller feed particle size, but gastrointestinal diseases such as LDA limit the extent to which this manipulation is profitable. Currently there is no adequate way to define the minimum level of large particle feedstuffs required to maintain normal forestomach and abomasal function.

LDA that occurs secondary to disease associated with endotoxic or febrile reactions in the cow (e.g., retained placenta or metritis and severe mastitis) may be the result of the depressant effect of endotoxin or endogenous pyrogen (interleukin-1) on gastric motility.[1223,1224] Extrinsic reticuloruminal contractions are abolished both by the stimulatory effects of inflammatory mediators on gastric smooth muscle tone, leading to reflex inhibition, and by a direct depressant effect on central vagal nuclei. Although reports of direct effects on the abomasum are lacking, data on the gastrointestinal effects of fever, endotoxin, and inflammatory mediators in a variety of species all suggest that abomasal motor and secretory functions would be inhibited by diseases that cause fever and inflammation. Endotoxemia and sepsis also result in hypocalcemia, which further depresses abomasal tone and motility. These effects would predispose the cow to abomasal displacement. Abomasal atony also occurs with hypocalcemia; thus cows with clinical or subclinical milk fever are prone to abomasal displacement.[1230] Many cows with LDA are also clinically ketotic, but the roles of cause and effect in this relationship are not clear.[1231] Severe ketonemia may depress gastrointestinal motility. However, the ketosis may have resulted from the reduction in nutrient availability secondary to the anorexia caused by the reduced forestomach emptying and the discomfort of LDA.

EPIDEMIOLOGY. Cows in early lactation are at greatest risk of developing LDA. In one prospective study of 3172 lactations in New York, 81% of 48 LDAs occurred in the first 30 days after calving.[1232] The overall incidence was 1.5% of lactations. An older study reported a lower incidence rate (0.35% from 1970 to 1972), but even within that period the rate increased each year.[1233] A higher incidence has been reported in late winter/early spring after the winter housing season.[1234] Cows in this study had LDA in association with parturition as expected, but a preponderance of cases occurred in cows calving in February to April. Increasing parity was associated with an increased incidence of LDA in studies from Ontario, Canada, New York, and Israel.[1233-1235] Milk production potential is not thought to be related to the risk of LDA.[1236] Most cows produce 300 to 500 kg less milk in lactations with LDA than would be expected if the disease did not occur.[1237] For unknown reasons, about 80% of recovered cases produce about 400 kg less milk, and 20% produce 2000 kg less milk. Herd life after correction of LDA is not af-

fected. The financial consequences of LDA for an individual cow suffering the smaller reduction in milk production favor maintaining the cow in the herd.

Energy and protein nutrition of the prepartum dry cow were suggested to be causally related to LDA in one study.[1238] On a herd basis, in cows fed levels of energy and protein above National Research Council recommendations, LDA was less likely to develop. Genetics factors may also play a role in the predisposition to LDA. In a retrospective case-control study, cows with LDA were $1\frac{1}{2}$ times more likely to be sired by bulls in one group than controls.[1234] Fox[1239] suggested that body depth had increased in dairy cattle since 1945 and that this may provide more room for the relatively empty abdominal viscera to move about at parturition. An experimental herd composed of two groups of Holstein cows, continuously mated and selected to produce large and small body sizes, had a 4.5% incidence of LDA in the large size group and a 1% incidence in the small cows during a 14-year period.[1240] Body weight was 514 kg versus 464 kg, wither height was 134 cm versus 129 cm, and fat-corrected milk production was 6163 kg versus 6135 kg for the two groups. Thus some evidence exists to support a genetic basis for predisposition to LDA, and perhaps this is mediated through body size or conformation.

TREATMENT AND PROGNOSIS. Treatment for LDA involves returning the abomasum to its normal anatomic location, occasionally treating the coincident electrolyte and acid-base abnormalities, and providing therapy for concurrent disease conditions. Several surgical and nonsurgical approaches to correcting LDA have been described. Nonsurgical approaches involve casting the cow on her right side, rolling her into dorsal recumbency, rocking back and forth, and then rolling the legs over the torso so she is on her left side. The cow is then allowed to stand. The gas in the abomasum causes it to float to a ventral location when the cow is in dorsal recumbency. Continuing the rolling motion may move the gas to the right side of the abdomen, but right displacement rarely occurs as a result. The usual result is only a temporary recovery with recurrence within a few days. Surgical approaches include blind-stitch abomasopexy[1241] and toggle pin fixation (bar suture),[1242] which do not involve celiotomy and are performed with the cow in dorsal recumbency. Other surgical techniques include left flank and right paramedian abomasopexies and right flank omentopexy.[1243] Most surgical procedures have a satisfactory outcome. Complications resulting from rolling the cow, such as torsion of the intestinal mass around the root of the mesentery, rarely occur. Redisplacement in a subsequent lactation has occurred in rare cases after all surgical procedures.

Right paramedian abomasopexy using nonabsorbable suture material has been suggested to lead to the most permanent fixation of the abomasum.[1244] There have been reports of serious complications involving abscess formation, herniation, suturing of the rumen, and pyloric obstruction after blind-stitch abomasopexy.[1245,1246] A success rate for toggle pin fixation equivalent to that of right paramedian open surgical abomasopexy was observed in a prospective clinical trial.[1247] Often the choice of procedure is dictated by the practitioner's preference, the available facilities, and other circumstances of the particular case. Specific correction of electrolyte and acid-base abnormalities is rarely necessary with LDA. After correction of the topographic anatomy, normal patterns of ingesta flow allow spontaneous correction of the alkalosis and hypochloremia.

PREVENTION AND CONTROL. The incidence of LDA has been reduced in problem herds by dietary manipulation that reduces the likelihood of forestomach and abomasal atony caused by high-concentrate rations. This includes slow introduction of concentrates after calving, prepartum introduction of ensiled and concentrate feeds, an increase in the particle size of the forage, and prevention of hypocalcemia. Reduction in other periparturient inflammatory diseases such as mastitis and metritis also reduces the incidence of LDA.

RIGHT DISPLACEMENT OF THE ABOMASUM

Simple right displacement of the abomasum (RDA) occurs at about 10% to 15% the frequency of LDA. The predisposing causes, pathophysiologic mechanisms, clinical pathologic conditions, and epidemiologic characteristics are the same as for LDA. The exception to this description is the reported higher incidence of RDA than LDA in Denmark.[1248] (See the discussion under Left Displacement of the Abomasum for information on the pathophysiologic, clinical pathologic, and epidemiologic characteristics of RDA.)

CLINICAL SIGNS AND DIFFERENTIAL DIAGNOSIS. The general systemic state of the cow with RDA is the same as that of the cow with LDA. An area of tympanitic resonance is heard on the right side with simultaneous auscultation and percussion. The ping usually is confined to an area under the last five ribs in the upper half of the abdomen. The condition must be differentiated from other causes of right-sided pings, such as cecal distention (with or without volvulus), gas in the spiral colon, pneumorectum after rectal examination, pneumoperitoneum, physometra (gas in the uterus), and abomasal volvulus.[1249,1250] Cecal and rectal pings usually are detectable in a linear pattern just below the transverse processes of the lumbar vertebrae extending to the tuber coxae. Rectal examination identifies the gas-filled structure. Pings heard with gas in the spiral colon typically have a variable pitch, depending on the location over the cranial paralumbar fossa and last three or four ribs. Generally the spiral colon may be palpated per rectum as a laterally flattened, mildly distended viscus adjacent to the right body wall. Gas in the uterus can be detected per rectum. Pneumoperitoneum creates a ping that is distributed all along the dorsal portion of the abdominal cavity and is usually heard on both sides. Abomasal volvulus is the most difficult to differentiate from RDA.

Determination of the difference by physical diagnosis in an early case of abomasal volvulus is probably impossible. With time the cow becomes progressively more dehydrated and more severely ill with volvulus than is usual with RDA. Advanced cases of volvulus also have a ping that has an arched dorsal border and a horizontal ventral border caused by the fluid level in the abomasum. This fluid is auscultable on succession of the abomasum. RDA is sometimes palpable per rectum, and advanced-stage abomasal volvulus is always palpable.

TREATMENT AND PROGNOSIS. Surgical treatment is required to correct RDA. Because of the difficulty of differentiating RDA from early volvulus, intervention should be as prompt as possible. Both right flank and right paramedian approaches are appropriate for RDA. Rolling for nonsurgical correction is contraindicated because of the perceived risk of creating abomasal volvulus from an RDA. The prognosis for a successful recovery after surgery is comparable to that for LDA.

ABOMASAL VOLVULUS

Abomasal volvulus, or right torsion of the abomasum, (RTA) leads to complete obstruction of the flow of ingesta through the duodenum and therefore is a surgical emergency. The condition occurs in all classes of cattle. Although RDA is thought to precede its development, unknown factors lead to RTA. RTA is much rarer than LDA and somewhat less rare than RDA. In my practice RTA is seen as a sporadic disease

that does not fit the epidemiologic picture for LDA (i.e., most cases do not occur in early postpartum cows).

CLINICAL SIGNS AND DIFFERENTIAL DIAGNOSIS. The systemic effects of the gastrointestinal obstruction that results from RTA progress to a much more severe degree than in LDA or RDA. Sunken eyes and loss of skin turgor accompany the dehydration that develops. The heart rate increases above 100 beats/min. The pulse is weak and thready. Abdominal distention is marked bilaterally. Complete rumen stasis develops, leading to bloat, and the abomasum greatly enlarges on the right. Despite the severe degree of gastric distention, colic rarely develops in RTA; it is much more likely with cecal distention. The skin is cool to the touch. Feces are absent or watery but scant. A large area of tympanitic resonance with uniform pitch throughout is detectable on the right, extending from the eighth rib to the middle of the paralumbar fossa.[1250] The ventral border of the ping is a horizontal line reflecting the fluid level in the greatly distended abomasum. Borborygmi are absent. Splashing fluid sounds can be heard when the abomasum is ballotted (succussed) behind the last rib.

Other causes of proximal intestinal obstruction and torsion of the intestinal mass around the root of the mesentery must be differentiated from RTA. On rectal examination the abomasum can be felt with RTA. With intestinal obstruction or intestinal volvulus, distended loops of small intestine can be palpated. Pings caused by gas in the intestines have a variable pitch over the area involved.

Cecal distention with rotation can produce a similar degree of abdominal distention high on the right, but the abdomen usually is less filled cranioventrally on the right. A ping extends to the tuber coxae, and the cecum can be palpated per rectum. Diffuse peritonitis leads to complete atony of the gastrointestinal tract, and the abdomen may become distended with gas in all parts of the tract; there is no discrete ping extending over a large area of the right side.

As RTA progresses, cattle become recumbent and depressed. Death occurs within hours of this stage, which occurs 1 to 3 days after the development of the volvulus.

CLINICAL PATHOLOGY. Dehydration and cardiovascular collapse eventually are seen in more prolonged cases of RTA. Earlier cases have profound acid-base and electrolyte abnormalities similar to those in cattle with LDA but more marked. Hypochloremic metabolic alkalosis with hypokalemia and paradoxic aciduria often is present early in the course of the disease. As the condition progresses, dehydration becomes more marked, and metabolic acidosis may eventually supersede the alkalosis terminally.

Under the influence of carbonic anhydrase, hydrogen ions are pumped into the abomasal lumen. A chloride ion follows into the lumen, whereas bicarbonate and sodium remain in the blood. Under normal circumstances the hydrochloric acid leaves the pylorus, where the hydrogen ions are neutralized by pancreatic and intestinal secretions and the chloride is resorbed. When RTA occurs, the hydrochloric acid is sequestered in the abomasum and regurgitated into the omasum and rumen. Rumen chlorides increase. The animal becomes alkalotic and hypochloremic. Because of shifts between intracellular and extracellular compartments, potassium moves intracellularly as hydrogen ions move extracellularly in response to the metabolic alkalosis. This, plus the total anorexia, leads to severe hypokalemia. The hallmarks of RTA are metabolic alkalosis, hypochloremia, and hypokalemia.

Paradoxic aciduria occurs in the face of metabolic alkalosis, when the cow should be retaining hydrogen ions. The overwhelming renal physiologic drive appears to be sodium retention. Dehydration and reduced cardiac output result in falling blood pressure. The animal must respond by volume expansion; thus sodium is resorbed in the renal tubules. Chloride is also resorbed. Because of the hypochloremia, the electrical gradient that must be corrected is high; if 140 mEq/L of sodium is resorbed and only 60 mEq/L of chloride is available, there is a net of 80 mEq/L (140 minus 60) of cations that must be secreted back into the tubules. This is normally accomplished by secretion of potassium. Because hypokalemia is severe, hydrogen gas ions are paradoxically secreted so that blood pressure can be maintained by means of maximum sodium resorption.

PATHOPHYSIOLOGY. At least some of the factors predisposing to LDA or RDA probably contribute to the paths of RTA. Whether true RDA precedes RTA is not known. Dissection of naturally occurring cases of RTA demonstrated that the structures involved in rotation can vary from the reticulum to the omasum at the orad end.[1248,1251,1252] The rotation probably occurs most frequently at the reticuloomasal junction. The duodenum is looped around the omasum, regardless of the degree of volvulus. Creating the condition manually in an anesthetized calf was easier if the gas-filled fundus ascended around the cranial surface of the omasum, pulling the reticulum with it.[1251] The ensuing displacement leads to a counterclockwise rotation of the abomasum and omasum as viewed from the right side. The duodenum is pulled medial to the body of the omasum and wraps around the neck of the omasum in the final configuration. The continued hydrochloric acid secretion of the abomasum and the gas produced in the omasum and abomasum further stretch and occlude the duodenum. The abomasal blood vessels and the ventral vagal trunk are compromised near the site at which the duodenum wraps around the omasum in long-standing cases. Thrombosis of vessels may occur.

The acid-base and electrolyte abnormalities of early RTA are the same as those of LDA. In cases of severe distention of the abomasum and omasum with vascular compromise, systemic cardiovascular insufficiency develops. Reduced perfusion of peripheral tissues may lead to metabolic acidosis terminally. Hemoconcentration develops, although bleeding into the abomasum may occur from devitalized mucosa, leading to a low hematocrit. These changes are compounded by the developing necrosis of the abomasum. The abomasum may physically leak contents through a weakened, overstretched wall. Endogenous inflammatory mediators and bacterial toxins may diffuse from the abomasum to viable surrounding tissues, where absorption occurs. In either case, the viability of the abomasum is lost, and death follows shortly.

TREATMENT AND PROGNOSIS. Immediate surgical intervention usually is necessary to save the animal's life. Simultaneously fluid, electrolyte, and acid-base abnormalities need correction. For early cases of hypokalemic, hypochloremic alkalosis and dehydration, intravenous fluids consisting of 20 to 80 L of 0.9% sodium chloride with 25 to 100 mEq/L of potassium chloride added are administered. Intravenous potassium should not be given at a rate greater than 1 mEq/kg/hr to prevent cardiotoxicity. For advanced cases with metabolic acidosis, balanced electrolyte solutions such as Ringer's solution are indicated. Broad-spectrum antibiotics are appropriate if the integrity of the abomasal mucosa is questionable. Corticosteroids or nonsteroidal antiinflammatory drugs may be indicated if shock has developed, or they may be used preoperatively to protect against acute toxemia when the abomasum is manipulated. Both standing right-sided and recumbent right paramedian approaches have been successful for correcting RTA.[1243,1253]

The prognosis for short-term recovery depends on the degree of damage to the abomasal mucosa and muscularis. Severely devitalized tissues do not tolerate surgical manipulation and may not recover after distention is relieved and perfusion restored. Classification of the severity of the RTA

has been made on the basis of surgical findings of the volume of fluid in the abomasum combined with serum chloride levels.[1254] More than 30 L of abomasal fluid or serum chloride less than 79 mEq/L was associated with a high rate of death or immediate salvage. Because salvage value is significantly decreased in a cow with evidence of recent surgery, preoperative clinicopathologic parameters have been evaluated as predictors of eventual outcome. Base-excess values greater than 0.0 were associated with a short-term survival rate of about 80%, even if markedly alkalotic.[1255] Values of −0.1 or lower (terminal acidosis) were associated with a survival rate of 50%. Anion gap calculation was the most efficient predictor of outcome when compared to base-excess and serum chloride in a group of hospitalized patients.[1251] The anion gap is calculated as follows:

$$\text{Anion gap} = (\text{Na}^+ + \text{K}^+) - (\text{Cl}^- + \text{HCO}_3^-)$$

An anion gap of less than 30 mEq/L had a sensitivity of 0.89 and a specificity of 0.92 for short-term survival with RTA. None of the clinicopathologic measures or surgical observations has been shown to predict long-term outcome for RTA. The subsequent vagal indigestion syndrome that occurs as a result of damage to the ventral vagal trunk affects 10% to 30% of survivors of RTA. This complication prevents profitable production levels in cattle and necessitates salvage at a later date.

EPIDEMIOLOGY. No data have been published on the epidemiologic factors associated with RTA in North America. In my experience, RTA does not have the same relationship to recent parturition as do LDA and RDA, but rather occurs sporadically. Further research is needed to clarify the predisposing factors leading to RTA.

NECROPSY FINDINGS. Cattle dying of RTA are grossly dehydrated, and the abomasum is greatly distended or ruptured. The omasum often is also greatly distended when torsion occurs at the reticuloomasal junction. If rupture has occurred, careful attention to the topography of the omasum, abomasum, and duodenum is critical. Usually it is not difficult to arrive at a correct diagnosis.

PREVENTION AND CONTROL. Because factors predisposing to atony of the forestomachs and abomasum probably are important in the genesis of RTA, prevention should be similar to that outlined for LDA.

REFERENCES

1221. Rebhun WC: Rumen collapse in cattle, *Cornell Vet* 77:244-250, 1987.
1222. Robertson JM: Left displacement of the bovine abomasum: laboratory findings, *J Am Vet Med Assoc* 149:1430-1434, 1973.
1223. Gingerich DA, Murdick PW: Paradoxic aciduria in bovine metabolic alkalosis, *J Am Vet Med Assoc* 166:227-230, 1975.
1224. McGuirk SM, Butler DG: Metabolic alkalosis with paradoxic aciduria in cattle, *J Am Vet Med Assoc* 177:551-554, 1980.
1225. Svendson P: Etiology and pathogenesis of abomasal displacement in cattle, *Nord Vet Med* 21(suppl 1):1-60, 1969.
1226. Becht JL, Whitlock RH, Chalupa W: Dietary effects on abomasal motility in cattle, *Bovine Proc* 15:140, 1983 (abstract).
1227. Tromp AM: Personal communication, 1988.
1228. Lohuis JACM et al: Pathophysiological effects of endotoxins in ruminants, *Vet Q* 10:109-116, 1988.
1229. Verheijden JHM et al: Pathophysiological aspects of *E. coli* mastitis in ruminants, *Vet Res Comm* 7:229-236, 1983.
1230. Hull BL, Wass WM: Abomasal displacement. II. Hypocalcemia as a contributing causative factor, *Vet Med Small Anim Clin* 68:412-417, 1973.
1231. Grymer J: Displaced abomasum: a disease often associated with concurrent diseases, *Compend Cont Educ* 2:S290-S295, 1980.
1232. Erb HN et al: Rates of diagnosis of six diseases of Holstein cows during 15-day and 21-day intervals, *Am J Vet Res* 45:333-335, 1984.
1233. Coppock CE: Displaced abomasum in dairy cattle: etiological factors, *J Dairy Sci* 57:926-933, 1974.
1234. Martin W: Left abomasal displacement: an epidemiological study, *Can Vet J* 13:61-68, 1972.
1235. Markusfeld O: Periparturient traits in seven high-producing dairy herds: incidence rates, association with parity, and interrelationships among traits, *J Dairy Sci* 70:158-166, 1987.

1236. Erb H: Interrelationships among production and clinical disease in dairy cattle: a review, *Can Vet J* 28:326-329, 1987.
1237. Martin SW, Kirby KL, Curtis RA: Left abomasal displacement in dairy cows: its relationship to production, *Can Vet J* 19:250-253, 1978.
1238. Curtis CR et al: Path analysis of dry period nutrition, postpartum metabolic and reproductive disorders, and mastitis in Holstein cows, *J Dairy Sci* 68:2347-2360, 1985.
1239. Fox FH: Abomasal disorders, *J Am Vet Med Assoc* 147:383-388, 1965.
1240. Mahoney CB et al: Health care of Holsteins selected for large or small body size, *J Dairy Sci* 69:3131-3139, 1986.
1241. Hull BL: Closed suturing technique for correction of left abomasal displacement, *Iowa State Univ Vet* 34:142-144, 1972.
1242. Grymer J, Sterner KE: Percutaneous fixation of left displaced abomasum using a bar suture, *J Am Vet Med Assoc* 180:1458-1461, 1982.
1243. St Jean GD et al: Comparison of the different surgical techniques for correction of abomasal problems, *Compend Cont Educ* 9:F377-F382, 1987.
1244. Smith DF: Treatment of left displacement of the abomasum. I, *Compend Cont Educ* 3:S415-S422, 1981.
1245. Rutgers LJE, Van Der Velden MA: Complications following the use of the closed suturing technique for correction of left abomasal displacement in cows, *Vet Rec* 113:255-257, 1983.
1246. Tithof PK, Rebhun WC: Complications of blind-stitch abomasopexy: 20 cases (1980-1985), *J Am Vet Med Assoc* 189:1489-1492, 1986.
1247. Kelton DF, Garcia J, Guard CL: Bar suture (toggle pin) vs open surgical abomasopexy for treatment of left displaced abomasum in dairy cattle, *J Am Vet Med Assoc* 193:557-559, 1988.
1248. Espersen G, Dilatatio ET: Dislocatio ad dextram abomasi bovis, *Nord Vet Med* 13(suppl 1):1-168, 1961.
1249. Grymer J, Ames NK: Bovine abdominal pings: clinical examination and differential diagnosis, *Compend Cont Educ* 3:S311-S318, 1981.
1250. Smith DF et al: The identification of structures and conditions responsible for right-side tympanitic resonance (ping) in adult cattle, *Cornell Vet* 72:180-199, 1982.
1251. Habel RE, Smith DF: Volvulus of the bovine abomasum and omasum, *J Am Vet Med Assoc* 179:447-455, 1981.
1252. Neal PA, Pinsent PJN: Dilatation and torsion of the bovine abomasum, *Vet Rec* 72:175-180, 1960.
1253. Robertson JT: Right-sided torsion of the abomasum in the cow, *Compend Cont Educ* 2:S105-S109, 1980.
1254. Smith DF: Right-side torsion of the abomasum in dairy cows: classification of severity and evaluation of outcome, *J Am Vet Med Assoc* 173:108-111, 1978.
1255. Simpson DF, Erb HN, Smith DF: Base excess as a prognostic and diagnostic indicator in cows with abomasal volvulus or right displacement of the abomasum, *Am J Vet Res* 46:796-797, 1985.
1256. Garry FB et al: Prognostic value of anion gap calculation in cattle with abomasal volvulus: 58 cases (1980-1985), *J Am Vet Med Assoc* 192:1107-1112, 1988.

ABOMASAL ULCERS

CHARLES GUARD

DEFINITION AND ETIOLOGY. Abomasal ulcers occur in cattle of all ages and rarely in sheep and goats. Signs of loss of gastric epithelium may range from no clinical signs, to hem-orrhage and subsequent melena, to peritonitis if the erosive processes penetrate all layers of the abomasum. The disease is associated with stress and in adults is associated with diets high in starch. Concurrent diseases are common with ulcers and include the common postpartum disorders of dairy cattle. Lymphosarcoma of the abomasum also may lead to clinical signs of ulcer disease.

CLINICAL SIGNS AND DIFFERENTIAL DIAGNOSIS. Smith, Munson, and Erb[1257] have classified abomasal ulcers into four types: (1) nonperforating, (2) nonperforating with severe blood loss, (3) perforating with local peritonitis, and (4) perforating with diffuse peritonitis (Table 30-12). These classifications are useful for describing the various clinical pictures that may be observed when examining an animal with abomasal ulceration. The mildest form is caused by nonperforating ulcers that do not result in extensive hemorrhage. The signs are mild abdominal pain, shown by partial anorexia, decreased rumen motility, and mild ruminal tympany. There is usually no febrile response. Manure may be normal or reduced in amount and stale because of prolonged transit. In some cases abdominal pain may be evident on manual pressure on the right ventral abdomen. Traumatic reticuloperitonitis or indigestion may be suspected. In one study about two thirds of such cows had a positive test finding for fecal occult blood.[1258]

In cattle with ulcers that erode into major gastric blood vessels, blood loss can be sufficient to cause signs of anemia and hemorrhagic shock. These animals have dark blood clots in their manure or tarry, black feces with the characteristic smell of partly digested blood. The mucous membranes may be pale, tachycardia may be pronounced, and the respiratory rate may be elevated. There are other possible sources of proximal gastrointestinal hemorrhage in cattle, but abomasal ulcers are by far the most common cause. Total anorexia and rumen stasis usually are present. The rumen may have a fluid consistency, and if the animal is able to stand, abdominal pain sometimes is evident. Melena must be differentiated from the very dark red feces sometimes seen with intussusception. The packed cell volume usually is increased with intussusception and decreased with a bleeding ulcer.

Abomasal ulcers that perforate the serosal surface lead to peritonitis from contamination with abomasal contents. If the lesion is small or the local inflammatory reaction sufficiently swift, localized peritonitis results. This condition is most like traumatic reticuloperitonitis in presenting signs. The animal may be moderately febrile and partly or totally anorectic, and milk production may decrease acutely. There is evidence of abdominal pain, usually localized to the right

TABLE 30-12

Abomasal Ulcers

Type	Lesions	Clinical Signs
Nonperforating	Mucosal and some submucosal tissue loss; focal mural thickening; local serositis	Partial anorexia; decreased rumen motility; positive fecal occult blood
Nonperforating with severe blood loss (bleeding)	Penetration of mucosa and submucosal blood vessel; hemorrhage into abomasum	Partial anorexia; decreased rumen motility; anemia; pale mucous membranes; melena; tachycardia; cool extremities
Perforating with local peritonitis	Penetration from mucosa to serosa; leakage of abomasal contents; localized peritoneal reaction with adhesion formation	Total anorexia; low-grade fever; decreased to absent rumen motility; localized abdominal pain; very similar to traumatic reticuloperitonitis
Perforating with diffuse peritonitis	Penetration from mucosa to serosa; widespread contamation of the peritoneal cavity with abomasal contents; significant exudate in peritoneal cavity; fibrin deposition of all serosal surfaces	Total anorexia; fever early, then hypothermia; ileus of entire gastrointestinal tract; tachycardia; shock; terminally recumbent with grunt on respiration

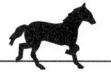

ventral quadrant. Rumen motility may be absent, and mild bloat may be present. As with hardware disease, the signs usually abate over the course of a few days if the infection is successfully contained. In some cases the infection is confined to the omental bursa, where extensive fluid and pus may accumulate. The course of omental bursitis is much more prolonged than that of simple localized peritonitis and usually results in death.

Major leakage from a perforating ulcer leads to acute diffuse peritonitis. The course of the disease usually is rapid, with signs of septic shock developing within 24 hours of the onset. Total anorexia and rumen stasis are accompanied by tachycardia with a weak, thready pulse and a heart rate over 100 beats/min. Pain may be evidenced by grinding of the teeth or groaning. The extremities are cool, and the animal generally becomes recumbent. Abdominal enlargement may be evident as a result of both ruminal tympany and the accumulation of peritoneal fluid. Dehydration is detectable by skin pinch or by observation of the position of the eye in the orbit. Septic shock from other causes may be difficult to distinguish from that caused by perforated abomasal ulcers in the terminal stages of the disease. Peritonitis from hardware disease, uterine rupture, and cecal rupture all have the same final course. Abomasal volvulus of more than a day's duration has similar characteristics but can be differentiated by the right-sided ping and fluid in the abomasum.

CLINICAL PATHOLOGY. The most useful diagnostic test for abomasal ulcer disease is the fecal occult blood test. In an evaluation of 296 hospitalized cattle with gastrointestinal disease, this test had a sensitivity of 0.77 and a specificity of 0.97 for ulcers confirmed at surgery or necropsy.[1258] The test is inexpensive and can be performed during the physical examination. Abdominocentesis confirms diffuse peritonitis (a large quantity of abdominal fluid is obtainable); centesis fluid may contain leukocytes with phagocytosed or free bacteria. In localized peritonitis the results of abdominocentesis may be normal. If peritonitis is present, leukocytosis usually is present, with neutrophilia predominating in many cases. The plasma fibrinogen is increased (over 700 mg/dl) in most cattle with peritonitis. This may be evaluated in the field with a glutaraldehyde coagulation test on whole blood. The hematocrit is normal or elevated with peritonitis, but plasma protein levels may be decreased as a result of protein accumulation in the peritoneal cavity or increased if dehydration is severe. If blood loss is severe, the packed cell volume is decreased. Cattle over 5 years of age with a bleeding abomasal ulcer should be tested for bovine leukosis virus.

PATHOPHYSIOLOGY. The specific events leading to erosion and ulceration of the abomasal mucosal epithelium are unknown but probably are similar to those in other species. (See Chapter 30).

EPIDEMIOLOGY. Abomasal ulceration occurs in cattle of all ages. At slaughter many calves are found to have clinically inapparent abomasal erosions and ulcers. In clinically affected calves, perforation with peritonitis (rather than hemorrhage) usually develops. In adult cattle with abomasal ulcers, approximately one third of clinical cases in a referral population had significant hemorrhage.[1259] Of these, half had lymphosarcoma and for the most part were older than 6 years of age. The age of the cattle with nontumor-associated bleeding ulcers was generally younger (7 of 12 were less than 5 years old). In the remaining two thirds of the cattle, ulcers had perforated, with about half having diffuse and half having localized peritonitis.[1260] Most adult cattle with abomasal ulcer disease are in the first month after calving and have a concurrent disease. Many cows have been discovered to have an abomasal ulcer at surgery for displaced abomasum. Metritis, mastitis, and ketosis are the other diseases commonly seen with abomasal ulcers. In my opinion, the incidence of

abomasal ulcers increased with the advent of heavy corn silage and high-moisture corn feeding. In the recent past, as feeding and management practices have addressed the most common abomasal displacements, the incidence of ulcer disease has also decreased.

NECROPSY. Cattle with bleeding abomasal ulcers resulting in death are very pale and may have blood or bloody fluid throughout the distal gastrointestinal tract. The lesion in the abomasum is typically small and involves an abomasal blood vessel in the submucosa. More bleeding and perforating ulcers were found in the fundic portion of the abomasum in the region of the proper gastric glands. The most ventral portion of the abomasum in its normal position is frequently affected.[1261-1263] Most animals have a single bleeding ulcer, but approximately 60% have one or more additional ulcers or erosions.[1261] Cattle with diffuse peritonitis have many liters of foul-smelling fluid in the peritoneal cavity. Fibrin usually covers the serosal surface of all abdominal organs. The defect in the serosal surface of the abomasum is usually nearly round and 3 to 6 cm in diameter. Abomasal fluid freely enters the peritoneal cavity. Omasal bursitis may be present, with the omental recess filled with purulent to fibrinous fluid. In these cases the remainder of the abdomen may not be grossly affected. Asymptomatic abomasal ulcers (often 50 to 200) may be found coincidentally in cattle that die of septic metritis or mastitis. These ulcers generally show no signs of hemorrhage and go undetected until necropsy.

TREATMENT AND PROGNOSIS. Treatment is aimed at correcting dietary problems, reducing stress, ameliorating concurrent disease problems, and initiating specific therapy for the clinical problems caused by the ulcer. Removal of very starchy feedstuffs and replacement with good-quality hay plus confinement to a stall are beneficial.[1264] Blood transfusions may be necessary for cattle that have lost enough blood to lower the hematocrit to 14% or below. Usually 4 L given once is adequate, but repeated transfusions occasionally may be necessary. Cross-matching usually is not necessary for cattle unless repeat transfusions are performed over a period of more than 3 days.

Broad-spectrum antibiotics are administered to cattle with signs of peritonitis and continued until 48 hours after such signs have subsided. The use of antacids and protectants is recommended by several authors but is of doubtful benefit because of dilution in the rumen and slow release into the abomasum. Preparations recommended include calcium carbonate, magnesium carbonate, bismuth subnitrate, and aluminum hydroxide gel. Oral medications administered after stimuli that induce reflex esophageal groove closure would be more likely to have the desired effect. Traditional stimuli have included copper sulfate solutions, and more recently vasopressin (0.25 IU/kg given intravenously) was shown to induce reliable abomasal deposition of materials given by drench to adult goats.[1265] Intravenous or oral fluids may be necessary to treat dehydration and metabolic or acid-base disturbances that occur concurrently. Animals with diffuse peritonitis must be given intravenous fluids with caution because of the risk of pulmonary edema associated with the low colloid osmotic pressure of their plasma.

The use of specific histamine H_2 antagonists has been of great benefit in treatment of gastric and duodenal ulcers in nonruminant species. Cimetidine, for example, reduces gastric secretion of hydrochloric acid, regardless of the nature of the stimulus. However, in cattle, experimental results with a range of cimetidine dosages from 4 to 16 mg/kg showed no effect on abomasal pH or chloride concentration.[1266]

The prognosis is good for ulcers that are not bleeding and not perforated. For those that stop bleeding and those with localized peritonitis, survival and eventual return to normal function can be expected. Many dairy cattle stop lactating during the acute course of the illness and do not return to milk until the next lactation. Because abomasal ulcers generally occur within the first month after calving, most of these animals are salvaged for slaughter. Most cattle with diffuse peritonitis die despite aggressive specific therapy. Early recognition and immediate surgery followed by antibiotic and fluid therapy may save some valuable individuals. Cattle with ulcers that occur secondary to lymphosarcoma should be euthanized or slaughtered.

PREVENTION AND CONTROL. Dietary management that reduces other abomasal diseases likewise reduces the incidence of abomasal ulcers. Avoiding abrupt changes in rations and including adequate fiber sources of sufficient particle size to facilitate normal rumen function also promote normal abomasal function. Minimizing stress caused by overcrowding, excessive competition, and adverse environmental conditions should also reduce problems with abomasal ulcers. Elimination of animals infected with the bovine leukosis virus from the herd eliminates lymphosarcoma as a cause of abomasal ulcers.

REFERENCES

1257. Smith DF, Munson L, Erb HN: Abomasal ulcer disease in adult dairy cattle, *Cornell Vet* 73:213-224, 1983.
1258. Smith DF, Munson L, Erb HN: Predictive values for clinical signs of abomasal ulcer disease in adult dairy cattle, *Prev Vet Med* 3:573-580, 1986.
1259. Palmer JE, Whitlock RH: Bleeding abomasal ulcers in adult dairy cattle, *J Am Vet Med Assoc* 183:448-451, 1983.
1260. Palmer JE, Whitlock RH: Perforated abomasal ulcers in adult dairy cows, *J Am Vet Med Assoc* 184:171-174, 1984.
1261. Aukema JJ, Breukink HJ: Abomasal ulcer in adult cattle with fatal haemorrhage, *Cornell Vet* 64:303-317, 1974.
1262. Hemmingsen I: Erosiones et ulcera abomasi bovis, *Nord Vet Med* 18:354-365, 1966.
1263. Hemmingsen I: Ulcur perforans abomasi bovis, *Nord Vet Med* 19:17-30, 1967.
1264. Rebhun WC: The medical treatment of abomasal ulcers in dairy cattle, *Compend Cont Educ Pract Med* 4:S91-S98, 1982.
1265. Mikhail M et al: Stimulated esophageal groove closure in adult goats, *Am J Vet Res* 49:1713-1715, 1988.
1266. Whitlock RH, Becht JL: Probantheline bromide and cimetidine in the control of abomasal acid secretion, *Proc Am Assoc Bov Pract* 15:140, 1982 (abstract).

ABOMASAL DILATION AND EMPTYING DEFECT OF SUFFOLK SHEEP

CHARLES GUARD

DEFINITION AND ETIOLOGY. A syndrome of abomasal dilation and mechanical transport failure has been described in adult Suffolk sheep.[1267-1269] The condition resembles but is uniquely different from abomasal impaction of cattle wintering on very poor-quality roughage. It has been reported only in Suffolks, even when other herds are held in the same circumstances. No hereditary pattern of disease has yet been found.[1267]

CLINICAL SIGNS AND DIFFERENTIAL DIAGNOSIS. The disease is primarily manifested by anorexia and weight loss. Most patients eventually die. Animals described in reports from several teaching hospitals were adults of both sexes.[1267-1269] Not all animals had all of these signs, but the following have been reported: watery green diarrhea or normal feces; ruminal tympany; pear-shaped abdominal distention; increased, normal, decreased, or absent rumen contractions; a palpable firm mass in the right lower abdomen; mild abdominal pain; tachycardia; duration of observed signs from days to months; partial to total anorexia; dullness and depression; marked to undetectable weight loss; ketonuria.

Wasting diseases of sheep include malnutrition, parasitism, dental problems, Johne's disease, caseous lymphadenitis, other chronic infections, and neoplasia. Abomasal emptying defect is distinguishable by the palpable abomasum in advanced cases and the exclusion of other possible problems. Other causes of abomasal enlargement or impaction resembling those reported in cattle must also be considered. However, when a mature Suffolk from a well-nourished flock shows weight loss and a palpable abomasum, this syndrome must be considered highly likely. Confirmation should involve response to therapy but may require necropsy or exploratory surgery.

CLINICAL PATHOLOGY. Reports on cases seen in North America have found hematologic and blood chemical determinations of little benefit in the diagnosis. The hypochloremic metabolic alkalosis common in cattle with abomasal problems has not been consistently observed in affected sheep. Elevated rumen chloride ion values have been the most consistent laboratory findings in published reports.[1267,1269,1270] The normal rumen chloride level in sheep is 8 to 15 mEq/L; affected sheep have had values ranging from 34 to 130 mEq/L. Mild hypocalcemia was observed in all cases in one report.[1267]

PATHOPHYSIOLOGY. The mechanisms underlying the dilation of the abomasum and the failure to transport ingesta to the intestines are unknown. None of the problems commonly associated with abomasal impaction and dilation in cattle have been identified in affected Suffolk sheep.

EPIDEMIOLOGY. The disease has been reported only in sheep of the Suffolk breed. In at least one affected flock a number of sheep of other breeds were present, but none were affected.[1267] The disease has mostly been seen in winter months in association with lambing and feeding of concentrates. Both rams and ewes have been affected. The incidence rate from one report was 11 of 92 mature ewes affected in the flock during one winter.[1267] Pedigree analysis of affected sheep in this flock showed no hereditary pattern. One report from a diagnostic laboratory in England described abomasal impaction in a Texel ewe and in a Suffolk ram that were simultaneously diagnosed as having scrapie.[1271] It remains to be seen if any causative connection exists between the two diseases. Because no antemortem tests exist for the diagnosis of scrapie, this relationship will be difficult to establish.

NECROPSY FINDINGS. The abomasum is greatly distended in sheep that die of this condition. The contents are either dry or liquid but most often have resembled normal ventral ruminal sac contents. The pylorus has always been patent. Normal ingesta has been observed throughout the remainder of the intestinal tract. Incidental findings have included aspiration of rumen contents and subsequent pneumonia, abomasal ulcer with local peritonitis, passive congestion of the liver, megaesophagus, and esophageal ulcers. Reports of histopathologic findings include no lesions other than thinning of the abomasal muscle layers[1267] (presumably as a result of stretching), mononuclear cell infiltration of the main muscle layers of the abomasum,[1268] and one case of myxomatous changes in the abomasal branches of the vagus nerve.[1269] No lesions consistent with a diagnosis of scrapie have been seen in any of the sheep examined in North America.

TREATMENT AND PROGNOSIS. Medical therapy alone with cathartics and laxatives has been of limited benefit. Mineral oil, dioctyl sodium sulfosuccinate, and magnesium sulfate have all been used. Neostigmine and calcium gluconate were not useful.[1268] Abomasotomy has led to death from complications in many affected sheep, but those that have survived more than 2 days and have been treated with metoclopramide (dosage not reported) shown varying degrees of recovery.

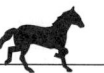

Metoclopramide is a dopamine antagonist that has been used in cattle at a dosage of 0.3 mg/kg given subcutaneously four to six times daily; it is believed to facilitate abomasal emptying. Despite these successes, most affected sheep die of cachexia. Because of the expense and risks associated with abomasotomy, this treatment is reserved for valuable breeding stock.

PREVENTION AND CONTROL. Until more is known about the pathogenesis of this specific defect in abomasal function in Suffolk sheep, no useful recommendations for prevention can be made.

REFERENCES

1267. Ruegg PL, George LW, East NE: Abomasal dilatation and emptying defect in a flock of Suffolk ewes, *J Am Vet Med Assoc* 193:1534-1536, 1988.
1268. Kline EE et al: Abomasal impaction in sheep, *Vet Rec* 113:177-179, 1983.
1269. Rings DM et al: Abomasal emptying defect in Suffolk sheep, *J Am Vet Med Assoc* 185:1520-1522, 1984.
1279. Kopcha M: Abomasal dilatation and emptying defect in a ewe, *J Am Vet Med Assoc* 192:783-784, 1988.
1280. Sharp MW, Collings DF: Ovine abomasal enlargement and scrapie, *Vet Rec* 120:215, 1987 (letter).

ABOMASAL IMPACTION

CHARLES GUARD

DEFINITION AND ETIOLOGY. Abomasal impaction is the accumulation of ingesta in the abomasum with failure of aboral transport. The usual cause is provision of poor-quality, coarse roughage as the sole feed; typically this feeding strategy is used for overwintering beef cows. Several animals in a herd may be affected over a short period during severely cold weather. Calves may also have impaction of the abomasum caused by eating bedding or indigestible objects when fed low-quality milk replacers. The distended abomasum is filled with a firm mass of fibrous ingesta. Animals on low-fiber diets may consume wood or baling twine. Hairballs occasionally may accumulate in the abomasum of calves. This indigestible material may accumulate in the abomasum, creating a mechanical outflow obstruction. Abomasal distention may occur with normal diets after correction of abomasal volvulus and may be due either to vagal nerve damage or to irreversible stretching of the abomasal musculature. Lymphosarcoma involving the abomasum or other space-occupying lesions adjacent to the pylorus may lead to abomasal distention. Abomasal emptying defects of Suffolk sheep are addressed in the previous section.

CLINICAL SIGNS AND DIFFERENTIAL DIAGNOSIS. In the beef cow with abomasal impaction, abomasal and ruminal enlargement slowly develop over a period of days to weeks. Closely monitored animals are observed to have reduced feed intake and reduced, firmer than normal feces. The animal may have bilateral ventral abdominal enlargement and bulging of the left paralumbar region. Ruminal contractions are of normal or increased frequency but often reduced in strength. In the later stages of the disease, rumen motility often is absent. Cattle with advanced abomasal impaction may be recumbent and groan with each respiration. The consistency of the ruminal ingesta, as judged by ballottement, may be more fluid than expected on the basis of the coarse diet. Other animals have a uniformly firm and distended rumen. The pulse and respiration usually are normal until the animal is near death, at which time tachycardia develops. The abomasum may be palpable as a firm mass following the right coastal arch. Rectal examination reveals a distended rumen; often the ventral sac extends to the right body wall. The pyloric part of the distended abomasum may be palpable in the right ventral quadrant. Wintering beef cows usually are pregnant, and thus the uterus prevents palpation of the abomasum. Feces are absent or very scant and dry. Mucus may be all that clings to the clinician's sleeve after rectal examination. In calves the abomasum may fill most of the abdomen and be doughy or firm on external palpation. The body condition of affected animals is invariably thin, because negative energy balance precedes and is amplified by the impaction. If the abomasum ruptures, signs of generalized peritonitis occur. Death usually follows within hours of rupture.

Conditions that cause dehydration and bilateral abdominal distention with absence of feces must be considered in the diagnosis. Hydropic conditions of the uterus are detectable on rectal palpation. The absence of a palpable fetus or cotyledons with a very large uterus is suggestive of hydrops. Ballottement of the abdomen usually produces a fluid wave from either side. Chronic peritonitis may produce ruminal distention and scant feces with progressive weight loss. Forestomach outflow problems caused by vagus indigestion or omasal impaction lead to ruminal distention without palpable abomasal enlargement. Chloride secreted in the abomasum normally flows into the intestine for resorption; thus hypochloremia and alkalosis do not develop with abomasal impaction. Intestinal obstruction usually is acute in onset and causes colic, distention of intestinal loops palpated per rectum, and auscultable pings.

Failure of abomasal transport may follow surgical correction of abomasal volvulus. Bradycardia often develops concurrently. The abomasum and rumen distend as with primary abomasal impaction, but the abomasal contents usually are of normal consistency. Progressive abdominal enlargement develops, and appetite gradually declines. Body weight might actually increase as a result of the enlargement of the stomach, but body condition is lost. When lymphosarcoma of the abomasum causes an outflow obstruction, other signs are similar to those that follow volvulus. However, bradycardia does not develop, and tumorous enlargement of palpable lymph nodes may exist to support the diagnosis.

Foreign body obstruction of the pylorus may occur as a result of accidental consumption of indigestible material such as scraps of plastic sheeting from the covering of a trench silo. Trichobezoars (hairballs) that could function as a ball valve in the pylorus have also been found in the abomasum of veal calves, but their significance is not certain. In these cases clinical signs resemble those after correction of abomasal volvulus. In many of these cases exploratory celiotomy is necessary to arrive at a definitive diagnosis.

CLINICAL PATHOLOGY. The hypochloremic, metabolic alkalosis typical of upper gastrointestinal obstruction in ruminants does not always develop in primary abomasal impaction. Initially some fluid ingesta may pass through the abomasum, preventing chloride sequestration. However, some cattle have metabolic alkalosis with chloride accumulated in the rumen. Terminally a metabolic acidosis from starvation may mask the metabolic alkalosis. Anemia and leukopenia can accompany the cachexia of chronic abomasal impaction in poorly fed animals. If abomasal rupture has occurred, profound hemoconcentration and leukopenia are present. Abdominocentesis generally is not useful in diagnosing abomasal impaction, because peritoneal fluid is only abnormal after abomasal rupture.

PATHOPHYSIOLOGY. Animals fed roughage that is poorly digestible and incapable of meeting their energy requirements consume as much as the rumen will physically permit. The flow of ingesta from the forestomachs to the abomasum normally contains only small, finely digested particles of forage material. With chronic engorgement of highly lignified, poorly digestible forage, larger particles escape the forestomach and accumulate in the abomasum. Once a mass of fiber

TABLE 30-13

Causes of Intestinal Obstruction in Ruminants

Disease	Animals Most Commonly Affected	Signs
Intestinal atresia or stenosis	Neonates	No feces; abdominal distention
Intestinal volvulus around mesenteric root	All ruminants; neonates more common	Colic; rapid abdominal distention; collapse; shock
Intussusception	All ruminants; LI or SI of neonates; SI of adults	Colic early, then chronic low-grade pain; dehydration; mucus plus blood in dark red feces; slow abdominal distention; decreased fecal output; mass palpated per rectum; distended loops of intestine per rectum.
Cecal dilatation and volvulus	Adult dairy cattle in early lactation	Mild to severe colic; distended abdomen, especially upper right; ping in right paralumbar fossa; distended cecum palpated per rectum
Intestinal tumors	Sheep; rare in cattle	Progressive weight loss; cattle—may palpate mass per rectum; sheep—identify for celiotomy or necropsy
Mesenteric fat necrosis	Cattle, especially Channel Island breeds	May discover masses on routine examination; progressive weight loss; scant or no feces; dilated loops of bowel per rectum
Intestinal incarceration	All ruminants	See Intussusception
Pseudoobstruction or ileus	All ruminants	Scant or no feces; right-sided ping; Succussable fluid on right; often associated with peritonitis

LI, Large intestine; *SI*, small intestine.

forms in the abomasum, further accumulation of particulate material is enhanced. With time, the mass fills the abomasum. Additional ingesta distends the abomasum to several times normal size. Some animals may not develop hypochloremic, metabolic alkalosis because channels through the abomasal mass may permit fluid to reach the intestine. Also, abomasal secretion may be inhibited by the cachexia and chronic distention of the organ.

Abomasal transport failure after correction of abomasal volvulus is typical of vagal indigestion syndrome. Presumably vagal nerve branches to the abomasum are damaged during the occurrence of the volvulus, or vascular thrombosis occurs, preventing the return of normal muscular activity of the abomasum. That vagal tone sometimes increases in these animals is indicated by the bradycardia that may develop concurrently. Hypochloremic, metabolic alkalosis does develop frequently, with chloride accumulating in the ruminoreticular contents. The abomasum distends moderately as a result of the forward pressure of the omasal pump. No specific measurements have been made, but presumably the abomasum becomes atonic.

Pyloric obstruction caused by foreign bodies or occlusion caused by lymphosarcoma leads to mechanical outflow obstruction. Chloride escapes into the rumen, and metabolic alkalosis develops. The abomasum retains motility, but it is ineffective in moving ingesta into the duodenum.

NECROPSY FINDINGS. Emaciation and a firm, grossly enlarged abomasum are consistent with primary abomasal impaction. The abomasal contents resemble normal, dry rumen contents. The rumen is also enlarged but either filled with homogenous, watery ingesta that lacks normal stratification or impacted with dry ingesta, similar to the abomasum. The abomasum is dilated, flaccid, and filled with watery ingesta if it becomes atonic after correction of abomasal volvulus. Intraluminal foreign body or tumor involvement of the abomasal wall is self-evident.

TREATMENT AND PROGNOSIS. Because most cases of primary abomasal impaction are quite advanced when brought to the attention of the veterinarian, treatment usually is unrewarding. The clinician must weigh the severity of the metabolic disturbances and the likelihood of recovery. Salvage by slaughter is often the most economic recommendation. If therapeutic measures do not resolve the impaction, death usually occurs within a few days of the onset of severe signs. Medical management includes correction of fluid and electrolyte abnormalities. Early cases may be resolved with easily digestible feeds, aggressive fluid therapy, and laxatives. Metoclopramide at a dosage of 0.3 mg/kg given subcutaneously four to six times daily may increase passage of ingesta through the pylorus. Pregnancy may be terminated by induction of parturition with corticosteroids or prostaglandin, leading to improved comfort. Surgical intervention by means of abomasotomy has not been successful in restoring abomasal function.[1272] Baker[1273] recommended rumenotomy followed by installation of a nasogastric tube inserted into the abomasum through the operator in the rumen. Through the indwelling tube laxatives and emulsifiers may be given during the postoperative days to aid in softening and removing the abomasal contents. Mineral oil (8 ml/kg/day), dioctyl sodium sulfosuccinate (50 mg/kg/day), magnesium hydroxide (1 g/kg/day), or magnesium sulfate (2.5 g/kg/day) have all been recommended. External massage may help break up the contents of the abomasum.

PREVENTION AND CONTROL. Prevention of primary abomasal impaction requires proper dietary management of cattle in cold weather. Because animals outside without shelter have substantially increased maintenance energy requirements in cold, windy weather, straw or corn stover is not adequate as the sole feed. Concentrates and better-quality forage prevent abomasal impaction. Monitoring body condition during winter weather alerts the good manager that supplemental feed is needed before abomasal impaction occurs.

REFERENCES

1272. Merritt AM, Boucher WB: Surgical treatment of abomasal impaction in the cow, *J Am Vet Med Assoc* 150:1115-1120, 1968.
1273. Baker JS: Abomasal impaction and related obstructions of the forestomachs in cattle, *J Am Vet Med Assoc* 175:1250-1253, 1979.

OBSTRUCTIVE INTESTINAL DISEASES

CHARLES GUARD

DEFINITION AND ETIOLOGY. Several conditions may lead to obstruction of the flow of ingesta through the intestinal tract. Congenital malformations may include atresia or constriction of portions of the gut. Mechanical accidents such as intussusception or volvulus obstruct the passage of ingesta. Tumors and in rare cases fibrous adhesions restrict the lumen of the gut. Functional obstructions caused by ileus or dilation of a segment may mimic mechanical problems. Each of the specific diseases is discussed in the following paragraphs and summarized in Table 30-13.

CLINICAL SIGNS AND DIFFERENTIAL DIAGNOSIS. Acute manifestations of the obstructive diseases include a reduced amount of feces or failure to pass feces, progressive abdominal enlargement with areas of tympanitic resonance on the right side of the abdomen, and sometimes colic. If pain is severe, forestomach atony reflexly occurs. Mechanical obstructions may lead to circulatory shock and collapse as a result of dehydration. Electrolyte abnormalities depend on the site of the obstruction; those near the duodenum or pylorus lead to sequestration of abomasal secretions and result in hypochloremic, hypokalemic metabolic alkalosis. Obstructions of the cecum, colon, or rectum may lead to dehydration without alkalosis. If bowel necrosis or rupture occurs, acidosis results from the circulatory collapse that accompanies peritonitis and the absorption of toxins.

INTESTINAL ATRESIA OR STENOSIS

A congenital condition, intestinal atresia or stenosis has been reported in calves and lambs.[1274-1276] Clinical signs usually are evident within a few days of birth. Animals with anal or distal rectal atresia usually have the slowest onset of signs, whereas obstructions farther orad lead to more rapid onset of signs. Malformations of the anus and rectum are believed to be hereditary,[1277] and breeding of surgically corrected survivors should be discouraged. Jejunal atresia in the Jersey cow has been reported to be inherited as an autosomal recessive trait.[1273] Colonic atresia is not thought to be caused by heritable factors.[1276] Hess, Leipold, and Muller[1278] have suggested that palpation of the amniotic vesicle at 42 days' gestation leads to colonic atresia. If the anus or distal rectum is atretic, animals strain or pump their tails in an attempt to defecate. A fistulous connection may exist between the rectum and the urogenital tract (i.e., either the vagina or the pelvic urethra). Visual and digital exploration of the perineum reveals the absence of feces and may permit definition of the specific defect. Stenosis or atresia of the intestinal tract may occur to any degree; narrowing, a membranous diaphragm with a perforation, an imperforate membrane, a cordlike remnant of the intestine, and blind-ended dilation all have been described.[1274] Affected neonates show depression and colic and progress to cardiovascular collapse after the intestine proximal to the obstruction becomes distended with fluid and gas. Tympany may be easily detected by percussion. Contrast radiography may be useful in defining the site of the obstruction but should be considered with caution because of the added stress and further distention of the gut. If the anus and rectum are normal, a digital examination usually reveals only mucus or blood (or both). Complete intestinal volvulus must be considered in young animals, but malformations always have the historic evidence of diminished or absent feces. In addition, such animals are presented for examination within hours to a few days of birth.

Surgical repair is indicated if the animal is to be salvaged. However, the prognosis for normal intestinal function is poor, even after surgical correction of the atresia. Many affected neonates appear to have poor intestinal motility. The development of bowel stasis and peritonitis after surgery is common. When registered animals are involved, a letter should be sent to the appropriate breed registry stating that the defect has been corrected.

VOLVULUS OF THE LARGE AND SMALL INTESTINE AROUND THE MESENTERIC ROOT

Volvulus of the large and small intestine around the mesenteric root leads to extremely painful colic and relatively rapid abdominal enlargement. Circulatory shock develops early, and the clinical course is short.[1274] Ruminants of any age are susceptible, but most cases are seen in preruminant neonates. In rare cases the condition is seen in adult ruminants after casting and rolling have been performed to correct a left displaced abomasum. Robertson[1275] reported that 1% to 2% of surgical abomasopexies were followed by torsion of the intestinal mass around the mesenteric root. Extremely violent signs of colic generally are seen, including kicking and vocalization. Affected animals soon become recumbent and develop rapid dehydration. The heart and respiratory rates increase greatly as shock develops. As in calves with congenital intestinal obstructions, variable-pitched resonant sounds may be heard bilaterally over the abdomen with simultaneous percussion and auscultation. In older cattle the tympany is restricted to the right side. Succussion reveals fluid splashing sounds, particularly on the right side. Rectal examination reveals a tense abdomen filled with distended loops of gut and the absence of normal topographic relationships. Surgical correction is the only successful treatment option. The prognosis depends on the degree of devitalization of bowel and the amount of venous thrombosis. Animals surgically corrected during the early stages characterized by violent colic have responded better than those that have progressed to recumbency and depression.

Volvulus of lesser portions of the intestinal tract leads to signs similar to those of complete intestinal volvulus around the root of the mesentery but often slower in onset. Colic with accompanying tachycardia, ruminal stasis, and anorexia is present to varying degrees. The abdomen is moderately distended on the right when the animal is viewed from the rear. Simultaneous auscultation and percussion on the right side reveal multiple-pitched, resonant pings from the gas accumulated proximal to the obstruction. Rectal examination may reveal scant feces, mucus, or blood. The affected bowel usually is palpable as grossly distended with gas and some fluid. Because of their relatively long mesentery, the spiral colon (or part of it), the distal jejunum, and the proximal ileum may develop an obstructive volvulus. Therapy requires correction of acid-base and electrolyte abnormalities and rapid surgical manipulation by means of celiotomy.

INTUSSUSCEPTION

In the development of an intussusception, the orad portion of gut (intussusceptum) usually is engulfed and propelled distally by peristaltic action of the enveloping portion (intussuscipiens). Intussusception of the small intestine is an uncommon cause of intestinal obstruction in cattle. The condition has been reported once in a goat[1281] and as a cause of multiple losses in three flocks of sheep.[1282] Intussusception may occur in either the large or small intestine of calves but is almost invariably in the jejunum of adults.[1283] Signs include early colic caused by the tension on the mesentery on the invaginating portion of the intestine. With time, ischemia of this portion leads to loss of sensation from tension receptors. Distention of the intestine with fluid and gas proximal to the obstruction leads to chronic pain. Thus a cow may show violent behavior or kicking at the abdomen in the first few hours, which is succeeded by treading and repeated lying and standing.[1284] Over the course of several days the intussusceptum may become totally devitalized and slough. This is accompanied by increasingly severe peritonitis, and in the event of bowel rupture, toxic shock probably will develop. Most cases of intussusception in adults are thought to be associated with an intermural mass or polyp. The mass is propelled into the intussuscipiens by normal peristaltic contractions. In contrast, in the young animal no such mass lesion is usually associated with intussusception, but enteritis often is. *Oesophagostomum columbianum* causes nodules in the intestinal wall of sheep but has not been proved to be linked to multiple deaths from intussusception.[1282]

Dehydration develops as gastrointestinal secretions accumulate in the gut lumen. In adults, hypochloremic, hypokalemic metabolic alkalosis develops gradually. The rumen becomes distended with fluid as its contents become more finely digested and abomasal reflux accumulates. The right side of the abdomen (or both sides) also enlarges as a result of the distention of the small intestine. Simultaneous auscultation and percussion of the right side of the abdomen reveals areas of variable-pitched resonance.[1285] Rectal examination reveals distended loops of small intestine. The intussusception may be palpable as a firm mass; the cow may demonstrate pain when the mass is palpated. Feces are absent within hours of the onset of signs. The examiner may find mucus and blood in the descending colon. In long-standing cases, the scant feces are very dark red and must be distinguished from the black feces (melena) associated with abomasal bleeding. Fluid obtained by abdominocentesis shows an increase in erythrocytes and leukocytes and an elevated protein level. Fever often is present. If the condition is long-standing and bowel rupture has occurred, bacteria may be present. The complete blood count may reveal neutrophilia and an elevated plasma fibrinogen level.

In neonates with enteritis, fecal output decreases as appetite is lost after intussusception. A fever may develop as peritonitis occurs. Calves and other neonates may not exhibit obvious signs of colic. Abdominal palpation using both hands in an attempt to detect a mass often is successful in delineating an intussusception in a neonate. When neutrophilia, hyperfibrinogenemia, and loss of appetite develop after "routine" enteritis, intussusception should be suspected.

Treatment requires both surgical correction of the obstruction and parenteral restoration of fluid and electrolyte balance. Because of the losses of chloride and potassium and the development of alkalosis, 0.9% sodium chloride solution with 30 mEq/L of added potassium chloride is recommended. Once intestinal patency has been restored, oral fluid and electrolyte supplementation usually allows the patient to achieve normal status. The prognosis usually is good if surgery is performed early in the course of the disease and complications such as peritonitis can be controlled. The surgical incision should be made high in the caudal right flank. The exceptions are animals with intestinal neoplasia that has metastasized[1286] or in which bowel rupture has occurred.

CECAL DILATION AND VOLVULUS

Dilation of the cecum in cattle occurs in the same epidemiologic circumstances as abomasal displacement and ulceration, although less often. Reports of hospitalized cases indicate that the postpartum interval to the development of cecal disease may be longer than that for left displacement of the abomasum; 57% of cases occurred within 2 months of parturition[1287] and 46% within 4 weeks.[1288] Dirksen and Doll[1289] described 19 cases in calves less than 6 months old. Of these, 84% were being raised for early slaughter, and the remainder for herd replacements; this suggests that feeding or management differences may predispose to cecal disease in calves. In adult cattle, cecal dilation generally is believed to precede volvulus or torsion. The presence of volatile fatty acids in the

cecum at concentrations above the normal range of about 1 mM/L leads to reduced motility.[1290,1291] Fermentable carbohydrates escape from the forestomach after a change to a more concentrate-rich diet or generally with inadequate feeding of roughage. Cecal flora metabolizes these carbohydrates into volatile fatty acids, methane, and carbon dioxide. Reduced motility plus increased production of gas may lead to pathologic distention of the cecum and proximal colon. Persistence of the dilation probably predisposes to volvulus.

Cattle with cecal dilation have a more gradual onset of illness than that noted with cecal volvulus, although the time required for dilation to develop into volvulus is unknown. With simple dilation, feed intake and milk production decrease. Mild abdominal pain may be evident. The right paralumbar fossa usually is distended without the ribs being sprung. A large area of resonance is auscultable from the tuber coxae a variable distance cranially.[1285] Manure usually is passed, but the consistency may be loose and the volume reduced. The apex of the gas-filled cecum can be felt in the pelvic canal or nearby on rectal examination.

Cattle with cecal volvulus show an abrupt onset of anorexia, agalactia, and marked abdominal pain. Tachycardia and forestomach stasis also are present. Manure usually is scant or absent. The abdominal distention usually exceeds that caused by simple cecal dilation. The area of resonance in the right paralumbar fossa is larger, and fluid usually can be detected in the cecum and proximal colon by ballottement. Although some cows with simple dilation have acid-base abnormalities, most with cecal volvulus have some degree of metabolic alkalosis with hypochloremia and hypokalemia. The apex of the cecum usually is not palpable per rectum; rather, the distended body of the cecum or proximal colon impinges on the pelvic canal because the apex is directed cranially. Distended small intestine may be palpated with either dilation or volvulus. Medical management of cecal dilation usually is successful with the use of antacid-laxatives such as magnesium hydroxide and intravenous or oral fluids to restore normal acid-base status, together with provision of a coarse, high-fiber diet. Intravenous or subcutaneous calcium therapy may also be helpful in lactating cows. Some cattle have recurrent episodes of cecal dilation, and preventive surgery such as typhlectomy may be indicated. The surgical incision should be made high in the caudal right flank. In two reports the recurrence rate after surgery was about 10% within a year of the first incident.[1287,1288] Cattle with cecal volvulus require surgical intervention and fluid management to correct the hypochloremic, hypokalemic metabolic alkalosis. The prognosis for surgical patients depends on the degree of ischemic injury to the cecum and other structures involved in the obstruction. There is a report of apparently benign chronic cecal distention after an acute episode of illness.[1292] The cow was repeatedly examined over 10 months and always had both a right-sided ping and rectally palpable gas-distended cecum. Appetite, milk production, and consistency of feces were reported as normal by the owner throughout the period.

INTESTINAL TUMORS

Intestinal carcinoma is very rare in cattle, but the incidence in sheep is relatively high in some areas of the world. Moulton[1293] cites Monlux and Monlux (1972) as reporting that 0.1% of cattle neoplasms in Denver abattoirs are intestinal carcinomas. Reports began accumulating that an unusually high incidence of intestinal tumors was seen in cull ewes in New Zealand beginning in the mid-1950s.[1294,1295] Certain breeds of British origin were observed to have a higher incidence than "fine wool" breeds. In subsequent studies in New Zealand, Australia, South Africa, and Iceland, the type of hus-

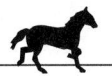

bandry practiced was linked by correlation analyses with a higher incidence of tumors. Details of which specific common factor or factors might be responsible await further research. No specific environmental or toxicologic exposures have been discovered in common among the major sheep-raising areas that have high rates of intestinal carcinoma. The rate of gross lesions in asymptomatic ewes going to slaughter ranged from 0.4% to 4.4%.[1296,1297]

Affected cattle or sheep may have a protracted course of weight loss with no other observable signs until near death. Alternatively there are reports of acute gastrointestinal disturbances manifested by colic, abdominal distention, and auscultable right-sided pings.[1298] Although these cases are rare, they must be differentiated from other causes of acute obstruction in cattle such as cecal volvulus, intussusception, or abomasal volvulus. In cattle in which rectal examination is possible, the lesion may be detected on routine examination as an intramural mass or annular constriction of the jejunum or ileum. In sheep, the diagnosis usually is made at necropsy. Signs in affected animals might include diarrhea, abdominal distention caused by the accumulation of gas and ingesta proximal to the obstruction, or ascites. The well-characterized lesions in sheep involve local spread of the tumor through the lymphatics and intraperitoneally. Ultimately cellular deposits occur on all visceral and parietal peritoneal surfaces, severely impairing lymphatic drainage from the abdomen. Attempts at surgical removal of affected tumors in cattle have not been successful because of undetected metastases.

MESENTERIC FAT NECROSIS

Mesenteric fat necrosis is a condition of cattle that is more common in dairy breeds of Channel Island region. However, it has occurred in all breeds and may be related to dietary factors such as consumption of feedstuffs high in long-chain, saturated fatty acids[1299]; cattle that are being fattened are at greatest risk. The lesions develop as an inflammatory response around degenerating adipose cells. The triglycerides in these cells are thought to undergo hydrolysis to glycerol and fatty acids. The longer the carbon skeleton and the greater the degree of saturation, the more resistant are the fatty acids to removal by normal cellular mechanisms. Remaining clumps or crystals of fatty acids serve as inflammatory foci for the subsequent necrotic masses. Affected cattle have subnormal free cholesterol and elevated free fatty acids in serum.[1300] Most cattle with fat necrosis eventually develop an intestinal obstruction as a result of the progressive nature of the mass lesions. The signs of clinical fat necrosis resemble those of progressive intestinal obstruction from other causes. Weight loss, anorexia, diarrhea, bloody stool, abdominal enlargement, and right-sided ping are all possible signs with partial obstruction. Fever, tachycardia, and signs of discomfort such as tenesmus, treading, and teeth grinding may be seen as the obstruction becomes more severe. Many affected cattle have no clinical signs, and the condition is discovered during rectal examination for other reasons. Rectal examination may be impossible because of stricture of the rectum, or dystocia may occur as a result of the necrotic fat masses in the pelvic canal. Fat necrosis usually affects mature cattle, but there is a report of a 6-month course of illness attributed to fat necrosis in a 13-month-old Black Angus heifer.[1301]

Animals with fat necrosis that causes clinical signs of intestinal obstruction usually are not treated. Recent experimental therapy of subclinical fat necrosis using a compound that alters lipid metabolism in fungi was successful.[1300] The fungicide isoprothiolane was given at the dosage of 20 g/day orally for 8 weeks. Approximately half of the treated cows had a 50% reduction in necrotic masses by 12 weeks; at follow-up evaluation in 1 year the masses were not detectable in half the surviving cows. The apparent success of this treatment suggests that treatment of mesenteric fat necrosis may be available at some future date.

INTESTINAL INCARCERATION

Intestinal obstruction may occur in ruminants as a result of accidental entrapment of loops, usually of jejunum, around remnants of embryonic structures or through acquired defects in mesentery or the abdominal wall. Intestinal adhesions caused by intraperitoneal injections of irritating substances can also lead to intestinal obstruction. Initial signs of colic followed by depression, anorexia, progressive abdominal distention, and absence of feces usually develop. Distended loops of small intestine usually are palpable per rectum. Remnants of the urachus,[1302] the omphalomesenteric duct,[1303] and the left umbilical vein[1304] in cows and of the ductus deferens[1305] in steers have been described as responsible for incarceration of the jejunum. The authors of one report indicated that 26% of cows examined had a persistent round ligament of the liver and falciform ligament.[1304] Thus tears in the falciform ligament leading to intestinal entrapment may be among the most common causes of the relatively rare problem of intestinal incarceration in cattle. Treatment of intestinal incarceration requires surgical intervention.

PSEUDOOBSTRUCTION OR ILEUS

Failure to pass feces usually is a sign of intestinal obstruction. However, in adult, lactating dairy cattle, a condition of ileus of the intestinal tract that mimics complete intestinal obstruction commonly occurs. The condition often resolves spontaneously; in rare instances surgical decompression of the affected bowel is required. In a series of 100 referred cases of intestinal obstruction, 39 were judged to be simple ileus.[1306] Cows are most often in early lactation, and treatment is sought for partial anorexia. Colic sometimes is the presenting sign. Clinical examination reveals a normal temperature, pulse rate, and respiratory rate. Rumen motility usually is normal in frequency but reduced in amplitude. In long-standing cases, with continued microbial digestion the rumen contents become more fluid in consistency. Slight right-sided abdominal enlargement may be seen early and may progress to extreme distention of the abdomen on the right. No borborygmi are heard on the right side, but fluid tinkling sounds may occur. Simultaneous auscultation and percussion reveal areas of variable-pitched resonance. Succussion produces sloshing sounds. On rectal examination a distended spiral colon, cecum, or small intestine may be palpated. Early in the course of the disease the distention is not extreme, and compression easily flattens the affected bowel. If abdominal distention is severe, introducing the arm into the abdominal cavity may be difficult because of the pressure of distended bowel at the pelvic inlet. No feces are passed, but the examiner's arm may be coated with sticky mucus and feces with a stale odor. Evaluation of serum electrolytes usually reveals no abnormalities. Differential diagnoses to consider include intussusception, intestinal incarceration, intestinal volvulus, and cecal dilation. There is no blood in the feces, and no masses are palpable per rectum with pseudoobstruction.

Because most obstructive lesions of the intestine in cattle are not immediately life-threatening, symptomatic therapy or simply close observation may be elected for 1 or 2 days if ileus is suspected. If surgery is elected, an approach high in the right flank gives the best access for exploration of the intestinal tract. In the absence of an obstructive lesion, the bowel may be decompressed and drained. This is a laborious procedure that requires multiple punctures unless the distention is restricted to the cecum and spiral colon. Despite the lack of correction of a specific underlying defect, many cows begin passing feces soon after an exploratory celiotomy. Manipulation of the intestinal tract alone seems to have beneficial effects.[1306] This response is difficult to differentiate from the spontaneous recovery that usually occurs without surgery in cows. Relief of distention of portions of the intestinal tract may remove reflex inhibition of motility that can occur in response to extreme stretching of mural tension and pain receptors. The cause of pseudoobstruction of the intestine is unknown, and little pathophysiologic information has been elucidated. Medical management often includes intravenous or subcutaneous administration of calcium, oral laxative-antacids such as magnesium hydroxide (0.5 to 1 g/kg repeated daily), and intravenous fluids if dehydration develops. Balanced electrolytes such as lactated Ringer's solution or 0.9% sodium chloride solution with 2.5% glucose added are adequate. Some patients may have hypochloremic, hypokalemic metabolic alkalosis; these require 0.9% sodium chloride solution with 30 mEq/L potassium chloride added. Many cases resolve without specific therapy.

REFERENCES

1274. van der Gaag I, Tibboel D: Intestinal atresia and stenosis in animals: a report of 34 cases, *Vet Pathol* 17:565-574, 1980.
1275. Steenhaut M et al: Intestinal malformations in calves and their surgical correction, *Vet Rec* 98:131-133, 1976.
1276. Ducharme N et al: Colonic atresia in cattle: a prospective study of 43 cases, *Can Vet J* 29:818-824, 1988.
1277. Barker IK, Van Dreumel AA: Congenital anomalies of the intestine. In Jubb KVP, Kennedy PC, Palmer N, eds: *Pathology of domestic animals*, vol 2, Toronto, 1985, Academic Press.
1278. Hess H, Leipold G, Muller W: Zur genese des angeborenen darmverschlusses des kalhes, *Monatshefte Veterinaermed* 37:89-92, 1982.
1279. Tulleners EP: Surgical correction of volvulus of the root of the mesentery in calves, *J Am Vet Med Assoc* 179:998-999, 1981.
1280. Robertson JT: Differential diagnosis and surgical management of intestinal obstruction in cattle, *Vet Clin North Am (Large Anim Pract)* 1:377-394, 1979.
1281. Mitchell WC: Intussusception in goats, *Vet Med (Small Anim Clin)* 78:1918, 1983.
1282. Osborne HG: Ileal intussusception causing multiple losses in sheep, *Aust Vet J* 34:42-43, 1958.
1283. Hamilton GF, Tulleners EP: Intussusception involving the spiral colon in a calf, *Can Vet J* 21:32, 1980.
1284. Smith DF: Intussusception in adult cattle, *Compend Cont Educ Pract Vet* 2:S49-S53, 1980.
1285. Smith DF et al: The identification of structures and conditions responsible for right side tympanitic resonance (ping) in adult cattle, *Cornell Vet* 72:180-199, 1982.
1286. Archer RM et al: Jejunojejunal intussusception associated with a transmural adenocarcinoma in an aged cow, *J Am Vet Med Assoc* 192:209-211, 1988.
1287. Whitlock RH: Cecal volvulus in dairy cattle, *Int Congr Dis Cattle* 1:69-73, 1976.
1288. Fubini SL et al: Cecal dilatation and volvulus in dairy cows: 84 cases (1977-1983), *J Am Vet Med Assoc* 189:96-98, 1986.
1289. Dirksen G, Doll K: Ileus and subileus in the young bovine animal, *Bovine Pract* 21:33-40, 1986.
1290. Svendsen P, Kristensen B: Cecal dilatation in cattle, *Nord Vet Med* 22:578-583, 1970.
1291. Svendsen P: Inhibition of cecal motility in sheep by volatile fatty acids, *Nord Vet Med* 24:393-396, 1972.
1292. Duelke BE, Whitlock RH: Persistent cecal dilatation in a lactating dairy cow, *Cornell Vet* 66:301-308, 1976.
1293. Moulton JE: *Tumors in domestic animals*, ed 2, Berkeley, Calif, 1978, University of California Press.
1294. Webster WM: Neoplasia in food animals with special reference to the high incidence in sheep, *NZ Vet J* 14:203-214, 1966.
1295. Webster WM: A further survey of neoplasms in abattoir sheep, *NZ Vet J* 15:51-54, 1967.
1296. Simpson BH, Jolly RD: Carcinoma of the small intestine in sheep, *J Pathol* 112:83-92, 1974.
1297. Ross AD: Small intestinal carcinoma in sheep, *Aust Vet J* 56:25-28, 1980.
1298. Bristol DG, Baum KH, Mezza LE: Adenocarcinoma of the jejunum in two cows, *J Am Vet Med Assoc* 185:551-553, 1984.
1299. Julian RJ: The peritoneum, retroperitoneum and mesentery. In Jubb KVF, Kennedy PC, Palmer N, eds: *Pathology of domestic animals*, ed 3, vol 2, New York, 1985, Academic Press.
1300. Oka A et al: Efficacy of isoprothiolane for the treatment of fat necrosis in cattle, *Br Vet J* 144:507-514, 1988.
1301. Johnson R, Ames NK, Dunstan R: Abdominal fat necrosis in a heifer, *Compend Cont Educ Pract Vet* 7:S103-S109, 1985.
1302. Baxter GM, Darien BJ, Wallace CE: Persistent urachal remnant causing intestinal strangulation in a cow, *J Am Vet Med Assoc* 191:555-558, 1987.
1303. Koch DB, Robertson JT, Donawick WJ: Small intestinal obstruction due to persistent vitelloumbilcal band in a cow, *J Am Vet Med Assoc* 173:197-199, 1978.
1304. Ducharme NG, Smith DF, Koch DB: Small intestinal obstruction caused by a persistent round ligament of the liver in a cow, *J Am Vet Med Assoc* 180:1234-1236, 1982.
1305. Wolfe DF et al: Incarceration of a section of small intestine by remnants of the ductus deferens in steers, *J Am Vet Med Assoc* 191:1597-1598, 1987.
1306. Pearson H, Pinsent PJN: Intestinal obstruction in cattle, *Vet Rec* 101:162-166, 1977.

DISEASES CAUSED BY *CLOSTRIDIUM PERFRINGENS* TOXINS (Enterotoxemia; Yellow Lamb Disease; Lamb Dysentery; Necrotic Enteritis)

PAUL G.E. MICHELSEN

DEFINITION AND ETIOLOGY. *Clostridium perfringens* is a toxin-producing, anaerobic, spore-forming rod. It is a variable species that causes a variety of diseases in human beings and animals. Some biotypes are normal inhabitants of soil, and some are commensal intestinal organisms of animals. A sometimes confusing nomenclature has evolved to organize the complexity of *C. perfringens* biology. Clinical isolates are assigned to one of the types (A through E) on the basis of possession of the major toxins (α, β, ϵ, ι) (Table 30-14). In addition to these four major toxins, strains of *C. perfringens* may produce any of at least eight other recognized soluble antigens, some of which have pathogenic importance and could be called toxins. Most of these antigens are named with Greek letters.[1307] The soluble *C. perfringens* toxin responsible for one type of food poisoning in humans has not received a Greek-letter name but is commonly known as enterotoxin (or CPE for *Clostridium perfringens* enterotoxin). Enterotoxin is also the general name for toxins that affect the intestines, and many of the *C. perfringens* antigens with Greek-letter names are also enterotoxins. In this discussion the toxin that causes food poisoning in human beings is denoted CPE to distinguish it from enterotoxin as a class of toxins. CPE is not recognized as the major component of classic *C. perfringens* disease in animals, but it may be important in some cases.[1308,1309]

The different biotypes of *C. perfringens* cause different diseases because they have different toxins, but a clear-cut assignment to one of the groups is not always possible, and overlap is considerable in the clinical signs caused by the various toxins. Many different diseases in many different animals have been ascribed to *C. perfringens*, but the ubiquitous nature of the organism and the fact that it rapidly overgrows into tissues after death makes the significance of its isolation questionable at times.

One additional potentially confusing bit of nomenclature concerns the term "enterotoxemia." Although this term is widely applied to various diseases caused by *C. perfringens*, it is strictly appropriate only for diseases in which the major signs are caused by systemic spread of the toxin in the blood.

One group of diseases caused by *C. perfringens* type C is commonly called "hemorrhagic enterotoxemia," even though the disease is not always hemorrhagic and, although the toxin may incidentally reach the circulation, it is produced in the

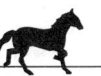

TABLE 30-14

Types of *Clostridium perfringens* by Toxin Type and Disease That Have Been Attributed to the Strain*

Type	Group Typing Toxins				Diseases Attributed
	Alpha	Beta	Epsilon	Iota	
A	XX	—	—	—	Gas gangrene (along with other organisms) Avian necrotic enteritis Hemorrhagic enteritis in cattle Yellow lamb disease Enterotoxemia of mink Type A enterotoxemia of horses Abomasal tympany and ulcers of calves[1313] Sudden infant death syndrome (crib death) Food poisoning in humans
B	X	XX	X	—	**Lamb dysentery**[1310] Enterotoxemia of sheep and goats (Iran) Enterotoxemia of foals (Britain)
C	X	XX	—	—	**Necrotic enteritis** (neonatal hemorrhagic enterotoxemia of calves, lambs, kids, foals, piglets)[1310,1315] Necrotic enteritis of fowl, Struck (enterotoxemia) of sheep (Britain) Necrotic enteritis of humans (pigbel, Darmbrand)[1310]
D	X	—	XX	—	**Enterotoxemia** ("overeating disease," "pulpy kidney disease") of sheep, goats, and cattle
E	X	—	—	X	Enteritis in rabbits Occasionally isolated from sheep and cattle Abomasal tympany and ulceration of calves[1313]

X, Toxin of minor importance; *XX*, toxin of major importance; —, not present.
*Disease of major veterinary importance in boldface.

intestine and exerts its major effects locally. A better descriptive name for this disease has been proposed to be necrotic enteritis.[1310] It is important to realize that many of the effects of other biotypes of *C. perfringens* are systemic and that enteric clinical signs may be entirely lacking with disease caused by *C. perfringens* types A and D. Each type is discussed in the following paragraphs. Type E is only occasionally isolated from livestock and is not discussed.

DIAGNOSIS OF DISEASE CAUSE BY *C. PERFRINGENS*. Meaningful diagnosis of *C. perfringens* as the cause of death or disease in an animal requires an integrative, open-minded approach. Type A is routinely isolated from soil and clinically normal animals. Types C and D are only rarely isolated from soil but can be isolated from asymptomatic individuals, especially those with neutralizing antibody to toxin. The bacterium proliferates after death, often crowding out other enteric organisms and invading tissues beyond the gut. The isolation of *C. perfringens* from a necropsied animal is not by itself sufficient basis for the diagnosis; however, if toxin is also demonstrated in gut contents and the history and lesions are compatible, a diagnosis of death from *C. perfringens* intoxication can be made.

Until recently, an isolate of *C. perfringens* was assigned to one of the five biotypes by demonstrating toxin production with mouse-protection assays or enzyme-linked immunosorbent assay (ELISA) techniques. This has been replaced by a multiplex polymer chain reaction (PCR) technique that detects the genes for toxin production in a clinical isolate.[1311] CPE, which causes food poisoning in human beings, can be detected with commercially available assays and is also detected by the multiplex PCR technique.[1312] Meaningful samples for bacterial isolation come from freshly dead animals. Samples of gut contents should be collected into sterile containers and cooled or frozen. In addition to typing bacterial isolates, demonstration of toxin itself in gut contents may aid in diagnosis. False negatives may occur in type C disease if proteases inactivate the β-toxin.

In the absence of definitive microbiologic evidence, a presumptive diagnosis of type C or D disease must be based on the history, clinical signs, pathologic findings, and differential diagnoses. Administration of toxoid vaccines is cheap and effective and may be recommended without conclusive evidence for causation. This "whole herd" protection test may be as close as one gets to definitive diagnosis in field situations. Examination of gut-content smears from various levels of the gastrointestinal tract to demonstrate large numbers of bacteria resembling *C. perfringens* may be a helpful piece of information, but the significance of such a finding, by itself, is questionable. Glucosuria in urine obtained from the bladder at necropsy is often seen in sheep (but not other species) afflicted with type D disease.

Type D disease should be distinguished from other causes of acute death (see Chapter 14). A history of sudden death in a rapidly growing, apparently healthy individual is characteristic. A single lamb is much more likely to be afflicted with overeating disease than is a twin. Other causes of acute disease in well-fed individuals include systemic pasteurellosis (lambs), acute bloat, grain overload, polioencephalomalacia, and thromboembolic meningoencephalitis (cattle). These generally have a longer disease course than type D enterotoxemia.

C. PERFRINGENS TYPE A (Yellow Lamb Disease)

C. perfringens type A can be found in many soils and is a normal inhabitant of the gut in many species. Although all five types of *C. perfringens* produce α-toxin, type A strains usually produce more than other types. The toxin is a phospholipase and causes lysis of red cells, platelets, and leukocytes (equine and caprine red cells are resistant to the hemolyzing effects of toxin). The toxin also causes vascular permeability through endothelial damage and can cause necrosis at the villous tips in the intestines.[1307]

Yellow lamb disease (so named because of the icteric nature of necropsied lambs) is an uncommon disease attributed to *C. perfringens* type A. Widespread hemolysis leads to anemia, weakness, hemoglobinuria, and icterus. The animals have a high temperature and usually die within 6 to 12 hours of onset. Differential diagnoses for yellow lamb disease include other causes of hemolytic disease, including leptospirosis and copper toxicosis. As with other type A infections, the diagnosis is always questionable, owing to the commensal nature of the organism and its rapid invasion after death. The finding of predominantly large gram-positive rods in impression smears from intestinal mucosa lends support to the diagnosis. No vaccine against type A disease is marketed in the United States, and types C and D toxoids are not expected to protect against type A unless they also contain α-toxoid.

One report implicates type A in neonatal calves with ruminal and abomasal tympany, abomasitis, and abomasal ulceration. The calves were 2 to 21 days old and died acutely or had signs of colic and depression of short duration.[1313] Type A is a relatively common cause of food poisoning in human beings. Speculation links this type to human sudden infant death syndrome ("crib death") as well.[1314]

C. PERFRINGENS TYPE B (Lamb Dysentery)

Lamb dysentery is a disease of young lambs in Britain and South Africa. Type B has not been isolated in North America. Its clinical course and presentation are similar to necrotic enteritis caused by *C. perfringens* type C. Lambs less than 1 week of age become depressed and die. A yellowish diarrhea becomes brown from blood as the disease progresses. Morbidity may be high, and mortality approaches 100%. Necropsy findings include ulcers (rarely perforating) in the small intestines and dehydration of the carcass and tissues. Sanitation and the use of type B vaccine aid in prevention and control. Types C and D toxoid cross-protect because of the overlap in toxin types.

C. PERFRINGENS TYPE C (Necrotic Enteritis; Neonatal Hemorrhagic Enterotoxemia; Pigbel; Struck)

DEFINITION AND ETIOLOGY. *C. perfringens* type C elaborates the α (hemolytic) toxin common to all types, in minor amounts, and the β-toxin in major amounts. The amount of β-toxin produced may determine the pathogenicity of a type C strain. In addition, type C strains produce the cytotoxic and hemolytic α-toxin, which is used to assign strains to group C if they have lost the ability to produce β-toxin in culture.[1305] β-toxin appears capable of producing all the signs of necrotic enteritis; the role of α-toxin or CPE in disease is unclear.[1310]

Necrotic enteritis is primarily a disease of neonates and occurs in calves, lambs, foals, and piglets. A similar disease in adult sheep, known as struck, has a very limited geographic range in Great Britain.

CLINICAL SIGNS AND DIFFERENTIAL DIAGNOSIS. Affected animals may die acutely without diarrhea, but this is rare. The diarrhea may be yellow or, in more hemorrhagic cases, brownish. Gray-red streaks of necrotic mucosa may be present in the stools. Foals with type C disease at first show acute abdominal pain, then explosive yellow diarrhea that becomes brown and hemorrhagic.[1315] Animals become dehydrated, anemic, weak, and moribund, despite intensive therapy. Morbidity and mortality are high, but the disease is quite sporadic in occurrence. Salmonellosis and coccidiosis should be considered in the differential diagnosis, but necrotic enteritis is the more common disease in very young animals.

PATHOPHYSIOLOGY. The causative β-toxin is readily destroyed by proteolytic enzymes such as trypsin. The neonate is especially predisposed to β-toxin attack by the presence of trypsin inhibitors in colostrum, the function of which is to prevent proteolytic degradation of immunoglobulins. Necrotic enteritis in humans is believed to be caused by decreased proteolytic activity arising from low-protein diets or the consumption of sweet potatoes, which contain heat-stable inhibitors of trypsin.[1310] The scattered cases of necrotic enteritis in adult animals may be the result of similar dietary factors. Type C disease has been reproduced experimentally in maturing lambs by dosing the sheep with type C cultures and soybean flour, which contains potent protease inhibitors.[1316]

Ingestion of a protein-rich diet into a protease-deficient intestinal tract allows rapid growth of *C. perfringens* organisms. The bacteria attach to the villi, and elaboration of the cytotoxic β-toxin results in necrosis and invasion of deeper intestinal layers. Death may result from the direct effects of the severe diarrhea or may be caused by secondary bacteremia or toxemia from the compromised gut barrier.

EPIDEMIOLOGY. Neonates that ingest type C organisms during the first few days of colostrum feeding are at risk. They pick up the organism from an environment contaminated by an asymptomatic shedder or from contaminated feed. Type C may be isolated from asymptomatic individuals on occasion, but it is not considered a normal commensal as is type A. Once established on a premise, the disease may become endemic. In foals the disease is significantly associated with housing in a stall or drylot during the first three days of life, previous presence of livestock on the farm, low amounts of grass hay fed postpartum, being born on dirt and having stock horse parentage (e.g., quarter horse, paint). Feeding smaller amounts of grain prepartum are associated with decreased incidence of the disease.[1317]

NECROPSY FINDINGS. Necrosis of the mucosa of the small intestine, especially the jejunum, is the consistent finding in all species. The large intestine may be normal except for intraluminal blood. The peritoneal cavity often contains excessive fluid, which clots when exposed to air. The mesenteric lymph nodes may be hemorrhagic. Microscopically, affected gut shows hemorrhage throughout the mucosa and submucosa. The tips of the necrotic villi are covered with numerous, large, gram-positive rods.

TREATMENT, PREVENTION, AND CONTROL. Once a case becomes clinically apparent, treatment generally is unsuccessful because of the fulminant nature of the disease. Foals can be treated with supportive intravenous broad-spectrum antibiotics (to cover gram-negative bacteremia caused by loss of gut integrity), fluids, plasma (intravenous and oral), withdrawal of milk for 24 hours, oral metronidazole, and intravenous *C. perfringens* types C and D antitoxin. Metronidazole (10 mg/kg PO or IV given twice daily) can be given to at-risk foals in the face of an outbreak, beginning at 8 to 12 hours of age and continuing for 5 days.[1318] Toxoid has been administered to horses[1319] to control the disease on an apparently endemic property, with good results. Antitoxin* may be given to animals at risk in an outbreak, and *C. perfringens* types C and D are common components of multivalent vaccines. The primary vaccination series consists of two injections 1 month apart, with the final dose given 2 weeks before parturition, and a yearly booster thereafter. Neonates should be vaccinated at 8, 12, and 16 weeks of age on problem farms.

C. PERFRINGENS TYPE D (Enterotoxemia; Overeating Disease; Pulpy Kidney Disease)

DEFINITION AND ETIOLOGY. Enterotoxemia caused by *C. perfringens* type D is a disease of major importance in sheep and of lesser importance in cattle and goats. It is caused by

---

*Dybelon *C. perfringens* types C and D antitoxin, Bio-Ceutic, St. Joseph, MO 64501.

strains of the bacterium that produces the epsilon toxin. This type is not a common soil organism, as is type A, but it may be isolated from the feces of apparently normal sheep and, less often, cattle.[1320] Most clinical disease occurs in animals fed a highly nutritious diet, especially grain-fed livestock.

CLINICAL SIGNS AND EPIDEMIOLOGY. The sudden death of a well-fed, rapidly growing animal is the most common presentation of enterotoxemia. The disease may run its course in 30 to 90 minutes, with affected lambs showing ataxia, trembling, stiff limbs, opisthotonus, convulsions, coma, and death. At the onset of clinical signs, the animal is hyperglycemic. At death it is glucosuric. The differential diagnoses should include other causes of neurologic signs and acute death: anthrax, botulism, black disease, leptospirosis, listeriosis, enterotoxigenic *Escherichia coli* infection, septicemia, polioencephalomalacia, toxic indigestion (grain overload), systemic pasteurellosis, and tetanus.

Sublethal doses may result in brain damage and *focal symmetric encephalomalacia* (see diseases of nervous system, Chapter 33). Affected lambs are dull and unresponsive to normal environmental stimulation. The major differential diagnosis is polioencephalomalacia.

PATHOPHYSIOLOGY. In some feedlot situations the animal ingests *C. perfringens* type D on a regular basis, but the acid environment of the abomasum and continuous peristalsis, as well as low amounts of fermentable substrate, conspire to keep bacterial numbers low and moving out of the animal. The intestinal environment also influences the amount of toxin produced.

Some factor of overnutrition, often heavy grain feeding or very rich pasture, provides substrate for rapid proliferation of the type D organism, leading to elaboration of the prototoxin. Cleavage of the prototoxin by proteases yields the active toxin. Epsilon toxin increases intestinal permeability, causing edema in a variety of organs, notably the lungs, kidney (hence the name "pulpy kidney disease") and brain (focal symmetric encephalomalacia). These lesions cause rapid deterioration and death. Hyperglycemia and glucosuria are the result of massive hepatic glycogen release caused by the epsilon toxin.

NECROPSY FINDINGS. Postmortem lesions are inconsistent. The "pulpy kidney" lesion may not be seen in freshly examined specimens. The epicardium, serosa, thymus, and diaphragm may have small areas of hemorrhage. The pericardial sac often contains excess fluid. The lungs may be edematous. Glucosuria is considered a hallmark of type D enterotoxemia.

TREATMENT, PREVENTION, AND CONTROL. If initiated at the first suspicion of overeating disease, type D antitoxin and oral antibiotics (sulfa) may have dramatic results.[1321] The diet should be adjusted downward in outbreaks to try to minimize the substrate, especially starch, that reaches the bacterium. Lambs on rich pasture should be moved to poorer pasture or corralled and fed hay until they have been vaccinated twice. Lambs and calves brought into a feedlot should have the concentrate ration increased slowly to minimize microfloral disruptions.

Antitoxin can be given in an outbreak, but previous vaccination is more effective. Vaccination with type D bacterin-toxoid is effective in preventing disease. Two doses are given 14 to 28 days apart, before heavy grain feeding or exposure to rich pasture begins. The aluminum hydroxide adjuvanted vaccines may cause raised subcutaneous lumps (most noticeable on goats) that may go on to abscess. Dairy goats fed continuous high-grain rations may need to be vaccinated more often for continuous protection. One study of three commercial vaccines found that one of the vaccines provoked no antibody response in goats 14 days after vaccination and that

at 28 days after vaccination, even the goats that had responded to the other two vaccines had titers no higher than unvaccinated controls.[1322] The vaccine is not licensed in the United States for use in goats but is routinely used. Bummer lambs may be protected by feeding bovine colostrum from cows vaccinated several times with the sheep vaccine to provide high titers in colostrum.[1323] Colostral titers from the dam are protective to 12 weeks of age, after which vaccination should be used to provide active immunity against the disease.[1324]

β₂-TOXIGENIC *C. PERFRINGENS* TYPHLOCOLITIS IN HORSES

β_2-Toxin is a newly described *C. perfringens* toxin that may play a role in intestinal diseases of adult horses, particularly typhlocolitis. Affected animals may have a history of recent stress or antibiotic administration and show hemorrhagic, profuse, watery diarrhea, low body temperature, severe leukopenia, and hypoproteinemia.[1325] The diagnosis depends on demonstration of the β_2-gene by PCR.[1326]

REFERENCES

1307. McDonel JL: Toxins of *Clostridium perfringens* type A, B, C, D and E. In Dorner F, Drews J, eds: *Pharmacology of bacterial toxins*, see Sec 119, pp. 477-517, International Encyclopedia of Pharmacology and Therapeutics, Oxford, England, 1986, Pergamon Press.

1308. Bueschel D et al: Enterotoxigenic *Clostridium perfringens* type A necrotic enteritis in a foal, *J Am Vet Med Assoc* 213:1305-1307, 1998.

1309. Donaldson MT, Palmer JE: Prevalence of *Clostridium perfringens* enterotoxin and *Clostridium difficile* toxin A in feces of horses with diarrhea and colic, *J Am Vet Med Assoc* 215:358-361,1999.

1310. Tzipori S: The relative importance of enteric pathogens affecting neonates of domestic animals, *Adv Vet Sci Comp Med* 29:103-206, 1985.

1311. Meer RR, Songer JG: Multiplex PCR method for genotyping *Clostridium perfringens*, *AJVR* 58:702-705, 1997.

1312. Songer JG: Molecular and immunological methods for the diagnosis of clostridial diseases. In Rood JI et al, eds: *The clostridia: molecular biology and pathogenesis*, London, 1997, Academic Press.

1313. Roeder BL, Chengappa MM, Nagaraja TG: Isolation of *Clostridium perfringens* from neonatal calves with ruminal and abomasal tympany, abomasitis and abomasal ulceration, *J Am Vet Med Assoc* 190:1550-1555, 1987.

1314. Lindsay JA: *Clostridium perfringens* type A enterotoxin (CPE): more than just explosive diarrhea, *Crit Rev Microbiol* 22:257-77, 1996

1315. Sims LD, Tzipori GH, Hazard GH: Haemorrhagic necrotizing enteritis in foals associated with *Clostridium perfringens*, *Aust Vet J* 62:194-196, 1985.

1316. Niilo L: Experimental production of hemorrhagic enterotoxemia by *Clostridium perfringens* type C in maturing lambs, *Can J Vet Res* 50:32-35, 1986.

1317. East LM et al: Foaling management practices associated with the occurrence of enterocolitis attributed to *C. perfringens* infection in the equine neonate, *Prev Vet Med* 46:61-74, 2000.

1318. Madigan JE: *Manual of equine neonatal medicine*, Woodland, Calif, 1997, Live Oak Publishing.

1319. Pearson EG, Hedstrom OR, Sonn R: Hemorrhagic enteritis caused by *Clostridium perfringens* type C in a foal, *J Am Vet Med Assoc* 188:1309-1310, 1986.

1320. Itado AE et al: Toxin types of *Clostridium perfringens* strains isolated from sheep, cattle, and paddock soils in Nigeria, *Vet Microbiol* 12:93-96, 1986.

1321. Blackwell TE: Enteritis and diarrhea, *Vet Clin North Am (Large Anim Pract)* 5:557-570, 1983.

1322. Green DS et al: Injection site reactions and antibody responses in sheep and goats after the use of multivalent clostridial vaccines, *Vet Rec* 120:435-439, 1987.

1323. Clarkson MJ, Faull WB, Kerry JB: Vaccination of cows with clostridial antigens and passive transfer of clostridial antibodies from bovine colostrum to lambs, *Vet Rec* 116:467-469, 1985.

1324. de la Rosa C, Hogue DE, Thonney ML: Vaccination schedules to raise antibody concentrations against epsilon toxin of *Clostridium perfringens* in ewes and their triplet lambs, *J Anim Sci* 75:2328-2334, 1997.

1325. Herholz C et al: Prevalence of β₂-toxigenic *C. perfringens* in horses with intestinal disorders, *J Clin Microbiol* 37:358-361, 1999.

1326. Garmory HS et al: Occurrence of *C. perfringens* β₂-toxin amongst animals, determined using genotyping and subtyping PCR assays, *Epidemiol Infect* 124:61-67, 2000.

OAK (ACORN) TOXICOSIS

BRADFORD P. SMITH

DEFINITION AND ETIOLOGY. Toxic signs can appear in ruminants[1327,1328] and occasionally in horses[1329] that ingest large quantities of oak buds, oak leaves (green or dried), or acorns. Most species of oak (*Quercus* spp.) cause similar signs when ingested, although there are marked differences in the amount of toxins among the 75 oak species.[1330] The metabolites of oak tannins and volatile phenols present in the buds, leaves, twigs, and acorns are responsible for causing toxicosis. The mouth, esophagus, gastrointestinal tract, and kidneys (renal tubular nephrosis) are the organs most affected. Because they are less selective in what they ingest, cattle seem to be the most frequently affected species. Signs begin shortly after ingestion of 50% or more of the diet as oak, and young cattle (under 300 kg) often appear to be more severely affected than adult cattle.

Factors leading to toxicosis include the presence of large acorn crops when forage is scarce, wind or hail that causes large numbers of acorns to drop suddenly, or the sudden presentation of oak buds and young leaves to hungry cattle, as in spring windstorms or snowstorms that cover the grass and break branches. In the southwestern United States, range cattle regularly consume some oak species, which are apparently highly palatable and nutritious.[1331] The condition has been described wherever oak grows, including most of the United States, France, Great Britain, Germany, Sweden, Australia, China, and South Africa.

Acorn calf syndrome is completely different from the oak toxicosis described in this section. Acorn calves are congenitally malformed calves born to dams that ingest large numbers of acorns under poor forage conditions during the second trimester of pregnancy. The cause appears to be a combination of poor nutrition and exposure to acorns. The calves have very short leg bones and may have abnormal hoof development and a short or long narrow head. In badly affected herds as many as 15% of calves are affected. The disease has been reproduced experimentally. Supplementation of the herd with adequate protein and energy eliminates the disease.

CLINICAL SIGNS AND DIFFERENTIAL DIAGNOSIS. The course of oak toxicosis usually is 1 to 12 days, but some cattle have a protracted, debilitating disease.[1327,1328] In the peracute stages cattle are recumbent, weak, anorectic, and listless.[1327] The rectal temperature is normal or below normal, and the heart and respiratory rates are elevated. Marked edema is present in the perineum and vulva (Fig. 30-57), and edema is obvious in the submandibular area, brisket, and ventral abdomen. Hydration appears adequate, but anuria is present. Firm, dark, mucus-covered feces usually are present. Evidence of hydrothorax, hydropericardium, and ascites may be noted on physical examination. Some cattle may simply be found dead.

A day or two after ingestion the animals appear anorectic and listless and have decreased rumen motility. Many calves have hemorrhagic diarrhea or dark diarrhea that tests positive for fecal occult blood. The feces may have a smell of phenol. Dehydration occurs rapidly, but vital signs may be remarkably normal until hypovolemia develops. As uremia progresses, scleral vessels become dark and engorged, and the breath may take on the smell of ammonia. The major differential diagnoses are other causes of renal failure and other toxins and clostridial diseases; viral diseases that cause ulceration of the alimentary tract should also be considered. Protracted cases most often result from renal failure and uremia, although some animals have chronic oral, esophageal, or gastrointestinal ulceration or perforation with abscessation.

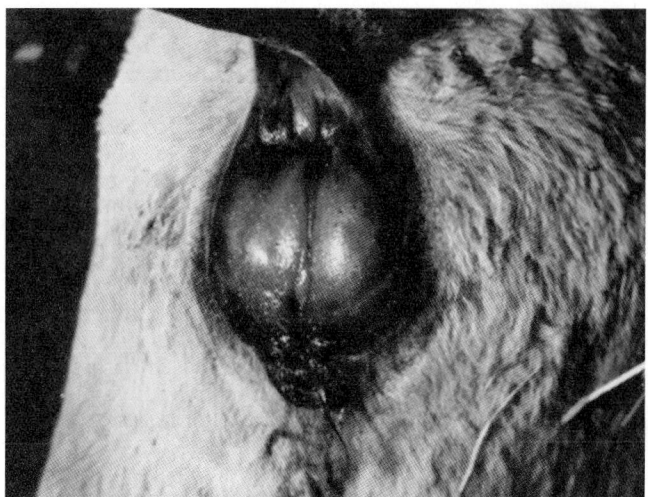

FIG. 30-57 ▮▮ Perirectal and vulvar edema in a 3-month-old calf with acute oak bud toxicity. Acute acorn or oak poisoning causes similar lesions.

In horses signs usually are peracute or acute; they include sudden death or colic, tenesmus, and hemorrhagic diarrhea.[1329] Acorn husks and shells may be noted in the feces. As with most colics, tachycardia, hyperpnea, and injected oral mucous membranes are seen. Increased abdominal borborygmi often are present, and hemoglobinuria may occur. Determination of serum or urinary phenolic (hydrolyzed tannin) content, based on a gallic acid standard, may be used in acute cases.[1329]

CLINICAL PATHOLOGY. In cattle with peracute and acute signs, the serum urea nitrogen and creatinine are elevated, whereas other laboratory values may show considerable variation.[1328,1329] Initially hyponatremia, hyperkalemia, hypochloremia, hyperphosphatemia, and a marked hypocalcemia (5.1 to 6.8 mg/dl) accompany a mild metabolic acidosis with a very high anion gap (29 to 32).[1327] Neutrophilia with a mild hyperfibrinogenemia may be present. Although sorbitol dehydrogenase and γ-glutamyltransferase may be elevated, biopsy does not indicate that significant hepatic disease occurs with oak toxicosis. Animals may be anuric. If urine is being produced, often isosthenuria, proteinuria, and glucosuria occur. The urinary fractional excretion of sodium was elevated in one steer.[1331]

In protracted cases the major findings are elevated serum urea nitrogen, creatinine, and anion gap, with variable hyponatremia, hypokalemia (versus hyperkalemia in acute stages), hypochloremia, and hyperphosphatemia. A mild metabolic alkalosis may be present. Hyperfibrinogenemia and an increase in total plasma proteins also are variable. An elevated white blood cell (WBC) count most often reflects chronic ulceration or abscessation (neutrophilia or monocytosis or both). Liver enzymes usually are normal in protracted cases. Urinalysis results are similar to those in acute cases; in addition, hematuria often is present. By 6 weeks after exposure, a normocytic, normochromic anemia may develop as a result of chronic inflammation and uremia, and hypoalbuminemia may result from chronic renal and gastrointestinal losses. By 8 weeks after exposure, surviving cattle have largely returned to normal renal function as determined by normal serum urea nitrogen and creatinine concentrations and by the ability to concentrate urine after a 24-hour water deprivation test.[1327]

Laboratory findings in horses are similar to those in ruminants, except that during the acute stages rapid hemoconcentration and marked increases in packed cell volume occur.[1329] Although protein, occult blood, and hemoglobin casts were present in the urine, the urine specific gravity was 1.052.

PATHOPHYSIOLOGY. The toxicity of oak is attributed to its high concentration of tannins, which are hydrolyzed in the rumen to gallic acid, pyrogallol, and other compounds. The tannins themselves may contribute to oral, esophageal, and gastrointestinal damage by binding to proteins, including those in epithelial cells. This results in oral, esophageal, and ruminal ulcers or perforations. Protein-bound tannins are liberated in the acidic abomasum, making them available once again to damage intestinal epithelium. Some hydrolyzed tannins are absorbed and bound to plasma proteins and endothelial proteins, resulting in hemorrhage and fluid loss from the vascular compartment into body cavities and tissues; this results in edema. The gallic acid and pyrogallols are extremely toxic to renal tubules, causing acute tubular necrosis, anuria, electrolyte abnormalities, and uremia. Ruminants are more susceptible than horses because of the hydrolysis of the gallotannins in the rumen.

EPIDEMIOLOGY. Young cattle in the 100- to 300-kg range seem to be particularly susceptible. In the southwestern United States oak toxicosis accounts for considerable economic loss in cattle.[1331] The disease is seen sporadically in other ruminants and in horses. The morbidity rate in cattle varies considerably, with several to many calves in a pasture usually affected, and case fatality rates frequently exceed 80%.[1328]

The disease is most often associated with ingestion of acorns in the fall and buds or young leaves in the spring. Cattle turned into a pasture with oak trees under which acorns have accumulated may have toxicosis even when adequate forage is available.[1328] In other cases windstorms have dropped numerous acorns or branches in a pasture to which cattle were already accustomed. In the early spring a heavy, unseasonable snowstorm may occur, covering the grass and bending young trees and breaking branches so that oak buds and young leaves are accessible.[1327] Young leaves and acorns are more palatable than older leaves and also contain more tannins (up to 10% dry matter in acorns). The seedlings, buds, and acorns of small scrub oak may be important forages for cattle in parts of the United States.[1331]

NECROPSY FINDINGS. In peracute and acute cases prominent edema is often the most striking lesion. Ascites, hydrothorax, hydropericardium, perirenal edema, and subcutaneous edema are found. The kidneys are normal in size with multiple diffuse hemorrhages on the surface and extending into the cortex. The liver is slightly swollen and pale or mottled. Digestive tract lesions vary from congestion to hemorrhage and deep ulceration or perforation with necrotizing inflammation. Mucosal ulceration is found in the pharynx, esophagus, rumen, abomasum, small intestine, cecum, and colon. Free blood or melena may frequently be observed.

Diffuse renal tubular damage is present. The changes include coagulation necrosis of cortical tubular epithelium and dilated tubules devoid of epithelium but with intact basement membranes. Many medullary tubules contain hyaline, granular, or cellular casts. The principal renal lesion is necrosis of the proximal convoluted tubules, but glomerular degeneration and fluid in Bowman's capsules are also seen.

By 3 to 6 weeks after exposure, the lesions include gastrointestinal ulceration, often with secondary infection; some healed ulcers; secondary bacterial bronchopneumonia; and slightly swollen, pale brown kidneys. Histologically, atrophy of the cortical tubular epithelium with a marked interstitial fibrosis and mononuclear infiltrate is seen. Evidence of tubular epithelial regeneration may be present. The liver appears normal.

TREATMENT AND PROGNOSIS. In acute stages intravenous fluid therapy aimed at promoting diuresis and cor-

recting acid-base and electrolyte abnormalities may be life-saving. Calcium, sodium, and chloride deficits should be replaced, and sodium bicarbonate should be given if needed to correct metabolic acidosis. In anuric animals furosemide (1 mg/kg given intravenously) can be administered every 12 hours, along with adequate fluid therapy. Corticosteroids and nonsteroidal antiinflammatory drugs are not likely to have a measurable effect on the course of the disease, because they are unlikely to alter the direct toxic effects of the toxic metabolites. The prognosis is guarded and must be considered poor in animals that remain anuric despite therapy. The case fatality rate undoubtedly depends more on the amount of toxic material ingested than on therapy. Antibiotics, given to prevent secondary pneumonia and abscessation, rumen transfaunation, and readily accessible grass hay and water are recommended components of nursing care.

If the animal survives the acute stage and begins to eat voluntarily, the prognosis for recovery is good unless secondary pneumonia or gastrointestinal abscessation after perforation occurs. Renal function can return to normal by 5 to 10 weeks, and weight gains as high as 1.76 kg/day may be recorded in recovered cattle.[1327]

Colicky horses can be treated as one would usually treat colic (intravenous fluids, analgesics, oral laxatives). Particular attention should be paid to diuresis, acid-base balance, and maintenance of serum calcium levels.

PREVENTION AND CONTROL. No specific antidote exists for oak toxicosis, but supplementation with calcium hydroxide (hydrated lime) immediately before anticipated exposure to oak has been effective under experimental conditions.[1332] Feed containing 10% or less calcium hydroxide is palatable. Consumption of 0.9 kg/head/day of cubed or pelleted supplement containing 10% hydrated lime is effective in preventing toxic manifestations.

Supplementation of cattle suddenly exposed to oak with any feed reduces death losses, apparently by allowing hungry cattle to consume the supplemental forage preferentially.[1327,1332] In an outbreak in California caused by spring snows in which 2700 cattle died of oak toxicosis, ranches where hay was immediately supplemented had minimum losses compared with ranches where feed supplementation was not offered.

REFERENCES

1327. Spier SJ et al: Oak toxicosis in cattle in northern California: clinical and pathological findings, *J Am Vet Med Assoc* 191:958-964, 1987.
1328. Kasari TR, Pearson EG, Hultgren BD: Oak *(Quercus garryana)* poisoning of range cattle in southern Oregon, *Compend Cont Educ Pract Vet* 8:F17-F24, 1986.
1329. Anderson GA et al: Fatal acorn poisoning in a horse: pathological findings and diagnostic considerations, *J Am Vet Med Assoc* 182:1105-1110, 1983.
1330. Basden KW, Dalvi RR: Determination of total phenolics in acorns from different species of oak trees in conjunction with acorn poisoning in cattle, *Vet Human Toxicol* 29:305-306, 1987.
1331. Merrill LB, Schuster JL: Grazing management practices affect livestock losses from poisonous plants, *J Range Manage* 31:351-354, 1978.
1332. Dollahite JW, Houshoulder BS, Camp BJ: Effect of calcium hydroxide on the toxicity of post oak *(Quercus stellata)* in calves, *J Am Vet Med Assoc* 148:908-912, 1966.

WINTER DYSENTERY IN CATTLE

CHARLES GUARD

DEFINITION AND ETIOLOGY. Winter dysentery is an acute, apparently contagious diarrheal disease of cattle that occurs in epizootic fashion in a herd, usually during the colder months of the year. It usually is recognized by the clinical syndrome that occurs in herds, with diagnosis by exclusion of other causes of epizootics of diarrhea. In the United States the disease is more common in the northern states; however, it has been reported in Australia, Sweden, the United Kingdom, Israel, France, Belgium, Japan, and Canada. The cause is unknown, but the rapid spread of the disease in a herd argues for an infectious cause. The period of illness in an individual is brief, and within a herd the outbreak usually lasts less than 2 weeks. Recovery is spontaneous in most individuals. The morbidity rate may be high in a herd that has not experienced winter dysentery for several years; regardless, mortality usually is rare. Although most reports indicate this to be a disease of adult cattle, in a herd outbreak mild diarrhea may be observed in animals as young as 4 months.

Investigations into the cause of winter dysentery have thus far been inconclusive. In early investigations, *Vibrio jejuni* was thought by many to be the infectious agent responsible for the syndrome. MacPherson[1333] demonstrated that a bacterial agent was not involved when he experimentally reproduced winter dysentery with feces passed through a Seitz filter. Since the demonstration that a virus-sized agent was involved, many investigators have unsuccessfully attempted to satisfy Koch's postulates for winter dysentery. Most recently attention has focused on a coronavirus that may be the same as or related to the coronavirus that causes diarrhea in neonatal calves. In Japan, France, Belgium, and the United States, investigators have identified a coronavirus or similar virus particle in the feces of cattle with winter dysentery.[1334-1338] The disease was reproduced by contaminating feed with untreated feces in one of two attempts.[1334] By immune electron microscopy, antigenic cross-reaction has been demonstrated between the original Nebraska calf coronavirus diarrhea agent and coronavirus isolated from field outbreaks of winter dysentery.[1336,1338] A rise in serum antibody titer to the calf coronavirus after an outbreak of winter dysentery in adult cattle was found.[1336]

CLINICAL SIGNS AND DIFFERENTIAL DIAGNOSIS. Winter dysentery is an explosive diarrheal disease accompanied by some degree of anorexia, dullness, and hypogalactia. In rare cases mild colic may be seen; others may appear weak and prefer to lie down. If the diarrhea is severe or persists longer than a day, dehydration may develop. Weight loss is apparent and is caused by loss of rumen fill and depletion of extracellular fluid. Rumen motility usually is reduced, but intestinal borborygmi may be increased. Thirst often is increased, and polydipsia follows the diarrhea. Rectal examination may reveal dilated intestinal loops. The feces vary from light tan to dark brown; bubbles commonly form in the puddles that are deposited several feet behind the cow. Blood may be present in the feces of several animals in a group, typically in the first lactation heifers. The amount of blood may range from just visible to large clots, or it may be uniformly mixed into the feces. Some animals may have thick mucus in the feces. The odor in a barn during an outbreak of winter dysentery has been described as musty, fetid, and sweet/nasty.[1340]

Fever usually is not present during the diarrheal phase of the disease but has been reported to precede it[1333] or have no consistent relation.[1341] Mild respiratory signs consisting of serous nasolacrimal discharge and a soft cough have been inconsistently observed before diarrhea. Diarrhea caused by the bovine virus diarrhea virus, coccidiosis, salmonellosis, Johne's disease, and dietary gastroenteritis must be considered in the differential diagnosis of winter dysentery. With winter dysentery no mucosal lesions are visible on physical examination. The absence of coccidial oocysts or parasite ova in the feces helps exclude these agents as responsible for the diarrhea. However, diarrhea caused by parasites may precede the shedding of detectable organisms in feces. The rapid occurrence of multiple cases within a herd, and often within herds in a locality, suggests winter dysentery. Fecal culture for *Salmonella* organisms yields negative results in uncomplicated cases of winter dysentery. Examination of feeds or the feeding history should elucidate the cause of an outbreak of dietary diarrhea associated with moldy or rancid feed.

CLINICAL PATHOLOGY. No consistent hematologic changes that would be of diagnostic benefit have been observed. If significant dysentery persists for longer than a day, signs of anemia develop.

PATHOPHYSIOLOGY. If the current contention that a coronavirus or coronavirus-like agent is causal in winter dysentery is correct, the pathophysiologic characteristics of the disease can be attributed to lesions of the colonic mucosa.[1337] Epithelial cells of colonic crypts are destroyed by viral action, leading to necrosis and hemorrhage. Even though histologic changes have been observed only in the colonic mucosa, blood was observed from the distal duodenum aborally in cattle that died of winter dysentery.[1339] Loss of intestinal mucosal epithelium from colonic crypts leads to transudation of extracellular fluid and blood. The exact mechanism leading to the voluminous, watery diarrhea has not been clarified but may be related to the inflammatory nature of the disease. Mediators of inflammation may lead to hypersecretion in the small intestine and colon.

EPIDEMIOLOGY. The incubation period is thought to be 2 to 8 days. The most susceptible animals are first and most severely affected. In a small, housed herd, the typical incidence of diarrhea during an outbreak begins with the explosive appearance of signs in 10% to 15% of animals on the first day. The second day another 20% to 40% are affected. On subsequent days similar proportions become ill. By the end of a week the first affected animals are completely recovered, and only a few new cases occur. Typically within 2 weeks of the onset of diarrhea, all animals have recovered. This period is marked by significant reduction in milk production. In large herds the outbreak may be prolonged for 6 to 8 weeks. Animals in their first lactation usually are most severely affected, but other cattle recently fresh or otherwise stressed may also have a longer clinical course. This scenario is typical of a herd that had not experienced an epizootic of winter dysentery during the preceding few years. In some herds milder outbreaks occur annually, with fewer animals showing diarrhea and with less severe clinical signs.

TREATMENT AND PROGNOSIS. Most animals with winter dysentery recover spontaneously in a few days without specific treatment. Many palliative treatments have been recommended and used over the years, including intestinal astringents, protectants, and adsorbents. On the basis of 30 years of observations, Roberts[1342] considered none of these treatments to alter the course of the disease. Provision of adequate fresh water, palatable feed, and free choice salt is the most useful nonspecific therapy. The occasional animal with prolonged or severe dysentery may need a transfusion of 4 to 8 L of whole blood.

REFERENCES

1333. MacPherson LW: Bovine virus enteritis (winter dysentery), *Can J Comp Med* 16:149-152, 1957.
1334. Takahashi E et al: Epizootic diarrhoea of adult cattle associated with a coronavirus-like agent, *Vet Microbiol* 5:151-154, 1980.
1335. Espinasse J et al: Winter dysentery: a coronavirus-like agent in the faeces of beef and dairy cattle with diarrhoea, *Vet Rec* 110:385, 1982.
1336. Broes A, Van Opdenbosch E, Wellemans G: Isolement d'un coronavirus chez des bovins atteints d'enterite hemorragique hivernale (winter dysentery) en Belgique, *Ann Med Vet* 128:299-303, 1984.
1337. Van Kruiningen HJ et al: Calfhood coronavirus enterocolitis: a clue to the etiology of winter dysentery, *Vet Pathol* 24:564-567, 1987.
1338. Saif LJ et al: Winter dysentery in adult dairy cattle: detection of coronavirus in the faeces, *Vet Rec* 123:300-301, 1988.
1339. Van Kruiningen HJ et al: Winter dysentery in dairy cattle: recent findings, *Compend Cont Educ Pract Vet* 7:S591-S599, 1985.

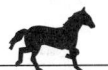

1340. Campbell SG, Cookingham CA: The enigma of winter dysentery, *Cornell Vet* 68:423-441, 1978.
1341. Kahrs RF, Scott FW, Hillman RB: Epidemiologic observations on bovine winter dysentery, *Bovine Pract* 8:36-39, 1973.
1342. Roberts SJ: Winter dysentery in dairy cattle, *Cornell Vet* 47:373-388, 1957.

SALMONELLOSIS IN RUMINANTS

BRADFORD P. SMITH

DEFINITION AND ETIOLOGY. Salmonellosis is one of the few diseases that are increasing in prevalence. Seventy-five percent of dairies sampled in California had evidence of *Salmonella* infection.[1343] More than 2200 *Salmonella* serotypes (serovars) have been identified, and many are potential animal and human pathogens. Multidrug-resistant *S. typhimurium* DT104 is particularly virulent to animals and human beings. Fortunately 10 serotypes of *Salmonella* in serogroups B, C, D, and E are responsible for most disease in cattle, therefore control programs can be aimed at these. Table 30-15 lists the 10 serotypes most commonly isolated from cattle in 1999 in the United States.[1344] *Salmonella* organisms are gram-negative enteric bacteria that are facultative intracellular parasites. Most serotypes are non–host-specific, but a few are host adapted. *Salmonella dublin* is host-adapted to cattle, *Salmonella abortus ovis* and *Salmonella arizonae* to sheep, and *Salmonella abortus equi* to horses. Host-adapted serotypes are found most often in their host species, where true long-term carriers exist.[1345] In contrast, non-host-adapted serotypes rarely achieve carrier status and usually infect an animal for a period of 3 to 16 weeks before infection is cleared.[1345] Infection with either host-adapted or non-host-adapted serotypes can be symptomatic or asymptomatic, depending on the dose, the virulence of the serotype, and the host's immune status. There appears to be an association between intensive management practices such as large farms, crowded conditions, and high-protein diets and an increased incidence of *Salmonella* infection.

Salmonella bacteria are grouped into serogroups (A to Z and 51 to 65), depending on their cell wall antigens (somatic antigens that comprise specific oligosaccharides, often called O antigens, lipopolysaccharides, or endotoxin). Thus, for example, local and regional laboratories often report that an isolate is a group D *Salmonella*. The most common group D isolate of cattle is *S. dublin* (Table 30-16). Final confirmation that the *Salmonella* isolated is indeed *S. dublin* comes from the National Veterinary Services Laboratory in Ames, Iowa, or from some other laboratory where antisera and facilities exist for identification of all 2200 serotypes on the basis of flagellar (H) antigens and somatic (O) antigens. Some serotypes also express capsular (Vi) antigens composed of mucopolysaccharide. Identification of the serotype is important in planning control strategies. In addition to the serotypes listed in Table 30-16, lambs may be infected with *S. arizonae*, which comes from several different serogroups. *Salmonella* organisms are relatively easy to culture from the feces or tissues of infected animals, using common enteric agar. Our laboratory currently prefers XLT4 and brilliant green (BG) agars, and tetrathionate and selenite as selective enrichment media.

CLINICAL SIGNS AND DIFFERENTIAL DIAGNOSIS. *Salmonella* infection can cause a variety of clinical signs. The most common signs are fever and diarrhea[1346] after an incubation period of 1 to 4 days after exposure or a recrudescence from the carrier state. Both adult animals and neonates may be affected.

The character of the diarrheic feces varies from watery to mucoid with fibrin and blood. Sheets of fibrin may appear to be sloughing mucosa. The feces often have a putrid, foul

TABLE 30-15

Most Frequently Identified *Salmonella* Serotypes From U.S. Cattle From July 1998 Through June 1999

Serotype	Serogroup
Typhimurium (Copenhagen)	B
Typhimurium	B
Kentucky	C3
Cerro	K
Montevideo	C1
Dublin	D1
Mbandaka	C1
Anatum	E1
Muenster	E1
Newport	C2

From National Veterinary Services Laboratory, U.S. Department of Agriculture, Ames, Iowa.

TABLE 30-16

Changing Incidence of *Salmonella* Serotypes on California Dairy Farms as Illustrated by the Percentage of Farms From Which Each Serotype Was Isolated in 1985 to 1986 Compared With 1987 to 1988

Serotype	*1985-1986* Percentage of Farm (No.)	*1987-1988* Percentage of Farms (No.)
S. *dublin*	78(29)	53(49)
S. *newport*	19(7)	36(33)
S. *typhimurium*	3(1)	7.6(7)
S. *montevideo*	0	6.5(6)
S. *infantis*	0	2.2(2)
S. *anatum*	0	1.1(1)
S. *arkansas*	0	1.1(1)

*Blanchard P, Anderson M: Unpublished data based on calves brought for necropsy from Tulare area farms, 1988.

odor because of the presence of plasma proteins associated with severe inflammatory bowel disease. Salmonellosis causes an acute protein-losing enteropathy. The systemic effects of endotoxins (and other toxic material) absorbed through the damaged bowel mucosa may be severe (fever, anorexia, depressed attitude, shock).

Bacteremia may occur rapidly, especially in neonates infected with *S. dublin* or *S. typhimurium*. Peracute to acute septicemia in calves may produce lesions in many organ systems. Affected calves usually are under 2 months of age (the range is 1 week to 6 months).[1342] Dyspnea, respiratory symptoms, sudden death, and occasionally diarrhea are the principal signs of *S. dublin* infection, the incidence of which usually peaks in 6-week-old calves. Blood culture results frequently are positive. Pure cultures of *S. dublin* often can be grown from specimens from the lungs of 4- to 8-week old calves with pneumonic (septicemic) salmonellosis. Calves infected with *S. typhimurium* are only 14 days of age on average (the range is 1 to 35 days) and have mainly enteric lesions, including enlarged mesenteric lymph nodes, abomasitis, fibrinonecrotic plaques in the ileum, and hemorrhage of Peyer's patches.[1347]

In adult cattle, diarrhea or abortion may occur.[1345] Abortion may occur by two mechanisms, because both culture-positive and culture-negative fetuses and placentae may be

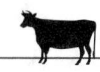
found in an outbreak. In the former, bacteremia in the dam results in infection of the placenta or fetus, with resulting fetal death and expulsion. Bacteremia or endotoxemia associated with diarrhea and damaged gut mucosa in cattle may result in release of prostaglandin F2$_\alpha$ (PGF) and subsequent lysis of the corpus luteum. Abortion follows in 2 to 3 days, and the fetus and placenta will have culture-negative findings. When the fetus has a culture-negative finding, many other causes of abortion must be considered. Many infectious agents that infect only the dam can act similarly to cause luteolysis and abortion.

Differential diagnoses for the enteric form of salmonellosis in neonates include all the common enteropathogens of neonates: *Escherichia coli*, rotaviruses and coronaviruses, clostridia, cryptosporidia, and other forms of coccidia. Concurrent infection with these agents is common. In older animals outbreaks should be differentiated from those caused by bovine virus diarrhea, winter dysentery, and feed-induced indigestion. Pneumonic and bacteremic salmonellosis in 4- to 8-week-old calves must be differentiated by culture from pneumonic pasteurellosis; in goats, from mycoplasmal infection; and in lambs from septicemic pasteurellosis.

CLINICAL PATHOLOGY. *Salmonella* enteritis often results in changes in the hemogram.[1343] Plasma fibrinogen frequently is elevated because of the inflammatory nature of the disease, and either neutrophilia or neutropenia may be seen. In severe cases a left shift may be present. Initial dehydration may result in an elevated packed cell volume and plasma protein level. The plasma protein level often drops over a period of days as protein is lost into the bowel lumen. Many other nonspecific abnormalities in clinical chemistry values are often seen, including elevated liver enzymes, decreased plasma calcium, and indications of prerenal azotemia if dehydration occurs.

Definitive diagnosis of salmonellosis requires culture of the organism from feces, blood, or tissues. Serologic evaluation to confirm the development of anti-*Salmonella* antibodies is useful[1349] but is not commonly performed and is not currently available in most laboratories.*

PATHOPHYSIOLOGY. Salmonellae are invasive organisms that may penetrate ocular, nasal, oral, or intestinal mucous membranes. *Salmonella* infection is most often transmitted by fecal-oral contamination from livestock or rodents, or by feeding of contaminated protein source animal by-products (e.g., fish meal, meat meal, bone meal, or feather meal, 40% of which are contaminated in the United States) or contaminated forages or plant proteins such as soybean or cottonseed. Recent research has also documented contaminated irrigation water as an important source of *Salmonella* organisms. On one dairy farm, river water used to sprinkler irrigate green chop contaminated the green chop, which was fed to cows. On another farm, *Salmonella*-contaminated river water was used to irrigate cotton. When the cottonseed from that gin was used as feed, cattle became infected. On a third dairy, contaminated irrigation water resulted in haylage containing *Salmonella* organisms.[1350] Unlike other serotypes, *S. dublin* may be carried as a chronic gut infection and passed in feces or carried as an intramammary infection and passed in contaminated milk.

Once eaten, salmonellae attach to mucosal cells, probably by means of a nonfimbrial adhesion.[1351] Attachment is increased if gastrointestinal stasis is present or the normal competitive flora has been disturbed. Salmonellae cause degeneration of nearby cells and penetrate both through microvilli and through tight junctions between cells.[1352] The

bacteria pass through the enterocytes to the lamina propria, where they stimulate an inflammatory response and are engulfed by macrophages and neutrophils.[1353] Intracellular bacteria reach regional mesenteric lymph nodes or beyond. The organism has a predilection for lymphoid tissues and is found in highest numbers in Peyer's patches and mesenteric lymph nodes.[1354] Thrombi form in vessels, and tissue damage can be severe. Virulent salmonellae are capable of surviving in host tissues and multiplying, often as facultative intracellular parasites in macrophages and reticuloendothelial cells.[1355] In the case of carrier animals, salmonellae survive in cells in the presence of high titers of specific extracellular (i.e., serum) immunoglobulins. Intracellular salmonellae can also avoid many antimicrobial drugs and complement. Stress may cause a latent infection to recrudesce, resulting in fecal or mammary gland shedding or clinical disease.

EPIDEMIOLOGY AND CONTROL. Infection with host-adapted *Salmonella* serotypes may occur as a cyclic endemic disease, especially in calves when *S. dublin* is involved. The disease is maintained by (1) carrier animals shedding *S. dublin* in the feces[1345] or milk,[1349] (2) infected calves, (3) rodents, and (4) environmental contamination. *Salmonella* carriers infected with a host-adapted serotype such as *S. dublin* may shed constantly or intermittently. Infected carriers that are not shedding are called latent carriers; stress may cause shedding in feces or milk to recrudesce. A single infected, asymptomatic fecal shedder may produce 1 billion *S. dublin* organisms per day to contaminate the environment (1 million organisms per gram of feces). Calving areas must be constantly cleaned and disinfected between calvings. Raw milk feeding to calves may be a source of *S. dublin* (100 to 100,000 organisms per milliliter of milk).[1349] Infected calves constantly amplify the number of organisms in the environment, causing exposure of other calves. Calves with clinical signs may shed billions of *S. dublin* into the environment daily.

Environmental contamination can be difficult to eliminate, because salmonellae survive for months in moist areas out of direct sunlight and in lagoons and drainage areas. *S. dublin* was recovered from feces dried for 41 months.[1356] Freezing feces at -20° C (-4° F) kills 85% of salmonellae in 2 days and over 95% by 1 month.[1357] Direct sunlight and drying in hot weather also are effective at eliminating salmonellae.

Feedlot cattle colonized by *Salmonella* organisms could pose a public health risk when meat is contaminated at slaughter. In a National Animal Health Monitoring System (NAHMS) study, 7.5% of cattle on feed the longest shed salmonellae, whereas 3.5% of cattle that had recently entered the feedlot were shedding salmonellae in the feces.[1358] Contamination of the animals before entry can cause the entering cattle to have a higher rate of shedding than was found in cattle that had been in the feedlot for several months[1359]; 1.4% of cattle, mostly from dairies, shed salmonellae when in a veterinary clinic.[1360]

Control of *Salmonella* infection requires an integrated herd approach. To detect herds infected with *S. typhimurium* or other serotype except *S. dublin* a herd serologic profile using ELISA can be used.[1361] Rectal swab sampling and culture of cull dairy cows was found not to be a satisfactory method of detecting *Salmonella*-infected herds.[1362] To control *S. dublin*, carrier cows and calves over 6 months of age are identified by serologic testing (enzyme-linked immunosorbent assay [ELISA]) for anti-*Salmonella* antibody.[1349,1363-1365] This test is not yet widely available but can be requested by contacting the livestock Salmonella Laboratory, VME, Tupper Hall, University of California at Davis, Davis, CA 95616 (phone: [530] 752-7135). Suspect animals are culled or tested further by serologic means or by multiple fecal cultures and milk cultures (five samples at weekly intervals). Animals with positive test results are culled. In infected herds, *S. dublin* carriers

---

*Contact Salmonella Laboratory, Department of Veterinary Medicine: Medicine and Epidemiology, University of California, Davis, CA 95616; Phone (530) 752-7135.

(fecal or mammary) usually make up 0.4% to 3% of a dairy herd. Animals that remain seropositive over a 2-month period should be considered carriers, even if a culture result is negative on five samples.[1349] A Danish study[1366] found that only 14 of 31 persistently seropositive animals were culture positive for *S. dublin* at postmortem and one seronegative animal was culture positive. Despite this low specificity, if culling more cattle than necessary by using serologic testing can help eradicate an endemic infection, it may be worth the price.

To control all non–host-adapted and host-adapted serotypes of *Salmonella*, calves are promptly treated when signs of illness occur, and strict procedures to prevent the spread of infection are instituted. A study of 14 farms infected with *S. typhimurium* DT104 showed that clinical disease ceased by 4 months, but widespread infection and contamination existed. Over time the number of infected farms gradually declined, and vaccination correlated positively with a herd remaining free of clinical illness from DT104.[1367] Control measures include the use of separate feeding utensils for each calf, washing of boots and hands by calf raisers between calves, isolation of ill calves to noncontact pens, and thorough disinfection of pens between calves. Decontamination of pens is most effectively accomplished if an all-in, all-out system is used. Pens are divided into four groups, with each group of pens used for calves born during a given week. When 3- to 4-week-old calves leave their pens as a group, these pens are cleaned and disinfected with a chlorine product such as bleach or a phenylphenolic disinfectant. This helps prevent continuous recycling of bacteria to each group of new calves. Environmental monitoring by frequent swab cultures of pens is the best way to check the effectiveness of the sanitation and disinfection program.

S. typhimurium and other non–host-adapted serotypes most often occur as epidemics after entering the farm by means of purchased cattle, rodents,[1368] rendering trucks, or feedstuffs. Even *S. dublin* may be maintained on a farm by mice.[1368] A case control study of farms infected with *S. typhimurium* DT104 found that the most effective interventions included purchasing cattle directly rather than through a sales yard, quarantining purchased cattle for 4 weeks, housing sick cattle in dedicated isolation areas, and preventing wild bird access to feed storage areas.[1369] Feeds may be contaminated by irrigation water[1350] or in manufacturing when by-product ingredients contain *Salmonella* organisms, on the farm, or in shipment by birds or rodents or contaminated trucks. When an epidemic involving an exotic serotype occurs, feedstuffs should be examined as a likely source. Exotic serotypes are uncommon serotypes; that is, all those not listed in Table 30-16. Feedstuff contamination with the serotypes not considered exotic may also occur. High-protein supplements, rumen by-pass protein, or calcium-phosphorus supplements of animal origin are sources of epidemics of various *Salmonella* serotypes in livestock. Forty percent of all animal by-product feedstuffs in the United States are contaminated with *Salmonella* organisms. Once a *Salmonella* serotype enters a herd, the bacteria are rapidly spread among livestock and into the environment, where they may cause a prolonged course of herd illness and can be difficult to eliminate. Such appeared to be the case with *Salmonella newport* and *Salmonella montevideo* in dairy cattle in California in the past several years (see Table 30-16). These and other group C *Salmonella* sp. tend to become endemic for years on a dairy farm once it has become infected. Culture of feeds before use on a farm currently is the only means of preventing the introduction of exotic *Salmonella* serotypes, because national and international controls currently appear to be inadequate.

Control by vaccination of dams using killed bacterins may be somewhat beneficial in protecting neonates under 3 weeks

of age through colostral and milk immunoglobulin. In neonates over 3 weeks of age, colostral immunity appears to play only a small role in protecting against salmonellosis. Because both humoral and cell-mediated immunity are important in protecting against salmonellosis,[1370-1372] active immunity is superior to passive. In the future, modified live, genetically altered vaccines that stimulate humoral and cell-mediated immunity may offer better protection for calves.[1373,1374] Modified live vaccines have been available in Europe for years. Such a vaccine recently became available in the United States. The role of increased nonspecific immunity to gram-negative core antigens (through immunization with rough mutants of *Escherichia coli* and salmonellae lacking complete cell walls) is being investigated. Some studies have been able to demonstrate an increased survival rate for salmonellosis after vaccination with a mutant stain of *E. coli* (J5),[1375] designed to produce antibodies to the common core antigens of gram-negative bacteria. Endovac-Bovi (remutant *Salmonella*) is marketed with the same goal.

Available commercial *Salmonella* vaccines are killed whole cell bacterins for use in cattle, and a new genetically altered modified live *S. dublin* vaccine for calves. The only products that are solely *Salmonella* vaccines contain *S. typhimurium* or *S. typhimurium* and *S. dublin* or live *S. dublin* organisms (see Chapter 44). Several other vaccines contain a *Salmonella* serotype in addition to other bacterial antigens. Autogenous bacterins can be made for serotypes not commercially available when they are isolated from animals on a farm and believed to be the causative agent of disease.

The two major problems associated with *Salmonella* bacterins are adverse reactions and lack of efficacy. Adverse reactions vary from fever, depression, and anorexia to collapse and death after vaccination. Animals may have severe reactions after the first, second, or third dose. The apparent cause of these severe reactions is a high degree of sensitivity to the presence of gram-negative endotoxin, which results in a rapid immune cascade leading to shock. This sensitivity is genetically controlled, possibly accounting for the high frequency of adverse reactions in one herd and their absence in a neighboring herd. High ambient temperatures also seem to increase sensitivity to the adverse effects of endotoxin. Adverse reactions usually can be reversed by using epinephrine (1 ml of 1:1000 [1 mg/ml] for every 50 kg of body weight given intramuscularly or intravenously) as soon as evidence of polypnea, dyspnea, or weakness appears.

Lack of efficacy of killed *Salmonella* bacterins in calves is evident in experimental studies. Commercial bacterin vaccines* in aluminum hydroxide administered directly to calves at 2 and 4 weeks of age failed to protect the calves when they were orally challenged at 6 weeks of age[1376] (the peak incidence of disease usually is 6 to 8 weeks of age). Other research has demonstrated protection in older vaccinated calves that were challenged intravenously.[1377] Recent work has shown that calves under 12 weeks of age do not serologically respond with antilipopolysaccharide antibodies after vaccination with two or three doses of killed bacterins in aluminum hydroxide.[1378] On the other hand, cows do respond serologically to two doses of the same vaccine.[1379] The ELISA titer in cows is short-lived (2 to 4 weeks), therefore the timing of vaccination before parturition is critical if the aim is to increase the anti-*Salmonella* colostral immunoglobulin G titer.[1379] Under experimental conditions, calves fed colostrum from vaccinated dams were not protected against oral challenge at 3 weeks of age.[1376] One report suggests that vaccination with killed *S. typhimurium* vaccine prevented reinfection and recrudescence of clinical signs after

---

Salmonella dublin-typhimurium bacterin, Colorado Serum Co., Denver, CO 80216.

an outbreak of DT104 and helped in eliminating the organism from the farm.[1369]

NECROPSY FINDINGS

Enteric Form. Calves often are emaciated and have serous atrophy of fat. Especially with *S. typhimurium*, the ileal, cecal, or colonic mucosae may be thickened and hemorrhagic with adherent fibrinonecrotic plaques. Fibrin may be found in sheets, especially pronounced in the areas of Peyer's patches. The abomasum, duodenum, and jejunum are often involved but less severely. The abomasum usually contains brown, fetid liquid. Bowel contents often are watery and may contain fibrin or blood or both.[1347] The mesenteric lymph nodes frequently are enlarged and dark. Chronically affected cows or calves may have discrete areas of necrosis in the cecum or colon that may involve the entire thickness of the wall.[1347]

Septicemic Form. Gross lesions of bacteremic *Salmonella* infection are acute and usually subtle. Serosal and subcutaneous petechiae are widespread. The spleen usually is enlarged. The lungs are edematous and fail to collapse and have random foci of hemorrhage or congestion.[1347] The wall of the gallbladder is thickened and may contain hemorrhages.[1347] The bile frequently is inspissated into a firm coagulum.[1347] Less common lesions include jaundice, cystitis, meningitis, osteomyelitis, and arthritis. Gastrointestinal lesions may or may not be present.

TREATMENT. The keys to successful treatment of bacteremia caused by gram-negative bacteria are (1) antimicrobial drugs, (2) fluids and electrolytes, and (3) nonsteroidal antiinflammatory drugs.[1375] *S. typhimurium* antiserum is available commercially. Adverse reactions by cattle to horse serum are common; care should be taken.

Early in the course of disease in calves, appropriate antimicrobial therapy often increases the survival rate markedly, because bacteremia frequently occurs. Appropriate antimicrobial therapy depends on culture and antimicrobial sensitivity patterns. In general, most *Salmonella* organisms are sensitive to florfenicol, ceftiofur (and other third-generation cephalosporins), trimethoprim-sulfa (TMS), gentamicin, amikacin, and fluoroquinolones such as enrofloxacin. Sulfas and fluoroquinolones may not be used extralabel in food animals in the United States. Aminoglycosides such as neomycin, gentamicin, and amikacin produce long-term tissue residues and should be avoided in animals intended for use as food. Susceptibility to ampicillin, amoxicillin, sulfas, and tetracycline varies considerably, whereas resistance to penicillin, streptomycin, erythromycin, and tylosin is anticipated. TMS combinations are relatively inexpensive, especially when given orally, but oral TMS should only be used in calves younger than 3 weeks of age. In calves over 3 weeks of age, trimethoprim should be given intravenously because it is destroyed in the rumen and not absorbed. Antimicrobial drugs such as fluoroquinolones, florfenicol, or trimethoprim-sulfas that achieve good intracellular levels and have a large volume of distribution appear to be more effective than those that do not achieve good intracellular levels (e.g., gentamicin and amikacin). Florfenicol or cephalosporins such as ceftiofur are good choices for therapy against many *Salmonella* isolates depending on susceptibility testing results. Antimicrobial drugs may not be effective at altering the clinical course of strictly enteric infections without bacteremia, but because bacteremia frequently accompanies salmonellosis, systemic antimicrobial therapy often is chosen.

Intravenous fluid therapy to maintain blood volume and pressure and correct acid-base or electrolyte abnormalities is important in any animal that is dehydrated or in shock (see Chapter 20, neonatal diarrhea, for neonates and Chapter 30, equine fluid therapy, for adults). Measurement of blood gases and electrolyte values is useful to assist in fluid therapy formulations. Fluids containing sodium, with supplementation of glucose, should be administered intravenously as needed. Metabolic acidosis with mixed water and electrolyte losses is most often seen. Oral fluids and electrolytes may also be effective supplements. The prognosis is good if animals are treated aggressively and early in the course of illness.

REFERENCES

1343. Smith BP et al: Prevalence of *Salmonella* on California dairies, *J Am Vet Med Assoc* 205:467-471, 1994.
1344. Ferris KE et al: *Salmonella* serotypes from animals and related sources: July 1998 to June 1999, *Proc US Animal Health Assoc* 1999.
1345. Wray C, Sojka WJ: Bovine salmonellosis, *J Dairy Res* 44:383-425, 1977.
1346. Gibson EA: *Salmonella* infection in cattle, *J Dairy Res* 32:97-133, 1965.
1347. Anderson M, Blanchard P: The clinical syndromes caused by *Salmonella* infection, *Vet Med* 84:816-819, 1989.
1348. Williams ML et al: Comparison of salmonellosis with bolus or slow infusion endotoxemia in calves, Conference of Research Workers in Animal Diseases, Chicago, November, 1984.
1349. Smith BP et al: Detection of *Salmonella* dublin mammary gland infection in carrier cows using an enzyme-linked immunosorbent assay for antibody in milk and serum, *Am J Vet Res* 50:1352-1360, 1989.
1350. Anderson RJ et al: *Biology of Salmonella in dairy herds*, 2000 (in press).
1351. Jones GW, Richardson LA: The attachment to and invasion of HeLa cells by *S. typhimurium*: the contribution of mannose-sensitive and mannose-resistant hemagglutinating antibodies, *J Gen Microbiol* 127:361-370, 1981.
1352. Takeuchi A: Electron microscope studies of experimental *Salmonella* infection. I. Penetration into the intestinal epithelium by *S. typhimurium*, *Am J Pathol* 50:109-119, 1967.
1353. Takeuchi A, Sprinz H: Electron microscope studies of experimental *Salmonella* infections in the preconditioned guinea pig. II. Response of the intestinal mucosa to invasion by *S. typhimurium*, *Am J Pathol* 51:137-146, 1967.
1354. Clarke RC: Virulence of wild and mutant strains of *S. typhimurium* in calves, doctoral dissertation, Ontario, Canada, University of Guelph.
1355. Collins FM, Campbell SG: Immunity to intracellular bacteria, *Vet Immunol Immunopathol* 3:5-66, 1982.
1356. Forshell LP, Ekesbo I: *Salmonella dublin* survival in dry feces in a cow barn and the implications thereof, *Deutsche Veterinaermed Gesellschaft* 229-232, 1990.
1357. Daniels EK et al: *Salmonella* viability in frozen bovine feces, *Bovine Pract* 27:166-167, 1993.
1358. Fedorka-Cray PJ et al: Survey of *Salmonella* serotypes in feedlot cattle, *J Food Protect* 61:525-530, 1998.
1359. Galland JC et al: Prevalence of *Salmonella* in beef feeder steers as determined by bacterial culture and ELISA serology, *Vet Microbiol* 76:143-151, 2000.
1360. Ravary B et al: Prevalence of *Salmonella* spp. infections in cattle and horses from the veterinary teaching hospital, University of Montreal, *Can Vet J* 39:566-572, 1998.
1361. Hoorfar J, Bitsch V: Evaluation of an O antigen ELISA for screening cattle herds for *S. typhimurium*, *Vet Rec* 137:374-379, 1995.
1362. Gay JM, Rice DH, Steiger JH: Prevalence of fecal *Salmonella* shedding by cull dairy cattle marketed in Washington state, *J Food Protect* 57:195-197, 1994.
1363. Smith BP, House JK: Prospects for *Salmonella* control in cattle, *Proc XVII World Buiatrics Congr* 67:73, 1992.
1364. House JK et al: Enzyme-linked immunosorbent assay for serologic detection of *Salmonella dublin* carriers on a large dairy, *Am J Vet Res* 54:1391-1399, 1993.
1365. Nielsen BB, Vestergaard EM: Use of ELISA in the eradication of *Salmonella dublin* infection, Proceedings of the International Symposium on *Salmonella*, Ploufragan, France, 1992.
1366. Hoorfar J, Wedderkopp A, Lind P: Comparison between persisting antilipopolysaccharide antibodies and culture at postmortem in *Salmonella*-infected cattle herds, *Vet Microbiol* 50: 81-94, 1996.
1367. Davies RH: A 2-year study of *S. typhimurium* DT104 infection and contamination on cattle farms, *Cattle Pract* 5:189-194, 1997.
1368. Tublante NL, Lane VM: Wild mice as potential reservoirs of *Salmonella* dublin in a closed dairy herd, *Can Vet J* 30:590-592, 1989.
1369. Evans SJ: A case control study of multiple-resistant *S. typhimurium* DT104 infection of cattle in Great Britain, *Cattle Pract* 4:259-263, 1996.
1370. Habasha F et al: Correlation of macrophage migration inhibition factor and protection from challenge exposure in calves vaccinated with *S. typhimurium*, *Am J Vet Res* 46:1415-1421, 1985.
1371. Johnson E, Hietala S, Smith BP: Chemiluminescence of bovine alveolar macrophages as an indicator of developing immunity in calves vaccinated with aro⁻ *Salmonella*, *Vet Microbiol* 10:451-464, 1985.
1372. Clarke RC, Gyles CL: Salmonella. In Gyles CL, Thoen CO, eds: *Pathogenesis of bacterial infections in animals*, Ames, Iowa, 1986, Iowa State University Press.

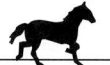

1373. Smith BP et al: Aromatic-dependent *Salmonella typhimurium* as modified live vaccines for calves, *Am J Vet Res* 45:59-66, 1984.
1374. Smith BP et al: Aromatic-dependent *Salmonella dublin* as parenteral modified live vaccine for calves, *Am J Vet Res* 45:2231-2235, 1984.
1375. Cullor J et al: Decreased mortality and severity of infection from salmonellosis in calves immunized with *E. coli* (J5), Conference of Research Workers in Animal Diseases, Chicago, November, 1985.
1376. Smith BP et al: Immunization of calves against salmonellosis, *Am J Vet Res* 41:1947-1951, 1980.
1377. Bairey M: Immunization of calves against salmonellosis, *J Am Vet Med Assoc* 173:610-613, 1978.
1378. Roden LD et al: Effects of calf age and *Salmonella* bacterin type on ability to produce immunoglobulins directed against *Salmonella* whole cells or lipopolysaccharide, *Am J Vet Res* 53:1895-1899, 1992.
1379. Spier SJ et al: Use of ELISA for detection of immunoglobulins G and M that recognize *Salmonella dublin* lipopolysaccharide for prediction of carrier status in cattle, *Am J Vet Res* 51:1900-1904, 1990.
1380. Smith BP: Understanding the role of endotoxins in gram-negative septicemia, *Vet Med* 81:1148-1161, 1986.

JOHNE'S DISEASE (Paratuberculosis)

ROBERT WHITLOCK

DEFINITION. Johne's disease is an insidious chronic infection of primarily ruminants is caused by *Mycobacterium paratuberculosis* (also called *M. avium* subsp. *paratuberculosis*). Lesions resembling paratuberculosis have been seen in a wild rabbit.[1381] The organism is taken up by phagocytic cells in the ileum and other sites along the jejunum and gradually spreads to regional lymph nodes and other body organs in the later stages of the disease, often 2 to 10 years later. The term "Johne's disease" usually refers to the clinical disease condition marked by weight loss and diarrhea, whereas the term "paratuberculosis" refers to the condition of being infected with the causative organism, *M. paratuberculosis*, but not necessarily having clinical signs.

CLINICAL SIGNS. Most infected animals appear clinically normal compared with herd mates. Only after a prolonged incubation period, typically longer than 2 years, do infected animals begin to develop subtle clinical signs, including gradual weight loss despite a normal appetite, usually with decreased milk production. Over a period of several weeks, concurrent with the weight loss, the manure consistency becomes more fluid and usually progresses to severe pipestream diarrhea without tenesmus. The diarrhea may be intermittent initially, with periods of normal manure consistency. During this time the animal continues to lose weight despite a normal appetite. In rare cases, diarrhea begins suddenly as a persistent loose manure or watery scours. Blood, excess mucus, and tenesmus are not present. Other than the loose consistency, the manure appears normal. As the disease progresses, the affected animals become increasingly lethargic and emaciated. Intermandibular edema caused by hypoproteinemia typifies advanced stages of the disease; cachexia and "waterhose" diarrhea characterize the terminal stages. Most animals are culled from the herd before this time because of decreased milk production or severe weight loss.

STAGES OF INFECTION AND DISEASE

Stage I: "Silent" Infection (Calves, Heifers, Young Stock, and Adult Cattle). Most cattle with Johne's disease are infected as young calves. The organism proliferates slowly in the jejunal and ileal mucosa and then slowly spreads to the regional lymph nodes. Animals in stage I of infection are rarely detected even with the most sensitive laboratory tests, such as fecal culture. The organisms in the intestinal tract may not be visible upon microscopic examination of tissues obtained at postmortem, but they may be detectable by culture of the tissues. This silent or eclipse phase of infection usually lasts at least 2 years and may last 10 years or longer.

Stage II: Inapparent Carrier Adults. These animals do not show weight loss or diarrhea, but they may have an altered immune response, with increased γ-interferon response by T cells sensitized to specific mitogens or increased antibody response to *M. paratuberculosis*.[1382] Some animals in stage II test positive on fecal culture. They shed organisms in the manure that contaminate the environment and serve as a source of infection for other animals on the farm. Animals may remain in stage II for several years, depending on an animal's age when infected, the dose of organisms, and the host's immune response.

Stage III: Clinical Disease. Animals at this stage show gradual weight loss and chronic diarrhea but have a normal appetite. Intermittent diarrhea often is present for a few weeks. The vital signs, heart rate, respiratory rate, and temperature are normal. Most animals at this stage test positive for *M. paratuberculosis* on fecal culture and have an increase in antibody, detectable by commercial ELISA and the agar gel immunodiffusion (AGID) test. The rate of progression in this stage varies considerably. Occasionally an animal reverts to normal with restoration of body weight and even tests negative on fecal culture.

Stage IV: Advanced Clinical Disease. Animals in the advanced stage of the disease are weak and emaciated and usually have a profuse, pipestream diarrhea. Intermandibular edema, or "bottle jaw," is characteristic of this phase. Animals can progress from stage II to stage IV in a few weeks. Once the diarrhea is profuse and hypoproteinemia (bottle jaw) occurs, the animal's condition deteriorates rapidly, often in a matter of days. Most animals are sent for salvage at slaughter and may not pass inspection for human consumption. Otherwise, death occurs as a result of dehydration and cachexia.

For every cow with advanced Johne's disease that was born on a farm, it is likely that 15 to 25 others on that farm are also infected.[1383-1385] Only 25% to 30% of these infected animals will be detected even by fecal culture, the most sensitive testing technique. The clinical animal is the "tip of the iceberg" (Box 30-10). As an example, consider a herd with 100 adult cattle and 100 young stock replacements. Two cows have clinical signs with weight loss and diarrhea, both were born on the farm several years earlier. It is likely that 30 to 50 other cattle are infected, but fewer than 30% of these will be detectable by fecal culture. It is also reasonable to conclude that if 25 to 30 of the adult cattle in a herd of 100 adult cattle test positive on a single herd fecal culture, most of the herd probably is infected.

CLINICAL PATHOLOGY. The clinicopathologic abnormalities reported with clinical Johne's disease are characteristic but not diagnostic. Stages I and II are not associated with any characteristic biochemical or enzymatic changes. Animals with clinical signs in stages III and IV typically are hypoproteinemic (total protein under 5.5 g/dl) with reductions in albumin (under 2 g/dl) and all classes of immunoglobulin. The marked muscle loss may be associated with elevated plasma phosphorous levels (up to 10 mg/dl), attributable to the catabolic state with phosphorus release from muscle wasting. The animals often are mildly anemic (packed cell volume under 25%) with

---

BOX 30-10

"The Iceberg Effect"

Stage IV	Advanced clinical disease	1	animal
Stage III	Clinical disease	1-2	animals
Stage II	Inapparent carrier adults	6-8	cattle
Stage I	Silent infection of calves—youngstock	10-15	cattle
		15-25	cattle

concurrent hypocalcemia (partly due to the hypoalbuminemia), hyponatremia, and hypokalemia.

Antibody-Based Diagnostic Tests

Agar Gel Immunodiffusion. The AGID test has significant diagnostic value if the animal is showing weight loss or diarrhea or both. A positive test result in an animal with clinical signs has high specificity (over 95%) for Johne's disease.[1386] The major drawback of the AGID test is lack of sensitivity, or failure to detect animals that test positive on fecal culture but are not showing clinical signs.[1386] The AGID test should be reserved for the individual cow with clinical signs compatible with Johne's disease. A small proportion of cattle with clinical signs (10% to 15%) have a positive result with the AGID technique but test negative on the ELISA.

ELISA. The advantages of the ELISA are the rapid turnaround time (2 to 4 days), the low unit cost, and the large number of samples that can be processed each day. The test detects and quantitates the host's serum antibody response to an antigen derived from *M. paratuberculosis*. The reported sensitivity and specificity of the ELISA are 45% and 99%, respectively.[1387,1388] Some cattle with clinical Johne's disease (about 15%) test negative with the ELISA but positive with the AGID technique, seemingly a paradox because the ELISA detects less antibody than the AGID test.

Animals with high ELISA antibody titers are more likely to be infected with *M. paratuberculosis*.[1388] The ELISA may be used to screen cattle to identify those at highest risk for Johne's disease.[1389] The high-risk animals would then be tested by fecal culture. This screening process would permit a much greater number of cattle to participate in a control and certification program for Johne's disease. An ELISA result should *not* be accepted as a definitive diagnostic test for the individual animal.

Recently a new, single-use ELISA, called the "tip-test," was approved by U. S. Department of Agriculture. This test's sensitivity and specificity are similar to those of other ELISAs for Johne's disease.[1390] The test can be done in the practitioner's office or in a small laboratory. It is best used to detect antibodies (infection) in cattle with clinical signs, which permits rapid culling of such animals. Cattle that test positive on the tip-test as they enter the dry period should also be culled, because they are at greater risk of passing the infection to their calves.

Complement Fixation Test. The complement fixation (CF) test often is required for export purposes, but it is not recommended for diagnostic purposes. The test is plagued with major faults, including false positive results and lack of sensitivity for detecting infected cattle.[1383]

Antigen or Organism Detection Tests

Deoxyribonucleic Acid Probe Test. Deoxyribonucleic acid (DNA) probe tests are used to identify specific DNA segments (IS900) in *M. paratuberculosis*. This is state-of-the-art technology for detecting this fastidious pathogen. The DNA probe approach potentially has the greatest sensitivity and exquisite specificity.[1391] A DNA probe test that quickly (within 4 days) detects *M. paratuberculosis* in a fecal sample when it is present in large numbers (10,000 to 100,000 organisms per gram of manure) has been developed.[1392,1393] At this stage most infected animals are showing clinical signs. The DNA probe test less frequently detects infected animals in the preclinical stages of infection. Currently, both commercial and research-based DNA probe tests have little field application because of the high cost, the technical expertise required, and the presence of inhibitors in bovine fecal tests. If the technical hurdles can be overcome and the expense reduced, this test has the potential to be 100% specific and relatively sensitive for detecting many animals in stage II and nearly all animals in stages III and IV of infection.

Histopathology. For the clinician, histopathologic examination of biopsies of the terminal ileum and ileocecocolic lymph node often offers the most definitive diagnosis of Johne's disease within a short time (48 to 72 hours). Microscopic examination of the tissues after acid-fast staining with Ziehl-Neelsen, Kinyoun, or auramine-O stain provides an accurate assessment of infection status if clinical signs of weight loss and diarrhea are present.[1394,1395] If acid-fast organisms are found in clumps in macrophages, the biopsy report is declared positive. If the biopsy report is negative, other causes for the weight loss and diarrhea should be explored. All infected cattle showing clinical signs should have a positive biopsy report. However, failure to demonstrate acid-fast organisms or to identify Langerhans' giant cells does not imply the absence of infection, especially in the early stages of the disease. Other, infected tissue sites may not have been selected for examination.

Rectal scraping in clinical cases may also be useful if it is positive. Mucus from the rectum is made into a thin smear on a slide and stained for acid-fast organisms. Using high magnification, the slide is searched for *clumps* of tiny acid-fast organisms (usually in the ghost outline of a macrophage). Single large saprophytic acid-fast organisms are ignored. This method has been sensitive in 50% of clinical Johne's cases seen at one teaching hospital.

Fecal Culture. Isolation of *M. paratuberculosis* from feces remains the "gold standard" for routine detection of individual infected animals in a herd suspected of having cattle with Johne's disease.[1393] Fecal culture techniques using both centrifugation and double incubation should detect 10 to 50 organisms per gram of manure[1383,1396] and identify two to three times as many infected animals as the ELISA.[1396] The organism can be detected in fecal samples of most infected cattle 1 to 2 years before the development of clinical signs.[1384] The major drawback of fecal culture is the prolonged incubation period of 12 to 16 weeks and the higher cost than the ELISA. Occasionally a positive result on fecal culture (low colony counts) is followed by several negative results. This may be due to passive excretion after consumption of contaminated feed materials[1397,1398] or intermittent detection by the laboratory. Fecal culture is a poor test for confirming the diagnosis in clinically suspicious cases when results are needed quickly. The strain of *M. paratuberculosis* that infects sheep was very difficult to grow in the laboratory until the recent development of new media formulations that facilitate growth.[1399]

Fecal culture tests are the most sensitive and specific test (100%) available to detect infection with *M. paratuberculosis* on a herd basis. However, fecal cultures detect fewer than 40% of all the currently infected adult cattle on a farm,[1384,1400] whereas the ELISA detects 15% to 20% of those infected animals. Whole herd fecal cultures, repeated annually, are recommended for infected herds to maximize detection of infected animals.[1401] This recommendation should be made only if the farm manager has agreed to implement the necessary biosecurity measures. Repeated use of any test is unwarranted unless the management changes necessary for reducing the spread of disease are made.

Cellular Immunity Tests: γ-Interferon. An ELISA for measuring γ-interferon, a mediator released by sensitized T lymphocytes in response to stimulation by specific mitogens, may be a useful diagnostic tool in the future. Reports suggest that the γ-interferon ELISA may be more sensitive than other currently available serologic tests.[1382]

Diagnostic Tests for Individual Animals without Clinical Signs. The usual reason for a request to test an animal without clinical signs is to determine if the animal is free of *M. paratuberculosis* infection before it is introduced into a herd. Confirming the absence of infection in an animal without clinical signs remains a challenge for even the seasoned clinician. A negative result on ELISA or the fecal culture test does not prove the absence of *M. paratuberculosis* infection. The early stages (I or II) of Johne's disease are nearly impossible to detect with any diagnostic test currently available. The clinician should obtain a complete history to determine if Johne's disease has been present in the herd in the previous 5 to 10 years. If both the herd owner and the herd veterinarian of record are willing to sign a statement that the disease has not been encountered in the herd in that time period, the risk of purchasing an infected animal from this herd is lower. Further evidence for the absence of Johne's disease may be obtained by finding negative results on ELISAs in a group of 30 second lactation or older cattle in the herd. Other diagnostic options are PCR DNA probe testing or culture testing of pooled fecal samples from groups of 10 cows in the herd; the latter approach offers the advantages of rapid turnaround, high sensitivity, and lower costs.

Diagnostic Tests for the Herd. The most cost-efficient method of determining if infection with *M. paratuberculosis* may be present in a herd is use of the ELISA, followed by fecal culture testing for each animal with a positive ELISA result, performed on all adult cattle in the herd. If the commercial ELISA detects one ELISA-positive animal and that is confirmed by fecal culture, the herd is likely to have many more infected animals, perhaps as many as five times the number that test positive on the ELISA and fecal culture. Although the ELISA is relatively specific, the sensitivity for detecting lightly infected cattle is less than 20%.[1388] Lightly infected animals (fewer than 10 colonies per tube) account for approximately 70% of the infected cattle in a herd. The DNA probe test is too costly to be used as a herd test. Fecal culture has the greatest specificity (100%) as well as a higher sensitivity than the ELISA. If paratuberculosis is to be eliminated from the herd, annual or semiannual whole herd fecal cultures are required to identify and cull animals that may be spreading the disease to other animals, along with implementation of a strict biosecurity program.

PATHOPHYSIOLOGY. *M. paratuberculosis* enters the intestinal tract and is taken up preferentially by the M cells of the ileum.[1402] The interval from infection to the onset of clinical signs is at least 12 months with heavy and repeated doses of *M. paratuberculosis*; with small doses more than 10 years may elapse before clinical signs appear. In heavily infected herds with many clinical cases, yearling heifers may show evidence of ill thrift and loose manure as a result of Johne's disease, but this is rare. Typically the first evidence of weight loss and diarrhea occurs within several months of calving or some other period of stress. In rare cases, uninfected adult cattle become infected when introduced to a heavily infected herd and develop clinical signs several years later.

The response of the animal's system to *M. paratuberculosis* infection is recruitment of macrophages and development of giant cells.[1395] As the organism multiplies over weeks and months, the thickened intestine becomes less able to absorb nutrients, and the animal loses weight despite a normal appetite. The thickened intestinal wall begins gradually to leak protein from the blood into the intestine, resulting in a direct nutrient loss from the bloodstream. Hypoproteinemia results from the malabsorption and protein-losing enteropathy.

TRANSMISSION AND EPIDEMIOLOGY. The fecal-oral route is the primary mode of transmission from an infected adult to the neonate. Most infections with *M. paratuberculosis* occur in the early neonatal period, and infection often is associated with the calf sucking a manure-contaminated teat and udder while ingesting colostrum. Multiple-use maternity pens serve as focal points for spreading the infection from one cow to a calf born to another cow. Although calves are most susceptible, older heifers and adult cattle can become infected by eating contaminated feedstuffs. Approximately 25% of calves born to cattle with clinical signs are infected in utero, but only 18% of calves born to asymptomatic cows are infected in utero.[1403,1404] *M. paratuberculosis* has been isolated from uterine flush fluids of infected cattle.[1405]

M. paratuberculosis may be passed though the colostrum and milk of cattle in the later stages of infection.[1401] Therefore feeding pooled waste milk from several cows or pooled colostrum spreads the infection from adults to calves during their most susceptible stage of life. Physical separation to calf hutches or better yet to another property, such as a commercial heifer raising facility, reduces the risk of transmission to young calves. Many small farms use manger sweepings from the adult cows as feed for older heifers, a practice that has proved to be a risk factor for spreading the disease. Semen from bulls kept in commercial bull studs represents a very low risk because these animals are tested twice yearly for paratuberculosis and must have a negative test result.

Because the organism survives in the environment for nearly a year, water and forages may become contaminated when nutrient wastes are applied to pastures or cropland if these are harvested soon after application. However, environmental contamination represents a much lower risk than direct fecal contamination of the feed for calves, heifers, or adult cows.

Johne's disease is widely distributed throughout the world. Reports suggest 7% to 18% of cattle in slaughterhouse surveys are infected.[1386,1407,1408] The 1996 dairy NAHMS study estimated that 3.4% of adult cattle and 22% of U. S. dairy herds were infected. The infection rate was 40% in herds with 300 or more cows,[1409] and 42% of dairy herds had at least one positive ELISA result. The 1997 beef NAHMS study indicated that 0.4% of adult beef cattle and 7.9% of beef herds were infected.[1410] Paratuberculosis is extensively distributed among other ruminants including sheep, goats, deer, elk, bison, and many exotic ruminant species kept in zoologic gardens. The apparent prevalence among cattle and other ruminant species is increasing, especially as herd size increases with the purchase of cattle of unknown infection status.

TREATMENT. No practical therapy for Johne's disease is available. However, for cattle with significant genetic or sentimental value, several therapeutic agents have been used to effect remission of clinical signs. Administration of isoniazid* (5 mg/kg daily given orally), rifampin† (5 mg/kg daily given orally), or clofazimine‡ (2.5 mg/kg daily given orally) has resulted in amelioration of clinical signs, facilitating collection of embryos and semen over an extended period.[1411,1412] The drugs must be given daily, and if therapy is stopped, clinical signs may reappear within a few weeks. No drug or combination of therapeutic agents has been shown to eliminate the infection to date. Treated animals continue to shed *M. paratuberculosis* in the manure, contaminating the environment, and have viable organisms in their tissues, indicating the possibility that semen and embryos from treated animals may be infected. If animals with Johne's disease are treated with chemotherapeutic agents, the owners should agree with the prescribing veterinarian that milk or meat from that animal will never be used for human consumption. Drugs used to treat Johne's disease can be used in an extralabel manner with an appropriate client-patient relationship, but no data are available regarding appropriate withdrawal times. For further information, refer to articles by Hoffsis[1411] and by St. Jean and Jernigan.[1412]

ECONOMIC LOSSES ATTRIBUTED TO PARATUBERCULOSIS. Economic losses associated with Johne's disease have been attributed to many factors including (1) decreased milk production, (2) increased susceptibility to other diseases, (3) loss of genetic potential, (4) loss of export market, (5)

---

*Available from several companies, including Henry Schein, Inc., Port Washington, NY; Barr Labs, Inc., Northvale, NY; and Eli Lilly & Co, Indianapolis, IN.

†Rifadin, Merrell Dow, Cincinnati, OH.

‡Lamprene, Geigy Pharmaceuticals, Summit, NJ.

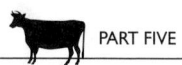

increased medical costs, (6) reduced weight at slaughter, (7) premature culling, (8) poor feed conversion, (9) decreased milk production, (10) increased calving interval, and (11) financial loss at auctions if animals are designated "exposed to Johne's disease."[1413] Johne's disease is a reportable disease in many states.

The estimated annual cost of paratuberculosis to Wisconsin farmers is more then $52 million. Buergelt and Duncan[1414] reported that clinically affected cows gave 2736 lb less milk for the 305-day lactation period than uninfected cows in the same herd. A slaughterhouse survey I conducted gave similar results. Infected cows produced 3400 lb less milk for the last lactation compared with uninfected cows.[1407] The 1996 dairy NAHMS survey estimated the economic loss to be $227 per adult cow in herds in which at least 10% of cull cows have clinical signs of Johne's disease. In herds in which the infection rate was low, the loss was estimated at $40 per adult cow, which for a 100-cow herd is $4000 a year.[1409]

BIOSECURITY PRACTICES AND CONTROL. The key to preventing, controlling, and eliminating Johne's disease in a herd is implementation of appropriate biosecurity measures as part of a herd plan, which should be written out.[1415-1419] Farm managers should adopt two fundamental control principles: (1) prevent *highly susceptible* newborn calves and young animals from ingesting manure from infected adults and (2) reduce total farm environmental contamination by *M. paratuberculosis* by culling infected animals shedding the bacteria. Calves should be separated from their dams at birth and fed single-source colostrum from culture-negative cows.[1420-1422] Cleaning of maternity pens after each use has been associated with a threefold reduction in the odds of a herd testing positive for *M. paratuberculosis* infection.[1417]

Fecal culture testing of the whole herd followed by aggressive culling of infected animals is very effective in reducing the prevalence of paratuberculosis in the herd.[1423] A method of eradicating Johne's disease from a heavily infected herd within 12 months has been described.[1424] In herds with low to moderate infection levels (1% or fewer clinical cases per year), wise use of a combination of testing, culling, and biosecurity measures may eliminate clinical disease within 1 to 3 years and most infected adults in 5 to 7 years, as the herd turns over. Complete elimination of infected cattle is likely to take many years after clinical Johne's disease is apparently gone from the herd. Biosecurity measures should remain in place, or Johne's disease is likely to recur.

Herds with more severe, widespread infection require aggressive control programs and many years to eliminate Johne's disease. However, a practical control program and sound herd management can eliminate clinical disease in these herds and reduce the economic impact of Johne's disease to a minimum. Many states offer assistance to cattle producers in their efforts to reduce and or eliminate Johne's disease on their farms. The National Johne's Working Group has developed a plan for states to adopt to help reduce the prevalence of this economically important disease.[1425] The plan, "Minimum Recommendations for Administering and Instituting State Voluntary Johne's Disease Programs for Cattle," was adopted by the U.S. Animal Health Association (USAHA) in 1999.[1426] Further information can be obtained at the association's Internet website (www.usaha.org/njwg.html).

Herds that have implemented biosecurity practices and have negative test results for Johne's disease may qualify for the U. S. Voluntary Johne's Disease Herd Status Program for Cattle, which was approved by the USAHA in 1998.[1426] The purpose of this program is to recognize herds at low risk for Johne's disease so that they may serve as resources for owners of other herds who want to expand their herd size yet maintain a low risk for Johne's disease.

VACCINATION. A killed Johne's disease vaccine is restricted for use in a few states by an accredited veterinarian with prior approval by the state veterinarian. The vaccine is effective in reducing the prevalence of the disease and delays the onset of clinical signs,[1427] but it does not eliminate infection. Animals must be less than 35 days old when vaccinated. Adverse reactions associated with use of the vaccine, which are common, include a granuloma or abscess at the injection site (the dewlap) and reactions to tuberculin skin tests or Johne's disease serologic tests. Some veterinarians have injected a finger, which resulted in severe, painful granulomas.[1428]

Paratuberculosis and Crohn's Disease

An increasing body of literature implicates mycobacteria as a factor in Crohn's disease, a chronic, smoldering inflammatory disease of the gastrointestinal tract in human beings.[1429,1430] Abundant evidence suggests that human exposure to *M. paratuberculosis* may occur from the milk[1406] and meat of infected cows or contaminated water supplies.[1427] Because most metropolitan water is not filtered and is collected from rural areas, drinking water may also represent a major potential source of the pathogen. Intestinal cohabitation may change parasitism to clinical disease after a long latency period. Genetic susceptibility, the coexistence of other enteric diseases, hormonal factors, and other, poorly understood stress factors may enhance the likelihood of clinical disease after a long incubation period. An association between Crohn's disease and paratuberculosis has been shown, but a causal relationship remains to be demonstrated.[1430-1432] A conference sponsored by the National Institutes of Health (NIH) in December 1998 reviewed current knowledge about a microbial etiology for Crohn's disease, including evidence for and against *M. paratuberculosis* as a possible cause. Further information about the findings of this conference are available at the NIH website (niaid.nih.gov/dmid/crohns.htm).

REFERENCES

1381. Angus KW: Intestinal lesions resembling paratuberculosis in a wild rabbit *(Oryctolagus cuniculus)*, *J Comp Pathol* 103:101-105, 1990.
1382. Stabel JR: Production of γ-interferon by peripheral blood mononuclear cells: an important diagnostic tool for detection of subclinical paratuberculosis, *J Vet Diagn Invest* 8:345-350, 1996.
1383. Whitlock RH: Laboratory diagnosis of Johne's disease, *Proceedings of the Third International Colloquium on Paratuberculosis*, Orlando, Fla, Sept 28–Oct 2, 1991.
1384. Whitlock RH et al: Pattern of detection of M. paratuberculosis–infected cattle in 10 dairy herds cultured every 6 months for 4 years, *Proceedings of the Fourth International Colloquium on Paratuberculosis*, Cambridge, England, 1994, pp 47-53.
1385. Whitlock RH, Buergelt C: Preclinical and clinical manifestations of paratuberculosis (including pathology), *Vet Clin North Am (Food Anim Pract)* 12:345-356, July, 1996.
1386. Sherman DM et al: Evaluation of the agar gel immunodiffusion test for diagnosis of subclinical paratuberculosis in cattle, *Am J Vet Res* 50:525-530, 1989.
1387. Collins MT et al: Reproducibility of a commercial enzyme-linked immunosorbent assay for bovine paratuberculosis among eight laboratories, *J Vet Diagn Invest* 5:52-55, 1993.
1388. Sweeney RW et al: Evaluation of a commercial enzyme-linked immunosorbent assay for the diagnosis of paratuberculosis in dairy cattle, *J Vet Diagn Invest* 7:488-493, 1995.
1389. McNabb WB et al: An evaluation of selected screening tests for bovine paratuberculosis, *Can J Vet Res* 55:252-259, 1991.
1390. Crabb JH et al: New rapid diagnostic test for Johne's disease in cattle, *Proceedings of the Thirty-second Annual Convention of the American Association of Bovine Practitioners*, 1999, pp 247-249.
1391. Vary PH et al: Use of highly specific DNA probes and the polymerase chain reaction to detect *Mycobacterium paratuberculosis* in Johne's disease, *J Clin Microbiol* 28:933-937, 1990.
1392. Whipple DL, Kapke PA, Andersen PR: Comparison of a commercial DNA probe test and three cultivation procedures for detection of *Mycobacterium paratuberculosis* in bovine feces, *J Vet Diagn Invest* 4:23-27, 1992.

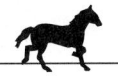
1393. Sockett DC, Carr DJ, Collins MT: Evaluation of conventional and radiometric fecal culture and a commercial DNA probe for the diagnosis of *M. paratuberculosis* infections in cattle, *Can J Vet Res* 56:148-153, 1992.

1394. Benedictus G, Bosha J: Paratuberculosis: a surgical method of diagnosis in practice, *Vet Q* 7:217-221, 1985.

1395. Buergelt CD et al: Pathological evaluation of paratuberculosis in naturally infected cattle, *Vet Pathol* 15:196-207, 1978.

1396. Whitlock RH, Rosenberger AE: Fecal culture protocol for *Mycobacterium paratuberculosis*: a recommended procedure, *Proceedings of the Ninety-fourth U S Animal Health Association Meeting*, 1990.

1397. Rosenberger AE et al: Environmental survey for *Mycobacterium paratuberculosis* on dairy farms with a history of Johne's disease, *Proceedings of the Third International Colloquium on Paratuberculosis*, Orlando, Fla, Sept 28-Oct 2, 1991.

1398. Sweeney RW et al: Isolation of *Mycobacterium paratuberculosis* after oral inoculation of uninfected cattle, *Am J Vet Res* 53:1312-1314, 1992.

1399. Whittington RJ et al: Evaluation of modified BACTEC 12B radiometric medium and solid media for culture of *Mycobacterium avium* ssp *paratuberculosis* from sheep, *J Clin Microbiol* 37:1077-1083, 1999.

1400. Whitlock RH et al: ELISA and faecal culture: sensitivity and specificity of each method, *Proceedings of the Sixth International Colloquium on Paratuberculosis*, Melbourne, Australia, 1999.

1401. Kalis CHJ et al: Factors influencing the isolation of *Mycobacterium avium* ssp *paratuberculosis* from bovine fecal samples, *J Vet Diagn Invest* 11:345-351, 1999.

1402. Momotani E et al: Role of M-cells and macrophages in the entrance on *Mycobacterium paratuberculosis* into dome of ileal Peyer's patches in calves, *Vet Pathol* 25: 131-137, 1988.

1403. Streeter RN et al: Isolation of *M. paratuberculosis* from colostrum and milk of subclinically infected cows, *Am J Vet Res* 56:1322-1324, 1995.

1404. Sweeney RW, Whitlock RH, Rosenberger AE: *Mycobacterium paratuberculosis* isolated from fetuses of infected cows not manifesting signs of the disease, *Am J Vet Res* 53:477-480, 1992.

1405. Rhode RF, Shulaw WP: Isolation of *Mycobacterium paratuberculosis* from the uterine flush fluids of cows with clinical paratuberculosis, *J Am Vet Med Assoc* 197:1482-1483, 1990.

1406. Sweeney RW, Whitlock RH, Rosenberger AE: *Mycobacterium paratuberculosis* cultured from milk and supramammary lymph nodes of infected asymptomatic cattle, *J Clin Microbiol* 30:166-171, 1992.

1407. Whitlock RH et al: Prevalence and economic considerations of Johne's disease in the northeastern United States, *Proceedings of the Eighty-ninth U S Animal Health Association Meeting*, Milwaukee, Wis, 1985.

1408. Merkal RS et al: Prevalence of *Mycobacterium paratuberculosis* in ileocecal lymph nodes of cattle culled in the United States, *J Am Vet Med Assoc* 190:676-680, 1987.

1409. National Animal Health Monitoring System: Johne's disease on U S dairy operations, #N245.1097, Fort Collins, Colo, 1997.

1410. National Animal Health Monitoring System: What do I need to know about Johne's disease in beef cattle? No N309.899, Fort Collins, Colo, 1999.

1411. Hoffsis GF et al: Therapy for Johne's disease, *Proceedings of the Twenty-fifth Annual Convention of the American Association of Bovine Practitioners*, 1990, pp 55-58.

1412. St Jean G, Jernigan AD: Treatment of *Mycobacterium paratuberculosis* infection in ruminants, *Vet Clin North Am (Large Anim Pract)* 7:793-804, 1991.

1413. Collins MT, Morgan ID: Economic decision analysis model of a paratuberculosis test and cull program, *J Am Vet Med Assoc* 199:1724-1729, 1991.

1414. Buergelt CD, Duncan JR: Age and milk production data of cattle culled from a dairy herd with paratuberculosis, *J Am Vet Med Assoc* 173:478-480, 1978.

1415. Rossiter CA: Four steps for a successful Johne's disease control plan: experience from the New York state paratuberculosis program, *Proceedings of the Seventy-fifth Annual Meeting of the Livestock Conservation Institute*, Minneapolis, Minn, 1991.

1416. Stabel JR: Johne's disease: a hidden threat, *J Dairy Sci* 81:283-288, 1998.

1417. Johnson-Ifearulundu Y, Kaneene JB: Management-related risk factors for *M. paratuberculosis* infection in Michigan, USA, dairy herds, *Prev Vet Med* 37:41-54, 1998.

1418. Johnson-Ifearulundu Y, Kaneene JB: Distribution and environmental risk factors for paratuberculosis in dairy cattle herds in Michigan, *Am J Vet Res* 60:589-596, 1999.

1419. Hansen D, Rossiter C: Tools to use against Johne's disease in cattle herds, *Proceedings of the Thirty-third Annual Convention of the American Association of Bovine Practice*, 1999, pp 88-191.

1420. Goodger WJ et al: Epidemiologic study of on-farm management practices associated with prevalence on *Mycobacterium paratuberculosis* infections in dairy cattle, *J Am Vet Med Assoc* 208:1877-1881, 1996.

1421. Rossiter CA: Approach for designing appropriate Johne's disease control programs on the farm, *Proceedings of the Twenty-ninth Annual Convention of the American Association of Bovine Practice*, 1996, pp 33-45.

1422. Rossiter CA et al: Johne's disease prevention/control plan for beef herds: manual for veterinarians, *Bovine Pract* 33:2, 194 (1)-194 (22), 1999.

1423. Rossiter CA et al: Johne's disease prevention/control plan for dairy herds: manual for veterinarians, *Bovine Pract* 33:2, 193 (1)-193 (22), 1999.

1424. Collins MT: Eradication of Johne's disease from a heavily infected herd in 12 months, *Proceedings of the Thirty-first Annual Convention of the American Association of Bovine Practice*, 1998, pp 241-244.

1425. Roussel AJ: What is the National Johne's Working Group? *Compend Cont Educ Pract Vet* 20:1281-1291, 1998.

1426. Bulaga LL: US Voluntary Johne's Disease Herd Status Program for Cattle, *Proc US Animal Health Assoc* 102:420-433, 1998.

1427. Larsen AB et al: Hypersensitivity and serologic responses in cattle vaccinated with disrupted *Mycobacterium paratuberculosis* cells and subsequently infected with *Mycobacterium bovis*, *Am J Vet Res* 30:2167-2172, 1969.

1428. Patterson CJ et al: Accidental self-inoculation with *Mycobacterium paratuberculosis* bacterin (Johne's bacterin) by veterinarians in Wisconsin, *J Am Vet Med Assoc* 192:1197-1199, 1988.

1429. Chiodini RJ: Crohn's disease and the mycobacteriosis: a review and comparison of two disease entities, *Clin Microbiol Rev* 2:90-117, 1989.

1430. Thompson DE: The role of mycobacteria in Crohn's disease, *J Med Microbiol* 41:74-94, 1994.

1431. Collins MT: *Mycobacterium paratuberculosis:* a potential food-borne pathogen? *J Dairy Sci* 80:3445-3448, 1997.

1432. Van Kruiningen HJ: Lack of support for a common etiology in Johne's disease of animals and Crohn's disease in humans, *Inflamm Bowel Dis* 5:183-191, 1999.

COPPER DEFICIENCY IN RUMINANTS

JOHN MAAS
BRADFORD P. SMITH

DEFINITION AND ETIOLOGY. Copper deficiency occurs when the diet contains an abnormally low amount of copper (primary copper deficiency) or when copper absorption or metabolism is adversely affected (secondary copper deficiency). If inadequate amounts of copper are available to tissues in the form of essential metalloenzymes, the signs of copper deficiency (hypocuprosis) may occur. Clinical signs include diarrhea, decreased weight gain, unthrifty appearance, anemia, changes in coat color (achromotrichia) or wool quality, anemia, spontaneous fractures (see Chapter 36), lameness (epiphysitis; see Chapter 36), and demyelinization (enzootic ataxia of sheep and goats, swayback; see Chapter 33). One of these syndromes usually predominates in a given herd.

The minimum recommended dietary copper concentration (dry matter basis) is 4 to 10 ppm (mg/kg) for cattle,[1433,1434] 5 ppm for sheep,[1435] and 7 ppm for merino sheep.[1435] Young animals and fetuses are more susceptible to copper deficiency than mature animals, and cattle are more susceptible than sheep.

Secondary copper deficiency is associated with high dietary levels of molybdenum, sulfates, zinc, iron, or other compounds. Secondary copper deficiency often manifests with clinical signs of diarrhea and weight loss or unthriftiness. It has been called teart, peat scours, renguerra, pine, and salt lick disease.[1436] Salt sickness in Florida appears to be the result of combined copper and cobalt deficiencies.

The cause of copper deficiency in clinical cases often is multifactorial and can be difficult to quantitate. In addition, unknown factors cause clinical expression of copper deficiency in ruminants to be manifested as a variety of syndromes.

CLINICAL SYNDROMES AND DIFFERENTIAL DIAGNOSIS. Profuse, watery diarrhea with poor weight gain or weight loss (or both) is a common syndrome in ruminants with copper deficiency.[1436] When it occurs on boggy pastures with high concentrations of molybdenum, the condition has been referred to as teart.[1436] Diminished weight gain or weight loss as a herd problem has many other causes, including parasitism, trace mineral deficiencies (selenium, cobalt), protein-calorie malnutrition, and Johne's disease.

A syndrome characterized by epiphyseal enlargement, stiffness, and unthriftiness is seen in young ruminants and is the result of copper deficiency.[1437] This disorder is sometimes called pine.[1436] Copper deficiency can result in spontaneous fractures in ruminants.

Enzootic neonatal ataxia (swayback) of lambs and kids is characterized by progressive incoordination and recumbency that begins with the hind limbs and progresses to the front limbs. It has also been reported in deer and pigs and is covered in the section on neurologic diseases (see Chapter 33).

Inadequate keratinization of wool and achromotrichia are the result of imperfect oxidation of free thiol groups during hair growth and keratinization. The wool fibers do not crimp normally and appear to be stringy or kinky. A copper-containing enzyme, tyrosinase (polyphenyloxidase), is needed to convert L-tyrosine to melanin. With copper deficiency this conversion is slow and hair is lighter in color than normal (achromotrichia). Loss of wool crimp and pigmentation changes in sheep or cattle, respectively, occur late in the course of copper deficiency.

In addition to the above clinical syndromes, which may occur alone or jointly, copper deficiency may be associated with anemia[1438] (altered iron metabolism) or infertility.[1439] Infertility probably is multifactorial and unlikely to respond to an increase in copper intake alone. Copper deficiency also seems to result in decreased immune function in ruminants.[1440,1441]

PATHOGENESIS. A frank dietary deficiency of copper results in hypocuprosis and eventually clinical signs. Also, a variety of conditions can reduce copper absorption from the gastrointestinal tract (the large intestine in sheep and the small intestine in cattle). The interactions between dietary copper and dietary molybdenum and sulfates (or sulfur) are important. Excess dietary molybdenum can lead to the formation of sparingly soluble cupric molybdates in the rumen that are not absorbed from the intestine. The addition of excess sulfur or sulfates in the diet or water can result in the formation of insoluble copper thiomolybdates in the rumen. The interactions among these three elements are complex (Fig. 30-58).[1442] The infertility seen with secondary copper deficiency may be due to excess circulating oxythiomolybdates, which interfere with the release of luteinizing hormone.[1443] It is important to note that with low sulfur concentrations in the diet, excess molybdenum has a minimum effect on reducing copper absorption. Even when no dietary molybdenum or sulfates are present, only about 5% of ingested copper normally is absorbed.

Excessive calcium in the diet, particularly limestone, reduces copper absorption. Excessive iron (30 mg/kg of body weight or 1200 ppm in the diet of calves) reduces copper absorption.[1444] Overgrazing, with the subsequent ingestion of excess soil, also reduces copper absorption. In addition, excess cadmium (3 to 7 ppm) or excess zinc (100 to 400 ppm) reduces hepatic copper concentration, probably through the combined effects of reduced absorption and competition with copper for hepatic metallothionein.[1445,1446] It had been suggested that excess dietary selenium might interfere with copper absorption or utilization or both, but recently this was shown not to occur in beef cattle[1447] or dairy cattle.[1448]

Copper is an essential component of a number of mammalian enzymes. Some of the medically important copper-containing enzymes are (1) the cytosol form of superoxide dismutase (copper and zinc), (2) cytochrome oxidase (c and aa$_3$), (3) lysyl oxidase, (4) ascorbic acid oxidase, and (5) ceruloplasmin.[1448]

In addition, normal copper nutrition appears to be essential for iron absorption and transportation of iron to the liver and reticuloendothelial system and thus is necessary for nor-

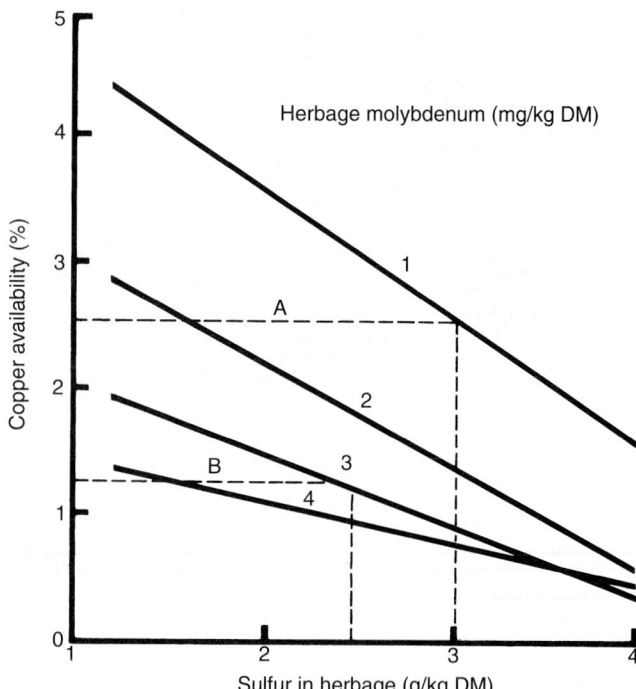

FIG. 30-58 ▌ Estimating the availability of copper in herbage from its molybdenum and sulfur concentration. The difference of 3 mg of molybdenum, and 0.5 g of sulfur per kilogram of dry matter between pastures A and B is sufficient to reduce availability from 2.6% to 1.3%, doubling the grazing animal's requirement of copper from the pasture. (From Suttle NF: *Vet Rec* 119:519-522, 1986.)

mal hemoglobin formation. The precise pathophysiology of most of the copper deficiency syndromes is not known. However, the central role of copper in preventing cellular oxidative damage and its role in iron and sulfur metabolism probably are important.

EPIDEMIOLOGY. Copper deficiency can occur when diets are inadequate in copper or contain excess amounts of interfering substances, particularly sulfates and molybdenum. This occurs in many parts of North America. Forages and water can be sources of molybdenum, sulfur, and sulfate.

To prevent primary copper deficiency, pasture (dry matter) should contain more than 5 ppm of copper, with 3 to 5 ppm considered marginal, and fewer than 3 ppm deficient. Soil copper concentrations generally are slightly lower than that of the harvested forage. Molybdenum adversely affects plant uptake of copper. Forage molybdenum concentrations greater than the copper concentrations often lead to secondary copper deficiency even when forage copper is adequate. Because the copper content of grasses and legumes can be different, forage samples must be randomly selected. Forage copper concentrations as high as 12 to 27 ppm have been associated with copper deficiency when molybdenum levels are high.[1436,1449] The critical ratio of copper to molybdenum in feeds is 2:1, with 5:1 recommended for sheep and 5:1 to 10:1 for grazing cattle.

CLINICAL PATHOLOGY. The primary site of copper reserves is the liver. Normal liver copper concentrations in cattle are approximately 60 to 120 μg/g (ppm) and in sheep 80 to 200 μg/g on a dry weight basis.[1436,1450] Hepatic copper concentrations as high as 250 μg/g are not unusual in ruminants fed supplements (the concentration may exceed 350 μg/g in sheep). Blood copper concentrations can be maintained near normal until the hepatic copper concentration falls below 35 μg/g, at which time the blood level invariably begins to decline (Fig. 30-59).[1451] When blood samples are used for copper determination, serum or plasma normally is preferred. The plasma copper concentration usually is about 5% higher than the serum copper concentration.[1452] The normal serum copper concentration is 0.7 to 1.2 μg/ml.[1436,1449] Serum or plasma copper concentrations of 0.4 μg/ml or less are considered evidence of frank deficiency. Values of 0.4 to 0.7 μg/ml are marginal and difficult to interpret.

Approximately 50% to 90% of the copper in serum or plasma is present in ceruloplasmin. The remainder is bound to albumin or amino acids. The correlation between serum copper and serum ceruloplasmin was found to be weak (0.5)[1452]; thus ceruloplasmin is not commonly used to aid in diagnosing copper deficiency.

The hepatic copper concentration is the preferred diagnostic sample and is easily secured at necropsy. Hepatic copper values below 35 μg/g (dry weight) are considered deficient.[1436,1450,1451] However, surgical biopsy is necessary for live patients, and because laboratories generally require 0.3 g or more of tissue, a biopsy instrument with an internal diameter of 3 to 5 mm is necessary. With smaller biopsy instruments, multiple biopsy samples may be needed. Liver biopsy can place the patient at increased risk for black disease or bacillary hemoglobinuria, the risk of which can be reduced by prior vaccination and administration of penicillin for 1 to 2 days after the biopsy.

The tissues of young animals (neonates) contain variable amounts of copper compared with adults of the same species. In sheep, serum and liver copper concentrations are the same for lambs (1 week of age) and adults.[1453] The plasma copper levels in lambs are low at birth but rise to adult values by 1 to 7 days of age. Plasma copper levels in the bovine neonate are lower than in mature cattle.[1453] In the bovine neonate the hepatic copper concentration changes little from birth to maturity; however, copper distribution in the liver is quite variable in the neonate.[1453,1454] Because of these differences, interpretation of neonatal serum copper concentrations is difficult. Milk is a poor source of copper, containing only 0.2 to 0.6 ppm in normal ewes and 0.01 to 0.02 ppm in severely copper-deficient ewes or cows. Milk copper in cattle is 0.05 to 0.2 ppm. To make matters worse, molybdenum is concentrated in milk.[1455]

Response trials using injectable copper are a valid means of diagnosis. However, adequate numbers of control animals are necessary for evaluation. Also, accurate measurement of clinical disease, production parameters such as feed efficiency, or other such objective criteria are necessary for interpretation.

TREATMENT AND CONTROL. Copper-deficient animals usually can be treated, and the prognosis is guarded to good, depending on the severity of the lesions. When excess molybdenum, sulfate, and other factors leading to secondary deficiency are present, they can be overcome to some extent by increasing dietary copper or by injecting copper.

Injectable copper glycinate (30% copper by weight) is given to adult cattle at the rate of 400 mg (120 mg copper) subcutaneously. Calves are given 100 to 200 mg of copper glycinate (30 to 60 mg of copper), depending on their age. One injection may be effective as a treatment or supplement for up to 4 to 6 months in cases of primary copper deficiency. However, in cases involving excess molybdenum, sulfates, or sulfur, repeat injections may be necessary every 4 to 6 weeks. Injections of copper glycinate frequently result in large swellings, granulomas, or abscesses and may be cosmetic considerations for show cattle. The reactions can be minimized by using sterile technique and selecting the subcutaneous tissue of the brisket as the injection site.

Copper can be supplemented to cattle in salt-mineral mixes when adequate consumption (28 to 56 g/cow/day) of the salt-mineral mix occurs. These mixes usually are 0.2% to

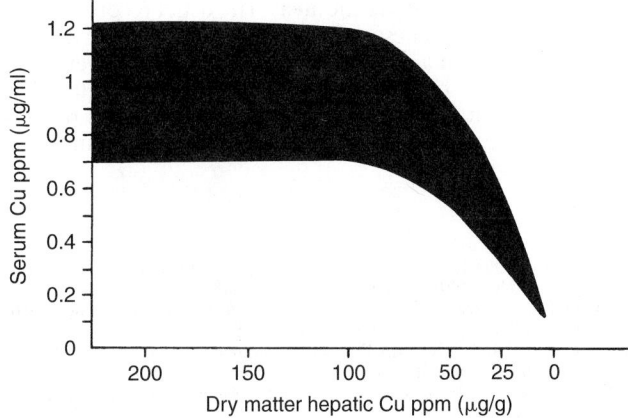

FIG. 30-59 ▦ Relationship between the serum and hepatic copper concentrations in ruminants.

0.6% copper. Feed-grade copper sulfate is 25% copper on an as-fed basis (40% copper on dry matter basis). Feed-grade copper oxide usually is 50% copper as fed (80% copper on a 100% dry matter basis). The copper in copper sulfate is more available than that in copper oxide. For a 0.4% copper-salt mixture, 7.2 g of copper sulfate or 3.6 g of copper oxide are added to each 454 g (1 pound) of salt. For large batches, 32 pounds of copper sulfate or 16 pounds of copper oxide are added per ton of salt. Salt mixtures for sheep usually should contain only 0.0625% to 0.13% copper (0.25% to 0.5% copper sulfate). Copper supplements can easily be added to a total mixed ration in the form of trace mineral–vitamin premixes or premix-containing pellets. Copper sulfate can be added to molasses or other sweet feed at 0.363 g/head/day for mature cattle and correspondingly less for calves. This would supply approximately 91 mg of copper to a 450-kg (1000-lb) cow per day or 10 ppm of the total diet (9.1 kg [20 lb] of dry matter).

In some countries, copper disodium edetate (copper EDTA) solutions are used as injectable copper supplements. The dosage of copper usually is the same as that recommended for copper glycinate solutions. However, acute death can occur after use of copper EDTA solutions in cattle.[1456] Another method of copper supplementation involves oral administration of copper oxide wires or needles (fine rods, 1 to 10 mm long) placed in gelatin capsules, which dissolve in the reticulorumen and liberate the copper oxide wires. The wires reside in the reticulum and abomasum and slowly release copper for absorption. These boluses currently are available in the United States* and contain either 25 g or 12.5 g per bolus. The usual recommended dosage is 25 g per animal weighing 272 kg (about 500 lb) or heavier. One 12.5-g bolus is recommended for calves, and the usual dose is 2 to 4 g for ewes and does,[1436,1457,1458] which is an extralabel recommendation for sheep and goats. The copper oxide needles are thought to provide copper supplementation for 4 to 12 months.

Sheep are particularly susceptible to copper toxicity (see Chapter 35), and appropriate care is necessary when supplementing them, because they require half or less as much dietary copper as cattle. Sheep therefore can become intoxicated when consuming cattle supplements or feeds. Continued monitoring of the hepatic copper concentration from slaughtered animals is an important tool in evaluating copper supplementation methods in cattle and sheep. Lambs can be given 35 mg of copper sulfate per head twice weekly to

---

*Capasure, Schering-Plough Corp., Kenilworth, NJ 07033.

prevent swayback in endemic areas. The usual recommendation by the National Research Council is 10 ppm (10 mg/kg) of the total diet on a dry matter basis for cattle. However, diets of 20 ppm are commonly fed to lactating dairy cattle. The most important goal of copper supplementation is to provide adequate dietary amounts without oversupplementing or risking toxicity.

REFERENCES

1433. National Research Council: *Nutrient requirements of beef cattle,* Washington, DC, 1976, National Academy of Sciences.
1434. National Research Council: *Nutrient requirements of dairy cattle,* Washington, DC, 1978, National Academy of Sciences.
1435. National Research Council: *Nutrient requirements of sheep,* Washington, DC, 1975, National Academy of Sciences.
1436. Blood DC, Radostits OM, Henderson JA: *Veterinary medicine,* ed 6, London, 1983, Baillière Tindall.
1437. Smith BP et al: Abnormal bone development and lameness associated with secondary copper deficiency in young cattle, *J Am Vet Med Assoc* 166:682-688, 1975.
1438. Schalm OW, Jain NC, Carrol EJ: *Veterinary hematology,* ed 3, Philadelphia, 1975, Lea & Febiger.
1439. Weiner G, Sales DI, Field AC: Libido and fertility in rams in relation to plasma copper levels, *Vet Rec* 19:115-116, 1976.
1440. Jones DG, Suttle NF: Some effects of copper deficiency on leukocyte function in sheep and cattle, *Res Vet Sci* 31:151-156, 1981.
1441. Boyne R, Arthur JR: Effects of molybdenum- or iron-induced copper deficiency on the viability and function of neutrophils from cattle, *Res Vet Sci* 41:417-422, 1986.
1442. Suttle NF: Copper deficiency in ruminants: recent developments, *Vet Rec* 119:519-522, 1986.
1443. Phillippo M et al: The effect of dietary molybdenum and iron on copper status, puberty, fertility and estrous cycles in cattle, *J Agri Sci Camb* 109:321-328, 1987.
1444. Campbell AG et al: Effect of elevated iron intake on the copper status of grazing cattle, *NZ J Agri Res* 17:393-399, 1974.
1445. Mills CF, Dalgarno AC: Copper and zinc status of ewes and lambs receiving increased dietary concentrations of cadmium, *Nature* 239:171-173, 1972.
1446. Brenner I, Young BW, Mills CF: Protective effect of zinc supplementation against copper toxicosis in sheep, *Br J Nutr* 36:551-561, 1976.
1447. Maas J et al: Safety, efficacy, and effects on copper metabolism of intrareticularly placed selenium boluses in beef heifer calves, *Am J Vet Res* 55:247-250, 1994.
1448. Buckley WT et al: Effect of selenium supplementation on copper metabolism in dairy cows, *Can J Anim Sci* 66:1009-1018, 1986.
1449. Lehninger AL: *Principles of biochemistry,* New York, 1982, Worth Publishers.
1450. Gay CC, Pritchett LC, Madson W: *Selenium and copper deficiencies in cattle,* Lenexa, Kan, 1988, Veterinary Medicine Publishing.
1451. Claypool DW et al: Relationship between the level of copper in the blood plasma and liver of cattle, *J Anim Sci* 41:911-914, 1975.
1452. Kincaid RL, Gay CC, Krieger RI: Relationship of serum and plasma copper and ceruloplasmin concentrations of cattle and the effects of whole blood sample storage, *Am J Vet Res* 47:1157-1159, 1986.
1453. Underwood EJ: Copper. In *Trace elements in human and animal nutrition,* ed 4, New York, 1977, Academic Press.
1454. Bingley JB, Dufty JH: Distribution of copper in the tissues of the bovine neonate and dam, *Res Vet Sci* 13:8-14, 1972.
1455. Huber JT, Price NO, Engel RW: Response of lactating dairy cows to high levels of dietary molybdenum, *J Anim Sci* 32:364-367, 1971.
1456. Bulgin MS et al: Death associated with parenteral administration of copper disodium edetate in calves, *J Am Vet Med Assoc* 188:406-409, 1986.
1457. Langlands JP et al: Copper oxide particles for grazing sheep, *Aust J Agri Res* 34:751-765, 1983.
1458. Inglis DM, Gilmour JS, Murray IS: A farm investigation into swayback in a herd of goats and the result of administration of copper needles, *Vet Rec* 118:657-660, 1986.

COBALT DEFICIENCY IN RUMINANTS

JOHN MAAS

DEFINITION AND ETIOLOGY. A number of syndromes occur in ruminants as a result of a primary cobalt (Co) deficiency in their diet. These include ill thrift or enzootic maras-

TABLE 30-17

Criteria Used to Determine Cobalt Deficiency in Sheep

Condition of Animal (Co/B$_{12}$ status)	Concentration of Vitamin B$_{12}$ (μg/g fresh liver)[1464]
Severe cobalt deficiency	<0.07
Moderate cobalt deficiency	0.07-0.10
Mild cobalt deficiency	0.11-0.19
Cobalt sufficiency	>0.19

mus and anemia. These conditions are characterized by decreased growth, weight loss, diarrhea, decreased feed efficiency, unthrifty appearance, anorexia, and anemia. Recently a Co deficiency syndrome referred to as ovine white liver disease has been described in sheep.[1459-1461] This syndrome is also characterized by ill thrift, weight loss, serous ocular discharge, and occasionally photosensitization.[1459-1461] Histopathologic lesions of this syndrome included accumulation of lipid droplets and lipofuscin particles, dissociation and necrosis of hepatocytes, and sparse infiltration by neutrophils, macrophages, and lymphocytes.[1461]

CLINICAL SIGNS AND DIFFERENTIAL DIAGNOSIS. Cobalt deficiency in ruminants is associated with the nonspecific signs of decreased growth, weight loss, diarrhea, ill thrift, pica, emaciation, pale mucous membranes (anemia), and lacrimation. Clinical disease is more common in young, growing animals. Sheep apparently are more susceptible to Co deficiency than cattle. Primary differential diagnoses include helminthic parasitism; protein-calorie malnutrition; coccidiosis; Johne's disease; nutritional deficiencies of selenium, copper, or vitamin D; and other causes of chronic disease that may be associated with weight loss.

Cobalt-deficient ruminants are commonly anorexic and fail to thrive on lush pasture or high-quality feeds. Anemia with cobalt deficiency is characterized as normocytic, normochromic and must be differentiated from other causes of anemia. Cobalt-deficient cattle are more susceptible to infestation with *Ostertagia ostertagi* and to the effects of parasitism.[1462] The primary differential diagnosis when considering Co deficiency is invariably internal parasitism.

CLINICAL PATHOLOGY AND DIAGNOSIS. Because the role of Co in ruminant nutrition is tied to the formation, absorption, and use of vitamin B$_{12}$, the most significant clinical chemistry analysis is the tissue vitamin B$_{12}$ concentration. However, the effects of starvation tend to increase vitamin B$_{12}$ concentrations in the liver and kidneys.[1463] If Co deficiency occurs with other conditions that cause anorexia, the tissue vitamin B$_{12}$ concentrations may appear falsely normal. Criteria used for sheep[1464] (and by extrapolation for cattle) are found in Table 30-17.

Serum vitamin B$_{12}$ analysis is advantageous in many clinical settings. Serum or plasma vitamin B$_{12}$ levels have a marked diurnal variation.[1465] The serum vitamin B$_{12}$ concentration more closely reflects short-term cobalt intake and can be decreased when adequate liver reserves of vitamin B$_{12}$ remain. In normal, cobalt-sufficient ruminants, the serum vitamin B$_{12}$ value usually is 1 to 3 ng/ml. When the serum vitamin B$_{12}$ value declines to 0.3 ng/ml, the threshold for clinical signs has been reached, and when values of 0.2 ng/ml or less are reached, marked signs of cobalt deficiency become evident.[1466]

Severe cobalt deficiency in ruminants results in the excretion of methylmalonic acid (MMA) and formiminoglutamic acid (FIGLU) in the urine.[1467] Urinary FIGLU levels of 0.08 to 0.2 μmol/ml would be presumptive evidence of cobalt defi-

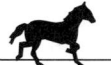

ciency, and the urinary FIGLU level should return to zero after vitamin B_{12} administration. Use of the urinary MMA level for diagnosis is best accomplished by loading the rumen with propionate and then comparing the urinary excretion of MMA with and without vitamin B_{12} supplementation. The fact that urinary MMA and FIGLU excretion occur very late in the course of cobalt deficiency limits the routine use of these methods for diagnosis.

PATHOPHYSIOLOGY. Cobalt deficiency in ruminants induces a deficiency of vitamin B_{12} (cyanocobalamin). It is the lack of vitamin B_{12} that is thought to cause most of the clinical signs and clinicopathologic abnormalities observed. Monogastric species need to ingest vitamin B_{12} preformed, whereas ruminants can manufacture adequate vitamin B_{12} if the rumen microorganisms are supplied with adequate cobalt in the diet. The rumen microorganisms incorporate Co into vitamin B_{12} and a number of physiologically inactive vitamin B_{12}–like compounds. The production of vitamin B_{12} from dietary cobalt was estimated to be about 15% in cobalt-deficient sheep and only about 3% in cobalt-sufficient sheep.[1468] About 50% of the vitamin B_{12} produced is absorbed in normal animals, but only 3% to 5% of vitamin B_{12} is estimated to be absorbed by cobalt-deficient sheep.[1469] Although the absorption of vitamin B_{12} formed in the rumen is not particularly efficient, with normal dietary Co there are usually no clinical problems, and interference by other dietary components does not appear to be important.

Ruminants use the volatile fatty acids acetate, propionate, and butyrate as their primary energy source. Propionate produced in the rumen is the precursor of glucose for ruminant metabolism. The general metabolic steps for conversion of propionate to glucose are shown[1470] in Fig. 30-60.

A primary defect in cobalt-deficient ruminants is the inefficient metabolism of propionate at the point in the pathway at which methylmalonyl-CoA mutase, an enzyme that requires vitamin B_{12}, catalyzes the conversion of methylmalonyl-CoA to succinyl-CoA.[1471] As cobalt deficiency becomes severe, the rate of propionate clearance from the blood decreases and the intermediate metabolite methylmalonyl-CoA accumulates.[1472] With severe cobalt deficiency, the amount of methylmalonic acid excreted in the urine increases.[1462] As the half-time for propionate clearance increases, the voluntary feed intake of cobalt-deficient sheep decreases.[1472] These changes correlate with the degree of anorexia and weight loss observed in severely cobalt-deficient sheep.

The decreased growth, weight loss, unthrifty appearance, and anorexia are closely correlated to the observed abnormalities of carbohydrate metabolism. The diarrhea commonly observed with cobalt deficiency is not well explained; however, an increase in susceptibility to parasitism[1459] may partly explain this clinical observation.

The anemia associated with cobalt deficiency occurs late in the development of the syndrome and is characterized as normocytic normochromic.[1473] Cobalt deficiency results in the depression of the vitamin B_{12}–containing enzyme 5-methyltetrahydrofolate homocysteine methyltransferase.[1474] This interference with the recycling of methionine has a marked influence on folate metabolism. In addition to possibly resulting in anemia through inefficient folate metabolism, the decreased activity of this methyltransferase could lead to a deficiency of methionine; this is a possible reason for nitrogen retention and decreased body growth and wool growth observed.

EPIDEMIOLOGY. Cobalt deficiency in ruminants occurs in selected regions throughout the world and in association with a variety of soil types. Clinically recognizable Co deficiency is reported in New Zealand, Australia, Brazil, the United Kingdom, Ireland, Scandinavia, and North America.

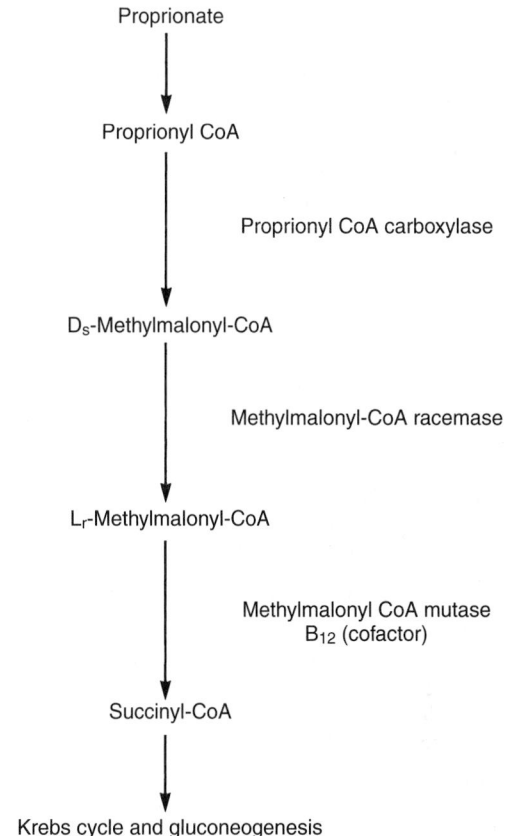

FIG. 30-60 ▌▌ Pathway for conversion of proprionyl CoA (from proprionate) to succinyl CoA.

In the United States, Co deficiency is most commonly seen in Florida, in the Northeast, along the Eastern seaboard, in the upper Midwest, and around the Great Lakes.[1475] Although various soil types are associated with Co deficiency, heavy fertilization with limestone reduces the cobalt available to plants and animals.[1476]

The dietary requirement of cobalt for ruminants generally is recommended as 0.1 mg/kg of dry matter (DM) of the complete ration.[1477-1479] The cobalt requirement of young, rapidly growing lambs is thought to be 0.2 mg/kg of DM of the diet.[1480] When pasture Co concentrations are less than 0.07 mg/kg of DM or 0.04 mg/kg of DM for sheep and cattle, respectively, signs of deficiency can be expected to develop. On a practical basis, diets with 0.1 mg/kg of DM are considered adequate. Legumes have relatively high Co concentrations. Rapidly growing grasses have much lower Co concentrations, and cereal grains are poor sources of cobalt.[1477] Oilseed meals generally are good sources.

TREATMENT AND CONTROL. Treatment is best accomplished in the short term with vitamin B_{12} injections. Ruminants absorb oral vitamin B_{12} poorly, therefore injections are the most efficient method. Lambs given 100 μg of vitamin B_{12} per week or 150 μg every other week show remission of clinical signs.[1481] Sheep given 300 μg weekly or cattle given 2000 to 3000 μg weekly would also be expected to regain normal status.

Rations with 0.1 to 0.2 mg/kg (ppm) of DM cobalt would be expected to prevent cobalt deficiency in ruminants. Salt-mineral mixes containing 0.1% Co also provide adequate supplementation. A mixture of 0.1% Co in salt can be made by mixing cobalt carbonate (which is 46% cobalt) at the rate of 4.35 pounds per ton of salt, or 1 g of cobalt carbonate per pound of salt.

Cobalt sulfate has been used as a top dressing for pastures to increase the Co concentration of pasture forage (1.5 kg/hectare every 3 to 4 years or 0.3 kg/hectare every 1 to 2 years). Heavily limed pastures[1476] and soils high in manganese oxide[1482] reduce Co availability, and cobalt top dressing of the pastures or cobalt–vitamin B_{12} supplementation to the animals should be considered.

A variety of rumen pellets containing cobalt are used to supplement grazing ruminants. These pellets have been successful in maintaining normal Co status in animals.[1480-1483] The pellets are not commercially available in the United States at this time.

The perennial grass *Phalaris tuberosa* can cause a syndrome in ruminants that is referred to as "phalaris staggers." Cobalt supplementation can aid in prevention of this syndrome, because it inactivates or reduces absorption of the neurotoxin contained in *P. tuberosa*, *Phalaris minor* (canary grass), or *Phalaris* hybrids (ronpha).[1484] The increased level of Co in the rumen is the important factor for preventing this condition; administration of oral or parenteral vitamin B_{12} is not effective.[1484] However, treatment of clinical phalaris staggers with cobalt is not effective.

Because cobalt is poorly absorbed, toxicity is an uncommon problem, and diets in excess of 30 mg/kg of DM are necessary for toxicosis to occur in most cases.[1477-1479]

REFERENCES

1459. Kennedy DG et al: Cobalt–vitamin B_{12} deficiency causes accumulation of odd-numbered, branched-chain fatty acids in the tissues of sheep, *Br J Nutr* 71:67-76, 1994.
1460. Kennedy DG et al: Cobalt–vitamin B_{12} deficiency causes lipid accumulation, lipid peroxidation, and decreased α-tocopherol concentrations in the liver of sheep, *Int J Vitam Nutr Res* 64:270-276, 1994.
1461. Kennedy S et al: Histopathologic and ultrastructural alterations of white liver disease in sheep experimentally depleted of cobalt, *Vet Pathol* 34:575-584, 1997.
1462. MacPherson A et al: Ostertagia infection and neutrophil function in cobalt-deficient and cobalt-supplemented cattle, *Br Vet J* 143:348-353, 1987.
1463. Andrews ED, Hart LI: A comparison of vitamin B_{12} concentrations in liver and kidneys from cobalt-treated and mildly cobalt-deficient lambs, *N Z J Agri Res* 5:403-408, 1962.
1464. Andrews Ed, Hart LI, Stephenson BJ: A comparison of the vitamin B_{12} and cobalt content of livers from normal lambs, cobalt-dosed lambs, and others with a recent history of mild cobalt deficiency disease. *N Z J Agri Res* 2:274-282, 1959.
1465. Somers M, Gawthorne JM: The effect of dietary cobalt intake on the plasma vitamin B_{12} concentration of sheep, *Aust J Exp Biol Med Sci* 47:227-223, 1969.
1466. Andrews ED, Stephenson BJ: Vitamin B_{12} in the blood of grazing cobalt-deficient sheep, *N Z J Agri Res* 9:491-507, 1966.
1467. Gawthrone JM: The excretion of methylmalonic and formiminoglutamic acids during the induction and remission of vitamin B_{12} deficiency in sheep, *Aust J Biol Sci* 21:789-794, 1968.
1468. Smith RM, Marston HR: Production, absorption, distribution and excretion of vitamin B_{12} in sheep, *Br J Nutr* 24:857-877, 1970.
1469. Kercher CJ, Smith SE: The response of cobalt-deficient lambs to orally administered vitamin B_{12}, *J Anim Sci* 14:458-464, 1955.
1470. Lehninger AL: *Biochemistry*, ed 2, New York, 1975, Worth Publishers.
1471. Marston HR, Allen SH, Smith RM: Primary metabolic defect supervening on vitamin B_{12} deficiency in the sheep, *Nature* 190:1085-1092, 1961.
1472. Marston HR, Allen SH, Smith RM: Production within the rumen and removal from the bloodstream of volatile fatty acids in sheep given a diet deficient in cobalt, *Br J Nutr* 27:147-157, 1972.
1473. Judson GJ, Gifford KE: Hematological values in vitamin B_{12}–responsive calves, *Aust Vet J* 55:504-505, 1979.
1474. Gawthorne JM, Smith RM: Folic acid metabolism in vitamin B_{12}–deficient sheep. Effects of injected methionine on methotrexate transport and the activity of enzymes associated with folate metabolism in liver, *Biochem J* 142:119-126, 1974.
1475. Kubota J: Distribution of cobalt deficiency in grazing animals in relation to soils and forage plants of the United States, *Soil Sci* 106:122-130, 1968.
1476. Poole DBR, Fleming GA, Kiely J: Cobalt deficiency in Ireland: soil, plant and animal, *Irish Vet J* 6:109-117, 1972.
1477. National Research Council: *Nutrient requirements of beef cattle*, ed 6, Washington, DC, 1984, National Academy of Sciences.
1478. National Research Council: *Nutrient requirements of sheep*, ed 5, Washington, DC, 1985, National Academy of Sciences.
1479. National Research Council: *Nutrient requirements of dairy cattle*, ed 5, Washington, DC, 1978, National Academy of Sciences.
1480. Lee HJ, Marston HR: The requirement for cobalt of sheep grazed on cobalt-deficient pastures, *Aust J Agri Res* 20:905-918, 1969.
1481. Andrews ED, Anderson JP: Responses of cobalt-deficient lambs to cobalt and to vitamin B_{12}, *N Z J Sci Tech* 35:483-488, 1954.
1482. Adams SN et al: Factors controlling the increase of cobalt in plants following the addition of a cobalt fertilizer, *Aust J Soil Res* 7:29, 1919.
1483. Poole DBR, Connolly JF: Some observations on the use of the cobalt heavy pellet in sheep, *Ir J Agri Res* 6:281-284, 1967.
1484. Lee HJ, Kuchel RE: The etiology of *Phalaris* staggers in sheep. I. Preliminary observations on the preventive role of cobalt, *Aust J Agri Res* 4:88-99, 1953.

RECTAL PROLAPSE IN RUMINANTS AND HORSES

SPRING K. HALLAND

DEFINITION AND ETIOLOGY. Rectal prolapse is the protrusion of the rectal mucous membranes through the anus. This evagination may be extensive and may include part of the small colon. Rectal prolapse occurs in all domestic animals, with the highest incidence in cattle, sheep, and swine. The age at which prolapse most commonly occurs is 6 to 12 months in sheep, 6 months to 2 years in cattle, and 6 to 12 weeks in swine.[1485] Rectal prolapse is much less common in horses and occurs more often in mares than males.[1486]

Rectal prolapse generally is the result of an increase in the pressure gradient between the abdominal or pelvic cavity and the anus. Factors that cause the increased pressure gradient can be divided into four categories: (1) factors that result in increased abdominal fill (e.g., excess fat, bloat, and large or multiple fetuses); (2) factors that cause tenesmus (e.g., enteritis, colitis, intestinal parasitism [coccidiosis], liver disease, constipation, proctitis, urinary obstruction, dystocia, aftermath of rectal examination, and false copulation); (3) conditions that result in chronic or excessive coughing (e.g., pneumonia, parasitism, and adverse environmental conditions); and (4) miscellaneous conditions (e.g., short tail docking [especially noted in sheep], use of growth implants, space-occupying lesions, and congenital or acquired sphincter tone problems). Certain toxicities such as from lead, fluoride, estrogen, and zinc have been implicated as playing a role in rectal prolapse.[1487] Any combination of factors may precipitate a rectal prolapse. Identification of predisposing factors becomes important in management of the case.

CLINICAL SIGNS. Four categories have been used to described rectal prolapse: type 1, mucosal prolapse; type 2, complete prolapse; type 3, complete prolapse with invagination of the colon; and type 4, intussusception of the peritoneal rectum or colon through the anus (Fig. 30-61).[1488] Types 1 and 2 are much more common and more amenable to correction. On physical examination, types 1, 2, and 3 are continuous with the mucocutaneous junction of the anus, whereas with type 4 a protrusion with a palpable trench inside the rectum is seen. Chronic cases can be seen and usually are type 1 or 2. Types 3 and 4 often cause loss of vascular integrity to the rectum or small colon and require more immediate intervention. Types 3 and 4 may accompany dystocias in mares.[1489]

TREATMENT AND PROGNOSIS. The first aim of therapy is identification and alleviation of the cause if possible. Early identification and correction of the prolapse is essential to saving tissues and the animal. The animal's value and intended use and the affected tissue's viability need to be considered when deciding on conservative or surgical options.

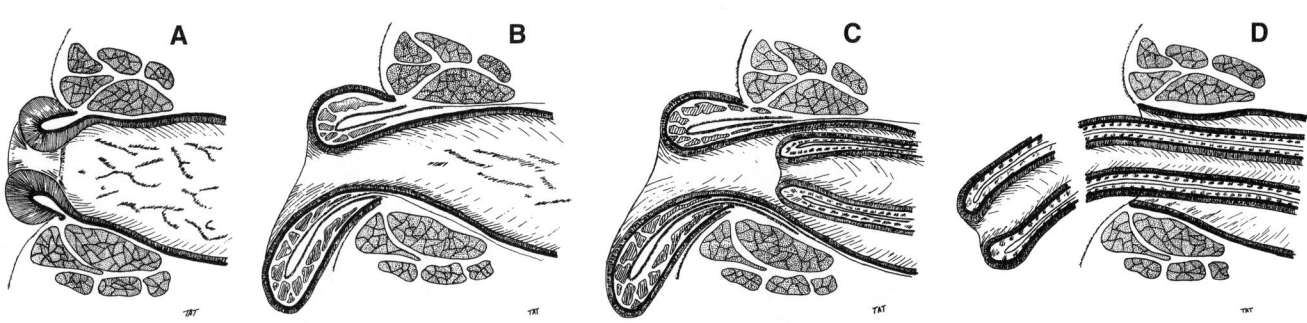

FIG. 30-61 ▓ **A,** Type I rectal prolapse. Mucosal prolapse, involving only muscosa and submucosa of the rectum. **B,** type II rectal prolapse. Complete prolapse involving full wall thickness of the rectum, **C,** Type III rectal prolapse. Complete prolapse plus intussusception of peritoneal rectum or small colon. **D,** Type IV rectal prolapse. Intussusception of the peritoneal rectum or small colon or both. (From Robinson NE, ed: *Current therapy in equine medicine,* ed 2, Philadelphia, 1987, WB Saunders.)

The color of the membranes is a good parameter for determining if the tissue is salvageable. In general, the rectum is a forgiving structure and attempts should be made to salvage the prolapsed tissue unless it is obviously cyanotic, necrosed, and devitalized.[1485] To prevent further damage, animals should remain standing and restrained in a small area until the prolapse can be corrected.

Types 1 and 2 usually are treated conservatively. A caudal epidural is necessary to reduce straining and facilitate correction of the prolapse. Sedation may also be necessary, depending on the individual animal. Effective conservative therapy includes thorough cleansing of the prolapse with warm water and mild soap to remove all debris. This allows evaluation for trauma, tears, necrosis, or sloughing. Edema can be removed by gentle kneading combined with topical application of glycerin or sugar. Generous lubrication and massage allows for reduction of the mass into the rectum. To ensure that the rectum is maintained in place, purse-string sutures using umbilical tape or other nonabsorbable suture are placed circumferentially around the anal sphincter, with care taken not to enter the rectum. The purse-string should not be so tight as to prohibit the passage of feces. If necessary, it should be loosened daily to expedite removal of accumulated fecal material. The purse-string should be removed in 3 to 4 days. In addition to purse-string sutures, counterirritants such as Lugol's iodine are often used.[1485] Two to 3 ml of these irritants are injected with a 7.5-cm needle at the 2, 6, and 10 o'clock positions around the rectum. The counterirritants create an inflammatory response that results in scar formation, which retains the prolapsed tissue after the purse-string has been removed. Broad-spectrum antimicrobial drugs should be administered if tissue compromise is a factor. When indicated, stool softeners and enemas may be used to ease the passage of feces through the rectum.

Surgical intervention often is necessary if type 1 or type 2 prolapse cannot be reduced, if tissue necrosis is extensive, or if prolapse recurs after conservative therapy.[1483] Submucosal resection, amputation, or the use of a prolapse ring are all accepted surgical options. Types 3 and 4 that cannot be manually reduced often require a celiotomy for surgical reduction of the intussusception or resection or both. An important fact to remember is that even with manual reduction of a type 4 prolapse, significant vascular compromise may have occurred, resulting in bowel leakage and peritonitis. Vascular damage encountered by the colon may necessitate a colostomy.[1486] Broad-spectrum antimicrobial drugs should be administered in these cases.

Unique problems are encountered when conservatively managing equine rectal prolapse versus ruminant prolapse. Equine patients may experience more hind limb ataxia with caudal epidurals, which can be prevented by using xylazine in the epidural. Another problem encountered is that horse feces often are too large and dry to readily pass through the purse-string in the anus. The use of enemas and stool softeners offers some assistance. The sutures tend to cause greater anal irritation than is seen in ruminants, causing the horse to strain against them.

The common complications after rectal prolapse include prolapse recurrence, rectal strictures, obstipation, formation of a pararectal abscess, and peritonitis. The prognosis for all types of rectal prolapse depends on early identification and reduction of the prolapse. Types 1 and 2 that can be managed conservatively have a favorable outcome. Surgical correction of types 1 and 2 also carries a good prognosis but with a higher incidence of postsurgical complications. Because of the cost of surgical repair, market animals often are slaughtered if conservative management fails. Rectal prolapse types 3 and 4 carry a fair to guarded prognosis, which depends on the extent of tissue involvement and viability, the surgeon's skill, and postsurgical complications

REFERENCES

1485. Welker B, Modransky M: Rectal prolapse in food animals. I. Cause and conservative management, *Compend Contin Educ* 13:1869-1873, 1991.
1486. Turner T: Rectal prolapse. In Robinson NE, ed: *Current therapy in equine medicine,* ed 2, Philadelphia, 1987, WB Saunders.
1487. Whitlock RH: Colitis and proctitis. In Howards JL, ed: *Current veterinary therapy: food animal practice,* ed 2, Philadelphia, 1986, WB Saunders.
1488. Fubini S: Surgery of the bovine large intestine, *Agri Pract* 14:40-42, 1993.
1489. Freeman DE, Martin BB: Rectum and anus. In Auer JA, ed: *Equine surgery,* Philadelphia, 1992, WB Saunders.

Diseases of the Hepatobiliary System

ERWIN G. PEARSON
Consulting Editor

DIAGNOSIS OF LIVER DISEASE

ERWIN G. PEARSON

The liver cannot be examined directly in large animals. The signs of liver disease are caused by failure of some of the liver's many functions, but these signs may not appear in the early stages of disease. Special tests may be needed to detect early damage or minor impairment of function that has not yet produced clinical signs.

LIVER DISEASE VERSUS LIVER FAILURE

Like many other organs, such as the heart and kidneys, the liver can be diseased long before it fails to function. For this reason, early cases of liver disease are not apparent to the owner or veterinarian through physical findings alone; such cases usually are detected by finding elevated levels of liver enzymes or bile acids in the serum. Pathologic changes in the liver may include biliary hyperplasia, death of hepatocytes, and fibrosis, and these may occur long before any signs of failure develop. Some functions may fail before others, and the onset of liver failure varies with the species and the disease process involved.

LIVER RESERVE AND REGENERATION

The liver has a large reserve capacity, and close to 80% of it can be removed before regeneration and recovery are no longer possible. It also has a remarkable capacity to regenerate. Regeneration can occur in areas receiving portal blood, but most cell division takes place in Rappaport zone 1 (the portal area), and the cells are pushed to the central lobular area. The liver undergoes constant repair; in human beings,

for example, it is estimated that the hepatocytes are renewed every 50 to 75 days.[1]

Normal regeneration does not occur in some cases. Antimitotic agents such as metabolites of pyrrolizine alkaloids or antineoplastic drugs can prevent cell division. Regeneration may be restricted by connective tissue. Once fibrosis has bridged the various lobules, additional regeneration is impaired because the fibrosis itself perpetuates the condition. Loss of a stroma to build on or lack of portal blood supply also reduces regeneration.

SIGNS OF LIVER DISEASE AND PATHOPHYSIOLOGY

Many signs may be present with liver disease, but none of these are pathognomonic, and none are present consistently. Table 31-1 lists some of the signs that may be present, as well as other possible causes of the same signs.[2]

The clinical history is useful in some cases, but consumption of plants containing pyrrolizine alkaloid may not be apparent because of the delay between consumption and the onset of clinical signs. Exposure to other hepatotoxins could be detected. Ruminants grazing on land infested with snails are more likely to have liver fluke disease. Administration of horse serum to Equidae 4 to 8 weeks previously makes acute serum hepatitis more likely.

Except for pain over the liver that is elicited with pressure and a change in liver size, most signs are related to failure of some function. Liver flukes may cause anemia and hypoproteinemia because of the effect of the parasite, its metabolites, or both. Liver abscesses and other infections may cause signs such as fever and anorexia because of the release of pyrogens and other mediators (caused by the organism and not necessarily related to the liver itself).

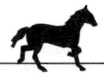

TABLE 31-1

Signs of Liver Disease or Failure

Sign	Pathogenesis	Other Causes
Icterus (E)	Failure of uptake, conjugation, or excretion of bilirubin	Massive hemolysis Bile blockage Fasting in the horse
Weight loss (E, B)	Energy demand greater than absorbed or metabolized	Poor nutrition, chronic inflammation, parasites, neoplasia, maldigestion, malabsorption
Ascites (B)	Portal hypertension and lymph leakage caused by cirrhosis or venoocclusion	Cardiac failure Hypoproteinemia Cushing's syndrome
Change in liver size	Nodular hyperplasia, tumor, cirrhosis Fatty degeneration	Right-heart failure Work hypertrophy Anemia
Diarrhea (B)	Bile deficit malabsorption Intestinal edema, portal hypertension	Gastrointestinal or systemic disease
Pruritus	Retention of bile salts	Dermatologic or central nervous system disorders
Dermatitis Unpigmented areas	Hepatogenic photosensitization	Primary phototoxic photosensitization

Central nervous signs
  Behavioral change, ataxia, dysmetria, circling, stupor, coma, tremors, bellowing
	Hepatic encephalopathy
	  (see text)
		Brain diseases
		Metabolic diseases
		Toxic diseases

Tenesmus (B)	Hepatic encephalopathy	Rectal or colonic disease Central nervous system disease
Rectal prolapse (B)	Tenesmus	Rectal or colonic disease
Change in feces color	Bile pigment deficit Undigested fat	Diet Gastrointestinal disease
Hemorrhage	Failure to synthesize clotting factors II, V, VII, IX, X	Other clotting factor or platelet deficit, trauma, disseminated intravascular coagulation
Pain over liver	Inflammation, swelling	Abscesses Traumatic reticulitis
Inspiratory stertor (E) Dyspnea	Hepatic encephalopathy	Upper airway obstruction

B, Frequent sign in cattle; *E,* frequent sign in horses.

Icterus is commonly seen in acute liver disease in horses but not in every case of chronic liver disease, and it is less commonly seen in ruminants unless biliary blockage occurs. Icterus is caused by failure of uptake, conjugation, or excretion of bilirubin. Excess production caused by hemolysis must also be considered when icterus is present; it is the most common cause of icterus in cattle. Horses are frequently icteric (up to 6 mg/dl of unconjugated bilirubin) from anorexia or fasting even when the liver is normal.

Weight loss is a common but not specific finding in some cases of chronic liver disease. It may be caused by anorexia or failure of metabolic functions of the liver and is probably not related to impaired fat absorption in the large herbivores. Diarrhea is also seen, especially in cattle with chronic liver disease. It is thought to be related to portal hypertension and increased hydrostatic pressure, although the exact mechanisms are not yet understood. It probably is not caused by fat malabsorption or steatorrhea, because the normal herbivore diet contains less than 3% fat.

Ascites is a common finding in calves with liver cirrhosis. The ascites is caused by portal hypertension that arises from venous blockage, which results in increased hydrostatic pressure, and to protein leakage into the peritoneal cavity. Production of hepatic lymph high in protein (over 3 g/dl) is increased. Because the liver sinusoids are permeable to plasma proteins, the protein-containing lymph leaks into the interstitial space and then into the peritoneal cavity.[3] Fluid moves into the abdominal cavity because of both osmotic and hydrostatic forces, according to Starling's law. The abdominal

fluid present with liver disease is a modified transudate, but the protein content may be relatively high (3 to 3.5 g/dl) because of leakage of protein from the liver. Hypoalbuminemia can aggravate the ascites, but if it occurs alone, it more likely will cause intramandibular and brisket edema.

Dermatitis of the white areas may occur because of hepatic photosensitization. The skin of the white areas first becomes erythematous, then thickened with keratin crusts, and finally necrotic. This is caused by the photodynamic agent phylloerythrin. Phylloerythrin is formed in the gastrointestinal tract of herbivores by the bacterial degradation of chlorophyll. After absorption into the portal circulation, it should be conjugated by the liver and excreted into the bile. With cholestasis the phylloerythrin may be carried to the skin, where it acts as a photodynamic agent. With bile duct ligation, the level of phylloerythrin steadily increases.[4] Although a small amount is removed by the kidneys, the rate is not fast enough to prevent accumulation in the plasma and skin. Phylloerythrin in the skin reacts to sunlight and emits energy that causes lesions of the white areas.[5]

Pruritus is seen in a few cases of liver disease in horses. In human beings this is assumed to be caused by accumulation in the skin of the bile acid that is not excreted by the liver. This same process may occur in horses, but pruritus is not commonly seen in large animals with liver disease.

A change in fecal color is not usually noted in adult herbivores with liver disease because other pigments such as chlorophyll contribute to the color. In a young animal or in animals with simple digestive tracts, much of the fecal color is from stercobilin, a metabolite of bilirubin. Therefore with cholestasis the feces may be a lighter color.

A few signs may be seen terminally in liver disease. hemorrhage may occur when the clotting factors are not synthesized in adequate amounts. Factors I, II, V, VII, IX, and X are all produced by the liver,[6] but disease usually is advanced before a deficit develops. Tenesmus, often followed by rectal prolapse, is seen in some cattle with liver disease. This may be associated with diarrhea or may be part of hepatic encephalopathy, or it may be aggravated by edema of the bowel caused by portal hypertension. Pharyngeal or laryngeal collapse with loud stertorous inspiratory noises and dyspnea has developed in some cases of hepatic failure, especially in ponies. The exact mechanism for this is not known, but it may also be part of hepatic encephalopathy.[7] Horses sometimes develop a terminal hemolytic crisis caused by increased fragility of red blood cells (RBCs). This has not been observed in ruminants.

HEPATIC ENCEPHALOPATHY

Hepatic encephalopathy is a clinical syndrome characterized by abnormal mental status that occurs secondary to hepatic insufficiency or shunting that allows portal blood to bypass the liver. It is considered a potentially reversible metabolic or neurotransmitter disorder, but it is associated with characteristic although not specific lesions in the central nervous system such as astrocytosis. The hepatic failure apparently causes some impairment of cerebral function.

Signs of hepatic encephalopathy are often subtle and nonspecific. Behavioral changes may be detected by the owner, who is more familiar with the patient's normal activity. Some docile animals become excitable and difficult to control, whereas other, normally unruly animals may become passive. Depression and lack of coordination are common manifestations, and some animals may walk aimlessly or even head press.[8,9] The animals eventually develop a stupor and may end up in hepatic coma. Yawning may be seen in horses, and ruminants sometimes vocalize excessively.

The pathophysiology of hepatic encephalopathy remains undefined and is controversial.[9] It occurs when portal blood bypasses the liver, as with congenital shunts in dogs and in human beings with shunts secondary to portal hypertension induced by alcoholic cirrhosis, or when the blood goes through an inadequately functioning liver. How neurologic function is altered has not been proven, but there is an abundance of uninhibited speculation.

Three basic mechanisms have been proposed.[6] It seems plausible to incriminate synergistic neurotoxins that bypass the liver. The blood ammonia level is elevated in most cases of hepatic encephalopathy because the liver is not metabolizing it to urea. Encephalopathy can be precipitated in cirrhotic patients by adding ammonia-generating substances, and these cause an increase in cerebrospinal glutamine, the product to which ammonia is detoxified. However, much higher concentrations of ammonia are needed to induce coma in normal animals, and the correlation between ammonia levels and the degree of encephalopathy is poor. Four cases of horses with hyperammonemia and encephalopathy without liver disease have been reported.[10] It has been proposed that other toxins such as mercaptans or short-chain fatty acids act synergistically with ammonia to cause the cerebral dysfunction.[11]

False neurotransmitters have been proposed as the cause of the abnormal nerve function. Increased amounts of tryptophan, phenylalanine, and tyrosine in the brain could cause more serotonin, a false neurotransmitter, to accumulate in the brain. Plasma amino acid ratios are altered in horses with pyrrolizine alkaloid–induced liver disease.[12] Concentrations of branched-chain amino acids (valine, isoleucine, and leucine) are decreased, and the concentration of aromatic amino acids (tyrosine, phenylalanine, and free tryptophan) are increased, partly because the liver is not adequately metabolizing the aromatic amino acids. Because the amino acids are transported across the blood-brain barrier by a common transport system, they compete for entry into the central nervous system. It has been suggested that higher levels of aromatic amino acids in the nervous system would lead to the formation of increased amounts of inhibitory neurotransmitters or to the alteration of catecholamine or monoamine neurotransmitters, such as γ-aminobutyric acid (GABA) or L-glutamate.

There may be an imbalance of true inhibitory and excitatory neurotransmitters. GABA is an inhibitory neurotransmitter, and 80% of it is metabolized by the liver.[6] The brains of animals with hepatic encephalopathy have an increased amount of GABA and an increased number of receptor sites.[13] Ammonia is believed to play a role in the metabolism of GABA in the brain and therefore could act synergistically.[11] Animals with hepatic encephalopathy also have a greater number of receptor sites for benzodiazepine.[13] Benzodiazepine augments the activity of GABA in stimulating the inhibitory neuron and causing sedation.

LABORATORY TESTS AND LIVER-DERIVED SERUM ENZYMES

Some blood constituents may be altered because of failure of some of the metabolic functions of the liver, but none of these changes are specific for liver disease. The blood glucose level is sometimes slightly lower in severe liver disease, especially in young animals, possibly because of decreased gluconeogenesis. A fourfold or more rise in the blood ammonia level can occur in some toxic liver diseases because the urease needed to convert ammonia to urea is found only in the liver. For the same reason blood urea nitrogen may decrease, especially in the terminal phases. In the later stages the blood clotting factors may be diminished, with delays in the partial thromboplastin time and clotting times.

Terminally the serum albumin concentration may decrease. A large amount of protein synthesis takes place in the liver; of the plasma proteins, all but the γ-globulins are produced by the liver. However, the amount of these proteins in the blood depends not only on the rate of synthesis but also on the rate of removal. The albumin half-life in cattle is about 16.5 days; in the horse, 19.4 days; and in sheep, 14 days.[14] Because of this, serum albumin is reduced mainly in chronic liver disease. With liver damage the synthesis of α-globulins and β-globulins is increased, so that the total plasma protein level is invariably normal, but the albumin/globulin (A/G) ratio may be decreased. The healthy liver has a large reserve for protein synthesis, and lost protein can be replenished. In a group from our teaching hospital, fewer than 5% of horses with hypoalbuminemia had liver disease. In a recent study, 18% of the horses with chronic liver disease and 6% of those with acute liver disease had albumin concentrations below the reference value.[15] It therefore is assumed that hypoproteinemia and hypoalbuminemia are not common features in horses with liver disease.

Amino acid ratios are altered in liver disease; the short branched-chain amino acids are decreased, whereas the aromatic amino acids are increased.[12]

LIVER ENZYMES

A number of enzymes are compartmentalized in the hepatocyte or in bile duct epithelium. This compartmentalization is useful for holding insoluble molecules close to the en-

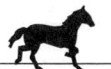

zymes for chemical reactions. Hepatocyte damage may result in release of the enzymes into the circulation, and cholestasis may cause increased release from bile epithelium. Serum levels of these enzymes therefore may be an indication of hepatocyte integrity or bile excretion. Table 31-2 lists some of the enzymes more commonly used for testing and their characteristics. Serum concentrations for some of these enzymes vary with the age of the animal and sometimes even with the type or use. Table 31-3 gives some approximate upper limits of normal for animals of various ages. Normal values, especially for the enzymes, should be established by each laboratory. Normal values of adult animals for one laboratory are given in Chapter 22.

γ-Glutamyltransferase (GGT) is one of the more commonly checked and fairly specific enzymes that is almost invariably elevated in chronic liver disease. It is found mainly in the biliary tract and indicates biliary damage (flukes) or hyperplasia (pyrrolizine alkaloid toxicity or aflatoxicosis). GGT also is present in the pancreas, mammary glands, lungs, kidney tubules, and other duct epithelium, but serum levels usually are not elevated with renal disease because the enzyme is lost in the urine. Serum concentrations are normally higher in neonatal calves (sometimes over 4000 IU/L after suckling)[15] because the enzyme is concentrated in colostrum.[16,17] They are also higher in foals than in adult horses, but the higher concentration may partly be the result of increased production.[18] An elevated GGT indicates cholestasis, but it often is elevated with histologic evidence of hepatocyte damage or biliary hyperplasia. GGT levels remain elevated for several weeks.

Alkaline phosphatase (ALP) usually is elevated in chronic liver disease of the horse and is a variable finding in ruminants. It can come from other sources, such as bone, intestines, placenta, and macrophages. Both ALP and GGT are

---

TABLE 31-2

Liver-Derived Enzymes

Enzyme	Specificity	Problems
GGT	Liver Kidney* Pancreas	High in young animals from colostrum
ALP	Liver Bone Intestine Macrophages Placenta	Not specific
SDH	Liver	Not elevated in chronic disease; short life; not stable
GLDH	Liver	Not elevated in chronic disease
AST (SGOT)	Liver Muscle Heart	Not specific
ALT (SGPT)	—	Low concentration in cattle and horses; not a good indicator
LDH	None unless isoenzymes	Not elevated in chronic disease; short life; not specific
Ar	Liver	Analysis not routinely available

ALT, Alanine aminotransferase; *ALP*, alkaline phosphatase; *Ar*, arginase; *AST*, aspartate aminotransferase; *GGT*, γ-glutamyltransferase; *GLDH*, glutamate dehydrogenase; *LDH*, lactate dehydrogenase; *SDH*, sorbitol dehydrogenase.
*Elevated in urine, not blood.

TABLE 31-3

Upper Limits of Normal for Selected Liver Function Tests*

Test	Horse				Cattle				Sheep	Goat
Age	<1 wk	1-4 wk	1-12 mo	Adult	<1 wk	1-4 wk	1-6 mo	Adult	Adult	Adult
Total bilirubin (mg/dl)	4.5	3	2	2	2.4	0.9	0.4	0.3	0.4	0.5
Direct bilirubin (mg/dl)	0.8	0.7	0.7	0.4	0.6	0.3	0.2	0.1	0.1	0.1
Total bile acids (μmol/L)	N/A	N/A	N/A	14	45	35	60	120	25?	N/A
BSP clearance (T$^{1}/_{2}$ min)	N/A	N/A	3.7	3.7	15	8	5	5	4	2.1
AST (IU/L)	600	540	700	270	60	60	60	60	110	80
GGT (IU/L)	170	170	40	30	4200	1300	N/A	24	55	50
ALT (IU/L)	2800	1200	840	194	1150	1000	N/A	81	188	386
SDH (IU/L)	8	8	N/A	5.8	N/A	N/A	N/A	15.3	28	23
GLDH (IU/L)	N/A	N/A	N/A	11	24	22	19	19		N/A
LDH (IU/L)	N/A	N/A	N/A	412	1380	2180	N/A	1445	440	392

N/A, Not available; *BSP*, bromsulphalein; *AST*, aspartate aminotransferase; *GGT*, γ-glutamyltransferase; *ALT*, alanine aminotransferase; *SDH*, sorbitol dehydrogenase; *GLDH*, glutamate dehydrogenase; *LDH*, lactate dehydrogenase.
*Values from various sources.

elevated with cholestasis.[19] The dehydrogenases, such as sorbitol dehydrogenase (SDH), lactate dehydrogenase (LDH), and glutamate dehydrogenase (GLDH), are found in hepatocytes and are elevated with acute hepatocyte damage, but serum concentrations may return to normal or drop below normal in chronic liver disease. SDH is liver specific and extremely useful in detecting active hepatocellular necrosis, but it is not as stable as some of the enzymes. LDH is found in many tissues other than liver and therefore is not specific unless isoenzymes are determined.

EXCRETION TESTS FOR FUNCTION

Because the liver excretes a number of endogenous compounds and foreign substances injected into the animal, the rate of excretion, or clearance, of these substances can be used to test the excretory function of the liver. Bilirubin itself can be used and, if it is elevated above normal, would indicate liver failure, bile blockage, or excess production from hemolysis. In the horse, bilirubin is also increased during fasting in animals without liver disease.[20] With liver damage in the horse or ruminant, most of the retained bilirubin is indirect reacting (unconjugated), and the direct to total ratio usually is less than 0.3. With bile blockage or intrahepatic cholestasis, the direct to total ratio may be over 0.3 in the horse or 0.5 in cattle.

Bilirubin, the main bile pigment, is produced from heme, 75% of which comes from RBCs.[21] When the erythrocytes are broken down, heme is converted first to biliverdin and then to bilirubin in the macrophage system. This unconjugated bilirubin is insoluble and must be bound to albumin for transfer, and this bound bilirubin is not removed by the kidneys. Unconjugated bilirubin is taken up by the hepatocytes with cytosolic binding proteins in the hepatocyte. In the hepatocyte some bilirubin is conjugated to the diglucuronide, but in the horse more than half of the bilirubin in bile is conjugated with glucose. Conjugated (direct reacting) bilirubin is water soluble, and some enters the general circulation; if it is in high enough concentration, it is filtered by the kidneys into the urine. Conjugated bilirubin is secreted into the bile canaliculi by an energy-dependent transport process. In most species this is the rate-limiting step, but this may not be true in the large herbivores. Conjugated bilirubin passes into the intestine through the bile ducts, and if they are blocked, both conjugated and unconjugated bilirubin increase in the plasma.

In the intestinal tract bilirubin is converted to urobilinogen by anaerobic bacteria. Some urobilinogen is absorbed and reexcreted by the liver, but a small fraction passes the normal liver and is excreted in the urine. Therefore with complete biliary blockage no urobilinogen is present in the urine, and with hemolysis urobilinogen may be increased in the urine. Urobilinogen is not very stable in the urine, therefore analysis must be done within 1 to 2 hours or the amount detected will be erroneously low.

Fasting diminishes the efficiency of plasma bilirubin removal in all species, but the horse shows a greater rise in plasma bilirubin, often reaching a plateau two to three times the normal state. This increase is caused by a decrease in the removal of bilirubin by the hepatic transport and not by an increase in production.[22,23]

The serum total bile acid concentration is a good test of liver function. The concentration of bile acids in the serum is increased with hepatocyte damage, blockage of bile flow, or shunting of portal blood to the systemic circulation, bypassing the liver. Bile acids are synthesized by the liver from cholesterol. Choleic and chenodeoxycholic acids are the primary bile acids conjugated with amino acids before excretion into the bile. Only conjugated bile acids are present in the intestine, are soluble, and form micelles with fat because of their detergent properties. Most of the bile acids excreted in the bile are resorbed by an active transport system in the ileum and carried by the portal circulation back to the liver for reexcretion. In most species more than 95% of the bile acids are resorbed and recirculated through the enterohepatic circulation.[24] The daily synthesis of bile acids is much less than the daily requirement, and one study in ponies showed that the bile acids secreted each day are about 38 times the total pool.[25]

In simple-stomached animals a postprandial increase in serum bile acid occurs because of the release of bile from the gallbladder during eating and subsequent resorption by the ileum. This does not seem to be important in the horse, which has no gallbladder, or in cattle, in which no relationship to feeding could be found.[26] Cattle have an hour to hour fluctuation in the bile acid level that can reach as high as 60 μmol/L (see Table 31-3).[26] In the horse, a serum concentration of bile acids above 14 μmol/L would indicate liver damage, bile blockage, or shunting.[27,28] In adult cattle, because of the hour to hour variations, the bile acid concentration on a single sample would have to be above 126 μmol/L in beef cattle and 88 μmol/L in dairy cattle to be specific for liver disease.[29] Levels are lower (under 64 μmol/L) in calves that are less than 6 months old. The serum bile acid concentration is a very specific test that has a high positive predictive value.[30]

A number of dyes are excreted primarily by the liver, and of these bromsulphalein (BSP) is the most commonly used. In large animals the BSP clearance (half-time) is used much more often than the retention test. In the clearance test, 500 to 1000 mg (approximately 2 mg/kg) of BSP is injected intravenously. Blood samples are taken before the injection and two to four times 5 to 12 minutes after the injection (i.e., at 5, 7, 9, and 11 minutes). These samples are analyzed for color produced by BSP, and a half-life is determined by plotting the points on semilog paper. For normal horses the half-life is less than $3^{1}/_{2}$ minutes, and for normal ruminants it is less than 5 minutes. This value may be increased in pregnant animals and in very young ones (see Table 31-3). Other dyes, such as indocyanine green, have some advantage (less renal excretion than BSP) but currently are too costly for use in large animals.

LIVER BIOPSY

Liver biopsy can be very useful not only in confirming the presence of liver disease but also in determining or ruling out some etiologies. It is a relatively safe and simple procedure but should not be performed when liver abscesses are suspected. A number of biopsy instruments are available, including aspiration punches, but the Precision Cut,* Temino,† or other similar notch-cutting needle seem to work quite well. In all species the skin over the biopsy site should be clipped and prepared for aseptic insertion of the needle. Local infiltration of 2% lidocaine helps reduce the patient's reaction, although the animal may still flinch when the pleura and peritoneum are penetrated. A small stab wound is made through the skin at the site of insertion with a No. 11 or a No. 15 Bard-Parker blade. Horses should have a twitch applied or be given chemical sedation if necessary.

The site of skin puncture for liver biopsy in the horse is the right fourteenth intercostal space at the intersection of a line drawn from the tuber coxae to the point of the shoulder. Some operators recommend more cranial insertion (twelfth or thirteenth space), but more lung is penetrated at points farther craniad. If a more cranial position is selected, it

---

*Becton Dickinson, Rutherford, NJ 07070.
†Bouer Medical, Clearwater, FL 34620.

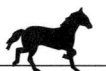

should also be more ventral. If the needle is directed slightly craniad and ventrad, it is more likely to remain in the liver parenchyma and not penetrate larger vessels on the visceral surface or pass through into the right kidney, pancreas, or colon. Ultrasound guidance increases the chances of obtaining liver specimens without penetrating other organs.

Cattle must be suitably confined for liver biopsy. A biopsy often can be performed on quiet dairy cows in a stanchion while the tail is elevated ("tailed"). The puncture site in cattle can be located by extending a horizontal line craniad from the middle of the paralumbar fossa. The needle is inserted where this line crosses the eleventh intercostal space on the right side. The lungs do not extend as far caudad as in the horse, thus the liver is more exposed. The needle is directed slightly craniad and ventrad, as in the horse.[2] Liver biopsy in sheep and goats is slightly more difficult. Additional sedation of sheep and goats usually is needed. A site at the ninth or tenth intercostal space at the level of the ventral end of the last rib has been recommended. The biopsy needle is advanced in a craniomedial direction until the liver is penetrated.

Diffuse or zonal lesions, such as are seen in most toxic, infectious, and metabolic liver diseases, usually can be diagnosed by liver biopsy. Focal lesions such as abscesses, granulomas, and neoplasias, as well as liver flukes, are easily missed by liver biopsy. If a liver abscess is suspected, biopsy is not indicated because of the danger of rupturing an abscess.

ULTRASOUND EXAMINATION

Ultrasound examination of the liver is useful in determining its size and situation and the diameter of its vessels. Liver abscesses often can be detected, and the circumference of the gallbladder can be determined in cattle.[31,32] Choleliths have been diagnosed in horses by ultrasound examination, and liver flukes have been identified in sheep. The parenchymal pattern of the liver is changed with diffuse fibrosis. An ultrasound examination is performed on cattle on the right side in the tenth to twelfth intercostal space. On sheep the examination is done on the right side in the seventh through twelfth intercostal spaces.[33] In horses the examination is performed below and caudal to the lung in the eighth to fourteenth intercostal spaces. The liver can also be visualized on the left side of the horse in the lower intercostal spaces.

PROGNOSIS

Indicators of a poor prognosis in liver disease include an albumin level below 2.5 g/dl in horses or an increased globulin level (or both), a prothrombin time over 30% of normal, and greatly elevated GGT and ALP with a normal or decreased SDH or GLDH. A markedly elevated BSP half-life (longer than 8 min in horses or 10 min in ruminants) and marked fibrosis that bridges the liver lobules on histopathologic examination are grounds for a poor prognosis. Severe pyrrolizine alkaloid toxicosis carries a particularly grave prognosis because the remaining hepatocytes are prevented from regeneration by mitotic arrest. Terminal clinical signs include development of a hemolytic crisis in the horse or marked hepatoencephalopathy in a patient with a fibrotic liver.

REFERENCES

1. Iber FL: Normal pathologic physiology of the liver. In Sodeman WA, Sodeman TM, eds: *Pathologic physiology,* ed 6, Philadelphia, 1979, WB Saunders.
2. Pearson EG, Craig AM: The diagnosis of liver disease in equine and food animals, *Mod Vet Pract* 61:233-237, 315-320, 1980.
3. Tennant BC: Hepatic function. In Kanedo JJ, Harvey JW, Bruss ML, eds: *Clinical biochemistry of domestic animals,* ed 5, San Diego, 1997, Academic Press.
4. Ford AJH, Gopinath C: The excretion of phylloerythrin and bilirubin by calves and sheep, *Res Vet Sci* 21:12-18, 1976.
5. Engelking LR, Anwer MS: Liver and biliary tract. In Anderson NV, ed: *Veterinary gastroenterology,* ed 2, Philadelphia, 1992, Lea & Febiger.
6. Galitzer SJ, Oehme FW: Photosensitization: a literature review, *Vet Sci Commun* 2:217-230, 1978.
7. Pearson EG: Liver failure attributable to pyrrolizine alkaloid toxicosis and associated with inspiratory dyspnea in ponies: three cases, *J Am Vet Med Assoc* 198:1651-1654, 1991.
8. Fowler ME: Clinical manifestations of primary hepatic insufficiency in the horse, *J Am Vet Med Assoc* 147:55-63, 1965.
9. Morris DD, Henry MM: Hepatic encephalopathy, *Compend Cont Educ* 13:1153-1160, 1991.
10. Peek SF, Divers TJ, Jackson CJ: Hyperammonemia associated with encephalopathy and abdominal pain without liver disease in four mature horses, *Equine Vet J* 29:70-74, 1997.
11. Maddison JE: Hepatic encephalopathy: current concepts of pathogenesis, *J Vet Intern Med* 6:341-353, 1992.
12. Gulick BA et al: Effect of pyrrolizine alkaloid-induced hepatic disease on plasma amino acid patterns in the horse, *Am J Vet Res* 41:1894-1898, 1980.
13. Tyler JW: Hepatoencephalopathy. I. Pathophysiology and treatment, *Compend Cont Educ* 12:1260-1270, 1990.
14. Kaneko JJ: Serum proteins and the dysproteinemias. In Kaneko JJ, ed: *Clinical biochemistry of domestic animals,* ed 3, New York, 1980, Academic Press.
15. Pearson EG et al: Evaluation of liver-derived serum enzymes and liver function tests in young calves, *J Am Vet Med Assoc,* 207:1466-1469, 1995.
16. Paraga ME, Carlson GP, Thurmond M: Serum protein concentrations in horses with severe liver disease: a retrospective study and review of the literature, *J Vet Int Med* 9:154-161, 1995.
17. Thompson JC, Pauli JV: Colostral transfer of γ-glutamyl transpeptidase in calves, *NZ Vet J* 29:223-226, 1981.
18. Gossett KA, French DD: Effect of age on liver enzyme activities in serum of healthy quarter horses, *Am J Vet Res* 45:354-366, 1984.
19. Kramer JW, Hoffman WE: Clinical enzymology. In Kaneko JJ, Harvey JW, Bruss ML, eds. *Clinical biochemistry of domestic animals,* ed 5, San Diego, 1997, Academic Press.
20. Tennant B et al: Clinical significance of hyperbilirubinemia in the horse, *Proceedings of the First International Symposium on Equine Hematology,* 1975, pp 246-254.
21. Gronwall R: Bilirubin metabolism, *Proceedings of the First International Symposium on Equine Hematology,* 1975, pp 237-241.
22. Gronwall RR, Mia AS: Fasting, hyperbilirubinemia in horses, *Am J Dig Dis* 17:241-249, 1972.
23. Gronwall R, Engelking RL, Noonan N: Direct measurement of biliary bilirubin excretion in ponies during fasting, *Am J Vet Res* 41:125-126, 1980.
24. O'Maille ER, Richards TG, Short AH: The influence of conjugation of cholic acid on its uptake and secretion: hepatic extraction of taurocholate and cholate in the dog, *J Physiol (Lond)* 189:337-350, 1967.
25. Gronwall R: Plasma bile acids, *Proceedings of the Twenty-first Annual Convention of the American Association of Equine Practitioners,* 1975, pp 255-257.
26. Pearson EG, Craig AM, Rowe K: Variability of serum bile acid concentrations over time in dairy cattle and effect of feed deprivation on the variability, *Am J Vet Res* 53:1780-1783, 1992.
27. West HJ: Evaluation of total plasma bile acid concentrations for the diagnosis of hepatobiliary disease in horses, *Res Vet Sci* 46:264-270, 1989.
28. Pearson EG, Craig AM: Serum bile acids for diagnosis of chronic liver disease in horses, *Proc Am College Vet Intern Med Forum* 10:71-76, 1986.
29. Craig Am, Pearson EG, Rowe K: Serum bile acid concentrations in clinically normal cattle: comparison by type, age, and stage of lactation, *Am J Vet Res* 53:1784-1786, 1992.
30. West HJ: Evaluation of total serum bile acid concentration for the diagnosis of hepatobiliary disease in cattle, *Proc XVI World Buiatric Congr* 16:531-536, 1990.
31. Braun U: Ultrasonographic examination of the liver and gallbladder in cows: normal findings, *Compend Cont Educ Pract Vet* 18:S61-S73, 1996.
32. Braun U: Ultrasonographic examination of the liver and gallbladder in cows: abnormal findings, *Compend Cont Educ Pract Vet* 18:1255-1269, 1996.
33. Braun U: Ultrasonographic examination of the liver in sheep, *Am J Vet Res* 53:198-202, 1992.

INFECTIOUS, TOXIC, AND PARASITIC LIVER DISEASE

ACUTE HEPATITIS IN HORSES

NAT T. MESSER IV

Idiopathic acute hepatic disease (IAHD) is the most common cause of acute hepatitis and hepatic failure in horses.[34] IAHD is also known as Theiler's disease,[35] serum hepatitis,[36] post-vaccinal hepatitis,[37] and acute liver atrophy.[38] The disease was first recognized by Theiler in large numbers of horses in South Africa after the animals had been immunized against African horse sickness with simultaneous administration of live virus and hyperimmune equine serum,[39] and the disorder since has been documented as a possible complication of the use of any equine serum product in horses. It is primarily a disease of adult horses[40] and recently has been most commonly associated with the use of tetanus antitoxin (TAT).[36,38,41-43] Mares appear to be affected more often than males, and recently parturient, lactating mares seem to be at greatest risk.[40,43] The seasonal nature of some IAHD epidemics[40,44] (most reported cases have occurred in the summer months) and the observation that some affected horses in outbreaks of the disease have not been treated with TAT[34,40,41,44] has raised the concern that a virus is involved, similar to the hepatitis B virus in human beings; however, this remains unproven.[35] IAHD also has been proposed to be a type III (immune complex–mediated) hypersensitivity reaction.[45]

The clinical effects of IAHD are associated with signs of acute hepatic failure; they include depression, jaundice, inappetence, pica, yawning, photoactive dermatitis, and hepatic encephalopathy.* Fever has been described as absent or rare in horses with IAHD.[37] Atypical signs that have been reported include progressive weight loss, ventral subcutaneous edema, jugular pulses, and acute respiratory distress.[43,47] Intravascular hemolysis has been reported to lead to hemoglobinuria in some terminal cases of IAHD.[35] Evidence of a subclinical or chronic component exists in some cases of IAHD,[43,48] but some horses that received TAT have clinicopathologic evidence of liver dysfunction without developing clinical signs, indicating that the severity of the disease may vary.[38,43,48]

The diagnosis of IAHD is based on the anamnesis, clinical signs, and findings from serum biochemical analysis, hepatic biopsy, or necropsy. High serum levels of unconjugated and total bilirubin and serum bile acids, coupled with high serum activity of GGT, SDH, aspartate aminotransferase (AST), LDH, and ALP are indicative of hepatic necrosis in horses. IAHD may be confirmed by hepatic biopsy or postmortem examination of hepatic tissue. A typical histopathologic change seen in biopsy specimens or those obtained at postmortem examination is widespread necrosis of hepatocytes that is most severe in the centrilobular and midzonal areas, with the few living cells confined to the periportal areas.[42] The normal architecture of the centrilobular and midzonal areas is replaced by a pale, eosinophilic, granular mass in which ghost outlines of necrotic hepatocytes are present.[42] A mild inflammatory cell infiltrate is seen in the portal areas, as are a number of spindle-shaped fibroblastic cells.[42] The histopathologic lesion often is more advanced than the clinical course of the disease would suggest.[42]

No specific treatment is available for IAHD.[49] Treatment should be aimed at supporting liver function and controlling abnormal behavior as described under treatment of liver diseases, pp. 820 to 821. Continuous intravenous administration of dextrose and balanced electrolyte solutions to reduce hepatic workload and maintain plasma volume is recommended.[48] If spontaneous bleeding occurs at injection sites or at sites of self-inflicted injury, plasma transfusions may be necessary to replace the deficient clotting factors.[35] The use of glucocorticoids for treating IAHD is controversial but may be indicated based on some histopathologic evidence of an immune-mediated etiology.[45]

Although the cause of IAHD is unknown, administration of TAT to recently parturient, lactating mares is associated with substantial risk for development of fatal IAHD.[40,43,48]

---

*References 35, 36, 40, 42, 45, and 46.

The susceptibility of postparturient mares to IAHD after TAT administration at foaling is not yet understood. Postparturient mares may be the most likely adult horses to receive TAT. The use of TAT, therefore, is not without risk, and it should be restricted to clinical situations requiring tetanus prophylaxis and in which a history of active tetanus (toxoid) immunoprophylaxis is absent or unknown. The risk of postvaccinal IAHD should be addressed with the owner before administration of TAT.

Routine administration of TAT to parturient mares should be strongly discouraged, and routine use of active tetanus immunoprophylaxis should be reemphasized. IAHD may be observed sporadically or may affect a group of horses. Recognition of the disease in one horse should necessitate careful observation of horses on the same premises for either clinical or serum biochemical signs of IAHD.[48] Based on recent case reports, it appears that not all cases of IAHD are clinically apparent and that screening for its presence using routine serum biochemical analysis is useful in detecting subclinical cases.[43,48]

REFERENCES

34. Tennant B: Acute hepatitis in horses: problems differentiating toxic and infectious causes in adults, *Proceedings of the Twenty-fourth Annual Convention of the American Association of Equine Practitioners*, 1978, pp 465-471.
35. Divers TJ: Hepatic disease. In Robinson NE, ed: *Current therapy in equine medicine*, Philadelphia, 1992, WB Saunders.
36. Howarth L, Shires M: Serum hepatitis in a horse, *Iowa State Vet* 38:28-32, 1976.
37. Blood DC, Radostits OM: *Veterinary medicine: a textbook of the diseases of cattle, sheep, pigs, goats, and horses*, ed 7, London, 1989, Baillière Tindall.
38. Hjerpe CA: Serum hepatitis in the horse, *J Am Vet Med Assoc* 144:734-740, 1964.
39. Theiler A: Acute liver atrophy and parenchymatous hepatitis of horses, Fifth and Sixth Report of the Director of Veterinary Research, Department of Agriculture, Union of South Africa 7-164, 1918.
40. Rose JA, Immenschuh RD, Rose EM: Serum hepatitis in the horse, *Proceedings of the Twenty-first Annual Convention of the American Association of Equine Practitioners*, 1975, pp 175-185.
41. Robinson M, Gopinath C, Hughes DL: Histopathology of acute hepatitis in the horse, *J Comp Pathol* 85:111-118, 1975.
42. Baker JC, Ames T: Equine serum hepatitis: a case report, *Minn Vet* 21:19-21, 1981.
43. Messer NT, Johnson PJ: Idiopathic acute hepatic disease in horses: 12 cases (1982-1992), *J Am Vet Med Assoc* 204:1934-1937, 1994.
44. Thomsett LR: Acute hepatic failure in the horse, *Equine Vet J* 3:15-19, 1971.
45. Smith HL, Chalmers GA, Wedel R: Acute hepatic failure (Theiler's disease) in a horse, *Can Vet J* 32:362-364, 1991.
46. Scarratt WK, Furr MO, Robertson JL: Hepatoencephalopathy and hypocalcemia in a miniature horse mare, *J Am Vet Med Assoc* 199:1754-1756, 1991.
47. Pearson EG: Liver failure attributable to pyrrolizine alkaloid toxicosis and associated with inspiratory dyspnea in ponies: three cases (1982-1988), *J Am Vet Med Assoc* 198:1651-1654, 1991.
48. Guglick MA et al: Hepatic disease associated with administration of tetanus antitoxin in eight horses, *J Am Vet Med* Assoc 206:1737-1740, 1995.
49. Pearson EG: Liver disease in the mature horse, *Equine Vet Educ* 11:87-96, 1999.

BLACK DISEASE

JOSEPH HOYT (JOE) SNYDER
STANLEY P. SNYDER

DEFINITION AND ETIOLOGY. Black disease (infectious necrotic hepatitis) is a disease of grazing animals, primarily sheep, that most often results in sudden death.[50-53] The disease is caused by toxins produced by the bacterium *Clostridium novyi* type B. *C. novyi* occurs in soil and is normally present in the digestive tracts and livers of animals grazing affected pastures. Disease occurs only when liver damage is sufficient to provide the anaerobic environment required for growth of the organism and subsequent toxin production. In practice, the liver insult almost always is caused by larval migration of the common liver fluke, *Fasciola hepatica*. The disease therefore is a seasonal one related to the liver fluke cycle and occurring in animals commonly infested by *F. hepatica*. Other liver parasites such as *Fascioloides magna, Dicrocoelium dendriticum,* and *Cysticercus tenuicollis* occasionally are implicated, as is damage to the liver by liver biopsy or trauma severe enough to result in localized anaerobiosis in the liver, but these cases are rare. Such a scenario should be considered when sudden deaths occur at times when flukes are not usually migrating or when they occur in equine species, which are not normal hosts for *F. hepatica*. The disease occurs worldwide where liver flukes are present. The *C. novyi* strains that cause black disease produce at least three potent exotoxins: the α-toxin, which is the classical lethal toxin; the β-toxin, which has both lethal necrotizing and hemolytic lecithinase activities; and the ζ-toxin, which is hemolytic.[54]

PATHOPHYSIOLOGY. *C. novyi* type B is widely distributed in soil, and its spores are continuously ingested and shed in the feces of grazing animals. Some of these organisms cross the intestinal mucosa and become disseminated throughout the animal's mononuclear macrophage system, including the Kupffer cells of the liver. When localized anaerobic conditions occur in the liver, as occurs with migration of liver fluke larvae, these resident spores may germinate and enter a vegetative state. As they proliferate, they release their toxins and create enlarging zones of coagulation necrosis in the liver. The exotoxins that are produced enter the general circulation, where they damage neurons, vascular endothelium, and other vital cells and tissues, eventuating in sudden death of the animal.

CLINICAL SIGNS. Clinical black disease consists almost entirely of animals found dead. In the unlikely instance that an affected animal is recognized before its demise, the signs are nonspecific. The animal often is off to itself and appears depressed, anorexic, and possibly in respiratory distress. The temperature is elevated initially to 40° to 41° C (104° to 106° F) but declines before death. Unlike with the closely related disorder bacillary hemoglobinuria, or "red water," affected animals do not show red urine or bleeding from the nose or rectum. The diagnosis of clinical black disease can often be accomplished at necropsy or with the help of simple laboratory tests. The history includes sudden death, usually in an endemic area during warmer weather when fluke transmission is active. Flock or herd vaccination is either overdue or absent. It is also helpful to know the history of fluke infestation on the farm and the timing of fluke control measures, if any have been taken. The time of death should be ascertained as closely as possible. The animal usually is presented in lateral recumbency without signs of struggle. It is severely bloated, even if death has occurred quite recently, and gives the impression of a carcass in a more advanced state of decomposition than the timing would suggest.

NECROPSY FINDINGS. Postmortem lesions often are obscured by rapid putrefaction of the tissues. Skinning the animal reveals engorgement and hemorrhage of subcutaneous blood vessels, resulting in "black" discoloration; hence the name of the disease. Once the body cavity has been entered, blood-tinged abdominal, thoracic, and pericardial fluids are seen. The urine is grossly normal. Subendocardial and subepicardial hemorrhages are present. There may be hemorrhages on serosal and pleural surfaces, but these are not always present. The tissues, especially solid organs such as the liver and kidneys, appear to be in a state of autolysis much more advanced than the time of death would suggest. In addition to the presence of migrating fluke channels, the liver is swollen and congested and has one or more small, pale areas of coagulative necrosis. These lesions typically are seen along the diaphragmatic surface of the liver, have hyperemic borders, and extend for a variable distance into the hepatic tissue. Careful slicing of the organ may be required to find them.[52]

DIAGNOSIS. If necropsy does not confirm the diagnosis or if additional documentation is needed, a simple Gram stain of an impression smear taken from the margin of the liver lesion or from any area of a liver without lesions will reveal numerous large, gram-positive rods typical of the clostridia. Because clostridial organisms proliferate rapidly after death, such findings must always be interpreted carefully, with consideration given to the time elapsed between death and necropsy. Further diagnostic measures include anaerobic culture and isolation of *C. novyi* type B, identification of the specific toxins, and fluorescent antibody identification of the organism. Characteristic histopathologic changes may also be seen in fixed sections of liver associated with necrotic lesions. Impression smears obtained from the liver lesions are ideal for fluorescent antibody identification of *C. novyi* type B. Specific toxin identification is impractical for most laboratory settings but is the confirming procedure of choice.

TREATMENT AND PREVENTION. Treatment of black disease is rarely undertaken because of its acute to peracute presentation, with animals usually found dead. *C. novyi* is highly sensitive to penicillin and the tetracyclines, but toxin production usually is too far advanced for antibiotics to be of value. If used, they should be administered at high doses, intravenously if possible for most rapid onset (20,000 IU/kg crystalline penicillin or 5 mg/kg oxytetracycline), followed by intramuscular or intravenous doses at appropriate intervals. Supportive intravenous and/or intraluminal fluid therapy should be initiated to correct dehydration. Antiserum is not available. Care should be exercised in handling affected animals because stress may result in sudden death. The chances of success are small. In the face of an "outbreak," vaccination should be initiated immediately, along with mass administration of penicillin or tetracycline, preferably in a long-acting form.

A good prevention program requires consideration of both the pathophysiology and immunology of the disease and the natural history of the liver fluke *(F. hepatica)* that is so intimately involved in expression of black disease. Efforts to clear the soil of the offending organism are unrewarding. However, it is recommended that the carcasses of animals that have died of black disease be burned, buried deeply, or removed from the premises. Commercial bacterin/toxoids against *C. novyi* are available in combination with other clostridial vaccines. These products generally are safe and highly efficacious. The duration of protection is short, however, and should not be relied on for more than 5 to 6 months. Field experience suggests that monovalent *Clostridium haemolyticum* vaccine is more effective than combination products in high-risk herds, and there may be some variation in efficacy among commercially available combination products. Animals vaccinated under 3 to 4 months of age require revaccination at weaning. Local reactions at the site of subcutaneous vaccination are common but primarily of cosmetic concern. Intramuscular vaccination should be avoided, because it frequently results in permanent damage to muscle tissue, with a resulting negative impact on meat marketing. The timing of vaccination must be determined by the local climate and liver fluke season. In more severe climates where the fluke season is relatively short, a single annual injection before fluke transmission season may suffice. In moderate climates with longer periods of fluke exposure, a second injection about 5 months later may be required. Control of liver fluke infestation is closely linked to prevention of black disease. Control measures include pasture or range management; control of water sources; limiting access to streams, canals, ponds, and marshes; and strategic treatment of animals with products effective against flukes. Appropriate disposal of infected carcasses is important. This is a complex subject, and the reader should refer to the section on liver flukes (p. 805) for more detail.

REFERENCES

50. Erwin BG: Clostridial hepatitis (black disease) and bacillary hemoglobinuria. In Howard JL, ed: *Current veterinary therapy: food animal practice,* ed 2, Philadelphia, 1986, WB Saunders.
51. Gay CC et al: Infectious necrotic hepatitis (black disease) in a horse, *Equine Vet J* 12:26-27, 1980.
52. Jubb KVF, Kennedy PC, Palmer N: *Pathology of domestic animals,* vol 2, New York, 1993, Academic Press, pp 278-280.
53. Kimberling CV: *Jensen and Swift's diseases of sheep,* Philadelphia, 1988, Lea & Febiger.
54. Eklund MW: The role of bacteriophages and plasmids in the production of toxins and other biologically active substances by *Clostridium botulinum* and *Clostridium novyi.* In Sebald M, ed: *Genetics and molecular biology of anaerobic bacteria,* New York, 1993, Springer-Verlag, pp 179-194.

BACILLARY HEMOGLOBINURIA (RED WATER)

JOSEPH HOYT (JOE) SNYDER
STANLEY P. SNYDER

DEFINITION AND ETIOLOGY. Bacillary hemoglobinuria (red water, icterohemoglobinuria) is a disease that causes sudden death in cattle and other ruminants and in rare cases in horses. It is caused by the toxins of *Clostridium haemolyticum* (*Clostridium novyi* type D). This organism is closely related to the etiology of black disease, in which toxin production is closely linked to bacteriophage infection of the clostridial organisms.[55] The major biologically active toxins in *C. novyi* type D (*C. haemolyticum*) are the β-toxin, which is a phospholipase C and has both lethal necrotizing and hemolytic lecithinase properties; the ζ-toxin, which is a tropomyosinase; and the θ-toxin, which is a lipase. Prominent actions of the toxins induce localized hepatic necrosis and intravascular hemolysis. *C. haemolyticum* occurs in soil, and its spores are routinely found in the liver and passed in the feces and urine of healthy animals grazing affected pastures. Disease occurs only when insult to the liver is sufficient to provide the anaerobic conditions required for bacterial growth and toxin production. In almost all cases the liver insult is caused by migration of *F. hepatica* (common liver fluke) larvae.[56-58] As in black disease, *F. magna, D. dendriticum* (the lancet liver fluke), and *Cysticercus cellulosae* occasionally have been implicated in bacillary hemoglobinuria, as has liver biopsy or trauma severe enough to result in bruising of the liver.[59] The disorder, then, for all practical purposes is a seasonal disease that occurs at the time of larval fluke migration.

Bacillary hemoglobinuria is a regionalized disease. It has been reported that *C. haemolyticum* is limited to alkaline soils, but the disease is also endemic in regions with acid soils. The factors affecting distribution of the disease are not well understood. Even in areas where it is common the distribution is erratic, with some farms severely affected and others nearby disease free. The disease is expanding from areas where it has traditionally been seen, probably in large part because of the shipment of cattle carrying *C. haemolyticum* and *F. hepatica.*

PATHOPHYSIOLOGY. Spores of *C. haemolyticum* are ingested by susceptible animals, cross the intestinal mucosa, and are transported to the liver and other organs, probably within the phagosomes of cells of the mononuclear macrophage series. The spores can persist for long periods in the liver in the Kupffer cells. Any localized area of anaerobiosis, as is caused by migrating fluke larvae, allows these spores to germinate and proliferate. Release of toxins from the vegetative cells further increases the anaerobic environment, favoring accelerated bacterial proliferation, toxin production, and hepatic necrosis. Absorption of toxins into the circulatory system rapidly leads to intravascular hemolysis, icterus, hemoglobinuria, and death.

CLINICAL SIGNS. In most cases of bacillary hemoglobinuria the animals are found dead. In the rare instances in which the disease is recognized antemortem, signs include malaise (the animal is by itself, "humped up," and reluctant to move), anorexia, and a fever of 40° to 41° C (104° to 106° F), which drops as death approaches. Breathing may be rapid and shallow, and blood or blood-tinged froth may be present in the nostrils. Rectal bleeding or bloody feces may also be observed. The eponymous sign is passage of dark red, "port wine"–colored urine (hemoglobinuria), but this sign is relatively infrequently seen. The blood is thin and watery and coagulates slowly, and the mucous membranes are pale and icteric. The severity of the signs increases as the disease progresses.

Bacillary hemoglobinuria usually is diagnosed at necropsy as a cause of sudden death. Historical concerns include occurrence in or origination of the animal from an endemic area, the season of the year, the last known sighting of the live animal, the approximate time of death (and the time from estimated death to necropsy), and the farm history of vaccination and liver fluke control. Frequently the animal has been seen apparently healthy 12 to 24 hours before death. Herd vaccination is either nonexistent or overdue. The animal usually is found in lateral recumbency, severely bloated, and without signs of struggle. Blood often is present in the nostrils, mouth, rectum, or vagina. The carcass appears to be in an advanced state of decomposition, even when it is actually quite fresh. A tentative diagnosis can be made on the basis of the history and observation of the carcass.

NECROPSY FINDINGS. On closer examination, the membranes and tissues are icteric. Skinning the animal reveals numerous subcutaneous petechial and ecchymotic hemorrhages, edema, and sometimes emphysema. Copious amounts of red-tinged abdominal and thoracic fluids are seen. Hemorrhages are present on all serosal surfaces. Dark red urine or traces of it are present in the bladder. The lymph nodes are congested and usually hemorrhagic, and there may be hemorrhage into the lumen of the bowel. The spleen is enlarged. The tracheobronchial tree usually is filled with blood-tinged froth or foam. The lungs show hemorrhages, edema, and frequently emphysema. The pericardial fluid is blood tinged, and hemorrhages are present on both the epicardium and endocardium. The solid organs, such as the liver and kidneys, appear to be in advanced stages of autolysis even in fresh carcasses. The confirming (pathognomonic) lesion is the so-called ischemic hepatic "infarct," which has a zone of hyperemia at its interface with viable liver tissue. This area of coagulative necrosis, sometimes partly liquefied at its center, can reach up to 30 cm in diameter and can have a very irregular outline.[57] Unlike a classic infarct, the lesion in bacillary hemoglobinuria results from the progressive enlargement of the focus of coagulative necrosis caused by the bacterial toxins. Any thrombosis seen in the lesion is secondary, with the vasculature being included in the necrotic process along with other hepatic tissue.[59] A thin coat of fibrin may cover the capsule of the liver where it overlies the necrotic lesion.

DIAGNOSIS. In most cases the diagnosis can be confirmed at necropsy. Some peracute cases may be less typical, or laboratory confirmation may be needed in certain unusual cases. A simple Gram-stained impression smear from the liver reveals numerous typical clostridial organisms. Smears may also be made from spleen, blood, or abdominal fluid, with the same outcome. The postmortem presence of clostridial organisms must be interpreted with caution, because they are always present and proliferate rapidly after death. It is important to have an accurate estimate of the time of death to determine the significance of these findings. Laboratory confirmation depends on

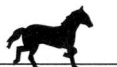

identification of the causative bacterium. Both fresh (refrigerated) and formalin-fixed liver lesions should be submitted. Fluorescent antibody tests on impression smears taken from a liver "infarct" test positive for *C. novyi* type D antigens. Extensive biochemical and toxin identification tests are confirmatory but are seldom used if lesions and fluorescent antibody tests are compatible. The histopathologic examination reveals numerous clostridial rods in the hepatic lesion, particularly immediately subjacent to the zone of neutrophils at the advancing margin of the lesion.

TREATMENT AND PREVENTION. Treatment of bacillary hemoglobinuria is seldom undertaken because of the acute nature of the disease. If the opportunity for treatment arises, penicillin at high dosages is the antibiotic of choice (at least 20,000 IU/kg IM twice a day), although tetracyclines are acceptable (5 mg/kg IV twice a day or 10 mg/kg IM daily). Because time is critical, initiating treatment with intravenous crystalline penicillin (20,000 U/kg) is indicated if available. Fluids are given intravenously or intraruminally to correct dehydration. Blood transfusion is advisable to counter the severe hemolytic anemia and should be repeated as necessary. Affected animals must be handled with great care, because stress or excitement may result in sudden death. In the rare instance of recovery, hematinics should be given to support RBC regeneration.

An effective prevention program requires consideration of both the pathophysiology and immunology of the disease and the natural history of the liver fluke *(F. hepatica)* that is so intimately involved in the expression of bacillary hemoglobinuria. Efforts to clear the soil of the offending organism are unrewarding. However, it is recommended that the carcasses of animals that have died of bacillary hemoglobinuria be burned, buried deeply, or removed from the premises. Commercial bacterin/toxoids against *C. haemolyticum* are available in both monovalent form and in combination with other clostridial vaccines. These products are generally safe and highly efficacious, but the duration of protection is short and should not be relied on for more than 5 to 6 months. Animals vaccinated under 3 to 4 months of age require revaccination at weaning. Local reactions at the site of subcutaneous vaccination are common but primarily of cosmetic concern. Intramuscular vaccination should be avoided, because it often results in permanent damage to muscle tissue, with a resulting negative impact on beef marketing. The timing of vaccination must be determined by the local climate and liver fluke season. In more severe climates where the fluke season is relatively short, a single annual injection before fluke transmission season may suffice. In moderate climates with longer periods of fluke exposure, a second injection about 5 months later may be required. Control measures include pasture or range management; control of water sources; limiting access to streams, canals, ponds, and marshes; and strategic treatment of animals with products effective against flukes. This is a complex subject, and the reader should refer to the section on liver flukes (p. 805) for more detail.

REFERENCES

55. Eklund MW: The role of bacteriophages and plasmids in the production of toxins and other biologically active substances by *Clostridium botulinum* and *Clostridium novyi*. In Sebald M, ed: *Genetics and molecular biology or anaerobic bacteria*, New York, 1993, Springer- Verlag.
56. Erwin BG: Experimental induction of bacillary hemoglobinuria in cattle, *Am J Vet Res* 38:1625-1627, 1977.
57. Jubb KVF, Kennedy PC, Palmer N: *Pathology of domestic animals*, vol 2, New York, 1993, Academic Press, p. 280.
58. Janzen ED, Orr JP, Osborne AD: Bacillary hemoglobinuria associated with necrobacillosis in a yearling feedlot heifer, *Can Vet J* 22:393-394, 1981.
59. Olander HJ, Hughes JP, Biberstein EL: Bacillary hemoglobinuria: induction by liver biopsy in naturally and experimentally infected animals, *Pathol Vet* 3:421-450, 1966.

HEPATIC FAILURE IN FOALS

THOMAS J. DIVERS

Hepatic failure in foals might result from infectious, parasitic, congenital, or toxic causes. Iron fumarate is the best documented of the toxic causes.[60] Iron toxicity most often occurs when newborn foals are given iron before nursing. Colostral-acquired glutathione or other protective substances may explain the great decrease in iron hepatotoxicity when the iron is administered after colostrum.[61] When the iron is given at birth and before colostrum, clinical signs develop 2 to 5 days later. In rare cases clinical signs may not develop until the foal is older. The initial clinical signs are associated with hepatoencephalopathy and include seizures, marked depression, ataxia, aimless wandering, head pressing, or any sign of abnormal behavior. Icterus is noted in most foals at the time neurologic signs are exhibited, although some foals may die so peracutely that icterus is not noticed. Although not documented in foals, nonsteroidal antiinflammatory drugs (NSAIDs) such as carprofen and mycotoxins are other possible toxic causes of hepatic failure.

Other causes of hepatic failure in foals include perinatal herpesvirus infection, leptospirosis, *Actinobacillus equuli* infection, Tyzzer's disease, other bacterial infections, systemic inflammatory response syndrome (SIRS) and multiple organ system dysfunction, septic portal vein thrombosis, chronic neonatal isoerythrolysis, cholangitis associated with duodenal ulcer disease, *Parascaris equorum* migration, congenital anomalies such as atresia of the bile duct, or portosystemic shunts and hyperammonemia in Morgan weanlings.

Infection of a near-term fetus with equine herpesvirus type 1 (EHV-1) may result in the birth of a nonviable foal with hepatic, respiratory, and/or gastrointestinal disease.[62] Generally a quick decline in the clinical condition occurs within 5 days after birth. Affected foals may have severe neutropenia and lymphopenia. Treatment with acyclovir (8 to 16 mg/kg given orally every 8 hours) may improve the chances for survival.[63]

Leptospirosis has been reported to cause jaundice and death in a 10-day-old foal.[64] Although *Leptospira pomona* is known to cause abortion and liver disease (giant cell hepatopathy) in the equine fetus, it is also apparently a rare cause of neonatal liver disease. *A. equuli* typically causes bacteremic embolic nephritis and acute death in very young foals (near 3 days of age). It may also cause widespread multifocal hepatitis in foals. Tyzzer's disease is the best documented cause of bacterial hepatitis in foals and is discussed briefly on the following pages. Other bacteria or bacterial toxins, or both, may initiate an exaggerated response to sepsis (SIRS), which may result in multiple organ dysfunction, including hepatic failure. A large number of vasoactive mediators are involved in this process; the hemodynamic system becomes ineffective and certain organs, such as the liver, may fail because of hypoxia. Diffuse hepatic necrosis and hepatocellular apoptosis are the characteristic lesions. The clinical signs may be identical to those of Tyzzer's disease except that the syndrome may affect a much wider age range. Prompt and aggressive treatment often is successful. Appropriate treatments include broad-spectrum antibiotics, fluids, oxygen, and antioxidants such as dimethyl sulfoxide and acetylcysteine. In rare cases bacterial sepsis may cause acute portal vein thrombosis. Variable degrees of hepatic hypoxemia and inflammation accompany the thrombosis. Unlike in adult horses, hepatoencephalopathy does not generally occur in foals with portal vein thrombosis. Diarrhea may occur in foals because of portal hypertension. The thrombus can be seen on ultrasound examination. A complete recovery may occur with long-term antimicrobial therapy.

Foals with severe and prolonged neonatal isoerythrolysis may develop liver failure. The failure may result from a combination of chronic hypoxia and iron overload from multiple transfusions. The levels of conjugated bilirubin generally are high enough to suggest that bile stasis also is present. With severe and persistent hemolysis, bile excretion may become the rate-limiting step in bilirubin clearance. Physical obstruction of bile flow may occur from duodenal scarring after a duodenal ulcer,[65] congenital biliary atresia, or parasitic obstruction.

Congenital portosystemic shunts occur infrequently in the equine and bovine.[66] Clinical signs may not be noted until foals are 2 to 3 months of age and begin ingesting large amounts of grain or grass. Waxing and waning signs of encephalopathy are the most common signs in foals. Encephalopathic signs and tenesmus are characteristic of the disease in calves. An elevation in plasma bile acids and ammonia in foals with encephalopathic signs and normal concentration of hepatic-derived serum enzymes should arouse suspicion of a portosystemic shunt. Shunts may be single or multiple and may be intrahepatic or extrahepatic. Positive contrast portography is the diagnostic technique of choice. Successful medical management followed by shunt ligation has been described in a foal.

Hepatic failure has been seen in Morgan foals.[67,68] The onset of clinical signs (depression and weight loss) occurs soon after weaning. Liver enzymes are elevated, and variable degrees of portal and bridging fibrosis with bile duct hyperplasia, karyomegaly, and cytomegaly often are seen on microscopic examination. The disease is fatal and may end with a terminal hemolytic crisis. The cause of the disease is unknown, but it may be inherited.

The best laboratory aids in confirming hepatic failure are abnormally high concentrations of serum bilirubin (both conjugated and unconjugated) and ammonia and a prolonged prothrombin time. An elevation in serum enzymes that are hepatic specific may indicate hepatic disease. Some foals with toxic hepatic failure have had normal or only modestly elevated SDH. GGT levels may be high in normal neonatal foals.[69] Plasma glucose concentrations are frequently abnormally low in neonatal hepatic failure. The measurement of bile acids may be useful in determining hepatic dysfunction in foals over 1 week of age.[70]

Treatment of these conditions is discussed on pp. 820 to 821 or under the specific chosen condition.

REFERENCES

60. Divers TJ et al: Toxic hepatic failure in newborn foals, *J Am Vet Assoc* 183:1407-1413, 1983.
61. Mullaney TP, Brown CM: Iron toxicity in neonatal foals, *Equine Vet J* 20(2):119-124, 1988.
62. Bryans JT et al: Neonatal foal disease associated with perinatal infection by equine herpesvirus I, *Equine Med Surg* 1:20, 1977.
63. Murray MJ et al: Neonatal equine herpes virus type 1 infection on a thoroughbred breeding farm, *J Vet Intern Med* 12:36-41, 1998.
64. Hodgin EC, Miller DA, Lozano F: *Leptospira* abortion in horses, *J Vet Diagn Invest* 1:283-287, 1989.
65. Orsini JA, Donawick WJ: Hepaticojejunostomy for the treatment of common hepatic duct obstructions associated with duodenal stenosis in two foals, *Vet Surg* 18:34-38, 1989.
66. Fortier LA et al: Guidelines for the diagnosis and surgical correction of equine and bovine congenital portosystemic shunts, *Vet Surg* 22(5):379, 1993.
67. Divers TJ et al: Unusual cases of liver disease in Morgan foals, *Gastroenterol View* 2:6, 1994.
68. McConnico R, Duckett WM, Wood PA: Persistent hyperammonemia in two related Morgan weanlings, *J Vet Intern Med* 11:264-266, 1997.
69. Patterson WH, Brown CM: Increase in serum γ-glutamyl transferase in neonatal standardbred foals, *Am J Vet Res* 47(11):2461-2463, 1986.
70. Clemmons RM et al: Reduced neonatal platelet function and serum bile acids, *Equine Vet J* 5(suppl):54, 1988.

TYZZER'S DISEASE IN FOALS

ERWIN G. PEARSON

Tyzzer's disease is a sporadic, acute, focal bacterial hepatitis that occurs in foals from 7 to 40 days of age.[71] The organism has been called *Bacillus piliformis*, but recent DNA sequencing evidence suggests that it should be reclassified as a *Clostridium* species.[72]

In many cases of Tyzzer's disease the foal is found dead with no previous signs of illness. The diagnosis in most cases is made at postmortem, and no method is available to make a definitive diagnosis except by postmortem examination. If clinical signs are detected, they may include fever, icterus, depression, anorexia, diarrhea, and seizures, none of which are specific for the disease.[73,74] Serum chemistry values show elevated liver enzymes, hyperbilirubinemia, hyperfibrinogenemia, and a severe hypoglycemia. Histopathologic examination of the liver reveals multifocal areas of necrosis in which the organism can be identified with special stains.

There are no reports of successful treatment of Tyzzer's disease in foals. Early antimicrobial therapy and intravenous fluids to correct the severe hypoglycemia and acidosis could be helpful.

REFERENCES

71. Peak SJ: Tyzzer's disease in foals. In Smith BP, ed: *Large animal internal medicine*, ed 2, St Louis, 1996, Mosby.
72. Duncan TJ et al: The agent of Tyzzer's disease is a *Clostridium* species, *Clin Infect Dis* 16(suppl 4):S422, 1993.
73. Hurber KA et al: Clinical and clinicopathologic findings in two foals affected with *Bacillus piliformis*, *J Am Vet Med Assoc* 193:1425-1428, 1988.
74. Brown CM et al: Serum biochemical and hematological findings in two foals with focal bacterial hepatitis (Tyzzer's disease), *Equine Vet J* 15:376, 1983.

CHRONIC ACTIVE HEPATITIS

ERWIN G. PEARSON

DEFINITION, ETIOLOGY, AND EPIDEMIOLOGY. Chronic active hepatitis represents a sustained inflammatory process in the liver. The diagnosis is made histologically when the principal features are infiltration of inflammatory cells into the portal areas, necrosis, and fibrosis.[75]

The etiology of chronic active hepatitis in large domestic animals is not currently known, but several factors probably are involved. Toxins may play a role.[76] In horses the histologic diagnosis usually is cholangiohepatitis.[77] Cholangiohepatitis that is not associated with liver flukes also has been confirmed in cattle. Bacterial infection through the portal drainage of the bowel or by ascending infection from the bile duct is a possible cause. Immune-mediated processes are thought to be possible causal factors in human beings and the dog, but no definitive work has been done in large animals.

CLINICAL SIGNS AND DIFFERENTIAL DIAGNOSIS. The signs of chronic active hepatitis are similar to those of other causes of chronic progressive liver failure described previously under diagnosis. Progressive weight loss associated with intermittent fever and icterus may be noted initially. Fever is most consistent with bacterial cholangiohepatitis. Other signs may develop progressively as liver functions begin to fail. Signs of concurrent intraabdominal diseases may be present, and some horses develop peculiar cutaneous lesions at the coronary band or areas of necrotic leathery skin.[78] These lesions usually appear as a moist, exfoliative dermatitis caused by an aseptic vasculitis. Differential diagnosis includes pyrrolizine alkaloid toxicity, bile stones, abdominal abscesses, and other chronic wasting diseases.

LIVER-DERIVED SERUM ENZYMES AND DIAGNOSTIC TESTS. Serum liver enzyme activities usually are elevated, reflecting active hepatocyte damage. ALP and GGT tend to be markedly elevated in the active stages of the disease process. Serum bile acid concentrations are increased, and the BSP clearance half-life is prolonged. In most cases serum bilirubin is elevated, especially direct-reacting (conjugated) bilirubin.

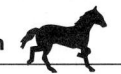

A definitive diagnosis is made from histopathologic examination of a liver biopsy (see following paragraphs). A part of the liver biopsy also should be submitted for bacterial culture and sensitivity testing.

PATHOPHYSIOLOGY. The exact pathophysiology is not known. The early stages are associated with inflammation of the bile ducts or the portal areas of the liver or both. Extension of bacterial infection through the bile duct or through the portal venous drainage may be responsible for the lesion distribution in animals with suppurative cholangiohepatitis. When lymphocytes and plasma cells are predominant in the cellular infiltrate, immune-mediated processes are more likely.

The liver responds by proliferation of bile ducts and bile duct epithelium, which may impair bile excretion. Because hepatocytes are destroyed more rapidly than they are replaced, connective tissue takes their place. Eventually areas are joined so that the fibrosis itself limits regeneration. At this stage some cholestasis may occur, along with failure of other metabolic functions.

Portal hydrostatic pressures could increase gradually, possibly leading to other clinical signs, such as ascites, but this has not been reported in large animals.

NECROPSY FINDINGS. Grossly the liver appears firm, is often pale brown to green in color, and the cut surface may have prominent irregular markings. Histologically most of the lesions are present in the periportal areas. Inflammatory cell infiltration consists primarily of mononuclear cells in some cases, whereas a neutrophilic infiltrate that may contain bacteria (often coliforms) is found in others. These infiltrates are believed to indicate the nature of the primary disease process. Biliary hyperplasia may be marked with cholangiohepatitis. Loss of hepatocytes and increased fibrous connective tissue may be pronounced in the periportal area.

TREATMENT AND CONTROL MEASURES. Supportive care is most important in these cases, especially maintaining proper appetite and nutrition (see Chapter 46).[79] General measures for treating liver disease apply in these cases (see pp. 820 to 821). Corticosteroids have been especially useful in horses with a lymphocytic plasmacytic hepatic infiltrate. They act to increase appetite, stabilize cell membranes, and reduce inflammation and connective tissue formation. Initial treatment with dexamethasone at a dosage of 20 to 40 mg a day for the first 4 to 7 days is followed by a gradual reduction in dosage over 2 to 3 weeks, depending on the response to therapy.[80] Low-level treatment with prednisolone at a dosage of 400 mg once a day may be required for an additional 2 to 4 weeks. Antibiotics are indicated when a bacterial cholangiohepatitis is suspected on the basis of the histologic features of the liver, the culture of the liver biopsy, and the presence of a persistent intermittent fever. Although data are limited, enteric organisms are likely to be encountered, and antibiotic therapy should be directed at the likely organism. Bacterial

culture and sensitivity testing of the biopsy specimen can guide appropriate antimicrobial therapy.

PROGNOSIS. Liver biopsy and the response to therapy are the best guides in formulating a prognosis. The prognosis for improvement and long-term survival is extremely poor in horses that have functional hepatic failure with widespread fibrosis and disruption of normal hepatic parenchyma. The prognosis is fair to good in patients with early (less severe) lesions, particularly those with a lymphocytic plasmacytic cellular infiltrate that responds well to corticosteroids.

REFERENCES

75. Ockaner RK: Chronic hepatitis. In Bennett JC, Plumb F, eds: *Cecil's textbook of medicine*, ed 20, Philadelphia, 1996, WB Saunders.
76. Byars TD: Chronic liver failure in horses, *Compend Cont Educ Pract Vet* 5:S423-S430, 1983.
77. Thornburg LP, Kintner LD: Cholangiohepatitis in a horse, *Vet Med Small Anim Clin* 75:1895-1896, 1980.
78. Carlson GP: Icterus in the horse. In Anderson NB, ed: *Veterinary gastroenterology*, ed 2, Philadelphia, 1992, Lea & Febiger.
79. Divers TJ: Liver disease and liver failure in horses, *Proceedings of the Twenty-ninth Annual Convention of the American Association of Equine Practitioners*, 1983, pp 29:213-223.
80. Carlson GP, Vivrette S: Chronic active hepatitis in horses, *Proc ACVIM Forum* 7:595, 1989.

PYRROLIZIDINE ALKALOID TOXICITY

ERWIN G. PEARSON

DEFINITION AND ETIOLOGY. Pyrrolizidine alkaloid (PA) toxicity is a chronic, progressive, often delayed intoxication that results when animals consume plants containing pyrrolizine alkaloids. The condition is manifested by signs of liver failure.[81] More than 350 pyrrolizine alkaloids have been identified in more than 6000 plant species.[82] Some of the more common plants that contain pyrrolizine alkaloids are listed in Box 31-1.

CLINICAL SIGNS AND DIFFERENTIAL DIAGNOSIS. The clinical signs of PA poisoning are basically those of liver failure, as described in the section on diagnosis of liver disease (p. 790). The most common signs of PA toxicity in the horse are weight loss, slight to moderate icterus, and/or abnormal behavior such as wandering and ataxia.[83] Signs seen less often in horses include photosensitization of the white areas and, in rare cases, diarrhea. A few cases in ponies have shown loud, stertorous inspiratory noises, possibly caused by pharyngeal-laryngeal paralysis.[7,84] Pruritus has been seen in two cases involving horses but never in cattle. Abortion may occur from ingestion of sublethal doses,[85] and PA has been shown to be teratogenic in rats.[86] Subtle signs such as poor performance (inability to race up to previous standards) may be seen in horses with pyrrolizine-induced liver damage before the onset of liver failure. Secondary gastric impaction has been reported in ponies.[87]

BOX 31-1

Common Plant Sources of Pyrrolizine Alkaloid

Tansy ragwort (*Senecio jacobaea*)	Salivation Jane (*Echium lycopsis*)
Common groundsel (*Senecio vulgaris*)	Common heliotrope (*Heliotropium europaeum*)
Threadleaf groundsel (*Senecio douglasii* var. *longilobus*)	Comfrey (*Symphytum officinale*)
Riddell groundsel (*Senecio riddellii*)	Hound's tongue (*Cynoglossum officinale*)
Tarweed (*Senecio trianularis*)	Bruner's trumpet (*Eupatorium maculatum*)
Alpenkreuzkraut (Europe) (*Senecio alpinus*)	Yerba de pasmo (*Baccharis pteronoides*)
Fiddleneck (*Amsinckia intermedia*)	Borage (*Borago officinalis*)
Rattlebox (*Crotalaria* spp.)	*Erechtites* spp.
Viper's bugloss (*Echium plantagineum*)	*Trichodesma* spp. (exotic)

Cattle more frequently show diarrhea, weight loss, tenesmus, prolapsed rectum, and ascites. Calves are much more susceptible than mature cattle. Behavioral changes or subtle neurologic signs may also be seen in cattle, but icterus is not common. Differential diagnosis includes other diseases causing liver failure (such as aflatoxicosis), and some chronic, debilitating diseases such as gastrointestinal parasites, liver flukes, and Johne's disease.[81]

Sheep and goats are more resistant to PA toxicosis but can be affected by certain alkaloids at doses 30 times or more the dose that affects cattle and horses. Certain microorganisms in the rumen of sheep metabolize the PA to less toxic metabolites before they are absorbed. PA injected directly into the portal vein is toxic in sheep, as is *Senecio* when put in the abomasum.[88]

DIAGNOSTIC TESTS. Liver-derived serum enzyme activities are elevated during periods of active hepatocyte destruction caused by PA poisoning. Although the dehydrogenases such as SDH, GLDH, and LDH are elevated initially, they may have returned to normal by the time the animal first shows clinical signs of functional failure. Because the lesions form largely in the portal region, the GGT and ALP levels tend to be consistently elevated.[89,90] In a study of sublethally poisoned horses, AST and the ratio of branched-chain to aromatic amino acids were persistently elevated.[85] Bile acids are elevated and increase early in some but not all horses.[91] Serum bile acid concentrations have a good predictive value, and levels above 50 μmol/L indicate a poor prognosis in the horse.[91] The serum protein concentration usually is normal, and only terminally does albumin decrease or blood clotting become altered. Bilirubin, both direct and indirect, tends to be increased in the horse in the later stages of the disease process.

Liver biopsy is useful in arriving at a definitive diagnosis, but other causes of chronic hepatitis such as aflatoxins may present a similar histologic appearance. The triad of fibrosis, bile duct proliferation, and megalocytosis is characteristic of PA toxicity. A more detailed description of the histologic lesions is given under Necropsy Findings in this section. Some of the changes can be used for prognosis. Modest changes in the hepatocytes and biliary hyperplasia are reversible. Fibrosis bridging portal areas indicates an eventually fatal condition, as does the extensive fibrosis of an end-stage liver.

Feed samples can be examined for PA-containing plants. Cubed or pelleted feeds can be analyzed for PAs, but this often is time-consuming and relatively expensive.* Recently a sulfur-bound pyrrolic metabolite was identified by thin-layer chromatography on the hemoglobin of horses exposed to pyrrolizine alkaloids.[92]

PATHOPHYSIOLOGY. There are a number of PAs, and many of the poisonous plants contain four to six different alkaloids. About 50% of the alkaloids are toxic, and some are more toxic than others. After absorption the portal circulation carries the alkaloids to the liver, where they are metabolized by microsomal enzymes of the hepatocyte to more toxic pyrroles.[93] The pyrroles may cross-link double-strand DNA. The more toxic pyrroles cross-link cellular DNA in a dose-dependent manner.[94] The cross-linking of DNA produces an antimitotic effect.[95] The hepatocytes cannot divide and often become megalocytes as cytoplasm expands without nuclear division. As cells die, they are replaced by connective tissue rather than new hepatocytes. This antimitotic effect may explain why megalocytosis (large hepatocytes and large nuclei)

*AM Craig Laboratory, c/o VDL, Oregon State University, Corvallis, OR 97331.

is seen with the disease. Besides cross-linking DNA, pyrroles, which are alkylating agents, may disrupt the hepatocyte in other ways.[96] They bind to protein and nucleic acid, thereby inhibiting enzymes and blocking protein synthesis. All these actions may lead to faster death of hepatocytes. With chronic doses hepatocyte death is more severe in the portal areas (Rappaport zone 1), although some islands of necrosis do occur.[89,90] Centrilobular necrosis may be seen with massive doses.

With progressive death of hepatocytes and subsequent fibrosis, liver function begins to fail. The blood supply through the hepatic lobule is disrupted by fibrosis, making regeneration impossible. This becomes a venoocclusive disease, resulting in marked portal hypertension. The increased portal hydrostatic pressure leads to diarrhea and ascites in ruminants. Why diarrhea and ascites are seen infrequently in horses with PA toxicity is not understood.

EPIDEMIOLOGY. PA toxicity is seen wherever plants containing the alkaloids are found. The plants are not very palatable and in most cases are not readily eaten, but animals may eat them when the growth of the toxic plant is so thick that the animal cannot separate it from normal forage or when other forage is sparse. The plants are toxic in hay, including pelleted and cubed hay. Some herbicides may make the plants more palatable as they begin to die. PAs also survive ensilage; oat silage contaminated with *Amsinckia* or other PA-containing plants has been responsible for illness in dairy cattle. Seeds of *Heliotropium* plants have poisoned feedlot cattle.[97]

The approximate toxic dose of dried *Senecio* plants as a percentage of body weight for each species is: horses, 5%; cattle, 2% to 5%; goats, 125% to 400%; and sheep, over 150%. Most tansy ragwort contains less than 0.2% PA by weight, but much higher levels have been reported in some of the other plants.[98] Horses were consistently poisoned when the dosage exceeded 250 mg of total PA per kilogram of body weight.[91] The PA in hound's tongue is extremely toxic to horses.[99] This dose does not have to be eaten all at once, because the effects are cumulative. Because signs often are delayed, some animals may not become ill until a year or more after removal from feed sources containing the toxins.[90,100] Signs do not occur until hepatocyte loss and replacement by fibrous tissue have caused failure of liver function.

NECROPSY FINDINGS. Cattle dying of PA poisoning have ascites and prolapsed rectums and are thin and emaciated. Horses usually are thin and may be icteric. In all species the liver tends to be small, pale brown to yellow, and firm and may appear to be scarred. Hepatic megalocytosis is considered the hallmark of PA poisoning, but it has also been seen in aflatoxicosis and is not always apparent in the earliest stages of PA poisoning. Biliary hyperplasia may occur fairly early in the disease. Nonspecific nuclear changes such as invaginations of cytoplasm into the nucleus have been seen.[89,90] Isolated hepatocyte necrosis is seen later, and finally portal or massive generalized fibrosis develops. Once bridging of connective tissue between the portal areas occurs, the disease is fatal. The condition is called a venoocclusive disease, because perivascular fibrosis sometimes occurs, but this is not a constant or characteristic feature.[101] Most of the vascular complications are caused by the generalized fibrosis and remodeling of the liver.

PROGNOSIS. Liver failure may occur with either acute or chronic liver disease; the two must be differentiated for prognosis, because end-stage fibrosis caused by PAs has virtually no chance for regeneration and recovery.

No satisfactory treatment for PA poisoning exists. Once obvious clinical signs of liver failure develop, the animal usually dies within 5 to 10 days. Horses with mild clinical signs and

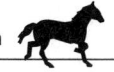

reversible histologic lesions have survived if they retained an appetite and were not exposed to any more PA-contaminated feed.[85] An accurate prognosis concerning mildly affected cases may best be obtained from a combination of consecutive liver biopsies and liver-derived serum enzyme activity,[85] as well as from the serum bile acid concentration.[91] Preventing further exposure to the toxic plants is indicated and may delay or stop the progression of the liver lesions, particularly if an uncontaminated feed source is provided before clinical signs develop.

TREATMENT. Therapy of liver failure is inappropriate if severe fibrosis has occurred, because regeneration is impossible. If the animal still has a reasonable appetite and only modest degrees of fibrosis histologically, treatment may be attempted by providing a low-protein, high-energy diet. The principles of treatment of hepatic disease should be followed (see pp. 820 to 821).

PREVENTION AND CONTROL MEASURES. PA poisoning can be prevented by keeping susceptible animals from pasture, hay, cubed hay, or seeds that contain PA plants. *Senecio vulgaris* tends to contaminate mainly first-cutting alfalfa, whereas *Amsinckia intermedia* often is found in planted fields of oat hay. *Senecio* plants can be controlled by cultivation because they are biennial or by herbicide spraying in the early rosette stage. Biologic controls for *Senecio jacobaea* include the cinnabar moth, *Tyria jacobae,* and the tansy flea beetle, *Longitarsus jacobae.* Sheep are sometimes used to graze *Senecio*-infested pastures to control the weed, because they are less susceptible to the poisoning.

REFERENCES

81. Muth OH: Tansy ragwort *(Senecio jacobaea)* a potential menace to livestock, *J Am Vet Med Assoc* 153:310-312, 1968.
82. Stegelmeier BL et al: Pyrrolizine alkaloid plants: metabolism and toxicity, *J Nat Toxins* 8:95-106, 1999.
83. Ford EJH: Clinical aspects of ragwort poisoning in horses, *Vet Ann* 14:86-88, 1973.
84. Byars TD: Chronic liver failure in horses, *Compend Cont Educ Pract Vet* 5:S423-430, 1983.
85. Lessard P et al: Clinicopathologic study of horses surviving pyrrolizine alkaloid *(Senecio vulgaris)* toxicosis, *Am J Vet Res* 47:1776-1780, 1986.
86. Peterson JE, Jago MV: Embryotoxicity and teratogenicity of pyrrolizine alkaloids and their metabolites in rats, Proceedings of the Symposium on Pyrrolizine Alkaloids: Toxicity, Metabolism, and Poisonous Plant Control Measures, Oregon State University, Corvallis, Ore, Feb 23-24, 1979, pp 57-60.
87. Milne EM, Pogson DM, Doxey DL: Secondary gastric impaction associated with ragwort poisoning in three ponies, *Vet Rec* 124:502-503,1990.
88. Craig AM, Blythe LL, Lassen ED: Resistance of sheep to pyrrolizine alkaloids, *Israel J Vet Med* 42:376-384, 1986.
89. Craig AM et al: Clinicopathologic studies of tansy ragwort toxicosis in ponies: sequential serum and histopathological changes, *J Equine Vet Sci* 11:261-271, 1991.
90. Craig AM et al: Serum liver enzyme and histopathologic changes in calves with chronic and chronic delayed *Senecio jacobaea* toxicosis, *Am J Vet Res* 52:1969-1978, 1991.
91. Mendel VE et al: Pyrrolizine alkaloid–induced liver disease in horses: an early diagnosis, *Am J Vet Res* 49:572-578, 1988.
92. Seawright AA et al: The identification of hepatotoxic pyrrolizine alkaloid exposure in horses by the demonstration of sulfur-bound pyrrolic metabolites on their hemoglobin, *Vet Hum Toxicol* 33(3):286-287, 1991.
93. Jago MB: Factors affecting chronic hepatotoxicity of pyrrolizine alkaloids, *J Pathol* 105:1-11, 1971.
94. Kim HY et al: Comparative DNA cross-linking by activated pyrrolizine alkaloids, *Food Chem Toxicol* 37:619-625, 1999.
95. McLean E: The toxic actions of pyrrolizine alkaloids, *Pharmacol Rev* 22:429-451, 1970.
96. Culvenor CCJ et al: Pyrrolidine alkaloids as alkylating and antimitotic agents, *NY Acad Sci* 163:837-847, 1969.
97. Hill BD, Baul KL, Noble JW: Poisoning of feedlot cattle by seeds of *Heliotropium europaeum, Australian Vet J* 75:360-361, 1997.
98. Roitman JN, Molyneux RJ, Johnson AE: Pyrrolizine alkaloid content of *Senecio* species, Proceedings of the Symposium on Pyrrolizine Alkaloids: Toxicity, Metabolism, and Poisonous Plant Control Measures, Oregon State University, Mountain Research Institute, Corvallis, Ore, 1979, pp 23-34.
99. Stegelmeier BL et al: Pyrrole detection and pathologic progression of *Cynoglossum officinale* (hound's-tongue) poisoning in horses, *J Vet Diagn Invest* 8:81-90, 1996.
100. Molyneux RJ, Johnson AE, Stuart LD: Delayed manifestation of *Senecio*-induced pyrrolizine alkaloidosis in cattle: case reports, *Vet Hum Toxicol* 30:201-205, 1988.
101. Jubb KVF, Kennedy PC: *Pathology of domestic animals,* ed 3, vol 2, New York, 1970, Academic Press.

OTHER HEPATOTOXINS

ERWIN G. PEARSON

The liver is particularly vulnerable to toxic insults because it is the first organ to receive toxins absorbed from the gastrointestinal tract. Enzymes in the hepatocyte may either activate a toxin or, in some cases, metabolize it before it can cause damage. Most hepatotoxic agents are described in more detail in Chapter 50. Some of the more common liver toxins are listed in Tables 31-4, 31-5, and 31-6, but these are not complete lists because many other plants and chemicals can damage the liver under the right conditions. Once a toxic liver disease has been diagnosed, possible sources of the toxin might be identified from these tables. A more detailed description of the toxin could then be found in Chapter 50.

TABLE 31-4

Hepatotoxic Plants

Name	Approximate Lethal Dose (% Body Weight)	Geographic Distribution	Liver Lesion
See Box 31-1 for a list of plants containing pyrrolizidine alkaloid.			
Lantana *(Lantana camara)*	1	Northern North America	Necrosis, canalicular collapse
Rabbitbush *(Tetradymia glabrata)*	0.5	Dry desert	Necrosis
Horsebrush *(Tetradymia* spp.)	Sheep	Western United States	Necrosis
Sacahuista *(Nolina texana)*	1.1	Southwestern United States	Fatty and centrilobular necrosis
Lechuguilla *(Agave lecheguilla)*	4-15	Southern United States, Mexico	Necrosis, photosensitivity
Puncture vine *(Tribulus terrestris)*	?	Warmer regions	Biliary fibrosis, necrosis (big head)
Whitebrush *(Lippia/Aloysia* spp.)	? Horses	Southern United States, Mexico	Fatty degeneration
Panic grasses *(Panicum* spp.)	?	Texas-California, South America	Biliary fibrosis, necrosis
Cocklebur *(Xanthium orientale)*	0.75-3	North America	Hemorrhagic centrilobular necrosis

?, Unknown.

Continued

TABLE 31-4

Hepatotoxic Plants—cont'd

Name	Approximate Lethal Dose (% Body Weight)	Geographic Distribution	Liver Lesion
Lupine (*Lupinus* spp.)	Varies	Western North America	Necrosis by mycotoxin
Cottonseed (*Gossypium* spp.) Gossypol pigment (improper preparation)	Varies with gossypol content	Southern United States	Necrosis (also cardiac effects)
Poisonous mushrooms (*Amanita phalloides, Galerina venenata*)	Few mushrooms	North America	Necrosis (also central nervous system effects)
Blue-green algae (*Microcystis aeruginosa, Nodularia spumgena*)	? 0.001	Ponds worldwide	Necrosis, dissociation
Alsike clover (*Trifolium hybridum*)	Varies	Cultivated	Portal fibrosis, biliary hyperplasia
Mexican firewood (*Kochia scoparia*)	?	Southwestern United States and South America	?
Cycad palm (*Cycas/Zamia* spp.)	?	South America, Australia	?
Yellow-wood (*Terminalia oblongata*)	?	Australia, Africa	Centrilobular necrosis
Sneezeweed (*Helenium* spp.)	0.25	Northern United States, Canada	?
Moldy alfalfa (*Medicago satiwa*)	?	Wet areas	Biliary hyperplasia and necrosis
Bitterweed (*Hymenoxys* spp.)	1	Southwestern United States	?

TABLE 31-5

Hepatotoxic Chemicals

Chemical	Source	Approximate Lethal Dose*	Liver Lesion
Carbon tetrachloride (CC1₄)	Tremacide Fumigant Solvent	10-40 mg/kg	Fatty degeneration, centrilobular necrosis, cirrhosis
C1-Hydrocarbons	Insecticides PCBP Solvents	Varies with species, chemical, and route	Necrosis
Pentachlorophenols	Wood preservative, herbicide, fungicide, molluscacide	100-200 mg/kg	Centrilobular fatty degeneration
Polybrominated biphenyl (PBB)	Fire retardant	100 mg/kg	Hemorrhagic necrosis, fatty degeneration
Carbon disulfide (CS₂)	Boticide Solvent Fumigant	100 mg/kg	Necrosis
Coal tar pitch	Clay pigeons Pipe sealer Tar paper	Swine 15 g/pig	Hemorrhagic necrosis
Phenol	Wood preservative	30 mg/kg	Hemorrhagic centrilobular necrosis
Iron	Iron supplements Injectable iron	>150 mg/kg	Portal necrosis
Copper	Species inappropriate supplements Fungicides, algicides Molluscacide Foot baths	Depends on species and molybdenum intake	Portal vacuolation and necrosis (hemolytic crisis)
Phosphorus	Fertilizer Matches Rodenticide	1-4 mg/kg	Portal necrosis and fatty degeneration
Tannic acid	Oak Skin astringent	20 mg/kg	Centrilobular necrosis (also renal damage)
Paraquat/diquat	Herbicide	4-10 mg/kg	Centrilobular necrosis (also lung damage)
Mycotoxins, aflatoxin B	Moldy feed	3 mg/kg	Centrilobular necrosis, biliary hyperplasia, megalocytosis
Rubratoxin B	Moldy feed	?	Necrosis
Sporidesmin	Moldy feed	?	Bile duct occlusion (big head)
Ochratoxin A	Moldy feed	?	Necrosis (also renal damage)
Phomopsin A	Lupine	?	Necrosis

?, Unknown.
*Lethal dose varies with individual, species, route of entry, rate or chronicity, enzyme induction, and many other factors.

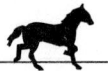

TABLE 31-6

Drugs Used in Large Animals That Could Damage the Liver

Drug	Lesion*	Drug	Lesion*
Carbon tetrachloride	Centrilobular necrosis or fatty degeneration	Fluothane	Active hepatitis/massive necrosis
Hexachloroethane	Centrilobular or massive necrosis	Isoflurane	Active hepatitis/massive necrosis
Carbon disulfide	Necrosis	Some diuretics	Cholestasis, icterus
Alcohol	Necrosis/cirrhosis	Diazepam	Cholestasis, icterus
Tetracycline	Fatty degeneration (also renal damage)	Phenobarbital	Necrosis/cholestasis icterus
Clindamycin	Cholestasis, icterus	Aspirin	Active hepatitis → cirrhosis
Erythromycin	Cholestasis, icterus	Oil of pennyroyal	Centrilobular necrosis
Isoniazid	Active hepatitis → cirrhosis/massive necrosis	Tannic acid	Centrilobular necrosis fatty degeneration (also renal damage)
Rifampin	Cholestasis, icterus	Dantrolene	Active hepatitis → cirrhosis
Nitrofurantoin	Active hepatitis → cirrhosis	Copper disodiumedetate	Massive centrilobular necrosis
Anabolic steroids	Cholestasis, icterus	Iron (injectable)	Necrosis, portal, cirrhosis, hemosiderosis
Phenothiazine tranquilizers	Cholestasis, icterus	Glucocorticoids	Hepatocellular vacuolization
Halothane	Active hepatitis → cirrhosis/massive necrosis		

*May vary with dose and time.

LIVER FLUKES IN RUMINANTS

JOHN B. MALONE

The common liver fluke *Fasciola hepatica* causes a disease of production in ruminants that mimics the production effects and clinical appearance of the gastrointestinal nematode parasite complex. The disease often has its maximum economic effect in late fall and winter, when animals are most likely to be under seasonal nutritional stress. *F. hepatic* is unique among the common helminths of ruminants in that it has an asexual multiplication phase of the life cycle in snail intermediate hosts that is highly sensitive to environmental conditions. *F. hepatica* is well-known for its exponential propagation of infective stages under favorable conditions, sometimes leading to explosive seasonal outbreaks of severe parasitism, especially in sheep. In addition, liver parenchyma migration forms leave necrotic tracts in their wake that are a primary predisposing factor in some areas for acute fatalities caused by *C. novyi* (black disease) and *C. haemolyticum* (bacillary hemoglobinuria).[102]

EPIDEMIOLOGY. The geographic distribution of *F. hepatica* in the United States is limited mainly to areas in the south central states and Florida and to the Pacific Northwest, where neutral, well-buffered soils are found and local hydrologic conditions provide suitable habitats for *Lymnaea* spp., the snail intermediate hosts. The important vector species in temperate climates are semiaquatic "mud" snails found in disturbed mud banks and hoofprints in shallow depressions in fields, drainage channels, and temporary water bodies in alluvial river basins, bottomlands, and coastal regions of the southeastern United States. Springs, small streams, seeps, and sloughs serve as habitats in areas of greater terrain relief in the western states. Most infections occur by grazing in and around water in fluctuating habitats that stay wet for more than half the year.

The life cycle development of both the snail host and the parasite in the snail occurs only when temperatures are above 10° C (50° F) and while snail habitats are wet. This leads to a distinct seasonal transmission in the mild, wet winter and spring of the south central states and Florida and a late spring to fall transmission in the cooler climates of the western states (Figs. 31-1 and 31-2). It takes a minimum of 42 days at 25° C

(77° F) or the accumulation of approximately 600 growing-degree days to complete intramolluscan development, with release of cercariae that encyst as infective metacercariae on pasture vegetation (600 growing-degree days = 25° C minus the base temperature of 10° C = 15 growing-degree days × 42 days; an equivalent value for the life cycle is 15° C or 5 growing-degree days × 120 days). Using soil water budget analysis to indicate the length of time habitats are wet and the accumulated sum of growing-degree days over 600, a climate forecast index can be calculated for use in describing the pattern of seasonal transmission at a given site and to provide an indicator of the risk of economic losses in a given climate year. Two weeks of sustained summer heat and drought ends the transmission season by killing pasture metacercariae and forcing snail populations to estivate in soil or perish. In the cooler climates of the western United States the season ends with drying of springs, seeps, sloughs, and other habitats or with the onset of sustained cold winter weather. Variation in the annual climate alone may lead to a 100-fold variation in fluke burdens in different climate years (Table 31-7).[103]

The amount of snail habitat present on individual farms related to pasture wetness conditions, such as premises with low-lying, heavy clay soils with a high water table, is also an important consideration in evaluating the need for fluke control. This factor has also been shown to lead to a 100-fold variation in the risk of fluke losses in the same year on different premises in otherwise ecologically similar areas.[104] The snail habitat area on most enzootic livestock operations typically is only 1% to 5% of the total land area; operations with over 5% habitat may be associated with a high risk of liver fluke losses.

CLINICAL SIGNS AND PATHOPHYSIOLOGY. Subclinical production effects of *F. hepatica* include reduced rate of gain and feed efficiency in growing stock. Economic effects have been experimentally demonstrated in calves on a marginal nutritional plane in the first 5 to 6 months after infection, resulting in an 8% loss in the rate of gain with a mean of 40 flukes and a 28% loss with 140 flukes. In cattle it is estimated that herd economic losses are negligible with a burden of less than 10 flukes per animal, possible at 10 to 40 flukes, and probable with over 40 flukes; clinical disease is seen with a burden of more than 200 flukes. In cow-calf operations flukes often act in concert with periods of nutritional stress

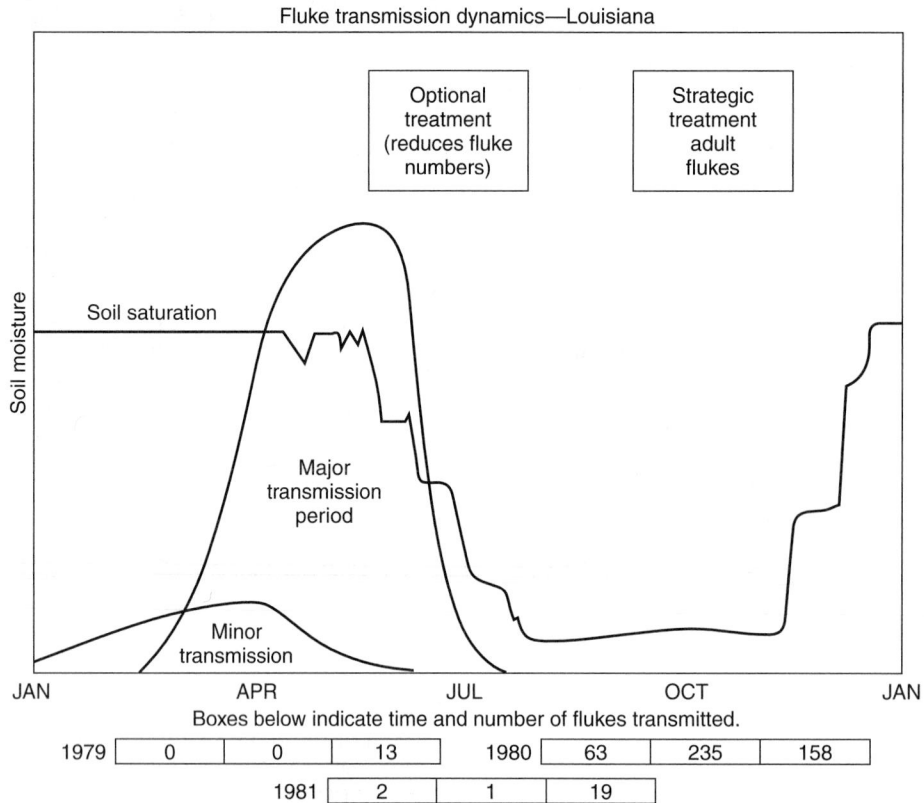

FIG. 31-1 ▦ Pattern of *Fasciola hepatica* transmission typical of the southern United States (based on 10 years of experimental data from Alexandria, Louisiana) and strategic treatment recommendations with adulticidal drugs. (Malone JB et al: *Prev Vet Med* 3:131-141, 1985.)

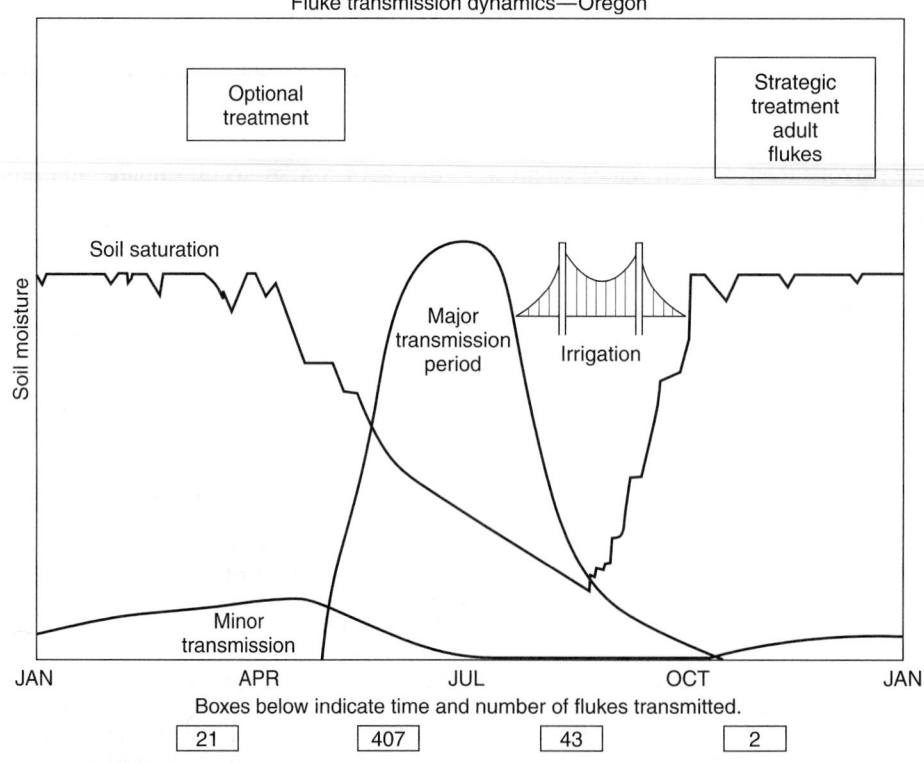

FIG. 31-2 ▦ Pattern of *Fasciola hepatica* transmission typical of the U.S. Pacific Northwest in natural rainfall and irrigated zones (based on experimental data from Langlois, Oregon) and strategic treatment recommendations with adulticidal drugs. (Rickard LG et al: *Vet Parasitol* 41:45-55.)

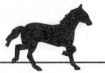

TABLE 31-7

Spring and Autumn Forecast Index Values and Observed *Fasciola* Risk at Dean Lee Research Station, Alexandria, Louisiana

Years	Spring Index	Autumn Index	Flukes Per Calf	Risk
1979	416	1423	2	Low
1980	757	2949	75	High
1981	326	956	5	Low
1982	370	1134	28	Moderate
1983	1304	3671	251	Very high
1984	549	1168	—	Moderate
1985	2899	3187	325	Very high
1986	2151	2470	146	High
1987	1619	2081	146	High
1988	669	1459	—	Low to moderate
1989	830	5741	124*	Very high
Average†	1081	2385	110	

From Malone JB, Zukowski SH: *Parasitol Today* 8:266-270, 1992.
*Average number of flukes despite subterranean drainage of half of the farm and improved preventive herd treatment in 1983. The neighboring farm averaged 189 flukes per calf.
†The 30-year-average reference value computed by the model was 579 for spring and 1978 for autumn.

and concurrent heavy gastrointestinal nematode infections, causing further reduction of body condition, poor milking ability, and slower return to estrus. This translates to reduced reproductive efficiency, prolonged calving interval, and light-weight calves at weaning.[105]

In cattle, flukes may lead to chronic disease or in rare cases subacute disease. When clinical signs occur, the typical population "overdispersion" (individual variation in parasite burdens) is manifested first in the 10% to 20% minority of the herd that harbor most of the parasite numbers. Signs may consist of weight loss, emaciation, depression, anorexia, rough hair coat, anemia, hypoproteinemia, submandibular edema and, in rare cases, mild icterus. The anemia associated with *F. hepatica* infections is more than can be accounted for by blood feeding by flukes. Evidence indicates that depression anemia and biliary hyperplasia result from high levels of proline, a product of fluke metabolism.[106] Cattle are able to mount a protective immune response, with partial acquired resistance to *F. hepatica* beginning at 5 to 6 months after initial exposure.[107] This and the short life span of flukes in cattle typically lead to a linear reduction of fluke numbers, with few surviving by the end of 1 year. Sheep and goats are more susceptible, and fatal acute disease with ascites, abdominal hemorrhage, pallor, and icterus can occur in association with massive entry to the bile ducts at 6 to 10 weeks after infection by 1000 to 5000 or more migrating immature forms from the liver parenchyma. Subacute disease has been associated with a burden of more than 800 flukes acquired over time. Chronic clinical disease in sheep with submandibular edema, ascites, and emaciation has been associated with fluke burdens above 200.[108]

NECROPSY FINDINGS. Necropsy findings attributable to migrating young flukes are due to tortuous tunnels of coagulative necrosis that organize and fibrose, ultimately leading to a diffusely fibrotic liver parenchyma, especially in the ventral lobe, which in severe cases undergoes marked atrophy. Fibrous tags may result from fibrinohemorrhagic deposits left by large numbers of flukes at liver penetration 3 to 4 days after infection. Inflammatory events associated with penetration of the bile ducts at 6 to 8 weeks after infection are especially pathogenic. Once in the bile ducts, flukes grow rapidly from 1 mm to 2.5 cm or more and induce a proliferative

cholangiohepatitis. The spines and suckers of flukes erode and denude the bile duct epithelium, leading to a fibrosed, thickened duct wall that is irregularly dilated and stenotic and begins to calcify in cattle (but not sheep) at about 20 weeks after infection. The bile becomes darkly discolored and laden with regurgitated fluke ingesta, plasma proteins, and inflammatory cells. The extent of pathologic change is generally proportional to the fluke burdens of current or recurring previous infections.[108]

DIAGNOSIS. Fecal sedimentation methods are the standard means of diagnosing liver flukes. A reusable commercial kit based on sieve-sedimentation of 2-g samples (Flukefinder, Visual Differences, Moscow, ID) reduces sample processing time by half and is suitable for use by practitioners for quantitative examination of an individual animal or of 10- to 15-animal herd composite samples. For herd or lot evaluations in cattle, egg counts of less than one egg per 2 g (EP2g) and 25% prevalence 2 to 4 months after the transmission season ends have a low probability of economic losses; 1 to 3 EP2g indicates possible economic loss and 10 EP2g or more indicates high probability of heavy infections and economic loss. It is important to differentiate *F. hepatica* eggs from the eggs of *Paramphistomum* spp., a nonpathogenic "rumen fluke" that is often found in the same herds in both the southern and western enzootic areas. Flukecides used against *F. hepatica* are ineffective against rumen flukes, and egg counts thus persist after treatment. *Paramphistomum* spp. eggs are grey (rather than amber), slightly smaller, and more pointed at the operculum end than *F. hepatica*. *Paramphistomum* egg counts can be used as a general indicator of the probable risk of *F. hepatica* in the absence of control in the southern states, because *Paramphistomum* flukes are known to be transmitted by the same snail vector in that region.[105]

Diagnostic enzyme-linked immunosorbent assays (ELISAs) have been developed to detect serum antibodies and coproantigen in the feces of infected animals[109] but have not yet found wide use outside of research or diagnostic laboratories. Blood and serum clinical pathologic results reflect the anemia, hypoproteinemia, and mild eosinophilia caused by *F. hepatica*. Pathologic changes in the liver bile ducts and parenchyma are reflected by an elevation in serum liver enzymes such as GGT, GLDH, and others.

TREATMENT AND CONTROL. Prevention is the key to control in foundation herds and flocks because even low numbers of eggs shed can multiply asexually in snails and lead to significant infection rates during the following transmission season. A single routine fall or late fall-winter treatment after the end of the transmission season with a highly effective drug is recommended to remove adult flukes before winter stress and to prevent egg shedding and snail infection in the next season (see Figs. 31-1 and 31-2). Most of the pathogenic and economic effects of flukes in cattle are reported to occur within the first 5 to 6 months after the major exposure period and may be related to metabolic products associated with the rapid growth and heavy egg production phases of the life cycle. This, coupled with linear loss of heavy fluke burdens in cattle and the onset of effective immunity at 20 weeks after exposure, suggests the value of early flukecide treatment, within 2 to 3 months after the transmission season ends. In some herds an optional curative treatment in spring may be needed in very high-risk years or on high-risk premises or as a second treatment to remove flukes acquired during late extended transmission on irrigation pastures or wet coastal areas in the west.

Flukecidal drugs available in the United States are effective against mature flukes in bile ducts (albendazole, 10 mg/kg; clorsulon 2 mg/kg). Closulon at a dosage of 7 mg/kg has added efficacy against juvenile flukes over 6 weeks old in the bile ducts. The optimum time to treat should be based on the estimated susceptibility of mature fluke populations (i.e., over 12 weeks old after the end of transmission season) but early enough to remove flukes while they are most pathogenic (under 6 months old). Triclabendazole, which is widely used in other countries, is more than 90% effective against migrating flukes over 2 weeks old and 99% effective against mature flukes and can be effectively given just after transmission ends. Worldwide, a number of other drugs are available, including oxyclozanide, niclofolan, bithionol, and hexochlorophene (80% to 99% of adult flukes), nitroxanil, closantel (over 90% of adult and 50% to 90% of juvenile bile duct flukes), rafoxinide (over 50% of late migratory flukes, over 90% of juvenile and adult flukes in bile ducts) and diamphenathide (over 90% of migratory flukes, 50% to 80% bile duct flukes).[110]

The economic benefit of routine flukecide treatment of feedlot calves from enzootic areas in the United States has not been consistently demonstrated industry-wide because of the high variability of fluke burdens in animals from enzootic areas or because lots are often of mixed origin. Fluke-related losses would be expected to be mainly absorbed by stocker operations, where lightweight calves are typically placed on small grain pastures for extended periods before feedlot, a common practice in the south central states. The economic return of treatment at feedlot should be evaluated on a case by case basis, because significant losses may occur if the lot originates from the same premises and the history suggests a high risk of recent, heavy infection rates such as in favorable climate years or use of irrigated pastures in fluke areas. Fecal egg counts on 10 to 15 randomly selected animals may aid in herd evaluation. An example case of the explosiveness of the life cycle is the greatly reduced feedlot performance and 100% liver condemnations of a lot from a stocker operation in the Pacific Northwest; animals originated from irrigated pastures where some habitats stayed wet year round, and untreated calves from fluke areas were allowed to contaminate pastures with eggs that translated to infection later in the grazing season and to the next stocker group rotated onto the premises.

OTHER FLUKES. *Fascioloides magna,* the large American liver fluke, may infect cattle and sheep that graze common areas with deer, the natural host. The life cycle is similar to that of *F. hepatica,* but with a wider variety of lymnaeid snail hosts and a broader geographic distribution in the Gulf states, the Great Lakes area, and the northwest. Cattle are abnormal, dead-end hosts that react with an intense encapsulation response, forming a closed cyst that does not allow escape of eggs and obviates diagnosis by fecal examination. The liver parenchyma and regional lymph nodes have a characteristic diffuse, black pigmentation. The major economic effect of *F. magna* in cattle is condemnation of livers and other organs, such as lungs, in which aberrant migration sometimes occurs. In sheep and goats, however, *F. magna* does not encyst and migrates uninterrupted. One or two *F. magna* kill sheep before flukes have time to mature, and this parasite limits sheep production in some areas. Albendazole given at high dose rates is moderately effective against *F. magna.*

In tropical regions *F. hepatica* is replaced by *Fasciola gigantica,* a similar species that is somewhat larger, has a longer prepatent period (10 to 12 weeks), and is of somewhat greater pathogenicity. *D. dendriticum* occurs worldwide but in North America is an unimportant species, mainly limited to areas of central New York, with smaller foci in Pennsylvania, New England, Quebec, and British Columbia. Albendazole (20 mg/kg) and high doses of thiabendazole (150 to 300 mg/kg) are effective treatments.[102]

REFERENCES

102. Malone JB: Fascioliasis and cestodiasis in cattle, *Vet Clin North Am Food Anim Pract* 2:261-275, 1986.
103. Malone JB et al: Fascioliasis in cattle in Louisiana: Development of a system to predict disease risk by climate, using the Thornthwaite water budget. *Am J Vet Res* 48:1167-1170, 1987.
104. Zukowski SH, Wilkerson G, Malone JB: Fascioliasis in cattle in Louisiana. II. Development of a system to use soil maps in a geographic information system to estimate disease risk on Louisiana coastal ranges, *Vet Parasitol* 47:51-65, 1992.
105. Malone JB, Craig TM: Cattle liver flukes: risk assessment and control, *Compend Cont Educ Pract Vet* 12:747-754, 1990.
106. Modavi S, Isseroff H: *Fasciola hepatica:* collagen deposition and other histopathology in the rat host's bile ducts caused by the parasite and by proline infusion, *Exp Parasitol* 58:239-244, 1984.
107. Mulcahy G, Joyce P, Dalton JP: Immunology of *Fasciola hepatica* infections. In Dalton JP, ed: *Fasciolosis,* Cambridge, 1999, CAB International Publications, pp 151-183.
108. Behm CA, Sangster NC: Pathology, pathophysiology, and clinical aspects. In Dalton JP, ed: *Fasciolosis,* Cambridge, 1999, CAB International Publications, pp 185-224.
109. Abdel-Rahman SM, O'Reilly KL, Malone JB: Evaluation of a diagnostic monoclonal antibody–based capture enzyme-linked immunosorbent assay for the detection of a 26-28kD *Fasciola hepatica* coproantigen in cattle, *Am J Vet Res* 59:533-537, 1998.
110. Fairweather I, Boray JC: Mechanisms of fasciolicide action and drug resistance in *F. hepatica.* In Dalton JP, ed: *Fasciolosis,* Cambridge, 1999, CAB International Publications, pp 228-229.

LIVER ABSCESSES

ERWIN G. PEARSON
JOHN MAAS

DEFINITION AND ETIOLOGY. Hepatic abscesses can be seen in any species but are more prevalent in ruminants, especially cattle. The primary etiologic agent of hepatic abscesses in cattle in 80% to 97% of cases is *Fusobacterium necrophorum.* Other bacteria occasionally isolated are *Arcanobacterium pyogenes* and *Streptococcus, Staphylococcus,* and *Bacteroides* organisms.[111] The liver is particularly susceptible to abscesses because it receives blood from several sources, including the hepatic artery, the portal system, and the umbilical vein in the fetus and neonate. Entry via the portal vein is the most common route.[112] In cattle, erosion of the ruminal epithelium secondary to grain overload, lactic acidosis, and ruminitis is thought to be the most common mechanisms allowing *F. necrophorum* colonization of the liver. *F. necrophorum* possesses a number of virulence factors, including leukotoxin, endotoxic lipopolysaccharide, and others, which are

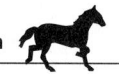

involved in the production of the abscesses.[113] Navel infections can spread (extend) to the liver in young animals, and foreign bodies could penetrate the liver.

CLINICAL SIGNS AND DIFFERENTIAL DIAGNOSIS. Most cases of liver abscesses in cattle are subclinical and are diagnosed at slaughter. Economic loss may still be significant, however, because the rate of gain may be reduced by 3% to 8% as a result of decreased feed intake, and feed efficiency may also be reduced.[114,115] Animals clinically affected most commonly exhibit weight loss, decreased gains, or decreased milk production. They may have periods of fever and anorexia. Some animals may exhibit pain when moving, lying down, or on physical examination with pressure over the right posterior rib cage.[114] Differential diagnosis includes other causes of weight loss that are discussed in Chapter 9, especially traumatic reticuloperitonitis, parasitism, malnutrition, Johne's disease, and lymphosarcoma.

A number of sequelae may occur with liver abscess in cattle. The abscess can erode into the caudal vena cava, producing caudal vena caval thrombosis (CVCT), which results in one of three clinical syndromes: (1) sudden death from septic or anaphylactic shock caused by rupture of the abscess; (2) epistaxis or hemoptysis and anemia caused by pulmonary thromboembolism and ruptured aneurysm[116,117] (some animals also have ascites because of portal hypertension); or (3) severe dyspnea, with open-mouth breathing and widespread rhonchi over the entire lung field, which may develop after rupture of an abscess that is not immediately fatal.[118] A variable fever and anorexia are common in these cases.

Cases have been seen in which liver abscesses enlarged to occlude the bile duct.[119] These cattle often show photosensitization and icterus. The abscesses may also rupture into the abdominal cavity, causing signs of diffuse peritonitis.

In the horse, signs may be similar to other abdominal abscesses and include intermittent colic, intermittent fever, and weight loss.[120,121] Liver abscesses cannot be palpated per rectum, but if several abscesses are present in the abdomen, some may be palpable.

CLINICAL PATHOLOGY AND DIAGNOSTIC TESTS. Laboratory findings vary and usually support a diagnosis but are not specific. A neutrophilia and a neutrophil to lymphocyte reversal may be seen. Plasma fibrinogen may be elevated after day 3 of experimentally induced hepatic abscesses in cattle.[122] The total plasma protein level is not usually affected, but the albumin concentration gradually decreases, along with a concurrent increase in serum globulin, which reduces the albumin/globulin (A/G) ratio. Cattle with acute dyspnea from CVCT may have globulin levels as high as 9 g/dl.[118] Anemia, manifested by decreases in the packed cell volume, hemoglobin, and RBC count, may be the result of loss of blood in hemoptysis or decreased erythropoiesis caused by chronic infection. Liver enzymes such as GGT and AST are elevated only if the abscess process is active. In general, hematologic and liver function tests are not reliable indicators of liver abscesses.[113] Total bilirubin is not increased unless the abscess obstructs the bile ducts, but the direct bilirubin concentration may be increased. Liver biopsy is not usually of value because the focal lesions are often missed, and biopsy should not be done if an abscess is suspected because of the risk of rupturing the abscess. Ultrasound examination could identify the abscess within 3 days of experimental induction of the abscess.[122] Older, coalesced abscesses appear as hyperechoic capsules enclosing an anechoic area of fluid and hyperechoic areas of inspissated pus.[122]

PATHOPHYSIOLOGY AND PATHOGENESIS. *F. necrophorum* is part of the normal ruminal and intestinal flora.[112] Liver abscesses occur secondary to the primary foci of infec-

tion in the ruminal wall. Acidosis-induced rumenitis occurs after a sudden change to a high-energy diet.[113] The starch in such diets is fermented to organic acids by *Streptococcus bovis* and other bacteria. Ruminal damage is often aggravated by sharp feed particles and hair. F. necrophorum invades the eroded wall of the rumen caused by rumenitis and subsequently is carried by the portal circulation to the liver. *F. necrophorum* produces a leukotoxin that destroys leukocytes and thus aids the pathogenic process.

Abscesses once formed tend to be encapsulated with connective tissue, but there is also a tendency for erosion of large veins. Abscesses may rupture into the vein or form a thrombus in the caudal vena cava, producing portal hypertension. This causes increased hydrostatic pressure, and both ascites and diarrhea may be seen. Emboli from this thrombus may be carried through the right heart to the lungs. In the lungs, massive hematogenous pneumonia with sepsis and pulmonary hypertension may result. Pulmonary thromboembolism may cause an aneurysm to develop. When the aneurysm ruptures, hemorrhage occurs into the airways, and blood is coughed up. An enlarged abscess in the liver may obstruct the common bile duct and block the excretion of bilirubin, bile acids, and phylloerythrin, a photodynamic agent produced by chlorophyll metabolism.

EPIDEMIOLOGY. The incidence of liver abscesses in grain-fed cattle can range from 1% or 2% to as high as 95%. The general incidence averages from 12% to 32%.[113] Liver abscesses are most common in beef and dairy cattle fed diets high in carbohydrate and low in roughage. Calves born in an unsanitary environment may be predisposed to navel infection, with possible liver abscess at a later time, although liver abscesses are not commonly found in calves with an umbilical abscess.

TREATMENT. Treatment is not usually undertaken in cattle because the condition is not diagnosed until slaughter. The prognosis would be poor for complete recovery in animals diagnosed with sequelae to the abscess. Most animals with abscess sequelae, such as CVCT, are more economically salvaged by slaughter. If antibiotic therapy is undertaken, the organism is most likely to be susceptible to penicillins, oxytetracycline, and macrolides (tylosin and erythromycin)[123] but they may not reach inhibitory concentrations within the abscess.[111] In the horse, some cases improve with long-term antibiotic therapy using penicillin or ampicillin, often in combination with rifampin or metronidazole.

PREVENTION. Slowly increasing the amount of grain (starch) over a 3- to 4-week period and supplying adequate long-stemmed or coarsely chopped hay (19 cm or longer) at a minimum of 1 kg/head/day may help reduce the incidence of abscesses. Feeding lactating dairy cattle excess concentrate (roughage to concentrate ratio of less than 45:55, dry matter basis) predisposes to liver abscesses. Feeding a total mixed ration with long-stemmed hay (2.3 kg/day or more) with or without rumen buffers (e.g., sodium bicarbonate, magnesium oxide) may aid in reducing liver abscesses.

Antibiotics can be added to cattle rations to reduce the incidence of liver abscesses (Table 31-8). Five antibiotics are currently approved for prevention of liver abscesses in feedlot cattle: bacitracin, chlortetracycline, oxytetracycline, tylosin, and virginiamycin. Tylosin seems to be the most effective, and continuous feeding did not induce resistance in F. necrophorum or A. pyogenes.[124] F. necrophorum isolates continue to exhibit extensive susceptibility to all approved antibiotics.[125] All feed additives must be fed at approved levels, and extra-label dosages are not permitted.

Leukotoxin-based *F. necrophorum* vaccines gave some protection to cattle against experimentally induced liver abscesses.[126] There are clinical reports that a *F. necrophorum*

TABLE 31-8

Antibiotic Feed Additives That Help Reduce the Incidence of Liver Abscess in Cattle

Antibiotic	Dosage	Applicable Class of Cattle	Comments
Chlortetracycline	70 mg/head/day	Beef	Increases rate of gain and feed efficiency
Oxytetracycline	75 mg/head/day	Beef	Increases rate of gain and feed efficiency
Tylosin	60-90 mg/head/day (8-10 g/ton of feed)	Beef	Can be used with monensin (10-30 g/ton of feed)
Monensin	50-360 mg/head/day (5-30 g/ton of feed)	Beef	Can be used with other antibiotic additives

bacterin* labeled for use in preventing foot rot may also help reduce the incidence of liver abscesses.

REFERENCES

111. Berg JN, Scanlan CM: Studies of *Fusobacterium necrophorum* from bovine hepatic abscesses: biotypes, quantitation, virulence, and antibiotic susceptibility, *Am J Vet Res* 43:1580-1586, 1982.
112. Nagaraja TG, Laudert SB, Parrott JC: Liver abscesses in feedlot cattle, *Compend Cont Educ* 18:S230-241, S264-273, 1996.
113. Nagaraja TG, Chengappa MM: Liver abscesses in feedlot cattle: a review, *J Anim Sci* 76:287-298, 1998.
114. Brink DR et al: Severity of liver abscesses and efficiency of feed utilization of feedlot cattle, *J Anim Sci* 68:1201-1207, 1990.
115. Deem DA: Liver abscesses in cattle, *Compend Cont Educ Pract Vet* 2:S268-S273, 1980.
116. Breeze RG, Pirie HM, Selman IE: Hemoptysis in cattle, *Bovine Pract* 11:64-71, 1976.
117. Selman IE et al: A respiratory syndrome in cattle resulting from thrombosis of the posterior vena cava, *Vet Rec* 94:459-466, 1974.
118. Rebuhn WC et al: Caudal vena cava thrombosis in four cattle with acute dyspnea, *J Am Vet Med Assoc* 176:1366-1369, 1980.
119. Pearson EG et al: Unpublished data, Ithaca, NY, 1982.
120. Rumbaugh GE, Smith BP, Carlson GP: Internal abdominal abscesses in the horse: a study of 25 cases, *J Am Vet Med Assoc* 172:304-309, 1978.
121. Sellon DC et al: Hepatic abscesses in three horses, *J Am Vet Med Assoc* 216:882-887, 2000.
122. Lechtenberg KF, Nagaraja TG: Hepatic ultrasonography and blood changes in cattle with experimentally induced hepatic abscesses, *Am J Vet Res* 52:803-809, 1991.
123. Lechtenberg KF, Nagaraja TG, Chengappa MM: Antimicrobial susceptibility of *Fusobacterium necrophorum* isolated from bovine hepatic abscesses, *Am J Vet Res* 59:44-47, 1998.
124. Nagaraja TG et al: Bacterial flora of liver abscesses in feedlot cattle fed tylosin or no tylosin, *J Anim Sci* 77:973-978, 1999.
125. Mateos E et al: Minimum inhibitory concentrations for selected antimicrobial agents against *Fusobacterium necrophorum* isolated from hepatic abscesses in cattle and sheep, *J Vet Pharmacol Ther* 20:21-23, 1997.
126. Saginala S et al: Serum neutralizing antibody response and protection against experimentally induced liver abscesses in steers vaccinated with *Fusobacterium necrophorum, Am J Vet Res* 57:483-488, 1996.

HEPATIC LIPIDOSIS

ERWIN G. PEARSON
JOHN MAAS

The conditions described in the following paragraphs can cause hepatic lipidosis. The pathophysiology and prevention measures are similar and are described at the end of this section.

FAT COW SYNDROME, LIPID MOBILIZATION SYNDROME

DEFINITION AND ETIOLOGY. Fat cow syndrome is a multifactorial condition that occurs in dairy cows after parturition. The syndrome is characterized by progressive depression and failure to respond to treatment of other predisposing diseases. It is associated with excessive mobilization of fat to the liver in well-conditioned cows. The mobilization of fat is induced by the negative energy balance and hormonal changes that occur during the periparturient period. This negative energy balance in most cases is aggravated by concurrent periparturient diseases that reduce feed intake and increase energy needs.[127-129]

CLINICAL SIGNS. The clinical condition occurs in the postparturient period. Most affected cows are either obese or very well conditioned with a large amount of omental and subcutaneous fat. Presenting signs usually include depression, anorexia, weight loss, and weakness that can lead to recumbency. Most cows have nonspecific signs such as decreased rumen motility and decreased milk production. Other signs vary and are related to concurrent diseases. The concurrent diseases most frequently seen are metritis, retained fetal membranes, mastitis, parturient paresis, and displaced abomasum.[127,128] It is important to look for these other diseases, because even if mild, they could be significant in these cases and must be treated.

CLINICAL PATHOLOGY AND DIAGNOSTIC TESTS. Most laboratory tests are poor indicators of hepatic lipidosis and are of little value in determining the severity of the disease.[130] Liver-derived enzymes are usually elevated above the level in the dry cow but are within normal ranges. Some serum enzyme levels increase in the periparturient period in normal cows. Many cows with hepatic lipidosis have a leukopenia and a degenerative left shift, but this is not specific. As expected, serum free fatty acids (FFAs) are increased, and triglycerides and cholesterol are decreased. Most of the total cholesterol is in lipoproteins. The serum total bile acids are not significantly increased in most cows with fatty livers.[131] The BSP dye excretion test may be useful prognostically, because animals with a clearance half-live over 9 minutes have a more guarded prognosis.[132] The more common abnormal laboratory findings are listed in Table 31-9.

Liver biopsy may confirm the fatty infiltration of the hepatocytes, but a moderate to high amount of fat (15% to 30%)* is present in the liver of all postparturient, high-producing dairy cows, even those that remain healthy.[133,134] Fat can be quantitated by histologic methods or by floating in copper sulfate solutions of various specific gravities.[135] However, there is little correlation between the amount of fat and signs of disease until the fat is above 34%, at which point the liver tissue will float in distilled water with a specific gravity of 1.

PATHOPHYSIOLOGY. See pp. 812, 814, 815.

EPIDEMIOLOGY. Fat cow syndrome occurs sporadically in dairy cows but more frequently in those with loose housing where the dry cows are managed with the lactating cows in one group. Cows commonly become overconditioned during late

---

*Fusogard, Immtech Biologics, LLC.

*Extraction by solvent and serologic estimation of fat volume.

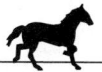

TABLE 31-9

Common Clinicopathologic Abnormalities in Fat Cow Syndrome

Test Parameter	Change From Normal	Amount	Normal ($\overline{X} \pm 2$ SD) Prepartum Dry	Normal ($\overline{X} \pm 2$ SD) Postpartum 1-2 wk
Ketonuria	↑	>(1+)	—	Trace +
FFA (µEq/L)	↑	>800	343-575	597-821
Triglycerides (mg/dl)	↓	<5		
BUN (mg/dl)	↑ or Normal	>20	16-24	16-24
BSP clearance (T$^{1/2}$ min)	↑	<5	4.4-4.8	4.7-5.5
GGT (IU/L)	↑	>16	9.1-10.7	10.3-16.1
AST (IU/L)	↑	>70	44-56	65-78
Insulin (U/ml)	↓ Variable		12-17	6.8-9.2
Glucose (mg/dl)	↓		52-57	48-52
White blood cells	↓	<4000	4000-12,000 bands <120	
	↑	Neutrophil/ lymphocyte ratio	Neutrophils < Lymphocytes	

FFA, Free fatty acid; *BUN,* blood urea nitrogen; *BSP,* bromsulphalein; *GGT,* γ-glutamyl transferase; *AST,* aspartate aminotransferase.

lactation and/or during the dry period. The overconditioning may be due to a poor breeding program associated with cows spending prolonged time in the low lactation strings and having excessive weight gain. Morbidity as high as 90% occurred in the original reports.[129] Mortality can be over 25%, and higher without intensive treatment and correction of concurrent diseases. Clinical disease in obese cows that enter the dry period can be minimized by carefully controlling their diets to meet NRC requirements and by preventing milk fever.

NECROPSY FINDINGS. Generalized obesity is noted unless the animal has been ill for longer than 1 to 2 weeks. Changes in the liver are most striking. The liver is enlarged, and the edges are swollen and rounded. It is pale yellow and may float in water. Histologically, fatty infiltration of the hepatocytes is noted, especially in the centrilobular and intermediate areas. However, these liver tissues are not markedly different from those of healthy, high-producing dairy cows in early lactation. The pathologist must make an extra effort to find lesions of other periparturient diseases even if mild.

TREATMENT AND PROGNOSIS. The prognosis must be guarded unless the concurrent diseases can be treated successfully and the liver fat mobilized. It is most important to treat the primary disease. Reduction of the negative energy balance and treatment of the hepatic lipidosis (as described on p. 815) must be tackled vigorously. Prevention is based on preventing overconditioning during the late lactation period and the dry period and treating periparturient diseases in a timely manner. General prevention of hepatic lipidosis is covered in more detail on p. 816.

PROTEIN-ENERGY MALNUTRITION/ PREGNANCY TOXEMIA OF BEEF COWS

ETIOLOGY. Protein-energy malnutrition (PEM)/pregnancy toxemia of beef cows is a condition of pregnant beef cattle on marginal diets. The disorder usually occurs in the winter and is manifested by weight loss, weakness, depression, and sometimes inability to rise. The condition is the result of the negative energy balance caused by decreased quality and quantity of feed when caloric requirements are increased by fetal development and cold weather. Growing, pregnant heifers are especially susceptible, because energy requirements for growth are superimposed on the other caloric requirements. A number of other factors such as unpalat-

able feed, snow cover, and diseases may reduce caloric intake (see Chapter 9). Fatty infiltration of hepatocytes occurs transiently in early PEM, and at necropsy the liver is smaller than normal.

CLINICAL SIGNS AND DIFFERENTIAL DIAGNOSIS. Animals are usually thin and have a long hair coat. In some cases they are down and unable to rise but still alert. The body temperature may be normal or subnormal. Occasionally the cows also develop diarrhea. Most cases die 7 to 14 days after becoming recumbent.[136] The differential diagnosis includes Johne's disease, lymphosarcoma, parasitism, chronic pulmonary disease, other deficiencies, and debilitating diseases.

CLINICAL PATHOLOGY AND DIAGNOSTIC TESTS. The diagnosis usually is based on demonstrating decreased caloric intake and ruling out other chronic diseases that could cause debility. Laboratory tests support but do not rule out the disease. The total serum calcium may be decreased. Packed cell volume also may be decreased, and serum insulin levels may be reduced. Ketonuria is not typical in PEM.

NECROPSY FINDINGS. Muscle mass usually is decreased. Serous (brown) atrophy of fat is often present, especially in the coronary groove, bone marrow, and perirenal areas. Lesions of concurrent disease also may be found if PEM is acute, and a fatty yellow liver may be noted.

TREATMENT AND PROGNOSIS. Treatment often is unrewarding. Efforts to reverse an advanced catabolic state may fail. A 454-kg cow requires 13 Mcal of metabolizable energy per day or approximately 6.5 L of 50% glucose solution by continuous drip. Alfalfa pellet gruels are helpful if force fed, and approximately 11 kg of alfalfa is recommended. Propylene glycol (150 to 200 ml) given orally twice a day can be helpful as a glucose precursor. Treatments include intravenous fluids, improving the energy balance as described below, and treating any concurrent disease. Prevention and control by nutrition are discussed on p. 816.

PREGNANCY TOXEMIA IN EWES AND DOES

DEFINITION AND ETIOLOGY. Pregnancy toxemia, also known as ketosis or twin-lamb disease, is a condition occurring in ewes and does during the last 2 to 4 weeks of gestation. It is characterized by anorexia, weakness, and depression. The condition is caused by a negative energy balance resulting from increased energy demands of rapid fetal growth in late gestation and insufficient intake.

CLINICAL SIGNS. Animals with pregnancy toxemia are usually separated from the rest of the flock or herd. They have a poor appetite, and many appear blind. They eventually become more depressed and recumbent. Neurologic signs such as tremors, star-gazing, incoordination, circling, and grinding the teeth may precede terminal depression. The differential diagnosis includes other periparturient diseases such as mastitis and hypocalcemia, as well as polioencephalomalacia, enterotoxemia type D, and toxicoses.

CLINICAL PATHOLOGY AND DIAGNOSTIC TESTS. Ketonuria is usually present and detected before ketonemia. Hypoglycemia is not a consistent finding but is sometimes present. The ewes and does often are acidotic and may have lowered serum calcium and potassium levels. The blood urea nitrogen and creatine levels are elevated terminally in some cases. The FFA concentration in the plasma usually is elevated above 500 μEq/L. Serum β-hydroxybutyrate (BHB) concentrations are elevated (above 1 mmol/L).[137] A nonspecific but marked neutrophilia may be found in some affected animals and is particularly dramatic in does, sometimes reaching 35,000 neutrophils per microliter.

PATHOPHYSIOLOGY. See Pathophysiology of Hepatic Lipidosis, below.

EPIDEMIOLOGY. The incidence of pregnancy toxemia is greater in ewes with more than one fetus, during the last 2 to 4 weeks of gestation,[138] and in does with three or more fetuses. Poor-quality feed, cold weather, lack of exercise, and stress of movement also may increase the incidence. Many ewes are overly fat to start with. Does seem to be more resistant to pregnancy toxemia than ewes in that three or more fetuses usually are required to produce the condition.

NECROPSY FINDINGS. These cases have a pale, swollen, friable, fatty liver. The animals may be somewhat dehydrated, and the uterus usually has more than one fetus.

PROGNOSIS AND TREATMENT. Mortality is high unless treatment is started early and the fetuses are removed. The most important step is removing the fetuses, either by inducing parturition or by cesarean section. Parturition can be induced in ewes with 15 to 20 mg of dexamethasone; in does the dose is either 10 mg of dexamethasone or 10 μg of prostaglandin F$_{2\alpha}$.[138] A cesarean section may be performed if the animal's value warrants it and there does not seem to be enough time to induce parturition. Besides removing the fetuses, the ketotic condition should be treated: 250 to 500 ml of 10% to 20% glucose is given intravenously, followed by a slow drip or 5% to 10% glucose intravenously. Acidosis and hypocalcemia must be corrected if present. Many practitioners use B vitamins in an attempt to stimulate appetite. Transfaunation of rumen liquor from a normal ruminant (a cow is acceptable) is useful in promoting voluntary feed intake and rumen motility. Cyanocobalamin (vitamin B$_{12}$) and biotin are particularly indicated as adjuncts to glucogenesis. The energy intake must be increased. Glucose precursors such as propylene glycol (15 to 30 ml every 12 hours) or sodium proportionate are often used, but excess propylene glycol may lead to acidosis or cause diarrhea, or both.

HYPERLIPEMIA/HYPERLIPIDEMIA IN PONIES

DEFINITION AND ETIOLOGY. Hyperlipemia occurs mainly in ponies and occasionally in horses and is characterized by a fatty liver and serum that is cloudy with accumulation of lipids. The triglyceride level usually is much higher than 500 mg/dl.[139] The condition is caused by decreased caloric intake, which causes fat mobilization and fat accumulation in the liver and accumulation in the plasma.[140] The decreased

food intake may develop secondary to other diseases. In horses, azotemia usually is also present and may block further triglyceride uptake by the liver.[139] Equine hyperlipemia is characterized by production of an abnormal very low density lipoprotein (VLDL) fraction (VLDL$_1$), which has a reduced content of apolipoprotein B-100 and an increased content of apolipoprotein B-48.[141] The substitution of B-48 for B-100 is thought to allow greater triglyceride content, because B-48 is the apolipoprotein of importance in chylomicrons. In one study the activities of lipoprotein lipase and hepatic lipase, the enzymes responsible for VLDL catabolism, were increased in hyperlipemic ponies.[141] It was concluded that overproduction of VLDL is the cause of hyperlipemia and that agents that reduce VLDL synthesis should be candidates for clinical investigation.[143]

Hyperlipidemia is a mild condition of ponies and horses characterized by mildly elevated triglyceride concentrations (over 500 mg/dl), clear plasma, and no evidence of hepatic dysfunction.[139] An increase in caloric intake usually is sufficient to reverse the condition. The more severe condition, hyperlipemia, is discussed further.

CLINICAL SIGNS. The clinical signs of hyperlipemia are not specific. Ponies usually are anorexic, depressed, weak, and uncoordinated. Diarrhea is a common clinical sign.[142]

CLINICAL PATHOLOGY AND DIAGNOSTIC TESTS. The diagnosis is based on examination of the blood and plasma to detect the white to yellow opacity caused by the presence of lipids. Bilirubin usually is elevated, as it is in most horses that are fasted. Triglycerides are elevated far above 500 mg/dl in hyperlipemia. FFAs are also increased. BSP clearances are delayed (see p. 794), and terminally there may be a large base deficit caused by metabolic acidosis.[139]

EPIDEMIOLOGY. The incidence of hyperlipemia is greater in ponies than in horses. It is seen more in the winter, especially from February to May, in animals on poor feed. Pregnant animals and those that are lactating are affected more often.

NECROPSY FINDINGS. Postmortem examination reveals fatty infiltration of the liver and kidneys, which are pale and swollen and have a greasy texture. In ponies the liver has sometimes ruptured, resulting in intraabdominal hemorrhage and death. Renal lesions may be seen histologically. A primary disease may be present that produced anorexia and secondarily resulted in hyperlipemia.

TREATMENT. It is most important to treat any primary disease to alleviate the cause of anorexia and to correct the negative energy balance as described in the following paragraphs. Insulin, along with 100 g of glucose given intravenously, has been used in some affected ponies.[142] The recommended dose of protamine zinc insulin (PZI)* is 30 IU IM twice a day with 100 g of glucose by mouth for a 200-kg pony. This is continued on odd days; on even days 15 IU of PZI and 100 g of galactose (orally) are given twice daily.[139] A slow intravenous drip of glucose for several days or until lipemia clears may be indicated. Heparin (100 to 250 IU/kg twice daily) has been used to alter the lipoprotein lipase activity and inhibit hormone-sensitive lipase of adipose tissue, but it may alter coagulation enough to cause hemorrhage. Glucose administration also stimulates insulin levels, but overdoses may result in a more severe acidosis.[139]

PATHOPHYSIOLOGY OF HEPATIC LIPIDOSIS (Fig. 31-3)

Storage of excess energy as fat and the periodic mobilization of fat for use as energy by the body is crucial.[143] The liver plays a major role in lipid metabolism and must process the absorbed

---

*Protamine zinc and iletin insulin, Lilly, Indianapolis, IN 46285.

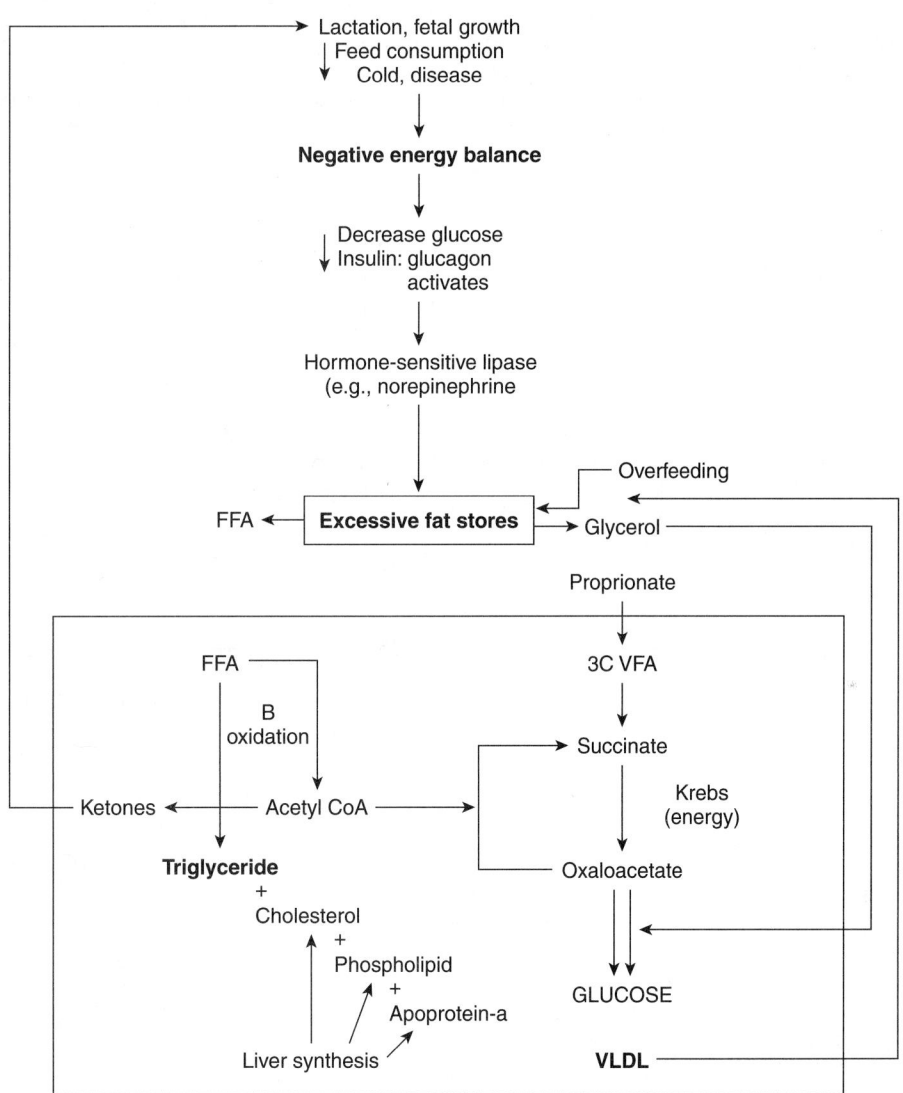

FIG. 31-3 ▓ Metabolism of fat in animals with hepatic lipidosis.

chylomicrons, the volatile fatty acids, and many of the FFAs and much of the glycerol obtained by mobilization of fat from adipose tissue. The liver of large herbivores has unique functions, because much of the dietary energy is absorbed as volatile fatty acids and not glucose. Glucose is still needed (in high amounts in lactating animals) and must be produced by gluconeogenesis, 85% of which takes place in the liver.[144]

Negative energy balance is induced by lactation, fetal growth, exercise, decreased feed consumption, environmental chilling, and diseases (Fig. 31-4). During these periods of negative energy balance and before lactation, the blood glucose level may drop slightly, the insulin to glucagon ratio drops, and these and other hormones (e.g., catecholamines, growth hormone) activate hormone-sensitive lipases that convert tissue fat to FFAs or nonesterified fatty acids (NEFAs) and glycerol (Fig. 31-5). In the liver the glycerol may be used to produce glucose, or it may be recombined with FFAs to make triglycerides. In addition to being recombined with glycerol to make triglycerides, the FFAs may be degraded through B oxidation, and the two carbon fatty acids converted to acetyl-CoA. The acetyl-CoA combines with oxaloacetate to enter the tricarboxylic acid cycle for the production of energy. This pathway is in competition with the use of oxaloacetate for gluconeogenesis.[128] If there is not enough oxaloacetate available, the acetyl-CoA is converted to ketone bodies, which in high concentrations can reduce feed consumption and perpetuate the negative energy balance.

When the liver is overwhelmed with mobilized FFAs, greater amounts of triglycerides are deposited within the hepatocytes. These triglycerides eventually leave the liver as VLDLs, which are plasma-soluble complexes of phospholipid, cholesterol, triglyceride, and apolipoprotein A. Hepatic lipidosis results when the rate of hepatic triglyceride formation exceeds oxidation of fatty acids and the formation and release

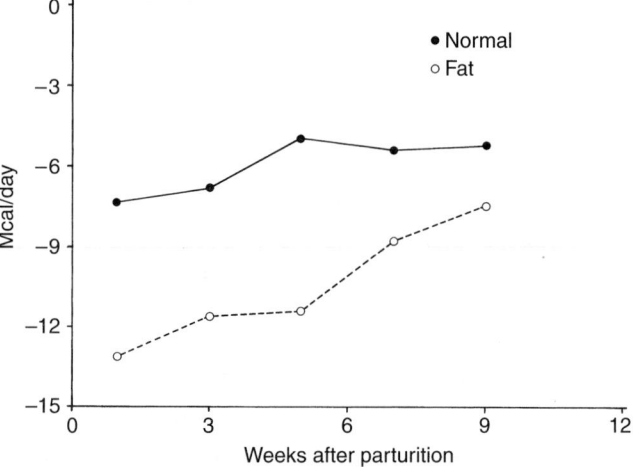

FIG. 31-4 ■ Energy balance (megacalories per day) in normal condition and obese dairy cows after parturition.

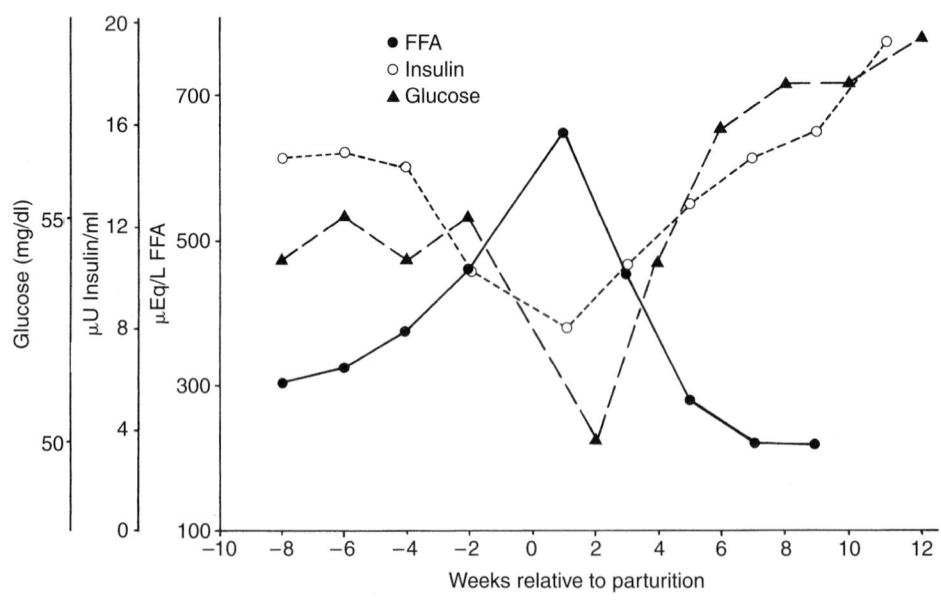

FIG. 31-5 ■ Plasma levels of glucose, insulin, and free fatty acids in dairy cows before and after parturition.

of VLDLs into the peripheral circulation. A number of factors have been incriminated in the inability of the liver to secrete adequate VLDLs to keep up with the deposition of triglycerides brought about by FFA mobilization from fat. Ruminants have a poor ability to export excess lipid from the liver as VLDLs. This is particularly true in bovine hepatic lipidosis,[145,146] and this is theorized to be due to a shortage of apolipoprotein-A. Hepatic lipidosis can be induced in cows by inhibiting the production of apolipoprotein,[147] and the lowest concentrations of lipoproteins occur in the serum of cows with the most severe hepatic lipidosis.[146] Cows on low-protein diets in the dry period are more likely to develop hepatic lipidosis than those on higher protein diets, regardless of the energy content.[145,148] Depression in dry matter intake in the final week before calving increases the liver triglyceride content after calving in dairy cows.[149] In the past, a lack of phospholipid or its precursor, choline, has been incriminated but never substantiated. However, in the face of an energy shortage, it seems redundant and a waste of energy to repackage fat and send it back to the tissues, even if the liver is being overwhelmed with FFAs. Some of the same endocrine hormones that activate hormone-sensitive lipase and inhibit lipogenesis and glycogen synthesis may also inhibit the production of VLDLs.

It has also been suggested that subclinical liver damage may inhibit the production of VLDLs, but experimental studies have indicated no significant elevation in liver-specific enzymes before lipid accumulation.[133,134] Function may eventually be impaired by the accumulation of fat, because fasted cows have a decrease in the surface area of rough endoplasmic reticulum and the number of mitochondria per unit volume.[150] Changes in the liver seem to be functional and not degenerative.[151] Hepatic lipidosis appears to be a reversible condition if the cause is removed and energy balance becomes positive (less negative). In cows fasted and refed, all major liver functions returned to normal within 18 days of refeeding,[149] and all lactating dairy cows with postparturient hepatic lipidosis had normal liver fat content (under 15%) at 6 months after calving.[134]

All high-producing dairy cows have increased amounts of fat (15% to 32% by weight) in the liver before calving and during the first few weeks after parturition (Fig. 31-6).[133,134,151] These fat accumulations in the liver begin before calving as the animal prepares for lactation, and the blood glucose concentration is actually lower before calving.[152] The amount of fat in the liver depends on the amount available and the extent of negative energy balance. Fatter cows tend to lose weight more rapidly and have more fat accumulation in the liver.[133,134] Serum cholesterol values (lipoprotein) are inversely related to loss in condition.[153]

TREATMENT OF HEPATIC LIPIDOSIS

The most important principle in treating hepatic lipidosis is the elimination of negative energy balance and the factors or diseases causing it. Continual intravenous glucose administered at a rate of approximately 100 to 200 mg/kg/hour may provide continuing energy and induce an insulin to glucagon ratio that will decrease hormone-sensitive lipase mobilization of FFAs and stimulate production of VLDLs. Insulin itself may be given to alter this ratio directly. In cattle, 200 U of protamine zinc (NPH or Lente) insulin is given every 12 hours per 1000 pounds of cow, along with glucose.

Precursors of lipoproteins, such as choline, a component of phospholipid, have been advocated to increase the rate at which triglycerides leave the liver as phospholipids (VLDLs), but no controlled studies have proved their efficacy. Choline is degraded in the rumen,[154] but theoretically choline chloride (25 g in 250 ml of sterile saline) given subcutaneously could have limited efficacy. Choline should *not* be given intravenously because it acts as a neuromuscular blocking agent. Addition of inositol both before and after birth did not reduce the incidence or severity of hepatic lipidosis.[155] Methionine given at a dosage of 40 to 50 g/day has been used for the same purpose. Nicotinic acid (niacin) fed at 6 to 12 g/head/day may help reduce lipolysis at the tissue level and thus reduce the amount of fat presented to the liver.[156] Treatment of hepatic lipidosis with nicotinic acid is often associated with a rebound of clinical signs, and its use as a preventive measure is recommended.

Corticosteroids as used for treating ketosis may be useful but should not be used repeatedly over a long period, because they may make the animal less resistant to infections.[155] Corticosteroids usually increase appetite, reduce milk production, and induce gluconeogenesis. Both vitamin E and selenium, which function as cellular antioxidants, have been found to be low in many of the cows with fatty liver syndrome[156]; therefore supplementation may be helpful in selected cases.

Digestion in the forestomachs can be enhanced by transfaunating with rumen fluid from a normal cow. This may increase the absorption of volatile fatty acids used for energy and for glucose precursors.

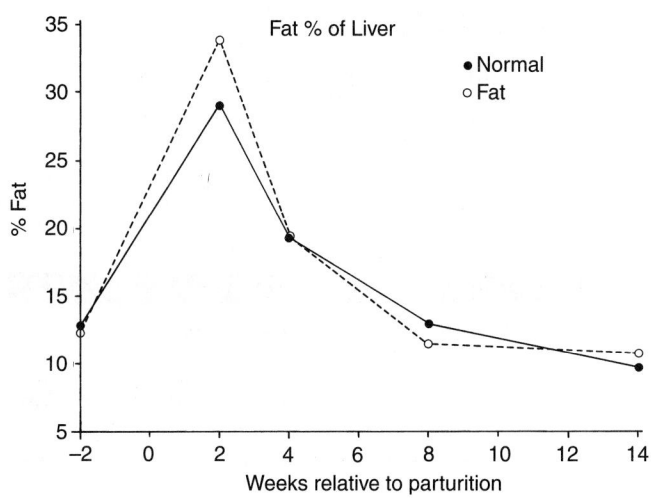

FIG. 31-6 ■ Liver fat as a percentage of total dry weight in normal condition and obese high-producing dairy cows before and after parturition.

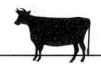

PREVENTION OF HEPATIC LIPIDOSIS AND HANDLING NEGATIVE ENERGY BALANCE AND OVERCONDITIONING

Hepatic lipidosis and associated conditions are most common in dairy cattle. Preventing obesity in cows during late lactation is an important factor in controlling this condition. This process involves a successful breeding program (maintaining a 12- to 13-month calving interval) and closely matching energy in the ration to the level of milk production during late lactation.[157] Once the cow reaches 7 months of pregnancy and the dry period, any dietary restriction below requirements for maintenance and pregnancy are sure to be counterproductive. The recommended nutrient requirements for a 600-kg cow are listed in Table 31-10.[158]

Adequate protein in the dry period is essential.[144,147,148] It has been shown that cows fed higher protein diets during the dry period perform better in the lactation that follows. Feeding good to excellent quality roughages (hay, silages) to meet most of these requirements is preferred. Additional grain (starch) 2 to 4 weeks before parturition is important to acclimate the ruminant to anticipated changes in the rations fed after calving. It must be stressed that high-quality dry cow rations be fed *but not overfed*. Dry matter consumption should be limited to approximately 2% of body weight per day while meeting requirements. Other factors in the dry cow ration also must be considered to prevent periparturient diseases such as milk fever and retained placenta.[159] Rations should be adequately supplemented with cobalt, the precursor of vitamin B_{12} that is a cofactor in the rate-limiting step in conversion of propionate (the primary glucose precursor) to succinyl-CoA. Nicotinic acid can be included in the rations of dry cows at 6 g/head/day and in the rations of early lactating cows at 12 g/head/day to help prevent hepatic lipidosis and ketosis. Recombinant bovine somatotropin has been used with diet changes to control fatty liver syndrome in dairy cattle.[160]

Nutrient requirements increase markedly for beef cattle during the third trimester of pregnancy; these requirements are listed in Chapter 9. As forage quality (digestibility) decreases, the time that feed material stays in the rumen increases (increased rumen turnover time). Therefore, as quality decreases, the maximum dry matter intake (DMI) decreases, which greatly decreases the maximum nutrient (energy) intake. This compounding effect of poor quality forage on maximum intake is particularly important for preventing hepatic lipidosis and the accompanying protein-energy malnutrition (PEM) of pregnant beef cattle in the winter. The approximate maximum DMI of forage of poor quality (oat straw, corn stover), medium quality (meadow grass hay), and excellent quality (alfalfa hay [25% crude fiber], corn silage) is 1% to 1.5%, 2%, and 2.5%, respectively. The environmental temperature can increase the energy needs of beef cattle on pasture or range; as the temperature falls from 20° C (68° F) to 10° C (50° F), approximately 10% more energy

is necessary for maintenance, and at freezing temperatures (0° C [32° F]), 20% additional energy is required. The key to preventing PEM and hepatic lipidosis in pregnant beef cattle is adequate body condition (body condition scores 5 to 7) entering the third trimester and availability of good to excellent quality forage in adequate amounts.

Preventing pregnancy toxemia and the associated severe hepatic lipidosis in ewes and does requires measures similar to those outlined for PEM in beef cattle. Both overconditioned and thin ewes and does in the third trimester of pregnancy are at increased risk. Because of the common occurrence of twins and triplets, nutrient requirements for pregnant ewes greatly accelerate during this period. Good to excellent quality forage for feeding sheep is very important. An additional tool for diagnosing underfeeding in ewes is measurement of plasma BHB. This test greatly facilitates assessment of nutritional inadequacy in pregnant ewes.[161] Plasma BHB concentrations of 0.8 mmol/L or higher are diagnostic of the need for increased energy consumption by pregnant ewes.[161] This clinicopathologic tool is of great benefit in diagnosing malnutrition before irreversible pregnancy toxemia develops.

The nutrient requirements of horses and ponies have been covered elsewhere (see Chapter 9). The presence of hyperlipidemia is readily detected and easily solved by increasing caloric intake. Although therapy of hyperlipemic ponies and horses is often unrewarding, the diagnosis is relatively straightforward, and prevention depends on providing adequate feed of good quality.

REFERENCES

127. Deem DA: Bovine fatty liver syndrome, *Compend Cont Educ Pract Vet* 11:S185-S191, 1985.
128. Stober M, Dirksen G: Lipomobilization syndrome (fatty degeneration syndrome) in the dairy cow, *Bovine Pract* 18:152-163, 1983.
129. Morrow DA: Fat cow syndrome, *J Dairy Sci* 59:1625-1629, 1976.
130. Cebra CK et al: Hepatic lipidosis in anorectic, lactating Holstein cattle: a retrospective study of serum biochemical abnormalities, *J Vet Intern Med* 11:231-237, 1997.
131. Gerry F: Serum bile acids as a test of liver function for cattle with hepatic lipidosis, *Proc ACVIM Forum* 7:672-675, 1989.
132. Rings DM: Hepatic lipidosis: mechanisms, diagnostics, and treatments, *Proceedings of the Twenty-second Annual Convention of the American Association of the Bovine Practice*, 1990, pp 19-23.
133. Reid IM: Incidence and severity of fatty liver in dairy cows, *Vet Rec* 107:281-284, 1980.
134. Perkins B: Body condition and fatty liver in dairy cows, PhD dissertation, Ithaca, NY, 1983, Cornell University.
135. Herdt TH et al: Test for estimation of bovine hepatic lipid content, *J Am Vet Med Assoc* 182:953-955, 1983.
136. Oetzel GR, Berger LL: Protein-energy malnutrition in domestic ruminants. II, Diagnosis, treatment, and prevention, *Compend Cont Educ Pract Vet* 8:S16-S21, 1986.
137. Hallford DM, Sansom DW: Serum profiles determined during ovine pregnancy toxemia, *Agri Pract* 4:27-33, 1983.
138. East NE: Pregnancy toxemia, abortions, and paraparturient diseases, *Vet Clin North Am (Large Anim Pract)* 5:601-603, 1983.
139. Naylor JM: Hyperlipemia and hyperlipidemia in horses, ponies, and donkeys, *Compend Cont Educ Pract Vet* 4:S321-S326, 1982.
140. Naylor JM, Kronfeld DS, Acland H: Hyperlipemia in horses: effects of undernutrition and disease, *Am J Vet Res* 41:899-905, 1980.

TABLE 31-10

Daily Nutrient Requirements for a 600-kg Cow During the Dry Period for Maintenance Plus the Last 2 Months of Gestation

Body Weight (kg)	NE$_1$ (Mcal)	TDN (kg)	Total CP (g)	Calcium (g)	Phosphorus (g)
600	12.61	5.55	<31	37	26

CP, Crude protein; *NE$_1$*, Net energy of lactation (same as net energy of maintenance) in dairy cows; *TDN*, total digestible nutrients.

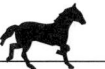

141. Watson TDG et al: Plasma lipids, lipoproteins, and lipases in ponies with hyperlipemia, *Equine Vet J* 24:341-346, 1992.
142. Thilstedt JP et al: Hyperlipemia in pony mares, *Mod Vet Pract* 63:467-470, 1982.
143. Cahill CF: Starvation, *Proc ACVIM Forum* 1:14-46, 1982.
144. Baird GD: Lipometabolism in the dairy cow: problems involved in meeting the demand of high productivity, *Bovine Pract* 17:147-149, 1982.
145. Holtenius P, Hjort M: Studies on the pathogenesis of fatty liver in cows, *Bovine Pract* 25:91, 1990.
146. Rayssinguier Y, Mazur A, Gueux E: Plasma lipoproteins and fatty liver in dairy cows, *Res Vet Sci* 45:389-393, 1988.
147. Uchida E, Katoh N, Takahashi K: Induction of fatty liver in cows by ethionine administration and concomitant decreases of serum apolipoproteins B-100 and A-1 concentrations, *Am J Vet Res* 53:2035-2042, 1992.
148. Van Saun R: Effects of undegradable protein supplementation fed prepartum on subsequent lactation, reproduction and health in Holstein dairy cattle, PhD dissertation, Ithaca, NY, 1992, Cornell University.
149. Berties SJ et al: Effect of prepartum dry matter intake on liver triglyceride concentration and early lactation, *J Dairy Sci* 75:1914-1922, 1992.
150. Reid IM, Stark HA, Isenor RN: Fasting and refeeding in the lactating dairy cow, *J Comp Pathol* 87:2141-2265, 1977.
151. Treachers RJ, Sansom BF: Liver function in dairy cows at parturition, *Res Vet Sci* 10:461-468, 1969.
152. West HJ: Liver function in dairy cows in late pregnancy and early lactation, *Bovine Pract* 25:127-130, 1990.
153. Ruegg PL et al: Relation among body condition score, milk production, and serum urea nitrogen and cholesterol concentrations in high-producing Holstein dairy cows in early lactation, *Am J Vet Res* 53:5-14, 1992.
154. Dawson RMC, Grime DW, Lindsay DB: On the insensitivity of sheep to the almost complete microbial destruction of dietary choline before alimentary tract absorption, *Biochem J* 196:499-505, 1981.
155. Gerloff BJ et al: Inositol and hepatic lipidosis. I. Effect of inositol supplementation and time from parturition on liver and serum lipids in dairy cattle, *J Anim Sci* 62:1682-1692, 1986.
156. Rings DM: Therapeutic consideration in ketosis and hepatic lipidosis in cattle, *Mod Vet Pract* 66:523-526, 1985.
157. Hidiroglou M, Hartin KE: Vitamins A, E, and selenium blood levels in the fat cow syndrome, *Can Vet J* 23:255-258, 1982.
158. National Research Council: *Nutrient requirements of dairy cattle*, ed 5, Washington, DC, 1978, National Academy Press.
159. Maas J: Prevention of retained placenta in dairy cattle, *Compend Cont Educ Pract Vet* 4:S519-S528, 1982.
160. Laven RA, Andrews AH: Control of fatty liver syndrome in a Jersey herd by a change of diet and the use of recombinant bovine somatotropin, *Vet Rec* 142:36-39, 1998.
161. Russel A: Nutrition of the pregnant ewe, *Vet Rec* 7(suppl):23-28, 1985.

CONGENITAL HYPERBILIRUBINEMIA

ERWIN G. PEARSON

GILBERT'S SYNDROME

Gilbert's syndrome is an unconjugated hyperbilirubinemia in the presence of normal erythrocyte life span. It occurs in 7% of human beings[162] and has been described in Southdown sheep.[163] Gilbert's syndrome involves a failure of unconjugated bilirubin to cross the liver cell membrane and be conjugated. This is most likely caused by a defect in carrier proteins or the conjugating enzyme or both.[164] Hepatic bilirubin clearance is about 30% of normal when tested with a loading dose of radiolabeled bilirubin.[165]

Affected Southdown sheep may have icterus or at least elevated plasma bilirubin levels, both conjugated and unconjugated. Affected sheep also cannot excrete BSP into the bile. No histopathologic lesions are present other than some pigment in the hepatocytes. The condition is inherited as an autosomal dominant trait in human beings.[162] The bile acid levels are normal in humans, but one sheep exhibited defects in hepatic bile acid clearance.[166]

DUBIN-JOHNSON SYNDROME

Dubin-Johnson syndrome is a failure of conjugated bilirubin to enter the bile canaliculi. This has been diagnosed sporadically in human beings and in Corriedale sheep.[167] There may be an impairment not only in bilirubin but also in the excretion of other conjugated organic anions. Sheep affected by this syndrome may be jaundiced or have hyperbilirubinemia. Both conjugated and unconjugated bilirubin are increased, and BSP clearance is delayed. Bile acids are reported to be normal in human beings, but delayed clearance was reported in three Corriedale sheep.[166] Histologically the hepatocytes contain a black, melanin-like pigment.[167]

PERSISTENT HYPERBILIRUBINEMIA IN THOROUGHBREDS

A persistent hyperbilirubinemia has been reported in a Thoroughbred race horse that had no evidence of liver damage, cholestasis, or hemolysis, and was not fasting.[168] The horse was persistently icteric, and had serum total bilirubin concentrations of 8.7 to 9.4 mg/dl. Ninety percent or more of the plasma bilirubin was the unconjugated form. The serum bile acid concentration, along with the liver enzymes GGT, AST, and SDH were within normal limits. The horse acted clinically normal, and the plasma FFA concentration was also within normal limits. The condition was similar to the human Crigler-Najjar type II syndrome, which involves a deficiency in the bilirubin-uridine diphosphate glucuronyl transferase needed to conjugate bilirubin, but this was not verified.

MISCELLANEOUS LIVER DISEASES

ERWIN G. PEARSON

TELANGIECTASIA

Telangiectasia, commonly known as "sawdust liver" in packing houses, is a focal degeneration in liver lobular circulation characterized by red-brown foci 1 to 5 mm in diameter. Microscopically hepatocytes are distorted, and sinusoids are congested.[169] It has been proposed that this may be caused by ischemia that occurs secondary to emboli or other vascular pathologic conditions, including part of the portal circulation, which supplies 60% to 80% of hepatic oxygen.[170] Clinical signs are not apparent with telangiectasia, but the condition results in condemnation of 1.7% to 2.1% of the livers of slaughtered cattle.

ISCHEMIA, HYPOXIA, AND CONGESTION

Ischemia and hypoxia can lead to death of hepatocytes, but less severe insults cause fatty infiltration, because lipoprotein synthesis depends on oxidative metabolism.[169] This damage is more apparent in the centrilobular areas that are the last to receive blood and oxygen.

Chronic passive congestion causes the grossly visible nutmeg liver. This is caused by the distention of the sinusoids and central veins with blood. The liver may be enlarged in these cases, but other signs related to the liver usually are not present. More significant findings are usually present in the cardiovascular system.

Portacaval shunts are rare in large domestic species but have been described in several foals.[171]

FETAL LIVER DAMAGE

The liver of the fetus may be damaged by infectious and toxic agents, but the result usually is abortion or birth of a weak neonate with signs related to other systems. The lesions in

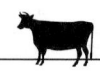

the liver may be diagnostic of the disease. Equine herpesvirus infection of the fetus causes hepatocyte necrosis with acidophilic intranuclear inclusion bodies in more than 50% of the hepatocytes. Cattle fetuses aborted because of infectious bovine rhinotracheitis may have some focal necrosis of the liver but not enough to be diagnostic.

NEOPLASIA

Neoplasia of the liver is uncommon in large domestic species. Metastasis of lymphosarcoma in cattle is the most common, but signs produced by growth in other organs such as the lymph nodes, abomasum, heart, uterus, or spinal cord are more predominant. Adenomas or adenocarcinomas of the liver have been reported, along with other metastatic tumors.[169] Only 0.011% of abattoir animals seen in one study had liver tumors.

FAILURE OF DRUG METABOLISM AND EXCRETION

A number of drugs are excreted by the liver and may have delayed clearance with hepatic insufficiency. These include antimicrobials such as chloramphenicol, erythromycin, and tetracycline. Chlorthiazide, most steroids, digitalis, morphine, many tranquilizers and anesthetic agents, and lecithin also are removed by the liver, and excretion may be reduced with hepatic insufficiency.[172]

REFERENCES

162. Berk PD: Bilirubin metabolism and the hereditary hyperbilirubinemias. In Berk JE, ed: *Bockus gastroenterology,* ed 4, vol 5, Philadelphia, 1985, WB Saunders.
163. Cornelius CE, Gronwall RR: Congenital photosensitivity and hyperbilirubinemia in Southdown sheep in the United States, *Am J Vet Res* 29:291-294, 1968.
164. Black M, Billing BH: Hepatic bilirubin UDP glucuronyltransferase activity in liver disease and Gilbert's syndrome, *N Engl J Med* 280:1266-1271, 1969.
165. Martin JF et al: Abnormal hepatic transport of indocyanine green in Gilbert's syndrome, *Gastroenterology* 70:385-391, 1979.
166. Engelking LR, Gronwall R: Bile acid clearance in sheep with hereditary hyperbilirubinemia, *Am J Vet Res* 40:1277-1280, 1979.
167. Arias IM, Bernstein L, Toffler R: Black liver disease in Corriedale sheep: a new mutant affecting hepatic excretory function, *J Clin Invest* 43:1249-1250, 1964.
168. Divers TJ et al: Persistent hyperbilirubinemia in a healthy thoroughbred horse, *Cornell Vet* 83:237-242, 1993.
169. Kelly WR: The liver and biliary system. In Jubb KVF, Kennedy PL, Palmer N, eds: *Pathology of domestic animals,* ed 3, vol 2, New York, 1985, Academic Press.
170. Jensen R et al: Ischemia: a cause of hepatic telangiectasis in cattle, *Am J Vet Res* 43:1436-1439, 1982.
171. Hillyer MH et al: Clinical signs and radiographic diagnosis of a portosystemic shunt in a foal, *Vet Rec* 132:457-460, 1993.
172. Iber FL: Normal pathologic physiology of the liver. In Sodman WA, Sodman TM, eds: *Sodman's pathologic physiology,* ed 6, Philadelphia, 1979, WB Saunders.

HEMOCHROMATOSIS

JOHN MAAS
ERWIN G. PEARSON

Hemochromatosis is a disorder caused by deposition of hemosiderin in the parenchymal cells, which causes tissue damage and dysfunction of the liver and other tissue. It is most commonly seen in human beings and mynah birds but has been described as a new disease of Salers cattle[173] and has been reported in three horses.[174] In humans there are a number of types, including idiopathic hemochromatosis, an autosomal recessive familial condition that involves increased iron stores, cirrhosis, and saturation of the iron transport capacity.[175] Both horses and cattle show increased

iron deposition in the liver. This is demonstrated on histopathologic examination of liver biopsy specimens by brown pigment that stains for iron in the hepatocytes and Kupffer cells. An increased concentration of iron can be measured in the liver, and fibrosis and liver-derived enzyme elevation are present.

In Salers cattle the condition appears to be a homozygous recessive condition more like the human familial type. Inappropriate absorption of iron (Fe) by the gastrointestinal tract occurs, with subsequent hepatic storage (Fe overload) and eventual loss of hepatic function. The primary clinical signs in cattle are decreased weight gains, poor body condition, dull hair coat, and diarrhea. Serum concentrations of liver enzymes are elevated, and marked hepatic fibrosis occurs, in addition to the hemosiderin deposits in the liver. The total serum Fe, Fe binding capacity (TIBC), and saturation of transferrin are increased similar to the familial disease in humans. The liver iron concentration rises above 5000 µg/g (ppm) on a wet basis (normal herd mates of affected cattle have a level of 84 to 100 ppm).[176]

Horses with hemochromatosis show evidence of liver disease as described on p. 790. Serum concentrations of the liver enzymes ALP, GGT, and AST are all elevated, and the serum total bile acid level is above 40 µmol/L. In the cases reported, the total serum iron level was not elevated, and unlike with the idiopathic human condition or the cattle cases, there is no saturation of the iron binding capacity. The total liver iron level has been as high as 6700 ppm (normal is 100 to 300 ppm).[174]

In human beings hemochromatosis is treated by reducing the iron stores by phlebotomies and removing blood. The one horse on which this was tried had very advanced disease and severe cirrhosis, and the animal succumbed a few days after the blood removal. Removal of 160 L of blood over 12 months failed to reduce the liver iron concentration in one heifer.[173] Deferoxamine is given to some human beings to induce a negative iron balance and reduce the rate at which iron accumulates, but there are no reports of its use in animals.

REFERENCES

173. House JK et al: Hemochromatosis in Salers cattle, *J Vet Intern Med* 8:105-111, 1994.
174. Pearson EG, Hedstrom OR, Poppengor RH: Equine hepatic cirrhosis associated with hemochromatosis, *J Am Vet Med Assoc* 204:1053-1056, 1994.
175. Holland KK, Spivak JL: Hemochromatosis, *Med Clin North Am* 73:831-845, 1989.
176. Smith BP: Idiopathic iron accumulation in the liver, *American Association of Bovine Practitioners Newsletter,* December, 1990.

GALLBLADDER AND BILIARY TRACT DISEASE

TERRY C. GERROS

Biliary tract disease in large animal medicine is rare and results from both intrahepatic and extrahepatic causes. Intrahepatic causes of cholestasis include cholangitis, cholecystitis, choledocholithiasis, or presence of a foreign body. Extrahepatic causes include abscess formation, inflammatory disease occurring near the common bile duct, or neoplasia.

CHOLEDOCHOLITHIASIS/CHOLELITHIASIS/ HEPATOLITHIASIS

By definition, cholelithiasis describes the presence of gallstones in either the bile ducts or gallbladder, whereas choledocholithiasis describes stones found in the common bile

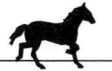

duct. Hepatolithiasis indicates the presence of gallstones in the intrahepatic bile ducts above the right and left hepatic ducts and are a variation of cholelithiasis. These conditions have been described in horses, cattle, sheep, and pigs; however, they do not seem to be recognized as a clinical problem in cattle and sheep.[177-195] Choledocholithiasis is the most common cause of biliary obstruction in large animals and occurs more frequently in horses.[177-188]

The pathogenesis of biliary stone formation is uncertain, but proposed mechanisms include ascariasis, ascending biliary infection or inflammation, biliary stasis, changes in bile composition, and presence of a foreign body.[180,194] Several pathogenic bacteria (*Salmonella* spp., *Escherichia coli*, *Aeromonas* spp., *Citrobacter* spp., group D *Streptococcus* spp.) have been cultured from the bile ducts of horses with cholelithiasis.[186,188,190,196] Whether these bacteria were the cause or the result of the stone formation remains unclear. In most reports the chemical analysis have shown that choleliths have a mixed composition containing bilirubin, bile pigments, cholesterol esters, esters of cholic and carboxylic acid, calcium phosphate, and sodium taurodeoxycholate.[178,180,186,188,190] In one study 80% of the choleliths contained less than 10% cholesterol.[190]

CLINICAL SIGNS, DIAGNOSTIC TESTS, AND DIFFERENTIAL DIAGNOSIS. Cholelithiasis should be suspected in horses when a triad of clinical signs exists, namely intermittent abdominal pain, pyrexia, and icterus. Hepatic encephalopathy, photosensitization, and weight loss are other, less common clinical features of cholelithiasis.[179-181,185,186,194,196] A subclinical presentation, caused by partial obstruction of the biliary tree, may be recognized only on postmortem examination.[191]

Elevations in the serum activity of ALP, AST, GGT, SDH (sorbitol dehydrogenase, also now named L-iditol dehydrogenase), and total bilirubin are associated with cholelithiasis.[179-181,186,190,194,196] The rise in total bilirubin is due to an elevation in both direct and indirect bilirubin. In the horse, cholestasis should be suspected if more than 30% of the total bilirubin is the direct type.[169] Serum bile acid concentrations also increase when bile flow is obstructed.[174] Other laboratory abnormalities that may be seen include hyperammonemia, increased urine bilirubin, and prolonged partial thromboplastin and thrombin times.[178,181,185,186,190] The most common alterations in the leukogram include a neutrophilic leukocytosis. Elevations in globulin and fibrinogen may also occur.[178-180,185]

Ultrasound examination of the liver is a safe, noninvasive tool for diagnosing cholelithiasis. Hepatomegaly and bile duct dilation are seen in horses with gallstones. The echogenicity of the hepatic parenchyma is increased compared with that of normal horses and may approach that of the spleen; the bile ducts are thick and distended.[188] The parallel channel sign (dilation of interhepatic biliary radicals adjacent to the portal vein) may also be seen.[188] Several choleliths generally are seen, but a single stone may be present. Choleliths may be hyperechoic, casting acoustic shadows, or they may be sonolucent.[188] The area of the liver where choleliths are most likely to be visualized is in the cranioventral part of the right hepatic lobe, especially in the sixth to eighth intercostal spaces.[188] Cholelithiasis can accurately be diagnosed by ultrasound in at least 75% of horses if an adequate scanning image of the liver is obtained and bile duct dilation and choleliths are visualized.[188]

The differential diagnosis for a horse with the clinical signs associated with cholelithiasis includes other causes of liver disease and mild, recurrent abdominal discomfort, including verminous arteritis, mesenteric abscesses, enterolithiasis, abdominal neoplasia, and urolithiasis.[179]

NECROPSY FINDINGS. At necropsy hepatomegaly is usually noted, although a shrunken liver may be observed. The liver is firmer than normal, has a consistent texture, and varies in color from red to green-brown. The hepatic ducts and common bile duct are generally dilated and may contain the calculi. Histologically periportal fibrosis is a common finding. Bile duct stasis and hyperplasia are usually noted; suppurative cholangitis is less common.[178,190,194,196]

Treatment of cholelithiasis includes relief of biliary flow obstruction and management of hepatitis and associated complications. Choledocholithotomy and choledocholithotripsy, described in horses, have had limited success.[185-187] Because the potential for bacteremia with surgical manipulation for cholelithiasis is high, treatment with potentiated sulfa drugs, ampicillin, tetracycline, or chloramphenicol before surgical intervention is warranted. In human beings chenodeoxycholate or ursodeoxycholate is used to dissolve cholesterol gallstones.[198] There are no reports of their use in animals. Dietary management for cholelithiasis has yet to be determined. The prognosis remains guarded for horses with cholelithiasis or choledocholithiasis.

DISEASES OF THE GALLBLADDER

TERRY C. GERROS

CHOLANGITIS

Clinical disease of the bovine gallbladder is rare. Obstructive gallbladder disease has been associated with abdominal fat necrosis, choleliths, fascioliasis, foreign bodies, hepatic abscesses, neoplasia, and suppurative cholecystitis.[199,200] Adenomas and adenocarcinomas, the most common tumors found in the gallbladder, papillomas, and lymphosarcoma, although rare, can cause obstruction.[199,201] Rupture of the gallbladder was found on necropsy of a cow in which icterus, anorexia, decreased milk production, and diarrhea were present.[202]

Cholangitis is considered the most common cause of bile duct obstruction in large animals and has also been observed in horses with chronic active liver disease. Clinical signs associated with cholangitis in the horse may include anorexia, subtle behavioral changes, chronic weight loss, colic, and icterus. Alterations in hepatic enzyme activity may indicate either hepatocellular damage or cholestasis or both. Histopathologic examination and bacterial culture are indicated to further identify the causative agent. In cases of suspected bacterial etiology, antibiotic therapy is indicated. The antibiotic choice should be based on bacterial sensitivity; however, in cases in which no bacterial organism is identified, an antibiotic that is secreted or cleared in the bile is warranted.

Several foreign bodies have been recovered from the biliary tract, including grain, nails, sticks, stones, and sand. Retrograde motion of the intestine may have allowed these foreign bodies to enter the duodenal papilla and become lodged.

CHOLANGIOHEPATITIS

Cholangiohepatitis has been reported both as a primary disease and as occurring secondary to cholelithiasis, duodenal inflammation, intestinal obstruction, neoplasia, parasitism, and certain toxins.[203] Sporidesmin, a fungal toxin from *Pithomyces chartarum*, causes cholangiohepatitis in cattle and sheep.[204] Horses with cholangiohepatitis, either primary or secondary, may show anorexia, icterus, pyrexia, and intermittent signs of colic.[194,203] Biochemical analysis revealing elevated cholestatic and hepatocellular enzyme activity and conjugated hyperbilirubinemia, combined with an inflammatory leukogram, support a diagnosis of cholangiohepatitis.

REFERENCES

177. Pearson EG: Clinical management of the icteric horse, *Compend Cont Educ Pract Vet* 4:S114-S122, 1982.
178. Traub JL et al: Cholelithiasis in four horses, *J Am Vet Med Assoc* 181:59-62, 1982.
179. Scarratt WK, Saunders GF, Fessler RL: Cholelithiasis and biliary obstruction in a horse, *Compend Cont Educ Pract Vet* 7:S428-S431, 1985.
180. McDole MG: Cholelithiasis in a horse, *Equine Pract* 2:37-40, 1980.
181. Roussel AJ, Becht JL, Adams SB: Choledocholithiasis in a horse, *Cornell Vet* 74:166-171, 1984.
182. Van der Luer RJT, Kroneman J: Three cases of cholelithiasis and biliary fibrosis in the horse, *Equine Vet J* 14:251-253, 1982.
183. Naus MJA, Jones BR: Cholelithiasis and choledocholithiasis in a cat, *NZ Vet J* 26:160-161, 1978.
184. Nelson NC, Piker JF, Welsh RA: Cholelithiasis in a dog, *J Am Vet Med Assoc* 152:47-50, 1968.
185. Tulleners EP et al: Choledocholithotripsy in a mare, *J Am Vet Med Assoc* 186:1317-1319, 1985.
186. Traub JL et al: Surgical removal of choleliths in a horse, *J Am Vet Med Assoc* 182:714-716, 1983.
187. Green DS, Davies JV: Successful choledocholithotomy in a horse, *Equine Vet J* 21:464-467, 1989.
188. Reef VB et al: Ultrasonographic findings in horses with cholelithiasis: eight cases (1985-1987), *J Am Vet Med Assoc* 196:1836-1840, 1990.
189. Dickson J, Nottle MC, White JB: Sand impaction of the bile duct of a sheep, *Aust Vet J* 60:64, 1983.
190. Johnson JK et al: Cholelithiasis in horses: ten cases (1982-1986), *J Am Vet Med Assoc* 194:405-409, 1989.
191. Petruzzi J et al: Spontaneous cholelithiasis in sheep: prevalence survey and analysis of gallstones and bile, *J Comp Pathol* 98:367-369, 1988.
192. Shumard RF, Eveleth DF: Choleliths in a ewe, *Vet Med* 50:217, 1955.
193. Holland PS, Schmitz DG, Read WK: Hepatolithiasis in an Arabian mare, *Equine Vet J* 23:229-232, 1991.
194. Gerros TC et al: Choledocholithiasis attributable to a foreign body in a horse, *J Am Vet Med Assoc* 202:301-303, 1993.
195. Ford EJH: A case of biliary calculus and jaundice in a cow, *Vet Rec* 67:634-635, 1955.
196. Moens Y: Cholelithiasis associated with partial liver atrophy in a horse, *Vlaams Diergeneeskd Tijdschr* 59:230-233, 1990.
197. Pearson EG, Craig AM: Serum bile acids for diagnosis of chronic liver disease in horses, *Proc Fourth Annu Vet Med Forum Am Coll Vet Intern Med* 2:71-75, 1986.
198. Malet PF, Soloway RD: Diseases of the gallbladder and bile ducts. In Wyngaarden JB, Smith LH, eds: *Cecil's textbook of medicine*, ed 18, Philadelphia, 1988, WB Saunders.
199. Haaland MA et al: Bovine leukosis involving the gallbladder in a dairy cow, *Vet Med Small Anim Clin* 78:403-405, 1983.
200. Tulleners EP: Empyema of the gallbladder in a cow, *J Am Vet Med Assoc* 182:410-412, 1983.
201. Anderson WA, Monlux AW, Davis CL: Epithelial tumors of the bovine gallbladder: a report of 18 cases, *Am J Vet Res* 19:58-65, 1958.
202. Grymer J, Coy CH: Ruptured gallbladder as the cause of bovine jaundice, *Vet Med Small Anim Clin* 78:947-948, 1983.
203. Schulz KS, Simmons TR, Johnson R: Primary cholangiohepatitis in a horse, *Cornell Vet* 80:35-40, 1990.
204. Kelly WR: Cholangiohepatitis. In Jubb KVF, Kennedy PC, Palmer N, eds: *Pathology of domestic animals*, ed 3, Orlando, Fla, 1985, Academic Press.

TREATMENT OF LIVER FAILURE

THOMAS J. DIVERS

Hepatic failure usually is treated medically and supportively, although in a few instances surgery may be indicated. Therapy is best indicated in cases of acute liver failure without chronic fibrosis, such as with serum hepatitis or suppurative cholangitis, because these animals have the best long-term prognosis for regeneration. The prognosis is generally poor if severe hepatoencephalopathy (HE) or hemolysis or severe acidosis or diarrhea is present. The initial therapy for hepatic failure should be directed toward any abnormal behavior (HE) the patient may be exhibiting.[205] HE is a metabolically induced, potentially reversible, functional disorder of the brain. The pathophysiologic mechanisms of HE are undoubtedly complex but are mostly due to abnormal protein metabolism.[206,207] Cerebral edema is characteristic of HE. Complex interactions of both excitatory and inhibitory neurotransmitters determine if the patient is depressed or maniacal.

If the animal is extremely agitated or convulsing, sedation should be accomplished before attempting further therapy. Xylazine provides adequate sedation in most cases and is the drug of choice for horses with maniacal behavior caused by HE. Most sedatives and tranquilizers are metabolized by the liver, therefore their use should be kept to a minimum and doses of xylazine that cause marked lowering of the head or abnormally low respiration should be avoided. Diazepam should be avoided with hepatoencephalopathy, because it may enhance the effect of GABA on inhibitory neurons and worsen the signs of hepatoencephalopathy.[208] The use of the benzodiazepine-receptor antagonist flumazenil has been reported to temporarily lessen the signs of hepatoencephalopathy in human beings.[209] The overall success of flumazenil in treating HE in humans and dogs has been low, and it has rarely been used in the horse. Sarmazenil, which has a different mechanism of action, appears to be more promising for reversing signs of HE in some humans.[210] After chemical restraint of the animal has been achieved, therapy can be directed at the physiologic events that may be causing the hepatoencephalopathy. If the blood glucose concentration is low, 0.2-0.4 ml/kg of a 10% glucose solution should be administered intravenously. This may result in a dramatic alleviation of the clinical signs of HE in a few cases (e.g., Theiler's and Tyzzer's diseases). Therapeutic measures directed toward decreasing the blood ammonia concentration also are indicated. These include oral administration of neomycin at a dosage of 10 to 30 mg/kg two or four times daily for 1 or 2 days, either alone or in combination with lactulose (90 to 120 ml PO per adult horse 3 or 4 times daily) or acetic acid (0.5 ml/kg PO two times daily).[211,212] Lactulose, a carbohydrate, is poorly absorbed from the small intestine and in the large intestine may reduce the colonic pH and enteric ammonia concentration. Vinegar (acetic acid) should do the same. Metronidazole (10 to 15 mg/kg twice daily) may also be used to reduce the number of ammonia-producing bacteria but is not preferred because it is metabolized by the liver and signs of toxicity may mimic HE. Nasogastric intubation should be performed with care, because excessive trauma to the nasal cavity, esophagus, or stomach may result in severe and prolonged hemorrhage, swallowing of blood, and worsening of the hepatoencephalopathy. For that reason, I prefer to administer oral drugs by dose syringe mixed with molasses and Karo syrup. Neomycin administration should not be prolonged, because this may have a toxic effect on the intestinal mucosa[213] and cause severe diarrhea in some horses. Some clinicians prefer not to treat with oral drugs that affect intestinal flora but rather to rely mainly on a low-protein diet.

Acidosis may be severe in many horses with hepatic failure, but attempts at correction must be made slowly.[211] Too rapid an increase in pH may exacerbate the hepatoencephalopathy. I recommend bicarbonate therapy only when the venous pH is below 7.1 and intravenous therapy with an alkalizing balanced electrolyte fluid has failed to improve the acidosis. The prognosis is poor in horses that maintain persistent acidosis. It is of utmost importance that dehydration be corrected with a balanced electrolyte solution (preferably without lactate), 20 to 50 g/L of dextrose, and supplemental potassium (20 to 40 mEq/L). Additional potassium should be given orally (5 to 20 g twice daily). Maintaining potassium intake is important because a low potassium level results in increased production and absorption of ammonia

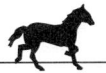

from the kidney.[214] Urine dipstick or plasma glucometer measurements (or both) should be used to monitor the glucose concentration. Although most adult horses with hepatic failure have a normal blood glucose concentration, it is important to supplement the fluids with glucose unless the animal is hyperglycemic. Glucose decreases the ammonia concentration, reduces the need for reliance on catabolic gluconeogenesis, decreases protein catabolism, and spares the hepatic energy consumed in hepatic gluconeogenesis. However, it is very important that glucose not be given as the sole source of fluid. Polycythemia may be relatively unresponsive in some cases of hepatic failure and should not be used as the primary guide for judging adequate fluid therapy. Fresh or fresh-frozen plasma can be used to increase colloidal oncotic pressure, clotting factor transport proteins, and antiproteases. Stored whole blood should not be used because the ammonia levels may be high. Hetastarch also should not be used in hepatic failure.

Antioxidant, antiinflammatory and antiedema therapy may be useful in some cases of acute hepatic disease and failure. Dimethyl sulfoxide (DMSO), acetylcysteine, vitamin E and mannitol are antioxidant or antiedema drugs that may be useful.[215] Antiinflammatory therapy should include flunixin meglumine and pentoxifylline (7.5 mg/kg PO every 12 hours). Horses with acute hepatic failure that cannot be controlled by the above therapy require extracorpeal liver support systems. Although these have not been used in the horse, dialysis, charcoal adsorption, or plasma exchange methods are available.[216]

Treatment of ponies with hyperlipemia is covered in the section on hepatic lipidosis on p. 812. If the hyperlipemia is thought to be associated with a pituitary adenoma, treatment with pergolide (1 to 5 mg/day) is warranted and may be successful. Hyperlipidemia may also occur in horses in late pregnancy associated with diarrhea or azotemia or both.[217] If the pony or horse is in late pregnancy, it may be advisable to abort the mare.[218] Fatty liver in ruminants is discussed on p. 810. Hepatic failure in cattle associated with septic metritis or mastitis and in those with biliary obstruction from hepatic abscesses often can be treated successfully by forced feeding (e.g., alfalfa gruel, electrolytes) and systemic antibiotics.[219] Treatment of hepatic fascioliasis is discussed on p. 808.

Animals with hepatic disease that maintain a fair appetite often are best treated by dietary management. Dietary management is important in the recovery of animals with acute hepatitis or hepatopathy and in prolonging life in cases with chronic hepatic disease. Energy and protein requirements (especially branched-chain amino acids in the horse) should be met. An example of a reasonable diet is one part beet pulp with one-quarter to one-half parts cracked corn mixed with molasses four to six times daily. Milo or sorghum may also be used as a grain mix. Small meals given frequently are ideal because of difficulties with gluconeogenesis and insulin regulation. Sorghum, oat hay, or grass hay may be substituted for beet pulp. If the horse will not eat, forced feeding should be considered, but nosebleeds should be avoided. An oral paste with a high branched-chain to aromatic amino acid ratio can be formulated or purchased for forced feeding.[220] Vitamin B_1, folic acid, vitamin K_1 or fresh plasma transfusion might be indicated with chronic biliary obstruction. Grazing of mixed grasses is permitted and should be encouraged as long as affected horses can be protected from sunlight. Spring-cut hay or grass should be limited, because these can be very high in protein. Alfalfa is generally high in protein and is best avoided except in cows that seem to be more tolerant of high-protein feeds. It is important that a horse with hepatic failure eat something, even if it is not one of the more desirable feeds mentioned above.

Bactericidal antibiotic therapy is indicated for horses with bacterial cholangitis and in cattle with liver abscesses. A diagnosis of suppurative bacterial cholangitis usually is made before the organism or its antibiogram is known. Therefore broad-spectrum aerobic drug therapy such as a combination of ampicillin and gentamycin, trimethoprim-sulfa, ceftiofur, or enrofloxacin is preferred for the initial therapy. Anaerobic organisms may also be involved, and metronidazole can be added to any of the above. Antimicrobial therapy can be adjusted if the offending organism can be identified from a liver biopsy. Gram-negative enteric organisms are usually the causative organisms, and in my experience only 50% or fewer are sensitive to trimethoprim/ sulfa. This is unfortunate, because prolonged antibacterial therapy (2 weeks to 3 months) usually is required for suppurative cholangitis.[221] Ultrasound examination is important in treating equine suppurative cholangitis, because some cases are associated with biliary stones, which makes the treatment more difficult and worsens the prognosis. If small obstructing stones or sludge is present, DMSO (0.5 to 1 g/kg given intravenously for 3 to 5 days) may help dissolve the calcium bilirubinate stones or debris.[222] Intravenously administered crystalloids may also thin secretions and promote bile flow. Ursodeoxycholic acid, a commercially prepared bile acid, is used for a variety of chronic biliary disorders in human beings and small animals and induces choleresis. The benefit of this drug in horses has not been proven, and safety is a concern because rabbits, which have a gastrointestinal system similar to that of the horse, metabolize this bile acid into noxious bile acids.[223] If a large obstructing stone is present, surgery is indicated.

Cattle with singular or multiple liver abscesses often respond to penicillin therapy, but long-term therapy is required, and there is a significant rate of recurrence of clinical signs after therapy is withdrawn. Small to medium abscesses that are echolucent have the best prognosis. Abscesses with an echodense appearance are difficult to treat. Single large abscesses are best treated by surgical drainage, especially those that interfere with vagal nerve function. High levels of intravenous penicillin and an aminoglycoside should be administered to foals suspected of having Tyzzer's disease. Penicillin in high dosages or metronidazole, or both, should also be used to treat suspected anaerobic abscesses of the liver. Foals with salmonellosis should be given antimicrobial therapy based on culture and sensitivity results from previously affected foals on the same farm and from the results of blood and fecal cultures of the affected foal.

Surgery may be indicated as part of the therapy for liver failure in foals with duodenal stricture or in horses with colonic displacements (usually 180 degrees volvulus) that result in biliary obstruction. Foals and calves with portosystemic shunts require surgical repair if desirable growth and performance are expected.[224] Surgery for cholelithiasis is indicated for an obstructing stone unless diffuse fibrosis is already present. Cattle with a single, large hepatic abscess or calves with an umbilical vein hepatic abscess are best treated by surgical drainage.

Horses thought to have chronic active hepatitis with bridging necrosis that is not believed to be associated with a bacterial infection may be given corticosteroids or colchicine (0.03 mg/kg PO every 24 hours), but the therapeutic benefits of these drugs appear to be variable. If steroids are used, 200 mg of prednisolone given orally daily for the adult horse is recommended.

REFERENCES
205. Tennant BC, Hornbuckle WE: Diseases of the liver. In Anderson NV, ed: *Veterinary gastroenterology*, Philadelphia, 1980, Lea & Febiger.

206. Hazell AS, Butterworth RF: Hepatic encephalopathy: an update of pathophysiologic mechanisms, *Proc Soc Exp Biol Med* 222(2):99-112, 1999.
207. Jones EA, Basile AS: Does ammonia contribute to increased GABA-ergic neurotransmission in liver failure? *Metab Brain Dis* 13(4):351-360, 1998.
208. Jones EA et al: The gamma-aminobutyric acid A (GABAA) receptor complex and hepatic encephalopathy, *Ann Intern Med* 110(7):532-545, 1989.
209. Grimm G et al: Improvement of hepatic encephalopathy treated with flumazenil, *Lancet* 2:1392-1394, 1988.
210. Meyer HP et al: Improvement of chronic hepatic encephalopathy in dogs by the benzodiazepine-receptor partial inverse agonist sarmazenil but not by the antagonist flumazenil, *Metab Brain Dis* 13(3):241-251, 1998.
211. Divers TJ: Liver disease and liver failure in horses, Proceedings of the Twenty-Ninth Annual Convention of the American Association of Equine Practitioners, Las Vegas, 1983.
212. Muting D: Therapy of hepatic insufficiency, *Fortschr Med* 95(32):1937-1941, 1997.
213. Ratnaike RN, Jones TE: Mechanisms of drug-induced diarrhea in the elderly, *Drugs Aging* 13(3):245-253, 1998.
214. Muting D, Reikowski J: Hepatic coma: principles of pathogenesis and treatment. II, Treatment, prognosis, *Fortschr Med* 101(39):1766-1773, 1983.
215. Buck R: The hydroxyl radical scavengers dimethylsulfoxide and dimethylthiourea protects rats against thioacetamide-induced fulminant hepatic failure, *J Hepatol* 31(1):27-38, 1999.
216. McLaughlin BE et al: Overview of extracorporeal liver support systems and clinical results, *Ann N Y Acad Sci* 875:310-325, 1999.
217. Naylor JM: Hyperlipemia. In Robinson NE, ed: *Current therapy in equine medicine*, Philadelphia, 1987, WB Saunders.
218. Jeffcott LB, Field JR: Current concepts of hyperlipaemia in horses and ponies, *Vet Rec* 116:461-466, 1985.
219. Sweeney RW et al: Hepatic failure in dairy cattle following mastitis or metritis, *J Vet Intern Med* 2(2):80-84, 1988.
220. Gulick BA et al: Effect of pyrrolizine alkaloid–induced hepatic disease on plasma amino acid patterns in the horse, *Am J Vet Res* 41:1894, 1980.
221. Peek SF, Divers TJ: Medical treatment of cholangiohepatitis and cholelithiasis in adult horses: nine cases (1991-1998), *Equine Vet J* 32:301-306, 2000.
222. Igimi H: DMSO as a direct solubilizer of calcium bilirubinate stones, *Hepatogastroenterology* 41(1):65-69, 1994.
223. Miyai K et al: Hepatotoxicity of bile acids in rabbits: urodeoxycholic acid is less toxic than chenodeoxycholic acid, *Lab Invest* 46:428, 1982.
224. Fortier LA et al: Guidelines for the diagnosis and surgical correction of equine and bovine congenital portosystemic shunts, *Vet Surg* 22(5):379, 1993.

PANCREATIC DISEASE

TERRY C. GERROS

Pancreatic disease is rare in both cattle and horses. In the horse, acute and chronic disease has been reported, whereas only chronic disease has been reported in cattle.

Recognized causes of pancreatitis include migrating parasites; bacterial and viral infections; immune-mediated damage; biliary or pancreatic duct inflammatory disease; deficiencies of vitamin E or A, selenium, and methionine; and vitamin D toxicity.[225-228] Drugs known to induce pancreatitis in human beings that are used frequently in horses include furosemide, tetracycline, estrogen, and certain corticosteroids and sulfonamides.[225-227] The cause of acute pancreatitis in the horse is unknown. The final common pathway may be due to autodigestion by activated enzymes, but the exact mechanism remains speculative.

The clinical signs associated with acute pancreatitis are not specific. The characteristic clinical features are moderate to severe abdominal pain, gastric reflux, hypovolemic shock, and cardiovascular compromise.[225,228-230] Gastric distension accounts for the pain and gastric reflux associated with acute pancreatitis. Hypovolemic shock, which occurs secondary to fluid losses into the peritoneal cavity and bowel lumen, is caused by release of vasoactive substances from the pancreas. Tachycardia, tachypnea, prolonged capillary refill, and congested mucous membranes result from hypovolemia and cardiovascular compromise.

Laboratory confirmation of pancreatic disease is difficult and not routinely attempted. Unfortunately the diagnosis usually is confirmed on histologic evaluation of the pancreas after necropsy. Laboratory tests that may be of value in the diagnosis of pancreatitis in the horse include measuring serum amylase and lipase activity, peritoneal fluid (PF) amylase concentrations, and fractional excretion of amylase.[228] Serum amylase values for normal horses range from 14 to 35 IU/L (mean 21 ± 6), whereas PF values range from 0 to 14 U/L (mean 5 ± 4).[231] Elevations of pancreatic enzyme activity are difficult to interpret, because the enzymes may be elevated in horses with proximal enteritis, colic, primary renal failure, and damage to intestinal mucosal cells, as well as in pancreatitis.[228,231,232] Clinical cases documented at necropsy had serum amylase activity over 700 IU/L; this magnitude of elevation may be helpful in differentiating acute pancreatitis from other causes. In acute pancreatitis, PF fluid amylase levels are higher than serum levels.[232]

Medical management of acute pancreatitis is symptomatic. Prevention of gastric rupture by continuous gastric decompression and control of abdominal pain are crucial in the treatment of pancreatitis.[227] Large volumes of balanced polyionic electrolyte solutions are necessary to maintain the circulating volume and prevent shock. Hypocalcemia is a possible problem, therefore the serum calcium concentrations should be monitored. Broad-spectrum antibiotics are warranted because of the potential for secondary bacterial infection.

Chronic interstitial pancreatitis (CIP) in horses and cattle seldom has clinical significance. In horses, *Strongylus equinus* and *Strongylus edentatus* are most commonly identified as the etiologic agent of CIP; however, *Parascaris equorum* has been identified in one case report.[227,233,234] In cattle CIP has been primarily associated with the trematodes *Eurytrema pancreaticum* and *Eurytrema coelomaticum*; these parasites have not been isolated in the United States.[232]

Reports of pancreatic disease in adult cattle have been limited to endocrine dysfunction.[235-237] The most commonly reported disorder is type I diabetes mellitus; however, the etiology in most cases is not determined.[235-237] Histopathologic examination generally reveals an absence of β-cells in the islet tissue. Foot-and-mouth disease virus has been associated with diabetes mellitus in cattle following convalescence.[232] Hypoplasia of the acinar pancreatic tissue has been described in calves.[232] Clinical signs include steatorrhea and diarrhea. Adenocarcinoma of the exocrine pancreas is reported in rare cases in the horse and should be considered in cases exhibiting the clinical signs of pyrexia, depression, weight loss, and icterus.[226,238,239]

Pancreatic calculi found in older cattle (over 5 years old) during necropsy are considered incidental findings.[232,240] The calculi are composed primarily of calcium carbonate and calcium phosphate. Their presence may be associated with grazing on silica-rich soil, vitamin A deficiency, or chronic inflammation of the pancreatic ducts.[232]

REFERENCES

225. Lilley CW, Beeman GM: Gastric dilatation associated with acute necrotizing pancreatitis, *Equine Pract* 3:8-15, 1981.
226. Furr MO, Robertson J: Two cases of equine pancreatic disease and a review of the literature, *Equine Vet Educ* 4:55-58, 1992.
227. Hamir AN: Verminous pancreatitis in a horse, *Vet Rec* 121:301-302, 1987.
228. McClure JJ: Acute pancreatitis. In Robinson NE, ed: *Current therapy in equine medicine*, Philadelphia, 1987, WB Saunders.
229. Nyack B et al: Abdominal crisis in a horse, *Equine Pract* 4:35-40, 1982.
230. Baker RH: Acute necrotizing pancreatitis in a horse, *J Am Vet Med Assoc* 172:268-270, 1978.
231. Parry BW, Crisman MV: Serum and peritoneal fluid amylase and lipase reference values in horses, *Equine Vet J* 23:390-391, 1991.

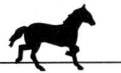

232. Jubb KVF: The pancreas. In Jubb KVF, Kennedy PC, Palmer N, eds: *Pathology of domestic animals,* ed 4, New York, 1993, Harcourt.
233. Bulgin MS, Anderson BC: Verminous arteritis and pancreatic necrosis with diabetes mellitus in a pony, *Compend Cont Educ* 5(suppl):482-485, 1983.
234. Collobert C et al: Chronic pancreatitis associated with diabetes mellitus in a standardbred racehorse, *Equine Vet Sci* 10:58-61, 1990.
235. Kaneko JJ, Rhode EA: Diabetes mellitus in a cow, *J Am Vet Med Assoc* 144:367-373, 1964.
236. Mostaghni K, Ivoghli B: Diabetes mellitus in the bovine, *Cornell Vet* 67:24-28, 1977.
237. Baker JS, Jackson HD, Sommers EL: Diabetes mellitus in a 4-year-old pregnant Holstein, *Compend Cont Educ* 5(suppl):328-331, 1983.
238. Kerr OM, Pearson GR, Rice DA: Pancreatic adenocarcinoma in a donkey, *Equine Vet J* 14:338-339, 1982.
239. Church S, West HJ, Baker JR: Two cases of pancreatic adenocarcinoma in horses, *Equine Vet J* 19:77-79, 1987.
240. Collins JP, Dromey MF: Pancreatic lithiasis in a shorthorn cow, *Irish Vet J* 30:69-71, 1976.

Diseases of the Renal System

HAROLD C. SCHOTT II
DAVID C. Van METRE
THOMAS J. DIVERS
Consulting Editors

EQUINE RENAL SYSTEM

ACUTE RENAL FAILURE

THOMAS J. DIVERS

Acute renal failure (ARF) in the horse is usually a consequence of exposure to nephrotoxins or vasomotor nephropathy (e.g., hypoperfusion or ischemia). The most common pathologic lesion with ARF is acute tubular necrosis (ATN).

TOXIC NEPHROPATHIES

Aminoglycosides

Administration of aminoglycoside antibiotics is one of the most common causes, if not the most common cause, of ATN in the horse. Neomycin is the most nephrotoxic of the aminoglycosides, followed by gentamicin, kanamycin, and amikacin (all three of similar toxicity), with streptomycin being the least nephrotoxic. The aminoglycoside antibiotics exert their toxic effect by accumulating within proximal tubular epithelial cells. Their entrance into the tubular epithelial cell is thought to be via urine, after filtration through the glomerulus.[1] Once toxic amounts are sequestered within the cell, cellular metabolism is disrupted and tubular cell swelling, death, and sloughing into the tubular lumen occur. Release of lysosomal enzymes and intracellular accumulation of calcium are likely involved in cell death.

Most cases of aminoglycoside nephrotoxicity are not the result of overdosing of the drug or administration of the to

drug to an azotemic patient.[2] The healthy kidney can usually tolerate a single major overdose (i.e., 10 times the normal amount) without detrimental effects. Toxicity is almost always the cumulative effect of repeated administration of aminoglycosides. Nephrotoxicity typically develops after several days of aminoglycoside administration to horses with diarrhea or septicemia that are not adequately hydrated[3] or because of other factors that may exacerbate a decrease in renal perfusion (e.g., concurrent treatment with nonsteroidal antiinflammatory drugs [NSAIDs]). Prolonged administration (>10 days) of aminoglycoside antibiotics without monitoring of aminoglycoside trough concentrations or serum creatinine concentration is a common history with aminoglycoside nephrotoxicity in the horse. Gentamicin or amikacin may be safely administered for longer than 10 days if the patient is adequately hydrated and appropriate trough concentrations and creatinine concentration are maintained. With regard to the latter, experimental induction of gentamicin nephrotoxicity in ponies was reflected by a rather small increase (0.3 mg/dl) in creatinine.[4] Although it has not been proven that the neonatal equine kidney is more susceptible to aminoglycoside toxicity than the adult kidney, sick foals appear to be at greater risk for aminoglycoside nephrotoxicity.[5] This apparently greater risk may simply reflect an increased incidence of septicemia in sick neonates and longer courses of treatment with aminoglycosides. Nevertheless, special attention (close monitoring of trough concentrations and creatinine) should be given to premature or young foals that are being treated with aminoglycoside antibiotics.[6]

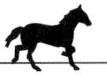

When aminoglycosides are administered to high-risk patients (those with concurrent dehydration or neonates), volume deficits must be replaced and serum trough concentrations or creatinine should be monitored frequently. It is rare for aminoglycoside nephrotoxicity to develop in horses receiving appropriate fluid therapy. Increased urinary sodium excretion and fluid diuresis appear to have a protective effect on the kidney. In contrast, hypokalemia (or total body potassium depletion) and low calcium intake may predispose horses to aminoglycoside nephrotoxicity by decreasing urine output.[7] Supplementation with oral electrolytes (e.g., 1 to 2 oz of NaCl and KCl daily) may be of benefit to horses being treated with aminoglycoside antibiotics by increasing water intake and urine output and by replacing potassium deficits in anorectic horses. In contrast, furosemide should not be administered prophylactically in an attempt to prevent aminoglycoside nephrotoxicity.[8] The recent shift to once daily aminoglycoside dosing, compared with previous dosing of aminoglycosides 2 to 3 times daily, has become a standard practice that likely reduces the potential for nephrotoxicity (by ensuring a longer period of the day with appropriate serum trough concentrations) but still provides a similar therapeutic response.[9-12] In patients with prerenal azotemia that receive aminoglycoside antibiotics, it is important to monitor creatinine closely and to consider prolonging the interval between drug administration until volume deficits are corrected. However, because nephrotoxicity is a cumulative effect of repeated dosing, delay of administration of the initial dose of an aminoglycoside pending rehydration of a critical patient (e.g., a septic neonate or a markedly dehydrated horse) is unwarranted.

Aminoglycoside nephrotoxicity should be considered in horses that become inexplicably depressed and inappetent while being treated with aminoglycosides or within a few days after aminoglycoside therapy is discontinued. Renal failure can develop even after the drug is withdrawn; thus monitoring renal function 2 to 4 days after discontinuing aminoglycoside therapy may be advised in high-risk patients. Polyuria may be observed before the onset of depression and anorexia or, if the patient becomes oliguric, mild stranguria and repeated posturing to urinate may be observed. A tentative diagnosis of nephrotoxicity is based on history of aminoglycoside use and supportive laboratory data. Abnormal laboratory findings associated with tubular damage that may be detected before onset of azotemia include enzymuria and cylindruria.[4,13] Although these parameters can be monitored for early detection of tubular injury, their finding does not necessarily indicate if or when aminoglycosides should be discontinued or to what degree the interval of administration should be prolonged.[14]

When ARF from aminoglycoside use develops, it is usually manifested as nonoliguric to polyuric renal failure and outcome is generally favorable as long as the duration of ARF is not prolonged and other underlying disease processes can be corrected. Peritoneal or pleural dialysis, plasmapheresis, or hemodialysis might be considered as methods to lower serum concentrations of nephrotoxic agents and uremic toxins; however, the amounts removed by a single use of some of these therapies are small and generally not worthy of pursuit in horses with nephrotoxic renal failure.[15]

Pigment Nephropathy

Acute tubular necrosis and development of ARF consequent to rhabdomyolysis is uncommon unless the tying-up episode is severe or the associated dehydration is prolonged.[16] Observation of grossly discolored urine is not a prerequisite for the development of renal failure. Hemolysis appears to be a less common cause of pigment nephropathy than myopathy, although ARF can occur sporadically. Horses with severe hemolysis or those with hemolysis accompanied by disseminated intravascular coagulation are at greater risk of developing pigment nephropathy.[17] Renal failure consequent to pigment nephropathy should be suspected in horses that become anorectic and more depressed during the week after an episode of tying-up or during a hemolytic crisis. Measuring serum activities of creatine kinase and aspartate aminotransferase may help confirm that ARF has developed in association with rhabdomyolysis. Because there is little preformed creatinine in muscle, rhabdomyolysis alone does not produce an increase in creatinine.[18]

Vitamin K_3

Vitamin K_3 (menadione sodium bisulfite) was a common cause of ATN and ARF in certain parts of the United States before its withdrawal from the market. The development of ARF was thought to be idiosyncratic.[19]

Nonsteroidal Antiinflammatory Drugs

Most horses do not experience appreciable adverse effects from NSAIDs as long as they are administered at the proper dose and animals are not dehydrated. However, NSAID use may produce ARF in an occasional horse when excessive doses are administered or when dehydration is not corrected promptly.[20,21] The lesion produced by NSAID toxicity is medullary crest necrosis, which can be manifested by gross hematuria.[20-24] Unless severe, this lesion rarely causes overt clinical signs and creatinine may actually decrease with fluid therapy in the face of medullary crest necrosis. An occasional horse may also develop chronic interstitial nephritis and nephrolithiasis after prolonged use (months to years) of NSAIDs at recommended doses.[25] Presence of concurrent gastrointestinal disease (ulceration) and protein-losing enteropathy would further support NSAID toxicity in both acutely and chronically affected horses.

When renal blood flow decreases as a consequence of dehydration or redistribution of cardiac output, counteracting vasodilatory mediators are produced and released within the kidney to attenuate the decrease in renal blood flow. The best studied of these vasodilatory mediators include renal prostaglandins (PGI_2 and PGE_2) and dopamine. Although the role of renal prostaglandins in control of basal renal blood flow is likely insignificant, renal prostaglandins are important mediators of vasodilation during periods of renal hypoperfusion.[26] Further, production of renal prostaglandins is severalfold greater in medullary tissue such that action of these mediators leads to a greater increase in inner cortical and medullary blood flow. Thus it should not be surprising that the lesion associated with NSAID toxicity is renal medullary crest necrosis (consequent to ischemia).[27] Similarly, it is important to remember that use of NSAIDs in dehydrated or hypovolemic patients increases the risk of acute nephrosis.[28]

Vitamin D

Vitamin D intoxication may result from ingestion of feed additives or plants (e.g., *Cestrum diurnum*) containing high amounts of vitamin D metabolites or parenteral administration of vitamin D.[29-31] Cholecalciferol (D_3) is thought to be more toxic in the horse than is ergocalciferol (D_2).[30] In general, horses do not need dietary supplementation with vitamin D as long as they are exposed to sunlight and have access to green forages. Further, because the effect of vitamin D supplementation is cumulative, signs of toxicity may not develop until several weeks after supplementation was started.

Clinical signs of vitamin D intoxication may be referable to the musculoskeletal, cardiovascular, or urinary systems.[31]

Calcification of tendons and ligaments results in lameness, and calcification of cardiac muscle and great vessels can lead to cardiovascular problems. Mineralization of tendons and ligaments may be detected directly by palpation or indirectly via ultrasonographic imaging. Heart murmurs may accompany calcification of the great vessels and ultrasonographic imaging of the heart and kidney may also reveal evidence of mineralization. Further clinical signs of renal toxicity include polyuria and weight loss.

Abnormal laboratory findings with vitamin D intoxication include azotemia, isosthenuria, hypochloremia, and elevations in both serum calcium and phosphorus concentrations. The latter combination of hypercalcemia and hyperphosphatemia is unusual for any other disease in the horse, although it may be seen with neoplasia on rare occasions. A definitive diagnosis of Vitamin D toxicosis can be made by measuring serum concentrations of 25-OHD$_3$, 25-OHD$_2$, and 1,25-(OH)$_2$D. Treatment of vitamin D intoxication includes removal of the inciting cause (feed or medication), fluid diuresis, and corticosteroid administration. Provision of feeds low in both calcium and phosphorus may be of benefit in less severely affected horses, but treatment is usually unrewarding once clinical signs attributable to tissue mineralization have developed.

Heavy Metals

Accidental ingestion of heavy metals may result in ATN and ARF in horses. Mercury, cadmium, zinc, arsenic, and lead are all nephrotoxic but are rare causes of renal failure in the horse. Mercury has been used experimentally to study renal failure in horses,[32,33] and there are reports of ARF in horses that have had legs "blistered" or "sweated" with products containing inorganic mercury.[34,35] Because inorganic mercury also causes severe damage to intestinal mucosa, signs of gastrointestinal irritation (e.g., increased salivation, oral erosions, colic, hemorrhagic diarrhea) predominate with mercury intoxication. Further evaluation may reveal oliguria. Exposure to excessive amounts of zinc and cadmium can result in nephrocalcinosis and renal failure but gait deficits (resulting from osseous effects, particularly in foals) and ill thrift are more likely presenting complaints than oliguria.[36]

Laboratory findings with heavy metal intoxication are characteristic for ATN (i.e., azotemia, isosthenuria to hyposthenuria, hyponatremia, and hypochloremia). In horses with ARF concurrent with gastrointestinal disease, as with mercury toxicity, severe hypocalcemia may be present. A tentative diagnosis of mercury intoxication may be made from history of exposure, clinical signs of erosive gastrointestinal disease, and oliguric renal failure. The diagnosis can be confirmed by measuring increased blood and tissue (kidney and liver) concentrations of the metal. In addition to judicious fluid therapy, treatment of ARF induced by exposure to heavy metals should include dimercaprol, 3 mg/kg every 4 hours parenterally and 1 lb of charcoal orally. Visceral analgesics (flunixin meglumine) and sedatives (xylazine or detomidine) are often necessary to control abdominal pain.

Acorn Poisoning

Acorn poisoning is less common in equids than cattle (see Chapter 30), but it has been reported in horses.[37] Death in horses is usually the result of erosive gastrointestinal disease, changes in vascular permeability, and resulting shock rather than a consequence of uremia. Immature leaves and green acorns are considered more toxic than mature acorns because the former have a higher tannin content. Clinical signs may include diarrhea, edema, and body cavity effusion, and lab-oratory evaluation usually reveals azotemia, isosthenuria to hyposthenuria, hyponatremia, and hypochloremia. Detection of increased urinary excretion of phenols may be useful to confirm the diagnosis.

Miscellaneous Drugs and Agents

Several other drugs and agents, particularly tetracycline, have been suspected of causing nephrotoxic ARF in horses.[38] When high doses of oxytetracycline (up to 70 mg/kg) are administered to neonatal foals for correction of limb contracture, ARF is a potential complication, especially if the foals are dehydrated or suffering from concurrent sepsis or hypoxic-ischemic encephalopathy.[39] With renewed interest in polymixin B as an adjunct treatment for endotoxemia, it is prudent to remember that this drug also has nephrotoxic potential. However, experimental studies have demonstrated that the risk of polymixin B nephrotoxicity is low, especially when it is conjugated with dextran 70.[40] Amphotericin B also has considerable nephrotoxic potential, but it is rarely administered systemically to horses. Ochratoxins have potential to produce ATN, but ARF caused by ochratoxins has not been documented in horses. Similarly, pyrrolizidine alkaloid poisoning may cause renal disease in horses, but failure is unlikely. Finally, blister beetle poisoning (cantharidin toxicosis) may cause abdominal pain, shock, hematuria, diaphragmatic flutter, dysuria, and renal dysfunction in horses fed alfalfa grown in regions where the beetles are prevalent.[41]

Vasomotor Nephropathy

Any condition that causes sustained, marked hypotension or release of endogenous pressor agents can initiate hemodynamically mediated (vasomotor) ARF. Although poorly documented, vasomotor ARF may be more common than nephrotoxic ARF in the horse. Hemorrhagic shock, severe intravascular volume deficit (e.g., as with enterocolitis), septic shock, and coagulopathy are important risk factors for vasomotor ARF in horses.[42] Another cause may be adverse drug reactions, including those accompanying intravenous administration of vitamin and mineral products or immunomodulators. The predominant lesion in vasomotor nephropathy is ATN, although diffuse renal cortical or renal medullary necrosis may occur in some cases.

Clinical signs with vasomotor ARF are nonspecific and are more often referable to the primary disease (e.g., hemorrhage or diarrhea). Additional subtle signs, including more marked depression and anorexia than would be expected with the primary disease, with or without signs of mild colic, may increase suspicion of ARF. If sedation for colic signs is deemed necessary, xylazine or detomidine can be administered as long as intravascular volume and blood pressure are not overly compromised. Occasionally, horses with severe ARF may also be ataxic or manifest neurologic signs similar to hepatoencephalopathy.

Oliguria (often manifested as a lack of expected urination in response to fluid therapy) is an important early indicator of vasomotor ARF and production of dilute urine (specific gravity <1.020) that may be discolored (hematuria or hemoglobinuria) may be observed when urine is eventually voided. If urine produced is clear, microscopic hematuria is usually present and will produce a positive result on reagent strip analysis of urine. Glucosuria may also be detected in an occasional horse with vasomotor ARF as a consequence of severe proximal tubular damage. Although the pathophysiologic relationship to ARF is not well defined, diarrhea and severe laminitis may develop in more serious cases of vasomotor ARF.

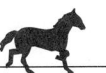

Acute Glomerulopathy

Although subclinical glomerular damage likely accompanies some diseases affecting horses, especially immune-mediated disorders (e.g., purpura hemorrhagica), acute glomerulonephritis is a rare clinical problem.[43] A syndrome of arteriolar microangiopathy and intravascular hemolysis causing distention of glomerular capillary loops with fibrin thrombi and accumulation of large amounts of proteinaceous debris in Bowman's capsule has also been described in a few horses.[44] Affected horses presented with oliguric ARF accompanied by hematuria, proteinuria, and intravascular hemolysis and response to treatment was poor. The cause of the syndrome is not known, although renal lesions resemble those found with the hemolytic-uremic syndrome in humans (caused by toxins of *Escherichia coli*). Bacterial toxins, a consumptive coagulopathy, immune-complex deposition, vasoactive amines, and hemodynamic alterations may all be contributors to this rare syndrome in horses.

Acute glomerulopathy should be also considered in horses with severe ARF that do not have a predisposing primary disease leading to vasomotor ARF and that have not been exposed to nephrotoxins. Gross hematuria, proteinuria, and oliguria would support an acute glomerulopathy and renal biopsy can be pursued to confirm the lesion. Recently a case of streptococcal toxic shock, caused by *Streptococcus mitis*, was described and ARF with glomerulopathy was one component of this syndrome.[45]

Acute Interstitial Nephritis

Acute interstitial nephritis is a rare syndrome of ARF accompanied by rapid elevations in creatinine and clinical signs of uremia. Renal lesions include interstitial edema with a mild inflammatory infiltrate. Although adverse drug reactions (idiosyncratic) may be a cause, the etiopathogenesis of this disease in horses is unknown. In humans, eosinophilic infiltrates in renal biopsy tissue are supportive of adverse drug reaction. Although there are no published reports of the syndrome in horses, I have examined three horses with apparent acute interstitial nephritis. Because of the pronounced interstitial edema that may accompany this disease, treatment with corticosteroids may be of benefit in suspect cases.

Leptospirosis

ARF attributable to infection with *Leptospira interrogans* serovar *pomona* has been documented in several foals and a stallion over the past decade.[46-49] Fever, partial anorexia, and depression were the presenting complaints, and gross hematuria was observed in one foal. Azotemia and low urine specific gravity (<1.020) without bacteriuria were common laboratory findings, although leptospiruria was detected in one foal. Leptospirosis should be included in the list of possible causes of ARF when an underlying primary disease leading to vasomotor nephropathy is not apparent and there has been no exposure to nephrotoxins. Seroconversion or high serum titers and positive fluorescent antibody test results on urine (air-dried sample on a microscope slide) can be used to establish the diagnosis. Successful treatment has been accomplished with intravenous fluids and penicillin administration.

Diagnosis

Acute renal failure should be suspected in patients showing more marked depression and anorexia than would be expected with the primary disease process and in patients that fail to produce urine within 6 to 12 hours of initiating fluid therapy. Rectal palpation in horses with ARF may reveal enlarged, painful kidneys in some cases and enlargement can be confirmed by renal ultrasonography. Renal ultrasonography may also reveal perirenal edema, loss of detail of the corticomedullary junction, or dilation of renal pelves.[50-52]

The diagnosis of ARF is confirmed on the basis of history, potential exposure to nephrotoxins, clinical signs, and laboratory findings. With regard to the latter, the increase in creatinine is often several-fold greater (e.g., to 5 to 15 mg/dl) than that for blood urea nitrogen concentration (BUN) (e.g., to 50 to 100 mg/dl) resulting in a BUN/creatinine ratio that is often less than 10:1. Hyponatremia, hypochloremia, and hypocalcemia are usually present, and, in more severe cases, hyperkalemia, hyperphosphatemia, and metabolic acidosis may also be detected.

In addition to assessment of the magnitude of azotemia and alterations in serum electrolyte concentrations and acid-base balance, urinalysis should be performed on all horses in which ARF is suspected. As mentioned previously, a low urine specific gravity (1.020 or less) in the face of dehydration and gross or microscopic hematuria are common findings with ARF. In addition, evidence of more substantial proximal tubular damage, including increased urinary enzyme activity and/or glucosuria may be detected in some horses and significant proteinuria (urine protein to creatinine ratio greater than 2:1, see Chronic Renal Failure) would support glomerular disease. Examination of urine sediment may reveal casts and increased numbers of erythrocytes and leukocytes, and the amount of urine crystals may be decreased. Increased fractional clearances of sodium and phosphorus are also common findings with ARF. It is important to remember that administration of intravenous fluids to healthy horses will also result in increased fractional clearances of sodium, chloride, and phosphorous[53]; thus electrolyte clearances are ideally determined using the initial urine sample voided after admission or a sample collected via catheterization (i.e., before urine may be substantially altered by fluid therapy).

The most accurate assessment of renal function involves measurement of glomerular filtration rate (GFR). GFR can be determined by performing timed urine collections (inulin and endogenous or exogenous creatinine clearances) or by assessing plasma disappearance of several compounds (sodium sulfanilate, phenolsulfonphthalein, or radiolabeled substances).[54] In a clinical setting, measurement of GFR in cases of ARF is rarely pursued because multiple measurements are required to assess changes in GFR and prognosis for recovery is more likely related to the duration of decreased GFR rather than the magnitude of the decrease. Further, because of the inverse relationship between GFR and creatinine, changes in GFR can be more practically assessed by daily creatinine measurement.

Glomerular injury and tubular necrosis can be further confirmed by performing a renal biopsy. However, biopsy is rarely indicated in cases of ARF because the diagnosis is usually evident. Further, correlation between light microscopic findings and functional changes in animals with ARF has not been well established; thus prognosis is often more dependent on response to treatment than results of renal biopsy. Immunofluorescent testing and electron microscopic examination are routinely performed on human renal biopsy samples to assess mechanisms of renal injury and extent of damage to glomerular and tubular basement membranes. If such detailed evaluation of renal biopsy tissue were also performed in horses with ARF, better information regarding etiopathogenesis and prognosis would likely be provided by the pathologist.

At present, renal biopsy is most indicated in the evaluation of horses with ARF for which exposure to nephrotoxins or another underlying primary disease process is not apparent. However, renal biopsy should be approached cautiously because life-threatening hemorrhage is a potential complication. Biopsy of the right kidney with ultrasonographic guidance, usually through the seventeenth intercostal space, is the preferred procedure for renal biopsy.[55] Use of proper instrumentation (automatic or spring-loaded biopsy instruments) and adequate restraint (stocks and sedation) are important considerations. Renal tissue collected should be placed in formalin for histopathologic examination as well as frozen (or placed into additional media specified by the testing laboratory) for immunofluorescent testing and electron microscopic examination. Although biopsy of the right kidney alone usually is adequate for assessment of the disease process affecting both kidneys, samples of the left kidney can also be collected by guiding the biopsy instrument through the spleen. Again, ultrasonographic guidance is important when collecting a biopsy from the left kidney or when biopsy of a specific area of either kidney is desired.

GENERAL PRINCIPLES OF TREATMENT IN ACUTE RENAL FAILURE

General principles of treatment of ARF in the horse are similar to those recommended for human patients.[56,57] Initial treatment should always focus on judicious fluid therapy to replace volume deficits and correct electrolyte and acid-base abnormalities. The magnitude of azotemia and serum concentrations of sodium, chloride, potassium, and bicarbonate should be monitored daily. Sodium and chloride replacement are often required in horses with polyuric ARF and can be accomplished by using 0.9% NaCl as the fluid administered or through electrolyte supplementation in grain feedings or as oral pastes. Serum potassium concentration in horses with nonoliguric ARF is often normal, and, except for postrenal problems (e.g., obstruction or rupture), therapy intended to lower serum potassium is usually not necessary. Similarly, it is usually unnecessary to correct the mild hypocalcemia that can accompany ARF in horses.

After correction of volume deficits and electrolyte and acid-base abnormalities, an attempt should be made to determine if the animal is oliguric or nonoliguric (polyuric) because the prognosis for recovery appears to be more favorable with nonoliguric ARF. This often becomes apparent by simple observation: oliguric horses fail to produce expected amounts of urine in the initial 12 to 24 hours of intravenous fluid therapy and the bedding remains dry while nonoliguric horses are observed to repeatedly void moderate volumes of dilute urine during the initial 6 to 12 hours of treatment. Further, edema can develop rapidly in horses with oliguric ARF. In horses with prerenal azotemia rather than intrinsic ARF, creatinine should decrease by at least 30% to 50% within the initial 24 hours of fluid therapy. In contrast, creatinine remains unchanged, or may even increase, with ARF.

In severely ill patients, especially those with vasomotor nephropathy, systemic blood pressure can be monitored to confirm that fluid therapy has been adequate to restore blood pressure. Some horses may remain hypotensive (systolic pressure <80 mm Hg) despite administration of large volumes of intravenous fluids because fluid may be accumulating extravascularly as edema or a third space fluid. If systemic blood pressure remains low, hypertonic saline, dobutamine, or other pressor agents may be needed to restore blood pressure and glomerular filtration. Fluid and sodium replacement in horses with oliguric renal failure and normal systemic blood pressure must be monitored closely because, as previously mentioned, overzealous fluid administration to horses with oliguric or anuric ARF will result in edema formation, which is often initially noticed in the conjunctiva (Fig. 32-1).

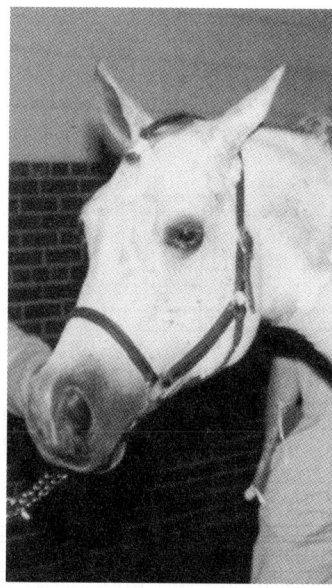

FIG. 32-1 ■ Severe conjunctival edema from intravenous fluid therapy in a 3-year-old Arabian with oliguric ARF. The ARF and a multifocal granulomatous pneumonia occurred after the intravenous administration of an approved immunomodulator.

In addition to regular assessment of attitude, vital parameters, packed cell volume, and total plasma protein concentration, monitoring should also include measurement of body weight once or twice daily (patients should not gain weight after rehydration) and comparison of fluid input with fluid (urine) output. Although there is no convenient method of collecting all urine voided by ambulatory foals or mares, urine output can be rather easily quantified in male horses by placing a urine collection device around the abdomen.[58] When monitoring urine output in critically ill foals and mares is desired, it can be accomplished by use of an indwelling Foley catheter and urine collection bag (closed system), but ascending infection is a risk. Finally, central venous pressure (CVP) can also be monitored as a more precise measure of fluid balance in critical patients. CVP is measured with a manometer, with the baseline at the level of the right atrium, attached to an intravenous catheter placed into the anterior vena cava via the jugular vein (normal CVP in horses is <8 cm H$_2$O).

In horses that remain oliguric after 12 to 24 hours of appropriate fluid and electrolyte replacement and restoration of systemic blood pressure, furosemide (1 mg/kg, IV, every 2 hours) should be administered. Unfortunately, furosemide treatment is often ineffective in increasing renal blood flow, GFR, and tubular flow in horses with ARF.[57,59] If urine is not voided after the second dose, administration of mannitol (1 mg/kg as a 10% to 20% solution) and/or a dopamine infusion (3 to 7 µg/kg/min IV) can be instituted. Dopamine administration should only be performed in a hospital setting in which heart rate and blood pressure can be monitored frequently to avoid development of tachycardia and hypertension. Use of dopamine for selective renal vasodilatory and natriuretic actions has recently been called into question because most studies in humans have not demonstrated prevention of ARF in high-risk patients or improved outcome in those with established ARF.[60] Further, the drug may precipitate serious cardiovascular and metabolic complications in critically ill patients. If these treatments are successful in converting oliguria to polyuria (may require 24 to 72 hours), they can be discontinued but maintenance of urine production must be monitored closely over the next few days. Fortunately, the majority of horses with ARF resulting from ATN are nonoliguric rather than oliguric, and administration of furosemide, mannitol, or dopamine is not needed in most of cases of nonoliguric ARF.

When this treatment approach to oliguria remains unsuccessful for more than 72 hours, the prognosis becomes grave. However, dialysis therapy may be a further treatment option in select patients. Hemodialysis has been successfully used to treat an adult horse with myoglobinuric ARF[61] and a neonatal foal with oxytetracycline-induced ARF.[39] Peritoneal dialysis has been attempted in a few horses with nephrotoxic-induced ARF; however, omental plugging of the catheter has limited its success and special dialysis catheters are needed for effective fluid exchange. Pleural dialysis is another option for which fluid exchange is less problematic. Hemodialysis or dialysis would likely be most effective in horses with nephrotoxic ARF, whereas vasomotor nephropathy is best treated by addressing the predisposing condition and instituting appropriate fluid therapy.

After volume deficits have been restored and polyuria has been achieved, patients usually require only continued fluid therapy (0.9% NaCl or another balanced electrolyte solution, 40 to 80 ml/kg/day) to promote a continued decrease in creatinine. Fluid therapy may need to be continued (20 to 40 ml/kg/day) for several days until creatinine returns to the normal range or a steady-state value and the horse is eating and drinking adequate amounts. Supplementation with oral electrolytes (1 to 2 oz of NaCl twice daily) will also promote greater fluid intake and diuresis. Potassium supplementation (1 oz of KCl twice daily) may also be required because the diuresis also results in kaliuresis. When horses remain anorectic during treatment, addition of 50 to 100 g of dextrose per liter of fluids can provide needed calories, and, if anorexia persists for several days, caloric intake may need to be provided by nasogastric tube feeding or total parenteral nutrition.

Within the week after fluid therapy is discontinued, creatinine should be measured again to ensure that it has not increased. Occasionally, creatinine may not decrease to below 2 to 3 mg/dl despite continued fluid therapy. As long as the horse is eating and drinking well, intravenous fluids can be discontinued. In some horses further recovery will be manifested as a return of creatinine to the normal range within the next couple of months while in other patients a persisting elevation in creatinine is indicative of a permanent loss of renal function.

REFERENCES

1. Humes HD et al: Clinical and pathophysiologic aspects of aminoglycoside nephrotoxicity, *Am J Kidney Dis* 11:5-28, 1982.
2. Bartol JM, Divers TJ, Perkins GA: Nephrotoxicant-induced acute renal failure in five horses, *Compend Cont Educ* 22:870-876, 2000.
3. Riviere JE, Traver DS, Coppoe GL: Gentamicin toxic nephropathy in horses with disseminated bacterial infection, *J Am Vet Med Assoc* 180:648-651, 1982.
4. Hinchcliff KW, McGuirk SM, MacWilliams PS: Gentamicin nephrotoxicity, *Proceedings of the Thirty-third Annual Convention of the American Association of Equine Practitioners*, New Orleans, 1987, pp 65-75.
5. Sojka JE, Brown SA: Pharmacokinectic adjustment of gentamicin dosing in horses with sepsis, *J Am Vet Med Assoc* 189:784-789, 1986.
6. Geor RJ, Brashier MK: Rational approach to gentamicin dosing in neonatal foals, *Proceedings of the Thirty-seventh Annual Convention of the American Association of Equine Practitioners*, San Francisco, 1991, pp 603-609.
7. Schumacher J et al: Effect of diet on gentamicin-induced nephrotoxicosis in horses, *Am J Vet Res* 52:1274-1278, 1991.
8. Hewitt WL: Reflections on the clinical pharmacology of gentamicin, *Acta Pathol Microb Scand* 241(suppl 1381):151-153, 1977.
9. Gilbert DN: Once-daily aminoglycoside therapy, *Antimicrob Agents Chemother* 35:399-405, 1991.
10. Godbar LM et al: Pharmacokinetics, nephrotoxicosis, and in vitro antibacterial activity associated with single versus multiple (three times) daily gentamicin treatments in horses, *Am J Vet Res* 56:613-618, 1995.
11. Magdesian KG et al: Pharmacokinetics of a high dose of gentamicin administered intravenously or intramuscularly to horses, *J Am Vet Med Assoc* 213:1007-1011, 1998.
12. Tudor RA, Papich MG, Redding WR: Drug disposition and dosage determination of once daily administration of gentamicin sulfate in horses after abdominal surgery, *J Am Vet Med Assoc* 215:503-506, 1999.
13. Adams R et al: Evaluation of a technique for measurement of γ-glutamyltranspeptidase in equine urine, *Am J Vet Res* 46:147-150, 1985.
14. Adams R, Brown M, Gronwall R: In defense of gentamicin, *Vet Rec* 120:277-278, 1987.
15. Sweeney RW et al: Kinetics of gentamicin elimination in two horses with acute renal failure, *Equine Vet J* 20:182-184, 1988.
16. Sprayberry KA et al: Renal failure, laminitis, and colitis following severe rhabdomyolysis in a draft horse-cross with polysaccharide storage myopathy, *Can Vet J* 39:500-503, 1998.
17. Long PH: Red maple-associated pulmonary thrombosis in a horse, *J Am Vet Med Assoc* 184:977-978, 1984.
18. Oh MS: Does serum creatinine rise faster in rhabdomyolysis, *Nephron* 63:255-257, 1993.
19. Rebhun WC et al: Vitamin K_3-induced renal toxicosis in the horse, *J Am Vet Med Assoc* 184:1237-1239, 1984.
20. MacKay RJ, French TW, Nguyen HT, et al: Effects of large doses of phenylbutazone administration to horses, *Am J Vet Res* 44:774-780, 1983.
21. MacAllister CG et al: Comparison of adverse effects of phenylbutazone, flunixin meglumine, and ketoprofen in horses, *J Am Vet Med Assoc* 202:71-77, 1993.
22. Read WK: Renal medullary crest necrosis associated with phenylbutazone therapy in horses, *Vet Pathol* 20:662-669, 1983.
23. Gunson DE: Renal papillary necrosis in horses, *J Am Vet Med Assoc* 182:263-266, 1983.
24. Behm RJ, Berg IE: Hematuria caused by renal medullary crest necrosis in a horse, *Compend Cont Educ* 9:698-703, 1987.
25. Ehnen SJ et al: Obstructive nephrolithiasis and ureterolithiasis associated with chronic renal failure in horses: eight cases (1981-1987), *J Am Vet Med Assoc* 197:249-253, 1990.
26. Dunn MJ, Zambraski EJ: Renal effects of drugs that inhibit prostaglandin synthesis, *Kidney Int* 18:609-622, 1980.
27. Clive DM, Stoff JS: Renal syndromes associated with nonsteroidal anti-inflammatory drugs, *New Engl J Med* 310:563-572, 1984.
28. Gunson DE, Soma LR: Renal papillary necrosis in horses after phenylbutazone and water deprivation, *Vet Pathol* 20:603-610, 1983.
29. Krook L et al: Hypercalcemia and calcinosis in Florida horses: implication of the shrub *Cestrum diurnium* as the causative agent, *Cornell Vet* 65:26-56, 1975.
30. Harrington DD, Page EH: Acute vitamin D_3 toxicosis in horses: case reports and experimental studies of the comparative toxicity of vitamins D_2 and D_3, *J Am Vet Med Assoc* 182:1358-1369, 1983.
31. McClure JJ et al: Vitamin D intoxication in a thoroughbred racehorse, *Compend Cont Educ* 9:573-578, 1987.
32. Roberts MC, Seawright AA: The effects of prolonged daily low-level mercuric chloride dosing in a horse, *Vet Human Toxicol* 20:410-415, 1978.
33. Bayly WM et al: A reproducible means of studying acute renal failure in the horse, *Cornell Vet* 76:287-298, 1986.
34. Markel MD et al: Acute renal failure associated with application of a mercuric blister in a horse, *J Am Vet Med Assoc* 185:92-94, 1984.
35. Schuh JCL et al: Concurrent mercuric blister and dimethyl sulphoxide (DMSO) application as a cause of mercury toxicity in two horses, *Equine Vet J* 20:68-71, 1988.
36. Gunson DE et al: Environmental zinc and cadmium pollution associated with generalized osteochondrosis, osteoporosis, and nephrocalcinosis in horses, *J Am Vet Med Assoc* 180:295-299, 1982.
37. Anderson GA et al: Fatal acorn poisoning in a horse: pathologic findings and diagnostic considerations, *J Am Vet Med Assoc* 182:1105-1110, 1983.
38. Schmitz DG: Toxic nephropathy in horses, 10:104-111, 1988.
39. Vivrette S et al: Hemodialysis for treatment of oxytetracycline-induced acute renal failure in a neonatal foal, *J Am Vet Med Assoc* 203:105-107, 1993.
40. Barton MH: Use of polymixin B for treatment endotoxemia in horses, *Compend Cont Educ* 22:1056-1059, 2000.
41. Schmitz DG: Cantharidin toxicosis in horses, *J Vet Intern Med* 3:208-215, 1989.
42. Divers TJ et al: Acute renal failure in six horses resulting from hemodynamic causes, *Equine Vet J* 19:178-184, 1987.
43. Roberts MC, Kelly WR: Renal dysfunction in a case of purpura haemorrhagica in a horse, *Vet Rec* 110:144-146, 1982.
44. Morris CF et al: Hemolytic uremic-like syndrome in two horses, *J Am Vet Med Assoc* 191:1453-1454, 1987.
45. Dolente BA, Seco OM, Lewis ML: Streptococcal toxic shock in a horse, *J Am Vet Med Assoc* 217:64-67, 2000.
46. Divers TJ, Byars TD, Shin SJ: Renal dysfunction associated with infection of *Leptospira interrogans* in a horse, *J Am Vet Med Assoc* 201:1391-1392, 1992.
47. Bernard WV et al: Hematuria and leptospiruria in a foal, *J Am Vet Med Assoc* 203:276-278, 1993.
48. Hogan PM et al: Acute renal disease due to *Leptospira interrogans* in a weanling, *Equine Vet J* 28:331-333, 1996.
49. Frazer ML: Acute renal failure from leptospirosis in a foal, *Aust Vet J* 77:499-500, 1999.
50. Kiper ML, Traub-Dargatz JL, Wrigley RH: Renal ultrasonography in horses, *Compend Cont Educ* 12:993-999, 1990.

51. Hoffman KL, Wood AKW, McCarthy PH: Sonographic-anatomic correlation and imaging protocol for the kidneys of horses, *Am J Vet Res* 56: 1403-1412, 1995.

52. Divers TJ, Yeager AE: The value of ultrasonographic examination in the diagnosis and management of renal diseases in horses, *Equine Vet Educ* 7:334-341, 1997.

53. Roussel AJ et al: Urinary indices of horses after intravenous administration of crystalloid solutions, *J Vet Int Med* 7:241-246, 1993.

54. Matthews HK et al: Measuring renal function in horses, *Vet Med* 88:349-356, 1993.

55. Barratt-Boyes SM et al: Ultrasound localization and guidance for renal biopsy in the horse, *Vet Radiol* 32:121-126, 1991.

56. Lieberthal W, Levisky NG: Treatment of acute tubular necrosis, *Semin Nephrol* 10:571-583, 1990.

57. Divers TJ: Treatment of acute renal failure in the horse, *Proceedings of the Thirty-first Annual Convention of American Association of Equine Practitioners*, Toronto, Canada, 1985, pp 673-679.

58. Divers TJ: Acute renal failure in the horse, *Proceedings of the 10th Bain Fallon Memorial Lectures*, Adelaide, Australia, 1988, pp 93-98.

59. Lindner A: Synergism of dopamine and furosemide in oliguric acute renal failure, *Nephron* 33:121-126, 1987.

60. Power DA, Duggan J, Brady HR: Renal-dose (low-dose) dopamine for the treatment of sepsis-related and other forms of acute renal failure: ineffective and probably dangerous, *Clin Exp Pharmacol Physiol Suppl*, 26:S23-8, 1999.

61. Thornhill JA et al: Hemodialysis in a horse with acute renal failure as induced by rhabdomyolysis, *Proceedings of the Conference of Research Workers in Animal Disease*, Chicago, 1983, p 16.

CHRONIC RENAL FAILURE

THOMAS J. DIVERS

Chronic renal failure (CRF) in the horse may be divided by clinical and pathologic findings into two broad categories: primary glomerular disease and primary tubulointerstitial disease.[62,63] However, pathology in one portion of the nephron usually leads to altered function and eventual pathology in the entire nephron. Thus CRF is an irreversible disease process characterized by a progressive decline in GFR. However, the rate of decline in GFR is variable between affected horses making the short-term (e.g., months to a couple of years) prognosis guarded to favorable while the long-term prognosis remains poor.

Primary glomerular diseases that can lead to CRF in horses include glomerulonephritis, nonspecific glomerulopathy, renal glomerular hypoplasia, and amyloidosis. Tubulointerstitial diseases causing CRF include incomplete recovery from acute tubular necrosis, pyelonephritis, nephrolithiasis, hydronephrosis, renal dysplasia and, rarely, papillary necrosis. Collectively, the latter disorders produce pathology categorized as chronic interstitial nephritis. Unfortunately, because renal disease is often advanced when horses are first presented for clinical evaluation, the inciting cause leading to CRF may be difficult to ascertain, and end stage kidney disease (ESKD) may be the pathologic diagnosis. The inciting cause may more likely be discerned from the history (long term) rather than clinical findings at presentation, especially for primary tubulointerstitial diseases. Adjunctive diagnostic evaluation including laboratory assessment, renal ultrasonography and renal biopsy may provide further evidence to document the inciting cause.

CAUSES

Proliferative Glomerulonephritis

Proliferative glomerulonephritis (GN), indicating increased cellularity of the glomerular tufts consequent to influx of inflammatory cells and proliferation of mesangium, is the most common glomerular disease causing CRF in horses. It is thought to result from deposition of circulating immune complexes along the glomerular capillaries or in situ formation along the glomerular basement membrane (Fig. 32-2). Deposition of immune complexes causes activation of complement and vasculitis (type III hypersensitivity response). In one study, deposits of immunoglobulin (IgG) and complement along the glomerular basement membrane (GBM) were found via immunofluorescent staining in a large percentage (22 of 53) of horses at necropsy.[64] However, only 1 of these 53 horses developed CRF. Thus, although immune (antigen-antibody) complex deposition and subclinical GN may be common in horses, progression to CRF appears to be an infrequent occurrence. In this necropsy survey the predominant immunofluorescent staining pattern was granular (patchy deposits of immune complexes and complement along the basement membrane), but linear deposits were found in 2 horses. The latter finding was supportive of true autoimmune disease with more diffuse deposition of anti-GBM antibodies (type II hypersensitivity response) along the basement membrane antibody. Streptococcal antigens have been suggested to be an important trigger for development of proliferative GN,[65] and in one horse with CRF streptococcal antigens were confirmed to be present in diseased glomeruli.[66] Although equine infectious anemia virus is the only other antigen that has been detected in glomeruli of horses with proliferative GN,[67] subclinical GN likely accompanies other chronic infections in horses. It has also been suggested that equine GN may also be associated with either mixed or monoclonal cryoglobulins forming antibody-antibody glomerular depositis.[68] Fortunately, GN in most patients is rarely of clinical significance.

Chronic Interstitial Nephritis

Chronic interstitial nephritis (CIN) and fibrosis may be the most common cause of CRF in horses. Interstitial nephritis (tubulointerstitial disease) usually develops as a sequela to acute tubular necrosis consequent to exposure to nephrotoxins or vasomotor nephropathy. Other causes include drug-induced interstitial nephritis, urinary obstruction, pyelonephritis, renal hypoplasia/dysplasia, and papillary necrosis. Although the majority of horses that develop ARF attributable to these causes recover with apparently normal renal function (they remain nonazotemic), a few may survive with significant loss of renal functional mass and subsequently (often ten years later) develop signs of CRF attributable to chronic interstitial nephritis.[69] In horses less than 5 years of age that develop CRF that cannot be attributed to other causes, anomalies of development including renal hypoplasia, dysplasia, or polycystic kidney disease should be strongly suspected (Fig. 32-3).[63,70-72]

Pyelonephritis

Bilateral septic pyelonephritis is a rare cause of CRF in horses.[73-75] Pyelonephritis is usually a result of an ascending infection and is often accompanied by nephrolithiasis or ureterolithiasis. Multiparous mares, especially those with a history of dystocia, and horses with bladder paralysis are at greater risk for bacterial colonization of the lower urinary tract and subsequent development of ascending infection. Chronic distention with bladder paralysis compromises the integrity of the ureteral orifices leading to vesiculoureteral reflux and pyelonephritis. With long-standing bladder paralysis, the ureteral orifices may appear wide open during cytoscopic examination, and in an occasional affected horse the endoscope can be advanced into the ureter with little resistance. With unilateral pyelonephritis, adequate renal function is usually maintained by the contralateral kidney; however, passage of small uroliths into the bladder can lead to recurrent urethral obstruction. Gram-negative organisms ap-

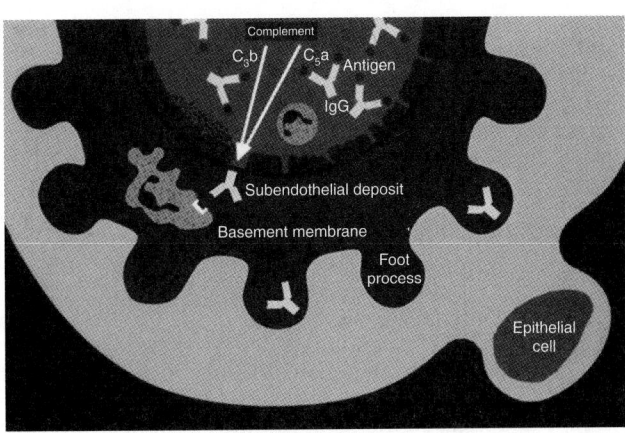

FIG. 32-2 ■ Depiction of a subendothelial immunologic reaction suspected to occur in horses with streptococcal antigen-antibody–associated glomerulonephritis.

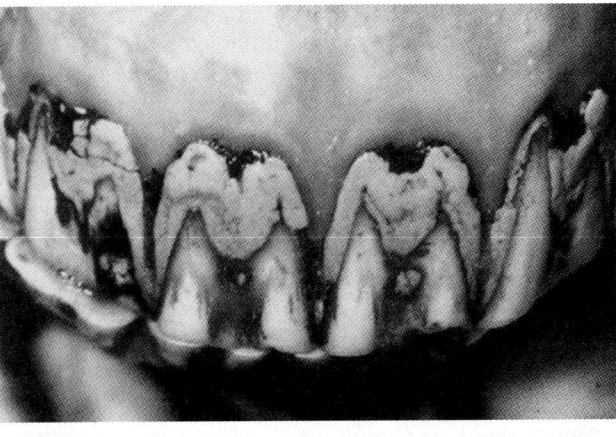

FIG. 32-4 ■ Dental tartar caused by chronic azotemia in a 5-year-old Standardbred with chronic renal failure.

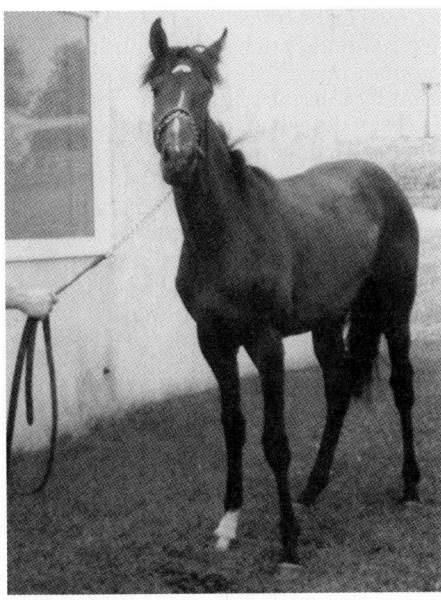

FIG. 32-3 ■ Yearling Thoroughbred with chronic renal failure caused by renal dysplasia. Failure to grow normally and lethargy were the primary complaints.

pear to be the most common causative agents, although *Staphylococcus* spp., *Streptococcus* spp., or *Corynebacterium* spp. may be isolated in some cases, and mixed bacterial infections are not uncommon.

Miscellaneous Causes

Other reported causes of CRF in horses include amyloidosis,[76] neoplasia,[77] focal glomerulosclerosis-like disease,[78] and chronic oxalate nephrosis.[79] Renal amyloidosis has only been reported in horses used for production of antiserum.[76] Further, oxalate nephropathy in horses is likely a misnomer because the presence of oxalate crystals in renal tissue of horses with CRF is typically a consequence, rather than the cause, of CRF.[79]

CLINICAL SIGNS AND LABORATORY FINDINGS. The most common clinical sign observed in horses with CRF is weight loss.[63] A small plaque of ventral edema, usually between the forelimbs, is another frequent finding in horses with CRF.[63,80] Moderate polyuria and polydipsia (PU/PD) are usually present at some stage of the disease process, but

PU/PD may not be noticed except by the astute owner or trainer.[63] Dysuria is generally not reported unless CRF is due to pyelonephritis, which may be associated with bladder paralysis, lithiasis, and lower urinary tract infection. Normal equine urine is rich in crystals and mucus, making a prediction of urine abnormalities on gross observation difficult. However, hematuria or pyuria (gross or microscopic) may be reported in some, but not all, horses with pyelonephritis, urinary calculi, or neoplasia. Often, urine produced by horses with CRF is light yellow and transparent because it is relatively devoid of crystals and mucus. Accumulation of dental tartar, especially on the incisors and canine teeth (Fig. 32-4); melena; and oral ulcers are other findings that may be detected in horses with CRF. Growth in horses with renal hypoplasia, dysplasia, or polycystic kidney disease may be stunted. Although abdominal pain would be expected in horses with obstructive nephroliths or ureteroliths, colic signs are not often reported in horses with lithiasis producing obstruction of the upper urinary tract.[69,81]

Clinicopathologic findings in horses with CRF vary depending on appetite, diet, and the cause and severity of renal damage. Most horses with clinical signs of CRF have moderate to severe azotemia (creatinine usually 5 mg/dl or greater). The BUN/creatinine ratio may vary, depending on protein intake, muscle mass, hydration, and degree of azotemia but is usually 10:1 or greater. Mild hyperkalemia, hyponatremia, and hypochloremia are commonly found in horses with CRF. Hypercalcemia, with serum concentrations sometimes exceeding 20 mg/dl, appears to be a laboratory finding with CRF that is unique to the equid. One early case series of CRF reported six of nine horses to be hypercalcemic[82]; however, others have found a lower percentage to be hypercalcemic.[83] Hypercalcemia in horses with CRF is not a consequence of hyperparathyroidism,[84] and its presence or absence appears to be more closely related to dietary intake than to the magnitude of azotemia. For example, four of four nephrectomized ponies fed alfalfa hay developed marked hypercalcemia,[85] whereas serum calcium concentration remained within the normal range in four of four nephrectomized ponies fed grass hay (although filterable calcium did increase).[62] Similarly, hypercalcemia in horses with spontaneously occurring CRF can resolve within a few days of changing diet from alfalfa to grass hay.[72] Serum phosphorus concentration in horses with CRF is usually normal to decreased and hypophosphatemia is more commonly detected with concurrent hypercalcemia. Hypermagnesemia may also be detected in some horses with CRF. Acid-base balance usually remains normal until CRF becomes advanced but metabolic acidosis is a common finding in horses with end-stage disease.

Many horses with CRF are moderately anemic (packed cell volume 20% to 30%) as a consequence of decreased erythropoietin production by the diseased kidneys. Those with CRF resulting from GN frequently have hypoalbuminemia and hypoproteinemia, and horses with advanced CRF of any cause may also have mild hypoproteinemia associated with intestinal ulceration. Hyperglobulinemia may be detected in horses with immune-mediated diseases or chronic pyelonephritis. Horses with CRF can also develop hypercholesterolemia and hypertriglyceridemia (hyperlipidemia) and an occasional horse with advanced CRF may have grossly lipemic plasma.[86]

Urinalysis findings may also vary depending on the cause of CRF. As mentioned, urine collected from horses with CRF is relatively devoid of normal mucus and crystals making samples transparent. Further, urine specific gravity is typically in the isosthenuric range (1.008 to 1.014), although heavy proteinuria in an occasional horse with GN may produce values up to 1.020. Quantification of urine protein concentration (as for cerebrospinal fluid) is required to accurately assess proteinuria. Urine protein concentration in normal horses is usually less than 100 mg/dl and the urine protein/creatinine ratio should be less than 1:1.[87,88] With significant proteinuria, urine protein/creatinine ratio is usually greater than 2:1.[66] In the earlier stages of GN, excessive urine protein is primarily albumin but with progression of glomerular pathology an increasing amount of globulin is also lost in the urine. Horses with CIN usually do not have significant proteinuria. Hematuria (gross or microscopic) may be present with pyelonephritis, urinary calculi, or neoplasia and can produce trace proteinuria but urine protein/creatinine ratio usually remains less than 2:1. Although horses with septic pyelonephritis would be expected to have pyuria (>5 leukocytes/high-power field) and significant bacteriuria on sediment examination, these findings are not consistently detected and a urine sample should be submitted for quantitative bacterial culture in all horses with CRF. Usually, more than 10,000 colony forming units per milliliter of urine are found with infection, although lower numbers do not always rule out septic pyelonephritis.

DIAGNOSIS. A diagnosis of CRF is most commonly made in horses with azotemia and isosthenuria that present with a complaint of weight loss or decreased performance. As discussed above, determining the inciting cause of CRF can be difficult because the disease has often advanced to ESKD when horses are initially presented for evaluation. Urinalysis does not often reveal the cause of CRF, except in some horses with pyelonephritis. In theory, assessment of urine protein concentration and urine protein/creatinine ratio should be helpful in separating glomerular disease from tubulointerstitial disease, but in practice these laboratory measures have not consistently been elevated in horses with histopathologic evidence of glomerulonephritis. However, detection of moderate to heavy proteinuria (urine protein/creatinine ratio >2:1) without hematuria provides support for glomerular disease.

Rectal examination may be helpful in determining the cause of CRF. Horses with pyelonephritis, as well as those with ureteral calculi, often have enlarged ureters that can be palpated dorsolaterally as they course through the retroperitoneal space. Although kidneys of horses with CRF are often small with an irregular surface, these changes are not always apparent on palpation of the caudal pole of the left kidney. The right kidney cannot usually be palpated in the horse unless it is markedly enlarged or displaced caudally by the liver or a mass. Ultrasonographic imaging is useful for evaluating kidney size and echogenicity and may reveal fluid distention (hydronephrosis, pyelonephritis, or polycystic disease) or presence of nephroliths.[89,90,91] Horses with significant renal parenchymal damage and fibrosis often have loss of detail of the corticomedullary junction and echogenicity of renal tissue may be similar or even greater than that of the spleen. In contrast, intravenous pyelography provides little information in adult horses and its use is generally limited to foals less than 50 kg. When hematuria or dysuria accompanies CRF, cystoscopic examination can be helpful in determining the side (e.g., right vs. left) from which renal hematuria is originating and further allows assessment of the ureteral orifices and urine flow from each kidney.

As described under Acute Renal Failure, measurement of GFR provides the most accurate assessment of renal function and repeated measurements at monthly or longer intervals can be useful to monitor rate of progression of CRF. It is also a useful measure to document a reduction in renal function in horses that are thought to be suffering from early CRF before significant azotemia has developed. GFR can be measured by several methods including urinary clearances of endogenous or exogenous creatinine, inulin, or ^{99m}TC-DTPA (all require timed urine collections) or plasma disappearance of sodium sulfanilate, phenolsulfonphthalein, or radiolabeled compounds (e.g., ^{99m}TC-DTPA).[92,72,93-95] Assessment of renal function by nuclear scintigraphic imaging of the kidneys has also been described, but in horses this technique appears to be better for documenting decreased individual kidney function (i.e., with unilateral or asymmetric disease) than for quantitative assessment of GFR.[96,97] In most clinical settings, performing a 24-hour endogenous creatinine clearance is the most practical and economical method for measuring GFR. The major challenge is application of a urine collection device for collection of all urine produced. Once urine has been collected, a well-mixed sample is submitted to the laboratory along with a sample of serum obtained during the collection period and GFR is estimated by the standard clearance formula:

$$\text{GFR } (ml \cdot kg^{-1} \cdot min^{-1}) = \{([Cr_{urine}]/[Cr_{serum}]) \times UF\}/bwt$$

where UF is urine flow ($ml \cdot min^{-1}$) and bwt is body weight in kg.[93] GFR in horses with normal renal function ranges from 1.5 to 3.0 $ml \cdot kg^{-1} \cdot min^{-1}$, and values less than 1.0 $ml \cdot kg^{-1} \cdot min^{-1}$ are indicative of a decrease in GFR. Although repeated measurement of endogenous creatinine clearance provides useful information about the rate of decline in GFR in horses with CRF, simply measuring creatinine and assessing body condition at monthly or longer intervals are the most common methods used to evaluate the progression of CRF in affected horses.

The inciting cause of CRF can be confirmed in some horses by renal biopsy. As was also discussed under Acute Renal Failure, renal biopsy should be approached cautiously and only be pursued if findings are likely to change treatment or prognosis. Treatment for CRF consists of supportive care and the long-term prognosis is poor; therefore renal biopsy is rarely indicated in horses with CRF. Further, most horses have rather advanced CRF at the time the disease is initially detected and biopsy results in these patients may not provide useful information regarding the inciting cause.

TREATMENT. Treatment of horses with CRF is most likely to produce improved renal function if there is an acute, reversible component exacerbating CRF (i.e., acute on chronic syndrome). Similar to ARF, sudden exacerbation can be caused by exposure to nephrotoxins or vasomotor nephropathy secondary to diseases producing hypovolemia (e.g., diarrhea or sepsis causing volume depletion). Ascending urinary tract infection or obstruction can also exacerbate CRF. If an acute component is detected, it should be corrected rapidly

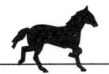

(as described for ARF) with the goal of minimizing further loss of functional nephrons. Further, surgical removal or fragmentation of stones may be indicated in horses with calculi that are thought to be causing a disruption in urine flow.

In horses with relatively stable CRF, management changes should be kept to a minimum and when necessary, they should be made gradually. Treatment of horses with stable CRF consists of supportive care: providing sufficient fluids, electrolytes, and nutritional support.[98] Water should be available at all times and salt can be provided freely as long as edema or hypertension are absent. If edema develops, salt should be restricted, even in the face of hyponatremia. In addition to creatinine, serum electrolyte concentrations and acid-base balance should be measured regularly (e.g., monthly or longer intervals). If serum sodium and chloride concentrations are decreased, 60 to 120 g (approximately 2 to 4 oz) of salt may be added to the feed, providing edema is not present. If metabolic acidosis is detected (e.g., blood pH <7.35 or serum bicarbonate concentration <20 mEq/L) and the patient is not edematous, sodium bicarbonate powder (100 to 200 g/day) or a mix of sodium bicarbonate and salt should be added to the diet. The goal of supplementation with salt and sodium bicarbonate is to maintain serum electrolyte concentrations and acid-base balance within reference ranges. However, the effect of electrolyte supplementation on progression of CRF is unclear because high-salt diets may actually hasten the decline in GFR and exacerbate proteinuria in human patients with CRF.[99]

Although no adverse effects of hypercalcemia in horses with CRF have been documented, decreasing calcium intake (e.g., replacing alfalfa or other legume hays with grass hay) may result in a return of serum calcium concentration to the normal range. The hypophosphatemia that commonly accompanies hypercalcemia in horses with CRF may prevent mineralization of soft tissues. There appears to be no need for vitamin D supplementation in horses with CRF but regular administration of vitamin B complex, and anabolic steroids may be helpful to stimulate appetite. If appetite remains good, anabolic steroids may further limit muscle wasting and may increase packed cell volume. Attenuation of anemia in human and canine patients with CRF by administration of recombinant erythropoietin has been one of the most significant advances in management of CRF because it has eliminated the need for blood transfusions, improved exercise capacity, and decreased morbidity associated with the uremic syndrome.[100] In an occasional horse with advanced CRF, marked hyperlipemia may develop and administration of heparin (40 to 100 IU/kg SC twice daily) may stimulate lipoprotein lipase and decrease plasma triglyceride concentration.[101] However, this treatment is not without risk because it may cause a further decline in packed cell volume and potentiate bleeding tendencies in a uremic patient. NSAIDs and corticosteroids are best avoided in horses with CRF attributable to primary tubulointerstitial disease. If these drugs are essential for treatment of a complicating problem, they should be used judiciously. Treatment of CRF consequent to GN appears to be even less rewarding than treatment of CRF caused by tubulointerstitial disease (CIN). Immunosuppressive therapy has been of limited benefit in slowing the progression of the disease and may even hasten weight loss. For patients with significant edema, treatment with diuretics may result in transient improvement, and plasma transfusions may be of temporary benefit to horses with edema and hypoalbuminemia.

As CRF progresses, partial anorexia and lethargy lead to more rapid loss of body condition. Thus nutritional management aimed at maintaining body condition is probably the most important aspect of supportive care of horses with CRF. Increasing carbohydrate (grain) intake and adding fat

to the diet are recommendations to increase caloric intake. Fat can be added by feeding corn oil (up to 16 ounces per day) or a commercial fat supplement. Increased intake of omega-3-fatty acids (e.g., available in linseed oil or flaxseed oil) has been demonstrated to slow the progression of renal failure in experimental models, but potential benefits in spontaneously occurring CRF are less clear.[102,103] Over the past couple of decades, restricting dietary protein intake by human and veterinary patients with CRF was thought to have beneficial effects[104]; however, the current recommendation is to provide adequate amounts of dietary protein and energy to meet or slightly exceed predicted requirements while maintaining a neutral nitrogen balance.[105] In horses with CRF, adequacy of dietary protein intake can be assessed by the BUN/creatinine ratio: values greater than 15:1 suggest excessive protein intake, and values less than 10:1 may indicate protein-calorie malnutrition. Finally, an important but often overlooked aspect of nutritional management of horses with CRF is provision of a highly palatable diet. Feeding smaller meals more frequently and varying the diet (e.g., offering various types of concentrate feeds as appetite may vary from day to day) are helpful methods to increase food intake.

Additional treatments for CRF in human patients include antihypertensive agents including diuretics, β-blockers, and angiotensin-converting enzyme inhibitors.[106] Use of the latter medications may have an additional benefit of limiting proteinuria.[107] Currently, little is known about the roles of systemic or intrarenal hypertension in progression of renal disease in horses, and there are no reports of potential benefits of use of antihypertensive medications in horses with CRF. Finally, efforts are under way to examine the roles of mediators of inflammation in development of renal fibrosis with the hope that future specific interventions may be developed to limit the progressive interstitial fibrosis that occurs in all patients with CRF.[108]

Horses with end-stage CRF often develop oliguria and uncontrollable metabolic acidosis. At this stage, CRF can only be managed by hemodialysis or peritoneal/pleural dialysis. However, pursuit of either hemodialysis or peritoneal dialysis in horses with CRF is impractical because, even when successful, dialysis prolongs the life of the patient for only a short time.

PROGNOSIS. The progressive loss of nephron function that is characteristic of CRF precludes successful long-term treatment in horses. However, many horses with early CRF may be able to continue in performance or live as a pet for quite some time (e.g., months to a few years). In general, as long as creatinine remains <5.0 mg/dl and the BUN/creatinine ratio is <15:1, affected horses seem to maintain a reasonably good attitude, appetite, and body condition. However, once creatinine exceeds 5.0 mg/dl, the rate of progression of CRF appears to accelerate and signs of uremia (e.g., anorexia, poor hair coat, and loss of body condition) become more apparent over a period of a few weeks to months. Although this threshold value for creatinine is a useful figure for offering an initial prognosis for most horses with CRF, it is important to remember that progression of CRF is highly variable between affected animals. Thus each case must be handled on an individual basis, with the emphasis on maintenance of body condition until humane euthanasia may become necessary.

REFERENCES

62. Divers TJ: Chronic renal failure in horses, *Compend Cont Educ* 5:S310-S317, 1983.
63. Schott HC et al: Chronic renal failure in 99 horses, *Proceedings of the Forty-third Annual Convention of the American Association of Equine Practitioners*, 1997, pp 345-346.
64. Banks KL, Henson JB: Immunologically mediated glomerulitis of horses. II, Antiglomerular basement membrane antibody and other mechanisms in spontaneous disease, *Lab Invest* 26:708-715, 1972.

65. Roberts MC, Kelly WR: Renal dysfunction in a case of purpura haemorrhagica in a horse, *Vet Rec* 110:144-146, 1982.

66. Divers TJ et al: Equine glomerulonephritis and renal failure associated with complexes of group C streptococcal antigen and IgG antibody, *Vet Immunol Immunopathol* 32:93-102, 1992.

67. Banks KL, Henson JB, McGuire TC: Immunologically mediated glomerulitis of horses. I, Pathogenesis in persistent infection by equine infectious anemia virus, *Lab Invest* 26:701-707, 1972.

68. Sabnis SG, Gunson DE, Antonovych TT: Some unusual features of mesangioproliferative glomerulonephritis in horses, *Vet Pathol* 21:574-581, 1984.

69. Ehnen SJ et al: Obstructive nephrolithiasis and ureterolithiasis associated with chronic renal failure in horses: eight cases (1981-1987), *J Am Vet Med Assoc* 197:249-253, 1990.

70. Andrews FM et al: Bilateral renal hypoplasia in four young horses, *J Am Vet Med Assoc* 189:209-212, 1986.

71. Ronen N et al: Renal dysplasia in two adult horses: clinical and pathological aspects, *Vet Rec* 132:269-270, 1993.

72. Bertone JJ et al: Monitoring the progression of renal failure in a horse with polycystic kidney disease: use of the reciprocal of serum creatinine concentration and sodium sulfanilate clearance half-time, *J Am Vet Med Assoc* 191:565-568, 1987.

73. Held JP, Wright B, Henton JE: Pyelonephritis associated with renal failure in a horse, *J Am Vet Med Assoc* 189:688-689, 1986.

74. Carrick JB, Pollitt CC: Chronic pyelonephritis in a brood mare, *Aust Vet J* 64:252-254, 1987.

75. Sloet van Oldruitenborgh-Oosterbaan MM, Klabec HC: Ureteropyelonephritis in a Fresian mare, *Vet Rec* 122:609-610, 1988.

76. Jakob W: Spontaneous amyloidosis of mammals, *Vet Pathol* 8:292-306, 1971.

77. Haschek WM, King JM, Tennant BC: Primary renal cell carcinoma in two horses, *J Am Vet Med Assoc* 179:992-994, 1981.

78. Wimberly HC, Antonovych TT, Lewis RM: Focal glomerulosclerosis-like disease with nephrotic syndrome in a horse, *Vet Pathol* 18:692-694, 1981.

79. Roberts MC, Seiler RJ: Renal failure in a horse with chronic glomerulonephritis and renal oxalosis, *J Equine Med Surg* 3:278-283, 1979.

80. Brown C: Equine nephrology, *Vet Annu* 26:1-16, 1986.

81. Macharg MA et al: Two methods for the treatment of ureterolithiasis in a mare, *Vet Surg* 13:95-98, 1984.

82. Tennant B et al: Chronic renal failure in the horse, *Proceedings of the Twenty-fourth Annual Convention of the American Association of Equine Practitioners*, 1978, pp 293-298.

83. Koterba AM, Coffman JR: Acute and chronic renal disease in the horse, *Compend Cont Educ Pract Vet* 3:S461-S469, 1981.

84. Brobst DF et al: Parathyroid hormone evaluation in normal horses and horses with renal failure, *Equine Vet Sci* 2:150-157, 1982.

85. Tennant B et al: Hypercalcemia and hypophosphatemia in ponies following bilateral nephrectomy, *Exp Biol Med* 167:365-368, 1981.

86. Naylor JM, Kronfeld DS, Acland H: Hyperlipemia in horses: effects of undernutrition and disease, *Am J Vet Res* 41:899-905, 1980.

87. Schott HC, Hodgson DR, Bayly WM: Haematuria, pigmenturia and proteinuria in exercising horses, *Equine Vet J* 27:67-72, 1995.

88. Kohn CW, Strasser SL: 24-hour renal clearance and excretion of endogenous substances in the mare, *Am J Vet Res* 47:1332-1337, 1986.

89. Kiper ML, Traub-Dargatz JL, Wrigley RH: Renal ultrasonography in horses, *Compend Cont Educ* 12:993-999, 1990.

90. Hoffman KL, Wood AKW, McCarthy PH: Sonographic-anatomic correlation and imaging protocol for the kidneys of horses, *Am J Vet Res* 56:1403-1412, 1995.

91. Divers TJ, Yeager AE: The value of ultrasonographic examination in the diagnosis and management of renal diseases in horses, *Equine Vet Educ* 7:334-341, 1997.

92. Matthews HK et al: Measuring renal function in horses, *Vet Med* 88:349-356, 1993.

93. Morris DD, Divers TJ, Whitlock RH: Renal clearance and fractional excretion of electrolytes over a 24 hour period, *Am J Vet Res* 45:2431-2436, 1984.

94. Brewer BD et al: A comparison of inulin, para-aminohippuric acid, and endogenous creatinine clearance as measures of renal function in neonatal foals, *J Vet Intern Med* 4:301-305, 1990.

95. Matthews HK et al: Comparison of standard and radionuclide methods for measurement of glomerular filtration rate and effective renal blood flow in female horses, *Am J Vet Res* 53:1612-1616, 1992.

96. Walsh DM, Royal HD: Evaluation of a single injection of ^{99m}Tc-labeled diethylenetriaminepentaacetic acid for measuring glomerular filtration rate in horses, *Am J Vet Res* 53:776-780, 1992.

97. Schott HC et al: Nuclear scintigraphy as a diagnostic aid in the evaluation of renal disease in horses, *Proceedings of Thirty-ninth Annual Convention of the American Association of Equine Practitioners*, 1993, pp 251-254.

98. Divers TJ: Management of chronic renal failure in the horse, *Proceedings of the Thirty-first Annual Convention of the American Association of Equine Practitioners*, 1985, pp 679-685.

99. Cianciaruso B et al: Salt intake and renal outcome in patients with progressive renal disease, *Miner Electrolyte Metab* 24:296-301, 1998.

100. Erslev AJ: Erythropoietin, *New Eng J Med* 324:1339-1344, 1991.

101. Watson TDG et al: Selective measurement of lipoprotein and hepatic triglyceride lipase in heparinized horses, *Am J Vet Res* 53:771-776, 1992.

102. Scharschmidt LA et al: Effects of dietary fish oil on renal insufficiency in rats with subtotal nephrectomy, *Kidney Int* 32:700-709, 1987.

103. Cappeli P et al: Lipids in the progression of chronic renal failure, *Nephron* 62:31-35, 1992.

104. Klahr S et al: The effects of dietary protein restriction and blood-pressure control on the progression of chronic renal disease, *New Engl J Med* 330:877-884, 1994.

105. Ikizler TA, Hakim RM: Nutrition in end-stage renal disease, *Kidney Int* 50:343-57, 1996.

106. Bretzel RG: Protecting the residual renal function: which drugs of choice? *Am J Hypertens* 10:159S-166S, 1997.

107. Porush JG: Hypertension and chronic renal failure: the use of ACE inhibitors, *Am J Kid Dis* 31:177-184, 1998.

108. Müller GA et al: Prevention of progression of renal fibrosis: how far are we? *Kidney Int* 49(suppl 54):S75-S82, 1996.

URINARY TRACT INFECTIONS

THOMAS J. DIVERS

Urinary tract infections (UTIs) can be anatomically divided into two categories: (1) those affecting the upper urinary tract: kidneys and ureters, and (2) those involving the lower urinary tract: bladder and urethra. Lower UTI in horses usually develops as a consequence of anatomical or functional causes of abnormal urine flow, especially bladder paralysis (see Urinary Incontinence, pp. 836 to 838). Although recognized less commonly, upper UTI is often a more serious, potentially life-threatening problem. In horses, UTI is also frequently accompanied by urolithiasis and partial obstruction. With the exception of single large cystoliths (that predispose affected horses to lower UTI), it is often difficult to determine whether development of nephroliths, ureteroliths, multiple small cystoliths, and urethroliths was a predisposing cause or a consequence of UTI.

RISK FACTORS AND CAUSES. The most common risk factors for development of UTI in horses are bladder paralysis, concurrent urolithiasis, and urethral damage (e.g., foaling trauma in mares, neoplasia or habronemiasis in stallions and geldings). The shorter urethra and its location near the anus also increase the risk of lower UTI in healthy females. For example, silent lower UTIs and pyelonephritis, resulting from infection with bacteria shed from the gastrointestinal tract, can develop in prepubertal girls and during pregnancy or after menopause in adult women.[109] This increased risk at certain times in women has been further attributed to a lack of estrogen, a hormone that appears to be important for production of glycosaminoglycans that cover uroepithelial surfaces and inhibit attachment of bacteria.[110] Whether or not fillies or pregnant mares are at increased risk for UTI has not been studied. However, horses with bladder paralysis (detrusor dysfunction) or decreased urethral sphincter tone (from trauma or neurologic disease) are clearly at greater risk of UTI than horses with normal detrusor and urethral sphincter function. Finally, because bladder catheterization cannot be performed in a sterile manner because of presence of normal bacterial flora of the vestibule and distal urethra, contamination of the lower urinary tract is an accepted risk of this procedure. Nevertheless, development of lower UTI is an unlikely complication of bladder catheterization in otherwise healthy animals because host defense mechanisms, including urine flow, are highly effective in eliminating contaminating bacteria. However, when urethral or bladder mucosa has been damaged or when urine stasis (bladder paralysis) is present, bladder catheterization has a greater risk of producing UTI.

In a group of horses with neurologic bladder dysfunction complicated by UTI, *Escherichia coli*, *Staphylococcus* spp.,

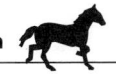

Corynebacterium spp., and *Pseudomonas aeruginosa* were the microbes isolated most frequently.[111] In my experience, *E. coli, Proteus mirabilis, Klebsiella* spp., and *Enterobacter* spp. are the most common pathogens isolated from individual horses with UTI. *P. aeruginosa* can cause lower UTI in some horses, but it can also be isolated from the urethra of many clinically normal horses. Gram-positive organisms are less frequent causes of UTI in horses, although *Staphylococcus* spp. and *Corynebacterium* spp. are occasionally identified pathogens.[112] In horses with abnormal urine flow (e.g., with uroliths) or instrumentation of the urinary tract (e.g., indwelling bladder catheters or ureteral stents), UTI with *Enterococcus* spp. (formerly *Streptococcus faecalis*) may also develop. Similarly, lower UTI with *Candida* spp. develop commonly in recumbent neonatal foals receiving broad-spectrum antibacterial therapy.

CLINICAL FINDINGS. Clinical signs with UTI usually reflect the location, severity, and duration of the infection. Lower UTI is typically characterized by recognizable disturbances in urine flow but seldom causes signs characteristic of a systemic infection (e.g., fever, weight loss). Dysuria, stranguria, pollakiuria, and incontinence are consistent with lower UTI. Urine scalding of the perineum may develop with chronic UTI in mares (but should not be confused with estrus), and the sheath opening and dorsal aspects of the hind limbs may be coated with urine crystals or blood in affected stallions and geldings. Gross hematuria may be observed if urinary calculi are present or if bladder or urethral mucosa has been eroded. Hematuria of bladder origin typically produces hematuria throughout urination but gross discoloration of urine is most obvious at the end of urination. In an occasional horse, gross pyuria may also be observed as passage of mucopurulent debris in otherwise clear urine. Horses with upper UTI are more likely to have signs characteristic of a systemic infection (e.g., fever, weight loss). However, because UTI is commonly accompanied by concurrent lower UTI, dysuria may also be present. As an example, recurrent urethral obstruction with small uroliths may be the presenting complaint for chronic upper UTI.

Rectal examination may help confirm a predisposing cause of lower UTI (e.g., enlarged and atonic bladder, cystic calculi, accumulation of sabulous urine sediment, or a bladder mass). Chronic cystitis also usually leads to bladder wall thickening; however, this change is not easily detected by rectal palpation. Although ureters are usually not found during rectal examination of the normal horse, careful palpation of the dorsolateral aspects of the caudal abdomen (retroperitoneal space) usually reveals enlarged ureters in horses with upper UTI. With pyelonephritis, palpation may further reveal kidneys that are either enlarged or shrunken and misshapen.

DIAGNOSIS. A diagnosis of UTI is based on clinical signs and laboratory analysis of blood and urine samples. With lower UTI, results of a CBC and serum biochemical profile are usually within reference ranges while CBC results with upper UTI often support a systemic inflammatory response. With chronic upper UTI, increased total protein and globulin concentrations are often detected, and when the UTI is bilateral, azotemia may also be present. Detection of greater than 20 organisms and more than 10 white blood cells (WBCs) per high-power field on sediment examination of a urine sample collected during midstream voiding or via bladder catheterization is highly supportive of UTI and growth of 10^4 or more organisms per milliliter of urine confirms the diagnosis.[113,114] When evaluating a horse for possible UTI, urine samples collected should be examined and processed for bacterial culture within 30 minutes after collection or they should be refrigerated because bacteria can continue to proliferate when urine is stored at room temperature.[113]

Detection of azotemia, low urine specific gravity, and WBC casts in urine sediment are indicative of bilateral upper UTI, especially when accompanied by signs of systemic illness. Ultrasonographic examination of the kidneys is useful for detecting abnormal renal size, shape, or consistency in horses with upper UTI.[115-117] Endoscopic examination of the lower urinary tract is another useful tool for evaluating the integrity of urethral and bladder mucosa, detecting small uroliths, and assessing urine flow from each ureteral orifice.[119,120] With long-standing cystitis, especially when bladder paralysis is the underlying cause, ureteral orifices may become dilated (and appear wide open) allowing for vesiculoureteral reflux and development of ascending pyelonephritis. When unilateral pyelonephritis is suspected on the basis of ultrasonographic findings and absence of azotemia, catheterization of each ureter to collect urine samples from each side of the upper urinary tract can be helpful to document unilateral disease. Ureters may be catheterized by passing a sterile polyethylene tubing through the biopsy channel of the endoscope during cystoscopy or can be accomplished in mares by directing blunt-ended catheters (e.g., 8-Fr polypropylene catheter) via the urethra into each ureteral orifice.[121]

TREATMENT. Treatment of UTI consists of proper antimicrobial therapy and correction, if possible, of predisposing anatomic or functional causes. Selection of the appropriate antimicrobial agent is best determined by prior knowledge of the following:

- Susceptibility patterns of the causative agent(s)
- Concentration of the antibiotic in renal tissue and urine
- Activity of the antibiotic at different pH values
- Ease of administration
- Toxicity
- Expense
- Compatibility with other antimicrobial drugs

Recommended antimicrobial agents for treatment of UTI in horses are discussed in the following paragraphs. It should be emphasized that in vitro resistance to a particular antibiotic may not preclude successful treatment with the drug as long as high concentrations are achieved in urine. Similarly, in vitro susceptibility does not always guarantee a successful response to treatment. For example, *Enterococcus* spp. are routinely found to be susceptible to trimethoprim-sulfa combinations; however, this pathogen is inherently resistant to these combinations in vivo.[122]

Trimethoprim/Sulfonamide Combinations. Trimethoprim-sulfonamide combinations have been highly successful in treating lower UTIs in some species.[123-125] Although sulfonamides alone can be effective in treating many lower UTIs,[126] addition of trimethoprim improves antibacterial spectrum without a prohibitive increase in expense or toxicity.[127] When selecting a trimethoprim-sulfonamide combination for treatment of horse with a UTI, metabolism of the sulfonamide should be considered. For example, sulfamethoxazole is largely metabolized to inactive products before urinary excretion, whereas sulfadiazine is excreted largely unchanged in urine.[128]

Penicillin and Ampicillin. Penicillin, administered parenterally, is effective for treating upper or lower UTIs caused by susceptible *Corynebacterium* spp., *Streptococcus* spp., and some *Staphylococcus* spp.[129] Ampicillin has also been used successfully for treatment of both upper and lower UTIs in animals and human patients.[123,130] Although many isolates of the Enterobacteriaceae family demonstrate resistance to ampicillin in vitro, this drug is highly concentrated in urine and many organisms that are resistant in vitro may be killed in the urine of treated animals.

Gentamicin and Amikacin. Gentamicin and amikacin, which can be nephrotoxic, should be reserved for treating lower UTIs caused by highly resistant organisms or acute, life-threatening upper UTIs caused by gram-negative organisms.

Pharmacokinetic studies in adults and foals are available.[131,132] Potentiated penicillins (ticarcillin or ticarcillin/clavulanic acid) may be considered as an alternative to aminoglycosides in horses with severely compromised renal function (e.g., creatinine >3.0 mg/dl).

Cephalosporins, Tetracyclines, and Chloramphenicol. Cephalosporins, tetracyclines, and chloramphenicol are frequently and effectively used for treatment of UTIs in other species.[130] Cephalosporins are concentrated in urine. Ceftiofur has broad-spectrum antimicrobial activity and could be selected when urinary pathogens demonstrate resistance to trimethoprim-sulfonamide combinations or penicillin. Tetracycline and chloramphenicol are predominantly metabolized in the liver with variable excretion in bile. However, when acceptable serum concentrations are achieved, excretion of active drug into urine may be high enough that either drug may be effective for treatment of UTIs caused by susceptible organisms.[133,134]

Other Antimicrobial Agents. Nitrofurantoin has an impressive in vitro spectrum, demonstrating activity against most common gram-negative organisms, including *Salmonella*.[126] The drug is inexpensive, is easily administered as an oral suspension, and achieves high concentrations in urine. Although this antimicrobial agent has not been well studied in horses, adverse effects and acquired resistance appear to be uncommon. However, nitrofurantoin does not attain high concentrations within renal parenchyma; thus, efficacy in treating upper UTI would be questionable. Further limitations of nitrofurantoin usage include decreased antimicrobial activity at an alkaline pH, and increased risk of toxicity has been described in other species as GFR falls (e.g., with chronic renal failure). Because urine concentration and antimicrobial activity of nitrofurantoin after oral administration have not been well substantiated in horses, use of this antibiotic should be reserved to select cases in which specific susceptibility of a gram-negative organism has been demonstrated or when expense precludes selection of another antibiotic for long-term therapy.

It is not unusual to find highly resistant organisms in urine of horses with chronic UTIs, especially those with bladder paralysis that have been repeatedly catheterized and have been on a variety of antibiotic agents. In some instances the organisms may be highly resistant to all drugs approved for use in the equine. The author has successfully treated a few adult horses and a yearling with UTI with enrofloxacin (2.5 mg/kg PO every 12 hours) without apparent adverse effects. Potential cartilage damage in younger horses should be considered and discussed with the owner before treatment with enrofloxacin would be pursued.

When treating UTIs in horses, antimicrobial therapy should be continued for at least 1 week for lower UTIs and for 2 to 6 weeks for upper UTIs. Ideally, a midstream-voided urine sample should be submitted for bacterial culture 2 to 4 days after initiation of therapy and again 1 to 2 weeks after treatment has been discontinued. If the UTI recurs and the same organism is isolated, a focus of upper UTI should be suspected. Ultrasonographic or nuclear scintigraphic examination of the kidneys should be considered in such cases to rule out a nephrolith or other parenchymal disease. Cystoscopy and ureteral catheterization can also be pursued to evaluate for unilateral or bilateral infection of the upper tract. In contrast, recurrence of UTI with a different pathogen suggests an anatomic or functional cause of abnormal urine flow as a predisposing cause of recurrent lower or upper UTI.

REFERENCES

109. Rubin RH, Tolkoff-Rubin NE, Cotran RS: Urinary tract infection. pyelonephritis, and reflux nephropathy. In Brenner BM, Rector FC, eds: *The kidney,* 4th ed, vol II, Philadelphia, 1991, WB Saunders, pp 1369-1429.

110. Mulholland SG et al: Effect of hormonal deprivation on the bladder defense mechanism, *J Urol* 127:1010-1013, 1982.

111. Adams LG et al: Cystitis and ataxia associated with sorghum ingestion, *J Am Vet Med Assoc* 155:518-524, 1969.

112. Roberts MC: Ascending urinary tract infection in ponies, *Aust Vet J* 55:191-193, 1979.

113. Farrar WE: Infections of the urinary tract: symposium on infections in office practice, *Med Clin North Am* 67:187-201, 1983.

114. Stamm WE: Measurement of pyuria and its relation to bacteriuria, *Am J Med* 28:53-58, 1983.

115. Kiper ML, Traub-Dargatz JL, Wrigley RH: Renal ultrasonography in horses, *Compend Cont Educ* 12:993-999, 1990.

116. Hoffman KL, Wood AKW, McCarthy PH: Sonographic-anatomic correlation and imaging protocol for the kidneys of horses, *Am J Vet Res* 56:1403-1412, 1995.

117. Divers TJ, Yeager AE: The value of ultrasonographic examination in the diagnosis and management of renal diseases in horses, *Equine Vet Educ* 7:334-341, 1997.

118. Deleted in proof.

119. Sullins KE, Traub-Dargatz JL: Endoscopic anatomy of the equine urinary tract, *Compend Cont Educ* 11:S663-S668, 1984.

120. Traub-Dargatz JL, McKinnon AO: Adjunctive methods of examination of the urogenital tract, *Vet Clin North Am (Equine Pract)* 4:339-358, 1988.

121. Schott HC, Hodgson DR, Bayly WM: Ureteral catheterisation in the horse, *Equine Vet Educ* 2:140-143, 1990.

122. Murray BE: Vancomycin-resistant Enterococcal infections, *New Engl J Med* 342:710-721, 2000.

123. Ling GV: Clinical use experience, *Proceedings of the Symposium on Trimethoprim/sulfadiazine,* Research Triangle Park, NC, 1978, Burroughs-Wellcome, pp 61-62.

124. Tolkoff-Rubin NE, Weber D, Fang LS, et al: Single-dose therapy with trimethoprim/sulfamethoxazole for urinary tract infections in women, *Rev Infect Dis* 4:444-448, 1982.

125. Divers TJ et al: Experimental induction of *Proteus mirabilis* cystitis in the pony and evaluation of therapy with trimethoprim/sulfadiazine, *Am J Vet Res* 42:1203-1205, 1981.

126. Keys TF: Antimicrobials commonly used for urinary tract infections, *Mayo Clin Proc* 52:680-682, 1977.

127. Bach MC et al: Susceptibility of recently isolated pathogenic bacteria to trimethoprim and sulfamethoxazole separately and combined, *J Infect Dis* 128(suppl):408-533, 1973.

128. Nouws JFM et al: Pharmacokinetics and renal clearance of sulfamethazine, sulfamerazine, and sulfadiazine and their N₄-acetyl and hydroxy metabolites in horses, *Am J Vet Res* 48:392-402, 1987.

129. Divers TJ: Urinary tract: horse, cow. In Johnston D, ed: *Bristol veterinary handbook of antimicrobial therapy,* Princeton, NJ, 1982, Veterinary Learning Systems, pp 84-91.

130. Sidor TA, Resnick MI: Urinary tract infections. In Speck, WT, Blumer JL: *Pediatric clinics of North America,* Philadelphia, 1983, WB Saunders, pp 322-332.

131. Cummings LE et al: Pharmacokinetics of gentamicin in newborn to 30-day-old foals, *Am J Vet Res* 51:1988-1992, 1990.

132. Sweeney RW, Divers TJ, Rossier Y: Disposition of gentamicin administered intravenously to horses with sepsis, *J Am Vet Med Assoc* 200:503-506, 1992.

133. Divers TJ: Serum levels of chloramphenicol after oral dosing and nasogastric administration in horses with acute *Salmonella* enteritis, *Proceedings of the Equine Colic Research Symposium,* Athens, Ga, 1982, pp 194-197.

134. Horspool LJI, McKellar QA: Disposition of oxytetracycline in horses, ponies and donkeys after intravenous administration, *Equine Vet J* 22:284-285, 1990.

URINARY INCONTINENCE

ELIZABETH A. CARR

Urinary incontinence in the horse can result from urolithiasis, congenital anomalies or defects of the lower urinary tract, trauma, neoplasia, neurologic diseases accompanied by bladder dysfunction, and decreased urethral tone. Bladder and urethral calculi frequently result in transient incontinence secondary to cystitis or partial obstruction. Ectopic ureter and other congenital malformations of the urinary tract generally produce incontinence from birth, although development of incontinence in adult horses has been described.[135-138] Traumatically induced incontinence may develop after breeding injury or dystocia in mares or in both sexes following sacral or spinal injury.[139] Incontinence has also been speculated to develop with long-standing lumbosacral or lower back problems that make it difficult for horses to posture to urinate. Over time, incomplete bladder emptying allows crystals normally present in equine urine to accumulate in the ventral aspect of the bladder. This crystalloid sediment becomes heavy and in some cases quite firm and further prevents complete bladder emptying. This condition, which has been termed sabulous urolithiasis,[140] can accompany bladder paralysis of any cause but may also be able to produce myogenic bladder dysfunction in the absence of an underlying neurologic problem. Horses with neoplasia of the lower urinary tract can also present with incontinence, but other complaints (e.g., stranguria or hematuria) are usually reported as well.

Neurologic disorders that commonly result in bladder paralysis and incontinence include equine herpes virus myelitis, cauda equina neuritis, and sorghum toxicosis. These diseases, along with other problems affecting gray matter of the sacral segments (e.g., an occasional horse with equine protozoal myelitis), result in loss of lower motor neuron function, whereas lesions of the lumbar or higher portions of the spinal cord result in loss of upper motor neuron function. Lower motor neuron damage leads to loss of detrusor function and overflow incontinence. A large, easily expressed bladder is found on rectal palpation. Initially, upper motor neuron disease is characterized by increased urethral resistance, leading to increased intravesicular pressure before voiding can occur. Voiding may occur as short bursts of urine passage with incomplete bladder emptying, and rectal examination may reveal a turgid bladder that is small to increased in size. Although upper motor neuron signs are initially different from those of lower motor neuron disease, incontinence is usually not recognized until overflow incontinence develops as a result of sabulous urolithiasis and progressive loss of detrusor function. The latter progression can explain why bladder paralysis and incontinence may occasionally be found in horses with other neurologic diseases such as cervical stenotic myelopathy, equine degenerative myelopathy, and even viral encephalomyelitis. Presence of other signs associated with lower motor neuron dysfunction (e.g., loss of anal or tail tone) or upper motor neuron dysfunction (e.g., ataxia) may aid in differentiating the inciting cause of bladder paralysis. Despite a large number of possible causes, the prognosis for recovery from incontinence resulting from bladder paralysis is generally poor because sabulous concretions and urinary tract infection (UTI) quickly complicate the problem.

A final syndrome of incontinence consequent to decreased urethral sphincter tone has been reported in a few mares.[141,142] This condition has been attributed to hypoestrogenism because incontinence improved after treatment with exogenous estrogen.

DIAGNOSIS. In addition to taking a complete history and performing physical and neurologic exams, it is helpful to observe the incontinence or any attempts made by the animal to urinate. Rectal palpation, transrectal ultrasonography of the bladder, and endoscopy of the lower urinary tract are useful to rule out uroliths, neoplasia, or congenital anomalies as causes of incontinence. Although most affected horses remain nonazotemic (unless significant obstruction or bilateral pyelonephritis has developed), laboratory analyses of blood and urine, including a quantitative urine culture, should be performed in all horses with incontinence because UTI is a common sequela of incontinence. Urethral and bladder pressure profiles can be pursued to assess urinary sphincter and detrusor muscle function. Normal values for both mares and geldings have been reported.[143-145] When an underlying neurologic problem is suspected, cerebrospinal fluid collection and analysis may also be of value.

A review of 21 horses presented to Michigan State University's Veterinary Teaching Hospital between 1995 and 2000 with a primary complaint of incontinence revealed that 15 horses had bladder paralysis, three had urolithiasis, and one foal had bilateral ureteral ectopia. Another horse had incontinence of undetermined cause that appeared to respond to treatment with phenylbutazone. The remaining horse had a urachal diverticulum, hydroureters, cystitis, pyelonephritis, an atonic bladder, and urethral sphincter dysfunction that was supported by an abnormal urethral pressure profile. Of the 15 horses with bladder paralysis, four developed the problem after foaling, two of which had dystocia. Fat necrosis around the urethra and bladder neck was found at postmortem examination in one of the latter mares. Bladder paralysis was attributed to equine protozoal myelitis (EPM) in two horses and to equine herpes virus myelitis, cauda equina neuritis, and cervical stenotic myelopathy in one horse each. One horse had segmental neuronal degeneration in the lumbosacral and caudal spinal cord, and another horse had histopathologic evidence of denervation atrophy of the detrusor that was attributed to prior spinal cord trauma. An underlying neurologic disease causing bladder paralysis could not be determined in the remaining four horses. Although originally presented for evaluation of acute-onset severe spinal ataxia and weakness, another mare developed signs of an upper motor neuron bladder dysfunction (squirts of urine and a turgid bladder on rectal palpation) during the course of hospitalization. Bladder function returned to normal as the neurologic disease improved over a period of 2 weeks.

TREATMENT. Treatment for incontinence varies with the underlying cause. Removal of calculi and appropriate antimicrobial therapy are effective treatments for urolithiasis. Surgical correction is generally needed for treatment of congenital anomalies but owners should be discouraged from using affected animals for breeding. Equine herpes virus myelitis and EPM carry the most favorable prognoses for recovery though bladder paresis may persist for several weeks. Removal of sabulous crystalloid material (via bladder lavage through a catheter or via cystotomy) and temporary placement of an indwelling bladder catheter is indicated in cases of recent onset of bladder paresis to prevent continued distension and further damage to the detrusor. Antimicrobial treatment, ideally based on urine culture results, is also indicated in all cases of bladder paralysis.

Bethanechol (0.25 to 0.75 mg/kg SQ or PO, every 8 to 12 hours), a parasympathomimetic agent that appears to have a somewhat selective effect on smooth muscle of the gastrointestinal tract and bladder, has been recommended for improving detrusor tone and strength of contraction in horses with bladder paralysis. However, response to treatment has usually been disappointing, perhaps because of long-standing paralysis before incontinence is recognized. Use of phenoxybenzamine (0.7 mg/kg PO, 4 times daily), an α-adrenergic blocker that decreases urethral sphincter tone, has also been recommended in combination with bethanechol in cases with upper motor neuron bladder dysfunction. In horses with evidence of urethral sphincter hypotonia, the sympathomimetic agent phenylpropanolamine (1 mg/kg PO, every 8 to 12 hours) has also been used but a successful response has not been reported. Dosing regimens for these autonomic drugs have been extrapolated from other species because no pharmacokinetic data is available for the equine species.

In general, treatment with these autonomic drugs has largely been ineffective in controlling incontinence resulting from bladder paralysis, and the long-term prognosis for recovery is usually poor. On a more positive note, treatment of a few mares with urethral sphincter hypotonia with estradiol cypionate or benzoate (5 to 10 µg/kg IM every other day) has been effective at resolving incontinence as long as detrusor function was normal. Estrogen may modulate the effect of norepinephrine on α-adrenergic receptor activity in the urethral sphincter, thereby improving urethral sphincter tone. Of further interest, incontinence in two mares with partial detrusor dysfunction was also reported to improve after treatment with estrogen,[142] although the mechanism by which estrogen would improve destrusor function is not clear.

REFERENCES

135. Pringle JK, Ducharme NG, Baird JD: Ectopic ureter in the horse: three cases and a review of the literature, *Can Vet J* 31:26-30, 1990.
136. Blikslager AT, Green EM: Ectopic ureters in horses, *Compend Cont Educ* 14:802-807, 1992.
137. Johnson PJ et al: Treatment of two mares with obstructive (vaginal) urinary outflow incontinence, *J Am Vet Med Assoc* 191:973-975, 1987.
138. Sponseller BA et al: Frontal septation of the bladder in a mare, *J Vet Intern Med* 12:313-315, 1998.
139. Watanabe T et al: High incidence of occult neurogenic bladder dysfunction in neurologically intact patients with thoracolumbar spinal injuries, *J Urol* 159:965-968, 1998.
140. Holt PE, Mair TS: Ten cases of bladder paralysis associated with sabulous urolithiasis in horses, *Vet Rec* 127:108-110, 1990.
141. Madison JB: Estrogen-responsive urinary incontinence in an aged pony mare, *Compend Cont Educ* 6:S390-S392, 1984.
142. Watson ED et al: Oestrogen responsive urinary incontinence in two mares, *Equine Vet Educ* 9:81-84, 1997.
143. Kay AD, Lavoie JP: Urethral pressure profilometry in mares, *J Am Vet Med Assoc* 191:212-216, 1987.
144. Clark ES et al: Cystometrography and urethral pressure profiles in healthy horse and pony mares, *Am J Vet Res* 48:552-555, 1987.
145. Ronen N: Measurements of urethral pressure profiles in the male horse, *Equine Vet J* 26:55-58, 1994.

ECTOPIC URETER

THOMAS J. DIVERS

Although rare, ectopic ureter is the most commonly reported developmental anomaly of the equine urinary tract. Of the cases reported, nearly 90% have been fillies and the primary complaint is urinary incontinence and perineal dermatitis (urine scalding).[146-149] However, this sex distribution may reflect easier recognition of urinary incontinence in females rather than a true sex predilection. In the male, intermittent urine dripping from the end of the penis is less easily recognized; further, urine entering the pelvic urethra may pass retrograde into the bladder.

DIAGNOSIS. Ectopic ureter should be suspected in young horses with incontinence observed shortly after birth. Renal function is usually normal but the affected ureter may be markedly dilated. In young foals (e.g., less than 50 to 75 kg) an excretory urogram (after intravenous administration of contrast agent) or pyelography (after percutaneous injection of contrast agent into the renal pelvis via ultrasonographic guidance) may aid in diagnosis of ectopic ureter.[149,150] Unfortunately, most patients are not presented until they are too large for this procedure to be performed (Fig. 32-5). Ultrasonographic examination may reveal mild dilation of the renal pelvis on the affected side. Vaginoscopic and cystoscopic examinations should also be pursued in older foals to determined whether the problem is unilateral or bilateral, and when unilateral, to determine which ureter is ectopic. In the latter instance, cystoscopic examination should reveal urine entering the bladder from only one normal ureteral opening, located at either 2 or 10 o'clock in the bladder neck. Urine can be seen squirting from normal ureteral openings every 20 to 30 seconds. Observation of normal bouts of voiding, in addition to incontinence, further supports a unilateral problem. To determine the location of the opening of the ectopic ureter, visual examination of the vestibule and vagina (using a blade speculum) should be performed initially to look for inter-

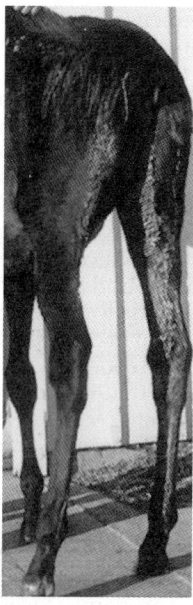

FIG. 32-5 ▓ Urine scalding in an 8-month-old Thoroughbred filly with a left ectopic ureter. The filly recovered after a nephrectomy.

mittent urine flow from the area of the urethral papilla. Ectopic ureteral openings are usually not apparent unless urine flow is seen. Intravenous administration of dyes including sodium fluorescein (10 mg/kg IV; yellow-green color), indigotindisulfonate (indigo carmine, 0.25 mg/kg IV; blue-purple color), azosulfamide (2.0 mg/kg IV; red color), or phenolsulfonphthalein (1.0 mg/kg IV; red color) to discolor the urine may aid in location of ectopic ureteral openings.[146,147]

TREATMENT. If the ectopic ureter is unilateral, creatinine is normal, and ultrasonographic examination of the opposite kidney appears normal, the preferred treatment may be to surgically remove the kidney on the affected side and ligate the ureter. Nephrectomy may produce an increase in creatinine (0.5 to 1 mg/dl) for a few days, but creatinine returns to the prenephrectomy value within a week. If both ureters are ectopic, which is not unusual, implantation of the distal ureters into the bladder neck should be attempted. Several surgical techniques have been described, but complications can include ascending infection, resulting from dilated ureters, and development of adhesions.[146-149]

REFERENCES

146. Pringle JK, Ducharme NG, Baird JD: Ectopic ureter in the horse: three cases and a review of the literature, *Can Vet J* 31:26-30, 1990.
147. Blikslager AT, Green EM: Ectopic ureters in horses, *Compend Cont Educ* 14:802-807, 1992.
148. Squire KRE, Adams SB: Bilateral ureterocystostomy in a 450-kg horse with ectopic ureters, *J Am Vet Med Assoc* 201:1213-1215, 1992.
149. Modransky PD, Wagoner PC, Robinette JD: Surgical correction of bilateral ectopic ureters in two foals, *Vet Surg* 12:141-147, 1983.
150. Blikslager AT et al: Ultrasonography and excretory urography in the diagnosis of bilateral ectopic ureters in a foal, *Vet Radiol* 33:41-47, 1992.

NEOPLASIA

THOMAS J. DIVERS

Neoplasia of the urinary tract is rare in horses. Primary kidney neoplasms include renal cell carcinoma and nephroblastoma, with the former being the most common tumor of the kidney.[151] Renal cell carcinoma (or adenocarcinoma) oc-

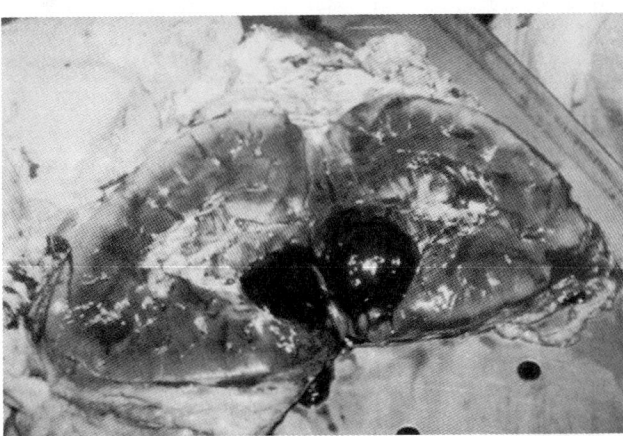

FIG. 32-6 Cut section of the left kidney from a 25-year-old horse with chronic weight loss, hematuria, and severe anemia. The kidney appeared normal, except for a small 4- by 5-cm carcinoma with surrounding hemorrhage.

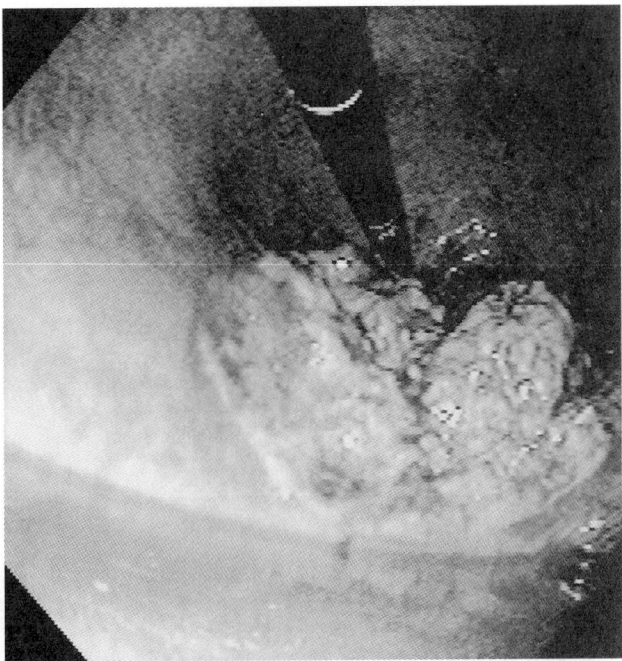

FIG. 32-8 Cystoscopic image of a squamous cell carcinoma of the bladder causing intermittent hematuria in a 14-year-old warmblood mare. The endoscope has been passed beyond the tumor and retroflexed to provide a view directed caudally; a pool of urine is in the foreground and the tumor can be seen in the ventral aspect of the bladder neck.

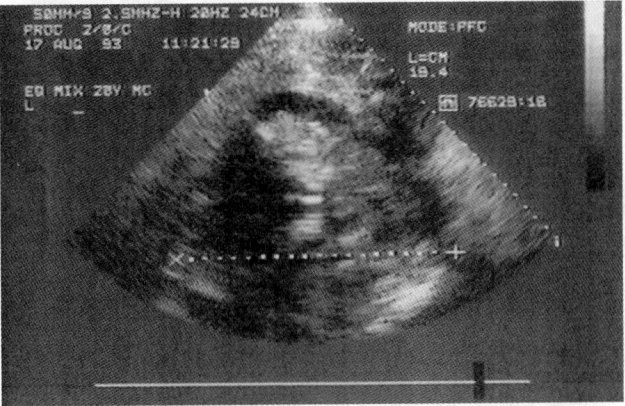

FIG. 32-7 Sonogram of the left kidney area of a 19-year-old horse with chronic hematuria. A 26- by 20- by 19-cm echocavitated mass (renal carcinoma) originates from the left kidney.

curs more frequently in older horses, but nephroblastomas may be detected in young horses. Squamous cell carcinoma is the most common bladder tumor, but horses may also develop transitional cell carcinoma.[152,153] Fibromatous polyps may also occur in younger horses, but bladder tumors usually develop in middle-age to older horses. Lymphosarcoma, hemangiosarcoma, and melanoma may also involve the kidneys and, on rare occasions, the bladder.[154,155]

CLINICAL SIGNS AND DIAGNOSIS. Clinical signs in horses with renal neoplasia include hematuria, weight loss, and recurrent colic. Sudden death may occur if the neoplasm hemorrhages into the abdomen or thorax. Renal tumors may result in marked enlargement of the kidneys such that both the left and right kidneys may be found on rectal palpation. In other cases, tumors may be small, circumscribed lesions within a kidney (Fig. 32-6) that cannot be felt during rectal palpation. Small tumors may also be difficult to visualize on ultrasonographic examination. The diagnosis is based on history, clinical signs, and ultrasonographic findings (Fig. 32-7). Affected horses usually are not azotemic, but mild anemia may be detected when gross hematuria is observed. Although neoplastic cells are unlikely to be found in urine, cytologic examination of urine sediment is warranted. Nephroblastoma usually remains limited to the kidney, but renal cell carcinomas commonly metastasize to the liver and lungs. Thoracic

radiographs are helpful in detecting pulmonary metastases. With ultrasonographic guidance, the tumor can usually be biopsied and a definitive diagnosis established.

In addition to hematuria and weight loss, horses with bladder tumors may also present with pollakiuria and stranguria. With bladder tumors, a mass can usually be palpated on rectal examination but it should not be confused with a cystolith or accumulation of sabulous concretions in the ventral aspect of the bladder. Horses with gross hematuria may be mildly anemic but usually are not azotemic. Other than hematuria and associated proteinuria, urinalysis results are often unremarkable; however, with bladder tumors, cytologic examination of urine sediment is more likely to reveal neoplastic cells than with renal tumors.[152,155] A diagnosis of bladder neoplasia may be confirmed by cystoscopic examination and biopsy (Fig. 32-8).

TREATMENT. The treatment of choice for unilateral renal neoplasia is nephrectomy. Unfortunately, most cases of renal cell carcinoma have metastasized by the time the diagnosis is made, and surgical intervention is of little benefit to horses with disseminated disease. Thus careful evaluation for metastatic disease should be pursued before contemplating a nephrectomy. Treatment of bladder tumors include surgical excision and/or topical chemotherapy using either 5-fluorouracil or triethylenethiophosphoramide.[152]

REFERENCES

151. Brown PJ, Holt PE: Primary renal cell carcinoma in four horses, *Equine Vet J* 17:473-477, 1985.
152. Fischer AT et al: Neoplasia of the equine urinary bladder as a cause of hematuria, *J Am Vet Med Assoc* 186:1294-1296.
153. Traub JL et al: Intraabdominal neoplasia as a cause of chronic weight loss in the horse, *Compend Cont Educ* 5:S526-S534, 1983.
154. Murray RC, Brodbelt DC: Hematuria due to renal hemangiosarcoma in a donkey. *Equine Pract* 21:14-17, 1999.
155. Sweeney RW, Hamir AN, Fisher RR: Lymphosarcoma with urinary bladder infiltration in a horse, *J Am Vet Med Assoc* 199:1177-1178, 1991.

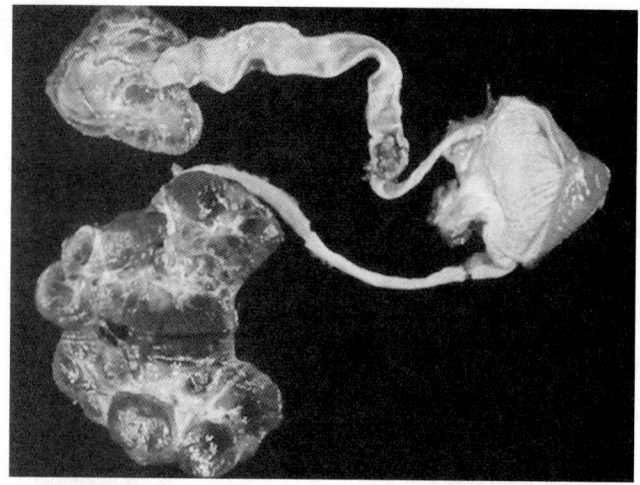

FIG. 32-9 ▮▮ Urinary tract removed from a 5-year-old Standardbred with chronic renal failure caused by intermittent or persistent obstruction by renal and ureteral stones. Note the location of the ureteral obstruction near the bladder. This is the most common site for the obstruction to occur.

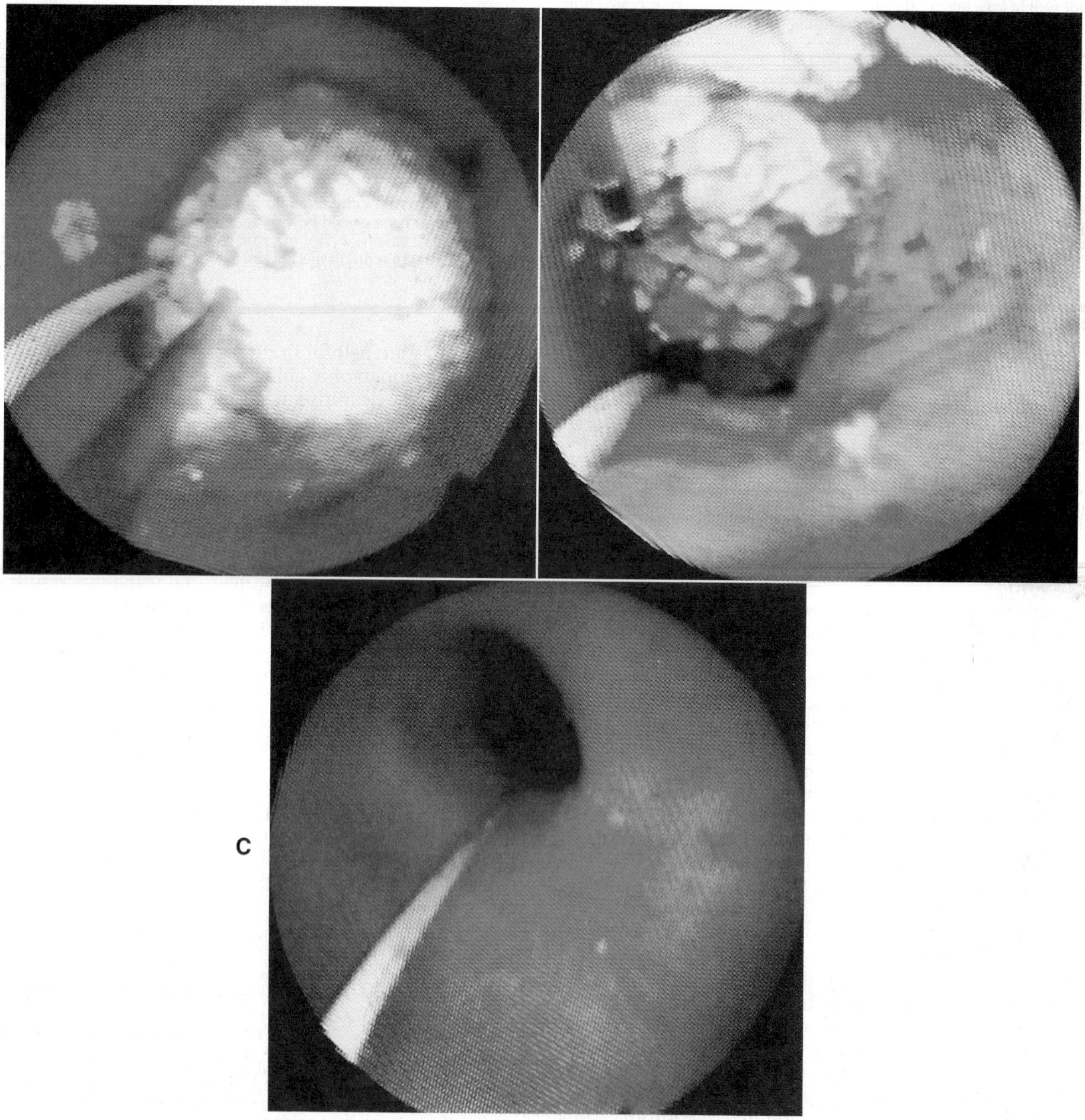

A

B

C

FIG. 32-10 ▮▮ Endoscopic images of a ureterolith completely obstructing the left ureter. **A,** Immediately before electrohydraulic lithotripsy. **B,** After partial fragmentation. **C,** After complete removal. White instrument is a ureteral stent placed to facilitate passage of the ureteroscope, and gray instrument (in **A** and **B**) is the lithotriptor touching the surface of the ureterolith.

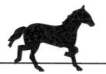

UROLITHIASIS AND OBSTRUCTIVE DISEASE

THOMAS J. DIVERS

RENAL AND URETERAL CALCULI

Renal and ureteral calculi can produce partial or complete obstruction of one or both sides of the upper urinary tract. Nephroliths usually develop within or adjacent to the renal pelvis, and obstruction can lead to hydronephrosis. Most ureteroliths likely originate as nephroliths that pass into the ureter, where they become lodged and enlarge over time. Ureteral stones have a propensity to lodge in the distal ureter and can sometimes be palpated per rectum dorsal and lateral to the bladder neck. Occasionally, small nephroliths may pass all the way down the ureter into the bladder; unlike their human counterparts, affected equine patients are rarely recognized to manifest renal colic.[156,157] Renal and ureteral calculi are most commonly composed of calcium carbonate crystals, although calcium phosphate stones may occasionally develop. Although usually not recognized clinically, a nidus of damaged tissue (e.g., interstitial inflammation, infection, or fibrosis or an area of medullary crest necrosis adjacent to the renal pelvis) is likely necessary for initiation of stone formation. Anomalies of development (e.g., renal hypoplasia, dysplasia, or polycystic disease) or prior exposure to nephrotoxins could also provide a nidus for stone formation.

Bilateral nephrolithiasis and ureterolithiasis has been best described in a series of young adult racehorses, and development of subclinical medullary crest necrosis as a consequence of NSAID use was a suggested risk factor.[158] When both sides of the upper tract are affected, the condition typically progresses to CRF before horses are presented for evaluation (Fig. 32-9). As described for CRF the most common presenting complaint is weight loss but polyuria or poor performance may be earlier complaints in competitive horses. Establishing a diagnosis of urolithiasis causing unilateral upper tract obstruction is more challenging because clinical signs are mild (recurrent colic) or nonexistent and azotemia is usually absent. In fact, unilateral upper tract stones may be detected as incidental necropsy findings in horses of all ages. In horses with clinical signs, careful palpation per rectum may reveal a turgid ureter and the presence of a ureterolith. When small uroliths are passed from the upper tract into the bladder, they may be voided without problem or they may cause urethral obstruction in males and horses with repeated bouts of urethral obstruction should be thoroughly evaluated for presence of upper tract disease.

In horses with bilateral disease leading to CRF, azotemia and isosthenuria are present. As already mentioned, azotemia is usually absent with unilateral obstruction. With either scenario, gross hematuria is uncommon unless stones have been passed into the bladder or urethra, but urinalysis usually reveals pigmenturia, and microscopic hematuria is confirmed by examination of urine sediment. Although UTI usually is not present with upper tract obstruction consequent to lithiasis at the initial evaluation, it may develop with catheterization or other instrumentation used for relief of the obstruction. Thus a quantitative urine culture should be considered part of the minimum database, especially if pyuria or bacteriuria are detected on sediment examination. Transabdominal ultrasonography is a valuable tool for detection of nephroliths, dilation of the renal pelvis (or complete hydronephrosis), and fibrosis (increased echogenicity) within the kidney.[159-161] However, small nephroliths (<1 cm in diameter) occasionally can be missed despite a complete ultrasonographic examination. Transrectal ultrasonography is also useful for detection of ureteral dilation and lithiasis.

If upper urinary tract obstruction is diagnosed before development of more severe azotemia (creatinine >5.0 mg/dl), surgical removal is recommended. A nephrotomy and/or ureterotomy may be required.[156,158] When equipment is available, electrohydraulic lithotripsy is the preferred technique for removal of ureteral stones.[162] This procedure involves passing an endoscope into the ureter until the stone can be seen and advancing a lithotriptor through the biopsy channel of the endoscope until the end touches the ureterolith (Fig. 32-10, *A*). An irrigating solution is pumped through the endoscope to distend the distal ureter, and delivery of an electrical impulse via the lithotriptor causes a shock wave at the surface of the stone. Because the majority of calcium carbonate stones are inherently fragile,[163] fragmentation via lithotripsy is usually rapid (Fig. 32-10, *B*), and remaining fragments are flushed distally by further infusion of irrigating solution (Fig. 32-10, *C*). Before surgical intervention is pursued, both kidneys should be thoroughly evaluated for evidence of other stones because upper tract lithiasis is often bilateral.

In addition to intermittent signs of mild colic, unilateral nephroliths may occasionally cause intermittent or persistent gross hematuria. In the absence of azotemia and evidence of disease of the contralateral kidney, unilateral nephrectomy is the treatment of choice for obstructing nephroliths and remains a reasonable alternative to lithotripsy for treatment of unilateral ureteroliths (Figs. 32-11 and 32-12).[164]

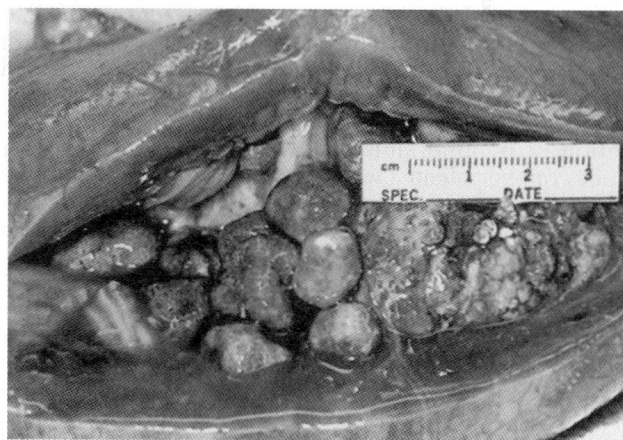

FIG. 32-11 ▓ The left kidney of a 12-year-old Thoroughbred that presented with a complaint of intermittent hematuria. The right kidney appeared normal on ultrasound examination, and renal function was normal.

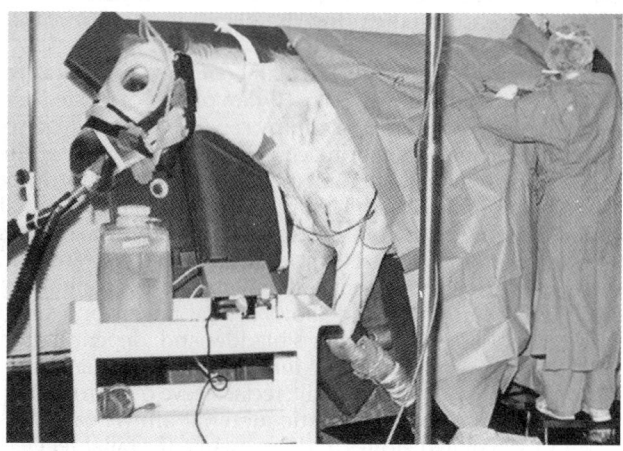

FIG. 32-12 ▓ The left kidney in Fig. 32-11 was removed with the horse anesthetized but strapped to the surgery table in an upright position. This is the preferred surgical position for nephrectomy or nephrotomy in adult horses.

CYSTIC CALCULI

Although occurrence is rare compared with other species, cystolithiasis is the most common form of urolithiasis in horses, and intact males appear to be at greater risk.[157,165] Calculi that develop in the bladder are usually single, large spiculated stones composed of calcium carbonate crystals.[163,165,166] Less commonly, stones are a mix of calcium carbonate and calcium phosphate crystals. The latter stones often have a smooth surface and are more resistant to fragmentation.[167] Risk factors for development of bladder stones in horses are not well understood, but anatomic defects (e.g., diverticuli) or suture material persisting from prior bladder surgery may predispose horses to cystic calculi. Although bacteria can often be detected by culture of the center of equine calculi, their role in stone formation is unclear.[157] Considering the fact that normal equine urine is rich in calcium carbonate crystals, it is surprising that cystoliths are not more common in horses than in ruminants or small animals. Their low occurrence can likely be attributed to the large amount of mucus that is also present in horse urine. Mucus, produced by glands in the renal pelvis and proximal ureter, appears to act as a lubricant to prevent adherence of crystals to uroepithelium.

The most common clinical sign exhibited by horses with cystic calculi is hematuria after exercise. Pollakiuria, stranguria, or incontinence may also be observed. Less commonly, dysuria may be caused by accumulation of urine sediment in the ventral aspect of the bladder. This condition, termed sabulous urolithiasis, usually develops as a consequence of bladder paralysis.[168] Urinary incontinence is usually present in horses with sabulous urolithiasis, and prognosis is guarded to poor because of underlying detrusor dysfunction.

Presence of a cystolith can be confirmed by rectal examination. It is important to remember that most bladder stones can be palpated with only the hand and wrist in the rectum. As a result of frequent urination, the bladder is usually small, and cystic calculi can be missed if the examiner passes quickly beyond the calculus during the rectal examination. Careful palpation may also allow discrimination between soft tissue masses of the bladder (neoplasia) and sabulous urolithiasis. With the latter, firm sediment is usually palpated well over the pelvic brim in the ventral aspect of a distended bladder. Manipulation of the bladder is accompanied by incontinence and sabulous uroliths may be indentable when palpated after the bladder has been emptied via catheterization. Although rarely needed to confirm the diagnosis, ultrasonographic examination of the entire urinary tract should be considered because calculi may be present in multiple locations. Because UTI can sometimes accompany cystolithiasis, urinalysis and a quantitative urine culture are warranted during the initial evaluation of all horses with bladder stones.

Treatment of cystic calculi usually consists of surgical removal accompanied by a 7- to 10-day course of postoperative antibiotic treatment. Cystotomy can be performed via celiotomy or a pararectal approach (Gökel's operation) or the stone can be removed after fragmentation with a lithotriptor passed via a perineal urethrotomy.[167,173,174] In mares, urethral sphincterotomy after epidural anesthesia with xylazine has been advocated as a practical method for stone removal. However, with sedation and epidural anesthesia, manual distention of the urethra often allows several fingers or a small hand to be passed into a mare's bladder and, depending on size, the stone can be retrieved intact or after fragmentation. Placing the cystolith into a sterile rectal sleeve or surrounding it with a similar smooth plastic material allows easier removal of spiculated stones and fragments. If available, electrohydraulic or pulsed dye laser lithotripsy may be the least traumatic method of fragmentation and removal of bladder stones in both sexes; however, success may be limited by the ability to effectively lavage all stone fragments out of the bladder.[175-179]

Historically, risk of recurrence after surgery has been considered low; however, in a series of 68 cases of urolithiasis (at all levels of the urinary tract), 12/29 horses (41%) with follow-up had recurrence from 1 to 32 months after surgery. Recurrence was more common with perineal urethrotomy than cystotomy and was attributed to inability to complete remove all fragments by lavage with the former approach.[157] This relatively high recurrence rate indicates that postoperative management changes are warranted to decrease risk of future stone formation. Changing from a legume to a grass hay is the most practical recommendation to decrease urinary calcium excretion. Urinary acidification with ammonium chloride (50 to 200 mg/kg/day PO) or ammonium sulfate (200 to 300 mg/kg/day PO) has also been recommended to decrease the amount of urine crystals in equine urine.[179,180] Unfortunately, these ammonium salts are rather unpalatable and should be administered as two or three doses daily for effective urinary acidification. Further, the actual benefit of urinary acidification in horses has never been established, and recurrence may be more likely related to inadequate mucus secretion or persistence of damaged uroepithelium in the upper or lower tract. A more practical recommendation may be to administer 2 to 4 oz of salt in the feed daily to increase water consumption and urine flow. The increase in urine flow is accompanied by a decrease in urine pH to near neutral values.

URETHRAL OBSTRUCTION

Calculi, neoplasms, congenital anomalies, and preputial edema and inflammation may all produce partial or complete obstruction of the urethra. Urethral calculi are most often calcium carbonate stones that lodge in the pelvic urethra in stallions or geldings,[181] and the most common neoplasm causing urethral obstruction is squamous cell carcinoma of the penis.[182] Preputial edema and inflammation may develop as a consequence of trauma or parasitism (habronemiasis). In addition, overweight horses may develop recurrent preputial inflammation and infection associated with fat deposition in the sheath. Horses affected with the latter condition may fail to drop the penis during urination and urine scalding within the sheath is likely a contributing factor to recurrent inflammation.

Complete urethral obstruction usually causes moderate to severe signs of colic, and an enlarged, turgid bladder is detected via rectal palpation. Careful palpation of the urethra below the anus may reveal the location of an obstructing urolith or frequent contraction of the urethralis muscle. Rarely, postrenal ARF may develop or the bladder may rupture. Partial urethral obstruction is usually accompanied by dysuria, incontinence, and urine scalding of the hindlimbs. A diagnosis of urethral obstruction is based on clinical signs, rectal examination findings, external examination of the penis and prepuce, and passage of a catheter or endoscope through the urethra to the bladder.

Treatment of urethral obstruction usually involves surgery. Urethral calculi can either be removed via a subischial urethrotomy over the site of obstruction or by hydropulsion through the urethrotomy incision. Excessive tissue trauma should be avoided because it may increase the risk of urethral stricture and recurrent urolithiasis. Laboratory assessment of fluid and electrolyte status is important for correction of dehydration, azotemia, and electrolyte alterations that may develop with sweating (caused by pain), bladder rupture, or anuria. With squamous cell carcinoma, aggressive surgical resection of involved tissues is warranted with larger lesions, whereas smaller lesions may be amenable to treatment with topical application of 5-fluorouracil ointment. However, because recurrence rate

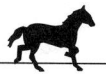

of squamous cell carcinoma of the penis and prepuce is 20% or greater,[182] surgical removal should be initially considered in all affected horses. Detrusor function may be decreased if bladder distention had been ongoing for several days and an indwelling bladder catheter (closed system) or treatment with bethanechol (0.25 to 0.75 mg/kg SQ or PO every 8 to 12 hours) may help with recovery of detrusor function.

REFERENCES

156. Macharg MA et al: Two methods for the treatment of ureterolithiasis in a mare, *Vet Surg* 13:95-98, 1984.
157. Laverty S et al: Urolithiasis in 68 horses, *Vet Surg* 21:56-62, 1992.
158. Ehnen SJ et al: Obstructive nephrolithiasis and ureterolithiasis associated with chronic renal failure in horses: eight cases (1981-1987), *J Am Vet Med Assoc* 197:249-253, 1990.
159. Kiper ML, Traub-Dargatz JL, Wrigley RH: Renal ultrasonography in horses, *Compend Cont Educ* 12:993-999, 1990.
160. Hoffman KL, Wood AKW, McCarthy PH: Sonographic-anatomic correlation and imaging protocol for the kidneys of horses, *Am J Vet Res* 56:1403-1412, 1995.
161. Divers TJ, Yeager AE: The value of ultrasonographic examination in the diagnosis and management of renal diseases in horses, *Equine Vet Educ* 7:334-341, 1997.
162. Rodger LD, Carlson GP, Moran ME, et al: Resolution of a left ureteral stone using electrohydraulic lithotripsy in a Thoroughbred colt, *J Vet Int Med* 9:280-282, 1995.
163. Neumann RD, Ruby AL, Ling GV, et al: Ultrastructure and mineral composition of urinary calculi from horses, *Am J Vet Res* 55:1357-1367, 1994.
164. Juzwiak JS, Bain FT, Slone DE, et al: Unilateral nephrectomy for treatment of chronic hematuria due to nephrolithiasis in a colt, *Can Vet J* 29:931-933, 1988.
165. DeBowes RM, Nyrop KA, Boulton CH: Cystic calculi in the horse, *Compend Cont Educ* 6:S268-S274, 1984.
166. Holt PE, Pearson H: Urolithiasis in the horse-a review of 13 cases, *Equine Vet J* 16:31-35, 1984.
167. DeBowes RM: Surgical management of urolithiasis, *Vet Clin North Am, (Equine Pract)* 4:461-471, 1988.
168. Holt PE, Mair TS: Ten cases of bladder paralysis associated with sabulous urolithiasis in horses, *Vet Rec* 127:108-110, 1990.
169. Deleted in proof.
170. Deleted in proof.
171. Deleted in proof.
172. Deleted in proof.
173. Kaneps AJ, Shires GMH, Watrous BJ: Cystic calculi in two horses, *J Am Vet Med Assoc* 187:737-739, 1985.
174. Mair TS, Holt PE: The aetiology and treatment of equine urolithiasis, *Equine Vet Educ* 6:189-192, 1994.
175. MacHarg MA et al: Electrohydraulic lithotripsy for treatment of a cystic calculus in a mare, *Vet Surg* 14:325-327, 1985.
176. Eustace RA, Hunt JM: Electrohydraulic lithotripsy for treatment of cystic calculus in two geldings, *Equine Vet J* 20:221-223, 1988.
177. Howard RD, Pleasant RS, May KA: Pulsed dye laser lithotripsy for treatment of urolithiasis in two geldings, *J Am Vet Med Assoc* 212:1600-1603, 1998.
178. Sertich PL et al: Medical management of urinary calculi in a stallion with breeding dysfunction, *J Am Vet Med Assoc* 213:843-846, 1998.
179. Johnson PJ, Crenshaw KL: The treatment of cystic and urethral calculi in a gelding, *Vet Med* 85:891-900, 1990.
180. Remillard RL et al: Dietary management of cystic calculi in a horse, *J Equine Vet Sci* 12:359-363, 1992.
181. Trotter GW, Bennett DG, Behm RJ: Urethral calculi in five horses, *Vet Surg* 10:159-162, 1981.
182. Mair TS, Walmsley JP, Phillips TJ: Surgical treatment of 45 horses affected by squamous cell carcinoma of the penis and prepuce, *Equine Vet J* 32:406-410, 2000.

IDIOPATHIC RENAL HEMATURIA

HAROLD C. SCHOTT II

Idiopathic renal hematuria is syndrome characterized by sudden onset of gross, often life-threatening hematuria.[183] Hemorrhage arises from one or both kidneys and is manifested by passage of large blood clots in urine. Endoscopic examination of the urethra and bladder usually reveals no abnormalities of these structures, but blood clots may be seen exiting one or both ureteral orifices. Although a definitive cause of renal hemorrhage may be established in some horses (e.g., renal adenocarcinoma, arteriovenous, or arterioureteral fistula),[184,185] the

disorder is termed idiopathic when a primary disease process cannot be found. Both sexes, a wide age range, and several breeds of horses (including a mammoth donkey and a mule) have been affected. However, more than 50% of animals with idiopathic renal hematuria (IRH) have been Arabians.

Use of the term idiopathic renal hematuria to describe this syndrome of horses was adopted from its use in human patients and dogs with severe renal hemorrhage.[186-190] Benign essential hematuria and benign primary hematuria are other terms that have been used to describe less severe hematuria that is not associated with trauma or other obvious causes of hematuria. In humans and dogs, hematuria is more commonly a unilateral than a bilateral problem, similar to what has been observed in the few affected horses. The pathophysiology remains poorly understood, but macroscopic hematuria has been associated with immune-mediated glomerular damage (e.g., acute postinfectious glomerulonephritis, membranoproliferative glomerulonephritis, and IgA nephropathy or Berger's disease), thin basement membrane nephropathy, and the loin pain-hematuria syndrome in human patients.

Although hematuria and/or pigmenturia can accompany several systemic diseases in horses,[191-194] patients affected with IRH appear to have spontaneous, severe hematuria in the absence of other signs of disease. Although one report suggested that severe renal hemorrhage was a consequence of pyelonephritis,[195] supportive data was lacking. In cases I managed, neither UTI nor lithiasis has been detected and the magnitude of hematuria often resulted in need for repeated blood transfusions. As with hemorrhage associated with guttural pouch mycosis, the syndrome may produce episodic hemorrhage. Initially, hemorrhage is noted by finding a large amount of clotted blood in stall bedding or in the pasture. However, other client complaints (e.g., depression, anorexia, weight loss, etc.) are typically absent. Examination may reveal dried blood at the end of the penis or in the sheath of males or on the vulvar lips and between the hind limbs of mares. In both sexes, neoplasia of the external genitalia or urinary tract is an important differential diagnosis, and in mares varicosities in the area of the vestibulovaginal sphincter also must be considered, especially in multiparous mares. When blood is not detected in the sheath or vulvar areas, further evaluation may be unrewarding because the renal bleeding may cease spontaneously. Bleeding has anecdotally been attributed to cystitis and pyelonephritis, in the absence of positive urine culture results because hemorrhage stops during a course of antimicrobial therapy. More likely, spontaneous resolution has occurred. Further, the magnitude of hematuria is considerably greater with IRH than with most urinary tract infections, pyuria is absent, and urine culture results are negative. In my experience, one or two initial episodes of hemorrhage are followed by a more severe hemorrhagic crisis within months to a couple of years after observation of the initial bleeding episode. Of interest, renal colic has been notably absent in the history of affected horses.

A diagnosis of IRH is made by exclusion of systemic disease, other causes of hematuria, and alterations in hemostasis. Physical examination may reveal tachycardia, tachypnea, and pale membranes consistent with acute blood loss. Rectal palpation may reveal an enlarged, irregular bladder resulting from the presence of blood clots. Azotemia is uncommon. Endoscopic examination is important to document that hematuria is originating from the upper urinary tract and to determine whether hemorrhage is unilateral or bilateral (Fig. 32-13). Repeated examinations may be required to answer the latter question. Ultrasonographic imaging is necessary to rule out nephrolithiasis or ureterolithiasis and may occasionally reveal a distended vascular space or renal vascular anomaly as the cause of hematuria. Renal scintigraphy can be a useful technique in affected horses because it may provide semiquantitative information about renal function

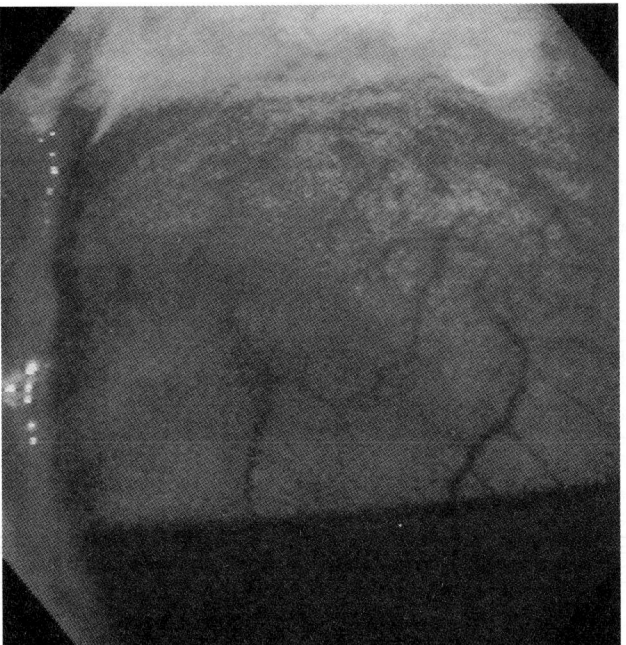

FIG. 32-13 ▌ Cystoscopic image of a 19-year-old Arabian mare with idiopathic renal hematuria. A large blood clot can be seen exiting the left ureter while the right ureteral opening appears normal.

when a nephrectomy is being considered. Renal biopsy and immunofluorescent staining may assist in documenting immune-mediated glomerular injury but the significance of such results is not well understood at this time.

Treatment for IRH consists of supportive care for acute blood loss, including blood transfusions. Medications intended to promote hemostasis (e.g., α-aminocaproic acid, formalin, etc.) have also been administered, but their efficacy has not been validated. Because the condition may be self-limiting in some patients, supportive care is warranted. With severe and recurrent hematuria of unilateral renal origin, a nephrectomy may be indicated but owners should be warned that there is a risk of hematuria developing in the contralateral kidney. In my experience, risk of contralateral renal bleeding appears to be greater in the Arabian breed.

REFERENCES

183. Schott HC, Hines MT: Severe urinary tract hemorrhage in two horses, *J Am Vet Med Assoc* 204:1320, 1994 (letter).
184. Latimer FG, Magnus R, Duncan RB: Arteriouretereal fistula in a colt, *Equine Vet J* 23:483-484, 1991.
185. Schott HC et al: Renal arteriovenous malformation in a Quarter Horse foal, *J Vet Int Med* 10:204-206, 1996.
186. Pardo V, Berian MG, Levi DF, Strauss J: Benign primary hematuria: clinicopathologic study of 65 patients, *Am J Med* 67:817-822, 1979.
187. Hughes JH et al: Massive nontraumatic hematuria: a challenging demand demanding immediate action, *Postgrad Med* 67:97-106, 1990.
188. Stone EA, DeNovo RC, Rawlings CA: Massive hematuria of nontraumatic renal origin in dogs, *J Am Vet Med Assoc* 183:868-871, 1983.
189. Holt PE, Lucke VM, Pearson H: Idiopathic renal hemorrhage in the dog, *J Small Anim Pract* 28:253-263, 1987.
190. Kaufman AC, Barsanti JA, Selcer BA: Benign essential hematuria in dogs, *Compend Contin Educ* 16:1317-1322, 1994.
191. Roberts MC, Kelly WR: Renal dysfunction in a case of purpura haemorrhagica in a horse, *Vet Rec* 110:144-146, 1982.
192. Morris CF et al: Hemolytic uremic-like syndrome in two horses, *J Am Vet Med Assoc* 191:1453-1454, 1987.
193. Dolente BA, Seco OM, Lewis ML: Streptococcal toxic shock in a horse, *J Am Vet Med Assoc* 217:64-67, 2000.
194. Bernard WV et al: Hematuria and leptospiruria in a foal, *J Am Vet Med Assoc* 203:276-278, 1993.
195. Kisthardt KK et al: Severe renal hemorrhage caused by pyelonephritis in 7 horses: clinical and ultrasonographic evaluation, *Can Vet J* 40:571-576, 1999.

URETHRAL HEMORRHAGE

HAROLD C. SCHOTT II

Although a recognized cause of hemospermia in stallions, defects or tears of the proximal urethra at the level of the ischial arch are a more recently described cause of hematuria in geldings.[196-198] Urethral defects typically result in hematuria at the end of urination, in association with urethral contraction. Affected horses generally void a normal volume of urine that is not discolored. At the end of urination, a series of urethral contractions results in squirts of bright red blood. Occasionally, a smaller amount of darker blood may be passed at the start of urination. In most instances the condition does not appear painful or result in pollakiuria. Interestingly, the majority of affected stallions with hemospermia and geldings with hematuria have been Quarter Horses or Quarter Horse crosses that have been free of other complaints.[199,200] Treatment with antibiotics for a suspected cystitis or urethritis has routinely been unsuccessful, although hematuria appears to resolve spontaneously in about 50% affected horses. Because the defects are difficult to detect without use of high resolution videoendoscopic equipment, previous reports of urethral bleeding have been attributed to urethritis or hemorrhage from "varicosities" of the urethral vasculature. However, vasculature underlying the urethral mucosa becomes quite prominent when the urethra is distended with air during endoscopic examination, especially in the proximal urethra (to the point that blood can be seen flowing in the submucosal vasculature). Thus it would be logical to suspect that hemorrhage could arise from an apparent urethritis or urethral varicosity, although these problems are poorly documented in horses.

Examination of affected horses is often unremarkable and laboratory analysis of blood reveals normal renal function, although mild anemia can be an occasional finding. Urine samples collected midstream or by bladder catheterization appear grossly normal. Urinalysis may have normal results or an increased number of red blood cells may be found on sediment examination, a finding that would also result in a positive reagent strip result for blood. Bacterial culture of urine yields negative results. The diagnosis is made via endoscopic examination of the urethra, during which a lesion is typically seen along the dorsocaudal aspect of the urethra at the level of the ischial arch. External palpation of the urethra in this area is usually unremarkable but can assist in localizing the lesion because external digital palpation can be seen via the endoscope. With hematuria of several weeks duration, there is little evidence of inflammation; rather the lesion appears as a fistula communicating with the vasculature of the corpus spongiosum penis (Fig. 32-14).

Although the pathophysiology of this condition remains unclear, it has been speculated that the defect is the result of a "blowout" of the corpus spongiosum penis (cavernous vascular tissue surrounding the urethra) into the urethral lumen.[198] Contraction of the bulbospongiosus muscle during ejaculation causes a dramatic increase in pressure in the corpus spongiosum penis, which is essentially a closed vascular space during ejaculation. The bulbospongiosus muscle also undergoes a series of contractions to empty the urethra of urine at the end of urination; thus the defect into the urethra may develop by a similar mechanism in geldings. Once the lesion has been created, it is maintained by bleeding at the end of each urination and the surrounding mucosa heals by formation of a fistula into the vascular tissue. An explanation for the consistent location along the dorsocaudal aspect of the urethra at the level of the ischial arch has not been documented but may be related to the anatomy of the musculature supporting the base of the penis and an enlargement of the corpus spongiosum penis in this area. Further, there is a

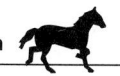

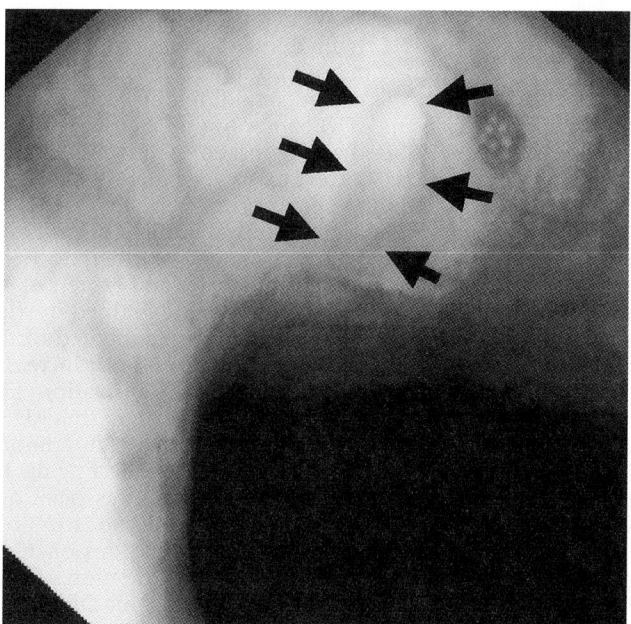

FIG. 32-14 ■ Endoscopic image of the proximal urethra of a gelding with hematuria at the end of urination. A urethral defect can be seen between the *arrows* along the caudal aspect of the urethra as it passes dorsocranially over the pelvic brim.

narrowing of the lumen of the urethra at the distal extent of the ampullar portion of the urethra, which may also contribute to the location of the defects. An anatomic predisposition in Quarter Horses has not been documented but could be speculated based on an apparent increased risk in this breed.

Because hematuria may resolve spontaneously, no treatment may be initially required. If hematuria persists for more than a month or if significant anemia develops, a temporary subischial "incomplete" urethrotomy has been successful in some affected geldings. After sedation and epidural or local anesthesia, a catheter is placed in the urethra and a vertical incision is made into the corpus spongiosum penis but not into the urethral lumen. The surgical wound requires several weeks to heal, and moderate hemorrhage from the corpus spongiosum penis is apparent for the first few days after surgery. Hematuria should resolve within a week after this procedure. Additional treatment consists of local wound care and prophylactic antibiotic treatment (typically a trimethoprim-sulfonamide combination) for 7 to 10 days.

REFERENCES

196. Sullins KE et al: Treatment of hemospermia in stallions: a discussion of 18 cases, *Compend Cont Educ* 10:1396-1403, 1988.
197. Lloyd KC et al: Ulceration in the proximal portion of the urethra as a cause of hematuria in horses: four cases (1978-1985), *J Am Vet Med Assoc* 194:1324-1326, 1989.
198. Schumacher J et al: Urethral defects in geldings with hematuria and stallions with hemospermia, *Vet Surg* 24:250-254, 1995.
199. Dunn MJ, Zambraski EJ: Renal effects of drugs that inhibit prostaglandin synthesis, *Kidney Int* 18:609-622, 1980.
200. Gunson DE, Soma LR: Renal papillary necrosis in horses after phenylbutazone and water deprivation, *Vet Pathol* 20:603-610, 1983.

POLYURIA AND POLYDIPSIA

HAROLD C. SCHOTT II

Polyuria and polydipsia (PU/PD) are defined as urine output in excess of 50 ml/kg/day and fluid intake of more than 100 ml/kg/day.[201,202] These values equate to production of 25 L of urine and consumption of 50 L of water for a 500-kg horse. It is important to remember that urine production and water consumption vary with age, diet, workload, environmental temperature, and gastrointestinal water absorption.[203,204] For example, urine production increases by 50% to 100% when the diet is changed from a grass to a legume hay.[205] Similarly, horses in heavy exercise, stabled in hot climates, or with chronic diarrhea may have a water intake in excess of 100 L/day yet produce normal volumes of urine. The major causes of PU/PD in horses include renal failure (discussed previously), pituitary adenoma (Cushing's disease), and primary or "psychogenic" polydipsia. Less common causes include excessive salt consumption, central and nephrogenic diabetes insipidus, diabetes mellitus, sepsis and/or endotoxemia, and iatrogenic causes (e.g., sedation with α_2-agonists, corticosteroid therapy, or diuretic use).[202]

POLYURIA/POLYDIPSIA WITH CUSHING'S DISEASE

Pituitary adenoma and the resulting syndrome of hyperadrenocorticism (Cushing's disease) is common in older horses.[206] Although the most consistent clinical sign is hirsutism, PU/PD may be reported in some horses. For example, in one review of 17 horses with Cushing's disease, PU/PD was found in 13 (76%).[207] However, in another series of 21 cases, PU/PD was not a historical complaint in any of the affected horses.[208] This discrepancy can be explained by the fact that PU/PD associated with Cushing's disease is generally of lesser volume than that observed with psychogenic polydipsia or diabetes insipidus.

Cushing's disease may lead to PU/PD by several mechanisms. First, polyuria may be the result of an osmotic diuresis. The renal threshold for glucose in horses (about 150 to 175 mg/dl) appears to be lower than in small animals.[209] When plasma glucose concentration exceeds the renal threshold, the resultant glucosuria can lead to an osmotic diuresis. Although commonly implicated as the cause of PU/PD in horses with Cushing's disease, glucosuria was found in only one of five affected horses in a recent report.[208] Further, horses with hyperglycemia and glucosuria may still be able to concentrate their urine in response to water deprivation.[210] A second mechanism implicated in the development of polyuria is antagonism of the action of antidiuretic hormone (ADH) on the collecting ducts by cortisol. Although frequently cited as the mechanism of polyuria in canine hyperadrenocorticism, experimental evidence to support this mechanism is lacking in both dogs and horses. Further, there is considerable species heterogeneity in the effects of corticoids on ADH activity and in some species a primary dipsogenic effect may be more important. Next, growth of the adenoma may lead to impingement on the posterior pituitary and hypothalamic nuclei (located immediately dorsal to the pituitary gland), the sites of ADH storage and production, respectively. Decreased ADH production and release would result in central diabetes insipidus as a third mechanism for polyuria.[206] All in all, PU/PD seen in some, but not all, horses with pituitary adenomas is likely the combined result of several mechanisms.

PSYCHOGENIC POLYDIPSIA

Although rare, primary or "psychogenic" polydipsia is probably the most common cause of PU/PD in adult horses for which clients will have a primary complaint of excessive urination.[204,211] Horses with this problem are generally in good body condition and are not azotemic. Further, the magnitude of polyuria is typically dramatic with owners reporting that horses drink two to three times more water than their stablemates, and stalls can be flooded with urine. In some horses, primary polydipsia appears to be a stable vice that reflects boredom, whereas in other cases it may develop after a change in environmental conditions, stabling, diet, or medication administration. Anecdotally, it has been reported to be more common in southern states during periods of high temperature and humidity.

The diagnosis of primary polydipsia is made by exclusion of renal failure and hyperadrenocorticism. In addition, other factors such as salt supplementation and medication administration must be excluded. Diabetes insipidus is excluded by demonstrating urinary concentrating ability after water deprivation.[212,213] Urine specific gravity should exceed 1.025 after water deprivation of sufficient duration (12 to 24 hours) to produce a 5% loss of body weight. In cases in which there has been long-standing polyuria, the osmotic gradient between the lumen of the collecting tubule and the medullary interstitium may be diminished (medullary washout). In these horses, ADH activity may not lead to an increase in urine specific gravity to values greater than 1.020. Consequently, in horses with primary polydipsia of several weeks duration that fail to concentrate their urine after 24 hours of water deprivation, a modified water deprivation test may be tried. This is performed by restricting water intake to approximately 40 ml/kg/day for 3 to 4 days. By the end of this period, urine specific gravity should exceed 1.025 in a horse that has had medullary washout. If urine specific gravity remains in the isosthenuric range (1.008 to 1.014), the polyuric horse should be further evaluated for early chronic renal failure in which urine concentrating ability may be compromised before the onset of significant azotemia. In theory, this could occur when between two-thirds and three-fourths of functional nephrons have been lost. Subtle signs of decreased performance and mild weight loss would also support early renal failure.

Management of horses with primary polydipsia is empirical. As it is a diagnosis of exclusion, once it has been established that the horse is not suffering from a significant renal disease, it is safe to consider restricting water intake to meet maintenance, work, and environmental requirements of the horse. In addition, steps should be taken to improve the attitude of the horse by reducing boredom. Increasing the amount of exercise or turning the horse out to pasture are possible options, as are providing a companion or diversions in the stall. Also, increasing the frequency of feedings or the amount of roughage in the diet may increase the time spent eating and thereby reduce the habitual drinking.

In an occasional case of primary polydipsia, PU/PD may be attributed to excessive salt consumption and is manifested by an increased fractional sodium clearance.[214] Such "psychogenic salt eaters" appear to be less common than "psychogenic water drinkers" because the former would have to consume a substantial amount of salt to develop polyuria. In fact, salt intake may have to exceed 5% to 10% of dry matter intake before PU/PD becomes apparent.[214,215] Successful management consists of limiting water intake and preventing access to excess salt.

DIABETES INSIPIDUS

Diabetes insipidus (DI) may occur because of inadequate secretion of ADH (neurogenic DI) or decreased sensitivity of the epithelial cells of the collecting ducts to circulating ADH (nephrogenic DI).[201,202,216] With both forms of DI, dramatic PU/PD may be reported and affected animals fail to concentrate urine in the face of water deprivation.

In human patients, neurogenic DI is the more common form of DI, with both hereditary and acquired forms described.[216] Two well-documented equine cases of neurogenic DI have been described.[217,218] Neither animal could concen-

trate urine in response to water deprivation, but administration of exogenous ADH resulted in an increase in urine specific gravity and decrease in urine volume. In a Welsh pony in which the condition was considered idiopathic, the absence of an increase in plasma ADH concentration after water deprivation further supported a diagnosis of neurogenic DI.[217] Acquired neurogenic DI secondary to encephalitis was confirmed histologically in the other horse.[218]

Nephrogenic DI is most commonly a familial disorder in man with an X-linked semirecessive mode of inheritance.[216] Therefore the disorder is carried by females and expressed in male offspring. Nephrogenic DI has been described in sibling Thoroughbred colts, suggesting that an inherited form may also occur in horses.[219] These colts could not increase urine specific gravity in response to water deprivation, although they did show appropriate increases in plasma ADH concentration. A lack of response to exogenous ADH administration further confirmed resistance of the collecting ducts to ADH. Nephrogenic DI can also develop in association with drug therapy or a variety of metabolic, infectious, or mechanical (postobstruction) disorders. Anomalous or neoplastic disorders resulting in structural deformation of the kidneys are other potential causes of nephrogenic DI.[216]

After determining that an equine patient with PU/PD is not azotemic, the initial diagnostic test to differentiate DI from primary polydipsia is a water deprivation test.[217,218] However, horses with suspected DI should be monitored closely during water deprivation because affected horses will continue to excrete excess water in the face of water deprivation. As a result, they may become substantially dehydrated (10% to 15%) within the first 12 hours of water deprivation. When a patient fails to concentrate urine during water deprivation, neurogenic DI can be differentiated from nephrogenic DI by measuring plasma ADH concentration or by administration of synthetic ADH (as illustrated by the cases described above). Currently, equine ADH cannot be measured at commercial laboratories, but synthetic ADH (60 IU, IM, or SC every 6 hours) can be administered in combination with monitoring urine specific gravity.

Treatment of DI is directed at managing PU/PD. With neurogenic DI, hormone replacement therapy with desmopressin (dDAVP, a potent ADH analog administered as eye drops) has been a successful treatment in small animal patients.[220] However, this treatment has not been described in horses and may be cost prohibitive. With nephrogenic DI, replacement hormone therapy is ineffective, and the only practical form of treatment for many years has been to restrict sodium and water intake and to administer thiazide diuretics. The latter treatment may reduce polyuria by 50% in human and canine patients.[216,221] Thiazide diuretics inhibit sodium reabsorption in the distal tubule (diluting segment of the nephron) and increase solute delivery to the collecting duct, but the mechanism by which such therapy benefits patients with nephrogenic DI is not well understood. Administration of prostaglandin inhibitors or amiloride may also decrease polyuria in patients with nephrogenic DI. The former agents probably work by decreasing renal blood flow and GFR while the latter drug, a sodium channel blocker, is thought to act in a manner similar to that of the thiazide diuretics.[216] No reports have documented the use of these treatments in horses.

DIABETES MELLITUS

Diabetes mellitus (DM) is a state of chronic hyperglycemia that is usually accompanied by glucosuria. The resultant osmotic diuresis is an occasional cause of PU/PD in horses and was described to result in a water intake in excess of 80 L/day in one report.[222] Type I, or insulin-dependent DM, results from of a lack of insulin, which in human patients is usually

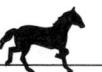

attributable to viral or autoimmune disease. Individuals with type II, or non–insulin-dependent DM have normal to high insulin concentrations but their tissues are insulin insensitive. The most common cause of equine type II DM is Cushing's disease, in which elevated plasma cortisol concentration appears to antagonize the effects of insulin. Although uncommon, there are a few reports of both types I and II DM that were not caused by a pituitary adenoma and that resulted in PU/PD as one of the presenting complaints.[222-224]

SEPSIS/ENDOTOXEMIA

PU/PD has been described in horses with sepsis or endotoxemia, although other clinical signs such as fever, abdominal pain, and weight loss predominate.[225] The mechanism of PU/PD is unclear but may be a consequence of endotoxin-induced prostaglandin production. Prostaglandin E_2 is a potent renal vasodilating agent that can antagonize the effects of ADH on the collecting ducts.[226] Perhaps some horses with chronic gram-negative bacterial infections (such as peritonitis or pleuritis) may have low-grade or intermittent endotoxemia as a mechanism for PU/PD, similar to the polyuria observed with canine pyometra.[227]

IATROGENIC POLYURIA

A final cause of PU/PD may be iatrogenic as a result of several treatments. The most obvious iatrogenic cause is fluid therapy for which polyuria is a desired response. Polyuria has also been observed with exogenous corticosteroid administration, although the mechanism remains unclear. Humans and dogs appear to experience a potent thirst response to exogenous corticosteroids; thus polydipsia may be an important cause of the polyuria observed. In horses on chronic dexamethasone treatment for immune-mediated disorders, profound glucosuria (2 to 3 g/dl) may be observed and could lead to an osmotic diuresis. Finally, a transient diuresis or polyuria accompanies sedation with the α_2-agonists xylazine and detomidine.[228] Although these agents also cause transient hyperglycemia and occasional glucosuria, a more likely mechanism for the polyuria is existence of α_2-adrenoreceptors on collecting duct epithelial cells. Activation of these receptors is another mechanism by which the action of ADH can be antagonized.[229]

REFERENCES

201. Hughes D: Polyuria and polydipsia, *Compend Cont Educ* 14:1161-1175, 1992.
202. Knotterbelt DC: Polyuria-polydipsia in the horse, *Equine Vet Educ AE* 2:237-248, 2000.
203. Sufit E, Houpt KA, Sweeting M: Physiological stimuli of thirst and drinking patterns of ponies, *Equine Vet J* 17:12-16, 1985.
204. Houpt KA: Thirst in horses: the physiological and psychological causes, *Equine Pract* 9:28-30, 1987.
205. Cymbaluk NF: Water balance of horses fed various diets, *Equine Pract* 11:19-24, 1989.
206. Love S: Equine Cushing's disease, *Br Vet J* 149:139-153, 1993.
207. Hillyer MH, Taylor FGR, Mair TS: Diagnosis of hyperadrenocorticism in the horse, *Equine Vet Educ* 4:131-134, 1992.
208. van der Kolk JH et al: Equine pituitary neoplasia: a clinical report of 21 cases (1990-1992), *Vet Rec* 133:594-597, 1993.
209. Link RP: Glucose tolerance in horses, *J Am Vet Med Assoc* 97:261-262, 1940.
210. Green EM, Hunt EL: Hypophyseal neoplasia in a pony, *Compend Cont Educ* 7:S249-S254, 1985.
211. Browning AP: Polydipsia and polyuria in two horses caused by psychogenic polydipsia, *Equine Vet Educ AE* 2:231-236, 2000.
212. Brobst DF, Bayly WM: Responses of horses to a water deprivation test, *Equine Vet Sci* 2:51-56, 1982.
213. Genetzky RM, Loparco FV, Ledet AE: Clinical pathological alterations in horses during a water deprivation test, *Am J Vet Res* 48:1007-1011, 1987.
214. Buntain BJ, Coffman JR: Polyuria and polydypsia in a horse induced by psychogenic salt consumption, *Equine Vet J* 13:266-268, 1981.
215. Schryver HF et al: Salt consumption and the effect of salt on mineral metabolism in horses, *Cornell Vet* 77:122-131, 1987.
216. Robertson GL: Differential diagnosis of polyuria, *Annu Rev Med* 39:425-442, 1988.
217. Breukink HJ, Van Wegen P, Schotman AJH: Idiopathic diabetes insipidus in a Welsh pony, *Equine Vet J* 15:284-287, 1983.
218. Filar J, Ziolo T, Szalecki J: Diabetes insipidus in the course of encephalitis in the horse, *Med Weterynaryjna* 27:205-207, 1971.
219. Schott HC II et al: Nephrogenic diabetes insipidus in sibling colts, *J Vet Intern Med* 7:68-72, 1993.
220. Harb MF et al: Central diabetes insipidus in dogs: 20 cases (1986-1995), *J Am Vet Med Assoc* 209:1884-1888, 1996.
221. Takemura N: Successful long-term treatment of congenital nephrogenic diabetes insipidus in a dog, *J Small Anim Pract* 39:592-594, 1998.
222. Muylle E et al: Non-insulin dependent diabetes mellitus in a horse, *Equine Vet J* 18:145-146, 1986.
223. Baker JR, Richie HE: Diabetes mellitus in the horse: a case report and review of the literature, *Equine Vet J* 6:7-11, 1974.
224. Ruoff WW et al: Type II diabetes mellitus in a horse, *Equine Vet J* 18:143-144, 1986.
225. Traver DS et al: Peritonitis in a horse: a cause of acute abdominal distress and polyuria-polydipsia, *J Equine Med Surg* 1:36-39, 1977.
226. Kinter LB, Huffman WF, Stassen FL: Antagonists of the antidiuretic activity of vasopressin, *Am J Physiol* 254:F165-F177, 1988.
227. Hardy RM, Osborne CA: Canine pyometra: pathophysiology, diagnosis and treatment of uterine and extra-uterine lesions, *J Am Anim Hosp Assoc* 10:245-268, 1974.
228. Thurmon JC et al: Xylazine causes transient dose-related hyperglycemia and increased urine volume in mares, *Am J Vet Res* 45:224-227, 1984.
229. Gellai M: Modulation of vasopressin antidiuretic action by renal α_2-adrenoceptors, *Am J Physiol* 259:F1-F8, 1990.

RENAL TUBULAR ACIDOSIS

MONICA R. ALEMAN

Renal tubular acidosis (RTA) is a syndrome characterized by abnormal renal tubular function, which results in a hyperchloremic metabolic acidosis.[230-232] Hyperchloremia develops as a result of enhanced renal conservation of chloride consequent to bicarbonate loss. RTA can be categorized as primary (genetic or idiopathic) or secondary when attributed to an underlying disease process or drug administration. Drug-induced RTA has been documented in human patients after administration of amphotericin B, trimethoprim-sulfamethoxazole, outdated tetracyclines, gentamicin, cephalosporins, carbonic anhydrase inhibitors, lithium carbonate, and other organic compounds.

Three types of RTA have been described: type I (distal), II (proximal) and IV (hyperkalemic distal).[230-232] Types I and II have been reported in dogs, cats, and horses. Type I develops when distal tubular excretion of hydrogen ions becomes compromised, and affected patients are unable to produce acidic urine. Type II results from decreased proximal tubular bicarbonate resorption and subsequent loss of bicarbonate in the urine. Because hydrogen ions are normally excreted as bicarbonate is reabsorbed in proximal tubules, acidosis with both type I and type II RTA results from decreased excretion of hydrogen ions. Type II RTA is often a self-limiting problem, but it commonly may be accompanied by more widespread proximal tubular dysfunction leading to defective resorption of glucose, amino acids, phosphate, potassium, sodium, calcium, magnesium, uric acid, and other organic acids. The latter disorder is known as Fanconi's syndrome and, as with RTA, it may be a primary (inherited) problem or it can develop secondary to kidney, metabolic, and autoimmune diseases or drug administration.[230-232] Although there are no well-documented reports, Fanconi's syndrome likely develops in an occasional horse as a sequela to nephrotoxic or vasomotor acute renal failure. To date, type IV or hyperkalemic distal RTA has only been described in human patients.[231]

RTA is a sporadically occurring metabolic disorder in horses.[233-236] There is no obvious breed or sex predilection, and to date there has been no indication that RTA is an inherited condition in horses. Typically, affected horses present with

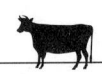

profound depression and anorexia and may have a history of poor performance, weight loss, and signs of abdominal pain. Vital parameters are generally within normal ranges, and horses do not appear clinically dehydrated. Hematologic and clinical chemistry findings are usually within reference ranges, with the exception of electrolyte concentrations and acid-base balance. A profound metabolic acidosis (plasma bicarbonate concentration <13 mEq/L and venous blood pH <7.25) and hyperchloremia (serum chloride concentration 105 to 120 mEq/L) are characteristic for horses with RTA. A compensatory decrease in $P\text{co}_2$ is also observed in most horses with RTA. Hypokalemia (and total body potassium depletion) is not uncommon in horses with RTA because of the combined effects of anorexia and ongoing loss of potassium in urine, especially in patients with type II RTA in which bicarbonaturia further increases urinary potassium excretion.

Mild to moderate azotemia may be detected in horses with RTA, especially when they are dehydrated at presentation. Affected horses may also have evidence of renal tubular damage detected on urinalysis (e.g., pigmenturia, glucosuria, and abnormal sediment), and urine specific gravity may be low. Despite profound metabolic acidosis, urine pH is generally neutral to alkaline. If pursued, renal biopsy results generally support tubulointerstitial disease (chronic interstitial nephritis).

Differentiation of type I from type II RTA in human and canine patients is most easily accomplished by assessing urine pH: it remains neutral to alkaline with type I and should be neutral to acidic with type II.[230-232] Most horses with RTA have had neutral to alkaline urine; however, because herbivores normally have alkaline urine, this distinction may be less useful in horses with RTA. A few reports have described horses with acidic urine,[235,237,238] supporting type II RTA, but urine pH values near neutral are difficult to interpret. Assessment of all laboratory abnormalities (Table 32-1) along with additional testing (e.g., ammonium chloride challenge and determination of urinary ammonium concentration) may allow further discrimination between type I and type II RTA[238,239]; however, this distinction may not be entirely necessary because the approach to treatment and prognosis is similar for both types of RTA in horses.

Treatment of RTA consists primarily of intravenous and oral administration of sodium bicarbonate. Response to treatment appears to be largely dependent on the rate of sodium bicarbonate administration. For initial correction of acidosis, intravenous sodium bicarbonate must be administered aggressively and large amounts (3000 to 9000 mEq) are often required to return plasma bicarbonate concentration to values above 20 mEq/L. Half of the estimated bicarbonate deficit is generally replaced with intravenous sodium bicarbonate over 6 to 12 hours, and the remaining deficit is replaced with a combination of intravenous and oral sodium bicarbonate (initial oral dose: 100 to 150 g twice daily; 1 g of sodium bicarbonate contains $\approx$12 mEq of $NaHCO_3$). Close monitoring of serum electrolyte concentrations and acid-base balance is required to adjust the rate of intravenous sodium bicarbonate replacement. Marked improvement in attitude and appetite usually accompanies correction of the acidosis but, unfortunately, relapse after discontinuation of intravenous bicarbonate therapy is not uncommon. Continued oral administration of sodium bicarbonate (baking soda) for months to years may be required for maintenance of a normal acid-base status in individual horses.

Because potassium excretion is proportional to the bicarbonate delivery to the distal tubule, initial correction of acidosis with sodium bicarbonate promotes kaliuresis and may exacerbate potassium depletion, especially when horses have been anorectic for several days. Therefore concurrent supplementation with intravenous or oral potassium chloride is usually also necessary during initial correction of the acidosis. Complications associated with rapid correction of acidosis have not been described, but transient diarrhea may develop if

---

TABLE 32-1

Classification of Type I and Type II Renal Tubular Acidosis

	Distal or Type I	Proximal or Type II
Acidosis	Severe	Self-limiting
Hypokalemia	Severe	Mild to moderate
Serum phosphate	Normal	Low
Urine pH	Neutral to alkaline	Neutral to acidic

---

large quantities of sodium bicarbonate (>200 g) are given via a nasogastric tube to horses that are completely anorectic.

Recurrence of metabolic acidosis is also not uncommon when oral sodium bicarbonate is discontinued. Relapses can be immediate or delayed by a few weeks to months, especially in horses that have RTA with evidence of renal damage. Reinstitution of sodium bicarbonate supplementation usually corrects the metabolic abnormalities and accompanying depression and anorexia. The short-term prognosis for horses with RTA is good, and although the long term prognosis has not been well documented, several horses have been reported to recover completely.[233-235]

REFERENCES

230. Battle D: Renal tubular acidosis, *Med Clin North Am* 67:859-878, 1983.
231. Rocher LL, Tannen RL: The clinical spectrum of renal tubular acidosis, *Ann Rev Med* 37:319-331, 1986.
232. Mueller DL, Jergens AE: Renal tubular acidosis, *Compend Contin Educ* 13:435-445, 1991.
233. Hansen TO: Renal tubular acidosis in a mare, *Compend Cont Educ* 8:864-866, 1986.
234. Trotter GW et al: Type II renal tubular acidosis in a mare, *J Am Vet Med Assoc* 188:1050-1051, 1986.
235. Ziemer EL et al: Clinical features and treatment of renal tubular acidosis in two horses, *J Am Vet Med Assoc* 190:294-296, 1987.
236. Van der Kolk JH, Kalsbeek HC: Renal tubular acidosis in a mare, *Vet Rec* 133:43-44, 1993.
237. MacLeay JM, Wilson JH: Type-II renal tubular acidosis and ventricular tachycardia in a horse, *J Am Vet Med Assoc* 212:1597-1599, 1998.
238. Ziemer EL et al: Renal tubular acidosis in two horses: diagnostic studies, *J Am Vet Med Assoc* 190:289-293, 1987.
239. Halperin ML et al: Urine ammonium: the key to the diagnosis of distal renal tubular acidosis, *Nephron* 50:1-4, 1988.

BLADDER RUPTURE IN ADULT HORSES

THOMAS J. DIVERS

On rare occasions, bladder rupture may occur in adult horses. The problem often develops in association with urethral obstruction, foaling, or prolonged recumbency.[240] As azotemia develops, affected horses become depressed and inappetent. Clinical signs may not be apparent for several days or stranguria may be observed, depending on the cause of the rupture. Abdominal distention is not as apparent in adult horses as in foals.

The diagnosis is based on history, rectal examination findings, laboratory results, and findings on ultrasonographic examination or cystoscopic examination. Postrenal azotemia develops within 24 hours after rupture and is accompanied by hyponatremia and hypochloremia. Unlike uroperitoneum in neonates, hyperkalemia is not a consistent finding. Transabdominal ultrasonographic examination of the abdomen reveals a large amount of peritoneal fluid (Fig. 32-15); abdominal fluid is easily recovered on abdominocentesis, and peritoneal fluid creatinine is twofold or greater than that of serum. Detection of calcium carbonate crystals on cytologic examination of peritoneal fluid is also diagnostic for uroperi-

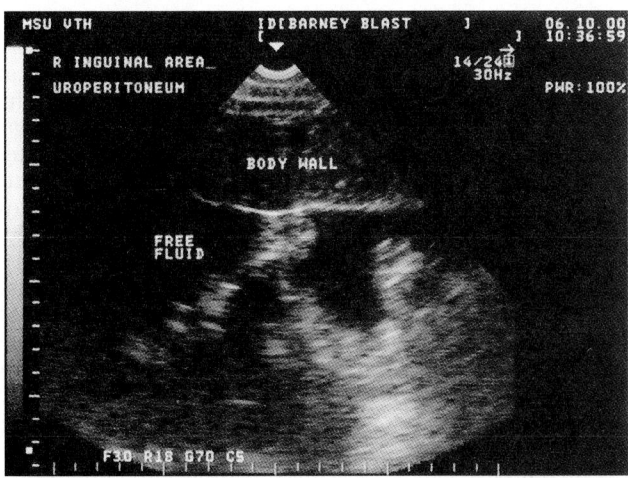

FIG. 32-15 ▓ Transabdominal ultrasonographic image of the right inguinal area of an adult horse with a ruptured bladder. A large amount of free hypoechoic fluid is apparent.

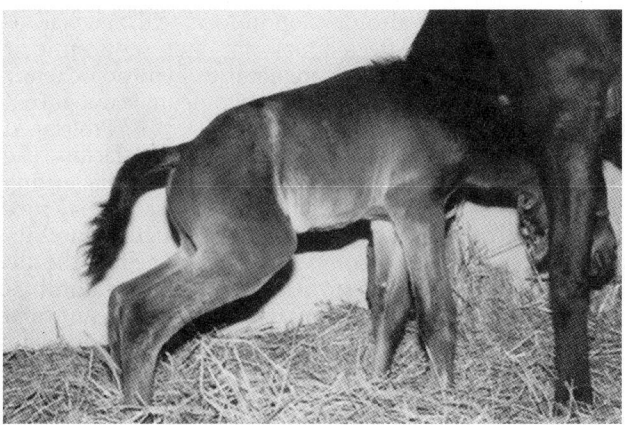

FIG. 32-16 ▓ A 2-day-old exhibiting stranguria caused by a ruptured bladder. Note the caudal position of the hind legs, suggesting that the foal is straining to urinate rather than defecate. Differentiating between stranguria and tenesmus (meconium impaction) is not always easy.

toneum. Endoscopic examination of the bladder should allow determination of the location and extent of the bladder tear. Rarely, uroperitoneum may also develop in some horses without full-thickness disruption of the bladder wall, and it is difficult to definitely establish the cause of uroperitoneum in these cases.

Surgical repair is indicated in horses with large tears in the ventral half of the bladder. In patients with small dorsal tears or incomplete tears, use of an indwelling bladder catheter (closed system) to keep the bladder small may allow the tear to heal without surgery.[241] Before surgery, intravenous fluids should be administered to correct dehydration, along with broad-spectrum antibiotics as prophylaxis against sepsis. If the abdomen is distended, urine accumulated in the abdomen should be removed (e.g., via placement of a chest tube or other large catheter through the ventral abdominal wall) before anesthesia is induced, to avoid further compromising respiration.

REFERENCES

240. Nyrop KA et al: Rupture of the urinary bladder in two post-parturient mares, *Compend Cont Educ* 6:S510-S513, 1984.
241. Gibson KT, Trotter GW, Gustafson SB: Conservative management of uroperitoneum in a gelding, *J Am Vet Med Assoc* 200:1692-1694, 1992.

URINARY SYSTEM DISORDERS IN THE FOAL

THOMAS J. DIVERS

UMBILICAL DISORDERS OF THE NEONATAL FOAL

Umbilical disorders of the neonatal foal, including patent urachus, urachal infections, and omphalitis, are discussed in Chapter 20.

UROPERITONEUM

Bladder Rupture

The most common disorder of the bladder of otherwise healthy newborn foals is bladder rupture.[242-244] It is more common in colts, and clinical signs include repeated posturing to urinate and stranguria during the first 2 days of life. As urine accumulates in the abdomen, depression and abdominal distention typically develop between 2 and 4 days of life. Repeated posturing and stranguria can easily be misinterpreted as tenesmus associated with meconium impaction (Fig. 32-16). Further, affected colts may continue to void small volumes of urine. Thus establishing a diagnosis of a ruptured bladder can initially be challenging until more obvious signs of uroperitoneum (e.g., decreased nursing and abdominal distention) develop.

Laboratory findings in foals with uroperitoneum include hyponatremia, hypochloremia, hyperkalemia, and azotemia.[242-245] An occasional foal may also develop intermittent fine muscle tremors or a cardiac arrhythmia consequent to these electrolyte alterations, especially hyperkalemia. Transabdominal ultrasonographic examination usually reveals a large quantity of free fluid in the abdominal cavity and peritoneal fluid creatinine/serum creatinine ratio greater than 2:1 confirms uroperitoneum.[242-245]

Treatment of bladder rupture includes surgical closure of the defect, supportive care, and broad-spectrum prophylactic antibiotics for 3 to 7 days postoperatively.[242,243,245,246] An emergency surgical procedure is usually not required, and in most cases surgery should be postponed for several hours until electrolyte abnormalities are partially corrected (most notably correction of hyperkalemia to a serum concentration <6.0 mEq/L). This can usually be accomplished by intravenous administration of 1 to 3 L of a 0.9% NaCl/5% glucose solution. Treatment with insulin should be avoided unless hyperkalemia is causing significant ECG abnormalities and response to initial fluid therapy is poor. With marked hyperkalemia or abdominal distention causing respiratory embarrassment, slow drainage of urine from the abdomen (e.g., via a chest tube or similar catheter) may be necessary before induction of anesthesia. Despite significant azotemia in some affected foals, use of aminoglycoside antibiotics is generally safe because the azotemia is postrenal rather than reflective of intrinsic renal disease. In most instances, placement of a urinary catheter to maintain an empty bladder for the initial couple of postoperative days is not necessary. However, uroperitoneum may recur after surgery in an occasional foal as a result of ongoing leakage from the bladder tear. When this complication occurs, it can usually be managed conservatively by placement of an indwelling bladder catheter (closed system) for 3 to 5 days. Rarely, a second celiotomy may be required.

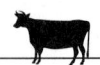

Urachal Urine Leakage

Uroperitoneum may also develop in foals with urachal infection or ischemia. Affected foals are often septicemic or hospitalized for treatment of prematurity, hypoxic-ischemic encephalopathy, or botulism and uroperitneum is recognized later (e.g., after 5 to 10 days of treatment).[246,247] Prolonged recumbency and bladder distention are likely risk factors. The umbilicus of many affected neonates appears normal during the first couple of days of life but, in some cases, it may subsequently become patent. Urine leakage through the umbilicus may or may not be accompanied by leakage into the abdominal cavity or subcutaneous tissues of the abdominal wall. In other affected foals the umbilicus remains normal and all urine leakage accumulates into the abdominal cavity. When monitored, inappropriate weight gain (e.g., greater than 2 kg in 24 hours) is another common finding in hospitalized neonates that develop uroperitoneum.

Laboratory abnormalities typical for uroperitoneum findings may be found in affected foals but are not consistently abnormal because these patients are often being treated with intravenous fluids. Correction of the problem includes surgical removal of the diseased urachus, closure of the bladder apex, and continued supportive care for the primary disease. The prognosis for a successful outcome for these foals is not as favorable as for simple bladder rupture because they often have a degree of peritonitis (increasing the risk for adhesions) and uroperitoneum is often only one of several complications of the underlying disease.[246,247]

In an occasional foal the urachus may also rupture more distally than usual and lead to subcutaneous accumulation of urine, ventral abdominal swelling, stranguria, signs of colic, and distress.[248] The swelling may be differentiated clinically from a hematoma or septic omphalitis because it may enlarge quickly and often becomes cold. Ultrasonographic examination and/or local aspiration of fluid and measurement of creatinine (twofold or greater than in serum) confirms the diagnosis. Prompt surgical removal of the leaking urachus is indicated.

Ureteral Defects

Ureteral defect(s) or disruption may also lead to development of uroperitoneum in foals of both sexes.[249-252] Stranguria is usually absent and urine initially accumulates in the retroperitoneal space, but with time the retroperitoneal tissue ruptures causing uroperitoneum. Affected foals may not be presented until 5 to 10 days of age because urine accumulation is slower than with a ruptured bladder. Clinical signs include decreased nursing, depression, and mild colic, and in fillies an external bulging of the vagina may be observed. Laboratory findings are typical for uroperitoneum and, with significant hyperkalemia, intermittent muscle fasciculations may be also noted.

If urine accumulation remains localized to the retroperitoneal space, ultrasonographic examination of the lower abdomen may be normal but a large amount of retroperitoneal fluid will be detected around the kidney and upper flank (within the retroperitoneal space) on the affected side(s). In addition the renal pelvis may be mildly dilated.[253] If the peritoneal membrane is ruptured, physical and ultrasonographic examination findings are similar to those that occur with a ruptured bladder but careful ultrasonographic examination may also reveal a full bladder or concurrent retroperitoneal fluid accumulation. As with a ruptured bladder the ratio of retroperitoneal or peritoneal fluid creatinine/serum creatinine is greater than 2:1. In small foals (e.g., less than 50 to 75 kg), excretory urography (after intravenous administration of contrast agent) or pyelography (after percutaneous injection of contrast agent into the renal pelvis via ultrasonographic guidance) may be useful for localizing the ureteral defect(s).

One or both ureters may be involved, and during surgical exploration one or more defects can usually be found in the proximal half of the ureter, often near the renal pelvis. During surgery the defects can be localized by placing a catheter into the ureter via a cystotomy and injecting dye (e.g., Evans blue dye or methylene blue dye). Successful correction of unilateral and bilateral defects can be accomplished by placing a stent in the affected ureter(s) for 7 to 10 days.[249,250]

A recent report describing bilateral ureteral defects adjacent to the renal pelves provided histopathologic evidence that the lesions were traumatic in origin, rather than developmental anomalies.[252] The foal in that report had previously been kicked by its dam. The editor has also seen three foals with similar ureteral defects, all of which also had multiple rib fractures. Ureteropelvic junction injuries and proximal ureteral tears are a recognized complication after blunt abdominal trauma in human patients.[254] Taken together, these observations suggest that many ureteral defects in foals may more likely be traumatically induced at foaling, rather than being developmental anomalies.

CYSTITIS

Cystitis is rare in foals but can develop in recumbent premature or neonatal foals being treated with broad-spectrum antibiotics. Voided urine may have a characteristic flocculent consistency. When cystitis is suspected, the bladder should be catheterized and a urine sample should be submitted for urinalysis and quantitative culture. Urinary tract infections with *Candida* spp. are fairly common in recumbent neonates. Specific antimicrobial therapy is not usually necessary for *Candida* cystitis as long as systemic antibiotics can be discontinued. If antibiotic therapy continues, dissemination of the yeast infection can spread to other sites (e.g., joints).

SERUM CREATININE ELEVATIONS IN NEWBORN FOALS

During the first 1 to 3 days of life, creatinine concentration in newborn foals is often 30% to 40% higher than in their dams.[255] The cause is unclear but is likely related to an inability of creatinine to rapidly equilibrate across placental membranes. This is supported by the fact that creatinine concentration of normal amniotic fluid (that contains fetal urine) at term is approximately 10 mg/dl (and may exceed 30 mg/dl in some mares).[256] This transient increase in creatinine, which may occasionally exceed 20 mg/dl in premature foals, has been called a "spurious" elevation, but this term should be discontinued because creatinine is truly increased. When an elevated creatinine is detected in an otherwise healthy foal (that has also been observed to urinate normally), there may be no cause for alarm. However, if creatinine does not decline rapidly after birth or remains greater than 2.5 mg/dl on day 3 of life, peritoneal or retroperitoneal accumulation of urine, renal hypoplasia, or other causes of renal failure should be considered. Unlike creatinine, blood urea nitrogen (BUN) values in foals are typically low (<10 mg/dl) after day 2 and remain low for the first several months of life. This finding can be attributed to the anabolic state of the growing foal.

Urinalysis results in normal neonatal foals are also different from those in adult horses. Specifically, normal foals may have marked proteinuria for 1 to 2 days after birth that is a consequence of filtration of small-molecular-weight proteins absorbed with colostrum. Next, water intake on a predominantly milk diet (approximately 250 ml/kg/day compared with intake of 50 ml/kg/day of water by adults) is high in

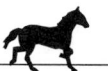

foals. As a result, after day 2 of life, urine is hyposthenuric (specific gravity 1.002 to 1.006) and remains that way for several months. Finally, urinary enzyme activity and sodium and chloride clearances may be greater than adult values, and urine pH is neutral to acidic in foals.[257]

ACUTE RENAL FAILURE

Acute tubular necrosis is the most common pathologic lesion causing ARF in neonatal foals. Many cases develop during or after episodes of diarrhea and are likely a consequence or poor perfusion (vasomotor nephropathy). Surprisingly the diarrheal disease in some affected foals does not appear to be serious, yet they may develop ARF. Similar to adult horses with ARF, the prominent clinical signs are depression and development of edema. Abnormal laboratory findings include azotemia, hyponatremia, hypochloremia, and hypocalcemia. Foals are more likely to develop significant hyperkalemia and hyperphospatemia than adult horses with ARF. A urine specific gravity less than 1.018 and microscopic hematuria are usually also found in foals with ARF. Urine output of sick neonates should be monitored closely because they may become oliguric to anuric 12 to 24 hours before significant depression or azotemia is recognized. In addition, fluid retention during incipient ARF is another cause of inappropriate weight gain (e.g., >2 kg in 24 hours) that can often be detected before obvious edema develops.

Nephrotoxicity, most often from administration of aminoglycoside antibiotics or tetracycline, is another important cause of ARF (usually nonoliguric) in neonatal foals. As in adult horses the recent change to once-daily aminoglycoside dosing appears to have decreased the incidence of hospital-acquired ARF in foals. However, it is important to remember that sick neonates are often more critically ill than many adult horses treated with aminoglycosides. Premature foals appear to be at even greater risk of nephrotoxicity than term foals. Judicious fluid therapy to correct dehydration and maintain blood pressure is an important precaution. Although there is a general impression that amikacin may be less nephrotoxic than gentamicin in foals, little supportive data exists. Regardless of which aminoglycoside antibiotic is selected, monitoring trough concentrations (below 2 mg/ml for gentamicin and below 4 mg/ml for amikacin) is warranted to decrease the risk of aminoglycoside toxicity in high-risk neonates. Dosage adjustment may be necessary in seriously ill neonates or premature foals because renal clearance may be decreased.[258]

The principles of treatment of ARF in neonates are essentially the same as those for adult horses. However, greater attention must be paid to monitoring responses to fluid therapy, including twice daily measurement of body weight. Although foals that suffer a bout of ARF in the neonatal period would seem at greater risk of developing chronic renal failure later in life, there has been no long-term follow-up study to corroborate this speculation.

SEPTIC RENAL DISEASE IN FOALS

Multifocal renal abscesses or infarct may be a complication of neonatal septicemia and can lead to ARF. *Actinobacillus equili* is the most common pathogen causing renal abscesses, but affected foals often die or are euthanatized as a consequence of overwhelming sepsis before clinical signs of ARF develop. Foals 2 to 4 days of age appear to be at greatest risk of developing acute *Actinobacillus* spp. septicemia; when this problem is suspected, intravenous therapy with penicillin and gentamicin (at a prolonged dosage interval) is recommended (see Chapters 18 and 20).

REFERENCES

242. Richardson DW, Kohn CW: Uroperitoneum in the foal, *J Am Vet Med Assoc* 182:267-271, 1983.
243. Hackett RP: Rupture of the urinary bladder in neonatal foals, *Compend Cont Educ* 6:S488-S494, 1984.
244. Hardy J: Uroabdomen in foals, *Equine Vet Educ* 10:21-25, 1998.
245. Behr MJ et al: Metabolic abnormalities associated with rupture of the urinary bladder in neonatal foals, *J Am Vet Med Assoc* 178:263-266, 1981.
246. Adams R et al: Exploratory celiotomy for suspected urinary tract disruption in neonatal foals: a review of 18 cases, *Equine Vet J* 20:13-17, 1988.
247. Kablack KA et al: Uroperitoneum in the hospitalised equine neonate: retrospective study of 31 cases, 1988-1997, *Equine Vet J* 32:505-508, 2000.
248. Lees MJ et al: Subcutaneous rupture of the urachus, its diagnosis and surgical management in three foals, *Equine Vet J* 21:462-464, 1989.
249. Robertson JT et al: Repair of a ureteral defect in a foal, *J Am Vet Med Assoc* 183:799-800, 1983.
250. Divers TJ, Byars TD, Spirito M: Correction of bilateral ureteral defects in a foal, *J Am Vet Med Assoc* 192:384-387, 1988.
251. Jean D, Marcoux M, Louf CF: Congenital bilateral distal defect of the ureters in a foal, *Equine Vet Educ* 10:17-20, 1998.
252. Cutler TJ et al: Bilateral ureteral tears in a foal, *Aust Vet J* 75:413-415, 1997.
253. Hoffmann-KL, Wood AK, McCarthy PH: Ultrasonography of the equine neonatal kidney, *Equine Vet J* 32:109-13, 2000.
254. Kawashima A et al: Ureteropelvic junction injuries secondary to blunt abdominal trauma, *Radiology* 205:487-492, 1997.
255. Bauer JE: Normal blood chemistry. In Koterba AM, Drummond WH, Kosch PC, eds: *Equine clinical neonatology*, Philadelphia, 1990, Lea & Febiger, p 608.
256. Schott HC, Mansmann RA: Biochemical profiles of normal equine amniotic fluid at parturition, *Equine Vet J Suppl* 5:52, 1988.
257. Edwards DJ, Brownlow MA, Hutchins DR: Indices of renal function: values in eight normal foals from birth to 56 days, *Aust Vet J* 67:251-254, 1990.
258. Geor RJ, Brashier MK: Rational approach to gentamicin dosing in neonatal foals, *Proceedings of the Thirty-Seventh Annual Convention of the American Association of Equine Practitioners*, San Francisco, 1991, pp 603-609.

RUMINANT RENAL SYSTEM

ULCERATIVE POSTHITIS AND VULVITIS

DAVID C. Van METRE
THOMAS J. DIVERS

Ulcerative posthitis and vulvitis (enzootic balanoposthitis, pizzle rot, sheath rot) is an ulcerative bacterial infection of the mucous membrane and surrounding skin of the prepuce and vulva of small ruminants. The causative organism, *Corynebacterium renale*, inhabits the mucosal surface of the prepuce and vulva, proliferating and inducing disease under conditions of high urea concentration in urine. Losses result from debilitation caused by pain, incapacitation of breeding animals, loss of breeding soundness, and deformation of external genitalia. Urinary tract obstruction is a serious sequela to the internal form of the disease in males and wethers. Predisposition caused by a high-protein ration, as well as the potential for venereal spread, make this disease a significant threat to breeding flocks and herds.

CLINICAL SIGNS. In rams, bucks, and wethers the infection begins as a moist ulcer, usually at or near the mucocutaneous junction of the prepuce. The ulcer surface is soon covered with a thin, loose, brownish, malodorous scab (Fig. 32-17). If the scabs are removed, little or no hemorrhage will occur from the underlying tissue.[259] Focal swelling is often noticeable at the cranial aspect of the prepuce, and the area is usually painful on palpation.

If unchecked, the infection may spread along the mucosal surface inside the prepuce, creating the more serious internal form of ulcerative posthitis. The entire prepuce may be swollen and elongated. A malodorous exudate, consisting of necrotic tissue and retained urine, is found within the preputial orifice. Palpation of the prepuce elicits extreme pain. Affected animals often show dysuria, and goats may vocalize during urine voiding. Weight loss may occur in chronic cases. As local inflammation progresses, ulceration of mucosal surfaces and fibrin deposition may result in fibrous adhesions between the penis and prepuce. Severe inflammation of the glans penis may cause stricture of the urethral process (pizzle), creating urinary tract obstruction. Loss of breeding soundness may result from penile adhesions, cicatricial scarring of the preputial orifice, urethral obstruction, or suppurative urethritis.

Ulcerative lesions of similar appearance develop on the vulva and perineum of affected ewes and does. Gross vulvar enlargement may be noticed from a distance. Involvement of the urethral orifice causes dysuria. The fibrosis and contracture that develop in chronic, severe cases may distort normal vulvar conformation to the point of impairment of fertility.

DIFFERENTIAL DIAGNOSIS. Ulcerative dermatosis (lip and leg ulcer) is a dermatitis of sheep caused by an unclassified poxvirus related to the parapox virus of contagious ecthyma.[260] Infection with this agent may manifest as balanoposthitis and vulvitis, and the crusted ulcers that develop closely resemble those induced by infection with *C. renale*. Removal of the crusts overlying ulcerative dermatosis lesions may reveal a granular lesion that bleeds readily. The genital form of ulcerative dermatosis occurs most commonly in the fall breeding season in the western United States. Ulcers on the lips, nares, coronets, and interdigital spaces may also be present.[260] Contagious ecthyma (orf) occasionally affects the genitalia and perineum, although lesions are much more commonly found on the lips, face, and udder. These lesions are raised, appear proliferative, and are covered with a thick,

durable scab. Urolithiasis must be considered strongly in the differential diagnosis of any dysuric male or castrated male small ruminant. Urethral rupture results in diffuse preputial swelling that involves the ventral abdomen and inguinal region as well. Although rare in small ruminants, preputial trauma, particularly if resulting from entrapped grass awns, can cause preputial swelling, pain, and exudation within the preputial cavity. External ulcerative lesions would not be expected in such cases.

PATHOPHYSIOLOGY. *C. renale* is an aerobic, gram-positive, short, rod-shaped bacterium[261] that is a normal inhabitant of the skin and external genitalia of small ruminants.[262] This organism is capable of surviving in wool and scabs from lesions for as long as 6 months and can survive freezing temperatures in lesion exudate.[263] *C. renale* is capable of hydrolyzing urea. The organism proliferates on the genital mucosal surface in response to elevated urinary concentration of urea. Experimental diversion of urine flow has demonstrated that the presence of urine is required for both induction of and maintenance of lesions on the genitalia.[261] Diets high in crude protein or nonprotein nitrogen increase the urinary urea content and are required for development of the disease.[259,263] *C. renale* hydrolyses urea to ammonia, which causes necrosis of surrounding epithelial cells.

EPIDEMIOLOGY. This condition appears to be more common in males and wethers than in females.[259] Lambs under 6 months of age can occasionally be affected,[263] but given the relatively short lifespan of market lambs, the disease is most commonly recognized in rams, Angora wethers, and pet wethers. Although all breeds are susceptible, higher rates of this disease are found in Merinos and Angoras.[259,264] Because of the dense wool and hair coat of these breeds, urine soaking near the preputial orifice may increase the local concentration of urea substrate for *C. renale*. Seasonal differences in the incidence of the disease are thought to reflect shearing schedules and changes in the availability of high-protein diets.[259]

Because the organism is part of the normal skin and genital flora, disease can occur in isolated individuals under proper dietary conditions. However, the disease is contagious, because transfer of necrotic debris from the ulcers of affected animals can induce the disease in normal animals.[259,263] Venereal transmission of the disease has been documented.[263] Several months may pass between the exposure of ewes to infected rams and the development of vulvitis in ewes.[263]

TREATMENT AND PREVENTION. Affected animals should be isolated to limit venereal or contact transmission. Wool or mohair should be removed from the skin surrounding the prepuce or vulva, and a topical antibiotic should be applied. Caustic antiseptic solutions should not be used. Treatment with systemic antibiotics is indicated for advanced cases or for outbreaks in which handling of several animals for topical therapy is not feasible. Penicillin is the antibiotic of choice, although tetracycline has provided favorable results. Treatment should continue until the lesions have dried and acute inflammation has subsided.

Reduction of protein and/or nonprotein nitrogen intake is crucial for successful treatment of affected animals and for prevention of additional cases.[259,263] Dietary crude protein levels of 16% to 18% (or higher) predispose sheep and goats to ulcerative posthitis and vulvitis.[259] Reduction of dietary protein alone may result in satisfactory cure if the lesions are early in development. Shearing, especially at the time of highest protein intake, may be efficacious in reducing disease incidence.[263] Incorporation of grass hay feeding into a program of legume pasture grazing may help limit protein intake.

Surgical treatment of advanced cases has been described.[265] The procedure involves resection of ventral preputial tissue to allow for normal urine flow, and, less commonly, successful return to breeding.

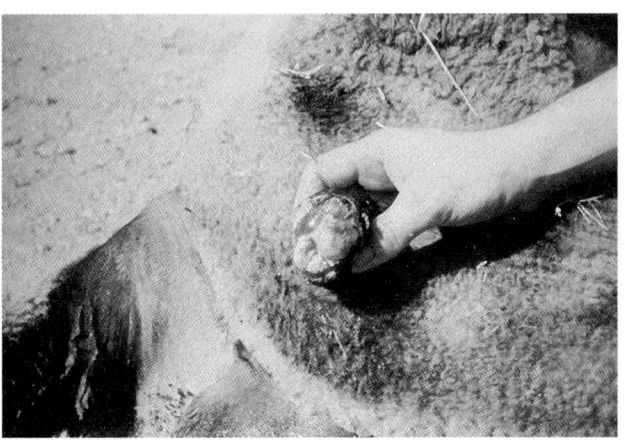

FIG. 32-17 ▪▪▪ Ulcerative posthitis in a Suffolk ram.

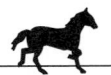

PROGNOSIS. Response to treatment is optimal early in the infection, before deformation of the prepuce and vulva as a result of fibrosis. The chances for full recovery without recrudescence are poor if dietary protein intake is not reduced. Complete recovery of breeding soundness is unlikely to occur with internal ulcerative posthitis.

REFERENCES

259. Kimberling CV, Arnold KS: Diseases of the urinary system of sheep and goats, *Vet Clin North Am (Large Anim Pract)* 5:637-655, 1983.
260. Scott DW: *Large animal dermatology*, ed 1, Philadelphia, 1988, WB Saunders, pp 102-104.
261. Southcott WH: Etiology of ovine posthitis: description of a causal organism, *Aust Vet J* 41:193-200, 1965.
262. Brook AH, Southcott WH, Stacy BD: Etiology of ovine posthitis: relationship between ovine posthitis and a causal organism, *Aust Vet J* 42:9-12, 1966.
263. Southcott WH: Epidemiology and control of ovine posthitis and vulvitis, *Aust Vet J* 41:225-233, 1965.
264. Shelton M, Livingston CW: Posthitis in angora wethers, *J Am Vet Med Assoc* 167:154-155, 1975.
265. Dent CHR: Ulcerative vulvitis and posthitis in Australian sheep and cattle, *Vet Bull* 41:719-723, 1971.

UROLITHIASIS

DAVID C. Van METRE
THOMAS J. DIVERS

Urolithiasis (urinary calculosis, obstructive urolithiasis) is a metabolic disease of intact and castrated male ruminants, swine, and camelids. Uroliths cause disease through trauma to the urinary tract and obstruction of urinary outflow. Calculi (uroliths) most commonly lodge in the urethra, although obstruction of the bladder trigone, ureter, and renal pelvis can occur. Sequelae to urinary tract obstruction include urethral perforation and rupture, urethral stricture, bladder rupture, ureteral rupture, hydroureter, hydronephrosis, and, rarely, rupture of the kidney(s). Although most often a sporadic disease, urolithiasis can occur in outbreaks or become an endemic problem. A definitive diagnosis of urolithiasis in a single animal suggests that all males in the population are at risk for the disease, because of the importance of dietary and environmental factors in its pathogenesis.[266] The clinical manifestations of urolithiasis in ruminants include acute urethral obstruction, urethral rupture, bladder rupture, chronic partial urethral obstruction, ureterolithiasis, and nephrolithiasis.

HISTORICAL FINDINGS. The clinical signs of urolithiasis can be quite variable, as the duration, extent (complete vs. partial), and the location of the obstruction determine the historical and examination findings. The early clinical signs of this disease can be remarkably subtle; in many cases the presenting complaint may be entirely unrelated to urinary system dysfunction. Anorexia, depression, and mild bloat are common chief complaints. A history of colic, stranguria, or tenesmus is more strongly suggestive of urinary tract obstruction. If possible, it is helpful to have potential urolithiasis cases placed in a dry, unbedded stall to allow for assessment of urine output.

Acute Urethral Obstruction

CLINICAL FINDINGS. Urethral trauma from impacted calculi and progressive bladder distention cause strangury and signs of abdominal pain. Affected animals are restless and may tread, swish their tails, and grind their teeth. Goats may vocalize. Stranguria is manifested as repetitive bouts of stretching and contraction of the abdominal muscles. Rectal prolapse may occur as a result of forceful voiding attempts. Rarely, affected calves may develop dilation of the urethra proximal to the obstruction, which manifests as a visible swelling localized to the midline of the perineum.[267] Tachycardia and tachypnea are common, but no consistent alteration in rectal temperature occurs. Mild bloat secondary to ruminal stasis is often present. Anuria occurs if urethral obstruction is complete, whereas urine may dribble from the urethral orifice in cases of partial obstruction. If a urine sample can be collected for dipstick analysis, proteinuria and occult hematuria are frequently detected. Crystals or blood may be found on the hairs of the preputial tuft; in cases of anuria the hairs are dry.

The lumen of the bovine urethra narrows at the distal aspect of the sigmoid flexure, near the level of insertion of the retractor penis muscles.[268,269] Calculi most frequently become lodged at this site in cattle,[268-271] and pain or focal swelling over this area may be appreciated. Rectal examination (digital rectal examination in small ruminants) often reveals pulsation of the pelvic urethra. In cattle, bladder distention is palpable per rectum in cases of complete obstruction uncomplicated by bladder rupture.

Abdominal palpation is useful in affected small ruminants. The examiner should place the fingertips of each hand into the ventral flank on each side of the abdomen. While slowly pressing the fingertips toward midline in the caudal abdomen, the examiner may encounter an orange- to grapefruit-size, firm, circular structure, which is the distended bladder (Fig. 32-18). Severe bladder distention will not be palpated in cases of incomplete urethral obstruction or bladder rupture.

The urethral process (pizzle) is the most common site of calculus impaction in sheep and goats and should be examined in suspected cases of urolithiasis.[271,272] Sedation facilitates extrusion of the penis for examination. Because of its diuretic effect, xylazine may exacerbate bladder distention and is not recommended. Diazepam (0.1 mg/kg IV slowly) or acepromazine (0.05 to 0.1 mg/kg IV or IM) have been used successfully.

An adjunct or alternative to sedation is administration of epidural anesthesia, which provides greater patient comfort and eliminates muscular resistance to penile extrusion. One ml of 2% lidocaine per 5 kg of body weight is injected into the epidural space at the lumbosacral junction,[273] although lower dosages may provide sufficient anesthesia. The total dose should not exceed 15 ml of 2% lidocaine in any small

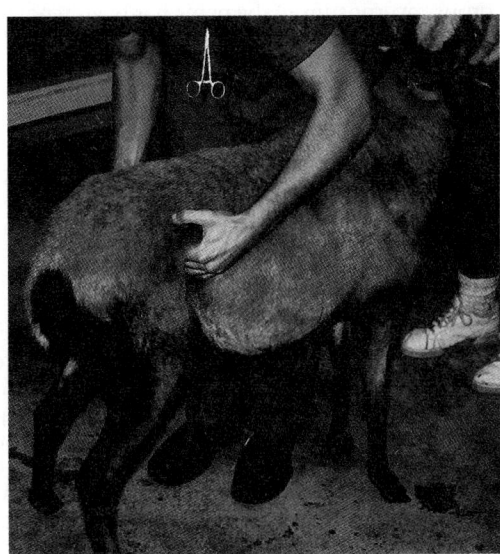

FIG. 32-18 ▦ Palpation of the bladder of a Barbados wether.

ruminant, regardless of size.[273] Hindlimb motor blockade, potentially lasting for several hours, is to be expected with this procedure.

The sheep or goat is then propped up on its rump. The examiner can exteriorize the penis by pushing the sigmoid flexure of the penis cranially from the base of the scrotum while pulling the sheath in a caudal direction. Small towel clamps or Allis tissue forceps can be used to apply traction to the penis. In many instances, preputial mucosa must be carefully grasped and extruded before the penis can be reached with a second pair of forceps. The urethral process can then be inspected and palpated for the presence of discrete uroliths or sandlike grit within the lumen. If the urethral process is obstructed, it can be amputated with scissors or a scalpel blade (see Surgical Treatment).

DIFFERENTIAL DIAGNOSIS. Tachycardia, colic, and anorexia are characteristic of gastrointestinal obstruction, but auscultation and percussion of the abdomen, abdominal succussion, and rectal examination should differentiate this condition from acute urethral obstruction. Goats suffering from grain overload will occasionally vocalize and show signs of colic.[274] Encephalopathies, salmonellosis, coccidiosis, or proctitis from rectal prolapse or trauma frequently cause tenesmus. Additional signs of primary neurologic or gastrointestinal dysfunction should be evident with these diseases.

Although rare in male ruminants, urinary tract infection may result in dysuria and pollakiuria. Bladder distention is uncommon with urinary tract infection, and large numbers of white blood cells and bacteria are present in the urine sediment. Occasionally an animal suffering from urolithiasis successfully voids the obstructing urolith(s). The resultant traumatic urethritis might cause dysuria, but the rate and ease of urination typically improve with time and antiinflammatory treatment. Another rare disease to consider in the differential diagnosis is ectopic ureter, which typically manifests as incontinence rather than dysuria or stranguria.

Urethral Rupture

The wall of the obstructed urethra may undergo pressure necrosis, resulting in leakage of urine into the subcutaneous tissue of the perineum and ventral abdomen. Urethral rupture is a common complication of urethral obstruction in cattle. Sequelae include cellulitis in the tissues exposed to urine, penile adhesions (possibly creating phimosis), and urethral stricture. Erection failure secondary to vascular obstruction of the corpus cavernosum of the penis has been reported as a sequela to urethral obstruction and rupture in a goat.[275]

CLINICAL FINDINGS. Affected animals are frequently depressed and inappetent. Pitting edema is present in the ventral perineum, inguinal region, prepuce, and ventral abdomen (Fig. 32-19). The affected areas are initially warm and painful on palpation but soon become cool, dark, and nonpainful as necrosis ensues. With time the ventral abdominal tissues become gangrenous and slough, and a fistula may develop to allow urine to escape. Pyrexia may occur if tissue necrosis is extensive. Rectal examination in steers and bulls reveals a small bladder.

DIFFERENTIAL DIAGNOSIS. Ventral abdominal swelling is found with umbilical, preputial, or subcutaneous infection and with abdominal or umbilical hernias. These conditions can be differentiated from urethral rupture by careful palpation of affected tissues. Pain and heat are more pronounced in local infection than in urethral rupture. Cytologic examination of aspirates are helpful in identifying primary infectious processes. Defects in the abdominal wall can be detected along the periphery of hernias. In bulls, penile hematomas may cause swelling of the prepuce. The swelling created by a penile hematoma is centered on midline and is

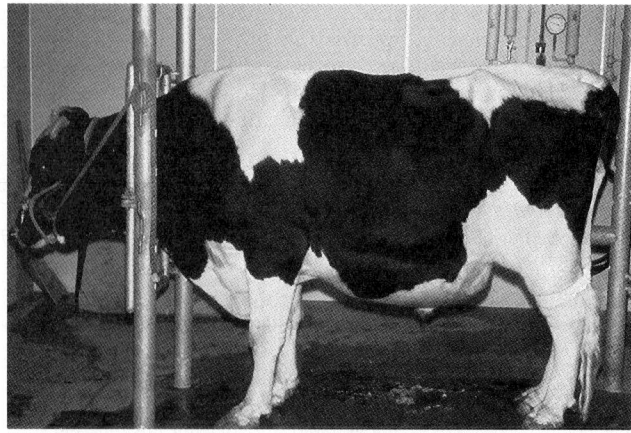

FIG. 32-19 ▌ Urethral rupture in a Holstein steer. Tissue swelling from urine accumulation may extend to the sternum and axillae.

usually localized to the prescrotal region and caudal sheath. Diffuse pitting edema of the ventral abdominal wall is not present in cases of penile hematoma. Aspiration of a suspected penile hematoma is not recommended because of the risk of iatrogenic infection.

Rupture of the Bladder (Water Belly)

Prolonged bladder distention secondary to urethral obstruction may result in pinpoint perforations, tears, or occasionally necrosis of large areas of the bladder wall. The dorsum of the bladder fundus may be the most common site for rupture,[271] but rupture in other bladder regions does occur.[276] Relief of bladder distention causes cessation of strangury. Uremia and dehydration result in debilitation and eventual death if medical and surgical treatment are not provided. In cows, bladder rupture may occur as a sequela to dystocia.[277,278]

CLINICAL FINDINGS. Bilateral distention of the ventral abdomen develops within 1 to 2 days after rupture. Ballottement of the abdomen may elicit a fluid wave. Rectal temperature may be normal,[279] but hypothermia is common in cases showing severe shock. Dehydration, depression, weakness, and injection of the scleral vessels may occur secondary to uremia.

The animal's breath may smell like ammonia. On rectal examination the bladder is small or is not palpable. Abdominocentesis yields a large volume of straw-colored, often blood-tinged fluid. The fluid may or may not smell like urine. The fluid may be warmed to aid in detection of the urine smell. Chemical analysis of the fluid can be used to confirm a diagnosis of uroperitoneum (see Clinical Pathology).

DIFFERENTIAL DIAGNOSIS. Ventral abdominal distention may develop with diffuse peritonitis, vagal indigestion, or ascites secondary to caudal vena caval thrombosis or hypoproteinemia. Marked peritoneal cavity effusion may be found in cases of mesothelioma. These conditions are differentiated from bladder rupture through rectal examination, cytologic and chemical analysis of peritoneal fluid, and evaluation of serum chemistry.

Chronic Partial Urethral Obstruction

An uncommon form of urolithiasis, chronic partial urethral obstruction occurs if calculi impair but do not completely obstruct urine outflow.[280] Chronic retention of urine elevates fluid pressure within the urinary tract lumen, potentially leading to hypertrophy of the bladder wall, hydroureter, and

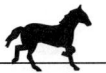

hydronephrosis. Azotemia, progressive renal failure, and uremia are evident in cases that develop hydronephrosis.

CLINICAL FINDINGS. Affected animals have been termed "dribblers" because of their characteristic slow or intermittent urine flow during voiding.[281] Lethargy, reduced appetite, or thin body condition are evident if renal failure has developed. On rectal examination the bladder may be small and thickening of the bladder wall may be palpated.[280]

DIFFERENTIAL DIAGNOSIS. Reduced rate of urine passage may occur with spinal cord disease or damage to the pelvic nerves that control bladder function. A careful neurologic examination is needed to detect other signs of spinal cord disease. Urethral stricture, a relatively uncommon complication of urolithiasis, may also cause impairment of urine flow. Contrast urethrography may be needed to identify the stricture. Small ruminants suffering from the internal form of ulcerative posthitis may dribble urine. In such cases, characteristic preputial lesions are present.

Ureterolithiasis and Nephrolithiasis

CLINICAL FINDINGS. Cattle with acute ureteral obstruction may show severe colic with stretching, kyphosis, treading, collapse, and vocalization.[271] However, intermittent ureteral obstruction with no evidence of colic has been described in a cow.[282] Rectal or vaginal examination may reveal ureteral enlargement secondary to buildup of urine proximal to the obstruction. If the left ureter is obstructed, enlargement of the left kidney may be palpable per rectum. Azotemia occurs if the obstruction is bilateral. Pyelonephritis may occur with ureteral[282] and renal[283] calculosis. With ureteral or renal rupture, uroperitoneum or retroperitoneal accumulation of urine occur.

DIFFERENTIAL DIAGNOSIS. Obstruction of the gastrointestinal tract may cause colic in cattle, particularly if the lesion results in strangulation of bowel. Auscultation and percussion of the abdomen and rectal examination findings of bowel distention allow for differentiation of gastrointestinal obstruction from ureteral or renal obstruction. Cases of ureteral or renal calculosis without colic may show nonspecific signs of illness, and serum chemistry, urinalysis, and ultrasound examination are required for diagnosis.[282]

ULTRASONOGRAPHY/RADIOGRAPHY. A presumptive diagnosis of urolithiasis can usually be made through historical and physical examination findings. Ultrasonographic or radiographic evaluation of the urinary tract may allow for confirmation of a diagnosis of urolithiasis.[284,285] In cases of prolonged urethral obstruction (48 hours) or urethral obstruction with severe azotemia, it is prudent to perform ultrasonographic examination of the kidneys before consideration of surgical treatment. Detection of hydronephrosis would warrant a grave prognosis for recovery.

Ultrasonographic evaluation of the bladder of small ruminants is most easily accomplished through transabdominal scanning with a 3.5- or 5.0-MHz sector array probe, directed caudodorsally from the right inguinal area. Both kidneys of small ruminants and the bovine right kidney can be examined from the right paralumbar fossa.[284] In cattle, transrectal examination of the pelvic urethra, bladder, ureters, and left kidney is performed with a 7.5-MHz linear array probe. Marked distention of the bladder, thickening of the bladder wall, and echogenic material within the bladder lumen may be seen with acute urethral obstruction. A large volume of free fluid in the abdomen is characteristic of uroperitoneum secondary to bladder rupture (Fig. 32-20).

Radiographic examination of the urinary tract is limited to small ruminants and young cattle. Radiodense calculi in the bladder may be most easily detected with lateral views of the abdomen, taken with the animal in lateral recumbency.

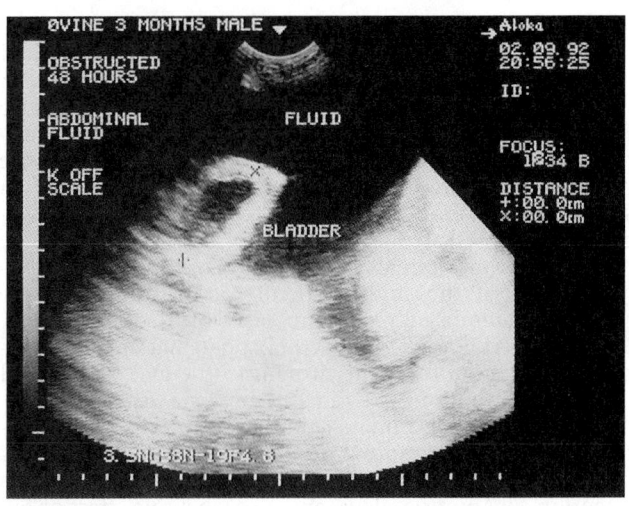

FIG. 32-20 ■ Transabdominal ultrasonogram of uroperitoneum secondary to bladder rupture in a ram. The ventral abdominal wall is at the top of the image, and the dorsal abdomen is at the bottom. Note the large volume of free abdominal fluid and the thickened bladder wall.

Positive contrast urethrography may allow for detection of radiolucent urethral calculi, urethral stricture, and urethral rupture. After catheter placement of approximately 5 cm into the penile urethra, injection of a volume of 10 to 30 ml of water-soluble contrast media has been used with success in adult bucks and rams. Accidental introduction of bubbles may complicate interpretation of urethrograms; thus the catheter should be completely filled with contrast material before insertion, and injection should be done slowly.

CLINICAL PATHOLOGY

Acute Urethral Obstruction. Hematologic and serum chemistry findings may be unremarkable in ruminants with acute urethral obstruction uncomplicated by urethral or bladder rupture.[272] Hyperglycemia and a stress leukogram may be present. With time, hemoconcentration and azotemia develop secondary to reduced water intake. Azotemia is severe in cases of hydronephrosis.

Hematuria and proteinuria are consistent abnormalities detected on urinalysis. Crystalluria may or may not be present.[286] Pyuria and bacteriuria are indicative of concurrent urinary tract infection.

Bladder Rupture. More profound alterations in hematologic and serum biochemical parameters occur with rupture of the bladder. Urine osmolality is normally two to three times that of extracellular fluid (ECF).[287] Ruminant urine contains higher concentrations of urea, creatinine, and potassium but lower concentrations of sodium and chloride than the ECF.[279,287,288] In cases of bladder rupture, uroperitoneum induces movement of water down an osmolar gradient from the ECF into the peritoneal cavity. This movement of water results in depletion of intravascular volume, manifested as an increased packed cell volume and serum protein concentration. Diffusion of sodium and chloride from the ECF into the peritoneal cavity results in eventual hyponatremia and hypochloremia. Urea and creatinine diffuse in the opposite direction, and azotemia results. Serum potassium concentration in ruminants with bladder rupture is variable. Potassium values tend to be normal or low in cattle with bladder rupture,[279,288] even if uroperitoneum exists for several days.[279] Anorexia may contribute to hypokalemia in these cases. Aldosterone release secondary to volume depletion results in dramatic increases in salivary potassium excretion, providing an alternative route of potassium excretion in

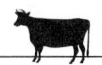
affected cattle.[277,288] Once in the gastrointestinal tract, potassium absorption may be diminished by ileus and preferential absorption of sodium over potassium.[277,288] Alkalosis, which occurs secondary to hypochloremia, may also serve to reduce ECF potassium concentration in cattle with bladder rupture.[288] However, hyperkalemia is an occasional consequence of bladder rupture in cattle[277] and small ruminants.[272] In such cases, metabolic acidosis may contribute to the development of hyperkalemia.[272]

Although only a small fraction (10% or less) of phosphorus excretion in the ruminant occurs via the urine,[277,288] hyperphosphatemia may occur in cases of bladder rupture. Potential mechanisms for hyperphosphatemia include phosphorus diffusion from the urine into the ECF,[279] reduced glomerular filtration,[288] and tissue hypoxia, causing breakdown of organic phosphate compounds in cells.[288] In addition, reduced salivary flow from anorexia may limit phosphorus excretion in the saliva, contributing to phosphorus retention.[278] Anorexia, ileus, and a competitive effect of hyperphosphatemia may contribute to reduction in serum calcium concentration in cases of uroperitoneum.[279,288]

Chemical analysis of peritoneal fluid is a useful means of documenting uroperitoneum. Peritoneal fluid creatinine concentration can be compared to serum creatinine concentration, with a ratio of 2:1 peritoneal fluid (creatinine)/serum (creatinine), indicating uroperitoneum.[279]

Experimentally induced bladder rupture did not cause peritonitis in steers, even after several days of uroperitoneum.[279] Nonetheless, white blood cell count and blood fibrinogen levels may increase in cases of ruptured bladder,[288] possibly reflecting more extensive tissue necrosis and inflammation in natural cases. With uremia, impairment of blood coagulation may become an important clinical consideration. Reduced platelet aggregation and alteration of coagulation factor function occur in uremic patients of other species.[289] Bleeding diathesis and elevation of partial thromboplastin time have been reported in azotemic cattle.[290]

Urethral Rupture. Leakage of urine into the subcutaneous space produces hematologic and serum biochemical alterations that are similar to but less severe than those seen with bladder rupture.[287] The muscles and subcutis holding the urine does not possess as large of a surface area as the peritoneal cavity. Therefore less rapid and less extensive fluxes of water, ions, and waste products occur in urethral rupture than in bladder rupture.[287] Tissue necrosis and secondary infection may result in neutrophilia, leukocytosis, and hyperfibrinogenemia in cases of urethral rupture.

Chronic Partial Obstruction. Hyponatremia, hypochloremia, hypocalcemia, hyperphosphatemia, and severe azotemia with isosthenuria are suggestive of extensive nephron damage due to hydronephrosis.[280]

NECROPSY FINDINGS. When the urethra is opened along the sagittal plane, hemorrhage and necrosis of the urethral mucosa are evident proximal to and at the site of obstruction. Particular attention should be paid to examination of the urethral process in sheep and goats and the sigmoid flexure in cattle. Calculi may be relatively large, discrete mineral aggregates or very fine, sandlike material. As much calculus material as possible should be collected for analysis of mineral composition. Occasionally no calculi can be found in the urinary tract, but mucosal trauma and necrosis of the bladder or urethra persist.

Urethral rupture is characterized by the subcutaneous accumulation of urine in the inguinal area, prepuce, and ventral abdomen. Hemorrhage surrounds the site of the urethral defect. In bladder rupture the abdominal cavity is filled with a large volume of straw-colored, possibly blood-tinged fluid. The site of the bladder tear is quite variable.[276] Hydronephrosis, hydroureter, and bladder wall hypertrophy may be present in cases of chronic partial urethral obstruction.[280]

TREATMENT AND PROGNOSIS

Salvage. Steers and feeder lambs may be sent for immediate slaughter if urethral obstruction is diagnosed before development of azotemia or urinary tract rupture.[291]

Medical Treatment. Medical treatment of urolithiasis involves the administration of tranquilizers early in the course of urethral obstruction.[270] The beneficial effect of these agents has been attributed to an antispasmodic effect.[266] Relaxation of the retractor penis muscle, which results in straightening of the sigmoid flexure, is another means by which these drugs may facilitate passage of calculi.[270] In small ruminants, however, medical treatment with intravenous fluids, nonsteroidal antiinflammatory agents, or tranquilizers has not met with much success.[272,292]

Surgical Treatment. Selection of a method of surgical treatment of urolithiasis is dictated by economic considerations, intended use of the animal, available facilities and equipment, and status of the patient. Removal or bypass of the obstruction and restoration of urine output are the goals of surgical treatment. The prognosis for both short- and long-term survival will vary according to the patient's status and the surgical procedure chosen. Acute renal failure is an occasional sequela to urinary tract obstruction and should be considered in the prognosis.

Preoperative Considerations. Ruminants with urinary tract obstruction, particularly those with uroperitoneum, often require preoperative stabilization of hypovolemia and electrolyte abnormalities. Surgical repair of the urinary tract should be delayed until the patient can withstand prolonged recumbency or general anesthesia. Whenever possible, fluid therapy should be guided by analysis of serum electrolyte concentrations. Physiologic (0.9%) saline solution is used to correct intravascular volume deficits, hyponatremia, and hypochloremia. Calcium salts can be added to the fluids if indicated. Empirical supplementation of intravenous fluids with potassium should be avoided, because the potential for hyperkalemia always exists. Hyperkalemia may induce fatal cardiac dysrhythmias, and this effect is augmented by concurrent hyponatremia.[293] Administration of dextrose or sodium bicarbonate reduces serum potassium concentration by promoting movement of potassium from the extracellular to the intracellular space. Uremic animals undergoing intravenous fluid therapy may develop pulmonary edema.[294] Attention must be paid to respiratory rate, auscultatory findings, and respiratory effort during fluid therapy in such cases. Slow drainage of urine from the abdominal cavity reduces pressure on the diaphragm and slows the progression of metabolic derangements caused by uroperitoneum.

Although bacterial infection is not considered to be a common primary cause of urolithiasis, secondary urinary tract infections may develop after surgical intervention. Loss of the flushing effect of urination, urinary mucosal damage, and impaired host cellular defenses secondary to uremia may contribute to the development of ascending urinary tract infection. Perioperative antibiotic therapy is therefore prudent, with due consideration of withholding times in animals intended for slaughter. Postoperative antibiotic therapy is discussed below.

Surgical Options. In sheep and goats, amputation of an obstructed urethral process is a simple procedure that may at least temporarily restore urethral patency. The urethral process can be removed without detrimental effects on breeding soundness.[295] Success rates for initial restoration of urine flow following urethral process amputation range from 37.5%[295] to 66%.[272] However, recurrence of urethral obstruction is extremely common, and urethral patency is usually maintained for only hours to days.[272,295] Failure of urethral process amputation results from additional calculi causing obstruction of the urethra, usually at or proximal to the sigmoid flexure. Therefore urethral process amputation

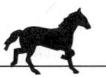

is palliative and may provide enough time to allow feeder lambs to survive until slaughter. For pet wethers, rams, and bucks, however, recurrence of urinary tract obstruction appears to be probable if this is the only procedure performed.

Urethral catheterization and retrograde flushing has been used to dislodge urethral calculi and restore urine flow in a ram.[296] However, successful clearance of the urethra is rarely achieved.[272] Retrograde passage of a catheter may allow for localization of the urethral obstruction, potentially guiding further surgical treatment. Passage of a catheter into the bladder of ruminants and camelids is difficult, because of the presence of a urethral recess located near the ischial arch.[297]

Penectomy is an option for animals intended for slaughter.[270] Perineal urethrostomy is a surgical option for ruminants not intended to be used for breeding. In small ruminants, postoperative urinary tract obstruction may result from stricture of the stoma or from recurrent obstruction with additional calculi.[272,286,298] Long-term restoration of urethral patency following perineal urethrostomy in sheep and goats may not be consistently achieved.

Ischial urethrostomy with placement of a Foley catheter into the bladder has been used as a treatment for urolithiasis in heavy feedlot steers[299] and bulls.[269] If urethral damage is not severe, this procedure allows the breeding ability of bulls to be maintained.[269]

Prepubic urethrostomy has been reported in a sheep and a goat.[300] In this procedure a midperineal penectomy is performed. The perineal segment of the penis and pelvic portion of the urethra are dissected free from the surrounding soft tissue via perineal and ventral celiotomy incisions, respectively. Bilateral ileal and/or ischiadic osteotomies may be required to free the pelvic urethra. The urethral mucosa is then sutured to the skin of the caudoventral abdomen to create a long-lasting stoma.

Urethrotomy, with removal of the obstructing calculi and primary closure of the urethra, is another option.[269,271,272] The calculi may be located, crushed with a towel clamp, and flushed from the urethral lumen, eliminating the need for a urethral incision.[269,271] Urethral stricture, adhesions resulting in phimosis in breeding males, and reobstruction with additional calculi are long-term complications associated with urethrotomy.

Cystotomy allows for maintenance of breeding soundness and removal of additional calculi from the bladder. In small ruminants, bidirectional (normograde and retrograde) flushing is used to restore urethral patency.[272,286]

Tube cystostomy allows urine to exit the bladder through a temporary Foley catheter, which is anchored in the bladder lumen and exits the ventral abdomen.[292] Urethral patency is apparently restored when calculi are spontaneously expelled from the urethra, dissolved, or are refluxed into the bladder. Contrast medium can be introduced into the bladder via the Foley catheter to monitor urethral patency, locate urethral obstruction, or identify urethral rupture.[285]

In cases of bladder rupture the urine should be drained from the abdominal cavity, and a surgical procedure should be performed to divert urine to the exterior. A catheter can be secured in the bladder via small abdominal incision[301] or via an ischial urethrotomy.[269,299] Alternatively, abdominal drainage may be combined with perineal urethrostomy or penectomy.[270,271] With these methods the bladder tear may be sealed by fibrin or by the omentum within a few days, and primary repair of the bladder defect may not be necessary. Tears are more likely to seal spontaneously if they are located on the dorsal aspect of the bladder[302]; however, it is generally difficult for the veterinarian to know the location of the bladder defect without performing a laparotomy. Depending on the size and location of the bladder defect, daily abdominal drainage may need to be performed until spontaneous sealing occurs.

Alternatively, the veterinarian may elect to suture the bladder defect in cases of bladder rupture. Laparotomy and primary repair of the bladder defect may be performed under local[276] or general anesthesia.[303] A tube cystostomy can be performed after the bladder defect is repaired.[292]

In bladder marsupialization, the apex of the bladder is exteriorized via a small paramedian incision, and the seromuscular layer of the bladder is circumferentially secured to the abdominal wall. A cystotomy is performed, and the bladder mucosa is secured to the skin, creating a permanent opening for urine drainage from the bladder to the exterior.[304]

Ureteral calculi may be removed via ureterotomy.[271] Nephrectomy may be performed in unilateral cases of obstructive nephrolithiasis.[305] If unilateral nephrectomy is under consideration, a biopsy of the apparently unaffected kidney should be done to evaluate remaining renal function.[306] Measurement of BUN, serum creatinine, and urine specific gravity is also essential in evaluating remaining renal function before unilateral nephrectomy.[306] Normal urine specific gravity, BUN concentration, and serum creatinine concentration indicates that the majority of nephrons in the remaining kidney are functional.

Multiple small stab incisions in the ventral abdominal wall may facilitate urine drainage in cases of urethral rupture.

Postoperative Considerations. Assessment of hydration and urine output and serum urea nitrogen, creatinine, and electrolyte concentrations may be necessary after surgery. Postobstruction diuresis has been reported in ruminants[296] and may result from tubular damage, accumulation of urea or natriuretic factors, or preoperative fluid therapy.[307] Induction of modest diuresis through fluid therapy after surgery may help to reduce azotemia and accumulation of blood clots and bacteria in the urethra.

Antimicrobial therapy with an antibiotic that achieves high urine concentrations (e.g., penicillin, ampicillin, sulfonamides) is warranted; the duration of therapy depends on the surgical procedure chosen, residue withholding considerations, and whether or not urinary tract infection exists at the time of surgery. For tube cystostomy, antimicrobial therapy is recommended while the tube is in place and for at least 1 week after the tube is removed.[292] Antimicrobial therapy should be maintained for at least 3 weeks after surgery in cases with active urinary tract infection.

Prompt initiation of preventive dietary and environmental management is critical for the long-term success of any surgical procedure for urolithiasis (see Prevention). In animals intended for slaughter, a period of at least 30 days is often required for resolution of tissue damage from urethral or bladder rupture.[299]

EPIDEMIOLOGY

Gender. Obstructive urolithiasis in ruminants is almost exclusively a disease of males and castrated males.[308] Urinary calculi appear to develop to a similar degree in female ruminants. However, most calculi can pass through the relatively short, distensible urethra of the female, making urethral obstruction uncommon.[308]

Calculi appear to form to a similar extent in the urinary tracts of bulls and steers.[268] Because of the trophic effect of testosterone, the urethral diameter of yearling bulls is approximately 25% greater than that of yearling steers.[268] Urethral obstruction therefore is more common in steers.[268] A similar predisposition for urethral obstruction may exist for wethers relative to buck goats.[309] However, because many wethers are kept as pets, factors such as diet, environment, and age are likely to differ in comparison to bucks.

Season. The incidence of urolithiasis increases in the late fall and winter in North America.[308] Limited water availability, increases in the silica content of range grasses, and a larger population of susceptible animals (young, growing males) during this time of year are factors that may be responsible for this trend. In warmer climates, urolithiasis is more frequently a problem in the arid months of the year, underscoring the role of water intake in the pathogenesis of the disease.[308]

Age. Cattle of a variety of ages may develop obstructive urolithiasis. The tendency for this disease to be seen in younger ruminants may be the result of dietary influences, because younger animals are more commonly fed concentrates for weight gain and eventual slaughter than are mature males kept for breeding. In addition, because relatively fewer mature males are kept for breeding, the apparent increased prevalence of urolithiasis in younger animals may simply reflect the fact that there are greater numbers of younger males and castrated males at risk.

Silica Urolithiasis. Estimates of annual death losses in steers in western North America range from 3%[299] to 5%[308] Deaths and treatment costs attributable to silica urolithiasis in cattle have been estimated to cost Canadian ranchers between $500,000 to $1 million per year.[308] Silica urolithiasis is a very common subclinical condition in certain areas. For example, in western North America, silica calculi can be found in the urinary tracts of 50% to 80% of range cattle, with urinary tract obstruction occurring in a variable percentage of these animals.[308,310]

Phosphatic Urolithiasis. In a recent study, the prevalences of urolithiasis were 0.5% and 0.35% for two Colorado lamb feedlots.[311] The calculus types in these lambs were not identified and are assumed to have been phosphatic calculi. Urolithiasis was the fifth most prevalent cause of death on each feedlot.[311] In beef feedlots, death losses from urolithiasis have been estimated at 0.6%.[312]

PATHOPHYSIOLOGY

Mechanisms of Calculogenesis. Multiple factors influence the development of urinary calculi, but of primary importance is the development of high urinary concentrations of soluble, ionized minerals (crystalloids) that, under appropriate conditions, may aggregate to form insoluble crystals. Supersaturation of urine with a calculus-forming crystalloid is a prerequisite for urolith development.[313] However, supersaturation alone is not solely responsible for urolith initiation because normal urine is typically supersaturated with a variety of calculogenic ions.[314] Urine contains variable concentrations of mucopolysaccharides, ions, and organic acids, which act as intrinsic inhibitors of crystallization. Through physical and electrochemical interactions, these compounds maintain calculogenic minerals in a colloidal suspension. Calculus formation is initiated if supersaturation of urine with appropriate crystalloids exceeds the protective capabilities of the crystallization inhibitors. The crystalloids are rendered insoluble and precipitate out of the aqueous phase of urine. Calculi enlarge as further mineral precipitation takes place on the crystal surfaces. Dietary, environmental, and management influences interact to determine the degree of supersaturation of urine with calculogenic minerals. Dehydration, with resultant concentration of urinary minerals, would appear to be a critical factor in the development of all types of uroliths.

Mucoproteins, which make up a variable fraction of most uroliths, may act as templates (matrices) on which calculogenic ions could initiate crystallization.[314] Urine mucoproteins may reduce the solubility of certain crystalloids or may be passively incorporated into developing uroliths.[315,316] Estrogenic substances in the diet may promote urolithiasis by increasing urinary mucoprotein concentration.[316,317] This was of particular concern in the past, when diethylstilbestrol was used as a growth promotant in sheep and cattle in North America.[317]

The solubility of some calculogenic crystalloids is influenced by urinary pH. Struvite (magnesium ammonium phosphate), calcium phosphate, and calcium carbonate uroliths

are less soluble in alkaline urine, whereas calcium oxalate solubility is not affected by changes in urine pH within the physiologic range.[314,318-320] The effect of urinary pH on silica calculi is debatable,[321] but recent findings show a trend toward reduction in calculi formation under conditions of mild aciduria.[322]

Primary urinary tract infection is considered to be an uncommon cause of ruminant urolithiasis.[319] Purulent debris within the urinary tract may serve as a nidus for crystal development, and bacterial ureases may increase urinary pH, thereby reducing the solubility of certain crystalloids. Pyelonephritis with presumed secondary urolithiasis has been reported in cattle.[282] Urolithiasis may be considered as both a cause[283] and a consequence[282] of urinary tract infection.

Although quite rare, vitamin A deficiency has been incriminated as a contributory factor for urolith development.[319] Metaplasia of urinary tract epithelium may create nidi for calculogenesis through desquamation of cells or altered cell surface characteristics.

Feeding patterns may influence the formation of urinary calculi. Providing a ration in one to two feedings per day to ruminants induces antidiuretic hormone release soon after feeding, resulting in a marked but transient decline in urine output and an increase in urine concentration.[271,308] These dramatic changes in urine composition can be limited through ad libitum feeding.[266]

Water hardness (dissolved mineral content) has not been considered to be a significant factor in ruminant urolithiasis.[308]

Phosphatic Urolithiasis. Ruminants consuming rations high in phosphorus, such as grain-based feedlot rations, commonly develop struvite (magnesium ammonium phosphate) calculi.[266,319,323,324] Increases in dietary phosphorus levels result in increased concentration of phosphate ion in ruminant urine.[323] Because calcium opposes phosphorus absorption from the gut, urinary excretion of phosphate is augmented by low dietary levels of calcium relative to phosphorus.[266,319,323,324] The interaction of magnesium with calcium and phosphorus is less clearly understood,[323] but experimental increases in dietary magnesium levels to 0.6% of dietary dry matter induced calcium phosphate and struvite urolithiasis in calves.[325]

Pelleting of rations has been associated with an increased incidence of phosphatic urolithiasis.[266] Ruminant saliva is rich in phosphorus, and the gastrointestinal tract is the primary route of phosphorus excretion in ruminants.[278] In theory, ruminants feeding on pelleted rations produce less saliva, which would reduce gastrointestinal phosphate losses and increase urinary phosphate excretion.[266]

Silica Urolithiasis. Silica urolithiasis is primarily a problem of sheep and cattle grazing native rangeland grasses of western North America. The silica fraction of these grasses tends to increase with maturity and may continue to increase even after growth ends. In some areas, 4% to 8% of total grass dry matter may be silicon compounds.[308] A fraction of dietary silica, as unpolymerized silicic acid, is dissolved in the ruminal fluid of the grazing animal, absorbed, and excreted in the urine. In sheep and cattle on range, water intake is usually intermittent. During periods of water deprivation, avid water and sodium resorption by the kidneys results in the formation of highly concentrated urine. Silicic acid may be concentrated to such an extent that it polymerizes to a less soluble form, polysilicic acid. Polysilicic acid, in turn, forms large micelles in solution that quickly become insoluble when bound to urinary mucoproteins.[315] The resultant calculi are usually composed of roughly 20% mucoprotein, 75% silicon dioxide, and variable amounts of calcium oxalate and calcium carbonate.[308]

Recently dietary deficiencies of copper and zinc have been identified as contributory factors in silica urolith forma-

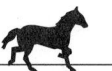

tion in rats.[326] The incidence of silica urolithiasis can be increased by feeding sheep rations that have a high calcium-to-phosphorus ratio (approximately 2.8:1) and induce more alkaline urine.[322,327] It is important to note that a high Ca:P ratio in the diet can help to prevent one type of urolith (struvite) but may be a contributory factor for another (silica). This underscores the importance of both ration and urolith mineral analyses in the formulation of preventive measures for this disease.

Calcium Carbonate Urolithiasis. Calcium carbonate calculi are common in sheep grazing lush, rapidly growing clover pastures in Australia.[320] These forages are rich in calcium and low in phosphorus and magnesium and have a high oxalate content. In the gut, oxalate avidly binds calcium and makes it unavailable for absorption. With gradual introduction of oxalate-rich diets, ruminal bacteria efficiently metabolize oxalate to bicarbonate.[320,328] Thus microbial metabolism of oxalate in the rumen may increase the availability of dietary calcium.[329] These factors may combine to increase urinary calcium excretion and alkalinize urine, thereby promoting calcium carbonate calculogenesis. Calcium carbonate urolithiasis has been reported in northern California.[330] Although many of the animals in this report had a history of being fed alfalfa hay, the relationship, if any, between alfalfa feeding and calcium carbonate urolithiasis remains unclear.[330]

Calcium Oxalate Urolithiasis. Oxalate is an end product of glycine and ascorbic acid metabolism and is a normal constituent of urine.[313,320] In humans, inherent defects in oxalate metabolism and calcium homeostasis contribute to calcium oxalate urolithiasis.[313] Dietary and metabolic factors that influence formation of this urolith type have not been elucidated in ruminants. Poisoning by oxalate-containing plants is not considered to be a cause of calcium oxalate urolithiasis.[319] Given its very low solubility, calcium oxalate crystals are often present in normal urine[319] and may be incorporated into other uroliths as a trace component.

PREVENTION. A preventive approach to a urolithiasis problem begins with a search for risk factors associated with the diet, management, and the environment. Whenever possible, ration analysis and mineral analysis of the urolith(s) should be performed to accurately identify causative dietary factors. Consult Box 32-1 for analysis laboratories. If uroliths are not obtained, ration analysis and/or a thorough dietary history may provide a strong suggestion of the urolith type. In light of the central role of urinary supersaturation in cal-

culogensis, the ultimate aim of preventive measures should be reduction of urinary concentration of calculogenic mineral ions. In addition the urine should be diluted to such an extent that the calculogenic ions are less prone to precipitate. Dilution of urine is achieved through increased salt and water intake.

Dietary Management of Phosphatic Urolithiasis. Prevention of phosphatic calculi requires adjustment of the dietary calcium/phosphorus ratio to a level of 2:1 or greater.[323] The magnesium content of the ration should be maintained at recommended levels. Abandoning pelleted feeds and increasing the quantity of long-stem forage in the ration may increase salivary flow and fecal phosphate excretion.[266]

Addition of salt to feedlot rations has proven effective in several studies. Sodium chloride, fed at a level of 3% to 5%, reduces the incidence of urolithiasis without adverse effects on feed intake or weight gain.[314] Cattle consuming such rations show variable increases in water intake and urine output, implying that some of the beneficial effect of salt feeding is due to diuresis.[308,331] Other studies show minimal effect of this level of salt supplementation on urine volume, and one investigator has suggested that the preventive effect is due to interruption of crystal development by chloride ion in urine.[317] Nonetheless, it is prudent to anticipate increased water intake after salt supplementation is initiated.

Ammonium chloride supplementation, fed at a level of 0.5% to 1% of ration dry matter, also reduces the incidence of struvite urolithiasis.[314,331,332] Ammonium chloride may increase the solubility of magnesium ammonium phosphate crystals through a modest reduction in urinary pH. The pH of the urine is likely to be influenced by the relative concentrations of strong cations (sodium and potassium) and strong anions (chloride and sulfate) of the entire ration, a relationship termed the dietary cation-anion difference.[333] Thus the efficacy of ammonium chloride in reducing urinary pH and therefore in reducing struvite urolithiasis may vary among different livestock operations because the concentration of these cations and anions may vary among rations.[330]

Dietary Management of Silica Urolithiasis. Restriction of dietary silica intake in ruminants grazing native grasses is not feasible; thus dietary preventive management is limited to salt (sodium chloride) supplementation. However, loose salt or lick salt is unlikely to be ingested in high enough quantities to affect water intake.[334] Sodium chloride supplementation of palatable creep feeds, at a level of 15% of dry matter, is an effective measure for range calves.[308] Creep feeding should begin at 4 months of age or earlier. Initially, lower salt concentrations may be required for young calves to become accustomed to the creep feed. The feeders should be located near a reliable source of palatable water.

Recently, ammonium chloride supplementation (1% of dry matter) has been demonstrated to significantly reduce silica urolith development in lambs.[327] In the same study, reduction of the dietary Ca:P ratio from 2:1 to near 1:1 resulted in a trend toward reduced silica calculi formation. The role of copper and zinc deficiencies in ruminant silica urolithiasis remains to be determined.

Dietary Management of Calcium Carbonate Urolithiasis. This type of urolith has been frequently recovered from small ruminants fed alfalfa hay.[330] In light of this observation and the risk factors identified in Australian sheep, reduction of dietary calcium levels could be beneficial. This may not be possible for sheep grazing legume pastures. Ammonium chloride supplementation may be an effective preventive measure, because calcium carbonate is more soluble in acidic solutions.[320]

Water Management of All Calculus Types. Maximizing water intake is an important aspect of urolithiasis prevention, regardless of the urolith type involved. Cleaning of water

---

BOX 32-1

Urolith Analysis Laboratories

Urinary Stone Analysis Laboratory
Department of Medicine and Epidemiology
School of Veterinary Medicine
University of California at Davis
Davis, CA 95616
1-530-752-3228
Dr. Carl Osborne
Department of Small Animal Clinical Sciences
College of Veterinary Medicine
University of Minnesota
1352 Boyd Avenue
St. Paul, MN 55108
1-612-625-7744
Urolithiasis Laboratory
PO Box 25375
Houston, TX 77265-5375
1-800-235-4846

containers should be a regular practice. Water palatability may also be improved through provision of shade for water containers during the summer. Dark liners (with sun exposure) or heaters for water containers will warm the water during the winter. Automatic waterers should be checked regularly for proper function. Shallow containers capable of rapid refilling provide higher rates of water turnover, resulting in less stagnation.[335]

In operations involving multiple animals or large pastures, placement of multiple watering sites might allow for more frequent water intake. This is especially true for sheep, whose banding instinct usually prevents individuals from traveling alone to distant watering sites.[335]

REFERENCES

266. Hay L: Prevention and treatment of urolithiasis in sheep, *In Pract* 12:87-91, 1990.
267. Gasthuys F, Martens A, DeMoor A: Surgical treatment of urethral dilatation in seven cattle, *Vet Rec* 138:17-19, 1996.
268. Bailey CB: Siliceous urinary calculi in bulls, steers, and partial castrates, *Can J Anim Sci* 55:187-191, 1975.
269. Wolfe DF, Moll HD, May KA: Urolithiasis. In Wolfe DF, Moll HD, eds: *Large animal urogenital surgery*, Baltimore, 1999, Williams & Wilkins, pp 349-359.
270. Oehme FW, Tillman H: Diagnosis and treatment of ruminant urolithiasis, *J Am Vet Med Assoc* 147:1331-1338, 1965.
271. Hofmeyr CFB: *Ruminant urogenital surgery*, Ames, 1987, Iowa State University Press, pp 15-28.
272. VanMetre DC, Smith BP: Clinical management of urolithiasis in small ruminants, *Proc ACVIM* 9:555-557, 1991.
273. Benson GJ, Thurmon JC: Regional anesthesia. In Howard JL, ed: *Current veterinary therapy 3: food animal practice*, Philadelphia, 1992, WB Saunders, pp 77-88.
274. House JK G et al: Assessment of ruminant digestive system, *Vet Clin North Am (Food Anim Pract)* 8:189-202, 1992.
275. Todhunter P, Baird AN, Wolfe DW: Erection failure secondary to obstructive urolithiasis in a male goat, *J Am Vet Med Assoc* 209:650-651, 1996.
276. Gera KL, Nigam JM: Urolithiasis in bovines: a report of 193 clinical cases, *Indian Vet J* 56:417-423, 1979.
277. Smith JA, Divers TJ, Lamp TM: Ruptured urinary bladder in a postparturient cow, *Cornell Vet* 73:3-12, 1983.
278. Carr EA et al: Ruptured urinary bladder after dystocia in a cow, *J Am Vet Med Assoc* 202:631-632, 1993.
279. Sockett DC et al: Metabolic changes due to experimentally induced rupture of the bovine urinary bladder, *Cornell Vet* 76:198-212, 1986.
280. Aldridge BM, Garry FB: Chronic partial obstructive urolithiasis causing hydronephrosis and chronic renal failure in a steer, *Cornell Vet* 82:311-317, 1992.
281. Blood DC, Radostits OM: *Veterinary medicine*, ed 7, London, 1989, Ballière Tindall, pp 402-409.
282. Divers TJ, Reef VB, Roby KA: Nephrolithiasis resulting in intermittent ureteral obstruction in a cow, *Cornell Vet* 79:143-149, 1989.
283. Ziemer EL, Smith BP: Pyelonephritis, glomerulonephritis, and urolithiasis in a Holstein bull with diarrhea, *Compend Cont Educ Pract Vet* 10:82-85, 1988.
284. Braun U, Schefer U, Fohn J: Urinary tract ultrasonography in normal rams and in rams with obstructive urolithiasis, *Can Vet J* 33:654-659, 1992.
285. Palmer JL et al: Contrast radiography of the lower urinary tract in the management of obstructive urolithiasis in small ruminants and swine, *Vet Radiol* 39:175-180, 1998.
286. Haven ML: Surgical management of urolithiasis in small ruminants, *Cornell Vet* 83:47-55, 1993.
287. Donecker JM, Bellamy JEC: Blood chemical abnormalities in cattle with ruptured bladders and ruptured urethras, *Can Vet J* 23:355-357, 1982.
288. Sockett DS, Knight AP: Metabolic changes associated with obstructive urolithiasis in cattle, *Compend Cont Educ Pract Vet* 6:S311-S315, 1984.
289. Harris CL, Krawiec DR: The pathophysiology of uremic bleeding, *Compend Cont Educ Pract Vet* 12:1294-1298, 1990.
290. Divers TJ et al: Acute renal disorders in cattle: a retrospective study of 22 cases, *J Am Vet Med Assoc* 181:694-699, 1982.
291. Larson BL: Identifying, treating, and preventing bovine urolithiasis, *Vet Med* 91:366-377, 1996.
292. Rakestraw PC et al: Tube cystostomy for treatment of urolithiasis in small ruminants, *Vet Surg* 24:498-505, 1995.
293. Surawicz B: Relationship between electrocardiogram and electrolytes, *Am Heart J* 73:814-834, 1967.
294. Vivrette S et al: Hemodialysis for treatment of oxytetracycline-induced acute renal failure in a neonatal foal, *J Am Vet Med Assoc* 203:105-107, 1993.
295. Smith MC: The reproductive anatomy and physiology of the male goat. In Morrow DA, ed: *Current therapy in theriogenology 2*, Philadelphia, 1986, WB Saunders, pp 616-618.
296. Murray MJ: Urolithiasis in a ram, *Compend Cont Educ Pract Vet* 7(suppl):269-273, 1985.
297. Garett PD: Urethral recess in male goats, sheep, cattle, and swine, *J Am Vet Med Assoc* 191:689-691, 1987.
298. Van Weeren PR, Klein WR, Voorhout G: Urolithiasis in small ruminants. I, A retrospective evaluation of urethrostomy, *Vet Q* 9:76-79, 1987.
299. Winter RB et al: Catheterization: an effective method of treating bovine urethral calculi, *Vet Med* 82:1261-1268, 1987.
300. Stone WC et al: Prepubic urethrostomy for relief of urethral obstruction in a sheep and a goat, *J Am Vet Med Assoc* 210:939-941, 1997.
301. Hastings DH: Retention catheters for treatment of steers with ruptured bladders, *J Am Vet Med Assoc* 147:1329-1330, 1965.
302. Noordsy JL: *Food animal surgery*, ed 3, Trenton, Veterinary Learning Systems, 1994, pp 501-510.
303. Tulleners EP, Hamilton GF, Farrow CS: Surgical repair of ruptured urinary bladder in a ram, *J Am Vet Med Assoc* 177:708-709, 1980.
304. May KA et al: Urinary bladder marsupialization for treatment of obstructive urolithiasis in male goats, *Vet Surg* 27:583-588, 1998.
305. Weaver AD: Nephrectomy and cystotomy in a bull, *Vet Rec* 76:191-193, 1964.
306. Tulleners EP et al: Indications for unilateral bovine nephrectomy: a report of four cases, *J Am Vet Med Assoc* 179:696-700, 1981.
307. Klahr, S: Pathophysiology of obstructive nephropathy, *Kidney Int* 23:414-416, 1983.
308. Bailey CB: Silica metabolism and silica urolithiasis in ruminants: a review, *Can J Anim Sci* 61:219-235, 1981.
309. Van Metre DC, Smith BP: Unpublished data, University of California at Davis, 1992.
310. Urinary calculi of beef cattle, Annual Report 1961, Montana Veterinary Research Laboratory, Montana Experimental Station, Bozeman, Mont, 1961.
311. Salman MD et al: Rates of diseases and their associated costs in two Colorado sheep feedlots (1985-1986), *J Am Vet Med Assoc* 193:1518-1523, 1988.
312. Jensen R, Mackey DR: *Diseases of feedlot cattle*, ed 3, Philadelphia, 1979, Lea & Febiger, pp 262-264.
313. Osborne CA, Klausner JS: Calcium oxalate urolithiasis. In Kirk RW, ed: *Current veterinary therapy VII*, Philadelphia, 1988, WB Saunders, pp 45-48.
314. Romanowski RD: Biochemistry of urolith formation, *J Am Vet Med Assoc* 147:1324-1326, 1965.
315. Bailey CB: The precipitation of polymerized silicic acid by urine protein: a possible mechanism in the etiology of silica urolithiasis, *Can J Anim Sci* 50:305-311, 1972.
316. Jubb KVF, Kennedy PC, Palmer N: *Pathology of domestic animals*, ed 4, San Diego, 1993, Academic Press, pp 525-531.
317. Udall RH, Seger CL, Chen-Chow, F: Studies on urolithiasis. VI, The mechanism of action of sodium chloride in the control of urinary calculi, *Cornell Vet* 55:198-203, 1965.
318. Hoar DW, Emerick RJ, Embry LB: Influence of calcium source, phosphorus level, and acid-forming effects of the diet on feedlot performance in lambs, *J Anim Sci* 31:118-125, 1970.
319. McIntosh GH: Urolithiasis in animals, *Aust Vet J* 54:267-271, 1978.
320. Manning RA, Blaney BJ: Epidemiological aspects of urolithiasis in domestic animals in Queensland, *Aust Vet J* 63:423-424, 1986.
321. Bailey CB: Effects of ammonium chloride on formation of siliceous urinary calculi in calves, *Can J Anim Sci* 56:359-360, 1976.
322. Stewart SR, Emerick RJ, Pritchard RH: Effects of dietary ammonium chloride and variations in calcium to phosphorus ratio on silica urolithiasis in sheep, *J Anim Sci* 69:2225-2229, 1991.
323. Bushman DH, Emerick RJ, Embry LB: Experimentally induced ovine phosphatic urolithiasis: relationships involving dietary calcium, phosphorus, and magnesium, *J Nutr* 87:499-504, 1965.
324. Hoar DW, Emerick RJ, Embry LB: Potassium, phosphorus, and calcium interrelationships influencing feedlot performance and phosphatic urolithiasis in lambs, *J Anim Sci* 30:597-600, 1970.
325. Kallfelz FA et al: Dietary magnesium and urolithiasis in growing calves, *Cornell Vet* 77:33-45, 1987.
326. Stewart SR, Emerick RJ, Kayongo-Male H: Silicon-zinc interactions and potential roles for dietary zinc and copper in minimizing silica urolithiasis, *J Anim Sci* 71:946-954, 1993.
327. Stewart SR, Emerick RJ, Pritchard RH: High dietary calcium to phosphorus ratio and alkali-forming potential as factors promoting silica urolithiasis in sheep, *J Anim Sci* 68:498-503, 1990.
328. Angus KW: Nephropathy in young lambs, *Vet Rec* 126:525-528, 1990.
329. Adair HS, Adams WH: Ascorbic acid as suspected cause of oxalate nephrotoxicosis in a goat, *J Am Vet Med Assoc* 197:1626-1628, 1990.
330. Van Metre DC et al: Obstructive urolithiasis in ruminants: surgical management and prevention, *Compend Cont Ed Pract Vet* 18:S275-S289, 1996.
331. Bushman DH, Emerick RJ, Embry LB: Effect of various chlorides and calcium carbonate calcium, phosphorus, sodium, potassium, and chloride balance and their relationship to urinary calculi in lambs, *J Anim Sci* 27:490-496, 1968.
332. Crookshank HR et al: Effect of chemical and enzymatic agents on the formation of urinary calculi in fattening steers, *J Anim Sci* 19:595-600, 1960.

333. Jardon PW: Using urine pH to measure anionic salt diets, *Compend Cont Ed Pract Vet* 17:860-862, 1995.
334. Bailey CB: Formation of siliceous urinary calculi in calves given supplements containing large amounts of sodium chloride, *Can J Anim Sci* 53:55-60, 1973.
335. East NE: Personal communication, University of California at Davis, 1994.

URACHAL ABSCESSES/ADHESIONS
LOREN G. SCHULTZ

Urachal abscesses and adhesions are commonly observed in calves during the first few weeks of life. However, onset of signs at several months of age may occur. The most common source of infection is contamination from the external environment leading to an ascending infection of the umbilicus (see Chapters 17 and 20) that can cause urinary tract infection or mechanical interference with bladder emptying.[336]

CLINICAL AND LABORATORY FINDINGS. Animals with large urachal abscesses are often unthrifty. Clinical signs may include fever, dysuria, perineal urine scalding, and pollakiuria.[336-338] During voiding, urine flow is often slow. The external umbilicus may or may not be enlarged and painful.[339] On deep abdominal palpation the infected urachus may be found to extend from the internal aspect of the umbilicus toward the apex of the bladder. When infected, this structure is relatively firm and is larger than the diameter of a pencil. In larger calves, rectal examination may reveal cranial displacement of the bladder, fixation of the bladder apex in a cranioventral position, and incomplete bladder emptying after urination. Transabdominal or transrectal ultrasonographic examination is often helpful in diagnosis. Normal values for the diameter of umbilical structures via ultrasound have been published.[340] Identification of a urachal remnant in calves is abnormal.

Leukocytosis, neutrophilia, and hyperfibrinogenemia are typical hematologic findings in ruminants with urachal abscesses.[338] Elevation of serum globulin concentration occurs with chronic infections. Hematuria and pyuria are found on urinalysis if secondary cystitis has developed.[339]

DIFFERENTIAL DIAGNOSIS. Neurologic disease may cause impairment of urine outflow in young ruminants, but concurrent signs of spinal cord dysfunction are expected. Urolithiasis in males and breeding trauma in females may result in dysuria from urethritis. Primary ascending infection of the urinary tract, although relatively rare in young animals, must be differentiated from a urachal abscess that communicates with the bladder lumen. Animals with developmental abnormalities of the urinary tract may also exhibit abnormal urine flow during micturition.

PATHOGENESIS. Urachal infections are established early in life, as a sequela to patent urachus or omphalitis. Organisms most commonly involved in umbilical remnant infections include *Arcanobacterium pyogenes, Escherichia coli, Proteus, Enterococcus, Staphylococcus,* and *Streptococcus* spp.[336] Anaerobic bacteria may also be isolated. The urachus is the most frequently infected umbilical reminant.[336] Abscesses may develop anywhere in its course to the apex of the bladder. The urachal abscess may communicate directly with the bladder lumen, resulting in suppurative cystitis. Adhesions may develop between the inflamed urachus and the omentum or viscera, including the bladder, which can cause mechanical interference with bladder emptying.[337]

TREATMENT AND PROGNOSIS. Surgical resection of the umbilicus and affected areas of the bladder apex is usually curative. If an abscess ruptures into the abdominal cavity or extensive intraabdominal adhesions occur, there is a poor prognosis for recovery. Perioperative antibiotic therapy is justified. Long-term, broad-spectrum antimicrobial therapy is effective in some cases but can be more expensive than surgical treatment.

Prevention of umbilical remnant infection is described in Chapter 20.

REFERENCES
336. Baxter GM: Umbilical masses in calves: diagnosis, treatment, and complications, *Compend Cont Educ Pract* 11:505-513, 1989.
337. Trent AM, Smith DF: Pollakiuria due to urachal abscesses in two heifers, *J Am Vet Med Assoc* 184:984-986, 1984.
338. Shearer AG: Internal navel abscesses in calves, *Vet Rec* 118:480-481, 1986.
339. Hassel DM et al: Urachal abscess and cystitis in a calf, *J Vet Int Med* 9:286-288, 1995.
340. Watson E et al: Ultrasonography of the umbilical structures in clinically normal calves, *Am J Vet Res* 55:773-780, 1994.

EVERSION OF THE BLADDER AND PROLAPSE OF THE BLADDER
DAVID C. Van METRE
THOMAS J. DIVERS

Eversion of the bladder is an uncommon event that occurs during or shortly after parturition in cows.[341-345] Forceful straining moves the bladder fundus caudally, eventually turning the bladder inside-out. The bladder is then forced out of the urethral orifice. Prolapse of the bladder is also a rare periparturient event in cattle, more commonly associated with dystocia.[341,342] In this condition a full-thickness tear of the vaginal wall occurs during delivery, allowing the bladder (and possibly other viscera) to be displaced from the abdominal cavity into the vagina.

CLINICAL FINDINGS AND DIFFERENTIAL DIAGNOSIS. Cows with either eversion or prolapse of the bladder present with a smooth, spherical mass within the vagina, usually protruding from the vulva. An affected cow may be alert and ambulatory, but if concurrent hypocalcemia, exhaustion, or peritonitis exist, the cow may be recumbent and depressed. Careful vaginal examination is required to differentiate these two conditions from each other and from vaginal prolapse, vaginal polyps, fat protrusion from a vaginal tear, vaginal neoplasia, fetal membranes, and uterine prolapse. Prevention of straining through epidural anesthesia is essential, because expulsive efforts can cause herniation of other viscera either through the urethra (bladder eversion) or through the vaginal tear (bladder prolapse).[341]

Eversion of the Bladder. The mucosal surface of the bladder is exposed. The ureteral openings may be visible on its dorsal aspect, although these may be occluded and difficult to see if the wall of the bladder is edematous.[344] Vaginal palpation reveals that the protruding tissue originates from the urethral orifice, ventral to the urethral fold. With time, constriction of the everted bladder by the narrow urethra may cause venous congestion, edema, thrombosis, and eventual necrosis of the bladder wall.[341] Palpation and ultrasonographic examination are required for detection of herniation of other viscera through the urethral orifice and into the interior of the everted bladder. Strangulation of incarcerated bowel may occur.[342,343] Careful fine-needle aspiration of the interior of the eversion has been used to differentiate eversion from prolapse of the bladder. With bladder eversion, aspiration may yield peritoneal fluid, but laceration of herniated bowel is a concern.[341]

TREATMENT AND PROGNOSIS. Manual reduction may not be possible if the everted bladder is edematous or if other viscera have herniated into its interior. The dorsal aspect of the urethra may be incised to widen the route through which the bladder is to be replaced.[341,342] Laparotomy is required for assessment of the viability of herniated bowel, and subtotal cystectomy may be performed if extensive bladder trauma or necrosis have occurred.[342] The viability of the involved structures is of primary concern for prognosis. Bladder paralysis and rupture are potential sequelae to ischemic damage that develops during eversion.[341] Cystitis and pyelonephritis may develop as well, and antibiotic therapy is warranted if repair is attempted. Chronic cases may develop hydroureter, hydronephrosis, and renal failure.[345]

Prolapse of the Bladder. The serosal surface of the bladder is exposed. The bladder protrudes from a full-thickness tear in the floor of the vagina, and other viscera may be present in the vagina as well. Fine-needle aspiration yields urine from the bladder lumen. A flexible catheter may be passed into the urethra to remove urine from the bladder, thereby confirming the diagnosis and facilitating bladder replacement.

TREATMENT AND PROGNOSIS. After catheterization and removal of urine, the bladder can be replaced into the abdominal cavity and the vaginal tear can be sutured. Severe contamination of the peritoneal cavity may render attempts at treatment unjustified. Antibiotic therapy is indicated for surgical candidates.

REFERENCES

341. Ducharme NG, Stem ES: Eversion of the urinary bladder in a cow, *J Am Vet Med Assoc* 179:996-998, 1981.
342. Peter AT, Arighi M, Gaines JD: Herniation of distal jejunum into the partially everted urinary bladder of a cow, *Can Vet J* 30:830-831, 1989.
343. Frazier GS: Uterine torsion followed by jejunal incarceration in a partially everted urinary bladder in a cow, *Aust Vet J* 65:24-25, 1988.
344. Hojbjerg A: Eversion of the bovine bladder, *Bovine Pract* 25:120-121, 1990.
345. Friesen CH, Theoret CL, Barber SM. Urinary bladder eversion with hydronephrosis and renal failure in a beef cow, *Can Vet J* 36:710-711, 1995.

PELVIC ENTRAPMENT OF THE BLADDER

DAVID C. Van METRE
THOMAS J. DIVERS

In pelvic entrapment of the bladder, the bladder is displaced caudodorsally into the pelvic cavity, resulting in impaired urine outflow. In one report the condition was diagnosed in two Holstein cows a few days after parturition had occurred, suggesting a potential role of delivery or postpartum straining in bladder displacement.[346] Entrapment of the bladder in a perineal hernia[347] or within a vaginal prolapse[348] may also occur.

CLINICAL FINDINGS. Bladder emptying is impaired, and the presence of the bladder in the pelvic inlet induces straining. An affected cow may show tenesmus, pollakiuria, and stranguria. On rectal examination a soft, fluctuant mass may be detected beside the vagina.[346] In calves, radiography has been used to demonstrate the pelvic position of the bladder.[349]

DIFFERENTIAL DIAGNOSES. Differential diagnoses include proctitis, vaginitis, retained placenta, bladder paralysis, cystitis, and perivaginal abscess. Needle aspiration of the bladder per vaginum has been used to make a definitive diagnosis,[346] although the danger of uterine puncture should be considered.[348] Ultrasonographic examination can also be useful for definitive diagnosis.[348] Draining the bladder via catheterization or needle aspiration facilitates replacement of the bladder by manipulation per vaginum. However, laparotomy was necessary in one cow to reset the bladder, because of the development of fibrinous adhesions between the bladder and vagina.[346] In cases of bladder entrapment within a vaginal prolapse, complete correction of the prolapse usually restores the bladder to its normal position.[346]

REFERENCES

346. Gaines JD: Postparturient pelvic entrapment of the bladder in two cows, *J Am Vet Med Assoc* 193:222-223, 1988.
347. Campbell SG, Fubini SL: External lumps on sheep and goats, *Vet Clin North Am (Large Anim Pract)* 5:457-476, 1983.
348. Scott PR, Gessert ME. Ultrasonographic examination of 12 ovine vaginal prolapses, *Vet J* 155:323-324, 1998.
349. Divers TJ: Assessment of the urinary system, *Vet Clin North Am (Food Anim Pract)* 8:373-382, 1992.

ENZOOTIC HEMATURIA

DAVID C. Van METRE
THOMAS J. DIVERS

Enzootic hematuria is a disease of chronic or intermittent hematuria in cattle and sheep and is associated with chronic ingestion of bracken fern *(Pteridium aquilinum)* (Fig. 32-21).[350-355] A different fern species, *Cheilanthes sieberi*, may induce this disease in Australian cattle.[350,351] Hemorrhagic cystitis is the initial consequence of exposure to the toxic compound(s) in the plant. With continued ingestion of bracken fern, cattle develop bladder neoplasms of epithelial, mesenchymal, or mixed origins. Bladder infection with bovine papillomavirus type 2 is involved in carcinogenesis.

CLINICAL FINDINGS. In most cases, several animals are affected in a group that is grazing a particular pasture or being fed a particular type or cutting of hay. Protracted, possibly intermittent, hematuria, is the first clinical sign detected in most cases.[350] Blood clots may be voided on occasion. Chronic blood loss eventually results in tachycardia, tachypnea, exercise intolerance, pale mucous membranes, and a decline in productivity and body condition. Bladder wall thickening and bladder tumors may be palpated per rectum. Proliferative changes or overt neoplasia of the bladder may cause dysuria, pollakiuria, and, rarely, obstruction of the bladder trigone. Occasionally blood clots may cause urethral obstruction. Depending on the magnitude and duration of bracken fern ingestion, hematuria may last for months to years before severe debilitation or death occurs.

The syndrome of enzootic hematuria is quite different from acute bracken poisoning, which occurs after ingestion of large quantities of bracken fern (roughly equivalent to the animal's body weight), usually over 1 to 3 months.[351,352] Acute bracken poisoning manifests as an acute coagulopathy or fulminant septicemic crisis associated with severe bone marrow suppression. Clinical signs include fever, profound weakness, epistaxis, hyphema, dysentery, and petechial hemorrhages of the mucosal surfaces and sclera.[351] Acute bracken poisoning is further described in Chapter 50.

CLINICAL PATHOLOGY. Severe anemia is commonly seen on hematologic examination of cattle and sheep with enzootic hematuria. Evidence of a regenerative response may not be present if bone marrow suppression is severe. The platelet, segmented neutrophil, and lymphocyte counts may

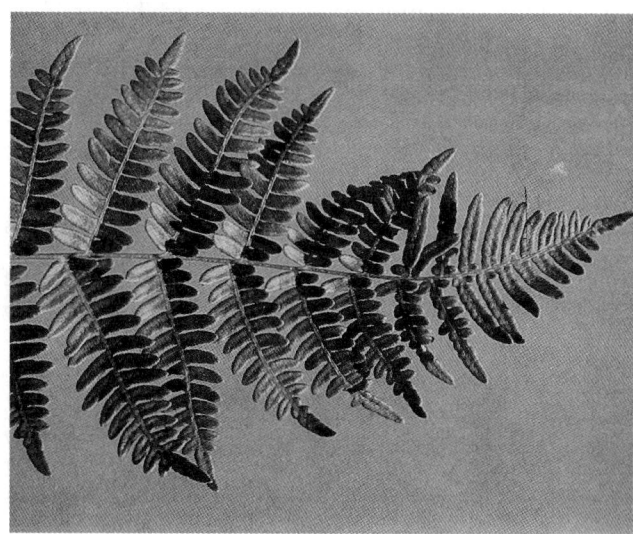

FIG. 32-21 ▪ Bracken fern *(Pteridium aquilinum)*.

be reduced.[351-353] Urinalysis reveals hematuria, proteinuria, and variable pyuria.[350]

DIFFERENTIAL DIAGNOSIS. Examination of serum for evidence of hemolysis and sediment from a freshly voided urine sample for intact red blood cells allow for differentiation of hematuria from the hemoglobinuria found in hemolytic diseases. Icterus, also characteristic of ruminant hemolytic disorders, is not found in cases of enzootic hematuria. Hematuria may be evident in urinary tract infection, but pyuria and bacteriuria are marked, and anemia, if present, is usually mild. Simultaneous involvement of several animals is uncommon with urinary tract infection but common in enzootic hematuria. Protracted, severe hematuria is rare in cases of urolithiasis, and anemia is also not expected. Without necropsy, a diagnosis of enzootic hematuria requires documentation of access to bracken fern in animals with characteristic clinical signs and laboratory data.

EPIDEMIOLOGY. Enzootic hematuria has a wide geographic distribution, with cases reported in North and South America, the United Kingdom, Australia, and several European countries.[350] Bracken fern is found in all areas of the United States except the Great Plains, with most livestock poisonings occurring in the Pacific Northwest and upper Midwest.[352] The plant grows best in well-drained, fertile soils and is often localized in open areas of forests.[354] Sheep and cattle are poisoned by grazing the plant or consuming contaminated hay.[354]

Enzootic hematuria is primarily seen in adult sheep and cattle. In field cases, cattle grazing infested pastures develop hematuria by 2 to 3 years of age.[350,355] Feeding adult cattle 1 to 2 kg bracken fern/head/day led to hematuria within 10 to 15 months in one trial.[350] Papillomas of the bladder occur as early as 1 year after bracken feeding begins, with invasive carcinomas arising 2 to 6 years later.[350,355]

PATHOPHYSIOLOGY. All parts of the plant are toxic to sheep and cattle.[351,352] Several compounds in bracken fern possess irritant, mutagenic, immunosuppressive or carcinogenic activities.[350,353] These include ptaquiloside (aquilide A), quercetin, and a-ecdysone.[356-359] The carcinogenic principle(s) are present in the milk of cows grazing bracken fern.[360,361] Bracken fern compounds may cause recrudescence of latent bovine papillomavirus-2 (BPV-2) infections through immunosuppression. Bladder infection with BPV-2 follows, and mutagenic compounds in bracken fern interact with BPV-2 in the bladder to induce local neoplasia.[350,353,356] Growth of the resultant neoplastic tissue may be enhanced by further exposure to mutagenic bracken compounds.[350,353,356] Similarly, bovine papillomavirus-4 and mutagens from bracken fern may act in synergy to induce neoplasia of the mucosa of the upper gastrointestinal tract.[356,358,359]

Immunosuppression occurs as a result of reduction in circulating neutrophil and lymphocyte counts. Neutropenia appears to be a reversible phenomenon that results from bone marrow suppression. Neutrophil counts may normalize within 1 to 2 weeks of cessation of bracken feeding.[353] Lymphopenia persists during periods of low-level ingestion.[353]

NECROPSY FINDINGS. Tissue pallor from anemia is often appreciated. The bladder wall is thickened and the mucosa is hemorrhagic and ulcerated. Microscopic examination of the bladder wall reveals capillary engorgement, intramural hemorrhage, and metaplasia of the bladder epithelium.[351] Several types of bladder tumors and mixed-origin neoplasms may be present. Metastasis of epithelial neoplasms to the regional lymph nodes or other organs can occur.[362] Pharyngeal, esophageal, or ruminal papillomas may be found as well, and carcinomas may develop in these same locations in cattle exposed to bracken fern over several years.[355]

TREATMENT AND PREVENTION. Treatment of enzootic hematuria is limited to reduction or elimination of bracken fern in the diet. Wooded areas that support growth of bracken fern can be fenced off, and forage improvement may help to limit incorporation of the plant into hay. If such measures are not feasible, a program of early culling may help to avoid low productivity from anemia and neoplasia. Hematuria will cease if bracken feeding is discontinued before the onset of tumor formation.

REFERENCES

350. Hopkins NCG: Aetiology of enzootic hematuria, *Vet Rec* 118:715-717, 1986.
351. Humphreys DJ: *Veterinary toxicology*, ed 3, London, 1988, Baillière Tindall, pp 258-262.
352. Osweiler GD, Ruhr P: Plants affecting blood coagulation. In Howard JL, ed: *Current veterinary therapy 3: food animal medicine*, Philadelphia, 1986, WB Saunders, pp 404-406.
353. Campo MS et al: Association of bovine papillomavirus type 2 and bracken fern with bladder cancer in cattle, *Cancer Res* 52:6898-6904, 1992.
354. Chick BF, Quin C, McCleary BV: Pteridophyte intoxication of livestock in Australia. In Seawright AA et al, eds: *Plant toxicology*, ed 1, Melbourne, 1985, Dominion Press, pp 453-464.
355. Madewell BR, Theilen GH: Tumors of the urinary tract. In Theilen GH, Madewell BR, eds: *Veterinary cancer medicine*, ed 2, Philadelphia, 1987, Lea & Febiger, pp 567-582.
356. Campo MS: Bovine papillomavirus and cancer, *Vet J* 154:175-188, 1997.
357. Bringuier P et al. Bracken fern-induced bladder tumors in guinea pigs, *Am J Pathol* 147:858-868, 1995.
358. Pennie WD, Campo MS: Synergism between bovine papillomavirus type 4 and the flavonoid quercetin in cell transformation in vitro, *Virology* 190:861-865, 1992.
359. Anderson RA et al: Viral proteins of bovine papillomavirus type 4 during the development of alimentary canal tumors, *Vet J* 154:69-78, 1997.
360. Panukcku AM et al: Carcinogenic and mutagenic activities of milk from cows fed bracken fern (*Pteridium aquilinium*), *Cancer Res* 38:1556-1560, 1978.
361. Alonso-Amelot ME et al: Bracken ptaquiloside in milk, *Nature* 382:587, 1996.
362. Jubb KVF, Kennedy PC, Palmer N: *Pathology of domestic animals*, ed 4, San Diego, 1993, Academic Press, pp 534-536.

URINARY TRACT INFECTION

DAVID C. Van METRE
THOMAS J. DIVERS

Cystitis, ureteritis, and pyelonephritis in ruminants most commonly result from ascending urinary tract infection (UTI) with *Corynebacterium renale* or *Escherichia coli*.[363] Less common causative organisms include various coliform species[364] and other members of the *C. renale* group.[365] Renal infection via the hematogenous route (suppurative embolic nephritis) is much less common but may result from bacteremia with such agents as *Salmonella* spp., *Actinomyces pyogenes*, or, in small ruminants, *Corynebacterium pseudotuberculosis*.[336]

CLINICAL SIGNS. Cystitis in cattle is typified by dysuria and pollakiuria, with or without gross hematuria and pyuria. During urination the rate of urine flow is often decreased. An affected cow may tread or swish her tail and retain an arched stance after voiding has ceased. Blood, purulent debris, or crystalline material may occasionally be found on the hairs of the ventral commissure of the vulva. Rectal palpation may reveal a thickened, painful bladder. If UTI is limited to the bladder, an affected cow usually does not show generalized signs of infectious disease, such as fever, anorexia, or depression.[363]

In contrast, cattle with acute pyelonephritis often have a history of an abrupt reduction in feed intake and milk production. Fever, depression, ruminal stasis, scleral injection, and occasional episodes of mild colic accompany the signs of cystitis described above.[363] With bilateral or left-sided pyelonephritis, renal enlargement, pain, and a loss of normal lobulation of the left kidney may be evident on rectal examination. Transabdominal ultrasonographic examination is useful for evaluation of the right kidney, because the right kidney usually cannot be reached during rectal examination unless it is markedly enlarged.[363] In an adult cow, ultrasound evaluation of the right kidney can be performed using a 3.5-MHz transducer at the 12th intercostal space.[367] This transducer can also be used to view the left kidney at the dorsocranial aspect of the right paralumbar fossa.[367] Alternatively, the left kidney can be imaged transrectally with a linear array transducer. Dilation of renal calyces; echogenic, flocculent material within the renal pelvis; abnormal renal shape; and renal enlargement are ultrasonographic findings suggestive of pyelonephritis. Vaginal palpation is usually necessary to detect ureteritis[363]; the ureters may be enlarged and painful when palpated through the vaginal wall.

The clinical signs of chronic pyelonephritis are relatively vague and inconsistent.[363] Weight loss, anorexia, and reduced milk production are common presenting complaints. Polyuria without gross urine abnormalities may be found in some cases. Diarrhea and pale mucous membranes may also be found during physical examination. Rectal and vaginal examination findings for chronic pyelonephritis are similar to those of the acute form, although the involved structures may not be painful or enlarged when palpated.

Urinalysis with chemical reagent strips appears to be a sensitive ancillary test for both acute and chronic pyelonephritis. In a study of 15 cases of bovine pyelonephritis, clinical signs suggestive of urinary tract disease were found in only three cows. However, evidence of hematuria or proteinuria was found through routine reagent strip urinalysis in all 15 cases.[363] Further examination and testing of the urinary tract confirmed a diagnosis of pyelonephritis.

DIFFERENTIAL DIAGNOSIS. Mild colic may result from a variety of gastrointestinal disorders, but urinalysis findings are normal in these conditions. Enzootic hematuria usually affects multiple animals in a particular locale, and access to bracken fern is usually demonstrable. Although dysuria and hematuria may be evident in enzootic hematuria, anemia is profound, whereas pyuria and bacteriuria are mild or nonexistent. Urolithiasis may induce colic, dysuria, and hematuria. However, urolithiasis is almost exclusively a disease of male ruminants, and UTI is more common in females. Bladder distention is a common finding in urolithiasis but rarely occurs in UTI. Other conditions that may cause dysuria include vaginitis, vulvar trauma, perivaginal abscesses, and pelvic entrapment of the bladder.

CLINICAL PATHOLOGY. Neutrophilic leukocytosis and hyperfibrinogenemia are evident on hematologic evaluation of cattle with pyelonephritis. Hyperglobulinemia may develop if the infection is established for several days.[363] Severe, protracted proteinuria may cause hypoalbuminemia, and the resultant low plasma oncotic pressure may contribute to the development of diarrhea in occasional cases. In chronic pyelonephritis, anemia may result from reduced erythropoietin production, chronic inflammatory disease, and blood loss through the urine.[363]

If azotemia is found on serum chemistry analysis, the clinician must consider renal and prerenal causes before formulation of a prognosis. Azotemia and isosthenuria would indicate bilateral renal involvement, lowering the chances for successful treatment.[363]

Urinalysis is required for definitive diagnosis of UTI, but careful collection technique is important for valid conclusions to be made. Concurrent metritis, vaginitis, or posthitis may result in contamination of urine with blood, bacteria, and inflammatory cells, particularly if the rate of voiding is slow. A midstream or end-stream catch is likely to provide the most accurate culture results.[368] Tentative identification of the organism may be obtained through Gram stain of the urine.

UTI consistently produces hematuria, proteinuria, and bacteriuria on urinalysis. Quantitative culture of a urine sample allows for confirmation of the diagnosis and identification of the causative organism. Although not present in all cases, leukocyte casts provide definitive evidence of pyelonephritis.[369]

PATHOPHYSIOLOGY. Factors involved in ascending UTI include the dose and virulence of the bacterial challenge, the presence of urogenital trauma (e.g., from calving injuries) or abnormal vulvar conformation, obstetric manipulation, bladder catheterization, and urine retention (as occurs with bladder paralysis or urethral obstruction). After cystitis is established, alterations in the contractility and thickness of the bladder wall may promote vesicoureteral reflux, spreading infection into one or both ureters.[370] Hemorrhage, fibrin deposition, and epithelial necrosis may result in intermittent ureteral or renal obstruction, which may be responsible for the episodic signs of colic occasionally seen in affected cows. Once pyelonephritis is established, necrosis of papillary and tubular epithelium leads to accumulation of necrotic debris in the renal pelvis, loss of functional nephron mass, abscess formation, fibrosis, and distortion of renal shape. Renal calculi, particularly struvite uroliths, may occasionally develop in cases of pyelonephritis. Crystal deposition on necrotic debris and the high local pH caused by bacterial urease activity may contribute to calculogenesis.

Members of the *C. renale* group of bacteria include *C. renale*, *C. cystitidis*, and *C. pilosum*.[365] These large, pleomorphic, club-shaped bacilli are aerobic, ureolytic, nonmotile, and gram-positive.[365] Of these, *C. renale* is most frequently isolated from cases of bovine UTI.[365] Pyelonephritis caused by *C. renale* has been reported in a sheep[370] and induced experimentally in goats.[371] *C. renale* is adapted to and maintained in the bovine and ovine urinary tract and is unlikely to be maintained in the external environment for prolonged periods of time.[365] Subclinical carriers and diseased animals transmit the organism through direct vulvar contact or by splashing urine droplets onto the vulvas of susceptible cows. Iatrogenic transmission through contaminated obstetric instruments or urinary catheters is also possible. Venereal transmission of *C. cystitidis*[365] and *C. renale*[372,373] from infected bulls may also occur.

Adherence of *C. renale* to urinary tract epithelium appears to be mediated by pili[374] in a pH-dependent manner.[375] Adherence is enhanced under alkaline conditions and inhibited by acidic conditions. This may explain the clinical improvements reported in infected cattle fed salts that promote urinary acidification.[372] Through ureolysis and ammonia production, the organism maintains urine alkalinity, thereby facilitating colonization of the epithelial surface. A serum antibody response develops after renal infection is established, but this response is rarely curative[363] and does not appear to impart resistance to reinfection with *C. renale*.[376]

Ruminant UTI is also commonly caused by *Escherichia coli*, a ubiquitous, gram-negative coliform bacterium.[363] The serotype(s) and virulence factors of *E. coli* involved in bovine pyelonephritis have not been identified. Clinical evidence suggests that UTI results from fecal contamination of the urogenital tract or loss of normal urinary tract defenses.

Congenital defects such as ectopic ureter occasionally result in urinary tract infection, presumably from ascending infection of an abnormally positioned ureter. Impairment of bladder emptying, as might occur with bladder adhesions, urachal remnant infection, or diseases of the spinal cord, may promote ascending infection of the urinary tract. Urethral trauma caused by urolithiasis, breeding injury, urogenital papillomas, or catheterization of the urethra may also be conducive to infection.

EPIDEMIOLOGY. In an Israeli study, the prevalence of pyelonephritis on a per-farm basis was found to vary between 0.3% and 2.7%.[377] UTI is far more common in female ruminants than in males, because of the relatively short urethral

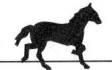

length in females[378] and the potential for urinary tract contamination and trauma during parturition. Seventy-three percent of pyelonephritis cases developed within the first 90 days after calving, suggesting that the postpartum period is a critical time for initiation of UTI.[377] Rebhun and colleagues[363] identified reproductive tract abnormalities such as pneumovagina, metritis, and poor perineal conformation in 7 of 15 cows with pyelonephritis.

C. renale has been regarded as the most common causative organism for bovine pyelonephritis.[364] However, the relative frequency of *E. coli* infections may be increasing, possibly because fewer practitioners today catheterize cows for urine sampling, a practice thought to be particularly conducive to *C. renale* infection.[363] Once *C. renale* infection exists in a herd, the number of subclinically infected cows increases over time, and the infection becomes difficult to eradicate.[365] Through increased frequency of contact, overcrowded cattle may experience more rapid transmission of infection.

NECROPSY FINDINGS. Hemorrhage, ulceration, and fibrin deposition are evident on the epithelium of the bladder and urethra. With chronic infection, polypoid growths may develop in the bladder mucosa; grossly these masses resemble tumors and must be definitively identified by histopathologic examination.[364] One or both ureters may be enlarged, with purulent debris occasionally occluding the ureteral lumen. Pyelonephritis cases may show gross renal enlargement in acute to subacute cases (Fig. 32-22). On sagittal sectioning of the kidney, viscous, gray, odorless exudate is found within the renal pelvis and extending into the medulla and cortex.[365] A Gram stain of the exudate is useful for differentiation of *C. renale* from *E. coli* infection. Renal abscesses, with gross distortion of renal size and shape, may be seen in cases of chronic pyelonephritis.

TREATMENT AND PROGNOSIS. Aggressive antibiotic therapy is essential for successful treatment of UTI. Penicillin is the treatment of choice for *C. renale* infection; recommended dosage regimens include procaine penicillin G (22,000 to 44,000 IU/kg IM twice daily) or ampicillin trihydrate (11 mg/kg IM twice daily).[363] For valuable animals, higher serum and urinary concentrations of penicillin may be achieved with intravenous administration of sodium or potassium penicillin (22,000 to 44,000 IU/kg IV every 6 hours) or sodium ampicillin (10 to 50 mg/kg IV every 8 hours). Treatment should be continued for a minimum of 3 weeks. Urinalysis and urine culture should be repeated 1 week after treatment is discontinued to ensure complete resolution. Af-

ter prolonged therapy with these extra-label dosages of antibiotics, residue withdrawal times for meat and milk must be extended appropriately. In addition, induction of diuresis through oral or parenteral fluid therapy may aid in removing necrotic debris and bacteria from the lumen of the urinary tract.

UTI with *E. coli* or other coliforms may also be successfully treated with high doses of penicillin or ampicillin.[363] Achievement of high urinary concentrations of these antibiotics may render them effective against many coliforms, even those that show in vitro resistance to the expected serum concentrations of the antibiotic.[363] Repeated assessment of appetite, attitude, rectal temperature, and reagent strip urinalysis is recommended for monitoring cows with coliform UTI that are receiving penicillin or ampicillin therapy. If these parameters do not improve after 96 hours of treatment, another antibiotic should be chosen.[363] Gentamicin (2.2 mg/kg IM twice daily) has been used to successfully treat refractory coliform UTI in a cow, but the nephrotoxicity of the drug and the current prolonged slaughter withdrawal period are important considerations.[363] Trimethoprim-sulfadiazine (15 mg/kg IV once daily)[364] and ceftiofur (3 mg/kg IV twice daily)[379] have also been used with success.

The prognosis for UTI in ruminants depends on the duration of infection, the extent of UTI (cystitis alone vs. unilateral or bilateral ureteritis and pyelonephritis), and the remaining renal function. The chances for successful treatment are improved if treatment is initiated early in the course of infection. In recent reports the combined case fatality and cull rate for pyelonephritis in dairy cattle varied between 18%[363] and 33%[377] for treated cases; however, antibiotic dose and duration varied markedly between these two studies. Cows with pyelonephritis and marked azotemia (BUN >100 mg/dl) were found to be at much greater risk for culling (odds ratio = 60) than nonazotemic cows with pyelonephritis.[377]

PREVENTION AND CONTROL. Isolation of animals infected with *C. renale* is recommended to limit spread of the organism, and disinfection of heavily contaminated areas is advised. Aseptic technique during urogenital procedures and disinfection of obstetric and surgical equipment will limit iatrogenic transmission. In herds using natural service, venereal transmission by subclinically infected bulls may be difficult to control over the long term. An artificial insemination or mass treatment program may be required to prevent further losses from UTI.

REFERENCES

363. Rebhun WC et al: Pyelonephritis in cows: 15 cases, *J Am Vet Med Assoc* 194:953-955, 1989.
364. Mills-Wallace LL et al: Polypoid cystitis, pyelonephritis, and obstructive nephropathy in a cow, *J Am Vet Med Assoc* 197:1181-1183, 1990.
365. Timoney JF et al: *Hagan and Bruner's infectious diseases of domestic animals*, ed 8, Ithaca, NY, 1988, Cornell University Press, pp 247-250.
366. Angus KW: Nephropathy in young lambs, *Vet Rec* 126:525-528, 1990.
367. Hayashi H et al: Ultrasonographic diagnosis of pyelonephritis in a cow, *J Am Vet Med Assoc* 205:736-738, 1994.
368. Divers TJ: Assessment of the urinary system, *Vet Clin North Am (Food Anim Pract)* 8:373-382, 1992.
369. Cotran RS, Kumar V, Collins T: *Robbins' pathologic basis of disease*, ed 6, Philadelphia, 1999, WB Saunders, pp. 931-996.
370. Higgins RJ, Weaver CR: *Corynebacterium renale* pyelonephritis and cystitis in a sheep, *Vet Rec* 109:256, 1981.
371. Elias S, Abbas B, El San-Ousi SM: The goat as a model for *Corynebacterium renale* pyelonephritis, *Br Vet J* 149:485-493, 1993.
372. Blood DC, Radostits OM: *Veterinary medicine*, ed 7, London, 1989, Baillière Tindall, pp 574-575.
373. Sheldon IM: Suspected venereal transmission of *Corynebacterium renale*, *Vet Rec* 137:100, 1995.
374. Honda E, Yanagawa R: Attachment of *Corynebacterium renale* to tissue culture cells by the pili, *Am J Vet Res* 36:1663-1666, 1975.
375. Takai S, Yanagawa R, Kitamura Y: pH-dependent adhesion of piliated *Corynebacterium renale* to bovine bladder epithelial cells, *Infect Immun* 28:669-674, 1980.

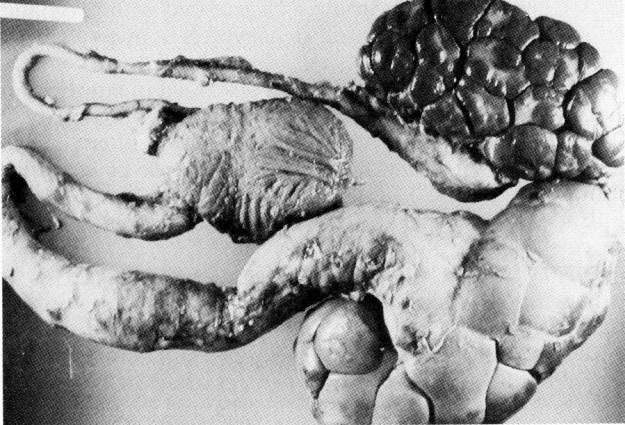

FIG. 32-22 ▮ Postmortem specimen of unilateral pyelonephritis and ureteritis in a cow. The affected kidney and ureter are markedly enlarged.

376. Campbell SG: Personal communication, 1994.
377. Markusfeld O et al: Observations on bovine pyelonephritis, *Br Vet J* 45:573-579, 1989.
378. Monoghan MLM, Hannan J: Abbatoir survey of bovine kidney disease, *Vet Rec* 113:55-57, 1983.
379. Tyler JW, Ruffin DC, Yu A: Probable ceftiofur-induced cutaneous drug reaction in a cow, *Can Vet J* 39:296-298, 1998.

AMYLOIDOSIS

DAVID P. GNAD

Amyloidosis in cattle is caused by deposition of insoluble protein fibrils in the kidney, gastrointestinal tract, liver, and adrenal glands. Renal amyloidosis in cattle is characterized as a sporadic, chronic wasting disease. Amyloid deposition in the kidney disrupts the normal glomerular structure, resulting in a protein-losing nephropathy.

CLINICAL SIGNS. The most common clinical signs of amyloidosis include chronic diarrhea, weight loss, and poor productivity in mature animals.[380,381] Generalized or ventral edema may be present as a result of hypoproteinemia. Alterations in appetite and attitude may be present, although this may be due to concurrent disease. Enlargement of the left kidney may be palpated during rectal examination. The enlarged kidneys generally are not painful and maintain normal lobular patterns. It may be noted that the urine develops stable foam after hitting the ground or being collected and shaken in a container, a result of high urine protein concentration.

CLINICAL PATHOLOGY. Cattle with renal amyloidosis consistently develop marked proteinuria and hypolbuminemia.[380] Serum creatinine and urea nitrogen levels may be elevated if renal damage is advanced. In cases of chronic, active inflammatory disease, hyperfibrinogenemia and hyperglobulinemia may occur.[380,381] Polarized light microscopy and electron microscopy have been used to examine urine sediment for the presence of amyloid protein in urine.[382]

DIFFERENTIAL DIAGNOSIS. Amyloidosis must be differentiated from other diseases causing chronic diarrhea, hypoproteinemia, weight loss, and poor productivity. Diseases to consider include Johne's disease, copper deficiency, salmonellosis, bovine viral diarrhea, gastrointestinal parasitism, and glomerulonephritis. Other than amyloidosis, glomerulonephritis is the only other differential diagnosis routinely displaying prolonged proteinuria. Renal biopsy can be performed to differentiate glomerulonephritis from amyloidosis in the live animal.

PATHOPHYSIOLOGY. Amyloidosis of cattle is classified as the reactive (AA) type,[383] which is frequently associated with chronic inflammatory disease in domestic animals and humans.[384] Concurrent inflammatory disease such as traumatic reticuloperitonitis, pneumonia, mastitis, and metritis have been found in some, but not all, cattle with amyloidosis.[380,381] Serum amyloid A protein (SAA) is synthesized in the liver and is a precursor of amyloid A (AA) fibril in tissues.[385] Serum concentrations of SAA increase dramatically in disorders such as trauma, neoplasia, and inflammatory disease. An elevation in SAA is apparently required for an animal to develop active amyloidosis.[384] Elevations in SAA as a result of abnormal catabolism by the reticuloendothelial system may also increase AA fibril formation.[384,386] AA fibrils are resistant to proteolysis, allowing for their accumulation in tissues over time.[383] Accumulation of amyloid in the glomerulus alters glomerular filtration. A resultant hypoalbuminemia develops, which in turn decreases intravascular oncotic pressure. Diarrhea develops as a result of edema or amyloid deposition in the gastrointestinal tract.[381] The protein-losing nephropathy and diarrhea result in weight loss. Glomerular filtration rate will be reduced if the glomeruli are obliterated by amyloid deposition. Renal or pulmonary thrombosis may develop as a result of the loss of low-molecular-weight anticoagulants through the compromised kidney.[387]

NECROPSY FINDINGS. Renal enlargement with yellow-tan discoloration is frequently present. A waxy quality of the renal parenchyma may be appreciated on cut surface of the kidney.[380] Generalized edema resulting from hypoalbuminemia may be present. Some cases will have renal or pulmonary thrombosis.[381] Other inflammatory lesions may be found in other sites. Histologic examination of the kidney may reveal amyloid deposition in the glomerulus, interstitium, and tubule lumen.

PROGNOSIS. Because the lesions of amyloidosis are irreversible, the prognosis for affected cattle is poor. The resilient nature of the amyloid protein results in its persistence in tissues, even if the underlying cause of inflammatory disease is treated successfully. Specific treatment for amyloidosis has not been reported in cattle.

REFERENCES
380. Johnson R, Jamison K: Amyloidosis in six dairy cows, *J Am Vet Med Assoc* 185:1538-1543, 1984.
381. Murray M, Rushton A, Selman I: Bovine renal amyloidosis: a clinico-pathologic study, *Vet Rec* 90:210-216, 1972.
382. Kim DH, Ono K et al: Urinary amyloids in bovine amyloidosis, *Jpn J Vet Sci* 47:129-132, 1985.
383. Gruys E, Timmermans HJF: Diagnosis of secondary amyloid in bovine renal amyloidosis, *Vet Sci Commun* 3:21-37, 1979.
384. DiBartola SP, Benson MD: The pathogenesis of reactive systemic amyloidosis, *J Vet Intern Med* 3:31-41, 1989.
385. Kawahara E, Shiroo M, Nakanishi I, Migita S: The role of fibronectin in the development of experimental amyloidosis, *Am J Pathol* 134:1305-1314, 1989.
386. Cotran RS, Kumar V, Robbins SL: Amyloidosis. In *Robbins' pathologic basis of disease*, ed 6, Philadelphia, 1999, WB Saunders, pp 251-259.
387. Cotran RS, Kumar V, Robbins SL: The kidney. In *Robbins' pathologic basis of disease*, ed 4, Philadelphia, 1989, WB Saunders, pp 1033-1047.

GLOMERULONEPHRITIS

DAVID C. Van METRE

THOMAS J. DIVERS

Glomerulonephritis (GN) is a rare clinical disorder of ruminants that may result from deposition of antigen-antibody complexes in the glomerular basement membrane or from binding of antibody to intrinsic or foreign antigens in the glomerulus. Glomerular injury occurs subsequent to targeting of glomerular tissues by the immune system. Nonimmune mechanisms may be involved in certain forms of the disease.

CLINICAL SIGNS. Cattle with GN may have a history of weight loss, poor productivity, and chronic diarrhea.[388,389] Lethargy and generalized edema may be detected on physical examination. Rectal palpation may reveal a mildly enlarged but nonpainful left kidney.[389] GN may be clinically occult in cattle persistently infected with bovine virus diarrhea (BVD) virus.[390] Ewes suffering from GN associated with pregnancy toxemia tend to show clinical signs typical of pregnancy toxemia (see Chapter 31).[391]

Mesangiocapillary GN has been described in Finnish Landrace lambs of specific lineage in Scotland and Canada.[392] The disease is heritable, but the exact mode of inheritance remains unknown. Clinical signs of this disease begin within hours after birth to 3 months of age. Affected lambs may be dull, ataxic, and appear blind. Fine muscle tremors, colic, and convulsions may also be seen.

DIFFERENTIAL DIAGNOSIS. The differential diagnosis for cattle with GN is similar to that for amyloidosis (see preceding section).

CLINICAL PATHOLOGY. Heavy proteinuria, mild anemia, and hypoalbuminemia have been reported in cattle with GN.[388,389] Granular casts, red blood cells, and leukocytes were found in the urine sediment of one affected cow.[388] Azotemia, proteinuria, and ketonuria are found in ewes with GN associated with pregnancy toxemia. Mesangiocapillary GN in Finnish Landrace lambs is characterized by uremia, hypoalbuminemia, proteinuria, hypocalcemia, and hyperphosphatemia.[392]

PATHOPHYSIOLOGY. In humans, GN may result from a variety of infectious, toxic, or autoimmune disorders, all of which induce eventual immunologic injury to the glomerulus.[388,393] Antibodies may be directed against host or foreign antigens located in the vascular endothelium, mesangial cells, or basement membrane. In addition, circulating immune complexes may deposit in the glomerulus. The ultimate consequences of antigen-antibody interaction in the glomerulus are activation of complement and chemotaxis of leukocytes, both of which result in direct glomerular injury and increased glomerular permeability.[393]

Filtration of plasma albumin through the damaged glomerulus results in chronic albuminuria, eventually leading to reduced plasma oncotic pressure and generalized edema. Passage of antithrombin III through the damaged glomerulus and into the urine may result in a hypercoagulable state.[394]

Immunohistochemical data suggest involvement of immune-mediated mechanisms for spontaneous GN in cattle[388,389] and sheep,[392] GN associated with persistent bovine diarrhea infection in cattle,[390] and mesangiocapillary GN of Finnish Landrace lambs.[392] In the last condition a heritable deficiency of the third component of complement has been documented, but the role of this deficiency in GN remains unclear.[391] Glomerulonephritis may also be an incidental histologic finding in animals suffering from acute septic disease.[392]

The clinical and histopathologic characteristics of GN of pregnancy toxemia in ewes resemble those of the preeclampsia syndrome of women.[391] Enlarged glomeruli with reduced blood content in glomerular capillaries are found throughout the renal cortex of affected ewes. The renal lesion in preeclampsic women may result from endothelial injury during disseminated intravascular coagulation or an excessive glomerular vasomotor response to angiotensin.[395] The lesion can be reversible in women, but the consequences of this condition in ewes have not been described.

TREATMENT AND PROGNOSIS. Treatment of GN in ruminants has not been described. Because most cases of GN are advanced at the time of diagnosis, the prognosis is poor. Mesangiocapillary GN in Finnish Landrace sheep is not invariably lethal, and some affected lambs may survive until adulthood.[391]

REFERENCES

388. White MR, Crowell WA, Blue JA: A nephrotic-like sydrome with an associated mesangio-proliferative glomerulopathy in a cow, *Vet Pathol* 23:439-442, 1986.
389. Wiseman A, Spencer A, Petrie L: The nephrotic syndrome in a heifer due to glomerulonephritis, *Res Vet Sci* 28:325-329, 1980.
390. Cutlip RC, McClurkin AW, Coria MF: Lesions in healthy cattle persistently infected with the virus of bovine viral diarrhea: glomerulonephritis and encephalitis, *Am J Vet Res* 41:1938-1941, 1980.
391. Ferris TF et al: Toxemia of pregnancy in sheep: a clinical, physiological, and pathological study, *J Clin Invest* 48:1643-1655, 1969.
392. Angus KW: Nephropathy in young lambs, *Vet Rec* 126:525-528, 1990.
393. Cotran RS, Kumar V, Collins T: *Robbins' pathologic basis of disease*, ed 6, Philadelphia, 1999, WB Saunders, pp 931-996.
394. Pusterla N et al: Antithrombin-III activity in plasma of healthy and sick cattle, *Vet Rec* 140:17-18, 1997.
395. Stratta P et al: Acute renal failure in pre- eclampsia-eclampsia, *Gynecol Obstet Invest* 24:225-231, 1987.

HEMOLYTIC UREMIC SYNDROME

DAVID G. RENTER

Hemolytic uremic syndrome (HUS) is classified within the group of thrombotic microangiopathy syndromes.[395] HUS is a set of symptoms characterized clinically by acquired nonimmune hemolytic anemia, thrombocytopenia, and acute renal failure.[396] Histologically, HUS is characterized by renal thrombotic microangiopathy.[397] HUS is the most common cause of acute renal failure in young children and infants, with prodromal diarrhea occurring in approximately 90% of the cases.[398] There is evidence that nearly all of the postdiarrheal human cases of HUS are caused by enterohemorrhagic (EHEC) or verotoxigenic *Escherichia coli* infections, and that the majority of the cases in the United States are caused by the EHEC serotype O157:H7.[398] Although three horses[399,400] and a heifer[401] have been reported with clinical syndromes very similar to HUS, an etiologic agent was not identified in any of these four animals.

CLINICAL FINDINGS. Horses with clinical signs indicative of HUS have exhibited fever, diarrhea, hematuria, hemoglobinuria, profound azotemia, oliguria, and ventral edema.[399,400] Hematologic findings included leukocytosis, anemia, and evidence of hemolysis.[399,400] The blood smear of one horse revealed the presence of poikilocytes and schistocytes.[400] All three horses were euthanatized following unsuccessful treatment of anuria and azotemia with fluid therapy and diuretics. The reported case in a heifer was fatal postparturient HUS demonstrated by severe progressive anuric renal failure, acute hemolytic anemia, and consumptive thrombocytopenia.[401]

In humans, HUS presents as pallor, oligoanuria, edema, seizures (rarely), or generalized hemorrhagic diathesis.[396] In prodromal human cases, this syndrome develops, on average, 1 week after the onset of diarrhea.[396] The classical clinical syndrome of HUS in people includes acute renal failure, hemolysis, thrombocytopenia, and manifestations of disseminated intravascular coagulation.[397] For the treatment of HUS in humans, there is insufficient evidence to support the use of specific therapies and some treatments, including certain antibiotics and motility modifying agents, may be detrimental.[396] Supportive therapy including fluid and/or plasma therapy and dialysis can be of paramount importance.

PATHOPHYSIOLOGY AND NECROPSY FINDINGS. In humans, HUS is the most common life-threatening complication of hemorrhagic colitis (HC) from EHEC infection.[402] The EHEC strains produce the exotoxins Shiga toxin 1 (Stx1) and Shiga toxin 2 (Stx2), also referred to as verotoxin 1 and verotoxin 2.[402] Although *E. coli* O157:H7 is the most widely publicized, as many as 100 different serotypes of *E. coli* (as well as *Shigella* and other Enterobacteriaceae) can carry the genes for Stx1 or Stx2 and are capable of causing disease.[395]

The EHEC, including serotype O157:H7, are noninvasive but attach to the intestinal mucosa and produce characteristic histologic attaching and effacing lesions.[395] The Shiga toxins (Stxs) released from the bacteria are believed to translocate across the mucosa, where they access the systemic circulation.[395] The Stxs bind to specific glycolipid receptors on the surface of vascular endothelial cells, are internalized by endocytosis, and induce cell death through inhibition of protein synthesis.[395] Activation of the coagulation cascade following exposure of subendothelial collagen may result in thrombosis of small vessels in the kidney and other organs. Acute oliguric or anuric renal failure can result from fibrin/platelet thrombi in renal vessels and glomeruli, fibrinoid necrosis of vessel walls, congestion of glomeruli, and tubular ischemia. Because the coagulation events may be localized to certain organs, the results of laboratory tests of coagulation (e.g. PT and PTT) are not consistently abnormal.[403]

Cattle feces are considered to be the major source of EHEC; however, these bacteria have been isolated from the feces of many other asymptomatic species, including humans. EHEC do not generally cause illness in cattle, although they do colonize the bowel. Fecal contamination of ground beef, other food sources, and water is thought to be the primary mode of transmission of the organisms. However, the small infectious dose makes person-to-person transmission a significant problem, especially in day care, nursing home, and outbreak situations.[395]

In the four large animals reported with HUS, the inciting cause was uncertain and the isolation of EHEC or other Stx-producing organisms was not attempted.[399-401] The heifer had a necrotizing endometritis, but during postmortem examination of the three horses no focus of infection was identified. Renomegaly, renal infarcts, and scattered petechial and ecchymotic hemorrhages within the renal parenchyma were apparent on gross necropsy. Acute tubular necrosis and fibrin thrombi within the glomerular capillaries were evident on histologic examination.

Although the etiology was not determined, the clinical signs and pathologic lesions reported in the four large animal cases are compatible with a diagnosis of HUS. Based on these reports the pathogenesis of HUS in large animal animals shares some features of the disease in humans.

REFERENCES

395. Keusch GT, Acheson DWK: Thrombotic thrombocytopenic purpura associated with shiga toxins, *Semin Hematol* 34:106-116, 1997.
396. Tarr PI: *Escherichia coli* O157:H7: clinical, diagnostic, and epidemiological aspects of human infection, *Clin Infect Dis* 20:1-10, 1995.
397. Cotran RS, Kumar V, Robbins SL: Thrombotic microangiopathies. In *Robbins' pathologic basis of disease*, ed 6, Philadelphia, WB Saunders, 1999, pp 985-986.
398. Siegler RL: The hemolytic uremic syndrome, *Pediatr Clin North Am* 42:1505-1529, 1995.
399. Morris CF et al: Hemolytic uremic-like syndrome in two horses, *J Am Vet Med Assoc* 191:1453-1454, 1987.
400. MacLachlan NJ, Divers TJ: Hemolytic anemia and fibrinoid change of renal vessels in a horse, *J Am Vet Med Assoc* 181:716-717, 1982.
401. Roby KW, Bloom JC, Becht JL: Postpartum hemolytic-uremic syndrome in a cow, *J Am Vet Med Assoc* 190:187-190, 1987.
402. Buchanan RL, Doyle MP: Foodborne disease significance of *Escherichia coli* O157:H7 and other enterohemorrhagic *E. coli*, *Food Technol* 51:69-76, 1997.
403. Cotran RS, Kumar V, Collins T: Thrombotic microangiopathies: thrombotic thrombocytopenic purpura (TTP) and hemolytic—uremic syndrome (HUS). In *Robbins' pathologic basis of disease*, ed 6, Philadelphia, WB Saunders, 1999, pp 636-637.

TUBULAR NECROSIS

DAVID C. Van METRE
THOMAS J. DIVERS

Tubular necrosis (TN) or tubular nephrosis is the disease condition that results from a variety of toxic, infectious, or hemodynamic insults to the kidneys. Compounds identified as nephrotoxins for ruminants are listed in Box 32-2. Hemodynamic causes of TN include diseases that reduce renal perfusion (blood loss, endotoxic shock) or that occlude the renal vasculature (disseminated intravascular coagulation, renal vein thrombosis). Bilateral bacterial infection of the kidneys may result in acute or chronic renal failure as a result of destruction of nephrons by bacterial toxins and the host inflammatory response. Renal infection may be established by ascending infection of the urinary tract or by hematogenous infection of the kidneys. Depending on the nature and duration of the primary insult, widespread dysfunction or necrosis of tubular epithelial cells may produce reversible renal injury, acute renal failure, or chronic renal failure.

CLINICAL SIGNS. The clinical signs of acute renal failure in ruminants are nonspecific and usually are not indicative of overt urinary tract dysfunction. Depending on the inciting cause, anuria, oliguria, or polyuria may exist. Cattle with acute renal failure frequently are presented for evaluation of poor appetite, diarrhea, or epistaxis.[404] Depression, nasal discharge, ileus, melena, and mild free gas bloat may also be present. If a concurrent septic condition exists, fever, tachycardia, and scleral injection may be present. The saliva may have a strong ammonia smell. Muscular weakness, even recumbency, may result from the acid-base and electrolyte imbalances and intravascular volume depletion that occur with severe acute TN. Rectal palpation findings are usually unre-

---

BOX 32-2

Nephrotoxic Agents

METALS
Arsenic
Mercury
Cadmium
Chromium
Lead
Zinc
Copper (secondary to hemolysis)

ANTIMICROBIALS
Aminoglycosides
Tetracyclines
Sulfonamides (rare)
Ionophores
Amphotericin B
Polymyxin B

ANALGESICS
Nonsteroidal antiinflammatory drugs

PLANTS
Amaranthus retroflexus (pigweed)
Lilium spp. (Easter lily)
Quercus spp. (oaks)
Philodendron spp. (philodendron)
Pinus ponderosa (Ponderosa pine; nephrosis occurs in conjunction with hepatocellular damage and abortion)
Xanthium spp. (cocklebur)
Cestrum diurnum (day-blooming jessamine)
Oxalate-containing plants: *Rumex* (curly dock), *Beta* (beets) *Rheum rhaponticum* (rhubarb), *Halogeton glomeratus* (halogeton), *Sarcobatus vermiculatus* (greasewood), *Oxalis* sp. (soursob), *Chenopodium album* (lamb's quarters), *Salsola pestifer* (Russian thistle)

ENDOGENOUS
Hemoglobin
Myoglobin
Calcium oxalate

MISCELLANEOUS
Ethylene glycol
Vitamin C (parenteral form) overdose
Pentachlorophenol
Mycotoxins: Ochratoxin, citrinin, fumonisin (high doses)
Cholecalciferol-based rodenticides
Parenteral vitamin D overdose

---

markable, although renal enlargement and perirenal edema may be found in occasional cases. Table 32-2 lists clinical criteria that may facilitate diagnosis of TN caused by nephrotoxins. If untreated, chronic renal failure may ensue, usually producing weight loss in addition to the signs listed above. In such cases a reduction in size of the left kidney may be appreciated on palpation per rectum of affected cattle.

DIFFERENTIAL DIAGNOSIS. Formulation of a differential diagnosis for a ruminant with TN may be difficult, because of the nonspecific nature of the clinical signs and the variety of primary disease conditions that may predispose cattle to secondary TN. Coagulopathies and pulmonary abscesses are common causes of epistaxis in ruminants. The differential diagnoses for diarrhea are listed in Chapter 7. Female ruminants suffering from advanced pregnancy toxemia may be depressed, azotemic, inappetent, and recumbent. Re-

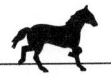

TABLE 32-2

Clinical Characteristics of Acute Toxic Nephrosis Caused by Common Nephrotoxins

Nephrotoxin	Clinical Findings*
Aminoglycosides	Usually nonoliguric, ototoxicosis possible; hematuria, glucosuria, proteinuria, increased serum trough concentration of drug
Tetracycline	Hematuria, glucosuria, proteinuria; possible hepatocellular enzyme elevation
Ionophores	Diarrhea, dark urine, dyspnea, cardiac dysrhythmias; elevated CK, AST, and indirect bilirubin
Ethylene glycol	Anuria or oliguria, tachypnea, ataxia, weakness; hemolysis, increased anion gap, increased serum osmolality, increased osmolar gap, acidosis, calcium oxalate crystalluria
Oxalate-containing plants, vitamin C	Hindlimb ataxia or paresis, apprehension, salivation; hypocalcemia, calcium oxalate crystalluria, aciduria, increased renal cortical echogenicity on ultrasonogram
Oak, acorns	Hemorrhagic diarrhea, ascites, hydrothorax, subcutaneous and perirenal edema; hyperfibrinogenemia, increased hepatic enzymes
Myoglobin	Muscle stiffness and weakness, dark urine; elevated serum CK and AST, positive reactions for blood and protein on urine chemistry strip, hemolyzed serum not present
Hemoglobin/ methemoglobin	Icteric to pale mucous membranes, tachycardia, tachypnea, red or brown urine; positive blood and protein reactions on urine chemistry strip, anemia, elevated serum total protein, hemolyzed serum (hemoglobin only)
Arsenic	Colic, hemorrhagic diarrhea, ataxia; elevated blood and liver arsenic levels

AST, Aspartate aminotransferase; *CK,* creatine kinase.
*Many general clinical characteristics of acute tubular necrosis are also present. See Clinical Signs and Clinical Pathology.

cumbent cattle should be evaluated for musculoskeletal injury, mastitis, metritis, peritonitis, spinal cord disease, and metabolic diseases. Cattle with TN are frequently misdiagnosed with milk fever, as a temporary improvement in muscular strength may be seen in cattle with TN following treatment with calcium salts.

CLINICAL PATHOLOGY. Elevation in serum urea nitrogen and creatinine levels occurs with clinical TN, and the azotemia is confirmed to be of renal origin by detection of isosthenuria on measurement of urine specific gravity. Proteinuria, hematuria, and granular casts may be found on urinalysis. Hypochloremia and metabolic alkalosis, resulting from abomasal atony or chloride loss in the urine, are commonly found in ruminants with acute renal failure.[404,405] Hyponatremia occurs after sodium loss in the urine. Because the kidney is the primary organ controlling magnesium excretion in ruminants, hypermagnesemia may occur in TN, particularly under conditions of high magnesium intake.[404,406] Hyperphosphatemia results from reduced phosphorus excretion in saliva during anorexia, reduced urinary phosphorus excretion, and tissue hypoxia.[407,408] Hypocalcemia is also common in TN in ruminants, because of reduced calcium intake, gastrointestinal stasis, and the competitive effect of hyperphosphatemia.[404] Metabolic acidosis may develop in juvenile ruminants with TN and concurrent diarrhea.[408,409]

Fractional clearance (fractional excretion) of sodium has been used to help document renal failure in cattle.[409] Values of near 0% to 4% have been described in normal cattle; age, ration, and metabolic status may affect FE values.[409] When applying this test, it is prudent to compare the patient's value for fractional clearance of sodium to that of an age-matched herdmate in a similar physiologic state and on a similar ration. The normal values for several urinary diagnostic indices in healthy calves have been reported.[410]

PATHOPHYSIOLOGY

Ischemic and Hypoxic Injury. Reduced blood flow to the kidneys most commonly occurs during generalized loss of vascular volume, as occurs with marked blood loss, septicemia, endotoxemia, or severe dehydration. Oliguria or anuria is seen initially, and urine output varies following intravenous fluid therapy. These conditions may also cause infarction of the renal cortex and renal vein thrombosis.[404] Severe ruminal gas distention may impair renal perfusion.[404] Prolonged, severe ischemia may destroy the tubular base-

ment membrane, thereby preventing tubular epithelial cell regeneration.[411]

Toxic Injury. The high metabolic demands of renal tubular epithelial cells render them susceptible to toxins that disrupt cellular enzymes. The injury caused by most nephrotoxins is compounded by dehydration, which concentrates the toxin in the tubular filtrate, slows toxin clearance, and, if severe, reduces renal perfusion. Because some nephrotoxins are therapeutic agents, it is vital that the veterinarian monitors appetite, body weight, water intake, urine output, routine urine chemistry, serum drug concentration, and/or serum creatinine concentration during administration of these agents. Young or elderly patients, patients with preexisting renal insufficiency or sepsis, those receiving other potentially nephrotoxic drugs, and patients on prolonged or high-dose therapy with these agents warrant the closest attention.[412]

TREATMENT AND PROGNOSIS. In cases of toxic nephroses, the animal should first be removed from the toxin source, or treatment with a nephrotoxic drug should be discontinued. Rumenotomy, with removal of toxic material, is most beneficial if performed soon (within 24 hours) after the animal has ingested a nephrotoxin. Activated charcoal (2 to 4 g/kg PO) may bind the agent in the gut lumen. The use of magnesium sulfate or other magnesium-containing laxatives should be avoided in such cases because severe hypermagnesemia may result in animals with concurrent compromise of renal function. If an animal is exposed to a potentially harmful quantity of a nephrotoxin, prophylactic diuresis through fluid therapy is warranted. In such cases, if the veterinarian were to wait for azotemia to appear before initiating fluid therapy, significant (>75%) loss of nephron function would be allowed to occur before medical intervention.

The cornerstone of treatment of TN is restoration of adequate renal perfusion and urine production. This is most effectively achieved through intravenous administration of isotonic, sodium-containing fluids, with calcium and potassium supplementation as indicated. If cost or facilities make IV fluid therapy impractical, repeated administration of water and electrolytes by stomach tube is an option. A small-bore stomach tube can be passed via the nasal cavity into the rumen and secured to the animal's halter to allow one person to administer fluids repeatedly without the need for repeated tube passage. Placement of a small rumenostomy or securing in place a nasogastric tube allows one person to repeatedly administer fluids with relative ease. Administration of intravenous or oral fluids at 1.5 to 2 times the adult maintenance level of 60 ml/kg/day may be adequate to induce diuresis. The patient should be monitored for chemosis or labored or rapid respiration, which may be indicative of overhydration. Fluid therapy should be continued until azotemia resolves, at which time the patient's voluntary fluid intake can be assessed. Oral supplementation of potassium and calcium salts may be necessary in some cases, because it is often not possible to add adequate yet safe levels of these salts to intravenous fluids in cases of refractory hypokalemia and hypocalcemia, respectively.

Restoration of urine production is necessary in anuric or oliguric animals. If fluid therapy does not promote diuresis, furosemide (1 mg/kg IV or IM) may be administered. Repeated administration (every 1 to 2 hours) may be necessary to induce urine production in oliguric or anuric patients. With repeated use of furosemide, the patient's serum sodium and potassium concentrations must be monitored. Mannitol (0.25 g/kg IV) or dopamine (2 to 5 µg/kg/min IV) may be required to initiate urine flow if the above measures are unsuccessful.

Lesions that occlude tubular blood flow (renal vein thrombosis, disseminated intravascular coagulation) warrant a grave prognosis, whereas renal failure resulting from toxic causes carries a more favorable prognosis with early diagnosis and aggressive therapy. Return of appetite and progressive reduction in serum urea nitrogen and creatinine levels are positive prognostic indicators.[413] Prolonged supportive treatment (2 to 3 weeks) may be necessary to allow for regeneration of tubular epithelium in cases of acute TN.

REFERENCES

404. Divers TJ et al: Acute renal disorders in cattle: a retrospective study of 22 cases, *J Am Vet Med Assoc* 181:694-699, 1982.
405. Fetcher A: Renal disease in cattle. II, Clinical signs, diagnosis, and treatment, *Compend Cont Educ Pract Vet* 8(suppl):338-345, 1986.
406. Kasari TR, Woodbury AH, Morcom-Kasari E: Adverse effects of orally administered magnesium hydroxide on serum magnesium concentration and systemic acid-base balance in adult cattle, *J Am Vet Med Assoc* 196:735-742, 1990.
407. Carr EA et al: Ruptured urinary bladder after dystocia in a cow, *J Am Vet Med Assoc* 202:631-632, 1993.
408. Brobst DF et al: Azotemia in cattle, *J Am Vet Med Assoc* 173:481-485, 1978.
409. Mechor GD, Cebra C, Blue J: Renal failure in a calf secondary to chronic enteritis, *Cornell Vet* 83:325-331, 1993.
410. Sommerdahl C et al: Urinary diagnostic indices in calves, *J Am Vet Med Assoc* 211:212-214, 1997.
411. Cotran RS, Kumar V, Collins T: *Robbins' pathologic basis of disease*, ed 6, Philadelphia, 1999, WB Saunders, pp 931-996.
412. Hinchcliff KW, Shaftoe S, Dubielzig RR: Gentamicin-induced nephrotoxicosis in a cow, *J Am Vet Med Assoc* 192:923-925, 1988.
413. Spier SJ et al: Oak toxicosis in northern California: clinical and pathologic findings, *J Am Vet Med Assoc* 191:958-964, 1987.

LEPTOSPIROSIS

DAVID C. Van METRE
THOMAS J. DIVERS

Multiple organ systems may be involved in infection of cattle with pathogenic serovars of *Leptospira interrogans* or *Leptospira borgpetersenii* (see Chapters 35 and 41); the renal manifestations will be emphasized in this section. Serovars *L. hardjo*, *L. pomona*, and *L. grippotyphosa* are most commonly implicated in renal infection of cattle.[414] Although data is scarce, renal disease caused by leptospirosis in small ruminants appears to be uncommon.[415,416] Sheep may serve as subclinical carriers of serovar *hardjo*.[417,418] Some serovars of Leptospira have zoonotic potential.[419]

In general, infection of cattle with the host-adapted serovar *hardjo* rarely results in acute, severe disease. If present, signs of disease are usually mild in acutely infected cattle. Persistent, latent urogenital infection usually follows acute infection, with most overt losses attributable to adverse effects on reproduction.[419] Acute, severe renal disease is more characteristic of incidental (often termed accidental) infection of cattle, particularly calves, with a nonadapted serovar of *Leptospira*. However, exceptions to this generalization do occur, because host immunity and virulence of the organism are variable.[418,419]

CLINICAL FINDINGS. Serovar *hardjo* is host-adapted to cattle. Infection of cattle may produce chronic interstitial nephritis of variable severity, but overt renal dysfunction rarely results.[420] Chronic infection of the genital tract is common.[421] Protracted shedding of the organism in the urine commonly results, possibly lasting for the life of the animal.[420] Infertility, stillbirth, abortion, and birth of weak calves are typical clinical manifestations of infection with serovar *hardjo* in cows.[421-423] Fever, agalactia, and mastitis may occasionally occur, and the resulting syndrome has been termed the milk-drop syndrome[418] or flabby udder.[419] The udder is uniformly soft, and the milk may be yellow- or red-tinged and thick, resembling colostrum.

In contrast, infection with the nonadapted serovars *pomona* or *grippotyphosa* can result in severe hemolytic disease, interstitial nephritis, and tubular nephrosis in calves and less commonly in adult cattle.[420,421] Meningitis is a rare manifestation.[416] Agalactia and mastitis (described above) commonly occur in lactating cows, and pregnant cows may abort. Shedding of these nonadapted serovars by infected cattle is of relatively short duration.[419,421,422] Renal lesions result from direct damage to the vascular endothelium during leptospiremia, hypoxia resulting from hemolysis, tubular epithelial damage from hemoglobin, and interstitial nephritis.[420]

PATHOPHYSIOLOGY. *Leptospira* spp. are a diverse genus of aerobic, motile, saprophytic spirochetes that are capable of survival in wet environments for prolonged periods, provided that freezing does not occur.[415] Contaminated surface water, wildlife, rodents, and domestic animals are potential sources of pathogenic serovars for cattle.[418,419] Leptospires penetrate external mucosal surfaces and scarified or macerated skin and disseminate in the bloodstream to invade multiple organs. After several days, opsonizing antibodies are generated which aid in clearing infection from most sites in the host. However, leptospires may become localized in the mammary gland, kidney, or genital tract, where they appear to be relatively protected from the immune response.[424] Chronic infection of the kidney or reproductive tract allows for transmission of the organism in urine, uterine and vaginal secretions, placenta, fetal tissues, and semen.[418,421,425] Depending on the virulence of the serovar involved, chronic renal infection may create few histologic changes; mild interstitial nephritis; or diffuse, severe, lymphocytic interstitial nephritis with fibrosis.[416] Nephritis may persist long after the host immune response has cleared the organism.[416]

DIAGNOSIS. The microscopic agglutination test (MAT) is the most widely used serologic test for the diagnosis of leptospirosis in cattle.[424] An increase in titer is expected following acute disease caused by nonadapted serovars such as *pomona*. Serologic detection of infection with serovar *hardjo* can be difficult because paired serum titers may be increasing, static, decreasing, or undetectable at the time of examination (e.g., at the time of abortion).[421,424] Antibodies to multivalent vaccines may complicate interpretation of titers[421,424]; consultation with a clinical immunologist affiliated with the laboratory performing the MAT is recommended for accurate interpretation of results.

Phase-contrast microscopy, dark-field microscopy, immunofluorescent antibody tests, and polymerase chain reaction tests can be performed on renal tissue, urine, or urine sediment.[414,424] Urine cultures are often unrewarding, be-

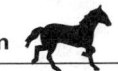

cause of the fastidious nature of the organism, and conclusive results may not be obtained for up to 6 months.[425] Administration of intravenous furosemide and collection of a midstream urine sample from the second voiding have been recommended for isolation attempts[415]; in theory, this procedure could improve the sensitivity of other urine tests. Biopsy or necropsy samples of renal tissue may be treated with Warrin-Starry or Levaditi silver stains before microscopic examination.[416]

EPIDEMIOLOGY. A recent abattoir study of over 5000 cattle in the United States determined that approximately 2% were renal carriers of *L. interrogans*. Serovar *hardjo* was the most common renal isolate, followed by serovar *pomona* and *grippotyphosa*.[414] Forty-nine per cent of cattle sampled were seropositive for *L. interrogans* serovars, with the highest seroprevalence found in cattle from the southeast, south central, and Pacific Coast states.[426] Because contact with urine from infected animals is a means of transmission within cattle populations, high stocking density or confinement may increase the rate of infection in a herd.

TREATMENT AND PROGNOSIS. For treatment of acutely infected cattle, oxytetracycline (10 to 15 mg/kg IM twice daily) and dihydrostreptomycin (12.5 mg/kg IM twice daily) have been recommended.[415] Nephrotoxicosis is a potential concern with this dosage of oxytetracycline in cattle with pre-existing renal disease, and dihydrostreptomycin is not currently available for use in cattle in the United States. Penicillin (25,000 IU/kg IM twice daily) and sodium ampicillin (20 mg/kg IM twice daily) have been suggested for treatment, but the efficacy of these regimens in cattle remains unproven.[415] In vitro susceptibility has been demonstrated for ampicillin, amoxicillin, penicillin G, erythromycin, tetracycline, and tylosin; data from human patients indicates that if penicillin G is selected for treatment, high dosages should be used.[422]

Chronic renal infection with *L. pomona* in cattle can be eliminated with a single injection of dihydrostreptomycin (25 mg/kg IM), although spontaneous clearance of this serovar often occurs in cattle.[415,422] Conflicting data exist on the efficacy of this treatment in clearing renal infection with *L. hardjo*.[3,427,428] Bolin and Prescott[418] have recommended long-acting oxytetracycline (20 mg/kg IM or SC, 2 doses 10 days apart) to treat chronic leptospiral infections or reduce the risk of introduction of infected animals into a herd. In the latter scenario, vaccination of newly introduced animals is also recommended.[418]

Prognosis for renal disease caused by leptospirosis is influenced by the virulence of the serovar involved, host immunity, and the extent of renal lesions. Cases with renal azotemia warrant a guarded prognosis, because more than 75% of nephrons are affected in such cases and chronic interstitial nephritis and fibrosis may occur after treatment of the acute disease.

PREVENTION. Vaccination (see Chapter 44) is currently regarded as the most effective means of preventing losses from leptospirosis. Draining or fencing off standing water may reduce transmission. Limiting rodent and wildlife contact with cattle and their feed and water is often difficult to accomplish, but it reduces the potential for transmission of leptospires.[421] As described above, oxytetracycline therapy of cattle entering a herd can be used to reduce the risk of introduction of leptospirosis into the population.[418]

REFERENCES

414. Miller DA, Wilson MA, Beran GW: Survey to estimate the prevalence of *Leptospira interrogans* infection in mature cattle in the United States, *Am J Vet Res* 52:1761-1765, 1991.
415. Thiermann AB: Leptospirosis: Current developments and trends, *J Am Vet Med Assoc* 184:722-725, 1984.
416. Jubb KVF, Kennedy PC, Palmer N: *Pathology of domestic animals*, ed 4, vol 2, San Diego, 1993, Academic Press, pp 503-511.
417. Ellis GR et al: Seroprevalence to *Leptospira interrogans* serovar *hardjo* in Merino stud rams in South Australia, *Aust Vet J* 71:203-206, 1994.
418. Bolin CA, Prescott JF: Leptospirosis. In Howard JL, Smith RA, eds: *Current Veterinary therapy 4: food animal practice*, 4th ed, Philadelphia, WB Saunders, 1999, pp 352-358.
419. Heath SE, Johnson R. Leptospirosis. *J Am Vet Med Assoc* 205:1518-1523, 1994.
420. Fetcher A: Renal disease in cattle. I, Causative agents, *Compend Cont Educ Pract Vet* 7(suppl):701-707, 1985.
421. Songer JG, Thiermann AB: Leptospirosis, *J Am Vet Med Assoc* 193:1250-1254, 1988.
422. Prescott J: Treatment of leptospirosis, *Cornell Vet* 81:7-12, 1991.
423. Ellis WA: Leptospirosis as a cause of reproductive failure, *Vet Clin North Am (Food Anim Pract)* 10:463-478, 1994.
424. Smith CR, Ketterer PJ, McGowan MR: A review of laboratory techniques and their use in the diagnosis of *Leptospira interrogans* serovar *hardjo* infection in cattle, *Aust Vet J* 71:290-294, 1994.
425. Bolin CA, Zuerner RL, Trueba G: Comparison of three techniques to detect *Leptospira interrogans* serovar *hardjo* subtype *hardjo-bovis* in bovine urine, *Am J Vet Res* 50:1001-1003, 1989.
426. Miller DA, Wilson MA, Beran GW: Relationships between prevalence of *Leptospira interogans* in cattle, and regional, climatic, and seasonal factors, *Am J Vet Res* 52:1766-1768, 1991.
427. Gerritsen MJ et al: Effective treatment with dihydrostreptomycin of naturally infected cows shedding *Leptospira interrogans* serovar *hardjo* subtype *hardjo-bovis*, *Am J Vet Res* 55:339-343, 1994.
428. Ellis WA, Montgomery J, Cassells JA: Dihydrostreptomycin treatment of bovine carriers of *Leptospira interrogans* serovar *hardjo*, *Res Vet Sci* 39:292-295, 1985.

CONGENITAL DEFECTS

DAVID C. Van METRE
THOMAS J. DIVERS

Most severe congenital defects of the urinary tract of ruminants manifest at an early age, although occasionally defects remain clinically occult until adulthood.[429] Congenital defects of the urinary system should be considered in the differential diagnosis for a young animal with renal disease or abnormal urination. However, tubular necrosis caused by severe volume depletion, nephrotoxins, and infectious diseases are far more common. If a congenital defect of the urinary tract is identified, a careful examination of other body systems should be performed; 73% of lambs with urogenital defects were found to have one or more defects in other organ systems.[430] Urogenital defects in ruminants are described in Chapter 47.

Renal Defects

Renal cysts are considered to be a common bovine renal defect[431] and have been described in sheep.[430] These are fluid-filled cavities within the renal parenchyma that are usually of no clinical significance unless they are large or numerous (polycystic kidneys).[429,431] Renal agenesis was found to be the most common renal defect in lambs, with hydronephrosis and renal dysgenesis occurring less frequently.[430]

Renal oxalosis is a metabolic disease of beefmaster calves that is suspected to have an inherited basis.[432] The calves show weakness, lethargy, and anorexia within days to several weeks of age. Alopecia over the head, neck, and extremities; dehydration; and diarrhea may also be seen. Evidence of renal failure is found on serum chemistry analysis. An inherited abnormality of glycine or glyoxalate metabolism may generate high levels of endogenous oxalate, which readily complexes with calcium. As a result, calcium oxalate crystals accumulate in the renal tubules, obstructing outflow of the tubular filtrate. Exposure to oxalate-containing plants and ethylene glycol must be ruled out in all cases of renal oxalosis.[432]

Ectopic Ureter

Ectopic ureter is a rare congenital defect in which one or both ureters terminate in an abnormal location. An ectopic ureter may terminate in the urethra, vagina, or cervix or caudal to the bladder trigone in females.[433] In males the ectopic ureter usually terminates in the urethra, vas deferens, or seminal vesicles.[433] Urinary incontinence is the most common presenting complaint for affected animals.[433] Urine dribbling results in scalding of the perineum and medial surfaces of the hindlimb in heifers, and scalding in males is usually located on the prepuce and ventral abdomen. Occasional episodes of normal micturition may be seen. Urinary tract infection, polycystic kidney(s), and hydronephrosis may exist concurrent to ectopic ureter(s).

Definitive diagnosis requires intravenous contrast urography or endoscopic examination of the urinary tract. Options for surgical correction include transposition of the ectopic ureter(s) or, in the case of unilateral involvement, ipsilateral nephrectomy. The latter option is valid only if the contralateral kidney is functional as determined by blood chemistry and structurally normal or near normal as determined by ultrasonography or intravenous pyelography. The use of affected animals for breeding should be discouraged.

REFERENCES

429. Deem DA, Whitlock RH: Renal cysts in a cow with anorexia, hypocalcemia, and abdominal pain, *Cornell Vet* 72:36-42, 1982.

430. Dennis SM: Urogenital defects in sheep, *Vet Rec* 105:344-347, 1979.
431. Fetcher A: Renal disease in cattle. I, Causative agents, *Compend Cont Educ Pract Vet* 7:S702-S707, 1985.
432. Rhyan JC et al: Severe renal oxalosis in five young beefmaster calves, *J Am Vet Med Assoc* 201:1907-1910, 1992.
433. Hammer EJ et al: Nephrectomy for treatment of ectopic ureter in a Holstein calf, Submitted, *Bov Pract* 34:101-103, 2000.

RENAL NEOPLASIA

DAVID C. Van METRE
THOMAS J. DIVERS

Other than those associated with ingestion of bracken fern, primary neoplasms of the urinary tract of ruminants are rare. Renal carcinoma has been described in cattle,[434] and nephroblastoma has been documented in a ewe and an aborted lamb.[435] Renal involvement may be seen in occasional cases of lymphosarcoma in ruminants.

REFERENCES

434. Sato S et al: Renal cell carcinoma in a cow, *Jpn J Vet Sci* 48:1007-1010, 1986.
435. Raperto F, Damiano S: Nephroblastoma in an ovine fetus, *Zendralbl Vet Med* 28(abstr):504-507, 1981.

Diseases of the Nervous System

MARY O. SMITH
Consulting Editor

CEREBROSPINAL FLUID

MARY O. SMITH
LISLE W. GEORGE

Cerebrospinal fluid (CSF) is partly derived from and in equilibrium with the extracellular fluid that bathes the brain and spinal cord parenchyma.[1-3] CSF has been shown to act as a "sink" for brain extracellular fluid,[4] and its composition is an indicator of the state of the intrathecal milieu. CSF is produced by a combination of ultrafiltration of plasma and active secretion.[5] The sites of CSF production are the choroid plexuses of the lateral, third, and fourth ventricles, the ependymal lining of the ventricular system, the pia arachnoid, and the meningeal blood vessels. The CSF in the ventricular system flows caudally and diffuses out of the lateral apertures in the fourth ventricle. It then circulates around the brain and the spinal cord. Circulation of cerebrospinal fluid is achieved through regional pressure changes caused by spinal motion and pulsations of blood vessels. The active flow of the CSF makes it possible to see subtle differences in fluid collected from the opposite end of the central nervous system (CNS) from a lesion.

COLLECTION OF CEREBROSPINAL FLUID

Cerebrospinal fluid may be collected from the lumbosacral cistern or the cisterna magna.[6]

Lumbosacral Spinal Tap

Collection of fluid from the lumbosacral cistern is preferred if the patient is unable to tolerate anesthesia or when the lesion is located in the spinal cord. Because the predominant flow of CSF is caudal, fluid collected from the cisterna magna reflects only changes within the brain and the most cranial parts of the spinal cord. However, fluid collected from the lumbosacral site is altered by either brain or spinal cord disease. Once a neuroanatomic diagnosis has been made, therefore, the site most suitable for collection can be chosen. For collection of CSF by lumbosacral puncture, the animal is lightly sedated, and the skin of the dorsal midline over the junction of the L6 and S1 vertebrae is surgically prepared (Fig. 33-1). A variety of standard sedative protocols are suitable, although xylazine has been shown to reduce CSF pressure.[7] Correct placement of the spinal needle is more easily achieved with the animal standing. The proper anatomic site for insertion of the spinal needle is between the dorsal spinous process of the L6 vertebra cranially and the S1 vertebra caudally and the two tuber sacrales laterally. The overlying skin forms a depression that can be recognized by palpation, although this may be difficult in well-muscled horses. Two alternative means of locating the correct site for needle placement include determining either the dorsal midline at the "highest point" of the quarters, or the point where a line drawn between the caudal aspects of the two tuber coxae intersects the midline.

The skin is anesthetized with 2% lidocaine, and a 1-cm incision is made with a No. 15 scalpel blade. A 6- to 9-inch, 18- to 20-gauge spinal needle is inserted perpendicularly through the incision and advanced until the tip punctures the lumbosacral cistern (a $3^{1}/_{2}$-inch needle can be used in small ruminants, foals, and most cattle). A "snapping" sensation sometimes is felt as the needle passes through the interarcuate ligament. The patient may reflexly contract the tail, anus, and gluteal muscles. Some patients, particularly horses, may respond with violent motor activity. For this reason, a lumbosacral spinal tap performed on a conscious horse should be done only when the animal is restrained in stocks; people have been severely injured when this rule was not followed. The average depth of insertion is 17.64 cm (7 inches) in horses, 8.26 cm ($3^{1}/_{3}$ inches) in ponies,[6] and about 7.5 cm (3 inches) in adult cattle.

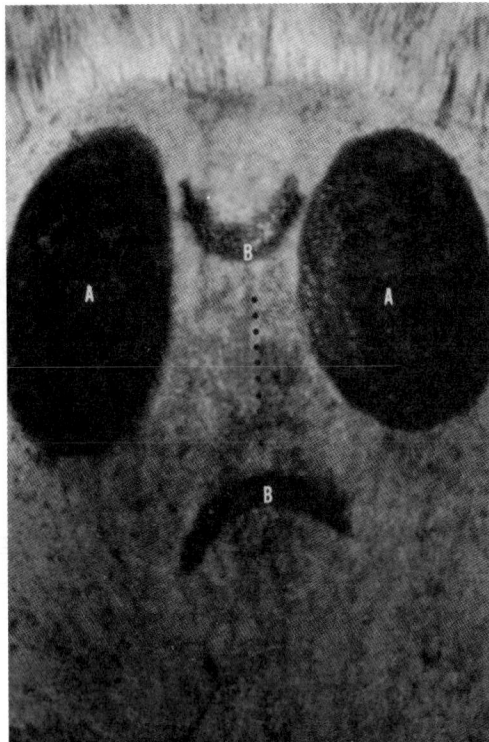

FIG. 33-1 ▓ Close-up view of landmarks for a lumbar cistern puncture in a horse. The large dark ovals *(A)* represent the position of the two tubers sacrale. The smaller curved lines *(B)* represent the respective caudal and cranial aspects of the L6 and S1 dorsal spinal processes. The dotted line represents the optimum area for placement of a skin stab.

The spinal needle is advanced gently to the floor of the spinal canal. Passage of the needle through the terminal spinal cord or the cauda equina does not cause subsequent neurologic abnormalities. When the needle is seated in the spinal canal, very gentle negative pressure can be applied by withdrawing spinal fluid into a series of 3-ml syringes. If frank blood is obtained, the tip of the needle probably is in one of the ventral vertebral sinuses. The needle should be withdrawn a few millimeters and a clean syringe attached to the hub. Compression of the jugular vein causes engorgement of the ventral vertebral plexus, which increases CSF pressure in the lumbosacral cistern. Failure of the CSF to flow from the needle after compression of the jugular vein could indicate incorrect needle placement or an obliterative lesion of the thoracolumbar spinal cord.

Cisterna Magna Tap

General anesthesia is required for a cisterna magna tap. After the patient has been anesthetized, the dorsal area of the neck overlying the atlantooccipital joint is surgically prepared. The patient's head is held flexed at a right angle to the neck, with the sagittal plane of the head parallel to the floor or table on which the patient is lying. The head must not be allowed to move while the needle is inserted. The needle is inserted at 1 to 2 cm caudal to a point corresponding to the intersection of the dorsal midline and a line drawn between the cranial aspects of the wings of the atlas. This point usually is 6 to 9 cm ($2^1/2$ to $3^1/2$ inches) from the poll (Fig. 33-2). A $3^1/2$-inch, 18-gauge spinal needle is inserted perpendicular to the skin and aimed toward the nose. The needle is advanced slowly with the stylet seated. After the needle has been ad-

vanced a few millimeters, the stylet is removed and the hub of the needle is examined for CSF flow. The stylet is replaced if it is dry and CSF is not spontaneously dripping from the hub, and the needle is advanced another few millimeters and checked again for CSF flow. Entry of the tip of the needle into the cisterna magna may be accompanied by the sensation of "popping" through a tissue plane or by a sudden decrease in resistance to the advancement of the needle. In other cases, however, no such sensation is perceived, hence the precaution of checking for CSF flow every time the needle is advanced a few millimeters.

In most large animals the needle is seated at approximately 5 to 8.75 cm (2 to $3^1/2$ inches). While advancing the needle, the heel of the hand should be held firmly against the animal's neck to minimize the possibility of spinal cord injury. The mean depth of insertion is 6.16 cm ($2^1/2$ inches) in horses[6] and 5.08 cm ($2^3/10$ inches) in cattle. In a cisterna magna tap, the needle entry site is close to the cervical spinal cord and the brainstem. To minimize the danger of CNS damage during a cisterna magna tap, the animal should be adequately anesthetized and ventilated, because an increased partial pressure of carbon dioxide (P_{CO_2}) results in elevated intracranial pressure.[8] Removal of fluid from the cisterna magna is contraindicated in a patient with increased intracranial pressure because a possibly fatal herniation of the brain through the foramen magnum and under the tentorium cerebelli may occur. Signs of increased CNS pressure include a moderate to marked decrease in mentation, mydriatic pupils, opisthotonos, extensor rigidity, ventrolateral strabismus, and papilledema.

Myelography

Contrast material for myelography is injected into the cisterna magna in large animal patients. Withdrawal of cerebrospinal fluid before injecting the contrast medium is unnecessary, and reinjection of CSF after it has been withdrawn is inadvisable. The turnover of CSF is rapid and under strict homeostatic control, therefore withdrawal of CSF through a spinal tap does not have deleterious effects that require its replacement.[9-11] In horses undergoing myelography, two spinal needles can be placed, one at the lumbosacral space and one into the cisterna magna. As the contrast medium is injected through the needle in the cisterna magna, CSF is allowed to drain freely from the lumbar needle. This technique facilitates injection of large volumes of contrast material but is not absolutely necessary to obtain a good-quality myelogram.

ANALYSIS OF CEREBROSPINAL FLUID

The color of the CSF should be noted as it flows from the hub of the spinal needle. Blood can originate from the tapping procedure (iatrogenic hemorrhage) or from a traumatic CNS lesion. Iatrogenic hemorrhage is unevenly mixed in the CSF and disappears as the fluid drips from the needle. Fluid collected immediately after placement of the spinal needle tends to be mildly contaminated with blood even when this is not apparent grossly. Successive aliquots are less contaminated, therefore the later aliquots are most suitable for cellular and protein analysis.[12] Blood resulting from CNS hemorrhage is evenly mixed with CSF even after a large amount has been removed. Hemorrhage that has occurred days previously may have a brownish rather than red discoloration. Prior hemorrhage also results in xanthochromia, a yellow discoloration of the CSF. Xanthochromia can be observed in the CSF for at least 10 days after the introduction of blood. Xanthochromic samples do not contain bilirubin.

Other abnormalities may be noted in the cerebrospinal fluid. For example, a black discoloration is diagnostic for a

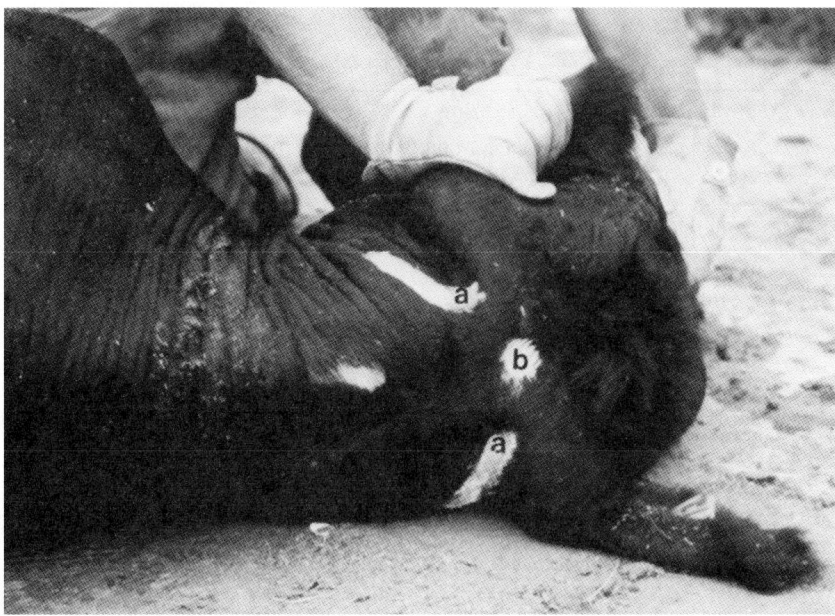

FIG. 33-2 ▨ View of the ideal area for a cisterna magna cerebrospinal fluid tap in a cow. The two lines *(a)* represent the wings of the atlas. The large spot in the center *(b)* is the optimum area for needle insertion. It is essential to prevent head movement by use of anesthesia and restraint.

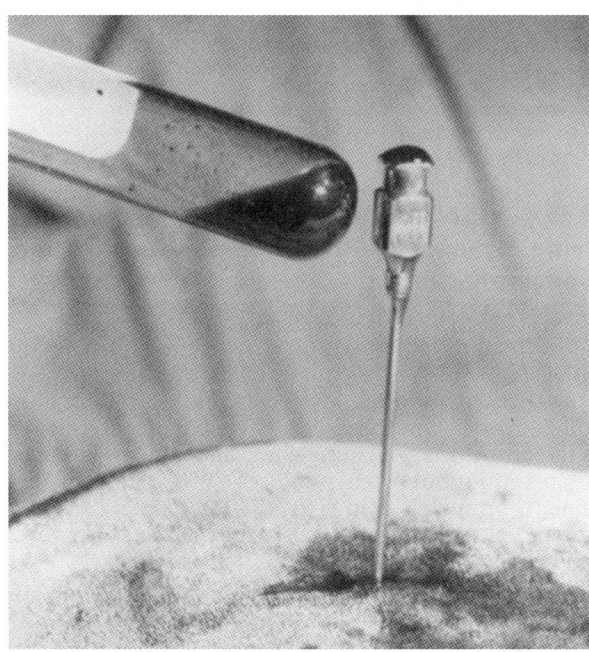

FIG. 33-3 ▨ Black cerebrospinal fluid from a lumbosacral tap of a gray horse with paraparesis. The animal had a melanoma that infiltrated the caudal spinal rootlets.

melanoma (Fig. 33-3). Foamy CSF denotes a protein concentration over 200 mg/dl, and turbid CSF usually denotes cell counts exceeding 400 mg/dl.

The normal values for cerebrospinal fluid are presented in Table 33-1. Cell counts should be determined in a noncentrifuged specimen as soon as the sample is collected. Morphologic examination of cells from CSF is most suitably done on cytospin preparations in an appropriately equipped laboratory,

but sedimentation and membrane filtration techniques for CSF cell preparations have been described.[13,14] Normal CSF from large animals contains fewer than 6 white blood cells (WBCs) per deciliter. Some reports have documented occasional WBC counts over 40/dl in the CSF of normal horses.[15] The refractive index of normal CSF is under 1.335. No visible reaction for protein should occur when the CSF is applied to a urine dipstick. The protein concentration of CSF in normal adult ruminants is under 50 mg/dl and in normal horses under 100 mg/dl, although reference values vary with the techniques used for protein measurement; reference values should be established for each laboratory.[16] The concentrations of glucose and protein in the CSF of newborn foals are almost twice those found in the CSF of adults, but they approximate adult normal values by 2 weeks of age.[17] The reference values for CSF proteins of normal horses and cattle are presented in Table 33-2. Neural tissue contains the BB isoenzyme of creatine kinase (CK), which increases after damage to the nerve cells.[18,19] The molecule does not cross the blood-brain barrier, therefore an increase in CK in the cerebrospinal fluid originates solely from neural tissue. In horses CK is often elevated in cases of protozoal myeloencephalopathy, often ranging as high as 115 IU/L. The level of CK activity in the cerebrospinal fluid is independent of the protein concentration or the WBC count.[20] The reference mean of CK in adult horses is 0 to 8 IU/L,[16] and that of foals ranges from 6 to 39 IU/L (the mean is 18.1 IU/L). Inflammation, anoxia, or trauma to the CNS results in an increased concentration of CK. A retrospective study indicated that high cerebrospinal fluid concentrations of CK indicate a poor prognosis regardless of the cause of the condition.[18,20]

The normal CSF concentration of glucose is approximately 80% of that in blood. A decline in the ratio of CSF to serum glucose occurs in animals with bacterial meningitis because of increased use of glucose by inflammatory cells.

Measurement of the sodium concentration of the CSF may be helpful for diagnosing salt poisoning in cattle. In animals that do not have salt poisoning, this value is always under 160 mmol/L; in animals with salt poisoning, the concentration usually is above 180 mmol/L.

TABLE 33-1

Normal Range of Values in Cerebrospinal Fluid for Large Animals[1,4,5]

Component	Unit	Equine	Bovine	Ovine	Caprine
Specific gravity		1.004-1.008	1.004-1.008	NA	NA
Refractive index		1.3343-1.3349	1.3343-1.3349	NA	NA
Protein	mg/dl	5-100	20-40	8-70	24-40
White blood cells (WBCs)	WBCs/dl	0-6	0-3	0-5	0-7
Glucose	mg/dl	30-70	35-70	48-109	45-87
Sodium	mEq/L	140-150*	132-144*	145-157*	NA
Potassium	mEq/L	2.5-3.5	2.7-3.2	3-3.3	3
Creatine kinase	IU/L	0-8	2-48	NA	NA
Magnesium	mEq/L	NA	1.7-2.7	NA	NA

NA, Result not available.
*Cerebrospinal fluid (CSF) sodium is the same as serum or plasma sodium when measured with ion-specific electrodes. When other measurements are used, the CSF sodium is usually higher than plasma sodium.

TABLE 33-2

Protein Composition* of Cerebrospinal Fluid in Horses and Cattle[3-6]

Factor	Horses	Cattle
Albumin	22.6-67.9* (55.1)	8.2-28.7 (15.7)
Total globulin	3.8-20.1 (10.5)	NA
Total alpha	0.51-12.8 (0.46)	9.7-24.3 (14.7)
Alpha$_1$	0.18-10.6 (0.48)	NA
Alpha$_{2a}$	0.1-0.76 (0.31)	NA
Alpha$_{2bc}$	0.23-1.44 (0.59)	NA
Beta$_1$	0.38-3.36 (1.59)	1.875-8.85 (3.8)
Beta$_2$	0.27-1.31 (7)	NA
Gamma	0.27-3.03 (1.35)	2.45-8.85 (4.8)

*Range of values for protein concentration is expressed in mg/dl; numbers in parentheses are mean values.
NA, Result not available.

REFERENCES

1. Davson H, Welch K, Segal M: *The physiology and pathophysiology of the cerebrospinal fluid,* Edinburgh, 1987, Churchill Livingstone.
2. Hochwald G, Wallenstein M: Exchange of albumin between blood cerebrospinal fluid and brain in the cat, *Am J Physiol* 212:1199-1204, 1967.
3. Hochwald G, Wallenstein M: Exchange of γ-globulin between blood cerebrospinal fluid and brain in the cat, *Exp Neurol* 19:115-126, 1967.
4. Olendorf W, Davson H: Brain extracellular space and the sink action of cerebrospinal fluid, *Arch Neurol* 17:196-205, 1967.
5. Frankhauser R: The cerebrospinal fluid. In Innes JRM, ed: *Comparative neuropathology,* New York, 1962, Academic Press.
6. Mayhew IG: Collection of cerebrospinal fluid from the horse, *Cornell Vet* 65:500-511, 1975.
7. Moore RM, Trims CM: Effect of xylazine on cerebrospinal fluid pressure in conscious horses, *Am J Vet Res* 53:1558-1561, 1992.
8. Moore RM, Trim CM: Effect of hypercapnia or xylazine on lateral ventricle and lumbosacral cerebrospinal fluid pressures in pentobarbital-anesthetized horses, *Vet Surg* 22:151-158, 1993.
9. Chodobski A, Szmydynger-Chodobska J, McKinley MJ: Cerebrospinal fluid formation and absorption in dehydrated sheep, *Am J Physiol* 275: F235-F238, 1998.
10. Boulton M et al: Raised intracranial pressure increases CSF drainage through arachnoid villi and extracranial lymphatics, *Am J Physiol* 275: R889-R896, 1998.
11. Silver I et al: Relationship between intracranial pressure and cervical lymphatic pressure and flow rates in sheep, *Am J Physiol* 277:R1712-R1717, 1999.
12. Sweeney CR, Russell GE: Differences in total protein concentration, nucleated cell count, and red blood cell count among sequential samples of cerebrospinal fluid from horses, *J Am Vet Med Assoc* 217:54-57, 2000.
13. Freeman KP, Brewer B, Slusher SH: Membrane filter preparations of cerebrospinal fluid from normal horses and horses with selected neurologic disease, *Compend Cont Educ Pract Vet* 11:1100-1108, 1989.
14. Mayhew IG, Beal CR: Techniques of analysis of cerebrospinal fluid, *Vet Clin North Am (Small Anim Pract)* 10:155-176, 1980.
15. Kirstensen F, Firth EC: Analysis of serum proteins and cerebrospinal fluid in clinically normal horses using agar rose electrophoresis, *Am J Vet Res* 38:1089-1092, 1977.
16. Mayhew IG, Whitlock RH, Tasker JB: Equine cerebrospinal fluid: reference values of normal horses, *Am J Vet Res* 38:1271-1274, 1977.
17. Furr MO, Bender H: Cerebrospinal fluid variables in clinically normal foals from birth to 42 days of age, *Am J Vet Res* 55:781-784, 1994.
18. Wilson JW: Clinical application of cerebrospinal fluid creatine phosphokinase determination, *J Am Vet Med Assoc* 171:200-202, 1977.
19. Welles EG et al: Composition and analysis of cerebrospinal fluid in clinically normal adult cattle, *Am J Vet Res* 53:2050-2057, 1992.
20. Furr MO, Tyler R: Cerebrospinal fluid creatine kinase activity in horses with central nervous system disease: 69 cases (1984-1989), *J Am Vet Med Assoc* 197:245-248, 1990.

DISEASES PRODUCING CORTICAL SIGNS

LISLE W. GEORGE
MARY O. SMITH

MAEDI–VISNA VIRUS INFECTION
(Ovine Progressive Pneumonia Virus Infection; Zwoegerziektie)

DEFINITION AND ETIOLOGY. Visna is a chronic, progressive encephalitis of sheep caused by a retrovirus (subfamily Lentivirinae).[21-30] Visna virus is related to the many lentiviruses that cause immunodeficiency and neurologic disease in other species; these viruses include equine arteritis virus, caprine arthritis-encephalitis virus, and simian, feline, and human immunodeficiency viruses.[31] The agent is an enveloped ribonucleic acid virus that contains reverse transcriptase.[32] The respiratory aspects of the viral infection are discussed in Chapter 29.

CLINICAL SIGNS. Nervous system signs of visna, which are characteristic of a diffuse encephalitis, include ataxia, twitching of the facial muscles, conscious proprioceptive deficits, normal gait along a straight path, staggering or stumbling when turned or forced to perform a complex maneuver, circling, and blindness. Coma, convulsions, and hyperexcitability may be seen terminally. Some sheep merely show emaciation without neurologic signs. The time between the onset of clinical signs and death may be as long as 1 to 2 years. Because of the slowly progressive nature of maedi–visna virus infection and the high probability that affected sheep eventually will develop chronic disorders of the nervous, musculoskeletal, mammary gland, or respiratory system, the presence of antibody in the serum usually is considered evidence of active infection.[33,34]

CLINICAL PATHOLOGY. The CSF of affected animals is characterized by pleocytosis, with the cell counts ranging from 1012 to 1478 for animals infected for 1 month and 4 years, respectively.[35] The protein concentrations of CSF range from 50 to 100 mg/dl for 30 days after infection. Antiviral antibody and virus can be detected in specimens of CSF. The CSF to plasma ratio of immunoglobulin G (IgG) in the CNS is normal (under 0.2) during the first month after infection but rises to over 0.4 after 1 month.[36]

PATHOPHYSIOLOGY. The lesions of maedi–visna virus infection are partly induced by the host's inflammatory response. Experimental immunosuppression of infected sheep ameliorates the severity of the clinical signs and reduces the pathologic lesions of the cerebral cortex without altering the amount of viral shedding.[37,38] The virus is immunosuppressive. Viral infections usually lead to a variety of secondary bacterial infections.[39] The chronic viremia may be caused by repeated antigenic changes of the virus; by intermittent expression of proteins by persistent proviral deoxyribonucleic acid (DNA) in cells; or by protection of the virus in circulating immune cells. Natural resistance to maedi–visna virus infection may be mediated partly by a nonimmunoglobulin inhibitory substance that is present in ovine plasma.[39]

PATHOLOGY. Gross lesions of visna infection are seen only rarely, when inflammation and malacia are very extensive. In such cases areas of yellowish tan discoloration are present in white matter.[40] The microscopic lesions of visna are predominantly those of a diffuse, nonsuppurative, perivascular inflammation throughout the neuraxis, affecting white matter in particular although gray matter also is involved. The lesions include demyelination, gliosis, lymphocytic choriomeningitis, round cell infiltration of the choroid plexus, and focal necrotic areas that are infiltrated by macrophages.[41,42] There is a predisposition for inflammatory lesions to develop in a periventricular location, including around the central canal of the spinal cord. After exposure to the virus, sheep develop an asymptomatic infection for as long as 6 weeks. During this time the virus can be isolated from the brain and other tissues; later the virus can be isolated from peripheral blood neutrophils but not from tissue homogenates, indicating that replication of the virus occurs in circulating cells during this stage of the infection.[43] Once the disease has been recognized, the affected sheep should be culled or slaughtered. Rigid control measures that may be partly successful[29] are discussed in Chapter 29.

DIAGNOSIS AND EPIDEMIOLOGY. The diagnosis of visna infection is made initially by recognition of the clinical neurologic disease in groups of animals in which the pulmonary form of the disease also is present. A specific diagnosis is made by a combination of agar gel immunodiffusion (AGID) testing and enzyme-linked immunosorbent assay (ELISA). [44,45] The diagnosis and epidemiology of maedi–visna virus infection are discussed in detail in Chapter 29.

TREATMENT. No effective treatment for maedi–visna virus infection is available for field use, although the disease is being used as an animal model system for the study of drugs effective against lentiviruses.[46]

REFERENCES

21. Gudnadottir M, Palsson PA: Successful transmission of visna by intrapulmonary inoculation, *J Infect Dis* 115:217-225, 1976.
22. Sigurdsson B, Palsson PA, Grimmson H: Visna, a demyelinating, transmissible disease of sheep, *J Neuropathol Exp Neurol* 16:389-395, 1957.
23. Sigurdsson B, Palsson PA, Von Bogaert L: Cultivation of visna virus in tissue culture, *Arch Gesamte Virusforsch* 10:368-378, 1960.
24. Gudnadottir M, Palsson PA: Host virus interaction in visna-infected sheep, *J Immunol* 95:1116-1123, 1965.
25. Thormar H, Helgadottir H: A comparison of visna and maedi viruses. II, Serological relationships, *Res Vet Sci* 6:456-465, 1965.
26. DeBoer GF: Zwoegerziektie virus, the causative agent for progressive interstitial pneumonia (maedi) and meningoleucoencephalitis (visna) in sheep, *Res Vet Sci* 18:15-25, 1975.
27. Stamp JT: Slow virus infections of the nervous system of sheep, *Vet Rec* 107:529-530, 1980.
28. Ressang AA, Stam FC, DeBoer GF: A meningoleucoencephalomyelitis resembling visna in Dutch Zwoeger sheep, *Pathol Vet* 3:401-411, 1966.
29. Petursson G et al: Pathogenesis of visna. I. Sequential virologic, serologic and pathologic studies, *Lab Invest* 35:402-412, 1976.
30. Sigurdsson B, Gunson H, Paulsson PA: Maedi, a chronic progressive pneumonia of sheep lungs, *J Infect Dis* 90:223-226, 1952.
31. Dawson M: Lentivirus diseases of domesticated animals, *J Comp Pathol* 99:401-419, 1988.
32. Harter DH et al: Visna virus: a slow neurotropic agent with tumor virus properties, *Trans Am Neurol Assoc* 96:249-251, 1971.
33. Molitor T, Schipper IA, Berryhill DL: Evaluation of the agar gel immunodiffusion test for the detection of precipitating antibodies against progressive pneumonia virus of sheep, *Can J Comp Med* 43:280-287, 1979.
34. Cutlip RA, Jackson TA, Laird GA: Immunodiffusion test for ovine progressive pneumonia, *Am J Vet Res* 38:1081-1084, 1977.
35. Georgsson G et al: An ultrastructural study of the cerebrospinal fluid in visna, *Acta Neuropathol (Berl)* 48:39-43, 1979.
36. Griffin DE et al: The cerebrospinal fluid in visna, a slow viral disease of sheep, *Ann Neurol* 4:212-218, 1978.
37. Narayan O, Griffin DE, Silverstein AM: Slow virus infection: replication and mechanisms of persistence of visna virus in sheep, *J Infect Dis* 135:800-806, 1977.
38. Nathanson N et al: Pathogenesis of visna. II. Effect of immunosuppression upon early central nervous system lesions, *Lab Invest* 35:444-451, 1976.
39. Haase AT, Varmus HE: Demonstration of a DNA provirus in the lytic growth of visna virus, *Nature (New Biology)* 245:237-239, 1973.
40. Summers BA, Cummings JF, De Lahunta A: *Veterinary neuropathology*, St Louis, 1995, Mosby.
41. Georgsson G et al: Experimental visna in foetal Icelandic sheep, *J Comp Pathol* 88:597-605, 1978.
42. Sigurdsson B, Palsson PA, Van Bogaert L: Pathology of visna: transmissible demyelinating disease in sheep in Iceland, *Acta Neuropathol (Berl)* 1:343-362, 1962.
43. Haase AT et al: Slow persistent infection caused by visna virus: role of host restriction, *Science* 195:175-177, 1977.
44. Saman E et al: A new sensitive serological assay for detection of lentivirus infections in small ruminants, *Clin Diagn Lab Immunol* 6:734-740, 1999.
45. Fevereiro M, Barros S, Fagulha T: Development of a monoclonal antibody blocking ELISA for detection of antibodies against maedi-visna virus, *J Virol Methods* 81:101-108, 1999.
46. Thormar H et al: Visna in sheep as a model for chemotherapy of lentiviral central nervous system infections, *Clin Microbiol Infect* 4:618-612, 1998.

CAPRINE ARTHRITIS-ENCEPHALITIS VIRUS INFECTION (Infectious Leukoencephalomyelitis)

DEFINITION AND CLINICAL SIGNS. The caprine arthritis-encephalitis (CAE) virus belongs to the retrovirus group. The systemic manifestations of the disease are thoroughly discussed in Chapter 36. The leukoencephalomyelitis form of CAE is predominantly seen in young goats but may occur in goats as old as 22 years.[47] The clinical signs of leukoencephalomyelitis include ataxia, paraparesis, paraplegia, tetraparesis, tetraplegia, hemiparesis, hemiplegia, head tilt, nystagmus, tremors, torticollis, trismus, salivation, depression, coma, and opisthotonos.[48-54] The neurologic deficits may be either symmetric or asymmetric. Goats with high cervical spinal cord lesions (L1 to L4) are recumbent and unable to raise their heads from the floor. They may show resistance to passive neck flexion. Vision and pupillary light reflexes may be diminished if the brainstem pathways are altered.[50-52] The specific gait disturbances depend on the areas of the spinal cord involved. Signs of neurologic dysfunction may range from paraparesis to tetraplegia. The spinal reflexes range from hypertonia and hyperreflexia to hypotonia and hyporeflexia.[48-53] This diversity of signs is related to the variable location of lesions in the central nervous system (CNS).

Other clinical signs also are variable. In one study affected goat kids remained afebrile, whereas in another study 61% of affected animals had rectal temperatures ranging from 38.9° to 41.3° C (103.6° to 106.4° F).[48-53] Other signs that could be associated with systemic viral infection include enlarged joints, vague and shifting leg lameness, weight loss, and tachypnea without significant auscultatory abnormalities.

The major differential diagnostic considerations for the neurologic form of CAE include listeriosis or chlamydial and mycoplasmal infections. The CAE virus causes neurologic lesions in numerous regions of the CNS, whereas the lesions of listeriosis are restricted to the brainstem. Mycoplasmal infections typically affect kids ranging from 1 to 6 months of age, and affected animals develop polyserositis. They are systemically ill, and the joints are hot, grossly swollen, and painful. Goats with a mycoplasmal infection show extreme pain when the neck is passively flexed because of meningeal and vertebral articular inflammation. Fluid from the body cavities of goats with mycoplasmal infection has a high protein concentration and an increased number of polymorphonuclear cells.

DIAGNOSIS. CAE can be diagnosed definitively using an agar gel diffusion (AGID) test. The antigen used for the test is a tissue culture–derived CAE virus.[55] However, demonstration of serum precipitins is not conclusive evidence that the clinical signs are virus related, because many goats are asymptomatically infected with CAE virus for life. Some chronically infected goats also may not show a serologic response to the virus proteins. Therefore accurate diagnosis of leukoencephalomyelitis must be based on a comparison of the pathologic lesions in the CNS and joints in conjunction with the clinical and serologic findings.

The changes in the CSF are characteristic only of a chronic granulomatous inflammation. Specific changes include an increased protein concentration and pleocytosis.[56] Cell counts in the CSF of affected goats range from 5 to 1800/dl, and the protein concentration ranges from 0 to 700 mg/dl.[47]

The CAE virus may be isolated by cocultivation of primary bovine testicular cells or sheep choroid plexus cells with infected caprine synovial cells. Isolation procedures are tedious, and the viremia may be intermittent. Consequently, virus isolation offers little advantage over serologic tests for detecting the infection unless the patient is a serologic nonresponder. One study has reported an increase in total plasma protein and hypergammaglobulinemia in affected goats.[49] The results of other hematologic and blood chemistry analyses are normal. Nucleic acid probes and polymerase chain reactions using viral DNA as primers have been produced. Such probes can be used to detect viral DNA in infected white blood cells, and additional development may allow rapid screening with high sensitivity and specificity (see Chapter 36).

PATHOGENESIS. Being a member of the retrovirus group, the CAE virus contains ribonucleic acid (RNA)–dependent DNA polymerase. When inoculated into goats, the virus causes a chronic infection characterized by demyelinating encephalomyelitis, arthritis, and interstitial pneumonia. The pathologic changes resemble those of an autoimmune process and are probably caused by interactions between the host's immunologic responses, denatured myelin, and the virus.[57] Macroscopic pathologic changes in the CNS of naturally infected goats include cloudiness of the meninges and tan discoloration of the white matter.[48] Microscopic changes include disseminated perivascular accumulations of mononuclear cells, demyelination originating in the subependymal region, astrocytosis, and mononuclear leptomeningitis.[48,52,55,57,58] The inflammatory foci are predominantly composed of macrophages containing material that tests positive on periodic acid–Schiff (PAS) staining. Neuronophagia and neuronal necrosis are not seen.[58] Lesions are most severe in the periductular, periventricular, and submeningeal regions of the white matter. Spinal cord lesions are most commonly observed in the thoracolumbar segments.[47]

TREATMENT. No treatment is available for goats with leukoencephalomyelitis. Control measures are discussed in Chapter 36.

REFERENCES

47. Norman S, Smith MC: Caprine arthritis-encephalitis: review of the neurologic form in 30 cases, *J Am Vet Med Assoc* 182:1342-1345, 1983.

48. Stavrou D, Deutschländer N, Dahme E: Granulomatous encephalomyelitis in goats, *J Comp Pathol* 79:393-397, 1969.
49. Dahme E et al: Klinik und pathologie einer ubertragbaren granulomatosen meningoencephalomyelitis (MEM) bei der hausziege, *Acta Neuropathol (Berl)* 23:59-76, 1973.
50. Cork LC, Hadlow WJ, Crawford TB: Infectious leukoencephalomyelitis of young goats, *J Infect Dis* 129:131-141, 1974.
51. Thomson RG: Viral leukoencephalomyelitis arthritis of goats, *Can Vet J* 22:358, 1981.
52. O'Sullivan BM et al: Leucoencephalomyelitis of goat kids, *Aust Vet J* 54:479-483, 1978.
53. Wilkie IW: Leukomyelitis in the goat: a report of three cases, *Can Vet J* 21:203-205, 1980.
54. Summers BA, Appel MJG, Griesen HA: Studies of viral leukoencephalomyelitis and swayback in goats, *Cornell Vet* 70:372-390, 1980.
55. Crawford TB, Adams DS: Caprine arthritis-encephalitis: clinical features and presence of antibody in selected goat populations, *J Am Vet Med Assoc* 178:713-719, 1981.
56. Cork LC: Differential diagnosis of viral leukoencephalomyelitis of goats, *J Am Vet Med Assoc* 171:1303-1306, 1976.
57. Cork LC, Narayan O: The pathogenesis of viral leukoencephalomyelitis-arthritis of goats. I. Persistent viral infection with progressive pathologic changes, *Lab Invest* 42:596-602, 1980.
58. Cork LC et al: Pathology of viral leukoencephalomyelitis of goats, *Acta Neuropathol (Berl)* 29:281-292, 1974.

BORDER DISEASE (Hairy Shaker Lambs; Hypomyelogenesis Congenita)

DEFINITION AND ETIOLOGY. Border disease is a congenital infection of sheep and goats caused by a noncytopathic togavirus (genus *Pestivirus*).[59] The border disease agent is antigenically similar to the bovine virus diarrhea (BVD) and hog cholera viruses. Once introduced into a flock, the border disease virus causes a devastating syndrome characterized by abortion, infertility, and deformed lambs. The virus infects naive ewes during pregnancy and causes a variety of fetal malformations, including early embryonic death, abortion and stillbirth, and small, malformed lambs. A seroprevalence rate as high as 29% has been seen in a newly infected flock; however, lambs infected in utero become immunotolerant and remain viremic.[60] In an infected flock the incidence of fetal malformations and abortions declines over time because of the growing population of ewes with persistent active immunity. Adult sheep that become infected with the border disease virus develop an inapparent, short-lived viremia and become immune to reinfection.

CLINICAL SIGNS. The severity of clinical signs in affected lambs varies. Changes are most marked in newborn lambs infected in early gestation (before 50 days). The central nervous system (CNS), skin, and skeleton are the most seriously affected. The hairs of congenitally affected lambs are coarse, straight, and elongated and stand out from the body like a halo.[61] The coat is abnormally pigmented and may have a dark gray appearance or hyperpigmented spots that are especially prominent over the top of the neck.[62] The combination of pigmentary abnormalities and long, coarse hair shafts gave rise to the descriptive term "steel wool coat." Animals that survive shed the abnormal hairs at 9 to 12 weeks of age and replace them with normal hair fibers. Affected lambs also have a short, thickened body, shortened legs, smaller orbital size, and doming of the frontal bone.[63,64] Arthrogryposis occasionally may be seen. Some infected lambs show neurologic symptoms such as ataxia and uncontrollable tremors. The tremors are coarse, involve the trunk and head, and disappear when the animal is asleep.[65,66] The lambs often are alert and appetent but initially need assistance to stand and nurse. Some animals walk normally but hop on the rear limbs when forced to run. Over time the lambs become stronger but continue to show impaired locomotion for months. The CNS signs usually disappear by 20 weeks of age, but the animals appear stunted. Affected animals have a markedly decreased viability compared with uninfected herd

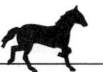

mates and may die suddenly without showing premonitory symptoms. Aside from neonatal death losses, economic burdens imposed by the viral infection include low birth weights, diminished weaning weights, lowered carcass quality, and infertility.[64,67]

Abortions that occur 9 to 106 days after inoculation are seen in 30% of experimentally infected sheep.[62,63,68] In field outbreaks the average gestational age of the aborted fetus is 63 days. Teratogenic effects are most commonly observed when lambs are infected between 50 and 90 gestational days of age.[69] Fetal mummification occasionally may be seen.

The border disease virus is also pathogenic in goats.[70] As in sheep, inoculation of pregnant does results in fetal mummification and abortion. The spinal cords of infected kids are hypomyelinated, but the characteristic hair changes usually observed in sheep fetuses are not seen in goat kids. The border disease virus has low pathogenicity for cattle. Abortions can be induced in cows inoculated with the virus at approximately 50 days of gestation, and affected calves have cerebral cavitations.[71] The condition is not recognized as naturally transmitted to cows.

DIAGNOSIS. Identification of the viral antigens in tissues using fluorescent antibody tests is the most accurate method of diagnosing border disease. Tissues that most consistently contain viral antigens are those of the abomasum, pancreas, kidneys, thyroid, and testicles.[72,73] Serodiagnostic methods, including serum neutralization, agar gel immunodiffusion (AGID), and complement fixation tests, have been developed.[74] In most cases the BVD virus has been used as the indicator antigen. Serodiagnosis of infected lambs is difficult, because the lambs tend to be immunotolerant and therefore do not develop strong serologic responses. Sheep infected as adults develop serum neutralization (SN) titers ranging from 1:20 to 1:320, whereas the SN titers of animals with congenital infections are consistently below 1:10.[68] The presence of viral antibodies in the CSF suggests border disease virus infection.

PATHOPHYSIOLOGY. Hypomyelination probably is caused by a combination of virus-induced degeneration of the oligodendroglial cells (dysmyelinogenesis), persistent viral infection, and diminished secretion of the thyroid hormones L-3,3',5'-triiodothyronine and thyroxine.[75] A deficiency of these hormones probably results in a lowered concentration of 2',3'-cyclic nucleotide-3'-phosphodiesterase, which contributes to the hypomyelination. The diminished production of thyroid hormones is thought to be related to direct inhibition of the thyroid gland, because the pituitary activity of these lambs appears to be normal. Hypomyelination appears at approximately the same time as specific antiviral delayed-type hypersensitivity, indicating that an immunopathologic event may be partly responsible. Morphometric measurements of the spinal cords of lambs infected in utero show a permanent reduction of both white and gray matter in a cross-sectional area as a result of the decreased myelin content.[76] Depressed blastogenic activity of lymphocytes, a decrease in T4 helper cell function, and an increase in T4 suppressor cell function have been demonstrated in affected lambs between 4 and 7 months of age, indicating a viral immunosuppression.[77-79] Such immunosuppressed lambs succumb to parasitism, diarrhea, and bronchopneumonia.

EPIDEMIOLOGY. Border disease is transmitted both vertically and horizontally.[77,80] The agent can efficiently infect sheep through the intact mucous membranes. The major reservoir in infected herds is the asymptomatic, congenitally infected seronegative animal.[60,81] Sheep exposed to the virus as adults develop antibody responses and are able to clear the infections within weeks. Asymptomatically infected animals may shed the virus through the placenta, infected offspring, saliva, respiratory secretions, urine, or feces.[68,77] In one sero-epidemiologic study of infected ewes in the western United

States, lambs were more often seropositive than ewes.[60] A large percentage of the seropositive lambs were born to seronegative ewes, indicating the presence of a large amount of virus cycling from asymptomatic carriers. Strain-related differences appear to exist in viral pathogenicity.[82]

NECROPSY FINDINGS. The macroscopic changes associated with border disease virus infection are hydranencephaly, porencephaly, microcephaly, cerebellar hypoplasia, abnormal curvature of the ribs, brachygnathia, doming of the frontal bones of the skull, narrowing of the distance between the orbits, a decrease in orbital size, shortening of the crown-to-rump and diaphyseal lengths, retention of secondary hair fibers, and abnormal skin pigmentation.

Microscopic changes in lambs with congenital infection include hypomyelinogenesis and hypercellularity of the white matter with abnormal-appearing glial cells.[83] The CNS shows dysmyelinogenesis, secondary demyelination, and a nodular periarteritis. Viral antigen can be demonstrated in the adventitia of the CNS arterioles.[75] The microscopic lesions of the placenta include endothelial swelling, thrombotic occlusion of the vessels, and fibrinonecrotic cellular debris in the fetomaternal space.[83]

TREATMENT AND CONTROL. In herd situations blood cultures and examination of skin biopsies by fluorescent antibody tests should be performed concurrently to identify carriers.[71] The serum neutralization test is not a reliable indicator of infection. Pregnant noninfected sheep should be kept separated from others in the flock for the first 60 days of gestation to ensure that in utero infections do not occur.

REFERENCES

59. Mathews REF: Classification and nomenclature of viruses, *Intervirology* 12:132-296, 1979.
60. Niemi SM, Evermann JF, Huffman EM: Border disease virus isolation from postpartum ewes, *Am J Vet Res* 44:86-88, 1982.
61. Plant JW, Acland HM, Gard GP: A mucosal disease virus as a cause of abortion, hairy birth coat, and unthriftiness in sheep. I. Infection of pregnant ewes and observations on aborted fetuses and lambs dying before 1 week of age, *Aust Vet J* 52:57-63, 1976.
62. Barlow RM et al: The definition of border disease: problems for the diagnostician, *Vet Rec* 104:334-336, 1979.
63. Terlecki S: Border disease: a viral teratogen of farm animals, *Vet Annu* 17: 74-79, 1977.
64. Nott JA, Shaw IG: Border disease in sheep: its effect on fertility, viability, and wool, *Vet Rec* 80:534-537, 1967.
65. Markson LM et al: Hypomyelinogenesis congenita in sheep, *Vet Rec* 71:269-271, 1959.
66. Sawyer MM et al: Border disease in a flock of sheep, *J Am Vet Med Assoc* 189:61-65, 1986.
67. Terpstra C: Border disease: virus persistence, antibody response, and transmission studies, *Res Vet Sci* 30:185-191, 1981.
68. Dickinson AG, Barlow RM: The demonstration of the transmissibility of border disease in sheep, *Vet Rec* 81:114, 1967.
69. Sawyer MM: Border disease of sheep: the disease in the newborn, adolescent, and adult, *Comp Immunol Microbiol Infect Dis* 15:171-177, 1992.
70. Gibbons DF, Winkler CE, Shaw IG: Pathogenicity of the border disease agent for the bovine fetus, *Br Vet J* 130:357-361, 1974.
71. Roeder PL, Drew TW: Persistence in tissues of border disease virus antigen demonstrable by immunofluorescence, *Res Vet Sci* 29:394, 1980.
72. Terpstra C: Detection of border disease antigen in tissues of affected sheep and in cell cultures by immunofluorescence, *Res Vet Sci* 25:350-355, 1978.
73. Huck RA, Evans DH, Woods DG: Border disease of sheep: comparison of the results of serological testing using complement fixation, immunodiffusion, neutralization, and immunofluorescence techniques, *Br Vet J* 131:427-435, 1975.
74. Gardiner AC, Zakarian B, Barlow RM: Periarteritis in experimental border disease of sheep. III. Immunopathological observations, *J Comp Pathol* 90:469-474, 1980.
75. Sweasey D, Patterson DSP: Congenital hypomyelinogenesis (border disease) of lambs: postnatal neurochemical recovery in the central nervous system, *J Neurochem* 33:705-711, 1979.
76. Westbury HA, Naphthine DV, Straube E: Border disease: persistent infection with the virus, *Vet Rec* 104:406-409, 1979.
77. Sweaseu D et al: Border disease: a sequential study of surviving lambs and an assessment of its effect on profitability, *Vet Rec* 104:447-450, 1979.

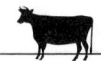

78. Burrells C et al: Lymphocyte subpopulations in the blood of sheep persistently infected with border disease virus, *Clin Exp Immunol* 76:446-451, 1989.

79. Woldehiwet Z, Sharma R: Effects of persistent infection with border disease virus on lymphocyte subpopulations of sheep, *Proceedings of the Eleventh International Symposium of the World Association of Veterinary Microbiologists, Immunologists, and Specialists in Infectious Diseases,* Perugia, Italy, 1989.

80. Harkness JW et al: Border disease of sheep: isolation of the virus in tissue culture and experimental reproduction of the disease, *Vet Rec* 100:71-72, 1977.

81. Clarke GL, Osburn BI: Transmissible congenital demyelination encephalopathy of lambs, *Vet Pathol* 15:68-82, 1978.

82. Nettleton PF et al: The production and survival of lambs persistently infected with a border disease virus, *Comp Immunol Microbiol Infect Dis* 15:179-188, 1992.

83. Barlow RM: Experiments in border disease. IV. Pathological changes in ewes, *J Comp Pathol* 82:151-157, 1972.

ENCEPHALITIC INFECTIOUS BOVINE RHINOTRACHEITIS VIRUS INFECTION

CLINICAL SIGNS. In most cases infection of calves with bovine herpesvirus type 1 (BHV-1) results in an acute, generally nonfatal upper respiratory tract disease characterized by fibrinonecrotic white plaques of the nasal, pharyngeal, and tracheal mucosa and abortions (see Chapter 29). Other clinical conditions associated with infectious bovine rhinotracheitis (IBR) infection include epizootic conjunctivitis (Chapter 37) and infectious balanoposthitis or vulvovaginitis (Chapter 41). Occasionally a specific strain of the IBR virus infects the CNS of calves, resulting in a meningoencephalitis. The clinical signs of this encephalitis include depression, mild nasal and ocular discharge, conscious proprioceptive deficit, head-pressing, aimless circling, bellowing, salivation, bruxism, paralysis of the tongue, head tilt, nystagmus, convulsions, blindness, coma, and death.[84,85] The seizural activity is characterized by a tonic-clonic convulsion with violent spasms or tremors of the head with all four legs flexed and the head in opisthotonos.[84,85] Rectal temperatures of 41° to 42° C (106° and 107° F) have been reported.[86] The case fatality rate of encephalitic IBR is nearly 100%; however, recovery occurs in rare case. Affected calves develop the full range of encephalitic signs within 1 to 2 days of infection and die by 5 days.[87]

EPIDEMIOLOGY. Epidemiologic factors that appear to favor dissemination of the virus among cattle include a high stocking rate, repeated introduction of animals from diverse backgrounds, and mass weaning of calves at a time when the passively acquired anti-IBR antibodies are waning.[84] Calves less than 6 weeks old are most susceptible to the encephalopathic effects of the virus. The case attack rate ranges from 15% to 37%.[85,86] The virus is shed from nasal secretions for 10 to 11 days after infection. Isolation of the virus from the brain or nasal secretions is the most accurate means of substantiating a clinical diagnosis of IBR encephalitis.[88]

The encephalitic viral strain grows in the nasal or ocular mucosa, where it produces fibrinonecrotic plaques three days after infection. The mucosal lesions disappear by 9 to 11 days, at which time the encephalitic signs become evident. Brainstem infections result from centripetal spread through the trigeminal nerve dendrites that originate in the pharynx and tonsils.[89] Hematogenous dissemination to the brain appears to be less important than retrograde migration of the virus along the axons. Intravenous inoculation of encephalitogenic IBR virus results in a viremia for 2 days but does not cause meningoencephalitis.

PATHOPHYSIOLOGY. The pathologic lesions of encephalitic IBR infection are widely distributed in the gray matter of the brain. They include marked perivascular cuffing with mononuclear cells, diffuse gliosis, and neuronal degeneration. Some neurons show chromatolysis. White matter lesions include myelitis with mononuclear cell infiltration and demyelination. Extensive lymphocytic meningoencephalitis is seen. Intranuclear inclusion bodies are rarely seen in the CNS form of IBR. The IBR virus usually can be isolated from brain homogenates of affected calves.

Strains of BHV-1 that cause encephalitis can be distinguished from mucosal isolates using molecular techniques.[89-92] One investigator has suggested that the differences between the encephalitic and respiratory isolates are significant enough to warrant assignment of the agents to different species.[93]

TREATMENT AND CONTROL. No adequate therapy exists for the encephalitogenic form of BHV-1 infection. Affected animals should be kept warm and, if convulsive, should be sedated with valium or phenobarbital (Table 33-3).

There are no known specific methods of preventing the encephalitogenic form of IBR. The close serologic relation-

TABLE 33-3

Recommended Drug Dosages for Treatment of Cerebrocortical Disease

	Dose	Route	Frequency
ANTICONVULSANT DRUGS			
Valium	0.01-0.4 mg/kg	IV or IM	Twice daily or as needed
Pentobarbital sodium	2-10 mg/kg	IV	Three times daily
Phenobarbital	Loading dose 20 mg/kg	IV	One time
	Maintenance dosage 1-4 mg/kg	IV, PO, or IM	Divided twice daily
ANTIINFLAMMATORY OR ANTIEDEMA DRUGS			
Methylprednisolone	1-30 mg/kg	IV	One time
Dexamethasone	1-4 mg/kg	IV or IM	Twice daily
Mannitol	0.25-0.5 g/kg 20% solution	IV	Twice daily
Furosemide	1 mg/kg	IV, IM, or SC	Twice daily
Flunixin meglumine*	1 mg/kg	IV or IM	Twice daily
Phenylbutazone†	2-4 mg/kg	IV or PO	Twice daily
Dimethyl sulfoxide (DMSO)	1-2 g/kg	IV	Twice daily
Acetylsalicylic acid (aspirin)	7-10 g/500 kg	PO	Twice daily

IM, Intramuscular; *IV,* intravenous; *PO,* oral; *SC,* subcutaneous.
*Monitor for signs of gastric or abomasal bleeding (fecal occult blood).
†An initial loading dose of 10 to 20 mg/kg, followed by 2.5 to 5 mg/kg daily to every other day thereafter has been recommended for cattle.[94] Because of the prolonged plasma half-life in ruminants, serial administration of the drug should be accompanied by careful monitoring of renal function and gastrointestinal bleeding.

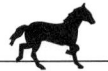

ship between the various herpes 1 viruses indicates that administration of the commercial vaccines just before weaning may be efficacious for preventing all clinical forms.

REFERENCES

84. Gardiner MR, Nairn ME, Sier AM: Viral meningoencephalitis of calves in western Australia, *Aust Vet J* 40:225-228, 1964.
85. Hill BD et al: Meningoencephalitis in calves due to bovine herpesvirus type 1 infection, *Aust Vet J* 61:242-243, 1984.
86. Carrillo BJ et al: Meningoencephalitis caused by IBR virus in calves in Argentina, *Zentralbl Veterinarmed* 30:327-332, 1983.
87. Johnston LAY, Simmons GC, McGavin MD: A viral meningoencephalitis in calves, *Aust Vet J* 38:207-214, 1962.
88. French EL: A specific virus encephalitis in calves: isolation and characterization of the causal agent, *Aust Vet J* 38:216-221, 1962.
89. Bagust TJ, Clark L: Pathogenesis of meningoencephalitis produced in calves by infectious bovine rhinotracheitis herpesvirus, *J Comp Pathol* 82:375-383, 1972.
90. Bagust TJ: Comparison of the biological, biophysical, and antigenic properties of four strains of infectious bovine rhinotracheitis herpesvirus, *J Comp Pathol* 82:365-374, 1972.
91. Mezler AE, Schudel AA, Engels M: Bovine herpesvirus 1: molecular and antigenic characteristics of variant viruses isolated from calves with neurological disease, *Arch Virol* 87:205-217, 1986.
92. Brake F, Studdert MJ: Molecular epidemiology and pathogenesis of ruminant herpes viruses including bovine, buffalo, and caprine herpes viruses 1 and bovine encephalitis herpesvirus, *Aust Vet J* 62:331-334, 1985.
93. Studdert MJ: Bovine encephalitis herpesvirus, *Vet Rec* 126:21, 1990.
94. Reference deleted in proof.

BOVINE SPONGIFORM ENCEPHALOPATHY ("Mad Cow" Disease)

CHRISTINE F. BERTHELIN-BAKER

DEFINITION AND ETIOLOGY. Bovine spongiform encephalopathy (BSE) is a transmissible spongiform encephalopathy (TSE) of cattle that was first described in 1987 in the United Kingdom.[95] The TSEs are a group of slowly progressing, invariably fatal neurodegenerative diseases that can affect human beings and animals. They are also called prion diseases because of the accumulation of prions (a specific protein marker of TSEs) in the central nervous system of affected animals and people. The prion PrPSc is widely accepted as the etiologic agent of the TSEs, although some research groups still dispute the "prion hypothesis," which holds that the infectious agent, PrPSc, an isoform of the normal prion protein PrPc, is a host-encoded membrane protein and does not carry any nucleic acid.[96-98] PrPSc replicates by inducing a posttranslational conformational change in the normal protein PrPc to form the abnormal prion PrPSc.

CLINICAL SIGNS. Like all transmissible spongiform encephalopathies, BSE has a long incubation phase. As a result, it occurs mostly in 4- to 6-year-old cattle (the age range is 20 months to 18 years). The clinical signs of BSE typically are insidious in onset.[99,100] They may be precipitated by stressful situations such as transportation, concurrent illnesses, or an increase in metabolic consumption of nutrients (e.g., late pregnancy and parturition). The closeness of observation may influence the array of clinical signs, the rate of progression, and the duration of the clinical signs noted. The initial clinical signs are subtle behavioral changes that are unlikely to be observed in large herds. Cattle with BSE may become apprehensive, stay apart from their herd mates, and become fearful of people. The changes are progressive. Cattle may panic or be extremely excited, especially in unfamiliar environments, during restraint, or when placed in confined quarters such as stocks. As a result, BSE cattle often are very difficult or impossible to restrain. Unprovoked aggressive behavior occurs infrequently. BSE cattle may be unwilling to move through previously familiar doorways. Hyperesthesia is common and most marked on approach to or touching of the head and

neck. Light touching of the hind limbs may induce forceful, "ballistic" kicking, which may be observed during milking. Animals may overreact, startle, or "panic" in response to visual, touch, or sound stimuli. The startle reaction may be gauged by using the hand test (the fist is thrown abruptly toward the animal's head without touching it), the flashlight test, or by a loud metallic "bang." Normal animals rarely startle in response to such stimuli or may startle once or twice when the stimulus is repeated. Cattle with BSE frequently startle violently and in a constant and repeatable fashion. There is no habituation to the stimulus, and in some cases the response may escalate. An extreme "aberrant" startle is seen in some BSE cattle with a transient but repeatable head shaking, seizurelike head bobbing, and in some cases running around or falling immediately after startling.

Other possible clinical signs of BSE are ptyalism, an increase in head rubbing, muscle fasciculations, and excessive vocalization. A relative bradycardia (approximately 60 beats/min) may be noted unexpectedly in animals that are very excited. Other behaviors seen in BSE may include frequent and repetitive head tossing, licking of the nostrils, yawning, flehmen, head tossing and head butting, and restlessness. Affected animals often lose weight and have reduced milk output. Ataxia and tremors are seen in more advanced cases. Tremors most often involve the head and neck and may become generalized, especially with exercise. Ataxia is most marked on turns, when going over steps, and on uneven terrain. It may also be accentuated with exercise. BSE cattle may become recumbent and unable to feed if the disease is left to run its course, because of an intercurrent illness, or as the result of an injury during a fall. Any of these causes may explain the finding of previously unsuspected cases of BSE in cattle during systematic targeted surveys of "fallen stock," such as those conducted in Switzerland in 1998-1999.[100a]

PATHOPHYSIOLOGY. The exact function of the prion protein and the mechanisms of the neurodegeneration and central nervous dysfunctions observed in the TSEs are unknown.

A major difference between BSE of cattle and TSEs in sheep is that the agent often is widespread in the lymphoid tissue in sheep, whereas in cattle BSE infectivity is seldom present in extraneural tissues. The presence of BSE infectivity in extraneural tissues in cattle has not been identified in natural disease. In a study of the pathogenesis of BSE, cattle were challenged by the oral route with 100 g of affected brain material. Cohorts were slaughtered every 4 to 6 months postinoculation up to 40 months postinoculation. The incubation period varied from 32 to 40 months. Infectivity was assessed by mouse bioassay and identified in the distal ileum from 6 months after challenge and in the CNS from 32 months after challenge.[101] PrPSc was detected in lymphoid tissue (Peyer's patches) of the distal ileum. It also was found in both the brain and spinal cord from 32 months after infection at the same time as infectivity was detected in these tissues. Infectivity was also identified in the dorsal root ganglia, trigeminal ganglia, and bone marrow.[102] The milk, placental tissue, tonsils, and lymph nodes of BSE-affected and incubating animals have not shown infectivity in mice bioassays. Further studies are underway to assess the infectivity of various tissues in the more sensitive cattle bioassay.

EPIDEMIOLOGY AND ZOONOTIC POTENTIAL. Epidemiologic studies have shown that the outbreaks of BSE in Europe were all linked to the transmission of BSE through the feeding of meat and bone meal that included recycled carcasses of BSE-infected cattle. BSE originally may have derived from feedstuffs containing rendered carcasses of scrapie-infected sheep. It is also possible that BSE was a sporadic and rare form of TSE that preexisted in the bovine population. The outbreak of BSE in the United Kingdom has been traced to the recycling of BSE infected carcasses into feed, mostly in the

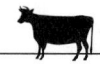

1980s.[103] Cattle in other countries were affected as a result of the importation of infected feedstuffs or cattle, followed by later recycling of the agent in rendered ruminant feedstuffs, similarly to the situation that occurred in the UK.

Dairy cattle predominantly have been affected, most likely because of their longer life span compared with beef cattle and because of the wider use of concentrate feeding in dairy herds. No clear genetic predisposition to BSE has been demonstrated in cattle, unlike scrapie infection in sheep. Calves born from dams in the later stages of the incubation of BSE are at most 10% more likely to develop BSE than their herd mates. This may be due to an unidentified genetic predisposition or to a low degree of vertical transmission. Mathematical modeling of the rate of reduction in the number of BSE cases in response to feed controls introduced in the UK shows that vertical and lateral transmission of BSE, if they do occur, do so at a very low rate. Such a low rate could not sustain an outbreak of BSE. On this basis experts have predicted that BSE will be eradicated from the UK by the year 2005.

From 1986 to June 2000, a total of 176,954 cases of BSE were confirmed in Great Britain on 35,051 farms, or 57.4 % of the farms that hold adult cattle.[104] The cattle cohorts born in 1986-89 had the highest incidence of BSE cases, and the peak of the outbreak occurred in 1992 (36,680 cases). A sustained and sharp decrease in the number of cases has occurred each year since 1993. In 1999 only 2,254 confirmed cases of BSE were reported in Great Britain. The initial ban on the feeding of ruminant-derived meat and bone meal to cattle took effect in 1989. This ban has been tightened and refined on several occasions since then, most recently in August 1996. A single case of BSE has been identified in a cow born in August 1996 in England, and no cases of BSE have been reported in cattle born in the UK after August 1996. Outside the United Kingdom, countries that have reported home-born cases of BSE include the Republic of Ireland (484 BSE cases identified since 1989), Portugal (365 cases since 1990), Switzerland (354 since 1990), France (101 since 1991), and a few other countries that reported only a very small number of cases (Statistics of the Office International Epizooties, OIE, October 2000).

Since the outbreak of BSE in the United Kingdom, new BSE-related TSEs have occurred in cats, in various exotic species, and in human beings.[104a] These new TSEs were caused by the BSE agent, as demonstrated by strain typing in mice.[105,106] The exact cause and route of infection of people by BSE is unknown. A new variant Creutzfeldt-Jakob disease (vCJD) was first identified in 1996 in the UK, where it has affected 80 people to date.[106a] Two cases of vCJD have been identified in France and one in the Republic of Ireland. The emergence of vCJD has put worldwide emphasis on the prevention and detection of TSEs in animals.

DIAGNOSIS. No in vivo test is available for the diagnosis of BSE. Clinical suspicion can be confirmed only by postmortem examination. The diagnosis of BSE is based on microscopic examination of the brain or on tests that identify PrPSc in brain or spinal cord tissue.[95,107] Neuronal degeneration and intraneuronal vacuolation are seen in specific brain areas. This vacuolation is accompanied or preceded by the accumulation of PrPSc.[103,108,109] The uniformity of the pathology among affected cattle along the epidemic and in various countries supports the notion that all BSE cases have been caused by a single strain of TSE agent. This has allowed the definition of a particular disease phenotype for BSE.[103,109-112] Prion detection is also possible by Western blot and paraffin embedded tissue blot (PET) testing and enzyme-linked immunosorbent assay (ELISA).[113-116] These tests are quicker than histopathologic techniques and are applicable to screening surveys. They are the only valuable assays when tissue autolysis has taken place.

DIFFERENTIAL DIAGNOSIS. Nervous system diseases that could be confused with BSE include pseudorabies, rabies, Borna encephalitis, bovine immunodeficiency virus (BIV) encephalitis, listeriosis, polioencephalomalacia, lead poisoning, CNS parasitic migration, brain tumors and abscesses, vitamin A deficiency, hepatic encephalopathy, and other metabolic imbalances. Because of the insidious nature of the illness, BSE cattle may appear to recover and later have relapses. This must be kept in mind whenever specific therapy for metabolic imbalances initially appears to be successful but later is followed by one or more relapses.

TREATMENT AND PROGNOSIS. BSE is a fatal disease for which no treatment is available. Because of the public health risk, the carcasses of animals suspected of having BSE should be incinerated.

CONTROL. Although BSE has not been identified in North American cattle, protective feed controls are enforced to eliminate the recycling of ruminants in ruminant feed. In countries that have had an outbreak of BSE, the complete exclusion of ruminant tissues from ruminant feed has aided progress toward eradication of BSE (see Epidemiology and Zoonotic Potential, above). In the UK the initial feed control measures were insufficient but have been refined through the years to prevent contamination of ruminant feed at feed mills. Because of the long incubation period of BSE there is a lag time in the effect of feed control measures, and the full effect of such measures can be assessed only when all animals born after a feed ban reach 4 to 8 years of age. Various other measures have been taken to protect public health by removing potentially infected animals and tissues from the food chain.

The disposal of BSE-infected tissues and the use of bovine tissues and body fluids in the preparation of medicinal products must take into account the extreme resistance of TSE agents. These agents are resistant to a wide range of inactivating treatments and environmental changes, such as autoclaving, rendering processes, storage at room temperature for months to years, exposure to ultraviolet light, freezing, thawing, prolonged boiling, and incubation with formalin.[117-120]

SCRAPIE

DEFINITION AND ETIOLOGY. Scrapie is the oldest known transmissible spongiform encephalopathy (TSE). It has affected sheep in various countries for more than 250 years. Despite this longevity, scrapie has shown no evidence of posing a danger to public health. Different scrapie agents have been identified by strain typing in mice. To date, no TSE agent directly isolated from sheep has ever been shown to be identical to the agent involved in bovine spongiform encephalopathy (BSE). Scrapie naturally affects sheep, goats, and mouflons.

CLINICAL SIGNS. Most cases of scrapie occur in animals 1 to 5 years of age. The clinical course varies but typically is slow and may last several months. Shepherds who work closely with and know their animals best recognize the early signs of scrapie. Early behavioral changes may be accompanied by weight loss. Withdrawal from the flock, nervousness, and restlessness are other signs.[121] Pruritus is a common feature of scrapie, and it increases in intensity over the course of the illness. It may be displayed through rubbing on fixed objects, scratching with the horns, and biting or licking of the head, flanks, back, rump, and limbs. Consequently there may be secondary wool loss, secondary dermatitis, skin infections, or excoriation of the skin. Such lesions are most commonly seen on the rump, at the base of the tail, on the withers and loins, on the head, or on the lower limbs.[121,122] Rubbing of the face and head may result also in corneal chemosis or aural hematomas. When the pruritic areas are stimulated by scratching, the animal may display a "scratch reflex" (also called nibble reflex); scratching induces nibbling, licking of the lips, or rhythmic head movements. This reflex is often but not always present in scrapie cases. It may also be observed in other CNS diseases and in pruritic skin diseases, especially ectoparasitism.

Some scrapie cases show leakage of ruminal fluid (cud) through the nostrils or the mouth. Tremors are present in some but not all cases. They often start with the head and generalize to the whole body. Other clinical signs of scrapie include bruxism (tooth grinding) and ptyalism. As the disease progresses, scrapie patients eventually develop apathy, exercise intolerance, and ataxia. Other signs seen in advanced cases include seizures, collapsing episodes, and depression. If scrapie is left to run its course, the animal may die while in a convulsion or succumb to starvation. The clinical signs of scrapie in goats are broadly similar to those in sheep.[121a,122-126] Scrapie has been identified in animals found dead. This may be an occurrence related to flocks that are not closely supervised.

PATHOPHYSIOLOGY. The exact mechanism of CNS degeneration has not been identified in the TSEs. The oral route is thought to be the most likely route of entry of the agent into the sheep.[127,128] The scrapie agent multiplies in the lymphatic tissues. Circulating lymphoid cells do not appear to be involved in scrapie replication.[129] Follicular dendritic cells are infected early in the course of the disease, and there may be an interface between the lymphoreticular system and the nervous system.[130] The scrapie agent probably enters the gastrointestinal tract and is transported to peripheral lymphoid tissue.[131,132] Transport to the CNS likely occurs along the vagus nerves from the gastrointestinal tract.[133] The suspected agent, PrPSc, has been identified by immunocytochemistry testing in the gastrointestinal tract (in Peyer's patches and in autonomic plexuses) and in various lymphoid tissues of sheep with scrapie.[134,135] Replication of the agent takes place in lymphoid tissues, including the spleen.[131,132]

EPIDEMIOLOGY. Scrapie occurs endemically in sheep flocks worldwide.[136-138] Sheep are the natural host of scrapie, but the infection can be maintained in goats that have no direct contact with sheep, indicating both lateral and vertical transmission of the agent in that species.[122,123,136,139] Scrapie cases usually occur sporadically in infected flocks. Only one or a few animals are affected at any given time. Outbreaks with up to 40% of animals affected in a flock have been linked to the use of infected vaccines[140] or to the introduction of scrapie by an infected animal in a previously uninfected and sensitive sheep population. The route of natural infection is presumed to be oral; the route of excretion and the means of transfer of the agent between sheep is unknown.[127] Lambing time is known to be a particularly high risk interval for infection for the young. Contamination of pastures with placentas from infected ewes probably is an important reservoir of the infectious agent in nature.[121,141,142]

Although there is no known breed predisposition to scrapie, the genetic make-up of the host controls differences in susceptibility and resistance to scrapie in various breeds.[120,143,144] The molecular basis of this resistance is largely controlled by the PrP gene.[145] The gene responsible originally was thought to determine the incubation period of scrapie and was called *sip.* This gene is now known to be the prion protein gene. Polymorphisms at three codons of this gene appear to be the main determinants of the susceptibility of sheep to scrapie.[146,147] According to current evidence, the genotype $VV_{136}RR_{154}QQ_{171}$ (or $AA_{136}RR_{154}QQ_{171}$ in some breeds) is most susceptible and the genotype $AA_{136}RR_{154}RR_{171}$ is totally resistant.[148] The potential relevance of other polymorphisms and other genetic factors is unknown. Selection of scrapie-resistant sheep flocks is possible, either on the basis of pedigree and phenotypic expression

of the disease[120] or by the selection of rams of "resistant" PrP genotypes.[148] "Genetic resistance" may confer resistance to disease and not resistance to infection, in which case some genotypes of sheep could act as asymptomatic carriers of scrapie.

TREATMENT AND PROGNOSIS. Scrapie is a fatal and irreversible disease.

DIAGNOSIS AND PATHOLOGY

In Vivo Diagnostic Tests. Immunohistochemistry testing may show PrPSc in biopsies of the lymphoid tissue of tonsils or nictitating membranes, allowing for diagnosis of infection in live animals.[149,150] However, these tests may show a negative result in scrapie cases, and their interpretation requires a high degree of experience. Further research is in progress to increase the sensitivity of PrPSc tests. Newer tests also are being developed to detect PrPSc in blood and cerebrospinal fluid (CSF).[151-153]

DIFFERENTIAL DIAGNOSIS. Nervous system diseases that could be confused with scrapie include pseudorabies, rabies, Borna encephalitis, listeriosis, polioencephalomalacia, lead poisoning, parasitic migration in the CNS (coenurosis), brain tumors, brain abscess, maedi–visna virus infection, vitamin A deficiency, pregnancy toxemia, and other metabolic imbalances. When pruritus is the only clinical sign, skin diseases such as psoroptic and sarcoptic mange, ringworm, myiasis, pediculosis, and atopy may be considered as differential diagnoses. A number of such alternate treatable conditions may be differentiated from scrapie by appropriate antemortem tests such as microscopic and microbiologic examination of skin scrapings, CSF analysis, and blood biochemistry profiles. An apparent response to therapy may be observed initially in early scrapie cases because of the insidious nature of the illness. Scrapie patients may appear to recover and later have relapses. This must be kept in mind whenever specific therapy for another suspected illness appears initially to be successful but is followed by relapse. When therapy of an alternate condition fails, the final diagnosis must rely on detailed examination of appropriate postmortem samples.

POSTMORTEM DIAGNOSIS. Microscopic examination of the brain and spinal cord is the classic diagnostic method for scrapie. It is possible only when tissues are collected soon after death, before autolytic changes take place. Neuronal vacuolation and PrP deposits are found in specific brain nuclei.[154-159] In autolyzed tissues, PrPSc can be identified by immunohistochemistry testing, Western blot tests, or ALISA.[114,115,159-161]

CONTROL. Because there is no effective treatment for scrapie, control measures designed to prevent the spread of the disease are especially important. Scrapie is a reportable disease. Eradication measures vary from country to country.[103,162] Animals suspected of having scrapie are slaughtered and destroyed, and contaminated pastures or paddocks may be left empty of livestock. However, it is not known if the scrapie agent is inactivated in the environment. Contaminated stalls, corrals, and sheds should be disinfected with sodium hypochlorite diluted at 4% available chlorine. In the United States and Canada, scrapie-affected animals and their families are destroyed, and their flocks are quarantined.[162] In countries that lack established control procedures, lines of sheep with natural resistance to the development of clinical scrapie have been selected.[163] These sheep do not develop the clinical signs of scrapie, but they may have a chronic asymptomatic infection that could spread to sheep of susceptible genotypes.[120,163,164]

PUBLIC HEALTH CONSIDERATIONS. Although scrapie has been endemic in various areas of the world for more than two centuries, epidemiologic studies have not shown any correlation between the incidence of Creutzfeldt-Jakob disease in human beings and that of scrapie in sheep.[165] It nevertheless is wise to take precautions to minimize the potential for

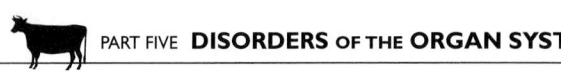

human exposure to scrapie. There is concern that BSE could have become endemic in sheep of certain countries as a result of consumption of infected feedstuffs and that BSE would be identical to scrapie in such populations.[166] In an ongoing study of BSE transmitted to sheep, the clinical signs of BSE in sheep of the Romney breed have been identical to those of scrapie in sheep of the most sensitive PrP genotype (the only genotype affected to date).[167]

REFERENCES

95. Wells GAH et al: A novel progressive spongiform encephalopathy in cattle, *Vet Rec* 121:419-420, 1987.
96. Prusiner SB: Molecular biology of prion diseases, *Science* 252:1515-1521, 1991.
97. Prusiner SB: Review article: prions and neurodegenerative diseases, *N Engl J Med* 317:1571-1598, 1987.
98. Prusiner SB et al: Transgenetic studies implicate interactions between homologous PrP isoforms in scrapie prion replication, *Cell* 63:673-686, 1990.
99. Braun U, Pusterla N, Schicker E: Bovine spongiform encephalopathy: diagnostic approach and clinical findings, *Compend Cont Educ Pract Vet* 20:S270-S278, 1998.
100. Berthelin-Baker C, Austin A: Transmissible spongiform encephalopathies: clinical features, *Proc ACVIM Forum* 17:277-280, 1999.
100a. Heim D: Personal communication, Bern, Switzerland, 1999.
101. Wells GAH et al: Preliminary observations on the pathogenesis of experimental bovine spongiform encephalopathy (BSE): an update, *Vet Rec* 142:103-106, 1998.
102. Wells GAH et al: Limited detection of sternal bone marrow infectivity in the clinical phase of experimental bovine spongiform encephalopathy, *Vet Rec* 144:292-294, 1999.
103. Wells GAH, Wilesmith JW: The neuropathology and epidemiology of bovine spongiform encephalopathy, *Brain Pathol* 5:91-103, 1995.
104. British Ministry of Agriculture, Fisheries, and Food: Bovine spongiform encephalopathy in Great Britain: a progress report, England, 2000, Ministry of Agriculture, Fisheries, and Food.
104a. Nettleton PF et al: The production and survival of lambs persistently infected with a border disease virus, *Comp Immunol Microbiol Infect Dis* 15:179-188, 1992.
105. Bruce ME et al: Transmissions to mice indicate that "new variant" CJD is caused by the BSE agent, *Nature* 389:498-501, 1997.
106. Hill AF et al: The same prion strain causes vCJD and BSE, *Nature* 389:448-450, 1997.
106a. Anonymous: Monthly Creutzfeldt-Jakob disease statistics, Oct 2, 2000, Department of Health, United Kingdom.
107. Haritani M, Spencer YI, Wells GAH: Hydrated autoclave pretreatment enhancement of prion protein immunoreactivity in formalin-fixed, bovine spongiform encephalopathy–affected brain, *Acta Neuropathol (Berl)* 87:86-90, 1994.
108. Wells GAH, Spencer YI, Haritani M: Configurations and topographic distribution of PrP in the central nervous system in bovine spongiform encephalopathy: an immunohistochemical study, *Ann NY Acad Sci* 724:350-352, 1994.
109. Simmons MM et al: BSE in Great Britain: consistency of the neuro-histopathological findings in two random annual samples of clinically suspect cases, *Vet Rec* 138:175-177, 1996.
110. Orge L et al: Similarity of the lesion profile of BSE in Portuguese cattle to that described in British cattle, *Vet Rec* 147:486-488, 2000.
111. Jeffrey M: Neurohistopathological observations on bovine spongiform encephalopathy submissions in Scotland, *State Vet J* 44:151-160, 1990.
112. Wells GAH, McGill IS: Recently described scrapielike encephalopathies of animals: case definitions, *Res Vet Sci* 53:1-10, 1992.
113. Collinge J et al: Molecular analysis of prion strain variation and the aetiology of "new variant" CJD, *Nature* 383:685-690, 1996.
114. Somerville RA et al: Biochemical typing of scrapie strains, *Nature* 386:564, 1997.
115. Grassi J et al: Specific determination of the proteinase K–resistant form of the prion protein using two-site immunometric assays: application to the postmortem diagnosis of BSE, *Proceedings of the Symposium on the Characterisation and Diagnosis of Prion Diseases in Animals and Man*, Tübingen, Germany, Sept 23-25, 1999.
116. Oesch B et al: Detection of disease-specific PrP for routine diagnosis of BSE and scrapie, *Proceedings of the Symposium on the Characterisation and Diagnosis of Prion Diseases in Animals and Man*, Tübingen, Germany, Sept 23-25, 1999.
117. Woodgate SL: Pilot plant studies in BSE/scrapie deactivation, *Proceedings of a Seminar in the CEC Agricultural Research Programme*, Brussels, 1990.
118. Gordon WS: Advances in veterinary research: louping ill, tick-borne fever, and scrapie, *Vet Rec* 58:516-520, 1946.
119. Hunter GD, Millson GC: Studies on the heat stability and chromatographic behavior of the scrapie agent, *J Gen Microbiol* 37:251-258, 1964.
120. Taylor DM et al: Effect of rendering procedures on the scrapie agent, *Vet Rec* 141:643-649, 1997.

121. Parry HB: Scrapie: a transmissible and hereditary disease of sheep, *Heredity* 17:75-103, 1962.
121a. D'Angelo A: Personal communication, Department of Pathology, School of Veterinary Medicine, Turin, Italy.
122. Brotherson JG et al: Spread of scrapie by contact to goats and sheep, *J Comp Pathol* 78:9-17, 1968.
123. Hadlow WJ et al: Virologic and neurohistologic findings in dairy goats affected with natural scrapie, *Vet Pathol* 17:187-199, 1980.
124. Harcourt RA: Naturally occurring scrapie in goats, *Vet Rec* 94:504, 1974.
125. Pattison IH: The spread of scrapie by contact between affected and healthy sheep, goats, or mice, *Vet Rec* 76:333-336, 1964.
126. Clark AM, Moar JAE: Scrapie: a clinical assessment, *Vet Rec* 130:377-378, 1992.
127. Hoinville LJ: A review of the epidemiology of scrapie in sheep, *Rev Sci Tech* 15:827-852, 1996.
128. Detwiler L: *Rev Sci Tech* 11:491-537, 1992.
129. Carp RI et al: Interaction of scrapie agent and cells of the lymphoreticular system, *Arch Virol* 136:255-268, 1994.
130. Brown KL et al: Scrapie replication in lymphoid tissues depends on prion protein-expressing follicular dendritic cells, *Nat Med* 5:1308-1312, 1999.
131. Kimberlin RH, Walker CA: Pathogenesis of mouse scrapie: dynamics of agent replication in spleen, spinal cord, and brain after infection by different routes, *J Comp Pathol* 89:551-562, 1979.
132. Somerville RA et al: Immunodetection of PrPSc in spleens of some scrapie-infected sheep but not BSE-infected cows, *J Gen Virol* 78:2389-2396, 1997.
133. Beekes M, Baldauf E, Diringer H: Sequential appearance and accumulation of pathognomonic markers in the central nervous system of hamsters orally infected with scrapie, *J Gen Virol* 77:1925-1934, 1996.
134. Van Keulen LJM et al: Immunohistochemical detection of prion protein in lymphoid tissues of sheep with natural scrapie, *J Clin Microbiol* 34:1228-1231, 1996.
135. Van Keulen LJM et al: Scrapie-associated prion protein in the gastrointestinal tract of sheep with natural scrapie, *J Comp Pathol* 121:55-63, 1999.
136. Pattison IH: Scrapie in the Welsh mountain breed of sheep and its experimental transmission to goats, *Vet Rec* 77:1388-1390, 1965.
137. Martin WB, Stamp JT: Slow virus infections in sheep, *Br Vet J* 136:290-295, 1980.
138. Zlotnik I, Katiyar RD: The occurrence of scrapie disease in sheep of the remote Himalayan foothills, *Vet Rec* 73:543-544, 1961.
139. Dickinson AG, Stamp JT, Renwick CC: Maternal and lateral transmission of scrapie in sheep, *J Comp Pathol* 84:19-25, 1974.
140. D'Angelo A et al: Scrapie in Italy: clinical aspects, *Proceedings of the Fourteenth Annual ESVN Symposium*, Turin, Italy, 2000.
141. Hourrigan JL, Klingsporn AL: Scapie: studies on vertical and horizontal transmission. In Gibbs CJ, ed: *Bovine spongiform encephalopathy: the BSE dilemma*, New York, 1996, Springer-Verlag.
142. Race RE, Jenny A, Sutton D: Scrapie infectivity and proteinase K–resistant prion protein in sheep placenta, brain, spleen and lymph node: implications for transmission and antemortem diagnosis, *J Infect Dis* 178:949-953, 1998.
143. Parry HB: Elimination of natural scrapie in sheep by sire genotype selection, *Nature* 277:127-129, 1979.
144. Kimberlin RH: Aetiology and genetic control of natural scrapie, *Nature* 278:303-304, 1979.
145. Carlson GA et al: Linkage of prion protein and scrapie incubation time genes, *Cell* 46:503-511, 1986.
146. Hunter N: Scrapie, *Mol Biotechnol* 9:225-234, 1998.
147. Hunter N, Cairns D: Scrapie-free Merino and poll Dorset sheep from Australia and New Zealand have normal frequencies of scrapie-susceptible PrP genes, *J Gen Virol* 79:2079-2082, 1998.
148. Dawson M et al: Guidance on the use of PrP genotyping as an aid to the control of clinical scrapie, *Vet Rec* 142:623-625, 1998.
149. O'Rourke KI et al: Preclinical detection of PrPSc in nictitating membrane lymphoid tissue of sheep, *Vet Rec* 142:489-491, 1998.
150. Schreuder BEC et al: Tonsillar biopsy and PrPSc detection in the preclinical diagnosis of scrapie, *Vet Rec* 142:564-568, 1998.
151. Schmerr MJ et al: Use of capillary eletrophoresis and fluorescent-labeled peptides to detect the abnormal prion protein in the blood of animals that are infected with a transmissible spongiform encephalopathy, *J Chromatogr A* 853:207-214, 1999.
152. Giese A et al: Putting prions into focus: ultrasensitive detection of pathological prion protein aggregates by fluorescence correlation spectroscopy, *Proceedings of the Symposium on Characterisation and Diagnosis of Prion Diseases in Animals and Man*, Tübingen, Germany, Sept 23-25, 1999.
153. Tshoeke S et al: Analysis of PrPSc deposition in human and animal prion diseases by PET blot, *Proceedings of the Symposium on Characterisation and Diagnosis of Prion Diseases in Animals and Man*, Tübingen, Germany, Sept 23-25, 1999.
154. Beck E, Daniel PM, Parry HB: Degeneration of the cerebellar and hypothalamoneurohypophyseal systems in sheep with scrapie and its relationship to human system degeneration, *Brain* 87:153-176, 1964.
155. Palmer AC: Wallerian-type degeneration in sheep scrapie, *Vet Rec* 82:729-731, 1968.
156. Summers BA, Cummings JF, De Lahunta A: *Veterinary Neuropathology*, St Louis, 1995, Mosby, pp 136-139.

157. Katz JB et al: Assessment of western immunoblotting for the confirmatory diagnosis of ovine scrapie and bovine spongiform encephalopathy (BSE), *J Vet Diagn Invest* 4:447-449, 1992.

158. Van Keulen LJM et al: Immunohistochemical detection and localization of prion protein in brain tissue of sheep with natural scrapie, *Vet Pathol* 32:299-308, 1995.

159. Mohri S et al: Immunodetection of a disease-specific PrP fraction in scrapie-affected sheep and BSE-affected cattle, *Vet Rec* 131:537-539, 1992.

160. Barnard G et al: The measurement of aggregated prion protein in bovine brain tissue by DELFIA, *Proceedings of the Symposium on Characterisation and Diagnosis of Prion Diseases in Animals and Man*, Tübingen, Germany, Sept 23-25, 1999 (poster).

161. Miller JM et al: Immunohistochemical detection of prion protein in sheep with scrapie, *J Vet Diagn Invest* 5:309-316, 1993.

162. US Department of Agriculture, Animal Disease Eradication Division: *Eradicating scrapie of sheep*, Washington, DC, 1965, US Government Printing Office.

163. Hoare M, Davies DC, Pattison IH: Experimental production of scrapie-resistant Swaledale sheep, *Vet Rec* 101:482-484, 1977.

164. Nussbaum RE, Henderson WM, Pattison IH: The establishment of sheep flocks of predictable susceptibility to experimental scrapie, *Res Vet Sci* 18:49-58, 1975.

165. Chatelan J et al: Epidemiologic comparisons between Creutzfeldt-Jakob disease and scrapie in France during the 12-year period 1968-1979, *J Neurol Sci* 51:329-337, 1981.

166. World Health Organization: Consultation on public health and animal-transmissible spongiform encephalopathies: epidemiology, risk, and research requirements, Geneva, Dec 1-3, 1999, WHO.

167. Berthelin-Baker CF et al: Unusual neurological diseases in ruminants: video presentations and discussion, *Proc ACVIM Forum* 18:248-249, 2000.

MURRURUNDI DISEASE

LISLE W. GEORGE

Murrurundi disease occurs in the sheep of New South Wales.[168] The condition is a spongiform encephalopathy that has some similarities to scrapie, humpyback, and Coonabarabran disease; however, the three conditions are pathologically differentiable. Murrurundi disease occurs in sheep between 1 and 5 years of age. The initial clinical sign is posterior paraparesis, with progression to paraplegia after several months. No wool breakage occurs in affected animals. Microscopic changes include multiple cytoplasmic vacuolation of the neurons and chromatolysis of Nissl substance. The cause of the disease is unknown.

REFERENCE

168. Harley WJ, Loomis LN: Murrurundi disease: an encephalopathy of sheep, *Aust Vet J* 57:399-400, 1981.

HUMPYBACK DISEASE

LISLE W. GEORGE

Humpyback disease affects Merino wethers of Australia. The neurologic signs of the condition are not usually observed until the sheep are gathered for shearing. The affected animals lag behind the flock and show posterior ataxia. They may fall or stand quietly with the head lowered and the back arched; hence the common name of the condition. The clinical signs include rear limb ataxia, stiffness of the rear limbs, knuckling of the fetlocks, arched back, and recumbency. After resting for several minutes, affected sheep arise and travel for a short distance but soon are immobilized again. Eventually the disease leads to recumbency and death. Affected animals worsen over several years.[169] Wallerian degeneration of the spinal cord is the major pathologic change seen in affected sheep; however, the severity of microscopic changes do not correlate well with the clinical signs. The cause of the condition is unknown.[170,171]

REFERENCES

169. O'Sullivan BM: Humpyback of sheep: clinical and pathological observations, *Aust Vet J* 52:414-418, 1976.

170. Pearse BHG, Peucker SKJ, Hoey WA: Hyperthermia in Merino wethers affected with humpyback disease, *Aust Vet J* 69:94-95, 1992.

171. Dunster PJ, McKenzie RA: Does *Solanum esuriale* cause humpyback in sheep? *Aust Vet J* 64:119-120, 1987.

EQUINE HERPES MYELOENCEPHALOPATHY

JOHN SCHLIPF

Eight types of herpesvirus affect horses, donkeys, and possibly other equids.[172,173] Of these, equine herpesvirus type 1 (EHV-1) is clinically important because it sometimes is associated with neurologic disease.[172] EHV-1 is more commonly associated with reproductive disorders, neonatal diseases, and respiratory disease.[172,174,175] Equine herpesvirus type 4 is primarily associated with respiratory disease and is discussed extensively in Chapter 29.[174] Equine herpes myeloencephalopathy is the result of ischemic damage to the spinal cord and not viral infection of neurons.[172]

CLINICAL SIGNS. Acute onset of ataxia and tetraparesis of variable severity most commonly characterizes the neurologic form of EHV-1.[175,176] Signs usually appear between 6 and 10 days after infection.[175] The severity of clinical signs can range from subtle neurologic deficits to complete recumbency. Other signs also may be seen, including nasal discharge, limb edema, colic, ocular lesions, and anorexia.[172,174-177] The animal may be febrile at presentation, but most are normothermic.[172,175] Coughing and nasal discharge sometimes accompany the neurologic deficits or may have been present in the preceding 2 weeks.[177]

The neurologic signs reflect damage to the white matter of the spinal cord, and they include ataxia, paresis, conscious proprioceptive deficits, urinary incontinence, flaccid tail and anal tone, and diminished perineal sensation.[172,175,176] Hind limbs are more severely affected, and deficits usually are symmetric. Bladder atony and dysuria frequently occur, and the associated dribbling of urine leads to secondary perineal scalding. Anal sphincter tone also is diminished, which may result in a distended rectum.

Cranial nerve deficits, including seizures, blindness, and vestibular signs, have been reported with EHV-1 infection.[177] Ocular lesions also may be present, such as mydriasis, hypopyon, uveitis, and optic neuritis.[172,175,178,179]

The clinical signs typically stabilize within 48 hours, although progression varies. Some patients continue to deteriorate and eventually die or are euthanized. Most horses begin to improve within the first 5 to 7 days and ultimately make a full recovery, although the recovery may take months. A patient that does not become recumbent has a much better prognosis.[176,178]

DIAGNOSIS. A tentative diagnosis can be made based on characteristic neurologic signs, the history, and supporting findings on the physical examination. A cerebrospinal fluid (CSF) analysis that shows an increase in protein and a normal or slightly increased nucleated cell count (albuminocytologic dissociation) is the classic CSF change seen with EHV-1 infection.[172,175,180] Cerebrospinal xanthochromia may also be seen.[176] The protein level may be normal, which does not necessarily rule out EHV-1. Occasionally, early in the disease the CSF may be normal or may show only mild abnormalities.[172]

A fourfold or greater increase between acute and convalescent serum neutralizing (SN) antibody titers is consistent with a diagnosis of EHV-1 infection.[180] SN titers usually are the easiest and most economic to perform. Because they rise quite rapidly and reach a level much higher with natural infection compared with vaccination, a fourfold rise in the SN titer may not be seen, especially if collection of the acute sample was delayed.[172,178] A single titer of 1:256 or higher is highly suggestive of recent infection.[175,180] Complement fixation (CF) titers decline quite rapidly after infection, requiring sample collection early in the course of the disease. A titer

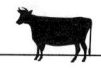
higher than 1:16 is consistent with recent infection.[180] It is important to know which assay the diagnostic laboratory uses, because interpretation of the results differs depending on the test performed.

Viral isolation attempts from the buffy coat of an ethylenediamine tetraacetic acid (EDTA) tube and nasopharyngeal swabs may yield a positive result for EHV-1 for approximately 10 to12 days after infection.[172] It is critical that samples be handled appropriately and transported to the laboratory as soon as possible. A viral transport medium is necessary and should be available from the diagnostic laboratory. Viral isolation from the CSF is unrewarding because there does not appear to be direct viral infection of neurons.[176]

PATHOPHYSIOLOGY. An apparent immune complex vasculitis and thrombosis in arterioles of the spinal cord lead to segmental spinal cord ischemia. Although the lesions are characteristic of a type III (Arthus) hypersensitivity, an immune-mediated pathogenesis has not been conclusively demonstrated.[175] However, the theory of an immune-mediated pathogenesis is supported by the finding that horses vaccinated within the previous 12 months were shown to be nine to 14 times more likely to develop the neurologic form of EHV-1 infection.[175] The vasculitis may be the result of viral infection of the CNS endothelium by circulating infected leukocytes.[176] The CNS vascular endothelium appears to be the primary sight for infection. Viral replication within neural tissue has not been definitively demonstrated.[172,175]

EPIDEMIOLOGY. Herpesvirus infection is enzootic in the horse population. Infection usually occurs via the respiratory or intestinal epithelium after the animal comes in contact with the virus in fluids from an abortion or in ocular, nasal, or respiratory tract secretions.[175,178] Most horses become infected before 1 year of age. As is the case in most herpesvirus infections, the virus is capable of evading the horse's immune system and can develop latency.[175,178,181] Sites considered likely for latency are the lymphoid tissue and the trigeminal ganglion.[181,182]

Equine herpes myeloencephalopathy is rare, but cases have been reported worldwide.[175] The existence of a neurovirulent form of the virus has been suspected, but the differences in the strains isolated from neurologic syndromes are not significant enough to warrant additional classification.[172] However, equine herpes myeloencephalopathy outbreaks have been reported, lending support to the idea of a neurovirulent form.[176,178]

Animals of any age or gender are susceptible; pregnant or lactating mares are most often affected.[172,175] Foals are rarely affected with the neurologic form of EHV-1 infection.[175] There appears to be some seasonal variation, because more cases are seen during the spring and winter months. Stress-associated recrudescence of latent infections and shedding without clinical signs are important in the development of equine herpes myeloencephalopathy in a closed population. The virus may be shed for 3 weeks or longer after infection. A morbidity rate of up to 90% and a mortality rate of up to 40% have been reported.[175,176] There are no reports of equine herpes myeloencephalopathy associated with any modified live virus vaccine currently approved for use in horses.[175]

NECROPSY FINDINGS. Gross and histologic lesions are not always limited to the central nervous system.[172,176] Ocular lesions have been reported, including hypopyon, iritis, and chorioretinitis. Cystitis and scrotal edema may be present.[172,175] Focal areas of hemorrhage may be found throughout the brain and spinal cord parenchyma and meninges. Vasculitis of the small arteries and veins of the spinal cord white matter and of the gray and white matter of the brain results in ischemic lesions in the CNS.[183,184] Equine herpesvirus is infrequently isolated from the CNS during a postmortem examination.[180]

TREATMENT. Supportive care is the most important aspect of treatment for equine herpes myeloencephalopathy.[172,175,176,180] Measures include bladder decompression twice a day for cases with bladder atony and urinary incontinence, evacuation of the rectum, enteral or parenteral nutritional support, and administration of intravenous or oral fluids. The horse may require support in a sling.

Administration of antiinflammatory drugs soon after the onset of neurologic signs may be beneficial. Corticosteroids have been used because of the possible immune-mediated pathogenesis, but no objective data are available evaluating the efficacy of these. Dexamethasone (0.05 to 0.1 mg/kg IV) can be given every 12 to 24 hours for 3 to 5 days, with the dosage then tapered for 1 to 3 days.[180] The possibility of viral reactivation is quite unlikely at the recommended dosage.[175] Dimethyl sulfoxide (DMSO) (0.25 to 0.1 mg/kg by slow intravenous infusion) given every 12 to 24 hours is routinely used when treating neurologic disease, although its efficacy has not been documented.[172]

Use of antibiotics should be considered if the horse is recumbent or has urinary tract involvement or if respiratory tract signs are present. Antiviral agents have been recommended based on their use in humans for herpes simplex virus encephalitis. There is insufficient evidence to recommend the use of antiviral agents for EHV-1 infection in horses.[180]

PREVENTION. Currently no prophylactic measures for or methods of preventing equine herpes myeloencephalopathy are available. The vaccines currently used to prevent EHV-1 respiratory and abortion syndromes do not claim to prevent equine herpes myeloencephalopathy. Vaccination may reduce the incidence of the other EHV-1–related diseases and thereby reduce exposure to the virus and the risk of developing equine herpes myeloencephalopathy. Vaccination in the face of an outbreak is very debatable[172]; viremia may be reduced or prevented as a result of vaccination, but an increase in antibody levels may be partly responsible for or may play a role in the development of the neurologic form.

Management practices may reduce the risk of introducing or disseminating EHV-1 infection. Such practices include isolating all new arrivals for at least 3 weeks and maintaining distinct herd groups based on age, gender, and occupation. Pregnant brood mares should be kept from the general population as much as possible. Minimizing stress may reduce the likelihood of recrudescence of a latent infection.

REFERENCES

172. Donaldson MT, Sweeney CR: Equine herpes myeloencephalopathy, *Compend Cont Educ Pract Vet* 19:864-882, 1997.
173. Borchers K, Frolich K: Antibodies against equine herpesviruses in free-ranging mountain zebras from Namibia, *J Wildl Dis* 33:812-817, 1197.
174. Ostlund EN: The equine herpesviruses, *Vet Clin North Am (Equine Pract)* 9:283-294, 1993.
175. Wilson WD: Equine herpesvirus 1 myeloencephalopathy, *Vet Clin North Am (Equine Pract)* 13:53-72, 1997.
176. Donaldson MT, Sweeney CR: Herpesvirus myeloencephalopathy in horses: 11 cases (1982-1996), *J Am Vet Med Assoc* 213:671-675, 1998.
177. Friday PA et al: Ataxia and paresis with equine herpesvirus type 1 infection in a herd of riding school horses, *J Vet Intern Med* 14:197-201, 2000.
178. McCartan CG et al: Clinical, serological and virological characteristics of an outbreak of paresis and neonatal foal disease due to equine herpesvirus 1 on a stud farm, *Vet Rec* 136:7-12, 1995.
179. Greenwood RES, Simson ARB: Clinical report of a paralytic syndrome affecting stallions, mares, and foals on a thoroughbred stud farm, *Equine Vet J* 12:113-117, 1980.
180. Scarratt WK, Friday PA: Diagnosis and management of equine herpesvirus 1 myeloencephalitis, *Proc ACVIM Forum* 18:178-179, 2000.
181. Edigton N, Welch HM, Griffiths L: The prevalence of latent equid herpesviruses in the tissues of 40 abattoir horses, *Equine Vet J* 26:140-142, 1994.
182. Welch HM et al: Latent equid herpesviruses 1 and 4: detection and distinction using the polymerase chain reaction and cocultivation from lymphoid tissues, *J Gen Virol* 73:261-268, 1992.
183. Whitwell KE, Blunden AS: Pathological findings in horses dying during an outbreak of the paralytic form of equid herpesvirus type 1 (EHV-1) infection, *Equine Vet J* 24:13-19, 1992.

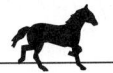

184. Charlton KM et al: Meningoencephalomyelitis in horses associated with equine herpesvirus 1 infection, *Vet Pathol* 13:59-68, 1976.

PSEUDORABIES (Mad Itch; Aujeszky's Disease)

DEFINITION AND ETIOLOGY. Pseudorabies is caused by a neurotropic α-herpes (deoxyribonucleic acid [DNA]) virus. The name is derived from the clinical resemblance of pseudorabies and rabies. Pseudorabies is an acute encephalitic disease of ruminants. The primary host of the virus probably is the pig, in which the infection frequently is asymptomatic.[185] Horses and human beings are resistant to pseudorabies virus infection.

CLINICAL SIGNS. Pseudorabies has an acute to peracute course in ruminants. The incubation period ranges from 90 to 156 hours, and the duration of illness ranges from 8 to 72 hours.[186] Because of the short incubation period, animals may die suddenly without premonitory signs.[187] In more slowly developing cases, the first clinical sign often is paresthesia. Dermal abrasions, swelling, pruritus, and alopecia occur at the site of virus inoculation.[186] Affected animals also have fever and may bellow, bloat, stamp their feet, salivate, and chew the tongue.[188] Other signs are ataxia, conscious proprioceptive deficits, circling, nystagmus, and strabismus. Aggression may be seen in some instances, but most affected animals become depressed.[188-190] Progression of the disease is associated with additional signs of diffuse cerebral dysfunction, which include twitching, hyperesthesia, tenesmus, wild, spasmodic kicking, licking of the nostrils, continuous mastication, sweating, vocalization, semicoma, coma, convulsions, opisthotonos, hyperpnea, tachypnea, or slow, irregular respirations.[191] Clinical disease lasts longest in animals with pruritus of the head.[192] Most affected animals die within 2 days of the onset of clinical signs. The clinical signs of pseudorabies in cattle closely resemble those of rabies, polioencephalomalacia, salt poisoning, meningitis, lead poisoning, hypomagnesemia, and enterotoxemia.

CLINICAL PATHOLOGY. The pseudorabies virus can be isolated from the pharyngeal or nasal secretions of affected animals and can be easily cultured from infected nervous tissues. Strains of pseudorabies virus are antigenically distinct from other herpesviruses, but they share common antigens with the infectious bovine rhinotracheitis (IBR) virus. Heterospecific antibodies to the IBR virus can cross-neutralize the pseudorabies virus and can confound serologic tests. For virus culture, tissues should be collected from the sensory parts of the spinal cord. Segments serving the pruritic sites should be collected preferentially because these areas contain the highest concentration of virus. The cerebrospinal fluid (CSF) changes of pseudorabies infection have not been reported; however, changes consistent with other encephalitic herpesvirus infections are likely. These include pleocytosis (50 to 200 mononuclear cells per deciliter) and an increased protein concentration (100 to 200 mg/dl).

PATHOPHYSIOLOGY. Ruminants are susceptible to pseudorabies infection after intradermal, subcutaneous, intranasal, or oral exposure to the virus. Intravenous injection of the virus into cattle produces an early infection of the autonomic ganglia, which apparently is followed by dissemination into the central nervous system (CNS). After subcutaneous, oral, or nasal infection, the virus spreads centripetally to the CNS by axonoplasmic transport. During the acute infection the virus may be present in the nasal mucosa, secretions, and saliva.

EPIDEMIOLOGY. Pseudorabies has a worldwide distribution and is economically important because of the regulatory quarantine and other restrictions imposed on animals from affected herds. Outbreaks have occurred in cattle in the United States, Europe, Australia, New Zealand, Latin America, and South America. The viral infection in cattle is perpetuated partly by the occurrence of latent infections in the trigeminal ganglia of pigs,[193] which can be recrudesced by stressful conditions.[193] Occasional spillover of the virus from swine into ruminants occurs because of the proximity of the two species in many livestock operations.[187,192] Sheep have been infected by modified live virus vaccines targeted for use in swine.[194] In one case a contaminated syringe used to administer modified live pseudorabies vaccine to swine transmitted the disease to sheep.[195]

Latency of the viral infection in ruminants is not an important mechanism for perpetuation of an outbreak. In ruminants the pseudorabies virus can be shed in the saliva, oral secretions, and mucous membranes for only 6 days after infection. For this reason, direct spread of the virus between infected and uninfected cattle is not likely.[192] Wild mammals such as raccoons may play a role in pseudorabies survival and transmission; rats, however, develop transient infections and do not appear to transmit or perpetuate the virus.[196-198] The pseudorabies virus may survive in contaminated meat products for up to 7 weeks. The role of this prolonged survival in perpetuating outbreaks in ruminants is unknown. Pathogenicity differences of the virus for cattle have been correlated with the type of syntcitium formation by the virus in tissue cultures.[198] The role of these strain differences in the perpetuation and dissemination of the disease is unclear.

NECROPSY FINDINGS. The macroscopic changes that occur in animals infected with the pseudorabies virus are alopecia, edema, and hemorrhage at the pruritic site. A mild congestion and edema of the regional lymph nodes and a generalized increase in the amount of CSF occur.[186] The microscopic changes include perivascular cuffing, interfascicular edema, nonsuppurative encephalitis, gliosis, neuronal degeneration, and eosinophilic intranuclear (Cowdry type A) inclusion bodies. The lesions are most pronounced in the dorsal nerve rootlets and the dorsal horn.

TREATMENT. There is no treatment for pseudorabies. Most affected ruminants die, but recoveries have been reported.[189]

PREVENTION. The most effective method of preventing pseudorabies virus infection is eliminating the exposure of ruminants to swine. Contaminated pens can be disinfected with 10% sodium hypochlorite solution, quaternary ammonium compounds, tamed iodines, or phenolics.[199] At least 5 minutes of contact time should be allowed before the disinfectant is rinsed from the contaminated surfaces. Fumigation with formaldehyde for 6 hours effectively kills the virus, as does 360 minutes of contact time with ultraviolet light.

REFERENCES

185. Aujeszky A: Uber eine neue infektionskrankheit bei haustieren (a new infectious disease in husbandry animals), *Zentralbl Bakteriol I Abt Orig* 32:353-357, 1902.
186. Dow C, McFerran JB: The pathology of Aujeszky's disease in cattle, *J Comp Pathol* 72:337-347, 1962.
187. Herweijer CH, De Jonge WK: De ziekte van Aujeszky bij de geit, *Tijdschr Diergeneeskd* 102:425-428, 1977.
188. Beasley TR et al: A clinical episode demonstrating variable characteristics of pseudorabies infection in cattle, *Vet Res Commun* 4:125-129, 1980.
189. Hagemoser WA, Hill HT, Moss EW: Nonfatal pseudorabies in cattle, *J Am Vet Med Assoc* 173:205-206, 1978.
190. Crandell RA: Selected animal herpesviruses: new concepts and technologies, *Adv Vet Sci Comp Med* 29:281-327, 1985.
191. Baker JC, Esser MB, Larson VL: Pseudorabies in a goat, *J Am Vet Med Assoc* 607:181, 1982.
192. Bitsch V: A study of outbreaks of Aujeszky's disease in cattle, *Acta Vet Scand* 16:420-433, 1975.
193. Van Oirschot JT, Gielkens ALJ: In vivo and in vitro reactivation of latent pseudorabies virus in pigs born to vaccinated sows, *Am J Vet Res* 45:567-571, 1984.
194. Benfield DA, Libal MC: Pseudorabies in a flock of lambs, *Compend Cont Educ Pract Vet* 8:F116-F118, 1986.
195. Van Alstine WG, Andersen TD, Reed DE: Vaccine-induced pseudorabies in lambs, *J Am Vet Med Assoc* 185:409-410, 1984.

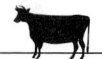

196. Wright JC, Thawley DG: Role of the raccoon in the transmission of pseudorabies: a field and laboratory investigation, *Am J Vet Res* 41:581-583, 1980.
197. Maes RK et al: Pseudorabies virus infections in wild and laboratory rats, *Am J Vet Res* 40:393-396, 1979.
198. Bitsch V: Correlation between the pathogenicity of field strains of Aujeszky's disease virus and their ability to cause cell fusion synctitia formation in cell cultures, *Acta Vet Scand* 21:708-710, 1980.
199. Brown TT: Laboratory evaluation of selected disinfectants as virucidal agents against porcine parvovirus, pseudorabies virus, and transmissible gastroenteritis virus, *Am J Vet Res* 42:1033-1036, 1981.

ALPHAVIRUS AND FLAVIVIRUS ENCEPHALITIS OF HORSES

(Western Equine Encephalomyelitis; Eastern Equine Encephalomyelitis; Venezuelan Equine Encephalomyelitis; Arboviral Encephalitis; Equine Viral Myeloencephalitis; Equine Encephalitis; Equine Sleeping Sickness)

JOHN SCHLIPF

DEFINITION AND ETIOLOGY. The Togaviridae family of arboviruses has been linked to severe and fatal encephalitis in equids for more than 150 years.[200] These viruses are distributed worldwide, but those occurring in the New World have the greatest impact in veterinary medicine.[201] The most prominent genus of the Togaviridae family is the alphaviruses, which cause eastern equine encephalitis (EEE), western equine encephalitis (WEE) and Venezuelan equine encephalitis (VEE).[202] An association between the flaviviruses (family Flaviviridae) and encephalitis has been reported. These viruses, which most often lead to asymptomatic infections,[200] include the Japanese B encephalitis, California encephalitis (snowshoe hare encephalitis), St. Louis encephalitis, Murray Valley encephalitis, Cache Valley, Main Drain, and West Nile viruses.[200,203-206]

Clinically the alphaviruses are most important. There is one EEE virus with two antigenic variants, North American and South American.[207] The VEE complex is one virus with six antigenic subtypes (I through VI). Subtypes IAB and IC are responsible for epizootics. The remaining variants and subtypes exist in sylvatic or enzootic cycles and apparently are nonpathogenic for equids.[200] The WEE complex has seven virus species: WEE, Highland J, Sindbis, Aura, Fort Morgan, Buggy Creek, and Y62-33.[201]

CLINICAL SIGNS. The clinical signs of EEE, WEE, and VEE are not pathognomonic and are indistinguishable from other encephalitides.[208] Fever (38.3° to 41.1° C [101° to 106° F]), anorexia, colic, or a generalized stiffness often is reported early in the course of the disease.[209] Animals infected with EEE, WEE, or VEE often are very obtunded. Signs attributable to spinal cord lesions sometimes are seen before generalized encephalitic signs.[209] A biphasic fever usually is associated with EEE and WEE, corresponding to the emergence of viremia approximately 2 days after infection and then a second fever spike 5 to 7 days later.[200] Initial febrile episodes are not always recognized. Animals with VEE have a consistently elevated temperature during the disease. Western equine encephalitis quite often does not progress beyond these non-specific signs. Eastern equine encephalitis differs in that it typically progresses to severe CNS deficits that occur secondary to diffuse cerebrocortical disease.[210] VEE may cause unapparent infections but does so less often than WEE.[201]

Neurologic signs related to diffuse encephalitis begin to develop approximately 5 days after infection. EEE and WEE have a similar clinical appearance; ataxia, somnolence, conscious proprioceptive deficits, a stiff neck, constant walking, constant chewing movements, and head-pressing may be seen. As the disease progresses, additional signs appear, including apparent blindness and circling, and excitement and aggressive behavior also may develop. As cortical damage worsens, laryngeal, pharyngeal, and tongue paralysis may occur, and loss of brainstem function ensues, leading to head tilt, nystagmus, strabismus, and pupil dilation. VEE may manifest signs similar to those caused by the other encephalitis viruses, or it may produce signs such as epistaxis, pulmonary hemorrhage, oral ulcers, and diarrhea that may be completely unrelated to CNS damage. Seizures may be observed with VEE, WEE, and EEE. The clinical signs may appear to be insignificant, but sudden death can occur.[211-216]

DIAGNOSIS. A definitive antemortem diagnosis is challenging. The clinical signs are often subtle and nonspecific and do not differentiate EEE, WEE, or VEE from other encephalitides.[208] Clinical signs, cerebrospinal fluid (CSF) analysis, clinical pathologic studies, serologic testing, and a corresponding related epidemiologic pattern support a diagnosis of viral encephalitis. Early in the disease peripheral lymphopenia and neutropenia may be detected. Postmortem results provide a definitive answer.

Leukocytosis (50 to more than 100,000 cells/μl) and an elevated protein level (up to 200 mg/dl) in the CSF reflect a generalized encephalitis. Segmented neutrophils usually predominate in cerebrospinal fluid early in the course of the disease. In more chronic disease a mononuclear pleiocytosis occurs.[208,217] CSF immunoglobulin G (IgG) and IgG index are elevated in most cases. The albumin quotient commonly is normal, although it may be elevated if inflammation and damage are sufficient to increase blood-brain or blood-CSF permeability.[208,218]

Serologic testing is helpful in diagnosing viral encephalitis. Antibodies rise rapidly after infection and often are present within 24 hours.[215] Hemagglutination inhibition, complement fixation, serum neutralization assay, and antibody-capture enzyme-linked immunosorbent assay (ELSIA) for IgM can be used to detect antibodies.[208,219] A fourfold rise is diagnostic of an infection. However, a fourfold rise may not be seen in many cases because of the rapid rise in the titer. The initial sample may actually be taken during the peak titer because of this rapid antibody rise, and the convalescent titer may be lower.[219,220] Horses with EEE do not usually live long enough for comparison of paired serum samples.[208] A single sample with an elevated neutralizing antibody, complement fixation, and hemagglutination titer is very likely positive for encephalitis. Comparing hemagglutination titers for WEE and EEE may help differentiate exposure and disease from vaccination. An eightfold difference is considered diagnostic for EEE.[209] If VEE is considered a likely differential diagnosis, an IgM ELISA is available that can identify a specific viral-induced IgM that is not seen in vaccinated horses.[221]

Reverse transcription–polymerase chain reaction assays that are specific for encephalitis viruses show promise for making a rapid diagnosis.[222] Viral isolation from the buffy coat or CSF is unrewarding.[208] Diagnosis in foals is difficult because the half-life of colostral antibodies may be longer than a month.

PATHOPHYSIOLOGY. Muscle tissue is the primary site of initial viral replication after inoculation by means of a mosquito bite. Low numbers of virus are shed after the virus reaches the regional lymph nodes and replicates in neutrophils and macrophages. This may be the extent of the disease progression if the immune system clears this low-level viremia. Viral particles that are not cleared have a predilection for endothelial cells and localize in the spleen and liver and begin to replicate. A resulting high-level viremia leads to CNS infection and initial neurologic signs. Encephalitis develops 3 to 5 days after initial exposure.[223,224]

EPIDEMIOLOGY. Epizootics of eastern and western equine encephalitis occur sporadically throughout the Americas

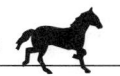

when environmental conditions are favorable. Characteristic geographic range differences exist between EEE, WEE, and VEE, but it is important to note similarities.[201] EEE, WEE, and VEE exist in enzootic cycles with avian or mammalian intermediate hosts. Epizootics involving horses and human beings occur when environmental conditions favor necessary vectors and intermediate hosts. The EEE and WEE viruses require an avian intermediate host in North America. VEE differs in that a genetic mutation of an enzootic viral strain into a virulent epizootic serotype must occur to cause an epizootic. VEE and EEE viruses use small mammals as intermediate hosts in the tropics.[201] Any suspected case should be reported to state health officials.

EEE is recognized primarily in southeastern Canada and the southeastern United States. The range also extends into the Midwest. Outside the United States, EEE has been reported in the Caribbean and in Central and South America.[201] Endemic regions for EEE correspond to those of the vector.[225] There is a seasonal variation, with the incidence peaking in late summer or early fall.[225] In temperate regions such as Florida and South America transmission may be continuous, although the mechanism for maintenance in temperate regions has yet to be identified.[210] Enzootic cycles are maintained by means of the mosquito *Culiseta melanura*. Epizootics are the result of feeding by *Aedes* and *Coquilletidia* spp. The species that transmits EEE varies between geographic regions.[201,226] Infected horses are a dead-end host because the level of viremia that develops is insufficient to infect epizootic hosts.[210]

WEE also occurs throughout most of the Americas. It has been identified in Canada and east of the Mississippi River. In South America extensive epizootics have been reported in Argentina and smaller ones outside of Argentina.[227] The principal enzootic vector is *Culex tarsalis* and the epizootic mosquito vector is an *Aedes* species. Summer epizootics occur when there is a large population of vectors (*Aedes* sp.) and a high level of infection in peridomestic birds. The horse is a terminal host for WEE.[200] Equine cases of WEE precede human cases by several weeks and act as a sentinel for humans.

VEE is the most important alphavirus. The geographic range is primarily South America extending into Central America. The last epizootic in the United States occurred in southern Texas in 1971. Enzootic cycles are maintained via *Culex* genus and small vertebrate hosts.[201] *Aedes* and *Psorophora* mosquito species transmit epizootic viruses IAB and IC.[201] Unlike with WEE and EEE, horses with VEE develop adequate viremia to act as an amplifier of the disease.[200] Respiratory tract secretions have high levels of virus, and direct contact can lead to infection.

NECROPSY FINDINGS. Gross lesions associated with the nervous system usually are not identified in horses euthanized for or dying from encephalitis. The brain may shown discoloration or congestion. Diffuse histopathologic changes include nonseptic suppurative and mononuclear inflammation, perivascular cuffing, astrogliosis, and neuronal degeneration.[228,229] The cerebral cortex, thalamus, and hypothalamus often are most severely affected.[229]

TREATMENT. No specific treatment is available. General supportive care is of utmost importance including providing protection from self-induced trauma. Good bedding reduces the formation of decubital ulcers in a recumbent animal. Antiinflammatory drugs, including flunixin meglumine (1.1 mg/kg SC, IM, or IV given every 12 to 24 hours) or phenylbutazone (4.4 mg/kg IV or PO given every 12 hours) should be administered. Dimethyl sulfoxide (DMSO) (1g/kg in 10% solution IV every 12 to 24 hours) may reduce nervous system inflammation.[230] Maintaining hydration with intravenous balanced electrolyte solutions or oral administration is critical. Depending on the patient's clinical status,

enteral or parenteral nutrition may be indicated, and the horse may need to be supported in a sling. A recumbent patient has a very grave prognosis.

The prognosis is grave to guarded for survival and complete recovery. The mortality rate for horses that develop neurologic signs ranges from 20% to 50% for WEE, 40% to 80% for VEE, and 75% to 100% for EEE.[210,215] Two thirds of animals that survive EEE have residual neurologic deficits,[201] although complete recovery without any neurologic deficits has been reported.[216] Horses with WEE less commonly develop permanent neurologic deficits.

PREVENTION. Vaccinating animals to maintain optimum immunity is the key to preventing viral encephalitis. Monovalent, bivalent, and trivalent vaccines are available. The bivalent vaccine is administered in the spring along with tetanus and the viral respiratory vaccines. Horses in temperate regions where the vectors are able to survive all year should be vaccinated semiannually. Just as important as a good vaccine program is limiting exposure to the vectors. This may be accomplished by eliminating mosquitoes or habitats where they thrive. Protecting horses from mosquitoes with repellents may help. Keeping horses off pastures at dawn and dusk, when mosquitoes are most active, reduces exposure.[231]

REFERENCES

200. Walton TE: Arborviral encephalomyelitis of livestock in the Western Hemisphere, *J Am Vet Med Assoc* 200:1385-1389, 1992.
201. Weaver SC et al: Molecular epidemiological studies of veterinary arborviral encephalitides, *Vet J* 157:123-138, 1999.
202. Calisher CH et al: Proposed antigenic classification of registered arborviruses. I. Togaviridae, alphavirus, *Intervirology* 14:229-232, 1980.
203. Parkin WE: The occurrence and effects of the local strains of the California encephalitis viruses in domestic mammals of Florida, *Am J Trop Med Hyg* 22:788-795, 1973.
204. Bailey CL et al: Isolation of St Louis encephalitis virus from overwintering *Culex pipiens* mosquitoes, *Science* 199:1346-1349, 1978.
205. Campbell J, Hore DE: Isolation of Murray Valley encephalitis virus from sentinel chickens, *Aust Vet J* 64:52-55, 1987.
206. Emmons RW et al: Main drain virus as a cause of equine encephalomyelitis, *J Am Vet Assoc* 183:555-558, 1983.
207. Casals J: Antigenic variants of eastern equine encephalitis virus, *J Exp Med* 119:547-565, 1964.
208. McFarlane D, Guy J, Cornish TB: Immunoperoxidase in formalin-fixed tissue to diagnose eastern equine encephalomyelitis, *Compend Cont Educ Pract Vet* 20:373-376, 1998.
209. Brewer BD, Mayhew IG: Clinicopathologic diagnosis of eastern equine encephalomyelitis, *Proc ACVIM Forum* 8:469-470, 1990.
210. Scott TW, Weaver SC: Eastern equine encephalomyelitis virus: epidemiology and evolution of mosquito transmission, *Adv Virus Res* 37:277-328, 1989.
211. Sponseller ML et al: Field strains of western encephalitis virus in ponies: virologic, clinical, and pathologic observations, *Am J Vet Res* 27:1591-1598, 1966.
212. Doby PB et al: Western encephalitis in Illinois horses and ponies, *J Am Vet Med Assoc* 148:422-427, 1966.
213. Kissling RE, Chamberlain RW: Venezuelan equine encephalitis, *Adv Vet Sci* 11:65-84, 1967.
214. Cox HR, Philip CB, Marsh H: Observations incident to an outbreak of equine encephalomyelitis in the Bitterroot Valley of western Montana, *J Am Vet Med Assoc* 94:225-232, 1938.
215. Gibbs EPJ: Equine viral encephalitis, *Equine Vet J* 8:66-71, 1976.
216. Devine EH, Byrne RJ: A laboratory confirmed case of viral encephalitis (equine type) in a horse in which the animal completely recovered from the disease, *Cornell Vet* 50:494-497, 1960.
217. Mayhew IG: Measurements of the accuracy of clinical diagnoses of equine neurologic disease, *J Vet Intern Med* 5:332-334, 1991.
218. Andrews FM: Cerebrospinal fluid analysis and blood-brain barrier function, *Compend Cont Educ Pract Vet* 20:376-383, 1998.
219. Calisher CH et al: Rapid and specific serodiagnosis of western equine encephalitis virus infection in horses, *Am J Vet Res* 47:1296-1299, 1986.
220. Calisher CH et al: Serodiagnosis of western equine encephalitis virus infections: relationships of antibody titer and test to observed onset of clinical illness, *J Am Vet Med Assoc* 183:438-440, 1983.
221. Coates DM et al: Assessment of assays for the serodiagnosis of Venezuelan equine encephalitis, *J Infect* 25:279-289, 1992.
222. Linssen B et al: Development of reverse transcription–PCR assays specific for detection of equine encephalitis viruses, *J Clin Microbiol* 38:1527-1535, 2000.

223. Binn LN et al: Efficacy of an attenuated western encephalitis vaccine in equine animals, *Am J Vet Res* 27:1599-1604, 1966.
224. Walton TE et al: Experimental infection of horses with enzootic and epizootic strains of Venezuelan equine encephalomyelitis virus, *J Infect Dis* 128:271-282, 1973.
225. Weaver SC, Scott TW, Lorenz LH: Detection of eastern equine encephalomyelitis virus deposition in *Culiseta melanura* following ingestion of radiolabeled virus in blood meals, *Am J Trop Med Hyg* 44:250-259, 1991.
226. Vaidyanathan R et al: Vector competence of mosquitoes (Dipters: Culicidae) from Massachusetts for sympatric isolate of eastern equine encephalitis virus, *J Med Entomol* 34:346-352, 1997.
227. Sabattini MS et al: Arborvirus investigations in Argentina 1977-1980. I. Historical aspects and descriptions of study sites, *Am J Trop Med Hyg* 34:937-944, 1985.
228. Monlux WS, Luedke AJ: Brain and spinal cord lesions in horses inoculated with Venezuelan equine encephalomyelitis virus (epidemic American and Trinidad strains), *Am J Vet Res* 34:465-473, 1973.
229. Roberts ED, Sanmartin C, Payan J: Neuropathologic changes in 15 horses with naturally occurring Venezuelan equine encephalomyelitis, *Am J Vet Res* 31:1224-1229, 1970.
230. Donaldson MT, Sweeney CR: Equine herpes myeloencephalopathy, *Compend Cont Educ Pract Vet* 19:864-882, 1997.
231. Wilson JH, Gibbs EPJ: Strategies for prevention of eastern equine encephalomyelitis, *Proc ACVIM Forum* 9:423-424, 1991.

BORNA DISEASE (Near Eastern Encephalitis)

Borna disease is an encephalitis of mammals caused by a member of the Flaviviridae family of viruses. Outbreaks of Borna disease have been reported from Europe and the Middle East. The virus is serologically distinct from those that cause eastern equine encephalitis, western equine encephalitis, St. Louis encephalitis, Venezuelan encephalitis, and Japanese B encephalitis, and it differs in host range. Natural infections of Borna disease virus can occur in sheep, goats, cattle, and rabbits.[232] The viruses of Borna disease and Near Eastern encephalitis are indistinguishable.[233]

The Borna disease virus is shed through nasal secretions and urine from infected animals. It is resistant to drying and other adverse environmental conditions. The virus is transmitted between birds by the tick *Hyalomma anatolicum*. Outbreaks in horses in the Middle East may represent transmission from a dense population of infected wild birds, and recurrent outbreaks in Germany have been thought to originate from birds that have migrated from the Near Eastern countries. Most outbreaks in horses occur in the early spring or autumn.

The clinical signs of Borna disease in horses are similar to those of the other equine encephalitides. In ruminants the clinical signs include head tremors, hyperesthesia, ataxia, anorexia, propulsive walking, coma, and convulsions. Antibodies to the agent may be found in the serum and cerebrospinal fluid of most but not all infected animals. The mortality rate is high. Pathologic abnormalities resemble those of a viral encephalomyelitis. The characteristic microscopic lesion of Borna disease is the Joest-Degen inclusion body in the neuronal nucleus.[233]

REFERENCES

232. Daubney R, Mahalu EA: Viral encephalomyelitis of equines and domestic ruminants in the Near East, I, *Res Vet Sci* 8:375-397, 1967.
233. Daubney R: Viral encephalitis of equines and domestic ruminants in the Near East. II, *Res Vet Sci* 8:419-439, 1967.

WEST NILE VIRUS MENINGOMYELOENCEPHALITIS

RICHARD BOWEN

DEFINITION AND ETIOLOGY. West Nile meningomyeloencephalitis is a mosquito-borne viral disease that affects a broad range of animals, including human beings, horses, mice, and many species of birds. Other animals, including dogs and cats, may be infected with the virus, but little if any work has been done to characterize their disease process. The West Nile virus is a positive-sense ribonucleic acid (RNA) virus that is closely related to the viruses that cause St. Louis encephalitis, Japanese encephalitis, and Murray Valley encephalitis.[234]

CLINICAL SIGNS. Clinical disease arising from infection with WNV has been best studied in horses and donkeys during natural outbreaks of disease or after experimental infection.[235-238] Most infections appear to result in subclinical or mild disease, but roughly 10% of animals develop severe disease. The incubation period typically ranges from 6 to 10 days, and some horses have been reported to show a secondary onset of disease approximately 20 days after infection. Some but not all equids develop a febrile response with the onset of clinical disease. Initial signs tend to occur abruptly and include depression, listlessness, ataxia, and paresis, particularly of the rear limbs. Some horses have been reported to show apprehension and anxiety. The disease progresses over 1 to 3 days to manifest such signs as head shaking and incessant chewing, paralysis of the lower lip or tongue, severe ataxia, ascending paralysis, and terminal recumbency. These clinical signs reflect a severe encephalomyelitis and widespread viral replication in the brain and spinal cord. Animals with less severe forms of the disease may recover fully within 5 to 15 days.

Clinical disease induced by infection of dogs and cats with WNV is virtually unstudied. It was reported that experimental infection of three dogs with a South African strain of WNV failed to induce overt clinical signs of disease within 2 weeks of inoculation.[239] Two of the three dogs were judged to have had a mild, recurrent myopathy based on elevations in serum concentrations of creatine kinase.

CLINICAL PATHOLOGY. Hematologic and biochemical profiles are reported to be essentially unaltered during the course of WNV infection in horses.[237,238] Similarly, no substantive alterations in hematologic or biochemical parameters were noted in three dogs infected with WNV, with the exception of transient rises in creatine kinase cited above.[239] Alterations in the characteristics of the cerebrospinal fluid have not yet been reported.

Several serologic assays are used to diagnose WNV infection, including serum neutralization tests and IgG- and IgM-capture enzyme-linked immunosorbent assay (ELISA).

PATHOLOGIC LESIONS. WNV induces in horses and other animals a non-suppurative meningomyeloencephalitis, with lesions concentrated in the brainstem and spinal cord.[238,240,241] Gross lesions in the CNS are typically absent, although meningitis and areas of focal hemorrhage may be evident. Histologically, the principle lesion is perivascular cuffing with lymphocytes and histocytes, with gliosis and some neuronophagia. In at least one case of experimentally-induced disease, vasculitis was prominent in the cord and brain. Significant lesions outside the CNS have not been reported. Immunohistochemistry can be used to confirm the presence of WNV antigens in tissues of suspect cases.

PATHOPHYSIOLOGY. Most of the research done to characterize the pathogenesis of WNV in mammals has focused on horses. Several published[235-237] and recent unpublished studies have demonstrated that horses experimentally infected with WNV develop a viremia of low magnitude (fewer than 1000 plaque-forming units per milliliter of serum) in the first week after infection. Viremia has not been demonstrated to persist past 1 week after infection and usually is of short duration (less than 2 days). The tentative conclusion from such studies is that horses are dead-end hosts and do not attain a level of viremia that serves as a significant source of virus for infecting mosquitoes. However, this conclusion must be tempered by acknowledgment of the small number of animals that have been investigated.

Single studies of WNV infection of dogs[239] and pigs[242] indicate that these animals also develop no or a very low-level viremia.

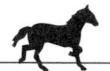

EPIDEMIOLOGY. West Nile meningomyeloencephalitis has been known for many years in several areas of Africa, southwestern Asia, and the Middle East, and periodic epizootics have occurred in European countries, including France and Italy. WNV was first recognized in North America in 1999 as the etiologic agent responsible for an outbreak of fatal disease in crows and human beings in New York.[243,244] Subsequently, several equine deaths that year were attributed to WNV infection. Continuing virus activity in New York, New Jersey, and adjoining states indicates that the virus overwintered in the northeastern United States and likely has become endemic in that area. As with other arboviruses, the peak period of transmission in temperate regions is the late summer and early fall, with cessation of cases during the winter months when mosquito populations disappear. However, WNV recently was isolated from a dead hawk in the middle of winter in New York, suggesting that non-vector transmission, possibly by predation, occasionally may occur.[245]

Birds are the principal natural host for WNV. Several species develop high-titer viremia and thus clearly have the potential to serve as important amplifying hosts. Identification of the virus in the United States was triggered by an outbreak of disease in crows. Subsequent research indicated that the avian host range for this virus is broad and that the mortality rate in infected birds often is very high. Mosquitoes of several genera (*Culex, Aedes,* and *Anopheles* spp.) become infected by feeding on viremic birds and after viral replication are able to transmit the virus to other birds and to a variety of mammalian hosts.

TREATMENT AND PROGNOSIS. No specific treatment is available for animals infected with WNV. The prognosis is very poor for horses that show clinical signs. However, some animals do recover, and standard supportive treatment may be indicated.

PREVENTION. The standard means for control during epidemics of West Nile is vector abatement via elimination of mosquito breeding sites and application of insecticides (larvacides and adulticides). There is no commercially available vaccine for West Nile, but several are being developed and are likely to be deployed in the near future.

REFERENCES
234. Monath TP, Heinz FX: Flaviviruses. In Fields BN, Knipe DM, Howley PM, eds: *Field virology*, ed 3, Philadelphia, 1996, Lippincott-Raven.
235. Schmidt JR, El Mansoury HK: Natural and experimental infection of Egyptian equines with West Nile virus, *Ann Trop Med Parasitol* 57:415-427, 1963.
236. Joubert L et al: Reproduction experimentale de la meningoencephalomyelite du cheval par l'arbovirus West Nile. III, Relations entre la virologie, la serologie, et l'evolution anatomoclinique: consequences epidemiologiques et prophylactiques, *Bull Acad Vet (France)* 44:159-167, 1971.
237. Oudar J et al: Reproduction experimentale de la meningoencephalomyelite du cheval par l'arbovirus West Nile. II. Etude anatomoclinique, *Bull Acad Vet (France)* 44:147-158, 1971.
238. Cantile C et al: Clinical and neuropathological features of West Nile virus equine encephalomyelitis in Italy, *Equine Vet J* 32:31-35, 2000.
239. Blackburn NK et al: Susceptibility of dogs to West Nile virus: a survey and pathogenicity trial, *J Comp Pathol* 100:59-66, 1989.
240. Guillion JC et al: Lesions histologiques du systeme nerveux dans l'infection a virus West Nile chez le cheval, *Ann Inst Pasteur* 114:539-550, 1968.
241. Joubert L et al: Epidemiologie du virus West Nile: etude d'un foyer en Camargue. IV, La meningoencephalomyelite du cheval, *Ann Inst Pasteur* 118:239-247, 1970.
242. Ilkal MA et al: Experimental studies on the susceptibility of domestic pigs to West Nile virus followed by Japanese encephalitis virus infection and vice versa, *Acta Virol* 38:157-161, 1994.
243. Briese T et al: Identification of a Kunjin/West Nile-like flavivirus in brains of patients with New York encephalitis, *Lancet* 354:1261-1262, 1999.
244. Lancioti RS et al: Origin of West Nile virus responsible for an outbreak of encephalitis in the northeastern United States, *Science* 286:2333-2337, 1999.
245. Garmendia AE et al: Recovery and identification of West Nile virus from a hawk in winter, *J Clin Microbiol* 38:3110-3111, 2000.

OVINE ENCEPHALOMYELITIS (Louping Ill)

DEFINITION AND ETIOLOGY. Louping ill is an acute, fatal encephalomyelitis of sheep that occasionally infects human beings, wild ruminants, horses, and cattle.[246-248] The disease has been reported in England, Scotland, Ireland, Norway, Turkey, and Bulgaria.[249-251] The etiologic agent of louping ill is a togavirus that is transmitted by the ticks *Ixodes ricinus* and *Rhipicephalus appendiculatus.* Most outbreaks occur in areas with dense populations of infected ticks and wild animals.

CLINICAL SIGNS. Sheep develop central nervous system (CNS) disorders. Infection in horses often is asymptomatic.[252] The initial clinical signs of louping ill include fever, anorexia, depression, constipation, and generalized muscular tremors. The ensuing signs are characteristic of CNS disease and include ataxia, conscious proprioceptive deficits, head tremors, hypermetria, and hyperexcitability. The hypermetria results in a characteristic "rabbit hopping gait," which gives the disease its name. Further progression of clinical signs is associated with cerebrocortical dysfunction; these signs include head-pressing, hyperesthesia, recumbency, convulsions, coma, and death. Survivors have residual deficits in intelligence. The duration of the illness is approximately 12 days.

CLINICAL PATHOLOGY. Both hemagglutination inhibition and serum neutralization tests have been described,[246,253] but the serum neutralization test is preferred.[252] High levels of virus-specific IgG and IgM can be detected in the cerebrospinal fluid (CSF) of affected animals.[253] Viremia peaks at approximately 3 days after inoculation and disappears by 7 days. Because animals usually are not viremic at the time the nervous system lesions develop, virus recovery is best done from the brain or spinal cord. Isolation of the louping ill virus from the CSF is difficult. For virus isolation from the brain, approximately 1 g of brainstem should be collected into a 50% glycerol saline solution.

PATHOPHYSIOLOGY. After inoculation into susceptible sheep, the louping ill virus migrates into the regional lymph nodes and spleen and then replicates. Viremia occurs 6 to 20 days after the invasion of the lymphatic tissues.[247] Viral replication in the brain causes non-supportive inflammation and neuronal degeneration.[247] Rapid antibody production is associated with recovery.[254] Concomitant infection of sheep with the agent of tick-borne fever (*Erlichia phagocytophila*) results in a greater level of viremia and increased mortality from the louping ill virus.[255]

EPIDEMIOLOGY. Louping ill principally affects yearling sheep in the spring, weeks to months after they have been placed on pastures infected by the tick *Ixodes ricinus.* In any outbreak the prevalence of clinical louping ill is low, but the seroprevalence of antibodies in adult sheep in endemic areas is high, indicating a continuous, low-level exposure to the virus, and many animals are asymptomatically affected. The case attack rate may reach 60% of the population, whereas the mortality rate is low, rarely exceeding 15%. The degree of susceptibility of neonatal lambs and adult sheep is similar. Adults tend to be more heavily parasitized by the host ticks and thus play a major role in virus survival and transmission.[256] Sylvatic cycles of virus transmission occur in which viral amplification takes place through rodents and red grouse.[246,257,258] Pigs, cattle, horses, and red deer also become infected with the virus and can develop clinical disease. These animals probably are dead-end hosts. The seroprevalence rate of the virus in horses from one endemic area was 10%.[252] Milk from infected goats can reach titers high enough to infect suckling kids.[259]

Mild occupational infections can occur in shepherds, veterinarians, or laboratory workers who cultivate the virus. The louping ill virus probably is maintained on pastures through infected sheep because grouse populations become unstable and die out whenever the virus is introduced.[260] The high incidence of louping ill in the spring and summer months probably corresponds to the peak activity of ticks. The virus may persist for long periods in the arthropod vector, but it is unclear if transovarial transmission of the agent occurs. *Ixodes ricinus* is a three-host tick with a life cycle of 3 years. The ticks do not walk, and dissemination over a range requires animal transport. After a blood meal, the tick molts and then rests on vegetation until the next meal, approximately 12 months later. The activity of the ticks tends to increase markedly in the spring whenever the ambient temperatures are above 7° C (43° F).

NECROPSY FINDINGS. The pathologic lesions of louping ill are similar to those seen with other togavirus infections, including perivascular cuffing with mononuclear cells and neutrophils, gliosis, neuronal necrosis, and mononuclear cell meningeal inflammation.[261,262] Microscopic lesions are most severe in the Purkinje cells, the motor nuclei, and the ventral horn cells. The forebrain is spared.[263]

PREVENTION. There is no treatment for louping ill encephalitis, but supportive care should be provided. A formalin-inactivated vaccine given in the last trimester has been recommended for preventing louping ill.[264] The vaccinal antibody titers (by hemagglutination inhibition tests) range from 1:10 to 1:640. A single dose of the vaccine provides responses that are protective for at least 2 years. Colostral antibody titers higher than 1:40 are considered protective.[256] Other methods of preventing the disease include frequent acaricidal dipping of sheep and clearing of pastures to reduce the population of infected intermediate hosts.

REFERENCES

246. Timoney PJ: Susceptibility of the horse to experimental inoculation with louping ill virus, *J Comp Pathol* 90:73-865, 1980.
247. Doherty PC, Smith W, Reid HW: Louping ill encephalomyelitis in the sheep. V, Histopathogenesis of the fatal disease, *J Comp Pathol* 82:337-344, 1972.
248. Svedmyr A et al: Infections with tick-borne encephalitis virus in the Swedish population of the elk *(Alces a. alces)*, *Acta Pathol Microbiol Immunol Scand* 65:613-620, 1965.
249. Pavlov P: Studies on tick-borne encephalitis of sheep and their natural foci in Bulgaria, *Zentralbl Bakteriol Parasitendk* 206:360, 1968.
250. Hartley WJ et al: A viral encephalitis of sheep in Turkey, *Pendik Inst J* 2:89, 1969.
251. Gao GF: Sequencing and antigenic studies of a Norwegian virus isolated from encephalomyelitic sheep confirm the existence of louping ill virus outside Great Britain and Ireland, *J Gen Virol* 74:109-114, 1993.
252. Timoney PJ et al: Encephalitis caused by louping ill virus in a group of horses in Ireland, *Equine Vet J* 8:113-117, 1976.
253. Reid HW, Doherty PC: Experimental louping ill in sheep and lambs. I, Viraemia and the antibody response, *J Comp Pathol* 81:291-298, 1971.
254. Reid HW, Doherty PC: Louping ill encephalomyelitis in the sheep. I, The relationship of viraemia and the antibody response to susceptibility, *J Comp Pathol* 81:521-529, 1971.
255. Reid HW et al: Response of sheep to experimental concurrent infection with tick-borne fever *(Cytoecetes phagocytophila)* and louping ill virus, *Res Vet Sci* 41:56, 1986.
256. Reid HW, Boyce JB: The effect of colostrum-derived antibody on louping ill virus infection in lambs, *J Hyg (Cambridge)* 77:349-354, 1976.
257. Reid HW et al: The response of three grouse species *(Tetrao urogallus, Lagopus mutus, Lagopus lagopus)* to louping ill virus, *J Comp Pathol* 90:257-263, 1980.
258. Timoney PJ: Recovery of louping ill virus from the red grouse in Ireland, *Br Vet J* 128:19-23, 1972.
259. Reid H: Louping ill, *Practice* 13:157-160, 1991.
260. Reid HW et al: Transmission of louping ill virus in goat's milk, *Vet Rec* 114:163-165, 1984.
261. Doherty PC, Vantsis JT, Hart R: Louping ill encephalomyelitis in the sheep. VI, Infection of the 120-day foetus, *J Comp Pathol* 82:385-388, 1972.
262. Doherty PC, Reid HW: Louping ill encephalomyelitis in the sheep. II, Distribution of virus and lesions in the nervous tissue, *J Comp Pathol* 81:531-536, 1971.
263. Doherty PC, Reid HW: Experimental louping ill in sheep and lambs. II, Neuropathology, *J Comp Pathol* 81:331-337, 1971.
264. Brotherson JG et al: Field trials of an inactivated oil-adjuvant vaccine against louping ill (arbovirus group B), *J Hyg (Cambridge)* 69:479-489, 1971.

RABIES

DEFINITION AND ETIOLOGY. Rabies is an invariably fatal neurologic disease that affects most warm-blooded animals. The rabies virus (genus *Lyssavirus*; family Rhabdovirus) contains ribonucleic acid (RNA) and is highly neurotropic. The major viral antigens are well conserved between heterologous isolates; however, strain differences in pathogenetic and host range have been identified. Serial propagation in laboratory animals results in loss of virulence for other species and increased virulence for the species in which the antigens have been passaged. Such laboratory strains of low virulence are called "fixed virus"; examples of these are the Flury and ERA strains. Isolates of rabies virus from field cases are called "street virus."[265-269]

CLINICAL SIGNS. The clinical signs of rabies virus infection in livestock are variable. The incubation period ranges from 3 weeks to 6 months. The shortest incubation periods are seen in animals bitten around the head and neck. Longer incubation periods are seen in animals bitten around the extremities and trunk. The early disease stage is associated with multifocal dysfunction of peripheral nerve rootlets, basal ganglia, or behavior centers in the rhombencephalon. Behavioral changes vary and range from extreme hyperexcitability, fear, or rage (furious rabies) to depression (dumb rabies) and flaccid tetraparesis or paraparesis (paralytic rabies). The paralytic form of rabies is especially common in cattle. Occasionally the affected animal is found dead without premonitory signs.

The early clinical signs of rabies in ruminants and horses may be nonspecific; they include anorexia, depression, and mild ataxia. As the disease progresses, animals may show repetitive twitching of muscular groups, hyperesthesia, hypermetria, and a mixture of conscious and unconscious proprioceptive deficits. Horses often appear colicky. In the early stages of the disease, animals may repeatedly attempt to mount inanimate objects or may show regional pruritus arising from a paresthesia. Rubbing of the pruritic area results in loss of hair or wool and deep skin ulcers. Less often, affected animals show belligerence or run frantically through fences and stall doors. Such behavior may be induced by mild tactile or auditory stimulation. The animals may charge at innocuous objects, resist restraint, or bite handlers or themselves. The episodes of violence may be interspersed with periods of normalcy or profound depression. Belligerent animals become recumbent but may retain many of their aggressive tendencies until they die in convulsions after 2 to 11 days.[268]

The spinal reflexes of infected animals range from normal to increased or diminished to absent. The animal may show an exaggerated response to tactile stimuli.[270] Furious rabies in cattle results in recumbency, coma, convulsions, bloat, tenesmus, ptyalism, pollakiuria, bellowing, hypersexuality, paraphimosis, and flaccidity of the tail and anus. Tetraplegic animals show frantic motor activity of the legs and bellow when stimulated.

Animals with the dumb form of rabies are depressed, inappetent, and febrile (temperature over 39.4° C [103° F]). These animals have a marked ataxia, drooped head and neck, ptosis, flaccid facial musculature, profuse salivation, yawning, repeated nibbling motions with the lips, tenesmus, and paraphimosis. If they are able to stand, the animals have a base-wide stance and may fall or have difficulty rising. Other clinical signs associated with the dumb form of rabies are flaccidity of the tongue, tail, anus, and urinary bladder. Odontoprisis, head-pressing, circling, blindness, strabismus, and nystagmus also may be seen before death.

The first clinical sign of the paralytic form of rabies is an unexplained ataxia or shifting leg lameness.[269] This is soon followed by paraparesis or paraplegia. Spinal reflexes and tone in the affected limbs may be decreased or absent.[269]

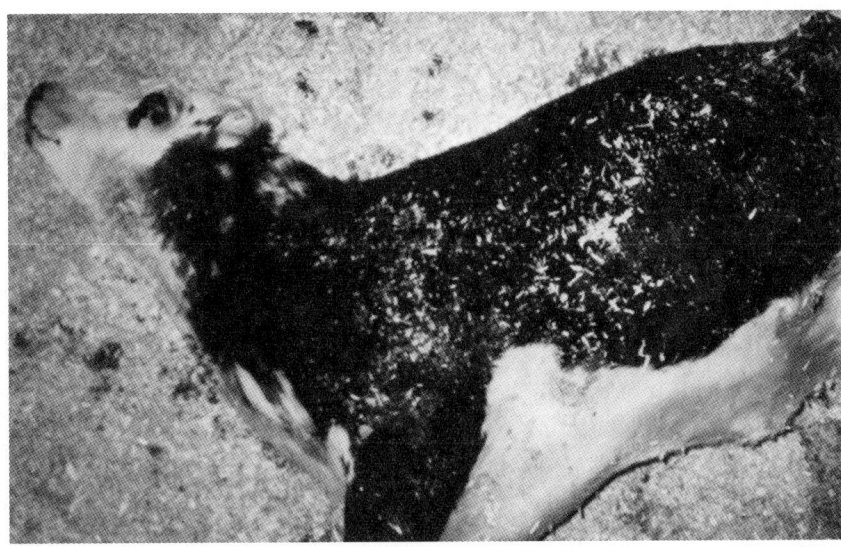

FIG. 33-4 ▮▮ A 10-month-old mixed-breed calf with terminal rabies virus encephalitis. The calf is comatose and showing opisthotonos.

TABLE 33-4

Occurrence of Particular Clinical Signs of Rabies in Horses

Clinical Signs	Frequency of Occurrence
Ataxia, paraplegia	11/21
Lameness	5/21
Pharyngeal paralysis	2/21
Recumbency	21/21
Colic	2/21
Hyperesthesia	17/21
Tail and anal paralysis	12/21
Fever	11/21

From Green S et al: *J Am Vet Med Assoc* 200:1133-1137, 1992.

Most affected animals become recumbent by 3 to 5 days. Initially the recumbent animal may eat and drink normally, but over several days it becomes anorectic and develops encephalopathic signs characterized by coma and grand mal seizures (Fig. 33-4).[271,272] Death usually occurs within 10 days. Irrespective of the clinical manifestations, rabies is rapidly progressive and uniformly fatal.

In all animals the clinical signs rapidly worsen over 1 to 3 days, until the patient becomes recumbent and comatose. The animal may develop a pharyngeal-laryngeal paralysis that results in stertorous breath sounds and regurgitation of saliva. Frothy saliva accumulates at the commissures of the lips, and the patient may be unable to drink. This last clinical sign has given rise to the common name of hydrophobia.[273]

One summary of 21 cases of rabies in horses enumerated the frequency of particular clinical signs seen as the presenting complaint; these are listed in Table 33-4. Differentiation of rabies from other encephalitic disorders is difficult. In horses the clinical signs of encephalitic rabies often are indistinguishable from other cerebral diseases, including hepatoencephalopathy, leukoencephalomalacia, togaviral encephalitis, equine herpesvirus type 1 (EHV-1) myeloencephalitis, space-occupying masses, meningitis, and protozoal myeloencephalitis. In ruminants rabies may resemble herpesvirus encephalitis, thromboembolic meningoencephalitis, nervous

ketosis, grass tetany, polio encephalomalacia, nervous coccidiosis, or even focal spinal cord or peripheral nerve diseases. Most horses die of fatal encephalopathy within 5 days of the onset of signs; however, more prolonged cases, lasting as long as 14 days, have been observed in our clinic.[274] The presence of pleocytosis and an increased protein concentration in the cerebrospinal fluid in conjunction with a progressive, diffuse central nervous system (CNS) disease and fever should indicate the possibility of rabies.

CLINICAL PATHOLOGY. The CSF may be normal or may show moderate increases in protein (60 to 200 mg/dl), mononuclear cells (5 to 30 cells/μl), and occasionally neutrophils. Eosinophils and xanthochromia have been reported. A definitive diagnosis of the disease is based on microscopic examination of cryostatically sectioned, fluorescent antibody–stained CNS tissues (hippocampus and cerebellum). Fluorescent antibody tests using monoclonal antibodies specific for epitopes of the rabies virus envelope proteins also are highly specific. Microscopic examination of hematoxylin and eosin-stained brain sections may reveal nonsuppurative encephalitis and Negri bodies, which also are diagnostic. Intracerebral inoculation of mice is considered an accurate method of confirming a rabies diagnosis. For mouse inoculation, weanlings are inoculated intracerebrally with brain homogenates from suspected cases and are killed after 5 days. The brains are removed and examined using fluorescence and light microscopy.

An antigen-capture enzyme immunodiagnostic technique has been developed. The test uses salivary gland specimens and captures antigen onto solid phase using purified polyclonal antibodies. The specificity and sensitivity of this method are similar to those of the direct immunofluorescence test. The antigen-capture test has not gained widespread clinical use in the United States.[275] An indirect fluorescent antibody test using slices of brain tissue accurately diagnoses 98% of all clinical cases and is considered the gold standard by public health departments.

PATHOLOGIC LESIONS. The pathologic lesions of rabies are characteristic of a nonsuppurative encephalitis. In horses a hemorrhagic poliomalacia of the spinal cord may be seen. The microscopic changes of rabies include brain edema, meningeal congestion, and focal areas of hemorrhage in the CNS. Microscopically perivascular cuffing by mononuclear cells, gliosis, glial nodules, neuronophagia, and neuronal degeneration are noted. These changes are most severe in the dorsal root ganglia but can be seen in all regions of the CNS. Examination of the dorsal root ganglia for nonsuppurative inflammation may be diagnostically helpful if no Negri bodies are visible or if the fluorescent antibody test for viral antigen shows a negative result.[276]

Negri bodies, which are intraneuronal eosinophilic cytoplasmic inclusions, are highly diagnostic for rabies virus infection but may not be seen in all cases, especially in patients euthanized early in the course of the disease. Other microscopic changes include poliomalacia, cytoplasmic hyalinization and vacuolations of neurons, and crenation of neuronal nuclei. Changes in the thymus, spleen, and lymph nodes include thymic atrophy, cortical effacement of thymus, depletion of periarticular lymphoid sheaths, and absent germinal centers of lymph nodes.[275]

PATHOPHYSIOLOGY. The structure of the rabies virus capsid proteins is similar to that of the neurotoxins of cobra venom and acetylcholine.[277] After subcutaneous or intradermal inoculation, the rabies virus replicates locally and after several days attaches to the acetylcholine receptors (and other receptors) of the peripheral nerves by a viral surface glycoprotein. The virus then migrates to the CNS through peripheral nerves, spinal rootlets, and the spinal cord. After entry into the nerve cell rootlets, the virus travels to the brain along nerve tracts and into CSF. From there it spreads antegrade along the rootlets of the cranial nerves to the salivary glands and the nasal epithelium. Shedding of the virus in the nasal secretions and saliva may precede the onset of clinical signs. The rabies virus has a predilection for replication in the cell bodies (gray matter) of the CNS. Dysfunction of these neurons results in behavioral changes and variable abnormalities of the cranial and the peripheral nerves (multifocal loss of lower motor neuron function). The cause of death is unclear. Affected animals may develop respiratory paralysis as a result of virus infection in the medulla. Before death, infected animals show a weight loss that is more severe than that caused by starvation and water deprivation alone. Such changes may be related to the failure of virus-infected pituicytes to produce growth hormone. The loss of this hormone results in a secondary alteration of the cellular immune response and degeneration of the cytoarchitecture of the thymus, lymph node, and spleen.[278]

EPIDEMIOLOGY. Rabies does not presently occur in Scandinavia, Great Britain, Ireland, Scotland, Australia, New Zealand, and the British Islands. The disease is endemic in other parts of the world, including the United States, Canada, and western Europe. The infection is epizootic in Central and South America and Malaysia, where a tropical climate and a high population of infected feral mammals favor viral propagation and transmission. The rabies virus is shed in the saliva and does not survive when dried. The most common method of viral transmission to domestic animals is through the bite of an infected feral mammal. Nevertheless, human beings and laboratory animals have developed fatal infections after respiratory exposure to viral aerosols. The rabies virus is shed in low levels in the milk of infected animals and may occasionally infect offspring nursing infected dams.[279,280] Laboratory animals, foxes, and skunks also can be infected experimentally by ingestion of infected tissues.[279,280] Survival of the virus in the wild may depend on cycling of infections in skunks, bats, or raccoons,[281] which also are common sources of livestock infections in the United States.[282]

Certain strains of rabies virus have low virulence in skunks and bats and, consequently, chronic asymptomatic infections in these species could serve as reservoirs over successive years. The rabies virus is also transmitted directly among bats through aerosols in caves, and during periods of high viral

contamination, die-offs due to encephalitic rabies occur in these bat populations. The fox is the most common wild reservoir in the northern United States, Europe, and Canada. In comparison, the raccoon is the most common source of rabies in the eastern and southern United States, and the skunk is the most common source of the virus in the western United States. Recent outbreaks of rabies in the eastern United States have been associated with proliferation of raccoons around metropolitan areas.[283] Because of the high level of prophylactic vaccination of dogs in North America, rabies transmission from domestic dogs to livestock is rare. In South America rabies outbreaks in cattle commonly occur as a result of bites from vampire bats, in which rabies virus infection is endemic. Death losses from rabies in these countries are estimated to exceed 50,000 cattle annually. Human rabies usually results from contact with infected pets; however, cases originating from contact with infected cattle and wild animals have been reported.[270]

Rabies virus infections are most common in the late summer. This may be because wild animals give birth to offspring during the early spring. The population density of the offspring remains high until they are reduced by selective forces such as predation, starvation, and hunting. Young animals become infected at that time and then spread the disease as they expand into new territory.

PREVENTION. Inactivated vaccines are the only licensed products for prevention of rabies in livestock in the United States.* Foals in rabies-endemic areas should be vaccinated at 4 to 6 months of age with two doses given 3 to 4 weeks apart and followed by a booster at 1 year of age.[284-287] Adults in endemic areas should receive yearly booster vaccinations.

Effective modified live vaccines are available for use in domestic dogs and cats, but these vaccines are either not approved for use in livestock or may produce fatal allergic or viral encephalitis when inoculated into large animals. Inactivated and attenuated vaccines produce similar peak titer responses, but the persistence of titers at 6 to 10 months is greater in horses vaccinated with the killed virus than with the modified live products. Numerous experimental vaccines and vaccine adjuvant combinations have been tested. Killed vaccines inactivated with binary ethylenimine or propionalactone have produced good seroconversion in horses.[288] Incorporation of aluminum hydroxide adjuvants or sapon into the inactivated virus vaccine also increased the antibody titer and persistency. The clinical usefulness of these enhancements is unknown.[286,289] The ERA modified live vaccine has been used for immunization of livestock in some countries. This attenuated virus vaccine protects cattle for 4 years when given to adults and for 2 years when given to animals under 2 months of age.[287]

The disposition of unimmunized livestock that have been bitten by rabid animals depends on the animal's vaccination history, local and national regulations, and the value of the bitten victim. In the United States and Canada, the disease must be reported to the state public health department. Management of exposed livestock should be conducted in conjunction with public health officials. A horse bitten by a wild animal should be considered to have been exposed to rabies regardless of the availability of the animal for testing. If the horse had been vaccinated, it should be revaccinated immediately and kept under observation for 90 days. Other exposed, unvaccinated animals with a low economic value should be euthanized. If the exposed animal is very valuable,

---

*Rabguard-TC and Defensor, SmithKline Beecham Animal Health, Exton, PA; Rabvac 3, Solvay Animal Health, Inc., Mendota Heights, MN; and Imbrab 3, Rhone Merieux, Inc., licensed by Pitman-Moore, Mundelein, IL 60060.

the bite wound should be washed with copious amounts of water and iodine or quaternary ammonium disinfectants.[290] Exposed animals should be quarantined for at least 6 months.

Vaccination of animals shortly after rabies virus infection is less effective than prophylactic vaccination. In one study postinoculation vaccination of experimentally infected sheep had no effect on the incubation period, clinical symptoms, or mortality rate. Moreover, antibody titers in the vaccinated animals had no predictive value for protection.[291] One other study indicated that cattle and horses exposed naturally did not develop clinical rabies after receiving four injections of a modified live virus vaccine.[292,293] For human exposure, the World Health Organization recommends vaccination at postexposure days 0, 3, 7, 14, and 30. Studies indicated that such postexposure vaccination of sheep had a minimal effect on survival unless the animals were immediately vaccinated and concomitantly treated with human antirabies immunoglobulin.[294,295] The clinical relevance of this information has not yet been determined. When human exposure to rabies virus is suspected, the suspected animal should be euthanized and the brain examined for evidence of infection. A valuable animal should be quarantined for 6 weeks under veterinary supervision, and the brain should be examined if it dies.

Control of rabies by immunization of susceptible wildlife using baits impregnated with modified live high egg passage virus vaccines has been successful in certain instances.[270,296] It has not been successful for immunization of all species, however, because of the difficulty of inducing protective responses through the oral route and because of the susceptibility of different species to the modified live viruses.[297] Orally administered recombinant vaccinia viruses containing inserts to rabies virus glycoproteins have successfully immunized fox cubs.[298] Such molecular approaches may provide a means for large-scale immunization of wildlife populations and for eventual eradication of the disease.

Island nations have been able to remain free of rabies by imposing a 6-month quarantine on imported dogs and cats. In one instance, however, a dog developed rabies 1 month after it was released from the quarantine. This outbreak demonstrated the highly variable incubation period of rabies and the necessity for constant vigilance against introduction of carriers into rabies-free areas.

REFERENCES

265. Fekadu M et al: Efficacy of rabies vaccines against Duvenhage virus isolated from European house bats (*Eptesicus serotinus*), classic rabies, and rabies-related viruses, *Vaccine* 6:533, 1988.
266. Tollis M et al: Antigenic characterization of twenty street rabies virus strains isolated in Italy using monoclonal antibodies, *J Vet Med* 34:317, 1987.
267. Webster WA et al: Antigenic variants of rabies virus in isolates from eastern, central, and northern Canada, *Can J Comp Med* 49:186, 1985.
268. Cran H: Some clinical observations on rabies, *Vet Rec* 118:23-24, 1986.
269. Marler RJ et al: Rabies in a horse, *J Am Vet Med Assoc* 175:293-294, 1979.
270. Steck F, Wandeler A: The epidemiology of fox rabies in Europe, *Epidemiol Rev* 2:71-96, 1980.
271. Ferris DH et al: A note on experimental rabies in the donkey, *Cornell Vet* 58:270-277, 1968.
272. Owen RR: Rabies in the horse, *Vet Rec* 191:69, 1978.
273. Glaes AM: Rabies in the equine, *Southwestern Vet*, 1974, pp 283-284.
274. Green SL: Equine rabies, *Vet Clin North Am* 9:337-347, 1993.
275. Perrin P, Rollin PE, Sureau P: A rapid rabies enzyme immunodiagnosis (RREID): a useful and simple technique for the routine diagnosis of rabies, *J Biol Stan* 14:217-222, 1986.
276. O'Toole D et al: Poliomyelomalacia and ganglioneuritis in a horse with paralytic rabies, *J Vet Diagn Invest* 5:95-97, 1993.
277. Lentz T: Structure-function relationships of curaremimetic neurotoxin loop 2 and of a structurally similar segment of rabies virus glycoprotein in their interaction with the nicotinic acetylcholine receptor, *Biochemistry* 30:10949-10957, 1991.
278. Torres-Anjel MJ et al: Failure to thrive, wasting syndrome, and immunodeficiency in rabies: hypophyseal/hypothalamic axis effect of rabies virus, *Rev Infect Dis* 10(suppl 4):S710-S725, 1988.
279. Fischman HR, Ward FE: Oral transmission of rabies virus in experimental animals, *Am J Epidemiol* 88:132-138, 1968.
280. Pablo Correa-Giron E, Allen R, Sulkin SE: The infectivity and pathogenesis of rabies virus administered orally, *Am J Epidemiol* 91:203-215, 1970.
281. Baer GM, Adams DB: Rabies in insectivorous bats in the United States, 1953-1965, *Public Health Rep* 85:637-645, 1970.
282. Constantine DG: Transmission experiments with bat rabies isolates: bite transmission of rabies to foxes and coyote by free-tailed bats, *Am J Vet Res* 27:20-23, 1966.
283. Uhaa IJ et al: Rabies surveillance in the United States during 1990, *J Am Vet Med Assoc* 200:920-929, 1992.
284. California Department of Health Services: Compendium of US-licensed animal rabies vaccines and their application in dogs under the California rabies control program, *Calif Vet* 47:16, 1993.
285. Prosperi S et al: Vaccination of cattle with live and inactivated rabies vaccines: a study of antibody responses, *Vet Res Commun* 8:181-185, 184.
286. Precausta P et al: Modalites de production et immunite conferee par un vaccin antirabique inactive provenant de culture cellulaire, *Comp Immunol Microbiol Infect Dis* 5:217, 1982.
287. Lawson KF, Crawley JF: The ERA strain of rabies vaccine, *Can J Comp Med* 36:339-344, 1972.
288. Flynn DV et al: Guidelines for vaccination of horses, *J Am Vet Med Assoc* 185:32-34, 1984.
289. Soulebot J et al: Immunisation of herbivores against rabies using an inactivated cell culture vaccine, In Juwert E, ed: *Proceedings of an International Conference on Rabies Control in the Tropics*, New York, 1983, Springer-Verlag.
290. Schroeder WG: Suggestions for handling horses exposed to rabies, *J Am Vet Med Assoc* 155:1842-1843, 1969.
291. Blancou J et al: Inefficacite de la vaccination antirabique du chien, du chat ou du mouton deja contamine par le virus dela rage, *Bulletin d'Information des Laboratoires des Services Veterinaires* 25:9-15, 1987.
292. Srisongmuang W, Pramayotin P, Pokmontri S: Veterinary viral diseases: their significance in southeast Asia and the western Pacific, *Proceedings of an International Seminar on Virus Diseases of Veterinary Importance in Southeast Asia*, CSIRO, Geelong, Australia, 1984.
293. Della-Porta AJ: Antibody responses in animals after inoculation with a modified live rabies virus vaccine: preliminary study, In Srisongmuang W, Pramayotin P, Pokmontri S, eds: *Antibody responses in animals in veterinary viral diseases: their significance in southeast Asia and the western Pacific*, Geelong, Australia, 1984, Academic Press.
294. Baltazar RS, Blancou J, Atrois M: Resultats de la vaccination antirabique chez des moutons deja infectes par le virus de la rage vulpino, *Recuil de Medicine Veterinaire* 163:573-577, 1987.
295. Blancou J et al: Effective postexposure treatment of rabies-infected sheep with rabies immune globulin and vaccine, *Vaccine* 9:432-437, 1991.
296. Lawson KF et al: Safety and immunogenicity of a vaccine bait containing ERA strain of attenuated rabies virus, *Can J Vet Res* 51:460-464, 1987.
297. Baer GM: Rabies in the tropics. In Juwert E, ed: *Proceedings of an international conference on rabies control in the tropics*, New York, 1983, Springer-Verlag.
298. Brocher BM et al: Use of recombinant vaccinia-rabies virus for oral vaccination of fox cubs (*Vulpes vulpes*) against rabies, *Vet Microbiol* 18:103-108, 1988.

SPORADIC BOVINE ENCEPHALOMYELITIS (Buss Disease; Polyserositis; Bovine Chlamydial Infection)

Sporadic bovine encephalomyelitis (SBE) is caused by chlamydiae (psittacosis-lymphogranuloma group), which produce a disseminated vasculitis and serositis. The host range of chlamydial SBE is limited to cattle and buffalo. The disease was first reported in the United States in 1940.[299] A similar but not identical viral disease occurs in cattle in Australia and has been named bovine ephemeral fever.[300-303] SBE occurs in Czechoslovakia, Hungary, and Japan.[304-307] Outbreaks of SBE are rare, but the case attack rate in an epizootic ranges from 5% in adults to 25% in calves.[308] The mortality is highest in calves and approximates 31% for all age-groups.[308]

Infected cattle shed the chlamydiae in urine, feces, nasal secretions, and milk, and chlamydiae can be found in the feces of asymptomatic calves exposed to clinically affected herd mates. However, the most common mode of transmission of chlamydiae is unknown. The chlamydial agent tends to remain endemic on a single farm, and sporadic outbreaks of disease may occur only on those premises. The pattern of these outbreaks varies, from a few cases annually to acute, recurrent epizootics with high case attack rates that subside after 3 to 4 weeks. Sheep and goats are resistant to the bovine agent. The serologic relationship between the chlamydial agent that infects calves and the chlamydia that infects sheep and goats is unclear. The chlamydial agent of ovine polyarthritis causes marked polyserositis when inoculated into calves but seems to be less pathogenic for cattle than the bovine chlamydial isolates.[308]

CLINICAL SIGNS. Affected animals show signs of a multisystemic disease. The initial clinical signs in cattle are fever (39° to 41.5° C [102.1° to 106.7° F]), anorexia, depression, and stiffness. The cattle also may show signs of a respiratory disease characterized by nasal discharge, dyspnea, and cough. These animals occasionally have a painful response to percussion of the hoof, as well as swelling of the coronary band or polyarthritis and tenosynovitis.[299] Auscultatory abnormalities may include high-pitched wheezes and crackles over the lung fields or pleural and pericardial friction rubs. Because of the fibrinous peritonitis and pleuritis, the clinical signs in some affected animals may resemble those of hardware disease. These animals may grunt or groan when sudden pressure is applied to the xiphoid region. Some animals may respond to soft percussion of the xiphoid region by striking or kicking at the examiner. There is an initial diarrhea. Progression of the disease is related to development of the meningoencephalitis and is characterized by ataxia and conscious proprioceptive deficits, circling, head tilt, opisthotonos, hyperesthesia, stiff neck, convulsions, and coma. Animals may die after 4 to 10 days.

DIAGNOSIS. The detection of elementary bodies in the exudate cells of pleural and peritoneal effusions is highly suggestive of SBE. The chlamydiae can be cultured from the blood and body fluids of early infections in guinea pigs inoculated intraperitoneally with fresh tissue specimens and held for 6 to 7 days. Inoculation of embryonated eggs is a less sensitive diagnostic technique than animal inoculation. A complement fixation test has been described but is not universally available. Cross-reactivity of the antibodies against the SBE agent with the antigens of *Chlamydia psittaci* has been detected, but the clinical usefulness of this reagent for diagnosis of the disease in cattle is unknown.

PATHOGENESIS AND PATHOLOGIC LESIONS. The mode of infection and the genesis of pathologic lesions are unknown in natural cases. Growth of the chlamydiae in the arteriolar endothelium causes vasculitis, hemorrhage, edema, and accumulation of fluid in the body cavities. Diffuse fibrinous pleuritis, peritonitis, and meningitis also are seen. Microscopic changes include perivascular mononuclear cell infiltration and neuronal degeneration. The lesions all are composed of networks of neutrophils and mononuclear cells enmeshed in fibrin. Some of the inflammatory cells contain elementary bodies.

TREATMENT. Early cases of SBE can be treated effectively with oxytetracycline. The chlamydial agent is also susceptible to penicillin and erythromycin, but the clinical efficacy of these drugs is unknown.

CONTROL. There are no known effective control measures for the prevention of SBE. The chlamydia agent is susceptible to a number of disinfectants, including 2% sodium hydroxide (NaOH), 5% cresol, and 0.3% quaternary ammonium compounds.

REFERENCES

299. Stearns TW, McNutt: Sporadic bovine encephalomyelitis: filtration of the causal agent, *Am J Vet Res* 3:253-257, 1942.
300. Egan AN: The occurrence of sporadic bovine encephalomyelitis in Australia, *Aust Vet J* 36:444, 1960.
301. French EL, Snowden W: The occurrence of sporadic bovine encephalomyelitis in Australia, *Aust Vet J* 36:444, 1960.

302. Harding WB: Transmissible serositis and its relationship to sporadic bovine encephalomyelitis, *Aust Vet J* 39:333, 1963.
303. Littlejohns IR, Harris ANA, Harding WB: Sporadic bovine encephalomyelitis, *Aust Vet J* 37:53, 1971.
304. Omori T et al: Studies on the disease of cattle caused by a psittacosis-lymphogranuloma group virus. IV. Identification of virus (*Shizouka* strain) as a causative agent of bovine encephalomyelitis, *Jpn J Exp Med* 24:257-273, 1974.
305. Omori T et al: Studies on the disease of cattle caused by a psittacosis-lymphogranuloma group virus. V. Experimental infection of laboratory animals with the *Shizouka* strain isolated from bovine encephalomyelitis, *Jpn J Exp Med* 24:313-323, 1974.
306. Kourad J, Bohac J: Encephalomyelitis in cattle, *Vet Casopsis* 8:228-234, 1959.
307. Csontos L, Szecky A: Bovine sporadic encephalomyelitis (myagawanellosis) in Hungary, *Magy Allatory Lap* 19:4-7, 1964.
308. Harshfield GS: Sporadic bovine encephalomyelitis, *J Am Vet Med Assoc* 156:466-477, 1970.

MORBILLIVIRUS ENCEPHALOMYELITIS OF CATTLE

A nonhemagglutinating paramyxovirus *(Morbillivirus)* has been isolated from a calf with encephalitis. The disease was first described in Germany, but subsequent cases have been identified in Switzerland.[309] The German *Morbillivirus* organism is serologically related to the subacute sclerosing panencephalitis virus of human beings but is unrelated to the parainfluenza virus of cattle. The clinical signs of *Morbillivirus* infection include pharyngeal paralysis, anorexia, salivation, hyperexcitability, intentional head tremors, aggressiveness, coarse muscle fasciculations, cutaneous analgesia, tonic-clonic seizures, dysphonia, and bellowing. The pathologic lesions include a diffuse, mononuclear cell encephalitis, perivascular cuffing with mononuclear cells, microglial cell proliferation, astrocytosis, neuronal loss, neuronophagia, and intraneuronal intranuclear (Cowdry type A) inclusion bodies.

REFERENCE

309. Bachmann PA et al: Sporadic bovine meningoencephalitis: isolation of a paramyxovirus, *Arch Virol* 48:107-120, 1975.

MENINGITIS (Suppurative Meningitis)

DEFINITION AND ETIOLOGY. Meningitis can occur either from direct extension of infectious agents into the calvarium or from hematogenous infection. Causes of suppurative meningitis include direct extension of pyogenic infections into the calvarium from infected skull fractures,[310] osteomyelitis from sinusitis or otitis, osteonecrosis caused by thermal cauterization during dehorning or by improper placement of trephination holes, cribriform plate fractures, and extension from infected coccygeal vertebrae. In horses septic meningitis is a common sequela to surgical removal of progressive ethmoidal hematomas. Centripetal migration of *Cryptococcus neoformans* along peripheral nerve rootlets results in suppurative meningoencephalitis.[311] Other bacterial species that cause suppurative meningitis are *Streptococcus zooepidemicus* in foals and goats,[312] *Streptococcus suis* in foals, and *Actinomyces* spp. in horses.[313] Embolic showers to the central nervous system (CNS) also occur in cases of left-sided endocarditis. *Pseudomonas aeruginosa* mastitis of cattle and goats may terminate with septicemia and meningitis.

Suppurative meningitis of hematogenous origin is common in neonates (see Chapter 18). Gram negative bacteria, *Escherichia coli*, and *Salmonella* spp. are the dominant species involved in neonatal infections. One survey reported a 43% prevalence of septic meningitis in necropsied calves.[314] Hematogenous meningitis is predisposed by deficient passive transfer of colostral antibodies to the neonate (see Chap-

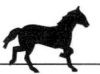

ter 49). *Mycoplasma mycoides* ssp. *mycoides* is a common cause of meningitis in goat kids.

CLINICAL SIGNS. The earliest clinical signs of meningitis are diarrhea, fever, anorexia, stiff neck, and hyperesthesia.[315,316] Passive manipulation of the head and neck causes sudden extension and hypertonicity of the limbs. Slight tactile stimulation of the skin may result in strong spasmodic extension of the limbs, fasciculations of the underlying musculature, or even generalized frantic motor activity. The patient's behavior may vary from extreme depression to hyperexcitability or mania. The animal may display trismus and may vocalize when the head and neck are flexed. Tetraparesis, hyperreflexia, and a tendency to circle or fall toward one side may be noted. A subtle intentional head tremor often is observed in foals. Dysfunction of one or more cranial nerves may result in facial muscular tremors, nystagmus, facial palsy, blindness, anisocoria, or strabismus. These deficits are inconstant. Progression of the clinical signs is associated with a decreased sensorium, propulsive walking, coma, and status epilepticus.

The clinical signs of purulent meningitis closely resemble those of hypomagnesemia and hypoglycemia, which may occur simultaneously with septic meningitis in neonates. The onset of clinical signs may be delayed in horses with *Cryptococcus neoformans* meningitis.[311]

CLINICAL PATHOLOGY. Septic meningitis should be differentiated from metabolic encephalopathies by measurement of the plasma concentrations of sodium, glucose, and magnesium and by laboratory evaluation of hepatic function. Diagnosis of meningitis is based on examination of the cerebrospinal fluid (CSF) (normal values are shown in Table 33-2). The CSF of animals with meningitis may be turbid and white-to-amber in color, may foam when shaken, and may clot. Xanthochromia may be observed in some specimens. The white blood cell (WBC) concentrations in the CSF of calves with purulent meningitis are typically over 100 neutrophils/μl (the mean WBC count is 4004 WBCs/ml), and protein concentrations range from 20 to 270 mg/dl.[315] The differential cell counts in the CSF are either predominantly neutrophilic or mononuclear with fewer neutrophils. The Pándy test result is strongly positive. The concentration of glucose in the CSF often is less than 50% of the corresponding concentration in the blood. Because of the lack of opsonic and bactericidal activity in the CSF, bacteria can proliferate to high titers and are commonly observed in Gram-stained smears of CSF. One study showed intracellular bacteria in 10 of 22 calves with meningitis.[317] Abnormalities in the blood are inconsistent and reflect secondary conditions such as septicemia, diarrhea, or overaggressive fluid therapy. These changes could include leukocytosis, left shift, toxic changes in the hemogram, hyperkalemia, respiratory acidosis, hypoglycemia, and hyponatremia or hypernatremia.

PATHOPHYSIOLOGY. Because there is little bactericidal or opsonic activity in the CSF, animals are highly susceptible to meningeal infection by low numbers of bacteria. After several days, inflammation of the arachnoid trabeculae and choroid plexus results in decreased CSF absorption and hypertensive hydrocephalus.

NECROPSY FINDINGS. The meningeal vessels appear to be congested, and the meninges are swollen, opalescent, and petechiated. The CSF is cloudy or amber and may contain fibrin clots. In cases associated with bacteremia, a fibrinopurulent iridocyclitis may be observed. Microscopic changes of the nervous tissues include infiltration of tissues by neutrophils and lymphocytes, endarteritis of the meningeal vessels, choroiditis, scattered leptomeningeal hemorrhages, and bacterial colonies around the blood vessels of the meninges and the brain parenchyma.

Concomitant pathologic lesions, including omphalo-

phlebitis, septic arthritis, anterior uveitis, and panophthalmitis, result from dissemination of the septic process. These lesions may be helpful in differentiating meningitis from metabolic encephalopathies. When meningitis occurs secondary to trauma, the site of organism entry may be detectable. Fungal meningitis caused by *C. neoformans* often is accompanied by granulomatous lesions of the lips, nasal mucosa, and peripheral nerves.

TREATMENT. Treatment of bacterial meningitis is difficult, and the mortality rate is high. Early recognition and treatment are essential for adequate recovery. Antimicrobial sensitivity tests performed on isolates from CSF may provide valuable information with respect to ideal drugs. However, these tests frequently are unavailable because of the difficulty of isolating primary pathogens from CSF in most cases of purulent meningitis. Because prompt treatment of meningitis is critical, antibiotic therapy usually must be based on the Gram-staining characteristics of sedimented bacteria and the initial 24-hour cultures.

Domestic animals have a well-defined blood-CSF barrier, and antibiotics that reach high plasma concentrations may not necessarily reach bactericidal concentrations in the brain. To ensure an adequate antibacterial efficacy, antibiotic concentrations in the CNS should range from 10 to 30 times the minimum inhibitory concentration of the infecting bacteria.[317-325] Antibiotics that are inherently bactericidal tend to produce superior responses compared with agents that are primarily bacteriostatic. The major factors influencing the CSF penetration of an antimicrobial agent are the lipid solubility, degree of ionization, and the molecular weight of the drug. In general, broad-spectrum drugs with a nonpolar basic character tend to have the greatest CNS penetration and efficacy for treatment of meningitis. Antibiotics tend to diffuse into cerebrospinal fluid to a greater extent when it is inflamed. The lists in Box 33-1 show the relative penetrability of antibiotics and antimicrobials into the CSF.

Antibiotic treatments should be administered by intravenous routes to attain maximum peak blood and CSF con-

---

BOX 33-1

Expected Penetration of Antibiotics and Antimicrobial Drugs into Cerebrospinal Fluid

GOOD PENETRATION
Minocycline
Doxycycline
Erythromycin
Sulfonamides
Chloramphenicol*
Metronidazole*
Quinolones
Ceftiofur
Cefotaxime
Moxalactam
Pyrimethamine
Isoniazid
Trimethoprim-sulfonamide

POOR PENETRATION
Cephaloridine
Gentamicin
Tetracycline
Penicillin G
Kanamycin
Streptomycin
Neomycin

*Prohibited in food-producing animals in the United States.

centrations and should be continued for 10 to 14 days. Table 33-5 presents the recommended dosages for each of the antibiotics.

The selection of the antibiotics should be based on the results obtained from Gram-stained smears and cultures of the CSF or from other infected areas. Penicillin G is a polar acidic drug that has limited distribution into the CSF. Because of this and the predominance of gram negative CNS infections in livestock, penicillin alone is a poor choice for initial therapy of uncharacterized purulent meningitis.[326-331] Nevertheless, administration of very high intravenous dosages of penicillin may be effective for the treatment of meningeal infections by highly susceptible bacteria such as *Streptococcus* or *Haemophilus* organisms. In these cases low but therapeutic concentrations of the drug can be achieved in the CSF. In human beings, intravenous dosages of 250,000 U/kg given daily are required to achieve CSF penicillin concentrations ranging from 0.3 to 0.8 μg/ml.[326] For infections caused by gram positive bacteria with intermediate susceptibility to penicillin, multiple daily intravenous dosages of ampicillin (15 to 20 mg/kg) may be useful.

Meningitis caused by the Enterobacteriaceae should be treated with aminoglycoside antibiotics or third-generation cephalosporins. Although aminoglycoside antimicrobials are highly effective against gram negative pathogens and are bactericidal, their efficacy for the treatment of purulent meningitis is diminished by their polar basic characteristics and low attainable CSF concentrations. The aminoglycosides used most commonly for the treatment of bacterial meningitis include gentamicin (3 mg/kg given IV or IM 3 or 4 times daily) or amikacin (6.6 mg/kg IM 3 or 4 times daily).[332]

Because of the difficulties associated with aminoglycoside penetration into the CSF and antimicrobial resistance, intrathecal therapy with preservative-free aminoglycoside antibiotics has been recommended for therapy of gram negative meningitis. Intrathecal or intraventricular administration of gentamicin (1 mg daily in smaller animals or 0.05 mg/kg of body weight in larger animals) has been recommended for the treatment of *P. aeruginosa* meningitis.[333] The safety of the procedure has been questioned, however, on the basis of reports of increased mortality in experimentally treated rabbits and in children with naturally acquired infections.[333,334]

The third-generation cephalosporins moxalactam, cefotaxime, and ceftazidime have a high efficacy against gram negative CSF pathogens and penetrate the blood-CSF barrier better than the penicillins or the aminoglycoside antibiotics.[335-337] They also are resistant to inactivation by the betalactamases of the gram negative bacteria and retain activity in purulent debris. Because of these characteristics, such drugs often are preferred over the aminoglycoside antibiotics for treating gram negative infections of the CNS. The recommended dosage for the third-generation cephalosporins is 40 to 50 mg/kg 2 to 4 times daily.[314,338]

The new fluorinated quinoline antibiotics have a reproducible penetration into the CNS; however, little quantitative information is available regarding the achievable CSF levels in cases of purulent meningitis. In laboratory animals, data show that the drugs reached CSF concentrations ranging between 4 and 8 mg/L.[339] The penetration of these drugs, their efficacy against a wide range of bacteria, and their bactericidal activities would recommend their use for treatment of bacterial meningitis, especially whenever the animal has failed to respond to more traditional drugs. The recommended dosage of enrofloxacin is 4 mg/kg, but experimental animals have

TABLE 33-5

Recommended Drug Regimens for Treatment of Bacterial Meningitis in Livestock

Antibiotic or Antimicrobial Drug	Dose, Route, and Frequency	Indication, Comments
Trimethoprim/sulfadiazine	30 mg/kg sulfa PO, twice daily	Staphylococci, *Klebsiella*, some coliforms; long-term medication, not for use during acute crises
Chloramphenicol*	100-200 mg/kg PO, four times daily *or* 100-200 mg/kg IV, six times daily	Staphylococci, streptococci, *Klebsiella, Actinobacillus, Corynebacterium*, some coliforms
Third-generation cephalosporins (moxalactam, ceftriaxone, cefotaxime)	40 mg/kg IV, four times daily	Staphylococci, streptococci, coliforms, *Klebsiella, Actinobacillus, Bordetella, Salmonella, Pseudomonas, Corynebacterium*; expensive
Isoniazid	5-20 mg/kg PO, two times daily	*Actinomyces pyogenes, Rhodococcus equi*; long-term oral therapy is indicated; combine treatments with penicillin, ampicillin, or erythromycin
Erythromycin (cattle only)	10 mg/kg IM, two times daily	Streptococci, some anaerobes, *Actinomyces pyogenes, Rhodococcus equi*; do not administer to horses or small ruminants; give to cattle only for 3 days; expect severe muscular swelling
Penicillin G, sodium	22,000-240,000 IU kg slow IV, four times daily	Some staphylococci, streptococci, anaerobes, *Pasteurella, Haemophilus, Actinomyces pyogenes, Rhodococcus equi*; rapid IV infusion may be acutely fatal to small ruminants
Ampicillin, sodium	15-20 mg/kg IV, four times daily	Some staphylococci, streptococci, anaerobes, *Pasteurella, Haemophilus, Actinomyces pyogenes, Rhodococcus equi*; safer for small ruminants than IV penicillin G
Ticarcillin/clavulanate	44-50 mg/kg IV, four times daily	Staphylococci, streptococci, anaerobes, *Pasteurella, Haemophilus, Actinomyces, Rhodococcus equi, Klebsiella*, coliforms
Tetracycline (100 mg/ml concentration)	6-12 mg/kg IV, two times daily	Some coliforms, staphylococci and streptococci, *Pasteurella, Haemophilus, Actinomyces, Rhodococcus equi* limited spectrum of activity
Amikacin sulfate	6.6-7.5 mg/kg IV or IM, two times daily	Coliforms, *Klebsiella, Pasteurella, Haemophilus*
Metronidazole*	22-25 mg/kg/day PO or IV	Anaerobes

Data regarding predicted susceptibility of bacteria to specific antimicrobials can be found in Prescott JF et al: *Can Vet J* 25:289-292, 1984.
IM, Intramuscularly; *IV,* intravenously; *PO,* orally.
*Use prohibited in food animals in the United States.

been given dosages as high as 50 mg/kg for some types of infections. A combination of the quinolones with aminoglycosides has been successful for the treatment of *P. aeruginosa* meningitis in human beings.

When the quinoline antibiotics or third-generation cephalosporins are too costly, trimethoprim-sulfonamide (TMS) combinations may be an effective substitute for horses.[340-344] TMS has good penetration into the CSF and may be useful for horses, foals, and preruminant calves, lambs, and kids. The drug is not useful for treating ruminating animals. In the ruminant the half-life of parenterally injected trimethoprim is short (60 minutes) compared with that of sulfonamide (11 hours). The short half-life of trimethoprim in the ruminant is caused largely by ruminal excretion and inactivation of the drug. The drug has a higher efficacy in preruminants and horses because the half-life of trimethoprim is significantly longer than in the adult ruminant. For horses and calves the recommended dosages are 15 to 24 mg/kg of the combined drugs given IV 2 to 4 times daily.[314,345,346]

Patients should be observed closely for the first 3 weeks after the start of therapy because clinical improvement is associated with decreased permeability of the blood-CSF barrier and reduced CSF concentration of the chemotherapeutic agent.[317,326-328] Bacteria remaining in the CNS may regrow as a result of the lowered antibiotic concentration, and clinical signs of meningitis may return after a period of initial improvement.[328] This recurrence of signs after 3 to 4 days of seemingly successful therapy should indicate the necessity for an increased antibiotic dosage or for a change in the type of antibiotic.

Although chloramphenicol has a nonpolar character and good lipid solubility, it is bacteriostatic and does not reach bactericidal concentrations in the CSF. Its efficacy for the treatment of gram negative meningitis is limited. Because of this and the current regulatory restrictions imposed by the U.S. Food and Drug Administration, chloramphenicol cannot be recommended for the treatment of purulent meningitis in large animals, especially ruminants. The tetracyclines do not appreciably cross the blood-brain barrier and also cannot be recommended for the treatment of bacterial meningitis except for certain highly susceptible infections such as *Haemophilus somnus*.

Cryptococcal meningitis of horses has been treated by intravenous administration of 100 to 150 mg of amphotericin B in 4000 ml of 5% glucose. The drug treatment was repeated every 48 hours for 23 days. One such treated horse improved with treatment but relapsed. Flucytosine* was recommended as an alternative treatment.

---

*Ancobon, Hoffman LaRoche, Inc.

Concomitant administration of dexamethasone phosphate may lessen the extent of neurologic sequelae in animals that survive purulent meningitis. The recommended dosage is 0.15 mg/kg given IM 15 minutes before the first dose of antibiotic and then every 6 hours thereafter for 4 days. Administration of the steroid 1 hour after initiation of the antibiotic treatment has little beneficial effect.[347] Supportive therapy for animals with suppurative meningitis should include protection from self-inflicted trauma, sedation, amelioration of pain, fluid therapy, and anticonvulsants.

Convulsions can be controlled by administration of diazepam (Valium) or phenobarbital at respective intravenous dosages of 0.01 to 0.4 mg/kg[332] and 20 mg/kg (Table 33-6). For intravenous administration of phenobarbital, the drug should be diluted in saline and administered slowly over 30 minutes. Repeated doses (1 to 9 mg/kg of body weight) are given 3 times daily.[348] After administration of 9 mg/kg to horses, plasma concentrations of phenobarbital range from 11.6 to 53 μg/ml.[346] Phenobarbital distributes slowly in the fat deposits. Because this could lead to drug accumulation, the trough drug concentrations should be measured frequently. The maximum desirable trough phenobarbital concentration is 40 μg/ml, and the minimum therapeutic level is 15 μg/ml.[348,349] After initial sedation long-term control of convulsions in horses can be maintained by oral administration of diphenylhydantoin (2.8 to 16 mg/kg of body weight PO 3 times daily) or phenobarbital (11 mg/kg IV once daily).[349-351] The trough plasma concentration of diphenylhydantoin should also be measured repeatedly during continuous drug therapy. The maximum desirable trough level of diphenylhydantoin is 10 to 20 μg/ml.[350] The optimum plasma concentration of the drug ranges from 5 to 10 μg/kg. Primidone is metabolically activated to phenobarbital. The drug is more expensive than phenobarbital and consequently is not commonly administered to large animals.

The concentration of plasma immunoglobulins should be measured in neonatal patients with bacterial meningitis. Neonates with a plasma protein concentration under 4.5 g/dl or an immunoglobulin G (IgG) concentration under 500 mg/dl should be given 1 to 2 L of plasma from a normal adult.

Nonsteroidal antiinflammatory drugs (flunixin meglumine or phenylbutazone) are useful analgesics in animals with suppurative meningitis. The suggested dosages and routes of administration of these drugs are listed in Table 33-5. Good nursing care is essential. Parenteral fluid therapy should be administered to animals that are unable to drink. Fluid dosages should be selected to replace insensitive water losses and existing deficits (40 to 80 ml/kg daily; balanced electrolytes). The blood pH, serum osmolality, and plasma concentrations of glucose, sodium, potassium, and magnesium should be closely monitored during the antimi-

---

TABLE 33-6

Suggested Anticonvulsant Drug Regimens for Treatment of Seizures in Horses and Cattle

Drug	Dose, Route, and Frequency	Comments
Diazepam (Valium)	0.01-0.2 mg/kg IV, every 30 min as needed to control convulsions	Effective for rapid control of status epilepticus; poor choice for long-term therapy because of cost and short plasma half-life
Phenobarbital	12-20 mg/kg IV initial dose, dilute in saline over 30 min 11 mg/kg PO, once daily (horses)	Begin treatment in convulsive neonates with intravenous drips; for long-term administration, give orally; monitor trough plasma concentrations of phenobarbital Therapeutic concentrations range from 15-40 μg/ml
Pentobarbital	2-20 mg/kg IV (approximately 2 ml/5 kg body weight); repeat every 4 hours as needed for control of status epilepticus; not good for long-term control of sporadic seizures	Must administer slowly and monitor depth of anesthesia carefully to prevent respiratory arrest; control of convulsions in adult horses and cattle often occurs at the lower intravenous dosages; use an intravenous catheter for repetitive administrations

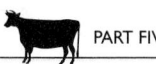
crobial therapy and measured repeatedly in animals having seizures.

REFERENCES

310. Fjeldborg J, Andresen PH, Svalastoga E: Osteomyelitis secondary to basilar skull fracture in a thoroughbred foal, *Equine Pract* 19:29-31, 1997.
311. Steckel RR et al: Antemortem diagnosis and treatment of cryptococcal meningitis in a horse, *J Am Vet Med Assoc* 180:1085-1089, 1982.
312. Gibbs HC, McLaughlin RW, Cameron HJ: Meningoencephalitis caused by *Streptococcus zooepidemicus* in a goat, *J Am Vet Med Assoc* 178:735, 1981.
313. Devriese LA et al: *Streptococcus suis* meningitis in a horse, *Vet Rec* 127:68, 1990.
314. Mosher AH, Helmboldt CF, Hayes KC: Coliform meningoencephalitis in young calves, *Am J Vet Res* 29:1483-1487, 1968.
315. Jamison JM, Prescott JF: Bacterial meningitis in large animals. I, *Compend Cont Educ Pract Vet* 9:399-406, 1987.
316. Green SL, Smith LL: Meningitis in neonatal calves: 32 cases, *J Am Vet Med Assoc* 201:125-128, 1992.
317. McCracken GH: The rate of bacteriologic response to antimicrobial therapy in neonatal meningitis, *Am J Dis Child* 123:547-553, 1972.
318. Jamison JM, Prescott JF: Bacterial meningitis in large animals. II, *Compend Cont Educ Pract Vet* 10:225-232, 1988.
319. Rahal JJ, Simberkoff MS: Host defense and antimicrobial therapy in adult gram negative bacillary meningitis, *Ann Intern Med* 96:468-474, 1982.
320. Strausbaugh LJ, Sande MA: Factors influencing the therapy of experimental *Proteus mirabilis* meningitis in rabbits, *J Infect Dis* 137:251-260, 1978.
321. Wright PF et al: The pharmacokinetics and efficacy of an aminoglycoside administered into the cerebral ventricles in neonates: implications for further evaluation of this route of therapy in meningitis, *J Infect Dis* 143:141-147, 1981.
322. Lorber J, Kalhan SC, Mahgrefte B: Treatment of ventriculitis with gentamicin and cloxacillin in infants born with spina bifida, *Arch Dis Child* 45:178-185, 1970.
323. Schaad UB et al: Clinical evaluation of a new broad-spectrum oxabetalactam antibiotic, moxalactam, in neonates and infants, *J Pediatr* 98:129-136, 1981.
324. Sande MA: Antibiotic therapy of bacterial meningitis: lessons we've learned, *Am J Med* 71:507-510, 1981.
325. Tauber MG, Zak O, Scheld WM: The postantibiotic effect in the treatment of experimental meningitis caused by *Streptococcus pneumoniae* in rabbits, *J Infect Dis* 149:575-583, 1984.
326. Heiber JP, Nelson JD: A pharmacologic evaluation of penicillin in children with purulent meningitis, *N Engl J Med* 297:410-413, 1977.
327. Beam TR, Allen JC: Blood, brain, and cerebrospinal fluid concentrations of several antibiotics in rabbits with intact and inflamed meninges, *Antimicrob Agents Chemother* 12:710-716, 1977.
328. Norrby R: A review of the penetration of antibiotics into CSF and its clinical significance, *Scand J Infect Dis* (suppl) 14:296-309, 1978.
329. Fishman RA: Blood-brain and CSF barriers to penicillin and related organic acids, *Arch Neurol* 15:113-124, 1966.
330. Scheld WM: Rationale for optimal dosing of betalactam antibiotics in therapy for bacterial meningitis, *Eur J Clin Microbiol* 3:579-591, 1984.
331. Sande MA et al: Factors influencing the penetration of antimicrobial agents into the cerebrospinal fluid of experimental animals, *Scand J Infect Dis* 14(suppl):160-163, 1978.
332. Morris DD: Bacterial infections of the newborn foal. II, Diagnosis, treatment, and prevention, *Compend Cont Educ Pract Vet* 6(suppl):436-449, 1984.
333. McCracken GH, Mize SG: A controlled study of intrathecal antibiotic therapy in gram negative enteric meningitis of infancy, *J Pediatr* 89:66-72, 1976.
334. Hodges GR et al: Central nervous system toxicity of intraventricularly administered gentamicin in adult rabbits, *J Infect Dis* 143:148-155, 1981.
335. Landesman S, Cherubin CE, Corrado ML: Gram negative bacillary meningitis, *Arch Intern Med* 142:939-940, 1982.
336. Rahal JJ et al: Prospective evaluation of moxalactam therapy for gram negative bacillary meningitis, *J Infect Dis* 149:562-5567, 1984.
337. Tauber MG, Hackbarth CJ, Kenyon G: New cephalosporins cefotaxime, cefpimizole, BMY 28142, and HR 810 in experimental pneumococcal meningitis in rabbits, *Antimicrob Agents Chemother* 27:340-342, 1985.
338. Morris DD, Rutkowski J: Therapy in two cases of neonatal foal septicaemia and meningitis with cefotaxime sodium, *Equine Vet J* 19:151-154, 1987.
339. Scheld WM: Quinoline therapy for infections of the central nervous system, *Rev Infect Dis* 11(suppl 5):S1194-S1201, 1989.
340. Svedhem A, Iwarson S: Cerebrospinal fluid concentrations of trimethoprim during oral and parenteral treatment, *J Antimicrob Chemother* 5:717-720, 1979.
341. Davitiyananda D, Rasmussen F: Half-lives of sulphadoxine and trimethoprim after a single intravenous infusion in cows, *Acta Vet Scand* 15:356-365, 1974.
342. Ardati KO, Thirumoothti MB, Dajani AS: Intravenous trimethoprim-sulfamethoxazole in the treatment of serious infections in children, *J Pediatr* 95:801-806, 1979.
343. Kim KS, Bascomb AF: Efficacy of trimethoprim/sulfamethoxazole in experimental *Escherichia coli* bacteremia and meningitis, *Chemotherapy* 29:428-435, 1983.
344. Mylotte JM et al: Trimethoprim-sulfamethoxazole therapy of experimental *Escherichia coli* meningitis in rabbits, *Antimicrob Agents Chemother* 20:81-87, 1981.
345. Hahn CN, Mayhew IG, MacKay RJ: The nervous system. In Colahan PT et al, eds: *Equine medicine and surgery*, ed 5, St Louis, 2000, Mosby.
346. Guard CL et al: Age-related alterations in trimethoprim-sulfadiazine disposition following oral or parenteral administration in calves, *Can J Vet Res* 50:342-346, 1986.
347. Odio CM et al: The beneficial effects of early dexamethasone administration in infants and children with bacterial meningitis, *N Engl J Med* 324:1525-1531, 1991.
348. Spehar AM et al: Preliminary study on the pharmacokinetics of phenobarbital in the neonatal foal, *Equine Vet J* 16:368-371, 1984.
349. Ravis WR et al: A pharmacokinetic study of phenobarbital in mature horses after oral dosing, *J Vet Pharmacol Ther* 10:283-289, 1987.
350. Duran SH et al: Pharmacokinetics of phenobarbital in the horse, *Am J Vet Res* 48:807-810, 1987.
351. Kowalczyk DF, Beech J: Pharmacokinetics of phenytoin (diphenylhydantoin) in horses, *J Vet Pharmacol Ther* 6:133-140, 1983.

PITUITARY ABSCESSES

Pituitary abscesses occur sporadically in ruminants. *Actinomyces pyogenes* is the most commonly isolated bacterium, but *Corynebacterium pseudotuberculosis*, as well as *Streptococcus, Staphylococcus, Actinomyces, Bacteroides, Fusobacterium, Acinetobacter, Pasteurella, Pseudomonas,* and *Actinobacillus* spp. occasionally have been isolated.[352] Pituitary abscesses are rare in horses.

The clinical signs of pituitary abscess occur suddenly and progress for 7 to 10 days before the affected animal dies.[352] The initial signs are ataxia, head-neck extension, base-wide stance, inappetence, depression, head-pressing, and recumbency.[352-354] Most affected animals have asymmetric deficits of one or more cranial nerves, resulting in dysphagia, blindness, anisocoria, absent pupillary light reflexes, mydriasis, flaccid tongue, nystagmus, facial paralysis, facial hypalgesia, ventrolateral strabismus, or head tilt.[352,355] Approximately 50% of the affected animals have bradycardia (pulse rate under 60 beats/min).

The cerebrospinal fluid (CSF) protein concentration in affected cattle ranges from 70 to 502 mg/dl, and nucleated cell counts range from 6 to 12,640/μl (6% to 84% neutrophils).[352] The antemortem diagnosis is based on the observation of bradycardia, blindness, and nonresponsive pupils in conjunction with evidence of pyogenic inflammation in the CSF.

Some authors[352] have postulated that the infectious agent gains entry to the sella turcica hematogenously and then localizes in the rete mirabile, which is the complex of blood vessels encircling the pituitary gland. There is a direct relationship between the complexity of the rete mirabile and the incidence of pituitary abscessation in different mammals. The horse and dog lack a well-defined rete and correspondingly have a low risk for developing a pituitary abscess, whereas the situation is reversed in cattle. One study reported that 55% of cattle with a pituitary abscess had pyogenic foci in other organ systems or in the sinuses, teeth, or soft tissues of the face,[352] indicating that the abscesses may result from a retrograde bacterial embolization through branches of the facial veins.

Ataxia is caused by interruption of extrapyramidal motor nuclei in the brainstem by the expanding abscess. Extension of the abscess into the communicating retroorbital rete may result in exophthalmos. Extradural extension of the abscess along the brainstem causes sequential loss of the cranial nerve function, with the nerves closest to the pituitary gland

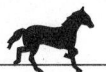

being the first to become dysfunctional. Bradycardia may be caused by interference with diencephalic cardioacceleratory centers. In animals that survive for several weeks, the abscess may extend into the dura mater and cause a suppurative meningoencephalitis.

Animals ranging in age from 9 months to 12 years have been affected, but most cases occur between 2 and 5 years of age.[356] There appears to be a slightly increased prevalence of the disease in castrated and intact males.[352] A high incidence of pituitary abscessation has been related to infections that developed in bulls after insertion of a nose ring. Prophylactic administration of penicillin and attention to aseptic procedure during insertion of the ring can reduce the incidence of the disease.[354] Because of the high mortality rate associated with pituitary abscesses, treatment usually is not attempted.

REFERENCES

352. Perdrizet JA, Dinsmore P: Pituitary abscess syndrome, *Compend Cont Educ Pract Vet* 8(suppl): 311-317, 1986.
353. Perl SH, Niska A, Tromp A: Abscess in the hypophysis of a cow, *Refuah Vet* 35:175-176, 1978.
354. Moriwaki M et al: Exophthalmos due to *rete mirabile* abscesses caused by infection with *Corynebacterium pyogenes* in cattle, *Natl Inst Anim Health Q* 13:14-22, 1973.
355. Espersen G: Hypofyseabsces-syndrom hos dvaeg I, Kliniske undersogelseer, *Nord Vet Med* 27:465-481, 1975.
356. Taylor PA, Meads EB: Pituitary abscessation and a "farcy like" condition in cattle due to *Corynebacterium pyogenes*, *Can Vet J* 4:208-213, 1963.

BRAIN ABSCESSES

Because of the high incidence of strangles, *Streptococcus equi* is the most common cause of brain abscesses in horses. *Actinomyces pyogenes* is a common cause of brain abscesses in cattle by means of extension of a sinus infection through the calvarium. Brain infections of cattle with *Bacteroides* spp. have also been reported.[357] The neurologic dysfunction caused by brain abscesses has a slower onset and is more asymmetric than that caused by meningitis, probably because most abscesses initially are extradural. The growing abscess compresses the cerebral cortex unilaterally, causing a caudal displacement of the brain and functional loss of one occipital lobe. Because of the high proportion of crossed fibers in the optic nerve decussation, unilateral cortical abscesses result in vision loss in the contralateral eye. Increased central nervous system (CNS) compression by the mass results in ipsilateral mydriasis caused by interference with the oculomotor nerve. Further increases in the size of the lesion cause more generalized cortical signs, including blindness, propulsive walking, circling, head tilt (toward the lesion side), depression, coma, head-pressing, or sudden unexplained mania. Abscesses at the base of the brain may cause additional abnormalities of cranial nerve function (Figs. 33-5 and 33-6). Ophthalmoscopic examination may reveal papilledema in the ipsilateral eye.

In later stages of the condition, animals may assume lateral recumbency and display a decerebrate posture characterized by hypertonicity, hyperreflexia, opisthotonos, coma, and convulsions. At this stage the disease is difficult to differentiate from septic meningitis. The cerebrospinal fluid (CSF) of animals with brain abscesses is normal, similar to CSF from patients with meningitis, or similar to CSF from patients with diffuse meningitis. Treatment of brain abscess includes antibiotics and supportive care (see Meningitis in this chapter). In one clinical report[358] a brain abscess in a horse was localized with computed tomography (CT scanning) and successfully drained via craniotomy.

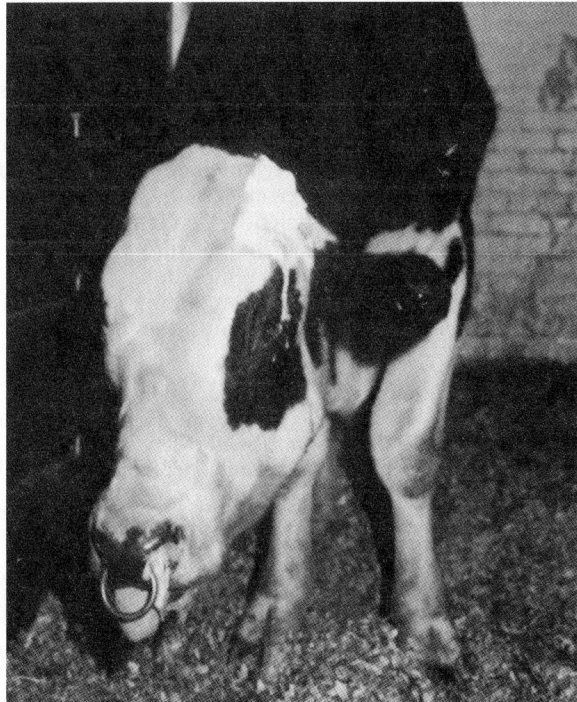

FIG. 33-5 Severely obtunded bull that developed a brain abscess from extension of a frontal sinusitis. The abscess extended to the base of the brainstem and affected cranial nerves V and XII, resulting in dropped jaw and tongue paralysis. The bull also was severely depressed, blind, and ataxic and had facial analgesia.

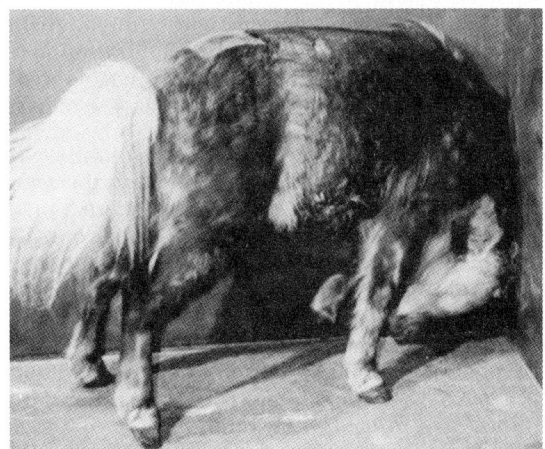

FIG. 33-6 Head-pressing in a pony caused an abscess in the right cerebral hemisphere. (Courtesy Dr. R.H. Whitlock.)

REFERENCES

357. McCormack JE: Papilledema related to left cerebral hemisphere abscess in a heifer, *Vet Med (Small Anim Clin)* 68:1249-1252, 1973.
358. Allen JR, Barbec DD, Boulton CR: Brain abscess in a horse: diagnosis by computerized axial tomography and successful surgical treatment, *Equine Vet J* 19:552-555, 1987.

MYCOTIC ENCEPHALITIS

Extension of a mycotic infection from the guttural pouch to the brain through the internal carotid artery has been reported.[359]

The infection caused disseminated necrosis and hemorrhage that was most severe in the thalamus, cerebral cortex, and hippocampus. The clinical signs were fever (38.3° C [100.9° F]), epistaxis, dysphagia, laryngeal hemiplegia, pharyngeal paralysis, circling, unilateral blindness, mydriasis, facial paralysis, and apprehension. Reports of a horse and a calf infected systemically with a phycomycete described recumbency and coma. Pathologic changes in the central nervous system consisted of cerebellar and occipital cortical infarction.[360,361] The cerebrospinal fluid (CSF) changes included a markedly increased Pándy test and an increased white blood cell (WBC) count (79 WBCs/μl). The cell population in the CSF was composed of 81% mononuclear cells and 19% neutrophils.

REFERENCES

359. Wagner PPA, Miller RA, Gallina AM: Mycotic encephalitis associated with a guttural pouch mycosis, *J Equine Med Surg* 2:355-358, 1978.
360. Austin JA: Disseminated phycomycosis in a horse, *Can Vet J* 17:86-89, 1976.
361. Juck F, Smith LL: Phycomycete meningoencephalitis in a neonatal calf, *Can Vet J* 19:75-78, 1978.

CEREBRAL TRAUMA

DEFINITION AND ETIOLOGY. Because of their size, behavior, and relatively thin calvarium, horses are more susceptible to head trauma than other livestock. Traumatic injuries of horses most commonly result from kicks, sharp blows, or falling over backward.[362] Blows to the poll of the horse result in fractures or displacements of the basisphenoid, occipital, and petrosal bones and the basioccipital and basisphenoid sutures.[363,364] The basisphenoid and basioccipital bones form a part of the foramen lacerum and the jugular foramen. Fractures around these foramina may result in dysfunction of cranial nerves IX, X, and XII.[365] Hematomas form at the fracture site and extend into the membranous labyrinths and basilar areas of the brain, where they cause vestibular and occipital cortex dysfunction. Blows to the forehead result in depression fractures of the dome of the calvarium and subsequent unilateral brain swelling.

Skull fractures occur in cattle from blows to the top of the calvarium. Most skull fractures are located in the center of the frontal bones where the internal and external plates of the frontal sinus are fused into a single-layer dorsal wall of the cranial vault. This position can be located on the skull as the imaginary cross found by intersecting lines drawn between the medial canthus of the eye and the horn of the opposite side. Injuries in this area compress the frontal and parietal lobes of the cerebral cortex. The pressure changes result in loss of sensorium, sensory deficits, blindness contralaterally, or convulsions.

In young goats and horned sheep under 4 to 6 months of age, the calvarium can be inadvertently opened by removal of excessive bone during disbudding or dehorning. In goats cerebrocortical burns can occur from overapplication of a hot iron or caustic dehorning paste. Cortical necrosis caused by bacterial infections after dehorning of calves has also been described.[366]

CLINICAL SIGNS. The clinical presentation of cerebral trauma depends on the area of the brain that has been damaged, the extent of the lesion, and the duration of the injury. Extreme brain swelling results in caudal displacement and herniation. Brainstem compression is characterized by serial dysfunction of cranial nerves, severe disturbance of consciousness, and abnormal respiratory rhythm. Compression of the mesencephalon and tectum results in decerebrate rigidity caused by loss of the reticulospinal tracts. Compression of the myelencephalon results in Kussmaul, Biot's, or Cheyne-Stokes respiratory patterns, hyperreflexia, tetraplegia,

and absence of pupillary reflexes. Compressive lesions of the mesencephalon in the region of the oculomotor nucleus result in mydriatic pupils on the ipsilateral side of unilateral brainstem lesions.

Basioccipital fractures of horses result in asymmetric signs of vestibular disturbance, including horizontal or rotary nystagmus, ipsilateral ventrolateral strabismus, contralateral dorsomedial strabismus, head tilt, and contralateral blindness. Horses that remain ambulatory lean or circle toward the side of the lesion. Additional signs of this syndrome include dysphagia, facial paralysis, conscious proprioceptive deficits, recumbency, depression, and coma. Horses that are recumbent struggle violently. Fracture of the petrous temporal bone may cause profuse bleeding from the ipsilateral nares, external ear canal, and guttural pouch.

Brain trauma caused by overaggressive dehorning in goats results in depressed sensorium, loss of menace response, increased extensor tonus on the contralateral side, ipsilateral mydriasis, sluggish pupillary reflex, and loss of conscious proprioceptive responses. The clinical syndrome may be delayed by several days in cases of cortical burns or trauma caused by caustic paste and may be complicated by brain abscess or bacterial meningitis (see preceding section).

PATHOLOGY AND PATHOGENESIS. The pathogenetic events leading to cerebral edema and increased intracranial pressure are complex. Intracranial hemorrhage or loss of vascular integrity and cerebral edema occur after concussive blows to the head. Displacement of the neural tissue is caused by cerebral swelling or hematoma formation. The increased pressure is transmitted to the cerebrospinal fluid (CSF) and interferes with normal flow through the cerebral arteries, resulting in cerebral hypoxia and interneuronal and intraneuronal edema. In tissue ischemia, hypoxia reduces mitochondrial oxidase activity. With the loss of this enzyme and decreased oxygenation of the tissues, xanthine dehydrogenase is converted to xanthine oxidase. This enzyme in turn produces large quantities of oxygen-derived free radicals during the conversion of adenosine monophosphate to hypoxanthine. When produced in sufficient quantities, these free radicles saturate the normally protective scavenger systems and attack the neuronal membranes. A major degree of the destruction therefore is the result of lipid peroxidation of the myelin and plasmalemma. During peroxidation, the free radical extracts a methylene hydrogen atom from an unsaturated fatty acid and forms alkyl radicals with the lipid. The specific products of these reactions include lipid peroxyl radicals, lipid alkoxyl radicals, and lipid hydroperoxides. Peroxidation of lipids results in fluid shifts across membranes. The net result of such movement of electrolytes and water is the formation of intraneuronal edema and brain swelling.

When the brain swelling becomes severe, the respiratory centers are depressed, resulting in hypoxemia and acidosis. The extra carbon dioxide diffuses into the brain, and water follows, which further swells the central nervous system. Acidosis and hypoxemia also worsen the vascular leakage and hypoxemia.

Extreme swelling of the cerebral cortex results in herniation through one or more anatomic sites of the calvarium. Four forms of brain herniation have been described in large animals.[367] These include cingulate gyrus herniation ventral to the falx cerebri, herniation of parts of the temporal cortex ventral to the tentorium cerebelli (caudal tentorial herniation), caudal cerebellar vermis herniation through the foramen magnum, and herniation of the rostral cerebellar vermis ventral to the tentorium cerebelli (rostral tentorial herniation). Compressed tissue becomes hypoxemic and edematous. Compression of the CNS causes more hypoxia, prompting a dramatic and rapid deterioration.

CLINICAL PATHOLOGY. Collection of CSF from the atlantooccipital cistern is contraindicated if signs of increased

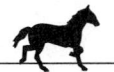

CNS pressure, uncontrolled hemorrhage from the ears or the nose, or dorsal sagittal sinus fractures are observed. Clinical signs that may suggest the presence of increased intracranial pressure include mydriasis, blindness, or papilledema. The CSF changes that occur from traumatic injuries are characteristic. For the first 24 hours, blood is admixed evenly in the CSF. Iatrogenic hemorrhage from the tapping procedure can be differentiated from that caused by trauma because in the former case, the CSF is irregularly streaked with blood; CNS hemorrhage usually results in an even admixture of blood through the CSF. During the first 24 hours, the protein concentration and white blood cell count of the cerebrospinal fluid are elevated and are in the approximate ratio as that of peripheral blood. By 48 hours after the traumatic episode, the amount of blood in the CSF decreases, and when centrifuged, the cell-free CSF appears xanthochromic. The white blood cell counts of the CSF are only marginally increased by 24 hours after hemorrhage, and the protein concentration may range from 500 to 1000 mg/ml (albuminocytologic dissociation). Thereafter the protein concentration gradually decreases, and the xanthochromia disappears by 14 days after the acute hemorrhage. The number of mononuclear inflammatory cells gradually increases as parts of the CNS degenerate. The creatine phosphokinase level of the CSF is elevated (10 to 100 IU/dl) for approximately 1 to 2 days after the acute traumatic episode.

TREATMENT. Successful treatment depends largely on early recognition and control of increased CSF pressure. Depression fractures of the frontal and parietal bones should be reduced surgically, and increased intracranial pressure should be treated medically. General medical principles for treating CNS trauma include establishment of proper respiratory function, administration of osmotic diuretics, control of seizures, nutritional and fluid support, and protection from decubitus and self-inflicted damage.

Administration of dexamethasone, methylprednisolone, mannitol, or dimethyl sulfoxide (DMSO) has been recommended for controlling CNS pressure caused by edema. The plasma half-life of dexamethasone in horses is 53 minutes and that of prednisolone is $99\frac{1}{2}$ minutes.[368] Prolonged adrenal suppression (3 to 4 days) occurs after administration

of dexamethasone at a dosage of 0.05 to 0.44 mg/kg of body weight[369,370] and for 24 hours after prednisolone treatment (dosage of 0.6 mg/kg). Controlled therapeutic trials in human beings have failed to show a beneficial effect of dexamethasone for the treatment of supratentorial intracerebral hemorrhage and edema.[371] The relationships between the pharmacologic half-life of these drugs and their antiedema effect in the CNS is unknown. An empiric recommendation for the treatment of horses is administration of dexamethasone at a dosage of 0.1 to 0.25 mg/kg of body weight by slow intravenous injection every 4 hours for 1 to 4 days or, for mature animals, 100 to 1000 mg of methylprednisolone by slow intravenous injection.[372] Similar dosages could be used in ruminants.

Experimental data indicate that administration of methylprednisolone early in the course of cerebral edema is beneficial. This benefit is thought to be derived from the stoichiometric antioxidant activity of the steroid. To attain the maximum benefit, the first dose of the drug must be administered intravenously at 30 mg/kg of body weight. Doses that fall outside this therapeutic margin either are ineffective or tend to worsen the amount of cerebral edema. A second and third dose (15 mg/kg each) should be given intravenously 2 and 6 hours later. Thereafter the drug should be given at a dosage of 2.5 mg/kg/hr for the next 48 hours.[373] The therapeutic efficacy of methylprednisolone for traumatic brain injuries in livestock is unknown. When treating livestock with corticosteroids, the possible benefits should be weighed against the deleterious effects, which include enhanced susceptibility to infection, muscular weakness, renal potassium and calcium loss, abortion in ruminants, and laminitis in horses. Table 33-7 presents a list of antiedema drugs that are commonly administered to large animals with traumatic brain disease.

Intravenous administration of a 20% solution of mannitol (2 g/kg) or oral administration of glycerol (20 ml/kg) has been used for the treatment of increased intracranial pressure. The physiologic activity of mannitol for lowering the CSF pressure may be related more to its vasoconstrictive effects than to its activity as an osmotic diuretic. Response to the treatment may occur as early as 1 hour after administration. Mannitol is expensive and usually only economically

TABLE 33-7

Recommended Drug Dosages for Treatment of Cerebrocortical Edema

Drug	Dose	Route	Frequency
Methylprednisolone	30 mg/kg	IV	Once
	15 mg/kg	IV	2 and 6 hours after 30-mg/kg dose
	2.5 mg/kg/hr	IV	Constant infusion, begin 6 hours after 30-mg/kg dose
Dexamethasone	1-4 mg/kg	IV or IM	Twice daily
Mannitol	0.25-2 g/kg	IV (20% solution)	Twice daily, monitor plasma osmolality, keep below 350 mOsm/L
Furosemide	1 mg/kg	IV, IM, or SC	Twice daily, monitor plasma, calcium, and potassium
Flunixin meglumine*	1 mg/kg	IV, IM, or SC	Twice daily
Phenylbutazone* (horse)	2-4 mg/kg	IV	Twice daily
Phenylbutazone† (cow)	10-20 mg/kg	PO	Initial dose
	2.5-5 mg/kg	IV	Alternate days
Dimethyl sulfoxide (DMSO)‡	0.5-2.5 g/kg	IV (20% solution)	Twice daily
Acetylsalicylic acid	31.2-62.4 g/500 kg	PO	Twice daily

IM, Intramuscular; *IV*, intravenous; *PO*, oral; *SC*, subcutaneous
*Monitor patient for gastrointestinal bleeding.
†The half-life of phenylbutazone in the plasma of the cow is prolonged. Continuous use of the drug in cattle should be accompanied by careful monitoring of renal function and gastrointestinal bleeding.
‡Doses of DMSO ranging from 0.5 to 1 g/kg are most commonly used. Use only in a well-ventilated area. If intravascular hemolysis develops, dilute DMSO to 5% final concentration. DMSO may be toxic for pregnant human beings, and therapeutic efficacy may be limited.

justifiable for use in neonates. If response to the initial mannitol dosage is noted, additional treatments should be given every 4 to 6 hours for the first day. Mannitol should be administered through blood administration filter sets to minimize the occurrence of microcrystalline emboli. The drug should not be given to animals with active CNS hemorrhage, because diffusion of mannitol into the center of a newly forming hematoma exerts an osmotic effect, enlarges the size of the lesion, and further attenuates the nervous tissues. Active CNS hemorrhage can be recognized by the presence of unclotted blood in the nose or ears, or parietal bone fractures that lacerate the dorsal sagittal sinus. Despite this provision, administration of mannitol is probably justified in an animal with rapidly worsening and potentially fatal deterioration in neurologic status, even in the likely presence of intracranial hemorrhage.

Intravenous use of DMSO has been recommended for the reduction of increased CSF pressure in large animals. The drug is administered intravenously at a dosage of 0.5 to 4 g/kg of body weight twice daily.[364,369,374,375] For administration, the drug is diluted fivefold to tenfold in saline (10% to 20% solution) to minimize the hemolytic and hyperthermic effects. The use of DMSO for cerebral trauma is controversial, and benefits may be species specific. For instance, anecdotal reports of benefit have been shown for horses, but controlled experiments in dogs have shown a limited clinical benefit when treating experimental CNS trauma.[370]

DMSO has several beneficial pharmacologic actions, including free-radical scavenging, interference with neutrophil chemotaxis, prevention of microthrombi, increased penetration of corticosteroids and antibiotics into the brain, and vasodilation.[376] A major effect of the drug is probably due to its diuretic action, which is greater than that of furosemide. In experimental situations, administration of DMSO to animals with experimentally induced CNS lesions resulted in more rapid neurologic recovery than did treatment with urea, corticosteroids, or mannitol.[376] The adverse effects of DMSO include muscular fasciculations, intravascular hemolysis, hemoglobinuria, and sweating.[375] Deaths have been reported in laboratory animals after intraperitoneal injections of 10 mg/kg and in dogs after intravenous dosages of 2.5 mg/kg.[377-379] The median lethal dosage of DMSO in large animals is unknown. The drug is teratogenic when administered to pregnant laboratory animals.[378,379] When the drug is administered intravenously, approximately 70% of the dosage is excreted through the respiratory tract.[380] These data indicate that DMSO should be administered only in well-ventilated areas. Exposure of pregnant human beings and animals should be avoided. In cattle DMSO is excreted rapidly and is essentially completely cleared from the plasma by 5 days.[380] A low-level residue of DMSO may persist in the fat tissues for at least 20 days. When administered intravenously to horses at dosages of 1 and 0.1 g/kg of body weight, the biologic half-life of DMSO is 8.6 and 9.8 hours, respectively.[375]

Convulsions may be controlled initially by intravenous administration of valium, phenobarbital, or pentobarbital. The recommended dosages and mode of administration of these drugs are presented in Table 33-6. Good nursing care is essential. These drugs are usually highly protein bound in plasma and can be displaced or functionally altered by other drugs. All anticonvulsant treatments should begin at the lowest possible dosage, which can be increased daily or every second or third day until the seizures have been controlled. If seizures cannot be controlled without causing depression or ataxia, a second anticonvulsant is added. The dosage of the second drug is increased gradually until the seizures stop. This combination treatment is continued for 2 to 4 weeks. Thereafter the dosage of the first anticonvulsant is tapered

until it is discontinued. If seizures reappear, the dosage of this drug is increased until the seizures disappear again. The trough blood concentration of all anticonvulsants is checked monthly. The suggested therapeutic trough concentration of phenobarbital ranges from 15 to 40 μg/ml of plasma and that of diphenylhydantoin from 5 to 20 μg/ml. Any attempt to withdraw anticonvulsant therapy should be done gradually over a 4-week period.

Horses with recurrent convulsions should not be ridden or used for sporting purposes. Infrequent seizures generally do not justify anticonvulsant treatment, and economic considerations often limit the amount of drug therapy that is possible. Status epilepticus can be treated with intravenous diazepam in 5-mg doses until seizures are controlled or by titrated doses of phenobarbital or pentobarbital. Mares with estral-related seizures may be treated with an ovariectomy.

REFERENCES

362. Little CB, Hilbert BJ, McGill CA: A retrospective study of head fractures in 21 horses, *Aust Vet J* 62:89-91, 1985.
363. Hahn CN, Mayhew IG, Mackay RJ: The nervous system. In Colahan PT et al, eds: *Equine medicine and surgery*, ed 5, St Louis, 2000, Mosby.
364. Fjeldborg J, Andresen PH, Svalastoga E: Osteomyelitis secondary to basilar skull fracture in a thoroughbred foal, *Equine Pract* 19:29-31, 1997.
365. Stick JA, Wilson T, Kunze D: Basilar skull fractures in three horses, *J Am Vet Med Assoc* 176:228-231, 1980.
366. Nation PN, Calder WA: Necrosis of the brain in calves following dehorning, *Can Vet J* 26:378-380, 1985.
367. Kornegay JN, Oliver JE, Gorgacz EJ: Clinicopathologic features of brain herniation in animals, *J Am Vet Med Assoc* 182:1111-1116, 1983.
368. Toutain PL, Brandon R, De Pomyers H: Dexamethasone and prednisolone in the horse: pharmacokinetics and action on the adrenal gland, *Am J Vet Res* 45:1750-1756, 1984.
369. McHarg MA et al: Effects of multiple intramuscular injections and doses of dexamethasone on plasma cortisol concentrations and adrenal responses to ACTH in horses, *Am J Vet Res* 46:2285-2287, 1985.
370. Goodnough J et al: The effect of dimethyl sulfoxide on gray matter injury in experimental spinal cord trauma, *Surg Neurol* 13:273-276, 1980.
371. Poungvarin N et al: Effects of dexamethasone in primary supratentorial intracerebral hemorrhage, *N Engl J Med* 316:1229-1233, 1987.
372. Beech J: Medical management and treatment of the horse with disease of the central nervous system, *Proceedings of the Thirty-first Annual Convention of the American Association of Equine Practitioners*, 1995, pp 33-36.
373. Brown SA, Hall ED: Role of oxygen-derived free radicals in the pathogenesis of shock and trauma, with focus on central nervous system injuries, *J Am Vet Med Assoc* 200:849-1859, 1992.
374. Brewer B: Therapeutic strategies involving antimicrobial treatment of the central nervous system in large animals, *J Am Vet Med Assoc* 185:1217-1220, 1984.
375. Blythe LL et al: Pharmacokinetic disposition of dimethyl sulfoxide administered intravenously to horses, *Am J Vet Res* 47:1739-1743, 1986.
376. De la Torre JC et al: Dimethyl sulfoxide in the treatment of experimental brain compression, *J Neurosurg* 38:345-354, 1973.
377. Rubin LF: Toxicity of dimethyl sulfoxide, alone and in combination, *Ann NY Acad Sci* 141:98-103, 1967.
378. Ferm VH: Teratogenic effect of dimethyl sulfoxide, *Lancet* 1:208-209, 1966.
379. Caujolle FME et al: Limits of toxic and teratogenic tolerance of dimethyl sulfoxide, *Ann NY Acad Sci* 141:110-125, 1967.
380. Tiews J et al: Metabolism and excretion of dimethyl sulfoxide in cows and calves after topical and parenteral application, *Ann NY Acad Sci* 141:139-150, 1967.

TRAUMATIC OPTIC NERVE BLINDNESS OF HORSES

Severe blunt trauma to the skull of young horses may result in a rapid caudal displacement of the brain and avulsion or stretching of the peripheral optic nerve. The condition often follows basisphenoid fractures or nonfracturing blows to the poll region (see preceding section). The clinical signs include blindness, loss of pupillary reflexes, and pupillary dilation. Ophthalmoscopic changes in the retina include pallor of the optic discs, reduction in the number and caliber of the retinal vessels, and linear peripapillary pigment disruptions. The condition is permanent.[381]

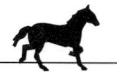

REFERENCE

381. Martin CL, Kaswan R, Chapman W: Four cases of traumatic optic nerve blindness in the horse, *Equine Vet J* 18:133-137, 1986.

NERVOUS COCCIDIOSIS

DEFINITION AND ETIOLOGY. Nervous coccidiosis is a neurologic syndrome of calves and yearling cattle, sheep, and goats that is associated with enteric infections by *Eimeria* spp. The condition is most commonly seen in western Canada and the northwestern United States and is especially prevalent in feedlots. The incidence of nervous coccidiosis is highest in the winter months. In contrast to enteric coccidiosis, the mortality rate of the nervous form of the disease can reach as high as 72%.[382] The pathogenesis of the encephalopathy may be related to the elaboration of a labile neurotoxin by the parasite.[383] The clinical signs and history of nervous coccidiosis are similar to those of other neurologic diseases that affect the function of the cerebral cortex.

CLINICAL SIGNS. The onset of the nervous signs is usually but not always preceded by diarrhea, tenesmus, and hematochezia. Some calves with severe diarrhea develop prolapsed rectums. Initial signs of central nervous system (CNS) dysfunction include depression, incoordination, twitching, and hyperesthesia. As the clinical signs worsen, the animal becomes recumbent and develops numerous cerebrocortical signs including opisthotonos, periodic tremors, horizontal nystagmus, frothing at the mouth, bellowing, snapping eyelids, and muscular fasciculations.[384-387] Blindness is rarely seen. Stimulation of the patient may precipitate a tonic-clonic seizure.[384-387] The animal may die after 1 to 5 days of encephalopathy. Convulsive calves may regain consciousness but relapse a week later.[388]

CLINICAL PATHOLOGY. Fecal flotations from the patient and herd mates show a large burden of coccidial oocysts. Fecal egg counts of affected animals may range from 5000 to 4 million/g. To exclude the possibility of other neurologic diseases, blood should be collected for measurement of electrolytes (calcium, magnesium, and potassium). The acid-base status, plasma glucose, and blood lead concentrations should be measured. Acute meningitis and salt poisoning may be ruled out by analysis of the cerebrospinal fluid (CSF). The plasma vitamin A concentration should be measured in any animal that has not had exposure to green forage. Polioencephalomalacia, ethylene glycol poisoning, lead poisoning, rabies, petroleum distillate poisoning, and clostridial enterotoxemia should be considered as possible differential diagnoses.

PATHOPHYSIOLOGY. The pathogenesis of the encephalopathy is unknown. The nervous form of coccidiosis cannot be transmitted to mice by injection of CSF from infected calves; however a heat-labile neurotoxin has been identified in the serum of calves with nervous coccidiosis.[383] The encephalotoxic activity is precipitable with 30% ammonium sulfate and may have an apparent molecular weight of 300,000 kDa.[389] The coccidia do not directly invade the CNS.

EPIDEMIOLOGY. Nervous coccidiosis occurs most commonly in feeder cattle, but dairy and pastured beef calves, lambs, and kids also may be affected occasionally. In one epidemiologic survey the prevalence of nervous coccidiosis was 0.3% of the calves that were affected with the intestinal form of the disease. Nevertheless, outbreaks with a large percentage of calves developing CNS disease have been reported.[384] In western Canada nervous signs have been reported in 21% of herd outbreaks of intestinal coccidiosis.[390] Approximately 90% of all cases of nervous coccidiosis occur in January, February, and March.

NECROPSY FINDINGS. No macroscopic lesions are seen in the CNS of calves afflicted with nervous coccidiosis. The microscopic lesions of the brain are mild and nonspecific and include edema, congestion, and occasional shrunken neurons. Parasitic invasion of the ileum, cecum, and colon results in lesions in these organs.

TREATMENT AND PREVENTION. Treatment should include 2 to 4 ml/kg of a commercially available calcium gluconate solution that contains magnesium, given subcutaneously. The coccidial infection should be treated with sulfamethazine (110 mg/kg PO for 5 days, or 1 pound/100 gallons of drinking water), or amprolium (50 mg/kg/day PO for 7 days). Diazepam, sodium pentobarbital, or phenobarbital may be used to control tonic-clonic convulsions (see Table 33-3). Slow intravenous administration of 50 to 100 ml of a 10% magnesium sulfate solution may also be useful as a sedative. The response to treatment is poor and the case fatality rate is high (approximately 90%) in calves that develop tonic-clonic seizures. Specific chemotherapeutic regimens and methods of preventing intestinal coccidiosis are described in Chapter 45.

REFERENCES

382. Eness P, Owen W: Bovine coccidiosis survey results, Ames, Iowa, 1984, Iowa State University Newsletter.
383. Isler CM, Bellamy JEC, Wobeser GA: Labile neurotoxin in serum of calves with nervous coccidiosis, *Can J Vet Res* 51:253-260, 1987.
384. Nillo L: Bovine coccidiosis in Canada, *Can Vet J* 11:91-98, 1970.
385. Julian RJ, Harrison KB, Richardson JA: Nervous signs in bovine coccidiosis, *Mod Vet Pract* 57:711-718, 1976.
386. Fanelli HH: Observations on nervous coccidiosis in calves, *Bovine Pract* 18:50-53, 1983.
387. Clayburg J: Neurological signs seen in coccidial infections, *Iowa State Vet* 2:85, 1970.
388. Tubb TF: Nervous disease associated with coccidiosis in young cattle, *Aust Vet J* 65:353-354, 1988.
389. Isler CM, Bellamy JEC, Wobeser GA: Characteristics of the labile neurotoxin associated with nervous coccidiosis, *Can J Vet Res* 51:271-276, 1987.
390. Radostits OM, Stockdale PHG: A brief review of coccidiosis in western Canada, *Can Vet J* 21:227-230, 1980.

SPOROZOAN INFECTIONS OF RUMINANTS (*Sarcocystis* Infection)

DEFINITION AND ETIOLOGY. The three recognized species of *Sarcocystis* that infect cattle, *Sarcocystis cruzi*, *Sarcocystis hominis*, and *Sarcocystis hirsuta* are sporozoan parasites with definitive hosts of dogs, primates, and cats, respectively.[391,392] Three other species, *Sarcocystis capricanus*, *Sarcocystis ovicanus*, and *Sarcocystis tenella*, have definitive hosts in dogs and secondary hosts in goats and sheep.[393]

When a carnivore ingests flesh from an infected cow, *Sarcocystis* cysts in muscle are broken down by digestive enzymes and motile bradyzoites are released. The bradyzoites infect the intestinal mucosal cell and differentiate into sexual stages called microgametes (male) and macrogamonts (female). The gametes fuse to form an oocyst, which is shed onto pastures as sporocysts. When eaten by a ruminant, the sporocysts hatch in the proximal small bowel and penetrate into the medium-sized mesenteric arteries, where they enter endothelial cells and form sporozoites. The sporozoites then mature in three successive waves. Each wave of development spreads downstream. The third-generation merozoites finally enter the soft tissues and encyst as sarcocysts. The total period of development in the ruminant requires 10 weeks. The life cycle is completed whenever a carnivore ingests uncooked meat containing viable sarcocysts. Chronic illness in the cow occurs during the maturation of the cyst in the muscles, at approximately 9 weeks after infection.

CLINICAL SIGNS. Most cases of *Sarcocystis* infestation are asymptomatic in both definitive and secondary hosts. However, if a large number of sporocysts are ingested by a nonimmune ruminant, clinical illness may develop. Clinical signs in cattle usually begin between 9 and 11 weeks after ingestion of infectious sporocysts. These signs include fever (temperature over 39.5° C [103.5° F]), anorexia, weight loss, symmetric lameness, and diarrhea. Neurologic signs include ataxia, muscular weakness, tremors, hyperexcitability, hypersalivation, recumbency, tonic-clonic seizures, leg biting, blindness, opisthotonos, and nystagmus.[394,395] Cattle may lose the hair of the tail switch ("rat tail"). Sheep may show a wool break.[391-405] Animals with chronic infections may develop edema of the limbs, poor weight gain, muscular atrophy, and pallor.[391-408] Second trimester abortions may occur in cattle and small ruminants beginning 28 days after ingestion of infectious sporocysts.[398] The fetuses may appear either normal or autolyzed. Lactating cows may have reduced milk production.[408]

CLINICAL PATHOLOGY AND PATHOGENESIS. Prolonged prothrombin times may be observed in some infected animals[391]; however, the activated clotting times and bleeding times are normal. The concentrations of plasma lactate dehydrogenase, alanine aminotransferase, sorbitol dehydrogenase, and blood urea nitrogen are increased. The packed cell volume and the serum protein concentration are decreased. During early infection there is a marked normocytic, normochromic anemia that is characterized by 75% reduction of the blood hemoglobin concentration and reduced packed cell volume.[409-411] The anemia is thought to be due to extravascular hemolysis.[412]

Antibodies to solubilized freeze-dried *Sarcocystis* antigens have been detected by indirect hemagglutination, enzyme-linked immunosorbent assay (ELISA), and an agar gel immunodiffusion (AGID) test.[413-415] Immunoglobulin M (IgM) responses first occur by 3 to 4 weeks after infection and peak by 11 to 15 weeks.[413-415] The concentrations of *Sarcocystis*-specific IgG begin to rise by 5 to 6 weeks and peak after 11 weeks after infection, with peak seroreactivity occurring by 39 days after infection. Background titers of normal cattle range from 1:54 to 1:486, and titers of infected cattle often exceed 1:10,000. There is no serologic cross-reactivity between *Sarcocystis* and *Toxoplasma gondii*, despite their physical similarities.[407]

PATHOPHYSIOLOGY. The pathogenesis of *Sarcocystis* is poorly understood. Pathologic changes in the skin and muscle and in serum chemistry probably are related to a combination of parasite-directed immunologic responses and diffuse vasculitis. Although toxins have not been identified, rabbits die acutely after parenteral administration of purified bradyzoites. The clinical signs exhibited by the inoculated rabbits resemble endotoxic shock. Other studies have indicated that chronic infections result in increased concentrations of somatostatin and decreased concentrations of somatomedin.[416] Abortions probably occur because of luteolysis that results from the increased concentrations of prostaglandin $F_{2\alpha}$ caused by vascular infection by the parasite.[417]

EPIDEMIOLOGY. Estimates of infection rates range from 70% to 98% in cattle in the United States.[391] The life cycle of the parasite is depicted in Fig. 33-7. When infected flesh is eaten by carnivores, the encysted sporozoites complete their life cycle.[391] The prepatent period of the parasite in the carnivore (primary host) ranges from 9 to 45 days. The primary host may shed the sporulated oocysts in the stool for as long as 2 months after a single infection. The oocysts withstand freezing but are rapidly killed by sunlight and drying.[391] Reexposure of previously infected canids results in a large fecal output of sporocysts. Ingestion of approximately 250 g of infected meat by a dog can result in an output of 100 to 6000

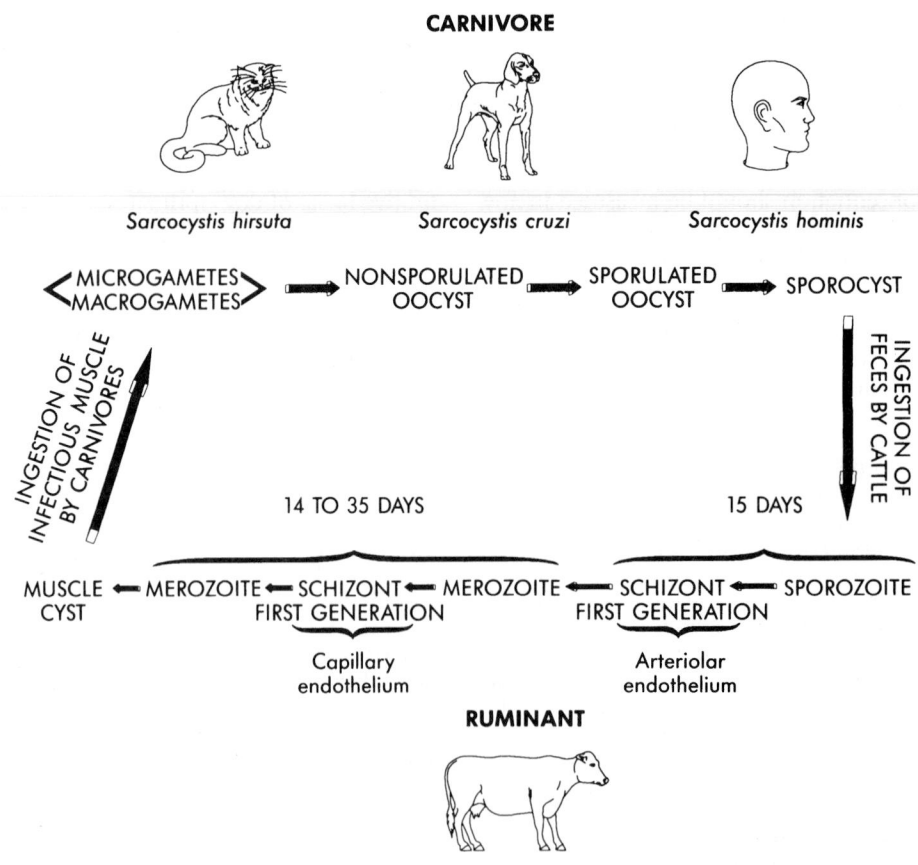

FIG. 33-7 ■ Life cycle of *Sarcocystis* parasite.

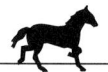

sporocysts per gram of feces. Wild canids are even more susceptible than domestic dogs and may serve as a major mechanism for propagation of *Sarcocystis* in range cattle in the western United States.

Most *Sarcocystis* infestations of cattle are asymptomatic; however, the disease may become clinically apparent with sudden, overwhelming exposure to the parasite in a nonimmune animal. Such conditions occur whenever there is an opportunity for extensive scavenging of ruminant carcasses by carnivores and contamination of feed bunks or pastures with infected carnivore feces.

The economic burden of *Sarcocystis* infection is unknown. One author has estimated an annual loss of $95 million in the United States alone.[391]

PATHOLOGIC LESIONS. The pathologic lesions of the CNS are similar for all species of sporozoans; they include granulomatous meningoencephalomyelitis, focal malacia, perivascular cuffing, neuronal degeneration, and gliosis. The changes are generally most severe in the cerebellum and midbrain but can occur anywhere in the CNS, including the spinal cord. The pathologic diagnosis is based on finding meronts and merozoites in the affected sections of neural tissue.[418,419]

Pathologic lesions elsewhere include hemorrhages on the sclera, serous surfaces, and muscles, fluid in the body cavities, and lymphadenopathy. The muscles have alternating light and dark stripes. Macroscopic changes may not be evident in animals with chronic sarcocystosis.[396,397] If changes are not evident, postmortem diagnosis is based on the finding of intravascular schizonts or intramuscular hemorrhages without significant inflammation. Ultrastructural examination of affected areas of CNS shows an intracellular colony with rosette orientation of agents in the cytoplasm of infected astrocytes.

TREATMENT. Feeding monensin (100 mg/kg daily for 30 days) during the incubation period is prophylactic; however, the efficacy of the drug in symptomatic cattle is unknown. For maximum effectiveness, monensin should be administered continuously for 2 to 5 weeks after exposure. Treatment of infected sheep with salinomycin (1 to 2 mg/kg of body weight) also has been recommended.[420] Administration of amprolium (100 mg/kg one time daily for 30 days) may reduce the severity of *Sarcocystis* infection[421] but may not completely eliminate the clinical disease.

CONTROL. The best method of controlling *Sarcocystis* infection is to protect the food supply of ruminants. Scavenging of carcasses by carnivores should also be prevented by deep burial or incineration. Feed bunks should be kept clean and raised approximately 1 to 3 feet off the ground. All carnivorous pets that have access to the feed or pastures should be fed cooked meat or processed dry food. In range pasture situations prophylactic feeding of monensin or elimination of predatory or scavenging carnivores may be necessary.

REFERENCES

391. Fayer R, Dubey JP: Bovine sarcocystosis, *Compend Cont Educ Pract Vet* 8:F130-F142, 1986.
392. Dubey JP, Fayer R: *Sarcocystis, Br Vet J* 139:371-377, 1983.
393. Dubey JP: Lesions in sheep inoculated with *Sarcocystis tenella* sporocysts from canine feces, *Vet Pathol* 26:237-252, 1988.
394. Jolley WR et al: Encephalitic sarcocystosis in a newborn calf, *Am J Vet Res* 44:1908-1911, 1983.
395. Dubey JP, Perry A, Kennedy MJ: Encephalitis caused by a *Sarcocystis*-like organism in a steer, *J Am Vet Med Assoc* 191:231-232, 1987.
396. Johnson AJ, Hildebrandt PC, Frayer R: Experimentally induced *Sarcocystis* infection in calves: pathology, *Am J Vet Res* 36:995-999, 1975.
397. Dubey JP, Spier CA, Epling GP: Sarcocystis in newborn calves fed *Sarcocystis cruzi* sporocysts from coyotes, *Am J Vet Res* 43:2147-2164, 1982.
398. Frayer R, Johnson AJ, Lunde M: Abortion and other signs of disease in cows experimentally infected with *Sarcocystis fusiformis* from dogs, *J Infect Dis* 134:624-628, 1976.
399. Reference deleted in proof.
400. Corner AH et al: Dalmeny disease: an infection of cattle presumed to be caused by an unidentified protozoan, *Can Vet J* 4:252-264, 1963.
401. Meads EB: Dalmeny disease: another outbreak, probably sarcocystosis, *Can Vet J* 17:271, 1976.
402. Ferguson HW: Toxoplasmosis in a calf, *Vet Rec* 104:392-393, 1979.
403. Landsverk T: An outbreak of sarcocystosis in a cattle herd, *Acta Vet Scand* 20:238-244, 1979.
404. Giles RC et al: Sarcocystosis in cattle in Kentucky, *J Am Vet Med Assoc* 176:543-548, 1980.
405. Frelier P et al: *Sarcocystis*: a clinical outbreak in dairy calves, *Science* 195:1341-1342, 1977.
406. Frayer R, Johnson AJ, Hildebrandt PK: Oral infection of mammals with *Sarcocystis fusiformis* bradyzoites from cattle and sporocysts from dogs and coyotes, *J Parasitol* 62:10-14, 1976.
407. Leek R, Frayer R: Sheep experimentally infected with *Sarcocystis* from dogs. II, Abortion and disease in ewes, *Cornell Vet* 68:108-123, 1978.
408. Hartley WJ, Blakemore WF: An unidentified sporozoan encephalomyelitis in sheep, *Vet Pathol* 11:1-12, 1974.
409. Mahrt JL, Frayer R: Hematologic and serologic changes in calves experimentally infected with *Sarcocystis fusiformis, J Parasitol* 61:967-969, 1975.
410. Prasse KW, Frayer R: Hematology of experimental acute *Sarcocystis bovicanis* infection in calves. II, Serum biochemistry and hemostasis studies, *Vet Pathol* 18:358-367, 1981.
411. Collery P: The pathogenesis of acute bovine sarcocystosis. IV, The effects of corticosteroid therapy on the course of anaemia, *Irish Vet J* 42:85-92, 1989.
412. Fayer R, Prasse KW: Hematology of experimental acute *Sarcocystis bovicanis* infection in calves. I, Cellular and serologic changes, *Vet Pathol* 18:351-357, 1981.
413. Lunde MN, Frayer R: Serologic tests for antibody to *Sarcocystis* in cattle, *J Parasitol* 63:222-225, 1977.
414. Frayer R, Lunde MN: Changes in serum and plasma proteins and in IgG and IgM antibodies in calves experimentally infected with *Sarcocystis* from dogs, *J Parasitol* 63:438-442, 1977.
415. Gasbarre LC, Frayer R: Humoral and cellular immune responses in cattle and sheep inoculated with *Sarcocystis, Am J Vet Res* 45:1592-1596, 1984.
416. Elasser TH et al: Hormonal perturbations in steers during infection with *Sarcocystis cruzi, Fed Proc* 44:760, 1985.
417. Dubey JP, Fayer R: Sarcocystosis: present and future, *J Vet Parasitol* 1:1-6, 1987.
418. Dubey JP, Speer CA, Douglass TG: Development and ultrastructure of first-generation meronts of *Sarcocystis cruzi* in calves fed sporocysts from dogs, *J Parasitol* 59:1135-1137, 1973.
419. Pacheco ND, Sheffield HG, Fayer R: Fine structure of immature cysts of *Sarcocystis cruzi, J Parasitol* 64:320-325, 1978.
420. Leek RG, Fayer R: Experimental Sarcocystis ovicanus infection in lambs, salinomycin chemoprophylaxis, and protective immunity, *J Parasitol* 69:271-276, 1983.
421. Fayer R, Johnson AJ: Effect of amprolium on acute sarcocystosis in experimentally infected calves, *J Parasitol* 61:932-936, 1975.

NEOSPORA INFECTION OF CATTLE (Protozoal Abortion)

DEFINITION AND ETIOLOGY. A cyst-forming protozoal parasite that closely resembles *Neospora caninum* has been identified in aborted fetuses from cattle in California. The condition is predominantly a disease of dairy cattle; however, sporadic abortions can occur in beef cows.[422-424] The predominant clinical sign of a *Neospora*-like agent is a midterm to late-term abortion (3 to 8 months of gestation). Fetal lesions consist of a focal nonsuppurative necrotizing encephalitis, nonsuppurative myocarditis and myositis, and mononuclear cell infiltrates disseminated in other tissues. Occasionally calves are mummified. The agent appears to have been responsible for as many as 24% of all abortions in northern California dairy cattle. Occasionally, however, a nonfatal infection may occur in the fetus. In this case the fetus is born with neurologic dysfunction (Fig. 33-8). The clinical signs of neurologic disease vary because of the randomly widespread distribution of the parasite within the central nervous system (CNS). Affected calves are often unable to stand and suckle and have abnormal spinal reflexes. Flexural contractions of the forelimbs, domed skull, and torticollis have also been reported in spontaneously occurring cases.[425,426] The calves are usually born with the CNS signs but initially they are mild and then progress after birth. Pathologic lesions

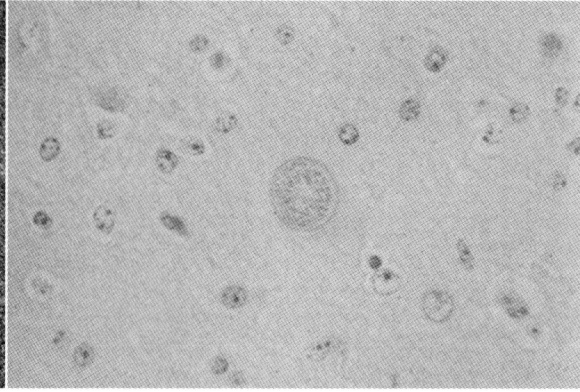

FIG. 33-8 ▥ Calf with congenital *Neospora* infection of the central nervous system *(left)* and a tissue cyst containing *Neospora* tachyzoites *(right)*.

associated with the fetal infection include focal areas of brain discoloration, focal cavitation with cyst formation, and reduction of gray matter. Microscopic changes of the CNS of affected calves include nonsuppurative inflammation of the gray and white matter, demyelination, perivascular cuffing, focal lymphocytic meningitis, and neuronal necrosis. Changes in other tissues include nonsuppurative myocarditis, myositis, and hepatitis. Protozoa can be seen in microscopic sections of the stained tissues.

Neospora organisms have been isolated in pure form using cultured cells.[427] Antibodies have been produced by intubation of laboratory animals, and the agent can be identified microscopically using immunoperoxidase staining on the fixed tissues. The cerebrospinal fluid (CSF) changes in affected calves range from normal to mild pleocytosis.[428] Similar conditions have been described in sheep[429,430] and goats.[431]

REFERENCES

422. Anderson M et al: Bovine protozoal abortions in California, *Bovine Pract* 26:102-104, 1991.
423. Anderson ML et al: *Neospora*-like protozoan infection as a major cause of abortion in California dairy cattle, *J Am Vet Med Assoc* 198:241-244, 1991.
424. Barr BC et al: Bovine fetal encephalitis and myocarditis associated with protozoal infections, *Vet Pathol* 27:354-361, 1990.
425. Barr BC: *Neospora*-like encephalomyelitis in a calf: pathology, ultrastructure, and immunoreactivity, *J Vet Diagn Invest* 3:39-46, 1991.
426. O'Toole D, Jeffrey M: Congenital sporozoan encephalomyelitis in a calf, *Vet Rec* 121:563-566, 1987.
427. Conrad PA et al: In vitro isolation and characterization of a *Neospora* species from aborted bovine foetuses, *Parasitology* 106:239-249, 1993.
428. Parish SM et al: Myelitis associated with protozoal infection in newborn calves, *J Am Vet Med Assoc* 191:1599-1600, 1987.
429. Hartley WJ, Bridge PS: A case of suspected congenital *Toxoplasma* encephalomyelitis in a lamb associated with a spinal cord anomaly, *Br Vet J* 131:380-384, 1975.
430. Dubey JP et al: Fatal congenital *Neospora caninum* infection in a lamb, *J Parasitol* 76:127-130, 1990.
431. Dubey JP, Acland H, Hamir AN: *Neospora caninum* (Apicomplexa) in a stillborn goat, *J Parasitol* 78:532-534, 1992.

EQUINE PROTOZOAL MYELOENCEPHALITIS (EPM; *Toxoplasma*-like Agent; Protozoal Encephalomyelitis; Segmented Myelitis)

WILLIAM J. A. SAVILLE

DEFINITION AND ETIOLOGY. Equine protozoal myeloencephalitis (EPM) is a multifocal, progressive disease of the central nervous system (CNS) that is primarily caused by infection with *Sarcocystis neurona*.[432] Recently another protozoal parasite (*Neospora caninum/Neospora hughesi*) was implicated as the cause of EPM in six cases.[433-438] The condition has been reported mostly from many states in the United States and from Canada, Panama, Brazil, and Argentina.[439-445] Several reports of the disease in countries other than those in the Western Hemisphere occurred primarily in horses that originated from the Americas.[446-448] Young standardbred, thoroughbred, and quarter horses are most often affected, although horses of any breed may develop the disease. There does not appear to be a gender predilection, and any age may be affected. The risk appears to be higher in young horses, but horses as old as 30 years of age have developed the disease. The parasite causes inflammation and necrosis of the brain, brainstem, and spinal cord. Under light microscopy, the structure of the EPM agents (*S. neurona* and *N. caninum*) resembles that of *Toxoplasma gondii*, but comparative electron microscopic analyses of the three agents show differences. The *Sarcocystis* agent responsible for infection in horses has been grown in explant cultures of monolayered bovine monocytes.[442,449] Antibodies in the sera or cerebrospinal fluid (CSF) can be detected using these specimens as probes of immunoblots of the cultured parasites.[450] Sera from clinically affected cases recognized eight *S. neurona*–specific antigens.[450]

Several of the unique *S. neurona*–specific antigens are the basis for the current diagnostic testing. Deoxyribonucleic acid (DNA) analysis has been very important in characterizing and classifying *S. neurona*. Using a random primed polymorphic DNA (RAPD) assay, a unique sequence of base pairs was identified that distinguished *S. neurona* from eight related coccidia, specifically two *Sarcocystis* species, one *Toxoplasma* species, and five *Eimeria* species.[451] This research demonstrated that unique DNA sequences could be used as a species-specific probe for *S. neurona* and that these probes allowe differentiation of *S. neurona* from other coccidia of equines.[451]

CLINICAL SIGNS. Descriptions of clinical signs of horses diagnosed with EPM may vary greatly because the organisms that cause this disease can affect any tissue in the central nervous system. Clinical signs recognized in the earliest studies of this disease still characterize the neurologic abnormalities in these cases. Early workers described horses with EPM as having an asymmetric ataxia and associated muscle atrophy.[452,453] Horses may have a sudden onset of clinical signs, or the disease may progress slowly over several months.[453] Vague, intermittent lameness that does not respond to therapy may be caused by EPM, and encephalitic signs typified by asymmetric cranial nerve deficits may also be seen.[453] Gait abnormalities include ataxia, tetraparesis, knuckling, circumduction, and crossing over. These abnormalities also may be asymmetric.

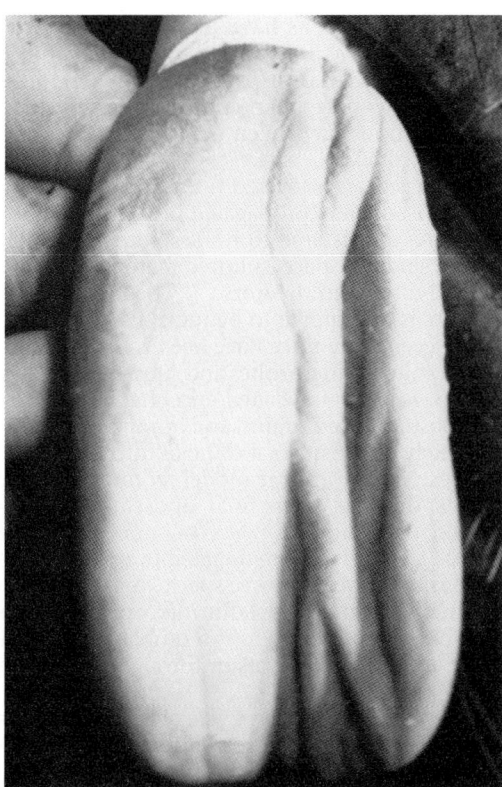

FIG. 33-9 ▦ Unilateral atrophy of the tongue in a Standardbred horse with protozoal myeloencephalitis. Atrophy also may occur in many other muscle groups of the head and the limbs. (Courtesy Dr. R.H. Whitlock.)

Depending on the location of the lesion in the spinal cord, areflexia, hyporeflexia, or hyperreflexia may be seen. Infections of the myelencephalon may result in head tilt, facial paralysis, circling, nystagmus, dysphagia, facial paralysis, and apparent blindness with or without abnormal pupillary reflexes. Parasitic invasion of the ventral spinal rootlets or the radicles of the maxillary branch of the trigeminal nerve may result in neurogenic atrophy of the tongue and masticatory muscles (Fig. 33-9). This often is accompanied by focal areas of desensitization. Regional sweating ("strip sweating") may be observed if the sympathetic tracts of the spinal cord are affected. Although EPM is typified by the presence of asymmetric, multifocal neurologic abnormalities, horses with EPM may have focal or symmetric signs.

Cerebral signs are rarely seen in horses with EPM. However, three horses with the disease brought to the Ohio State University Veterinary Teaching Hospital displayed seizure activity and evidence of cortical electrical activity abnormalities on electroencephalographic (EEG) examination.[454] Horses with cerebral neurologic signs often have a poor prognosis. However, seizure activity in horses with EPM may be treatable. Visual deficits and behavioral abnormalities have been reported in horses with EPM.[455] Head shaking was also reported in a recent case series describing three horses diagnosed with EPM.[456] Head shaking resolved in these horses after treatment for EPM.

The differential diagnoses of the most common neurologic diseases of horses that resemble EPM are equine degenerative myelopathy, cervical spinal injuries, cervical vertebral stenosis or malformation, equine herpes virus type 1 (EHV-1) infection, and equine lower motor neuron disease.

CLINICAL PATHOLOGY. A Western blot analysis for the diagnosis of EPM has been described and commercially mar-

keted.[450] Macrophage-cultured *S. neurona* is used as the antigen. After electrophoresis the blots are probed with suspect CSF or serum. Reactions are seen as bands developing on the blotted membrane. The sensitivity and specificity of the Western blot test has been reported as 89% based on 295 postmortems.[457] However, these figures probably are based on more severe cases. Although the test is promising, exhaustive examinations of its sensitivity and specificity in clinical cases are not yet available. Some recent research suggests that the sensitivity is excellent but the specificity in current clinical cases is much lower than originally reported.[458] There is no apparent serologic cross-reactivity between the parasites of EPM (*S. neurona* and *N. caninum*) and *T. gondii*.

Use of the Western blot test for antibody to *S. neurona* differs depending on the prevalence of the disease in the population being studied.[459] If the test is applied in the normal horse population, in which the prevalence of EPM probably is less than 1%, the predictive value of a positive test result is extremely low (under 8%), based on the 89% sensitivity and specificity. However, given the presence of neurologic signs, the prevalence increases dramatically (50% at Ohio State), leading to a positive predictive value of ~90%. This suggests that the test should not be applied in normal horses.[459] A recent report attempted to demonstrate increased specificity of the Western blot test for *S. neurona* antibody detection by blocking the reaction using *S. cruzi* antibody.[460] However, in a double-blind investigation conducted by the author, that increased specificity was questionable (unpublished data).

One of the difficulties in diagnosing EPM is the large number of horses that have detectable quantities of antibody to *S. neurona* in the CSF for several months after therapy or in horses that do not show neurologic signs. *S. neurona*–specific IgG found in the CSF is assumed to be produced locally because the blood-brain barrier should prevent large molecules from freely entering the cerebrospinal space. However, antibody detected in the CSF could have been produced systemically if the blood-brain barrier is compromised by disease or if peripheral blood contaminates the spinal fluid during sampling.

To help determine whether IgG in CSF was produced locally or was present due to peripheral blood contamination, a series of tests were modified from those used in human patients with neurologic diseases. For these tests, the albumin quotient (AQ) and the IgG index are calculated using concentrations of albumin and IgG found in serum and CSF of the patient.[461] The AQ is a measure of blood-brain barrier integrity, and the IgG index is a measure of intrathecal antibody production.[461] Some reports suggest that horses with EPM usually have a normal CSF albumin concentration and a normal AQ, but the IgG index usually is elevated.[462] It has been suggested that these indices, specifically an elevated AQ, can be used to distinguish a true positive result on a Western blot test from a false positive result caused by blood contamination during sampling.[462] False positive test results caused by blood contamination may alter the AQ and the IgG index by increasing the albumin and IgG concentrations in the CSF.[462]

It has also been recommended that the CSF indices may be used to monitor the response to therapy by identifying a decrease in the IgG index, which would mark a decrease in intrathecal antibody production over time.[463] However, a small number of horses were used in the initial evaluation of these tests, and the reported results show some inconsistencies.[463] Although the IgG index did decrease in 9 of 12 horses that were treated for EPM, it increased in 3 of 12 horses.[463] The reliability of the CSF indices has been questioned by others.[464,465] One controlled investigation suggests that the CSF indices are inconsistent and therefore, if used, should be interpreted with caution.[458]

Polymerase chain reaction (PCR) testing is available to aid in diagnosing EPM.[466,467] The sensitivity and specificity of

PCR testing of the cerebrospinal fluid has been reported to be 83% and 100%, respectively, when histologically confirmed cases of EPM were used to validate the assay.[468] However, other research suggests that the sensitivity of the PCR may be only approximately 40%.[469] The PCR test requires that parasite DNA be intact.[468] A strong inflammatory response favors enzymatic degradation of parasite DNA, and this process may affect the sensitivity of the PCR test.[468] It therefore has been suggested that the PCR test may be useful early in the course of the disease and in chronic cases.[468] In addition, PCR analysis of the CSF may be insensitive because the parasite most often is found in tissues and not floating freely in the CSF. For this reason, parasite DNA may not be present in CSF even when adjacent tissue is infected.[469] *T. gondii* infections are difficult to detect in human beings for the same reasons.[470] A recent study of clinical cases found that PCR testing alone was not useful for antemortem diagnosis of EPM because of the low sensitivity.[464]

S. neurona DNA has been detected in blood samples.[468] The presence of DNA in blood samples is thought to indicate recent ingestion of *S. neurona* sporocysts and subsequent infection.[468] However, it is not known how long detectable amounts of DNA remain in the bloodstream after infection.[468] Controlled investigations of PCR testing in horses with neurologic deficits and in normal horses are required to define the usefulness of this procedure.

CSF analysis has been used to aid in determining the etiology of neurologic diseases in the horse. Early studies suggested that horses with EPM had a mildly elevated CSF protein concentration, an increase in the number of mononuclear cells, and mild elevations in CSF enzyme activity, specifically creatine kinase (CK) and aspartate aminotransferase (AST).[471] Two early studies reported marked elevations in CK activity in horses diagnosed with EPM.[472,473] However, more recent studies suggest that neurologic disease of horses cannot be reliably differentiated based on the CSF leukocyte counts, CK or AST activity, or protein concentration.[458,474,475]

Several serologic tests have been developed for detecting *N. caninum* antibodies in animal species.[476] The three methods currently used are the enzyme-linked immunosorbent assay (ELISA), the indirect fluorescent antibody test (IFAT), and the direct agglutination test.[476] However, these antibody tests are only measures of exposure to the organism.

PATHOGENESIS. Little is known about the pathogenesis of EPM. It is assumed that the affected horses ingest *S. neurona* and that the course of infection and disease are then similar to those observed in other host species infected with other *Sarcocystis* spp. Because the sporocysts of *S. neurona* are passed in the feces of the opossum, infective oocysts probably are introduced into the feed and water supply of intermediate hosts.[477] Once ingested, the sporocysts excyst and release sporozoites, which penetrate the gut and enter the arterial endothelial cells of various organs.[477] Meronts develop and rupture the host cell, releasing merozoites into the bloodstream.[477] This probably is followed by a second round of merogony throughout the body.[477] In most diseases resembling *Sarcocystis* infection, this process results in the formation of sarcocysts in the muscle.[477] Subsequent ingestion of the infected muscle tissue by a predator or the definitive host completes the life cycle.[477] Sarcocysts of *S. neurona* have not been found in affected horses, indicating that the horse probably is an aberrant, dead-end host.[480]

The life cycle of *N. caninum/N. hughesi* in horses is not well known. Recent reports have demonstrated that the definitive host of *N. caninum* probably is the dog.[478] Currently it is not known if the dog is the definitive host of *N. hughesi*. The dog is the definitive host and also can be an intermediate host, which is similar to the situation with *T. gondii* in cats.[476] Unlike with EPM caused by *S. neurona*, tachyzoites have been

found in horse tissues, as have tissue cysts, in two of the horses reported to have EPM caused by *Neospora* infection.[476] In addition, in one case of neosporosis in a foal, the animal was determined to have been congenitally infected.[436] No congenital infections have been demonstrated in horses infected with *S. neurona*.

S. neurona has been recovered from CNS lesions in several horses and subsequently propagated in culture in the laboratory.[479] When administered to horses parenterally or introduced via the epidural space, cultured merozoites have not induced clinical disease in the horse.[479] The merozoite stage of *Sarcocystis* spp. is not known to be transmissible to other animals.[479] However, nude mice have been inoculated intraperitoneally with cultured merozoites and subsequently developed evidence of *S. neurona*-associated encephalitis.[480] These mice were immunosuppressed strains, and intraperitoneal injection would not likely be the normal route of infection with *S. neurona* in horses. A better mouse model recently was developed by feeding sporocysts from feral opossums to IFN-γ/KO mice.[481] These procedures in IFN-γ/KO mice also help differentiate *Sarcocystis* spp. that are excreted in opossum feces, because it appears that at least three species are present in the feces.[481] The mechanism by which the merozoites enter the CNS currently is unknown. The organism probably enters the CNS by means of infected leukocytes or through the cytoplasm of endothelial cells.[479]

Specific details about the life cycle of *S. neurona* are mostly unknown, although recent research has demonstrated that the opossum probably is the definitive host. The geographic distribution of opossums is similar to that of EPM, and areas with a lower seroprevalence of *S. neurona* appear to coincide with regions outside the natural range of opossums.[482] Further evidence that the opossum is the definitive host for *S. neurona* was obtained by experimental induction of EPM.[483] When sporocysts from feral opossums were fed to horses, neurologic disease developed.[483] This study has been repeated by other research groups.[484] However, induction of clinical EPM by feeding *Sarcocystis falcatula* sporocysts was not successful.[485] More recent work has demonstrated that, as was mentioned previously, at least three species of *Sarcocystis* sporocysts can be found in feces from the opossum.[486] Development of DNA probes that distinguish among *Sarcocystis* spp. in opossum feces has enhanced researchers' understanding of this organism.[487,488] Some recent work suggests that in fact four species of *Sarcocystis* sporocysts may be present in opossum feces.[487,488] The probes will allow researchers to better characterize sporocysts from opossum feces, which will help in additional induction studies to develop a reliable equine model for EPM.

Unlike most *Sarcocystis* spp., *S. neurona* may aberrantly infect a large number of intermediate hosts. Although the full range of intermediate hosts for *S. neurona* has not yet been identified, several species of animals and birds have been reported to show symptoms similar to those seen in horses with EPM. Several reports indicate that an *S. neurona*–like organism has infected and caused neurologic disease in dogs, sheep, cats, a mink, raccoons, a striped skunk, a golden hawk, rhesus monkeys, Pacific harbor seals, sea otters, and chickens.[489-500] The harbor seals and the sea otter showed evidence of sarcocysts in the muscle that tested positive for *S. neurona*.[499,500] To this author's knowledge, this is the first evidence of possible *S. neurona* sarcocysts to date; however, the significance of this finding is not well understood. This positive reaction to anti-*S. neurona* antibody could be due to cross-reactivity to other *Sarcocystis* spp. The wide host range is atypical for *Sarcocystis* spp, and the host range behavior is similar to that of *T. gondii*, which is phylogenetically close to *S. neurona*.[501,502]

Based on the estimated number of opossums in North America, the poor survival rate of these animals, and the small areas in which they travel, there is speculation that this organism may be transmitted by methods other than direct contact with opossum feces. Experiments performed by researchers in the 1980s indicated that some transmission by birds may occur.[503] In experiments attempting to characterize the life cycle of *S. falcatula*, birds apparently were infected by aerosol spread.[503] Vector transmission also was demonstrated by the recovery of sporocysts after budgerigars, canaries, white mice, and chickens were fed opossum feces.[504] The recovered sporocysts were then fed to budgerigars to assess the viability of the sporocysts.[504] Four of six budgerigars died, demonstrating that the sporocysts were viable.[504] These experiments suggest that sporocysts might be transmissible between intermediate hosts.[504] Considering the apparent wide range of natural and aberrant intermediate hosts for *S. neurona* and *S. falcatula*, transmission of infectious organisms between intermediate hosts implies that control of disease caused by these organisms may be extremely difficult.

Insects such as flies and cockroaches may also be transport vectors for *S. neurona*. Early work demonstrated that flies may act as transport vectors for *T. gondii*.[505] Subsequently, the same group found that cockroaches may also act as transport vectors for *T. gondii*.[506] In addition, fatal pulmonary disease developed in psittacine birds that were fed cockroaches after the cockroaches had been fed opossum feces.[507] Although this suggests that insects may play a role in the transmission of *S. neurona*, further investigation is necessary to determine which insects are actually involved in the life cycle of the organism.

It has been postulated that stress may play a role in the development of EPM,[477,501] but limited evidence is available to support this hypothesis. The severity of EPM may be related to the size of the infective dose, the immune competency of the host, and the environmental stressors to which the horse is exposed.[479] A similar association between immunosuppression and disease has been documented in other species with EPM-like symptoms. For example, recent mouse models for the disease have been developed using nude mice and IFN-γ/KO mice, both of which are immune-compromised strains.[480,481] Raccoons have been identified that were concurrently infected with a *Sarcocystis*-like protozoan and canine distemper virus.[498,508] This is interesting because the canine distemper virus is known to be immunosuppressive and often has been associated with cerebral toxoplasmosis in dogs, foxes, and raccoons.[508]

Sarcocystis infection of the CNS was also identified with a concurrent simian immunodeficiency virus (SIV) infection in a monkey that developed asymmetric neurologic signs similar to those seen in EPM.[496] Immunocompromised human beings are often infected with *T. gondii*, and it has been demonstrated that stress plays a major role in the recrudescence of the clinical signs of *T. gondii*–associated encephalitis.[509] Infection with either *N. caninum* or *T. gondii* can cause T cell hyporesponsiveness to the parasite antigen.[510]

It has also been demonstrated that an intact T cell response (specifically, appropriate production of interleukin-12 and interferon-γ) is necessary for resistance against either *N. caninum* or *T. gondii*. The parasite may therefore facilitate further infection by compromising host immune responses.[510] Recent evidence suggests that neuropeptides (neuroimmune proteins [NIP]) are released from the CNS when an animal is stressed, which may lead to suppression of lymphocyte production and function.[511] It has also been demonstrated that stress leads to high circulating glucocorticoid concentrations, which are also immunosuppressive.[511] The combination of high resting concentrations of glucocorticoids and an increase in NIP release may result in immunosuppression and facilitate development of clinical disease in horses infected with *S. neurona*.

Recent evidence from a controlled investigation performed at Ohio State University demonstrated that health events before diagnosis of EPM were strongly associated with the disease.[458] Further controlled investigations are needed to examine the role of stress in the development of clinical signs of EPM in horses.

PATHOLOGIC LESIONS. Diagnosis of EPM has been difficult because of a lack of understanding of the pathogenesis of the disease and because of the variety of clinical signs. Postmortem examination was the first method used to definitively diagnose EPM and is still considered by many to be the gold standard for diagnosis. Grossly, the CNS lesions identified at postmortem are described as multifocal areas of hemorrhage to light discoloration of the brain or spinal cord.[477] Histologic examintion often reveals a marked mononuclear perivascular cuffing with necrosis and loss of neurons and with infiltration of monocytes, lymphocytes, some eosinophils, and in rare cases, neutrophils.[452,471] Protozoal organisms can be seen in some of the lesions but are often difficult to detect.[471] Difficulty in detecting the organisms increases if the animal has been treated with antiprotozoal medications.[512] Immunohistochemical staining techniques can be used to definitively identify parasites in situ.[513,514]

Postmortem examination is also the definitive diagnostic test for EPM caused by *N. caninum (N. hughesi)*.[476] Immunohistochemistry testing is a useful tool for identifying the *Neospora* organisms.[476] A significant problem with this method of diagnosis is that by definition, it cannot be applied in horses antemortem and therefore cannot be applied to most clinical cases. A reliable diagnostic test that could be used for antemortem diagnosis is needed to better understand EPM and appropriately manage horses with this disease.

EPIDEMIOLOGY. Little is known about the epidemiology of EPM, although knowledge about this disease is increasing. A small study from one county in Pennsylvania indicated that the seroprevalence was approximately 45% of the horse population, along with an increase in prevalence with age.[515] Another report found an overall seroprevalence of 45% among horses in Oregon with differences in seroprevalence among geographic regions.[482] In Oregon, the seroprevalence ranged from 22% in the eastern arid region of the state to 65% in the coastal region. A third study reported a prevalence of serum antibodies to *S. neurona* in Ohio horses at 53.6%.[516] The Ohio study demonstrated an increase in prevalence with the increase in age, and greater prevalence in the southwestern part of the state than in the northeastern part.[516] The location differences in prevalence in Ohio may have been related to climatic differences based on freezing days in various regions of the state.[516]

These studies suggest that in many areas of the United States, approximately 50% of the horses may have serum antibodies to *S. neurona*.[455] Another study suggested that horses are exposed to *S. neurona* in the eastern half of the United States at a rate 10% to 15% higher than in the western half of the country.[468] Two recent reports suggest that the seroprevalence of *S. neurona* antibody in horses in Argentina and Brazil is 35.5% and 35.6%, respectively.[444,445] Little work has been done regarding the prevalence of antibody to *N. caninum* in horses; however, recent work found a seroprevalence of 23.3% in sera examined from two horse slaughterhouses in the United States and a lack of antibody detection in Argentina and Brazil.[444,445,517] Because these studies involved small numbers of horses, they may not reflect the true prevalence of *N. caninum* antibody in horses.[444,445,517] The results suggest that exposure to *S. neurona* is common but that geographic differences may exist. Much more work needs to be done regarding *N. caninum* exposure.

There were no formal studies of the incidence or prevalence of EPM in the United States until recently. Based on the number of cases diagnosed at postmortem at the University of Kentucky, it appears that the incidence of EPM may be increasing.[479] The number of samples submitted to the University of Kentucky for immunoblot analysis suggests that several hundred new cases of EPM may be diagnosed in the United States each year.[479] An estimate of the incidence of EPM based on accessions to the University of Kentucky diagnostic laboratory was 1% or fewer of all horses each year.[477] The U.S. Department of Agriculture (USDA) recently monitored the number of cases in the United States, which provided approximate incidence rates and a baseline for future reference. According to that study, the average incidence of EPM was 14 cases per 10,000 horses per year.[518] The incidence was examined based on the primary use of the horse and found that the lowest incidence was in farm and ranch horses (1 case per 10,000 horses per year).[518] In pleasure horses the rate was 6 cases per 10,000 horses per year.[518] A marked increase occurred in breeding horses (17 cases per 10,000 horses per year), racing horses (38 cases per 10,000 horses per year) and competition and show horses (51 cases per 10,000 horses per year).[518] The racing horses did not include horses at racetracks.[518] The estimates reflect an incidence of the disease similar to that previously reported, if not lower. No controlled investigations of neosporosis in horses have been done. There have been six reports of neosporosis in horses reportedly caused by *N. caninum (N. hughesi)*.[433-438] However, only four of the reports were in horses with neurologic signs, one was in an aborted fetus, and the other was related to an intestinal problem.[433-438]

EPM has been reported from a number of states in the United States, as well as from Canada, Mexico, Panama, Argentina, and Brazil.* EPM has also been reported in England among horses imported from the eastern United States.[446] EPM was diagnosed in an 8-month-old Arabian horse in South Africa that had been imported from the United States approximately 5 months before the onset of signs.[447] The most recent report was a California horse that developed clinical signs of EPM after 10 months in Hong Kong.[448] EPM thus is primarily a disease of the Western Hemisphere.

Several authors have suggested that the prevalence of disease may be high among standardbred horses.[452,454,512,520] However, two authors suggested that this apparent predilection may be due to the environment in which horses were kept rather than to breed characteristics.[453,512] Another case series reported that the disease was most common in thoroughbreds.[441] A recent controlled investigation into risk factors for the development of EPM did not find a breed predilection, but occupations such as racing and showing demonstrated increased risk compared to breeding and pleasure horses.[521] This finding was corroborated by a recent study by the National Animal Health Monitoring System (NAHMS).[518]

Early reports on EPM suggested that young horses had an increased risk of the disease.[441,452,512] A consistent theme in the reports was that at least 60% of the affected horses were 4 years of age or younger.[441,452,512] This finding was corroborated by the Ohio State study, which also showed an increased risk in horses over 13 years of age.[521]

Historically EPM has been reported as a sporadic disease; more than one case is rarely reported on farms.[453,522] There are reports of EPM cases from Panama in which all affected horses were stabled at the same location, although this is not a common occurrence.[442] There is also a report of an outbreak on a farm in Kentucky.[523] A recent finding in Ohio suggested that the risk of EPM was increased (more than two and one half times higher) if the disease had been previously diagnosed on the farm, which suggests that clustering of cases may occur.[521]

Several other risk factors for the development of EPM have been reported. The Ohio State study found an increased risk if opossums were seen on the farm and if woods were present on the farm; it also noted a seasonal effect or the occurrence of a health event before the development of clinical signs of EPM.[521] The seasonal effect increased the risk of EPM as the temperature increased, with the highest risk in the fall.[521] The Ohio State study also found a decreased risk if a creek or river was present on the farm and if the feed was kept protected from wildlife access.[521]

The NAHMS study also found a higher in risk if opossums were seen on the premises compared with never seeing an opossum on the premises, and an even higher risk if the opossums were seen frequently.[518] An increase in risk was also seen with increased numbers of horses, purchased versus home-grown grain, use of wood chips or shavings as bedding, the presence of rats and mice on the premises, and increased human population density.[518] A lower risk was seen where there were woods within 5 miles of the premises and where surface water was used as the primary drinking source.[518] As was seen in the Ohio State study, the highest risk for disease was in the fall.[518] It is difficult to explain some of the findings from both studies, but it appears that management practices play a role in the development of clinical EPM.

TREATMENT. Because no consistent equine model for induction of EPM has been developed and because clinical patients require medication due to the severity of the disease, treatment regimens have evolved empirically. Until recently, the recommended therapy had not changed since the disease was originally identified. However, recent use of liquid combination therapies with questionable stability led to a perceived lack of response and consistently longer durations of treatment. This has led to the development of novel treatments.

The standard therapy for horses with EPM is a combination of sulfadiazine and pyrimethamine, both antifolate medications. Based on the description of the pathologic lesions of EPM and identification of organisms that resemble *T. gondii*, the first recommendations for treatment of EPM were extrapolated from therapy used to treat toxoplasmosis in human beings.[524,525] Numerous changes have since been made with regard to dosage and duration of the therapy.[522,526-528] Most of these recommendations were empirically based on clinical impression rather than controlled clinical trials.[528] More recently, some therapeutic recommendations have been based on pharmacokinetic data.[529,530]

In a very recent study, the activity of pyrimethamine, trimethoprim, sulfonamides, and combinations of the medications were tested against *S. neurona* merozoites in tissue cultures.[531] Pyrimethamine was demonstrated to be completely inhibitory and coccidiocidal at 1 µg/ml.[531] The same was true for trimethoprim at 5 µg/ml.[531] None of the sulfonamides by themselves had activity when administered at 100 µg/ml.[531] When sulfonamides at either 5 or 10 µg/ml were used in combination with pyrimethamine at 0.1 µg/ml, the activity against *S. neurona* was improved.[531] However, these findings are based on in vitro studies, and further work is needed in controlled clinical trials in horses.

The duration of therapy required to effectively treat horses with EPM has been a controversial issue. Initially recommendations regarding duration of therapy were based on clearing of specific IgG from the CSF as indicated by a negative result on the Western blot test. However, many horses remain CSF positive for antibody to *S. neurona* for months after therapy. One author's recommendation that the medications should be continued at least 2 weeks past resolution of the signs or 4 weeks past a plateau of the clinical signs has been adopted by many clinicians. The current recommendation for the pyrimethamine-sulfadiazine combination is 20 mg/kg of sulfadiazine PO once or twice daily and 1 mg/kg

*References 439, 440, 442, 443, 446, and 519.

of pyrimethamine PO once daily for at least 150 to 180 days. Horses with EPM are often treated for long periods with medications that act by inhibiting folate metabolism. Some authors have suggested that complete blood counts should be monitored in horses treated for EPM for signs of folic acid deficiency. Potential side effects of treatment with antifolate medications include bone marrow suppression, anemia, colitis, and even teratogenesis. Most of the anemias are mild and improve after withdrawal of the medication.

One other side effect of the use of a combination of trimethoprim-sulfamethoxazole and pyrimethamine, a commonly used combination in the past, is its effect on reproductive function in pony stallions.[532] Although it may not affect the semen quality, testicular volume, sperm production efficiency, erection, or libido of healthy stallions, it may induce changes in copulatory form and agility and alter the pattern and strength of ejaculation.[532] Therefore caution should be used when treating stallions for neurologic disease believed to be EPM.

Recently triazine-derivative drugs have been used to treat EPM. These drugs (diclazuril and toltrazuril) originally were designed for use as herbicides and have been used in other countries in the prophylaxis of coccidiosis in poultry and swine. The response to therapy in horses with EPM was slightly better than the response documented for the standard therapy.[533] The pharmacokinetics of both diclazuril and toltrazuril have been demonstrated.[534] Currently diclazuril is available only as a ration premix, therefore large volumes must be given daily. Another disadvantage is the poor palatability of diclazuril in its present form. One advantage to the use of these compounds is an appreciably shorter duration of therapy. Diclazuril is administered at the rate of 5 mg/kg for a minimum of 28 days.[535] Recent in vitro testing for activity of diclazuril against *S. neurona* has been demonstrated.[536] It may have to be administered by nasogastric tube daily.[535]

Toltrazuril is another coccidiostat that is becoming very popular because of its ease of use and good absorption orally in horses.[535] Toxicity studies of toltrazuril in horses at 50 mg/kg for 10 days resulted in mild anorexia and depression.[535] The current recommended dosage is 5 to 10 mg/kg for a minimum of 28 days.[535] Nitazoxanide (NTZ) is another novel treatment that has recently been used in the treatment of EPM. NTZ is a 5-nitrothiazole with a broad spectrum of activity against bacterial, protozoal, and helminthic parasites.[535] It has been shown to kill *S. neurona* in cell cultures.[535] Toxicity studies were performed in horses, and when horses were given twice the recommended dosage, they became lethargic after 1 week of daily dosing.[535] When horses were given NTZ at four times the recommended dosage, they became significantly ill and one died.[535] Currently the suggested treatment schedule is 25 mg/kg PO once daily for the first week and 50 mg/kg PO once daily for the next 23 days.[535] None of these three new EPM medications have been approved by the U.S. Food and Drug Administration (FDA); however, field trials are underway to gain FDA approval.

The prognosis for horses diagnosed with EPM is similar regardless of the treatment used. Most reports suggest an approximate improvement rate of 70% when using the standard therapy,[455,537,538] but earlier work suggested the success rate was about 50%.[526] Fewer than 25% of affected horses may return to their original function, although little objective information is available about this issue.[455] A recent study with diclazuril resulted in approximately 75% improvement in horses severely affected with EPM.[533] In the diclazuril study, approximately 30% of the horses treated (11/36) either returned to their original level of performance before EPM diagnosis or improved their level of performance.[533] An efficacy study of 70 horses given NTZ found that 63% of the horses met the criteria for success after treatment.[535]

A growing concern is the percentage of horses that have a relapse in clinical disease after cessation of therapy. Some horses relapse days, weeks, or even months after treatment stops, but the mechanism of relapse is unknown.[528] It may be due to recrudescence of a truly latent stage of the parasite, the presence of a small persistent focus of infection, or perhaps reexposure to the parasite.[528] Anecdotal estimates of the relapse rate range from 10% to 28% of treated horses.[455,537,538] The relapse rate when diclazuril was used was less than 5%.[533]

Before the recognition of EPM as a disease, corticosteroids were widely recommended for treatment of neurologic diseases in horses. However, corticosteroids should be used with caution in suspected cases of EPM because of the possibility of adversely affecting the host immune response to the organism.[440,446,524,525] Nonsteroidal antiinflammatory drugs and dimethyl sulfoxide (DMSO) also have been routinely used in the treatment of horses with EPM since the mid-1980s.[446,455]

Based on the persistence in the cerebrospinal fluid of the antibody to *S. neurona* for long periods in some horses with EPM, one author has recommended the use of immune stimulants.[455] This recommendation was also based on the observation that some horses may not mount a sufficient immune response to clear the organism.[455] Several nonspecific T cell stimulating compounds have been recommended for this purpose.[455] Unfortunately, no controlled trials have been undertaken to examine the efficacy of these treatments.

Supplementation with folic acid, folinic acid, and/or brewer's yeast has been recommended for treatment of presumed folic acid deficiency, particularly in pregnant mares.[446,526] However, folic acid supplementation has been discouraged by other investigators because of poor absorption and the potential for toxic effects on the bone marrow activity.[455] Toxicity has also been reported in newborn foals born to mares treated for EPM with antifolate medications and concurrently supplemented with folic acid.[539] These foals showed evidence of bone marrow aplasia and hypoplasia, renal nephrosis or hypoplasia, and skin lesions.[539] A cause-and-effect relationship between folic acid supplementation and these developmental abnormalities has not been conclusively demonstrated. However, folic acid supplementation should not be used, particularly in pregnant mares, until controlled clinical trials can be performed to corroborate or refute these findings.

Several authors have recommended the use of additional supplements, such as vitamin E and thiamine, that may facilitate healing of nervous tissue for the treatment of horses with EPM.[455,538] However, clinical trials have not been performed to establish the efficacy of this supplementation.

REFERENCES

432. Dubey JP et al: *Sarcocystis neurona* (protozoa Apicomplexa), the etiologic agent of equine protozoal myeloencephalitis, *J Parasitol* 77:212-218, 1991.
433. Daft B et al: *Neospora* encephalomyelitis and polyradiculoneuritis in an aged mare with Cushing's disease, *Equine Vet J* 28:240-243, 1996.
434. Dubey J, Porterfield M: *Neospora cannier* (Apicomplexa) in an aborted equine fetus, *J Parasitol* 76:732-734, 1990.
435. Hamir A et al: *Neospora caninum*-associated equine protozoal myeloencephalitis, *Vet Parasitol* 79:269-274, 1998.
436. Lindsay D et al: Central nervous system neosporosis in a foal, *J Vet Diagn Invest* 8:507-510, 1996.
437. Marsh AE et al: Neosporosis as a cause of equine protozoal myeloencephalitis, *J Am Vet Med Assoc* 209:1907-1913, 1996.
438. Gray M et al: Visceral neosporosis in a 10-year-old horse, *J Vet Diagn Invest* 8:130-133, 1996.
439. Clark EG, Townsend HGG, McKenzie NT: Equine protozoal myeloencephalitis: a report of two cases from western Canada, *Can Vet J* 22:140-144, 1981.
440. De Barros CSL, De Barros SS, Dos Santos MN: Equine protozoal myeloencephalitis in southern Brazil, *Vet Rec* 117:283-284, 1986.

441. Fayer R et al: Epidemiology of equine protozoal myeloencephalitis in North America based on histologically confirmed cases, *J Vet Intern Med* 4:54-57, 1990.

442. Granstrom DE et al: Equine protozoal myelitis in Panamanian horses and isolation of *Sarcocystis neurona, J Parasitol* 78:909-912, 1992.

443. Masri MD, Lopez de Alda J, Dubey JP: *Sarcocystis neurona*–associated ataxia in horses in Brazil, *Vet Parasitol* 44:311-314, 1992.

444. Dubey J, Kerber C, Granstrom D: Serologic prevalence of *Sarcocystis neurona, Toxoplasma gondii,* and *Neospora caninum* in horses in Brazil, *J Am Vet Med Assoc* 215:970-972, 1999.

445. Dubey J et al: Prevalence of antibodies to *Sarcocystis neurona, Toxoplasma gondii,* and *Neospora caninum* in horses from Argentina, *Vet Parasitol* 86:59-62, 1999.

446. Mayhew IG, Greiner EC: Protozoal diseases, *Vet Clin North Am (Equine Pract)* 2:439-459, 1986.

447. Ronen N: Putative equine protozoal myeloencephalitis in an imported Arabian filly, *J S Afr Vet Assoc* 63:78-79, 1992.

448. Lam K, Watkins K, Chan C: First report of equine protozoal myeloencephalitis in Hong Kong, *Equine Vet Educ* 11:54-56, 1999.

449. Davis SW, Speer CA, Dubey JP: In vitro cultivation of *Sarcocystis neurona* from the spinal cord of a horse with equine protozoal myelitis, *J Parasitol* 77:789-792, 1991.

450. Granstrom DE et al: Equine protozoal myeloencephalitis: antigen analysis of cultured *Sarcocystis neurona* merozoites, *J Vet Diagn Invest* 5:88-90, 1993.

451. Granstrom DE et al: Differentiation of *Sarcocystis neurona* from eight related coccidia by random amplified polymorphic DNA assay, *J Mol Cell Probes* 8:353-356, 1994.

452. Rooney JR et al: Focal myelitis-encephalitis in horses, *Cornell Vet* 60:494-501, 1970.

453. Mayhew IG et al: Equine protozoal myeloencephalitis, *Proceedings of the Twenty-second Annual Convention of the American Association of Equine Practitioners,* 1976, pp 107-114.

454. Dunigan CE et al: Seizure activity associated with equine protozoal myeloencephalitis, *P Vet Neuro* 6:50-54, 1995.

455. MacKay RJ: Equine Protozoal Myeloencephalitis, *Vet Clin North Am (Equine Pract)* 13:79-96, 1997.

456. Moore L et al: Management of head shaking in three horses by treatment for protozoal myeloencephalitis, *Vet Rec* 141:264-267, 1997.

457. Granstrom DE: Equine protozoal myeloencephalitis: parasite biology, experimental disease, and laboratory diagnosis, International Equine Neurology Conference, Ithaca, NY, 1997.

458. Saville W: The epidemiology of equine protozoal myeloencephalitis (EPM), *Vet Prev Med* 458:223, 1998.

459. Cohen N, MacKay R: Interpreting Immunoblot testing of cerebrospinal fluid for equine protozoal myeloencephalitis, *Compend Cont Educ Pract Vet* 19:1176-1181, 1997.

460. Rossano M et al: Improvement of Western blot specificity for detecting equine serum antibodies to *Sarcocystis neurona, J Vet Diagn Invest* 12:28-32, 2000.

461. Andrews FM, Maddux JM, Faulk D: Total protein, albumin quotient, IgG and IgG index determinations for horse cerebrospinal fluid, *P Vet Neuro* 1:197-204, 1991.

462. Andrews FM, Granstrom DE, Provenza M: Differentiation of neurologic diseases in the horse by the use of albumin quotient and IgG index determinations, *Proceedings of the Forty-first Annual Convention of the American Association of Equine Practitioners,* 1995, pp 215-217.

463. Andrews F et al: CSF indices after repeated spinal taps in horses diagnosed with equine protozoal myeloencephalitis, *Proceedings of the Forty-third Annual Convention of the American Association of Equine Practitioners,* 1997, pp 10-12.

464. Miller MM, Bernard WV: Usefulness of cerebrospinal fluid indices and the polymerase chain reaction for *Sarcocystis neurona* in diagnosing equine protozoal myeloencephalitis *Proceedings of the Forty-second Annual Convention of the American Association of Equine Practitioners,* 1996, pp 82-84.

465. Miller M et al: Effects of blood contamination of cerebrospinal fluid on Western blot analysis for detection of antibodies against *Sarcocystis neurona* and on albumin quotient and immunoglobulin G index in horses, *J Am Vet Med Assoc* 215:67-71, 1999.

466. Fenger C et al: Detection of *Sarcocystis neurona* in blood, cerebrospinal fluid, and feces by polymerase chain reaction, *Am Assoc Vet Parasitol* 1995.

467. Fenger CK: Update on the diagnosis and treatment of equine protozoal myeloencephalitis (EPM), *Proc Am Coll Vet Intern Med Forum* 13:597-599, 1995.

468. Granstrom DE: Recent advances in the laboratory diagnosis of equine parasitic diseases, *Vet Clin North Am (Equine Pract)* 486:437-442, 1995.

469. Marsh AE et al: Sequence analysis and polymerase chain reaction amplification of small subunit ribosomal DNA from *Sarcocystis neurona, Am J Vet Res* 57:975-981, 1996.

470. Parmley S, Goebel F, Remington J: Detection of *Toxoplasma gondii* in cerebrospinal fluid from AIDS patients by polymerase chain reaction, *J Clin Microbiol* 30:3000-3002, 1992.

471. Mayhew IG et al: Spinal cord disease in the horse, *Cornell Vet* Suppl 6:1-207, 1978.

472. Furr MO, Tyler RD: Cerebrospinal fluid creatine kinase activity in horses with central nervous system disease: 69 cases (1984-1989), *J Am Vet Med Assoc* 197:245-248, 1990.

473. Green EM, Kroll RA, Constantinescu GM: Equine cerebrospinal fluid: analysis, *Compend Cont Educ Pract Vet* 15:288-300, 1993.

474. Reed SM et al: Clinical findings and cerebrospinal fluid analysis, including Western blot analysis, on horses presented for neurologic disease at Ohio State University, *Proc Am Coll Vet Intern Med Forum* 13:739-741, 1995.

475. Jackson C et al: The diagnostic utility of cerebrospinal fluid creatine kinase activity in the horse, *J Vet Intern Med* 10:246-251, 1996.

476. Dubey J: Recent advances in *Neospora* and neosporosis, *Vet Parasitol* 84:349-367, 1999.

477. Granstrom DE, Saville WJ: Equine protozoal myeloencephalitis In Reed SM, Bailey WM, eds: *Equine internal medicine,* Philadelphia, 1998, WB Saunders.

478. McAllister M et al: Dogs are definitive hosts of *Neospora caninum, Int J Parasitol* 28:1473-1478, 1998.

479. Granstrom DE: Diagnosis of equine protozoal myeloencephalitis: Western blot analysis, *Proc Am Coll Vet Intern Med Forum* 11:587-590, 1993.

480. Marsh A et al: Experimental infection of nude mice as a model for *Sarcocystis neurona*–associated encephalitis, *Parasitol Res* 83:706-711, 1997.

481. Dubey J, Lindsay D: Isolation in immunodeficient mice of *Sarcocystis neurona* from opossum *(Didelphis virginiana)* faeces and its differentiation from *Sarcocystis falcatula, Int J Parasitol* 28:1823-1828, 1998.

482. Blythe LL et al: Seroprevalence of antibodies to *Sarcocystis neurona* in horses residing in Oregon, *J Am Vet Med Assoc* 210:525-527, 1997.

483. Fenger CK et al: Experimental induction of equine protozoal myeloencephalitis using *Sarcocystis* sp. sporocysts from the opossum *(Didelphis virginiana), Vet Parasitol* 68:199-213, 1997.

484. Cutler T et al: Experimental challenge of horses with characterized *S. neurona* sporocysts, *Am Coll Vet Intern Med Forum,* Abstract No 17, 1994.

485. Cutler T et al: Are *Sarcocystis neurona* and *S. falcatula* synonymous? A horse infection challenge, *J Parasitol* 85:301-305, 1999.

486. Dubey J, Speer C, Lindsay D: Isolation of a third species of *Sarcocystis* in immunodeficient mice feces from opossums *(Didelphis virginiana)* and its differentiation from *Sarcocystis falcatula* and *Sarcocystis neurona, J Parasitol* 84:1158-1164, 1998.

487. Tanhauser S et al: Multiple DNA markers differentiate *Sarcocystis neurona* and *Sarcocystis falcatula, J Parasitol* 85:221-228, 1999.

488. Tanhauser S et al: Multiple DNA markers differentiate *Sarcocystis neurona* and *Sarcocystis falcatula* and identify two additional *Sarcocystis* spp. shed by opossums, *Am Assoc Vet Parasitol,* Abstract No 27, 1999.

489. Dubey JP et al: Fatal necrotizing encephalitis in a raccoon associated with a *Sarcocystis*-like protozoan, *J Vet Diagn Invest* 2:345-347, 1990.

490. Dubey JP et al: Development of a *Sarcocystis*-like apicomplexan protozoan in the brain of a raccoon *(Procyon lotor), J Helminthol Soc Wash* 58:250-255, 1991.

491. Dubey JP, Speer CA: *Sarcocystis canis* n. sp. (Apicomplexa: Sarcocystidae): the etiologic agent of generalized coccidiosi in dogs, *J Parasitol* 77:522-527, 1991.

492. Dubey JP et al: Sarcocystosis-associated clinical encephalitis in a golden eagle *(Aquila chrysaetos), J Zoo Wildl Med* 22:233-236, 1991.

493. Dubey JP, Hedstrom OR: Meningoencephalitis in mink associated with a *Sarcocystis neurona*–like organism, *J Vet Diagn Invest* 5:467-471, 1993.

494. Dubey JP: *Sarcocystis*-associated meningoencephalomyelitis in a cat, *J Vet Diagn Invest* 6:118-120, 1994.

495. Dubey JP et al: A *Sarcocystis neurona*–like organism associated with encephalitis in a striped skunk *(Mephitis mephitis), J Parasitol* 82:172-174, 1996.

496. Klumpp SA et al: Encephalomyelitis due to a *Sarcocystis neurona*–like protozoan in a rhesus monkey *(Macaca mulatta)* infected with simian immunodeficiency virus, *Am J Trop Med Hyg* 51:332-338, 1994.

497. Mutalib A et al: Sarcocystosis-associated encephalitis in chickens, *Av Dis* 39:436-440, 1995.

498. Thulin JD et al: Concurrent protozoal encephalitis and canine distemper virus infection in a raccoon *(Procyon lotor), Vet Rec* 130:162-164, 1992.

499. Lapointe J et al: Meningoencephalitis due to a *Sarcocystis neurona*–like protozoan in Pacific harbor seals *(Phoca vitulina richardsi), J Parasitol* 84:1184-1189, 1998.

500. Rosonke B et al: Encephalomyelitis associated with a *Sarcocystis neurona*–like organism in a sea otter, *J Am Vet Med Assoc* 215:1839-1842, 1999.

501. Dubey JP, Speer CA, Fayer R: *Sarcocystosis of animals and man,* Boca Raton, Fla, 1989, CRC Press.

502. Fenger CK et al: Phylogenetic relationship of *Sarcocystis neurona* to other members of the family Sarcocystidae based on the sequence of the small ribosomal subunit gene, *J Parasitol* 80:966-975, 1994.

503. Box ED, Smith JH: The intermediate host spectrum in a *Sarcocystis* species of birds, *J Parasitol* 68:668-673, 1982.

504. Box E: Recovery of *Sarcocystis* sporocysts from feces after oral administration, *Proc Helminthol Soc Wash* 50:348-350, 1983.

505. Wallace G: Experimental transmission of *Toxoplasma gondii* by filth flies, *Am J Trop Med Hyg* 20:411-413, 1971.

506. Wallace G: Experimental transmission of *Toxoplasma gondii* by cockroaches, *J Infect Dis* 126:545-547, 1972.

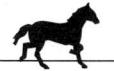

507. Clubb SL, Frenkel JK: *Sarcocystis falcatula* of opossums: transmission by cockroaches with fatal pulmonary disease in psittacine birds, *J Parasitol* 78:116-124, 1992.
508. Stoffregen DA, Dubey JP: A *Sarcocystis* spp–like protozoan and concurrent distemper virus infection associated with encephalitis in a raccoon (*Procyon lotor*), *J Wildl Dis* 27:688-692, 1991.
509. Weiss L et al: The association of the stress response and *Toxoplasma gondii* bradyzoite development, *J Eukaryot Microbiol* 43:120s, 1996.
510. Khan I et al: *Neospora caninum:* role for immune cytokines in host immunity, *Exp Parasitol* 85:24-34, 1997.
511. Fan S, Shao L, Ding G: A suppressive protein generated in peripheral lymph tissue induced by restraint stress, *Adv Neuroimmunol* 6:279-288, 1996.
512. Boy MG, Galligan DT, Divers TJ: Protozoal encephalomyelitis in horses: 82 cases (1972-1986), *J Am Vet Med Assoc* 196:632-634, 1990.
513. Granstrom DE, Giles RC, Tuttle PA: Immunohistochemical diagnosis of protozoan parasites in lesions of equine protozoal myeloencephalitis, *J Vet Diagn Invest* 3:75-77, 1991.
514. Hamir AN et al: Immunohistochemical study to demonstrate *Sarcocystis neurona* in equine protozoal myeloencephalitis, *J Vet Diagn Invest* 5:418-422, 1993.
515. Bentz BG, Granstrom D, Stamper S: Seroprevalence of antibodies to *Sarcocystis neurona* in horses residing in a county of southeastern Pennsylvania, *J Am Vet Med Assoc* 210:517-518, 1997.
516. Saville WJ et al: Prevalence of serum antibodies to *Sarcocystis neurona* in horses residing in Ohio, *J Am Vet Med Assoc* 210:519-524, 1997.
517. Dubey J et al: Prevalence of antibodies to *Neospora caninum* in horses in North America, *J Parasitol* 85:968-969, 1999.
518. National Animal Health Monitoring System: Equine protozoal myeloencephalitis in the United States, Fort Collins, Colo, 2000, US Department of Agriculture.
519. Dorr TE et al: Protozoal myeloencephalitis in horses in California, *J Am Vet Med Assoc* 185:801-802, 1984.
520. Traver DS et al: Protozoal myeloencephalitis in sibling horses, *J Equine Med Surg* 2:425-428, 1978.
521. Saville WJA et al: Analysis of risk factors for the development of equine protozoal myeloencephalitis in horses, *J Am Vet Med Assoc* 217:1174-1180, 2000.
522. MacKay RJ, Davis SW, Dubey JP: Equine protozoal myeloencephalitis, *Compend Cont Educ Pract Vet* 14:1359-1366, 1992.
523. Fenger CK et al: Epizootic of equine protozoal myeloencephalitis on a farm, *J Am Vet Med Assoc* 210:923-927, 1997.
524. Beech J, Dodd DC: *Toxoplasma*-like encephalomyelitis in the horse, *Vet Pathol* 11:87-96, 1974.
525. Beech J: Equine protozoan encephalomyelitis, *VM SAC* 69:1562-1566, 1974.
526. Welsch BB: Update on equine therapeutics: treatment of equine protozoal myeloencephalitis, *Compend Cont Educ Pract Vet* 13:1599-1602, 1991.
527. Reed SM, Granstrom DE: Equine protozoal encephalomyelitis, *Proc Am Coll Vet Intern Med Forum* 11:591-592, 1993.
528. Granstrom DE et al: Equine protozoal myeloencephalitis: biology and epidemiology, *Proceedings of the Seventh International Conference on Equine Infective Disorders*, 1994.
529. Clarke CR et al: Pharmacokinetics, penetration into cerebrospinal fluid, and hematologic effects after multiple oral administrations of pyrimethamine to horses, *Am J Vet Res* 53:2296-2299, 1992.
530. Clarke CR et al: Pharmacokinetics of intravenously and orally administered pyrimethamine in horses, *Am J Vet Res* 53:2292-2295, 1992.
531. Lindsay D, Dubey J: Determination of the activity of pyrimethamine, trimethoprim, sulfonamides, and combinations of pyrimethamine and sulfonamides against *Sarcocystis neurona* in cell cultures, *Vet Parasitol* 82:205-210, 1999.
532. Bedford S, McDonnell S: Measurements of reproductive function in stallions treated with trimethoprim-sulfamethoxazole and pyrimethamine, *J Am Vet Med Assoc* 215:1317-1319, 1999.
533. Granstrom D et al: Diclazuril and equine protozoal myeloencephalitis, *Proceedings of the Forty-third Annual Convention of the American Association of Equine Practitioners*, 1997, pp 13-14.
534. Tobin T et al: Preliminary pharmacokinetics of diclazuril and toltrazuril in the horse, *Proceedings of the Forty-third Annual Convention of the American Association of Equine Practitioners*, 1997, pp 15-16.
535. Furr M: Treatment and management of equine protozoal myeloencephalitis, *Proceedings of the North American Veterinary Conference*, Orlando, Fla, 2000, pp 137-138.
536. Lindsay D, Dubey J: Determination of the activity of diclazuril against *Sarcocystis neurona* and *Sarcocystis falcatula* in cell cultures, *J Parasitol* 86:164-166, 2000.
537. Fenger CK: Equine protozoal myeloencephalitis: early detection means more successful treatment, *Large Anim Vet*, 1996, pp 14-20.
538. Reed SM, Saville WJA: Equine protozoal encephalomyelitis, *Proceedings of the Forty-second Annual Convention of the American Association of Equine Practitioners*, 1996, pp 75-79.
539. Toribio R et al: Congenital defects in newborn foals of mares treated for equine protozoal myeloencephalitis during pregnancy, *J Am Vet Med Assoc* 212:697-701, 1998.

BABESIA ENCEPHALITIS (Babesiosis; Piroplasmosis; Texas Cattle Fever; Tick Fever; Red Water)

Parasitemia of cattle caused by the protozoans *Babesia bovis, Babesia argentina,* and *Babesia bigemina* usually is subclinical. The disease is transmitted to cattle by the cattle fever ticks *Boophilus annulatu, Boophilus microplus,* or *Boophilus decoloratus.* Babesiosis occurs in the Americas, Europe, Africa, Asia, and Australia. Ticks acquire *Babesia* infection from an infected animal and then pass the agent to their offspring through the ovaries. The protozoan is passed to susceptible cattle by nymphs and adults. Most infections result in intravascular and extravascular hemolysis and kidney and liver failure. A small proportion of *Babesia* infections cause acute encephalitis.[540] The central nervous system (CNS) signs begin suddenly and include fever (41.7° C [107° F]), anorexia, depression, ataxia, conscious proprioceptive deficits, mania, convulsions, and coma. Sudden death occasionally is observed. The nervous signs are accompanied by engorgement of the scleral vessels, icterus, proteinuria, and hemoglobinuria. Encephalopathic diseases that closely resemble babesiosis include rabies, coccidiosis, polioencephalomalacia, lead poisoning, infectious bovine rhinotracheitis virus encephalitis, theileriasis, heartwater disease, salt poisoning, and chlorinated hydrocarbon toxicity.

The pathogenesis of the CNS signs are unclear; however, possible causes include capillary thrombosis and infarction, disseminated intravascular coagulation (DIC), anoxic encephalopathy, and direct invasion of the CNS by the parasite. Thrombi are disseminated throughout the CNS. This finding and the observation of increased prothrombin times, partial thromboplastin times, thrombocytopenia, and decreased fibrinogen concentrations indicate that DIC plays an important role in the pathogenesis of the CNS disease.[541-543]

The condition is a reportable disease in the United States. Suspect cases should be referred to the appropriate state and federal authorities.

REFERENCES

540. Rogers RJ: Observations on the pathology of *Babesia argentina* infections in cattle, *Aust Vet J* 47:242-247, 1971.
541. Dalgliesh RJ et al: *Babesia argentina:* disseminated intravascular coagulation in acute infections in splenectomized calves, *Exp Parasitol* 40:124-131, 1976.
542. Wright IG: An electron microscopic study of intravascular agglutination in the cerebral cortex due to *Babesia argentina, Int J Parasitol* 2:209-215, 1972.
543. Mahoney DF, Goodger BV: *Babesia argentina:* serum changes in infected calves, *Exp Parasitol* 24:375-382, 1969.

COWDRIA (RICKETTSIA) RUMINANTIUM INFECTION (Heartwater Disease)

DEFINITION AND ETIOLOGY. *Cowdria ruminantium* is a rickettsial parasite that causes a fatal encephalitis in goats, sheep, and cattle.[544] The disease originated in sub-Saharan Africa and has spread to cattle in the West Indies (Guadeloupe, Antigua, and Marie Galante),[545] where it has become an economically important tick-borne disease of cattle. *C. ruminantium* is transmitted by *Amblyomma* spp. ticks.[546] Although a number of *Amblyomma* species have been implicated in the transmission of heartwater disease, the most important agents are *Amblyomma hebraeum* and *Amblyomma variegatum.* The intermittent feeding behavior of the tick makes it particularly resistant to treatment with acaricides. *Amblyomma* ticks require three separate blood meals to complete their life cycle. The gravid females fall from the host and lay the eggs in rotting vegetation, particularly in areas where the hosts are bedded for the evening. Recently hatched larvae crawl onto foliage and await a host. After their first feed the larvae detach, molt into nymphs, and await a second host. After refeeding, the nymphs detach and molt into adults. The adults remain under rotting vegetation until they are activated by carbon dioxide exhaled by a large mammal. They are further attracted to the host by pheromones from male ticks that remain permanently attached to the host. Animals that do not have male tick infestations are poor attractants for nongravid females. Once attached to the proper host, the females seek the male, breed, feed, and fall from the host when it lies down for the evening. Ticks that feed from *Cowdria*-infected hosts develop ovarian infections and transmit the agent to their offspring. This serves to perpetuate the agent over successive seasons.[547]

Many species of vertebrates, including snakes, iguanas, lizards, and birds, are reservoirs for *C. ruminantium* because these animals may serve as the first two hosts for the *Amblyomma* tick.[548]

CLINICAL SIGNS. After inoculation into a ruminant, the rickettsial agent infects reticuloendothelial cells and proliferates by binary fission within membrane-bound vacuoles.[549,550] Release of the parasite from degenerating macrophages and neutrophils causes successive waves of parasitemia that infect endothelial cells and cause vasculitis.[550,551] In the cell the developmental stages of the *Cowdria* organism resemble those of chlamydia; they include elementary, reticulate, and intermediate bodies, which can be differentiated microscopically.[552] Nervous lesions may be caused by permeability changes in the cerebral capillaries. Changes in the other soft tissues include hydropericardium, hydrothorax, and subcutaneous edema.[544]

Except for Angora goats, which are highly susceptible to *Cowdria* infection, animals reared in indigenous areas usually have a high level of immunity and do not succumb to the infection.[553] Animals that survive the initial infection become asymptomatic but remain rickettsemic for as long as 223 days (sheep), 246 (cattle), and 8 days (goats). Calves under 3 weeks of age, lambs under 8 days of age, and kids under 6 weeks of age are inherently resistant to *C. ruminantium* infection, regardless of the amount of colostral protection they have received.[554,555]

PATHOLOGY. Pathologic changes of cowdriosis include hydropericardium, hydroperitoneum, hydrothorax, pulmonary edema, perirenal edema, hemorrhages in the pleura and peritoneum, and hemorrhagic enteritis. Microscopic changes include microgliosis, necrotizing vasculitis in the brain, hemorrhage, edema of the neuropil, microcavitation, and focal necrosis of the granular layer of the cerebellum. In clinical cases the parasite can only be definitively diagnosed by biopsy of the cerebral cortex or by collection of the cortical tissues at postmortem examination.[556] Simple techniques for collection of such biopsy specimens have been described.[557-559] Squash preparations of the biopsied material should be stained with either methyl green pyronine or Giemsa stains before microscopic examination of the tissues.[560,561] A cloned DNA probe that identified *C. ruminantium* DNA has been developed, but the clinical usefulness of the test is unknown.[562]

NECROPSY FINDINGS. Animals with the peracute form of heartwater disease die suddenly without premonitory signs. The acute form of the disease is characterized initially by fever, anorexia, depression, and respiratory distress. Cyanosis also may be noted. Nervous signs, which may appear within a few days, include hyperesthesia, snapping closure of the eyelids, rapid extension of the tongue, behavioral changes, muscular fasciculations, hypermetria, ataxia, conscious proprioceptive deficits, and head-pressing. As the disease progresses, the animals become recumbent and comatose. Convulsions may occur terminally. These episodes

are characterized by opisthotonos, nystagmus, chewing movements, and frothing at the mouth. Mild forms of the disease are characterized by transient diarrhea, malaise, and fever, with no CNS involvement. The mortality rate in sheep ranges from 6% to 80%. Animals that recover are immune to reinfection for at least 58 months.[563] Losses may reach 60% of susceptible cattle and 40% of goats. The mortality rate among Angora goats may exceed 90%.

An indirect fluorescent antibody (IFA) test using infected bovine aortic endothelial cells for indicators has been described.[564] The specificity of the test was thought to be greater than that of previous IFA tests using macrophage-derived antigen. Laboratory-infected animals seroconverted by day 13 and retained a detectable titer for 30 weeks after infection. The presence of antibodies in the serum of sheep had a partial correlation to resistance to challenge with virulent rickettsiae.[565] Antibodies induced to *Anaplasma marginale*, *Theileria parva*, *Babesia bigemina*, or *Rickettsia conorii* did not cross-react with the *Cowdria*-infected endothelial cells. Cloned deoxyribonucleic acid (DNA) probes from *Cowdria* organisms have been developed. The probes recognize DNA from the plasma of infected sheep and are specific for *Cowdria* DNA.[566]

TREATMENT. The administration of oxytetracycline (6 to 10 mg/kg IV twice daily for 3 to 4 days) may be beneficial for treatment of the early stages of the disease. The long-acting formulation of oxytetracycline also is effective, but for best results it should be administered as soon as the animal becomes febrile. Treatment usually is futile if the first dose of oxytetracycline is administered after the onset of neurologic symptoms.[567] Despite the depository nature of the long-acting formulation, two or more administrations 48 hours apart are needed to achieve a good clinical response. Cattle should be retreated if they develop a fever after the first dosage has been administered.[568] Animals with nervous system signs frequently die despite intensive antibiotic therapy. Angora goats are highly susceptible to heartwater disease. In South Africa Angora producers routinely treat all animals every 14 days during the summer with oxytetracycline. Nevertheless, the number of deaths caused by heartwater disease is directly related to the number of antibiotic treatments administered. Animals that remain essentially tick free never develop adequate immunity to the *Cowdria* organism.

It would seem that a small degree of tick infestation and exposure of the animals to low numbers of the agent, combined with judicious oxytetracycline therapy, would favor the development of immunity over time.[569] A method of immunization using a controlled infection of a virulent strain (Onderstepoort Ball 3 strain) of the *Cowdria* organism and treatment with long-acting oxytetracycline (800 mg per adult goat) at the beginning of clinical disease and 10 days later has been described.[570] Vaccination with this isolate produces immunity against exposure to homologous but not heterologous strains of *Cowdria*.[571-573] Despite this strain difference, immunoblotting of *C. ruminantium* proteins with heterologous and heterologous antiserum has not resolved the antigenic differences between strains.[574] An attenuated live strain of *Cowdria* has been isolated. When inoculated in sheep and goats, the agent proved to be nonpathogenic, yet it stimulated protective antibody responses. The effectiveness and safety of the vaccine under field conditions is still unknown.[575] The immunity against *C. ruminantium* may be short-lived, and animals that have been affected by the agent and treated with oxytetracycline may be susceptible within 2 years after the treatment is administered.

PREVENTION AND CONTROL. Control of ticks on cattle pastures is the most desirable means of controlling heartwater disease. Complete eradication of the ticks in most regions of sub-Saharan Africa is neither possible nor desirable. Cattle that are reared in areas where *Cowdria* infection is endemic develop acquired immunity over time. In these areas the ticks should be sufficiently abundant to permit a low level of heartwater infections in most cattle, yet not so populous as to introduce severe, overwhelming infections. Integrated methods for tick control have been recommended. These include exclusion of wildlife from paddocks, artificial induction of host resistance to ticks, application of insecticidal ear tags, and conventional acaracide application.

Insecticides currently used for tick control include Taktic Dairy Collar and Taktic EC,* Permectrin,† coumaphos, chlorovinphos, and dimethoate. Application of insecticides as the sole method of tick control has not proved highly effective. Resistance to the acaricides may develop with prolonged use. The dips are expensive and frequently are used at improper concentrations. Moreover, some species are not highly attracted to ruminants unless other ticks are already attached. Treatment of these animals would be ineffective and wasteful. A novel osmotic pump loaded with ivermectin that delivers 60 μg/kg/day kills *A. hebraeum* and reduces the number of fertile eggs shed. The efficacy of the drug under field conditions has not yet been examined.

REFERENCES

544. Cowdry EV: Studies on the etiology of heart water. I, Observation of a rickettsia, *Rickettsia ruminantium* (n. sp.), in the tissues of infected animals, *J Exp Med* 42:231-251, 1925.
545. Camus E, Barre N, Iemvt C: Epidemiology of heart water in Guadeloupe and in the Caribbean, *Onderstepoort J Vet Res* 54:419-426, 1987.
546. Cowdry EV: Studies on the etiology of heart water. II, *Rickettsia* (n. sp.) in the tissues of ticks transmitting the disease, *J Exp Med* 42:253-272, 1925.
547. Bezuidenhout JD, Jacobsz CJ: Proof of transovarial transmission of *Cowdria ruminantium* by *Amblyomma hebraeum*, *Onderstepoort, J Vet Res* 53:31-34, 1986.
548. Kocan KM et al: Demonstration of colonies of *Cowdria ruminantium* in midgut epithelial cells of *Amblyomma variegatum*, *Am J Vet Res* 48:356-360, 1987.
549. Du Pleiss JL: Electron microscopy of *Cowdria ruminantium*–reticuloendothelial cells of the mammalian host, *Onderstepoort J Vet Res* 42:1-14, 1975.
550. Pienaar JG: Electron microscopy of *Cowdria (Rickettsia) ruminantium* (Cowdry, 1926) in the endothelial cells of the vertebrate host, *Onderstepoort J Vet Res* 37:67-78, 1970.
551. Du Pleissis JL: Pathogenesis of heartwater. I, *Cowdria ruminantium* in the lymph nodes of domestic ruminants, *Onderstepoort J Vet Res* 37:89-96, 1970.
552. Jongejan F, Zanderbergen PA, Van De Wiel: The tick-borne rickettsia *Cowdria ruminantium* has a chlamydia-like developmental cycle, *Onderstepoort J Vet Res* 58:227-237, 1991.
553. Norval RAI et al: Biological processes in the epidemiology of heartwater. In Fivaz B, ed: *Tick vector biology: medical and veterinary aspects*, New York, 1992, Springer-Verlag.
554. Andrew, Norval: The carrier status of sheep, cattle, and African buffalo recovered from heartwater, *Vet Parasitol* 34:261-266, 1989.
555. Barre N, Camus E, Iemvt-Craag BP: The reservoir status of goats recovered from heartwater, *Onderstepoort J Vet Res* 54:435-437, 1987.
556. Schreuder BEC: A simple technique for the collection of brain samples for the diagnosis of heartwater, *Trop Anim Health Prod* 12:25-29, 1980.
557. Johnston LAY, Callow LL: Intracerebral inoculation and brain biopsy in cattle, *Aust Vet J* 39:22-24, 1963.
558. Synge BA: Brain biopsy for the diagnosis of heartwater, *Trop Anim Health Prod* 10:45-48, 1978.
559. Malika J et al: A simple method for collection of brain samples for the diagnosis of heartwater, *Bull Animal Health Prod Afr* 40:157-159, 1992.
560. Burdin ML: Selective staining of *Rickettsia ruminantium* in tissue sections, *Vet Rec* 74:1371-1372, 1962.
561. Purchase HS: A simple and rapid method for demonstrating *Rickettsia ruminantium* (Cowdry, 1925) in heartwater brains, *Vet Rec* 36:413-414, 1945.
562. Waghela SD et al: A cloned DNA probe identifies *Cowdria ruminantium* in *Amblyomma variegatum* ticks, *J Clin Microbiol* 29:2571-2577, 1991.
563. Neitz WO: The immunity in heartwater, *Onderstepoort J Vet Sci Anim Ind* 13:245-283, 1939.
564. Semu SM et al: Development and persistence of *Cowdria ruminantium*: specific antibodies following experimental infection in cattle as detected by the indirect fluorescent antibody test, *Vet Immunol Immunopathol* 333:339-352, 1992.
565. Du Plessis JL, Van Gas L: Immunity of tick-exposed seronegative and seropositive small stock challenged with two stocks of *Cowdria ruminantium*, *Onderstepoort J Vet Res* 56:185-188, 1989.
566. Mahan SM et al: A cloned DNA probe for *Cowdria ruminantium* hybridizes with eight heartwater strains and detects infected sheep, *J Clin Microbiol* 30:981-986, 1992.
567. Uilenberg G: Heartwater (*Cowdria ruminantium* infection): current status, *Adv Vet Sci Comp Med* 27:427-479, 1983.
568. Gueye A, Vassilaides G: Traitment et perspectives de chimioprophylaxie de la codriose ovine pare une oxytetracycline a longue duree, *Rev Elev Med Vet Pays Tropic* 38:428-432, 1985.
569. Spickett AM, Fivaz BH: A survey of small stock tick control practices in the eastern Cape province of South Africa, *Onderstepoort J Vet Res* 59:197-201, 1992.
570. Erasmus JA: Heartwater: the immunization of Angora goats, *J S Afr Vet Med Assoc* 47:143, 1976.
571. Duplessis JL, Potgieter FT, Van Gas L: An attempt to improve the immunization of sheep against heartwater by using different combinations of three stocks of *Cowdria ruminantium*, *Onderstepoort J Vet Res* 57:205-208, 1990.
572. Brown CC et al: Protection of goats against Caribbean and African heartwater isolates by the ball 3 heartwater vaccine, *Trop Animal Health Prod* 21:100-106, 1989.
573. Jongejan F, Uilenberg G, Franssen FFJ: Antigenic differences between stocks of *Cowdria ruminantium*, *Res Vet Sci* 44:186-189, 1988.
574. Rossouw M et al: Identification of the antigenic proteins of *Cowdria ruminantium*, *Onderstepoort J Vet Res* 57:215-221, 1990.
575. Jongejan F: Protective immunity to heartwater (*Cowdria ruminantium* infection) is acquired after vaccination with in vitro–attenuated rickettsiae, *Infect Immun* 59:729-731, 1991.

CEREBRAL THEILERIASIS (Turning Sickness; Draaisiekte; East Coast Fever, Corridor Disease, January Disease, Tropical Fever)

DEFINITION AND ETIOLOGY. Cerebral theileriasis is an encephalitic disease of cattle caused by the piroplasma parasites *Theileria annulata* and *Theileria parva*. theileriasis is seen mainly in Africa (Kenya and Tanganyika) and India, where it is characterized by a high mortality rate and is known as East Coast Fever. *Theileria mutans*, a parasite of cattle in the southwestern United States, is relatively nonpathogenic.[576] A mild form of theileriasis, locally called January disease, occurs in cattle in Mozambique. This condition is caused by the subspecies *Theileria parva bovis*. Corridor disease is caused by *Theileria parva Lawrence*, and *Theileria annulata* is the cause of Mediterranean Coast fever or tropical theileriasis.

East Coast fever probably originated in buffalo in eastern Africa and later spread to cattle. Spread of the disease to southern Africa probably occurred through introduction of infected cattle from eastern Africa. European breeds of cattle (*Bos taurus*) develop a more severe disease than do comparably infected Indian breeds (*Bos indicus*). *Theileria* organisms are transmitted to susceptible cattle by the ticks *Hyalomma anatolicum* and *Amblyomma hebraeum*.

CLINICAL SIGNS. The clinical signs of *Theileria* infections include lymphadenopathy, nasal discharge, lacrimation, tachycardia, fever, subcutaneous edema of the face, gangrenous dermatitis, sloughing of facial skin, dyspnea, pallor, central nervous system (CNS) disorder, and emaciation.[577] The neurologic syndrome is characterized by ataxia, hypermetria, conscious proprioceptive deficits, depression, headpressing, hyperesthesia, blindness, nystagmus, circling, and aggressiveness. Terminally the animals become recumbent and develop opisthotonos, tonic-clonic seizures, and coma. In rare cases the parasite may localize in the spinal cord. The CNS signs occur as a result of vasculitis and lymphocytic inflammation of the brain.[578-580] Clinically recovered animals become persistently infected.

NECROPSY FINDINGS. The postmortem lesions of theileriasis include capillary engorgement, scattered punctate

---

*Hoescht Roussel, Somerville, NJ.

†Bio-Ceutic, Boehringer-Ingelheim, St. Joseph, MO 64501.

hemorrhages on the surface of the brain, thrombosis of the meningeal vessels, hemorrhage in the cerebral ventricles, pulmonary edema, peripheral lymphadenopathy, and infarctions of the kidney and spleen. The brain of affected animals appears to have a yellow hue.[580] Microscopically blue cytoplasmic inclusion bodies (Koch's blue bodies) are seen in the lymphocytes adjacent to the hemorrhagic areas.

The nervous form of theileriasis is difficult to diagnose definitively because the parasite is only sporadically visible in sections of nervous tissue from the infected animals. Parasitemia occasionally can be detected by microscopic examination of blood smears from infected calves. Reliable blood tests currently are not available. Biopsy of the cerebral cortex has been recommended as a confirmatory test for the disease. The cerebrospinal fluid (CSF) of affected animals is normal or has an increased protein concentration ranging from 1400 to 12,452 mg/dl, with normal numbers of white blood cells.[579]

TREATMENT. Parvaquone (Clexon),* administered at a dosage of 10 to 20 mg/kg IM by two injections 48 hours apart, is effective for the treatment of experimentally infected animals. This treatment resulted in clinical cures in as many as 92% of patients, providing it was administered early in the course of the disease.[581] Posttherapeutic relapses were common but could be controlled by administering a single dose of parvaquone (20 mg/kg of body weight) or halofuginone† (1.2 mg/kg of body weight PO 1 to 4 times).[582,583]

Menoctone (10 mg/kg IV or IM) also is curative. Single doses were effective, but repeating the treatment daily for 5 days eliminated posttherapeutic recrudescence.[584] A single dose of buparvaquone (2.5 mg/kg) also is effective. The disease is exotic to the United States.

PREVENTION. Prevention of *Theileria* infection is difficult. Recovered animals tend to be immune to rechallenge with *T. parva parva*, indicating the development of immune responses. Because strain differences in immunogenicity have been identified, the feasibility of immunization of cattle with heterologous strains currently is being explored.[585] Animals have been successfully immunized against *T. annulata* with an attenuated, tissue culture–derived vaccine.[586]

The development of an analogous vaccine for *T. parva* is more difficult. Most vaccinal strategies involve some form of infection by virulent *Theileria*, usually in a blood stabilate. After a period of time in which the parasites are allowed to develop into sporocysts, the vaccinated animals are treated with an antiprotozoal drug to prevent the development of clinical signs. Immunity to East Coast fever develops only after establishment of infection with schizonts in the host. Consequently, the immunizing infection must be allowed to proceed to that stage but must not be allowed to reach a state of serious illness. Because the stabilates are highly virulent, the timing of chemoprophylaxis is critical. Initial experiments indicated that exposure to blood stabilates containing virulent parasites combined with oxytetracycline injections (10 mg/kg, nondepot formulation) on postinoculation day 0 produced some protection, but a number of vaccinated animals became sick and succumbed to East Coast fever.[587,588] Other combinations of tetracycline dosage and formulation have been examined. However, none has provided consistent immunity to heterologous *Theileria* infections or offered complete protection against heterologous strains of the protozoa.

More recent studies have used the napthoquinones as the preferred chemotherapeutic agents in vaccinated animals. The three drugs (listed under Treatment, above) are parvaquone, halofuginone lactate, and buparvaquone. Of these, buparvaquone (Butalex)* was most promising. Vaccinated animals given a single dose (2.5 mg/kg) of buparvaquone had mild or inapparent signs of *Theileria* infection, yet were subsequently immune to rechallenge.[589]

CONTROL. Tick control is vital. Weekly spraying with coumaphos and insertion of cypermethrin (Decum)†–impregnated ear tags has been effective for controlling ticks and preventing *Theileria* infections in calves in Tanzania. The calves became infected with *Theileria parva* by 3 months after the tags were removed. The authors of the study suggested that the intensive tick control could minimize the incidence of theileriasis until the calves could be successfully vaccinated.[590]

REFERENCES

576. Kuttler KL, Craig TM: Isolation of a bovine *Theileria*, *Am J Vet Res* 36:323-325, 1975.
577. De Kock G et al: Bovine theileriasis in South Africa with special reference to *Theileria mutans*, *Ondosterpoort J Vet Sci Anim Ind* 8:9-70, 1937.
578. Khanna BM, Kharole MU, Shruti D: Histopathological studies in cerebral theileriasis of calves experimentally infected with *Theileria annulata*, *Indian J Parasitol* 6:91-94, 1982.
579. Van Amstel SR: Bovine cerebral theileriosis: some aspects of its clinical diagnosis, *Proceedings of the Twelfth World Congress on Diseases of Cattle*, Amsterdam, 1982.
580. Van Rensburg IBJ: Bovine cerebral theileriosis: a report on five cases with splenic infarction, *J S Afr Vet Assoc* 47:137-141, 1976.
581. Mbwambo HA, Mkonyi PA, Chua RB: Field evaluation of parvaquone against naturally occurring East Coast fever, *Vet Parasitol* 23:161-168, 1987.
582. Chema S et al: Clinical trial of halofuginone lactate for treatment of East Coast fever in Kenya, *Vet Rec* 120:575-577, 1987.
583. Chema S et al: Clinical trial of parvaquone for the treatment of East Coast fever in Kenya, *Vet Rec* 118:588-589, 1986.
584. McHardy N, Haigh AJB, Dolan TT: Chemotherapy of *Theileria parva* infection, *Nature* 261:698-699, 1976.
585. Irvin AD et al: Immunization of cattle with a *Theileria parva bovis* stock from Zimbabwe protects against challenge with virulent *T. p. parva* and *T. p. lawrencei* stocks from Kenya, *Vet Parasitol* 32:271-278, 1989.
586. Pipano E: Schizonts and tick stages in immunization against *Theileria annulata* infection. In Irvin AD, Cunningham MP, Young AS, eds: *Advances in the control of theileriosis*, The Hague, 1981, Martinus Nijhoff.
587. Morzaria SP, Nene V: Bovine theileriosis: progress in immunisation methods, *Int J Anim Sci* 5:1-4, 1990.
588. Mutugi JJ et al: Responses to a vaccine trial for East Coast fever in five cattle herds at the Kenyan coast, *Prev Vet Med* 10:173-183, 1991.
589. Mutugi JJ et al: Immunization of cattle using varying infective doses of *Theileria parva lawrencei* sporozoites derived from an African buffalo (*Syncerus caffer*) and treatment with buparvaquone, *Parasitology* 69:391-402, 1988.
590. Woodford JD: The use of cypermethrin-impregnated ear tags as an adjunct to East Coast fever immunization in theileriosis in eastern, central, and southern Africa. In TT Dolan, ed: *Proceedings of a Workshop on East Coast fever Immunization*, Lilongwe, Malawi, Sept 20-22, 1988.

CEREBRAL TRYPANOSOMIASIS
(Sleeping Sickness)

DEFINITION, ETIOLOGY, AND CLINICAL SIGNS. Trypanosomiasis is a hemoprotozoan disease of African cattle that also infects the central nervous system (CNS). The disease is transmitted to cattle by the bite of the tsetse fly (*Glossina* spp.). The agents that infect cattle include *Trypanosoma vivax*, *Trypanosoma congolense*, and *Trypanosoma brucei*. An especially severe neurologic form of the disease has been caused by the inoculation of cattle with *T. congolense* followed 1 year later by infection with *T. brucei* or by simultaneous inoculation with the two agents.[591] The encephalitic signs develop $2\frac{1}{2}$ to 5 months after infection. They include ataxia, conscious proprioceptive deficits, knuckling, depression, circling, and head-pressing. Some animals may show signs of behavioral change, lose the herd instinct, and develop hyperesthesia and constant repetitive movements. Other signs associated with

---

*Coopers Animal Health, Inc., Mundelelin, IL 50050.
†Terit, Hoescht, Germany.

*Burroughs-Wellcome, United Kingdom.
†Decum Tearina, USA.

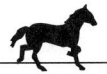

progression of trypanosomiasis are semicoma, coma, recumbency, opisthotonos, and intermittent tonic-clonic convulsions, which occur 2 to 3 days before death. Affected animals are emaciated, anemic, and icteric at the time of death.[592]

Experimental infection with trypanosomes causes a marked fever (as high as 40.5° C [105° F]). Other common nonneurologic signs are anemia, petechiation of the mucous membranes, occult fecal blood, melena, and epistaxis. Chronic weight loss without other clinical signs may be seen in some animals. Hematologic abnormalities include anemia, hypoalbuminemia, hyperbilirubinemia, and increased plasma concentrations of glutamic oxalic transaminase and urea nitrogen.

Acutely infected animals may develop a thrombocytopenia and prolongation of the prothrombin and partial thromboplastin times, indicating that disseminated intravascular coagulopathy may be responsible for the vascular changes that occur before death. The anemia is characterized by increased mean corpuscular volume and mean corpuscular hemoglobin, with increased serum iron concentrations early in the infection.[593,594] One study did not demonstrate a change in the concentration of white blood cells or protein in the cerebrospinal fluid (CSF) of animals with the encephalitic form of trypanosomiasis[591]; however, another study showed significant alterations in cattle infected with *T. bruceii*.[595] These included an increase in total protein (range of 37 to 44 mg/dl) and pleocytosis (range of 0 to 3060 mononuclear cells per microliter). The abnormalities in the CSF may be present in infected cattle not currently displaying clinical neurologic signs. Antitrypanosomal antibody may be found in the CSF of affected cattle using indirect fluorescent antibody tests.

PATHOLOGY. The pathologic lesions of trypanosomiasis are a nonsuppurative encephalomyelitis, serosanguinous pericardial fluid, serosal hemorrhages, pulmonary edema, centrilobular coagulative necrosis, splenomegaly, necrotizing myocarditis, and glomerulonephritis.[596] Macroscopic lesions of the CNS include subtle thickening and grayish discoloration of the meninges. The meningeal vessels are congested. Microscopic lesions of the CNS include mild to moderate diffuse meningoencephalitis, plasmacytic and lymphocytic perivascular cuffing, nodular gliosis, and mononuclear choroiditis. The pathogenesis of the encephalitis is not understood.

Trypanosomes may be cultured from the blood and CSF of infected cattle. The number of hematogenous parasites is highest in animals with a dual infection by *T. congolense* and *T. brucei*. The clinical diagnosis of trypanosomiasis may be confirmed by inoculating blood or CSF specimens into laboratory mice and observing the recipients for parasitemia with direct dark field examination of the patient's blood. Identification of motile trypanosomes in the buffy coat zone of a microhematocrit capillary tube using dark field illumination apparently is the most accurate of all diagnostic methods. Trypanosomes can be differentiated by their morphologic features, manner of attachment to erythrocytes, and type of motility.[597] Species-specific antibodies can be detected in serum using either an antigen-capture enzyme-linked immunosorbent assay (ELISA) or an indirect fluorescent antibody (IFA) test wherein the column-purified trypanosomal antigen is fixed with acetone or formalized saline. Titers of 1:200 to 1:2000 were consistent with acute infection. The test is not commonly used for field diagnosis of trypanosomiasis.[598,599] Infected cattle develop acquired resistance to homologous but not heterologous isolates of trypanosomes.

TREATMENT AND CONTROL. Of the drugs available for the treatment of trypanosomiasis, isometamidium chloride* is most commonly used. The recommended dosage ranges from 0.25 to 1 mg/kg IM; a single dose of 1 mg/kg exerts a protective effect for up to 6 months.[600] The higher dosage (1 mg/kg) was required to obtain increased weight gain and prevent recurrent infection. The treatment was particularly effective when combined with weekly surveillance, followed by treatment of confirmed infected animals.[601] Side effects of isometamidium chloride include tachycardia, salivation, lacrimation, pollakiuria, muscle fasciculations, convulsions, diarrhea, and in rare cases death. The drug apparently does not cause abortion in pregnant cows or otherwise affect the calf.[602]

Other drugs used include suramin sodium,* diminazene aceturate† (7 mg/kg), quinapyramine sulfate and homidium chloride‡ (1 mg/kg). These drugs provide residual protection from reinfection for approximately 2 months; however, recurrent infection and resistance, especially to diaminazene, have been reported.[603-606] Combinations of these drugs (e.g., diaminazene followed by isometamidium) reduce the number of resistance-related therapeutic failures. Relapses also undoubtedly occur because many of the chemoprophylactic drugs are unable to penetrate the blood-brain barrier in sufficient concentrations to eliminate the parasite in the CNS tissues.

Because of the variable responses to treatment and the ability of *Trypanosoma* organisms to develop drug resistance, all control programs must include methods of controlling the tsetse fly.[605] Current recommendations for fly control include application of insecticides with residual pyrethroids. Several methods of pyrethroid application have been investigated, including inclusion in a visual baited target (deltamethrin)[607] or application of a pyrethroid pour-on formulation (Bayticol pour on, 10 ml/100 kg of body weight).§ Both methods have been highly effective for reducing the tsetse fly population and trypanosome infection rates. Animals can be dipped in Deltamethrin dip every 2 weeks. A single dip application of the chemical has residual activity for as long as 52 days after application; however, to ensure maximum killing, application every 14 days is recommended. The tsetse fly prefers to feed from the ventral torso or the legs; for this reason, insecticide-impregnated ear tags have been ineffective for preventing infection.[608] Other fly control methods include aerial spraying with endosulfan, ground-based spraying with 4% dichloro-diphenyltrichloroethane (DDT), or use of scented insecticidal traps.[607] However, cost and environmental concerns have limited the usefulness of these techniques.

Selection of resistant lines of cattle is possible. The taurine N'Dama and West African shorthorn breeds have innate resistance to trypanosomiasis and are the sole breeds of cattle in areas of tsetse fly range.[609] Resistant breeds of small ruminants include the Djallonke, Red Maasai, Blackhead Persian, and East African sheep and goats.[610] Imported breeds of livestock usually cannot be maintained even in areas of low tsetse fly risk without intensive drug therapy.[611]

REFERENCES
591. Masake RA, Nantulya GWO: Cerebral trypanosomiasis in cattle with mixed *Trypanosoma congolense* and *T. brucei brucei* infections, *Acta Trop* 41:237-246, 1984.
592. Wellde B et al: *Trypanosoma congolense.* I, Clinical observations of experimentally infected cattle, *Exp Parasitol* 36:6-19, 1974.
593. Wellde BT et al: *Trypanosoma vivax:* disseminated intravascular coagulation in cattle, *Ann Trop Med Parasitol* 83:177-183, 1989.
594. Wellde BT et al: *Trypanosoma congolense:* erythrocyte indices, plasma iron turnover, and effects of treatment in infected cattle, *Ann Trop Med Parasitol* 83:201-206, 1989.

---

*Samorin, May & Baker; Trypamidium, Specia.

---

*Naganol, Bayer Ag Division, Animal Health, Shawnee Mission, KS 66201-0390.
†Berenil, Hoescht, Germany.
‡Novidium, May & Baker.
§Bayer AG, Germany.

595. Wellde BT et al: Cerebral trypanosomiasis in naturally infected cattle in the Lambwe Valley, South Nayanza, Kenya, *Ann Trop Med Parasitol* 83:151-160, 1989.

596. Olubayo RO, Mugera GM: The pathogenesis of hemorrhages in *Trypanosoma vivax* infection II. Pathomorphological changes, *Bull Anim Health Prod Africa* 35:286-292, 1987.

597. Murray MM, Murray PK, McIntyre WIM: An improved parasitological technique for the diagnosis of African trypanosomiasis, *Trans R Soc Trop Med Hyg* 71:325-326, 1977.

598. Katende JM et al: A new method for fixation and preservation of trypanosomal antigens for use in indirect immunofluorescence antibody test for diagnosis of bovine trypanosomiasis, *Trop Med Parasitol* 38:41-44, 1987.

599. Nantulya VM, Lindqvist KJ: Antigen detection enzyme immunoassays for the diagnosis of *Trypanosoma vivax, T. congolense,* and *T. brucei* infections in cattle, *Trop Med Parasitol* 40:267-272, 1989.

600. Holmes PH et al: The association between samorin chemoprophylaxis and immune responses in cattle under experimental metacyclic *Trypanosoma congolense* challenge, Pub No 113, *Proceedings of the Eighteenth Meeting of the International Scientific Council for Trypanosomiasis Research Control,* Harare, Nairobi, Kenya, 1985.

601. Munstermann S et al: Trypanosomiasis control in Boran cattle in Kenya: a comparison between chemoprophylaxis and a parasite detection and intravenous treatment method using isometamidium chloride, *Trop Anim Health Prod* 24:17-27, 1992.

602. Dowler ME, Schillinger D, Connor: Notes on the routine intravenous use of isometamidium in the control of bovine trypanosomiasis on the Kenya coast, *Trop Anim Health Prod* 21:3-10, 1989.

603. ILRAD Reports: *Improved trypanosomiasis control: studies on drug treatment,* vol 5, Nairobi, 1987, ILRAD.

604. Rowlands GJ et al: Epidemiology of bovine trypanosomiasis in the Ghibe valley, southwest Ethiopia. II, Factors associated with variations in trypanosome prevalence, incidence of new infections, and prevalence of recurrent infections, *Acta Tropica* 53:135-150, 1993.

605. Codjia V et al: Epidemiology of bovine trypanosomiasis in the Ghibe valley, southwest Ethiopia. III, Occurrence of populations of *Trypanosoma congolense* resistant to diminazene, isometamidium, and homidium, *Acta Tropica* 53:151-163, 1993.

606. Mwambo HA, Mella PNP, Lekaki KA: Trypanosomiasis chemotherapy: further observations on a strain of *Trypanosoma congolense* resistant to diminazene aceturate, *Tanz Vet Bull* 8:45-51, 1988.

607. Hursey BS, Whittingham GW, Chadenga V: The integration of insecticidal techniques for the control and eradication of *Glossina morsitans* in northeast Zimbabwe, *Proceedings of the Nineteenth Meeting of the International Scientific Council for Trypanosomiasis Research and Control,* 1987.

608. Thompson M: The effect on tsetse flies (*Glossina* sp.) of deltamethin applied to cattle either as a spray or incorporated into ear tags, *Trop Pest Manag* 33:329-335, 1987.

609. Leak SGA, Paling RW, Moloo SK: The trypanotolerance network. II, A study on health and productivity of N'Dama Nguni and their crosses under quantified levels of tsetse challenge in Gabon. II, Tsetse survey, *Proceedings of the Eighteenth Meeting of the International Science Council on Trypanosomiasis Research and Control,* Nairobi, 1985.

610. Paling RW et al: Susceptibility of N'Dama and Boran cattle to sequential challenges with tsetse-transmitted clones of *Trypanosoma congolense, Parasite Immunol* 13:427-445, 1991.

611. Murray M, Trail JCM, D'ieteren GDM: Trypanotolerance in cattle and prospects for the control of trypanosomiasis by selective breeding, *Rev Sci Tech Off Int Epiz* 9:369-386, 1990.

POLIOENCEPHALOMALACIA
(Cerebrocortical Necrosis)

GUY LONERAGAN
DANIEL GOULD

DEFINITION AND ETIOLOGY. Polioencephalomalacia (PEM) is a common and important neurologic disease of ruminants[612,613] with a worldwide distribution. An animal with clinical manifestations of PEM often is referred to as suffering "polio" or as a "sleeper" or "brainer."

Polioencephalomalacia is a descriptive term for histologic lesions[612,614] that may have multiple etiologies. Literally, the name means softening or necrosis (malacia) of regions of the gray matter (polio) of the brain (encephalo). Thus a definitive diagnosis of PEM requires appropriate histologic examination of brain tissue. Although PEM is a nonspecific diagnosis with regard to etiology, many authors assume that the disease results solely from an altered thiamine metabolism.[615] In fact, there are multiple possible etiologies of PEM, including but not limited to excessive sulfur consump-

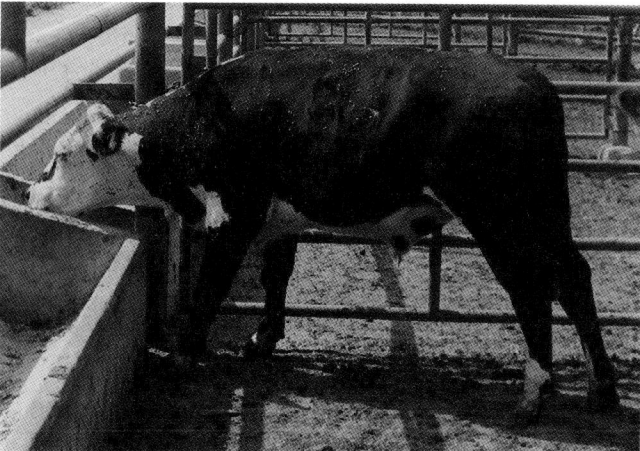

FIG. 33-10 ■ Feedlot steer with clinical manifestations of polioencephalomalacia. The steer has adopted a sawhorse posture.

tion,[616,617] presumably manifested through elevated ruminal sulfides[619-620]; altered thiamine metabolism[621]; so-called salt poisoning or water deprivation[622]; and lead toxicity.[623]

Most recent published reports describing outbreaks of PEM have associated occurrence of the disease with consumption of excessive sulfur, either from feedstuffs or water. When attempts have been made to estimate the patient's thiamine status, rarely if ever are alterations demonstrated,[620,624,625] although it is not clear that a diagnostically practical set of tests is available. Regardless of the etiology, patients with PEM generally respond favorably to therapies that include large doses of thiamine, possibly because administration of thiamine at concentrations above maintenance requirements might be beneficial to the metabolically impaired brain.

CLINICAL SIGNS. PEM appears to have both a subacute and an acute manifestation.[612,620] In the subacute form clinical manifestations may develop within hours or over several days. In the early stages of the disease, the affected animals detach from the herd or flock, become anorectic, and stagger. They often appear blind, walk with the head held erect, and demonstrate a slight hypermetric gait. Occasionally, affected animals are excitable and charge around their enclosure, which may present a significant hazard to the veterinarian and animal handlers. Other early signs of PEM can include diarrhea, hyperesthesia, and muscle tremors, which are most obviously observed as ear flicking or facial twitching. Progression of the condition is associated with cortical blindness, head-pressing, opisthotonos, dorsomedial strabismus, miosis, repetitive chewing, profuse ptyalism, and odontoprisis (Figs. 33-10 and 33-11.)[612,617,626-628] Despite the defective menace response, the animals usually have normal palpebral reflexes. Affected animals may also develop a variable nystagmus, strabismus (Fig. 33-12), and head tilt. The rectal temperature is normal unless excessive muscular fasciculations have developed. The pulse and respiratory rates are usually increased but not always. An odor of hydrogen sulfide may be detected on the breath if the PEM is associated with excessive sulfur consumption.

Although most of these animals respond favorably to aggressive therapeutic intervention, clinical signs may progress to recumbency, tonic-clonic convulsions, and death. In facilities with certain types of fencing, such as cables, affected animals may push or press with sufficient force that they die of asphyxiation.

In the acute form of PEM, animals are found recumbent and comatose.[612,620] These animals often experience episodic

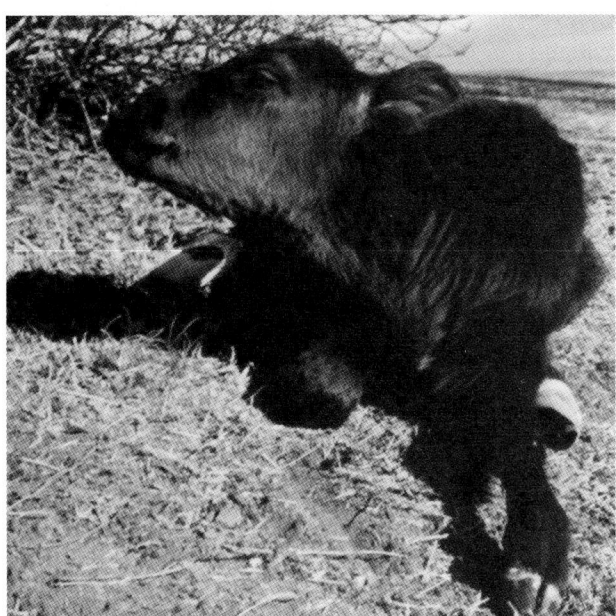

FIG. 33-11 ■ Calf with advanced signs of polioencephalomalacia showing abnormal head posture and depressed sensorium.

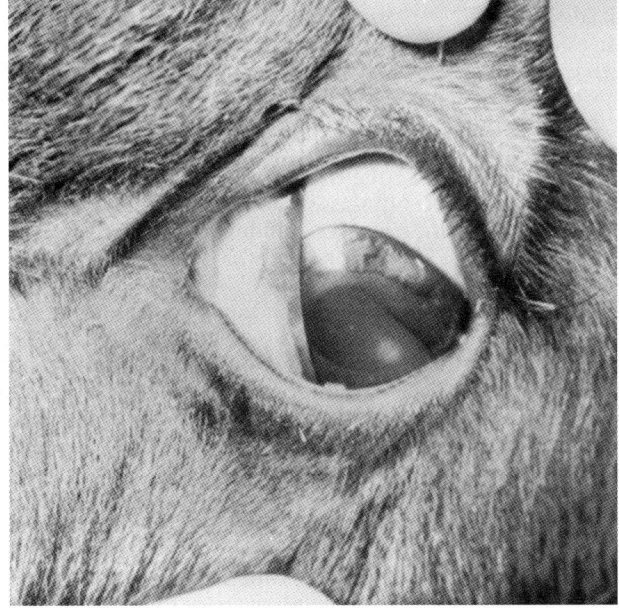

FIG. 33-12 ■ Abnormal pupillary angle associated with strabismus in a calf with polioencephalomalacia. Because the calf's head is tied upward, the eye has rotated ventrally, although this is actually dorsomedial strabismus.

tonic-clonic convulsions, and they remain recumbent and hypertonic between seizures. The prognosis is grave for acutely affected animals or those with advanced subacute manifestations. Survivors may remain irreversibly decorticated and are culled because of poor performance, chronic anorexia and ataxia, or blindness. However, mildly affected animals may remain as productive members of the herd.

Because the clinical manifestations of PEM may be subtle and nonspecific, they can be confused with other disorders. PEM often is temporarily associated with lactic acidosis that develops after consumption of excessive amounts of readily fermentable carbohydrates. Animals with lactic acidosis may appear ataxic and obtunded in addition to having a foul-smelling, watery stool and a distended, fluid-filled rumen. Concurrent PEM may not be diagnosed, or producers may confuse PEM for lactic acidosis or primary ruminal tympany in acutely affected animals that have remained laterally recumbent for some time.

The major differential diagnoses for PEM include enterotoxemia type D (focal symmetric encephalomalacia form), *Haemophilus* meningoencephalitis (thrombotic meningoencephalitis), coccidiosis with nervous involvement, listeric meningoencephalitis, vitamin A deficiency, ethylene glycol poisoning, rabies, and infectious bovine rhinotracheitis encephalitis (calves only).

CLINICAL PATHOLOGY. Although a definitive diagnosis depends on histologic confirmation, a presumptive diagnosis may be made antemortem based on the history and clinical signs or on a definitive diagnosis in herd mates of affected animals. If a diagnosis of PEM is made, either presumptive or definitive, attention should be focused on identifying the likely causes so that exposure of herd mates to etiologic agents can be mitigated or eliminated. The investigation may proceed at the animal, herd, and environmental level to identify evidence supportive of sulfide toxicity, thiamine deficiency, lead toxicity, or water deprivation–salt toxicosis.

Sulfide concentrations in the ruminal fluid and gas cap in experimentally induced sulfur-associated PEM have been shown to be elevated.[625,629] However, unpublished data supported a finding of a decrease in gas cap sulfide concentrations in naturally developing PEM associated with increased sulfur consumption.[630] This probably is due to the rapid metabolism of sulfate to sulfide in the rumen and resultant absorption or eructation of hydrogen sulfide (H_2S). Animals with naturally developing PEM are likely to have been anorectic for some time, resulting in a decrease in oxidized and reduced forms of ruminal sulfur concentrations.

Estimation of the rumen gas cap H_2S concentration in clinically healthy pen mates of affected cattle is an effective chuteside diagnostic procedure that can indicate excessive sulfur consumption.[620] This method provides real-time results that may aid direction of further animal and environmental investigations. In short, an area in the left paralumbar fossa is prepared for ruminocentesis. An 18-gauge, $3^1/_2$-inch spinal needle is inserted through the body wall and into the rumen gas cap. A modified gas sampler is attached to the spinal needle by means of an extension set, and a known amount of gas is drawn through an H_2S detector tube.[629] It is important to adjust the values to account for any dead space of the sampling instrument such as the extension set and other modifications. Hydrogen sulfide concentrations above 1000 ppm are indicative of excessive sulfur consumption.[631]

Appropriate blood samples may be analyzed for lead concentration and possibly estimation of thiamine status. Thiamine status generally is evaluated using one of several available methods, including determining the total blood thiamine concentration using a thiamine-dependent *Lactobacillus* bioassay.[632] The erythrocyte thiamine pyrophosphate concentration may be measured by means of high-performance liquid chromatography.[633] The value of estimating all phosphorylation forms of thiamine (free, diphosphate, and triphosphate forms) is questionable. Table 33-8 shows the reference ranges for the total thiamine concentration in normal and affected cattle.

Another method of evaluating thiamine status is determining erythrocyte transketolase activity. This is a sensitive and specific measurement of active thiamine status.[634] Transketolase catalyzes the reaction between xylulose-5-P and ribose-5-P to form sedoheptulose-7-P and 3-phosphoglyceraldehyde in the pentose phosphate pathway. Normal mean transketo-

TABLE 33-8

Mean Concentration of Thiamine in Tissues*: 95% Confidence Intervals in Clinically Normal Cattle and Sheep and in Patients with Polioencephalomalacia

Tissue	Species	Normal	Polioenceph-alomalacia
Liver, wet	Cattle	2.81±0.515	0.613±0.102
	Sheep	2.07±0.474	0.421±0.06
Liver, dry	Cattle	11.1±2.11	2.51±0.428
	Sheep	7.34±1.73	1.42±0.197
Heart, wet	Cattle	2.81±0.46	0.549±0.118
	Sheep	3.1±0.432	0.581±0.093
Heart, dry	Cattle	13.18±2.12	2.45±0.558
	Sheep	13.5±1.75	2.44±0.416
Brain, wet	Cattle	1.4±0.248	0.301±0.061
	Sheep	1.21±0.101	0.592±0.111
Brain, dry	Cattle	7.67±1.52	1.8±0.366
	Sheep	5.81±0.566	3.22±0.558

From Edwin EE et al: *Vet Rec* 104:4-8, 1979.
*Values given in μg/g (ppm).

TABLE 33-9

Mean and 95% Confidence Range* Values of Erythrocyte Transketolase as a Percentage of Thiamine Pyrophosphate Effect in Erythrocytes of Normal Cattle and Sheep and in Patients with Polioencephalomalacia

Species	Normal (%)	Polioenceph-alomalacia (%)
Cattle	15	172
	(2-114)	(120-247)*
Sheep	23	122
	(12-41)	(96-158)

From Edwin EE et al: *Vet Rec* 104:4-8, 1979.
*Value given in parentheses.

lase activity has been reported to range from 0.301 to 2.9 mmol pentose/hr/10^9 red blood cells (mean is 0.782). Transketolase assays often are reported as the mean thiamine pyrophosphate effect (Table 33-9). This test compares the specific activity in the active (holoenzyme) and inactive (apoenzyme) forms with the activity of the two forms after addition of thiamine to the homogenates. A large increase in specific transketolase activity after addition of the thiamine pyrophosphate is suggestive of thiamine deficiency. Theoretically, in animals with thiamine-associated PEM, the concentration of holoenzyme is decreased and that of the apoenzyme is increased. Thiaminase may be detected in the rumen and feces of affected animals, but its value is questionable.[621,633,635,636] It is important to note that, as mentioned previously, recent papers investigating PEM have not been able to identify altered thiamine status. Even if a thiamine deficiency is identified in an affected animal, caution should be used in interpreting the results because a period of anorexia may result in a decrease in ruminal de novo synthesis[637,638]; thus affected animals may have a thiamine deficiency that develops secondary to PEM.

Changes in the cerebrospinal fluid (CSF) of affected animals usually are vague. They include mild pleocytosis (5 to 50 WBCs/dl) and increased protein concentrations (over 50 mg/dl).[621,639]

Electrophysiologic studies of affected animals show a normal latency and decreased amplitude of the late peaks of the visual-evoked potentials. These changes reflect a decreased population of neurons capable of responding to the photic stimulation.[640] Electroencephalographic changes in some animals include constant high amplitude (50 to 60 mV) and slow activity (1 to 4 Hz). Another change is diffuse lowered activity, which is consistent with diffuse necrosis.[641]

Environmental investigations should include evaluation of all practical feed and water sources for sulfur concentrations.

PATHOGENESIS

Sulfur Metabolism. Dietary sulfur and sulfates are an important factor in the development of PEM. Beef cattle require 0.15% to 0.20% sulfur on a dry matter basis.[642] Sources of sulfur include elemental sulfur[616]; feed additives, such as gypsum and ammonium sulfate[617,643]; feedstuffs, such as corn processing by-products,[642] cruciferous crops,[644,645] molasses[646]; and fertilizers. Water can be an important contributor to sulfur intake, usually in the form of sulfates.[619,647,648]

There are two primary metabolic pathways of sulfur in the rumen.[649-653] The assimilatory pathway involves reduction of sulfate to sulfides and incorporation into sulfur-containing organic compounds such as cysteine and methionine.[651] These are ultimately incorporated into microbial crude protein. The dissimilatory pathway is an energy-producing pathway in which microorganisms use sulfate as a terminal electron acceptor is a manner similar to that in which mammals use oxygen.[654] The end product is liberated sulfide ion. At a ruminal pH of 5.2, 97.2% of sulfide ions are in the form of hydrogen sulfide and move freely to the rumen gas cap.[650,655] Hydrogen sulfide is readily absorbed and transported to the liver and oxidized to sulfate.[656,657] Some of the hydrogen sulfide may be lost via eructation,[625,655] but the significance of this route has been questioned.[658] Excess sulfur is excreted in the urine and large intestine[656,659] or recycled to the rumen.[660,661] A period of adaptation is required for maximum hydrogen sulfide production after exposure to sulfur.[652,659,662-664]

Because sulfur and sulfate demonstrate low cellular toxicity, it is unlikely that sulfur-associated PEM results from a sulfate or sulfur toxicity. However, sulfides are highly toxic.[665,666] Sulfur-associated PEM is more likely to occur secondary to a sulfide toxicity.[618,620,625]

It has been proposed that the pathogenesis of sulfur-induced PEM involves inhibition of cytochrome C oxidase, an enzyme in the electron transport chain involved in adenosine triphosphate (ATP) production. For highly toxic sulfide to reach the brain, it must escape hepatic oxidation. This could possibly be achieved by two mechanisms. A surge in ruminal sulfide generation usually follows a period of adaptation to high-sulfur diets. This may overwhelm the hepatic detoxification capacity. As an alternative possibility, cattle inhale a significant amount of eructated ruminal gas.[667] These inhaled gases can contain significant amounts of hydrogen sulfide, and if absorbed via the pulmonary route, the hydrogen sulfide would completely bypass the hepatic circulation. However, this concept has been questioned.[668]

In feedlot cattle a summer peak in PEM occurrences was associated with consumption of water sulfate containing 2500 mg/L.[619] The total sulfur intake of these steers was estimated to be 0.6% on a dry matter basis during the hottest days of the year. Most PEM cases occurred between 15 and 35 days after arrival in this feedlot. In another investigation, 11% of weaners consuming a diet containing 0.9% sulfur on a dry matter basis developed clinical manifestations of PEM.[620] Lesions were confirmed in one steer that died. Addition of gypsum (calcium sulfate) to feeder steer rations at a final concentration of over 2% organic sulfate results in a significantly greater risk of developing PEM. The addition of sodium sulfate (0.6% to 0.8%) to diets may induce PEM within 11 days.[625,662,669,670] High sulfur concentrations in well water in combination with accumulation in forage has been traced to an outbreak of PEM

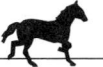

in Canada.[620] One survey described an outbreak of cerebrocortical necrosis in cattle eating diets containing 7200 mg/kg of sodium sulfate.[648]

The recommended maximum tolerance level of sulfur is 0.4% of dry matter intake (NRC, 1980). Other effects of excessive sulfur intake are decreases in feed intake and weight gains (NRC, 1980). Accurate diagnosis of sulfur toxicity requires measurement of sulfur in all food and water sources. Sulfur from water must be included when calculating total sulfur intake. One third of the molecular weight of sulfate is sulfur. Hence, if an animal drinks 30 L of water a day containing 2000 mg/L of sulfate, this contributes 60,000 mg of sulfate, or 20 g of sulfur. Furthermore, if this animal consumes an average of 10 kg of dry matter daily at 0.15% sulfur, the feed or forage contributes 15 g of sulfur, making the total sulfur intake 35 g, or 0.35% on a dry matter basis. Water therefore may be a substantial source of sulfur.

Some have suggested that sulfides result in thiamine destruction, thereby directly implicating a thiamine deficiency in the pathogenesis of sulfur-associated PEM. Rumen thiamine production was slightly reduced by the inclusion of excessive sulfur in the ration.[671] However, the authors deemed the reduction clinically insignificant. It would appear that sulfur-associated PEM occurs independent of thiamine status.

PEM induced by feeding of molasses and urea is thought to be related to the high sulfur content of the molasses and to the depletion of propionate and other glucogenic precursors induced by the foodstuff.[646] It is not considered to be caused by an underlying thiamine destruction. The tissue thiamine concentrations of animals with molasses-related PEM are normal,[672] and signs are preventable by concomitant feeding of glycerol, which is converted to glucose in the rumen. Outbreaks of PEM in range cattle have been associated with ingestion of the plant *Kochia scoparia*.[673,674] The pathogenesis of this condition is unknown; however, some have suggested that the plant has the capacity to accumulate sulfur in the forage.[648]

Thiamine Metabolism. Although the role of thiamine deficiency in the pathogenesis of PEM is increasingly being questioned, a brief description of its metabolism is warranted. Thiamine diphosphate is a cofactor for transketolase, which is the rate-limiting enzyme in the pentose phosphate pathway in the erythrocytes and brain cells.[675] The pentose phosphate pathway (hexose monophosphate shunt) is the major metabolic pathway for glucose metabolism in the brain. Thiamine also serves as a coenzyme for pyruvate decarboxylase, pyruvate dehydrogenase, and oxoglutarate dehydrogenase, which are part of the Krebs cycle. Loss of transketolase results in increased concentrations of lactate, oxoglutarate, and pyruvate in the plasma. The overall result of such changes in the CNS is to reduce the activity of the ATP-dependent sodium and water transport mechanisms in the neurons. Inward water fluxes result in a net intraneuronal swelling, which in turn results in increased intracranial pressure and neuronal necrosis. As the neuronal necrosis increases, swelling and proliferation of the capillary endothelium and infiltration of the cerebral cortex by macrophages occurs. The combination of thiamine-related cell death, increased intracranial pressure, and intraneuronal edema causes laminar cortical necrosis and the pathologic change of PEM.

Thiamine also may play an important role in the metabolism of neurotransmitters. Studies have indicated that synaptosomal preparations of thiamine-deficient mice had decreased uptake of serotonin, aspartate, and glutamate[676] and lower concentrations of acetylcholine and cyclic guanosine monophosphate. However, the relationship between these biochemical changes and the clinical syndrome is unclear.[676] Thiamine is stored primarily in the liver and muscles and, because of its water solubility, has a short half-life in the body.[677,678] The daily requirement of thiamine for sheep has

been estimated at 2 to 4 mg, which is slightly less than the daily production in the rumen. Therefore conditions that inactivate thiamine in the rumen or reduce the thiamine synthetic activity rapidly result in acute thiamine deficiencies.[679]

Other mechanisms that cause low ruminal thiamine concentrations in affected animals include production of bacterial thiaminases, production or ingestion of inactive thiamine analogs, ingestion of preformed plant thiaminases, decreased intake of preformed thiamine by preruminants, impaired absorption or phosphorylation of thiamine by rumen bacteria, increased fecal excretion of thiamine, or decreased ruminal production of thiamine diphosphate.[633,680-682] Two types of bacterial thiaminases have been described. Thiaminase I, which is produced by *Bacillus thiaminolyticus* or *Clostridium sporogenes*,[683] catalyzes the cleavage of thiamine at the methylene bridge between the pyrimidinyl and the thiazole ring. A basic cosubstrate is required to combine with the pyrimidinyl derivative to form a new compound[684] (Fig. 33-13).

Thiaminase II is produced by *Bacillus aneurinolyticus*, which proliferates in response to excessive grain intake.[685]

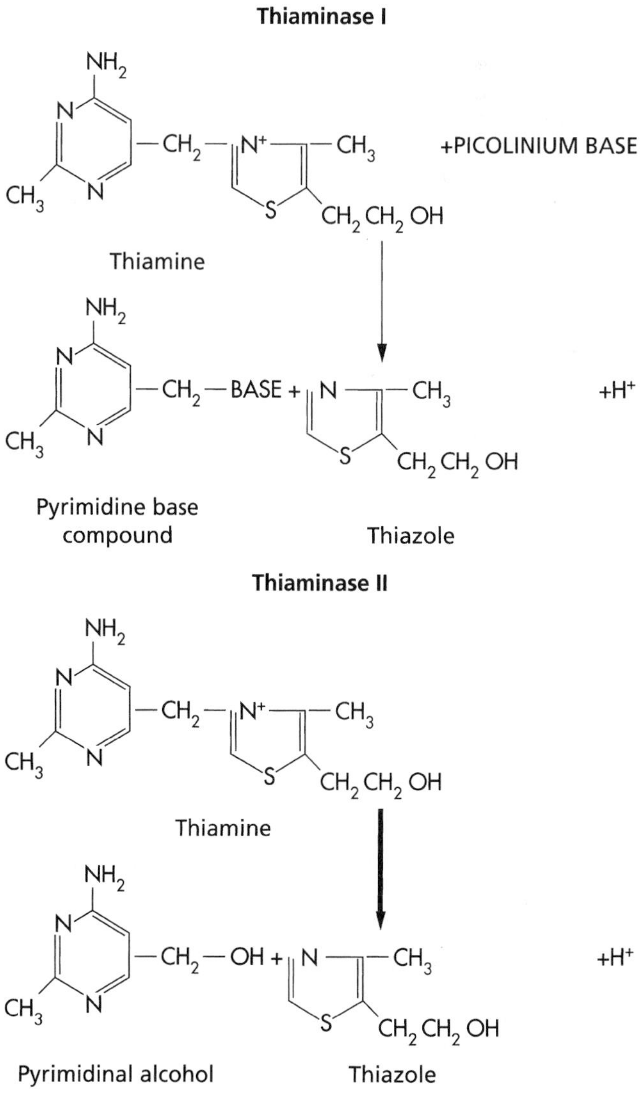

FIG. 33-13 ▮ Enzymatic cleavage of thiamine by thiaminase I and II. Thiaminase I attaches a picolinium base to the pyrimidine ring structure, whereas thiaminase II catalyzes the hydrolysis of thiamine at the methylene bridge. (From Edwin EE, Jackman R: *J Sci Food Agric* 25:357-368, 1974.)

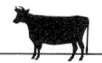

The enzyme catalyzes the hydrolysis of the methylene bridge between the two ring structures of the thiamine molecule. The specific relationship of this thiaminase to the clinical syndrome of PEM as seen in the field is unclear.

Complete correlation has not been established between the production of ruminal and fecal thiaminase, the tissue and plasma concentration of thiamine, and the development of clinical encephalopathy.[635,675] Some affected animals may show normal amounts of thiamine in the plasma but have markedly decreased levels in the erythrocytes and other tissues, indicating the existence of other causes of PEM.[676]

EPIDEMIOLOGY. PEM has a worldwide distribution.* The condition is seen both in individuals and as herd outbreaks. In one instance, approximately 2000 of 2200 sheep grazing were clinically affected with PEM.[616] No predilection by gender or breed is seen, although anecdotal reports suggest that heifers are less likely to develop PEM than steers in a feedlot environment. The condition affects cattle, sheep, goats, deer, camels, and camelids.[615,617,687-690] Although PEM is seen predominantly in animals that eat a high concentrate supplement, the condition also can occur in unsupplemented animals on pasture. The inciting cause of PEM sometimes can be identified and other times not.

One report from the United States indicated a predominance of cases in the summer in range cattle.[612] The age range for susceptibility to PEM has been reported to be 3 weeks to 5 years in sheep, 3 weeks to 8 years in cattle, and 2 months to 2½ years in goats. The peak age of incidence is 18 months or younger in cattle and sheep, but this depends on the production system.[612,620,691] The incidence of PEM has been reported to be as high as 90% in some sheep flocks, and the mortality rate has been reported to be 1% to 10%.[616] The incidence of PEM is high in sheep exported by sea from Australia to the Middle East. In these cases the underlying disturbance was thought to be associated with a thiamine deficiency caused by a lack of rumen synthesis that occurred secondary to the shipboard conditions.[692]

NECROPSY FINDINGS. In cases of sulfur-associated PEM, rumen contents may have an odor of hydrogen sulfide. The macroscopic pathologic lesions of PEM include cortical swelling, softening, flattening, and yellowish discoloration of the gyri. Necrotic areas of the cerebral cortex autofluoresce under ultraviolet light (365 nm).[693,694] Severe cases show herniation of the cerebellum through the foramen magnum or the occipital cortex under the tentorium cerebelli. Recovered animals that are necropsied months after recovery may show cerebral atrophy and submeningeal cortical cysts. The major microscopic lesion is a diffuse laminar necrosis. Other changes include intracellular and intercellular edema, neuronal necrosis, gliosis, and neuronophagia.[614,627]

TREATMENT AND PROGNOSIS. Regardless of the underlying cause, animals suffering the subacute form of PEM often respond favorably to parenteral administration of thiamine hydrochloride. These animals may remain blind and may have depressed sensorium for weeks or months.[695] Thiamine should be administered at a dosage of 10 to 20 mg/kg IM or SC 3 times daily. If given intravenously, it should be diluted in 5% dextrose or other isotonic fluid and administered slowly to avoid adverse reactions. If no improvement occurs initially, the treatment should be continued for at least 3 days. In some patients recovery may take as long as 7 days, but most patients show improvement by 24 hours. A single administration of sodium dexamethasone at a dosage of 1 to 2 mg/kg of body weight intramuscularly or intravenously may be beneficial in reducing cerebral edema. Anecdotal reports indicate that feedlot animals that have recovered from

PEM are at increased risk of respiratory disease, therefore prophylactic antimicrobial administration may be indicated.

Animals with the acute form of PEM usually have more severe cortical and deep gray matter lesions than animals with the acute form.[620] These animals generally do not respond to therapeutic regimens.

Convulsions may be controlled with phenobarbital, pentobarbital, or diazepam. Specific dosing regimens are listed in Tables 33-6 and 33-7. Other medical treatments that have been recommended to reduce cerebral edema and the amount of pressure-related neuronal necrosis include dimethyl sulfoxide (DMSO), furosemide, and mannitol.

PREVENTION AND CONTROL. Thiamine supplementation may not prevent outbreaks of PEM. Ultimately, the best way to prevent outbreaks is to manage the dietary intakes of susceptible animals appropriately. Ruminants should be allowed an adequate period of adaptation to high-concentrate rations. All feedstuffs and water sources should be carefully analyzed on a routine basis and an estimate of total sulfur intake made. If excess sulfur consumption is a factor, steps should be taken to remove sources such as high-sulfur hay, ammonium sulfate, and molasses. If the excess sulfur intake is unavoidable, steps can be taken to limit its effects. Older members of the cow herd could be used to graze the high-sulfur pastures and younger, more susceptible animals could be kept to lower sulfur pastures or given hay supplementation. Attempts should be made to train personnel so that animals with PEM can be identified early in the disease and treated appropriately.

Thiamine may be supplemented (3 to 10 mg/kg of feed) in rations in which the concentrate to fiber ratio is high, but this has little or no effect in preventing PEM. Other recommendations for preventing PEM include addition of brewer's yeast to the ration and gradual adaptation of ruminants (at least 2 weeks) to high-concentrate diets. If present as a feed-limiting additive, gypsum should be removed from the diet. Elimination of supplementation and rotation of pastures have been sufficient for controlling some outbreaks.[691] Supplementation with cobalt in trace mineral salt mixes may be necessary in deficient areas.

REFERENCES

612. Jensen R, Griner LA, Adams OR: Polioencephalomalacia of cattle and sheep, *J Am Vet Med Assoc* 129:311-321, 1956.
613. Terlecki S, Markson LM: Cerebrocortical necrosis in cattle and sheep, *Vet Rec* 43:23-28, 1961.
614. Jubb KVF, Huxtable CR: The nervous system. In Jubb KVF, Kennedy PC, Palmer N, eds: *Pathology of domestic animals*, ed 4, New York, 1993, Academic Press.
615. Beck C et al: Polioencephalomalacia in two alpacas, *Aust Vet J* 74:350-352, 1996.
616. Bulgin MS, Lincoln SD, Mather G: Elemental sulfur toxicosis in a flock of sheep, *J Am Vet Med Assoc* 208:1063-1065, 1996.
617. Raisbeck MF: Is polioencephalomalacia associated with high-sulfate diets? *J Am Vet Med Assoc* 180:1303-1305, 1982.
618. McAllister MM, Gould DH, Hamar DW: Sulphide-induced polioencephalomalacia in lambs, *J Comp Pathol* 106:267-278, 1992.
619. McAllister MM et al: Evaluation of ruminal sulfide concentrations and seasonal outbreaks of polioencephalomalacia in beef cattle in a feedlot, *J Am Vet Med Assoc* 211:1275-1279, 1997.
620. Lonergan GH et al: Association of excess sulfur intake and an increase in hydrogen sulfide concentrations in the ruminal gas cap of recently weaned beef calves with polioencephalomalacia, *J Am Vet Med Assoc* 213:1599-1604, 1571, 1998.
621. Pill AH: Evidence of thiamine deficiency in calves affected with cerebrocortical necrosis, *Vet Rec* 81:178-181, 1967.
622. Padovan D: Polioencephalomalacia associated with water deprivation in cattle, *Cornell Vet* 70:153-159, 1980.
623. Wells GAH, Howell JM, Gopinath C: Experimental lead encephalopathy in calves: histological observations on the nature and distribution of the lesions, *Neuropathol Appl Neurobiol* 2:175-190, 1976.
624. Sager RL, Hamar DW, Gould DH: Clinical and biochemical alterations in calves with nutritionally induced polioencephalomalacia, *Am J Vet Res* 51:1969-1974, 1990 (published erratum appears in *Am J Vet Res* 52:514, 1991).

*References 615, 617, 645, 646, 648, and 686.

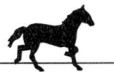

625. Gould DH et al: High sulfide concentrations in rumen fluid associated with nutritionally induced polioencephalomalacia in calves, *Am J Vet Res* 52:1164-1169, 1991.
626. Colontino J, Bulmer WS: Polioencephalomalacia in a dairy cow, *Can Vet J* 18:356-357, 1997.
627. McHowell J: Polioencephalomalacia in calves, *Vet Rec* 75:1165-1167, 1961.
628. Claes-Goran L: Cerebrocortical necrosis (CCN) in a calf and experimental reproduction of the disease, *Acta Vet Scand* 14:464-473, 1973.
629. Gould DH, Cummings BA, Hamar DW: In vivo indicators of pathologic ruminal sulfide production in steers with diet-induced polioencephalomalacia, *J Vet Diagn Invest* 9:72-76, 1997.
630. McAllister MM, Gould DH: Decreased H$_2$S concentrations in gas caps of PEM affected animals, personal communication, 1998.
631. Loneragan GH et al: The effect of varying water sulfate content on H$_2$S generation and health of feedlot cattle, American Society of Animal Science Eighty-Ninth Annual Meeting, Nashville, 1997.
632. Olkowski AA, Gooneratne SR: Microbiological methods of thiamine measurement in biological material, *Int J Vitam Nutr Res* 62:34-42, 1992.
633. Edwin EE, Jackman R: Ruminal thiaminase and tissue thiamine in cerebrocortical necrosis, *Vet Rec* 92:640-641, 1973.
634. Edwin EE et al: Diagnostic aspects of cerebrocortical necrosis, *Vet Rec* 104:4-8, 1979.
635. Linklater KA, Dyson DA, Morgan KT: Faecal thiaminase in clinically normal sheep associated with outbreaks of polioencephalomalacia, *Res Vet Sci* 22:308-312, 1977.
636. Edwin EE, Jackman R: A rapid radioactive method for determination of thiaminase activity and its use in the diagnosis of cerebrocortical necrosis in sheep and cattle, *J Sci Food Agric* 25:357-368, 1974.
637. Gupta GC, Joshi BP, Rai P: The levels of thiamine in the rumen fluid and blood serum in the spontaneous bovine rumen dysfunctions, *Acta Vet Brno* 45:205-210, 1976.
638. Thornber EJ et al: Induced thiamin deficiency in lambs, *Aust Vet J* 57:21-26, 1981.
639. Loew FM, Dunlop RH, Christian RG: Biochemical aspects of an outbreak of bovine polioencephalomalacia, *Can Vet J* 11:57-61, 1970.
640. Strain GM et al: Visual evoked potentials and electroretinograms in ruminants with thiamine-responsive polioencephalomalacia or suspected listeriosis, *Am J Vet Res* 51:1513-1517, 1990.
641. Suzuki M et al: Electroencephalogram of Japanese Black calves affected with cerebrocortical necrosis, *Nippon Juigaku Zasshi* 52:1077-1087, 1990.
642. National Research Council: *Nutrient requirements of beef cattle*, ed 7, Washington, DC, 1996, National Academy of Sciences.
643. Jeffrey M et al: Polioencephalomalacia associated with the ingestion of ammonium sulphate by sheep and cattle (see comments), *Vet Rec* 134:343-348, 1994.
644. Loneragan GH, Gould DH, Garry FB: Field investigations of sulfur-associated polioencephalomalacia (PEM), Ninetieth Annual Meeting of the American Society of Animal Science, Denver, 1998.
645. Hill FI, P.C. E: Polioencephalomalacia in cattle in New Zealand fed chou moellier (*Brassica oleracea*), *N Z Vet J* 45:37-39, 1997.
646. Mella CM, Perez-Oliva O, Loew FM: Induction of bovine polioencephalomalacia with a feeding system based on molasses and urea, *Can J Comp Med* 40:104-110, 1976.
647. Hamlen H, Clark E, Janzen E: Polioencephalomalacia in cattle consuming water with elevated sodium sulfate levels: A herd investigation, *Can Vet J* 34:153-158, 1993.
648. Beke GJ, Hironaka R: Toxicity to beef cattle of sulfur in saline well water: a case study, *Sci Total Environ* 101:281-290, 1991.
649. Bird PR, Moir RJ: Sulphur metabolism and excretion studies in ruminants. I, The absorption of sulphate in the sheep after intraruminal or intraduodenal infusions of sodium sulphate, *Aust J Biol Sci* 24:1319-1328, 1971.
650. Bray AC, Till AR: Metabolism of sulfur in the gastrointestinal tract: digestion and metabolism in the ruminant, *Proceedings of the Fourth International Symposium on Ruminant Physiology*, Tamworth, Australia,1975.
651. Goodrich RD et al: *Sulfur in ruminant nutrition*, West Des Moines, Iowa, 1978, National Feed Ingredients Association.
652. Lewis D: The reduction of sulphate in the rumen of the sheep, *Biochem J* 56:391-399, 1954.
653. Cummings BA et al: Identity and interactions of rumen microbes associated with dietary sulfate-induced polioencephalomalacia in cattle, *Am J Vet Res* 56:1384-1389, 1995.
654. Macy JM et al: Growth of *Wolinella succinogenes* on H$_2$S plus fumarate and on fomate plus sulphur as energy sources, *Arch Microbiol* 144:147-150, 1986.
655. Bray AC: Sulphur metabolism in sheep. II, The absorption of inorganic sulphate and inorganic sulphide from the sheep's rumen, *Aust J Agric Res* 20:739-748, 1969.
656. Bray AC. Sulphur metabolism in sheep III, The movement of blood inorganic sulphate across the rumen wall of sheep. *Aust J Agric Res* 1969;20:749-58.
657. Bray AC: Sulphur metabolism in sheep. IV, The effect of a varied dietary sulphur content on some body fluid sulphate levels and on the utilization of urea-supplemented roughage by sheep, *Aust J Agric Res* 20:759-773, 1969.
658. Kandylis K, Bray AC: Loss of volatile sulfur from sheep, *Aust J Agric Res* 33:585-589, 1982.
659. Bird PR, Hume ID: Sulfur metabolism and excretion studies in ruminants. IV, Cystine and sulphate effects upon the flow of sulphur from the rumen and upon sulphur excretion by sheep, *Aust J Agric Res* 22:443-452, 1971.
660. Kennedy PM, Milligan LP: Quantitative aspects of the transformations of sulphur in sheep, *Br J Nutr* 39:65-84, 1978.
661. Kandylis K: Transfer of plasma sulfate from blood to rumen: a review, *J Dairy Sci* 66:2263-2270, 1983.
662. Alves de Oliveira L et al: Use of a semicontinuous culture system (RUSITEC) to study the effect of pH on microbial metabolism of thiamin (vitamin B$_1$), *Arch Tierernahr* 49:193-202, 1996.
663. Cummings BA et al: Ruminal microbial alterations associated with sulfide generation in steers with dietary sulfate-induced polioencephalomalacia, *Am J Vet Res* 56:1390-1395, 1995.
664. Doyle PT, Adams NR: Toxic effects of large amounts of DL-methionine infused into the rumen of sheep, *Aust Vet J* 56:331-334, 1980.
665. Beauchamp RO Jr et al: A critical review of the literature on hydrogen sulfide toxicity, *Crit Rev Toxicol* 13:25-97, 1984.
666. Evans CL: The toxicity of hydrogen sulphide and other sulphides, *Q J Exp Physiol Cogn Med Sci* 52:231-248, 1967.
667. Dougherty RW et al: Pulmonary absorption of eructated gas in ruminants, *Am J Vet Res* 23:205, 1962.
668. Olkowski AA: Neurotoxicity and secondary metabolic problems associated with low to moderate levels of exposure to excess dietary sulphur in ruminants: a review, *Vet Hum Toxicol* 39:355-360, 1997.
669. Rousseaux CG et al: Ovine polioencephalomalacia associated with dietary sulphur intake, *Zentralbl Veterinarmed [A]* 38:229-239, 1991.
670. Olkowski AA et al: Role of thiamine status in sulphur-induced polioencephalomalacia in sheep, *Res Vet Sci* 52:78-85, 1992.
671. Alves de Oliveira L et al: Effect of a high sulfur diet on rumen microbial activity and rumen thiamine status in sheep receiving a semi-synthetic, thiamine-free diet, *Reprod Nutr Dev* 36:31-42, 1996.
672. Thomas KW: Oral treatment of polioencephalomalacia and subclinical thiamine deficiency with thiamine propyl disulphide and thiamine hydrochloride, *J Vet Pharmacol Ther* 9:402-411, 1986.
673. Dickie CW et al: Polioencephalomalacia in range cattle, *J Am Vet Med Assoc* 175:460-462, 1979.
674. Dickie CW, Berryman JR: Polioencephalomalacia and photosensitization associated with *Kochia scoparia* consumption in range cattle, *J Am Vet Med Assoc* 175:463-465, 1979.
675. Edwin EE, Jackman R: Elevation of blood keto acids in cerebrocortical necrosis, *Vet Rec* 109:75-76, 1981.
676. Plaitakis A et al: Effect of thiamine deficiency on brain neurotransmitter systems, *Ann NY Acad Sci* 378:367-381, 1982.
677. Rammell CG, Hill JH: A review of thiamine deficiency and its diagnosis, especially in ruminants, *N Z Vet J* 34:202-204, 1986.
678. Naga MA et al: Suspected B-vitamin deficiency of sheep fed a protein free urea–containing purified diet, *J Anim Sci* 40:1192-1198, 1975.
679. Breves G et al: Thiamine balance in the gastrointestinal tract of sheep, *J Anim Sci* 51:1177-1181, 1980.
680. Markson LM et al: The aetiology of cerebrocortical necrosis: the effects of administering antimetabolites of thiamine to preruminant calves, *Br Vet J* 128:488-499, 1972.
681. Markson LM et al: The production of cerebrocortical necrosis in ruminant calves by the intraruminal administration of amprolium, *Br Vet J* 130:9-16, 1974.
682. Evans WC et al: Induction of thiamine deficiency in sheep, with lesions similar to those of cerebrocortical necrosis, *J Comp Pathol* 85:253-267, 1975.
683. Shreeve JE, Edwin EE: Thiaminase-producing strains of *Cl. sporogenes* associated with outbreaks of cerebrocortical necrosis, *Vet Rec* 94:330, 1974.
684. Edwin EE, Jackman R: Thiaminase I in the development of cerebrocortical necrosis in sheep and cattle, *Nature* 228:772-774, 1970.
685. Murata K: Actions of two types of thiaminase on thiamine and its analogs, *Ann NY Acad Sci* 378:146-155, 1982.
686. Loew FM: A thiamine-responsive polioencephalomalacia in tropical and nontropical livestock production systems, *World Rev Nutr Diet* 20:168-183, 1975.
687. Smith MC: Polioencephalomalacia in goats, *J Am Vet Med Assoc* 174:1328-1332, 1979.
688. Seimiya Y, Itoh H, Ohshima K: A case of cerebrocortical necrosis in a sheep, *Nippon Juigaku Zasshi* 51:1075-1077, 1989.
689. Kurtz HJ, Karns PD: Polioencephalomalacia in a white-tailed deer (*Odocoileus virginianus borealis*), *Pathol Vet* 6:475-480, 1969.
690. Wernery U, Haydn-Evans J, Kinne J: Amprolium-induced cerebrocortical necrosis (CCN) in dromedary racing camels, *Zentralbl Veterinarmed [B]* 45:335-343, 1998.
691. Gabbedy BJ, Richards RB: Polioencephalomalacia of sheep and cattle, *Aust Vet J* 53:36-38, 1977.
692. Thomas KW et al: Thiamine deficiency in sheep exported live by sea, *Aust Vet J* 67:215-218, 1990.
693. Edwin EE, Jackman R: Nature of the autofluorescent material in cerebrocortical necrosis, *J Neurochem* 37:1054-1056, 1981.

694. Little PB: Identity of fluorescence in polioencephalomalacia, *Vet Rec* 103: 76, 1978.
695. Spicer EM, Horton BJ: Biochemistry of natural and amprolium-induced polioencephalomalacia in sheep, *Aust Vet J* 57:230-235, 1981.

THIAMINE DEFICIENCY OF HORSES

Horses may develop thiamine deficiency when fed diets that contain thiaminases. Common sources of thiaminases are bracken fern *(Pteridium aquilinum)*, horsetails, *(Equisetum arvense)*, and amprolium (400 to 800 mg/kg). The clinical signs of thiamine deficiency are ataxia, conscious proprioceptive deficits, heart block, bradycardia, blindness, weight loss, dysuria, hypothermia of the extremities, and periodic muscular fasciculations. Terminally, affected horses develop convulsions. Electrolyte changes include hyperkalemia, hyperphosphatemia, hyperglycemia, and decreased glucose tolerance. Parenterally administered thiamine is effective for the treatment of this condition.[696,697]

REFERENCES

696. Carpenter KJ, Phillipson AT, Thomson W: Experiments with dried bracken *(Pteris aquilina)*, *Br Vet J* 106:292-308, 1950.
697. Cymbaluk NF, Fretz PB, Loew FM: Amprolium-induced thiamine deficiency in horses: clinical features, *Am J Vet Res* 39:225-261, 1978.

SALT POISONING

DEFINITION AND ETIOLOGY. Salt poisoning is a common central nervous system (CNS) disease of livestock. Salt-rich solutions ingested over time can cause production-related losses and even death. Ingestion of water containing more than 7000 mg/L of total dissolved salts is likely to result in acute salt poisoning.[698] Water that contains less than 3000 mg/L of total dissolved salts is considered safe for consumption. Salt poisoning can be associated with water deprivation. Provided that access to free water is constantly available, animals may tolerate as much as 13% dietary salt intake.[699] The total dietary salt concentration should never exceed 4%. The acute toxic dose of oral sodium chloride (NaCl) for cattle and horses has been reported to be approximately 2.2 g/kg of body weight and that for sheep has been reported to be approximately 6 g/kg of body weight.[699] With water restriction the toxic dose of salt is considerably less, and poisonings have resulted from ingestion of 0.9% NaCl in water-restricted cattle.[700] Ingestion of water with salt concentrations above 1% uniformly results in toxicosis if no other source of ion-free water is provided.[701,702] Ingestion of water containing 0.7% salt lowers the fertility of females,[702] and water containing 0.25% salt suppresses milk production in cattle.[703] Dairy calves have been poisoned by daily feeding of 4 L of milk replacer containing 2.6% NaCl.[704] Animals are most susceptible to salt poisoning during the summer because of the increased insensitive loss of water that occurs at that time.

CLINICAL SIGNS. Rapid ingestion of large amounts of salt causes gastrointestinal and neurologic signs,[701,704-709] including mucohemorrhagic diarrhea and colic, head-neck extension ("star gazing"), blindness, aggressiveness, hyperexcitability, psychomotor seizures (paddling and loss of consciousness), vocalization, ataxia, proprioceptive deficits, head-pressing, constant chewing movements, nystagmus, muscle twitching, and coma. Death occurs as a result of respiratory failure. Before the onset of the nervous signs, cattle with chronic salt toxicosis may appear to be depressed and dehydrated. Table 33-10 summarizes the spectrum of clinical syndromes associated with different levels of salt intake.

Excessive salt intake also may interfere with productivity in the absence of acute neurologic signs. In one study cattle were given either tap water (196 ppm of dissolved salts) or saline (2500 ppm NaCl), and their milk production was measured.[703] Cows given tap water had a greater fluid intake and a significantly greater lactational persistence and daily milk production than did cows given saline. The serum concentrations of sodium and potassium were normal in the animals fed saline.

The clinical diagnosis of salt poisoning depends on the demonstration of exposure to toxic concentrations (over 7000 ppm of sodium), the presence of water deprivation, or the determination of serum or cerebrospinal fluid (CSF) sodium concentrations over 160 mEq/L. CSF to serum sodium ratios greater than 1 are also suggestive of salt poisoning. The serum sodium concentration may vary, depending on whether the patient had recently been given ion-free water before measurement. Some animals with acute neurologic lesions may be normonatremic if they have recently drunk to repletion with ion-free water, whereas others that have not had ion-free water may be hypernatremic. The CSF sodium concentration in salt-poisoned animals is consistently elevated and may exceed 200 mEq/L.[705] Ruminal sodium concentrations above 0.36% to 0.5% or brain sodium concentrations over 150 mEq/g or 1800 ppm[710] are also suggestive of salt poisoning in cattle.[705,706,711]

The concentration of acetyl cholinesterase in plasma and red blood cells is decreased in animals that have been ingesting excessive salt (more than 0.49% of the diet).[712] The decrease is first seen after 4 months of continuous ingestion of the high-salt diet.

PATHOPHYSIOLOGY. The pathogenesis of salt poisoning involves the deposition of sodium ions in the CNS parenchyma and the CSF, which occurs either acutely from ingestion of a large quantity of salt or chronically after long periods of reduced water consumption. The ionic sodium accumulates in the CSF and neurons by passive diffusion. The resulting hyperosmolality reduces energy-dependent sodium

TABLE 33-10

Effects of Different Salt Concentrations in Drinking Water on Performance in Cattle

Salt Concentration (mg/L or ppm)	Clinical Effect
<1000	No effect
1000-3000	Temporary diarrhea; reduced milk production
3000-5000	May reduce milk production and feed intake; may produce reproductive failures (failure to conceive)
5000-7000	Conception failures (abortion, infertility), reduced appetite
>7000	Unsafe, especially in hot weather, may produce encephalopathic signs, abdominal pain, mucoid diarrhea, thirst, salivation, polyuria, central nervous system signs, include knuckling, blindness, convulsions, coma, and abdominal pain

From McCoy CP, Edwards WC: *Bovine Pract* 15:152-154, 1980.

transport mechanisms and the anaerobic glycolytic pathways.[713] These mechanisms normally provide energy by which the sodium ion is removed from the cell cytoplasm.[708] The thirst receptors are triggered in response to the hyperosmolality. The animal is permitted to drink ion-free water to repletion, the fluid is absorbed from the gastrointestinal tract, resulting in expansion of the extracellular fluid and a return to normal plasma osmolality. Water then diffuses from the blood into the relatively hyperosmolar CSF and neurons, resulting in CNS edema, increased intracranial pressure, and acute encephalopathy. If the patient has had sudden access to a large quantity of salt, the hyperosmolality in the intestine results in saline catharsis and diarrhea.

EPIDEMIOLOGY. Animals are tolerant of high dietary salt levels if they have concomitant access to fresh drinking water. Feedstuffs that are common sources of excessive salt include whey, saline-preserved fish or fish meals, bakery by-products, and certain milk replacers.[714] Confined calves may be poisoned by improperly formulated milk replacers or oral electrolyte replacements.[705,714] Cattle eagerly ingest large amounts of oil well sludge, which is a potential source of salt for cattle in the western and southwestern United States.[709,715] Brine is used extensively as a flush during the drilling of oil wells. Effluents from drilling rigs may contain as much as 100,000 ppm of salt. The effluents are also contaminated by heavy metals and magnesium salts that complicate the clinical syndrome of salt poisoning. Salt poisoning caused by water restriction may occur either inadvertently from freezing of water sources in northern climates or from intentional water restriction of veal calves.[705] Ingestion of brackish or tidal water is a cause of salt poisoning in cattle pastured on the coastal regions of the world.

NECROPSY FINDINGS. The pathologic changes of salt poisoning include cerebral edema and softening and flattening of the cortical gyri. Microscopic lesions include laminar cortical necrosis, poliomalacia, and occasionally meningeal or perivascular infiltration of eosinophils. Perivascular infiltration of eosinophils is not as reliable an indicator of salt poisoning in ruminants as in pigs because most affected ruminants show perivascular cuffing of mononuclear cells.

TREATMENT. Treatment of animals affected by salt poisoning is difficult. Most of these animals die even after intensive medical treatment. Therapy should be aimed at limiting the ingestion of nonionic water and attempting to slowly remove intracellular solutes from the brain while simultaneously controlling cerebral edema and attendant CNS signs. To prevent brain swelling and herniation of the brain through the foramen magnum or the tentorium cerebelli, slow reduction of the CSF and plasma sodium is imperative.

In calves this can be accomplished by administration of hypertonic saline concomitantly with feeding of 2 to 4 L of fresh milk daily. First, the plasma sodium concentration is measured, and the calf then is given 1 to 2 L of a hypertonic saline solution intravenously. The molar strength of the sodium ion in the intravenous fluid should be equal to or slightly greater than that of the plasma. If the hypotonicity of the whole milk is not counterbalanced by treatment with hypertonic saline, the CNS will rapidly expand as a result of absorption of free water. The plasma electrolyte concentration is measured twice daily. If the plasma sodium concentration declines too rapidly, 1 L of hypertonic saline solution is infused over several hours. The concentration of sodium in this fluid should be greater than the most recent plasma sodium measurement and less than the beginning plasma sodium concentration. If the calf develops nervous twitching, salivation, head-neck extension, stiff forelimbs, or convulsions, 0.5 to 1 g/kg of mannitol is immediately infused intravenously. A blood administration set is used to filter insoluble mannitol crystals. The calf should have no access to fresh water.

The use of solutions containing 5% glucose is dangerous and probably contraindicated because this represents ion-free extracellular fluid, which can exacerbate brain edema. Administration of corticosteroids (dexamethasone, 0.4 to 0.8 mg/kg by slow intravenous injection given twice daily for 2 to 3 days) may be helpful in animals with acute cerebral edema. However, potential benefits should be weighed against the possibility of inducing extrarenal sodium retention. If the nervous signs diminish and the plasma sodium level returns to normal, the animal may be given fresh ion-free drinking water.

CONTROL. Cattle should be fenced away from polluted ponds and oil wells. Cattle on coastal pastures should have access to fresh well water. The total daily dietary salt intake should not exceed 4% of dry matter intake. Drinking water must contain less than 7000 ppm of sodium unless the dietary sodium load is reduced correspondingly. Oral rehydrating fluids for calves should be dissolved in strict accordance with the manufacturer's recommendations and should not be administered for longer than 3 consecutive days.

REFERENCES

698. Beke GJ, Hironaka R: Toxicity to beef cattle of sulfur in saline well water: a case study, *Sci Total Environ* 101:281-290, 1991.
699. Meyer JH et al: The influence of high sodium chloride intakes by fattening sheep and cattle, *J Anim Sci* 14:412-418, 1955.
700. Pistor W, Nesbitt JC, Cardon BP: The influence of high salt intake on the physiology of ruminants, *Proceedings of the Annual Meeting of the American Veterinary Medicine Association,* Seattle, 1954.
701. Sandals WCD: Acute salt poisoning in cattle, *Can Vet J* 19:136-137, 1978.
702. McCoy CP, Edwards WC: Sodium ion poisoning in livestock from oil wastes, *Bovine Pract* 15:152-154, 1980.
703. Jaster EH, Schuh JD, Wegner TN: Physiological effects of saline drinking water on high-producing dairy cows, *J Dairy Sci* 61:66-71, 1978.
704. Ratliff RD: Sodium chloride poisoning in cattle, *Vet Med* 37:438-439, 1942.
705. Pearson EG, Kallfelz FA: A case of presumptive salt poisoning (water deprivation) in veal calves, *Cornell Vet* 72:142-149, 1982.
706. Bohosiewicz M: Laboratory research on sodium chloride poisoning in cattle, *Weterynaria Wroclaw* 4:91-101, 1958.
707. Jones TH: Salt poisoning in a cow, *Vet Rec* 10:10, 1930.
708. Ballantyne EE: Drinking waters toxic for livestock, *Can J Comp Med* 21:254-257, 1957.
709. Trueman KF, Clague DC: Sodium chloride poisoning in cattle, *Aust Vet J* 54:89-91, 1978.
710. Thilsted JP et al: Sodium salt toxicosis in beef cows resulting from the consumption of saline water, *Proc Am Assoc Vet Lab Diagn* 81:229-236, 1981.
711. Osweiler GD, Hurd JW: Determination of sodium content in serum and cerebrospinal fluid as an adjunct to diagnosis of water deprivation in swine, *J Am Vet Med Assoc* 165:165-167, 1974.
712. Assad F, Bayoumi MT: Response of sheep to selective drinking of fresh and saline water, *World Rev Anim Prod* 26:39-42, 1991.
713. Utter MI: Mechanism of inhibition of anaerobic glycolysis of brain by sodium ions, *J Biol Chem* 185:499-517, 1950.
714. Pringle JK, Berthiaume LM: Hypernatremia in calves, *J Vet Intern Med* 1:66-70, 1988.
715. Monlux AW et al: The effects of oil field pollutants on vegetation and farm animals, *J Am Vet Med Assoc* 158:1379-1390, 1971.

VITAMIN A DEFICIENCY

DEFINITION AND ETIOLOGY. Vitamin A (retinol) is found in green plants and can be synthesized by the small intestinal mucosal cells from plant carotenoid precursors. Precursors of vitamin A are usually fed in cattle rations as β-carotene or as retinoids (retinyl palmitate or acetate). Carotenoid in forage is converted to retinol in the liver and gut. Vitamin A deficiency occurs primarily in growing ruminants in feedlots. Deficiency develops under these conditions because the growing animal has a higher requirement for the vitamin, and feedlot-reared animals may have limited access to succulent plants. The vitamin is labile in foodstuffs and is essentially depleted after several years of storage. Diets that are naturally low in vitamin A include cereal grains, beet pulp, and cottonseed hulls.

The clinical signs of vitamin A deficiency in cattle are related to increased intracranial pressure and ill thrift caused by secondary infections. The clinical signs include intermittent convulsions, depression, and blindness. The usual dietary or management conditions that favor the vitamin deficiency include grazing on dry pastures or cereal grains other than corn, exclusive feeding of cereal grains that have been stored at high temperature and humidity, or prolonged feeding of mineral oil as a preventive for frothy bloat.

CLINICAL SIGNS. The neurologic signs of vitamin A–depleted animals are age dependent. The signs in deficient calves include anorexia, ill thrift, blindness, diarrhea, and pneumonia. The syndrome in adults is characterized by stargazing attitude, blindness, diarrhea, anasarca, nystagmus, strabismus, exophthalmos, loss of pupillary light reflexes, and intermittent tonic-clonic convulsions. The seizures last for only a few minutes and are followed by partial recovery.[716-718] Animals may die while convulsing. Stimulation of the animals frequently precipitates tonic-clonic convulsions.[719,720] Death often is preceded by hyperesthesia and coma.[716,717] Vitamin A–deficient adults appear to be in good body condition unless parasitism or some other nutritional deficiency is superimposed on the low vitamin A intake.[716,721] Secondary factors that could influence the appearance of the animals include concomitant nutritional deficiencies, parasitism, and pneumonia.

The ophthalmoscopic changes of vitamin A deficiency are characteristic. The pupils become dilated and unresponsive. The border of the optic disk becomes indistinct, particularly in the upper quadrants,[716,718,722] giving the appearance of an inverted heart. The swollen disk may cast a shadow on the adjacent retina. The blood vessels become tortuous or appear to be occluded as they course over the disk. The color of the disk becomes faded. In advanced cases the disk may become atrophic and appear dull, gray, flattened, and smaller than normal. Corneal changes are an uncommon clinical finding.[716,717]

Reproductive disturbances can occur. These include malformed fetuses, abortions, loss of libido, testicular degeneration, and decreased sperm counts. Calves born to vitamin A–deficient dams show blindness, domed foreheads, thickened carpal joints, and weakness at birth.[723]

Vitamin A deficiency can be clinically differentiated from polioencephalomalacia and salt poisoning by comparing the menace response with the pupillary light reflex. Calves with lead poisoning and polioencephalomalacia generally have intact pupillary light reflexes because of the proper functioning of the mesencephalon and optic nerves, whereas vitamin A–deficient cattle have absent pupillary light responses because of retinal degeneration and constriction of cranial nerve II at the level of the optic foramen.

CLINICAL PATHOLOGY. Assay of vitamin A and carotene concentrations in the plasma and feed is the most direct method of diagnosing the dietary deficiency. The concentration of plasma vitamin A and β-carotene in normal animals ranges from 25 to 85 μg/dl and 150 and 397 μg/dl, respectively.[717] Plasma concentrations of vitamin A– and β-carotene–deficient animals usually are below 7 and 70 μg/dl, respectively. Papilledema first occurs when plasma concentrations of the vitamin fall below 18 μg/dl.[724] Ataxia and blindness occur when the serum vitamin A concentration ranges from 4.87 to 8.88 μg/dl.[719] The hepatic concentration of vitamin A and carotene in normal calves ranges from 60 to 200 and from 4 to 800 μg/g of tissue, respectively. In deficient calves the hepatic concentrations of the vitamin A and carotene nutrients range from 2 to 14 and from 0.5 to 32 μg/g, respectively.[721,724] There are no consistent changes in the blood chemistry analysis or the hemogram of deficient animals. Increased cerebrospinal fluid (CSF) pressure (over 200 mm) may occur; however, standardization of the measurement for all forms of anesthesia and methods of measurement is difficult.[725] Changes in the CSF of vitamin A–deficient animals include a mononuclear cell pleocytosis (40 to 50 nucleated cells per deciliter) and an increased protein concentration (140 mg/dl).[726]

PATHOPHYSIOLOGY. Vitamin A is responsible for the regeneration of rhodopsin in the retina and the maintenance of tissue integrity. The vitamin has effects on osteoblasts and osteoclasts, epithelial tissues, the choroid plexus, and reproductive tissues. The arachnoid villi and the retina are most sensitive to a deficiency of the vitamin. Vitamin A deficiency causes a thickening of the dura mater, resulting in diminished CSF absorption from the arachnoid granulations and the nerve rootlets. Narrowing of all the bony foramina of the skull occurs. The combined effects cause an increase in CSF pressure.[721] In severe cases the brain may herniate through the foramen magnum. Closure of the optic foramen may lead to transection of the optic nerve. The high CSF pressure is transmitted into the optic nerves and results in papilledema.

Three causes of blindness have been associated with vitamin A deficiency. One cause is nyctalopia, presumably caused by the decreased formation of vitamin A aldehyde in the regeneration of the visual pigment rhodopsin; this type of blindness usually is reversible. Another cause of blindness results from the degenerative changes in the outer retinal layers; this is reversible if treated in the early stages. The third cause is associated with stenosis of the optic foramen and compression of the optic nerve; this condition is irreversible.[727] An experimental study has shown that humoral immune function also is impaired in sheep with vitamin A deficiency. The pathogenesis of this condition is unclear.[728]

EPIDEMIOLOGY. The vitamin A requirement of all species ranges from 40 to 80 IU/kg of body weight daily.[729-731] The minimum recommended daily dose of vitamin A for growing calves up to 1 year of age, for pregnant sheep, and for growing horses is 40 IU/kg of body weight. Pregnant cattle and pregnant or lactating horses require 40 to 50 IU (13.76 to 17.2 μg/kg) of vitamin A daily.[729] Lactating cattle require 80 IU (27.5 μg/kg) of vitamin A daily. Horses are susceptible to vitamin A deficiency, but the condition is rarely seen in that species. This is thought to be the result of differing conditions of management rather than an inherent resistance to the deficiency. The daily dietary requirement for carotene is 0.12 mg/kg.[729] Pasture forage, silage, and properly cured hay (less than 1 year old) contain large amounts of carotene. Common constituents that have low concentrations of vitamin A are sorghum, brewer's grain, and wheat straw. Livestock are protected from short-term deprivation of vitamin A by their ability to accumulate the vitamin in the liver; however, it is estimated that the intake required to initiate storage is at least three times the minimum daily intake.[729] Vitamin A–replete cattle fed a diet devoid of vitamin A require approximately 180 days before they begin to show clinical signs. During that time the cattle grow and fatten normally and show no adverse effects. Offspring born to these animals may show severe deficiencies. Papilledema and blindness develop rapidly after the hepatic stores are depleted.[729]

Vitamin A deficiency may be categorized as a primary or a secondary condition. Primary deficiencies of vitamin A develop in cattle confined in dry-lot corrals or pasture on dry grass forage for prolonged periods or when cattle are kept indoors and fed unsupplemented, vitamin-depleted cereals and dry forage in which the activity of carotene has been destroyed. Also, there is a seasonal difference in the concentration of vitamin A in feedstuffs. For example, cattle grazed on green pastures are consistently replete with the vitamin, whereas those grazed on dry pastures at the end of summer may become marginally deficient. Approximately 80% of the vitamin A concentration of hay is lost during field curing.[732]

Destruction of carotene is hastened by many environmental and physical factors, including heat, sunlight, trace mineral supplements, and humidity. In one study exposure of nine different supplements to trace minerals in a humidified atmosphere (60% relative humidity) at 28° C (82.2° F) resulted in depletion of 47% to 92% of the total vitamin A after 1 week of incubation.[733] Improper storage has been implicated as the cause of the depletion of vitamin A in one field case.[729] Other factors that affect the stability of vitamin A in feedstuff include pelleting and exposure to rancid fat in the feed. The addition of gelatin to vitamin premixes has been recommended to stabilize the vitamin A activity in feed.[724,734]

Secondary deficiencies of vitamin A result from interference with vitamin absorption, inhibition of the conversion of β-carotene to retinol (vitamin A) in the small intestine, or an increased requirement in the face of limited vitamin intake. The conversion of carotene to retinol is impaired in vitamin A–deficient patients.[735] Sheep may be more resistant to vitamin A deficiency because they convert β-carotene more efficiently than cattle.[735] Extensive destruction of preformed vitamin A by microflora appears to occur in the rumen and the abomasum.[734,736-738] Microbial destruction, fever, lactation, high ambient temperatures, and inadequate dietary energy may increase the daily requirement for vitamin A.[739] Females are slightly more resistant to the vitamin deficiency than males, presumably because of the interconversions of estrogenic hormones into vitamin A.

Secondary deficiencies of vitamin A may be caused by impaired vitamin absorption, which may occur from long-term feeding of mineral oil. Ingestion of highly chlorinated naphthalenes (X disease) causes severe vitamin A deficiency as a result of interference with the conversion of carotene to vitamin A. Some in vitro evidence indicates that a high level of dietary nitrates inactivates intraruminal vitamin A by oxidation. This may not be clinically important, however, because studies performed in vivo failed to show a greater requirement for the vitamin when animals were fed subtoxic doses of nitrates.[738,740-743]

NECROPSY FINDINGS. The major pathologic changes in the fundus of vitamin A–deficient calves include papilledema; small, flame-shaped hemorrhages around the optic disk; venous congestion in the area of the swollen optic disk; degeneration of the retinal ganglion cells; focal retinal thinning; and fusion of parts of the retina to the choroid plexus.[722] Other changes associated with vitamin A deficiency include doming of the frontal bones, enlargement of the carpi, cerebellar and cerebral compression, partial transtentorial herniation of the cerebellum, cystic dilation of the hypophyseal cleft, focal ruminal hyperkeratosis, and increased keratinization of the squamous epithelium of the penile and the preputial mucous membrane.[744,745] Corneal ulceration and clouding have been observed in the eyes of calves with naturally occurring deficiencies.[717,725] Other changes of vitamin A deficiency include anasarca, squamous metaplasia of the salivary ducts, and degeneration of the germinal testicular epithelium.[745]

Microscopic changes in the CNS include attenuation of the optic nerve with necrosis and demyelination. Focal accumulations of phagocytic cells containing lipofuscin and hemosiderin are present in the necrotic area. The optic nerve is attenuated along its entire length. Gliosis and focal vacuolization of the nerve also are seen, as is a focal loss of granular and molecular layers and Purkinje cells in the cerebellum. The meninges are thickened by fibrosis and mononuclear cell inflammation. The microscopic changes in the bones include wider than normal spacing of the central canals and reduction of osteoclastic lacunae.

TREATMENT AND CONTROL. Cattle with severe blindness caused by damage to the retina or optic nerves do not regain their vision when treated with vitamin A; however, cattle with acute encephalopathy and simple papilledema may respond favorably after a short period of vitamin supplementation.[729] Affected cattle should receive 440 IU/kg of body weight (1 IU = 0.4 μg) of vitamin A parenterally and then 6000 IU/kg parenterally every 50 to 60 days until the diet has been enriched. High-dose oral therapy is important because carotene and oil suspensions of vitamin A are not efficiently used when administered by parenteral injection.[746] Administration of large doses orally is important because conversion of β-carotene to vitamin A is inhibited in deficient calves.[735]

Prophylactic dietary supplementation of vitamin A should be considered in all cattle that lack access to green feed. Dietary supplements could include leafy, freshly cured hay, green pasture, or 0.5 to 2 kg of alfalfa meal daily. Concentrate feeds formulated with exogenous, stabilized vitamin A are commercially available. Vitamin A powder* may be added to the drinking water at a rate of 425,000 U/50 gallons. This treatment should be continued for as long as the dietary deficiency exists.

Subclinical deficiencies in ewes have been treated with a vitamin-mineral premix containing 0.3 kg to 0.27 kg iodine, 20.6 kg zinc, 7.9 kg copper, and 1644.5 million IU vitamin A per ton of feed. Addition of this premix to the diet of a group of sheep increased the productivity as measured by viability, birth weights and rate of gain of lambs, and amount and quality of wool.[747]

REFERENCES

716. Divers TJ et al: Blindness and convulsions associated with vitamin A deficiency in feedlot steers, *Am J Vet Res* 189:1579-1582, 1986.
717. Shlosberg A, Levinsohn M, Nagel N: Severe hypovitaminosis A in two herds of beef calves, *Refuah Vet* 34:25-27, 1977.
718. Moore LA: Some ocular changes and deficiency manifest in mature cows fed a ration deficient in vitamin A, *J Dairy Sci* 24:843-902, 1941.
719. Booth A, Reid M, Clark T: Hypovitaminosis A in feedlot cattle, *J Am Vet Med Assoc* 190:1305-1308, 1981.
720. Sustonck B, Deprez Muylle E: Nervous disorders associated with hypovitaminosis A in beef cattle, *Vlaams Diergeneeskd Tijdschr* 62:95-97, 1993.
721. Eaton HD: Chronic bovine hypo- and hypervitaminosis A and cerebrospinal fluid pressure, *Am J Clin Nutr* 22:1070-1080, 1969.
722. Barnett KC et al: Ocular changes associated with hypovitaminosis A in cattle, *Br Vet J* 126:561-573, 1970.
723. Van Der Lugt JJ, Prozesky L: The pathology of blindness in newborn calves caused by hypovitaminosis A, *Onderstepoort J Vet Res* 56:99-109, 1989.
724. Eaton HD et al: Association of plasma or liver vitamin A concentrations with the occurrence of parotid duct metaplasia or of ocular papilledema in Holstein male calves, *J Dairy Sci* 53:1755-1779, 1970.
725. Dbanapalan P et al: Cerebrospinal fluid pressure measurement as a diagnostic aid for hypovitaminosis A in calves, *Indian Vet J* 69:917-918, 1992.
726. Anderson WI et al: The ophthalmic and neuroophthalmic effects of a vitamin A deficiency in young steers, *Vet Med* 86:1143-1148, 1991.
727. Van Der Lugt JJ, Prozesky L: The pathology of blindness in newborn calves caused by hypovitaminosis A, *Onderstepoort J Vet Res* 56:99-109, 1989.
728. Brans NJ et al: Humoral immunity in vitamin A–deficient and vitamin A–repleted lambs, *FASEB J* 3:A663, 1989.
729. Guilbert HR, Miller RF, Hughes EH: The minimum vitamin A and carotene requirement of cattle, sheep, and swine, *J Nutr* 13:543-564, 1937.
730. Guilbert HR, Howell CE, Hart GH: Minimum vitamin A and carotene requirements of mammalian species, *J Nutr* 19:91-103, 1940.
731. National Research Council: *Nutrient requirements of beef cattle*, ed 5, Washington, DC, 1975, National Academic Press.
732. Shepherd JB: Experiments in harvesting and preserving alfalfa for dairy cattle feed, USDA Technical Bulletin 1954, Baltimore, US Department of Agriculture.
733. Myburgh SJ: The stability of vitamin A in synthetic vitamin A concentrates (acetate or palmitate). I. In phosphatic salt licks with and without trace elements, *Onderstepoort Vet J* 29:269-278, 1962.

*Vitamin AD 500, Butler, Inc., Dublin, OH 43017.

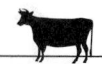

734. Mitchell GE: Vitamin A nutrition of ruminants, *J Am Vet Med Assoc* 151:430-436, 1967.
735. Diven RH, Erwin ES: Utilization of vitamin A and carotene by normal and deficient sheep, *Proc Soc Exp Biol Med* 97:601-603, 1958.
736. Keating EF, Hale WH, Hubbert F: In vitro degradation of vitamin A and carotene by rumen liquor, *J Anim Sci* 23:111-119, 1964.
737. King TB, Lohman TG, Smith GS: Evidence of rumenoreticular losses of vitamin A and carotene, *J Anim Sci* 21:1002-1008, 1962.
738. Hoar DW, Embry LB, Emerick RJ: Nitrate and vitamin A interrelationships in sheep, *J Anim Sci* 27:1727-1733, 1968.
739. Anderson TA, Hubbert F, Roubicek CB: Influence of protein depletion on vitamin A and carotene utilization by vitamin A deficient sheep, *J Nutr* 78:341-347, 1962.
740. Davison KL, Hansel W, Krook L: Nitrate toxicity in dairy heifers. I. Effects on reproduction, growth, lactation, and vitamin A nutrition, *J Dairy Sci* 47:1065-1073, 1964.
741. Hale WH, Hubbert F, Taylor RE: Effect of energy level and nitrate on hepatic vitamin A and performance of fattening steers, *Proc Soc Exp Biol Med* 109:289-290, 1960.
742. Cline TR, Hatfield EE, Garrigus US: Effects of potassium nitrate, alpha-tocopherol, thyroid treatments, and vitamin A on weight gain and liver storage of vitamin A in fattening lambs, *J Anim Sci* 22:911-913, 1963.
743. Davison KL, Seo J: Influence of nitrate upon carotene destruction during in vitro fermentation with rumen liquor, *J Dairy Sci* 46:862-864, 1963.
744. Nielsen SW et al: The pathology of marginal vitamin A deficiency in calves, *Res Vet Sci* 7:143-150, 1966.
745. Helmbolt CF, Jungherr EL, Eaton HD: The pathology of experimental hypovitaminosis A in young dairy animals, *Am J Vet Res* 14:343-354, 1953.
746. Page HM et al: Effect of hepatic vitamin A and carotene concentration on the biological value of carotene in the bovine, *Am J Physiol* 194:313-320, 1958.
747. Podshibyakin AE et al: Use of a complex of vitamin A and trace elements to prevent vitamin A deficiency in sheep, *Soviet Agric Sci* 2:52-55, 1988.

HYDROCEPHALUS AND HYDRANENCEPHALY OF CATTLE

DEFINITION AND ETIOLOGY. Hydrocephalus/hydranencephaly is a common occurrence in large ruminants. It is underdiagnosed because many of the affected animals die of complications, and the primary condition is overlooked during clinical and pathologic examinations. One study reported that 97 of 155 calves with central nervous system (CNS) lesions had hydrocephalus.[748] Hydrocephalus may be classified as being either hypertensive or normotensive.[749]

Normotensive Hydrocephalus (Hydranencephaly). Normotensive hydrocephalus that develops as a result of a failure of cell growth or cellular necrosis is called hydranencephaly.[749] Most cases of hydranencephaly in domestic livestock are caused by in utero infection of the fetus by the bluetongue, bovine virus diarrhea (BVD), akabane, Cache Valley, aino, or border disease virus.[748,750-756] The pathogenesis and epizootiology of the multisystemic virus infections bluetongue and BVD are discussed in detail in Chapter 30. The neurologic effects of border disease virus infection are discussed in detail elsewhere in this chapter.

The loss of neurons results in flexural contractions of the limbs (arthrogryposis) and inability to nurse. The calves appear blind and are unaware of their surroundings. They usually are unwilling to stand and display a weak suckle. They may exhibit a dysphonia, which resembles a bark. Neonates that are unable to nurse are deprived of colostrum and die of septicemia by 4 days after birth.

Akabane Virus Infection. The akabane virus is a member of the Sindbis serologic subgroup of the Bunyaviridae family of the Arboviridae.[750] It has been isolated from cattle in Africa, Japan, Israel, Korea, and Australia.[751-756] The host range of the virus includes sheep, cattle, and goats. Infection of pregnant, nonimmune dams results in hydranencephaly of the fetus. The disease is thought to be transmitted to the cow by various *Culicoides* species. Experimentally infected calves develop porencephaly and encephalitis when exposed to the akabane virus between gestational days 62 and 96.[757] Lambs are susceptible when exposed to the virus on gestational days 30 to

36.[756] Fetuses that survive the in utero infection are born with arthrogryposis. The CNS lesions apparently are the result of a direct necrotizing effect the virus has on the developing neurons. The pathologic changes of the CNS in experimentally infected calves and lambs are similar to those of naturally acquired infections.[753,756] Adults occasionally abort when infected by the virus but do not develop clinical disease.

Aino Virus. The aino virus causes arthrogryposis and hydranencephaly in calves of Japan and Australia.[758,759] This virus is antigenically and biologically distinct from the akabane virus, but the clinical syndromes of fetal infection by the two viruses are indistinguishable.

Chuzan Virus. Hydrocephalus, hydranencephaly, and cerebellar hypoplasia have been attributed to infection of pregnant cattle with the Chuzan virus.[760,761] This virus is a relative of the akabane and aino viruses and is classified as a new member of the Palyam subgroup of the genus *Orbivirus*. The virus has been isolated from *Culicoides oxystoma*, which may serve as the major vector. The clinical signs are characteristic of hydrocephalus.

Cache Valley Virus. A flock outbreak of arthrogryposis and hydranencephaly in newborn lambs in the southwestern United States was attributed to in utero infection with the Cache Valley virus (family Arboviridae).[762] Cache Valley virus was first isolated from mosquitoes from Utah and has since been isolated from caribou, horses, sheep, and cattle elsewhere. Antibodies have been found in white-tailed deer in the southwestern United States, but the role of this mammal in the survival of the virus and the transmission of the disease to livestock is unknown.[763] In one survey of sheep in the western United States, the seroprevalence for the Cache Valley virus was 19.1%.[762]

Bluetongue Virus Infection. The bovine fetus is most susceptible to the development of hydranencephaly from bluetongue virus when the dam is infected at approximately 125 days of gestation.[764,765] Abortions occur when nonimmune dams are infected at other times of gestation. Serotype 11 or serotype 17 of the virus is most commonly isolated from calf and lamb neonates in field epizootics.[765] Calves infected in utero may develop one or more associated birth defects, including hydranencephaly, arthrogryposis, brachygnathia, prognathia, and excessive gingival tissue. Some surviving calves that are infected at an early gestational age remain persistently infected and shed the bluetongue virus for as long as 5 years. These calves remain immunologically incompetent to the viral antigens[766] and serve as a reservoir for the virus. (See Chapter 30 for additional information.)

Bovine Virus Diarrhea Virus Infection. Hydranencephaly, hydrocephalus, and cerebellar hypoplasia have been associated with fetal infection of cattle with the BVD virus.[767-770] Precolostral serum antibody titers for the virus in affected calves vary; some titers range from 1:32 to 1:256, but other calves may have persistent viremias yet no demonstrable antibody. The BVD antibody titer in the cerebrospinal fluid (CSF) may range from 1:4 to 1:32. The virus can be isolated from approximately 12% of affected calves.

Hypertensive Hydrocephalus. An increase in CSF volume that results from compressive or obstructive lesions in the ventricular system or from decreased CSF absorption is called hypertensive hydrocephalus.[749] Obstructive lesions of the ventricular system trap the CSF in the ventricles, causing an increase in CSF volume and pressure. Ischemia and degeneration of the central nervous system results from the high CSF pressure. The sites of obstruction most commonly include the lateral apertures, the mesencephalic aqueduct, the lateral ventricles, the interventricular foramina, and the fourth ventricle. The obstructions may be either congenital or acquired. Causes of acquired obstructive hydrocephalus include cerebral abscesses, cholesteatomas (equines), equine infectious

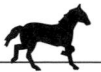

anemia, *Coenurus cerebralis* infestation, pachymeningitis, or lymphosarcoma. Hypertensive hydrocephalus also may be caused by acute inflammatory disease such as meningitis or vitamin A deficiency. In these diseases the increased pressure is the result of impaired CSF resorption.

Congenital Hypertensive Hydrocephalus. Congenital hypertensive hydrocephalus is a hereditary condition seen in Hereford, Charolais, Ayrshire, Dexter, Holstein, and Jersey calves.[771-773] The condition also has been recognized in Arabian foals.[774]

At least six forms of congenital hypertensive hydrocephalus (types I through VI) have been identified in cattle. Type I is a communicating hydrocephalus that is unrelated to dwarfism and apparently has a hereditary basis.[771] The mode of inheritance is thought to be a single autosomal recessive character. In highly inbred herds the prevalence of heterozygotes may exceed 20%. Pathologic lesions of this form of hydrocephalus included cranial doming and enlargement of the cerebral cortex and the choroid plexus. All affected calves die by 5 weeks of age.

Type II occurs in Herefords and is characterized by dorsal kinking of the mesencephalon and stenosis of the sylvian aqueduct, without cranial doming. Ventricular dilation is less than that described for type I hydrocephalus.

Type III also occurs in horned Hereford cattle. This type is similar to type II, except that cerebellar hypoplasia, microphthalmia, and muscular degeneration are observed. These are not characteristics of the type II hydrocephalus.

Type IV occurs in white shorthorn calves. The disease is considered to be heritable through either an autosomal recessive gene or a dominant gene with incomplete penetrance. Affected animals develop an obstructive hydrocephalus, microphthalmia, and scoliosis of the thoracolumbar spinal column. Ocular lesions associated with the disease include persistent pupillary membranes, retinal detachment, retinal dysplasia, vitreous hemorrhage, and hypoplasia of the optic tracts. A misshapen sylvian aqueduct apparently causes the fluid accumulation.

Type V is a form of hydrocephalus with congenital achondroplasia that has been reported in Dexter and Jersey calves. The disease is considered to result from a recessive genetic trait. The calves are either aborted or stillborn. Animals that survive to term have arrested development of the nasal bones and maxillae. Anasarca, achondroplasia, kyphosis, and cleft palate also are seen.

Type VI is a form of internal hydrocephalus of Holstein-Friesian calves. The animals are born dead or die shortly after birth. The pathologic abnormalities include fluid enlargement of the lateral ventricles with normal cranial development.[774] The condition is thought to be hereditary.

CLINICAL SIGNS. Hydrocephalic animals often are born dead or are weak and die shortly after birth. The most obvious signs in animals that survive include failure to bond to the dam, depression, diminished learning ability, partial failure of suckling, droopy head and ears, muscular fasciculations, head tremor, conscious proprioceptive deficits, blindness, ventrolateral strabismus, nystagmus, dysphonia, tongue flaccidity or paralysis, retention of food material in the cheeks and lips, limb spasticity, hyperreflexia, psychomotor seizures, recumbency, and coma. Occasionally doming of the calvarium or protrusion of fluid-filled cystic structures through an open fontanelle is seen.[775] Affected neonates often do not ingest sufficient amounts of colostrum and frequently die of septicemia.

In virally induced cases of hydranencephaly, associated skeletal deformities, including abnormally curved ribs, kyphoscoliosis, flexural deformities of the limbs, domed skulls, and brachygnathia, may be observed. Patients with hydrocephalus caused by compressive lesions around the ventricular system may show unilateral or bilateral signs of increased intracranial pressure. The clinical signs of unilateral lesions include head tilt (toward the lesion side), ipsilateral mydriasis, and contralateral menace deficit. Signs of hydrocephalus in foals are similar to those in calves. The cause of the condition in horses is unknown.

CLINICAL PATHOLOGY. The diagnosis of hydrocephalus in calves and lambs is commonly based on the presence of characteristic clinical signs and a domed skull. Whenever hydranencephaly is suspected, blood should be collected for virus isolation, serologic testing, and quantitative immunoglobulin determination. Presuckle serum samples from bovine fetuses that have been infected by the akabane or bluetongue virus in the latter part of gestation may be seropositive. Immunologically competent calves that are infected with the bluetongue virus have serum neutralization indices ranging from 2.5 to 4.[763]

NECROPSY FINDINGS. The pathologic lesions of hydranencephaly are similar regardless of the etiologic agent. They include microcephaly, cerebellar hypoplasia, hydrocephalus, hydranencephaly, and porencephaly of the cerebral and the cerebellar cortex. Microscopic lesions of hydranencephaly include segmental loss of dorsolateral ventricular ependyma, thinning of the periventricular white matter, porencephalic cysts, and nonsuppurative meningoencephalitis. Lesions in other parts of the CNS may include loss of ventral horn cells in the spinal cord and demyelination in the spinal cord. Nonsuppurative inflammatory changes may be seen in cases caused by viral infections. Polymyositis has been described in affected calves; however, it is unclear if these lesions are caused by viral infection or occur secondary to the denervation. The skeletal deformities associated with virally induced hydranencephalies include rigid extension or contraction of one or more limbs (arthrogryposis), abnormally curved ribs, domed skull, thickening of the calvarium, kyphoscoliosis, and brachygnathia.

TREATMENT. Except for one report of successful surgical intervention in a calf with a meningocele, no satisfactory therapy is available for the treatment of hydrocephalus or hydranencephaly in large animals.

REFERENCES

748. De Lahunta A: *Veterinary neuroanatomy and clinical neurology,* Philadelphia, 1977, WB Saunders.
749. Greene HJ et al: Congenital defects in cattle, *Irish Vet J* 27:37-45, 1973.
750. Doherty RL et al: Virus strains isolated from arthropods during an epizootic of bovine ephemeral fever in Queensland, *Aust Vet J* 48:81-86, 1972.
751. Blood DC: Arthrogryposis and hydranencephaly in newborn calves, *Aust Vet J* 32:987-999, 1969.
752. Hartley WJ, Wanner RA, Della-Porta AJ: Serological evidence for the association of akabane virus with epizootic bovine congenital arthrogryposis and hydranencephaly syndromes in New South Wales, *Aust Vet J* 51:103-104, 1975.
753. Hartley WJ, De Saram WG, Della-Porta AJ: Pathology of congenital bovine epizootic arthrogryposis and hydranencephaly and its relationship to akabane virus, *Aust Vet J* 53:319-325, 1977.
754. Whittem JH: Congenital abnormalities in calves, arthrogryposis and hydranencephaly, *J Pathol Bacteriol* 73:357-387, 1957.
755. Inaba Y, Kurogi H, Omori T: Akabane disease: epizootic abortion, premature birth, stillbirth, and congenital arthrogryposis-hydranencephaly in cattle, sheep and goats caused by akabane virus, *Aust Vet J* 51:584-585, 1975.
756. Parsonson IM, Della-Porta AJ, Snowdon WA: Congenital abnormalities in newborn lambs after infection of pregnant sheep with akabane virus, *Infect Immun* 15:254-262, 1977.
757. Kurogi H et al: Congenital abnormalities in newborn calves after inoculation of pregnant cows with akabane virus, *Infect Immun* 17:338-343, 1977.
758. Cybinski DH, St George TD: A survey of antibody to aino virus in cattle and other species in Australia, *Aust Vet J* 54:371-373, 1978.
759. Kitano Y et al: Congenital abnormalities in calves suggesting aino virus infection in Kagoshima prefecture, *J Jpn Vet Med Assoc* 46:469-471, 1993.
760. Miura Y et al: Chuzan disease as congenital hydranencephaly cerebellar hypoplasia syndrome in calves, *Jpn Agric Res Q* 25:55-60, 1991.

761. Miura Y et al: Hydranencephaly cerebellar hypoplasia in a newborn calf after infection of its dam with chuzan virus, *Jpn J Vet Sci* 52:689-694, 1990.

762. Livingston CW et al: Foreign animal disease report, No 15-2, Washington, DC, 1987, US Department of Agriculture, Animal and Plant Health Inspection Services.

763. Jochim M, Luedke AJ, Chow TL: Bluetongue in cattle: immunologic and clinical responses in calves inoculated in utero and after birth, *Am J Vet Res* 35:517-522, 1974.

764. Osburn BI et al: Experimental viral-induced congenital encephalopathies. II. The pathogenesis of bluetongue vaccine virus infection in fetal lambs, *Lab Invest* 25:206-210, 1971.

765. Luedke AJ, Jochim MM, Jones RH: Bluetongue in cattle: effects of *Culicoides variipennis*–transmitted bluetongue virus in pregnant heifers and their calves, *Am J Vet Res* 38:1687-1695, 1977.

766. Luedke AJ, Jochim MM, Jones RH: Bluetongue in cattle: effects of vector-transmitted bluetongue virus on calves previously infected in utero, *Am J Vet Res* 38:1697-1704, 1977.

767. Badman RT, Mitchell G, Jones RT: Association of bovine viral diarrhea virus infection to hydranencephaly and other central nervous system lesions in perinatal calves, *Aust Vet J* 57:306-307, 1981.

768. Axthelm MK et al: Congenital microhydranencephalus in cattle, *Cornell Vet* 71:164-174, 1981.

769. Trautwein G et al: Cerebellar hypoplasia and hydranencephaly in cattle associated with transplacental BVD virus infection. In Harkness JW, ed: *Agriculture pestivirus infections of ruminants*, Brussels, 1985, Commission of the European Communities.

770. Trautwein G et al: Studies on transplacental transmissibility of a bovine virus diarrhoea (BVD) vaccine virus in cattle. III. Occurrence of central nervous system malformations in calves born from vaccinated cows, *J Vet Med* 33:260-268, 1986.

771. Urman HK, Grace OD: Hereditary encephalomyopathy: a hydrocephalus syndrome in newborn calves, *Cornell Vet* 54:229-249, 1964.

772. Axthelm MK, Leipold HW, Howard D: Hereditary internal hydrocephalus, *Proc Am Assoc Vet Lab Diagn*, 1980, pp 115-126.

773. Baker M, Payne LC, Baker GN: The inheritance of hydrocephalus in cattle, *J Hered* 52:135-138, 1961.

774. Gilman JPW: Congenital hydrocephalus in domestic animals, *Cornell Vet* 45:487-499, 1956.

775. Mouli SP: Surgical correction of congenital external hydrocephalus in an Ongole bull calf, *Indian Vet J* 64:696-698, 1987.

AMMONIATED FORAGE TOXICOSIS
(Cow Bonkers)

Exposure of poor-quality forage to anhydrous ammonia improves the nutritional density of the material and reduces certain toxic fungal metabolites, specifically the prolactin-like toxins of the endophytic fungus *Acremonium coenophialum*.[776] Ammoniation increases dry matter intake, enhances digestibility, and increases the relative value of the protein content of the feed. However, overammoniation of the forage, at a rate exceeding 3% of the forage on a dry matter basis, may result in toxicosis because of the formation of 4-methylimidazole. Ammoniated foodstuffs containing high levels of molasses are more toxic than similarly treated grass hay. The toxin may be concentrated in milk; consequently, calves suckling from normal-appearing dams may show clinical signs of intoxication.

Affected animals are hyperesthetic and ataxic. At rest the animals assume a sawhorse stance, but when excited, they become hyperactive, appear to be blind, and circle propulsively. Other clinical signs include vocalization, dysphonia, and walking or running into objects. The periods of frenzy may result in recumbency and convulsions. The spasmodic episodes last for 15 to 20 minutes. Afterward the animals rest quietly, with occasional muscle tremors. Repeated occurrences of the mania may be precipitated by loud noises or other frightening experiences. The concentrations of ammonia in the cerebrospinal fluid (CSF) and blood may be increased. In one report, blood and CSF concentrations of ammonia were 8.16 and 1.05 μg/ml, respectively. Although specific treatments have not been identified, one report indicated that affected calves benefited from treatment with acepromazine (0.045 mg/kg IV) and thiamine (1.14 mg/kg IM).[777]

REFERENCES

776. Kerr LA, McCoy CP, Boyle CR: Effects of ammoniation of endophyte fungus–infested fescue hay on serum prolactin concentration and rectal temperature in beef cattle, *Am J Vet Res* 51:76-78, 1990.

777. Kerr LA, Groce AW, Kersting KW: Ammoniated forage toxicosis in calves, *J Am Vet Med Assoc* 191:551-552, 1987.

LEAD POISONING

DEFINITION AND ETIOLOGY. Lead poisoning in ruminants is characterized by an acute encephalopathy. In contrast, lead poisoning in horses is characterized by chronic polyneuritis. Blindness, ataxia, and depressed sensorium are significant clinical signs in cattle, sheep, and goats, whereas in horses the poisoning is associated with weight loss, dysphagia, and secondary aspiration pneumonia. Cattle most often are poisoned because of their tendency to lick or chew on foreign objects, their access to lead-containing materials, and their propensity to drink contaminated petroleum distillates.[778]

CLINICAL SIGNS. The signs of lead poisoning in ruminants are characteristic of central nervous system (CNS) derangement. During the first stages of lead poisoning, affected cattle stand alone and are depressed.[779] They may show hyperesthesia, muscular fasciculations, and rapid, spastic twitching of the eyelids or other facial muscles. Progression of the disease is associated with ataxia, conscious proprioceptive deficits, blindness, head-pressing, odontoprisis, coma, and convulsions.[780,781] Despite the blindness, the pupillary reflexes usually are normal. Some animals may display episodic running, hyperesthesia, and bellowing.[780,781] Others may die suddenly without premonitory signs. Affected cattle may accumulate frothy salvia at the commissures of the lips. Bloat and diarrhea may be observed, depending on other substances that have been ingested with the lead.

The clinical signs of lead poisoning in horses include weight loss, lack of coordination, laryngeal or pharyngeal paralysis, dysphonia, roaring, conscious proprioceptive deficits, loss of anal tone, facial paralysis, and difficulty with mastication. Aspiration of pharyngeal debris caused by dysphagia may result in pneumonia. Fine muscular tremors occur intermittently. The poisoned animals die in psychomotor seizures. Horses suffering from lead poisoning are emaciated at the time of death.[782]

In cattle, lead produces microscopic changes of the myocardium that result in arterial hypertension (120 to 150 mm Hg) and electrocardiographic abnormalities. These electrical changes, which occur by 30 days after exposure, include increased duration and amplitude of the p wave (0.16 sec and 0.06 mV, respectively), prolongation of the PR interval (0.14 to 0.16 sec), decreased Q-T interval (0.32 sec), and inverted T wave in lead II.[783]

CLINICAL PATHOLOGY. Diagnosis of lead poisoning is based on measurement of increased blood and tissue concentrations of lead. Tissue levels of lead in naturally poisoned cattle can reach 20 to 100 ppm in the liver, 30 ppm in the kidneys, and 5000 ppm in bone. Reported reference blood lead concentrations vary considerably, ranging from 0.05 to 2.5 ppm.[780,781,784] Suggested toxic ranges also vary considerably among laboratories. Reference values derived from earlier colorimetric studies are consistently higher than those obtained from tests performed later using atomic absorption spectrophotometry.[785] Modern techniques usually report 0.3 ppm as the maximum normal blood lead concentration. When interpreting the results of a lead measurement, consideration of the reference ranges obtained with similar methodology is essential. Table 33-11 compares the lead concentrations of various tissues of experimentally poisoned and control calves. The lead concentration of ruminal fluid from acutely poisoned cattle ranges from 0 to 11,875 ppm.[780]

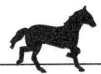

TABLE 33-11

Mean Lead Concentration* in Calf Tissues After Exposure to Different Dosages of Lead Acetate for 7 to 20 Days

Tissue	Dosage of Lead Administered		
	Control ± SD	2.7 mg/kg (ppm) ± SD	5 mg/kg (ppm) ± SD
Bone	0.22±0.07 (0.18-0.32)	49.2±14.15 (30-75.34)	54.92±20.15 (32.63-105.81)
Kidney	0.11±0.02 (0.09-0.13)	49.49±32.54 (20.72-90.36)	88±19.5 (51.55-114.24)
Liver	0.13±0.04 (0.09-0.18)	19±11.76 (5.42-29.96)	30.51±11.67 (15.13-54.98)
Cerebrum	0.07±0.02 (0.06-0.1)	0.66±0.16 (0.54-0.89)	0.81±0.27 (0.5-1.18)
Blood	0.03±0.01 (0.03-0.04)	0.47±0.29 (0.3-0.9)	1.57±0.62 (1.08-3.21)

Data from Zmudski J et al: *Bull Environ Contam Toxicol* 30:435-441, 1983.
SD, Standard deviation.
*Data in parentheses show the range of concentrations.

TABLE 33-12

Urine and Blood Lead Concentrations* in Horses With Chronic Lead Poisoning Before and After Intravenous Treatment With Calcium Disodium EDTA†

Tissue	Status	0 Hours	6 Hours	16 Hours	24 Hours
Urine	Poisoned	0.1-1.2	3.8-4.6	1.1-5.5	1.1-0.05
Urine	Normal	0.04-0.05	0.11-0.17	0.05-0.06	0.03-0.05
Blood	Poisoned	0.2-0.25	0.3-0.47	0.3-0.37	0.3-0.37
Blood	Normal	0.15-0.2	0.2-0.3	0.2-0.25	0.1-0.2

From Knight HD, Burau RG: *J Am Vet Med Assoc* 162:781-786, 1973.
*Values given in ppm; numbers reflect the range of observations.
†Dosage of 75 mg/kg of body weight.

Livestock that are chronically poisoned with low concentrations of lead may have a normal blood lead concentration but a high concentration in the bone. In these cases the poisoning can be diagnosed by administration of calcium disodium ethylenediamine tetraacetic acid (EDTA), which solubilizes the bone lead stores and increases the concentration of lead in the plasma. The soluble lead-EDTA complexes are excreted in the urine. The urinary lead concentration may rise by 40-fold over pretreatment levels within a few hours. Table 33-12 shows the lead concentrations in the urine and blood of naturally exposed horses and the temporal changes that occur after treatment with calcium disodium EDTA (75 mg/kg of body weight).

When blood lead concentrations are normal in chronically poisoned animals, measurement of free erythrocyte porphyrins and erythrocyte concentrations of α-aminolevulinic acid (ALA) are the preferred methods of diagnoses. The concentration of porphyrins is increased in the blood, urine, and feces of animals with lead poisoning. The reference range of blood porphyrin concentrations in normal calves is 21.6 ± 11.6 to 45.6 ± 10.3 μg/dl for whole blood and 113 and 142.8 ± 32.4 μg/dl for erythrocytes.[781,786,787] In chronically exposed, asymptomatic cattle, the free erythrocyte porphyrin concentrations frequently are over 2000 μg/dl. A field test has been developed for determining blood porphyrins.[787]

Reference ranges for ALA dehydrase are 45.8 ± 20.6 U, whereas activities ranging from 28 to 33 U have been reported in naturally exposed calves.[782] The urinary concentration of δ-aminolevulinic acid (δ-ALA) is increased and range above 500 μg/ml.[783,788,789] Measurement of ALA in the erythrocytes is more reliable than measurement of urine.[790]

Environmental sources of lead can be detected by direct measurement of the lead concentration of the soil or pasture forage. Forage from toxic pastures contains more than 30 ppm of lead, and in some cases the level may exceed 300 ppm.[789,791]

The hematologic abnormalities of lead poisoning are subtle. Most poisoned livestock have a normal hemogram. If present, lead-related changes are characteristic of a hemolytic anemia with an inappropriately large bone marrow response. The morphologic abnormalities of erythrocytes include anisocytosis, poikilocytosis, polychromasia, hypochromia, Howell-Jolly bodies, metarubricytes, and basophilic stippling.[780,792] The shape changes begin within hours after ingestion of the lead and become maximal by 100 days.[780,792] Blood changes do not occur in all cases of the disease and are not necessarily specific indicators of lead poisoning in cattle, but they tend to be more suggestive in horses.

In poisoned animals the concentrations of protein and white blood cells in the cerebrospinal fluid are increased, ranging from 50 to 100 mg/μl of protein and 5 to 50 mononuclear cells per milliliter, respectively.

PATHOPHYSIOLOGY. Lead enters the body through the gastrointestinal or respiratory tracts. Metallic lead and the sulfide form are less well absorbed than the acetate, phosphate, carbonate oxide, and hydroxide salts. Metallic lead is poorly absorbed and causes toxicity only when a lead foreign body becomes entrapped in the stomach for prolonged periods. Interaction between lead and other minerals may occur. For example, high levels of dietary calcium reduce the gastrointestinal absorption of lead. Concomitant exposure to lead and cadmium results in a worsening of the clinical signs of lead poisoning.[793]

Acute toxic single doses of lead range from 200 to 600 mg/kg for calves and 600 to 800 mg/kg for adults.[794,795] Although intestinal absorption of lead is relatively inefficient, significant amounts can cross into the blood if sufficient quantities are ingested. Approximately 1% to 2% of the total oral dose of lead is absorbed by 24 hours.[780] Increases in the blood lead concentration are observed as early as 3 hours after dosing. Most of the lead absorbed from the digestive tract (90%) is bound irreversibly to erythrocyte proteins, resulting in a low lead concentration in the plasma but higher concentrations in whole blood specimens.[796] At the end of the erythrocytes' life span, the cell-bound lead is metabolized from the erythrocyte proteins and deposited in the bone as the triphosphate salt. A smaller amount of dissolved lead is deposited into the soft tissues as the diphosphate. A portion of the soft tissue lead is excreted through the gastrointestinal tract via the secretions (pancreatic juices, bile) and direct diffusion. The approximate half-life of blood lead in adult cattle is 9 days; however, increased blood lead concentrations may persist for as long as 38 weeks after a single exposure to lead.[797]

Lead also crosses the placental barrier and accumulates in fetal bone, liver, and kidneys but does not substantially accumulate in milk. The concentration of lead in milk from lactating cattle fed a daily dose of 13 mg of lead acetate remains less than 5.9 ppb.[798] In one study a logarithmic relationship between blood and milk lead concentrations was found. At blood concentrations below 3.6 μg/dl, milk lead concentrations were 0.8 μg/ml. However, cattle with higher blood lead levels (4.8 μg/dl) had exponentially greater concentrations in milk (2.2 μg/kg).[797] Lead cannot be detected in milk by 7 months after exposure.[799]

The toxic effects of lead include inhibition of free sulfhydryl groups of enzymes, interference with zinc-containing metalloproteins, and steric inhibition of enzyme activity.[792] Enzymes of heme synthesis are particularly susceptible to injury. These include δ-ALA dehydratase and ferrochelatase. Interference with ferrochelatase inhibits the formation of heme from protoporphyrin, resulting in a buildup of unmetabolized porphyrins, including protoporphyrin I, uroporphyrins, and coproporphyrins. The last two molecules are excreted in the urine and feces, respectively.[779] Protoporphyrin I is retained in the erythrocyte.

Interference with the activity of ALA dehydrase may be partly responsible for the brain damage associated with lead poisoning. The enzyme δ-ALA dehydrase combines two molecules of δ-ALA into a single porphobilinogen molecule. This enzyme is exquisitely sensitive to lead. Inhibition of the enzyme leads to accumulation of ALA, which is excreted into the urine. Concentrations of the synthetic product, porphobilinogen, in the erythrocytes are reduced.[787,788,790,800]

Because of the interference with heme metabolism and the altered function of other erythrocyte proteins, the erythrocyte half-life is shortened, which may result in a normochromic, normocytic anemia in a small proportion of chronically poisoned animals.[800] Iron is not adequately used and is stored in sideroblasts in the bone marrow.[787] Lead also interferes with the activity of pyrimidine-specific 5'-nucleotidase.[801] Loss of activity of this enzyme results in basophilic stippling.

After absorption lead rapidly enters the brain at a dose-dependent rate. The lead deposition in the CNS results in acute cerebellar hemorrhage and edema from capillary dysfunction.[796] Abnormalities of brain cerebroside content and catecholamine metabolism have also been described in animals with lead poisoning; however, the role of these changes in the pathogenesis of the clinical signs is unknown. The pathogenesis of lead encephalopathy is multifactorial. Encephalitic signs probably originate from a combination of decreased microvasculature, cellular necrosis, brain swelling, neurotransmitter dysfunction, and decreased glucose uptake by the brain.[802]

The molecular effects of lead on the myocardium are unknown. Hypertension that arises from chronic poisoning is thought to result from an inhibition of sodium-potassium adenosine triphosphatase or an alteration of the juxta-glomerular apparatus.[803]

Ingestion of lead also results in aberrations of other minerals. For example, long-term exposure to lead diminishes the absorption of selenium by as much as 26%.[795] If selenium intake is marginal, lead toxicosis could manifest as an outbreak of white muscle disease.

EPIDEMIOLOGY. Common sources of lead include lead arsenate defoliants, batteries, used motor oil, linoleum, roofing felt, paint, machinery grease, caulking compounds, and foliage near lead smelters.[779,782,789,804,805] High concentrations of lead in grasses near busy roadways have been reported, but the danger these pose to livestock is unclear.[806] The single lethal dose of lead for cattle is estimated to range from 220 to 600 mg/kg for calves and 600 to 800 mg/kg for adults.[794] Poisonings from cumulative intake are associated with substantially lower daily doses. Lead poisoning has been induced in cattle by feeding 5 to 6 mg of lead per kilogram of body weight per day for 3 years or 6 mg/kg of lead (lead acetate) for 7 days.[789,807] Lead poisoning has been reported in cattle exposed naturally to 6 to 7 mg/kg/day of lead on foliage and in calves given oral lead acetate at dosages ranging from 2.7 to 20 mg/kg/day.[807] The interval for development of clinical signs ranges from 5 to 20 days and is related to the dose and the ionic form of lead administered.[807] Ensiling of contaminated forage results in percolation and concentration of lead at the bottom of the silo.[808]

The toxicity of lead is apparently influenced by dietary factors. Calves on a milk diet are more susceptible to lead poisoning than are calves fed hay and grain.[784] There appears to be a direct correlation between high levels of vitamin D and enhanced lead absorption, which may explain the greater occurrence of the poisoning during the summer.

The estimated cumulative toxic dose of lead for horses is 2.9 mg/kg/day.[809] Poisonings have been reported in horses grazing pastures contaminated with 320 to 440 ppm of lead from a metal smelter; this amounted to a daily intake of 2 g (approximately 6.4 mg/kg of body weight). Metallic lead and the "galena" (insoluble sulfide salt) are less toxic than the acetate and carbonate lead salts.[810]

NECROPSY FINDINGS. The macroscopic brain lesions of lead poisoning are mild; they include brain edema, congestion of vessels of the cerebral cortex, and yellowish discoloration and flattening of the cortical gyri. Lesions tend to be most severe in the occipital lobes. Microscopic changes in the brain include capillary prominence, endothelial cell swelling, edema of the Purkinje cell layer of the cerebral cortex, laminar cortical neuronal necrosis, and edema of the white matter.[811] The lesions are predominantly located on the tips of the gyri. Whether these lesions are caused by a direct effect of lead on the neurons or from vascular damage is unclear.[796] Intranuclear acid-fast inclusion bodies in the renal tubular epithelial cells have been described in experimentally poisoned cattle. Chronic lead exposure also may interfere with normal functioning of the immune system, resulting in an increased susceptibility to infections.[812]

TREATMENT. Therapy for lead poisoning should include removal of the lead from the digestive tract, chelation therapy with calcium disodium EDTA, and fluid and nutritional support of the patient. Treatment with calcium disodium EDTA has been shown to be superior to treatment with penicillamine or dimercaprol (BAL). The EDTA chelates osseous but not soft tissue–bound lead.[793] After chelation the unsaturated bone stores reequilibrate with the lead remaining in the soft tissues. In cases of acute lead poisoning, several days are required before reequilibration results in a decreased blood lead concentration. Calcium disodium EDTA may be administered by a slow intravenous drip at a dosage of 73 mg/kg of body

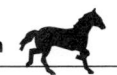

weight[813] daily for 3 to 5 days. After five daily treatments, a 2-day nontreatment period is recommended to reequilibrate the soft tissue and bone lead. After the 2 days' rest, daily treatments are given for another 5 days. The decision to continue therapy with EDTA should be based on the results of post-treatment blood lead analyses and renal function tests.

Another author has recommended administration of two intravenous injections of calcium disodium EDTA (110 mg/kg per dose) given 12 hours apart for 2 days.[814] Therapy then is withheld for 2 days, after which the EDTA treatments are re-instituted for 2 more days. The comparative efficacy of this regimen is unknown.

The EDTA also chelates other divalent cations. Consequently, prolonged administration of the drug results in trace mineral deficiencies, especially of zinc. For this reason, after prolonged EDTA therapy oral supplementation with zinc should be considered to prevent the development of parakeratosis.

Reports have indicated that thiamine therapy is an effective adjunctive treatment with EDTA in cases of acute lead poisoning of cattle.[794,815,816] Administration of 2 mg/kg of thiamine daily was more effective than treatment with disodium EDTA (62 mg/kg given twice daily for 4 days) or thiamine plus disodium EDTA in inducing remission of clinical signs of experimentally induced lead poisoning.[817] For clinical treatment of lead poisoning, thiamine dosages of 500 mg for small ruminants and 1 g for cattle weighing 300 kg or 5 mg/kg have been recommended.[815] Administration of daily doses of thiamine (100 mg/calf/day or 5 mg/kg of body weight) has protected experimentally exposed calves from clinical signs of lead poisoning and reduced lead deposition in the soft tissues.[816,818,819] The nature of the protective effects of thiamine is unclear. Apparently either lead interferes with thiamine synthesis or the tissue distribution and deposition of lead are reduced by the formation of rapidly excreted lead-thiamine complexes.

In ruminants, ingested lead is best removed from the digestive tract by means of a rumenotomy.[794] Magnesium sulfate laxatives are administered concomitantly to form insoluble lead sulfides. Because of the possibility of additional lead absorption from the gastrointestinal tract, oral administration of chelators is contraindicated.

Patients that respond slowly to chelation and thiamine therapy should be given supportive care. These measures should include provision of 40 to 80 ml of free water per kilogram per day for maintenance, oral hyperalimentation, and administration of diazepam or phenobarbital for convulsions (see Table 33-8).

PREVENTION AND CONTROL. Toxic pastures can be made safe by removing contaminated forage. This is best done by cutting, baling, and burying native grasses, burning the stubble, and applying agricultural lime at the rate of 1 ton per acre where the lead concentration of topsoil exceeds 175 ppm.[787] In the case of negligent poisonings, vigorous attempts at laboratory confirmation of the clinical diagnosis should be made. The source of the lead should be established, and the affected animals should be carefully documented. In the United States insurance liability responsibilities may be covered under homeowners or farm insurance.

REFERENCES

778. Priester WA, Hayes HM: Lead poisoning in cattle, horses, cats, and dogs as reported by 11 colleges of veterinary medicine in the United States and Canada from July 1968 through June 1972, *Am J Vet Res* 35:567-572, 1974.
779. Christian RG, Tryphonas L: Lead poisoning in cattle: brain lesions and hematologic changes, *Am J Vet Res* 32:203-216, 1971.
780. Buck WB: Toxins and neurologic disease in cattle, *J Am Vet Med Assoc* 166:222-226, 1975.
781. Osweiler GD, Ruhr LP: Lead poisoning in feeder calves, *J Am Vet Med Assoc* 172:498-500, 1978.
782. Knight HD, Burau RG: Chronic lead poisoning in horses, *J Am Vet Med Assoc* 162:782-786, 1973.
783. Dey S, Swarup D, Singh GR: Effect of experimental lead toxicity on cardiovascular function in calves, *Vet Hum Toxicol* 35:501-503, 1993.
784. McSherry BJ, Willoughby RA, Thompson RG: Urinary delta aminolevulinic acid (ALA) in the cow, dog, and cat, *Can J Comp Med* 35:136-140, 1971.
785. George JW, Duncan JR: Erythrocyte protoporphyrin in experimental chronic lead poisoning in calves, *Am J Vet Res* 42:1630-1637, 1981.
786. Ruth GR, Schwartz S, Stephenson B: Bovine protophorphyria: the first nonhuman model of this hereditary photosensitizing disease, *Science* 198:199-201, 1977.
787. Green RA, Monlux AW, Randolph TC: Blood porphyrin determination: a rapid field test for lead poisoning in cattle, *Bovine Pract* 5:30-35, 1973.
788. Kelliher DJ, Hilliard EP, Poole DBR: Chronic lead intoxication in cattle: preliminary observations on its effects on the erythrocyte and on porphyrin metabolism, *Irish J Agric Res* 12:61-69, 1973.
789. Zmudzki J et al: The influence of milk diet, grain diet, and method of dosing on lead toxicity in young calves, *Toxicol Appl Pharmacol* 76:490-497, 1984.
790. Bolton CE, Horton BJ, Pass DA: Evaluation of tests for the diagnosis of lead exposure in sheep, *Aust Vet J* 54:392-397, 1978.
791. Schmitt N, Brown G, Devlin EL: Lead poisoning in horses: an environmental health hazard, *Arch Environ Health* 23:185-195, 1971.
792. George JW, Duncan JR: The hematology of lead poisoning in man and animals, *Vet Clin Pathol* 8:23-30, 1979.
793. Burrows GE, Borchard RE: Experimental lead toxicosis in ponies: comparison of the effects of smelter effluent–contaminated hay and lead acetate, *Am J Vet Res* 43:2129-2133, 1982.
794. Gudmundson J: Lead poisoning in cattle, *Agric Pract* 14:43-47, 1993.
795. Neathery MW et al: Influence of high dietary lead on selenium metabolism in dairy calves, *J Dairy Sci* 70:645-652, 1987.
796. Goldstein GW, Asbury AK, Diamond I: Pathogenesis of lead encephalopathy uptake of lead and reaction of brain capillaries, *Arch Neurol* 31:382-389, 1974.
797. Oskarsson A et al: Lead poisoning in cattle: transfer of lead to milk, *Sci Total Environ* 111:83-94, 1992.
798. Lynch GP, Cornell DG, Smith DF: Excretion of cadmium and lead into milk. In Hoekstra WG, ed: *Trace element metabolism in animals*, Baltimore, 1974, University Park Press.
799. Galey F et al: Lead concentrations in blood and milk from periparturient dairy heifers seven months after an episode of acute lead toxicosis, *J Vet Diagn Invest* 2:222-226, 1990.
800. Hilliard EP, Poole DBR, Collins JD: Accidental lead intoxication of cattle: further evidence of an interference in heme biosynthesis, *Br Vet J* 129:82-85, 1973.
801. George JW, Duncan JR: Pyrimidine-specific 5' nucleotidase activity in bovine erythrocytes: effect of phlebotomy and lead poisoning, *Am J Vet Res* 43:17-20, 1982.
802. Ahrens FA: Effects of lead on glucose metabolism, ion flux, and collagen synthesis in cerebral capillaries of calves, *Am J Vet Res* 54:808-812, 1993.
803. Dey S, Swarup D, Singh GR: Effect of experimental lead toxicity on cardiovascular function in calves, *Vet Hum Toxicol* 35:501-503, 1993.
804. Every RR, Nicholson SS: Bovine lead poisoning from forage contaminated by sandblasted paint, *J Am Vet Med Assoc* 178:1277-1278, 1981.
805. Leary SL et al: Epidemiology of lead poisoning in cattle, *Iowa State U Vet* 3:112-117, 1970.
806. Aronson AL: Lead poisoning in cattle and horses following long-term exposure to lead, *J Am Vet Med Assoc* 33:627-629, 1972.
807. Zmudski J et al: Lead poisoning in cattle: reassessment of the minimum toxic oral dose, *Bull Environ Contam Toxicol* 30:435-441, 1983.
808. Coppock RW, Wagner WC, Reynolds RD: Migration of lead in a glass-lined bottom-unloading silo, *Vet Hum Toxicol* 30:458-459, 1988.
809. Hammond PR, Aronson AL: Lead poisoning in cattle and horses in the vicinity of a lead smelter, *Ann NY Acad Sci* 3:595-611, 1964.
810. Allcroft R: Lead poisoning in cattle and sheep, *Vet Rec* 63:583-590, 1951.
811. Semiya Y, Itoh H, Oshima K: Brain lesions of lead poisoning in a calf, *J Vet Med Sci* 53:117-119, 1991.
812. Hemphill FE, Kaeberle ML, Buck WB: Lead suppression of mouse resistance to *Salmonella typhimurium*, *Science* 172:1031-1032, 1971.
813. Holm LW, Wheat JD, Rhode EA: The treatment of chronic lead poisoning in horses with calcium disodium ethylenediaminetetraacetate, *J Am Vet Med Assoc* 123:383-388, 1953.
814. Hammond PB, Sorensen DK: Recent observations on the course and treatment of bovine lead poisoning, *J Am Vet Med Assoc* 130:23-25, 1957.
815. Bratton GR, Zmudzki J, Kincaid N: Thiamine as treatment of lead poisoning in ruminants, *Mod Vet Pract* 62:441-446, 1981.
816. Bratton GR et al: Thiamine (vitamin B₁) effects on lead intoxication and deposition of lead in tissues: therapeutic potential, *Toxicol Appl Pharmacol* 59:164-172, 1981.
817. Coppock RW et al: Evaluation of EDETATE and thiamine for treatment of experimentally induced environmental lead poisoning in cattle, *Am J Vet Res* 52:1160-1165, 1991.
818. Swarup D, Upadhyay AK: Chemoprophylactic efficacy of thiamine hydrochloride in experimental lead toxicosis in calves, *Indian J Anim Sci* 61:1170-1173, 1991.

819. Maiti SK, Swarup D, Chandra SV: Therapeutic potential of thiamine hydrochloride in experimental chronic lead intoxication in goats, *Res Vet Sci* 48:377-378, 1990.

GASOLINE AND PETROLEUM DISTILLATE TOXICOSIS

Ingestion of natural gas condensate or petroleum distillates can cause neurologic disease in livestock. Affected animals appear to be anesthetized and fail to respond to auditory or visual stimuli. The clinical signs of petroleum distillate poisoning include depression, ataxia, diarrhea, recumbency, coma, semicoma, absent menace response, decreased palpebral reflex, and muscular hypotonia. The feces and rumen contents have a strong odor of petroleum or gasoline. Some animals may die suddenly without premonitory signs.

Necropsy findings in poisoned animals include diffuse serosal hyperemia of the bowel and forestomachs and diffuse serosal ecchymotic hemorrhages. The lungs are firm and mottled, especially in the middle and cranial lobes. These pulmonary changes may be associated with moderate amounts of serofibrinous pleural exudates. Microscopic changes in poisoned animals include myocardial degeneration and necrosis, enteritis, mild renal tubular degeneration, and granular eosinophilic casts. Affected livers develop periacinar fatty degeneration and periportal infiltrations of lymphocytes and plasma cells.

Gas chromatography of the intestinal contents usually reveals peaks of aromatic hydrocarbons. For identification of the source of hydrocarbons, gas chromatographic profiles of the environmental specimens can be compared to those of the rumen liquor.

In early cases of petroleum distillate poisoning, removal of the hydrocarbons by means of a rumenotomy should be considered. Treatment usually is futile when the animal becomes recumbent and unresponsive.[820]

REFERENCE

820. Adler R et al: Toxicosis in sheep following ingestion of natural gas condensate, *Vet Pathol* 29:11-20, 1992.

ETHYLENE GLYCOL TOXICOSIS (Antifreeze Poisoning)

Antifreeze poisoning occurs primarily in ruminants.[821,822] When ingested, ethylene glycol is enzymatically converted to a number of acidic intermediate compounds, especially glycolic acid, which is further metabolized to oxalic acid. This acid combines with calcium in the kidneys to precipitate as calcium oxalate. Ruminants are thought to be more resistant to the toxic effects of ethylene glycol than monogastric animals because of their ability to metabolize large quantities of oxalate in the rumen. The acute toxic dose of ethylene glycol for adult ruminants ranges from 5 to 10 ml/kg, whereas the dose for preruminant calves amounts to 2 ml/kg.

Animals that have ingested sufficient amounts of ethylene glycol become ill by 3 to 4 days after ingestion. Clinical signs of ethylene glycol toxicity include blindness, progressive hind limb ataxia, salivation, depressed sensorium, nystagmus, tonic-clonic seizures, and status epilepticus. Pupillary reflexes usually are intact. Hemolytic anemia and hemoglobinuria occasionally may be seen.[821] The clinicopathologic changes of ethylene glycol toxicosis include azotemia (448 mg/dl), increased serum creatinine, hypophosphatemia, hypocalcemia, acidosis, hyperosmolality, and increased γ-glutamyl transaminase.

The pathologic lesions include slight swelling of the kidneys and pulmonary edema. Oxalate crystals can be demonstrated by microscopic examination of the kidney tissues using polarized light. Ethylene glycol can be detected in the rumen for at least 4 days after ingestion. Mass spectrometry of body fluids may show increased urinary and ocular fluid concentrations of glycolic acid (4.3 μg/ml and 2.3 μg/ml, respectively).

Treatment with 20% ethanol at a rate of 50 ml/hr has been recommended but is unsuccessful in advanced stages of the disease. Some authors have suggested that ruminants also be given an oral dose of activated charcoal, but the effect of this treatment on long-term survival is unknown.[822]

REFERENCES

821. Crowell WA, Whitlock RH, Stout RC: Ethylene glycol poisoning in cattle, *Cornell Vet* 69:272-279, 1979.
822. Boermans HJ, Ruegg PL, Leach M: Ethylene glycol toxicosis in a pygmy goat, *J Am Vet Med Assoc* 193:694-695, 1988.

NARDOO FERN POISONING

LISLE W. GEORGE

Sheep that graze extensively on the Nardoo fern (*Marsilea drummondii*) develop a condition that is indistinguishable from polioencephalomalacia. Death losses of 2200 of 57,000 sheep have been reported.[823] The clinical signs are indistinguishable from those of polioencephalomalacia. Neuronal necrosis, malacia, perivascular cuffing, vacuolation of the neuropil, vascular dilation and endothelial hypertrophy, and gliosis occur in the central nervous system. The condition responds to a single subcutaneous injection of thiamine (200 mg). The fern is thought to contain a form of thiaminase I.

REFERENCE

823. Pritchard D, Eggleston GW: Nardoo fern and polioencephalomalacia, *Aust Vet J* 54:204, 1978.

HELICHRYSUM ARGYROSPHAERUM POISONING

LISLE W. GEORGE
MARY O. SMITH

Both naturally occurring and experimental poisoning of sheep and cattle in South Africa by plants of the genus *Helichrysum* results in blindness and a variety of central neurologic signs.[824,825] The clinical signs of intoxication include progressive tetraparesis, depression, nystagmus, mydriasis, blindness, intentional head tremor, and star-gazing attitude. Older sheep may develop lens cataracts 2 to 3 months after eating the plants. The case attack rate ranges from 1% to 29%. *Helichrysum* plants are toxic only in the flowering stage.

Pathologic findings include widespread status spongiosis of brain white matter, particularly in subependymal areas and in the cerebellar peduncles and brainstem.[825] Myelin edema is present in some cases. Edematous swelling of the optic nerve causes compression of the nerve in the optic canal, with secondary damage to nerve axons and myelin. The toxic principle in *Helichrysum* plants also causes a primary retinopathy in some animals.

REFERENCES

824. Basson PA et al: Blindness and encephalopathy caused by *Helichrysum argyrosphaerum* DC (compositae) in sheep and cattle, *Onderstepoort J Vet Res* 42:135-148, 1975.
825. Van der Lugt JJ et al: Status spongiosis, optic neuropathy, and retinal degeneration in *Helichrysum argyrosphaerum* poisoning in sheep and a goat, *Vet Pathol* 33:495-502, 1996.

FLATPEA (LATHYRUS SYLVESTRIS, LATHYRUS COLLIS) POISONING

LISLE W. GEORGE

MARY O. SMITH

Ingestion of flatpea (*Lathyrus sylvestris, Lathyrus collis*) results in a central nervous system (CNS) disorder. The condition may be seen by 5 days after consumption of a diet composed of 50% flatpea vines. Toxicosis has been induced in sheep ingesting forage of 35% flatpea vines.[826] Livestock can develop a tolerance for the plant through rumen microbial detoxification. Nevertheless, acclimatized animals can be rendered susceptible by treatment with monensin or by a change in rumen microflora.[827]

The toxic constituent of the plant, 2,4,diaminobutyric acid, is known to inhibit ornithine transcarbamylase, an enzyme responsible for urea detoxification. Consequently the blood ammonia concentration in clinically affected animals ranges from 189 to 263 mmol/ml (the normal range is 108 to 185 mmol/ml). Diaminobutyric acid also interferes with the uptake of γ-aminobutyric acid (GABA) and inhibits GABA transaminase activity.

The clinical signs of flatpea intoxication are depression, muscular tremors, and spasmodic torticollis. Affected animals become recumbent and are reluctant to rise. When stimulated to move, they display circling, head-pressing, and odontoprisis. The urine may appear dark brown. The clinical disorder often culminates fatally in a seizure. During the interictal periods, the animals may rest, rise, and resume normal behavior and gait. Treatment is empiric and supportive and could include administration of 1 to 2 L of vinegar given orally, intravenous diazepam, and removal from the offending forage.

L. sylvestris is a leguminous plant with a high protein content that might be an adequate substitute for alfalfa in areas where the latter grows poorly. When fed as part of a mixed silage in which the concentration of diaminobutyric acid was approximately 1%, *L. sylvestris* produced an acceptable weight gain in cattle without signs of toxicity.[828]

REFERENCES

826. Rowe LD, Ivie GW, DeLoach JR: The toxic effects of mature flatpea (*Lathyrus sylvestris* CV Lathco) on sheep, *Vet Hum Toxicol* 35:127-133, 1993.
827. Rasmussen M, Allison MJ: Flatpea intoxication in sheep and indications of ruminal adaptation, *Vet Hum Toxicol* 35:123-127, 1993.
828. Foster JG et al: Performance of feeder cattle offered a diet containing early bloom–stage flatpea silage, *J Prod Agric* 9:415-418, 1996.

LEUKOENCEPHALOMALACIA (Moldy Corn Disease; Equine Encephalomalacia; Pesta de Cegare; Pen Yan Disease; Moldy Cornstalk Disease; Blind Staggers)

DEFINITION AND ETIOLOGY. Leukoencephalomalacia is an intoxication of horses caused by ingestion of corn contaminated with the fungus *Fusarium moniliforme*.[829-832] Fumonisin toxins (B1, B2, and B3) produced by *F. moniliforme* interfere with sphingolipid metabolism, disrupting endothelial cell walls and basement membranes.[833] Outbreaks of multifocal neurologic signs and hepatic disease occur in groups of horses exposed to tainted feedstuffs.

CLINICAL SIGNS. The clinical signs of leukoencephalomalacia occur suddenly. Occasionally animals die acutely, without other overt signs,[834] but most affected horses show a variety of neurologic signs before death. These include somnolence, flaccidity of the facial and pharyngeal muscles, muscle fasciculations over the neck and withers, ataxia, conscious proprioceptive deficits, head-pressing, mania, facial desensi-

tization, pharyngeal paralysis, blindness, seizures, and a tendency to circle or lean to one side.[834,835] Most animals die while convulsing.[829] The few horses that recover usually have permanent neurologic dysfunction. Hepatic involvement occurs in many cases, as evidenced by elevated serum liver enzymes, although hepatic failure is uncommon. Signs of liver disease include icterus, petechiation on mucous membranes, and swelling of the muzzle or lips. Gastrointestinal disease caused by fumonisin toxins has been reported and may manifest as signs of colic.

Unique constellations of clinical signs may predominate within any one outbreak of the disease. Fumonisin toxins cause a variety of clinical syndromes in other species, but horses appear to be particularly susceptible and can show signs when exposed to toxin concentrations as low as 5 to 10 ppm, almost 10 times less than the concentration needed to cause mild signs of inappetence and decreased weight gain in cattle.

CLINICAL PATHOLOGY AND DIAGNOSIS. Fumonisin toxicosis has no unique clinicopathologic findings, therefore antemortem diagnosis relies on recognition of the clinical signs with a history of exposure to moldy corn. Specific changes in the cerebrospinal fluid of affected horses have not been reported. Serum liver enzymes (aspartate aminotransferase [AST], γ-glutamyl transferase [GGT], and sorbitol dehydrogenase [SDH]) and bilirubin may be elevated. Nonspecific changes in serum chemistry associated with dehydration (increased hematocrit, prerenal azotemia) and recumbency (elevated serum creatine kinase) also may be present. Anemia, leukocytosis, and leukopenia all have been reported, but none is a consistent finding.

Differential diagnoses include craniocerebral trauma, the arboviral encephalitides, hepatic encephalopathy, equine protozoal myeloencephalitis, Theiler's disease, and botulism.

EPIDEMIOLOGY. Leukoencephalomalacia occurs worldwide.[831,836] Corn becomes contaminated during growth rather than in storage, and climatic factors that stress the plants, such as drought, excess moisture, or heat, contribute to the likelihood of mold development. Most cases of equine disease occur during the winter and early spring.[830,834] In experimental studies the toxic dose of infected corn ranged from 5 to 15 kg (10 to 30 lb), but the amount of corn required to cause the disease is likely to vary considerably depending on the amount of toxin in the grain.[832] A direct link between the onset and severity of clinical signs and the dose of toxin has not been established in naturally occurring cases, but experimental data suggest a dose-related effect.[837] Repeated exposure to the toxin, rather than a single large dose, seems to be associated with the development of clinical signs.[838] Experimental studies with infected corn demonstrated an onset of clinical signs on the ninth day after the beginning of the feeding period. Older animals develop clinical signs of leukoencephalomalacia more rapidly than younger animals and thus appear to be most susceptible to the effects of the mycotoxin.[832]

The rates of disease in exposed horses vary widely, from 14% to 100% in some reports.[839-842] Ruminants apparently are more resistant than horses to the effects of the neurotoxin, but this is not a complete resistance because camels and water buffalo have died after ingesting toxic corn. Diplodiosis, a similar neuromycotoxicosis of cattle caused by ingestion of *Diplodia maydis*, occurs in Africa; however, the toxicologic relationship between these conditions is unknown.

PATHOLOGY. The major pathologic features in the central nervous system (CNS) are a consequence of the vascular damage caused by fumonisin toxins. They include liquefactive necrosis and degeneration or malacia of the white matter of one or both cerebral hemispheres.[843,844] The size of the le-

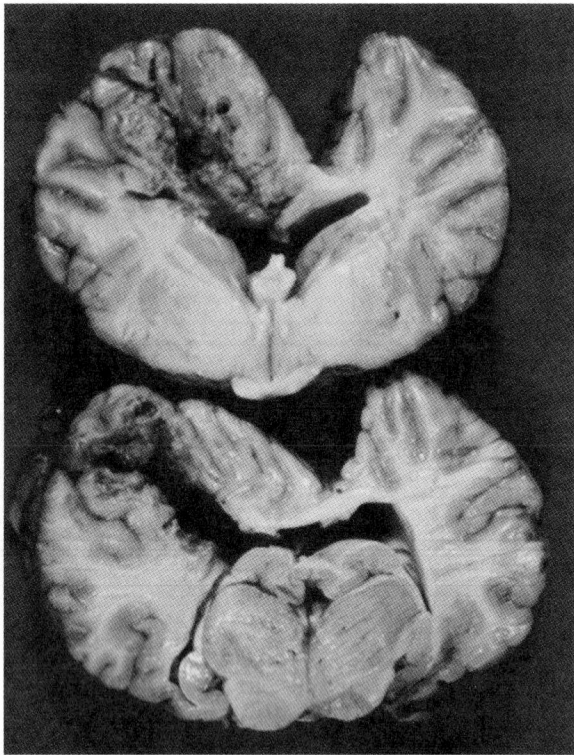

FIG. 33-14 ◼ Characteristic appearance of a malacic lesion in the brain of a horse that died of moldy corn poisoning. (Courtesy Dr. R.H. Whitlock.)

sions may vary from 0.5 cm in diameter to complete necrosis of the entire cerebral cortex.[829] Flattening of the cortical gyri, enlargement of the cerebral cortex, vascular congestion, cortical softening, yellowish discoloration of the white matter, hemorrhage, and cavitation of the cerebral cortex may be present (Fig. 33-14).[829,834,836] A gelatinous fluid can be seen in many of the cavitary lesions.[834] Hemorrhage in the CNS also has been reported.[839] Lesions in the visceral organs, including hepatic congestion, centrilobular hepatic necrosis, hemorrhagic enteritis, and cystitis are found in some horses. The relationship between these lesions in the CNS and those in the liver, urinary bladder, and gastrointestinal tract is unknown.

TREATMENT. There is no known specific treatment for leukoencephalomalacia, but there has been a report of successful treatment of horses using antiinflammatory medications such as dimethyl sulfoxide (DMSO) (1 g/kg given as a 10% solution by slow intravenous infusion once daily for 3 days) or flunixin meglumine (0.25 to 1 mg/kg), as well as antibiotics and supportive care (thiamine 5 g IV every 12 hours).[845] In other cases survivors usually have permanent neurologic dysfunction.

REFERENCES
829. Graham R: Cornstalk disease investigation, *Vet Med* 31:46-50, 1936.
830. Wilson TM, Nelson PE, Ryan TB: Linking leukoencephalomalacia to commercial horse rations, *Vet Med (Equine Pract)* 80:63-69, 1985.
831. Cole RJ: Toxin from *Fusarium moniliforme:* effects on plants and animals, *Science* 179:1324-1326, 1973.
832. Wilson BJ, Maronpot RR: Causative fungus agent of leucoencephalomalacia in equine animals, *Vet Rec* 88:484-486, 1971.
833. Ramasamy S et al: Fumonisin alters sphinglolipid metabolism and disrupts the barrier function of endothelial cells in culture, *Toxicol Appl Pharmacol* 133:343-348, 1985.
834. Schwarte LH, Biester HE, Murray C: A disease of horses caused by feeding moldy corn, *J Am Vet Med Assoc* 90:76-85, 1937.
835. MacCallum WG, Buckley SS: Acute epizootic leucoencephalitis in horses, *J Exp Med* 6:65-74, 1901.
836. Biester HE, Schwarte LH, Reddy CH: Further studies on moldy corn poisoning (leukoencephalomalacia) in horses, *Vet Med* 35:636-639, 1940.
837. Ross PF et al: Experimental equine leukoencephalomalacia, toxic hepatosis and encephalopathy caused by corn naturally contaminated with fumonisins, *J Vet Diagn Invest* 5:69-74, 1993.
838. Brownlie CF, Cullen J: Characterization of experimentally induced equine leukoencephalomalacia (LEM) in ponies *(Equus caballus):* preliminary report, *Vet Hum Toxicol* 29:34-38, 1987.
839. Buck WB et al: Equine leukoencephalomalacia: comparative pathology of naturally occurring and experimental cases, *Proc Am Assoc Vet Lab Diagn* 22:239-258, 1979.
840. Knight AP: Mycotoxicoses of food animals, *Compend Cont Educ Pract Vet* 3:S112-S118, 1981.
841. McCue P: Equine leukoencephalomalacia, *Compend Cont Educ Pract Vet* 11:646-651, 1989.
842. Uhlinger C: Clinical and epidemiological features of an epizootic of equine leukoencephalomalacia, *J Am Vet Med Assoc* 198:126-128, 1991.
843. Graham R: Results of inoculating laboratory animals with equine brain tissue suspensions and equine brain tissue filtrates from spontaneous cases of so-called cornstalk disease, *J Am Vet Med Assoc* 86:778-780, 1935.
844. Wilson TM, Maronpot RR: Causative fungus agent of leukoencephalomalacia in equine animals, *Vet Rec* 88:484-485, 1971.
845. Wilkins PA et al: A herd outbreak of equine leukoencephalomalacia, *Cornell Vet* 84:53-59, 1994.

BLUE-GREEN ALGAE TOXICOSIS

DEFINITION AND ETIOLOGY. Ingestion of stagnant pond water containing certain species of blue-green algae may result in a peracute intoxication of livestock. Blue-green algae poisoning is characterized by convulsions, ataxia, bloody diarrhea, and sudden death.[846-848] The algal toxins have been responsible for high losses of livestock and illness in human beings and for deaths of domestic dogs.[849] The algal toxins may also be responsible for occasional die-offs of fish and aquatic birds. Toxic algal species include *Microcystis aeruginosa, Anabaena flos-aquae, Aphanizomenon flos-aquae, Anacystis cyanea, Gloeotrichia echinulata, Nodularia sphaerocarpa,* and *Oscillatoria agardhii.* Of these, the first three are most toxic.[850] Blue-green algae poisoning most commonly results in sudden death. Affected animals rarely move far from the source of the toxin. Some of the algae produce hepatotoxins, and animals develop liver failure, diarrhea, and photosensitivity. The development of toxic stands of blue-green algae requires specific environmental conditions, including a water pH above 6, organic pollution, and a water temperature ranging from 15° to 30° C (59° to 86° F).

CLINICAL SIGNS. Clinical syndromes of blue-green algae poisoning in livestock may be separated into acute and chronic forms. In the acute form affected animals may show signs resembling those of milk fever,[851] including muscle tremors; reluctance to rise or move; ataxia; cold extremities; weak, rapid pulse; mydriasis; muscle tremors; salivation; colic; rumen atony; mild bloat; pallor; increased capillary refill time; vomiting; ataxia; conscious proprioceptive deficits; and bloody diarrhea. Some of the toxins are absorbed through the oral mucosa. Consequently the full range of clinical signs, culminating in death from respiratory arrest, can occur within minutes of ingestion of the toxic water. If clinical signs are seen before death, affected animals tend to be afebrile but have significantly increased pulse and respiratory rates. Many animals die suddenly without premonitory symptoms.[852,853] The deaths often occur in the vicinity of the pond, and dead animals may be covered by the green scum.

In the chronic form of blue-green algae intoxication, affected animals show ataxia, depression, anorexia, hemorrhagic diarrhea, icterus, and photosensitization, which occur secondary to hepatic necrosis.[853] Death from respiratory arrest and circulatory shock may occur within 2 to 72 hours after the toxin is ingested.

CLINICAL PATHOLOGY. The diagnosis of blue-green algae poisoning depends on recognition of a relationship between livestock deaths and ingestion of pond water, identification of toxic algae in the pond water, recognition of hepatic disease in chronically affected animals, and elimination of the possibility of similar clinical conditions such as cyanide or acute poisoning. Diseases that kill animals suddenly should be considered as differential diagnoses (see Chapter 14). Blue-green algae poisoning should be considered whenever a group of cattle simultaneously develop marked massive hepatic necrosis.

The vegetative cells of the algae can be identified by microscopic examination of rumen contents. The intestinal contents should be split. Half the contents should be placed in 10% neutral buffered formalin for microscopic analysis, and the other half should be refrigerated (not frozen) for mouse bioassay tests or chromatographic identification of the toxin using high-pressure liquid chromatography. The blood of animals poisoned by microcystin, the toxic principle of *M. aeruginosa*, shows changes characteristic of hepatic necrosis, including increased concentrations of bilirubin, AST, GGT, alkaline phosphatase (ALP), and arginase. The animals may be secondarily hypocalcemic, which complicates the clinical picture.[851]

PATHOPHYSIOLOGY. Blue-green algae grow more slowly than other algae in cold water; consequently, highly flushed systems cannot achieve a toxic bloom. The blue-green algae can fix atmospheric nitrogen dissolved in the water, and they have intracellular gas vesicles that accumulate the nitrogen when photosynthesis decreases. If mixing occurs because of the wind, the amount of light reaching the algae decreases because of the turbulence. The buoyancy of the cells increases because of the decreased photosynthetic activity. At night the winds become calmer, and the algae lose their ability to regulate density. The cells float to the surface of the water and form a scum, which is concentrated on the leeward side. For these reasons, poisonings tend to occur in the period of stable weather just after a frontal system has passed.

All species of blue-green algae probably produce toxins, which can be classified into three groups:

- *Aphanizomenon, Oscillatoria,* and *Anabaena* spp.: *Aphanizomenon* produces two alkaloid toxins that have a structure resembling that of saxitoxin, the agent of paralytic shellfish poisoning. Toxins from *Anabaena* spp. are named anatoxin-a and anatoxin-a(s) and are structural analogs of cocaine. Toxins from *Oscillatoria* spp. resemble those of *Anabaena* spp.[852-856]; these toxins can be absorbed unchanged through the mucous membranes and kill by depolarizing blockade of the neuromuscular junction.[852-856]
- *Peptide hepatotoxins:* These substances are produced by strains of *Microcystis, Oscillatoria,* and *Anabaena* algae. Microcystin-LR is the most commonly isolated hepatotoxin.[857-861] On a weight basis, this toxin is 20 times more active than cyanide or strychnine. A single intraperitoneal injection of 1 to 2 μg in a mouse is lethal. At least nine structural variants of microcystin have been identified. The toxins can cross the placenta and cause lesions in the fetus.
- *Lipopolysaccharides:* These substances may be produced by most species of blue-green algae.

NECROPSY FINDINGS. The pathologic lesions of blue-green algae poisoning are either severe centrilobular hepatic necrosis in animals that die of the chronic poisoning or generalized petechiation and body cavity effusions in animals that die peracutely.[852]

EPIDEMIOLOGY. Blue-green algae intoxication occurs worldwide and affects mammals, birds, and fish. The bloom is most abundant during the late summer and early autumn when warm, sunny conditions favor algal growth. Growth is most abundant in ponds with an alkaline pH and in high concentrations of nitrogen, phosphates, carbonates, or organic matter. Release of the toxin is associated with death of the algae and production of a "rotting fish" odor. Most poisonings occur on the leeward side of the pond, where the algae are concentrated by the action of the prevailing wind. Ingestion of approximately 1080 to 1500 ml of heavily contaminated water can be fatal for cattle.[846] Toxicity varies daily and in different parts of the pond or lake.

TREATMENT. The treatment of blue-green algae poisoning is symptomatic and usually unsuccessful. Experimentally poisoned calves have not recovered, even after 30 hours of artificial respiration.[855]

PREVENTION. Methods for control of the disease include restriction of access to infested ponds and treatment of the pond with copper sulfate or algacides.[848] Prevention of blue-green algae poisoning depends on the proper construction of farm ponds and the prophylactic treatment of the water with bluestone (copper sulfate) to achieve a final concentration ranging from 0.5 to 1 ppm in acid water and 1.5 to 2 ppm in alkaline water. The bluestone is either dissolved in water and sprayed over the pond or dragged through the pond in a burlap sack in lanes that are 5 to 10 feet apart.[848] This amounts to 1.22 kg/acre foot in alkaline water. Cattle should be fenced from the pond for several days after the copper sulfate treatment. The treatment should be repeated whenever the toxic bloom recurs. To prevent algal bloom without application of copper sulfate, farm ponds should be constructed so that they are 80 × 20 feet in length and width and 10 feet in depth. Surrounding drainage areas should be fenced from the livestock. Water should be pumped from the pond to the cattle in polyethylene pipes and delivered into raised water troughs. The water for the troughs should be pumped from the center and bottom of the pond.

REFERENCES

846. Zin LL, Edwards WC: Toxicity of blue-green algae in livestock, *Bovine Pract* 14:151-153, 1979.
847. Kerr LA, McCoy CP, Eaves D: Blue-green algae toxicosis in five dairy cows, *J Am Vet Med Assoc* 191:829-830, 1987.
848. Flint EA: Toxic algae in some New Zealand freshwater ponds, *N Z Vet J* 14:181-185, 1966.
849. National Rivers Authority: Toxic blue-green algae: a report by the National Rivers Authority, England, 1990, Stanley Hunt.
850. Hammer UT: Toxic blue-green algae in Saskatchewan, *Can Vet J* 9:221-229, 1968.
851. Galey FD et al: Blue-green algae (*Microcystis aeruginosa*) hepatotoxicosis in dairy cows, *Am J Vet Res* 48:1415-1420, 1987.
852. Main DC et al: Sheep mortalities associated with the blue-green alga *Nodularia spumigena, Aust Vet J* 53:578-581, 1977.
853. Macdonald DW: Algal poisoning in beef cattle, *Can Vet J* 1:108-110, 1960.
854. Carmichael WW, Biggs DF, Gorham PR: Toxicology and pharmacological action of *Anabaena flos-aquae* toxin, *Science* 187:542-544, 1975.
855. Carmichael WW, Gorham PR, Biggs DF: Two laboratory case studies on the oral toxicity to calves of the freshwater cyanophyte (blue-green algae) *Anabaena flos-aquae* NRC-44-1, *Can Vet J* 18:71-75, 1977.
856. Alam M et al: Purification of *Aphanizomenon flos-aquae* toxin and its chemical and physiological properties, *Toxicon* 11:65-72, 1973.
857. Elleman TC et al: Isolation, characterization, and pathology of the toxin from a *Microcystis aeruginosa (Anacystis cyanea)* bloom, *Aust J Biol Sci* 31:209-218, 1978.
858. Gorham PR: Laboratory studies on the toxins produced by waterblooms of blue-green algae, *Am J Public Health* 52:2100-2105, 1962.
859. Konst BH et al: Symptoms and pathology produced by toxic *Microcystis aeruginosa* NRC-1 in laboratory and domestic animals, *Can J Comp Med Vet Sci* 29:221-228, 1965.
860. Hughes EO, Gorham PR, Zehnder A: Toxicity of a unialgal culture of *Microcystis aeruginosa, Can J Microbiol* 4:225-235, 1958.
861. Done SH, Bain M: Hepatic necrosis in sheep associated with ingestion of blue-green algae, *Vet Rec* 133:600, 1993.

NITROFURAZONE TOXICOSIS

Nitrofurazone is an antimicrobial that has been fed to cattle for the treatment and control of respiratory or gastrointestinal diseases. Treatment of food-producing animals with the nitrofurans currently is prohibited by the U.S. Food and Drug Administration (FDA). Nervous system signs of nitrofurazone toxicosis occur after 1 to 3 weeks of continuous feeding at dosages exceeding 15 to 30 mg/kg of body weight.[862,863] Lower dosages (7.1 mg/kg) reduce feed intake but do not result in neurologic signs. The nitrofurans inhibit enzymes of the oxidative glycolytic pathways and are thought to interfere with brain metabolism of carbohydrates.

Clinical signs of nitrofurazone toxicosis include hyperirritability, propulsive running, muscular tremors, blindness, convulsions, and death. At lower doses the convulsions may appear intermittently, but as the condition progresses, the signs become continuous.

REFERENCES

862. Buck WB: Toxic materials and neurologic disease in cattle, *J Am Vet Med Assoc* 166:222-226, 1975.
863. Lister EE, Fisher LJ: Establishment of the toxic level of nitrofurazone for young liquid-fed calves, *J Dairy Sci* 53:1490-1495, 1970.

INTRACAROTID DRUG INJECTION

DEFINITION AND ETIOLOGY. Intracarotid drug injection is common in horses because the jugular vein and the common carotid artery are closely apposed in the caudal third of the neck. The condition is rarely seen in cattle because the omohyoideus muscle lies between the carotid artery and the jugular vein in the posterior part of the neck. Hypertonic or caustic drugs, including phenothiazine tranquilizers, chloramphenicol, chloral hydrate, barbiturate anesthetics, phenylbutazone, calcium gluconate, sodium iodide, and chloramphenicol, cause cortical necrosis when injected into the carotid artery.[864,865]

CLINICAL SIGNS. The onset is peracute. When the drug is injected into the carotid artery, the animal recoils backward and falls over. Some horses strike or rear violently or run wildly without regard to obstructions. Other animals fall down and become comatose without showing severe motor activity. Severely affected animals may die after a variable period of time, but others regain their footing and recover completely. Residual neurologic deficits may occur in surviving animals. These deficits include contralateral blindness, facial hypalgesia, head tilt (toward the side of the lesion), and a largely contralateral conscious proprioceptive deficit. If the injection has damaged the ascending vagosympathetic pathways, the animal may display Horner's syndrome. Specific signs of this syndrome include ptosis, miosis, and enophthalmos. Horses with Horner's syndrome also sweat profusely over the head and neck of the ipsilateral side, whereas cattle with the syndrome fail to sweat on the planum nasale on the ipsilateral side of the lesion.

PATHOPHYSIOLOGY. The central nervous system (CNS) lesions are caused by vascular endothelial damage. Intracarotid drug injection results in intense vasospasm and profound alterations of the blood-brain barrier. The vascular damage causes endothelial cell swelling, increased vascular permeability, mural necrosis, hemorrhage, intercellular edema, and thrombosis.[864]

NECROPSY FINDINGS. Pathologic lesions include diffuse cerebral edema and brain swelling. Microscopic lesions include arteriolar hyalinization, hemorrhage, edema, necrobiosis, and status spongiosis. Vacuolation of the neuropil, perivascular hemorrhage, fibrin, and edema are also commonly seen.

TREATMENT. There is no effective treatment for an accidental intracarotid drug injection. Violent horses should be placed in a padded stall, sedated with diazepam, and treated with dexamethasone (1 to 2 mg/kg of body weight). Administration of mannitol or other osmotic diuretics should be avoided in the first 24 hours because of active bleeding in the CNS and loss of the blood-brain barrier. Administration of a hypertonic dehydrating agent at that time may result in distribution of the osmotically active drugs into the CNS parenchyma, resulting in a large increase in intracranial pressure. Although most animals eventually recover from the effects of an intracarotid injection, fatalities have been reported.[864-866]

PREVENTION. Intracarotid injection of drugs is best prevented by the use of large-bore needles or catheters for intravenous injections. This allows better visualization of pulsating oxygenated blood when the carotid artery has been accidentally punctured. In the horse, venipunctures should be performed in the anterior one third of the jugular furrow because the artery and vein are separated by the omohyoideus muscle in this area. Needles should be inserted into the vein while they are separated from the syringe.

REFERENCES

864. Gabel AA, Koestner A: The effects of intracarotid artery injection of drugs in domestic animals, *J Am Vet Med Assoc* 142:1397-1403, 1963.
865. Christian RG, Mills JHL, Kramer LL: Accidental intracarotid artery injection of promazine in the horse, *Can Vet J* 15:29-33, 1974.
866. Rosseaux CG, Wenkoff M: Fatal intracarotid artery injection of chloramphenicol in a cow, *J Am Vet Med Assoc* 184:1287-1288, 1984.

COENUROSIS (Sheep Gid; *Coenurus cerebralis* Infestation; *Taenia multiceps* Infestation)

Coenurosis is caused by invasion of the central nervous system (CNS) by *Coenurus cerebralis*, the intermediate stage of the tapeworm *Taenia multiceps*. The adult worms live in the canine intestine and shed eggs into the feces. Ruminants eat the eggs from contaminated pastures. The eggs hatch in the small intestine of the ruminant and travel via the blood to the CNS, where they mature into *C. cerebralis*. The life cycle is completed when the ruminant dies and the brain is eaten by a scavenging carnivore. *Coenurus* cysts then develop into sexually mature adults in the bowel of the canine host. Many animals, including sheep, goats, cattle, horses, wild ruminants, and human beings, are susceptible to *C. cerebralis* infestation.[867-869] Outbreaks of coenurosis may occur in previously uninfected sheep that are suddenly exposed to contaminated fecal matter from carnivores. Cases initially occur as early as 2 weeks after the sheep are exposed and continue for as long as 4 months.

The clinical presentation of coenurosis is that of a space-occupying cranial lesion; signs include depression, anorexia, ataxia, unilateral or asymmetric loss of vision, facial hemiplegia, head tilt, circling, high-stepping forelimb gait, and hyperesthesia. As the disease progresses, the sheep assume lateral recumbency and become comatose.[870,871] In advanced cases the calvarium directly over the parasite enlarges and softens.[869]

Lesions of the CNS may occur as a result of three separate pathogenic mechanisms. These include encephalitis from invasion of the CNS by large numbers of immature worms, hypertensive hydrocephalus resulting from interference with cerebrospinal fluid (CSF) drainage, and development of large cerebral cysts that increase intracranial pressure. Full development of the *Coenurus* cyst requires 6 to 7 months. Mature cysts may reach 5 cm in diameter and displace the bones of the calvarium.

The condition can be diagnosed on the basis of a characteristic clinical syndrome in an endemic area. Radiographs in the lateral and posteroanterior planes may detect radiolucent areas in the calvarium. The optimum diagnostic views in the posteroanterior projection occur whenever the base of the nose is level with the upper margin of the orbit.

TREATMENT. Praziquantel* (100 mg/kg of body weight given orally daily for 5 days) is effective for the treatment of

---

*Droncit, Miles Laboratories, Shawnee, KS 66201.

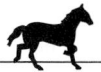

coenurosis in sheep.[872] Concomitant administration of a nonsteroidal antiinflammatory drug and dexamethasone may enhance the posttreatment survival rate.

The cyst can also be removed surgically. Success rates as high as 90% have been reported.[873] For surgery the patient is anesthetized, and the skull is trephined over the frontal bone. Approximately 70% of the cysts are located extradurally and can be removed easily with no further dissection. The other cysts are located on the surface of the pia arachnoid, in which case the dura mater is incised. The cyst usually bulges from under the incised dura and can be removed. When the cyst is located in the cerebral cortex, ultrasound probes placed on the surface of the brain may be used to locate the pocket of fluid.[874-876]

PREVENTION. In endemic areas the carcasses of affected animals should not be fed to dogs, and dogs in endemic areas should be treated repeatedly with a vermifuge to minimize the possibility of pasture contamination. Lyophilized antigens from in vitro–cultured larvae have protected sheep; however, this preparation is not commercially available.

REFERENCES

867. Greig A: Coenurosis in cattle, *Vet Rec* 100:266, 1977.
868. Soulsby EJL: *Textbook of veterinary clinical pathology,* vol 1, Oxford, England, 1965, Blackwell Scientific Publications.
869. De Villers: Treatment of gid in sheep, *S Afr Vet Med Assoc J* 21:155-157, 1950.
870. Doherty ML et al: Outbreak of acute coenuriasis in adult sheep in Ireland, *Vet Rec* 125:185, 1989.
871. Yoshino T, Momotani E: A case of bovine coenurosis *(Coenurus cerebralis)* in Japan, *Jpn J Vet Sci* 50:433-438, 1988.
872. Verster A, Tustin RC: Treatment of cerebral coenuriasis in sheep with praziquantel, *J S Afr Vet Assoc* 61:24-26, 1990.
873. Harwood DG: Metacestode disease in goats, *Goat Vet Soc J* 7:35-37, 1986.
874. Tirgari M, Howard BR, Boargob A: Clinical and radiographical diagnosis of coenurosis cerebralis in sheep and its surgical treatment, *Vet Rec* 120:173-178, 1987.
875. Doherty ML, McAllister H, Healy A: Ultrasound as an aid to *Coenurus cerebralis* cyst localization in a lamb, *Vet Rec* 124:591, 1989.
876. Skerritt GC, Stallbaumer MF: Diagnosis and treatment of coenuriasis (gid) in sheep, *Vet Rec* 115:399-403, 1984.

CEROID LIPOFUSCINOSIS (Batten's Disease)

DEFINITION AND ETIOLOGY. Ceroid lipofuscinosis is a lysosomal storage disease that occurs in South Hampshire and Rambouillet sheep, Nubian goats, and Devon cattle.[877-880] The disease is inherited through an autosomal recessive trait[881] and is characterized by the intracellular accumulation of abnormal autofluorescent lipopigments in lysosomes of neurons and other cells throughout the body. The storage material has been shown to consist predominantly of the subunit c of mitochondrial c synthase.[882,883] The mechanism of neuronal dysfunction is hypothesized to be mediated by N-methyl-D-aspartate (NMDA) receptor excitotoxicity.[884] Affected animals display progressive ataxia, blindness, sensory depression and, terminally, coma. Lesions seen on computed tomography (CT) scans include enlargement of the lateral ventricles and reduced thickness of the cerebral cortex.[885]

Gross pathologic lesions in the central nervous system include moderate enlargement of the lateral ventricles and a yellowish discoloration of the brain parenchyma. Accumulation of protein storage material in neuronal lysosomes is evident on microscopic examination and is accompanied by neuronal necrosis and astrocytosis, which may be severe. The lesions sometimes have a lamellar appearance.[884] The disease is ultimately fatal, and no practical method of treatment is currently available.

REFERENCES

877. Read WK, Bridges CH: Neuronal lipodystrophy: occurrence in an inbred strain of cattle, *Vet Pathol* 6:235-243, 1968.
878. Harper PA et al: Neurovisceral ceroid lipofuscinosis in blind Devon cattle, *Acta Neuropathol (Berl)* 75:632-636, 1988.
879. Edwards JF et al: Juvenile-onset neuronal ceroid lipofuscinosis in Rambouillet sheep, *Vet Pathol* 31:48-54, 1994.
880. Fiske RA, Storts RW: Neuronal ceroid lipofuscinosis in Nubian goats, *Vet Pathol* 25:171-173, 1988.
881. Jolly RD, Janmaat DM, West DM: Ovine ceroid lipofuscinosis: a model of Batten's disease, *Neuropathol Appl Neurobiol* 6:195-209, 1980.
882. Jolly RD: Comparative biology of the neuronal ceroid lipofuscinoses (NCL): an overview, *Am J Med Genet* 57:307-311, 1995.
883. Martinus RD et al: Bovine ceroid lipofuscinosis (Batten's disease): the major component stored is the DCCD-reactive proteolipid, subunit c, of mitochondrial ATP synthase, *Vet Res Commun* 15:85-94, 1991.
884. Jolly RD, Walkley SU: Ovine ceroid lipofuscinosis (OCL6): postulated mechanism of neurodegeneration, *Mol Genet Metab* 66:376-380, 1999.
885. Woods PR et al: Computed tomography of Rambouillet sheep affected with neuronal ceroid lipofuscinosis, *Vet Radiol Ultrasound* 34:259-262, 1993.

CITRULLINEMIA

LISLE W. GEORGE
MARY O. SMITH

Citrullinemia is a rare genetic defect of Holstein calves that has been reported in Australasia, Europe, and India.[886-888] The genetic defect has been found in one carrier bull in the United States.[889] The mutation responsible has been traced to offspring of a North American sire named Greyview Crisscross and his son Linmack Kriss King.[890] Approximately 8% of all bulls used for artificial insemination in Australia are heterozygous for the gene, but the gene prevalence appears to be much lower in the United States.[891,892]

Citrullinemia is caused by a defect of arginosuccinate synthetase, an enzyme that processes citrulline in the pathway for the formation of urea. The condition is fatal. Affected calves are normal at birth but become clinically depressed by 24 hours after birth. By 2 to 3 days after birth, affected calves show head-pressing, drooling of saliva, bellowing, muzzle twitching, tongue protrusion, and odontoprisis. Convulsions are first seen at 1 to 4 days of age, and death rapidly follows.

The diagnosis may be made by observing an increased concentration of citrulline in the plasma. The concentration of citrulline in normal calves is 0.16 mM and in affected calves is over 1.5 mM by the third day after birth. The plasma arginine concentration is decreased to less than 0.02 mM at death.[893] There is a marked hyperammonemia because of the inactivity of the hepatic ornithine-citrulline cycle. The brain concentrations of the transmitter amino acids glutamate, aspartate and γ-aminobutyric acid are decreased. Affected calves also have a reduced affinity of postsynaptic glutamate N-methyl-D-aspartate (NMDA) receptors in the brain.[894] The genetic deficit has been traced to the insertion of a chain termination codon for arginine in the argininosuccinate synthetase genome, which causes a complete loss of enzymatic activity. A polymerase chain reaction (PCR) test for detection of heterozygotes has been developed.[891] The microscopic changes of the brain include astroglial edema, and mild to severe spongiform change of the deep laminae of the cerebral cortex.[895]

REFERENCES

886. Harper PAW et al: Citrullinaemia as a cause of neurological disease in neonatal Friesian heifers, *Aust Vet J* 63:378-379, 1986.
887. Grupe S, Dietl G, Schwerin M: Population survey of citrullinemia in German Holsteins, *Livestock Prod Sci* 45:35-38, 1996.
888. Muraleedharan P et al: Incidence of hereditary citrullinemia and bovine leucocyte adhesion deficiency syndrome in Indian dairy cattle *(Bos taurus, Bos indicus)* and buffalo *(Bubalus bubalis)* population, *Arch fur Tierzucht* 42:347-352, 1999.
889. Robinson JL et al: Low incidence of citrullinemia carriers among dairy cattle of the United States, *J Dairy Sci* 76:853-858, 1993.
890. Healy PJ et al: Bovine citrullinaemia traced to the sire of Linmack Kriss King, *Aust Vet J* 68:4, 1991.
891. Dennis JA et al: Molecular definition of bovine argininosuccinate synthetase deficiency, *Proc Natl Acad Sci (USA)* 86:7947, 1989.

892. Robinson JL et al: Low incidence of citrullinemia carriers among dairy cattle of the United States, *J Dairy Sci* 76:853-858, 1993.
893. Thornton R: Citrullinaemia in Friesian calves, *Surveillance* 19(4):23-24, 1992.
894. Dodd PR et al: Glutamate and -Aminobutyric acid neurotransmitter systems in the acute phase of maple syrup urine disease and citrullinemia encephalopathies in newborn calves, *J Neurochem* 59:582-590, 1992.
895. Harper PAW, Healy PJ, Dennis JA: Animal model of human disease, Citrullinemia (arginosuccinate synthetase deficiency), *Am J Pathol* 135:1213-1215, 1989.

BRAIN TUMORS

Nervous system tumors of ruminants include medulloblastoma, ependymoblastoma, neurofibrosarcoma, angioblastoma, meningioma, meningeal hemangioma, neurofibroma, schwannoma, and reticulosis.[896,897] Central nervous system (CNS) tumors of horses include pituitary adenomas, microgliomas, medulloepithelioma, choroid plexus papilloma, ependymoma, neurofibroma, meningioma, meningeal carcinoma, and reticulosis.[896,898-902] Secondary tumors that invade the CNS include melanoma, lymphosarcoma, adenocarcinoma, squamous cell carcinoma, hemangioma, and osteoma.[896,902-904] Of these, lymphosarcoma is most commonly encountered.[905-907] Metastatic invasion to the CNS occurs either by vascular routes or by extension along the peripheral nerve rootlets.

Clinical signs of most brain tumors are the result of compression of the brainstem at the cerebellopontine angle. Neurologic structures that often become denervated include cranial nerve nuclei V, VII, and VIII and the cerebellum.[908] Clinical signs include hypermetric gait, ataxia, depression, facial paresis or paralysis, facial anesthesia or analgesia, head tilt, strabismus, nystagmus, and unilateral loss of menace. Migration of facial tumors (squamous cell carcinomas) into the cranial vault through the cranial nerve foramina may also result in facial swelling, exophthalmos, Horner's syndrome, or asymmetric airflow through the nares.[907] Pituitary adenomas of aged horses (see Chapter 39) rarely cause neurologic disease, but they secrete melanocyte-stimulating hormone, which stimulates the adrenal cortex and causes Cushing's disease.

REFERENCES

896. Braund K: Neoplasia of the nervous system, *Compend Cont Educ Pract Vet* 6:717-722, 1984.
897. Guarda F, Biolatti B: Cerebral medulloblastoma in two calves, *Summa* 4:33-35, 1987.
898. Jolly RD, Alley MR: Medulloblastoma in calves: a report of three cases, *Pathol Vet* 6:463-468, 1969.
899. Saunders GK: Ependymoblastoma in a dairy calf, *Vet Pathol* 21:528-529, 1984.
900. Finn JP, Tennant BC: A cerebral and ocular tumor of reticular tissue in a horse, *Vet Pathol* 8:458-466, 1971.
901. Brobst DF, Dulac GC: Meningeal tumors induced in calves with the bovine cutaneous papilloma virus, *Pathol Vet* 6:135-145, 1969.
902. Wright JA, Giles CJ: Diffuse carcinomatosis involving the meninges of a horse, *Equine Vet J* 18:147-150, 1986.
903. Hodgin EC: Meningeal hemangioma and renal hamartoma in a heifer, *Vet Pathol* 22:420-421, 1985.
904. Guard CL, Rebhun WC, Perdrizet JA: Cranial tumors in aged cattle causing Horner's syndrome and exophthalmos, *Cornell Vet* 74:361-365, 1984.
905. Williams G, Feldman R, Baldwin E: Malignant lymphoma of the thoracic spinal canal of a bull, *Texas Vet*, 1972, pp 227-229.
906. Shamis LD, Everitt JI, Baker GJ: Lymphosarcoma as the cause of ataxia in a horse, *J Am Vet Med Assoc* 184:1517-1518, 1984.
907. Sweeney RW et al: Intracranial lymphosarcoma in a Holstein bull, *J Am Vet Med Assoc* 189:555-556, 1986.
908. Baloh RW, Konrad HR, Honrubia V: Cerebellar-pontine angle tumors, *Arch Neurol* 33:507-512, 1976.

CHOLESTEROL GRANULOMAS

MARY O. SMITH

LISLE W. GEORGE

Cholesteatomas are common lesions in the brains of older horses and frequently are incidental findings at necropsy.

Cholesteatomas usually are found in the lateral ventricles.[909] It has been suggested that they form secondary to chronic hemorrhage into the choroid plexuses, but their exact pathogenesis is unknown. Clinical signs of cerebral dysfunction, such as seizures, result only when the masses grow large enough either to obstruct cerebrospinal fluid (CSF) flow from the lateral ventricles or to attenuate the surrounding neuropil directly. Antemortem diagnosis of cholesteatomas in horses can be done by computed tomography (CT) scanning of the brain.[910]

Cholesteatomas appear grossly as brownish nodular thickenings in the choroid plexuses, or, less commonly, as large masses filling the ventricle. Under light microscopy they are found to consist of abundant cholesterol crystals interspersed with empty clefts, hemosiderin, and an inflammatory reaction consisting both of macrophages and giant cells.

There is no specific treatment for cholesteatomas, and relief of clinical signs should be symptomatic, including anticonvulsants as appropriate.

REFERENCES

909. Summers BA, Cummings JF, De Lahunta A: *Veterinary neuropathology*, St Louis, 1995, Mosby, pp 52-53.
910. Vink-Nooteboom M et al: Computed tomography of cholesterolinic granulomas in the choroid plexus of horses, *Vet Radiol Ultrasound* 39:512-516, 1998.

EPILEPSY

GEORGE M. STRAIN

LISLE W. GEORGE

Epilepsy is a condition of recurrent seizures not attributable to other neurologic or metabolic disorders.[911] A seizure (ictus) may be generalized, involving the entire cortex and accompanied by loss of consciousness, or partial (focal). Partial seizures involve a limited cortical region but do not render the patient unconscious. Partial seizures may in turn become generalized. Seizures may result from trauma, infection, tumors, electrolyte disturbances, or cerebral swelling. Some seizures are idiopathic. Seizures may be preceded by a prodromal aura, usually consisting of a stereotyped sensory disturbance and followed by a postictal depression of variable duration. Seizures in very young or old animals frequently are not of epileptic origin.

Seizure activity results from the synchronization of large aggregates of neurons that are driven, at least in the case of partial seizures, by abnormal epileptic neurons in a seizure focus that recruit increasing numbers of connected neurons.[912] Generalized epileptic seizure activity may result from subcortical pacing neurons acting through the excitatory amino acid system.[913] These neurons probably are heavily dependent on aspartate and glutamate for facilitation.[914]

Microscopic abnormalities of the brain may be detectable in focal epilepsies but usually are not in generalized epilepsies. Status epilepticus, a condition of repetitive seizures with little or no intervening recovery that requires immediate emergency treatment, may be the first detected clinical manifestation of epilepsy. Status epilepticus may result if antiepileptic medication is abruptly discontinued.

CLINICAL SIGNS. Generalized seizures may consist of muscle contractions that are tonic, clonic, or alternating between tonic and clonic. Affected animals may fall and display various autonomic signs such as salivation, urination, and defecation. During the seizure there may be dorsiflexion of the head and neck and rotation of the eyes. Postictal depression may last minutes to days. Partial seizures may consist of tonic or clonic contractions of isolated muscle groups without loss of consciousness. Seizure disorders have been described in Romagnola,[915] Swedish Red,[916] Brown Swiss[917] Hereford,[918] Angus,[919] Brahman,[920] and crossbred cattle.[921] Attacks in a 6-month-old Brown Swiss bull were prompted by undue excitement and declined in number with age.[922] Young progeny exhibited similar attacks, suggesting that the trait was transmitted as an autosomal dominant genetic character.

Epilepsy has been poorly documented in horses but probably occurs in Arabians and in some ponies.[923] There is anecdotal evidence of the existence of the condition in Paso Fino horses of the western United States. A condition known as benign epilepsy is seen in foals of many breeds, especially Arabians, but unlike true epilepsy, is usually outgrown. Idiopathic epilepsy in mares associated with elevated levels of estrogen has been reported.[924]

An epileptic condition in an 8-year-old Hereford cow has been described.[918] The seizures began at 6½ years of age. Tonic-clonic convulsions could be elicited by administration of pentylenetetrazol at doses of 4 mg/kg, which was well below the convulsant dose for normal animals. The electroencephalogram showed high-frequency spike bursts, spike and wave, and polyspike and sinusoidal wave abnormalities (Fig. 33-15). No microscopic abnormality could be found in the central nervous system of the affected animal. Partial epilepsy has been described in a 5-year-old Nubian goat with a 3½-year history of episodic convulsions. Between episodes the goat appeared to be healthy. The seizures appeared more often at times of peak endogenous plasma estrogen concentrations and could be induced by administration of ketamine. The clinical signs included repetitive tremors of the fore and rear limbs, head tremors, and mastication without loss of consciousness. The postictal depression lasted for several hours.[925]

Electroencephalographic evaluation of seizure disorders may be performed using evocative drug challenges with pentylenetetrazol, ketamine, or other seizure-inducing agents and established techniques, but care must be taken to prevent injury to the animal. Because of the rarity of epilepsy in large animals, specific drug therapies have not been established; however, Table 33-8 presents several drugs that could be administered. These drugs usually are highly protein bound in plasma and can be displaced or functionally altered by other drugs, including tetracycline and chloramphenicol. Because of these potential interactions, these agents should not be used concomitantly with the anticonvulsants.

All anticonvulsant treatments are begun at a low dose, which is increased daily or every second or third day until the seizures have been controlled. If seizures cannot be controlled without causing depression or ataxia, a second anticonvulsant is added. The dose of the second drug is gradually increased until the seizures stop. This combination treatment is continued for 2 to 4 weeks. Thereafter the first anticonvulsant is tapered until it is discontinued. If seizures reappear, the dose of this drug is increased until they disappear again. After 1 month the trough blood concentration of all anticonvulsants is monitored. The suggested therapeutic trough concentration of phenobarbital ranges from 15 to 40 µg/ml of plasma; that of diphenylhydantoin ranges from 5 to 20 µg/ml. Any attempt to withdraw anticonvulsant therapy should be made gradually over 4 weeks.

In many animals epilepsy may be incurable because of its genetic basis. In these cases treatment is rarely indicated. Horses with epilepsy should not be ridden or used for sporting purposes. Specific methods of control other than breeding selection against affected animals are unavailable.

Mares with estral-related seizures may be treated with an ovariectomy. All ruminants experiencing seizures should also immediately be treated with thiamine in gram doses (10 to 20 mg/kg IM or SC 3 times daily or diluted in 5% dextrose or isotonic fluid and given slowly intravenously [see also p. 924]) in case the seizural problem is due to polioencephalomalacia. The plasma sodium, magnesium, potassium, and calcium levels should be measured in all animals experiencing seizures of unknown origin. Infrequent seizures generally do not justify anticonvulsant treatment, and economic considerations often limit the amount of drug therapy possible. Status epilepticus can be treated with intravenous diazepam given in 5-mg doses until the seizures are controlled or by titrated doses of phenobarbital or pentobarbital.

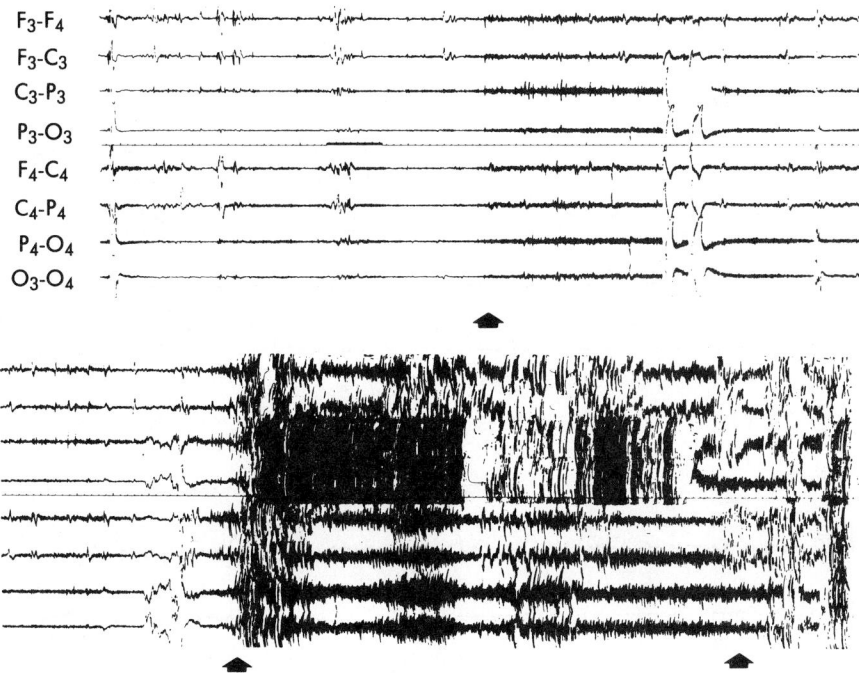

FIG. 33-15 ▥ Electroencephalographic (EEG) recording of a tonic-clonic seizure in an epileptic cow elicited by injection of pentylenetetrazol (6 mg/kg given IV, marker on time channel). High-frequency EEG changes began at the first arrow, the convulsion began at the second arrow, and vocalization began at the third arrow. Electrodes: Left and right frontal (F_3, F_4), central (C_3, C_4), parietal (P_3, P_4), and occipital cortex (O_3-O_4). Calibration: 10 sec and 1 mV; recording bandwidth: 1 to 75 Hz. (From Strain GM, Olcott BM, Turk MAM: *J Am Vet Med Assoc* 191:833-836, 1987.)

REFERENCES

911. Russo ME: The pathophysiology of epilepsy, *Cornell Vet* 71:221-247, 1981.
912. Jeffreys JGR: Basic mechanisms of focal epilepsies, *Exp Physiol* 75:127-162, 1990.
913. Faingold CL: The role of the brainstem in generalized epileptic seizures, *Metab Brain Dis* 2:81-112, 1987.
914. Cook CJ et al: Contribution of amino acid transmitters to epileptiform activity and reflex suppression in electrically head-stunned sheep, *Res Vet Sci* 52:48-56, 1992.
915. Lombardi L: Quadro clinico di epilessia traumatica osservato in uno bovina, *Nuova Vet* 16:86-88, 1938.
916. Isaksson A: Genuin epilepsi hos notkreatur, *Skand Veterinar Bakteriol Patol, Kottoch Mjolkhugien* 33:1-27, 1943.
917. Hill CB: Tetaniform convulsions in newborn calves, *North Am Vet* 37:31, 1956.
918. Strain GM, Olcott BM, Turk MAM: Diagnosis of primary generalized epilepsy in a cow, *J Am Vet Med Assoc* 191:833-836, 1987.
919. Barlow RM, Linklater KA, Young GB: Familial convulsions and ataxia in Angus calves, *Vet Rec* 83:60-65, 1968.
920. Palen NO: Communication sobre dos casos de epilepsia en toros Brahman puros de pedigree, *Gac Vet* 3:158-159, 1970.
921. Lazarus AE: Idiopathic epilepsy in calves, *Livestock Advis* (Bangalore, India) 6:47-49, 1981.
922. Atkeson FW, Ibsen HL, Eldridge F: Inheritance of an epileptic-type character in Brown Swiss cattle, *J Hered* 35:45-48, 1944.
923. Mittel L: Seizures in the horse, *Vet Clin North Am (Equine Pract)* 3:323-332, 1987.
924. Sweeney CR, Hansen TO: Narcolepsy and epilepsy. In Robinson NE, ed: *Current therapy in equine medicine 2*, Philadelphia, 1987, WB Saunders.
925. Olcutt BM, Strain CM, Kreeger JM: Diagnosis of partial epilepsy in a goat, *J Am Vet Med Assoc* 19:837-840, 1987.

NARCOLEPSY AND CATAPLEXY

GEORGE M. STRAIN
LISLE W. GEORGE

DEFINITION AND ETIOLOGY. Narcolepsy is a central nervous system (CNS) disorder characterized by excessive daytime sleepiness, episodes of muscular weakness (cataplexy), and rapid eye movement (REM)-onset sleep.[926,927] Narcoleptic attacks differ from convulsions in that they do not involve tonic-clonic muscular activity.[926] Cataplexy, a sudden episode of paralysis of the voluntary muscles, frequently is induced by stimulation of the patient and can range from atonic, areflexic paralysis of all nonrespiratory muscles to weakness of facial neck and forelimb muscles. Episodes of cataplexy last seconds to minutes. Environmental factors that can stimulate cataplectic attacks include active restraint, feeding, or changing the stall environment.[926,928,929] Excessive daytime sleepiness and REM-onset sleep are difficult to document in large animals. The disorder is considered an intrusion of aspects of REM sleep into the waking stage, especially the active descending paralysis of skeletal muscle. This intrusion results in indistinct boundaries between wakefulness and REM and non-REM sleep. Cataplectic attacks result from sequential activation of pontine α_1-adrenergic and muscarinic cholinergic systems. The numbers of muscarinic and dopaminergic receptors also are increased.[927,930]

Attacks of narcolepsy and cataplexy are considered a paradoxic form of sleep because the electroencephalogram is characteristic of an alert, awake animal, yet the rapid eye movement is characteristic of deep sleep.[926] Narcolepsy has been reported in quarter horses, a Shetland pony, thoroughbreds, Morgans, paints, Arabians, Appaloosas, standardbreds, Welsh ponies, Suffolk sheep, Spanish fighting bulls, a Guernsey bull, and a Brahman bull.[929,931-936] A familial occurrence has been reported in American miniature horses.[937]

CLINICAL SIGNS. The clinical signs of narcolepsy include staggering, drooped head, kneeling posture, flaccidity of the lips, closure of the eyes, loss of the menace reflex, stertorous breathing, and proprioceptive deficits. During severe narcoleptic attacks the animal assumes lateral recumbency and appears comatose. The sensorium returns to normal after a period of time. In the periods between attacks, the patient appears normal.

Electroencephalographic changes of narcolepsy and cataplexy have been reported in cattle.[931] The wave forms vary between low-voltage high-frequency (LVHF) and high-voltage low-frequency (HVLF) patterns, with LVHF corresponding to the actual period of narcoleptic attack (Fig. 33-16). The

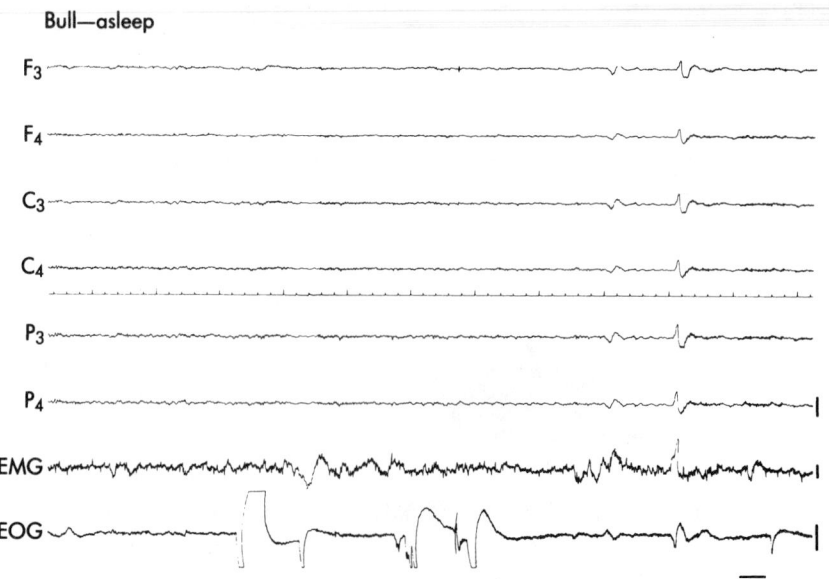

Bull—asleep

F₃
F₄
C₃
C₄
P₃
P₄
EMG
EOG

FIG. 33-16 ■ Electrophysiologic examination of a narcoleptic Brahman bull. The electroencephalogram shows low-voltage, high-frequency waves in all leads (i.e., left and right frontal [F_3, F_4], central [C_3, C_4], and parietal [P_3, P_4]). The electrooculogram *(EOG)* shows bursts of activity characteristic of rapid eye movement (REM) sleep, and the electromyogram *(EMG)* reflects data from extrinsic ocular muscles.

normal electroencephalographic sleep patterns of the horse are usually unavailable; consequently, the technique has limited application for diagnosis of the condition in that species.

Cataplexy can be induced by intravenous administration of centrally acting cholinomimetics such as physostigmine salicylate (0.05 to 0.1 mg/kg of body weight) or α_1-adrenergic blockers such as prazocin (0.02 to 0.06 mg/kg), but attacks cannot be evoked in all animals. Signs can be reversed for several hours by antimuscarinic drugs such as atropine sulfate (0.02 to 0.1 mg/kg IV once for acute signs). Diagnostic drugs must be used with caution because of the possibility of inducing colic, especially in horses. Pathologic lesions have not been reported in narcolepsy of large animals. In human beings narcolepsy can be caused by lesions in the rostral brainstem.[926]

TREATMENT AND PREVENTION. Administration of imipramine (0.5 mg/kg of body weight PO for life), a tricyclic antidepressant, or amphetamine sulfate may counteract excessive sleepiness.

REFERENCES

926. De Lahunta A: *Veterinary neuroanatomy and clinical neurology,* ed 2, Philadelphia, 1983, WB Saunders.
927. Aldrich MS: The neurobiology of narcolepsy-cataplexy, *Prog Neurobiol* 41:533-541, 1993.
928. Zarcone V: Narcolepsy, *N Engl J Med* 288:1156-1166, 1973.
929. Sheathers AL: Fainting in foals, *J Comp Pathol Ther* 37:106-113, 1924.
930. Mignot E et al: Role of central α_1-adrenoceptors in canine narcolepsy, *J Clin Invest* 82:885-894, 1988.
931. Strain GM, Olcott B, Archer RM: Narcolepsy in a Brahman bull, *J Am Vet Med Assoc* 185:538-541, 1984.
932. Sweeney CR et al: Narcolepsy in a horse, *J Am Vet Med Assoc* 183:126-128, 1983.
933. Jordano D, Cardenas GG: Investigationes sobre la caida de los toros de lidia (research on bulls falling during bullfights), *Archivos de Zootecnia* 3:3-52, 1954.
934. Palmer AC, Smith GF, Turner SJ: Cataplexy in a Guernsey bull, *Vet Rec* 106:421, 1980.
935. Hines MT, Schott HC, Byrne BA: Adult-onset narcolepsy in the horse, *Proceedings of the Thirty-eighth Annual Convention of the American Association of Equine Practitioners,* 1992, pp 289-296.
936. Rodero A et al: Simple autosomic recessive inheritance of cataplexy in fighting bulls, *Archivos de Zootecnia* 32:123, 1983.
937. Lunn DP et al: Familial occurrence of narcolepsy in miniature horses, *Equine Vet J* 25:483-487, 1993.

HEAD SHAKING IN HORSES

JOHN E. MADIGAN

Head shaking in the horse is a well-recognized problem that shows no predilection for age, breed, or gender.[938-949] Some horses head shake at rest, whereas most manifest head shaking shortly after the onset of exercise. Head shaking may be vertical, horizontal, or both and often is accompanied by agitation. Suggested causes have included middle ear disorders, ear mites, *Trombicula autumnalis* (harvest mite) larval infestation, cranial nerve abnormalities, ocular disease, guttural pouch mycosis, dental abnormalities, and allergic vasomotor rhinitis. Diagnosis has been difficult, and therapy until recently has been largely unsuccessful. The onset of the disorder occurs most often in spring and early summer, although some cases have been reported to have started in the fall and winter.[947] In many horses sneezing, snorting, and nose rubbing accompanies head shaking. Most horses continue head shaking for many years, often at the same time of year each year.

A recent paper found that five of seven horses with head shaking improved when treated with cyproheptadine (0.3 mg/kg of body weight PO twice daily).[950] Before treatment these horses improved when they were blindfolded or worked in darkness. Neuropharmacologic alterations associated with photoperiod mechanisms leading to optic trigeminal summation (similar to photic sneezing in human beings) are suggested as possible reasons for the spring onset of head shaking. Some of the horses were also treated with melatonin (12 mg total dosage given on a sugar cube at 5 to 6 PM) beginning in the fall and continuing all year.

Examination of horses with head shaking included a complete physical examination; ophthalmic, otoscopic, neurologic, and dental examinations; endoscopic examination of nasal passages, pharynx, and guttural pouches; radiography of the skull, and a complete blood count and chemistry panel. No abnormalities were noted in these examinations.[950]

One author demonstrated that intraorbital neurectomy eliminated head shaking in three to seven horses.[951] These results would seem to support the idea that some cases of head shaking are due to a tingling (or other uncomfortable sensation) in the muzzle area. It is postulated that light may play a role in stimulating the response and that exercise may lower the threshold for onset in some horses.[950] It is important to note that infraorbital neurectomy has a number of complications and is not indicated for the treatment of this condition. The infraorbital branch of the trigeminal nerve is just one branch from of that nerve, and it is believed the problem may reside higher up, at the trigeminal ganglia area.

The etiology of head shaking is not known in most cases. Most horses have not had any physical abnormalities on comprehensive physical examination, and no lesions have been seen in at necropsy. It is my opinion that the symptoms seen in most such horses are best explained by the presence of neuropathic pain involving the trigeminal nerve. Neuropathic pain is a burning, tingling, itching, or electriclike pain that can be intermittent or continuous. The symptoms these horses manifest are sharp, quick movements of the head; occasional striking at the face with a front hoof; excessive snorting and rubbing of the head on objects; carrying the head very low during exercise; and sometimes dragging the nose in the dirt. These behaviors could be manifestations of neuropathic pain. The cause of the assumed dysfunction of the trigeminal nerve is not known. The average age of onset of head shaking is 9 years, and most affected horses are geldings, although about 10% to 20% are mares. Often a period of inactivity precedes the onset of head shaking, which can occur quite abruptly.[952]

As noted previously, cyproheptadine, a type I histamine and serotonergic (5-hydroxytryptamine) blocking agent, was chosen for treating head shaking in horses because of serotonin's role in pain sensations in human beings[951] and because of photoperiod-induced increases in serotonin in the central nervous system in the spring. The dosage used in horses is 0.3 mg/kg of body weight PO twice daily. Side effects are few, but mild colic and lethargy have been reported. The drug cannot be used in show or performance horses because it is not an approved medication. Because cyproheptadine appears to be effective only when the horse has an adequate blood level of the drug, it often is not possible to treat a horse and then withdraw the medication before a show and have the head shaking controlled during the event. Other medications such as corticosteriods, antihistamines, nonsteroidal antiinflammatory drugs, and chiropractic and acupuncture have not met with success. A few horses respond to the presence of something applied to the nose area, such as a heavy hair net or a dangling device that makes contact with the nose area or upper forehead (Fig. 33-17). It is suspected that this type of contract my prevent the nerve from "firing," similar to when a person attempts to block a sneeze by placing a finger under the nose and applying pressure.

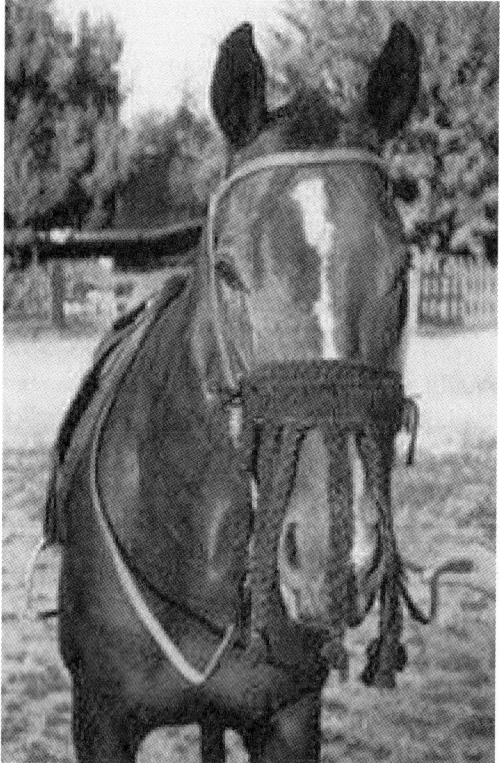

FIG. 33-17 ▌ Head shake device.

REFERENCES

938. Williams WL: Involuntary twitching of the head relieved by trifacial neurectomy, *J Comp Med Vet Arch* 18:426-428, 1897.
939. Tutt JFD: Head shaking in horses, *Vet Rec* 58:374, 1946.
940. Cook WR: Head shaking in horses. I, *Equine Pract* 1:9-17, 1979.
941. Cook WR: Head shaking in horses. II, History and management tests, *Equine Pract* 1:36-39, 1979.
942. Cook WR: Head shaking in horses. III, Diagnostic tests, *Equine Pract* 2:31-40, 1980.
943. Cook WR: Head shaking in horses. IV, Special diagnostic procedures, *Equine Pract* 2:7-15, 1980.
944. Cook WR: Head shaking in horses: an afterward, *Compend Cont Educ Pract Vet* 14:1369-1372, 1992.
945. Kold SE, Ostblom LC, Philipsen HP: Head shaking caused by a maxillary osteoma in a horse, *Equine Vet J* 14:167-169, 1982.
946. Lane JG, Mair S: Observations on head shaking in the horse, *Equine Vet J* 19:331-336, 1987.
947. Mair T, Lane G: Head shaking in horses, *In Pract* 9:183-186, 1990.
948. Mayhew J: How I treat head shakers, *Proc North Am Vet Conf* 1991, 6:453-454, 1992.
949. McGorum BC, Dixon PM: Vasomotor rhinitis with head shaking in a pony, *Equine Vet J* 22:220-222, 1990.
950. Madigan JE et al: Photic head shaking in the horse, *Equine Vet J* 27:306-311, 1995.
951. Cady RK et al: Efficacy of subcutaneous sumatriptan in reported episodes of migraine, *Neurology* 43:1363-1368, 1993.
952. Madigan JE, Bell SA: Characterization of head shaking syndrome: 31 cases, *Equine Vet J* 27:28-29, 1998.

DISEASES PRESENTING PRINCIPALLY WITH BRAINSTEM AND CRANIAL NERVE DYSFUNCTION

LISLE W. GEORGE

LISTERIOSIS (Circling Disease; Silage Disease; *Listeria monocytogenes* Infection)

DEFINITION AND ETIOLOGY. Listeriosis is an acute meningoencephalitis caused by the gram positive bacterium *Listeria monocytogenes*. The disease has a worldwide distribution but occurs most often in temperate climates. Listeriosis commonly affects ruminants, fowl, and human beings but is rare in horses. The prevalence of listeric meningoencephalitis in infected herds does not usually exceed 1% of the adult animals at risk.[953]

Clinical forms of listeriosis include septicemia of neonates, abortion, neonatal death, ophthalmitis, septicemia and diarrhea of ewes, and neurologic disease.[954] Usually only one clinical form is recognized during an outbreak, and only one serovar can be isolated from the clinically affected animals. Neurologic listeriosis may manifest as a multifocal brainstem disorder, as a diffuse meningoencephalitis, or as a spinal cord myelitis. The condition usually affects individual animals but occasionally can affect several members of a herd.[955] Asymptomatic intramammary infections apparently occur and may be responsible for outbreaks of listeriosis in human beings. Repeated intramammary inoculation of 10^6 million to 10^7 colony-forming units of *L. monocytogenes* into cattle resulted in 500 to 50,000 colony-forming units of *Listeria* in the milk for as long as 12 months.[956]

CLINICAL SIGNS. The neurologic signs of listeriosis in adults reflect dysfunction of the caudal brainstem, cerebellar peduncles, or spinal cord.[957] Signs common to most *Listeria* infections of the central nervous system (CNS) include fever, anorexia, depression, conscious proprioceptive deficits, head-pressing, and centrally located cranial nerve deficiencies. Depressed consciousness is the result of lesions of the reticular activating system. Conscious proprioceptive deficits are caused by interference with the descending motor pathways and the ascending proprioceptive fibers in the brainstem and may precede or occur simultaneously with cranial nerve dysfunction. The fever occurs early in the course of the disease and often disappears after 3 to 5 days. Head-pressing and propulsive walking or compulsive circling are caused by lesions of the basal ganglia.

Cranial nerves (CNs) V through XII usually are dysfunctional in listeric animals. Patients with loss of the trigeminal nerve (CN V) show dropped jaw or asymmetric jaw closure and facial analgesia or anesthesia. Facial analgesia is best detected by stimulation of the nasal septum with a pencil or piece of straw. Animals with lesions of CN VI exhibit a medial strabismus on the ipsilateral side of the lesion. Animals with lesions of CN VII have ptosis, loss of menace response, absent palpebral reflex, drooped ear, loss of levator nasolabialis muscle function, and decreased lip tone (Fig. 33-18). Small ruminants with CN VII loss have a deviated philtrum. The paralysis of the orbicularis oculi muscle results in exposure keratitis and, in chronic cases, in panophthalmitis.[958] The loss of levator nasolabialis function is best detected by observation of the muscular contraction on the dorsum of the nose during inspiration. Loss of lip and cheek muscle tone is best detected by observation of drooling of saliva from the ipsilateral side of the mouth and by palpation of the lips and nostrils.

Animals with CN VIII lesions display a nystagmus that changes as the position of the head is altered. Other signs include a head tilt toward the side of the lesion and a tendency to circle or fall to the lesion side. The nystagmus may be horizontal, vertical, or rotatory and usually is inconstant. Goats may lie on their backs with the head curved toward the trunk and tilted with the lesion side toward the ground. If the spinal reflexes can be tested, the affected animals show a mild to moderate hypertonia and hyperreflexia in the limbs opposite the side of the lesion. Lesions of the cerebellar peduncles (juxtarestiform body) may cause paradoxic vestibular signs in which the head tilt and the circling are directed away from the side of the lesion and proprioceptive deficits that are on the same side as the lesion.[959] This should be suspected whenever the head tilt is directed toward the side opposite that of the other dysfunctional cranial nerves. Animals with acute loss of CNs IX, X, and XII develop stertorous breathing and dyspha-

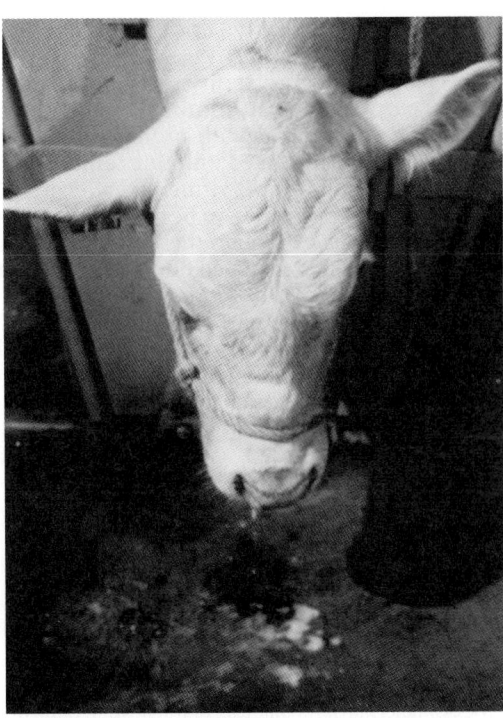

FIG. 33-18 ▇ Clinical appearance of the neurologic form of listeriosis in a Charolais bull. Note the dropped right eye and ear and the drooling of saliva from the right side of the mouth. (Courtesy Dr. W.D. Wilson.)

gia. Animals with dysfunctional cranial nerve XII have paresis or paralysis of the tongue. With unilateral lesions the tongue protrudes from the side of the mouth ipsilateral to the lesion. Progression of listeriosis is associated with decreased consciousness, coma, and convulsions.

Lambs may selectively develop spinal myelitis without brainstem disease. This condition results in flaccid paraparesis or hemiparesis without attendant signs of brainstem dysfunction.[960] The clinical signs of myelitis include tetraparesis, tetraplegia, paraparesis paraplegia, conscious proprioceptive deficits, and recumbency. The sensorium and appetite are normal in some of the affected animals and are markedly depressed in others.[961]

CLINICAL PATHOLOGY. The clinical signs of multifocal brainstem disease with fever in a ruminant are suggestive of listeriosis, *Haemophilus somnus* infection (cattle), or aberrant parasite migration. Examination of the cerebrospinal fluid (CSF) should be helpful for confirming a diagnosis of listeriosis, but the cell and protein concentrations of the specimens do not correlate with the severity of the clinical signs or the prognosis. The protein concentration in the CSF may be over 40 μg/dl, and the CSF white blood cell counts may be over 12 mononuclear cells per microliter.[953,962,963] Many cattle with advanced signs of listeriosis develop metabolic acidosis as a result of salivary bicarbonate loss.

PATHOLOGY. Pathologic confirmation of listeriosis is based on identification of multifocal microabscesses in the brainstem and isolation of *L. monocytogenes* from infected brain tissue. The agent is only rarely isolated from cerebrospinal fluid and is best recovered from refrigerated nervous tissues. Enrichment of the *Listeria* organisms may be accomplished by refrigerating slices of brain at 4° C (39.1° F) for 3 months while culturing the tissues weekly. In contrast to septicemic listeriosis of monogastric animals, peripheral monocytosis is not observed in infected ruminants.

PATHOPHYSIOLOGY. *Listeria* organisms produce a hemolysin, listeriolysin-O, a thiol-activated toxin (MW 58 kDa) that is correlated with pathogenicity. The molecular role of the toxin in dissemination of the infection and in cell death is not known.

It is unclear whether infection of the brain by *L. monocytogenes* occurs hematogenously or by ascent from the cranial nerve rootlets.[964] Morphologic studies of naturally occurring cases of encephalitic listeriosis have demonstrated the bacterium in the axons of the trigeminal nerve rootlets, indicating a possible centripetal migration.[964,965] Similar findings have been reported in animals that were infected experimentally.[966] Younger animals may be susceptible because eruption of the permanent teeth may expose trigeminal nerve rootlets. A model for experimental induction of listeriosis by inoculation of the bacterium into the pulp cavity of sheep has been described.[967] Infection of the CNS without bacteremia has been detected, indicating that centripetal migration of the bacterium is possible.[968] Some investigators have considered axonal migration to be an unlikely mode of pathogenesis. Reasons for this include a lack of nutritional dependency of *L. monocytogenes* for nervous tissue and the ready ability to produce multifocal brain microabscesses by intravenous inoculation of the bacteria into susceptible hosts.[964,969]

EPIDEMIOLOGY. *L. monocytogenes* has 16 major serologic types based on comparison of somatic and flagellar antigens. Most clinical infections are caused by serovars 1/2a, 1/2b, 4a, and 4b. *Listeria ivanovii*, a bacterium that usually is associated with abortions in sheep, also has been classified as *L. monocytogenes* serovar 5. The serovar 1/2 (a and b subtypes) is most prevalent in livestock. The 1/2b subtype appears to be exclusively related to encephalitic infections, whereas other subtypes, including 1/2a, can be associated with any of the clinical forms of listeriosis.[970] The pathogenicity of serovar 1/2a is hemolysin dependent. Serogroup 1/2 (a or b type) is most often isolated from feedstuffs. Serovar 4b is responsible for most infections in human beings.[971]

The case attack rate in ruminants may reach 9% but rarely is greater than 2%.[972] Listeriosis occurs sporadically in weaned lambs confined to a dry lot and appears in only a small proportion of the lambs at risk. The encephalitis usually occurs from 4 to 32 days after weaning and at 6 to 12 weeks of age. Between 0.7% and 1.6% of all lambs at risk may develop the infection.[973] In untreated cases the fatality rate is almost 100%.[957] The survival rate in treated animals is considerably higher than in untreated patients. The disease in sheep and goats tends to be more acute and results in a higher case fatality rate than in cattle. Occasional outbreaks of listeriosis may occur in sheep without access to silage.[957,974] In these cases the source may be the feces of carrier animals or rotting vegetation on the pastures or feed bunks. During an outbreak of listeriosis, the bacterium can be isolated from the feces of a large percentage of normal animals.[975] It is unclear whether this high rate of asymptomatic infections represents a true carrier state or is simply the result of a high environmental contamination by nonpathogenic isolates.[975] The agent infects the udder but rarely causes clinical mastitis. In sheep, excretion of the bacterium in the milk is greatest during the immediate postlambing period.[976,977]

L. monocytogenes can survive for long periods in the environment and in asymptomatic carriers. The bacterium can multiply at low environmental temperatures and is resistant to environmental influences. *L. monocytogenes* is shed in the feces of asymptomatic carriers, especially at the end of pregnancy and at lambing. Once in the environment, the bacterium can survive for 2 years in dry soil. It is resistant to freezing and thawing in the soil but does not survive for more than 1 to 2 weeks in properly preserved silage. The bacterium proliferates in rotting vegetation in which aerobic conditions exist and the pH is above 5.4.[978-980] Common sources of contaminated forage include spoiled silage at the ends of trench silos, decaying forage at the bottom of feed bunks, or rotting hay at the periphery of hay stacks.[978,981] The incidence of listeriosis may be increasing because of the greater use of trench silos and bulk handling methods that result in a greater amount of spoilage than in conventional upright silos. Although *L. monocytogenes* can be isolated from silage with a pH below 4, fewer bacteria are found in well-preserved forage.[982]

A selective enrichment medium has been developed for identifying and enumerating the *Listeria* organisms in silage. This medium permits semiquantitative enumeration of *Listeria* bacteria in 10 g of silage. Hemolysin production is measured by overlaying the colonies with bovine blood agar and reincubating the plates. Using this method, outbreaks of listeriosis have been correlated with silage containing 1 million *Listeria* organisms and more than 1 million enterobacteria per gram of silage. The pH of such silage characteristically is above 7.8.[983]

There is a significant public health concern about *Listeria* contamination of milk products. The 4b serotype of *L. monocytogenes* is most often responsible for infections in human beings.[984] Outbreaks have been traced to ingestion of pasteurized milk, cole slaw, and soft, ripened cheese. The occurrence in cheese has led to concerns that the bacterium may survive the pasteurization process[985]; however, heat resistance by *Listeria* organisms does not appear to be a significant factor in milk-related human exposures. One study indicated that intracellular *Listeria* bacteria survived after exposure to temperatures as high as 73.9° C (165° F) for 16.4 sec. Complete killing of the *Listeria* organisms required temperatures as high 76.4° C (169.5° F) for 15.4 sec. These temperatures exceeded the minimum temperatures required by the U.S. Food and Drug Administration (71.7° C [161° F] for 15 sec).[986] The public health implications of these findings are unclear.

PATHOLOGIC LESIONS. The lesions of listeric meningoencephalitis are most common in the pons and the trapezoid bodies, but they can be located anywhere in the brainstem. Neurologic structures that are most commonly affected include the reticular formation and CNs V and VII through X. Macroscopic lesions are limited to mild meningeal congestion and clouding of the CSF. Microscopic lesions include perivascular cuffing with mononuclear cells, multifocal asymmetric brainstem microabscesses, and mononuclear cell meningoencephalitis.[987] The microabscesses are composed predominantly of neutrophils. Other microscopic changes include degeneration of the neuropil and neuronophagia. To enhance the speed and accuracy of pathologic diagnosis, a peroxidase-antiperoxidase method has been developed for use with formalin-fixed nervous tissue. The test detects degraded bacterial proteins, as well as intact bacteria in the suspect tissue. Bacterial antigen is exclusively located in areas of malacia or in the microabscesses.[988]

TREATMENT. The recovery rate is best if treatment is administered early in the course of the disease. Animals that are recumbent, comatose, or convulsive rarely survive despite intensive antibiotic and supportive therapy. In most instances treatment must be administered for a prolonged period because recovery may take as long as 1 month. *L. monocytogenes* is susceptible to most commonly used antimicrobial drugs. Recommended treatments are either oxytetracycline (10 mg/kg of body weight given intravenously twice daily), or penicillin G.[958] Specific recommendations for penicillin therapy include an initial dosage of 40,000 IU/kg of body weight (intravenous potassium penicillin G) given 3 to 4 times daily for 7 days and then 22,000 IU/kg of body weight (procaine penicillin) IM once daily for 14 to 21 additional days.[958]

The plasma concentrations of bicarbonate and potassium should be measured, and specific corrective fluid therapy should be administered. Maintenance fluids also may be administered by gavage. Good footing and nursing care are helpful in the short-term but may not influence the overall recovery rate.[989]

PREVENTION. Serologic responses to flagellin and listeriolysin-O develop after oral administration of virulent *L. monocytogenes* and correlate with protection against listerial bacteremia.[968] Cell-mediated immune responses also are important in protection against virulent challenge. Vaccines of attenuated or killed bacteria have been used to successfully protect sheep and goats. Although these vaccines reduce the incidence of listeriosis in vaccinated flocks, they are not commercially available in the United States.

Although the case attack rate of listeriosis is low, occasional epizootics may occur in cattle, sheep, or goat herds; these are invariably associated with high rates of environmental contamination. In such cases the hay and silage should be examined culturally for *L. monocytogenes*. Rotten vegetation should be discarded, and cattle should be fenced from contaminated areas.

REFERENCES

953. Scott PR: A field study of ovine listerial meningoencephalitis with particular reference to cerebrospinal fluid analysis as an aid to diagnosis and prognosis, *Br Vet J* 149:165-170, 1993.
954. Gitter M: Veterinary aspects of listeriosis, *PHLS Microbiol Dig* 6:38-42, 1983.
955. Akpavie SO, Ikheloa JO: An outbreak of listeriosis in cattle in Nigeria, *Revue d'Elevage et de Medecine Veterinaire des Pays Tropicaux* 45:263-264, 1992.
956. Bryner J, Wesley I, Van der Maaten M: Research on listeriosis in milk cows with intramammary inoculation of *Listeria monocytogenes*, *Acta Microbiol Hung* 36:137-140, 1989.
957. Vandegraaff R, Borland NA, Browning JW: An outbreak of listerial meningoencephalitis in sheep, *Aust Vet J* 57:94-96, 1981.
958. Rebhun WC, De Lahunta A: Diagnosis and treatment of bovine listeriosis, *J Am Vet Med Assoc* 180:395-398, 1982.
959. Roeder B, Johnson J, Cash WC: Paradoxic vestibular syndrome in a cow with a metastatic brain tumor, *Compend Cont Educ Pract Vet* 12:1175-1181, 1990.
960. Gates GA, Blenden DC, Kintner LD: Listeric myelitis in sheep, *J Am Vet Med Assoc* 150:200-204, 1967.
961. Seaman JT, Carrigan MJ, Cockram FA: An outbreak of listerial myelitis in sheep, *Aust Vet J* 67:142-143, 1990.
962. Scarratt WK: Ovine listeric encephalitis, *Compend Cont Educ Pract Vet* 9:F28-F33, 1987.
963. Grottker S: Liquor-Untersuchungen bei der listerienbedingten meningoenzephalitis des rindes, *DTW* 92:257-259, 1985.
964. Charlton KM, Garcia MM: Spontaneous listeric encephalitis and neuritis in sheep: light microscopic studies, *Vet Pathol* 14:297-313, 1967.
965. Otter A, Blakemore WF: Observation on the presence of *Listeria monocytogenes* in axons, *Acta Microbiol Hung* 36:125-131, 1989.
966. Otter A, Blakemore WF: Observations on the neural transport of *Listeria monocytogenes* in a mouse model, *Neuropathol Appl Neurol* 15:590, 1989.
967. Barlow M, McGorum B: Ovine listerial encephalitis: analysis, hypothesis, and synthesis, *Vet Rec* 116:233-236, 1985.
968. Low JC, Donachie W: Clinical and serum antibody responses of lambs to infection by *Listeria monocytogenes*, *Res Vet Sci* 51:185-192, 1991.
969. Osebold JW: *Second symposium on listeric infection*, Bozeman, Mont, 1963, Artcraft Printers.
970. Low JC et al: Serotyping and distribution of Listeria isolates from cases of ovine listeriosis, *Vet Rec* 133:165-166, 1993.
971. Menudier A, Bosiraud C, Nicholas JA: Virulence of *Listeria monocytogenes* serovars and *Listeria* spp in experimental infection of mice, *J Food Protect* 54:917-921, 1991.
972. Reiter R, Bowden M, Palmer M: Ovine listeriosis in south coastal western Australia, *Aust Vet J* 66:223-224, 1989.
973. Green LE, Morgan KL: Descriptive epidemiology of listerial meningoencephalitis in housed lambs, *Prev Vet Med* 18:79-87, 1994.
974. Du Toit IF: An outbreak of caprine listeriosis in the western Cape, *J S Afr Vet Assoc* 48:39-40, 1977.
975. Gronstol H: Listeriosis in sheep: *Listeria monocytogenes* excretion and immunological state in sheep in flocks with clinical listeriosis, *Acta Vet Scand* 20:417-428, 1979.
976. Gronstol H: Listeriosis in sheep: *Listeria monocytogenes* excretion and immunological state in healthy sheep, *Acta Vet Scand* 20:168-179, 1979.
977. Gronstol H: Listeriosis in sheep: isolation of *Listeria monocytogenes* from organs of slaughtered animals and dead animals submitted for postmortem examination, *Acta Vet Scand* 21:11-17, 1980.

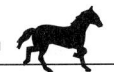

978. Killinger AH, Mansfield ME: Epizootiology of listeric infection in sheep, *J Am Vet Med Assoc* 157:1318-1324, 1970.

979. Irvin AD: The effect of pH on the multiplication of *Listeria monocytogenes* in grass silage media, *Vet Rec* 131:115-116, 1968.

980. Gronstol H: Listeriosis in sheep: isolation of *Listeria monocytogenes* from grass silage, *Acta Vet Scand* 20:492-497, 1979.

981. Green LE, Morgan KL: Descriptive epidemiology of listerial meningoencephalitis in housed lambs, *Prev Vet Med* 18:79-87, 1994.

982. Gronstol H: Listeriosis in Norway, *Annu Proc Sheep Vet Soc* 9:54-55, 1985.

983. Vazquez-Boland JA et al: Epidemiologic investigation of a silage-associated epizootic of ovine listeric encephalitis using a new *Listeria*-selective enumeration medium and phage typing, *Am J Vet Res* 53:368-371, 1992.

984. Fleming DW et al: Pasteurized milk as a vehicle of infection in an outbreak of listeriosis, *N Engl J Med* 312:404-407, 1985.

985. Moore RM, Zehmer RB: Listeriosis in the United States, *J Infect Dis* 127:610-611, 1973.

986. Doyle MP et al: Survival of *Listeria monocytogenes* in milk during high-temperature, short-time pasteurization, *Appl Environ Microbiol* 53:1433-1438, 1987.

987. Ladds PW et al: Pathology of listeric infection in domestic animals, *Vet Bull* 44:67-74, 1974.

988. Marco A et al: Immunocytochemical detection of *Listeria monocytogenes* in tissue with the peroxidase-antiperoxidase technique, *Vet Pathol* 25:385-387, 1988.

989. Kumper H: Therapieversuche bei der zentralnervosen Listeriose der Schafe, *Tierarztl Prax* 19:369-372, 1991.

THROMBOEMBOLIC MENINGOENCEPHALITIS (*Haemophilus somnus* Infection; Sleeper Calves)

DEFINITION AND ETIOLOGY. Thromboembolic meningoencephalitis (TEME) is a fulminant neurologic disease of cattle that arises from septicemia caused by the pleomorphic, nonencapsulated, gram negative bacterium *Haemophilus somnus*.[990] The disease was first reported in Colorado in 1956,[991] but characterization of the etiologic agent, *H. somnus*, was not completed until 1960.[992] The disease is economically significant for livestock owners. One study in feedlots of western Canada indicated that the average economic loss from TEME resulted in 15 sick animals and five deaths annually, amounting to $3190 in lost revenue.[993] In addition to TEME, disease syndromes that have been associated with *H. somnus* infection include pneumonia, infertility, metritis, vulvitis, orchitis, conjunctivitis, otitis, and mastitis.[994-996] The bacterium has been isolated from unthrifty calves, but its causative relationship to that syndrome is unclear.

Cross-agglutination, complement fixation tests and countercurrent immunoelectrophoresis have shown the existence of common surface antigens among isolates of *H. somnus*.[997] Nevertheless, differences in the susceptibility of heterologous isolates of *H. somnus* to antibody and complement have been identified.[998] Isolates from septicemic animals are serum resistant, whereas those from preputial or vaginal mucosa of healthy animals tend to be serum susceptible.

CLINICAL SIGNS. Only the neurologic syndrome (TEME) is discussed here. Descriptions of other clinical syndromes of *H. somnus* infection are discussed in Chapters 29, 37, and 41. The neurologic signs of TEME occur peracutely and may be preceded for 1 to 2 weeks by a dry, harsh cough and dyspnea.[999] Death may occur within 36 hours after the onset of neurologic signs. The initial signs of TEME are fever (40° to 41.6° C, [104° to 107° F]), anorexia, depression, and ataxia.[1000-1002] In addition to depression, affected animals show a number of conscious proprioceptive deficits, including knuckling, circumduction, crossing over, and interference.[1002] Affected animals may fall while attempting to walk. Signs specifically associated with lesions of the cerebellum and caudal brainstem include head tilt, nystagmus, strabismus, blindness, muscular tremors, opisthotonos, coma, and convulsions.[1003] Auscultatory abnormalities in the chest include harsh bronchovesicular sounds and pleural friction rubs. Localization of the bacterium in the joints or lungs may result in lameness, joint swelling, and fluctuant swellings over the joint surface. Other signs that have been observed in some animals include retinal hemorrhages, hyphema, and hypopyon.[1001,1004]

After recovery from the pneumonia, some affected animals may develop pleuritis, necrotic laryngitis, and weight loss.[1005] Some symptomatic animals and as many as 10% of inapparently infected cattle may develop suppurative arthritis of the hock and the stifle joints.

CLINICAL PATHOLOGY. Examination of the cerebrospinal fluid (CSF) may be helpful in substantiating a clinical diagnosis of TEME. Specific CSF changes are characteristic of hemorrhage; they include high erythrocyte counts, xanthochromia, and increased concentrations of protein (over 100 mg/dl), and neutrophils (more than 500 white blood cells [WBCs] per microliter). In untreated cases of TEME, the bacterium may be isolated from pleural fluid, lung sections, aspirated tracheal exudate, urine, blood, and preputial washings. The bacterium can be isolated from approximately 25% to 34% of all fatally infected cattle.[1003] *Haemophilus* organisms die rapidly on swabs or transport media; therefore specimens should be inoculated directly onto a growth medium as soon as they are collected from the patient.[996] The inoculated medium should be incubated in an atmosphere containing 5% carbon dioxide. Isolation of *H. somnus* from joint fluid and cerebrospinal fluid usually is unsuccessful.[1006] The kidneys and brain should be collected at postmortem examination because these tissues contain the highest concentrations of *H. somnus*.[1006]

Initial changes in the peripheral WBC count include neutropenia, left shift, and the appearance of toxic changes in the neutrophils. A test for serum agglutinins has been developed. Cattle that develop acute TEME invariably have antibody titers above 1:400 and show a fourfold increase by 2 to 4 days after infection.[1007] Serum agglutination titers above 1:1024 are seen in convalescent cattle; lower titers may be seen with inapparent infection or vaccination.[1008]

PATHOPHYSIOLOGY. Infection of cattle by *H. somnus* probably occurs through the respiratory tract. Bacterial proliferation in the lungs and other soft tissues by serum-resistant isolates results in bacteremia. Circulating *Haemophilus* organisms are phagocytosed by neutrophils but are not killed. Blood-borne bacteria also adhere to and may be phagocytosed by the cells of the vascular endothelium. The infected endothelial cells then degenerate and desquamate, exposing the subendothelial collagen and initiating the blood-clotting cascade and thrombosis.[1009] Death of neutrophils in the tissues is thought to enhance the tissue damage.[1010,1011] The sites of the body most affected by the thrombosis are the brainstem, spinal cord, synovial membranes, pleura, and lungs. Although the name "thromboembolic meningoencephalitis" implies the presence of disseminated coagulopathy, there probably is only a local thrombus formation at the specific vascular lesion. Immunologic mechanisms may play a role in the vascular lesion. Thrombosis occurs most commonly in animals with high levels of specific agglutinating antibodies and is not seen in colostrum-deprived calves with *H. somnus* septicemia, indicating the importance of antigen-antibody complexes for the development of vasculitis.[1012]

Cattle probably develop immunity to *H. somnus* infection; however, the presence of serum antibodies does not always confer substantial protection against challenge exposure by virulent bacteria.

EPIDEMIOLOGY. Most cattle develop *Haemophilus* infection by inhalation of contaminated respiratory secretions from carrier animals. Although TEME occurs most commonly in feedlot cattle,[1002] outbreaks in the western United States and Canada have been reported in both pasture and dry lot environments.[1000,1013] The disease occasionally may occur in adult cattle.[993] Outbreaks of the neurologic form of TEME tend to occur in the winter months, after shipment or overcrowding, or after additions to the herd in the past 7 months. Outbreaks usually are preceded by a poorly defined respiratory infection.[993] In feedlot outbreaks the disease frequently is restricted to herd mates in a single pen or pasture.

Transmission of *H. somnus* from asymptomatic carriers to uninfected calves may be enhanced by concomitant infection with infectious bovine rhinotracheitis virus.[1001] The anatomic site of bacterial infection in the carrier animals is unknown. *Haemophilus* organisms can be readily isolated from the vaginal and urethral epithelium and from urine, the preputial cavity, and accessory sex glands, but the relationship between these isolates and those found in TEME is unknown.[1014] Although random bacteriologic surveys of cattle indicated that 71% of bulls may have *H. somnus* in the preputial orifice, the concentration in the nasal secretions and upper respiratory tract epithelium in cattle with TEME is low.[1014] Consequently, some investigators have suggested that the urogenital tract may constitute the primary colonization site in chronically infected cattle.[1014] There are some differences in serum susceptibility of isolates from the central nervous system (CNS) and those from the urogenital tract.[998]

The seroprevalence rate may be as high as 100% in some endemic herds and may range from 25% to 56% in herds in which the CNS disease is uncommon. In comparison, the case attack rate of TEME ranges from 2% to 7.4%.[1015] Repeated annual outbreaks can occur in some herds. Estimates of the proportion of carrier animals in feedlots range from 3.2% to 8.8%.

NECROPSY FINDINGS. Cattle with the neurologic lesions do not tend to develop fibrinous pneumonia. Macroscopic pathologic lesions of the CNS include disseminated multifocal hemorrhages and 0.1- to 0.3-cm infarctions in the spinal cord, brainstem, and cerebral cortex. Bacterial colonies frequently are observed in thrombosed blood vessels and the surrounding infarcted tissues. Ocular lesions are characterized by conjunctivitis, multifocal retinal hemorrhages, and areas of retinal edema. The CSF is cloudy and xanthochromic. A focal fibrinous meningitis is seen, and suppurative otitis may be seen in some cases.

The earliest microscopic lesion of TEME is a vasculitis that progresses to septic infarction and abscessation. The lesions usually are found in the CNS, but in severe cases they may be disseminated throughout the body.

Nonneurologic lesions of *H. somnus* infection include suppurative arthritis, synovitis, suppurative pleuritis, and bronchopneumonia. Changes associated with the bronchopneumonia include infarction, cranioventral pulmonary consolidation, and hemorrhagic interstitial pneumonia. Simultaneous pulmonary infections with *H. somnus* and *Pasteurella multocida* result in particularly severe pathologic changes.[1016] These lesions include ecchymotic to petechial hemorrhages over the serous surfaces, purulent exudate in the joints, and ulceration of the laryngeal and tracheal mucosa with pseudodiphtheritic membrane formation.[1017]

TREATMENT AND PROGNOSIS. During an outbreak, cattle must be examined frequently and should be treated when the neurologic signs first appear. *H. somnus* is susceptible to many antibiotics and antimicrobial drugs. Drugs that have been reported to be effective for the treatment of TEME include tetracyclines, penicillin, aminoglycosides, and ampicillin. Parenteral oxytetracycline is regarded as the most cost-effective treatment for infected commercial cattle. Dosages of 10 mg/kg of a conventional formulation given intravenously twice daily for 3 days or 20 mg/kg of a long-acting formulation given intramusculary every other day for three treatments should be administered. After that therapy, daily treatment with procaine penicillin (10,000 to 20,000 IU/kg IM) should be continued until complete recovery is observed. Some authors have advocated the addition of chlortetracycline (2.2 mg/kg) to the feed for 10 successive days.[1018] This

method of mass therapy for a TEME epizootic is considered more efficacious than vaccination when the mortality rate is below 2%.[1018]

PREVENTION AND CONTROL. Antibody responses protective against respiratory challenge have been generated by vaccinating cattle with anionic, heat-stable proteins derived from the bacterial cell wall.[1019] In comparison, cattle vaccinated with cationic cell wall proteins developed precipitating antibodies but were not protected against challenge exposure.[1019] Bactericidal antibodies may constitute important mechanisms for host resistance against *H. somnus*.[1011,1016] Vaccination of cattle with commercial products affords substantial protection from experimentally induced *H. somnus* septicemia and neurologic disease[999,1020] for as long as 95 days after vaccination.[999] (See Chapter 44 for more information about vaccines.)

Mass prophylactic treatment of affected cattle with a parenterally administered, long-acting oxytetracycline formulation may be efficacious for preventing TEME in cattle that have been stressed and exposed to carrier animals.[1021] Oxytetracycline feed additives also may be useful for preventing *H. somnus* infection.[1017] One field study has indicated that administration of modified live virus vaccines for infectious bovine rhinotracheitis and bovine virus diarrhea at the time of arrival at a feedlot significantly increased the incidence of TEME.[1016] Such data indicate that modified live virus vaccines should be administered cautiously to cattle exposed to *H. somnus*.

REFERENCES

990. Stephens LR, Little PB: Ultrastructure of *Haemophilus somnus*, causative agent of bovine infectious thromboembolic meningoencephalitis, *Am J Vet Res* 42:1638-1640, 1981.
991. Griner LA, Jensen R, Brown WW: Infectious embolic meningoencephalitis in cattle, *J Am Vet Med Assoc* 129:418-421, 1956.
992. Kennedy PC, Biberstein EL, Howarth JA: Infectious meningoencephalitis in cattle caused by a *Haemophilus*-like organism, *Am J Vet Res* 21:403-404, 1960.
993. Saunders JR, Thiesen WA, Janzen ED: *Haemophilus somnus* infections. I, A 10-year (1969-1978) retrospective study of losses in cattle herds in western Canada, *Can Vet J* 21:119-123, 1980.
994. Hazlett MJ, Little PB: Experimental production of mastitis with *Haemophilus somnus* in the lactating bovine mammary gland, *Can Vet J* 24:135-136, 1983.
995. Klavano GG: Observations of *Haemophilus somnus* infection as an agent producing reproductive diseases: infertility and abortion, *Proceedings of the Annual Meeting of the Society of Theriogenology,* Omaha, 1980.
996. Keister MD: *Haemophilus somnus* infections in cattle, *Compend Cont Educ Pract Vet* 3:260-264, 1981.
997. Canto J et al: Cross-reactivity of *Haemophilus somnus* antibody in agglutination and complement fixation tests and in enzyme-linked immunosorbent assay, *J Clin Microbiol* 17:500-506, 1983.
998. Corbeil LB et al: Serum susceptibility of *Haemophilus somnus* from bovine clinical cases and carriers, *J Clin Microbiol* 22:192-198, 1985.
999. Williams JM, Smith GL, Murdock FM: Immunogenicity of a *Haemophilus somnus* bacterin in cattle, *Am J Vet Res* 39:1756-1761, 1978.
1000. Panciera RJ, Dahlgren RR, Rinker HB: Observations on septicemia of cattle caused by a *Haemophilus*-like organism, *Pathol Vet* 5:212-226, 1968.
1001. Crandell RA, Smith AR, Kissil M: Colonization and transmission of *Haemophilus somnus* in cattle, *Am J Vet Res* 38:1749-1751, 1977.
1002. MacDonald DW, Christian RG, Chalmers GA: Infectious thromboembolic meningoencephalitis: literature review and occurrence in Alberta, 1969-71, *Can Vet J* 14:57-61, 1973.
1003. Bailie WE et al: Infectious thromboembolic meningoencephalomyelitis (sleeper syndrome) in feedlot cattle, *J Am Vet Med Assoc* 148:162-166, 1966.
1004. Dukes TW: The ocular lesions in thromboembolic meningoencephalitis (TEME) of cattle, *Can Vet J* 12:180-182, 1971.
1005. Pritchard DG, Shreeve J, Bradley R: The experimental infection of calves with a British strain of *Haemophilus somnus*, *Res Vet Sci* 26:7-11, 1979.
1006. Nayar PSG et al: Diagnostic procedures in experimental *Haemophilus somnus* infection in cattle, *Can Vet J* 18:159-163, 1977.
1007. Stephens LR et al: Humoral immunity in experimental thromboembolic meningoencephalitis in cattle caused by *Haemophilus somnus*, *Am J Vet Res* 42:468-473, 1981.
1008. Beeman K: *Haemophilus somnus* of cattle: an overview, *Compend Cont Educ Pract Vet* 7:S259-S263, 1985.
1009. Little PB: *Haemophilus somnus* complex: pathogenesis of the septicemic thrombotic meningoencephalitis, *Can Vet J* 27:94-96, 1986.

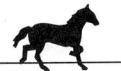

1010. Czuprynski CJ, Hamilton: Bovine neutrophils ingest but do not kill *Haemophilus somnus* in vitro, *Infect Immun* 50:431-436, 1985.
1011. Pennell JR, Renshaw HW: *Haemophilus somnus* complex: in vitro interactions of *Haemophilus somnus*, leukocytes, complement, and antiserums produced from vaccination of cattle with fractions of the organism, *Am J Vet Res* 38:759-769, 1977.
1012. Thompson KG, Little PB: Effect of *Haemophilus somnus* on bovine endothelial cells in organ culture, *Am J Vet Res* 42:748-754, 1981.
1013. Dewey KJ, Little PB: Environmental survival of *Haemophilus somnus* and influence of secretions and excretions, *Can J Comp Med* 48:23-26, 1984.
1014. Humphrey JD, Little PB, Stephens LR: Prevalence and distribution of *Haemophilus somnus* in the male bovine reproductive tract, *Am J Vet Res* 43:791-795, 1982.
1015. Saunders JR, Janzen ED: *Haemophilus somnus* infections. II. A Canadian field trial of a commercial bacterin: clinical and serological results, *Can Vet J* 21:219-224, 1980.
1016. Corstvet RE et al: Survey of tracheas of feedlot cattle for *Haemophilus somnus* and other selected bacteria, *J Am Vet Med Assoc* 163:870-873, 1973.
1017. Jensen R et al: Laryngeal contact ulcers in feedlot cattle, *Vet Pathol* 17:667-671, 1980.
1018. Davidson JN, Carpenter TE, Hjerpe CA: An example of an economic decision analysis approach to the problem of thromboembolic meningoencephalitis (TEME) in feedlot cattle, *Cornell Vet* 71:383-390, 1981.
1019. Stephens LR, Little PB, Wilkie BN: Isolation of *Haemophilus somnus* antigens and their use as vaccines for prevention of bovine thromboembolic meningoencephalitis, *Am J Vet Res* 45:234-239, 1984.
1020. Stephens LR et al: Vaccination of cattle against experimentally induced thromboembolic meningoencephalitis with a *Haemophilus somnus* bacterin, *Am J Vet Res* 43:1119-1342, 1982.
1021. Janzen ED, McManus RF: Observations on the use of a long-acting oxytetracycline for in-contact prophylaxis of undifferentiated bovine respiratory disease in feedlot steers under Canadian conditions, *Bovine Pract* 15:87-90, 1980.

BACTERIAL OTITIS MEDIA-INTERNA OF RUMINANTS

Otitis media-interna is a common disease of cattle and sheep. The condition usually occurs as a sequel to severe respiratory infections caused by *Pasteurella haemolytica, Pasteurella multocida, Corynebacterium pseudotuberculosis, Pseudomonas aeruginosa, Haemophilus somnus,* or *Mycoplasma* spp.[1022-1027] Bacterial ear infections are common in feedlot-reared lambs. The incidence may range from 2.9% to 12% of all animals raised under those conditions, and in those animals the condition usually is subclinical.[1022-1031]

Suppurative bacterial otitis is characterized by thickened mucosae of the vestibular membranes and accumulation of thick fluid in the labyrinths. The infection enters the ear through the eustachian tube. The tympanum may be intact in sheep.[1025] In calves, however, it usually is ruptured, and a clear, yellow, proteinaceous fluid is discharged through the external ear canal; the fluid then accumulates at the base of the ear.[1024,1032] In chronic cases of bacterial otitis, invasion of the local bone of the skull may result in bone remodeling and hyperostosis.[1027]

Vestibular disease results from infections that extend into the inner ear. Patients with vestibular signs display heat tilt (toward the side of the lesion), continuous horizontal nystagmus (fast phase away from the side of the lesion), and a tendency to stumble or fall toward the side the lesion. Head shaking with development of an aural hematoma may precede the clinical vestibular signs. Animals may become recumbent[1027] and lie with the lesion side toward the ground; if turned, they return to the same position. If the lesion involves the cerebellar peduncles, the animal develops paradoxic signs. In this case the head tilt is away from the lesion side, the fast phase of the nystagmus is toward the lesion side, and the patient circles away from the lesion side. Many animals with otitis media also develop facial nerve dysfunction, which results in ptosis, drooped ear, and flaccid lips and nostrils. In small ruminants facial nerve paralysis results in deviation of the philtrum toward the normal side. Deviation of the philtrum does not occur in cattle because of the large amount of connective tissue surrounding the planum nasale. Sheep with *Pseudomonas* otitis may develop necrotizing dermatitis of the ear canal. Some affected sheep also develop signs of cortical or brainstem disease, including unilateral blindness and contralateral mydriasis. These signs occur when the infection extends from the middle ear into the meninges.

Although the clinical signs of peripheral vestibular disease are characteristic, it is important to differentiate this condition from that of central vestibular disturbance. Animals with peripheral vestibular disease usually are appetent, alert, and aware of their surroundings and do not have a significant deficit of postural placement. The nystagmus of these animals is constantly horizontal. In comparison, animals with central vestibular disturbances are systemically depressed, have a nystagmus that varies in direction, and show marked conscious proprioceptive abnormalities.

Treatment of bacterial otitis with oxytetracycline (6 mg/kg IM or IV daily or 20 mg/kg of a long-acting formulation IM every other day) or procaine penicillin (40,000 IU/kg IM daily) may be effective. Drug therapy should be continued for several weeks to prevent relapses. Treatment is very effective in obtaining a complete cure in animals with acute otitis but is less so in the chronic form. Otic instillation of aminoglycoside antibiotics is contraindicated. Lincomycin (6.5 mg/kg), and spectinomycin (10 mg/kg) have been used successfully when oxytetracycline or trimethoprim-sulfonamide therapy has failed.[1024] Other drugs that have been beneficial for the treatment of otitis include ampicillin, gentamicin, and enrofloxacin. Animals that do not respond should be examined for an abscess or squamous cell carcinoma invading the calvarium or osteomyelitis of the petrous temporal bone.

REFERENCES
1022. Jensen R et al: Middle ear infection in feedlot lambs, *J Am Vet Med Assoc* 181:805-807, 1982.
1023. Nation PN et al: Otitis in feedlot cattle, *Can Vet J* 24:238, 1983.
1024. Jensen R et al: Cause and pathogenesis of middle ear infection in young feedlot cattle, *Am J Vet Res* 182:967-972, 1983.
1025. Davies IH, Done SH: Necrotic dermatitis and otitis media associated with *Pseudomonas aeruginosa* in sheep following dipping, *Vet Rec* 132:460-461, 1993.
1026. Davies IH, Done SH, Clarkson M: Necrotic dermatitis and otitis media associated with *Pseudomonas aeruginosa* in sheep following dipping, *Proc Sheep Vet Soc 1993-1994* 18:23-24, 1995.
1027. Walz PH et al: Otitis media in preweaned Holstein dairy calves in Michigan due to *Mycoplasma bovis, J Vet Diagn Invest* 9:250-254, 1997.
1028. Wilson J, Brewer BD: Vestibular disease in a goat, *Compend Cont Educ Pract Vet* 6:S179-S182, 1984.
1029. Ladds PW et al: *Raillieta auris* and otitis media in cattle in northern Queensland, *Aust Vet J* 48:532-533, 1972.
1030. Olsen OW, Bracken FR: Occurrence of the ear mite *Raillieta auris* (Leidy, 1872) of cattle in Colorado, *Vet Med* 43:320-321, 1950.
1031. Macleod NS, Wiener G, Barlow RM: Factors involved in middle ear infection (otitis media) in lambs, *Vet Rec* 91:360-361, 1972.
1032. Henderson JP, McCullough WP: Otitis media in suckler calves, *Vet Rec* 132:24, 1993.

EAR MITE INFESTATIONS

The ear mite of cattle is *Raillieta auris,* and that of small ruminants is *Psoroptes cuniculi.* Cattle that become infected with the ear mite develop a hearing impairment. Severe infestations perforate the tympanum and result in vestibular disease.[1033-1035] Infected sheep and goats shake their heads vigorously and develop aural hematomas.[1036] Infestation of cattle can be recognized by observation of ulceration and purulent debris in the auditory canal next to the tympanum. In cattle, mites may be entrapped between the plug and the tympanum and may not be visible during an otoscopic examination. All infested cattle have pus and ulceration of the ear canal.[1037] A foul-smelling discharge on the side of the face under the ear canal may be seen in some affected animals. Chronically affected cattle develop a hearing loss of high-frequency sounds.

The psoroptic ear mite of small ruminants does not spread over the remainder of the body. The accumulation of purulent debris and swelling of auricular tissues block the transmission of sound to the tympanum.

Ear mite infestations in cattle are common and in some herds may affect most of the adults. One study in the United States reported a prevalence rate of 66% (29 of 44 cattle).[1033] The biologic importance of the infestation may be related to changes in the herding or mothering behavior of range cattle. The economic significance of the infestation is unknown. The parasite can complete a full life cycle by 8 days.

Ear mites have been successfully treated in goats using ear drops containing rotenone* once daily for 5 to 10 days. Good clinical responses can be obtained in cattle with the same treatment. Fenthion (Spotton,† 0.2 ml) drops also have been used successfully. In cases of parasitic otitis in which the discharge has been inspissated, lateral resection of the ear canal should be considered to establish adequate ventral drainage.[1038] The addition of nicotine to final concentrations of 2 ppm in dip tanks containing 0.25% toxaphene has been 95% effective in some outbreaks.[1039] Plunge-dipping in diazonon, propetamphos, or flumethrin, pour-on preparations of synthetic pyrethroids, and oral dosing with ivermectin all are ineffective.[1039] A single subcutaneous injection of ivermectin at a dosage of 0.2 mg/kg of body weight has been shown to be an effective treatment for *P. cuniculi* otitis in both sheep and goats.[1039,1040]

The life cycle of the mite involves two free living stages, the proto and the deuto nymphs. These forms molt in the vegetation and reinfest cattle as they graze or bed during the evening.[1041] Because of this, tilling the soil of the infested pastures or retreating cattle every 14 to 21 days with insecticide should be considered as part of an eradication scheme.

REFERENCES

1033. Heffner RS, Heffner HE: Effect of cattle ear mite infestation on hearing in a cow, *J Am Vet Med Assoc* 182:612-613, 1983.
1034. Ladds PW et al: *Raillieta auris* and otitis media in cattle in northern Queensland, *Aust Vet J* 48:532-533, 1972.
1035. Olsen OW, Bracken FK: Occurrence of the ear mite *Raillieta auris* (Leidy, 1872) in cattle in Colorado, *Vet Med* 45:320-321, 1950.
1036. Morgan K: Parasitic otitis in sheep associated with *Psoroptes* infestation: a clinical and epidemiological study, *Vet Rec* 130:530-532, 1992.
1037. Heffner RS, Heffner HE: Ear mites in cattle, *Cornell Vet* 73:193-199, 1983.
1038. Msolla P, Fatafu EPM, Monrad J: Epidemiology of bovine parasitic otitis, *J Trop Anim Health Prod* 18:51-52, 1986.
1039. Bates PG: Epidemiology of subclinical ovine psoroptic otoacariasis in Great Britain, *Vet Rec* 138:388-393, 1996.
1040. Kambarage DM, Kusiluka LJM: Parasitic otitis associated with *Psoroptes* infestation in goats, *J Appl Anim Res* 12:173-176, 1997.
1041. Da Costa LA, Cerqueira Leite R, Faccini H: Preliminary investigations on transmission and life cycle of the ear mites of the genus *Raillietia trouessart* (Acari: Gamasida) parasites of cattle, *Mem Inst Oswaldo Cruz* 87(suppl 1):97-100, 1992.

SPACE-OCCUPYING LESIONS OF CRANIAL NERVES IN CALVES

LISLE W. GEORGE

An epizootic disease of Groningse Blaarkop calves characterized by facial paralysis and vestibulocochlear disease has been identified.[1042] The calves showed drooped ear, loss of vision with normal pupillary reflexes, head tilt, dorsolateral strabismus, circling, and depression. One calf had a mild fever, dysphagia, and mandibular paralysis. The cerebrospinal fluid (CSF) contained a high white blood cell count and an increased total protein level. The disease was caused by multifocal space-occupying lesions that surrounded the cranial nerves at the entrance of the calvarium. The microscopic lesions consisted of granulomatous inflammation of the nerves at the internal acoustic meatus and the facial canal. The inflammatory cells in the lesions consisted of histiocytes, lymphocytes, multinucleated giant cells, and plasma cells. The specific etiologic agent was not identified. The granulomas did not contain acid-fast bacilli, fungal elements, or *Listeria monocytogenes*. The microscopic appearance of the lesions and their location in the nervous system were similar to those of cauda equina neuritis in horses. The disease in the calves was nonprogressive, and some of the calves recovered, which differentiates the calf disease from the progressively fatal cauda equina neuritis in horses.

REFERENCE

1042. Maenhout D, Ducatelle R, Coussement W: Space-occupying lesions of cranial nerves in calves with facial paralysis, *Vet Rec* 115:407-410, 1984.

PERIPHERAL VESTIBULAR DISEASE OF HORSES

DEFINITION AND ETIOLOGY. Vestibular disease of horses is an acute, asymmetric condition with one of several causes: extension of pyogenic bacterial infections from the guttural pouch, polyneuritis equi, viral labyrinthitis, and traumatically induced skull fractures.[1043,1044] Idiopathic labyrinthitis probably represents an acute viral inflammation of the vestibular system that is severe,[1044] but spontaneous recovery is common.

Vestibular disease may also be caused by pyogenic inflammation of the petrous temporal bone or membranous labyrinths. Staphylococci, streptococci, and *Aspergillus* spp. have been isolated from cases of suppurative otitis in horses.[1043,1045] Two forms of suppurative otitis media-interna have been identified.[1043,1045] In the least severe form the pyogenic inflammation localizes in the petrous temporal bone but does not spread into the calvarium or rupture the tympanum. This infection results in vestibular signs. This mild form of otitis media-interna also causes dysfunction of cranial nerves VII and VIII.

CLINICAL SIGNS. The clinical course of the disease may be chronic with acute exacerbations. Recovery is common with appropriate therapy. The more severe form of the disease occurs when the pyogenic inflammation extends outward into the temporohyoid joint and stylohyoid bone.[1045] The inflammatory process fuses the tympanohyoid joint, which fractures during strong contractions of the muscles of the pharynx and neck. The fracture line extends into the calvarium, resulting in hematoma formation in the central nervous system (CNS). Pyogenic agents from the original septic site may then gain access to the CNS and cause meningitis. The clinical signs are peracute, and the mortality rate is high. Extension of the fracture lines along the cranial vault and osteomyelitis result in dysfunction of cranial nerves VII and VIII and the cerebrum. Affected horses show a rapid deterioration in mental status immediately after the initial onset of clinical signs. Involvement of the temporohyoid bone can be recognized by radiographic examination of the head and pharynx. The radiographic changes include thickening and pathologic fracture of the stylohyoid bone and tympanosclerosis.

Early clinical signs may appear to be unrelated to the CNS. The horse may appear to be uncomfortable and may shake the head or rub the affected ear for 2 to 3 weeks before the onset of vestibular signs. Otorrhea is not usually observed. The neurologic signs appear suddenly. Horses with mild dis-

---

*Ear Miticide, Vedco Laboratories, St. Joseph, MO 64504 *or* Phoenix Pharmaceutical, St. Joseph, MO 64506.

†Miles Laboratories, Shawnee, KS 66201.

ease develop ataxia, head tilt, facial paralysis, and nystagmus. The nystagmus is not changed by movement of the head (rapid phase away from the side of the lesion). There also is a ventrolateral strabismus on the side of the lesion. The affected animals circle or more commonly lean against the stall walls for support. There often is a mild conscious proprioceptive deficit that is worse on the affected side. Horses with severe calvarium fractures fall and become recumbent. They lie with the side of the lesion facing the floor. Because of the proximity of the facial nerve to the vestibular apparatus in the petrous temporal bone, most affected horses also show signs of facial palsy, including drooped ear and lips, drooling of saliva, ptosis, exposure keratitis, and deviation of the philtrum toward the opposite side of the lesion (Fig. 33-19). If extensive bleeding into the calvarium has occurred, the animal becomes blind in the eye contralateral to the side of the hematoma. Pressure in the cerebral cortex may result in mydriatic pupils on the ipsilateral side. Lesions located central to the geniculate ganglion denervate the lacrimal glands and result in keratitis sicca.

Horses with lesions of the peripheral vestibular system remain appetent and alert. In comparison, animals with vestibular disease accompanied by petrous temporal bone fractures and meningitis tend to be depressed, febrile, and inappetent. Animals that develop septic meningitis secondary to a temporal bone fracture show rapid deterioration of mental status, rigidity, or flailing of the limbs with mild stimulation, stiffness of the neck, hyperesthesia, fever, otorrhea, and dysphagia.[1046]

DIAGNOSIS AND TREATMENT. Ancillary diagnostic measures for vestibular disease in horses include skull radiographs and endoscopic examination of the guttural pouch to exclude the possibility of tympanosclerosis, fractured hyoid bone, or a fungal otitis. The rate of tear secretion may be tested with a Schirmer tear test strip. The normal rate of tear secretion is approximately 21 mm/min, whereas deficient tear production is less than 17 mm/min.

Antibiotic treatment of peripheral vestibular disease should include high doses of penicillin (20,000 to 40,000 IU/kg IV 4 times daily) or, as an alternative, a third-generation cephalosporin or trimethoprim-sulfonamide combination. The alternative drugs should be considered when infection by penicillin-resistant bacteria is suspected. One study reported clinical improvement in patients treated with chloramphenicol (10 mg/kg PO 4 times daily).[1045]

Patients with early cases of vestibular disease may benefit from treatment with nonsteroidal antiinflammatory drugs. Administration of corticosteroids in the acute stages of the disease may ameliorate the clinical signs, but the beneficial antiinflammatory effects of these drugs should be weighed against the potential for nonspecific immune suppression and ultimate extension of pyogenic foci into the CNS along cracks in the calvarium.

Affected horses should be kept in a quiet, heavily bedded stall with good footing. Exposure keratitis may be treated by performing a tarsorrhaphy or by repeatedly administering petrolatum ophthalmic-lubricating ointments. Horses with keratoconjunctivitis sicca may be treated by administration of 0.25% pilocarpine eye drops 4 times daily.[1047]

Horses that recover after long-term antibiotic therapy should be used cautiously because subtle neurologic deficits that interfere with coordinated motor activities could precipitate catastrophic accidents. Relapses may occur in some seemingly recovered patients.

REFERENCES

1043. Firth EC: Vestibular disease and its relationship to facial paralysis in the horse: a clinical study of 7 cases, *Aust Vet J* 53:560-565, 1977.
1044. Hahn CN, Mayhew IG, Mackay RJ: The nervous system. In Colahan PT et al, eds: *Equine medicine and surgery*, ed 5, St Louis, 2000, Mosby.
1045. Blythe LL et al: Vestibular syndrome associated with temporohyoid joint fusion and temporal fracture in three horses, *J Am Vet Med Assoc* 185:775-781, 1984.
1046. Power HT, Watrous BJ, De Lahunta A: Facial and vestibulocochlear disease in six horses, *J Am Vet Med Assoc* 183:1076-1080, 1983.
1047. Spurlock SL, Spurlock GH, Wise M: Keratoconjunctivitis sicca associated with fracture of the stylohyoid bone in a horse, *J Am Vet Med Assoc* 194:258-259, 1989.

EXOPHTHALMOS AND STRABISMUS OF CATTLE

LISLE W. GEORGE

A heritable exophthalmos and strabismus of Jersey, Holstein, Brown Swiss, and shorthorn cattle has been described.[1048-1051] The defect is characterized by protrusion of the eyeballs and anteromedial rotation of the eye around the axis (cross-eyed). The defect does not become evident until the animals are over 6 months of age. Affected animals have defective vision and show difficulty walking in unfamiliar environments. Both genders are affected. The condition in Holsteins is thought to be related to a decreased number of nerve cells in the abducens motor nucleus.

REFERENCES

1048. Holmes JR, Young GB: A note on exophthalmos with strabismus in shorthorn cattle, *Vet Rec* 31:148-149, 1957.
1049. Regan WM, Gregory PW, Mead SW: Hereditary strabismus in Jersey cattle, *J Hered* 35:233-234, 1944.
1050. Schutz-Hanke VW, Stober M, Drommer W: Klinische, genealogische und pathomorphologische untersuchungen an schwerzbunten ringern mit beiderseitigem exophthalmisch konvergierendem schielen, *DTW* 86:185-191, 1979.
1051. Distl VO, Wenninger A, Krausslich H: Zur erblichkeit von strabismus convergens mit exophathalmus bein rind, *DTW* 98:354-356, 1991.

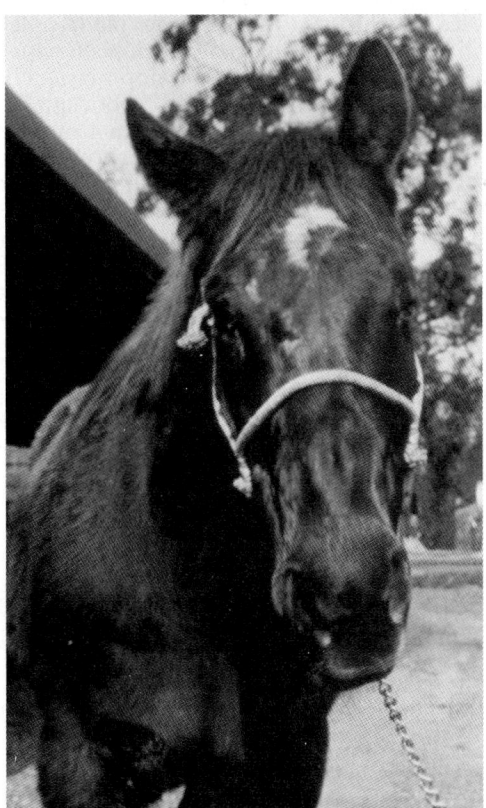

FIG. 33-19 ▮▮ Head tilt and right-sided facial paresis in a horse with peripheral vestibular disease. (Courtesy Dr. W.D. Wilson.)

NIGROPALLIDAL ENCEPHALOMALACIA
(Yellow Star Thistle Poisoning; Russian Knapweed Poisoning)
LISLE W. GEORGE
MARY O. SMITH

DEFINITION AND ETIOLOGY. Nigropallidal encephalomalacia is a disease of adult horses characterized by facial dystonia, variable ataxia, mild depression, and food retention in the mouth. The disease is caused by ingestion of large quantities of the plants *Centaurea solstitialis* (yellow star thistle) or *Centaurea repens* (Russian knapweed).[1052-1055]

CLINICAL SIGNS. The signs appear suddenly but always after long-term ingestion of large quantities of the plants. Characteristic signs of nigropallidal encephalomalacia common to all cases include weight loss, mild to moderate depression, conscious proprioceptive deficits, yawning, lowered head, protruding tongue, tremor of the tongue and lips, and facial hypertonicity when feed is offered. The facial hypertonicity causes a retraction of the lips, resulting in a fixed grimace with the mouth and lips held half open (Fig. 33-20). The patient may display constant chewing movements, and prehension, mastication, and deglutition of food are uncoordinated and inefficient. Affected horses can grasp food in their incisors but are unable to adequately chew and propel the food to the back of the mouth. Food retained in the mouth and cheek pouches may protrude from the commissures of the lips. Affected animals may attempt to drink by immersing their muzzles deeply into the bucket to force the water into the back of the pharynx. Once the food or water is in the posterior part of the pharynx, the animal is able to swallow. Affected animals die of starvation or dehydration. Horses that appear to be depressed usually can be aroused by mild stimulation. Motor and sensory deficits include hypertonicity, ataxia, conscious proprioceptive deficits, and occasionally hypermetria. There also may be a transient tendency to walk propulsively or to circle. Occasionally the animals are hyperexcitable. After several days the signs stabilize, and the disease does not progress. Affected animals usually do not recover.

CLINICAL PATHOLOGY. The cerebrospinal fluid of affected horses may show increases in the white blood cell (WBC) count (75 WBCs/dl).[1054] There are no characteristic changes in the complete blood count or the serum chemistries.

PATHOPHYSIOLOGY. The toxic principle in the plants has been isolated and chemically characterized. The toxic molecule is called repin, a sesquiterpene lactone with high affinity for neural tissue.[1056-1059] Long-term feeding of alcoholic extracts containing repin to monkeys has resulted in collapse, convulsions, and death.[1060] Studies in rats suggest that repin exerts its neurotoxic effects by inhibiting dopamine release.[1059] Additional neurotoxic compounds, including aspartic and glutamic acids, also have been isolated from *Centaurea* plants.[1061]

NECROPSY FINDINGS. At necropsy sharply demarcated areas of yellowish malacia are visible grossly in the substantia nigra and globus pallidus (extrapyramidal system). Lesions are bilaterally symmetric in more than 50% of cases but are asymmetric in a substantial proportion of affected animals. Lesions in other brainstem nuclei are found in a small number of animals.[1053,1062] Microscopic lesions include neuronal necrosis, vacuolation with gliosis, liquefactive necrosis, and cavitation in well-developed lesions.[1056]

EPIDEMIOLOGY. Nigropallidal encephalomalacia has been reported in horses of the United States, Australia, and South America. Yellow star thistle is a common plant in unirrigated pastures in the arid regions of the western United States. The plant is resistant to the effects of saline or alkaline soil conditions and has a minimum moisture requirement. Russian knapweed belongs to the sunflower family and grows predominantly on flood plains, where it can extract deep subterranean moisture. In the United States the plants tend to remain green during the dry months; consequently, most poisonings occur during the summer or late autumn. Most horses are reluctant to eat *Centaurea* plants unless other vegetation is unavailable, but some develop a craving and selectively seek it out. Horses that develop nigropallidal encephalomalacia usually are being fed a poor-quality, high-roughage diet. Affected horses range from 4 months to 10 years of age, with a median age of occurrence of 2 years.[1056] The case attack rates of yellow star thistle poisoning range from 3% to 31% of horses on infested pastures.[1056] Feeding studies have reported that as much as 59% to 200% of the body weight of yellow star thistle and 59% to 63% of Russian knapweed must be eaten over 3 to 11 weeks to cause clinical disease.[1053,1056] Continuous protracted exposure to the weeds seems to be important for expression of clinical disease. The dried plants retain their toxicity.

TREATMENT AND PREVENTION. There is no known treatment for the poisoning. Prevention is best aimed at correcting the nutritional problem by daily supplementation with 10 to 15 lb of alfalfa hay and by not pasturing horses in areas where the thistle grows.

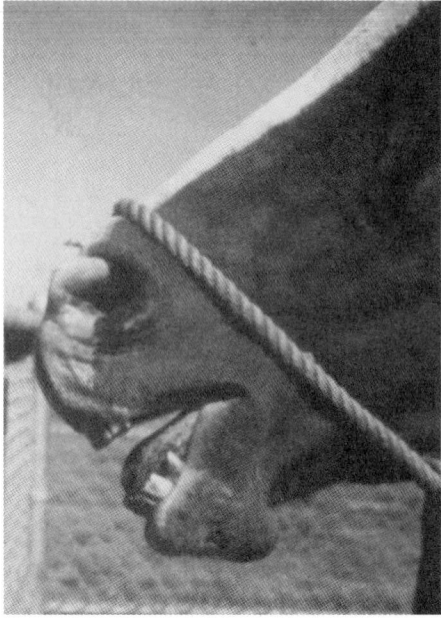

FIG. 33-20 ▉ Characterisitc facial expression of a horse with nigropallidal encephalomalacia. When the animal is offered feed, the marked dystonia of the facial muscles, caused by loss of upper motor neuron inhibition, becomes obvious. (Courtesy Dr. G.P. Carlson.)

REFERENCES

1052. Larson KA, Young S: Nigropallidal encephalomalacia in horses in Colorado, *J Am Vet Med Assoc* 156:626-627, 1970.
1053. Young S, Brown WW, Klinger B: Nigropallidal encephalomalacia in horses caused by ingestion of weeds of the genus *Centaurea*, *J Am Vet Med Assoc* 157:1602-1605, 1970.
1054. Farrell RK, Sande RD, Lincoln SD: Nigropallidal encephalomalacia in a horse, *J Am Vet Med Assoc* 158:1201-1204, 1971.
1055. Fowler ME: Nigropallidal encephalomalacia in the horse, *J Am Vet Med Assoc* 147:607-616, 1965.
1056. Cordy DR: Nigropallidal encephalomalacia in horses associated with ingestion of yellow star thistle, *J Neuropathol Exp Neurol* 13:330-342, 1954.
1057. Stevens KL et al: Sesquiterpene lactone from *Acroptilon repens* possessing exceptional biological activity, *J Biol Sci* 53:218-221, 1990.

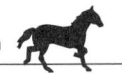

1058. Riopelle RJ et al: Neurotoxicity of sesquiterpene lactones. In James LF et al, eds: *Poisonous plants: proceedings of the third international symposium*, Ames, Iowa, 1992 Iowa State University Press.

1059. Robles M et al: Repin-induced neurotoxicity in rodents, *Exp Neurol* 152:129-136, 1998.

1060. Stern GM: Observations on the toxic effects of yellow star thistle, *J Neuropathol Exp Neurol* 22:164-169, 1963.

1061. Roy DN, Peyton DH, Spencer PS: Isolation and identification of two potent neurotoxins, aspartic acid and glutamic acid, from yellow star thistle (*Centaurea solstitialis*), *Nat Tox* 3:174-180, 1995.

1062. Cordy CR: *Centaurea* spp and equine nigropallidal encephalomalacia. In Keeler RF, Van Kampen KR, James LF, eds: *Effects of poisonous plants on livestock*, New York, 1978, Academic Press.

RUPTURED RECTUS CAPITIS VENTRALIS MUSCLES (Trauma to Cranial Nerves IX through XI)

LISLE W. GEORGE

Traumatic avulsion of the rectus capitis ventralis muscle is seen exclusively in equids. The condition causes dysphagia. The muscle is ruptured when horses fall over backward and hyperextend the neck and head. Tearing of the tendinous insertion of the muscle damages cranial nerves IX through XI. The clinical signs include mild transitory epistaxis, laryngeal hemiplegia, dysphagia, and pharyngeal paralysis. Endoscopic abnormalities of the pharynx and larynx include mucoid discharge from the guttural pouch, pharyngeal and laryngeal paralysis, atonic proximal esophagus, and food particles in the trachea and bronchi.

Radiographic examination of the head and neck may be helpful for substantiating a clinical diagnosis. The radiologic lesions include irregular radiopaque lesions in the guttural pouch and fracture of sclerotic occipital and petrous temporal bones. These cases usually are associated with a preexisting mycotic lesion that results in bone weakness and pathologic fractures. The neurologic lesion usually is reversible, but affected horses may die of aspiration pneumonia before neurologic resolution.[1063]

REFERENCE

1063. Knight AP: Dysphagia resulting from a unilateral rupture of the rectus capitis ventralis muscles in a horse, *J Am Vet Med Assoc* 170:735-738, 1977.

HORNER'S SYNDROME

DEFINITION AND ETIOLOGY. Horner's syndrome results from interruption of ocular sympathetic pathways. Sympathetic fibers originate from neuronal cell bodies located in the mesencephalic tectum. Axons descend to the T1 to T3 segments of the spinal cord, where they enter the gray matter, synapse, and exit through the ventral spinal nerves. From there the nerves pass through the cervicothoracic and middle cervical ganglia (stellate ganglia) and ascend in the cranial vagosympathetic trunk.[1064] The nerves enter the cranial ganglion in the petrous temporal bone, where they synapse. The postganglionic fibers are distributed to the sweat glands of the head, the ciliary muscles, the periorbital smooth muscles, and the periarteriolar musculature. Fibers of the vagosympathetic trunk or the cranial cervical ganglion can be injured as they pass through the neck or over the caudodorsal aspect of the guttural pouch.

Specific causes of Horner's syndrome include mycotic guttural pouch infections, traumatic lesions of the basisphenoid area, cervical trauma, abscesses, tumors, or space-occupying lesions in the anterior aspect of the thorax, periorbital abscesses or tumors, esophageal rupture, and complications associated with surgical ligation of the carotid artery. Horner's syndrome also has occurred after intravenous injection of certain drugs, including xylazine, vitamin E/selenium, or phenylbutazone.[1065-1067] Horner's syndrome has also been seen in horses with polyneuritis equi (cauda equina neuritis) syndrome and equine protozoal myeloencephalitis of the cervical spinal cord.[1068,1069] Tumors that have resulted in Horner's syndrome include sclerosing respiratory epithelial carcinoma, squamous cell carcinoma, and melanoma.[1065,1070]

CLINICAL SIGNS. The clinical signs of Horner's syndrome in horses vary but include miosis, enophthalmos, ptosis, regional hyperthermia, excessive sweating on the ipsilateral side of the face, congested mucous membranes, inspiratory stridor, and dermatitis caused by chronic sweating. Ptosis may be detected by palpation of decreased eyelid tone. The palpebral reflex and the menace response are normal. Facial sweating often disappears 6 to 14 days after sympathectomy. If concomitant damage to the cervical sympathetic nerves is present, sweating of the skin of the neck also may be seen. This is not observed in animals with lesions solely in the tectotegmentospinal pathway. Regional hyperthermia is caused by vasodilation, which results from deficient vasomotor tonus. Sweating is thought to be caused by vasodilation and increased cutaneous blood flow.[1071,1072] Increased sweating can be induced by β_2-agonists, including intravenous clenbuterol (200 µg) or isoprenaline (2 mg) or local application of 10% phenylephrine.[1073] Dysfunction of adjacent neurologic structures may result in simultaneous facial nerve paralysis and laryngeal hemiplegia.

In contrast to the disease in horses, cattle do not sweat on the planum nasale of the affected side. This can be explained by the mediation of normal sweat gland secretion by α-adrenergic receptors in the bovine.[1072] The other signs seen in cattle are similar to those in horses. The clinical signs of experimentally induced Horner's syndrome in sheep and goats are limited to a mild ptosis.[1072] Retrobulbar tumors may cause Horner's syndrome, but in these cases the eyeball proptosis is due to the excessive retrobulbar pressure.[1070]

DIAGNOSIS. The specific site of the denervation of the ocular sympathetic system usually can be located by physical examination and instillation of epinephrine in the eye. In animals with a postganglionic lesion, topical administration of 0.1 ml of 1:1000 epinephrine solution produces mydriasis by 20 minutes, whereas the onset of dilation is 30 to 50 minutes in animals with preganglionic lesions. Parenteral administration of 1 ml of 1:1000 epinephrine solution causes affected horses to sweat profusely over the affected side of the face.[1065] However, this latter test does not differentiate between preganglionic and postganglionic lesions. The guttural pouches of horses and the pharynx of all patients should be examined endoscopically to exclude the possibility of pharyngeal or laryngeal paralysis or guttural pouch disease. The jugular furrows should be palpated for swellings. Insertion of a nasogastric tube during palpation may be helpful for detecting subtle lesions on the left side of the neck. The cervical vertebrae should be radiographed to exclude the possibility of a spinal cord disease. The thorax should be examined using auscultation and percussion and, if indicated, should be radiographed. The gait and proprioceptive responses should be examined to evaluate the function of the spinal cord. The skin temperature may be measured using thermography.[1074] The skin temperature on the affected side is 1° to 2.5° C (33.4° to 37.5° F) higher than normal.

TREATMENT. The treatment for Horner's syndrome depends on the underlying cause of the denervation. Except for Horner's syndrome related to intravenous injection of xylazine, the neurologic signs often are irreversible, even if the primary cause of the condition has been eliminated. When xylazine is administered intravenously, the condition disappears spontaneously. The situation is different in the case of inadvertent perivascular drug injections, wherein permanent neurologic sequelae may occur. The necrotizing effects of

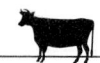
perivascular drug injections can be minimized if treatment is administered immediately. These treatments should include aseptic infusion of large volumes of saline at the site of the perivascular injection and systemic administration of nonsteroidal antiinflammatory drugs or dexamethasone, or both. Abscesses should be drained, and fungal infections of the guttural pouch should be treated as described in Chapter 29.

REFERENCES

1064. De Lahunta A: *Veterinary neuroanatomy and clinical neurology,* Philadelphia, 1977, WB Saunders.
1065. Firth EC: Horner's syndrome in the horse: experimental induction and a case report, *Equine Vet J* 10:9-13, 1978.
1066. Green SL, Cochrane SM, Smith-Maxie L: Horner's syndrome in 10 horses, *Can Vet J* 33:330-333, 1992.
1067. Sweeney RW, Sweeney CR: Transient Horner's syndrome following routine intravenous injections in two horses, *J Am Vet Med Assoc* 185:802-803, 1984.
1068. Mayhew IG: Horner's syndrome and lesions involving the sympathetic nervous system, *Equine Pract* 2:44-47, 1980.
1069. White PL et al: Neuritis of the cauda equina in a horse, *Compend Cont Educ Pract Vet* 6:S217-S237, 1984.
1070. Guard CL, Rebhun WC, Perdrizet JA: Cranial tumors in aged cattle causing Horner's syndrome and exophthalmos, *Cornell Vet* 74:361-365, 1984.
1071. Robertshaw D, Taylor CR: Sweat gland function of the donkey (*Equus asinus*), *J Physiol* 205:79-89, 1969.
1072. Smith JS, Mayhew IG: Horner's syndrome in large animals, *Cornell Vet* 67:529-542, 1977.
1073. Simoens P et al: Horner's syndrome in the horse: a clinical, experimental, and morphological study, *Equine Vet J* 10(suppl):62-65, 1990.
1074. Purohit RC, McCoy MD, Bergfield WA: Thermographic diagnosis of Horner's syndrome in the horse, *Am J Vet Res* 41:1180-1182, 1980.

GUTTURAL POUCH MYCOSIS, NEUROLOGIC SIGNS (Damage to Cranial Nerves IX through XII)

DEFINITION AND ETIOLOGY. In one retrospective survey mycotic infections of the guttural pouch were the third most common disease of the upper respiratory tract of horses.[1075] The clinical signs occur because fungal infections in the medial part of the pouch extend dorsally and damage cranial nerves (CNs) IX through XII and the internal carotid artery. Mycotic guttural pouch infection usually occurs in older animals; however, horses as young as 3 months of age have been affected.[1076]

CLINICAL SIGNS. The clinical signs of mycotic guttural pouch infection are mild. Initially the horse may display head shaking and unilateral nasal discharge. Additional clinical signs are nasal catarrh, dysphagia, head shyness, head shaking, roaring, dysphonia, protrusion of the tongue from the mouth, and epistaxis (Fig. 33-21).[1076-1078] Other clinical signs that have been described include parotid pain, abnormal head posture, facial sweating, shivering, Horner's syndrome, colic, and facial paralysis.[1076-1081] Epistaxis may be fulminant and life threatening. The abnormal head posture is characterized by a tendency to hold the head in extension or lower to the ground than normal. Atrophy of the brachiocephalicus and trapezius muscles occurs secondary to denervation of the accessory spinal nerve. Horner's syndrome occurs secondary to damage of the cranial cervical ganglion and sympathetic trunk. The sensorium is intact unless aspiration pneumonia develops or unless the fungus embolizes into the basal ganglia and limbic system.[1082] Occasionally affected horses die peracutely as a result of exsanguination from a ruptured internal carotid artery. Endoscopic examination of the larynx of affected horses may reveal dorsal displacement of the soft palate, inability to swallow, and unilateral or bilateral laryngeal hemiplegia. Mycotic guttural pouch infection can be definitively diagnosed by endoscopically identifying the characteristic fungal mass in the dorsomedial

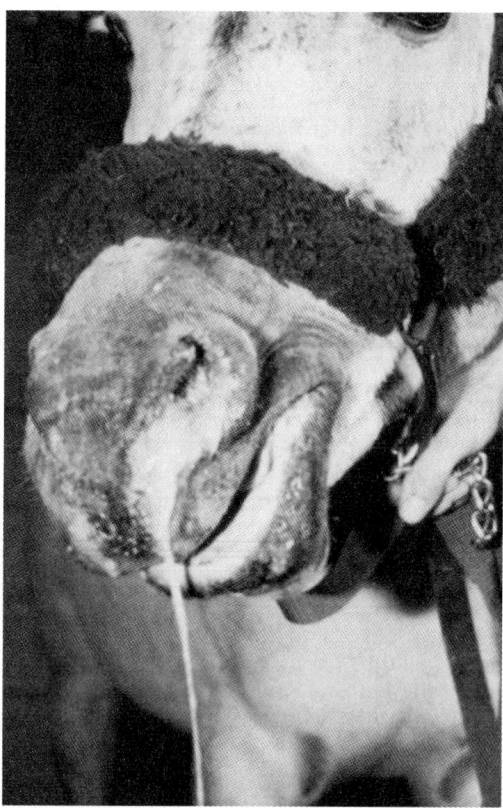

FIG. 33-21 ▓▓ Regurgitation of food material from the nose of a dysphagic horse with pharyngeal paralysis. The horse had a mycotic infection of the guttural pouch.

compartment (Fig. 33-22). Radiographic examination of the pouches shows a poorly defined border of the pouch in the abnormal area.

PATHOPHYSIOLOGY. The guttural pouch is separated into two compartments by the stylohyoid bone and the occipitohyoideus muscle. CNs IX through XII and the internal carotid artery are located in the dorsomedial aspect of the medial compartment and are susceptible to damage from mycotic infections. Extension to the cranial nerves occurs because of inflammation and direct destruction of these structures by the fungal elements. Pathologic studies have shown swelling of the myelin sheaths and Schwann cells. Some sections demonstrate necrosis of the nerves and invasion by fungal elements.[1083]

In chronic infections the fungal lesion may extend into the tympanic bulla and cause vestibular disease. Extensive growth of the lesion also results in temporomandibular osteoarthropathy and fusion of the temporomandibular joint or osteoarthritis of the atlantooccipital joint. Excessive muscular force on the fused joint can result in avulsion fractures of the petrous temporal bone and calvarium. Hemorrhage or spread of infection into the vestibular apparatus and calvarium results in acute vestibular disease, cerebral hemorrhage, and septic meningitis. These complications are discussed more completely under Vestibular Disease, p. 952. In rare cases fungal elements may reach into the lateral compartment, invade the wall of the internal maxillary artery, and affect the facial nerve. Facial nerve paralysis also has been observed as a result of abscessation of the parotid lymph nodes that occurred secondary to a fungal guttural pouch infection.[1077] In rare cases Horner's syndrome may be caused by

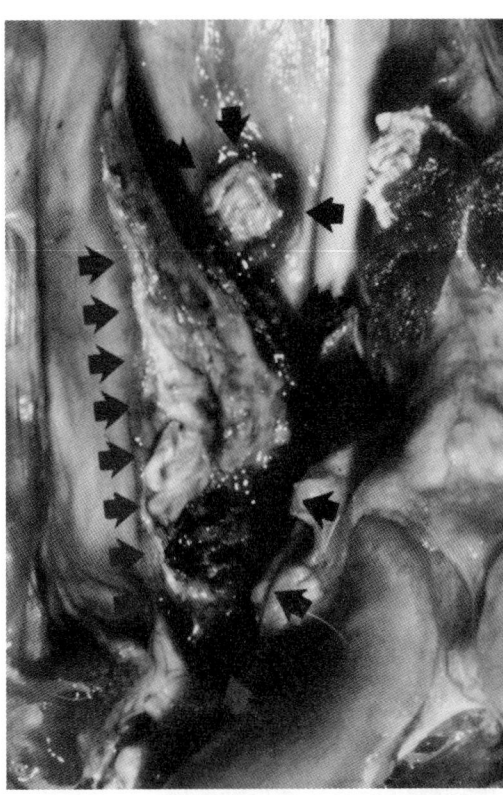

FIG. 33-22 ▨ Appearance of a mycotic lesion in the dorsomedial compartment of the guttural pouch. The mycotic plaque is outlined by *arrows*.

mycotic lesions in the cranial cervical ganglion. The syndrome also may occur iatrogenically during surgical ligation of the external carotid artery.[1084] On occasion, the mycotic infection may extend into the brain and cause encephalitic signs.[1082]

TREATMENT. Before the onset of neurologic disturbances, the internal carotid artery may be occluded using a ligature or by insertion of a balloon-tipped catheter.[1085] During the exploration the fungal mass is debrided surgically. The surgical procedure is effective for preventing fatal epistaxis but may not reduce the potential for nerve deficits or extension of the infection to the central nervous system. Moreover, optic neuropathy and blindness of the ipsilateral eye are common postsurgical sequelae.[1086] There is no effective therapy for the condition once functional loss of CNs IX through XII has occurred. Affected horses often are euthanized for humane reasons. (See Chapter 29 for treatment of guttural pouch mycosis.)

REFERENCES
1075. Cook WR: The clinical features of guttural pouch mycosis in the horse, *Vet Rec* 83:336-345, 1968.
1076. Ryan JA, Modransky PD, Welker B: Guttural pouch mycosis in a 3-month-old foal, *Equine Pract* 14:21-22, 1992.
1077. Hilbert BJ, Huxtable CR, Brighton AJ: Erosions of the internal carotid artery and cranial nerve damage caused by guttural pouch mycosis in a horse, *Aust Vet J* 57:346-347, 1981.
1078. Johnson JH, Merriam JG, Attleberger M: A case of guttural pouch mycosis caused by *Aspergillus nidulans*, *Vet Med (Small Anim Clin)* 68:771-774, 1973.
1079. Boucher WB, Elliott GA, Schmucker B: Epistaxis due to rupture of an aneurysm in a horse, *J Am Vet Med Assoc* 145:1004-1006, 1964.
1080. Lingard DR, Gosser HS, Monfort TN: Acute epistaxis associated with guttural pouch mycosis in two horses, *J Am Vet Med Assoc* 164:1038-1040, 1974.
1081. Bjorkland NE, Palsson G: Luftsacksmykos hos hast, en oversikxt over 7 fall och ett hasuistisk meddelande, *Nord Vet Med* 22:65-74, 1970.
1082. McLaughlin BG, O'Brien JL: Guttural pouch mycosis and mycotic encephalitis in a horse, *Can Vet J* 27:109-111, 1986.
1083. Cook WR, Campbell RSF, Dawson C: The pathology and aetiology of guttural pouch mycosis in the horse, *Vet Rec* 83:422-428, 1968.
1084. Owen RR, McKelvey WAC: Ligation of the internal carotid artery to prevent epistaxis due to guttural pouch mycosis, *Vet Rec* 104:100-101, 1979.
1085. Lane JG: The management of guttural pouch mycosis, *Equine Vet J* 21:321-324, 1989.
1086. Hardy J, Robertson JT, Wilkie DA: Ischemic optic neuropathy and blindness after arterial occlusion for treatment of guttural pouch mycosis in two horses, *J Am Vet Med Assoc* 196:1631-1634, 1990.

DISEASES PRODUCING TREMORS AND ATAXIA—CEREBELLAR DISEASES

CEREBELLAR HYPOPLASIA CAUSED BY CONGENITAL BOVINE VIRUS DIARRHEA VIRUS INFECTION

A complete discussion of bovine virus diarrhea–mucosal disease (BVD-MD) can be found in Chapter 30. BVD virus infection of susceptible pregnant cattle from 90 to 170 days of gestation results in abortion or stillbirth, hydranencephaly, or cerebellar hypoplasia in the fetus.[1087,1088] These signs are also seen in calves born to susceptible dams vaccinated during gestation with a modified live BVD vaccine.[1089] The BVD virus infects the developing germinal cells of the cerebellum and kills the Purkinje cells in the granular layer, resulting in necrosis and inflammation.[1090] Such cerebellar lesions tend to be most severe by 21 days after inoculation of the pregnant susceptible dams.[1087] The microscopic lesions include necrosis of the external germinal cells, focal parenchymal hemorrhages, and folial edema. After infection the acute inflammatory responses subside by 42 days, at which time the microscopic changes include cavities ranging from 1 to 7 mm in diameter, thinning of the neuropil, atrophy of the cerebellar folia, axonal torpedoes, and mild reactive astrocytosis. Calves infected with vaccine virus between 90 and 118 days of gestation may develop hydrocephalus and hydranencephaly.[1091]

The signs of cerebellar dysfunction usually are present at birth. They include truncal ataxia, falling backward, opisthotonos, base-wide stance, coarse intentional head tremors, hypermetria, hyperreflexia, and nystagmus or strabismus (Fig. 33-23).[1092,1093] If severely affected, the animal may be unable to stand or lie in sternal recumbency. Excitatory stimuli in these animals precipitate wild oscillations and side-to-side movements of the head, which can be mistaken for convulsions. The affected calves may have a deficient menace response and appear to be blind, especially with concomitant hydranencephaly or microphthalmia. The neurologic condition rarely improves after birth. Other fetal changes that may be induced by the BVD virus include thymic atrophy, retinal degeneration, corneal opacity, failure to grow, and abortion.[1087,1092] The diagnosis of cerebellar hypoplasia is based on identification of the specific clinical signs and the recognition of BVD antibodies in precolostral blood specimens. The virus may be cultured from the blood of some affected calves. Viral antigen has been detected in the spleen, kidneys, and lymph nodes of aborted fetuses.[1093] The virus cannot usually be isolated from immunocompetent calves after antiviral antibody responses develop but may be recovered repeatedly from immunoincompetent, seronegative calves. Bluetongue virus may also occasionally cause cerebellar lesions in calves and lambs.

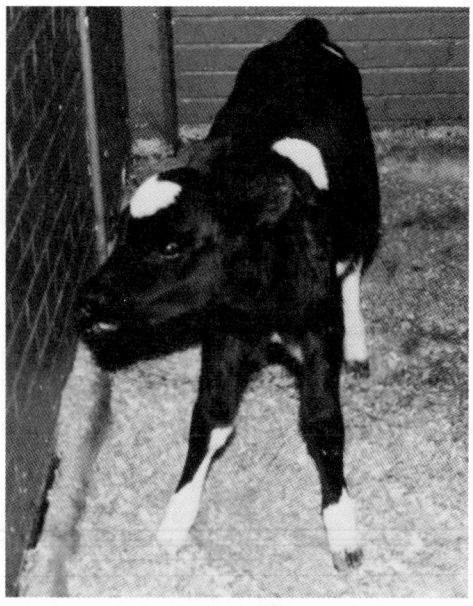

FIG. 33-23 ▮▮ Characteristic head position and base-wide stance of a calf with cerebellar hypoplasia.

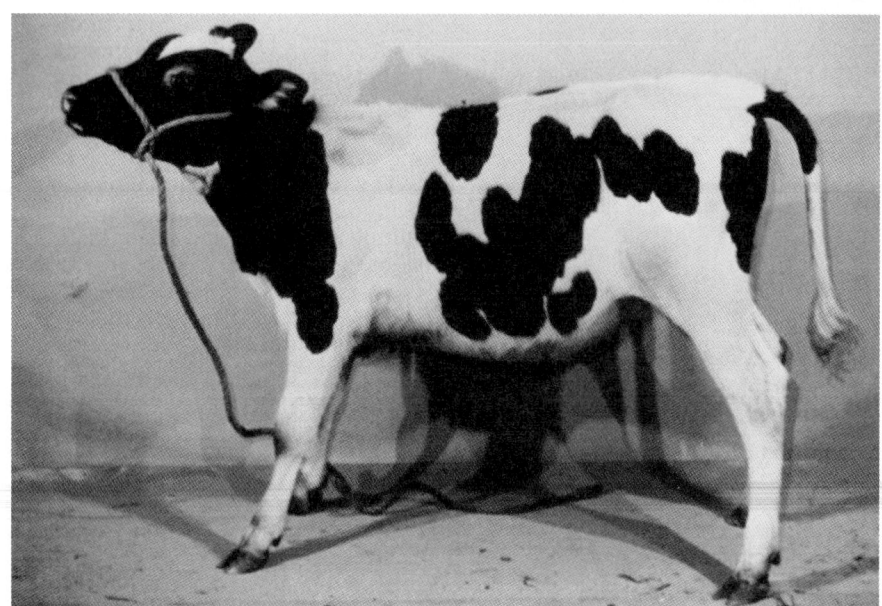

FIG. 33-24 ▮▮ Characteristic head posture and stance of a calf with cerebellar abiotrophy. (Courtesy Dr. R.H. Whitlock.)

REFERENCES

1087. Brown TT et al: Pathogenetic studies of infection of the bovine fetus with bovine viral diarrhea virus, *Vet Pathol* 11:486-505, 1974.

1088. Done JT et al: Bovine virus diarrhoea-mucosal disease virus: pathogenicity for the fetal calf following maternal infection, *Vet Rec* 106:473-479, 1980.

1089. Trautwein G et al: Studies on transplacental transmissibility of a bovine virus diarrhoea (BVD) vaccine virus in cattle. III. Occurrence of central nervous system malformations in calves born from vaccinated cows, *J Vet Med B* 33:260-268, 1986.

1090. Straver PJ, Journee DLH, Blinkhorst GJ: Neurological disorders, virus persistence, and hypomyelination in calves due to intrauterine infections with bovine virus diarrhea virus, *Vet Q* 5:156-164, 1983.

1091. Trautwein G et al: Cerebellar hypoplasia and hydranencephaly in cattle associated with transplacental BVD virus infection. In Harkness JW, ed: *Pestivirus infections of ruminants, CEC programme of coordination of research on animal husbandry,* Conference proceedings, Brussels, September 10-11, 1985, 1987, Commission of the European Communities.

1092. Ohmann BH: An oculocerebellar syndrome caused by congenital bovine viral diarrhoea virus-infection, *Acta Vet Scand* 25:36-49, 1984.

1093. Wilson TM, De Lahunta A, Confer L: Cerebellar degeneration in dairy calves: clinical, pathologic, and serologic features of an epizootic caused by bovine viral diarrhea virus, *J Am Vet Med Assoc* 183:544-547, 1983.

CEREBELLAR ABIOTROPHY OF CATTLE

Abiotrophy is defined as a degeneration of formed elements of the nervous system. Cerebellar abiotrophy occurs in 3- to 9-month-old Holstein, Angus, and Limousin heifers. The condition has been reported in the United States, Canada,[1094-1096] and Australia.[1097] In Holstein calves the condition has implicated a recessive mode of genetic inheritance, which can be traced to a single sire. The etiology of the condition in other breeds of cattle is uncertain. The calves may be normal at birth and remain so for 3 to 9 months or may show signs intermittently.[1097] Animals may be presented for treatment because they are in lateral recumbency and unable to rise. Nystagmus and opisthotonos are commonly seen in these calves. During the physical examination, signs of cerebellar dysfunction may be observed (Fig. 33-24); these include intentional head tremors, base-wide stance, hypermetria, hyperesthesia, hyperreflexia, and lack of menace with preservation of eyesight. The clinical condition of affected animals may remain static or

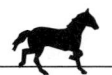

progress slowly until the animals become recumbent and unable to rise. The biochemical lesion of the disease is unknown. There are no macroscopic abnormalities of the cerebellum of affected calves. The microscopic pathologic changes of abiotrophy include noninflammatory focal loss of Purkinje cells and cerebellar nuclear neurons and gliosis in the Purkinje cell layer.

REFERENCES

1094. Johnson KR et al: Hereditary congenital ataxia in Holstein-Friesian calves, *J Dairy Sci* 41:1371-1375, 1958.
1095. White ME, Whitlock RH, De Lahunta A: A cerebellar abiotrophy of calves, *Cornell Vet* 65:476-491, 1975.
1096. Mitchell PJ et al: Cerebellar abiotrophy in Angus cattle, *Aust Vet J* 70:67-68, 1993.
1097. Woodman MP et al: Selective cerebellar degeneration in a Limousin-cross heifer, *Vet Rec* 132:586-587, 1993.

HEREDITARY HYPERMETRIA IN SHORTHORN CATTLE

A neurologic disease characterized by symmetric cerebellar signs was reported in 15 shorthorn cattle of Brazil. The animals were affected at birth, and the clinical disorder was not progressive. The affected animals had no pathologic changes in the central nervous system that differentiated the condition from cerebellar hypoplasia and cerebellar abiotrophy. Examination of the relatives of the affected animals indicated a familial distribution. Pedigree analysis suggested an autosomal recessive mode of inheritance.[1098]

REFERENCE

1098. Schild AL et al: Hereditary hypermetria in shorthorn cattle, *J Vet Diagn Invest* 5:640-642, 1993.

CEREBELLAR MALFORMATIONS OF AYRSHIRE CALVES

Cerebellar malformations have been reported in two Ayrshire calves from Great Britain.[1099] The calves appeared to be normal at birth but displayed characteristic signs of cerebellar dysfunction by 24 hours of age. A similar condition has been reported in Jersey calves.[1100] The clinical signs included opisthotonos, base-wide stance, truncal ataxia, hypermetria and hypertonia of all four limbs, and head tremors. The pathologic lesions in the calves were restricted to the cerebellum and the pons. The amount of cerebellar white matter was reduced. The cause of the condition was not definitely determined, but it initially was described as a hereditary condition. The relationship of this disease to bovine virus diarrhea virus infection is unclear.

REFERENCES

1099. McHowell J, Ritchie HE: Cerebellar malformations in two Ayrshire calves, *Pathol Vet* 3:159-168, 1966.
1100. Saunders LZ et al: Hereditary congenital ataxia in Jersey calves, *Cornell Vet* 42:559-591, 1952.

BOVINE FAMILIAL CONVULSIONS AND ATAXIA

Bovine familial convulsions and ataxia is a disease of Angus cattle characterized by multiple tetanic tonic-clonic convulsions and a spastic ataxia that persists for several months.[1101-1103] A similar condition was reported in a 9-month-old Charolais calf in the United States.[1104] Some authors have suggested that a defective autosomal dominant gene with incomplete penetrance is responsible for the condition, although others have identified affected animals that did not have a close relationship to affected blood lines.[1103] A similar condition has been reported in polled Hereford calves of Australia.[1105]

CLINICAL SIGNS. The onset of clinical signs ranges from 2 to 3 hours after birth to 3 months of age. Calves may be born dead at or near term or may be aborted. Some aborted calves show a dorsiflexion of the spine. Calves usually are born alive and subsequently show intermittent signs of cerebellar dysfunction and have multiple "tetaniform seizures" that last 3 to 12 hours. Two forms of seizures have been described. One form is characterized by a generalized stiffness and inability to protract the legs, elevation of the tail head, and head-neck extension with mild head tremor. The animals are hyperesthetic. A more severe form is characterized by lateral recumbency, loss of consciousness, opisthotonos, hypertonicity, tonic-clonic seizures, and trismus. The animals may improve markedly if supported during the tetaniform activity. The frequency of the seizures declines over several months, but the animal is left with a permanent ataxia that is characterized by classic cerebellar signs. The attacks may be precipitated by sudden violent auditory, olfactory, visual, or tactile stimuli. These could include driving by dogs, shipment, flashing light, loud sounds, or painful tactile stimulation. The animals do not respond to treatment with electrolytes, mineral supplements, or B-complex vitamin injections. The seizural activities can be controlled by administration of barbiturates or inhalational anesthetics.

Most animals improve when they are turned onto grass pastures, but episodic relapses associated with excitement may occur for as long as 2 years. Affected animals gradually recover and by 2 years of age either show only mild cerebellar signs or are completely normal. There are no specific diagnostic tests for the disease.

PATHOLOGY. It is difficult to explain the tetaniform seizures based on the pathologic findings. The gross appearance of the brain is normal. Microscopic lesions are restricted to the cerebellar cortex; they include swelling and vacuolation of the Purkinje cells, chromatolysis, loss of neurofibrils, and the formation of axonal torpedoes. The axonal structures have been defined as argyrophilic axonal swellings. They are located in the granular layer of the lingula, uvula, and adjacent parts of the vermis. The lesions may not be directly related to the onset of clinical signs because they are not seen in affected animals under 6 weeks of age or in recovered cases.[1106]

TREATMENT AND CONTROL. There is no known effective treatment. Affected animals can be fattened and slaughtered but should not be used as breeding stock because of the possibility that the disease is genetically transmitted.

REFERENCES

1101. Barlow RM: Morphogenesis of cerebellar lesions in bovine familial convulsions and ataxia, *Vet Pathol* 18:151-162, 1981.
1102. Barlow RM, Linklaeter KA, Young GB: Familial convulsions and ataxia in Angus calves, *Vet Rec* 83:60-65, 1968.
1103. Barlow RM: Further observations on bovine familial convulsions and ataxia, *Vet Rec* 105:91-94, 1979.
1104. Cho DY, Leipold HW: Cerebellar cortical atrophy in a Charolais calf, *Vet Pathol* 15:264-266, 1978.
1105. Whittington, Morton AG, Kennedy DF: Cerebellar abiotrophy in cross-bred cattle, *Aust Vet J* 66:12-15, 1989.
1106. Barlow RM et al: *Genetic cerebellar disorders in cattle in animal models of neurological disease*, London, 1980, Pittman Medical.

CEREBELLAR ABIOTROPHY (HYPOPLASIA) IN ARABIAN HORSES

MARY O. SMITH
LISLE W. GEORGE

Cerebellar abiotrophy occurs in purebred Arabian or Arabian crossbred horses.[1107-1112] Clinical signs may be present at birth or may develop after several weeks to months of postnatal life. Signs most commonly develop between 2 and 4 months of age and almost always occur before 6 months of age. The disease was initially reported as a cerebellar hypoplasia, but most descriptions suggest that the degeneration begins in the postnatal animal, prompting some authors to classify the condition as an abiotrophy.[1113] Other investigators have suggested that the clinical and pathologic course of the disease is not always consistent with a progressive postnatal degeneration of the nervous system.[1109]

The signs of cerebellar abiotrophy appear suddenly and range from subtle ataxia to complete diffuse cerebellar dysfunction. Head tremor is a commonly recognized sign and may occur in either a vertical or a horizontal direction. Some horses show no progression, whereas others have a slow progression for a time, followed by a plateau. The initial clinical sign in most foals is mild conscious proprioceptive deficits. As the deficits worsen, affected animals show hypertonia and stiff, hypermetric gaits that are accentuated by stimulation. In the most severe cases the animal may rear and fall over backward when suddenly startled. More severely affected animals have marked intentional head tremor, truncal ataxia, and hypermetria of all four limbs, often more pronounced in the forelimbs. These deficits are exaggerated by turning the animal sharply, by having the foal step up and down a curb, or by walking the foal on an incline. Most affected animals have a decreased to absent menace response despite normal visual acuity and facial nerve function; however, two affected foals with normal menace responses have been described.[1108,1110] Rotary nystagmus occurs in rare cases.

Diagnosis generally is made on the basis of typical clinical signs in an Arabian horse under 6 months of age. Differential diagnoses include head trauma (particularly associated with basisphenoid bone fracture) and atlantooccipital malformation. In the former case other evidence of head trauma usually is apparent, and signs of vestibular dysfunction often are present. In the latter case, foals are ataxic and somewhat weak but do not have intentional head tremors. Muscular strength is preserved in cerebellar abiotrophy. The cerebrospinal fluid (CSF) values in affected foals usually are normal, although creatine kinase occasionally is elevated.

The major histologic finding is a degeneration and loss of Purkinje cells in the cerebellum accompanied by gliosis and thinning of the molecular and granular layers of the cerebellum. Mineral deposits in the thalamus also are found in Arabian horses with cerebellar abiotrophy, but their significance and relationship to the cerebellar changes are unknown.[1112]

The cause of cerebellar hypoplasia in Arabians is unknown, but there is a familial pattern of occurrence. One survey has reported an 8% prevalence rate in one family of 36 foals and a 6% rate in another family of 67 foals.[1107] Two of four full sibling colts from a mare were affected.[1107] Pedigree analysis of 19 affected animals showed a high degree of relationship between the patients.

There is no effective treatment for cerebellar abiotrophy of Arabian foals. Occasional animals are reported to have shown gradual mild improvement, with considerable resolution of the head tremor. They remain unsafe for riding, however, and are not suitable as breeding stock because the disease probably is inherited. When recognized, the owners should be counseled about the probable hereditary nature of the disease and should be encouraged to discontinue use of the parent lineage as breeding stock.

REFERENCES

1107. Sponseller ML: Equine cerebellar hypoplasia and degeneration, *Proceedings of the Thirteenth Annual Convention of the American Association of Equine Practitioners*, 1967, pp 122-126.
1108. Fraser H: Two dissimilar types of cerebellar disorders in the horse, *Vet Rec* 78:1-5, 1966.
1109. Palmer AC, Blakemore WF, Whitwell KE: Cerebellar hypoplasia in degeneration in the young Arab horse: clinical and neuropathological features, *Vet Rec* 93:62-66, 1973.
1110. Beatty MT et al: Cerebellar disease in Arabian horses, *Proceedings of the Thirty-First Annual Meeting of the American Association of Equine Practitioners*, Toronto, 1985.
1111. Riber C, Blanco A, Castejon FM: Cerebellar abiotrophy: diagnosis of an Arabian horse in southern Spain, *J Equine Vet Sci* 11:178-179, 1991.
1112. DeBowes RM, Leipold HW, Turner-Beatty M: Cerebellar abiotrophy, *Vet Clin North Am (Equine Pract)* 3:345-352, 1987.
1113. De Lahunta A: Comparative cerebellar disease in domestic animals, *Compend Cont Educ Pract Vet* 8:8-19, 1980.

FAMILIAL ATAXIA IN HEREFORD CALVES

A central nervous system (CNS) disorder characterized by lateral recumbency, ataxia, incoordination, pupillary dilation, and abnormal head posture has been reported in Hereford calves.[1114] The disease occurred at 24 hours of age. The pathologic lesions could be differentiated from those of hereditary neuraxial edema and familial convulsions and ataxia of Angus cattle. The lesions in the Hereford calves included hypomyelination of the cerebellum, cerebral cortex, medulla, and midbrain and vacuolation of the white matter. No necrosis of the CNS or inflammatory lesions were seen, and the neurons of the cerebellum appeared to be normal. The cause of the condition was not identified, but the dams were highly related, and a genetic etiology was postulated.

REFERENCE

1114. Abid HN: Familial ataxia in Hereford calves, *Calif Vet* 37:28-29, 1983.

MICROGNATHIA AND CEREBELLAR HYPOPLASIA IN ANGUS CALVES

Micrognathia was observed in Angus calves of a small herd in western Missouri. These animals were born dead. The calves had severe brachygnathia and cerebellar hypoplasia. Other somatic changes included hepatomegaly and patent foramen ovale. A pedigree analysis indicated that an autosomal recessive genetic trait derived from a common ancestor may have been responsible for the condition.[1115]

REFERENCE

1115. Edmonds L, Crenshaw D, Shelby L: Micrognathia and cerebellar hypoplasia in an Aberdeen-Angus herd, *J Hered* 64:62-64, 1973.

STORAGE DISEASES AND INBORN ERRORS OF METABOLISM

Storage diseases and inborn errors of metabolism are characterized by intraneuronal accumulation of indigestible metabolic products. The material accumulates in the cells because of a deficient activity of one of several lysosomal catabolic enzymes. Neurons have a long life span and are rich in gangliosides and glycolipids, which are continuously degraded and resynthesized. In normal animals the metabolic products are internalized by the intraneuronal lysosomes and are degraded into constituent amino acids, monosaccharides, fatty acids, alcohols, and simple lipids by acidic catabolic enzymes. Disturbances of ganglioside metabolism result in accumulation of the degraded by-products in the neurons and other cells.[1116] Overloading of the lysosomes by the undigested material produces profound neurologic dysfunction.

Storage diseases can be classified as either genetic or acquired. Acquired storage diseases are caused by ingestion of plants that contain specific inhibitors of one or more lysosomal catabolic enzymes. Genetic storage diseases are caused by the production of an inactive lysosomal enzyme. One such storage disease, ceroid lipofuscinosis (see p. 941), was described earlier.

The genetic storage diseases are named according to the metabolic by-product that accumulates in the lysosomes.

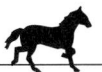

When tissues of affected animals are sectioned, processed, and examined microscopically, the metabolic storage product is dissolved from the tissue sections by the normal dehydrating and fixative agents. The spaces that contain the product appear as intraneuronal vacuoles when examined by light microscopy. Special fixation and staining procedures may be used to preserve and identify the metabolic product.[1116]

α-MANNOSIDOSIS (Pseudolipidosis)

α-Mannosidosis is a genetic defect of the enzyme α-mannosidase. The condition occurs in Angus, Murray Gray, Simmental, Galloway, and Holstein cattle.[1117] The disease is inherited as an autosomal recessive genetic trait. In animals deficient in α-mannosidase, the final cleavage between N-acetylglucosamine and mannose cannot occur, and the oligosaccharide accumulates in the lysosomes of the macrophages, neurons, and reticuloendothelial cells.[1116] The granules in the neuronal cell bodies contain mannose and N-acetylglucosamine tetrasaccharides at an equimolar ratio. These oligosaccharides can be detected using thin-layer chromatography of tissue extracts.

The clinical signs first appear by 1 week to 15 months of age. Affected calves tend to be less well developed than age-matched herd mates.[1118,1119] The first symptom usually is a mild ataxia of the pelvic limbs that develops after exercise. Other signs include mild intentional head tremor, hypermetria, base-wide stance, and unwarranted aggressiveness.[1118] When galloping the rear limbs are overflexed, and the animal's hindquarters appear to be sunken. The nervous signs become markedly worse when the animals are excited. Most patients develop diarrhea, become recumbent after 3 to 4 months, and die shortly thereafter. A few affected animals survive for as long as 4 years. The neurologic signs of these animals remain constant, but they usually fail to grow normally. Other clinical manifestations in calves include premature delivery, abortion, stillbirth, and superior brachygnathia. Mannosidosis in Galloway calves is associated with somatic abnormalities such as arthrogryposis, hydrocephalus, and hepatic and renal enlargement.[1117,1120] Phenotypic variations affect the severity and onset of the neurologic signs.

The concentration of α-mannosidase in the plasma can be measured with an enzymatic assay. Heterozygotes have less activity than genetically normal animals; however, occasional overlapping between the phenotypes of homozygotes and heterozygotes can confound attempts at classification. Three isoenzymes of α-mannosidase exist, but only one form is inactive in diseased animals. Delays in separation of the plasma from the cells or the use of serum for enzymatic assays results in a leakage of other isoenzymes from tissue compartments and causes uncertainty in interpretation of the results. In most cases two populations of animals usually are evident, the homozygous normal and the heterozygote. The mean plasma concentration of α-mannosidase in heterozygotes is 6.6 nmol/min/ml, whereas the mean plasma enzyme activity in homozygotes is 29.1 nmol/min/ml. The test is most accurate at detecting heterozygotes over 18 months of age.

The brain enzyme activity of heterozygotes ranges from 0.03 to 0.05 IU/g of tissue; the reference range of enzyme activity is 1.8 to 3.1 IU/g. Heterozygotes also may be detected by measuring the relative concentration of α-mannosidase and hexosaminidase in purified peripheral blood neutrophils. This test has been recommended for confirmation of a carrier animal whenever the plasma mannosidase assay is questionable.

PATHOLOGY. The diagnosis of a clinical case of mannosidosis can be substantiated pathologically by observation of cytoplasmic vacuolation in the neurons of the cerebrum, cerebellum, brainstem, and spinal cord.[1117] There is also a mild to marked internal hydrocephalus. The microscopic appearance of the brain of affected calves is characterized by vacuolation of the neurons and astrocytes and by reactive astrocytosis.[1117] The vacuolation is not restricted to the nervous system, however, and can be seen in the Kupffer cells, pancreatic exocrine cells, fibrocytes, and macrophages of the spleen and lymph nodes.[1121] The vacuoles are lined by a single membrane and are thought to be part of the Golgi apparatus.[1121] Associated neuronal changes include axonal swelling and spheroids.

Because of the hereditary nature of the disease, the ancestry of affected animals should be traced, and the biochemical phenotypes of related individuals should be tested. Heterozygotes are recognized by measuring a plasma α-mannosidase concentration below 30% to 40% of respective controls.[937] There is no effective treatment for α-mannosidosis of cattle.

REFERENCES

1116. Jolly RD, Blakemore WF: Inherited lysosomal storage diseases: an essay in comparative medicine, *Vet Rec* 92:391-400, 1973.
1117. Embury DH, Jerrett IV: Mannosidosis in Galloway calves, *Vet Pathol* 22:548-551, 1985.
1118. Jolly RD: Mannosidosis and its control in Angus and Murray Grey cattle, *N Z Vet J* 26:194-198, 1978.
1119. Healy PH, Harper PAW, Dennis JA: Phenotypic variation in bovine α-mannosidosis, *Res Vet Sci* 49:82-84, 1990.
1120. Borland NA, Jerrett IV, Embury DH: Mannosidosis in aborted and stillborn Galloway calves, *Vet Rec* 114:403-404, 1984.
1121. Jolly RD, Thompson KG: The pathology of bovine mannosidosis, *Vet Pathol* 15:141-152, 1978.

β-MANNOSIDOSIS

β-Mannosidosis is an autosomal recessive genetic trait of Anglo-Nubian goats and Salers calves. Mannosidosis in goats has a worldwide distribution, with reported cases occurring in Australia, Canada, and the United States.[1122-1126] The frequency of the condition is estimated to be approximately 1 of every 2000 births of purebred Salers calves. The disease is seen in both the red and black phenotypes of Salers.

The lesions of mannosidosis have been identified in aborted fetuses, and clinical signs are often present at birth.[1127-1130]

The clinical signs in goats include recumbency at birth, deafness, shortened sternum, narrowed palpebral fissures, decreased muscle mass, intentional head tremor, carpal contractures, pastern joint hyperextension, thickened skin, shortened head, excessive gingival tissue, short, curled ears, and domed-shaped skull.[1122,1131] Numerous ocular changes are seen, including pendular nystagmus, ventrolateral strabismus, thickened immovable eyelid, hazy vitreous humor, ptosis, and Horner's syndrome.[1132] The head movements are described as wide circular motions that culminate with the animal in lateral recumbency. Pupillary and corneal reflexes are intact, and the affected animals appear to have some vision. In comparison to goats, affected calves respond to aural and visual stimuli. Other neurologic abnormalities include recumbency, depression, loss of suckle reflex, spontaneous chewing activity, head tremors, depression, and nystagmus.

The diagnosis of β-mannosidosis is based on observation of characteristic microscopic lesions in the central nervous system (CNS), demonstration of decreased tissue β-mannosidase activity, and demonstration of mannose-based oligosaccharides (Nanβ1-4G1cNAc and Manβ1-4G1cNAcβ1-4G1cNAc) in the CNS.[1133] The concentration of serum thyroid hormones is decreased.[1134] Some affected calves have concomitant colisepticemia or bovine virus diarrhea infection.

In contrast to α-mannosidase, β-mannosidase has no isoenzymes.[1135] The mean concentration of β-mannosidase in the plasma of normal goats ranges from 66 to 222 nmol/hr/ml of plasma.[1128] There is no detectable β-mannosidase activity in the plasma of affected goats, and the activity in heterozygotes is intermediate between these ranges. The plasma concentrations of β-mannosidase in heterozygotes range from 43 to 64 nmol/hr/ml. These tests cannot be interpreted rigidly because there is significant variability among assays, storage conditions, and different age-groups of cattle.[1126]

In addition to the CNS abnormalities, cardiomegaly, thyromegaly, and pathologic fractures have been described in affected goats. Calves show a cerebral ventricular dilation and green discoloration of the renal cortices. Microscopic pathologic changes in the CNS include hypomyelination, axonal spheroids, and foamy-appearing neuronal cytoplasm.[1135] The heat shock protein ubiquitin has been detected in the CNS of affected calves.[1136] Cytoplasmic vacuolation also is present in the visceral organs.[1137,1138] There is no treatment for animals with β-mannosidosis.

REFERENCES

1122. Kumar K et al: Caprine β-mannosidosis: phenotypic features, *Fed Proc* 44:1592, 1985.
1123. Jolly RD et al: β-mannosidosis in a Salers calf: a new storage disease of cattle, *N Z Vet J* 38:102-105, 1990.
1124. Abbitt B et al: β-Mannosidosis in twelve Salers calves, *J Am Vet Med Assoc* 198:109-113, 1991.
1125. Healy PJ et al: β-mannosidosis in Salers calves in Australia, *Aust Vet J* 69:145, 1991.
1126. Cavanagh KT et al: Bovine plasma β-mannosidase activity and its potential for use for β-mannosidosis carrier detection, *J Vet Diagn Invest* 4:434- 440, 1992.
1127. Cavanagh MZ, Dawson G: Caprine β-mannosidosis inherited deficiency of β-D-mannosidase, *J Biol Chem* 256:5185-5188, 1981.
1128. Cavanagh K, Dunstan RW, Jones MZ: Plasma α- and β-mannosidase activities in caprine β-mannosidosis, *Am J Vet Res* 43:1058-1059, 1982.
1129. Jones MZ, Laine RA: Caprine oligosaccharide storage disease, *J Biol Chem* 256:5181-5184, 1981.
1130. Cavanagh K, Dunstan RW, Jones MZ: Measurement of caprine plasma β-mannosidase with a *p*-nitrophenyl substrate, *Am J Vet Res* 44:681-689, 1983.
1131. Kumar K et al: Caprine β-mannosidosis: phenotypic features, *Vet Rec* 118:325-327, 1986.
1132. Render JA et al: Ocular pathology of caprine β-mannosidosis, *Vet Pathol* 26:444-446, 1989.
1133. Jones MZ et al: Oligosaccharides accumulated in the bovine β-mannosidosis kidney, *J Inher Metab Dis* 15:57-67, 1992.
1134. Boyer PJ et al: Caprine β-mannosidosis, abnormal thyroid structure and function in a lysosomal storage disease, *Lab Invest* 63:100-106, 1990.
1135. Patterson JS et al: Neuropathology of bovine β-mannosidosis, *J Neuropathol Exp Neurol* 50:538-546, 1991.
1136. O'Toole DO et al: Ubiquinated inclusions in brains from Salers calves with β-mannosidosis, *Vet Pathol* 30:381-385, 1993.
1137. Lovell KL, Jones MZ: Axonal and myelin lesions in β-mannosidosis: ultrastructural characteristics, *Acta Neuropathol (Berl)* 65:293-299, 1985.
1138. Lovell KL, Jones MZ: Prenatal dysmyelogenesis in caprine β-mannosidosis: morphometric and ultrastructural studies of the optic nerve, *J Neuropathol Exp Neurol* 45:362, 1986.

GENERALIZED GLYCOGENOSIS (GM1 Gangliosidosis; β-Galactosidase Deficiency)

Generalized glycogenosis is a rare heritable defect of Holstein cattle and Suffolk sheep.[1139-1142] The condition in cattle is seen principally in Ireland. Generalized glycogenosis results from deficient activity of β-galactosidase, resulting in accumulation of the GM1 ganglioside, asialo-GM1, and neutral long-chain oligosaccharides in the tissues (Fig. 33-25).[1140]

A combined deficiency of β-galactosidase and α-neuraminidase has also been described.[1143] This condition is thought to result from a defect of the structural gene of β-galactosidase. The loss of α-neuraminidase occurs because of an inability of the β-galactosidase molecule to dimerize with α-neuraminidase, leading to deactivation of both molecules.

The clinical signs of all forms of β-galactosidase deficiency are similar. Affected animals tend to show lethargy and anorexia by 1 month of age. The head and neck are held low and rigidly extended. The animals are depressed, stiff, and ataxic, have a base-wide stance, appear to be blind, and eventually become recumbent. The animals tend to fall whenever the head is moved. The blindness is the result of dysmyeli-

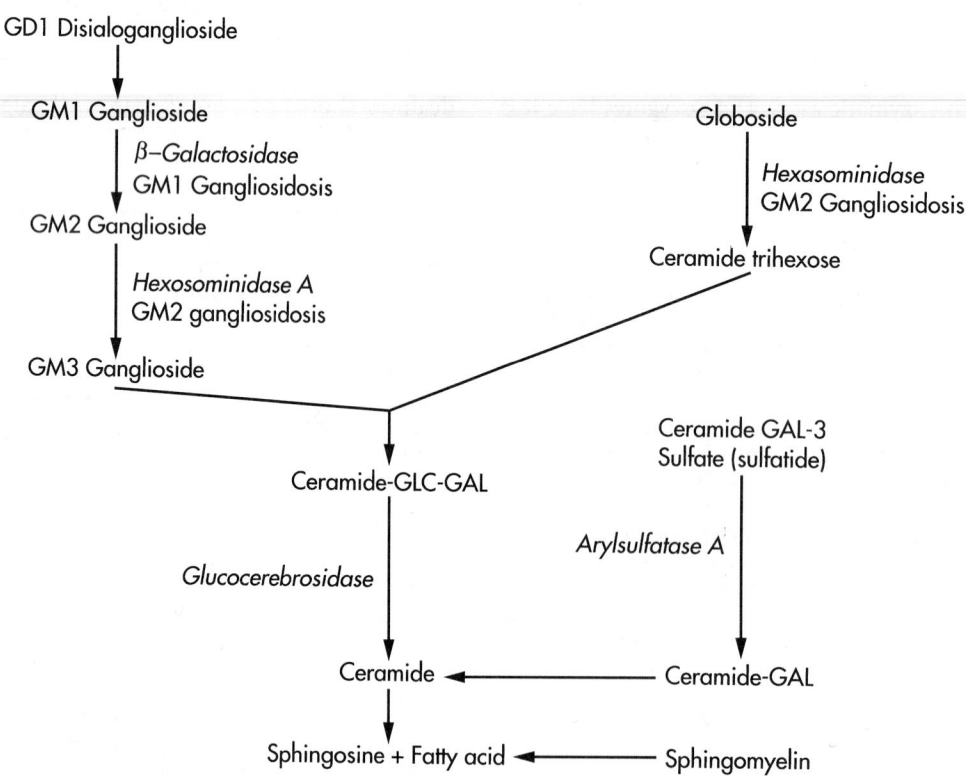

FIG. 33-25 ▥ Catabolic pathways for gangliosides. Relevant enzymes and diseases caused by enzyme deficiencies are shown in italics.

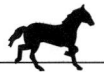

nation in the optic nerve, which can be detected by observation of numerous small white spots on the retina.

The genetic disorder is thought to be caused by an autosomal recessive gene. A biochemical test for β-galactosidase using centrifugally purified bovine neutrophils has been described.[1140] Animals with fewer than 3 U of heat-stable activity are considered deficient. In herds in which GM1 gangliosidosis has already been substantiated, observation of slowness in feeding and lack of alertness has proved to be diagnostically significant.

Pathologic changes of glucogenosis include neuronal enlargement, vacuolation, accumulation of granular material in the nerve cells, spheroids, and loss of neurons without gliosis.[1144] The material stains strongly with periodic acid-Schiff (PAS)/alcian blue, Sudan black, and oil red O. The vacuolar contents are composed of complex lipopolysaccharides, including β-galactose, N-acetylneuraminic acid and N-acetylgalactosamine.[1145]

REFERENCES

1139. Jolly RD, Hartley WJ: Storage diseases of domestic animals, *Aust Vet J* 53:1-8, 1977.
1140. Donnelly WJC, Kelly M, Sheahan BJ: Leukocyte β-galactosidase activity in the diagnosis of bovine GM1 gangliosidosis, *Vet Rec* 100:318-319, 1977.
1141. Murnane RD, Hartley WJ, Prieur DJ: Similarity of lectin histochemistry of a lysosomal storage disease in a New Zealand lamb to that of ovine GM1 gangliosidosis, *Vet Pathol* 28:332-335, 1991.
1142. Ahern AJ, Murnane RD, Prieur DJ: β-Galactosidase activity in fibroblasts and tissues from sheep with a lysosomal storage disease, *Biochem Gen* 26:733-846, 1988.
1143. Murnane RD, Ahern-Rindell AJ, Prieur DJ: Ovine GM1 gangliosidosis, *Small Rum Res* 6:109-118, 1991.
1144. Murnane RD et al: The lesions of an ovine lysosomal storage disease: initial characterization, *Am J Pathol* 134:263-270, 1989.
1145. Murnane RD, Ahern-Rindell AJ, Prieur DJ: Lectin histochemistry of an ovine lysosomal storage disease with deficiencies of β-galactosidase and α-neuraminidase, *Am J Pathol* 135:623-630, 1989.

BOVINE GENERALIZED GLYCOGENOSIS
(Type II Glycogenosis; Pompe's Disease)

Generalized glycogenosis results from a dysfunction of α-glucosidase. The condition occurs in shorthorn and Brahman cattle[1146,1147] and is controlled by a single recessive allele.[1148] Two separate clinical entities have been described, the cardiac (infantile) form and the late onset form. The clinical signs of the infantile form, which are first seen at approximately 2 to 3 months of age, include growth failure, weakness, hyperesthesia, muscle tremors, ataxia, conscious proprioceptive deficits, and recumbency.[1148] The cardiac form is characterized by right-sided heart failure at 3 to 5 months of age. Brahman calves with the late onset form die at 8 to 9 months of age, whereas affected shorthorn calves may survive for more than a year. The tissues of affected cattle contain only 2% to 5% of the normal α-glucosidase activity.[1148,1149] The concentration of glycogen in the liver and muscles is increased.

The pathologic lesions of the central nervous system (CNS) in both forms are similar to those of cattle with α-mannosidosis; they include cytoplasmic swelling and foamy cytoplasm in the neurons of the CNS. Lesions are found in the myocardium and skeletal muscle. These include vacuolation and swelling of the Purkinje cells and myofibers.[1150] Because of a gene dilution effect, the activity of α-glucosidase in peripheral blood lymphocytes can be used to detect asymptomatic heterozygotes.[1151] However, the test result may be falsely positive if the animals are ingesting seeds of *Castanospermum australe* (Moreton Bay chestnut trees). The seeds of this tree have an α-glucosidase antagonist.

REFERENCES

1146. O'Sullivan BM et al: Generalized glycogenosis in Brahman cattle, *Aust Vet J* 57:227-229, 1981.

1147. Richards RB et al: Bovine generalized glycogenosis, *Neuropathol Appl Neurobiol* 3:45-46, 1977.
1148. McHowell J et al: Infantile and late onset form of generalized glycogenosis type II in cattle, *J Pathol* 134:266-277, 1981.
1149. Cook RD et al: Bovine generalized glycogenosis: a model for human disease, *J Neuropathol Exp Neurol* 37:603, 1978.
1150. Di Marco PN, McHowell J, Dorling PR: Bovine glycogenosis type II: biochemical and morphological characteristics of skeletal muscle in culture, *Neuropathol Appl Neurobiol* 10:379-395, 1984.
1151. McPhee CP, Reichmann KG: A genetic analysis of lysosomal enzyme activities in Brahman cattle, *Aust J Agric Res* 41:205-211, 1990.

GLOBOID CELL LEUKODYSTROPHY
(Krabbe's Disease)

LISLE W. GEORGE

Globoid cell leukodystrophy has been reported in polled Dorset sheep.[1152] The genetic defect is the result of a lack of galactocerebrosidase, which produces a high concentration of galactocerebroside in myelin. The clinical signs are seen by 4 months of age. Affected animals show depression, hypersensitivity, conscious proprioceptive deficits, slight tremor of the head and neck, exaggerated patellar reflex, incoordination, and tetraplegia. The activity of the tissue galactocerebrosidase can be measured to substantiate the clinical diagnosis.

REFERENCE

1152. Pritchard DH, Bapthine DV, Sinclair AJ: Globoid cell leukodystrophy in polled Dorset sheep, *Vet Pathol* 17:399-405, 1980.

NEURONAL LIPODYSTROPHY

Neuronal lipodystrophy occurs in Angus and Beefmaster calves and in sheep.[1153-1155] The biochemical lesion of the condition is unknown. The clinical signs, which are first seen at approximately 10 months of age, include depression, blindness, ataxia, circling, coma, and tonic-clonic convulsions. The pathologic lesions include neuronal vacuolation with eosinophilic and sudanophilic inclusions. The inclusions are cytoplasmic and perinuclear and are located in the axonal and dendritic zones. As with other neurovisceral storage diseases, the inclusions are bound by a single membrane. Involvement of the spleen and lymph nodes also can be demonstrated. The mode of inheritance is unknown. There is no effective treatment for the disease.

REFERENCES

1153. Read WK, Bridges CH: Neuronal lipodystrophy occurrence in an inbred strain of cattle, *Pathol Vet* 6:235-243, 1969.
1154. Hartley WJ, Kater JC: Observations on diseases of the central nervous system of sheep in New Zealand, *N Z Vet J* 10:128-142, 1962.
1155. Whittem JH, Walker D: "Neuronopathy" and "pseudolipidosis" in Aberdeen-Angus calves, *J Pathol Bacteriol* 74:281-288, 1957.

SHAKER CALF SYNDROME

Shaker calf syndrome is an inherited neurodegenerative disorder of newborn horned Hereford calves.[1156] The condition is characterized by recumbency, fine tremors of the neck and hind limbs, and hypermetria. The amplitude and frequency of the tremors are increased by stimulation. Other clinical signs include aphonia, loss of fine motor control of the tongue, hyperesthesia, exaggerated spinal reflexes, and hypertonia. Most affected calves die of starvation by 5 days of life; however, one case of remission followed by relapse after 2 weeks has been described. The cause of the disease is unknown. Limited breeding trials indicate a 12.5% inbreeding factor in affected calves, suggesting a hereditary etiology. The pathologic lesions include a neurofilamentous neuronal degeneration of multiple cell groups of the central nervous system and of ganglion cells of the peripheral and autonomic nervous systems. The spinal cord is most severely affected.

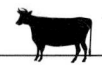

Neuronal degenerative changes include distention of axons and dendrites by a faintly fibrillar material, neuronophagia, and reactive gliosis. Wallerian degeneration of the spinal rootlets, spheroids, and empty fiber tracts in the spinal cord are noted. The pathologic appearance of the tissues differs from that of calves with hereditary neuraxial edema.

REFERENCE
1156. Rousseaux CG et al: Shaker calf syndrome: a newly recognized inherited neurodegenerative disorder of horned Hereford calves, *Vet Pathol* 22:104-111, 1985.

MAPLE SYRUP URINE DISEASE (Spongiform Encephalopathy)

MARY O. SMITH
LISLE W. GEORGE

Maple syrup urine disease is a hereditary spongiform encephalopathy characterized by severe central nervous system (CNS) disturbance in newborn Hereford and polled shorthorn calves.[1157] The disease has been reported in Australia and Canada and possibly has been seen in the United States.[1158] The biochemical lesion is a deficiency of branched-chain 2-oxo acid dehydrogenase, which results in accumulation of the 2-oxo acids 4-methyl-2-oxopentanoate, 3-methyl-2-oxobutanoate, (S)-(S-KMV), and (R)-3-methyl-2-oxopentanoate, and their precursors leucine, valine, isoleucine and alloisoleucine.[1157,1159,1160] The urine becomes highly viscous, discolored, and malodorous because of the excretion of these substances through the kidneys. The buildup of the transamination product of isoleucine, α-keto-β-methylvaleric acid, probably gives the urine the odor of burnt maple syrup. The toxic metabolite in the CNS is likely to be α-keto-isocaproic acid, which interferes with pyruvate production, although high levels of leucine also have been shown to be directly neurotoxic and result in behavioral abnormalities.[1161] Pyruvate is a vital constituent of the Krebs cycle, which is important for the production of transmitter amino acids. The CNS hyperactivity probably is related to a decrease in γ-aminobutyric acid–mediated inhibitory transmission. The genetic defect in polled shorthorns and polled Herefords has been shown to be a thymidine to cytidine transition in the cDNA coding for a subunit of the branched-chain amino acid dehydrogenase, resulting in a substitution of leucine for proline.[1162] Polymerase chain reaction (PCR) testing now can be used to detect both affected and carrier animals.

Affected calves are born normal but are depressed by 2 to 3 days. They also are febrile (temperature of 39.5° to 42° C [103.1° to 107.6° F]). They initially show ataxia and depression and become recumbent by the second to third day of life. At that time, they show hyperesthesia, opisthotonos, muscular rigidity, myoclonic limb jerks, nystagmus, repetitive head tremors, stimulus-induced tetanic spasms, blepharospasm, generalized decrease of spinal reflexes, and convulsions. The urine has the characteristic color and odor reminiscent of burnt maple syrup. The calves usually die by 5 to 10 days of age. The presence of ketoacids can be detected by mixing urine with dinitrophenylhydrazine and observing a faint yellow precipitate.[1163]

The clinical presentation of maple syrup urine disease differs from that of hereditary neuraxial edema.[1158] Calves with neuraxial edema have extensor rigidity but tend to be bright and alert, whereas calves with maple syrup urine disease have rigid extensor tonus and obtundation. These differential features appear to be significant because it is likely that the original reports of hereditary neuraxial edema included calves with maple syrup urine disease.[1164]

Spongiform changes caused by intramyelinic vacuolation are present in the brains of affected calves in both white and gray matter.[1165] The disorder can be definitively diagnosed by measuring the ratio of isoleucine, leucine, and valine to α-aminobutyric acid in fixed tissues and finding increased concentrations of these amino acids or their corresponding branched chain 2-keto acids in urine or blood.[1165] Heterozygotes have normal blood and urine levels of both amino acids and keto acids. PCR analysis of DNA extracted from hair root samples can identify both homozygote affected animals and the clinically normal heterozygote carriers of the disease.[1166-1168] Pharmacologic dosages of thiamine are beneficial for treatment of the disease in some human beings, probably by increasing mitochondrial thiamin diphosphate, which promotes the activity of the branched-chain α-keto acid dehydrogenase complex.[1169] However, there is no known effective treatment for maple syrup urine disease in calves.[1157,1158]

REFERENCES
1157. Elsas LJ, Danner DJ: The role of thiamine in maple syrup urine disease, *Ann NY Acad Sci* 77:404-419, 1982.
1158. Harper PAW, Healy JA, Dennis JA: Maple syrup urine disease as a cause of spongiform encephalopathy in calves, *Vet Rec* 119:62-65, 1986.
1159. Harper PAW et al: Maple syrup urine disease in calves: a clinical, pathological and biochemical study, *Aust Vet J* 66:46-49, 1989.
1160. Schadewaldt P et al: Renal clearance of branched-chain L-amino and 2-oxo acids in maple syrup urine disease, *J Inher Metab Dis* 22:706-722, 1999.
1161. Mello CF et al: Chronic early leucine administration induces behavioral deficits in rats, *Life Sci* 65:747-755, 1999.
1162. Dennis JA, Healy PJ: Definition of the mutation responsible for maple syrup urine disease in poll shorthorns and genotyping poll shorthorns and polled Herefords for maple syrup urine disease alleles, *Res Vet Sci* 67:1-6, 1999.
1163. Chuang DT, Shih V: Disorders of branched-chain amino acid and ketoacid metabolism. In Stanbury JB, Wyngaarden JB, Frederickson DS, eds: *The metabolic basis of inherited disease*, ed 4, New York, 1995, McGraw Hill.
1164. Cordy DR, Richards WPC, Stormont C: Hereditary neuraxial edema of calves, *N Z Vet J* 23:181, 1975.
1165. Harper PAW, Healy PJ, Dennis JA: Ultrastructural findings in maple syrup urine disease in polled Hereford calves, *Acta Neuropathol (Berl)* 71:316-320, 1986.
1166. Baird JD et al: Maple syrup urine disease in five Hereford calves in Ontario, *Can Vet J* 28:505-511, 1987.
1167. Healy PJ, Dennis JA: Heterozygote detection for maple syrup urine disease in cattle, *Aust Vet J* 72:392, 1995.
1168. Healy PJ, Dennis JA, Moule JF: Use of hair root as a source of DNA for the detection of heterozygotes for recessive defects in cattle, *Aust Vet J* 72:346-348, 1995.
1169. Blair PV et al: Dietary thiamine level influences levels of its diphosphate form and thiamine-dependent enzymatic activities of rat liver, *J Nutr* 129:641-648, 1999.

HEREDITARY NEURAXIAL EDEMA (Congenital Myoclonus; Doddler Syndrome)

LISLE W. GEORGE

Neuraxial edema is an inherited neurologic disease of newborn calves. Polled and horned Herefords and Hereford-Friesian crossbred cattle are affected.[1170-1177] An autosomal recessive genetic trait is thought to be responsible for the condition. The disease is well defined clinically and pathologically[1174,1177]; however, some investigators have reported a disease of polled Hereford calves that has similar neurologic signs yet does not result in status spongiosis or edema of the central nervous system (CNS). These calves had a high frequency of bilateral slippage of the capital femoral epiphysis, subluxation of the femoral head, and acetabular articular cartilage fractures.[1175] The authors named the condition congenital myoclonus to differentiate it from hereditary neuraxial edema. Calves with congenital myoclonus have a shorter gestational length than normal.

The earliest reports of hereditary neuraxial edema also described two clinical forms in which some calves were bright, alert, and responsive and others had a severely depressed sensorium. Subsequent studies suggested that the calves with systemic depression probably had maple syrup urine disease, and those with normal sensorium had hereditary neuraxial edema.

The clinical signs of hereditary neuraxial edema include hyperesthesia and myoclonic discharges of skeletal musculature that occur either spontaneously or in response to tactile, visual, or auditory stimuli. The calves are stillborn or are affected at birth. Affected calves are of normal size but are unable to rise; they lie quietly without lifting the head.[1170-1173] These calves develop marked extensor tonus and clonic spasms of the limbs and head when stimulated. During the spasm the animals become transiently apneic and remain dyspneic for several minutes afterward.[1174] The spasms are less severe after repeated stimulation. Between spasms the patients can stand with assistance, but the proprioceptive responses are markedly altered, and the animals fall when support is withdrawn.[1173] The sensorium and suckling reflexes are unaltered when the calves are not in a spasmodic episode. Some authors have reported that vision and cranial nerve function are unimpaired, but others have reported nystagmus in some calves.[1170,1174] Administration of anticonvulsant drugs does not ameliorate the clinical signs. Pathologic lesions usually are not seen in the CNS of affected calves.[1171] The condition has an autosomal recessive mode of inheritance. Recent studies have indicated that the hereditary neuraxial edema is caused by a defect in the postsynaptic glycinergic receptors in the inhibitory interneurons of the spinal cord.[1178]

REFERENCES

1170. Duffell SJ: Neuraxial oedema of Hereford calves with and without hypomyelinogenesis, *Vet Rec* 118:95-98, 1986.
1171. Harper PAW, Healy PJ, Dennis JA: Inherited congenital myoclonus of polled Hereford calves (so-called neuraxial oedema): a clinical, pathological and biochemical study, *Vet Rec* 119:59-62, 1986.
1172. Cho DY, Leipold HW: Hereditary neuraxial edema in polled Hereford calves, *Pathol Res Pract* 163:158-162, 1978.
1173. Davis GB, Thompson EJ, Kyle RJ: Hereditary neuraxial oedema of calves, *N Z Vet J* 23:181, 1975.
1174. Cordy DR, Richards WPC, Stormont C: Hereditary neuraxial edema in Hereford calves, *Pathol Vet* 6:487-501, 1969.
1175. Healy PJ, Harper PAW, Bowler JK: Prenatal occurrence and mode of inheritance of neuraxial oedema in polled Hereford calves, *Res Vet Sci* 38:96-98, 1985.
1176. Blood DC, Gay CC: Hereditary neuraxial edema in calves, *Aust Vet J* 47:520, 1971.
1177. Jolly RD: Congenital brain oedema of Hereford calves, *J Pathol* 114:199-204, 1974.
1178. Gundlach AL et al: Deficit of spinal cord glycine/strychnine receptors in inherited myoclonus of polled Hereford calves, *Science* 241:1897-1801, 1988.

INHERITED MYOCLONUS OF PERUVIAN PASO FOALS

LISLE W. GEORGE

Inherited myoclonus is a disorder of Peruvian Paso foals that is characterized by myoclonic contractions of the musculature in response to auditory or tactile stimuli.[1179] These contractions are sustained with repeated stimulation. Some animals are ambulatory but have a "rabbit hopping" gait. Some animals are recumbent. If assisted, the foals can rise and walk, and the animals are not depressed. Analeptic drugs and tranquilizers are ineffective for controlling this condition. Inherited myoclonus is associated with a specific deficiency of spinal glycine receptors, which are responsible for synaptic inhibition in the central nervous system. Glycine is a major inhibitory transmitter and works through the Ia afferent neurons in the ventral columns and the Renshaw cells. Loss of the receptors results in uninhibited synaptic transmission.

REFERENCE

1179. Gundlach AL et al: Deficit of inhibitory glycine receptors in spinal cord from Peruvian Pasos: evidence for an equine form of inherited myoclonus, *Brain Res* 628:263-270, 1993.

CONGENITAL ENCEPHALOMYELOPATHY IN QUARTER HORSES

Congenital encephalomyelopathy has been described in quarter horse foals.[1180] The condition occurred in three foals born to two different mares and three unrelated stallions. The condition was seen at birth, and clinical signs include recumbency and coarse tremors of the rear limbs. When assisted into a standing position, the rear quarters bounced off the ground. The forelimb function appeared normal; however, the patellar reflexes were exaggerated. Affected foals are bright, alert, and responsive and have intact pain perception. There are no macroscopic lesions of the central nervous system. Microscopic lesions include spongiform degeneration and axonal swelling of the white matter of the medulla, spinocerebellar, and spinothalamic tracts. The lesions extend through the entire length of the ventral funiculi of the spinal cord.

REFERENCE

1180. Seahorn TL et al: Congenital encephalomyelopathy in a quarter horse, *Equine Vet J* 23:394-395, 1991.

LOCOWEED POISONING (*Astragalus* and *Oxytropis* Poisoning; Locoism)

DEFINITION AND ETIOLOGY. Chronic ingestion of plants of the *Astragalus* and *Oxytropis* genera (Table 33-13) results in an acquired neurovisceral storage disease.[1181,1182] Horses are most susceptible to the intoxication, but cattle, sheep, and goats also can be affected. Locoweeds grow in the western United States, Canada, Mexico, and Australia. In Australia, poisoning by the darling pea (*Swainsona* spp.) causes a disease similar to locoweed intoxication.[1183]

Conditions that promote locoweed poisoning are hot, dry weather and a scarcity of alternative forage. Chronically exposed livestock become habituated and feed selectively on the plant over successive grazing seasons.[1184]

Several toxic components have been identified:
- Locoine, swansonine n-oxide, and indolizidine alkaloids,[1182,1183] which interfere with α-mannosidase activity
- Aminonitrile, a compound that caused abortion and teratogenesis
- Miserotoxin, a compound that causes a respiratory disease complex
- Selenium accumulation (selenium toxicity may contribute to the neurotoxicity and fetal deformities)

Oxytropis and *Astragalus* plants are legumes that have herbaceous stems and alternate pinnately compound leaves.[1185] The fruits are characteristic leguminous pods that contain kidney-shaped seeds with pods marked by characteristic longitudinal grooves.[1185] The plant is eaten because it is the first

---

TABLE 33-13

Species of *Astragalus* and *Oxytropis* Found in the Western United States

Scientific Name	Common Name
Oxytropis sericea	White locoweed, point locoweed
Oxytropis lambertii	Purple locoweed
Oxytropis campestris	Yellow locoweed
Astragalus argillophilus	Halfmoon locoweed
Astragalus bisculatus	Two-grooved milk vetch
Astragalus earlei	Earles locoweed
Astragalus lentiginosus	Speckled, spotted locoweed
Astragalus mollissimus	Wooly locoweed
Astragalus mothoxys	Sheep locoweed
Astragalus wootnii	Wooton locoweed

From Knight AP: *Compend Cont Educ Pract Vet* 9:F418-F420, 1987.

vegetation available in the spring. The *Oxytropis* and *Astragalus* species found in the United States are listed in Table 33-13. Symptoms do not usually develop in cattle until 3 weeks after the animals first begin grazing the plant and may not occur until long after ingestion of the plant has stopped. The toxicity of the locoweed may vary from year to year. Despite its relative unpalatability, some sheep may become habituated to the plant and selectively eat forage containing up to 20% *Astragalus* plants.[1184]

CLINICAL SIGNS. Experimentally poisoned horses show clinical signs by 21 days after continuous ingestion of the plant. The clinical signs include ataxia, conscious proprioceptive deficits, and depression, with alternating periods of frenzied or maniacal activity. At rest the horses show intentional head tremor, flaccidity of the nose and lips, repetitive movements with the lips and tongue, and dysphagia.[1186] High-stepping, stringhalt-like gaits have been described in some horses.[1186] The clinical signs worsen markedly when affected horses are handled or transported. Tranquilization usually is ineffective for controlling the apparent hyperexcitability. Horses that survive locoweed poisoning retain an altered behavior.

Neurologic signs in adult cattle include conscious proprioceptive deficits, hypermetria, weakness, depression, dull, staring eyes, and loss of herding instinct. Heavy losses from abortions or malformed calves have also been described. The indolizidine alkaloids are secreted in the milk and may cause unthriftiness and weak suckling behavior in calves. Calves that have been exposed to the toxin in utero are weak and fail to thrive. Some may have flexural contractions of the limbs and lateral rotation of the carpus.[1187-1190] Ingestion of locoweed by certain cattle at high altitudes may result in the development of cor pulmonale.[1187,1188]

Poisoned sheep have a star-gazing attitude and appear to be blind, nervous, and stiff. The normal flocking behavior is absent.[1183] Affected sheep may exhibit ptyalism. Testicular atrophy in rams has been reported.[1191] Affected animals have intercurrent pyogenic infections such as pneumonia, keratoconjunctivitis, and footrot. This is thought to be related to the immunosuppressive effect of the plant on the T lymphocytes.[1192] Many cattle with mild signs of locoweed poisoning recover completely by 60 days after removal from the offending pastures. Ruminants with advanced chronic intoxication apparently have permanent loss of neural tissue.

CLINICAL PATHOLOGY. Microscopic examination of stained blood smears may reveal the presence of vacuolation in the cytoplasm of the lymphocytes. These changes are diagnostic in animals with characteristic clinical signs and historic evidence of exposure.

PATHOLOGY. The microscopic abnormalities of the soft tissues of acutely poisoned animals are similar to those of the lysosomal storage diseases of cattle; they include cytoplasmic vacuolation of the neurons and other cells.[1186] Vacuolation of renal tubular epithelial cells may occur as early as 4 days after the start of daily feeding of 0.34 kg of locoweed to horses.[1193] Pulmonary lesions that have been associated with chronic ingestion of locoweeds and that may predispose the patient to high altitude disease (brisket disease) in cattle (see Chapter 29) include alveolar emphysema, bronchiolar constriction and hypertrophy, and interlobular edema and fibrosis. In animals that have been chronically poisoned by locoweed, the vacuolation disappears in all tissues except the cytoplasm of the cerebellar Purkinje cells. Pyloric or gastric ulcers have been reported in affected cattle.[1190,1193] Placental edema, fetal ascites, and hydrops allantois have been described in pregnant exposed cattle.

TREATMENT. There is no known effective long-term therapy for locoweed poisoning. Animals remain affected for a prolonged period after removal from the plants. Some authors have recommended the use of either tranylcypromine, a monoamine oxidase inhibitor, (60 mg PO) and protryptyline (60 mg PO) or reserpine (3.125 g/500 kg IM once or 1.25 mg PO per animal once daily) for treatment of chronically affected animals.[1194] However, the efficacy of these treatments is unknown.

PREVENTION. Nonaddicted livestock normally do not eat locoweed if other forage is available. The intoxication may be prevented by supplemental feeding during the early spring and late summer.

REFERENCES

1181. Van Kampen KR, James LF: Pathology of locoweed *(Astragalus lentiginosus):* sequential development of cytoplasmic vacuolation in tissues, *Pathol Vet* 7:503-508, 1970.
1182. Molyneux RJ, James LF: Loco intoxication: indolizidine alkaloids of spotted locoweed *(Astragalus lentiginosus), Science* 216:190-191, 1982.
1183. Dorling RR, Huxtable CR, Colegate SM: Inhibition of lysosomal α-mannosidase by swainsonine, and indolizidine alkaloid isolated from *Swainsona canescens, Biochem J* 191:649-651, 1980.
1184. Ralphs MH, Panter KE, James LF: Feed preferences and habituation of sheep poisoned by locoweed, *J Anim Sci* 68:1354-1362, 1990.
1185. Knight AP: Locoweed poisoning, *Compend Cont Educ Pract Vet* 9:F418-F420, 1987.
1186. Haries WN, Baker FP, Johnston A: An outbreak of locoweed poisoning in horses in southwestern Alberta, *Can Vet J* 13:141-145, 1972.
1187. James LF, Van Kampen KR, Binns W: Sequence in the abortive and teratogenic effects of locoweed fed to sheep, *Am J Vet Res* 30:377-380, 1969.
1188. James LF et al: Locoweed *(Oxytropis sericea)* poisoning and congestive heart failure in cattle, *J Am Vet Med Assoc* 189:1549-1556, 1986.
1189. James LF, Hartley WJ: Effects of milk from animals fed locoweed on kittens, calves, and lambs, *Am J Vet Res* 38:1263-1265, 1977.
1190. James LF, Van Kampen KR, Staker GR: Locoweed *(Astragalus lentiginosus)* poisoning in cattle and horses, *J Am Vet Med Assoc* 155:525-530, 1969.
1191. James LF, Van Kampen KR: Effects of locoweed intoxication on the genital tract of the ram, *Am J Vet Res* 32:1253-1256, 1971.
1192. Sharma RP, James LF, Molyneux RJ: Effect of repeated locoweed feeding on peripheral lymphocytic function and plasma proteins in sheep, *Am J Vet Res* 45:2090-2093, 1984.
1193. James LF, Van Kampen KR: Acute and residual lesions of locoweed poisoning in cattle and horses, *J Am Vet Med Assoc* 158:614-618, 1971.
1194. Staley EE: An approach to treatment of locoism in horses, *Vet Med Small Anim Clin* 73:1205-1206, 1978.

GRASS STAGGERS

Grass staggers is caused by a number of related products of plant or fungal metabolism. These compounds appear to have a universal activity at the γ-aminobutyric acid (GABA) receptor of the internuncial neurons, therefore intoxication causes clinical signs characteristic of released inhibition. The structural backbone of these toxins permits the molecules to bind to GABA receptors, thereby inactivating them. Some associated plant or fungal toxins also induce other physiologic effects, including agalactia, fever, and low productivity because of a prolactin-like effect.

RYEGRASS STAGGERS

Perennial Ryegrass Staggers

Ingestion of toxic stands of perennial ryegrass *(Lolium perenne)* results in ataxia and tremors in horses, cattle, and sheep. The condition is recognized in livestock of New Zealand, Australia, Northern Europe, the United States, South America, and Great Britain.[1195-1210] The case attack rate may reach 100%, but the mortality rate is typically less than 50%.[1204] Conditions that favor toxicity include late seasonal growth, ambient temperatures over 23° C (73.4° F), and closely grazed pastures. For these reasons, the disease is seen

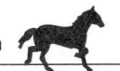

exclusively between June and September and between December and June in the northern and southern hemispheres, respectively. The condition may appear 5 to 10 days after grazing on highly toxic pastures. For a pasture to develop toxicity, the ryegrass must constitute a majority of the forage growth.

Perennial ryegrass produces tremorgenic toxins when infested with the endophytic fungus *Acremonium loliae* or *Acremonium coenophialum*. The fungal infection confers resistance to the Argentine stem weevil; therefore there is a selective pressure for toxigenic cultivars. Strains of *Acremonium*-resistant ryegrass have been propagated but are difficult to maintain because of the devastating effects of the stem weevil infestation. The chemicals produced by *Acremonium*-infected plants are classed as indole terpenes. These compounds are chemically related to the fungal tremorgens, penitrem A and fumotremogen. A number of separate toxic compounds have been isolated. These include lolitrems A and B, paxilline, and peramine. Paxilline is a biosynthetic precursor of lolitrem B. Lolitrem B is related chemically to peramine. Peramine has the major antagonistic effects against the Argentine stem weevil. The lolitrems have the greatest tremorgenic effect on livestock.[1211] Concentrations of more than 2000 ppb of lolitrem B in forage or 1.68 mg/kg of forage have been associated with toxicity for sheep and cattle, respectively.[1212] The concentration of lolitrem varies seasonally in the same grass, and toxic pastures may become nontoxic over the course of the grazing season.[1213]

There also is a relationship between the frequency of poisonings and the proportion of plants infested by the *Acremonium* fungus. Infection rates below 25% are associated with sporadic cases, whereas plots containing 90% infection rates are associated with large outbreaks of staggers. Intoxication is most common on dry pastures where the perennial ryegrass is growing slowly under relatively low ambient temperatures. The *Acremonium* fungus can be identified by microscopic examination of boiled leaves. The fungus is in greatest prevalence in the summer and is found in the uppermost part of the leaf. To identify the fungus, the ryegrass leaves are immersed in a stain containing 0.06 g aniline blue in 50 ml of lactic acid in 250 ml of distilled water, 50 ml of glycerine, and 50 g of phenol. The mixture is boiled 5 minutes and mounted in lactophenol (20 g of phenol, 16.7 ml of lactic acid, 40 ml of glycerine, and 20 ml of water). For biologic assay of lolitrem, chloroform: methanol extracts of suspect plants are injected into mice. The recipients are then examined every few hours for tremors.

The endophyte-infested grasses also produce ergovaline or other ergopeptine alkaloids that exert prolactin-like activity. The resulting clinical signs are diarrhea, fever, tachypnea, and reduced live weight gains.

High peramine, low lolitrem cultivars of *Lolium** have been propagated. Such cultivars have partial protection against the stem weevil but do not cause staggers in pastured animals.[1214]

Annual Ryegrass Staggers

Annual ryegrass toxicity is caused by corynetoxin, which is manufactured in the seed heads of annual ryegrass *(Lolium rigidium)* and related grasses. The seed head is infested by the nematode *Anguina agrostis (Anguina funesta)*. The parasitic infestation forms a gall that becomes secondarily infected by the bacterium *Clavibacter toxicus (Corynebacterium rathayii)*.[1215,1216] The *Corynebacterium* organisms produce a

neurotoxin called corynetoxin. This toxin has been purified using high-performance liquid chromatography and can be detected using an enzyme-linked immunosorbent assay (ELISA). The structure of corynetoxin is similar to that of the antibiotic tunicamycin.[1217] The corynetoxin is a glycolipid that inhibits the synthesis of lipid-linked oligosaccharides and blocks protein glycosylation.[1218,1219] Bacterial proliferation in the gall results in the formation of a yellow to orange exudate, which contains the toxin. The toxic material usually leaks out over the seed but occasionally remains encapsulated within the gall and cannot be detected by external examination. Galls that have a normal external appearance are toxic if the interior of the defect maintains a deep orange color. Loss of color is associated with a decrease in the amount of toxicity. A method of evaluating toxic pastures based on enumeration of contaminated seed heads and an ELISA test to detect the presence of the corynetoxin has been developed.

Outbreaks of staggers may occur in animals that have been on the same pasture for months; this may be due to several factors. The toxin is not inactivated by the rumen microflora, and daily doses may accumulate in sheep for as long as 9 weeks.[1220] Thus repeated exposure leads to an accumulation of the toxin and delayed onset of clinical disease. The concentration of the toxin increases in the seed heads during the summer and is greatest as the plant dries and the seeds ripen.[1221,1222] Finally, toxic ryegrass may occur only in patches in the pastures, and the grazing patterns of the animals is altered by changes in the climatic conditions, the growth of the ryegrass, or introduction of new sheep. This could explain the observation of outbreaks that occur shortly after the onset of inclement weather or after introduction of new sheep to the pastures.

Pathologic changes associated with annual ryegrass staggers include hemorrhage in the cerebellum, liver, and spleen. Ultrastructural changes include swelling of the capillary endothelial cells, dilation of the endoplasmic reticulum in the endothelial cells, mitochondrial degeneration, swelling of the astrocytic end feet, protein leakage across the blood-brain barrier, pyknosis and death of granular cell nuclei of the cerebellum, and changes in the neuropil adjacent to the damaged capillaries. These changes indicate that the toxin may access the central nervous system (CNS) by damaging the blood-brain cerebrospinal (CSF) barrier. Effects on neurons in the CNS could occur because of vascular damage or direct activity of the toxins.[1223]

CLINICAL SIGNS AND PATHOLOGIC LESIONS. The clinical signs of annual and perennial ryegrass staggers are similar. For both disorders the case attack usually is high, but the mortality rate varies and can range from 0 to over 90%. The clinical signs may occur within 48 hours to several weeks after cattle are introduced to toxic pastures. The animals appear normal at rest but tremble when they are excited. The gait is stiff, and limbs are hypermetric. There are fine and coarse tremors of all major muscle groups, especially those of the shoulder and flank areas. The tremors worsen as the animal becomes excited. Other clinical signs include intentional head tremor, truncal sway, and base-wide stance. With continued stimulation, affected animals kneel and then fall over. While down, affected animals have stiff extension of the legs with occasional flailing and may display opisthotonos or convulsions. Frothy exudate from the mouth also has been described. After approximately 10 to 20 minutes of struggle, the animal recovers, stands, and walks back to the herd or flock. New cases and deaths can continue for as long as 1 week after the animals have been removed from the toxic pasture.

DIFFERENTIAL DIAGNOSIS. Grass staggers is easily recognized by clinical signs. The specific plant involved must be identified by examination of the pasture forage. Tremorgenic diseases of adult cattle are common throughout most

---

*Nui Endosafe, Dairying Research Corp., Hamilton, New Zealand.

of the world. In addition to ryegrass pastures, tremorgenic plants include *Swainsona luteola* and *Swainsona galegifola*; *Solanum dimidiatum* and *Solanum fastigatum*; *Astragalus* spp.; red buckeye; *Phalaris* spp. (canary and reed canary grass); *Eupatorium rugosum* (white snakeroot); *Cynodon dactylon* (Bermuda grass); Dallis grass infested with the fungus *Claviceps paspali*; *Polypogon monospeliensis* (annual beard grass); *Pennisetum clandestinum* (kikuyu grass); and the mycotoxins of *Penicillium cyclopium*.[1222] Hypomagnesemia has been reported to cause cerebellar degeneration under some circumstances. The storage diseases (α- and β-mannosidosis, generalized glycogenosis, globoid cell leukodystrophy, and neuronal lipodystrophy) may also be important differential diagnoses for ataxic animals with tremor and cerebellar signs.

TREATMENT. There is no specific treatment for grass staggers. If the animals are removed from toxic pastures as soon as signs are first seen, the mortality rate is low despite the high number of affected animals. Several months may elapse before the neurologic signs resolve completely. Treatment with high doses of magnesium chloride have been recommended but have been shown by others to be ineffective for controlling the muscular spasms.[1224] Pastures may lose toxicity after rain and growth of new grass. In subtropical regions cattle should not be introduced to toxic pastures until the late fall or winter, when less toxic growth becomes abundant.

PREVENTION. Ammoniation of dried feed has been recommended as a method of reducing the toxicity of hay. This treatment simultaneously increases the digestibility and protein equivalency of the forage.[1225] For preventing annual ryegrass staggers, high-risk pastures can be identified by visually examining seed heads for infected galls. The ELISA test is sufficiently sensitive to identify one infected seed gall per 100 g of dried seed heads and also can accurately predict toxicity in pastures.[1226] The most practical strategy for controlling annual ryegrass toxicity is to break the nematode's life cycle by killing the ryegrass for two or three growing seasons. Otherwise, pastures remain perpetually toxic. Integrated control measures that have been recommended for prevention of annual ryegrass toxicity include applying herbicides in the spring, seeding the pastures with legumes, burning the infected pasture grasses during early autumn, and applying ryegrass-selective herbicides in the summer months, combined with heavy winter grazing.[1227]

Prevention of perennial ryegrass staggers using endophyte-free cultivars has been recommended. Such resistant biotypes of ryegrass lack resistance to the Argentine stem weevil and consequently are less productive than other biotypes. The most convenient solution has been to minimize exposure of the animals until fall rains stimulate less toxic pasture growth. Newer cultivars containing fewer tremorgens may be useful in the future.

REFERENCES

1195. Wilson AD, Gay CC, Fransen SC: An acremonium endophyte of *Lolium perenne* associated with hyperthermia of cattle in Pacific County, Washington, *Plant Dis* 76:212, 1992.

1196. Aasen AJ et al: Alkaloids as a possible cause of ryegrass staggers in grazing livestock, *Aust J Agric Res* 20:71-86, 1969.

1197. Stynes BA et al: The production of toxin in annual ryegrass, *Lolium rigidum*, infected with a nematode, *Anguina* spp, and *Corynebacterium rathayii*, *Aust J Agric Res* 30:201-209, 1979.

1198. Gallagher RT, Keogh RG, Latch GCM: The role of fungal tremorgens in ryegrass staggers, *N Z J Agric Res* 20:431-440, 1977.

1199. Production of tremorgenic toxins by *Penicillium janthinellum biourge*: a possible etiological factor in ryegrass staggers, *Aust J Exp Biol Med* 57: 31-37, 1979.

1200. Day JB, Mantle PG: Tremorgenic forage and ryegrass staggers, *Vet Rec* 106:463-464, 1980.

1201. Peterson AJ, Bass JJ, Byford MJ: Decreased plasma testosterone concentrations in rams affected by ryegrass staggers, *Res Vet Sci* 25:266-268, 1978.

1202. Stynes BA, Wise JL: The distribution and importance of annual ryegrass toxicity in western Australia and its occurrence in relation to cropping rotations and cultural practices, *Aust J Ag Res* 31:557-569, 1980.

1203. Berry PH et al: Central nervous system changes in sheep and cattle affected with natural or experimental annual ryegrass toxicity, *Aust Vet J* 56:402-403, 1980.

1204. Lunday BL, Mason RW: Lesions in ryegrass staggers in sheep, *Aust Vet J* 43:598-599, 1967.

1205. Berry PH, Wise JL: Wimmera ryegrass toxicity in western Australia, *Aust Vet J* 51:525-530, 1975.

1206. Mason RW: Axis cylinder degeneration associated with ryegrass staggers in sheep and cattle, *Aust Vet J* 44:428, 1968.

1207. Berry PH et al: Lesions in sheep and guinea pigs pen-fed parasitized annual ryegrass (*Lolium rigidum*), *Aust Vet J* 52:540-541, 1976.

1208. Odriozola E et al: Ryegrass staggers in heifers: a new mycotoxicosis in Argentina, *Vet Hum Toxicol* 35:144-146, 1993.

1209. Huizing HJ et al: Detection of lolines in endophyte-containing meadow fescue in the Netherlands and the effect of elevated temperature on induction of lolines in endophyte-infected perennial ryegrass, *Grass Forage Sci* 46:441-445, 1991.

1210. Galey FD et al: Staggers induced by consumption of perennial ryegrass in cattle and sheep from northern California, *J Am Vet Med Assoc* 199:466-470, 1991.

1211. Rowan E: Lolitrems, peramine, and paxilline: mycotoxins of the ryegrass/endophyte interaction, *Agric Ecosys Environ* 44:103-122, 1993.

1212. Gallagher RT et al: Tremorgenic neurotoxins from perennial ryegrass causing ryegrass staggers disorder of livestock: structure elucidation of lolitrem B, *J Chem Soc Chem Commun* 111:614-666, 1984.

1213. Blythe LL, Tor-Agbidye J, Craig AM: Correlation of quantities of lolitrem B toxin to clinical field cases of ryegrass staggers, *N Z Vet J* 41: 217-219, 1993.

1214. Clark DA: Beating ryegrass staggers, *Proc Ruakura Farmers Conf* 44:87-92, 1992.

1215. Edgar JA et al: Corynetoxins, causative agents of annual ryegrass toxicity: their identification as tunicamycin group antibiotics, *J Chem Soc Chem Comm* 4:222, 1982.

1216. Riley IT, Ophel KM: *Clavibacter toxicus* spp: the bacterium responsible for annual ryegrass toxicity in Australia, *Int J Sys Bacteriol* 42:64, 1992.

1217. Brown AGP, Vogel P: Annual ryegrass toxicity research update, *J Agric W Aust* 27:3-6, 1986.

1218. Jago MV et al: Inhibition of glycosylation by corynetoxin, the causative agent of annual ryegrass toxicity: a comparison with tunicamycin, *Chem Biol Interaction* 45:223, 1983.

1219. Tkacz JS, Lampen JO: Tunicamycin inhibition of polyisoprenyl N-acetylglucosaminyl pyrophosphate formation in calf liver microsomes, *Biochem Biophys Res Com* 65:248, 1975.

1220. Vogel P, McGrath MG: Corynetoxins are not detoxicated by in vitro fermentation in ovine rumen fluid, *Aust J Agric Res* 37:523-526, 1986.

1221. Jago MV, Culvenor CC: Tunicamycin and corynetoxin poisoning in sheep, *Aust Vet J* 64:232-235, 1987.

1222. Finnie JW: Corynetoxin poisoning in sheep in the southeast of South Australia associated with annual beard grass, *Aust Vet J* 68:370, 1991.

1223. Finnie JW, Mukherjee TM: Ultrastructural changes in the cerebellum of nursing rats given corynetoxin, an etiological agent of annual ryegrass toxicity, *J Comp Pathol* 96:205-216, 1986.

1224. Allsop TF, Watters SJ: Magnesium for the treatment of ryegrass staggers, *N Z Vet J* 32:39-40, 1984.

1225. Khan MFU: Ammoniation of moldy straw and hays to improve nutritive value and (or) alleviate mycotoxicosis when fed to ruminants, Sciences and Engineering, vol 50, Las Cruces, New Mexico, 1990, New Mexico State University.

1226. McKay A, Riley IT: Sampling ryegrass to assess the risk of annual ryegrass toxicity, *Aust Vet J* 70:241-243, 1993.

1227. Burdass WJ: Control strategies for annual ryegrass toxicity, *J Agric W Aust* 27:7-10, 1986.

BERMUDA GRASS STAGGERS

Bermuda grass (*Cynodon dactylon*) occasionally may become toxic for livestock.[1228] Cattle are most susceptible, followed by sheep, goats, and horses. Although the nature of the toxic principle in Bermuda grass is unknown, several associated factors, including sooty mold (*Pullularia* sp.), endogenous basic alkaloids, and leaf hopper infestation, have been associated with toxic pastures.[1228]

Animals may develop clinical signs as early as 36 hours after consuming toxic forage. Experimentally poisoned goats have developed clinical signs 8 days after being fed 772 g/

head/day of toxic hay.[1228] The toxin survives drying. Hay that is cut from offending pastures may remain toxic for as long as 9 years.[1229] The pharmacologic nature of the toxin is unknown; however, the sclerotia of *Claviceps purpurea* have been identified on the seed heads of toxic pastures.[1230] Pastures that are toxic remain so for successive seasons unless the vegetation is burned off and the ground is tilled and reseeded.

The clinical signs of Bermuda grass intoxication occur suddenly, usually simultaneously, in several animals in the herd. In some cases most of the animals on a single pasture may be affected, whereas animals on an adjacent pasture remain normal. The clinical disease is indistinguishable from ryegrass staggers described in the preceding sections. The electroencephalograms of affected animals are normal, indicating that the biochemical lesion is below the cortical level.[1231] The mortality rate is low, and deaths usually occur from self-inflicted trauma. Affected animals recover 2 days to 2 months after they are removed from the pasture. Tremors may be controlled using intravenous diazepam (0.1 to 1.0 mg/kg 2 to 3 times a day as needed).

REFERENCES

1228. Killebrew RL et al: Bermuda grass tremors: a research report by the Louisiana Cooperative Extension Service, Baton Rouge, 1972.
1229. Whitehair CK et al: A nervous disturbance in cattle caused by a toxic substance associated with mature Bermuda grass, Feeder's Day Report, Oklahoma Agricultural Experimental Station Pub No 22, Stillwater, Okla, 1951.
1230. Conway KE, Taliaferro CM, Shelby RA: First report on formation of sclerotia of *Claviceps purpurea* on Bermuda grass *(Cynodon dactylon)*, *Plant Dis* 76:1077, 1992.
1231. Strain GM, Segere CL, Flory W: Toxic Bermuda grass tremor in the goat, an electroencephalographic study, *Am J Vet Res* 43:158-162, 1982.

KIKUYU GRASS POISONING

A nervous system disease characterized by depression, ataxia, drooling of saliva, and ruminal distention occurs in cattle and sheep of northern New Zealand that are grazing kikuyu grass *(Pennisetum clandestinum)*.[1046]

REFERENCE

1232. Martinovich D, Smith D: Kikuyu poisoning in sheep, *N Z Vet J* 20:169, 1972.

DALLIS GRASS STAGGERS (*Paspalum* Staggers; *Claviceps paspali* Toxicity; Nervous Ergotism)

Ingestion of Dallis grass that has been infected with the ergot fungus *Claviceps paspali* produces a tremorgenic disease similar to that of Bermuda and ryegrass staggers. Other *Paspalum*-type grasses that may become toxic include Argentine bahia grass *(Paspalum dilatatum)* and water couch grass *(Paspalum distichum)*. Horses are susceptible to the toxin, but the condition occurs most commonly in cattle. The disease has been recognized in the United States, Great Britain, Australia, and New Zealand.[1233-1237] *C. paspali* first attacks the pistil of the grass flower and replaces the ovary with fungal tissue. The fungus secretes a sticky fluid, the "honeydew," which contains a large number of spores but little toxin. The fluid hardens into a mature sclerotia containing large amounts of toxin. Toxic stands of Dallis grass can be recognized by the presence of numerous small, reddish-brown or black sclerotia measuring 3 to 5 mm in diameter on the seed head of the plant. The fungus produces a number of neurologically active agents. Some of the products resemble lysergic acid diethylamine in structure and activity, whereas others may act as dopaminergic agonists. Animals apparently develop a craving for the infested seed heads and graze them selectively. The

toxin remains active in cured hay. Toxin production is greatest when there is a wet period following formation of the seed heads. Mowing the toxic pastures and removing or burning the infested seed heads are effective for preventing further outbreaks of the disease. If the amount of rainfall diminishes after mowing, the new growth usually is nontoxic.

The clinical signs of Dallis grass staggers are similar to those described above for ryegrass; they include coarse and fine muscular fasciculations, head tremors, spastic, hypermetric gait, and falling. The clinical signs are exacerbated by fright or external stimulation. Clinical diagnosis is made by visible detection of the toxic agent in the feed or by using thin-layer chromatography. Animals recover spontaneously within 1 to 3 months after being removed from the pasture.

REFERENCES

1233. Brown HB: Life history and poisonous properties of *Claviceps paspali*, *J Agric Res* 7:401-406, 1916.
1234. Grayson AR: *Paspalum* ergotism in cattle, *J Dept Agric* 39:441-442, 1941.
1235. Hopkirk CSM: *Paspalum* staggers, *N Z J Agric* 53:105-108, 1936.
1236. Simms BT: Dallis grass poisoning, *Auburn Vet* 76:64-65, 1945.
1237. Simpson CF, Erdman W: Ergot poisoning in cattle, Bulletin of the Florida Agricultural Experimental Station, 1952.

CANARY GRASS STAGGERS (*Phalaris* Staggers)

Cattle or sheep that graze on certain species of canary grass *(Phalaris arundinacea, Phalaris tuberosa, Phalaris acquatica, Phalaris angusta, Phalaris caroliniana, Phalaris brachystachys)* grown under specific environmental conditions may develop neurointoxication.[1238-1243] *Phalaris* poisoning has been reported in Australia, New Zealand, South Africa, Norway,[1244] South America,[1245] and the United States.[1246] In the United States the plant can be found in Virginia, Colorado, Oregon, Florida, Texas, Georgia, Mississippi, Alabama, and California.[1247] The case attack rate may reach 80%,[1241] and the mortality rate ranges from 4% to 40%.[1239,1241] Acute deaths may occur as early as 4 to 12 hours after commencement of grazing on a toxic pasture.[1239,1242] Animals usually recover by 8 days after removal from offending pastures, but signs can persist for as long as 1 month after removal, and relapses can occur for up to 5 months.[1238,1239,1242]

Continuous exposure to low concentrations of alkaloid (less than 0.001% of dry matter intake) over 40 days has resulted in severe toxicosis in sheep on a drylot.[1248]

The toxic principles of canary grass are tryptamine alkaloids (dimethylated indolealkyl amines), which are found in one or more species of the genus *Phalaris (P. tuberosa, P. minor,* and *P. arundinacea)*.[1241] The most potent of the toxins is the alkylamine 5-methoxydimethyltryptamine. Intravenous doses of this compound as low as 0.1 mg/kg can cause severe neurologic signs in sheep in 16 sec.[1243] The toxins competitively inhibit the initial step in the breakdown of serotonin by monoamine oxidase and act on midbrain and medullary nuclei via presynaptic serotonin type 1 cholinergic receptor sites. The overall activity of the toxin is to enhance response to excitatory inputs.[1249]

The dynamics of toxin production have been examined.[1250] The concentration of alkaloid in the plant is increased by a reduction of light intensity (shade) but not by a decrease in length of the daylight.[1250] If light intensities are high, the grass is unlikely to be toxic unless soil nitrate levels are also high.[1250] Rapid growth of the grass also favors the formation and accumulation of toxin. Other factors that enhance the toxicity of a pasture include fog, humidity, or rain followed by sunny, warm weather or sunshine on nitrogen-fertilized pastures.[1250] Although there is no specific age-related susceptibility to the toxin, only weaned animals tend to be affected during an outbreak. Many outbreaks occur when hungry sheep ingest large amounts of toxic grass over a short period.[1239] The disease has also occurred 3 to 5 days after a rainfall has ended a period of drought.[1245]

Electromyographic studies have indicated that the tremors and spasms probably originate from the spinal cord and the peripheral nervous system. Excitation leads to increased muscle tone and extensor rigidity.[1251]

There are at least two distinct clinical forms of the intoxication: acute death from cardiovascular collapse and a more chronic nervous form.[1240] The cardiovascular form of the disease occurs by 12 to 72 hours after animals are placed on a toxic pasture.[1240,1242] Affected animals die suddenly from heart failure while being herded off toxic pastures. Animals also may be found dead with the head fixed in opisthotonos and the legs in rigid extension. The ground surrounding the limbs is disturbed, indicating that the animal died in convulsions. Signs that are associated with cardiac collapse include acute dyspnea, cyanosis, pounding heart sounds, irregular heart rate with alternating periods of extreme tachycardia (170 to 240 beats/min), and then bradycardia.[1243,1248]

The nervous form of the disease is more prolonged and occurs after repeated exposures of 2 to 33 weeks' duration. Signs may be delayed for as long as 4 months after removal from the toxic grass.[1246] The clinical signs include hyperexcitability, exaggerated responses to auditory or tactile stimuli, fine muscular fasciculations, particularly of the masseter muscles, licking of the lips, wrinkling of the facial muscles, repetitive chewing, inability to swallow, flaring of the nostrils, ptyalism, nystagmus, intentional head tremor, ear and tail twitching, base-wide stance, reduced menace response, and deficient pupillary reflexes.[1243,1251] The gait of affected sheep is described as stiff legged, with both rear limbs moving in unison ("rabbit hopping"). Affected sheep buckle at the knees and assume sternal recumbency with the rear quarters elevated. They then fall into lateral recumbency and flail wildly while attempting to regain a standing posture.[1240] Poisoned cattle also show incoordination and repeated stabbing movements with the tongue and are unable to adequately grasp the forage. They salivate profusely and drop feed from the mouth. Eventually the animals die of starvation. There may be an increased protein concentration (40 to 100 mg/ml) and white blood cell count (4 to 50 mononuclear cells per deciliter) in the cerebrospinal fluid of affected animals.[1238] Animals may survive the initial signs but have neurologic symptoms for as long as 10 months.[1252]

For confirmation of a diagnosis, the amount of tryptamine alkaloids in suspect grasses can be measured. Alkaloid concentrations above 30 to 50 mg/100 g dry weight of forage are considered toxic for sheep.[1250,1251]

The pathologic lesions in the central nervous system of affected animals include focal, demarcated greenish or slate gray discoloration in the pons, medulla, and corticomedullary junction of the kidney; intracytoplasmic accumulations of greenish brown pigment in the dorsal root ganglia and medullary nuclei; neuronal loss; focal gliosis; and swelling of the axonal sheaths in the ventromedial aspect of the spinal cord.[1238,1241] The pigment is thought to originate from metabolism and deamination of the toxic alkylamines but is not thought to play a direct role in the development of the neurologic deficits.[1247,1251] Other lesions in cattle that have died acutely include ulcerative abomasitis, jejunitis, and ileitis; subcapsular renal hemorrhage; and ecchymoses of the pericardium and epicardium.

Administration of cobalt to animals on toxic grass pastures is protective. The biochemical function of cobalt is thought to be related to increased ruminal inactivation of the toxins. Weekly administration of 28 mg of cobalt to each animal has been recommended to prevent clinical signs in exposed sheep.[1246,1247,1252-1254] This dosage is much higher than that delivered by standard supplementation. Additional rec-

ommendations include removal of affected animals from the offending pasture, sedation with a phenothiazine tranquilizer, and administration of sodium pentobarbital or diazepam to convulsive sheep. *Phalaris* plants may also contain potentially toxic concentrations of nitrate or cyanide. In any outbreak of suspected *Phalaris* toxicosis when the acute death signs have been encountered, cyanide and nitrate poisonings should also be considered.[1255]

To prevent *Phalaris* poisoning, animals should be removed from the toxic grasses. The concentration of dimethylindolealkyl amines may be reduced by curing the forage as hay. Ensiling the canary grass does not reduce the amount of toxins.[1256]

REFERENCES

1238. East NE, Higgins RJ: Canary grass (*Phalaris* spp) toxicosis in sheep in California, *J Am Vet Med Assoc* 192:667-669, 1988.
1239. Gallagher CH, Koch JH, Hoffman H: Deaths of ruminants grazing *Phalaris tuberosa* in Australia, *Aust Vet J* 43:495-500, 1967.
1240. Mendel VE et al: Staggers in pastured cattle, *J Am Vet Med Assoc* 154:769-772, 1969.
1241. Simpson BH, Jolly RD, Thomas SHM: *Phalaris arundinacea* as a cause of deaths and incoordination in sheep, *N Z Vet J* 17:240-244, 1969.
1242. Kerr DR: Rapid death of cattle grazing recently irrigated *Phalaris tuberosa*, *Aust Vet J* 48:421, 1972.
1243. Gallagher CH et al: Toxicity of *Phalaris tuberosa* for sheep, *Nature* 204:542-545, 1964.
1244. Ulvund MJ: Chronic poisoning in a lamb grazing *Phalaris arundinacea*, *Acta Vet Scand* 26:286-288, 1985.
1245. Odriozola E et al: Neuropathological effects and deaths of cattle and sheep in Argentina from *Phalaris angusta*, *Vet Hum Toxicol* 33:465-467, 1991.
1246. Nicholson S et al: Delayed *Phalaris* grass toxicosis in sheep and cattle, *J Am Vet Med Assoc* 195:345-346, 1989.
1247. Gould FW: *The grasses of Texas,* College Station, Texas, 1975, Texas A&M University Press.
1248. Lean IJ et al: Tryptamine alkaloid toxicosis in feedlot sheep, *J Am Vet Med Assoc* 195:768-771, 1989.
1249. Bourke CA, Carrigan MJ, Dixon RJ: The pathogenesis of the nervous syndrome of *Phalaris aquatica* toxicity in sheep, *Aust Vet J* 67:356-358, 1990.
1250. Moore RM, Williams JD, Chia J: Factors affecting concentrations of dimethylated indolealkylamines in *Phalaris tuberosa*, *Aust J Biol Sci* 20:1131-1140, 1967.
1251. Gllagher CH, Koch JH, Hoffman H: Diseases of sheep due to indigestion of *Phalaris tuberosa*, *Aust Vet J* 42:279-286, 1966.
1252. Lee HJ, Kuchel RD: The aetiology of *Phalaris* staggers in sheep. I. Preliminary observations of the preventative role of cobalt, *Aust J Agric Res* 4:88-89, 1953.
1253. Lee HJ et al: The aetiology of *Phalaris* staggers in sheep. III, The preventative effects of various oral dose rates of cobalt, *Aust J Agric Res* 8:494-501, 1957.
1254. Lee HJ et al: The aetiology of *Phalaris* staggers in sheep. IV, The site of preventative action and its specificity to cobalt, *Aust J Agric Res* 8:502-511, 1957.
1255. Bourke CA, Carrigan MJ: Mechanisms underlying *Phalaris aquatica* "sudden death" syndrome in sheep, *Aust Vet J* 69:165-167, 1992.
1256. Tosi HR, Wittenberg KM: Harvest alternatives to reduce the alkaloid content of reed canary grass forage, *Can J Anim Sci* 73:373-380, 1993.

PENICILLIUM CYCLOPIUM (TREMORGEN) INTOXICATION

Ruminants that ingest toxic species of *Penicillium* develop clinical signs that are indistinguishable from those of Dallis, ryegrass, *Phalaris*, and Bermuda grass staggers.[1257-1260] The tremors are caused by mycotoxins,[1260] which can be classified into four major groups: the aflatrem-paxilline group, the verruculogen-fumotremo-gen group, the territrem group, and the tryptoquivaline group. Of these the most important fungal tremorgens are aflatrem, penitrem A, fumotremogen B, and verruculogen. Verruculogen and fumotremogen B can be isolated from cultures of *Penicillium estingogenum*. Penitrem A is elaborated from *Penicillium nigricans, Penicillium anitellum, Penicillium cyclopium, Penicillium clavigerum,* and *Aspergillus canescens*. Verriculogen has also been identified in pure cultures of *Aspergillus fumigatus*.[1261,1262]

Ingestion of moldy cornstalks constitutes the most common source of fungal tremors in livestock. The fungi pro-

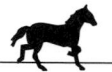

liferate in the corn but do not produce tremorgens until the stalks touch the ground. After production at or near the soil surface, the toxins translocate in plants through root absorption.[1260]

The pathophysiologic mechanisms by which mycotoxins affect the central nervous system are unknown, but there is increased release of the transmitter amino acids aspartate, glutamate, and γ-aminobutyric acid in the corpus striatum, indicating the presence of a reversible biochemical lesion.

Diagnosis is based on the clinical signs, demonstration of the mycotoxin in the feed, and identification of the fungal elements in the feces. There is no specific treatment for the intoxication. Affected animals recover completely when they are removed from infected pastures. The diagnosis of tremorgenic fungal intoxication is difficult. The mycelial elements survive degradative conditions in the gastrointestinal tract and can be isolated from the feces of intoxicated animals. Penitrem A and verriculogen can be demonstrated in the forage by thin-layer chromatography or by mouse assay.

REFERENCES

1257. Cysewski SJ: *Paspalum* staggers and tremorgen intoxication in animals, *J Am Vet Med Assoc* 163:1291-1292, 1973.
1258. Gallagher RT et al: The role of fungal tremorgens in ryegrass staggers, *N Z J Agric Res* 20:431-440, 1977.
1259. Lanigan GW, Payne AL, Cockrum PA: Production of tremorgenic toxins by *Penicillium janthinellum biourge:* a possible etiological factor in ryegrass staggers, *Aust J Exp Biol Med Sci* 57:31-37, 1979.
1260. Day JB, Mantle PG: Tremorgenic forage and ryegrass staggers, *Vet Rec* 106:463-464, 1980.
1261. Mantle PG et al: Tremorgenic mycotoxins and incoordination syndromes, *Vet Rec* 103:403, 1978.
1262. Penny RHC et al: Clinical studies on tremorgenic mycotoxicoses of sheep, *Vet Rec* 105:392-393, 1979.

DISEASES PRODUCING SPINAL CORD OR PERIPHERAL NERVE SIGNS

CERVICAL STENOTIC MYELOPATHY (Wobbler Syndrome; Cervical Vertebral Instability)

BONNIE R. RUSH

CLINICAL SIGNS. Cervical stenotic myelopathy (CSM) is a common cause of symmetric spinal ataxia in horses 6 months to 3 years of age. Neurologic gait deficits are caused by spinal cord compression by stenotic and malformed cervical vertebrae.[1263] A neurologic examination is performed to assess the symmetry of deficits and the severity of weakness, ataxia, and spasticity.[1264] Gait analysis is performed at the walk; neurologic deficits can be accentuated by circling, elevation of the head, and maneuvering over obstacles and inclines. Ataxia or proprioceptive loss is manifested by circumduction of the hind limbs, posting (pivoting on the inside hind limb during circling), and truncal sway. Moderately to severely affected horses have lacerations on the heel bulbs (wobbler heels) and medial aspect of the forelimbs from overreaching and interference. Stumbling and toe dragging indicate weakness. The hooves of horses with prolonged clinical signs of CSM are chipped, worn, or squared at the toe. At rest affected horses may have a base-wide stance and may demonstrate delayed responses to proprioceptive positioning. When prompted to back, the horses may stand base wide, lean backward, drag their hind limbs, and/or step on their hind foot with a forelimb. The musculature of the neck may appear disproportionately thin compared to the rest of the body, and in some horses prominent

articular processes of the fifth and sixth cervical vertebrae may be evident.[1265]

CSM has been reported in most light and draft breeds.[1266] Thoroughbreds are particularly predisposed to the condition, which affects approximately 2% of the population. Approximately 10% to 50% of thoroughbreds have characteristic developmental malformations of the cervical vertebrae without spinal cord compression.[1267,1268] Male horses are more frequently affected than females. Most horses with CSM are under 3 years of age at presentation, although, middle-aged horses occasionally are diagnosed with the condition. Neurologic gait deficits typically progress for a short time and then stabilize.[1266]

PATHOPHYSIOLOGY. CSM appears to be a manifestation of developmental orthopedic disease. Developmental orthopedic disease of the appendicular skeleton, such as physitis, joint effusion, osteochondrosis, and flexural limb deformities, occurs more often in young horses with CSM.[1269] A direct cause-and-effect relationship between osteochondrosis and CSM has not been identified; however, the association between the frequency of occurrence of osteochondrosis and CSM indicates that the two conditions have a similar pathophysiology.

The etiology of osteochondrosis and CSM probably likely multifactorial, consisting of genetic and environmental influences. It is unlikely that CSM is heritable by simple mendelian dominant-recessive patterns.[1270] The mode of inheritance more likely involves multiple alleles and variable penetrance, which determine genetic predisposition to CSM. A high plane of nutrition, micronutrient imbalance, rapid growth, trauma, and abnormal biomechanical forces probably contribute to the development of CSM in genetically predisposed animals.

Dietary copper, zinc, and carbohydrates are thought to play a role in the pathogenesis of osteochondrosis and CSM. Low dietary copper (12 ppm) and high dietary zinc (1000 to 2000 mg/kg of dry weight) concentrations cause osteochondrosis in foals, whereas copper supplementation (55 ppm) reduces the incidence of osteochondrosis of the axial and appendicular skeleton.[1271,1272] Copper supplementation does not eliminate developmental orthopedic disease, suggesting the existence of other etiologic factors. Excessive carbohydrate in the diet is hypothesized to contribute to the pathogenesis of osteochondrosis through endocrine imbalance.[1273,1274]

Spinal cord compression can be dynamic or static in horses with CSM.[1275] Dynamic compression occurs because of vertebral instability and causes intermittent spinal cord compression during ventroflexion of the neck; spinal cord compression is relieved when the neck is in the neutral position. Pathologic changes most commonly observed in horses with dynamic compression are instability between adjacent vertebrae, malformation of the caudal vertebral epiphysis (caudal epiphyseal flare), and malformation or malarticulation of the articular processes. Osteochondrosis of the articular processes is not always present at the site of spinal cord compression in horses with dynamic compression.[1269] The intervertebral sites most commonly affected by dynamic compression are C3-C4 and C4-C5.

Static compression is defined as continuous spinal cord impingement regardless of cervical position. It occurs predominantly in the caudal cervical region, C5-C6 and C6-C7. Static spinal cord compression is exacerbated by thickening of the dorsal lamina, hypertrophy of the ligamentum flavum, and degenerative joint disease of the articular processes. Static and dynamic spinal cord compression are both associated with narrowing of the vertebral canal from C3-C6, regardless of the site of spinal cord compression, indicating that generalized vertebral canal stenosis is an important factor in the pathophysiology of CSM.[1276]

Histopathologic examination of the spinal cord identifies myelin degeneration (ventral and lateral funiculi), malacia, focal neuronal loss, and fibrosis at the sites of spinal cord

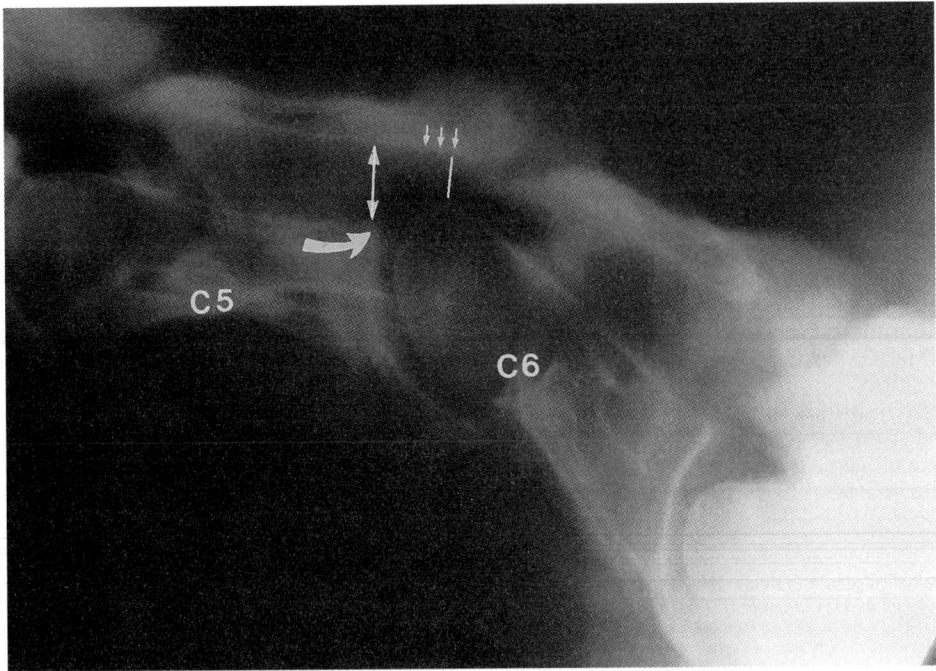

FIG. 33-26 ■ Survey radiograph of the fifth and sixth cervical vertebrae. Bony malformations depicted in this radiograph include flare of the caudal physis (*curved arrow*—C5), caudal extension of the dorsal lamina (*small arrows*—C5), and subluxation and malalignment of the C5-C6 articulation. Measurement of the intervertebral canal diameter of the C5-C6 articulation is indicated by the *solid line,* and the determination of the intravertebral canal diameter of C5 is indicated by the *double arrow.*

compression. Wallerian degeneration occurs in ascending white matter tracts cranial to the affected site and in descending tracts distal to the site of spinal cord compression.[1277]

DIAGNOSIS. Radiographic examination and cerebrospinal fluid (CSF) analysis are indicated in horses with symmetric tetraparesis and ataxia to differentiate CSM from other spinal cord disorders. Differential diagnoses for horses with symmetric tetraparesis and ataxia include equine herpesvirus myeloencephalitis, equine protozoal myeloencephalitis, equine degenerative myeloencephalopathy, occipitoatlantoaxial malformation, vertebral fracture, vertebral abscess, and verminous myelitis. Cytologic findings in the cerebrospinal fluid usually are unremarkable in horses with CSM. When the findings of CSF analysis are abnormal, the alterations are consistent with acute spinal cord compression, such as mild xanthochromia or mild increases in protein concentrations.

Survey radiographs of the cervical spine are obtained in standing, sedated horses. Cervical radiographs are evaluated by subjective assessment of vertebral malformation and objective determination of vertebral canal diameter.[1276] The five categories of cervical vertebral malformation that are subjectively assessed in horses with CSM are degenerative joint disease of the articular processes, subluxation between adjacent vertebrae, flare of the caudal physis of the vertebral body, abnormal ossification patterns, and caudal extension of the dorsal laminae (Figs. 33-26 and 33-27).[1276,1278] Although the presence of characteristic vertebral malformations supports the diagnosis of CSM, subjective evaluation of survey radiographs does not reliably discriminate between horses affected by CSM and those that are not.[1267,1276] Degenerative joint disease of the articular processes of the caudal cervical vertebrae is the most common and severe malformation observed in affected horses.[1276] However, degenerative arthropathy occurs in 10% to 50% of nonataxic horses and is the most common and severe vertebral

malformation in horses without CSM.[1268,1276] Subjective evaluation of degenerative arthropathy of the articular processes may lead to a false positive diagnosis of CSM.[1267]

The vertebral canal diameter is objectively assessed by determining the sagittal ratio.[1276] The sagittal ratio is obtained by dividing the minimum sagittal diameter of the vertebral canal by the width of the corresponding vertebral body. The minimum sagittal diameter is measured from the dorsal aspect of the vertebral body to the ventral border of the dorsal laminae, and the vertebral body width is measured perpendicular to the vertebral canal at the widest point of the cranial aspect of the vertebral body (Fig. 33-28). The sagittal ratio eliminates error caused by magnification because the vertebral canal and vertebral body are in the same anatomic plane. The sagittal ratio should exceed 52% from C4 through C6 and 56% at C7 in horses weighing more than 320 kg. The sensitivity and specificity of the sagittal ratio for identification of CSM-affected horses is approximately 89% for vertebral sites C4 through C7.[1279] Accurate measurement of the sagittal ratio requires a precise, lateral radiograph of the cervical vertebrae. Oblique views yield indistinct margins of the ventral aspect of the vertebral canal, resulting in erroneous values for minimum sagittal diameter and vertebral body width.

The semiquantitative scoring system developed by Mayhew[1278] should be used in foals under 1 year of age to assess cervical radiographs for diagnosis of CSM. The scoring system combines objective measurement of the vertebral canal diameter and subjective evaluation of vertebral malformation. Stenosis of the vertebral canal is assessed by determining the intervertebral and intravertebral minimum sagittal diameters. These values are corrected for radiographic magnification by dividing them by the length of the vertebral body. (see Fig. 33-26). Foals that measure below the mean are assessed 5 points, and foals that measure 2 standard de-

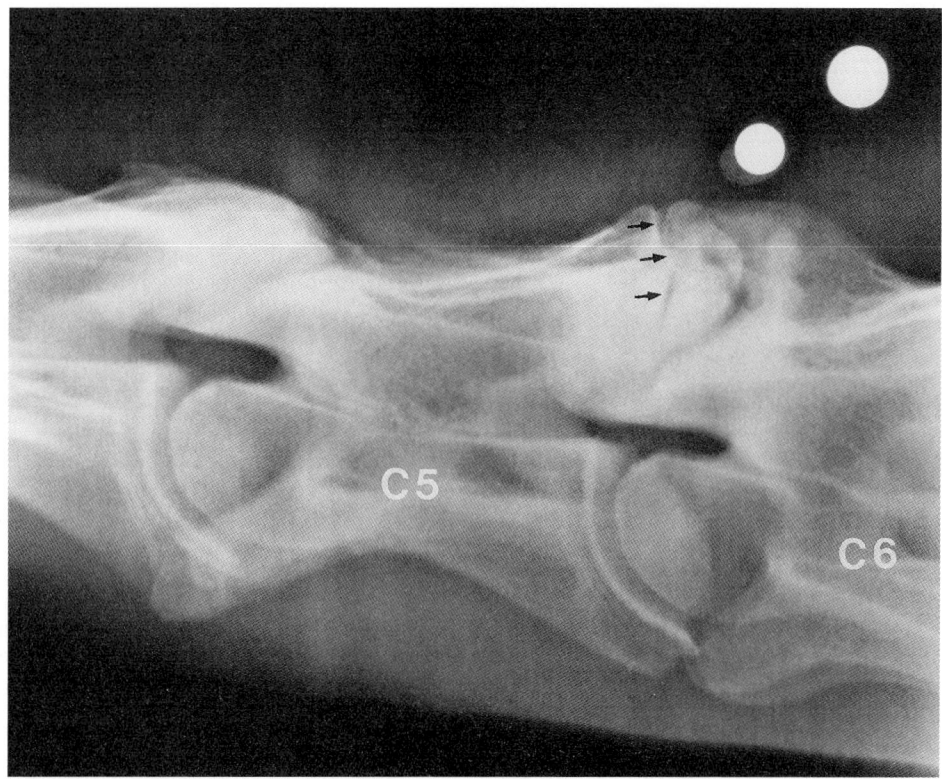

FIG. 33-27 ▌▌ Survey radiograph of the fifth and sixth cervical vertebrae. Degenerative joint disease, bony proliferation, and a facet fracture *(arrows)* can be seen on the articular processes of the C5-C6 articulation.

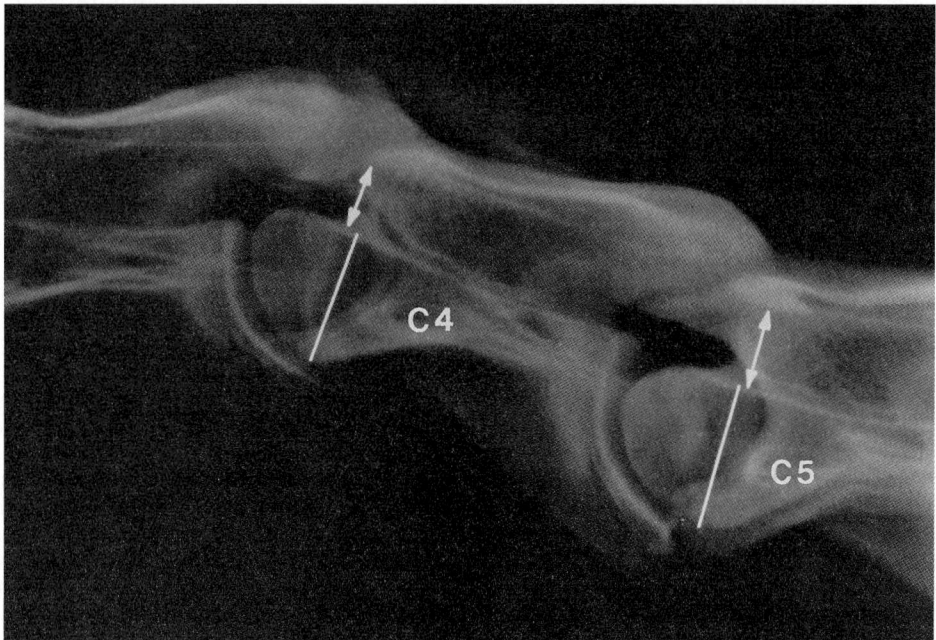

FIG. 33-28 ▌▌ Survey radiograph of the fourth and fifth cervical vertebrae. The sagittal ratio is determined by dividing the minimum sagittal diameter *(double arrows)* by the width of the corresponding vertebral body *(lines)*.

TABLE 33-14

Mean Minimum Sagittal Diameters* and Corrected Minimum Sagittal Diameters of Cervical Vertebrae in Foals without Neurologic Disease

Cervical Vertebral Site	Minimum Sagittal Diameter (mm) ± SD	Corrected Minimum Sagittal Diameter (%) ± SD
C2	23±1	18±1
C2-3	28±4	33±2
C3	20±1	24±2
C3-4	25±2	30±2
C4	20±1	24±2
C4-5	25±2	31±2
C5	21±1	25±2
C5-6	26±3	34±3
C6	21±1	27±2
C6-7	31±5	46±5
C7	23±1	35±2

From Mayhew IG et al: *Equine Vet J* 25(5):435-440, 1993.
SD, Standard deviation.
*Intravertebral and intervertebral.

viations below the mean or fall below the mean at multiple sites are assessed 6 to 10 points (Table 33-14). Cervical vertebral malformation is determined by subjective assessment of five categories: encroachment of the caudal epiphysis of the vertebral body dorsally into the vertebral canal; caudal extension of the dorsal lamina to the cranial physis of the next vertebra; angulation between adjacent vertebral bodies; abnormal ossification of the physis; and degenerative joint disease of the articular processes. The maximum score allotted for each category of bony malformation is 5 points. A total score of 12 or higher (the maximum total score is 25) confirms the radiographic diagnosis of CSM. Stenosis of the vertebral canal and malalignment between adjacent vertebrae are the most discriminating parameters in this semiquantitative scoring system to differentiate CSM-affected foals from normal foals.

Survey radiographic examination of the cervical vertebrae determines the likelihood of spinal cord compression. Myelographic examination is required for definitive diagnosis of CSM, identification of the location of affected vertebral sites, and classification of spinal cord compressive lesions. The clinician should use radiographic interpretation to classify the patient into one of the following categories:

1. Low sagittal ratio (under 48% at C4 through C6), moderate to severe bony malformation: A myelographic examination is performed to identify sites of spinal cord compression and to classify lesions as static or dynamic.
2. Marginal sagittal ratio (48% through 56%), mild to moderate bony malformation: A myelographic examination is performed to confirm or rule out CSM.
3. High sagittal ratio (over 56%), minimal bony malformation: Other differential diagnoses are pursued.

Myelographic examination is performed under general anesthesia with the patient in lateral recumbency.[1280] The landmarks for cisternal puncture at the atlantooccipital site are the cranial border of the wings of the atlas, the caudal border of the occipital protuberance, and the dorsal midline. The poll region is aseptically prepared and the head flexed at a 90-degree angle to the cervical vertebral column. The spinal needle (3½-inch, 18-gauge needle with stylet) is introduced and directed toward the lower jaw. The needle is advanced until the dura mater is penetrated, which often produces a "popping" sensation. Clear cerebrospinal fluid should drip rapidly or flow from the hub with success-

ful placement of the needle. An equal volume (20 to 40 ml) of CSF is removed before injection of a contrast agent. Twenty to 40 ml of contrast medium produces sufficient positive-contrast opacity to identify spinal cord compression in adult horses.[1280] The bevel of the spinal needle is directed caudally, and contrast medium is injected at a constant rate over 5 minutes. The head and neck are elevated under a wedged platform for 5 minutes at 30 to 45 degrees to facilitate caudal flow of the contrast medium. Iohexol (350 mg iodine/ml) and iopamidol (370 mg iodine/ml) are the most popular nonionic, water-soluble contrast media used for equine myelographic studies.[1281-1283] These second-generation agents cause less neurotoxicity and meningeal irritation than metrizamide.[1284]

The diagnosis of CSM is defined myelographically by a 50% or greater decrease in the sagittal diameter of the dorsal and ventral contrast columns.[1280] The decrease in the sagittal diameter of the contrast column is determined by comparing the value at the intervertebral space to a midvertebral site cranial or caudal to the suspected intervertebral space. The ventral contrast column often is obliterated at the intervertebral space in normal myelographic studies, particularly when the neck is in the flexed position. Therefore a decrease of 50% or greater of the dorsal and ventral columns must be present for definitive diagnosis of CSM. Some investigators prefer to use a diagnostic criterion of less than 2 mm of dorsal contrast column (or smaller) to reduce the occurrence of false positive results on myelographic studies.[1263]

A complete myelographic examination should include neutral and stressed (flexed and extended) views of the cervical vertebrae.[1263,1280] Horses with dynamic spinal cord compression show obliteration of the dorsal and ventral contrast columns during ventroflexion of the neck (Fig. 33-29), whereas spinal cord compression is not apparent with the neck in the neutral position. Static vertebral canal stenosis is characterized by constant spinal cord compression regardless of cervical position (Fig. 33-30). In some cases of static compression, ventroflexion of the neck stretches the ligamentum flavum and relieves spinal cord compression, whereas hyperextension exacerbates compression. In horses with obvious sites of spinal cord compression on neutral myelographic views, excessive flexion and extension of the neck should be avoided while obtaining dynamic views to prevent exacerbation of spinal cord injury.

Horses should be monitored for 24 hours after the myelographic procedure for depression, fever, seizure, and worsening of neurologic status.[1285] Worsening of neurologic status after myelography may result from spinal cord trauma during hyperflexion, iatrogenic puncture of the spinal cord, or chemical meningitis. Administration of phenylbutazone (4.4 mg/kg PO every 24 hours) 1 day before through 1 day after myelographic examination attenuates fever and depression associated with chemical meningitis.

TREATMENT. Conservative management of CSM-affected horses consists of administration of antiinflammatory therapy (glucocorticoids, dimethyl sulfoxide [DMSO], and nonsteroidal antiinflammatory drugs) and exercise restriction. Antiinflammatory therapy alone may reduce the edema associated with spinal cord compression; however, full recovery is unlikely without dietary or surgical intervention.

The most successful conservative treatment option for CSM-affected foals (those under 1 year of age) is the "paced diet" program.[1286] This program is designed to correct endocrine imbalance associated with high-carbohydrate diets. After a carbohydrate meal, high serum insulin and low serum thyroxine concentrations promote cartilage proliferation and retention without promoting maturation. This dietary program is restricted in energy and protein (65% to 75% of the National Research Council [NRC] recommendations) but

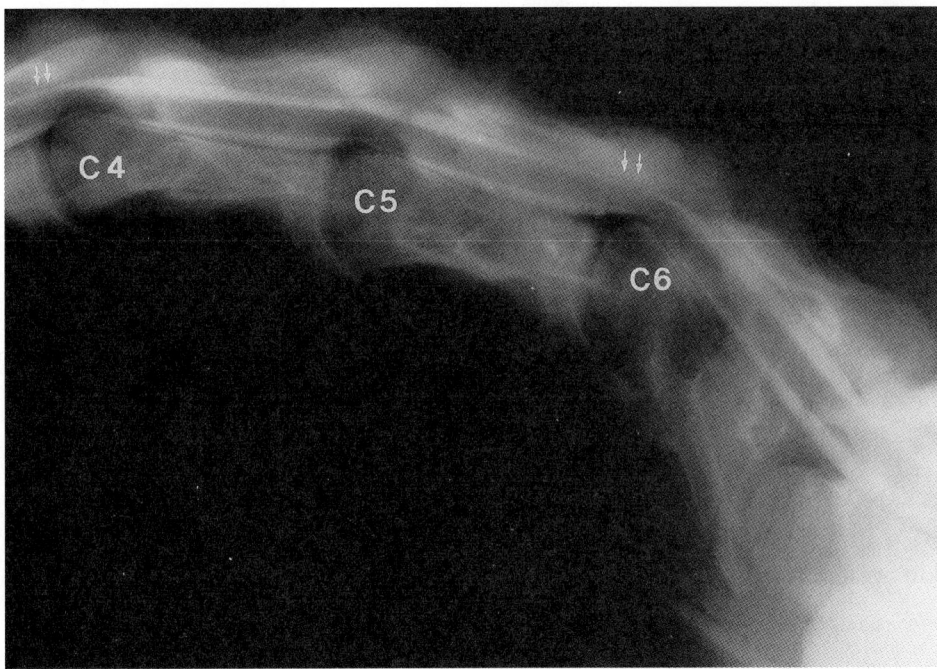

FIG. 33-29 ▓ Myelographic examination of C3 through C6 with the cervical spine in ventroflexion. Dynamic instability and spinal cord compression are present at the C3-C4 and C5-C6 articulations. The ventral contrast columns are obliterated and the dorsal contrast columns are narrowed (to less than 2 mm) at C3-C4 and C5-C6 *(arrows)*.

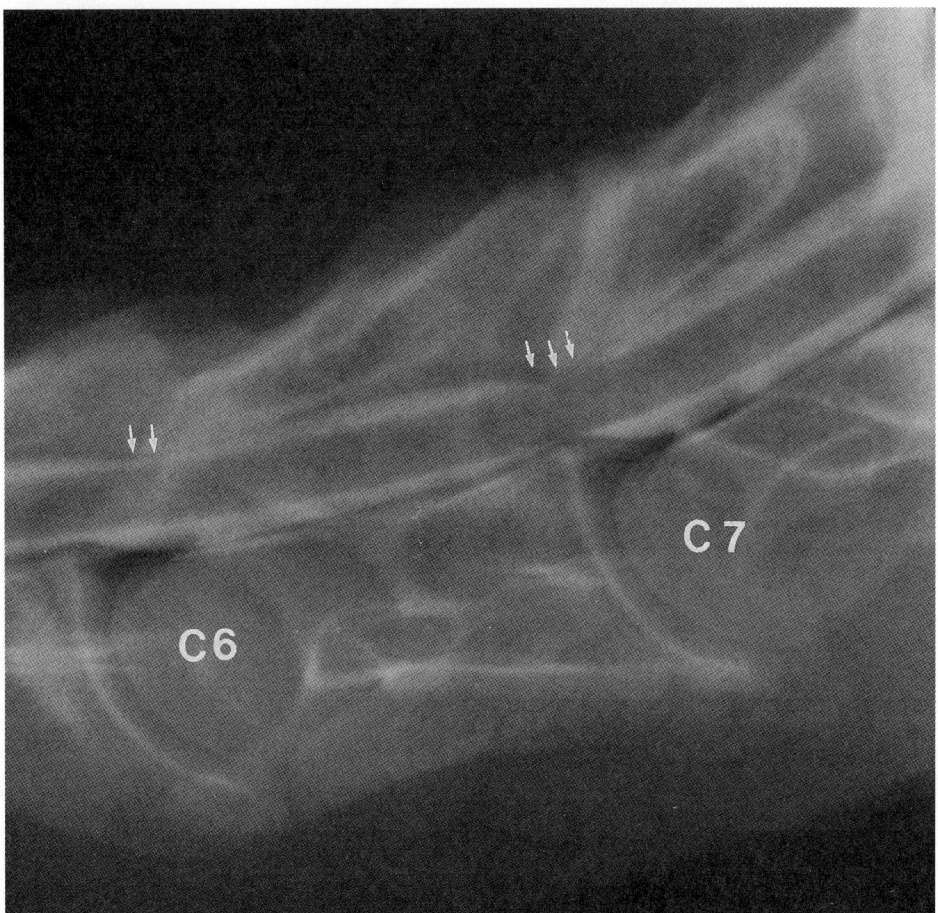

FIG. 33-30 ▓ Myelographic examination of C5 through C7 with the cervical spine in neutral position. Static spinal cord compression is demonstrated by obliteration or narrowing (to less than 2 mm) of the dorsal and ventral contrast columns at C5-C6 and C6-C7 *(arrows)*.

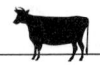

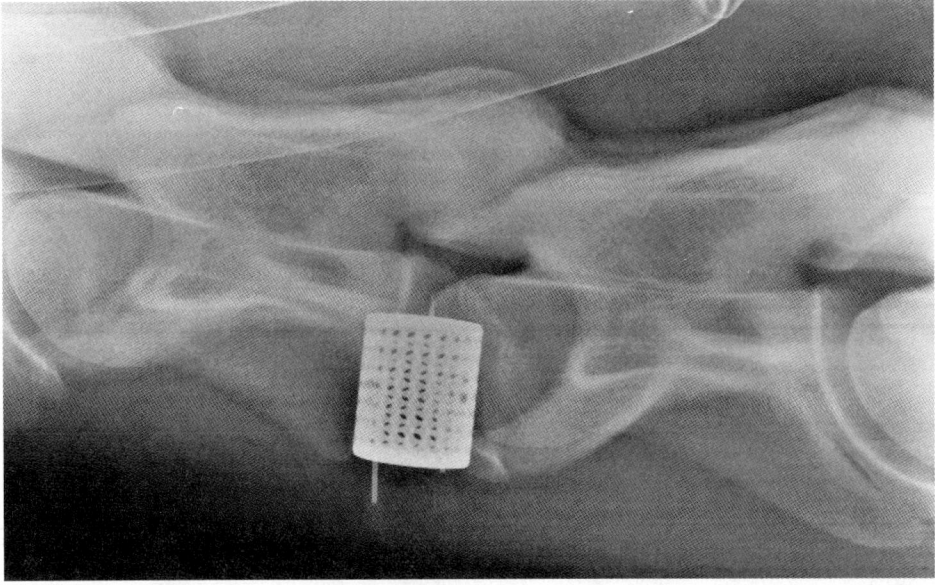

FIG. 33-31 ▌ Intraoperative radiograph of the third and fourth cervical vertebrae during cervical vertebral interbody fusion. The stainless steel basket is placed in the ventral aspect of the vertebral bodies, spanning the intervertebral disk and vertebral end plates, at the C3-C4 articulation.

maintains a balanced vitamin and mineral intake (minimum 100% of the NRC recommendations). Vitamins A and E are provided at 3 times the NRC recommendations, and selenium is supplemented to 0.3 ppm. Roughage is provided by pasture or low-quality grass hay (6% to 9% crude protein). Solitary stall confinement is recommended to minimize repetitive spinal cord compression from dynamic instability.

Surgical intervention is the most widely reported treatment for CSM.[1287-1290] The goals of surgical intervention are to stabilize the cervical vertebrae and decompress the spinal cord. Cervical vertebral interbody fusion (ventral stabilization) provides intervertebral stability for horses with dynamic spinal cord compression. The affected cervical vertebrae are fused in the extended position to provide immediate relief of spinal cord compression and prevent repetitive spinal cord trauma (Fig. 33-31).

Dorsal laminectomy (subtotal Funkquist type-B) is performed to decompress static lesions by removing portions of the dorsal lamina, ligamentum flavum, and joint capsule at the compressed site.[1288] This procedure provides immediate decompression of the spinal cord; however, fatal postoperative complications may occur.[1289] Interbody fusion in horses with static compression causes remodeling and atrophy of the articular processes, resulting in delayed decompression of the spinal cord over a period of weeks to months.[1291] Decompression is immediate with dorsal laminectomy; however, because of its relative safety, interbody fusion is believed by some surgeons to be the technique of choice for both dynamic and static compressive lesions.[1289]

Cervical vertebral interbody fusion improves the neurologic status in 44% to 90% of horses with CSM, with 12% to 62% of horses returning to athletic function.[1287,1289] Dorsal laminectomy results in improvement in neurologic status in 40% to 75% of horses with static compression.[1288,1289] The most important patient factor for determining the postoperative prognosis is the duration of clinical signs before surgical intervention; horses that have had clinical signs for less than 1 month before surgery are more likely to return to athletic function than are horses that have had clinical signs for longer than 3 months.[1289] Subtotal laminectomy and cervical vertebral interbody fusion for static compression of the caudal cervical vertebrae are associated with fatal postoperative complications, including vertebral body fracture, spinal cord edema, and implant failure.[1289]

Postoperatively, horses should be maintained on strict stall rest for 3 weeks and fed from a hay net to minimize motion at the surgery site. The duration of convalescence and rehabilitation after cervical vertebral interbody fusion is approximately 6 to 12 months. An individualized exercise program, determined by the projected use of the horse and the animal's neurologic status, should be designed to promote muscular strength. Extended exercise at slow speed, including ponying and lunging on inclines, is recommended during rehabilitation. A neurologic examination should be performed to determine the horse's ability to return to athletic function after surgery. It is unlikely that significant improvement in neurologic status will occur beyond the 1-year postoperative period.[1289]

REFERENCES

1263. Mayhew I, De Lahunta A, Whitlock R: Spinal cord disease in the horse, *Cornell Vet* 68(suppl 6):44-105, 1978.
1264. Reed S, Bayly W, Traub J: Ataxia and paresis in horses. I. Differential diagnosis, *Compend Cont Educ Pract Vet* 3:S88-S99, 1981.
1265. Moore BS et al: Contrast-enhanced computed tomography in six horses with cervical stenotic myelopathy, *Equine Vet J* 24:197-202, 1992.
1266. Wagner PC, Grant BD, Reed SM: Cervical vertebral malformations, *Vet Clin North Am (Equine Pract)* 3:385-396, 1987.
1267. Papageorges M et al: Radiographic and myelographic examination of the cervical vertebral column in 306 ataxic horses, *Vet Radiol* 28:53-59, 1987.
1268. Whitwell KE, Dyson S: Interpreting radiographs. VIII. Equine cervical vertebrae, *Equine Vet J* 19:8-14, 1987.
1269. Stewart R, Reed S, Weisbrode S: The frequency and severity of osteochondrosis in cervical stenotic myelopathy in horses, *Am J Vet Res* 52:873-879, 1991.
1270. Wagner P et al: A study of the heritability of cervical vertebral malformation in horses, *Proceedings of the Thirty-first Annual Convention of the American Association of Equine Practitioners*, 1987, pp 43-51.
1271. Gabel A et al: Comparison of incidence and severity of developmental orthopedic disease on 17 farms before and after adjustment of ration, *Proceedings of the Thirty-third Annual Convention of the American Association of Equine Practitioners*, 1987, pp 33:163.
1272. Knight D et al: The effects of copper supplementation on the prevalence of cartilage lesions in foals, *Equine Vet J* 22:426-432, 1990.

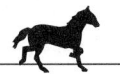

1273. Kronfeld D: Dietary aspects of developmental orthopedic disease, *Vet Clin North Am (Equine Pract)* 6:451-465, 1990.

1274. Glade MJ, Reimers TJ: Effects of dietary energy supply on serum thyroxine, triiodothyronine, and insulin concentrations in young horses, *J Endocrinol* 104:93, 1985.

1275. Rantanen NW, Gavin PR: Ataxia and paresis in horses. II. Radiographic and myelographic examination of the cervical vertebral column, *Compend Cont Educ Pract Vet* 3:S161-S171, 1981.

1276. Moore BR et al: Assessment of vertebral canal diameter and bony malformations of the cervical part of the spine in horses with cervical stenotic myelopathy, *Am J Vet Res* 55:5-13, 1994.

1277. Yovich JV, LeCouteur RA, Gould DH: Chronic cervical compressive myelopathy in horses: clinical correlations with spinal cord alterations, *Aust Vet J* 68:326-334, 1991.

1278. Mayhew IG et al: Diagnosis and prediction of cervical vertebral malformation in thoroughbred foals based on semiquantitative radiographic indicators, *Equine Vet J* 25:435-440, 1993.

1279. Moore BR, Granstom DE, Reed SM: Diagnosis of equine protozoal myelitis and cervical stenotic myelopathy, *Compend Cont Educ Pract Vet* 17:419-426, 1995.

1280. Neuwirth L: Equine myelography, *Compend Cont Educ Pract Vet* 14:72-79, 1992.

1281. Burbidge HM et al: Iohexol myelography in the horse, *Equine Vet J* 21:347-350, 1989.

1282. May SA, Wyn-Jones G, Church S: Iopamidol myelography in the horse, *Equine Vet J* 18:199-203, 1986.

1283. Maclean A et al: Use of iohexol for myelography in the horse, *Equine Vet J* 20:286-290, 1988.

1284. Widmer WR, Blevins WE: Veterinary myelography: a review of contrast media, adverse effects, and technique, *J Am Anim Hosp Assoc* 27:163-177, 1991.

1285. Hubbell J et al: Sequelae of myelography in the horse, *Equine Vet J* 20:438-440, 1988.

1286. Donawick WJ et al: Results of a low-protein low-energy diet and confinement on young horses with wobbles, *Proceedings of the Thirty-ninth Annual Convention of the American Association of Equine Practitioners*, 1993.

1287. Grant B, Barbee D, Wagner P: Long-term results of surgery for equine cervical vertebral malformation, *Proceedings of the Thirty-first Annual Convention of the American Association of Equine Practitioners*, 1985, pp 91-96.

1288. Nixon A, Stashak T, Ingram J: Dorsal laminectomy in the horse. III, Results in horses with cervical vertebral malformation, *Vet Surg* 12:184-188, 1983.

1289. Moore B, Reed, S, Robertson, J: Surgical treatment of cervical stenotic myelopathy in horses: 73 cases (1983-1992), *J Am Vet Med Assoc* 203:108-112, 1993.

1290. Wagner PC, Grant BD, Gallina AM: Ataxia and paresis in horses. III. Surgical treatment of cervical spinal cord compression, *Compend Cont Educ Pract Vet* 3:S192-S202, 1981.

1291. DeBowes RM et al: Cervical vertebral interbody fusion in the horse: a comparative study of bovine xenografts and autografts supported by stainless steel baskets, *Am J Vet Res* 45:191-199, 1984.

EQUINE DEGENERATIVE MYELOENCEPHALOPATHY

DEFINITION AND ETIOLOGY. Equine degenerative myeloencephalopathy (EDM) is a symmetric, noncompressive spinal cord disease of young horses characterized by demyelination of the dorsal funiculi of the cervical spinal cord and brainstem.[1292] Foals may be born with the condition, but horses ranging from 6 to 8 months of age are most often affected (the mean age of onset is about 5 months).[1292] The incidence of EDM in Arabian horses is disproportionately high.[1292] The disease has been recognized in zebras, donkeys, Welsh ponies, and horses of the Przewalski, thoroughbred, standardbred, Appaloosa, quarter horse, Paso Fino, paint, Haflinger, Norwegian Fjord, and Morgan breeds.[1293-1298] It has also been observed in Mongolian wild horses.[1294]

Myeloencephalopathy may be related to a dietary deficiency of vitamin E, but it also has a familial pattern of distribution. These observations suggest a genetic etiology, but the mode of inheritance is not clear.[1299]

CLINICAL SIGNS. Affected horses show a symmetric proprioceptive (sensory) ataxia characterized by knuckling, stumbling, circumduction, abduction, interference, abnormal limb protraction, spasticity, hypermetria, and inability to turn sharply or lift the inside forefoot during sharp turns.

When the animal is forced to turn sharply in a circle, the inside rear foot pivots instead of lifting off the ground. Affected animals appear clumsy and cannot stop rapidly from a gallop. When stopped suddenly, they step on the rear of the forelimbs and end in a dog-sitting posture. Affected animals usually have severe conscious proprioceptive deficits that can be detected by postural placement tests. Some patients are unable to back or move easily down an incline. They may fall or stumble when light pressure is applied to the tuber coxae or withers. In most cases the neurologic abnormalities in the fore and rear limbs are of similar severity. This observation may aid in the differentiation between degenerative myeloencephalopathy and cervical stenotic myelopathy, both of which result in more severe lesions in the rear limbs than in the forelimbs.

Other clinical signs characteristic of equine degenerative myeloencephalopathy are a deficit of the local cervical and the cervicoauricular reflexes and paralysis of the laryngeal adductor muscles. A test of laryngeal function that detects lesions of the dorsal cervical funiculi or the vagosympathetic trunk has been described.[1300] The horse is restrained in stocks, and the larynx is visualized with an endoscope. The horse is struck three times sharply on the saddle area. Normal horses respond to each slap by closing the rima glottis symmetrically. Unilateral lesions of the dorsal spinal cord funiculi are associated with paralysis of the contralateral arytenoid.[1293] This test is not completely accurate, however. The predictive value of a positive test result could increase the index of suspicion by 50% to 70%. Negative results, however, do not completely exclude the possibility of a cervical spinal cord disease.[1301] In rare cases animals with EDM may present in acute recumbency without a prior history of neurologic disease (Smith MO: unpublished data).

CLINICAL PATHOLOGY AND RADIOGRAPHIC FINDINGS. EDM is best differentiated from cervical stenotic myelopathy by plain and contrast radiographic examination of the spinal column. The cervical spinal canal, the cerebrospinal fluid (CSF) protein concentration, and the white blood cell count of horses with degenerative myeloencephalopathy are normal. The plasma vitamin E concentration may be below the reference range (300 to 1050 µg/dl) in some but not all unsupplemented affected horses.[1294,1295] For analysis, optimal methods of blood collection include collection of unhemolyzed blood in a clot tube and storage in an upright position in a refrigerator. The refrigerated specimens should not be allowed to contact rubber stoppers and should not be stored for longer than 72 hours unless the red cells are removed and the plasma is gassed with nitrogen and frozen at −16° C (3.2° F). The concentration of vitamin E in specimens handled in this manner remains constant for at least 3 months.[1302]

PATHOPHYSIOLOGY. Some authors have suggested that the disease is associated with a low plasma concentration of vitamin E from 6 weeks to 10 months of age.[1295,1303,1304] Oral absorption of vitamin E does not appear to be deficient in affected horses.[1304] Vitamin-replete, clinically normal horses have a plasma concentration ranging from 1.7 to 9.5 µg/ml. The plasma concentration of vitamin E is approximately 2 µg/ml higher in the spring and summer than in winter. Horses fed diets that lack fresh green forage have a low plasma concentration of vitamin E. Such diets include poor-quality, sun-baked hay and pelleted rations.

Myeloencephalopathy occurs most often in related horses, indicating the possibility of a genetic predisposition to the deficiency.[1304] In one dietary study in which vitamin E supplementation was tested, the case attack rate declined from 40% to 10% in the first year after supplementation, and the severity of disease in subsequent foal crops was diminished. Moreover, supplementation of five affected horses with 6000 IU of vitamin E daily resulted in an improvement in their neurologic condition. Horses' susceptibility to development of low vitamin E concentrations also appears to be age related. Foals sired by affected stallions tend to have lower plasma α-tocopherol concentrations than those sired by normal stallions. These lower concentrations are first noted by 6 weeks of age, but the differences disappear by 10 months. The causes of the differences in the two groups of animals are unknown. An alternative explanation for the role of vitamin E in EDM is a defect in vitamin E metabolism. The nature of such a defect has yet to be elucidated.

Vitamin E deficiency is apparently not the sole etiologic factor in the condition, however, because one report documented normal vitamin E levels in the serum of 40 affected horses examined at a veterinary hospital.[1305] Subsequent epidemiologic studies indicated that risk factors for the disorder include heredity, application of insecticides on foals, exposure to dirt lots without pasture, and exposure to wood preservatives. Access to green pasture had a protective effect on foals.[1304] This study may indicate that the changes in the central nervous system are related to the patient's inability to respond adequately to oxidative stress such as phenols, anthelmintics, and insecticides.

PATHOLOGY. The microscopic lesions are present in the dorsolateral and ventromedial tracts of the white matter funiculi and in the sensory nuclear relay areas of the spinal cord and the medulla.[1294] These lesions include moderate-to-severe diffuse fiber degeneration of ascending and descending spinal cord funiculi, variable astrogliosis, and prominent myelin loss. Large eosinophilic "spheroids" can be seen in the gray matter of the spinal cord at all levels. Other gray matter lesions include astrocytosis, vesicle formation (from loss of cell bodies), and accumulation of pigments in macrophages that stain positively for lipofuscin. These lesions are diffuse and extend to all levels of the spinal cord and the caudal brainstem.

TREATMENT AND CONTROL. EDM usually is chronically progressive, although the clinical signs may stabilize for an indefinite period. The clinical signs are irreversible, and most patients eventually are euthanized because they become hazardous to other livestock and human beings.

The current recommended vitamin E level for horse feed is 80 to 100 IU/kg/day.[1306] In suspected cases of EDM, supplementation with 6000 IU of d,1,- α-tocopherol acetate in feed is recommended, a level that appears to be safe. It is suggested that this dose be mixed with 60 ml of corn oil and fed in 1 L of concentrate ration daily.[1306] Once clinical signs are present, the prognosis for complete recovery is guarded to poor.

REFERENCES

1292. Mayhew IG, De Lahunta A, Whitlock RH: Spinal cord disease in the horse, *Cornell Vet* 6(suppl 68):11-206, 1978.
1293. Montali RJ et al: Spinal ataxia in zebras: comparison with the wobbler syndrome of horses, *Vet Pathol* 11:68-78, 1974.
1294. Liu S-K et al: Myelopathy and vitamin E deficiency in six Mongolian wild horses, *J Am Vet Med Assoc* 11:1266-1268, 1983.
1295. Mayhew IG et al: Equine degenerative myeloencephalopathy: a vitamin E deficiency that may be familial, *J Vet Intern Med* 1:45-50, 1985.
1296. Scarratt WK et al: Degenerative myelopathy in two equids, *Equine Vet Sci* 5:139-141, 1985.
1297. Mayhew IG et al: Equine degenerative myeloencephalopathy, *J Am Vet Med Assoc* 170:195-201, 1977.
1298. Baumgartner W, Frese K, Elmadfa I: Neuroaxonal dystrophy associated with vitamin E deficiency in two Haflinger horses, *J Com Pathol* 103:113-119, 1990.
1299. Blythe LL et al: Clinical, viral, and genetic evaluation of equine degenerative myeloencephalopathy in a family of Appaloosas, *J Am Vet Med Assoc* 198:1005-1013, 1991.
1300. Greet TRC et al: The slap test for laryngeal adductory function in horses with suspected cervical spinal cord damage, *Equine Vet J* 12:127-131, 1980.
1301. Newton-Clarke MS, Divers TJ, De Lahunta A: Evaluation of the thoracolaryngeal reflex (slap test) as an aid to the diagnosis of cervical spinal cord and brainstem disease in horses, *Equine Vet J* 26:358-361, 1994.
1302. Craig AM et al: Variability of α-tocopherol values associated with procurement, storage, and freezing of equine serum and plasma samples, *Am J Vet Res* 53:2228-2234, 1992.
1303. Blythe LL, Craig Am, Lassen ED: Vitamin E in the horse and its relationship to equine degenerative myeloencephalopathy, Proceedings of the Seventh Annual ACVIM Forum, San Diego, 1989.
1304. Blythe LL et al: Serially determined plasma α-tocopherol concentrations and results of the oral vitamin E absorption test in clinically normal horses and in horses with degenerative myeloencephalopathy, *Am J Vet Res* 52:908-911, 1991.
1305. Dill SG et al: Serum vitamin E and blood glutathione peroxidase values of horses with degenerative myeloencephalopathy, *Am J Vet Res* 50:166-168, 1989.
1306. Blythe LL, Graig AM: Equine degenerative myeloencephalopathy. II. Diagnosis and treatment, *Compend Cont Educ Pract Vet* 14:1633, 1992.

EQUINE MOTOR NEURON DISEASE

THOMAS J. DIVERS
MARY O. SMITH

In 1990 an acquired neurodegenerative disease of adult horses was first described.[1307] The equine disease appeared to be very similar to human motor neuron disease (amyotrophic lateral sclerosis, known as ALS or Lou Gehrig's disease). Equine motor neuron disease (EMND) is the only naturally occurring animal model for ALS. Recent experimental studies have revealed that the disease occurs secondary to chronic vitamin E deficiency. Reports of this disorder are now almost worldwide.

CLINICAL SIGNS. Affected animals are adults with a mean age of 9 years (the range is 2 to 23 years).[1308] Clinical signs vary depending on the stage or duration of the disorder. For this reason, the signs are best summarized by dividing the disease into subacute and chronic forms. A subclinical form also probably occurs, although definitive evidence of this currently is lacking.

Subacute Form. Horses develop acute onset of trembling, fasciculations, lying down more than normal, frequent shifting of weight in the rear legs, and abnormal sweating. Head carriage may be abnormally low. Appetite and gait usually are not noticeably affected. The owner may mention that the horse had been losing weight (loss of muscle mass) for a month before the other signs appeared.

Chronic Form. The trembling and fasciculations subside, and the horse's condition stabilizes, but with varying degrees of muscle atrophy. In some cases the atrophy is so severe, the horse looks emaciated. In other cases muscle mass or fat deposition (or both) show noticeable improvement. The tail head frequently is in an abnormally high resting position.

Subclinical Form. Experimental research has proved that horses maintained on prolonged diets low in vitamin E may have subclinical disease. This could have significant implications, because unknown to the rider or owner, the affected horse would have diminished strength.

CLINICAL PATHOLOGY. Horses with EMND have mildly elevated levels of creatine kinase and aspartate aminotransferase. The serum vitamin E is low (under 1 μg/ml) in almost all acute and subacute cases. Superoxide dismutase (SOD) activity in red blood cells also is severely decreased, which is believed to be due to increased consumption of SOD. Various other clinicopathologic abnormalities may be present in particular individuals, including elevated serum γ-glutamyl transferase activity; low vitamin A, beta-carotene, or ascorbic acid; and high liver iron levels. Many horses have been found to have abnormal glucose absorption, but the relationship of this finding to vitamin E deficiency and EMND is unknown.

The protein level of the cerebrospinal fluid is elevated in almost half of affected horses, and intrathecal IgG is increased in many. The latter effect is thought be a response to neuronal death rather than a primary pathophysiologic event.

PATHOPHYSIOLOGY. The sites of lesions in EMND are the ventral horn cells (lower motor neurons) of the spinal cord gray matter; the nuclei of cranial nerves V, VII, XII; and the nucleus ambiguus, which undergo noninflammatory degeneration. Neurogenic atrophy occurs in muscles innervated by degenerate neurons, particularly those with predominantly type 1 myofibers, which have a higher oxidative requirement than type 2 fibers and thus are more susceptible to oxidative damage. The dysfunction and death of motor neurons is an oxidative disorder, presumably caused by vitamin E deficiency and the resulting inability to protect against oxidative (prooxidant) stress. Clinical signs occur when approximately 30% of the motor neurons are affected. Some of these neurons may regain function with vitamin E treatment, offering an explanation of why some horses do not have continual progression of clinical signs as occurs in ALS in human beings. Human motor neuron disease, although an oxidative disorder, is more complex that EMND and the cause or causes have yet to be determined.

PATHOLOGY. Gross lesions are limited to pallor of the medial head of the triceps brachii and vastus intermedius muscles. Severe atrophy is present in these muscles and many others, including the sacrocaudalis dorsalis medialis muscle of the tail, which shows severe denervation atrophy and fibrosis. Scattered areas of myofiber necrosis are present in many muscles. A pigment retinopathy and deposition of lipopigment in the vasculature of the spinal cord are found in horses with EMND, and these appear to be related to similar pigment depositions in other species with vitamin E deficiency. Provision of a vitamin E–supplemented diet may result in resolution of pigment deposition.

EPIDEMIOLOGY. EMND is a sporadic disease, with only single animals in a barn being affected in most cases, although a few outbreaks of the disease have been reported. All breeds of horse can be affected, as can ponies. The apparent prevalence of the disease in certain breeds probably is a reflection of the prevalence of the breed in specific populations of horses, and no familial or heritable predisposition has been identified. Affected horses usually are housed in facilities with little or no access to pasture for over a year before signs appear.[1308,1309] The diet of affected animals is deficient in green foodstuffs and frequently consists of pelleted or sweet feed and poor-quality grass hay, without alfalfa or other sources of vitamin E supplementation.[1310,1311] No other management practices, such as worming and vaccination regimens, insecticide use, amount of exercise, and type of bedding, have been related to development of the disease. The highest prevalence of EMND in North America occurs in the northeastern United States and Canada, although sporadic cases have been reported across the continent. This regional distribution is believed to relate to the frequency of predisposing management practices in high incidence areas rather than other environmental factors.

DIAGNOSIS. The diagnosis can be made from the following observations and test.
1. Epidemiologic information:
   a. Previous cases in the stable
   b. Historic information that suggests the horse might have been without green forage for an extended period
2. Clinical signs (see above)
3. Measurement of plasma vitamin E and muscle enzyme levels

Muscle or Nerve Biopsy. Biopsy of the sacrocaudalis dorsalis muscle is the invasive test of choice, having almost 90% sensitivity and specificity.[1312] The biopsy specimen should be placed in 10% formalin for submission to the laboratory. A positive result is the finding of characteristic abnormalities, including denervation atrophy of myofibers and scattered myofiber necrosis. Biopsy of the spinal accessory nerve is more technically demanding but is a more sensitive test in chronic cases.[1312,1313] Nerve biopsy requires general anesthesia, whereas muscle biopsy can be performed using a local block in the sedated horse.

Differential diagnoses for EMND include equine protozoal myeloencephalitis, colic, laminitis, botulism, and tying-up.

TREATMENT. Oral vitamin E supplementation at a dosage of 5000 to 7000 IU daily may result in improvement in some clinically affected horses, although full recovery is unlikely. It cannot reverse the neuronal death, and all affected horses are permanently weakened. Acute death has been reported in some horses treated for EMND that appeared to have recovered. Use of a source of pure vitamin E is preferable to a multivitamin-mineral supplement.

PREVENTION. All horses without green forage (grass of good quality or green hay) for prolonged periods (longer than 1 year) should be routinely tested for the plasma vitamin E concentration and/or supplemented with vitamin E. If this were a standard policy, most if not all cases of EMND could be prevented.

REFERENCES
1307. Cummings JF et al: Equine motor neuron disease: a preliminary report, *Cornell Vet* 80:357-379, 1990.
1308. Mohammed HO et al: Risk factors associated with equine motor neuron disease: a possible model for human MND, *Neurology* 43:966-971, 1993.
1309. Divers TJ et al: Equine motor neuron disease: findings in 28 horses and proposal of a pathophysiological mechanism for the disease, *Equine Vet J* 26:409-415, 1994.
1310. De la Rua-Domenech R et al: Incidence and risk factors of equine motor neuron disease: an ambidirectional study, *Neuroepidemiol* 14:54-64, 1995.
1311. De la Rua-Domenech R et al: Association between plasma vitamin E concentration and the risk of equine motor neuron disease, *Br Vet J* 154:203-213, 1997.
1312. Divers TJ et al: Simple and practical muscle biopsy test for equine motor neuron disease, *Proceedings of the Forty-second Annual Convention of the American Association of Equine Practitioners*, 1996, pp 180-181.
1313. Jackson CA et al: Spinal accessory nerve biopsy as an antemortem diagnostic test for equine motor neuron disease, *Equine Vet J* 28:215-219, 1996.

SPINAL FRACTURES AND LUXATIONS AND SPINAL CORD TRAUMA

DEFINITION AND ETIOLOGY. Vertebral fractures are common causes of spinal cord injury in large animals. Because of the relative differences in management, temperament, and regional strength of the spine, the pathogenesis and predominant anatomic location of spinal injury sites differ among the livestock species.

Horses. In one study from the United Kingdom in which 26 horses with spinal lesions were examined, 16 had lesions of the cervical spine, 17 had fractures of the thoracic spine, and 5 and 4 had fractures of the lumbar and sacrococcygeal spine, respectively.[1314] The vertebrae that were most commonly injured were C1, T12, and L5.[1314] Horses with lesions of the thoracic dorsal spinous processes did not show neurologic deficits, whereas a high proportion of horses that had lesions in the lumbar and cervical spine had ataxia or other associated neurologic deficits.

Ruminants. Fractures of the vertebral column in ruminants may result from abnormal bone mineralization. The common sites of spinal fractures in calves are C2 to C4, T10 to T13, and L3 to L6 vertebrae. Spinal fractures are especially common in 3- to 6-month-old ruminants as a result of nutritional deficiencies. These deficiencies could include vitamin D, calcium, or copper. Differentiation of nutritional osteodystrophies from traumatic vertebral fractures is essential, because different preventive measures must be taken for the two conditions. Traumatic cervical vertebral fractures of cattle and small ruminants may be caused by injuries sustained in falls, roadway accidents, butting of other animals, predation, or squeeze chutes.[1315] Spontaneous fractures of vertebrae weakened by developmental defects (hemivertebrae) or spinal abscesses also are common problems in calves.

Traumatic luxations or fractures of the atlantooccipital and atlantoaxial joints of pygmy goats may occur when the horns are held during restraint.

Fractures of the lumbosacral spine of cattle are commonly caused by slipping in cemented areas.[1315] Many of the spinal fractures occur during mounting by herd mates exhibiting estral behavior. Thoracolumbar fractures may occur in calves during correction of a dystocia.[1316] The occurrence of spinal fractures during delivery is mostly related to excessive traction and rotational force during the assisted delivery.[1317] Luxation of the sacroiliac joint in the dam may occur with the use of excessive force during manual extraction of a calf. Traumatic lumbar vertebral fractures occur secondary to chronic ankylosing spondylosis in mature bulls and rams.[1318]

CLINICAL SIGNS. The clinical presentation of a spinal fracture varies, depending on the site of the traumatic lesion, the severity of the spinal cord compression, and the involvement of specific anatomic tracts.

Cervical Spine. Vertebral fractures are painful, and the patient usually shows some distress in the early stages. Goats may bleat or cry when the spine is manipulated. Horses groan and, if recumbent, thrash wildly. Cattle and sheep may lie on their sides and groan. Animals with noncompressive cervical spinal column lesions maintain a stiff neck (weather vane attitude), refuse to lower the head, and eat from the ground while kneeling. To prehend food, they often keep the head away from the ground and extend the tongue. These animals have stiff necks and resist passive flexion of the head.[1319] Similar signs may be seen with meningitis.

Animals with severe lesions may be recumbent. Depending on the amount of pain and the secondary complications associated with the disease, the sensorium varies from bright, alert, and responsive to depressed and obviously painful. Recumbent animals may not be able to lift the head from the floor if a high cervical lesion (C1 to C4) is present.[1320] Crepitation may be palpable in some cases. Luxation of the atlantooccipital joint results in asymmetry of the wings of the atlas. These animals often have a wry neck as a result of the twisting forces on the displaced atlas.[1321] Patients with mild lesions of the cervical spine may be able to stand and show varying degrees of ataxia and conscious proprioceptive deficits. Specific gait abnormalities include circumduction, interference, knuckling, incomplete limb protraction, crossing over, and excessive body sway. Animals with high partial cervical spinal cord lesions show hypalgesia of the entire body. Bilateral compressive lesions of the cervical spinal cord result in rapid death caused by respiratory paralysis. The neurologic injury causes paralysis of the phrenic nerve. If the spinal cord lesion is above the C6 segment (C6 to C7 vertebrae), the muscular tone and spinal reflexes (panniculus, triceps, and biceps) are normal to increased in all limbs. If the lesion is located at the sixth to eighth cervical spinal cord segments, the forelimb reflexes are diminished or absent and those of the rear limbs are normal to increased.

Conscious pain perception in the limbs often is diminished or absent, depending on the amount of damage in the sensory spinal cord tracts. In long-standing cases in which the ventral rootlets or motor neurons of C6 to C8 have been destroyed, the muscles of the neck and forelimbs may become atrophic. Regional or strip sweating may be observed in some horses. The anal and tail tone are normal. The bladder may be distended, but the tone of the urethral musculature is normal.

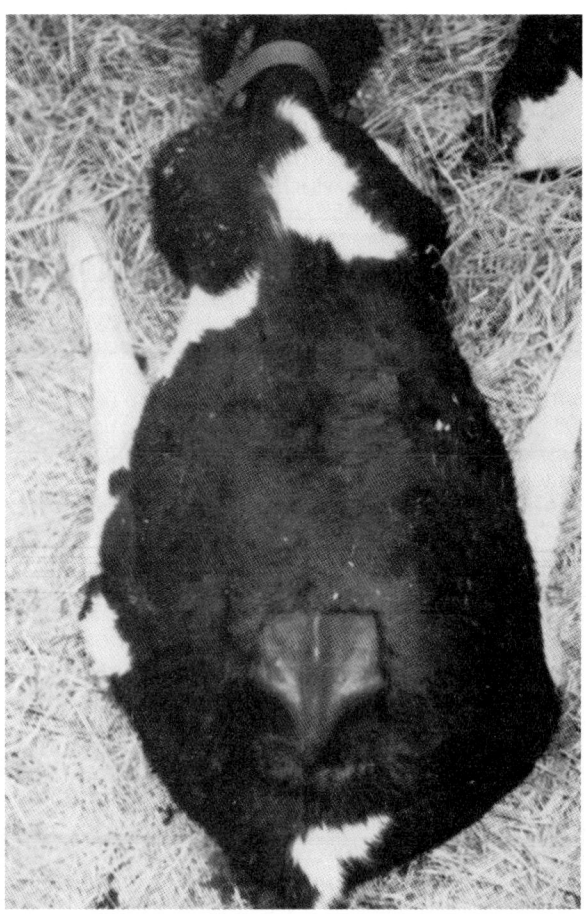

FIG. 33-32 ▓ Characteristic posture of a calf with a compressive fracture of the L6 vertebra and hematomyelia. The calf was fed a diet of grass hay and corn and developed nutritional osteodystrophy. (Courtesy Dr. R.H. Whitlock.)

Thoracic Spine. Affected animals have an attitude similar to those with cervical spinal cord lesions, except that thoracic limbs are normal. Animals with severe spinal cord lesions intermittently lie on their sides and then arise to assume a dog-sitting posture. When lying in sternal recumbency, the rear limbs of these animals are held extended rather than in the normal tucked-up position. The spinal reflexes of the forelimbs are normal. A crossed extensor reflex may be observed in the rear limbs. Depending on the amount of damage to the sensory tracts, conscious perception of pain in the rear limbs may be decreased or absent. The tail and anal tone are normal. The bladder is distended, but the tone of the urethral sphincter and penis is normal. Animals with acute lesions of the thoracic spine (less than 2 days' duration) may display Schiff-Sherrington syndrome,[1322] which is characterized by hypertonia and normoreflexia of the forelimbs and flaccidity and normoreflexia or hyperreflexia of the rear limbs.[1322] The animals are able to move the forelimbs normally. Schiff-Sherrington syndrome is rare in large animals. Most animals with thoracic spinal cord injury have normal to exaggerated spinal reflexes and hypertonia of the rear limbs.

Lumbar Spine. Affected animals have an attitude, gait, and posture similar to those with thoracic spinal cord lesions. Fig. 33-32 shows the characteristic posture of a calf with a vertebral fracture at the L6 vertebra. Fig. 33-33 illustrates myelographic findings of cord compression at L6. The forelimbs are usually normal. Lesions at the L1 to L3 spinal cord segments result in normal or hypertonic and hyperreflexic rear limbs.

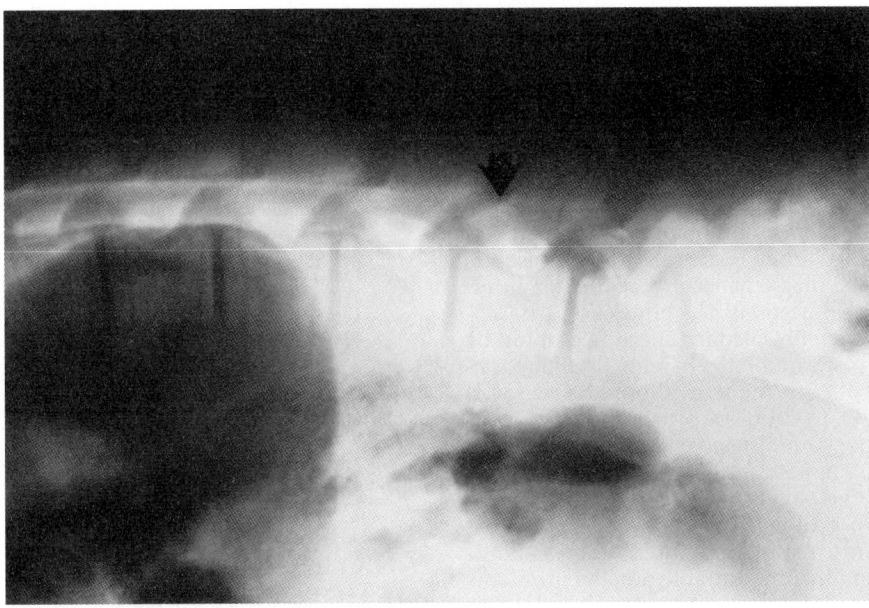

FIG. 33-33 ▓ Myelogram of a calf with nutritional osteodystrophy showing a mild compression fracture of the L6 vertebra and complete obstruction of dye flow posterior to L5 *(arrow).*

Conversely, hypotonia and hyporeflexia of the rear limbs may be seen in animals with lesions at spinal cord segments L4 to S2.[1323] Marked spasm of the longissimus dorsi muscle has been described in horses with a lesion between the T11 and T12 spinal cord segments.[1324] Lesions of spinal cord segments L4 to L6 result in cutaneous desensitization of the medial surface of the rear leg and diminished or absent patellar reflex because of dysfunction of the femoral and saphenous nerves. Lesions of spinal cord segments L6 to S2 result in desensitization of the rear limb and diminished withdrawal (flexor) reflexes. The panniculus response is absent when the skin posterior to the lesion is stimulated. Damage to the spinal rootlets may cause regional swelling. The tail and anal tone are normal. The bladder is distended, but the sphincter tone is normal.

Sacrococcygeal Spine. Lesions of spinal cord segments S1 to S2 result in decreased conscious proprioceptive responses of the rear limbs[1325] and diminished flexor reflexes of those limbs. Anal tone is diminished to absent, and the bladder is distended and hypotonic. The patient is incontinent as a result of atonia of the urethral sphincter, and urine scalding may be seen over the perineum. The tail is flaccid and paralyzed. The anal sphincter is dilated, and the rectum is filled with dry fecal matter. There may be palpable abnormalities of the pelvis or sacrococcygeal joint. Crepitus of the pelvic bones may be noted when the animal is moved.

CLINICAL PATHOLOGY AND RADIOGRAPHIC FINDINGS. Plain radiographs are the most definitive method of diagnosing a spinal fracture. In young horses slipped physeal plates are commonly seen in the atlas.[1324,1326] Shortening of the lumbar vertebrae is consistent with either an oblique overriding fracture of the vertebral body or a compression fracture.[1323,1326] Abnormally shaped vertebrae may signify an anomalous vertebral arch. A myelographic examination may detect stenosis in segments distant from the fracture site.

Examination of cerebrospinal fluid (CSF) collected through a lumbosacral puncture may be useful for ancillary diagnosis of a spinal fracture. Fracture-induced changes in the CSF may be classified as either acute (0 to 1 day) or chronic (longer than 1 day). The acute changes include diffuse blood contamination, a high red blood cell (RBC) count, a normal to high white blood cell (WBC) count, and a high protein concentration. The CSF changes in patients with more chronic injuries include a normal to slightly increased WBC count, normal to increased RBC count, increased protein concentration, and xanthochromia. Assuming that motor neuron units have been denervated, fibrillation potentials may be seen in muscles by 5 days after injury.

PATHOLOGY AND PATHOPHYSIOLOGY. Neurologic dysfunction is caused by traumatic compression. Over time neural transmission over a large number of spinal segments is reduced. This represents the so-called spinal shock syndrome, during which the spinal neurons become unresponsive. Leakage of potassium ions from the injured cells combined with a defect in neurotransmitter activity is thought to result in reduced neurologic function. Local vasogenic reflexes, mostly mediated by α-adrenergic receptors, result in decreased blood flow in the gray and white matter. Platelets aggregate in the hypoperfused capillaries and form microthrombi and infarcts. Regional ischemia caused by hypoperfusion results in lipid peroxidation of the axons, myelin degradation, and demyelination.[1327]

TREATMENT AND PROGNOSIS. It is important to recognize that the radiographic appearance of a spinal fracture is not a reliable prognostic indicator, because the vertebral components are likely to be in a different position than at the time of injury. Not all vertebral body fractures result in neurologic disease. The prognosis is best judged on the basis of repeated neurologic examinations. Provided the animal is not suffering inhumanely and the pain can be adequately controlled, repeated neurologic examinations should be made over the first several hours. The longer the patient remains recumbent and neurologically impaired, the more unfavorable the prognosis. Most recoveries from spinal cord contusion occur spontaneously and are not appreciably influenced by drug administration. Nevertheless, some authors have recommended treating acutely affected animals with dimethyl sulfoxide (DMSO) (0.25 to 1 g/kg IV in 5% dextrose as a 40% DMSO solution) and dexamethasone (0.1 to 0.2 mg/kg of body weight given 4 times daily for 2 to 4 days). Analgesics or tranquilizers should be administered with care to ambulatory patients that have thoracolumbar spinal lesions because an ataxic patient may slip and worsen the spinal cord contusion. If signs of pain are severe, nonsteroidal antiinflammatory agents or narcotic analgesics (morphine, 0.2 to 0.4 mg/kg) may be administered. Lumbar epidural injection of 0.1 mg/kg of body weight of morphine in 10 to 20 ml of normal saline also may provide analgesia. In animals with pelvic lesions, the bladder should be evacuated either by manual palpation per rectum or by insertion of a catheter and use of a closed urinary drainage system. Addition of 1% hydrogen peroxide to the urinary collection bag and attention to aseptic procedure during catheter maintenance may reduce the number of iatrogenic bacterial infections. The urine should be cultured and examined repeatedly. Bladder infections should be treated with an appropriate antibiotic. In animals with paralysis of the rectal musculature, the feces should be removed manually. Lubricants (1 to 2 quarts of warm detergent or methyl cellulose) may be administered with an enema.

If the spinal fracture appears stable and the animal can stand with assistance, the patient may be placed in a water tank and supported for prolonged periods. Goats are most amenable to treatment for spinal fractures, whereas adult horses and cattle present insurmountable nursing problems and should be euthanized if they are unable to rise after several days or are suffering intractable pain. Slings are commercially available or can be fashioned from canvas or burlap and wool or cotton. The time that the patient should spend in the sling varies, depending on its temperament and the degree of neurologic dysfunction. Some horses become frantic while suspended in the device and cannot be supported without the risk of severe injury to the patient and the handlers. The sling should not be used for recumbent animals that cannot support themselves while harnessed. Such animals can suffer severe (even fatal) respiratory compromise or secondary myositis. Nevertheless, daily prolonged slinging of animals with mild neurologic signs may minimize secondary medical complications and improve extensor muscle tone.

Recumbent cattle should be floated in a tub of warm water. Watertight tubs for use with large cattle are commercially available* (see Down Cows, p. 1017).

Cervical fractures and luxations of small ruminants may be stabilized by incorporation of the head, neck, and anterior thorax in a fiberglass cast. The cast should extend from the middle part of the thorax to the tip of the nose. The feed and water supply of all animals with cervical fractures should be placed so that the animal can reach it without bending the neck. Although surgical methods for stabilization of atlantoaxial fractures have been described in horses, the effectiveness of such treatments for restoration of neurologic function after traumatic injury or fracture of the spinal column is unclear.[1328]

The dietary intake of copper, molybdenum, and calcium should be measured in cattle. If the daily intake is inadequate, the minerals should be fed via supplements. Animals with metabolic bone disease should not be restrained because of the possibility of inducing additional pathologic fractures.

REFERENCES

1314. Jeffcott LB, Whitwell KE: Fractures of the thoracolumbar spine of the horse, *Proceedings of the Twenty-second Annual Convention of the American Association of Equine Practitioners,* 1976, pp 91-102.
1315. Julian RJ, Maxwell TW: Fracture of the cervical vertebrae in a heifer, *Can Vet J* 4:29-30, 1963.
1316. JoAnn CL, Killeen JR: A retrospective study of dystocia-related vertebral fractures in neonatal calves, *Can Vet J* 29:830-833, 1988.
1317. Schuijt G: Iatrogenic fractures of ribs and vertebrae during delivery in perinatally dying calves: 235 cases (1978-1988), *J Am Vet Med Assoc* 197:1196-1202, 1990.

*Aqualift, Kirby Manufacturing Co., Merced, CA 95341.

1318. Thompson RG: Vertebral body osteophytes in bulls, *Pathol Vet* 6(suppl):1-47, 1969.
1319. Funk KA, Erickson ED: A case of atlantoaxial subluxation in a horse, *Can Vet J* 9:120-123, 1968.
1320. Guffy MM, Coffman JR, Strafuss AC: Atlantoaxial luxation in a foal, *J Am Vet Med Assoc* 155:754-757, 1969.
1321. Baker GJ: Comminuted fracture of the axis, *Equine Vet J* 2:37-38, 1970.
1322. Chiapetta C, Baker JC, Feeny DA: Vertebral fracture, extensor hypertonia of thoracic limbs, and paralysis of the pelvic limbs (Schiff-Sherrington syndrome) in an Arabian foal, *J Am Vet Med Assoc* 186:387-388, 1985.
1323. Mason JE: A case of spinal cord compression causing paraplegia of a foal, *Equine Vet J* 3:155-157, 1971.
1324. Whitwell KE, Dyson S: Interpreting radiographs. VIII. Equine cervical vertebrae, *Equine Vet J* 19:8-14, 1987.
1325. Moyer WA, Rooney JR: Vertebral fracture in a horse, *J Am Vet Med Assoc* 159:1022-1024, 1971.
1326. Ramey DW, Selcer BA: Radiographic diagnosis, *Vet Radiol* 25:218-219, 1984.
1327. Hahn CN, Mayhew IG, McKay R: The nervous system. In Colahan PT et al, eds: *Equine medicine and surgery,* ed 5, St Louis, 2000, Mosby.
1328. Owen R ap R, Smith LL: Repair of fractured dens of the axis in a foal, *J Am Vet Med Assoc* 173:854-856, 1978.

ANKYLOSING SPONDYLITIS OF HOLSTEIN BULLS

LISLE W. GEORGE

Ankylosing spondylitis is an inflammatory disease of joint tissue associated with fusion of lumbar vertebrae in Holstein bulls. Approximately 4% of all Holstein bulls used for artificial insemination are culled each year because of spondylitis.[1329] The clinical onset of the condition is insidious. The first signs of the disorder are a stilted gait, reluctance to move, and dragging of the toes of the rear limbs. Affected bulls are slow to mount teaser dummies for collection. The condition is progressive, and over several months the animals develop paraparesis and ataxia. With mounting, the ankylosed area of the spine may fracture, leading to acute recumbency. Pathologic changes associated with the condition include calcification of the ventral vertebral ligaments between the T11 and L3 vertebrae. The condition appears to be hereditary. All bulls with the condition possess the class I MHC-BoLA A8 phenotype. In comparison, the phenotypic frequency of BoLA A8 in the general population of normal Holstein bulls is only 44%.[1330]

REFERENCES

1329. Monke DR, Parker WG, Hillman R: Progressive posterior paralysis, Proceedings of the Ninth Technical Conference on Artificial Insemination and Reproduction, National Association of Artificial Insemination Breeders, Columbia, Mo, 1982.
1330. Park CA et al: Association between the bovine major histocompatibility complex and chronic posterior spinal paresis—a form of ankylosing spondylitis—in Holstein bulls, *Anim Genet* 24:53-58, 1993.

SPINAL ABSCESSES

DEFINITION AND ETIOLOGY. Most abscesses of the spinal cord originate from a preexisting vertebral body osteomyelitis. The bone usually is infected hematogenously. Extension of bacteria from the lungs, the heart, or a septic injection site is common. Neonates frequently develop vertebral abscesses secondary to septicemia.[1331] Bone lesions may develop from sequestra broken from fractured vertebrae. Epizootics of spinal abscesses can occur as a result of injection of contaminated vaccines or mineral supplements near the spinal column. This is especially common in lambs given selenium–vitamin E injections and cattle vaccinated with *Vibrio* vaccines. Infectious agents isolated from spinal abscesses of ruminants include *Corynebacterium pseudotuberculosis, Actinomyces pyogenes, Pasteurella haemolytica, Staphylococcus aureus,* and *Fusobacterium necrophorum.*[1331-1334] Agents commonly found in vertebral infections of foals include *Salmonella* spp., *Actinobacillus equuli,*

Escherichia coli, β*-hemolytic streptococci, Rhodococcus equi,* and *Klebsiella pneumoniae.*[1334-1336] Agents less commonly associated with vertebral body osteomyelitis of horses and cattle include *Mycobacterium bovis, Mycobacterium avium, Aspergillus* spp., *Eikenella corrodens,* and *Brucella abortus.*[1337-1339] In rare cases septic arthritis of the atlantooccipital joint may develop as a result of extension of a mycotic guttural pouch lesion.[1340,1341]

If the infectious agent remains localized in the vertebral body, the patient usually shows signs consistent with occlusion of the spinal canal. If the infection erodes through the dura mater, the animal develops signs of septic meningitis. If the bone infection is extensive, the vertebrae may fracture suddenly, resulting in signs characteristic of spinal trauma.

CLINICAL SIGNS. The neurologic deficits of animals with vertebral body abscesses without pachymeningitis are similar to those described previously for spinal fractures.[1333] Animals with mildly compressive cervical spinal abscesses show a characteristic "weather vane" attitude, appear stiff, and are reluctant to eat food from the ground.[1333,1335,1336] Ruminants with this lesion hold the neck in extension and attempt to prehend the food with the tongue while the head is held more than 12 inches from the ground.[1333] Additional signs of spinal abscess include heat, pain, swelling, or crepitus over the affected areas and associated signs of bacteremia. Animals with pachymeningitis show characteristic signs of meningeal inflammation such as hyperesthesia, intermittent spasmodic muscle contractions, and recurrent profuse sweating (see the section on meningitis earlier in this chapter).[1335,1337]

CLINICAL PATHOLOGY AND RADIOGRAPHIC FINDINGS. Plain film radiographs are the best method of obtaining a definitive diagnosis of spinal abscessation. A random pattern of hyperlucency and increased bone density characteristic of osteomyelitis is seen in the affected vertebrae (Fig. 33-34).[1338] Discospondylitis usually results in detectable osteolysis in the intervertebral joints.[1335] Occasional cases of extradural abscesses without radiographic evidence of osteomyelitis have been described in calves and lambs.[1331] Nuclear scintigraphy can be used when the bone lesions are not well defined in plain film radiography.[1339] In addition, myelography can be used to detect the specific site of the spinal cord compression.

A complete blood count (CBC) may indicate the presence of a chronic inflammatory focus. Specific changes in the CBC include hyperfibrinogenemia, neutrophilia, monocytosis, nonresponsive anemia, and left shift. The plasma globulin levels are increased in adults but may be increased or decreased in neonates, depending on the adequacy of colostral immunoglobulin transfer.

The changes in the cerebrospinal fluid (CSF) depend on the location of the abscess in the nervous tissue and the meninges. In most instances the abscess does not infiltrate through the pachymeninges, and the CSF is normal or shows xanthochromia and mild increases in the protein concentration (60 to 120 mg/dl). The CSF of animals with pachymeningitis contains high numbers of white blood cells (more than 100 neutrophils/dl) and a markedly increased protein concentration (over 200 mg/dl). The CSF may clot after collection because of high concentrations of fibrinogen. Bacteria may be observed in a Gram-stained smear of CSF sediment. Horses with spinal brucellosis may have a rising serum agglutination titer or one above 1:160.[1337] Because of a high number of nonspecific reactions in equine sera, titers below 1:40 are considered nondiagnostic.[1342] Horses with spinal tuberculosis may be identified by an intradermal skin test using purified protein derivative or tuberculin.[1338]

PATHOPHYSIOLOGY. Hematogenously derived abscesses arise because of embolization of septic thrombi into the metaphyseal arteries. These vessels have a sluggish blood flow because they become torturous as they approach the physis. The metaphyseal vessels communicate with the ventral vertebral plexus, which in turn drains into the post cava, the portal vein, and the pulmonary veins. The ventral vertebral plexus does not have valves; blood flow reverses with an increase in abdominal or pleural pressure. Regurgitated blood from infected sites in the body cavities showers the vertebrae and spinal cord with bacteria.[1332,1339]

NECROPSY FINDINGS. The most common sites of involvement are the costovertebral and intervertebral articula-

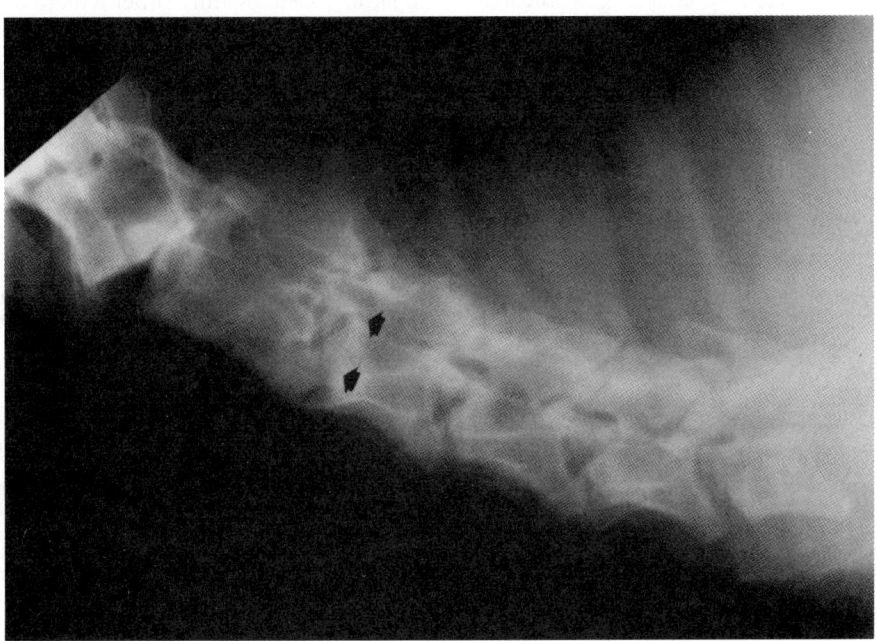

FIG. 33-34 ▦ Cervical radiograph of a sheep with osteomyelitis and discospondylitis at the C2-C3 intervertebral space *(arrows).* The sheep recovered fully after application of a full-length cast of the head, neck, and trunk and after continuous therapy with parenteral penicillin G for 1 month.

tions and the vertebral body epiphyses.[1343] Lumbar vertebrae commonly are involved. The bone is uneven, deformed, and softened. The abscessed area is interspersed with calcified trabeculae and pockets of necrotic debris. Sequestration of necrotic bone may be seen in some cases. The meninges may be adherent to the abscessed site, and occasionally a fistulous tract may be seen from the center of the abscess pocket to the subarachnoid space. In other cases the abscess is compartmentalized away from the CSF, but the proliferating bone impinges on the spinal cord.

TREATMENT AND PREVENTION. If spinal abscessation is recognized early, prolonged antimicrobial therapy generally is effective. Selection of the appropriate antimicrobial agents should be based on the results of cultures from the patient's blood, urine, feces, and CSF. When bacteriologic culturing is inconclusive, a broad-spectrum antimicrobial should be chosen. Amikacin (7.5 to 10 mg/kg IM 4 times daily) or gentamicin (1 mg/kg IM 3 times daily) combined with potassium penicillin G (10,000 IU/kg IV 3 or 4 times daily) should be administered. One or 2 weeks of therapy with these drugs could be followed by a 2- to 3-month treatment with a trimethoprim-sulfonamide combination in horses (2 to 3 mg/kg of trimethoprim and 10 to 15 mg/kg of sulfadiazine PO twice daily) or procaine penicillin G in cattle (10,000 to 20,000 IU/kg SC or IM daily).

Small ruminants with cervical discospondylitis may show a good response after 2 to 4 weeks of intramuscular procaine penicillin G (10,000 IU/kg given twice daily). Phenylbutazone, flunixin meglumine, or aspirin may be administered for pain relief. Immobilization of the head and neck in a fiberglass cast extending from the thorax to the nose may provide support to smaller patients with a cervical abscess. Some authors have recommended surgical drainage of the abscess and curettage of the necrotic bone, but such surgical intervention is difficult because of the size of the epaxial musculature and the inaccessibility of the spine in large animals.

REFERENCES
1331. Dodd DC, Cordes DO: Spinal abscess and cord compression syndrome in lambs, *N Z Vet J* 12:1-5, 1964.
1332. Finley GG: A survey of vertebral abscesses in domestic animals in Ontario, *Can Vet J* 16:114-117, 1975.
1333. Sherman DM, Ames TR: Vertebral body abscesses in cattle: a review of five cases, *J Am Vet Med Assoc* 188:608-611, 1986.
1334. Chladek DW, Ruth GR: Isolation of *Actinobacillosis lignieresii* from an epidural abscess in a horse with progressive paralysis, *J Am Vet Met Assoc* 168:64-66, 1976.
1335. Adams SB, Steckel R, Blevins W: Diskospondylitis in five horses, *J Am Vet Med Assoc* 186:270-272, 1985.
1336. Richardson DW: *Eikenella corrodens* osteomyelitis of the axis in a foal, *J Am Vet Med Assoc* 188:298-299, 1986.
1337. Collins JD, Kelly WR, Twomey T: *Brucella*-associated vertebral osteomyelitis in a thoroughbred mare, *Vet Rec* 88:321-326, 1971.
1338. Kelly WR, Collins JD, Farrelly BT: Vertebral osteomyelitis in a horse associated with *Mycobacterium tuberculosis* var. *bovis* (*M. bovis*) infection, *Am J Vet Rad Soc* 13:59-69, 1972.
1339. Markel MA et al: Vertebral body osteomyelitis in the horse, *J Am Vet Med Assoc* 188:632-634, 1986.
1340. Dixon PM, Rowlands AC: Atlantooccipital joint infection associated with guttural pouch mycosis in a horse, *Equine Vet J* 13:260-262, 1981.
1341. Walmsley JP: A case of atlantooccipital arthropathy following guttural pouch mycosis in a horse: the use of radioisotope bone scanning as an aid to diagnosis, *Equine Vet J* 20:219-220, 1988.
1342. Denny HR: A review of brucellosis in the horse, *Equine Vet J* 5:121-125, 1973.
1343. Evans LH, Dodd D, Walton FN: Clinicopathologic conference, *J Am Vet Med Assoc* 153:1085-1093, 1968.

SPINAL TUMORS

With the exception of lymphosarcoma, spinal tumors in domestic animals are rare. Tumors that have been reported to invade the spinal cord of horses include lymphosar-

coma, plasma cell myeloma, meningioma, ependymoblastoma, fibrosarcoma, schwannoma, melanoma, carcinoma, angioma, angioblastoma, ganglioglioma, and neurofibroma.[1344-1355] The most common tumor of the spine of ruminants is lymphosarcoma.

CLINICAL SIGNS. The clinical signs of tumorous invasion are indistinguishable from those described previously for spinal fractures. The onset of the neurologic dysfunction varies. Some neurofibromas, melanomas, and lymphosarcomas invade centripetally along the peripheral nerve rootlets. In these cases the patient develops slowly progressive dysfunction of the peripheral nerve or spinal cord, which eventually leads to tetraplegia or paraplegia (Figs. 33-35 and 33-36). In rare instances the onset of tetraplegia in cattle with a neurofibroma or lymphosarcoma may be peracute and unaccompanied by prodromal neurologic symptoms. Lymphosarcoma has a predilection for the lumbar segments of the spinal cord and the cauda equina in cattle over 5 years of age. A diagnosis of tumorous spinal invasion should be considered in cases of progressive neurologic disease characterized by flaccid tail and anus, dysuria, urine scalding, distended bladder, perineal analgesia or anesthesia, and/or paraparesis.

CLINICAL PATHOLOGY. Examination of the cerebrospinal fluid (CSF) may be useful in cases in which the tumor has infiltrated the cauda equina and is located in the lumbosacral cistern. In these cases tumor cells may be biopsied as the needle is inserted into the lumbosacral space. In other cases the CSF is normal or shows signs of mild hemorrhage (xanthochromia, high protein concentration, and normal white blood cell count).

TREATMENT. There is no effective treatment for spinal tumors of large animals. One study reported a prolonged survival of 57 days with three treatments with L-asparaginase. The drug was administered at a dosage of 10,000 IU/mm². The body surface area was estimated using the following formula:

$$\text{Surface area (m}^2) = \text{Body weight (g)}^{2/3} \times 10^b/10^4$$

where 10;kb is a constant that is routinely used for the calculation of surface area in dogs.

The nearly 2-month period of survival allowed the investigators to successfully superovulate the cow. When treating food animals with L-asparaginase, the benefits of the antimetabolite drug must be weighed against the potential for teratogenicity of the fetus, toxicity for human beings, and the certainty of relapse in the patient.[1356]

REFERENCES
1344. Traver DS et al: Epidural melanoma causing posterior paresis in a horse, *J Am Vet Med Assoc* 170:1400-1403, 1977.
1345. Drew RA, Greatorex JC: Vertebral plasma cell myeloma causing posterior paralysis in a horse, *Equine Vet J* 6:131-134, 1974.
1346. Reinertson EL: Fibrosarcoma in a horse, *Cornell Vet* 64:617-621, 1974.
1347. Palmer AC, Hichman J: Ataxia in a horse due to angioma of the spinal cord, *Vet Rec* 72:611-613, 1960.
1348. Helfer DH, Stevens DR: Spinal neurofibroma in a sheep, *Vet Pathol* 15:784-786, 1978.
1349. Luginbuhl H: Comparative aspects of tumors of the nervous system, *Ann NY Acad Sci* 108:702-721, 1963.
1350. Baker JR: A case of an invasive melanoma in a newborn lamb, *Vet Rec* 97:496-497, 1975.
1351. Shamis LD, Everitt JI, Baker GJ: Lymphosarcoma as the cause of ataxia in a horse, *J Am Vet Met Assoc* 184:1517-1518, 1984.
1352. Rebhun WC et al: Compressive neoplasms affecting the bovine spinal cord, *Compend Cont Educ Pract Vet* 6:S396-S400, 1984.
1353. Saunders GK: Ependymoblastomas in a dairy heifer, *Vet Pathol* 21:528-529, 1984.
1354. Williams G, Feldman R, Baldwin E: Malignant lymphoma in the thoracic spinal canal of a bull, *Southwestern Vet* 25:227-230, 1972.
1355. Roth L et al: Ganglioglioma of the spinal cord in a calf, *Vet Pathol* 24:188-189, 1987.
1356. Masterson MA, Hull BL, Vollmer LA: Treatment of bovine lymphosarcoma with L-asparaginase, *J Am Vet Med Assoc* 192:1301-1302, 1988.

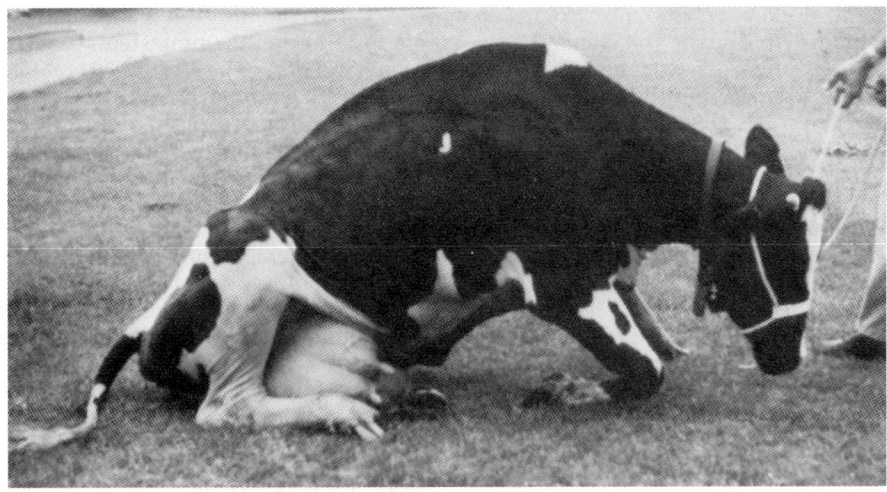

FIG. 33-35 ▓ Characteristic appearance of a paraplegic cow with lymphosarcoma of the L6 to cauda equina spinal rootlets and the cauda equina. (Courtesy Dr. R.H. Whitlock.)

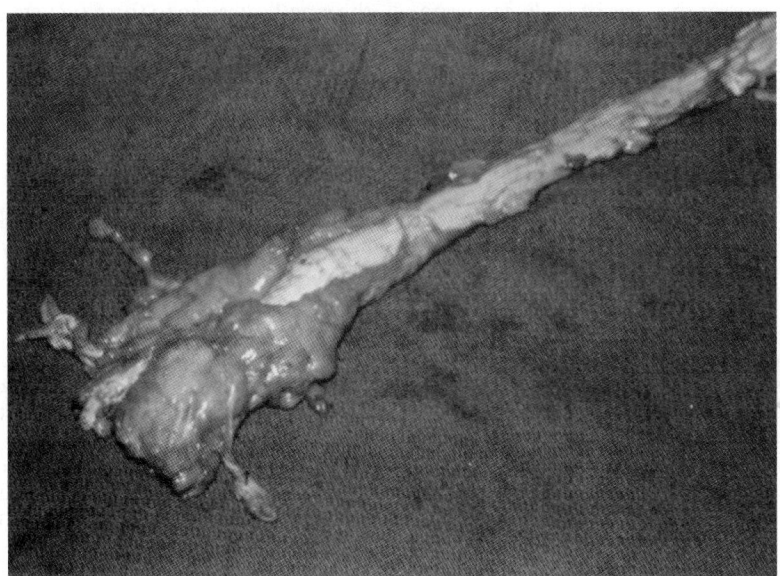

FIG. 33-36 ▓ Spinal cord from a cow with lymphosarcoma. The mass is an accumulation of neoplastic lymphocytes that surround the spinal rootlets, filum terminale, and cauda equina.

CEREBROSPINAL NEMATODIASIS

Migration of nematodes and insect larvae through the central nervous system (CNS) can cause acute CNS disease in all species of domestic livestock. The condition occurs in most countries. Parasitic agents that have been reported in the CNS of horses include *Micronema deletrix, Hypoderma lineatum, Hypoderma bovis, Strongylus vulgaris, Draschia megastoma,* hydatid cysts, and *Setaria* spp.[1357-1382] In cattle the condition is caused principally by *Setaria* spp. and *Hypoderma bovis*. Small ruminants that share pastures with the white-tailed deer may become infected with the meningeal worm *Parelaphostrongylus tenuis*.[1367-1369]

These parasites can attack any region of the CNS, but most clinical cases are the result of lesions of the brainstem and spinal cord. The clinical signs are similar for all parasitic infestations of the CNS; they include tetraplegia, tetraparesis, paraplegia, paraparesis, asymmetric deficit of conscious proprioception, hyperreflexia, areflexia, anesthesia or analgesia of dermatomes, and neurogenic atrophy. Cranial nerve deficits may be seen if the parasites migrate through the brainstem. Specific parasitic syndromes in livestock are detailed in the following paragraphs.

▓ HORSES

Strongylus vulgaris Migration

S. vulgaris migration in the CNS causes two major clinical syndromes: acute embolization of parasitic emboli and slow perivascular migration of living parasites in the central nervous system. The two forms have a common pathogenesis. Aberrantly migrating fourth- or fifth-stage larvae in the intima of the aorta or left ventricle damage the endothelium, stimulate the clotting cascade, and cause formation of a thrombus that often contains the parasitic larva.[1374] Embolization of the thrombus to the brain results in fulminating encephalitic signs.[1363] As the embolus is degraded, the parasite migrates from the blood vessel into the CNS, resulting in the progressive brainstem disease. The cranial brainstem (diencephalon) is most often affected. The thrombosis and migration are accompanied by multifocal infarction, edema, hemorrhage, and necrosis (Fig. 33-37).[1361] Microscopic findings include linear tracts of hemorrhage lined by neutrophils, macrophages, eosinophils, and reactive glial cells. Anesthesia of the rear quarters has been described in some affected horses.[1364] Donkeys are also susceptible to the aberrant migration.[1383] Cerebrospinal fluid (CSF) changes that have been associated with *S. vulgaris* migration in equids include xanthochromia, a refractive index over 1.3353, a protein concentration ranging from 32 to 550 mg/dl, and an increased white blood cell (WBC) count (42 to 10,000/μl). The differential counts range from 70% to 80% neutrophils, 12% to 19% mononuclear cells, and 1% to 2% eosinophils.

Hypoderma lineatum and *Hypoderma bovis* (Warble Flies)

H. lineatum and *H. bovis* are parasites that commonly affect cattle but occasionally migrate aberrantly in the horse. Warble flies hatch from pupae in the early spring and mature during the summer. The flies deposit the eggs of *H. lineatum* on the lips, where they hatch and are swallowed. The ingested worms burrow through the intestine and along the adventitia of blood vessels until they reach the CNS.[1362] The flies deposit the eggs of *H. bovis* on the legs, where they hatch and burrow into the skin. The subcutaneous parasites then migrate as first instar larvae to the spinal column, where they penetrate the epidural space along the peripheral nerves.[1358] Peroneal nerve paralysis from a local parasitic invasion has been reported in a pony.

Micronema deletrix

M. deletrix is thought to be a free-living rhabditid nematode that gains access to the CNS by penetration through the skin of the face and the lips, gums, and tongue.[1359,1360] The parasites migrate into the brain through the vascular system and cause diffuse encephalitis. Nematodes are found in the tunica adventitia and tunica media of blood vessels.[1359] Clinical signs of *M. deletrix* depend on the localization of the para-

site. Spinal cord invasion is apparently less common than migration through the brainstem, cerebellum, thalamus, forebrain, and deeper layers of the cerebral cortex. Clinical signs that have been reported include asymmetric ataxia, loss of conscious proprioception, depression, behavioral changes, propulsive walking, head-pressing, head tilt, circling, nystagmus, recumbency, convulsions, and coma. Affected animals may have granulomatous masses in the nares, pharynx, and maxilla. These could be helpful in formulating a differential diagnosis when parasitic migration is suspected. CSF changes in affected horses have been described,[1357] including pleocytosis (25 to 80 nucleated cells/μl), a normal to high protein concentration (69 to 114 mg/dl), and xanthochromia. The cellular types were mostly lymphocytes and macrophages ranging from 78% to 91% of the nucleated cells. Eosinophils were observed in the CSF of one horse.

Draschia megastoma

D. megastoma has been found in the brainstem of a horse from the southern United States.[1365] The adult worm is embedded in a pyogranulomatous lesion of the equine stomach, and the eggs are shed into the stomach. They hatch in the small intestine to form first-stage larvae, which are passed in the feces and ingested by the larvae of *Musca* flies. The third-stage larvae migrate to the mouth parts of the fly and are deposited on the mucous membranes of the host as the fly feeds.

Setaria

Setaria parasites are common filarid parasites of cattle that migrate aberrantly when they infect horses, sheep, or goats. These parasites have a worldwide distribution, and clinical cases are especially common in India and the Orient, where the common name for the disease is kumri (weak back).[1379] There are at least four different genera, of which *Setaria equina*, *Setaria digitata*, and *Setaria labiotopapillosa* are most common. The parasite is found in the connective tissues and peritoneal cavity of cattle, where it produces circulating microfilariae. Mosquitoes and possibly other bloodsucking insects become infected by the microfilariae and thus transmit the parasite.[1378] The parasite has a predilection for the spinal cord in horses.

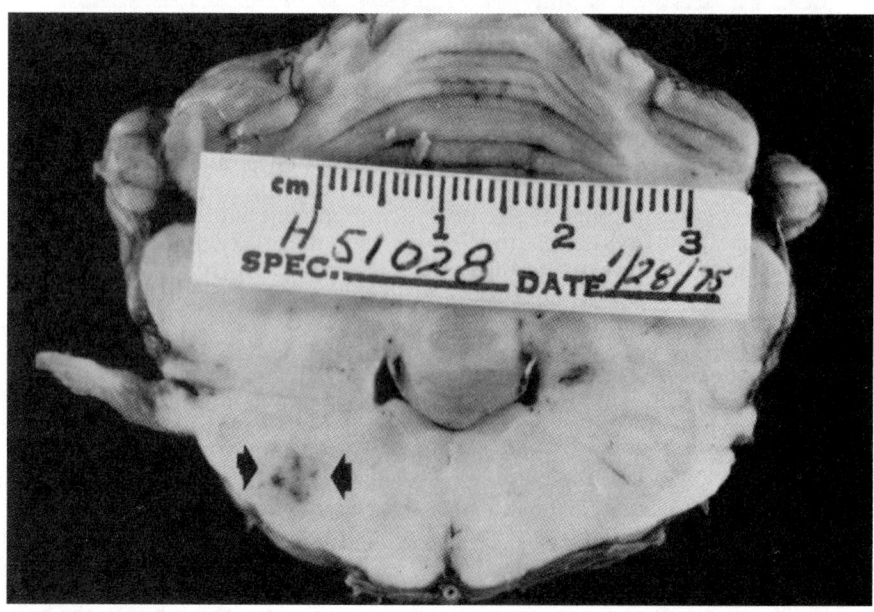

FIG. 33-37 ▓ Parasitic lesions in the brainstem of a horse. The arrows indicate the major lesion, but other, smaller lesions are distributed over the entire brainstem. (Courtesy Dr. R.H. Whitlock.)

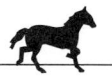

The clinical signs of reported cases include hypotonic tail, bladder paralysis, ataxia, and conscious proprioceptive deficits.[1366] Changes in the CSF that have been associated with *Setaria* infestation include xanthochromia, pleocytosis (25 to 84 cells/dl), and a slightly increased protein concentration (approximately 114 mg/dl). The cells of one horse contained a small proportion of eosinophils and basophils, but this finding was inconsistent with other reports.[1357]

■ *SHEEP AND GOATS*

Setaria

The infection caused by *Setaria* spp. in sheep and goats is similar to that described previously for horses.

Parelaphostrongylus tenuis

Disease caused by *P. tenuis* occurs predominantly in sheep and goats of the northeastern United States and western Canada.[1367,1370,1372,1373] The case attack rate ranges from 10% to 59%.[1368] The disease appears to be spreading because of the increased range of the primary host, the white-tailed deer. Migration of the parasite in the CNS of deer is relatively innocuous, but aberrant migration occurs in domestic small ruminants. The result of this migration is severe signs of spinal cord and brainstem disease.[1368] The life cycle of the worm is complex. Adult worms are found in the cranial subarachnoid space, venous sinuses, and spinal subarachnoid space of the deer, where they reproduce.[1369] Eggs are deposited into the venous blood and migrate into the lungs, where they embryonate. The larvae penetrate into the airways and are coughed into the pharynx, swallowed, and passed in the feces. They then penetrate into snails and slugs. Sheep and goats are infected when they eat the snails. After ingestion by the ruminant, the larvae penetrate the gastrointestinal wall and enter the CNS by migration along the nerve rootlets. Because of the complex life cycle of the parasite and the indirect life cycle in invertebrate hosts, the neurologic disease in sheep and goats is seen exclusively in late fall and winter. The pathologic lesions of the CNS of affected animals include asymmetric irregular tracts of disrupted necrotic tissue with macrophage infiltration. Coiled larvae occasionally may be seen in the tissues of some affected animals and may be excreted in the feces; however, these are difficult to distinguish from the larvae of *Müllerius* worms.

The clinical signs of *P. tenuis* infection are acute. In untreated animals the disease is progressive. The CSF of animals with *Parelaphostrongylus* infection contains increased concentrations of protein (56 to 157 mg/dl), red blood cells (RBCs) (300 to 41,000/μl), and WBCs (17 to 700/μl). The differential cell counts contain a large number of eosinophils (7% to 97%).[1384]

■ *CATTLE*

Hypoderma bovis

After hatching, the larvae of *H. bovis* burrow through the skin and migrate along the peripheral nerves to the spinal canal. When the larvae reach the spinal canal, they lie dormant for approximately 2 to 3 months in the epidural fat. Most of the larvae lodge in the lumbosacral part of the spinal cord; very few are found in the cervicothoracic region. If the larvae are killed while lodged in the epidural fat, the host mounts a marked inflammatory response. The swelling and inflammation caused by the dead worms results in spinal cord disease. In clinical practice these signs most often occur by 2 days after administration of a systemic organophosphate grub treatment.[1381,1382] Other drugs that kill *Hypoderma* larvae in the spinal cord could cause a similar problem. In most of North America the grub is located in the epidural space between the months of July and October.

The clinical signs of hypodermiasis include stiffness of the rear limbs, ataxia, paraparesis, and paraplegia, hemiparesis, or hemiplegia, or tetraparesis and tetraplegia. The conscious proprioceptive responses are markedly altered in the affected limbs. Reflex activity varies, depending on the level of the lesion in the spinal cord.

The CSF changes of hypodermiasis vary. Because of the epidural location of the grub, most affected animals have normal CSF values. If pressure changes induce vascular damage, CSF changes might include mild xanthochromia and slight increases in WBCs and the protein concentration.

Setaria digitata

Infection of the spinal cord of cattle by *S. digitata* has been described in India.[1371]

DIAGNOSIS OF PARASITIC INFESTATION OF THE CENTRAL NERVOUS SYSTEM. Parasitic myeloencephalopathy must be considered in all cases of acute asymmetric disease of the spinal cord, cerebellum, or brainstem. Identification of eosinophils in the CSF may be helpful; however, this pattern is not seen in every neuroparasitic diseases. For example, *Hypoderma* infestations often are extradural, and CSF changes reflect only increased pressure. The CSF of horses with acute *S. vulgaris* migration could be normal or could show xanthochromia, increased concentrations of RBCs or WBCs, and an increased protein concentration.[1363]

TREATMENT. Although severe reactions often are associated with death of the CNS parasites, administration of parasiticides in conjunction with heavy antiinflammatory therapy is recommended. Such treatment prevents further migration of the parasite yet mitigates the host inflammatory responses.

The recommended treatment for neural *S. vulgaris* infection is either thiabendazole (440 mg/kg PO given daily for 2 days) or mebendazole (30 mg/kg given daily for 2 days). Horses should also be given a combination of corticosteroids and nonsteroidal antiinflammatory drugs for 10 days after administration of the parasiticides. Some experts speculate that ivermectin may be a valuable broad-spectrum treatment for all CNS parasitic infections. The drug has a prolonged plasma half-life after parenteral or oral administration (2.7 days) and may exert an antiparasitic effect for as long as 14 to 21 days after subcutaneous administration.[1385-1387] Although the drug diffuses across the blood-brain barrier, the plasma concentrations after oral administration are low, and the drug should be administered parenterally to achieve optimum efficacy. Unfortunately, significant side effects occur (0.92% overall adverse reaction rate) after parenteral administration of the drug to horses.[1388-1389] Consequently, until the drug is proven to be effective by pharmacologic and clinical studies, alternative parasiticides should be considered for initial treatment of parasitic CNS disease in horses.

Hypoderma bovis. Systemic organophosphate insecticides formulated for oral administration or pour-on application have been recommended for eliminating *H. bovis* from the CNS. These one-time include crufomate (75 mg/kg as 13.5% Ruelene), trichlorfon (40 mg/kg PO), famphur* (13.2% 1 fluid ounce 90 kg of body weight, not to exceed a total dosage of 4 oz for cattle), ronnel (100 mg/kg PO for cattle or horses), and ivermectin 0.5% solution (1 ml per 10 kg of body weight). Although ivermectin kills the cattle grub in the subcutaneous tissues, the safety and efficacy of this drug for the treatment of clinical neurologic disease is unclear.

It is important to remember that the treatment of affected animals with any of the systemic parasiticides may aggravate neurologic disturbances through release of toxic factors or the

---

*American Cyanimid, Wayne, NJ 07470.

development of local immunologic responses to the dying worms.[1373,1390] Concomitant treatment with corticosteroids (dexamethasone 0.1 to 0.25 mg/kg of body weight IV given every 6 hours) on the day preceding the treatment and for 5 days thereafter is recommended to reduce the inflammation. Dying cattle grubs also release a systemic toxin that lowers blood pressure and causes acute dyspnea and collapse. The systemic toxic effects of the dying grubs can be ameliorated by concomitant administration of phenylbutazone (4 mg/kg IV or PO given 2 times daily in horses; 10 mg/kg given once every 36 hours IV or PO in the cow), aspirin (100 mg/kg PO given 2 or 3 times daily for cattle), or flunixin meglumine (1 to 2.2 mg/kg IV given 2 times daily for horses or cattle). Naproxen (10 mg/kg IV given 2 times daily for horses) may be a useful alternative to phenylbutazone therapy.

Hypoderma infestation can be controlled by prophylactic administration of the pour-on insecticides before the time the worms have migrated into the nervous tissues. The appropriate time for application of the grubicide depends on the time of pupation and the emergence of adults. In most of North America, the flies emerge by May and the larvae reach the nervous tissues by November. Therefore prophylactic treatment of cattle or horses with organophosphorus compounds should be completed by August or September in warmer climates and October in colder areas.

Parelaphostrongylus tenuis. A number of drugs, including levamisole (7 mg/kg PO in a single dose), diethylcarbamazine (40 to 100 mg/kg given 2 times at a 72-hour interval), and thiabendazole (250 to 440 mg/kg of body weight PO on two consecutive days) may be effective for eliminating *P. tenuis* from the CNS.[1367,1391] Ivermectin has been administered to some affected goats, but only one of three treated animals recovered.[1384] The lack of response to ivermectin was related to the poor distribution of the drug into the CNS. Administration of the drug to animals before exposure protects them from the larval migrans for periods ranging from 7 to 14 days.[1392] All patients that are to be treated with anthelmintics should be given corticosteroids and nonsteroidal antiinflammatory drugs concomitantly.

Setaria spp. Administration of a single dose of diethylcarbamazine (80 to 100 mg/kg PO) may be effective for the treatment of migrating *Setaria* larvae and adults. The drug also has been shown to effectively prevent infection in sheep and goats when given at 20-day intervals (40 mg/kg PO) during the vector season. The drug's efficacy for the treatment and prevention of *Setaria* infection in horses is unclear. As with the treatment of other parasitic nervous system infections, patients should be given corticosteroids and antiinflammatory drugs concomitantly with the parasiticide therapy.

REFERENCES

1357. Darien BJ, Belknap J, Nietfeld J: Cerebrospinal fluid changes in two horses with central nervous system nematodiasis *(Micronema deletrix)*, *J Vet Intern Med* 2:201-205, 1988.
1358. Hadlow WJ, Ward JK, Krinsky WL: Intracranial myiasis by *Hypoderma bovis* (Linnaeus) in a horse, *Cornell Vet* 67:272-281, 1977.
1359. Jordan WH, Gaafar SM, Carlton WW: *Micronema deletrix* in the brain of a horse, *Vet Med (Small Anim Clin)* 70:707-709, 1975.
1360. Stone WM, Stewart TB, Peckham JC: *Micronema deletrix* in the central nervous system of a pony, *J Parasitol* 56:986-987, 1970.
1361. Pohlenz VJ, Schulze D, Eckert J: Spinale nematidosis beim pferd, verursachy durch *Strongylus vulgaris*, *DTW* 72:510-511, 1965.
1362. Olander HJ: The migration of *Hypoderma lineatum* in the brain of a horse, *Pathol Vet* 4:477-483, 1967.
1363. Little PB: Cerebrospinal nematodiasis of equidae, *J Am Vet Med Assoc* 160:1407-1413, 1972.
1364. Swanstrom OG, Rising JL, Carlton WW: Spinal nematodosis in a horse, *J Am Vet Med Assoc* 155:748-753, 1969.
1365. Mayhew IG et al: Migration of a spiruroid nematode through the brain of a horse, *J Am Vet Med Assoc* 180:1306-1311, 1982.
1366. Fraunfelder HC, Kazacos KR, Lichtenfels JR: Cerebrospinal nematodiasis caused by a filarid in a horse, *J Am Vet Med Assoc* 177:359-362, 1980.
1367. Mayhew IG, De Lahunta A, Georgi JR: Naturally occurring cerebrospinal parelaphostrongylosis, *Cornell Vet* 66:56-72, 1976.

1368. Jortner BS et al: Lesions of spinal cord parelaphostrongylosis in sheep: sequential changes following intramedullary larval migration, *Vet Pathol* 22:137-140, 1985.
1369. Anderson RC: The development of *Pneumostrongylus tenuis* in the central nervous system of white-tailed deer, *Pathol Vet* 2:360-379, 1965.
1370. Alden C et al: Cerebrospinal nematodiasis in sheep, *J Am Vet Med Assoc* 166:784-786, 1975.
1371. Mohiyuddeen S: Enzootic bovine paraplegia in some malnad tracts (hilly and heavy rainfall region) of Mysore state with particular reference to cerebrospinal nematodiasis as its probable cause, *Indian J Vet Sci* 26:1-19, 1956.
1372. Kennedy PC, Whitlock JH, Roberts SJ: Neurofilariosis, a paralytic disease of sheep. I. Introduction, symptomatology, and pathology, *Cornell Vet* 42:118-124, 1952.
1373. Whitlock JH: Neurofilariosis, a paralytic disease of sheep. II. *Neurofilaria cornellensis* ng, n sp (Nematoda, Filariodea): a new nematode parasite from the spinal cord of sheep, *Cornell Vet* 42:125-132, 1952.
1374. Little PB, Lwin S, Fretz P: Verminous encephalitis of horses: experimental induction with *Strongylus vulgaris* larvae, *Am J Vet Res* 35:1501-1510, 1974.
1375. Ferris DH, Levine ND, Beamer PD: *Micronema deletrix* in the equine brain, *Am J Vet Res* 33:33-38, 1972.
1376. Powers RD, Benz GW: *Micronema deletrix* in the central nervous system of a horse, *J Am Vet Med Assoc* 170:175-177, 1977.
1377. Alstad AD, Berg IE: Disseminated *Micronema deletrix* infection in the horse, *J Am Vet Med Assoc* 174:264-266, 1979.
1378. Innes JRM, Shoho C, Pillai CP: Epizootic cerebrospinal nematodiasis or setariasis, *Br Vet J* 108:71-78, 1952.
1379. Innes JR, Pillai C: Kumri: so-called lumbar paralysis of horses in Ceylon (India and Burma) and its identification with cerebrospinal nematodiasis, *Br Vet J* 111:223-235, 1955.
1380. Wood AP: Cerebrospinal nematodiasis in a horse, *Equine Vet J* 185:185-190, 1970.
1381. Cox DD, Mozier JO, Mullee MT: Posterior paralysis in a calf caused by cattle grubs *(Hypoderma bovis)* after treatment with a systemic insecticide for grub control, *J Am Vet Med Assoc* 157:1088-1090, 1970.
1382. Brown FG: Toxicological hazards in warble fly eradication programmes, *Vet Parasitol* 3:265-270, 1977.
1383. Mayhew IG et al: Verminous *(Strongylus vulgaris)* myelitis in a donkey, *Cornell Vet* 74:30-37, 1984.
1384. Kopcha M et al: Cerebrospinal nematodiasis in a goat herd, *J Am Vet Med Assoc* 194:1439-1442, 1989.
1385. Lo PA et al: Pharmacokinetic studies of ivermectin: effects of formulation, *Vet Res Commun* 9:251-268, 1985.
1386. Wilkinson PK, Pope DG, Baylis FP: Pharmacokinetics of ivermectin administered intravenously to cattle, *J Pharm Sci* 74:1105-1107, 1985.
1387. Bennett DG: Clinical pharmacology of ivermectin, *J Am Vet Med Assoc* 189:100-102, 1986.
1388. Anderson RR: The use of ivermectin in horses: research and clinical observations, *Compend Cont Educ Pract Vet* 6:S516-S520, 1984.
1389. Karns PA, Luther DG: A survey of adverse effects associated with ivermectin use in Louisiana horses, *J Am Vet Med Assoc* 185:782-783, 1984.
1390. Anderson PH, Kirkwood AC: A reaction in cattle to toxins of *Hypoderma bovis* (warble fly) larvae, *Br Vet J* 124:569-575, 1968.
1391. Shoho C: Prophylaxis and therapy in epizootic cerebrospinal nematodiasis of animals by I-diethylcarbamyl-4-methyl-piperazine dihydrogen citrate: report of a second field trial, *Vet Med* 49:459-464, 1954.
1392. Kocan AA: The use of ivermectin in the treatment and prevention of infection with *Parelaphostrongylus tenuis* (Doughterty) nematoda metastrongyloidia in white-tailed deer *(Odocoileus virginanus,* Zimmerman), *J Wildlife Dis* 21:454-455, 1985.

FIBROCARTILAGINOUS EMBOLIZATION

LISLE W. GEORGE
MARY O. SMITH

Fibrocartilaginous embolization has been described in two horses and mixed-breed lambs.[1393-1396] The clinical signs are those of an acute to peracute onset of myelopathy that usually is asymmetric. Paresis to paralysis of the limbs caudal to the lesion occurs, as does hyperreflexia (if the lesion is above the brachial or lumbosacral intumescences) or hyporeflexia to areflexia (if the lesion is in an intumescence). Lambs may develop diffuse tremors that resemble the truncal ataxia of cerebellar disease. There is no effective treatment for the condition, and affected animals have not recovered. In dogs, however, in which a similar or identical condition is common, partial to complete recovery over several weeks to months is common and might be anticipated in some milder cases of this problem in large animals, particularly when the signs are the upper motor neuron type.[1397,1398]

The emboli are believed to originate from the nucleus pulposus of the intervertebral disks and can be identified pathologically using an alcian blue stain.[1396] The exact cause of the embolization and the mechanisms by which it occurs are unknown. Pressure changes or lesions associated with degenerative arthropathy might result in herniation of disk material into the marrow cavity of a vertebral body. From there the material is hypothesized to enter the basivertebral veins and to pass retrograde along the valveless basivertebral plexus to the spinal veins, where it gains access to the vertebral arterial circuit. The manner in which the material enters the arteries is unknown, but some authors have postulated the presence of arteriovenous shunts in the vertebral vasculature.[1393] Once the material has embolized, the neurologic signs are related to swelling, infarction, necrosis, and hemorrhage of the neuropil. The emboli occur exclusively in the brainstem, spinal cord, and cerebellum. The cerebrospinal fluid (CSF) of affected animals has been reported to be normal,[1394] but mild to pleocytosis and elevations in the protein concentration could be expected in some cases.

REFERENCES

1393. Abid HN, Holscher MA: Acute necrotizing myelopathy in lambs, *Vet Med (Small Anim Clin)* 78:1615-1616, 1983.
1394. Taylor HW, Vandevelde M, Firth E: Ischemic myelopathy caused by fibrocartilaginous emboli in a horse, *Vet Pathol* 14:479-481, 1977.
1395. Fuentealba IC et al: Spinal cord ischemic necrosis due to fibrocartilaginous embolism in a horse, *J Vet Diagn Invest* 3:176-179, 1991.
1396. Jeffrey M, Wells GAH: Multifocal ischaemic encephalomyelopathy associated with fibrocartilaginous emboli in the lamb, *Neuropathol Exp Neurobiol* 12:415-424, 1986.
1397. De Lahunta A, Alexander JW: Ischemic myelopathy secondary to presumed fibrocartilaginous embolism in nine dogs, *J Am Anim Hosp Assoc* 12:37-48, 1976.
1398. Gilmore DR, De Lahunta A: Necrotizing myelopathy secondary to presumed or confirmed fibrocartilaginous embolism in 24 dogs, *J Am Anim Hosp Assoc* 23373-376, 1987.

OCCIPITOATLANTOAXIAL MALFORMATION

Occipitoatlantoaxial malformation appears to consist of a spectrum of cervical spinal abnormalities rather than a single specific anatomic defect.[1399] It occurs in cattle, sheep, goats, and horses.[1400-1402] At least five different types of defects have been reported in horses[1403-1410]:

1. A heritable condition in Arabians characterized by symmetric atlantooccipital fusion, atlantalization of the axis, and hypoplasia of the atlantal wings.[1404,1408,1411]A similar disorder has been reported in an Arabian-cross colt.[1412]
2. A nonfamilial disease of quarter horses with spinal lesions similar to the lesions in Arabians.
3. Asymmetric malformations of the occipitoatlantoaxial area in Morgan horses and standardbred foals.[1399]
4. Atlantal duplication of Arabian crossbred horses.[1413]
5. Asymmetric occipitalization of the atlas and symmetric atlantalization of the axis.

Macroscopic pathologic lesions common to the five forms include loss or flattening of the occipital condyles, asymmetric flattening of the articular surfaces of the axis, and shortened dens. The pathogenesis of the vertebral defects is unknown, but the disease has been shown to be heritable in the Arabian horse.[1414]

The clinical signs vary considerably and range from normal neurologic function with or without torticollis to brainstem compression, sudden unexpected death, and stillbirth.[1399] In typical cases signs of tetraplegia or tetraparesis begin at or shortly after birth and progress at a variable rate. Foals may become suddenly tetraplegic, appear to stabilize for several days, but then die suddenly.[1408] In rare instances horses may not show nervous signs until they are 3 years of age.[1407]

The signs are symmetric in most affected animals and include conscious proprioceptive deficits, tetraplegia, hyperreflexia, and hypertonia. Some affected animals may show a reluctance to move the neck and head and resist vigorously when the proximal cervical area is passively flexed. A clicking, creaking, or crepitation may be palpated over the cervical spine when the head is moved.[1399,1403] Animals with asymmetric bone lesions often show torticollis, whereas patients with symmetric lesions hold their heads in extension and frequently display the "weather vane" attitude. Neurologic deficits may not be seen despite moderate torticollis.

The bone lesions are readily apparent by radiographic examination (Figs. 33-38 and 33-39). Affected animals may show subluxation of the atlantoaxial joint, ventral displace-

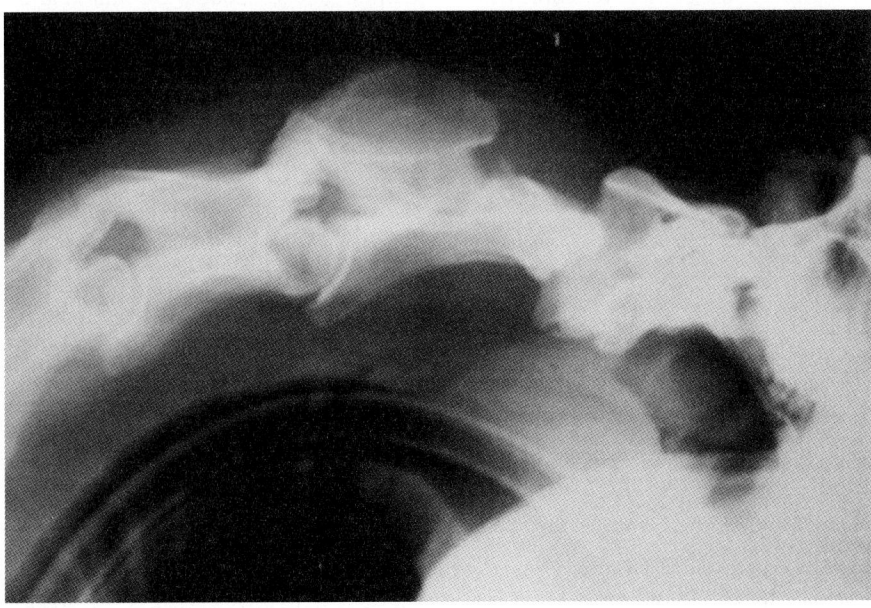

FIG. 33-38 ▓ Lateral radiographic view of a 2-month-old foal with occipitoatlantoaxial malformation. The atlas is occipitalized, and the axis is subluxated dorsally. The odontoid process of the dens is hypoplastic and is not anchored to the floor of the atlas. (Courtesy Dr. W.D. Wilson.)

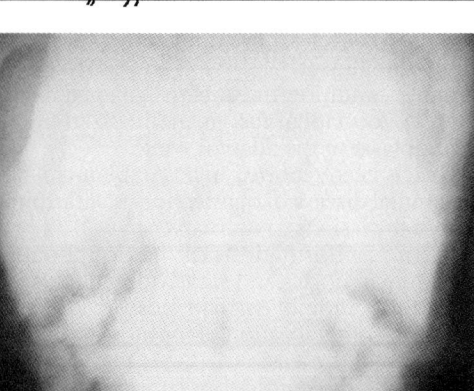

FIG. 33-39 ▮ Dorsoventral myelogram of a foal with occipitoatlantal malformation showing spinal compression and attenuation of the contrast column at the C1-C2 vertebral junction *(arrow)*.

ment of C2 in relation to C1, ununited ossification center of the dens, shortened or elongated dens, shortened transverse process of the atlas, fusion of C1 with the occipital condyles, atlantal duplication, and deviation of the basilar bone.[1415] In sheep additional malformations of the cervical vertebrae have been seen concomitantly.

Some authors have suggested that treatment could include surgical fusion of the atlantoaxial joints with or without a laminectomy.[1404,1407,1416-1418] Laminectomy alone has been used to alleviate spinal cord compression and clinical signs caused by occipitoatlantoaxial malformation.[1419]Arabian horses should not be treated because of the hereditary nature of the disease in that breed.

REFERENCES

1399. Mayhew IG, Watson AG, Heissan JA: Congenital occipitoatlantoaxial malformations in the horse, *Equine Vet J* 10:103-113, 1978.
1400. Schmidt SP et al: A case of congenital occipitoatlantoaxial malformation (OAAM) in a lamb, *J Vet Diagn Invest* 5:458-462, 1993.
1401. Engelken TJ et al: Atlantooccipital fusion in two polled Hereford calves, *Zentralbl Veterinarmed* 39:236-238, 1992.
1402. Boyd JS, McNeil PE: Atlantooccipital fusion and ataxia in the calf, *Vet Rec* 120:34-37, 1987.
1403. Watson AG et al: Occipitoatlantoaxial malformation with atlantoaxial subluxation in an ataxic calf, *J Am Vet Med Assoc* 187:740-742, 1985.
1404. McCoy DJ et al: Stabilization of atlantoaxial subluxation secondary to atlantooccipital malformation in a Devon calf, *Cornell Vet* 76:277-286, 1986.
1405. Leipold HW et al: Congenital defect of the atlantooccipital joint in a Holstein-Friesian calf, *Cornell Vet* 62:646-653, 1972.
1406. Van Nie CJ, Folkerts JF: Occipitalization of the atlas in a sheep, *Schweiz Arch Tierheilkd Anat Histol Embryol* 6:99, 1977.
1407. Wilson WD et al: Occipitoatlantoaxial malformation in two non-Arabian horses, *J Am Vet Med Assoc* 187:36-40, 1985.
1408. Leipold HW et al: Congenital atlantooccipital fusion in a foal, *Vet (Small Anim Clin)* 69:1312-1316, 1974.
1409. Von Schmaltz: Ebildung des occipitale und des atlas beim fohlen, *Berl Munch Tierarztl Woschenschr* 31:169-172, 1915.
1410. Robinson WF et al: Atlantoaxial malarticulation in Angora goats, *Aust Vet J* 58:105-107, 1982.
1411. Whitwell KW: Craniovertebral malformations in an Arab foal, *Equine Vet J* 10:125-129, 1978.
1412. Blikslager AT et al: Atlantoaxial malformation in a half-Arabian, *Cornell Vet* 81:67-75, 1991.
1413. De Lahunta A, Hatfield C, Dietz A: Occipitoatlantoaxial malformation with duplication of the atlas and axis in a half-Arabian foal, *Cornell Vet* 79:185-193, 1989.
1414. Watson AG, Mayhew IG: Familial congenital occipitoatlantoaxial malformation in the Arabian horse, *Spine* 11:334-339, 1986.
1415. White ME, Pennock PW, Seiler RJ: Atlantoaxial subluxation in five young cattle, *Can Vet J* 19:79-82, 1978.
1416. Slone DE, Bergfeld WA, Walker TL: Surgical decompression for traumatic atlantoaxial subluxation in a weanling filly, *J Am Vet Med Assoc* 174:1234-1236, 1979.
1417. McCoy DJ, Shires PK, Beadle R: Ventral approach for stabilization of atlantoaxial subluxation secondary to odontoid fracture in a foal, *J Am Vet Med Assoc* 185:545-549, 1984.
1418. Owen R ap R, Smith Maxie LL: Repair of fractured dens of the axis in a foal, *J Am Vet Med Assoc* 173:854-856, 1987.
1419. Nixon AJ, Stashak TS: Laminectomy for relief of atlantoaxial subluxation in four horses, *J Am Vet Med Assoc* 193:677-682, 1988.

SYSTEMIC NEUROAXONAL DYSTROPHY

Systemic neuroaxonal dystrophy is seen in purebred Suffolk sheep.[1420] The animals are born normal but show a rear limb ataxia beginning at 1 to 5 months of age. The disease is progressive, and eventually the animals become recumbent and either die or are euthanized after 8 to 10 weeks. Pedigree analyses have indicated that an autosomal recessive genetic trait may be responsible for the condition.

REFERENCE

1420. Cordy DR, Richards WPC, Bradford GE: Systemic neuroaxonal dystrophy in Suffolk sheep, *Acta Neuropathol (Berl)* 8:133-140, 1967.

WEAVER SYNDROME (Bovine Progressive Degenerative Myeloencephalopathy)

Weaver syndrome is a progressive hereditary central nervous system (CNS) disease of 5- to 10-month-old Brown Swiss and Angler cattle.[1421,1422] The disease has been reported in the United States, Canada, Denmark, and Switzerland. The incidence of Weaver syndrome in some countries may be as high as 563 per 100,000 registered Brown Swiss cattle.[1423,1424] The disease affects both genders, but males are more commonly affected than females.[1423] Affected animals develop clinical signs between 5 and 8 months of age. The animals are easily pushed around by herd mates and when forced to move show marked proprioceptive deficits. The clinical signs worsen until the animals become recumbent by 18 to 36 months of age.[1421,1425,1426] The pelvic limbs are most severely affected. Specific signs include weakness, ataxia, conscious proprioceptive deficits (circumduction, crossing over, interference, knuckling), muscle tremors, and recumbency. In early stages attempts to move rapidly may result in cessation of movement of gait in the rear limbs while the animal continues to pull with the fore limbs, causing the rear limbs to be pulled too far caudally. Some animals may show varying degrees of hypermetria ("goose stepping" gait) in the limbs. The spinal reflexes and cranial nerve function are normal. Anestrus in females and aspermatogenesis of affected bulls have been described.[1426] The disease is progressive and leads to irreversible recumbency. The sensory nerve conduction velocity is reduced in affected calves, but motor nerve conduction velocity is normal. Electromyograms and electroencephalograms are normal in affected calves.[1427] The cerebrospinal fluid of affected cattle may show an increased concentration of protein (range of 0 to 127 mg/dl) and creatine phosphokinase (range of 2 to 89 mg/dl).[1428]

Except for muscular atrophy of the pelvic limbs in long-standing cases, the small ovaries, and hypoplastic testicles, macroscopic lesions are not seen.[1423,1429,1430] Severe muscular changes are not observed.[1431] The primary microscopic abnormalities include degeneration of the rubrospinal spinocerebellar tracts, particularly in the ventral funiculi of the thoracic spinal cord. The lesions include axonal degeneration, vacuolation of the white matter, spheroids, phagocytosis of myelin debris, gliosis, and status spongiosus.[1423] Axonal swellings have been observed in the brainstem nuclei and medulla oblongata. An ultrastructural study has shown a reduction of the height of the paramembranous densities of the synaptic junctions of affected cattle,[1432] indicating impairment of transmitter releases, dysfunction of the synaptic end plates, or losses of specific cell populations from the motor cortex. Other ultrastructural changes include axonal swelling and vesiculation, swelling of the mitochondria of the Schwann cells, and membrane-bound vesicles.[1426,1433] Cerebellar lesions include degeneration and loss of Purkinje cells and swelling of Purkinje cell axons.[1429]

The disease is thought to be transmitted by a simple autosomal recessive genetic trait. Apparent association between the Weaver condition and genetic predisposition for high milk yield would favor retention of Weaver carriers in situations in which intense genetic pressure for production is exerted.[1434] Recent development of a genetic test for the disease offers the possibility of genetic screening to eliminate this disease. However, the effect on milk yield when this trait is eliminated is not yet known.[1435]

Carrier bulls identified by the American Brown Swiss registry are designated by the suffix "W" as an integral part of their registry name.[1436]

REFERENCES

1421. Leipold HW et al: Weaver syndrome in Brown Swiss cattle: clinical signs and pathology, *Vet Med (Small Anim Clin)* 68:645-647, 1973.
1422. Braun U, Ehrensperger F, Bracher V: Das Weaver Syndrom beim Rind, *Tierarztl Prax* 15:139-144, 1987.
1423. Stuart LD, Leipold HW: Lesions in bovine progressive degenerative myeloencephalopathy "weaver" of Brown Swiss cattle, *Vet Pathol* 22:13-23, 1985.
1424. Baird JD, Sarmiento UM, Basrur P: Bovine progressive degenerative myeloencephalopathy (weaver syndrome) in Brown Swiss cattle in Canada: a literature review and case report, *Can Vet J* 29:370-377, 1988.
1425. Stuart LD, Leipold HW: Bovine progressive degenerative myeloencephalopathy "weaver" of Brown Swiss cattle. I. Epidemiology, *Bovine Pract* 18:129-132, 1983.
1426. Stuart LD, Leipold HW: Bovine progressive degenerative myeloencephalopathy "weaver" of Brown Swiss cattle. II. Clinical and laboratory findings, *Bovine Pract* 18:133-146, 1983.
1427. Oyster R et al: Electrophysiological studies in bovine progressive degenerative myeloencephalopathy of Brown Swiss cattle, *Prog Vet Neurol* 4:243-251, 1993.
1428. Oyster R et al: Laboratory studies of bovine progressive degenerative myeloencephalopathy in Brown Swiss cattle, *Bovine Pract* 26:77-83, 1991.
1429. Leipold HW, El-Hamidi ME, Troyer D: Pathogenic studies of bovine progressive degenerative myeloencephalopathy (weaver) of Brown Swiss cattle, *Bovine Pract* 24:145-146, 1989.
1430. Oyster R et al: Electron microscopic studies of bovine progressive degenerative myeloencephalopathy in Brown Swiss cattle, *Zentralbl Veterinarmed A* 39:600-608, 1992 (abstract).
1431. Oyster R et al: Histochemical and morphometric studies of peripheral muscle in bovine progressive degenerative myeloencephalopathy of Brown Swiss cattle, *Zentralbl Veterinarmed [A]* 39:321-327, 1992.
1432. Aitchison CS et al: Ultrastructural alterations of motor cortex synaptic junctions in Brown Swiss cattle with weaver syndrome, *Am J Vet Res* 46:1733-1736, 1985.
1433. El Hamidi ME, Leipold HW, Cook JE: Ultrastructural changes in Brown Swiss cattle affected with bovine progressive degenerative myeloencephalopathy (weaver syndrome), *Zentralbl Veterinarmed [A]* 37:729-736, 1990.
1434. Hoeschele I, Meinert TR; Association of genetic defects with yield and type traits: the weaver locus effect upon yield, *J Dairy Sci* 73:2503-2515, 1990.
1435. Georges M et al: Microsatellite mapping of the gene causing weaver disease in cattle will allow the study of an associated quantitative trait locus, *Proc Natl Acad Sci* 90:1058-1062, 1993.
1436. Anonymous: We need more weaver reports, *Brown Swiss Bulletin* 64:44, 1985.

PROGRESSIVE SPINAL MYELINOPATHY OF BEEF CATTLE

LISLE W. GEORGE
MARY O. SMITH

Spinal myelinopathy of beef cattle has been reported in Australia.[1437] The condition occurs mainly in animals of the Murray Grey breed and is inherited in an autosomal recessive manner.[1438] Most of the affected animals are unable to stand at birth. Less severely affected calves usually exhibit severe deficiencies of conscious proprioception. The muscular tone of the rear limbs is increased. The condition is progressive, and affected animals die or are euthanized by 12 months of age.

The pathologic changes are restricted to the white matter of the spinal cord. These included swollen axons, dilated myelin sheath, wallerian degeneration, and ballooning of the axonal sheaths. There is mild chromatolysis. The animals have normal hepatic copper concentrations, indicating that the condition is not related to enzootic ataxia.[1437]

REFERENCES

1437. Richard RB, Edwards JR: A progressive spinal myelinopathy in beef cattle, *Vet Pathol* 23:35-41, 1986.
1438. Edwards JR, Richards RB, Carrick MJ: Inherited progressive spinal myelinopathy in Murray Grey cattle, *Aust Vet J* 65:108-109, 1988.

BOVINE SPINAL MUSCULAR ATROPHY

LISLE W. GEORGE
MARY O. SMITH

Bovine spinal muscular atrophy (SMA) is a heritable disorder of Brown Swiss cattle characterized pathologically by degeneration of motor neurons in the ventral horn of the spinal cord gray matter (equivalent to human anterior horn cells). The sensory neurons are unimpaired in calves with the spinal muscular atrophy.[1439,1440] The SMA-determining gene has recently been mapped to chromosome 20q12 → q13 in Brown Swiss cattle and is 85% homologous to the equivalent gene in human beings.[1441] Although this condition resembles weaver syndrome, the two diseases can be clinically differentiated. Signs of spinal muscular atrophy usually are first seen between 2 and 5 weeks of age. Calves with weaver syndrome first show signs at 5 months of age. The degree of muscular wastage is much greater in calves with spinal muscular atrophy than with weaver syndrome.[1442]

REFERENCES

1439. El Hamidi M et al: Spinal muscular atrophy in Brown Swiss calves, *J Vet Med* 36:731-738, 1989 (abstract).
1440. Troyer D et al: Upper motor neuron and descending tract pathology in bovine spinal muscular atrophy, *J Comp Pathol* 107:305-317, 1992.
1441. Pietrowski D et al: Description and physical location of the bovine survival of motor neuron gene (SMN), *Cytogenet Cell Genet* 83:39-42, 1998.
1442. Dahme E, Hafner A, Schmidt P: Spinal muscular atrophy in German Braunvieh calves: comparative neuropathological evaluation, *Neuropathol Appl Neurobiol* 17:517, 1991.

SPINAL DYSMYELINATION OF BRAUNVIEH–BROWN SWISS CALVES

A congenital spinal condition characterized by dysmyelination of the dorsal tracts of the spinal cord has been described in Braunvieh–Brown Swiss crossbred calves.[1443] Test matings have shown that the disease is inherited in an autosomal recessive manner.[1444] Calves are recumbent from birth. They have a coarse tremor of the head, neck, and body when stimulated and generalized muscular atrophy. Necropsy findings

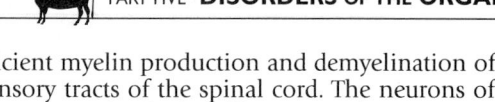
included deficient myelin production and demyelination of the dorsal sensory tracts of the spinal cord. The neurons of these calves are normal, which differentiates the condition from weaver syndrome and spinal muscular atrophy.

REFERENCES

1443. Hafner A et al: Spinal dysmyelination in newborn Brown Swiss-Braunvieh calves, *J Vet Med* 40:413-422, 1993.
1444. Agerholm JS, Andersen O: Inheritance of spinal dysmyelination in calves, *Zentralbl Veterinarmed [A]* 42:9-12, 1995.

PROGRESSIVE ATAXIA OF CHAROLAIS CALVES

Progressive ataxia occurs in pure and mixed breed Charolais calves 6 to 36 months of age.[1445-1450] The condition has a worldwide distribution. Affected calves develop posterior paresis and become recumbent by approximately 2 years of age. The disease is thought to be caused by a recessive genetic defect. The clinical signs begin with posterior ataxia and end in lateral recumbency. Other neurologic signs of progressive ataxia include stiffness of the neck, aggressiveness, dragging of the rear toes, stumbling, and loss of conscious proprioception (abduction, knuckling, circumduction, abnormal leg placement at rest).[1451] In the initial stages of the disease the gait deficits worsen with exercise and improve after a period of rest. Muscular tremors or a jerking movement of the limbs and tail may be seen when the affected animal attempts to rise.[1447,1452] Some animals may be found down acutely and show primarily signs of central vestibular disturbance.[1451] Difficulty in assuming and maintaining a urination posture and prolonged pulsatile micturition are characteristic abnormalities in affected animals.[1445,1449,1453] The major pathologic lesion is eosinophilic plaques in the white matter of the brain. Plaques also extend into the white matter of the cerebellar folia and peduncles. Ultrastructural changes include hypertrophied tongues of oligodendrocytes and dysmyelination.[1454]

REFERENCES

1445. Palmer AC et al: Progressive ataxia of Charolais cattle associated with a myelin disorder, *Vet Rec* 91:592-593, 1972.
1446. Patton CS: Progressive ataxia in Charolais cattle, *Vet Pathol* 14:535-537, 1977.
1447. Palmer AC, Blakemore WF: Progressive ataxia of Charolais cattle, *Bovine Pract* 10:84-85, 1975.
1448. Cordy DR: Progressive ataxia of Charolais cattle: an oligodendroglial dysplasia, *Vet Pathol* 23:78-80, 1986.
1449. Daniel RCW, Kelly WR: Progressive ataxia in Charolais cattle, *Aust Vet J* 58:32, 1982.
1450. Zicker SC et al: Progressive ataxia in a Charolais bull, *J Am Vet Med Assoc* 192:1590-1592, 1988.
1451. Montgomery DL, Mayer JC: Progressive ataxia of Charolais cattle, *Southwestern Vet* 37:247-250, 1986.
1452. Ogden AL, Palmer AC, Blakemore WF: Progressive ataxia in Charolais cattle, *Vet Rec* 94:555, 1974.
1453. Blakemore WF, Palmer AC, Barlow RM: Progressive ataxia in Charolais cattle associated with disordered myelin, *Acta Neuropathol (Berl)* 29:127-139, 1974.
1454. Zicker SC et al: Progressive ataxia in a Charolais bull, *J Am Vet Med Assoc* 192:1590-1592, 1988.

SPASTIC PARESIS (Elso Heel)

Spastic paresis is characterized by marked asymmetric spasticity and hypertonia of the rear limbs. The etiology is uncertain; it may be genetic. Breeds in which the condition has been recognized include the Holstein, Brahman, Angus, shorthorn, Charolais, Red Danish, crossbred shorthorn, Gelbvieh, Ayrshire, polled Hereford, Hungarian red spotted, Kankrej, Belgian blue, and other rare European breeds.[1455-1466] The clinical signs of this condition are clinically similar to inherited periodic spasticity (p. 993), except that spastic paresis is seen in young animals (onset at 3 weeks to 1 year of age) and occurs at all times when the animal stands.[1455-1458] In comparison, inherited periodic spasticity occurs in adults in episodic fashion, with normal gait between episodes. Spastic paresis has been recognized in pygmy goats.[1467]

CLINICAL SIGNS. Spastic paresis is characterized by intermittently increased extensor tonus in the pelvic limb as the animal attempts to walk.[1455,1459,1464,1468] The gastrocnemius and superficial digital extensor muscles are spastically contracted in all calves, whereas the biceps femoris, adductor, quadriceps, semitendinosus, and semimembranosus muscles are less often affected.[1456,1459,1468,1469] The extensor tone is normal when the calf is recumbent and relaxed but becomes excessive when the animal stands and attempts to bear weight. The excessive extensor motor activity results in an inability to flex the hock during protraction of the pelvic limb. To prevent the toes from dragging, the limb is circumducted, resulting in a pendulum-like motion.[1469] At rest the limb is held stiffly abducted and is repeatedly circumducted. The foot is held off the ground, and the gastrocnemius muscles appear to be underdeveloped. The tail is elevated from the ischiorectal fossa as the animal attempts to move. Eventually there is atrophy of the rear quarters. The spasticity is progressive, and affected animals experience difficulty rising and grazing. If untreated, the animals are stunted and usually are culled.

The excessive pull of the extensor tendons produces radiographically detectable changes in the bones of the hock, including osteoporosis, lipping of the dorsal aspect of the tibial epiphysis, plantar displacement of the proximal part of the tibial diaphysis and epiphysis, and excessive straightening of the tuber calcis.[1455,1456,1470]

The etiology and pathogenesis of spastic paresis is unknown. Some investigators have documented the presence of subtle demyelinating lesions of the red nucleus but were unclear about the contribution of these changes to the clinical syndrome.[1460,1462] Changes observed in affected calves include nonsuppurative encephalitis and reduced concentrations of dopamine and 5-homovanillic acid in the cerebrospinal fluid.[1471] There are no histologic or biochemical alterations of the myofibrils.[1472] Neuropharmacologic studies have indicated that the disease may be related to overstimulation of the gamma motoneurons of the spinal cord.[1473] The disease has been postulated to have a genetic basis, because affected offspring tend to have a common paternity[1455,1458,1460]; however, breeding experiments and progeny evaluation of cattle have not demonstrated a genetic deficit. Consequently, some authors do not recommend culling a bull merely because an offspring has developed the condition.[1474] Others have expressed disagreement with these findings.[1475]

TREATMENT. Surgical techniques for correction of the spasticity include sectioning of the spinal afferents at segments L4 through L6, neurectomy of the tibial nerve rootlets supplying the medial and lateral heads of the gastrocnemius muscle, and superficial digital flexor tenotomy proximal to the tuber calcis.[1457,1468,1476-1478] The tenotomy procedure is performed by incising proximal to the tuber calcis and transecting the superficial head of the gastrocnemius tendon completely (this tendon twists around the superficial digital flexor tendon from medial to lateral coursing distally) and partly nicking the superficial digital flexor tendon.[1477,1479]

To perform a tibial neurectomy, an incision is made in the groove separating the heads of the biceps femoris. The tibial nerve is identified as the more caudal of the branches off the ischiatic nerve. Some surgeons have recommended a concomitant sectioning of the caudal cutaneous sural nerve.

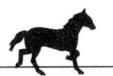

Success rates of 82% for the neurectomy technique and 40% for the tenotomy procedure have been reported.[1476,1480] Although recurrences have been reported to be common, some authors found high rates of sustained improvement over several months with the neurectomy technique.[1476] Results are poorer when animals under 2 months of age are treated.

Despite the reported success of these procedures, these treatments are not routinely performed in most countries because of the possible hereditary nature of the condition and the need for specialized instruments and general anesthesia. Administration of lithium gluconate (4 g/100 kg of body weight IM daily for 10 to 30 days) has been reported to be efficacious when used to treat calves in the early stages of the condition.[1463]

REFERENCES

1455. Leipold HW et al: Spastic paresis in beef shorthorn cattle, *J Am Vet Med Assoc* 151:598-601, 1967.
1456. Browning GF, Rawlinson RJ, Begg AP: Spastic paresis in a polled Hereford heifer, *Aust Vet J* 63:367-369, 1986.
1457. Bouckaert JH, De Moor A: Treatment of spastic paralysis in cattle: improved denervation technique of the gastrocnemius muscle and postoperative course, *Vet Rec* 79:226-229, 1966.
1458. Gadgil BA, Agarwal SP, Patel UG: Spastic paresis in adult Indian cattle, *Vet Rec* 86:694-697, 1970.
1459. Love J, Weaver AD: Spastic paresis in a crossbred shorthorn steer, *Vet Rec* 75:395-397, 1963.
1460. Chomiak M, Milart Z: Neurohistological changes in the central nervous system of the bull "Bosfor" affected with paresis spastica, *Zentralbl Veterinarmed [A]* 18:48-54, 1971.
1461. Wheat JD: Spastic lameness of the hind limbs of an Aberdeen-Angus heifer, *J Am Vet Med Assoc* 660:659-660, 1960.
1462. Chomiak M, Milart Z, Hoppe R: Alterations du systeme nerveux chez un taureau atteint de paresis spastica chronique, *Rev Med Vet* 122:8-9, 1971.
1463. Arnault GA: Bovine spastic paresis: an epidemiologic, clinical and therapeutic study in a Charolese practice with efficacy of lithium therapy, Proceedings of the XII World Congress on Diseases of Cattle, vol II, Utrecht, Netherlands, 1982, World Association for Buiatrics.
1464. Goetze R: Spastiche parese der hinteren extremitat bei kalbern und jungrindern, *DTW* 40:197-200, 1932.
1465. Thomason KJ, Beeman KB: Spastic paresis in Gelbvieh calves: an examination of two cases, *Vet Med* May:548-553, 1987.
1466. Browning GF, Rawlinson RJ, Begg, AP: Spastic paresis in a polled Hereford heifer, *Aust Vet J* 63:367-369, 1986.
1467. Baker J et al: Spastic paresis in pygmy goats, *J Vet Intern Med* 3:113, 1989.
1468. Denniston JC et al: Spastic paresis syndrome in calves, *J Am Vet Med Assoc* 152:1138-1149, 1968.
1469. Baird JD et al: Spastic paresis in Friesian calves, *Aust Vet J* 50:239-245, 1974.
1470. Van Gastel-Jansen A, Frederick GH: Pathological changes in the tarsi of cattle suffering from paresis spastica examined by means of x-rays, *Vet Rec* 74:1260-1263, 1962.
1471. De Ley G, De Moor A: Bovine spastic paralysis: cerebrospinal fluid concentrations of homovanillic acid and 5-hydroxyindoleacetic acid in normal and spastic calves, *Am J Vet Res* 36:227-228, 1975.
1472. De Ley G, De Moor A: Bovine spastic paralysis: a comparative study of serum enzymes and biopsies of the gastrocnemius muscle, *Zentralbl Veterinarmed A* 23:89-96, 1976 (abstract).
1473. De Ley G, De Moor A: Bovine spastic paralysis: results of selective efferent suppression with dilute procaine, *Vet Sci Commun* 3:289-298, 1980.
1474. Dawson PLL: The economic aspect of spastic paresis of the hind legs of Friesian cattle, *Vet Rec* 97:432-433, 1975.
1475. Wijeratne WVS: Heritability of spastic paresis, *Vet Rec* 98:139-140, 1976.
1476. Vlaminck L et al: Partial tibial neurectomy in 113 Belgian blue calves with spastic paresis, *Vet Rec* 147:16-19,2000.
1477. Formston C, Jones EW: A spastic form of lameness in Friesian cattle, *Vet Rec* 68:624-627, 1956.
1478. De Ley G, De Moor A: Bovine spastic paralysis: results of surgical dysafferentiation of the gastrocnemius muscle by means of spinal dorsal root resection, *J Am Vet Med Assoc* 38:1899-1900, 1977.
1479. Weaver AD: Modified gastrocnemius tenectomy: a procedure to relieve spastic paresis in dairy calves, *Vet Med*, 1991, pp 1234-1239.
1480. Mulville P, Curran N: Spastic paresis in cattle, *Irish Vet News*, November 9-11, 1992.

INHERITED PERIODIC SPASTICITY (Crampy Syndrome; Stretches; Barn Cramps; Krampfigkeit)

Inherited periodic spasticity is seen commonly in Holstein, Ayrshire, Jersey, Brown Swiss, and Guernsey cattle of either gender.[1481] Beef cattle are rarely affected. The condition is thought to be transmitted by a single autosomal recessive factor.[1482] Affected cattle are normal until they reach 3 to 7 years of age, at which time they develop marked muscular spasms of the hip and upper limb.[1481] The disease is mild for the first 2 to 3 years but progressively worsens with time. Eventually affected animals are culled early because of weight loss or chronic foot problems.

CLINICAL SIGNS. During the attack the leg may be held spastically in flexion, but more commonly it is held in rigid extension. The attacks are episodic, which differentiates them from the spasms of spastic paresis. The two diseases are otherwise similar in appearance. Each spasm is accompanied by kyphosis, which initially lasts 15 to 30 sec and which often is terminated by a fine tremor in the rear quarters or the digit. The intensity and duration of the spasms progressively increase over time. Both rear limbs are affected. During a spasm the animal usually extends or flexes only one leg at a time. Some animals with advanced disease arch the neck and back dorsally and lift the contralateral forelimb during an attack.[1481] At first the signs appear to typify a response to a painful focus, and affected animals may be misdiagnosed as having laminitis, colic, or peritonitis. Gait and proprioceptive responses appear normal.

TREATMENT. There is no specific treatment for the condition, but one author has recommended the use of mephenesin. A total 3-day dosage of the drug is calculated to be 100 to 120 mg/kg of body weight PO.[1483] Although the pharmacologic effect of the drug lasts only 6 to 8 hours, the same author has reported a reduction of severe symptoms for as long as several months after a single course of therapy.[1483]

REFERENCES

1481. Furie WS: Inherent nervous system disorders of cattle. III. Disorders lacking light microscopic lesions, *Agric Pract* 4:25-28, 1983.
1482. Becker RB, Wilcox CJ, Pritchard WR: Crampy or progressive posterior paralysis in mature cattle, *J Dairy Sci* 54:542-547, 1964.
1483. Roberts SJ: Hereditary spastic diseases affecting cattle in New York state, *Cornell Vet* 55:637-644, 1965.

DODDLER SYNDROME (Hereditary Lethal Spasms)

Doddler syndrome is a rare congenital lethal trait of Jersey cattle.[1484] The calves are down but appear bright and alert and usually are able to suckle. When stimulated, they develop severe intermittent spasms of the head and neck and convulsions. The animals can stand with assistance but are very ataxic and fall easily. They have a severe head tremor when forced to stand. The signs improve when the animal is allowed to rest but worsen again with restimulation.[1485] Calcification of multiple neurons and small vessels in the brainstem and cerebellum is observed at necropsy. The condition probably is inherited as a autosomal recessive lethal trait.

REFERENCES

1484. Gregory PW, Mead SW, Regan WM: Hereditary congenital lethal spasms in Jersey cattle, *J Hered* 35:195-200, 1944.
1485. High JW, Kincaid CM, Smith HJ: Doddler cattle, *J Hered* 49:250-252, 1958.

CONGENITAL VERTEBRAL ANOMALIES
(Spina Bifida; Butterfly Vertebrae; Hemivertebrae; Arnold-Chiari Syndrome)
(see also Chapters 47 and 48)

A large number of spinal deformities have been reported in domestic livestock, including the following:

■ *Spina bifida:* Failure of closure of a vertebral neural arch; spina bifida usually occurs concomitantly with one of the forms of myelodysplasia.[1486,1487]

■ *Spina bifida cystica:* Spina bifida associated with a cerebrospinal fluid cyst at the site of the bony defect.

■ *Hemivertebra:* A unilaterally incomplete vertebral segment; spina bifida and hemivertebrae have been described in calves, and spina bifida also has been reported in sheep and foals.[1486-1495]

■ *Arnold-Chiari syndrome:* A complex disorder that occurs in lambs and calves[1497] and is characterized by a number of pathologic changes, including herniation of cerebellar tissue through the foramen magnum, caudal overgrowth and displacement of the brainstem, internal hydrocephalus, polymicrogyria of the cerebral cortex, malformation of the base of the skull, and enlargement of the foramen magnum. There is a strong correlation between the occurrence of spina bifida and Arnold-Chiari syndrome of calves, indicating that the pathogenesis of the two conditions may be interrelated.[1486,1497]

Animals with spina bifida may be asymptomatic or may show paraparesis and paraplegia or tetraparesis and tetraplegia. If the spina bifida is associated with syringomyelia, the calves may have a peculiar "rabbit hopping" gait. The clinical signs often are present at birth or develop in the first 2 postnatal months.[1493,1498] Kyphoscoliosis and abnormalities of the rib cage may be seen at birth in some animals.[1493] The skin over the abnormal vertebrae may be smooth and hairless. When examined microscopically, this tissue resembles meninges or ependyma.[1487,1488]

Spina bifida and hemivertebrae are easily diagnosed by examination of plain radiographs. The specific site of central nervous system stenosis can be detected by performing a myelogram. The etiology of spina bifida is unknown, but some authors have suggested that it may have either genetic[1488-1490] or toxic etiologies.[1499,1500]

Arthrogryposis occurs secondary to the spinal cord changes. Spina bifida and myelodysplasias are not the only causes of arthrogryposis, however, and clinicians should attempt to differentiate between these and other diseases that interfere in utero with motor neuron development in the spinal cord. Nongenetic arthrogrypotic conditions of cattle include perosomus elumbis, hydranencephaly, manganese deficiency, and ingestion of lupines or *Nicotiana glauca* (40 to 60 days of gestation).[1501-1505]

REFERENCES

1486. Cho DY, Leipold HW: Spina bifida and spinal dysraphism in calves, *Zentralbl Veterinarmed A* 24:680-695, 1977 (abstract).
1487. Cho DY et al: Diagnosis of bovine congenital central nervous system defects, *Am Assoc Vet Lab Diagn* 21:103-116, 1978.
1488. McFarland LZ: Spina bifida with myelomeningocele in a calf, *J Am Vet Med Assoc* 134:32-34, 1959.
1489. Goss LJ, Hull FE: Spina bifida (calf), *Cornell Vet* 29:239-240, 1939.
1490. Nes AN: Spina bifida ledsaget av muskelkontraktur og andre defekter hos kalv, *Nord Vet Med* 11:33-54, 1959.
1491. Leipold HW: Spinal dysraphism, arthrogryposis and cleft palate in newborn Charolais calves, *Can Vet J* 10:268-273, 1969.
1492. Bollard JF: Syringomyelia in a Jersey calf, *J Am Vet Med Assoc* 87:575-576, 1935.
1493. Dodge CE: Spina bifida, *Can Vet J* 16:22-25, 1975.
1494. Keens JA: A case of spina bifida in a lamb, *Tijdschr Diergeneeskd* 70:307-308, 1945.
1495. Uberreiter O: Spina bifida occulta bei einen fohlen, *Tierarztl Umsch* 7:341-355, 1952.
1496. Reference deleted in proof.
1497. Gruys E: Dicephalus, spina bifida, Arnold-Chiari malformation, and duplication of thoracic organs in a calf, *Zentralbl Veterinarmed [A]* 20:789-800, 1973.
1498. Greene HJ et al: Bovine congenital defects: arthrogryposis and associated defects in calves, *Am J Vet Res* 34:887-891, 1973.
1499. Rokos J, Cekanova E, Kitheirova E: Pathogenesis of trypan blue-induced spina bifida, *J Pathol* 118:25-34, 1976.
1500. Rokos J: Pathogenesis of diastematomyelia and spina bifida, *J Pathol* 117:155-161, 1975.
1501. Leipold HW et al: Arthrogryposis and associated defects in newborn calves, *J Am Vet Med Assoc* 31:1367-1374, 1970.
1502. Keeler RF et al: *Nicotiana glauca*–induced congenital deformities in calves: clinical and pathologic aspects, *Am J Vet Res* 42:1231-1234, 1981.
1503. Leipold HW, Husby F, Brundage AL: Congenital defects of calves on Kodiak island, *J Am Vet Met Assoc* 170:1408-1410, 1977.
1504. Keeler RF: Lupine alkaloids from teratogenic and nonteratogenic lupines. III. Identification of anagyrine as the probable teratogen by feeding trials, *J Toxicol Environ Health* 1:887-898, 1976.
1505. Whittem JH: Congenital abnormalities in calves: arthrogryposis and hydranencephaly, *J Pathol Bacteriol* 73:375-386, 1957.

MYELODYSPLASIAS (Syringomyelia; Spinal Dysraphism; Hydromyelia)

The types of myelodysplasia that occur in livestock are[1506-1508]:

1. *Spinal dysraphism:* A general term denoting arrested development of the spinal cord before complete differentiation of gray and white matter; the areas of agenesis form longitudinal cystic structures instead of differentiated nervous tissue
2. *Syringomyelia:* Longitudinal canalicular cavitations of the spinal cord
3. *Hydromyelia:* Abnormal dilation of the central canal
4. *Diastematomyelia:* Duplication of the gray matter at one or more segments
5. *Rachischisis:* Complete failure to close the neural tube; the central canal remains open and communicates with the integument
6. *Meningocele:* Herniation of the dura mater through a spinal column defect
7. *Meningomyelocele:* Herniation of the meninges through a spinal column defect and a concomitant myelodysplasia

Myelodysplasias are most often seen in Charolais calves, in which the condition is associated with palatoschisis and arthrogryposis.[1506,1509] The condition has also been recognized in 5-month-old Thoroughbred foals and an Arabian foal.[1510,1511]

The neurologic deficits of myelodysplasia are difficult to differentiate from other spinal diseases unless the disorder is accompanied by spina bifida. Clinical recognition of myelodysplasia usually is based on the historic findings of paraplegia in a newborn calf without radiographic evidence of spinal fractures and with no myelographic evidence of spinal cord compression.

REFERENCES

1506. Leipold HW et al: Spinal dysraphism, arthrogryposis, and cleft palate in newborn Charolais calves, *Can Vet J* 10:268-273, 1969.
1507. Cho DY et al: Diagnosis of bovine congenital central nervous system defects, *Am Assoc Vet Lab Diagn* 21:103-116, 1978.
1508. Cho DY, Leipold HW: Spina bifida and spinal dysraphism in calves, *Zentralbl Veterinarmed A* 24:680-695, 1977 (abstract).
1509. Singh UM, Little PB: Arthrogryposis and cleft palate in a Charolais calf, *Can Vet J* 13:21-24, 1972.
1510. Cho DY, Leipold HW: Syringomyelia in a thoroughbred foal, *Equine Vet J* 9:195-197, 1977.
1511. Doige CE: Congenital cleft vertebral centrum and intra- and extraspinal cyst in a foal, *Vet Pathol* 33:87-89, 1996.

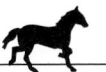

COYOTILLO POISONING

LISLE W. GEORGE

MARY O. SMITH

Ingestion of the fruit of the coyotillo plant, *Karwinskia humboldtiana*, by domestic animals produces a stiff, stilted gait, hypotonia, and hyperreflexia to areflexia.[1512,1513] The neurotoxin identified in and purified from the plant has been named tullidora toxin, after another name for the plant itself.[1514] Goats are susceptible to the effects of the intoxication. Daily doses of the fresh plant amounting to 0.04% to 0.05% of the body weight are sufficient to produce central nervous system disease by 60 days. The intoxication results in a peripheral polyneuropathy characterized by degenerative changes in both axons and myelin.[1514] Higher dosages may result in neuroaxonal dystrophy characterized by axonal swelling and gliosis. The condition occurs in the southwestern United States.

REFERENCES

1512. Charlton KM et al: A neuropathy in goats caused by experimental coyotillo *(Karwinskia humboldtiana)* poisoning. V. Lesions in the central nervous system, *Pathol Vet* 7:435-447, 1970.
1513. Charlton KM, Pierce KR: A neuropathy in goats caused by experimental coyotillo *(Karwinskia humboldtiana)* poisoning. IV. Light and electron microscopic lesions in peripheral nerves, *Pathol Vet* 7:420-434, 1970.
1514. Munoz-Martinez EJ, Cueva J, Joseph-Nathan P: Denervation caused by tullidora *(Karwinskia humboldtiana)*, *Neuropathol Appl Neurobiol* 9:121-134, 1983.

CYCAD PALM POISONING (*Zamia* Paralysis)

LISLE W. GEORGE

MARY O. SMITH

Ingestion of the palm cycad *Cycas circinalis* L., *Bowenia serrulata*, *Macrozamia lucida*, and *Cycas media* is associated with the development of posterior paresis in cattle and sheep.[1515-1517] The condition is seen exclusively in the tropics. The toxic principles of the cycad palm are glycosides and methylazoxymethanol (aglycone). The clinical signs include curvature of the spine, elevation of the tail head, paraparesis, and paraplegia. The anal sphincter and tail tone are normal. Cattle develop ataxia by 50 days after feeding of the plant (3.9 kg wet weight total intake). The cerebrospinal fluid of affected cattle is normal. The pathologic lesions include demyelination, spheroids, and cavitation of the spinal cord white matter. Changes relating to hepatic disease have also been reported.[1518] These lesions included coagulative centrilobular hepatic necrosis, icterus, and petechial hemorrhages on the serous surfaces.

REFERENCES

1515. Hooper PT, Best SM, Campbell A: Axonal dystrophy in the spinal cords of cattle consuming the cycad palm *Cycas media*, *Aust Vet J* 50:146-149, 1974.
1516. Mason MM, Whiting MG: Caudal motor weakness and ataxia in cattle in the Caribbean area following ingestion of cycads, *Cornell Vet* 58:541-554, 1968.
1517. Hall WT: Cycad *(Zamia)* poisoning in Australia, *Aust Vet J* 64:149-151, 1987.
1518. Reams RY et al: Cycad *(Zamia puertoriquensis)* toxicosis in a group of dairy heifers in Puerto Rico, *J Vet Diagn Invest* 5:488-494, 1993.

ACQUIRED TORTICOLLIS

Primary acquired torticollis with or without neurologic disease occurs in all species of domestic livestock. Causes include fracture or subluxation of the cervical vertebrae, basilar skull fractures, dystrophic muscle degeneration, unilateral cicatricial muscular contracture from injections, lupinosis, traumatic rupture of the cervical muscles, hydranencephaly, asymmetric neurodegeneration, or congenital vertebral deformity.[1519-1523] Calves with torticollis have a deviated head and neck. Physical constraint of late in utero development by narrow tips of uterine horns were hypothesized to be the cause of acquired torticollis and a variety of other deformities, such as head scoliosis and limb malformations, in more than 200 foals in one study.[1525] Draught horses may be predisposed to this problem, which frequently results in severe dystocia in horses. Provided the spinal cord is intact, no neurologic deficits result.

TREATMENT. Treatment of traumatic torticollis should be directed at reducing the edema, relieving pain, and immobilizing the damaged structures. Muscular tears may be treated by incorporating the head, neck, and proximal thorax in a fiberglass cast. Ancillary supportive treatment may include dexamethasone (0.04 to 0.08 mg/kg given daily for 2 to 3 days), methocarbamol (8 mg/kg IV daily for 5 days), and nonsteroidal antiinflammatory drugs (phenylbutazone PO or IV or flunixin meglumine administered IV for 3 to 5 days after injury). A method of surgical correction of cervical muscular contractures using a muscle splitting procedure has been described[1526]; however, this seems unnecessary because most animals recover with only medical treatment. When torticollis is the cause of equine dystocia, delivery of the foal by cesarean section often is followed by rapid and complete anatomic and functional recovery.[1525]

REFERENCES

1519. McKelvey WAC, Owen ap R R: Acquired torticollis in eleven horses, *J Am Vet Med Assoc* 175:295-297, 1979.
1520. Whittem JH: Congenital abnormalities in calves: arthrogryposis and hydranencephaly, *J Pathol Bacteriol* 73:375-386, 1957.
1521. Keeler RF: Lupin alkaloids from teratogenic and nonteratogenic lupins. III. Identification of anagyrine as the probable teratogen by feeding trials, *J Toxicol Environ Health* 1:887-898, 1976.
1522. Gruys E: Dicephalus, spina bifida, Arnold-Chiari malformation and duplication of thoracic organs in a calf, *Zentralbl Veterinarmed [A]* 20:789-900, 1973.
1523. Leipold HW, Husby F, Brundage AL: Congenital defects of calves on Kodiak Island, *J Am Vet Med Assoc* 170:1408-1410, 1977.
1524. Keeler RF: Lupine alkaloids from teratogenic and nonteratogenic lupines: crooked calf disease incidence with alkaloid distribution determined by gas chromatography, *Teratology* 7:23-30, 1973.
1525. Vandeplasscne M et al: Aetiology and pathogenesis of congenital torticollis and head scoliosis in the equine foetus, *Equine Vet J* 16:419-424, 1984.
1526. Smith RG: Operation for torticollis (congenital wry neck), *Vet Rec* 53:189-191, 1941.

TETANUS (Lockjaw)

DEFINITION AND ETIOLOGY. Tetanus is characterized by muscular rigidity and death from respiratory arrest or convulsions. The disease is caused by the exotoxins produced by the anaerobic, spore-forming, gram positive bacterium *Clostridium tetani*. Tetanus has a worldwide distribution, and all species of domestic livestock are susceptible. The bacterium is commonly isolated from the bowel contents of herbivores, but fecal contamination is considered to be only partly responsible for soil contamination.[1527] The agent also can be found in dirt that has had no documented contact with domestic livestock. This indicates that *C. tetani* should be considered a primary soil contaminant. Tetanus usually is a disease of individual animals; however, herd outbreaks of tetanus after tail docking or castration have been described.[1528,1529] During outbreaks of tetanus, *C. tetani* can be isolated from the feces of a large proportion of the cattle, indicating that in some cases the disease may be caused by proliferation of *C. tetani* in the patient's gastrointestinal tract.[1528,1529]

CLINICAL SIGNS. The incubation period of tetanus varies and depends on the size of the wound, the redox potential in the contaminated tissue, the number of bacteria inoculated, and the host's antitoxin titer. In most susceptible animals the signs occur from 2 weeks to 1 month after the bacterial inoculation. During the first 24 hours horses may develop intractable colic, and ruminants may bloat.[1530] The first signs in some animals may be a vague stiffness and lameness of the infected limb, which are related to a local effect of the absorbed toxin (localized tetanus). By 24 hours, generalized spasticity usually is evident. Affected animals display a stiff gait and an extended head posture.[1531] The hypertonia is most evident in the antigravity muscles. Thus the limbs are held in a characteristic posture that resembles the legs of a sawhorse (sawhorse stance). The lips are retracted toward the poll, and the ears are pulled slightly down and caudal. The tail is elevated from the ischiorectal fossa. There is excessive muscle tone of all facial musculature. The jaws are clamped tightly shut (trismus), and the legs are held rigidly extended.

Muscular spasms can be elicited by auditory, ocular, or tactile stimulation. The limbs and head are very resistant to passive flexion. Retraction of the eye and a rapid flashing of the third eyelid across the cornea occurs after a menacing gesture or a slap over the neck.[1530,1532] This sign is more consistently observed in horses than in ruminants. Aspiration pneumonia may develop as a result of impaired deglutition. Severely affected animals become recumbent and lie on their side with the head and legs in full extension and the ears held almost parallel to the thoracic spinal cord (Fig. 33-40). Progression of the disease is associated with increased tonic muscular activity, which results in pyrexia in all species and profuse sweating in horses.[1529,1533] Frothy saliva accumulates at the commissures of the lips because the animals are unable to swallow, and respiratory incursions whip the mucinous saliva into a foam. The respiratory muscles (diaphragm and intercostals) are affected, and the animals develop hypoxia. Ventrolateral strabismus and dilated, fixed pupils may occur in advanced tetanus of cattle. Animals die while in a terminal convulsion. Death is attributable to hypoxemia and heart failure that occur secondary to systemic hypertension and aspiration pneumonia. Survivors begin to show some improvement after 2 weeks, but the clinical signs may persist for as long as 1 month, and lameness may be permanent.

CLINICAL PATHOLOGY. There are no reliable useful clinicopathologic tests for confirmation of a diagnosis of tetanus. Attempts should be made to culture *C. tetani* from the suspected site of entry.

PATHOPHYSIOLOGY. In horses puncture wounds of the foot or the soft tissues are the most frequent sites of infection, whereas dairy cattle are infected most commonly through the uterus. Other sites for growth of *C. tetani* include lesions induced by elastrator bands, tail docking, dehorning, bull rings, or infected umbilical stalks.[1534] Proliferation of *C. tetani* in the forestomachs of normal cattle may produce sufficient concentrations of toxin to result in clinical signs.[1535,1536] Outbreaks of tetanus have been correlated with ingestion of millet. This diet has been postulated to promote the growth of *C. tetani* in the large bowel[1537] and probably accounts for the lack of visible wounds in some animals affected with tetanus.[1528,1532]

When inoculated into the anaerobic site, *C. tetani* spores germinate into the vegetative form. Factors that enhance the sporulation and growth of *C. tetani* include necrotic tissue, pus, concomitant bacterial infection, and foreign bodies. Spores inoculated into the tissues are highly resistant to normal host defenses and may remain dormant for months or years before developing into the vegetative state. The production of the tetanus toxins occurs at the end of the logarithmic growth phase of the vegetative form and is governed by a plasmid-associated gene.[1538,1539] The bacterium produces at least three toxic proteins: tetanospasmin, tetanolysin, and a nonspasmogenic toxin. Tetanolysin promotes the spread of the infection by increasing the amount of local tissue necrosis.[1533] Tetanospasmin is a lipoprotein exotoxin that diffuses from the site of production into the vascular system, where it is distributed hematogenously to the presynaptic part of the motor end plates. Once bound to the nerves, the toxin is internalized and transported to the central nervous system along the axons of the alpha motoneurons through the

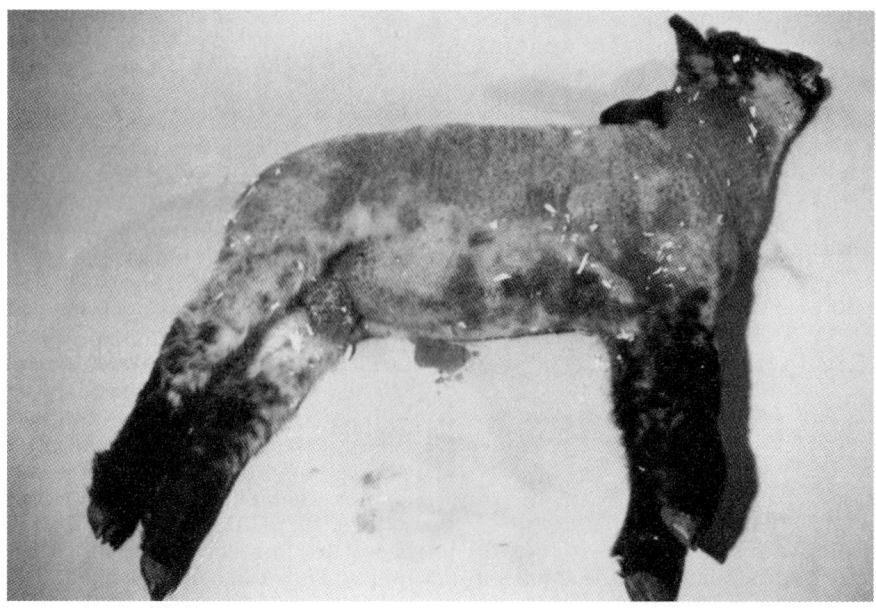

FIG. 33-40 ■ Characteristic appearance of tetanus in a lamb. This condition developed subsequent to application of an elastrator band to the scrotum.

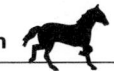

membrane-bound smooth endoplasmic reticulum.[1531,1540,1541] After the toxin reaches the ventral horn of the spinal cord, it crosses the synaptic cleft to presynaptic inhibitory interneurons (Renshaw cells) in the intermediate gray column.[1542] The toxin probably inhibits the release of glycine and γ-aminobutyric acid (GABA) from the Renshaw cells, resulting in disinhibition of the gamma motoneurons. The inhibition of these cells results in hypertonia and muscular spasms.

The nonspasmogenic toxin is thought to produce overstimulation of the sympathetic nervous system. Systemic hypertension seen in tetanus can be related to excessive catecholamine production by the adrenal medulla. Other physiologic changes that have been identified in humans and laboratory animals include increased plasma cortisol concentrations and neuromuscular blockade. Whether these are due to the effects of the toxin or are secondary changes occurring in response to a painful and life-threatening problem is unclear. There are no characteristic postmortem lesions associated with tetanus.

TREATMENT. The six general medical principles for treating tetanus in large animals are:
1. Provide muscular relaxation.
2. Ensure good footing.
3. Eliminate the infection.
4. Neutralize the unbound toxin.
5. Maintain hydration and nutritional status.
6. Establish active antitoxic immunity.

Provide Muscular Relaxation. The patient should be sedated and placed in a quiet, darkened stall. Drugs are administered that may reduce the muscular spasms. These include promazine (0.5 to 1 mg/kg IV) or acetylpromazine (0.05 to 0.1 mg/kg IV) given at 4- to 6-hour intervals. Predictable muscular relaxation may be obtained inexpensively by concomitant intravenous administration of acetylpromazine (0.06 mg/kg) and 5% sodium pentobarbital (2 to 4 ml/50 kg). An intravenous catheter may be placed to minimize treatment-associated stimulation. Mephenesin (10 to 20 mg/kg IV given 3 times daily) and guaifenesin have also been recommended. These drugs interfere with the internuncial neurons of the spinal cord that participate in reflex muscle activities. They do not have a high therapeutic efficacy for tetanus. Diazepam (0.01 to 0.4 mg/kg IV 2 to 8 times daily) effectively reduces muscular spasms in large animals by enhancing GABA, but prolonged administration of this drug to a large ruminant or horse is expensive because of the short duration in the plasma and CNS. In addition to its enhancement of GABA, the drug is efficacious because of its glycine-mimetic effects.[1530] Packing the ears with cotton to minimize auditory stimulation also can help reduce muscle spasms.

Ensure Good Footing. Excellent footing is essential. Tetanic animals have difficulty rising because of increased spasms and muscular tone. The stall should be bedded deeply in shavings or straw to minimize decubital ulcers. Horses and small ruminants that cannot stand should be supported in a sling, provided they do not become frantic while suspended.

Eliminate the Infection. C. tetani grows in nonvascularized sites, therefore the infection is best eliminated by surgical debridement of the affected area. Concomitant infiltration of penicillin G around the wound and parenteral administration of either potassium penicillin G (22,000 IU/kg given 3 or 4 times daily) or procaine penicillin G (22,000 IU/kg IM 2 times daily) also may be beneficial.

Neutralize the Unbound Toxin. Before the tetanus antitoxin has bound to the nerve cells, it is susceptible to neutralization with antitoxin. Although administration of antitoxin to animals several days after the onset of clinical signs seems to have little benefit in horses, increased survival rates have been documented in human patients who have received high dosages of tetanus antitoxin in the early phase of the disease.

Infiltration of the area with 3000 to 9000 IU of tetanus antitoxin may effectively neutralize toxin that has not yet reached the peripheral vasculature. Although specific dosages have not been determined for domestic animals, suggested doses range from 1000 to 5000 IU/500-kg animal to 1000 to 5000 IU/kg.[1543-1545] The limited therapeutic benefits of intravenously administered antitoxin must be compared to the cost of the biologic, the potential side effects of hepatic necrosis (see Chapter 31) or anaphylaxis, and the economic value of the animal.

Some have claimed that administration of 50 ml antitoxin (1000 IU/ml) intracysternally to horses resulted in stabilization of the clinical signs. However, this treatment did not reverse the condition.[1546] The antitoxin is administered after slow removal of 30 ml of cerebrospinal fluid (CSF). Although a survival rate of 77% has been claimed,[1546] the study failed to consider several cysternally injected horses that died of intercurrent diseases. When all cases were considered, there appeared to be no statistically significant difference between cysternally injected horses and conventionally treated controls. Complications of this procedure included iatrogenic CSF infections, anesthesia-related deaths, and sepsis from indwelling catheters. Because of severe reactions to intrathecal equine serum in ruminants, intrathecal administration of equine-origin tetanus antitoxin is contraindicated.

Maintain Hydration and Nutritional Status. The patient's hydration and food intake should be monitored daily. The food should be placed off the ground in an elevated feed bunk or hay net to allow easier access. Intravenous fluids should be administered as needed to correct dehydration and electrolyte abnormalities. Alimentation with a nasogastric tube may be attempted in anorectic horses, but severe adverse reactions to this procedure in some tetanus patients may limit its usefulness. A rumenostomy in anorectic cattle relieves the chronic ruminal tympany and provides a convenient means of administering oral fluids and feed.

Establish Active Antitoxic Immunity. The concentration of tetanus toxin necessary to cause neurologic symptoms is less than that required to stimulate an active immunologic response. Affected animals should be immunized with tetanus toxoid at the time of treatment and given a second dose 1 to 2 months later. Concomitant injections of tetanus antitoxin and toxoid should be made at different sites of the body and should not be admixed before administration.

PROGNOSIS. The mortality rate may reach 50% in cattle and 80% in horses. The rate of progression of clinical signs is indirectly related to the prognosis. Animals that survive for longer than 7 days have a fair to good chance of complete recovery.

PREVENTION. Because cattle appear to be more resistant to tetanus than horses and small ruminants, they are not routinely immunized against the disease unless outbreaks have occurred previously. Colostral antibodies may interfere with the active immunization of neonates. One report has indicated that most foals from immunized dams (82.9%) lose passively acquired specific antitoxic antibodies by 4 months of age. However, other studies have suggested that passive immunity may last as long as 6 to 12 months of age. Because some animals have low titers and others have high, persistent titers, a general recommendation might include vaccination of livestock at 2, 3, and 6 months of age, followed by a booster after 1 year. To ensure protective levels of colostral antibodies, mares, does, or ewes should receive an annual booster dose of the toxoid 1 to 2 months before the anticipated date of parturition. One study indicated that tetanus prophylaxis was not cost-effective for sheep, but recommendations about vaccination would differ, depending on the economic value of the animal at risk.[1547]

Acute hepatic necrosis of horses (Theiler's disease) has been associated with administration of certain lots of commercially prepared tetanus antitoxin (see Chapter 31) 1 to 3 months previously. Such findings indicate that administration of tetanus antitoxin should be limited to unvaccinated horses with tetanus-prone wounds. The recommended dosages of tetanus antitoxin are 1500 IU SC or IM for adult horses or cattle[1548] and 500 IU SC or IM for sheep and goats. Tetanus toxoid should be administered concomitantly. The antitoxin and the toxoid should not be mixed in the same syringe and should be administered at different sites of the body; a second toxoid dose should be given in 1 month.[1548,1549] Previously immunized horses with tetanus-prone lesions should be given a booster dose of tetanus toxoid and should not be given antitoxin. Foals from unvaccinated dams should receive 1500 IU of tetanus antitoxin at birth.[1548]

Tetanus toxoid is effective, but not all horses develop protective immunity. Historic information citing a previous vaccination should not completely exclude the possibility of tetanus.[1550]

REFERENCES

1527. Wilkins CA et al: Occurrence of *Clostridium tetani* in soil and horses, *S Afr Med J* 73:718-720, 1987.
1528. Herd RP, Riches WR: An outbreak of tetanus in cattle, *Aust Vet J* 40:356-357, 1964.
1529. Ramsay WR: An outbreak of tetanus-like disease in cattle, *Aust Vet J* 49:188-189, 1973.
1530. McGuirk SM: Tetanus in a prepartum dairy heifer, *Compend Cont Educ Pract Vet* 5:594-597, 1983.
1531. Seib UC et al: Supporting evidence for a role of neural ascent of toxin in the pathogenesis of general tetanus in cats, *Naunyn-Schmiedeberg's Arch Pharmacol* 276:403-411, 1973.
1532. Puckett LW: Idiopathic tetanus in a horse, *Vet Med (Small Anim Clin)* 59:963-964, 1964.
1533. Ansari MM, Matros LE: Tetanus, *Compend Cont Educ Pract Vet* 4:S473-S478, 1982.
1534. Robinson NE: Clinicopathologic conference, *J Am Vet Med Assoc* 152:1158-1164, 1968.
1535. Wallis AS: Some observations on the epidemiology of tetanus in cattle, *Vet Rec* 75:188-191, 1963.
1536. O'Connor B, Leavitt S: Tetanus in feeder calves associated with elastic castration, *Can Vet J* 34:311-312, 1993.
1537. Ellison RS: Tetanus epidemic in a mob of dairy heifers, *Surveillance (Wellington)* 19:14, 1992.
1538. Finn CW et al: The structural gene for tetanus neurotoxin is on a plasmid, *Science* 224:881-884, 1984.
1539. Laird WJ, Aaronson W, Silver RP: Plasmid-associated toxogenicity in *Clostridium tetani, J Infect Dis* 142:623, 1980.
1540. Stoeckel K, Schwab M, Thoenen H: Role of gangliosides in the uptake and retrograde axonal transport of cholera and tetanus toxin as compared to nerve growth factor and wheat germ agglutinin, *Brain Res* 132:273-385, 1977.
1541. Wellhoner HH, Hensel B, Seib UC: Local tetanus in cats: neuropharmacokinetics of 125I-tetanus toxin, *Naunyn-Schmiedeberg's Arch Pharmacol* 276:375-386, 1973.
1542. Habermann E, Dimpfel W, Raker KO: Interaction of labeled tetanus toxin with substructures of rat spinal cord in vivo, *Naunyn-Schmeideberg's Arch Pharmacol* 276:361-373, 1973.
1543. Hahn CN, Mayhew IG, McKay R: The nervous system. In Colahan PT et al, eds: *Equine medicine and surgery,* ed 5, St Louis, 2000, Mosby.
1544. Blood DC et al: *Veterinary medicine,* ed 6, Philadelphia, 1985, Bailliére Tindall.
1545. Hoyt H: Tetanus treatment and prophylaxis, *Am Assoc Equine Pract* 1:261-265, 1963.
1546. Muyle E et al: Treatment of tetanus in the horse by injections of tetanus antitoxin into the subarachnoid space, *J Am Vet Med Assoc* 167:47-48, 1975.
1547. Maru A, Kumar K, Arora AL: A note on the cost-effectiveness of tetanus vaccination in sheep flocks, *Indian J Anim Health* 25:193-194, 1986.
1548. Radvila VP, Lohrer J: Passive und aktive tetanusim-munitat und ihr verlauf, *Schweiz Arch fur Tierheilkd* 107:124-157, 1965.
1549. Le Metayer E, Nicol L: Prophylaxie specifique inter-rompue du tetanos realise chez des la naissance, Stockholm, *Proc Int Vet Congr* 1:57-61, 1953.
1550. Green SL: Equine tetanus: a review of the clinical features and current perspectives on treatment and prophylaxis, *Proceedings of the Thirty-eighth Annual Conference of the American Association of Equine Practitioners,* 1993, pp 229-306.

TRIARYL PHOSPHATE POISONING (Chronic Organophosphate Poisoning; Dying Back Axonopathy)

LISLE W. GEORGE
MARY O. SMITH

Ingestion of lubricants containing triaryl phosphates causes a neurologic disturbance of livestock characterized by a delayed neuropathy resulting in incoordination and paralysis. Common sources of the triaryl phosphate esters include turbojet lubricants, hydraulic oils, industrial solvents, plasticizers, and automotive brake fluid. Chronic organophosphate poisoning also occurs in some families of sheep after treatment with organophosphorus anthelmintics.[1551] At least six different phenotypes of sheep have been identified with respect to their ability to metabolize carboxylic acid esters.[1552,1553] These are designated as Esa/a, Esa/b, Esa/c (high enzyme groups) and Esa/c, Esb/b, and Esc/c (low enzyme groups). This genetically determined inability to inactivate organophosphates governs the appearance of demyelination after administration of therapeutic dosages of the drugs.

Triaryl phosphates have few effects on the glial cells,[1554] but they have profound neurotoxicity for the longest axons.[1555] These fibers degenerate first at the distal, nonterminal areas. The degenerative lesions then spread proximally from the terminal nerve rootlets into the spinal cord until the cell body dies (dying back axonopathy). Dosages of triaryl phosphate ranging from 5 to 10 g/kg cause paralysis by 19 to 36 days after exposure.[1556] Cats may be poisoned by a single topical application of tri-O-cresyl phosphate ester at 1000 mg/kg or by daily application of 1 to 100 mg/kg,[1557] and massive topical exposure may cause toxicity in livestock. The poisoning may be cumulative, because in some outbreaks compounds containing as little as 0.4% triorthocresyl phosphaester have been found in toxic materials. Animals belonging to the low enzyme groups are much more susceptible than their high-enzyme herd mates.

CLINICAL SIGNS. The onset of slowly progressive neurologic signs occurs about 10 days to a few months after exposure.[1558-1560] The clinical signs of chronic organophosphate intoxication are rough hair coat, bloat, dyspnea, muscular weakness, and incoordination of the rear legs. The animals may slip on their rear limbs and assume a dog-sitting posture. The limbs are circumducted and lack normal conscious proprioceptive responses. Affected animals become recumbent, attempt to rise, but do so incompletely and fall. Muscular tone and flexor reflexes may be normal, or flaccid paralysis may be evident.[1559] The tail, bladder, and rectum often are paralyzed; and affected animals show signs of incontinence, constipation, and perineal scalding. Slight ventrolateral strabismus has been described, and some animals have been reported to become mute.[1560,1561] Most animals retain a normal appetite and sensorium during the development of the paralysis. Electromyographic changes in experimentally poisoned animals include increased insertional activity, positive sharp waves, and fibrillation potentials in the muscles of the hind limb, consistent with denervation of affected muscles.[1562]

PATHOLOGY. Laboratory confirmation of the condition usually is based on histopathologic detection of a dying back axonopathy in the peripheral nervous tissues. Clinical pathologic parameters usually are normal. The red blood cell cholinesterase is low or undetectable at the time of clinical onset but may return to normal concentrations by the time the animals display profound paralysis. The specific concentration of cholinesterase depends largely on the type of organophosphate and the patient's genetic ability to metabolize the toxic compounds. Whole blood cholinesterase concentrations in haloxon-treated esterase A–deficient animals remain significantly lower than in controls for at least 27 days after administration of 375 mg. In comparison, the enzyme concentrations in the plasma of normal sheep do not decrease after drug treatment.[1563] Cholinesterase levels in exposed animals are not predictive of the later onset of delayed neurotoxicity.[1560]

Macroscopic lesions are not usually seen. Microscopic lesions are found exclusively in the central nervous system, and their severity appears to be dose dependent. The lesions begin distally and progress retrograde along the long, unsynapsed proprioceptive and motor tracts. The dorsospinal, cerebellar, gracile, and cuneate tracts are most susceptible to the effects of the toxins.[1562] Specific lesions include demyelination, internodal axonal swelling, and wallerian degeneration. There also is a vacuolation of the large neurons of the ventral motor nucleus of the spinal cord. The mechanism of neurotoxicity is unknown, but alteration of a cell membrane protein found in neurons and some other cells has been implicated.[1563-1565] This protein has been designated a neuropathy target esterase and is thought to be "aged" by phosphorylation induced by the toxicosis.

Newer compounds in the triaryl phosphate group are less capable of causing delayed neurotoxicity, which gives some hope that the incidence of this type of toxicity may decline in the future.[1565] Delayed organophosphate toxicity is not treatable and is irreversible.

REFERENCES

1551. Williams JF, Dade AW: Posterior paralysis associated with anthelmintic treatment of sheep, *J Am Vet Med Assoc* 169:1307-1309, 1976.
1552. Malone JC: Toxicity of haloxon, *Res Vet Sci* 5:17-31, 1964.
1553. Baker NF et al: Neurotoxicity of haloxon and its relationship to blood esterases of sheep, *Am J Vet Res* 31:865-871, 1970.
1554. Seung UK, Rizzuto N: Neuroaxonal degeneration induced by sodium diethyldithiocarbamate in cultures of central nervous tissue, *J Neuropathol Exp Neurol* 34:531-541, 1975.
1555. Patton SE et al: Changes in brain and spinal cord protein phosphorylation after a single oral administration of tri-O-cresyl phosphate to hens, *J Neurochem* 45:1567-1577, 1985.
1556. Dollahite JW, Pierce KR: Neurologic disturbances due to triaryl phosphate toxicity, *Am J Vet Res* 30:1461-1464, 1969.
1557. Abou-Donia MB, Trofatter LP, Graham DG: Electromyographic, neuropathologic, and functional correlates in the cat as the result of tri-O-cresyl phosphate-delayed neurotoxicity, *Toxicol Appl Pharmacol* 83:126-141, 1986.
1558. Beck BE, Wood CD, Whenham GR: Triaryl phosphate poisoning in cattle, *Vet Pathol* 14:128-137, 1977.
1559. Prantner MM, Sosalla MJ: Delayed organophosphate neurotoxicosis in four heifers, *J Am Vet Med Assoc* 203:1453-1455, 1993.
1560. Coppock RW et al: A review of nonpesticide phosphate ester-induced neurotoxicity in cattle, *Vet Hum Toxicol* 37:576-579, 1995.
1561. Perdrizet JA, Cummings JF, De Lahunta A: Presumptive organophosphate-induced delayed neurotoxicity in a paralyzed bull, *Cornell Vet* 75:401-410, 1985.
1562. Spencer PS, Schaumburg HH: Ultrastructural studies of the dying back process. IV. Differential vulnerability of PNS and CNS fibers in experimental central-peripheral distal axonopathies, *J Neuropathol Exp Neuropathol* 36:300-320, 1977.
1563. Richardson RJ: Neurotoxic esterase: research trends and prospects, *Neurotoxicol* 4:157-162, 1983.
1564. Johnson MK: Organophosphates and delayed neuropathy: Is NTE alive and well? *Toxicol Appl Pharmacol* 102:385-399, 1990.
1565. Weiner ML, Jortner BS: Organophosphate-induced delayed neurotoxicity of triaryl phosphates, *Neurotoxicol* 20:653-673, 1999.

MOTOR UNIT AND CAUDA EQUINA DISEASES

MARY O. SMITH

ELECTROMYOGRAPHY AND NERVE CONDUCTION TESTING IN MOTOR UNIT DISEASE

A number of electrodiagnostic techniques now are commonly applied to the diagnosis of neurologic disease in animals. They are particularly useful when clinical signs of generalized weakness, muscle atrophy, tremors, or obscure

lameness are present. Electromyography (EMG) and peripheral nerve conduction testing (NCT) are of great value for diagnosing diseases that affect the motor unit, for assessing the prognosis, and for determining the effects of therapy. EMG and NCT are simple, relatively noninvasive techniques. They provide objective information on the functional status of the nerves and muscles that cannot be determined by other means.

Motor Unit

In muscles in which very precise control of movement is necessary, each motoneuron innervates only a few muscle fibers, whereas in large postural muscles in which fine control is not required, a single motoneuron innervates many hundreds of muscle fibers. The cell body of the alpha motoneuron lies in the ventral horn of the spinal cord or, in the case of cranial nerves, in cranial nerve nuclei in the brainstem. The myelinated axon of the motoneuron runs within the ventral root to the spinal nerve and peripheral nerves and finally terminates in small unmyelinated terminal arborizations (Fig. 33-41). Enlargements of the ends of the terminal arborizations form the presynaptic components of the neuromuscular junctions. The postsynaptic part of the neuromuscular junction consists of a specialized region of the muscle fiber membrane. When acetylcholine release from the nerve terminal is sufficient to provoke an action potential in the myofibers, all the myofibers of the motor unit respond equally, an "all or nothing" response. Motor unit disease (lower motoneuron disease) may result from damage to any one of the following: the alpha motoneuron cell body or axon, the Schwann cells that form the myelin sheath of the alpha motoneuron, the neuromuscular junction, or the muscle fiber.

Although they are not part of the motor unit, the neurons that provide the sensory supply to the skeletal muscles may

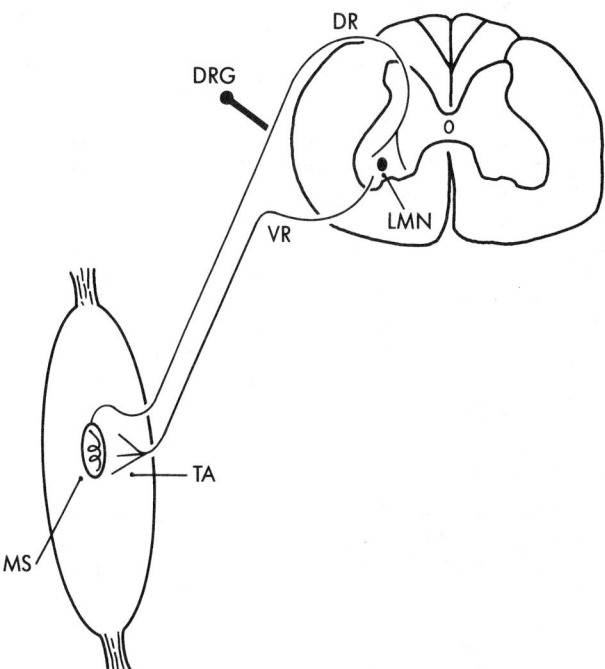

FIG. 33-41 ■ Components of the motor unit. *DR*, Dorsal root of the spinal nerve; *DRG*, dorsal root ganglion; *LMN*, lower motor neuron; *MS*, muscle spindle; *TA*, terminal arborizations of the lower motor neuron axon; *VR*, ventral root of the spinal nerve.

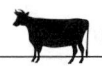
be involved in motor unit diseases in animals. Dysfunction of the peripheral sensory nerves causes clinical signs similar to those seen with motor unit disorders, even when all the components of the motor unit are normal.[1566] The cell bodies of sensory neurons lie in the dorsal root ganglia or in the sensory nuclei of cranial nerves. Their axons extend centrally to synapse with lower motoneurons and interneurons in the spinal cord and brainstem and distally in peripheral nerves to the stretch receptors in the muscle spindles of skeletal muscles and to proprioceptors in joints (see Fig. 33-41).

Instrumentation

The recording of the electrical activity of nerve and muscle cells requires an electrode system, an amplifier, and a device to display the recording. An electrical stimulator is needed for NCT. A variety of units are now available for EMG and NCT, with a range of specifications to supply the different needs of investigators and clinicians. The components of a system may be purchased individually, but most clinicians prefer to use a complete unit.

For recording, three electrodes are required: an active or exploring electrode, a reference electrode, and a ground electrode. A number of different arrangements are possible, but one that is commonly used is the coaxial needle electrode. The central wire of the coaxial electrode is the active component, and the surrounding hollow needle is the reference component. The wire is insulated from the needle along its length by a material such as Teflon, except at its tip, where it is exposed. This type of electrode is particularly suited to use in large animals because it minimizes the problem of poor electrical contact encountered with the use of surface electrodes and does not seem to cause the patient excessive discomfort. For similar reasons a subcutaneous needle electrode usually is chosen for the ground electrode, which is placed a short distance from the recording and reference electrodes, usually over a bony prominence.

The signal recorded by the electrodes must be amplified. Amplifiers available today offer a wide range of specializations to improve signal amplification while minimizing interference. These include high- and low-frequency filters, common mode rejection (to reduce 60 Hz interference from nearby electricity sources), and signal-averaging capabilities to facilitate the recording of nerve action potentials.

The display unit most commonly used is the cathode ray oscilloscope (CRO). In the CRO a "pen" that has essentially zero inertia, the electron beam, is able accurately to display rapidly changing low voltage potentials. Most systems have specializations that permit permanent storage of information on magnetic tape or a paper printout. An audioamplifier is a useful addition to the system, because many of the potentials recorded by EMG produce characteristic sounds when converted to an audible signal. It often is easier for an experienced electromyographer to make a diagnosis by listening to the audio EMG than by trying to follow a series of very rapidly changing potentials displayed on the CRO screen.

Electromyography

EMG usually can be carried out in a conscious animal. Some restraint is necessary, such as placing the animal in stocks and administering a sedative agent. Commonly used sedatives such as xylazine and acepromazine do not interfere with EMG. An electromyographic examination should include testing of many muscles over the whole body, with special concentration on those thought to be involved in the disease process. The recording electrode must be inserted into four or five sites in each muscle tested to ensure that focal abnormalities are not missed.

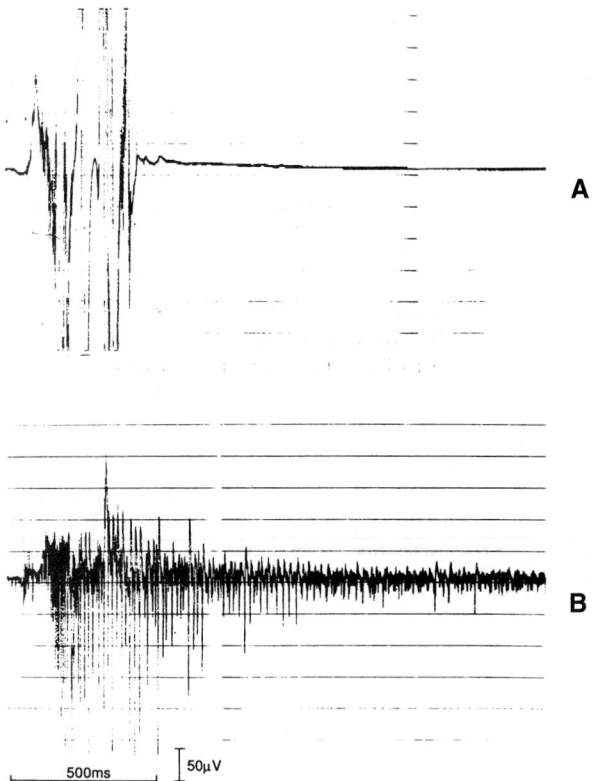

FIG. 33-42 ■ Electromyogram insertion activity. **A,** Normal: insertion activity ends abruptly when movement of the exploring electrode stops. **B,** Abnormal: insertion activity persists after the exploring electrode is at rest.

EMG alone usually does not provide a definitive diagnosis of the disease process present. It helps to localize the lesion and provides information that can then be used in selecting further diagnostic modalities such as nerve conduction velocity testing and choice of the most suitable site for muscle or nerve biopsy.

Normal Muscle

INSERTION ACTIVITY. Insertion of the recording electrode into a muscle or its movement in the muscle results in a burst of electrical activity that stops abruptly when movement of the electrode stops (Fig. 33-42). It is accompanied by a harsh, crackling sound. This "insertion activity" is the result of direct stimulation of muscle fibers by the moving electrode.

ELECTRICAL SILENCE. When the electrode is motionless in a normal resting muscle (one that is not actively contracting), no electrical activity is seen on the electromyograph. The electron beam of the CRO traces a straight line, and the audio electromyograph is silent. Electrical silence is the normal state in resting muscle except in the end plate zone.

MOTOR UNIT ACTION POTENTIAL (MUAP). A MUAP is the electrical activity of a single motor unit (Fig. 33-43). Only the activity of the fibers lying within approximately 1 mm of the electrode tip is recorded.[1567] MUAPs may be observed during EMG of normal active muscle. The parameters of a MUAP vary with the nature of the motor unit that has produced it, with the type of electrode arrangement and electromyograph used, and with the position of the electrodes in relation to the electrical event itself. The important characteristics of the MUAP are the amplitude, duration, and number of phases. Normal motor unit potentials are biphasic or triphasic potentials with amplitudes of 500 to 3000 μV and durations of 3 to 15 msec.[1567,1568] In very

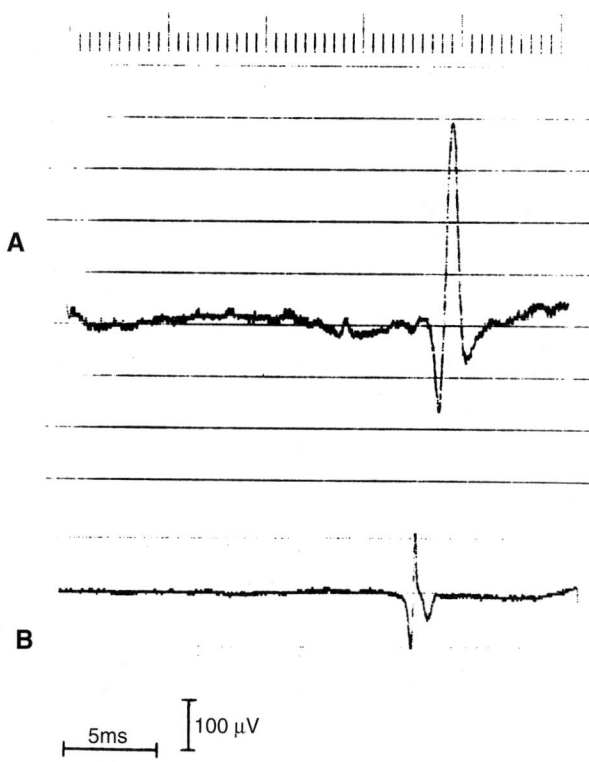

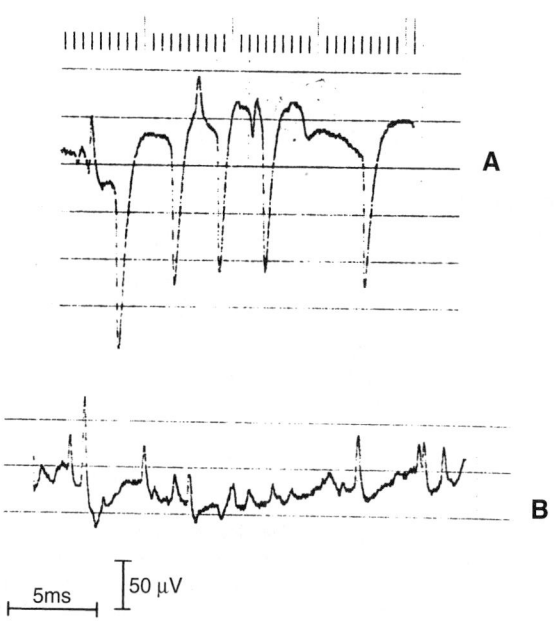

FIG. 33-45 ■ Abnormal electromyographic potentials. **A,** Positive sharp waves. **B,** Fibrillation potentials.

FIG. 33-43 ■ Motor unit action potentials. **A,** Normal: amplitude is approximately 550 μV. **B,** Abnormal: amplitude is decreased approximately 200 μV.

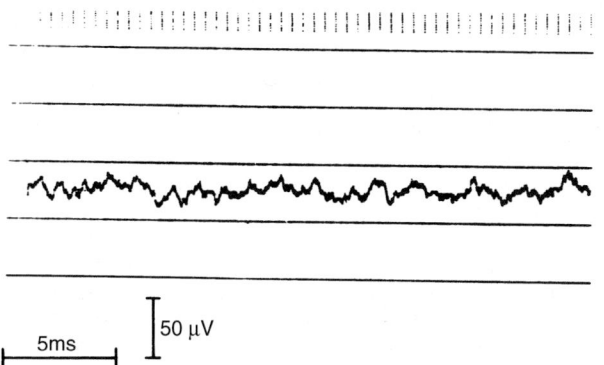

FIG. 33-44 ■ Miniature end plate potentials (MEPPs). MEPPs are a normal electromyographic finding.

active muscles many MUAPs are superimposed, producing "interference patterns." This may be observed in the limb muscles of a standing animal.

MINIATURE END PLATE POTENTIALS (MEPPs). The neuromuscular junctions of the myofibers of one muscle tend to lie in a band across the midpoint of the muscle fibers; this region is called the end plate zone. The spontaneous release of quanta of acetylcholine from the nerve terminal at a neuromuscular junction results in local electrical responses in the muscle fiber. This activity can be recorded when the recording electrode lies close to the neuromuscular junction in the end plate zone (Fig. 33-44). MEPPs are monophasic-negative potentials having amplitudes of 10 to 20 μV and durations of 0.5 to 1 msec.[1569] They are local electrical responses in the muscle fiber that are not propagated throughout the whole fiber and thus do not result in fiber contraction.

MEPPs are present even in resting muscle and are normal. MEPPs may be absent in disorders in which there is a lack of acetylcholine release from the nerve (neuropathies), in those in which there is an abnormality in transmission across the neuromuscular junction (junctionopathies), and in some myopathies. MEPPs cannot be detected when the recording electrode is not close to a neuromuscular junction.

Abnormal Muscle

INSERTION ACTIVITY. In both neuropathic and myopathic diseases, insertion activity may be prolonged or occasionally reduced (see Fig. 33-42). Either of these findings is evidence of abnormality. Abnormalities in EMG recordings caused by neuropathic disease do not begin to appear until approximately 5 days after the onset of the neuropathy.

MOTOR UNIT ACTION POTENTIALS. In both myopathies and neuropathies changes in the characteristics of MUAPs occur. These include reductions in amplitude, polyphasia, temporal dispersion, and even absence of MUAPs.

After damage to some nerve fibers, others may undergo collateral sprouting, wherein new terminal arborizations grow and innervate denervated myofibers. The net result of this process is an increase in the size of the motor unit. The MUAPs of these large motor units have correspondingly larger amplitudes and hence are called giant MUAPs (see Fig. 33-43).

FIBRILLATION POTENTIALS AND POSITIVE SHARP WAVES. These activities result from the electrical activity of single muscle fibers (Fig. 33-45). The muscle activity may be spontaneous or the result of mechanical stimulation of the fiber by the electrode. It is thought that the occurrence of spontaneous individual fiber contraction is a manifestation of an increase in the excitability of the muscle fiber membrane. Fibrillation potentials and positive sharp waves occur in both neuropathies and myopathies. The presence of either activity is not pathognomonic for the type of pathologic condition present.

Fibrillation potentials are biphasic spikes with an initial positive phase. Their peak to peak amplitude is less than 1 mV and their duration less than 5 msec.[1569] Fibrillation potentials are recorded when the recording electrode lies a short distance from the muscle fiber whose activity is being recorded.

Positive sharp waves have an initial positive phase with amplitude of up to 1 mV and duration under 5 msec, followed by a negative phase with lower amplitude and a duration of 10 to 100 msec.[1569] They are recorded when the recording electrode tip lies close to the electrically active myofiber.

Nerve Conduction Testing

Nerve conduction studies usually require that the animal be sedated or under general anesthesia, because the procedure is somewhat painful. Routinely used sedatives and anesthetic agents do not interfere with the results of testing. Two stimulating needle electrodes, the anode and cathode, are placed on or close to the nerve to be stimulated. A short pulse of current is applied to the nerve. A compound nerve action potential (CNAP) is evoked in the nerve by the applied current and is propagated along the nerve in the same manner as a naturally occurring action potential. Either the CNAP is recorded directly from the nerve itself, or the compound muscle action potential (CMAP) evoked in the muscle innervated by that nerve is recorded. To ensure that all the nerve fibers are stimulated, the stimulus intensity is varied to determine the maximum stimulus (i.e., the current that just evokes the maximum CNAP or CMAP). A supramaximum stimulus (150% to 200% of the maximum stimulus) is applied when making recordings.[1568,1570]

MOTOR NERVE CONDUCTION (MNC). MNC is determined by stimulating a mixed peripheral nerve such as the radial or median nerve and recording the CMAP evoked in a muscle innervated by that nerve. By recording the CMAP evoked by stimulating the nerve, only the activity of the alpha motoneurons in that nerve is evaluated. The latency between the application of the stimulus and the onset of contraction of the muscle can be broken down into three components: the time for conduction of the action potential in the nerve, the time for neuromuscular transmission, and the time for conduction of the muscle action potential from the neuromuscular junction to the vicinity of the recording electrode. By stimulating the nerve at two or more points, the latter two variables can be eliminated from the calculation and the velocity of conduction of the nerve action potential between the stimulus points determined.

SENSORY NERVE CONDUCTION (SNC). SNC is determined by stimulating a purely sensory nerve peripherally (e.g., the palmar digital nerves)[1570] and recording the CNAP from the same nerve at a more proximal point. Because the amplitude of the CNAP is relatively small, (usually less than 1 mV), the technique of signal averaging is used. In signal averaging, the responses to repeated stimuli are recorded and electrically averaged, eliminating background electrical activity that otherwise would obscure the evoked potential.

Physiologic alterations in nerve conduction must be differentiated from pathologic changes. Cooling of the nerve results in a slowing of conduction velocity.[1571] Therefore it is important to monitor limb temperature when doing nerve conduction studies to avoid erroneous interpretation of results. Heating pads and lamps can be used to maintain normal temperature. Conduction velocity of the action potential in the nerve is proportional to fiber diameter. In ponies and dogs, nerve conduction velocity is faster in the proximal portion of the nerve. This is thought to be because of the greater diameter of the proximal regions of peripheral nerves.[1572] SNC velocity is slower in horses than in ponies, which is thought to be due to distal tapering of peripheral nerves.[1571] Nerve conduction velocity is slower in young and aged dogs than it is in mature adults.[1573] This finding is probably true for all species.

Specific techniques for peripheral nerve testing in the horse have been described, and normal values for both MNC and SNC velocities have been determined for a number of peripheral nerves.[1570,1571,1574] Nerve conduction velocity, amplitude, and waveform characteristics all provide valuable information on the functional status of the nerve. In pathologic conditions changes in nerve function occur that depend only on the nature of the pathologic process in the nerve, not on its etiology.

SLOWING OF NERVE CONDUCTION. Reduction in the velocity of nerve conduction is the result of segmental demyelination, which may occur in sensory or motor fibers or both. Demyelination may be present as the sole pathologic change or may be accompanied by other neuropathologic processes. No pathologic significance has been attributed to increased conduction velocity; it is the result of technical error.

INCREASED TEMPORAL DISPERSION. Increased temporal dispersion of an action potential is also due to segmental demyelination and is the result of differences in the rate of conduction in individual nerve fibers. For example, if some fibers are normal and some are undergoing demyelination, increased dispersion of the action potential is recorded, be it a nerve or a muscle action potential. In this case, because some nerves are normal, the nerve conduction velocity calculated will be normal.

REDUCTION IN AMPLITUDE. The amplitudes of the CNAP and the CMAP depend on the number of functional neurons stimulated. The CMAP also depends on the number of functional myofibers in the motor unit and on the functional integrity of the neuromuscular junctions. Because different complements of neurons are present in different nerves and in the same nerve in different animals, and also because the size of muscles themselves varies, it is not possible to determine absolute parameters for the amplitude of CNAP or CMAP. However, qualitative evaluations of amplitude can be made. Reduced amplitude of nerve action potentials is seen as a result of primary axonopathy (wallerian degeneration), junctionopathy (e.g., botulism), and nerve conduction block in some demyelinating diseases.[1575] Reduction in the amplitude of the CMAP also may be caused by primary muscle disease, resulting in a reduction in the number of functional myofibers.

POLYPHASIA. In cases in which collateral sprouting has occurred, the larger motor units that result are distributed more widely in the muscle. Some of the nerve terminal arborizations are longer than others; therefore the nerve action potential does not arrive at all the neuromuscular junctions at the same time. A polyphasic waveform in the CNAP results.

EMG and NCT are valuable aids to the diagnosis of motor unit disease in animals. Although they provide considerable information about the nature, extent, and progress of pathologic changes, they do not define the etiology of those changes. Further diagnostic procedures such as muscle or nerve biopsy, cerebrospinal fluid analysis, serologic testing, and other studies are required to arrive at a specific diagnosis.

REFERENCES

1566. Duncan ID, Griffiths IR: A sensory neuropathy affecting long-haired Dachshund dogs, *J Small Anim Pract* 23:381-390, 1982.
1567. Sims MH: Electrodiagnostic techniques in the evaluation of diseases affecting skeletal muscle, *Vet Clin North Am (Small Anim Pract)* 13:145-162, 1973.
1568. Mechelse K: The motor unit. In Notermans SLH, ed: *Current practice of electromyography,* Amsterdam, 1984, Elsevier Science Publishers.
1569. American Association of Electromyography and Electrodiagnostics: Glossary of terms in clinical electromyography, *Muscle Nerve* 10:G1-G60, 1987.
1570. Blythe LL et al: Sensory nerve conduction velocity in forelimb of ponies, *Am J Vet Res* 44:1419-1426, 1983.
1571. Blythe LL, Engel HN, Rowe KE: Comparison of sensory nerve conduction velocities in horses versus ponies, *Am J Vet Res* 49:2138-2142, 1988.
1572. Henry RW, Diesem CD: Proximal equine radial and median motor nerve conduction velocity, *Am J Vet Res* 42:1819-1822, 1981.
1573. Swallow JS, Griffiths IR: Age-related changes in the motor nerve conduction velocity in dogs, *Res Vet Sci* 23:29-32, 1977.

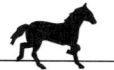

1574. Henry RW, Diesem CD, Wiechers DO: Evaluation of equine radial and median nerve conduction velocities, *Am J Vet Res* 40:1406-1410, 1979.
1575. Griffiths IR, Duncan ID: The use of electromyography and nerve conduction studies in the evaluation of lower motor neurone disease or injury, *J Small Anim Pract* 19:329-340, 1978.

BOTULISM (Shaker Foals; Forage Poisoning)

ROBERT H. WHITLOCK

DEFINITION AND ETIOLOGY. The clinical signs of botulism result from the effect of the neurotoxin (an exotoxin) produced by *Clostridium botulinum* on the myoneural junction, leading to muscular weakness.[1576-1581] Botulism spores, which can be found in the soil in most of the United States, cause isolated occurrences of botulism in human beings, birds, fish, and other animals.[1582] Eight toxin types have been identified: A, B, C_1, C_2, D, E, F, and G.[1583,1584] In North America, horses are most commonly affected by type B toxin (more than 85% of cases) and occasionally by type C or type A.[1585] Type C toxin invariably is associated with a decomposing carcass[1586] or with cases in which ravens or crows fed off a decomposing carcass and then transported the toxin to the feed buckets or feed troughs of horses.[1587,1588] Types A and B botulism are associated with forage; that is, spores and or toxin in the hay. Type A cases have been reported in California, Utah, Idaho, Oregon, and Ohio but almost never in the mid-Atlantic region.[1589] Types C and D cases occur sporadically in cattle fed poultry litter[1589,1560] and have caused serious outbreaks in beef cattle in Israel[1591-1593] and Australia.[1594] Type E botulism typically is associated with fish and may cause clinical signs in human beings[1583,1584] but is rarely reported in other animals. Types F and G have only rarely been reported in human beings.[1584]

Clinical botulism occurs by one of three routes: (1) ingestion of the preformed toxin (the most common form in cattle and adult horses); (2) ingestion of spores, leading to toxicoinfectious botulism (shaker foal syndrome); and (3) contamination of wounds with botulism spores, with subsequent production and absorption of toxin. Wound botulism may occur in horses, most often in castration sites,[1595] umbilical hernia repairs, or deep puncture wounds such as may occur with injection of counterirritants.[1596] If forage containing *C. botulinum* is fed to both horses and cattle, the horses invariably develop clinical signs first, and more horses are affected than cattle.[1597] Horses are much more susceptible to botulinum toxin than cattle. This probably is because rumen microbes degrade the toxin,[1598] whereas horses have more time to absorb it from the intestinal tract before the it reaches the colon, the site of microbial degradation.

CLINICAL SIGNS IN FOALS. In foals the owner's chief complaint frequently is that the foal is found lying down more often than normal. When forced to rise, it stands for a few moments, develops generalized muscle tremors (thus the term shaker foal) and drops to the ground, usually in lateral recumbency.[1599,1600] Closer physical examination reveals a well-nourished foal that is bright and alert, usually with normal vital signs and normal clinical pathologic findings that help differentiate it from other diseases. Affected foals often drool milk from the mouth when suckling the mare. The tongue is easier to pull from the mouth than normal, and the foal slowly retracts the tongue when released.[1601] Mild mydriasis and weak eyelid tone may be detected in most foals. Progressive symmetric myasthenia with absence of fever and other signs of systemic disease that lead to recumbency remains the predominant clinical sign. Constipation and ileus are consistent findings.[1602] As the disease progresses, the heart and respiratory rates increase, conditions that may progress to inhalation pneumonia and terminate in respiratory failure. In a small proportion of foals the condition stabilizes at a certain level of neuromuscular weakness, and the foal gradually recovers over

a period of 10 to 14 days with intensive nursing care. The disease can occur at any age, but the peak age is 4 weeks, with 70% of cases occurring between 2 and 5 weeks.[1603]

CLINICAL SIGNS IN ADULT HORSES

History. Generalized muscle weakness (myasthenia) or dysphagia, or both, typically is the first clinical sign of botulism detected by an alert horse owner. Some owners may not seek veterinary attention until the horse is recumbent. Astute individuals may detect a change in the horse's attitude (slight depression), decreased exercise tolerance, slowness to eat hay or grain, and diminished ability to swallow hay and water as subtle early signs. This is especially true after a few cases have occurred on the premises.[1604] Colic may be the initial clinical sign in some cases of botulism, presumably the result of ileus and accumulation of gas.[1605-1608]

Reduced Tongue Strength. Characteristic early signs of botulism include reduced tongue strength and slow tongue retraction. Tongue strength is best assessed by the following technique. The jaws are kept closed by putting the left arm under the jaw and placing the hand on the top of the nasal bones. Using the right hand the tongue is gently retracted through the interdental space and allowed to hang down and is then slowly released. If performed properly, this procedure, the "tongue stress test," is one of the most sensitive methods of detecting an early clinical sign of botulism in horses. Most normal horses quickly retract the tongue into the mouth after release with one or two tugs or attempts.[1605] The strength of the normal tongue retraction response varies significantly from horse to horse, and this fact must be considered when assessing tongue strength in a horse suspected of having botulism. In more advanced stages of the disease but before recumbency, the horse retracts the tongue very slowly if at all (Fig. 33-46).

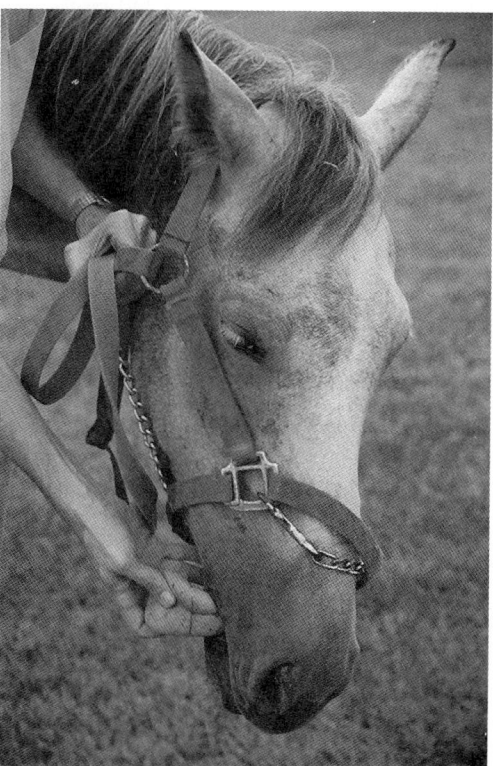

FIG. 33-46 Horse with very weak tongue. The tongue may hang over the lips for several seconds, up to a minute or longer in severe cases. This test is not specific for botulism, but is characteristic, and with other compatible clinical signs, strongly suggests botulism.

Grain Test. For this test the horse is offered 8 oz of sweet feed in a large, flat feeding tube on the floor, and the animal's ability to consume the feed is observed and timed. Most normal horses can eat 8 oz of grain (sweet feed) in less than 2 minutes, many in less than 1 minute.[1608] As the ability to retract the tongue diminishes, the horse eats sweet feed more slowly than usual, and grain mixed with saliva often falls out of the mouth through the lips; this is very characteristic of botulism and one of the earliest clinical signs[1608] (Fig. 33-47). In outbreaks of equine botulism, owners can be taught to perform the grain test and the tongue stress test to detect these early signs.

Horses with beginning dysphagia may attempt to eat hay but have difficulty swallowing it. Inability to swallow water occurs after loss of the ability to swallow hay. Horses seem to respond differently to the inability to drink water; many refuse to attempt to drink, whereas others immerse their muzzles below the surface. Decreased tongue strength and dysphagia typically occur before the onset of obvious muscle weakness. Recumbent horses with botulism are very difficult to assess with regard to swallowing ability because the struggle to stand takes priority over eating and drinking.

Decreased eyelid and tail tone may be detected, but the variation in tail tone from horse to horse makes this assessment problematic. Moderately affected horses walk with a shuffling gait, occasionally dragging their toes, and show evidence of muscle weakness. As the disease progresses, the dysphagia becomes more complete and the myasthenia more obvious, often with muscle tremors leading to recumbency and difficulty rising. Clinical signs of botulism are always symmetric and gradually progressive, often to recumbency followed by death caused by respiratory paralysis or euthanasia for humane considerations.

Vital signs, including capillary refill, are normal in the early stages of the disease. Once the horse is recumbent, both the heart and respiratory rates increase in proportion to the intensity of the struggle to rise and the severity of the disease. Borborygmal sounds are gradually diminished as the horse eats less. In the early phases of type C botulism, the character of the respiratory effort changes. The respiratory rate does not increase, but the expiratory effort becomes more exaggerated, with a prolonged abdominal lift. This unusual respiratory effort rarely occurs with other types of botulism, which helps differentiate type C from types A and B in horses.[1608]

Moderate mydriasis is an early sign that persists for several days, with a sluggish pupillary response to light persisting for several weeks. Muscle trembling and inability to lift the head are two additional but inconsistent signs of type C botulism. The muscle trembling often starts in the triceps and extends to other large muscle groups. As the disease progresses, some horses have difficulty lifting the head, and head carriage becomes lower and lower. Massive edema of the muzzle and face may interfere with breathing, primarily in type C botulism. Supporting the head in a sling several hours at a time may give some relief. Affected horses regain the strength to lift the head over 7 to 14 days.[1608]

During examination of the 40 horses affected by type C botulism in a California outbreak, dysphagia was not readily apparent or detected.[1609] The absence of dysphagia in these horses with confirmed type C botulism is unexplained. Horses in Canada,[1606] a Florida foal,[1610] and horses with experimentally induced type C botulism[1608] all had evidence of dysphagia. Some California horses that recovered from botulism had unusual prominent muscle atrophy of the supraspinatus and gluteal muscles. The atrophy was still apparent after 2 months but had healed by 5 months in four of the

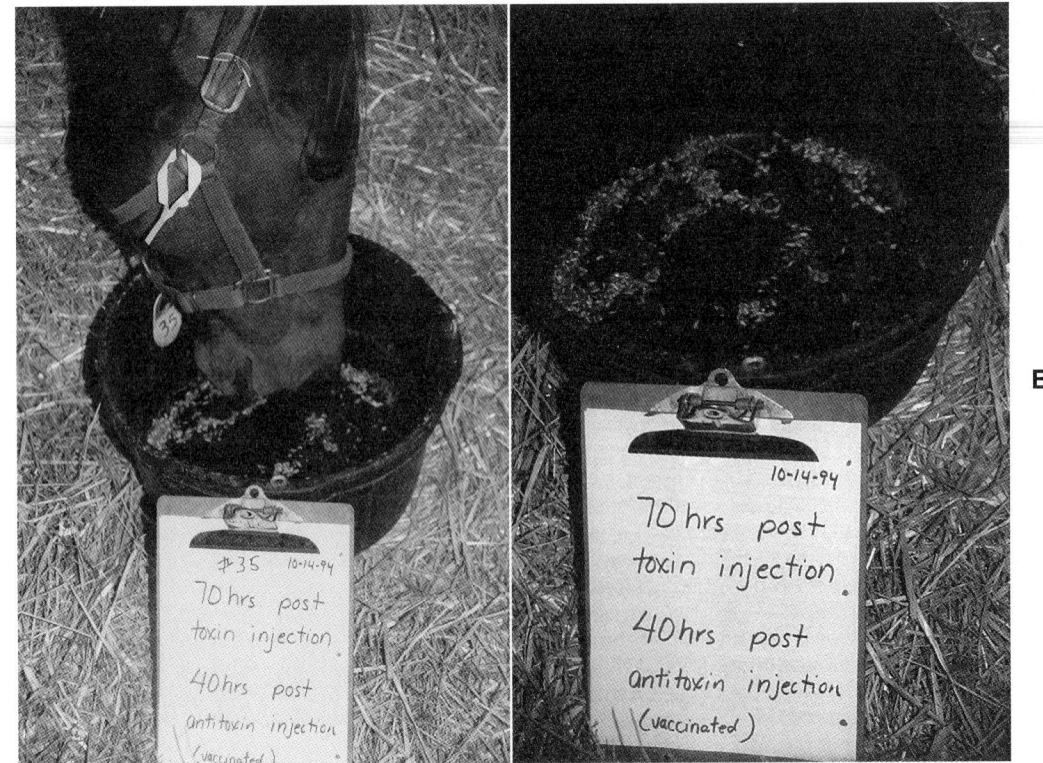

FIG. 33-47 ■ **A,** Abnormal "grain test," showing sweet feed mixed with saliva falling out of the side of the mouth. **B,** Note the trail of grain on the bottom of the bucket.

seven surviving horses[1609]; this type of muscle atrophy has not been reported previously or since.

The higher the dose of botulinum toxin at the neuromuscular junction, the more rapidly progressive the clinical signs and the poorer the prognosis for survival. Low levels of toxin (1000 units) result in a more gradual onset of clinical signs (3 to 7 days) and reduced severity of signs. Mildly affected horses may have only transient dysphagia and may recover with minimal treatment. Larger doses of toxin (100,000,000 units) result in peracute, rapidly progressive illness. These horses may become recumbent within 8 to 12 hours of the onset of the first detectable signs.

Adult recumbent horses are more difficult to manage medically than foals, consequently the prognosis for survival is much worse for recumbent adults. Once an adult horse is recumbent because of botulism and unable to rise, the prognosis for recovery becomes grave despite the most intensive care, including mechanical ventilation.[1596] However, some horses quickly learn to adjust to their muscular weakness and do not object to being recumbent. The condition of these horses may stabilize at a certain point and gradually improve over time. Terminally ill horses paddle their legs in an intermittent struggling manner and die of respiratory paralysis. Euthanasia is recommended if the horse is recumbent, unable to rise, and has respiratory compromise.

CLINICAL SIGNS IN CATTLE

History. Most clinical cases of botulism in cattle occur as a herd outbreak, in contrast to horses, in which single cases are most common. In cattle the referring veterinarian is called to evaluate several down cows that may have initially responded to treatment for hypocalcemia but then relapsed.[1589] These downer cows often are not associated with recent parturition. Many outbreaks of botulism in cattle are typified by the presence of several cattle in a herd with clinical signs similar to those of milk fever and evidence of progressive muscular weakness. Affected cattle are anorectic and hypogalactic and may develop paraparesis, which leads to recumbency. Affected cows have diminished strength, decreased frequency of rumen contractions, and firm feces.[1611]

Further investigation of the herd outbreak usually finds a point source of botulinum toxin. Feeding of small grain silage (e.g., ryelage or oatlage) that had been stored in large plastic bags often has occurred 3 to 4 days before the onset of clinical signs. Clearly, storage of ryelage and haylage in plastic bags or a long plastic tube is a major risk factor for botulism in cattle.[1589] In some outbreaks the plastic covering may be damaged, permitting mold and spoilage, which may lead to anaerobic conditions that allow botulism spores to produce toxin.

Occasionally incorporation of an animal carcass during the silage making process may lead to an outbreak of botulism. Cats, dogs, and poultry carcasses are typical villains that lead to type C botulism. In one California outbreak, total mixed ration (TMR) contaminated by a cat carcass was responsible for the death of more than 420 adult cattle over 1 week.[1586] Poultry litter containing decomposing chicken carcasses predisposes cattle to type C or type D botulism.[1590,1593,1594,1612] Repeated occurrences of type C and type D botulism in beef cattle have occurred in West Virginia, Arkansas, and other states associated with the feeding of poultry litter–based rations.[1589]

Tongue Stress Test. In cattle a tongue stress test assesses three aspects of tongue muscular strength. The test is performed in the following manner. The right hand and fingers are inserted through the interdental space while the left arm and hand keep the jaws closed. The tongue muscular tone is assessed by reaching back in the mouth and putting pressure on the base of the tongue. Normally the tongue is firm and relatively turgid; softness and lack of tongue turgor indicate

weakness. Next, the tongue is grasped and pulled out the side of the mouth. Normally it is not easy to grasp or pull the tongue out of a cow's mouth, therefore this is another assessment of tongue strength. In the last step, the tongue is slowly released and allowed to hang out the side of the cow's mouth. Normally when the tongue is pulled out the side of the mouth with the jaws closed, cows quickly retract the tongue. If the tongue rests limply over the lip, even for a few seconds, this is very abnormal and suggests a very weak tongue. However, cattle in herds experiencing botulism will appear normal but have decreased tongue strength and reduced jaw tone. Tongue weakness is not specific for botulism but is characteristic.

If tongue strength is normal, some other cause for the weakness should be considered. Decreased lingual strength may occur with listeriosis and other causes of hypoglossal nerve injury. In cases of botulism, tongue weakness is symmetric and often associated with dysphagia and progressive muscle weakness, with several animals typically involved.

Jaw Movement and Muscle Tone. In addition to tongue weakness, masseter muscle strength should be assessed. This is best done by grasping the mandible in the area of the symphysis and moving it laterally. In cattle with botulism little resistance is encountered, and the jaw seems very loose compared with normal cattle.

Pupillary Response and Dysphagia. In cattle with botulism the pupils tend to be dilated and poorly responsive to light. The animals may drool small amounts of saliva because they are unable to swallow. These cattle rarely develop severe acidosis, as may occur with listeriosis. Often cattle with botulism appear to prehend hay or grass, chew, and then swallow. On closer examination the affected animal is seen to chew the same cud for hours without swallowing. Examination of the pharynx or oral cavity may reveal evidence of chewed hay cud or a forage bolus resulting from the inability to swallow.

Affected cattle are dull, depressed, and lethargic and often become dehydrated because of the inability to swallow. They closely resemble cattle with milk fever except that with botulism, several cows are involved at the same time. Animals may show muscle tremors and truncal ataxia, even to the point of dribbling urine, before becoming recumbent. When recumbent they remain in sternal recumbency in the initial phases and in the more advanced stages become laterally recumbent with evidence of respiratory failure.

CLINICAL COURSE.

The rate of progression of clinical signs after ingestion of toxin-contaminated forage depends on the dose of toxin. Massive concentrations of toxin may lead to clinical signs within 12 to 24 hours of ingestion (an unusual event). Low toxin concentrations may not yield any clinical signs for 7 to 10 days or longer after toxin ingestion.[1589] Typically cattle that absorb a moderate amount of botulinum toxin exhibit evidence of weakness 24 to 48 hours before becoming recumbent, then are unable to rise for 2 to 3 days before death. Physical activity has a major influence on the progression of clinical signs. Physically active cattle or cattle that are stimulated to walk some distance are more likely to be affected by lower doses of toxin. The physical activity results in depletion of acetylcholine reserves, then muscle weakness and recumbency in the next 12 to 24 hours.

Most cattle that become recumbent after absorption of botulinum toxin die of respiratory failure, dehydration, or complications of recumbency. Cattle with a more gradual progression of clinical signs before becoming recumbent often are able to eat, drink, and swallow, maintaining homeostatic mechanisms, and may recover. Typically, botulism-affected down cattle that recover are down for 5 to 10 days and then gradually regain muscular strength until they are able to rise. In the author's experience, in a typical herd outbreak, many cattle have subclinical signs, such as a weak tongue and decreased jaw tone, and possibly mild dysphagia and never become recumbent. These animals should have a detectable antibody response to botulinum toxin 3 to 4 weeks after recovery from subclinical botulism.[1613-1616] The clinical course ranges from 2 to 30 days, depending on the dose of toxin absorbed and the treatment provided.

DIFFERENTIAL DIAGNOSES IN HORSES. Diagnostic rule-outs for horses include any disease associated with muscular weakness and dysphagia, including equine protozoal myelitis (EPM), rhinopneumonitis (spinal cord myeloencephalopathy), white muscle disease, azoturia, eclampsia, guttural pouch mycosis, leukoencephalomalacia (moldy corn poisoning), eastern and western equine encephalitis, yew poisoning (*Taxus* sp.), rabies, white snake root poisoning, yellow star thistle toxicosis, hypocalcemia, organochlorine toxicosis, and pharyngeal ulceration. EPM with brainstem involvement is one of the most difficult diseases to differentiate from early botulism. Most horses with EPM have asymmetric neurologic deficits, which rarely occurs with botulism. Ionophorous antibiotics (monensin, salinomycin, and narasin) may cause signs of profound muscular weakness similar to those seen in botulism, but dysphagia and the absence of an increase in muscle enzymes distinguish botulism. The absence of systemic signs of illness also helps differentiate botulism from sepsis and more generalized infectious diseases.

Hyperkalemic periodic paralysis (HYPP) should be included in the diagnostic rule-out list for myasthenic quarter horses. HYPP, a dominant inheritable condition of quarter horses, is characterized by episodes of muscular fasciculations, weakness, myotonia, and/or recumbency.[1617] These episodes are associated with hyperkalemia attributable to a defect in sodium channels. Electromyographic examination, plasma potassium determination, and demonstration of a DNA marker help confirm HYPP.[1618]

DIFFERENTIAL DIAGNOSES IN CATTLE. Hypocalcemia and hypokalemia resemble botulism but are easy to differentiate, because most cases of hypocalcemia occur in the periparturient period, and hypokalemia is most common in early lactation. Most herd outbreaks of botulism involve several cows at the same time. Listeriosis almost always shows localized cranial nerve involvement, which is not present with botulism. Organophosphate toxicosis results in sailosis, nervousness, and constricted pupils, not mydriasis, as occurs with botulism. Spinal cord compression, as may occur with lymphosarcoma or a vertebral body abscess, are single animal diseases, not herd problems.

CLINICAL PATHOLOGY AND DIAGNOSTIC APPROACH. Laboratory support for a diagnosis of botulism requires one of the following: (1) demonstration of preformed toxin in the patient's serum or gastrointestinal contents or in a wound; (2) demonstration of *C. botulinum* spores in the gastrointestinal contents or feed materials (or both); or (3) detection of an antibody response to *C. botulinum* in patients recovering from suspected botulism. A definitive diagnosis may be obtained by demonstration of preformed toxin in the plasma or intestinal contents, but this is rarely possible in horses. Preformed toxin has been identified in about 20% of the intestinal contents of shaker foals but rarely in adult horses. Finding *C. botulinum* spores in the intestinal or ruminal contents in addition to the presence of clinical signs compatible with botulism is strongly supportive of a diagnosis of botulism, because these spores are rarely present in the rumen or intestinal contents of normal cattle or horses.

Botulinum toxin is relatively stable in tissues or plasma frozen at −20° C (−4° F) for several weeks. The mouse bioassay, the most sensitive test for botulism yet devised, requires a minimum of 5 ml of plasma or serum from an affected animal as early in the clinical course of the disease as possible.

Detection of toxin in the serum is likely only in animals with peracute onset and rapidly progressive clinical signs (onset to death in less than 48 hours). The serum (1 ml) is injected into two ICR Swiss Webster mice. If clinical signs of botulism occur in the mice (waist wasping), four additional mice are injected with the suspect serum. Two of the mice receive either monovalent or polyvalent botulism antiserum along with the test serum. If mice are protected by a specific antitoxin, the test is definitive for the presence of botulinum toxin of that type.[1619] Because horses are very susceptible to botulinum toxin, the level of circulating toxin in an affected horse often is below the threshold of detection of the mouse bioassay. There have been few reports of demonstration of preformed toxin (type B) in plasma or serum from an acutely affected foal or horse.[1620,1621]

A tentative diagnosis may be based on the presence of botulinum spores and toxin in feedstuffs recently consumed by animals with clinical signs compatible with botulism.[1622] Spores of *C. botulinum* type B are found in the feces of approximately 34% of adult horses (three fecal samples per horse) with clinical signs compatible with botulism. *C. botulinum* toxin can be found in the feces of approximately 30% of foals affected with botulism, and spores can be found in the feces of about 70% of affected foals. Spores are rarely detected in fecal samples from normal foals or adult horses.[1605] The presence of neutralizing botulinum antibody is a recently recognized indicator of botulism in unvaccinated animals.[1613-1616] The polymerase chain reaction (PCR) test for detecting botulinum neurotoxin gene type B was reported to be more sensitive than the mouse bioassay in a natural case of type B botulism in Australia.[1622,1623] Currently this technique remains a research tool that is not readily available for routine diagnostic purposes. Electromyographic evaluation has not been very rewarding, in the author's experience, for confirming a diagnosis of botulism in horses.[1597]

Botulism typically is a diagnosis by exclusion. Other diseases that may result in similar clinical signs must be ruled out. Both the hematologic and routine plasma biochemical findings in early to moderate cases of botulism show few abnormalities. If significant changes are present, a disease other than botulism should be strongly considered. Gradually progressive clinical signs over 1 to 4 days of muscular weakness leading to recumbency with dysphagia and tongue weakness are fully compatible with botulism.

PATHOPHYSIOLOGY. Botulinum toxin acts primarily presynaptically at the peripheral cholinergic neuromuscular junction by blocking evoked release of acetylcholine.[1577] The three steps involved in the neuromuscular blockage include (1) a primary step in which toxin binds rapidly and irreversibly to receptors on the presynaptic nerve terminal, (2) an internalization process involving receptor-mediated endocytosis, and (3) a final blocking step to prevent the release of acetylcholine from the vesicle,[1581] leading to a flaccid paralysis. Once toxin is bound at the motor end plate, improved neuromuscular function is achieved only by regeneration of new end plates, thus the prolonged time (4 to 10 days) for clinical improvement after antitoxin therapy. Each neurotoxin serotype has its own specific receptor, an endopeptidase,[1624-1626] which may explain differences in species susceptibility to different toxin types. (For more detailed information about neurotransmission, the reader is referred to a text by Das Gupta.[1578])

Toxicoinfectious botulism occurs in foals and was initially reported as "shaker foal syndrome." Foals may ingest botulinum spores with their food material as "normal" contaminants. The spores produce toxin in the gastrointestinal tract, resulting in neurologic disease.[1599,1600,1610] The toxin is detectable in the feces of approximately 30% of shaker foals but

only in the acute clinical phase of the condition.[1605] The normal intestinal flora of adult horses, human beings, and other animals inhibits intraintestinal growth of botulism spores, limiting the occurrence of toxicoinfectious botulism to neonates.[1626] In human infants under 6 months of age, *C. botulinum* may colonize the gastrointestinal tract, which lacks competing microbial microflora. After ingestion, botulism spores vegetate to produce botulinum toxin, which may be detectable in the stool for several weeks.[1627]

Most cases of type B equine botulism are associated with spores in the hay and in rare cases with commercial grain contaminated by decomposed animal carcasses. Commercial feeds (grains) are seldom proven to be the source of botulinum toxin for horses. The origin of botulism that affects only one or two horses on a farm often is not identified. When several horses are involved, the source typically is found to be the forage, as was the case in outbreaks in California (hay cubes),[1609] Ohio (contaminated wheat fed to work horses),[1605] North Carolina (baled alfalfa hay),[1604] England (big baled hay),[1620,1628] Sweden (big bale ensilage,[1629] and Australia (oaten chaff).[1630] Silage and hay contaminated with type B botulinum toxin and spores are the typical sources of exposure for horses.[1605] Hay stored in plastic bags or tubes has become a common factor in many outbreaks of botulism in the United States and England. Spoiled hay or poorly fermented silage also are potential sources of botulism exposure for horses.[1589]

The forage pH is critical for germination of botulism spores. An acid environment (a pH below 4.5) inhibits sporulation, whereas an alkaline environment favors toxin production. Silage with a high pH (over 4.5) is a notorious source of botulism for horses and is not a recommended equine feed, because horses are much more susceptible to botulism toxin than cattle.[1597] In cattle, ryelage seems to be more frequently associated with botulism than other types of forage.

NECROPSY FINDINGS. Typically, no obvious gross or histologic lesions are associated with botulism in most species. Inhalation pneumonia may be present in some foals and adult horses because the deglutition reflex is abnormal.

TREATMENT AND PROGNOSIS. Equine botulism usually is fatal unless the animal is treated promptly with the specific antitoxin.[1605] In a series of 91 foals, yearlings, and adults with presumed type B botulism, none were treated with antitoxin, and only two animals survived.[1631] Neutralization of circulating toxin with specific or multivalent botulinum antiserum should be the first and immediate therapeutic objective. Every hour between initial examination and antitoxin treatment worsens the prognosis for survival. Only one dose of antitoxin is needed, because the half-life of botulinum antitoxin of equine origin is about 12 days in normal horses. Unfortunately the antitoxin has no effect on the toxin after it has bound to the cell receptor.[15790] Once the foal or horse is recumbent, the prognosis for survival is greatly diminished.

The recommended dose of antitoxin is 200 ml (30,000 IU) for a foal and 500 ml (70,000 IU) for an adult horse. A single dose of antitoxin should provide passive protection for more than 60 days. Horses with mild, slowly progressive disease may survive without antitoxin. The patient should be confined to a stall to restrict muscular activity as much as possible. Frequent attempts to force the horse to rise also are contraindicated in order to prevent further depletion of acetylcholine stores and exacerbation of the clinical signs. Antimicrobial drugs may be given for specific secondary complications such as aspiration pneumonia. If such drugs are used, those that may potentiate neuromuscular weakness, such as the aminoglycosides, should be avoided.[1632,1633] Metronidazole, which often is effective against anaerobic bacteria,[1634] is not effective against botulism and has predisposed laboratory animals and human patients to developing botulism.[1635] Mineral oil often is recommended as a cathartic for horses with ileus to prevent impaction colic. Parasympathomimetics (neostigmine) and 4-aminopyridine are contraindicated for the treatment of botulism in animals.[1605]

Because most equine patients cannot swallow, supportive alimentation is required. To support a 450-kg horse, a high-quality protein slurry composed of 4 lb of alfalfa meal and up to 12 L of water should be administered twice daily by nasogastric tube using a bilge pump. Hydration should be monitored by daily determinations of the packed cell volume and total plasma protein (TPP). Alfalfa meal gruel with adequate water was shown to maintain dysphagic horses for more than 2 weeks.[1608] Expensive mixtures of electrolytes and semipurified nutrients are not necessary for oral alimentation.[1636] If the horse or foal is recumbent, it should be fed in a sternal position and supported during gastric emptying. Recumbent foals are prone to developing ileus and may accumulate a large amount of fluid in the stomach, which must be relieved by nasogastric intubation. Additionally, a recumbent male horse must have its bladder catheterized several times daily because it will be unable or unwilling to urinate. If the animal is not catheterized, severe cystitis or bladder necrosis may result. Most animals continue to attempt to eat, and muzzling may be necessary to prevent aspiration of food or bedding, which can lead to aspiration pneumonia.

Foals often require intragastric feeding with mare's milk, goat's milk, or a commercial milk replacer (Foal-Lac, Borden, Inc., Illinois) through an indwelling nasogastric tube (Levin Tube, 16 Fr, 1.27 m; Davol Inc., Rhode Island). Additional therapy often includes histamine receptor (H_2) blockers such as ranitidine or cimetidine, along with sucralfate, to help prevent gastric ulcers, which occur frequently in shaker foals.[1603] Ophthalmic lubricating ointments (Lacri-Lube; Allergan Pharmaceuticals, Inc., California) often are needed to prevent corneal abrasions, which may result from decreased eyelid tone. Recumbent foals must be turned frequently to help prevent decubital ulcers and muscle necrosis. Parenteral antibiotics, such as potassium penicillin, are indicated to help reduce secondary infections, especially inhalation pneumonia.

Recovery from botulism depends on the toxin dose and the resulting severity of the clinical disease. Dysphagic horses able to stand gradually regain the ability to swallow over 3 to 7 days. The more complete the dysphagia, the longer the time required for recovery. An occasional horse remains dysphagic for longer than 2 weeks. Most adult horses are able to eat hay and swallow grain and water by 7 to 10 days after treatment with antitoxin. Return to full strength often takes longer than 1 month. Very few adult horses that become recumbent and unable to rise for 24 hours recover unless they are provided meticulous nursing care. Decubital ulcers and secondary respiratory problems are the major complications. Recumbent foals usually are able to stand after 7 to 10 days of intensive nursing care.[1603]

PREVENTION. A toxoid is available for *C. botulinum* type B (Bot Tox B, ELISA Technology Co., Lexington, Kentucky). According to current recommendations, three doses of vaccine 1 month apart are required to successfully immunize horses.[1637] Three vaccinations given at 10- to 12-day intervals may provide protective antibody after 3 weeks if necessary for emergency situations such as outbreaks.[1638] Annual revaccination of mares 4 to 6 weeks before foaling is highly recommended. Horses from an endemic area should be revaccinated annually. The colostrum from vaccinated mares boostered 6 to 8 weeks before foaling should contain adequate antibody to protect the foal for 8 to 12 weeks.[1639] Foals vaccinated with toxoid in the first few days of life should be immunoresponsive and should develop antibodies to the toxoid even in the presence of passive antibody.[1638]

Botulism toxoid is considered highly efficacious when administered properly, one of the safest and most effective vaccines for horses. The occurrence of clinical botulism in fully immunized horses has not been reported. No multivalent vaccine or licensed type C toxoid for horses is available in North America at this time. However, horses have been vaccinated and immunized with a type C toxoid approved for use in mink. This vaccine has been used for several years in endemic type C areas, such as the southwestern United States.

REFERENCES

1576. Critchley MR: A comparison of human and animal botulism: a review, *J Roy Soc Med* 84:295-298, 1991.
1577. Oguma K, Fujinga Y, Inoue K: Structure and function of clostridial toxins, *Microbiol Immunol* 39:161-168, 1995.
1578. Das Gupta BR: *Botulinum and tetanus neurotoxins: neurotransmission and biomedical aspects*, New York, 1993, Plenum Press.
1579. Simpson LL: Molecular pharmacology of botulinum toxin and tetanus toxin, *Annu Rev Pharmacol Toxicol* 26:427-453, 1986.
1580. Sugiyama H: *Clostridium botulinum* neurotoxin, *Microbiol Rev* 44:419-448, 1980.
1581. Hambleton P: *Clostridium botulinum* toxins: a general review of involvement in disease, structure, mode of action, and preparation for clinical use, *J Neurol* 239:16-20, 1992.
1582. Smith LDS: *Clostridium botulinum*: characteristics and occurrence, *Rev Infect Dis* 1:637-641, 1979.
1583. Hatheway CL: Toxigenic clostridia, *Clin Microbiol Rev* 3:66-98, 1990.
1584. Hatheway CL: Botulism: the present status of the disease, *Curr Top Microbiol Immunol* 195:55-75, 1995.
1585. Whitlock RH, Buckley C, Messick J: Investigations of herd outbreaks of botulism in cattle and horses, *Proc Am Assoc Vet Lab Diagn* 40:38, 1989.
1586. Galey FD et al: Type C botulism in dairy cattle from feed contaminated by a dead cat, *J Vet Diagn Invest* 12:204-209, 2000.
1587. Whitlock RH et al: Type C botulism in New Mexico horses: an outbreak, *Proc Am Assoc Vet Lab Diagn*, 1997, p 61 (abstract).
1588. Schoenbaum MA et al: An outbreak of type C botulism in 12 horses and a mule, *JAVMA* 217:365-368, 2000.
1589. Whitlock RH, Williams JM: Botulism toxicosis of cattle, *Bovine Proc* 32:45-53, 1999.
1590. Jean D et al: *Clostridium botulinum* type C intoxication in feedlot steers being fed ensiled poultry litter, *Can Vet J* 36:626-628, 1995.
1591. Savir D: Mass outbreaks of botulism in ruminants associated with ingestion of feed containing poultry waste. III, Epidemiologic findings, *Refuah Vet* 35:105-108, 1978.
1592. Egyed MN et al: Mass outbreaks of botulism in ruminants associated with ingestion of feed containing poultry waste. II, Experimental investigation, *Refuah Vet* 35:93-104, 1978.
1593. Egyed MN: Outbreaks of botulism in ruminants associated with ingestion of feed containing poultry waste. In Eklund MW, Dowell Jr VR, eds: *Avian botulism*, 1987.
1594. Trueman KF et al: Suspected botulism in three intensively managed Australian cattle herds, *Vet Rec* 130:398-400, 1992.
1595. Bernard W et al: Botulism as a sequel to open castration in a horse, *J Am Vet Med Assoc* 191:73-74, 1987.
1596. Mitten LA et al: Mechanical ventilation and management of botulism secondary to an injection abscess in an adult horse, *Equine Vet J* 26:420-423, 1994.
1597. Divers TJ et al: *Clostridium botulinum* type B toxicosis in a herd of cattle and a group of mules, *J Am Vet Med Assoc* 188:382-386, 1986.
1598. Allison MJ, Maloy SE, Matson RR: Inactivation of *Clostridium botulinum* toxin by ruminal microbes from cattle and sheep, *Appl Environ Microbiol* 32:685-688, 1976.
1599. Swerczek TW: Toxicoinfectious botulism foals and adult horses, *J Am Vet Med Assoc* 176:348-350, 1980.
1600. Swerczek TW: Experimentally induced toxicoinfectious botulism in horses and foals, *Am J Vet Res* 41:348-350, 1980.
1601. Whitlock RH, Messick JB: Foal botulism (shaker foal syndrome): clinical signs, diagnosis, treatment, and prevention, *Proceedings of the Thirty-third Annual Convention of the American Association of Equine Practitioners*, 1987, pp 359-366.
1602. Crane SA: Field management of two foals with suspected botulism, *Equine Vet Educ* 3:184-186, 1991.
1603. Vaala WE: Diagnosis and treatment of *Clostridium botulinum* infection in foals: a review of 53 cases, *Proc 9th Am Coll Vet Med Forum* 9:379-381, 1991.
1604. Wichtel JJ, Whitlock RH: Botulism associated with feeding alfalfa hay to horses, *J Am Vet Med Assoc* 199:471-472, 1991.
1605. Whitlock RH, Buckley CA: Botulism, *Vet Clin North Am (Equine Pract)* 13:107-128, 1997.
1606. Heath SE, Bell RJ, Harland RJ: Botulism type C intoxication in a mare, *Can Vet J* 29:530-531, 1988.

1607. Heath SE et al: Feed trough dirt as a source of *Clostridium botulinum* type C intoxication in a group of farm horses, *Can Vet J* 31:13-19, 1990.
1608. Whitlock RH: Botulism type C: experimental and field cases in horses, *Equine Pract* 18:11-17, 1996.
1609. Kinde H et al: *Clostridium botulinum* type C intoxication associated with consumption of processed hay cubes in horses, *J Am Vet Med Assoc* 199:742-746, 1991.
1610. MacKay RJ, Berkhoff GA: Type C toxicoinfectious botulism in a foal, *J Am Vet Med Assoc* 180:163-164, 1982.
1611. Kelch WJ et al: Fatal *Clostridium botulinum* toxicosis in eleven Holstein cattle fed round bale barley haylage, *J Vet Diagn Invest* 12:453-455, 2000.
1612. McLoughlin MF, McIlroy SG, Neill SD: A major outbreak of botulism in cattle being fed ensiled poultry litter, *Vet Rec* 122:579-581, 1988.
1613. Thomas RJ: Detection of *Clostridium botulinum* types C and D toxin by ELISA, *Aust Vet J* 68:111-113, 1991.
1614. Jubb TF, Ellis TM, Gregory AR: Diagnosis of botulism in cattle using ELISA to detect antibody to botulinum toxins, *Aust Vet J* 70:226-227, 1993.
1615. Main DC, Gregory AR: Serological diagnosis of botulism in dairy cattle, *Aust Vet J* 73:77-78, 1996.
1616. Gregory AR et al: Use of enzyme-linked immunoassay for antibody to types C and D botulinum toxins for investigations of botulism in cattle, *Aust Vet J* 73:55-61, 1996.
1617. Rudolf JA et al: Periodic paralysis in quarter horses: a sodium channel mutation disseminated by selective breeding, *Nat Genet* 2:144-147, 1992.
1618. Naylor JM et al: Electromyography in the diagnosis of equine hyperkalemic periodic paralysis, *J Vet Intern Med* 3:116-119, 1989.
1619. Hatheway CL: Laboratory procedures for cases of suspected infant botulism, *Rev Infect Dis* 1:647-651, 1979.
1620. Ricketts SW et al: Thirteen cases of botulism in horses fed big bale silage, *Equine Vet J* 16:515-518, 1984.
1621. Haagsma J et al: An outbreak of botulism type B in horses, *Vet Rec* 127:206, 1990.
1622. Szabo EA, Pemberton JM, Desmarchelier PM: Detection of the genes encoding botulism neurotoxin types A-E by the polymerase chain reaction, *Appl Environ Microbiol* 59:3011-3020, 1993.
1623. Szabo EA et al: Application of PCR to a clinical and environmental investigation of a case of equine botulism, *J Clin Microbiol* 32:1986-1991, 1994.
1624. Montecucco C, Schiavo G: Mechanism of action of tetanus and botulinium neurotoxins, *Mol Microbiol* 13:1-8, 1994.
1625. Montecucco C, Schiavo G: Structure and function of tetanus and botulinium neurotoxins, *Q Rev Biophys* 28:423-472, 1995.
1626. Arnon SS et al: Intestinal infection and toxin production by *Clostridium botulinum* as one cause of sudden infant death syndrome, *Lancet* 1:1273-1277, 1978.
1627. Arnon SS: Infant botulism: anticipating the second decade, *J Infect Dis* 154:201-206, 1986.
1628. Ricketts SW et al: Botulism-like signs in horses fed "big bale" silage, *Vet Rec* 114:51, 1984.
1629. Franzen P, Gustafsson A, Gunnardsson A: Botulism hos hast relaterad till utfodring med rundbalsensilage (botulism in horses associated with feeding big bale silage), *Svensk Veterinar Tidning* 44:555-559, 1992.
1630. Kelly AR et al: Outbreak of botulism in horses, *Equine Vet J* 16:519-521, 1984.
1631. Thomas RJ, Rosenthal DV, Rogers RJ: A *Clostridium botulinum* type B vaccine for prevention of shaker foal syndrome, *Aust Vet J* 65:79-80, 1988.
1632. L'Hommedieu C et al: Potentiation of neuromuscular weakness in infant botulism by aminoglycosides, *Pediatr Pharmacol Ther* 95:1065-1070, 1979.
1633. Wang Y et al: Acute toxicity of aminoglycoside antibiotics as an aid in detecting botulism, *Appl Environ Microbiol* 48:951-955, 1984.
1634. Sweeney RW et al: Pharmacokinetics of metronidazole given to horses by intravenous and oral routes, *Am J Vet Res* 47:1726-1729, 1986.
1635. Wang Y, Sugiyama H: Botulism in metronidazole-treated conventional adult mice challenged orogastrically with spores of *Clostridium botulinum* type A or B, *Infect Immun* 46:715-719, 1984.
1636. Sweeney RW, Hanson TO: Use of a liquid diet as the sole source of nutrition in six dysphagic horses and as a dietary supplement in seven hypophagic horses, *J Am Vet Med Assoc* 197:1030-1032, 1990.
1637. Lewis GE Jr: Approaches to the prophylaxis, immunotherapy, and chemotherapy of botulism. In Lewis GE, ed: *Biomedical aspects of botulism*, New York, 1981, Academic Press.
1638. Crane SA et al: *Clostridium botulinum* type B toxoid for vaccination of adult horses, pregnant mares, and foals: a study of vaccination protocols, *Proceedings of the Thirty-seventh Annual Convention of the American Association of Equine Practitioners*, 1991, pp 611.
1639. Lewis GE et al: Evaluation of a *Clostridium botulinum* toxoid, type B, for the prevention of shaker foal syndrome, *Proceedings of the Twenty-seventh Annual Convention of the American Association of Equine Practitioners*, 1981, pp 233-237.

NEURITIS OF THE CAUDA EQUINA

DEFINITION AND ETIOLOGY. The etiology of neuritis of the cauda equina in horses is unknown. Inflammatory changes occur in various nerve roots, particularly those of the cauda equina and cranial nerves. All nerve roots may be affected to a greater or lesser degree, which has led to the suggestion of polyneuritis equi as a more descriptive name for the condition.[1640,1641]

The disease usually occurs in adult horses,[1640-1644] although it has been described in a yearling filly.[1642] No breed or gender predilection has been noted.[1643]

A number of hypotheses have been proposed for the cause of this disease. The lesions it causes bear some histopathologic resemblance to experimental allergic neuritis of rats, coonhound paralysis of dogs, and Guillain-Barré syndrome in human beings, all of which are suspected of having an autoimmune basis.[1644,1645] Other etiologies that have been proposed are a hypersensitivity reaction after a systemic infection, aberrant migration of helminth larvae, and association with equine herpes virus type 1 and equine viral arteritis infections.[1642,1643,1646-1648] However, conclusive evidence supporting any of these theories is lacking.

CLINICAL SIGNS AND DIFFERENTIAL DIAGNOSES. The clinical signs of cauda equina neuritis reflect the involvement of the lower motoneurons and sensory neurons at the level of the nerve roots. In the initial stages of the acute form, horses show signs of hyperesthesia, particularly around the tail head, and rub and chew at this area.[1644] Sometimes pain is apparent, and horses become apprehensive of handling.[1649] The condition can progress to hypoesthesia or anesthesia of the affected areas.[1640,1641,1646] In the chronic form a gradually progressive paresis of the tail, bladder, rectum, and anal sphincter develops, which may terminate in paralysis.

Commonly the signs include weakness or paralysis of the tail.[1650,1651] The anus may be hypotonic or atonic and distended.[1640,1649-1652] Fecal retention or incontinence is sometimes a feature.[1640,1641,1646,1649,1653] Urinary incontinence occurs in many horses as a result of involvement of parasympathetic fibers in the sacral nerves and is of the lower motoneuron type (i.e., the bladder is atonic, distended, and easily expressed manually). In severe cases overflow incontinence develops, and urine dribbling may cause vaginal hyperemia and scalding of the perineum in mares and scalding of the thighs in animals of either gender.[1640,1641,1646,1650-1654] Retention of urine predisposes to urinary tract infections.[1652] In males the penis may be relaxed and protruding, with decreased sensation in the perineal skin.[1640,1641,1652] Impotence due to incomplete erection and inability to achieve intromission was the presenting complaint in one stallion with cauda equina neuritis.[1655] The preputial skin, which derives its innervation from spinal cord segments L2 to L4 through the genitofemoral nerve, usually retains normal sensory function.[1656] When the nerve roots of the lumbosacral enlargement of the spinal cord are involved, hind limb weakness with ataxia is seen.[1643,1644,1646,1649] Weakness and ataxia have been observed in all four limbs of some horses.[1641,1644,1650,1653] The gait may be stiff,[1649,1652] and denervation atrophy of muscles may result.[1649]

Cranial nerves can be involved. The signs depend on the individual nerves affected and the severity of the disease. The motor branch of the trigeminal nerve is reported to be the most commonly involved, resulting in atrophy of the temporal and masseter muscles, with drooling and dysphagia.[1650,1653,1654,1657] Involvement of the facial nerve results in unilateral or bilateral facial paralysis, which can cause keratitis and corneal ulceration.[1644,1646,1650,1653,1657] Head tilt and other signs of cranial nerve dysfunction may also occur.[1641,1650,1657]

Any disorder that affects the cauda equina may cause similar signs. These include instabilities of the caudal spine caused by luxations or fractures, equine herpesvirus myelitis, and sorghum intoxication.

CLINICAL PATHOLOGY. Cerebrospinal fluid (CSF) may have a mononuclear and neutrophilic pleocytosis, sometimes with more than 100 cells/μl.[1642] The CSF protein concentration usually is moderately to markedly increased.[1643,1653,1657] Electromyographic abnormalities occur in cauda equina neuritis as a result of denervation of affected muscles. A recent study suggests that the presence of circulating antibodies to P2 myelin protein may prove to be a useful diagnostic test, but further research is required to confirm this.[1658,1659]

PATHOPHYSIOLOGY. The finding that some horses with cauda equina neuritis possess antibodies to P2 myelin protein supports the theory that this disease has an autoimmune etiology.[1658,1659] An initial traumatic or infectious insult might cause the release of autoantigens from nerve tissue and disrupt the blood-nerve barrier so as to permit an autoimmune reaction.[1649] Experimental inoculation of P2 protein in rats produces an antibody response and an allergic neuritis that has some pathologic features in common with cauda equina neuritis.[1660] However, it is possible that such autoantibodies represent an epiphenomenon and are not central to the pathogenesis of the disease.

NECROPSY FINDINGS. The main lesions are in the nervous system. The cauda equina is thickened, discolored, and covered with edematous tissue and fibrous material.[1644,1654,1661] There may be adhesions of the nerve roots or the spinal cord to the meninges and the periosteum of the vertebral canal.[1640,1652] Subdural or epidural petechiation and hemorrhage are sometimes seen.[1640,1646,1649]

At the microscopic level the major finding is a granulomatous inflammation that is most intense in the extradural part of the nerve roots. On rare occasions microabscesses are found at the center of the granulomatous lesions.[1640,1644] The epineuria, perineuria, and endoneuria are thickened and are infiltrated to varying degrees by lymphocytes, plasma cells, lymphoblasts, macrophages, giant cells, eosinophils, and in rare cases neutrophils.* Intraneural inflammation, necrosis, and endoneurial thickening can obliterate nerves.[1640,1646,1649] Axonal degeneration and demyelination are present.[1644] Often myelinated axons are absent in the affected nerves. Mildly affected nerves have axonal swelling and ballooning of myelin sheaths. Nerve bundles are separated by large amounts of fibrous tissue. There is minimum to moderate evidence of nerve regeneration.[1644]

Lesions can also be found in the spinal cord itself, having occurred secondary to the nerve root lesions such as wallerian degeneration in the dorsal columns and axonal reaction in the ventral horn cells.[1649] Inflammatory lesions in dorsal root ganglia and in trigeminal ganglia have been found in some horses with this disease.[1650]

TREATMENT AND PROGNOSIS. It has been suggested that treatment with corticosteroids at antiinflammatory doses early in the course of the disease may be helpful.[1642,1646,1654,1662] However, no therapy has consistently been shown to be effective. General supportive care should be given, including fluid therapy when necessary, and the bladder and bowels should be manually evacuated. Because of the slow progression of signs in some horses, these animals may be maintained on supportive care for a long time. Because of the severity of the clinical signs, the gradual deterioration, and the poor prognosis, euthanasia usually is the eventual choice.

REFERENCES

1640. Milne FJ, Carbonell PL: Neuritis of the cauda equina of horses: a case report, *Equine Vet J* 2:179-182, 1970.

*References 1640, 1644, 1646, 1650, 1651, and 1654.

1641. Eustis S, Rings M: Polyneuritis in the equine, *Minn Vet* 14:28-30, 1974.
1642. Scarratt WK, Jortner BS: Neuritis of the cauda equina in a yearling filly, *Compend Cont Educ Pract Vet* 7:S197-S202, 1985.
1643. Fankhauser R et al: Clinical aspects and pathology of neuritis of the cauda equina in the horse, *Schweiz Arch Tierheilkd* 117:675-699, 1975.
1644. Cummings JF, De Lahunta A, Timoney JF: Neuritis of the cauda equina: a chronic idiopathic polyradiculoneuritis in the horse, *Acta Neuropathol (Berl)* 46:17-24, 1979.
1645. Leibowitz S, Hughes RAC: *Immunology of the nervous system*, London, 1983, Edward Arnold.
1646. White PL et al: Neuritis of the cauda equina in a horse, *Compend Cont Educ Pract Vet* 6:S217-S223, 1984.
1647. Little PB, Moran K: Virus involvement in equine paresis, *Vet Rec* 95:575, 1974.
1648. Innes JRM, Saunders LZ: *Comparative neuropathology*, New York, 1962, Academic Press.
1649. Greenwood AG, Barker J, McLeish I: Neuritis of the cauda equina in a horse, *Equine Vet J* 5:111-115, 1973.
1650. Rousseaux CG et al: Cauda equina neuritis: a chronic idiopathic neuritis in two horses, *Can Vet J* 25:214-218, 1984.
1651. Manning JP, Gosser HS: Neuritis of the cauda equina in horses, *Vet Med (Small Anim Clin)* 68:1162-1165, 1973.
1652. Rimaila-Parnanen E: Neuritis of the cauda equina in a horse, *Nord Vet Med* 28:464-467, 1976.
1653. Martens R, Stewart JS, Eicholtz D: Clinicopathologic conference from the School of Veterinary Medicine, University of Pennsylvania, *J Am Vet Med Assoc* 156:478-487, 1970.
1654. Beech J: Neuritis of the cauda equina, *Proceedings of the Twenty-second Annual Convention of the American Association of Equine Practitioners*, 1976, pp 75-76.
1655. Held JP et al: Impotence in a stallion with neuritis cauda equina: a case report, *Equine Vet Sci* 9:67-68, 1989.
1656. De Lahunta A: *Veterinary neuroanatomy and clinical neurology*, Philadelphia, 1983, WB Saunders.
1657. Bilinski J, Sprinkle T, Lee J: A case of cauda equina neuritis, *Vet Med (Small Anim Clin)* 72:597-598, 1977.
1658. Fordyce PS et al: Use of an ELISA in the differential diagnosis of cauda equina neuritis and other equine neuropathies, *Equine Vet J* 19:55-57, 1987.
1659. Kadlubowski M, Ingram PL: Circulating antibodies to the neuritogenic myelin protein P2 in neuritis of the cauda equina of the horse, *Nature* 293:299-300, 1981.
1660. Hughes RAC et al: Immune responses in experimental allergic neuritis, *J Neurol Neurosurg Psychiatry* 44:565-569, 1981.
1661. Edington N et al: Equine adenovirus 1 isolated from cauda equina neuritis, *Res Vet Sci* 37:252-254, 1984.
1662. Rooney JR: Cauda equina neuritis, *Mod Vet Pract* 60:228-230, 1979.

SORGHUM TOXICITY

DEFINITION AND ETIOLOGY. A syndrome of ataxia and cystitis in horses, cattle, and sheep has been linked to the feeding of *Sorghum* spp.[1663-1667] The underlying mechanism is probably toxic damage to the central nervous system, but the precise toxin responsible is not known. This disease does not appear to be linked to the breed, gender, or age of an animal.[1663]

CLINICAL SIGNS. The first sign observed usually is ataxia of the hind limbs, commonly followed by urinary incontinence. Affected animals have a swaying rear limb gait and a tendency to knuckle over. Occasionally affected horses may walk with a hopping gait, in which both rear limbs are lifted off the ground simultaneously (Fig. 33-48). Signs in horses tend to worsen on backing, and animals may fall or even become recumbent.[1663] During an outbreak of the disease in cattle, three of 54 affected cows became recumbent, and two of these died.[1664] The perineal muscles are relaxed, and urine dribbles from a flaccid, distended bladder.[1663,1664] In mares the vulva opens and closes repeatedly; in stallions and geldings the penis is relaxed and protrudes from the prepuce.[1663] Paresis of the tail may be present in both horses and cattle. Loss of skin sensation over the hindquarters has been described in a cow, suggesting involvement of both the sensory and motor nervous pathways.[1664]

Cystitis in affected animals may be severe and occurs secondary to urine retention. Dribbling of urine onto the skin of the perineum and hind limbs results in scalding of the skin and dermatitis. Pyelonephritis is a common sequela to chronic cystitis and may be fatal.[1663,1665] Sometimes the clinical signs may be chronic; in one outbreak horses had been showing signs for as long as 3 years.[1663]

Abortion in mares and arthrogryposis as a congenital deformity of foals have also been linked to the feeding of *Sorghum* plants.[1663]

CLINICAL PATHOLOGY. Diagnosis of sorghum toxicity is made by the presence of typical clinical signs in association with a history of feeding *Sorghum* plants. No specific diagnostic test is available. Cystitis and pyelonephritis are identified by typical findings on routine urinalysis, serum biochemistry, and urine culture.

PATHOPHYSIOLOGY. The precise nature of the toxic substance in *Sorghum* plants that causes this syndrome is unknown. Most *Sorghum* spp. are cyanogenetic plants that contain hydrocyanic acid at potentially toxic concentrations.[1667] Chronic exposure to cyanide has been suggested as the cause of the neuropathologic changes found in animals suffering

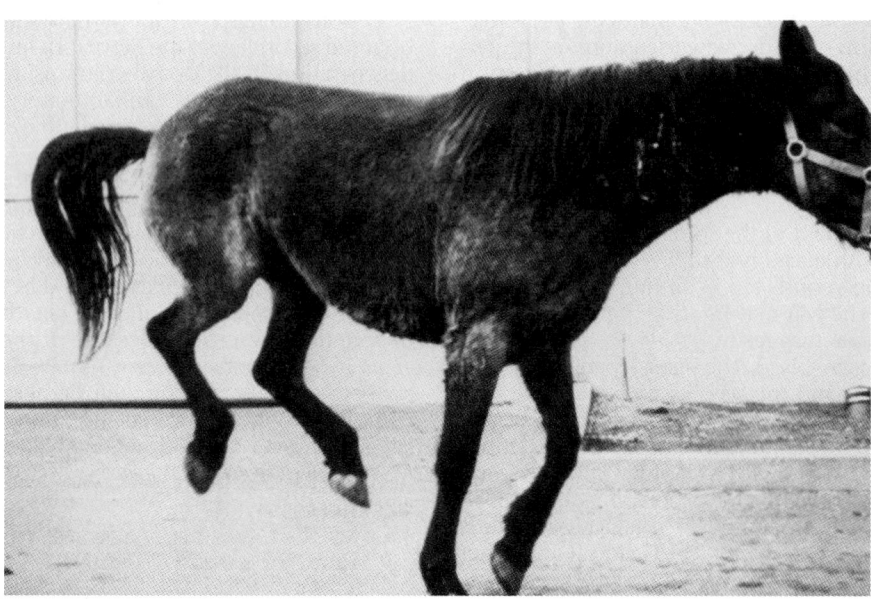

FIG. 33-48 ■ Characteristic "rabbit hopping" gait of a horse with lathyrism. This horse was believed to have eaten sweet peas (*Lathyrus* spp.). Horses may also simply show ataxia and paraparesis. (Courtesy Dr. G. P. Carlson.)

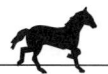

from this disease.[1663] Similarities in the clinical signs of this syndrome and those of neurolathyrism in human beings have led one author to suggest that the toxic principle in *Sorghum* plants may be a lathyrogen-like substance.[1668]

EPIDEMIOLOGY. The cyanide content of *Sorghum* plants is increased by drought or freezing and also is higher in new shoots and wet plants.[1667,1668] In one survey of the disease in horses, most cases occurred during the wet season and involved young, growing plants.[1663] The period of grazing before the onset of signs ranges from 1 week to many months.[1663,1664]

NECROPSY FINDINGS. Wallerian degeneration, swelling of axons and myelin sheaths, and demyelination in a small number of nerve fibers throughout the length of the spinal cord, in the cerebellum, cerebellar peduncles, and the pons have all been described, together with the presence of phagocytic gitter cells.[1663,1664] These changes are not associated with specific tracts.[1664]

TREATMENT AND PROGNOSIS. Withdrawal of *Sorghum* plants from the diet of affected animals results in a gradual improvement in the clinical signs over weeks to months, although recovery may not be complete.[1664] There is no specific treatment for affected animals. Supportive therapy includes antibiotics for treatment of bacterial urinary tract infections.

CONTROL. Avoiding the feeding of *Sorghum* plants as a predominant part of the diet or the sole diet is the only method of control. This plant has considerable feed value and should not present a major hazard when used as part of a diversified feeding regimen.

REFERENCES

1663. Adams LG et al: Cystitis and ataxia associated with *Sorghum* ingestion by horses, *J Am Vet Med Assoc* 155:518-524, 1969.
1664. Everist SE: *Poisonous plants of Australia*, ed 3, Sydney, 1981, Angus & Robertson.
1665. Van Kampen KR: Sudan grass and *Sorghum* poisoning of horses: a possible lathyrogenic disease, *J Am Vet Med Assoc* 156:629-630, 1970.
1666. Knight PR: Equine cystitis and ataxia associated with grazing of pastures dominated by *Sorghum* species, *Aust Vet J* 44:257, 1968.
1667. McKenzie RA, McMicking LI: Ataxia and urinary incontinence in cattle grazing *Sorghum*, *Aust Vet J* 53:496-497, 1977.
1668. Gaggino OP, Carillo BJ: Ataxia de bovinos en pastoro de Sorgo (bovine ataxia due to *Sorghum* feeding), *IDIA (Argentina)* 197:28-30, 1944.

STRINGHALT

DEFINITION AND ETIOLOGY. Stringhalt is a disorder of unknown etiology that produces a characteristic hyperflexion of one or both hock joints in affected horses. It occurs in both sporadic and epidemic forms. Traumatic injury has been suggested as the cause of some sporadic cases; plant toxicity may be the cause of the epidemic form of stringhalt.

CLINICAL SIGNS. Affected horses appear normal at rest but have a characteristic involuntary hyperflexion of the tarsocrural joint when moving. The disorder may be unilateral or bilateral and can vary in severity from a slight exaggeration of normal movement to a motion wherein the rear foot strikes the belly. The signs generally worsen on turning or backing and may also be more severe when the animal is frightened, after a period of rest, or in cold weather.[1669-1671] The clinical signs in the sporadic form usually are unilateral, whereas the epidemic form more commonly manifests with bilateral signs.

CLINICAL PATHOLOGY. No abnormal clinical pathologic findings are associated with this disease. Electromyography of affected muscles reveals increased insertion activity and abnormal spontaneous activity such as fibrillation potentials and positive sharp waves, which is consistent with denervation.

PATHOPHYSIOLOGY. The etiology and pathophysiology of stringhalt are unknown. The sporadic form occurs in individual animals. In some sporadic cases a history of traumatic injury to the limb, particularly to the dorsoproximal metatarsus, precedes the development of stringhalt by several months,[1672,1673] although in other cases the cause is unknown. Explanations advanced to account for the development of stringhalt after traumatic injury include tendinous adhesions and alterations in the function of nervous or muscular components of the myotactic reflex in the affected muscles.[1670,1674-1676] Outbreaks of stringhalt among horses in Australia and the western United States have been associated with ingestion of certain plants, particularly *Hypochoeris radicata*, but a causal role for a plant toxin has not been proven.[1677-1680] Detailed pathologic studies of horses affected by the epidemic form of stringhalt have revealed that the lesion is a distal axonopathy in peripheral nerves that selectively affects large-diameter myelinated axons.[1678,1681] The pathologic changes are widespread and involve nerves of the forelimb and the recurrent laryngeal nerves, as well as those supplying the hind limbs. Neurogenic myofiber atrophy is present in muscles innervated by the affected nerves, with type II fibers being more severely affected than type I fibers. Recovery in affected horses is presumed to be due to axonal regeneration, a process that requires an intact neuronal cell body.[1678]

EPIDEMIOLOGY. The sporadic form of stringhalt occurs in individual animals worldwide and at any time of year. The epidemic form occurs in outbreaks in which several horses in the same location are affected; it has a seasonal incidence, being most prevalent in the late summer or early autumn after a period of very dry weather. Outbreaks have been reported in Australia (hence the alternative name for the epidemic form, "Australian stringhalt") and in the western United States.[1679,1680]

NECROPSY FINDINGS. Lesions are limited to the peripheral nerves and muscles.[1678] There is a loss of large-diameter myelinated fibers in a number of peripheral nerves, especially those innervating the hind limbs and the recurrent laryngeal nerves. The pathologic changes in the nerves include demyelination, fibrosis, and proliferation of Schwann cells. Longer nerves are more severely affected. Muscles innervated by the affected nerves show evidence of denervation atrophy, particularly of type II myofibers.

TREATMENT AND PROGNOSIS. Individual cases rarely recover spontaneously. Surgical therapy by tenotomy or tenectomy of the lateral digital extensor tendon has been the treatment of choice in sporadic cases, resulting in a guarded to favorable prognosis for recovery.[1669,1670] Conservative treatment using gradually increasing exercise or intraarticular administration of corticosteroids also has been advocated for animals with a history of trauma to the affected limb.[1672,1673] Steroid therapy was successful in the one case reported, whereas exercise alone resulted in improvement in two out of four horses but complete recovery in only one horse.[1672]

In the epidemic form most horses recover in weeks to months without treatment.[1677] Because a toxic etiology is suspected, it usually is recommended that the horses be removed from the pasture they were grazing when they developed signs. Administration of phenytoin (10 to 15 mg/kg PO once or twice daily) resulted in clinical improvement and reduced abnormal electromyographic activity within 24 hours of starting therapy and reached full effect by 1 week.[1682] Horses that did not recover spontaneously while receiving phenytoin showed reappearance of signs within a few days. Mild sedation is a possible side effect of this treatment.

CONTROL. Because plant toxicity is suspected as the cause of the epidemic form of stringhalt, control is best effected by not grazing horses on weed-infested pasture and by using weed control and good pasture management where horses are being grazed. Judicious exercise regimens may be helpful in reducing the likelihood of stringhalt in horses that have sustained traumatic injuries to the dorsoproximal region of the metatarsus.[1672]

REFERENCES

1669. Hahn CN, Mayhew IG, MacKay RJ: Stringhalt and shivering. In Colahan PT et al, eds: *Equine medicine and surgery*, ed 5, St Louis, 2000, Mosby.
1670. Stashak ES: *Adams' lameness in horses*, ed 4, Philadelphia, 1987, Lea & Febiger.
1671. Wheat JD: Stringhalt. In Catcott EJ, Smithcors JF, eds: *Equine medicine and surgery*, ed 2, 1972, Wheaton, Ill, American Veterinary Publications.
1672. Crabill MR et al: Stringhalt secondary to trauma to the dorsoproximal region of the metatarsus in horses: 10 cases (1986-1991), *J Am Vet Med Assoc* 205:867-869, 1994.
1673. Herbert C, Jann HW: Intraarticular corticosteroid treatment for stringhalt in a quarter horse: a case report, *J Equine Vet Sci* 14:53-54, 1994.
1674. Cahill J, Goulden B, Pearce H: A review and some observations of stringhalt, *N Z Vet J* 33:101-104, 1985.
1675. Huntington PJ et al: Australian stringhalt: epidemiological, clinical and neurological investigations, *Equine Vet J* 21:266-273, 1989.
1676. Mayhew IG: *Large animal neurology*, Philadelphia, 1989, Lea & Febiger.
1677. Pemberton DH, Caple IW: Australian stringhalt in horses, *Vet Annu* 20:167-171, 1980.
1678. Slocombe RF et al: Pathological aspects of Australian stringhalt, *Equine Vet J* 23:174-183, 1992.
1679. Galey FD, Hullinger PJ, McCaskill J: Outbreaks of stringhalt in northern California, *Vet Hum Toxicol* 33:176-177, 1991.
1680. Gay CC et al: Hypochoeris-associated stringhalt in North America, *Equine Vet J* 25:456-457, 1993.
1681. Cahill JI, Goulden BE, Jolly RD: Stringhalt in horses: a distal axonopathy, *Neuropathol Appl Neurobiol* 12:459-475, 1986.
1682. Huntington PJ, Seneque S, Slocombe RF: Use of phenytoin to treat horses with Australian stringhalt, *Aust Vet J* 68:221-224, 1991.

TICK PARALYSIS

DEFINITION AND ETIOLOGY. An ascending lower motoneuron paralysis has been described in horses, sheep, cattle, and goats in Australia, associated with infestation by the tick *Ixodes holocyclus*.[1683-1688] In the United States a similar disease occurs in dogs, human beings, cattle, and wild animal species as a result of infestation with *Dermacentor* spp.[1689]

CLINICAL SIGNS. The clinical signs are those of progressive generalized paresis that terminates in recumbency and death from respiratory paralysis in as little as 24 hours.[1683] The disease usually is fatal when caused by *I. holocyclus*, but animals affected by *Dermacentor* spp. recover if the ticks are removed before the animals are moribund. Diagnosis is made on the basis of the clinical signs and finding ticks on the affected animal. The major differential diagnosis is botulism.

CLINICAL PATHOLOGY. There are no pathognomonic findings in the clinical pathology of affected animals. Electromyography in tick paralysis in dogs in North America reveals minimal spontaneous activity and lack of evoked compound muscle action potentials in response to motor nerve stimulation.[1690] Findings in large animals can be expected to be similar.

PATHOPHYSIOLOGY. The cause of tick paralysis is believed to be a neurotoxin in the saliva of female ticks that is inoculated into the host when the tick feeds. Nymphs and larvae may also cause the disease.[1684,1686,1687] In the case of *I. holocyclus* the toxin has been named holocyclotoxin. The toxin elaborated by *Dermacentor* spp. has been less well characterized. The pathogenesis of the disease is blockage of transmission at the neuromuscular junction as a result of reduced release of acetylcholine. Mortality is common in tick paralysis caused by *I. holocyclus* despite tick removal.

EPIDEMIOLOGY. The disease occurs worldwide, associated with different tick species in different areas. In North America the region from the Pacific coastal range to the Continental Divide provides especially favorable conditions for the proliferation of *Dermacentor andersoni*.[1689]

NECROPSY FINDINGS. There are no pathognomonic findings at necropsy. Death usually is due to respiratory paralysis.

TREATMENT AND PROGNOSIS. Treatment is symptomatic after removal of the ticks, which is essential. Spraying or dipping affected animals facilitates tick removal. In small animals shaving the hair coat may be necessary to ensure detection and removal of all ticks. The prognosis is good in the case of *Dermacentor*-induced paralysis when tick removal and supportive care are instituted before animals are moribund. Fatalities frequently occur in the case of *Ixodes*-induced paralysis despite removal of ticks.

Because resistance to paralysis may occur in dogs and wild host species due to the development of humoral immunity to holocyclotoxin, administration of hyperimmune serum has been shown to be beneficial in the treatment and prevention of this disease in dogs.[1688] No report of such treatment in large animal species was found.

CONTROL. Environmental control to reduce tick populations may reduce the incidence of the disease.

REFERENCES

1683. Sloan CA: Mortality in sheep due to *Ixodes species*, *Aust Vet J* 44:527, 1968.
1684. Legg J: Note on the infestation of sheep with ticks, *Aust Vet J* 3:12-14, 1927.
1685. Bootes BW: A fatal paralysis in foals from *Ixodes holocyclus neumann* infestation, *Aust Vet J* 38:68-69, 1962.
1686. Seddon HR: *Diseases of domestic animals in Australia*. III. Tick and mite infestations, Canberra, Australia, 1951, AJ Arthur.
1687. Roberts FHS: *Insects affecting livestock*, Sydney, 1952, Angus & Robertson.
1688. Malik R, Farrow BRH: Tick paralysis in North America and Australia, *Vet Clin North Am (Small Anim Pract)* 21:157-171, 1991.
1689. Schofield LN, Saunders JR: An incidental case of tick paralysis in a Holstein calf exposed to *Dermacentor andersoni*, *Can Vet J* 33:190-191, 1992.
1690. Chrisman CL: Differentiation of tick paralysis and acute idiopathic polyradiculoneuritis in the dog using electromyography, *J Am Anim Hosp Assoc* 11:455-458, 1975.

GRASS SICKNESS

Grass sickness is a disorder of unknown etiology that occurs in horses, ponies, and donkeys in Great Britain and northern Europe.[1691-1697] A disease with similar clinical signs has been described in horses in Colombia.[1698] The major clinical finding is a decrease in or cessation of gut motility. The signs of grass sickness, which are mainly caused by intestinal stasis, include colic, bloat, constipation, inappetence, weight loss, and dehydration. Esophageal dysfunction may be manifested by dysphagia. Paralysis of the urinary bladder occurs in some animals, and in males the relaxed penis may protrude from the prepuce. Significant cardiac functional disturbance has been documented in horses with grass sickness.[1699] The course of the disease varies from peracute with sudden death to chronic; some animals survive for many months despite alimentary dysfunction.[1692,1693] More recently, survival and return to function has been documented in some horses that received good nursing care.[1700] Risk factors for developing the disease include younger age, male gender, location on premises that had previously experienced the disease, and dry weather. The peak incidence of the disease occurs from April to June.[1701]

Histologic examination reveals characteristic degenerative changes in peripheral autonomic ganglia, in the myenteric and submucous plexuses, cardiac ganglia, and in certain central nervous system nuclei.[1694,1695,1699] These neuronal changes are the major pathologic lesion.[1702] Some degree of esophageal dysfunction occurs in all horses with grass sickness.[1697] The histopathology of autonomic ganglia in horses that showed complete clinical recovery from grass sickness was virtually normal, with normal morphology in four of four horses studied and normal cells numbers in three of four.[1702]

Studies suggesting an association between grass sickness and *Clostridium perfringens* type A enterotoxin have been disputed.[1692,1703] The presence of a neurotoxic factor in the plasma of affected horses was suggested by induction of typical neuropathologic lesions in ponies by intraperitoneal inoculation of plasma and serum from horses with acute disease. Clinical illness was not observed in the ponies.[1704] Recent studies support the hypothesis that the disease is caused by toxicoinfection with *Clostridium botulinum* type C.[1705] Growth of the organism in the gastrointestinal tract is hypothesized to be the source of the botulinum toxin.

Treatment is supportive and includes supplementary feeding and fluid therapy. The indirect-acting cholinergic cisapride (0.5 to 0.8 mg/kg PO given every 8 hours for 1 week) facilitates release of acetylcholine from the myenteric plexus and increases gut motility in chronic grass sickness. Colic signs may increase shortly after administration of this drug.[1706] Many affected animals die, but recovery has been reported in some chronic cases, and a recent report documents recovery in 50% to 70% of chronic cases that receive appropriate treatment.[1694] Analgesia with intravenously administered flunixin meglumine or intravenously or orally administered phenylbutazone is appropriate in some cases, and diazepam (0.05 mg/kg given every 2 hours) may be helpful as an appetite stimulant. Factors associated with a better prognosis include willingness to eat concentrates and milder signs of dysphagia.[1707]

REFERENCES

1691. Gilmour JS: Grass sickness. In Robinson NE, ed: *Current therapy in equine medicine,* Philadelphia, 1983, WB Saunders.
1692. Keith NW: The clinical features of grass sickness in horses, *Proceedings of the Second Annual Congress of the British Equine Veterinary Association,* 1963, pp 36-42.
1693. Begg GW: Grass disease in horses, *Vet Rec* 48:655-662, 1936.
1694. Barlow RM: Neuropathological observations in grass sickness of horses, *J Comp Pathol* 79:407-411, 1969.
1695. Gilmour JS: Observations on neuronal changes in grass sickness of horses, *Res Vet Sci* 15:197-200, 1973.
1696. Greet TRC, Whitwell KE: Barium swallow as an aid to the diagnosis of grass sickness, *Equine Vet J* 18:294-297, 1986.
1697. Gilmour JS, Jolly GM: Some aspects of the epidemiology of grass sickness, *Vet Rec* 95:77-81, 1974.
1698. Ochoa R, De Velandia S: Equine grass sickness: evidence of association with *Clostridium perfringens* type A enterotoxin, *Am J Vet Res* 39:1049-1051, 1978.
1699. Perkins JD et al: Functional and histopathological evidence of cardiac parasympathetic dysautonomia in equine grass sickness, *Vet Rec* 146:246-250, 2000.
1700. Doxey DL et al: Prediction of long-term outcome following grass sickness (equine dysautonomia), *Vet Rec* 144:386-387, 1999.
1701. A case control study of grass sickness (equine dysautonomia) in the United Kingdom, *Vet J* 156:7-14, 1998.
1702. Doxey DL et al: Histology in recovered cases of grass sickness, *Vet Rec* 146:645-646, 2000.
1703. Gilmour JS, Brown R, Johnson P: A negative serologic relationship between cases of grass sickness in Scotland and *Clostridium perfringens* type A enterotoxin, *Equine Vet J* 13:56-58, 1981.
1704. Gilmour JS, Mould DL: Experimental studies of neurotoxic activity in blood fractions from acute cases of grass sickness, *Res Vet Sci* 22:1-4, 1977.
1705. Hunter LC, Miller JK, Poxton IR: The association of *Clostridium botulinum* type C with equine grass sickness: a toxicoinfection? *Equine Vet J* 31:492-499, 1999.
1706. Milne EM et al: An evaluation of the use of cisapride in horses with chronic grass sickness (equine dysautonomia), *Br Vet J* 152:537-549, 1996.
1707. Milne E: Grass sickness: an update, *In Pract* 19:128-133, 1997.

PERIPHERAL NERVE DISORDERS

LISLE W. GEORGE

Most peripheral nerve disorders of large animals are traumatically induced, but injections, abscesses, tumors, or parasitic invasion of the nerves may occur in rare instances. The peripheral nerves that are most commonly damaged in large animals are discussed in the following paragraphs.

PERIPHERAL NERVES

Suprascapular Nerve

Mechanical damage to the suprascapular nerve results in paralysis of the infraspinatus and supraspinatus muscles.[1708] Early denervation is characterized by a slight outward bowing of the scapulohumeral joint as weight is placed on the limb. Neurogenic atrophy develops after several months, and the scapular spine becomes prominent (Fig. 33-49). The common name for this condition is "Sweeney."

Brachial Plexus

Damage to the brachial plexus may result in any combination of dysfunction of the biceps and coracobrachialis muscles (musculocutaneous nerve), as well as the pectoral, subscapularis, and triceps muscles.

Lesions of the brachial plexus are caused by trauma to the shoulder, deep penetrating axillary wounds, or traction on the forelimbs of a fetus during relief of a dystocia. Because of their tendency to rear and jump over objects, horses are most susceptible to brachial plexus injuries. The condition may occur in small ruminants after automobile accidents, carnivore attacks, or blows from larger animals.

MOTOR DEFICITS. Severe lesions of the brachial plexus result in complete flaccidity of the fore limb. The animals are unable to bear weight. Triceps reflexes are absent. Loss of pectoral nerve function results in abduction of the elbow. Subscapular muscle paralysis results in dropped shoulder.[1709] Musculocutaneous nerve paralysis results in a hyperextension of the elbow at rest and an inability to flex the joint. There is loss of the biceps reflex. The clinical signs of radial nerve paralysis are described in the following paragraphs.

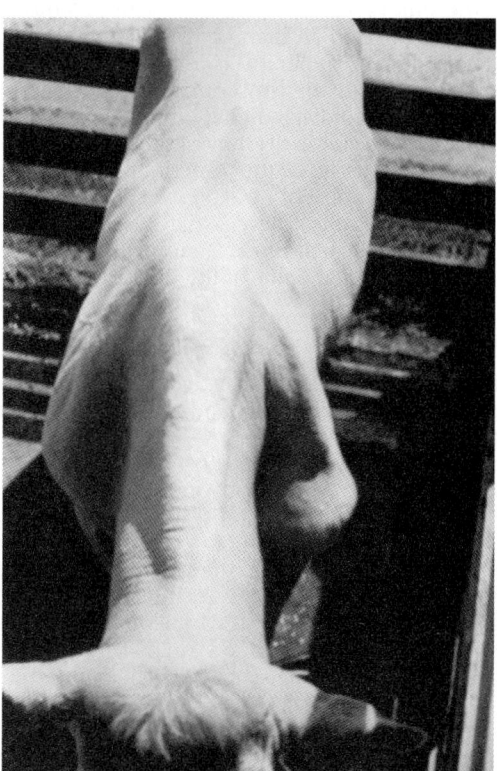

FIG. 33-49 ▓ Sweeney (neurogenic atrophy) of the left supraspinatus and infraspinatus muscles in a Charolais bull. The lesion was caused by trauma related to running through a cattle chute.

SENSORY DEFICITS. Avulsions of the brachial plexus result in complete desensitization of the entire forelimb.

Radial Nerve

The radial nerve is motor to the extensor muscles of the forelimbs. The nerve courses over the lateral aspect of the elbow joint and is vulnerable to traumatic insult at that point. Radial nerve paralysis most commonly arises from direct trauma to the nerve, during prolonged anesthesia, or during restraint in lateral recumbency with inadequate padding of the forelimb.[1710,1711] Degeneration of the triceps muscles also plays a significant role in many cases of radial nerve paralysis.[1710]

The limb position varies, depending on the location of the lesion in the radial nerve. Lesions at or near the elbow joint result in high radial nerve paralysis, which is characterized by a dropped elbow, failure of limb protraction with scuffing of the toe, and flexion of all distal limb joints (Fig. 33-50). The foot is knuckled over at rest, and the animal is unable to bear weight on the leg. Lesions of the distal radial nerve result in knuckling of the carpus, fetlock, and pastern joints. The animal can support weight on the affected limb if the metacarpus and distal limb are held in extension. The triceps reflex is depressed to absent. Chronic dysfunction of the radial nerve results in neurogenic atrophy of the extensor muscles of the forelimb. Detectable sensory deficits resulting from radial nerve paralysis tend to be vague and probably vary from patient to patient.

Femoral Nerve

The femoral nerve is distributed to the quadriceps femoris muscles and the skin of the rear limb extending from the medial thigh to the medial part of the coronet (saphenous nerve). Traumatic overextension of the hip and stifle joint from a fall or other injury or forced posterior delivery can damage the femoral nerve. The clinical signs of femoral nerve paralysis are related to an inability to extend and fix the stifle.[1708] The reciprocal apparatus is unable to fix the hock, resulting in collapse of the limb during weight bearing and constant flexion of all distal digital joints. Chronic lesions of the femoral nerve result in atrophy of the quadriceps femoris muscles and the muscles of the posterior part of the gluteals. The patellar reflex is absent or depressed, and the patella often is displaced laterally. There is analgesia to anesthesia of the medial part of the rear limb extending from the proximal thigh to the medial malleolus of the tibia.

Sciatic Nerve

The sciatic nerve innervates the extensor muscles of the hip, the flexor muscles of the stifle, and most of the muscles of the distal limb.

Sciatic nerve paralysis occurs most commonly in postpartum cows after forced fetal extraction. Loss of function of the lumbar branches of the nerve most likely plays a major role in the so-called calving or obturator paralysis syndrome.[1712] Injection of irritating drugs into the space between the greater trochanter and the ischial tuberosity may cause a sciatic neuritis. This occurs most commonly in neonates but can occur in rare cases in adult cattle and small ruminants. Other causes of sciatic nerve damage are pelvic fractures, tumors, or abscesses located along the course of the nerve.

The sciatic nerve innervates most of the musculature of the rear limb, therefore the motor deficits associated with denervation are profound. At rest the limb is hanging behind the animal. The stifle is dropped and extended (Fig. 33-51). The foot is constantly knuckled. If the limb is positioned properly, the animal usually can bear weight for a limited period be-

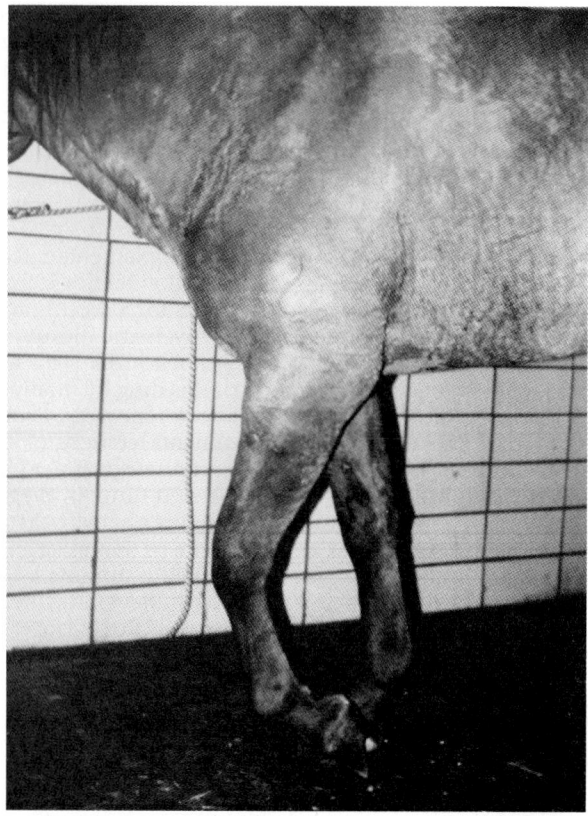

FIG. 33-50 ▮▮ High radial nerve paralysis in a horse showing knuckling of the carpus and digit and dropped elbow. (Courtesy Dr. R.H. Whitlock.)

cause of the normal function of the quadriceps muscles and the action of the reciprocal apparatus. Chronic denervation of the sciatic nerve results in neurogenic atrophy of the caudal thigh muscles and all of the muscles distal to the stifle.

The sciatic nerve divides into the tibial and the peroneal nerves in the distal limb. Therefore except for the medial part of the thigh and rear limb, there is analgesia and anesthesia of the entire limb distal to the stifle.

Peroneal Nerve

The peroneal branch of the sciatic nerve is distributed to the flexor muscles of the hock joint and the extensor muscles of the digit. The nerve becomes superficial and is exposed to damage as it crosses over the lateral condyle of the fibula.[1713] The condition is commonly seen in all species of large animals and is very common in postpartum dairy cattle that have been recumbent as a result of hypocalcemia or other causes and in horses because of postanesthetic myopathy. Neurologic deficits of the peroneal nerve result in a hyperextended hock joint and flexion of the fetlock and pastern (Fig. 33-52).[1708,1713,1714] Many cows knuckle at the fetlock even when the foot is flat on the ground, and others may be able to bear weight only when the limb is manually placed in the proper position.

There is desensitization of the skin over the craniolateral aspect of the limb extending from the stifle to the hoof.

Tibial Nerve

The tibial nerve supplies the extensor muscles of the hock joint (gastrocnemius) and the digital flexors.

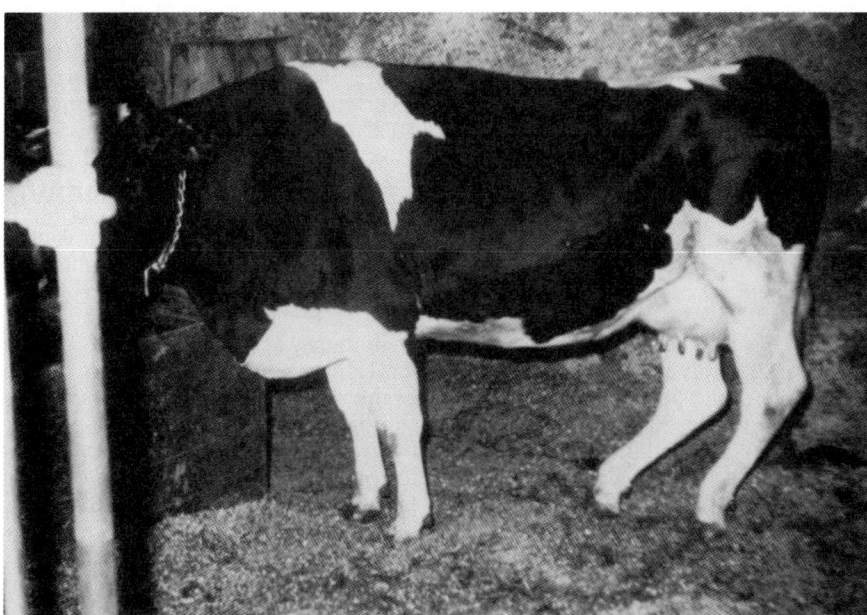

FIG. 33-51 ▌▌ Characteristic posture of a cow with partial sciatic nerve paralysis. The condition pictured here was induced during correction of a severe dystocia. Note the flexion of the hocks, fetlocks, and stifle. These signs differentiate the condition from peroneal paralysis. (Courtesy Dr. R.H. Whitlock.)

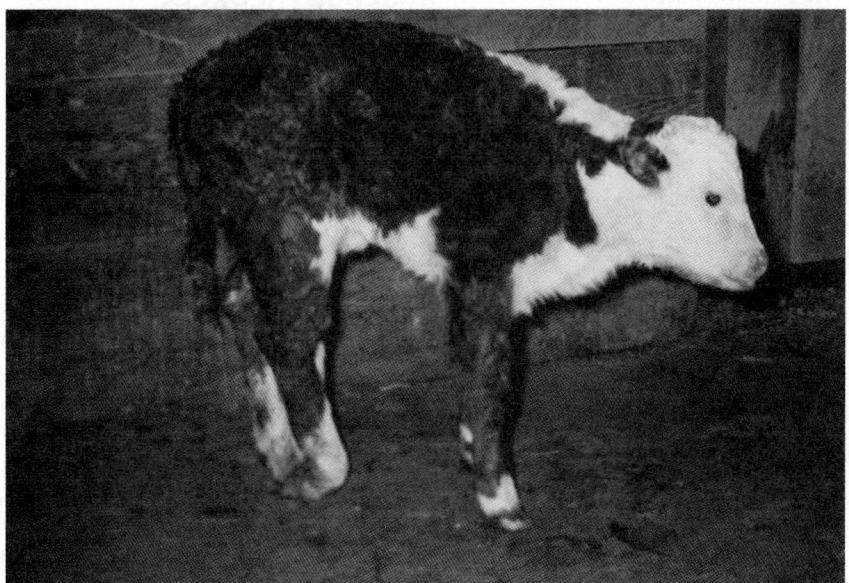

FIG. 33-52 ▌▌ Calf with peroneal nerve paralysis. Note the flexed fetlock and digit and the hyperextended carpus. This condition was caused by injection of antibiotics into the peroneal nerve on the caudolateral aspect of the leg. (Courtesy Dr. R.H. Whitlock.)

Tibial paralysis is most commonly observed in periparturient cattle or neonates that have been given an injection of an irritant drug in the caudal leg at the level of the stifle. Tibial paralysis also is seen in sheep and goats and is a common sequela to dog-bite injuries. With tibial paralysis the hock is overflexed and is pulled higher than normal when the limb is protracted. The toe does not drag on the ground, and the limb is dropped suddenly perpendicularly to the ground at the end of the stride. At rest the pelvis is asymmetric, with the affected side held lower than normal.[1708]

Chronic loss of tibial nerve function results in atrophy of the gastrocnemius and digital flexor muscles. There is anesthesia to analgesia of the skin of the caudomedial aspect of the leg.

Obturator Nerve

The obturator nerve supplies motor impulses to the adductor muscles. The nerve is well protected in the equine and small ruminants, and therefore damage is rare in these species. The cow has a shallow acetabulum and a poorly developed round ligament. Consequently, the condition is seen commonly in peripartum cows. Reports of obturator nerve paralysis of cattle accompanied by knuckling and inability to support weight on the rear limbs probably represent a combination of sciatic and obturator nerve deficits. Coxofemoral luxation is a common complication of obturator paralysis in cattle housed in stalls with slippery flooring. Such luxation can be recognized by the identification of crepitus during passive manipulation of the hip joint. There may be a difference in the length of the rear limbs.

Obturator nerve paralysis is most common in cattle and is nearly always a result of dystocia. The nerve injury is located in the pelvis at the level of the obturator foramen. Approximately 9.2% of all dystocias result in paraplegia.[1715]

The obturator nerve innervates the adductor, pectineus, and gracilis muscles. Only minimum deficits are observed if the cow is placed on a surface that has good traction. Clinical signs of an obturator nerve deficit include a hopping gait when the animal attempts to run and severe abduction or splay-leggedness when the animal is placed on a slippery surface (Fig. 33-53). In severe cases the cow may be sternally recumbent with the rear limbs extending laterally to each side. Experimental studies have indicated that the so-called calving paralysis syndrome is actually a result of a combination of lesions of the lumbar root (L6) of the sciatic nerve and the obturator nerve. Experimental sectioning of the obturator nerve alone does not produce paralysis, provided the animal has a nonslip footing.[1708,1712,1716] Obturator nerve paralysis does not result in a cutaneous sensory deficit.

Damage of one or more peripheral nerves during parturi-tion or milk fever may play a large role in the so-called downer cow syndrome (see p. 1017).[1717,1718] The incidence of the condition ranges from 4% to 28% of all cases of milk fever and is associated with a mortality rate ranging from 20% to 67%.[1437]

PERIPHERAL FACIAL NERVE PARALYSIS

The facial nerve becomes superficial as it courses across the lateral aspect of the mandibular ramus and the masseter muscle. It is most susceptible to blunt trauma or laceration at that site. Horses are most commonly injured from prolonged recumbency or from trauma caused by a poorly designed halter. Halters with large brass rings in the caudodorsal aspect of the cheek pouch are most likely to result in iatrogenic facial palsy. Similar conditions occur in goats and are caused by excessive pull on neck chains while the animal is being led onto the milk stand or tied with the neck chain. In cattle, facial nerve deficits usually are the result of space-occupying masses at the caudal aspect of the mandibular ramus.

Most cases caused by trauma recover after 1 to 10 days of treatment, but in some several months may be required before resolution is observed. Occasionally the nerve deficits are permanent. In chronic cases food should be removed from the cheek pouches twice daily, and the tongue and fauces should be routinely examined for ulcers. If oral ulcers develop, they should be treated by flushing the mouth.

TREATMENT OF PERIPHERAL NERVE DISEASES

Medical management of peripheral nerve injuries consists of reduction of inflammation in the nerves; relief of musculoskeletal pain; prevention of secondary medical complications such as mastitis, fractures, and joint and ligament tears; and prevention of malnutrition and dehydration. Medical treatment for reduction of neurologic inflammation should be instituted as soon as possible after the injury.[1717] Dexamethasone (0.05 mg/kg IV given daily for the first 3 to 5 days after the injury) may be beneficial. Plasma concentrations of calcium, magnesium, and potassium should be measured repeatedly, because low levels of these electrolytes may aggravate the muscular weakness, increase the animal's struggling, and enhance the severity of the musculoskeletal lesions. Calcium gluconate can be given empirically to down cows (500 ml SC daily), as may potassium chloride (100 g in 20 L of water given daily by stomach tube). Concomitant administration of phenylbutazone by intravenous injection and application of cold water or ice packs to the affected part also may be beneficial during the first 24 hours after injury. Appendicular pain may be controlled by administration of nonsteroidal antiinflammatory drugs (e.g., banamine, phenylbutazone, or salicylic acid), and/or narcotic analgesics, including Demerol (1 to 2 mg/kg IV) or morphine (0.07 to 0.14 mg/kg IV).

Affected patients should be placed in a dry soil stall that has been deeply bedded. Concrete-floored stalls should be avoided because the poor footing may promote an accidental fall that worsens the musculoskeletal lesions. Recumbent animals should be turned six to eight times daily to prevent decubital ulcers and pressure myopathy. Support of some patients in slings may be useful for minimizing decubitus and maintaining strength in the opposite limbs. Goats tolerate dog slings well, but care must be used when lifting cattle in a hip sling, because the instrument may cause severe contusions of the muscles at the point or attachment to the tuber coxae. The instrument should not be used repeatedly to support cattle that fail to support weight when lifted. Abduction of the rear limbs may be prevented in cattle by application of a hobble around the metatarsus. The distance between the

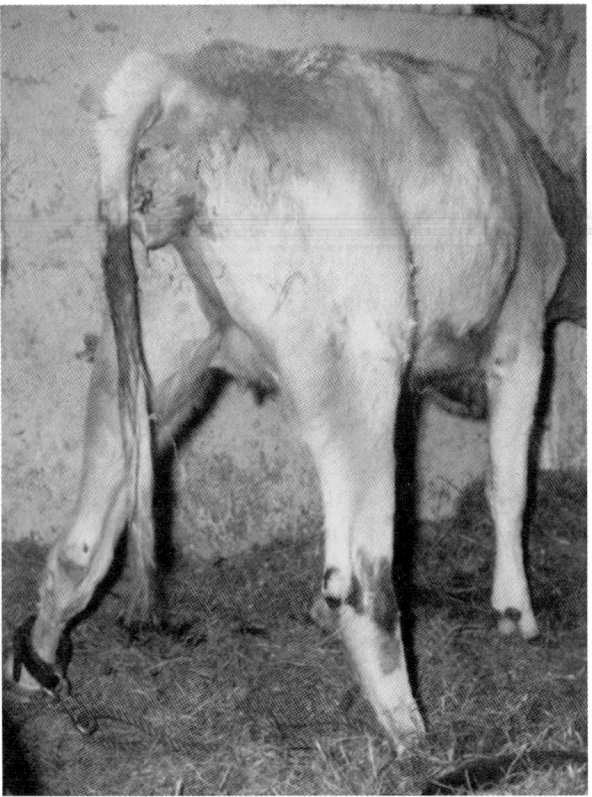

FIG. 33-53 ■ Cow with obturator nerve paralysis caused by relief of a difficult dystocia. Note the base-wide stance, yet the apparent ease with which the cow is able to stand on the deep bedding. Note also that rope hobbles are being applied to prevent further abduction and possible luxation of the coxofemoral joint.

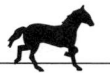

legs should be approximately 35.6 to 50.8 cm (14 to 20 inches) when the legs are tied together and are held abducted. It is important to apply the hobbles with a nontightening bowline knot to prevent strangulation of the foot. The prognosis is poor for animals with neurologic dysfunctions lasting longer than 2 weeks.

REFERENCES

1708. Vaughan LC: Peripheral nerve injuries: an experimental study in cattle, *Vet Rec* 76:1293-1305, 1964.
1709. Kaneps AJ, Blythe LL: Diagnosis and treatment of brachial plexus trauma resulting from dystocia in a calf, *Compend Cont Educ Pract Vet* 8:S4-S6, 1986.
1710. Trim CM, Mason J: Postanaesthetic forelimb lameness in horses, *Equine Vet J* 5:71-76, 1973.
1711. Rooney JR: Radial paralysis in the horse, *Cornell Vet* 53:328-338, 1963.
1712. Cox VS, Breazile JE, Hoover TR: Surgical and anatomic study of calving paralysis, *Am J Vet Res* 36:427-430, 1975.
1713. Keown GH: Peroneal nerve damage, *Can J Comp Med* 20:445-448, 1956.
1714. Cox VS: Peroneal nerve paralysis in a heifer, *J Am Vet Med Assoc* 167:142-143, 1975.
1715. Sloss VA: Clinical study of dystocia in cattle, *Aust Vet J* 50:294-297, 1974.
1716. Cox VS, Breazile JE: Experimental bovine obturator paralysis, *Vet Rec* 93:109-110, 1973.
1717. Cox VS: Understanding the downer cow syndrome, *Compend Cont Educ Pract Vet* 3:S472-S478, 1981.
1718. Curtis RA, Cote JF, Willoughby RA: The downer cow syndrome: a complication not a disease, *Mod Vet Pract* 51:25-28, 1970.

DOWN COWS (Alert Downers)

BRADFORD P. SMITH
JOHN ANGELOS
LISLE W. GEORGE

Alert cows that are unable to rise to a standing position but will eat and drink are referred to as down cows, downer cows, or downers. The alert downer cow is in sternal recumbency and often presents a diagnostic and therapeutic challenge.

Such conditions as hypocalcemia, hypophosphatemia,[1719] primary musculoskeletal injuries, pelvic swelling from dystocia (calving paralysis or obturator paralysis), and spinal cord compression may result in an alert downer. The alert downer cow often is a result of secondary muscle or nerve damage (or both) associated with recumbency, particularly if the animal was down on a hard surface in one position for several hours. Heavy cows down on concrete are particularly susceptible to pressure ischemia of the muscles and nerves and to muscle and ligament tears that occur secondary to struggling and slipping. The degree of pressure damage depends on regional anatomic factors and the duration of compression.

Periparturient downer cows should be treated for hypocalcemia with one or more doses of calcium. Those that fail to respond by standing after one or two doses are classified as alert downer cows. It is reported that 3.8% to 28.2%[1720-1723] of all milk fever cases become alert downers, with a mortality rate of 20% to 67%.[1720,1721,1723,1724] The incidence of downers (24 hours or longer) was 21.4 cases per 1000 cow years in Minnesota dairy herds, with a 33% recovery rate.[1725] Fifty-eight percent of downers occurred within a day of calving, and 97% occurred within the first 100 days after calving.[1725]

Because the pressure damage done to muscles and nerves is aggravated by recumbency, it is desirable to have the animal on soft bedding or grass and to have the animal stand as soon as possible. Eight of 16 normal cows anesthetized for 6 to 12 hours in sternal recumbency with the right hind limb under the body were unable to stand on recovery and became alert downers.[1726] Those that could stand exhibited swelling and stiffness and/or peroneal nerve deficits and paresis in the right hind limb.[1726] These signs are commonly seen in cows that have been recumbent for several hours on a hard surface. As pressure applied to a nerve increases, nerve conduction is im-

paired and eventually lost.[1727] Serum creatine kinase (CK) values in experimental downer cows rose, starting at 12 hours and continuing up for the first 48 hours, and then decreased, even though the cow remained down.[1726] The CK values at 12 and 24 hours did not differ statistically for the cows that could rise after anesthesia and the downers. After 48 hours and 96 hours, the downers had higher mean CK values than the ambulatory group, but there was a great range in values.[1726] In another study of downers, aspartate amino transferase levels were markedly elevated on days 4 to 7, even after CK levels fell.[1728] The clinical difference between cows that recovered and those that remained downers was attributed to damage to the sciatic nerve or its branches, particularly the peroneal nerve.[1726] Peroneal nerve damage results in knuckling over at the fetlock.

Devices that aid and promote standing traditionally include hip lifters (hip clamp), slings, and inflatable bags. Although these devices help less severely affected animals to stand temporarily, they frequently fail to allow for hours of comfortable standing, and they may even induce additional trauma in struggling animals. For these reasons, the use of water flotation has been explored as a tool in the management of downer cows.[1729] Rasmussen[1730] reported on the use of a warm water flotation system in Denmark in 1982. Commercial flotation systems practical for cows, such as the Aqualift (Kirby Manufacturing Co., Merced, CA 95341) are now marketed.

Use of a device such as the Aqualift proceeds in the following manner. First the animal is examined to determine that it is a candidate for flotation and to rule out fractures, severe spinal cord compression, and severe systemic illness. The procedure then is: (1) the Aqualift is brought up near the down cow; (2) the wheels and tongue are detached, and both ends of the tub are removed; (3) a mat is pulled from the tub to a position beside the cow, and the down cow is rolled or slid onto the mat; (4) the mat is winched or otherwise pulled into the tub, and the ends of the tub are put in place; they easily seal with rubber gaskets and large turnbuckles; (5) the cow's head is held up a few inches by a rope halter, and a hose is inserted into the tub, which is filled with water as quickly as possible; the water temperature should be 37.7° to 38.7° C (100° to 102° F). Cows in lateral recumbency on the mat become sternal when 12 to 24 inches of water fills the tub and usually attempt to stand beginning when the tub is one-half to two-thirds full. If a cow is still not trying to stand when the tub is full, pushing her nose briefly under water usually stimulates her to stand. If no hot water is available near the cow or if the tub is not next to dirt or grass suitable for the cow to exit on, the wheels can be put back on and the cow easily trailered to a better location.

Once the cow is standing in warm water, it often is obvious by observation which limb or limbs are paretic or painful. Most cows calm down and relax in a standing position within 5 minutes. Most will eat hay, and even first calf heifers that haven't been handled much seem to be remarkably calmed by the warm water. Unlike horses, cattle do not panic or attempt to jump out. It appears that the hot water may even have some beneficial therapeutic effects on improving peripheral circulation. The cow can be left in the water for 6 to 8 hours, but cows have been left in it for longer than 24 hours. If the water temperature drops below 35° C (95° F), some water should be released from the discharge valve and replaced with hot water. This is especially important in cold weather. When the decision is made to remove the cow from the tub, the water is drained, and the end of the tub facing the dirt, sand, or grass is opened. The cow is encouraged to *slowly* exit into a pen with good footing. Some cows fall as the water is let out, and others collapse as they try to walk. Careful observation as the cow moves can be very helpful in trying to locate anatomic or functional problems.

The animal that collapses can be pulled out on the mat and left on suitable bedding, dirt, sand, or grass until refloated the next day. Advance planning on location is important to the success of using flotation. Cows that can walk out into a pen may or may not be able to stand by the next day and may be refloated. Cows may need to be floated for up to 10 days in a row before they can get up by themselves. If cases are carefully selected to rule out fractures, severe traumatic stifle injuries, septic arthritis, and spinal cord compression, a recuperative success rate of up to 90% can be expected.[1730]

Flotation is most effective if applied early, before a downer cow develops serious myopathy and neuropathy. Studies have shown that flotation using the Aqualift is practical and effective, even when cattle have been down for 24 hours or longer and have a variety of serious problems.[1730]

REFERENCES

1719. Barlet JP, Davicco MJ: α-Hydroxycholecalciferol for treatment of the downer cow syndrome, *J Dairy Sci* 75:1253-1256, 1992.

1720. Bjorsell KA, Holtenius P, Jacobson SO: The downer cow syndrome in milk fever, *Acta Vet Scand* 10:36-43, 1969.

1721. Curtis RA, Cote JF, Willoughby RA: The downer cow syndrome: a complication, not a disease, *Mod Vet Pract* 51:25, 1975.

1722. Hallgren W: Studies of parturient paresis in dairy cows, *Nord Vet Med* 7:433, 1955.

1723. Waage S: Milk fever and the downer cow syndrome: prognostic factors at first treatment, Proceedings of the International Congress on Disease in Cattle, Tel Aviv, 1980.

1724. Jonsson G, Pehrson B: Studies on the downer syndrome in dairy cows, *Zentralbl Veterinarmed A* 16:757, 1969 (abstract).

1725. Cox VS al: Downer cow occurrence in Minnesota dairy herds, *Prev Vet Med* 4:249, 1982.

1726. Cox VS, McGrath CJ, Jorgensen SE: The role of pressure damage in the pathogenesis of the downer cow syndrome, *Am J Vet Res* 43:26-31, 1982.

1727. Gelberman RH et al: Tissue pressure threshold for peripheral nerve viability, *Clin Orthop* 178:285-291, 1983.

1728. Prasad B, Rathor SS, Wadhwa DR: A note on serum creatine phosphokinase and transaminases in downer cows, *Indian J Vet Med* 8:159-160, 1988.

1729. Smith BP et al: Down cows and hot tubs, *Proc ACVIM Forum* 12:652-655, 1994.

1730. Rasmussen AJ: Fysiurgisk behandling of lammelser hos Kvaeg, *Dansk Vet Tidsskr* 65:1018, 1982.

Mammary Gland Health and Disorders

JEFF W. TYLER

JAMES S. CULLOR

The modern dairy farm is a "food manufacturing facility." Every day it produces raw milk, dairy beef, and liquid and solid nutrients. Therefore, we must learn how to manage the facility on a daily basis for animal health and well-being, public health, environmental health, and its financial well-being. It is in the spirit of this philosophy that we present the information contained herein. We will begin by giving an overview of bovine mastitis and traditional approaches to diagnosis, treatment, and prevention. Then we will review information on colostrum and lactation itself.

BOVINE MASTITIS

The overall process of milk synthesis and secretion involves the supply of suitable precursors to the mammary gland, their transformation into milk, and its expulsion from the mammary gland. The immune defense mechanisms must respond in the face of changing mammary gland conditions between milkings and throughout lactational stages. This is a difficult task and must be met with optimal conditions for the dairy cow to reach high production levels on a consistent basis. Nutrition, hygiene, genetics, and environmental conditions influence the host's ability to respond to mastitis challenges.[1]

Mastitis is the single most common disease syndrome in adult dairy cows, accounting for 38% of all morbidity.[2] On an annual basis 3 of every 10 dairy cows have clinically apparent inflammation of the mammary gland. Of the affected cattle, 7% are culled and 1% will die as a consequence of the disease. The same survey presented data suggesting that more than 25% of all disease-related economic losses of dairy cattle can be directly attributed to mastitis. Although similar data are not available for goats, infections of the mammary gland are common problems in dairy animals and occur in all livestock species.

Mastitis may result from the introduction of microorganisms through the teat sphincter. The clinical course of the disease varies with the ability of bacteria to colonize and thrive in the mammary gland secretions; their inherent virulence; and the type, magnitude, and duration of the host response to the bacterial invasion. The resulting inflammation of the mammary gland is indicated by a wide variety of clinical signs. However, common pathogenic mechanisms may permit the development of systematic treatment, control, and preventive measures. The National Mastitis Council (http://www.nmconline.org) recommends a time-proven five-point control program to solve this disease problem: (1) milking machine maintenance, (2) teat dipping, (3) early treatment of clinical cases, (4) dry cow therapy, and (5) culling of cows with chronic mastitis.

In general, mastitis can be subdivided into two broad and overlapping categories (contagious and environmental) on the basis of the source of the infectious inoculum.

Contagious mastitis has the infected mammary gland quarter as its primary reservoir. Thus this type of mastitis results when bacteria are transferred from an infected mammary gland to a healthy one by contaminated milking equipment, a nursing calf, or the hands of dairy employees. *Streptococcus agalactiae, Corynebacterium bovis, Staphylococcus aureus,* and *Mycoplasma* spp. comprise the most commonly noted bacteria for this category. *S. agalactiae* is the pathogen that best falls under this classification, being an obligate parasite of the ruminant mammary gland. *S. aureus* and *Mycoplasma* spp. are capable of colonizing and persisting in alternate host sites (skin, respiratory, and genitourinary tracts). Nevertheless, the most important mode of transmission of these organisms involves the cow-to-cow transfer of bacteria-laden milk. As mentioned above, an overall strategy to control contagious

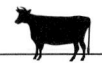

mastitis includes teat dipping, dry cow and lactating cow therapy, culling, and proper maintenance of milking machine equipment.

MASTITIS CONTROL PRINCIPLES

Postmilking Disinfectant Teat Dips

The single most important procedure in the prevention of contagious mastitis is the consistent use of postmilking disinfectant teat dips. Teat dips are superior to spray applications because they provide optimal coverage and contact on the teat skin. Isolation of *C. bovis* from either bulk milk samples or samples collected from individual cows should be considered presumptive evidence of inadequate teat dip procedures. This particular minor pathogen is restricted to the streak canal, and consequently these infections are readily eliminated by disinfectant teat dips.

Predips (Barrier Dips)

Predipping is often employed as a measure of contagious mastitis control and as a means to meet the guidelines of the Pasteurized Milk Ordinance (PMO) that require milking a clean, dry, presanitized mammary gland. The predip contact time is usually recommended to be at least 30 seconds before the teat is wiped dry and the milking machine attached.[3]

Traditional teat dips will not decrease the incidence of clinical gram-negative mastitis. Most disinfectants function by killing potential pathogens that are transmitted to the streak canal during the milking act. Killing these bacteria will halt transmission of contagious pathogens like *S. agalactiae* and *S. aureus*. Because the bulk of environmental transmission occurs between milkings rather than at the time of milking, this short-term disinfection will not prevent environmental mastitis. Noteworthy among these novel teat dip preparations are the premilking application of disinfectants with residual activity and postmilking teat dips that function as a physical barrier and have the potential to decrease the incidence of environmental mastitis. These procedures are widely practiced in the dairy industry, but the evidence supporting these practices is less compelling than that supporting the use of postmilking disinfectant teat dips to control contagious mastitis. Each year the Research Committee of the National Mastitis Council helps provide a bibliography of research publications available on teat dips. It is recommended that you obtain this information for annual updates in the scientific literature.

Intramammary Dry Cow Antibiotic Therapy

The second critical procedure in controlling contagious mastitis pathogens is the use of intramammary dry cow therapy. Preparations used generally contain high doses of slow-release antibiotic preparations. This type of treatment is highly efficacious against *Streptococcus* spp., including *S. agalactiae*, and *Staphylococcus* spp. Efficacy against *S. aureus* is limited; approximately 50% of such infections will be cured by dry cow therapy. Dry cow therapy has no efficacy against gram-negative or *Mycoplasma* spp. infections.

In summary, the best control for contagious mastitis is to break the chain of transmission for the infectious agent. This may be accomplished by eliminating the source of infection (the infected mammary gland), by treatment, or by isolation and strict sanitation at the time of milking.

Environmental mastitis results when bacteria with reservoirs of infection distinct from the mammary gland (the environment of the cow, i.e., bedding, corrals) gain entrance to the gland and cause disease. This type of mastitis occurs at an in-creasing rate when contagious mastitis is brought under control. Thus clinical mastitis caused by environmental pathogens becomes most prevalent in well-managed herds with low somatic cell counts (SCCs). Organisms that cause environmental mastitis do not require the presence of an infected gland to perpetuate within a herd. Contaminated bedding, water, fecal material, or fomites may all harbor and nurture bacterial populations capable of causing disease if introduced into the mammary gland. Gram-negative coliform bacteria that are representative of this category of mastitis pathogens include *Escherichia coli*, *Klebsiella* spp., and *Enterobacter* spp. Other gram-negative organisms of clinical significance include *Pseudomonas*, *Serratia*, and *Proteus*. Several species of environmental streptococci may be involved in this category of mastitis; however, *Streptococcus uberis* is the one most commonly isolated and identified. The presence of an environmental reservoir does not preclude cow-to-cow transfer; however, this mode of infection is probably minor.

Control of Environmental Mastitis

Environmental mastitis control is more problematic and does not respond to contagious mastitis control programs. Therefore, reducing the exposure of the teat ends to environmental pathogens and maximizing the resistance of the cow to intramammary infections are the critical strategies to be implemented for the control of environmental mastitis. Populations of environmental bacteria and their contact with the mammary gland may be restricted but never eliminated. In direct contrast to contagious mastitis syndromes, transmission typically occurs between milkings, rather than at the time of milking. Additionally, the source or reservoir of infectious bacteria is not the mammary gland of infected cows, but rather the farm environment. The vast majority of environmental pathogens will thrive, multiply, and persist in the environment with or without the presence of cattle. Consequently, prevention of environmental mastitis is premised upon prevention of the transmission of potential pathogens from the environment to the mammary gland, rather than the identification and treatment or isolation of infected cows. This is most often accomplished by optimal sanitation: clean housing, clean bedding, and use of free stall housing designs.

Complicating matters is the existence of pathogens occupying the space where contagious and environmental pathogens overlap. This group contains the bacteria that are shed in appreciable numbers in the milk of infected cows and maintain alternate niches (either within the host or the environment). Either may serve as the source of an infectious inoculum. Representative bacteria include *S. uberis* and *S. dysgalactiae*.

Economic Considerations

Clinical mastitis cases that occur early in lactation result in the greatest economic losses. Subclinical and clinical mastitis cause significant and appreciable economic losses through decreased milk production, discarded milk, treatment costs, and replacement of dead or nonproductive individuals.[4,5] Although several investigators have reported varying relationships between increased milk SCCs, Raubertas and Shook[6] observed that each doubling of the average lactation SCC above 50,000 is associated with a 400-lb production loss per lactation in mature cows and a 200-lb production loss in first lactation cows.

Milking Hygiene and Milking Practices

Because contagious mastitis infections are spread between cows at the time of milking, particular attention and focus must be placed on how cows are handled at that time. Any

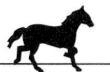

object which moves among cows can potentially function as a fomite. This includes milkers' hands, towels used for premilking disinfection, milking machine liners, and strip cups. As a general rule, no object or surface should be carried from cow to cow without prior disinfection. Improperly functioning milking machines, which permit reverse milk flows, have the potential to transmit infections from cow to cow. Detailed discussions of milking hygiene are available from the National Mastitis Council.

Although milking hygiene is not a primary component of environmental mastitis control programs, specific failures in milking hygiene are occasionally responsible for outbreaks of environmental mastitis. Excessive water use in the premilking preparation of the mammary gland will mobilize skin contaminant bacteria and increase contamination of teat ends during milking. Additionally, water sources or low-flow wash-water delivery systems can become colonized by bacteria, which may function as environmental mastitis pathogens. Noteworthy among these bacteria are *Serratia* spp., which have been associated with point-source outbreaks of clinical mastitis when wash water or teat dips become heavily contaminated. It should be noted that the practice of washing teats and the mammary gland before each milking is required by the PMO as a food safety and aesthetic precaution.

Feeding Strategies

Feeding strategies are an important component of environmental mastitis control programs. The streak canal remains open for a variable but relatively short time period after each milking, closing within two hours postmilking.[7] Consequently, strategies which will maintain hygiene of the teat ending immediately after milking will reduce the incidence of environmental mastitis. Providing fresh, palatable feedstuffs after each milking will increase the interval that cows remain standing and enhance teat-end hygiene.[8]

Nutrition

Proper nutrition is critical for the cow to maintain optimal immune function and disease resistance. In particular, vitamin E and selenium deficiencies have been associated with an increased incidence of clinical gram-negative mastitis.[9] This pattern of increased disease susceptibility does not appear to hold true for gram-positive mastitis. When environmental mastitis is present in a herd, all of the cows should receive a balanced diet including micronutrient supplementation. This includes those that are dry or non-lactating. Blood selenium and vitamin E concentrations can be measured during late gestation and early lactation.[10,11]

Bedding and Housing Management

Bedding materials used in free stall and stanchion or tie stall barns should be comfortable, dry, and biologically inert. Organic materials, such as wood shavings or straw, are both comfortable and dry; however, bacteria will actively grow in these materials when they are inevitably inoculated and contaminated by dirt or fecal material. Wood shavings are often blamed for *Klebsiella* spp. mastitis outbreaks; however, dry wood products are acceptable as bedding, particularly if the product has been kiln dried before use. Straw or chopped straw is often blamed for *Streptococcus* spp. mastitis outbreaks. Sand is probably an optimal bedding material, but many waste handling systems are susceptible to the abrasive properties of sand bedding. Regardless of the bedding material used care should be taken to maintain clean, comfortable stalls. Stalls should be sized in such a manner that urine and fecal material are deposited outside, rather than within the stall area. Feces and soiled bedding should be removed from stalls once or twice per day. Removal of feces will remove a ready source of nutrients for bacterial growth and the source of bacterial inoculation of bedding materials. Fecal material has a relatively low bacteria load (10^3 to 10^5 bacteria per gram). Aged bedding material will often have bacterial concentrations exceeding 10^7 bacteria per gram.

Milking Machine Function

The milking machine can serve as a fomite for the transmission of contagious mastitis.[12] Additionally, improperly functioning milking systems will damage teats and increase cow susceptibility to mastitis-causing bacteria. Milking machines should provide an appropriate and stable teat-end vacuum. Adequate pulsation rates should be maintained to permit a regular rest or massage phase of adequate length.[13] Plastic or rubber parts, particularly liners, must be replaced frequently. Stray voltage should not be permitted in the milking environment. The topic of milking machine function and maintenance exceeds the scope of this chapter. The reader is referred to alternative sources for detailed discussions of this topic. The National Mastitis Council provides readily accessible articles for this on its website at http://www.nmconline.org/. Veterinarians and farmers unfamiliar with this topic should ensure that dairy equipment company personnel service milking machines on a routine basis.

Prevention of Opportunistic Infections

This intermediate family of mastitis pathogens can function either as environmental or contagious pathogens. Consequently, control programs for these bacteria will typically include the components of both environmental and contagious mastitis control programs described in following sections. In contrast with environmental mastitis control programs, neither vaccines nor optimal vitamin E and selenium nutrition has been demonstrated to reduce the incidence of these infections. In contrast to contagious mastitis syndromes, efforts at case finding and treatment should be avoided in lactating cows.

GENERAL CLASSIFICATIONS OF CONTAGIOUS AND ENVIRONMENTAL MASTITIS

Inflammation of the mammary gland, mastitis, is almost always infectious and can be classified as either subclinical or clinical. Microbial infections involving *S. aureus*, *S. agalactiae*, *S. dysgalactiae*, *S. uberis*, coliform organisms, *Pseudomonas* spp., *Mycoplasma* spp., and other pathogens cause serious problems for the dairy industry. Faulty milking machine function, poor environmental sanitation, improper milking procedures, or teat trauma frequently lead to infection because of reduced natural defenses and/or increased exposure to infectious agents that can overwhelm the defense capability.

Subclinical mastitis occurs when the mammary gland is infected and the number of leukocytes (somatic cells) is increased. In this condition the milk appears grossly normal, and there is no visible sign of inflammation in the mammary gland. Subclinical mastitis is detected by routine tests such as the California Mastitis Test (CMT), SCCs reported in Dairy Herd Improvement Association (DHIA) records, or routine culturing of all quarters. With time, most types of subclinical infections result in fibrosis of mammary tissue, a firmer and larger gland, and decreased milk production. Subclinical mastitis is most commonly associated with *S. agalactiae* and *S. aureus*.

Clinical mastitis is characterized by grossly abnormal milk and evidence of varying degrees of mammary gland inflam-

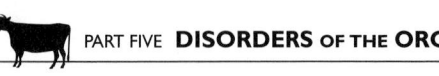

mation (redness, heat, swelling, pain). The milk can vary from having a few milk clots (garget) to serum with clumps of fibrin in the secretion. Clinical mastitis can be further categorized into acute mastitis, acute gangrenous mastitis, and chronic active mastitis.

Acute Mastitis

Acute mastitis is often characterized by a swollen, painful gland that may be edematous or very hard, making it difficult for the patient to walk normally. If some mild flare-ups of *S. agalactiae* or *S. aureus* occur, the milk can be abnormal, but no other abnormalities may be noted. Systemic signs may be slight or severe, with a sudden onset. Anorexia, depression, and elevated rectal temperature are often associated with this clinical event. Severe, toxic cases may have low serum calcium and paraplegia resembling milk fever. The associated hypocalcemia is largely nonresponsive to parenteral calcium administration. The secretions might contain flakes or clots of milk and can be watery, serous, or purulent. Acute mastitis cases can be new infections or exacerbations of chronic infections. Most new infections with environmental pathogens (gram-negative bacteria, *S. dysgalactiae*, and *S. uberis*) are generally eliminated in a few days to 3 weeks, whereas some pathogens (e.g., *Klebsiella*) tend to persist for longer periods. Contagious pathogens tend to persist as subclinical infections.

Acute Gangrenous Mastitis

Fortunately, gangrenous mastitis is not a common event. The patient exhibits anorexia, dehydration, depression, fever, and signs of toxemia. The etiologic agent is primarily staphylococci, with involvement of one to four quarters. Infections caused by *Clostridium, Staphylococcus,* and coliforms sometimes result in gangrenous mastitis. The gland is red, swollen, and warm early in the disease. However, within a few hours the teat becomes cold, and the secretions watery and sanguineous. The gland soon exhibits an area of sharply delineated blue discoloration in the region extending from the teat to various parts of the gland. Sloughing of this area occurs within 10 to 14 days and is followed by secondary bacterial infections, necrosis, and continued sloughing of most of the glandular tissue in the affected quarter(s). The organisms most commonly associated with gangrenous mastitis are *S. aureus* and *Clostridium perfringens.*

Chronic Mastitis

Patients with this form of mastitis may exhibit no clinical signs for prolonged intervals. Events that are not well characterized may, from time to time, exacerbate the chronic infection, causing clinical signs of an acute infection. SCCs are generally chronically elevated, and the mammary gland secretions periodically contain flakes, clots, or shreds of fibrin. In the chronic type of mastitis, prolonged destruction of mammary gland alveoli and ducts, with replacement by scar tissue, results in reduced milk-producing capabilities. The bacteria that are commonly associated with this type of infection are coliforms, *S. agalactiae,* and *S. aureus. Salmonella dublin* mastitis has also been shown to persist in this manner.

MICROBIOLOGIC TECHNIQUES FOR DIAGNOSIS OF MAMMARY GLAND INFECTION

Implementation of routine culturing of mammary gland secretions is supported for the following reasons:
1. The prevalence of subclinical mastitis in dairy herds is often a surprise to the owner or veterinarian and may have

significant impact on the productivity and profitability of the herd.
2. Determining the etiology of individual animal or herd outbreaks of clinical mastitis is important for developing management strategies to reduce the number of new mastitis cases and to improve the prognosis for the patients already affected by the pathogens. It is important to initiate a program of routine milk culturing when one or more of the following benchmarks occur:
   - Bulk tank SCCs are >250,000.
   - DHIA-SCCs reveal that >15% of lactating cows in the herd have a linear score (LS) >4.5.
   - New clinical cases in the herd are >2% per month.
   - Acutely ill cows in the herd are >1% per year.

Although the precise etiology of the infection may be difficult to ascertain, accurate microbiologic determination is most appropriately obtained through milk cultures and not by variations in the discoloration of the milk. The results of milk culture are no better than the sample; and the sample is no better than the manner in which it is collected, transported, and processed. Useful references for microbiologic procedures for the diagnosis of bovine mastitis are readily available for implementation in veterinary practice.[14,15]

Sample Collection

1. Prepare sterile glass or plastic tubes of at least 15-ml capacity. The tubes must have appropriate tight-fitting caps to minimize contamination and leakage once the container has been sealed.
2. Collect samples just before milking (foremilk) to enhance the detection of intramammary infections. Foremilk usually contains more mastitis organisms than milk taken during milking.
3. After washing the udder and teats, dry the mammary gland thoroughly with a single-use paper towel. Before drying, excessive wash water should have time to run off the mammary gland. Stripping each teat two or three times initiates milk letdown and helps to rid the streak canal of chance contaminants.
4. Sample each quarter individually, or take milk from all four quarters to obtain a single (composite) sample. The latter method is often used for herd tests to identify infected cows. Scrub each teat end and orifice thoroughly with a separate absorbent cotton ball or cloth gauze section moistened with 70% alcohol (ethyl or isopropyl). Repeat this procedure if the wipe is visibly soiled after adequate teat scrubbing. A practical tip is to clean and disinfect the teats on the far side of the gland first and to sample in reverse order; this reduces the potential for contamination.
5. Grip the tube in a manner that allows it to be held close to a horizontal plane during filling, and hold the cap with its inside facing downward. Do not allow the teat end to contact the container. The container should be filled approximately half full (5 to 10 ml) and then sealed.
6. Rinse the hands, preferably gloved, in a germicidal solution and thoroughly dry them after each animal sampled. Alternatively, one can change to clean disposable gloves after sampling each animal.

Sample Transport

In situations where the interval from collection to processing of samples may exceed 15 to 30 minutes, the samples should be cooled to 4° to 5° C until culture procedures are performed. Freezing of milk samples precludes their use to determine SCCs; however, they may still be used for culture as-

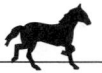

says. Gelation-based assays, the CMT, or the Wisconsin Mastitis Test may be performed following frozen storage. Each freeze-thaw manipulation of a sample reduces the numbers of recoverable bacteria, especially coliform bacteria. Samples should not be repeatedly frozen and thawed. Recovery of staphylococci, however, might be enhanced by a single freeze-thaw cycle. Isolation of most of the common mastitis pathogens is not affected when samples are stored at 4° C for one week or stored frozen. A decline in survival of some bacterial species can be expected with samples handled in this manner, impeding estimates of original bacterial concentrations.

Routine Culture of Clinical Samples

One of the most useful infection-monitoring systems is to culture all quarters with clinical mastitis. Samples are taken before therapy is given. This is the only way to determine the true causes of clinical mastitis in the herd and their relative importance. Because coliform infections are of short duration and often result in clinical mastitis, they often cause most of the cases, even in herds that have a high rate of chronic staphylococcal or streptococcal infections. Culture of all clinical cases often reveals the presence of *S. agalactiae, S. aureus,* or mycoplasma infections in herds believed to be free of infection due to these organisms.

Routine culture of all clinical cases also provides an opportunity for antibiotic susceptibility testing to guide future treatment recommendations for the herd. Samples for culture should be taken before the first treatment and refrigerated or frozen until taken to the laboratory. If clinical samples are not cultured routinely, certainly they should be cultured as often as possible, especially whenever mastitis with an unusual clinical course is encountered. Approximately 25% to 30% of clinical samples will show negative culture results. It is probable that many of these come from cows with coliform infections that have already been controlled by the animal's own defenses.

Herd Test Cultures

Culture of milk from all cows in a herd is indicated most often when *S. agalactiae, S. aureus, Mycoplasma bovis,* or some other contagious pathogen is known to be a problem in the herd. The object is to identify infected cows for segregation and/or treatment (e.g., *S. agalactiae*). Because each cow is handled as a unit, diagnosis by individual quarters may not be important in such cases, at least not initially. The task of sample collection, culturing, and record keeping is substantially reduced by collection of composite samples (i.e., a sample from each quarter in one collection tube).

Selected Survey Cultures

Microbiologic testing of cattle selected on the basis of elevated SCCs is sometimes done by producers or veterinarians when the DHIA-SCC linear score for an individual animal is >4.5. This may be interpreted that the animal has an SCC of >300,000. Although SCC targeted testing may increase the chances of obtaining positive cultures, such a selection procedure will fail to identify all infected cattle. The range of SCCs from healthy and infected cattle markedly overlap, particularly in the case of *S. aureus* mastitis.

An alternate procedure that may be beneficial at the inception of a mastitis control program is microbiologic screening of: (1) all cows that have recently freshened, (2) all clinical cases of mastitis, and (3) bulk tank cultures at least once per month. Information regarding mastitis prevalence and etiology of the herd problem permits the rational design of control or eradication programs with an economy of effort.

Bulk Tank Milk Cultures

Monitoring the herd health status of a dairy by routine monthly culturing of bulk tank milk has become an important management tool for the dairy producer to assess the milk bacterial profile in the herd. This screening method should be used on four consecutive days to account for the daily variation in shedding rates of *S. aureus*.[16] This technique provides the herd health team with an additional convenient and inexpensive means to monitor the parameters of milk quality and the mastitis status in a herd on a monthly basis.[17] The approach of bulk tank monitoring at the herd level can enable the investigator to recognize new or emerging problems and to identify the possibility of a milk residue accumulation in the milking equipment.

PLATING OF MILK SAMPLES

1. Gently invert or shake sample to thoroughly mix the milk. Those samples to be submitted for SCCs should not be vortexed because the procedure can rupture white cells.
2. After removing the container cap, insert a sterile swab and swirl it to the bottom of the tube. Discard any milk-laden swab that makes contact with any item such as the exterior of the container, the counter top, a hand, or clothing. If an estimate of bacteria numbers is desired, a calibrated loop may be used.
3. Many techniques are described for streaking the sample onto the test plate. One pattern for use with quarter samples is to mark the plate into four quadrants on the bottom exterior of the 5% washed bovine blood agar (BBA) plate and label them by quarter sample (right front = A, right rear = B, left front = C, left rear = D). Remove the lid of the BBA plate, and streak a line of milk down the center of the quadrant. Next, streak in a side-to-side motion across the quadrant up to but not across quadrant borders. The CAMP test may be performed in conjunction with initial isolation procedures. Sterile *S. aureus* hemolysin is dotted or streaked across each quadrant of the blood agar plate before plating, thus permitting presumptive identification of *S. agalactiae*. Half plates should be used for composite samples, and entire plates for bulk tank samples.
4. The same streaking procedure can be applied to samples being examined for growth on mycoplasma plates. Remember, mycoplasma agar may have inhibitors (penicillin, ampicillin, thallium acetate) that may interfere with organism growth on BBA plates. It is therefore advisable to streak the BBA plates first; then the same swab can be used on the mycoplasma agar.
5. Identification of specific pathogens should proceed according to the flow chart (Fig. 34-1).

Interpretation of Milk Microbiology Results

Assuming the sample has been handled in a manner that would eliminate contamination, interpretation of the bulk tank culture results must be carefully considered before recommendations are given to the producer. For instance, the absence of a positive culture result on a single sample must not be interpreted to mean that a pathogen is not present in the herd, although the rate of shedding would be low. If *S. agalactiae* and *S. aureus* are present in the bulk tank sample, it can be interpreted to mean that they originate from infected cows. The shedding of these organisms is highly variable among animals; therefore the percentage of infected cows in a herd does not consistently correlate well with the number of organisms recovered from the bulk tank sample. Strepto-

1. Cocci

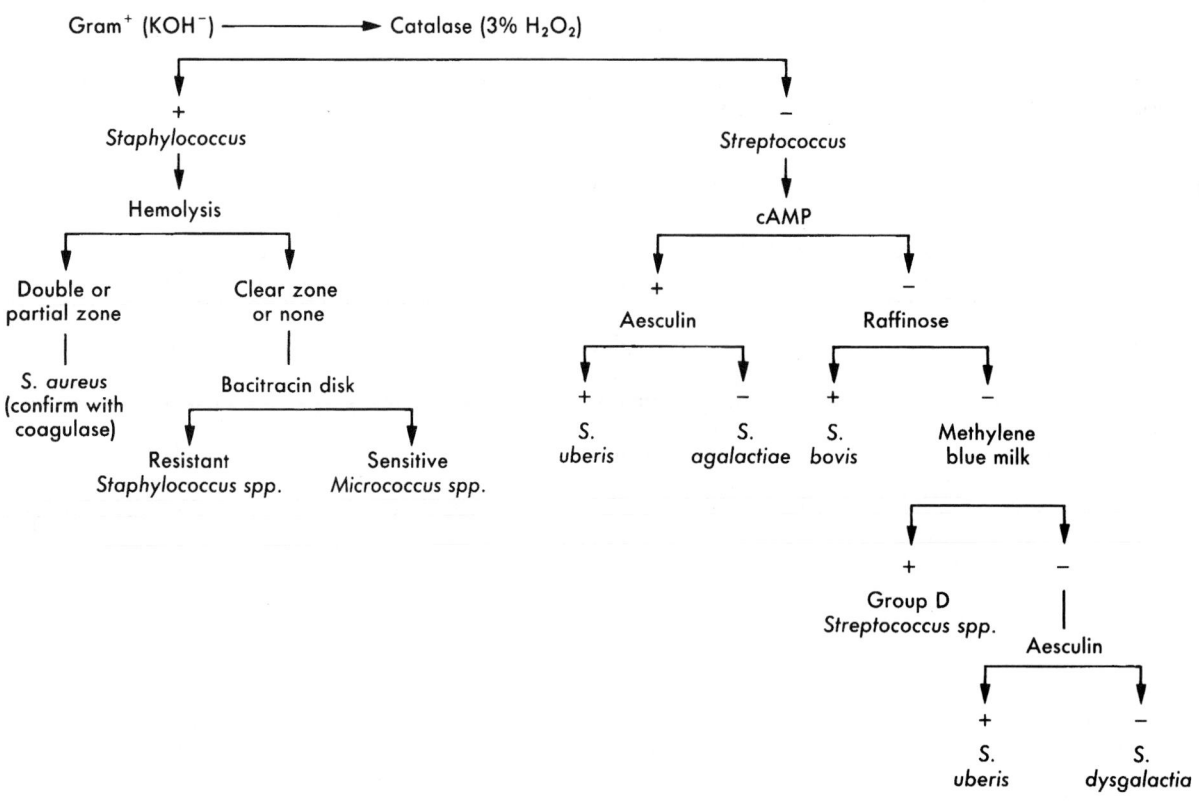

2. Rods

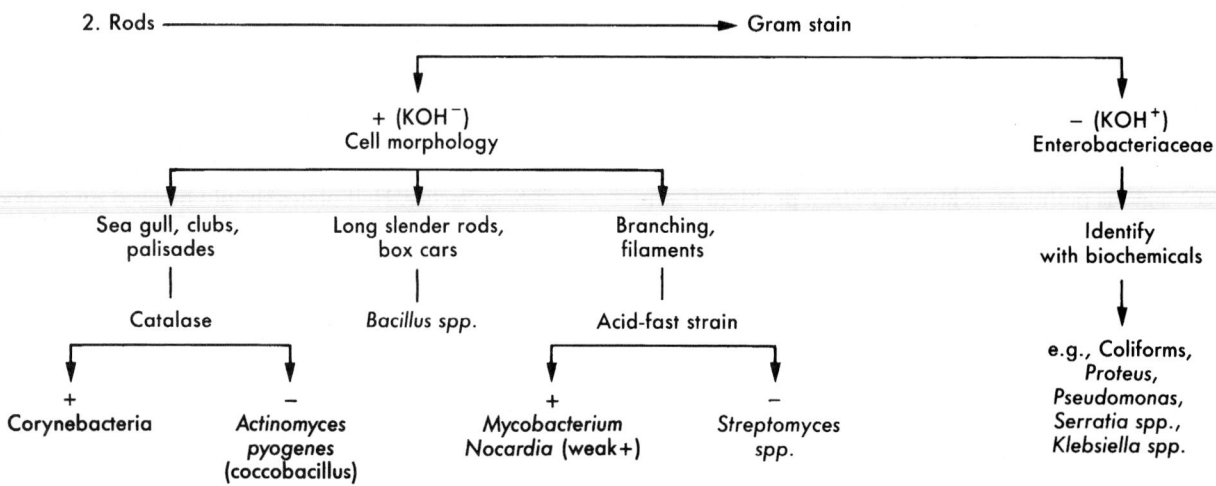

3. Large, irregular forms ⟶ Gram⁺ (KOH⁻) ⟶ Barrel-shaped or football-shaped
wet mount = reproductive structure, budding yeast

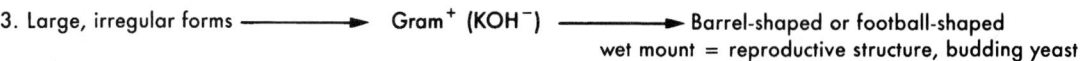

FIG. 34-1 ▌ Identification key for microorganisms from bovine mammary gland secretions. (Modified from Thurmond MC: *Laboratory procedures for the examination of milk quality,* ed 2, David, Calif, 1987, published by the author.)

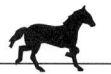

cocci other than *S. agalactiae* and coagulase-negative *Staphylococcus* spp. are found in the cow's environment; thus the teat skin may be the primary source of these organisms. The degree of bedding contamination and/or poor milking hygiene tends to correlate well with bulk tank numbers of coliform bacteria.

The isolation of a single colony of *S. agalactiae, S. aureus,* or *Mycoplasma* spp. is generally considered diagnostic of intramammary infection. This high degree of diagnostic significance is dictated by (1) the intimate relationship of these organisms with the mammary gland, rather than the farm environment as a whole, and (2) their potential for rapid cow-to-cow transmission. Both of these factors tend to place a premium on diagnostic sensitivity (assay detection limit). The remaining isolates often associated with intramammary infection have significant environmental reservoirs. Consequently, isolation of these organisms may result either from a sampling contaminant or from actual intramammary infection. The diagnostic significance of bacteria with environmental reservoirs is premised on four criteria: (1) concentration of bacteria in the milk sample, (2) purity of culture, (3) evidence of intramammary inflammation (elevated CMT), and (4) presence of the organism on repeated sampling.

In summary, the organisms cultured from bulk tank sampling methodologies thought to come almost exclusively from the mammary gland are *Mycoplasma* spp., *S. aureus,* and *S. agalactiae.* Problems with refrigeration of the milk, poor milking hygiene, or samples obtained from the hose port of the bulk tank generally result in increased bacterial counts in bulk tank milk samples. Coagulase-negative staphylococci cultured from bulk tank samples may be contaminants from the environment or from infection. Other organisms that come from the environment or the wash water are Corynebacteria, bacilli, and yeasts and may cause some bulk tank samples to show positive culture results. A nonchlorophyll-forming algae, *Prototheca,* commonly thrives in standing water and may infect the mammary gland. It is spread from cow to cow via infected quarters.

Most bulk tank samples yield a negative or trace reading when using the CMT; thus it is considered not adequately sensitive for routine evaluation. Automated SCC determination is the assay of choice for bulk tank milk. The procedures used for bulk tank milk interpretation are discussed by Guterbock and Blackmer.[18]

SPECIFIC MASTITIS INFECTIONS

Staphylococcal Infections

The main source of staphylococcal infection is the milk secreted by adult cows with infected quarters. Contaminated milking equipment and milkers' hands are common sources of transmission. Staphylococci have also been cultured from the skin of the udder, the teats, and other parts of the body. Introduction of mastitis-causing *Staphylococcus* spp. into uninfected herds generally takes place when infected animals are aquired or from handling by attendants previously in contact with infected cows. One or more quarters generally become subclinically infected, with severe mastitis developing only occasionally.

CLINICAL SIGNS. Most *S. aureus* infections are chronic subclinical infections with occasional clinical flare-ups that are usually mild or moderate. *S. aureus* can also produce severe mastitis with systemic signs of illness, particularly at parturition or during the first month of lactation. Systemic signs include anorexia, depression, toxemia, elevated body temperature, and recumbency. Swelling, firmness, subcutaneous edema, redness, heat, and pain may extend along the mammary vein. Alterations in the appearance of the mammary se-

cretions begin with the presence of flakes and clots. The degree of abnormal milk characteristics can vary. The secretion can become creamy or pus-like as the disease progresses, at which point it may then become watery. The most common form of staphylococcal mastitis is a chronic, relatively mild disease characterized by an occasional acute or subacute flare-up at parturition, which reverts to a subclinical state.

In a few cases of *S. aureus* infection, particularly those that occur in the immediate postpartum period, a gangrenous mastitis may occur due to the staphylococcal α–toxin. This form of the disease has also been reported in sheep and goats. Vasoconstriction, ischemia, and death of the tissue occur. The quarter becomes markedly swollen, followed within hours to days by cold areas, and the teat and adjacent areas of the udder become blue or black. Although arterial flow remains intact, thrombosis of large veins generally leads to a moist gangrene with continuous dripping of blood-tinged serum from the teat and the skin around the base of the teat. Amputation of the affected teat facilitates drainage and sloughing. Although mortality can often be prevented by aggressive treatment, the cow loses weight and will have decreased milk production in the unaffected quarters. In most cases convalescence is protracted, and sloughing of tissue occurs for many weeks. Subsequent lactations with two or three functional quarters may result in partial recovery of milk production. Recovered cows are often sold for slaughter.

PREVENTION AND CONTROL. Staphylococcal mastitis must be considered a herd problem. Ignoring the infection will damage the productive capacity of the farm. The treatment of isolated clinical cases is of little or no value; the efficacy of current lactating cow antimicrobial therapy is clearly limited. Although intramammary dry cow therapy offers improved cure rates, the high incidence of treatment failures prevents this procedure from forming the basis for an effective control program. Dry cow therapy is useful in reducing the incidence of new infections. Staphylococcal mastitis is a contagious disease spread from cow to cow at the time of milking. Although skin or fomites may harbor the organism, milk from an infected cow must be considered the principal source of new infections. Control measures logically target the transmission from diseased to noninfected cattle in the milking parlor or barn. Effective procedures can be broadly categorized as either sanitation or segregation.

Using single-service paper towels and cleaning milkers' hands and milking units in germicidal solutions between cows are commonly used procedures. Automatic backflush equipment is an integral component of many newer milking facilities. Properly functioning milking equipment minimizes the reverse flow of potentially contaminated milk and reduces trauma to the teat end. A thorough analysis of milking machine performance, including vacuum levels, vacuum reserve, pulsation rates, and pulsation ratios must be considered an integral part of any mastitis control program. The use of germicidal teat dip solutions immediately after milking reduces the potential for skin or teat canal contamination from progressing to intramammary infection.

The physical separation of infected and noninfected cattle eliminates the source and spread of infection from diseased cows, resulting in a decrease in the rate of new infections. Such isolation procedures can be accomplished either by culling infected cattle or segregating the herd into culture-positive and culture-negative management groups or some combination thereof. The decision as to whether one should cull an infected cow or manage it by isolation is influenced by the prevalence of infection in the herd, the availability of replacement stock, physical makeup of the facility, and the level of management expertise. At the present time, culling chronically infected cows or segregating the herd into staphylococci-positive and staphylococci-negative groups following culture of composite milk samples from all cows, together with improved milking hygiene, is an effective approach to reducing the rate of new infections. Often infected cows are segregated from the clean cows permanently and culled as their economic value dictates. Infected cows are always milked after the uninfected cows.

Herds need to be screened to identify new cases of S. aureus infection. This requires the testing of composite milk samples from cows with high SCCs and group samples from penned stock. A sampling frequency of every six weeks should be considered. Many variations of sampling schedules can be arranged to suit the situation. All clinical cases of mastitis, all purchased cows, and all fresh cows and heifers should be routinely cultured, also. Cows with one or more quarters exhibiting scarring, fibrosis, and decreased milk production should be dried off and culled when they are no longer profitable. Dry cow therapy of infected cattle with currently available agents is of limited value in eliminating chronic Staphylococcus infection but should be followed in all cows because the procedure is useful in eliminating S. agalactiae and preventing some other new infections.

PUBLIC HEALTH SIGNIFICANCE. Certain strains of Staphylococcus may produce an enterotoxin that causes food poisoning. The enterotoxin is not formed within the mammary gland. It is produced when milk, milk products, or food prepared with milk products containing strains of bacteria associated with food poisoning is stored at temperatures that enhance rapid multiplication of the organisms. Some staphylococci that cause mastitis may also produce the enterotoxin.

Streptococcal Infections

S. agalactiae is a highly contagious, obligate infector of mammary glands that, in general, causes subclinical mastitis with periodic acute local inflammation. It remains on the epithelial surfaces, creating tissue damage during growth and multiplication and stimulating an inflammatory response. This organism does not invade the glandular tissue and survives for only short periods of time outside the mammary gland on the teat skin or other locations. It is transmitted from quarter to quarter and from cow to cow by fomites, calves, milking machines, or on the hands of personnel who have been contaminated with milk from infected glands.[19]

The pathology associated with this organism is similar to that previously described in chronic mastitis caused by S. aureus. In clinical flare-ups, polymorphonuclear neutrophils (PMNs) and serum proteins cause the formation of fibrin clots that block the ducts and prevent drainage of that area of the gland. The inflammatory response causes necrosis of the secretory tissue and replacement by fibrosis, resulting in decreased milk production.

The development of herd intervention strategies involves a balancing of long- and short-term benefits and costs. Rigorous application of milking hygiene procedures, teat dipping, and dry cow antimicrobial therapy will effectively reduce, if not eliminate, S. agalactiae infections over a period of time. Alternatively, whole herd cultures followed by intramammary treatment of infected cows with an effective antimicrobial drug have been reported to be efficacious in the initial phases of control programs. More aggressive programs entail additional costs in terms of culture procedures, antibiotics, and discarded milk. However, treatment during the first half of lactation has been found to be cost effective during that lactation. Benefits of more active control programs will include increased milk production following elimination of infection and elimination of reservoirs of infection.

S. dysgalactiae has a herd infection rate that is generally lower than S. agalactiae because S. dysgalactiae is not as contagious and is not an obligate pathogen. This organism is found in the environment and can live there for prolonged periods of time. Mammary infections with S. dysgalactiae often follow teat injury. Affected quarters may be rendered partially or completely nonfunctional. Treatment is somewhat less effective than treatment for S. agalactiae.

S. uberis, like S. dysgalactiae, is not an obligate mammary pathogen. It is resistant to cold temperatures and has been recovered from soil, bedding, bovine skin, udders, teats, lips, nostrils, and vagina. Mastitis caused by this organism is usually subclinical and transitory, but it can be an important cause of mastitis in a herd. A variety of other streptococci have been isolated from individual cases of bovine mastitis. These other streptococcal infections are generally environmental in origin and sporadic in incidence.

THERAPEUTIC CONSIDERATIONS. Always review the Animal Medicinal Drug Use Clarification Act (AMDUCA) guidelines before recommending antibiotic use. Streptococcal mastitis may be caused by S. agalactiae; however, other Streptococcus spp. may be present. Therefore adequate diagnostic evaluations must be performed before any treatments are prescribed. For S. agalactiae, intramammary administration of penicillin G is used at 100,000 units per quarter per dose. This is highly effective against this pathogen. Infections due to other streptococci usually respond to penicillin therapy, but sensitivity patterns are variable. Higher doses have been used in S. agalactiae eradication efforts; however, extended withholding times for milk and meat will result. Bulk tank milk should be checked for penicillin residues via laboratory methods that may include High Performance Liquid Chromatography (HPLC). Streptococcus spp. (other than S. agalactiae) are less amenable to eradication efforts because of the existence of environmental reservoirs. Control programs for these infections typically involve lactating cow therapy for clinical cases, routine dry cow therapy, and rigorous application of milking sanitation procedures.

PREVENTION AND CONTROL. S. agalactiae infections can be eliminated from most herds because this organism is an obligate inhabitant of the mammary gland, does not invade the tissues, and is susceptible to antibiotics. S. agalactiae is very susceptible to lactating or dry cow intramammary therapy. Milking sanitation previously detailed is an integral part of any control and eradication program.

Coliform Infections

Coliforms are an important group of environmental organisms that cause mastitis. The most frequent mastitis pathogens in this group are E. coli, Enterobacter aerogenes, and Klebsiella pneumoniae. Less common isolates include Pseudomonas aeruginosa, Pasteurella multocida, and Serratia marcescens.[20] Clinical manifestations by infections of one or more of the coliform group include acute, sometimes peracute, disease with high fevers, toxemia, and occasionally death due to generalized toxemia. Chronic active forms with periods of quiescence punctuated by periodic acute flare-ups may also occur.

Unlike in S. aureus or S. agalactiae mastitis, cow-to-cow transmission at the time of milking has minimum impact on the incidence of coliform mastitis. The source of infections is the environment. Infections can occur either at milking, between milking times, or during the dry period. The focus of control efforts centers not on the infected cow, but on general environmental sanitation and prevention of contamination of the teat end during the variable interval that the streak canal remains open following milking.

Improperly executing premilking sanitation procedures, particularly milking cows with wet udders, may dramatically increase the incidence of coliform mastitis. Contaminated wash water dripping off either the cow's back or udder carries bacteria to the teat end. If udders are hand washed, individual paper towels should be used, both to wash and dry the udder. If automatic wash pens are used, careful attention must be paid to their design and function. Sprinkler head angle should be sufficiently low, and cow density in the wash pen must be adequate to ensure that water is applied only to the cow's udder. Individual paper towels should be used to dry the udder before attaching the milking unit. In either case, excessive use of water should be avoided. Traditional postmilking teat dipping procedures have minimum efficacy in the prevention of coliform mastitis. Dipping teats in germicidal solutions before milking has been reported to reduce the population of contaminant skin flora and consequently reduce the incidence of infections of environmental origin. Further investigation will determine whether this procedure is an effective management technique. The potential for disinfectant residues in milk may limit predipping use in the future.

Coliform mastitis is related to exposure to bacterial populations in the environment. Bedding populations in excess of 1×10^6 bacteria per gram have been associated with increased clinical cases of coliform mastitis. Aesthetic cleanliness should not be confused with microbiologic hygiene. Apparently clean and wholesome bedding sources may have bacteria counts exceeding those found in fresh fecal material. In general, ideal bedding materials are comfortable, dry, relatively inert, and, consequently, fail to support the proliferation of bacteria following inevitable contamination. Bedding composed of sawdust and shavings may harbor unsafe levels of coliform bacteria, whereas inorganic bedding materials such as sand harbor a much lower bacterial population. Provision of fresh, palatable feedstuffs immediately following milking helps to ensure that cows will remain standing until the closure of the streak canal, thereby reducing the incidence of coliform mastitis.

In the event that a unique isolate is consistently recovered from several clinical cases, a common source of exposure should be suspected. Procedures available to characterize such isolates include antimicrobial sensitivity, biochemical reactions, and serologic assays. These procedures may exceed the capability of laboratories in many practices. Contamination of wash water or teat dip solutions and the colonization of teat cup inflations by these organisms has led to point source coliform mastitis outbreaks. However, most herd problems are related to the general level of farm sanitation rather than to a single source of infection.

THERAPEUTIC CONSIDERATIONS. Spontaneous recovery without treatment is a common course for most cases of coliform mastitis. However, some cases become very severe, with acute toxicity and sometimes death of the patient. Therapeutic regimens in severe cases of coliform mastitis must be initiated early in the disease process.[21] No published regimen has emerged as clearly superior to all others. Frequent milking (i.e., every two hours) to eliminate toxins, inflammatory mediators, and bacteria is the most important measure in the treatment of coliform mastitis.

The cow exhibiting clinical toxic shock requires additional symptomatic support beyond antimicrobial therapy. Various regimens of normal electrolyte therapy administered via intravenous drip, hypertonic saline administration, corticosteroid therapy, and nonsteroidal antiinflammatory compounds administered via the intravenous route have been recommended. *Warning:* If corticosteroids are used, the chances of bacteremia are increased.[22] Data strongly suggest that mammary gland health status can be altered by sudden exposure of blood neutrophils to glucocorticoids because these steroid hormones cause profound down-regulation of the adhesion molecules that direct neutrophil margination and migration through the vascular endothelium. The total volume of fluids for supportive therapy (40 to 110 ml/kg) should be given to the adult bovine at the initial rate of 5 to 10 L/hr during the

first two hours, followed by a rate of 5 L/hr. Metabolic acidosis may be present in severe cases. Sodium bicarbonate therapy should not be used unless serum acid-base balance is measured and base deficit can be calculated. Administration of large amounts of bicarbonate in the absence of severe metabolic acidosis can result in severe metabolic alkalosis. Calculation of the amount of bicarbonate needed is based on bicarbonate space volume being approximately 50% of body weight (0.50 × body weight in kg × base deficit = mEq of bicarbonate required). The total dosage of sodium bicarbonate should not exceed 250 g in a concentration not greater than 5% (1.3% $NaHCO_3$ is isotonic), followed by isotonic fluids.

Some patients become hypocalcemic during the course of the disease. Careful administration of calcium solutions may be undertaken if serum biochemistry values warrant such therapeutic measures. These patients are very susceptible to cardiac dysrhythmias and subsequent cardiac failure if intravenous calcium is administered too rapidly. Therefore, either subcutaneous administration or dilution in large volumes of intravenous fluids are considered the safest routes.

ENDOTOXIC MEDIATOR SHOCK. In most cases the severe systemic manifestations of acute coliform mastitis are not related to the presence of a circulating bacteremia. Cattle with acute gram-negative mastitis have uniformly negative blood culture results. Rather, generalized clinical signs are referable to the endotoxin-mediated release of endogenous inflammatory mediators (e.g., eicosanoids, histamine, serotonin). Involvement of vasoactive amines such as histamine and serotonin in the early phases of acute inflammation is clearly documented. Elevated concentrations of histamine are present in the milk of cows with mastitis and in rabbits with mastitis, resulting from *E. coli* inoculation. Increases in concentrations of prostaglandin (PG) $F_{2\alpha}$, PGE_2, and thromboxane B_2 (TXB_2) are present in the milk of cows with clinical and experimental *E. coli* mastitis. An experimental intramammary challenge with varying doses of live *K. pneumoniae* produced increased levels of milk serotonin, histamine, PGF_2, PGE_2, TXB_2, and a subsequent elevated level of plasma PGF_2. The clinical signs following endotoxin-induced release of eicosanoids is responsible for many pathophysiologic changes including shock, pulmonary hypertension, elevated temperature, abortion, diarrhea, and inflammation. These effects may be ameliorated to some degree by nonsteroidal antiinflammatory compounds (acetylsalicylic acid, flunixin, phenylbutazone, indomethacin, and ibuprofen) if administered early in the course of disease.

Mycoplasma Infections

Causative organisms of Mycoplasma mastitis in the United States has been reported to include at least five different species of this organism (*M. bovis, M. californicum, M. canadensis, M. bovigenitalium,* and *M. alkalescens*). The clinical course of mycoplasma mastitis differs from other common mastitis syndromes in the probable existence of a systemic phase of the disease process. This finding has been confirmed by the rapid spread of the disease to unaffected quarters and joints and the isolation of organisms from a variety of tissues and body fluids coincidental with intramammary infection. The systemic phase of mycoplasma mastitis raises the possibility for modes of infection other than milk-borne transmission. The epidemiology and pathogenesis of mycoplasma mastitis are poorly understood at present. The concentration of reports in the southwestern United States and Florida (outbreaks have also been noted in New York, Massachusetts, Connecticut, and other states) and the common isolation of mycoplasma from the respiratory tract in herds with no history of mycoplasma mastitis suggest that unknown environmental or management factors promote the establishment and transmission of intramammary infections.[15]

Mastitis due to *M. bovis* is usually severe with marked changes in the secretions from watery to purulent. Clinical signs often are first noted in a single quarter and may spread until all four quarters produce grossly abnormal secretions. Clinical cases do not respond to currently available therapeutic agents, either by systemic or intramammary delivery. Milk secretion may cease until the next lactation. The patients are not systemically ill and continue to eat well. Mild forms of this exceptionally contagious disease occur. Clinical signs can be indistinguishable from mastitis caused by either staphylococci, streptococci, or gram-negative bacteria. Mycoplasma mastitis should be suspected in herds with a history of nonresponsive mastitis and negative milk cultures using standard microbiologic methods. Formulation of bulk mastitis treatments, where one syringe is used to inject multiple cows, and poor intramammary treatment hygiene have been associated with herd epidemics of mycoplasma mastitis. Particular care should be taken in the design of mastitis culture and treatment protocols in herds in which there is the history or suspicion of mycoplasma mastitis.

THERAPEUTIC CONSIDERATIONS. Although *Mycoplasma* spp. are susceptible in vitro to many antimicrobial agents, including tetracyclines, kanamycin, neomycin, gentamicin, and novobiocin, intramammary infusion of these agents has not effectively altered the expected course of the disease. Consequently, treatment has little beneficial effect and may only delay slaughter or sale of milk because of extended antibiotic residues.

PREVENTION AND CONTROL. Although mycoplasma mastitis is not amenable to therapeutic intervention, control measures used to control *S. agalactiae* and *S. aureus* will limit the spread of mycoplasma to nonaffected herdmates. If rigorously adhered to, teat dipping and proper milking procedures will reduce the incidence of new cases. Segregation and culling procedures previously described for *S. aureus* mastitis should also be considered and adopted if possible. Given the potential for explosive outbreaks, herdsmen and veterinary practitioners often opt for eradication programs involving monthly or bimonthly serial herd cultures that include testing of bulk tanks, groups, and pens.

Routine cultures of bulk tank samples, fresh cows, and new cows can provide an early warning system and ensure that the herd management team can respond to the introduction of mycoplasma mastitis in a timely fashion. Maintenance of negative herd status depends on culturing of milk from all additions to a closed herd. Heifers purchased from herds that have previously experienced mycoplasma mastitis may carry the organisms in the nasal passages as well as in the mammary glands. The mycoplasma organisms responsible for bovine mastitis can be readily identified by culture if they are given access to media meeting the more rigorous growth requirements of mycoplasma and microaerophilic incubation facilities (a candle jar may be adequate). Positive growth on defined media can be considered only a presumptive test. Nonpathogenic organisms, *Acholeplasma laidlawii*, are common contaminants in milk samples. Differentiation on an individual sample basis necessitates more laborious serologic or biochemical growth requirement characterization.

Salmonella Infections

Several species of *Salmonella* have been isolated from the mammary glands of cows, including *S. typhimurium*, *S. newport*, *S. muenster*, *S. enteriditis*, and *S. dublin*. *Salmonella* infection causes a chronic, active subclinical mastitis with occasional flare-ups of clinical mastitis. In this regard it is very similar to chronic coliform mastitis. *S. dublin* infections in

humans have been linked to consumption of contaminated dairy and beef products and have resulted in a high rate of mortality.[23,24] *S. dublin* is an invasive pathogen that causes septicemia with high morbidity and mortality in calves, whereas its most common clinical manifestations in adult cattle are severe enteritis and abortion. Animals that recover from acute infections shed the organism in their feces for four to six weeks after the clinical event. A small percentage of infected animals recover clinically but maintain chronic mammary gland and/or enteric infections without overt clinical signs of the disease. Carrier animals can shed in feces and milk billions of *S. dublin* organisms per day for years, thus presenting a substantial challenge for susceptible hosts and serious environmental concerns.[25] A combination of routine serology plus bacterial culture of milk and feces from suspect animals can help identify persistently infected cattle so they can be culled from the herd. Mice and rats can also be infected with *S. dublin* and must be eradicated as part of the overall control program.[26] *Salmonella* is widespread in the dairy cow's environment; thus it will be difficult to eradicate the organism. However, ongoing research is providing insights into effective control measures that can be economically implemented on the farm.[27]

Corynebacterium bovis Infections

Corynebacterium bovis can colonize the teat canal, producing mild elevation of the SCC but little or no gland pathology. Routine teat dipping prevents these infections. Consistent isolation of this organism from individual or bulk tank samples should be considered presumptive evidence that teat dipping is either not practiced or is ineffective. The mild increases in SCCs associated with infection have been postulated to protect against infection by major pathogens, but there is some evidence that this is not usually the case because *C. bovis* infections rarely elevate the SCC to protective levels. It should be noted that SCCs exceeding values as low as 50,000 cells per milliliter have been associated with decreased production.

Other Mastitis Etiologic Agents

There is a large list of other bacteria and close to 30 yeasts that occasionally cause mastitis cases or mastitis outbreaks. This list includes *Cryptococcus neoformans*, *Bacillus cereus*, *Actinomyces pyogenes* (summer mastitis), *Clostridium* spp., *Nocardia* spp., *Prototheca* spp., *Mycobacterium* spp., serotypes of *Leptospira interrogans*, various *Candida* spp., and others. These organisms are considered atypical but may become herd problems under unique circumstances, especially when mastitis preparations are contaminated, or when animals are kept in muddy conditions and proper milking hygiene is not performed on a daily basis.[28] Many of these organisms, such as *C. neoformans*, *Nocardia* spp., and *Leptospira* spp. have potential to cause zoonotic disease, and care should be taken when handling infected samples or tissues. *A. pyogenes* may cause abscessed quarter, usually with minimal systemic signs of illness.

MASTITIS THERAPY

Legal Concerns

The AMDUCA of 1994 spells out the rules and regulations veterinarians must follow when using drugs in an extralabel manner (ELDU):

- ELDU is permitted only by and under the supervision of a veterinarian.
- ELDU is allowed only for FDA-approved animal and human drugs.

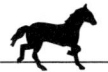

- A valid veterinarian-client-patient relationship is a prerequisite for all ELDU.
- ELDU is used for therapeutic purposes, only in cases when an animal's well being is threatened, and not for production use (i.e., feed supplements).
- Rules apply to dosage-form drugs and drugs administered in water. ELDU in feed is prohibited.
- ELDU is not permitted if it results in a violative food residue or any residue which may present a risk to public health.
- FDA prohibition of a specific ELDU precludes such use.

Treatment Record Requirements

- Identification of the animals, either as individuals or a group
- Animal species treated
- Numbers of animals treated
- Condition being treated
- Established name of the drug and its active ingredient
- Dosage prescribed or used
- Duration of treatment
- Specified withdrawal, withholding, or discard time(s), if applicable, for meat, milk, eggs, or animal-derived food
- Records to be kept for 2 years

FDA may have access to these records to estimate the risk to public health.

Label Requirements

- Name and address of the prescribing veterinarian
- Established name of the drug
- Specified directions for use, including the class/species or identification of the animal or herd, flock, pen, lot, or other group; the dosage frequency and route of administration; and the duration of therapy
- Cautionary statements

The use of illegal drugs must be avoided. Strictly prohibited or illegal treatments include chloramphenicol, glycopeptide antibiotics (vancomycin), sulfonamides other than sulfadimethoxine, phenylbutazone, and dipyrone. Additionally, the use of enrofloxacin in dairy cattle is an illegal act. The use of aminoglycoside antibiotics, although not illegal per se if AMDUCA guidelines are followed, is strongly discouraged by the American Association of Bovine Practitioners. The use of aminoglycoside antibiotics could be reasonably and rationally argued to fall outside of the accepted standard of care. Consequently, use of these compounds by the veterinary practitioner creates unwarranted legal exposure and potential liability.

The goals of antimicrobial therapy in the treatment of mastitis are: (1) prevention of mortality in peracute cases, (2) return of normal milk composition and production, (3) elimination of sources of infectious microorganisms, and (4) prevention of new infections during the dry period. The elimination of invading microorganisms would appear to support these goals. Practitioners have traditionally administered mastitis medications by the intramammary route, attempting to concentrate the chemotherapeutic agent in the active site of infection. Clinical efficacy of an antibiotic is very difficult to quantify because there are large variations in response from cow to cow and among herds due to the type of organism involved, location of infected sites, degree of mammary gland induration, duration of infection, and other undefined factors.[29,30]

In general, the choice of an antimicrobial agent and the route of administration will be dictated by antibiotic sensitivity, drug distribution, and the pharmacokinetics-clearance of the active drug[31,32] (Box 34-1).

Passive diffusion is thought to be the major mode of

BOX 34-1

FDA/CVM Approved Antibiotics for Bovine Mastitis (1994)

PRESCRIPTION REQUIRED (Rx)
Pirlimycin
Hetacillin
Cloxacillin
Amoxicillin
Novobiocin
Sulfamethazine*

OVER-THE-COUNTER (OTC)
Penicillin G
Dihydrostreptomycin
Cephapirin
Erythromycin
Novobiocin

*Not approved for use in lactating cows.

transport of the pharmacologic agent from the general circulation into the mammary gland. Thus agents that are predicted to reach the mammary gland more efficiently are nonionized, nonprotein-bound, and lipid soluble. When the pH of milk is weakly acidic (pH 6.4 to 6.8), antibacterial agents that are weak bases (trimethoprim, aminoglycosides, polymyxin B, macrolides, lincosamides) are thought to be preferentially concentrated in the mammary gland by ion trapping. Milk from animals with clinical mastitis can have a pH in the physiologic range found in serum; in this scenario antimicrobial agents that are weak acids (sulfonamides, penicillins, cephaloridine, rifampin) may reach effective antimicrobial concentrations in milk.

Intramammary administration of antibacterial agents for the treatment of clinical or subclinical mastitis has developed as a preferred route used by the dairy industry. The same properties governing the transfer of antibiotic from serum to the mammary gland will dictate the behavior of a potential therapeutic agent following intramammary administration. Weakly basic or lipid-soluble antibiotics tend to remain in the mammary gland following treatment. Intramammary administration permits delivery of small amounts of antimicrobial agents directly to the site of infection. Many can be used in this manner because several antibiotics possess inherent physiochemical properties that often preclude effective parenteral therapeutic modalities. Products used in lactating cows are generally designed for rapid clearance and reduced milk-withholding restrictions. Extended milk withdrawal times are associated with the usage of antibiotics with extensive tissue binding (polymyxin B and aminoglycosides). Dry cow formulations using higher dosages of antibiotics, oils or repository vehicles, or benzathine antibiotic salts are designed to produce prolonged intervals of effective antibiotic concentrations.

Treatment of Subclinical Mastitis and Clinical Mastitis With Local Clinical Signs Only

The use of antibiotics in the treatment of subclinical mastitis and mastitis with local clinical signs should be restricted to cattle in herds in which the predominant pathogen is *S. agalactiae*. These infections are readily cured in more than 90% of the cows that receive commercially available intramammary antibiotic preparations. Treated cows are removed as a potential reservoir of infection, their milk SCCs return to normal or nearly normal, and their milk production in-

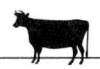
creases. Generally, these benefits will outweigh the costs of treatment, drugs, and milk discards when cows are treated during the first half of lactation. More aggressive treatment strategies may be developed in those herds with illegally high milk somatic cell or bacteria counts. Similar definitive evidence is not available to support antimicrobial therapy of *Mycoplasma* spp., *S. aureus*, gram-negative, *Staphylococcus* spp., and non–*S. agalactiae Streptococcus* spp. mastitis.

Only single-use commercially available preparations should be used for intramammary therapy. Compounded preparations have no advantages relative to approved, commercially available products and do not fit within AMDUCA requirements (Box 34-2). The illegality of compounding, the potential for product liability due to potential pathogen contamination, and the increased potential for violative drug residues provide clear contraindications for a practitioner who might consider compounding for intramammary therapy.

Treatment of Acute Clinical Mastitis With Systemic Disease

Cattle with evidence of acute systemic clinical signs should be targeted for more aggressive treatment regimens. Clinical signs suggestive of acute systemic disease include anorexia, rectal temperature >103.5° F, dehydration, and recumbency. These treatment regimens will generally include fluid therapy, antiinflammatory therapy, systemic antibiotics, and intramammary antibiotics. Some practitioners may choose to recommend frequent stripping of the affected gland; however, no clear evidence regarding the efficacy of this procedure has been published.

Large volume intravenous fluid therapy should be performed unless economic considerations preclude this type of therapy. Near-isotonic sodium chloride solutions supplemented with potassium and calcium salts should be considered the fluids of choice for treatment of cows with acute mastitis. Both hypokalemia and hypocalcemia are common in cattle with acute mastitis. Untreated, these electrolyte disorders can be life threatening. Extensive use of dextrose-containing solutions should be avoided because most cows with acute mastitis are in fact hyperglycemic. Additional glucose supplementation will act as an osmotic diuretic, potentiating hypovolemia and shock. Likewise, there is little justification for the administration of bicarbonate or bicarbonate equivalent to most cows with acute mastitis with systemic clinical signs. Severe acidosis is rarely present in most cows with acute mastitis.

The antiinflammatory agent most frequently used to treat cows with acute mastitis is flunixin meglumine, 1 mg/kg q 12 hr. Ketoprofen and glucocorticoids are advocated by some practitioners; however, the potential abortifacient effects of glucocorticoids should be considered before their administration.

Although no clear evidence exists which demonstrates a benefit to systemic antibiotic therapy in cows with acute mastitis, most practitioners choose to administer antibiotics to these cows. One study has documented that bacteremia in cows with acute mastitis may benefit from systemic use of antibiotics.[21] The use of antiinflammatory agents in these cows sets a minimum milk and meat withdrawal time, effectively eliminating a major consideration in the decision making process. The optimal antibiotic would be concentrated in milk and have a favorable sensitivity pattern against bacteria associated with acute mastitis. In the absence of any legal antibiotic which fulfills these criteria, most practitioners choose to treat systemically ill cows suffering from acute mastitis with either oxytetracycline or ceftiofur. Oxytetracycline is often chosen because of its favorable distribution to the mammary gland and its low cost. Ceftiofur is chosen because systemic therapy does not necessitate extensive milk or meat withholding times.

Frequent Milkings

Potential mastitis pathogens that invade the mammary gland must overcome the ebb and flow of frequent milkings. The flushing effect of milkings is a notable mechanism for shortening the clinical course of coliform mastitis. It appears that bacteria attempt to resist the repulsion either by adhering to tissue linings or by increasing their replication rates. Repeated milkings throughout acute coliform mastitis events can be useful in removing inflammatory mediators that may be harmful if allowed to persist for extended periods.

The use of exogenous oxytocin, 20 IU at each milking, has been reported to enhance milk production.[33] In this study, the oxytocin group produced 849 kg more milk during the lactation than the control group, with a significant difference occurring after peak milk yield. No significant differences were reported for milk fat or protein percentages. The use of exogenous oxytocin at milking increased milk production with no apparent adverse effect on health. The use of this compound provides an opportunity for enhancing milk letdown and therefore the ability to flush the mammary gland. The efficacy of oxytocin therapy in clinical mastitis has not been established under controlled research conditions. Although potentially useful in *E. coli* mastitis for reasons mentioned above, this approach has not demonstrated a significant level of clinical efficacy against contagious mastitis pathogens.[29] It should be noted that the routine use of oxytocin in healthy cattle to increase milk production is illegal in the United States.

Antibiotic Residues

Antibiotic contamination of dairy and meat products poses a potential health risk to a small percentage of the human population. Specific on-farm residue avoidance programs aid in reducing health risks to the consumer (Box 34-3). Antibiotic contamination of the milk supply is of additional concern to creameries because antibiotic residues are capable of inhibiting the growth and activity of bacterial cultures used in the processing of many dairy products. Mastitis therapy should be administered according to label instructions and the latest policies and recommendations of state and federal governing bodies. Every consideration concerning dosage and withholding periods for milk and meat of treated animals or neonates consuming milk or colostrum containing antibiotics must be followed. Rational administration of antibiotics is further complicated by the limited number of agents approved for use in lactating dairy cattle. When careful and considered appraisal of a clinical situation indicates a need for extralabel (nonapproved host species, dose, or route of administration) use of antibiotics, the veterinarian assumes direct responsibility for safety of the prescribed treatment and potential contamination of the human food chain. Such extralabel antibiotic usage presumes a current and active practitioner-client relationship, knowledge of pharmacokinetics and drug clearance times, adequate patient identification, and permanent treatment records.

Numerous reports over the years describe problems with antibiotic residue assays.[34-36] These reports indicate that antibiotic residue assays cannot be used to determine antibiotic withdrawal times under field conditions. If one tests a quarter of the composite samples from the following time periods: pretreatment, milking after the last treatment, and at the labeled withdrawal time from treated and an additional group of untreated animals, there will be sufficient data to properly interpret the tests. If the assay findings are positive before the animal has been treated or if findings are positive on normal lactating cows, it will be difficult to interpret the test results on the later samples.

Health departments or milk cooperative laboratories test samples for antibiotic residues. Descriptions and information on these tests are available from extension veterinarians, creameries, and other sources.

Mastitis Vaccines

Many strategies to develop vaccination measures against bovine mastitis continue to be explored by researchers around the world.[37] A major hurdle is the number and heterogeneity of mastitis pathogens; thus we must be aware of just what can be accomplished by immunization strategies. Little is known regarding optimal dose, route, and duration of immunization strategies at this point[38]; however, more research is being completed each year that should help us enhance this valuable tool against mastitis.

Attempts to reduce the incidence and severity of bovine mastitis through immunization with various antigens have been made throughout the last several decades with little documented benefit for either the cow or the producer. For a mastitis immunization program to be of value to the dairy producer, the vaccine(s) must do one or more of the following: (1) eliminate chronic mammary gland infections, (2) prevent new intramammary infections, or (3) reduce the incidence and severity of new intramammary infections. None of the past or current vaccines has proven effective in eliminating chronic intramammary infections (e.g., *S. aureus*). Vaccines might reduce the numbers of bacteria being shed in the milk, but no data has been presented to indicate that immunizing with these products will clear the mammary gland of this pathogen. Also, no immunogens have proven effective in pre-

venting potential mammary gland infectious organisms from colonizing the teat ends. However, the last approach, that of reducing the incidence or severity of the infections, has been demonstrated to be an effective strategy, at least for *E. coli* mastitis. All dairy cows should be vaccinated with an R-mutant bacterin. These vaccines provide cross-protective immunity which targets homologous or highly conserved antigens present in the lipopolysaccharide layer of the gram-negative cell wall.[39,40] Cows with low antibody titers to gram-negative core antigens are at greater risk for clinical gram-negative bacterial mastitis,[41] and vaccinated cows have a dramatically lower incidence of clinical gram-negative mastitis.[42] Economic analysis of reported responses to vaccination suggests that herds which experience more than one episode of clinical gram-negative mastitis per 100 complete lactations will benefit from vaccination.[43] This break-even incidence is less than 10% of the average rate of clinical mastitis. Consequently, all dairy cows should be vaccinated using an R-mutant bacterin.[40,42-47]

Although inconsistent outcomes are reported, a variety of experimental and commercial vaccines have been used for *S. aureus* mastitis.[48-50] A growing series of efforts has been put forth toward developing vaccines for *Streptococcus* spp. The research literature is beginning to document increased work in this area.[51,52]

Feeding Waste Milk to Calves

Selim et al.[53] undertook a cross-sectional prospective study to assess the number of bacteria and presumptive antibiotic residues in milk fed to calves and to identify those bacteria and the antibiotic susceptibility of selected bacterial strains. They employed 189 samples obtained from 12 local dairies and examined samples of waste milk and milk-based fluids (e.g., milk replacer, colostrum, and bulk-tank milk). Standard aerobic bacteria counts (cumulative number of viable bacteria was determined) and antibiotic susceptibility testing of selected strains were performed. Presumptive antibiotic residues were detected by use of antibiotic residue screening test kits.

We found that the mean of the cumulative number of bacteria for waste milk samples was significantly higher than for other types of milk or milk-based products. *Streptococcus* spp. (84/165 samples) and *Enterobacteriaceae* spp. (83/165 samples) were the predominant bacteria identified, followed by *Staphylococcus* spp. (68/165 samples). *E. coli* was the gram-negative species most commonly isolated (52/165 samples, 32%); however, none was strain O157. *Salmonella* spp. and *Mycoplasma* spp. were not isolated. Of 189 samples, 119 (63%) tested positive for beta-lactams or tetracycline by use of two commercially available assays. In vitro, some bacteria were resistant to commonly used antibiotics.

This study indicates waste milk that has not been effectively treated (e.g., pasteurization) to reduce microbial load before use as calf feed should be used with caution, because it may contain a high number of bacteria that may be pathogenic to cattle and human beings. Presence of antibiotic residues that would constitute violative amounts and multiple antibiotic-resistant bacterial strains are concerns in calf health management and dairy food safety.

HEIFER MASTITIS IN DAIRY CATTLE

Studies in recent years have reminded us that we cannot assume that young replacement stock are free of intramammary infections.[54-60] Microbiologic examination of prepartum samples of mammary gland secretions have indicated that 2% to 7% of quarters of first-lactation heifers may have mastitis pathogens. The organisms isolated include coliforms, strep-

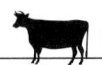

tococci, and *Staphylococcus* spp., including *S. aureus, C. bovis,* and others.

Specific control practices for the prevention of intramammary infections in prepartum heifers are not known. The standard control measures recommended are separating preweaned calves to prevent suckling, controlling flies, and segregating pregnant heifers from dry cows. Several investigations have reported some success with different regimens of antibiotic therapy. Although these findings are encouraging, further studies of the efficacy of such therapy in prepartum primigravid heifers must be performed before general recommendations can be provided.

EQUINE MASTITIS

The mammary gland of the equine consists of paired mammae separated by a fascial septum, each with a glandular body and teat. The glandular part of each half is divided into two or occasionally three lobes by fibroelastic capsules. The narrower teat canal and shorter teat cistern are significantly different from those in the bovine mammary gland. Each teat has two separate openings.

Mastitis in the equine has a profoundly lower incidence than in the bovine. Accounts of equine mastitis are uniquely limited to individual case reports, and no reports of herd outbreaks are presented in the literature. In addition to the obvious fact that mares are not exposed to mammary handling and milking machines is the reality that the mammary gland of the mare occupies a more concealed position, with the teats less exposed to environmental trauma and possible infection. Mastitis has been documented in mares at all stages of lactation; however, clinical cases are most often observed within a few weeks after weaning the foal. The clinical signs most repeatedly observed are mammary swelling, heat, pain, and ventral edema, with some patients exhibiting depression and anorexia. Mild lameness may infrequently occur in the hindlimb proximal to the affected mammary gland. Lameness and swelling may be severe when draining lymph nodes become involved; these may abscess when infected with *Corynebacterium pseudotuberculosis*.

The organisms isolated from milk of equine mastitis cases represent almost a balanced grouping between gram-positive and gram-negative bacteria. *Streptococcus zooepidemicus* is the most frequent isolate recovered from equine mastitis milk or exudate. Other isolates associated with equine mammary gland inflammation include *S. equi, Streptococcus equisimilis, S. agalactiae, Streptococcus viridans, Actinobacillus* spp. including *Actinobacillus suis, Pasteurella ureae, E. aerogenes, C. pseudotuberculosis, Staphylococcus* spp., *P. aeruginosa, K. pneumoniae,* and *E. coli.* It is essential to obtain clean samples from the mare. The shorter teats and multiple openings in the teat provide ample opportunities for contamination of specimens. Therefore exceptional care in obtaining milk samples for microbiologic examination must be undertaken.

Since antimicrobial susceptibility patterns of clinical isolates are inconsistent, culture and antimicrobial susceptibility tests should be done in each case. On the basis of laboratory data acquired from the records of 28 mares that suffered from acute inflammation of the mammary gland, McCue and Wilson[61] suggest using trimethoprim-sulfonamide (5 mg/kg, based on the trimethoprim portion orally bid) or penicillin (20,000 IU/kg IM bid) and gentamicin sulfate (2 mg/kg IV or IM tid) while awaiting results of culture and antimicrobial susceptibility assays. All of these therapies can result in meat residue problems if proper withdrawal times are not observed. Nursing care that includes frequent milking and hot-packs or hydrotherapy may be of additional benefit.

Although clinical case reports describe the use of commercial bovine intramammary infusion products (lactating and dry cow) in the mare, no efficacy data are available on this subject. It has been reported that most horses, including one treated without antibiotics, exhibited clinical improvement within three to five days, with the mammary gland appearing clinically normal within one week.

SMALL RUMINANT MASTITIS

Most of the milk produced in the dairy goat and the ewe is consumed without prior pasteurization. This brings to the forefront the potential risks to consumers of goat and sheep milk that can contain bacterial organisms from subclinical or clinical mastitis or environmental contaminants. Although not addressed in this section, caprine arthritis-encephalitis (CAE) virus and ovine progressive pneumonia (OPP) virus cause severe fibrosis and agalactia, a syndrome known as hard udder or hard bag.

MASTITIS ISOLATES OF SHEEP

Although few sheep are raised as dairy animals in developed countries, mastitis control is an important component of flock health programs. Losses are referable to acute clinical disease of the ewe and decreased milk production associated with subclinical mastitis, leading to increased lamb mortality and decreased rate of gain. The bacteria most commonly isolated from ewes' milk include *S. aureus,* coagulase-negative *Staphylococcus* spp., *Streptococcus* spp., *C. bovis, Pasteurella haemolytica,* and *E. coli. S. aureus* and *P. haemolytica* are often responsible for an acute mastitis characterized by severe, life-threatening systemic toxemia. These organisms may cause gangrenous changes in the udder. Lameness is often the first clinical sign noted. Systemic and local therapy decisions are typically based on extrapolation of information available from work performed on the cow. Routine udder palpation is a typical component of flock management programs. Ewes with evidence of scarring or fibrotic changes of the udder are typically culled. This relatively simple procedure tends to remove less productive ewes and reduce the infectious reservoir within the flock. The prevalence of subclinical mastitis is increased when sheep are reared in close confinement, probably relating to the function of lambs as mechanical vectors that carry mastitis pathogens from infected to healthy ewes.

MASTITIS ISOLATES OF THE DAIRY GOAT

As with the bovine, a variety of mammary gland isolates have been reported from goat milk.[62,63] However, only a few species of bacteria are associated with herd outbreaks in this species. East, Birnie, and Farver,[62] and East and Birnie,[64] in a quite comprehensive study, reported on an investigation that included 16 herds composed of 2,522 lactating does with culture results on 4,662 composite milk samples gathered from the does over a nine-month period. Gram-negative bacteria were isolated from 2% of the does; coagulase-negative *Staphylococcus* spp. totaled 17.5% of the isolates from milk of the does, *S. aureus* from 3.1%, *Mycoplasma* spp. from 1.2%, and *Streptococcus* spp. from 0.3%. A number of previous reports mentioned gram-positive cocci, including coagulase-

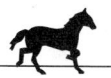

negative staphylococci and *S. aureus*, as the most frequently encountered mammary gland pathogens. It appears that dairy goats have a much lower prevalence of *Streptococcus* spp. isolated from milk than dairy cattle.

BACTERIA

Staphylococcus aureus

As with cows, *S. aureus* mastitis is difficult to eliminate from the caprine mammary gland. All of the clinical signs associated with this infection are described in the section on bovine mastitis. Infections can manifest as acute gangrenous mastitis, nongangrenous mastitis, or a chronic subclinical mastitis with fibrosis of the gland and a gradual decrease in milk production. Unlike cows, goats frequently develop large nodular abscesses within the affected gland. Segregating does infected with staphylococci into a separate milking herd or culling these animals is strongly recommended. Strict hygienic measures at the time of milking limits the spread of the disease. Teat dipping is a critical component of any control program. Current antibiotic therapy on a herd basis that treats both lactating and dry does will not eliminate the problem.

Coagulase-Negative Staphylococci

Coagulase-negative staphylococci organisms have been isolated in pure cultures from subclinical, acute, and chronic caprine mastitis cases. Coagulase-negative staphylococci are thus considered to be mastitis pathogens in goats. Elevated SCCs in milk can result from the presence of these organisms. Many researchers report them to be less prevalent than *S. aureus* as a cause of clinical mastitis. The caprine isolates are sensitive to procaine penicillin in vitro.

Mycoplasma mycoides

The isolate, *Mycoplasma mycoides* spp. *Mycoides*, has been identified with mastitis, decreased milk production, systemic illness, and peracute death in kids and adult goats. Transmission of this pathogen through colostrum and milk to caprine neonates has been associated with subsequent pneumonia and arthritis in the kids. This organism is easily spread by milking machines and milkers' hands. New intramammary infections can allow shedding of the organisms for weeks before decreased milk production is noted. Present antimicrobial agents are not effective in vivo against this pathogen. Herd culture and culling programs similar to those used in the cow are recommended.

Mycoplasma putrefaciens

Although not as prevalent as *M. mycoides*, *Mycoplasma putrefaciens* is noted as a major cause of sudden agalactia in dairy goats. This pathogen is highly contagious, self-limiting, and is not associated with clinical signs of systemic illness. Normal levels of lactation may return within 90 days after elimination of the pathogen.

Streptococcus

Streptococci other than *S. agalactiae* have been isolated from the milk of does with subclinical and clinical caprine mastitis. Clinical cases may have elevated temperatures and a warm, firm, agalactic, enlarged mammary gland. An extralabel therapeutic regimen of administration of penicillin (10,000 IU/kg SC bid for 5 to 7 days) or intramammary infusion of a product formulated for use in cattle ($\frac{1}{2}$ dose) may be effective in eliminating the pathogen. However, antibiotic residues will remain in the meat and milk for an unknown period of time. Please consult the Food Animal Residue Avoidance Data Bank (FARAD) before using extralabel therapeutic regimens (http://www.farad.org/).

Caprine Arthritis-Encephalitis and Ovine Progressive Pneumonia

In addition to systemic signs of illness, caprine arthritis-encephalitis (CAE) and ovine progressive pneumonia (OPP) viruses cause fibrosis of the mammary gland and agalactia. This syndrome is known as hard udder or hard bag.

LABORATORY PROCEDURES FOR CAPRINE MASTITIS

Microbiologic methods used in the diagnosis of bovine mastitis are generally applicable to samples obtained from small ruminants. SCCs, a common component of bovine mastitis control programs, are probably less useful in goats. Reported cell count ranges for normal and infected goat milk overlap. Interpretation of cell counts is further complicated by the presence of lipid-protein particles in normal milk. Assay systems based on the gelation of DNA are probably more reliable and are clinically relevant. Some high cell counts are associated with very long lactations. It has been reported that several of the antibiotic residue assays may yield an assay-positive outcome on normal, noninfected mammary gland secretions. It is not recommended to use these assays to establish antibiotic withdrawal times after therapeutic intervention.

MAMMARY GLAND EDEMA

Physiologic udder edema is common in mares and in prepartum dairy cattle. It is usually noted in either high-producing cows or first-calf heifers. The primary importance of this condition is the need to differentiate it from the pathologic edema associated with intramammary infection. Unless the condition is serious, treatment is unnecessary.

The development of an excessively heavy and pendulous udder may threaten the integrity of the udder suspensory apparatus. Under these circumstances therapeutic intervention may be indicated, and salt intake should be limited. Corticosteroids have been prescribed in the past but appear not to alter the clinical course of the disease process.

Diuretics, primarily thiazide derivatives and furosemide, have been used, but their potential benefits may be offset by serious side effects if used for more than 48 hours. Electrolyte imbalances are a particular concern, particularly in older high-producing cows predisposed to milk fever. Prepartum milking may be initiated as early as two weeks prepartum. If this approach is used, an alternate source of colostrum should be made available to the calf at birth. Following calving, the frequency of milking may be increased. Prolonged massage and hydrotherapy of the mammary gland will be of benefit either prepartum or following parturition. In the mare, hand walking to increase exercise, salt deprivation, and diuretics have proven beneficial in reducing the swelling of this tissue.

BLOODY MILK

Blood contamination of mammary gland secretions predominantly results from trauma or may appear as a sequelae to prepartum udder edema and rupture of small mammary vessels. Milk discoloration will vary in degree and typically disappear within one week of parturition, although shorter clinical courses are more common. Frequently the streak canal may be blocked by blood clots, necessitating frequent and prolonged hand stripping. Specific antibiotic treatments are neither efficacious nor indicated. The use of antibiotic residue tests on individual animals may indicate that a patient with bloody milk is being given antibiotics, even though antibiotic therapy was not administered. Potential adverse influences of bloody milk in the bulk tank are unknown and are not covered in the PMO. Certain antibiotic residue assay procedures that require milk to be centrifuged may reveal blood in the milk.

COLOSTRUM SECRETION IN CATTLE

Mammary gland growth, the appearance of a lobuloalveolar structure, and the secretion of colostrum and lactogenesis occur when precise endocrine equilibrium takes place during gestation and lactation. The formation of alveoli requires hormonal sequences, including the ovarian and fetal-placental hormones, estrogens and progesterone, anterior pituitary prolactin, and adrenal corticoids. These hormone sequences appear during pregnancy and foster the complete development of the mammary gland at parturition in the bovine.

Synthesis of casein and lactose remains low through pregnancy and increases sharply after calving. Secretion of colostrum takes place near parturition, coincidental with a decreased plasma progesterone concentration and increased plasma estrogen concentration. During the last month of gestation, fluid accumulates in the mammary gland.[65,66] In the goat, this lacteal secretion has a higher content of sodium, chloride, and protein and a lower content of potassium and lactose than does milk.[67]

Immunoglobulins (Igs) represent the most consequential class of proteins in bovine milk. In cattle, IgG1 is the Ig present in the highest concentration in colostrum and milk.[68] IgG1 concentrations decrease in maternal plasma 2 to 3 weeks before calving; from this time until parturition, maximum concentrations of IgG1 are present in lacteal secretions. The higher levels of IgG1 in colostrum than in serum correspond to a selective transfer which becomes active two to three weeks before parturition.[69] This selective transfer occurs at a much lower level during lactation. Maximum transfer of IgG1 occurs one to three days before calving and coincides with the appearance of IgG1 receptors in epithelial cells. A class of IgG1 receptors having higher affinity are present during the last 15 days of gestation.[70] Presence of these receptors supports the selective transfer of IgG1 through the epithelial cell.

The Ig content of colostrum is reduced immediately after the first suckling, and the selective transfer of IgG1 ends during the first two days of lactation. The passive transfer of immunity to the young is required to provide the neonate with the ability to target potential pathogens recognized by the dam. Synthesis of IgG1 in the calf is limited in the first few weeks of life.[70]

LACTATION CONTROL MECHANISMS

The seemingly simple process of producing milk on a daily basis requires an enormous regulatory effort by the dam. Milk consists of a solution of salts, carbohydrates, and other compounds in which protein molecules and aggregates, ca-

sein micelles, accessory immune effector cells, and fat globules are dispersed. Milk synthesis alone, at peak lactation, may require up to 80% of the dam's net energy intake. A shift in nutrient partitioning requires a number of adaptations within the animal. The balance between homeostatic and homeorrhetic mechanisms must be orchestrated to attempt maintenance of metabolic and physiologic equilibrium in the face of a large energy expenditure during peak lactation. A complex series of hormonal regulatory signals attempt to control this energy-expensive process.[71]

LACTOGENESIS

Lactogenesis is a process under hormonal and neural controls in which the mammary alveolar cells are stimulated to secrete milk. The secretory activity of the mammary gland is not under the direct control of afferent innervation. Completely denervated mammary glands can still secrete milk. However, prepartum milking commonly initiates lactation by transmitting neural impulses from the teat to the hypothalamus, where secretion of the prolactin-inhibiting factor is suppressed and the corticotrophin-releasing factor is stimulated. Secretion of prolactin and adrenocorticotropic hormone (ACTH) induces the mammary cell to secrete. In addition, the hypothalamus affects milk secretion by regulation of processes involved in feed intake and water consumption.[72]

For milk ejection to occur, resistance of the streak canal in the teat must be overcome, and contraction of the myoepithelial cells must ensue to force milk from the alveoli through the ducts. A neurohormonal reflex involving pressure-sensitive nerve receptors in the skin of teats activates release of oxytocin to cause the contraction of myoepithelial cells, resulting in milk ejection. Oxytocin binds specifically and with high affinity to protein receptors located on the myoepithelial cells.[73]

Increased activity of the sympathetic nervous system caused by diverse stimuli may inhibit milk ejection. This inhibition may be a consequence of elevated levels of epinephrine and norepinephrine, resulting from stressful stimuli. Epinephrine directly blocks oxytocin from binding to myoepithelial cells. Catecholamine compounds increase the tone of smooth muscles in the mammary ducts and blood vessels, causing a partial occlusion of the mammary ducts. Exogenous administration of oxytocin does not reverse milk ejection deficits in animals exhibiting such peripheral inhibition.

Milk production in the bovine reaches a peak two to eight weeks after parturition and then gradually declines over the next several months. In simplified terms, the hormonal regulatory complex controls lactation. However, unless milk is extracted frequently from the mammary gland, synthesis of milk will not continue at maximum levels, despite a satisfactory hormonal status. Although oxytocin is essential for milk removal, the hormones thought to be required for maintenance of milk synthesis include ACTH (or glucocorticoids), insulin, prolactin, growth hormone, thyroid-stimulating hormones, and parathyroid hormone.

Lactation requires a precise interaction among several hormones. Therefore it is not surprising that exogenous administration of hormones to induce or maintain lactation has not been met with uniform success. The empiric methodologies used consist of administering (by injection or implants) either estrogen alone or a combination of estrogen and progesterone from one dose to periods of administration of up to two to four months. In practically every report, some undesirable effects are observed (e.g., cystic ovaries, poor milk yields), and none of these procedures has been approved in the United States for use in the bovine. It should be noted that pharmacologic induction of lactation is illegal in the United States.

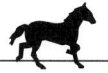

MAMMARY GLAND DEFENSE MECHANISMS

The attributes that make the mammary gland unique contribute to both the protective mechanisms from infectious disease and the opportunity for challenge of normal homeostasis. The mammary gland of the bovine consists of irregular lobes provided with excretory ducts radiating from the teat cistern and the gland cistern or from the mammary papillae. The secretory parts, the alveolar ducts and alveoli, consist of a basement membrane, a layer of myoepithelial cells, and on the internal surface of the resting gland a row of columnar glandular cells. This biologic membrane separates the extracellular fluid from the mammary gland secretion. It is important to note that water and some compounds in the extracellular fluid can pass through this membrane, in which active synthesis of milk takes place. Milk is a suspension of fat droplets in an aqueous phase in which lactose, inorganic salts, and proteins (mainly casein) are dissolved. During various stages of lactation, the mammary gland secretions are a media suitable for supporting bacterial growth.

Intramammary infection results when an agent successfully penetrates the teat canal and reaches the milk-producing tissues. This cannot be accomplished without overcoming many defense mechanisms designed to prevent penetration of the organisms, suppress bacterial growth, and counteract the potentially detrimental effects of bacterial cell wall products being released into the milk matrix.

The maximum functional capability of the cells responsible for mammary gland defense may be influenced by stage of lactation, length of the dry period, genetic background, composition of the secretion, types of antimicrobials used, and antiinflammatory agents administered to the patient. Alternatively, functional properties of these cells may influence the integrity of milk-synthesizing tissues. Known soluble chemical defense mechanisms in milk include lactoferrin, complement, and Igs. The role of inflammatory mediators (e.g., serotonin, histamine, PGs, and leukotrienes) in mammary gland defense is poorly understood.

COMMENSAL ORGANISMS

Biologic control of intramammary infections by nonpathogenic organisms that colonize the teat end or the gland may provide protection against major mastitis pathogens. Udder infections caused by coagulase-negative staphylococci or *C. bovis* may deter establishment of coagulase-positive staphylococcal species *(S. aureus)* by elevating SCCs. However, final resolution of the role which teat canal infections by *C. bovis* and coagulase-negative *Staphylococcus* spp. may play in preventing infections with mastitic pathogens is not complete. Some research workers feel that colonization by nonpathogenic organisms is not protective against infection by environmental pathogens, because it rarely results in SCC elevations sufficiently high to be protective.

STREAK (TEAT) CANAL

Streak (teat) canal and its associated tissues form a primary barrier to mastitis pathogens. The teat canal can be an efficient valve guarding the entrance to the teat cistern. Studies have demonstrated that the ability of bacteria to infect the mammary glands is intimately related to the proportion of the canal bypassed by the inoculation procedure.[74-76]

An additional defense mechanism of the streak canal is its keratin lining. Keratin is a unique compound having both physical and chemical properties that facilitate its role as a barrier to intramammary infections. It has been proposed that there are three primary defense mechanisms provided by the streak canal: (1) adsorption of bacteria to keratin, (2) desquamation of bacteria-coated keratin, and (3) desiccation of the canal lumen allowing for resealing of keratinized surfaces. The predominant fatty acid types composing teat canal keratin in extracellular and intracellular lipids are C16, C18:1, and C18. Data suggest that milk fat may represent a part of the extracellular lipid components. Polyene C18:2 and C18:3 acids possess in-vitro bactericidal activity against *S. aureus, Staphylococcus hyicus, S. agalactiae,* and *C. bovis.*[77,78]

PHAGOCYTES OF THE MAMMARY GLAND

PMNs and macrophages constitute >80% of the nonspecific immune defense cells found in milk. An average of 50,000 to 200,000 of these cells per milliliter is found in the milk of an uninfected gland. Oddly enough, the milk is considered a hostile environment for these phagocytic cells. Both cell types have reduced phagocytic and bactericidal capabilities when present in milk. More than 500,000 cells per milliliter are required to protect the lactating gland against bacterial infection. Consequently phagocytic cells may not provide an effective barrier to infection of a normal, quiescent mammary gland in the early stages following bacterial challenge.

The mammary gland macrophage in milk functions as an early detection system in the initiation of the inflammatory process. These cells produce interleukin-1 (IL-1) and lipid-type mediators on stimulation and are strategically placed at the primary defense locations such as the milk ducts. Stimulatory agents include microorganisms, microbial toxins, inflammatory agents, antigen-antibody complexes, and lymphokines. The macrophage-PMN host defense circuit is promoted by the mechanism involving IL-1 stimulation of membrane events leading to increased phospholipase activity.[79] The subsequent release of arachidonic acid makes this substrate available for PG or leukotriene synthesis. Leukotriene B_4 (LTB_4) produced by the macrophage is known to be one of the most potent in-vitro neutrophil chemoattractants.

Mastitic milk is rich in PMNs.[80] PMN function is mediated by protein receptors for Ig, complement, enzymes, chemotactic factors, and hormones. A negative correlation has been reported between the presence of clinical mastitis and the ability of milk to support phagocytosis. The decreased killing capacity of milk PMNs compared to that of blood PMNs has been attributed to: (1) absence of glucose in milk, (2) decreased amounts of glycogen in milk PMNs, (3) deficiency of opsonins and complement in milk, (4) coating of the surface of the neutrophil with casein, (5) loss of PMN pseudopods due to ingestion of fat, and (6) a decrease in the supply of hydrolytic enzymes within the PMNs following ingestion of fat and casein. PMN function of the oxygen-dependent killing pathway may be critically down-regulated during the last month of gestation and extending into the first month of lactation, making the gland more susceptible to infection.

The diapedesis of PMN into infected glands is delayed in cows that have recently freshened. This contributes to the well-documented increased susceptibility of cows in early lactation to peracute coliform mastitis. Recent evidence indicates that increasing dietary selenium to optimal levels markedly improves the ability of the mammary PMNs to kill ingested bacteria.

Two general antimicrobial systems contribute to PMN-mediated killing of microorganisms.[81-84] These antimicrobial processes are distinguished by their relationships to the postphagocytic metabolism of oxygen by the PMNs and are designated O_2-dependent or O_2-independent. Many investigators have demonstrated that PMNs are microbicidal for various organisms under anaerobic conditions. Fractionation of granule extract proteins by size and/or electrophoretic mobility has led to the identification of four major microbicidal protein activities. One of these, myeloperoxidase (MPO), requires hydrogen peroxide and halide ions for activity and thus fits into the O_2-dependent category.

Accordingly, the three other granule protein activities are presumed to be capable of functioning independently of the products of oxidative burst. An intermediate size microbicidal protein (25,000 to 30,000 daltons) has been isolated from human and bovine PMN extract and is referred to as cathepsin G or chymotrypsin-like cationic protein (CLCP). A relatively large antibacterial protein, BPI (50,000 to 60,000 daltons) has been purified from rabbit, human, and bovine PMNs.

An entirely separate family of bactericidal and bacteriostatic polypeptides have been isolated from the neutrophils of several species, including the rabbit, guinea pig, human, and bovine. These compounds comprise between 5% and 7% of the total protein content of the PMN and account for most of the microbicidal activity of crude PMN extracts against bacteria, viruses, and yeast. These defensins have been characterized as small (3,000 to 4,000 daltons) cystine and arginine-rich antimicrobial peptides found in the azurophil granules of the PMN.[85-87]

On the surface, the use of antibiotics in the mammary gland would not seem to influence defense mechanisms used by the host. However, in vitro studies indicate that some serious consequences may indeed exist.[88,89] These reports indicated that the potential for enhanced PMN phagocytosis exists through the use of macrolides, and that depressed phagocytosis results from the administration of chloramphenicols and aminoglycosides.

HUMORAL IMMUNE RESPONSE

In general, antibodies found in the mammary gland appear to serve as toxin neutralizers, bacteriocidins, and opsonins for PMNs and macrophages. Ig-mediated bacterial killing is used either in direct lysis via antibody plus complement (considered to be of minor importance) or in phagocytosis via opsonization by antibody (with or without complement). Phagocytosis of invading pathogens is the major defense mechanism preventing establishment of intramammary infections. Macrophages are the predominant cell type in normal lacteal secretions, and IgG_1 is the predominant Ig. However, bacteria that have been opsonized with IgG_2, but not IgG_1, enhance bovine PMN phagocytosis, whereas both IgG_1 and IgG_2 enhance phagocytosis by macrophages.[90,91] It is suggested that IgG_1 is more important to the defense of the mammary gland in early stages of infection, and the importance of IgG_2 increases as PMNs enter the gland during inflammation. Recent results using flow cytometry indicate that bovine PMNs bind IgM to a greater extent than other Ig isotypes. The exact influence on the outcome of mastitic events has not been elucidated. Intracellular pathogens such as *S. dublin* have been shown to survive in the mammary gland

(and be shed in milk) for periods of over one year in the face of high levels of anti-*S. dublin*–specific IgG.[92]

IgA in the mammary gland may function by: (1) neutralizing bacterial toxins, (2) agglutinating bacteria and thereby facilitating their removal during milking, (3) preventing bacterial multiplication, and (4) preventing bacterial adherence to epithelial surfaces.

CELL-MEDIATED IMMUNE RESPONSE

Development of cell surface markers delineating various subpopulations of bovine lymphocytes in the mammary gland is in its infancy. It should be noted that advances in knowledge of cell surface markers and flow cytometry may make the following information incomplete and will most likely change as specific infectious disease manifestations are evaluated.[93] Nevertheless, it appears that the lymphocyte population of bovine peripheral blood may consist of 73% T lymphocytes and 27% B lymphocytes. In bovine milk T lymphocytes comprise 31% to 65% of the population, in which B lymphocyte percentages are approximately 22% to 42%.[94]

Taylor, Dellinger, Cullor, et al.[95] report that T lymphocytes traffic selectively into bovine milk, whereas B lymphocytes represent a minor population in milk compared to peripheral blood. The vast majority of T cells in milk express α-β T cell receptors and are predominantly CD8+. T cells in milk express two-fold higher levels of CD^2 and five-fold lower levels of CD45R, characteristics that are associated with memory T cells. Grouping of cows by lactational stage and analysis of lymphocyte subpopulation percentages indicated that CD4+ T cells are present in relatively low numbers in milk of cows during the first 50 days of lactation and have a significant tendency to increase in number as lactation progresses.

Observations of lymphocytes recovered from quarters infected with *S. aureus* demonstrated that in vitro lymphocyte blastogenesis is markedly depressed during infection.[94] This suggests that in vivo lymphocyte function is compromised, possibly contributing to the chronicity of staphylococcal mastitis. It is quite likely that cell-mediated immune response has an influence on mammary gland defense mechanisms that has yet to be clearly delineated. Taylor and colleagues[96] observed that naturally occurring mastitis had significant effects on mammary gland subpopulations of T cells and cytokine expression. This information may give us our first insight into more specific cytokine treatments that may become available in the future.

LACTOFERRIN

Apolactoferrin, the iron-deficient form of lactoferrin (LF), is an iron-binding glycoprotein with antibacterial properties. It is found in mammary gland secretory cells, in high concen-

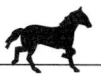

trations in milk during intramammary infection and involution, and in PMN granules. The resultant iron binding makes this essential element unavailable to bacteria that require iron for growth. The concentration of LF increases 100-fold during mammary involution.

RESISTANCE TO MASTITIS

Dairy breeds of cattle have undergone intense selective pressure over the decades. The literature indicates that both the structure and function of the bovine mammary gland have been impacted by the selective pressures to increase milk production.[97,98] In addition, associations between Major Histocompatibility Complex (MHC) BoLA antigens are beginning to give insight into genetic disease resistance in cattle against clinical and subclinical mastitis.[99,100]

Box 34-4 lists websites related to mammary gland health.

REFERENCES

1. Wilson DJ et al: Association between management practices, dairy herd characteristics, and somatic cell count of bulk tank milk, *J Am Vet Med Assoc* 210(10):1499-1502, 1997.
2. Sischo WM et al: Economics of disease occurrence and prevention in California dairy farms: A report and evaluation of data collected for the National Animal Health Monitoring System, *Prev Vet Med* 8:141-155, 1990.
3. Ruegg PL, Dohoo IR: A benefit to cost analysis of the effect of premilking teat hygiene on somatic cell count and intramammary infections in a commercial dairy herd, *Can Vet J* 38(10):632-636, 1997.
4. DeGraves FJ, Fetrow J: Economics of mastitis and mastitis control, *Vet Clin North Am Food Anim Pract* 9(3):421-434, 1993.
5. Berry SL et al: Effects of antimicrobial treatment at the end of lactation on milk yield, somatic cell count, and incidence of clinical mastitis during the subsequent lactation in a dairy herd with a low prevalence of contagious mastitis, *J Am Vet Med Assoc* 211(2):207-211, 1997.
6. Raubertas RF, Shook GE: Relationship between lactation measures of somatic cell concentration and milk yield, *J Dairy Sci* 65:419, 1982.
7. McDonald JS: Streptococcal and staphylococcal mastitis, *J Am Vet Med Assoc* 170(10 Pt 2):1157-1159, 1977.
8. Tyler JW et al: Modification of postmilking standing time by altering feed availability, *J Dairy Res* 65 (4):681-683, 1998.
9. Smith KL, Hogan JS, Weiss WP: Dietary vitamin E and selenium affect mastitis and milk quality, *J Anim Sci* 75(6):1659-1665, 1997.
10. Erskine RJ et al: Effects of parenteral administration of vitamin E on health of periparturient dairy cows (see comments), *J Am Vet Med Assoc* 211(4):466-469, 1997.
11. Weiss WP et al: Effect of vitamin E supplementation in diets with a low concentration of selenium on mammary gland health of dairy cows, *J Dairy Sci* 80(8):1728-1737, 1997.
12. Saran A: Disinfection in the dairy parlour, *Rev Sci Tech* 14(1):207-224, 1995.
13. Osteras O et al: Field studies show associations between pulsator characteristics and udder health, *J Dairy Res* 62(1):1-13, 1995.
14. Sears PM et al: Procedures for mastitis diagnosis and control, *Vet Clin North Am Food Anim Pract* 9(3):445-468, 1993.
15. Jasper DE: Bovine mycoplasmal mastitis, *Adv Vet Sci Comp Med* 25:121-157, 1981.
16. Gonzalez RN et al: Relationship between mastitis pathogen numbers in bulk tank milk and bovine udder infections in California dairy herds, *J Am Vet Med Assoc* 189(4):442-445, 1986.
17. Farnsworth RJ: Microbiologic examination of bulk tank milk, *Vet Clin North Am Food Anim Pract* 9(3):469-474, 1993.
18. Guterbock WM, Blackmer PE: Veterinary interpretation of bulk-tank milk, *Vet Clin North Am (Large Anim Pract)* 6(2):257-268, 1984.
19. Keefe GP: Streptococcus agalactiae mastitis: a review, *Can Vet J* 38(7):429-437, 1997.
20. Ruegg PL et al: Microbiologic investigation of an epizootic of mastitis caused by *Serratia marcescens* in a dairy herd, *J Am Vet Med Assoc* 200(2):184-189, 1992.
21. Cebra CK, Garry FB, Dinsmore RP: *Naturally occurring acute coliform mastitis in Holstein cattle*, *J Vet Intern Med* 10(4):252-257, 1996.
22. Burton JL, Kehrli ME, Jr: Regulation of neutrophil adhesion molecules and shedding of *Staphylococcus aureus* in milk of cortisol- and dexamethasone-treated cows, *Am J Vet Res* 56(8):997-1006, 1995.
23. Ferris KE, Miller DA: Salmonella serotypes from animals and related sources reported during 1991-1992. In Proceedings of the U.S. Animals Health Association, San Diego, 1992.
24. Lammerding AM et al: Prevalence of *Salmonella* and thermophillic *Campylobacter* in fresh pork, beef, veal, and poultry in Canada, *J Food Prot* 51:47-52, 1988.

25. Smith BP et al: Detection of *Salmonella dublin* mammary gland infection in carrier cows, using an enzyme-linked immunosorbent assay for antibody in milk or serum (published erratum appears in *Am J Vet Res* 50(10):1799, 1989). *Am J Vet Res* 50(8):1352-1360, 1989.
26. Tablante NL, Dubose DA: Field investigations of sporadic *Salmonella dublin* outbreaks in a closed dairy herd. In Proceedings of the Eighth Annual Western Conference for Food Animal Disease, Boise, Idaho, 1987.
27. House JK et al: Enzyme-linked immunosorbent assay for serologic detection of *Salmonella dublin* carriers on a large dairy, *Am J Vet Res* 54(9):1391-1399, 1993.
28. Da Costa EO et al: An increased incidence of mastitis caused by *Prototheca* species and *Nocardia* species on a farm in Sao Paulo, Brazil, *Vet Res Commun* 20(3):237-241, 1996.
29. Guterbock WM et al: Efficacy of intramammary antibiotic therapy for treatment of clinical mastitis caused by environmental pathogens, *J Dairy Sci* 76(11):3437-3444, 1993.
30. Wilson DJ et al: Comparison of seven antibiotic treatments with no treatment for bacteriological efficacy against bovine mastitis pathogens, *J Dairy Sci* 82(8):1664-1670, 1999.
31. Ziv G: Drug selection and use in mastitis: systemic vs local therapy, *J Am Vet Med Assoc* 176(10 Spec No):1109-1115, 1980.
32. Ziv G: Practical pharmacokinetic aspects of mastitis therapy—3: intramammary treatment, *Vet Med Small Anim Clin* 75(4):657-670, 1980.
33. Nostrand SD et al: Effects of daily exogenous oxytocin on lactation milk yield and composition, *J Dairy Sci* 74(7):2119-2127, 1991.
34. Sischo WM, Burns CM: Field trials of four cowside antibiotic-residue screening tests, *J Am Vet Med Assoc* 202:1249-1254, 1993.
35. Cullor JS et al: Performance of various tests used to screen antibiotic residues in milk samples from individual animals, *J AOAC Inter* 77:862-870, 1994.
36. Angelidis AS, Farver TB, Cullor JS: Evaluation of the Delvo-X-Press assay for detecting antibiotic residue in milk samples from individual cows, *J Food Prod* 62:1183-1190, 1999.
37. Yancy RJ Jr: Vaccines and diagnostic methods for bovine mastitis: fact and fiction, *Adv Vet Med* 41:257-273, 1999.
38. Tomita GM et al: Immunization of dairy cows with an *Escherichia coli* J5 lipopolysaccharide vaccine, *J Dairy Sci* 78(10):2178-2185, 1995.
39. Tyler JW et al: Humoral response in neonatal calves following immunization with *Escherichia coli* (strain J5): the effects of adjuvant, age and colostral passive interference, *Vet Immunol Immunopathol* 23(3-4):333-344, 1989.
40. Tyler JW et al: Effect of passive transfer status and vaccination with *Escherichia coli* (J5) on mortality in commingled dairy calves, *J Vet Intern Med* 13(1):36-39, 1999.
41. Tyler JW et al: Relationship between serologic recognition of *Escherichia coli* 0111:B4 (J5) and clinical coliform mastitis in cattle, *Am J Vet Res* 49(11):1950-1954, 1988.
42. Gonzalez RN et al: Prevention of clinical coliform mastitis in dairy cows by a mutant *Escherichia coli* vaccine, *Can J Vet Res* 53(3):301-305, 1989.
43. DeGraves FJ, Fetrow J: Partial budget analysis of vaccinating dairy cattle against coliform mastitis with an *Escherichia coli* J5 vaccine, *J Am Vet Med Assoc* 199(4):451-455, 1991.
44. Hogan JS et al: Field trial to determine efficacy of an *Escherichia coli* J5 mastitis vaccine, *J Dairy Sci* 75(1):78-84, 1992.
45. Hogan JS et al: Efficacy of an *Escherichia coli* J5 bacterin administered to primigravid heifers, *J Dairy Sci* 82(5):939-043, 1999.
46. Hogan JS et al: Effects of an *Escherichia coli* J5 vaccine on mild clinical coliform mastitis, *J Dairy Sci* 78(2):285-290, 1995.
47. Tomita GM et al: Antigenic crossreactivity and lipopolysaccharide neutralization properties of bovine immunoglobulin G, *J Dairy Sci* 78(12):2745-2752, 1995.
48. Calzolari A et al: Field trials of a vaccine against bovine mastitis. 2. Evaluation in two commercial dairy herds, *J Dairy Sci* 80(5):854-858, 1997.
49. Giraudo JA et al: Field trials of a vaccine against bovine mastitis. 1. Evaluation in heifers, *J Dairy Sci* 80(5):845-853, 1997.
50. Watson DL, McColl ML, Davies HI: Field trial of a staphylococcal mastitis vaccine in dairy herds: clinical, subclinical and microbiological assessments, *Aust Vet J* 74(6):447-450, 1996.
51. Leigh JA et al: Vaccination with the plasminogen activator from *Streptococcus uberis* induces an inhibitory response and protects against experimental infection in the dairy cow, *Vaccine* 17(7-8):851-857, 1999.
52. Finch JM et al: Further studies on the efficacy of a live vaccine against mastitis caused by *Streptococcus uberis*, *Vaccine* 15(10):1138-1143, 1997.
53. Selim SA, Cullor JS: Number of viable bacteria and presumptive antibiotic residues in milk fed to calves in commercial dairies, *J Am Vet Med Assoc* 211(8):1029-1035, 1997.
54. Oliver SP, Mitchell BA: Intramammary infections in primigravid heifers near parturition, *J Dairy Sci* 66(5):1180-1183, 1983.
55. Matthews KR, Harmon RJ, Langlois BE: Prevalence of *Staphylococcus* species during the periparturient period in primiparous and multiparous cows, *J Dairy Sci* 75(7):1835-1839, 1992.
56. Trinidad P, Nickerson SC, Alley TK: Prevalence of intramammary infection and teat canal colonization in unbred and primigravid dairy heifers, *J Dairy Sci* 73(1):107-114, 1990.

57. Fox LK et al: Survey of intramammary infections in dairy heifers at breeding age and first parturition, *J Dairy Sci* 78(7):1619-1628, 1995.
58. Nickerson SC, Owens WE, Boddie RL: Mastitis in dairy heifers: initial studies on prevalence and control, *J Dairy Sci* 78(7):1607-1618, 1995.
59. Roberson JR et al: Sources of intramammary infections from *Staphylococcus aureus* in dairy heifers at first parturition, *J Dairy Sci* 81(3):687-693, 1998.
60. Waage S et al: Bacteria associated with clinical mastitis in dairy heifers, *J Dairy Sci* 82(4):712-719, 1999.
61. McCue PM, Wilson WD: Equine mastitis—a review of 28 cases, *Equine Vet J* 21(5):351-353, 1989.
62. East NE, Birnie EF, Farver TB: Risk factors associated with mastitis in dairy goats, *Am J Vet Res* 48(5):776-779, 1987.
63. Ryan DP, Greenwood PL: Prevalence of udder bacteria in milk samples from four dairy goat herds, *Aust Vet J* 67(10):362-363, 1990.
64. East NE, Birnie EF: Diseases of the udder, *Vet Clin North Am (Large Anim Pract)* 5(3):591-600, 1983.
65. Delouis C: Physiology of colostrum production, *Ann Rech Vet* 9(2):193-203, 1978.
66. Tucker HA: Physiological control of mammary growth, lactogenesis, and lactation, *J Dairy Sci* 64(6):1403-1421, 1981.
67. Holt C: Interrelationships of the concentrations of some ionic constituents of human milk and comparison with cow and goat milks, *Comp Biochem Physiol Comp Physiol* 104(1):35-41, 1993.
68. Butler JE: Immunoglobulins of the mammary secretions, In Butler JE: *Lactation*, New York, 1974, Academic Press.
69. Brandon MR, Watson DL, Lascelles AK: The mechanism of transfer of immunoglobulin into mammary secretion of cows, *Aust J Exp Biol Med Sci* 49(6):613-623, 1971.
70. Sasaki M, Larson BL, Nelson DR: Kinetic analysis of the binding of immunoglobulins IgG1 and IgG2 to bovine mammary cells, *Biochem Biophys Acta* 497(1):160-170, 1977.
71. Bauman DE, Currie WB: Partitioning of nutrients during pregnancy and lactation: a review of mechanisms involving homeostasis and homeorrhesis, *J Dairy Sci* 63(9):1514-1529, 1980.
72. Delouis C et al: Relation between hormones and mammary gland function, *J Dairy Sci* 63(9):1492-1513, 1980.
73. Soloff MS: Oxytocin receptors and mammary myoepithelial cells, *J Dairy Sci* 65(2):326-337, 1982.
74. Nickerson SC: Resistance mechanisms of the bovine udder: new implications for mastitis control at the teat end, *J Am Vet Med Assoc* 191(11):1484-1488, 1987.
75. Comalli MP et al: Changes in the microscopic anatomy of the bovine teat canal during mammary involution, *Am J Vet Res* 45(11):2236-2242, 1984.
76. Capuco AV et al: Increased susceptibility to intramammary infection following removal of teat canal keratin, *J Dairy Sci* 75(8):2126-2130, 1992.
77. Hogan JS, Pankey JW, Duthie AH: Growth responses of *Staphylococcus aureus* and *Streptococcus agalactiae* to *Corynebacterium bovis* metabolites, *J Dairy Sci* 70(6):1294-1301, 1987.
78. Hogan JS, Pankey JW, Duthie AH: Growth inhibition of mastitis pathogens by long-chain fatty acids, *J Dairy Sci* 70(5):927-934, 1987.
79. Jensen DL, Eberhart RJ: Macrophages in bovine milk, *Am J Vet Res* 36(5):619-624, 1975.
80. Paape MJ et al: Leukocytes—second line of defense against invading mastitis pathogens, *J Dairy Sci* 62(1):135-153, 1979.
81. Root RK, Cohen MS: The microbicidal mechanisms of human neutrophils and eosinophils, *Rev Infect Dis* 3(3):565-598, 1981.
82. Elsbach P, Weiss J: A reevaluation of the roles of the O_2-dependent and O_2-independent microbicidal systems of phagocytes, *Rev Infect Dis* 5(5):843-853, 1983.
83. Spitznagel JK: Bacteriocidal mechanisms of the granulocyte, In Spitznagel JK: *The granulocyte: function and clinical utilization*, New York, 1977, Alan R. Riss.
84. Mandell GL: Bactericidal activity of aerobic and anaerobic polymorphonuclear neutrophils, *Infect Immun* 9(2):337-341, 1974.
85. Selsted ME, Szklarek D, Lehrer RI: Purification and antibacterial activity of antimicrobial peptides of rabbit granulocytes, *Infect Immun* 45(1):150-154, 1984.
86. Selsted ME et al: Primary structures of six antimicrobial peptides of rabbit peritoneal neutrophils, *J Biol Chem* 260(8):4579-4584, 1985.
87. Selsted ME et al: Indolicidin, a novel bactericidal tridecapeptide amide from neutrophils, *J Biol Chem* 267(7):4292-4295, 1992.
88. Selsted ME et al: Purification, primary structures, and antibacterial activities of beta-defensins, a new family of antimicrobial peptides from bovine neutrophils, *J Biol Chem* 268(9):6641-6648, 1993.
89. Nickerson SC, Paape MJ, Dulin AM: Effect of antibiotics and vehicles on bovine mammary polymorphonuclear leukocyte morphologic features, viability, and phagocytic activity in vitro, *Am J Vet Res* 46(11):2259-2265, 1985.
90. Ziv G, Paape MJ, Dulin AM: Influence of antibiotics and intramammary antibiotic products on phagocytosis of *Staphylococcus aureus* by bovine leukocytes, *Am J Vet Res* 44(3):385-388, 1983.
91. Guidry AJ, Miller RH: Immunoglobulin isotype concentrations in milk as affected by stage of lactation and parity, *J Dairy Sci* 69(7):1799-1805, 1986.
92. Spier SJ et al: Persistent experimental *Salmonella dublin* intramammary infection in dairy cows, *J Vet Intern Med* 5(6):341-350, 1991.
93. Yang #387-1997.
94. Nonnecke BJ, Harp JA: Effect of chronic staphylococcal mastitis on mitogenic responses of bovine lymphocytes, *J Dairy Sci* 68(12):3323-3328, 1985.
95. Taylor BC et al: Bovine milk lymphocytes display the phenotype of memory T cells and are predominantly CD8+, *Cell Immunol* 156(1):245-253, 1994.
96. Taylor BC et al: T cell populations and cytokine expression in milk derived from normal and bacteria-infected bovine mammary glands, *Cell Immunol* 182(1):68-76, 1997.
97. Sordillo LM, Shafer-Weaver K, DeRosa D: Immunobiology of the mammary gland, *J Dairy Sci* 80(8):1851-1865, 1997.
98. Akers RM: Selection for milk production from a lactation biology viewpoint, *J Dairy Sci* 83(5):1151-1158, 2000.
99. Aarestrup FM, Jensen NE, Ostergard H: Analysis of associations between major histocompatibility complex (BoLA) class I haplotypes and subclinical mastitis of dairy cows, *J Dairy Sci* 78(8):1684-1692, 1995.
100. Sharif S et al: Associations of the bovine major histocompatibility complex DRB3 (BoLA-DRB3) with production traits in Canadian dairy cattle, *Anim Genet* 30(2):157-160, 1999.

Diseases of the Hematopoietic and Hemolymphatic Systems

GARY P. CARLSON
Consulting Editor

DISEASES ASSOCIATED WITH BLOOD LOSS OR HEMOSTATIC DYSFUNCTION

DEBRA DEEM MORRIS

Blood loss may be acute or chronic, and the clinical and laboratory manifestations are widely different because physiologic adaptation occurs in the chronic state.

ACUTE BLOOD LOSS

Common causes for acute blood loss include trauma (e.g., severe lacerations), surgical procedures (e.g., dehorning, castration), and erosion of the carotid artery by guttural pouch mycosis in horses. External hemorrhage is immediately obvious, but hemorrhage into a major body cavity may be occult (e.g., spontaneous rupture of the middle uterine artery, splenic rupture resulting from trauma or erosion of a major vessel by abscess, aneurism, or neoplasia). Hemoperitoneum may induce signs of colic, and hemothorax is generally attended by dyspnea. Acute massive blood loss induces hypovolemic shock characterized by tachycardia, tachypnea, cold extremities, pale mucous membranes, muscle weakness, and eventual death resulting from cardiovascular collapse.

Acute blood loss does not initially cause a change in the packed cell volume (PCV) or total plasma protein (TPP), although rapid mobilization of extracellular fluid to maintain circulating blood volume causes the PCV and TPP to decline within 12 to 24 hours. The severity of blood loss may be partially masked by splenic contraction because shock causes activation of the sympathetic nervous system. Icterus is absent, and bone marrow erythroid hyperplasia is delayed by 3 to 4 days. Peripheral signs of erythroid regeneration in horses are limited to mild anisocytosis with a variable increase in mean corpuscular volume. Ruminants show erythrocyte polychromasia, basophilic stippling, Howell-Jolly bodies, and occasionally nucleated erythrocytes within 4 days of the onset of hemorrhage.

DIAGNOSIS. Diagnosis of acute blood loss is based on clinical signs, evidence of recent hemorrhage, and anemia accompanied by hypoproteinemia. Hemoperitoneum and hemothorax may be suggested by ultrasound and abdominocentesis and thoracocentesis respectively.

TREATMENT. Treatment of acute blood loss should initially be aimed at stopping the hemorrhage. External hemorrhage may be managed by pressure wraps or appropriately placed ligatures; however, it may be inadvisable to attempt to control internal hemorrhage when the patient is a poor risk for general anesthesia, and the source of hemorrhage may not be found. Hypovolemic shock should be treated by prompt intravenous administration of 40 to 80 ml/kg of sodium-containing crystalloid solutions. Studies indicate that a small volume of hypertonic saline (4 to 6 ml/kg, 7.2% sodium chloride) may permanently reverse the pathophysiologic sequelae of severe hemorrhagic shock.[1,2] The total volume of necessary crystalloid solution is usually much greater than the volume of blood lost because crystalloid solutions distribute throughout the extracellular space. The clinical response to fluid administration should be evaluated in light of ongoing losses to determine the necessary replacement volume.

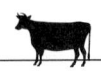

If anemia becomes life-threatening, whole blood transfusion must be considered. A PCV less than 20% in an animal with acute blood loss suggests depletion of erythrocyte reserves, and persistent reduction of the PCV over a period of 24 to 48 hours to 12% or less indicates the need for blood transfusion. A low but stable PCV (12% to 20%) does not necessitate transfusion because transfusion should be reserved for instances in which oxygen delivery to the tissues is inadequate to support life. Blood transfusion can only be viewed as a temporary therapeutic procedure because even cross-match–compatible, allogeneic erythrocytes are removed from the circulation by the mononuclear phagocyte system (MPS) within 2 to 4 days of transfusion.[3] Horses and cattle display a high degree of blood type polymorphism, and minor antigenic incompatibilities are only delineated by blood typing (see Chapter 49).[4] Serum antibodies against nonhost erythrocyte antigens (erythrocyte alloantibodies) probably mediate the short life span of transfused erythrocytes. Compatibility testing is used to avert life-threatening antigen-antibody reactions caused by major blood group mismatching.

The routine cross-match involves incubating washed erythrocytes from donor (major) and recipient (minor) with serum from the other. Gross and microscopic examination for clumping demonstrates serum agglutinins in horses. Sensitized cattle erythrocytes do not become clumped in saline solution but do lyse in the presence of rabbit complement, so only a hemolytic crossmatch can be performed in this species. Not all equine erythrocyte alloantibodies act as agglutinins, and hemolysins must be detected by adding complement to the reaction mixture. Pooled rabbit serum must first be absorbed with equine erythrocytes to remove naturally occurring antibodies. The need for special handling and storage of rabbit serum makes hemolytic cross-match procedures impractical for most veterinarians. These tests are best performed by veterinary hematology laboratories (e.g., Veterinary Genetics Laboratory, School of Veterinary Medicine, University of California, Davis), which usually require serum and whole blood in sodium citrate or acid-citrate-dextrose (ACD) to cross-match.

The first transfusion of whole blood to a horse or ruminant that has not been previously transfused or sensitized by immunization or pregnancy is usually well tolerated because natural alloantibodies are of low concentration and weak activity. After incompatible transfusions, alloantibodies develop rapidly, making subsequent transfusions more hazardous.

Blood for transfusion should be collected aseptically into sterile containers containing sodium citrate (2.5% to 4%) or ACD solution and used immediately. The necessary dosage can only be estimated, but in most instances replacing 20% to 40% of the calculated blood loss is sufficient to maintain life until the bone marrow can respond. A drop in PCV from 36% to 12% in a 500-kg animal (8% body weight blood) represents a loss of 27 L of blood. In this case, 6 to 8 L of whole blood would be therapeutic and easily donated by another 500-kg individual. Blood warmed to 37° C (98.6° F) should be administered through an in-line filter to remove clots. After pretransfusion vital parameters have been recorded, 0.1 ml of blood per kilogram of body weight is given over 5 to 10 minutes and the evaluation is repeated. If parameters and attitude are unchanged, the transfusion can be continued at a rate not to exceed 20 ml/kg/hr. The recipient should be continuously monitored so the transfusion can be stopped if there are adverse reactions such as tachypnea, dyspnea, restlessness, defecation, tachycardia, piloerection, muscle fasciculations, or sudden collapse. Although these signs may not indicate anaphylaxis, severe reactions should be treated with epinephrine (0.01 to 0.02 ml/kg, 1:1000). Mild signs may respond to a slowed transfusion rate or administration of corticosteroids or flunixin meglumine. Because it is often not possible to delineate the cause of transfusion reactions, the safest approach is to discontinue the blood and administer isotonic crystalloid solutions.

The prognosis is good for most cases of acute blood loss if hypovolemic shock is quickly treated and the bleeding stops. The normal bone marrow begins to replace lost cells within 5 days. Sequential analysis of the PCV will be necessary to determine whether blood loss is controlled.

CHRONIC BLOOD LOSS

A number of diseases can result in chronic loss of blood that is insidious until clinical signs of anemia develop. Physiologic adaptation to gradually developing tissue hypoxia generally masks signs of anemia until the PCV is less than 15%. Causes for chronic blood loss include bleeding gastrointestinal lesions, certain renal diseases, hemostatic dysfunction, bloodsucking external parasites, and hemonchosis (especially in goats and sheep).

Gastrointestinal hemorrhage is usually caused by neoplasia (especially gastric squamous cell carcinoma in horses and abomasal lymphosarcoma in cattle), parasitism, or mucosal ulceration (e.g., abomasal ulcers in cattle and nonsteroidal antiinflammatory drug toxicity in horses). Significant hemorrhage may occur in ruminants heavily infested with *Haemonchus contortus* shortly after they are treated with an anthelmintic. Generally gastrointestinal hemorrhage is best detected by chemical determination of fecal occult blood because melena rarely occurs in horses, and bleeding abomasal ulcers cannot be excluded in cattle when melena is absent. Because of the low specificity of tests for fecal occult blood, the diagnosis of chronic gastrointestinal blood loss is usually supported by strong clinical suspicion and ruling out of other sources of hemorrhage.

Although renal papillary necrosis, caused by nonsteroidal antiinflammatory drug therapy, and urinary calculi cause hematuria, anemia rarely results. Renal neoplasia or congenital renal vascular anomalies rarely may be associated with chronic blood loss anemia.

Disorders of hemostasis may cause internal or external hemorrhage that leads to anemia if enough blood is lost. Qualitative or quantitative abnormalities of blood vessels, platelets, or coagulation factors result in hemostatic dysfunction (see next section). Loss of erythrocyte iron secondary to chronic severe blood loss may result in iron deficiency anemia. Hypoferremia or reduced serum ferritin develops with increased total iron-binding capacity and reduction in marrow iron. The degree of iron depletion can be qualitatively evaluated by Prussian blue iron staining of a bone marrow aspirate or biopsy. Iron deficiency produces an inadequate marrow response and compounds chronic blood loss anemia.

The aim in management of chronic blood loss is to determine the primary cause. Treatment of the anemia per se is rarely indicated. Iron deficiency may be alleviated by oral supplementation with ferrous sulfate, although good-quality forages contain more than adequate amounts of iron. Parenteral iron supplementation as iron dextran should be avoided because it has been associated with anaphylactoid reactions in large animals. If iron must be given parenterally, iron cacodylate is approved for intravenous administration in horses but is not readily available except from some compounding pharmacies.

HEMOSTATIC DYSFUNCTION

Basic Physiology of Normal Hemostasis

The basis for understanding the pathogenesis and manifestations of hemostatic disorders is a thorough understanding of the normal physiologic mechanism of hemostasis (Fig. 35-1). Hemostasis can be viewed as two interrelated components, coagulation and fibrinolysis (both with their respec-

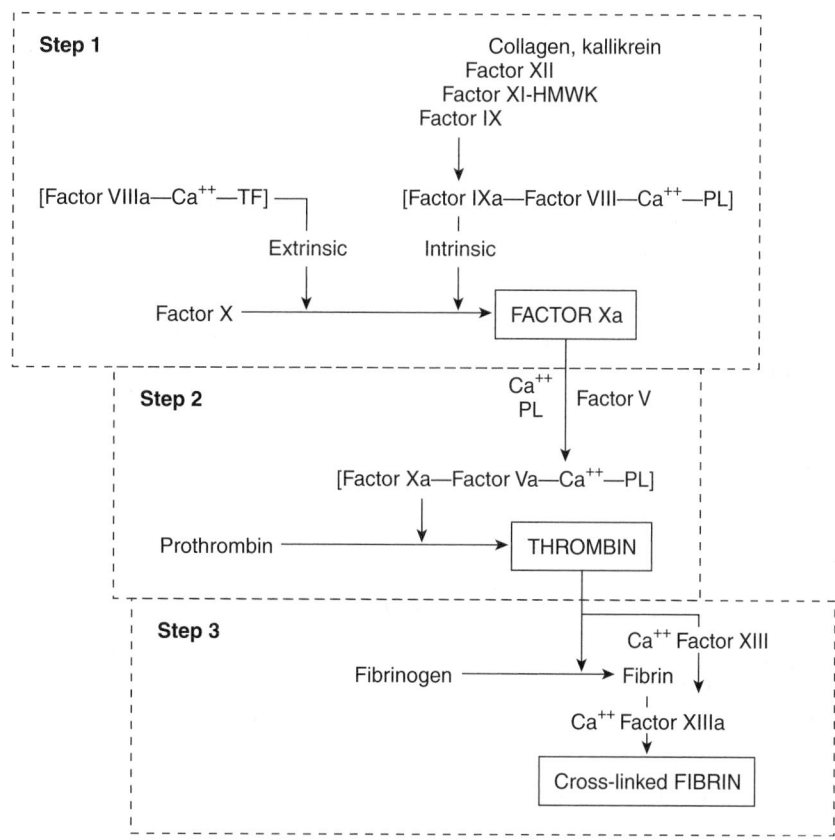

FIG. 35-1 ▓ Normal blood coagulation sequence: formation of activated factor X; formation of thrombin; formation of fibrin.

tive inhibitors), which function to arrest bleeding from a damaged blood vessel and to maintain nutrient blood flow.

Coagulation is mediated by blood vessels, platelets, and blood procoagulant proteins. When a blood vessel is damaged, vasoconstriction occurs, followed by rapid adherence of platelets to subendothelial collagen. Platelet adhesion causes membrane conformational changes that trigger aggregation, contraction, and granule secretion (the basic platelet reaction). Platelet phospholipoprotein (platelet factor 3) provides the necessary surface to catalyze interactions among the activated coagulation proteins that result in thrombin formation. Coagulant proteins are localized to this hemostatic plug because the platelet surface protects them from plasma anticoagulants. Through some incompletely understood mechanism, platelets also prevent spontaneous hemorrhage into the skin and mucous membranes by maintaining "vascular integrity."

Procoagulant proteins circulate in the blood as precursive forms (zymogens) that must be altered during coagulation to become active. Numerous communications exist between the traditional extrinsic and intrinsic pathways, although initiating mechanisms remain distinct.[5] The extrinsic system is initiated when lipoprotein tissue factor (TF) gains access to the bloodstream. TF is widely distributed in most tissues, including endothelial cells and monocytes, and it may be increased or secreted in response to numerous pathologic stimuli such as bacterial endotoxin. Intrinsic coagulation is initiated when blood is exposed to a negatively charged surface such as activated platelets. Because of reciprocal activation between factor XII and prekallikrein, the intrinsic coagulation pathway stimulates formation of numerous inflammatory mediators such as kinins and complement. Both coagulation pathways culminate in the formation of activated factor X (Xa) by which

thrombin is generated. In addition to catalyzing the conversion of fibrinogen to fibrin, thrombin promotes platelet aggregation, enhances cofactor activities of factors V and VIII, and activates factor XIII and protein C.[6] Mechanisms to localize coagulation to the site of vascular injury are critical to protect against generalized thrombosis.[7] Plasma anticoagulant proteins include the serpins, which inhibit activated coagulation factors, and the protein C system, which is directed against cofactors V and VIII.[8] Antithrombin III (AT III), the main physiologic inhibitor of thrombin and Xa, normally provides 70% of the anticoagulant activity of plasma. Although not absolutely needed, heparin accelerates AT III action by 2000-fold.[9] Activated protein C destroys factors V and VIII, ultimately limiting its own activation, which depends on thrombin and endothelial cofactor, thrombomodulin. Protein S enhances the anticoagulant ability of protein C.

The fibrinolytic system is activated simultaneously with coagulation and functions to prevent tissue ischemia by limiting the extent of fibrin clot formation. Plasmin, primarily responsible for degradation of fibrin, exists in the plasma as the zymogen, plasminogen. Plasminogen has a high affinity for fibrin, as does tissue plasminogen activator (tPA); therefore clots contain the necessary components to allow lysis from within and systemic plasmin formation is avoided. α-2-Antiplasmin (α-2-AP), the main physiologic inhibitor of plasmin, competes with the binding of plasminogen to fibrin, and the clot contains equal amounts of both glycoproteins. Because of this molar balance between α-2-AP and plasminogen, a normal blood clot does not lyse spontaneously, despite fixation of tPA. Physiologic inhibitors of tPA (PAIs) are found in plasma, platelets, and endothelial cells; and platelet-derived PAI also protects a blood clot against premature lysis. Clot lysis is initiated if additional tPA is

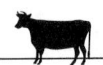

taken up from the surrounding tissues; stasis upstream from the occluded vessel is a potent stimulus for release of endothelial tPA. Conversion of plasminogen to plasmin allows partial digestion of fibrin and exposure of additional plasminogen binding sites. When this additional plasminogen is converted to plasmin, the inhibitory effect of α-2-AP is overcome, and clot lysis is accelerated. Plasmin hydrolyzes fibrinogen and fibrin with equal affinity, as well as numerous other procoagulants, and it can activate complement and kininogen. The physiologic actions of plasmin are limited to the fibrin clot by the affinity between the latter and plasminogen and the presence of α-2-AP in blood. Because of multiple interactions between the coagulation and fibrinolytic systems, the most important factor that determines the rate of fibrinolysis is the rate of fibrin formation.[10]

Inherited Coagulation Disorders

Inherited deficiencies of factors VIII,[11] IX, XI,[12] and prekallikrein[13] have been described in horses. Holstein cattle may have inherent factor XI deficiency.[14] Congenital factor VIII deficiency (hemophilia A) is sex linked and recessive, occurring only in males. Factor XI deficiency in cattle is transmitted as an autosomal recessive trait.[14] The inheritance pattern of the other deficiencies has not been proven.

Clinical signs of clotting factor deficiency reflect the tendency for abnormal hemorrhage from larger vessels (e.g., subcutaneous hematomas; hemarthroses; epistaxis; melena; hematuria; and prolonged bleeding after trauma, diagnostic procedures, or surgery). Petechiae are a feature of vascular or platelet disorders (see next section) and are not caused by clotting factor deficiency. Clinical signs do not always result from inherited clotting factor deficiencies. Cattle deficient for factor XI and horses with prekallikrein deficiency have complete in vivo coagulation competency. Prekallikrein appears to perform an accelerating rather than required role in activation of factor XII.[5] Activated factor XII activates factor XI, which then catalyzes the remainder of the clotting sequence. Factor XII is also capable of activating factor VII in the extrinsic pathway,[5] and this may explain why deficiency of factor XI does not cause a hemorrhagic diathesis. Values for the coagulant part of factor VIII (VIII:C) or factor IX must be reduced to less than 5% of normal before spontaneous hemorrhage occurs. Less severe deficiencies may result in excessive hemorrhage only after trauma.

The major differential diagnoses for heritable factor deficiencies include the acquired coagulation factor–deficient states, disseminated intravascular coagulation (DIC), warfarin toxicosis (horses), moldy sweet clover toxicosis, and acute hepatic disease. The heritable clotting factor deficiencies involve proteins in the intrinsic pathway; thus a prolonged activated partial thromboplastin time (APTT) is the only hemostatic abnormality. Acquired coagulation factor deficiencies involve proteins in the extrinsic or common pathways as well, causing a trend toward prolongation of both the prothrombin time (PT) and APTT. The definitive diagnosis of heritable clotting factor deficiency must be based on specific quantitative assays of intrinsic clotting factors. The only possible treatment for heritable clotting factor deficiency is replacement of clotting factors through the administration of fresh plasma. Specific clotting factor concentrates are not commercially available for large animals, and the rarity of specific factor-deficiency states that produce clinical signs makes the development of these products unlikely. Because of the expense of therapy and the potential for complications, the long-term prognosis for horses with hemophilia A or multiple congenital coagulation factor defects is poor. Cattle with factor XI deficiency apparently live a normal life but may be more susceptible to secondary diseases.[14]

Acquired Coagulation Disorders

Acquired defects of hemostasis may be divided into those involving blood vessels, platelets, and coagulation factors, although some diseases affect more than one component.

VASCULITIS. Vasculitis is a clinicopathologic process that involves inflammation and necrosis of blood vessels walls, regardless of size, location, or cause.[15] Vasculitis in large animals is generally a secondary manifestation of a primary infectious, toxic, or neoplastic disorder and has characteristics of hypersensitivity vasculitis in humans. The predominant involvement of small vessels in the skin such as venules and arterioles is the hallmark of hypersensitivity vasculitis.

The clinical manifestations of vasculitis include demarcated areas of dermal or subcutaneous edema, which may progress to skin infarction, necrosis, and exudation.[16] Hyperemia, petechial and ecchymotic hemorrhages, and ulceration of mucous membranes are common. Although the skin and mucous membranes are predominantly involved, hemorrhage and necrosis may occur in any organ system, resulting in conditions such as lameness, colic, dyspnea, and ataxia. Subclinical renal disease is not uncommon. Vasculitis is often attended by a number of adverse sequelae such as cellulitis, thrombophlebitis, laminitis, and pneumonia. Characterized vasculitis syndromes with predominant cutaneous involvement include equine purpura hemorrhagica (EPH), equine viral arteritis (EVA), equine infectious anemia (EIA), and equine ehrlichiosis (EE). In addition, there are a number of vasculitis syndromes in horses for which the cause, pathogenesis, and clinical course are poorly defined.[17,18] Vasculitis is apparently uncommon in ruminants but may accompany certain septicemic diseases such as malignant catarrhal fever of cattle and bluetongue of sheep.[19] Hematologic and serum biochemical findings in vasculitis are determined by the underlying disease, length of illness, organ involvement, and secondary complications. Chronic inflammation may be attended by neutrophilia, mild anemia, hyperglobulinemia, and hyperfibrinogenemia. Some horses with EPH develop a moderate anemia (PCV 20% to 25%) that is thought to be caused by increased erythrocyte destruction.[20] The platelet count is generally normal. Muscle damage may be reflected by increased serum concentrations of creatine phosphokinase (CPK) and aspartate aminotransferase (AST). The creatinine may be elevated, and urinalysis may rarely show trace hematuria or proteinuria if there is glomerulonephritis.

The definitive diagnosis of vasculitis is made by demonstration of the characteristic histopathology of involved vessels. Full-thickness punch biopsies (at least 6 mm in diameter) of skin in an affected area should be obtained and preserved in 10% formalin and Michel's transport medium. Multiple biopsies from different sites may be necessary to reach the diagnosis. The most common inflammatory pattern is neutrophilic infiltration of venules in the dermis and subcutaneous tissue, with nuclear debris in and around involved vessels (leukocytoclasis) and fibrinoid necrosis. Immunofluorescence on biopsies preserved in Michel's medium may reveal immune complexes. Considerable evidence suggests that most vasculitis syndromes are mediated by immunologic mechanisms, that is, an allergic reaction to a microbe, drug, toxin, or protein.[15] In some instances an exogenous stimulus cannot be identified, and an autoimmune pathogenesis is suspected. Immune complex deposition in vessel walls, with subsequent complement activation and chemoattractant production seems to be the major pathogenic mechanism. Infiltrating neutrophils and macrophages release proteolytic enzymes that cause vessel wall necrosis with subsequent edema, hemorrhage, and infarction of supplied tissues. Size and physiochemical properties of immune

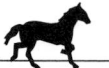

complexes, blood flow turbulence in sites of vessel bifurcation, and hydrostatic forces in dependent areas account for preferential formation of lesions in certain disease states and anatomic locations.

Equine Purpura Hemorrhagica. Although the etiology remains unproven, EPH is believed to represent an allergic reaction that follows respiratory tract infections. EPH has been seen in horses that have recovered from *Streptococcus equi* infection and are vaccinated with *S. equi,* and in horses vaccinated excessively against *S. equi* (situations attended by high levels of both antibody and antigen). Typically respiratory infection by *S. equi* (strangles) precedes clinical signs of EPH by 2 to 4 weeks[21]; however, EPH rarely may follow infections with *Streptococcus zooepidemicus,* equine influenza, or *Rhodococcus equi.* EPH may occur in a previously sensitized horse that does not develop strangles but is exposed to other horses infected with *S. equi.*[16] Clinical signs of EPH include well-demarcated areas of cutaneous edema, usually on head, ventral abdomen, or extremities with mucosal petechial or ecchymotic hemorrhages. The edema is often sensitive, with affected horses being depressed and reluctant to move. Diagnosis of EPH is usually based on history and clinical signs. Documentation of leukocytoclastic venulitis in skin biopsies adds support to the diagnosis. Some cases are refractory to therapy, and death may result from secondary septic processes.

Treatment of hypersensitivity vasculitis (purpura hemorrhagica and other syndromes) is directed at (1) removing the antigenic stimulus, (2) reducing the immune response, (3) reducing vessel wall inflammation, and (4) supportive care. Edema can be minimized by aggressive hydrotherapy and pressure wraps where possible. Fluids, administered through nasogastric tube or intravenously, may be necessary for animals that become severely depressed and fail to drink or those that develop dysphagia from pharyngeal edema. Stridor and dyspnea may indicate the need for tracheostomy. Nonsteroidal antiinflammatory drugs such as phenylbutazone or flunixin meglumine reduce inflammation and provide analgesia. Antimicrobial therapy may reduce the incidence or severity of cellulitis and other septic sequelae.

Any medication being given when signs occurred should be discontinued, and a thorough search for an underlying infection is necessary. Horses with a known streptococcal infection should receive penicillin (22,000 U/kg of procaine penicillin G IM, twice daily; or potassium penicillin G IV every 6 hours) for at least 2 weeks. Any accessible abscesses must be drained. Although EPH seems to be an allergic response to streptococcal antigen, the sensitizing infection has resolved in most cases, except when mesenteric abscessation has occurred. The use of immunosuppressive therapy is controversial,[15] but clinical experience suggests that systemic corticosteroids are indicated in the treatment of hypersensitivity vasculitis such as EPH and other undefined vasculitis syndromes. Dexamethasone (0.05 to 0.2 mg/kg IV or IM once daily, given in the morning) followed by prednisolone (0.5 to 1 mg/kg IM twice daily) should be administered at the dosage and rate necessary to effect reduction in edema. Some clinicians have found dexamethasone to be much more effective than prednisolone. Once edema starts to resolve, the dosage of corticosteroids should be gradually reduced (10% daily) over 7 to 21 days, as long as signs do not recur. Some cases require more than 4 weeks of corticosteroid therapy, and relapse may occur in spite of treatment, particularly if therapy is changed from dexamethasone to prednisolone too soon in the course of the disease (before 10 days). Antimicrobials should be used throughout the period of corticosteroid administration because the incidence of secondary sepsis is high.[16] The prognosis for EPH is fair with early aggressive therapy and supportive care. Skin sloughing,

laminitis, cellulitis, pneumonia, and diarrhea are not uncommon and may significantly prolong the convalescence. Horses and cattle with idiopathic vasculitis may have incomplete response to therapy, with an unpredictable poor prognosis.[19,20] Failure to identify the antigenic stimulus or eliminate it from the body is the usual cause for inadequate resolution of hypersensitivity vasculitis.[15] Host factors that define immunoregulatory mechanisms probably determine which individuals develop vasculitis and clinical progression of their disease. There is no means of prevention, other than avoiding exposure of previously sensitized horses to *S. equi* antigen.

Equine Viral Arteritis. EVA is caused by an RNA virus, classified in the genus *Arterivirus.*[22] Although usually transmitted through inhalation of aerosolized secretions from an acutely infected horse, stallions can transmit the virus venereally. Infection is much more common than clinical disease, although pregnant mares seem to be more susceptible. The virus proliferates in the media of small muscular arteries throughout the body. Fever, anorexia, serous ocular and nasal discharge, and edema of the limbs, ventral abdomen, and conjunctivae may develop 1 to 10 days after infection. Pregnant mares in late gestation may abort 3 to 8 weeks later. Diagnosis of EVA is based on isolation of the virus or seroconversion after infection. Affected horses usually recover within 4 weeks with only supportive care, but a persistent viral carrier/shedder state may exist.

Equine Infectious Anemia. Necrotizing vasculitis, affecting a variety of organ systems, may accompany EIA.[23] Classic signs of acute EIA include fever, anemia, icterus, ventral edema, and weight loss. Infected horses carry the EIA retrovirus for life. Infection may be inapparent or cause periodic flareups of clinical disease. Diagnosis is confirmed by the agar-gel immunodiffusion (Coggins) test for serum antibodies to the EIA virus.

Equine Ehrlichiosis. The rickettsia *Ehrlichia equi* is the etiologic agent for EE, which causes a necrotizing vasculitis in many parts of the body. The disease is most common in northern California, but is not geographically restricted.[24] Clinical signs are more severe in horses over 3 years and include fever, depression, anorexia, limb edema, mucosal petechiae, ataxia, and reluctance to move. Diagnosis of EE can be made by identification of characteristic cytoplasmic inclusions in neutrophils and eosinophils.[25] In the absence of inclusions, diagnosis is made by seroconversion using an indirect fluorescent antibody test. Recovery usually occurs within 10 days with supportive care, although oxytetracycline therapy may shorten the clinical course.

Other systemic diseases may be characterized histologically by vasculitis. A discussion of malignant catarrhal fever (MCF) and bluetongue is found in Chapter 30. Other vasculitis syndromes in horses are poorly defined with an unpredictable clinical course. Clinical signs without or in addition to edema and hemorrhages include cutaneous alopecia, erythema, hyperkeratosis, and hypopigmentation. Diagnosis must be based on histopathologic findings in skin biopsies.

THROMBOCYTOPENIA. Thrombocytopenia (platelet count <100,000/μl) can result from one or more of three basic mechanisms: (1) decreased or ineffective platelet production; (2) abnormal sequestration (usually in the spleen); or (3) shortened platelet survival (consumption or destruction). Thrombocytopenia causes a hemorrhagic diathesis characterized by multiple sites of small vessel bleeding. Petechial hemorrhages with or without ecchymotic hemorrhages are generally found on the oral, nasal, or vaginal mucous membranes, as well as on the nictitans and sclera. Epistaxis, melena, hyphema, or microscopic hematuria may occur, but spontaneous hemorrhage is unusual unless the platelet count is less than 10,000/μl. Prolonged bleeding from wounds, injections, or surgical procedures and the propensity to form hematomas after minor trauma are quite common when the platelet count drops below 40,000/μl. The platelet count below which bleeding occurs varies among individuals and seems to be determined by concurrent diseases.

The interaction of blood platelets with a discontinuous vascular surface constitutes the basis for primary hemostasis. In addition, platelets provide the phospholipoprotein surface necessary to catalyze interactions among the activated coagulation proteins that culminate in fibrin formation. The platelet surface also protects activated clotting factors from destruction by plasma anticoagulants, thereby localizing coagulation to the hemostatic plug. Finally, platelets maintain "vascular integrity" through obscure mechanisms and prevent spontaneous hemorrhage into the skin and mucous membranes. Severe thrombocytopenia produces prolonged bleeding time and abnormal clot retraction without affecting clotting times or plasma fibrinogen.

Persistent life-threatening hemorrhage caused by thrombocytopenia may be treated with a transfusion of compatible fresh whole blood or, preferably, platelet-rich plasma. The latter may be produced by centrifugation thrombocytopheresis[26] or by centrifugation of freshly collected blood, 3 to 5 minutes at 250 × g.[27] Blood or plasma must be used immediately and contact with glass must be prevented to avoid platelet adhesion and activation. Platelet transfusion is a very transient life-saving measure, and the ultimate prognosis for thrombocytopenia depends on the cause.

Decreased production of platelets may occur secondary to replacement of the normal marrow architecture by neoplastic or inflammatory tissue (myelophthisic disease) or bone marrow aplasia. Both conditions are characterized by peripheral pancytopenia of variable severity and are extremely unusual in large animals. Myelophthisic disease with thrombocytopenia has been described in horses with various forms of myelogenous neoplasia[28-30] and eosinophilic myeloproliferative disorder.[31]

Hypoplastic anemia with leukopenia and thrombocytopenia has been reported in horses and cattle and is discussed later in the chapter in the section on aplastic anemia. Shortened platelet life span is by far the most common cause of thrombocytopenia in large animals. Increased platelet consumption accompanies disseminated intravascular coagulation (DIC; discussed in the next section) and rare cases of vasculitis. Immune-mediated mechanisms result in platelet destruction.

Immune-mediated thrombocytopenia (IMTP) may be primary (idiopathic) or secondary to the administration of drugs, infections, neoplasia, or other immunologic disorders.[27] This disease is most common in horses and has been reported secondary to EIA,[32] lymphosarcoma,[33] and autoimmune hemolytic anemia.[34] The clinical signs of IMTP include mucosal hemorrhages and the propensity to bleed from small blood vessels. Horses with idiopathic IMTP are usually bright, afebrile, and without overt hemorrhage despite severely reduced platelet numbers. Thrombocytopenia in a horse with obvious primary disease should prompt a thorough hemostatic workup to rule out DIC.

Alloimmune thrombocytopenia of neonates has been recognized as a spontaneous disease of human infants, piglets, foals, and possibly mule foals.[35] Clinical signs include depression, loss of suckle, a bleeding tendency, blood loss, and rapidly developing anemia because of a profound thrombocytopenia. The condition occurs in multiparous dams and immunoglobulins may be found in the mare's plasma, serum, and milk that bind to the foal's platelets. Alloimmune thrombocytopenia should be considered in neonates with severe thrombocytopenia when other causes can be excluded, and platelet antibody assays should be used to support this diagnosis. Differential

considerations include neonatal sepsis, neonatal maladjustment syndrome, and neonatal isoerythrolysis. Laboratory findings of IMTP include severe thrombocytopenia (<40,000/μl), prolonged bleeding time, and abnormal clot retraction with normal thrombin time (TT), PT, APTT, and plasma fibrinogen. Fibrin(ogen) degradation products (FDPs) may be mildly increased, and anemia accompanied by hypoproteinemia develops if there is ongoing blood loss. In most cases of IMTP and other causes for shortened platelet life span, megakaryocytic hyperplasia is evident on examination of bone marrow aspirates or biopsies. Megakaryocytic destruction by the immunologic process could induce megakaryocytic hypoplasia, although this is apparently rare in horses. The definitive diagnosis of IMTP requires demonstration of increased quantities of platelet-associated IgG or C3 or antiplatelet activity in the serum. Unfortunately methods to detect platelet-associated immunoreactants have not been adapted for horses, although it appears they affect platelet function.[36] Therefore the diagnosis of IMTP must be based on small-vessel hemorrhagic diathesis and severe thrombocytopenia in a horse with normal coagulation times and no other evidence of DIC. Response to therapy (see next section) supports the diagnosis. A tentative diagnosis of IMTP in the horse should prompt a thorough search for an underlying disorder, especially lymphosarcoma.

Platelet destruction in IMTP is apparently mediated by antibodies coating the platelet surface that cause premature platelet removal from circulation by the mononuclear phagocyte system (MPS).[37] In primary IMTP the platelet-associated immunoglobulin (Ig) is directed against a membrane antigen, is usually of the IgG class, produced in the spleen, fixes complement, and can be absorbed from serum by platelets from a normal individual of the same species. Autoantibodies may attach to megakaryocytes, but the latter are not necessarily destroyed because they do not circulate through the spleen or liver. In secondary IMTP the Ig bound to the platelet surface is part of an immune complex composed of antibody directed against a drug, microbe, or neoplastic antigen that is nonspecifically attached to the platelet Fc receptor. For secondary IMTP to be perpetuated, the foreign antigen must be constantly replenished or difficult to excrete. Drug-induced IMTP generally subsides within a few days of drug discontinuation, although thrombocytopenia secondary to chrysotherapy (gold therapy) may persist for weeks to years. Because gold is occasionally used to treat pemphigus foliaceus in horses, thrombocytopenia should be considered as a potential side effect. The spleen is the major site of platelet phagocytosis because (1) much antiplatelet antibody is secreted locally, (2) more than 30% of circulating platelets are normally stored there, and (3) the stagnant splenic blood flow allows sensitized platelets to pass slowly through a dense network of phagocytic cells. The mean cell life of circulating platelets and the platelet count are inversely proportional to the quantity of platelet-associated IgG. In some humans with chronic IMTP, antiplatelet antibody also impairs platelet production.[36]

When any unexplained case of thrombocytopenia is treated, all current medication should be stopped. If a drug is absolutely necessary, it must be replaced by the chemically most-dissimilar substitute. Drug-induced IMTP usually responds within 14 days of drug withdrawal. Most animals with suspected IMTP improve when treated with corticosteroids. Although their precise mechanisms of action are speculative, corticosteroids improve capillary integrity, impair clearance by the MPS, decrease the number and avidity of macrophage Fc receptors, impair antiplatelet antibody production, impede platelet-antibody interactions, and increase thrombocytopoiesis.

Dexamethasone (0.05 to 0.2 mg/kg IV or IM) given once daily generally results in an elevation in the platelet count within 4 to 7 days. Once the platelet count is greater than 100,000/μl, the dose of dexamethasone can be reduced by 10% to 20% daily, while the platelet count is monitored for a relapse. Occasionally animals with IMTP are refractory to dexamethasone, in which case prednisolone (1 mg/kg IM twice daily) may be tried. Most animals respond best to dexamethasone, but some may be uniquely sensitive to prednisolone. Treatment with corticosteroids can usually be discontinued after a period of 10 to 21 days, provided the platelet count has been normal for at least 5 days. Most horses with IMTP have a favorable prognosis, and the disease resolves within 14 to 21 days. This suggests that many cases may be secondary, yet the initiating cause is rarely found. Chronic or recurrent IMTP requiring prolonged corticosteroid therapy has been reported.[38] Chronic refractory IMTP suggests an underlying disease.

Alternative treatment modalities for IMTP are largely unproven in horses because most cases are responsive to corticosteroids. Splenectomy has been variably successful for refractory IMTP in humans and dogs.[39] Although technically feasible, splenectomy is not routinely performed in horses. A single dose of vincristine (0.01 to 0.025 mg/kg or 0.5 mg/m²) combined with corticosteroids may effect remission of IMTP in dogs; however, released platelets may be nonfunctional.[40] Remission of IMTP for variable periods has occurred in humans given large doses of intravenous Ig (200 to 1000 mg/kg) daily for 5 days.[40] Large-dose Ig therapy may interfere with macrophage immune clearance and enhance suppressor T-cell function.[41] A 6- to 50-L amount of plasma would be a necessary daily dose for a 500-kg horse, depending on the plasma Ig content. Although expensive, high-dose Ig therapy presents less risk than splenectomy or cytotoxic drugs to the patient that is refractory to corticosteroids.

DISORDERS OF COAGULATION FACTORS. Normal blood coagulation proceeds in an integrated sequence that can be simplistically viewed as three key reactions: the formation of activated factor X; the formation of thrombin; and the formation of fibrin (see Fig. 35-1). Other protein interactions serve to accelerate or inhibit the reaction rate of the coagulation factors.[5] Excessive use or inhibition of these proteins produces a relative deficiency that causes hemorrhagic diathesis.

Disseminated Intravascular Coagulation. The most common form of hemostatic dysfunction in large animals is a syndrome known variously as DIC, consumption coagulopathy, defibrination syndrome, or intravascular coagulation fibrinolysis. The pathologic process is characterized by widespread fibrin deposition in the microcirculation, with subsequent ischemic damage, and by the development of a hemorrhagic diathesis caused by the consumption of procoagulants and hyperactivity of fibrinolysis.[42] Never a primary disease entity, DIC represents an intermediary mechanism of underlying disease. In large animals, DIC has been described in association with forms of localized or systemic septic processes,[43-46] neoplasia,[43] gastrointestinal disorders,[20,47] renal disease,[47] and hemolytic anemia.[46,48] Diffuse activation of the hemostatic system is particularly prevalent in horses with acute gastrointestinal disorders that cause colic[10,46,47] and is a likely initiating factor for laminitis.[49,50] Because of the dynamic nature of DIC, clinical manifestations may fall anywhere in the spectrum from diffuse thrombosis leading to ischemic organ failure to severe hemorrhagic diathesis. The most important determinants are the rate of thrombin generation, which depends on the triggering disease, the adequacy of fibrinolysis, and the functional state of the MPS, which is largely determined by peripheral circulation. Coagulopathy usually occurs in a compensated form in horses and cattle and is rarely attended by overt hemorrhage; however, microvascular thrombosis and subsequent ischemia to vital

tissues leads to organ malfunction (e.g., renal failure), which contributes to the morbidity and mortality of the primary disease process.

Renal involvement is common in DIC, which produces ischemic cortical necrosis followed by acute tubular necrosis. Renal disease may be manifested by oliguria, depression, and ileus caused by azotemia and electrolyte imbalances. Gastrointestinal microthrombosis may induce colic as a result of submucosal necrosis and superficial ulceration. Spontaneous gastrointestinal hemorrhage caused by DIC may cause melena in ruminants and occult fecal blood loss in horses. Pulmonary function may rarely be compromised by microvascular thrombosis in DIC, causing tachypnea and variable hypoxemia. Altered consciousness, delirium, convulsions, or coma may follow cerebral microvascular thrombosis, although these signs are not common in DIC in large animals. Although reported in both horses[51] and cattle,[48] microangiopathic hemolysis is rare in large animals with DIC because of their small erythrocyte size.

Digital ischemia frequently accompanies DIC in horses and plays a key role in the development of acute laminitis. Laboratory evidence of DIC has been documented during the developmental phase of equine laminitis,[50] and digital microvascular thrombosis occurs in horses that develop laminitis with colic or septic conditions.[49] The tendency for thrombosis of major peripheral veins is another prominent manifestation of coagulopathy in horses. Venous thrombosis occurs in horses and is associated with needle- or catheter-induced intimal trauma, nonsterility during catheterization, blood sampling or treatment procedures, and thrombogenic catheter materials. However, the strong clinical impression remains that severely ill horses with diseases known to induce coagulopathy have a greater tendency toward venous thrombosis. Spontaneous thrombosis of smaller cutaneous vessels also occurs.

As the thrombotic stimulus continues or intensifies, the tendency for hemorrhage develops because of clotting factors and platelet depletion or generation of excessive fibrinolytic byproducts (FDPs). Petechial or ecchymotic hemorrhages on mucosae and sclerae and a tendency to bleed from venipuncture or after minor trauma are the principal signs. Spontaneous life-threatening hemorrhage is very rare; however, trauma or surgery may induce uncontrollable hemorrhage. Once signs of blood incoagulability develop, the prognosis is poor.

Horses may develop a chronic, compensated form of DIC that is attended by few or no clinical signs. This entity develops in patients with illnesses that produce a low-grade or intermittent procoagulant stimulus that allows used coagulant proteins and platelets to be partially or totally replenished and activated clotting factors and FDPs to be cleared by the MPS. Localized sepsis (e.g., pleuritis), neoplasia, protein-losing enteropathy, and immune-mediated disorders (vasculitis, anemia) are common initiating diseases. This compensated state may become imbalanced by stress, concurrent diseases, or worsening of the primary process, resulting in clinically obvious DIC. Diseases that must be differentiated from DIC include IMTP, warfarin toxicosis (horses), moldy sweet clover toxicosis, and inherited coagulation abnormalities.

Numerous laboratory tests of hemostasis may be abnormal during DIC; however, no one test consistently or specifically provides a definitive diagnosis. Lack of test sensitivity results from the dynamic nature of DIC, the laboratory reflection of which is determined by the balance between coagulation and fibrinolytic forces, as well as MPS integrity at the time of blood sampling. The plasma concentrations of proteins and cells that are measured by hemostatic function tests are influenced by their synthetic rate, catabolism, and losses by other routes, in addition to utilization rate so no pattern is uniquely specific for DIC.

The most widely used hemostatic function tests in large animals include the platelet count, plasma fibrinogen, PT, APTT, and serum FDPs. Other data, including TT, bleeding time, activated coagulation time, the protamine sulfate test and plasma concentrations of proteins involved in coagulation (e.g., factors V, VIII, and antithrombin III), and fibrinolysis (e.g., plasminogen, soluble fibrin monomer) have been used on a limited basis. Because clinical manifestations of DIC vary widely, clarification of the most frequent laboratory abnormalities in large animals with DIC is hindered by lack of a definitive diagnosis in most instances. A disseminated coagulopathy is manifested by multiple hemostatic abnormalities, and serial analyses should reveal reduced platelet numbers and a trend toward prolongation of the PT, APTT, and TT, with reduction in plasma AT III. Repeated hemostatic testing is advised when there is a strong suspicion for DIC. Serum FDPs are most often elevated by DIC, but they are usually normal in the early or compensated form of the disease. Hypofibrinogenemia is an uncommon manifestation of DIC in large animals and, when present, should strongly suggest concomitant liver dysfunction. Hemostatic function tests are totally unreliable unless blood samples are collected and handled properly. If the laboratory does not have a normal reference interval for the patient species, samples should be submitted from at least two normal individuals along with the patient.

Criteria used for diagnosis of DIC are extremely arbitrary, and laboratory results must be interpreted in light of the patient's underlying disease. The combination of thrombocytopenia with mild to moderate prolongation of the PT or APTT strongly suggests DIC. The clinician should seek laboratory assistance when considering the diagnosis of DIC but appreciate that the findings are often not helpful. Clinical signs and specific situations suggest the possibility of DIC, and laboratory tests are only used to provide support.

Diseases initiate DIC by two major mechanisms: (1) generation of excessive procoagulant activity within the blood, or (2) contact of blood with abnormal surfaces. Many diseases act by more than one mechanism to induce the overwhelming stimulus needed to trigger DIC. The nature and intensity of the procoagulant force (which determines the rate of thrombin formation), the concentration of natural coagulation inhibitors, and the functional capacity of the MPS determine (1) whether an individual with a given disease process develops DIC, and (2) the clinical manifestations of DIC. Many diseases that produce DIC have the propensity to cause endotoxemia. The intestinal tract in large animals normally contains large quantities of endotoxins, only a small part of which is absorbed through the portal vein and removed by the liver. Conditions that cause intestinal mucosal edema or disruption allow endotoxins to gain access to the peripheral circulation and initiate many morbid sequelae, one of which is DIC. Intestinal strangulating obstruction, thromboembolic infarction, and severe colitis induce mucosal abnormalities, allowing endotoxemia to occur. The proliferation of gram-negative bacteria within tissues and the blood is also accompanied by endotoxemia.

Gram-negative endotoxins are capable of direct factor XII activation. However, most studies indicate that the procoagulant effects of endotoxin are primarily mediated by cytokine production by mononuclear phagocytes.[6,52] After endotoxin stimulation, phagocytes produce a PAF, tissue factor, prostaglandins, interleukins, tumor necrosis factor (TNF), and other mediators with procoagulant activity.[6,53] A PCA with actions identical to tissue thromboplastin is produced by endothelial cells, monocytes, and macrophages in response to endotoxins, and hepatic Kupffer cells produce a PCA that acts similar to factor VII. Thus any disease associated with endotoxemia has a great potential to induce DIC.

The net result of any triggering mechanism for DIC is the exaggerated generation of systemic thrombin, which causes widespread microcirculatory thrombosis. In addition to the cleavage of fibrinogen to produce fibrin monomers, thrombin activates factor XIII to render fibrin more resistant to fibrinolysis, enhances the cofactor activity of factors V and VIII, and induces platelet aggregation and exposure of platelet phospholipid. Circulatory obstruction produces organ hypoperfusion, leading to ischemic necrosis. The byproducts of fibrinogen activation, fibrinopeptides A and B, can produce systemic vasoconstriction that compounds hypoperfusion and eventual end-organ failure. Polymerized fibrin entraps platelets (enhancing thrombocytopenia) and damages erythrocytes. Microangiopathic hemolysis provides ADP and phospholipids to intensify DIC. Natural inhibitors of thrombin, the most important of which are AT III and protein C, reduce procoagulant forces; however, they too may be consumed during DIC, resulting in a greater propensity for thrombosis.

The counterbalance fibrinolytic system is also activated by DIC and plasmin contributes to factor consumption by destroying factors V, VIII, XIIa, IX, and XI, in addition to fibrin and fibrinogen. FDPs contribute greatly to the hemorrhagic manifestations of DIC because they have antithrombin activity, interfere with fibrin monomer polymerization, and cause platelet dysfunction.[7] Paradoxically the combination of consumption and anticoagulation predisposes to hemorrhage at the same time that disseminated thromboses occur.

The MPS plays a vital role in the pathogenesis of DIC. The tissue-fixed macrophages of the spleen and liver normally remove FDPs and activated clotting factors from the peripheral circulation, and FDPs only increase when their rate of formation exceeds the ability of the MPS to clear them. Shock and hypoperfusion of the liver and spleen or diseases associated with excessive tissue debris that must be removed by MPS (e.g., sepsis, metastatic neoplasia) reduce the function of the MPS and predispose to or perpetuate DIC.

Therapy for DIC is highly controversial, and the only noncontended modalities are those directed toward identification and treatment of the primary disorder, along with general supportive measures to combat shock and maintain tissue perfusion.[5,40,54,55] Intravenous fluid administration helps to prevent organ dysfunction after microvascular thrombosis and can correct existing acid-base or electrolyte imbalances. Septic conditions should be treated with appropriate antimicrobial agents, and necrotic tissue or purulent exudate removed whenever possible. Any animal with a strangulating intestinal obstruction requires immediate surgical intervention to resect nonviable bowel. Flunixin meglumine mitigates the deleterious effects of endotoxin caused by eicosanoids and is used in horses at a dosage of 0.25 mg/kg IV every 8 hours).[20] Corticosteroids may worsen DIC because they reduce the phagocytic action of the MPS and potentiate the vasoconstrictor effects of catecholamines.

Significant life-threatening hemorrhage is rare in large animals with DIC; however, if it occurs, fresh plasma should be administered (15 to 30 ml/kg) to replace used coagulant and anticoagulant proteins. The use of heparin in DIC has been recommended in various regimes to stall the disseminated microvascular thrombosis that precipitates organ failure; however, there is still controversy regarding its efficacy.[40,55] In dogs, minidose heparin therapy (5 to 10 U/kg SQ three times daily) is commonly used with blood products in treatment of DIC.[40,54] Efficacy of heparin for DIC in horses is unproven. Heparin in all species can predispose to hemorrhage, thrombosis, and thrombocytopenia[56] and causes anemia and erythrocyte agglutination in horses.[57] If heparin therapy is considered, one must ensure there is adequate plasma AT III, which is necessary for heparin action. Because AT III is often depleted by DIC, plasma may be necessary. Heparin has been suggested for the prevention or control of laminitis in

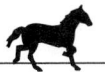

horses.[57] Clinical trials in humans have not indicated therapeutic benefit of anticoagulants in chronic DIC.

The prognosis for DIC in large animals depends largely on the nature and severity of the underlying disease and how effectively the latter is treated. Once DIC has progressed to the stage at which signs of blood incoagulability predominate, the prognosis is generally very poor.

Warfarin Toxicosis. Horses may develop a hemorrhagic diathesis after warfarin toxicosis.[58] This coumarin derivative anticoagulant is used by some to treat horses with navicular disease.[59] Rarely horses and other animals may be exposed to coumarins used as rodenticides in grains or other feedstuffs. Therapeutic concentrations of warfarin can have a cumulative toxic effect if the diet is altered to contain less vitamin K or if there is concurrent protein-bound drug therapy. The clinical signs of warfarin toxicosis include hematomas, ecchymoses of mucous membranes, epistaxis, and hematuria. Lack of petechial hemorrhages should help rule out DIC. The earliest laboratory indication of warfarin toxicosis is a prolongation of the PT because the plasma half-life of factor VII is shorter than the other clotting factors.[60] As the disease progresses, the APTT becomes prolonged, and the animal may develop blood-loss anemia and hypoproteinemia. The diagnosis of warfarin toxicosis is based on a history of exposure, clinical signs of large-vessel hemorrhagic diathesis, and prolonged PT with or without APTT and with no other abnormalities of the clotting profile.

Warfarin acts through competitive inhibition of vitamin K, which is necessary for liver production of clotting factors II, VII, IX, and X.[59] Factor activity is reduced in the blood at a rate dependent on its individual half-life. In most species, factors VII, IX, X, and XI have increasingly greater half-lives, accounting for the greater sensitivity of PT for the early diagnosis of warfarin toxicosis. The gastrointestinal absorption of warfarin is rapid and warfarin is highly bound to plasma proteins. The unbound pharmacologically active component remains fairly constant in plasma, with the protein-bound warfarin acting as a reservoir. Drugs such as phenylbutazone and chloral hydrate that are normally protein-bound can enhance the toxicity of warfarin by allowing a greater proportion of the administered drug to be unbound.[61] In the same manner, hypoalbuminemia may increase the likelihood of warfarin toxicosis. Corticosteroids and thyroxin can lower the necessary therapeutic dose of warfarin by increasing both the receptor affinity and the clotting factor catabolism. Drugs such as barbiturates, rifampin, and chloramphenicol that induce hepatic microsomal enzyme activity can accelerate warfarin metabolism and reduce therapeutic response to a given dose. Finally, any reduction in hepatic function or content of vitamin K in the diet can precipitate warfarin toxicosis.

Treatment of warfarin toxicosis depends on clinical signs. Warfarin therapy should be stopped if the PT exceeds twice the pretherapeutic value. Vitamin K1 (0.5 to 1 mg/kg SC) must be given every 6 hours until the PT is again normal and stable. Significant hemorrhage can be controlled by the administration of fresh plasma to provide necessary clotting factors. If the anemia is life-threatening, whole blood transfusion should be considered. Although warfarin is eliminated rapidly, some potentiated coumarins have a prolonged half-life, requiring a longer course of vitamin K therapy. The prognosis for warfarin toxicosis is good, provided there is early diagnosis and prompt administration of vitamin K. It is imperative that vitamin K3 not be used because it has poor therapeutic action and is highly nephrotoxic for horses.

Prevention of warfarin toxicosis is based on limiting access of livestock to rodenticides and carefully monitoring the therapeutic use of warfarin in horses. The benefits of warfarin in horses are highly controversial, and many question whether advantages outweigh the risks. A history or clinical/laboratory evidence of hepatic disease is a strong contraindication for warfarin use. The administration of other drugs (particularly phenylbutazone) should be limited during warfarin therapy, and the dosage of warfarin reevaluated if the dosage or rate of other medications is changed. The potential for trauma must be minimized and the PT should be monitored daily until a dosage of warfarin has been found to effect doubling of the baseline PT. During warfarin therapy the PT should be evaluated twice weekly or more often if there is a change in diet, concurrent disease, or other medication.

Sweet Clover Toxicosis. Sweet clover (*Melilotus* spp.) toxicosis is caused by the ingestion of moldy sweet clover hay or silage containing dicoumarol. Natural coumarins in sweet clover can be converted to dicoumarol when hay or silage is improperly cured and mold forms. The toxin persists in moldy hay or silage and is palatable. This disease can occur in all species but is most commonly seen in cattle fed sweet clover hay in the northern plains states. Early signs include epistaxis and melena, with the development of subcutaneous hematomas and periarticular swellings as the disease progresses. Visible swellings occur at points of trauma such as the brisket, tuber coxae, or carpi and are not hot or painful, although they may cause stiffness and disinclination to move. Accidental and surgical wounds cause severe hemorrhage and may precipitate fatal blood-loss anemia.

Clinical pathology is similar to that described for warfarin toxicosis, with prolonged PT being the earliest abnormality (detected before clinical evidence of hemorrhage). As the disease progresses, the APTT and activated clotting time become prolonged, and blood loss anemia develops. The platelet count remains normal, which differentiates this syndrome from DIC and bracken fern toxicosis. Other diagnostic rule-outs include mycotoxicosis, and toxicosis from trichloroethylene-extracted soybean meal.[62] In the absence of fever and anorexia, coagulopathy should make moldy sweet clover toxicosis a strong tentative diagnosis in animals with a history of access. A prolonged PT, with or without prolonged APTT, with no other clotting abnormalities, lends support. Chemical analysis for dicoumarol in suspected feed or in the blood and liver of affected animals aids in the diagnosis[63]; however, the disease cannot be excluded if dicoumarol is not detected.

The pathogenesis of moldy sweet clover toxicosis is identical to that of warfarin toxicosis. Dicoumarol interferes with hepatic synthesis of clotting factors II, VII, IX, and X by inhibiting vitamin K. Usually the syndrome appears in cattle 2 to 7 days after they ingest the moldy hay. Lower levels of dicoumarol (<70 mg/kg) in feed may prolong the onset of signs for up to 3 months.[62]

The succulent nature of sweet clover creates a high incidence of molding in hay. Grazing the crop is not dangerous. Because of its high forage yield, sweet clover is usually harvested as silage, which should carry less danger of molding when properly cured. The toxic level of dicoumarol in sweet clover feed samples is 10 mg/kg of feed.[63] Newborn calves may die of the disease when dams have been fed affected hay.[62] Lesions of moldy sweet clover toxicosis include extravasation of blood or suffusive hemorrhages in any tissue or organ No evidence of hemolytic disease exists, although large hematomas may result in mild icterus.

Treatment of sweet clover toxicosis involves discontinuing the use of contaminated feed and administering vitamin K1.[61] Dosages between 1.1 and 3.3 mg/kg of body weight should be administered intramuscularly; response occurs within 24 hours. The efficacy of vitamin K3 in cattle is controversial. Vitamin K3 should not be administered parenterally in horses because there have been reports of acute tubular nephrosis and death of horses after receiving the drug.[64] Animals with severe blood-loss anemia or ongoing hemorrhage should be treated with plasma or whole fresh blood.

Sweet clover toxicosis can be prevented by careful forage preparation, followed by the inspection of hay and silage before feeding. When the disease is suspected, questionable feed should be removed from the diet.

REFERENCES

1. Schmall LM, Muir WW, Robertson JT: Haemodynamic effects of small volume hypertonic saline in experimentally induced haemorrhagic shock, *Equine Vet J* 22:273-277, 1990.
2. Bertone JJ, Shoemaker KE: Effects of hypertonic and isotonic saline solutions on plasma constituents of conscious horses, *Am J Vet Res* 53:1844-1849, 1992.
3. Kallfelz FA, Whitlock RH, Schultz RD: Survival of 59Fe-labeled erythrocytes in cross-transfused equine blood, *Am J Vet Res* 39:617-620, 1978.
4. Stormont CJ: Blood groups in animals, *J Am Vet Med Assoc* 181:1120-1124, 1982.
5. Mosher DF: Disorders of blood coagulation. In Bennett JC, Plum F, eds: *Cecil textbook of medicine*, ed 20, Philadelphia, 1996, WB Saunders, pp 987-1003.
6. Weiss DJ, Rashid S: The sepsis-coagulant axis: a review, *J Vet Int Med* 12:3217-3324, 1998.
7. Collen D, Lijner HR: Basic and clinical aspects of fibrinolysis and thrombolysis, *Blood* 78:3114-3124, 1992.
8. Clouse LH, Camp PC: The regulation of hemostasis: the protein C system, *N Engl J Med* 314:1298-1304, 1986.
9. Moore BR, Hinchcliff KW: Heparin: a review of its pharmacological therapeutic use in horses, *J Vet Intern Med* 48:26-35, 1994.
10. Collates CA et al: Intravascular and peritoneal coagulation and fibrinolysis in horses with acute gastrointestinal tract diseases, *J Am Vet Med Assoc* 207):405-470, 1995.
11. Archer RK, Allen BV: True hemophilia in horses, *Vet Rec* 91:655-656, 1972.
12. Hinton M et al: A clotting defect in an Arab colt foal, *Equine Vet J* 9:1-3, 1977.
13. Turrentine MA et al: Prekallikrein deficiency in a family of miniature horses, *Am J Vet Res* 47:2464-2467, 1986.
14. Gentry PA, Ross ML: Failure of routine coagulation screening tests to detect heterozygous state of bovine factor XI deficiency, *Vet Clin Pathol* 15:12-16, 1986.
15. Rosenwasser LJ: The vasculitic syndromes. In Bennett JC, Plum F, ed: *Cecil textbook of medicine*, ed 20, Philadelphia, 1996, WB Saunders, pp 1490-1493.
16. Morris DD: Cutaneous vasculitis in horses: 19 cases (1978-1985), *J Am Vet Med Assoc* 191:460-464, 1987.
17. Morris DD et al: Chronic necrotizing vasculitis in a horse, *J Am Vet Med Bick* 183:579-582, 1983.
18. Werner LL, Gross TL, Hillidge CJ: Acute necrotizing vasculitis and thrombocytopenia in a horse, *J Am Vet Med Assoc* 185:87-90, 1984.
19. Blood DC, Radostits OM: *Veterinary medicine*, ed 7, London, 1989, Baillière Tindall, pp 841-857, 871, 873-877.
20. Morris DD: The haemolymphatic system. In Higgins AJ, Wright IM, eds: *The equine manual*, London, 1995, WB Saunders, pp 409-451.
21. Logus DB, Barbet JL: Diseases characterized by ulceration, exudation and crusting of the distal extremities. In Colahan PT et al, eds: *Equine medicine and surgery*, ed 5, St Louis, 1999, Mosby, pp 500-502.
22. Aiello SE: *The Merck veterinary manual*, ed 8, pp 500-502.
23. Tashjian RJ: Transmission and clinical evaluation of an equine infectious anemia herd and their offspring over a 13-year period, *J Am Vet Med Assoc* 184:282-288, 1984.
24. Ziemer EL, Keenan DP, Madigan JE: *Ehrlichia equi* infection in a foal, *J Am Vet Med Assoc* 190:199-200, 1987.
25. Madigan JE, Gribble D: Equine ehrlichiosis in northern California: 49 cases (1968-1982), *J Am Vet Med Assoc* 190:445-448, 1987.
26. Gordon BJ et al: Evaluation of leukapheresis and thrombocytapheresis in the horse, *Am J Vet Res* 47:997-1001, 1986.
27. Morris DD: Idiopathic thrombocytopenia. In Robinson NE, ed: *Current therapy in equine medicine 3*, Philadelphia, 1992, WB Saunders, pp 507-510.
28. Searcy GP, Orr JP: Chronic granulocytic leukemia in a horse, *Can Vet J* 22:148-151, 1981.
29. Brumbaugh GW et al: Myelomonocytic myeloproliferative disease in a horse, *J Am Vet Med Assoc* 180:313-316,1981.
30. Burkhard E, Saldern FV, Haskamp B: Monocytic leukemia in a horse, *Vet Pathol* 21:394-398, 1984.
31. Morris DD et al: Eosinophilic myeloproliferative disorder in a horse, *J Am Med Assoc* 185:993-996,1984.
32. Cohen ND, Carter KG: Persistent thrombocytopenia in a case of equine infectious anemia, *J Am Vet Med Assoc* 199:750-752,1991.
33. Reef VB, Dyson SS, Beech J: Lymphosarcoma and associated immune-mediated hemolytic anemia and thrombocytopenia in horses, *J Am Vet Med Assoc* 184:313-317, 1984.
34. Sockett DC, Traub-Dargatz J, Weiser MG: Immune-mediated hemolytic anemia and thrombocytopenia in a foal, *J Am Vet Med Assoc* 190:308-310, 1987.
35. Buechner-Maxwell V et al: Neonatal alloimmune thrombocytopenia in a quarter horse foal, *J Vet Internal Med* 11:304-308, 1997.
36. Ramirez S et al: Detection and effects on platelet function of anti-platelet antibody in mule foals with experimentally induced neonatal alloimmune thrombocytopenia, *J Vet Int Med* 13:534-539, 1999.
37. Shuman M: Hemorrhagic disorders: abnormalities of platelets and vascular function. In Bennett JC, Plum F, eds: *Cecil textbook of medicine*, ed 20, Philadelphia, 1996, WB Saunders, pp 997-987.
38. Morris DD, Whitlock RH: Relapsing idiopathic thrombocytopenia in a horse, *Equine Vet J* 15:73-75, 1983.
39. Jans HE, Armstrong J, Price GS: Therapy of immune-mediated thrombocytopenia, *J Vet Int Med* 4:4-7, 1990
40. Nelson RW, Couto GC, eds: *Small animal internal medicine*, ed 2, St Louis, 1998, Mosby, pp 1192-1206.
41. Blanchette V: Randomized trial of intravenous immunoglobulin G, intravenous anti-D and oral prednisone in childhood acute immune thrombocytopenic purpura, *Lancet* 344:703-707, 1994.
42. Gando S et al: Disseminated intravascular coagulation as a frequent complication of systemic inflammatory response syndrome, *Thromb Haemost* 75:224-228, 1996.
43. Morris DD, Beech J: Disseminated intravascular coagulation in six horses, *J Am Vet Med Assoc* 183:1067-1072, 1983.
44. Vestweber JGE, Krukenberg SM, Spencer H: Disseminated intravascular coagulation in a cow with coliform mastitis, *Compend Cont Educ Pract Vet* 5:S185-S189, 1983.
45. Buntain B: Disseminated intravascular coagulopathy (DIC) in a cow with left displaced abomasum, metritis, and mastitis, *Vet Med Small Anim Clin* 75:1023-1026, 1980.
46. Morris DD, Vaala WE, Sartin E: Protein-losing enteropathy in a yearling filly with subclinical disseminated intravascular coagulation and autoimmune hemolytic anemia, *Compend Cont Educ Pract Vet* 4:S542-S546, 1982.
47. Johnstone IB, Crane S: Hemostatic abnormalities in equine colic, *Am J Vet Res* 47:356-358, 1986.
48. Roby KAW, Bloom JC, Becht JL: Postpartum hemolytic-uremic syndrome in a cow, *J Am Vet Med Assoc* 190:187-190, 1987.
49. Baxter GM: Equine laminitis caused by distal displacement of the distal phalanx:12 cases (1976-1985), *J Am Vet Med Assoc* 189:326-329, 1986.
50. Weiss DJ, Trent AM, Johnston GI: Prothrombotic events in prodromal stages of acute laminitis in horses, *Am J Vet Res* 56:986-991, 1995.
51. MacLachlan NJ, Divers TJ: Hemolytic anemia and fibrinoid change of renal vessels in a horse, *J Am Vet Med Assoc* 181:716-717, 1982.
52. Dosquet C, Weill D, Wautier JL: Cytokines and thrombosis, *J Cardiovasc Pharmacol* 25: 513-519, 1995.
53. Morris DD: Endotoxemia in horses: a review of cellular and humoral mediators involved in its pathogenesis, *J Vet Int Med* 5:167-181, 1991.
54. Couto CG: Disseminated intravascular coagulation in dogs and cats, *Vet Med* June 1999, pp 547-554.
55. Bick RL: Disseminated intravascular coagulation. In Bick RL, ed: *Disorders of thrombosis and hemostasis: clinical and laboratory practice*, Chicago, 1992, ASCPP Press, pp 137-173.
56. Silver D, Kapsch D, Tsoi E: Heparin-induced thrombocytopenia, thrombosis and hemorrhage, *Ann Surg* 198:301-306, 1983.
57. Moore JN, Mahaffey EA, Zboran M: Heparin-induced agglutination of erythrocytes in horses, *Am J Vet Res* 48:68-71, 1987.
58. Broom TA: Warfarin toxicosis. In Robinson NE, ed: *Current therapy in equine medicine 3*, Philadelphia, 1992, WB Saunders, pp 502-504.
59. Turner TA: Management of navicular disease in horses: an update, *Mod Vet Pract* 1:24-27, 1996.
60. Vrins A, Carlson G, Feldman B: Warfarin: a review with emphasis on its use in the horse, *Can Vet J* 24:211-213, 1983.
61. Scott EA, Byars TD, Lamar AM: Warfarin anticoagulation in the horse, *J Am Vet Med Assoc* 177:1146-1150, 1980.
62. Blood DC, Radostits OM, eds: *Veterinary medicine*, ed 7, London, 1989, Bailliere Tindall, pp1332-1335.
63. Casper HH et al: Dicoumarol levels in sweet clover toxic to cattle, *Proc 25th Annu Conv Vet Lab Diagn* 25:41-48, 1982.
64. Rebhun WC, Tennant BC, Dill SG, et al: Vitamin K3-induced renal toxicosis in the horse, *J Am Vet Med Assoc* 184:1237-1239, 1984.

DISEASES ASSOCIATED WITH INCREASED ERYTHROCYTE DESTRUCTION (Hemolytic Anemia)

GARY P. CARLSON

Hemolytic disorders are characterized by an increased rate of red cell destruction. Anemia occurs when the rate of red cell destruction exceeds the bone marrow capacity for increased proliferative response. Although intravascular hemolysis occurs in some circumstances, these anemias are primarily

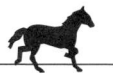

caused by an increased rate of extravascular erythrocyte destruction and shortened intravascular life span.

Hemolytic anemias are associated with a wide range of systemic disease processes. The mechanisms responsible for the enhanced red cell destruction also vary markedly. A list of differential considerations of possible causal factors for hemolytic anemia in large animals is presented in Box 35-1. Clinical manifestations of hemolytic anemia vary with the degree of anemia, the rate of red cell destruction, and the primary or underlying disease process. However, several common clinical signs are seen in animals with a severe hemolytic anemia, regardless of the cause. These signs include pallor of the mucous membranes, fatigue, depression, and anorexia. Clinical icterus can be quite variable, depending on the rate of red cell destruction and the ability of the liver to excrete bilirubin. Icterus is a characteristic feature in hemolytic anemia, but intense icterus is noted only after massive red cell destruction and often is transient. With continued low-level hemolytic processes, the liver may be able to excrete bilirubin at a rate that is sufficient to avoid clinical icterus. Hemolytic icterus must be differentiated from other potential causes such as liver disease or anorexia in horses. If icterus is caused by hemolytic processes, clear clinical and hematologic evidence of anemia should exist. Massive intravascular hemolysis may result in an orange-to-reddish discoloration of the mucous membranes. Modest-to-marked and often variable febrile responses are frequently encountered in hemolytic anemias that are caused by infectious agents and during periods of active erythrocyte destruction. With advanced anemia the pulse and respiratory rates are elevated at rest. Death losses may occur, and neurologic abnormalities ranging from bizarre behavior to mania, collapse, and death may be associated with handling animals with a severe anemia.

The hematologic manifestations of hemolytic anemia also vary with the rate of red cell destruction, the time course of the anemia, and the primary or underlying disease process. The anemia may be modest to severe; and, after the first few days in all species except the horse, there is usually hematologic evidence of enhanced erythropoietic response as manifested by increased anisocytosis, polychromasia, reticulocytosis, and the presence of nucleated red blood cells in the circulation. Morphologic abnormalities of diagnostic significance such as intracellular or epicellular parasites, granulocytic inclusion bodies, Heinz bodies, spherocytes, schistocytes, or poikilocytes may be noted on examination of stained blood smears. Responsive anemias often are accompanied by a neutrophilia and regenerative left shift. The bone marrow usually shows an active erythropoietic response with a decreased myeloid/erythroid (M/E) ratio. The serum concentration of haptoglobin is decreased, and serum lactate dehydrogenase enzyme activity may be elevated during acute hemolytic episodes. An increase in serum bilirubin concentration caused primarily by an increase in indirect reacting bilirubin is a reflection of active red cell destruction. Specific serologic diagnostic procedures are available for many of the infectious causes of hemolytic anemia. Immunohematologic procedures such as the direct and indirect Coombs' tests provide an indication that immune-mediated processes contribute to enhanced erythrocyte destruction. It should be noted that the principal mechanisms responsible for increased rate of red cell destruction associated with many of the infectious causes of hemolytic anemia (parasitic, bacterial, and viral) are immunologically mediated, and affected animals may be transiently Coombs' positive.

ANAPLASMOSIS

GUY H. PALMER
STUART LINCOLN

DEFINITION AND ETIOLOGY. Anaplasmosis is an infectious, transmissible disease of cattle, sheep, and goats caused by bacterial pathogens of the genus Anaplasma and characterized by progressive anemia. *Anaplasma* spp. are genetically and antigenically most closely related to ehrlichiae, notably *Ehrlichia phagocytophila, Ehrlichia platys,* and *Ehrlichia bovis,* within the order Rickettsiales. Taxonomic unification of this group of pathogens into the genus Anaplasma is likely to be adopted in the near future. As presently classified, the two primary pathogenic Anaplasma species are *Anaplasma marginale* and *Anaplasma ovis.* Both species infect mature erythrocytes within a relatively wide range of ruminant hosts; however, disease is usually manifested only by *A. marginale* infection in cattle and by *A. ovis* infection in sheep and goats. Historically, a third species, *Anaplasma centrale,* has been described as causing mild disease in cattle and has been used as a live vaccine to induce partial protection against *A. marginale.*[65] Whether *A. centrale* is truly a distinct species, a subspecies of *A. marginale,* or simply a specific strain of *A. marginale* has not been resolved to date.

CLINICAL SIGNS AND DIFFERENTIAL DIAGNOSIS. Clinical signs are highly variable, from acute severe disease to subclinical infection, and reflect variation in virulence among pathogen strains and age- and breed-related differences in host susceptibility. Age at the time of initial infection is a primary determinant of host susceptibility. Disease is often mild in calves in the first 6 to 9 months of life and increasingly severe in older cattle. The incubation period ranges from 21 to 45 days, with an average of about 30 days. Infec-

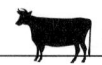

tions in young calves often are asymptomatic. Occasionally, however, one may observe mild lethargy and partial anorexia for 24 to 48 hours. In contrast, the early stage of acute anaplasmosis in adult cattle is typified by fever, with rectal temperatures ranging from 39.5° to 41° C (103° to 106° F). Within 12 to 24 hours the fever subsides, and the temperature may drop to normal and become subnormal before the animal dies. Anorexia and, in dairy cows, a dramatic decrease in milk production can usually be observed soon after a fever is detected. Concurrently there is suppression of rumination, dryness of the muzzle, and lethargy. Some cattle may become aggressive, possibly as a result of cerebral hypoxia associated with anemia. Care must be taken not to overstress severely anemic cattle because this may result in collapse and death. Cattle that stagger are usually anemic and hypoxic. Early, the mucous membranes are pallid, but they may be icteric if an animal has survived for 2 to 3 days past the acute crisis. Constipation is a consistent sign, with the feces dark brown and covered with mucus, and pollakiuria is characterized by dark yellow urine. Hemoglobinuria does not occur. Abortion may occur when infection occurs late in gestation. If an animal survives the acute crisis, the convalescent period is protracted and depends on the severity of the anemia. Icterus and weight loss are more commonly observed in the convalescent period, which may last for 3 to 4 weeks.

Although *A. ovis* infection in sheep and goats is often asymptomatic, anemia occasionally becomes severe enough to produce signs similar to those seen during *A. marginale* infection of cattle.

The differential diagnosis requires consideration of the diseases that can produce anemia or icterus, including leptospirosis, bacillary hemoglobinuria, and babesiosis. In pastured cattle, hepatotoxic plant poisonings *(Senecio)* and other causes of liver disease that produce icterus also have to be considered (see Chapter 7, Causes of Icterus, and Chapter 31, Liver Disease). Copper poisoning must be considered in sheep.

CLINICAL PATHOLOGY. Because acute bovine anaplasmosis is characterized by anemia, a falling hematocrit is an excellent criterion for prognostic purposes and for determining the severity of infection. The packed cell volume (PCV) drops below 30% when the first clinical signs are observed and may drop precipitously within 24 to 48 hours. Death can occur during this period despite a PCV above 20%. Conversely, the PCV may decease to 6% to 10% before death. During this acute phase, *A. marginale* can be detected within the erythrocytes by microscopic examination of blood smears stained with Wright's, new methylene blue, or Giemsa stain. The inclusion is composed of a small morula of 2 to 8 individual organisms and >5% and as many as 20% to 70% of the erythrocytes may be infected. Later, after several days of anemia, the percentage of infected erythrocytes decreases dramatically and evidence of erythrocyte regeneration can be detected. There is anisocytosis, basophilic stippling, poikilocytosis, polychromatophilia, and reticulocytosis. Although some cattle with acute anaplasmosis are icteric, the icterus index is variable, ranging from normal to 100 U. After recovery from acute disease, cattle and sheep remain persistently infected with 0.000001% to 0.1% of erythrocytes being infected.[66] These very low levels cannot be reliably detected by microscopic examination and these persistently infected animals, which serve as reservoirs for transmission, are usually detected serologically. In contrast, serologic tests are of minimal value in the diagnosis of acute anaplasmosis.

PATHOPHYSIOLOGY. *Anaplasma* spp. are transmitted by ixoid species ticks, most commonly *Dermacentor* in the mainland United States and by *Boophilus* spp. in tropical and subtropical regions worldwide. However, direct transfer of infected blood by either hematophagous flies or iatrogenically

(contaminated needles, dehorning, castrating, hormone implanting, and ear-tagging instruments) can result in transmission. After transmission, sequential rounds of bacterial invasion of mature erythrocytes, replication, and egress result in a progressively increasing rickettsemia, with a doubling time of approximately 24 hours. Clinical signs appear when greater than 1% of erythrocytes are infected and the severity roughly correlates with the percentage of infected erythrocytes. Anemia is, at least in part, caused by splenic and hepatic macrophage-mediated phagocytosis of both infected and uninfected erythrocytes. This appears to reflect both induction of autoantibodies against the erythrocyte surface[67] as well as induction of acute phase reactants, including complement activation, during high level rickettsemia. The regenerative response to anemia can be vigorous and does not appear to be affected by the *Anaplasma* organisms.

Protective immunity appears to require induction of both antibody against the outer membrane proteins and macrophage activation for enhanced phagocytosis and bacterial killing.[68] This coordinated induction is mediated by CD4+ T cells that secrete interferon-γ. Although the immune response controls the acute rickettsemia, organisms are not completely cleared from the blood because of emergence of antigenic variants. These variants are responsible for persistent infection, characterized by recurring waves of rickettsemia that reflect sequential emergence and then immune control of antigenically variant organisms.[69]

EPIDEMIOLOGY. Anaplasma is the most prevalent of the tick-borne diseases of cattle worldwide and remains as a serious constraint to livestock production in tropical and subtropical regions. However, anaplasmosis is also a significant problem in temperate regions. In the United States, infection is endemic in southeastern states and much of the west. In addition, anaplasmosis occurs episodically in many historically nonendemic regions and has been detected in at least 40 states. Endemic regions reflect a high tick infection rate and are maintained by the prevalence of both competent arthropod vectors and persistently infected carrier cattle. These carrier cattle, which are typically asymptomatic, are efficient reservoirs for tick-borne transmission.[70] Outbreaks of acute disease are often related to the vector activity and the number of susceptible animals in a herd. Although vector activity varies by region, in general, outbreaks of anaplasmosis occur most frequently in the late spring and summer when arthropod activity is highest.[71] However, it should be emphasized that the determinants of tick- and fly-borne transmission are not well understood and transmission is often unpredictable. In contrast, iatrogenic transmission can occur at any time and can be controlled by avoiding blood contamination during veterinary medical procedures. Although wild ruminants (deer, elk, bison) rarely have clinical disease and generally are asymptomatic carriers, their overall importance in the epidemiology of infection is unclear. Currently, wild ruminants are thought to play at most only a minor role in natural transmission.

PATHOLOGY. At necropsy there are no specific lesions that can be used to unequivocally diagnose anaplasmosis. In acute anaplasmosis the blood is thin and watery and fails to clot readily. Mucous membranes, subcutaneous tissues, and skeletal musculature are pale (anemic pallor). However, in later stages of acute disease the same tissues exhibit varying degrees of icterus. Splenomegaly is a consistent finding while hepatomegaly and distention of the gallbladder are commonly but less frequently observed. Urine is deep yellow, but hemoglobinuria or hematuria does not occur. The absence of hemoglobinuria helps differentiate anaplasmosis from other hemolytic diseases (bacillary hemoglobinuria, leptospirosis, onion toxicity, copper poisoning in sheep). Occasionally petechiae may be found in the subepicardium,

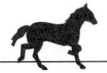

subendocardium, and other serous membranes. Detection of *Anaplasma*-infected erythrocytes within capillaries of Giemsa-stained histologic sections can be used to confirm a diagnosis of anaplasmosis.

TREATMENT. Tetracyclines are the antibiotic of choice for treating acute disease and resistance has not been reported. In acute anaplasmosis, oxytetracycline administered intravenously at 11 mg/kg once daily for 3 to 5 days is effective. One to two administrations of long-acting oxytetracycline at 20 mg/kg IM at 72-hour intervals is also an effective treatment. In addition to antibiotic therapy, supportive therapy is important. If the PCV is 12 or below, whole blood transfusion may be indicated in order to prevent death and to shorten the convalescence period. Four to 8 L of whole blood is usually administered to an adult animal. A PCV of 8 or below indicates an unfavorable prognosis and death often occurs despite appropriate antibiotic and supportive therapy. Importantly, the oxytetracycline regimen used to treat acute anaplasmosis is not effective in completely clearing the animal of the organism and recovered animals become persistently infected carriers. To obtain complete clearance, long-acting oxytetracycline must be administered at 20 mg/kg every 3 days for four successive treatments.[72] However, not all cattle treated with this regimen will clear the infection and, if required for exportation, clearance should be confirmed by conversion to seronegative status or by a negative polymerase chain reaction (PCR) test.

PREVENTION AND CONTROL. The control measures used vary depending on the geographic region and type of livestock production system. In endemic regions with high transmission rates, such as those in tropical countries, beef cattle are often allowed to become naturally infected at a young age and remain asymptomatic carriers with minimal risk of later acute disease. In regions with lower transmission rates, live blood-based vaccines may be used to ensure infection of cattle at a young age. This is exemplified by the use of over 1.5 million doses of trivalent (*A. marginale, Babesia bovis, Babesia bigemina*) live vaccine in Australia since 1990. Similarly, live vaccines based on *A. centrale* or weakly virulent strains of *A. marginale* are commonly used in Africa, Asia, and Central and South America. However, these are not licensed for use in the United States, largely because of the risk of transmitting known or newly emergent pathogens contaminating the blood-based vaccine. The exception to this is the provisional licensing of a live vaccine for use in California.* Importantly, these live vaccines should only be used in young animals and are contraindicated for use in older and especially in pregnant animals. Killed vaccines are less efficacious and require multiple immunizations; however, these can induce at least partial protection against severe morbidity and mortality. Unfortunately, none of the killed vaccines previously marketed in the United States are currently available. Experimental vaccines based on recombinant outer membrane proteins have shown efficacy in controlled trials but have not been commercially developed at present.[67] In the absence of immunoprophylaxis, control of anaplasmosis is limited to preventing transmission. Although it is difficult to completely prevent the contact of ticks and blood-sucking insect vectors with cattle grazing on open ranges or farm pastures, strategic use of acaricides and insecticides can reduce transmission during periods of high vector activity. Periodic spraying for tick control and the use of insecticide-impregnated ear tags or insecticide dust bags for biting fly control are cost effective, not only for control of anaplasmosis but for control of pinkeye and for directly reducing irritation and increasing weight

gain. Because blood-contaminated instruments and needles can mechanically transmit infection, appropriate sanitary measures should be implemented when injections or surgical procedures are performed. Because persistently infected carrier cattle can be cleared by administration of tetracyclines, the elimination of all carriers by this means can be an effective control procedure in a herd. As noted previously, this requires intramuscular administration of long-acting tetracycline at 20 mg/kg every 3 days for four successive treatments[72] and requires confirmation of clearance. After elimination of persistent infection, animals become susceptible to reinfection.[73] Thus success of this strategy depends on effective vector control and preventing introduction of new carrier cattle into the herd. However, serologic screening using the complement fixation (CF) test has poor sensitivity for detecting persistently infected carriers. Although the specificity of the CF test, which is the currently approved United States Department of Agriculture (USDA) procedure, is high (98%), the sensitivity in detecting carriers is unacceptably low (20%).[74]

Consequently, relying on the CF test to screen incoming cattle into a negative herd is risky and *Anaplasma*-free herds can likely be maintained only in areas of very low transmission. The recent development of a competitive ELISA based on a conserved recombinant *A. marginale* antigen (MSP5) should allow better identification of carriers, as this test has a reported sensitivity of 96% and a specificity of 95%.[74] The MSP5 CI-ELISA also detects *A. ovis* infections.[75] This test* is commercially available and is currently undergoing evaluation by the USDA for approval as an official test.

REFERENCES

65. Losos GJ: Anaplasmosis. In Losos G, ed: *Infectious tropical diseases of domestic animals*, Harlow, UK, 1986, Longman Press, p 742.
66. French DF et al: Expression of *Anaplasma marginale* major surface protein 2 variants during persistent cyclic rickettsemia, *Infect Immunol* 66:1200-1207, 1998.
67. Cox FR, Dimopoullos GT: Demonstration of an antoantibody associated with anaplasmosis, *Am J Vet Res* 33:73-76, 1972.
68. Palmer GH et al: Molecular basis for vaccine development against the ehrlichial pathogen *Anaplasma marginale, Parasitol Today* 15:281-286, 1999.
69. French DM, Brown WC, Palmer GH: Emergence of *Anaplasma marginale* antigenic variants during persistent rickettsemia, *Infect Immunol* 67:5834-5840, 1999.
70. Eriks IS, Stiller D, Palmer GH: Impact of persistent *Anaplasma marginale* rickettsemia on tick infection and transmission, *J Clin Microbiol* 31:2091-2096, 1993.
71. Zaugg JL: Seasonality of natural transmission of bovine anaplasmosis under desert mountain range conditions, *J Am Vet Med Assoc* 196:1106-1109, 1990.
72. Magonigle RA, Newby MS: Elimination of naturally acquired chronic *Anaplasma marginale* infections with a long-acting oxytetracycline injectable, *Am J Vet Res* 43:2170-2172, 1982.
73. Zaugg JL, Lincoln SD: How susceptible are anaplasmosis-cleared cattle to reinfection? *Vet Med* 82:184-190, 1987.
74. Bradway DS et al: Sensitivity and specificity of the complement fixation test for detection of *Anaplasma marginale* persistently infected carriers, *J Vet Diagn Invest* 13:77-79, 2001.
75. Ndung'u LW et al: Detection of Anaplasma ovis infection in goats using the MSP5 competitive inhibition ELISA, *J Clin Microbiol* 33:675-679, 1995.

BABESIOSIS

JERRY L. ZAUGG

Babesiosis is a tick-borne intraerythrocytic disease of domestic and wild mammals and humans caused by protozoan parasites of the genera *Babesia* and *Theileria*. The acute disease is characterized by fever, hemolytic anemia, icterus, hemoglo-

---

*AnaVac, Poultry Health Laboratories, Inc., Davis, CA.

*VMRD Inc., Pullman, WA.

TABLE 35-1

Babesia (babesiosis)

Organism	Livestock Affected	Principal Geographic Distribution	Morphology of Organism	Tick Vectors
B. bigemina	Cattle	Americas, Europe, Africa, Australia, Middle East	4.5 × 2.5 μm (large, round, and pyriform; acute angle)	Boophilus annulatus, B. decoloratus, B. microplus spp.
B. bovis (syn. B. berbera, B. argentina)	Cattle	Americas, Europe, Russia, Africa, Asia, Australia	2.4 × 1.5 μm (small and more rounded; obtuse angle)	B. annulatus, B. microplus, Ixodes spp.*(?)
B. divergens	Cattle	Europe	1.5 × 1.4 μm (small, narrow and obtuse angle)	Ixodes ricinus
B. major	Cattle	Europe, Russia, North Africa, Middle East	2.6 × 1.5 μm (similar to B. bigemina, but smaller)	Haemaphysalis punctata
B. jakimovi	Cattle	USSR, Asia	2-4.6 × 1.5-2.1 μm (large, round, and pyriform)	I. ricinus
B. ovata	Cattle	Japan	4.5 × 2.5 μm (large, round, and pyriform)	Haemaphysalis longicornis
B. caballi	Horses	Americas, Europe, Russia, Asia, Africa, Middle East	3 × 2 μm (large, pyriform; acute angle)	Dermacentor, Hyalomma, and Rhipicephalus spp.
T. equi (B. equi)	Horses	Americas, Europe, Russia, Asia, Africa, Middle East	1-2 μm (small and rounded; maltese cross is characteristic)	Dermacentor, Hyalomma, and Rhipicephalus spp.
B. motasi	Sheep and goats	Europe, Russia, Asia, Middle East	3 × 2 μm (large, pyriform; acute angle)	D. silvarum (?), Haemaphysalis spp., R. bursa
B. ovis	Sheep and goats	Europe, Russia, Asia, Middle East	1.5 × 1 μm (small and more rounded; obtuse)	I. ricinus (?), R. bursa, D. reticulatis (?)
B. trautmanni	Swine	Europe, Africa, Russia	3.5 × 2 μm (large, narrow, and long; acute angle)	R. sanguineus (?), Dermacentor spp. (?) Boophilus spp. (?) Hyalomma spp. (?)
B. perroncitoi	Swine	Europe, Africa, Asia	0.7-2 μm (small and more rounded)	Vectors unknown

From Kuttler, KL: *Foreign animal diseases*, Richmond, Va, 1984, United States Animal Health Association, p 77.
?, Suspected vector.

binuria, and death. Although both morphologic and serologic differentiation is needed for specific identification of the various disease-producing species, all can be categorized as being either "large" or "small" in size. A list of the commonly encountered *Babesia* spp., and *Theileria equi*, their usual biologic vectors, and livestock hosts is presented in Table 35-1. Babesiosis has a wide geographic distribution, particularly in the tropics and subtropics, largely related to the distribution of vector ticks. Of the different diseases the economically most important infections of livestock are those of cattle and horses.

Bovine Babesiosis

ETIOLOGY. Known variously by such names as bovine babesiosis, piroplasmosis, Texas fever, redwater, tick fever, and tristeza, the disease may be caused by at least six *Babesia* species (see Table 35-1). Some animals other than cattle known to be susceptible to agents of bovine babesiosis include white-tailed deer, American bison, water buffalo, reindeer, and the African buffalo. Infections in these species are nominal and, except under unusual conditions, such hosts are probably not significant reservoirs.

Of greatest concern in the Western Hemisphere are *B. bigemina* and *B bovis*. *B. bigemina* is a large *Babesia* species characteristically appearing within mature erythrocytes as nonpigmented, paired, pear-shaped bodies joined at an acute angle. Irregularly shaped, round, or amoeboid forms are also seen. *B. bovis* is a small, pleomorphic *Babesia* species often identified as a single round body or as paired, pear-shaped bodies joined at an obtuse angle within mature erythrocytes. Of the two species, *B. bovis* is usually considered the most virulent.

Natural transmission of both species occurs primarily by the feeding of various stages of the one-host ticks of the genus *Boophilus*. Ticks are most commonly infected transovarially (vertically). The female tick becomes infected by the ingestion of parasites during engorgement. After it drops off the host, the babesial organisms reproduce within the tick's tissues. Some of the reproducing organisms are incorporated within developing tick embryos, and the disease agents are transmitted to new vertebrate hosts by the feeding of ensuing tick larvae, nymphs, or adults. Larval ticks may transmit *B. bovis*, but *B. bigemina* is not transmitted until the larvae have molted into the nymphal or adult stages.

Both *Babesia* spp. may also be transmitted iatrogenically through blood-contaminated fomites, as described under anaplasmosis.

CLINICAL SIGNS. Clinical signs are manifest 2 to 3 weeks after tick infestation. The incubation period after blood inoculation may be less than 5 days to more than 3 weeks, depending on the volume of inoculum. Clinical signs of fever (40° to 42° C, 104° to 107.6° F), depression, icterus, anorexia, tachycardia, tachypnea, anemia, hemoglobinemia, hemoglobinuria, abortion, and death are seen. Anemia is caused by intravascular destruction of erythrocytes by escaping merozoites after intraerythrocytic reproduction of the babesias by binary fission. In addition, the osmotic fragility of the whole erythrocyte population increases terminally, such that massive lysis occurs even though the parasitemia may be less than 1%.[76] Additionally, as also seen with anaplasmosis, an autoimmune condition may result in which the spleen removes damaged and apparently healthy erythrocytes from circulation. Thus the degree of anemia may exceed that which might be expected with a low parasitemia. The anemia may occur

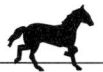

very rapidly, with 75% or more of the erythrocytes being destroyed in just a few days. The exit of *B. bigemina* and *B. bovis* parasites from infected erythrocytes releases two or more parasite-associated proteolytic enzymes into the plasma. These enzymes and other parasite metabolic products are believed to interact with blood components and are responsible for such clinical signs as metabolic acidosis and anoxia. Tachycardia may be dramatic. The noise of the accentuated heartbeat can become so pronounced that it may be heard at a distance of a few meters from the animal.

Cerebral babesiosis (also see Chapter 33), characterized by hyperexcitability, convulsions, opisthotonos, coma, and death may be observed in cattle infected with either *B. bigemina* or *B. bovis,* but especially with the latter. Central nervous system signs are caused by brain anoxia resulting from severe anemia or erythrocyte blockage of cerebral capillaries.

Death is caused by a shocklike syndrome associated with the accumulation of toxins, release of vasoactive substances, and anemic anoxia. Most cases with cerebral involvement are fatal; however, mortality is extremely variable, depending on the species of *Babesia* concerned, susceptibility of the host, and management and environmental stress factors. Many cattle that survive the acute phase recover but become chronic carriers. Other survivors often experience episodes of recrudescence, eventually succumbing to the disease, or they may die as a result of secondary infections contracted during their debilitated state.

Cattle of all breeds are susceptible to babesiosis. However, *Bos indicus* breeds exhibit a definite degree of resistance to both of the *Babesia* spp. and the tick vectors.[77] Calves possess a natural immunity to babesiosis. Such immunity was believed to be reinforced by colostral antibodies for calves born to previously infected dams.[77] However, erythrocytes of young bovines may contain factor(s) independent of antibody that provide an innate resistance to severe babesiosis.[79] Thus calves infected up to the age of 9 months experience a minimum reaction to the disease, becoming asymptomatic carriers. Carriers remain resistant to clinical disease for at least 4 years.[80] The carrier state can be overcome, however, by such stresses as calving, malnutrition, or concurrent disease.[81]

CLINICAL PATHOLOGY. Clinical signs observed in cattle located in enzootic areas where *Boophilus* ticks occur may provide sufficient data for a presumptive diagnosis. Other conditions that may exhibit some of the same signs as babesiosis are anaplasmosis, trypanosomiasis, theileriosis, leptospirosis, chronic copper toxicity, and bacillary hemoglobinuria. The cerebral signs may be confused with rabies and other encephalitides. A positive diagnosis requires identification of the *Babesia* organisms on Giemsa-stained thin blood smears, positive serologic tests, or inoculation of splenectomized calves with infective blood. In acute infection, *Babesia* spp. can usually be detected in smears made from peripheral blood. In chronic cases the numbers of parasitized erythrocytes diminish, becoming so sparse as to make detection difficult. This is especially true with *B. bovis,* which shows a marked tendency to accumulate in capillaries, particularly those of the brain. *B. bovis* may favor capillaries in the brain and kidney because the major energy-producing pathway of *Babesia* appears to be anaerobic glycolysis. The blockage of cerebral and renal capillaries by parasitized erythrocytes results in an anaerobic condition that enables the parasites to absorb preformed substrates by pinocytosis and diffusion through their surface membranes.[87] PCV values drop rapidly from a normal of 35% to below 10% in less than a week after the first onset of clinical signs.[82] Serum potassium levels decrease in some infected animals whereas urine potassium levels increase in nearly all cases.[83]

Specific anti-*Babesia* antibodies are detectable in cattle sera in fewer than 7 days after infection.[84] Such antibodies also exist for at least 252 days after the disappearance of detectable parasites.[85] The CF and IFA tests are the most widely used.[84] The CF test follows the same basic procedure used in anaplasmosis CF testing[86] with a *Babesia* antigen.[87] The test is effective, but approximately 100 days after infection the CF antibodies drop below a reliable diagnostic level.[84] The IFA test uses the whole intraerythrocytic parasite as antigen rather than an extract and commercially prepared rabbit antibovine gamma-globulin conjugated to fluorescein.[84] Other serologic tests include gel precipitation,[88] latex particle agglutination,[89] rapid card agglutination,[90] and enzyme-labeling immunoassay (EIA).[91] The immunologic assays, however, are indirect methods and do not detect the causal organisms in samples obtained from a suspected infected animal. Recombinant DNA techniques using selected clones containing inserts of *Babesia* genomic DNA sequences are now available to be utilized as specific, highly sensitive DNA or RNA probes to detect the presence of the hemoparasite DNA in an infected animal, or tick vector.[92]

NECROPSY FINDINGS. Postmortem findings in cattle that die peracutely are caracteristic of an acute hemolytic crisis. Such findings include a generalized pallor or icterus throughout the carcass; an enlarged, icteric liver; gallbladder distended with thick, dark green bile; and a markedly enlarged, dark soft spleen. Hydropericardium and subepicardial/subendocardial petechiation may be seen. The blood is thin and watery. The urinary bladder is frequently distended with dark red urine. There may be subserosal ecchymotic hemorrhages in abomasal and intestinal mucosa, and the lymph nodes are edematous.

The carcass of an animal that dies after a prolonged illness is generally emaciated and icteric. The blood is thin and watery, and the intermuscular fascia is edematous. The kidneys are pale and edematous, and the bladder may contain pink-tinged or normal urine. The liver is enlarged and jaundiced, and the bile may contain flakes of semisolid material.

TREATMENT AND PROGNOSIS. After the onset of hemoglobinuria or cerebral signs, the prognosis is poor. Acute cases with PCV values above 12% usually respond well to treatment. The prognosis decreases for cases with PCV values below 10%. Successful treatment depends on early diagnosis and prompt therapy. In addition to specific treatment, supportive therapy such as blood transfusions (4 L of whole blood per 250 kg of body weight), fluids, hematinics, and prophylactic antibiotics are important. However, wild, excitable cattle may best be left alone. With severe hemolytic anemias, any exertion associated with restraint and treatment may precipitate an anoxic crisis. The small *Babesia* spp. are more resistant to chemotherapy and may require increased dosages or additional treatments. The most commonly used, effective, and relatively less toxic specific babesiacides are diminazine diaceturate (Berenil or Ganeseg*) at 3 to 5 mg/kg; phenamidine diisethionate (Lomdine†) at 8 to 13 mg/kg: imidocarb dipropionate (Imizol‡A) at 1 to 3 mg/kg; and amicarbalide diisethionate (Diampron§) at 5 to 10 mg/kg.[93] Generally, treated cattle become chronic carriers and are resistant to further clinical episodes of the disease. However, treatment of *B. bigemina* may be so effective that sterilization occurs, eventually leaving the animal susceptible to reinfection. Imidocarb has both therapeutic and prophylactic activities. In enzootic areas, its use prevents clinical infection for as long as 2 months but at the same time allows mild, subclinical infections to occur, resulting in premunition immunity.[94,95]

---

*Farbwerke-Hoechst AG, Frankfurt, West Germany.
†ER Squibb and Sons de Mexico, Mexico, D.F., Mexico.
‡May & Baker, Ltd, Deganham, England.
§Burroughs Wellcome & Co, Ltd, London, England.

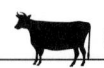

PREVENTION AND CONTROL. Eradication of *Boophilus* tick vectors has provided effective control in the United States. Other such projects attempted elsewhere have not been successful because of such diverse reasons as tick resistance to acaricides; ability of some ticks to infest alternative, nonbovine hosts; failure to obtain 100% cooperation of cattle producers; and lack of financial resources to sustain a prolonged program.

Most procedures aimed at reducing tick infestations (i.e., acaricide applications [on host or over environment], controlled range burning, cultivation, prolonged pasture rest, and use of repellents) are beneficial. Care should be taken to prevent accidental transfer of blood from one animal to another in routine surgery (e.g., dehorning, castration, ear marking, hormone implanting) and vaccination procedures.

The most common form of immunization consists of inoculating live organisms (virulent or attenuated) into susceptible calves to induce a state of premunition. Inoculation of older animals is followed by nonsterilizing chemotherapy as needed to modify clinical effects.[96] Although a premunition approach is useful in endemic areas, it is less desirable in areas with low infection rates because the premunized carriers provide a large reservoir of infection.

Some killed adjuvant vaccines have proven successful in limited trials.[97] In vitro cell cultivation techniques have yielded highly immunogenic soluble antigens of *B. bovis*.[98] Subunit vaccines derived from monoclonal technologies were proven effective in protecting against severe clinical disease.[99] The monoclonal antibodies apparently inhibit merozoite invasion of the erythrocytes. Vaccines of such noninfectious material generally do not prevent disease, but they do moderate the effects of infection and do not directly produce carriers. To date, none of the killed preparations, soluble cell culture products, or subunit vaccines are commercially available.

Equine Babesiosis

ETIOLOGY. Babesiosis/theileriosis of the horse (piroplasmosis) is a febrile, tick-borne disease of equids caused by *Babesia caballi* and *T. equi*. Until recently *T. equi* was known as *B. equi*. However, because the organism more closely resembles members of the genus *Theileria* with its exoerythrocytic (lymphocytic) stages within the vertebrate host with the development of microschizonts and macroschizonts, it is now classified as *T. equi*[100] (see Table 35-1). *B. caballi* is a large *Babesia* resembling *B. bigemina* and affecting cattle. Although *T. equi* is not a member of the genus *Babesia*, for practical purposes it is still considered a "small" parasite somewhat like *B. bovis* in stained thin blood smears. However, a unique characteristic of *T. equi* is that the intraerythrocytic parasites divide into four cells to form a Maltese cross.[101]

Equine piroplasmosis is widely distributed throughout the tropics and subtropics and to a lesser extent in temperate regions. The distribution roughly corresponds to those of the tick vectors. Both species are naturally transmitted by ticks of the genera *Dermacentor*, *Hyalomma*, and *Rhipicephalus*. *B. caballi* is passed transovarially (vertically) from one tick generation to the next. Transmission of *T. equi* apparently only occurs transstadially (horizontally) that is, one tick stage (larvae or nymphs) becomes infected and the disease agent is passed to the next vertebrate host in the next tick stage (nymph or adult). Because of the widespread prevalence of potential tick vectors in the United States (*Dermacentor albipictus*, *Dermacentor iteus*, and *Dermacentor variablis*), it is unknown why equine piroplasmosis is not a problem in the United States.

CLINICAL SIGNS. Apparently all equids are susceptible to both parasite species. The zebra in Africa is naturally infected with *T. equi* but not with *B. caballi*. Once infected, survivors remain chronic carriers. *T. equi* is known to be transmitted transplacentally.

Clinical features occurring after an incubation period of 5 to 28 days are fever (39° to 42° C [102° to 107.6° F]), hemolytic anemia, jaundice, hemoglobinuria, and death. Generalized signs of depression, anorexia, incoordination, lacrimation, mucous nasal discharge, swelling of the eyelids, and frequent lying down are seen. *T. equi* is considered the most pathogenic of the two species and is responsible for a greater incidence of hemoglobinuria and death. *B. caballi* causes a more persistent fever and anemia.

Differential diagnoses include equine monocytic ehrlichiosis, equine infectious anemia, liver failure with hemolytic anemia, and other hemolytic anemias of the horse.

CLINICAL PATHOLOGY. A fever associated with anemia, jaundice, and hemoglobinuria, with the detection of parasite-infected erythrocytes in Geimsa-stained blood smears, is diagnostic. A significant increase in relative and absolute numbers of monocytes and an absence of eosinophils may be observed in horses infected with *T. equi*. Hemoglobinuria is rare in animals infected with *B. caballi*, but urine is often dark yellow in color. The most commonly used serologic tests are the complement fixation (CF) and indirect fluorescent antibody (IFA) tests. Blood from spleen-intact horses can become CF-positive within 14 days after parasite exposure. There is also a competitive ELISA test for *T. equi* and a polymerase chain reaction (PCR) test for both equine diseases. Further, as with the bovine infections, both *B. caballi* and *T. equi* infections can be specifically detected with nucleic acid probes.[92]

NECROPSY. Postmortem features are similar to those seen in bovine babesiosis, but jaundice is even more prominent throughout the carcass. There is excessive fluid in the body cavities, especially the pericardial sac. Pulmonary edema is evident. The liver is swollen, and hepatic vessels contain large, yellowish clots. The spleen in enlarged with rounded edges.

TREATMENT AND PROGNOSIS. Generally both *B. caballi* and *T. equi* respond to the same babesiacidal drugs used to treat bovine babesiosis, but *T. equi* is more refractory to treatment than *B. caballi*. If diagnosed early and treated promptly, recovery is the rule. The drug of choice for eliminating the carrier state of infected animals is imidocarb. Imidocarb, at the level of 2.2 mg/kg given 2 times at a 24-hour interval, is effective against *B. caballi*. A 4 mg/kg amount given 4 times at a 72-hour interval is effective against *T. equi* of eastern hemisphere origin.[93] However, donkeys receiving similar treatment died from drug toxicosis.[77] The higher doses of imidocarb often produce transient side effects in horses similar to the signs seen in colic. To date, attempts to consistently eliminate the carrier state of *T. equi* of Eastern European origin have been unsuccessful.[102] However, as was earlier proposed,[103] irregular chemical sterilization success has been obtained with concurrent IV administration of buparvaquone (Butalex) at 4 mg/kg and IM imidocarb at 4 mg/kg.

PREVENTION AND CONTROL. Control of the tick infestations does much to reduce disease incidence, as does care to prevent blood transfer during such routine surgical procedures as castration.

No vaccines effectively prevent equine babesiosis. Although premunition as used in bovine babesiosis is of limited value in some enzootic areas, it is not widely practiced. This is because early treatment without sterilization is effective and the resulting chronic carriers resist further disease challenge.

REFERENCES

76. Wright IG: Biochemical characteristics of *Babesia* and physicochemical reactions in the host. In Ristic M, Kreier JP, eds: *Babesiosis*, New York, 1981, Academic Press, pp 171-205.

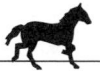

77. Francis S: Resistance of zebu and other cattle to tick infestation and babesiosis with special reference to Australia: a historical review, *Br Vet J* 122:301-307, 1966.
78. Mahoney DF: Studies on the protection of cattle against *Babesia bovis* infection. In Dunsmore, JD, ed: *Tropical parasitoses and parasitic zoonoses*, Perth, Australia, 1983, World Association for the Advancement of Veterinary Parasitology, pp 93-104.
79. Levy MG, Clabaugh G, Ristic M: Age resistance in bovine babesiosis: role of blood factors in resistance to *Babesia bovis, Infect Immunol* 37:1127-1131, 1982.
80. Mahoney, DF, Wright IG, Mirre GB: Bovine babesiosis: the persistence of immunity to *Babesia argentina* and *B. bigemina* in calves *(Bos taurus)* after naturally acquired infection, *Ann Trop Med Parasitol* 67:197-302, 1973.
81. Robertson A: *Handbook on animal diseases in the tropics*, ed 3, London, England, 1976, British Veterinary Association, pp 166-170.
82. Kuttler KL: Babesiosis. In Trevono GS, Hyde JL, eds: *Foreign animal diseases*, Richmond, Va, 1984 Committee on Foreign Animal Diseases of the United States Animal Health Association, pp 76-96.
83. Wright IG: Studies on the pathogenesis of *Babesia argentina* and *Babesia bigemina* infections in splenectomized calves, *Z Parasitenkd* 39:85-102, 1972.
84. Kuttler KL, Adams LG, Todorovic RA: Comparisons of the complement-fixation and indirect fluorescent antibody reactions in the detection of bovine babesiosis, *Am J Vet Res* 38:153-156, 1977.
85. Madruga CR et al: Antibody levels anti-Babesia bigemina and *Babesia bovis* in calves of Nelore and Ibage breeds and Nelore crosses, *Pesq Aqropec Gras Brasilia* 19:1163-1168, 1984.
86. Anonymous: *Microtiter technique for the complement-fixation test for anaplasmosis*, Beltsville, MD, USDA, APHIS, p 6, 1974.
87. Mahoney DF: Bovine babesiosis: preparation and assessment of complement fixing antigens, *Exp Parasitol* 20:232-241, 1967.
88. Todorovic RA, Adams LG: Serodiagnosis of babesiosis, *Proc XIX World Vet Congr* 3:1114-1116, 1971.
89. Zuckerman A, Ristic M: Blood parasite antigens and antibodies. In Weinman D, Ristic M. eds: *Infectious blood diseases of man and animals*, New York, 1968, Academic Press, pp 79-122.
90. Todorovic RA, Kuttler KL: A babesiosis card agglutination test, *Am J Vet Res* 35:1347-1350, 1974.
91. Barry DN, Rodwell BJ, Timms P, et al: A microplate enzyme immunoassay for detecting and measuring antibodies to *Babesia bovis* in cattle serum, *Aust Vet J* 59:136-140, 1982.
92. Fiqueroa JV, Buening GM: Nucleic acid probes as a diagnostic method for tick-borne hemoparasites of veterinary importance, *Vet Parasitol* 75:75-92, 1994.
93. Kuttler KL: Chemotherapy of babesiosis: a review. In Ristic M, and Dreier JP, eds: *Babesiosis*, New York, 1981, Academic Press, pp 65-85.
94. Kuttler KL, Graham OH, Trevino JL: The effect of imidocarb treatment on *Babesia* in the bovine and the tick *(Boophilus microplus)*, *Res Vet Sci* 18:198-200, 1975.
95. Todorovic Ra et al: Chemoprophylaxis (imidocarb) against *Babesia bigeminia* and *Babesia argentina* infections, *Am J Vet Res* 39:1153-1161, 1974.
96. Todorovic RA, Gonzales Ed, Adams LG: *Babesia bigemina, Babesia argentina, Anaplasma marginale*: coinfectious immunity in bovines, *Exp Parasitol* 37:179-192, 1975.
97. Kuttler KL, Johnson LW: Immunization of cattle with a *Babesia bigemina* antigen in Freund's complete adjuvant, *Am J Vet Res* 41:536-538, 1980.
98. Montenegro-James S et al: Heterologous strain immunity in bovine babesiosis using a culture-derived soluble *Babesia bovis* immunogen, *Vet Parasitol* 19L:321-337, 1985.
99. Wright IG et al: Protective vaccination against virulent *Babesia bovis* with a low-molecular-weight antigen, *Infect Immunol* 48:109-113, 1985.
100. Mehlhorn H, Schein E. Redescription of *Babesia equi* Lavern, 1901 as *Theileria equi* Mehlhorn, Scheim 1998, *Parasitol Res* 84:467-475, 1998.
101. Frerichs MW, Allen PC, Holbrook AA: Equine piroplasmosis *(Babesia equi)*: therapeutic trials of imidocarb dihydroshloride in horses and donkeys, *Vet Rec* 93:73-75, 1973.
102. Kuttler KL, Zaugg JL, Gipson CA: Imidocarb and parvaquone in the treatment of piroplasmosis *(Babesia equi)* in equids, *Am J Vet Res* 48:1613-1616, 1987.
103. Zaugg J: Buparvaquone in the treatment of equine piroplasmosis *(Babesia equi)* of European origin, *Equine Pract* 15:19-22, 1993.

HEMOBARTONELLOSIS (Eperythrozoonosis)

GARY P. CARLSON

Haemobartonella bovis is an epicellular organism that is closely associated with the surface of erythrocytes. It may appear as a rod shape, an ovoid shape, or in chains with conventional stains. Haemobartonellosis is primarily of academic interest in North America because it is rarely a cause of anemia.[104] The organism has been found in association with other rickettsial diseases and has been experimentally transmitted in splenectomized calves. The agent may be visualized as delicate ovoid, rod, or dumbbell forms that are arranged in chains or in tight groups or are randomly distributed epicellularly throughout appropriately stained blood smears.

Eperythrozoonosis in Cattle

The causal agent in eperythrozoonosis is *Eperythrozoon wenyoni.* Infection is usually latent, producing no clinical signs in normal cattle, but it may become apparent in animals that have been severely stressed by some other systemic disease. The disease can be produced experimentally if infected blood is administered to splenectomized calves. Even under experimental circumstances, clinical signs consist of mild depression, fever, and modest anemia. The disease in cattle is of little clinical consequence, except for the potential for confusion should the organism be seen on stained blood films. Occasionally cattle may have swollen and tender teats and legs.[104]

Eperythrozoonosis in Sheep and Goats

The causal organism of eperythrozoonosis in sheep and goats is *Eperythrozoon ovis*, which appears to be very similar morphologically and serologically to that found in cattle. The disease can produce more prominent clinical signs in sheep with profound depression, anemia, and significant death losses in young lambs.[105] Red cell destruction is thought to be caused by intravascular hemolysis and erythrophagocytosis.

THEILERIASIS

GARY P. CARLSON

Theileriasis is caused by small hemoparasite of the genus *Theileria* that infect lymphocytes and erythrocytes of ruminants and is most common in tropical and subtropical climates. The organism is spread by bloodsucking arthropods, particularly ticks of the Ixodidae family. *Theileria parva* is the cause of East Coast fever, a highly fatal disease occurring in cattle in Africa. Other members of the genus *Theileria (T. annulata, T. mutans, T. hirci, and T. ovis)* tend to be less pathogenic and produce diseases with a wider geographic distribution.[105] *T. cervi* has been seen in North American deer. *T. mutans* has been seen in erythrocytes of both cattle and deer in North America. Theileriosis caused by an agent indistinguishable from *Theileria buffeli* has been described in cattle from Texas and North Carolina with parasitemia, but clinical signs were not reported.[106] Recently *T. buffeli* was reported as the cause of a hemolytic anemia in a 6-month-old Simmental calf.[107] There was serologic evidence of a high herd prevalence of *Theileria* infection, and the agent was transmitted to splenectomized calves that developed mild anemia. The organism produces a brief illness that is characterized by mild fever, anorexia, and modest anemia, followed by rapid recovery.

TRYPANOSOMIASIS

GARY P. CARLSON

Trypanosomes are flagellated protozoal organisms that can produce a variety of serious diseases of humans and animals, although many are nonpathogenic. Nagana, a disease of cattle in Africa, is caused by *Trypanosoma congolensi. Trypanosoma evansi* is the cause of surra, a disease occurring in cattle in India, and *Trypanosoma equiperdium* produces dourine in horses. In North America, *Trypanosoma theileri (Trypanosoma americanum)* is the only agent reported and is principally of academic interest because it is relatively nonpathogenic. The organism is occasionally seen free in the plasma in small numbers on stained blood films from cattle as a large flagellated protozoa with an undulating membrane.[105] The organism is best visualized in buffy coat smears that tend to concentrate it. *T. theileri* rarely produces clinical signs, but occasionally a fulminating parasitemia may develop, resulting in fever, depression, and decreased milk production.

REFERENCES

104. Smith JA et al: Eperythrozoon wenyoni infection in dairy heifers, *Proc ACVIM* 1989, pp 698-701.
105. Jain NC: *Schalm's veterinary hematology*, ed 4, Philadelphia, 1986, Lea & Febiger, pp 606-615.
106. Chae J et al: Nucleotide sequence heterogeneity in the small subunit ribosomal RNA gene variable (V4) region among and within geographic isolates of *Theileria* from cattle, elk and white-tailed deer, *Vet Parasitol* 75:42-52, 1998.
107. Stockman SL et al: Theileriosis in a Missouri beef herd caused by *Theileria buffeli*: case report, herd investigation, ultrastructure, phylogenetic analysis, and experimental transmission, *Vet Pathol* 37:11-21, 2000.

LEPTOSPIROSIS

GARY P. CARLSON

Leptospira species infections produce disease in cattle, sheep, and swine, but the acute hemolytic syndrome that is associated with these infections is seen most commonly in calves and lambs. *Leptospira pomona* and *Leptospira icterohaemorrhagiae* are the serotypes usually involved in the hemolytic syndrome. Clinical signs of the hemolytic syndrome vary, but they generally include fever, depression, icterus, anemia, and petechial hemorrhages. The anemia is brought about, at least in part, by immune-mediated mechanisms. Cold-reacting IgM antibodies have been implicated in the hemolytic anemia that is seen in lambs. The degree of anemia is variable but can be severe with evidence of erythropoietic response apparent in the peripheral blood within a period of 4 to 7 days. A moderate leukocytosis and elevation in plasma fibrinogen are often associated with the hemolytic anemia. The diagnosis is generally made on the basis of demonstration of the organism in the urine and an increase in serum antibody titer. Discussion of leptospirosis as a reproductive problem can be found in Chapter 41, as a renal problem in Chapter 32, and as an ocular problem in Chapter 37.

BACILLARY HEMOGLOBINURIA (RED WATER)

GARY P. CARLSON

Bacillary hemoglobinuria is an acute hemolytic disorder that is caused by *Clostridium novyi* type D. Also known as "Nevada Red Water," it has been reported as a naturally occurring disease in cattle and has been experimentally produced in sheep. Clinical signs develop rapidly and affected animals may manifest severe depression, anorexia, fever, hemoglobinemia, and/or hemoglobinuria; death losses often are seen. The disease is endemic in certain poorly drained areas of the western United States and is caused by ingestion of infectious spores. The organism finds a favorable environment for development in areas of preexisting liver damage that most often have been produced by migrating liver flukes. The hemolytic syndrome is produced by toxins elaborated by the organism, which also produce a characteristic focal liver lesion. The anemia produced may be marked, and both icterus and evidence of erythropoietic response may be seen in animals that survive for more than a few days. For a more complete discussion of the diagnosis and management of this disease, see Chapter 31.

EQUINE INFECTIOUS ANEMIA

GARY P. CARLSON

DEFINITION AND ETIOLOGY. Equine infectious anemia (EIA) is a viral disease that is limited to horses, donkeys, and mules and is characterized by recurrent episodes of fever, hemolytic anemia, icterus, depression, edema, and chronic weight loss.[108] The anemia and the widespread lesions that may involve the kidney, liver, spleen, lymph nodes, and bone marrow are largely the result of immunologically mediated processes.[109-111] The disease is associated with a persistent viral infection and infected animals remain carriers for life.[112]

CLINICAL SIGNS AND DIFFERENTIALS. The clinical and hematologic manifestations of EIA vary with the dose and virulence of the virus, host resistance factors, and environmental stressors. Clinical staging usually is divided into the acute form, subacute-to-chronic intermittent form, and chronic inapparent form of the disease.[113] The acute form is associated with the first exposure of the animal to the virus; clinical signs may include fever, depression, and petechial hemorrhages. Occasionally horses develop fulminant processes that can result in death within a few days. In some horses, onset of the disease after the initial exposure may produce only mild clinical signs. This may represent exposure to less virulent strains of the EIA virus. The subacute to chronic stage of the disease presents with more classic signs of EIA. These consist of recurrent episodes of fever, depression, anemia, icterus, lymphadenopathy, petechial hemorrhages, edema, and weight loss. These episodes are associated with recrudescence of the virus and viremia. Both the frequency of these episodes and the severity of clinical signs tend to decrease with time. Over 90% of these episodes occur within the first year of infection.[113] Neurologic disturbances have been reported in association with EIA in some horses. Chronically infected horses may manifest few clinical or hematologic indications of the disease. Periodic exacerbations of clinical disease and associated viremia can develop unpredictably in these horses. Recrudescence of the viremia and clinical manifestation can occur in response to corticosteroid administration and may be associated with other stresses such as transport, hard work, intercurrent disease, or adverse environmental factors.

In the acute and subacute stages of the disease, the differential considerations include equine viral arteritis, equine ehrlichiosis, purpura hemorrhagica, and autoimmune hemolytic anemia. With the chronic form of the disease, additional differential considerations include causes of chronic weight loss, including internal abscesses, chronic active hepatitis, and some forms of lymphoreticular neoplasia. Conducting of complete and thorough clinical and clinicopathologic investigation may be necessary to resolve these differential considerations. The diagnosis of EIA is usually based on the results of serologic testing using the EIA ELISA test or the Coggins' test.

CLINICAL PATHOLOGY. The clinicopathologic features of EIA are quite variable and depend largely on the stage of the disease process. During active febrile episodes a moderate to severe hemolytic anemia is noted. The anemia may be marked and rapidly progressive because it is the result of immune-mediated hemolysis and reduced intravascular

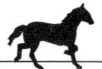

erythrocyte survival time, as well as decreased bone marrow erythrocyte production.[114,115] The Coombs' test may be positive during these episodes, particularly if complement-specific reagents are used. Thrombocytopenia is a common feature during febrile episodes and contributes to the petechial hemorrhages noted at this time. Although a leukopenia is often expected in the acute phases of the disease, the leukocyte count can be quite variable, and a mild lymphocytosis and monocytosis often are associated with active disease. The blood picture of chronic inapparent carrier horses is often within normal limits, except for marginally low erythrocyte parameters.

The gold standard for the diagnosis of EIA has for many years been the Coggins' test, an agar gel immunodiffusion procedure, which is a specific indicator of antibodies directed against EIA p26 viral antigens. There is now several highly sensitive ELISA procedures; the competitive ELISA (CELISA), which tests for core protein (p26), and the synthetic antigen or SA-ELISA, which tests for transmembrane glycoprotein gp45, available for the diagnosis of EIA. These procedures are approved tests for determination of the EIA status of horses for health certificates for interstate transport within the United States. At present the Coggins' test is still required for international health certificates. The advantage of the EIA ELISA test is that it can be performed rapidly for a fast turn-around time from submission to result. These tests are highly sensitive and there may be some false-positive results. For this reason all positive CELISA results are required to be confirmed by the Coggins' test. If discrepant results (positive by CELISA, but negative by Coggins' test) occur, testing by Western blot is recommended. These tests may be negative in the early stages of the disease process before specific antibody production. The test may be falsely positive in foals born to infected dams because of the absorption of antibodies from the colostrum. For this reason the Coggins' status of test-positive foals should be reevaluated after 4 to 6 months of age when essentially all maternally derived antibodies are gone.[116] There is some indication that the highly sensitive EIA ELISA test may remain positive in these foals until nearly a year of age. With these exceptions in mind, the EIA ELISA and the Coggins' test are highly specific and accurate indicators of EIA virus infection, even in horses in the chronic inapparent carrier state. This disease has such important ramifications that the Coggins' test is sometimes conducted first to rule out EIA in a horse with fever, anemia, edema, or chronic weight loss before a full investigation of other differential considerations is undertaken.

PATHOPHYSIOLOGY. There are no other natural hosts for the EIA virus, and transmission involves the transfer of blood from an infected to a susceptible animal. Viral titers in the blood are particularly high during febrile episodes, and it is at these times that the potential for transmission to unaffected horses is highest. Biting insects of the Tabanus species, deer flies *(Chrysops flavidus)*, stable flies *(Stomoxis calcitrans)*, and mosquitoes have been incriminated.[117,118] Transmission can occur as a result of blood or blood product transfusion, use of blood-contaminated instruments or needles, or transplacental passage to the fetus; and the virus may be found in milk or semen. The EIA agent is a nononcogenic retrovirus that possesses an RNA-directed DNA polymerase that infects macrophages and endothelial cells throughout the body and integrates into the host genome.[119] The agent has been the subject of intense investigation with regard to its relationship to other retroviral agents of comparative interest. This viral disease elicits brisk humoral and cellular immune responses. Clinical signs are associated with recrudescence of viremia, which results in immunologically mediated damage to red blood cells and a variety of other tissues. The disease consists of a series of recurrent episodes that are thought to be the result of sequential production and release of antigenically novel strains of the virus that temporarily escape the host's immunosurveillance system.[119,120,121] The absence of clinical signs in the chronic inapparent state is thought to be caused by the host's eventual immune response against antigenic epitomes common to all EIA viruses.[119] Viral persistence in these animals is the result of latent or nearly latent infected cells that are maintained by integrated DNA intermediates.[119] Despite the absence of overt clinical signs in these horses, the persistently elevated globulins and the change in lymphocyte populations are indicators of persistent if low-grade infection and response to infection.

NECROPSY FINDINGS. Pathologic features vary with the stage of the disease process. Gross lesions in animals necropsied during active stages of the disease consist of splenomegaly, generalized lymphadenopathy, anemia, widespread hemorrhages, and edema. Histologic lesions are largely the result of immune-mediated processes, with initial lymphoid necrosis giving way to lymphoproliferative changes characterized by perivascular lymphocytic infiltration of most organs and tissues. Hemosiderosis is widespread, especially in the liver.

TREATMENT AND PROGNOSIS. There is no effective treatment or vaccination for this disease. The prognosis for horses with EIA is unfavorable, but rest and supportive care may aid clinical recovery.

PREVENTION AND CONTROL. The disease must be reported, and state and federal regulations determine the disposition of infected animals. A recent negative EIA ELISA or Coggins' test is required for nearly all interstate or international health certificates as discussed earlier. Most racing and horse show associations require serologic evidence that horses are negative for EIA in order to participate in their events. Many chronically affected horses are poor doers, are incapable of regular work, or are banned from participation in their regular athletic events. Even the relatively normal chronic inapparent carrier horses pose a serious health risk to other horses.[108,112] Thus it is generally recommended, and indeed required in some states, that Coggins'-positive horses be euthanatized to prevent the spread of the disease. Although nothing can be done at present to effect a cure for this disease, it may be possible in selected circumstances, if regulations permit, to maintain infected horses in isolation so that they do not serve as a source of infection to other horses. This approach might be taken to maintain a valuable breeding animal. Because interrupted feeding of biting insects is the principal means of disease transmission, strict insect control and double screening of stalls may be effective in some circumstances. Simply separating infected horses from healthy horses by 200 yards, even in open pens, is sufficient to prevent spread of the disease. Of course, absolute attention must be taken to avoid blood contamination of needles or surgical and dental instruments.

REFERENCES

108. Issel CJ, Coggins L: Equine infectious anemia: current knowledge, *J Am Vet Med Assoc* 174:727-733, 1979.
109. Gorham JR et al: Pathogenesis of equine infectious anemia, *J Equine Med Surg* 1:71-73, 1977.
110. Henson JB, McGuire TC: Immunopathology of equine infectious anemia, *Am J Clin Pathol* 50:306-313, 1971.
111. Squire RA: Equine infectious anemia: a model of immunoproliferative disease, *Blood* 32:157-169, 1968.
112. Kemen MJ: Equine infectious anemia: the controversy continues, *Cornell Vet* 67:177-189, 1977.
113. Roberts DH, Lucas MH: Equine infectious anaemia, *Vet Annu* 27:147-150, 1987.

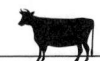
114. McGuire TC, Henson JB, Quist SE: Impaired bone marrow response in equine infectious anemia, *Am J Vet Res* 30:2091-2097, 1969.
115. McGuire TC, Henson JB, Quist SE: Viral-induced hemolysis in equine infectious anemia, *Am J Vet Res* 30:2099-2104, 1969.
116. Issel CJ, Adams WV Jr, Foil LD: Prospective study of progeny of inapparent equine carriers of equine infectious anemia virus, *Am J Vet Res* 46:1114-1116, 1985.
117. Foil L et al: Tabanid (*Diptera*) populations associated with an equine infectious anemia outbreak in an inapparently infected herd of horses, *J Med Entomol* 21:28-30, 1984.
118. Tashjian RJ: Transmission and clinical evaluation of an equine infectious anemia herd over a 13-year period, *J Am Vet Med Assoc* 3:282-288, 1984.
119. Cheevers WP, McGuire TC: Equine infectious anemia virus: immunopathogenesis and persistence, *Rev Infect Dis* 7:83-88, 1985.
120. Montelaro RC et al: Antigenic variation during persistent infection by equine infectious anemia virus: a retrovirus, *J Biol Chem* 259:10539-10544, 1984.
121. Sellon DC, Fuller FJ, McGuire TC: The immunopathogenesis of equine infectious anemia virus, *Virus Res* 32:111-38, 1994.

AUTOIMMUNE HEMOLYTIC ANEMIA

GARY P. CARLSON

DEFINITION AND ETIOLOGY. Autoimmune hemolytic anemia is associated with the production of autologous antibodies that are directed against the patient's own red cells. These antibodies combine with complement and antigens on the red blood cell membrane, leading to the rapid removal of affected red blood cells from the circulation and their accelerated destruction. Autoimmune hemolytic anemia occurs rarely as a primary idiopathic disorder[122,123] but more commonly is found secondarily associated with some other primary disease process.[122] An idiopathic immune-mediated hemolytic anemia was recently reported in a calf[123] and pony.[124]

CLINICAL SIGNS AND DIFFERENTIAL DIAGNOSIS. The presenting clinical signs of animals with autoimmune hemolytic anemia are quite variable, depending on the degree of anemia and the primary disease. Animals with marked anemia (packed cell volume less than 15%) manifest signs typical of those seen in any animal with a severe hemolytic anemia (i.e., depression, pale mucous membranes, variable icterus, elevated heart and respiratory rate, and variable to intermittent fever). Secondary autoimmune hemolytic anemia in horses has been associated most often with some other primary problem such as purpura hemorrhagica, lymphosarcoma, other neoplasms, protein-losing enteropathy, or chronic bacterial infections.[125,126] Clinical features are typical of the primary problem, with additional findings of a hemolytic anemia. In humans, exposure to a wide variety of drugs has been causally associated with the development of autoimmune hemolytic anemia. There are a number of reports of an association between procaine penicillin and autoimmune hemolytic anemia in horses.[127-132] Autoimmune hemolytic anemia was recently reported in a 10-year-old horse that was treated with trimethoprim-sulfamethoxazole.[133] This apparently occurs rarely, perhaps only in specific individuals, but drug history should be ascertained in all animals with an otherwise unexplained hemolytic anemia.

It should be noted that the anemia in cattle with anaplasmosis and babesiosis or that in horses with equine infectious anemia, piroplasmosis, or ehrlichiosis is largely the result of an immune-mediated hemolytic process. These diseases are discussed fully elsewhere in this book.

CLINICAL PATHOLOGY. The hemolytic process often is rapid and persistent, leading to a pronounced anemia. The hematologic features are those typically expected for a responsive hemolytic anemia. The anemia often is progressive and may become severe, even life threatening (i.e., PCV less than 10%). Erythrophagocytosis and autoagglutination may be noted on blood smears. Spherocytosis may be difficult to recognize in large animals because of the relatively small cell size and lack of a clear area or central pallor of the erythrocytes from these species. If the process has gone on for 4 days or more, hematologic evidence of active erythropoietic response may be seen in the peripheral blood of all species except the horse. This evidence of bone marrow response is a favorable prognostic indicator, even when the anemia is quite advanced. A moderate neutrophilic leukocytosis is a common feature, and thrombocytopenia may be noted in some individuals if the autoimmune process is directed at platelets and megakaryocytes, as well as the erythrocytes. Documentation of the presence of antierythrocyte antibodies or complement on the red cell membrane is based on the direct Coombs' test. The indirect Coombs' test detects antierythrocyte antibody in the serum. It is important to remember that the Coombs' test is based on species-specific reagents. These reagents are commercially available in the United States for small animals and horses, and not all diagnostic laboratories will have suitable Coombs' reagents for other species. Special procedures may be necessary to adsorb these reagents to avoid nonspecific reactions. Multivalent Coombs' reagent directed against IgG, IgM, and complement is most commonly used. The Coombs' test usually is conducted at body temperature and also in the cold. A positive reaction at body temperature indicates that the antibodies are primarily IgG. These warm antibodies are associated more commonly with anemia, generally produce a more severe anemia, and tend to be more responsive to corticosteroids than the cold-reacting antibodies. The cold-reacting antibodies detected with the saline agglutination test run at 25° and 4° C are primarily of the IgM class. Exposure to a cold environment may be necessary to produce clinical signs associated with cold agglutinin disease. Both the warm- and cold-reacting antibodies are capable of fixing complement. Unfortunately the Coombs' test is not always positive in affected animals. In humans and dogs, approximately one third of patients with autoimmune hemolytic anemia have a negative direct Coombs' test, possibly because of low concentrations of antibody or low binding to the red cell membrane. The diagnosis in these cases is contingent on ruling out other causes of a responsive hemolytic anemia and on the response to administration of corticosteroid therapy. Recently, direct immunofluorescence flow cytometry was used to determine the classes of antibody bound to erythrocytes in 3 horses and 12 dogs with immune-mediated hemolytic anemia. The horses had surface-bound IgG, including a horse with suspected penicillin-induced IMHA, a foal with neonatal isoerythrolysis, and a foal with clostridial septicemia.[134]

A substantial proportion of otherwise normal horses have small amounts of cold-reacting Coombs' antibodies, and spontaneous agglutination may be noted in blood sample tubes exposed to the cold. In most instances, these cold agglutinins appear to occur naturally and in low levels are of little clinical significance. Prior treatment with corticosteroids may inhibit antibody production and could lead to a false-negative Coombs' test.

PATHOPHYSIOLOGY. Autoimmune hemolytic anemia rarely has been reported as a primary or idiopathic process in large animals; however, immune-mediated anemia occurs more commonly as a secondary problem (1) in association with certain types of neoplasia; (2) with a variety of viral, bacterial, rickettsial, and protozoal infections; (3) after exposure to certain drugs; or (4) in association with other immune-mediated disorders such as systemic lupus erythematosus.[135] The initiating factors for this autoimmune disorder are not completely understood but may be related to alterations in the red cell membrane through direct or indirect injury, which elicits an abnormal response by the immune

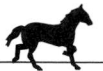

system. The red blood cell membrane is no longer recognized as self but is treated as a foreign antigen. Alternatively, alterations in the immune system or stimulation by some other antigenic source may result in production of antibodies with a misdirected cross-reactivity with the patient's own normal red blood cells. Structural and functional changes in the red blood cell membrane are induced by the antigen-antibody reaction and complement fixation. The complement-fixing IgG or IgM antigen-antibody reaction may produce sufficient erythrocyte damage to result in intravascular lysis of erythrocytes, but, more commonly, affected cells are removed from the circulation at a rapid rate by the reticuloendothelial system of the liver and spleen. Partial phagocytosis of affected cells may result in spherocyte formation. Although the presence of spherocytes on blood smears is a characteristic diagnostic feature in human and canine patients with autoimmune hemolytic anemia, the relatively small size of red cells of most large domestic animals may make it difficult to recognize spherocytes.

TREATMENT AND PROGNOSIS. The approach to treatment of autoimmune hemolytic anemia depends on the causal factors. If the animal has a history of drug therapy, it is advisable to discontinue medication or to change to another class of drug. Patients with primary or idiopathic autoimmune hemolytic anemia may be the best candidates for treatment. Immune-mediated hemolytic anemias that are secondary to other diseases can only be managed if the primary problem is amenable to treatment. Thus treatment of an immune-mediated hemolytic anemia in a patient with extensive lymphoreticular neoplasia is likely to be unrewarding, and thorough diagnostic efforts should precede case selection for treatment. Although immune-mediated processes are responsible for hemolytic anemia in a number of infectious diseases, therapy must be directed at the primary agent, and corticosteroids are contraindicated in these diseases. Corticosteroids can cause recrudescence of viremia in horses with equine infectious anemia, and a negative Coggins' test should be a prerequisite to treatment of horses with an autoimmune hemolytic anemia of undetermined cause.

Treatment of autoimmune hemolytic anemia is directed at providing supportive care and interrupting the immune response that is responsible for antibody production. This is usually accomplished with the administration of systemic glucocorticoids. For a 450-kg horse dexamethasone is recommended at an initial dosage rate of 30 to 40 mg/day given parenterally. This dosage rate is continued for 3 to 5 days and then is decreased gradually over a period of 7 to 14 days, depending on the response to therapy. The hematologic response to therapy should be closely monitored. If there has been no response in 5 to 7 days, the diagnosis of autoimmune hemolytic anemia should be reviewed, and potential causes of bone marrow suppression should be evaluated. Once the hemolytic process is well under control, oral prednisolone can be administered at a dosage rate of 400 to 500 mg daily. Human patients and small animals with immune-mediated hemolytic anemia that is unresponsive to corticosteroids are often treated with cyclophosphamide. There is one report of successful management of a horse with cyclophosphamide and azathioprine when the anemia failed to respond to corticosteroids.[136] Supportive care consists of providing a quiet, restful environment and good nutrition, including vitamin supplementation. Iron- and copper-containing hematinics are generally of little benefit because neither of these elements is lost with hemolytic anemia. Blood transfusion is also of little benefit because it is often impossible to find a compatible donor and the transfused cells are rapidly removed from the circulation. Blood transfusion should not be administered unless the anemia is life threat-

ening and the immune response can be controlled with corticosteroids.

REFERENCES

122. Beck DJ: A case of primary autoimmune haemolytic anaemia in a pony, *Equine Vet J* 22:292-294, 1990.
123. Fenger CK et al: Idiopathic immune-mediated hemolytic anemia in a calf, *J Am Vet Med Assoc* 201:97-99, 1992.
124. Ford RB: Immune-mediated hemolytic anemia: a clinical review, *Calif Vet* 34:13-16, 1980.
125. Mair TS, Taylor FG, Hillyer MH: Autoimmune haemolytic anaemia in eight horses, *Vet Rec* 126:51-53, 1990.
126. Collins JD: Autoimmune haemolytic anemia in the horse, *Proc First Internatl Symp Equine Hematol* 1:342-348, 1975.
127. Sockett DC, Traub-Dargatz J, Weiser MG: Immune-mediated hemolytic anemia and thrombocytopenia in a foal, *J Am Vet Med Assoc* 190:308-310, 1987.
128. Blue JT, Dinsmore RP, Anderson KL: Immune-mediated hemolytic anemia induced by penicillin in horses, *Cornell Vet* 77:263-276, 1987.
129. Lokhurst HM, Breukink HJ: Auto-immune hemolytic anemia in two horses, *Tijdschr Diergeneesk* 100:752-756, 1975.
130. Step DL, Blue JT, Dill SG: Penicillin-induced hemolytic anemia and acute hepatic failure following treatment of tetanus in a horse, *Cornell Vet* 81:13-18, 1991.
131. McConnico RS, Roberts MC, Tompkins M: Penicillin-induced immune-mediated hemolytic anemia in a horse, *J Am Vet Med Assoc* 201:1402-1403, 1992.
132. Robbins RL et al: Immune-mediated haemolytic disease after penicillin therapy in a horse, *Equine Vet J* 25:462-465, 1993.
133. Thomas HL, Livesey MA: Immune-mediated hemolytic anemia associated with trimethoprim-sulphamethoxazole administration in a horse, *Can Vet J* 39:171-173, 1998.
134. Wilkerson MJ et al: Isotype-specific antibodies in horses and dogs with immune-mediated hemolytic anemia, *J Vet Int Med* 14:190-196, 2000.
135. Geor RJ et al: Systemic lupus erythematosus in a filly, *J Am Vet Med Assoc* 197:1489-1492, 1990.
136. Messer NT, Arnold K: Immune-mediated hemolytic anemia in a horse, *J Am Vet Med Assoc* 198:1415-1416, 1991.

HEINZ BODY HEMOLYTIC ANEMIA

GARY P. CARLSON

DEFINITION AND ETIOLOGY. An acute hemolytic anemia can develop after an animal's exposure to a variety of oxidizing agents. These agents include drugs such as phenothiazine or methylene blue[137] and acetylphenyl hydrazine[138] or plants such as wild or domestic onions,[139] members of the Brassica family (rape or kale), and wilted or dried leaves of the red maple *(Acer rubrum).*[140-143] Heinz body hemolytic anemia also occurs in sheep on specially formulated diets that are low in molybdenum, which results in chronic copper toxicity; as herd problems in cattle grazing rye grass *(Secale cereale)*[144] or selenium-deficient pastures in Florida[145]; and in association with selenium deficiency as a contributing factor in postparturient hemoglobinuria in cattle in New Zealand.[146] These agents produce or allow oxidative denaturation of hemoglobin and resultant aggregation of the protein globin, which appears as Heinz body inclusions within the red blood cells. Heinz body anemia has been seen in association with lymphosarcoma in a horse, possibly because of failure of the reticuloendothelial system to remove the Heinz bodies, as has been reported in horses with EIA.[147]

CLINICAL SIGNS AND DIFFERENTIAL DIAGNOSIS. Clinical signs vary with the species involved, the specific toxin or toxic metabolites, the amount of toxin ingested, the time course of the disease process, and the occurrence of complicating secondary factors such as hemoglobin nephrosis and acute renal failure. Weakness, depression, anorexia, and exercise intolerance are the usual presenting complaints, and death losses can occur. Mucous membranes are generally pale with variable to marked icterus. The heart and respiratory rates are generally elevated, but rectal temperature is usually within normal limits. Many horses with red maple leaf toxicity develop methemoglobinemia with a resultant brown discoloration of the blood, mucous membranes, and urine.

The high mortality rate in horses affected by red maple toxicity may relate to the combination of a rapidly progressive hemolytic anemia and the formation of methemoglobin. Urine output may be reduced, and the urine may be dark because of the presence of hemoglobin, methemoglobin, or bilirubin.

It is not possible to differentiate Heinz body hemolytic anemia from other potential causes of hemolytic anemia without the aid of laboratory evaluation. The absence of fever may help to differentiate these anemias from infectious causes of hemolytic anemia. History of exposure to potential oxidizing agents and the fact that these toxic plants may produce death losses or clinical signs in multiple animals at the same time should help to differentiate these cases from autoimmune hemolytic anemia.

CLINICAL PATHOLOGY. Poisoning or intoxication resulting in Heinz body formation usually causes acute and profound anemia. In the early stages a very high percentage of erythrocytes may have Heinz body inclusions. Later, as these cells are removed from the circulation and replaced by young cells from the bone marrow, the relative number of affected cells may decrease markedly. Heinz bodies are round, oval to serrated refractile granules that are usually located near the cell margin or protruding from the cell and are best visualized with vital stains such as crystal violet or new methylene blue applied to unfixed blood smears. Heinz bodies appear as bluish-green inclusions with the new methylene blue stain. Fixing of blood smears with methanol in preparation for staining with the classic Wright's stain interferes with stain uptake, and Heinz bodies appear as a pale area within or projecting from the cell margin and can easily be missed. After the first 3 or 4 days the anemia is usually associated with hematologic evidence of an active erythrogenic response in all species except the horse. The total plasma proteins usually remain within normal limits, and the Coombs' test is negative. Red maple poisoning also results in depletion of red cell-reduced glutathione, methemoglobinemia, increased osmotic fragility, and modest elevations of liver-derived serum enzyme activities.

The rapid and profound erythrocyte destruction may lead to hemoglobinemia and hemoglobinuria. The development of renal failure secondary to hemoglobin nephrosis is a definite risk in these animals and is reflected by modest to marked increases in the BUN and creatinine, as well as changes in the urinalysis.[142,143] These parameters should be monitored in severely affected animals. As with other causes of hemolytic anemia, serum bilirubin, particularly the indirect-reacting bilirubin, is elevated.

PATHOPHYSIOLOGY. Heinz bodies are formed by the precipitation of oxidatively denatured hemoglobin. The hemoglobin contained within the red blood cell is constantly undergoing mild oxidative stress associated with oxygen transport, as well as generation of superoxide radicals and hydrogen peroxide within the cell. There are a number of reducing mechanisms within the red cell to counteract these oxidative processes through production of NADPH and reduced glutathione. The occurrence of Heinz body hemolytic anemia could be viewed as a consequence of exposure to oxidative stresses that simply overwhelmed the cells' reductive capacity. Selenium deficiency results in a decrease in glutathione peroxidase, a selenium-containing enzyme; and selenium deficiency may in special circumstances contribute to Heinz body formation by impeding the ability of the cells to respond to oxidative stress. There are substantial species variations in the rate of Heinz body formation that relate to the chemical structure of hemoglobin and the efficacy of erythrocyte-reducing mechanisms in the face of oxidative stress.[137] Red cells with Heinz bodies are less deformable than normal cells and are rapidly removed from the circulation by

the reticuloendothelial system in the spleen, where they are phagocytized and broken down. Old or senescent erythrocytes are thought to be more prone to develop Heinz bodies. Splenectomy or corticosteroid therapy may alter Heinz body clearance mechanisms, allowing significant numbers of affected red cells to remain in the circulation of otherwise normal animals.

The toxins involved in red maple poisoning are somewhat unusual in that they often result in production of methemoglobin, as well as Heinz body hemolytic anemia.[141,142] Methemoglobin is the result of oxidative change of hemoglobin iron to the nonfunctional ferric state (see discussion of nitrate poisoning, Chapter 50). This is normally prevented by glutathione reductase, ascorbic acid, and reduced glutathione. Methemoglobin cannot load or transport oxygen and, when present in sufficient quantities, results in a brown color of peripheral blood and mucous membranes. An estimation of methemoglobin concentration in a blood sample can be made by comparing the hemoglobin concentration measured by the cyanmethemoglobin method, which measures all forms of hemoglobin, and the oxyhemoglobin method, which only measures oxyhemoglobin but not other forms such as methemoglobin. Methemoglobinemia and hemolytic anemia have been reported in a mare and her dam in association with decreased levels of red cell glutathione and glutathione reductase, presumably as a result of an inherited enzymatic defect.[148]

TREATMENT AND PROGNOSIS. Treatment is largely a matter of removal from the source of toxicity and provision of supportive care. Blood transfusion can be very beneficial in severely anemic patients, particularly when there is insufficient evidence of active erythropoietic response. Iron-containing hematinics are of little benefit. Intravenous fluid therapy is indicated in animals with hemoglobinuria or azotemia in order to reduce the potential for further renal damage. High doses of vitamin C (ascorbic acid), together with fluids and transfusion, were thought to aid recovery in two horses with red maple poisoning.[149] A recent report suggest that vitamin C therapy may have little impact on survival of affected horses, and, when methylene blue was used to treat the associated methemoglobinemia in two horses, both died.[150]

Prognosis in animals with modest anemia with evidence of response is good if the inciting factor can be controlled or eliminated. The mortality rate of experimental and naturally occurring cases of red maple leaf toxicity in horses is said to be 60% to 65%.[150] In animals with rapidly progressive and profound anemia, prognosis is poor unless blood transfusion is undertaken. The occurrence of renal failure is an unfavorable complication, although many animals regain normal function with appropriate fluid therapy and supportive care.

REFERENCES

137. Harvey JW, Kaneko JJ: Interactions between methylene blue and erythrocytes of several mammalian species in vitro, *Proc Soc Exp Biol Med* 147:245-249, 1974.
138. Easley JR: Erythrogram and red cell distribution width of equidae with experimentally induced anemia, *Am J Vet Res* 46:2378-2384, 1985.
139. Pierce KR, Joyce JR, Jones LP: Acute hemolytic anemia caused by wild onion poisoning in horses, *J Am Vet Med Assoc* 160:323-327, 1977.
140. Divers TJ, George LW, George JW: Hemolytic anemia in horses after the ingestion of red maple leaves, *J Am Vet Med Assoc* 180:300-302, 1982.
141. George LW, Divers TJ, Mahaffey EA, et al: Heinz body anemia and methemoglobinemia in ponies given red maple (*Acer rubrum*, L.) leaves, *Vet Pathol* 19:521-533, 1982.
142. Tennant B et al: Acute hemolytic anemia, methemoglobinemia, and Heinz body formation associated with ingestion of red maple leaves by horses, *J Am Vet Med Assoc* 179:143-150, 1982.
143. Warner A: Methemoglobinemia and hemolytic anemia in a horse with acute renal failure, *Compend Cont Educ* 8:S465-S468, 1984.
144. Simpson CF, Anderson B: Heinz body anemia in cattle grazing rye pastures, *Florida Vet J* 9:26-29, 1980.
145. Morris JG et al: Selenium deficiency in cattle associated with Heinz bodies and anemia, *Science* 223:491-493, 1984.

146. Ellison RS, Young BJ, Read DH: Bovine post-parturient haemoglobinuria: two distinct entities in New Zealand, *N Vet J* 34:7-10, 1986.
147. Rollins JB, Wigton DH, Clement TH: Heinz body anemia associated with lymphosarcoma in a horse, *Equine Pract* 13:20-23, 1991.
148. Dixon PM, McPherson EA: Familial methaemoglobinaemia and haemolytic anaemia in the horse associated with decreased erythrocytic glutathione reductase and glutathione, *Equine Vet J* 9:198-201, 1977.
149. McConnico RS, Brownie CF: The use of ascorbic acid in the treatment of 2 cases of red maple (*Acer rubrum*)-poisoned horses, *Cornell Vet* 82:293-300, 1992.
150. Corriher CA et al: Equine red maple leaf toxicosis, *Compend Cont Educ* 21:74-80, 1999.

L-TRYPTOPHAN–INDOLE INTOXICATION

Experimental studies in ponies have demonstrated an acute hemolytic process associated with orally administered L-tryptophan, which is converted to indole in the gastrointestinal tract.[151] Intoxication was associated with an acute onset of restlessness, tachypnea, intravascular hemolysis, and hemoglobinuria. At necropsy examination there was evidence of hemoglobinuric nephrosis and bronchiolar degeneration in some ponies. Similar clinical signs were noted after the oral administration of tryptophan at dose rate of 0.35 to 0.60 g/kg and indole at 0.1 to 0.2 g/kg.[151,152] Intravascular hemolysis was associated with increased osmotic fragility and with Heinz body formation in a few of the experimental ponies.

REFERENCES

151. Paradis MR et al: Acute hemolytic anemia after oral administration of L-tryptophan in ponies, *Am J Vet Res* 52:742-747, 1991.
152. Paradis MR et al: Acute hemolytic anemia induced by oral administration of indole in ponies, *Am J Vet Res* 52:748-753, 1991.

WATER INTOXICATION

GARY P. CARLSON

Massive water intake may produce marked hypotonicity of the body fluids with subsequent intravascular hemolysis of erythrocytes.[153] This problem has been described as a naturally occurring entity in milk-reared calves when first given access to unlimited quantities of water.[154,155] Severe neurologic signs may be observed, including depression, convulsions, and coma; respiratory distress, hemoglobinuria, and death losses occur in some cases. Clinicopathologic features include hemolytic anemia, hypoproteinemia, hyponatremia, hypochloremia, hyposmolality, hemoglobinuria, and hyposthenuria. A sudden decrease in serum osmolality is believed to result in osmotic lysis of erythrocytes.[156] It is worthy of note that the fragility of the erythrocytes to osmotic shock is greatest in calves between 4 and 5 months of age. Treatment is primarily a matter of temporarily restricting intake of water and providing supportive care. Calves with marked hyponatremia (sodium < 110 mEq/L) that are manifesting neurologic signs may benefit from hypertonic saline, mannitol, and corticosteroids. The goal of treatment is the rapid restoration of serum sodium to 120 to 125 mEq/L without overcorrection. Death losses can occur in as little as 2 hours, but most calves recover without long-term adverse effects.

REFERENCES

153. Shimizu Y, Naito Y, Murakami D: The experimental study on the mechanism of hemolysis on paroxysmal hemoglobinemia and hemoglobinuria in calves due to excessive water intake, *Jpn J Vet Sci* 41:583-592, 1979.
154. Hannan J: Water intoxication of calves, *Irish Vet J* 19:211-214, 1965.

155. Wright MA: Haemaglobinuria from excessive water drinking, *Vet Rec* 73:129-130, 1961.
156. Kirkbride CA, Frey RA: Experimental water intoxication in calves, *J Am Vet Med Assoc* 151:742-746, 1967.

POSTPARTURIENT HEMOGLOBINURIA

GARY P. CARLSON

A syndrome consisting of intravascular hemolysis, hemoglobinuria, and anemia has been recognized in postparturient dairy cattle around the world.[157] The disease occurs sporadically, and the incidence is relatively low. Affected animals are most often high-producing multiparous cows that develop clinical signs during the first month after calving.[158] Depression, decreased feed consumption, and decreased milk production are associated with hemoglobinuria, anemia, and icterus. The anemia is often marked and after 4 or 5 days is associated with evidence of a marked erythropoietic response. The precise mechanism by which the intravascular hemolysis occurs has not been fully defined. The condition has been related to the marked hypophosphatemia commonly found in affected cows and moderately low phosphate levels in unaffected herd mates. Hypophosphatemia is brought about by inadequate dietary phosphorus intake in animals grazing phosphorus-deficient soils or fed fodder grown on phosphorus-deficient soil. Low intracellular phosphate concentration may interfere with energy metabolism, thus affecting cell viability and the ability of the red cells to deal with potential hemolysins such as saponins from sugar beets or alfalfa. A postparturient hemolytic problem has been described as a herd problem in New Zealand associated with copper deficiency and Heinz body formation (see previous section).[159]

Blood transfusion and supportive intravenous fluids are indicated in valuable cows with severe life-threatening anemia. Treatment of hypophosphatemia consists of provision of phosphate, initially as sodium acid phosphate ($NaH_2PO_4H_2O$), 60 g/300 ml of water intravenously followed by oral phosphorus supplementation. Correction of dietary imbalances is indicated.

REFERENCES

157. MacWilliams PS, Searcy GP, Bellamy JEC: Bovine post-parturient haemoglobinuria: a review of the literature, *Can Vet J* 23:309-312, 1982.
158. Parkinson B, Sutherland AK: Post-parturient haemoglobinuria of dairy cows, *Aust Vet J* 30:232-236, 1954.
159. Ellison RS, Young BJ, Read DH: Bovine post-parturient haemoglobinuria: two distinct entities in New Zealand, *N Z Vet J* 34:7-10, 1986.

COPPER TOXICOSIS

LISLE W. GEORGE
GARY P. CARLSON

An acute, highly fatal hemolytic crisis has been described primarily in sheep,[160] but it also has been produced in calves,[161] associated with the sudden release of massive hepatic copper stores that have accumulated over a long period of excessive copper intake. Growing lambs appear to be the most susceptible to this problem. Liver damage secondary to copper accumulation precedes the onset of signs; and stress, shipping, or starvation may serve as triggering events to the release of copper from the liver.[162] The massive hemolysis that occurs is thought to be the result of the direct interaction of copper with sulfhydryl groups of red blood cell membrane proteins, peroxidation of membrane lipids, interactions of cuprous ions with oxygen to produce superoxide radicals, and the inhibition of a number of important red blood cell enzymes.[163] Clinical signs are depression, anorexia, weakness, hemoglobinemia, hemoglobinuria, anemia, and high death losses within 1 to 2 days.[160] Icterus and evidence of active erythropoiesis may be noted in sheep surviving for longer periods.

The single toxic dose of copper for sheep ranges between 20 and 110 mg/kg, whereas the toxic dose for cattle ranges between 220 to 880 mg/kg. Chronic copper poisoning can occur in sheep after several months of a daily dosage of 3.5 mg/kg of copper. The condition has occurred after ingesting feed containing as little as 20 ppm for several months. Increased dietary molybdenum levels make animals more tolerant to dietary copper levels (at least 1 part molybdenum to 6 parts of copper is needed).

Goats are more resistant to copper poisoning than are sheep and may not show signs until 144 days after ingesting as much as 80 mg/kg/day of copper sulfate. Although cattle are most resistant of all ruminants, calves have been poisoned after 6 to 8 weeks of feeding copper-supplemented milk replacer (115 ppm of copper). Adult cattle may be poisoned by an intake of 5 g of copper sulfate daily for approximately 4 months.

Sources of copper that have been responsible for the occurrence of toxicosis in sheep include trace mineralized salt (formulated for dairy cattle), rations containing greater than 20% dried poultry waste, diets richly supplemented with palm oil by-products, pastures fertilized with chicken litter, forages from fruit orchard pastures that are contaminated by copper sulfate fungicides, parasiticides for gastrointestinal helminths, copper sulfate foot baths, fungicide-treated fence posts, corroded overhead cables, copper-treated seed grains, and therapeutic parenterally administered copper salts (commercially marketed for treatment of copper deficiency).

Horses tend to be resistant to high concentrations of the element and remain normal despite daily ingestion of diets containing 791 ppm of copper. This resistance appears to be related to factors other than a lack of absorptive capacity because liver concentrations of the exposed animals may exceed 4000 ppm on a dry matter basis. Adult ponies treated with single oral dosages of 40 mg/kg did not show signs of acute copper intoxication.

During the acute hemolytic crisis the concentration of copper in the blood is significantly increased and ranges between 240 and 2000 g/dl (2.4 to 20 ppm). The reference range for blood copper is considered to be 20 to 100 g/dl (0.2 to 1 ppm). Fecal copper concentration may exceed 10,000 ppm. Concentrations of the element in livers of poisoned animals are usually greater than 150 ppm (wet weight) and 900 ppm (dry weight). Concentrations of copper in the kidney of poisoned sheep may exceed 15 ppm (wet weight) and 50 ppm (dry weight).

Therapy for acute poisonings includes large volumes of intravenous fluids, oxygen insufflation, and whole blood if the packed cell volume is less than 8%. Chelator therapy with D-penicillamine (Cuprimine,* 52 mg/kg of body weight daily for 6 days) and daily oral administration of 100 mg of ammonium molybdate and 1 g of anhydrous sodium sulfate per sheep may help to mobilize excessive hepatic copper. Dietary supplementation of sheep with ammonium molybdate may reduce blood copper levels, but hepatic copper concentrations of exposed animals may remain high. Sheep that have been exposed to copper and treated with ammonium molybdate may suffer decreased reproductive performance in the subsequent breeding season. Specific reproductive-related problems include dystocia caused by lack of cervical dilation, placental retention, persistent postpartum fevers, and hypolactia. Whether these problems arise from the copper poisoning or from the treatment is unknown. Ammonium tetrathiomolybdate (orally at a dosage of 50 to 100 mg per adult sheep two times weekly) is a drug that shows some promise for the treatment of copper poisoning. Treatment of affected cattle with daily oral doses of 3 g of sodium molybdate and 5 g of sodium thiosulfate has been effective in a field outbreak.

Molybdenum-deficient pastures can be fertilized with molybdenum superphosphate at a rate of 113 g of molybdenum per acre. When sheep are treated prophylactically for copper deficiency, the occurrence of acute toxicity from the therapeutic compounds may be minimized by use of copper methionate administered at doses less than 6 mg/kg of body weight.

REFERENCES

160. Pierson RE, Aanes WA: Treatment of chronic copper poisoning in sheep, *J Am Vet Med Assoc* 133:307-311, 1958.
161. Asano R, Kaseda M, Hokari S: The effect of copper and copper-O-phenanthroline complex on cattle erythrocytes, *Jpn J Vet Sci* 45:77-83, 1983.
162. Jain NC: *Schalm's veterinary hematology,* ed 4, Philadelphia, 1986, Lea & Febiger, pp 608-610.
162. Hochstein P, Kumar KS, Forman SJ: Mechanisms of copper toxicity in red cells, *Prog Clin Biol Res* 21:669-681, 1978.

HEMOLYTIC SYNDROME IN HORSES WITH LIVER FAILURE

GARY P. CARLSON

A fulminant, intravascular hemolytic syndrome has been reported as a near-terminal event in horses with either acute or chronic liver failure.[164] Marked hemoglobinemia and hemoglobinuria are associated with intense icterus. The sclerae and conjunctivae often take on a distinctive, deep reddish-orange color. The onset of intravascular hemolysis is sudden and rapidly progressive. The prognosis is highly unfavorable because nearly all horses that develop this syndrome die or must be euthanatized because of clinical deterioration.[165] Intravenous fluids, corticosteroids, and supportive care do not appear to alter the clinical course or the unfavorable outcome.

The cause of this syndrome has not been determined, but apparently it is not related to a release of hepatic copper stores. The hemolysis appears to be associated with increased erythrocyte osmotic fragility. Human patients with liver cirrhosis develop a hemolytic syndrome that is associated with alterations in the exchangeable lipoproteins of the red cell membrane. It is not known if a similar mechanism is responsible in horses, but morphologic alterations in the red cells of these horses resemble the "burr cells" described in human patients.[166] Bile acids and their salts are markedly increased in liver failure and could play a contributing role in the hemolytic process. At necropsy, widespread hemorrhagic lesions that resemble those described for disseminated intravascular coagulation (DIC) are often present.[166] It may be that DIC and the activation of various mediators may play a role in the terminal stages of this almost invariably fatal process.

REFERENCES

164. Tennant BC et al: Intravascular hemolysis associated with hepatic failure in the horse, *Calif Vet* 26:15-18, 1972.
165. Carlson GP: The liver. In Anderson NV, ed: *Veterinary gastroenterology,* ed 2, Philadelphia, 1992, Lea & Febiger, pp 688-702.

*Merck Sharp & Dohme, Rahway, NJ 07065.

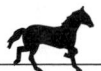

166. Schalm OW, Carlson GP: The blood and blood-forming organs. In Mansmann RA, McAllister ES, eds: *Equine medicine and surgery*, ed 3, vol 1, Santa Barbara, 1982, American Veterinary Publications, pp 377-414.

CONGENITAL ERYTHROPOIETIC PORPHYRIA

GARY P. CARLSON

A rare congenital disorder of hemoglobin production that is inherited as an autosomal-recessive condition has been recognized primarily in Holstein cattle, but has also been reported in Shorthorns and Jamaican cattle.[167,168] This disorder is commonly called "pink tooth" and is characterized by slow growth rates in calves, photosensitization and exfoliation of nonpigmented skin when exposed to sunlight, reddish-brown teeth, and modest anemia. The teeth and bones exhibit a pink fluorescence under ultraviolet light, and the urine is a brownish-red as a result of the presence of uroporphyrin. The condition is present at birth and the metabolic defect in these cattle is a hereditary deficiency of the enzyme uroporphyrinogen III cosynthetase, which catalyzes an essential step in the synthesis of the porphyrin structure of hemoglobin.[168] This leads to the accumulation of uroporphyrin and coproporphyrin, which deposit in the teeth, where it is concentrated in the dentine, bones, and other tissues. The anemia seen in these cattle is variable among individuals, and several factors contribute to it. A reduced intravascular red blood cell life span is related to the high concentration of uroporphyrin and coproporphyrin within the cells. Porphyrins may induce hemolysis and also delay maturation of the red blood cell series in the bone marrow, although there is often evidence of active erythropoietic response in the peripheral blood.[168]

Currently, there is no treatment for this inherited disorder, but genetic counseling is advisable. Substantial efforts have been made to reduce the incidence of this disease in the Holstein breed. It may be possible to detect carrier animals. Affected cattle have much lower levels of uroporphyrinogen III cosynthetase than normal cattle and carrier animals have intermediate levels of this enzyme. Despite their rather serious problems, cattle with this condition do reasonably well if housed indoors out of direct sunlight. The principal differential consideration is chronic fluorosis, which also produces brown discoloration of the teeth. However, the teeth of cattle with chronic fluorosis do not fluoresce under ultraviolet light.

An additional form of altered porphyrin metabolism, erythropoietic porphyria, has been described in humans and cattle.[168] In humans the mode of inheritance is autosomal-dominant, whereas in cattle the disorder appears to have a recessive pattern of inheritance and may be sex linked because it is only seen in females. The disease does not produce anemia, porphyrinuria, or discoloration of the teeth. This disorder is caused by a deficiency of ferrochelase (heme synthase) that leads to high concentrations of erythrocyte and fecal protoporphyrins. Porphyria has also been reported in swine, where it is inherited as a dominant.[168] There is little effect on the health of the pigs. There is no photosensitivity, but the teeth have reddish brown discoloration. Although there are similarities with bovine congenital erythropoietic porphyria, the precise deficit has not been found. Finally, animals may develop acquired toxic porphyrias. This can occur with heavy metal poisonings, principally lead, but has also been produced experimentally with hexachlorobenzene and other chemicals. Lead inhibits several key enzymes of heme synthesis. Inhibition of aminolevulinate dehydrase leads to an accumulation of aminolevulinic acid and decreased in aminolevulinate dehydrase activity is a sensitive indicator of lead poisoning. Lead also inhibits ferrochelase leading to

marked elevation of erythrocyte zinc protoporphyrin IX. For these reasons, the measurement of zinc protoporphyrin IX provides a means of monitoring lead exposure.[168]

REFERENCES

167. Rhode EA, Cornelius CE: Congenital porphyria (pink tooth) in Holstein-Freisian calves in California, *J Am Vet Med Assoc* 132:112-116, 1958.
168. Kaneko JJ: Porphyrins, heme erythrocyte metabolism: the porphyrias. In Kaneko JJ, Harvey JW, Bruss ML, eds: *Clinical biochemistry of domestic animals*, ed 5, Academic Press, New York, 1997, pp 205-221.

DEPRESSION ANEMIA

GARY P. CARLSON

The most common form of anemia in domestic animals is associated with inadequate erythropoiesis or bone marrow depression. Depression anemia can be caused by (1) deficiencies of vitamins or minerals that are essential for erythrocyte production, (2) systemic disease processes that interfere with normal erythropoiesis, or (3) processes that damage or displace normal bone marrow elements. Some of the common causes of depression anemia are listed in Box 35-2. Depression anemia is often mild to moderate in severity and generally is only slowly progressive. Depressed erythropoiesis is occasionally associated with processes that also result in blood loss or an increased rate of erythrocyte destruction. When this occurs a profound rapidly progressive and potentially life-threatening anemia can develop. With the possible exception of chronic iron or copper deficiency, depression anemia tends to be normocytic and normochromic. Bone

---

BOX 35-2

Causes of Depression Anemia

NUTRITIONAL DEFICIENCY
Iron deficiency
Copper deficiency
Cobalt deficiency
Vitamin B_{12} deficiency
Folic acid deficiency

ANEMIA OF INFLAMMATORY DISEASE
Chronic infection
Chronic inflammation
Fractures and severe trauma
Neoplasia

ANEMIA SECONDARY TO ORGAN DYSFUNCTION
Chronic liver disease
Chronic renal disease
Chronic gastrointestinal disease
Parasitism (trichostrongylosis)

BONE MARROW DAMAGE OR DYSPLASIA
Myeloid and megakaryocytic bone marrow hypoplasia in Standardbred horses
Aplastic anemia
Bracken fern poisoning
Congenital dyserythropoiesis and keratosis in polled Hereford calves
Trichloroethylene-extracted soybean meal toxicity
Myelophthistic disorders (myeloproliferative disease, lymphosarcoma)

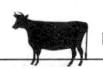

marrow evaluation is an extremely useful diagnostic tool in animals with nutritional deficiencies or when bone marrow damage or dyscrasia is suspected. A thorough clinical evaluation and vigorous application of appropriate diagnostic procedures are necessary to establish a diagnosis of depression anemia and to determine the factors responsible for the anemia.

IRON DEFICIENCY ANEMIA

Iron deficiency most commonly is associated with chronic blood loss as the result of internal or external parasitism, bleeding gastrointestinal lesions, or hemostatic defects.[169] Dietary iron deficiency is seldom the sole cause of anemia, even in neonates on an all-milk diet, unless they are raised on cement or in barns or hutches with no access to the soil. A modest anemia is anticipated in veal calves. The anemia seen in some young calves during the first few days to weeks of life is apparently the result of congenital iron deficiency,[170] but the causal factors have not been determined. Altered immune functions, high incidences of infection, and reduced growth performance are reported in veal calves on low iron diets.[171]

The circulating erythrocytes account for approximately two thirds of the total iron reserves found in the body. The remaining iron stores are distributed in the liver, spleen, and bone marrow. With chronic blood loss anemia, iron depletion is first indicated by decreased marrow iron, which can be appreciated with special staining of the bone marrow with Prussian blue stain for iron. As blood loss continues and iron deficiency progresses, serum iron is decreased, whereas iron-binding capacity actually may increase. It is only late in this whole process that iron-deficient erythropoiesis results in the typical microcytic, hypochromic erythrocytes that generally are thought to be characteristic of iron deficiency anemia.[169,172] The normal serum iron and iron-binding capacity for most domestic animals is 100 and 300 g/dl, respectively. Serum ferritin also is reported to decrease in animals with iron deficiency anemia. Treatment of iron deficiency anemia is contingent on evaluation of the cause and the correction or resolution of the process responsible for the chronic blood loss. Iron is usually supplied as an oral supplement or as a feed additive, and a wide variety of commercial preparations are available. Injectable iron dextran intended for use in baby pigs should be avoided in horses and cattle because it can induce an anaphylaxis, especially if administered repeatedly.[171] Iron cacodylate was a safe parenteral iron preparation for use in horses but is no longer readily available. An injectable iron preparation intended for use in horses was reported to result in acute iron overload, massive hepatic necrosis, and severe death losses in a group of young cattle.[174] Iron overload has resulted in acute death losses in neonatal foals fed an iron-containing microbial supplement. Iron accumulation resulting in hemochromotosis with extensive liver damage has also been reported in adult horses, although the mechanism responsible for the iron accumulation has not been explained.[175]

COPPER DEFICIENCY

Copper deficiency can occur as a primary problem in milk-fed animals or in pastured animals in copper-deficient areas. More commonly, copper deficiency occurs secondarily in association with other trace mineral imbalances such as dietary molybdenum excess and is influenced by the sulfur and zinc content of the diet. Copper is an essential cofactor for a wide variety of enzymatic reactions, and copper deficiency produces a constellation of clinical signs related to impairment of these reactions.[176] Clinical signs of copper deficiency are most prominent in young, growing animals and may include reduced growth rate, rough and depigmented hair, diarrhea,

osteoporosis with spontaneous fractures, and anemia. In lambs, copper deficiency can produce a demyelinating syndrome known as "swayback" or "enzootic ataxia." Copper deficiency has also been associated with hemolytic anemia in postparturient dairy cattle in New Zealand.[174] Copper plays an important role in the transport of iron from the gut to the marrow and in the incorporation of iron into the heme moiety. The anemia produced by copper deficiency is generally moderate, slowly progressive, and closely resembles iron deficiency in that it is usually a microcytic, hypochromic anemia. Bone marrow evaluation often reveals intracellular accumulations of iron known as "sideroblasts." This finding indicates that the principal problem is a function of altered incorporation of iron into the erythrocyte hemoglobin rather than an actual deficiency of iron. Copper deficiency can be documented by measuring serum copper as ceruloplasmin, erythrocyte superoxide dismutase, or the copper content of hair, liver, or kidney. Serum iron tends to be low in animals with copper deficiency. Copper can be supplied as a dietary supplement or as an injectable copper glycinate preparation. See Chapter 30 for a more complete discussion of copper deficiency and its treatment.

VITAMIN B$_{12}$ AND FOLIC ACID DEFICIENCY

Nearly all the vitamins are necessary for normal erythropoiesis, but in ruminants and horses only deficiencies of vitamin B$_{12}$ and folate have been associated with the development of anemia.[169] These two vitamins play essential roles in deoxyribonucleic acid (DNA) synthesis. When deficiency of both vitamins coexists, as has been experimentally produced in pigs, a marked macrocytic anemia with hypersegmented circulating neutrophils and giant metamyelocytes and neutrophils in the bone marrow may be found. In ruminants, vitamin B$_{12}$ deficiency has been associated with grazing cobalt-deficient pastures. A macrocytic-to-normocytic anemia may be noted in these animals. Folate deficiency has been reported as a cause of a mild seasonal decline in erythrocyte parameters in horses.

ANEMIA OF INFLAMMATORY DISEASE

A depression anemia that is associated with characteristic disturbances of iron metabolism is often found in animals with conditions that result in a chronic inflammatory response.[177,178] These conditions include chronic internal or cutaneous infections, infectious diseases, or immune-mediated processes that result in chronic inflammation, severe traumatic injury or fractures, and active malignant neoplasia. The anemia tends to be mild, slowly progressive, and, of itself, of little clinical consequence. Clinical signs relate to the primary disease process and hematologic features are those of a mild, nonresponsive anemia, often with indications of a chronic inflammatory response (neutrophilic leukocytosis, as well as monocytosis with elevated fibrinogen, total protein, and globulin). Serum iron and iron-binding capacity are decreased, but marrow iron reserves and serum ferritin are increased.[169,178] Anemia in these animals is partially the result of a modest decrease in the circulating red cell life span, but it is primarily caused by major alterations in iron metabolism and depressed bone marrow response to the anemia. These alterations represent part of the body's response to inflammation, which includes the release of interleukin and other mediators and the production and release of a variety of "acute phase" proteins from the liver. The body tends to sequester iron from the circulation into storage forms primarily in the liver and bone marrow, where it is retained and is relatively unavailable for erythropoiesis. This general reaction may play a protective role by denying readily available

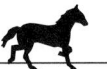

iron to potential bacterial pathogens that require iron for rapid growth and multiplication. Iron supplementation is not indicated for the treatment of the anemia of chronic inflammation, and therapeutic effort should be directed at resolution of the primary disease process.

ANEMIA SECONDARY TO ORGAN DYSFUNCTION

A mild to moderate nonresponsive anemia can develop in patients with chronic endocrine, hepatic, renal, or gastrointestinal diseases. These disorders can produce bone marrow depression by reducing the production or absorption processing and the distribution of elements essential for erythropoiesis, by allowing the elaboration or accumulation of toxic compounds, or by interfering with the production or action of erythropoietin.[179,180] These effects can occur independent of alterations in iron metabolism that characterize the anemia of inflammatory disease.[178] However, should inflammatory processes be responsible for the specific organ damage or dysfunction, the same pattern of anemia as described in the previous section would apply. Specific therapy for the anemia in these patients is not indicated, and resolution of the anemia depends on successful management of the primary disease process.

Internal parasitism, particularly that associated with *Trichostrongylus* spp. in ruminants, can result in a marked anemia. The anemia in these animals is primarily the result of bone marrow depression in which failure to absorb iron, copper, and essential amino acids plays a major role.

Myeloid and Megakaryocytic Bone Marrow Hypoplasia

Myeloid and megakaryocytic bone marrow hypoplasia has been reported in 8 young Standardbred horses sired by the same stallion.[181] Clinical signs were variable and included in some individual horses nonhealing wounds, nonresponsive fevers, pleuritis, pneumonia, ataxia, hemoperitoneum, and bleeding into the bowel. Seven of eight horses died or were euthanized. The principal laboratory findings were a variable red cell count from normal to modest to marked anemia, moderate to profound neutropenia and an intermittent thrombocytopenia in most of the horses. There appeared to be a cyclic variation in neutrophil and platelet counts. A bone marrow microenvironment or growth factor defect is suspected as the cause of this problem as myeloid progenitor cells were present and these cells were able to respond to exogenous growth factors. A familial basis for the disease is suspected.[181]

REFERENCES

169. Jain NC: *Schalm's Veterinary hematology*, ed 4, Philadelphia, 1986, Lea & Febiger, pp 655-675.
170. Tennant B et al: Hematology of the neonatal calf. III, Frequency of congenital iron deficiency anemia, *Cornell Vet* 65:543-556, 1975.
171. Gygax M et al: Immune functions of veal calves fed low amounts of iron, *Zentralbl Veterinarmed (A)* 40:345-358, 1993.
172. Easley JR: Erythrogram and red cell distribution width of equidae with experimentally induced anemia, *Am J Vet Res* 46:2378-2384, 1985.
173. Hartikka P, Dahlbom M, Westermark H: Effect of iron-saccharate injections of Finnish horses, *Nord Vet Med* 35:251-256, 1983.
174. Ruhr LP et al: Acute intoxication from a hematinic in calves, *J Am Vet Med Assoc* 182:616-618, 1983.
175. Pearson EG et al: Hepatic cirrhosis and hemochromatosis in three horses, *J Am Vet Med Assoc* 204:1053-6, 1994.
176. Smith B: The effects of copper supplementation on stock health and production, *N Z Vet J* 23:73-75, 1975.
177. Lee GR: The anemia of chronic disease, *Semin Hematol* 20:61-80, 1983.
178. Feldman BF, Kaneko JJ: The anemia of inflammatory disease in the dog. I, The nature of the problem, *Vet Res Commun* 4:237-252, 1980.
179. Lavoie J-P et al: Pancytopenia caused by bone marrow aplasia in a horse, *J Am Vet Med Assoc* 191:1462-1464, 1987.
180. Weiss DJ, Miller DC: Bone marrow necrosis associated with pancytopenia in a cow, *Vet Pathol* 22:90-92, 1985.
181. Kohn C W et al: Myeloid and megakaryocytic hypoplasia in related standardbreds, *J Vet Intern Med* 9:315-323, 1995.

APLASTIC ANEMIA

DEBRA DEEM MORRIS

Aplastic anemia is a stem cell disorder characterized by reduced marrow production of all blood components in the absence of a primary disease process infiltrating the bone marrow or suppressing hematopoiesis.[182,183] Peripheral pancytopenia secondary to marrow aplasia is apparently very uncommon in horses, although idiopathic hypoplastic anemia has been reported,[184-186] as well as rare cases associated with the use of phenylbutazone.[187,188] Hemorrhagic diathesis caused by thrombocytopenia is often the first indication of disease, manifested by epistaxis, mucosal petechiae, or prolonged hemorrhage after trauma or injections. Pallor may be present, with other signs of anemia such as reduced exercise tolerance, depending on the severity and rapidity in which aplasia progresses. Neutropenia causes increased susceptibility to infections, which may result in intermittent fever or weight loss. The production of lymphocytes is reportedly not impaired; however, absolute lymphopenia is not uncommon in aplastic anemia. Circulating lymphocytes are often highly reactive, producing the suspicion of neoplasia or a preleukemic syndrome.[188]

Marrow aplasia in humans is most always termed idiopathic, although some cases are associated with exposure to a drug, chemical, ionizing radiation, or presence of another disease.[183] However, association is not equivalent to cause, nor does it define that mechanism. Marrow failure results from damage to the hematopoietic stem cell compartment. This may be in the form of DNA damage to stem cells or depletion of later progenitor cells by a cycle-active agent. Some cases of marrow aplasia appear to be immune-mediated, either genetically determined or incited by a particular viral infection or drug exposure.

The diagnosis of aplastic anemia is based on the combination of peripheral pancytopenia and bone marrow hypoplasia with fatty replacement. Because the normal erythrocyte life span in horses is approximately 140 days and in cattle exceeds 160 days,[189] neutropenia with no left shift and thrombocytopenia are earlier hematologic manifestations.

The major aims in treatment of aplastic anemia are to remove the animal from suspected causative agents and to provide supportive care, in the hope that spontaneous remission will occur. Broad-spectrum antimicrobials are necessary to control infections. Blood transfusions are rarely indicated, and platelet transfusion should be reserved for severe bleeding episodes, which rarely occur. Bone marrow transplantation is used with some success in humans, although graft-versus-host disease poses significant risk. The latter would presumably limit this therapy in horses and too few horses with aplastic anemia have been studied to give a clear indication of prognosis.

Bracken fern toxicosis in ruminants causes bone marrow depression and subsequent pancytopenia.[189,190] Most field outbreaks of the disease occur in cattle. The toxic effects of the plant are cumulative, and clinical signs occur suddenly 2 to 8 weeks after cattle gain access to the plant. Clinical signs include fever, melena, epistaxis, hematuria, mucosal petechiae, hyphema, and bleeding from the eyes and vagina. Hematology reveals a platelet count less than $40,000/\mu l$, and profound leukopenia with essentially no neutrophils present. Death may follow in 1 to 3 days as a result of the combined effects of multiple internal hemorrhages and bacteremia. The aplastic anemia factor in bracken fern has not been identified, although ptaquiloside has been suggested.[189] Necropsy of cattle with bracken fern toxicosis reveals multiple hemorrhages throughout most tissues, necrotic gastrointestinal tract ulcers, and pale bone marrow. DL-batyl alcohol as a bone marrow stimulant is rarely successful. Antibiotics and blood and platelet transfusions may be appropriate but cattle with advanced bracken fern toxicosis (platelet count less than 50,000/µl and leukocyte count less than 2000/µl) usually die.

REFERENCES

182. Erslev AJ: Hemopoietic stem cell disorders: aplastic. In Williams WJ et al, eds: *Hematology*, ed 3, New York, 1983, McGraw Hill, pp 151-170.
183. Keitt AS: Anemia due to failure of progenitor cells. In Bennett JC, Plum F, eds: *Cecil textbook of medicine*, ed 20, Philadelphia, 1996, WB Saunders, pp 831-837.
184. Archer RK, Miller WC: A case of idiopathic hypoplastic anaemia in a two-year-old thoroughbred filly, *Vet Rec* 77:538-541, 1965.
185. Berggren PC: Aplastic anemia in a horse, *J Am Vet Med Assoc* 179:1400-1402, 1981.
186. Ward MV, Moutan PC, Dodds WJ: Severe idiopathic refractory anemia and leukopenia in a horse, *Calif Vet* 34:19-23, 1980.
187. Dunavant ML, Murry ES: Clinical evidence of phenylbutazone-induced hypoplastic anemia, *Proc First Int Symp Equine Hematol* 1:383-385, 1975.
188. Lavoie JP et al: Pancytopenia caused by bone marrow aplasia in a horse, *J Am Vet Med Assoc* 191:1462-1464, 1987.
189. Aiello SE, ed: *The Merck veterinary manual*, ed 8, Whitehouse Station, NJ, 1998, Merck & Co, Inc, pp 2026-2028.
190. Blood DC, Radostits OM: *Veterinary medicine*, ed 7, London, 1989, Baillière Tindall, pp 1320-1322.

ERYTHROCYTOSIS (POLYCYTHEMIA)

DEBRA DEEM MORRIS

Absolute erythrocytosis is caused by increased erythropoiesis that creates a circulating erythrocyte mass above normal for the species. Relative erythrocytosis caused by hemoconcentration, endotoxemia, and splenic contraction (horses) must be ruled out because these conditions are much more common in large animals than absolute erythrocytosis. Diagnosis of absolute erythrocytosis is based on persistently elevated packed cell volume (PCV), hemoglobin, and erythrocyte count without clinical evidence of shock or dehydration and without response to intravenous fluid therapy. Primary erythrocytosis is associated with normal arterial oxygen tension and reduced plasma erythropoietin, whereas secondary erythrocytosis is caused by increased production of erythropoietin.

Irrespective of underlying etiology, all disorders characterized by an absolute erythrocytosis share clinical manifestations caused by expanded blood volume and increased blood viscosity. Generalized vascular expansion and venous engorgement cause the characteristic "muddy" hyperemia of mucous membranes. A marked decrease in cardiac output accompanies blood hyperviscosity and ultimately impairs tissue oxygenation, producing the vague signs of lethargy and weight loss. There may be an increase in thrombotic complications such as laminitis and renal failure.

CONGENITAL ERYTHROCYTOSIS

Familial erythrocytosis, described in cattle[191] and humans,[192] is caused by autonomous erythropoietin production without a demonstrable lesion. Congenital erythrocytosis is thus a form of inappropriate secondary erythrocytosis. Chronic hypoxia should be ruled out by measuring the arterial oxygen concentration. The only way to definitively differentiate secondary erythrocytosis from primary erythrocytosis is by determination of serum erythropoietin.

ACQUIRED ERYTHROCYTOSIS

Primary Erythrocytosis

Polycythemia vera is an idiopathic myeloproliferative disorder characterized by excessive proliferation of erythroid, myeloid, and megakaryocytic elements, resulting in elevated peripheral erythrocyte, granulocyte, and platelet counts. Apparently this hematologic malignancy is rare in large animals because there are no reported cases. The diagnosis of polycythemia vera is based on demonstration of increased erythrocyte mass that is not associated with excessive erythropoietin production, as well as increased bone marrow production of granulocytes and platelets. A recently described syndrome in humans has been designated "primary erythrocytosis" and differs from polycythemia vera by involving only autonomous erythrocyte proliferation.[192] Examination of the bone marrow is indicated in the evaluation of all cases of erythrocytosis; however, the marrow may appear normal, and erythroid hyperplasia is not specific for primary or secondary erythrocytosis.

Secondary Erythrocytosis

PHYSIOLOGICALLY APPROPRIATE ERYTHROCYTOSIS. In domestic animals, absolute erythrocytosis is usually secondary to chronic diseases that produce tissue hypoxia. Chronic tissue hypoxia that attends residence at high altitude, congenital heart defects that produce right to left shunting, and some forms of chronic pulmonary disease induce a compensatory increase in plasma erythropoietin that results in absolute secondary erythrocytosis.[193]

The partial pressure of oxygen (PO_2) in capillaries must be maintained close to 40 mm Hg to ensure adequate off-loading of oxygen to tissues. At elevated altitudes diminished atmospheric oxygen tension produces a much smaller alveolar capillary PO_2 gradient and an inadequate driving force for tissue oxygenation. Erythropoietin production in response to hypoxia causes erythrocytosis to increase the oxygen-carrying capacity of circulating blood. Cattle are most susceptible to the effects of high altitude, and some develop polycythemia at 1800 m above sea level.[194] Horses develop an increased erythrocyte mass above 2200 m, especially when in training. Sheep are similar to cattle, but goats are apparently least susceptible to elevation hypoxia.

Congenital cardiac disorders that produce right-to-left shunts are a common cause for absolute erythrocytosis in large animals. Tetralogy of Fallot is the most common defect to cause shunting of unoxygenated blood into the peripheral circulation, although a number of other defects, including the most common ventricular septal defect,may eventually result in right-to-left shunting and secondary erythrocytosis.[195]

Chronic impairment of alveolar ventilation may eventually cause erythrocytosis, although most chronic pulmonic diseases in large animals are not associated with significant hypoxemia. Chronic obstructive pulmonary disease in horses may produce enough ventilation to perfusion mismatching to reduce the pressure of arterial oxygen below normal; however, the resultant hypoxemia is insufficient to induce erythrocytosis. Physiologically appropriate erythrocytosis can be diagnosed by determination of arterial PO_2 and documenting hypoxemia. Thoracic radiographs, transtracheal aspiration, and echocardiography may more thoroughly delineate cardiorespiratory function.

PHYSIOLOGICALLY INAPPROPRIATE ERYTHROCYTO-SIS. Inappropriate elaboration of erythropoietin (i.e., normal PO_2 and secondary erythrocytosis) may rarely accompany renal, hepatic, or endocrine disorders, especially those caused by neoplasia. In humans, carcinomas of the liver, kidney, adrenal gland, and ovary may produce erythropoietin, although the development of erythrocytosis is highly variable. Secondary erythrocytosis may accompany nonmalignant renal disorders, in which local intrarenal ischemia is believed to mediate increased erythropoietin production. Some humans with paraneoplastic erythrocytosis have normal serum erythropoietin. Tumor production of androgenic steroids or a protein with erythropoietin-like action has been suggested.[196] Increased plasma erythropoietin and secondary erythrocytosis has been identified in horses with hepatocellular carcinoma.[193,197] Erythrocytosis was recently described in a horse with hepatoblastoma, and serum erythropoietin was within reference range.[198] The diagnosis of inappropriate secondary erythrocytosis is based on elevated serum erythropoietin in the absence of hypoxemia. Unfortunately it may not be possible to demonstrate the elevation of erythropoietin because of the nature of the assay or other compounds causing erythrocytosis.

TREATMENT OF ERYTHROCYTOSIS

When erythrocytosis is not in response to an appropriate physiologic stimulus (e.g., primary erythrocytosis and inappropriate secondary erythrocytosis), phlebotomy to keep the PCV less than 50% is the mainstay of the treatment to control hypervolemia and blood hyperviscosity. Initially 2 to 4 L of blood may have to be removed every 2 to 3 days; but as iron deficiency supervenes the frequency of phlebotomy may be reduced. The myelosuppressive drug hydroxyurea has been used in humans and dogs with polycythemia vera.[192,199] This drug has not been tried in large animals.

The management of appropriate secondary erythrocytosis is more complex because there is a need for increased oxygen-carrying capacity of the blood. The beneficial effect of expanded red cell mass is ultimately offset by the detrimental effect of increased blood viscosity on oxygen delivery. Oxygen delivery is impaired when the PCV exceeds 60%, although continued erythropoietin output may result in overcompensation. Phlebotomy is indicated when the PCV is greater than 60%, but the optimum PCV for patients residing at high altitudes or those with right-to-left cardiac shunts must be determined by trial and error.

The long-term prognosis for patients with erythrocytosis is determined by the severity and cause of the disorder. Congenital cardiac defects, neoplastic diseases, and chronic organ insufficiency carry a guarded to poor prognosis. Familial or primary erythrocytosis may be managed by phlebotomy, although there are no long-term follow-ups for large animals with these disorders.

REFERENCES

191. Tennant B et al: Familial erythrocytosis in cattle, *J Am Vet Med Assoc* 150:1493-1509, 1967.
192. Silverstein MN, Tefferi A: Erythrocytosis and polycythemia vera. In Bennett JC, Plum F, eds: *Cecil textbook of medicine*, ed 20, Philadelphia, 1996, WB Saunders, pp 920-922.
193. Beech J, Bloom JC, Hodge TG: Erythrocytosis in a horse, *J Am Vet Med Assoc* 184:986-989, 1984.
194. Blood DC, Radostits OM: *Veterinary medicine*, ed 7, London, 1989, Baillière Tindall, pp 1231-1233.
195. Bayly WM et al: Multiple congenital heart anomalies in five Arabian foals, *J Am Vet Med Assoc* 81:684-689, 1982.
196. John WJ, Foon KA, Patchell RA: Paraneoplastic syndromes. In DeVita VT, Hellman S, Rosenberg SA, eds: *Cancer: principles and practice of oncology*, ed 5, Philadelphia, 1997, Lippincott-Raven Publishers, pp 2397-2418.
197. Roby KAW et al: Hepatocellular carcinoma associated with erythrocytosis and hypoglycemia in a yearling filly, *J Am Vet Med Assoc* 196:1106-1108, 1990.
198. Lennox TJ et al: Hepatoblastoma with erythrocytosis in a young female horse, *J Am Vet Med Assoc* 216:718-721, 2000.
199. Campbell KL: Diagnosis and management of polycythemia in dog, *Comp Contin Educ Pract Vet* 12:543-550, 1990.

BOVINE LYMPHOSARCOMA

MARK C. THURMOND

Bovine lymphosarcoma (LS) has been categorized in terms of the frequency of occurrence (sporadic or endemic/enzootic), age at onset, organ system(s) involved, and the etiologic agent. Lymphosarcoma occurs sporadically as a generalized lymphadenopathy in calves (calf or juvenile form), as thymic involvement in cattle between 6 months and 2 years of age (thymic or adolescent form), and as cutaneous lesions in cattle between 1 and 3 years of age. No etiologic agent has been associated with sporadic forms of LS. The most common form of LS appears endemically in adult cattle more than 2 years of age. This form usually involves multiple organ systems and is associated with bovine leukemia virus (BLV) infection.

Another condition, not yet shown to have a neoplastic component, but which has been characterized by lymphadenopathy and lymphocytosis, has been reported in calves infected with a lentivirus.[200]

SPORADIC LYMPHOSARCOMA

Calf or Juvenile Form

The prevalence rate of juvenile LS is unknown but appears to be extremely rare, and multiple cases are seldom seen in the same herd.[201] The cause of juvenile LS also is unknown, and it does not appear to be associated with BLV.[202] Dairy breeds may be predisposed to developing this form of LS.[203]

The age at onset ranges from 3 to 6 months, but cases may occasionally be seen in calves as young as 1 month or in cattle as old as 3 years. There have been reports of fetal involvement with the calf form.[204] Calves are generally presented with a history of slight to moderate depression, weight loss, weakness (mainly in older calves and in spite of a good appetite), or lymphadenopathy (mainly in younger calves).[205] The onset of signs is often sudden (within a week).

Physical examination may reveal generalized bilateral enlargement of lymph nodes, particularly the deep cervical and parotid nodes and occasionally the popliteal and hemonodes. Moderate to marked enlargement may be noted for the iliac and mandibular nodes. Rarely, node enlargement is not generalized but is restricted to a regional anatomic site.[202,205] Enlarged nodes tend to be smooth, firm, and not hot or painful. Mucous membranes are usually pale, as a result of anemia. Tachycardia, tachypnea (>30 breaths/min), hyperpnea, cough, and harsh respiratory sounds may be evident on auscultation. Less commonly reported signs include fever, ruminal tympany, an enlarged liver, ataxia, and diarrhea.[205]

Hematologic features tend to include a microcytic hypochromic anemia, a low hemoglobin (<7 g/100 ml),[206] a low packed cell volume (typically in the mid 20s), and a leukocytosis primarily caused by a lymphocytosis.[201,202,205-207] Bone marrow examinations may reveal an elevated myeloid/erythroid ratio,[201] with massive neoplastic infiltration in some calves.[206] Affected calves also tend to have low serum globulin and elevated AST. Neoplastic involvement of a variety of organs, including the spleen, heart, kidney, liver, pancreas, uterus, and thymus, may occur.[202,205,206] The thymus is less involved than in the thymic form of LS; neoplastic tissue is

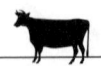
found only as small, microscopic nodules.[206] Subperiosteal neoplastic infiltration may produce spinal cord compression and result in paresis.[206] The disease is rapidly progressive and is usually fatal within 2 to 8 weeks of onset.

Thymic or Adolescent Form

The thymic form of LS is very rare. The disease is usually seen in cattle 6 to 24 months of age but may occur in newborn calves and in cattle up to 4 years of age.[205] Beef breeds, particularly Hereford cattle, may be predisposed to develop this form of LS.[203] Clinical signs are produced by space-occupying lesions in the neck or thorax.[208] Affected cattle are generally presented with an enlargement or swelling in the presternal area of the brisket, which is firm and associated with pitting edema. Loss in condition, rumen tympany, and dysphagia are commonly seen. Bloat may occur as a result of interruption of eructation by the space-occupying lesion around the esophagus.[208] Although generalized lymphadenopathy is uncommon, superficial cervical and prescapular nodes are usually enlarged. The jugular veins tend to be distended and nonpulsating, and there may be muffling of heart sounds and diminished resonance on percussion of the thorax. Tachycardia, dyspnea, coughing, or respiratory distress may be present. Hematologic features generally are unremarkable. Anemia is not a consistent feature, and lymphocytosis is only seen occasionally. The course of the disease from the time of recognition is generally from 2 to 9 weeks, but poor condition may have been present for several months before presentation.[200] The disease is fatal, often as an immediate consequence of bloat.

Cutaneous Form

Cutaneous LS is not as age-specific as the other forms of sporadic LS and may affect cattle between 1 and 3 years of age. The history may reveal an initial period of 1 to 3 months, during which cutaneous swellings are observed around the anus, vulva, escutcheon, shoulders, or flank. These signs may regress and subsequently recur.[209] Lesions tend to be raised and ulcerated. They are generally about 2 to 3 cm in diameter with necrotic centers and may be painful on palpation. Other signs depend on the organ system involvement of the tumor and may include cardiac insufficiency, with brisket edema extending along the ventral abdomen and with a jugular pulse. Pulse and respiration may be elevated as a result of anemia. Hematologic features include anemia and presence of atypical lymphocytes. The mandibular, prescapular, prefemoral, and supramammary lymph nodes are usually enlarged.[210]

At necropsy, a variety of organs may be involved, including heart, brain, skin, spinal cord, liver, lung, kidney, and abomasum. The massive lymphoid infiltration of the skin resembles the clinical manifestations of mycotic fungoides of humans.[204]

Hemonode Enlargement (Hemal Lymph Node)

A lymphoproliferative condition associated with hemonode enlargement and some generalized lymphadenopathy has been described for cattle infected with a lentivirus.[200] It has been proposed that the virus be called bovine immunodeficiency-like virus (BIV)[211] because of its molecular similarity to human immunodeficiency virus. Infected calves may develop enlarged superficial nodes (hemonodes), mainly in the cervical region anterior and dorsal to the prescapular lymph node, over the spine of the scapula, in the paralumbar fossa, and dorsal to the prefemoral lymph node. Lymphocytosis has been reported and is possibly related to an increase in B

lymphocytes. It is not known what, if any, detrimental effect infection with this virus may have on cattle.

ADULT LYMPHOSARCOMA (BLV)

OCCURRENCE. The adult, or enzootic, form of LS is the most common neoplastic disease of cattle and is associated with BLV infection. Rates of LS in cattle may vary considerably, probably reflecting variation in BLV infection rates. In 1978 the US condemnation of carcasses because of lymphoma was reported to be 170 per 100,000 head slaughtered.[212] A very high condemnation rate, sometimes exceeding 1%, was reported for slaughtered California dairy cows,[213] and about 1.73% of BLV-infected cattle had LS.[214] The rate of cattle condemnations because of LS appears to have increased markedly in recent years.[213]

EPIDEMIOLOGY. The epidemiology of adult LS is not completely understood. Herd size might be positively correlated with a high rate of LS, which may reflect higher rates of BLV infection in large herds or a preponderance of susceptible pedigrees in some of the herds studied.[214,215] Susceptibility to BLV infection has been found to be associated with BoLA type,[216,217] which may explain why higher rates of LS are found in certain families of cattle. The progression of disease to lymphocytosis in some BLV-infected cows may be influenced also by BoLA type, suggesting that there may be a genetic predisposition to development of LS through the antigens of the major histocompatibility complex encoded at closely linked loci. Other potentially contributing factors such as nutrition, concurrent infections, and environmental/meteorologic stressors have not been explored sufficiently. No evidence exists for a seasonally associated pattern to appearance of clinical lymphosarcoma.[213]

ECONOMICS. The economic importance of adult lymphosarcoma has several dimensions applicable to different segments of the cattle industry and to different producers.[218] Producers suffer losses from LS associated with death of cattle (particularly genetically valuable livestock), loss of milk production, costs incurred in treatment and diagnosis, and premature replacement costs for cattle dying or culled as a result of LS. The latter may explain, in part, an observed increased rate of culling found for BLV-infected dairy cattle.[219] In addition to premature culling and replacement, losses are incurred because of failure to retain salvage value of cows condemned for LS at slaughter.[213] A hidden cost of LS also may be in the perpetuation of BLV-infected cattle via in utero infection of calves born to cows with LS.[220,221]

DIAGNOSIS. Cattle presented with the adult or enzootic form of LS usually are older than 4 years of age but may be as young as 2 years. Cattle are often presented with a history of loss in condition, an abrupt drop in milk production (over a period of a few days), enlarged peripheral nodes, exophthalmos, or partial to complete anorexia, particularly with regard to grain or concentrates. Because dry cows are not observed as closely as lactating cows and are not monitored for milk yield, LS is less likely to be recognized until they freshen. Subclinical LS may be diagnosed in cows submitted for routine reproduction examinations; other signs may include diarrhea, ataxia, paresis, ketosis, and infertility.

Physical examination often reveals an organ system failure resulting from tumor involvement. Cattle with LS may be immunosuppressed,[221] and clinical signs may be related to the extent of secondary infection. Thoracic auscultation may reveal cardiac dysrhythmia, tachycardia, tachypnea, and hyperpnea.[222] Dependent, pitting edema is a common finding when cervical or supramammary lymph nodes are involved. Involvement of the intestinal lymphatics is often associated with generalized dependent edema anterior to the udder. Peripheral nodes commonly found to be enlarged are the

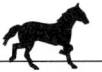

prescapular, femoral, and supramammary nodes. Feces may be scant, sticky, or watery, sometimes with melena. The fecal consistency may reflect ulcerative or obstructive lesion within the gastrointestinal tract.

Rectal palpation of the abdominal cavity is the most useful diagnostic procedure in cases lacking peripheral node enlargement or exophthalmos. Tumor masses palpated in the abdomen typically are multiple and range in size from only slightly enlarged lymph nodes to massive lesions of half a meter in diameter. The internal iliac nodes are involved in most cattle with abdominal tumors. Other internal organs involved include the uterus, rumen, colon, and kidney. Tumors tend to be firm but not hard and may feel slightly lobulated. Differentiation by palpation of LS tumors from other masses is highly subjective. Carcinomas tend to be of similar consistency but are seldom larger than 15 cm in diameter and are usually associated with intestinal tissue. Lymph nodes of cows with a carcinoma are not usually enlarged unless a secondary infection is present. Melanomas are generally less than 15 cm in diameter and hard, sometimes with protrusions 1 to 2 cm high along the surface. They usually are not found associated with lymph nodes. Masses of fat necrosis tend to be softer and smaller and are usually associated with omental tissue. Internal abscesses are often single and associated with the uterus, as a consequence of uterine tear and infection during parturition, or with gluteal muscles of the pelvic ceiling, as a consequence of injection-related infection. Exploratory laparotomy may be indicated as an additional diagnostic tool in difficult cases, particularly in valuable cattle.

The hemogram of cattle with LS often is generally unremarkable. Anemia, characterized as microcytic and hypochromic, may be present in cattle with gastrointestinal hemorrhage. Lymphocytosis is not usually associated with LS, although presence of a large number of bizarre, immature-appearing lymphocytes is seen in some cases. Fibrinogen levels have been inconsistent in LS, and therefore its measurement may be helpful only in differentiating an abscess.

Cytology of aspirates of tumors or tumorous nodes is not a reliable diagnostic tool, although it can be helpful. Discrimination cannot be made between a normal node responding to an infectious agent and a node involved with neoplastic lymphocytes, because in both situations cells resembling young, poorly differentiated lymphocytes may be present. Examination of nontumorous active lymph nodes may reveal elevated proportion of large, young lymphocytes that could resemble those of lymphosarcoma. Histopathologic examination of biopsied tumors or nodes may be more useful than aspirates in diagnosis. However, cytology and culture of aspirates could be helpful in differentiating a tumor from an abscess.

Lymphosarcoma is very rare in cattle without BLV infection (1.55 cases per 10,000 noninfected cattle),[224] and serology may be helpful in some diagnoses. The standard serologic test for BLV is the agar gel immunodiffusion test using the gp-51 antigen of BLV available commercially as a kit.* Presence of antibodies to BLV gp-51 antigen generally is considered to be a prerequisite to a diagnosis of LS, except for cows during the periparturient period when circulating antibodies may fall below the level detectable by a serologic test.[224] Mere presence of BLV antibodies does not necessarily mean that an animal has LS, which is found in only about 1.7% of BLV-infected cattle.[201] However, serology can be helpful in predicting the chance of LS in cattle seropositive to the gp-51 antigen. Sera from cattle with LS generally have high titers to the gp-51 antigen (a score of 3 or 4 on agar gel im-

munodiffusion), compared with those of infected cattle without LS (score of 1 or 2). In addition, cattle that do not have LS tend not to have antibodies to the p-24 antigen of BLV, as detected by agar gel immunodiffusion. The percentage of cattle with histologically confirmed LS but in which LS was not diagnosed by a gp-51-positive and p-24-negative test result (false-negative rate of the diagnostic test) has been found to be only 0.21%, using the agar gel immunodiffusion test.[214] Unfortunately most diagnostic laboratories do not have the capability to perform the test using the p-24 antigen.

At necropsy tumors are found enclosed in a capsular-like tissue that, when sectioned with a knife, results in an eversion of tumor stroma. Cut tumor tissue is cream-colored and friable, with little binding structure. Centers of tumors may appear necrotic and mushy, whereas peripheral regions are firmer and pink to white. Histopathology provides the only definitive diagnosis. Tissue should be biopsied by surgical removal of as much of the node (or mass) as possible.

Sensitivity and specificity of the AGID test to detect BLV infection have been estimated to be 0.985 and 0.998, respectively.[225] Thus, depending on the prevalence, the AGID can be expected to have good negative and positive predictive values. For example, the positive predictive value for the test on herd with a prevalence of 5% would be 0.84, indicating that the probability of infection for a positive test result would be 84%. The negative predictive value for the same herd would be 99.9%. Although estimates of sensitivity and specificity of the ELISA test for BLV have not been reported, the test is probably of comparable sensitivity and specificity to the AGID,[226] with the ELISA perhaps being more capable of detecting new infections earlier than the AGID.

CONTROL. No curative treatment for LS exists. However, supportive therapy may be indicated to reduce discomfort and prolong life long enough to remove valuable ova/embryos or calves or to harvest semen.

Until more information is available on the epidemiology of LS, control and eradication hinge on success of efforts to eradicate BLV from a herd. Presently there are no vaccines that offer effective protection from BLV infection.[225,227-229] Control and eradication of BLV require reduction of blood transmission through iatrogenic means and through physical contact among cattle.[230] Transmission associated with physical contact between infected and susceptible cattle can be reduced by segregating infected and noninfected cattle.[231-233] Separation of cattle by 10 feet is preferred, but a single fence may reduce sufficiently the degree of contact necessary for transmission. Transmission after physical contact may be via inhalation of BLV shed in nasal secretions.[234-237] Experimental studies have found that under extreme conditions of blood contamination and mucosal irritation, BLV can be transmitted per rectum.[238-241] Under conditions typical of routine palpation during pregnancy examination; however, BLV appearance may not necessarily be transmitted to any measurable degree.[240,241] If potential for rectal transmission is a concern, palpation sleeves may be rinsed or replaced between cows. Although insect transmission of BLV is theoretically possible,[244] studies of natural infection have not been able to link flies, particularly horse flies, with new natural infections.[245,246] Several studies have been unable to demonstrate transmission after use of a common needle.[247-249] However, infection after use of a Tb needle dipped in blood of a BLV-infected animal could be prevented by wiping the needle with cotton before injection.[250] Although data have not shown the use of common needles to be an important means of BLV transmission, it would be prudent to use individual sterile needles for treatment, testing, or vaccination. Although transmission has not been shown in cows inseminated artificially using commercially prepared frozen semen,[251-255] infection resulting from the use of an infected bull in natural

---

*Leukassay B, Pitman Moore Co, Washington Crossing, NJ.

breeding may be possible.[256-258] Embryo transfer using non-infected recipients offers a means of producing phenotypically preferred cattle from BLV-infected cows and controlling in utero infection[255,259-261] because at the time of harvesting embryos are not infected.[252] For most herds, control and eradication of the infection would require modification of facilities, alteration of management practices, and serologic surveillance at least annually. Planning a control program should include a cost/benefit analysis to evaluate potential return on the investment.

REFERENCES

200. van der Maaten MJ, Boothe ED, Seger CL: Isolation of a virus from cattle with persistent lymphocytosis, *J Natl Cancer Inst* 49:1649-1657, 1972.
201. Hugoson G: Juvenile bovine leukosis, *Acta Vet Scand* 22(suppl):5-115, 1967.
202. Bundza A et al: Sporadic bovine leukosis: a description of eight calves received at Animal Diseases Research Institute from 1974-1980, *Can Vet J* 21:280-283, 1980.
203. Theilen GH et al: Bovine lymphosarcoma in California. I, Epizootiologic and hematologic aspects, *Health Lab Sci* 1:96-106, 1964.
204. Theilen GH, Madewell BR: Hematopoietic neoplasms, sarcomas and related conditions. In Theilen GH, Madewell BR, eds: *Veterinary cancer medicine*, Philadelphia, 1987, Lea & Febiger, pp 408-430.
205. Grimshaw W et al: Bovine leucosis (lymphosarcoma): a clinical study of 60 pathologically confirmed cases, *Vet Rec* 105:267-272, 1979.
206. Theilen GH, Dungworth DL: Bovine lymphosarcoma in California. III, Calf form, *Am J Vet Res* 26:696-709, 1965.
207. Chander S et al: Bovine lymphosarcoma in twin calves, *Can J Comp Med* 41:274-278, 1977.
208. Dungworth DL, Theilen GH, Lengyl J: Bovine lymphosarcoma in California. II, The thymic form, *Vet Pathol* 1:323-350, 1964.
209. Clegg FG, Moss B: Skin leukosis in a heifer: an unusual clinical history, *Vet Rec* 77:271-272, 1965.
210. Marshak RR et al: Observations on a heifer with cutaneous lymphosarcoma, *Cancer* 19:724-734, 1966.
211. Gonda M et al: Characterization and molecular cloning of a bovine lentivirus related to human immunodeficiency virus, *Nature* 330:388-391, 1987.
212. Sorenson D, Beal VC: Prevalence and economics of bovine leukosis in the United States, *Proceedings of the Bovine Leukosis Symposium*, College Park, Md, 1979, pp 33-50.
213. Thurmond MC et al: Retrospective study of four years of carcass condemnation rates for malignant lymphoma in California dairy cows, *Am J Vet Res* 46:1387-1391, 1985.
214. Thurmond MC, Holmberg CA, Picanso JP: Antibodies to bovine leukemia virus and presence of malignant lymphoma in slaughtered California dairy cattle, *J Natl Cancer Inst* 74:711-714, 1985.
215. Cypress R et al: Epidemiologic and pedigree study of the occurrence of lymphosarcoma from 1953 to 1971 in a closed herd of Jersey cows, *Am J Epidemiol* 99:37-44, 1974.
216. Lewin HA, Bernoco D: Evidence for BoLA-linked resistance and susceptibility to subclinical progression of bovine leukaemia virus infection, *Anim Genet* 17:197-207, 1986.
217. Palmer C et al: Susceptibility of cattle to bovine leukemia virus associated with BoLA type, *Proceedings of the Ninety-first Annual Meeting of the United States Animal Health Association*, Salt Lake City, 1988, pp 218-228.
218. Thurmond MC: Economics of enzootic bovine leukosis. In Burny A, Mammerick M, eds: *Enzootic bovine leukosis and bovine leukemia virus*, Boston, 1987, Martinus Nijhoff, pp 71-84.
219. Thurmond MC, Maden CB, Carter RL: Cull rates in dairy cattle with antibodies to bovine leukemia virus, *Cancer Res* 45:1987-1989, 1985.
220. Kono Y et al: Studies of foetuses from cows clinically affected with bovine leucosis, *Vet Microbiol* 8:505-509, 1983.
221. Lassauzet M-L, Johnson W, Thurmond M: Transmission of bovine leukemia virus in calves on a California dairy (in preparation).
222. Jacobs R, Valli V, Wilkie B: Inhibition of lymphocyte blastogenesis by sera from cows with lymphoma, *Am J Vet Res* 41:372-376, 1980.
223. Grimshaw WTR et al: A confirmed clinical case of enzootic bovine leukosis in Britain, *Vet Rec* 107:110, 1980.
224. Burridge M et al: Fall in antibody titer to bovine leukemia virus in the periparturient period, *Can J Comp Med* 46:270-271, 1982.
225. Monke D et al: Estimation of the sensitivity and specificity of the agar gel immunodiffusion test for bovine leukemia virus, *J Am Vet Med Assoc* 200:2001-2004, 1992.
226. Roberts D, Lucas M, Swallow C: Comparison of the agar gel immunodiffusion test and ELISA in the detection of bovine leukosis virus antibody in cattle persistently infected with bovine virus diarrhea virus, *Vet Immunol Immunopathol* 11:275-281, 1989.
227. Ohishi K et al: Augmentation of bovine leukemia virus BLA0-specific lymphocyte proliferation responses in ruminants by inoculation with BLV ENV-recombinant vaccinia virus: their role in the suppression of BLV replication, *Microbiol Immunol* 36:1317-1323, 1992.
228. Ohishi K et al: Protective immunity against bovine leukaemia virus (BLV) induced in carrier sheep by inoculation with a vaccinia virus-BLV ENV-recombinant: association with cell-mediated immunity, *J Gen Virol* 71:1887-1892, 1991.
229. Fukuyam S et al: Protection against bovine leukemia virus infection by use of inactivated vaccines in cattle, *J Vet Med Sci* 55:99-106, 1993.
230. DiGiacomo RF, Darlington RL, Evermann JF: Natural transmission of bovine leukemia virus in dairy calves by dehorning, *Can J Comp Med* 49:340-342, 1985.
231. Miller J, Van Der Maaten M: Attempts to control spread of bovine leukemia virus infection in cattle by serologic surveillance with the glycoprotein agar gel immunodiffusion test. In Ressang AA, ed: *The serological diagnosis of enzootic bovine leukosis*, Luxembourg, 1978, Commission of European Communities, pp 127-135.
232. Johnson R, Gibson CD, Kaneene JB: Bovine leukemia virus: a herd-based control strategy, *Prev Vet Med* 3:339-349, 1985.
233. Thurmond MC et al: A prospective investigation of bovine leukemia virus infection in young dairy cattle, using survival methods, *Am J Epidemiol* 117:621-631, 1983.
234. Lucas M, Roberts D, Banks J: Shedding of bovine leukosis virus in nasal secretions of infected animals, *Vet Rec* 132:276-278, 1993.
235. Roberts D, Lucas M, Wibberley G: To compare the incubation period following intratracheal and subcutaneous inoculation of bovine leukosis virus infected lymphocytes and to study their clearance from the circulation, *Vet Immunol Immunopathol* 11:351-359, 1986.
236. Roberts D et al: Detection of bovine leukosis virus in bronchoalveolar lung washings and nasal secretions, *Vet Rec* 111:501-503, 1982.
237. Roberts D et al: An investigation into the susceptibility of cattle to bovine leukosis virus following inoculation by various routes, *Vet Rec* 110:222-224, 1982.
238. Henry E, Levine J, Coggins L: Rectal transmission of bovine leukemia virus in cattle and sheep, *Am J Vet Res* 48:634-636, 1987.
239. Hopkins S et al: Experimental transmission of bovine leukosis virus by simulated rectal palpation, *Vet Rec* 122:389-391, 1988.
240. Hopkins S et al: Trauma and rectal palpation of dairy cows, *J Infect Dis* 158:1133-1134, 1988.
241. Wentink G et al: Experimental transmission of bovine leukosis virus by rectal palpation, *Vet Rec* 132:135-136, 1993.
242. Hopkins S et al: Rectal palpation and transmission of bovine leukemia virus in dairy cattle, *J Am Vet Med Assoc* 199:1035-1038, 1991.
243. Lassauzet M, Thurmond M, Walton R: Lack of evidence of transmission of bovine leukemia virus by rectal palpation of dairy cows, *J Am Vet Med Assoc* 195:1732-1733, 1989.
244. Perino L et al: Bovine leukosis virus transmission with mouthparts from *Tabanus abactor* after interrupted feeding, *Am J Vet Res* 51:1167-1169, 1990.
245. Thurmond M, Carter R, Burridge M: An investigation for seasonal trends in bovine leukemia virus infection, *Prev Vet Med* 1:115-123, 1982.
246. Wilesmith J, Straub O, Lorenz R: Some observations on the epidemiology of bovine leucosis virus infection in a large dairy herd, *Res Vet Sci* 28:10-16, 1980.
247. Lassauzet M-L et al: Effect of brucellosis vaccination and dehorning on transmission of bovine leukemia virus in heifers on a California dairy, *Can J Vet Res* 54:184-189, 1990.
248. Thurmond M: Epidemiology of the natural transmission of bovine leukemia virus, PhD dissertation, Gainesville, 1982, University of Florida.
249. Weber A et al: Failure to demonstrate transmission of enzootic bovine leukemia virus infection from cows to sheep by use of common injection needles, *Am J Vet Res* 49:1814-1816, 1988.
250. Roberts D et al: Investigation of the possible role of the tuberculin intradermal test in the spread of enzootic bovine leukosis, *Vet Res Commun* 4:301-305, 1980.
251. Eaglesome MD, Hare WCD, Singh EL: Embryo transfer: a discussion of its potential for infectious disease control based on a review of studies on infection of gametes and early embryos by various agents, *Can Vet J* 21:106-112, 1980.
252. Eaglesome MD et al: Transfer of embryos from bovine leukemia virus-infected cattle to uninfected recipients: preliminary results, *Vet Rec* 111:122-123, 1982.
253. Hare WCD: Embryo transfer and disease transmission in farm animals. *Proceedings of the Eighty-seventh Annual Meeting of the US Animal Health Association*, 1988, pp 303-324.
254. Olson C, Rowe RF, Kaja R: Embryo transplantation and bovine leukosis virus: preliminary report. In Straub OC, ed: *Fourth International Symposium on Bovine Leukosis*, Bologna, The Hague, 1980, Martinus Nijhoff, pp 361-368.
255. DiGiacomo RF et al: Embryo transfer and transmission of bovine leukosis virus in a dairy herd, *J Am Vet Med Assoc* 188:827-828, 1986.
256. van der Maaten MJ, Miller JM: Susceptibility of cattle to bovine leukemia virus infection by various routes of exposure. In Bentvelzen P et al, eds: *Advances in comparative leukemia research*, Amsterdam, 1978, Elsevier/North-Holland, pp 29-32.
257. Lucas MH et al: Enzootic leucosis virus in semen, *Vet Rec* 106:128, 1980.
258. Lorton SP et al: Leukosis-negative status of calves produced by embryo splitting, *Theriogenology* 27:250, 1987.
259. Jacobsen KL et al: Transmission of bovine leukemia virus: prevalence of antibodies in precolostral calves, *Prev Vet Med* 1:265-272, 1982/1983.

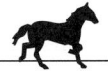

260. Thurmond MC, Carter RL, Burridge MJ: An investigation for seasonal trends in bovine leukemia virus infection, *Prev Vet Med* 1:115-123, 1983.
261. Thurmond MC et al: An epidemiological study of natural in utero infection with bovine leukemia virus, *Can J Comp Med* 47:316-319, 1983.

LYMPHOMA (LYMPHOSARCOMA) IN HORSES

GARY P. CARLSON

The common term used in the past for this class of neoplasia in horses has been lymphosarcoma. However, none of the lymphatic neoplasms are benign and the preferred terminology is lymphoma.[262] Lymphoma is a sporadic disease and one of the more common neoplasms of the horse. Clinical signs depend on lesion location and the organ systems involved. Hematologic features of lymphoma are variable, and frank leukemia is rare.[263,264] Although leukemia was first described in horses in 1858, the number of systematically evaluated and well-documented cases is limited. Viral etiologic agents have not been documented as causal factors in the development of lymphoma in horses, although virus-like particles were described in a lymph node from a foal with lymphoma that died shortly after birth.[265] The system used in cattle may not be appropriate for classification of lymphoma in the horse.

Despite recent attempts to classify equine lymphomas based on morphologic and immunohistochemical characteristics,[266] there is considerable confusion in the present literature regarding the nature of these tumors with regard to cell type involved. Both T cell and B cell lymphomas have been described. Frequently, lesions are described as the T cell rich B cell lymphoma or vice versa. It would appear that at this point in time adequate tools may not be available to accurately assess which cells types in these lesions are truly neoplastic and which represent a reactive inflammatory response. At present this may appear to be a largely academic issue. However, when we are able to accurately determine the cell types in these lesions we will be in a much better position to design rational and more effective therapeutic intervention as well as to provide a more accurate prognostic assessment of these patients.

The disease is usually found in adult horses from 5 to 10 years of age, with a range from birth to over 20 years.[267-269] Lymphoma has been reported at necropsy of an aborted equine fetus. Some forms of lymphoma such as the alimentary form appear to be more common in younger horses.[270-273] There is no clear sex or breed predisposition. It has been suggested that some horses with lymphoma have compromised humoral or cellular immunologic defense mechanisms.[273-277] This may contribute to the development of secondary infections seen in some patients.

The most commonly encountered clinical signs are depression, weight loss, and lymphadenopathy and may be associated with ventral edema, respiratory distress, fever, anemia, mild colic, or diarrhea.[268,272,278-280] A variety of neurologic disturbances may be associated with lymphoma with signs related to lesion location.[281-285] The lymphadenopathy may be generalized or involve only a few regional lymph nodes. Affected lymph nodes tend to be firm, cool, and nonpainful. Splenic enlargement or internal tumor masses may be palpated on rectal examination. Ultrasound can be a useful diagnostic tool for evaluation of internal organ involvement.[286] In one recent report, ocular manifestations of lymphoma were identified either in the eye or ocular adnexa in 21 of 79 horses with lymphoma in which a careful ocular examination was conducted.[287] A paraneoplastic pruritus and alopecia has been described in a horse with diffuse lymphoma.[288]

The diagnosis of lymphoma depends on the demonstration of neoplastic cells. This is occasionally possible on routine examination of blood smears in the rare instance when there is a frank leukemia. However, in most cases the diagnosis is based on cytologic evaluation of bone marrow or pleural or peritoneal fluid or histologic examination of biopsies of enlarged lymph nodes, tumor masses, or infiltrated tissues. Cytologic evaluation of needle aspirates of lymph nodes or tumors is often nondiagnostic in the horse, and biopsy specimens are much preferred. Histologic classification of lesions have prognostic implications. Lymphoblastic lymphomas tend to affect younger horses and are often rapidly progressive.[289]

SERUM CHEMISTRY. Serum chemistry profiles may provide an indication of internal organ involvement. Many patients with lymphoma have alterations in serum protein concentration that frequently include a polyclonal gammopathy and hypoalbuminemia. Some horses with lymphoma are reported to have a low serum IgM,[277] but this has not been a consistent feature. Hypercalcemia has been reported in a number of horses with lymphoma.[290,291]

HEMATOLOGY. The hematologic features of lymphoma are quite varied. Frank leukemia is rare, but there are reports of lymphocyte counts as high as 150,000/L in a few cases. When leukemia is present, neoplastic cells are generally found in the bone marrow. More often the lymphocyte count is within the normal range or even decreased. Atypical lymphocytes may be noted in the blood smears of 20% to 30% of affected horses, particularly late in the course of the disease. A modest neutrophilic leukocytosis with an elevated fibrinogen is often seen. This hematologic reflection of an inflammatory response may be appropriate in patients with rapidly growing or invasive tumors, but it can cause confusion when trying to differentiate lymphoma from internal abscessation.[292]

Anemia is a relatively common feature of lymphoma. Anemia in these circumstances is generally thought to be caused by suppression of erythropoiesis or bone marrow infiltration. In some cases, Coombs'-positive immune-mediated hemolytic anemia, thrombocytopenia, or blood loss may play a role in the development of anemia.[293] The immune-mediated hemolytic anemia and thrombocytopenia in many of these patients may be transiently responsive to corticosteroids.

GENERALIZED OR MULTICENTRIC FORM

The generalized or multicentric form is the most common form of lymphoma. Horses often present with severe depression, emaciation, generalized lymphadenopathy, and ventral edema.[268,272,294] Additional clinical signs may be associated with internal organ involvement and dysfunction.[269,273] Anemia is common, and, although leukemia is rare, it is generally associated with this form of lymphoma when it does occur. At necropsy widespread lesions are noted in most lymph nodes, liver, spleen, and other internal organs.

INTESTINAL OR ALIMENTARY FORM

The intestinal or alimentary form of lymphoma is most often seen in horses less than 5 years of age. Affected horses are often very thin, appear to have intestinal malabsorption, and may have a history of mild recurrent colic or recurrent febrile episodes.[270-272] Peripheral lymph nodes generally are not enlarged, but intestinal lymphadenopathy may be noted on rectal palpation. Altered stool character may be noted, but profuse diarrhea is not common. The oral glucose absorption test may indicate malabsorption, and the fecal occult blood may be positive. Anemia is common and, when present, is frequently associated with an immune-mediated hemolytic process. The leukogram often reflects an inflammatory response, and leukemia occurs very rarely. Albumin is often low, and the globulins are frequently elevated. Intestinal lesions are largely confined to the small bowel; and the intestinal, splenic, and hepatic lymph nodes are usually involved.

MEDIASTINAL OR THYMIC FORM

The mediastinal or thymic form of lymphoma is usually seen in adult horses and is associated with respiratory signs, pleural effusion, edema of the ventral thorax, and regional lymphadenopathy at the thoracic inlet and in the retropharyngeal areas.[272,295,296] Temperature, pulse, and respiratory rates are often elevated. Horses may develop respiratory distress. Neoplasia is often evident on examination of pleural fluid.

CUTANEOUS FORM

There is considerable question whether the cutaneous form of the disease truly represents a malignant neoplastic process. The lesions are generally confined to the skin and regional lymph nodes. The lesions tend to wax and wane and some have reported that this waxing and waning may be modulated by hormonal influences either seasonally or during the estrus cycle. There is one report of complete regression of cutaneous lymphoma lesions after the surgical removal of an ovarian tumor.[297] Although not prominently reported in published surveys, in my experience this is one of the most common forms of lymphoma in horses. Multiple subcutaneous nodules ranging from less than 1 cm to greater than 10 to 20 cm in diameter can develop regionally or over most of the body surface.[298] These nodules may appear suddenly, frequently regress, and then reappear. They tend to gradually increase in size but may remain static for years. Local lymph nodes may become involved, but generalized lymphadenopathy and internal organ involvement seldom, if ever, occur. Horses may live and function well for many years with these lesions. The hemogram in most of these horses is normal.

This form of lymphoma is responsive to corticosteroids. Lesions often regress almost completely over 1 to 2 weeks in response to dexamethasone given at a dosage rate of 20 mg daily. Unless gradually tapering doses of corticosteroids are continued for long periods, the lesions tend to recur, often in a more vigorous and rapidly expanding form. For this reason, and because of the generally benign and slowly progressive nature of the disease, these lesions are usually left untreated. See section on dermatology for a more complete description of cutaneous lymphoma (lymphosarcoma) (Chapter 38).

REFERENCES

262. Savage CJ: Lymphoproliferative and myeloproliferative disorders, *Vet Clin North Am (Equine Pract)* 14:563-578, 1998.
263. Madewell BR et al: Lymphosarcoma with leukemia in a horse, *Am J Vet Res* 43:807-812, 1982.
264. Kramer J et al: Large granular lymphocyte leukemia in a horse, *Vet Clin Pathol* 22:126-128, 1993.
265. Haley PJ et al: Lymphosarcoma in an aborted equine fetus, *Vet Pathol* 20:647-649, 1983.
266. Kelley LC, Mahaffey EA: Equine malignant lymphomas: morphologic and immunohistochemical classification, *Vet Pathol* 35:241-252, 1998.
267. Neufeld JL: Lymphosarcoma in a mare and review of cases at the Ontario Veterinary College, *Can Vet J* 14:149-152, 1973.
268. Neufeld JL: Lymphosarcoma in the horse: a review, *Can Vet J* 14:129-135, 1973.
269. Seahorn TL et al: Lymphosarcoma in a foal: a case report, *J Equine Vet Sci* 8:317-319, 1988.
270. Platt H: Alimentary lymphomas in the horse, *J Comp Pathol* 97:1-10, 1987.
271. Wilson RG et al: Alimentary lymphosarcoma in a horse with cutaneous manifestations, *Equine Vet J* 17:148-150, 1985.
272. van den Hoven R, Franken P: Clinical aspects of lymphosarcoma in the horse: a clinical report of 16 cases, *Equine Vet J* 15:49-53, 1983.
273. Dopson LC et al: Immunosuppression associated with lymphosarcoma in two horses, *J Am Vet Med Assoc* 182:1239-1241, 1983.
274. Perryman LE, McGuire TC: Evaluation for immune system failures in horses and ponies, *J Am Vet Med Assoc* 176:1374-1377, 1980.
275. Furr MO et al: Immunodeficiency associated with lymphosarcoma in a horse, *J Am Vet Med Assoc* 201:307-309, 1992.
276. Ahmed SA et al: Immunologic studies of a horse with lymphosarcoma, *Vet Immunol Immunopathol* 38:229-239, 1993.
277. Perryman LE et al: Biochemical and functional characterization of lymphocytes from a horse with lymphosarcoma and IgM deficiency, *Comp Immunol Microbiol Infect Dis* 7:53-62. 1984.
278. Rebhun WC, Bertone A: Equine lymphosarcoma, *J Am Vet Med Assoc* 184:720-721, 1984.
279. Staempfli HR et al: An unusual case of lymphoma in a mare, *Equine Vet J* 20:141-143, 1988.
280. Mair TS, Brown PJ: Clinical and pathological features of thoracic neoplasia in the horse, *Equine Vet J* 25:220-223, 1993.
281. Kannegieter NJ, Alley MR: Ataxia due to lymphosarcoma in a young horse, *Aust Vet J* 64:377-379, 1987.
282. Rousseaux CG, Doige CE, Tuddenham TJ: Epidural lymphosarcoma with myelomalacia in a seven-year-old Arabian gelding, *Can Vet J* 30:751-753, 1989.
283. Zeman DH et al: Vertebral lymphosarcoma as the cause of hind limb paresis in a horse, *J Vet Diag Invest* 1:187-188, 1989.
284. Williams MA et al: Lymphosarcoma associated with neurological signs and abnormal cerebrospinal fluid in two horses, *Prog Vet Neurol* 3:51-56, 1992.
285. Lester GD et al: Primary meningeal lymphoma in a horse, *J Am Vet Med Assoc* 201:1219-1221, 1992.
286. Chaffin MK et al: Ultrasonographic characteristics of splenic and hepatic lymphosarcoma in three horses, *J Am Vet Med Assoc* 201:743-747, 1992.
287. Rebhun WC, Del Piero F: Ocular lesions in horses with lymphosarcoma: 21 cases (1977-1997), *J Am Vet Med Assoc* 212:852-854, 1998.
288. Finley MR et al: Paraneoplastic pruritus and alopecia in a horse with diffuse lymphoma, *J Am Vet Med Assoc* 213:102-104, 1998.
289. Platt H: Observations on the pathology of non-alimentary lymphomas in the horse, *J Comp Pathol* 98:177-194, 1988.
290. Marr CM, Love S, Pirie HM: Clinical, ultrasonographic and pathological findings in a horse with splenic lymphosarcoma and pseudohyperparathyroidsim, *Equine Vet J* 21:221-226, 1989.
291. Mair TS, Yeo SP, Lucke VM: Hypercalcaemia and soft tissue mineralisation associated with lymphosarcoma in two horses, *Vet Rec* 126:99-101, 1990.
292. Zicker SC, Wilson WD, et al: Differentiation between intra-abdominal neoplasms and abscesses in horses, using clinical and laboratory data: 40 cases (1973-1988), *J Am Vet Med Assoc* 196:1130-1134, 1990.
293. Reef VB, Dyson SS, Beech J: Lymphosarcoma and associated immune-mediated hemolytic anemia and thrombocytopenia in horses, *J Am Vet Med Assoc* 184:313-317, 1984.
294. Mackey VS, Wheat JD: Reflections on the diagnostic approach to multicentric lymphosarcoma in an aged Arabian mare, *Equine Vet J* 17:467-469, 1985.
295. Adams R et al: Malignant lymphoma in three horses with ulcerative pharyngitis, *J Am Vet Med Assoc* 193:674-676, 1988.
296. Sweeney CR, Gillette DM: Thoracic neoplasia in equids: 35 cases (1967-1987), *J Am Vet Med Assoc* 195:374-377, 1989.
297. Henson KL et al: Regression of subcutaneous lymphoma following removal of an ovarian granulosa–theca cell tumor in a horse, *J Am Vet Med Assoc* 212:1419-1422, 1998.
298. Johnson PJ: Dermatologic tumors (excluding sarcoids), *Vet Clin North Am (Equine Pract)* 14:625-658, 1998.

MYELOPROLIFERATIVE DISEASE

GARY P. CARLSON

A rare form of myelogenous neoplasia associated with abnormal proliferation of bone marrow elements has been recognized in the horse.[299-306] The myelophthisic changes in bone marrow result in failure of normal erythrocyte, thrombocyte, and leukocyte production. Affected animals are often relatively young (i.e., less than 5 years of age, with a range 10 months to 9 years). Variable clinical signs may develop over a period of weeks to months and often include poor performance, depression, weight loss, intermittent fever, lymphadenopathy, splenomegaly, edema, petechial and ecchymotic hemorrhages, and anemia. These signs largely relate to the failure of normal production of marrow elements, resulting in blood loss caused by thrombocytopenia or infections secondary to neutropenia. Hematologic features generally include anemia, thrombocytopenia, and neutropenia. Atypical cells may be found in the peripheral blood, and frank leukemia (granulocytic,[302-304] myelomonocytic,[299-301,304,306] or eosinophilic[303]) may be noted. Bone marrow aspiration or biopsy reveals neoplastic infiltration and disruption of marrow architecture with loss of normal marrow elements. Special staining procedures are often required to determine neoplastic cell type.

Myeloproliferative disease should be considered in animals with vague signs of depression, recurrent fever, and petechial hemorrhages that have hematologic evidence of thrombocytopenia, neutropenia, and nonregenerative anemia. The presence of abnormal cells in the circulation and neoplastic infiltration of the bone marrow confirm the diagnosis. At necropsy neoplastic infiltration may be confined largely to the bone marrow, but the spleen, lymph nodes, and other internal organs often are involved. Intravascular leukostasis may contribute to thrombus formation and blood loss,[299] and local infections or bacteremia may be noted.[300] The prognosis for these animals is highly unfavorable and no effective treatment is available at present.

REFERENCES

299. Boudreaux MK et al: Intravascular leukostasis in a horse with myelomonocytic leukemia, *Vet Pathol* 21:544-546, 1984.
300. Brumbaugh GW et al: Myelomonocytic myeloproliferative disease in a horse, *J Am Vet Med Assoc* 180:313-316, 1982.
301. Burkhardt E, Saldern F, Huskamp B: Monocytic leukemia in a horse, *Vet Pathol* 21:394-398, 1984.
302. Lewis HB: A case of granulocytic leukemia in the horse, *Proc Intern Symp Equine Hematol Am Assoc (Equine Pract)* 1:141-143, 1975.
303. Morris DD et al: Eosinophilic myeloproliferative disorder in a horse, *J Am Vet Med Assoc* 185:993-996, 1984.
304. Searcy GP, Orr JP: Chronic granulocytic leukemia in a horse, *Can Vet J* 22:148-151, 1981.
305. Bienzle D, Hughsin SL, Vernau W: Acute myelomonocytic leukemia in a horse, *Can Vet J* 34:36-37, 1993.
305. Mori T et al: Acute myelomonocytic leukemia in a horse, *Vet Pathol* 28:344-346, 1991.

VETERINARY INFECTIONS WITH GRANULOCYTOTROPIC EHRLICHIEAE (*E. PHAGOCYTOPHILIA* and *E. EQUI*)

JOHN E. MADIGAN

Ehrlichia phagocytophila is a tick-borne, granulocytotropic *Ehrlichia* organism known to infect goats, sheep, and cattle in Europe.[307,308] The disease caused by this agent was first recognized in 1932[309] and is called tick-borne fever (TBF). The etiologic agent was identified in 1939 as a rickettsia[310] and later was classified as *E. phagocytophila* (*Cytoecetes phagocytophila*). The organisms can be identified in circulating granulocytes,[311,312] but histopathologic examinations have not revealed specific clues to pathogenesis.[307,313,314] The ultrastructural morphology of the bacterium is identical to that of other species of *Ehrlichia*.[311,315] The infection is transmitted by nymphal or adult *Ixodes ricinus* ticks, and although transstadial transmission of infectivity is well documented, transovarial transmission has not been demonstrated.[316] In fact, *E. phagocytophila* persists in blood after recovery in untreated hosts for up to 2 years.[311] The peak incidence of the disease coincides with emergence and activity of ticks in the spring and fall.[317] Prevalence estimates are scarce, but some authors suggest that TBF may be a dominant factor in the development of fatal staphylococcal pyemia,[318-320] which results in the death of between 1% to 2% of the entire sheep population of Great Britain per year.[317]

The infection in sheep is characterized by an incubation period of between 3 to 13 days, and, if untreated, the febrile phase lasts approximately 10 days.[311,316] During this febrile phase, the animals appear dull and listless, lose body weight, develop thrombocytopenia, develop leukopenia from decreases in both absolute neutrophil and lymphocyte counts,[308,318,321,322] and have increasing numbers of infected neutrophils.[311] The illness resolves after 1 to 12 days, but relapse occasionally occurs after primary untreated infection. Splenectomy and other inflammatory disturbances have resulted in recrudescence up to 1 year after infection.[311] Tickborne fever in sheep is a strong risk factor for severe concurrent or secondary bacterial, fungal, and viral infections,[323-327] as well as hemorrhages.[314] Although TBF is benign if uncomplicated, the mortality rate in complicated cases has been reported as being as high as 24%.[316,317] TBF may be easily treated with tetracyclines.[317]

EQUINE GRANULOCYTIC EHRLICHIOSIS

Equine granulocytic ehrlichiosis (EGE) is a rickettsial disease of horses first reported in the late 1960s in the foothills of northern California. The etiologic agent is *Ehrlichia equi*, a coccobacillary gram-negative organism with a tropism for neutrophils. Clinical manifestations include fever, lethargy, anorexia, limb edema, thrombocytopenia, and petechial hemorrhages. The vector of EGE is *Ixodes* spp. ticks. The disease is being diagnosed with increasing frequency in the United States with cases confirmed in California, Washington, Oregon, New Jersey, Colorado, Illinois, Minnesota, Connecticut, Florida, Wisconsin, and outside the United States, in Canada, Brazil and northern Europe.

ETIOLOGIC AGENT. *Ehrlichia equi* belongs to the *E. phagocytophila* complex of ehrlichial agents, which includes *E. phagocytophila*, the agent of tick-borne fever of ruminants in Europe and the recently reported agent of human granulocytic ehrlichiosis (HGE) in the United States and Europe. The members of this genogroup have similar morphology and neutrophil cell tropism, and they are very closely related serologically and genetically to one another.[328,329] The DNA sequences of the 16S rRNA gene from the peripheral blood of naturally infected horses in Connecticut and California are identical with that of the HGE agent and differ only slightly from the published 16S rRNA gene sequences of *E. equi*.[329,330] Moreover, infected human blood from HGE patients injected into horses causes typical equine ehrlichiosis, which can be transmitted to other horses. It induces protection in horses to subsequent challenge with *E. equi*.[332,333] Recently, granulocytic *Ehrlichia* organisms from horses and from humans have been grown in HL60 human leukemia cell cultures.[334]

CLINICAL MANIFESTATIONS. Clinical signs of EGE include fever, lethargy, partial anorexia, limb edema, mild petechiation, icterus, ataxia, and reluctance to move.[335,336] Cases of the disease occur in the fall, winter, and spring in the western United States and are associated with tick exposure. The incubation period is 10 to 20 days; this is based on the time of onset of clinical signs in horses that had presumptive exposure to ticks while on a trail ride before returning to a nonendemic area for EGE.[337] The initial stage of the disease is characterized by the development of a fever and may be mistaken for a viral infection. Limb edema and more severe signs of disease develop by days 3 to 5, with fever and illness lasting 10 to 14 days in untreated horses. Rarely, there is cardiac involvement with development of premature ventricular beats that may be associated with myocardial vasculitis.[338] The disease is normally self-limiting in untreated horses; fatalities can occur, however, from injury secondary to trauma caused by incoordination, and from secondary infection, presumably resulting from *E. equi*-induced immunosuppression.[336] Clinical signs can vary in severity depending on the age of the infected animal, with horses less than 3 to 4 years of age experiencing milder signs with minimal limb edema. Abortion has not been observed in pregnant mares nor has laminitis been a reported feature of the clinical syndrome.[336]

HEMATOLOGIC FINDINGS. Anemia, leukopenia, thrombocytopenia, and inclusion bodies within neutrophils or eosinophils are the characteristic hematologic findings in EGE affected horses.[335,336] The inclusion bodies are pleomorphic, blue-gray to dark blue in color, and often have a spokewheel appearance.[337]

DIAGNOSIS. Confirmation of a provisional clinical diagnosis of EGE is based on the clinical signs, hematological abnormalities (i.e., leukopenia and thrombocytopenia, and demonstration of the characteristic inclusion bodies representing morulae of *E. equi* in at least three neutrophils in a blood smear. The number of cells containing these inclusions varies from less than 1% of cells initially, to 20% to 30% of the neutrophils by day 3 to 5 of infection. The inclusions can readily be detected in buffy-coat smears of peripheral blood stained with Giemsa or Wright's stain. Alternatively, a diagnosis of EGE may be confirmed by demonstrating a significant (fourfold or greater) rise in antibody titer to *E. equi* using the indirect fluorescent antibody test.[338] Recently, a polymerase chain reaction (PCR) assay has been developed for *E. equi* and found to be highly sensitive and specific.[339] The differential diagnosis for EGE includes purpura hemorrhagica, liver disease, equine viral arteritis, and encephalitis.

EPIDEMIOLOGY. In recent years, EGE has been successfully transmitted by the tick *Ixodes pacificus*.[339] Ticks are commonly found on clinical patients, and the seasonality of the disease strongly supports *Ixodes* spp. tick transmission.[335] There is no information on the vector competence of other tick vectors at this time. Horses from endemic areas have a higher seroprevalence of antibody to *E. equi* than horses from nonendemic areas, suggesting the occurrence of subclinical infection in some animals.[336] Subclinical infection may be rather common in endemic areas based on studies of horse farms where a single case of clinical *E. equi* may occur yearly and yet nearly 50% of horses on that farm had evidence of antibody to *E. equi*.[336] Persistence of *E. equi* has not been demonstrated in naturally or experimentally infected animals.

TREATMENT AND PREVENTION. The intravenous administration of oxytetracycline at a rate of 7 mg/kg body weight once daily for 5 to 7 days has been an effective treatment for EGE. Defervescence occurs quickly, within 24 hours of the onset of treatment. On rare occasions, horses treated for less than 7 days relapse within the following 30 days. A chronic form of E. equi infection has not been reported. At the present time there is no vaccine available against EGE and prevention is limited to observance of tick control measures.

Equine granulocytic ehrlichiosis should be considered in a differential diagnosis for horses presenting with a febrile illness and known or presumptive tick exposure in many areas of North America and Europe. Studies have failed to demonstrate persistence of *E. equi* in horses, suggesting that horses are an unlikely reservoir host. It appears horses acquire infection in the same manner as humans, by exposure to infected ticks. No direct transmission of *E. equi* from horses to humans has been reported nor would it be expected to occur based on the epidemiologic features of the infection.

REFERENCES

307. Gordon WS et al: "Tick-borne fever" (a hitherto undescribed disease of sheep), *J Comp Pathol Ther* 65:301-307, 1932.
308. Hudson JR: The recognition of tick-borne fever as a disease of cattle, *Br Vet J* 106:3-17, 1950.
309. Gordon WS et al: Studies in louping-ill, *J Comp Pathol Ther* 45:106-140, 1932.
310. Gordon WS, Brownlee A, Wilson DR: Studies in louping-ill, tick-borne fever and scrapie. In *Program and Abstracts of the Third International Conference on Microbiology*, New York, 1940, pp 362-363.
311. Foggie A: Studies on the infectious agent of tick-borne fever in sheep, *J Pathol Bacteriol* 63:1-15, 1951.
312. Tuomi J, von Bonsdorff CH: Electron microscopy of tick-borne fever agent in bovine and ovine phagocytizing leukocytes, *J Bacteriol* 92:1478-1492, 1966.
313. Munro R et al: Pulmonary lesions in sheep following experimental infection by *Ehrlichia phagocytophila* and *Chlamydia psittaci, J Comp Pathol* 92:117-129, 1982.
314. Foster WNM, Foggie A, Nisbet DI: Haemorrhagic enteritis in sheep experimentally infected with tick-borne fever, *J Comp Pathol* 78:255-258, 1968.
315. Rikihisa Y: The tribe Ehrlichieae and ehrlichial diseases, *Clin Microbiol Rev* 4:286-308, 1991.
316. MacLeod JR, Gordon WS: Studies in tick-borne fever of sheep. I, Transmission by the tick *Ixodes ricinus*, with a description of the disease produced, *Parisitology* 25:273-285, 1933.
317. Brodie TA, Holmes PH, Urquhart GM: Some aspects of tick-borne diseases of British sheep, *Vet Rec* 118:415-418, 1986.
318. Foggie A: The effect of tick-borne fever on the resistance of lambs to staphylococci, *J Comp Pathol* 66:278-285, 1956.
319. Foggie A: Further experiments on the effect of tick-borne fever infection on the susceptibility of lambs to staphylococci, *J Comp Pathol* 67:369-377, 1957.
320. Webster KA, Mitchell GBB: Experimental production of tick pyaemia, *Vet Rec* 119:186-187, 1986.
321. Taylor AW, Holman HH, Gordon WS: Attempts to reproduce the pyaemia associated with tick-bite, *Vet Rec* 53:337-344, 1941.
322. Foster WNM, Cameron AE: Thrombocytopenia in sheep associated with experimental tick-borne infection, *J Comp Pathol* 78:251-254, 1968.
323. Gilmour NJL, Brodie TA, Holmes PH: Tick-borne fever and pasteurellosis in sheep, *Vet Rec* 111:512, 1982.
324. Overas J: Disease in sheep kept on Ixodes ricinus infected pastures, *Norsk Veterinaer Tidzskrift* 83:561-567, 1972.
325. Gronestol H, Ulvund MJ: Listerial septicaemia in sheep associated with tick borne fever (*Ehrlichia ovis*), *Acta Vet Scand* 18:575-577, 1977.
326. Batungbacal MR, Scott GR: Tick-borne fever and concurrent parainfluenza-3 virus infection in sheep, *J Comp Pathol* 92:415-428, 1982.
327. Jamieson S: Some aspects of immunity to tick-borne fever in hogs, *Vet Rec* 59:201-202, 1947.
328. Chen S et al: Identification of a granulocytotropic *Ehrlichia* species as the etiologic agent of human disease, *J Clin Microbiol* 32:589-595, 1994.
329. Dumler JS et al: Serologic cross-reactions among *Ehrlichia equi, Ehrlichia phagocytophila*, and human granulocytic *Ehrlichia, J Clin Microbiol* 33:1098-1103, 1995.
330. Chae JS et al: Comparison of the nucleotide sequences of 16S rRNA, 444 Ep-ank, and groESL heat shock operon genes in naturally occurring *Ehrlichia equi* and human granulocytic ehrlichiosis agent isolates from northern California, *J Clin Microbiol* 38:1364-1369, 2000.
331. Madigan JE et al: Identification of an enzootic diarrhea "Shasta River crud" in northern California as Potomac horse fever, *J Equine Vet Sci* 17:270-272, 1997.
332. Barlough JE et al: Protection against Ehrlichia equi is conferred by prior infection with the human granulocytotropic *Ehrlichia* (HGE agent), *J Clin Microbiol* 33:3333-3334, 1995.
333. Madigan JE et al: Evidence for a high rate of false-positive results with the indirect fluorescent antibody test for *Ehrlichia risticii* antibody in horses, *J Am Vet Med Assoc* 207:1448-1453, 1995.
334. Goodman JL et al: Direct cultivation of the causative agent of human granulocytic ehrlichiosis, *N Engl J Med* 334:209-215, 1996.
335. Gribble DH: Equine ehrlichiosis, *J Am Vet Med Assoc* 155:462-469, 1969.
336. Madigan JE et al: Seroepidemiologic survey of antibodies to *Ehrlichia equi* in horses of northern California, *J Am Vet Med Assoc* 196:1962-1964, 1990.
337. Madigan J: Personal communication.
338. Gribble DH: Equine ehrlichiosis PhD thesis. Davis, Ca, University of California, Davis, 1970.
339. Madigan JE et al: Transmission and passage in horses of the agent of human granulocytic ehrlichiosis, *J Infect Dis* 172:1141-1144, 1995.
340. Barlough JE et al: Nested polymerase chain reaction for detection of *Ehrlichia equi* genomic DNA in horses and ticks (*Ixodes pacificus*), *Vet Parasitol* 63:319-329, 1996.
341. Rikihisa Y et al: Serosurvey of horses with evidence of equine monocytic ehrlichiosis, *J Am Vet Med Assoc* 197:1327-1332, 1990.

ANTHRAX

ARLENA B. PIPKIN

DEFINITION AND ETIOLOGY. Anthrax, also known as "splenic fever," "charbon," "milzbrand," and "woolsorter's disease," is an acute, contagious, and usually fatal septicemia affecting a wide range of mammalian species, including humans. Most commonly affected are cattle and sheep and, less

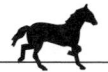

commonly, horses and goats. Although all ages are susceptible, older animals are more commonly affected. This may reflect grazing habits rather than susceptibility. Also, bulls are more at risk than cows.[342] The causative bacterium, *Bacillus anthracis,* is a nonmotile, capsulated, blunt, spore-forming, aerobic bacilli.[343] *B. anthracis* survives as part of the normal bacterial flora found in many alkaline soils.

CLINICAL SIGNS AND DIFFERENTIALS. Anthrax can occur as an acute, subacute, or rarely, as a chronic disease. The incubation period is usually 3 to 7 days but can range from 1 to 14 days. The clinical signs of anthrax vary, but the most common sign is sudden death. Although the ultimate outcome is usually death, reports of chronic anthrax exist.[344]

The clinical signs in ruminants include marked pyrexia, rumen stasis, anorexia, hematuria, bloody diarrhea, abrupt decrease in milk production, and possibly blood-tinged or yellow milk. A period of stimulation and aggression is usually followed by depression, muscle tremors, respiratory distress, and convulsions. Death usually occurs in 1 to 3 days. Nonautolyzed carcasses typically exude bloody discharges from body orifices and show marked splenic swelling. Chronic anthrax in ruminants may be characterized by localized edematous swellings on the shoulders, ventral neck, and thorax.[345]

The clinical signs of anthrax in the horse include marked pyrexia, colic, enteritis, dyspnea, and subcutaneous edematous swellings on the ventral neck, thorax, and abdomen and may extend to the prepuce and mammary gland. Death usually occurs in 2 to 4 days.

Differential diseases include most causes of sudden death: acute fatal bloat, malignant edema, blackleg, Black's disease, acute poisonings, enteritis, lightning strike, and death after epistaxis caused by vena caval syndrome. Anthrax should be considered in the list of differential considerations when an animal is suddenly found dead after having been observed in apparent good health during the preceding 24 hours.[343]

PATHOPHYSIOLOGY. Anthrax infections occur by spore ingestion, inhalation, or cutaneous penetration. The most common route of infection is by ingestion, which may be facilitated by the grazing of abrasive forages allowing penetration of the spore through breaks in the oral mucosa. *B. anthracis* possesses two primary virulence factors: a poly D-glutamic acid capsule, which protects the organism from phagocytosis and lytic antibodies, and a toxin composed of edema factor (EF), protective antigen (PA), and lethal factor (LF). These factors are independently innocuous, but the combination of PA and LF produces lethality in some species.[345] Because of these factors, lesions produced by anthrax involve the widespread damage of the reticuloendothelial system and vasculature. Death results from secondary changes, including diffuse edema formation, tissue damage, acute renal failure, anoxia, and shock.

EPIDEMIOLOGY. Anthrax is distributed worldwide. South Dakota, Arkansas, Missouri, Louisiana, Texas, and California have the highest incidence and recurrence rates in the United States. Outbreaks are irregular and may be traced back to a previous occurrence on that premise. Typically anthrax occurs during the warm, dry summer months of July, August, and September, when grass is short and dusty conditions prevail. However, anthrax has been known to occur in cold climates. Epizootics tend to follow periods of marked climatic or ecologic changes such as a heavy rainfall or flooding preceded by drought or dusty conditions.

In the unopened carcass, the vegetative organisms are rapidly destroyed (1 to 2 hours) at ambient temperatures often experienced during the summer. Recontamination of the soil develops as a result of the bloody exudates that occur at death, on-site necropsies, and predation. On exposure to oxygen the bacteria form spores that are highly resistant to chemical and physical agents and to the adversity of the environ-

ment for as long as 37 years.[346] However, bacterial regrowth followed by new spore formation undoubtedly occurs.

Biting flies and insects have been found to harbor anthrax, but the incidence of this type of vector transmission is unclear. Although the main reservoir of anthrax spores is alkaline soils, spores can be found in animal-origin feed, fertilizer, water contaminated by animal-product processing wastes, and wool products.

NECROPSY FINDINGS. It is recommended that a necropsy not be performed on a carcass suspected of having anthrax. At the onset of a disease outbreak, a carcass may be necropsied, but subsequent carcasses should remain unopened to reduce environmental contamination and health risk to personnel.[346] A necropsy can be safely performed using simple precautions such as gloves and a facial mask and in an area that can be easily and thoroughly disinfected.

The hallmark features of anthrax include black tarry exudates from body orifices, failure of blood to clot, incomplete rigor mortis, and splenomegaly. A variety of other necropsy findings include serosal and mucosal hemorrhages on the abdomen, thorax, epicardium, pericardium, and alimentary tract and erosions of Peyer's patches. Areas of gelatinous edema in skeletal muscles, organs, subcutis, and especially in the lymph node at the site of entry into the body, as well as serosanguinous peritoneal and pericardial effusions, may be present. The spleen can be enlarged two to four times and may appear dark and soft from rapid liquefaction. Red pulpy exudates appear from splenic capsule incisions.

A diagnosis of anthrax can be confirmed without a complete necropsy if appropriate tests are performed. Various laboratory tests can be performed to determine the presence of *B. anthracis*: bacterial staining and culture, string-of pearls test,[347] ELISA test, fluorescent antibodies, and animal inoculation. The organisms may be detected in blood collected from a superficial vessel (ear or jugular vein) and transported to the laboratory through sealed syringe, sterile swab, or blood smear. Also, an intact eyeball or section of spleen sealed in a leak-proof bag can be used for bacterial isolation. Postmortem samples should be collected from untreated animals dead less than 12 hours. Antemortem identification of *B. anthracis* is often unrewarding because bacteremia occurs shortly before death.

Perhaps the simplest and quickest determination of anthrax is through the use of staining techniques in combination with clinical signs, history of endemic areas, and necropsy findings. Various stains can be used, including Giemsa, Loeffler's, methylene blue, or Wright's stain. Using Giemsa staining, the bacilli should appear in single or short chains with purplish-pink capsules. With a Gram stain, young bacteria will appear gram-positive, but older organisms may appear gram-negative. Early sample collection is necessary because other motile, capsulated bacilli such as *Clostridium perfringens* and other *Bacillus* spp. rapidly contaminate the carcass. Retrospective diagnosis using ELISA for detection of anticapsule antibodies has been described.[348]

TREATMENT AND PROGNOSIS. Because of the rapid onset and high mortality rate (90%) associated with anthrax, there is often insufficient time to initiate treatment before death. If anthrax is suspected, immediate segregation of infected animals is advised. Early supportive and antimicrobial therapy may be useful. *B. anthracis* is highly susceptible to a wide range of antimicrobials, including penicillin, streptomycin, and tetracycline. The first dose of antimicrobials should be administered intravenously and can be continued intramuscularly for at least 5 days. In some countries an anthrax antiserum is available and can be administered at 50 to 100 ml SQ 2 to 4 times per day.[349] Because of limited availability and cost, this antiserum is not commonly used. Regardless of therapy, the prognosis is guarded in most cases, but survival has been documented.[349]

PREVENTION AND CONTROL. Economic losses result from animal deaths, property depreciation, quarantine enforcement, and the cost of immunization programs, treatment practices, and dead animal disposal.[345] Prevention and control are paramount in limiting the disease incidence and economic losses that occur with an anthrax outbreak. The perpetuation of anthrax in a livestock population is commonly a sequential cycle involving spores, a susceptible host, disease, death, dissemination of organisms from the carcass, and spore development.[343] Because of the survivability of spores in the environment, the elimination of the susceptible host should disrupt the disease cycle. This can be accomplished through the use of a viable, avirulent, noncapsulated spore vaccine (Stern-strain spore vaccine).[344] Immunity is established within 1 week, and, although a repeated dose in 4 to 5 weeks is recommended for initial vaccination, a single annual dose should provide sufficient protective immunity for subsequent seasons.[344] The vaccine is approved for horses, cattle, sheep, and pigs.

Annual vaccination in endemic areas is recommended for cattle and sheep 2 to 4 weeks before the onset of summer and during disease outbreaks in endemic areas. There is a 60-day slaughter withdrawal after administration of live spore vaccines. Because the vaccine is a viable spore product, the spore must germinate and grow to stimulate host immunity. If antibiotics are administered before and during the first week after vaccination, immunity may be minimal, and revaccination is recommended in 4 to 5 weeks. Two vaccine doses may also produce more solid immunity in the face of an outbreak.[350]

Before vaccinating dairy cattle, official regulatory advice should be sought. Milk should be discarded for 2 to 3 days after vaccination because a human health hazard may exist through the remote possibility of spore passage into milk. However, one study suggests that dairy cattle recently vaccinated do not shed detectable levels of spores in the milk and therefore do not pose a human health risk.[351]

Outbreaks of anthrax must be reported to the local regulatory and public health officials. The control of anthrax depends on two factors: hygiene and carcass disposition. Both the animal population and the farm should be quarantined from the onset of anthrax identification and remain quarantined for 2 weeks after the last diagnosed case. All susceptible animals should be vaccinated, and all animals submitted for salvage slaughter should be condemned.

Necropsies should not be performed in the pasture or pen areas. All contaminated carcasses, bedding, and feedstuff should be burned or buried at least 2 meters below ground surface to decrease environmental contamination. The use of quicklime (calcium oxide) applied on top of the buried debris has been recommended. If contamination occurs, everything exposed should be disinfected, including the soil, walls, and equipment. Most ordinary disinfectants kill the vegetative form; but, once the bacteria is exposed to oxygen, it sporulates in 1 to 2 hours, and the spores are difficult to kill. Cleansing with a pressurized spray of 5% aqueous lye solution or exposing spores to 10% formaldehyde for 15 minutes usually eliminates the spores. The incidence of anthrax appears to be decreasing. Some reasons for this may include: (1) use of a safe and effective vaccine, (2) indiscriminate use of antibiotics in the animal population, and (3) enforcement of regulations by animal health personnel that require reporting, quarantine measures, vaccination, and proper disposal of dead carcasses.[352]

REFERENCES

342. Kaufmann AF: Anthrax. In Howard JL, ed: *Current veterinary therapy (food animal practice)*, ed 2, Philadelphia, 1986, WB Saunders, pp 566-567.
343. Whitford HW: Factors affecting the laboratory diagnosis of anthrax, *J Am Vet Med Assoc* 173:1467-1469, 1978.
344. Turnbull PCB: Anthrax vaccines: past, present and future, *Vaccine* 9:533-539, 1991.
345. Jensen R, Swift BL: Diseases of the blood and blood-forming system: anthrax. In Kimberling CV, ed: *Diseases of sheep*, ed 3, Philadelphia, 1988, Lea & Febiger, pp 359-364.
346. Whitford HW: Anthrax: update and overview, *Proceedings of the Twenty-sixth Annual Meeting of the Association of Veterinary Laboratory Diagnosticians*, 1983, pp 1-12.
347. Balie WE, Stowe EC: A simplified test for identification of *Bacillus anthracis*, Abstract of the Seventy-seventh Annual Meeting, American Society for Microbiology, 1977, Washington, DC, C-80:48.
348. Harrison LH et al: Evaluation of serologic tests for diagnosis of anthrax after an outbreak of cutaneous anthrax in Paraguay, *J Infect Dis* 160:706-710, 1989.
349. Gill IJ: Antibiotic therapy in the control of an outbreak of anthrax in dairy cows, *Aust Vet J* 58:214-215, 1982.
350. Salmon DD, Ferrier GR: Postvaccination occurrence of anthrax in cattle, *Vet Rec* 130:140-141, 1991.
351. Tanner WB et al: Public health aspects of anthrax vaccination of dairy cattle, *J Am Vet Med Assoc* 173:1465-1466, 1978.
352. Blood DC et al: *Veterinary medicine*, ed 6, London, 1983, Baillière Tindall, pp 531-535.

LYME DISEASE (*BORRELIA BURGDORFERI* BORRELIOSIS)

JOHN E. MADIGAN

Lyme borreliosis is caused by a bacteria that is a member of the family Spirochaetaceae. Many *Borrelia* spp. have caused disease in human beings and domestic animals.[353,354] Lyme borreliosis is caused by *Borrelia burgdorferi*, first identified as a causative agent of an epidemic of juvenile inflammatory arthritis in children and adults in Old Lyme, Lyme, and East Haddam, Connecticut.[355,356] Hence, medical references commonly site "Lyme disease" when referring to infection with *B. burgdorferi*.[357,358]

EPIZOOTIOLOGY OF LYME BORRELIOSIS

B. burgdorferi is widely distributed in the northern hemisphere all over the world. Lyme borreliosis has been reported extensively in Europe, England, the Soviet Union, China, Japan, Southeast Asia, and South Africa.[358] *B. burgdorferi* is transmitted from ticks to humans and animals by ticks belonging to the *Ixodes ricinus* complex.[359] These ticks each feed three times during the larval, nymphal, and adult stages.[355] The larvae and nymphs feed on wild animals, and adults are found most commonly on deer.[359] On the east coast *Ixodes scapularis* ticks are the principle vector, whereas on the west coast *Ixodes pacificus*, the western black-legged tick, is the main vector identified.[360] *I. scapularis* is seen from the Atlantic coast to Oklahoma and Texas.[361] A much higher percentage of *I. scapularis* ticks (12% to 99%) will carry the spirochete compared with *I. pacificus*, in which the maximum number of infected ticks is 4% to 5%.[360,361] *I. scapularis* larval ticks acquire the spirochete principally from *Peromycus leucopus*, the white-footed mouse, and the nymphal stages are the major transmitters of disease to animals and humans.[362] With *I. pacificus* the California kangaroo rat, *Dipodomys californicus*, and the dusky-footed wood rat, *Neotoma fusicipes*, are the likely enzootic reservoirs of *B. burgdorferi*.[363]

B. burgdorferi is found in many arthropods, but the major route of transmission to animals and humans is believed to be limited to the *Ixodes* sp. ticks. Experimental studies have demonstrated that ticks may harbor and transmit several pathogens, the human granulocytic ehrlicheal agent, and *B. burgdorferi*, at the same time.[364] Exposure to ticks infected with *B. burgdorferi* produced seroconversion without detectable histopathologic changes except for skin lesions in experimental horses.[365] Most transmissions of *B. burgdorferi* oc-

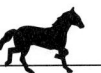

cur after the tick has been attached for 24 hours.[364] Birds are frequently infected with *B. burgdorferi* and may be responsible for the spread of the disease to new areas.[359]

PUBLIC HEALTH CONSIDERATIONS

Surveillance for Lyme disease was initiated by the Centers for Disease Control and Prevention in 1982, and in January 1991 it became nationally reportable. Cases have been reported from 46 states, and the annual number of Lyme disease cases has increased eighteenfold from 497 to 8803. It is now the most common tick transmitted disease in the United States.

B. burgdorferi organisms have been recovered from the urine of feral white-footed mice, *Peromyscus leucopus*.[367] Contact transmission has been reported between white-footed mice,[367] further complicating the understanding of transmission. Because of lack of any proof to the contrary, it is generally believed at this time that any potential increased risk to humans from infected animals is attributable to animals bringing ticks into areas of human habitation rather than any animal transmission.[368]

MOLECULAR BIOLOGY. Immunochemical analysis of North American strains of *B. burgdorferi* reveal two abundant surface proteins termed outer surface protein A (OspA) 30 to 32 kd and another outer surface protein B (OspB) that is 34 to 36 kd.[369] The 41-kd antigen is located on the flagellum and is similar to the flagellar antigens of other spirochetes.[370] All isolates to date have four to nine pieces of extrachromosomal plasmid DNA. Plasmid may code for proteins that are important in pathogenicity because the loss of infectivity of isolates that have been heavily passaged in the laboratory correlates with the loss of particular plasmid in culture.[371] Recent work suggests that *B. burgdorferi* can vary its antigenicity like the relapsing fever–causing Borrelia such as *Borrelia hermsii* do, although by a different mechanism and by using subtle alterations in the genome.[372]

Clinical Reports of Lyme Borreliosis

EQUIDS. Horses from endemic areas have serologic evidence of exposure.[373-376] Attempts have been made to correlate individual cases of arthritis, uveitis, or brain infection with this organism.[377-379] Experimental infection has produced seroconversion and shedding of the organism in the urine and seroconversion in contact controls.[380] In the United Kingdom, most seropositive horses do not show clinical signs of disease.[381]

RUMINANTS. Although there are some reports in the literature of seropositive animals with arthritis, the evaluation performed on the patients makes it difficult to determine if *B. burgdorferi* was a cause of the symptoms.[382] It appears at this time that many ruminants are seropositive to *B. burgdorferi* but do not have clinical signs. Whether these tests lack specificity in the ruminant or represent a host-adapted strain of the Borrelia organism is unknown.[383] A recent report correlates exposure of *I. scapularis* ticks in dairy cattle with titers to *B. burgdorferi*.[384] An attempt to develop a more specific test in cattle using the 41-kd flagellin antigen has recently been reported.[385]

Diagnosis

Definitive diagnosis is difficult in animals from endemic areas with signs referable to the organ systems often affected by *B. burgdorferi* borreliosis. Apparently many animals with lameness or joint disorders respond well to antimicrobial treatments and are seropositive and therefore suspected of having Lyme disease.

Culture of the organism requires special media (BSK) and is difficult but may be possible from blood, urine, or CSF. Polymerase chain reaction technology may aid the diagnosis in the future. It is quite clear that a positive serology is no grounds for treatment when no clinical signs are present. Clinical diagnosis is probably the most important component after a careful history, examination, and laboratory and radiographic evaluation.

Testing for *B. burgdorferi* Antibodies

A number of methods are available, including IFA, ELISA, and western blot.[384] Although numerous reports have found poor correlation with interlaboratory agreement,[386] I found IFA and indirect complement fixation testing to have good correlation among three laboratories.[387]

Recent evaluation of several kits for Lyme testing in offices have found very poor correlation. I would suggest finding a laboratory that has performed quality control on the assay and has the expertise to perform the assay. Quality control involves testing over 100 negative control animals from nonendemic areas and standardization of the assay at a particular titer or ELISA to eliminate false-positive results, as well as verification of positive sera.

Treatment

Antibiotic susceptibility of *B. burgdorferi* has been reported but may lack appropriate standardization.[388] *B. burgdorferi* is sensitive to tetracycline and moderately sensitive to penicillin. Amoxicillin, ceftriaxone, and imipenem are highly active against *B. burgdorferi*. Aminoglycosides, ciprofloxacin, and rifampin lack activity.[389] Doxycycline twice daily in humans has been frequently used. Probenecid and ampicillin or amoxicillin also have been used.[388] When central nervous system involvement is present, ceftriaxone or intravenous penicillin G has been used. The appropriate duration of therapy is unknown but is related to the stage of infection. Early infections are generally treated for 2 to 3 weeks.

Experimental studies have shown that vaccination with recombinant *B. burgdorferi* outer-surface protein A (eospA) protected ponies against infection from experimental challenge with ticks infected with *B. burgdorferi*.[390]

REFERENCES

353. Barbour AG, Hayes SF: Biology of *Borrelia* species, *Microbiol Rev* 50:381-400, 1986.
354. Southern PM, Sanford JP: Relapsing fever, *Medicine* 48:129-149, 1969.
355. Burgdorfer W et al: Lyme disease: a tick borne spirochetosis? *Science* 216:1317-1319, 1982.
356. Steere AC et al: Lyme arthritis: an epidemic of oligoarticular arthritis in children and adults in three Connecticut communities, *Arthritis Rheum* 20:7-17, 1979.
357. Barbour AG: Isolation and cultivation of Lyme disease spirochetes, *Yale J Biol Med* 57:521-525, 1984.
358. Schmid GP: The global distribution of Lyme disease, *Rev Infect Dis* 7:41-49, 1985.
359. Anderson JF: Epizootiology of Lyme borreliosis, *Scand J Infect Dis* 77(suppl):23-34, 1991.
360. Anderson JF: Epizootiology of *Borrelia* in *Ixodes* tick vectors and reservoir hosts, *Rev Infect Dis* 11(suppl 6):S1451-S1459, 1989.
361. Lane RS, Burgdorfer W: Spirochetes in mammals and ticks (Acari: Ixodidae) from a focus of Lyme borreliosis in California, *J Wildlife Dis* 24:1-9, 1988.
362. Donahue JG, Piesman J, Spielman A: Reservoir competence of white-footed mice for Lyme disease spirochetes, *Am J Trop Med Hyg* 36:92-96, 1987.
363. Lane RS, Brown RN: Wood rats and kangaroo rats: potential reservoirs of the Lyme disease spirochete in California, *J Med Entomol* 28:299-302, 1991.
364. Chang YF et al: Human granulocytic ehrlichiosis agent infection in a pony vaccinated with a *Borrelia burgdorferi* recombinant OspA vaccine and challenged by exposure to naturally infected ticks, *Clin Diagn Lab Immunol* 7:68-71, 2000.

365. Chang YF et al: Experimental infection of ponies with *Borrelia burgdorferi* by exposure to Ixodid ticks, *Vet Pathol* 37:68-76, 2000.

366. Piesman J et al: Duration of tick attachment and *Borrelia burgdorferi* transmission, *J Clin Microbiol* 25:557-558, 1987.

367. Burgess EC et al: Experimental inoculation of *Peromyscus* spp. with *Borrelia burgdorferi*: evidence of contact transmission, *Am J Trop Med Hyg* 35:355-359, 1986.

368. Eng TR A, et al: Greater risk of *Borrelia burgdorferi* infection in dogs than in people, *J Infect Dis* 158:1410-1411, 1988.

369. Barbour AG, Tessier SL, Hayes SF: Variation in a major surface protein of Lyme disease spirochetes, *Infect Immunol* 45:94-100, 1984.

370. Barbour AG et al: A *Borrelia*-specific monoclonal antibody binds to a flagellar epitope, *Infect Immunol* 52:549-554, 1986.

371. Hyde FW, Johnson RC: Characterization of a circular plasmid from *Borrelia burgdorferi*, etiologic agent of Lyme disease, *J Clin Microbiol* 25: 2203-2205, 1988.

372. Barbour AG: Molecular biology of antigenic variation in Lyme borreliosis and relapsing fever: a comparative analysis, *Scand J Infect Dis* 77(suppl):88-93, 1991.

373. Marcus LC et al: Antibodies to *Borrelia burgdorferi* in New England horses: serologic survey, *Am J Vet Res* 46:2570-2571, 1985.

374. Bernard WV et al: Serologic survey for *Borrelia burgdorferi* antibody in horses referred to a mid-Atlantic veterinary teaching hospital, *J Am Vet Med Assoc* 196:1255-1258, 1990.

375. Magnarelli LA, Anderson JF: Class-specific and polyvalent enzyme-linked immunosorbent assays for detection of antibodies to *Borrelia burgdorferi* equids, *J Am Vet Med Assoc* 195:1365-1368, 1989.

376. Madigan JE: Veterinary Lyme borreliosis, Abstract 59, *Proceedings of the American Association of Advancement of Science*, 1991.

377. Magnarelli LA et al: Borreliosis in equids in northeastern United States, *Am J Vet Res* 49:359-362, 1988.

378. Burgess EC, Gillette D, Picket JP: Arthritis and panuveitis as manifestations of *Borrelia burgdorferi* infection in a Wisconsin pony, *J Am Vet Med Assoc* 189:1340-1342, 1986.

379. Burgess EC, Mattison M: Encephalitis associated with *Borrelia burgdorferi* infection in a horse, *J Am Vet Med Assoc* 191:1457-1458, 1987.

380. Patterson WH: Lyme spirochetosis in equine: bacteriologic, epidemiologic, and clinical aspects of *Borrelia burgdorferi* infection in equine, *Proc ACVIM* 8:677-680, 1990.

381. Carter SD et al: *Borrelia burgdorferi* infection in UK horses, *Equine Vet J* 26:187-190, 1994.

382. Burgess EC, Gendron-Fitzpatrick A, Wright WO: Arthritis and systemic disease caused by *Borrelia burgdorferi* infection in a cow, *J Am Vet Med Assoc* 191:1468-1470, 1987.

383. Ryder JK: Lyme disease in dairy cattle: serologic and clinical presentations. *Proc ACVIM* 8:673-676, 1990.

384. Benxiu J, Collins MT: Seroepidemiologic survey of *Borrelia burgdorferi* exposure in dairy cattle in Wisconsin, *Am J Vet Res* 55:1228-1231, 1994.

385. Benxiu J, Thomas CB, Collins MT: Evaluation of an enzyme-linked immunosorbent assay that uses the 41-kd flagellin as the antigen for detection of antibodies to *Borrelia burgdorferi* in cattle, *Am J Vet Res* 55:1213-1219, 1994.

386. Corpuz M et al: Problems in the use of serologic tests for the diagnosis of Lyme disease, *Arch Intern Med* 151:1837-1840, 1991.

387. Lane RS, Lennette ET, Madigan JE: Interlaboratory and intra-laboratory comparisons of indirect immunofluorescence assays for serodiagnosis of Lyme disease, *J Clin Microbiol* 28:1774-1779, 1990.

388. Philipson A: Antibiotic treatment in Lyme borreliosis, *Scand J Infect Dis* 77(suppl):145-150, 1991.

389. Steere AC: Medical progress: Lyme disease, *N Engl J Med* 31:586-596, 1989.

390. Chang YF et al: Vaccination against lyme disease with recombinant *Borrelia burgdorferi* outer-surface protein A (rOspA) in horses, *Vaccine* 14:540-548, 1999.

TULAREMIA

BRADFORD P. SMITH

Tularemia is an infectious disease of humans, wild animals, livestock, and pets caused by *Pasteurella (Francisella) tularensis*. The organism is a nonspore-forming, gram-negative rod that survives frozen or in mud and water for long periods (over a year)[391] but only survives for hours in carcasses. The natural hosts are rabbits and rodents, and transmission to livestock occurs chiefly through ticks, fleas, deerflies, and other insects.[392] Sheep are the most commonly affected livestock species. Massive epidemics with a high mortality in range sheep have been reported.[392] Humans are stricken with a plaguelike illness when bitten by infected ticks, fleas, or insects and from handling infected rabbits. Sheep shearers may become infected by bites of parasites from the sheep.[390] Disease in horses has also been documented.[393] Oral infection from contaminated water occurs; thus fresh water should be provided.[392]

The disease causes an acute septicemia, with localization and granulomatous lesions in the organs (particularly the liver and spleen). Signs are very nonspecific, as expected with bacteremia, and include fever, anorexia, depression, and in some cases cough, rapid respiration, or diarrhea. Stiffness and edema of the limbs may be seen. The course of disease is usually 2 to 14 days.

Agglutination titers in recovered affected sheep range from 40 to 5000. Agglutination titers persist for very short periods (21 days) in horses,[392] probably because they measure mainly IgM. Diagnosis is based on culture of the organism from blood or organs.

Necropsy usually reveals ticks on the carcass. Often reddened or necrotic areas appear in and under the skin at the site of infected bites. Regional lymph nodes may be swollen and congested. Congestion and edema of the lungs are common. Differentials include other bacteremias such as *Pasteurella haemolytica* in sheep, *Hemophilus somnus* in cattle, *Mycoplasma mycoides* subsp. *mycoides*, in goats, and anthrax in all livestock. Treatment early in the course of infection is effective. Aminoglycosides, tetracyclines, or cephalosporins all would probably be beneficial initially until results of antimicrobial susceptibility testing are available. Insecticide removal of ticks from affected animals and herdmates is important. No vaccine is currently available; thus insect and tick control in endemic areas remains the major prevention. Because oral infection from contaminated water has also been documented, fresh water should be provided.

REFERENCES

391. Bell JF et al: Enigmatic resistance of sheep *(Ovis aries)* to infection by virulent *Francisella tularensis, Can J Comp Med* 42:310-315, 1978.

392. Jellison WL: *Tularemia in North America,* 1929-1974, Missoula, 1974, University of Montana.

393. Klaus KD, Newhall HJ, Mee D: Isolation of Pasteurella tularensis from foals, *J Bacteriol* 78:294-295, 1959.

CORYNEBACTERIUM PSEUDOTUBERCULOSIS INFECTION

MONICA R. ALEMAN
SHARON J. SPIER

DEFINITION. *Corynebacterium pseudotuberculosis* infections occur worldwide, and cause external and internal caseous lymphadenitis in sheep and goats, cutaneous excoriated granulomas, mammary, visceral or mixed infection in cattle, and ulcerative lymphangitis and external and internal abscesses in horses.[394-397] Subacute to chronic lymphadenitis and pneumonia have been reported in humans handling infected sheep.[398,399] Several zebras in the United States developed multiple internal abscesses and died weeks after being exposed to horses in California.[400] There have been reports of the disease in camels and buffalo.[401,402]

MICROBIOLOGY. *C. pseudotuberculosis* infection is caused by a 2-μm gram-positive intracellular, nonmotile, pleomorphic rod-shaped, facultative anaerobe.[394,403] *C. pseudotuberculosis* grows well at 37° C on blood agar in 24 to 48 hours, and it forms small, pinpoint, whitish, opaque colonies that are surrounded by a weak zone of hemolysis. Because of the high content of lipids in the bacterial cell wall, particularly corynomycolic acid, the colonies spatter in a flame can be pushed across the agar surface.[394] The high content of lipids may fa-

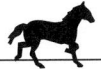

cilitate survival of the organism in macrophages.[404] Two species specific biotypes of *C. pseudotuberculosis* have been identified based on differences in nitrate reduction,[398] and DNA fingerprinting techniques.[405-406] Strains isolated from small ruminants are nitrate negative, strains from horses are nitrate-positive, whereas both strains have been isolated from cattle.[398,408] From the result of DNA studies, the terms "biovar *equi*" for nitrate-positive and "biovar *ovis*" for the nitrate-negative strains were proposed.[405] Two horses with ulcerative lymphangitis from different studies had a nitrate-negative isolate[395,406]; through ribotyping in 1 of the 2 horses, the isolate resembled the nitrate-positive isolates of equine origin rather than the nitrate-negative isolates from equine sheep and goats.[406] Recent studies revealed that there is more heterogeneity of the isolates of *C. pseudotuberculosis* from small ruminants and horses,[406,407,409] and concluded that nitrate reduction may not absolutely distinguish between the isolates as does ribotyping.[406] On the basis of ribotyping, sheep and goats have specific isolates throughout the world, and horses and cattle have two distinct groups of isolates depending on geographic location, one from the United States and the other from South Africa and Kenya.[406] Natural cross-species transmission does not seem to occur.[394]

C. pseudotuberculosis produces various exotoxins such as phospholipase D (PLD), sphingomyelinase, inhibitory factor of staphylococcal β hemolysin, hemolysis factor, dermanecrotoxins, and mouse lethality toxins.[410] Phospholipase D and sphingomyelinase are important in the pathogenesis of the disease because they hydrolyze lysophosphatidylcholine and sphingomyelin respectively, thus degrading the endothelial cell wall and increasing vascular permeability.[411] The synergistic activity of sphingomyelinase with the exotoxin of *Rhodococcus equi* in lysing red blood cells in agar forms the basis for the synergistic hemolysis inhibition (SHI) test.[412]

CLINICAL SIGNS AND DIFFERENTIAL DIAGNOSIS

Sheep and Goats. *C. pseudotuberculosis* causes caseous lymphadenitis (CLA) in sheep and goats worldwide. Caseous lymphadenitis is a major cause of poor production, premature culling, and mortality. There are two forms of CLA: external and internal abscesses.[413] The infection in small ruminants is primarily characterized by suppuration and necrosis of the large superficial lymph nodes. The external abscesses are found more commonly involving the mandibular, parotid, prefemoral, or prescapular lymph nodes and are often referred to as boils. The exudate present in those abscesses is thick or inspissated, and may appear white in sheep and greenish in goats.[394] A breed association with the type of CLA cutaneous lesions was observed in an outbreak in a commercial ram stud in Scotland.[414] Differential diagnosis should include abscesses caused by other organisms, trauma, seroma, hematoma, foreign body, injection reaction, and, less commonly, tumors. Because *C. pseudotuberculosis* infection represents a major herd health problem, culturing of the abscess to determine the causative agent is important. Mastitis occasionally develops.[396]

Internal abscesses, less common than external abscesses, can be found in the lungs, mediastinal, bronchial, kidneys, and mesenteric and lumbar lymph nodes.[413] Chronic weight loss is the most common presenting complaint. Other clinical signs are related to the organ or tissues affected. Other diagnostic procedures may be necessary for the differentiation of internal abscesses as the cause of weight loss. Signs of spinal cord compression by vertebral abscesses have been seen in lambs born in unsanitary conditions.[394] Knowledge of the local prevalence can help in the diagnosis of the infection when uncommon anatomic locations are affected. The prevalence of the infection (external and internal abscesses) in large breeding operations in endemic areas is estimated to be between 5% to 10%. In sheep and goats, humoral and cel-

lular immune responses develop after infection, and macrophages acquire the ability to kill the organism.[399]

Cattle. The infection in cattle occurs as a herd problem with a sporadic incidence. The most common clinical form affecting cattle is cutaneous excoriated granulomas. Other forms are mastitis and visceral and mixed infections.[396] In the most common form, the lesions appear as ulcerative granulomatous lesions as large as 20 cm in diameter and exuding pus and serum, with necrotic areas that are easily surgically removed, leaving granulation tissue underneath.[394,397] The location of the lesions is usually in the lateral exposed areas of the body: face, neck, thorax, and flanks (Fig. 35-2). The exudate varies from bloody to thick greenish in color. The lesions heal spontaneously in 2 to 4 weeks and do not appear to cause significant illness or decreased milk production in cattle in California.[394] However, monthly milk production was decreased by 6% in Israeli cattle.[395] The prevalence of the infection has been reported to be up to 10% in dairies of California.[394] The morbidity was reported to be up to 35% in Israeli herds.[397]

Management problems, such as broken posts or exposed wires, traumatize the skin of cattle and allow penetration of the organism. Young cattle appeared to be less susceptible to the disease than older cattle in Israel.[397] Seventy percent of the affected Israeli cattle were lactating cows.[397] The differential diagnoses include trauma, foreign body, and other masses such as tumors. Cutaneous lesions and mastitis were seen in 6%, and cutaneous lesions with concurrent visceral involvement in 1.6% of the Israeli cases.[397] The rest of the cows (92%) only had the cutaneous form.[397] The most affected organ in the visceral form was the lung.[397] The infection has been reported in bison from Egypt, resulting in severe emaciation and edema in the ventral areas and flanks.[401] Severe lymphadenitis was reported in camels in Asia.[402]

Horses. Three forms have been described in horses: ulcerative lymphangitis and external and internal abscesses. In a recent study of *C. pseudotuberculosis* infection in horses from California, ulcerative lymphangitis was diagnosed in 1%, external abscesses in 91%, and internal abscesses in 8% of the cases.[415] There appears to be no breed or sex predilection for the development of the infection. Ulcerative lymphangitis appears as a severe cellulitis, where the lymphatics are affected in one or more limbs with multiple draining ulcerative

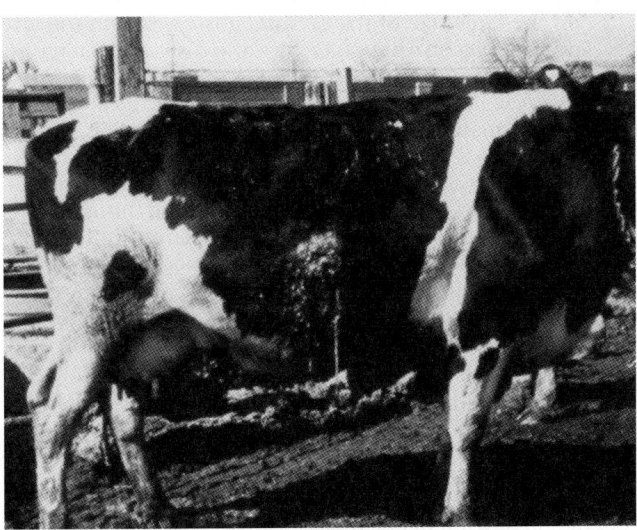

FIG. 35-2 ■ Typical presentation of *C. pseudotuberculosis* abscess in a dairy cow. Note open weeping sore on lateral body.

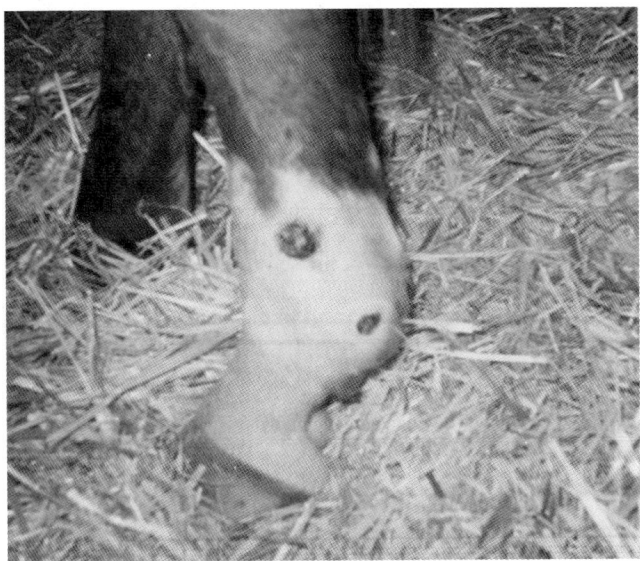

FIG. 35-3 ▪ Chronic sores and enlarged limb associated with ulcerative lymphangitis (*C. pseudotuberculosis*) in a horse.

lesions (Fig. 35-3). Horses often develop a non–weight-bearing lameness, fever, lethargy, and anorexia. This form of the disease has a worldwide distribution and often becomes chronic resulting in limb edema, lameness, weakness, and weight loss.[394] The differential diagnosis should include blunt trauma, fracture, foreign body, puncture wounds, nonseptic cellulitis, staphylococcal cellulitis, other septic cellulitis, and glanders.

The median age for horses with external abscesses is 5 years, with a range from 3 months to 28 years.[415] Young horses appear to be predisposed to infection as 52% of the cases in a large retrospective study were 5 years or younger.[415] Only a low number of cases involved foals under 6 months of age, suggesting that foals born to mares in endemic areas may be protected for several months by colostral antibodies.[415] The external abscesses located primarily in the pectoral and ventral abdominal regions are common in geographically restricted areas of the Western United States (Texas, New Mexico, Nevada, and California) and Brazil.[394,395,415,416] This form of infection is commonly known as "pigeon fever" because of the large size of the pectoral abscesses with the appearance of a pigeon's breast, or "dryland distemper," a name given in relation to its geographic distribution in the most arid areas (Fig. 35-4). Other common anatomic locations are the prepuce, mammary gland, axilla, inguinal region, limbs, and head (Fig. 35-5).[415] Abscesses involving the head include the ears, eyelids, forehead, and maxillary and mandibular regions.[415] Other less common areas are the thorax, neck, parotid gland, guttural pouches, larynx, flanks, umbilicus, tail, and rectum (see Fig. 35-5).[415] Septic joints and osteomyelitis have been reported to occur.[415] A large area of edema develops in the region of abscess formation. As the abscess matures the area becomes hard and painful, and some abscesses get very large, particularly in the pectoral area. The abscesses typically have a thick capsule, measuring up to 10 cm, and can cause severe lameness if located in the axillary or inguinal region.[395,415] Maturation can be slow and drainage difficult to establish if the abscess lies deep to muscle. Once drainage is established by either spontaneous rupture or lancing, the majority of the cases resolve within 10 to 14 days without complications. The abscesses may contain from 5 to 400 ml of thick tan purulent exudate.[395] The majority of the horses present with a single abscess, rather than multiple abscesses.[415] Around 25% of the cases develop fever up to 40° C. Other signs are nonhealing wounds, lameness, ventral dermatitis, and less commonly depression, anorexia, mastitis, and other problems, depending on the abscess location.[415] In the majority of horses (91.4%), complete recovery occurs with no recurrence of infection in subsequent years, implying a long-lasting immunity. However, 8.6% of the infections persisted for more than 1 year, or recurred as external or internal abscesses.[415] The case fatality for horses with external abscesses is very low (0.8%).[415] The differential diagnosis for an external abscess, particularly pectoral, should include trauma, seroma, hematoma, foreign body or abscess caused by a different organism.

In a recent study of *C. pseudotuberculosis* infection in horses, almost half of the horses that were presented with internal abscesses also had external abscesses.[415] The location of the internal abscesses was mainly in the liver; other locations included in the mesentery, mediastinum, lungs, diaphragm, pericardium, kidneys, and uterus.[415] The organism has been isolated from blood.[415] The most common clinical signs were fever up to 41.1° C, and weight loss. Other signs may include colic, pale mucous membranes, depression, ventral or limb edema, ventral dermatitis, ataxia, anorexia, hematuria, nasal discharge, and abortion.[415] The median age was 7 years with a range of 1 to 23 years old.[415] The case fatality for horses with internal abscesses was reported to be 40%.[415] The differential diagnosis should include other causes of internal abscesses such as infection by *Streptococcus* spp., *Actinomyces* spp., *Staphylococcus* spp., and *R. equi* in foals, *Coccidioides immitis*, anaerobes, neoplasia, and other causes of weight loss. The clinical signs and differential diagnosis will depend on the location of the abscess.

Humans. Human infection may result from the consumption of unpasteurized infected milk or milk products, continued close contact with infected animals, handling contaminated equipment, and exposure of wounds with exudates.[399,417] Human infection has been reported from strains of small ruminants.[399] Transmission from horses to humans has not been reported, but precautions must be taken when handling infected horses. The infection in humans occurs as a subacute to chronic lymphadenitis and pneumonia.[399]

CLINICAL PATHOLOGY AND LABORATORY DIAGNOSIS. In a recent study, almost half of the horses with external or internal abscesses had anemia of chronic disease.[415] Leukocytosis with neutrophilia and elevated fibrinogen are common features of developing bacterial infections, particularly in the case of internal abscesses.[415] Leukocytosis with neutrophilia was seen in 36% and 76% of the horses with external and internal abscesses, respectively.[415] Hyperproteinemia, caused by increased globulins, was observed in 38% and 59% of the horses with external and internal abscesses, respectively.[415] Similarly, infected cattle and small ruminants had increases in white blood cell counts.[397,414]

Peritoneal fluid from 93% of the horses with abdominal abscesses was abnormal. The remainder of the horses with abdominal abscesses and normal peritoneal fluid had abscesses located retroperitoneally in the kidneys without involvement of other abdominal structures. *C. pseudotuberculosis* was isolated in 32% of the samples of peritoneal fluid.[415] Intracellular and extracellular bacteria could be seen on Gram's stain. Failure to isolate the organism from peritoneal fluid does not rule out the disease. The organisms could be located retroperitoneally, or sequestered within a thick capsule, or suppressed by local factors or nucleated cells.[418]

Reportedly, the use of ELISA for the detection of cell wall antigens is not very accurate in horses.[394,410] The ELISA test appears to be more useful for detection of infection in sheep.[419-422] The most useful diagnostic aid is the synergistic

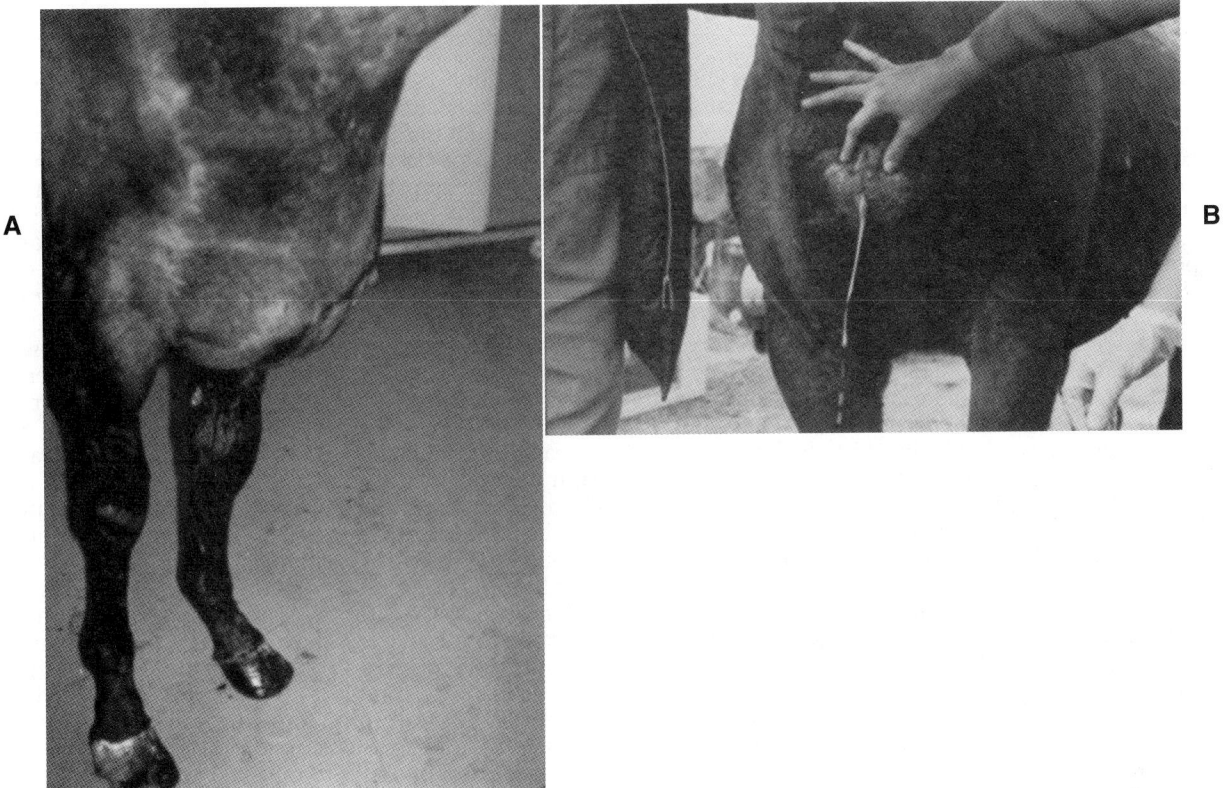

FIG. 35-4 ▓ Abscesses seen in equine infection with *C. pseudotuberculosis*. **A,** Markedly enlarged, painful pectoral abscess caused by *C. pseudotuberculosis* in a horse. **B,** Typical liquid, light tan, nonodorous pus from *C. pseudotuberculosis* infection in a horse.

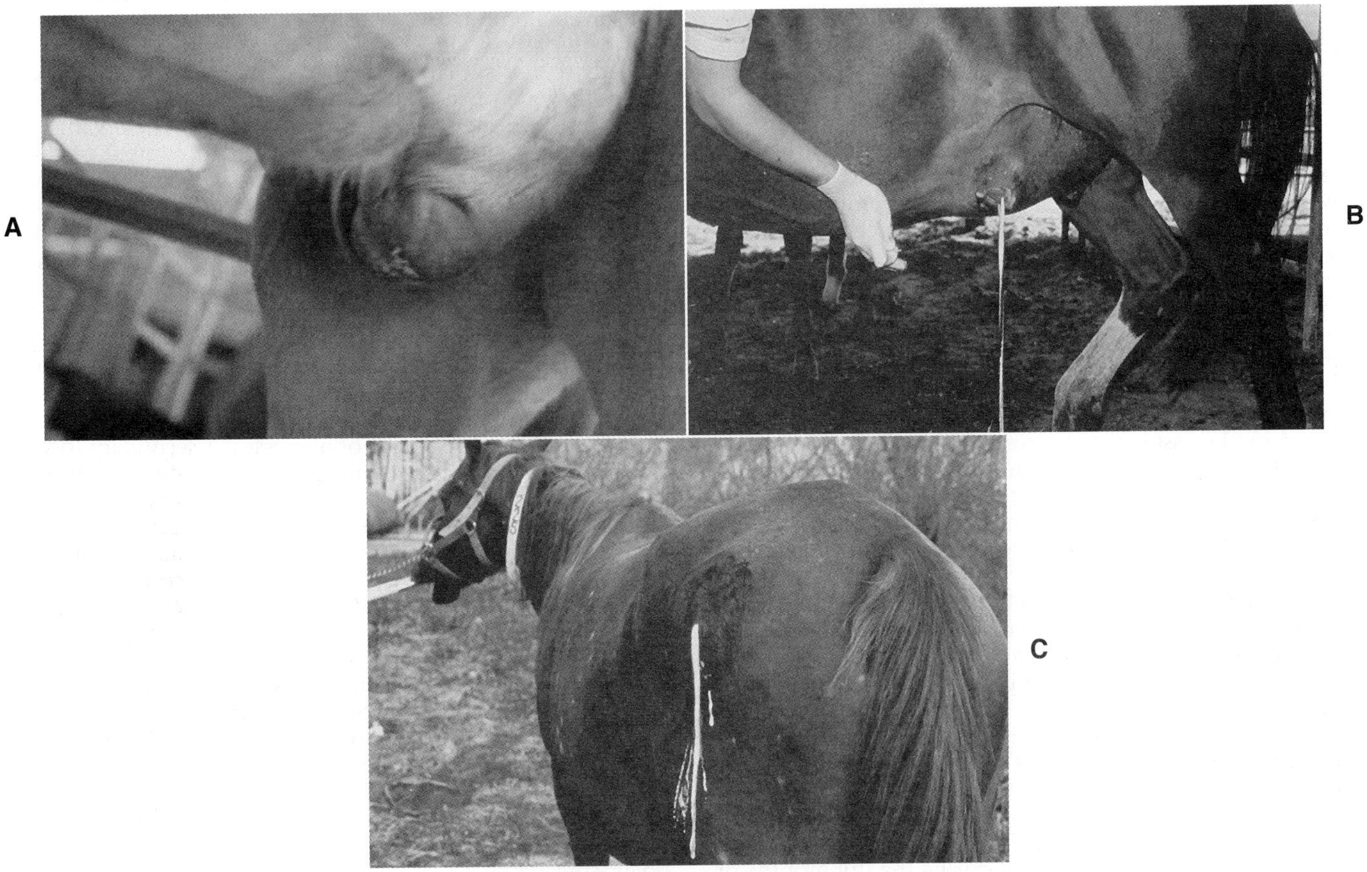

FIG. 35-5 ▓ Abscesses caused by *C. pseudotuberculosis* in horses. **A,** Marked swelling associated with an inguinal abscess. **B,** Draining abscess located near the mammary gland. **C,** Less common site for abscess formation on the hip of a horse. (**B** and **C** courtesy WD Wilson.)

hemolysis inhibition (SHI) test, which measures IgG response to the exotoxin in the patient's serum by detecting the highest dilution that will prevent hemolysis of *R. equi* exotoxin-sensitized bovine red cells when mixed with *C. pseudotuberculosis* exotoxin of a known concentration.[412,423] The IgG response to the exotoxin depends on the chronicity and severity of the infection and antibody availability.[394] It has been reported that a serum antibody titer of 1:128 indicates exposure, whereas 1:512 or higher indicates the presence of infection.[394] Studies in goats have demonstrated that most animals have serum antibody titers that correlate with bacterial culture results.[424] The SHI test has been used in sheep and goats to monitor prevalence and exposure of incoming animals, and to detect subclinical infections.[394,423] Only 40% of the horses with external abscesses, in which the infection was confirmed by culture, had serum antibody titers greater than 1:256. However, the absence or presence of a low SHI titer does not rule out the disease. Possible reasons for lack of elevated titers in infected animals are the acute onset of infection and rapid maturation of the abscess before developing an immunoglobulin response, presence of a thick capsule isolating the organisms and preventing a serologic response, or consumption of antibody during active infection.[394,415] Many horses that are seronegative at the time of drainage of an external abscess will seroconvert at a later date. In contrast, all horses with confirmed *C. pseudotuberculosis* internal abscesses had titers greater than 1:512.[415] The high titers in horses with internal abscesses probably reflect the chronicity of the disease and the resulting prolonged immune stimulation. Prolonged seropositivity has been observed in horses and goats.[415,423,425] The SHI test appears to be a reliable ancillary diagnostic aid for the diagnosis of internal abscesses in horses caused by *C. pseudotuberculosis*.[415] Presence of a SHI titer greater than 1:512 can occasionally be found in horses with external abscesses and exposed herdmates. Other serodiagnostic tests used in sheep and goats are tube agglutination, complement fixation, and gel immunodiffusion.[410,426]

A presumptive diagnosis of *C. pseudotuberculosis* infection can be made based on the history, local prevalence, time of the year, and clinical signs and characteristics of the exudate.[394] For the diagnosis of internal abscesses, the previous features coupled with clinical signs of fever and weight loss must be considered in addition to the presence of an inflammatory leukogram with elevated fibrinogen, serum chemistry abnormalities, abnormal peritoneal fluid or transtracheal wash, SHI titer greater than 1:512, and ultrasonographic or radiographic evidence of masses.[415] Ultrasound is a valuable diagnostic aid for the localization, quantification, and characterization of the abscesses. Typically the ultrasonographic appearance of the exudate caused by *C. pseudotuberculosis* contained in abscesses from horses is anechoic, in contrast to other types of exudates. The definitive diagnosis is established through the isolation of the organism from abscesses or draining wounds. The organism is readily isolated and grows well in blood agar in 24 to 48 hours, even when contaminant bacteria are present.[415]

PATHOPHYSIOLOGY AND EPIDEMIOLOGY. Little epidemiologic and immunologic data are available on *C. pseudotuberculosis* infection. *C. pseudotuberculosis* is a soil-borne organism that survives for long periods of time, months to years, even in direct sunlight.[399,427,428] The incidence of infection in horses varies considerably from year to year. External and internal abscesses in horses can occur at any time of the year, but are more commonly observed during the fall and early winter months, with the highest incidence in September, October, and November.[415] The largest numbers of equine cases have been observed during the dry months of the year, after years of heavy rainfall, which may result in optimal breeding conditions for insects.[395,415,416] The seasonal incidence in horses has been associated with the presence of biting insects such as *Haematobia irritans* (horn fly) that causes ventral midline dermatitis because of its feeding pattern. Other insects that have been incriminated but not confirmed in the transmission of the disease in horses are *Culicoides* spp., *Musca domestica*, and *Stomoxys calcitrans*.[394,395] The results of a recent study suggest that the disease could be transmitted through horse-to-horse contact, vectors, or contaminated soil.[429] The disease in cattle from Israel occurred during the spring and summer dry season, from March to October, when the housefly population is high.[397] *C. pseudotuberculosis* was isolated from houseflies collected over an Israeli cow lesion.[430] The infection in cattle may spread by direct contact, or indirectly by houseflies or fomites.[397,430] The disease in sheep and goats is not seasonal and the transmission is through contact of exudate from a draining abscess from animal to animal or via contaminated equipment.[395,428] Lambs born in contaminated surroundings can be infected through the umbilicus, mouth, or via inhalation.[394] Sheep that have exposure to the organism orally or from shearing wounds tend to have parotid, submandibular, prefemoral, or thoracic abscesses.[394] Goats can get the infection when wounds are exposed to contaminated milking equipment. The incubation period is long and variable. In experimental infections in small ruminants, the incubation period was from 2 weeks to several months. The incubation period in horses is not known, but appears variable from weeks to months. There is no breed or sex predilection.[415] Horses housed outside or with access to an outside paddock appeared to be at higher risk than stabled horses.[429]

The pathogenesis of the disease is not clear in horses, but it is speculated that the organism enters the equine host through skin or mucous membrane abrasions or wounds, as was confirmed in sheep.[431,432] Experimentally induced infections in small ruminants revealed that once *C. pseudotuberculosis* gains access via wounds or abrasions, the organism spreads to the subcutaneous or submucosal lymphatics, where they are phagocytosed by macrophages that migrate to the invasion site to engulf the organism.[433] The organism survives intracellularly because of its high content of the lipid, corynomycolic acid, that resists the action of lysosomal enzymes.[404,433] *C. pseudotuberculosis* replicates in the phagolysosome, and if large numbers of organisms are engulfed, phagocytic cells die. Experimental inoculation of the organism in sheep revealed a massive infiltration with polymorphonuclear leukocytes,[434] which are believed to carry the bacteria to regional lymph nodes.[394] A phospholipase D (PLD) toxin of approximately 31.5 kD, produced by all *C. pseudotuberculosis* isolates, increases the vascular permeability, causing spread of the organism regionally and systemically.[399,424,435] Development of abscesses at secondary locations in horses can occur in up to 25% of the cases.[415] Phospholipase D toxin can cause necrosis and thrombosis of the lymphatics, and may enhance survival and multiplication of the organism via complement depletion and inhibitory effects on phagocytic cells.[399] The corynomycolic acid and PLD toxin contribute to the inflammation, edema, and pain during the abscess development.[436] The profound reaction of these compounds is probably responsible for the formation of a thick abscess capsule that develops as phagocytes accumulate in the abscess core. The abscess eventually matures and drains, but if removal of infected material is incomplete, recurrence may be expected, particularly in small ruminants.[394]

The development of internal abscesses in horses is unclear but has been postulated to result from hematogenous or lymphatic spread of bacteria from more superficial sites.[394] Forty-three percent of the horses with internal abscesses had concurrent external abscesses.[415]

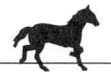

TREATMENT AND PROGNOSIS. Important features to consider when treating external abscesses are as follows:

- Allow the abscess to mature
- Establish drainage and collect and dispose of the infective exudate
- Lavage the wound with an antiseptic solution
- Control flies around the wound.

In a retrospective study in horses, the majority of the external abscesses were incised to establish drainage and some horses received antimicrobials after drainage in effort to decrease cellulitis.[415] Many horses received no treatment and the abscesses broke and drained on their own. Other horses were only treated with antimicrobial agents. The outcome was successful for 99% of the horses with external abscesses.[415] Horses with abscesses in the axillary region or deep within muscles have considerable pain, necessitating incision and drainage. The use of ultrasound is useful for the detection of deep abscesses.

A study revealed that the median resolution time for horses with external abscesses that did not receive antimicrobial therapy before drainage of the abscess was 18 days versus 30 days for horses that received antimicrobials.[415] These data suggest that systemic antimicrobial therapy before abscess drainage in horses with external abscesses may prolong the course of the disease.[415] However, when abscesses recur, drainage and concurrent antimicrobials may improve the chance of resolution. Conversely, long-term (minimum 4 to 6 weeks) antimicrobial therapy is necessary for the treatment of internal abscesses and ulcerative lymphangitis. The median resolution time for horses with internal abscesses treated with antimicrobials was 42 days.[413] The case fatality for horses with internal abscesses treated with antimicrobials was 40%, and, if not treated, fatality was 100%.[415] In vitro, *C. pseudotuberculosis* is susceptible to nearly all commonly used antimicrobials, including penicillin, trimethoprim-sulfonamide, tetracycline, cephalosporin, chloramphenicol, erythromycin, and rifampin.[437,438] Most isolates are resistant to nitrofurans, cycloheximide, and nalidixic acid.[438] Bacitracin has marked activity against the bacterium.[439] In selecting an antimicrobial agent, the following features must be considered: the intracellular location of the organism, presence of a thick abscess capsule and presence of pus, that a lengthy course of treatment may be required, risk of complications (e.g., diarrhea), and cost. Antimicrobial-associated diarrhea was seen in 6% of the horses receiving antimicrobials for *C. pseudotuberculosis* infection in a retrospective study.[415] The antimicrobials included rifampin, trimethoprim-sulfa, and penicillin.[415] In a study in cattle the skin lesions on individual cows healed on average in 23 days after local or parenteral treatment.[397] Seventeen percent of severely affected cattle were culled.[397]

Additional therapies include marsupialization of internal abscesses if location allows. The abscess is located and the capsule sutured to the skin before the capsule is penetrated. This prevents contamination of surrounding tissues. Nonsteroidal antiinflammatory drugs such as phenylbutazone or flunixin meglumine may be used to control the pain or fever. Nonsteroidal agents are often used to control pain while waiting for external abscess maturation.

Simple drainage in small ruminants does not usually result in resolution of the disease and open lesions become potential sources of infection. Complete excision of the abscess with the animal under general anesthesia may be necessary to keep the abscess from draining and to prevent spread of the infection to other animals.[394] Treatment of choice in small ruminants is surgical removal of the affected lymph nodes. If lesions are simply lanced, the animal should be isolated until the wound heals.

The prognosis for external abscesses is good. Most resolved in 3 weeks from the day of drainage.[394] The prognosis for horses with internal abscesses and ulcerative lymphangitis is guarded. The prognosis improves if infection is detected early and appropriate therapy is administered.

PREVENTION AND CONTROL. Even though *C. pseudotuberculosis* infection is one of the most commonly diagnosed infectious diseases in California, little is known about its prevention and control. General recommendations to prevent the spread of the infection are isolation of infected animals, fly control, good sanitation, careful shearing practices, disinfection of contaminated fomites, and careful disposal of bedding. In small ruminants the morbidity can reach 100%, with depopulation being the most economic option. The potential of environmental contamination from a ruptured abscess or dripping of infected milk is very high.[427,430]

Immunization trials, applying whole cells, cell wall, toxoids, and bacterin-toxoid combinations have been used on the prevention of CLA in small ruminants.[440-444] These trials have provided a high degree of protection, decreasing the number of infected sheep and the number of abscesses per sheep.[440-444] *C. pseudotuberculosis* toxoids are commercially available for sheep* and goats.† The use of autogenous bacterin-toxoid in horses resulted in fewer abscesses and less postchallenge pain in experimentally inoculated horses, but did not reduce the incidence of infection on one farm because of low prevalence of disease.[445] The efficacy of bacterins in a clinical study in horses remains to be proven.

REFERENCES

394. Davis WE: *Corynebacterium pseudotuberculosis* infections in animals. In Smith BP, ed: *Large animal internal medicine*, ed 2, St Louis, 1996, Mosby, pp 1251-1257.
395. Miers KC, Ley WB: *Corynebacterium pseudotuberculosis* infection in the horse: study of 117 clinical cases and consideration of etiopathogenesis, *J Am Vet Med Assoc* 177:250-253, 1980.
396. Shpigel NY et al: An outbreak of *Corynebacterium pseudotuberculosis* infection in an Israeli dairy herd, *Vet Rec* 133:89-94, 1993.
397. Yeruham I et al: *Corynebacterium pseudotuberculosis* infection in Israeli cattle: clinical and epidemiological studies, *Vet Rec* 140:423-427, 1997.
398. Biberstein EL, Knight HD, Jang S: Two biotypes of *Corynebacterium pseudotuberculosis*, *Vet Rec* 89:691-692, 1971.
399. Songer JG, Prescott JF: Corynebacterium. In Gyles CL, Thoen CO, eds: *Pathogenesis of bacterial infections in animals*, Ames, Iowa, 1993, Iowa State University Press, pp 57-62.
400. Hietala SK: California Veterinary Diagnostic Laboratory, Davis, California, 1995, personal communication.
401. Anon A: *Second Annual Report of the US Agricultural Research Program*, Cairo, 1980, Animal Health Research Institute.
402. Afzal M, Sakir M, Hussain MM: *Corynebacterium pseudotuberculosis* and lymphadenitis (taloa or mala) in the camel, *Trop Anim Health Produc* 28:158-162, 1996.
403. Coyle MB, Lipsky BA: Coryneform bacteria in infectious diseases: clinical and laboratory aspects, *Clin Microbiol Rev* 3:227-246, 1990.
404. Hard GC: Comparative toxic effect of the surface lipid of *Corynebacterium ovis* on peritoneal macrophages, *Infect Immunol* 12:1439-1449, 1975.
405. Songer JG et al: Biochemical and genetic characterization of *Corynebacterium pseudotuberculosis*, *Am J Vet Res* 49:223-226, 1988.
406. Sutherland SS, Hart RA, Buller NB: Genetic differences between nitrate-negative and nitrate-positive *C. pseudotuberculosis* strains using restriction fragment length polymorphisms, *Vet Microbiol* 49:1-9, 1996.
407. Costa LRR, Spier SJ, Hirsh CH: Comparative molecular characterization of *Corynebacterium pseudotuberculosis* of different origin, *Vet Microbiol* 62:135-143, 1998.
408. Barakat AA, Selim SA, Atef A: Two serotypes of *Corynebacterium pseudotuberculosis* isolated from different animal species, *Rev Sci Tech Office Int Epizoo* 3:151-163, 1984.
409. Sutherland SS, Hart RA, Buller NB: Ribotype analysis of *Corynebacterium pseudotuberculosis* isolates from sheep and goats, *Aust Vet J* 70:454-456, 1993.
410. Menzies PI, Muckle CA, Hwang YT, Songer JG: The evaluation of an enzyme-linked immunosorbent assay using an *Escherichia coli* recombinant phospholipase D antigen for the diagnosis of *Corynebacterium pseudotuberculosis* infection, *Proceedings of the American Dairy Goat Association National Convention*, 1993, pp 13-20.

---

*Caseous D-T, Colorado Serum Co., Denver, CO 80206.

†Glanvac TM, Parkville, 3052, Victoria, Australia.

411. Yozwiak ML, Songer JG: Effect of *Corynebacterium pseudotuberculosis* phospholipase D on viability and chemotactic responses of ovine neutrophils, *Am J Vet Res* 54:392-397, 1993.

412. Knight HD; A serologic method for the detection of *Corynebacterium pseudotuberculosis* in horses, *Cornell Vet* 68:220-237, 1978.

413. Piontkowski MD, Shivvers DW: Evaluation of a commercially available vaccine against *Corynebacterium pseudotuberculosis* for use in sheep, *J Am Vet Med Assoc* 212:1765-1768, 1998.

414. Scott PR, Collie DDS, Hume LH: Caseous lymphadenitis in a commercial ram stud in Scotland, *Vet Rec* 141:548-549, 1997.

415. Aleman M et al: Retrospective study of *Corynebacterium pseudotuberculosis* infection in horses: 538 cases, *J Am Vet Med Assoc* 209:804-809, 1996.

416. Welsh RD: *Corynebacterium pseudotuberculosis* in the horse, *Equine Pract* 12:7-16, 1990.

417. Henderson A: Pseudotuberculosis adenitis caused by *Corynebacterium pseudotuberculosis*, *J Med Microbiol* 12:147-149, 1979.

418. Rumbaugh GE, Smith BP, Carlson GP: Internal abdominal abscesses in the horse: a study of 25 cases, *J Am Vet Med Assoc* 172:304-309, 1978.

419. Gezon HM et al: Epizootic of external and internal abscesses in a large goat herd over a 16-year period, *J Am Vet Med Assoc* 2:257-263, 1991.

420. Holstad G: *Corynebacterium pseudotuberculosis* infection in goats: evaluation of two serological diagnostic tests, *Acta Vet Scand* 27:575-583, 1986.

421. Ter Laak EA et al: Double-antibody sandwich enzyme-linked immunosorbent assay and immunoblot analysis used for control of caseous lymphadenitis in goats and sheep, *Am J Vet Res* 53:1125-1132, 1992.

422. Sutherland SS et al: Evaluation of an enzyme-linked immunosorbent assay for the detection of *Corynebacterium pseudotuberculosis* infection in sheep, *Aust Vet J* 64:263-266, 1987.

423. Brown CC, Olander HJ: Caseous lymphadenitis of goats and sheep: a review, *Vet Bull* 57:1-12, 1987.

424. Hodgson ALM et al: Rational attenuation of *Corynebacterium pseudotuberculosis*: potential cheesy gland vaccine and live delivery vehicle, *Infect Immunol* 60:2900-2905, 1992.

425. Cameron CM, Fuls WJP: Studies on the enhancement of immunity to *Corynebacterium pseudotuberculosis*, *J Vet Res* 40:105-114, 1973.

426. Ellis JA et al: Differential antibody responses of *Corynebacterium pseudotuberculosis* in sheep with naturally acquired caseous lymphadenitis, *J Am Vet Med Assoc* 196:1609-1613, 1990.

427. Augustine JL, Renshaw HW: Survival of *Corynebacterium pseudotuberculosis* on common barnyard fomites. In *Proceedings of the Third International Conference on Goat Production and Disease*, 1982, pp 525-526.

428. Knight HD: Corynebacterial infections in the horse: problems of prevention, *J Am Vet Med Assoc* 155:446-452, 1969.

429. Doherr MG et al: Risk factors associated with *Corynebacterium pseudotuberculosis* infection in California horses, *Prev Vet Med* 35:229-239, 1998.

430. Yeruham I et al: Mastitis in dairy cattle caused by *Corynebacterium pseudotuberculosis* and the feasibility of transmission by houseflies, *Vet Q* 18:87-89, 1996.

431. Nagy G: Caseous lymphadenitis in sheep: methods of infection, *J S Afr Vet Med Assoc* 47:197-199, 1976.

432. Serikawa S et al: Seroepidemiological evidence that shearing wounds are mainly responsible for *Corynebacterium pseudotuberculosis* infection in sheep, *J Vet Med Sci* 55:691-692, 1993.

433. Ashfaq MK, Campbell SG: Experimentally induced caseous lymphadenitis in goats, *Am J Vet Res* 41:1789-1792, 1980.

434. Pepin M et al: Experimental *Corynebacterium pseudotuberculosis* infection in lambs: kinetics of bacterial dissemination and inflammation, *Vet Microbiol* 26:381-392, 1991.

435. Muckle CA, Gyles CL: Relation of lipid content and exotoxin production to virulence of *Corynebacterium pseudotuberculosis*, *Am J Vet Res* 44:1149-1153, 1983.

436. Bernheimer AW, Campbell BJ, Forrester LJ: Comparative toxicology of Loxosceles reclusa and *Corynebacterium pseudotuberculosis*, *Science* 228:590-591, 1985.

437. Adamson PJW et al: Susceptibility of equine bacterial isolates to antimicrobial agents, *Am J Vet Res* 46:447-450, 1985.

438. Judson R, Songer JG: *Corynebacterium pseudotuberculosis*: in vitro susceptibility to 39 antimicrobial agents, *Vet Microbiol* 27:145-150, 1991.

439. Zhao HK et al: Antimicrobial susceptibility of *Corynebacterium pseudotuberculosis* isolated from lesions of caseous lymphadenitis in sheep in Hokkaido, Japan, *J Vet Med Sci* 53:355-356, 1991.

440. Menzies PI et al: A field trial to evaluate a whole cell vaccine for the prevention of caseous lymphadenitis in sheep and goat flocks, *Can J Vet Res* 55:362-366, 1991.

441. Eggleton DG et al: Immunisation against ovine caseous lymphadenitis: efficacy of monocomponent *Corynebacterium pseudotuberculosis* toxoid vaccine and combined clostridial-corynebacterial vaccines, *Aus Vet J* 68:320-321, 1991.

442. Eggleton DG et al: Immunisation against ovine caseous lymphadenitis: correlation between *Corynebacterium pseudotuberculosis* toxoid content and protective efficacy in combined clostridial-corynebacterial vaccines, *Aust Vet J* 68:322-325, 1991.

443. Eggleton DG et al: Immunisation against ovine caseous lymphadenitis: comparison of Corynebacterium pseudotuberculosis vaccines with and without bacterial cells, *Aust Vet J* 68:317-319, 1991.

444. Hodgson ALM et al:vEfficacy of an ovine caseous lymphadenitis vaccine formulated using a genetically inactive form of the *Corynebacterium pseudotuberculosis* phospholipase D, *Vaccine* 17:802-808, 1999.

445. Davis EW, Spensley MJ: Use of autogenous bacterin-toxoid and toxoid to prevent *Corynebacterium pseudotuberculosis* infection in horses, *J Vet Int Med* 6:137, 1992.

Diseases of the Bones, Joints, and Connective Tissues

SUSAN M. STOVER
Consulting Editor

PHYSITIS (EPIPHYSITIS)

HAROLD F. HINTZ

DEFINITION AND ETIOLOGY. *Developmental orthopedic disease* is a term used to describe a set of skeletal problems, including osteochondrosis, physitis (epiphysitis), and flexural deformities. Physitis is a disturbance of the endochondral ossification that affects the metaphyseal physes of young horses. It is closely related to osteochondrosis (see p. 1086). The disease has been associated with secondary copper deficiency (molybdenosis) in young growing cattle on pasture[1] and with calves raised on slatted floors.[2] It is occasionally seen in yearling rams being heavily fed for show. The only report in sheep or goats appears to be the syndrome of pregnancy-associated epiphysitis, and angular limb deformities in yearling does, which spontaneously regress after parturition.[3] It appears in about 1% of all yearling dairy does. The etiology of physitis is complex. Some of the following factors have been suggested in horses:

1. Genetic capacity for a rapid growth rate, as physitis is found much more commonly in foals that are growing rapidly than in slower-growing animals.[4]
2. Genetic predisposition for conformation that causes greater stress on the physis[5] (e.g., toe-in conformation and upright conformation in fetlock joints have been associated with physitis).
3. Overweight as a result of excessive intake of a high-energy diet; excessive weight that increases the mechanical loading of the physis has long been considered to be a factor; Thompson et al[6] studied the incidence of radiographic bone aberrations in foals gaining more or less than 1.05 kg/day

when suckling and more or less than 0.67 kg/day after weaning. They reported an increased incidence of aberrations in the high-gaining group and more involvement of the distal bones than the more proximal bones of the limb. A link between above-average weight gains and the onset of physitis was determined.

4. Growth spurts or compensatory growth spurts after periods of skeletal stunting caused by malnutrition seem to increase the incidence of physitis,[7] but the mechanism has not been established.
5. Stimulation of physes caused by hormone changes in response to a high intake of carbohydrate.[8]
6. Trace mineral deficiencies (such as of copper or zinc) leading to improper maturation and retention of cartilage.[9]
7. Calcium malnutrition:[9] Calcium deficiency causes poor ossification of bone; excessive calcium could cause reduced trace mineral absorption and increased release of calcitonin.
8. Exercising of young foals on hard surfaces; anecdotal reports by practitioners indicate that the incidence of physitis may be greater during a dry summer when the ground is hard than during a wet summer when the ground is softer.
9. Excessive exercise causing increased mechanical stress to the growing cartilage.[10]

CLINICAL SIGNS. Horses most likely to be affected are foals ranging from 4 to 8 months of age, yearlings, and horses in early training up to about 2 years of age.[7] Affected cattle are 5 to 12 months of age.[1] It is most commonly characterized by enlargement and abnormal shape of the distal physes of the radius, tibia, third metacarpal and metatarsal bones, and the proximal physis of the first phalanx. The enlarge-

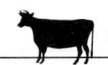

ments may be generally symmetric throughout the entire circumference of the physis rather than in one area.[4] Diagnosis is based on clinical signs and radiographic findings of a widened irregular zone of cartilage with a squashed lipping appearance. Figure 36-1 illustrates the radiographic appearance of abnormal epiphyseal growth.

PATHOPHYSIOLOGY. Enlargements may result because overloading of poorly formed metaphyseal bone leads to loss of structural integrity, microfracture, pain, and callus formation[10] (see Osteochondrosis, below).

NECROPSY FINDINGS. Sclerosis, widening of the growth plate, irregularity, and perhaps some swelling of the soft tissue can be found. Poulos,[11] however, pointed out that it is often difficult to confirm an inflammatory response. He stated that in the majority of cases there is no inflammatory process; thus the use of the "itis" is of some concern. Some believe that the term *physosis* might be a more accurate nomenclature.

TREATMENT AND PROGNOSIS. Turner[5] concluded that the first step in treating physitis is to evaluate the animal's feed; however, considerable controversy persists as to which dietary recommendations should be followed. For example, dietary recommendations could include a reduction of soluble carbohydrate intake (grain). Lewis[12] suggests that, to prevent alterations in endochondral ossification caused by excessive energy intake, the total concentrate intake be limited to 0.5 kg to 0.75 kg/100 kg of body weight for nursing foals, 1 kg to 1.5 kg/100 kg for weanlings, and 0.5 kg to 1 kg/100 kg for yearlings. He stated that a good rule of thumb is to feed a maximum of 0.45 kg of concentrate/day for each month of age up to a maximum of 3.5 to 4.5 kg/day. These values, however, are less than those recommended by the National Research Council[13] and could hamper normal development. Furthermore, many growing horses fed high grain intakes do not develop physitis; thus energy restriction is not always recommended.

Total dietary calcium concentrations of 0.8% and phosphorus concentrations of 0.6% seem reasonable. High intakes of calcium could reduce trace mineral absorption and perhaps induce malformation of bone because of hypercalcitonism. The maximum tolerable level of calcium, however, has not been established.

Wide variations exist in the recommended amounts of copper. Gabel et al[9] recommend that weanlings be fed a total dietary copper concentration of 25 to 30 ppm or a total of 150 to 175 mg of copper daily and that yearlings be fed 20 to 25 ppm or 150 to 175 mg of copper daily. These values are about three times the level recommended by the National Research Council,[13] but are well below the maximum tolerable level (800 ppm) of copper. In neonatal foals plasma copper concentrations are 16% to 20% of adult values.[14] These values increased threefold to eightfold within a week and were at or above adult normals by 6 to 12 months of age.[14]

Further studies are needed to establish the level of copper needed and particularly to define the effects of other nutrients on copper use. Secondary copper deficiency caused by interactions with molybdenum, zinc, and sulfates has been reported in cattle.[1] The bone abnormalities include a widened zone of cartilage lipping of the medial and lateral areas of the physeal plate and zones of uncalcified cartilage.[1] See Chapter 30 for treatment of secondary copper deficiency and its prognosis in ruminants.

Turner[5] suggests that nonsteroidal antiinflammatory drugs are indicated to help diminish pain and prevent further development of flexural deformities in certain cases in which the animal is stiff. He also states that cases of physitis usually resolve spontaneously, but the horse is left with a residual problem that can be severe enough to limit future athletic soundness.

REFERENCES

1. Smith BP, Fisher GL, Poulos PW, et al: Abnormal bone development and lameness associated with secondary copper deficiency in young cattle, *J Am Vet Med Assoc* 166:682-688, 1975.
2. White SL, Rowland GN, Whitlock RH: Radiographic, macroscopic and microscopic changes in growth plates of calves raised on hard flooring, *Am J Vet Res* 45:633-639, 1984.
3. Anderson KL, Adams WM: Epiphysitis and recumbency in a yearling prepartum goat, *J Am Vet Med Assoc* 183:226-228, 1983.
4. Pool RR: Developmental orthopedic disease in the horse: normal and abnormal bone formation. Proceedings of the 33rd American Association of Equine Practitioners, 1987, pp 143-158.
5. Turner AS: Diseases of bone and related structures. In Stashak TS, editor: *Adam's lameness in horses*, ed 4, 1987, Philadelphia, Lea & Febiger.
6. Thompson KN, Jackson SG, Rooney JR: The effect of above average weight gains on the incidence of radiographic bone aberrations and epiphysitis in growing horses. Proceedings of the Tenth Equine Nutrition and Physiology Society, 1987, pp 5-11.
7. Hintz HF, Schryver HF, Lowe JE: Delayed growth response and limb conformation in young horses. Proceedings of the Cornell Nutrition Conference, 1976, pp 94-96.
8. Glade M: The role of endocrine factors in equine developmental orthopedic disease. Proceedings of the 33rd American Association of Equine Practitioners, 1987, pp 171-190.
9. Gabel AA, Knight DA, Reed SM, et al: Comparison of incidence and severity of developmental orthopedic disease on 17 farms before and after adjustment of ration. Proceedings of the 33rd American Association of Equine Practitioners, 1987, pp 163-170.
10. Bramlage LR: Clinical manifestations of disturbed bone formation in the horse. Proceedings of the 33rd American Association of Equine Practitioners, 1987, pp 135-138.
11. Poulos P: Radiologic manifestations of developmental problems. Proceedings of the AQHA Developmental Orthopedic Disease Symposium, 1986, pp 1-3.
12. Lewis L: Nutrition. In Stashak ED, ed: *Adam's lameness in horses*, ed 4, Philadelphia, 1989, Lea & Febiger.
13. National Research Council: *Nutrient requirements of horses*, Washington DC, 1989, NRC-NAS.
14. Cymbaluk NF, Bristol FM, Christensen DA: Influence of age and breed of equid on plasma copper and zinc concentrations, *Am J Vet Res* 47:192-195, 1986.

OSTEOCHONDROSIS

ANDREW T. FISCHER, JR.

DEFINITION AND ETIOLOGY. Osteochondrosis (OCD) is a developmental disease characterized by a defect in endochondral ossification that leads to a dissecting cartilage flap (i.e., osteochondrosis dissecans), subchondral bone cysts, or physitis. Because the primary defect appears to be with cartilage maturation, the term chondrodysplasia or dyschondroplasia may be more appropriate. Osteochondrosis has been recognized more commonly in horses than in cattle, sheep, or goats, although a very severe hereditary dyschondroplasia of Suffolk and Suffolk crossbred sheep known as spider lamb syndrome (see p. 1094) is now commonly recognized.

CLINICAL SIGNS AND DIFFERENTIAL DIAGNOSIS. Osteochondrosis is manifested in a variety of ways and is most frequently diagnosed in young animals. Physitis is seen in young, actively growing horses; osseous enlargements occur at the physeal plates, and inflammation in the area may cause lameness. Physitis may be isolated to one limb, but more commonly it is bilateral. Osteomyelitis and septic physitis should be considered in the differential diagnosis.

Osteochondrosis dissecans may be diagnosed in weanling or adult horses, but is most commonly recognized when horses are first placed in training. The onset of clinical signs may be insidious or acute. The severity of lameness varies from nonexistent to severe. Typically, joint effusion is present, particularly in the tarsocrural, femoropatellar, metacarpophalangeal, and metatarsophalangeal joints, although virtually any joint may be affected. In young animals septic arthritis, trauma, and synovitis should be considered in the differential diagnosis. In the adult the important differentials are secondary joint disease, trauma, and synovitis. In young

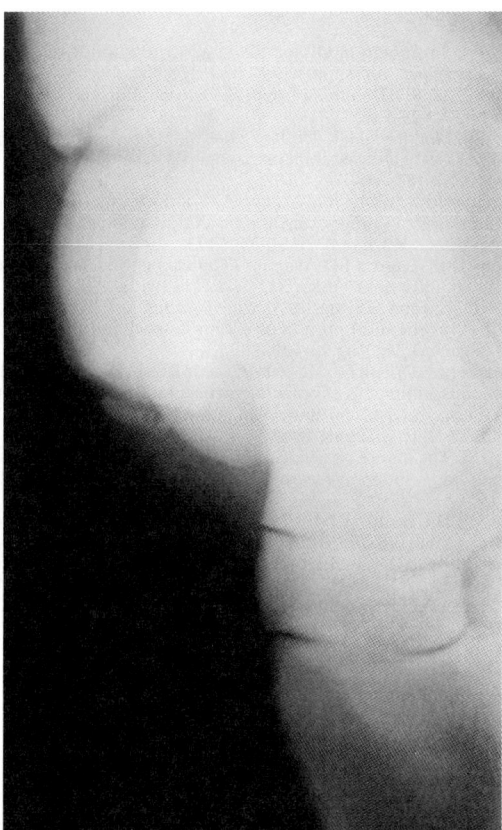

FIG. 36-1 ▓ Osteochondrosis of the tarsocrural joint. Note the osteochondral fragments located at the distal intermediate ridge of the tibia and the distal aspect of the lateral trochlear ridge of the talus.

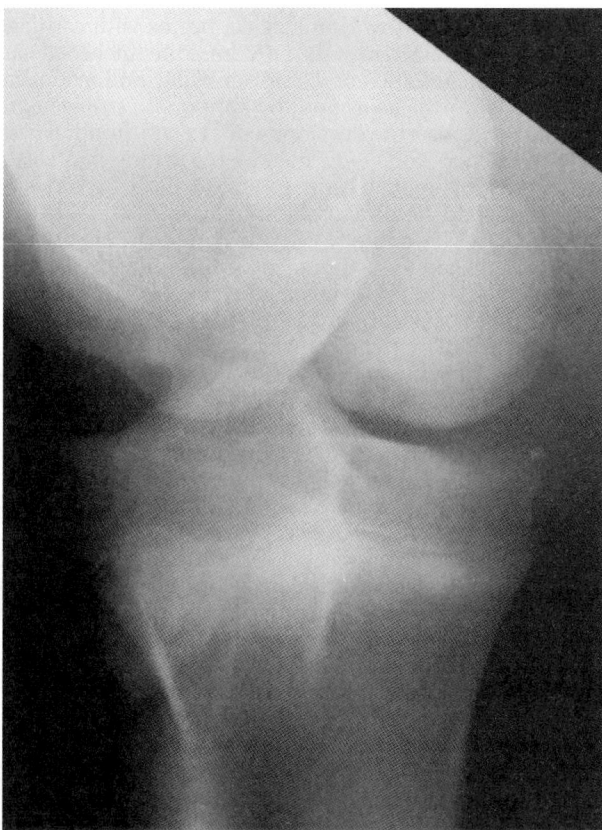

FIG. 36-2 ▓ Osteochondrosis of the medial part of the femoral condyle, exemplified by the subchondral cystic lesion typical in this location.

growing cattle the lateral trochlear ridge of the distal femur is most commonly affected.[15-17] Subchondral bone cysts occur while animals are still growing; clinical signs often are noticed first when horses start training. Joint effusion is not as common as in osteochondrosis dissecans.

DIAGNOSTIC TESTS. Lameness of any type is best evaluated by careful physical examination, observation of the animal at different gaits, local or intraarticular anesthetic, and radiography (Fig. 36-1). Osteochondrosis of physeal growth plates should be evaluated radiographically. If a complete blood count suggests physeal infection or osteomyelitis, biopsy and culture of the affected growth plate are warranted. Radiographic signs may differ from clinical signs. Clinical signs and joint effusion may precede radiographic evidence of femoropatellar OCD. Typical radiographic lesions may be evident several months later.[18] Juvenile spavin (tarsal osteoarthritis) has been linked to osteochondrosis.[19]

Lameness associated with osteochondrosis dissecans of the femoropatellar, tarsocrural, metacarpophalangeal, metatarsophalangeal, and scapulohumeral joints can be improved by intraarticular anesthesia. After the lameness has been localized by physical examination and local anesthesia, radiographic examination of the affected area is warranted.

Because joint effusion is atypical with subchondral bone cysts, the cysts are commonly localized by intraarticular anesthesia and demonstrated radiographically (Fig. 36-2). In horses with subchondral bone cysts of the medial part of the femoral condyle, deep palpation of the femorotibial joint with the leg in a flexed position may elicit pain.

The contralateral joint always should be radiographed because of the frequently bilateral nature of osteochondrosis.

For example, osteochondrosis dissecans of the distal sagittal ridge of the metacarpus or metatarsus indicates the need for radiographs of the contralateral fetlock joint.

PATHOPHYSIOLOGY. The zone of cartilage closest to the epiphysis is termed the zone of resting chondrocytes. In normal cartilage growth and subsequent endochondral ossification, these cells—under the control of somatotropin—undergo mitosis and form organized columns of cells in the zone of proliferating cells. They differentiate and become larger, rounded, and vacuolated in the zone of hypertrophy. Here the intercellular matrix calcifies under the influence of thyroxine. Capillaries invade this area, bringing in osteogenic cells. The osteogenic cells lay down a matrix on the calcified cartilage cores, which becomes mineralized, forming the primary spongiosa. The primary spongiosa is then replaced by secondary spongiosa.

In osteochondrosis, cartilage cells fail to differentiate normally. The hypertrophied zone of cartilage cells is retained, and calcification of this area fails to occur. Capillaries do not invade the abnormal cartilage, and endochondral ossification does not proceed. The net result is an area of thickened cartilage. Because nutrients now must diffuse a great distance from the synovium to the basal layers of cartilage cells, necrosis of these cells is thought to develop. Further, the thickened cartilage is biomechanically inferior to normal and is susceptible to fissuring. Fissuring leads to dissecting flaps that are present in osteochondrosis dissecans. The liberation of cartilage debris into the joint probably is responsible for lameness and effusion. Osteochondrotic cartilage differs biochemically, morphologically, and immunohistochemically from normal cartilage.[20] Subchondral bone cysts may de-

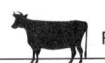

velop by a similar pathway; the defect begins with cartilage thickening. Normal stress and strain cause the thickened cartilage to become infolded or to cease growing. Endochondral ossification of cartilage around the abnormal cartilage continues normally with the development of a subchondral cyst.

Physitis is associated with marked thickening and weakening of the growth plate cartilage. The cartilage becomes irregular, and endochondral ossification is arrested.

ETIOLOGY. The etiology of osteochondrosis is unclear and may be related to factors such as hormone levels or dietary minerals. Heritability is considered to be a factor in the development of osteochondrosis and has been demonstrated in the tarsocrural, metacarpophalangeal, and metatarsophalangeal joints of Swedish trotters.[21] Males may be more commonly affected with osteochondrosis than females because they have a larger body mass and a faster rate of growth. Dietary influences have been investigated extensively. Animals fed for higher rates of growth develop osteochondrosis with increased frequency compared with animals fed for normal or decreased rates of growth.[22] For example, high-energy rations fed to bulls have caused an increased frequency and severity of osteochondrosis lesions. Copper deficiency may be implicated in the development of osteochondrosis[23]; lysyl oxidase depends on copper for normal cross-linking of collagen molecules. In ponies chronic administration of glucocorticoids, which inhibit lysyl oxidase activity, has induced lesions typical of osteochondrosis.[23] By decreasing copper absorption, zinc intoxication induces lesions grossly similar to osteochondrosis.[23]

Alterations in hormone concentrations have been demonstrated to cause osteochondrosis in various species. Hypercalcitonism and increases in exogenous somatotropin, corticotropin, thyrotropin, and corticosteroids have induced osteochondrosis dissecans. Trauma is suspected of being involved in osteochondrosis because lesions tend to occur at specific anatomic sites. The usually bilateral nature of the disease, however, is not consistent with trauma. It is more likely that abnormal cartilage in certain sites is mechanically inferior to normal cartilage and that mechanical stresses lead to cartilage fissuring or the development of cysts.

TREATMENT AND PROGNOSIS. Most horses with osteochondrosis dissecans are managed either by conservative treatment (e.g., extended periods of rest and dietary management) or by surgery.[24] The diet should be examined carefully for levels of macronutrients and micronutrients. Osteochondrosis dissecans of the scapulohumeral, femoropatellar, tarsocrural, metacarpophalangeal, and metatarsophalangeal joints are best treated with arthroscopic surgery. If signs of degenerative joint disease are present before surgery, the prognosis is guarded. Surgery is not always indicated, particularly if lameness or effusion has not been associated with the lesion. Osteochondrosis dissecans may be an incidental finding on survey radiographs.

Treatment of subchondral bone cysts is more controversial. Cysts of the medial part of the femoral condyle that do not respond to conservative therapy within 3 to 6 months should be treated using arthroscopy. Subchondral bone cysts of the glenoid cavity have been treated successfully by arthroscopic surgery. Cysts of the proximal interphalangeal joint are usually treated by arthrodesis. Return to activity is more likely when arthrodesis is performed in the hind limbs than the forelimbs, and convalescence can take 1 year. Cysts in other locations have been managed either surgically or conservatively, but the number of cases is insufficient to make definite recommendations.

Osteochondrosis that results from nutrient or mineral imbalances is treated best by balancing the diet and correcting any preexisting deficiencies. If multiple joints are affected by nutritional problems, surgery probably is not indicated.

REFERENCES

15. Reiland S, Stromberg B, Olsson SE, et al: Osteochondrosis in growing bulls, *Acta Radiol* 358 (suppl):179-195, 1978.
16. Jensen R, Park RD, Lauerman LH, et al: Osteochondrosis in feedlot cattle, *Vet Pathol* 18:529-535, 1981.
17. Weisbrode SE, Monke DR, Dodaro ST, et al: Osteochondrosis, degenerative joint disease and vertebral osteophytosis in middle-aged bulls, *J Am Vet Med Assoc* 181:700-705, 1982.
18. Dabareiner RM, Sullins KE, White NA II: Progression of femoropatellar osteochondrosis in nine young horses: clinical, radiographic and arthroscopic findings, *Vet Surg* 22:515-523, 1993.
19. Watrous BJ, Hultgren BD, Wagner PC: Osteochondrosis and juvenile spavin in equids, *Am J Vet Res* 52:607-612, 1991.
20. Lillich JD, Bertone AL, Ruggles AJ, et al: Biochemical, histochemical, and immunohistochemical profiles of equine osteochondrotic articular cartilage (abstract), *Vet Surg* 23:407, 1994.
21. Grondahl AM, Dolvik NI: Heritability estimations of osteochondrosis in the tibiotarsal joint and of bony fragments in the palmar/plantar portion of the metacarpo- and metatarsophalangeal joints of horses, *J Am Vet Med Assoc* 203:101-104, 1993.
22. Olsson SE: The nature of osteochondrosis in animals: summary and conclusion with comparative aspects in man, *Acta Radiol* (suppl) 358:123-137, 1978.
23. Glade MJ: The control of cartilage growth in osteochondrosis: a review, *Equine Vet Sci* 6:175-187, 1986.
24. McIlwraith WC: Disease of joints, tendons, ligaments, and related structures. In Stashak TS, editor: *Adams' lameness in horses*, ed 4, Philadelphia, 1987, Lea & Febiger, pp 396-419.

RICKETS IN RUMINANTS

JOHN MAAS

DEFINITION AND ETIOLOGY. Rickets (occasionally referred to as osteodystrophy) is a disease of young, growing animals characterized by defective mineralization of developing bones. Nutrient accumulation by the fetus is invariably adequate for normal bone formation, and ruminants on a milk diet rarely experience nutrient deficiencies that would predispose them to rickets. Weaned, rapidly growing animals are occasionally managed in such a way that rickets might develop. Rickets primarily affects rapidly growing animals and is most commonly associated with phosphorus or vitamin D deficiency, although calcium deficiency can result in rickets. Protein-calorie malnourished animals are generally not at risk.

CLINICAL SIGNS AND DIFFERENTIAL DIAGNOSIS. Clinical signs of rickets include stiffness, reluctance to move, lameness, joint enlargement, arching of the back, and enlargement of the costochondral junctions (i.e., rachitic rosary). The long bones of the limbs become curved forward and outward (i.e., bow-legged). Tooth eruption is delayed and irregular, and the teeth are mottled and poorly calcified. Patients are often partially anorexic and have decreased growth, decreased weight gain, and poor feed efficiency from the underlying causes. Differential diagnoses include fluorosis, arthritis from any cause, copper deficiency, epiphysitis (physitis), manganese deficiency, and hyperparathyroidism (e.g., primary or renal secondary).

PATHOPHYSIOLOGY. The underlying sequence of events in the pathogenesis of rickets includes the following: (1) failure of cartilage to mineralize, (2) failure of growing cartilage to degenerate, (3) irregular persistence of cartilage, (4) formation of osteoid on persistent cartilage that forms an irregularity of osteochondral junctions, (5) overgrowth of fibrous tissue in the metaphysis, and (6) bone deformity.[25] Clinically, the primary abnormality to consider is the lack of mineralization. In young animals, rapidly growing bones that fail to mineralize properly are probably predisposed to developing rickets.

The most common cause of rickets in young ruminants is a deficiency of phosphorus or vitamin D. Rickets has been associated with calcium deficiency and excess dietary phosphorus, either of which may be causing nutritional secondary hyperparathyroidism. Dietary deficiencies of magnesium, zinc, manganese, and vitamin A have also been associated with rickets.[26] Animals that do not receive direct sunlight (e.g., because of winter grazing, confinement) or vitamin D supplements are at increased risk. Young animals grazing green cereal crops during cloudy seasons are particularly at risk for vitamin D deficiency. Animals grazing *Brassica* spp. (e.g., turnips, swedes, rape) are prone to hypophosphorosis and rickets.[27] Elevated dietary iron may raise serum phosphorus and inhibit 1,25-dihydroxycalciferol production in the kidney, resulting in rickets.[28] Similarly, the conditions that cause osteomalacia in adult ruminants would be expected to cause rickets in growing ruminants.

DIAGNOSIS. The clinical diagnosis depends on an accurate and complete dietary history and appropriate clinical signs. Important radiographic findings include cortical thinning, bowing of the long bones of the limbs, enlargement and widening of the physeal plates, increased metaphyseal bone density parallel to the physeal plate, an irregular radiolucent band at the junction of the metaphysis with the epiphysis, and physeal "lipping." Cattle with copper deficiency exhibit similar physeal lipping; however, not all ruminants with rickets show classic radiographic lesions.

Histologic examination of affected bone may be diagnostic.[25] Samples and biopsies of costochondral junctions are practical in the live patient; examination of the distal metatarsus or metacarpus is preferred at necropsy.

CLINICAL PATHOLOGY. Serum alkaline phosphatase activity is greater than in normal growing animals of a similar age and breed. Serum calcium and phosphorus concentrations are often normal; however, abnormal serum calcium and/or phosphorus concentrations are not diagnostic of a specific cause. With hypophosphorosis, hypophosphatemia is expected. With inadequate dietary calcium or vitamin D, hypocalcemia is usually only seen during terminal stages. Trace mineral or vitamin concentrations in blood or tissue may be helpful retrospectively; however, published data regarding the interpretation of trace mineral status to field cases of rickets are lacking. Determination of bone ash can be helpful. In normal bone, the ratio of ash to organic matter is about 3:2; however, in rickets the ratio ranges from 1:2 to 1:3. A thorough analysis of the diet is usually essential to confirm the cause of rickets and to institute appropriate therapeutic changes. The nutrient requirements for growth of various ruminant species and classes are published by the National Research Council, National Academy of Sciences. Management factors that predispose to rickets occasionally can predispose animals to urolithiasis in certain cases, such as high concentrate (grain) diets.

TREATMENT, PROGNOSIS, AND PREVENTION. The prognosis is fair to good for ambulatory patients. The first therapeutic step is to provide adequate dietary calcium and phosphorus. Supplements such as dicalcium phosphate (23% Ca, 18.5% P), bone meal, or limestone plus a phosphorus source (monoammonium phosphate), are all acceptable. Injectable vitamin D (10,000 to 30,000 IU/kg bodyweight, intramuscularly) often is given. Providing vitamin D parenterally without adequate dietary calcium and phosphorus in cases of rickets, however, does not restore effective bone mineralization. Prevention of rickets is straightforward and easily accomplished by providing a balanced diet with appropriate supplements to young, growing ruminants.

REFERENCES

25. Jubb KVF, Kennedy PC, Palmer N: *Pathology of domestic animals,* ed 3, Orlando, 1985, Academic Press, pp 42-44.
26. Mahin L, Chadli M, Marzou A: Osteodystrophy in growing lambs fed a diet rich in wheat bran, *Vet Rec* 115:355-357, 1984.
27. Thompson KG, Cook TG: Rickets in yearling steers on a swede (*Brassica napus*) crop, *NZ Vet J* 35:11-13, 1987.
28. Hidiroglow M, Dukes TW, Ho SK, et al: Bent limb syndrome in lambs raised in total confinement, *J Am Vet Med Assoc* 173:1573-1574, 1978.

ANGULAR LIMB DEFORMITIES

JEFFREY P. WATKINS

DEFINITION, ETIOLOGY, AND CLINICAL SIGNS. Angular limb deformities are deviations in the axis of the forelimbs or hind limbs in the frontal plane. *Valgus* deformity denotes a lateral deviation of the limb distal to the origin of the deformity; deformity *varus* denotes a medial deviation. The deformity is further described by naming the joint adjacent to the origin of the deformity; for example, carpus valgus describes an angular deformity arising in the carpal region with lateral deviation of the metacarpus (knock-kneed conformation) (Fig. 36-3).

Angular limb deformities may be either congenital or acquired.[29-31] In general, they are caused by laxity of periarticular supporting structures, incomplete ossification, or asynchronous growth rate. Although the underlying cause of these abnormalities remains an enigma, etiogenic considerations include intrauterine malpositioning, relative immaturity, hereditary predisposition, rapid growth, dietary imbalances, osteochondrosis, and trauma.[29-33]

Congenital angular deformities frequently are attributed to intrauterine malpositioning and laxity of periarticular supporting structures. They commonly originate in the region of the carpus and tarsus, resulting in bilateral valgus deformity. It is also common to identify a "windswept" foaling in which valgus deformity of one limb is accompanied by varus defor-

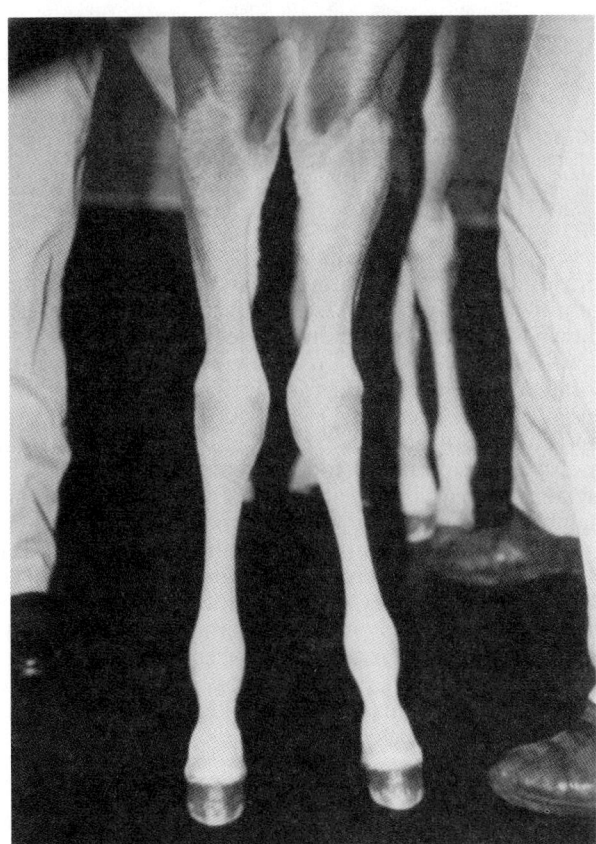

FIG. 36-3 ▌ Carpus valgus deviation.

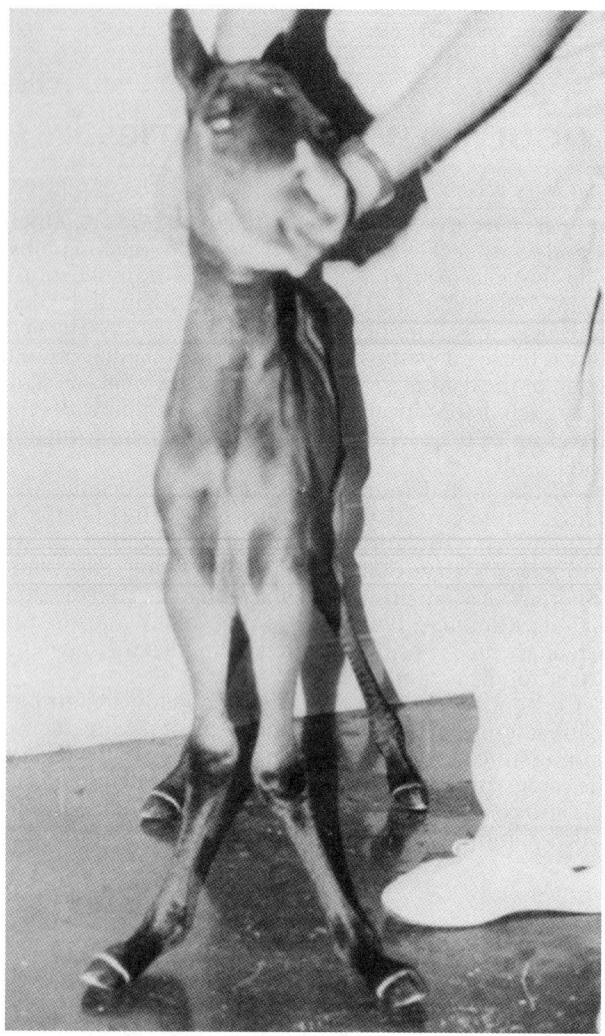

FIG. 36-4 ▮▮ Premature foal with incomplete ossification of the cuboidal carpal bones showing marked bilateral carpus valgus.

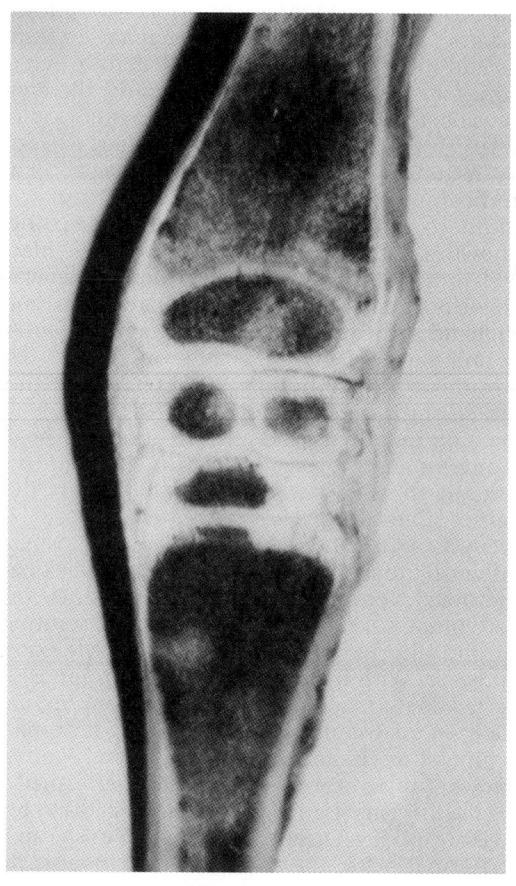

FIG. 36-5 ▮▮ Specimen from a foreleg of the premature foal in Figure 36-4, cut in the frontal plane. Note the thick cartilage surrounding the centers of ossification of the cuboidal carpal bones.

mity of the contralateral limb. A hereditary angular limb deformity of Suffolk, Suffolk crossbred, and Hampshire sheep is known as spider lamb syndrome (see p. 1094).

PATHOPHYSIOLOGY. Incomplete ossification is an important cause of angular deformity that originates at the carpus and tarsus. The epiphyses and cuboidal bones of the carpus (ulnar, third, and fourth carpal bones) and tarsus (central and third tarsal bones) and the proximal epiphysis of the metatarsus are primarily affected.[29] Ossification of the cartilaginous precursors of these bones occurs in late gestation; prematurity or relative immaturity often results in the birth of a foal before these precursors are completely ossified (Figs. 36-4 and 36-5). If laxity of the periarticular supporting structures accompanies incomplete ossification, the deformity is congenital and may progressively worsen with weight bearing. If laxity is not present, the foal may be born with straight legs and acquire an angular deformity following deformation of the precursors of the cuboidal bones during weight-bearing activity.

Foals that grow rapidly appear predisposed to developing angular limb deformities as a result of asynchronous growth at the metaphyseal and epiphyseal growth cartilages.[30,31] An important cause of asynchronous growth is trauma to a portion of the growth cartilage.[34] In many foals this trauma is in the form of nonphysiologic compression of the growth cartilage resulting from asymmetric weight bearing in the affected limb. This asymmetry may arise when a foal with a mild pre-existing angular deformity is allowed uncontrolled exercise. Trauma to the growth cartilage occurs, and the angular deformity progressively worsens. When the angular deformity is greater than 15 degrees, normal weight-bearing activity may cause sufficient trauma to the growth cartilage to cause progressive deformity.

Asymmetric loading also occurs when severe lameness is present. With the change from a rectangular stance with four weight-bearing limbs to a triangular stance with three weight-bearing limbs, asymmetric, nonphysiologic loading of the weight-bearing limb occurs, which predisposes it to develop an angular deformity. Because compressive forces are concentrated along the medial aspect of the growth cartilages, a varus deformity usually develops in the overloaded limb. Abnormalities of the growth cartilage that affect ossification, such as osteochondrosis, also may be responsible for angular deformities caused by asynchronous growth. Foals with a predisposition for rapid growth or those that are exposed to nutritional imbalances appear to be at greatest risk for developing the disease. Rapid growth also may result in a foal with a large body size disproportionate to its skeletal structures. This condition may cause increased compressive forces, nonphysiologic loading of the growth cartilages, and angular deformity.[34]

Ruminants raised in confinement may experience endochondral dysplasia and angular limb deformities if dietary iron is high or dietary vitamin D is low[35] (see Rickets, p. 1088). Elevated dietary iron results in elevations in serum phosphorus, which may in turn inhibit synthesis of 1,25-dihydroxycholecalciferol production by the kidney, resulting in rickets.[35] Pregnancy-associated epiphysitis in primiparous dairy goats[36] also may result in angular limb deformities.

EVALUATION AND RADIOGRAPHIC FINDINGS. In the evaluation of a foal with an angular deformity, important historical information includes age, onset and progression of the deformity, and intended use of the foal. The foal should be observed carefully while standing and walking to characterize the degree of deformity and determine the presence of compensatory problems or lameness. Physical examination includes careful palpation of the affected limb and a determination of whether the deformity can be corrected by manual manipulation of the limb. If the foal is examined before ossification has progressed, deformities resulting from laxity of periarticular supporting structures and incomplete ossification can be corrected manually. On the other hand, if deformities in foals born with incomplete ossification are left untreated and the cuboidal bones are in a collapsed configuration, or if deformities are the result of asynchronous growth, they cannot be corrected manually.

An arthropathy should be suspected if lameness is present. Collapse of incompletely ossified cuboidal bones may result in deformation of articular surfaces and subsequent degenerative joint disease. When lesions are in the carpus the prognosis is guarded to poor for athletic performance; however, if the cuboidal bones of the tarsus are affected, even though there may be lameness, these foals often perform their intended function once fusion of the affected distal intertarsal and tarsometatarsal joints occurs. A less common cause of lameness in foals with angular limb deformity is osteochondrosis. The prognosis for athletic performance in foals with osteochondrosis-associated angular limb deformities is guarded, depending on the severity of the cartilage lesions.

The importance of early radiographic evaluation of foals with angular limb deformities cannot be overemphasized. If a diagnosis of incomplete ossification is delayed, irreparable damage, as described previously, may occur. In fact, a strong argument can be made for radiographic evaluation of all foals shortly after birth before uncontrolled exercise is allowed. Radiographic evaluation is mandatory to determine the degree of ossification in premature foals, twins, foals that appear to be relatively immature at birth, and foals born with angular deformities.

Radiography also is important to identify the origin of the deformity and determine its severity in foals. Dorsopalmar views for the carpus and fetlock using 7 × 17-inch film cassettes and a lateromedial view of the tarsus are recommended. In the carpus and fetlock the origin of the deformity may be subjectively determined by two geometric methods (Fig. 36-6). One is to draw longitudinal lines bisecting the long bones above and below the joint. Where these lines intersect is the pivot point, which is considered the origin of the deformity. In addition, the angle of incidence of these lines is an estimation of the degree of deformity. Another method, which I prefer for the carpus, is to draw lines through the carpal joints and the distal radial physis. These lines should be parallel to each other and perpendicular to the long axis of the radius and metacarpus. The origin and

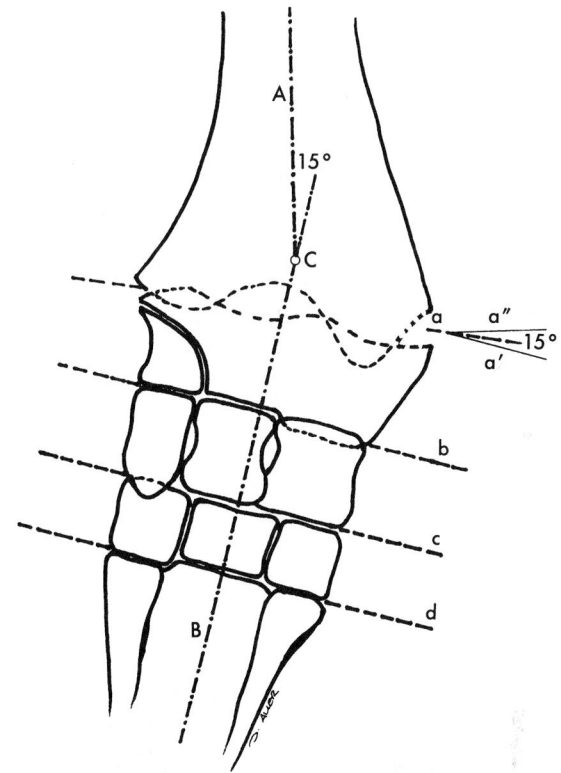

FIG. 36-6 ▓ Two methods for geometric evaluation of an angular deformity at the carpus. Lines *A* and *B* are drawn through the long axis of the radius and metacarpus, respectively. The angle of incidence is 15 degrees. Lines *a, b, c,* and *d* are drawn through the distal radial physis, antebrachiocarpal (radiocarpal), middle, and carpometacarpal joints, respectively. Line *a'* is drawn parallel to line *b,* and line *a* is perpendicular to *A.* Their angle of incidence is 15 degrees. (Reprinted with permission from *Compend Cont Educ Pract Vet* 4:S330-S339, 1982.)

degree of deformity are estimated by determining where and by what degree these lines deviate from normal. Both asynchronous growth and incomplete ossification can occur concurrently, and is most easily determined with the latter method of geometric evaluation[29] (Fig. 36-7).

Radiographic examination of foals with incomplete ossification reveals a rounded contour to the affected bones instead of their normal angular appearance. The width of the radiolucent cartilage is increased, appearing radiographically as an increase in the width of the joint space (Fig. 36-8). As ossification progresses, the bones may appear wedge-shaped or crushed because of deformation of the cartilage during weight bearing. This phenomenon often is noted in the ulnar, fourth, and lateral aspect of the third carpal bones in the forelimb and the central and third tarsal bones in the hind limb. In severe cases the affected bones may be grossly deformed and appear to be partially extruded from the joint (Fig. 36-9). Geometric evaluation of an angular deformity at the carpus as a result of incomplete ossification reveals that the deformity originates in the proximal or distal row of carpal bones.

In the tarsus, lateromedial radiographs are used to determine whether ossification is complete (Fig. 36-10). Geometric examination of the tarsus for varus and valgus deformity by the methods described previously is not performed because the tibia and third metatarsus are not in the same frontal plane. The severity of the angular deformity is best

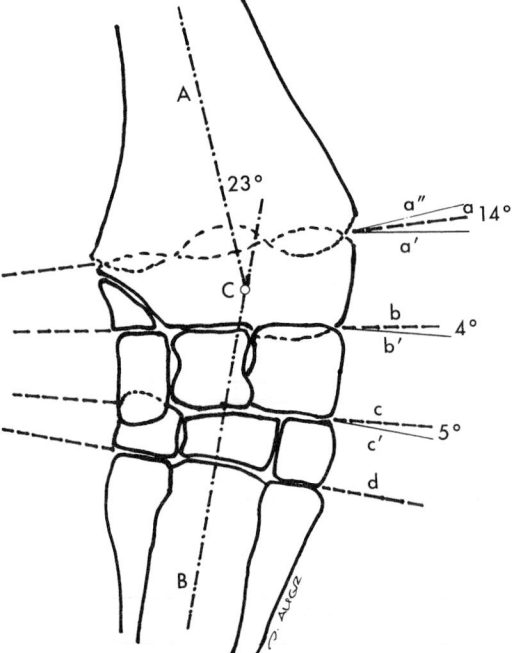

FIG. 36-7 ▮▮ Geometric evaluation of an angular deformity at the carpus caused by a combination of asynchronous growth and incomplete ossification. The pivot point, *C,* identified by lines *A* and *B,* indicates that the origin of the deformity is in the distal radial epiphysis. However, lines *a, b, c,* and *d* are not parallel to each other; and lines *a, b,* and *c* are not perpendicular to the long axis of the metacarpus and radius. Their orientation indicates that the deformity is in the distal radial physis and the cuboidal carpal bones as well. Note that the sum of angles of *a-a', b-b',* and *c-c'* equals the angle of incidence of lines *A* and *B.* (Reprinted with permission from *Compend Cont Educ Pract Vet* 4:S330-S339, 1982.)

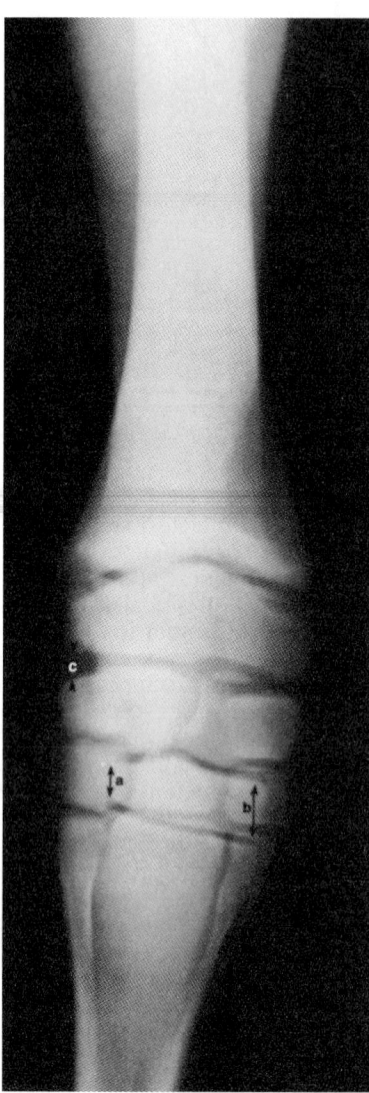

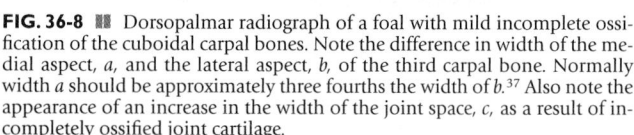

FIG. 36-8 ▮▮ Dorsopalmar radiograph of a foal with mild incomplete ossification of the cuboidal carpal bones. Note the difference in width of the medial aspect, *a,* and the lateral aspect, *b,* of the third carpal bone. Normally width *a* should be approximately three fourths the width of *b.*[37] Also note the appearance of an increase in the width of the joint space, *c,* as a result of incompletely ossified joint cartilage.

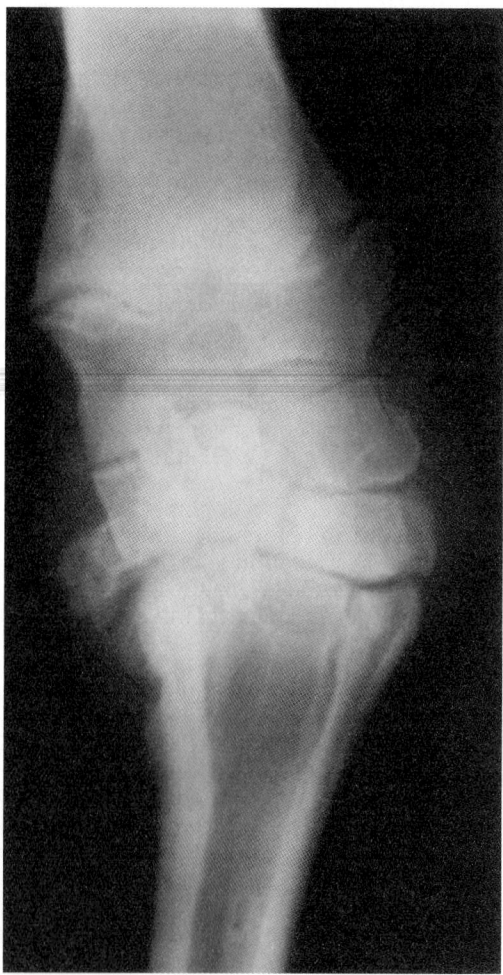

FIG. 36-9 ▮▮ Dorsopalmar radiograph of a foal with incomplete ossification that was not externally supported. Severe deformation and collapse of the fourth and third carpal and proximal fourth metacarpal bones have occurred.

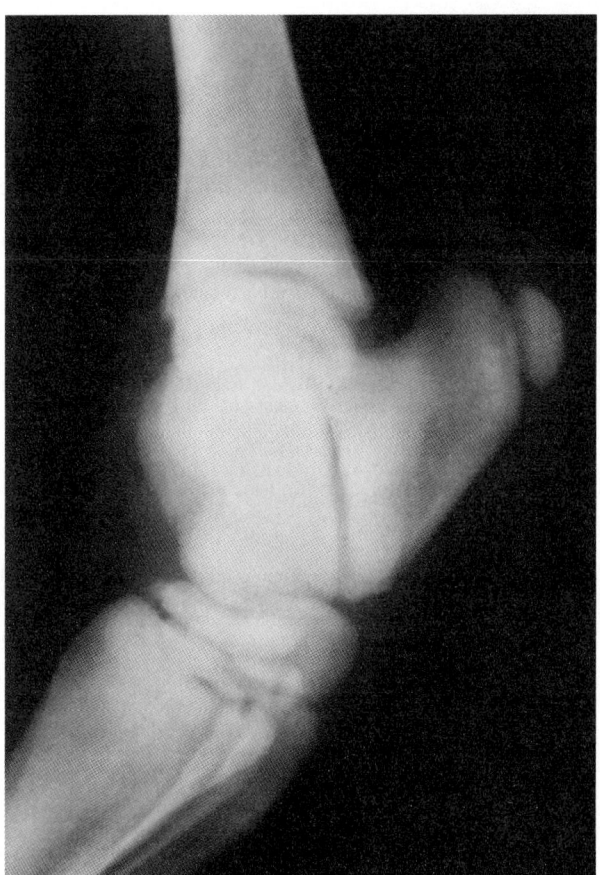

FIG. 36-10 ▍▍ Lateral-to-medial radiograph of a tarsus from a foal with incomplete ossification. Note the lack of an angular appearance of the central tarsal bone and incomplete ossification of the third tarsal bone.

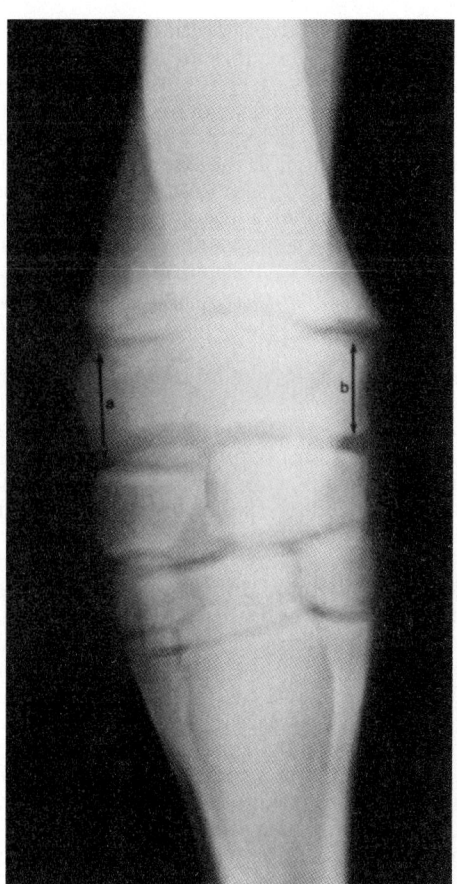

FIG. 36-11 ▍▍ Dorsopalmar radiograph of a foal with angular deformity caused by wedging in the distal radial epiphysis, the result of asynchronous growth of the epiphyseal growth cartilage.

determined by a careful visual assessment. Radiographic evaluation of foals with angular deformity caused by asynchronous growth may show wedging of the epiphysis (Fig. 36-11), widening of the physis, and sclerosis adjacent to the physis. In the carpus, geometric evaluation places the deviation in the metaphysis or the epiphysis of the distal radius. The carpal joints parallel each other and are perpendicular to the long axis of the metacarpus.

TREATMENT AND PROGNOSIS. Once an angular deformity is recognized, the mare and foal should be confined to a stall until clinical and radiographic examinations are completed. If the deformity is equal to or less than 10 degrees and radiographs reveal normal ossification, stall confinement with periods of controlled exercise is recommended. This regimen promotes continued development of the supporting structures while minimizing trauma to growth cartilages that could result if the foal is allowed uncontrolled exercise. Foals with angular deformity resulting from asynchronous growth also should be confined to a stall and allowed only controlled exercise to minimize the magnitude of asymmetric loading at the growth cartilages. In foals less than 2 to 3 months of age, with angular deformities of the carpus and tarsus of less than 10 degrees, correction may occur spontaneously. In these instances, reducing the magnitude of the forces acting asymmetrically at the growth cartilage may allow compensatory growth to occur and correct the deformity. Additional therapy consists of corrective hoof trimming. Because foals with valgus deformity typically have a toe-out conformation, emphasis in the past has been to lower the lat-

eral hoof wall of the affected limb. If this mode of therapy is vigorously pursued, compensatory varus deformity has developed in the fetlock region. This form of corrective trimming concentrates forces asymmetrically on the medial aspect of the distal metacarpal and proximal phalangeal growth cartilages. Currently, trimming the hoof level and squaring the toe to promote breakover at the toe are recommended. If the lateral hoof wall is to be lowered, only a few millimeters should be removed each week.

The affected limb in foals with a congenital angular deformity of more than 10 degrees accompanied by incomplete ossification or failure to improve with controlled exercise for 3 to 5 days should be externally supported. If incomplete ossification is present and the limb is not supported and axially aligned, continued weight bearing results in deformation of the cartilaginous structures. Subsequent ossification results in a permanent deformity of the affected bones (see Fig. 36-9).

Methods of externally supporting the carpus and tarsus vary from the application of tube casts or rigid splints to orthotic devices that have been adapted from human medicine. The introduction of a commercial brace developed for foals has renewed interest in the use of orthotic devices. Success with this device has been reported anecdotally; however, an objective evaluation of its use in foals has not yet appeared in the scientific literature. Tube casts have been recommended and used successfully for several years.[29-31] Although they provide the rigid external support needed to maintain axial alignment while ossification progresses, several potential complications are associated with their use. Most serious of these complications is the potential for the occurrence of coxofemoral luxation when they are used on the hind limbs. In addition, foal skin is easily traumatized by an ill-fitting cast, and deep ulcerations may occur. Other considerations include the cost of materials and need for constant monitoring to detect signs of an ill-fitting cast. In my experience monitoring the status of a cast requires at least evaluations twice a day by a trained individual, and owners are seldom capable or willing to take on this responsibility. Therefore hospitalization is recommended. An alternative method of supporting the carpus is with the use of rigid splints. A 4-inch-diameter polyvinyl chloride pipe can be split in half longitudinally or in thirds to form a splint that extends from the distal metacarpus to the proximal radius. The leg is protected with a padded support bandage, and the splint is applied with nonelastic tape while the limb is held in axial alignment by an assistant. These splint bandages are changed every third or fourth day. Care still must be taken to avoid developing pressure sores beneath the splint bandage. A splint for the tarsus may be fashioned from synthetic casting material molded lengthwise over the cranial aspect of a padded bandage centered at the joint. Once the material has dried, the splint is taped to the dorsal surface of the bandage.

Regardless of the means of external support used for the carpus or tarsus, it should not extend beyond the distal metacarpus or metatarsus. This approach allows weight bearing by the suspensory apparatus and helps prevent the development of fetlock hyperextension after removal of the external support. However, some degree of carpal hyperextension is usually present immediately after removal of external support from the forelimb. In affected foals, exercise should be limited until the tendons and periarticular supporting structures regain their normal tone.

Acquired 10-degree angular limb deformities of the carpus or tarsus or those not responding to stall confinement within 4 to 6 weeks are candidates for surgical therapy. In addition, deformities at the fetlock in foals 4 to 6 weeks of age should be considered for surgery. Although it was previously believed that angular deformities arising distal to the physis were not candidates for surgical therapy, it has been shown recently that they do respond favorably to surgery.[37,38]

To be effective, surgical therapy aimed at modulating growth at the physis must be accomplished during a period of active physeal growth. The most rapid rate of growth occurs from birth to 10 weeks of age.[39] In the distal radius, continuous though declining growth occurs until 60 weeks of age. In the distal third metacarpal and metatarsal bones, growth nearly ceases by 10 weeks of age. Therefore timing of surgery should consider these periods of growth. In general, surgery for correction of angular deformities of the carpus and tarsus is best performed before the foal is 3 months old. Angular limb deformities of the fetlock, however, must be approached more aggressively and, in general, should be treated surgically before 6 weeks of age.

Growth at the physis may be modulated in two ways. Historically, the preferred treatment was growth retardation by bridging the physis with metallic implants on the convex side of the bone. Techniques of transphyseal bridging include stapling, screw and wire implants, and the use of a small bone plate. These techniques are still used in certain instances, but in routine cases have been replaced by periosteal transection. In foals approaching the end of physiologic growth or with very severe angular deformity, the two techniques may be combined.

Periosteal transection (stripping) is aimed at accelerating growth on the concave side of the bone.[40] It has the advantage of rapid correction without the potential for overcorrection.[37,40] Periosteal transection does not require implants;

therefore the potential for infection, implant failure, and excessive fibrosis is reduced. In addition, a second surgery for implant removal is not required. The procedure does not require specialized equipment and is technically easy to perform. In one series of foals, correction of the deformity occurred in 22 of 25 limbs treated with periosteal transection.[40] In a second series of 23 foals, 83% had straight limbs and were sound for their intended use at long-term follow-up.[37] The success rate was not affected by the origin of the deformity, degree of deviation, or the presence of mild-to-moderate morphologic changes of the involved bones.[40]

REFERENCES

29. Auer JA, Martens RJ, Morris EL: Angular limb deformities in foals. Part I. Congenital factors, *Compend Cont Educ Pract Vet* 4:S330-S339, 1982.
30. Auer JA, Martens RJ, Morris EL: Angular limb deformities in foals, Part II. Developmental factors, *Compend Cont Educ Pract Vet* 5:S27-S40, 1983.
31. Leitch M: Angular limb deformities arising at the carpal region in foals, *Compend Cont Educ (Pract Vet)* 1:S39-S43, 1979.
32. McLaughlin BG, Doige CE, Fretz PB, et al: Carpal bone lesions associated with angular limb deformities in foals, *J Am Vet Med Assoc* 178:224-230, 1981.
33. Pharr JW, Fretz PB: Radiographic findings in foals with angular limb deformities, *J Am Vet Med Assoc* 179:812-817, 1981.
34. Turner AS: Diseases of bones and related structures. In Stashak TS, editor: *Adams' lameness in horses,* ed 4, Philadelphia, 1987, Lea & Febiger, pp 293-338.
35. Hidiroglou M, Dukes TW, Ho SK, et al: Bent-limb syndrome in lambs raised in total confinement, *J Am Vet Med Assoc* 173:1572-1574, 1978.
36. Anderson KL, Adams WM: Epiphysitis and recumbency in a yearling prepartum goat, *J Am Vet Med Assoc* 183:226-228, 1983.
37. Bertone AL, Turner AS, Park RD: Periosteal transection and stripping for treatment of angular limb deformities in foals: clinical observations, *J Am Vet Med Assoc* 187:145-152, 1985.
38. Bertone AL, Park RD, Turner AS: Periosteal transection and stripping for treatment of angular limb deformities in foals: radiographic observations, *J Am Vet Med Assoc* 187:153-156, 1985.
39. Fretz PB, Cymbaluk NK, Pharr JW: Quantitative analysis of long-bone growth in the horse, *Am J Vet Res* 45:1602-1609, 1984.
40. Auer JA, Martens RJ, Williams EH: Periosteal transection for correction of angular limb deformities in foals, *J Am Vet Med Assoc* 181:459-466, 1982.

SPIDER LAMB SYNDROME (OVINE HEREDITARY CHONDRODYSPLASIA)

NANCY E. EAST

By the mid-1980s, multiple reports from all areas of the United States were documenting the occurrence of Suffolk lambs with skeletal abnormalities, commonly called *spiders, spider lambs, corkscrew lambs, monkey lambs, crooked lambs,* and *bent lambs* by producers. Simultaneously in several university-owned Suffolk sheep flocks, lambs were born affected with the spider syndrome, and research began to describe and characterize the syndrome.[41]

DEFINITION AND ETIOLOGY. Spider lamb syndrome is characterized by generalized chondrodysplasia and is apparently a semilethal autosomal-recessive trait. Variable expressivity of the trait may occur in the homozygous animal.[42-44] It has been seen in Suffolk, Suffolk crossbred, and Hampshire sheep (Hampshire sheep often have some Suffolk breeding). At this time no chondrodysplastic lambs from any white face breeds of sheep have been reported.

CLINICAL SIGNS. Lambs affected with spider lamb syndrome are characterized by overall appendicular and axial deformities, including one or more of the following conditions[42,44]: kyphosis, scoliosis, concavity of the sternum, lateroventral deviation of the maxilla (crooked nose and roman nose), and angular limb deformities. The limb deformities usually include a "knock-kneed" appearance at the carpus (carpus valgus) and lateral deviation with rotation of the metacarpus or metatarsus (Fig. 36-12). In addition, these lambs show extreme height, fineness of bone, poor muscling, and failure to thrive (Fig. 36-13).

The number and severity of the deformities seen in individual lambs vary widely. Spider lamb syndrome can occur in two types of lambs: those that are obviously abnormal at birth and, more commonly, those that develop abnormali-

ties at 3 to 8 weeks of age. Lambs that are abnormal at birth may have kyphosis, scoliosis, facial deformities, deformed sternum, and angular limb deformities.[42] Lesions may be present as early as day 100 of gestation, but are not detectable by radiographic or ultrasound examination.[44] The lambs may be stillborn or die within a few days of birth because of their inability to stand or nurse. If these lambs are maintained by good nursing care, they fail to gain weight normally and usually die of secondary problems such as scours or pneumonia by 4 weeks of age. In lambs that are apparently normal at birth but develop angular limb deformities at 3 to 8 weeks of age, from one to four limbs may be affected; and on close examination curvature of the spine and concavity of the sternum is present. Often these lambs are unusually tall, long necked, fine boned, and poorly muscled. The growth rate of these spider lambs decreases after 4 to 8 weeks of age, and the various deformities become more marked until the lambs can no longer walk; chronic bacterial pneumonia and pathologic fractures are common.

Attempts to maintain spider lambs for research are rarely successful beyond 6 months to 1 year of age. In Illinois an affected ram lamb was able to breed seven ewes before he died, but in California two affected ram lambs failed successive semen evaluations from 7 to 12 months of age and were euthanized because of their poor condition.

RADIOGRAPHIC FINDINGS. Currently spider lamb syndrome is diagnosed on the basis of appearance, radiographic changes, and pathology (gross and microscopic). Radiographic changes are diagnostic; however, serial radiographs may be necessary in some cases. Radiographically, there are widened irregular growth plates with retained islands of cartilage in the olecranon, sternum, shoulder, long bones, and spine (Fig. 36-14). The most constant radiographic lesion is in the olecranon, which exhibits multiple islands of ossifica-

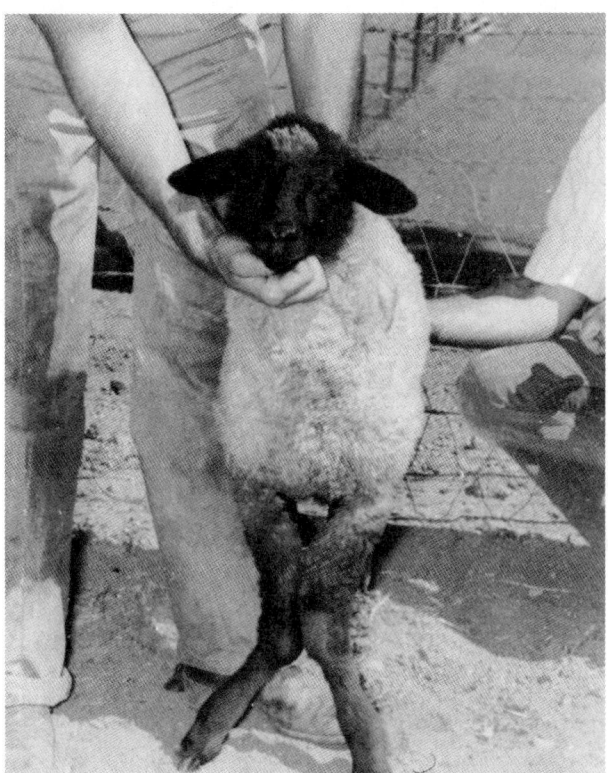

FIG. 36-12 ▮▮ Rotation and deviation of front legs (carpus valgus) characteristic of spider lamb syndrome in a 16-week-old Suffolk lamb.

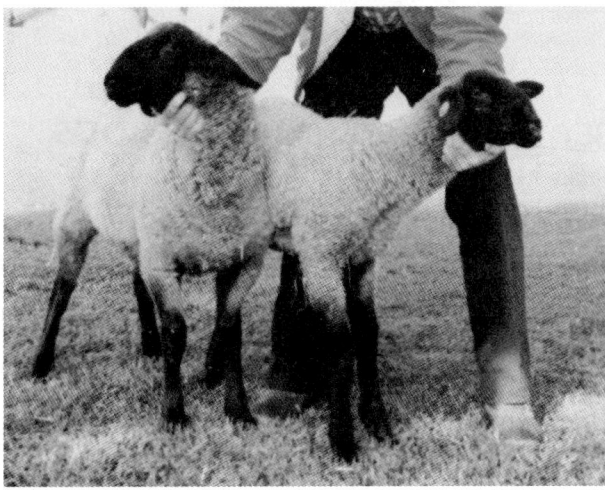

FIG. 36-13 ▮▮ Normal (78 pounds) *(left)* and lambs with spider syndrome (37 pounds) *(right)*. Twin Suffolks (12 weeks old); note extreme height, narrow chest, scoliosis, kyphosis, and facial deformity of affected lamb.

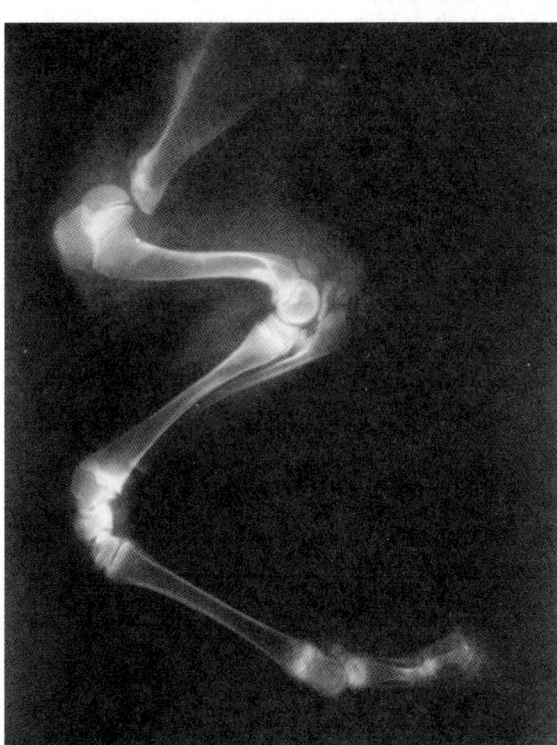

FIG. 36-14 ▮▮ Lateral radiograph of front leg of a lamb with spider syndrome. Note thick, irregular growth plates and multiple ossification centers near the olecranon and distal humerus.

tion instead of the uniform nonmineralized cartilage surrounded by dense bone in a normal lamb[42,45] (Fig. 36-14). The olecranon should be radiographed lateral to medial with the elbow flexed. The changes in the olecranon usually begin by 1 to 3 weeks of age and are progressive. Lambs that are stillborn or die in the first week of life may not exhibit radiographic abnormalities in growth plates associated with spider syndrome. Chromosome evaluation, hematology, and standard serum chemistry, as well as morphologic and biochemical evaluations of growth plate, have not been abnormal in spider lambs.[44-46] Circulating levels of insulin-like growth factor-I and its associated hepatic mRNA are increased in very young spider lambs. The proliferative zone of the growth plate is a major target of insulin-like growth factor-I.[47] Differential diagnosis includes other diseases that result in congenital defects (scoliosis, kyphosis, and arthrogryposis, often associated with hydranencephaly), including Cache Valley virus, bluetongue virus, lupine ingestion, and the bent leg syndrome.[42,45] The bent leg syndrome is believed to be a dietary problem in young lambs suckling ewes on unimproved pasture; chondrodysplasia of the elbow is not present.

EPIDEMIOLOGY. Limited breeding trials, pedigree analysis of breeding stock producing spiders, and the wide geographic distribution of spider lambs indicates that the spider syndrome is an inherited defect and is probably an autosomal-recessive gene.[43,44] Some workers believe that the selection for very tall sheep within the Suffolk breed resulted in selection for the recessive trait. Affected lambs are double recessive (ss), and both of the parents must be carriers (heterozygotes Ss) to produce a spider lamb (Fig. 36-15). Carrier sheep appear to be fairly common within the seed stock of the Suffolk breed and presently can be identified only when they produce a spider lamb. The appearance of a clinically affected lamb may lag years behind the introduction of carrier breeding stock, especially if a carrier ram is crossed into a ewe flock free of the trait. It is important that the diagnosis of a spider lamb is made correctly and with care, particularly in lambs that die before 3 weeks of age, because the condition may be confused with other congenital defects causing scoliosis, kyphosis, and arthrogryposis. Not all lambs suspected as being spider lambs can be confirmed as such.

NECROPSY FINDINGS. Gross postmortem examination findings are similar to radiographic changes (generalized chondrodysplasia). Joint cartilage may show erosion, and excess cartilage is evident in thickened irregular growth plates and in the olecranon. Retained cartilage cores are apparent on the metaphyseal side of affected growth plates. Dysplastic growth plates of spider lamb syndrome are characterized by thickened proliferative and hypertrophic zones and a failure to form organized columns. Histologically, chondrocytes exhibit a chaotic pattern of ossification, with chondrocyte pro-liferation in areas of maturation and loss of normal pattern and direction.[42,46]

PREVENTION AND CONTROL. Carrier rams should be destroyed, but carrier ewes can be used to produce market lambs or to progeny test rams for the spider trait. Ram lambs produced from carrier ewes must not be used for crossbreeding on commercial ewes of any breed except for terminal cross-market lambs because crossbred Suffolk lambs can carry the trait into the commercial sheep industry. A ram can be progeny tested by breeding to ewes that have produced spider lambs or by breeding to its own daughters. If a ram produces 16 normal offspring from matings with known carrier ewes or 32 normal offspring from mating with his own daughters, the probability that he is a carrier is less than 1 in 100. This procedure is costly to the breeder, and the temptation to retain a ram without an adequate number of test progeny is great. Rams that have enough normal progeny to reduce the probability of being a carrier to less than 5 out of 100 have produced spider lambs from the next test breedings needed to complete the progeny test.* Within the purebred industry, breeding stock is classified as white (no known spider progeny), gray (sire or dam or sibling has produced a spider lamb, but this individual has not), or carrier or black (individual has produced a spider lamb). Inaccuracies in sheep pedigrees make prediction of the genetic makeup of any individual risky, and classification without proper testing may be potential grounds for legal action. If parentage of a spider lamb is in question, blood-typing of the sire, dam, and offspring may be helpful.†‡

REFERENCES

41. Culham A: The spider lamb syndrome: where are we today, where shall we go tomorrow? *Suffolk Banner* 11:54-56, 70, 1988.
42. Rook JS, Trapp AL, Krehbiel J, et al: Diagnosis of hereditary chondrodysplasia (spider lamb syndrome) in sheep, *J Am Vet Med Assoc* 193:713-718, 1988.
43. Berg PT, Alstad AD, Moore BL, et al: The mode of inheritance of the "spider" lamb syndrome in Suffolk sheep, *Sheep Industry Res Dig* Fall 1987.
44. Oberbauer AM, East NE, Pool R et al: Developmental progression of the spider lamb syndrome, *Small Rumin Res* 18:179-184, 1995.
45. Troyer DL, Thomas DL, Stein LE: A morphologic and biochemical evaluation of the spider syndrome in Suffolk sheep, *Anat Histol Embryol* 17:289-300, 1988.
46. Vanek JA, Bleier WJ, Whited DA, et al: Comparison of G-banded chromosomes from clinically normal lambs and lambs affected with ovine hereditary chondrodysplasia (spider syndrome), *Am J Vet Res* 49:1164-1168, 1988.
47. Osborne JM, Thomas DL, White ME: Insulin-like growth factor-I levels and gene expression in ovine hereditary chrondrodysplasia (spider lamb syndrome), *Dom Anim Endocrinol* 9:25-35, 1992.

SEPTIC ARTHRITIS (INFECTIOUS ARTHRITIS)

JAMES A. ORSINI

DEFINITION AND ETIOLOGY. Septic, infectious, or suppurative arthritis is an inflammatory disease confined to the joints as a result of sequestered bacteria, fungi, or viral microorganisms.[48,49] One or more joints may be involved. Suppurative arthritis (SA) can arise in one of four ways: (1) hematogenous, (2) trauma, (3) extension, and (4) iatrogenic infections.[50,51] Hematogenous infection is seen most frequently in septicemic foals. *Actinobacillus equuli*, *Streptococcus* spp., *Salmonella* spp.,

---

*Bob Rutherford: Personal communication, 1988.

†Stormont Laboratories, 1237 East Beamer Street, Woodland, CA 95695.

‡Genetics Lab, School of Veterinary Medicine, University of California, Davis, CA 95616.

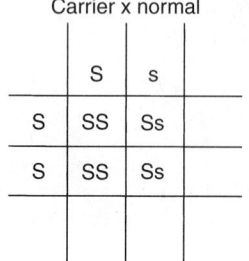
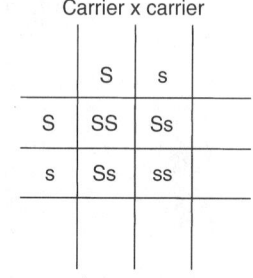

Carrier x normal				Carrier x carrier		
	S	s			S	s
S	SS	Ss		S	SS	Ss
S	SS	Ss		s	Ss	ss

FIG. 36-15 ■ Spider syndrome is believed caused by an autosomal recessive. This figure illustrates probable mode of inheritance in two possible matings that could produce spider lambs. *SS,* Normal; *Ss,* carrier; *ss,* affected.

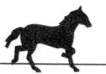

and *Escherichia coli,* and other enterobacteriaceae are frequently implicated in these cases.[51-53] In older horses, SA often follows intraarticular injections, particularly of corticosteroids. Staphylococci are the most frequently reported isolates in iatrogenic infections.[53] Not unexpectedly, multiple organisms may be isolated in SA related to traumatic wounds, commonly including enterobacteriaceae and anaerobes.[53,54]

In SA in cattle *Actinomyces pyogenes* is the most commonly identified pathogen.[55] *Chlamydia psittaci* polyarthritis occurs endemically or epidemically in sheep, goats,[53] and calves.[54] It is characterized by stiffness, shifting leg lameness, and fever. Keratoconjunctivitis may accompany the disease. *C. psittaci* abortion (enzootic abortion of ewes) is caused by a different serotype and is not associated with polyarthritis and/or keratoconjunctivitis.

Chlamydial polyarthritis is of major importance to the U.S. sheep industry. It occurs mainly in 1- to 8-month-old lambs.[55] *Mycoplasma mycoides* polyarthritis in goats also must be considered (see p. 1099). In lambs, *Erysipelothrix rhusiopathiae* commonly causes polyarthritis. It is found in soil and manure and gains entrance through the umbilical stump, freshly docked tail, or castration site. Most cases appear 1 to 5 weeks after processing of lambs. Prevention is by use of hot iron tail-docking techniques, disinfection of instruments and hands during castration, and keeping lambs in a clean environment (ample clean pasture) after processing.[55] *Actinobacillus seminis* is a cause of septic polyarthritis in lambs and rams 4 to 8 months old and is often associated with epididymitis in the latter group. Blood cultures should be obtained in all neonates and under all circumstances in which systemic involvement is present (e.g., fever, leukocytosis, plasma hyperfibrinogenemia). Septic arthritis in neonates is discussed further in Chapters 19 and 20.

CLINICAL SIGNS AND DIFFERENTIAL DIAGNOSIS. Localizing signs in SA include lameness, which progresses to nonweight bearing in the advanced stages of the disease. Classic signs of inflammation are usually present: heat, pain, swelling, and redness involving the periarticular soft tissues, accompanied by a synovial effusion. However, a transient inflammatory response to intraarticular injections may mimic the clinical signs of SA, including synovial fluid changes. Given that microorganisms are not always successfully isolated from synovial fluid or membrane, if any uncertainty exists, the joint should be treated as if it were infected.[53-59] Fever, especially in the neonate, is not a consistent finding unless polyarthritis is present. The physical examination, laboratory analysis (e.g., complete blood count, synovial fluid cytology, and culture), ultrasonography, and radiography are useful procedures to aid

in a definitive diagnosis. When *C. psittaci* is the cause of the polyarthritis, follicular conjunctivitis often accompanies the lameness.[55] Corneal vascularization and edema may be present. Lambs with erysipelothritic polyarthritis are stiff and lame and show marked weight loss. Death usually occurs from starvation or secondary disease such as pneumonia. Arthritis in lambs caused by *Chlamydia* and *Erysipelothrix* spp. must be carefully differentiated.

CLINICAL PATHOLOGY AND DIAGNOSTIC TESTS. The importance of early and accurate diagnosis of joint infection cannot be overemphasized because of the severity of cartilage and connective tissue destruction associated with infection. Generally, systemic examination of peripheral blood for leukocytosis and hyperfibrinogenemia and synovial fluid for bacteria leads to a diagnosis of SA. Joint fluid cytology indicating inflammation can suggest infection without positive cultures or histopathologic findings to substantiate bacterial invasion. Significant findings include a nucleated cell count in excess of 10,000 cells/μl, a >80% neutrophilia, and a total protein count >40 g/L.[53,59,60] Adjunctive techniques that help to confirm joint infection include synovial fluid and tissue bacterial and fungal cultures, joint fluid analysis (Table 36-1), radiographic evaluation, and gas chromatography.[48,50,54] Bacteria often localize in the synovial membrane, and joint fluid cultures may be negative when a biopsy of synovium results in bacterial growth. If *Chlamydia* or *Mycoplasma* spp. are suspected, special culture techniques must be used.

Joint fluid from lambs with either *C. psittaci* or *Erysipelothrix insidiosa* polyarthritis is off-color with flakes of fibrin but is not purulent in appearance, and mononuclear cells predominate.[55]

Elementary inclusion bodies may be seen on Giemsa-, Gimenez-, or Macchiavellos-stained smears of joint fluid when *Chlamydia* spp. are present.[55] Fluorescent antibody (FA) techniques on joint fluid (or synovial tissue or conjunctiva at necropsy) is a useful diagnostic aid. The FA technique is applicable to both serotypes of *Chlamydia* spp. A rising titer from acute to convalescent sera is diagnostic.

Samples for aerobic and anaerobic bacteria should be obtained, together with synovial fluid samples collected for immediate Gram stain. The sediment obtained after centrifugation of synovial fluid yields a higher number of organisms for Gram stain and culture. Rapid identification of bacteria is possible based on short-chain and total cellular fatty acid composition of the bacteria and their metabolic byproducts.[50] This method may become more useful in the early diagnosis of suppurative arthritis.

Radiology in the diagnosis of SA is useful after 2 to 3 weeks, when extensive destruction of cartilage has occurred.

TABLE 36-1

Characteristics of Synovial Fluid According to Condition in Large Animals

Characteristic	Normal	Septic	Degenerative Joint Disease	Inflammatory*
Color	Clear	Yellow/green	Yellow	Yellow to irridescent
Clarity	Transparent	Turbid	Transparent	Translucent
Fluid volume	Low	Increased	Low	Increased (usually)
Viscosity	High	Low	Variable	Low (usually)
WBC/μl	<200	30,000-100,000	200-2000	2000-10,000
PMN (%)	<25	>75	25	>75
Glucose	Equal to blood	<25 mg/dl	Equal to blood	25 to 50 mg/dl lower than blood
Gram or other stain	No bacteria seen	Bacteria observed frequently	No bacteria seen	No bacteria seen

WBC, White blood cell; *PMN,* polymorphonuclear cell.
*May include some low-grade septic conditions in which bacteria are not found.

In reality, diagnostic radiology plays a minor role in the clinical management of acute joint infection. In specific cases, if its limitations and drawbacks are understood, the application of radiology may be useful (Fig. 36-16).

PATHOPHYSIOLOGY. The specific pathophysiologic changes that occur intraarticularly as a result of infection and the reaction of joints to a given infection can vary markedly. The progression of septic arthritis includes (1) bacterial invasion, (2) polymorphonuclear cells (PMNs), (3) synovitis, and (4) cartilage destruction. If multiplication of the invading organism is limited and the reaction is confined to a small area in the synovium, there will be minimum tissue destruction with slight-to-moderate effusion.[49,50,52,54]

The detrimental effect of inflammation and infection on the absorptive function of synovial membrane is debated. Particle size is important because of different routes available for absorption (i.e., lymphatics, capillaries). Absorption increases during acute inflammation and decreases during chronic inflammation.[50] This is of particular importance when considering antimicrobial penetration.

The host inflammatory response is thought to be the primary cause of joint damage in SA. During inflammation, specifically in response to infection, fibrin clots are a principal component of the inflammatory exudate. Fibrin deposited in the synovium contributes substantially to permanent joint damage and maintains a vicious cycle of inflammation. Intraarticular fibrin disrupts normal cartilage function by adhering to articular cartilage and altering the flow of nutrients to cartilage and the flow of metabolic byproducts from cartilage.[50] Leukocytes are chemotactically attracted to the fibrin, where they self-destruct and release enzymes into the synovial fluid. Cartilage destruction may be the result of collagenase enzymatic attack on cartilage matrix. Joint damage can be minimized if fibrin deposition can be reduced or fibrin accumulation is efficiently removed.

PATHOLOGY. Gross findings at necropsy in SA include intracapsular fibrinous-to-purulent exudate. The articular surfaces may be eroded with edematous periarticular tissues. In chlamydial polyarthritis the joint is slightly enlarged, the amount of fibrin is remarkably large, and there is synovitis and often tendon sheath involvement. In goats this must be differentiated from *M. mycoides* polyarthritis. Chlamydial polyarthritis results in villus proliferation, focal necrosis of synovial cells, edema, fibrin deposition, and mononuclear cell infiltration.[55] Lesions caused by *E. rhusiopathiae* are similar to those of *Chlamydia* spp.[55]

TREATMENT. Successful treatment of SA depends on an accurate clinical and microbiologic diagnosis. A successful treatment regimen for horses with suppurative arthritis must neutralize lysosomal enzymes, drain the joint of purulent exudate,

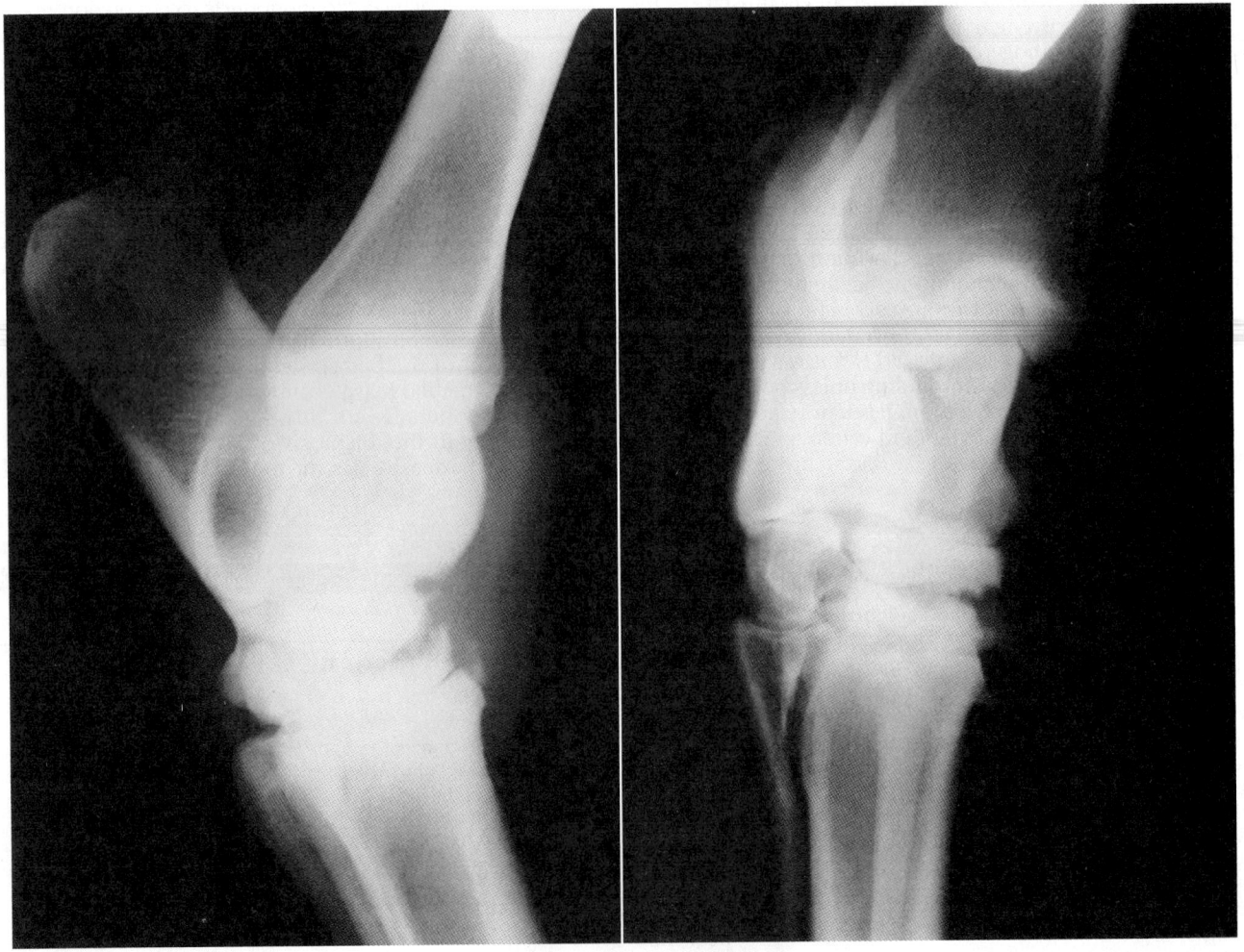

A

B

FIG. 36-16 ▮▮ Tarsal joint with infectious (septic) arthritis. **A,** Lateral projection of the tarsus. **B,** Dorsal plantar anterior view. Medial oblique with periosteal proliferative changes with osteolysis.

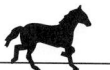

and eliminate fibrin clots. For management to be successful, it is mandatory that horses with a positive culture from a joint aspirate be treated with antimicrobial drugs.[48,51,54]

Systemic use of antimicrobial agents relies on appropriate antimicrobial penetration across the synovial membrane. Antimicrobial agents of large molecular size do not cross the synovial membrane with the same rapidity as those of smaller-sized molecules. All presently known antimicrobial agents, however, cross the synovial membrane when administered in therapeutic concentrations. The intraarticular injection of antimicrobial agents to attain high and prolonged therapeutic concentrations in joint fluid may be another consideration. Chemical synovitis is the primary disadvantage of intraarticular administration.[50] Specific antimicrobial agents that attain therapeutic concentrations in joint fluid after systemic administration are penicillin G, β-lactamase-resistant penicillins, cephalosporins, ticarcillin, ticarcillin-clavulanic acid, erythromycin, and aminoglycosides. A combination of amikacin and a cephalosporin has been recommended for empiric therapy of SA in horses, based on in vitro susceptibility studies of bacterial isolates from horses with musculoskeletal infection.[54] A 4- to 6-week course of antibiotics is advisable to reduce the risk of recurrence.

Several methods of joint drainage have been used, including needle aspiration, through-and-through lavage, distention irrigation, and arthrotomy/arthroscopy with or without synovectomy.[48-50,57] Good results have been obtained with the use of closed suction drainage for SA of the tarsocrural joint in horses.[61] A combination of open drainage arthrotomy, joint lavage, and systemic and intraarticular antibiotics (primarily amikacin) also has been used with success.[62] In one study of experimental SA, arthrotomy with lavage provided better drainage and more rapid clinical response than the combination of arthroscopy, synovectomy, and lavage; however, horses treated by arthrotomy had a higher risk of contamination through the incisions.[63] Other supportive treatments include immobilization of the affected limb, analgesics, and intraarticular injections of sodium hyaluronate.

Chlamydial polyarthritis must be vigorously treated with tetracycline (20 mg/kg of long-acting tetracycline intramuscularly or subcutaneously every 48 hours for three treatments), tylosin (label dose), or erythromycin (label dose). Animals should not be medicated through feed or water, because they are reluctant to eat and drink when they are in pain. *E. rhusiopathiae* is sensitive to most antibiotics; penicillin is commonly used. Many animals fail to respond to treatment if joint damage is advanced. Chlamydial vaccines are available (see Chapter 44).

PROGNOSIS. Variables that have a direct relationship on the outcome of SA include duration of the infection before treatment, the identity of the offending organism, and host factors such as immunocompetence and anatomic properties of the joint. SA in foals generally has a poor prognosis unless treated very early. In a number of cases, early and aggressive treatment of SA in mature horses has resulted in full return to athletic function. Of 13 horses treated with systemic antibiotics and closed-suction drainage, 10 returned to good health or to previous level of competition.[61] In humans clinical studies have shown a direct relationship between the duration of infection before treatment and outcome.[53] A retrospective review of 192 horses with aggressively treated SA or tenosynovitis found a hospital discharge rate of 45% for foals and 85% for horses, with 56% returned to racing to make at least one start.[53]

REFERENCES

48. Koch DB: Management of infectious arthritis in the horse, *Compend Cont Educ Pract Vet* 1:S45-S50, 1979.

49. McIlwraith CW: Infectious arthritis. In Stashak TS, editor: *Adam's lameness in horses*, Philadelphia, 1987, Lea & Febiger, pp 423-432.

50. Orsini JA: Strategies for treatment of bone and joint infections in large animals, *J Am Vet Med Assoc* 185:1190-1193, 1984.

51. Martens RJ: Pathogenesis, diagnosis and therapy of septic arthritis in foals, *J Vet Orthop* 2:49-58, 1980.

52. Martens RJ, Auer JA, Carter KC: Equine pediatrics: septic arthritis and osteomyelitis, *J Am Vet Med Assoc* 188:582-585, 1986.

53. Schneider RK, Bramlage LR, Moore RM, et al: A retrospective study of 192 horses affected with septic arthritis/tenosynovitis, *Equine Vet J* 24:436-442, 1992.

54. Moore RM, Schneider RK, Kowalski J, et al: Antimicrobial susceptibility of bacterial isolates from 233 horses with musculoskeletal infection during 1979-1989, *Equine Vet J* 24:450-456, 1992.

55. Trent AM, Plumb D: Treatment of infectious arthritis and osteomyelitis, *Vet Clin North Am (Food Anim Pract)* 7:747-778, 1991.

56. Bulgin MS: Diagnosis of lameness in sheep, *Compend Cont Educ Pract Vet* 8:F122-F128, 1986.

57. Perez-Martinez JA, Storz J: Chlamydial infections in cattle. Part 1, *Mod Vet Pract* 66:517-522, 1985.

58. Jensen R, Swift BL: *Diseases of sheep*, ed 2, Philadelphia, 1982, Lea & Febiger.

59. Tulamo RM, Bramlage LR, Gabel AA: Sequential clinical and synovial fluid changes associated with acute infectious arthritis in the horse, *Equine Vet J* 21:325-331, 1989.

60. Madison JR, Sommer M, Spencer PA: Relations among synovial membrane histopathologic findings, synovial fluid cytologic findings, and bacterial culture results in horses with suspected infectious arthritis: 64 cases (1979-1987), *J Am Vet Med Assoc* 198:1655-1661, 1991.

61. Ross MW, Orsini JA, Richardson DW, et al: Closed suction drainage in the treatment of infectious arthritis of the equine tarsocrural joint, *Vet Surg* 20:21-29, 1991.

62. Schneider RK, Bramlage LR, Mecklenburg LM, et al: Open drainage, intraarticular and systemic antibiotics in the treatment of septic arthritis/tenosynovitis in horses, *Equine Vet J* 24:443-449, 1992.

63. Bertone AL, Davis DM, Cox HU, et al: Arthrotomy versus arthroscopy and partial synovectomy for treatment of experimentally induced infectious arthritis in horses, *Am J Vet Res* 53:585-591, 1992.

MYCOPLASMA MYCOIDES POLYARTHRITIS OF GOATS

NANCY E. EAST

DEFINITION AND ETIOLOGY. *Mycoplasma mycoides* ssp. *mycoides* is a pathogenic mycoplasma that causes a variety of clinical syndromes in goats. Although the organism was formerly considered exotic to the United States, several large herd outbreaks have been described.[64,65] In most outbreaks the predominant clinical signs are polyarthritis and pneumonia in goat kids, occurring concurrently with mastitis in does. Abortions also may occur in pregnant does. Overwhelming generalized infection can occur in kids or adults, resulting in death.

CLINICAL SIGNS AND DIFFERENTIAL DIAGNOSES. Affected kids are from a few days of age to weaning age and have multiple warm swollen joints, elevated body temperatures of 40.8° C to 41.5° C (105.4° F to 106.7° F), pneumonia, conjunctivitis, and weight loss. They may have conjunctivitis. Many kids are unable to get up or are very reluctant to move. The acute febrile phase lasts from 1 to 3 days, after which polyarthritic kids will be bright and alert and continue to eat. In addition, a few very young kids may exhibit central nervous system (CNS) signs (opisthotonos) or sudden death. Failure to respond to conventional antibiotic treatment or rapid relapse after treatment also characterizes outbreaks. Acute mastitis caused by *M. mycoides* ssp. mycoides is characterized initially as an agalactia with a firm, hot gland(s); the milk is brownish and watery with some sandy clots present. The affected doe is febrile, depressed, and anorexic; has diarrhea; may abort; and may have swollen joints or pneumonia. Some does develop a toxic shocklike syndrome and die rapidly, whereas others make an apparent clinical recovery with variable amounts of udder fibrosis and atrophy remaining. The milk becomes normal in appearance, but intermittent chronic shedding of *M. mycoides* ssp. *mycoides* may occur.

Differential diagnosis in kids includes septic arthritis caused by bacteria, chlamydial polyarthritis, or white muscle disease, whereas in adult does the mastitis must be differentiated from that caused by *Mycoplasma putrefaciens* and other bacteria. Other *Mycoplasma* spp., particularly *M. putrefaciens*, occasionally cause polyarthritis in goat kids.

CLINICAL PATHOLOGY AND LABORATORY AIDS. Most affected kids have an increased white blood cell (WBC) count (>13,000 WBCs/mm^3 with neutrophilia >7200 cells/mm^3, monocytosis >530 cells/mm^3) and plasma fibrinogen >400 mg/dl. Peracutely affected kids and does have a complete blood count (CBC) typical of toxic shock, with neutropenia and a degenerative left shift. The joint fluid is increased in volume and contains large fibrin clots with increased numbers of neutrophils and lymphocytes. The organism is usually cultured on mycoplasma media from the most applicable affected site (i.e., joint fluid, milk, or tracheal wash).

PATHOPHYSIOLOGY. *M. mycoides* ssp. *mycoides* infection leads to mycoplasmemia and multiple organ involvement of varying degrees, with pyrexia, fibrinopurulent polyarthritis, pneumonia, pleuritis, pericarditis, peritonitis, mastitis, abortion, and encephalitis being the most common clinical expressions of infection. Recovery is accompanied by the conversion to carrier status in many animals with intermittent shedding of *M. mycoides* ssp. *mycoides* in milk and in ocular and nasal secretions. Pathogenic mycoplasmas are thought to produce toxins, but little is known of the pathogenesis of mycoplasma diseases.

EPIDEMIOLOGY. *Mycoplasma mycoides* ssp. *mycoides* is usually a milkborne infection that enters herds through inapparent carriers (usually adult milking does). The organism is an obligate intracellular parasite and survives poorly in the environment. It is easily transmitted to other does during normal milking operations and to young stock by ingestion. One milliliter of infected milk contains enough organisms (10^6) to cause polyarthritis in kids.[66] In reported outbreaks the morbidity is high (60% to 90%), and the mortality is 15% to 91%. The morbidity and mortality are highest in young animals. Transmission by contact occurs in conjunction with high density stocking rates. Environmental and other stressors (transport, kidding, kid processing, changes within herd grouping) induce shedding in chronic carrier animals and may facilitate herd outbreaks. The goat ear mite (genus *Psoroptes*) may play a role in maintaining a reservoir for *M. mycoides* ssp. *mycoides*.[67] Numerous isolations have been made from the external ear canals of clinically normal goats infected with mites.

NECROPSY FINDINGS. Gross necropsy findings may include fibrinopurulent polyarthritis, with erosions of articular surfaces, fibrinous pleuritis, fibrinous pericarditis, pneumonia, mastitis, peritonitis, and conjunctivitis. Subcutaneous edema often extends into soft tissues above and below the joint. In addition, meningoencephalitis may be appreciated on gross examination. Histologically, affected tissues exhibit neutrophilic infiltration with perivascular infiltration of plasma cells and lymphocytes.[64,65]

TREATMENT AND PROGNOSIS. There is no effective treatment for *M. mycoides* ssp. *mycoides*. Treatment with antibiotics may result in complete or transient remission followed by relapse. Naturally recovered animals are considered to be carriers, although the number of exposed-recovered kids that remain carriers is not well understood. Treatment with tylosin (10 to 50 mg/kg tid) may result in apparent clinical improvement, but the associated risk of producing carrier animals weighs against treatment. Newly developed antibiotics may make successful treatment possible in the future.

PREVENTION AND CONTROL. *M. mycoides* ssp. *mycoides* can be prevented from entering goat dairies by isolating and performing milk cultures on new herd additions. Milk cultures should be performed at the time of purchase and 2 and 4 weeks later, before the doe is declared free of *M. mycoides* ssp. *mycoides*. If the doe is dry at the time of purchase, isolation should be maintained until she is cultured at kidding and 2 and 4 weeks fresh. Herd outbreaks are controlled by feeding cow colostrum, cows' milk, or milk replacer to kids and by performing milk cultures on individual does. Initially each doe should have a composite milk sample cultured for mycoplasma.

Does with positive cultures are culled to slaughter or are housed together and milked last until they can be sold to slaughter. At weekly intervals after the milk tank has been emptied, a culture is taken after each string is milked, and the identity of each doe that contributed to the can or tank string sample is recorded. If a positive culture occurs in a string, individual cultures must be performed on that string to identify the doe(s) shedding *M. mycoides* ssp. *mycoides*. After 1 to 2 months of weekly cultures, monthly string cultures are adequate, combined with individual cultures for all does kidding. After 6 to 8 months, monthly bulk tank samples and fresh doe samples are monitored for 1 more year. The majority of infected lactating does are identified in the first 4 weeks of milk culturing. Some does infected with *M. mycoides* spp. *mycoides* may remain undetected for years even with intensive surveillance, thereby leading to sporadic disease. All kids that were being fed milk on the dairy during the outbreak should be sold for meat if they are in satisfactory condition, whereas clinically affected kids should be euthanized because, even with treatment, they may become carriers.

REFERENCES

64. Rosendal S, Erno H, Wyand DS: *Mycoplasma mycoides* subspecies *mycoides* as a cause of polyarthritis in goats, *J Am Vet Med Assoc* 175:378-380, 1979.
65. East NE, DaMassa AJ, Logan LL, et al: Milkbone outbreak of *Mycoplasma mycoides* subspecies *mycoides* infection in a commercial goat dairy, *J Am Vet Med Assoc* 182:1338-1341, 1983.
66. DaMassa AJ, Brooks DL, Holmberg CA: Introduction of mycoplasmosis in goat kids by oral inoculation with *Mycoplasma mycoides* subspecies *mycoides*, *Am J Vet Res* 47:2084-2089, 1986.
67. DaMassa AJ: Preliminary report: prevalence of mycoplasma and mites in the external auditory meatus of goats, *Calif Vet* 37(12):10-13, 1983.

CAPRINE ARTHRITIS ENCEPHALITIS

NANCY E. EAST

Caprine arthritis encephalitis virus (CAEV) is a lentivirus in the family Retroviridae. Infection with CAEV results in a low-level persistent viral replication followed by a delayed onset (years) of clinical disease. The virus infects cells of the monocyte-macrophage series, resulting in the production of large amounts of nonneutralizing antibody produced against both viral core protein (p28) and envelope glycoproteins (gp90 and gp125). The disease has a major impact on lifetime productivity of dairy goats and on the eligibility of the United States to export dairy goats.

CLINICAL SIGNS. CAEV infection causes two major recognized forms of disease.[68] The first is a leukoencephalomyelitis of kids 2 to 6 months of age characterized by a rear leg paresis that progresses to paralysis and may ascend to the front legs. A mild viral interstitial pneumonia may precede or accompany the leukoencephalomyelitis. Affected kids eat normally and are alert and afebrile, except in the more severe progressive cases, in which urinary retention and bloating result in discomfort. Copper deficiency (enzootic ataxia), lumbar cord abscesses, white muscle disease, septic arthritis, or spinal cord injury may result in similar clinical signs. This leukoencephalitic form is uncommon. Occasional cases of neurologic disease caused by CAEV in adult goats have been reported.[68]

The most common clinical presentation of CAEV is a polysynovitis-arthritis of goats 6 months of age and older, with most cases occurring in mature adults. The onset of the disease is insidious, with brief inflammatory episodes followed by apparent remission. The carpal joints are most commonly involved, followed by the stifle, hock, hip, and atlantooccipital joints. Over time, chronic joint enlargement is evident and is accompanied by weight loss. The joint fluid increases in volume during inflammatory episodes, but the majority of the swelling is caused by hyperplasia of the synovial tissue of the joints and tendon sheaths associated with the joints. The affected joints are painful and show a decreased range of motion. The goats have a stiff gait, and severely affected animals may remain recumbent or walk on their knees, resulting in a soft tissue contraction of the carpus. In addition to polyarthritis, most does infected with CAEV have some mammary gland involvement, which may result in decreased milk production. The mammary gland is firmer than normal, and the appearance of the milk is normal. The milk production decrease can be mild to moderate or result in agalactia ("hard udder"). Differential diagnosis of arthritis initially includes chlamydial polyarthritis and mycoplasma polyarthritis. These are acute inflammatory conditions and are usually accompanied by systemic illness, both of which differentiate them from CAEV; however, adult-onset degenerative joint disease may follow juvenile infectious arthritis.

A chronic interstitial viral pneumonia resulting in progressive respiratory distress and weight loss also may occur with CAEV infection with or without evidence of polysynovitis-arthritis. This chronic form of pneumonia is similar to viral ovine progressive pneumonia (see Chapter 29). It must be differentiated from lungworm infestation, chronic bacterial pneumonia, and pulmonary abscessation.

CLINICAL PATHOLOGY AND LABORATORY AIDS. The joint fluid in affected joints may be normal but is usually increased in volume, brown-to-red tinged in color with decreased protein and increased cell count (1000 to 20,000 cells/mm³ with 90% mononuclear cells, of which 60% to 70% are lymphocytes). The cerebrospinal spinal fluid (CSF) from kids affected with leukoencephalomyelitis also shows increased numbers of mononuclear cells. The complete blood count (CBC) and blood chemistry panels are unremarkable. Radiographs of early affected joints reveal soft tissue swelling dorsal to the carpus and sometimes the tarsus. This is followed by the appearance of calcified deposits in periarticular tissue, joint capsules, ligaments, tendons, and tendon sheaths. The atlantal and supraspinous bursae may become radiographically prominent as a result of fluid distention and mineralization. Bony changes include mild periosteal reaction, periarticular mineralization, and roughening of bone surfaces proximal and distal to the joint.

An agar gel immunodiffusion (AGID) test using ovine progressive pneumonia virus as antigen is the official USDA test for serum antibodies to CAEV. Enzyme-linked immunosorbent assay (ELISA) tests have been developed using recombinant envelope or core proteins as well as whole CAEV as antigen. In general ELISA tests are more sensitive and slightly less specific than the AGID test.[69] Either AGID or ELISA tests are adequate for herd surveillance and control programs. Polymerase chain reaction techniques have been developed to detect proviral DNA present in blood, milk, and tissues. A positive serologic test indicates that the individual animal is infected with the virus. Most goats become seropositive 4 to 16 weeks after infection. The infection is lifelong, and virus is shed by these individuals, regardless of clinical appearance. Many seropositive goats are asymptomatic for

years. A few goats have been reported to shed virus for long periods of time without seroconversion.[70]

PATHOPHYSIOLOGY. CAEV infects cells of the monocyte-macrophage lines with localization in tissue-associated macrophages primarily in the synovium, mammary gland, central nervous system (CNS), and lung. Large amounts of virus nonneutralizing antibodies are produced by lymphocytes associated with the virus-infected macrophage. These large immune complexes are thought to be the basis for the chronic inflammatory changes seen in the associated tissues.

EPIDEMIOLOGY. CAEV is transmitted primarily via milk and colostrum to nursing goat kids.[71,72] The feeding of pooled milk has resulted in a high prevalence of infection in goat dairies. Seroprevalence in U.S. goats ranged from 38% to 80% (n = 2826) in one study, and 81% (n = 1160) were found to be seropositive in another study.[68,73] Contact is also important in transmission of CAEV.[71-74] High-density stocking rates common to goat dairies favor contact transmission.[72] There is some evidence that intramammary, in utero, or immediate periparturient transmission also may occur. Current work has demonstrated virus-infected cells in estrual mucus, preputial swab, lochia postkidding, and from semen aspirated from the tail of the epididymis.* The epidemiologic implications of these findings are unknown but may explain some of the continued transmission in herds with good pasteurization and segregation programs.

NECROPSY FINDINGS. The most striking gross necropsy finding is the chronic hyperplastic synovitis associated with affected joints. Some joints may contain a white, chalky exudate whereas others exhibit synovial folding and thickening. Histologic changes consist of chronic hyperplastic synovitis with subsynovial mononuclear cell infiltrates of lymphocytes, macrophages, and plasma cells. Synovial villi exhibit cellular necrosis and necrobiosis of collagen, with fibrinous concentrations in synovial spaces.[68]

Goat kids with leukoencephalomyelitis may have mild interstitial pneumonia at gross necropsy with no other apparent lesions. Histologic CNS lesions consist of perivascular infiltration of lymphocytes, macrophages, and plasma cells, accompanied by loss of myelin and malacia in the brain and spinal cord. Degenerative changes may occur in gray matter.[75]

TREATMENT AND PROGNOSIS. There is no treatment for CAEV. The prognosis is variable, with many infected individuals having little or no clinical disease for most of their lives, whereas in others the arthritis and weight loss are rapidly progressive. A genetically determined predisposition for the development of CAEV-induced arthritis has been identified using DNA fingerprinting.[76] Stress appears to speed the development of clinical disease. The myelitis in kids and the occasional encephalitis seen in mature goats have an unfavorable prognosis, and affected individuals are usually euthanized.

PREVENTION AND CONTROL. Control programs are based on prevention of milk transmission, isolation from seropositive goats, and serologic monitoring.[74] Current work indicates that eradication of the disease is difficult under field conditions; however, the prevalence can be greatly reduced. Dairy goat kids must be prevented from any contact (licking) with the dam and nursing the dam. This requires that someone is present at the birth because goat kids can be up and nursing less than 15 minutes after birth. The kids are then fed goat colostrum that has been held at 45° C (131° F) for 1 hour or cow colostrum followed by pasteurized goats' milk or cows' milk. There are a few reports of neonatal isoerythrolysis in goat kids fed cow colostrum related to single-source colostrum. After the kids reach 2 to 3 weeks of age, a high-

---

*JD Rowe, DVM, PhD, University of California, Davis School of Veterinary Medicine; personal communication, 1993.

quality milk replacer can be fed. The use of goats' always carries some risk from failure to pasteurize properly or other mismanagement. Feeding goat colostrum may result in a CAEV-seropositive kid as a result of passive antibody transfer. These titers are usually gone by 8 to 16 weeks of age but do interfere with early testing. Under no conditions should milk or colostrum from seronegative does be used as a substitute for heat-treated products, because virus shedding precedes seropositive status. Periodic serologic testing of kids is required to detect and remove seropositive kids. Management factors and herd prevalence determine the testing schedule. Negative goats must be permanently isolated by a minimum of a 6-foot alley from seropositive goats, and no sharing of feeders or waters should be allowed. Negative does should be bred to CAEV negative bucks, or they can be hand-mated to positive bucks at minimal risk, but they should not be housed with them. Individual disposable sterile needles should be used for all injections.

REFERENCES

68. Crawford TB, Adams DS: Caprine arthritis-encephalitis: clinical features and presence of antibody in selected goat populations, *J Am Vet Med Assoc* 178:713-719, 1981.
69. Rimstad E, East N, DeRock E, et al: Detection of antibodies to caprine arthritis-encephalitis virus using recombinant gag proteins, *Arch Virol* 134:345-356, 1994.
70. Rimstad E, East NE, Torten M, et al: Delayed seroconversion following naturally acquired caprine arthritis-encephalitis virus infection in goats, *Am J Vet Res* 54:1858-1862, 1993.
71. Adams DS, Kevljer-Anderson P, Carlson JL, et al: Transmission and control of caprine arthritis-encephalitis virus, *Am J Vet Res* 44:1670-1675, 1983.
72. East NE, Rowe JD, Dahlberg JE, et al: Modes of transmission of caprine arthritis-encephalitis virus infection, *Small Ruminant Res* 10:251-262, 1993.
73. East NE, Rowe JD, Madewell BR, et al: Serologic prevalence of caprine arthritis-encephalitis virus in California goat dairies, *J Am Vet Med Assoc* 190:182-186, 1987.
74. Rowe JD, East NE, Frant CE, et al: Risk factors associated with the incidence of seroconversion to caprine arthritis-encephalitis virus in goats on California dairies, *Am J Vet Res* 53:2396-2403, 1992.
75. Cork LC, Hadlow WJ, Gorham RC, et al: Pathology of viral leukoencephalomyelitis goats, *Acta Neuropathol* 29:281-292, 1974.
76. Dolf G, Ruff G: A DNA fingerprinting band associated with the susceptibility to CAE virus–induced arthritis in goats, *Br Vet J* 150:349-353, 1994.

OSTEOARTHRITIS

MELINDA H. MacDONALD

DEFINITION. The term osteoarthritis (OA) encompasses a large group of joint disorders that are characterized by progressive permanent deterioration of the articular cartilage.[77-80] Cartilage damage is often accompanied by changes in the adjacent bone and soft tissue structures including subchondral bone sclerosis, periarticular new bone formation, and synovial inflammation. Unfortunately, there is some confusion and debate regarding the best term to use for this broad group of disorders. Osteoarthritis, degenerative joint disease (DJD), osteoarthrosis, and secondary joint disease have been used almost interchangeably in veterinary medicine.[77,78] However, osteoarthritis emphasizes the characteristic synovial inflammation detected in most patients, and that term will be used here.

Interestingly, OA is one of the oldest documented orthopedic conditions. In fact, the fossilized remains of early dinosaurs suggest that OA predates the evolutionary development of mammals. Unfortunately, despite its long-standing existence, there are still a number of questions regarding the etiopathogenesis of OA, and this condition is still regularly diagnosed in most large animal species including horses, cattle, and small ruminants. In goats OA is frequently associated with caprine arthritis encephalomyelitis virus (CAEV),[81,82] and in pigs it is a common debilitating sequela of infectious arthritis or osteochondrosis.[83] Although OA is not routinely diagnosed in sheep, it has been reported to develop in individuals infected with ovine progressive pneumonia.[81] In contrast, joint disease is a common and expensive problem in the equine industry, and a wide variety of athletic injuries can progress to a common end point with stereotypic features of chronic OA.[77-79]

ETIOLOGY AND CLASSIFICATION. Many factors, including athletic performance, repetitive trauma, and age, are thought to influence cartilage homeostasis and contribute to degenerative changes in the joint. Contrary to the traditional view of articular cartilage as a passive bystander subjected to overexertion and traumatic wear-and-tear damage, it is now recognized that both resident and infiltrating articular cells have a critical role in the development of OA. Cartilage degeneration is an active process ultimately resulting from the inability of resident cells to maintain a normal balance between matrix synthesis and degradation. This occurs when chondrocytes and synovial cells are exposed to various nonphysiologic stimuli including trauma and inflammation. Once the balance is disrupted, proteoglycans within the hyalin cartilage matrix are depleted and reduced in size, while the collagen meshwork progressively deteriorates. These changes in turn alter the mechanical properties of articular cartilage. A variety of different joint problems can initiate an imbalance between the rate of cartilage degradation and repair and, if left untreated, will ultimately progress to a common end point of OA.

Although a number of initiating and predisposing conditions have been identified, it is generally felt that trauma, either a single severe injury or low-grade repetitive damage, is the most important basis for the development of OA in large animal species.[77-79] In many instances, the traumatic damage is augmented by abnormal weight bearing, poor quality cartilage, or congenital joint instability such as that seen with hip dysplasia in calves. In addition, OA frequently develops in joints that have unresolved or untreated osteochondrosis, subchondral bone collapse, or septic arthritis. In all of these cases, the link between the cause and the end result of OA is a series of complex biochemical and metabolic events that are not yet fully understood. Regardless of the inciting etiology, advanced OA is characterized by fibrillated and ulcerated cartilage, eburnation and sclerosis of the subchondral bone, hyperplasia of the synovial membrane, and development of periarticular osteophytes.

Several classification schemes have been proposed to group clinical OA conditions in both human and veterinary medicine. One useful classification developed for equine OA defines three main categories of disease based on predisposing causes and clinical findings.[82] The categories include: OA associated with synovitis and capsulitis (Type-1), OA secondary to other identified injuries or disorders (Type-2), and incidental or nonprogressive articular cartilage erosion (Type-3).[78] For example, Type-2 OA would include the chronic degenerative changes typically associated with intraarticular fractures, septic arthritis, osteochondrosis, traumatic cartilage or ligamentous injuries. All three categories are routinely identified in equine athletes, but this simple scheme can easily be applied to other large animal species as well. For example, cattle most commonly develop Type-2 OA as a consequence of septic arthritis, cruciate rupture, osteochondrosis, or nutritional deficiencies.[83]

A second way of classifying OA is based on the possible deleterious effects of biomechanical forces on normal and abnormal joints.[79] According to this scheme, the first of two major causes of OA is the concentration of abnormal forces on a previously normal joint. For example, OA can develop when there is increase weight bearing on one limb to protect a painful contralateral limb. The second cause of OA defined in this scheme is the concentration of normal forces on an abnormal articulation. This second category would include the joint damage that occurs when normal weight-bearing forces are applied to cartilage previously exposed to infection.

PATHOLOGY AND PATHOGENESIS. Despite the many pathways by which OA may develop, the resulting changes in the joint are essentially indistinguishable regardless of the initiating cause. By definition this condition has a characteristic picture of cartilage damage with variable amounts of hypertrophic cartilage and bone remodeling.[77-79] Pathologic features include different degrees of cartilage splitting and fragmentation extending to complete erosion and loss of articular cartilage.[77-79] Typically, the rate of disease progression and severity of OA are related to the nature and severity of the primary insult, the age of the animal at the time of the initial insult, the joint location, and the type/level of activity the animal participates in.

The pathogenesis of these changes is only partially understood. Several explanations have been proposed for the failure of resident chondrocytes to maintain the extracellular matrix. Mechanical trauma to the joint surface could initiate matrix damage, and repetitive microtrauma could damage chondrocytes and physically disrupt the joint surface. Leukocytes in an inflamed joint release destructive enzymes, which can degrade the cartilage surface. Recent work has also demonstrated that various polypeptide mediators released in inflamed joints can stimulate chondrocytes to degrade their surrounding matrix. Regardless of the initiating factor, once the balance of chondrocyte matrix-turnover is shifted toward degradation, proteoglycans are rapidly depleted from the extracellular matrix, and collagen fibers are exposed to direct traumatic and enzymatic breakdown. Unfortunately, hyaline cartilage has no effective intrinsic repair mechanism.

Articular cartilage damage is accompanied by changes in the adjacent subchondral bone (e.g., sclerosis), joint capsule (e.g., synovial hyperplasia, thickening of the fibrous joint capsule), and joint margin (e.g., osteophyte formation, enthesophyte formation at joint capsule and ligament insertions).[79] Subchondral bone sclerosis may develop from an abnormal distribution of forces under damaged articular cartilage, or it may actually precede the cartilage damage. It is now known that bone remodeling and subchondral bone sclerosis occur in response to repetitive cyclic compression during exercise, and in certain instances could result in trauma to the overlying articular cartilage and predispose to the development of OA (e.g., third carpal bone disease in horses). Joint margin changes occur as a result of progressive cartilage deterioration and subchondral remodeling (osteophytes) or joint instability (enthesophytes).

CLINICAL SIGNS. History and occupation are important for identifying animals at risk for developing OA. Typically, the first sign that an owner or caretaker recognizes in an affected animal is lameness or stiffness. Whereas the pain and dysfunction may develop insidiously, the owner will often report a sudden onset of clinical signs. Flexion and extension of an involved joint frequently exacerbates the lameness or elicits a pain response. Because articular cartilage is aneural, pain is thought to result from joint inflammation and secondary changes in adjacent tissues. Pain receptors are abundant in joint capsule, articular ligaments, and subchondral bone. Joint stiffness may be associated with guarding of a painful joint. Decreased range of motion with joint capsule inflammation is also common. Osteophytes and enthesophytes may be palpable in chronic cases of bone spavin and ringbone. A postural deformity may be evident if articular degeneration progresses to ankylosis. It is also important to remember that OA may exist in the absence of any clinical signs.

Gait abnormalities compatible with OA include shortened stride length, limb abduction, and dragging the toe. Increased lameness after sustained flexion of a single joint suggests that the joint is involved. Horses with OA often present early in the course of disease with a primary complaint of poor performance. These individuals can warm out of the lameness, or temporarily improve with rest and are often difficult to diagnose. In contrast, food animals typically present in the advanced stages of OA. Rams and bulls may stand post-legged and appear weak in the rear when the hind limbs are severely affected. In all species the severity of signs varies with the joint affected, stage of disease, amount of inflammation, cartilage degeneration, and periarticular changes.

DIAGNOSIS. Regional nerve blocks and intraarticular anesthesia can be useful for determining the origin of lameness. Unfortunately, standard synovial fluid analysis typically shows only minimal nonspecific changes. Although not useful for determining the severity of cartilage destruction, cytology is often useful for differentiating OA from other causes of synovial inflammation (e.g., septic arthritis). A variety of synovial fluid markers have been evaluated as possible diagnostic aids for evaluation of equine synovitis and joint disease (e.g., cytokines, eicosanoids, glycosaminoglycan concentrations, immune complexes, collagen type-specific antibodies and propetptides, cartilage wear fragment, free radical oxidation products, polymerization of hyaluronate, chondroitin sulfate epitopes). Current detection techniques for cytokines and eicosanoids may prove useful diagnostically and prognostically.

After identification of an involved joint, radiographs are used to determine the severity and extent of disease. Articular cartilage is not visualized, but may be indirectly assessed by evaluating joint space width. In contrast, the associated subchondral and periarticular bone reaction can be directly evaluated. Radiographic signs of OA develop gradually, affect opposing joint surfaces, and may include destructive as well as productive lesions. Changes typical of advanced OA include marginal osteophyte proliferation, periosteal new bone production at sites of joint capsule and ligamentous attachments (enthesophytes), narrowing or obliteration of the joint space, subchondral bone sclerosis, and occasionally subchondral lysis. Early in the disease no bony lesions may be detected, and clinical findings from the entire examination must be considered. Radiographic changes associated with OA must be differentiated from similar bone reactions caused by active infection, fractures, osteochondrosis, and invasive tumors. Infectious arthritis classically causes rapid, widespread osteochondral destruction. Minimally displaced fractures may mimic OA, but are usually discrete, isolated lesions. Knowledge of the characteristic site distribution and site-respective appearances of ostechondroses in each species is useful for differentiation from OA. The presence of OA in joints with osteochondrosis usually worsens the prognosis.

Scintigraphy is particularly valuable in early disease states when conventional diagnostic methods have not revealed bone or soft tissue changes. Increased scan activity is associated with soft tissue inflammation or increased bone remodeling, but alone, is not diagnostic for OA. Arthroscopy is the best method for gross evaluation of articular cartilage and is most useful when lameness has been localized to a specific joint but no bony changes are detected radiographically. This technique provides the added therapeutic benefit of simultaneous joint lavage. Although arthroscopy was initially promoted for diagnostic and therapeutic use in equine patients, these techniques are gaining popularity in food animal practice as well.[84]

TREATMENT. The choice and efficacy of treatment depend on the inciting cause of OA, stage of cartilage degradation, joint involved, and degree of active inflammation. In general terms, the treatment of OA should be directed at eliminating any primary causes, reducing active joint inflammation, and treating articular cartilage loss or degeneration.[77,78,85] Early treatment of primary problems minimizes the extent of secondary joint damage. For example, fractures and osteochondritis dissecans can often be managed successfully with arthroscopic surgery; however, early intervention is essential to avoid the secondary changes of OA.

Many therapeutic options are designed to treat active soft tissue inflammation and prevent progression of articular cartilage damage. Rest is the simplest but often the most difficult recommendation to enforce, especially when dealing with elite performance horses. There are also valid concerns that complete rest may result in resorption of subchondral bone and predispose the horse to subsequent injury. Other treatments for soft tissue disturbances in the joint include physical therapy and controlled exercise, systemic nonsteroidal antiinflammatory agents (e.g., phenylbutazone, flunixin meglumine), joint lavage, and topical application of antiinflammatory products.

Numerous medications have been specifically designed and marketed for treating OA in human and veterinary patients. However, many of these products remain controversial in terms of their safety and efficacy in large animals. The most popular formulations include intraarticular corticosteroids, intraarticular and intramuscular polysulfated glycosaminglycan, intraarticular and intravenous hyaluronan, and oral glycosaminoglycan supplements.

Intraarticular steroids are the most potent antiinflammatory agents available; however, they have historically been associated with progressive cartilage damage.[85,86] Nevertheless, recent investigations critically evaluating the effects of corticosteroids in equine joints suggest that when administered at physiologic doses, these drugs may have beneficial protective effects.[85,86] Current recommendations emphasize the need for appropriate caution and encourage the use of low doses of steroids in conjunction with other antiinflammatory medications. Hyaluronan (sodium hyaluronate) is currently used both intravenously and intraarticularly to treat synovial inflammation and OA in the horse.[85,87] The intraarticular products vary in molecular weight and cost and include cross-linked hylans, which may prolong intraarticular retention. Clinical reports document the efficacy of hyaluronan for mild to moderate synovitis, and some research supports an inhibition of proteoglycan degradation and inhibition of synoviocyte release of various inflammatory mediators. Other studies failed to demonstrate beneficial effects in joints with significant articular cartilage damage or osteochondral fragmentation.

The intraarticular administration of polysulfated glycosaminoglycan has been reported to reduce progressive degenerative changes in articular cartilage, but is controversial in terms of its ability to augment the chondrocyte repair response.[85,88] Intramuscular use is advocated because intraarticular use has been associated with adverse reactions and potentiates the risk of iatrogenic joint infection.[85,88]

There is currently a great deal of interest in the use of nutritional supplements to prevent and treat OA, and there has been a dramatic proliferation of products on the market being promoted as beneficial to joint health and cartilage regeneration.[89] Among the most popular are the oral glucosamine sulfate and chondroitin sulfate preparations. However, oral absorption of chondroitin sulfates has not been documented in the horse, and although clinical reports suggest a beneficial effect from these supplements, additional controlled studies are needed to confirm these effects. Methylsufonylmethane (MSM), a dietary derivative of dimethylsulfoxide (DMSO), is also being utilized as a dietary supplement to control the inflammation associated with OA. Again, there is very little documentation of its value in treating joint disease in large animals. Other compounds being sold for treatment of OA include S-Adenosine-L-methionine and various vitamins known to provide antioxidant protection.

The most challenging aspect of OA management is treatment of existing articular cartilage degeneration and loss. Partial thickness cartilage defects do not heal, and full-thickness defects heal with inferior fibrocartilaginous tissue. Some surgical techniques (e.g., curettage, subchondral bone drilling, and microfracture) facilitate defect repair by enhancing fibrocartilage ingrowth from the underlying subchondral bone; however, fibrocartilage is biomechanically inferior to normal hyaline cartilage. Grafting cartilage defects with periosteum, perichondrium, and sternal cartilage has not been encouraging. Recent work focuses on transplantation resurfacing using chondrocyte grafts and growth factors to stimulate repair.[90]

PROGNOSIS. Prognosis depends on the initiating factors, extent of the secondary disease, joint affected, and intended use of the animal. With early and aggressive treatment, many animals can return to soundness and athletic performance. In other cases salvage in the form of surgical arthrodesis may provide the most favorable outcome.

REFERENCES

77. McIlwraith CW, Vachon A: Review of pathogenesis and treatment of degenerative joint disease, *Equine Vet J* S6:3-11, 1988.
78. McIlwraith CW: General pathobiology of the joint and response to injury. In McIlwraith CW, Trotter GW, editors: *Joint disease in the horse*, Philadelphia, 1996, WB Saunders Co, pp 40-70.
79. Pool RR: Pathologic manifestations of joint disease in the athletic horse. In McIlwraith CW, Trotter GW, editors: *Joint disease in the horse*, Philadelphia, 1996, WB Saunders Co, pp 87-104.
80. Bulgin MS: Ovine progressive pneumonia, caprine arthritis-encephalitis, and related lentiviral diseases of sheep and goats, *Vet Clin North Am Food Anim Pract* 6:691-704, 1990.
81. Phelps SL, Smith MC: Caprine arthritis-encephalitis virus infection, *J Am Vet Med Assoc* 203:1663-1666, 1993.
82. Hill MA: Causes of degenerative joint disease (osteoarthrosis) and dyschondroplasia (osteochondrosis) in pigs, *J Am Vet Med Assoc* 197:107-113, 1990.
83. Vailey JV: Bovine arthritides: classification, diagnosis, prognosis and treatment, *Vet Clin North Am Food Anim Pract* 1:39-51, 1985.
84. Gaughan E: Arthroscopy in food animal practice, *Vet Clin North Am Food Anim Pract* 1:233-247, 1996.
85. McIlwraith CW: Intra-articular and systemic medications for the treatment of equine joint disease. *Proceedings of the Forty-second Annual Convention of the American Association of Equine Practitioners*, 1996, pp 101-125.
86. Trotter GW: Intra-articular corticosteroids. In McIlwraith CW, Trotter GW, editors: *Joint disease in the horse*, Philadelphia, 1996, WB Saunders, pp 237-256.
87. Howard RD, McIlwraith CW: Hyaluronan and its use in the treatment of equine joint disease. In McIlwraith CW, Trotter GW, editors: *Joint disease in the horse*, Philadelphia, 1996, WB Saunders Co, pp 257-269.
88. Trotter GW: Polysufated glycosaminoglycan (Adequan). In McIlwraith CW, Trotter GW, editors: *Joint disease in the horse*, Philadelphia, 1996, WB Saunders, pp 270-280.
89. Jones WE: A nutritional approach to osteoarthritis. *J Equine Vet Sci* 20:160-218, 2000.
90. Nixon AJ: Advances in promoting cartilage healing. *Proc Am College Vet Surg* 9:221-224, 1999.

SPRAINS, SUBLUXATIONS, AND LUXATIONS

KEVIN HAUSSLER

DEFINITIONS. Sprains are periarticular injuries caused by overstretching or tearing of a ligament (desmitis) or its bony insertions (enthesitis). Sprains differ from strains, which are injuries to musculotendinous units, although they often occur simultaneously.[91] Ligaments function to maintain joint stability while allowing for joint motion. Partial ligamentous tearing to complete rupture produces disorders varying from subluxation (altered bony alignment) to luxation (complete separation of articular surfaces).

ETIOPATHOGENESIS. Sprains are initiated by overloading of collagen fibers beyond the limits of normal deformation,[92] caused by direct trauma, a fall, or an abnormally restrained movement. Sprains are classified as mild (collagen fiber stretching, intraligamentous hemorrhage, inflammatory exudate), moderate (significant fiber damage, prominent hemorrhage, and inflammation), and severe (ligament rupture, extensive hemorrhage and inflammation, joint instability).[91]

Tissue disruption increases with larger forces and with longer duration or repetitive forces.[93] In horses, poor riding techniques may create repetitive microtrauma and induce a chronic back sprain syndrome. Muscle fatigue lessens joint stability and may predispose to ligamentous injury. Sprains are more common in underconditioned horses working maximally.[92] Aging, degenerative joint disease, and disuse predispose to ligamentous failure.[94] Secondary inflammation is accompanied by pain, swelling, heat, hyperesthesia, and altered function (lameness). Complete ligament disruption results in joint instability and luxation.

Ligamentous healing and regain of function are typically slow. Delayed ligamentous repair may lead to excessive fibrosis, predisposition to injury recurrence, chronic joint instability, and degenerative joint disease. Aberrant neurologic reflexes and proprioception caused by damaged articular afferent and efferent nerves also may predispose to further injury.[95,96] Vertebral subluxation may produce spinal cord compression.

CLINICAL SIGNS AND DIFFERENTIAL DIAGNOSIS. Clinical signs include localized pain, ligament laxity, localized muscle guarding, heat, swelling, and altered gait. Mild sprains with localized swelling or pain may be difficult to detect by palpation and joint manipulation.[97] Moderate sprains are associated with noticeable lameness, obvious pain and swelling, and ligamentous laxity. Complete ligamentous rupture may result in non-weight-bearing lameness, edema, and extraligamentous hemorrhage, joint crepitus, and joint instability. Acute sprains are characterized by signs of inflammation, but lameness may vary from none to non-weight-bearing. Chronic sprains have minimal acute inflammatory signs, but are characterized by joint capsule thickening and joint instability. Subluxation and luxation result in loss of joint function and mobility and postural deformities.[98] Common sites of subluxation or luxation include the pastern, shoulder, coxofemoral, and upper cervical vertebral articulations.

Differential diagnoses include soft tissue contusion, musculotendinous strain, fracture, inflammatory joint disease, osteomyelitis, neoplasia, and congenital malformation.

DIAGNOSIS. Careful and thorough joint and ligament palpation may elicit a pain response and signs of joint instability.[99] Joint manipulation under anesthesia reduces secondary muscle spasm and allows an accurate assessment of joint instability. Trauma-induced synovial effusion may be present. Although local anesthesia and regional nerve blocks can help to localize a sprain, horses should be moved cautiously to avoid exacerbating the injury. Ultrasonography and magnetic resonance imaging are useful for assessing ligamentous damage. Radiographs assist in the diagnosis of soft tissue swelling, avulsion fracture, increased joint space, subluxation, and luxation. Stress radiographs are useful for evaluation of ligament and joint integrity. Scintigraphy or thermography may be useful for detecting bony changes at ligament insertions that may not be detected with radiography. Arthroscopy or arthrotomy may provide direct visualization of intraarticular ligamentous and capsular injury.[99,100]

TREATMENT. Mild sprains are treated symptomatically, with physical therapy (cold or hydrotherapy) and antiinflammatory medication to reduce inflammation.[91] Support bandages reduce swelling and may help stabilize the affected articulation. Rest or confinement is indicated for a few days, with length of time depending on severity of injury and response to treatment.

Moderate sprains require more intensive treatment and treatment of longer duration. Splints and casts can be used to provide short-term joint immobilization. Muscle relaxants help to alleviate secondary muscle spasms. Stall confinement (2 to 3 weeks) followed by limited exercise and gradual return to full activity should be recommended.

Severe sprains or joint instability requires immediate external coaptation or surgical intervention to minimize secondary degenerative joint disease. Immobilization (4 to 6 weeks) and rest (3 to 4 months) are recommended. Conservative treatment with a cast and stall confinement may compromise long-term joint integrity by restricting joint motion. Arthrodesis may provide early return to weight bearing and can maintain most function when used in low motion joints (e.g., pastern joint). Cervical vertebrae subluxation may require laminectomy or vertebral body fusion to decompress the spinal cord or stabilize vertebrae.

Joint luxations require immediate reduction (either manually, under anesthesia, or surgically) to avoid additional muscle and soft tissue injuries or contractures that would prevent future reduction or return to function.[101] Support and stall rest are indicated after reduction. Arthrodesis may be necessary to stabilize a joint with severe ligamentous damage.

PROGNOSIS. Complete recovery depends on the severity of injury, response to therapy, and owner compliance to treatment protocols. Avulsion fractures may have a better prognosis than intraligamentous injury because of bone's superior repair ability. Mild sprains usually resolve within 1 to 2 weeks, may have residual periarticular fibrosis, and heal with minimal loss of function.[91,100] Moderate sprains heal in 6 to 10 weeks, may have residual periarticular fibrosis, with functional stability regained in 3 to 6 months. Severe injuries often produce fibrosis, joint stiffness, and chronic lameness. Joint subluxation or luxation have a poor prognosis for return to athletic activities and often predispose to secondary degenerative joint disease or ankylosis.

REFERENCES

91. Farrow CS: Sprain, strain, and contusion, *Vet Clin North Am (Small Anim Pract)* 8:169-182, 1978.
92. Goodship AE, Birch HL, Wilson AM: The pathobiology and repair of tendon and ligament injury, *Vet Clin North Am (Equine Pract)* 10:322-349, 1994.
93. Denoix JM: Functional anatomy of tendons and ligaments in the distal limbs (manus and pes), *Vet Clin North Am (Equine Pract)* 10:273-322, 1994.
94. Johnson JM, Johnson AJ: Cranial cruciate ligament rupture, *Vet Clin North Am (Small Anim Pract)* 23:717-733, 1993.
95. Bullock-Saxton JE: Local sensation changes and altered hip muscle function following severe ankle sprain, *Phys Ther* 74:17-31, 1994.
96. Brunt D, Anderson JC, Huntsman B, et al: Postural responses to lateral perturbation in healthy subjects and ankle sprain patients, *Med Sci Sports Exercise* 24:171-176, 1992.
97. Nelson DR, Smith RM: Intermittent lameness in two cows from detachment of the anterior horn of the medial meniscus, *Vet Rec* 127:133, 1990.
98. Tulleners EP, Nunamaker DM, Richardson DW: Coxofemoral luxations in cattle: 22 cases (1980-1985), *J Am Vet Med Assoc* 191:569-574, 1987.
99. Prades M, Grant BD, Turner TA, et al: Injuries to the cranial cruciate ligament and associated structures: summary of clinical, radiographic, arthroscopic and pathological findings from 10 horses, *Equine Vet J* 21:354-357, 1989.
100. McIlwraith CW: Tearing of the medial palmar intercarpal ligament in the equine midcarpal joint, *Equine Vet J* 24:267-271, 1992.
101. Malark JA, Nixon AJ, Haughland MA, et al: Equine coxofemoral luxations: 17 cases (1975-1990), *Cornell Vet* 82:79-90, 1992.

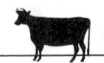
ANKYLOSIS

KEVIN HAUSSLER

DEFINITION AND ETIOPATHOGENESIS. Ankylosis is the naturally occurring bony fusion of a joint. Congenital ankylosis (absence of an articulation) occurs rarely (e.g., block vertebrae). Inherited multiple ankylosis of Holstein calves affects intervertebral and limb joints and is a cause of dystocia related to fetal musculoskeletal inflexibility. Ankylosis can be acquired after degenerative joint disease, septic arthritis, and severe articular or periarticular trauma.[102,103] Biomechanical or biochemical mechanisms induce joint instability, subsequent degeneration and, eventually, stabilization via osseous proliferation. Stages of development include (1) joint immobility from chronic muscle spasm, periarticular contracture, or capsular fibrosis; (2) synovitis and articular cartilage destruction; (3) periarticular soft tissue ossification with partial osseous bridging of the joint; and (4) complete joint obliteration with trabecular bone bridging adjacent bones.

Prolonged joint immobilization through bandaging, splinting, casting, or surgical procedures (arthrodesis) predisposes joints to ankylosis. Vertebral ankylosis may produce neurologic deficits because of direct bony impingement of nerve roots at intervertebral foramina, the spinal cord, or cauda equina or indirectly, from dynamic compression related to abnormal motion or spinal ligament hypertrophy at adjacent vertebrae. Similar mechanisms occur in cervical malformation and instability syndromes in horses. Ankylosed joints are susceptible to fracture because biomechanical forces are no longer dissipated in a physiologic manner. Ankylosed joints also induce nonphysiologic stresses on adjacent joints and increase their risk for degenerative joint disease at an age earlier than normal.[104]

CLINICAL SIGNS AND DIFFERENTIAL DIAGNOSIS. Lameness and local inflammation may be present during the initial development of ankylosis. Complete ankylosis manifests as a nonpainful, immobile articulation. Postural or conformational abnormalities, regional muscle wasting, fibrotic or enlarged periarticular structures, and gait stiffness may be present. Reduced range of motion will be most notable in joints with a large physiologic range of motion (e.g., upper limbs, cervical vertebrae), or if multiple adjacent joints are involved (e.g., lumbar vertebrae).[105] Altered gait may not be evident in animals with an ankylosed joint with a small physiologic range of motion (distal carpal and tarsal joints).

Differential diagnoses include arthrodesis, spondylosis, soft tissue contracture, intraarticular or periarticular adhesions, joint luxation, osseous neoplasia, and an intraarticular mass. Diagnosis is based on restricted joint motion and radiographic evidence of articular obliteration and osseous bridging.

TREATMENT AND PROGNOSIS. Joint immobilization, antiinflammatory medication, and restricted activity may be indicated to reduce periarticular pain and inflammation associated with the development of ankylosis.[103] Residual lameness and disability range from none to severe, and vary with the anatomic alignment of the affected structures and the degree of compensatory joint movement. Complete ankylosis is a nonpainful, irreversible process.

REFERENCES

102. Honnas CM, Schumacher J, Kuesis BS: Ankylosis of the distal interphalangeal joint in a horse after septic arthritis and septic navicular bursitis, *J Am Vet Med Assoc* 200:964-968, 1992.
103. Honnas CM, Welch RD, Ford TS, et al: Septic arthritis of the distal interphalangeal joint in 12 horses, *Vet Surg* 21:261-268, 1992.
104. Gorse, MJ, Early TD, Aron DN: Tarsocrural arthrodesis: long-term functional results, *J Am Anim Hosp Assoc* 27:231-235, 1991.
105. Fowler JD, Presnell KR, Holmberg DL: Scapulohumeral arthrodesis: results in seven dogs, *J Am Anim Hosp Assoc* 24:667-672, 1988.

ARTHROGRYPOSIS

K.C. KENT LLOYD
BRADFORD P. SMITH

Arthrogryposis is one of the most frequently encountered congenital diseases affecting calves; foals, goat kids, and lambs are less frequently affected (see also Chapters 47 and 48). The condition is characterized commonly by flexural deformity of the interphalangeal, metacarpophalangeal, carpal, and/or metatarsophalangeal joints (Fig. 36-17). Beef breeds are typically affected (e.g., Charolais, Herefords, Simmental), and the incidence is greater in bull calves. The disease is multifactorial in origin and thus often is accompanied by other anatomic and neurologic defects, including hydranencephaly, scoliosis, and cleft palate.

Arthrogrypotic diseases can be categorized on the basis of their suspected etiology: infectious (e.g., epizootic bovine and ovine congenital arthrogryposis-hydranencephaly caused by Akabane virus, bluetongue virus, border disease virus, and the Cache Valley virus), genetic[106,107] (e.g., arthrogryposis and palatoschisis of Charolais calves and arthrogryposis and other abnormalities in Norwegian Fjord horses, Welsh Mountain,[108] Merino[109] and inbred sheep flocks), and toxic[110] (e.g., arthrogryposis in foals associated with sudan pasture and crooked calf and lamb disease associated with lupine alkaloid). Lambs also may have scoliosis, kyphosis, brachygnathism, and cleft palate.

CVV is widespread in the western United States and has been isolated in Wisconsin and Michigan. Nineteen percent of young sheep from 50 flocks in the western United States were seropositive. CVV appears capable of causing arthrogryposis-hydranencephaly in fetal lambs.[111] Experimentally infected gnotobiotic lambs developed head tremors and convulsions. Other toxins, together with lamb manganese deficiency, poisonous plants such as Solanum dimidiatum, and sporadic genetic accidents resulting in maldevelopment also are associated with arthrogryposis and related defects.

Despite numerous causes, the clinical features of arthrogryposis are similar. Varying degrees of irreducible and rigid flexural deformity of both carpi and forelimb fetlock joints

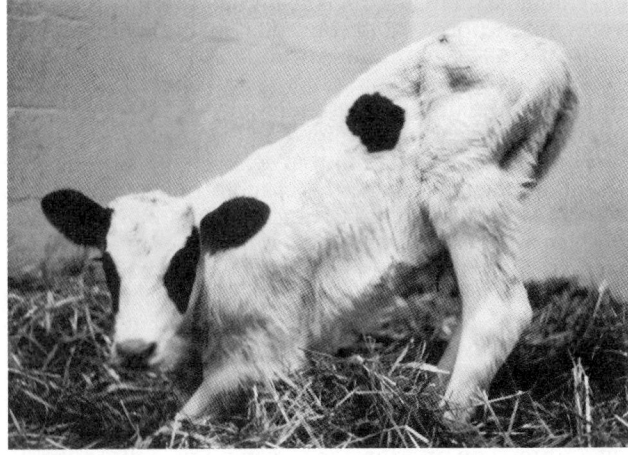

FIG. 36-17 ▊ Two-day-old heifer calf with bilateral congenital arthrogryposis of the carpus.

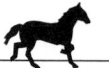

are more frequently observed than hyperextension of the tarsus, flexural deformity of the hind limb fetlocks, or tetramelic arthrogryposis. In contrast, flexural deformities caused by contracted tendons are not associated with improper articular alignment or rotational deformity, and the limb often can be straightened manually. Flexural deformities that could be confused with arthrogryposis may be secondary to septic arthritis or fracture (Box 36-1).

Rigid flexural deformity is a common cause of dystocia in cattle and horses. Failure to straighten a flexed limb manually through the vagina usually indicates the need either for cesarean section or fetotomy if the fetus is dead. Forced extraction is dangerous to the dam, because during the procedure the flexural deformity may cause damage to the uterus, cervix, and vagina. Depending on the etiology, other defects are observed in association with arthrogryposis (Table 36-2). The most commonly observed triad of signs is arthrogryposis, scoliosis, and cleft palate in Charolais calves.[106,112]

The pathogenesis of arthrogryposis is speculated to be related to restricted fetal movement in utero as a result of mechanical limitations, agenesis of α-motoneuron cell bodies in the ventral horn of the sixth cervical segment of the spinal cord, and radial nerve dysfunction.[106] Agenesis of some motoneuron cell bodies may result in lack of normal fetal movement, hypoplastic musculature, and frozen joints.[113] The cause for agenesis of motor horn cells in the spinal cord in unknown, but in virus-associated outbreaks it is probably virally induced. Treatment of mildly rigid flexural deformities may be effective if joint mobility and the ability to stand progressively improve over several days. Passive stretching and flexing of the affected limbs, bandages, and splints, and later casts may be beneficial. Vitamin E and selenium supplementation is suggested by some, but the only mineral deficiency associated with arthrogryposis is that of manganese.[112] Surgical techniques also have been described for transection of the flexor retinaculum and flexor tendons and for excision of the carpal bones with arthrodesis of the joint, depending on the location and severity of the deformity. These procedures are intended to salvage the animal for rearing to market weight.

BOX 36-1

Mechanisms of Joint Immobility and Arthrogryposis

Agenesis of ventral motor horn cells of spinal cord
Fractures involving one or more joints
Severe joint or tendon swelling
Contracture of muscles or tendons
Septic arthritis
Ankylosis
Skeletal neoplasia
Agenesis or dysgenesis of joint structures

Calves with suspected inherited deformities should not be returned to breeding stock.

REFERENCES

106. Russell RG, Doige CE, Oteruleo FT, et al: Variability in limb malformations and possible significance in the pathogenesis of Charolais cattle (syndrome of arthrogryposis and palatoschisis), *Vet Pathol* 22:2-12, 1985.
107. Nes N, Lomo OM, Bjerkas I: Hereditary lethal arthrogryposis ("muscle contracture") in horses, *Nord Vet Med* 34:425-430, 1982.
108. Morley FHW: A new lethal factor in Australian merino sheep, *Aust Vet J* 30:237-240, 1954.
109. Roberts JAF: The inheritance of a lethal muscle contracture in the sheep, *J Genet* 21:57-69, 1929.
110. Pritchard JT, Voss JL: Fetal ankylosis in horses associated with hybrid sudan pasture, *J Am Vet Med Assoc* 150:871-873, 1967.
111. Livingston CW, Crandell RA, Collisson E, et al: Sheep arthrogryposis and hydranencephaly, *Foreign Anim Dis Rep* 15(2):2-3, 1987.
112. Van Huffel X, De Moor A: Congenital multiple arthrogryposis of the forelimbs in calves, *Compend Cont Educ Pract Vet* 9:F333-F339, 1987.
113. Mayhew IG: Neuromuscular arthrogryposis multiplex congenita in a thoroughbred foal, *Vet Pathol* 21:187-192, 1987.

OSTEOMYELITIS

PATRICIA A. HOGAN
CLIFFORD M. HONNAS

DEFINITION AND ETIOLOGY. Osteomyelitis is an infectious inflammatory disease of the substance of bone and its marrow cavity. Most large animal bone infections are of bacterial origin; mycotic infections rarely occur. Osteomyelitis may be acute or chronic, and involve the epiphyseal, metaphyseal, or diaphyseal regions of a bone. Osteomyelitis can originate hematogenously, secondary to a contiguous focus of infection, or by direct bacterial inoculation (e.g., trauma, orthopedic surgery).[114,115]

CLINICAL SIGNS AND DIFFERENTIAL DIAGNOSIS. Diagnosis is based on history, physical examination findings, microbiologic culture results, and radiographic findings. Clinical signs vary with the length and severity of infection and the organism involved.

Animals with acute osteomyelitis usually exhibit localized inflammation and soft tissue swelling, may resent palpation of the affected area, and often have an obvious lameness. Fever, anorexia, depression, and general malaise may be observed. Acute bacterial osteomyelitis is seen most commonly in very young animals and is usually of hematogenous origin.[114,116] In the neonate it is frequently secondary to other foci of infection such as the respiratory or gastrointestinal tracts, or umbilical remnant.[116] There is often a history of prematurity, failure of passive transfer of colostral immunoglobulins, or peripartum difficulties. Osteomyelitis in foals, calves, kids, and lambs is typically associated with septic arthritis and may or may not involve infection of the epiphyseal, physeal, and metaphyseal regions of the long bones.[116]

TABLE 36-2

Other Defects Associated With Arthrogryposis Syndromes (see Chapters 47 and 48)

Disease	Related Signs
Epizootic bovine congenital arthrogryposis—hydranencephaly (Akabane virus—exotic)	Incoordination, hydranencephaly, blindness, abortion, microencephaly
Arthrogryposis and palatoschisis (genetic in Charolais breed)	Cleft palate, hydrocephalus, kyphosis, scoliosis, hypoplastic patella
Crooked calf disease (lupine toxicity)	Scoliosis, torticollis, cleft palate
Hereditary arthrogryposis	Kyphosis, torticollis, scoliosis, cleft palate

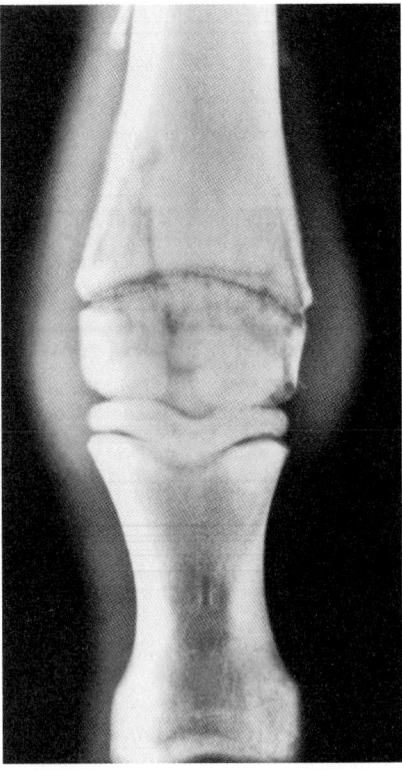

FIG. 36-18 ■ Osteomyelitis of the distal metaphyseal, physeal, and epiphyseal regions of the third metacarpal bone of a 3-week-old foal that did not receive colostral immunity at birth. Bony destruction is advanced. Note the associated soft tissue swelling.

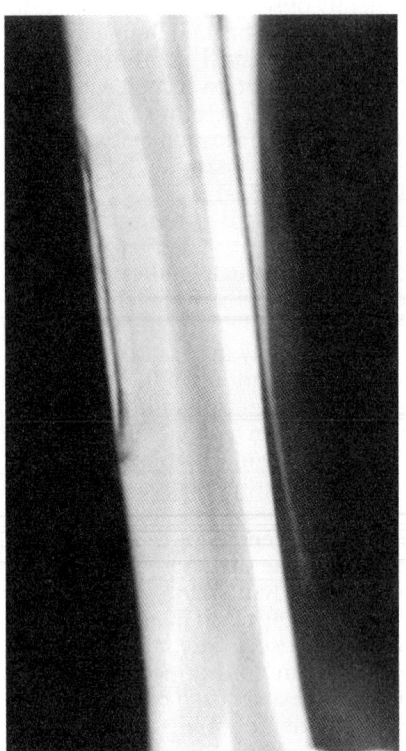

FIG. 36-19 ■ Cortical sequestration of the dorsal aspect of the third metatarsal bone in a horse 4 weeks after blunt trauma to the region.

The acute form of osteomyelitis is rare in adults and usually is associated with direct bacterial inoculation during trauma or open reduction of a fracture. Clinical signs of fever, localized pain, inappetence, and soft tissue swelling often make differentiation between infection and postoperative inflammation difficult. Persistent elevation in rectal temperature for more than 48 hours may be more indicative of an acute infectious process.

Fever and depression are usually not observed in chronically affected animals. In adults, infection is usually localized and the result of direct trauma to bone. Clinical signs commonly observed in chronic osteomyelitis include firm swelling of the affected area, reluctance to bear weight on the limb, mild-to-moderate lameness, and the presence of a draining fistulous tract. Drainage may be constant or intermittent and is usually purulent.

Radiographic signs of acute osteomyelitis are often subtle and can be difficult to interpret. Soft tissue swelling adjacent to the affected area may be the only radiographically visible abnormality during the initial signs of infection. Osteolysis may be observed as early as 3 days; however, serial radiography is often necessary to visualize bony changes, which may lag 7 to 14 days behind the evolution of infection.[116] Destruction of cortical bone initially appears as focal radiolucent holes that subsequently enlarge and coalesce to involve a region of bone (Fig. 36-18). Radiographic changes frequently noted in animals with chronic osteomyelitis include sclerotic bone, cortical resorption and thinning, and periosteal proliferation that may be smooth, expansile, or spiculated.[114] A sequestrum, a necrotic portion of cortical bone that is devoid of an osseous blood supply, is a classic radiographic observation. It appears radiodense and is surrounded by an area of cortical lysis[117] (Fig. 36-19). As the body's defenses attempt to isolate the area of infection, periosteal new

bone forms an involucrum or bony sheath around the sequestrum with a cloaca that allows inflammatory debris an avenue to egress through a fistulous tract to the skin[117] (Fig. 36-20).

Osteomyelitis at a fracture repair site delays healing and fracture instability is often noted clinically. Radiographically, lysis or bone resorption around implants may be observed, and fracture gap widening or nonunion is frequently observed.[114] Implant loosening and fixation collapse may occur with progression of bone lysis.

A definitive diagnosis of osteomyelitis is made by microbiologic culture of the suspected focus of infection. Samples for culture may be obtained from deep needle aspirates, sequestra, and necrotic tissue removed during surgical debridement or metallic implants removed from the affected area. It is not recommended to culture draining tracts because tract organisms are not usually the pathogen(s) responsible for bone infection. Blood cultures are advisable in the neonate. Culture for both aerobic and anaerobic bacterial pathogens is indicated. Clinical characteristics suggestive of, but not limited to, anaerobic infection include a fetid odor, presence of bony sequestra, and purulent discharge. Anaerobic infection should be suspected if bacteria were identified on cytologic analysis but routine aerobic cultures had no bacterial growth.[114] Anaerobes are frequently associated with infection after surgical repair of an open fracture. Culture results will most accurately reflect the causative bacteria if samples have been collected and transported properly.

CLINICAL PATHOLOGY. The white blood cell count is usually elevated in animals with acute osteomyelitis. A degenerative left shift in the leukogram is often present. In neonates an initial leukopenia may be observed as the result of a primary disorder such as generalized septicemia or enteritis. Plasma fibrinogen also may be elevated in acute

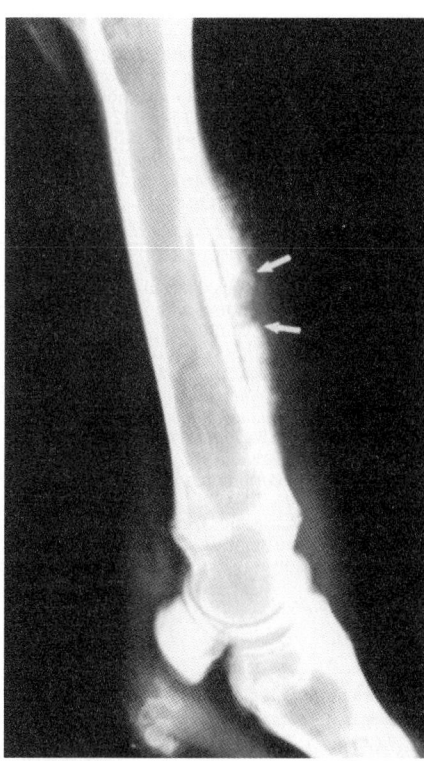

FIG. 36-20 ▊▊ Lateral radiograph of the third metacarpal bone of a cow with chronic osteomyelitis. A sequestrum is visible surrounded by an area of osteolysis. An involucrum formed by medullary sclerosis and periosteal new bone and a cloaca *(arrows)* are evident.

infection. The leukogram tends to return to normal with chronicity.

Osteomyelitis is frequently associated with septic arthritis in the neonate.[115,116] Synovial fluid of affected joints has an elevated leukocyte count and total protein concentration. Gram stain of synovial fluid can be helpful initially in determining the type of bacteria present to aid in the selection of appropriate antimicrobial therapy before the results of microbiologic culture are known. Blood cultures also may be helpful for identification of causative organism(s) in the neonate.

PATHOPHYSIOLOGY. Sequestration of cortical bone results from mechanical trauma to the periosteum and overlying soft tissues, which compromises the defenses of normal cortical bone and leads to regional vascular injury and venous stasis.[114,115,117] Increased capillary permeability permits inflammatory cells to infiltrate the injured area and engulf bacteria. Lysed neutrophils release proteolytic lysosomal enzymes that induce local tissue and bone necrosis; and an exudate composed of serum, neutrophils, bacteria, and nonviable tissue accumulates.[115] If host defense mechanisms are inadequate to contain the infection, bacterial colonization of adjacent periosteal, cortical, and medullary regions ensues.[115] Antibodies and antibiotics cannot easily penetrate the infected area because of the compromised blood supply. The necrotic cortical bone or sequestrum is enveloped by granulation tissue and new bone forming an involucrum in an effort to contain the infection.[115] Draining sinus tracts may eventually form during the progression of the disease. Acute hematogenous osteomyelitis has historically been attributed to sluggish blood flow in the metaphyseal region of long bones in young, growing animals.[114,115] It was thought that vascular stasis in the capillary loops of the primary spongiosa resulted in localization of blood-borne bacteria in the meta-

physis. Recently it has been shown that the endothelial lining of the capillaries pervading the primary spongiosa of neonates is incomplete and allows extravasation of bacteria and erythrocytes.[114] Because leukocytes are absent from this location in the young animal, macrophages provide the sole defense against bacterial colonization in this region.[114] The inability of these macropohages to effectively eliminate bacteria appears to be a critical factor in the development of hematogenous osteomyelitis in young animals.

TREATMENT. Selected cases of acute osteomyelitis may respond to aggressive antimicrobial treatment in the early stages, but once infection is established in bone it is difficult to resolve without surgical intervention. Broad-spectrum antimicrobial administration in combination with surgical management constitutes the hallmark of treatment for osteomyelitis.[114,115]

The goal of surgical treatment is to facilitate the penetration of blood-borne antibiotics to the site of infection by eliminating necrotic debris and encouraging vascular access to compromised tissues. The most important precepts are careful and thorough debridement of all nonviable tissue and sequestrated bone fragments, establishment of open drainage, and removal of foreign material implants.[114,115] Certain bacteria such as staphyloccci are capable of producing a viscous substance that enshrouds bacterial colonies and facilitates adhesion of bacteria to necrotic bone and foreign implants.[114] When combined with host-derived matrix proteins and cellular debris, this biofilm protects bacteria from host defenses and may actually alter bacterial susceptibility to certain antibiotics.[114]

The exception to implant removal arises when the implant is required for fracture stabilization. Although healing is delayed, stable fractures can heal in the presence of infection.[114] Therefore it is advisable to maintain implants until they are no longer necessary for fracture stability while treating the infection. However, delayed healing can lead to excessive cycling of the implant and fixation failure.

Initially the choice of appropriate antibiotic is based on known susceptibilities of the organism suspected to be responsible for infection. Antibiotic therapy may require modification after a definitive organism(s) is isolated and in vitro susceptibilities determined. The ideal antibiotic demonstrates the greatest bacteriocidal activity against the offending organism, the least toxicity to the patient, and is economically feasible. Duration of antibiotic therapy is empirical and depends on clinical response. Because compromised bone requires 4 to 6 weeks for revascularization, this time frame has generally been accepted for treatment duration in cases of chronic osteomyelitis.[114,118]

The most common aerobic bacterial groups isolated from musculoskeletal infections in horses include Enterobacteriaceae, streptococci, and staphylococci.[119] *Actinomyces pyogenes* is the most frequent isolate recovered from adult cattle, sheep, and goats. Neonates appear particularly susceptible to infection from *Escherichia coli* and *Salmonella* spp.[116] *Bacteroides* spp. is the most predominant obligate anaerobic genus encountered; however, most infections include a mixture of anaerobes or a combination of aerobes and anaerobes.

Parenteral administration of antibiotics constitutes the mainstay of antimicrobial therapy in the treatment of osteomyelitis.[118] Localized antibiotic therapy, however, is a useful adjunct to systemic antibiotic treatment. Regional limb antibiotic perfusion, local implantation of polymethylmethacrylate (PMMA) antibiotic-impregnated beads, and use of autogenous cancellous bone grafts enhance the resolution of osteomyelitis.[120-122]

Regional limb perfusion delivers a systemic dose of antibiotic to an isolated area of infected tissue,[120-121] subjecting the tissue to antibiotic concentrations in excess of the minimum

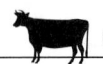

inhibitory concentration (MIC) for the infectious agent. This technique is particularly useful for cases of septic arthritis where vascular compromise of synovial membrane may prevent adequate antimicrobial distribution.[120] A tourniquet is placed proximal to the site of infection. A systemic dose of antibiotic is administered through a catheterized vein distal to the site of infection[120,121] or through a single 4.5-mm-diameter hole into the medullary cavity and allowed to perfuse the isolated area for 30 minutes. In horses, cattle, and rabbits synovial antibiotic concentrations are significantly greater than peak serum concentrations associated with systemic administration.[120,121] We have used regional limb perfusion as an adjunct treatment in selected cases of septic tenosynovitis and navicular bursitis and osteomyelitis of the calcaneus, phalanges, and distal sesamoid bone.

Antibiotic-impregnated PMMA beads are an effective drug delivery system for bone and soft-tissue infections in human medicine.[114,122] Although this treatment is gaining popularity in large animal orthopedics, there are no published reports of its efficacy in veterinary medicine. Gentamicin is the traditional antibiotic impregnated in beads and elutes over time to yield local concentrations well above the therapeutic concentration range for as long as 80 days postimplantation.[122] Aminoglycoside toxicity does not appear to be a problem, with human serum and urine concentrations below those associated with systemic administration.[122] Gentamicin-impregnated PMMA beads are used routinely in our hospital in the repair of open fractures and in the internal fixation of closed fractures that incurred significant soft tissue trauma.

The use of autogenous cancellous bone graft has been advocated as an ancillary treatment in some cases of septic navicular bursitis and osteomyelitis of the navicular bone in horses.[123] Placement of the graft in a surgically created defect underlying the navicular bone may reduce dead space, provide protection of the deeper tissues from environmental contamination, and afford a temporary scaffold for the ingrowth of capillaries and precursor cells of granulation tissue.[122] We believe this modality has merit for continued clinical application and routinely use it for deep-seated infections of the foot.

PREVENTION AND CONTROL. Early and aggressive medical therapy for neonates suspected to be at risk for developing septicemia is prudent in the prevention of acute hematogenous osteomyelitis. Therapy may include administration of prophylactic antibiotics and hyperimmune plasma in cases where failure of passive transfer of colostral antibodies has occurred. Prompt and meticulous debridement of avascular and necrotic tissue in treatment of soft tissue wounds and repair of open fractures cannot be overemphasized. Delayed wound closure may be desirable in select cases of overwhelming contamination or infection.

Many infections associated with fracture repair occur during open reduction and internal fixation of closed fractures.[114] Strict adherence to the principles of aseptic technique is imperative to a successful outcome. Prophylactic antibiotics are commonly used because the risk of infection increases with metallic implants. The timing of antibiotic administration is crucial for efficacy and should achieve sufficient blood antibiotic levels while the amount of bacteria in the exposed tissues exceeds the host's ability to eliminate the organisms and allow tissue healing to commence.[115] For elective uncomplicated orthopedic procedures, antibiotics should be administered 1 to 2 hours before surgery and continued for no more than 72 hours after surgery.[115] For long bone fracture repair, the risk of infection is much greater because of increased operative time, the presence of metallic implants, and the soft tissue trauma incurred during the injury and the subsequent fixation.[119] In this instance, administration of the most effective broad-spectrum antibiotic combination for an extended period of time is advisable.

REFERENCES

114. Johnson KA: Osteomyelitis in dogs and cats, *J Am Vet Med Assoc* 205: 1882-1887, 1994.
115. Rudd RG: A rational approach to the diagnosis and treatment of osteomyelitis, *Compend Cont Educ Pract Vet* 8:225-234, 1986.
116. Wagner PC, Watrous BJ, Darien BJ: Septic arthritis and osteomyelitis. In Robinson NE, editor: *Current therapy in equine medicine,* ed 3, Philadelphia, 1992, WB Saunders, pp 455-462.
117. Clem MF, Yovich JV, Douglass JP: Osseous sequestration in horses, *Compend Cont Educ Pract Vet* 9:1219-1224, 1987.
118. Mader JT, Landon GC, Calhoun J: Antimicrobial treatment of osteomyelitis, *Clin Orthop Rel Res* 295:87-95, 1993.
119. Moore RN, Schneider RK, Kowalski J, et al: Antimicrobial susceptibility of bacterial isolates from 233 horses with musculoskeletal infection during 1979-1989, *Equine Vet J* 24:450-456, 1992.
120. Whitehair KJ, Adams SB, Parker JE, et al: Regional limb perfusion with antibiotics in three horses, *Vet Surg* 21:286-292, 1992.
121. Murphey ED, Santschi EM, Papich G: Local antibiotic perfusion of the distal limb of horses, *Proceedings of the Fortieth Annual Convention of the American Association of Equine Practitioners,* 1994, pp 141-142.
122. Calhoun JH, Henry SL, Anger DM, et al: The treatment of infected nonunions with gentamicin-polymethylmethacrylate antibiotic beads, *Clin Orthop Rel Res* 295:23-27, 1993.
123. Honnas CM, Crabill MR, Mackie JT, et al: Use of autogenous cancellous bone grafting in the treatment of septic navicular bursitis and distal sesamoid osteomyelitis in horses, *J Am Vet Med Assoc* 206:1191-1194, 1995.

NAVICULAR DISEASE

MICHAEL A. LIVESAY

The distal sesamoid (navicular) bone was first implicated as a cause of lameness in 1701, when an unknown author described erosions of the cartilage covering the bone and recommended neurectomy for pain relief. Today it is probably the most common diagnosis made in chronic forelimb lameness of the riding horse. Applied to animals with pain isolated to the palmar third of the hoof, the term navicular syndrome is preferred to navicular disease because a specific etiology and treatment are usually not known. Disorders encompassed by navicular syndrome include distal interphalangeal joint synovitis, deep digital flexor tendinitis, desmitis of the collateral or distal impar sesamoidean ligaments, navicular bursitis, and degenerative changes of the navicular bone.

DIAGNOSIS. Navicular syndrome is a clinical diagnosis based on history, physical findings, selective regional and intraarticular anesthesia, and diagnostic imaging. The condition is species specific to Equidae, affecting all breeds and work types of horse; but it is seldom seen in ponies, Arabians, and heavy breeds and is absent in donkeys and mules. The highest reported incidence is in the quarter horse, probably reflecting the geographic origins of the authors. There is no sex predisposition. These disorders usually become apparent in horses 3 to 12 years of age, with a peak incidence at 7 to 9 years. Warmblood breeds may be affected at a younger age. There is little evidence for a hereditary component.

The most common clinical sign is a chronic, progressive forelimb lameness of insidious onset, which in the early stages improves with exercise. Hind feet also may be affected. Occasionally, animals will present with an acute onset. As the condition progresses and becomes persistent, lameness is exacerbated by exercise and improves with rest. The condition is generally bilateral, with the majority of cases being asymmetric. As a result, a frequent presenting complaint (22% of cases) is unilateral lameness, without a limb predisposition. Lameness is usually mild to moderate at initial presentation, often worsening with time. With chronicity, however, lameness may plateau at a level permitting comfortable pasture retirement and seldom warranting euthanasia.

The first presenting signs often are shortening of the anterior phase of stride and increasing lameness that improves with rest. Riders often complain that gait is short and choppy or that the horse trips, stumbles, or will not take one's lead.

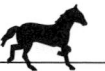

Lack of forelimb extension frequently leads people to falsely implicate the shoulder. Bilateral lameness may be difficult to observe in animals trotted in a straight line, but lameness usually can be accentuated unilaterally by circling. The toe may contact the ground before the heel. Lameness may be more apparent on a hard surface, particularly if the feet are unshod. At rest, the horse may point the affected limb with the heel raised off the ground, or pack shavings under the foot. Chronic reduced weight bearing frequently leads to an upright boxy foot with atrophy of the frog and narrow contracted heels. The toe of the hoof wall or shoe may be excessively worn.

Compression of the navicular bone and adjacent structures by hoof tester application over the middle third of the frog produces a positive pain response in 11% to 73% of cases. Forced flexion of the distal limb may exacerbate lameness, but is not specific for structures affected by navicular syndrome. The distal interphalangeal joint can be selectively extended by toe elevation with a wedge-shaped block while holding the contralateral limb off the ground for 1 minute. Increased lameness indicates a positive pain response.

Diagnostic regional anesthesia is useful for localizing pain. The medial and lateral palmar digital nerves supply the navicular bone and adjacent structures. Many nerve endings are closely associated with the attachment of the collateral sesamoidean ligaments to the proximal border of the navicular bone and with the deep digital flexor tendon. Myelinated fibers run under the synovial lining of the distal interphalangeal joint and over the distal impar sesamoidean ligament before entering the navicular bone.

Medial and lateral palmar digital analgesia, performed immediately proximal to the collateral cartilages, usually produces at least 80% improvement in lameness, with frequent enhancement of lameness in the contralateral limb. Complete resolution of lameness does not usually occur because of (1) incomplete local analgesia as a result of aberrant nerves, (2) fibrous adhesions between the flexor surface of the navicular bone and the deep digital flexor tendon that mechanically limit extension of the distal interphalangeal joint, and (3) other concurrent problems in the foot or limb. More diffuse foot pain secondary to landing on the toe requires additional analgesia. Lameness in many horses with navicular syndrome is improved with intrasynovial anesthesia of (1) the distal interphalangeal joint, (2) the navicular bursa, or (3) both. Often used to localize the cause of lameness when radiographic findings are inconclusive, these blocks are not specific for the joint or bursa. Dye injected into the distal interphalangeal joint will diffuse into the navicular bursa, the medullary cavity of the navicular bone, the synovial lining of the collateral sesamoidean ligaments, and the distal impar sesamoidean ligament. Peptidergic nerves, believed to be thinly myelinated or unmyelinated nerves that convey pain sensation, are present in synovial linings overlying the collateral and distal impar sesamoidean ligaments. In contrast, dye injected into the navicular bursa does not diffuse into the distal interphalangeal joint, other than the rare cases where there is direct communication. These studies suggest that response to distal interphalangeal joint analgesia indicates that pain may originate from (1) articulating surfaces of the middle and distal phalanges or navicular bone, (2) collateral or distal impar sesamoidean ligaments, (3) navicular bone or central portion of the distal phalanx, or (4) periarticular soft tissues. Response to navicular bursa analgesia indicates that the pain may originate from the (1) deep digital flexor tendon, (2) palmar surface of the collateral sesamoidean ligaments, (3) flexor surface of the navicular bone, or (4) adjacent soft tissues.

Navicular bursa injection is not usually a routine procedure because it is difficult to adequately disinfect the skin at the site for needle puncture. It should be performed with radiographic guidance because of close proximity of the bursa to the deep digital flexor tendon sheath and the distal interphalangeal

joint capsule. A logical approach to local anesthesia of the foot is to perform the following blocks in sequence, on different occasions: (1) palmar digital perineural analgesia, and when necessary, palmar perineural analgesia at the abaxial, proximal sesamoid bone site; (2) distal interphalangeal joint analgesia; and (3) navicular bursa analgesia in those cases where a specific diagnosis is necessary and has not been made.

Radiographic examination has an important role in confirming a diagnosis of navicular syndrome. A minimum of three radiographic projections are taken, including (1) lateromedial (LM), (2) dorsoproximal-palmarodistal oblique (DPr-PaDiO), and (3) palmaroproximal-palmarodistal oblique (PaPr-PaDiO, flexor, or caudal tangential) views. Radiographic features considered to be of diagnostic relevance for navicular syndrome are the following (Fig. 36-21):

1. The size, shape, number, and position of synovial fossae in the distal border of the navicular bone. Lucencies in

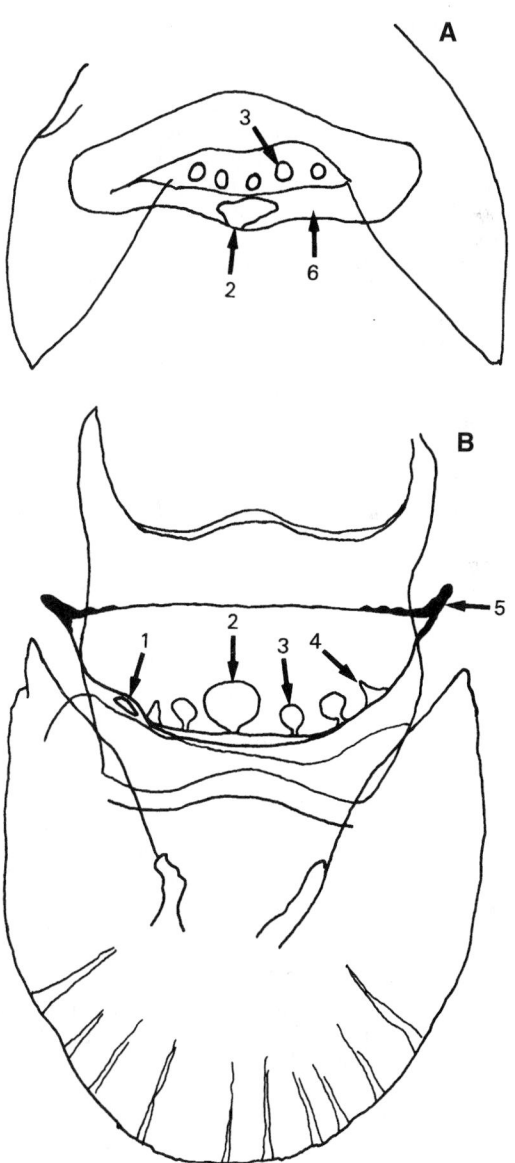

FIG. 36-21 ■ Drawing of **A,** dorsoproximal-palmarodistal oblique (DPr-PaDiO), and **B,** palmaroproximal-palmarodistal oblique (PaPr-PaDiO) projection radiographs of the navicular bone, showing abnormalities associated with navicular syndrome. *1,* Fracture of the distal border with associated concavity; *2,* large-sagittal flexor cortex defect; *3,* "inverted flask"–shaped synovial invagination extending from the distal border; *4,* "cone-shaped" invagination on the sloping distal border; *5,* proximal border enthesiophytes; and *6,* thickened flexor cortex, with loss of corticomedullary demarcation.

the distal border of the navicular bone are attributed to nutrient foraminae (vascular channels, synovial fossa, synovial invaginations). Up to seven invaginations of triangular outline, with a height approximately 1.5 times base width are normally found on the distal border of the bone. Increase in size, change in shape to an "inverted flask," "mushroom," or "lollipop," or the presence of any invagination on the sloping, abaxial portion of the distal border of the bone, is considered abnormal.

2. Osteophyte (enthesiophyte) formation on the proximal and distal borders, or the wings of the navicular bone (spurs). Enthesiophytes on the proximal border or extremities (wings) of the navicular bone occur in the attachment of the collateral sesamoidean ligaments; those on the distal border occur in the distal impar sesamoidean ligament. They are indicative of normal aging and inflammation secondary to strain. "Spurs" of the wings occur bilaterally or unilaterally. If unilateral, they are more commonly lateral and have been associated with foot imbalance.

3. Radiolucent areas within the body of the navicular bone. Radiolucencies within the bone are frequently described as "cysts." Cysts visualized on the DPr-PaDiO view are usually flexor cortex defects, which vary greatly in size; most involve the sagittal ridge. The PaPr-PaDiO view is useful for differentiating subchondral cystic lesions.

4. Fragmentation of the distal border. Osseous bodies adjacent to the distal border of the navicular bone are associated with the distal impar sesamoidean ligament. They may be fractures of the distal margin, separate centers of ossification within the distal impar sesamoidean ligament, ossification secondary to ligamentous damage, or ossification of cartilage particles in adjacent synovial tissue. The presence of a defect in the distal margin adjacent to the fragment supports the diagnosis of a fracture. Visualization of these fragments depends on good radiographs, with the distal margin of the navicular bone projected away from the distal interphalangeal joint and the middle phalanx.

5. Loss of flexor corticomedullary demarcation. Poor flexor corticomedullary demarcation, medullary trabecular disruption, and medullary sclerosis are changes visualized on the caudal tangential view, indicative of navicular bone remodeling.

6. Dystrophic calcification. Calcification in the collateral and distal impar sesamoidean ligaments represents injury to the suspensory apparatus of the navicular bone and may or may not be accompanied by other signs of degeneration. Mineralization of the deep flexor tendon is usually accompanied by pathology in the flexor cortex of the navicular bone. It is an indication of degeneration and possibly fibrillation or adhesion formation between the tendon and the flexor surface of the bone. New bone formation associated with the proximal and the distal borders of the navicular bone, frequently referred to as bone "spurs," often can be differentiated into enthesiophytes and periarticular osteophytes. The latter are present at the articular margins of the navicular bone, adjacent to the middle phalanx. Whereas enthesiophytes are considered indicative of navicular syndrome, osteophytes are more likely an indication of distal interphalangeal joint arthrosis.

Although radiographic findings are essential to the diagnosis of navicular syndrome, interpretation of findings is less clear because the same radiologic changes can be seen in both lame and sound animals. The radiographic findings of greatest significance are lucencies associated with defects in the flexor cortex, proximal border remodeling, and medullary trabecular disruption and sclerosis. Perhaps the most contentious radiographic feature is the appearance of synovial invaginations on the distal border of the navicular bone. A radiographic scoring scheme classified synovial invaginations into seven types. Significant differences were observed among the radiographs of sound horses, those with a clinical diagnosis of navicular disease, and animals with a forefoot lameness of unknown etiology.

Scintigraphy is useful when radiographic findings do not support clinical findings. The specificity of radiography and scintigraphy clinical signs of the syndrome are similar, whereas the sensitivity of scintigraphy is greater than that of radiography. The greatest sensitivity and specificity is obtained by concurrently evaluating soft tissue and bone phase scintigraphy with radiographic findings.

Because horse owners are often aware of the chronic, irreversible nature of navicular syndrome, the condition carries a powerful negative connotation. It is imperative therefore that all other possible diagnoses are explored before labeling an animal with the condition. Unless there are advanced radiographic changes, it is wise not to make the diagnosis until the animal has been lame for at least 3 months.

ETIOLOGY. Many theories have been proposed to explain the cause or causes of navicular syndrome, but the condition is still poorly understood. Most theories can be classified as either vascular or biomechanical in nature.

Arterial thrombosis could disturb intraosseus circulation of the navicular bone and result in ischemic necrosis. Increased vascularization around nutrient arteries could appear osteoporotic, compatible with radiographic changes on the distal border of the bone. Resorption of necrotic bone could result in areas of subchondral lysis beneath the flexor surface. This theory is not widely accepted because the presence of thrombosed vessels has not been confirmed by other investigators, and experimental reduction in blood flow by occlusion of blood vessels failed to reproduce the clinical, radiographic, and histologic changes associated with navicular syndrome.

Increased intraosseous bone marrow pressure is associated with continuous pain in human patients with degenerative joint disease. Horses with clinical evidence of navicular syndrome have increased intramedullary navicular bone pressure and a prolonged reduction time after an experimental increase in pressure. Pain is presumed to result from distention of sinusoids and venules in the subchondral spongiosa.

Biomechanically, the navicular bone is compressed between the deep digital flexor tendon and the distal extremity of the middle phalanx. Corresponding pathology could include navicular bursitis, degeneration of fibrocartilage overlying the flexor cortex, and ultimately, hyperemia and bone rarefaction. It is hypothesized that concussion, poor conformation, and improper trimming and shoeing may be predisposing factors. Flat soles, fast work on hard surfaces, a large body weight/foot size ratio, and an upright pastern angle will all increase concussive forces. A common predisposing conformation is a flat foot, low underrun heels, and a "broken back" foot/pastern axis. In animals with a long toe or low heel, the deep digital flexor tendon bends more acutely around the navicular bone before inserting on the distal phalanx. Similarly, a broken-back foot/pastern axis (associated with distal interphalangeal joint hyperextension) may produce greater pressure on the navicular bone. Increased pressure between the navicular bone and deep digital flexor tendon is compatible with histologic evidence of increased bone remodeling and vascularization demonstrated in trabecular bone of the distal and central parts of the navicular bone and in the subchondral bone of the flexor surface in animals with navicular syndrome.

Both vascular and biomechanical factors likely participate in the etiopathogenesis of navicular syndrome. Injury may

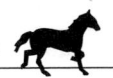

be initiated by excessive or sustained compressive forces exerted against the flexor surface of the navicular bone. If the rate of injury exceeds the physiologic rate of repair (remodeling), fibrocartilaginous and bony tissues degenerate. Accompanying stromal fibrosis may entrap sinusoids and venules, slowing venous drainage and increasing intraosseous pressure and pain. Conversely, vascular compromise could initiate the pathologic process. Venous drainage could be impaired by poor conformation and excessive tension on veins associated with the distal impar sesamoidean ligament, or by synovial effusion and increased distal interphalangeal intraarticular pressure, causing intracapsular vein compression.

Ischemic necrosis and mechanical damage could be expected to initiate similar repair processes. Active hyperemia induced by the repair and remodeling processes activates osteoclasts lying beneath the synovial lining of the synovial fossae, along the distal aspect of the bone. Osteoclasts resorb the thin shell of cortical bone separating the fossa from the medullary cavity and follow the course of the nutrient artery for a variable distance. The fossae then vary in size, shape, and penetration into the bone. The synovial membrane follows, lining the tunnel, thus creating the "synovial invaginations" seen radiographically on the distal border of the bone. Bone changes are most severe in the flexor cortex, particularly in the central region of the sagittal ridge. With chronic remodeling of the flexor cortex, granulation tissue may fill the synovial fossa of the sagittal ridge and enhance adhesion formation to the deep digital flexor tendon. The ensuing bone lucency is visible radiographically as a "cyst" on the dorsal view and as an erosion on the caudal tangential view.

DIFFERENTIAL DIAGNOSES. The differential diagnosis should include sheared heels, broken bars, corns, quarter cracks, fractures of the navicular bone or distal phalanx, pedal osteitis, sole bruising, and coffin joint arthrosis.

TREATMENT. Numerous treatments are directed toward slowing or arresting progressive degeneration of the navicular bone or providing palliative pain relief. In general, conservative treatments are applied to younger animals with minor radiographic abnormalities in the initial stages of the disease. Initial management should begin with correction of any foot abnormalities, rest, and nonsteroidal antiinflammatory medication for 7 to 14 days. Other medical treatments should be considered if clinical signs accompany return to work. Surgical options are considered with chronicity, marked radiographic changes, and lack of response to medical therapy. Medical treatment options include the following:

1. *Corrective shoeing.* The goal of balancing the feet is to reestablish normal foot/pastern axis and mediolateral balance, with even heel heights during weight bearing. Corrective shoeing traditionally involves shortening the toe and elevating the heels to increase hoof angle by 2 to 4 degrees. The toe of the shoe is "rolled" or rounded in a vertical plane to enhance breakover. These changes are speculated to decrease deep digital flexor tendon tension and loads exerted by the collateral and distal impar sesamoidean ligaments on the navicular bone. Changes in hoof wall angle may be made by trimming, applying wedge shoes, or inserting wedge pads between the shoe and hoof. Concussion may be reduced by applying commercial shock-absorbing rim or full pads and packing the space between a full pad and the sole with silicone rubber. A bar shoe may provide added protection to the frog. Shoes should extend as far in a palmar direction as the bulbs of the heels. Egg-bar shoes may be used to extend the weight-bearing surface of the foot in a palmar direction. Heel expansion may be enhanced by rasping the hoof wall from the quarters to the heels, 1 cm distal to the coronary band, by grooving the wall with a series of vertical lines, or by "slippering" the branches of the shoe so that the upper surface of the shoe slopes distally in an abaxial direction. Good hoof management is tailored to the conformation and use of the horse and is continued indefinitely.

2. *Nonsteroidal antiinflammatory drugs.* Nonsteroidal antiinflammatory drugs are frequently used palliatively for their analgesic, antiinflammatory, and platelet aggregation inhibitory effects. Phenylbutazone is most commonly used; however, flunixin meglumine,* naproxen, and meclofenamic acid can be effective. The primary goal is to maintain comfort with the minimum effective dose to avoid toxicity. Dosage can be tailored to work schedules, with the maximum recommended dose of phenylbutazone 4.4 mg/kg twice a day for no more than 5 consecutive days. Dosages for prolonged use should not exceed 3 mg/kg/day.

3. *Corticosteroids.* Intrabursal or intraarticular methylprednisolone acetate or triamcinolone, alone or in combination with hyaluronic acid, may provide short-term relief when these synovial structures are inflamed. In one study this treatment had no effect in 19% of cases, provided relief for less than 1 month in 14%, and for up to 12 months in 60% of cases. This treatment can mask signs of lameness and has potential for abuse.

4. *Polysulfated glycosaminoglycans.* This chondroprotective medication (Adequan), given by repeated intramuscular injection, has been reported to have beneficial effects.

5. *Isoxsuprine hydrochloride.* A peripheral vasodilator, this β-agonist and α-antagonist causes a reduction in blood viscosity and has demonstrated efficacy in the treatment of navicular syndrome. The drug presumably relaxes the vasculature, increasing local blood flow and relieving venous congestion of the navicular bone. This effect is supported by thermographic evidence of increased temperature and is compatible with lower limb vasodilation. The original recommended dose is 0.6 mg/kg twice a day for 6 to 12 weeks. Some animals respond to higher dosages, but a dose-related effect (up to 1.8 mg/kg twice a day) was not demonstrated. One dosing method is to begin treatment at 0.6 mg/kg twice a day for 3 weeks. If the animal does not become sound, the dose is increased by 0.3 mg/kg twice a day every 3 weeks, until the level of 1.2 mg/kg is reached. If there is no response after 3 weeks, the drug is discontinued. If improvement is maintained for 2 weeks, the dosage is reduced to once a day for 2 weeks, then every other day for 2 weeks, and finally discontinued after a further 2 weeks. Animals that become sound on the drug may have recurrence of the lameness after several months. For this reason, some clinicians will continue alternate-day treatment. No adverse effects or changes in hematologic or serum biochemical values have been reported in horses receiving oral isoxsuprine hydrochloride, which is often combined with phenylbutazone in a treatment program. In general, the response to therapy and the longevity of the effect are reduced with increasing duration of lameness.

6. *Pentoxifylline.* This hemorrheologic drug is a methylxanthine derivative that may increase blood flow to hypoxic tissues by changing the deformability and stickiness of blood cells and by inhibiting thrombus formation. Although the clinical efficacy has not been documented, it is widely used in Canada for the treatment of navicular syndrome (Navicon, Sanofi†).

---

*Banamine, Schering Plough Animal Health, Union, NJ 07083.
†Sanofi, Animal Health, Inc., Overland Park, KS 62210.

Recommended dose is 6 g a day for 6 weeks. Clinical investigation of a related compound, propentofylline (7.5 mg/kg twice a day for 6 weeks), significantly improved lameness, but complete soundness was not obtained in any horse.

Surgical options for treatment of navicular syndrome include the following:

1. *Navicular suspensory desmotomy.* The navicular bone is suspended at the palmar aspect of the distal interphalangeal joint by three ligaments: the paired collateral sesamoidean (suspensory) ligaments and the distal impar sesamoidean ligament. Tension in these ligaments during weight bearing is increased with distal interphalangeal hyperextension (e.g., "broken-back" foot/pastern axis). The goal of suspensory ligament desmotomy is to reduce forces on the navicular bone and ligaments. Concurrent sensory denervation may contribute to clinical improvement. Clinical success has been variable. In one study, at 6 and 36 months after surgery 76% and 43% of 118 horses, respectively, were sound. Some horses had radiographic evidence of diminished flexor cortex defects after surgery. Factors that worsen prognosis include increasing horse age, lameness severity and duration, angular limb deformity, and radiographic evidence of flexor cortex defects, deep digital flexor tendon mineralization, and proximal border enthesiophytes.

2. *Palmar digital neurectomy.* Palmar digital neurectomy provides palliative pain relief by eliminating sensation from the palmar aspect of the foot. It is usually used only when medical therapies are not effective. Although foot proprioception and toe sensation should be retained, potential complications include (1) incomplete loss of sensation because of aberrant nerve distribution, (2) recurrence of sensation and pain after reinnervation, (3) painful neuroma formation, (4) deep digital flexor tendon rupture with uninhibited exercise, and (5) sloughing of the hoof wall. Approximately 65% of horses are sound 1 year after neurectomy. A major complication of surgical resection is neuroma formation; alternative neurectomy techniques include (1) perineural injection of cytotoxic agents contained in cobra venom or an extract of a pitcher plant (Serapin) and (2) percutaneous cryotherapy. Clinical improvement with these techniques is of short duration, with reinnervation within 2 to 4 months.

SUGGESTED READINGS

Bowker R, Linder K, Sonea I, et al: Sensory innervation of the navicular bone and bursa in the foal, *Equine Vet J* 27:60-65, 1995.
Bowker R, Rockershouser S, Sonea I, et al: Immunocytochemical and dye distribution studies of nerves potentially desensitized by injections into the distal interphalangeal joint or the navicular bursas of horses, *J Am Vet Med Assoc* 203:1708-1714, 1993.
Dyson S, Kidd L: A comparison of responses to analgesia of the navicular bursa and the intra-articular analgesia of the distal interphalangeal joint in 59 horses, *Equine Vet J* 25:93-98, 1993.
Field J, Dobson H, Bonnett B: Navicular syndrome: preliminary assessment of radiographic scoring, *Vet Comp Orthop Traumatol* 8:36-39, 1995.
Hickman J: Navicular disease—what are we talking about? *Equine Vet J* 21: 395-398, 1989.
Kaser-Hotz B, Uettschi G: Radiographic appearance of the navicular bone in sound horses, *Vet Radiol* 33:9-17, 1992.
Kirker-Head CA, Fackelman GE, Hoogasian JJ, et al: Studies on propentofylline for the treatment of navicular disease, *Equine Vet Sci* 13:106-113, 1993.
MacGregor CM: Radiographic assessment of navicular bones, based on changes in the distal nutrient foramina, *Equine Vet J* 18:203-206, 1986.
Ostblom L, June C, Melsen F: Histological study of navicular bone, *Equine Vet J* 14:199-202, 1982.
Pleasant R, Baker G, Foreman J, et al: Intraosseous pressure and pathologic changes in horses with navicular disease, *Am J Vet Res* 54:7-12, 1993.

Pool RR, Meagher DM, Stover SM: Pathophysiology of navicular syndrome, *Vet Clin North Am (Large Anim Pract)* 5:109-129, 1989.
Poulos PW: Correlation of the radiographic signs and histologic changes in navicular disease, *Proc Am Assoc Equine Pract* 29:241-255, 1983.
Poulos PW, Brown A: On navicular disease in the horse:A roentgenological and patho-anatomic study. Part 1. Evaluation of the flexor central eminence, *Vet Radiol* 30:50-53, 1989.
Poulos PW, Brown A, Brown E, et al: On navicular disease in the horse: a roentgenological and pathoanatomic study. Part II. Osseous bodies association with the impar ligament, *Vet Radiol* 30:54-58, 1989.
Stashak TS: Lameness. In Stashak TS, editor: *Adams' lameness in horses*, ed 4, Philadelphia, 1987, Lea & Febiger, pp. 499-514.
Trout DR, Hornof WJ, O'Brien TR: Soft tissue- and bone-phase scintigraphy for diagnosis of navicular disease in horses, *J Am Vet Med Assoc* 198:73-77, 1991.
Turner ST, Tucker CM: The evaluation of isoxsuprine hydrochloride for the treatment of navicular disease: a double blind study, *Equine Vet J* 21:338-341, 1989.
Turner TA, Kneller SK, Baderscher RR, et al: Radiographic changes in the navicular bones of normal horses, *Proc Am Assoc Equine Pract* 32:309-313, 1986.
Verschooten F, Desmet P, Peremans K, et al: Navicular disease in the horse: the effect of controlled intrabursal corticosteroid injection, *Equine Vet Sci* 10:316-320, 1990.
Wright IM: A study of 118 cases of navicular disease: clinical features, *Equine Vet J* 25:488-492, 1993.
Wright IM: A study of 118 cases of navicular disease: radiological features, *Equine Vet J* 25:493-500, 1993.
Wright IM: A study of 118 cases of navicular disease: treatment by navicular suspensory desmotomy, *Equine Vet J* 25:501-509, 1993.
Wright IM, Douglas, J: Biomechanical considerations in the treatment of navicular disease, *Vet Rec* 133:109-114, 1993.

SPONDYLITIS

KEVIN HAUSSLER

DEFINITION. Spondylitis (vertebral osteomyelitis) is an infectious or inflammatory degenerative disease of one or more adjoining vertebrae. Discospondylitis is a concurrent infection of the vertebral body and the adjacent intervertebral disc. Vertebral osteomyelitis and discospondylitis are rare but life-threatening conditions in large animals. Vertebral osteomyelitis occurs in foals and calves, whereas discospondylitis is more prevalent in the cervical or upper thoracic region of adult horses.[124]

ETIOPATHOGENESIS. Vertebral osteomyelitis is caused by bacterial and occasionally fungal infection that extends from local wounds or, most commonly in the newborn, hematogenously from a distant infection or septicemia. Tail docking wounds in sheep; omphalitis in foals, calves, and sheep; and bacterial endocarditis or traumatic reticulitis in adult ruminants are possible sources of infection for vertebral osteomyelitis.[125,126] Vertebral infection usually progresses to a paravertebral abscess, meningitis, vertebral collapse, and spinal cord compression. Cervical intervertebral disk protrusion may also be a sequela.[127] Discospondylitis may result from direct injury to a vertebral end plate or intervertebral disc, which causes vascular disruption and increased susceptibility to infection. Pathogens include *Aspergillus* spp., *Mycobacterium tuberculosis* var *bovis*, and *Brucella abortus* in horses and *Rhodococcus equi*, *Streptococcus* spp., *Staphylococcus* spp., *Escherichia coli*, *Salmonella* spp., *Actinobacillus* spp., and *Eikenella corrodens* in foals.[128-131] Vertebral osteomyelitis isolates in cattle include *Actinomyces pyogenes*, *Fusobacterium necrophorus*, *Streptococcus* spp., *Staphylococcus* spp., *Pseudomonas* spp., and *E. coli*.[125]

CLINICAL SIGNS AND DIFFERENTIAL DIAGNOSES. An early sign of spondylitis is acute, localized spinal pain; however, the diagnosis is usually not made until signs of meningitis or spinal cord compression occur.[132] Vertebral osteomyelitis produces malaise, fever, stiffness, sensory deficits in the limbs, and variable degrees of paresis that progress to recumbency. Discospondylitis often affects cervical or cervicothoracic intervertebral discs in horses.[128] Signs of discospondylitis include severe neck pain, ataxia, or tetraplegia.

Differential diagnoses for spinal pain or stiffness include paraspinal muscle strain, vertebral fracture, spondylosis, impinged spinous processes, vertebral or sacroiliac subluxation or luxation, vertebral infarcts, and aberrant parasitic migration.

DIAGNOSIS. Diagnosis is based on history, clinical signs, and positive findings on plain film radiography, scintigraphy, computed tomography, or ultrasonography.[129,132,133] Radiographic signs of vertebral osteomyelitis include the following: bony proliferation, lysis, sclerosis, and local soft tissue swelling; however, lesions may not be visible radiographically until 2 to 8 weeks after onset of clinical signs.[124] Abnormal hematologic findings in horses include hyperfibrinogenemia, leukocytosis with neutrophilia, and mild anemia.[132] Serum globulin values, cranial nerve examination, and cerebrospinal fluid analysis are often normal. Cytology and culture and sensitivity of a fine-needle aspirate, blood, and feces are important for determining an etiologic agent and selecting appropriate antimicrobial therapy. Suspected animals also should have a *B. abortus* titer taken if direct culture of the lesion is not possible.

TREATMENT AND PROGNOSIS. Successful treatment depends on early diagnosis and appropriate antibiotic or antifungal therapy.[133] Surgical curettage is recommended to debride infected bone or disc material with subsequent lavage and drainage if possible.[147] Long-term antibiotic therapy (2 to 6 months) is usually required to eliminate the infection but relapses are common.[133] Antibiotic choices in horses include trimethoprim-sulfamethoxazole, rifampin, or the newer cephalosporins, depending on culture and sensitivity results. Subsequent neurologic disorders and meningitis are often associated with a poor prognosis for recovery.

REFERENCES

124. Markel MD, Madigan JE, Lichtensteiger CA, et al: Vertebral body osteomyelitis in the horse, *J Am Vet Med Assoc* 188:632-634, 1986.
125. Finley GG: A survey of vertebral abscesses in domestic animals in Ontario, *Can Vet J* 16:114-117, 1975.
126. Gerro TC: Challenging cases in internal medicine: what's your diagnosis? [Discospondylitis in a goat], *Vet Med* 94:83-90, 1999.
127. Furr MO, Anver M, Wise M: Intervertebral disk prolapse and diskospondylitis in a horse, *J Am Vet Med Assoc* 198:2095-2096, 1991.
128. Adams SB, Steckel R, Blevins W: Discospondylitis in five horses, *J Am Vet Med Assoc* 186:270-272, 1985.
129. Giguere S, Lavoie JP: *Rhodococcus equi* vertebral osteomyelitis in 3 quarter horse colts, *Equine Vet J* 26:74-77, 1994.
130. Olchowy TWJ: Vertebral body osteomyelitis due to *Rhodococcus equi* in two Arabian foals, *Equine Vet J* 26:79-82, 1994.
131. Richardson DW: *Eikenella corrodens* osteomyelitis of the axis in a foal, *J Am Vet Med Assoc* 188:298-299, 1986.
132. Markel MD, Ryan AM, Madigan JE: Vertebral and costal osteomyelitis in a foal, *Compend Cont Educ Pract Vet* 10:856-861, 1988.
133. Hillyer MH, Innes JF, Patteson MW, et al: Discospondylitis in an adult horse, *Vet Rec* 139:519-521, 1996.

SPONDYLOSIS

KEVIN HAUSSLER

DEFINITION. Spondylosis is an ankylosing or degenerative disease of the intervertebral joints. Spondylophytes are osteophytes associated with intervertebral disc thinning and degenerative joint disease in the vertebral column.[134] An enthesophyte is an ossification within the transition zone between bone and ligament or tendon[135] and, more specifically, a syndesmophyte if associated with a spinal ligament. Syndesmophytes usually partially bridge a vertebral joint, but occasionally completely bridge, or ankylose, a joint without significant loss of intervertebral disc width. The general term

vertebral enthesophyte describes spinal changes seen in large animal medicine that do not have well-defined diagnostic criteria. Various veterinary medical syndromes characterized by vertebral enthesophyte formation include vertebral osteophytosis, ankylosing spondylitis, and spondylosis deformans.[136-139] The clinical, pathologic, and radiographic criteria for diagnosis of proliferative spinal arthropathies in veterinary medicine vary dramatically from those used in human medicine.[134] Pain and neurologic abnormalities associated with spinal arthropathies in animals may not correlate with the severity of osseous pathology. In aged cattle and horses the thoracolumbar vertebrae are commonly predisposed to the chronic, progressive development of vertebral enthesophytes at the ventrolateral peripheral margins of the anulus fibrosus or within the ventral longitudinal ligament. Bone proliferation (exostosis) is continuous with the cortex of the vertebral body and bridges apparently normal vertebral end plates and intervertebral discs. Secondary degenerative joint disease may develop in the dorsal articular processes because of local chemical mediators and restricted joint mobility, with subsequent articular degeneration or ankylosis.

ETIOPATHOGENESIS. The exact cause of vertebral enthesophytes is unknown, but biomechanical and biochemical mechanisms have been proposed.[140] Excessive joint loading produces microtrauma and degeneration of the anulus fibrosus and periarticular tissues. Abnormal mechanical stresses further stimulate inflammation and alter chondrocyte function. Altered joint biomechanics and chemical mediators act on the periarticular ligaments and joint capsule to induce metaplastic changes and propagate articular cartilage destruction. Portions of the anulus fibrosis and ventral longitudinal ligament become ossified and produce partial bridging of the involved joints. As enthesophytes increase in size, nerve roots may be compressed at the intervertebral foramen. Spinal cord compression occurs if proliferation extends dorsally into the vertebral canal. The cycle of altered joint biomechanics and inflammatory mediators perpetuates the production of fibrous and osseous adhesions until complete ankylosis and joint obliteration occur. Eventually, bone and tissue remodeling yields trabecular bone in a continuous medullary cavity between the two ankylosed bones at the site of the previous articulation.

The forming vertebral enthesophytes and the ankylosed vertebral bodies are susceptible to fracture because of a decreased ability to absorb or transfer normal locomotor forces through the ossified ligaments and fused vertebral articulations. The prevalence of vertebral fractures in bulls in artificial insemination centers is about 3%.[141] Clinical signs usually appear suddenly with varying severity, depending on the amount of tissue damage or neurologic injury. Neurologic signs may result from direct nerve root or spinal cord compression from the vertebral fractures or expanding enthesophytes.[141,142]

Bulls older than 8 years of age used in artificial insemination centers show a high predilection (>49%) for vertebral enthesophytes,[141,143,144] but bulls less than 5 years of age also have significant bone production.[145] Vertebral enthesophytes are not related to frequency of semen collection, intensity of pelvic thrust,[145] or a high calcium diet.[141]

CLINICAL SIGNS AND DIFFERENTIAL DIAGNOSIS. Vertebral enthesophytes are initially insidious and subclinical unless inflammation, impingement, or fracture of spondylophytes occurs to produce pain. Horses present with reduced performance, vague lameness, or altered gait. Affected bulls usually have a good appetite and are afebrile. Mild signs include difficulty in rising, general body stiffness, reluctance to move, and difficulty in mounting. Vertebral fractures or acute inflammation of the enthesophytes result in local pain and paraspinal muscle guarding. Once clinical signs are present they usually slowly progress to severe

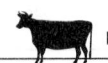

lameness and neurologic deficits.[158] Bilateral neurologic deficits of the rear limb resulting from altered conscious proprioception include the following: hoof dragging, excessive hind limb flexion, and incoordination.[142,146]

The differential diagnoses for spinal pain or stiffness include paraspinal muscle strain, vertebral fracture, discospondylitis, impinged spinous processes, vertebral or sacroiliac subluxation or luxation, vertebral infarct, and aberrant parasitic migration. Additional differential diagnoses for cattle that have rear limb neurologic deficits include downer cow syndrome, encephalopathy, progressive degenerative myeloencephalopathy, lymphosarcoma, hereditary ataxia, and cerebellar hypoplasia.[142]

DIAGNOSIS. In bulls, diagnosis is based on lameness and inability to mount or breed. Signs of pain or stiffness are usually elicited on palpation of the paraspinal tissues and spinous processes of the involved region. Vertebral enthesophytes located on the vertebral bodies of the lower lumbar vertebrae are palpated rectally. A thorough neurologic examination is indicated if neurologic signs or vertebral fractures are suspected. Cerebrospinal fluid analysis is usually normal. Variably sized ventrolateral vertebral enthesophytes may be noted on plain film radiography or scintigraphy. Peak predilection sites in bulls occur in the mid-cervical (C3-C5), cranial thoracic (T2-T6), and the thoracolumbar (T11-L5) regions with the largest vertebral enthesophytes forming in older bulls and in the region of the thoracolumbar junction.[143,145] Several vertebral bodies are usually involved, especially in advanced stages. Enthesophytes have smooth contours that blend with the vertebral body cortex and bridge apparently normal end plates and intervertebral discs. In contrast, intervertebral disk disease is characterized by subchondral sclerosis and narrowing of the intervertebral disc. Radiographs may not be as sensitive as direct visualization of the vertebral enthesophytes at necropsy because of variable degrees of enthesophyte ossification, a ventrolateral location, and the inability to obtain quality radiographs of the thoracolumbar vertebrae in cattle and horses.

A study of 21 bulls showed a significant association between bovine lymphocyte antigen (BoLA)-A8 and hind limb neurologic deficits associated with vertebral enthesophytes.[146] The authors suggest that a chronic posterior spinal paresis syndrome is analogous to inflammatory joint disease of ankylosing spondylitis in humans. Many clinical, radiographic, and pathologic criteria, however, are not met and several different seropositive arthropathies affect humans in addition to ankylosing spondylitis.[134]

TREATMENT AND PROGNOSIS. Treatment of symptomatic vertebral enthesophytes involves palliative care for pain and stiffness. Systemic antiinflammatory medication (NSAIDs, corticosteroids, DMSO), cryotherapy (ice packs), and confinement are recommended until inflammation subsides, or until ankylosis forms a stable, nonpainful joint. Altered spinal function and multiple vertebral involvement predispose the animal to the recurrence of clinical signs. If vertebral fractures or neurologic signs are present, supportive care will probably be ineffective and the prognosis is poor.

REFERENCES

134. Rowe LJ, Yochum TR: Arthritic disorders. In Yochum TR, Rowe LJ, editors: *Essentials of skeletal radiology*, Baltimore, 1987, Williams & Wilkins, pp 539-698.
135. Widmer WR, Blevins WE: Radiographic evaluation of degenerative joint disease in horses: interpretive principles, *Compend Cont Educ Pract Vet* 16:907-918, 1994.
136. Morgan JP: Spondylosis deformans in the dog: a morphologic study with some clinical and experimental observations, *Acta Orthop Scand* 96 (suppl):1-88, 1967.
137. Morgan JP: Spondylosis versus spondylitis, *Scientif Proc Semin Synopses 37th Ann Meet*, Am Anim Hosp Assoc 37:402-403, 1970.
138. Morgan JP, Stavenborn M: Disseminated idiopathic skeletal hyperostosis (DISH) in a dog, *Vet Radiol* 32:65-70, 1991.
139. Weisbrode SE, Monke DR, Dodaro ST, et al: Osteochondrosis, degenerative joint disease, and vertebral osteophytosis in middle-aged bulls, *J Am Vet Med Assoc* 181:700-705, 1982.
140. Clyne MJ: Pathogenesis of degenerative joint disease, *Equine Vet J* 19:15-18, 1987.
141. McEntee K, Hall CE, Dunn HO: The relationship of calcium intake to the development of vertebral osteophytosis and ultimobrachial tumors in bulls. Proceedings of the Eighth Technical Conference on AI and Reproduction, NAAB 45-47, NAAB, Columbia, Missouri, 1980.
142. Monke DR, Parker WG, Hillman R: Progressive posterior paralysis. Proceedings of the Ninth Technical Conference on AI and Reproduction, NAAB 89-93, NAAB, Columbia, Missouri, 1982.
143. Thompson RG: Vertebral body osteophytes in bulls, *Pathol Vet* 6 (suppl):1-47, 1969.
144. Bane A, Hansen HT: Spinal changes in the bull and their significance in serving ability, *Cornell Vet* 52:362-384, 1962.
145. Almquist JO, Thompson RG: Relation of sexual behavior and ejaculatory frequency to severity of vertebral body osteophytes in dairy and beef bulls, *J Am Vet Med Assoc* 163:163-168, 1973.
146. Park CA, Hines HC, Monke DR, et al: Association between the bovine major histocompatibility complex and chronic posterior spinal paresis—a form of ankylosing spondylitis—in Holstein bulls, *Anim Genet* 24:53-58, 1993.

LAMINITIS (Founder)

ROBERT L. LINFORD

DEFINITION. Laminitis, literally, "inflammation of the laminae," is a disease that causes degeneration, necrosis, and inflammation of the dermal and epidermal laminae in the hoof wall of horses and ruminants.

ETIOPATHOGENESIS. Because the epidermal laminae suspend the distal phalanx and therefore the body weight of a horse, laminar degeneration destroys the suspension mechanism and permits weight-bearing forces to push the distal phalanx ventrally. Failure of the laminar suspending mechanism causes a painful and potentially crippling lameness. Laminitis is commonly a sequela of digestive disturbances and other disorders that cause endotoxemia and elaboration of inflammatory mediators. Unless preventive measures are taken, laminitis often occurs after colonic torsion, enteritis, grain overload, pleuropneumonia, and septic metritis (i.e., postparturient retention of the placenta).[147-151] In horses it is sometimes seen following changes in feed, excess intake of cold water after hard exercise, grazing on lush spring grasses containing highly available carbohydrates, or persistent feeding of a high-concentrate ration.[147,148] Laminitis also may be precipitated in horses by administration of high levels of corticosteroids,[152] which decrease protein synthesis and potentiate digital vasconstriction and microthrombosis.[153] Excessive weight bearing in the support limb during severe lameness of the contralateral limb can produce laminitis, as can hard work on hard ground or extreme exhaustion and dehydration.[147,150,151] A water-soluble toxin in black walnut shavings also has been shown to induce laminitis in horses.[154] In cattle it is most commonly seen right after calving in fat heifers that have been fed excess concentrates and kept on concrete surfaces.[155]

PATHOPHYSIOLOGY. The pathophysiology of laminitis has not been totally elucidated; however, laminitis is often considered a local manifestation of a variety of disorders that cause a generalized metabolic disturbance. Several factors may produce laminar degeneration. The integrity of the laminar suspending mechanism depends on maintenance of proteins in the cytoskeletal networks and intercellular junctions of the epidermal laminar cells. This process is energy-dependent and disorders that decrease laminar perfusion or decrease protein synthesis have the potential to initiate laminar degeneration. In addition, laminar degeneration may be initiated by disorders that cause the elaboration of factors that are cytotoxic to the epidermal laminae, or by disorders that increase the tension on the laminae. Because the laminae and their sustaining vasculature are confined within the rigid hoof wall, factors that cause tissue swelling, such as inflammation and edema, can theoretically increase the interstitial tissue pressure beyond critical capillary closing pressure, producing a compartment syndrome and functional ischemia of the corium. Opening of arteriovenous shunts within the corium occurs during carbohydrate-overload laminitis, but such shunting has not conclusively been shown to be the major factor producing laminar degeneration.

Laminitis is often a sequela of diseases producing gram-negative sepsis and endotoxemia, but experimental administration of endotoxin has failed to produce laminitis. Overingestion of grain or of other feeds containing large amounts of highly available carbohydrates, however, is thought to produce endotoxemia and is the most common cause of acute laminitis. Carbohydrate overload results in bacterial overgrowth in the colon, lactic acidosis, decreased colonic pH, colonic mucosal slough, and death of colonic bacteria with concomitant liberation of endotoxin. Degeneration of the colonic mucosa is thought to allow endotoxin to gain access to the portal circulation. The mechanistic link between endotoxemia and laminar degeneration is not totally understood; however, hyperimmune serum to gram-negative core antigens has a strong protective effect on horses at high risk of developing laminitis as a result of intestinal crises or carbohydrate overload.[156]

Sequential biopsies of the epidermal laminae and corium during the development of grain overload laminitis indicated that initial laminar degeneration was most compatible with ischemic or cytotoxic injury and that inflammation, edema, and microthrombosis did not precede laminar degeneration but occurred later and were likely to accelerate the degeneration.[157]

Because perfusion of the most dorsal laminae depends on vessels that course through vascular canals in the distal phalanx, distal migration of the distal phalanx because of laminar degeneration may compromise laminar perfusion and result in a cycle that intensifies the laminar lesion. It is also theorized that the pain associated with laminar degeneration may cause release of catecholamines that potentiate peripheral vasoconstriction and further diminish laminar perfusion.

CLINICAL SIGNS. The signs of acute laminitis are lameness, depression, anorexia, and reluctance to move. Early in the disease affected animals often paddle or shift weight from one foot to the other. Increased pulsations can be palpated and sometimes visualized in the digital arteries. Hoof tester examinations reveal sensitivity over the sole at the toe, and tapping on the hoof wall at the toe may elicit pain. Severely affected animals may be unwilling to pick up a forefoot or hindfoot because of a reluctance to bear full weight on the contralateral foot (Obel grade III lameness[158]). The forefeet are usually affected more often and more severely than the hind feet in horses, and the most dorsal laminae are more severely involved than laminae in the heel regions. Therefore horses with laminitis commonly draw the hind limbs under the body and place the forelimbs forward to shift weight to the hindquarters and load the heels more than the toes. In ruminants the hind limbs are most commonly involved, and affected animals characteristically become recumbent. In severe cases, when laminar degeneration circumferentially involves the foot, a noticeable depression can be palpated along the coronary band. In such cases exudation is sometimes noted in the coronary region, and the skin may separate from the hoof wall. These signs indicate that the distal phalanx has shifted distally with respect to the hoof wall (i.e.,

severe rotation or sinking of the distal phalanx) and suggest a grave prognosis. With dislocation of the distal phalanx, the sole loses its normal cupped appearance and is flat or bulges between the toe and apex of the frog. Pulse and respiration rates are usually increased, and other clinical signs reflect underlying disease processes.

Signs of chronic laminitis are lameness and abnormal conformation of the foot. The sole is flat or dropped, the white line is widened, and the hoof wall shows signs of uneven growth. Irregular rings of horn, closely spaced at the toe and more widely spaced near the heels, encircle the hoof wall. In ruminants the sole softens and assumes a light yellow discoloration. Hemorrhages can often be identified in the abaxial white line region, and fissures that are parallel to the coronary band may be seen in the hoof wall. The signs of subsolar abscessation sometimes mimic those of laminitis; however, abscesses most commonly involve only one foot and rarely cause anorexia, depression, or elevation of the pulse and respiratory rates.

CLINICAL PATHOLOGY AND RADIOLOGY. Clinical pathologic findings during the development of acute laminitis most commonly represent alterations associated with underlying disease processes, such as enteritis or metritis, and are not pathognomonic for laminitis. During the onset of alimentary laminitis, packed cell volume, total plasma protein, heart rate, respiratory rate, rectal temperature, and blood glucose level are commonly elevated. Arterial blood pressure is usually elevated in horses but depressed in ruminants.[159] Neutrophilia and eosinopenia also are often seen. These changes are thought to reflect compartmental fluid shifts and a stress response consistent with release of adrenal glucocorticoids and catecholamines. Horses with chronic severe laminitis, in which euthanasia was deemed necessary, had total white blood cell (WBC) counts that were significantly elevated (total WBC 15,000 to 18,000/μl) over control horses and horses that recovered from less severe bouts of laminitis.[160] The persistent neutrophilia was presumably a response to infection and was thought to signify an unfavorable prognosis.

Radiographic examinations should be performed for the affected digits of horses suspected to be developing laminitis. The initial examinations should include lateromedial and 65-degree dorsoproximal-palmarodistal projections. These views should be taken to assess the appearance of the distal phalanx, the soft tissues of the hoof wall and corium, and their relationship. Lateromedial examinations are periodically repeated to check the progression of the disease. Radiographic signs of laminitis include ventral displacement of the extensor process with respect to the coronary groove of the hoof wall, increased distance between the dorsal cortex of the distal phalanx and the surface of the hoof wall, and ventral rotation of the tip of the distal phalanx. Linear radiolucencies are noted interior to the hoof wall in cases where the corium has separated from the epidermal laminae. Increasing degrees of rotation of the distal phalanx and increases in the distance between the dorsal surface of the distal phalanx and the hoof wall indicate progression of the disease (Fig. 36-22).

Because variations in technique affect subsequent radiographic distance and angle measurements, it is essential to standardize the radiographic procedure to detect small changes between examinations. For the lateromedial radiograph, the foot is cleaned and placed on a wooden block approximately 3 inches thick. A radiopaque marker can be embedded in the dorsal surface of the block and along the dorsal surface of the hoof wall to aid in determining the amount of rotation of the distal phalanx. If the same marker or a marker of known length is placed along the hoof wall for each examination, it can be used to calculate the amount

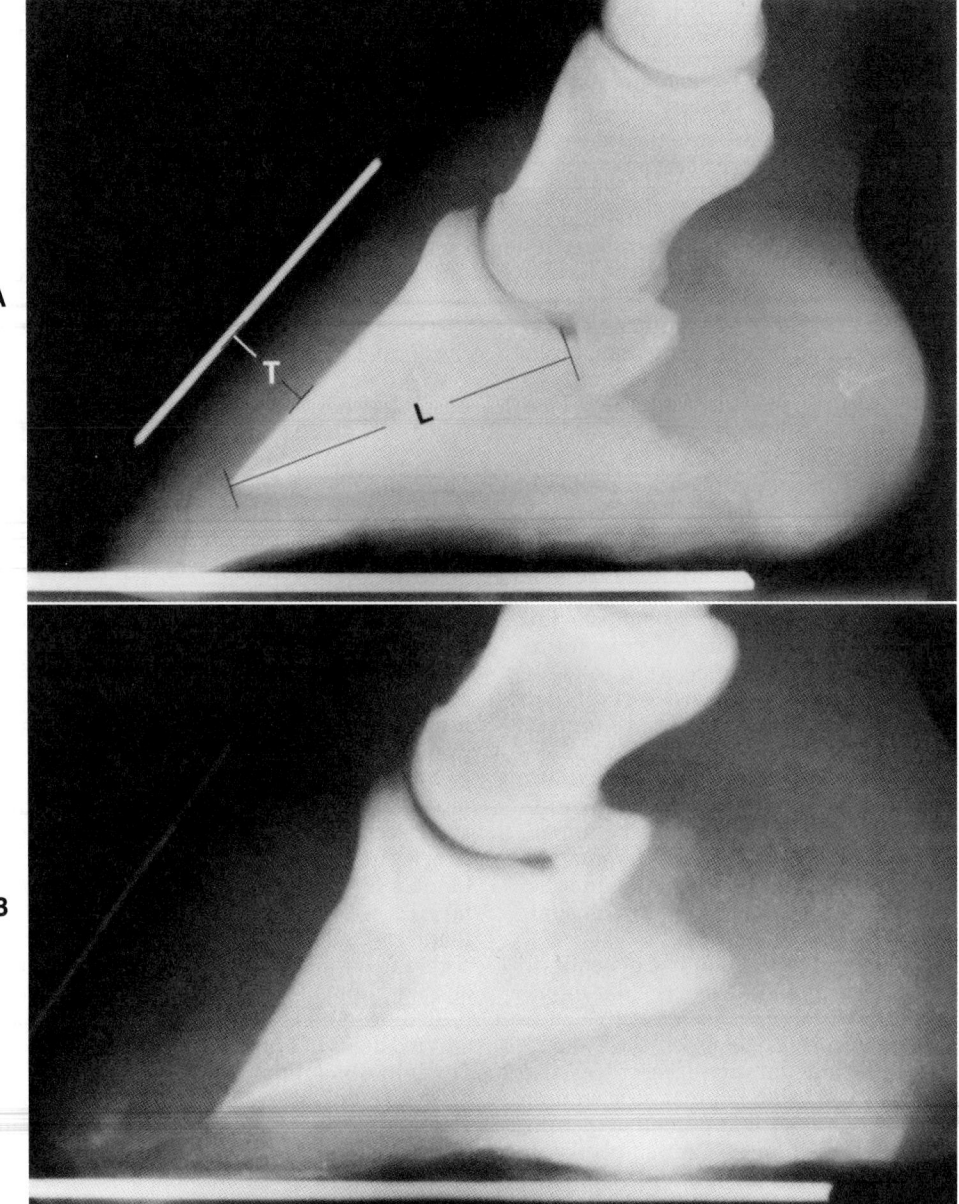

FIG. 36-22 ▮▮ **A,** Lateromedial radiograph of a normal digit. Two radiopaque markers can be seen. One has been placed on the block below the foot to mark the bearing surface of the wall, and the other marker identifies the location of the dorsal surface of the hoof wall. Notice that the dorsal surface of the hoof wall and the dorsal cortex of the distal phalanx are parallel and that the distance between them, the soft tissue thickness *(T),* is approximately 25% of the distance from the tip of the distal phalanx to the articulation of the distal phalanx and the navicular bone, that is, the length of the distal phalanx *(L).* **B,** Lateromedial radiograph of a digit from a horse with severe laminitis. The distal phalanx has dropped ventrally without rotating. This phenomenon is seen in some horses with laminitis. The most consistent radiographic manifestation in such cases is an increased distance between the dorsal cortex of the distal phalanx and the dorsal surface of the hoof wall. The soft tissue thickness as measured between the dorsal cortex and the dorsal surface of the hoof wall in this case is 45% the length of the distal phalanx. The soft tissue thickness is normally less than 28% of the distal phalanx length for Thoroughbred racehorses.   *Continued*

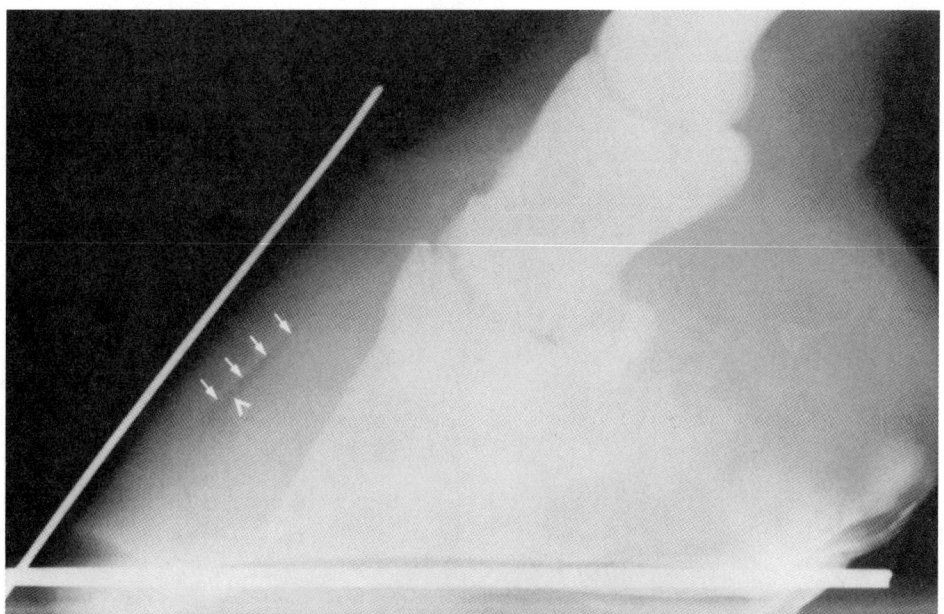

C

FIG. 36-22, cont'd ■ C, Lateromedial radiograph of a digit from a horse with severe laminitis. Note the linear radiolucency dorsal to the distal phalanx *(arrowhead)*. The presence of this lucency indicates that there has been a separation between the corium and primary epidermal laminae, and the lucency marks the inner aspect of the hoof wall *(arrows)*. The dorsal cortex of the distal phalanx is rotated approximately 14 degrees with respect to the inner surface of the hoof wall. Note that the dorsal and inner surfaces of the hoof wall are not parallel. This is the result of rasping along the distal portion of the dorsal surface of the hoof wall. The soft tissue thickness in this case is markedly increased to nearly 42% of the distal phalanx length.

of radiographic magnification to permit an accurate comparison of measurements among radiographs with different magnification factors. A tack, screw, or groove can be placed in the proximal dorsal hoof wall as a reference for measuring vertical displacement of the distal phalanx in repeated radiographs.

The radiographic beam should be perpendicular to a sagittal plane through the digit and should be centered midway between the toe and heels, 2 to 3 cm above the bearing surface of the wall. The radiographic cassette should be parallel to the sagittal plane through the digit and should be placed as close to the foot as possible. Using consistent focus-object and object-film distances or correcting for radiographic magnification and performing the examination in this standardized manner permit straight lateral radiographs to be produced and allow accurate quantification of radiographic parameters so that subtle changes may be identified.

EPIDEMIOLOGY. A survey of the risk factors associated with laminitis indicated that intact mares and stallions were at greater risk of developing laminitis than geldings. Ponies also accounted for a significantly greater number of laminitis cases than was expected on the basis of their proportion of the caseload. The peak incidence of new cases also corresponded with growth of lush spring grasses, suggesting that ingestion of large quantities of fresh grass is also a significant risk factor for pastured horses.[161]

Other risk factors include diseases that cause overweight bearing or trauma in the digit, and diseases that produce endotoxemia. Persistent feeding of a high concentrate ration, stabling on concrete surfaces, long van trips, and exposure to, or ingestion of, black walnut wood products are also thought to be associated with an increased risk of laminitis. In addition, horses that have previously had laminitis are at greater risk of developing it again than are other horses.

NECROPSY FINDINGS. Peracute cases may have total degeneration of the secondary epidermal laminae, which causes a separation between the primary epidermal laminae of the hoof wall and the collagen fibers of the corium. Abscessation may occur in the necrotic laminae or subsolar tissues. The distal phalanx may sink or be rotated ventrally with respect to the hoof capsule, and the tip may penetrate the sole (Fig. 36-23). Severe cases are accompanied by fractures of the solar margin, osteomyelitis, or severe resorption of the distal phalanx. The necropsy findings generally demonstrate a variable degree of elongation of the epidermal laminae, which depends on the severity and duration of the problem (Fig. 36-24).

TREATMENT. Treatment of animals developing acute laminitis should be considered an emergency. Laminar degeneration is under way by the time clinical signs of lameness appear, and even a few hours of delay in treatment can mean the difference between success and failure. Therapy should be initiated before the development of clinical signs in circumstances in which the untreated animal is at high risk of developing laminitis (e.g., animals that have recently ingested a large quantity of grain, mares with retention of the placenta, and horses with strangulating colon torsions).

General principles of therapy are aimed at eliminating the cause, promoting digital circulation, reducing tension on the laminae, and administering nonsteroidal antiinflammatory agents to minimize digital inflammation and necrosis and to relieve pain.

ELIMINATION OF CAUSE. A laxative or purgative should be administered to animals that have ingested a large quantity of grain. In such cases 3 to 4 L of mineral oil are usually given through a nasogastric tube. Intravenous administration of balanced electrolyte solution is indicated for horses with laminitis resulting from exhaustion, dehydration, and hypovolemia. Retained placentas should be treated appropriately

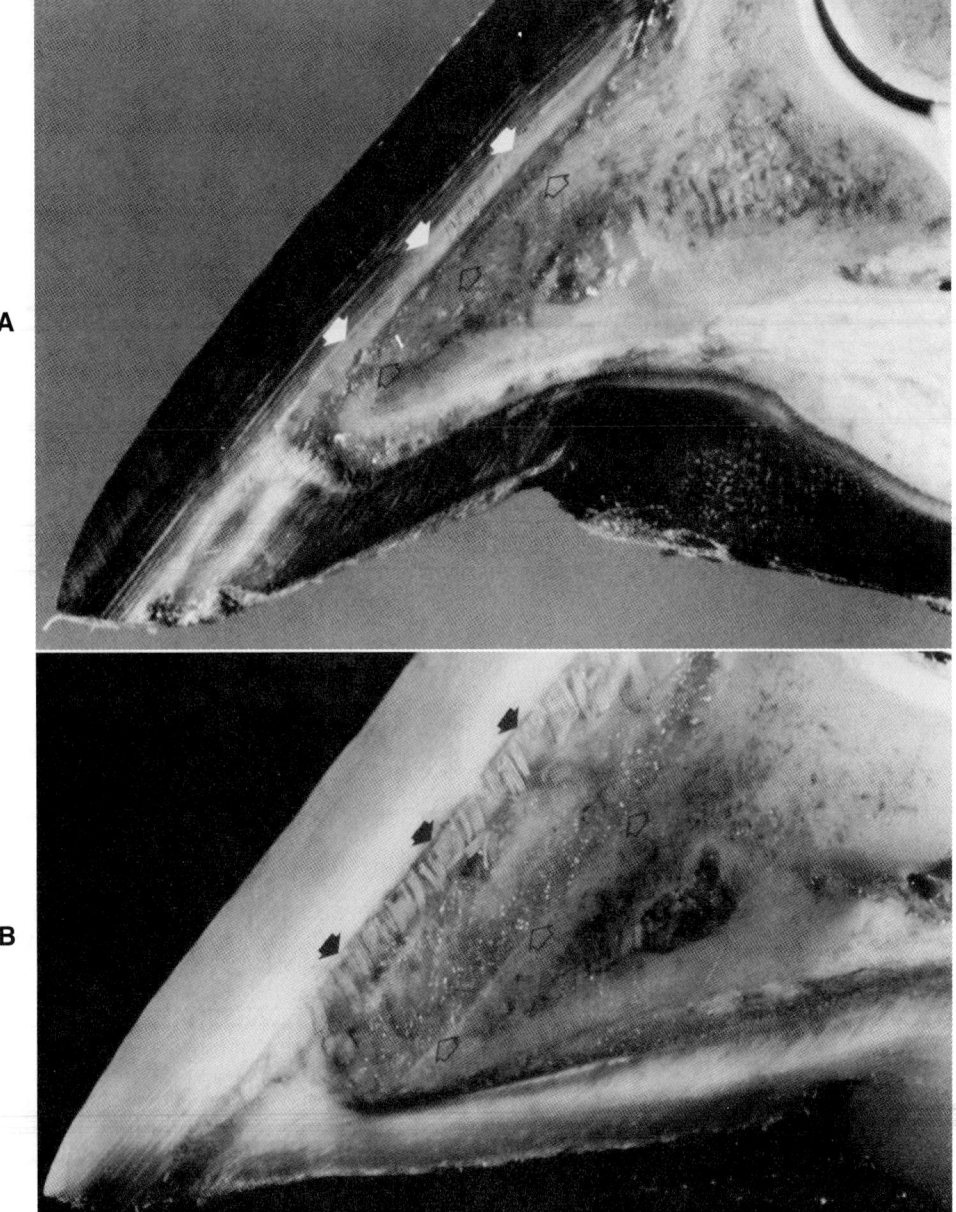

FIG. 36-23 ▓ **A,** Midsagittal section from the foot of a horse with a normal digit. Note the distance between the dorsal surface of the dorsal cortex of the distal phalanx *(open arrows)* and the inner surface of the hoof wall *(arrows).* The dorsal surface of the hoof wall and dorsal cortex of the distal phalanx are parallel. Compare with Fig. 36-22, *A.* **B,** Midsagittal section from the foot of a horse with severe laminitis, a "sinker." Note the increased distance between the dorsal surface of the dorsal cortex of the distal phalanx *(open arrows)* and the inner surface of the hoof wall *(arrows).* Also note that the distal phalanx has not rotated with respect to the hoof wall. Compare with Fig. 36-22, *B.*

Continued

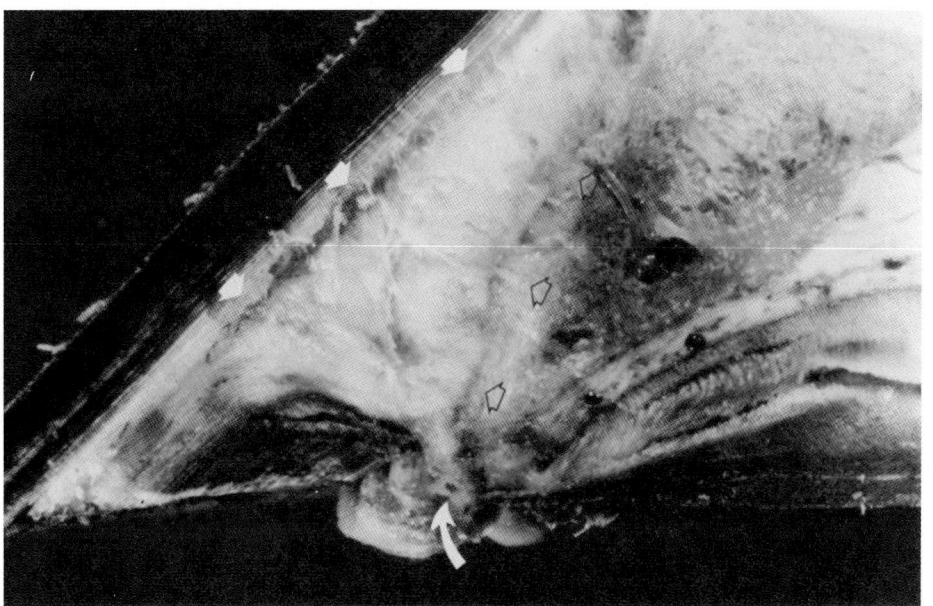

FIG. 36-23, cont'd ▓ C, Midsagittal section from the foot of a horse with severe laminitis. There is approximately an 18-degree rotation of the distal phalanx, and its tip has penetrated the sole *(curved arrow)*. Note the increased distance between the dorsal surface of the dorsal cortex of the distal phalanx *(open arrows)* and the inner surface of the hoof wall *(arrows)*. Compare with Fig. 36-22, *C.*

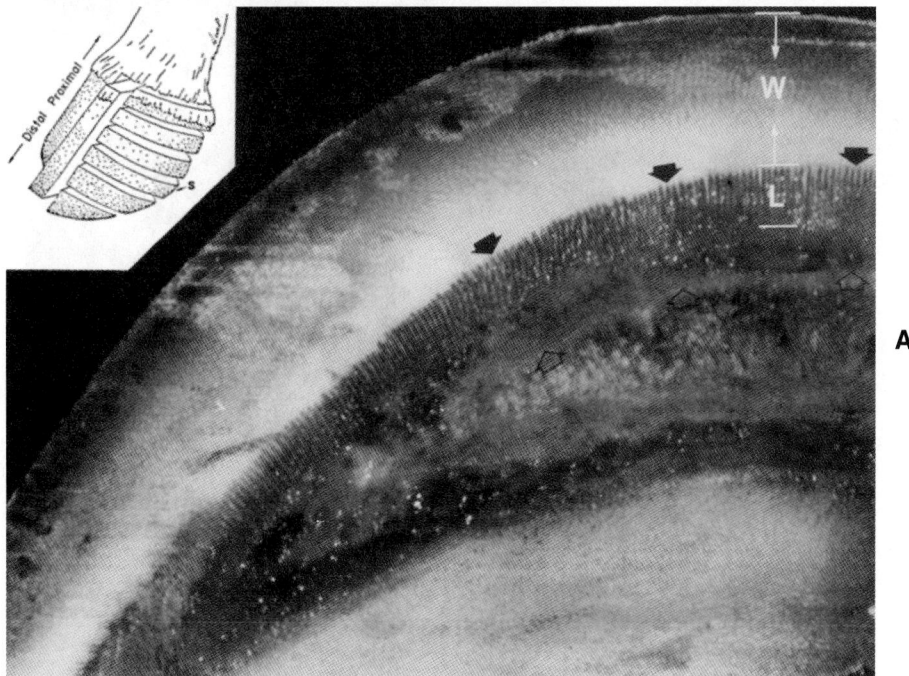

FIG. 36-24 ▓ A, Section of a healthy foot. The section was cut parallel to the coronary band, midway between the coronary band and the bearing surface of the hoof wall *(inset, S)*. The length of the epidermal laminae (L) is approximately 33% of the thickness of the hoof wall *(W)* in normal horses. The distance between the dorsal cortex of the distal phalanx *(open arrows)* and the inner surface of the hoof wall *(arrows)* is normally less than 75% of the thickness of the hoof wall. *Continued*

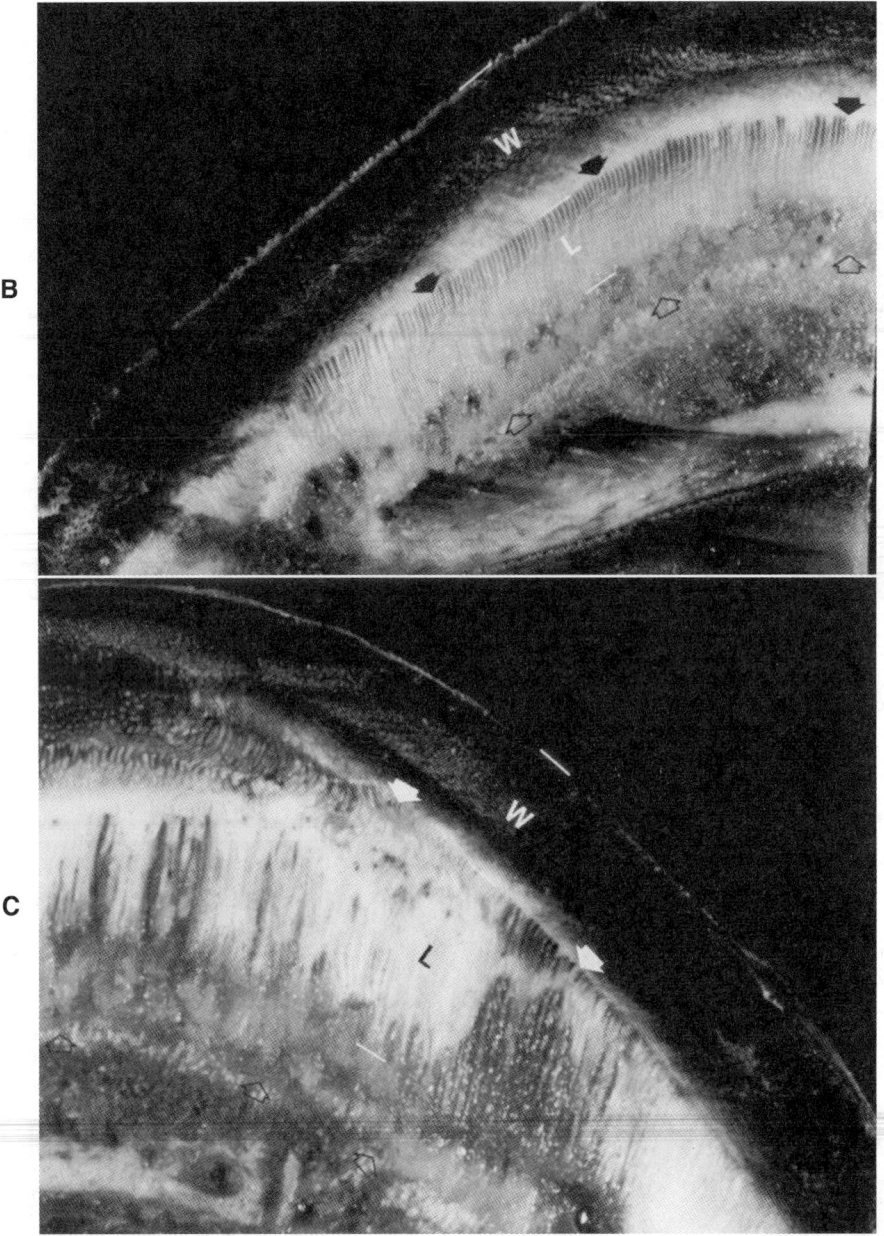

FIG. 36-24, cont'd ▌ **B,** Foot section, cut in a manner similar to that of *A,* from a foot of a horse with moderate laminitis. Note the increased length of the epidermal laminae *(L).* The increase in epidermal laminar length has allowed the distance between the dorsal cortex of the distal phalanx *(open arrows)* and the inner surface of the hoof wall *(arrows)* to become nearly as large as the thickness of the hoof wall *(W).* **C,** Foot section, cut in a manner similar to that of A, from a foot of a horse with severe laminitis. Note the marked increase in length of the epidermal lamina *(L).* The distance between the dorsal cortex of the distal phalanx *(open arrows)* and the inner surface of the hoof wall *(arrows)* is abnormally increased to nearly three times the thickness of the hoof wall *(W).*

if the placenta has not been expelled within 3 hours after parturition in mares. Antiendotoxin hyperimmune serum may be indicated for horses at risk of developing endotoxemia as a result of colon torsion, toxic diarrhea, toxic proximal enteritis, septic metritis, grain overload, or other disorders.

NONSTEROIDAL ANTIINFLAMMATORY AGENTS. Phenylbutazone is the recommended antiinflammatory agent, and at the onset of the syndrome it may be given once at a dose of up to 8.8 mg/kg intravenously. It is then usually given at a dose of 4.4 mg/kg (orally, twice a day) for several days. The dose should be tapered to 2.2 mg/kg (orally, twice a day) as soon as possible. Flunixin meglumine* is sometimes given concurrently for the first 3 to 4 days in severe cases (1.1 mg/kg intravenously, once a day). Dimethylsulfoxide (DMSO) also may be given daily (0.2 to 1 g/kg) for 2 to 3 days. To administer it intravenously in a 450-kg horse, 250 ml of the 90% solution is mixed in 3 L of balanced electrolyte solution of 5% dextrose and given slowly. DMSO should be diluted to less than 20% concentration to avoid hemolysis when it is given intravenously. The use of aspirin

*Banamine, Schering Plough Animal Health, Union, NJ 07083.

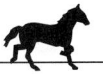

(10 mg/kg, orally, once a day) is sometimes advocated for its antiinflammatory and antiplatelet activities. Corticosteroids and adrenocorticotropic hormone (ACTH) are contraindicated because they decrease protein synthesis, and they may potentiate peripheral vasoconstriction and microthrombosis.

REDUCTION OF TENSION ON THE LAMINAE. The force related to suspending the weight of the horse by the attachment between the hoof wall and the distal phalanx is likely to be a major factor producing laminar deformity in horses with laminitis. Reduction of laminar tension may be achieved by focusing the forces of weight bearing more on the frog and sole and reducing the amount of weight taken by the hoof wall. This can be accomplished by using frog support bandages or shoes, sole casts, or sand stalls. Recently, elevation of the heel with an 18-degree wedge has been advocated to reduce the pull of the deep flexor tendon and decrease the tension on the laminae.[162] This elevation can be achieved with a plastic-cuff shoe* that is taped, glued, or screwed to the hoof wall and used with a frog support pad† and an 18-degree heel wedge.

For horses with severe acute laminitis, do not lower the heel in the acute stage and avoid shoes that require the horse to bear full weight on one foot for a prolonged period while the shoe is being nailed on the other. Avoid using shoes that increase laminar tension by transferring more weight-bearing forces to the hoof wall. A plastic-cuff heel-wedge shoe can be taped temporarily to the hoof with minimal trauma and effort. If it is makes the horse more comfortable, the shoe can be glued in place. Frog support shoes continue to put pressure on the frog when the horse is recumbent and may predispose to subsolar necrosis. Frog support bandages or Lilly Pads† provide satisfactory support and avoid the complications associated with shoeing. The toe should be dubbed off to decrease the lever arm effect that a long toe has on prying the wall away from the distal phalanx during break over.

Affected horses should be encouraged to lie down to reduce laminar tension. This goal usually can be accomplished with sedation. The stall should be heavily bedded with straw and pine chip shavings to a depth of 30 to 60 cm for comfort and to reduce the risk of pressure sores.

PROMOTION OF DIGITAL CIRCULATION. Walking with frog supports in soft ground for 5 to 10 minutes every 3 to 4 hours is beneficial for nonlame horses during the developmental stages of laminitis. It may increase the amount of laminar deformity when used in horses with lameness, or in nonlame horses that have a depression at the coronary band, indicating that laminar degeneration has already begun. Perineural anesthesia of the palmar digital nerves, at the level of the apex of the proximal sesamoid bones, may decrease pain-related peripheral vasoconstriction and thereby promote digital circulation. A 3- to 4-ml dose of 0.75% bupivacaine hydrochloride (Marcaine HCl)‡ may be used at each site at approximately 12-hour intervals for 1 to 2 days. Severely lame horses should not undergo nerve blocking because it may prompt them to put more stress on tenuous laminar attachments. α-Adrenergic blocking drugs such as acetylpromazine, phenoxybenzamine, and prazosin also have been advocated to decrease peripheral vasoconstriction and promote digital circulation. Acetylpromazine (0.02 to 0.04 mg/kg intramuscularly, four times a day) may be given for its theoretic effect on digital circulation and for the sedative effect that encourages the horse to lie down and reduce laminar tension. Before lameness develops, heparin may be administered (40 to 100 U/kg, SC, two to three times a day) to provide laminitis prophylaxis by atten-

uating potential microthrombosis. This therapy significantly reduced the number of horses developing laminitis after proximal enteritis when given before the onset of laminitis.[163]

OTHER TREATMENTS. Antibiotics may be indicated in severe cases to reduce the risk of secondary sepsis in the foot. Methionine (20 to 60 mg/kg, PO sid) and biotin 0.03 to 0.2 mg/kg PO sid) have been used for their effect on keratinization.

PROGNOSIS. Owners should be advised that it is often hard to arrive at an accurate prognosis for up to 6 weeks after the original insult. Redden[164] has suggested the following general guidelines regarding prognosis:

Horses that become sound within 24 to 48 hours of the onset of treatment remain sound, demonstrate no radiographic changes, and have no palpable increased pulsation of the digital arteries after they have been off all medication for 5 days have a good prognosis. They should be given 10 additional days of stall rest, after which they can be vanned or put back to regular work.

Horses that develop 2 to 5 degrees of rotation within the first 30 days of onset but then become sound, remain sound, and show no further radiographic progression after an additional 45 days without treatment have a good prognosis. They may resume light exercise, but they should not be shipped long distances for several months, and they should be considered to have an increased risk of recurrence.

Horses that develop 5 to 10 degrees of rotation in the first 6 weeks but then have no further radiographic progression should receive an additional 90 days of stall rest. If they remain sound without medication, they may resume light exercise with caution after they have been turned to pasture for an additional 12 months. Such horses will not return to their previous level of performance and are not suited for racing or endurance, but may function as pleasure horses.

Horses that develop 10 to 15 degrees of rotation within the first 4 to 6 weeks have a poor prognosis. The tip of the distal phalanx often penetrates the sole. Necrosis of the dermal and epidermal laminae and subsolar tissues usually occurs. Drainage commonly is noted at the coronary band or heels and is an indication of subcapsular abscessation. Gas or fluid pockets may develop between the hoof wall and the dorsal surface of the distal phalanx. Such cases require drainage and debridement of the necrotic tissue, which may be accomplished through an anterior hoof wall resection. If the keratinized sole is underrun, it is thinned enough to be elevated off the underrun areas so that necrotic debris can be curetted and the area flushed with antiseptic solution. Daily bandage changes and antiseptic flushing or soaking are required. If it is possible to access all necrotic subsolar tissue without removing the keratinized sole, a thin layer of keratinized tissue should be left in place. Horses with a thin layer of keratinized sole are usually more comfortable than those in which the sole has been completely removed. Leaving a thin layer of keratinized tissue reduces the potential for exuberant granulation and seems to increase the rate of reepithelialization across granulating wounds in the sole.

Horses with this degree of laminitis require several months of stall rest and will be chronically crippled, at best. They will require several thousand dollars of care and bandaging just to stabilize the foot. The foot usually remains chronically painful, and, if so, euthanasia is justified on humane grounds. Tenotomy of the deep digital flexor tendon is beneficial in these cases. It seems to permit such severely affected horses to become more comfortable, enhances reepithelialization of defects in the sole, and permits the anterior hoof wall to grow better.

Horses that have circumferential laminar necrosis where the distal phalanx drops 2 cm or rotates 15 to 20 degrees with respect to the hoof capsule within the first 4 to 6 weeks of onset carry a grave prognosis.

---

*Fort Dodge Animal Health, Inc, Fort Dodge, IA 50501.
†Lilly Pad, Therapeutic Equine Products, Inc, Indianapolis, IN.
‡Marcaine HCl, Abbott Labs, N. Chicago, IL 60064.

PREVENTION AND CONTROL. Prevention should be aimed at controlling as many risk factors as possible. Unrestricted grazing on lush spring grasses should be avoided, especially in areas where horses have developed laminitis in preceding years and especially for horses with a history of laminitis. Horses should not be allowed unrestricted access to grain or concentrates, nor should they be fed a ration that primarily consists of concentrates. Factors that cause gastrointestinal upsets should be avoided; for example, changes in the ration should be made slowly, and overheated horses should not be allowed to engorge on cold water. Retained placenta in the mare should be treated within 3 hours after parturition.

Preventive measures should be instituted before the development of clinical signs for horses that are at high risk of developing laminitis from conditions such as metritis, torsion of the colon, pleuropneumonia, or severe diarrhea. Preventive therapy should include frequent walking, frog support bandages or stabling on soft surfaces, and administration of nonsteroidal antiinflammatory agents and antiendotoxin hyperimmune serum.

REFERENCES

147. Adams OR: *Lameness in horses*, ed 3, Philadelphia, 1974, Lea & Febiger, pp 247-260.
148. Garner HE: Update on equine laminitis, *Vet Clin North Am (Large Anim Pract)* 2:25-32, 1980.
149. Hood DM: Current concepts of the physiopathology of laminitis, *Proceedings of the Twenty-fifth Annual Convention of the American Association of Equine Practitioners*, 1979, pp 13-20.
150. Colles CM, Jeffcott LB: Laminitis in the horse, *Vet Rec* 100:262-264, 1977.
151. Farrow CS, Payne RM: Equine laminitis: clinicoradiologic considerations, *California Vet* 35:25-30, 1981.
152. Muylle E, Oyaert W: Lung function tests in obstructive pulmonary disease in horses, *Equine Vet J* 5:37-44, 1973.
153. Eyre P, Elmes PJ, Strickland S: Corticosteroid-potentiated vascular responses of the equine digit: a possible pharmacologic basis for laminitis, *Am J Vet Res* 40:135-138, 1979.
154. Minnick PD, Brown CM, Braselton WE, et al: The induction of equine laminitis with an aqueous extract of the heartwood of black walnut (juglans nigra), *Vet Human Toxicol* 29:230-233, 1987.
155. Greenough PR, MacCallum FJ, Weaver AD: *Lameness in cattle*, ed 2, Bristol, England, 1981, Wright Scientechnica, pp. 219-227.
156. Garner HE, Sprouse RF, Green EM: Active and passive immunization for blockade of endotoxemia, *Proceedings of the Thirty-first Annual Convention of the American Association of Equine Practitioners*, 1985, pp 525-532.
157. Linford RL: A radiographic, morphometric, histological, and ultrastructural investigation of lamellar function, abnormality, and the associated radiographic changes in sound and footsore thoroughbreds, and horses with experimentally induced traumatic and alimentary laminitis. Doctoral dissertation, Davis, 1987, University of California, Davis.
158. Obel N: Studies on the histopathology of acute laminitis. Doctoral dissertation, Uppsala, Sweden, 1948, Almqvist & Wiksells Boktryckeri.
159. Nilsson SA: Laminitis in cattle in comparison with equine laminitis. In Espinasse J, editor: *Fourth international symposium on disorders of the ruminant digit*, Maisons-Alfort, 1982, Societe Francaise De Buiatrie.
160. Coffman JR, Hammond LS, Garner HE, et al: Haematology as an aid to prognosis of chronic laminitis, *Equine Vet J* 12:30-31, 1980.
161. Dorn CR, Garner HE, Coffman JR, et al: Castration and other factors affecting the risk of equine laminitis, *Cornell Vet* 65:57-64, 1975.
162. Redden RF: Eighteen-degree elevation of the heel as an aid to treating acute and chronic laminitis in the equine, *Proc Annu Meet Am Assoc Equine Pract* 38:375-379, 1992.
163. Cohen ND, Parson EM, Seahorn TL, et al: Prevalence and factors associated with development of laminitis in horses with duodenitis/proximal jejunitis: 33 cases (1985-1991), *J Am Vet Med Assoc* 204:250-254, 1994.
164. Redden RF: Laminitis, Second Annual Charles Heumphreus Memorial Lecture, Davis, Calif, 1988.

FLUOROSIS

JOHN MAAS

DEFINITION AND ETIOLOGY. Ingestion of excessive fluoride by cattle, sheep, and horses can result in toxicosis. Acute fluoride toxicosis is relatively rare and is the result of accidental massive ingestion of fluoride compounds such as sodium fluoride or sodium fluorosilicate. Signs of acute fluoride toxicosis include restlessness, stiffness, anorexia, agalactia, salivation, vomiting or regurgitation, urinary incontinence, diarrhea, clonic convulsions, hyperemia, weakness, severe depression, and cardiac failure. Necrosis of the gastrointestinal mucosa and high concentrations of fluoride in plasma and urine are present in acute fluoride toxicosis. Chronic fluoride toxicosis is most commonly referred to as *fluorosis*, a general term that includes osteofluorosis and dental fluorosis. The most common sources of excess fluorides in the diet are (1) water with a naturally high fluoride content, (2) forages contaminated with fluorides from nearby (upwind) industrial plants (e.g., phosphate-processing plants, aluminum plants, smelters), (3) mineral (nondefluorinated rock phosphorus) and feed supplements with excessive fluoride content, (4) forages contaminated by soil or water (particularly sprinkler irrigation water) with a high fluoride content, or (5) volcanic activity, which can deposit fluoride-containing ash on soil, plants, or in water used for agriculture.

CLINICAL SIGNS, DIFFERENTIAL DIAGNOSIS, AND PATHOPHYSIOLOGY. Clinical signs of fluorosis are usually first recognized as either dental fluorosis or osteofluorosis. Developing teeth are very sensitive to the ingestion of excess fluorides. The deciduous teeth rarely show signs of dental fluorosis because a partial placental barrier to the accumulation of fluorides appears to be present in the fetus. During tooth development excess fluorides cause ameloblasts to prematurely reduce in size and the enamel epithelium to form an irregular matrix. This matrix does not calcify normally, producing defects in the mature teeth. Cattle are susceptible to dental fluorosis during enamel matrix formation occurring from approximately 6 months to 3 years of age. Excess fluoride intake after 3 years of age does not result in the typical fluoride-induced dental lesions. Changes in incisor teeth are observed most commonly and include chalkiness, mottling (striations or patches in the enamel), hypoplasia (defective enamel), and hypocalcification. Clinical lesions can be graded from normal to excessive.[165] Factors that influence dental fluorosis include the amount of fluoride ingested, the animal's age, the duration and consistency (intermittent vs. continuous) of exposure to fluoride, and the source and chemical form of fluoride ingested. Although diagnostically useful, dental lesions should not be used as the sole criterion to determine the degree of fluorosis.

Fluoride accumulation in bone occurs over a prolonged time; osteofluorosis can eventually develop if excessive fluoride is ingested. In cattle the first palpable lesions occur on the medial surface of the proximal third of the metatarsal bones. Later, lesions can be palpated on the mandible, metacarpal bones, and ribs. Radiographically, osteofluorotic bones are thickened with a chalky, roughened, and irregular periosteal surface.

The presence of osteoporosis, osteosclerosis, hyperostosis, osteophytosis, or osteomalacias depends on the amount of fluoride ingested and the duration of exposure to fluorides. The articular surfaces are not involved in osteofluorosis and can be used to differentiate osteofluorosis from osteomyelitis, osteoarthritis, and septic arthritis. The osseous lesions eventually cause intermittent lameness and stiffness, which may affect feed intake, body condition, milk production, and reproduction. Severe dental fluorosis causes reduced feed intake and efficiency, and affected animals are sometimes reluctant to drink cold water.

CLINICAL PATHOLOGY AND DIAGNOSIS. Diagnosis of fluorosis is difficult and complicated by many factors that affect fluoride intake and deposition. Fluorosis may be suspected by history, clinical signs, and physical examination. Radiographic findings of bone disease without evidence of joint involvement is highly suggestive of fluorosis in the live animal. The fluoride concentration in the urine of cattle may help to approximate recent fluoride exposure. The diagnostic value of urine fluoride analysis increases as the duration of

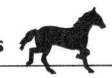

excess fluoride ingestion increases. Normal cattle have a urine fluoride concentration of about 2 to 6 ppm. Cattle exhibiting moderate fluorosis have urine fluoride concentrations of about 15 to 20 ppm. Cattle with urine fluoride concentrations of 40 ppm or greater or a urinary fluoride/creatinine ration of 0.025:1 or greater could be suspected of ingesting a diet with a fluoride concentration of 60 ppm or greater.[165,166] The concentration of fluoride in bone is quite helpful in the diagnosis of fluorosis (Table 36-3). Fluoride content in cancellous bone (e.g., rib, pelvis) is greater than in cortical bone. In addition, fluoride concentrations may vary in different areas of the same bone.

Fluoride concentration of bone is usually expressed as ppm (mg/kg) of dry, fat-free bone; however, some bone samples are ashed before fluoride determination. Therefore, it is critical to note precisely which bone was sampled, how it was prepared, and what part of the bone was analyzed. The metatarsus and metacarpus are commonly analyzed for fluoride content. For all practical purposes, fluoride concentration is equal in either of these bones from the same patient.[177] Using sawdust from longitudinal section of bovine metatarsus (either dividing the bone into lateral and medial halves or dorsal and palmar halves) yields virtually the same fluoride concentration as the whole bone.[167] The fluoride concentration of the fourteenth coccygeal vertebrae (ash basis) is approximately twice that of the metacarpus (dry, fat-free weight basis).[168] This is a practical tool for clinical diagnosis.

Analysis of dietary fluoride is a valuable adjunct to the diagnosis of fluorosis. The upper safe limit of fluoride in water for livestock is 2 mg/L (ppm).[169,170] This safe limit may not protect against fluorosis in all field situations because of the large number of variables involved in the pathogenesis of fluorosis. The long-term dietary tolerances for cattle are listed in Table 36-4. Under field conditions the clinician must consider all possible sources of fluoride ingestion in evaluating total intake. In addition, because fluoride intake may be intermittent, a low dietary intake at one time may not necessarily eliminate a diagnosis of fluorosis.

TREATMENT AND PROGNOSIS. A specific treatment is unknown for ruminants with severe fluorosis, and the prognosis is poor for cattle lame from extensive bony lesions. Animals removed from the offending diet or water may lose 50% of the fluoride from bone within 2 to 5 years[171]; however, severe dental damage is irreversible.

PREVENTION AND CONTROL. Prevention involves avoiding feeds, water, and supplements with excessive fluoride concentrations. Feeding aluminum sulfate at 0.5% of the total diet reduces bone fluoride storage by 30% to 40%. Additional phosphorus, however, must be supplied in the diet, or osteoporosis and possibly spontaneous fractures may occur. Aluminum chloride or calcium aluminate also can be fed to cattle to reduce fluoride absorption. Calcium carbonate added to soils high in fluorides aids in reducing fluoride in forages. Cereal grains do not accumulate fluorides and thus can be helpful in reducing overall fluoride consumption. In circumstances of high fluoride concentrations in water, use of flood irrigation rather than sprinkler irrigation decreases the fluoride content of crops such as alfalfa hay.

REFERENCES

165. Shupe JL, Miner ML, Greenwood DA, et al: The effect of fluorine on dairy cattle. II. Clinical and pathologic effects, *Am J Vet Res* 24:964-979, 1963.
166. Shupe JL, Harris LE, Greenwood DA, et al: The effect of fluorine on dairy cattle. V. Fluorine in the urine as an estimator of fluorine intake, *Am J Vet Res* 24:300-305, 1963.
167. Suttie JW, Kolstad DL: Sampling of bones for fluoride analysis, *Am J Vet Res* 35:1375-1376, 1974.
168. Suttie JW: Vertebral biopsies in the diagnosis of bovine fluoride toxicosis, *Am J Vet Res* 28:709-712, 1967.
169. National Research Council: *Nutrients and toxic substances in water for livestock and poultry*, Washington DC, 1974, National Academy of Science, p 63.
170. National Research Council: *Mineral tolerance of domestic animals*, Washington DC, 1980, National Academy of Science, pp 184-226.
171. Shupe JL, Olson AE, Sharma RP: Fluoride toxicity in domestic and wild animals, *Clin Toxicol* 5:195-213, 1972.

HYPERTROPHIC OSTEOPATHY

JAMES A. ORSINI

DEFINITION AND ETIOLOGY. Hypertrophic osteopathy (HO), also called hypertrophic pulmonary osteopathy (HPO), or Marie's disease refers to the formation of subperiosteal new bone on the distal diaphyses of the long bones or on the axial skeleton or facial bones, with nonedematous swelling of the extremities and occasional swelling and tenderness of joints. Although these changes are most often associated with pulmonary disease, it has become clear that other infectious and neoplastic processes may induce this group of lesions. It is considered an infrequently occurring disease in the horse and a rare disease in cattle. The term hypertrophic osteopathy is preferred to HPO because pulmonary disease is not a consistent finding, and to hypertrophic pulmonary osteoarthropathy (HPOA) because articular surface involvement has not been reported in domestic animals.

In horses HO has been associated with pulmonary abscesses,[172-174] chronic suppurative pneumonia,[175] pulmonary or intrathoracic neoplasms,[172,175-177] pituitary adenoma,[178] rib fracture with adhesions,[179] granular cell tumor (myoblastoma),[172] primary intraabdominal disorders,[180] and dysgerminoma and other ovarian neoplasms.[175,181,182] One case in-

TABLE 36-3

Fluoride Concentration (ppm–Dry, Fat-Free Basis) in Bones of Dairy Cattle Fed Various Levels of Sodium Fluoride

Fluoride in Feed (ppm, Dry Basis)	Fluoride in Bone (ppm—Dry, Fat-Free Basis)		
	2 years	4 years	6 years
0-15 (Normal conditions)	401-714	706-1138	653-1221
15-30 (No adverse effects)	714-1605	1138-2379	1221-2794
30-40 (Borderline fluorosis)	1605-2130	2379-3138	2794-3788
40-60 (Moderate fluorosis)	2130-3027	3138-4504	3788-5622
60-109 (Severe fluorosis)	3027-4206	4504-6620	5622-8676

TABLE 36-4

Long-Term Tolerances of Dietary Fluoride for Cattle

Animal	Dietary Fluoride (ppm—Dry Basis)
Dairy or beef heifers	30-40
Mature dairy cattle	40
Mature beef cattle	40-50
Fattening cattle	100

volving the limbs proximal to the carpus and tarsus in a 10-year-old bull was associated with pulmonary lymphosarcoma,[183] and another case involving the metacarpal and metatarsals (also in a 10-year-old bull) was associated with reticuloperitonitis and widespread abscessation.[184]

CLINICAL SIGNS AND DIFFERENTIAL DIAGNOSIS. In the early stages of disease the distal limbs are swollen, warm, and throbbing. Limbs are affected asymmetrically. The skin overlying the dorsal metacarpal and metatarsal regions is taut. There may be a decreased range of motion and pain on manipulation of the affected joints, with a stiff gait and a reluctance to move. If there is an associated pulmonary lesion, signs such as coughing, inspiratory difficulty, or decreased lung sounds may be present.

Radiographically generalized soft tissue swelling and periostitis are present. Irregular new bone growth is seen predominantly at the proximal and distal ends of the long bones, often involving the metacarpal and metatarsal bones (Fig. 36-25).

Differential diagnosis should include fluorosis and, for the primary underlying disease process, intrathoracic and intraabdominal masses (abscess, neoplasm). With the absence of dental changes, the gross appearance of bones, and low concentration of fluorine in blood and urine, fluorosis can be ruled out with relative ease. A complete physical examination, ultrasonography, and radiography assist in establishing the presence of a primary pulmonary or intraabdominal lesion.

PATHOPHYSIOLOGY. Humoral, hypoxic, and neural mechanisms all have been proposed to explain HO. Given the number of disorders associated with HO, a nonspecific response to neural or humoral stimuli is the most plausible hypothesis at this time. The primary lesion is associated with increased blood flow to the affected limbs, followed by proliferation of vascular connective tissue around the bone. New bone formation then occurs on the inner aspect of the periosteum, separating the periosteum from the cortical bone.

NECROPSY FINDINGS. Post mortem examination findings vary with the primary disease process. The long bones of the extremities have marked periosteal proliferation oriented perpendicular to the surface of the cortices, especially the cranial, medial, and lateral aspects. The forelimbs and hind limbs may be affected to different degrees.

TREATMENT AND PROGNOSIS. When HO is recognized early and the underlying primary disease process is treated appropriately, periosteal reactions disappear. Prognosis is affected by the primary disorder and by the severity of HO. The presence of an ovarian or pulmonary neoplasm should be considered a poor prognosis because of the advanced stage at which these are typically recognized. If a primary respiratory infection (e.g., abscess) is successfully treated medically or surgically while HO is not yet advanced, a favorable outcome may be possible.

REFERENCES

172. Turner S: Diseases of bones and related structures. In Stashak TS, editor: *Adams' lameness in horses,* Philadelphia, 1987, Lea & Febiger, pp 316-318.
173. Messer NT, Powers BE: Hypertrophic osteopathy associated with pulmonary infarction in a horse, *Compend Cont Educ Pract Vet* 5:S636-S641, 1983.
174. Chaffin MK, Ruoff WW, Schmitz DG, et al: Regression of hypertrophic osteopathy in a filly following successful management of an intrathoracic abscess, *Equine Vet J* 22:62-65, 1990.
175. LaVoie J, Carlson GP, George L: Hypertrophic osteopathy in three horses and a pony, *J Am Vet Med Assoc* 210:1900-1904, 1992.
176. Leach MW, Pool RR: Hypertrophic osteopathy in a Shetland pony attributable to pulmonary squamous cell carcinoma metastases, *Equine Vet J* 24:247-249, 1992.
177. Godber LM, Brown CM, Mullaney TP: Polycystic hepatic disease, thoracic granular cell tumor and secondary hypertrophic osteopathy in a horse, *Cornell Vet* 83:227-235, 1993.
178. Sweeney CR, Stebbins KE, Schelling CG, et al: Hypertrophic osteopathy in a pony with a pituitary adenoma, *J Am Vet Med Assoc* 195:103-105, 1989.
179. McClintock S, Hutchins DR: Case report: hypertrophic osteopathy in a stallion with minimal thoracic pathology, *Aust Vet Pract* 11:115-120, 1981.
180. Brody RS: Aspects of hypertrophic osteoarthropathy, *Vet Annu* 19:178-187, 1979.
181. McLennan MW, Kelly WR: Hypertrophic osteopathy and dysgerminoma in a mare, *Aust Vet J* 53:144-146, 1977.
182. Meuten DJ: Hypertrophic osteopathy in a mare with a dysgerminoma, *J Equine Med Surg* 2:445-450, 1978.
183. Laszlo P: Marie's disease in cattle, *Allatorv Lap* 16:191, 1929.
184. Hofmeyr CFB: Hypertrophic osteo-arthropathy (acropachia, Marie's disease) in a bull, *Berl Munch Tierarztl Wochenschr* 77:319, 1964.

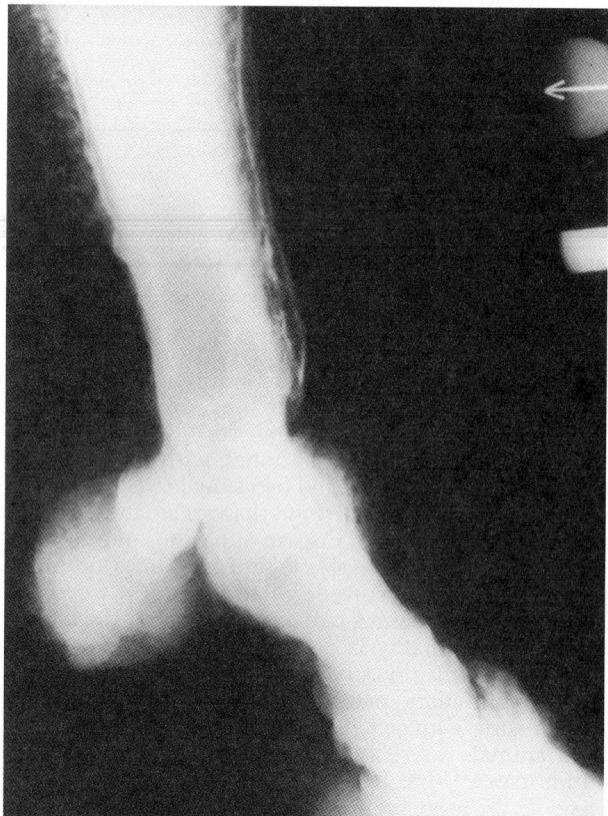

FIG. 36-25 ■ Hypertrophic osteopathy. Lateral projection (bovine) with characteristic new bone growth involving the metacarpal bones, proximal-sesamoid bones, first, second, and third phalanges.

FESCUE FOOT

ERIC W. DAVIS

DEFINITION AND ETIOLOGY. Fescue foot is a toxicosis of cattle grazing pastures that contain tall fescue grass (Festuca arundinaceae schreb). The condition is characterized by lameness, particularly of the rear limbs, progressing to dry gangrene of the feet and lower legs. The end of the tail and the ear tips occasionally may be affected.

Fescue pastures also cause three other syndromes. "Summer slump" is characterized by reduced gain and milk production, dull hair coat, and poor heat tolerance. Abdominal fat necrosis also has been reported in cattle on fescue pasture.[185] Equine reproductive problems, including prolonged gestation and agalactia, as a result of grazing tall fescue late in gestations have been described.[186]

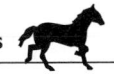

The earliest description of "fescue foot" appeared in 1949 in Australia. It has been reported in Europe, New Zealand, and the United States, particularly in the southeast. The etiologic agents in fescue have not been definitely established, although several toxins have been identified.[185,187-191] Although chemicals produced by the grass itself, such as loline, perloline, and several organic acids, could be toxic agents contributing to fescue foot and other syndromes, mycotoxins produced by endophytic fungi, which infect tall fescue, are generally accepted as being the most important agents. The endophytic fungus of tall fescue, *Acremonium coenophialum* (formerly *Epichloe typhina*), produces ergovaline, ergonine, ergosine, and lysergamide.[185,187,191] All these toxins are capable of producing vasoconstriction similar to that caused by ingestion of the ergot fungus *Claviceps purpurea*. In fact, the symptoms of fescue foot are identical to gangrenous ergotism. Pastures not infected with *Acremonium* do not produce any of the symptoms of fescue toxicosis in animals.[191]

Environmental factors play a part in the development of fescue foot. Although the disease can occur over a range of seasons, symptoms usually occur during colder months. Another factor is the level of pasture fertilization. High levels of nitrogen in soil, regardless of the form applied, increase pasture toxicity. Certain strains of fescue, particularly Kj-31, seem to be more toxic.[192] Finally, because the endophyte imparts a selective advantage on the infected plant by increasing growth rate and disease resistance, the number of toxic plants in a pasture increases. The infestation rate of the fescue endophyte is high; over half the forage samples from states in which fescue foot occurs are infected with *A. coenophialum*.[193]

CLINICAL SIGNS AND DIFFERENTIAL DIAGNOSIS. Clinical signs of fescue foot usually begin as hind limb lameness. Affected cattle also are underweight and have a dull, "rough" hair coat. The feet and pasterns become cold to palpation, and the coronary bands become reddened and swollen. Hair may be rubbed from the pastern area with the fingers, and limb edema may be present. As the condition progresses, the classic signs of fescue foot appear, including a sharp line of demarcation at the level of the pastern or fetlock, distal to which the skin becomes dry and gangrenous and eventually sloughs. The tips of the ears and tail also may necrose. Affected animals lose condition initially and eventually are unable to stand or to walk. There seems to be considerable variation in the susceptibility of animals on a given pasture to the toxin. Generally, morbidity is low, although 20% to 30% of the herd may be affected in some circumstances.[194]

The diagnosis is made on the basis of characteristic signs and gross lesions, as well as on the presence of tall fescue in the pasture. As mentioned earlier, gangrenous ergotism is identical clinically, except that it occurs in the presence of the easily recognizable "ergot" fungus, *C. purpurea*, which grows on rye grass. Similarly, "alkali-disease" or chronic selenium toxicosis mimics fescue foot, except that this disease does not occur on fescue pastures, and affected animals have elevated tissue selenium concentrations. Both ergot and selenium poisoning affect animals other than cattle, whereas fescue foot has been described only in the bovine.

Early in the course of the disease, mechanical foot injury, foot rot, or laminitis can resemble fescue foot, especially as only a few animals in a herd are affected. Close inspection of the foot, however, reveals lesions that are typical of these diseases. Necrosis as a result of freezing may be difficult to distinguish from fescue toxicosis, as both occur at the same time of year.

PATHOPHYSIOLOGY. Pastures that contain tall fescue infected with *A. coenophialum* produce toxins responsible for vasoconstriction. Peripheral vasoconstriction causes blood stasis, endothelial damage, and thrombosis in peripheral vessels. As a result of impaired circulation, tissues of the distal extremities become ischemic and gangrenous. By decreasing peripheral circulation, cold ambient temperatures exacerbate the condition.

NECROPSY FINDINGS. At necropsy the principal finding is a characteristic line of demarcation between normal and gangrenous tissues. Generalized loss of condition also is found because of the animal's inability to ambulate and eat. Vascular thrombosis and necrosis of the tissues of the lower limbs are found microscopically.

TREATMENT AND PROGNOSIS. When animals with fescue foot are recognized early in the course of the disease, they should be removed from pasture as soon as possible. Antibiotic treatment to prevent bacterial invasion of injured skin and hooves is valuable; recovery can occur in 2 weeks. Once the extremities have necrosed, however, treatment is unsuccessful and euthanasia is recommended.

CONTROL. Unlike *C. purpurea*, which grows only on the seed head of grasses, the toxins causing fescue foot are contained in the leaves and stems. As a result, mowing contaminated pastures is not an effective control measure. Growing strains of tall fescue with low toxicity mixed with legume forage plants seems to be the best management technique for controlling the disease. In cold weather, feeding hay to cattle when the pasture contains tall fescue decreases the ingestion of toxins.

REFERENCES
185. Bacon CW, Lyons PC, Porter JK, et al: Ergot toxicity from endophyte-infected grasses: a review, *Agronomy* 78:106-116, 1986.
186. Putnam MR, Bransby DI, Schumacher J, et al: Effects of fungal endophyte *Acremonium coenophialum* in fescue pasture on pregnant mares and foal viability, *Am J Vet Res* 52:2071-2074, 1992.
187. Lyons PC, Plattner RD, Bacon CW: Occurrence of peptide and clavine ergot alkaloids in tall fescue grass, *Science* 232:487-489, 1986.
188. Garner GB, Cornell CN, Yates SG, et al: Fescue foot: assay of extracts and compounds identified in extracts of toxic tall fescue herbage, *J Anim Sci* 55:185-193, 1982.
189. Yates SG: Tall fescue toxins. In Rechcigl M, Jr: *Handbook of naturally occurring food toxicants*, Chicago, 1983, CRC Press, pp 249-273.
190. Davis CB, Camp BJ: The vasoactive potential of halostachine on alkaloid of tall fescue in cattle, *Vet Human Toxicol* 25:408-411, 1983.
191. Strickland JR, Oliver JW, Cross DL: Fescue toxicosis and its impact on animal agriculture, *Vet Human Toxicol* 35:454-464, 1993.
192. Cornell CN, Garner GB, Yates SG, et al: Comparative fescue foot potential of fescue varieties, *J Anim Sci* 55:180-183, 1982.
193. Shelby RA, Dalrymple LW: Incidence and distribution of the tall fescue endophyte in the United States, *Plant Dis* 71:783-786, 1987.
194. Groodman AA: Fescue foot in cattle in Colorado, *J Am Vet Med Assoc* 122:289-290, 1952.

INTERDIGITAL NECROBACILLOSIS (FOOTROT) OF CATTLE

ANITA J. EDMONDSON

DEFINITION AND ETIOLOGY. Interdigital necrobacillosis (footrot, "foul-in-the-foot," interdigital pododermatitis, phlegmona interdigitalis) is an infectious disease of cattle characterized by lameness and inflammation of the subcutaneous tissues of the interdigital space. It is caused by interdigital trauma and infection with two nonmotile, anaerobic, gram-negative bacteria acting synergistically, *Fusobacterium necrophorum* and *Bacteroides melaninogenicus*.[195] *Bacteroides nodosus*, the agent causing ovine footrot, also may be involved.[196]

CLINICAL SIGNS. There is usually a sudden onset of mild-to-severe lameness in one or more limbs, with the hind limbs being affected most frequently. The fetlock and pastern are usually held in a flexed position, and only light weight placed on the toe. The interdigital space is swollen and painful and may cause the toes to spread apart. The coronet and bulbs become swollen, and more proximal spread of the swelling to the pastern and fetlock may occur. The interdigital space is often necrotic and fissured, with a characteristic foul odor but little pus. In severe cases the body temperature is elevated, appetite is reduced, milk yield drops, and body condition is lost, resulting in loss of production.

Interdigital necrobacillosis usually can be diagnosed by the characteristic lesion and odor. Foreign bodies in the interdigital space, interdigital dermatitis, interdigital hyperplasia (corns), and other causes of lameness in cattle must be differentiated from it.

CLINICAL PATHOLOGY. Biopsy material usually reveals *F. necrophorum* and *B. melaninogenicus.*[197] *B. nodosus* and spirochetes may be found; these organisms are more commonly associated with interdigital dermatitis or chronic infections. Lesions are also highly contaminated with fecal flora.

PATHOPHYSIOLOGY. The bacteria are thought to enter the skin in the interdigital region after trauma to the skin from straw, stones, hardened mud, or wet conditions underfoot causing softening of the skin. *F. necrophorum* produces a leukocidal exotoxin that reduces phagocytosis and causes suppurative necrosis.[198] *B. melaninogenicus* produces powerful proteases, including collagenases, which may damage the subcutaneous connective tissue and tendons.[199]

Initially there is a mild cellulitis and swelling, and a fine diphtheritic membrane appears on the skin between the hooves. Subsequent cellulitis and liquefactive necrosis produce longitudinal fissuring and scabby exudate. Extensive necrosis of the interdigital area may follow before the lesion starts to organize and heal by fibrosis.[200] Complications may occur in severe cases, resulting in septic arthritis, tenosynovitis, or other deep infections of the foot. Interdigital hyperplasia and distortion of the horn also may occur as chronic sequelae.

EPIDEMIOLOGY. Interdigital necrobacillosis is one of the most common foot lamenesses seen in cattle, affecting the dermal and subdermal tissues of one or more of the digits. It is usually a sporadic problem affecting one or two animals in a herd at a time, although epizootics have been reported. All ages and all breeds of cattle can be affected, although dairy cattle appear to be affected more commonly than beef cattle, and Bos taurus breeds more than Bos indicus breeds.[201] The disease is seen year round, but the prevalence is usually higher in the wet seasons. The same animals may be affected repeatedly, and because the susceptibility to footrot changes only slightly with age, acquired immunity to the bacteria appears to be poor.[202] Factors predisposing to interdigital infection are those affecting skin integrity such as stubble, stones, frozen or dried mud, and standing in wet pens, which may soften, macerate, or traumatize the skin and allow the infecting organisms to enter. Interdigital dermatitis, caused by *B. nodosus*, also may play a role in initiating interdigital necrobacillosis.[203] Cattle with a widespread interdigital space may be more susceptible. Nutritional deficiencies affecting the integrity of the interdigital skin also influence disease susceptibility but are poorly defined; zinc deficiency has been suspected in several countries. The etiologic agents are present in the normal digestive tract, the environment (*F. necrophorum* may survive in soil for up to 10 months), and the digits of affected animals but are not skin invasive. The disease is not fatal, but animals may be culled because of severe lameness.

NECROPSY FINDINGS. Necropsy examinations are rarely performed. Pathology reveals a dermatitis and necrosis of the skin and subcutaneous tissues. Suppurative changes in the joints and tendon sheaths may be found in severe cases.

TREATMENT AND PROGNOSIS. Systemic antimicrobials and local treatment of the interdigital area usually result in rapid healing (2 to 4 days). Sulfonamides (e.g., sulfadimidine or sulfamethazine at 130 mg/kg/day IV) or antibiotics

(e.g., oxytetracycline, 10 mg/kg/day intravenously, or procaine penicillin, 20,000 to 40,000 IU/kg/twice a day IM or SC) may be used systemically. One treatment is often sufficient, but the response should be evaluated and animals retreated as necessary. Oral sulfonamides (e.g., sulfamethazine in the drinking water) or tetracyclines (e.g., chlortetracycline in feed) may be used in feedlot outbreaks.

Local wound cleaning, curettage of the necrotic tissue, and the application of antiseptics or antimicrobials (e.g., copper sulfate, sulfonamide powder, or oxytetracycline aerosol spray) used in conjunction with the systemic therapy may improve the rate of healing. Lame cows also may be stood in foot baths of 10% zinc sulfate, 2.5% formalin (1% formaldehyde), or 5% copper sulfate for approximately 20 minutes twice a day.[195] If the lesion is severe, a dressing may be applied to the foot after local treatment to reduce further mechanical trauma. The digits are bandaged together, leaving the interdigital space free of dressings to drain and heal. Alternatively, the digits may be wired together to protect the interdigital area. Oral zinc supplements have been recommended for treatment; 5 to 7 mg of $ZnSO_4$ mZ $7H_2O$ per kilogram of live-weight supplement when feeding 30 to 56 µg of zinc per gram of dry matter in the diet of bulls resulted in rapid recovery.[204] Zinc deficiencies, however, have not been shown.

If left untreated, spontaneous recovery after several weeks of lameness may occur. The lesion generally heals rapidly (2 to 4 days) if it is treated before infection of deeper structures of the foot has occurred. If the joint space or tendon sheaths are involved, the prognosis for recovery is poor, as suppurative arthritis or tenosynovitis may result.

PREVENTION AND CONTROL. Prevention involves removing factors predisposing to interdigital trauma and cleaning areas where the pathogenic organisms survive. For example, cattle should be moved off stubble and stones, paths rerouted to avoid problem areas, or the regions causing injury removed. Areas where the pathogenic organisms survive should be eliminated by draining or cleaning wet zones and removing manure slurry more frequently. Nutritional deficiencies affecting the skin quality should be corrected, and efforts made to keep the feet dry. Foot baths of 10% copper sulfate, 5% formalin, or 10% zinc sulfate (which is the least toxic) may be used weekly throughout the year to inhibit or destroy the bacteria involved in the interdigital skin disease.[205] Frequent changes of the solutions or another footbath to clean the feet before entering the treatment bath increase the effectiveness. Treatment of feedlot litter with paraformaldehyde has significantly reduced the incidence of interdigital necrobacillosis in feedlot cattle.[206]

Feeding chlortetracycline to feedlot cattle (500 mg/head/day for 28 days and 75 mg/head/day for 90 days during the fattening period) has reduced the incidence of infection.[207] Ethylenediamine dihydroiodide (EDDI) at 50 to 60 mg/head/day fed continuously has been used widely in beef cattle, and its efficacy shown in experimental infections.[208] Cattle must be observed for tolerance, however, because of the variation in susceptibility to iodides. Oral zinc has been used both for prevention and treatment with good results.[204] *F. necrophorum* vaccines are available in some countries, but their efficacy is based mostly on clinical impressions, although a degree of protection against experimental infection has been shown.[209] Immunization with *B. nodosus* vaccine appears to reduce the severity of interdigital dermatitis but not that of interdigital necrobacillosis.[210]

REFERENCES

195. Weaver AD: Interdigital necrobacillosis. In Chandler EA, Bedford PGC, Sutton JB, editors: *Bovine surgery and lameness,* Oxford, 1986, Blackwell Scientific Publications, p 179.

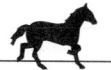

196. Edgerton JR, Laing EA: Characteristics of *Bacteroides nodosus* isolated from cattle, *Vet Microbiol* 3:269-279, 1979.

197. Berg JN, Loan RW: *Fusobacterium necrophorum* and *Bacteroides melanino-genicus* as etiologic agents of foot rot in cattle, *Am J Vet Res* 36(8):1115-1122, 1975.

198. Roberts DS: The pathogenic synergy of *Fusiformis necrophorus* and *Corynebacterium pyogenes*. I. Influence of the leucocidal exotoxin of *F. necrophorus*, *Br J Exp Pathol* 48:665-673, 1967.

199. Biberstein EL, Knight HD, England K: *Bacteroides melaninogenicus* in diseases of domestic animals, *J Am Vet Med Assoc* 153 (8):1045-1049, 1968.

200. Greenough PR, MacCallum FJ, Weaver AD: Interdigital necrobacillosis. In Weaver AD, editor: *Lameness in cattle*, ed 2, Philadelphia, 1981, JB Lippincott, p 151.

201. Frisch JE: The comparative incidence of foot rot in Bos taurus cattle and Bos indicus cattle, *Aust Vet J* 52:228-229, 1976.

202. Rowlands GJ, Russell AM, Williams LA: Effects of stage of lactation, month, age, origin, and heart girth on lameness in dairy cattle, *Vet Rec* 117:576-580, 1985.

203. Egerton JR, Laing EA: Bacterial infections in the aetiology of foot disease of ruminants. In Andersson L, editor: *Report on the second symposium on bovine digital diseases*, Skara, Sweden, Sept. 25-28, 1978, Veterinary Institute.

204. Demertzis PN, Mills CF: Oral zinc therapy in the control of infectious pododermatitis in young bulls, *Vet Rec* 93:219-222, 1973.

205. Amstutz HE: Prevention and control of lameness in dairy cattle. In Ferguson JG, editor: Bovine lameness and orthopedics, *Vet Clin North Am (Food Anim Pract)* 1:25-37, 1985.

205. Greenfield J, Bigland CH, Milligan JD: Control of bovine foot rot by treatment of feedlot litter with paraformaldehyde, *Br Vet J* 128:578-583, 1972.

207. Johnson WP, Algeo J, Kleck J: The efficacy of chlortetracycline supplementation on the incidence of footrot and feedlot performance in cattle, *Vet Med* 52:375-378, 1957.

208. Berg JN, Maas JP, Paterson JA, et al: Efficacy of ethylenediamine dihydroiodide as an agent to prevent experimentally induced bovine foot rot, *Am J Vet Res* 45 (6):1073-1078, 1984.

209. Clark BL, Emery DL, Stewart DJ, et al: Studies into the immunization of cattle against interdigital necrobacillosis, *Aust Vet J* 63 (4):107-110, 1986.

210. Clark BL, Stewart DJ, Emery DL, et al: Immunization of cattle against interdigital dermatitis (foot-rot) with an autogenous *Bacteroides nodosus* vaccine, *Aust Vet J* 63 (2):61-63, 1986.

CONTAGIOUS FOOT ROT OF SHEEP

NANCY E. EAST

Contagious foot rot of sheep is a universally distributed, economically important disease caused by *Bacteroides nodosus* and resulting in the separation of the hoof wall from the basal epithelium and dermis.

CLINICAL SIGNS AND DIFFERENTIAL DIAGNOSIS. The disease occurs in all age groups and is characterized by lameness in one or more feet. The disease is progressive, with initial signs occurring 10 to 20 days after exposure. First the interdigital skin becomes reddened and swollen, followed by slight undermining of the sole at the heels. Eventually, undermining progresses to the sole and wall. Some sheep improve and rid themselves of infection spontaneously, some are resistant to infection, and others become chronic carriers. Infected feet have a characteristic foul odor. Differential diagnosis includes foot abscess, strawberry foot rot, and bluetongue (lameness associated with myopathy and coronitis).

CLINICAL PATHOLOGY AND LABORATORY AIDS. Diagnosis is generally made on the basis of clinical signs; however, stained smears of material from areas of hoof separation can be examined for *B. nodosus* (*Fusobacterium necrophorum* also will be found in large numbers in the smear). The organism also may be cultured from infected feet.

PATHOPHYSIOLOGY. *F. necrophorum* and *B. nodosus* are synergistic pathogens of the foot. *F. necrophorum* colonizes moist or damaged epithelium of the interdigital skin, followed by attachment of *B. nodosus*. There are at least 20 serotypes of *B. nodosus*, with pathogenicity determined by amounts of pili and protease production. Large amounts of pili and protease production correlate with high pathogenicity (i.e., rapid undermining of the sole and walls of the hoof). *F. necrophorum* and sometimes *Actinomyces* (*Corynebacterium*) *pyogenes* continue to be involved in the pathogenic process of hoof tissue invasion and destruction.

EPIDEMIOLOGY. *B. nodosus* has a finite survival period of less than 2 weeks outside the hoof. The usual source of the bacteria is chronic carrier sheep or a surface (corral, truck, trailer) contaminated in the last few days by infected sheep. The tendency for sheep to walk over the same area repeatedly contributes to the spread of the disease. Moisture, warmth, foot injuries, and interdigital skin penetration by the larvae of *Strongyloides papillosus* are the major risk factors associated with transmission of contagious foot rot.[211] Sheep infected with foot rot have lower body condition scores and increased mortality when compared with noninfected sheep. The morbidity may reach 70%, and outbreaks may last weeks to months, depending on environmental conditions, and the serotype of *B. nodosus* involved in the outbreak.

TREATMENT AND PROGNOSIS. Treatment is based on foot trimming, foot bathing, segregation, vaccination, and culling chronically infected sheep.[211-214] The feet of all sheep should be trimmed carefully to remove all necrotic tissue, but extreme trimming that causes severe bleeding should be avoided because it leads to chronic hoof deformity and may produce carrier sheep. On the basis of observation when trimming, the sheep should be divided into "clean" (unaffected) and infected groups. After trimming, the sheep are put through a foot bath (10% zinc sulfate or 10% to 20% copper sulfate or 5% to 10% formalin). The disadvantages of copper sulfate are that it stains wool and its use may lead to accumulations of toxic levels of copper in the environment. Formalin is highly irritating to the skin and respiratory tract, and it is not available for use in some states. Thirsty or salt-deprived sheep should not have access to foot baths because the materials are highly toxic if ingested. As an alternative to a foot bath, a foot soak of 1 hour may be a more successful treatment, particularly with severely affected sheep. To increase penetration, sodium dodecyl sulfate (Tide, $^2/_3$ cup/gallon of H_2O) is added to foot solutions. Individual sheep may be treated with a product such as Kopertox* that contains copper naphthenate following trimming if a foot bath is not available. Sheep are then turned onto separate clean pastures. Paint-branding of infected sheep is recommended to maintain identification through the treatment period in case sheep are mixed or stray. The sheep are then run through the foot bath weekly for 3 weeks, with recovered sheep going to a new separate pasture. Lame sheep or sheep with deformed feet should be culled after 4 weeks of treatment. The segregation of infected sheep and the culling of chronic carrier sheep are essential for a successful outbreak control program. Vaccination with Footvax† (*B. nodosus* bacteria) has some therapeutic value and speeds the recovery of about 50% of the infected sheep; however, the cost is fairly high. Systemic or topical antibiotics (tetracyclines or penicillin) may aid in treatment of valuable individual sheep.[212]

PREVENTION. Proper maintenance of feet (trimming wall overgrowth), isolation, examination of incoming sheep for foot rot, and vaccination are all applied in a total program to prevent foot rot. In addition, sheep should not be confined in muddy areas, and water tanks should be maintained so that water does not leak around them.

Vaccination has both a therapeutic and prophylactic effect. In one study 53% of vaccinated footrot-infected sheep recovered versus 19% of the nonvaccinated sheep.[213] The

---

*Kopertox, Fort Dodge Laboratories, Fort Dodge, IA.

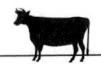

prophylactic effect was demonstrated by a prevalence of foot rot of 9% in vaccinated sheep and 53% in nonvaccinated sheep at the end of 18 weeks. Injection site reactions (lumps) are common and vary widely, with the most severe reactions seen in the blackface breeds of sheep. For this reason show sheep or sheep going to sales should not be vaccinated within 3 months of the anticipated date. Generally, these reactions are only of cosmetic importance. Vaccination should be completed about 4 weeks before the onset of conditions conducive to foot rot transmission. Under prolonged wet conditions in high rainfall or humid areas, biannual booster vaccination may be required (see Chapter 44). One study based on epidemiologic modeling concludes that vaccination is not cost effective and that the most cost-effective treatment is the use of 10% zinc sulfate foot solution.[214,215]

REFERENCES

211. Cross RF: Influence of environmental factors on transmission of ovine contagious foot rot, *J Am Vet Med Assoc* 173:1567-1570, 1978.
212. Bagley CV, Healey MC, Hurst RL: Comparison of treatments for ovine foot rot, *J Am Vet Med Assoc* 191:541-546, 1987.
213. Glenn J, Carpenter TE, Hird DW: A field trial to assess the therapeutic and prophylactic effect of a foot rot vaccine in sheep, *J Am Vet Med Assoc* 187:1009-1012, 1985.
214. Bulgin MS, Lincoln SD, Lane MV, et al: Comparison of treatment methods for the control of contagious ovine foot rot, *J Am Vet Med Assoc* 189:194-196, 1986.
215. Salman MD, Dargatz DA, Kimberling CV, et al: An economic evaluation of various treatments for contagious foot rot in sheep, using decision analysis, *J Am Vet Med Assoc* 193:195-204, 1988.

OTHER INFECTIOUS CONDITIONS OF THE FOOT

DENNIS M. MEAGHER

Infectious processes in the foot of horses and cattle are common and are almost always caused by contamination gaining access to the soft tissue structures of the foot deep to the horny outer covering. The most common clinical sign, acute lameness, may be so severe that the animal is almost non–weight bearing on the affected limb. There is an increase in the digital pulse pressure, and the foot is warm to touch and sensitive to hoof tester pressure over the affected area. Regional nerve blocks localize the lameness to the foot. Frequently, if the foot is thoroughly cleaned and trimmed, a hole or crack leading to the area of infection can be identified. Because the foot is encased in a shell of horny tissue, exudate from an infectious process often accumulates between the soft tissue and horn. The exudate then spreads or dissects along that plane until it reaches a soft tissue surface such as the coronary band, especially near the bulbs of the heels, where rupture and drainage can occur.

SUBSOLAR ABSCESS (SOLE ABSCESS)

Subsolar abscess is one of the most common causes of lameness in the horse and cow, but it is relatively rare in sheep and goats. In one study in cattle, 88% of cases of lameness were caused by problems in the hoof.[216] Most often lameness is caused by a hole or crack in the horny sole, which then becomes packed with dirt, and eventually contamination extends to and is trapped within the sensitive soft tissue beneath the sole. Animals that are housed in filthy or muddy conditions and have inadequate hoof care or overgrown feet are more prone to this problem. Horses that go from a very dry environment to a very wet one and vice versa also tend to have a higher incidence of sole abscesses, apparently because of the sudden change in the moisture content of the hoof and the resultant cracking of the sole. Cattle with corkscrew

claw (a hereditary condition) or other growth deformity in the claw are more prone to sole abscess. Puncture wounds or any form of trauma that introduces contamination to the soft tissue of the sole also may result in abscessation.

Clinical signs (e.g., lameness, heat, swelling, point-pressure pain) are caused by an acute inflammation of the foot that often lasts 24 hours or less. Careful cleaning, paring the sole, application of a hoof tester, inspection, and examination of the foot should always be part of a lameness examination.

The entry site of contamination is not always apparent, even after careful cleaning and trimming of the foot. If signs point to an infection, additional trimming, hot water soaks, or the use of a poultice is necessary. Radiographic examination of the foot is useful if there is joint or bone involvement, but should not be used in place of a careful clinical examination. The principles of treating infectious processes in the foot are adequate drainage, removal of separated sole or wall, local disinfection, protective covering, and tetanus prophylaxis. If the area of abscessation is small, all that may be required is drainage, packing the area with iodine or povidone-iodine–soaked gauze for a few days, and a protective bandage to keep the foot clean and dry. Abscesses that are more extensive or that have dissected between the horny sole and the soft tissue must be treated more aggressively.[217,218] The area of separated sole should be pared away completely to expose the affected area. A local nerve block may be required.

Regional intravenous anesthesia (Bier block) using a tourniquet is the method of choice for producing local anesthesia in cattle. Paring should be performed carefully so that the solar corium is not injured with the hoof knife. Because the corium of the foot represents the horn-producing epithelial covering of the foot, injuries to it heal the same way as skin injuries. The epithelium cornifies after the corium has healed. In severe cases a large section of the horny sole (and frog in horses) may have to be removed, and occasionally the entire horny sole will need to be removed if separated. The foot can then be packed with povidone-iodine–soaked sponges daily and protected with a bandage. In horses the use of thick cotton on the bottom of the foot covered with plastic and elastic tape, and resting the horse in a deeply bedded stall, provides protection and allows the horse to bear more weight on its affected foot. In cattle simple sole abscesses may heal quite satisfactorily without bandaging. Use of a wooden block on the unaffected claw of the affected foot elevates the affected claw to a non–weight-bearing level and markedly reduces lameness. The block is attached with an epoxy such as Technovit* and allowed to wear off over a period of weeks.

If granulation tissue becomes excessive or epithelialization and cornification is slow, 2% tincture of iodine should be used in place of povidone-iodine. Depending on the severity of the lameness, the animal may require a nonsteroidal antiinflammatory drug such as phenylbutazone (4 mg/kg twice a day in horses; 10 mg/kg once a day in cattle) to reduce pain and lameness in the initial stages. Once a thin layer of cornified tissue has covered the defect, the foot of a horse may be protected with a full pad and shoe. Packing such as pine tar and oakum is applied under the pad to reduce contamination and provide added protection for the sensitive tissue. The horse may be returned to work as soon as the lameness subsides, but may need to wear a full pad for 6 to 12 weeks until the sole has gained sufficient thickness to protect the bottom of the foot.

Foot infections also may result from a horseshoe nail that is placed too close to the soft tissue.[217,219] This condition is referred to as the horse being "quicked." Clinically acute lameness appears 1 to 3 days after the horse has been shod. The foot

---

*Technovit, Jorgensen Labs, Veterinary Equipment, 4950 Oakland St, Denver, CO 80239.

shows signs of acute inflammation; but the history, combined with careful inspection and hoof tester examination over the nails, usually identifies the problem. Often removal of the nail is all that is required; removal may be followed by flushing the hole with 2% tincture of iodine. If the nail has contaminated the edge of the soft tissue, a small local abscess results, requiring drainage and treatment as described for a foot abscess.

ASCENDING INFECTION UNDER THE HOOF WALL (GRAVEL)

Gravel is a layman's term for an ascending infection starting at the white line and breaking out just above the coronary band or bulbs of the heel.[217] This infection is thought to be caused by a grain of sand or small pebble that becomes imbedded in the white line and subsequently migrates to the soft tissue above the coronary band, resulting in a small abscess. In fact, the only requirement for "gravel" is the trapping of contamination in the sensitive tissue above the white line. The exudate from the ensuing infection then takes the line of least resistance and abscesses above the coronary band. Often acute lameness and signs of foot inflammation precede the appearance of the abscess above the coronary band by 1 to 2 days.[220] In some instances the site of infection can be identified under the hoof wall and above the white line when the foot is trimmed, and the area that is sensitive to hoof testers is explored. In these cases the abscess is drained from the bottom of the foot, flushed with a disinfectant, and treated like a sole abscess. The drainage hole needs to be large enough to allow the affected tissue to heal from the inside out. If an ascending infection is suspected but cannot be identified, the foot should be soaked in a warm, saturated solution of magnesium sulfate; a poultice should be applied for 2 to 4 days until the abscess appears or inflammation subsides. When abscessation occurs above the coronary band, the abscess should be drained and flushed directly over the swelling.

The bottom of the hoof is trimmed in an attempt to identify a tract from the white line under the hoof wall that extends up to the abscess. If a tract is identified, it is flushed daily with dilute povidone-iodine until it becomes sealed. In chronic cases in which a large area of separation has occurred under the hoof wall, it may be necessary to remove a portion of the hoof wall to provide adequate drainage and to debride the necrotic soft tissue. It may be necessary to trephine a hole in the hoof wall at the lowest point of the infection to provide drainage. If a section of hoof wall must be removed, the coronary band should be left intact to avoid a chronic hoof wall defect. This procedure may require regional nerve block or general anesthesia if the infection is extensive. The hoof is treated with povidone-iodine or iodine packs and covered with a bandage that is changed daily. When practical, the hoof of a horse is protected with a shoe and pad. If a section of hoof wall has been removed, large clips on the horseshoe are applied to both sides of the hoof until the defect has grown out. This helps to stabilize the hoof wall and prevent the development of a chronic hoof crack.

In cattle use of a wooden block on the unaffected claw of the affected limb allows increased mobility by reducing painful weight bearing and also allows the damaged hoof wall to heal.

FOREIGN BODIES

Foreign bodies (e.g., wood or metal) may become imbedded in the foot. They occur most commonly in the bottom of the foot[221,222] or, in the horse, under the hoof wall from above the coronary band. The animal presents with acute lameness and signs of acute foot inflammation. Regional nerve blocks localize the lameness in the foot. Often careful examination and inspection of the foot are needed to find the point of entry of

the foreign body, particularly for small splinters of wood that have become driven beneath the coronary band. This problem may occur when horses are housed in plywood stalls or transported in vans that have plywood partitions. The foreign body is removed, and the tract is debrided and flushed with a disinfectant solution until it heals by granulation. In long-standing cases it may be necessary to remove a portion of the sole or hoof wall that has become separated to provide adequate drainage and allow for debridement of the infected area. The foot is then treated as described for extensive subsolar abscess or hoof wall removal for ascending infections.

OSTEOMYELITIS AND SEQUESTRATION OF THE DISTAL PHALANX

Infection of the distal phalanx or coffin bone may result from an extension of any foot infection through the soft tissue into the bone. Frequently it results from a foot infection that has gone undetected or one that has not responded to treatment,[219,223,224] often because of inadequate drainage or debridement. The history usually is one of a long-standing foot lameness, which may be accompanied by locally recurring episodes of drainage or multiple abscesses that tend to recur in the same area. Careful and deep trimming of the foot may reveal a draining tract leading to bone. Sequestration may occur as a result of the initial injury, but in the coffin bone more frequently it is the result of osteomyelitis. As the bone infection progresses, the blood supply to local areas of bone is disrupted, and the area of avascular bone becomes separated from the parent bone, forming a sequestrum. Good-quality radiographs following careful trimming and preparation of the foot are important for detecting deep-seated osteomyelitis and for identifying sequestra.

Treatment includes surgical drainage, removal of any sequestra, and careful curettage of the infected bone. The opening in the sole or hoof wall should be large enough that the wound will granulate from its deepest site to the surface, allowing adequate drainage during the healing process. After surgical debridement of the infected bone, the area is packed daily with povidone-iodine–soaked sponges, and the foot is covered with a soft protective bandage. The wound should be dressed as aseptically as possible until the exposed bone is covered with granulation tissue. When the granulation bed has reached the surface of the surrounding cornified layer, the packing is changed to 2% tincture of iodine until the surface is completely cornified. At that time the foot of the horse is supported with a protective shoe and pad. Depending on the severity of the osteomyelitis, the animal may need to remain on a course of nonsteroidal antiinflammatory drugs for several days to weeks to encourage weight bearing on the affected foot. This regimen is particularly important in horses when a forefoot is involved to help avoid the occurrence of laminitis in the contralateral foot. In cattle a wooden block can be attached with Technovit to the other digit of the affected limb to relieve weight bearing on the affected digit.[225]

PUNCTURE WOUNDS OF THE FOOT

Puncture wounds of the foot are relatively common and are usually caused by nails. They are treated by pulling the nail and debriding the puncture wound to the full depth, being sure to make the hole large enough in the sole to maintain drainage during the healing process. If the nail has penetrated to the coffin bone, that area of bone should be curetted to prevent the development of local osteomyelitis. Aftercare is the same as described for sole abscess. In horses nail punctures that enter the sulcus of the frog or the frog itself have a tendency to end up directed toward the navicular bursa because of the concavity of the ventral surface of the coffin bone. Extreme care must be taken to ensure that the puncture wound has been traced to the deepest point of penetration.[223] If the puncture wound has extended into the deep digital flexor tendon or the navicular bursa, the horse will be non–weight-bearing on the affected leg. Surgical drainage of the navicular bursa (street nail procedure) should be performed without delay.[226]

A basic rule in dealing with all foot infections and puncture wounds of the frog area in particular is that if the lameness has not improved significantly 48 to 72 hours after drainage of the infected area, the process is probably more extensive than first identified and additional exploration of the area is needed. If swelling proceeds up the leg following sole abscess or a puncture wound and septic tenosynovitis or septic arthritis occurs, the prognosis is guarded to poor. Septic arthritis of the distal interphalangeal (coffin) joint in cattle can be treated by amputation of the affected claw. Cattle may ambulate well on one claw for only months before breaking down or may last for years if the animal is light and protects the affected limb. The prognosis is poor when concurrent septic tenosynovitis is present.

QUITTOR. Quittor is a term that has been used for chronic infection of the medial or lateral collateral cartilage of the distal phalanx in the horse. This condition is characterized by local inflammation and necrosis of the affected cartilage, with subsequent formation of draining tracts occurring proximal to the coronary band. The infection is usually caused by a wound, and the horse often presents with moderate to severe lameness and a history of chronic or recurrent drainage.[227] Although this condition occasionally responds to medical treatment, the treatment of choice is surgical debridement with the horse under general anesthesia, the foot in full extension, and a tourniquet around the pastern. An elliptic section that includes the draining tract should be incised above the coronary band and discarded. All underlying infected soft tissue and necrotic cartilage should be excised. If the case has not become chronic and only a small amount of cartilage has to be removed, the wound may be packed and partially sutured. The pack can be removed in 24 to 48 hours, and the wound flushed twice a day until it has healed. If the condition is chronic with extensive cartilage necrosis or multiple draining tracts, the infectious process usually extends below the level of the coronary band. In this event it is best to trephine a hole in the hoof wall at the lowest point of the infection. This procedure provides better drainage, facilitates debridement of the necrotic cartilage, and allows for complete closure of the surgical incision above the coronary band. The wound should be packed through the trephine hole and treated as an open wound until it heals. In cases with extensive cartilage necrosis, care should be taken to avoid accidental opening of the coffin joint. If debridement is complete, the prognosis for the return to soundness is fair to good.

REFERENCES

216. Baggot DG, Russel AM: Lameness in cattle, *Br Vet J* 137:113-132, 1981.
217. Johnson JH: Septic conditions of the equine foot, *J Am Vet Med Assoc* 161:1276-1279, 1972.
218. Johnson JH: Puncture wounds of the sole and subsolar abscesses. In Catcott EJ, Smithcors JF, editors: *Equine medicine and surgery,* ed 1, Wheaton, Ill, 1972, Veterinary Publications, pp 534-535.
219. Johnson JH: Puncture wounds of the foot, *Vet Med Small Anim Clin* 65:147-152, 1970.
220. Stashak TS: *Adams' lameness in horses,* ed 4, Philadelphia, Lea & Febiger, pp 496-538.
221. Johnson JH: Puncture wounds of the sole. In Mannsman RH, McAllister ES, Pratt PW, editors: *Equine medicine and surgery,* ed 3, Santa Barbara, 1982, American Veterinary Publishing Co, pp 1040-1041.
222. Fessler JF: Surgical management of equine foot injuries, *Mod Vet Pract* 52:41-46, 1971.
223. Richardson GL, Pascoe JR, Meagher DM: Puncture wounds of the foot in horses: diagnosis and treatment, *Compend Cont Educ Pract Vet* 8:S379-S387, 1986.
224. Steckle RR, Fesler JF: Surgical management of severe hoof wounds in the horse: a retrospective study of 30 cases, *Compend Cont Educ Pract Vet* 5:S435-S443, 1983.
225. Greenough PR, MacCallum FJ, Weaver AD: Treatment and control of digital disease. In Weaver AD: *Lameness in cattle,* ed 2, Philadelphia, 1981, JB Lippincott, pp 228-262.
226. Richardson GL, O'Brien TR, Pascoe JR, et al: Puncture wounds of the navicular bursa in 38 horses: a retrospective study, *Vet Surg* 15:156-160, 1986.
227. Honnas CM, Ragle CA, Meagher DM: Necrosis of the collateral cartilage of the distal phalanx: 16 cases, *J Am Vet Med Assoc* 193:1303-1307, 1988.

FISTULOUS WITHERS

STEVEN C. ZICKER

DEFINITION AND ETIOLOGY. Fistulous withers is an inflammatory condition of the supraspinous bursa in the horse. The bursa is variable in location and size, but usually overlies the second through fifth thoracic vertebrae and may extend ventrolaterally to the margin of the scapular cartilage. The majority of clinical cases are thought to be primarily infectious in origin, but most cases are not seen until the bursa is fistulated and secondary contamination is prevalent. Microorganisms incriminated in the primary infectious process are *Brucella abortus* and *Actinomyces bovis.*[228,229] Secondary contamination with environmental microorganisms such as *Streptococcus* spp., *Escherichia coli,* and anaerobic bacteria have been elucidated. Primary trauma to the bursa or underlying thoracic vertebra may also cause bursal swelling. Migration and encystment of *Onchocerca cervicalis* larvae through the ligamentum nuchae and into the bursa have been incriminated as a cause of fistulous withers.[230]

CLINICAL SIGNS AND DIFFERENTIAL DIAGNOSIS. Fistulous withers may develop abruptly or insidiously, depending on the etiologic agent. Initially, the most common clinical signs are pain, heat, and swelling of the supraspinous bursa overlying the second through fifth thoracic vertebrae.[228,229] Lethargy, fever, and generalized stiffness may also be present.[231,232] After several days to weeks the bursa ruptures, resulting in drainage of fluid, which may be serous or purulent in consistency, through a cutaneous fistula. If untreated, apparent healing, fibrosis, and refistulation may occur. The list of differentials should include atypical infection causing abscessation, tumors, and external trauma not involving the bursa. Contact with *Brucella*-infected cattle is suggestive for a diagnosis of fistulous withers caused by *B. abortus.*

CLINICAL PATHOLOGY. Percutaneous aspiration and microbiologic culture of fluid from the bursa before it ruptures are useful diagnostically. Unopened bursal effusion contains few cells and occasional flecks of fibrin. Special media and growth conditions are needed to culture *Brucella* and *Actinomyces* spp. After the bursa ruptures, secondary bacterial contaminants may interfere with isolation of pure cultures of the primary organism and result in a purulent discharge.

In all suspected cases of fistulous withers, a serum agglutination titer for *Brucella* should be performed. Any rise in paired serum titers 2 weeks apart is considered diagnostic for *Brucella* infection.[231] If paired serum titers are not performed, a single titer of 1:40 and above is evidence of concurrent *Brucella* infection.[231,232] Intradermal or subcutaneous testing with *Brucella* antigen is not as reliable as serology.

PATHOPHYSIOLOGY. Many factors are implicated in the pathophysiology of fistulous withers. Bursitis can be reproduced by inoculations into the supraspinous bursa of mixed, but not individual, cultures of *B. abortus* and *A. bovis* organisms.[228] Trauma to the soft tissue or thoracic vertebrae also may be a contributing cause of the disease and therefore radiographs of the dorsal processes of the thoracic vertebrae are recommended. Careful evaluation of some surgically excised bursa have revealed necrotic foci containing encysted and calcified larvae of *Onchocerca* spp. in Australia.[230]

EPIDEMIOLOGY. *B. abortus* has been identified in as many as 80% of clinical cases by serum agglutination titer and culture.[229] Similarly, *A. bovis* often is isolated from the bursa of *Brucella*-positive reactors.[228] Cattle are the major reservoir of infection for horses. A 1985 survey from Great Britain, which is currently considered a *Brucella*-free country, demonstrated a serum agglutination reactor-rate of 3% to 10% in horses.[233] Similar results were found in a 1982 serologic survey performed in horses from Florida.[234] A 1992 retrospective study of horses with fistulous withers in Texas revealed that 37.5% of the subjects had a *Brucella* titer greater than 1:100.[235] The same study revealed that horses with a higher titer had a significant association with pastured cattle. It is thought that horses in endemic areas are more likely to have Brucella-positive sera and a higher incidence of fistulous withers.

NECROPSY FINDINGS. Intact supraspinous bursae have an enlarged and thickened capsule containing a clear, straw-colored, viscid transudate; open bursa usually contain exudate. Infection may extend to and involve the dorsal spinous processes of the thoracic vertebrae and cause osteomyelitis and necrosis. Multiple tracts, severe fibrosis, and scarring may be seen in chronic cases.

TREATMENT AND PROGNOSIS. In *Brucella*-confirmed cases, an effective treatment regimen using a killed Brucella vaccine has ranged from a single subcutaneous injection to a series of three subcutaneous injections given 10 days apart.[232,233] Controlled studies have not been performed to assess the efficacy of this treatment, and severe swelling and systemic illness may result.[231] Intravenous injection of the vaccine has been associated with a high mortality rate and should not be performed.[235]

In unfistulated, non-Brucella cases, use of appropriate antimicrobial and antiinflammatory agents has been suggested. Fistulated bursae may be treated by flushing the open tract with dilute betadine solution or mild oxidizing agents in conjunction with parenteral antimicrobial treatment. Radiographs are indicated to assess thoracic vertebrae for fracture and osteomyelitis that extended from bursal infection. Cases of fistulous withers that are refractory to conservative medical treatment may require surgical excision and drainage.[236]

PREVENTION AND CONTROL. Clients should be made aware of the public health implications of brucellosis.[237] Public health authorities may require isolation and possible disposal of *Brucella*-positive horses. Effective parasite control programs that eliminate *Onchocerca* spp. and flies, and separation of horses from known *Brucella*-positive cattle are recommended. Properly fitted saddles and harnesses minimize trauma to the area of the withers and may help to reduce the incidence of the disease.

REFERENCES
228. Roderick LM, Kimball A, McLeod WM, et al: A study of equine fistulous withers and poll evil, *Am J Vet Res* 9:5-10, 1948.
229. Duff HM: Fistulous withers and poll evil due to Brucella abortus, *Vet Rec* 16:175-181, 1936.
230. Ottley ML, Dallemagne L, Moorhouse DE: Equine onchocerciasis in Queensland and the Northern Territory of Australia, *Aust Vet J* 60:200-203, 1983.
231. Denny HR: A review of brucellosis in the horse, *Equine Vet J* 5:121-125, 1973.
232. Cosgrove JSM: Clinical aspects of equine brucellosis, *Vet Rec* 73:1377-1382, 1961.
233. MacMillan AP: A retrospective study of the serology of brucellosis in the horse, *Vet Rec* 117:638-639, 1985.
234. Nicolletti PL, Mahler JR, Scarrett WK: Study of agglutinins to *Brucella abortus*, *B. canis* and *Actinobacillus equuli* in horses, *Equine Vet J* 14:302-303, 1982.
235. Cohen ND, Carter GK, McMullan WC: Fistulous withers in horses: 24 cases (1984-1990), *J Am Vet Med Assoc* 201:121-124, 1992.
236. Rashmir-Raven A, Gaughn EM, Modransky P: Fistulous withers, *Compend Cont Educ Pract Vet* 12:1633-1640, 1990.
237. Vaughn JT: Fistulous withers. In Catcott EJ, Smithcors FJ, editors: *Equine medicine and surgery*, ed 2, Wheaton, Ill, 1972, Veterinary Publications, p 828.

FLEXURAL LIMB DEFORMITIES (CONTRACTED TENDONS)

PAMELA WAGNER VON MATTHIESSEN
ANDRIS J. KANEPS

Flexural limb deformities or "contracted tendons" commonly occur in young horses and calves and are less common in sheep, goats and camelids.[238-242] Although the tendons may not be "contracted," this term has been used historically to describe the condition. Soft tissue structures responsible for flexion of the distal limb are mechanically or functionally shorter than the osseous structures, resulting in some degree of flexion in one or more joints. Flexural deformities may be congenital or acquired and may affect the carpal, metacarpophalangeal, or distal interphalangeal joint. These syndromes have distinctly different clinical manifestations and prognoses and must be differentiated before treatment is begun. The condition sometimes occurs simultaneously with joint contractures (arthrogryposis), and this possibility must be strongly considered if joints are not mobile.

CONGENITAL FLEXURAL DEFORMITIES

ETIOLOGY. The cause of congenital flexural deformities is unknown. Both intrauterine malpositioning and osseous hypoplasia with subsequent distortion of the fetal limb and ingestion by the pregnant mare of toxic substances such as *Astragalus* (locoweed) have been reported.[238,243] More severe deformities are often associated with spinal and skull abnormalities and thus may represent a teratogenic insult during early development of the fetal skeleton. The condition is believed to be inherited in Jersey and shorthorn cattle,[243] but occurs sporadically in other dairy breeds without access to known teratogens. Carpal and distal limb flexural contractures in foals may be associated with rupture of the common digital extensor tendon over the carpus.[244]

CLINICAL SIGNS. Congenital flexural deformities are present at birth.[239] In severe cases dystocia results because of the inability of the foal or calf to straighten its limbs during delivery. Milder cases may be unnoticed until the foal attempts to rise. Deformities may affect either the fetlock or carpus (and, rarely, the tarsus). Congenital fetlock and carpal flexural deformities may be different entities, as they differ in their response to therapy. Further, the prognosis in fetlock flexural deformity is generally more favorable than carpal flexural deformity.

FETLOCK. Many foals and calves are born with mild tendon contracture, causing fetlock flexion that resolves spontaneously in the first few hours of life. In these cases the flexural deformity is bilateral or affects all four limbs. Contracture affecting the superficial digital flexor tendon results in upright fetlocks; if the deep digital flexor tendons also are affected, the heels are elevated as well. In severe cases the fetlock cannot be straightened manually (Fig. 36-26).

CARPUS. Congenital flexural abnormalities of the carpus range from very mild ("bucked knees") to very severe. If the limb can be straightened manually, the prognosis for resolution is good. If not, the deformity probably involves more than the musculotendinous unit; the joint capsule and intercarpal ligaments may be the constricting elements (Fig. 36-27). In newborn foals with carpal contracture the common digital extensor tendon should be evaluated. Rupture of the tendon is evident as a fluid swelling within its carpal sheath. The rupture may cause flexural deformity by inhibiting full extension of the limb or may be a consequence of moderate to severe congenital limb contractures. Radiographic evaluation of the carpus in these cases is recommended before undertaking therapy to ascertain whether osseous abnormalities, such as inadequate mineralization of the cuboidal bones, are present.

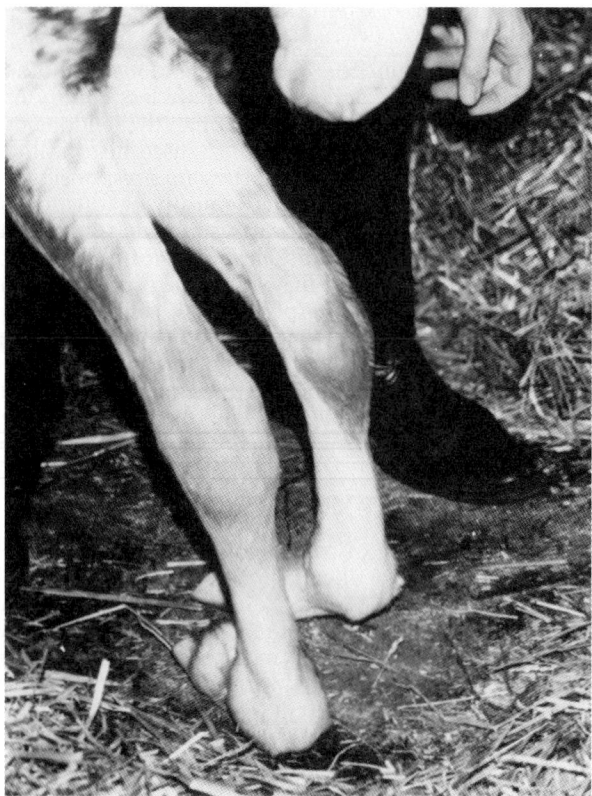

FIG. 36-26 ▓ Severe congenital fetlock flexural deformity. This foal could not stand without assistance.

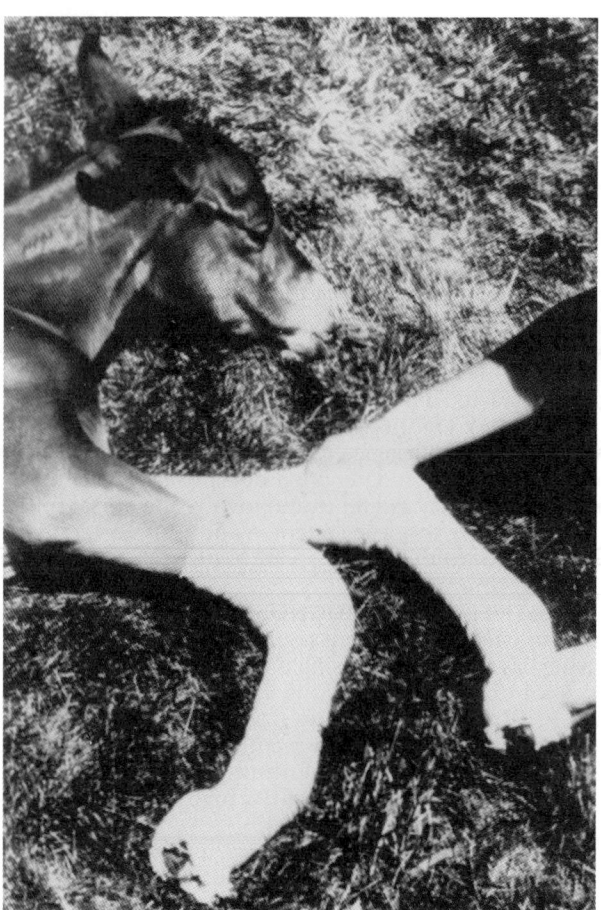

FIG. 36-27 ▓ Severe carpal flexural deformities cannot be straightened manually, but the carpus can be flexed.

PATHOPHYSIOLOGY. Congenital flexural deformities often are accompanied by osseous defects that have led to speculation on the pathophysiology of contracted tendons.[245] Multiple joint defects leading to joint instability initiate inappropriate neurologic signals and muscle responses, which result in contracture of the soft tissues that reinforce the abnormal angulation. Fetuses of less than 9 months' gestation have been observed with such defects, suggesting that the original abnormality may be bony in nature. Therefore the foal should be examined for skull malformations, scoliosis, kyphosis, and abnormalities in other than the obviously affected joint(s). Foals with severe carpal flexural deformities often show severe prognathism and laxity of the fetlock joints. Alternatively, lack of normal development of motor horn cells in the spinal cord could lead to abnormal musculotendinous development, resulting in contracted tendons or arthrogryposis.

NECROPSY FINDINGS. Foals with severe flexural deformities in which the limb cannot be straightened show abnormal alignment of the limb, even when all the tendons and muscles are removed after death. The joint capsules and intraarticular ligaments appear to be the constricting influence. In many cases the cuboidal bones are misshapen, and ossification is incomplete. Abnormalities in the articulations of the spinal column have been described.[245]

In mild cases of flexural deformity, severing of tendons or check ligaments may allow manual straightening of the limb. In these cases the bones of the carpus or tarsus are usually not radiographically or grossly defective.

TREATMENT
Fetlock

If the animal can stand and the limb can be straightened manually, the prognosis for resolution is good. If the flexion is so severe that the animal cannot stand alone or if standing results in abrasion to the dorsum of the fetlock, immediate therapy is recommended to avoid limb trauma. In mild-to-moderate cases, manual stretching and splinting are often successful. The limb may be manually stretched for 5 minutes 2 to 3 times daily. The splint should be heavily padded and placed on the palmar or plantar surface of the bandaged leg, including the entire limb on the foreleg or to the tarsus on the rear limb. Pneumatic splints specifically designed for use in foals also have been used successfully to treat flexural deformities. The pneumatic splints uniformly distribute pressure over the entire limb, minimizing pressure points, and are much lighter in weight than conventional splints or casts.[243] More severe flexural deformities that can be manually straightened can be cast for 10 to 14 days. The cast should include the foot, fetlock, and carpus or tarsus. In contractures in foals that are unresponsive to external coaptation, distal check desmotomy and full limb casting have been successful. In calves partial-to-complete tenotomy (until the limb can be straightened) is necessary if splinting fails to allow sufficient improvement to make walking possible. Both the superficial and deep digital flexor tendons may be cut if necessary. A firm support bandage and confinement to a small, clean area are necessary after surgery. Nonsteroidal antiinflammatory medications should be administered to reduce the discomfort associated with stretching of the contracted tissues. The prognosis in these cases is good.

A single dose of oxytetracycline (3 g in 250 ml saline administered intravenously) has been used to treat severe flexural deformities in foals.[246] The drug is effective in increasing fetlock hyperextension in normal foals and may act by chelating calcium, making it less available for muscle contraction, and thereby relaxing the musculotendinous unit.[247]

Carpus

Splinting of the limbs in mild cases may be helpful and should be undertaken immediately. If there is no change in 3 to 4 days, the prognosis for resolution is poor. Severe congenital flexural deformity of the carpus in the foal and calf is believed to be the result of contracture of the caudal carpal fascia, joint capsule, and the palmar carpal ligament. Transection of tendons crossing the palmar aspect of the carpus is not successful in relieving the contracture. Recently, transection of the palmar aspect of the joint capsule has been performed to salvage foals for breeding purposes and has been successful in selected cases.[248] If rupture of the common digital extensor tendon is recognized, splints or casts should be applied for 10 to 14 days. Casts for carpal contracture should end just proximal to the fetlock to prevent excessive distal limb laxity.

PROGNOSIS. It is advisable to radiograph the most severely affected joints to rule out carpal or tarsal bone hypoplasia. Underdeveloped carpal or tarsal bones carry a poor prognosis.

ACQUIRED FLEXURAL DEFORMITIES

Acquired flexural deformities occur during the growth phase; two distinct clinical presentations are recognized.

Flexural Deformity of the Distal Interphalangeal Joint (Deep Digital Flexor Tendon Contracture)

ETIOLOGY. There are probably several causes of deep digital flexor (DDF) tendon contracture, and more than one cause may be present in the same animal. Genetic predisposition to rapid bone growth, faulty nutrition caused by unbalanced dietary minerals or excessive feeding, pain from other skeletal disorders, and lack of exercise have all been implicated. Histologic studies of muscle bellies, tendons and check ligaments have been unrewarding in identifying specific causes.

CLINICAL SIGNS. This condition occurs in foals and weanling horses (rarely in cattle) and is characterized by flexion of the distal interphalangeal joint, resulting in a raised heel or "club foot."[239,240,245] The distal check ligament modulates the stretch in the long tendon of the DDF; it originates at the back of the carpus and inserts on the DDF tendon in the mid-metacarpal area. If this musculotendinous unit becomes functionally too short, flexion of the distal interphalangeal joint occurs. The heel is elevated, and a boxy foot develops (Fig. 36-28) or the distal phalanx is pulled palmarly giving a dished appearance to the hoof (Fig. 36-29). The subdivision of this contracture into stage 1 (dorsal hoof wall less than vertical) and stage 2 (dorsal hoof wall past vertical) has been used to grade the severity of the deformity.

TREATMENT. Initial therapy in mild cases of DDF tendon contracture should include dietary management (i.e., reducing caloric intake and balancing mineral content in feed). Heavy milk production by a mare resulting in overfeeding by a foal warrants early weaning. Heavy wraps and splints slacken soft tissue structures and allow proper realignment of the limb. Other measures that may be helpful are trimming the heels to increase the stretch on the deep digital flexor tendon and shoeing to elevate the toe. Glue-on shoes or hoof acrylic may be used to extend the toe in foals and calves, thereby causing stretching of the contracted structures. Nonsteroidal antiinflammatory drugs and analgesics may be helpful if pain is an underlying cause.

Surgical therapy is most successful when performed early[239,249,250]; therefore repeated assessment of the progress

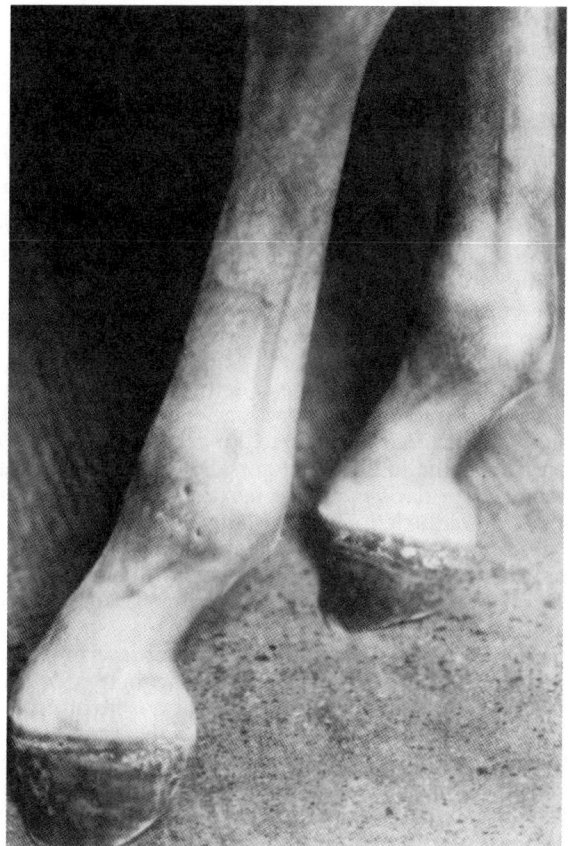

FIG. 36-28 ■ Typical appearance of an acute case of flexural deformity of the distal interphalangeal joint (deep digital tendon contracture). The "boxy" appearance of the hoof indicates that the hoof wall and distal phalanx have maintained attachment.

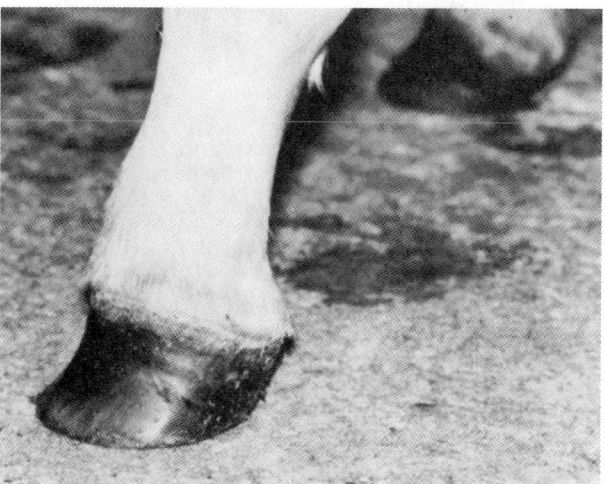

FIG. 36-29 ■ Flexural deformity of the distal interphalangeal joint (deep digital flexor tendor contracture) also can present as a "dished" foot.

of the affected limb should be made if initial therapy is conservative. If substantial improvement is not seen in 3 to 4 weeks, surgical intervention is advised. Distal check desmotomy and corrective shoeing have been successful in allowing over 80% of affected horses to pursue their intended work[250] when the deformity is classified as stage 1. In stage 2 deformities check desmotomy and shoeing are often helpful. If the horse does not respond, however, deep digital flexor tenotomy may be required.

Flexural Deformity of the Metacarpophalangeal Joint (Superficial Digital Flexor Tendon Contracture)

ETIOLOGY. Horses with this condition are often being prepared for show at halter, are on an elevated plane of nutrition, and are growing rapidly. Horses most severely affected have a tendency to experience rapid growth spurts. The condition occurs in growing ruminants secondary to limb disuse associated with recumbency.

CLINICAL SIGNS. This type of deformity occurs in young animals from 8 to 18 months of age.[239] The fetlocks at first appear upright and then begin to dorsally subluxate. In stage 1 deformities the fetlock may dorsally subluxate but intermittently "pop" back into place; in stage 2 deformities dorsal subluxation of the fetlock is constant (Fig. 36-30).

It is important to determine all involved structures to formulate therapy and determine a prognosis. Superficial digital flexor (SDF) tendon contracture may involve only the SDF tendon or both DDF and SDF tendons, and in some cases the suspensory ligament. Flexion of the distal interphalangeal joint seen on lateral radiographs may help determine whether the deep digital flexor tendon also is involved. With the toe on a board, differential palpation of the SDF and DDF tendons to determine the structures that tighten most when the foot is extended aids in the identification of the involved tendons.

TREATMENT. Mild cases may be treated initially with corrective shoeing, bandaging, and splinting of the limb; balancing and reducing the diet; nonsteroidal antiinflammatory medication; and increasing exercise. Mild cases appear to improve when the heel is elevated, relieving pressure on the DDF tendon and forcing the SDF tendon and suspensory ligament to assume the support of the fetlock. If this therapy does not result in sufficient axial limb realignment within 3 to 4 weeks, surgery is indicated. If only the SDF tendon is involved, accessory ligament of the SDF (AL-SDF; proximal check) desmotomy is recommended. Moderate cases in which the SDF and DDF tendons are involved are best treated by AL-SDF and accessory ligament of the DDF (AL-DDF; distal check) desmotomies.[251] In ruminants it is often necessary to sever flexor tendons to achieve realignment.

Foal owners are at times reluctant to have desmotomies performed because of their concerns regarding the future strength of the limb. AL-DDF desmotomy does not prevent a foal from becoming a successful athlete. In a study of 23 Standardbred foals with DDF tendon contracture, 6 of 11 treated with AL-DDF desmotomy successfully entered racing careers, whereas none of 12 foals treated conservatively did.[252] Foals less than 8 months of age at the time of surgery had a better prognosis for racing than did older foals.[252]

PROGNOSIS. Severely affected horses have a poor prognosis.[251] Even if both check ligaments are transected, contracture may recur 2 to 4 months after surgery. Salvage for breeding may be achieved by suspensory desmotomy; however, subluxation at the proximal interphalangeal joint is the usual consequence. The prognosis is good in ruminants if the limb can be straightened after tenotomy.

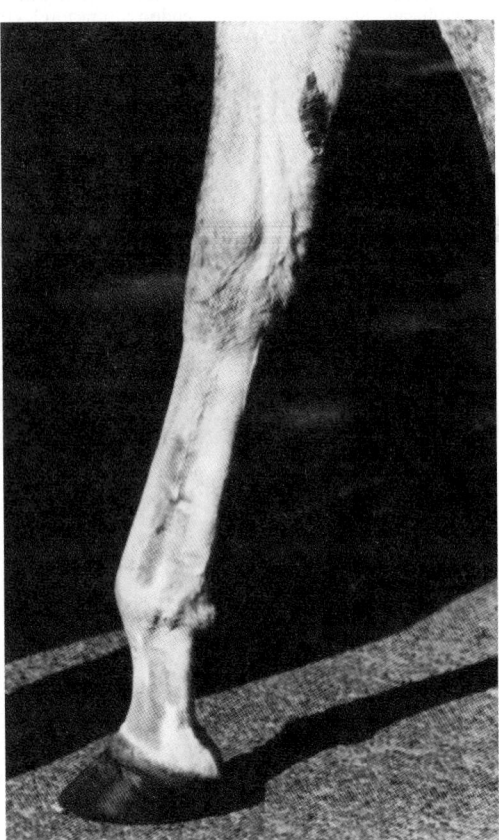

FIG. 36-30 ■ Flexural deformity of the metacarpophalangeal joint (superficial digital flexor tendon contracture).

REFERENCES

238. McIlwraith CW: Diseases of joints, tendons, ligaments and related structures. In Stashak TS, editor: *Adam's lameness in horses,* ed 4, Philadelphia, 1987, Lea & Febiger, pp 458.
239. Wagner PC, Reed SM, Hegreberg GA: Contracted tendons (flexural deformities) in the young horse, *Compend Cont Educ Pract Vet* 4(3):5101-5111, 1982.
240. Owen JM: Abnormal flexion of the corono-pedal joint or "contracted tendons" in the unweaned foal, *Equine Vet J* 7(1):40-45, 1975.
241. Greenough PR, MacCallum FJ, Weaver AD: *Lameness in cattle,* ed 2, Philadelphia, 1981, JB Lippincott, pp 381-383.
242. Cashman T, Dart AJ, O'Shea A, Hodgson DR: Management of bilateral flexural deformity of the metacarpophalangeal joints in three alpaca crias, *Aust Vet J* 77(8):508-510, 1999.
243. Jones PA: The use of pneumatic splints for treatment of congenital flexural deformities in foals. Proceedings of the 37th Annual Convention of the American Association of Equine Practitioners, 1991, pp 519-524.
244. Kaneps AJ, Smith BL: Management of distal limb lameness in foals, *Compend Cont Educ Pract Vet* 20(9):1060-1067.
245. Rooney JR: Forelimb contracture in the young horse, *J Equine Med Surg* 1:350-351, 1977.
246. Lokai MD, Meyer RJ: Preliminary observations on oxytetracycline treatment of congenital flexural deformities in foals, *Mod Vet Pract* 237-239, 1985.
247. Madison JB, Garber JL, Rice B, et al: Effect of oxytetracycline on metacarpophalangeal and distal interphalangeal joint angles in newborn foals, *J Am Vet Med Assoc* 104:246-249, 1994.
248. Wagner PC: Caudal carpal capsule release as a treatment for severe congenital contractures in foals. Proceedings of the Fourteenth Annual Conference of the Veterinary Orthopedic Society, 1987.
249. McIlwraith CW, Fessler JF: Evaluation of inferior check ligament desmotomy for treatment of acquired flexor tendon contracture in the horse, *J Am Vet Med Assoc* 172(3):293-298, 1978.
250. Wagner PC, Grant BD, Kaneps AJ, et al: Long-term results of desmotomy of the accessory ligament of the deep digital flexor tendon (distal check ligament) in horses, *J Am Vet Med Assoc* 187(12):1351-1353, 1985.
251. Wagner PC, Shires GMH, Watrous BJ, et al: Management of acquired flexural deformity of the metacarpophalangeal joint in *Equidae, J Am Vet Med Assoc* 187(9):915-918, 1985.
252. Stick JA, Nickels FA, Williams A: Long-term effects of desmotomy of the accessory ligament of the deep digital flexor muscle in standardbreds: 23 cases (1979-1989), *J Am Vet Med Assoc* 200:1131-1132, 1992.

TENDINITIS

CAROL L. GILLIS

DEFINITION AND ETIOLOGY. The superficial digital flexor (SDF) tendon is the most frequently injured tendon in the horse and the mid-metacarpal region of the forelimbs is the most common site of injury. The deep digital flexor tendon, which is infrequently injured, usually develops tendinitis in the pastern region. Extensor tendon injuries are seen most frequently just distal to the carpus or the tarsus. In cattle, rupture of the gastrocnemius (Achilles) tendon or of its muscle is the most frequent tendon injury.

Tendons act to transmit muscle contraction force to bone, and have developed to withstand large tensile forces, yet they are of small size or cross-sectional area, thus occupying a relatively small space as they traverse the bones and joints of the limbs. In large animals virtually no muscle exists distal to the carpus and tarsus; joint motion is accomplished by tendon transmission to bone of contraction forces generated by the more proximal large muscle groups. When muscle becomes fatigued, changes in contractile force and pattern contribute to cyclic overloading of the tendon. Tendinitis occurs most frequently in equine athletes that either perform at high speed, as in racing or polo, or strenuously load one limb as in jumping, to the point of fatigue and beyond. Tendinitis also occurs infrequently as a result of a fall or other single traumatic event.

The pathophysiology of tendinitis involves stretching of the parallel collagenous fibers beyond the physiologic limit, resulting in fiber tearing, accompanied by vessel rupture and hemorrhage. Initially a clot forms to fill the damaged space(s), and inflammatory products cause edema, pain, heat, and swelling. A compartment syndrome may occur, in which more tendon fibers undergo necrosis as a result of compression by the expanding clot and inflammation. Neovascularization and granulation tissue replace the clot and fibroblasts infiltrate to begin producing new tendon collagen. Initially new collagen is primarily Type III, which is relatively weak; gradually Type I, or normal tendon collagen replaces, but never completely, the less functional Type III collagen. Finally, the collagen fibers reorient along primary stress lines, resulting in a repaired tendon that can withstand the forces incurred in athletic work. The entire process of inflammation, repair, and functional remodeling requires 8 to 11 months; remodeling may continue for several years.

CLINICAL SIGNS. Tendinitis causes lameness occurring either immediately in cases of severe tendon disruption, or within 48 hours in less severe cases, as edema and expanding clot cause compression and pain. In mild to moderate cases, lameness resolves with 3 to 5 days of rest, recurring when the horse is returned to full work. Pain, heat, and swelling are present in the affected tendon regions. In cases of very proximal tendinitis, involving the carpal sheath (tenosynovitis), the horse may stand with the carpus in partial flexion and distention of the carpal sheath may be palpated. In the mid-metacarpal region, the flexor tendons are enclosed by peritenon rather than a sheath; this thin vascular membrane often becomes thick and painful in cases of tendinitis. Tendinitis at the level of the palmar annular ligament may be complicated by compression of the affected tendon by this constricting structure, resulting in a characteristic bulging of the tendon at the proximal border of the annular ligament, and notching where the ligament is compressing the swollen tendon. Tendinitis occurring within the digital sheath is often accompanied by inflammation and effusion of the sheath, causing pain on fetlock flexion. Tendinitis of the distal branches of the SDF tendon causes pastern swelling and pain on palpation of the branches, particularly at insertion on P2. Deep digital flexor tendinitis results in swelling and pain on palpation over the palmar aspects of P1 and P2. Pain, heat, and swelling subside at the end of the inflammatory phase, but long before significant tendon repair has occurred, often resulting in a return to work and recurrent tendinitis. In human athletes the term tendinitis refers to a primary injury, and is differentiated from tendinosis, which results from recurrent injury. In tendinosis, the fibroblasts degenerate through repeated trauma, resulting in the inability to produce normal new repair collagen; these patients have a poorer prognosis for return to athletic endeavors. The same syndrome probably occurs in horses, therefore it is important to detect primary tendinitis and to allow sufficient time for primary tendon injury to be repaired before return to work.

DIAGNOSIS. Until tendinitis is severe, clinical signs of lameness, heat, and swelling often resolve if the patient is given a few days of rest, particularly when accompanied by such antiinflammatory therapy as NSAIDs and local cold application. Lameness, if present, can be eliminated with a proximal metacarpal nerve block. Careful palpation of the affected tendon will often reveal localized pain and swelling, even in the absence of lameness. Because tendinitis often results in subtle clinical signs, any change should be viewed with suspicion. Definitive diagnosis is provided by ultrasonographic examination of the affected structures. Cross-sectional and longitudinal images should be obtained to detect changes in tendon size, echogenicity, and fiber pattern, as well as the presence of discrete core lesions.[253-259] Acute core lesions will present as black or anechoic areas within the affected tendon, representing hemorrhage and loss of fibers; over time, as healing occurs, tendon swelling will decrease, and core lesions will become more echoic. Some cases of tendinitis will present as diffuse, hypoechoic, and swollen tendon regions without discrete core lesions. Progression of tendon healing may also be monitored with ultrasound. As lesions resolve, tendon size decreases, and fiber pattern improves toward normal, linear array.

TREATMENT. Medical treatment is initially aimed at reduction of inflammation and prevention of further tendon damage. For cases of mild to moderate tendon damage, treatments include stall rest and gradually increasing hand walking, NSAIDs, and local cold application. One or two doses of short-acting systemic corticosteroids may be useful to limit swelling of the affected tendon. A course of systemic polysulfated glycosaminoglycan, 500 mg administered at 4-day intervals for a total of 7 doses, has been shown to be of value in treatment of acute tendinitis.[260]

Surgical treatment is useful for several types of tendon injury. Acute core lesions can be decompressed through stab incisions (tendon splitting). Incisions should be oriented to penetrate the core hematoma, yet disturb as little normal tendon as possible; ultrasound guidance is helpful to achieve this aim. Tendon splitting is useful from 1 to 21 days postinjury; after this time the lesion clot is organized and attempts at decompression are ineffective. Severe tendinitis in the distal metacarpal region may be exacerbated by tendon compression by the palmar annular ligament. This syndrome can cause severe pain and impede tendon healing. Transection of the ligament increases patient comfort and allows tendon healing to proceed at a normal pace.[261]

Based on the theory that tendon damage results in functional shortening of the affected tendon through scar formation, proximal check ligament desmotomy can be performed to attempt to allow tendon lengthening during work. Reports indicate an improvement in prognosis for return to athletic use with reduced incidence of recurrent tendinitis following surgery in Standardbred racehorses.[262] However, other surveys have indicated that superior check desmotomy did not appear to offer an advantage over nonsurgical treatment in preventing recurrent or new injuries in Thoroughbred racehorses. Also, horses undergoing superior check desmotomy appeared to be at 5.5 times greater risk of developing suspensory ligament injuries than horses managed nonsurgically.[263]

For severe cases of tendinitis, in which sufficient tendon damage has occurred to permit partial dropping of the fetlock, a support shoe that extends caudally can be helpful. To be effective, such a shoe should extend to the level of the fetlock and can be elevated 2 to 4 cm. An elevated shoe without caudal extension to the level of the fetlock increases tension on the superficial digital flexor tendon and is contraindicated. For deep digital flexor tendon injuries, heel elevation can be helpful to reduce tendon tension initially. Healing progress should be carefully monitored and elevation decreased accordingly to prevent long-term functional shortening of the deep flexor tendon.

Stall rest with hand walking should be continued for 60 days; at that time, if ultrasonographic examination reveals a reduction in tendon size, partial resolution of core lesion(s), and an improvement in fiber pattern, exercise can be gradually increased. Ultrasonographic examinations at 60-day intervals will allow the amount of exercise to be tailored to tendon healing and provide the best opportunity for return to athletic use. Time to return to full work averages 7 to 9 months. Pasture turnout is contraindicated until a substantial amount of healing has occurred and tendon strength is judged to be nearly normal; if turnout is initiated too soon, incomplete tendon healing (caused by repetitive damage) may persist indefinitely.

PROGNOSIS. Return to athletic use depends on the severity of tendon injury. Reported incidence of successful (5 race starts) return to racing was 58% for severe injuries, 66% for moderate injuries, and 64% for mild tendinitis.[264] Another survey revealed that 70% of horses with SDF tendon branch lesions were able to return to previous use without reinjury.[265] Although severe tendinitis may prevent a return to uses such as racing or eventing, which require maximal effort on the part of the horse, many such patients will heal with tendon scar that can withstand the stress of pleasure riding. A potential complication of moderately severe to severe SDF tendinitis is the long-term formation of adhesions between the SDF tendon and the accessory ligament of the deep flexor tendon; this occurrence results in a poor prognosis for soundness.[266]

Whatever athletic use is desired, it is important to bear in mind that the initial injury is often the result of fatigue and that the repaired tendon will always contain a varying amount of scar and result in less than optimal tendon function. Because of these considerations, future training should be conducted in a manner designed to prevent excessive fatigue, meaning graduated exercise programs without sudden, marked increases in speed or in amount of work.

REFERENCES

253. Palmer SE, Genovese R, Longo KL, et al: Practical management of superficial digital flexor tendinitis in the performance horse, *Vet Clin North Am (Equine Pract)* 10:425-480, 1994.
254. Marr CM, McMillan I, Boyd JS, Wright NG, Murray M: Superficial digital flexor tendon injuries in National Hunt and Point-to-Point racehorses: factors affecting the clinical outcome, *Vet Rec* 132:476-479, 1993.
255. Genovese RL, Rantanen NW, Simpson BS, et al: Clinical experience with quantitative analysis of superficial digital flexor tendon injuries in Thoroughbred and Standardbred racehorses, *Vet Clin North Am (Equine Pract)* 6:129-147, 1990.
256. Genovese RL: Prognosis of superficial flexor tendon and suspensory ligament injuries, *Proc 39th Ann Am Assoc Equine Pract* 39:17-19, 1993.
257. Dyson SJ: Ultrasonographic examination of the metacarpal and metatarsal regions in the horse, *Eq Vet Ed* 4:139-144, 1992.
258. Genovese RL, Rantanen NW, Hauser ML, et al: Diagnostic ultrasonography of equine limbs, *Vet Clin North Am (Equine Pract)* 2:145-226, 1986.
259. Dyson SJ, Dik, KJ: Miscellaneous conditions of tendons, tendon sheaths, and ligaments, *Vet Clin North Am (Equine Pract)* 11(2):315-337, 1995.
260. Dow SM, Wilson AM, Goodship AE: Treatment of acute superficial digital flexor tendon injury in horses with polysulphated glycosaminoglycan, *Vet Rec* 139(17):413-416, 1996.
261. Dik KJ, Dyson SJ, Vail TB: Aseptic tenosynovitis of the digital flexor tendon sheath, fetlock and pastern annular ligament constriction, *Vet Clin North Am (Equine Pract)* 11(2):151-162, 1995.
262. Hogan PM, Bramlage LR: Transection of the accessory ligament of the superficial digital flexor tendon for treatment of tendinitis: long-term results in 61 standardbred racehorses (1985-1992), *Equine Vet J* 27(3): 221-226,1995.
263. Gibson KT, Burbidge HM, Pfeiffer DU: Superficial digital flexor tendinitis in thoroughbred race horses: outcome following non-surgical treatment and superior check desmotomy, *Aust Vet J* 75(9):631-635, 1997.
264. Genovese RL, Rantanen NW, Simpson BS, et al: Clinical experience with quantitative analysis of superficial digital flexor tendon injuries in Thoroughbred and Standardbred racehorses, *Vet Clin North Am (Equine Pract)* 6:129-145, 1990.
265. Gibson KT, Burbidge HM, Anderson BH: Tendinitis of the branches of insertion of the superficial digital flexor tendon in horses, *Aust Vet J* 75(4):253-256, 1997.
266. McDiarmid A: Acquired flexural deformity of the metacarpophalangeal joint in five horses associated with tendinous damage in the palmar metacarpus, *Vet Rec* 144(17):475-478, 1999.

SUSPENSORY LIGAMENT DESMITIS

CAROL L. GILLIS

DEFINITION AND ETIOLOGY. The suspensory ligament, also named the interosseous muscle, originates on the proximal palmar aspect of the third metacarpal (metatarsal) bone and divides into medial and lateral branches, which insert on the respective proximal sesamoid bones. The suspensory ligament acts to limit the range of extension of the fetlock. Desmitis is the result of inflammation and tearing of ligament fibers. The pathophysiology of suspensory ligament damage and repair is similar to that of the superficial digital flexor tendon (see preceding section on Tendinitis). Severe desmitis or disruption of the ligament results in partial dropping of the fetlock and severe lameness. Twenty-five percent of horses with suspensory ligament (SL) desmitis also have apical fractures of the sesamoid bones, avulsion fractures of the proximal palmar third metacarpal bone, or fractures of the distal third of the small metacarpal bones.[267]

The SL branches are more frequently affected than the body. Left and right limbs are equally likely to sustain damage. Forelimb injuries are more common than those in the hindlimb. Equine athletes that perform at a sustained rapid trot, such as Standardbred racehorses and endurance horses, injure the suspensory ligament more frequently than other tendons or ligaments. Horses in other athletic pursuits that involve galloping injure the superficial digital flexor tendon most often, apparently because of stress increases; however, all types of performance horses are susceptible to SL injury.[268,269]

CLINICAL SIGNS. Mild to moderate SL desmitis causes clinical signs of lameness, average Grade II/V, which often persists over months duration if the horse is continued in work or tried at work intermittently. Suspensory ligament branch lesions demonstrate swelling, heat, and pain on palpation, which are readily detected on clinical examination. Lesions of the SL body are more difficult to diagnose because of the location of the SL, surrounded by the metacarpal bones, and deep to other soft tissue structures. Deep palpation for 1 to 2 minutes followed by observation of the horse in motion is a useful stress test to detect SL body desmitis. Lameness caused by SL body desmitis, particularly near the site of origin, may not be abolished by a high metacarpal nerve block; either infiltration of local anesthetic directly around the SL origin, or local anesthesia of the median and ulnar (or tibial) nerves may be required for proximal SL anesthesia.[270,271]

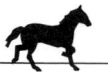

Severe SL desmitis results in extensive swelling in the metacarpal region, Grade IV/V to V/V lameness, and partial fetlock dropping, or hyperextension. Fractures of the apical portions of the proximal sesamoid bones are associated with extensive SL desmitis and acute, marked lameness. Fractures of the small metacarpal bones, in association with SL branch desmitis, produce local swelling, often in the form of pitting edema, pain on palpation, and acute, moderate lameness. Proximal palmar third metacarpal avulsion fractures are often of small size and are buried deep to the SL origin; they often produce clinical signs dependent primarily on the extent of associated SL injury.

DIAGNOSIS. Ultrasonography is the most useful tool to diagnose SL desmitis. Cross-sectional and longitudinal views should be obtained to evaluate the SL body and branches, from the SL origin on proximal palmar MCIII to branch insertions on the respective sesamoid bones, for changes in size, echogenicity, and fiber pattern.[270,272-274] Generalized diffuse desmitis, detected ultrasonographically as an increase in ligament size and a loss of echogenicity and normal parallel fiber pattern, is more common than are discrete core lesions, particularly in the SL branches. Fractures of the sesamoid bones and small metacarpal bones can also be seen on ultrasonographic examination and confirmed radiographically. Conversely, whenever these fractures are detected radiographically, an ultrasonographic examination should be performed to evaluate the suspensory ligament because severity of SL desmitis affects fracture prognosis. Proximal palmar MCIII avulsion fractures are more readily diagnosed ultrasonographically than radiographically because they are often small in size. Nuclear scintigraphy can be used to confirm the diagnosis and to monitor fracture healing. Ultrasound will also provide fracture healing information, as callus forms and is remodeled.

TREATMENT. Suspensory ligament desmitis therapy should include an initial period of 3 weeks of NSAIDs, local cold therapy, and stall rest with hand walking. If inflammation is severe, a short course of systemic steroids may be helpful. If an acute (1- to 14-day duration) core lesion is detected with ultrasonographic examination as an anechoic or very hypoechoic region, decompression of the lesion hematoma by percutaneous ligament splitting is indicated. Small stab incisions that disturb as little normal ligament as possible will result in an optimal outcome. Ultrasound examinations at 60-day intervals allow evaluation of SL healing progress as evidenced by decreasing ligament size and improvement in echogenicity and fiber pattern. Exercise is tailored to ligament healing to provide the best chance to return to full work without recurrence of desmitis. In general, 7 to 9 months are required for suspensory ligament damage to heal sufficiently such that the animal can withstand the forces generated by full work.

Surgical treatment is indicated for apical sesamoid fractures and for some small metacarpal bone fractures. Apical sesamoid fractures involving one third or less of the sesamoid body should be carefully removed, traumatizing the remaining SL branch attachment as little as possible. An initial period of stall rest is followed by hand walking; exercise is gradually increased based on ultrasonographic evidence of SL branch healing. Proximal palmar MCIII fractures respond to conservative treatment and tend to heal at a similar rate to the SL origin. Fractures of the distal third of the small metacarpal bones can be surgically removed; concomitant SL branch desmitis is then monitored for healing. Proximal small metacarpal bone fractures are occasionally encountered in association with SL body desmitis; these must be approached with caution as removal of proximal portions may result in instability of the carpus or tarsus.

PROGNOSIS. Approximately 55% of all horses with SL desmitis return to their original use. Of these, most racehorses compete at a lower level than before the injury whereas horses in other athletic uses usually return to their previous level of competition. Sesamoid fractures that involve a large part of the SL branch attachment carry a poor prognosis for return to racing; 28% of Thoroughbred racehorses in one retrospective study of 19 cases were able to do so.[267] Standardbred racehorses have a better prognosis for return to racing following apical sesamoid fracture.[275] Suspensory ligament body desmitis located in the hind limb adversely affects prognosis; 38% of these cases returned to their prior use. It has been proposed that the large size of proximal MTIV restricts swelling of the damaged SL body, creating compression necrosis of the ligament and chronic pain. Hind limb lameness caused by SL body desmitis may not be diagnosed until the ligament damage is severe or chronic, which also contributes to a decreased chance for successful return to performance. Earlier diagnosis combined with aggressive antiinflammatory therapy may improve the percentage of patients that are able to compete as intended.

The method of rehabilitation has a significant impact on the prognosis for return to performance. Follow-up on 230 cases of SL desmitis revealed that 68% of horses in a controlled exercise program returned to their intended use whereas only 50% of those with 2 to 3 months of stall confinement followed by pasture turnout were able to do so.[267]

REFERENCES

267. Gillis CL, Meagher DM, Balesdent A: Suspensory ligament desmitis and associated fractures, *Proc 40th Ann Am Assoc Equine Pract* 40:187-188, 1994.
268. Biewener AA: Muscle-tendon stresses and elastic energy storage during locomotion in the horse, *Comp Biochem and Physiol Part B, Biochem Molec Biol* 120(1):73-87, 1998.
269. Patterson-Kane JC, Firth EC, Parry DA, Wilson AM, Goodship AE: Effects of training on collagen fibril populations in the suspensory ligament and deep digital flexor tendon of young thoroughbreds, *Am J Vet Res* 59(1):64-68, 1998.
270. Dyson SJ: Proximal suspensory ligament desmitis: clinical, ultrasonographic and radiographic features, *Equine Vet J* 25:25-31, 1991.
271. Keg PR, Schamhardt HC, van Weeren PR, Barneveld A: The effect of the high palmar nerve block and the ulnar nerve block on lameness provoked by acollagenase-induced tendinitis of the lateral branch of the suspensory ligament, *Vet Q* 18 (Suppl) 2:S103-105, 1996.
272. Genovese RL, Rantanen NW, Hauser Ml, et al: Diagnostic ultrasonography of equine limbs, *Vet Clin North Am (Equine Pract)* 2:145-226, 1986.
273. Marr CM: The differential diagnosis of soft tissue swelling of the palmar aspect of the metacarpal region, *Eq Vet Ed* 4:292-300, 1992.
274. Dyson SJ: Ultrasonographic examination of the metacarpal and metatarsal regions in the horse, *Eq Vet Ed* 4:139-142, 1992.
275. Spurlock GH, Gabel AA: Apical fractures of the proximal sesamoid bones in 109 Standardbred horses, *J Am Vet Med Assoc* 1:76-79, 1983.

FRACTURES

LAURIE A. McDUFFEE
K.C. KENT LLOYD

The practicing veterinarian plays an important role in the treatment of fracture patients. Knowledge of the fundamentals of fracture diagnosis, available treatment options, and prognostication are essential to advise clients appropriately. Proficiency in emergency treatment of the patient and temporary stabilization of the fracture enhances the prognosis. Surgical principles and strategies are not discussed here but can be found in other texts specializing in these areas.

DEFINITION AND ETIOLOGY. This section is concerned with (1) acute catastrophic long bone fractures that result in non–weight-bearing lameness and that often are life threatening, and (2) nondisplaced or incomplete fractures that may become complete fractures if undiagnosed and untreated. A single traumatic event is a common cause of acute complete and incomplete fractures. Stress fractures, which are also incomplete fractures, are the result of fatigue and microdamage associated with the cyclic loading of rigorous training schedules (e.g., race training). Concurrent nutritional, infectious, and neoplastic factors can play a role in other types of fractures (e.g., pathologic fractures).

CLINICAL SIGNS AND DIFFERENTIAL DIAGNOSES. Fracture should be considered a differential diagnosis for any horse with a non-weight-bearing lameness. The fracture configuration may be complete and displaced, complete and nondisplaced, or incomplete. A complete systemic examination is important to assess the animal's overall condition and to identify all areas of trauma. Many complete catastrophic fractures of a distal extremity are readily identified by postural deformation and limb instability. Limbs should be examined closely for evidence of soft-tissue trauma, including trauma to vessels and nerves. Luxation or subluxation should be considered with instability and/or deformation near an articulation. Physeal fractures should be considered in young animals.

Complete displaced fractures of a proximal extremity or incomplete fractures may not be immediately obvious. Complete fractures of bones surrounded by a large muscle mass such as the humerus or femur result in non–weight-bearing lameness, soft-tissue swelling, and crepitus during limb manipulation. Nondisplaced or incomplete fractures as a result of an acute traumatic event may be associated with a wound, and pain may be elicited during manual palpation. Horses having a history of trauma to a long bone, such as being kicked by another horse, require radiographs of the bone to determine the presence of an incomplete fracture. Undiagnosed incomplete fractures in such cases often become complete displaced fractures if the animal is allowed unrestricted exercise.

Stress fractures may result in moderate to severe lameness or intermittent lameness that improves with rest. Pain is often elicited from discrete areas of the bone when it is manually palpated. Sites of stress fractures in race horses include the metacarpus (dorsal, middiaphyseal, and distolateral cortices), humerus (proximocaudal and distal craniomedial cortices), tibia (proximolateral, caudal middiaphyseal, and distolateral cortices), pelvis (wing of the ilium near the tuber sacrale), and the scapula (neck). Stress fractures may be diagnosed by radiographs or nuclear scintigraphy.

CLINICAL EVALUATION. Radiography is useful to confirm the presence of a fracture; however, it may be unnecessary if a fracture is evident and the owner has no intention of treating the animal. Radiographs provide information about the fracture, which is essential for determining an accurate prognosis including: fracture position, configuration, and degree of comminution; articular involvement; physeal involvement; and cortical bone loss that may impede anatomic reduction. An open fracture, of a nondiaphyseal location with comminution, articular involvement, and bone loss, has the worst prognosis. Complete nondisplaced or incomplete fractures may not be visible on radiographs at the time of injury. Radiographs taken 10 to 14 days after injury enhance the likelihood of visualization of these fractures.

Stress fractures are recognized radiographically by the presence of either an incomplete cortical fracture, endosteal callus, or periosteal callus; however, they may not be visible on conventional radiographs until either resorption occurs along the fracture line or callus formation is substantial. Scintigraphy (bone scanning) is useful for the identification of acute stress fractures, which appear as a "hot spot" or focal concentration of a bone-seeking radiolabel in an area of active inflammation or bone remodeling. Scintigraphy can be performed with the animal under sedation and is available at large referral and university hospitals.

PATHOPHYSIOLOGY OF BONE HEALING. Fractured bones can heal by primary or secondary bone healing. Absolute anatomic reduction and stability, which are necessary for primary bone healing, are difficult to achieve in large animal fracture repair. Because of the weight of the animal, there is often micromovement at the fracture site even when rigid internal fixation is attained; therefore primary bone healing in large animals is uncommon.

Secondary bone healing proceeds in several stages: development of a hematoma, formation of granulation tissue, and a transition to cartilaginous tissue that undergoes endochondral ossification. The progression of these stages depends on a viable vascular supply as well as stability and stiffness at the fracture gap. If the soft tissues and blood supply are devitalized or stability is inadequate, healing will not progress. Local infection is potentiated by a poor blood supply and will impede healing and cause loosening of implants, leading to instability. It is essential that soft tissues are preserved, infection is prevented or treated aggressively, and stabilization is adequate for fracture healing.

TREATMENT AND PROGNOSIS. Treatment options currently available for large-animal fracture repair include conservative, nonsurgical treatment including external coaptation and stall rest or surgical stabilization including external fixation and internal fixation. Incomplete and stress fractures are treated with stall rest, but these fractures must be recognized and appropriately managed to prevent progression to catastrophic fracture. Some nondisplaced complete humeral and femoral fractures in foals and calves may heal with stall rest. Most other fractures require some form of stabilization. Ruminants are more amenable to fracture repair with nonrigid methods of stabilization including external coaptation. Horses of any size tend to require external or internal fixation for adequate stability.

In general, fractures in ruminants have more treatment options and a better prognosis compared to those in horses. Most ruminants have a temperament amenable to immobilization, are less susceptible to secondary problems such as laminitis, and do not require complete soundness for a successful outcome.[276] The successful use of external fixation for ruminant fracture repair is increasing. External fixation provides improved stability compared to external coaptation, while remaining more economical than internal fixation.[276a-279] Open fractures and comminuted fractures occur less commonly in ruminants than in horses; but when they are present, they carry the poorest prognosis.

In general, horses have a significantly lower survival rate than ruminants because they are less likely to protect the injured limb, are predisposed to complications in the contralateral limb, and have fractures that are often not amenable to external coaptation alone or in conjunction with internal fixation; in addition, internal fixation is often associated with infection, which impedes bone healing.[280] Because horses often are used as athletes, fracture repair that results in survival but not in soundness may not be a desirable treatment option.

Young, light-weight animals have a better prognosis than heavy adult animals because of the propensity toward simple fracture configurations, suitable strength of implants, and more rapid bone healing. Fractures in adult horses are often comminuted as a result of high-energy trauma. Severely comminuted fractures that cannot be anatomically reduced in the proximal aspect of the limb of adult horses are not amenable to treatment. Available implants cannot withstand the weight of an adult horse without load sharing by the reconstructed bone or additional support from external coaptation.

Recently, intramedullary interlocking nails are being used as a type of internal fixation for large animal fracture repair.[281,282] Interlocking nails can be placed in a manner similar to intramedullary pins with little disruption to the soft tissues; however, biomechanically interlocking nails are superior to intramedullary pins in resisting torsional and com-

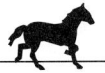

pressive forces placed on the bone. Expanded use of interlocking nails in large animal fracture repair may result in improved prognosis for certain fractures such as humeral, femoral, and third metacarpal bone fractures.

Treatment options and prognosis for fracture of the individual bones are mentioned below (Table 36-5). The likelihood for survival and for soundness usually varies with treatment method for each fracture.

Humerus. The humerus often fractures in a long oblique or spiral configuration. In cattle and horses, humeral frac-

tures have been treated conservatively and surgically. Surgical repair includes internal fixation with one or two dynamic compression plates (DCPs), intramedullary (IM) pins, and interlocking nails. Small ruminants and foals can be treated conservatively with stall confinement and/or Thomas splints when there is minimal displacement or overriding associated with the fracture.

The prognosis for ruminant humeral fractures is variable, depending on size and age of the animal. A calf or goat will have a better prognosis with any option compared to a large

TABLE 36-5

Splinting Techniques, Treatment Options and Prognosis for Common Fractures in Large Domestic Animals

Species/ Age	Fracture Configurations	Emergency Splint	Treatment Options	Prognosis
HUMERUS				
Horse	Comminuted, physeal (young adult)	Not applicable	Stall confinement, sling, IM stacked pins	Poor
Foal	Long oblique or spiral	Not applicable	Stall confinement	Fair
			DCPs	Fair to good
			IM pins and cerclage	Not reported
			Interlocking nail	Fair
Cattle	Spiral or oblique	Not applicable	Pen confinement	Fair to poor
			DCPs	Fair to poor
			Interlocking nail	Fair to poor
Calf	Spiral or oblique	Not applicable	Pen confinement	Fair to good
			Thomas-Schroeder splint	Fair to good
			DCPs	Fair to good
			IM pins	Fair to good
			Interlocking nail	Fair to good
RADIUS				
Horse	Comminuted	Robert-Jones bandage with a caudal splint up to the elbow and a lateral splint up to the withers	DCPs	Poor
	Oblique nondisplaced	Not applicable	Tie stall	Good
Foal	Transverse or short oblique	Robert-Jones bandage with a caudal splint up to the elbow and a lateral splint up to the withers	DCPs	Good
Cattle, calf	Transverse or short oblique	Robert-Jones bandage with a caudal splint up to the elbow and a lateral splint up to the withers	External coaptation, external fixation, internal fixation	Good
ULNA				
Horse	Transverse, oblique, comminuted	Splint carpus in extension	Stall confinement (nondisplaced)	Good
			Tension band plate	Good
Foal	Physeal, transverse, oblique	Splint carpus in extension	Tension band plate, screws and Figure 8 wire	Good
LARGE METACARPAL/METATARSAL BONES				
Horse	Diaphyseal	Wrap with dorsal (forelimb) or planter (hindlimb) splint and cast material	DCPs, Nunamaker external skeletal fixator, cast, cast and transfixation pins	Poor
Foal	Diaphyseal	Wrap with dorsal (forelimb) or planter (hindlimb) splint and cast material	DCPs, cast, cast and transfixation pins	Fair to poor
Cattle	Diaphyseal		Cast, cast and transfixation pins	Good
Calf	Diaphyseal		Cast, cast and transfixation pins	Excellent
PROXIMAL PHALANX				
Horse	Simple	Wrap with dorsal (forelimb) or planter (hindlimb) splint and cast material, Kimsey splint	Lag screw fixation	Good
	Comminuted	Wrap with dorsal (forelimb) or planter (hindlimb) splint and cast material, Kimsey splint, cast	DCP, Nunamaker external skeletal fixator, cast and transfixation pins	Poor
Cattle	Simple, comminuted	Definitive treatment	Block on opposite claw, cast	Good

DCP, Dorsal compression plate; *IM*, intramedullary.

Continued

TABLE 36-5

Splinting Techniques, Treatment Options and Prognosis for Common Fractures in Large Domestic Animals—cont'd

Species/ Age	Fracture Configurations	Emergency Splint	Treatment Options	Prognosis
MIDDLE PHALANX				
Horse	Palmar/plantar eminence	Wrap with dorsal (forelimb) or planter (hindlimb) splint and cast material, Kimsey splint, cast	Lag screw fixation, cast	Poor
	Comminuted	Wrap with dorsal (forelimb) or planter (hindlimb) splint and cast material, Kimsey splint, cast	Arthrodesis Cast, cast and transfixation pins, Nunamaker external skeletal fixator	Good Poor
DISTAL PHALANX				
Horse, foal	Simple	Definitive treatment	Bar shoe with clips	Good (nonarticular)
			Cast	Fair to good (articular)
Cattle, calf	Simple, comminuted	Definitive treatment	Lag screw (adult) Wooden block on opposite claw, amputation, cast	Fair to good Good
FEMUR				
Horse		Not applicable	DCPs	Grave
Foal	Proximal physeal	Not applicable	IM pins, cancellous bone screws, dynamic hip screw plate, femoral head and neck ostectomy	Poor
	Diaphyseal	Not applicable	DCPs	Fair to poor
	Distal physeal	Not applicable	Stall confinement	Fair
Cattle	Proximal physeal	Not applicable	Femoral head and neck ostectomy	Good
	Diaphyseal	Not applicable	DCP	Good
Calf	Proximal physeal	Not applicable	Pen confinement, IM pins, Cancellous bone screws, femoral head and neck ostectomy	Good
	Diaphyseal	Not applicable	DCPs, IM pins Interlocking nail	Good Fair
TIBIA				
Horse	Simple or comminuted diaphyseal	Robert-Jones bandage with medial splint up to stifle and lateral splint up to the hip	DCPs	Grave
Foal	Proximal physeal	Robert-Jones bandage with medial splint up to stifle and lateral splint up to the hip	Stall confinement (nondisplaced), DCP	Good
	Diaphyseal	Robert-Jones bandage with medial splint up to stifle and lateral splint up to the hip	Cross pin fixation DCPs	Fair Good
Cattle, calf	Diaphyseal	Modified Thomas splint	Modified Thomas splint, cast, external fixation; DCPs	Good

adult cow or bull. A larger number of successful cases have been reported for ruminants than for horses.

In horses the prognosis depends on the fracture configuration, age and weight of the animal, and method of repair.[283,284] In general the prognosis for young horses with simple fractures is fair to guarded. Adult horses with humeral fractures are not amenable to treatment with current fixation techniques.

Radius and Ulna. Radial and ulnar fractures in young and old ruminants repaired with external or internal fixation have a reported 86% survival rate.[285] These fractures have been repaired with a modified Thomas splint, external fixator and cast,[279] bone plates, cast alone, or cast and transfixation pins.

Radial fractures in horses less than 2 years old have been repaired with two DCPs with a success rate of 80%, but in adult horses these fractures tend to be comminuted and are more difficult to stabilize, resulting in a poor prognosis.[286]

Ulnar fractures are the most common traction physeal fracture seen in foals.[287] Ulnar fractures vary in configuration; however, most are treated with internal fixation with a bone plate applied as a tension band. The prognosis for repair of ulnar fractures is good, with 62% to 76% of horses of all ages returning to function.[288]

Femur. Femoral fractures in calves are most commonly diaphyseal fractures, whereas those in foals are more often proximal physeal fractures. Calves subjected to forced extrac-

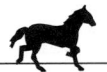

tion from the cow are predisposed to both fracture configurations. Proximal femoral physeal fractures in calves have been treated with IM pins and by femoral head and neck ostectomy, with both resulting in functional animals. Diaphyseal femoral fractures in calves have been repaired with internal fixation using IM pins with or without cerclage wires or with bone plates. Neonatal calves treated with IM pins healed with an 83% success rate.[279]

Proximal femoral physeal fractures are the most common pressure physeal fractures in foals. These fractures have been repaired with IM pins, cancellous bone screws, and dynamic hip screw plates and by femoral head and neck ostectomy, but the prognosis remains poor. Diaphyseal fractures in foals repaired with two DCPs have a 50% survival rate, with only 65% of the survivors having athletic potential.[289]

Recently, experimental diaphyseal femoral fractures in foals have been repaired with interlocking nails with reasonable success.[281]

Although internal fixation with two bone provides the greatest stability for fracture repair at this time, this technique is difficult to use for femoral fracture stablization in heavily muscled adult horses.

Tibia. Tibial fractures in ruminants have been repaired successfully with a modified Thomas splint, external fixator, cast with transfixation pins, and DCPs with good results. Calves with tibial fractures repaired with transfixation pins and cast material had an 81% success rate.[278] Adult cattle with tibial fractures repaired with external fixation had a 64% success rate, while those treated conservatively had a 44% success rate.[290] In foals with diaphyseal fractures, DCP-repaired tibia have the best prognosis, but complications and prolonged hospitalization are common.[291] An external fixator has been used to repair diaphyseal osteotomies in research foals successfully.[292] Proximal physeal fractures have a good prognosis when repaired with internal fixation.

In adult horses DCPs can be used successfully with simple anatomically reducible tibial fractures. Nonreconstructable comminuted fractures cannot be repaired with current techniques. Because the tibia lacks circumferential soft-tissue coverage, fractures are often open and contaminated. Coupled with a limited extraosseous blood supply and the presence of implants, they are particularly susceptible to infection. Accordingly, the prognosis for adult horses is currently poor.

Metacarpus and Metatarsus. Third and fourth metacarpal and metatarsal (cannon) bone fractures are common in ruminants and have a good prognosis. Distal physeal fractures may result from forced extraction of calves during a dystocia. These fractures can be reduced closed and immobilized with a half limb cast with excellent results. Closed fractures in adult ruminants can be treated with cast immobilization alone or combined with transfixation pins, or DCPs.[277,293]

In horses third metacarpal and metatarsal fractures are often open with devitalized soft tissues, limiting the prognosis. Infection rates have been reported as high as 68% postoperatively.[294] In young lightweight animals a cast, cast with transfixation pins, or cast with transfixation pins and a walking bar may be successful.[295] If closed, the fracture is best repaired with DCPs and a cast. Adult cannon bone fractures have been repaired using DCPs combined with a cast and with external fixation. In one study of 25 in horses of all ages, cannon bone fractures repaired with internal fixation or external fixation had a 67% success rate.[294]

Phalanges. Fractures of a proximal or middle phalanx are easier to treat in cattle than in horses because weight on the limb can be supported by the remaining digit in ruminants. A wooden block applied to the claw of the intact digit or cast immobilization share good success. In horses phalangeal fractures vary in configuration, which greatly influences the prognosis. Proximal phalangeal fractures with an intact strut

of bone are amenable to internal fixation with large screws alone or combined with a DCP. Rate of patient survival is good; however, athletic function is related to the ability to achieve articular surface congruency and minimize subsequent degenerative joint disease. In a review of 59 cases of simple sagittal fractures in racehorses, 61% of standardbred racehorses and 75% of thoroughbred racehorses returned to racing.[296]

Comminuted proximal phalangeal fractures without an intact strut of bone result in collapse of the bony column of the limb with compressive forces. The fracture fragments traumatize the soft tissue and blood supply in the area, predisposing the bone and soft tissue to infection. Comminuted proximal phalangeal fractures have been repaired using external fixation, including casts and transfixation pins or the Nunamaker external skeletal fixator, and with DCPs. The repair can result in survival of the animal with pasture soundness.[297]

Fractures of the middle phalanx are usually either palmar/plantar eminence fractures or comminuted fractures. Palmar/plantar eminence fractures may be treated successfully by arthrodesis of the proximal interphalangeal joint using internal fixation. Return to intended use is reported as 50% and 80% for front and hind limb fractures, respectively. Comminuted middle phalangeal fractures often collapse and incur soft-tissue trauma; however, these fractures may heal with a cast alone, unlike similar proximal phalangeal fractures. Resistance to axial loading is best achieved by stabilization with a cast and transfixation pins or with the Nunamaker external skeletal fixator. The probable outcome for horses with comminuted fractures is salvage only.

EMERGENCY TREATMENT. If the fracture and soft tissues are deemed amenable to repair, institution of emergency treatment can prevent further bone and soft tissue damage and optimize the success of treatment. Treatment for shock should be instituted if necessary. Broad-spectrum antibiotics and analgesics should be initiated, and local debridement of the wound, when dealing with open fractures, completed if the animal is tractable.

Immobilization is essential to preserve the vasculature to the distal extremity. Splinting techniques for immobilization are designed to neutralize the damaging forces acting on the fractured limb and can usually be accomplished with the standing animal. General recommendations[298] for splinting fractures in different regions of the limb are delineated in Table 36-5.

Shoulder and Arm. Fractures of the scapula, humerus, and elbow region are protected by muscle coverage, reducing the need for a splint to protect the fracture site. If the triceps muscle apparatus is disabled, a splint that supports the carpus in an extended position can aid the horse in controlling the limb.

Forearm Region. Fractures of the mid and proximal radius should be stabilized with a Robert Jones bandage and a lateral splint that extends from the ground to the withers. The extension of this splint proximal to the elbow is critical to prevent the splinted limb distal to the fracture site from acting as a pendulum around a fulcrum at the fracture site, causing additional damage to the fracture site. A caudal splint should also be applied.

Carpal Region. Fractures in the area of the distal radius to the distal metacarpus are best immobilized with a Robert Jones bandage and external splints. The bandage and splints should span the length of the forelimb from the elbow to the hoof. Two splints, placed caudal and lateral, provide adequate support.

Distal Extremity. Splinting of the distal extremity for fractures of the distal portion of the metacarpus and phalanges can consist of a light wrap, splint, and cast material. A splint along the dorsal (metacarpus) or plantar (metatarsus) aspect

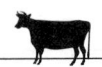

of the limb should align the bones in a straight column, neutralizing the bending forces at the fracture and at the fetlock joint. In young animals a heavy wrap and splint may be applied without cast material.

Femur. Fractures of the femur, like those of the humerus, are protected by the musculature of the proximal limb and do not require splinting.

Tibia. Fractures of the tibia tend to result in overriding fragments with flexion of the stifle because of the reciprocal apparatus. Because the muscles covering the tibia are located cranially and laterally, muscle contraction results in limb abduction and penetration of bone fragments through soft tissues on the medial aspect of the tibia. To counteract these forces, a lateral splint should be placed over a Robert Jones bandage. The splint should extend proximally to the hip to prevent the fracture site from acting as a fulcrum and the splinted distal limb from acting as a pendulum. If materials are available, a double metal splint that follows the contour of the limb is the most stable splint configuration.

Proximal Metatarsal Region. Fractures of the mid and proximal metatarsus should be splinted with lateral and plantar splints over a Robert Jones bandage. The Robert Jones bandage should be less extensive than that on the forelimb, as this will facilitate application of the splints on the metatarsus. Splints applied to the lateral and caudal aspect of the limb should reach the level of the calcaneal tuber.

Fractures of the mid and proximal metatarsus should be splinted with lateral and plantar splints over a Robert Jones bandage. The Robert Jones bandage should be less extensive than that on the forelimb, as this will facilitate application of the splints on the metatarsus. Splints applied to the lateral and caudal aspect of the limb should reach the level of the calcaneal tuber.

TRANSPORTATION. Transportation of fracture patients is best accomplished with strict confinement, using chest and rump bars and partitions that assist the horse in maintaining balance. Horses with fractured forelimbs should be transported facing rearward, and those with fractured hindlimbs facing forward. This allows the horse to control his weight with his sound limbs during acceleration and deceleration of the trailer.

REFERENCES

276. Tulleners EP: Management of bovine orthopedic problems. Part 1. Fractures, *Compend Cont Educ Pract Vet* 8:69-79 (suppl), 1986.
276a. Bramlage LR: Long bone fractures, *Vet Clin North Am* 5:285-310, 1983.
277. Kaneps AJ, Schmotzer WB, Huber MJ, et al: Fracture repair with transfixation pins and fiberglass cast in llamas and small ruminants, *JAVMA* 195:1257-1261, 1989.
278. Anderson DE, St-Jean G, Vestweber JG, et al: Use of a Thomas splint-cast combination for stabilization of tibial fractures in cattle: 21 cases (1973-1993), *Agri-Practice* 15:16-23, 1994.
279. St Jean G, DeBowes RM: Transfixation pinning and casting of radial-ulnar fractures in calves: a review of three cases, *CVJ* 33:257-262, 1992.
280. Turner AS: Long bone fractures in horses. Part 1. Initial management, *Compend Cont Educ Pract Vet* 13:S347-S353, 1981.
281. McClure SR, Watkins JP, Ashman RB: In vivo evaluation of intramedullary interlocking nail fixation of transverse femoral osteotomies in foals, *Vet Surg* 27:29-36, 1998.
282. Herthel DJ, Lauper L, Mark CR, et al: Comminuted MC3 fracture treatment using titanium static interlocking intramedullary nails, *Equine Practice* 18:26-34, 1996.
283. Carter BG Schneider RK Hardy J, et al.: Assesment and treatment of equine humeral fractures: retrospective study of 54 cases (1972-1990), *EVJ* 25:203-207, 1993.
284. Zamos DT, Parks AH: Comparison of surgical and nonsurgical treatment of humeral fractures in horses: 22 cases (1980-1989), *JAVMA* 201:114-116, 1992.
285. Adams SB, Fessler JF: Treatment of radial-ulnar and tibial fractures in cattle, using a modified Thomas splint- cast combination, *JAVMA* 183:430-433, 1983.
286. Sanders-Shamis M, Bramlage LR, Gable AA: Radius fracture in the horse: a retrospective study of 47 cases, *EVJ* 18:432-437, 1986.
287. Embertson RM, Bramlage LR, Herring DS, et al: Physeal fractures in the horse 1. Classification and incidence, *Vet Surg* 15:223-229, 1986.
288. Denny HR, Barr ARS, Waterman A: Surgical treatment of fractures of the olecranon in the horse: a comparative review of 25 cases, *EVJ* 19:319-325, 1987.
289. Hance SR, Bramlage LR, Schneider RK, et al: Retrospective study of 38 cases of femur fractures in horses less than one year of age, *EVJ* 24:357-363, 1992.
290. Martens A, Steenhaut M, Gasthuys F, et al: Conservative and surgical treatment of tibial fractures in cattle, *Vet Rec* 143:12-16, 1998.
291. Young DR, Richardson DW, Nunamaker DM, et al: Use of dynamic compression plates for treatment of tibial diaphyseal fractures in foals: nine cases (1980-1987), *JAVMA* 194:1755-1760, 1989
292. Sullins, KE McIlwraith CW: Evaluation of 2 types of external skeletal fixation for repair of experimental tibial fractures in foals, *Vet Surg* 16:255-264, 1987.
293. Steiner A, Iselin U, Auer JA: Shaft fractures of the metacarpus and metatarsus in cattle, *VCOT* 6:138-145, 1993.
294. McClure SR, Watkins JP, Glickman NW, et al: Complete fracture of the third metacarpal or metatarsal bone in horses: 25 cases (1980-1996), *JAVMA* 213:847-850, 1998.
295. Nemeth F, Back W: The use of the walking cast to repair fractures in horses and ponies, *EVJ* 23:32-36, 1991.
296. Holcombe SJ, Schneider RK, Bramlage LR: Lag screw fixation of noncomminuted sagittal fractures of the proximal phalanx in racehorses: 59 cases (1973-1991), *JAVMA* 206:1195-1199.
297. McClure SR, Honnas CM, Watkins JP: Managing equine fractures with external skeletal fixation, *Compend Contin Educ* 17:1054-1062, 1995
298. Bramlage LR: Current concepts of emergency treatment and transportation of equine fracture patients, *Compend Cont Educ Pract Vet* 5:S594, 1983.

SPONTANEOUS FRACTURES IN RUMINANTS

JOHN MAAS

DEFINITION AND ETIOLOGY. Spontaneous fracture of bone is a syndrome that occurs when underlying bone disease weakens bone(s) to the point where otherwise normally applied stresses result in bone failure. The terms *spontaneous fracture* and *pathologic fracture* are synonymous for clinical usage. Fractured bones commonly include (1) long bones of the limbs, (2) vertebrae, (3) ribs, and occasionally (4) the mandible or pelvic bones.

CLINICAL SIGNS AND DIFFERENTIAL DIAGNOSIS. Clinical signs of postural deformity, swelling, and lameness are observed, with bone fracture occurring as a result of minimum or no apparent stress. Thorough physical examination often reveals additional fractures that are in the process of healing, particularly of the ribs and long bones. A fracture that occurs in normal bone in response to applied stress is the main differential diagnosis.

PATHOPHYSIOLOGY, EPIDEMIOLOGY, AND CLINICAL PATHOLOGY. The specific causes of spontaneous fractures in ruminants are varied and include pathologic processes that affect the tensile strength of bone. Although spontaneous fractures are not common, certain disease processes predispose animals to this condition, including (1) tumors affecting individual bones, (2) osteomyelitis, (3) rickets (osteodystrophy) in young ruminants, (4) osteomalacia in adult ruminants, and (5) osteoporosis associated with copper deficiency (see Chapter 30).

The effect of localized infection or tumor growth is to weaken bone tissue by dissolution of the mineral matrix. More common tumors causing bone weakness and fracture include lymphosarcoma and primary bone tumors in ruminants. Osteomyelitis as a primary condition or as an extension from septic arthritis can severely affect the strength of bone over a period of time. Osteomyelitis causing pathologic fractures can be wound-associated or can occur in diseases such as actinomycosis.

Rickets in young growing animals occasionally can result in spontaneous fractures of long bones and vertebrae and has been discussed previously. Osteomalacia in adult ruminants

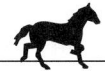

is caused by the same factors that result in rickets in young, growing livestock. As in young ruminants, the cause of osteomalacia is most commonly a deficiency of phosphorus or vitamin D. Calcium deficiency (primary or secondary), however, can be involved in the pathogenesis. Individual uremic animals may develop osteomalacia and spontaneous fractures from a lack of active vitamin D (1,25-dihydroxycholecalciferol). The pathogenesis of osteomalacia in the adult differs from that of rickets, in that mature and well-mineralized bone is removed and replaced by inadequately mineralized organic matrix. Therefore, radiographic and histologic examination of osteomalacic bone occasionally reveals signs of osteoporosis. Osteomalacia of the metaphysis and epiphysis is less prominent than with rickets. Spontaneous fractures associated with osteomalacia are usually accompanied by pica, skeletal deformities, and hypophosphatemia.

Copper deficiency (see Chapter 30) can be caused by a lack of adequate dietary copper (primary) or a relative excess of sulfates and molybdenum (secondary), which bind copper and make it unavailable for metabolism, resulting in osteoporosis.[299] The biochemical mechanism of bony lesions in copper deficiency is unknown; however, lysyl oxidase, a copper-containing metalloenzyme, may be involved. Copper deficiency can be a significant cause of lameness even without spontaneous fractures.[300-301] Radiography and histology of affected bones in lame, copper-deficient ruminants are similar to that seen with rickets.[302] Copper-deficient ruminants can also exhibit signs of anemia, achromotrichia, alopecia, diarrhea, poor growth, decreased feed efficiency, osteoporosis, and sudden death. Diagnosis of copper deficiency can be made when serum or plasma copper concentration is less than 0.5 μg/ml (ppm) or when hepatic copper concentration is less than 35 μg/g on a dry weight basis. Differentiating primary from secondary copper deficiency requires the analysis of diet and water. In my experience with spontaneous fractures associated with copper deficiency two additional findings are commonly seen: (1) concurrent selenium deficiency and (2) hypophosphorosis with adequate dietary calcium. It is possible that syndromes seen in the field are more complicated than we currently understand.

There are a number of possible causes of spontaneous fractures in ruminants. Factors that might affect a group of animals include dietary deficiencies of phosphorus, calcium, copper, trace minerals (Se, Mn, Zn); mineral (Ca, P, Mg) imbalances; indoor housing (vitamin D deficiency); protein deficiency (osteoporosis); rapid growth; lactation; and advanced pregnancy. The differentiation of spontaneous fractures from other causes of bone fractures is made by history, physical examination, and identification of one or more associated conditions mentioned previously.

TREATMENT AND PREVENTION. Treatment of spontaneous fracture is similar to that of commonly seen orthopedic problems caused by trauma. In addition, the underlying condition(s) must be corrected. Although the prognosis must be considered guarded or poor, I have examined recovered and ambulatory cattle with multiple healing rib fractures and two healing long-bone fractures. With spontaneous fractures associated with osteomalacia, rickets, and osteoporosis caused by copper deficiency, the animals' ability to heal is remarkable. Prevention of spontaneous fractures depends on identifying and correcting all underlying problems.

REFERENCES

299. Suttle NF, Angus KW, Nibet DI, et al: Osteoporosis in copper-depleted lambs, *J Comp Pathol* 82:93-97, 1972.
300. Cymbaluk NF, Schryver HF, Hintz HF: Copper metabolism and requirement in mature ponies, *J Nutr* 111:87-96, 1981.
301. Smith BP, Fisher GL, Poulos PW, et al: Abnormal bone development and lameness associated with secondary copper deficiency in young cattle, *J Am Vet Med Assoc* 166:682-688, 1975.
302. Irwin MR, Poulos PW, Smith BP, et al: Radiology and histopathology of lameness in young cattle with secondary copper deficiency, *J Comp Pathol* 84:611-621, 1974.

BUCKED SHINS AND STRESS FRACTURES OF THE METACARPUS IN THE HORSE

SUSAN M. STOVER

DEFINITION AND ETIOLOGY. Bucked shins and stress fractures are the acute and chronic manifestations of disease of the dorsal cortex of the third metacarpal bone. Bucked shins is a painful condition most commonly involving the mid-diaphyseal dorsal cortex of 2-year-old and occasionally 3-year-old horses in their first year of race training.

Stress or fatigue fractures are incomplete fractures located in the mid-diaphyseal dorsal cortex and, less commonly, in the distal diaphyseal dorsal or dorsolateral cortex. These fractures are seen most commonly in 3-year-old horses, but can affect 2-year-old horses later in the racing season and, with decreasing numbers, older horses.

Bucked shins and stress fractures are occupational diseases of horses in race training. They are more prevalent in young horses training at fast speeds on dirt surfaces than in older horses or horses training on grass surfaces.

CLINICAL SIGNS AND DIFFERENTIAL DIAGNOSIS. A general pattern of clinical signs was observed in one study of 2-year-old thoroughbred horses in race training.[303] Bucked shins usually occurred bilaterally. Both metacarpi usually were affected simultaneously, although occasionally one was affected several days before signs were observed in the contralateral metacarpus. In most horses the first clinical indication of bucked shins was a painful response to palpation of the metacarpus. Subtle pain often was found before the detection of an unwillingness of the horse to work at fast speed. Lameness was not necessarily manifested by affected horses.

Pain usually was localized to the dorsal aspect of the mid-diaphysis or near the junction of the proximal and middle thirds of the diaphysis. Initially, pain was mild and elicited from a diffuse area. With continued training, soft-tissue thickness became palpable, and diffuse swelling became visible on the dorsum of the metacarpus. Later, soft-tissue thickness and swelling became more focal unless hard work was continued. Approximately 2 to 3 weeks after pain first was detectable, discrete hard swellings could be palpated on the dorsum of the metacarpus. Radiographic abnormalities often are absent in horses with acute bucked shins.[304] The dorsal cortex thickens during adaptation to the stresses associated with training,[305] but indistinct periosteal proliferation, subperiosteal demineralization,[304] or subperiosteal radiolucencies support a diagnosis of bucked shins. Even in the absence of radiographic abnormalities, bone scintigraphy demonstrates a diffuse region of intense radiopharmaceutical uptake in the dorsal cortex of affected horses[306] (Fig. 36-31).

Differential diagnoses include cellulitis, periostitis, and osteitis of traumatic or infectious origin, although these conditions are much less common in the racehorse population. Signs of external trauma or infection (e.g., elevated temperature or wound drainage) may be present with these other conditions.

Incomplete cortical fractures occur approximately five times more frequently in the left than in the right metacarpus.[303,307] Left metacarpal fractures occur more commonly in the mid-diaphysis than in the distal diaphysis; however, in one study[303] a large proportion of right metacarpal fractures occurred in the distal diaphysis. Horses with incomplete

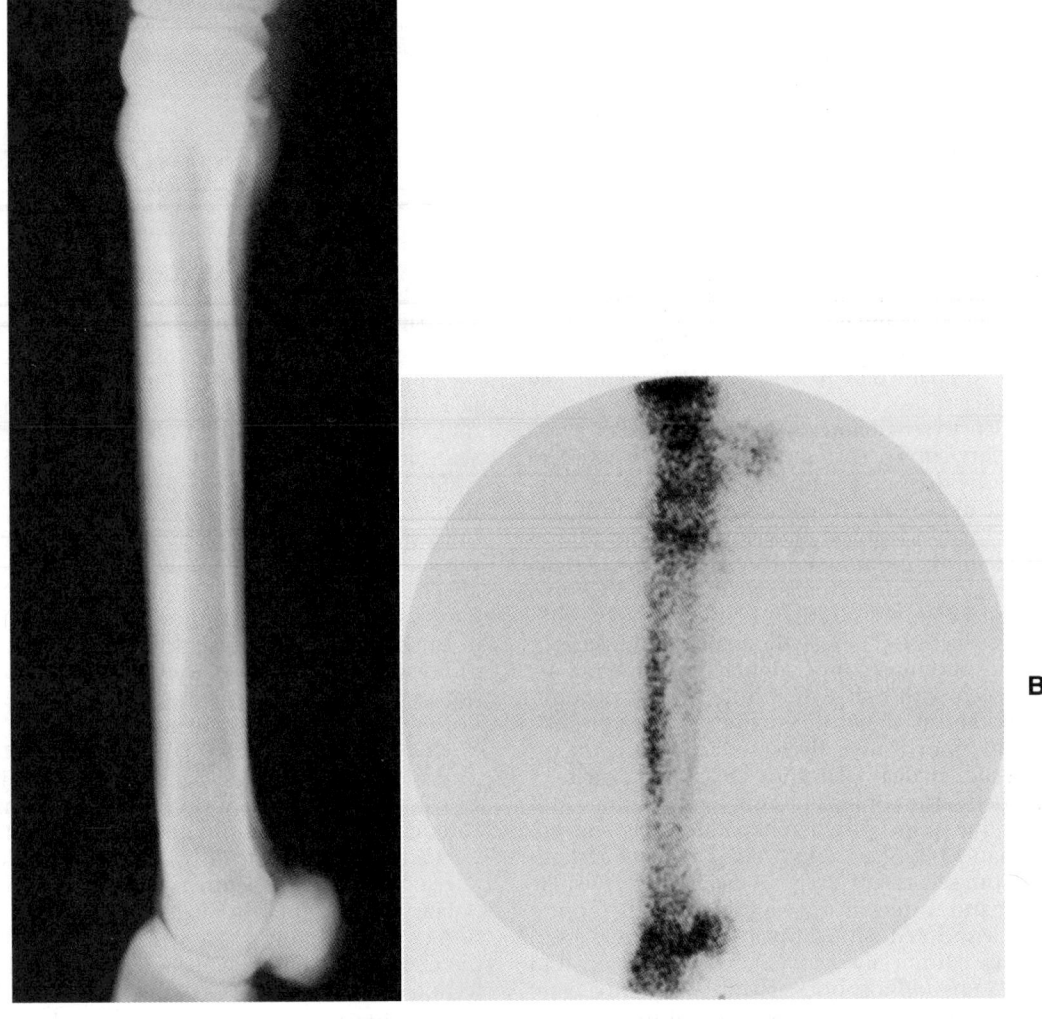

FIG. 36-31 ■ **A**, Lateromedial radiograph and **B**, lateral scintigram of the third metacarpal bone of a horse with bucked shins. Although dorsal cortical thickening is present, distinct radiographic changes associated with acute metacarpal disease cannot be detected. However, diffuse exaggerated radiopharmaceutical uptake is demonstrated in the dorsal cortex. (Courtesy PD Koblik.)

cortical fractures are more likely to be examined because of lameness of the affected leg(s) than horses with bucked shins. Lameness, which may be marked after activity, usually subsides within a few days.[307,308] With chronicity a discrete, hard tissue enlargement is visible and palpable overlying the fracture. Focal pain usually can be elicited by digital palpation of the enlargement.

Incomplete cortical fractures may be detected radiographically; however, not all fractures can be visualized. Fracture lines usually extend in a proximopalmar direction from the periosteal surface of the dorsal cortex at a 30- to 45-degree angle to the dorsal cortical surface (Fig. 36-32, A). Occasionally, fractures extend in a distopalmar direction from the periosteal surface, and less commonly a saucer-shaped fragment is noted within the dorsal cortex. Fractures rarely appear to course completely to the endosteal surface of the dorsal cortex. In the absence of a radiolucent fracture line, a localized periosteal or endosteal reaction is highly indicative of an incomplete cortical fracture. Alternatively, occult fractures may be identified with bone scintigraphy by intense focal accumulation of radiopharmaceutical[306] (Fig. 36-32, B). Differential diagnoses for stress fractures include traumatic periostitis or osteitis and osteomyelitis. Radiographic findings and clinical signs of external trauma are helpful diagnostically.

PATHOPHYSIOLOGY. Bucked shins are believed to result from cumulative microscopic damage within the dorsal cortex of the third metacarpal bone. Microdamage results from excessive strain (i.e., deformation) of young, developing metacarpal bones during training at fast speeds on hard surfaces.

Although third metacarpal bones of 2- to 3-year-old horses have attained adult length, the bone continues to adapt to the increased stresses of race training by enlarging in diameter and replacing intracortical bone through internal remodeling. These processes strengthen the metacarpal bone by increasing its resistance to deformation, decreasing its susceptibility to microdamage with repeated loading, and repairing microdamage. Adaptation usually is completed by 3 to 4 years of age and accounts for the lower incidence of bucked shins and stress fractures in older horses.

If accumulated microdamage with continued training exceeds adaptive and remodeling processes of the metacarpal cortex, bucked shins or chronically incomplete cortical fracture may become clinically and radiographically evident. Because fractures result from accumulation of damage caused by repetitive loading, they are often referred to as "fatigue" fractures. Evidence indicates that the direction of maximum strain on the surface of metacarpal bones changes with a shift from training to racing gaits.[309] Because bone adapts by re-

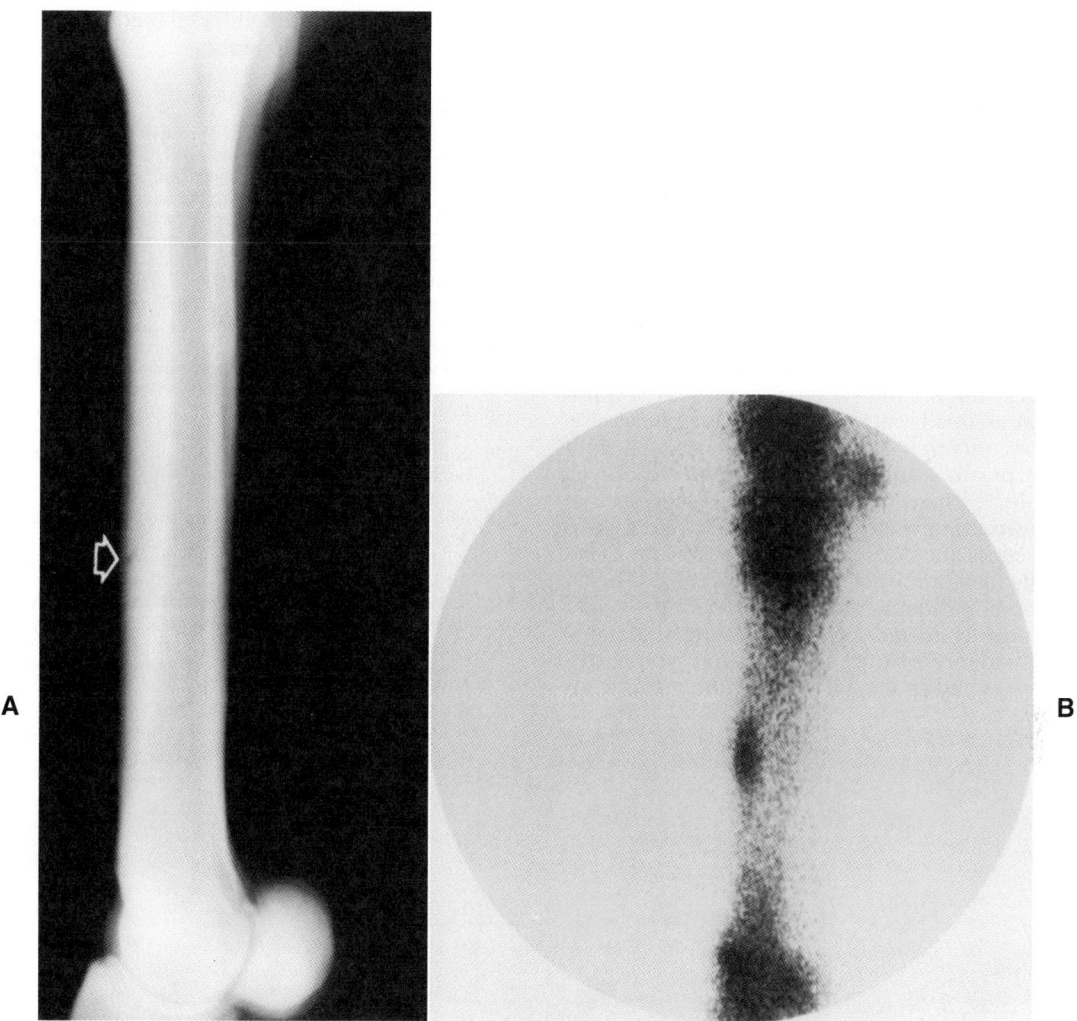

FIG. 36-32 ▓ **A,** Lateromedial radiograph and **B,** lateral scintigram of the third metacarpal bone of a horse with an incomplete cortical fracture *(arrow)* associated with focal intense radiopharmaceutical uptake. (Courtesy PD Koblik.)

sponding to the magnitude and direction of strain encountered, adaptation during training (i.e., trot and slow gallop) is probably different from that which would occur during racing (i.e., racing gallop). Thus metacarpal bones that have adapted to training may not adapt well to the strains of racing and may incur significant microdamage during initial exercise at racing speeds.[305]

EPIDEMIOLOGY. The incidence of bucked shins in 2-year-old Thoroughbred racehorses is approximately 70%,[307] occurring most commonly during the first year of race training. With continued training, horses with cortical microdamage develop stress fractures that are most common in 3-year-old horses.

The incidence of bucked shins and stress fractures is lower in quarter horse and Standardbred racehorses than in Thoroughbreds. The high incidence in Thoroughbred horses may be associated with running long distances at the racing gallop.[310] Thoroughbred horses are subjected to more high-stress loading cycles than Quarter Horses running shorter distances or than Standardbred horses trotting or pacing. Therefore Thoroughbred horses are more likely to accumulate clinically significant amounts of cortical microdamage.

NECROPSY FINDINGS. Bucked shins and incomplete cortical fractures may be found incidentally on postmortem ex-

amination of racehorses. Callus may be evident on the periosteal surface. Cross-sections of the bone may disclose an incomplete cortical fracture or endosteal bony proliferation. Histologic examination usually reveals an indistinct fracture line characterized by marked bone resorption.[311]

TREATMENT AND PROGNOSIS. Treatment of bucked shins varies with the degree of pain and the decrease in the performance of affected horses. On palpation, mildly and moderately affected horses exhibit resentfulness and mild soreness, which disappears within 2 to 4 days.[312] Training should be continued but at a slower pace to promote continued adaptation of bone to the stress of racing and to prevent the accumulation of additional microdamage. In severely affected horses, pain remains evident after 1 week of rest. These horses may require complete rest for a minimum of 3 months before they can be returned to training. After a horse has recovered from bucked shins, the prognosis is good for return to training, although the condition will recur in severely affected horses that were not rested for long enough before their return to training or horses whose exercise intensity was accelerated too rapidly on return to training.

Many adjunct therapies, including pinfiring, cold therapy, and electrostimulation, also are commonly used. Their effectiveness, however, is difficult to assess without considering concurrent training or rest therapy. Horses with incomplete cortical fractures must be rested for a minimum of 3 to 6 months. Most rested horses show radiographic evidence of bone healing and can be returned to training. Some chronic fractures are refractory to rest alone. Occasionally, returning these horses to light exercise stimulates fracture healing. Alternatively, interfragmentary drilling has resulted in better healing of fractures with fewer adverse affects than lag screw fixation. After interfragmentary drilling and adequate rest (e.g., 3 to 6 months), the prognosis is good for return to racing. Without an apparent relationship to type of treatment, however, incomplete fracture recurs in some horses.

PREVENTION. Factors considered important in the prevention of bucked shins and stress fractures include training regimen, racetrack surface, and shoeing. In general, a training program that gradually increases the degree of exercise, allowing time for concurrent bone adaptation, and that subjects the metacarpus to similar strains encountered during racing is desirable.[305] Experimental evidence[313] suggests that the metacarpus would have to encounter the strain associated with racing stress only for short duration a few times per week to stimulate the appropriate adaptive response. The effect of exercise on bone adaptation and remodeling is under active investigation. Hard racetrack surfaces are associated with a higher incidence of bucked shins than softer surfaces.[314] The stresses and strains incurred by the metacarpus

probably can be modified by changing the character of the racing surface or the horseshoe.

REFERENCES

303. Stover SM: Dorsal metacarpal disease in thoroughbred horses: relationship to the development of the third metacarpal bone. Doctoral dissertation, Davis, 1987, University of California, Davis.
304. Norwood GL, Haynes PF: Dorsal metacarpal disease. In Mansmann RA, McAllister ES: *Equine medicine and surgery*, ed 3, Santa Barbara, Calif, 1982, American Veterinary Publications, pp 1110-1114.
305. Nunamaker DM: Personal communication, 1987.
306. Koblik PD, Hornof WJ, Seeherman HJ: Scintigraphic appearance of stress-induced trauma of the dorsal cortex of the third metacarpal bone in racing thoroughbred horses: 121 cases (1978-1986), *J Am Vet Med Assoc* 192:390-395, 1988.
307. Norwood GL: The bucked-shin complex in thoroughbreds, *Proc Am Assoc Equine Pract* 24:319-336, 1978.
308. Richardson DW: Dorsal cortical fractures of the equine metacarpus, *Compend Cont Ed* 6:S248-S254, 1984.
309. Nunamaker DM, Butterweck DM, Black J: Fatigue fractures in thoroughbred racehorses: relationship with age and strain, *Trans Orthop Res Soc* 33:72, 1987.
310. Nunamaker DM: The bucked shin complex, *Proc Am Assoc Equine Pract* 32:457-460, 1987.
311. Pool RR: Personal communication, 1987.
312. Arthur R: Personal communication, 1988.
313. Rubin CT, Lanyon LE: Regulation of bone mass by mechanical loading: the effect of peak strain magnitude, *Calcif Tissue Int* 37:411-417, 1985.
314. Moyer W, Spencer PA, Kallish M: Relative incidence of dorsal metacarpal disease in young thoroughbred racehorses training on two different surfaces, *Equine Vet J* 23:166-168, 1991.

Diseases of the Eye

CECIL P. MOORE
Consulting Editor

OPHTHALMOLOGIC HISTORY AND EXAMINATION

CECIL P. MOORE
ERIN CHAMPAGNE

Before pursuing a detailed ophthalmic history, it is imperative to document the species, breed, age, sex, coat color, and use of the animal(s) to be examined and to obtain a general medical history. Because ophthalmic diseases of large animals may be genetic, an awareness of breed-related ocular abnormalities is important.

The primary complaints of the owner regarding the animal's eye(s) or vision may generally be categorized into one of the following areas of concern (also see Chapter 8):

- Abnormal appearance of one or both eyes (i.e., asymmetry or color change)
- Presence of ocular discharge
- Presence of ocular pain
- Reduced vision or blindness

Additional reasons for obtaining a thorough ophthalmic history and performing a detailed ocular examination are to follow up on a preexisting or previously treated eye condition or to examine the eyes as part of a prepurchase examination. Examinations for inherited eye diseases in horses may be performed by board-certified veterinary ophthalmologists and registration forms submitted to the Equine Eye Registration Foundation.[1]

OPHTHALMIC HISTORY

A series of questions should be directed to the owner or responsible person regarding the signs observed, the duration and clinical course of the condition, the animal's ability to function in its normal environment, the existence of previous eye problems, and whether related animals or other animals on the premises have been affected. Potential causes for an ophthalmic or visual problem, including any possible relationship to neurologic or iatrogenic (e.g., drug-induced) disease, toxin exposure, or systemic illness, should be explored. To ensure that the necessary questions are asked in a reasonable sequence, a history form (Fig. 37-1) is suggested.

OPHTHALMIC EXAMINATION PROCEDURES

General Inspection

It is optimal to observe the animal's activities and movements in its normal environment. Before restraining the animal, the examiner should study the animal's unencumbered movements, its posture, coordination, and head carriage. During this initial inspection the animal's vision and its response to visual stimuli should also be observed.

As the animal is approached, closer inspection reveals whether facial and ocular symmetry and normal eye movements are present. Signs of ocular pain (i.e., blepharospasm, photophobia, or epiphora) are noted. Size and position of the globes and the presence of ocular and nasal discharge, opacities, or masses are also noted.

Restraint

Adequate restraint is an essential prerequisite to performing a detailed ophthalmic examination in large animals. Manual restraint of small ruminants and neonates is usually adequate. For most cattle restraint with a chute, head catch, and halter is essential; restraining the horse with a halter in stocks is recommended. Chemical restraint may be necessary in cattle and horses before a thorough examination can be performed. This may consists of a combination of injectable sedative (e.g., xylazine or detomidine for horses), with or without an injectable analgesic (e.g., butorphanol for horses), with auriculopalpebral (and occasionally frontal) nerve blocks using a local anesthetic agent such as 2% lidocaine. A neuroophthalmologic assessment, including menace and palpebral and papillary light reflexes, should be done before administration of sedatives, analgesics, or local anesthetics.

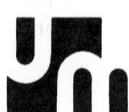

UNIVERSITY
OF MISSOURI-COLUMBIA
Veterinary Teaching Hospital

OPHTHALMOLOGY
HISTORY

Case Number _____

Species _____ Breed _____

Color _____ Sex _____ Age _____

Name or identification _____

Owner's name _____

Address _____

Telephone _____

1. What led you to believe your animal has an eye problem?
   ☐ Loss of vision
   ☐ Eye discharge
   ☐ Abnormal appearance
   ☐ Ocular pain
   ☐ Veterinarian noted problem
   ☐ Other (explain, i.e., observed injury) _____

2. How long has this problem been present? _____

3. Which eye(s) is(are) affected?   RIGHT   LEFT   BOTH

4. Has the character of the eye(s) changed since you first noticed it? .... NO   YES   UNKNOWN
   If YES, how? _____

5. Have the eyes been treated? .... NO   YES
   If YES, how, and with what? _____

6. How well do you believe your animal sees?
   ☐ Excellent   ☐ Poor in regard to moving objects
   ☐ Poor on all occasions   ☐ Poor in regard to stationary objects
   ☐ Poor especially in dim light or dark   ☐ Poor when turning to the right
   ☐ Poor especially in bright light   ☐ Poor when turning to the left
   ☐ Poor in regard to near objects   ☐ Poor when jumping or climbing down
   ☐ Poor in regard to far objects   ☐ Poor when jumping or climbing up

7. Do you think your animal sees well in familiar surroundings? .... YES   NO   UNKNOWN
   Strange surroundings? .... YES   NO   UNKNOWN

8. Has your animal had any other eye problems? .... NO   YES   UNKNOWN
   If YES, what type? _____   NO   YES

9. Has your animal experienced seizures, loss of balance, weakness, incoordination, or personality change? ... NO   YES   UNKNOWN

10. Is your animal receiving medication? .... NO   YES
    If YES, what? _____

11. Do you have other animals? .... NO   YES
    If YES, do they have eye problems? .... NO   YES
    If YES, what type? _____

12. Do you know your animal's dam, sire, or other related animals? .... NO   YES
    If YES, do any of them have eye problems? .... NO   YES   UNKNOWN

13. Has your animal been exposed to house or farm chemicals (cleaners, agricultural, industrial, or automotive
    chemicals) or building supplies? .... NO   YES   UNKNOWN

14. Has your animal had previous or present illness? .... NO   YES   UNKNOWN
    If YES, what type? _____

15. Is your animal consuming water and food normally? .... YES   NO   UNKNOWN

16. Is your animal urinating more frequently than normal? .... NO   YES   UNKNOWN

Date _____   _____
                        Signature of Person Completing This Form

FIG. 37-1 ▮▮ Example of an ophthalmologic history form that may be completed by the owner, an animal caretaker, veterinary technician, or clinician.

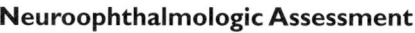

Neuroophthalmologic Assessment

An evaluation of the integrity of cranial nerves associated with normal ocular function is conducted (see Chapter 8). This includes a rapid assessment aimed at determining the animal's ability to do the following:

- Perceive tactile stimuli of the facial and ocular surfaces
- Blink effectively
- Move and position the eyes normally
- Constrict or dilate pupils in response to background and focal illumination
- Respond to visual stimuli such as hand motions or moving objects

Instruments and Materials

After a general inspection, restraint, and neuroophthalmologic assessment, a detailed ophthalmic examination is performed. A few basic instruments and materials should be available to permit an efficient, thorough examination. Necessary instruments are a focused light source (a 3.5-V halogen rechargeable light source with a Finoff transilluminator is preferred), a direct ophthalmoscope, magnifying loupes, and thumb forceps (blunt-tipped forceps with shallow serrations are recommended).

Important diagnostic supplies and drugs are sterile fluorescein dye strips, tear test strips, culture swabs, physiologic saline solution (flushing solution), topical anesthetic (0.5% proparacaine), and mydriatic solution (1% tropicamide). For irrigating nasolacrimal ducts, polyethylene tubing (French scale No. 5) should also be available.

Detailed Examination

For recording results of the ophthalmic examination, use of a standard form (Fig. 37-2, p. 1152) is recommended. The detailed examination begins with palpation of the boundaries of orbit for irregularities, asymmetry, masses, or fractures. Next, the globe is retropulsed to assess for increased resistance (indicating a space-occupying mass) and to inspect the anterior aspect of the third eyelid. Then, by digital tonometry (gently indenting the globe through the upper eyelid), an evaluation of the intraocular pressure is made and is characterized as hypotensive, normotensive, or hypertensive. Retropulsion and digital tonometry should not be done if the cornea is compromised by a deep ulcer or laceration.

At this point the examiner determines if ocular cultures or tear measurements are desired because these procedures should be completed before further manipulations are performed and before topical pharmacologic agents are instilled.[2] Depending on the clinical signs, severity of ocular disease, and species being examined, viral, bacterial (including *Chlamydia* and *Mycoplasma*), or fungal cultures may be indicated. Sterile swabs, moistened with saline, an appropriate enrichment broth, or transport media, are applied to the tissue to be cultured (usually cornea or conjunctiva). The moistened tip is placed in direct contact with the tissue surface and the swab is rotated by spinning the end of the stem with the finger tips.

The rest of the ophthalmic examination is performed in a darkened area and is initiated by directing a focused light through each pupil to establish the presence of a fundus reflex (light reflected from the back of the eye that normally fills the pupil space). By evaluating the fundus reflex in each eye, the examiner may compare pupil sizes, characterize pupillary light reflexes, and assess clarity of the ocular media.

Examination of ocular structures should be performed in a set pattern (i.e., anterior to posterior [internal]).[3-6] Use of an ophthalmic examination form (see Fig. 37-2) is helpful in systematically guiding the clinician through the examination and providing a record of examination findings.

The eyelids are inspected for integrity, position, and movements. Each lid is digitally everted for inspection of the margins, the meibomian gland openings, and the palpebral conjunctiva. Paresis, malposition (entropion, ectropion), defects, masses, inflammation (swelling, ulceration, exudates), alopecia, foreign bodies, or abnormal lashes are noted.

The third eyelids are examined for normal position, integrity of surfaces and margin, degree of pigmentation, and the presence of follicles or masses. To inspect for foreign bodies possibly concealed by the third eyelid, topical anesthetic solution (0.5% proparacaine) is instilled repeatedly onto the ocular surface. Two drops every 20 to 30 seconds for four applications is generally adequate. After topical anesthesia is applied, the third eyelid is grasped and manipulated with blunt-tipped, slightly serrated thumb forceps, and both sides are examined for foreign bodies.

Normally the conjunctiva appears moist, glistening, and semitransparent. Signs of conjunctivitis are chemosis, hyperemia, and ocular discharge. Color changes of the conjunctiva commonly accompany anemia (blanched, pale) and icterus (yellow, amber). Chemosis may indicate severe hypoproteinemia. Conjunctival lesions noted include focal swellings, follicles, adhesions, or masses. The sclera underlying the conjunctiva is inspected for color, contour, swellings, masses, pigmented areas, or surface irregularities.

The avascular cornea should be smoothly contoured and transparent with a moist, reflective surface. The cornea is examined for irregularities and opacities and for the presence of blood vessels and pigmentation. Corneal edema is characterized as localized or diffuse hazy blue corneal opacity. When severe corneal edema is present, the surface may bulge, or epithelial bullae (vesicles) may be noted. With corneal suppuration and necrosis, the cornea becomes more densely opaque and acquires a beige, green, or milky appearance. Infectious keratitis is characterized by suppuration and necrosis. Corneal abscesses occur as focal areas of suppuration within the stroma of either ulcerated or nonulcerated cornea.

Corneal opacities may also result from focal or diffuse scarring, areas of corneal degeneration or dystrophy, or stretching of Descemet's membrane from previous elevation of intraocular pressure or previous trauma. Inflammatory products clustered on the corneal endothelium (keratitic precipitates) appear as multiple beige or brown foci usually located on the ventral aspect of the corneal endothelial surface. This finding indicates the presence of anterior uveitis.

Nasolacrimal system examination entails evaluation of both secretory and excretory components. Normal secretions result in a moist, glistening ocular surface. Although not commonly performed in large animals, tear test strips may be used to quantify the volume of aqueous tear secretion (see Ancillary Diagnostic Procedures, p 1155). To examine the excretory components, the upper and lower puncta and nasal openings are identified. Any overflow of tears onto the face (epiphora) is noted. Causes of increased ocular secretions (e.g., frictional irritants, foreign bodies, corneal ulcers, and ocular inflammation) must be ruled out. Causes for stimulation of lacrimal secretions must be differentiated from causes of outflow occlusion such as congenital atresias and acquired obstructions of the nasolacrimal duct system.

Fluorescein dye instillation determines if corneal ulceration is present and aids in assessment of nasolacrimal patency. Passage of dye from the nasal opening of the nasolacrimal duct within 5 minutes confirms patency. Retrograde irrigation of the nasolacrimal duct by inserting a flexible tubing (French scale No. 5) into the nasal punctum and flushing with physiologic saline solution may be necessary to differentiate insufficient drainage from excessive secretions.

Intraocular examination begins with evaluation of the clarity and depth of the anterior chamber. Opacities within the anterior chamber include inflammatory products (cells

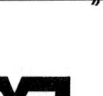
University of Missouri-Columbia
Veterinary Medical Teaching Hospital
OPHTHALMOLOGY EXAMINATION

T_____ P_____ R_____ Wt_____

History_____
_____
_____
_____

Case number _____

Species _____ Breed _____

Color _____ Sex _____ Age _____

Name or identification _____

Owner's name _____

Address _____

Telephone _____

Pupillary Light Reflexes: OD   direct _____ consensual _____   OS   direct _____ consensual _____

                                              (left to right response)   (right to left response)

Vision (menace response):   OD _____   OS _____

Schirmer Tear Test: OD _____ mm/60 seconds   OS_____ mm/60 seconds

Tonometry: OD _____mmHg   OS_____ mmHg

Right Eye

P   A

Lens   P   A

Fundus

Left Eye

A   P

A   P   Lens

Fundus

Diagnosis: _____   Treatment: _____
_____   _____
_____   _____

Comments: _____
_____
_____

Clinician Signature:_____ Date_____

FIG. 37-2 ▌ Use of an ophthalmologic examination form allows the clinician to perform a complete systematic ocular examination.

and fibrin), proteins (flare), red blood cells (hyphema), or white blood cells (hypopyon). Suspended or clustered inflammatory materials in the anterior chamber indicate intraocular inflammation (anterior uveitis). Besides the presence of exudates, loss of anterior chamber transparency may result from lens luxation, anterior synechia, or intraocular masses (neoplasia or foreign bodies). Loss of normal anterior chamber depth may result from flattening of the cornea, leakage of aqueous humor, staphyloma formation (protrusion of uvea through the cornea), iris bombe (forward bulging of the iris caused by iris-lens adhesions), or forward displacement of the lens. Increased depth of the anterior chamber may be caused by a protruding cornea (keratoconus) or posterior displacement of the iris or lens.

Each iris is inspected for contour, pigmentation, mobility, neovascularization, pupil size and shape, and the presence of iridal masses (including the normal granula iridica). Transillumination of iris masses allows differentiation of solid iridal masses (e.g., melanoma) from iris cysts. In animals with lightly colored or spotted hair coats, multicolored irides should be recognized as normal variants. Although uncommon, congenital iris thinning (hypoplasia) may be noted as dark, flat, or translucent areas. The lens-iris interface is best evaluated when the pupil is dilated and free of adhesions. Iris membranes, adhesions, or strands should be characterized as congenital (persistent pupillary membranes) or acquired (synechiae or remnants of iris atrophy).

Pupillary openings are evaluated for size, shape, symmetry, movements, and opacities. Pupil movements are observed as direct and indirect (consensual) pupillary light reflexes are assessed. The examiner must recall that pupillary light reflexes are not a test for vision (i.e., abnormal responses may be observed in visual animals and normal reflexes may occur in avisual animals). Pupillary abnormalities that should be noted are inequality in size (anisocoria), abnormal movements (hippus), abnormal location (corectopic), or abnormal shape (dyscoria).

Opacities of the pupil usually result from loss of lens transparency or from the presence of intraocular exudates. Obscuration of the pupil space may occur with severe miosis (from acute anterior uveitis), condensation of anterior chamber exudates, or synechiae formation (from chronic uveitis). In animals with normal pupillary light reflexes, complete examination of the lens and structures posterior to the lens (i.e., the vitreous and fundus) may be achieved only after dilation with a mydriatic agent such as 1% tropicamide, which usually occurs 20 to 30 minutes after instillation.

Using a focused light, the lens is inspected for a smooth, transparent, convex anterior capsule and normal position (no part of the equator should be visible). When evaluating for lens opacities (cataracts), the examiner should direct the focused light through the axial part of the lens to establish the presence of a fundus reflex. Cataracts may be classified according to the extent to which a fundus reflex occurs (i.e., a partial reflex indicates an incomplete cataract, whereas an absent reflex indicates a complete cataract). Focal cataractous changes are observed as dark areas seen within the area of reflected light.

An ophthalmoscope must be used to examine the vitreous and fundus; in general practice the monocular direct ophthalmoscope is most commonly used for this purpose. The vitreous should be in focus with a dioptric setting between +6 to +1, and the fundus is usually in focus between +1 and −2 diopters. The vitreous is examined for congenital remnants (retained hyaloid structures) and opacities, including degenerative materials or exudates.

Examination of the fundus begins with identifying the optic disc (papilla) and studying its size and shape. In ruminants the optic disc margin typically appears irregular and fluffy, indicating myelination of axons entering the optic disc. The shape, location, and vascular pattern of the optic disc and the appearance of the fundus vary considerably among species.

In ruminants the optic disc is horizontally elliptic and kidney-shaped and is located in the tapetal portion of the fundus.[4] An optic disc with extensive myelination may be elevated above the surface of the fundus; the term *pseudopapilledema* is used to describe this appearance. The major retinal arterioles are large and are accompanied by venules that anastomose on the surface of the optic disc. The dorsal arteriole and venule usually intertwine as they course away from the disc over the mid-tapetum (Fig. 37-3).

By contrast, the equine fundus is characterized by a large, pink or salmon-colored elliptic or oval disc located in the nontapetum (Fig. 37-4).[5] In equids, multiple small retinal blood vessels extend radially from the margin of the disc and no anastomotic venules are visible over the optic disc.

In both ruminants and horses the fibrous tapetum is penetrated by choroidal capillaries; thus the fundi are typified by dark, stippled foci termed *stars of Winslow*. Coloration of the tapeta of large animals also varies considerably and may range from gold to bluish-green. In animals with heterochromia irides, areas of the fundi may characteristically be void of pigmentation and may lack a tapetum. These areas may appear orange or red, reflecting the choroidal vasculature.

Abnormal funduscopic findings of the optic disc include hypoplasia (micropapilla), elevation (papilledema), depression (cupping), degeneration (atrophy; Fig. 37-5), and vascular changes (e.g., congestion, attenuation, or hemorrhage). The tapetal fundus is evaluated for clarity, coloration, pigmentation (Fig. 37-6), and integrity of the retinal vessels (Fig. 37-7). The nontapetal fundus is evaluated for uniformity of pigmentation. Both tapetal and nontapetal areas are assessed

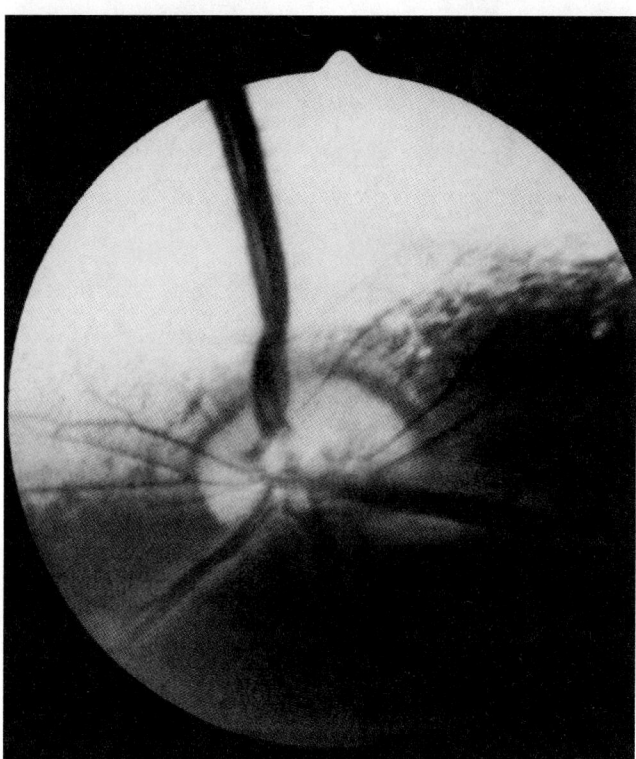

FIG. 37-3 ▓ Normal ruminant fundus characterized by a large, kidney-shaped, myelinated optic disc. Note that the large retinal arteriole and venule intertwine as they course dorsally.

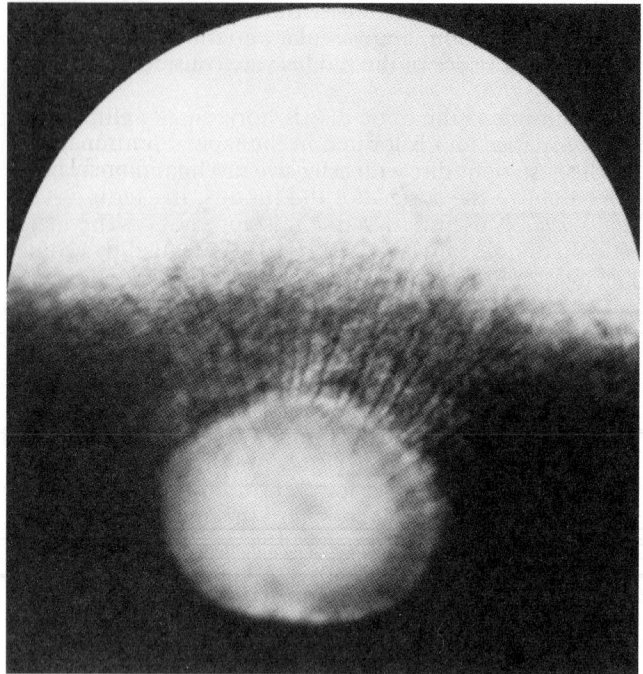

FIG. 37-4 ▮ The normal equine fundus characterized by a large horizontally elliptic optic disc with numerous small retinal vessels entering (arterioles) and exiting (venules) the margin of the optic disc. Note that the optic disc lies in the nontapetal portion of the fundus.

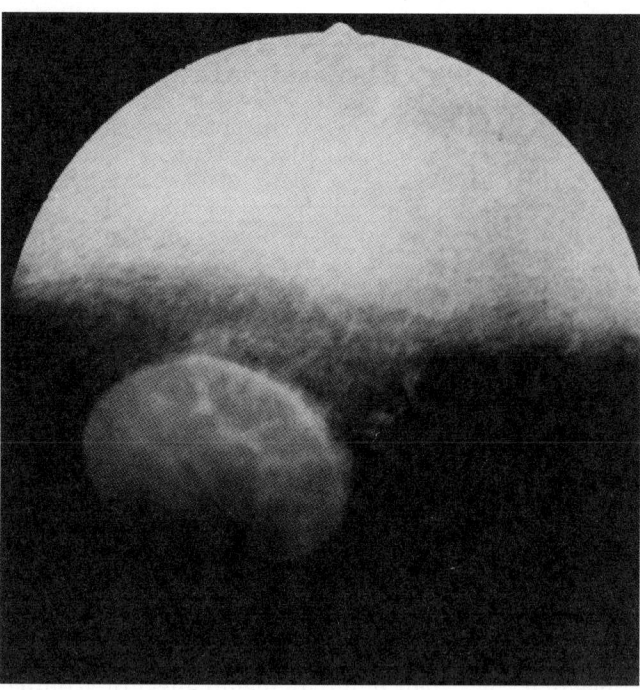

FIG. 37-5 ▮ Optic nerve atrophy (equine). The margin of the disc is quite distinct because of myelin loss, which is characteristic of optic nerve atrophy. Note absence of blood vessels.

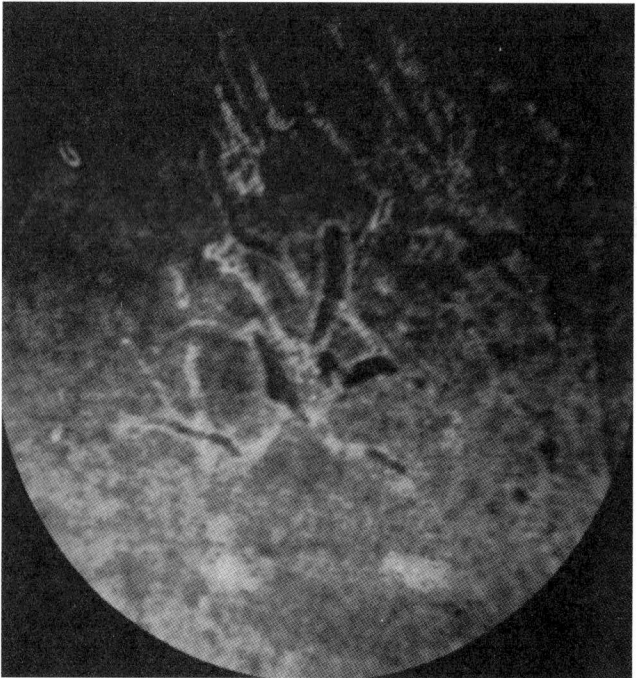

FIG. 37-6 ▮ Pigmentary changes after traumatic chorioretinopathy. Irregular linear areas of hypopigmentation and hyperpigmentation are present in the tapetal fundus of a horse following ocular trauma. Pigmentary changes reflect retinal pigment epithelial disturbance from previous hemorrhage and edema. (Courtesy Dr. K.N. Gelatt.)

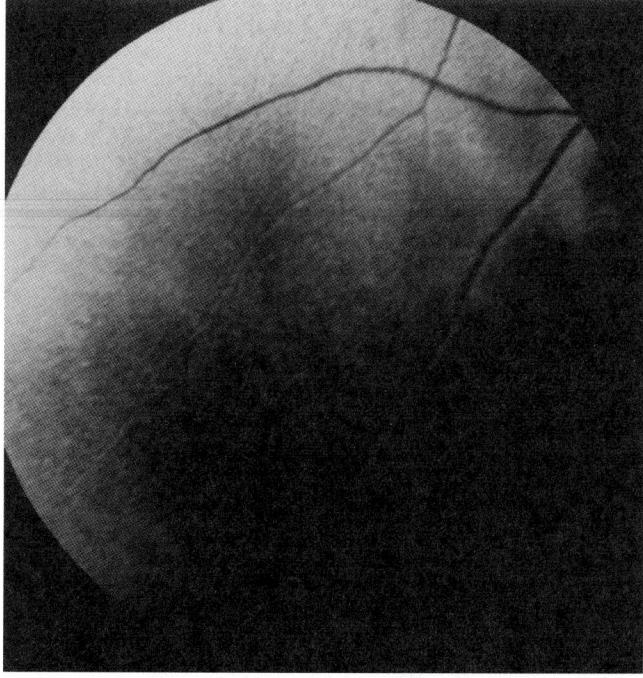

FIG. 37-7 ▮ Retinal degeneration (bovine). Peripheral retinal vessels are markedly attenuated near the tapetal-nontapetal junction. The attenuation is accompanied by hyperreflection of the tapetal region. These changes are consistent with generalized retinal atrophy.

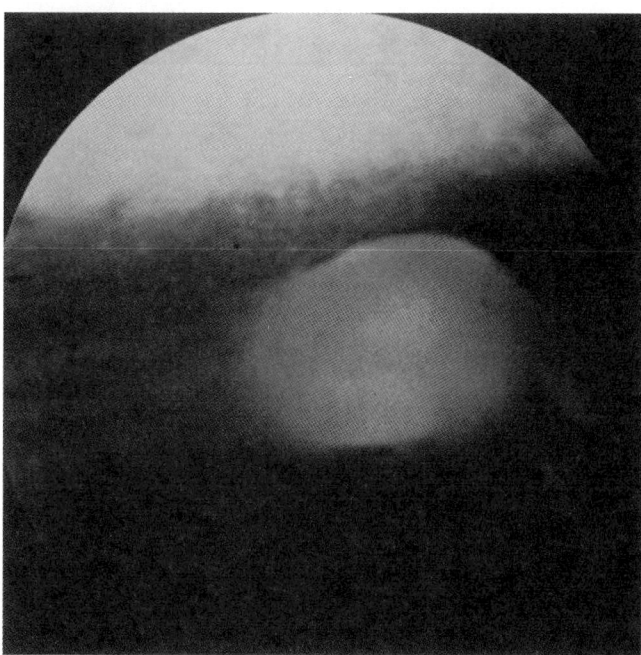

FIG. 37-8 ▉ Retinal separation (equine). Gray, linear areas radiate from the optic disc into the nontapetal region of the fundus. Note that the margin of the disc is quite indistinct in the affected area. An absence of retinal vessels indicates concurrent retinal degeneration.

for retinal elevations or separations (Fig. 37-8), hemorrhages, degenerations, disorganization (dysplasia), or scleral defects (colobomata).

ANCILLARY DIAGNOSTIC PROCEDURES

Several additional procedures may be important diagnostic aids that supplement the complete ophthalmologic examination. Although some ancillary procedures require specialized equipment and expertise, many of them may be performed in general practice.

Fluorescein and rose bengal are ocular surface stains most often used as aids in diagnosing conjunctival and corneal diseases. The tip of a sterile dye-strip is moistened with saline or eye-irrigating solution, and a drop of the stain is instilled onto the eye. Fluorescein is a water-soluble dye used to detect exposed corneal stroma resulting from an epithelial defect (erosion), stromal ulceration, or descemetocele. The pattern of fluorescein staining for a descemetocele is characterized by a donut-shaped area of positive fluorescence with the perimeter retaining stain and the center or deepest area (Descemet's membrane) not retaining stain. Fluorescein may also be used to evaluate the patency of nasolacrimal ducts because an open duct allows the transmission of stain, which may be observed exiting the duct system at the nasal orifice. Rose bengal is retained by devitalized surface cells and is therefore useful in detection of subtle abnormalities such as hyperplastic or desquamating cells associated with ocular surface drying.

Although tear deficiencies are uncommon in large animals, tear test strips may be beneficial to quantitate aqueous tear production in selected cases. A sterile filter paper strip (40 mm by 5 mm with a notched end) is inserted into the lower conjunctival fornix. In large animals it is sufficient to measure the amount of wetting in 30 seconds (20 mm or greater is normal).

Cytologic evaluation of ocular surface scrapings or intraocular aspirates may differentiate between inflammatory and neoplastic diseases or in some cases may provide a definitive diagnosis. Orbital aspirates may be diagnostic in cases of exophthalmos caused by neoplasia (e.g., lymphosarcoma). Immunofluorescent testing of cytologic specimens may confirm viral (e.g., infectious bovine rhinotracheitis) or chlamydial infections.

Bacterial cultures taken from the ocular surface or from ocular aspirates, with subsequent antimicrobial susceptibility testing, may be necessary for definitive diagnosis and appropriate treatment of ocular infections. The diagnostic laboratory performing ocular cultures may offer suggestions on culture procedures, including preferred transport media and handling of samples. It is especially important to consult with the laboratory in advance when anticipating culturing for fungi, *Mycoplasma*, *Chlamydia*, or viral agents.

Tonometry, a means of measuring the intraocular pressure, is useful in diagnosing glaucoma (elevated pressure) and uveitis (low pressure) and in assessing response to therapy for these conditions. Applanation tonometry provides accurate and reproducible intraocular pressure readings in large animals and is routinely performed at referral institutions or specialty practices. Schiotz tonometry is not applicable to large domestic species.

Biomicroscopy, using a portable handheld slit-lamp, is quite useful for identifying the location and nature of anterior ocular opacities. Focal irritants (e.g., ectopic cilia and small foreign bodies) may only be visible with the magnification provided using biomicroscopy. In addition, subtle opacities of the lens and anterior vitreous may only be detected with the use of a slit-lamp biomicroscope.

Funduscopic examination may be performed relatively quickly and easily using the technique of indirect ophthalmoscopy. Monocular indirect ophthalmoscopy is performed using a handheld light source and a separate 20- or 28-diopter focusing lens. Binocular indirect ophthalmoscopy uses a light source mounted on a head band with an incorporated prism and binocular viewing apertures. Binocular indirect ophthalmoscopy provides a stereoscopic, panoramic view of the fundus and is routinely performed by veterinary ophthalmologists. The light sources used for indirect ophthalmoscopy may be adjusted to relatively high intensities and therefore enhance visualization of the fundus through partially opacified or hazy ocular media.

Other ancillary diagnostic procedures include electroretinography, visual-evoked cortical responses, and imaging procedures (i.e., radiography, ultrasonography, and computerized tomography). Although plain skull radiographs and some contrast studies (e.g., dacryocystorhinography) may be performed in a general practice setting, the remaining procedures require techniques and equipment usually only available at referral centers.

REFERENCES

1. ACVO Genetics Committee: *Ocular disorders presumed to be inherited in purebred horses,* West Lafayette, Ind, 1999, Equine Eye Registration Foundation.
2. Whitley RD, Moore CP: Ocular diagnostic and therapeutic techniques in food animals, *Vet Clin North Am (Large Anim Pract)* 6:553-575, 1984.
3. Betts DM: Ophthalmic examination techniques for food and fiber animals. In Howard JL, ed: *Current veterinary therapy food animal practice 3,* section 15, Philadelphia, 1993, WB Saunders, pp 829-834.
4. Hakanson NE, Merideth RE: Ocular examination and diagnostic techniques in the horse. I, Examination of the adnexa and extraocular structures, *Equine Pract* 9:7-10, 1987.
5. Hakanson NE, Merideth RE: Ocular examination and diagnostic techniques in the horse. II, Assessment of vision and examination of the intraocular structures, *Equine Pract* 9:6-9, 1987.
6. Cooley PL: Normal equine ocular anatomy and eye examination, *Vet Clin North Am: (Equine Pract)* 8:3:427-450, 1992.

TABLE 37-1

Causes of Important Ocular Signs in Large Animals

Signs/Findings	Cause(s)		
	All Species (Ruminants and Horses)	Ruminants	Horses
RED EYES (SURFACE REDNESS)			
Hemorrhage	Trauma		
	Clotting disorders		
Hyperemic mass	Granulation/healing corneal ulcer		Habronema granuloma
	OSCC		
	Hemangiosarcoma		
Diffuse redness			
Conjunctivitis/keratitis	Entropion	Moraxella (IBK)	Fungal keratitis
	Foreign body	Mycoplasma (O, C)	Pseudomonas
	Chemical irritation	Chlamydia (O)	Streptococcus
		Herpes virus (IBR) (B, C)	Coliforms
		Branhamella (O, C)	
		Bluetongue (B)	
Uveitis	Septicemia	Mycoplasma (C)	Immune-mediated uveitis (ERU)
	Trauma	MCF (B)	
Glaucoma	Trauma	IBK (B)	ERU
Hemorrhage	Trauma		
CLOUDY EYE (OCULAR OPACITIES)			
Cornea	Keratitis	Infectious keratoconjunctivitis (see causative agents above under Conjunctivitis/keratitis by species)	
	Trauma		
	Ulcers		
	Scars (healed ulcers)		
	Uveitis (see Red eyes, column 1)	IBK (B)	ERU
	Glaucoma		
Anterior chamber			
Exudates blood	Trauma	Mycoplasma (C)	ERU
	Uveitis (see Red eyes, column 1)	Septicemias (B, C, O)	
	Glaucoma		
Lens luxation (anterior)	Trauma		ERU
Lenses (cataracts)	Trauma		ERU
	Congenital (see Chapters 47 and 48)		
	Genetic		
	Uveitis (see Red eyes, column 1)		
Vitreous			
Exudates/blood	Trauma (hemorrhage, detached retina)	Congenital hyaloid vascular remnants (B)	ERU
	Uveitis (see Red eyes, column 1)		
Lens luxation (posterior)	Trauma		ERU
OCULAR DISCHARGE			
Watery (serous)			
Painful eye	Ectopic or misdirected cilia	Conjunctivitis/keratitis (see specific etiologies above)	
	Foreign body (plant awn)		
	Entropion		
	Uveitis (see Red eyes, column 1)		ERU
	Trauma (ulcer, uveitis)		
	Chemical irritation		
Nonpainful eye	Nasolacrimal atresia		
	Nasolacrimal obstruction (acute blockage)		
Thick (mucoid or mucopurulent)	Foreign body	Infectious keratoconjunctivitis (see causative agents above under Conjunctivitis/keratitis by species)	
	Surface tumors		
	Dacryocystitis		
	Chronic nasolacrimal blockage		
	Foreign body		
	Sinusitis		
	Bacterial infections		
Hemorrhagic	Trauma		
	Foreign body		
	Ulcerative conjunctivitis		
	Tumor		

B, Bovine; *BVD,* bovine viral diarrhea (significance as a primary cause of conjunctivitis not established); *C,* caprine; *ERU,* equine recurrent uveitis; *IBK,* infectious bovine keratoconjunctivitis; *IBR,* infectious bovine rhinotrachetitis; *MCF,* malignant catarrhal fever; *O,* ovine; *OSCC,* ocular squamous cell carcinoma.

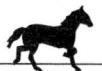

SIGNS OF OCULAR DISEASE

CECIL P. MOORE
DAVID J. MAGGS

The five major signs of eye disease are:
1. Ocular or periocular asymmetry
2. Ocular color change
3. Ocular discharge
4. Ocular pain
5. Visual deficits or blindness

Although any one of these signs alone may be the most obvious evidence of ocular disease, they frequently occur in various combinations. This chapter provides a general description of the signs and examples of ocular diseases in which a particular sign predominates. Some common signs of ocular disease in large animals are summarized in Table 37-1.

OCULAR OR PERIOCULAR ASYMMETRY

Ocular or periocular asymmetry results from the presence of an ocular surface mass, or unilateral changes in anatomy of the orbit, orbital contents, globe, eyelids, or pupils. Reduction in tissue volume is associated with congenital hypoplasia, cicatricial shrinkage, atrophy, or dehydration. Increase in tissue volume may involve the whole globe (buphthalmos) or be characterized by irregular enlargement as seen with inflammatory or neoplastic lesions involving the globe, orbit, or lids. Asymmetry may also result from neurologic dysfunction. Common examples include reduced palpebral fissure size (secondary to facial nerve paralysis), strabismus, third eyelid protrusion, and anisocoria (see Localization and Differentiation of Neurologic Diseases).

Forward displacement of the eye (exophthalmos) is commonly associated with a space-occupying orbital lesion or, less commonly, a congenitally shallow, underdeveloped orbit. Posterior malposition of the globe (enophthalmos) may result from active globe retraction caused by pain or occur secondary to loss of supporting retrobulbar soft tissues. Congenital strabismus is a developmental abnormality that results in ocular asymmetry and is commonly seen in Jersey, Shorthorn, and Holstein cattle.[7]

Unequal globe size can also account for ocular asymmetry. A congenitally small globe (microphthalmia) occurs as a genetic defect in cattle and horses.[7,8] Microphthalmia is frequently accompanied by multiple ocular anomalies and sometimes is associated with multiple organ involvement. Acquired variations in ocular size usually result from fibrosis and shrinking (phthisis bulbi) secondary to chronic uveitis, or stretching of the globe (megaloglobus; buphthalmos) because of glaucoma.

Asymmetry of the upper or lower lid may occur as a result of entropion, ectropion, blepharitis, conjunctivitis, or facial nerve paralysis (ptosis). Third eyelid protrusion is commonly seen secondary to active retraction of the globe in response to ocular pain, presence of third eyelid masses, orbital disease, or neurologic disorders (e.g., Horner's syndrome and tetanus). Pupillary asymmetry, or anisocoria, may occur for a variety of reasons, including Horner's syndrome, intraocular diseases (uveitis, glaucoma, unilateral retinal lesions), diseases involving the optic nerve or brainstem, and previous use of pharmacologic agents such as atropine that alter iris smooth muscle function.

The presence of an ocular mass may be the primary cause of ocular asymmetry. Ocular surface neoplasms are quite common in horses and cattle. Ocular squamous cell carcinomas commonly arise from nonpigmented tissues of the third eyelid, the lateral limbal region, or the eyelid margin. They may appear as irregularly raised surface masses or, less commonly, as smooth, vascularized lesions that invade the globe.

Ulceration, exudation, and mucopurulent ocular discharge are frequent concurrent findings (see Ocular Neoplasia). Periocular sarcoids are also common in horses and appear as firm, raised, nonulcerative lesions.[9] Other ocular tumors, such as adenomas, adenocarcinomas, angiomas, angiosarcomas, mastocytomas, and melanomas occur in large domestic animals but are relatively uncommon. Dermoids and orbital cysts are congenital masses involving the eye or orbit. Other nonneoplastic ocular masses seen in large animals include firm parasitic and foreign body granulomas and soft fluctuant subconjunctival swelling characteristic of prolapsed periorbital fat. Ocular and orbital pseudotumors have also been described in the horse.[10]

OCULAR COLOR CHANGE

Changes in the color of the ocular or periocular tissues or the presence of opacities in the clear ocular media (cornea, aqueous humor, lens, or vitreous) are important features of ocular disease. Such changes must be differentiated from normal congenital differences in ocular pigmentation. Developmental color dilution or absence of ocular pigmentation results in light or multicolored irides (heterochromia iridis). When this occurs unilaterally, the resulting appearance may be striking. Examples of abnormal coloration include hyperemia of conjunctival (superficial) or episcleral (deep) blood vessels associated with ocular inflammation (see Red eyes in Table 37-1), hemorrhage secondary to trauma or coagulopathies, pallor of the conjunctiva, which reflects severe anemia, and yellowing of the sclera and sometimes iris, indicating icterus.

Opacities of the ocular media may occur either as surface (corneal) or intraocular (anterior chamber, lens, or vitreous) phenomena. Sources of corneal opacification include pigmentation (melanosis) secondary to chronic exposure, grayish scars from previous episodes of ulcerative keratitis, neovascularization secondary to chronic inflammation, and bluish discoloration caused by corneal edema. These color changes frequently occur in various combinations in more severe keratitis, especially those of infectious origin such as chronic keratoconjunctivitis caused by chlamydia, mycoplasma, or *Moraxella bovis*. Cataracts are the most frequent cause of intraocular opacities in large animals. However, the presence of exudates within the aqueous humor or vitreous, congenital vascular remnants in the vitreous, or retinal detachment may also account for intraocular opacities (see Table 37-1).

OCULAR DISCHARGE

Ocular discharges are characterized as serous (watery), mucoid (catarrhal), mucopurulent, or hemorrhagic. The type of discharge present may suggest the severity of the eye disease. For example, serous discharge generally indicates milder forms of eye disease, whereas mucopurulent or hemorrhagic discharge indicates more serious disorders. A notable exception to this generalization is equine recurrent uveitis (ERU), which is a serious and potentially blinding disease but is usually associated with serous discharge. The nature of the discharge may also change as the disease progresses or improves. This is most notable in inflammatory or infectious ocular diseases. Initially, the discharge is predominantly serous; however, it tends to become mucopurulent with chronicity. Causes for abnormal ocular discharges in large animals are summarized in Table 37-1.

Epiphora describes facial wetting and results from overflow of tears over the eyelid margin. This may result from excessive secretion of tears or from obstruction of the nasolacrimal system. In large animals reflex lacrimation with an associated overabundance of tears is the typical response to ocular inflammation (e.g., conjunctivitis, keratitis, or uveitis).

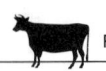

When epiphora is noted, careful digital and visual examination for foreign bodies within the conjunctival fornix or under the third eyelid is indicated. Epiphora is generally one of the earliest signs of conjunctivitis, ulcerative keratitis, or anterior uveitis. In cattle with keratoconjunctivitis caused by *Moraxella bovis*, epiphora is present several days before visible corneal ulceration occurs.[11]

Developmental defects or malformations of the nasolacrimal duct system (e.g., imperforate puncta) may account for ineffectual outflow of tears in neonates. In these instances the presence of epiphora may be misinterpreted as an overproduction of lacrimal fluid. Previously undiagnosed congenital defects may also be the cause of persistent ocular discharge in adult animals. Acquired obstructions of the nasolacrimal ducts may result from infections, foreign bodies, facial trauma, nasal tumors, or sinusitis that involve the duct system. When nasolacrimal obstruction is present, the nature of the ocular discharge depends on the chronicity of the lesion and the presence or absence of infection within the duct system. Whether congenital or acquired, simple nonseptic obstructions are characterized by epiphora. Occlusions with concurrent sepsis result in mucopurulent discharge from the eye or nostril on the affected side. Excessive mucus production is a feature of follicular conjunctivitis, possibly as a result of the rubbing of elevated lymphoid follicles on apposing conjunctival surfaces. Lymphoid follicles are noted in subacute or chronic forms of chlamydial conjunctivitis in sheep and with Onchocerca larval migration in horses. Mucoid ocular discharge may be observed concurrently with epiphora in acute ocular surface infections caused by viral or chlamydial agents. Excessive, tenacious mucus may also result from inadequate secretion of the aqueous component of tears (i.e., keratoconjunctivitis sicca or KCS). Although KCS is not diagnosed as commonly in large animals as it is in dogs, it has been reported in horses, sometimes as a complication of guttural pouch pathology.[12]

Mucopurulent material is the characteristic ocular discharge when bacterial organisms, including *Mycoplasma* spp., are the primary infectious agents or in cases of secondary bacterial infections. Bacterial conjunctivitis occurs frequently in large domestic species and manifests as red eyes with copious amounts of mucopurulent ocular exudate. Ocular foreign bodies and surface masses (e.g., squamous cell tumors) commonly have associated bacterial infections. Mucopurulent discharge in the absence of ocular inflammation suggests infection of the nasolacrimal sac (dacryocystitis) or ducts, with reflux of exudate from the lacrimal puncta.

Hemorrhagic discharge most commonly occurs after blunt or penetrating trauma to the eye. Foreign body penetration may damage the eyelid, conjunctiva, or globe, resulting in bleeding onto the ocular surface. Corneal ulcers may rupture and result in uveal prolapse and subsequent hemorrhage on the ocular surface. Ulcerative conjunctivitis from abrasion or infection may result in bleeding into the tear fluids. Similarly, ocular surface tumors may become ulcerative and cause bloody ocular discharge. Whenever blood is noted on the surface of the eye, it is imperative that a thorough ophthalmic examination be performed to determine the cause and to evaluate integrity of the globe.

OCULAR PAIN

Blepharospasm, epiphora, photophobia, and periocular hyperesthesia are signs of ocular pain. Animals with severe ocular pain usually resist manipulation of the eyelids or any form of ocular examination by persistently jerking the head away from the examiner and by closing the eyelids tightly. In cases of persistent ocular inflammation, discomfort and pruritus may be manifested by rubbing and self-trauma to ocular or periocular structures.

Ocular pain may result from blunt or penetrating trauma. Corneal ulceration and uveitis are painful sequelae to ocular trauma. Limbal (scleral) ruptures from blunt injury or penetrating lacerations of the fibrous tunic may result in uveal prolapse (staphyloma), which is extremely painful. Periocular trauma may cause eyelid swelling or paresis with exposure and drying of ocular surface tissues, resulting in painful ulcerative keratitis. Inflammatory diseases of nontraumatic origin such as infectious keratoconjunctivitis or ERU may also cause severe ocular pain in an affected animal. Other causes of ocular pain include frictional irritation caused by entropion, trichiasis, distichia, or ectopic cilia, or by direct irritation of the ocular surface by foreign material. Foreign bodies causing ocular irritation in large animals are typically plant materials such as seeds, hay stems, straw, twigs, bark, or thorns, although particles of sand or soil can also cause severe ocular irritation. Nonembedded particulate matter is usually entrapped by mucus and washed out of the eye by reflex tearing; therefore it typically results only in transient discomfort. By contrast, embedded foreign material (i.e., between ocular surface layers or within ocular tissues) causes persistent ocular pain.

BLINDNESS

Visual deficits in large animals are manifest in a variety of ways. Obvious signs include bumping into objects in the path of locomotion and being unable to respond to visual stimuli such as light or hand motions. Other signs of blindness are reliance on stationary objects, such as fences, railings, or other animals to maneuver within the environment. Behavioral changes include reluctance to move or to venture into unfamiliar areas. The nonvisual animal is frequently found standing isolated from the group.

Nonvisual animals attempt to compensate for the loss of vision with their other senses, resulting in behaviors that seem peculiar. For example, as an apparent overcompensation for visual deficits, the blind animal may raise its head extremely high with the ears erect at the slightest auditory stimuli. A similarly dramatic response to olfactory stimuli may be noted in affected animals when snorting or intensive sniffing associated with nervousness and maximum neck extension is observed. Frequently, blind animals will show exaggerated elevation of the limbs while walking. This must be differentiated from true hypermetria (see Localization and Differentiation of Neurologic Diseases). Partial loss of vision may be difficult to determine, and detection depends on observing more subtle behavioral changes such as slight head cocking or tilting, a searching nystagmus, difficulty maneuvering in dim light, or shying and startling from objects on one side or objects present in some specific part of the visual field. Animals may effectively compensate for congenital blindness or slow diminution of vision, particularly when they remain with other unaffected animals in a familiar environment. Visual disturbance may not be apparent until an affected animal is isolated or moved to an unfamiliar area.

There are numerous causes of blindness in large animals including those that involve only the visual system and some that involve other nervous system tissues or are multisystemic (Box 37-1). A functional approach to blindness involves anatomically classifying the cause as one of the following:
- Obstruction of the ocular media (light does not reach the retina)
- Failure of the retina to process the light appropriately
- Failure of the central nervous system, including the optic nerve, to transmit or assimilate the visual stimuli appropriately.

Assessment of the pupillary light reflexes (PLRs) will assist with the localization of the lesion. Animals with lesions in-

Lesions and Diseases Causing Visual Deficits or Blindness

OBSTRUCTION OF THE OCULAR MEDIA
(see Ocular Opacities in Table 37-1)
Cornea
Scarring, edema, pigmentation, inflammatory cell infiltration

Anterior Chamber
Hyphema, hypopyon

Vitreous
Retinal detachment, vitreal exudation, vitreal hemorrhage

RETINOPATHIES
Degenerative
Glaucoma
Retinal degeneration

Congenital
Retinal dysplasia
Microphthalmia
Retinal detachment

Inflammatory
Retinitis/chorioretinitis
Phthisis bulbi
Retinal detachment

EXTRAOCULAR/CENTRAL NERVOUS SYSTEM DISEASE
Congenital/Inherited
Optic nerve hypoplasia
Storage diseases (e.g., ceroid lipofuscinosis in sheep)

Inflammatory
Optic neuritis
Meningitis/encephalitis
Trauma
Neoplasia

Toxic/Nutritional
Toxic optic neuropathy (Male fern)
Vitamin A deficiency (optic neuropathy/hydrocephalus

volving the retina, optic nerves, optic chiasm, or optic tracts will generally not have a PLR, whereas more central ("higher") lesions involving the lateral geniculate bodies, optic radiations, or occipital (visual) cortex are likely to exhibit a normal PLR (see Localization and Differentiation of Neurologic Diseases).

REFERENCES

7. Leipold HW: Congenital ocular defects in food-producing animals, *Vet Clin North Am (Large Anim Pract)* 6:577-595, 1984.
8. Munroe GA, Barnett KC: Congenital ocular disease in the foal, *Vet Clin North Am (Large Anim Pract)* 6:519-537, 1984.
9. McConaghy FF, Davis RE, Hodgson DR: Equine sarcoids: a persistent therapeutic challenge, *Compend Contin Educ* 16:1022-1031, 1994.
10. Moore CP et al: Equine conjunctival pseudotumors, *Vet Ophthalmol* 3:51-63, 2000.
11. Brown MH et al: Infectious bovine keratoconjunctivitis: a review, *J Vet Intern Med* 12:259-266, 1998.
12. Moore CP: Eyelid and nasolacrimal disease, *Vet Clin North Am (Eq Pract)* 8:499-519, 1992.

OCULAR TRAUMA

R. DAVID WHITLEY
KRISTINA R. VYGANTAS

CAUSES OF TRAUMA

The eye is anatomically prominent in food animals and horses and therefore is prone to blunt and sharp trauma. Injuries result from a variety of causes: foreign materials such as soil, sand, or stones, which may be thrown into the eye by wind or during running; trauma from disciplinary action; scratches by vegetable matter such as hay, weed stems, tree limbs, or thorns; exposure to chemical irritants; and sudden, violent head movements during grooming, training, or working. Other sources of ocular injury include trailer or stanchion latches, hooks, protruding nails, fencing, bucket handles, and other animals, particularly horned ruminants.

Recumbent neonates and animals with central nervous system disease or severe illnesses causing depressed mentation often suffer eye injuries from abrasion by debris such as sand, straw, hay, or wood shavings. Such injuries can be prevented by protecting the eye from trauma through use of a padded hood or soft mats under the head, keeping the cornea lubricated in dehydrated or nonblinking animals, and administering sedation to prevent thrashing. Following ocular trauma, opportunistic or pathogenic organisms may become established and cause superficial or deep corneal infections.[13] Normal ocular flora include potential pathogens that can cause severe infections.[14]

OCULAR EXAMINATION IN CASES OF HEAD TRAUMA

The goals of examination are to determine the degree of ocular trauma and offer a prognosis for recovery of vision and preservation of the eye. The history should elicit information as to the cause and duration of the injury, previous ocular and systemic disease or therapy, previous sedation, and anesthesia.

Ophthalmic examination (see pp. 1149 to 1155) can be performed after adequate restraint of the head. Intravenous sedation; sensory and motor nerve blocks; topical anesthesia; and use of a halter, twitch (in horses), or nose tongs (in cattle) are often necessary for adequate examination of the traumatized eye.

Blunt facial trauma frequently results in damage to the orbit and globe and may include fractures or soft-tissue injuries of the orbit, corneal abrasions and edema, hyphema, traumatic uveitis, lens luxation, traumatic cataract, vitreal hemorrhage, retinal laceration or detachment, corneal or scleral rupture, or proptosis. Therefore the orbit and globe should be examined as thoroughly as possible when evaluating a patient with facial trauma.

TRAUMA TO THE ORBIT

Orbital injuries in domestic animals frequently include fractures of the orbital rim and zygomatic arch and damage to the supraorbital process of the frontal bone.[15] Fractures of the orbit may be identified by palpation and radiography. Contusions or lacerations of orbital soft tissues and temporary or permanent neurologic dysfunction may also be present.

Radiographic examination of the bony orbit in large animals is technically difficult and often unrewarding. Standard lateral and dorsoventral views require powerful radiographic equipment for penetration of bony structures in horses and cattle.[16] Large fractures may be identified; however, distinct delineation of the bony orbit is difficult because of overlying sinus and nasal structures. An oblique view of the frontal bone is often the most helpful projection.[16] This view may be taken with a portable radiographic machine because only minimum penetration of skull structures is required. Outlining the orbit and surrounding bony structures allows identification of fractures; osteomyelitis, with or without bony sequestra; and soft-tissue abnormalities, including swelling and radiopaque foreign bodies. If a periorbital sinus is involved in the fracture, subcutaneous emphysema may be present. Computerized tomography or magnetic resonance imaging may also be available at some referral centers.[17,18]

Immediate evaluation for orbital fractures should include careful examination of the globe. In cases with substantial swelling, ice packs applied to the fracture site may reduce swelling. Systemic antiinflammatory therapy such as aspirin, phenylbutazone, or flunixin meglumine may also be given. Systemic antibiotics should be used if sinus involvement is suspected. If the fracture fragments are only minimally displaced, surgical intervention may not be required. Surgical repair should be considered with severe fragment displacement or entrapment of extraocular muscles. Neurologic dysfunction, particularly immobility of the eyelids, is not uncommon.

If eyelid movement is impaired, the globe must be adequately protected and lubricated until neurologic function returns. If the globe is only minimally exposed, a sterile ophthalmic lubricant may be used 3 or 4 times daily. In more severe cases a third-eyelid flap or temporary tarsorrhaphy may be required. If neurologic dysfunction is permanent and results in significant exposure conjunctivitis or keratitis, partial or complete permanent tarsorrhaphy should be performed.[3] Enucleation may be the treatment of choice in severely affected eyes.

Traumatic puncture wounds of the eyelids and conjunctiva may result in orbital cellulitis and exophthalmos in food animals and horses. The onset of swelling may be sudden. Pyrexia and leukocytosis may be present. If retrobulbar abscess occurs, temporomandibular movement causes extreme pain; the animal may have the eyes partially closed, be off feed, and stand with the head extended. The client may observe a relatively sudden onset of exophthalmos, eyelid swelling, severe chemosis, and exposure keratitis.[19] Therapy should consist of systemic and topical antibiotics. Ophthalmic ointments and lubricants should be used to provide protection from desiccation for the exposed cornea and conjunctiva. With time, the cellulitis may organize into a discrete abscess that can be located by palpation or ultrasound. The wound or abscess should be debrided or drained to facilitate healing.

Although traumatic proptosis is uncommon, it can occur in horses and food animals. The prognosis for return of vision is guarded to poor, depending on the extent of the damage to the optic nerve and retina. If the globe is ruptured or the extraocular muscles avulsed, the eye should be enucleated. If the extent of the damage cannot be evaluated initially, the globe should be repositioned, a temporary tarsorrhaphy performed, and the globe reevaluated after 7 to 10 days of therapy. Treatment should include topical broad-spectrum antibiotics and atropine. With severe fractures or serious ocular damage, consultation with the appropriate specialist is advised.

TRAUMA TO THE EYELID

Eyelid trauma is frequently accompanied by injuries to other ocular structures. Careful ocular examination should be part of the evaluation of animals with eyelid trauma. Injuries may range from simple swelling (blepharoedema) or orbital cellulitis to extensive lacerations and avulsion. Blepharoedema may be accompanied by hemorrhage and usually resolves quickly without therapy; however, recovery may be hastened by use of ice packs and systemic use of aspirin, phenylbutazone, flunixin meglumine, or corticosteroids.

Horses are particularly prone to eyelid lacerations because of the prominence of the eye and their tendency toward sudden head movements. Lacerations may be divided into those without eyelid margin involvement, those with eyelid margin involvement, and avulsions of part or all of the eyelid. For all types of eyelid injury, several basic principles should be followed. Lacerations should be treated promptly to avoid distortion from excessive swelling, infection, scarring, and loss of function. Lacerated or displaced tissue should not be excised. All foreign material should be removed with copious saline flushing. Cold compresses may assist in decreasing swelling. In suturing an eyelid laceration, it is essential to preserve the eyelid margin, therefore eyelid lacerations should be repaired with minimal debridement. In cases of avulsion of part or all of the eyelid, a variety of blepharoplastic procedures may be performed to restore functional eyelid margin.[20,21] For a more detailed description of the principles of surgical repair of the eyelids, an ophthalmic surgical text is recommended.

Postoperative care of all eyelid lacerations should include standard wound hygiene, application of fly repellent and topical ophthalmic antibiotics, and prevention of self-trauma. In contaminated wounds, systemic antibiotic therapy is indicated for 5 to 7 days. Tetanus prophylaxis should be administered.

Improper repair of eyelid lacerations can lead to abnormal function and secondary problems, including chronic epiphora and associated dermatitis, exposure keratitis, ulcerative keratitis, cicatricial entropion or ectropion, conjunctivitis, and pigmentary keratitis.

TRAUMA TO THE THIRD EYELID

Lacerations involving the third eyelid should be repaired to avoid irritation and damage to the cornea. This appears to be more important in horses than in ruminants. The margin should be realigned as precisely as possible, and the lacerated conjunctiva should be repaired with absorbable, small suture material such as No. 5-0 polyglactin.* Topical ophthalmic antibiotics should be used 3 times a day for 7 to 10 days. The third eyelid should only be removed if irreparably damaged.

TRAUMA TO THE CONJUNCTIVA

Conjunctival lacerations result in swelling (chemosis) and hemorrhage. The cornea and sclera should be examined carefully for evidence of lacerations or perforation. If the globe is excessively soft on digital palpation or the anterior chamber is shallow or flat, a concurrent scleral laceration is probable.

Chemosis and hemorrhage frequently resolve without therapy; however, if the chemosis is severe enough to cause exposure and drying of tissues, topical sterile ophthalmic lubricants or antibiotic ointments are indicated to prevent secondary irritation. Conjunctival lacerations rarely require closure unless they are extensive. Subconjunctival hemorrhage sustained during parturition is common in foals and calves and requires no therapy.

TRAUMA TO THE CORNEA

Corneal injuries in horses and food animals include blunt compressive trauma, foreign body penetration, ulcerative keratitis, and lacerations. Corneal perforation often results in iris

---

*Vicryl, Ethicon, Inc., Somerville, NJ 08876.

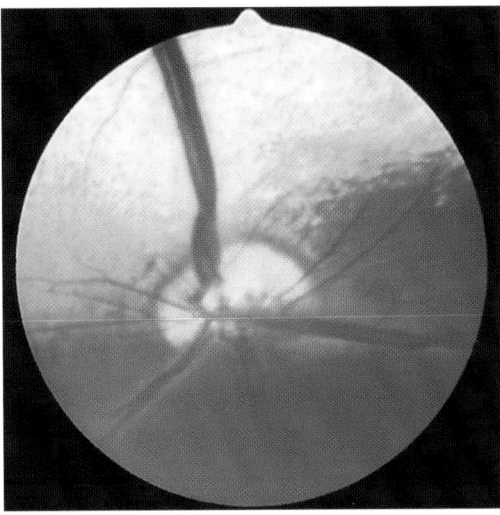

PLATE 13 ▮ Normal ruminant fundus characterized by a large, kidney-shaped, myelinated optic disc. Note that the large retinal arteriole and venule intertwine as they course dorsally.

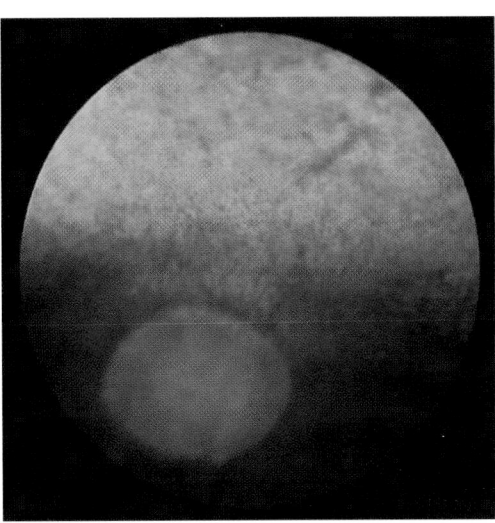

PLATE 14 ▮ The normal equine fundus characterized by a large, horizontally elliptic optic disc with numerous small retinal vessels entering (arterioles) and exiting (venules) the margin of the optic disc. Note that the optic disc lies in the nontapetal portion of the fundus.

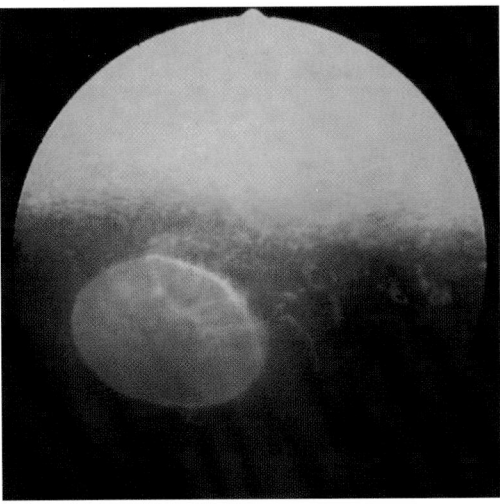

PLATE 15 ▮ Optic nerve atrophy (equine). The optic disc is avascular. The margin of the disc is quite distinct because of myelin loss, which is characteristic of optic nerve atrophy.

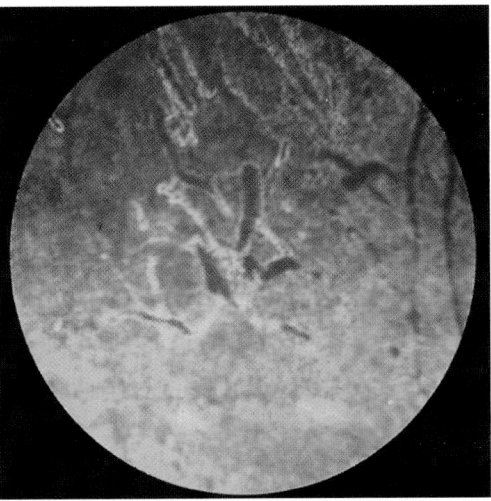

PLATE 16 ▮ Pigmentary changes following traumatic chorioretinopathy. Irregular linear areas of hypopigmentation are present in the tapetal fundus of a horse following ocular trauma. Pigmentary changes reflect retinal pigment epithelial disturbance from previous hemorrhage and edema.

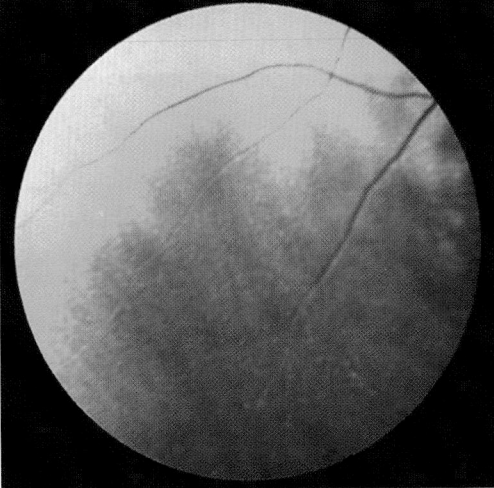

PLATE 17 ▮ Retinal degeneration (bovine). Peripheral retinal vessels are markedly attenuated near the tapetal-nontapetal junction. The attenuation is accompanied by hyperreflection of the tapetal region. These changes are consistent with generalized retinal degeneration.

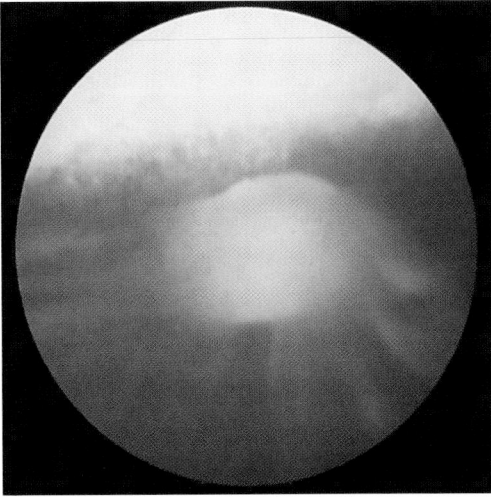

PLATE 18 ▮ Retinal separation (equine). Grey, linear areas radiate from the optic disc into the nontapetal region of the fundus. Note that the margins of the disc are quite indistinct in the affected area. An absence of retinal vessels indicates concurrent retinal degeneration.

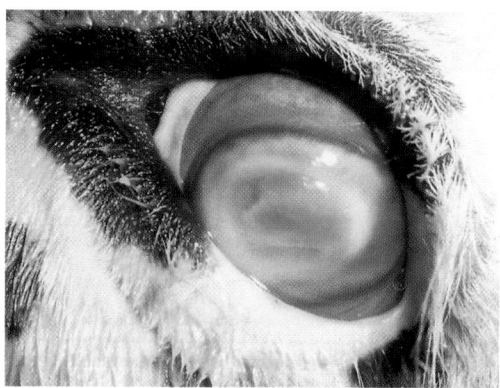

PLATE 19 ▮▮ Appearance of severe, acute infectious bovine keratoconjunctivitis *Moraxella bovis* in a calf.

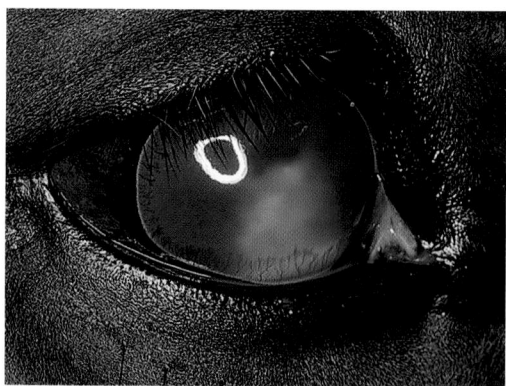

PLATE 20 ▮▮ Recurrent uveitis in a 7-year-old Thoroughbred. Intraocular structures are obscured by corneal edema and hypopyon.

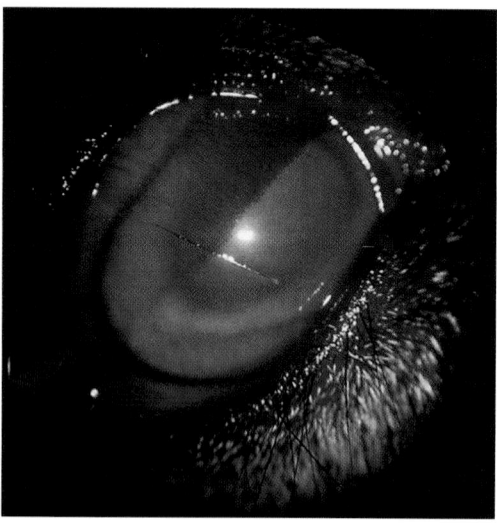

PLATE 21 ▮▮ Left eye of goat with mycoplasma keratoconjunctivitis. Note the corneal neovascularization.

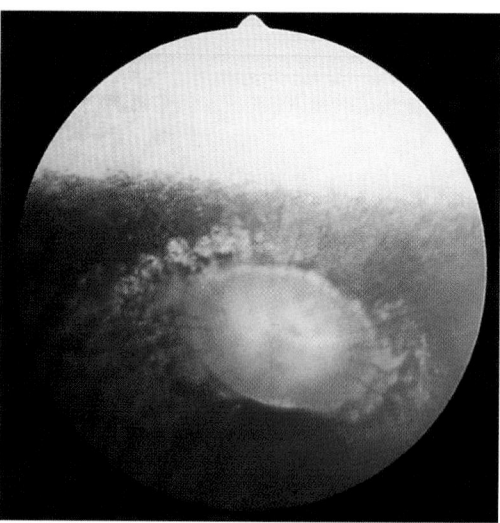

PLATE 22 ▮▮ Peripapillary retinal and choroidal depigmentation after recurrent episodes of equine uveitis. These inactive chorioretinal scars are also referred to as "butterfly" lesions.

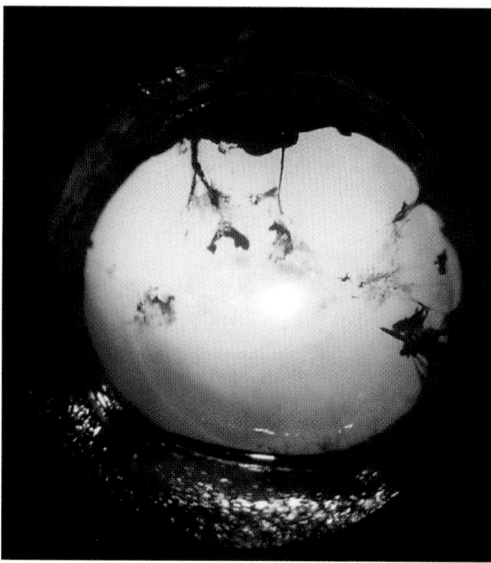

PLATE 23 ▮▮ Pigmented iridial tissue adheres to the anterior lens capsule after an episode of uveitis. Focal cataracts may develop at the adhesion site.

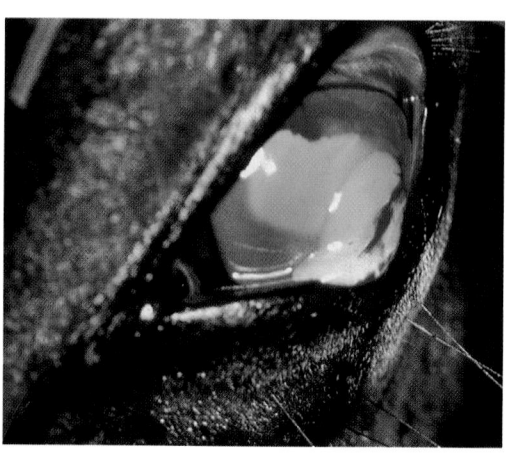

PLATE 24 ▮▮ Right eye of horse with a melting corneal ulcer caused by *Pseudomonas* spp. Corneal stroma has liquefied and is lying on the lower lid.

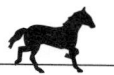

(uveal tissue) prolapse. Therapy is dictated by the type and extent of corneal injury, the complications encountered, the intended use and economic value of the animal, and other financial considerations.

Blunt Trauma to the Cornea

Blunt trauma to the globe from whips, lead shanks, and other objects can result in corneal endothelial injury and subsequent edema. Signs of traumatic uveitis may also accompany such an injury. The corneal edema that results from blunt trauma to the globe may be focal, linear, or diffuse. Therapy for blunt trauma includes a topical hypertonic saline solution or ointment* 2 to 4 times a day.[22] A linear keratopathy, characterized by a nonedematous deep striate refractile opacity in the cornea may represent a focal thinning or break in Descemet's membrane that has resulted from blunt trauma to the cornea. This type of lesion must be distinguished from Haab's striae, which are linear breaks in Descemet's membrane that result from high intraocular pressures in glaucoma.

Corneal Foreign Bodies

Plant matter embedded in the epithelium or superficial stroma is the most commonly encountered corneal foreign body. Foreign bodies usually are easily removed with a moistened cotton-tipped applicator or ophthalmic forceps. Sedation, motor or sensory nerve blocks, and topical anesthesia facilitate removal. Culture and sensitivity tests and cytologic examination of corneal samples are recommended before therapy is initiated. The cornea is stained with fluorescein† to evaluate the extent of corneal ulceration. While awaiting laboratory results, medical therapy should include a topical ophthalmic antibiotic (gentamicin 3 or 4 times a day) and atropine (twice a day or as needed). The prognosis is guarded until the cornea heals; the eye should be reevaluated in 24 to 48 hours.

Complications of corneal foreign bodies include bacterial and fungal infection, corneal perforation, and severe corneal scars that may restrict vision. Subpalpebral lavage systems are used in severe injuries when frequent, prolonged therapy is needed or when treating intractable animals.[23]

Corneal Ulcers

Corneal ulcers in horses are usually initiated by trauma and should be considered contaminated. Trauma may play a lesser role in food animals in which primary infectious etiologies are more common. The conjunctival fornices and eyelids should be carefully examined for foreign material. Diagnosis is based on cytologic examination, culture and sensitivity testing of corneal samples, and fluorescein staining of the cornea. Material for bacterial and fungal culture is collected from the ulcer with rayon-tipped swabs. The eyelid margins should be avoided, and cultures are obtained before application of topical anesthetics. Better culture results are obtained if the swab is moistened with a sterile solution before specimen collection. Use of a culture tube with transport medium in an enclosed, breakable ampule‡ is useful.[24] The ampule is crushed, and transport medium is allowed to moisten the swab before specimen collection.[13] Immediately after collection, the swab is replaced in the tube or inoculated

onto blood agar, Mycosel, and Sabouraud dextrose medium or MacConkey and thioglycolate broth.

Corneal scrapings for microscopic examination are collected with the use of topical anesthesia. The eyelids are retracted, and the margin of the corneal ulcer gently rubbed with a spatula or the blunt edge of a Bard-Parker scalpel blade until a small droplet of material is collected. This material is transferred to 2 to 4 clean glass slides, spread over a 1-cm area and allowed to air dry. One smear is stained with Diff-Quik, one with new methylene blue, one with Giemsa or PAS, and one with Gram stain.

Therapy of corneal ulcers is based on removal of the cause if still present; control of infection with topical antimicrobials; use of topical atropine for pain relief and prevention of synechia; and, in horses, systemic use of nonsteroidal antiinflammatory drugs such as flunixin meglumine or phenylbutazone. The initial choice of topical antibiotic should be based on the results of cytologic evaluation and later modified, if necessary, according to the results of culture and sensitivity testing. One study showed that oxytetracycline combined with polymixin B had an in vitro efficacy against isolates from infectious keratitis that was comparable to gentamicin and superior to chloramphenicol.[25] Should fungal hyphae be demonstrated on cytology, initial therapy with a topical antifungal agent should be immediately instituted. A recent study showed natamycin,* miconazole, itraconazole, and ketoconazole to be superior to fluconazole† based on the results of in vitro susceptibility testing.[26] Initially the ulcer may be cleaned with povidone-iodine solution‡ diluted 50:50 with sterile saline or collyrium. Subpalpebral lavage systems greatly facilitate delivery of topical medication to the equine eye.[23]

Surgical intervention should be considered in cases of deep corneal ulceration and exposure of Descemet's membrane. Surgical procedures most commonly used for corneal ulceration include conjunctival pedicle flap, keratoplasty, and tarsorrhaphy.[13,27,28] Ophthalmic tissue adhesives and soft contact lenses may also be used as nonsurgical therapy for deep corneal ulcers. Perforating ulcers with iris prolapse in cases of mixed bacterial and fungal keratitis or in cases of ulcers of greater than 2 weeks duration usually have a poor visual outcome.[29]

Corneal Lacerations

Corneal lacerations may be caused by sharp, protruding objects or projectories. Corneal lacerations can occur with or without scleral laceration, and, if nonperforating, are frequently treated as corneal ulcers. By contrast, perforating corneal lacerations are repaired surgically. Preoperative preparation includes tetanus prophylaxis (horses and goats), systemic antibiotics, and sample collection for corneal culture and sensitivity. Ocular ultrasonography may be quite useful to determine the integrity of intraocular structures. Care must be exercised during ocular examination and during anesthesia because extrusion of the intraocular contents can occur if excessive pressure is exerted on the globe or if the eyelids are forced open. Complete examination may have to be delayed until the animal is anesthetized.

General anesthesia, adequate magnification, proper instrumentation, appropriate suture material and needles, and adequate postoperative care are necessary to successfully repair a corneal laceration. Specific surgical considerations and

*AK-NaCl, Akorn Inc, Buffalo Grove, IL 60089.
†Ful-glo, Akorn, Inc, Albita Springs, LA 70420.
‡Culturette, Becton Dickenson Microbiology Co, Cockneysville, MD 21030.

*Natacyn, Alcon Laboratories, Inc, Fort Worth, TX 76134.
†Diflucan, Pfizer, Inc, New York, NY 10071.
‡Betadine, Purdue Frederick, Norwalk, CT 06850-3590.

techniques are discussed elsewhere. Postoperative therapy must include topical antibiotics, mydriatic/cycloplegics, and systemic antiinflammatory agents.[27,30] The prognosis for recovery of vision and preservation of the globe is generally guarded. Complications that may occur following repair of corneal lacerations include phthisis bulbi, corneal fibrosis, synechiation, blindness, retinal detachment, cataract formation, uveitis, endophthalmitis, bacterial or mycotic keratitis, and wound dehiscence with subsequent iris prolapse.

The prognosis after surgical repair of corneal or corneoscleral lacerations is best when the animal is presented immediately with a small wound in which the cornea or sclera is sealed and the anterior chamber has reformed. Minimum hyphema, clear intraocular media, a clearly visible fundus, and laceration length of less than 15 mm are additional findings that indicate a favorable prognosis.[27,29] In horses the success rate when only the cornea is involved is about 70% for recovery of vision and 90% for a cosmetically acceptable globe.[27] With corneoscleral lacerations the prognosis is much worse. In our experience, the success rate in such cases is 20% for recovery of vision and 70% for a cosmetically acceptable globe. Most phthisical globes are not considered cosmetically acceptable. Enucleation should be considered initially with severe corneoscleral lacerations because the prognosis is poor for return of vision and guarded for preservation of the globe.

TRAUMA TO THE UVEAL TRACT

Trauma to the globe can damage the iris, ciliary body, and choroid. The resulting inflammatory response may range from very mild with rapid recovery to loss of vision and chronic discomfort. Signs of inflammation of the iris and ciliary body include ocular pain, miosis, aqueous flare, corneal edema, fibrin in the anterior chamber, hyphema, hypopyon, low intraocular pressure, and synechiae formation. Damage involving the choroid may also affect the retina and lead to retinal detachment or degeneration. Concurrent damage to the corneal epithelium may be present and must be evaluated with fluorescein dye.

Traumatic uveitis is treated similarly to uveitis of other etiologies. Therapy is directed toward dilating the pupil to prevent synechiation, cycloplegia to prevent painful ciliary spasm, and controlling the intraocular inflammatory response.[16,28] Topical atropine is instilled to maintain mydriasis and provide cycloplegia. Topical corticosteroids and prostaglandin inhibitors such as 0.03% flurbiprofen* are used to decrease inflammation of the anterior segment. The topical corticosteroids of choice are 1% prednisolone acetate or 0.1% dexamethasone.[13,31] Subconjunctival injection of corticosteroids may also be quite beneficial in controlling inflammation. However, topical and subconjunctival corticosteroid use must be avoided in the presence of corneal ulceration or abrasion. Systemic medication should include flunixin meglumine, phenylbutazone, or oral corticosteroids. In horses, prednisolone is given by mouth at 0.5 to 2 mg/kg for 7 to 21 days. Care must be taken to avoid secondary complications from systemic corticosteroids.

Trauma-induced hyphema usually has a good prognosis if the blood has clotted and fills less than half the anterior chamber. Stall rest, topical 1% atropine, topical corticosteroids, and systemic antiinflammatory therapy should be instituted to control the associated uveitis. If a penetrating wound is suspected, topical and systemic antibiotic therapy should be included with periodic fluorescein staining. Surgi-

cal intervention to remove large blood clots is rarely indicated because it may result in rebleeding or worsen the uveitis. Lavage with urokinase of the anterior chamber with total hyphema of over 24 to 48 hours' duration has been beneficial in selected equine cases.[30] Dilute tissue plasminogen activator* may be injected to dissolve fibrin in the anterior chamber.[32]

Chronic uveitis following ocular trauma may be associated with lens damage or introduction of infectious or foreign agents into the eye and carries a poor prognosis. If the lens is ruptured, surgical removal of the lens material is advocated. Ocular perforation is a frequent cause of panophthalmitis in food animals and horses. Although therapy consists of systemic and topical antibiotics, as well as tetanus prophylaxis in susceptible species, panophthalmitis usually necessitates enucleation (see below).

TRAUMA TO THE LENS

Blunt or sharp trauma to the eye may damage the lens by causing lens opacity (cataract), rupturing the lens capsule, or, less commonly, may cause a shift in position (subluxation or luxation). A luxated lens should be removed if it causes obstructive glaucoma or chronic corneal edema from endothelial contact or if it becomes cataractous and reduces vision.

Release of lens protein into the eye following lens capsule rupture can induce severe granulomatous uveitis. In such cases the eye should be treated vigorously for lens-induced uveitis with topical atropine and topical and systemic antiinflammatory drugs. If the globe has been penetrated, topical and systemic antibiotics are indicated. The prognosis for preservation of vision is poor. Lens removal is often required to control the inflammatory response.

Cataracts (lens opacities) associated with ocular trauma may occur acutely or develop weeks after the initial injury. The opacity may be only focal and not hinder vision significantly, or it may be complete and cause a visual deficit. If the remainder of the eye is normal, surgical removal of the cataractous lens may improve vision.[33] Removal of cataracts secondary to uveitis is not currently recommended; however, with the advent of new surgical techniques, procedures such as combined vitrectomy (to possibly remove the immunologic stimulus in recurrent uveitis) and lensectomy may become more commonplace.[34]

TRAUMA INVOLVING THE VITREOUS

Trauma to the eye may result in hemorrhage into the vitreous or release of inflammatory products that cause vitreal degeneration. Either circumstance can result in vitreal syneresis (liquefaction), formation of vitreal traction bands, and subsequent retinal detachment. Treatment for the inflammation is generally adequate; however, vitrectomy may be beneficial in the management of severe vitreal hemorrhage.[16] Foreign material that becomes entrapped in the vitreous can initiate endophthalmitis. If infectious endophthalmitis is suspected, diagnostic paracentesis of the vitreous or anterior chamber should be performed to obtain samples for cytologic examination and culture and sensitivity testing. After the samples are obtained but before removing the needle from the globe, 200 g of gentamicin or 2.2 mg of cefazolin may be injected into the vitreous.[35] Further therapy should be based on culture and sensitivity results, as well as cytologic findings. If a foreign body can be identified, removal and vitrectomy may be beneficial, but the prognosis for successful treatment is poor.

---

*Ocufen, Allergan American, Hormigueros, Puerto Rico 00660.

*Activase, Genentech, South San Francisco, CA 94080.

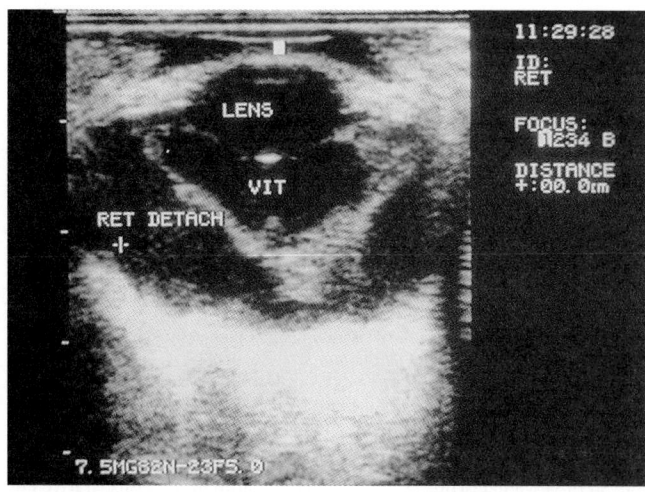

FIG. 37-9 ◼ Ocular ultrasound of a horse eye after blunt trauma to the globe. Note the characteristic V-shaped retinal detachment.

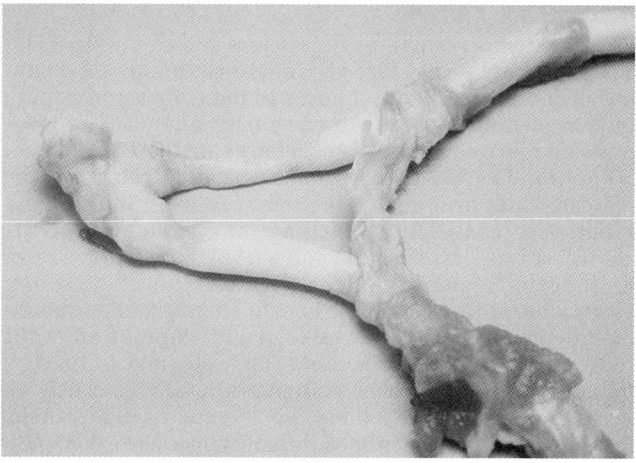

FIG. 37-10 ◼ Optic nerves and chiasm of a foal that was blind due to head trauma. Note the constrictions of the optic nerves due to necrosis and degeneration. (Courtesy Dr. C.L. Martin.)

TRAUMA TO THE RETINA

Retinal tears, hemorrhage, edema, and detachment may be caused by trauma.[36] In cases of opaque ocular media, retinal separations may be diagnosed by ocular ultrasonography (Fig. 37-9). Retinal degeneration may also occur following ocular trauma. Retinal hemorrhage and edema may be treated with systemic and topical corticosteroids. With current technology, surgical repair of retinal tears, lacerations, or detachments in food animals and horses may be feasible in selected cases.

TRAUMA TO THE OPTIC NERVE

The pathogenesis of damage to the optic nerve is not well understood but is considered to be the result of shearing forces at the optic foramen from displacement of the brain following severe head trauma[37] (Fig. 37-10). Direct contusion or concussion to the optic nerve can also occur. Loss of blood supply to the nerve and subarachnoid hemorrhage may also play a role. Early examination may reveal only a dilated pupil that may be partially responsive or completely unresponsive to light. Later changes may include optic nerve atrophy (Fig. 37-11) and peripapillary retinal pigmentation changes. Therapy with systemic antiinflammatory drugs may be of benefit, but severe damage is often irreversible.

Traumatic optic nerve atrophy is usually characterized by a unilateral or bilateral sudden onset of blindness; dilated, fixed pupils; and a lack of menace reflex. In horses the traumatic episode is frequently characterized by damage to the poll from rearing over backwards and striking the back of the head, from rearing up and hitting a ceiling beam, or from blunt trauma (blows) to the side or front of the face. The animal usually stands without loss of consciousness, and the injury is not considered serious by the owner at the time. Initially blindness with a normal-appearing fundus is observed.

At 3 to 4 weeks following trauma, examination of the fundus reveals a pale optic disc (see Fig 39-11). Later, loss of peripapillary retinal vessels is usually evident. The optic disc often appears depressed, with increased prominence of the lamina cribrosa. Confirmation of optic nerve or optic tract lesions causing blindness may be made by the absence of a direct pupillary light reflex and by a normal electroretinogram. The pathologic lesion is a rupture of the nerve axons

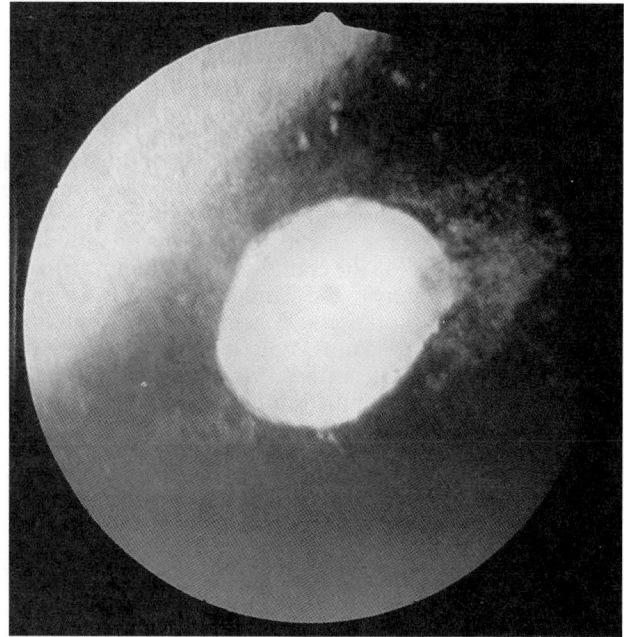

FIG. 37-11 ◼ Appearance of the optic nerve 3 months after head trauma in a horse. Note the pale optic disc and peripapillary retinal degeneration. (Courtesy Dr. C.L. Martin.)

from stretching forces produced by movement of the brain.[37] Chiasmal hemorrhage and fractures of the basisphenoid bone may be present at necropsy. Although therapy includes systemic corticosteroids (dexamethasone 1 mg/kg) and intravenous dimethyl sulfoxide,[37] medical therapy has not generally been successful. The lack of response to medical therapy appears to be related to the severity of the injury.

A segmental optic nerve atrophy involving one to three quadrants of the optic disc occurs in horses. The appearance is characterized by pallor, loss of normal vasculature, and increased prominence of the lamina cribrosa in the affected quadrants. The etiology is unknown; however, traumatic injury is suspected in most cases. Response to medical therapy is poor.

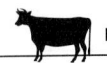

CHEMICAL INJURY

Ocular irritation caused by insecticides and disinfectants inadvertently applied to the eye is not uncommon in the farm or ranch setting. Chemical burns to the cornea and adnexa can have serious consequences and may warrant a poor prognosis for salvage of the eye. Alkali burns are more severe than acid burns. Corneal burns from acids tend to be sharply demarcated and nonprogressive, whereas alkali burns cause progressive coagulation, melting, and sloughing of the corneal stroma.[16] Chemically induced melting of the cornea must be differentiated from bacterial and fungal infections. Treatment for a suspected or known chemical burn should include lavage of the affected area with copious amounts (500 to 2000 ml) of sterile saline. Tap water may be used by the owner until veterinary assistance is available. It may be necessary to sedate the animal. No attempt should be made to neutralize the substance because this may cause precipitation within the cornea. The damage should then be evaluated with the aid of local nerve blocks.

Treatment should include appropriate topical antimicrobials, atropine, and acetylcysteine. Hourly application of a collagenase inhibitor (acetylcysteine)* may be needed. Systemic antiinflammatory drugs should be used to control the associated uveitis. Therapeutic soft contact lenses have also been used to protect the corneal stroma in cases with extensive corneal ulcerations.

THERMAL INJURY

Thermal injuries can damage the eyelids, conjunctiva, and cornea. Anterior uveitis and exfoliation of the lens capsule can also occur. Therapy for minor burns to the eyelids is directed toward keeping the injured area moist with antibiotic dressings, and protecting the cornea if eyelid dysfunction occurs. Treatment for injury to the conjunctiva or cornea should include topical antibiotics and systemic antiinflammatory drugs in horses. Full-thickness eyelid burns may require immediate grafting to protect the cornea and minimize scarring.[8] Third-eyelid or conjunctival flaps may be required to protect the cornea until eyelid function returns.

REFERENCES

13. Whitley RD, Turner LM: Management of ocular trauma in horses. I, Cornea and sclera, *Mod Vet Pract* 67:233-238, 1986.
14. Whitley RD, Moore CP: Microbiology of the equine eye in health and disease, *Vet Clin North Am (Large Anim Pract)* 6:451-466, 1984.
15. Caron JP et al: Periorbital skull fractures in five horses, *J Am Vet Med Assoc* 188:280-284, 1986.
16. Turner LM, Whitley RD, Hager D: Management of ocular trauma in horses. I, Orbit, eyelids, uvea, lens, retina, and optic nerve, *Mod Vet Pract* 67:341-347, 1986.
17. Morgan RV, Daniel GB, Donnell RL: Magnetic resonance imaging of the normal eye and orbit of the horse, *Prog Vet Comp Ophthalmol* 3:127-134, 1993.
18. Boroffka S, van den Belt A: CT/ultrasound diagnosis: retrobulbar hematoma in a horse, *Vet Radiol Ultrasound* 37:441-443, 1996.
19. Rebhun WC: Diseases of the bovine orbit, *J Am Vet Med Assoc* 175:171-175, 1979.
20. Wilkie DA: Repair of superior palpebral defect in a horse by use of a silicone subdermal implant, *J Am Vet Med Assoc* 200:821-824, 1992.
21. Welker B: Ocular surgery, *Vet Clin North Am (Food Anim Pract)* 11:149-157, 1995.
22. Rebhun WC: Conditions of the cornea, uvea, and lens. In White NA, Moore JN, eds: *Current techniques in equine surgery and lameness*, Philadelphia, 1998, WB Saunders, p 185.
23. Sweeney CR, Russell GE: Complications associated with use of a one-hole subpalpebral lavage system in horses: 150 cases (1977-1996), *J Am Vet Med Assoc* 211:1271-1274, 1997.
24. Whitley RD, Moore CP: Ocular diagnostic and therapeutic techniques in food animals, *Vet Clin North Am (Large Anim Pract)* 6:553-575, 1984.

25. Moore CP et al: Antimicrobial agents for treatment of infectious keratitis in horses, *J Am Vet Med Assoc* 207:855-862, 1995.
26. Brooks DE et al: Antimicrobial susceptibility patterns of fungi isolated from horses with ulcerative keratitis, *Am J Vet Res* 59:138-142, 1998.
27. Lavach JD, Severin GA, Roberts SM: Lacerations of the equine eye: a review of 48 cases, *J Am Vet Med Assoc* 184:1243-1248, 1984.
28. Millichamp NJ: Ocular trauma, *Vet Clin North Am (Equine Practice)* 8:521-536, 1992.
29. Chmielewski NT et al: Visual outcome and ocular survival following iris prolapse in the horse: a review of 32 cases, *Equine Vet J* 29:31-39, 1997.
30. Lavach JD: *Large animal ophthalmology*, St Louis, 1990, Mosby, pp 134-141, 172-175.
31. Ward DA: Comparison of the blood-aqueous barrier stabilizing effects of steroidal and non-steroidal anti-inflammatory agents in the dog, *Prog Vet Comp Ophthalmol* 2:117-124, 1992.
32. Martin C et al: Ocular use of tissue plasminogen activator in companion animals, *Prog Vet Comp Ophthalmol* 3:29-36, 1993.
33. Dziezyc J, Millichamp NJ, Keller CB: Use of phacofragmentation for cataract removal in horses: 12 cases (1985-1989), *J Am Vet Med Assoc* 198:1774-1778, 1991.
34. Heidbrink V: First experiences with endoscopic surgery on the equine eye, *Praktische Tierarzt* 79:824-836, 1998.
35. Stern GA, Engel HM, Driebe WT: The treatment of postoperative endophthalmitis: results of differing approaches to treatment, *Ophthalmology* 96:62-67, 1989.
36. Mätz-Rensig K et al: Retinal detachment in horses, *Equine Vet J* 28:111-116, 1996.
37. Martin CL, Kaswan R, Chapman W: Four cases of traumatic optic nerve blindness in the horse, *Equine Vet J* 18:133-137, 1986.

INFECTIOUS OCULAR DISEASES

JOAN DZIEZYC

NICHOLAS J. MILLICHAMP

The major infectious ocular diseases in large animals are listed in Table 37-2.

MYCOPLASMAL KERATOCONJUNCTIVITIS IN GOATS AND SHEEP

DEFINITION AND ETIOLOGY. *Mycoplasma conjunctivae* has been frequently isolated from epidemics of keratoconjunctivitis, respiratory disease, and/or arthritis in goats and sheep.[38-40] *Mycoplasma mycoides* var. *mycoides* has been isolated from an epidemic of mastitis, arthritis, and keratoconjunctivitis in goats.[41] *Acholeplasma oculusi (oculi)* has been isolated from sheep and goats in epidemics of keratoconjunctivitis.[42,43] *Mycoplasma agalactiae* and *Mycoplasma arginini* have also been described as causing keratoconjunctivitis and systemic disease.[44]

CLINICAL SIGNS AND DIFFERENTIAL DIAGNOSES. Clinical signs of mycoplasmal keratoconjunctivitis include lacrimation, conjunctival vessel injection, and occasionally follicular conjunctivitis. Later in the disease, keratitis with neovascularization (Fig. 37-12) and occasionally anterior uveitis can be seen.[38,45] One case of choroiditis and hyalitis has been described.[46] Signs can be seen in individuals, as well as in herd or flock outbreaks. The disease is usually unilateral, but it can be bilateral. Differential diagnoses include other infectious causes of keratoconjunctivitis such as *Chlamydia* spp. (sheep), *Branhamella (Neisseria)* spp., aerobic bacteria, parasites, and infectious bovine rhinotracheitis (goats), as well as noninfectious causes such as trauma.

CLINICAL PATHOLOGY. In conjunctival scrapings taken early in the disease many neutrophils are seen; later lymphocytes predominate. Plasma cells and necrotic epithelial cells are also seen.[47] Organisms can be seen occasionally in epithelial cell cytoplasm as coccobacillary or varied forms.[48] Pigment granules can be mistaken for organisms.[42,47]

Mycoplasmal organisms can be cultured and identified from conjunctival swabs. Recent experimental work has been performed using polymerase chain reaction (PCR) to identify *Mycoplasma conjunctivae* in conjunctival smears.[49] Egwu

*Acetylcysteine 10% solution, American Reagent Laboratories, Inc., Shirley, NY 11967.

TABLE 37-2

Major Infectious Ocular Diseases of Large Animals

Agent	Common Name/ Disease	Major Sign(s)	Cattle	Sheep	Goats	Horses
Mycoplasma conjunctivae	Pinkeye	Keratoconjunctivitis		++	++	
Mycoplasma mycoides ssp. *mycoides*	Pinkeye	Keratoconjunctivitis			+	
Acholeplasma oculusi	Pinkeye	Keratoconjunctivitis		+	+	
Chlamydia psittaci	Pinkeye	Keratoconjunctivitis		++		
Branhamella (Neisseria)	Pinkeye	Keratoconjunctivitis		+	+	
Mycoplasma agalactiae		Keratoconjunctivitis		+	+	
Mycoplasma arginini		Keratoconjunctivitis		+	+	
Listeria monocytogenes		Keratoconjunctivitis	+	+		
Infectious bovine rhinotracheitis		Keratoconjunctivitis	++		+	
Colesiota (Rickettsia) conjunctivae	Pinkeye	Keratoconjunctivitis		+		
Equine viral arteritis		Keratoconjunctivitis				+
Equine herpes virus serotype 2		Keratoconjunctivitis				+
Mycoplasma bovoculi		Conjunctivitis	+			
Ureaplasma ssp.		Conjunctivitis	+			
Equine adenovirus		Conjunctivitis				+
Moraxella spp.		Conjunctivitis				+
Streptococcus equi	Strangles	Conjunctivitis				+
Moraxella bovis	Pinkeye	Corneal ulcer	++			
Equine herpes virus serotype 1	Rhinopneumonitis	Keratitis				+
Malignant catarrhal fever		Uveitis, keratitis	+			
Neonatal septicemia		Uveitis	+	+	+	+
Mycobacterium bovis	Tuberculosis	Uveitis	+			
Salmonella spp.		Uveitis				+
Borrelia burgdorferi	Lyme disease	Uveitis				+
Leptospira interrogans		Recurrent uveitis				+
Brucella abortus		Recurrent uveitis				+
Scrapie		Retinitis		+		
Hemophilus somnus	Infectious thromboembolic meningoencephalitis	Retinitis	+			
Bovine virus diarrhea		Retinal dysplasia, cataracts	+			
Bluetongue		Chorioretinitis conjunctivitis	+	+		
Toxoplasma gondii		Chorioretinitis				+
Rhodococcus (Coryne-bacterium) equi		Panophthalmitis				+
Bovine leukemia virus	Bovine leukosis/ lymphosarcoma	Exophthalmos	+			
Cryptococcus neoformans		Exophthalmos				+

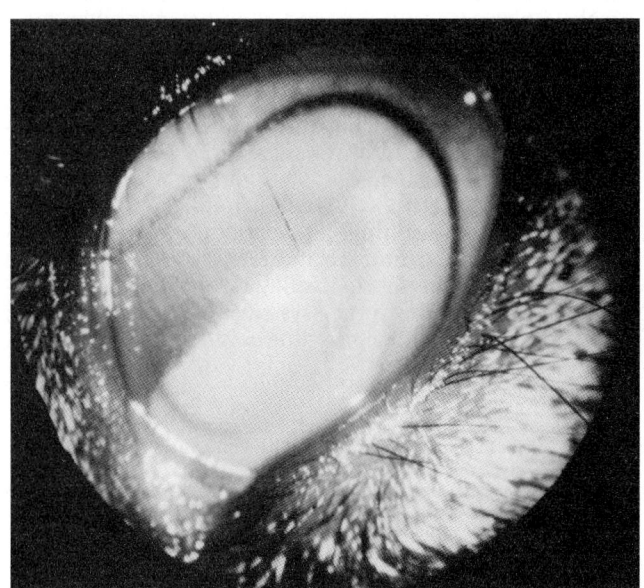

FIG. 37-12 ▦ Left eye of goat with mycoplasmal keratoconjunctivitis. Note diffuse corneal edema and dorsally the marked corneal neovascularization.

and Faull[50] describe rising serum and lacrimal antibody titers in sheep topically inoculated with *M. conjunctivae.* However, Trotter and colleagues report low serum titers to *M. conjunctivae* in normal animals and no rise in titer in animals inoculated with *M. conjunctivae* subconjunctivally that subsequently developed signs of disease.[39]

EPIDEMIOLOGY. Mycoplasmal infections apparently are transmitted directly from animal to animal as evidenced by herd or flock outbreaks. The presence of carrier animals is postulated and *M. conjunctivae* can be cultured from unaffected animals.[51,52] Animals can become reinfected. Keratoconjunctivitis can be induced in sheep with topically applied *M. conjunctivae.*[50,53,54] Clinical signs were identical to natural outbreaks and spread to uninoculated sheep. The organism was cultured from eyes long after clinical signs abated. See Chapter 36 for more details on *M. mycoides.*

TREATMENT AND PROGNOSIS. In most animals, mycoplasmal keratoconjunctivitis associated with *M. conjunctivae* is transient. The animal usually recovers spontaneously in 10 days, although some animals seem to have recurring episodes that last for several weeks. In one controlled clinical trial, one dose (200 mg/10 kg) of long-acting oxytetracycline was given to experimentally inoculated lambs. This treatment seemed to hasten the cessation of clinical signs although the results were not analyzed statistically.[55] The treatment did not, however, eliminate the *M. conjunctivae* infection. Other drugs recommended for the ocular disease include topical oxytetracycline or oxytetracycline and polymyxin B,[38] and subconjunctival oxytetracycline[43] (which should be diluted). Subconjunctival oxytetracycline is not currently recommended because it may cause a severe inflammatory reaction. In vitro antibiotic testing of *M. conjunctivae* shows that tylosin, oxytetracycline, streptomycin, and chlortetracycline are suitable for treatment.[56]

PREVENTION AND CONTROL. Introduction of new animals into a herd or flock has been implicated in starting an outbreak of keratoconjunctivitis. Therefore isolation and, if necessary, treatment of new animals are important before contact with the herd. Otherwise no specific recommendations have been made for prevention and control of *M. conjunctivae.* See Chapter 36 for control of *M. mycoides* spp. *mycoides.*

REFERENCES

38. Baas EJ et al: Epidemic caprine keratoconjunctivitis: recovery of *Mycoplasma conjunctivae* and its possible role in pathogenesis, *Infect Immunol* 8:806-815, 1977.
39. Trotter SL et al: Epidemic caprine keratoconjunctivitis: experimentally induced disease with a pure culture of *Mycoplasma conjunctivae, Infect Immunol* 18:816-822, 1977.
40. Rodriguez JL et al: High mortality in goats associated with the isolation of a strain of *Mycoplasma mycoides* subsp. *mycoides* (large colony type), *J Vet Med* 42:587-593, 1995.
41. Bar-Moshe B, Rapapport E: Observations on *Mycoplasma mycoides subsp. mycoides* infection in Saanen goats, *Israel J Med Sci* 17:537-539, 1981.
42. Al-Aubaidi JM et al: Identification and characterization of *Acholeplasma oculusi spec. nov.* from the eyes of goats with keratoconjunctivitis, *Cornell Vet* 63:117-129, 1973.
43. Arbuckle JBR, Bonson MD: The isolation of *Acholeplasma oculi* from an outbreak of ovine keratoconjunctivitis, *Vet Rec* 106:15, 1980.
44. Jones GE: Mycoplasmas of sheep and goats: a synopsis, *Vet Rec* 113:619-620, 1983.
45. McCauley EH, Surman PG, Anderson DR: Isolation of *Mycoplasma* from goats during an epizootic of keratoconjunctivitis, *Am J Vet Res* 32:861-870, 1971.
46. Whitley RD, Albert RA: Clinical uveitis and polyarthritis associated with *Mycoplasma* species in a young goat, *Vet Rec* 115:217-218, 1984.
47. Surman PG: Cytology of "pink-eye" of sheep, including a reference to trachoma of man, by employing acridine orange and iodine stains, and isolation of *Mycoplasma* agents from infected sheep eyes, *Aust J Biol Sci* 21:447-467, 1968.
48. Dagnall GJR: Use of exfoliative cytology in the diagnosis of ovine keratoconjunctivitis, *Vet Rec* 135:127-130, 1994.
49. Giacometti J et al: Detection and identification of *Mycoplasma conjunctivae* in infectious keratoconjunctivitis by PCR based on the 16S rRNA gene, *J Vet Med* 46:173-180, 1999.
50. Egwu GO, Faull WB: Humoral immune responses in lambs following ocular experimental infection with a pure cloned culture of *Mycoplasma conjunctivae,* Bull Anim Health Prod Afr 39:333-337, 1991.
51. Egwu GO et al: Ovine infectious keratoconjunctivitis: a microbiological study of clinically unaffected and affected sheep's eyes with special reference to *Mycoplasma conjunctivae, Vet Rec* 125:253-256, 1989.
52. Dagnall GJR: An investigation of colonization of the conjunctival sac of sheep by bacteria and mycoplasmas, *Epidemiol Infect* 112:561-567, 1994.
53. ter Laak EA et al: Ovine keratoconjunctivitis experimentally induced by instillation of *Mycoplasma conjunctivae, Vet Q* 10:217-224, 1988.
54. Dagnall GJR: Experimental infection of the conjunctival sac of lambs with *Mycoplasma conjunctivae, Br Vet J* 149:429-435, 1993.
55. Hosie BD, Greig A: Role of oxytetracycline dihydrate in the treatment of *Mycoplasma*-associated ovine keratoconjunctivitis in lambs, *Br Vet J* 151:83-88, 1995.
56. Egwu GO: In vitro antibiotic sensitivity of *Mycoplasma conjunctivae* and some bacterial species, *Small Rumin Res* 7:85-92, 1992.

CHLAMYDIAL KERATOCONJUNCTIVITIS IN SHEEP

DEFINITION AND ETIOLOGY. Chlamydial agents have been isolated from outbreaks of keratoconjunctivitis in sheep flocks. The agent has been identified as *Chlamydia psittaci,* which may also cause abortion (see Chapter 41) and polyarthritis (see Chapter 36).

CLINICAL SIGNS AND DIFFERENTIAL DIAGNOSES. Early clinical signs consist of epiphora, chemosis, and conjunctival hyperemia. Later in the disease, follicle formation in the conjunctiva becomes prominent. Still later, corneal neovascularization may be seen. Most cases are bilateral and symmetric.[57,58] In some flock outbreaks of keratoconjunctivitis, outbreaks of polyarthritis are also noted. Most lambs that develop chlamydial polyarthritis will also develop conjunctivitis.[57,58] Differentials include other infectious causes of keratoconjunctivitis such as *Mycoplasma* spp. and *Branhamella (Neisseria)* spp. aerobic bacteria, and parasites, as well as noninfectious causes such as trauma.

CLINICAL PATHOLOGY. Early in the disease conjunctival smears show numerous neutrophils and some lymphocytes. Later there are more neutrophils and fewer mononuclear cells. Cytoplasmic chlamydial inclusions are occasionally seen in up to a third of the eyes scraped. Conjunctival epithelial cells are often necrotic. Chlamydial organisms can be cultured from conjunctival scrapings and from blood taken from sheep with polyarthritis and conjunctivitis.[57-59] In one study, titers to chlamydial antibodies were found at 1:16 or higher in a number of the affected lambs, although titers on normal lambs were not reported.[58]

EPIDEMIOLOGY. Chlamydial organisms are apparently transmitted by direct contact, as evidenced by flock outbreaks. *Chlamydia psittaci* caused conjunctivitis when topically administered to five lambs.[60] An uninoculated lamb housed with the five lambs also developed conjunctivitis. Lambs subsequently developed follicular conjunctivitis.[59] In another study chlamydial organisms were injected intraarticularly, intravenously, and intramuscularly and caused polyarthritis and conjunctivitis.[59]

TREATMENT AND PROGNOSIS. In uncomplicated cases the disease is self-limiting, and eyes are normal in 2 to 3 weeks.[58] The same treatments indicated for *M. mycoides* var. *mycoides* are also effective in treating chlamydial conjunctivitis polyarthritis of sheep (i.e., systemic oxytetracycline and, when possible, a topical tetracycline ophthalmic preparation).

REFERENCES

57. Stephenson EH, Storz J, Hopkins JB: Properties and frequency of isolation of chlamydiae from eyes of lambs with conjunctivitis and polyarthritis, *Am J Vet Res* 35:177-180, 1984.
58. Hopkins JB et al: Conjunctivitis associated with chlamydial polyarthritis in lambs, *J Am Vet Med Assoc* 163:1157-1160, 1973.
59. Storz J et al: Isolation of psittacosis agents from follicular conjunctivitis of sheep, *Proc Soc Exp Biol Med* 125:857-860, 1967.

60. Wilsmore AJ et al: Experimental conjunctival infection of lambs with a strain of *Chlamydia psittaci* isolated from the eyes of a sheep naturally affected with keratoconjunctivitis, *Vet Rec* 127:229-231, 1990.

BRANHAMELLA (NEISSERIA) OVIS KERATOCONJUNCTIVITIS IN SHEEP AND GOATS

Branhamella ovis is a gram-negative diplococcus that is similar to *Moraxella* spp. This agent has been cultured from sheep and goats with keratoconjunctivitis[61]; however, it can also be cultured from normal eyes.[62] Clinical signs include lacrimation, injected conjunctival vessels, corneal edema, and neovascularization and secondary uveitis.

In one outbreak,[63] neutrophils and gram-negative coccobacilli were seen on conjunctival scrapings. *B. ovis* was cultured from the initial outbreak and was then instilled into the conjunctival sac of experimental goats with or without UV radiation. The experimental goats developed lacrimation and conjunctivitis, but no keratitis.[63] In another study, *B. ovis* instilled into the conjunctival sac of lambs induced reddened conjunctiva and follicle formation. *B. ovis* could be cultured from these eyes for up to 20 days after inoculation.[64]

In one outbreak, animals were treated with parenteral tylosin and topical neomycin, polymyxin B, and a corticosteroid, and all 10 recovered.[61] Bankemper and colleagues[63] used subconjunctival penicillin to treat her affected goats.

B. ovis has been cultured from cattle with serous conjunctivitis and rarely keratitis.[65]

REFERENCES

61. Bulgin MS, Dubose DA: Pinkeye associated with *Branhamella ovis* infection in dairy goats, *Vet Med (Small Anim Clin)* 77:1791-1793, 1982.
62. Spradbrow PB: The bacterial flora of the ovine conjunctival sac, *Aust Vet J* 44:117-118, 1968.
63. Bankemper KW et al: Keratoconjunctivitis associated with *Neisseria ovis* infection in a herd of goats, *J Vet Diagn Invest* 2:76-78, 1990.
64. Dagnall GJR: The role of *Branhamella ovis, Mycoplasma conjunctivae,* and *Chlamydia psittaci* in conjunctivitis of sheep, *Br Vet J* 150:65-71, 1994.
65. Nagy A et al: Further data to the aetiology, pathogenesis and therapy of infectious bovine keratoconjunctivitis, *Comp Immunol Microbiol Infect Dis* 12:115-127, 1989.

SCRAPIE-ASSOCIATED RETINOPATHY IN SHEEP AND GOATS

The scrapie agent causes a degenerative central nervous system disease in sheep and less commonly in goats (see Chapter 33 for more information on scrapie). Barnett and Palmer[66] described two sheep with scrapie that also had multifocal hyperreflective areas in the tapetum, histologically seen as small areas of retina raised by accumulation of eosinophilic material between photoreceptors and retinal pigment epithelium. The eosinophilic material was characterized as a complex lipid. It was not shown that scrapie had caused the lesions.[66]

REFERENCES

66. Barnett KC, Palmer AC: Retinopathy in sheep affected with natural scrapie, *Res Vet Sci* 12:383-385, 1971.

BLUETONGUE-INDUCED RETINAL DYSPLASIA IN SHEEP

Bluetongue is a disease of ruminants caused by an arbovirus that is transmitted by *Culicoides* gnats. Clinical signs include fever and vasculitis that leads to oral lesions, lameness, swollen face, pulmonary edema, and death (see Chapter 30). In pregnant ewes vaccinated with modified live virus (MLV)

on day 40 of gestation, fetuses developed cerebral anomalies.[67] These anomalies have also been described in clinical cases in which ewes had been vaccinated with MLV at about 5 or 6 weeks' gestation. In addition, when the fetus was vaccinated with MLV vaccine between days 50 and 75 of gestation, lesions of retinitis and choroiditis were noted that appeared to center around retinal vessels. In some eyes, inflammatory lesions produced persistent areas of retinal dysplasia.[68]

REFERENCES

67. Young S, Cordy DR: An ovine fetal encephalopathy caused by bluetongue vaccine virus, *J Neuropathol Exp Neurol* 23:635-659, 1964.
68. Silverstein AM et al: An experimental, virus-induced retinal dysplasia in the fetal lamb, *Am J Ophthalmol* 72:22-34, 1971.

LISTERIA MONOCYTOGENES KERATOCONJUNCTIVITIS IN SHEEP AND CATTLE

Listeria monocytogenes has been cultured from conjunctival smears taken from sheep and cattle with keratoconjunctivitis.[69] In most of the sheep, *B. (Neisseria) ovis* was also cultured. Clinical signs included hyperemic conjunctiva, lacrimation, photophobia, and cloudy cornea. Treatment with topical chlortetracycline was curative. Walker and Morgan[70] provide a description of two experimental sheep that developed unilateral anterior uveitis. *L. monocytogenes* was cultured from the conjunctiva of each animal that recovered after treatment with parenteral ampicillin and topical antibiotics.

REFERENCES

69. Kummeneje K, Mikkelsen T: Isolation of *Listeria monocytogenes* type 04 from cases of keratoconjunctivitis in cattle and sheep, *Nord Vet Med* 27:144-149, 1975.
70. Walker JK, Morgan JH: Ovine ophthalmitis associated with *Listeria monocytogenes, Vet Rec* 132:636, 1993.

INFECTIOUS BOVINE RHINOTRACHEITIS KERATOCONJUNCTIVITIS IN GOATS

Goats are susceptible to infectious bovine rhinotracheitis (IBR) virus, which may in some cases result in ocular disease. In one goat with ocular signs, conjunctivitis and keratitis with keratoconus were seen 5 days after the onset of severe respiratory illness. IBR virus was isolated from ocular and nasal discharge.[71]

REFERENCES

71. Mohanty SB et al: Natural infection with infectious bovine rhinotracheitis in goats, *J Am Vet Med Assoc* 160:879-880, 1972.

COLESIOTA (RICKETTSIA) KERATOCONJUNCTIVITIS IN SHEEP

Colesiota (or *Rickettsia*) *conjunctivae* has been described as the cause of infectious keratoconjunctivitis in sheep, but documentation is sparse. The organism has not been cultured, only identified on conjunctival scrapings. Clinical signs include lacrimation, hyperemic conjunctiva, and neovascularization of the cornea.[72] Several authors have since suspected that this organism is the same as *Chlamydia psittaci*.[73,74]

REFERENCES

72. Beveridge WIB: Investigations on contagious ophthalmia of sheep, with special attention to the epidemiology of infection by *Rickettsiae conjunctivae, Aust Vet J* 18:155-164, 1942.
73. Cello RM: Ocular infections in animals with PLT (Bedsonia) group agents, *Am J Ophthalmol* 63:1270-1272, 1967.
74. Bulgin MS, Dubose DA: Pinkeye associated with *Branhamella ovis* infection in dairy goats, *Vet Med (Small Anim Clin)* 77:1791-1793, 1982.

INFECTIOUS BOVINE KERATOCONJUNCTIVITIS (IBK, pinkeye)

ETIOLOGY. Infectious bovine keratoconjunctivitis (IBK, pinkeye) is an infectious and contagious ocular disease of cattle characterized by conjunctivitis and ulcerative keratitis. The only organism recovered from clinical cases that has repeatedly been shown to fulfill Koch's postulates is the gram-negative coccobacillus *Moraxella bovis*.[75-77]

CLINICAL SIGNS AND DIFFERENTIAL DIAGNOSES. The earliest signs of disease are excessive lacrimation, blepharospasm, and photophobia. Simultaneously or within 24 hours, conjunctival injection and chemosis develop. Two to 4 days after onset of the disease, keratitis is detected. Initially an area of central or pericentral corneal opacification (edema) is seen. This stains with fluorescein, indicating the presence of superficial corneal ulceration. Multiple small ulcers (1 to 4 mm) may be seen, and epithelial vesicles may occur. The ulcers become wider and deeper over the next few days, and signs of anterior uveitis (aqueous flare, miosis) secondary to the keratitis may be seen. The ocular discharge becomes mucopurulent. Circumlimbal corneal vascularization begins to invade the cornea 4 to 7 days after ulceration is first seen (Fig. 37-13). Typically by 7 to 9 days a radiating network of blood vessels will have grown into the corneal stroma toward the ulcer, which appears yellowish as a result of necrosis and infiltration of the corneal stroma by white blood cells adjacent to the lesion. The corneal blood vessels gradually reach the edges of the ulcer, and granulation tissue begins to fill in the defect (Fig. 37-14). Two to 3 weeks after onset of the disease the cornea is often reepithelialized.

After the cornea heals, a faint corneal scar may be detected. In younger cattle the disease is often more severe, with deepening of the corneal ulcer through the stroma and eventual corneal perforation. In such cases, anterior uveitis with hypopyon is marked. The perforated cornea usually becomes plugged with iris, resulting in anterior synechiation in the healed eye, although in some cases panophthalmitis or glaucoma may occur that eventually results in phthisis bulbi.

The central corneal ulceration typical of IBK clinically differentiates this disease from conjunctivitis caused by infectious bovine rhinotracheitis (IBR). It has been shown that IBK is more severe in cattle concurrently infected with IBR and may be more prevalent in cattle that have received modified live IBR intranasal vaccine before *Moraxella* infection.[78-80] Several other infectious agents (i.e., adenovirus,[81] *Mycoplasma*,[82,83] *Branhamella [Neisseria]*,[84] and *Listeria*[85]) have been recovered from eyes showing clinical signs similar to those seen in *Moraxella*-induced IBK. None of these organisms have been demonstrated to cause corneal lesions when reinoculated in eyes of susceptible animals. However, it is probable that these infectious agents may predispose the eye to subsequent infection by *M. bovis* or complicate concurrent infections.

CLINICAL PATHOLOGY. Although diagnosis is usually based on the clinical signs, affected eyes can be cultured to isolate the *M. bovis* strain for antibiotic sensitivity testing. *Moraxella* is most readily recovered during the acute stage of the disease.

PATHOPHYSIOLOGY. Pathogenic strains of *M. bovis* are piliated strains. Two types of pili, I and Q, have been identified. It is suggested that the Q pili are specific for binding to corneal epithelium.[86,87] There are at least seven distinct serogroups of piliated *M. bovis*.[88] After adhering to the epithelium, virulent strains of *M. bovis* release enzymes that damage corneal epithelial cells to gain access to the corneal stroma.[88-94] β-Hemolysin appears to have some importance in this damage.[95] Several factors may enhance the access of the bacteria to the corneal stroma by damaging the epithelial barrier. Ultraviolet light has been shown to be capable of

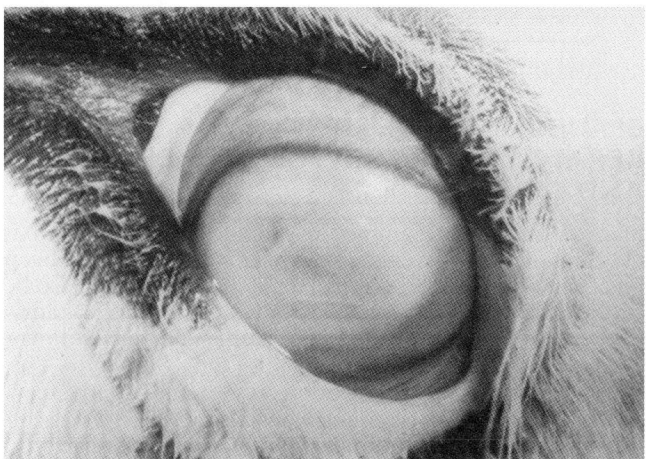

FIG. 37-13 ▓ Appearance of severe, acute infectious bovine keratoconjunctivitis *(Moraxella bovis)* in a calf.

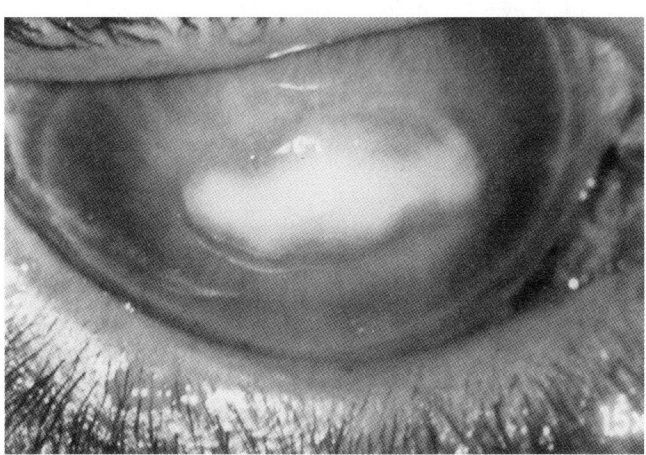

FIG. 37-14 ▓ Corneal neovascularization and granulation in the cornea of a cow recovering from infectious bovine keratoconjunctivitis *(Moraxella bovis)*.

damaging the corneal epithelium and enhancing entry of *Moraxella* to the corneal stroma and probably is an important factor in the increased incidence of the disease in summer.[96,97] Other factors that allow entry of *M. bovis* by damaging the corneal epithelium include dust, plant seeds, and other mechanical irritants. Lactoferrin and secretory IgA in tears probably contribute to the defense of the eye against *M. bovis*.[98]

Progression of the ulcer is a result of disruption and breakdown of stromal collagen by hydrolases and proteases released by the bacteria, polymorphonuclear leukocytes, and corneal cells.[89,90] Healing of the ulcerated site is the result of vascularization reaching the area and subsequent remodeling of corneal collagen to produce a corneal scar.

EPIDEMIOLOGY. *M. bovis* causes the most severe disease in young cattle. The disease is transmitted by direct contact, aerosols, and fomites. Nasal and ocular secretions are a source of the bacteria and recovered, nonclinically affected cattle may act as carriers, shedding the bacteria in nasal secretions.[99,100] The disease most commonly occurs as a summer epidemic from which hemolytic strains are recovered.[75] Flies may serve as mechanical vectors of the bacteria.[101] Several studies have shown that the economic impact of the disease can be significant because of decreased weight gain in young animals, re-

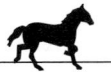

duced milk yield, costs of treatment and labor, decreased value of calves, reduced value of purebred cattle as a result of disfigurement of the eyes, or losses in slaughter cattle.[102]

TREATMENT AND PROGNOSIS. Numerous treatments have been suggested for IBK in cattle. The bovine cornea has a tremendous capacity to overcome infection and heal deep ulcers (even if untreated) that would have a very grave prognosis in other domestic species. This fact, combined with the wide range of antibiotic sensitivities of *M. bovis*, enables most treatments to be effective if administered promptly and frequently. But the practical problem of treating several individuals within a herd 2 or 3 times daily has stimulated several studies to determine alternative, more cost-effective therapies for both treating the ulcerative keratitis and eliminating *M. bovis* from carrier animals.[94,103-105]

In large herd outbreaks, antibiotics should ideally be chosen on the basis of in vitro sensitivity testing and establishment of minimum inhibitory concentration (MIC) data. This is especially true in younger animals that are affected with severe ulcerative keratitis, which could result in loss of the eye.

Antibiotics that can be recommended for topical treatment include erythromycin, ceftiofur, tylosin, ampicillin, bacitracin, neomycin, nitrofurazone, oxytetracycline, penicillin, gentamicin, kanamycin, triple sulfonamides, and a combination of neomycin, polymyxin B, and gramicidin or bacitracin.[106,107] Kanamycin and gentamicin should probably be reserved for treating resistant strains rather than as first-choice therapy. Two topical doses of benzathine cloxacillin (375 mg suspended in mineral oil to a final volume of 1 ml) administered 72 hours apart resulted in reduced severity and shedding of organisms.[108] When antibiotic treatment is instituted early in the course of the disease, the subsequent corneal damage should be less severe.

In instances in which topical medications cannot be applied frequently, subconjunctival injections may offer an alternative and are frequently recommended for treating IBK. Subconjunctival injection usually maintains a higher corneal drug concentration than does topical treatment. Penicillin (procaine penicillin G 300,000 U) used subconjunctivally in the bulbar conjunctiva, used twice 48 to 72 hours apart, reduced healing times in naturally occurring IBK.[109] However, a similar regimen of subconjunctival penicillin put into palpebral conjunctiva did not affect the severity or healing times of naturally occurring IBK.[110] Although subconjunctival oxytetracycline is effective in eliminating the infection, it is severely irritating to the conjunctiva and this route is best avoided.

To administer a subconjunctival injection, the animal is first restrained and then the nose is raised to tilt the head with the affected eye directed upward. The upper bulbar conjunctiva of the globe is then exposed. Topical local anesthetic (proparacaine hydrochloride)* is applied to the eye, and the antibiotic is injected beneath the bulbar conjunctiva using a 23- or 25-gauge needle. When penicillin G is used, the drug cost is low and milk withdrawal time is short.

Either topical or subconjunctival therapy is effective if used properly. However, because of the labor intensiveness of local treatments, these options may be unattractive to veterinarians and clients. Recent studies have shown that intramuscular administration of oxytetracycline is an effective means of controlling the disease and is especially valuable in a large herd where frequent handling of stock is impractical. Although the drug does not reach MIC values in the lacrimal gland or tears, it appears to be concentrated on the epithelial cell surface of the cornea, which is the site first damaged by the bacteria.[111] Alternate-day therapy with long-acting oxytet-

racycline (Liquamycin LA-200)* at a dose of 20 mg/kg is recommended until clinical improvement is apparent. In mildly affected animals one dose may be sufficient, whereas two or more treatments may be needed in younger animals or in cases with severe keratitis.[112] Two doses of Liquamycin LA-200 at 72-hour intervals are effective at eliminating carriers. Liquamycin LA-200 should not be used in lactating cattle. Another treatment regimen of oxytetracycline consists of a single intramuscular injection of LA-200 (20 mg/kg) followed by feeding calves alfalfa pellets with oxytetracycline (1 g/lb fed at 2 g/calf).[109] This was shown to be more effective than subconjunctival penicillin at decreasing the prevalence of IBK.[109]

Florfenicol has also been shown to be effective in experimentally,[113] as well as naturally occurring cases of IBK.[114] Florfenicol (Nuflor), which is not approved for this use, was used either subcutaneously once at 40 mg/kg or intramuscularly once and then 2 days later at 20 mg/kg/treatment.[114]

In selected cases of IBK (i.e., when frequent medication of one eye is impractical or when subconjunctival or intramuscular antibiotic injections may produce drug residues in milk or tissues after slaughter), third-eyelid flaps have been recommended as an alternative means of therapy. Eye patches or a temporary tarsorrhaphy may be used in place of a third-eyelid flap to achieve a similar effect. Unfortunately, third-eyelid flaps are time consuming and relatively inconvenient to perform, they prevent effective examination of the eye, and they limit access of topical antibiotics to the corneal surface. There is a belief, for which no experimental evidence exists, that third-eyelid flaps are indicated to save deeply ulcerated eyes. If poorly placed, the flap may exert pressure on the cornea and precipitate corneal rupture. Flaps can probably be safely used in cases of moderate ulceration, although such ulcers usually heal as readily with the achievement of appropriate antibacterial drug concentrations at the corneal surface. In such cases, they may provide some protection from the environment.

Corticosteroids are occasionally recommended for topical treatment of IBK. Steroidal antiinflammatory drugs should not be used during the acute ulcerative phase of the disease and are of doubtful value later in the healing stages to reduce vascularization and granulation. Although corticosteroids may reduce some of the inflammation associated with the disease, they potentiate corneal perforation and increase the rate of shedding of *M. bovis* in ocular secretions. There is no evidence to show that ultimate regression of corneal vascularization and granulation after IBK is substantially improved by using steroids in affected eyes compared with eyes that do not receive steroids.

The prognosis for vision is good in most cases of IBK, provided that the diagnosis and treatment is begun early. The prognosis in younger calves depends on the disease severity.

PREVENTION AND CONTROL. At present no vaccine is available that completely and reliably prevents IBK.[115-117] At best vaccines reduce the incidence and severity of the disease within the herd. Vaccines are composed of *M. bovis* or *M. bovis* pili. The rationale for basing the vaccine on bacterial pili reflects the mode of adherence and initial damage to corneal epithelial cells by the bacteria. Unfortunately, if the challenge *M. bovis* is heterologous to the bacteria used to produce the vaccine, there is little protection from the vaccine.[118] Also some research suggests that *M. bovis* may be able to switch pilus gene expression.[119] Work continues on finding a more efficacious vaccine.[120]

Control of flies is important in reducing the incidence of the disease in a herd. Perhaps the most convenient and

---

*Alcaine, Alcon, Fort Worth, TX 76134.

*Liquamycin LA-200, Pfizer, NY 10017.

effective technique is the use of ear tags impregnated with 10% permethrin attached to both ears of all cattle before the fly season begins.[121] Alternatively, insecticide-charged face rubbers or dust bags containing 5% coumaphos may be used. This must be done on an area-wide basis to be effective.[94] Other control measures that may be helpful include segregating clinically affected animals from the rest of the herd to reduce direct transmission; segregating the younger, more susceptible animals from older cattle; mowing overgrown pastures to reduce the chance of ocular trauma; minimizing dust and pollen in the animals' environment; and providing shade and ample space for animals when housed and fed together. To avoid spread of infection while treating affected animals, hands should be washed or disposable gloves changed between animals. Vaccination with modified live IBR vaccine should not be performed during a herd outbreak of IBK.

REFERENCES

75. Pugh GW, Hughes DE: Infectious bovine keratoconjunctivitis: *Moraxella bovis* as the sole etiologic agent in winter epizootic, *J Am Vet Med Assoc* 161:481-486, 1972.
76. Chandler RL et al: Virulence of *Moraxella bovis* in gnotobiotic calves, *Vet Rec* 106:364-365, 1980.
77. Aikman JG, Allan EM, Selman IE: Experimental production of infectious bovine keratoconjunctivitis, *Vet Rec* 117:234-239, 1985.
78. Pugh GW Jr, Hughes DE, Packer RA: Bovine infectious keratoconjunctivitis: interactions of *Moraxella bovis* and infectious bovine rhinotracheitis virus, *Am J Vet Res* 31:653-662, 1970.
79. Webber JJ, Selby LA: Risk factors related to the prevalence of infectious bovine rhinotracheitis, *J Am Vet Res* 179:823-826, 1981.
80. George LW et al: Enhancement of infectious bovine keratoconjunctivitis by modified-live infectious bovine rhinotracheitis virus vaccine, *Am J Vet Res* 49:1800-1806, 1988.
81. Wilcox GE: Isolation of adenoviruses from cattle with conjunctivitis and keratoconjunctivitis, *Aust Vet J* 45:265-270, 1969.
82. Friis NF, Pedersen KB: Isolation of *Mycoplasma bovoculi* from cases of infectious bovine keratoconjunctivitis, *Acta Vet Scand* 20:51-59, 1979.
83. Rosenbusch RF, Ostle AG: *Mycoplasma bovoculi* infection increases ocular colonization by *Moraxella bovis* in calves, *Am J Vet Res* 47:1214-1216, 1986.
84. Wilcox GE: Bacterial flora of the bovine eye with special reference to the *Moraxella* and *Neisseria*, *Aust Vet J* 46:253-257, 1970.
85. Morgan JH: Infectious keratoconjunctivitis in cattle associated with *Listeria monocytogenes*, *Vet Rec* 100:113-114, 1977.
86. Annuar BO, Wilcox GE: Adherence of *Moraxella bovis* in cell cultures of bovine origin, *Res Vet Sci* 39:241-246, 1985.
87. Ruehl WW et al: Q pili enhance the attachment of *Moraxella bovis* to bovine corneas in vitro, *Molec Microbiol* 7:285-288, 1993.
88. Ruehl WW et al: Infection rates, disease frequency, pilin gene rearrangement, and pilin expression in calves inoculated with *Moraxella bovis* pilin-specific isogenic variants, *Am J Vet Res* 54:248-253, 1993.
89. Pedersen KB, Fronholm LO, Bovre K: Fimbriation and colony type of *Moraxella bovis* in relation to conjunctival colonization and development of keratoconjunctivitis in cattle, *Acta Pathol Microbiol Scand (B)* 80:911-918, 1972.
90. Moore LJ, Rutter JM: Attachment of *Moraxella bovis* to calf corneal cells and inhibition by antiserum, *Aust Vet J* 66:39-42, 1989.
91. Kagonyera GM, George LW, Munn R: Light and electron microscopic changes in corneas of healthy and immunomodulated calves infected with *Moraxella bovis*, *Am J Vet Res* 49:386-395, 1988.
92. Frank SK, Gerber JD: Hydrolytic enzymes of *Moraxella bovis*, *J Clin Microbiol* 13:269-271, 1981.
93. Ostle AG, Rosenbusch RF: *Moraxella bovis* hemolysin, *Am J Vet Res* 46:1011-1014, 1984.
94. George LW, Kagonyera G: Pathogenesis and clinical management of infectious bovine keratoconjunctivitis, *Proceedings of the Twentieth Annual Convention of the American Association of Bovine Practitioners*, 1988, pp 26-32.
95. Beard MKM, Moore LJ: Reproduction of bovine keratoconjunctivitis with a purified haemolytic and cytotoxic fraction of *Moraxella bovis*, *Vet Microbiol* 42:15-33, 1994.
96. Hughes DE, Pugh GW, McDonald TJ: Ultraviolet radiation and *Moraxella bovis* in the etiology of bovine infectious keratoconjunctivitis, *Am J Vet Res* 26:1331-1338, 1965.
97. Vogelweid CM et al: Scanning electron microscopy of bovine corneas irradiated with sun lamps and challenge exposed with *Moraxella bovis*, *Am J Vet Res* 47:378-384, 1986.
98. Brown MH et al: Infectious bovine keratoconjunctivitis: a review, *J Vet Intern Med* 12:259-266, 1998.
99. Powe TA et al: Prevalence of nonclinical *Moraxella bovis* infections in bulls as determined by ocular culture and serum antibody titer, *J Vet Diagn Invest* 4:78-79, 1992.

100. Pugh GW, McDonald TJ, Kopecky KE: Infectious bovine keratoconjunctivitis: effects of vaccination on *Moraxella bovis* carrier state in cattle, *Am J Vet Res* 41:264-266, 1980.
101. Gerhardt RR et al: The role of the face fly in an episode of infectious bovine keratoconjunctivitis, *J Am Vet Med Assoc* 180:156-159, 1982.
102. George LW: Clinical infectious bovine keratoconjunctivitis, *Compend Cont Educ Pract Vet* 6:S712-S721, 1984.
103. Buswell JF, Hewett GR: Single topical treatment for bovine keratoconjunctivitis using benzathine cloxacillin, *Vet Rec* 113:621, 1983.
104. Hughes DE et al: Comparison of vaccination and treatment in controlling naturally occurring infectious bovine keratoconjunctivitis, *Am J Vet Res* 40:241-261, 1979.
105. George LW: Antibiotic treatment of infectious bovine keratoconjunctivitis, *Cornell Vet* 80:229-235, 1990.
106. Webber JJ, Fales WH, Selby LA: Antimicrobial susceptibility of *Moraxella bovis* determined by agar gel diffusion and broth microdilution, *Antimicrob Agents Chemother* 21:554-557, 1982.
107. Shryock TR, White DW, Werner CS: Antimicrobial susceptibility of *Moraxella*, *Vet Microbiol* 61:305-309, 1998.
108. George LW et al: Effectiveness of two benzathine cloxacillin formulations for treatment of naturally occurring infectious bovine keratoconjunctivitis, *Am J Vet Res* 50:1170-1174, 1989.
109. Eastman TG et al: Combined parenteral and oral administration of oxytetracycline for control of infectious bovine keratoconjunctivitis, *J Am Vet Med Assoc* 212:560-563, 1998.
110. Allen LF, George LW, Willits NH: Effect of penicillin or penicillin and dexamethasone in cattle with infectious bovine keratoconjunctivitis, *J Am Vet Med Assoc* 206:1200-1203, 1995.
111. George LW, Smith JA, Kaswan R: Distribution of oxytetracycline into ocular tissues and tears of calves, *J Vet Pharmacol Ther* 8:47-54, 1985.
112. Smith JA, George LW: Treatment of acute ocular *Moraxella bovis* infections in calves with a parenterally administered long-acting oxytetracycline formulation, *Am J Vet Res* 46:804-807, 1984.
113. Dueger EL et al: Efficacy of Florfenicol in the treatment of experimentally induced infectious bovine keratoconjunctivitis, *Am J Vet Res* 60:960-964, 1999.
114. Angelos JA et al: Efficacy of Florfenicol for treatment of naturally occurring infectious bovine keratoconjunctivitis, *J Am Vet Med Assoc* 216:62-64, 2000.
115. Miller RB, Fales WH: Infectious bovine keratoconjunctivitis: an update, *Vet Clin North Am (Large Anim Pract)* 6:597-608, 1984.
116. Pugh GW, Hughes DE, Booth GD: Experimentally induced infectious bovine keratoconjunctivitis: effectiveness of a pilus vaccine against exposure to homologous strains of *Moraxella bovis*, *Am J Vet Res* 38:1519-1522, 1979.
117. Smith PC et al: Effectiveness of two commercial infectious bovine keratoconjunctivitis vaccines, *Am J Vet Res* 51:1147-1150, 1990.
118. Smith PC et al: Effectiveness of two commercial infectious bovine keratoconjunctivitis vaccines, *Am J Vet Res* 51:1147-1150, 1990.
119. Lepper AWD et al: The protective efficacy of cloned *Moraxella bovis* pili in monovalent and multivalent vaccine formulations against experimentally induced infectious bovine keratoconjunctivitis (IBK), *Vet Microbiol* 45:129-138, 1995.
120. Lepper AWD et al: A *Moraxella bovis* pili vaccine produced by recombinant DNA technology for the prevention of infectious bovine keratoconjunctivitis, *Vet Microbiol* 36:175-183, 1993.
121. Williams RE et al: Use of insecticide-impregnated ear tags for the control of face flies and horn flies on pastured cattle, *J Anim Sci* 53:1159-1165, 1981.

INFECTIOUS BOVINE RHINOTRACHEITIS CONJUNCTIVITIS

ETIOLOGY. IBR is a herpes virus that may involve the respiratory or reproductive tracts, nervous system, or conjunctiva or may cause widespread systemic disease (also see Chapter 29). Conjunctivitis is the most common ocular manifestation of the disease; it may occur as an isolated clinical entity or with involvement of other body systems.[122-124]

CLINICAL SIGNS AND DIFFERENTIAL DIAGNOSES. Although conjunctivitis is frequently bilateral, it can be unilateral. Excessive lacrimation, initially serous and later becoming mucopurulent, is usually seen without blepharospasm. Chemosis may be severe, especially by 1 week after infection. Both the palpebral and bulbar conjunctivae are injected, and petechial hemorrhages may occur. Multiple 0.2- to 0.5-mm-diameter, white plaques may develop on the palpebral and, to a lesser extent, the bulbar conjunctival surfaces at 1 to 2 weeks after the onset of clinical signs. These may coalesce later in the disease (5 to 9 days). Vascularization and perilimbal edema and opacification occur in severe cases. Iridocyclitis (miosis accompanying the corneal vascularization) can be present in occasional severe cases.

Corneal changes of IBR are differentiated from those of infectious bovine keratoconjunctivitis caused by *Moraxella bovis* by their peripheral rather than central distribution and the lack of corneal ulceration in IBR, unless IBR and IBK occur concurrently in the same eye. Corneal vascularization and opacification in malignant catarrhal fever accompany marked signs of anterior uveitis[125] and other signs of generalized vasculitis.

Although ocular disease may occur as an isolated entity, ocular signs may be found in animals with upper respiratory tract signs, including rhinitis and dyspnea. Affected animals may be pyrexic, and a fall in milk yield may occur. Abortion in pregnant animals may occur following ocular manifestations of the disease.

DIAGNOSTIC PROCEDURES. Herpesvirus can be recovered from infected eyes during the first 7 to 9 days of the disease but infrequently thereafter. Swabs may be taken for viral isolation in cell culture, which is probably the most reliable means of making a definite diagnosis. Fluorescent antibody techniques may be used on conjunctival scrapings, and serology may be helpful if blood samples can be collected during the acute and convalescent stages of the disease. Polymerase chain reaction is also being used. Histopathology to detect intranuclear inclusions is not likely to allow reliable diagnosis of the disease.[125,126]

PATHOPHYSIOLOGY. Specific strains of the virus cause mainly one form of the disease (such as the ocular form) in a herd. Ocular infection results in lymphoid hyperplasia, visible as white plaques. These are comprised histologically of plasma cells and lymphocytes in the conjunctival stroma and subepithelial area. Mild conjunctival epithelial ulceration may occur histologically. During the recovery phase of the disease, diphtheritic membranes develop on the conjunctival surface secondary to conjunctival necrosis.

TREATMENT AND PROGNOSIS. Recovery from the conjunctival form of the disease is spontaneous within 10 to 20 days. In certain situations palliative treatment may be helpful. This is achieved by cleaning the ocular discharge from the lids and applying a topical broad-spectrum antibiotic to prevent secondary bacterial infection. Treatment of the conjunctival form of the disease with topical antiherpetic agents has not been studied and would rarely be practical or cost effective.

PREVENTION AND CONTROL. Vaccination of susceptible animals is the most effective means to prevent and control the disease. IBR vaccination programs are discussed in Chapter 44.

REFERENCES

122. Abinanti FR, Plumer GJ: The isolation of infectious bovine rhinotracheitis virus from cattle affected with conjunctivitis: observations on the experimental infection, *Am J Vet Res* 86:13-17, 1961.
123. Hughes JP, Olander HJ, Wada EM: Keratoconjunctivitis associated with infectious bovine rhinotracheitis, *J Am Vet Med Assoc* 145:32-39, 1964.
124. Mohanty SB et al: Effects of an experimentally induced herpesvirus infection in calves, *J Am Vet Med Assoc* 161:1008-1011, 1972.
125. Rebhun WC et al: An outbreak of the conjunctival form of infectious bovine rhinotracheitis, *Cornell Vet* 68:297-307, 1978.
126. Crandell RA: Infectious bovine rhinotracheitis. In Howard JL, ed: *Current veterinary therapy: food animal practice*, ed 2, Philadelphia, 1986, WB Saunders, pp 470-472.

MALIGNANT CATARRHAL FEVER KERATOCONJUNCTIVITIS

Malignant catarrhal fever (MCF) is a sporadic disease characterized by fever, lymphadenopathy, and generalized vasculitis resulting in inflammation of the mucosa of the mouth, nose, and eye; the skin; and the gastrointestinal and nervous systems, with variable but usually high mortality. The African form is caused by alcelaphine herpesvirus 1. The North American form is believed to be caused by a similar virus, although none has yet been isolated.[127-129]

Various forms of the disease are described on the basis of clinical signs (see Chapter 30). Ocular involvement is seen in the acute "head and eye" form, which is the most common presentation of the disease. Ocular signs include photophobia, excessive lacrimation, episcleral injection and scleritis, severe conjunctivitis, keratitis (corneal opacification caused by edema and vascularization appearing perilimbally), and anterior uveitis. Less significantly, and difficult to diagnose clinically, retinal vasculitis may develop. Bullous keratopathy may develop as a result of edema in the anterior cornea, with subsequent rupture of bullae to form painful corneal erosions.[130] The absence of central corneal ulceration distinguishes the disease from IBK, whereas the severity of the ocular lesions is worse than would be expected in IBR, bovine virus diarrhea/mucosal disease (BVD/MD), or bluetongue. Differentiating this disease from Rinderpest could be clinically difficult in areas where both are endemic in cattle.

No specific diagnostic tests are available for MCF. The ocular lesions are those of a nonsuppurative uveitis and vasculitis. The lesions involve the conjunctiva, cornea, anterior uvea, and retinal blood vessels; the choroid is rarely involved. Serofibrinous and cellular infiltrates develop in the uvea and retina as a result of vasculitis and thrombosis. Perivascular cuffing and optic neuritis may be detected histologically.[131-133]

Prognosis for the eyes and the animal's recovery is poor.[130] Most importantly, cattle should be kept away from sheep in endemic areas that may act as a reservoir for the disease and affected animals should be isolated. Vaccination is not available.[128]

REFERENCES

127. Mebus CA, Kalunda M, Ferris DH: Malignant catarrhal fever, *Bovine Pract* 14:130-132, 1979.
128. Castro AE: Malignant catarrhal fever. In Howard JL, ed: *Current veterinary therapy: food animal practice*, ed 2, Philadelphia, 1986, WB Saunders, pp 473-474.
129. Bridgen A, Reid HW: Derivation of a DNA clone corresponding to the viral agent of sheep-associated malignant catarrhal fever, *Res Vet Sci* 50:38-44, 1991.
130. Rebhun WC: Viral diseases of the bovine eye, *Bovine Pract* 14:139-142, 1979.
131. Pierson RE et al: Clinical and clinicopathologic observations in induced malignant catarrhal fever of cattle, *J Am Vet Med Assoc* 173:833-837, 1978.
132. Jubb KVF, Kennedy PC: *Pathology of domestic animals*, ed 2, New York, 1970, Academic Press, p 34.
133. Jubb KV, Saunders LZ, Stenius PI: Die histologische augenveranderungen bein bosartigen katarhalfieber des rindes, *Schweiz Arch Tierheilkd* 102:393-400, 1960.

BOVINE MYCOPLASMAL CONJUNCTIVITIS

Mycoplasma bovoculi and *Ureaplasma* spp. have been isolated from cattle with conjunctivitis and IBK. Inoculation of normal calves with *M. bovoculi* or *Ureaplasma* spp. isolates produced conjunctivitis characterized by serous discharge and localized to diffuse conjunctival hyperemia. Experimentally induced conjunctivitis ran a course of over 1 month. Suspected cases should be cultured using swabs moistened with *Mycoplasma* broth.[134] *Mycoplasma* may predispose the animals to development of *Moraxella* IBK.[135] Although treatment of mycoplasmal conjunctivitis per se may not be warranted, it may be advisable in areas where IBK is endemic. Topical oxytetracycline ointment applied 3 times daily or intramuscular injection of long-acting oxytetracycline is recommended.

REFERENCES

134. Rosenbusch RF, Knudtson WU: Bovine mycoplasmal conjunctivitis: experimental reproduction and characterization of the disease, *Cornell Vet J* 70:307-320, 1980.

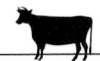

135. Pugh GW, Hughes DE, Schulz VD: Infectious bovine keratoconjunctivitis: experimental induction of infection in calves with mycoplasmas and *Moraxella bovis, Am J Vet Res* 37:493-495, 1976.

HEMOPHILUS SOMNUS CONJUNCTIVITIS AND RETINITIS

Thromboembolic meningoencephalitis (TEME) is a fatal septicemia caused by infection with *Hemophilus somnus* (see Chapter 33). Calves and young adult cattle can be affected, but the disease most commonly occurs in feedlot cattle less than 1 year of age. The organism is capable of damaging vascular endothelial cells and activating blood clotting. Therefore most of the ocular histologic signs are referable to thrombosis of retinal vessels.

Although conjunctivitis may be seen, the main ocular findings are in the fundus. Retinal hemorrhages and exudates may be focal or diffuse. Retinal infiltrates may elevate the retina and involve the vitreous. Retinal edema, hemorrhage and necrosis, vascular thrombosis, and infiltration of the retina and vitreous with neutrophils are seen histologically. Eosinophilic cytoid bodies (swollen axons) are seen in the nerve fiber layer of the retina. Retinal detachments may result from retina edema. Later in the disease, areas of chorioretinitis result in chorioretinal scars. The anterior segment is less involved in the disease than in MCF in which keratitis and anterior uveitis is usual.[136,137]

REFERENCES

136. Dukes TW: The ocular lesions in thromboembolic meningoencephalitis (TEME) of cattle, *Can Vet J* 12:180-182, 1971.
137. Little PB, Sorensen DK: Bovine polioencephalomalacia, infectious embolic meningoencephalitis, and acute lead poisoning in feedlot cattle, *J Am Vet Med Assoc* 155:1892-1903, 1969.

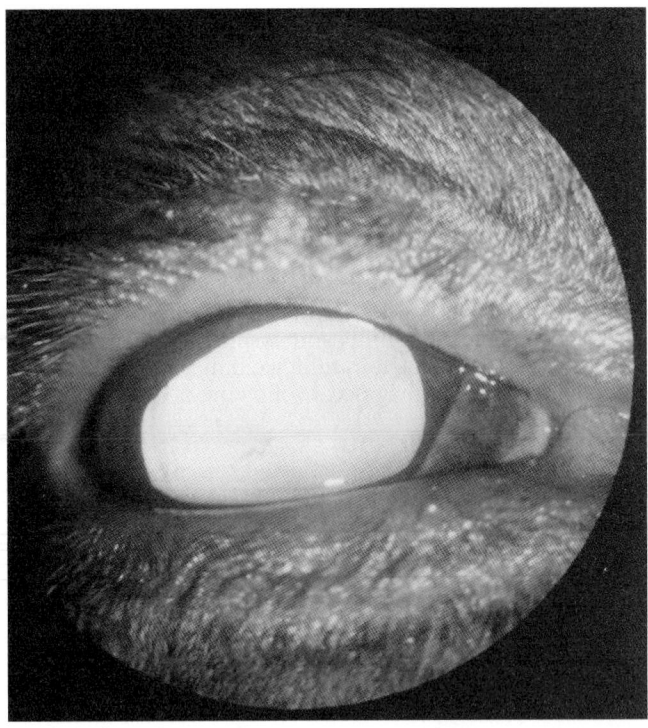

FIG. 37-15 ■ Leukocoria (white pupil) in a Simmental calf caused by inflammatory debris in the vitreous and on the posterior capsule of the lens after intrauterine infection with bovine viral diarrhea.

BOVINE VIRUS DIARRHEA–INDUCED RETINAL DYSPLASIA, CATARACTS, MICROPHTHALMIA, OPTIC NEURITIS, AND LEUKOCORIA

The causative agent of bovine virus diarrhea (BVD) is a pestivirus (part of the togaviruses) that, in congenitally affected animals, causes retinal inflammation and necrosis. Cattle infected between days 75 and 150 of gestation may produce calves with cerebellar hypoplasia or ocular lesions. Calves with ocular signs may be blind, and nystagmus may be present. Pupillary light reflexes may or may not be absent. Other abnormalities may include microphthalmia, cataract, leukocoria (either as a result of cataract or dense white inflammatory infiltrate in the anterior vitreous) (Fig. 37-15), retinal hemorrhages, chorioretinitis, retinal dysplasia (retinal folds), retinal detachment, or optic neuritis or atrophy.[138-141] Retinal dysplasia that is clinically characterized by retinal folds, rosettes, and detachment ensues. The optic disc may appear atrophic, and areas of tapetal color change and hyperreflectivity may be seen, with retinal vascular attenuation. In some cases inflammatory debris may persist in the vitreous after birth, precluding adequate fundus examination (Fig. 37-15). Congenital cataracts also occur in this disease, and, although the pathophysiology of their development is unknown, they probably develop secondary to the intraocular inflammation and necrosis. Cataracts mainly involve the lens cortex.

Transplacental infection may occur when the dam is infected during pregnancy. The severity of the disease is related to the age of intrauterine infection. Severe fetal disease and often fetal death occur in cattle infected between 100 and 200 days of gestation. Infected fetuses can also survive and become persistently infected with the virus. In these cattle viral antigens can be found in neurons of the retina and CNS in the absence of clinical signs.[142] Ocular discharges have been reported in cases of acute or chronic cases of BVD, although the significance of these observations is uncertain.[141,143]

Precolostral serum samples from affected calves can be submitted for serologic diagnosis (serum-virus neutralization test), or virus isolation can be attempted from buffy coat cells of a whole blood sample taken in EDTA. More details of BVD are found in Chapter 30.

REFERENCES

138. Baker JC: Bovine viral diarrhea virus: a review, *J Am Vet Med Assoc* 190: 1449-1458, 1987.
139. Bistner SI, Rubin LF, Saunders LZ: The ocular lesions of bovine viral diarrhea-mucosal disease, *Pathol Vet* 7:275-286, 1970.
140. Scott FW et al: Virus-induced congenital anomalies of the bovine fetus, *Cornell Vet* 63:536-560, 1973.
141. Olafson P, MacCallum AD, Fox FH: An apparently new transmissible disease of cattle, *Cornell Vet* 36:205-213, 1946.
142. Fernandez A et al: Viral antigen distribution in the central nervous system of cattle persistently infected with bovine viral diarrhea, *Vet Pathol* 26:26-32, 1989.
143. Perdrizet JA et al: Bovine viral diarrhea: clinical syndromes in dairy herds, *Cornell Vet* 77:46-74, 1987.

OCULAR SIGNS OF LISTERIOSIS

Listeriosis in ruminants is manifested mainly as either an encephalitis or as a septicemia in neonates, or as a reproductive problem manifested as abortions.[144] Listeriosis is caused by *Listeria monocytogenes.* Ocular signs with the neural form include facial paralysis and ptosis, often unilateral, on the side of the central lesion, medial strabismus (often on the ipsilateral side because of involvement of the abducens nucleus), nystagmus, and amaurosis.[144] Uveitis with hypopyon has been described in chronic cases.[145] Diagnosis is usually achieved by isolation of *L. monocytogenes* from tissues at necropsy. Early treatment with broad-spectrum antibiotics may be effective in some cases.

REFERENCES

144. Cooper J, Walker RD: Listeriosis. *Vet Clin North Am (Food Anim Pract)* 14:113-125, 1998.
145. Rebhun WC, De Lahunta A: Diagnosis and treatment of bovine listeriosis, *J Am Vet Med Assoc* 180:395-398, 1982.

BLUETONGUE CONJUNCTIVITIS

Conjunctivitis and mucopurulent ocular discharge may be found in cattle chronically infected with bluetongue virus. Although topical antibiotics could be applied to reduce secondary bacterial infection and reduce the ocular discharge, this would rarely be necessary.[146]

REFERENCE

146. Bowne JG et al: Bluetongue disease in cattle, *J Am Vet Med Assoc* 153: 662-668, 1968.

BOVINE LEUKOSIS AS A CAUSE OF EXOPHTHALMOS

Lymphosarcoma in adult cattle is usually caused by bovine leukemia virus, although noninfectious sporadic cases are reported in young animals. Lymphosarcoma may result in progressive unilateral or bilateral exophthalmos.[147,148] This is the most common orbital neoplasm in cattle. If undiagnosed, exposure keratitis and chemosis develop. Intraocular involvement can occur, although it is less common than orbital neoplasia. Generalized lymphadenopathy or other signs of generalized lymphosarcoma usually accompany the orbital involvement. Specific serologic tests will confirm the diagnosis. Enucleation or exenteration is rarely indicated because of the poor prognosis for affected animals. Differentials for progressive exophthalmos include frontal or maxillary sinusitis or nasal neoplasia, actinomycosis, and actinobacillosis.

REFERENCES

147. Rebhun WC: Diseases of the bovine orbit and globe, *J Am Vet Med Assoc* 175:171-175, 1979.
148. Rebhun WC: Orbital lymphosarcoma in cattle, *J Am Vet Med Assoc* 180:149-152, 1982.

OCULAR MANIFESTATIONS OF TUBERCULOSIS

Tuberculosis caused by *Mycobacterium bovis* may cause granulomatous lesions in the eye of affected cattle. The uvea (posterior or anterior) is initially affected, with later expansion of granulomas into other ocular structures. Uveitis, keratitis, and retinal detachment and chorioretinitis are seen clinically.[149]

REFERENCE

149. Saunders LZ, Rubin LF: *Ophthalmic pathology of animals,* Basel, 1975, S Karger, p 52.

OCULAR MANIFESTATIONS OF NEONATAL SEPTICEMIA

Neonatal septicemia in calves, foals, lambs, and kids may occur in the first few weeks after birth and may arise from umbilical infection or oral intake of bacteria (see Chapter 19). Septicemia is especially common in colostrum-deprived neonates. Secondary meningitis, polyarthritis, uveitis, and chorioretinitis may develop. Ocular signs include miosis, aqueous flare with fibrin deposition, hypopyon or hyphema,

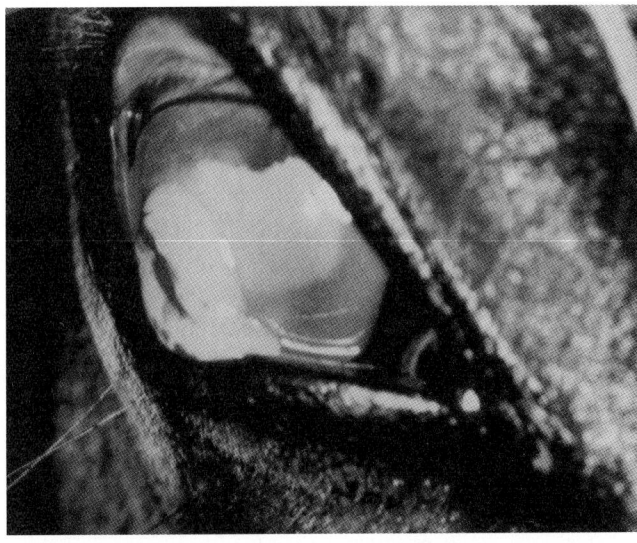

FIG. 37-16 Right eye of horse with a melting corneal ulcer caused by *Pseudomonas* spp. Corneal stroma has liquefied and is overlying the lower lid.

and in severe cases panophthalmitis. Bacteria involved include *Escherichia coli, Streptococcus* spp., *Pasteurella* spp., *Salmonella* spp., *Rhodococcus equi, Corynebacterium pyogenes,* and *Klebsiella* spp. The incidence of infection with different bacteria varies among the domestic species. Therapy should include systemic antibacterial agents (based when possible on sensitivity testing) and treatment for the uveitis. Prognosis for cases treated early is still guarded.[150-153]

REFERENCES

150. Latimer CA, Wyman M: Neonatal ophthalmology, *Vet Clin North Am (Equine Pract)* 1:235-259, 1985.
151. Rubin LF: *Atlas of veterinary ophthalmoscopy,* Philadelphia, 1974, Lea & Febiger, p 302.
152. Williams LW, Gelatt KN: Ocular manifestations of systemic disease: food animals. In Gelatt KN, editor: *Veterinary ophthalmology,* Philadelphia, 1981, Lea & Febiger, p 746.
153. Stiles J: Ocular manifestations of systemic disease. III, The horse. In Gelatt KN, ed: *Veterinary ophthalmology,* Philadelphia, 1999, Lippincott Williams & Wilkins, p 1481.

BACTERIAL KERATITIS IN HORSES

DEFINITION AND ETIOLOGY. Bacterial keratitis occurs when a traumatic corneal ulcer becomes infected with opportunistic bacteria. The most devastating clinical manifestations are associated with *Pseudomonas* spp. and *Streptococcus* spp. Additional bacteria isolated from infected corneas include nutritionally variant streptococci,[154] *Staphylococcus* spp., *E. coli, Acinetobacter* spp., *Clostridium* spp.,[155] and others.[156,157]

CLINICAL SIGNS AND DIFFERENTIAL DIAGNOSES. Whether corneal ulcers are infected or not, they cause signs of pain (i.e., blepharospasm, lacrimation, and photophobia). The conjunctiva is hyperemic, and the ulcerated area of the cornea stains with fluorescein. Signs that make one suspect that the corneal ulcer is infected include a deep ulcer; that is, one that looks like a crater in the corneal stroma. Superficial ulcers, on the other hand, are usually not infected and the cornea maintains its normal curvature in the ulcerated area. Other signs of an infected ulcers are a white or yellowish opacity of the cornea (signifying influx of neutrophils and bacterial colonization) and a rapid progression. An ulcer that is rapidly becoming wider or deeper or a "melting" ulcer in which corneal stroma liquefies (Fig. 37-16) is highly suggestive of a bacterial infection. Fungal keratitis can appear similar, but most cases of bacterial keratitis present more acutely and have a much more rapid course. A cornea with fungal keratitis can become secondarily infected with a bacteria. Bacterial keratitis can also present as a stromal abscess.[158] In these cases a cellular infiltrate is seen in the corneal stroma over which the initially damaged epithelium has healed. Such lesions do not stain with fluorescein.

CLINICAL PATHOLOGY. A diagnosis of a bacterial keratitis is made using gram-stained corneal scrapings. Stained scrapings usually show many bacteria, some intracellular bacteria, and many neutrophils, some of which are degenerate. Bacterial organisms are definitively identified following culture of the corneal ulceration.

PATHOPHYSIOLOGY. Bacterial keratitis is the result of pathogenic or opportunistic organisms colonizing a damaged cornea. The cornea is most likely to be damaged by mechanical trauma, but chemical damage is seen occasionally. In a normal eye many different types of bacteria can be cultured. These include *Corynebacterium* spp., *Streptococcus* spp., *Staphylococcus* spp., *Bacillus* spp., and rarely *Pseudomonas* spp. or other gram-negative bacteria.[159] Damage to the epithelium enables bacteria to adhere to the exposed corneal stroma and begin replicating.[160] Some bacteria such as *Pseudomonas* elaborate collagenase and proteoglycanolytic enzymes,[161] which result in corneal melting. Also involved in the melting are proteases and collagenases found in degenerating white blood cells and possibly in corneal epithelial and stromal cells. In this way, what begins as a small wound to the cornea can progress to a corneal perforation within 24 to 48 hours.

TREATMENT AND PROGNOSIS. Prognosis is grave for any corneal ulcer that is rapidly progressing or melting. These ulcers can easily progress to corneal perforation and loss of the eye despite timely appropriate treatment. On the other hand, with vigorous therapy some eyes with infected ulcers can be saved, leading to a visual, although usually scarred, eye.

In any eye in which a bacterial component is suspected, a culture and sensitivity of the ulcer and a corneal scraping for Gram staining and cytology should be taken. The horse is restrained or sedated, a palpebral block performed (see p. 1179), topical anesthetic is applied to the cornea, and a culture of the ulcer taken with a moistened swab. Then a scraping of the ulcer margins is performed with a Kimura spatula or the blunt, handle-end of a scalpel blade.

In cases of equine bacterial keratitis, including stromal abscesses, the therapeutic goals are to eliminate the bacteria and treat the concurrent uveitis. In a cornea with rapidly developing keratitis or melting ulcer, one should always suspect the presence of *Pseudomonas* organisms, although other organisms such as *Streptococcus* spp. have also been described. Treatment should be started with an appropriate antibiotic used every 1 to 2 hours.[162] Aminoglycosides recommended for gram-negative bacteria include gentamycin, tobramycin, or amikacin and/or ticarcillin.[163] When we use gentamicin, we use a fortified gentamicin solution (adding 30 mg gentamicin sulfate to a 5-ml bottle of Gentocin Ophthalmic* increases gentamicin concentration to 0.9%). Tobramycin comes as an ophthalmic solution (Tobrex†). Amikacin can be mixed as a 10-mg/ml solution and ticarcillin as a 6.3-mg/ml solution.[163] Fluoroquinolones such as ciprofloxacin (Ciloxan) and ofloxacin (Ocuflox) can also be used.

If gram-positive organisms are seen on the corneal scraping, ticarcillin, cefazolin,‡ penicillin, or ampicillin can be used.[163,164] Cefazolin is mixed to a concentration of 50 mg/ml, ampicillin to 10 mg/ml,[163] and penicillin G to 100,000 U/ml. Subpalpebral lavage systems are the best means of delivering the drug (see pp. 1179 to 1181).

If the ulcer continues to worsen, antibiotics should be changed on the basis of the initial sensitivity results, and corneas should always be recultured in these cases, because organisms can become resistant to the first antibiotic that was used. For resistant organisms, sensitivity testing that gives MIC may be very useful because it is possible to safely attain higher drug concentrations in the cornea than in the systemic circulation.

In the past, melting of the cornea has been treated with collagenase and protease inhibitors such as acetylcysteine. Experimentally these drugs were not always effective in reducing melting,[150] and these drugs are used far less commonly now. This emphasizes that the main goal of therapy should be to kill bacteria that elaborate the enzymes. There are currently no inhibitors of neutrophil accumulation. When these become available, they may be helpful in reducing the elaboration of collagenase plus other hydrolases by neutrophils.

As well as medical therapy, surgical therapy can also be used and may improve prognosis. Conjunctival pedicle flaps can be used to bring a blood supply to deep corneal ulcers and possibly slow progression[164] while still allowing medication to reach the site of the ulcer. A conjunctival flap allows observation of the cornea; treatment can be changed if the cornea continues to deteriorate. A nictitans flap should not be used in rapidly progressing or deep ulcers because it does not allow observation of the cornea. In such a case, worsening of the ulcer would go unnoticed, reculturing would not be performed, and appropriate changes in therapy would not be instituted.

A corneoconjunctival transposition using autologous tissue or a corneal graft (after a lamellar keratectomy) or a penetrating keratoplasty using donor cornea are the treatments of choice to repair very deep ulcers, descemetoceles, and perforations if melting has ceased.[156,165,166] These procedures require microsurgical instruments and techniques. Keratectomies with conjunctival flaps or penetrating keratoplasties can also be used to treat stromal abscesses.[167]

The typical response to appropriate therapy is initially a failure of worsening of the ulcer. Bacteria have been killed and tissue destruction is halted. Blood vessels will be seen to begin growing into the cornea from the limbus and epithelium will begin to grow down the sides of the ulcer covering the stroma. Once epithelialization is complete new infection with microorganisms is unlikely. If surgery has not been performed, however, the area that had been ulcerated will be thinner than the surrounding stroma. Thickening of this area will only happen when neovascularization fills the old ulcer bed. This can take weeks and until this happens the cornea is susceptible to traumatic rupture.

The third goal of therapy is to decrease the reflex uveitis seen secondarily to the ulcer. Atropine is used to decrease pain and keep the pupil dilated to reduce the chance of posterior synechia formation. Often atropine must be used every hour or two initially. Atropine is absorbed into the systemic circulation, and gastrointestinal motility should be assessed frequently. Topical or systemic nonsteroidal antiinflammatory drugs can be used to decrease inflammation. However, these drugs will probably slow corneal neovascularization, which is necessary for complete healing of the defect.[168,169] Corticosteroids are sometimes recommended for treatment once epithelialization is complete. Although topical steroids may hasten regression of granulation tissue, no evidence exists to indicate that steroid administration decreases the final size of the scar, and steroids may compromise healing and predispose to corneal rupture.

*Schering, Kenilworth, NJ 07033.
†Tobrex Ophthalmic, Alcon, Forth Worth, TX 76134.
‡Ancef, Smith, Kline & French, Philadelphia, PA 19101.

REFERENCES

154. da Silva Curiel JMA et al: Nutritionally variant streptococci associated with corneal ulcers in horses: 35 cases (1982-1988), *J Am Vet Med Assoc* 197:624-626, 1990.
155. Rebhun WC et al: Presumed clostridial and aerobic bacterial infections of the cornea in two horses, *J Am Vet Med Assoc* 214:1519-1522, 1999.
156. Chmielewski NT et al: Visual outcome and ocular survival following iris prolapse in the horse: a review of 32 cases, *Equine Vet J* 29:31-39, 1997.
157. Moore CP, Collins BK, Fales WH: Antibacterial susceptibility patterns for microbial isolates associated with infectious keratitis in horses: 63 cases (1986-1994), *J Am Vet Med Assoc* 207:928-933, 1995.
158. Rebhun WC: Corneal stromal abscesses in the horse, *J Am Vet Med Assoc* 181:677-679, 1982.
159. Hamor RE, Whelan NC: Equine infectious keratitis, *Vet Clin North Am (Equine Pract)*15:623-646, 1999.
160. Ramphal R, McNiece MT, Polack FM: Adherence of *Pseudomonas aeruginosa* to the injured cornea: a step in the pathogenesis of corneal infections, *Ann Ophthalmol* 13:421-425, 1981.
161. Brown SI, Bloomfield SE, Tam WI: The cornea-destroying enzyme of *Pseudomonas aeruginosa*, *Invest Ophthalmol* 13:174-180, 1974.
162. Sweeney CR, Irby NL: Topical treatment of *Pseudomonas* sp–infected corneal ulcers in horses: 70 cases (1977-1994), *J Am Vet Med Assoc* 209:954-957, 1996.
163. Moore CP et al: Antimicrobial agents for treatment of infectious keratitis in horses, *J Am Vet Med Assoc* 207:855-861, 1995.
164. Nasisse MP, Nelms S: Equine ulcerative keratitis, *Vet Clin North Am (Large Anim Pract)* 8:537-555, 1992.
165. Brown SI, Weller CA: The pathogenesis and treatment of collagenase-induced diseases of the cornea, *Trans Am Acad Ophthalmol Otolaryngol* 74:375-382, 1970.
166. Hendrix DV et al: Corneal stromal abscesses in the horse: a review of 24 cases, *Equine Vet J* 27:440-447, 1995.
167. Hamilton HL et al: Histological findings in corneal stromal abscesses of 11 horses: correlation with cultures and cytology, *Equine Vet J* 26:448-453, 1994.
168. Robin JB et al: The histopathology of corneal neovascularization: inhibitor effects, *Arch Ophthalmol* 103:284-287, 1985.
169. Ezra DB: Neovasculogenesis: triggering factors and possible mechanisms, *Surv Ophthalmol* 24:167-176, 1979.

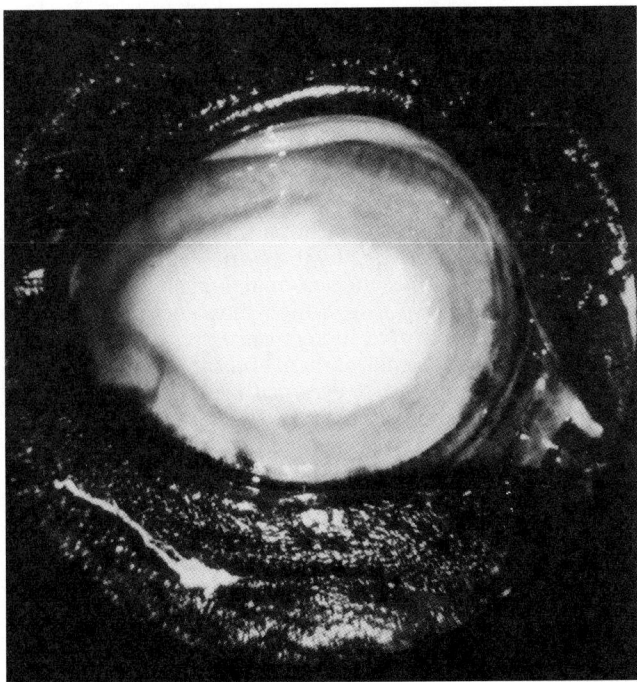

FIG. 37-17 Right eye of horse with fungal keratitis. Note corneal neovascularization and dense cellular infiltrates in the cornea.

FUNGAL KERATITIS IN HORSES

DEFINITION AND ETIOLOGY. Fungal keratitis occurs when an ulcerated cornea becomes infected with a mycotic organism. The most common genera isolated in cases of equine fungal keratitis are *Aspergillus* and *Fusarium* spp., but *Cylindrocarpon destructans*, *Phycomycetes* spp., *Penicillium* spp., *Paecilomyces* spp., *Candida* spp., *Mucor* spp., *Alternaria* spp., and others have been cultured.[170-174] Horses seem to be uniquely susceptible to fungal keratitis when compared to the other domestic species.

CLINICAL SIGNS AND DIFFERENTIAL DIAGNOSES. Fungal keratitis has various manifestations.[175] A common presentation is a corneal ulcer, often with a history of chronicity. Typical history is a nonhealing or worsening ulcer despite antibiotic and/or antiinflammatory therapy. The eye is painful; the conjunctiva is hyperemic; and blepharospasm, lacrimation, and photophobia are also present. Corneal edema and cellular infiltrates surround the ulcer. Sometimes the cellular infiltrates can be very dense and appear as a white or yellow area throughout the corneal ulcer. Corneal neovascularization is usually seen (Fig. 37-17). The secondary uveitis present can be very severe and fluorescein stains the ulcerated cornea.

In some cases of fungal keratitis the epithelium heals over the fungal infection, forming a stromal abscess. In these cases the cornea will not stain with fluorescein. The cellular infiltrate can be deep in the cornea, and on the endothelial surface of the cornea protruding into the anterior chamber. Other ocular signs such as cellular infiltrate, neovascularization, and severe secondary uveitis are similar to the fungal ulcers.

Fungal keratitis can also present as a chronic mild corneal disease. Small multifocal, superficial opacities can be seen. Sometimes there are small focal areas of fluorescein stain, sometimes there is no uptake of stain. Horses are usually in

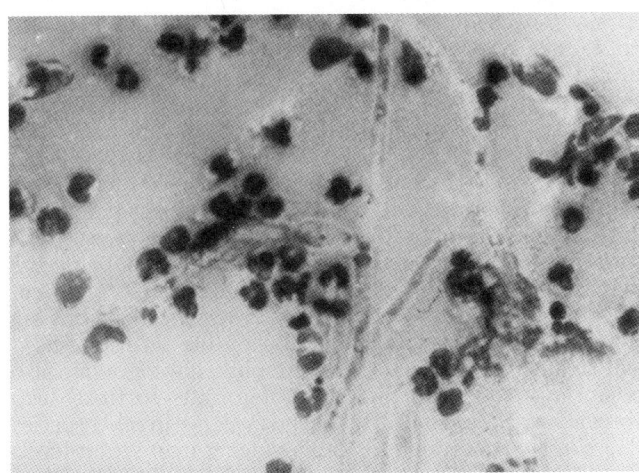

FIG. 37-18 Corneal scraping from horse with fungal keratitis. Note septate hyphae and surrounding inflammatory cells.

mild pain with some lacrimation; usually there in neither corneal neovascularization nor uveitis.

Differential diagnoses include keratouveitis and other causes of corneal ulceration.

CLINICAL PATHOLOGY. A diagnosis of superficial fungal keratitis is made when fungal hyphae or yeast are seen on cytology from corneal scrapings. A diagnosis of deep keratitis may only be made with a corneal biopsy (Fig. 37-18). The fungus can be identified from a culture of the material. If the culture is positive when scrapings or biopsy do not show hyphae, the possibility of an incidental finding must be considered, especially if only one or two colony-forming units are cultured. Unfortunately some diagnoses of fungal keratitis are

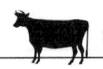
only made after enucleation. Fungal hyphae may have a predisposition for Descemet's membrane, which makes a preenucleation diagnosis difficult.[176] Because treatment is prolonged and expensive, a definitive diagnosis of fungal colonization ideally should be made before treatment is initiated.

PATHOPHYSIOLOGY. Fungal hyphae do not colonize intact cornea. Damage to epithelium is necessary for pathogenic or opportunistic fungi to begin growth in the corneal stroma. This usually results from a traumatic incident that may or may not be noticed by the owner. The use of antibiotics and corticosteroids alters normal flora and decreases the normal immune response, which may encourage fungal growth. Fungi implicated in keratomycoses are commonly present in the horse's environment and can be cultured from over 90% of normal horse eyes, with *Aspergillus* spp. again being the most common isolate.[170] There is one report in the literature of keratomycosis caused by *Candida albicans* secondary to disseminated candidiasis.[177]

EPIDEMIOLOGY. This disease is sporadic. Various author have reported varying seasonal distribution.[171,174]

TREATMENT AND PROGNOSIS. Treatment consists of eliminating the fungus from the cornea. This can be accomplished medically by using antifungal agents. These must be used frequently, and the course of treatment usually lasts for a number of weeks. Healing is usually not complete until corneal neovascularization has reached the infected area. Medical therapy is most effective for treating superficial disease. For deep disease, surgical therapy can also be used with the medical therapy. Lamellar and penetrating keratoplasties probably carry the best prognosis,[176,178] although superficial keratectomies with a conjunctival flap can also be used for more superficial lesions.

A number of antifungal agents are available.[179-182] Miconazole, used as the undiluted intravenous preparation, was the drug of choice for many ophthalmologists; unfortunately it is in no longer on the market. Natamycin* is manufactured as an ophthalmic suspension and is the drug of choice for treating fungal keratitis in humans. Its biggest drawback is its relatively high cost. Fluconazole† is now often recommended as a replacement for miconazole. The intravenous preparation is a 2 mg/ml solution, which is used undiluted as a topical preparation. Subpalpebral lavage systems are probably the best means of delivering these drugs. Both penetrate intact epithelium when given topically, but drug concentrations are higher if epithelium is absent.[183] Fluconazole can also be used subconjunctivally or intravitreally. Ophthalmologists are also beginning to use fluconazole systemically to treat deep corneal fungal disease. There is good evidence in other species that corneal concentrations can be higher than serum levels when fluconazole is given orally.[184] No toxicity studies have been performed on the horse, but anecdotal evidence does not report toxicities and does report resolution of deep disease. One study reported that fluconazole had lower in vitro activity levels than a number of other antifungal drugs.[185]

Another drug used topically is an itraconazole/dimethyl sulfoxide (DMSO) ointment. High concentrations can be reached in intact cornea with this preparation, and it has been used successfully in clinical cases.[186]

Other drugs that have been suggested as treatment for fungal keratitis include miconazole skin cream‡ or vaginal cream.§ These seem to work best for mild, superficial disease; however, no clinical trials on their efficacy and safety for ocular use have been reported. Amphotericin B has good antifungal properties but can be very irritating and is probably not the drug of choice.

In addition, topical mydriatic/cycloplegics such as atropine should be used to combat the accompanying uveitis, and topical antibiotics are indicated to prevent superinfection with bacteria. Topical and systemic nonsteroidal antiinflammatory drugs should be used for the secondary uveitis, especially at the beginning of treatment when fungal death can exacerbate the uveitis. NSAIDs probably slow neovascularization of the cornea, and treatment with these drugs should be decreased as the uveitis is controlled.[187]

Prognosis is guarded to poor in most cases of fungal keratitis. Usually the best possible outcome is a visual eye with some degree of residual scarring. Because there is no evidence to suggest that corticosteroids decrease the eventual size of the scar and the possibility exists that they promote the presence of residual hyphae, the use of steroids is not recommended in a healing fungal ulcer. Complications of fungal keratitis include perforation of the ulcer with loss of the eye, superinfection with a bacteria, and phthisis bulbi.

REFERENCES

170. Whitley RD, Moore CP: Microbiology of the equine eye in health and disease, *Vet Clin North Am (Large Anim Pract)* 6:451-466, 1984.
171. Coad CT, Robinson NM, Wilhelmus KR: Antifungal sensitivity testing for equine keratomycosis, *Am J Vet Res* 46:676-678, 1985.
172. Moore CP et al: Bacterial and fungal isolates from equidae with ulcerative keratitis, *J Am Vet Med Assoc* 182:600-603, 1983.
173. Hendrix DVH et al: Keratomycosis in four horses caused by *Cylindrocarpon destructans*, *Vet Comp Ophthalmol* 6:252-257, 1996.
174. Andrew SE et al: Equine ulcerative keratomycosis: visual outcome and ocular survival in 39 cases (1987-1996), *Equine Vet J* 30:109-116, 1998.
175. Gaarder JE et al: Clinical appearances, healing patterns, risk factors, and outcomes of horses with fungal keratitis: 53 cases (1978-1996), *J Am Vet Med Assoc* 213:105-112, 1998.
176. Grahn B et al: Equine keratomycosis: clinical and laboratory findings in 23 cases, *Prog Vet Comp Ophthalmol* 3:2-7, 1993.
177. Hendrix DVH, Ward DA, Guglick MA: Disseminated candidiasis in a neonatal foal with keratomycosis as the initial sign, *Vet Comp Ophthalmol* 7:10-13, 1997.
178. Whittaker CJG et al: Therapeutic penetrating keratoplasty for deep corneal stromal abscesses in eight horses, *Vet Comp Ophthalmol* 7:19-28, 1997.
179. Bistner S: Clinical diagnosis and treatment of infectious keratitis, *Compend Cont Educ* 3:1056-1066, 1981.
180. Lavach JD, Roberts SM, Severin GA: Current concepts in equine ocular therapeutics, *Vet Clin North Am (Large Anim Pract)* 6:435-449, 1984.
181. Kern TJ, Brooks DE, White MM: Equine keratomycosis: current concepts of diagnosis and therapy, *Equine Vet J* 2(suppl):33-38, 1983.
182. Beech J, Sweeney CR: Keratomycosis in 11 horses, *Equine Vet J* 2(suppl): 39-44, 1983.
183. Yee RW et al: Ocular penetration and pharmacokinetics of topical fluconazole, *Cornea* 16:64-71, 1997.
184. O'Day DM et al: Ocular uptake of fluconazole following oral administration, *Arch Ophthalmol* 108:1006-1008, 1990.
185. Brooks DE et al: Antimicrobial susceptibility patterns of fungi isolated from horses with ulcerative keratomycosis, *Am J Vet Res* 59:138-142, 1998.
186. Ball MA et al: Corneal concentrations and preliminary toxicological evaluation of an itraconazole/dimethyl sulphoxide ophthalmic ointment, *J Vet Pharmacol Therap* 20:100-104, 1997.
187. Robin JB et al: The histopathology of corneal neovascularization: inhibitor effects, *Arch Ophthalmol* 103:284-287, 1985.

UVEITIS ASSOCIATED WITH LEPTOSPIROSIS IN HORSES AND COWS

Leptospirosis is caused by a filamentous bacteria, a spirochete. Disease is seen in most domestic animals as well as humans. Various serovars of *Leptospira interrogans sensu stricto* and *L. kirschneri* have been shown to affect various organs such as kidneys, liver, spleen, muscles, CNS, and eyes and has been associated with abortions.[188] These organisms primarily cause a vasculitis and endotheliitis in these organs.[189]

Because leptospirosis causes vasculitis, it is reasonable to assume that uveitis might be present in an acute infection.

*Monistat IV, Janssen, Piscataway, NJ 08854.
†Diflucan, Pfizer, Exton, PA 19341.
‡Monistat-Derm, Ortho, Raritan, NJ 08869.
§Monistat vaginal cream, Ortho, Raritan, NJ 08869.

This has been reported in horses during the acute phase of leptospirosis (serovar *pomona*).[190] Uveitis has also been seen experimentally in a calf during acute disease with serovar *pomona*.[191] However, it is far more interesting that leptospirosis is associated with uveitis that is seen weeks to months after the acute disease. In domestic species this has mostly been associated with the horse, in which uveitis and periodic ophthalmia has been described.[190,192,193] Uveitis in these horses was bilateral or unilateral, and frequently was recurrent, leading to loss or decrease in vision.[192] Uveitis was not seen until 18 to 24 months after the acute outbreak of leptospirosis. Treatment with systemic antibiotics did not seem to affect the uveitis. In this study, serum titers to serovar *pomona* often remained high for at least 6 years.[193] In another study, uveitis was seen in 22 eyes of 18 ponies experimentally infected with serovar pomona. The earliest sign of uveitis was seen at 1 year postinoculation. Anterior uveitis with cataract formation and posterior synechiae were also seen, as were recurrences.[194]

More recently, in preliminary work 33 out of 50 horse eyes with recurrent uveitis were positive for *Leptospira* antigen in the aqueous, via the PCR technique.[195] Interestingly, treatment with antibiotics in some of these horses did not decrease the inflammation.[196] In another report, serum titers for leptospires by microscopic agglutination test (MAT) were similar in horses with or without uveitis, but vitreous titers were 1:100 in 217 of 324 (67%) eyes with uveitis and 0 of 30 eyes without uveitis, the assumption being that intraocular synthesis of antibodies is occurring.[197] In this same study, leptospiral cultures were positive in 41 of 104 (39.4%) vitreous samples in eyes with uveitis (taken at the time of vitrectomy). Four of these horses had negative serum titers, and in 23 of these horses serum titers were lower than vitreous titers.[197] In several other studies, intraocular synthesis of antibodies to several serovars were shown in horses with uveitis.[198,199] (See also Equine Recurrent Uveitis on pp. 1148 to 1188).

REFERENCES

188. Bernard WV: Leptospirosis, *Vet Clin North Am (Equine Pract)* 9:435-444, 1993.
189. Wong ML et al: Leptospirosis: a childhood disease, *J Pediatr* 90:532-537, 1977.
190. Roberts SJ, York CJ, Robinson JW: An outbreak of leptospirosis in horses on a small farm, *J Am Vet Med Assoc* 121:237-242, 1952.
191. Hoag WG, Bell WB: Isolation of *Leptospira pomona* from a bovine eye, *J Am Vet Med Assoc* 125:381-382, 1954
192. Roberts SJ: Sequelae of leptospirosis in horses on a small farm, *J Am Vet Med Assoc* 133:189-194, 1958.
193. Williams RD et al: Experimental chronic uveitis, *Invest Ophthalmol* 10:948-954, 1971.
194. Riecke JA, Rhoades HE: *Brucella canis* isolated form the eye of a dog, *J Am Vet Med Assoc* 166:583-584, 1975.
195. Faber NA et al: Detection of *Leptospira* spp. in the aqueous humor of horses with naturally acquired recurrent uveitis, *J Clin Microbiol* 38:2731-2733, 2000.
196. Faber N: Personal communication.
197. Gerhards H, Wollanke B, Brem S: Vitrectomy as a diagnostic and therapeutic approach for equine recurrent uveitis (ERU), *Proceedings of the Forty-fifth Annual Convention of the American Association of Equine Practitioners*, 1999, pp 89-93.
198. Davidson MG, Nasisse MP, Roberts SM: Immunodiagnosis of leptospiral uveitis in two horses, *Equine Vet J* 19:155-157, 1987.
199. Halliwell RE et al: Studies on equine recurrent uveitis. II, The role of infection with *Leptospira interrogans* serovar *pomona*, *Curr Eye Res* 4:1033-1040, 1985.

OCULAR MANIFESTATIONS OF EQUINE ADENOVIRUS

Equine adenovirus is a DNA virus that causes bronchopneumonia in foals, especially if they are immunodeficient. Mucopurulent nasal and ocular discharges accompany the respiratory system disease. Histologically there is swelling and necrosis of conjunctival cells with intranuclear inclusions, together with accumulation of neutrophils in the lumens and adventitia of uveal blood vessels.[200]

REFERENCE

200. McChesney AE, England JJ, Rich LJ: Adenoviral infection in foals, *J Am Vet Med Assoc* 162:545-549, 1973.

OCULAR MANIFESTATIONS OF SALMONELLOSIS IN HORSES

Salmonella spp. cause one of the more common and serious of bacterial enteritides in foals and adult horses. It is often accompanied by septicemia in foals. Salmonellosis can also be seen as a cause of enteritis in adult horses. Anterior uveitis and hypopyon have been seen in animals with salmonellosis, and *Salmonella* spp. can sometimes be cultured from these eyes.[201]

REFERENCE

201. Whitley RD, Gelatt KN: Ocular manifestations of systemic disease. II, Horse. In Gelatt KN, ed: *Textbook of veterinary ophthalmology*, Philadelphia, 1981, Lea & Febiger, pp 724-741.

MORAXELLA CONJUNCTIVITIS IN HORSES

Two authors have described a *Moraxella* spp. recovered from several horses in herd outbreaks of conjunctivitis, ocular discharge, and erosions of eyelid epithelium at the canthi.[202,203] The organism was similar but not identical to *M. bovis*, and the disease was reproduced experimentally in horses by instillation of the organism into the conjunctival sac. One author[203] described successful treatment of the lesions with chloramphenicol ointment, whereas the other[202] described the lesions as healing spontaneously.

REFERENCES

202. Hughes DE, Pugh GW: Isolation and description of a *Moraxella* from horses with conjunctivitis, *J Am Vet Med Assoc* 31:457-462, 1970.
203. Huntington PJ et al: Isolation of a *Moraxella* sp. from horses with conjunctivitis, *Aust Vet J* 64:118-119, 1987.

OCULAR MANIFESTATIONS OF EQUINE VIRAL ARTERITIS

Equine viral arteritis is a rare disease caused by an RNA virus classified as a toga virus. Clinically ocular and nasal discharges, palpebral, periorbital, or peripheral edema, skin rash, pyrexia, leukopenia, and abortions are seen.[204] Corneal opacity and photophobia have also been described.[205] The virus characteristically causes a panvasculitis.

REFERENCES

204. Traub-Dargatz JL et al: Equine viral arteritis, *Compend Cont Ed* 7:5490-5496, 1985.
205. Jones TC: Clinical and pathologic features of equine viral arteritis, *J Am Vet Med Assoc* 155:315-317, 1969.

OCULAR MANIFESTATIONS OF *RHODOCOCCUS (CORYNEBACTERIUM) EQUI* IN HORSES

Rhodococcus equi is a gram-positive coccobacillus that causes bronchopneumonia in young foals. One report of *R. equi* from the eye of a foal with bilateral panophthalmitis and pneumonia can be found.[206] Clinically the foal was seen to have bilateral miosis and hypopyon.

REFERENCE

206. Blogg JR et al: Blindness caused by *Rhodococcus equi* infection in a foal, *Equine Vet J* 2(suppl):25-26, 1983.

OCULAR MANIFESTATIONS OF BORRELIOSIS IN HORSES

Borrelia burgdorferi, the agent of Lyme disease, has been described as causing predominantly polyarthritis in horses, cows, and dogs. One case has been reported of a pony infected with *B. burgdorferi.*[207] Unilateral anterior and posterior uveitis was noted, and spirochetes were found in the anterior chamber. Other clinical signs included arthritis and synovitis of both carpal joints.

REFERENCE

207. Burgess EC, Gillette D, Pickett JP: Arthritis and panuveitis as manifestations of *Borrelia burgdorferi* infection in a Wisconsin pony, *J Am Vet Med Assoc* 189:1340-1342, 1986.

OCULAR MANIFESTATIONS OF CRYPTOCOCCOSIS IN HORSES

Exophthalmia and blindness caused by *Cryptococcus neoformans* have been described in a horse.[208] The frontal sinus and retrobulbar area were involved with a fungal granuloma, but the eye itself was normal. The chorioretinitis seen in other species associated with *C. neoformans* has not been described in the horse.

REFERENCE

208. Scott EA, Duncan JR, McCormack JE: Cryptococcosis involving the postorbital area and frontal sinus in a horse, *J Am Vet Med Assoc* 165:626-627, 1974.

OCULAR MANIFESTATIONS OF EQUINE HERPESVIRUS TYPE 2 (EHV-2)

Equine herpesvirus serotype 2 (EHV-2) has been isolated from eyes in herd outbreaks of keratoconjunctivitis in horses.[209,210] Clinical signs in one outbreak included photophobia, lacrimation, corneal neovascularization, corneal color change, and pinpoint ulcerations; eyes healed within 2 weeks.[209] In the other outbreak, conjunctivitis, and multifocal superficial corneal opacities were seen; eyes healed within 2 weeks on topical idoxuridine.[210] Experimental inoculation of EHV-2 intranasally in two ponies pretreated with dexamethasone caused conjunctivitis, as well as lymphadenopathy and coughing.[211] Conjunctiva from both ponies was positive for virus by PCR 6 months after inoculation.

Miller[212] confirmed EHV-2 by fluorescent antibody staining after isolating virus from the cornea of a thoroughbred mare with multiple superficial punctate corneal lesions. The keratitis was successfully treated with topical 1% trifluridine ophthalmic solution.*

REFERENCES

209. Thein P: The association of EHV-2 infection with keratitis and research on the occurrence of equine coital exanthema (EHV-3) of horses in Germany, *Proceedings of the Fourth International Conference of Equine Infectious Diseases,* Lyon, France, 1976, pp 33-41.
210. Collinson PN et al: Isolation of equine herpesvirus type 2 (equine gamma herpesvirus 2) from foals with keratoconjunctivitis, *J Am Vet Med Assoc* 205:329-331, 1994.
211. Borchers K et al: Virological and molecular biological investigations into equine herpes virus type 2 (EHV-2) experimental infections, *Virus Res* 55:101-106, 1998.
212. Miller TR et al: Herpetic keratitis in a horse, *Equine Vet J* 17(suppl 10):15-17, 1990.

---

*Viropic, Burroughs-Wellcome, Research Triangle Park, NC 27709.

OCULAR MANIFESTATIONS OF STRANGLES (*Streptococcus equi*)

Strangles is a respiratory infection caused by *Streptococcus equi* that can have an accompanying ocular discharge.[213] In one group of horses clinically diagnosed as having strangles, chorioretinal depigmentation was noted in the nontapetal fundus of several horses. Because these lesions pigmented with time, it was suggested that they were caused by seeding of the choroid during bacteremia.[214] One case of panophthalmitis in a horse caused by *S. equi* has been described.[214] Ten days after a bout of strangles this horse developed anterior uveitis, which progressed to corneal stromal abscesses and panophthalmitis. *S. equi* was cultured from the eye at the time of enucleation.

REFERENCES

213. Yelle MT: Clinical aspects of *Streptococcus equi* infection, *Equine Vet J* 19:158-162, 1987.
214. Roberts SR: Chorioretinitis in a band of horses, *J Am Vet Med Assoc* 158:2043-2046, 1971.
215. Barratt-Boyes SM et al: *Streptococcus equi* infection as a cause of panophthalmitis in a horse, *J Equine Vet Sci* 11:229-231, 1991.

OCULAR MANIFESTATIONS OF EQUINE HERPESVIRUS TYPE 1 (EHV-1)

Equine herpesvirus serotype 1 (EHV-1) is a cause of rhinopneumonitis in horses. It has been cultured from cases of superficial punctate keratitis in the horse; the significance of these isolations is unknown.[216]

Six foals were experimentally inoculated intranasally with EHV-1.[216] All developed typical mild signs of upper respiratory infection. One foal developed vision problems 1 month postinoculation. Bilateral chorioretinitis was diagnosed. On necropsy, chorioretinal degeneration with mononuclear cell infiltration in some areas was seen, as well as demyelination of the optic nerve and mononuclear cell infiltrate in parts of the CNS.[217] These findings are not surprising in that EHV-1 causes a vasculitis and CNS disease in horses.[218]

REFERENCES

216. Riis RC: Equine ophthalmology. In Gelatt KN, ed: *Textbook of veterinary ophthalmology,* Philadelphia, 1981, Lea & Febiger, p 574.
217. Slater JD et al: Chorioretinopathy associated with neuropathology following infection with equine herpesvirus-1, *Vet Rec* 131:237-239, 1992.
218. McCartan CG et al: Clinical, serological and virological characteristics of an outbreak of paresis and neonatal foal disease due to equine herpesvirus-1 on a stud farm, *Vet Rec* 136:7-12, 1995.

OCULAR MANIFESTATIONS OF BRUCELLOSIS IN HORSES

Brucella abortus has been suggested as a cause for equine recurrent uveitis (ERU),[219] although serum agglutination titers for *B. abortus* in normal horses and horses with ERU are similar.[220]

REFERENCES

219. Whitley RD, Gelatt KN: Ocular manifestations of systemic disease. II, Horse. In Gelatt KN, ed: *Textbook of veterinary ophthalmology,* Philadelphia, 1981, Lea & Febiger, pp 724-741.
220. Jones TC: The relation of brucellosis to periodic ophthalmia in equidae, *Am J Vet Res* 1:54-57, 1940.

OCULAR MANIFESTATIONS OF *MYCOBACTERIUM AVIUM* IN HORSES

A case of anterior uveitis and bilateral chorioretinitis with retinal detachments has been described in a horse from Denmark. Acid-fast organisms were seen in both eyes as well as in

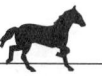

numerous other organs. *Mycobacterium avium* was cultured from these organs.[221]

REFERENCE
221. Leifsson PS, Olsen SN, Larsen S: Ocular tuberculosis in a horse, *Vet Rec* 141:651-654, 1997.

INSTALLATION OF A SUBPALPEBRAL LAVAGE SYSTEM

Subpalpebral lavage systems in horses are excellent means of providing frequent ocular therapy over an extended period of time. Medication is certain to enter the eye and there is no risk of damaging the cornea with an ointment tube. Because the painful eye is not manipulated, most horses do not become head-shy.

On the negative side, poorly placed tubing or tubing that is not carefully monitored can rapidly produce a corneal ulcer. Misplaced tubing can also cause leakage of topical medication subcutaneously, leading rapidly to a swollen and inflamed eyelid. The following equipment is necessary:

- 12-gauge needle with hub removed
- Silastic tubing (Dow Corning Silastic medical-grade tubing, Cat. No. 602-175; 0.03-inch ID ×0.065-inch OD*— this is much softer than polyethylene and causes less damage if it migrates)
- Feline in-dwelling catheter, 20-gauge; needle, 22-gauge†
- Intermittent injection cap (prn), if needed for catheter‡
- Gauze sponges
- White tape
- Applicator stick
- Lidocaine
- Topical anesthetic such as proparacaine (Ophthaine)§
- Needle holder
- Scissors
- Monofilament nonabsorbable suture on a cutting needle (optional)
- Tetanus toxoid

The horse should be tranquilized and/or twitched. The auriculopalpebral nerve is blocked over the zygomatic arch to paralyze the orbicularis oculi muscle to allow eyelid manipulation. The supraorbital (frontal) nerve is blocked at its exit from the supraorbital process to anesthetize the upper eyelid (Fig. 37-19). Topical anesthesia is then flushed into the upper conjunctival fornix with a small syringe with a broken-off 25-gauge needle.

The blunt end of the 12-gauge needle is used to probe the lateral conjunctival fornix to establish the placement of the needle. The needle is reversed and pushed through the eyelid in a lateral direction. The tip of the needle enters the dorsalmost aspect of the fornix and exits near the orbital rim. A folded gauge sponge is used to help force the needle through (Fig. 37-20). The ring end of a pair of scissors or open needle holders can be used to help keep the skin from tenting as the needle is pushed through (Fig. 37-21). After the needle is pushed through the skin (Fig. 37-22), the Silastic tubing is pushed through the needle, starting at the blunt end. When the tubing appears at the sharp end of the needle, the needle and tubing are pulled through the eyelid (Fig. 37-23). Needle holders can be used to help pull out the needle. During the manipulations the needle must not be pushed against the cornea.

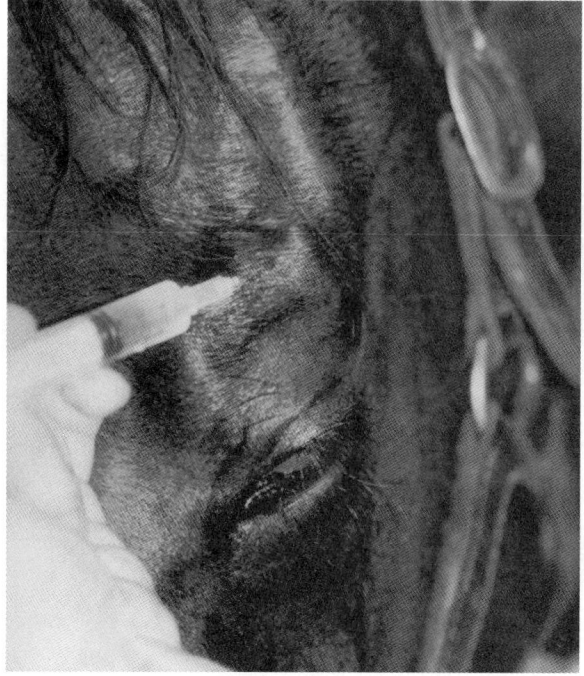

FIG. 37-19 ▌▌ Frontal (supraorbital) nerve block in horse. A 25-gauge needle is inserted into the supraorbital foramen, and 5.0 ml of lidocaine injected alongside the nerve.

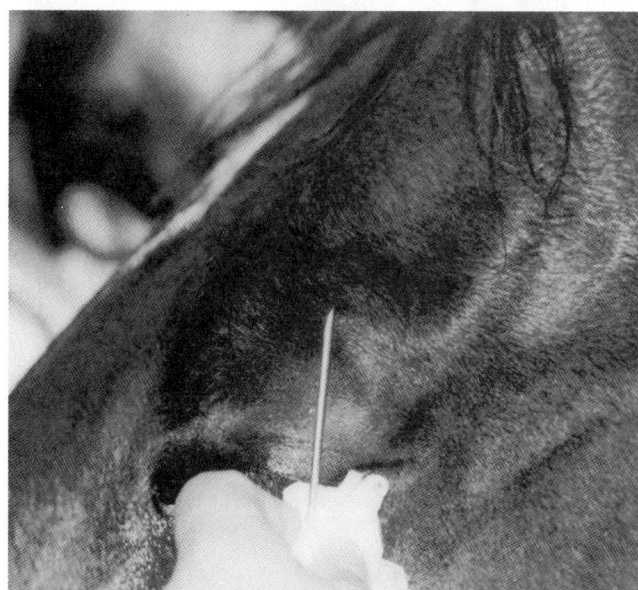

FIG. 37-20 ▌▌ Preparing to push the 12-gauge needle with a gauze sponge before placing a palpebral lavage system.

This procedure is then repeated medially, with the exit holes 4 to 5 cm apart (Figs. 37-24 and 37-25). The medial end of the tubing is knotted several times (Fig. 37-26). To measure the tubing for hole placement, the medial (knotted) end is pulled out and laid on the eyelid skin (Fig. 37-27). Two to three holes are made in the center of the tubing with

---

*Storz Instrument Co, St. Louis, MO 63122.
†Sherwood Medical, Ireland.
‡Critikon, Tampa, FL 33630.
§ER Squibb & Sons, Inc, Princeton, NJ 08543.

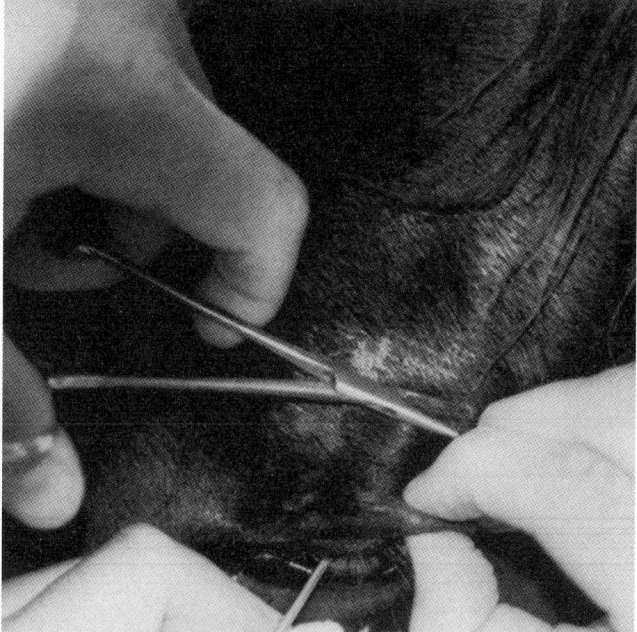

FIG. 37-21 ▮▮ Pushing the needle through the eyelid with open needle holders to keep the skin from tenting.

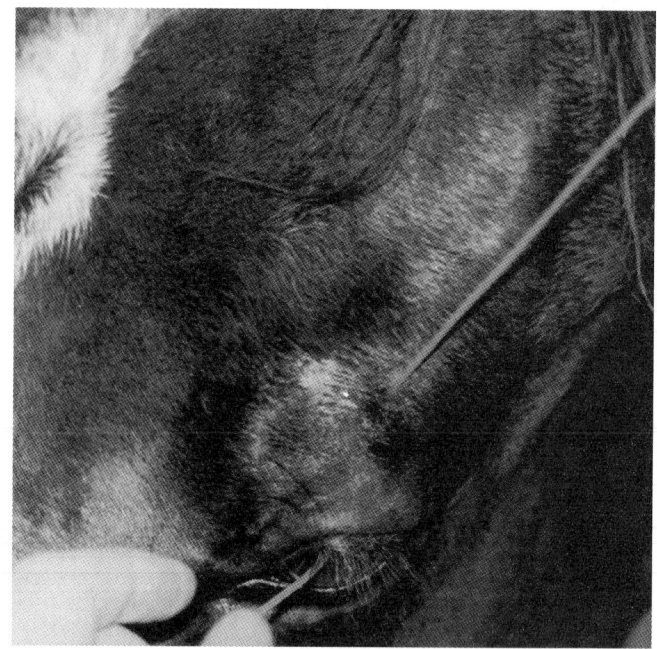

FIG. 37-23 ▮▮ Silastic tubing placed through the eyelid laterally.

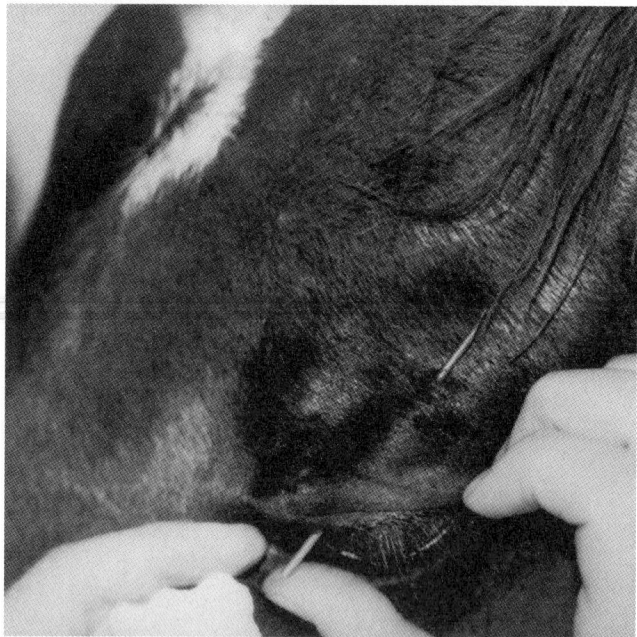

FIG. 37-22 ▮▮ Needle pushed through the eyelid laterally. Note that the needle was inserted at 45 degrees to the eyelid margin.

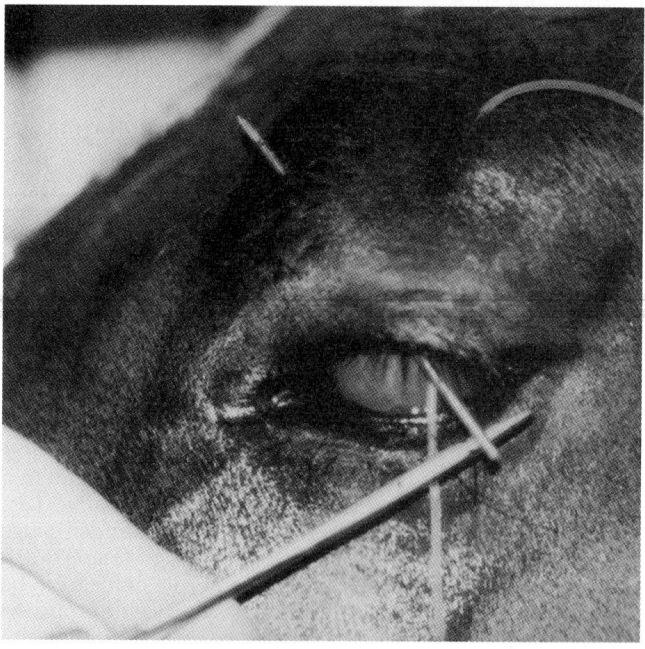

FIG. 37-24 ▮▮ Needle pushed through the eyelid medially. Note that the needle is prevented from rubbing the cornea. The needle was again inserted at 45 degrees to the eyelid margin.

a 25-gauge needle (Fig. 37-28). The holes should be close together because widely spaced or uncentered holes cause the subcutaneous leakage of medication. The tubing is then repositioned (Fig. 37-29).

Tape secures the tubing laterally, and sutures can be used to secure the tape to the skin (Fig. 37-30). Additional tape and skin sutures can be placed several centimeters from the first tape, or tubing can be braided through the forelock (Fig. 37-31). Silastic tubing is then run down the neck through several braids to keep it secure. The feline in-dwelling catheter is run into the end of the tubing, a prn is taped into the end of the catheter if necessary, and catheter and tubing are taped to an applicator stick to prevent bending. The stick is then taped to a braid of the mane.

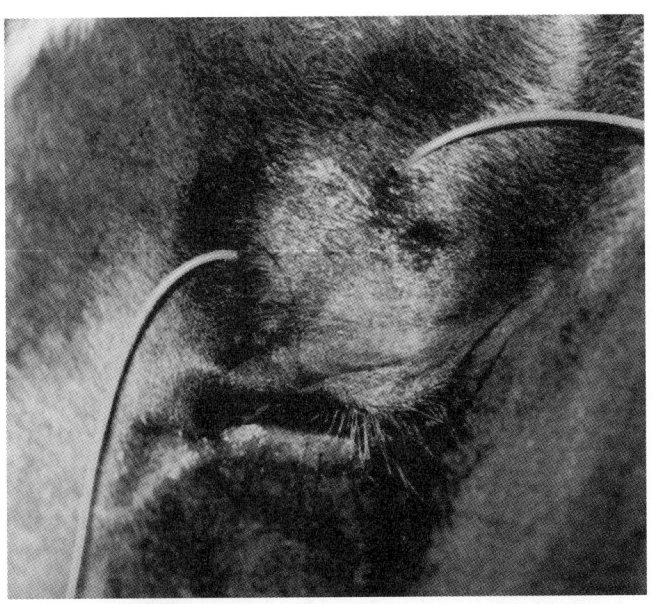

FIG. 37-25 ■ Silastic tubing through the eyelid medially.

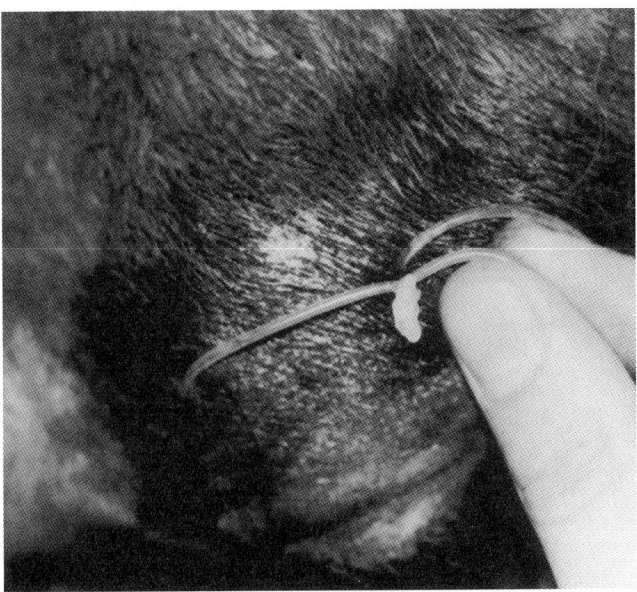

FIG. 37-27 ■ The tubing is measured before fenestrating.

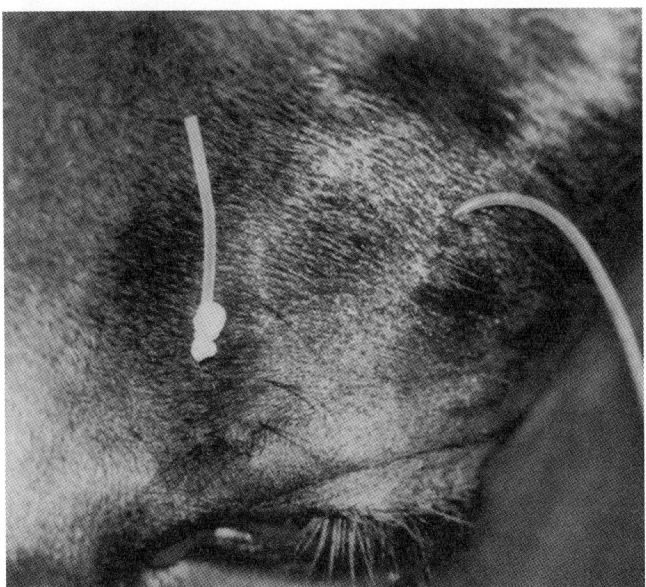

FIG. 37-26 ■ Several knots are tied on top of one another in the medial end of tubing to prevent the tube from pulling back through the skin into the conjunctival fornix.

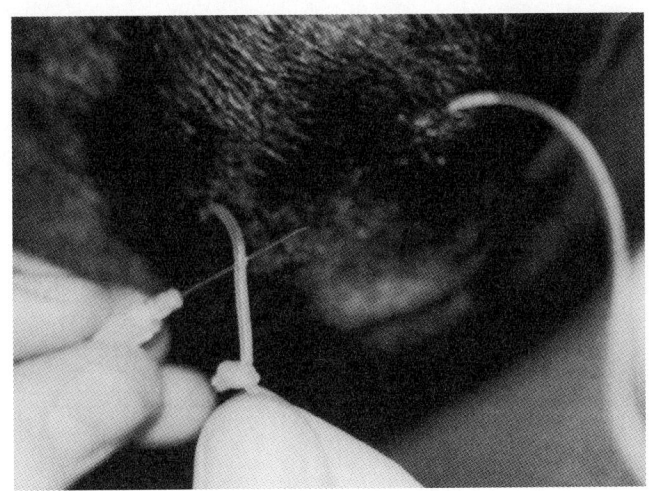

FIG. 37-28 ■ Holes are created in the Silastic tubing with a 25-gauge needle.

The most common problem with this system is that the tape that secures the Silastic tubing laterally loses its stickiness within a day or two. This is easily repaired by putting a new piece of tape medial to the first. Before administering any medication, one should always make sure the tubing has not slipped medially.

An alternative to this system is the Mila Subpalpebral Eye Lavage Kit.* This kit comes complete with a large-gauge needle, a prn, a plastic device to secure the tubing to the skin

(which eliminates the piece of tape) and Silastic tubing with a very soft footplate. This tubing is placed identically to the above system, but only one (lateral) hole is needed in the upper eyelid. For this reason, the Mila system is easier to use. This tubing does not plug easily because the hole in the footplate is relatively large. This system is a little more difficult to remove than the previously mentioned system; we had one footplate migrate subconjunctivally, necessitating general anesthesia to remove.

Most horses tolerate this system well, and we have kept the tubing in place for up to 6 weeks. Occasionally horses try to rub out the tubing; neck cradles prevent this in such horses.

*Mila International, Florence, KY 41042.

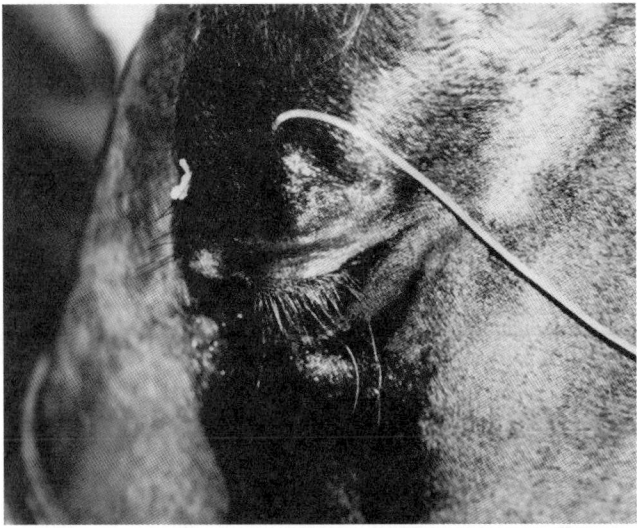

FIG. 37-29 ▮▮ Silastic tubing in place.

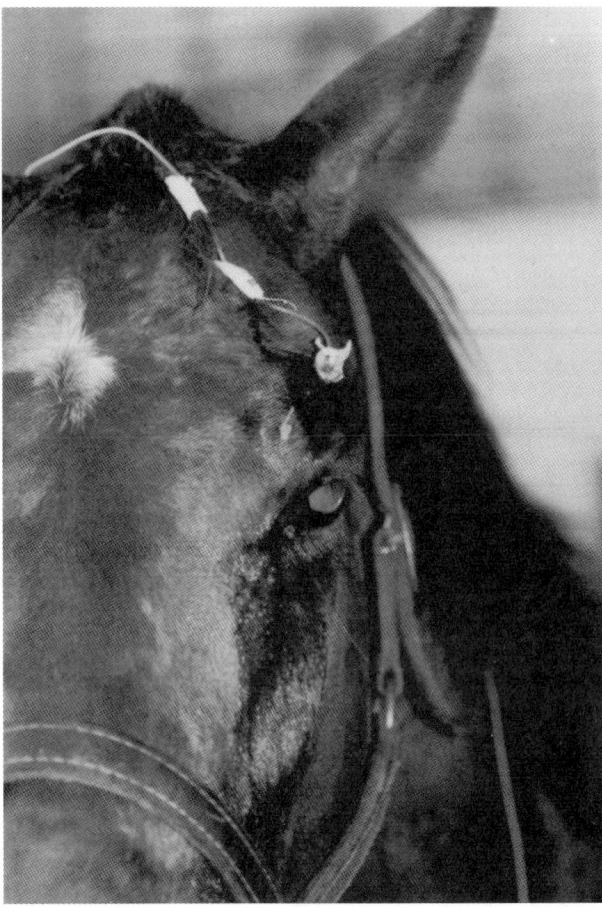

FIG. 37-31 ▮▮ Front view of lavage tubing secured to skin in two places and taped to braided forelock. The tubing is run back to the halter or neck to expedite treatment.

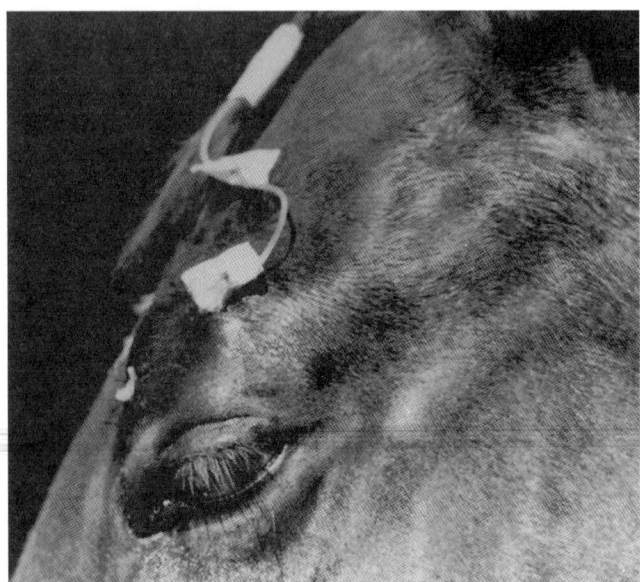

FIG. 37-30 ▮▮ A tape butterfly is applied to the tubing at the lateral exit from the eyelid. The tape has been sutured to the skin.

IMMUNE-MEDIATED OCULAR DISEASES

MARY BELLE GLAZE

Except for the conjunctiva, the eye has no lymphatic drainage. The access of antigens to potentially reactive lymphoid tissue is also restricted by the avascularity of the cornea and the presence of selective blood-ocular barriers. As unlikely as immunologically mediated abnormalities might seem under these circumstances, immune-related inflammation remains a leading cause of blindness in the horse. In contrast, immune-mediated ocular disease is rare in ruminants.

OCULAR IMMUNOLOGY

The conjunctiva processes ocular surface antigens with the help of regional lymph nodes. Antigen is first bound by specialized lymphoid tissue within the conjunctiva or by limbal Langerhans' cells. The bound antigen is delivered to the regional node by circulating lymphocytes or is transmitted directly through adjacent lymphatic channels. Stimulated lymphocytes migrate back to the conjunctiva (T-cells) and lacrimal gland (B-cells), where they participate in cell-mediated reactions and local production of IgA, respectively.[222,223]

Because the globe itself is without lymphatic drainage, intraocular antigens must be processed at a distant site. These antigens pass into the systemic circulation, stimulating the spleen, bone marrow, and other distant lymphoid organs. After an interval of 5 to 7 days, sensitized lymphocytes migrate back to the eye and localize within the uvea and limbal conjunctiva. Like those on the ocular surface, these immunologically competent cells are capable of antibody production and can participate in cell-mediated reactions. Further exposure to the same antigen provokes an anamnestic response, endowing the uveal and limbal tissues with behavior comparable to that of a regional lymph node.[224]

Each of the four major types of immunologic reactions occurs within the eye.[225] Type I (immediate) hypersensitivity is usually manifest as conjunctivitis, an acute local inflammatory reaction that follows IgE-mediated release of histamine, proinflammatory cytokines, and chemotactic mediators from

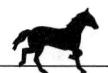

tissue mast cells and synthesis of a variety of cytokines, leukotrienes, prostaglandins, thromboxane, platelet-activating factor (PAF), and kinins.[226] These mediators of the IgE/mast cell inflammatory pathway increase vascular permeability, constrict smooth muscle, dilate blood vessels, and activate leukocyte chemotaxis and the complement cascade. Allergic reactions of the lids and conjunctiva undoubtedly occur in all domestic species. Type II (cytotoxic/cytolytic) hypersensitivity is an antibody-mediated cytolytic reaction in which the antigen is a cell surface or basement membrane component. Three basic effector pathways lead to cell destruction: opsonization, with increased efficiency of phagocytic destruction; antibody-dependent cellular cytotoxicity, inducing the release of enzymes capable of destroying cells and digesting basement membranes; and lysis of immunoglobulin-bearing cells.[227] Conjunctival damage resulting from autoantibodies directed against epithelial basement membranes is described in equine ocular pemphigoid. Type III (immune-complex) hypersensitivity may share similar effector mechanisms with those described for cytolytic reactions, but antigen locale accounts for dissimilar disease manifestations in these two pathways.[226] This reaction may explain the clinical signs of pemphigus foliaceus[228] and the intraocular inflammation observed in horses following influenza vaccination or contact with infected animals.[229] Antibody-mediated cell destruction has also been implicated in uveitis.[225] Type IV (cell-mediated/delayed) hypersensitivity is an important factor in contact allergy of the lids and conjunctiva and may also play a role in ocular toxoplasmosis. The tissue destruction associated with herpetic keratoconjunctivitis in the horse has been attributed to a cell-mediated response.[225] Increasing evidence implicates delayed hypersensitivity in the pathogenesis of equine recurrent uveitis.[230,231] The reaction requires an initial antigen exposure that results in sensitization of antigen-specific T lymphocytes. Reintroduction of antigen induces interleukin production, with subsequent T-cell activation, proliferation, and cytokine production. Once activated by cytokines, recruited leukocytes display increased activity to many antigens.[232]

ALLERGIC BLEPHAROCONJUNCTIVITIS

In humans, several forms of allergic conjunctivitis are mediated by IgE, and histamine receptors (specifically H₂-receptors) have been discovered on the human ocular surface.[233] The ubiquitous presence of H₂-receptors in domestic animals implies a similar distribution[222] and the potential for immediate hypersensitivity reactions of the eyelids and conjunctiva.

Affected animals demonstrate acute swelling of the eyelids and conjunctiva, accompanied by serous ocular discharge, mild conjunctival hyperemia, and pruritus. If the stimulus persists, multiple subconjunctival aggregates of lymphocytes appear as tiny, semitransparent follicles within the conjunctival cul-de-sac. In contrast to bacterial conjunctivitis, crusting and purulent discharge are not conspicuous in allergic conjunctivitis.

Diagnosis of allergic blepharoconjunctivitis is often presumptive, so other causes of lid and conjunctival swelling must be ruled out. Trauma, orbital inflammation, mechanical irritants, conjunctival parasites, and other infectious agents (both ocular and systemic) should be considered. Conjunctival cytology may reveal eosinophils in response to mast cell degranulation.

The offending allergen may be difficult to identify. Insect stings and toxic plants (e.g., nettle) are possible causes, as are molds and pollens. Allergic conjunctivitis was described in 17 of 187 cows pastured adjacent to a field of blossoming cotton.[234] A group of Angus cross Holstein cattle demonstrated

excessive lacrimation and ocular pruritus associated with familial allergic rhinitis. Several inhaled allergens have been incriminated, including caperweed, clover, dock, lucerne, pepper tree, paspalum, wattle, ryegrass, sorrel, and fungal extracts.[235] New feeds and certain drugs (including oxytetracycline, penicillin, and sulfas) may produce generalized urticaria, with accompanying eyelid and conjunctival edema.[236] Similar findings have been reported in cattle with milk allergy. Agents directly inducing mast cell degranulation via osmotic or charge interactions include hypertonic saline, nonsteroidal antiinflammatory agents, thiopental, opiates, neuromuscular blocking agents, mannitol, radiocontrast agents, polymyxin B, and vancomycin.[237] Occasionally allergic conjunctivitis may be associated with a topical medication such as neomycin. Clinical signs exacerbate with continued application and diminish when the medication is discontinued.

Ocular signs subside with removal of the offending allergen, but this is often impractical. Individual animals may be treated with a topical ophthalmic corticosteroid preparation such as 0.5% dexamethasone ointment* to hasten resolution of swelling and redness. An agent with antiprostaglandin activity such as oral or parenteral flunixin meglumine† (1 mg/kg) may be of benefit in the horse. Signs associated with urticaria respond to a decreasing regimen of oral prednisone or prednisolone, initiated at a dosage of 1 mg/kg once daily in the nonpregnant animal.[238] Single parenteral doses of short-acting corticosteroids, epinephrine, or antihistamines have also been used with reported success in food animals.[235]

OCULAR MANIFESTATIONS OF PEMPHIGUS

Pemphigus refers to a group of chronic blistering diseases that affect healthy skin and mucous membrane. Although these disorders are of presumed autoimmune origin, their exact pathogenesis is unknown. Pemphigus foliaceus and bullous pemphigoid have been described in the horse.[239,240]

Ocular manifestations may include ulceration or crusting of the periocular skin and erosions of the conjunctiva. Chemosis and hyperemia are likely; secondary corneal disease may follow that of the mucous membrane. Diagnosis is based on clinical findings, cytology, histopathology, and positive immunofluorescence of affected skin. See the discussion of immune-mediated dermatologic disorders for therapeutic recommendations and prognosis.

EOSINOPHILIC KERATOCONJUNCTIVITIS

DEFINITION AND ETIOLOGY. Eosinophilic keratoconjunctivitis is an uncommon disorder characterized clinically by corneal ulceration and plaque formation in one or both eyes.[241,242] Its name is derived from the predominance of eosinophils found in cytologic samples. The specific cause of this disorder is still unknown.

CLINICAL SIGNS. Clinical signs may be unilateral or bilateral and include nonspecific signs of blepharospasm, ocular discharge, and conjunctival hyperemia. Perilimbal corneal ulcers appear as raised, white corneal plaques because of adherent caseous exudates, often accompanied by corneal edema and superficial vascularization.

DIAGNOSTIC AIDS. Differential diagnoses include mycotic keratitis, onchocercal keratoconjunctivitis, neoplasia, foreign body granuloma, traumatic keratitis, and calcific degeneration. Definitive diagnosis is based on clinical signs and

---

*Maxidex, Alcon Laboratories, Inc, Fort Worth, TX 76134.
†Banamine, Schering Corp, Kenilworth, NJ 07033.

cytologic findings. Eosinophils and segmented neutrophils predominate in corneal scrapings, with fewer mast cells, plasma cells, and lymphocytes. Light microscopy of corneal tissue reveals coalescing foci of degenerated collagen fibers in the corneal plaques.

PATHOPHYSIOLOGY. The exact cause of the disorder is unknown. The finding of eosinophils in equine ocular surface disease is usually attributed to parasitic infection by *Onchocerca* sp. or *Habronema* sp.,[243] although neither has been identified in the eight reported cases to date. One proposed mechanism for eosinophilic keratoconjunctivitis is an allergic or inflammatory response to long-term use of ivermectin as an anthelmintic, triggering the complement cascade and cellular chemotaxis in patients with ocular onchocerciasis.[242] Similarities to vernal keratoconjunctivitis in humans suggest that eosinophil granule major basic protein may play a significant role in the equine disease, inhibiting corneal epithelial migration and protein synthesis and promoting collagen degeneration.[244] Eosinophil collagenase also has been reported to degrade type-1 collagen, the predominant collagen in cornea.[241]

TREATMENT AND PROGNOSIS. Treatment consists of topically applied 0.05% dexamethasone and prophylactic topical antibacterial ointments every 6 hours until clinical signs resolve. Lesions remodel with minimal corneal scarring but mean duration of treatment in one series of patients was 64 days (range, 45 to 105 days).[241] Use of ophthalmic nonsteroidal antiinflammatory preparations may increase the severity of clinical signs of eosinophilic keratoconjunctivitis in horses because of potentiation of leukotrienes, the primary promoter of eosinophilic inflammation in horses.[241] Excision of the corneal plaques by superficial keratectomy appears to enhance healing, attributable to removal of the eosinophil granule major basic protein.[241,242]

EQUINE RECURRENT UVEITIS (Periodic Ophthalmia; Moon Blindness)

DEFINITION AND ETIOLOGY. Equine recurrent uveitis (ERU) is a leading cause of blindness in the horse and mule. Although the exact prevalence is unknown, estimates as high as 10% to 25% have been reported.[245,246] The disorder is characterized by a specific clinical pattern of intraocular inflammation in which recurring episodes of acute uveitis are separated by periods of clinical quiescence. Anterior uveitis (iridocyclitis) predominates in the early stages; repeated episodes damage other structures, including the cornea, lens, vitreous, retina, and optic nerve.

Despite extensive clinical research, the etiology of ERU is still unknown. The pathogenesis is undoubtedly immune-mediated, and characterization of T-lymphocyte populations in affected horses document a delayed hypersensitivity reaction as the basic immunologic mechanism underlying the recurrent inflammatory episodes.[231] Identification of the triggering antigen has proven more elusive, suggesting the disease does not result from the persistence of or repeated exposure to a single antigen but rather to a variety of circulating antigens or native ocular antigens. Two infectious pathogens most frequently incriminated are *Leptospira interrogans* serovar *pomona*[246] and *Onchocerca cervicalis*,[247] but diversification of T-cell responses to a particular antigen or group of antigens over time may result in evolution of the immune response to encompass endogenous ocular self-antigens.[228]

CLINICAL SIGNS. The lesions observed in ERU vary, depending on the severity and duration of the disease.[245,248-250] Acute episodes are painful, characterized by blepharospasm and excessive tearing. Affected eyes appear red and cloudy because of changes in the conjunctiva and cornea (Fig. 37-32). Ciliary flush refers to dilation of subconjunctival vessels near

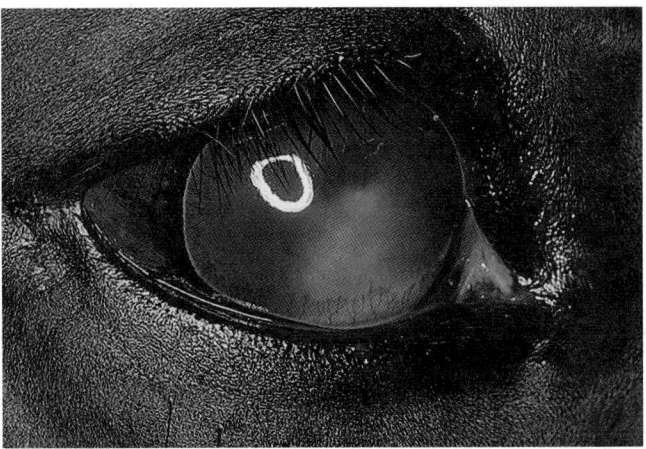

FIG. 37-32 ▦ Equine recurrent uveitis in a 5-year-old Quarter horse mare. The cornea is diffusely edematous and peripherally vascularized. A large yellow fibrin clot rests above a smaller accumulation of neutrophils (hypopyon). The bright circular reflection is a flash artifact.

the limbus, which may intensify the hyperemia. As corneal endothelial function decreases, generalized corneal edema gives the eye a blue-white appearance. The cornea may also exhibit peripheral, circumferential vascularization, cellular precipitates on its inner surface, and linear stromal opacities.

Increased uveal vessel permeability causes the aqueous to appear cloudy following the influx of protein (flare), inflammatory cells (hypopyon), erythrocytes (hyphema) or fibrin into the anterior chamber. The iris appears edematous and lackluster. Prostaglandins and other inflammatory mediators cause pupillary constriction, favoring the formation of adhesions between the iris and lens (posterior synechiae) and distortion of the pupillary shape. Even without adhesions, the inflamed iris responds poorly to mydriatic agents. Intraocular pressure is usually decreased owing to diminished aqueous production by the inflamed ciliary body, but intermittent pressure elevations can occur.[251] The ciliary body can also deposit cellular exudates within the anterior vitreous.

Active chorioretinitis causes dullness and loss of detail in affected tissues. Retinal detachment may follow choroidal exudation (Fig. 37-33). Multifocal depigmented or hyperpigmented foci on either side of the optic disc are the inactive sequelae of chorioretinitis, commonly referred to as peripapillary "butterfly" lesions (Fig. 37-34).

Intraocular damage increases as inflammation recurs. If the corneal endothelium is severely damaged, permanent corneal opacity results. Chronic recurrent uveitis is characterized by widespread posterior synechiae, iris depigmentation/hyperpigmentation, and iris atrophy. The anterior chamber may appear shallow if aqueous trapped in the posterior chamber by extensive iris to lens adhesions causes the iris to balloon forward (iris bombé). Most lens changes occur weeks or months after uveitis begins. Abnormalities may range from pigment flecks on the anterior lens capsule (Fig. 37-35) to dense cataracts. Lens luxation often follows zonular and vitreal degeneration. Retinal detachment may also follow vitreous liquefaction or may result from traction by fibrous tissue bands within the vitreous. If retinal degeneration is substantial, the optic disc atrophies. Permanent hypotony is followed by shrinkage of the globe (phthisis bulbi). Conversely, chronic uveitis may result in secondary glaucoma. The combination of these acute and chronic ocular lesions determines the degree of vision loss in the affected animal.

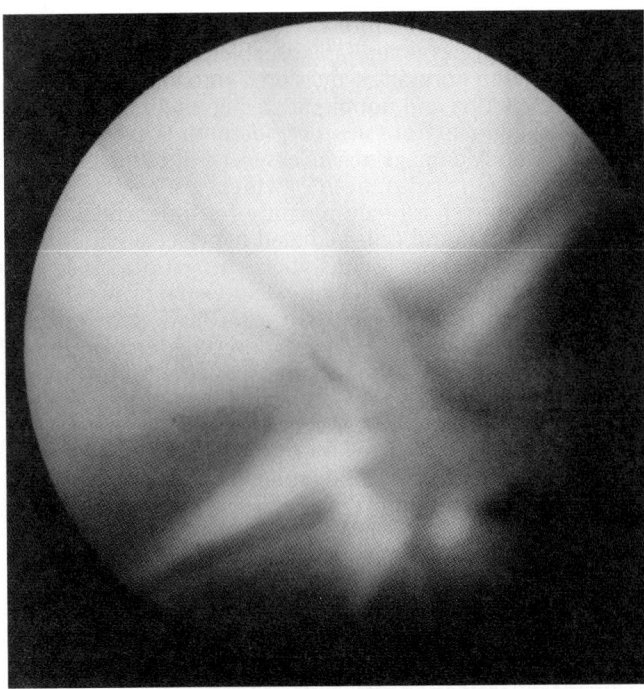

FIG. 37-33 ▌ Retinal detachment and subretinal exudation associated with ERU in a 5-year-old Quarter horse.

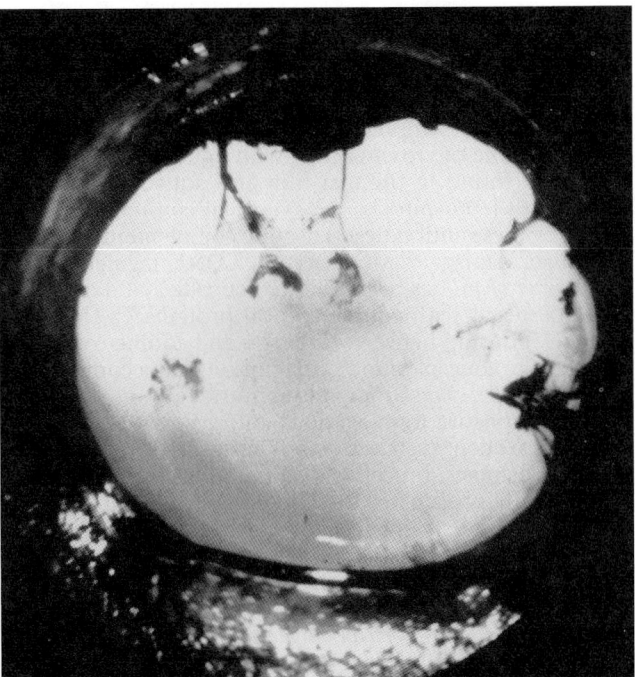

FIG. 37-35 ▌ Pigmented iridal tissues adhere to the anterior lens capsule after an episode of uveitis. Focal cataracts may develop at the adhesion site.

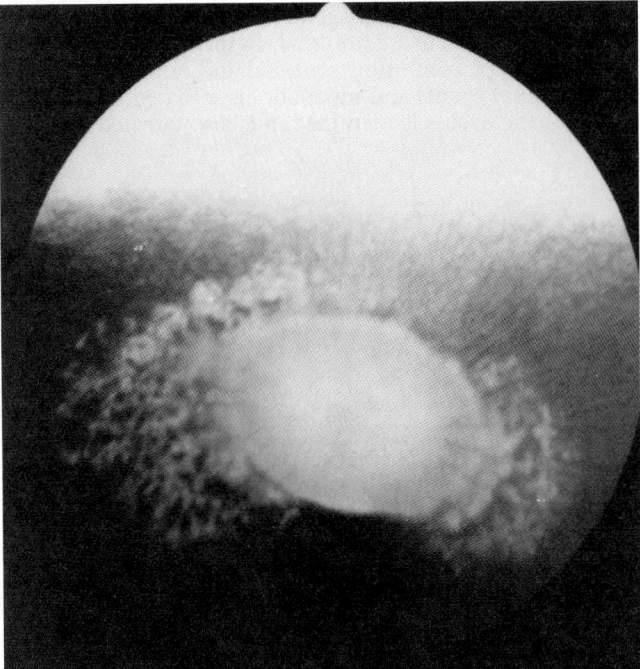

FIG. 37-34 ▌ Peripapillary retinal and choroidal depigmentation following recurrent episodes of equine uveitis. These inactive chorioretinal scars are also referred to as "butterfly" lesions.

DIAGNOSTIC AIDS. Diagnosis is based on a chronic, recurrent history of ocular disease and the presence of characteristic ocular lesions. Other causes of a red, painful eye that can mimic acute anterior uveitis include conjunctivitis, corneal ulceration, and glaucoma.

Serologic testing of paired serum samples for *Leptospira*, *Brucella*, or *Toxoplasma* spp. may be contributory, but negative titers do not exclude a diagnosis of ERU. A positive leptospiral titer for serovars at dilutions of 1:400 or greater are of clinical importance.[245] A higher titer in the aqueous than in the serum is indicative of intraocular antibody production and further supports a leptospiral cause for the uveitis.[252] *Onchocerca* microfilariae may be identified in conjunctival biopsies, although detection of live microfilaria does not necessarily indicate a causal relationship.[253]

PATHOPHYSIOLOGY. Experimental findings in ERU patients indicate that a T-cell-mediated autoimmune mechanism underlies the recurrent episodes of inflammation. T-lymphocytes are the predominant cell type to infiltrate the anterior uvea of horses with ERU[230] and cell-mediated immunity to uveal antigens has been demonstrated in affected horses.[254,255] Recent analysis of mRNA collected from horses with uveitis demonstrates elevated levels of IL-2 and IFN-mRNA,[231] indicating a Th1 response in the disease process.[256] In the absence of bacteria or viruses, this Th1 response by CD4+ uveal T-lymphocytes suggests a delayed-type hypersensitivity reaction to self or sequestered antigens in the uveal tract.[231,257] The observation of a deviant MHC class II antigen expression on resident ocular cells indicates that aberrant immune regulation may also play a role in ERU.[230,258]

Both exogenous and endogenous antigens have been proposed as stimuli for these basic immunologic responses. One theory suggests that an infectious agent such as *Leptospira* (or another, perhaps noninfectious, exogenous antigen) causes the initial iridocyclitis. Sensitized immunocompetent cells enter the uvea during this first inflammatory episode, imparting immunologic memory that is specific for the inciting antigen. Subsequent challenge of these cells by the immunogen causes recurrence of the inflammatory reaction.[225,259]

All major serogroups of *Leptospira interrogans* have been isolated from the horse and implicated as initiating factors in ERU.[246,260-262] Anti-*Leptospira* antibodies are found in the

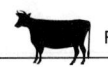

serum, tears, and aqueous humor of infected horses.[261,263] Horses seropositive to *Leptospira interrogans* serovar *pomona* are reportedly 13.2 times more likely to have signs of uveitis than seronegative horses.[246]

Interestingly, complement-binding, anti-*Leptospira* antibodies capable of cross-reacting with equine corneal tissue have been found in the tear film and aqueous humor of horses with leptospirosis.[262,263] Corneal epithelial cells are bound by these antibodies, activating complement and initiating tissue damage.[264] More recently, a DNA fragment of *Leptospira interrogans* has been found to encode a 90-kd protein that crossreacts with equine corneal proteins.[265] This antigenic relationship between *Leptospira* and equine cornea introduces the concept of molecular mimicry as a contributing factor in ERU, whereby an autoimmune response is stimulated by exposure to exogenous antigens with molecular structural sequences shared by self-antigens.[228]

Toxoplasmosis, brucellosis, salmonellosis, streptococcal hypersensitivity, *Escherichia coli, Rhodococcus equi*, borreliosis,[266] intestinal strongyles, and viral infections have also been implicated as causes of ERU, with no consistency in culture or serology results in affected horses.[246] More recent studies on vitreous and serum samples from affected horses discount the role of *Borrelia burgdorferi*, Borna disease virus, and *Toxoplasma* in ERU.[267]

An autoimmune phenomenon in response to damaged uveal tissue has also been proposed in the pathogenesis of ERU.[268] In general, autoimmunity may occur when a normally sequestered component is exposed to lymphoid cells or when the antigenicity of a component increases as a result of structural alterations.[269] Investigators have demonstrated sensitized cells and antibodies to antigens from the lens, uvea, and retina in human patients with uveitis.[270] Of particular interest is a soluble retinal glycoprotein called S-antigen that appears to play a major role in the pathogenesis of human autoimmune uveoretinitis.[271] The isolation of S-antigen in the horse and the subsequent finding of anti-S antibodies in the aqueous humor of horses with uveitis support the theory that this species is similarly capable of local production of antibodies to normally sequestered autoantigens.[254,255,272] Because the retina and nonpigmented epithelium of the ciliary body originate from neuroectoderm, it is even possible that ciliary body damage may release an S-like antigen or another uveitogenic substance.[273] Evidence suggests that response to S-antigen is predominantly T-cell-dependent.[274]

Both humoral and cell-mediated hypersensitivities have been implicated in the lesions of ocular onchocerciasis. Immunoelectrophoretic studies have demonstrated an influx of IgG and complement (C_3) into the tears of affected horses in response to larval death.[275] The resulting chemotaxis of mast cells, eosinophils, and lymphocytes perpetuates the inflammatory response and facilitates destruction of the parasite. Human patients with onchocerciasis have demonstrated deficiencies in suppressor T-cell function that may interfere with the normal control of antibody function.[276]

Regardless of etiology, the ocular inflammatory process may attract other reactive lymphocytes to the eye. During primary uveitis only 10% of the ocular immunoglobulin-secreting cells are specific for the inciting antigen. The remaining cells produce antibodies against immunogens that may not have entered the eye but with which the host has had previous contact. As a consequence, the eye may develop recurrent inflammation after systemic exposure to any one of a multiplicity of antigens. It is therefore conceivable that subsequent episodes of uveitis may differ etiologically, creating a perplexing clinical picture.[277]

TREATMENT AND PROGNOSIS (FIG. 37-36). Traditionally, reduction of intraocular inflammation is the primary therapeutic objective in acute uveitis. Preservation of vision depends on successful management at this stage, when sight-threatening sequelae are minimal. In most instances, symptomatic therapy combining steroidal and nonsteroidal anti-inflammatory agents and mydriatics is initiated. If a specific cause for the uveitis is identified, it is also targeted pharma-

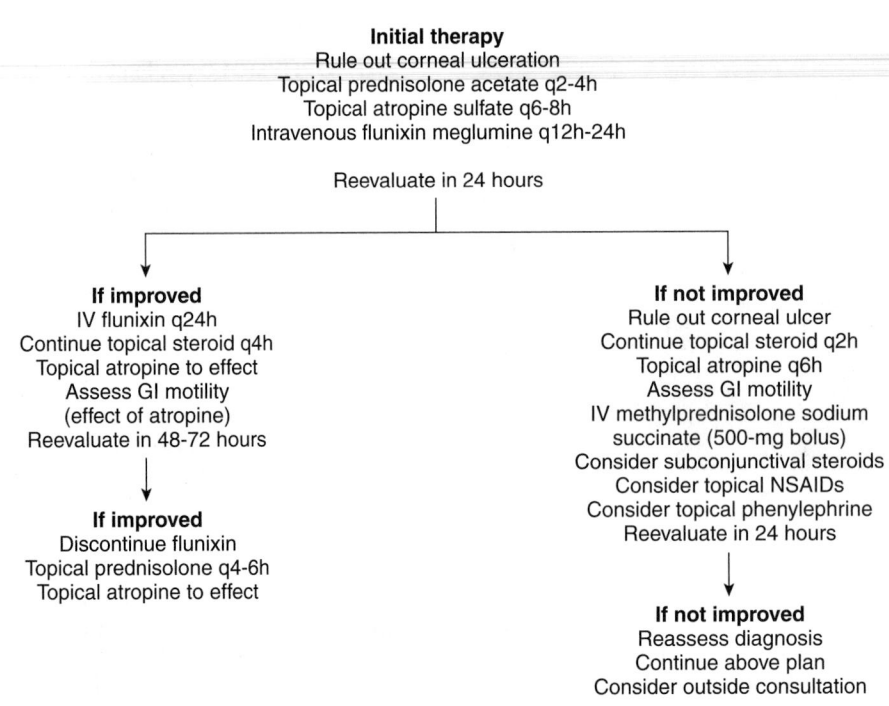

FIG. 37-36 ▦ Treatment algorithm for acute uveitis.

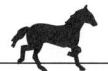

cologically. Because the triggering antigen is seldom if ever documented, a more effective strategy may be the nonspecific suppression of T-lymphocyte activation.[231]

No therapy is indicated in nonpainful eyes with lesions of chronic end-stage uveitis. Those eyes that remain painful or are nonresponsive to therapy are candidates for enucleation or evisceration, followed by silicone prosthesis implantation in the orbit or sclera, respectively.

Corticosteroids. The severity of the uveitis dictates the routes and frequency of corticosteroid administration. Although topical therapy is most often used, efficacy is limited by the agents' relatively short contact time with the eye. As a consequence, topical corticosteroids must be applied 3 to 4 times per day even in eyes with mild clinical signs. In more severe uveitis, topical preparations should be applied every 2 to 4 hours and combined with other routes of therapy. Consideration should be given to the use of a subpalpebral or nasolacrimal lavage system when such frequent application is indicated.

Both ophthalmic solutions and ointments are acceptable for topical use in the horse. Prednisolone acetate* has excellent intraocular penetration and is considered the solution of choice. Potent dexamethasone preparations† are also effective. In general, therapy should be continued for at least 2 weeks after clinical signs have resolved.

An alternative or supplement to frequent topical therapy is the subconjunctival injection of corticosteroids. Repositol corticosteroids are most beneficial in treating recurrent uveitis. Methylprednisolone acetate‡ 10 to 40 mg is injected in a 0.5- to 1-ml volume beneath the superior bulbar conjunctiva. Duration of effect depends on the severity of the uveitis. Subconjunctival triamcinolone acetonide§ (20 to 40 mg) is effective for 1 to 3 weeks, but nonocular use of the drug has been linked to equine laminitis.

Topical and subconjunctival corticosteroids are contraindicated in the therapy of corneal ulcers because they delay healing; potentiate collagenase, a devastating endogenous corneal enzyme; and predispose the cornea to fungal infection. Evaluation of inflamed eyes should always include a fluorescein dye test to rule out ulcerative keratitis.

Nonsteroidal Antiinflammatory Drugs. Parenteral corticosteroids may be used when topical and subconjunctival agents are ineffective in controlling inflammation, but nonsteroidal antiinflammatory drugs (NSAIDs) are usually preferred in such cases. Use of these antiprostaglandin agents nullifies an important mediator of intraocular inflammation and has minimized the role of parenteral steroids in uveitis therapy. This is desirable because systemic corticosteroid therapy in the horse has been linked to laminitis.

Three NSAIDs are currently used in the management of equine uveitis. Flunixin meglumine‖ is the drug of choice. A 1 mg/kg amount may be administered orally, intravenously, or intramuscularly once or even twice daily in cases of severe uveitis. Ketoprofen,¶ administered intravenously once daily at a dosage of 2.2 mg/kg for up to 5 days, is also beneficial in the treatment of equine uveitis. Frequency should be reduced as clinical response occurs because antiprostaglandins may cause gastric ulceration and renal dysfunction. Oral phenylbutazone,** at a dosage of 3 mg/kg twice a day, is best

indicated in cases of mild uveitis or in animals requiring chronic low-dose oral prophylaxis for recurrent disease. Dosage requirements for aspirin make it less practical in acute cases, but prolonged oral administration of 15 mg/kg twice a day has been used to avert relapses.

Topical ophthalmic NSAIDs are more costly and not as potent as corticosteroids but may be useful supplements in cases of acute or resistant uveitis. Although once considered a safe alternative to topical corticosteroids in horses with concurrent corneal ulceration, topical NSAIDs have recently been implicated in the development of melting corneal ulcers and are no longer recommended in ulcerated eyes. Available solutions include flurbiprofen sodium* and diclofenac sodium.† Suprofen has been withdrawn from the market in response to its adverse corneal effects. Dosage frequency is empiric, with intervals ranging from 6 to 12 hours.

Mydriatics-Cycloplegics. A parasympatholytic mydriatic-cycloplegic agent must be used if equine uveitis is to be managed successfully. By dilating the pupil and decreasing iris-lens contact, the chance of posterior synechia formation—and secondary glaucoma—is reduced. An adequately dilated pupil may also promote vision during the acute episode. Ciliary spasm is relieved, making the horse more comfortable, and the iridociliary vessels return to a more normal state of permeability.

Topical application of 1% atropine solution or ointment is indicated 2 to 4 times daily until the pupil dilates. The ultimate goal is to maintain mydriasis with the least frequent application possible, keeping in mind the resistance of the inflamed iris to the effects of atropine. Horses on an intensive parasympatholytic regimen should be strictly monitored for signs of reduced gut motility and colic because systemic effects occur with frequent topical atropine administration. Pupillary dilation may persist for up to 4 weeks after cessation of therapy.

If mydriasis is slow or incomplete, 10% phenylephrine hydrochloride‡ may be used topically in conjunction with atropine.[278] Although a study in the horse suggests that phenylephrine is ineffective when combined with a parasympatholytic agent, investigators did not rule out a possible benefit if dosage or duration of therapy were increased.[279] However, frequently applied phenylephrine has been associated with the development of corneal ulcers, corneal endothelial toxicity, and increased uveal exudation, so response to the drug should be carefully monitored.

Antibiotics. Because current evidence suggests an immune rather than an infectious basis for recurrent uveitis, antibiotics have assumed a secondary role in ERU management. Topical antibiotic preparations such as chloramphenicol, neomycin-polymyxin B, or gentamicin may discourage opportunistic bacteria during intensive corticosteroid therapy. Horses with increasing leptospiral titers may benefit from parenteral penicillin-streptomycin therapy.

Other Agents. The precise role of *Onchocerca* spp. in the pathogenesis of ERU is not yet determined, and considerable controversy exists regarding the necessity or benefit of microfilaricidal therapy in cases of ocular onchocerciasis. The treatment of ocular onchocerciasis is discussed elsewhere. If leptospiral infection has been well documented in a group of horses with uveitis, periodic vaccination against the disease

---

*Pred-Forte, Allergan Pharmaceuticals, Irvine, CA 92713.
†Maxidex and Maxitrol, Alcon Laboratories, Inc, Fort Worth, TX 76134.
‡Depo-Medrol, Upjohn Co, Kalamazoo, MI 49001.
§Kenalog, Westwood-Squibb Pharmaceuticals, Buffalo, NY 14213.
‖Banamine, Schering Corp, Kenilworth, NJ 07033.
¶Ketofen, Fort Dodge Laboratories, Fort Dodge, IA 50501.
**Butazolidin, Cooper's Animal Health, Inc, Kansas City, MO 64141.

*Ocufen 0.03%, Allergan Pharmaceuticals, Irvine, CA 92713.
†Voltaren 0.1%, Ciba Vision Care, Atlanta, GA 30360.
‡Neo-Synephrine, Winthrop-Breon Laboratories, New York, NY 10016.

may be considered, although the efficacy and implications of vaccinating to prevent ERU have not been investigated. The long-term prognosis for vision in horses with recurrent uveitis is guarded.

Experimental Treatment Modalities. Cyclosporine A is a noncytotoxic immunosuppressive drug that blocks the transcription of IL-2 production and decreases the responsiveness of the T-cell during the initiation of inflammation,[280] properties that could block the nonspecific activation of T-cells in recurrent episodes of ERU. Though topical application of cyclosporine fails to achieve effective intraocular levels,[281] implantation of a cyclosporine-impregnated device into the anterior vitreous of horses with experimental uveitis significantly decreased the duration and severity of inflammation, cellular infiltration, tissue destruction, protein concentrations, and the level of transcription of pro-inflammatory cytokines.[282] Ongoing studies of cyclosporine include development and evaluation of a subconjunctival delivery device that would circumvent the need for intraocular surgical skills.

Pars plana vitrectomy has been used successfully to remove vitreal debris to improve vision and delay progression of clinical signs in affected horses.[283,284] Proponents theorize that removal of uveitis-induced "immunologic memory" in the vitreous may reduce adverse interactions between the vitreous and the uveal tract, thereby reducing the recurrence of ERU. In one study recurrence of ERU was prevented in 85% (29/34) of treated eyes followed for intervals ranging from 5 months to 5 years.[284]

BOVINE-SPECIFIC OPHTHALMIA

A recurrent uveitis of cattle has been described and compared to that of the horse.[285,286] Like equine recurrent uveitis, its definitive etiology is unknown, although a viral infection was originally incriminated. Clinical signs include conjunctival hyperemia, corneal edema and vascularization, inflammatory cells and hemorrhage within the anterior chamber and uveal tract, and retinal and choroidal edema and hemorrhage. The disorder is uncommon and does not share the notoriety of its equine counterpart. Therapy is directed at reducing inflammation, as described for the horse.

REFERENCES

222. Eichenbaum JD et al: Immunology of the ocular surface, *Compend Cont Educ Pract Vet* 9:1101-1109, 1987.
223. English RV: Regulation of intraocular immune responses, *Prog Vet Comp Ophthalmol* 2:41-49, 1992.
224. Rahi AHS, Garner A: *Immunopathology of the eye*, Oxford, England, 1976, Blackwell Scientific, pp 77-93.
225. Hines MT: Immunologically mediated ocular disease in the horse, *Vet Clin North Am (Large Anim Pract)* 6:501-512, 1984.
226. Swiderski CE: Hypersensitivity disorders in horses, *Vet Clin North Am (Equine Pract)* 16:131-151, 2000.
227. Frank MM, Lawley TJ: Immune complexes and allergic disease. In Middleton E et al: *Allergy: principles and practice*, ed 5, St Louis, 1998, Mosby, pp 702-712.
228. McClure JJ: Equine autoimmunity, *Vet Clin North Am (Equine Pract)* 16:153-164, 2000.
229. Matthew AG, Handscombe MC: Uveitis in the horse: a review of the aetiological and immunopathological aspects of the disease, *Equine Vet J Suppl* 2:61-64, 1983.
230. Romeike A, Brugmann M, Drommer W: Immunohistochemical studies in equine recurrent uveitis (ERU), *Vet Pathol* 35:515-526, 1998.
231. Gilger BC et al: Characterization of T-lymphocytes in the anterior uvea of eyes with chronic equine recurrent uveitis, *Vet Immunol Immunopathol* 71:17-28, 1999.
232. Askenase P: Effector and regulator molecules and mechanism in delayed type hypersensitivity. In Middleton E et al, eds: *Allergy: principles and practice*, ed 5, St Louis, 1998, Mosby, pp 323-341.
233. Abelson MB, Udell IJ: H$_2$-receptors in the human ocular surface, *Arch Ophthalmol* 99:302-304, 1981.
234. Severin GA, Hazel SJ, Kainer RA: The eye. In Amstutz HE, ed: *Bovine medicine and surgery*, ed 2, Santa Barbara, Calif, 1980, American Veterinary Publications, p 939.
235. Krahwinkel DJ et al: Familial allergic rhinitis in cattle, *J Am Vet Med Assoc* 192:1593-1596, 1988.
236. Rebhun WC: Ocular manifestations of systemic disease in the bovine. In Howard JL, ed: *Current veterinary therapy: food animal practice*, ed 2, Philadelphia, 1986, WB Saunders, pp 836-840.
237. Swiderski C: Hypersensitivity reactions. In Reed S, Bayly W, eds: *Equine internal medicine*, Philadelphia, 1997, WB Saunders, pp 19-47.
238. Evans AG: Recurrent urticaria due to inhaled allergens. In Robinson NE, ed: *Current therapy in equine medicine*, ed 2, Philadelphia, 1987, WB Saunders, pp 619-621.
239. Scott DW et al: Immune-mediated dermatoses in domestic animals: ten years after. I, *Compend Cont Educ Pract Vet* 9:423-435, 1987.
240. George LW, White SL: Autoimmune skin disease of large animals, *Vet Clin North Am (Large Anim Pract)* 6:79-86, 1984.
241. Ramsey DT et al: Eosinophilic keratoconjunctivitis in a horse, *J Am Vet Med Assoc* 205:1308-1311, 1994.
242. Yamagata M, Wilkie DA, Gilger BC: Eosinophilic keratoconjunctivitis in seven horses, *J Am Vet Med Assoc* 209:283-1286, 1996.
243. Moore CP et al: Equine ocular parasites: a review, *Equine Vet J Suppl* 2:76-85, 1983.
244. Trocme SD et al: Eosinophil major basic protein deposition in corneal ulcers associated with vernal keratoconjunctivitis, *Am J Ophthalmol* 115:640-643, 1993.
245. Schwink KL: Equine uveitis, *Vet Clin North Am (Equine Pract)* 8:557-574, 1992.
246. Dwyer AE, Crockett RS, Kalsow CM: Association of leptospiral seroreactivity and breed with uveitis and blindness in horses: 372 cases (1986-1993), *J Am Vet Med Assoc* 207:1327-1331, 1995.
247. Schmidt GM et al: Equine ocular onchocerciasis: histopathologic study, *Am J Vet Res* 43:1371-1375, 1982.
248. Rebhun WC: Diagnosis and treatment of equine uveitis, *J Am Vet Med Assoc* 175:803-808, 1979.
249. Abrams KL, Brooks DE: Equine recurrent uveitis: current concepts in diagnosis and treatment, *Equine Pract* 12:27-35, 1990.
250. Brooks DE: Equine ophthalmology: equine recurrent uveitis. In Gelatt KN, ed: *Veterinary ophthalmology*, ed 3, Philadelphia, 1999, Williams & Wilkins, pp 1101-1105.
251. Miller TR et al: Equine glaucoma: clinical findings and response to treatment in 14 horses, *Vet Comp Ophthalmol* 5:170-182, 1995.
252. Davidson MG, Nasisse MP, Roberts SM: Immunodiagnosis of leptospiral uveitis in 2 horses, *Equine Vet J* 19:155-157, 1987.
253. Attenburrow DP, Donnelly JJ, Soulsby EJL: Periodic ophthalmia (recurrent uveitis) of horses: an evaluation of the aetiological role of microfilariae of *Onchocerca cervicalis* and the clinical management of the condition, *Equine Vet J Suppl* 2:48-56, 1983.
254. Hines MT, Halliwell REW: Autoimmunity to retinal S-antigen in horses with equine recurrent uveitis, *Prog Vet Comp Ophthalmol* 1:283-290, 1991.
255. Hines MT, Jarpe A, Halliwell REW: Equine recurrent uveitis: immunization of ponies with equine retinal S-antigen, *Prog Vet Comp Ophthalmol* 2:3-11, 1992.
256. Horohov DW: Equine T-cell cytokines, *Vet Clin North Am (Equine Pract)* 16:1-14, 2000.
257. Caspi R, Silver P, Chan C: Genetic susceptibility to experimental autoimmune uveoretinitis in the rat is associated with an elevated Th1 response, *J Immunol* 157:2668-2675, 1996.
258. Caspi R et al: T cell mechanisms in experimental autoimmune uveoretinitis: susceptibility is a function of the cytokine response profile, *Eye* 11:209-212, 1997.
259. Shimada K, Silverstein AM: Local antibody formation within the eye: a study of immunoglobulin class and antibody specificity, *Invest Ophthalmol Vis Sci* 14:573-583, 1975.
260. Halliwell RE et al: Studies on equine recurrent uveitis. II, The role of infection with *Leptospira interrogans* serovar pomona, *Curr Eye Res* 4:1033-1040, 1985.
261. Sillerud CL et al: Serologic correlation of suspected *Leptospira interrogans* serovar pomona-induced uveitis in a group of horses, *J Am Vet Med Assoc* 191:1576-1578, 1987.
262. Parma AE et al: Tears and aqueous humor from horses inoculated with *Leptospira* contain antibodies which bind to cornea, *Vet Immunol Immunopathol* 14:181-185, 1987.
263. Parma AE et al: Experimental demonstration of an antigenic relationship between *Leptospira* and equine cornea, *Vet Immunol Immunopathol* 10:215-224, 1985.
264. Parma AE et al: C3 fixed in vivo to cornea from horses inoculated with *Leptospira interrogans*, *Vet Immunol* 34:181-187, 1992.
265. Lucchesi PMA, Parma AE: A DNA fragment of *Leptospira interrogans* encodes a protein which shares epitopes with equine cornea, *Vet Immunol Immunopathol* 71:173-179, 1999.
266. Hahn CN et al: A possible case of Lyme borreliosis in a horse in the UK, *Equine Vet J* 28:84-88, 1996.
267. Wollanke B et al: Studies on vitreous and serum samples from horses with equine recurrent uveitis (ERU): the role of *Leptospira*, *Borrelia burgdorferi*, Borna disease virus and *Toxoplasma* in the etiology of ERU, *Proceedings of the American College of Veterinary Ophthalmologists*, Seattle, 1998, p 31.

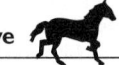

268. Morter RL: Equine leptospirosis, *J Am Vet Med Assoc* 155:436-442, 1969.
269. Eisen HN: *Immunology*, Philadelphia, 1980, Harper & Row, pp 509-512.
270. Muller-Ruchholtz W: Fundamentals of immunology and their application to uveitis. In Kraus-Mackiw E, O'Connor GR, ed: *Uveitis: pathophysiology and therapy*, New York, 1986, Thieme Medical, pp 19-27.
271. Nussenblatt RB, Silverstein AM: Ocular diseases of presumed autoimmune origin. In Rose NR, Mackay IR, ed: *The autoimmune diseases*, London, 1985, Academic Press, p 371.
272. Maxwell SA et al: Humoral responses to retinal proteins in horses with recurrent uveitis, *Prog Vet Comp Ophthalmol* 1:155-161, 1991.
273. O'Connor GR: Overview of ocular autoimmune diseases. In Helmsen RJ et al, eds: *Immunology of the eye, workshop II: Autoimmune phenomena and ocular disorders, immunology abstracts* (special suppl), Washington, DC, 1981, Information Retrieval, p 7.
274. Banga JP et al: Antigenicity and uveogenicity of partially purified peptides of a retinal autoantigen, S-antigen, *Immunology* 61:357-362, 1987.
275. Glaze MB et al: Immunoglobulin levels in tears and aqueous humor of horses before and after diethylcarbamazine (DEC) therapy, *Vet Immunol Immunopathol* 7:185-198, 1984.
276. Greene BM, Taylor HR, Aikawa M: Cellular killing of microfilariae of *Onchocerca volvulus*: eosinophil and neutrophil-mediated immune serum-dependent destruction, *J Immunol* 127:1611, 1981.
277. Shimada K, Silverstein AM: Induction of booster antibody formation without specific antigen drive, *Cell Immunol* 18:484-488, 1975.
278. Lavach JD: *The handbook of equine ophthalmology*, Fort Collins, Colo, 1987, Giddings Studio, p 19.
279. Hacker DV et al: Effect of topical phenylephrine on the equine pupil, *Am J Vet Res* 48:320-322, 1987.
280. Granelli-Piperno A: Cellular mode of action of cyclosporin A. In Bach Jf, ed: *T-cell directed immunointervention*, Oxford, 1993, Blackwell Scientific, pp 3-24.
281. Gilger BC, Allen JB: Cyclosporine A in veterinary ophthalmology, *Vet Ophthalmol* 1:181-187, 1998.
282. Gilger BC et al: Effect of an intravitreal cyclosporine implant on experimental uveitis in horses, *Proceedings of the American College of Veterinary Ophthalmologists*, 1999, p 50.
283. Gerhards H et al: Technique for and results with surgical treatment of equine recurrent uveitis, *Proceedings of the American College of Veterinary Ophthalmologists*, Seattle, 1998.
284. Fruhauf B et al: Surgical management of equine recurrent uveitis with single port pars plana vitrectomy, *Vet Ophthalmol* 1:137-151, 1998.
285. Marolt J et al: Specific ophthalmia of cattle, *Zentralb Veterinarmed* 10:286-294, 1963.
286. Davidson HJ, Blanchard GL, Coe PH: Idiopathic uveitis in a herd of Holstein cows, *Prog Vet Comp Ophthalmol* 2:113-116, 1992.

OCULAR PARASITES

ROBERT V. ENGLISH
MARK P. NASISSE

Parasites are an often overlooked cause of ocular disease in large animals. Many ocular parasitic diseases can threaten vision and can reduce the economic value of the animal through decreased function, decreased production, or both. The mechanisms by which parasites damage ocular tissues are extremely varied and range from direct tissue effects of aberrant parasite migration to complex immunopathologic responses to parasite antigens. In the following discussion the major ocular parasites of large animals are reviewed with reference to the ocular tissue of primary importance.

ADNEXAL PARASITISM

Parasitic eyelid diseases are covered in the dermatology section of the text (see Chapter 38).

CORNEAL AND CONJUNCTIVAL PARASITISM

Ocular Onchocerciasis

Ocular disease caused by *Onchocerca cervicalis* is the result of aberrant migration of noninfective microfilaria into the palpebral, conjunctival, and corneal tissues.[287] The larvae do not appear to have a predilection for ocular tissues; instead the eye is involved merely as part of a generalized subcutaneous migration. Approximately 50% of the horses with cutaneous onchocerciasis will have ocular involvement.[288]

The pathogenesis of ocular onchocerciasis remains unclear. In humans, keratoconjunctivitis and uveitis associated with the local presence of *Onchocerca volvulus* microfilaria occurs only after the microfilaria die. Because *Onchocerca* microfilaria are commonly found in equine ocular tissues without evidence of inflammation, a similar mechanism is probably involved. Therefore some change in the parasite, the host's immune response, or both must occur to incite an inflammatory response.

Ocular onchocerciasis occurs mostly in adult horses. The older the host, the greater is the exposure to the vector and the parasite and presumably the greater the potential for ocular migration of microfilaria. Furthermore, increased immune sensitivity may occur with increased exposure to dead microfilaria.

CLINICAL SIGNS. Conjunctivitis and keratoconjunctivitis concentrated at the temporal limbus are the most common manifestations of ocular onchocerciasis. Acutely there is chemosis and hyperemia of the conjunctiva, accompanied by increased lacrimation and blepharospasm. Small, raised, white nodules (0.5 to 2 mm in diameter) in the limbal conjunctiva and similar-sized, punctate, subepithelial corneal opacities are commonly present. Corneal lesions are often wedge shaped, with the base of the triangle at the limbus, and are characterized by varying degrees of superficial and deep neovascularization and cellular stromal infiltrates. Untreated, the lesions progressively enlarge, although the rate of progression and the severity of the disease varies. With chronicity, patches of depigmentation (vitiligo) occur in the perilimbal bulbar conjunctiva. Recurrent episodes of keratoconjunctivitis are common.

Migration and subsequent death of microfilaria in the uveal tract result in uveal inflammation. Both the anterior and the posterior uveal tracts may be involved. The clinical signs of *Onchocerca* uveitis include photophobia, epiphora, miosis, aqueous flare, inflammatory cells in the anterior chamber, and globe hypotonicity. However, these signs are not specific for onchocerciasis, and other etiologies must be considered (see Table 37-1).

Chorioretinitis is a reportedly common manifestation of posterior segment involvement. Active lesions are recognized ophthalmoscopically by hyporeflective areas, representing edema and inflammation, which are commonly observed around the optic papilla in a "butterfly-shaped" pattern.[289] However, aqueous and vitreous opacification often preclude accurate assessment of the fundus.

DIAGNOSIS. Characteristic clinical signs are highly suggestive of *Onchocerca* keratoconjunctivitis; but definitive diagnosis requires corneal or conjunctival biopsy. Conjunctival biopsy may be collected following topical anesthesia, whereas general anesthesia is necessary for partial-thickness lamellar keratectomies to obtain corneal biopsies. A single 3- to 5-mm biopsy is divided into two samples. One sample is placed on a slide with physiologic saline, minced, and warmed to 37° C (98.6° F) to stimulate larvae movement and therefore enhance their detection. Slides are examined repeatedly over the next hour for migrating microfilaria (see Chapter 11). The organisms are 200 to 240 mm long and 4 to 5 mm in diameter, with a short, unsheathed tail. The other half of the biopsy specimen is placed in 10% buffered neutral formalin for histopathologic examination.

The presence of microfilaria in ocular tissue does not substantiate a diagnosis of *Onchocerca* keratoconjunctivitis unless evidence of a host inflammatory response exists. The cytologic response is usually pleomorphic, with neutrophils, lymphocytes, plasma cells, and eosinophils present. Varying degrees of neovascularization, pigmentation, lamellar disorganization, collagen degeneration, and calcification are present in the cornea. The overlying epithelium becomes thickened and keratinized. The presence of eosinophils in corneal and conjunctival scrapings is suggestive of a parasite etiology; however, *Onchocerca* microfilaria are rarely found. Definitive diagnosis of *Onchocerca* as the cause of uveitis is rarely possible.

The differential diagnosis for equine keratoconjunctivitis also includes squamous cell carcinoma, habronemiasis, and mycotic infections. Because horses with ocular *Onchocerca* have a generalized larval migration, they may also demonstrate a dermatitis, especially of the ventral thorax.

TREATMENT. In humans chronically infected with *O. volvulus*, systemic ivermectin therapy decreases ocular microfilaria burden and improves associated ocular disease. In horses, however, microfilaricide therapy has been associated with increased ocular inflammation. Therefore treatment is directed at controlling the inflammatory reaction and then eliminating the parasite.[290,291] Corticosteroids are the mainstay of *Onchocerca* treatment and may be given topically, subconjunctivally, or systemically, depending on the severity of the inflammation, the extent of ocular and dermal involvement, and the temperament of the horse.

Because of superior solubility, prednisolone acetate* and dexamethasone alcohols† are the preferred topical corticosteroid preparations. Mild lesions without concurrent uveitis are treated 4 to 6 times daily. When keratoconjunctivitis is severe or when uveitis is present, hourly application may be indicated. Subconjunctivally administered corticosteroids are also beneficial but must be used with caution if corneal ulceration exists. Therapy is tapered as the inflammation is controlled.

Systemic corticosteroids are indicated for severe uveitis with concurrent *Onchocerca* dermatitis or before larvicidal therapy. Prednisolone, at an initial dose of 0.5 to 1 mg/kg of body weight daily for 5 to 7 days, is tapered as the inflammation decreases. Refractory cases have been treated for extended periods of time with 0.25 mg of prednisone per kilogram of body weight every other day.[292] The antiprostaglandin activity of nonsteroidal antiinflammatory drugs such as phenylbutazone and flunixin meglumine is also beneficial, especially when corneal ulceration prohibits the use of corticosteroids.

When inflammation is controlled, elimination of the microfilaria is recommended (Chapter 38). The use of topical antibiotics is also recommended in cases in which epithelial ulceration is present to prevent bacterial infection. With uveal involvement, topical cycloplegics such as atropine are indicated to relieve ciliary spasm and reduce the chance of posterior synechia formation.

Ocular Habronemiasis

Equine ocular habronemiasis occurs when larva from *Habronema muscae*, *Habronema microstoma*, or *Draschia megastoma* are deposited on ocular tissues. Flies serving as intermediate hosts for *Habronema* are attracted for feeding to moist areas of the body, including the conjunctiva. Ocular discharge and periocular wounds provide increased attraction for the flies. As the flies feed, *Habronema* larvae are deposited on the surface of ocular tissues, migrate into the tissues, and produce a local granulomatous inflammatory reaction. Equine habronemiasis occurs worldwide.

CLINICAL SIGNS. Ocular lesions commonly consist of raised, proliferative, nonhealing wounds present at the me-

dial canthus. The lesions are friable and pruritic and bleed easily. Lesions often contain small (1 to 2 mm), yellow, caseated nodules (so-called "sulfur granules"). Fistulous tracts and subdermal nodules may develop below the medial canthus. Corneal neovascularization, edema, and ulceration can occur as a result of altered lid function and irritation to the cornea from contact with the rough, irregular surface of the lesion. Corneal involvement increases the degree of ocular pain and blepharospasm.

Habronemiasis lesions are typically seasonal, occurring in the warm summer months when there is an increased fly population. Certain horses appear to have a predilection for developing cutaneous and ocular habronemiasis, so recurrence may be seen in these animals each summer.

DIAGNOSIS. Demonstration of the larvae in the granulomatous lesions or fistulous tracts is diagnostic. Biopsies of the affected tissue are directly examined for *Habronema* larvae and may also be submitted for histopathologic examination. Cytologic examination of conjunctival scrapings reveals a mixed inflammatory response, with neutrophils, eosinophils, and macrophages predominating; however, *Habronema* larvae are usually not seen. The differential diagnosis for these lesions includes neoplasia (especially squamous cell carcinoma), sarcoids, phycomycosis, onchocerciasis, foreign body reaction, and exuberant granulation tissue.

TREATMENT. Until recently, treatment was routinely topical, with systemic therapy reserved for severe or refractory cases. However, oral ivermectin (0.2 mg/kg of body weight) has become the treatment of choice. Lesions begin to regress in 7 days and are usually healed by 4 to 6 weeks following treatment. Other effective larvicides include trichlorfon, ronnel, and diethylcarbamazine.

Topical, intralesional, and systemic corticosteroids may be used to decrease the inflammatory response to the larvae, but with ivermectin larvicidal treatment they are often not needed. Topical antibiotics are indicated, and topical corticosteroids avoided if corneal ulceration dermatitis is present. Debridement and drainage of granulomatous areas and fistulous tracts may increase topical drug penetration and prevent abscess. Fly control and prompt treatment of disorders causing ocular discharge or exposure of fresh tissue are important in prevention of habronemiasis.

Ocular Thelaziasis

The presence of *Thelazia* nematodes in the conjunctival sac of large animals is considered commensal but can cause clinical ocular disease. *Thelazia* have a worldwide distribution, with *Thelazia lacrymalis* found more commonly in horses and *Thelazia gulosa*, *Thelazia rhodesii*, and *Thelazia skrjabini* found more commonly in cattle. The infection rate for cattle and horses in the United States is estimated at 15% to 38%, with horses under 3 years of age affected more commonly than adult horses. The complete life cycle of the parasite is unknown, but *Muscae autumnalis* (face fly) and other *Muscae* spp. serve as the intermediate hosts.

CLINICAL SIGNS. Most horses and ruminants infested with *Thelazia* are asymptomatic. However, chronic conjunctivitis, conjunctival cysts, and superficial keratitis can occur, especially in the summer months when flies are active. The disease is often mild but can progress to cause corneal neovascularization, edema, and ulceration. Dacryocystitis from parasite migration in the nasolacrimal system occurs and is more common in cattle than horses. Migration into the lacrimal gland and its ducts is seen and may theoretically lead to keratoconjunctivitis sicca.[293]

DIAGNOSIS. Direct visualization of the adult *Thelazia* worms in the conjunctival sac or nasolacrimal flushings is diagnostic. The parasites are motile unless topical anesthetic is

---

used. Adult *Thelazia* are 8 to 18 mm long and milky white, and their cuticle contains prominent transverse striations.

TREATMENT. In cattle, both ivermectin and doramectin given systemically at 200 mg/kg are effective in eliminating *Thelazia*.[294,295] It is unclear if ivermectin therapy is effective in eliminating *Thelazia* in horses.[295] Alternatively, the parasites may be removed manually with saline flushes or forceps after topical anesthetic is administered, followed by topical ophthalmic organophosphate therapy.*[296]

Ocular Elaeophoriasis

Elaeophoriasis or "sore head" is a disease of sheep that is caused by the nematode *Elaeophora schneideri*. Adult *Elaeophora* are found in the common carotid and internal maxillary arteries of deer, where microfilaria are produced and migrate into the capillaries of the face and head. Biting flies of the genera *Hybomitra* and *Tabanus* transmit the microfilaria to new hosts. The disease is most prevalent in the fall and winter in the western parts of the country where sheep are grazed at high altitudes. *Elaeophora* infections in deer are usually asymptomatic. In small domestic ruminants and elk, however, the migrating microfilaria can cause a hypersensitivity reaction in facial and ocular capillaries.

CLINICAL SIGNS. Migration of *Elaeophora* microfilaria in ocular capillaries leads to local inflammation. Although the uveal tract is affected more often, sheep with elaeophoriasis may develop a chronic keratoconjunctivitis evidenced by epiphora, blepharospasm, conjunctival hyperemia, chemosis, and corneal opacities. Clinical signs of anterior uveitis caused by *Elaeophora* are nonspecific and include epiphora, blepharospasm, miosis, clouding of the anterior chamber, and cataract formation. Funduscopic changes indicative of chorioretinitis and optic neuritis are common and include retinal edema, pigment changes in the tapetal and nontapetal fundus, optic disc edema, and optic disc atrophy.[297]

DIAGNOSIS AND TREATMENT. Diagnosis depends on demonstrating the microfilaria in skin or conjunctival biopsies. Treatment of heavily parasitized animals may cause death by occlusion of the carotid arteries with *Elaeophora* adults. Drugs used in treatment include piperazine (50 mg/kg of body weight orally), diethylcarbamazine (DEC, 100 mg/kg of body weight), and stibophen (35 ml IV). The efficacy of ivermectin to treat *Elaeophora* is unknown, but it is poor against other filarides. Symptomatic treatment of keratitis and uveitis is indicated.

Ocular Manifestations of Nasal Bots

Larva of the arthropod *Oestrus ovis*, the sheep botfly, can aberrantly migrate up the nasolacrimal duct and enter the conjunctival sac, causing local inflammation. Conjunctival migration is accompanied by epiphora, conjunctival erythema, and chemosis. Finding the larva within the conjunctival sac is diagnostic. Treatment consists of mechanical removal and topical or systemic organophosphates. The nasal botfly *Gedoelstia hassleri* is reported to cause ocular lesions in horses in South Africa.

Ocular Manifestations of Trypanosomiasis and Piroplasmosis

Many species of the protozoal blood parasite *Trypanosoma* can infect horses and ruminants, causing edema, hyperemia, and petechiation of the conjunctiva. Sheep infected with *Try-*

panosoma brucei can develop keratoconjunctivitis and panuveitis, including chorioretinitis and optic neuritis. Demonstration of the organism in blood smears is diagnostic.

Other blood protozoans, *Babesia* and *Theileria*, can also cause conjunctival edema, petechiation, icterus, swollen eyelids, and blood-stained tears.

UVEAL AND RETINAL PARASITISM

Onchocerciasis, Elaeophoriasis, and Trypanosomiasis

Onchocerca cervicalis causes equine parasitic uveitis and chorioretinitis, and *Elaeophora* and *Trypanosoma* cause uveitis in sheep. Ocular manifestations of these diseases were discussed previously with corneal and conjunctival parasites.

Toxoplasma Iridocyclitis and Retinitis

The intracellular protozoan parasite *Toxoplasma gondii* can cause ocular disease in large animals. Invasion and replication in the retina and uveal tract leads to retinitis, chorioretinitis, and anterior uveitis. The acquired form of toxoplasmosis in ruminants, however, is often asymptomatic, and ocular lesions are uncommon. Toxoplasmosis is rare in horses.

CLINICAL SIGNS. The most common ocular findings with ocular toxoplasmosis are iridocyclitis and retinitis.[298] Retinitis is the primary posterior segment lesion, with secondary involvement of the chorioid. Retinal degeneration, clumping of pigment in the retinal pigment epithelium and chorioid, and optic disc avascularity are seen ophthalmoscopically; however, these lesions are not pathognomonic for toxoplasmosis. Orbital pain and swelling may result from parasitic invasion of extraocular muscles and orbital fat.

DIAGNOSIS AND TREATMENT. Diagnosis and treatment of toxoplasmosis is discussed in the central nervous system section of the text (see Chapter 33, p. 908).

MISCELLANEOUS INTRAOCULAR PARASITES

The most common intraocular parasite in horses is *Setaria*, with *Setaria digitata* found more frequently within the eyes of horses than *S. equina*. Ocular infestation is presumed to result from aberrant migration of the larval stage. Although *Setaria* causes minimum inflammation in the peritoneal cavity, it can cause serious intraocular inflammation. Diagnosis is by visualizing the parasite in the aqueous humor. Treatment involves symptomatic antiinflammatory therapy and surgical removal.

Other filarides found free within the anterior chamber of horses' eyes include *Dirofilaria immitis* and *Onchocerca cervicalis*. Diagnosis and treatment are the same as for *Setaria*. Severe endophthalmitis caused from intraocular infection with the free-living nematode *Halicephalobus* has been reported in a horse.[299] The ocular disease was accompanied by a fatal encephalopathy. Diagnosis was based on finding the parasite during microscopic examination of intraocular tissues.

The canine cestodes, *Echinococcus granulosa* and *Echinococcus multilocularis*, may form intraocular hydatid cysts in horses and ruminants, thereby producing extensive inflammation and retinal detachment. There is no treatment because surgical removal is often impossible. Diagnosis is made on histopathologic examination of affected tissues.

Coenurus cerebralis, the intermediate form of *Taenia multiceps* and *Taenia serialis*, can develop in the central nervous system of sheep, causing a disease known as "sturdy" or "gid." Besides having abnormal gait, affected animals are often centrally blind. No treatment exists.

---

*Echothiophate iodide: Phospholine iodide, Ayerst Labs, New York, NY 10017.

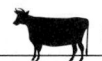

REFERENCES

287. Cello RM: Ocular onchocerciasis in the horse, *Equine Vet J* 3:148-154, 1971.
288. Moore CP et al: Equine ocular parasites, *Equine Vet J* 2(suppl):76-85, 1985.
289. Gelatt KN: *Textbook of veterinary ophthalmology,* Philadelphia, 1982, Lea & Febiger.
290. Herd RP, Donham JC: Efficacy of ivermectin against *Onchocerca cervicalis* microfilarial dermatitis in horses, *Am J Vet Res* 44:1102-1105, 1983.
291. Schmidt GM et al: Observations of three horses with ocular onchocerciasis before and after treatment with diethylcarbamazine therapy, *Transactions of the American College of Veterinary Ophthalmology,* Chicago, 1980, pp 73-84.
292. McMullan WC: Onchocerciasis filariasis. In McMullan WC: *Equine dermatology,* Texas, 1977, Texas AM University Press, pp 17-30.
293. Patton S, Marbury K: *Thelazia* in cattle and horses in the United States, *J Parasitol* 64:1147-1148, 1978.
294. Kennedy MJ, Phillips FE: Efficacy of doramectin against eyeworms (*Thelazia* spp.) in naturally and experimentally infected cattle, *Vet Parasitol* 49:61-66, 1993.
295. Lyons ET et al: Apparent inactivity of several antiparasitic compounds against the eyeworm *Thelazia lacrymalis* in equids, *Am J Vet Res* 42:1046-1047, 1981.
296. Soll MD et al: The efficacy of ivermectin against *Thelazia rhodesii* (Demaret, 1828) in the eyes of cattle, *Vet Parasitol* 42:67-71, 1992.
297. Abdelbaki YZ, Davis RW: Ophthalmoscopic findings in elaeophoriasis of domestic sheep, *Vet Med (Small Anim Clin)* 67:69-74, 1972.
298. Piper RC et al: Natural and experimental ocular toxoplasmosis in animals, *Am J Ophthalmol* 69:662-668, 1970.
299. Rames DS et al: Ocular *Halicephalobus* (syn. *Micronema deletrix*) in a horse, *Vet Pathol* 32:540-542, 1995.

OCULAR NEOPLASIA

STEVEN M. ROBERTS

A wide variety of tumor types may involve the ocular or periocular tissues of food animals. Except for the most common neoplasms, limited information is available regarding treatment modalities, drug dosages, overall prognosis, and prevention or control. The tendency has been to adapt information and methods used in other areas of medicine for use in large animals. Table 37-3 lists potential presenting signs and corresponding ocular neoplastic conditions or related differential diagnoses for horses, cattle, sheep, and goats. Table 37-4 categorizes ocular neoplasms that have been reported in the literature for each of these species. The greatest breadth and depth of information pertains to the horse.

Despite the wide variety of primary and secondary neoplasms affecting the ocular and periocular tissues, most tumors produce similar effects on the eye, with tissue distortion and loss of function being the initial concerns. Strategic therapy and management goals may vary from curative or palliative (e.g., eliminating discomfort by enucleation) for individuals to elimination of the problem (e.g., culling from the herd) for a population. Specific tumor treatment options are often similar for neoplasms involving a particular ocular region or location, yet when designing a management plan, the specific histologic tumor type is important in determining prognosis. Classification of a tumor as benign versus malignant or localized (e.g., equine sarcoid) versus systemic (e.g., lymphosarcoma) greatly influences treatment options and management approaches. The following discussion addresses the major tumors of concern in large animals and briefly surveys miscellaneous tumors that have been associated with ocular signs.

OCULAR SQUAMOUS CELL CARCINOMA

DEFINITION AND ETIOLOGY. Bovine ocular squamous cell carcinoma (OSCC), also commonly called "cancer eye," represents the most economically important neoplasm of large animals. It is the most common tumor affecting cattle in North America, and, according to estimates from federally inspected slaughter houses in the United States, 12.5% of all bovine carcass condemnations were caused by OSCC.[300] The economic impact includes carcass condemnations, production losses, treatment expenditures, and management costs.

OSCC arises from the epithelial surfaces of the conjunctiva (corneoscleral junction, nictitating membrane, and palpebra) or cornea. The etiology is probably multifactorial, with genetic, environmental, and viral factors being proven or suspected.[300-302] In particular, increasing levels of solar irradiation and decreasing amounts of circumocular pigmentation are linked to an increased prevalence of OSCC.[303-304]

Equine squamous cell carcinoma is the most prevalent equine ocular neoplasm (equine sarcoid is second) and commonly occurs in horses with unpigmented eyelids.[302,305] The amount of perilimbal and nictitans pigmentation represents another important causal factor in cattle and horses that has received little attention but should be considered on prepurchase and health examinations (see Chapters 1 and 2).

CLINICAL SIGNS AND DIFFERENTIAL DIAGNOSES. The gross appearance depends not only on the anatomic tumor site (because this determines the overall interaction between epithelium and underlying connective tissue elements) but also the stage of malignancy. In general, premalignant squamous cell tumors are small, white, elevated, hyperplastic plaques or papilloma-like structures with verrucous surfaces (Fig. 37-37). In contrast, malignant tumors are more irregular, nodular, pink, erosive, and necrotic in nature (Fig. 37-38). Necrotic tumors often have a characteristic foul odor. Squamous cell carcinomas that invade the orbit may become massive and eventually aggressively invade bone. Often the gross appearance allows a diagnosis to be established, but at times cytology or histology is necessary to differentiate between benign tumors, carcinoma in situ, and invasive squamous cell carcinoma. Bovine OSCC typically involves (in decreasing order of frequency) the lateral limbus, eyelid margins (especially the lower), nictitans, and medial canthal regions.[300,301] Similar tissues are involved in horses, although some reports suggest that the nictitans is more frequently involved than the corneoscleral junction.[302,306] Clinical signs resulting from metastatic lesions are not common, although lymphatic tissues may become infiltrated with neoplastic cells. Despite characteristic lesion appearance, other differential considerations (especially in the horse) include adenocarcinoma, adenoma, angiosarcoma, basal cell tumor, conjunctival follicular hyperplasia, dermoid, fibroma, fibrosarcoma, granulation tissue, habronemic blepharoconjunctivitis, lymphosarcoma, mastocytoma, plasma cell tumors, sarcoid, and schwannoma (see Tables 37-3 and 37-4).

PATHOPHYSIOLOGY. The tumor in all species develops through a series of premalignant stages (i.e., hyperplastic plaques or epidermal plaques and papillomas) to progress over the course of months and years to a carcinoma in situ and finally an invasive squamous cell carcinoma. Neoplastic lesions may arise without notable precursor stages. It is unlikely that tumors arise in the cornea unless previous vascularization has occurred.[307] Spontaneous regression of 30% to 50% of bovine precancerous lesions may occur,[300] and in rare instances early OSCC may regress spontaneously. Tumors arising at the limbus are confounded by the dense and poorly vascularized sclera and cornea, thus retarding metastasis to extraocular sites. Nictitans tumors extend to the base of the membrane and cartilage more rapidly, with spread into the orbit and surrounding bones occurring much sooner than with tumors involving the globe. Although metastasis will eventually occur, extensive extraocular spread is limited in cattle by the practice of sending most affected animals to slaughter. Horses demonstrate multiple tumor locations and local invasion in up to 50% of the cases.[306,307] Metastasis beyond extraocular sites is rare in horses.

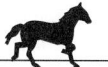

TABLE 37-3

Ocular Neoplasia and Differential Diagnoses by Species Based on Presenting Clinical Signs

Clinical Sign	Equine	Bovine	Caprine	Ovine
Ocular pain	*Habronema* blepharoconjunctivitis* Brain stem neoplasia Ocular dermoid Ocular trauma Squamous cell carcinoma* Sarcoid	Brain stem neoplasia Ocular dermoid Orbital lymphosarcoma* Sporadic bovine leukosis Squamous cell carcinoma*	Brain stem neoplasia Ocular dermoid Squamous cell carcinoma	Brain stem neoplasia Ocular dermoid Squamous cell carcinoma
Exophthalmos	Optic nerve neuroepithelial tumor Lymphosarcoma Retrobulbar neoplasia	Enzootic adult lymphosarcoma* Nasal and paranasal sinus neoplasia Nonprogressive bilateral exophthalmos Oral, maxillary, and mandibular neoplasia Retrobulbar neoplasia Sporadic bovine leukosis Squamous cell carcinoma*	Nasal and paranasal sinus neoplasia Oral, maxillary, and mandibular neophasia Squamous cell carcinoma	Adenocarcinoma of the nasal cavity Nasal and paranasal sinus neoplasia Squamous cell carcinoma
Intraocular mass	Exudative optic neuritis Mastocytoma Medulloepithelioma Ocular melanoma Optic disc astrocytoma Optic nerve neuroepithelial tumor Squamous cell carcinoma Proliferative optic neuropathy Uveal or iris cyst	Ectopic lacrimal gland Ocular melanoma Squamous cell carcinoma	Ocular trauma Squamous cell carcinoma	Ocular trauma Squamous cell carcinoma
Nictitans protrusion	Horner's syndrome Ocular trauma Orbital neoplasia Nasal and paranasal sinus neoplasia	Horner's syndrome Lymphosarcoma Ocular trauma Nasal and paranasal sinus neoplasia	Ocular trauma Nasal and paranasal sinus neoplasia	Ocular trauma Nasal and paranasal sinus neoplasia
Nasolacrimal duct obstruction	Cutaneous squamous cell carcinoma* *Habronema* blepharoconjunctivitis Nasal and paranasal sinus neoplasia	Nasolacrimal duct occlusion Nasal and paranasal sinus neoplasia	Nasolacrimal duct occlusion Nasal and paranasal sinus neoplasia	Nasolacrimal duct occlusion Nasal and paranasal sinus neoplasia
Ocular discharge	Conjunctivitis Ocular trauma Lymphosarcoma Nasal and paranasal sinus neoplasia Retrobulbar neoplasia	Conjunctivitis Ocular trauma Lymphosarcoma Nasal and paranasal sinus neoplasia Retrobulbar neoplasia	Conjunctivitis Lymphosarcoma Nasal and paranasal sinus neoplasia	Conjunctivitis Lymphosarcoma Nasal and paranasal sinus neoplasia
Periorbital or eyeball mass	Adenocarcinoma Angiosarcoma Hemangioma Hemangiosarcoma Lipoma Lymphosarcoma Mastocytoma Melanoma Nasal and paranasal sinus neoplasia Ocular dermoid Reticulum cell sarcoma Retrobulbar neoplasia Sarcoid* Squamous cell carcinoma* Warts	Ectopic lacrimal gland Fibroma Fibrosarcoma Ocular dermoid Ocular melanoma Retrobulbar neoplasia Squamous cell carcinoma*	Fibroma Fibrosarcoma Melanoma Nasal and paranasal sinus neoplasia Ocular dermoid Papillomatosis Squamous cell carcinoma	Fibroma Fibrosarcoma Melanoma Nasal and paranasal sinus neoplasia Ocular dermoid Papillomatosis Squamous cell carcinoma

*Denotes the most prevalent and important differential diagnostic considerations.

Continued

TABLE 37-3

Ocular Neoplasia and Differential Diagnoses by Species Based on Presenting Clinical Signs—cont'd

Clinical Sign	Equine	Bovine	Caprine	Ovine
Buphthalmia	Glaucoma Ocular melanoma Ocular trauma Medulloepithelioma Infectious bovine 　keratoconjunctivitis* Ocular melanoma Ocular trauma	Ocular trauma Ocular melanoma Ocular trauma		
Corneal mass	Angiosarcoma Hemangioma Hemangiosarcoma Keratomycosis Ocular dermoid Squamous cell carcinoma*	Enzootic adult 　lymphosarcoma Infectious bovine 　keratoconjunctivitis* Interstitial keratitis Ocular dermoid Squamous cell carcinoma*	Keratomycosis Ocular dermoid Squamous cell carcinoma	Keratomycosis Ocular dermoid Squamous cell carcinoma
Facial mass	Angiosarcoma Cutaneous habronemiasis Cutaneous squamous cell 　carcinoma Hemangioma Hemangiosarcoma Lymphosarcoma Mastocytoma Nasal and paranasal sinus 　neoplasia Ocular dermoid Ocular melanoma Oral, mandibular, and 　maxillary neoplasia Retrobulbar neoplasia Salivary gland neoplasia Sarcoid* Schwannoma of the eyelids Sialoadenitis	Enzootic adult 　lymphosarcoma Fibroma Fibrosarcoma Melanoma Nasal and paranasal sinus 　neoplasia Ocular dermoid Ocular melanoma Papillomatosis Retrobulbar neoplasia Sebaceous cyst Sporadic bovine leukosis Squamous cell carcinoma*	Fibroma Fibrosarcoma Histiocytoma Lymphosarcoma Melanoma Nasal and paranasal sinus 　neoplasia Papillomatosis Squamous cell carcinoma Fibroma Fibrosarcoma Lymphosarcoma Nasal and paranasal sinus 　neoplasia Ocular melanoma Papillomatosis Squamous cell carcinoma	

TABLE 37-4

Ocular Neoplasms Reported in Large Animal Species

Neoplasm	Equine	Bovine	Caprine	Ovine
Adenocarcinoma	+			+
Angiosarcoma	+			
Basal cell tumor	+			
Chondroma rodens	+			
Equine sarcoid	+			
Hemangioma	+			
Lymphangioma	+			
Lymphosarcoma	+	+	+	+
Mastocytoma	+	+	+	+
Medulloepithelioma	+			
Nasal, paranasal sinus, neoplasia	+			+
Ocular melanoma	+			
Optic nerve astrocytoma	+			
Optic nerve neuroepithelioma	+	+		
Papilloma	+			
Reticulum cell sarcoma	+			
Retrobulbar neoplasia	+	+	+	+
Schwannoma	+			
Squamous cell carcinoma	+	+	+	+

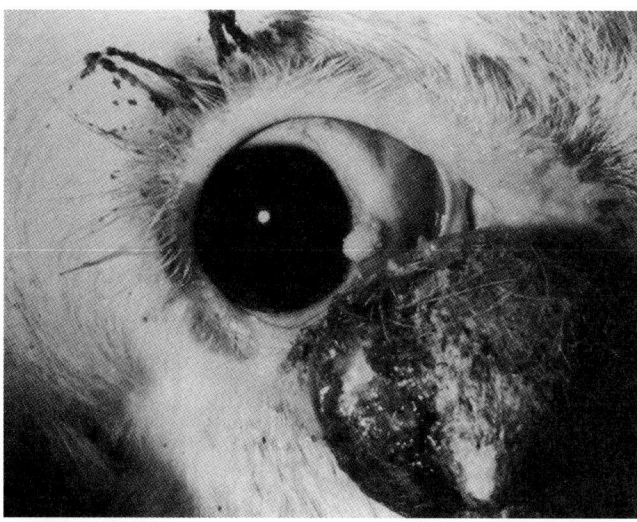

FIG. 37-37 ▓ Bovine ocular squamous cell carcinoma. Note the small pre-malignant, hyperplastic plaque involving the medial limbus and the large malignant nodular mass on the lower eyelid. The large mass is becoming ulcerated and necrotic.

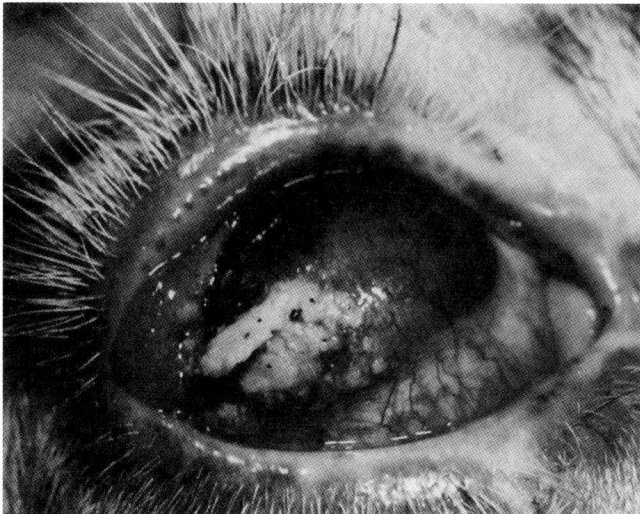

FIG. 37-38 ▓ Bovine ocular squamous cell carcinoma involving the cornea and conjunctiva. Note the irregular and invasive growth into the cornea. The surface is rough and necrotic.

EPIDEMIOLOGY. Although OSCC has been reported in a wide variety of cattle breeds, the Hereford breed (either pure-bred or crossbred) is most often diagnosed with this tumor as a result of the common use of this breed as a range animal and the strong genetic trait for a white face. Thus selective breeding for partially to fully pigmented periocular skin greatly reduces the occurrence of this tumor.[300] The tumor is more common in older cattle, with the peak age prevalence being 7 to 8 years. Exposure to increasing levels of actinic radiation raises the prevalence of bovine OSCC.[303] The prevalence of ocular squamous cell tumors, including nonmalignant tumors, involving Hereford herds in regions with abundant sunlight can range from 20% to 40%. Research performed in cattle herds suggests that a high plane of nutrition or a lower-than-normal body weight in cows for the first 2 years acts to increase the prevalence.[300] The intriguing pos-

sibility that bovine OSCC may be induced by viruses (e.g., papillomavirus) warrants further research.

Equine OSCC in North America demonstrates an increased prevalence with increasing longitude (°W), altitude, and mean solar irradiation.[305] Breeds with a greater risk of developing OSCC include draft breeds, especially the Belgian (odds ratio [OR] = 21.7), Appaloosa (OR = 7.9), paint and pinto (OR = 4.5), and grade horses (OR = 3.1). Coat colors showing an increased risk include white (OR = 26.7), creamello/palomino (OR = 13.7), gray (OR = 6.7), red/white and strawberry/white (OR = 4.7), buckskin (OR = 4.4), and chestnut/sorrel (OR = 3.8).[305]

NECROPSY FINDINGS. Depending on the extent of involvement, gross changes are noted that involve the globe, conjunctiva and nictitans, orbit, bones of the orbit, and regional cervical lymph nodes. In rare instances, metastasis to thoracic and abdominal organs can occur.

TREATMENT AND PROGNOSIS. Numerous modalities are available, and applications depend on availability of instrumentation, location and extent of the tumor, and value and intended function of the animal. Choices include radiofrequency hyperthermia,* cryonecrosis, intralesional injection of biologic response modifiers (e.g., allogeneic OSCC extract, mycobacterial cell wall fraction,† and *Propionibacterium acnes*‡) intralesional chemotherapy with cisplatin§ (with or without initial debulking),[308,309] radiotherapy (cesium-137, cobalt-60, gold-198, iridium, and strontium-90), and surgical removal (local excision, enucleation, and exenteration with or without salivary gland and lymph node resection). Intralesional use of cisplatin (1 mg/cm³ of tumor volume) is highly effective, but multiple injections are necessary (4 times at 2- to 3-week intervals). Handling of the drug and animal after treatment must adhere to OSHA guidelines,[310] and animals must not be used for food consumption. Appropriate precaution should be followed with extralabel use of cytotoxic drugs. Surgical debulking with adjunctive cryonecrosis or radiofrequency hyperthermia is an effective and affordable treatment modality. Cryonecrosis is achieved with liquid nitrogen, using a probe or spray delivery system to freeze the tissues to −30° C twice with complete thawing between freeze cycles. Radiofrequency hyperthermia is performed with piercing or surface probes to heat the tissues to 50° C for 30 seconds. Multiple treatment sites are necessary for lesions larger than 0.5 cm in diameter.

Because recurrence rates range between 30.4% to 42.4%,[302,306] the willingness of the owner to return the animal for follow-up treatment is a significant determinant in overall survival. Financial constraints were the most common reason for cessation of treatment. Many horses that die as a consequence of OSCC are euthanized at the owner's request. The overall prognosis is determined by the degree of neoplastic involvement of normal tissue, but a guarded prognosis is warranted. If treatment is to be undertaken, intervention should begin at the earliest stages of tumor development. In animals destined for slaughter, the guidelines for condemnation of bovine carcasses affected with OSCC shown in part A of Box 37-2 should be considered.

PREVENTION AND CONTROL. In cattle, factors such as genetics, ultraviolet light, and environmental factors (e.g., wind and dust) are known to be involved in OSCC. Ocular viral infection may also be contributory. If possible, affected animals should be culled as soon as possible because most production situations preclude environmental factor

---

*RDM Hypertherm, RDM International, Inc, Phoenix, AZ 85027.
†Normagen, Fort Dodge Laboratories, Inc, Fort Dodge, IA 50501.
‡ImmunoRegulin, ImmunoVet, Inc, Tampa, FL 33630.
§Platinol, Bristol-Myers Co, Wallingford, CT 06492.

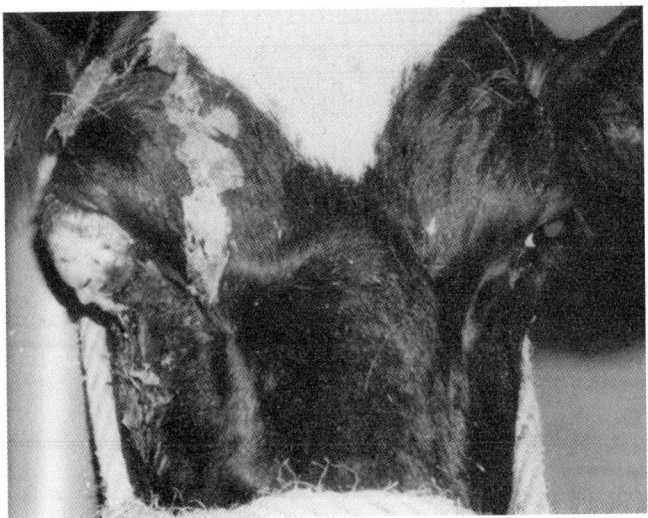

FIG. 37-39 ■ Orbital lymphosarcoma. Diffuse orbital involvement causing exophthalmos and secondary exposure keratitis of the right eye.

modification. Specific preventive measures have not been systematically evaluated in horses, but recommendations include reducing ultraviolet light exposure, using protective fly masks in horses (to decrease solar irradiation and environmental irritants), tattooing lightly pigmented periocular skin, and avoiding breeds thought to have an increased risk of tumor development.

OCULAR MANIFESTATIONS OF LYMPHOSARCOMA

DEFINITION AND ETIOLOGY. Lymphosarcoma is a fatal systemic neoplastic disease of the lymphoreticular tissue. The adult or enzootic form of bovine lymphosarcoma is likely the most devastating and common neoplasm of dairy cattle. This is a systemic disease with ocular manifestations rather than a pure ophthalmic problem. See Chapter 35 for specific information regarding bovine lymphosarcoma and the bovine leukemia virus. Lymphosarcoma represents the most common cause of orbital neoplasia in cattle,[311] excluding OSCC that involves the orbit by local extension. It may affect horses[312] and goats. The etiology in horses and goats is unknown.

CLINICAL SIGNS AND DIFFERENTIAL DIAGNOSES. Clinical signs are usually associated with exophthalmos caused by orbital disease. Neoplastic lymphoid cell infiltra-

tion behind the globe results in exophthalmos, subsequent exposure keratitis, and eventual proptosis[311] (Fig. 37-39). One report has documented intraocular lymphosarcoma in a Holstein cow as the presenting sign of generalized lymphosarcoma.[313] Subtle exophthalmos is often overlooked because of the natural exophthalmic state of some dairy breeds. Typically these animals present with a history that suggests an acute onset of exophthalmos, when actually orbital involvement has been present for a period of time. Clinical signs associated with the exophthalmos and exposure keratitis include corneal edema, vascularization, ulceration, epidermalization, conjunctival hemorrhage, chemosis, and ocular discharge. These signs may develop, progress, and change quickly once corneal protection is compromised. Other physical examination findings are discussed in Chapter 35. Differential considerations for exophthalmos include orbital cellulitis, trauma, retrobulbar hemorrhage, retrobulbar soft tissue masses, chronic sinusitis, and sinus neoplasia (see Tables 37-3 and 37-4).

CLINICAL PATHOLOGY. Definitive diagnosis is achieved by cytologic samples obtained with a spatula following topical anesthesia[300] or specimens excised for biopsy and fixed in formalin. Benign lesions typically contain superficial, anucleated, keratinized squamous cells and deeper epithelial cells with enlarged nuclei and coarse chromatin clumping. Biopsies of these lesions show that the basal layer or basement membrane has not been invaded. Malignant OSCC lesions are comprised of pleomorphic cells with bizarre shapes, large hyperchromatic nuclei containing large clumps of chromatin, and prominent nucleoli. On biopsy examination, invasion across the basement membrane is noted, and keratin-pearl formation or marked anaplasia is usually present.[307] In the event of regional lymphatic involvement, fine-needle aspiration or, preferably, a biopsy may demonstrate neoplastic infiltration.

Equine lymphosarcoma involving the eye also represents a systemic disease with ocular manifestations. Other systemic manifestations are discussed in Chapter 35. Ocular lesions include uveitis, nictitans masses, chemosis and conjunctivitis, and neoplastic infiltration of the eyelids and orbit.[313] Differential considerations should include any chronic inflammatory disease, equine infectious anemia, equine piroplasmosis, and infectious causes of uveitis (see Table 37-2, Infectious Ocular Diseases).

NECROPSY FINDINGS. As with the clinical signs, necropsy findings are variable. In cattle, orbital involvement is common, with lymphoid tumors being firmly attached to the periorbita and walls of the orbit. Extraocular muscles are frequently infiltrated with tumor cells. The globe itself is typically not involved.[307] Ocular lesions in horses are less frequent than in cattle. In the horse the globe (uveal tract) can be involved, in addition to extraocular tissues. As with other systemic neoplastic diseases, multiple organ involvement is expected with lymphosarcoma.

TREATMENT AND PROGNOSIS. This systemic disease may be treated palliatively or systemically to attempt to achieve remission for a time. Enucleation provides palliative treatment and chemotherapy with corticosteroids, vincristine, and L-asparaginase may induce remission. Extralabel use of these cytotoxic drugs must be approached with extreme caution, and treated animals must not be used for food consumption. Most cattle with orbital lymphosarcoma either die or are euthanized in terminal stages of disease within 6 months of the original diagnosis.[311] Horses can have a much more protracted course of disease, with many presenting because of chronic illness of up to 12 months' duration.[312] The overall prognosis is unfavorable, regardless of the species involved.

PREVENTION AND CONTROL. Control of bovine lymphosarcoma depends on efforts to eradicate bovine leukemia virus, a monumental task in most instances. In other large animal species, prevention and control recommendations for lymphosarcoma are not possible until the etiology can be identified. If animals are destined for slaughter, the guidelines for condemnation of bovine carcasses affected with lymphosarcoma as shown in part B of Box 37-2 should be followed.

OCULAR MANIFESTATIONS OF EQUINE SARCOID

DEFINITION AND ETIOLOGY. Equine sarcoid is a locally aggressive, nonmalignant, fibroblastic tumor of the equine skin (see Chapter 38). It appears to be the most common equine neoplasm, with 14.7% of ocular and adnexal tumors in the horse being sarcoids (all involved the eyelids).[314] This neoplasm develops more frequently in sites predisposed to trauma and areas that come into contact with existing sarcoids and does not metastasize to internal organs.

CLINICAL SIGNS AND DIFFERENTIAL DIAGNOSES. Sarcoids involving the eyelids are classified according to the scheme used for cutaneous lesions (verrucous, fibroblastic, mixed, or occult). Tumors of the eyelids may appear smooth and nodular, crusted and nodular, ulcerated, or pedunculated (Figs. 37-40 and 37-41). Regardless of their appearance, the tumors are nonregressing. Periocular sarcoids are subject to trauma; thus the verrucous type frequently transforms into the fibroblastic type with surface ulceration. It is difficult to differentiate this tumor from the following neoplasms: fibroma, fibrosarcoma, neurofibroma, neurofibrosarcoma, schwannoma, and nonneoplastic granulation tissue (see Tables 37-3 and 37-4).

TREATMENT AND PROGNOSIS. Problematic lesions can be treated by a variety of modalities, none of which is uniformly successful. Often multiple treatment sessions are required for tumor control. Treatment modalities used include surgical excision (50% success rate), cryonecrosis (30% success rate), radiofrequency hyperthermia,* intralesional injection of biologic response modifiers (bacille Calmette-Guérin),[314] chemotherapy with intralesional cisplatin† (with

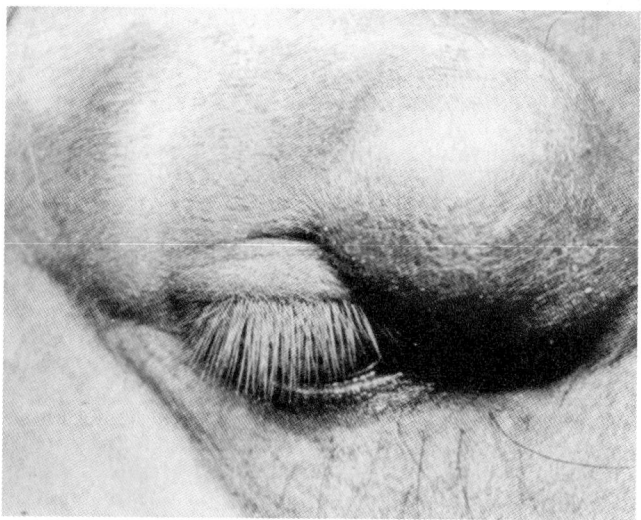

FIG. 37-40 ■ Equine sarcoid. The upper eyelid exhibits a smooth, nodular mass typical of many periocular sarcoids.

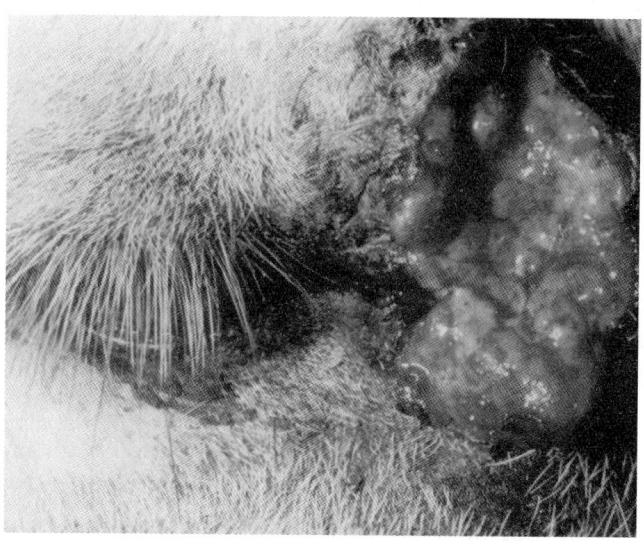

FIG. 37-41 ■ Equine sarcoid involving the medial eyelid. At the time of examination or during the course of treatment, sarcoids may become ulcerated. This tumor became ulcerated after one injection of a *Mycobacterium* cell wall preparation and subsequently resolved.

or without initial debulking),[307,308] radiation therapy (cesium-137, cobalt-60, gold-198, iridium, and strontium-90), and chemotherapy (5-fluorouracil) combined with surgical excision. Biologic response modifier therapy has not proven as successful for sarcoids located at other body sites. An available commercial *Mycobacterium* product,* can be used, but it does not demonstrate the clinical efficacy seen with previously used research preparations. If the sarcoid is static, flat, and hairless, it may be best left alone because any trauma, surgical or otherwise, could increase the growth rate and invasiveness of the lesion. Response to therapy varies on the basis of

*RDM Hypertherm, RDM International, Inc., Phoenix, AZ 85027.
†Platinol, Bristol-Myers Co, Wallingford, CT 06492.

*Normagen, Fort Dodge Laboratories, Inc., Fort Dodge, IA 50501.

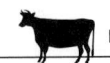

tumor location, duration, severity, and previous therapeutic measures.

Treatment of periocular sarcoid with biologic response modifiers shows particular promise but has the disadvantage of requiring a potentially long course of treatment, involving a series of intralesional injections. Intratumoral use of cisplatin is highly effective (see Chapter 38). Successful treatment measures exist for this disease, and if a complete treatment protocol is followed, the prognosis is favorable. As with any neoplastic disease, at the first evidence of recurrence the animal should be reevaluated.

MISCELLANEOUS TUMORS WITH OCULAR INVOLVEMENT

The aforementioned tumors represent the most significant ocular or periocular neoplasms of large animals. However, to the individual animal or owner, any tumor type represents a significant problem. Thus clinicians must remember that numerous primary and secondary neoplastic processes can involve the eye and surrounding tissues. Secondary tumors may be either metastatic masses or locally invasive masses extending from sites near the eye. The greatest variety of ocular neoplastic diseases have been reported in the horse (see Table 37-4).

Adnexal tumors that have been reported include adenoma, adenocarcinoma, basal cell carcinoma, fibroma, fibrosarcoma, hemangioma,[315] hemangiosarcoma,[316] lymphosarcoma, melanocytoma, melanoma, papilloma, plasma cell tumors, and schwannoma. Few reports address treatment of these tumors thoroughly.

Surgical excision of small lesions, cryosurgery, radiation therapy, intralesional cisplatin,[308,309] and medical treatment with cimetidine[317,318] have been used successfully on select tumors. Oral cimetidine (2.5 mg/kg 3 times daily for an initial 3-month period) is useful as a means of melanoma control. If lesions are progressively enlarging, cimetidine has been particularly successful in arresting or resolving tumor lesions. This treatment is also a useful adjunct to cryonecrosis, surgical excision, or chemotherapy. The prognosis is poor for malignant masses because metastatic disease or local recurrence usually results. This is especially true with angiosarcomas[306] that involve primarily the conjunctiva but may also involve the corneoscleral junction. Limited success with angiosarcoma treatment has been achieved in a case of equine orbital lymphangiosarcoma through enucleation and chemotherapy with intravenous vincristine (four doses of 1.3, 1.3, 1.2, and 1 mg/m^2 of body surface area on days 0, 7, 14, and 51, respectively) and prednisone. Seven years after treatment, the horse has shown no signs of recurrence. An additional case of conjunctival and nictitans malignant hemangiosarcoma was treated by local excision and perioperative intratumoral cisplatin. Follow-up demonstrated tumor lysis and no recurrence after 6 months.

Any tumor involving the nasal and paranasal cavities has the potential to involve the ocular structures as the result of orbital spread. Enzootic adenocarcinoma in sheep is an example of this type of process. Although not commonly noted, exophthalmos secondary to orbital invasion of this tumor has been reported.[319] Primary orbital neoplasia in the form of a multilobular osteoma (chondroma rodens) has been reported in the horse[320] and reminds one that a space-occupying mass (neoplasia) can affect the eye by causing progressive exophthalmos.

Neoplasia involving the central nervous system, diencephalon, or occipital cortex can result in a central blindness, abolished pupillary light responses, and mydriasis. Other forms of intracranial neoplasia can secondarily involve the eye as a result of cranial nerve dysfunction. For example, an intracranial schwannoma caused exposure ulcerative keratitis in a cow that presented with left facial paresis.[321]

Reports of neoplasia involving the globe, all in horses, describe the clinical, histologic, and treatment aspects of the following tumors: epibulbar melanocytoma,[322] intraocular melanoma,[323,324] and medulloepithelioma.[325] Optic nerve tumors that have been noted include neuroepithelial tumors and meningiomas. In the intraocular cases the globe was rendered nonfunctional by the neoplastic process, and the involved eye was subsequently enucleated. An optic nerve neuroepithelial tumor displayed metastatic spread as a result of extension into the brain through the optic foramen, causing brain compression.[326] Although documented cases of these miscellaneous ocular neoplasia are not widespread, they must be taken into consideration as possible causes of large animal ocular neoplasia.

Other than vascular tumors, most ocular tumors do not display a severe metastatic threat. Although enucleation may be curative, histologic evaluation of excised tissues and long-term patient follow-up are necessary if accurate epidemiologic and prognostic data are to be available. Once an accurate diagnosis has been made, the clinician and owner must determine in light of all available medical information and the proposed use of the animal whether treatment should be curative or palliative or whether elimination of the problem from the herd should be of greater concern than care of the individual animal.

REFERENCES

300. Heeney JL, Valli VEO: Bovine ocular squamous cell carcinoma: an epidemiological perspective, *Can J Comp Med* 49:21, 1985.
301. Roberts SM, Kainer RA: Food animal ocular neoplasia. In Howard JL, ed: *Current veterinary therapy: food animal practice 3*, Philadelphia, 1993, WB Saunders, p 846.
302. Schwink K: Factors influencing morbidity and outcome of equine ocular squamous cell carcinoma, *Equine Vet J* 19:198, 1987.
303. Anderson DE, Badzioch M: Association between solar radiation and ocular squamous cell carcinoma in cattle, *Am J Vet Res* 52:784, 1991.
304. Bailey CM, Hanks DR, Hanks MA: Circumocular pigmentation and incidence of ocular squamous cell tumors in *Bos taurus* and *Bos indicus* × *Bos taurus* cattle, *J Am Vet Med Assoc* 196:1605, 1990.
305. Dugan SJ et al: Epidemiologic study of ocular/adnexal squamous cell carcinoma in horses, *J Am Vet Med Assoc* 198:251, 1991.
306. Dugan SJ et al: Prognostic factors and survival of horses with ocular/adnexal squamous cell carcinoma: 147 cases (1978-1988), *J Am Vet Med Assoc* 198:298, 1991.
307. Wilcock BP: The eye and ear. In Jubb KVF, Kennedy PC, Palmer N, eds: *Pathology of domestic animals*, New York, 1985, Academic Press, p 386.
308. Théon AP, Pascoe JR, Meagher DM: Perioperative intratumoral administration of cisplatin for treatment of cutaneous tumors in Equidae, *J Am Vet Med Assoc* 205:1170, 1994.
309. Théon AP et al: Intratumoral chemotherapy with cisplatin in oily emulsion in horses, *J Am Vet Med Assoc* 202:261, 1993.
310. Yodaiken MD, Bennett D: OSHA work-practice guidelines for personnel dealing with cytotoxic (antineoplastic) drugs, *Am J Hosp Pharm* 43:1193, 1986.
311. Rebhun WC: Orbital lymphosarcoma in cattle, *J Am Vet Med Assoc* 180:149, 1982.
312. Rebhun WC, Bertone A: Equine lymphosarcoma, *J Am Vet Med Assoc* 184:720, 1984.
313. Meek LA, Cooley AJ, Whitley RD: Intraocular lymphosarcoma as the presenting sign of generalized lymphosarcoma in a Holstein cow, *Compend Cont Educ* 9:F239, 1987.
314. Lavach JD et al: BCG treatment of periocular sarcoid, *Equine Vet J* 17:445, 1985.
315. Crawley GR, Bryan GM, Gogolewski RP: Ocular hemangioma in a horse, *Equine Pract* 9:11, 1987.
316. Hacker DV, Moore PF, Buyckmihci NC: Ocular angiosarcoma in four horses, *J Am Vet Med Assoc* 189:200, 1986.
317. Goetz TE et al: Cimetidine for treatment of melanomas in three horses, *J Am Vet Med Assoc* 196:449, 1990.
318. Goetz TE, Long MT: Treatment of melanomas in horses, *Compend Cont Educ* 15:608, 1993.
319. Rings MD, Rojko J: Naturally occurring nasal obstructions in 11 sheep, *Cornell Vet* 75:269, 1985.
320. Richardson DW, Acland HM: Multilobular osteoma (chondroma rodens) in a horse, *J Am Vet Med Assoc* 182:289, 1983.

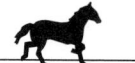

321. Mitcham SA et al: Intracranial schwannoma in a cow, *Can Vet J* 25:138, 1984.
322. Hirst LW et al: Benign epibulbar melanocytoma in a horse, *J Am Vet Med Assoc* 183:333, 1983.
323. Murphy J, Young S: Intraocular melanoma in a horse, *Vet Pathol* 16:539, 1979.
324. Neumann SM: Intraocular melanoma in a horse, *Mod Vet Pract* 66:559, 1985.
325. Szymanski CM: Malignant teratoid medulloepithelioma in a horse, *J Am Vet Med Assoc* 190:301, 1987.
326. Bistner S et al: Neuroepithelial tumor of the optic nerve in a horse, *Cornell Vet* 73:30, 1983.

Diseases of the Skin

STEPHEN D. WHITE
Consulting Editor

IMMUNE-MEDIATED SKIN DISORDERS

STEPHEN D. WHITE
ANNE G. EVANS

PEMPHIGUS FOLIACEUS

DEFINITION AND ETIOLOGY. The term pemphigus is derived from the Greek word for blister and is used to describe a group of autoimmune vesiculobullous disorders characterized histologically by intraepidermal acantholysis and immunologically by intercellular deposition of immunoglobulin. Pemphigus foliaceus is among this group of autoimmune diseases. It affects the skin and has been recognized in horses[1-3] and goats[1,4,5] as well as humans,[6,7] dogs, and cats.[8] In humans, pemphigus foliaceus has been associated with administration of certain drugs, exposure to ultraviolet radiation, malignancy, and other autoimmune diseases,[6,7] although the majority of cases are idiopathic. The factors precipitating the development of pemphigus foliaceus in large animals are unknown. The clinical lesions recognized in horses and goats are primarily scaling and crusting.

PATHOPHYSIOLOGY. Pemphigus foliaceus is characterized by the production of autoantibodies directed (in humans and in dogs) against a transmembrane protein (desmoglein 1) that results in immunoglobulin-mediated detachment of epidermal cells. The pemphigus antibody binds to the desmoglein, resulting in the release or activation of one or more enzymes. These enzymes (proteases) destroy the attachments between adjoining epidermal cells. The result is acantholysis; the epidermal cells assume a rounded shape and separate from one another, leading to the formation of intraepidermal clefts and vesicles. Complement components and inflammatory cells may be found in lesional skin but are not necessary to cause cellular damage.[7,9-11]

CLINICAL SIGNS. Pemphigus foliaceus is characterized clinically as a generalized exfoliative dermatitis (Fig. 38-1). Appaloosas appear to be predisposed to this condition, although there is no recognized age or sex predilection.[1] In the horse lesions are usually first noted on the head, limbs, or ventrum.

Initial lesions may be associated with ventral and rear limb edema, fever, depression, coronary band erosions, or, rarely, urticaria. The disease progresses to involve the entire body over a period of days to weeks. The primary lesion is a vesicle, but vesicles are fragile and hence transient lesions. They rupture soon after formation, resulting in erosions, epidermal collarettes (rings of exfoliating superficial epidermis), scale, and crust. The lesions may or may not be associated with pruritus or pain.[1,3,12]

In the goat, pemphigus foliaceus also presents as a generalized exfoliative dermatitis. In the limited number of cases described, lesions were initially noted on the limbs, perineal region, and ventrum. The lesions consisted of crusting and scaling that formed secondary to rupture of vesicles and bullae. Pruritus and malaise appear to be variable findings.

CLINICAL PATHOLOGY. Diagnosis of pemphigus foliaceus in large animals is typically based on biopsy of lesions submitted for routine histopathology. Characteristic histologic findings include intragranular to subcorneal cleft and vesicle formation associated with acantholysis. Both follicular and surface epithelia are frequently involved. Neutrophils tend to predominate in the inflammatory infiltrate, although eosinophils may also be present.[1,4,5] In some equine cases, acantholysis is restricted to uppermost layers of the epidermis, so that acantholytic cells are only recognizable in surface crusts.[13]

Direct immunofluorescence as an aid in the diagnosis of pemphigus foliaceus in large animals is relatively new. In humans, characteristic immunofluorescent findings of lesional and perilesional skin include the presence of an autoantibody (usually IgG) with or without complement in the epidermal intercellular spaces.[6] Two investigators[1,2] report this as a consistent immunopathologic finding in horses as well, although direct immunofluorescence can be negative in the face of strong clinical and histologic support for a diagnosis of equine pemphigus foliaceus. Intraepidermal deposits of immunoglobin[4,5] and complement[4] were observed in both of the goats reported with pemphigus foliaceus. Positive direct immunofluorescence results depend on finding an early active lesion in a patient that has not received corticosteroid therapy for at least 3 weeks.

Indirect immunofluorescence testing of serum is reported to be unreliable for the diagnosis of pemphigus foliaceus in

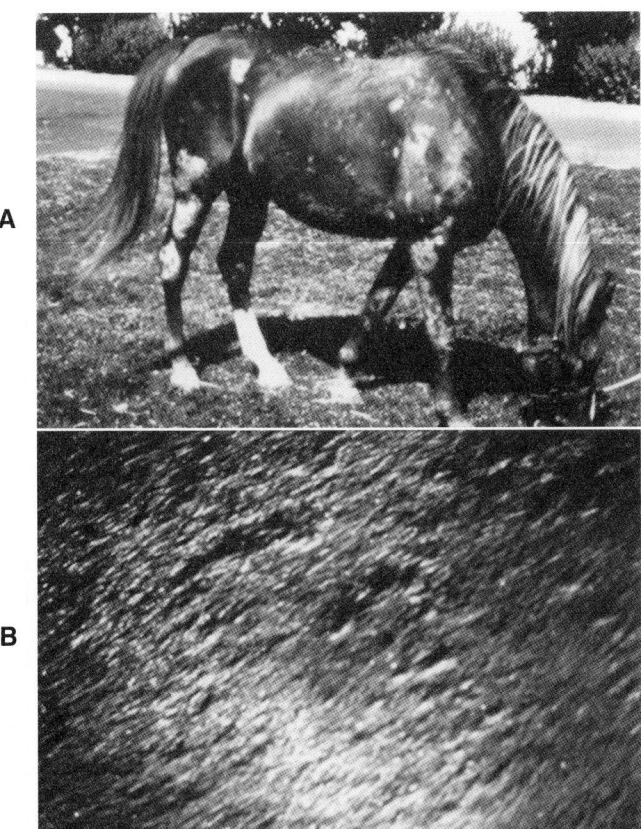

FIG. 38-1 ■ Pemphigus foliaceus in a horse. **A,** Advanced case with hair loss. **B,** Close-up view showing scaling and crusting.

domestic animals. In one study, four of nine horses with pemphigus foliaceus had negative indirect serum immunofluorescence.[1] In addition, normal horses or horses with skin disease other than pemphigus foliaceus have been demonstrated to have positive indirect immunofluorescent findings (pemphigus-like serum antibodies) consistent with a diagnosis of pemphigus foliaceus.[14] Thus both false-positive and false-negative indirect immunofluorescent test results are possible in horses. In one of the reported cases of caprine pemphigus foliaceus, indirect immunofluorescence was negative[4]; the second was positive at a dilution of 1:5.[5]

THERAPY. Treatment of equine pemphigus foliaceus involves the use of immunosuppressive doses of glucocorticoids with or without the concurrent use of chrysotherapy (treatment with gold compounds). Initially horses should receive oral prednisone or prednisolone, 2 mg/kg/day, until all signs of active disease disappear (usually 10 to 14 days). If a response is not observed within 24 to 48 hours, dexamethasone is substituted (0.05 to 1 mg/kg twice daily) until complete remission occurs. Alternatively, dexamethasone may be utilized first. The dose of glucocorticoids is gradually reduced until the minimum daily dose is reached, which will keep the disease in remission. This dose is then doubled and administered on alternate mornings. Ideally a maintenance dosage of oral prednisone or prednisolone at 0.5 mg/kg given on alternate mornings should be established.

In horses that are at risk for steroid-induced laminitis or that do not respond to treatment with glucocorticoids alone, gold (aurothioglucose) may be given therapeutically.[3] The recommended induction dose is 20 mg administered intramuscularly, followed by a dose of 50 mg 1 week later and 1 mg/kg

administered at weekly intervals thereafter until the disease is in remission (usually 6 to 8 weeks). Once the clinical signs have abated, administration of aurothioglucose is decreased in frequency to bimonthly and then monthly injections. It is advisable to inject large doses of aurothioglucose divided into multiple intramuscular sites.

One case of caprine pemphigus foliaceus was brought into remission with an induction dose of aurothioglucose of 5 mg, followed 1 week later with 10 mg. The disorder was kept in remission for 6 months with monthly dosing. The goat relapsed when therapy was discontinued but was brought back into remission when aurothioglucose administration was resumed.[1,4] Aurothioglucose is an experimental treatment in the horse and goat and is not an approved therapy. Gold therapy should be discontinued if any unforeseen reactions occur.

PROGNOSIS. The response to therapy in equine pemphigus foliaceus varies from patient to patient. Many horses require lifelong administration of medication to control the symptoms; others may be gradually weaned from medication without further relapse. One investigator found that horses less than 1 year of age manifesting the disease carry a much better prognosis for cure, with eventual discontinuation of therapy.[13] A sufficient number of reported cases of caprine pemphigus foliaceus have not been reported to reliably establish a prognosis.

REFERENCES

1. Scott DW, Smith CA: Immune-mediated dermatoses in domestic animals: ten years after. I, *Compend Cont Educ Pract Vet* 9:423-437, 1987.
2. George LW, White SL: Autoimmune skin diseases of large animals, *Vet Clin North Am (Large Anim Pract)* 6:79-96, 1984.
3. Manning TO: Pemphigus foliaceus. In Robinson NE, ed: *Current therapy in equine medicine*, 1983, WB Saunders, pp 541-542.
4. Scott DW et al: Pemphigus foliaceus in a goat, *Agri-Pract* 5:38-45, 1984.
5. Jackson PGG, Lloyd S, Jeffries AR: Pemphigus foliaceus in a goat, *Vet Rec* 114:479, 1984.
6. Moscella SL, Hurley, HJ: *Dermatology*, ed 2, Philadelphia, 1985, WB Saunders, pp 557-566.
7. Sams WM, Gammon WR: Mechanisms of lesion production in pemphigus and pemphigoid, *J Am Acad Dermatol* 6:431-448, 1982.
8. Muller GH, Kirk RW, Scott DW: *Small animal dermatology*, ed 3, Philadelphia, 1983, WB Saunders, pp 557-566.
9. Jordon RE: Complement activation in pemphigus, *J Invest Dermatol* 74:357-358, 1980.
10. Schiltz JR: Pemphigus acantholysis: a unique immunological injury, *J Invest Dermatol* 75:359-362, 1980.
11. Singer KH et al: Proteinase activation: a mechanism for cellular dyshesion in pemphigus, *J Invest Dermatol* 74:363-367, 1980.
12. Manning TO, Sweeney C: Immune-mediated equine skin diseases, *Compend Cont Educ Pract Vet* 8:979-988, 1986.
13. Stannard AA: Personal communication, 1987.
14. Scott DW et al: Pitfalls in immunofluorescence testing in dermatology. III, Pemphigus-like antibodies in the horse and direct immunofluorescence testing in equine dermatophilosis, *Cornell Vet* 74:305-311, 1984.

BULLOUS PEMPHIGOID

Bullous pemphigoid is an autoimmune, vesiculobullous, and ulcerative disorder that affects the cutaneous basement membrane zone (BMZ). In rare instances it has been recognized in horses.[15,16] Factors leading to the development of bullous pemphigoid in the horse are unknown.

The pathophysiology of bullous pemphigoid in horses is assumed to be similar to that described in humans. Complement-activating anti-BMZ antibodies bind to a glycoprotein antigen in the lamina lucida of the BMZ. In two horses, this has been shown to be similar to bullous pemphigoid antigen II of persons, dogs, and cats. Complement activation results in degranulation of mast cells and chemotaxis of neutrophils and eosinophils. Eosinophils release tissue-destructive enzymes with resultant injury to the BMZ, loss of dermoepidermal adherence, and subsequent blister formation.[17]

Equine bullous pemphigoid is characterized clinically by painful, ulcerative lesions of the skin (face and axillae), mucous membranes, and mucocutaneous junctions.[15,16] The diagnosis is based on histopathologic, and when available, immunofluorescent findings. In one reported case of equine bullous pemphigoid, therapy involved the use of glucocorticoids. The horse failed to respond clinically while receiving a dose of 1.1 mg/kg prednisolone daily and was euthanized when it developed laminitis and pleuritis.[15] A second horse died 24 hours after the initial examination without attempted therapy.[16]

REFERENCES

15. George LW, White SL: Autoimmune skin diseases of large animals, *Vet Clin North Am (Large Anim Pract)* 6:79-96, 1984.
16. Scott DW, Smith CA: Immune-mediated dermatoses in domestic animals: ten years after. I, *Compend Cont Educ Pract Vet* 9:423-437, 1987.
17. Sams WM, Gammon WR: Mechanisms of lesion production in pemphigus and pemphigoid, *J Am Acad Dermatol* 6:431-448, 1982.

HYPERSENSITIVITY DISORDERS

STEPHEN D. WHITE
ANNE G. EVANS

URTICARIA

DEFINITION AND ETIOLOGY. Urticaria is characterized by transient focal swellings in the skin or mucous membranes called wheals, which represent localized areas of dermal edema. Angioedema is essentially identical but involves the subcutaneous tissues. The swelling of angioedema is diffuse, often involving the entire face and neck of the animal.

Urticaria is more frequently recognized in the horse than in ruminants, with the most common causes in all species being drugs and ingestants (Box 38-1). Urticaria is a recognized manifestation of milk allergy in cattle; and inhaled allergens such as pollens, molds, and dusts can result in urticaria in horses.[18] Insect bites are commonly incriminated, although they rarely cause urticaria. Dermatophytes and pemphigus foliaceus can also be associated with urticaria.

PATHOPHYSIOLOGY. The wheals result from vasodilation and transudation of fluid from capillaries and small blood vessels. Thus the basic underlying disorder in urticaria involves an imbalance in factors that control small blood vessel permeability. Both immunologic and nonimmunologic factors can trigger the release of mediators from mast cells and blood basophils that will ultimately produce the characteristic wheals. Figure 38-2 is a simplified diagram of the flow of pathophysiologic events in the development of urticaria.

The most commonly cited immunologic mechanism of urticaria is type I hypersensitivity (IgE). Non-IgE-dependent, immune-mediated urticaria may be induced by either type II (cytotoxic, involving antibody and complement) or type III (immune complex) hypersensitivity reactions. Complement-activated urticaria may involve either immunologic or nonimmunologic mechanisms and may occur through either the classic or alternative pathways. Complement activation produces the anaphylatoxins C3a and C5a, leading to release of histamine and other mediators, which results in wheal formation. Urticariogenic materials can induce wheal formation without involving immunologic mechanisms by being ingested, injected, or contacting the host. Physical agents, including mechanical injury, thermal changes, and solar radiation, may induce urticaria. The most common type of mechanically induced urticaria is dermatographism (whealing after blunt scratch injury to the skin). Local or generalized exposure to heat or cold may induce urticarial lesions in certain individuals. Urticaria may be induced by a drug. Dermatophytes, pemphigus foliaceus, and erythema multiforme may also initially present with urticaria.

> **BOX 38-1**
>
> **Possible Causes of Urticaria in Horses and Ruminants**
>
> **ALLERGIC URTICARIA**
> **Inhalants**
> Pollens, animal danders, mold spores, feather down, aerosols, smoke, dust, and volatile chemicals
>
> **Injectants**
> Drugs, diagnostic agents, vaccines, insect stings, serums, and blood
>
> **Ingestants**
> Drugs, various food items, beverages, and occult additive materials found in foods
>
> **Infections**
> Foci of bacteria, fungal, viral, and parasitic infections
>
> **Contactants**
> Animal products, plant materials, cosmetics, plastic, and other chemicals
>
> **Drugs**
> Penicillin, aspirin, quinine, sulfonamides, insulin, and many others
>
> **Milk Proteins**
> Milk retention (cattle)
>
> **URTICARIA CAUSED BY URTICARIOGENIC MATERIALS**
> **Drugs**
> Cocaine, morphine, codeine, atropine, quinine, thiamin, pilocarpine, polymyxin B, D-tubocurarine, dextran, dehydrocholate sodium (Decholin), and other drugs
>
> **Foods**
> Certain citrus fruits, strawberries, and certain fish
>
> **Toxins**
> Cobra venoms, jellyfish toxin, and certain plant and insect toxins
>
> **PHYSICAL URTICARIA**
> Dermographic (induced by blunt-scratch injury)
> Heat
> Cold
> Light
> Erythema multiforme
> Pemphigus foliaceus
>
> **SECONDARY URTICARIA**
> Infections
> Collagen vascular disease
> Neoplasia
> Psychogenic

MEDIATORS. Many mediators (especially histamine) are released from mast cells and basophils by the triggering factors mentioned previously, resulting in increased vascular permeability and leading to wheal formation. Kinins, SRS-A, PGE$_1$, PGE$_2$, and increased sensitivity to acetylcholine can be involved in urticaria.

CLINICAL SIGNS AND DIFFERENTIAL DIAGNOSES. Wheals range from 1 to 10 cm in diameter and tend to involve the cervical and craniolateral thorax (Fig. 38-3). The an-

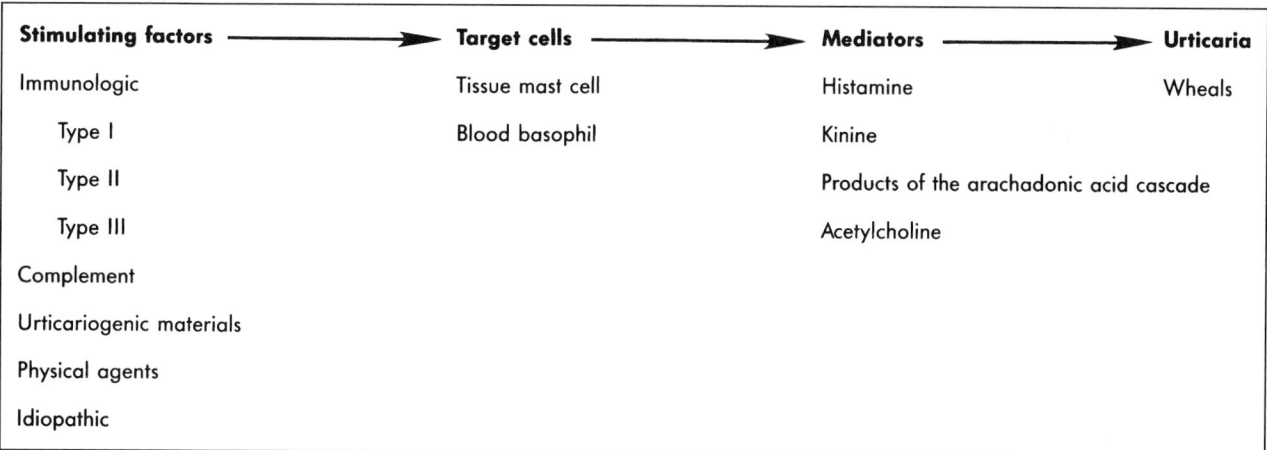

FIG. 38-2 ▐▐ Flow of pathophysiologic events in the development of urticaria.

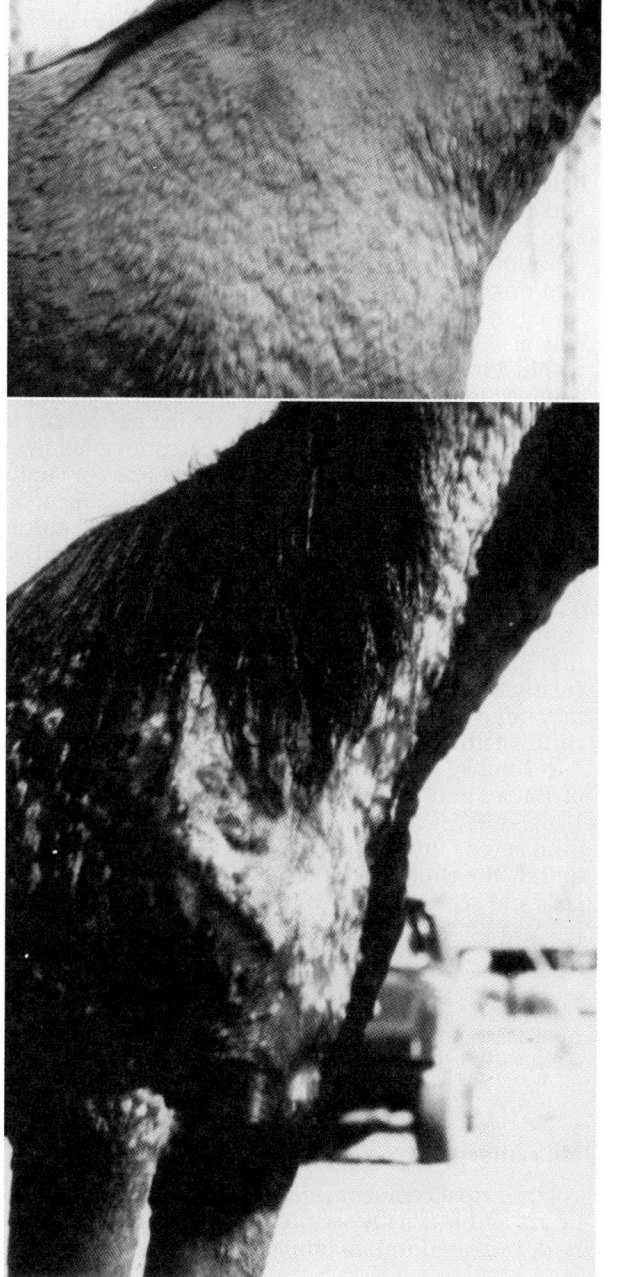

A

B

FIG. 38-3 ▐▐ Chronic urticaria in horses. **A,** Moderately severe case. **B,** Severe case.

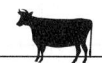

imal may or may not be pruritic. Hair loss is not usually a feature of urticaria unless there has been serum leakage to the surface.

The most important factor in distinguishing urticaria from other nodular diseases is that the individual lesions pit with pressure. This is easily demonstrated in the early stages of wheal formation when the lesions consist primarily of dermal edema. In the later stages when there is cellular infiltration into the dermis, the pitting is less apparent.

CLINICAL PATHOLOGY. A biopsy of a lesion submitted for routine histopathologic study may lend support to a clinical diagnosis of urticaria. The diagnostic dilemma is to determine the cause of the urticarial eruption. Clinical trials should be performed sequentially to determine whether insects, feeds, or environmental factors (such as inhaled animal danders, dusts, or pollens) are responsible for the urticarial eruption. Intradermal skin testing may be of value in identifying an allergic inhalant cause for recurrent urticaria and in determining the offending allergen(s).[18] The test involves making a series of intradermal injections of aqueous allergen extracts along with a positive (histamine) and negative (saline) control. The injections are usually performed over the lateral cervical or thoracic region. The injection sites are then observed for a period of 30 minutes to 24 hours for evidence of wheal formation associated with the injection sight. A positive reaction does not necessarily mean that the patient's urticaria is caused by the reacting allergen. Instead, a positive reaction indicates that the patient has skin-sensitizing antibody to the allergen. False-negative skin test reactions may also occur; the most important factor is the use of corticosteroids, antihistamines, or phenothiazine tranquilizers before testing.

THERAPY. Avoiding the allergens is the best therapy. When this is not possible or when the allergens cannot be identified, medical therapy should be used.

Corticosteroids are the most commonly used medical therapy for urticaria. For a 450-kg horse, a dose of 500 to as much as 1000 mg of prednisone or prednisolone orally may be required every morning to induce clinical remission. After remission, the dose is gradually decreased over a period of weeks to the lowest possible daily dose that will keep the urticaria from recurring. The regimen is then modified so that twice the daily maintenance dose is given on alternate mornings. An attempt may be made to further decrease this alternate-morning dose. Ideally the urticaria should be controlled with 200 to 300 mg of prednisolone every other morning. Short-acting oral corticosteroids such as prednisone and prednisolone are preferable to dexamethasone or triamcinolone because they are less immunosuppressive and less likely to produce laminitis. Other agents that have been tried with minimum benefits include diethylcarbamazine, levamisole, and antihistamines. Of the antihistamines, hydroxyzine HCl has the most promise for treatment of urticaria, and, although not FDA-approved for use in horses and ruminants, it has been beneficial at a dose of 200 to 400 mg 2 to 3 times daily. A tricyclic antidepressant with antihistaminic effects, doxepin has also been helpful at a dose of 300 to 600 mg twice daily.

Hyposensitization is only a therapeutic option for the animal that has urticaria resulting from inhaled allergens. Selection of allergens to be used for hyposensitization is based on the results of intradermal skin testing, together with historic information that suggests exposure of the animal to the allergen(s) demonstrating positive skin test reactions. The allergen extracts are combined in solution and administered by subcutaneous injections in gradually increasing doses. The dose and frequency of allergen injections is varied according to each patient's clinical response. If hyposensitization benefits the patient, it is continued for life. Therapy should be monitored by a veterinary allergist or dermatologist.

REFERENCE
18. Evans AG: Recurrent urticaria due to inhaled allergens. In Robinson NE, ed: *Current therapy in equine medicine,* ed 2, Philadelphia, 1986, WB Saunders, pp 619-621.

OTHER SYNDROMES ASSOCIATED WITH HYPERSENSITIVITY REACTIONS

Anaphylaxis

Anaphylaxis is an acute, transient, life-threatening alteration in vascular permeability and smooth muscle contraction that occurs rapidly following a variety of possible stimuli.[19] Anaphylactic reactions are allergic and follow antigenic challenge, whereas anaphylactoid reactions differ in that they are initiated by nonallergic mechanisms such as chemical or physical stimuli. Both reactions result in the release of chemical mediators, including histamine, kinins, and products of the arachidonic acid cascade, with the end clinical result being the same.

Typically, anaphylaxis involves a number of organ systems, including the respiratory and cardiovascular systems. It may or may not be associated with cutaneous manifestations such as urticaria. Initial clinical signs are evident within 2 to 20 minutes after challenge with a stimulus. In the horse, anaphylaxis initially manifests as anxiety, tachycardia, colic, and dyspnea, which may be followed by sweating, piloerection, and diarrhea. Ultimately, severe respiratory distress, recumbency, convulsions, and typically death occur. Cattle, sheep, and goats manifest a sudden onset of severe dyspnea associated with anxiety and muscle shivering that may result in an elevation of body temperature. There may be profuse salivation or gastrointestinal signs such as bloat or diarrhea followed by collapse and death. Palpebral and vulvar edema may also be seen. If recovery occurs, it is usually complete within 2 hours. Necropsy findings in ruminants are typically confined to the lungs and include vascular engorgement, pulmonary edema, and emphysema. Similar pulmonary lesions are noted in the horse and may be accompanied by edema and hemorrhage of the large bowel or lesions of lamini.[20]

Diagnosis is based on clinical signs, and treatment must be administered immediately to prevent death. In life-threatening situations, epinephrine diluted 1:10,000 (0.1 mg/ml) should be given slowly intravenously (0.01 mg/kg [approximately 5 ml] for a mature horse or cow). In less acute situations or if an intravenous injection cannot be administered, epinephrine 5 to 10 ml of 1:1000 [1 mg/ml] may be given intramuscularly or subcutaneously.[21] Repeated doses of epinephrine may be given as needed at 15-minute intervals. In addition, a corticosteroid such as methylprednisolone sodium succinate 1 to 2 mg/kg IV or IM or dexamethasone 0.25 to 1 mg/kg IV or IM, an antihistamine such as diphenhydramine 0.25 to 1 mg/kg IV or IM, and intravenous polyionic fluids are administered. Prognosis is guarded and depends on how quickly the clinician recognizes the clinical signs of anaphylaxis and acts to treat them medically.

REFERENCES
19. Moschella SL, Hurley HJ: *Dermatology,* ed 2, Philadelphia, 1985, WB Saunders, pp 255-275.
20. Blood DC, Radostits OM, Henderson JA: *Veterinary medicine,* ed 6, London, 1983, Baillière Tindall, pp 79-82.
21. Robinson NE: *Current therapy in equine medicine,* ed 2, Philadelphia, 1987, WB Saunders, p 731.

Milk Allergy

The principal cutaneous manifestation of milk allergy is urticaria and is usually seen in cows during the drying-off period. Increased intramammary pressure presumably causes milk proteins to gain access to the circulation, where they induce a type I hypersensitivity reaction.[22] The disorder is believed to be hereditary, with cattle of the Channel Island breeds demonstrating increased susceptibility.[23]

The urticarial reaction can be localized or generalized. Other clinical signs that may be noted include muscle tremors, respiratory distress, restlessness, ataxia, dullness, and even maniacal behavior. Diagnosis is made by observing an edematous swelling at the sight of an intradermal injection of the cow's milk or the milk protein-casein diluted 1:1000, in combination with the appropriate clinical symptoms.[24]

Treatment involves the use of antihistamines early in the course of the disease, and prevention requires avoiding milk retention. An affected cow is likely to suffer recurrences of milk allergy, so culling is usually recommended.

REFERENCES

22. Campbell SG: Milk allergy, an autoallergic disease of cattle, *Cornell Vet* 60:684, 1970.
23. Blood DC, Radostits OM, Henderson JA: *Veterinary medicine,* ed 6, London, 1983, Baillière Tindall, pp 1205-1206.
24. Campbell SG: The milk proteins responsible for milk allergy, an autoallergic disease of cattle, *J Allergy Clin Immunol* 48:230, 1971.

Erythema Multiforme

Erythema multiforme (EM) has been recognized clinically in the horse but not in ruminants. Drugs are probably the most common identifiable cause of EM, although the majority of cases in both humans and horse are idiopathic. The pathogenesis of EM is unknown. Evidence in humans indicates that the disorder is immune mediated.[25] Circulating immune complexes have been identified, and immunoglobulins and complement have been found in and around dermal microvasculature.

In the horse, EM consists of an acute onset of asymptomatic skin lesions that form a raised annular and polycyclic pattern (Fig. 38-4). Usually the lesions remain haired unless there is serum exudation, resulting in a secondary alopecia.

Histopathologically a biopsy of an early lesion of EM minor demonstrates individual necrotic keratinocytes identified by their homogeneous eosinophilic cytoplasm and pyknotic or absent nuclei. There may be hydropic degeneration of basal cells and epidermal spongiosus. A superficial perivascular infiltrate is present in the dermis that is primarily lymphohistiocytic. There may be endothelial swelling, superficial dermal edema, exocytosis, and extravasation of red blood cells.[26]

The primary clinical differential diagnosis in the horse is urticaria. However, individual urticarial lesions tend to re-solve over a matter of hours, whereas the lesions of EM remain fixed for as long as a week.

The most important aspect of treatment is elimination of suspected etiologic factors. Use of unnecessary medications should be discontinued, and concurrent infections should be treated. Thereafter the treatment is symptomatic. Controlled studies concerning the value of corticosteroid treatment for EM in the horse are lacking. Because spontaneous resolution is the rule, if the symptoms are mild, it is probably best to avoid overuse of systemic steroids.

EM may be a mild, asymptomatic disorder resolving in 2 to 3 weeks, or it more rarely may be a severe ulcerative disease. The tendency for recurrence has not been established in the horse.

REFERENCES

25. Huff JC et al: Erythema multiforme: a critical review of characteristics, diagnostic criteria, and causes, *J Am Acad Dermatol* 8:763-775, 1983.
26. Lever WF, Schaumburg-Lever G: *Histopathology of the skin,* ed 6, JB Lippincott, 1983, Philadelphia, pp 122-123.

Vasculitis

Vasculitis is a histopathologic term that implies the presence of inflammatory changes in the walls of blood vessels and is associated with a broad spectrum of disorders. *Cutaneous vasculitis* is recognized in horses, although it has not yet been described in ruminants. Affected vessels may be limited to the skin or may involve other organs, resulting in systemic disease. The cutaneous lesions are characterized by purpura, necrosis, and ulceration—most commonly affecting the head and extremities (Fig. 38-5). Vasculitis is discussed thoroughly in Chapter 35.

Drug Eruption

A drug eruption is a cutaneous reaction to any agent that enters the circulation either by ingestion, injection, inhalation, or percutaneous absorption. Drug eruptions may or may not be associated with systemic symptoms. Many drug eruptions are thought to be immunologically mediated hypersensitivity reactions, although on occasion they may occur with the initial administration of a drug and therefore without any prior sensitizing exposure characteristic of an immunologic reaction. Drug eruptions may also occur after years of repeated asymptomatic exposure to a drug. Any chemical compound can potentially trigger a drug eruption, but the classes of compounds most commonly incriminated include antibacterial agents (especially penicillin and the sulfas), phenothiazine tranquilizers, nonsteroidal antiinflammatory agents and antipyretics (especially aspirin and phenylbutazone), local anesthetics, and anticonvulsants.

Because drug eruptions can result in a wide variety of cutaneous manifestations, they must be considered in the differential diagnosis of all skin disorders. Certain clinical symptoms are more commonly associated with drug eruptions. Urticaria and angioedema, diffuse erythema, papular rashes, intense pruritus that is poorly responsive to corticosteroids (Fig. 38-6), sharply demarcated ulcers secondary to vasculitides, vesicular and bullous eruptions, and photosensitization should arouse clinical suspicion of a drug eruption. Typically, cutaneous lesions are noted 24 to 48 hours after drug administration, although there may be a longer lag interval. The eruption usually subsides within 24 to 48 hours after exposure ceases, although lesions may persist up to 6 months after the offending agent is eliminated.[27]

A diagnosis of drug eruption is based on clinical suspicion associated with an incriminating history of drug administration and by ruling out other possible causes. In a suspected

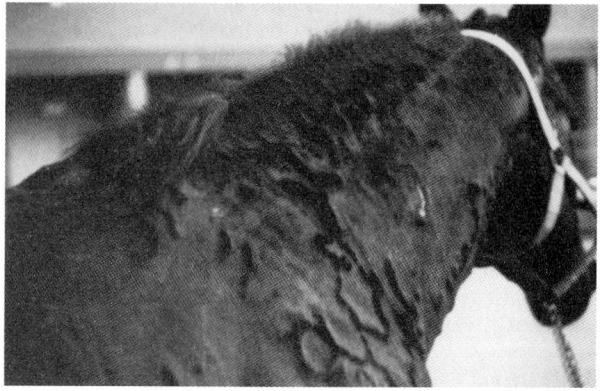

FIG. 38-4 ▓ Erythema multiforme in a horse.

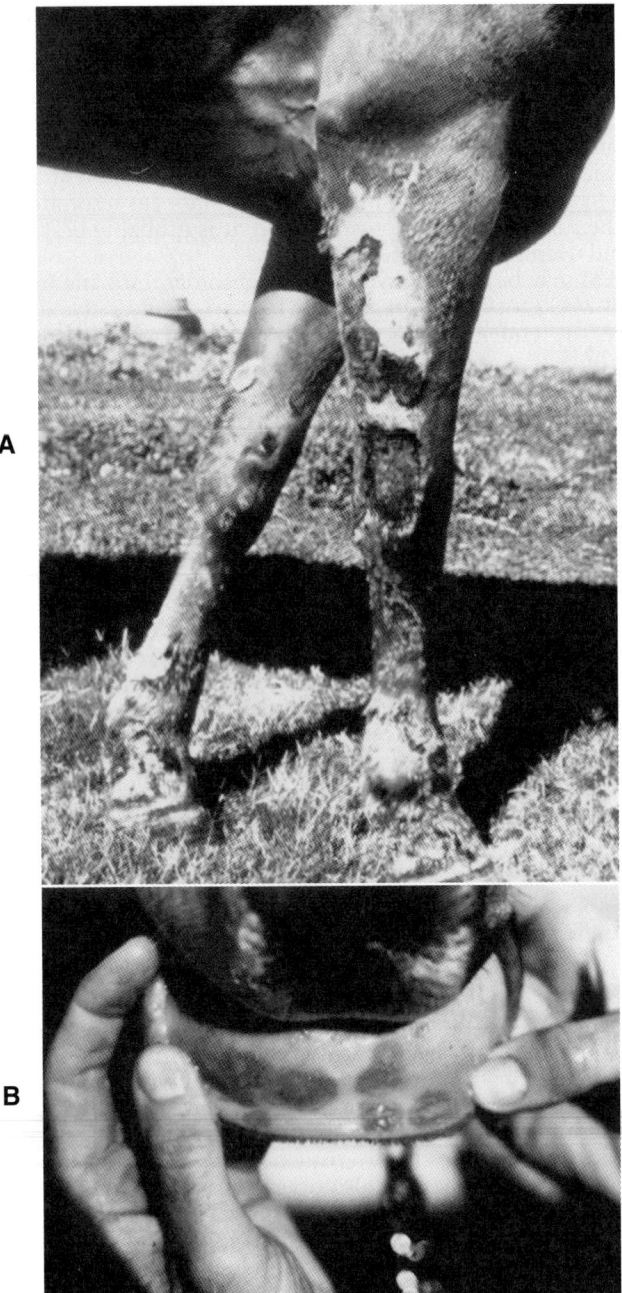

FIG. 38-5 ■ Cutaneous vasculitis in a horse. **A,** Vasculitis involving the forelimbs. **B,** Vasculitis involving the mucous membranes of the inner lip.

case, all medications should be discontinued. If lifesaving medications are being administered, a chemically unrelated compound with similar pharmacologic effects should be substituted. Administration of corticosteroids may provide some relief, but typically drug eruptions are minimally responsive to corticosteroids. Although development of a cutaneous reaction following readministration of the suspected agent would support a diagnosis of drug eruption, readministration is not advisable because it can be fatal. Future exposure to any implicated compounds and chemically related substances should be avoided.[28]

REFERENCES

27. Stannard AA: Modern veterinary practice seminars: equine dermatology, Oct 1 and 2, 1984, Santa Barbara, Calif.

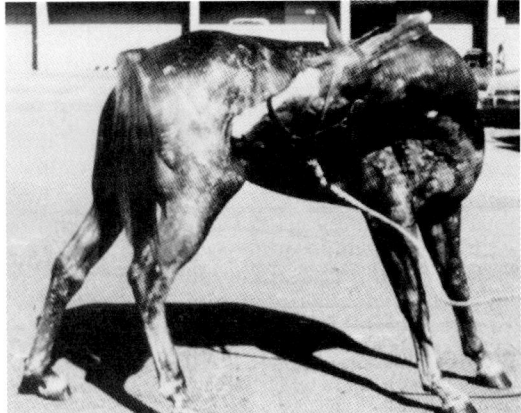

FIG. 38-6 ■ Drug eruption in a horse. Note pruritus.

28. Moschella SL, Hurley HJ: *Dermatology,* ed 2, Philadelphia, 1985, WB Saunders, pp 425-463.

CONTACT DERMATITIS

DEFINITION AND ETIOLOGY. Contact dermatitis is recognized in both horses and ruminants and can be subdivided into irritant and allergic contact dermatitis. Irritant contact dermatitis occurs more commonly and is defined as a cutaneous reaction to an irritating concentration of an offending agent. The substance chemically damages the skin without immunologic mediation. The reaction may occur after a single contact with a strong irritant or after repeated contacts with a milder irritant. Allergic contact dermatitis represents a cutaneous reaction in a sensitized animal to a nonirritating concentration of the offending agent. Tissue damage is immunologically mediated by delayed-type hypersensitivity (type IV); thus prior exposure is required to sensitize the skin to the material eliciting the dermatitis.[29,30]

CLINICAL SIGNS. The clinical lesions associated with allergic and irritant contact dermatitis are very similar. Predisposed areas include the muzzle, the extremities, and the areas contacted by tack. Early lesions include erythema, edema, and vesiculation, which progress to erosions, ulcerations, and crusting and ultimately to lichenification and hyperpigmentation.

PROVOCATIVE EXPOSURE. Patch testing is sometimes used, but it is usually impractical. Provocative exposure is the most useful test for diagnosis of contact dermatitis, although it does not reliably distinguish between allergic and irritant contact dermatitis. Provocative exposure requires avoiding contact with all suspected agents for a 7- to 10-day period to permit clearing of the skin lesions. The patient is then reexposed to these agents on an individual basis at 7- to 10-day intervals while being observed for recurrence of the dermatitis. When a positive reaction is observed, challenge with the suspected agent should be repeated to confirm the diagnosis. The process is time consuming, requiring patience and cooperation on the part of the owner.

THERAPY. An animal with a suspected or confirmed diagnosis of acute or irritant contact dermatitis should be placed in an environment where there is negligible chance of exposure to contactants that might have produced the dermatitis. Symptomatic treatment pending spontaneous resolution includes gently washing the affected regions with water.

REFERENCES

29. Moschella SL, Hurley HJ: *Dermatology,* ed 2, Philadelphia, 1985, WB Saunders, pp 289-322.

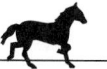

30. Ihrke PJ: Contact dermatitis. In Robinson NE, ed: *Current therapy in equine medicine,* Philadelphia, 1983, WB Saunders, pp 547-548.

BACTERIAL DISEASES

ANNE G. EVANS
STEPHEN D. WHITE

DERMATOPHILOSIS (Streptothricosis, Rain Scald, Lumpy Wool, Strawberry Footrot)

DEFINITION AND ETIOLOGY. Dermatophilosis is a superficial bacterial dermatitis caused by the actinomycete *Dermatophilus congolensis* and is characterized by exudation and crust formation. The organism is a gram-positive, nonacid fast, branching, filamentous, aerobic bacteria that divides longitudinally and then transversely to form parallel rows of coccoid zoospores. Dermatophilosis affects horses, cattle, sheep, and goats, as well as a wide host range of other mammals.[31-34] In horses the disease is often called "rain scald." In cattle and goats the term "cutaneous streptothrichosis" is frequently used. In sheep the condition is referred to as "lumpy wool" or "mycotic dermatitis" when wooled areas are affected and "strawberry footrot" when the distal extremities are involved. Although the distribution is worldwide, the frequency of occurrence of dermatophilosis varies with geographic location. There is no apparent age, breed, or sex predilection.

PATHOPHYSIOLOGY. Infection occurs when the motile, coccoid zoospores germinate in a moist defect of the stratum corneum to form a mycelium that proliferates within the living layers of the epidermis. The resulting inflammatory response is primarily neutrophilic and forms a barrier that the organisms are unable to penetrate. The organisms are eliminated as the epidermis reepithelializes, and the serocellular crusts containing the organisms are lost. Healing requires both a cell-mediated and humoral antibody response on the part of the host.

The exact origin of the disease is unknown. The organism is suspected of having a saprophytic existence in soil, although attempts to isolate it from soil have been unsuccessful. Chronically infected carrier animals are believed to be the primary source of infection. The organism can be transmitted following direct contact with a reservoir host, by contaminated fomites, or by both biting and nonbiting flies and ticks. *D. congolensis* has been shown to persist in crusts in the environment for up to 42 months, thus accounting for repeated herd outbreaks in contaminated areas.

CLINICAL SIGNS AND DIFFERENTIAL DIAGNOSES. The characteristic lesions of dermatophilosis in large animal species include proliferative, suppurative crusts and matted hair (Fig. 38-7), resulting in a "paintbrush" appearance. In sheep, crusts bound by wool fibers lead to accumulations of dense keratinized masses. Removal of crusts reveals a moist, gray-to-pink surface, with the roots of the hairs protruding through the under surface of the crust. These findings are characteristic of, although not specific for, dermatophilosis. In areas of shorter hair length, crusted papules and scale may be noted with less significant matting of the hair. These lesions are more obvious with palpation than they are visually. The affected regions are typically painful and not pruritic.

Body areas predisposed to infection include those that are most susceptible to maceration and trauma. The distal extremities, muzzle, and entire length of the dorsum are frequently the initial sites of infection. Nonpigmented skin is also reported to be more susceptible to infection. Horses develop lesions in areas rubbed by tack, and cattle often have involvement of the udder and scrotum. Goat kids reportedly

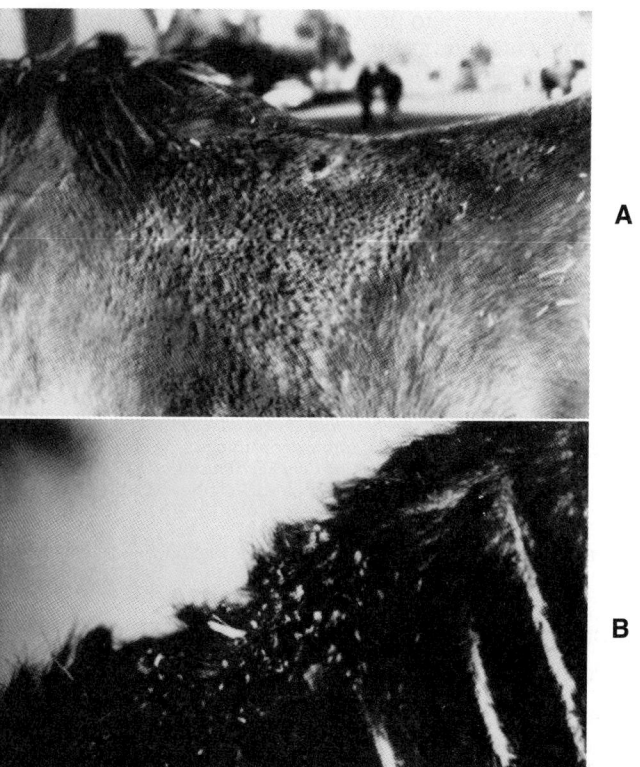

FIG. 38-7 ■ Dermatophilosis *(D. congolensis).* **A,** Horse with suppurative crusts and matted hair on the back. **B,** Scaling and crusting over withers and neck of a bovine.

have a tendency to develop lesions on the pinnae and under the surface of the tail. Sheep may develop a form of dermatophilosis that begins as a proliferative dermatitis at the coronet region, which is known as strawberry footrot. Removal of the external crusts reveals a pink-to-red granulation bed that resembles the surface of a strawberry. Lesions can extend from the hoof to the hock, and, with loss of the crusts, ulceration occurs. Under appropriate conditions dermatophilosis can become generalized in any infected animal.

CLINICAL PATHOLOGY. In the acute stages of the disease, when suppuration underlies the crusts, direct smears of the exudate on a glass slide should be stained and examined for the characteristic bacteria. If bacteria are not seen or if lesions are limited to dry crusts, a dermatophilosis preparation should be made (see Chapter 11). *D. congolensis* can be recognized as gram-positive, branching, filamentous bacteria that form parallel rows of cocci; it is commonly described as resembling "railroad tracks." If a *Dermatophilis* preparation is negative in an animal that is suspected clinically of having the disease, the diagnosis should not be ruled out without first culturing crusts for the organism.

In chronic cases the organism is most successfully isolated by submitting crusts to a microbiologist for specialized culture techniques.

THERAPY. The most important aspect of therapy involves removal of factors predisposing to infection. Moist conditions that result in cutaneous maceration must be avoided to give the skin an opportunity to dry out. External parasites that cause skin damage and transmission of the bacteria should be eliminated.

Infected animals must be carefully groomed to remove crusts that contain the organisms. The crust must be appropri-

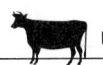

ately disposed of to prevent further contamination of the environment, and the area where the infected animal(s) have been kept should be either disinfected or abandoned. Topical treatment includes bathing with a povidone-iodine shampoo or chlorhexidine solution daily for 7 days, followed by treatment one to two times weekly until there is clinical resolution.

Systemic therapy is generally reserved for severe and generalized cases. Penicillin 22,000 IU/kg IM twice daily for 3 to 5 days is beneficial. In severe cases, it should be given at this dose twice daily. Long-acting oxytetracycline given as a single 20-mg/kg intramuscular dose has been reported to be effective for bovine and ovine dermatophilosis.

REFERENCES
31. Scanlan CM, Garrett PD, Geifer DB: Dermatophilus congolensis infections of cattle and sheep, *Compend Cont Educ Pract Vet* 6:S4-S8, 1984.
32. Scott DW, Manning TO: Caprine dermatology. I, Normal skin and bacterial fungal disorders, *Compend Cont Educ Pract Vet* 6:S197-S199.
33. Scheidt VJ, Lloyd DH: Dermatophilosis. In Robinson NE, ed: *Current therapy in equine medicine*, ed 2, Philadelphia, 1987, WB Saunders, pp 630-632.
34. Blood DC, Radostits OM, Henderson JA: *Veterinary medicine*, ed 6, London, 1985, Baillière Tindall, pp 655-658.

FOLLICULITIS/FURUNCULOSIS AND IMPETIGO

Bacterial folliculitis is defined as inflammation of the hair follicles secondary to a bacterial infection. Less severe, more superficial bacterial infection that does not involve the hair follicles is called impetigo. Impetigo is diagnosed and treated similarly to the more severe processes. When the inflammatory process ruptures the hair follicle and extends into the surrounding dermis and subcutis, the process is called furunculosis. Coalescing areas of furunculosis that form a fistulous tract are described as a carbuncle or boil.[35] Folliculitis and furunculosis are commonly recognized in horses[35-38] and goats[39]; they are an uncommon problem in cattle and sheep. Impetigo is common in cattle and goats. In addition to *D. congolensis*, bacteria that have been found to cause folliculitis and furunculosis in the horse include *Staphylococcus* spp., *Corynebacterium pseudotuberculosis* (Canadian horsepox),[35,36,38] *Corynebacterium equi*, and in rare instances other bacteria such as *Bacillus* spp.[37] In the goat, causative agents include *Staphylococcus* spp., *C. pseudotuberculosis*, *Actinomyces (Corynebacterium) pyogenes*, and *Pseudomonas aeruginosa*.[39] When grains or granules are present, infection may be called botryomycosis. In cattle, furunculosis caused by *C. pseudotuberculosis* manifests as a locally extensive, raised, raw lesion that is frequently hemorrhagic. The lesion(s) are almost constantly covered with a serosanguineous exudate, and palpation of the lesion(s) usually elicits a pain response.

Factors that predispose to the development of bacterial folliculitis and furunculosis include mechanical trauma from tack or insect bites, heat, and moisture—either environmental or from heavy work, poor sanitation, and poor grooming. Stress from parturition is also an important predisposing factor in goats. Clinical signs in horses are typically first noted in the saddle and harness regions, neck, or dorsal lumbosacral region, although any haired region is susceptible. The primary lesion is a follicular papule. Pustules are rarely found. The initial sign may be multiple 2- to 3-mm foci of erect hairs. Close inspection reveals that each hair projects from the center of a papule. These areas may spontaneously regress or enlarge, exude serum, and scab. Hair loss is a common sequela. The lesions are painful rather than pruritic. In goats, lesions commonly begin on the udder and spread to the abdomen, thigh, perineum, and face.

Pastern folliculitis is a specific form of folliculitis and furunculosis recognized in the horse. *Staphylococcus* spp. or hemolytic streptococci are usually cultured. The lesions are limited to the posterior aspects of the pastern or fetlock of one or more limbs. The initial papular lesions may coalesce, resulting in large areas of ulceration and suppuration if left untreated.[40]

Gram stain smears of pustular contents, bacterial culture and sensitivity tests, and biopsies for routine histopathology should be performed. The most important aspect of treatment is to correct any predisposing factors. Mild cases of folliculitis may resolve without treatment. More severe cases require topical therapy with antibacterial solutions containing chlorhexidine or iodophors. Small areas may respond to topical application of silver-sulfadiazine cream, or mupirocin ointment. In addition to topical treatment, furunculosis requires systemic antibiotic therapy, which should be based on the results of a bacterial culture and sensitivity. The affected areas of pastern folliculitis should be lightly clipped as part of the initial treatment before cleansing with antibacterial solutions. It is advisable to sedate the horse because the lesions are painful. The prognosis for cure of bacterial folliculitis and furunculosis is good, provided that predisposing causes are eliminated. The exception is chronic pastern folliculitis and furunculosis when long-term infection has become deep, resulting in the formation of scar tissue and fissures.

REFERENCES
35. Scott DW: Folliculitis and furunculosis. In Robinson NE, ed: *Current therapy in equine medicine*, Philadelphia, 1983, WB Saunders, pp 542-545.
36. Mullowney PC, Fadok VA: Dermatologic diseases of horses. II, Bacterial and viral skin diseases, *Compend Cont Educ Pract Vet* 6:S16-S22, 1984.
37. Pascoe RR: Infectious skin diseases of horses, *Vet Clin North Am (Large Anim Pract)* 6:27-58, 1984.
38. Scott DW, Manning TO: Equine folliculitis and furunculosis, *Equine Pract* 2:11-32, 1980.
39. Scott DW, Manning TO: Caprine dermatology. I, Normal skin and bacterial and fungal disorders, *Compend Cont Educ Pract Vet* 6:S190-S211, 1984.
40. Stannard AA: Modern veterinary practice seminars: equine dermatology, Oct 1 and 2, 1984, Santa Barbara, Calif.

EQUINE STAPHYLOCOCCAL CELLULITIS

Cellulitis is a severe, deep, suppurative process in which a poorly defined area of infection tends to dissect through tissue planes. Although many organisms are capable of producing cellulitis, staphylococcal cellulitis has been recognized as a specific disease entity in thoroughbred racehorses.[41] Coagulase-positive staphylococci have been isolated from all reported cases and, when speciated, the isolants were classified as *Staphylococcus aureus*.[41] Other studies of pathogenic *Staphylococcus* spp. from horses have suggested that *S. aureus* and *Staphylococcus intermedius* are the major cutaneous pathogens,[42,43] with no significant difference in their susceptibility patterns.[42] The cause of staphylococcal cellulitis is uncertain. Management practices may be associated with the condition because bathing, grooming devices, and handlers can be a source of the organism.[41]

The initial symptom is acute swelling and lameness that involves one or more limbs. Lesions progress rapidly by dissection along tissue planes. The overlying skin becomes devitalized and frequently sloughs. Accompanying systemic signs include increased rectal temperature and heart rate. Laminitis of either the affected or contralateral limbs, osteomyelitis, and bacteremia are possible sequela.[41] Diagnosis is based on the results of bacterial culture and biopsies for routine histopathology.

Treatment must be aggressive and initiated early in the course of the disease. Pending the results of bacterial culture and sensitivity, treatment should include broad-spectrum antibiotics such as potassium penicillin G and gentamicin sulfate or trimethoprim-sulfamethoxazole. To decrease edema, promote weight bearing, and reduce the chance of laminitis,

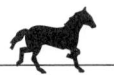

therapy should include nonsteroidal antiinflammatory agents, hydrotherapy, and support wraps.[41] The prognosis for complete recovery is guarded.

REFERENCES

41. Markel MD, Wheat JD, Spenser SJ: Cellulitis associated with coagulase-positive staphylococci in racehorses: nine cases (1975-1984), *J Am Vet Med Assoc* 189:1600-1604, 1986.
42. Biberstein EL, Spencer SJ, Hirsh DC: Species distribution of coagulase-positive staphylococci in animals, *J Clin Microbiol* 19:610-615, 1984.
43. Devriese LA, Nzuambe D, Godard C: Identification and characteristics of staphylococci isolated from lesions and normal skin of horses, *Vet Microbiol* 10:269-277, 1985.

PAPILLOMATOUS DIGITAL DERMATITIS (Digital Dermatitis, Foot Warts, Heel Warts, Hairy Foot Warts, Mortellaro's Disease, Strawberry Heel Warts)

STEVEN L. BERRY

Papillomatous digital dermatitis (PDD) of cattle is an infectious, contagious dermatitis of the digital skin of cattle. It is primarily a disease of housed dairy cattle. Digital dermatitis, a less consistently papillomatous form of the same disease, was first described in Italy in 1974.[44] The first documented cases of PDD in the United States occurred in New York in 1980.[45] During the early 1990s the reported first observations of PDD increased dramatically in the United States,[46,47] and this disease is a major cause of lameness in dairy cattle in many countries.[48-50] Financial losses from reduced milk production, reduced reproductive efficiency, and costs of treatment are enormous, estimated at $1.25 to $5 million per year in California alone.[48]

CLINICAL SIGNS. Roughly 80% of PDD lesions occur on the plantar aspect of the hind foot, immediately proximal to the heel bulbs and adjacent to or extending into the interdigital space.[49,51] Less common sites for lesions are the plantar aspect of a forefoot and the dorsal aspect of any foot.[49,51] Multiple lesions may exist on a single animal, even on a single foot, but lesions are confined to the digital skin and have not been reported to occur above the level of the dewclaws.[49]

The gross appearance of the lesions, predilection for hind limbs and skin-horn junctions, especially those bordering the heel bulbs and interdigital space, distinguish this disease from other bovine dermatitides.[49] Lesions are most often 2 to 6 cm across at their greatest dimension, circular or oval, and have clearly demarcated, raised borders.[49] Lesion borders are often surrounded by hairs that are 2 to 3 times normal length. Lesion surfaces may have filiform papillae varying in length from 1 mm to 3 cm and 0.5 to 1 mm in diameter, hence the name "hairy foot warts."[49,50] Lesions lacking the filiform papillae ("hairs") may have a granular surface.[49] Lesions vary in color and appearance. Washed surfaces are generally very painful and either red and granular, or may be composites of white-yellow, gray, brown, or black papillary areas with red, granular areas interspersed.[49,50] The lesions bleed easily if traumatized. When PDD lesions develop in the interdigital space, they frequently occur on a preexisting fibroma.

The time required for these lesions to progress to the mature ("hairy" or papillomatous) form appears to vary. The lesions slowly enlarge and become raised masses 2 to 6 cm in diameter that are red, gray, or black; and oval, spherical, or U shaped.[49] Proliferative or papillomatous lesions are seen less often in Europe than in the United States.[50]

A foul odor may or may not be present.[52-55] This odor appears to be caused by secondary bacterial growth in the exudate covering the PDD lesion. Swelling of the pastern and fetlock regions is not present in uncomplicated cases. Lameness is a herd characteristic on dairies where PDD has a high prevalence but is an inconsistent finding on individual, infected cat-

tle and is not consistently related to lesion size or maturity. If PDD lesions remain untreated, the claws of feet with plantar or palmar lesions may develop a clubbed appearance because the cow prefers to bear weight on (and wear down) the toes.[48]

DIFFERENTIAL DIAGNOSES. Differential diagnoses for an individual case of PDD include interdigital necrobacillosis (footrot, foul in the foot, or interdigital phlegmon), interdigital hyperplasia (corns or interdigital fibroma), interdigital dermatitis, and traumatic injury with granulation tissue. For herd problems of lameness localized to the digit, the differential diagnosis list should include PDD, interdigital necrobacillosis, interdigital dermatitis, laminitis, excessive sole wear from caustic or abrasive flooring, and improper or no foot trimming. If signs of polysystemic disease exist, coronitis from viral diseases (e.g., bovine virus diarrhea) should also be considered.

EPIDEMIOLOGY. Once introduced into a herd, PDD spreads rapidly within adult cows, often affecting the majority of adults within the first year of infection. When established in a herd, lameness is most commonly seen in first and second lactation cows, usually after entry into the milking string.[48,50] Lesions are typically present in a significant proportion of older cows, but lameness is commonly less than that in the younger cows. Bulls and yearling heifers can also be affected but usually comprise a small fraction of clinical cases. In California the disease appears to be most severe during the spring and summer months,[48] but it is most severe in the winter months in Europe.[50,52] Freestall herds tend to be more commonly affected than stanchion (tie stall) herds.[48,52] Cattle confined to pasture are rarely affected.[56,57] PDD is almost exclusively seen in dairy cattle, with no breed predilection yet demonstrated. Eradication of PDD from an affected herd has been documented on one small university herd.[58]

Retrospective epidemiologic studies in the United States indicated that two risk factors are significant in high prevalence herds: (1) muddy or wet conditions, and (2) purchasing replacement cattle from off premises.[46,47,59] Attempts to transmit the disease experimentally were successful when scrapings from active lesions were applied to feet of calves that were subjected to constant moisture and low oxygen tension.[60,61] Constant moisture and low oxygen tension are present on confinement dairies if manure management and hygiene are not adequate. Poor freestall or bedding area management will exacerbate the problem by forcing cows to stand in manure slurry for longer periods and will not allow the feet of cattle to dry out periodically. Other risk factors identified were the use of outside hoof trimmers and not washing hoof trimming equipment between cows.[59]

PATHOGENESIS. Numerous obligate anaerobic organisms have been associated with PDD.[62-72] Spirochetes from the genus *Treponema* have been identified the most consistently, comprise the bulk of the colonizing bacterial mat found on active lesions, and are the organism found to invade the epidermis and dermis.[63-69,71,72] These spirochetes also produce a humoral response in cows with active lesions.[58] Read and Walker[48] have hypothesized that the disease occurs as a result of exposure of digital skin to oxygen-depleted, wet organic material containing the causative organism(s). PDD lesions show gross and histological similarities to viral papillomas; however, bovine papilloma viruses have not been found in lesions.[45,48-50]

Current evidence indicates that PDD is multifactorial involving environmental, microbial, host, and management factors.[46,49,50,59,73-75] Factors such as rough flooring; poor drainage; accumulation of feces and urine on floors; dirty, wet, or uncomfortable bedding areas; and overcrowding have an adverse effect on digital skin health and could increase the risk of PDD. The mode of transmission between cows and between herds is currently unclear. Clinically and subclini-

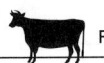

cally affected cows and fomites such as foot-trimming instruments, livestock trailers, and farm equipment may be sources of infection for naive herds.

A California study found that antibodies against two antigenically distinct spirochetes were increased on dairies with PDD compared with PDD-free dairies.[58] Also, cattle with PDD on a high-prevalence dairy were much more likely to have antibodies to the spirochetes than were cattle without lesions on the same dairy.[58] There was no cross-reactivity between the two spirochetes or to other spirochetal diseases of cattle.[58] The concentration of clinical disease in the younger animals of a chronically affected herd suggests that some degree of immunity may develop in older cows.[48] Nonetheless, chronic and recurrent cases in otherwise healthy adult cattle have been reported, and immunity to PDD, if it does develop, may be incomplete or temporary. Preliminary studies on large California dairies indicate that up to 60% of successfully treated cows may develop recurrent lesions in 7 to 15 weeks.[48,76] Spontaneous regressions of lesions and resolution of lameness have also been observed but appear quite rare.

PATHOLOGIC FINDINGS. Histopathologic criteria to establish a diagnosis of PDD are as follows[49]:

- Circumscribed plaque of eroded acanthotic epidermis attended by parakeratotic papillomatous proliferation profusely colonized by spirochete-dominant bacterial flora
- Loss of stratum granulosum
- Invasion of stratum spinosum by spirochetes
- Infiltration of neutrophils, plasma cells, lymphocytes, and eosinophils in the dermis

If biopsies are performed, they should be full-thickness 4- or 6-mm punch biopsies, washed off with sterile saline, and placed in buffered formalin. Histopathology is helpful to confirm a diagnosis of PDD but is not necessary because lesions have such a characteristic appearance and location.[49,53,76]

Preliminary results of a biopsy study on treatment and recurrence of PDD indicate that the clinical and histopathologic diagnoses were in agreement for active lesions before treatment.[77] Histopathology on day 28 posttreatment with lincomycin or oxytetracycline, however, found a high percentage (55%) of lesions that appeared to be healed but still had microscopic evidence of infection.[77] It could not be determined if lesions were incompletely healed or recurrent infections.

TREATMENT AND PREVENTION. The most common treatments for PDD involve the use of topical antibiotics.[49,50,52,53,76-90] There are limited reports of nonantibiotic products being efficacious[82,86] although research and development continues.[81] There are currently no antibiotics labeled for treatment of PDD; therefore, adherence to extralabel drug use regulations is imperative. Laws regarding the use and disposal of certain chemicals, as well as *where* on the dairy such medications can be used, often vary among locales. Consultation with local regulatory agencies is prudent before initiation of a control program on a dairy.

The most commonly used treatments for PDD are topical oxytetracycline, lincomycin, or lincomycin/spectinomycin used as a spray or applied with a bandage.* For topical spray treatments, oxytetracycline or lincomycin are mixed with deionized or distilled water in a 2- to 4-L agricultural sprayer (25 g/L oxytetracycline, 8 g/L lincomycin) and applied directly to the heels of PDD-affected cattle. The recurrence rate is high enough that topical treatments will need to be repeated every 45 to 60 days on affected cattle to control the disease. There have been no reported antibiotic residue violations resulting from topical application of antibiotics.[50,94,95] Parenteral antibiotics (Ceftiofur or procaine penicillin G)

have been reported to be efficacious by U.S. researchers[49,85] but require milk withholding. European researchers have not found parenteral antibiotics efficacious.[50,53]

Footbaths containing 5% formalin,[50,51,53] lincomycin (1 to 4 g/L),[50] oxytetracycline (1 to 4 g/L),[50,51,84] copper sulfate (0.25 to 1 g/L), or zinc sulfate (20%)[51] provide effective control of the disease in infected herds. On large dairies, footbaths may be more effective at controlling PDD when the disease is at a low prevalence (<10%). When the disease has a high prevalence, individual topical treatment is probably more efficacious at reducing the prevalence. The efficacy of footbaths is reduced if feces and debris are allowed to accumulate in the treatment solution. This problem can be limited by placing two footbaths in tandem, with the first containing water or a mild detergent solution for cleaning the feet and the second containing the antibiotic or antiseptic solution. The footbath solution should be changed every 150 to 300 cow passages. Footbaths should be a minimum of 8 feet long and 2 to 3 feet wide, with a depth of 5 to 6 inches. The baths should be covered to limit dilution by rain and should be located in an exit alley off of the milking parlor to avoid splash contamination of the teat ends before milking. Additional footbaths can be placed in other locations to treat bulls, dry cows, and heifers. Treatments should occur every 3 to 7 days.[84]

Improvement of stall, corral, and alley hygiene; provision of dry and comfortable bedding; reduction of stocking rate; and improved ventilation to allow drying of stalls and alleys may result in reduction of the incidence or severity of clinical cases. Foot-trimming equipment, mobile tilt tables, and livestock trailers should be thoroughly cleaned and disinfected to prevent potential transmission of the agent(s) of PDD between dairies.

INTERDIGITAL DERMATITIS
(Nonpapillomatous Interdigital Dermatitis)

Interdigital dermatitis is a condition of acute or chronic inflammation of the interdigital skin, characterized by none to moderate lameness.[52,84,94,96] Inflammation is confined to the epidermis. Diffuse epidermal erosion in the interdigital cleft may be seen in early cases. More chronic cases show hyperkeratosis, which creates a roughened appearance to the interdigital skin and dorsal and palmar commissural skin folds.[52,84,94,96] A malodorous, gray, serous exudate may be present and there is mild sensitivity to pressure. This condition is frequently accompanied by cracks in the heel (heel horn erosion), with potential under-running of the heel horn.[84,96]

Several investigators have hypothesized that interdigital dermatitis and PDD are forms of the same disease complex.[48,94] *Dichelobacter nodosus* may be a primary or a contributory pathogen.[52,84,96] Interdigital dermatitis and PDD share several histological characteristics (including spirochetal involvement),[52,53,97] and both can be successfully treated and prevented with the same topical antibiotics or footbaths.[52,53] However, interdigital dermatitis can persist on dairies that practice regular footbathing.[84] The causative organisms may survive within deep heel cracks that are not permeated by footbath solutions; hence heel cracks must be trimmed away to allow for exposure.[84]

Interdigital dermatitis differs from interdigital necrobacillosis (footrot), in which infection extends into the dermis, leading to fissure formation, infection of deeper structures, and cellulitis of the pastern and fetlock regions.[52,96]

REFERENCES

44. Cheli R, Mortellaro C: La Dermatite Digitale Del Bovino, *Proceedings of the VIII International Meeting on Diseases of Cattle* 1974, pp 208-213.
45. Rebhun WC et al: Interdigital papillomatosis in dairy cattle, *J Am Vet Med Assoc* 137:437-440, 1980.

*References 49, 50, 76-78, 81, 82, 84, 86, 88-93.

46. Rodriguez-Lainz A eta al: Papillomatous digital dermatitis in 458 dairies, *J Am Vet Med Assoc* 209:1464-1464, 1996.

47. Wells SJ et al: Papillomatous digital dermatitis on U.S. dairy operations (footwarts), *National Animal Health Monitoring System (NAHMS)*, 1997, pp 1-28.

48. Read DH, Walker RL: Papillomatous digital dermatitis of dairy cattle in California: clinical characteristics, *Proceedings of the Eighth International Symposium of Disorders of the Ruminant Digit*, Banff, Canada, 1994, pp 159-163.

49. Read DH, Walker RL: Papillomatous digital dermatitis (footwarts) in California dairy cattle: clinical and gross pathologic findings, *J Vet Diagn Invest* 10:67-76, 1998.

50. Brizzi A: Bovine digital dermatitis, *Bovine Pract* 27:33-37, 1993.

51. Mortellaro CM: Digital dermatitis, *Proceedings of the Eighth International Symposium of Disorders of the Ruminant Digit*, Banff, Canada, 1994, pp 137-141.

52. Blowey RW: Interdigital causes of lameness, *Proceedings of the Eighth International Symposium of Disorders of the Ruminant Digit*, Banff, Canada, 1994, pp 142-154.

53. Blowey RW, Sharp MW: Digital dermatitis in dairy cattle, *Vet Rec* 122:505-508, 1988.

54. Gourreau JM, Scott DW, Rousseau JF: La Dermatite digitee des bovins (bovine digital dermatitis), *Le Pointe Vet* 24:49-57, 1992.

55. Van Amstel SR, Van Vuuren S, Tutt CLC: Digital dermatitis: report of an outbreak, *J S Afr Vet Assoc* 66:177-181, 1995.

56. Frankena K et al: Prevalence of lameness and risk indicators for dermatitis digitalis (Mortellaro disease) during pasturing and housing of dairy cattle, *Proceedings of the Society of Veterinary Epidemiology and Preventive Medicine*, London, UK, 1991, pp 107-118.

57. McLennan MW, McKenzie RA: Digital dermatitis in a Friesian cow, *Aust Vet J* 74:314-315, 1996.

58. Walker RL et al: Humoral response of dairy cattle to spirochetes isolated from papillomatous digital dermatitis lesions, *Am J Vet Res* 58:744-748, 1997.

59. Wells SJ, Garber LP, Wagner BA: Papillomatous digital dermatitis and associated risk factors in US dairy herds, *Prev Vet Med* 38:11-24, 1999.

60. Read D, Walker R: Experimental transmission of papillomatous digital dermatitis (footwarts) in cattle, *Vet Pathol* 33:607-607, 1996 (abstract).

61. Read DH:. Pathogenesis of experimental papillomatous digital dermatitis (PDD) in cattle: bacterial morphotypes associated with early lesion development, *Proceedings of the Seventy-eighth Conference of Research Workers on Animal Disease*, 1997, p 78.

62. Blowey RW et al: *Borrelia burgdorferi* infections in UK cattle: a possible association with digital dermatitis, *Vet Rec* 135:577-578, 1994.

63. Borgmann IE, Bailey J, Clark EG: Spirochete-associated bovine digital dermatitis, *Can Vet J* 37:35-37, 1996.

64. Choi BK et al: Spirochetes from digital dermatitis lesions in cattle are closely related to treponemes associated with human periodontitis, *Intl J Systematic Bacteriol* 47:175-181, 1997.

65. Collighan RJ, Woodward MJ: Spirochaetes and other bacterial species associated with bovine digital dermatitis, *FEMS Microbiol Lett* 156:37-41, 1997.

66. Demirkan I et al: The frequent detection of a treponeme in bovine digital dermatitis by immunocytochemistry and polymerase chain reaction, *Vet Microbiol* 60:285-292, 1998.

67. Demirkan I et al: Serological evidence of spirochaetal infections associated with digital dermatitis in dairy cattle, *Vet J* 157:69-77, 1999.

68. Doherty ML et al: Severe foot lameness in cattle associated with invasive spirochetes, *Irish Vet J* 51:195, 1998.

69. Döpfer D et al: Histological and bacteriological evaluation of digital dermatitis in cattle, with special reference to spirochaetes and *Campylobacter fecalis*, *Vet Rec* 140:620-623, 1997.

70. Ohya T et al: Isolation of *Campylobacter sputorum* from lesions of papillomatous digital dermatitis in dairy cattle, *Vet Rec* 145:316-318, 1999.

71. Read DH et al: An invasive spirochaete associated with interdigital papillomatosis of dairy cattle, *Vet Rec* 130:59-60, 1992.

72. Walker RL et al: Spirochetes isolated from dairy cattle with papillomatous digital dermatitis and interdigital dermatitis, *Vet Microbiol* 47:343-355, 1995.

73. Rodriguez-Lainz A et al: Case-control study of papillomatous digital dermatitis in Southern California dairy farms, *Prev Vet Med* 28:117-131, 1996.

74. Rodriguez-Lainz A et al: Farm- and host-level risk factors for papillomatous digital dermatitis in Chilean dairy cattle, *Prev Vet Med* 42:87-97, 1999.

75. Zemljic B: Current investigations into the cause of dermatitis digitalis in cattle, *Proceedings of the Eighth International Symposium on Disorders of the Ruminant Digit*, Banff, Canada, 1994, pp 164-167.

76. Berry SL et al: The efficacy of *Serpens* spp bacterin combined with topical administration of lincomycin hydrochloride for treatment of papillomatous digital dermatitis (footwarts) in cows on a dairy in California, *Bovine Pract* 33:6-11, 1999.

77. Berry SL, Read DH, Walker RL: Topical treatment with oxytetracycline or lincomycin HCl for papillomatous digital dermatitis: gross and histological evaluation, *Proceedings of the Tenth International Symposium on Lameness in Ruminants*, Lucerne, Switzerland, 291-292, 1998.

78. Berry SL, Maas J, Reed BA, Schechter A: The efficacy of 5 topical spray treatments for control of papillomatous digital dermatitis in dairy herds, *Proceedings of the Twenty-ninth Annual Convention of the American Association of Bovine Practitioners*, 1996, p 188.

79. Berry SL, Maas J: Clinical treatment of papillomatous digital dermatitis (footwarts) on dairy cattle, *Proceedings of the 1997 Hoof Health Conference*, Batavia, New York, 1997, pp 4-7.

80. Berry SL, Read DH, Walker RL: Recurrence of papillomatous digital dermatitis (footwarts) in dairy cows after treatment with lincomycin HCl or oxytetracycline HCl, *J Dairy Sci* 82:34, 1999.

81. Britt JS et al: Comparison of topical application of three products for treatment of papillomatous digital dermatitis in dairy cattle, *J Am Vet Med Assoc* 209:1134-1136, 1996.

82. Britt JS, McClure J: Field trials with antibiotic and non-antibiotic treatments for papillomatous digital dermatitis, *Bov Pract* 32:25-28, 1998.

83. Graham PD: A survey of digital dermatitis treatment regimes used by veterinarians in England and Wales, *Proceedings of the Eighth International Symposium of Disorders of the Ruminant Digit*, Banff, Canada, 1994, pp 205-206.

84. Guard C: Recognizing and managing infectious causes of lameness in cattle, *Proceedings of the Twenty-seventh Annual Convention of the American Association of Bovine Practice*, 1995, pp 80-82.

85. Guterbock W, Borelli C: Footwart treatment trial report, *West Dairyman* 76:17, 1995.

86. Hernandez J, Shearer JK, Elliott JB: Comparison of topical application of oxytetracycline and four nonantibiotic solutions for treatment of papillomatous digital dermatitis in dairy cows, *J Am Vet Med Assoc* 214:688-690, 1999.

87. Deed B et al: Comparison of 5 topical spray treatments for control of digital dermatitis in dairy herds, *J Dairy Sci* 79:189-189, 1996.

88. Shearer JK, Elliott JB: Preliminary results from a spray application of oxytetracycline to treat, control, and prevent digital dermatitis in dairy herds, *Proceedings of the Eighth International Symposium on Disorders of the Ruminant Digit*, Banff, Canada, 1994, p 182.

89. Shearer JK, Elliott JB: Papillomatous digital dermatitis: treatment and control strategies. I, *Compend Cont Educ Pract Vet* 20:S158-S173, 1998.

90. Shearer JK, Hernandez J, Elliot JB: Papillomatous digital dermatitis: treatment and control strategies. II, *Compend Cont Educ Pract Vet* 20:S213-S223, 1998.

91. Berry SL: Footwarts: what do we know about the epidemiology and treatment? *Proceedings of the 1999 Hoof Health Conference*, Modesto, Calif, 1999, pp 41-44.

92. Shearer JK, Elliott JB, Injoque RE: Control of digital dermatitis in dairy herds using a topical spray application of oxytetracycline, *J Dairy Sci* 78:170, 1995.

93. Shearer JK et al: Effect of oxytetracycline topical spray treatment on prevalence of digital dermatitis, *J Dairy Sci* 78:257, 1995.

94. Blowey RW: Studies on the pathogenesis and control of digital dermatitis, *Proceedings of the Eighth International Symposium on Disorders of the Ruminant Digit*, Banff, Canada, 1994 pp 168-173.

95. Britt JS et al: Antibiotic residues in milk samples obtained from cows after treatment for papillomatous digital dermatitis, *J Am Vet Med Assoc* 215:833-836, 1999.

96. Bergsten C: Identifying diseases of the bovine foot and their causes, *Proceedings of the 1999 Hoof Health Conference*, Modesto, Calif, 1999 pp 28-33.

97. Read DH, Walker RL: Papillomatous digital dermatitis and associated lesions of dairy cattle in California: pathologic findings, *Proceedings of the 8th International Symposium on Disorders of the Ruminant Digit*, Banff, Canada, 1994 pp 156-158.

VIRAL DISEASES

BRADFORD P. SMITH

PAPILLOMATOSIS (Warts, Fibropapillomas)

DEFINITION AND ETIOLOGY. Cutaneous papillomas or warts occur (in decreasing order of frequency) in cattle, horses, goats, and sheep. The growths usually occur in young animals (also on teats of mature cattle and goats) and are white, tan, or gray, firm, harmless protruding masses with a dry, horny surface. They vary in size from 1 to 500 mm and may be single or multiple. Species-specific papilloma viruses (subgroup of papova virus) are responsible for causing warts. There is some evidence that the bovine papilloma virus (BPV) genome is found in naturally occurring equine sarcoids. There are at least six BPV strains, designated BPV-1 through BPV-6 (Table 38-1),[98] and there are probably many more. Only one strain of virus is recognized in horses, goats, and sheep, but little research on papillomas has been done in these species, and two horse and two goat strains are likely.

TABLE 38-1

Distribution and Appearance of Bovine Warts by Type of Virus[98]

Virus Strain	Usual Site	Appearance	Comments
BPV-1	Nose, teats, glans penis	Filamentous or frondlike	Can prevent breeding when on penis
BPV-2	Head, neck, brisket, occasionally alimentary tract	Pedunculated or broad-based mass	Most common typical warts
BPV-3	Atypical warts, head, neck, possibly interdigital*	Nonpedunculated protruding growths, delicate fronds with hair between	Persist for years
BPV-4	Alimentary tract, urinary bladder	Pedunculated mass	See Chapters 30 and 32
BPV-5	Teat	Smooth, white	Persist for years; other types may also occur on teats
BPV-6	Teat	Round and either flat or frondlike	Similar in appearance to BPV-1 when frondlike

BPV, Bovine papilloma virus.
*Suspected, but BPV-3 not yet isolated from interdigital warts. Some authors speculate that interdigital warts may be caused by yet another new BPV strain.

CLINICAL SIGNS. Warts are usually small, benign growths that appear on young animals under 2 years of age, persist for 3 to 12 months, and then spontaneously regress without causing clinical signs (other than a blemish). In cattle, warts on the teats, penis, or interdigital skin[99] or in the alimentary tract may produce clinical signs of pain or occlusion. Warts commonly develop in the ears of young cattle following tagging or tattooing, especially if instruments are not disinfected between individuals. They are not age related. Teat warts also predispose to environmental mastitis. Occasionally individuals with defective cellular immunity may develop multiple extremely large warts that may result in weight loss.

In horses, warts on the face are rather common (Fig. 38-8) but rarely cause a significant problem. The equine sarcoid is much more likely to cause clinical signs.

Warts are relatively rare in goats. They occur mainly on teats and may spread throughout the herd. One herd outbreak involving the head, neck, shoulders, and forelegs was seen in milking goats.[100] Adult Saanens develop persistent mammary gland warts that may undergo transformation to become squamous cell carcinomas.[101] There are probably at least two different strains of goat papilloma virus (head/neck and mammary forms).

Warts are rare in sheep, but they may occur on the face or legs. Differential diagnosis in sheep and goats includes contagious ecthyma, ulcerative dermatosis, strawberry footrot, and sheep and goat pox.

TREATMENT AND CONTROL. Small warts can be crushed, pinched off, or surgically removed. Cryosurgery can be used on larger warts. Many regress spontaneously within a few months, even without treatment.

When show animals are involved or when animals have multiple large papillomas, tissue can be removed and made into crude autogenous vaccine (2 ml intradermally 3 times at weekly intervals) by homogenizing, grinding, freeze-thawing twice, filtering, and killing virus with 0.5% formalin. Autogenous wart vaccines are sometimes very effective,[102] but failures have also been reported.[103] Autogenous vaccines are capable of preventing new lesions caused by the same BPV strain in a herd. Commercial wart vaccines for cattle rarely seem to effectively result in regression of existing warts, but they may be capable of preventing the development of new lesions if the same BPV strain is involved. There is no indication that cattle vaccines have any efficacy in other species. No wart vaccines for horses, sheep, or goats are currently marketed.

Because the viruses can be directly or fomite transmitted, prevention involves isolation; preventing animals from rubbing on each other; and not sharing halters, brushes, and other equipment. Dipping of dehorning, tagging, and tattooing instruments in a viricidal solution between animals will also slow spread of the virus.

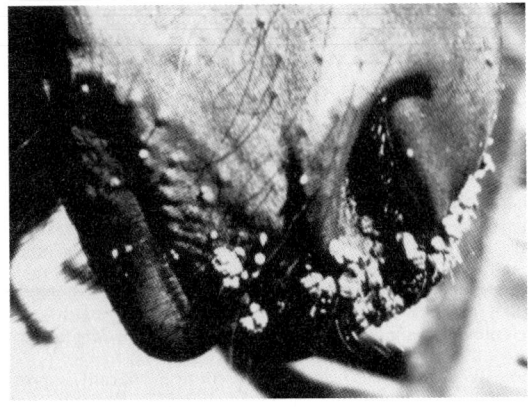

FIG. 38-8 Typical warts (papillomas) on the nose of a yearling horse.

REFERENCES

98. Hunt E: Infectious skin diseases of cattle, *Vet Clin North Am (Large Anim Pract)* 6:163-167, 1984.
99. Rebhun WC: Interdigital papillomatosis in dairy cattle, *J Am Vet Med Assoc* 177:437-440, 1980.
100. Davis CL, Kemper HE: Warts in goats, *J Am Vet Med Assoc* 88:175-179, 1936.
101. Smith MC: Caprine dermatologic problems: a review, *J Am Vet Med Assoc* 178:724-729, 1981.
102. Olson C, Robl MG, Larson, LL: Cutaneous and penile bovine fibropapillomatosis, *J Am Vet Med Assoc* 153:1189-1194, 1968.
103. Barthold SW et al: Atypical warts in cattle, *J Am Vet Med Assoc* 165:276-280, 1974.

AURAL PLAQUES

Aural plaques are gray-to-white keratinous crusts that occur on the inner surface of the pinna of the ear of horses (Fig. 38-9). They do not appear to cause discomfort to the horse, although they persist indefinitely. The etiology of the lesions is unknown, but it appears that they may be caused by a variant of the equine papilloma virus.[104] The condition is common in both sexes and all breeds. The crust can be dislodged, revealing a pink nonulcerated base. No effective treatment has been found.

REFERENCE

104. Scott DW: *Large animal dermatology*, Philadelphia, 1988, WB Saunders.

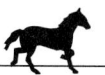

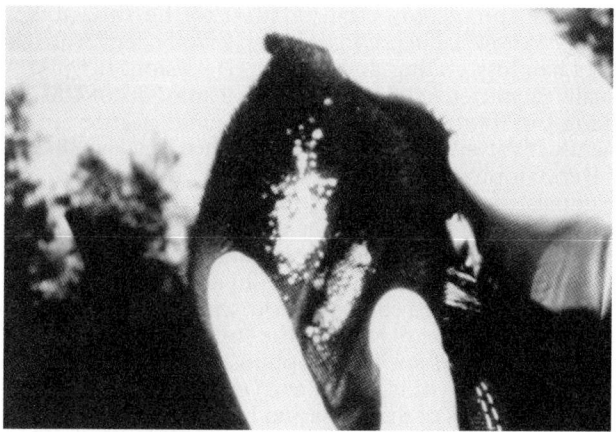

FIG. 38-9 ▍▍ Aural plaques on the inner surface of the pinna of the ear in a horse.

PSEUDOCOWPOX

Pseudocowpox is a common parapox virus of cattle related to the viruses of contagious ecthyma (soremouth) of sheep and goats and bovine papular stomatitis (see Chapter 30 for these diseases). All three parapox viruses may cause nodular lesions on humans. The lesions of pseudocowpox are usually confined to the teats of cattle and the disease is common worldwide. Cyclic waves of reinfection occur in a herd, where it causes minor teat lesions characterized initially by a small papule 2- to 3-mm in diameter, followed by crusting and circular spread of the lesion. Approximately 10 days later the 15- to 20-mm lesion appears as a ring or horseshoe-shaped scab.[105] Lesions occasionally involve the udder, medial thighs, or scrotum. Deep ulceration is rare. The major problem associated with the teat lesions is an increased incidence of mastitis. The most important and common differential diagnoses are bovine herpes mammillitis and papillomatosis. Rare viruses involving the teat include vaccinia, cowpox, and horsepox.[105] Cowpox is a rare disease of cattle in Europe that causes ulcers and that may also produce lesions in humans.

REFERENCE

105. Gibbs EPJ: Viral diseases of the skin of bovine teat and udder, *Vet Clin North Am (Large Anim Pract)* 6:187-202, 1984.

BOVINE HERPES MAMMILLITIS (Bovine Herpes II Virus, Bovine Ulcerative Mammillitis)

Bovine mammillitis teat lesions are caused by bovine herpes virus II, which is widely disseminated in most cattle populations.[106] The disease may be epidemic or endemic. The virus may also cause oral lesions, udder lesions, or generalized skin disease in cattle. The teat lesions start as swollen, edematous teats that are tender. Vesicles may appear in some lesions, whereas others ulcerate almost immediately. The teats become painful, and ulcers require 3 to 10 weeks to heal.[106] Mastitis is increased because the scabs on the teats are laden with bacteria. Therapy consists of segregation of affected animals from the rest of the herd, and affected cows should be milked last. Handwashing between cows should be practiced by milkers. In severe cases, secondary infection may be controlled by topical antibiotic creams or parenteral antibiotics, with proper residue avoidance precautions in place.

REFERENCE

106. Gibbs EPJ: Viral diseases of the skin of bovine teat and udder, *Vet Clin North Am (Large Anim Pract)* 6:187-202, 1984.

SHEEPPOX AND GOATPOX

Sheeppox and goatpox are caused by capripoxviruses.[107] Both occur in Africa, Asia, and the Middle East; goatpox also occurs in parts of Europe and the United States. The two diseases are clinically similar, except that sheeppox has the most severe systemic signs of the animal pox diseases. The diseases affect all ages, causing pyrexia, anorexia, conjunctivitis, rhinitis, and skin lesions. Morbidity is high. Mortality may reach 80% with sheeppox, but usually is low with goatpox. Humans may develop skin lesions from goatpox.

REFERENCE

107. Scott DW: *Large animal dermatology*, Philadelphia, 1988, WB Saunders, pp 97-100.

MYCOTIC DISEASES

ANTHONY A. STANNARD
STEPHEN D. WHITE

DERMATOPHYTOSIS

Dermatophytosis refers to infections of the keratinized tissues of the skin (the horny cell layer of the epidermis, hairs, and potentially the nails, hoof, and horns) by *Microsporum* and *Trichophyton* spp. Dermatomycosis is a more general term simply referring to fungal infections of the skin.

ETIOLOGY AND PATHOGENESIS. Although several genera are involved in the production of dermatophytosis, the vast majority of lesions are caused by either *Microsporum* or *Trichophyton* spp.

In the horse the most common agent involved is *Trichophyton equinum*. To a lesser extent, *Trichophyton mentagrophytes*, *Microsporum gypsum*, *Microsporum equinum*, and *Microsporum canis* are implicated. Because *M. equinum* has only recently been recognized as a unique species distinctive from *Microsporum canis*, the relative prevalence of those two species in the horse is not known. In ruminants the vast majority of dermatophytosis lesions are caused by a single species, *Trichophyton verrucosum*. The transmission of the disease is usually from animal by direct contact or indirectly through fomites such as grooming instruments, tack, housing, fencing, or feed bunks. The incubation period may range from 1 to 6 weeks. In animals, invasion of the hair shafts is far more common than involvement of the epidermal horny cell layer; the opposite is true in humans.

Several factors influence the susceptibility of an animal to dermatophyte infection. Probably the most important is the age of the animal, with young animals being far more susceptible to infection. The susceptibility of young animals is probably related to lack of prior exposure/infection and thus no immunity. Other factors that may be operative on occasion are crowding together of young animals and conditions that decrease resistance to infection such as poor nutrition, concurrent disease, and the prior use of immunosuppressive drugs. Environmental factors may also play a role because the prevalence of the disease is increased in hot, humid climates. Calves kept indoors or exposed to foggy weather with little or no sunlight have an increased incidence.

Under normal circumstances, dermatophytes only invade fully keratinized nonliving tissues.[108] Thus the only clinical sign of their presence is alopecia, which results from breaking of the weakened hair shafts. For inflammation to occur, the fungi must elaborate some soluble substances that reach the dermal vasculature and act either as irritants (toxins) or on occasion as allergens.

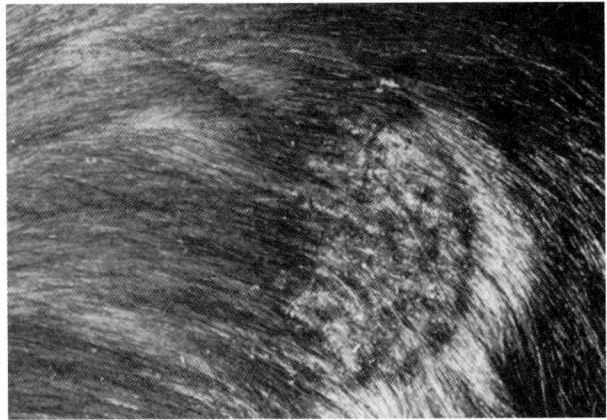

FIG. 38-10 ■ Ringworm lesion in flank area of a horse (*Tricophyton* spp).

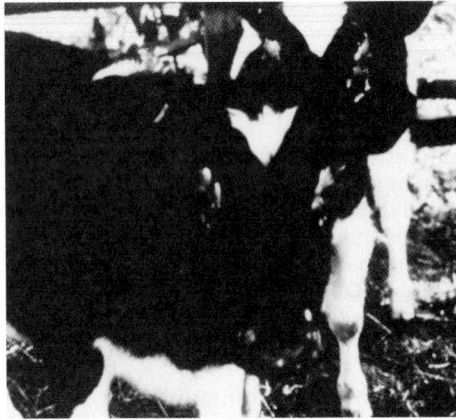

FIG. 38-11 ■ Ringworm lesions around the eyes of two calves, caused by *Tricophyton verrucosum*.

In most instances, dermatophytosis is a self-limiting disease, with the duration of infection ranging from 1 to 4 months. The spontaneous regression is probably at least partly related to the development of immunity, of which cell-mediated immunity is thought to be the most important. The immunity that develops is probably not complete, and its duration is unknown.

CLINICAL FEATURES. A variety of dermatoses characterized by alopecia or scaling and crusting are sometimes erroneously ascribed to dermatophyte infections. Dermatophytosis is relatively common in the horse and in cattle (Figs. 38-10 and 38-11) and relatively rare in sheep and goats.[109] The primary clinical characteristic of dermatophytosis is the multifocal nature of the lesions. Except initially, dermatophytosis is rarely manifested as a single solitary lesion; and, except under very unusual circumstances, generalized body involvement is also very rare. In addition to the multifocal nature of the disease, the individual lesions usually vary considerably in size. The primary changes that are observed clinically are alopecia, scaling, and crusting.

The degree of associated pruritus varies, but pruritus is usually either mild or absent. Frank clinical evidence of inflammation such as erythema is usually absent or obscured by pigmented skin. In horses and cattle, lesions are usually located on the head, neck, shoulders, and sides of the thorax. Rarely in the horse, dermatophytoses may be limited to the posterior aspect of the pastern region. In the horse the initial manifestation of the disease may be urticaria-like, with the hairs in the affected areas standing erect. This may be fol-

lowed by some serum transudation to the surface. Very quickly, however, the lesions develop sharply demarcated areas of hair loss, scaling, and crusting. The lesions in cattle are usually characterized by very excessive amounts of crusting, taking on an almost wartlike appearance. Cattle are frequently involved around the eyes and face (see Fig. 38-11).

Dermatophytosis must be considered in the differential diagnosis of any dermatoses characterized by multifocal alopecia or scaling and crusting. In the case of multifocal areas of alopecia without any scaling and crusting, diseases of the hair follicle such as telogen effluvium must be considered. In the case of a solitary lesion, the "flat sarcoid" is the primary differential diagnosis. The two most important differential diagnoses are dermatophilosis and pemphigus foliaceus. Alopecia or scaling and crusting involving the long-haired areas of the mane and tail are rarely involved.

DIAGNOSIS IN ITS MOST TYPICAL FORM. Direct microscopic examination of infected hairs is of value, but in general the most commonly used and most reliable method of diagnosing dermatophytosis is the use of fungal cultures (see Chapter 11 for techniques). Broken hairs at the periphery of lesions are most satisfactory for this purpose. Large crusts and areas of separation should be avoided. The use of specialized indicator media is preferred. On occasion, dermatophytosis is diagnosed histopathologically.

CLINICAL MANAGEMENT. Because dermatophytosis is a spontaneously regressing disease, controlled studies on the efficacy of therapeutic agents are difficult to obtain. Nevertheless, fungistatic and fungicidal products are widely used topically to decrease the spread of the disease. Topical therapy is generally curative. In the United States the most common treatment is to sponge the horse's tack with 50% captan (2 Tbs of the powder form in 1 gallon of water) 1 to 2 times per week for either 1 month or until 2 weeks after clinical cure. Miconazole shampoos may be practical for small areas. Alternatively, 20% NaI may be given (250 ml/500 kg horse IV every 7 days, 1 to 2 times). This is contraindicated in pregnant mares because it may cause abortion. In Europe and Canada an enilconazole rinse (Imaveral) is highly effective. Griseofulvin's efficacy in horses (as well as an effective dose) has not been convincingly demonstrated. However, a dosage of 100 mg/kg daily for 7 days has been advocated. Vaccination to *T. equinum* may reduce the incidence of new infections and protect a high percentage (>80%) of vaccinates from infection. This data is based on results with an inactivated vaccine containing both conidia and mycelial elements.

REFERENCES
108. Stannard AA: *Syllabus for veterinary dermatology*, Davis, Calif, 1988, University of California.
109. Scott DW: *Large animal dermatology*, Philadelphia, 1988, WB Saunders, pp 172-182.

MYCETOMAS AND ZYGOMYCOSIS (Phycomycosis, Fungal Tumors, Swamp Cancer, Gulf Coast Fungus, Florida Horse Leech, Bursattee)

BRADFORD P. SMITH

Mycetomas and phycomycosis are terms that denote subcutaneous fungal or actinomycotic infections. They occur most commonly in tropical areas and are caused by a variety of fungal agents or by members of the bacterial genera *Actinomyces*, *Nocardia*, and *Actinobacillus*.[110] The lesions are usually

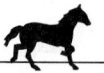

localized on the limbs, abdomen, neck, or head (including nasal cavity, lips, and trachea) and are characterized by granulation tissue, necrotic draining tracts, and pruritus. It is believed that the fungus invades through a break in the skin. Biopsy material contains diagnostic fungal hyphae. Fungi can also be isolated on Sabouraud's dextrose agar. Mixed infections with cutaneous habronemiasis are common.

Intravenous therapy with amphotericin B in conjunction with surgical debridement is most effective, starting with a total daily dose of 150 mg of amphotericin B given intravenously in 1 L of 5% dextrose. The dose is increased by 50 mg every 2 days until a maximum of 400 mg/day is given for up to 30 days.[110] Amphotericin B is nephrotoxic, and kidney function must be monitored. Oral potassium iodide (20 g/day) is also recommended. Ketoconazole therapy may be less toxic than amphotericin B. Topical therapy with etisazole in dimethyl sulfoxide (DMSO) or amphotericin B in DMSO has been reported to be effective.

REFERENCE

110. Blackford J: Superficial and deep mycoses in horses, *Vet Clin North Am (Large Anim Pract)* 6:47-58.

SPOROTRICHOSIS

BRADFORD P. SMITH

Sporotrichum schenckii is a yeastlike fungus that causes a sporadic infection (usually chronic) of the skin and lymphatics.[111] Other tissues are rarely involved. Horses are most frequently affected. The organism is a ubiquitous saprophyte that enters through wounds or thorn punctures. It is most common in warm, moist climates. Hard nodules 1 to 5 cm in diameter form, often in lines along lymphatics; these may ulcerate and discharge a creamy exudate and become encrusted. Diagnosis is by culture on Sabouraud's dextrose agar and biopsy for histopathology. Treatment is often effective. Sodium iodide 40 mg/kg IV as 20% solution for 2 to 5 days, followed by orally administered organic iodides, such as ethylenediamine dihydroiodide, or potassium iodide (either is given at 2 mg/kg PO daily for up to 60 days).[112] Systemic iodides may cause abortion in pregnant mares and cows.

REFERENCES

111. Blackford J: Superficial and deep mycoses in horses, *Vet Clin North Am (Large Anim Pract)* 6:47-58, 1984.
112. Scott DW: *Large animal dermatology,* Philadelphia, 1988, WB Saunders, pp 188-190.

PARASITIC SKIN DISEASES

STEPHEN D. WHITE
ANNE G. EVANS

PEDICULOSIS

Lice are obligatory ectoparasites that are generally host specific. Adults and nymphs are seldom able to live more than a few days away from their host. Large domestic animals suffer from infestation with several species of lice that belong to the orders *Mallophaga* sp., the biting lice, and *Anoplura* sp., the sucking lice (Table 38-2).[113]

Clinical infestations are most apparent during the winter months and reflect efficient louse reproduction during the late fall and the fact that summertime temperatures on body areas exposed to sunlight are too high for lice. Apparent "car-

TABLE 38-2

Lice Associated With Large Domestic Animals[113]

Host	Mallophaga (Biting)	Anoplura (Sucking)
Horse	Bovicola (Damalinia) equi	Haematopinus asini
Cattle	Bovicola (Damalinia) bovis	Haematopinus eurysternus
		Haematopinus quadripertusus
		Haematopinus tuberculatus
		Linognathus vituli
		Solenopotes capillatus
Goats	Bovicola (Damalinia) caprae	Linognathus stenopsis
	Bovicola (Damalinia) limbatus	Linognathus africanus
	Bovicola (Damalinia) crassipes	Linognathus vituli
Sheep	Bovicola (Damalinia) ovis	Linognathus pedalis
	Bovicola (Damalinia) capre	Linognathus ovillus
		Linognathus africanus

rier" animals within a herd maintain populations during the "off" season and serve as a source for reinfestation of the herd during the fall.[113] The hallmark of infestation is pruritus, and many of the clinical changes are secondary to self trauma. The neck and tail are typically affected first,[114] but infestation and symptoms may become generalized. The coat becomes dry and scaly. There is patchy alopecia and crusted ulcerations resulting from excoriation. A heavily infested animal may become anemic. Significant hide damage occurs as a result of excoriation, and hairballs may accumulate in the gastrointestinal tract from self-grooming. Reduced productivity and weight loss result from decreased feed intake associated with restlessness.

There are several possible therapeutic approaches. Application of an appropriate topical insecticide to infested animals and to all contact animals at 2-week intervals for two to three treatments is curative. Repetition of treatment is necessary to break the louse life cycle because eggs are not killed by insecticides and will hatch despite therapy. Effective topical agents include coumaphos, crotoxyphos, malathion, pyrethrins, methoxychlor, and lindane.[115] Few pesticides are licensed for use on the goat, but some have been recommended for controlling lice in adult goats; these pesticides include rotenone or flea powders approved for use in cats, dichlorvos-impregnated flea collars on clipped animals, and sprays or dips of coumaphos, crotoxyphos, and crotoxyphos-dichlorvos.[116] The organophosphate compounds (malathion, toxaphene, and methoxychlor) must be used with caution and should never be used on lactating dairy goats. Blankets, brushes, and rope halters are soaked in boiling water; and leather articles, including saddles, can be rubbed with the pesticide solution. Articles should be retreated in 2 weeks. Ivermectin is said to be effective given orally at 0.2 mg/kg twice over a 2-week interval to treat lice on horses.[117] Ivermectin may be administered subcutaneously to ruminants at 0.2 mg/kg at 2-week intervals for treatment of the sucking lice *Haematopinus eurysternus* and *Linognathus vituli*.[118]

REFERENCES

113. Butler JF: Lice affecting livestock. In Williams RE et al, eds: *Livestock entomology,* New York, 1985, Wiley-Interscience, pp 101-127.
114. Loomis EC: Common ectoparasites and their control. In Robinson NE, ed: *Current therapy in equine medicine,* ed 1, vol 6, Philadelphia, 1983, WB Saunders, pp 529-533.
115. Fadok YA: Parasitic skin diseases of large animals, *Vet Clin North Am (Large Anim Pract)* 6:3-26, 1984.
116. Manning TO, Scott DW: Caprine dermatology. III. Parasitic, allergic, hormonal, and neoplastic disorders, *Compend Cont Educ Pract Vet* 7: S437-S452, 1985.
117. Fadock VA: Ectoparasites. In Robinson NE, ed: *Current therapy in equine medicine,* ed 2, Philadelphia, 1987, WB Saunders, pp 622-624.

118. Campbell WC, Benz GW: Ivermectin: a review of efficacy and safety, *J Vet Pharmacol Ther* 7:1-16, 1984.

ACARIASIS

Trombiculidiasis

Trombiculidiasis is caused by the larval stages of several species of mites commonly known as "harvest mites" or "chiggers." Important species that infest horses and other large animals include *Eutrombicula alfreddugesi* and *Trombicula* species. The adults and nymphs are free living. As the larvae feed on their hosts, they secrete substances in their saliva that hydrolyze the epidermis and allow extraction of tissue fluids. Infestation is recognized most commonly during the late summer and early fall in pastured animals or in animals that have been taken through infested fields or wooded areas.[119,120]

The clinical symptoms associated with trombiculidiasis include a crusted papular eruption on the face, neck, extremities, and thorax. Pruritus is variable.[119] Diagnosis may be made early in the course of infestation by careful inspection and finding the minute, red larvae in the center of a papule. The six-legged larvae have round bodies and may be identified specifically on skin scrapings.[121] Trombiculid larvae only remain on the animal host for several days, but clinical symptoms may persist longer. Thus trombiculidiasis should be suspected even in the absence of mites in an animal with appropriate symptoms in the summer and fall.

Because the larvae remain on the host for only a short period, the disorder is self-limiting. Reinfestation is possible if the animal remains in an infested pasture. Topical applications of 5% lime sulfur may be beneficial in eliminating mites still present on the host.[120] Coumaphos, dioxathion, malathion, and toxaphene are also effective.[122]

Psoroptic Mange

Psoroptic mange has been recognized in all the large domestic species. It is common in cattle and is recognized in goats, but it has been eradicated from horses and sheep in the United States. The mites are relatively host specific and contagious among members of the same species, but they do not affect people. *Psoroptes ovis* infests cattle and sheep, and *Psoroptes equi* infests horses.[123] *Psoroptes cunniculi*, the rabbit ear mite, also infests goats.[120] The mites have a 2-week life cycle on their host but can live away from the host for up to 3 weeks. *Psoroptes* spp. live on the surface of the epidermis and do not burrow. Symptomatic infestation tends to be more prevalent during the cooler months.[120]

The hallmark of infestation in all species is pruritus. In cattle, crusted papular lesions are typically first apparent on the withers but then generalize, resulting in weight loss, secondary infections, and decreased production.[124] Horses develop papules at the base of the mane and tail and under the forelock, with subsequent alopecia secondary to excoriation. Occasionally symptoms are limited to a pruritic otitis externa.[119] In sheep, typical lesions include papules and crusts in wooled areas. The intense pruritus can be debilitating. Goats usually have lesions restricted to the ears, although infestation and symptoms may spread to the neck and body.[120] Diagnosis is based on demonstrating mites in skin scrapings and ear swabs from affected animals. Psoroptic mites are recognized by their round bodies and long, segmented pedicles.[121]

Several topical insecticides have been recommended for treatment and should be applied to all affected and contact animals at 5- to 7-day intervals at least twice. These include lindane, coumaphos, diazinon, malathion, toxaphene, and lime sulfur.[120,122,125] The contaminated environment should also be treated. Ivermectin is approved for treatment of *P. ovis* in cattle at a dose of 0.2 mg/kg administered subcutaneously,[126] but treatment does not immediately eliminate live mites from infested cattle. It has been recommended that *P. ovis*-infested cattle be isolated for a minimum of 14 days after treatment to prevent transmission to susceptible contact cattle.[125] Psoroptic mange is a reportable disease.

Chorioptic Mange

Chorioptic mange, also known as foot or leg mange, is common in cattle and sheep, uncommon in goats and is seen with variable frequency in horses, dependent on geographical area. Draft horses may be more susceptible than other equids. The species are relatively host specific and include *Chorioptes bovis, Chorioptes ovis, Chorioptes equi*, and *Chorioptes capre*. The mites do not affect humans. They have a life cycle that spans 2 to 3 weeks and can only live off of the host for a few days.[120]

The primary symptom is extreme pruritus. Secondary lesions consisting of scaling, crusting, ulceration, and alopecia result from self-trauma. In cattle the lower aspects of the hindlimbs, the perineum (particularly the perianal fossa), tail, and scrotum are usually affected. Sheep typically demonstrate involvement of the lower limbs and scrotum. Goats have involvement of the lower limbs, hind quarters, and abdomen; and lesions in horses are typically restricted to the lower rear limbs, although they can progress up the limbs to involve the abdomen. In all species, infestation can become generalized.[120]

Mites are usually numerous and readily demonstrated with skin scrapings. They are distinguished from other mites by their rounded body, long legs, and short unsegmented pedicles.[121] It has been stated that mites may be found normally on cattle and sheep without accompanying clinical signs.[120] Chorioptic mange will respond to treatments described for psoroptic mange. In most cases, lesions and pruritus are mild, and the condition may be left untreated.

Sarcoptic Mange

Sarcoptic mange is an uncommon, contagious disease of horses, cattle, sheep, and goats. The etiologic agent is *Sarcoptes scabeii*. There are several species variations that are relatively host specific but capable of being transmitted to humans. The mite burrows in the epidermis where the egg is deposited, and its life cycle is complete in 10 to 17 days. Transmission is usually by direct contact; but the mite has a variable survival time off the host; therefore environmental and fomite transmission are possible.[120]

The hallmark of infestation is pruritus. There is often an associated papular eruption. Other lesions, including scaling, crusting, ulceration, and alopecia, are all secondary to self-trauma. The head (especially the ears) and neck are usually the initial areas of involvement, although lesions generalize.[119] Sheep tend to have initial involvement of the non-wool areas. The ears should always be scraped for mites; the mite is identified by its rounded body, terminal anus, short legs, and long unsegmented pedicles.[121] Because mites may be present only in small numbers, negative skin scrapings do not rule out the disease. Diagnosis should be based on clinical suspicion and response to therapy.[119] Several topical insecticides have been recommended for treatment and are applied to all affected and contact animals at 10-day intervals for six treatments. These include lindane, coumaphos, diazinon, malathion, toxaphene, and lime sulfur.[120,122,125] Ivermectin is approved for treatment of sarcoptic mange in cattle at a dose of 0.2 mg/kg SC and repeated in 2 weeks.[126] The medication should be effective in other large animal species, but it is not approved for this purpose. The contaminated environment must also be treated. It is recommended

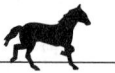

that the state regulatory agency for livestock disease control be consulted for methods of treatment and products to use.[120] Sarcoptic mange is a reportable disease.

Demodectic Mange

Demodectic mange is a rare disorder, although it has been recognized in all the large domestic species. The mites live in the hair follicles and sweat glands and are host specific. They are not contagious between members of the same species, but *Demodex* spp. are transmitted from mother to offspring during the first few days of life by direct contact with the dam. Little else is known regarding the life cycle of the mite.[120] Two species of *Demodex* are recognized in the horse.[127,128] *Demodex caballi* is a normal inhabitant of the pilosebaceous apparatus of the eyelids and muzzle and may be found in skin scrapings of these areas on horses in the absence of skin lesions. *Demodex equi* inhabits the pilosebaceous apparatus of the rest of the body and is the only one of the two species found on horses that has been associated with disease. The species found on cattle, sheep, and goats are *Demodex bovis*, *Demodex ovis*, and *Demodex caprae*, respectively.[120] Clinical signs are variable, depending on the species affected. Horses usually develop alopecia and scaling of the head, neck, and withers. Pruritus and secondary pyoderma are variable. Goats and cattle usually develop nodular lesions that involve the face, shoulder, and neck. In goats the nodular contents may be white and caseous; these nodules must be differentiated from *Corynebacterium pseudotuberculosis* abscesses by microscopic examination for mites. Sheep tend to develop periocular nodular lesions.[120] Diagnosis is based on recognizing mites with microscopic examination of skin scrapings or exudates obtained from nodular lesions. The mites are elongated and have short, stubby legs.[121]

No treatment has been proven to be effective in large animals.[120] Amitraz, currently used to treat canine generalized demodicosis, should not be used on horses. Horses sprayed with 0.025% amitraz developed somnolence, depression, ataxia, muscular weakness, and progressive large intestinal impaction.[129] In ruminants that have a limited number of nodular lesions, excision followed by applications of topical iodine solutions has been reported to be beneficial.[125] Spontaneous resolution may occur in all species.[120]

REFERENCES

119. Fadock VA: Ectoparasites. In Robinson NE, ed: *Current therapy in equine medicine*, ed 2, Philadelphia, 1987, WB Saunders, pp 622-624.
120. Fadock VA: Parasitic skin diseases of large animals, *Vet Clin North Am* 6:3-26, 1984.
121. Georgi JR: *Parasitology for veterinarians*, ed 4, Philadelphia, 1985, WB Saunders.
122. Loomis EC: Common ectoparasites and their control. In Robinson NE, ed: *Current therapy in equine medicine*, ed 1, Philadelphia, 1983, WB Saunders, pp 529-535.
123. Hall RD: Mites of veterinary importance. In Williams RE et al, eds: *Livestock entomology*, New York, 1985, Wiley-Interscience, pp 174-175.
124. Stromberg PC et al: Systematic pathologic responses in experimental *Psoroptes ovis* infestation in Hereford calves, *Am J Vet Res* 47:1326-1328.
125. Fraser CM: *Merck veterinary manual*, ed 6, Rahway, NJ, 1986, Merck, pp 784-788.
126. Campbell WC, Benz GW: Ivermectin: a review of efficacy and safety, *J Vet Pharmacol Ther* 7:1-16, 1984.
127. Bennison JC: Demodicosis of horses with particular reference to equine members of the genus *Demodex*, *J Royal Army Vet Corps* 14:34, 1943.
128. Scott DW: Demodicosis. In Robinson NE, ed: *Current therapy in equine medicine*, ed 2, Philadelphia, 1987, WB Saunders, pp 626-627.
129. Auer DE et al: Illness in horses following spraying with amitraz, *Aust Vet J* 61:247, 1984.

CULICOIDES HYPERSENSITIVITY

DEFINITION AND ETIOLOGY. *Culicoides* hypersensitivity (Queensland itch, equine sweet itch, kasen, dhobie itch) is an intensely pruritic dermatitis affecting horses that is recognized in many parts of the world. It is seen primarily in adult horses during the warmer months of the year. The tendency to develop *Culicoides* hypersensitivity may be inherited. The disorder is caused by a hypersensitivity reaction to the saliva of the small (1 to 4 mm), dorsally feeding, female *Culicoides* gnats (punkies, no-see-ums, biting midges).[130,131] The gnats possess piercing mouth parts specialized for blood feeding and attack humans, as well as livestock. *Culicoides* spp. are a problem primarily between April and November. Maximum feeding activity occurs on windless days in the morning and early evening hours, although midges may be a problem throughout the day when it is humid or overcast.[132] In general, *Culicoides* spp. breed in standing water as is found in lakes, marshes, swamps, and stagnant watering troughs. The midges are not capable of flying farther than 0.25 to 0.5 mile from their breeding areas.[133] Icelandic horses may have a higher incidence of allergic reactions to the *Culicoides* insects than other breeds.

CLINICAL SIGNS. *Culicoides* hypersensitivity tends to be a dorsally distributed, seasonal, pruritic dermatitis. It may become nonseasonal as the animal ages, particularly in areas where an ideal climate for midge activity exists year round. *Culicoides* hypersensitivity is rarely seen in horses less than 1 year of age. Lesions are primarily the result of self-trauma and include alopecia, crusting, and scaling; erythematous papules may be noted early in the course of the disease. The lesions have a dorsal distribution; the forehead, neck, withers, shoulder, rump, and tail are most severely affected (Fig. 38-12). Chronic excoriation results in marked lichenification and scarring. Mane and tail hairs are usually broken and matted as a result of self-trauma. *Culicoides* hypersensitivity varies in severity from horse to horse but tends to worsen with age. Diagnosis is based on seasonality, history of exposure, distribution of lesions, and response to therapy.

THERAPY. The most important aspect of therapy for *Culicoides* hypersensitivity is the reduction of insect exposure. This is most effectively achieved by moving the sensitized horse to a new area at least 0.5 mile from *Culicoides* breeding habitats such as ponds, marshes, and irrigation canals. Small breeding sources of stagnant water such as water troughs should be cleaned frequently. When the horse cannot be relocated, stabling during the peak feeding hours, primarily at dusk, is advisable, particularly when the humidity is high. The stall must be completely enclosed to prevent insect exposure and should be screened with a fine wire mesh that is sprayed frequently with insect repellents. Placing ceiling fans in barns can be helpful because increased air circulation discourages the insects.[133]

Frequent applications of insect repellents to the horse are necessary to further decrease *Culicoides* exposure. Products

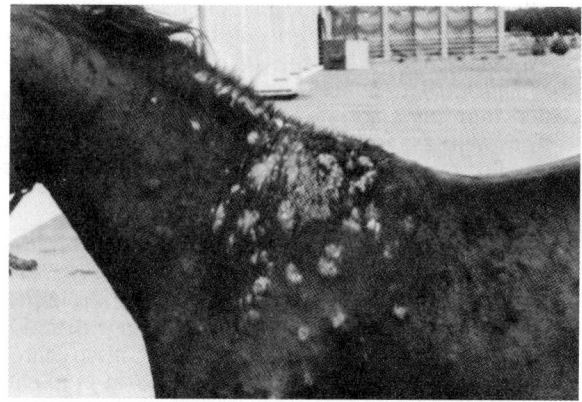

FIG. 38-12 ■ Severe *Culicoides* hypersensitivity in a horse, showing typical distribution of withers, shoulders, and head (not visible).

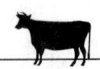

that contain pyrethrins with synergists and repellents are of most value and should be applied in the late afternoon before the insect's peak feeding time. Frequent bathing of affected regions help to decrease scale and crust formation and provide some relief from pruritus.[133]

Corticosteroid therapy is required for management of many horses with *Culicoides* hypersensitivity. Short-acting oral corticosteroids such as prednisone or prednisolone should initially be administered at a dose of 1 mg/kg/day until the horse is nonpruritic (usually 7 to 10 days). The dose is then slowly tapered and adjusted to the lowest alternate-morning dose that will control the clinical symptoms.

Hyposensitization is controversial; success may vary with the presence of an adjuvant.[134]

REFERENCES

130. Townley P, Baker KP, Quinn PJ: Preferential landing and engorging sites of *Culicoides* species landing on a horse in Ireland, *Equine Vet J* 16: 117-120, 1984.
131. Fadok VA, Greiner EC: Equine insect hypersensitivity: skin test and biopsy results correlated with clinical data, *Equine Vet J* 22:236-240, 1990.
132. Baker KP: The rational approach to the management of sweet itch, *Vet Ann* 18:163-167, 1978.
133. Fadok VA: Culicoides hypersensitivity. In Robinson NE, ed: *Current therapy in equine medicine*, ed 2, Philadelphia, 1987, WB Saunders, pp 624-626.
134. Anderson GS et al: Immunotherapy trial for horses in British Columbia with *Culicoides* hypersensitivity, *J Med Entomol* 33:458-466, 1996.

VENTRAL DERMATITIS OF HORSES

Single or multiple punctate ulcers with areas of alopecia, leukoderma, crusts, and thickened skin develop on the ventral thorax or abdomen of some horses as a result of fly or gnat bites.[135] Serum or blood exudation from the ulcers is usually present. Pruritus is variable, possibly reflecting the degree of hypersensitivity to fly salivary antigens. The lesions occur during the fly season and are most commonly seen in horses over 4 years of age. No breed predilection exists.

Treatment consists of diligent application of fly repellents around the lesions and topical application of antibiotic-corticosteroid creams on the lesion surface. Severely pruritic animals may require systemic corticosteroids for a period of a few days.[135] If tolerated by the horse, fly-repellent ear tags for cattle can be hung on loops of gauze that encircle the horse's girth. Thick layers of petroleum jelly applied to the abdomen may also limit fly bites, although dirt buildup is a potential problem. Reduction of fly populations on the premises through environmental management (sprays, baits, manure removal) is often helpful.

OTHER FLYING INSECTS

Stable flies (*Stomoxys calcitrans*), black flies (Simuliidae), horn flies (*Lyperosia* or *Haematobia irritans*), horse flies (*Tabanus* spp. and *Hypbomitra* spp.), deer flies (*Chrysops* spp.), house flies (*Musca domestica*), face flies (*Musca autumnatis*), and mosquitos are commonly associated with irritant and allergic skin disease, as well as being vectors of many parasites. They must be controlled by limiting breeding areas and by chemicals.

SCREWWORM INFESTATION

Screwworm flies cause primary myiasis; the species of importance in the Americas is *Cochliomyia hominivorax* (*Callitroga americana*). The fly is found throughout the American tropics and subtropics from the southern United States to northern Chile.[135] The Southwest Screwworm Eradication Program has greatly restricted the range of this fly so that within the United States there are presently only occasional attacks in areas bordering Mexico.[136] The adult fly is about

three times the size of a house fly with a metallic bluish or blue-green color.[135,137] Females are attracted to fresh wounds (castration, dehorning, branding and shearing sites), abraded body orifices, areas soiled by discharges or excretions, and navels of newborns. They lay batches of 150 to 500 white eggs on the margin of damaged tissue in rows that overlap like shingles. Eggs hatch within 24 hours, and the larvae begin to feed in a head-downward position. Larvae are obligate parasites that require living tissue as feed stuff. They cannot develop in carrion. Larval development continues for 4 to 10 days, and at the time of their maturation they may have created a cavity 10 to 12 cm in diameter.[137] Mature larvae are about 2 cm in length, pink in color, pointed anteriorly, and blunt posteriorly. The larvae then drop to the soil and pupate. The life cycle averages about 21 days and is favored by hot, humid weather. Screwworms do not have a dormant stage in their life cycle and cannot overwinter in cold climates.[135] Thus the susceptible stage of development is the pupae, which will not survive soil temperatures below 15° C (59° F).[98] The feeding larvae burrow deeply, creating a cavernous lesion characterized by liquefaction necrosis, profuse brownish exudate, and an objectionable odor. The syndrome is self-perpetuating in that wounds infested by screwworm larvae become increasingly attractive to gravid females. The end result is often death of the host as a result of secondary bacterial infection, toxemia, and fluid loss.[137]

Treatment of wounds requires clipping and cleansing, as well as destroying all larvae. Dressings containing larvicides and antiseptics should be applied. Preparations containing 5% lindane or 3% coumaphos in an ointment or gel base have been recommended. The treatment is repeated twice weekly. When large numbers of animals are affected, a 0.25% solution of coumaphos, chlorfenvinphos, or fenchlorfos may be applied to herds with a power sprayer. Calves may become ill from the spray; thus applications should be restricted to the ventral abdomen.[137] Subcutaneous injection of ivermectin has been shown to clear wounds of larvae within 3 days and to prevent reinfestation for 14 days following injection.[138] Control of screwworm flies in the United States has been achieved largely through the release of sterile males, because of the single mating tendency of the female fly. The eradication program has proceeded through Mexico south to the twenty-first-degree parallel.[135] Screwworm myiasis is a reportable disease in the United States, and suspect larvae should be preserved in 70% alcohol for positive identification.[139]

REFERENCES

135. Williams RE, Hall RD, Broce AB, et al, eds: *Livestock entomology*, New York, 1985, Wiley-Interscience.
136. Loomis EC: Common ectoparasites and their control. In Robinson NE, ed: *Current therapy in equine medicine*, Philadelphia, 1983, WB Saunders, pp 529-535.
137. Blood DC, Radostits OM, Henderson JA: *Veterinary medicine*, ed 6, London, 1983, Baillière Tindall, pp 949-954, 960-962.
138. Fraser CM, editor: *Merck veterinary manual*, ed 6, Rahway, NJ, 1986, Merck, pp 804-806.
139. Fadock VA: Parasitic skin diseases of large animals, *Vet Clin North Am* 6:3-26, 1984.

BLOW FLY STRIKE (Fleeceworms, Woolmaggots, Secondary Screwworms)

Blow flies are found throughout the western hemisphere. The species of importance include *Cochliomyia macellaria* (secondary screwworm), *Phaenicia sericata* (green bottle fly), and *Phormia regina* (black blow fly). The flies tend to be most common in the warmer regions, with the exception of *P. regina*, which is widespread throughout the cooler parts of North America and Europe.[140] Blow flies cause serious loss of sheep and wool in many countries.[141] Female flies are attracted to decaying animal matter such as wounds infested by primary screwworms, infected sores, carcasses, and fleeces

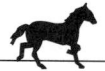

that are dampened with feces, urine, or bloody fluids.[140,141] They lay eggs in batches of up to 300 that hatch within hours after being laid. The larvae feed on necrotic tissue, but they may invade healthy tissue. Larvae develop for 3 to 5 days and, when fully mature, are white and 6 to 12 mm in length. The larvae then drop to the ground for pupation. As soil temperatures fall, larvae fail to pupate and may overwinter until the following spring.[125] The entire life cycle is generally complete in 2 to 4 weeks under ideal conditions of warm temperatures and high humidity.[142]

Unlike primary screwworms that feed in pocketlike aggregations, secondary screwworms tend to be dispersed throughout the infested tissue. In the case of wool infestation the larvae may remain on the skin surface, feeding on the decomposing wool, or they may penetrate the skin through small abrasions. The most common site of involvement is the breech. Infested tissue attracts more ovipositing females, and thus the syndrome is perpetuated.[143] Affected sheep are restless and do not feed. They move with their heads close to the ground, bite or kick at their wounds, and continually wriggle their tails. Affected wool is moist and brown with an obvious odor. Animals may become systemically ill and die.[144]

Treatment of individual wounds is as described for screwworms. Control involves management practices that decrease the incidence of wounds or skin irritations. Sheep are often clipped below the tail and between the hind limbs ("crutched"), where wool is likely to become saturated with urine or feces. Castration, shearing, docking, and lambing are avoided during the summer season.[140]

REFERENCES

140. Williams RE et al, eds: *Livestock entomology,* New York, 1985, Wiley-Interscience.
141. Blood DC, Radostits OM, Henderson JA: *Veterinary medicine,* ed 6, London, 1983, Baillière Tindall, pp 949-954, 960-962.
142. Loomis EC: Common ectoparasites and their control. In Robinson NE, ed: *Current therapy in equine medicine,* Philadelphia, 1983, WB Saunders, pp 529-535.
143. Williams RE, Hall RD, Broce AB, et al, editors: *Livestock entomology,* New York, 1985, Wiley-Interscience.
144. Fadock VA: Parasitic skin diseases of large animals, *Vet Clin North Am* 6:3-26, 1984.

CUTANEOUS ONCHOCERCIASIS

DEFINITION AND ETIOLOGY. Cutaneous onchocerciasis is a common filarial dermatitis with a worldwide distribution that is of clinical importance in the horse. The disease is caused by the microfilaria of *Onchocerca cervicalis* and is seen primarily in adult horses.[145] Adults typically are found coiled in the funicular part of the ligamentum nuchae, where they produce calcified nodules. Viviparous females may live for up to 5 years and produce large numbers of microfilaria that migrate through connective tissues to the superficial layers of the dermis. Preferential areas of microfilarial localization include the ventral midline, lower eyelid, and lateral limbus of the eye.[145] The infection is transmitted by *Culicoides,* which act as an intermediate host. The larvae are ingested by the vector and undergo development into the third-stage larvae (L_3) in approximately 2 weeks. The L_3 enter the animal host through lesions created by the feeding vector.[146] Surveys of the prevalence of infection have been conducted in many areas of the world; microfilaria are found in 48% to 96% of horses surveyed.[106] Many horses are infected with the parasite without demonstrating clinical disease.[145,147]

PATHOPHYSIOLOGY. Pathogenesis is believed to involve a hypersensitivity reaction to antigens released by dying microfilaria.[145-148] This theory is supported by the fact that not all infected horses demonstrate disease, that neither the presence nor the severity of the dermatitis is correlated with the number of organisms present, and that treatment with

filaricides often causes a temporary exacerbation of clinical signs.

CLINICAL SIGNS AND DIFFERENTIAL DIAGNOSES. Clinical signs occur most commonly in older horses and can include both ocular and cutaneous lesions.[145,147] Ocular lesions include uveitis, conjunctivitis, keratitis, and depigmentation of the lateral limbus.[149] Cutaneous lesions include diffuse or patchy alopecia, erythema, and scaling. Focal cutaneous depigmentation is common. Lesions tend to occur in regions where microfilaria are typically present in highest concentrations such as the ventral midline, face (Fig. 38-13), base of the mane, anteriomedial proximal forelimbs, and anterior pectoral region. A "bull's eye" lesion in the center of the forehead is highly suggestive of the disorder.[147] The dermatitis is generally reported as being nonseasonal and nonpruritic,[146,147] although one investigator reports otherwise.[148]

Because many normal horses have microfilaria without disease, the finding of microfilaria does not prove that they are the cause of the cutaneous lesions. In addition, because microfilaria tend to "nest" in the dermis, there is a tremendous difference in the number of microfilaria recovered from adjacent skin samples.[145] Thus, although the absence of microfilaria makes cutaneous onchocerciasis unlikely, it does not definitively exclude it as a diagnosis. Differential diagnoses should include ventral midline dermatitis caused by the hornfly *Lyperosia irritans,* hypersensitivity reaction to *Culicoides,* dermatophytosis, and infestation with mange mites. Ultimately, diagnosis should be based on history, supportive clinical findings, exclusion of other differential diagnoses and, most important, response to therapy.

CLINICAL PATHOLOGY. Onchocerca microfilarial saline preparation (see Chapter 11). A positive preparation demonstrates slender, delicate microfilaria that are approximately 8 m by 220 m.

BIOPSIES FOR ROUTINE HISTOPATHOLOGY. Typical histopathologic changes include an eosinophilic and lymphocytic perivascular dermatitis, a finding that is nonspecific and common to many other equine parasitic dermatoses (see Chapter 11). Clumps of microfilaria may be found in the superficial dermis or perifollicular region.[145,147]

THERAPY. Ivermectin is the treatment of choice and is administered at 0.2 mg/kg PO.[150] Most horses improve within 2 to 3 weeks. Minor adverse reactions, including fever and swelling of the periorbital, facial, and ventral midline regions, may occur in up to 25% of infected horses treated with ivermectin. Severe reactions may benefit from treatment with antiinflammatory medications, but most reactions resolve within 24 to 72 hours, irrespective of whether horses are treated with corticosteroids.[150] Because there is no effective adulticide, recurrence may be noted within 2 months of therapy. Most

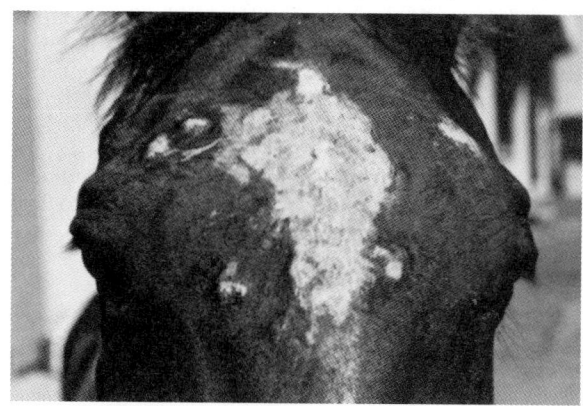

FIG. 38-13 ▌ Cutaneous onchocerciasis in a horse.

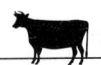

animals remain symptom free for 6 to 12 months.[147] Re-treatment is recommended at 4-month intervals. Previous therapeutics have included administration of either diethyl-carbamazine or levamisole but, because of the ease of ad-ministration and effectiveness of ivermectin, these medica-tions have become outmoded.

REFERENCES

145. Stannard AA, Cello RM: Onchocerca cervicalis infection in horses from the western United States, *Am J Vet Res* 36:1029-1031, 1975.
146. Foil CS: Cutaneous onchocerciasis. In Robinson NE, ed: *Current therapy in equine medicine*, ed 2, Philadelphia, 1987, WB Saunders, pp 627-629.
147. Fadock VA: Parasitic skin diseases of large animals, *Vet Clin North Am* 6:3-26, 1984.
148. McMullan WC: Onchocerca filariasis, *Southwestern Vet* 25:179-190, 1972.
149. Cello RM: Ocular onchocerciasis in the horse, *Equine Vet J* 3:148-154, 1971.
150. Herd RP, Donham JC: Efficacy of ivermectin against Onchocerca cervi-calis microfilarial dermatitis in horses, *Am J Vet Res* 44:1102-1105, 1983.

OTHER FILARIAL DERMATOSES

Stephanofilariasis

Cutaneous stephanofilariasis is a filarial dermatitis that is of clinical importance in cattle. The disease is caused by organ-isms of the genus *Stephanofilaria* and has been observed in cattle in many countries.[151] Within the United States the dis-ease is most prevalent in the western and southwestern re-gions, where it is caused by *Stephanofilaria stilesi*.[152,153] Adults and microfilaria inhabit the epidermis. The parasite is trans-mitted by the female horn fly *(Lyperosia irritans)* when it feeds on lesions on the ventral midline. The microfilaria are in-gested and develop to the third-stage infective larvae (L_3) in 2 to 3 weeks. The L_3 is introduced into the animal host on sub-sequent feedings.[153]

Clinical signs of cutaneous stephanofilariasis include a ven-tral midline dermatitis initially associated with a papular erup-tion. The lesions progress to nodules, alopecia, and crusted ul-cers. There may be mild pruritus.[152] Diagnosis is based on history and appropriate clinical signs, excluding differential di-agnosis and demonstration of the nematode. Biopsies may be taken as described for equine onchocerciasis, or the crust can be removed from an acute lesion, and deep skin scrapings per-formed to recover the parasite. The tissues should be minced in isotonic saline and then examined microscopically. Multiple skin scrapings may be required to demonstrate the parasite. Ei-ther adults or microfilaria may be found. The adult male is about 3 mm in length, and the adult female 6 mm in length.[151] Microfilaria are 50 m in length.[153] Characteristic histopathologic findings include a perivascular dermatitis as-sociated with an eosinophilia. Microfilaria may be noted in the dermis, and adults in epithelial-lined cysts at the base of the hair follicles, although both may be difficult to find.[151,152]

Topical 6% to 10% trichlorfon in petroleum jelly applied daily for 7 days is reported to be beneficial,[137] as is 4% feni-trothion applied once daily for 30 days.[154] Because iver-mectin is effective against microfilaria of *Onchocerca cervicalis* in the equid, it may also be effective against microfilaria of *S. stilesi*. But it has not been approved for this purpose, and it has not been shown to be effective against adults that also contribute to the cutaneous lesions. Adults persist 2 to 3 years if untreated.[155] To prevent reinfection, exposure to vectors must be controlled.

REFERENCES

151. Kral F, Schwartzman RM: *Veterinary and comparative dermatology*, Phila-delphia, 1964, JB Lippincott, pp 328-330.
152. Fadock VA: Parasitic skin diseases of large animals, *Vet Clin North Am* 6:3-26, 1984.
153. Fraser CM, ed: *Merck veterinary manual*, ed 6, Rahway, NJ, 1986, Merck, pp 783-784.
154. Blood DC, Radostits OM, Henderson JA: *Veterinary medicine*, ed 6, Lon-don, 1983, Baillière Tindall, p 944.
155. Smith JP: Fly infestations. In Howard JL, ed: *Current therapy 2: food ani-mal practice*, Philadelphia, 1986, WB Saunders, pp 915-916.

HYPODERMA (Warbles)

DEFINITION AND ETIOLOGY. Infestation with the larvae of *Hypoderma* spp. is a common and serious economic problem in cattle and is recognized sporadically in horses that are pas-tured near cattle. Occurrences have also been reported in sheep, goats, and humans.[156] Warble flies are present in the Northern Hemisphere between 25 and 60 degrees latitude in more than 50 countries of North America, Europe, Africa, and Asia. *Hypoderma* spp. are not established south of the equa-tor.[156,157] The annual losses to the U.S. cattle industry because of cattle grubs was estimated to be $360 million in 1976.[158]

Two species of *Hypoderma* parasitize cattle: *Hypoderma bo-vis* and *Hypoderma lineatum*. The latter prefers warmer cli-mates and is the only species present in the southern United States. Each of the species occurs in the northern United States and in Canada.[157] *H. lineatum* and *H. bovis* have very similar life cycles, but the stages of *H. lineatum* tend to occur 3 to 8 weeks earlier than those of *H. bovis*. There is also some variation with timing of the life cycle in accordance with lo-cal geographic and climatic factors.[156,157]

The adult flies are beelike in appearance, covered with dense hair, 12 to 188 mm in length, and have nonfunctional mouth parts.[158] They are short lived, surviving for only 1 week. Adult flies are active in the spring to early summer, with *H. lineatum* appearing 3 to 4 weeks before *H. bovis*. Fe-male *H. lineatum* deposit eggs on the hairs of the legs or lower body, whereas *H. bovis* tends to deposit eggs on the rump or upper parts of the hindlimbs. Total egg production by a single female has been estimated to range from 500 to 800.[158] The eggs hatch in 3 to 7 days, after which the larvae penetrate the skin and begin their migration through the con-nective tissues. *H. lineatum* larvae migrate to the subcuta-neous connective tissues of the esophageal wall, whereas *H. bovis* larvae migrate toward the spinal canal. The first-stage larvae remain in this location for 2 to 4 months, during au-tumn and early winter. Between January and February the lar-vae begin a final migration through the connective tissues to the subdermal tissue of the back of the host, where they form a breathing hole through the skin. Cysts (warbles) develop around the first-stage larvae. Within the cyst the larvae un-dergo two molts over a 4- to 6-week period. The third-stage larvae (grub) emerges from the breathing pore, falls to the ground, and pupates. Adult flies emerge from the pupae in 1 to 3 months, and emergent adults are ready to mate almost immediately.[158] The life cycle is complete in 1 year.[117,118] Most larvae fail to reach normal size and complete their life cycle in the horse.[159]

CLINICAL FINDINGS

Cattle. During the spring and summer when adult flies are active, "fly worry" may be a serious problem. Cattle exhibit a stampeding behavior called "gadding" when chased by ovipositing females even though the flies do not bite or sting. This fear reaction results in self-injury and decreased feeding and production.[158]

Clinical lesions are not usually observed in association with migration of the first-stage larvae unless the larvae die along the migratory path.[156] Lesions that have been associ-ated with infestation of the first-stage larvae of *H. bovis* in-clude fat necrosis and inflammation of the connective tissues surrounding the spinal canal. Secondary periostitis, os-teomyelitis, and, rarely, paralysis or other nervous disorders may occur. Similarly, infestation with the first-stage larvae of

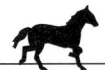

H. lineatum in the submucosa of the esophagus may cause inflammation and edema in the surrounding tissues. Swallowing and eructation may be hindered, resulting in bloat and subsequent respiratory failure.[156]

Lesions most commonly observed with *Hypoderma* infestation are attributed to the third-stage larvae. Warbles occur along the back from the shoulders to the tail head and from the dorsal midline to a point about one third the distance down the sides. The lesions may be firm to fluctuant, raised, and painful to the touch. They measure approximately 3 cm in diameter and contain a breathing pore that usually exudes a yellowish serum. Excisional biopsy of a nodular lesion reveals the larvae within a cystlike structure that contains yellow fluid. The surrounding tissue is necrotic. Secondary infection of the cysts can result in large, suppurating abscesses. The number of warbles in an infested animal may range from 1 to 300. Infestations are most serious in younger animals and become progressively lighter with age. Emergence of the grub results in healing, although carcasses retain evidence of infestation and are devalued at slaughter.[156,157]

Horses. Most horses have only one or two grubs, but in rare instances heavy infestations are present. Lesions associated with the third-stage larvae include small nodular swellings that develop dorsally and frequently in the region of the withers. Most lesions have a breathing pore.[159] Differential diagnosis most commonly include nodular collagenolytic granuloma (nodular necrobiosis); but mastocytoma, sterile nodular panniculitis, and amyloidosis should also be considered. Posterior paralysis associated with involvement of the spinal cord has been reported in both horses and cattle.[157]

The season, location of the lesion(s), and the presence of a breathing pore are usually diagnostic. Larvae can be recovered by enlarging the breathing pore with a scalpel and extracting the grub.

THERAPY. When small numbers of cattle are affected with just a few grubs, manual removal of the grubs is possible by simply enlarging the breathing pore. This is usually the preferred treatment in horses as well, if only 1 or 2 lesions are typically present. Care must be taken to remove the larvae in their entirety because breaking the larvae and rupturing the cyst during removal can result in a severe systemic reaction.[156,157]

Systemic insecticides are the only means of eliminating the migrating larvae. Several organophosphates, including trichlorphon, crufomate, fenthion, phosmet, bromophos, coumaphos, and fenchlorphos, have been used for this purpose. They may be applied by spray, pour-on, spot-on, oral dosing, or impregnated slow-release strips to the legs.[157] It is essential to use these insecticides in strict accordance with the manufacturer's recommendations to avoid toxicity and to observe withdrawal periods before slaughter or freshening (see Table 38-1). Organophosphates are not permitted for use on lactating dairy cattle. Ivermectin has been shown to be effective against *Hypoderma* spp. as well.[160] Administration of insecticides should be timed to provide treatment in early autumn after all eggs have hatched and larvae are in the early stages of their connective tissue migration. Third-stage larvae are less susceptible to insecticides, and destruction of larvae in later stages of migration increases the risk of serious secondary illness. It is advisable not to administer systemic insecticides later than 8 to 12 weeks before the anticipated first appearance of grubs along the back.[157,159] In the northern United States and Canada, treatment of cattle with systemic insecticides is not recommended between October 1 to March 1 because this is the time period when *H. bovis* larvae are located in the epidural space and *H. linneatum* larvae reside in the esophages.[157,159]

Rotenone has been used to kill larvae already located in the subcutaneous tissues along the back when systemic in-

secticides cannot be used. Treatment requires direct contact with the grub to be effective, and it does not reverse the damage that has already occurred as a result of presence of the larvae. In regions with extended seasons, applications must be repeated at 4-week intervals.[156,157]

REFERENCES

156. Fraser CM, editor: *Merck veterinary manual*, ed 6, Rahway, NJ, 1986, Merck, pp 752-754.
157. Blood DC, Radostits OM, Henderson JA: *Veterinary medicine*, ed 6, London, 1983, Baillière Tindall, pp 947-949.
158. Williams RE et al, eds: *Livestock entomology*, New York, 1985, Wiley-Interscience, pp 87-90, 195-196, 215-216, 233-234.
159. Stannard AA: *Modern veterinary practice seminars: equine dermatology*, Santa Barbara, Calif, Oct 1 and 2, 1984.
160. Campbell WC, Benz GW: Ivermectin: a review of efficacy and safety, *J Vet Pharmacol Ther* 7:1-16, 1984.

SHEEP KEDS

The sheep ked, *Melophagus ovinus*, is a wingless fly approximately 6 to 7 mm in diameter with a ticklike appearance. Sheep keds have a worldwide distribution. They primarily parasitize sheep and occasionally goats that are kept under poor management conditions.[161,162]

The entire life cycle is spent on the host. Females live for 4 to 5 months, during which time they lay 10 to 15 larvae individually that are cemented to the wool or hair. The larvae pupate in 12 hours, and the adult emerges 3 weeks later. Adults feed on blood and do not survive longer than a few days off of the host. Transmission is by direct contact, and infestation is more common in the winter months.[162-164]

Clinical signs of infestation include pruritus with subsequent self-trauma, wool stains from the fly's fecal material, and, in severely parasitized animals, anemia. Multiple firm nodules (cockles) develop as a result of repeated puncture of the skin as the keds feed.[162,164] Infestation results in economic loss from reduction of dressed carcass weights of lambs, reduced clean dry weight of fleece, wool staining, and reduced value of sheep skins because of nodular defects.[161-164] Diagnosis is based on demonstration of the parasite.

Therapy involves shearing all sheep in the affected flock, followed by two topical applications of malathion, diazinon, or coumaphos at 14- to 21-day intervals to kill emerging adults.[162] Because the larvae are attached to the wool or hair some distance above the skin surface, many larvae and pupae are removed by shearing.[162,164] All new animals should be isolated and treated before introduction to prevent reinfestation. A control program includes annual treatment of the entire flock.

REFERENCES

161. Manning TO, Scott DW: Caprine dermatology. III, Parasitic, allergic, hormonal and neoplastic disorders, *Compend Cont Educ Pract Vet* 7:S437-S452, 1985.
162. Blood DC, Radostits OM, Henderson JA: *Veterinary medicine*, ed 6, London, 1983, Baillière Tindall, pp 954-955.
163. Lloyd JE: Arthropod pests of sheep. In Williams RE et al, eds: *Livestock entomology*, New York, 1985, Wiley-Interscience, pp 253-267.
164. Fraser CM, ed: *Merck veterinary manual*, ed 6, Rahway, NJ, 1986, Merck, pp 574, 775-776.

CUTANEOUS HABRONEMIASIS
(Equine Summer Sore)

Cutaneous habronemiasis (summer sores) is a granulomatous dermatitis restricted to horses that occurs throughout the United States, although the prevalence varies considerably in different parts of the country.[165] The disease results from aberrant intradermal migration of the larvae of the adult nematodes *Habronema muscae*, *Draschia megastoma*, and *Habronema microstoma.* Adults normally reside in the stomach, where they cause little tissue reaction, with the exception of *D. megastoma,* which produces gastric nodules of varying sizes near the margo plicatus.[166] Females are viviparous, and larvae are passed in the feces, where they are then ingested by the larvae of flies acting as intermediate hosts. *H. muscae* and *D. megastome* develop in the house fly, *Musca domestica;* and *H. microstoma* develops in the stable fly, *Stomoxys calcitrans.* The third-stage larvae are then deposited around the horse's mouth and swallowed to pass to the stomach, where they mature to adults.[127] Cutaneous lesions occur when the larvae are deposited in damaged skin or areas of natural body moisture. The larvae cannot penetrate normal healthy skin.[165,167] In these aberrant locations, they are unable to mature to adults, and the proliferative lesions that result are believed to represent a type of hypersensitivity reaction to antigens released by the dead or dying larvae.[165,167]

Cutaneous habronemiasis is a seasonal disorder corresponding with the occurrence of the fly that acts as the vector. There is a tendency for lesions to recur in subsequent years. Lesions associated with cutaneous habronemiasis are usually found on the lower limbs (a common location for wounds), at the medial canthus of the eye (possibly related to maceration from ocular discharge), and on the urethral process.[165,167,168] They consist of ulcerative, nodular, and tumorous masses with multiple yellow, necrotic foci containing mineralized, dead larvae. Diagnosis is based on history and clinical findings and on biopsies of lesions submitted for histopathology. Characteristic histopathologic findings include granulation tissue with a diffuse infiltration of eosinophils and an ulcerative epithelial surface. The granulation tissue usually contains focal areas of coagulation necrosis surrounded by a dense eosinophilic infiltrate. Cross sections of larvae can often be identified within some of the necrotic foci. Rarely larvae are found in scrapings from the lesions.[161] Cutaneous habronemiasis must be considered in the differential diagnosis of all nonhealing ulcerative lesions, particularly those involving mucocutaneous junctions. Squamous cell carcinoma, sarcoids, exuberant granulation tissue, botryomycosis (bacterial granuloma), and fungal infections are the major differential diagnoses. Any ulcerative lesion may be complicated by secondary habronemiasis, and the primary cause may be overlooked if biopsies for histopathology do not contain adequate tissue.

Treatment of cutaneous habronemiasis includes four objectives: reduction of the size of lesions, reduction of inflammation associated with the lesions, elimination of the adult *Habronema* from the stomach, and reduction of vector populations.[165] When possible, lesions are reduced by surgical debridement. If they are located in areas that are inaccessible to surgery, cryosurgery may be a viable alternative.[168] Several treatments have been proposed to reduce inflammation. When multiple lesions are present, prednisone or prednisolone should be given at 1 mg/kg for 10 to 14 days, followed by 0.5 mg/kg for another 10 to 14 days. If there are only one or two isolated lesions, intralesional triamcinolone at 5 to 15 mg/lesion, not to exceed a total dosage of 20 mg, may be injected. This may be repeated at 10- to 14-day intervals if necessary.[165] For lesions involving the conjunctiva, frequent topical applications of a corticosteroid ophthalmic preparation are of benefit. Topical DMSO-corticosteroid preparations may be of value in other regions as well.[165] Several topical and systemic insecticidal therapies, including ivermectin, have been recommended for cutaneous lesions,[168-170] although their benefit for cutaneous lesions already present is controversial as the pathogenesis of cutaneous habronemiasis is believed to be related to larval death, which occurs soon after they gain entrance to the skin.[165,167] Systemic insecticidal therapy is important for elimination of adult *Habronema*

from the stomach, which decreases potential for reinfection, and ivermectin at 0.2 mg/kg is effective.[171] Dichlorvos and carbon disulfide also have known efficacy against *Habronema,* and all horses on the premises should be treated. Predosing by 30 minutes with 8 quarts of 2% Na HCO₃ increases anthelmintic efficacy by helping to dissolve the mucous plugs of *D. megasoma* nodules.[158] To prevent reinfection of lesions it is important to wrap and protect the existing wounds and to control vector populations. Prompt removal and disposal of droppings and soiled bedding are vital to eliminate vector breeding habitats. Insect repellents should be applied to affected horses. Face guards (fly masks) will also prevent infection. In general, the prognosis for resolution of individual lesions is good if the therapeutic ideals are achieved. Owners should be aware of the likelihood of recurrence if effective wound care and fly control are not practiced.

REFERENCES

165. Stannard AA: Modern veterinary practice seminars: equine dermatology. Presented Oct 1 and 2, 1984, Santa Barbara, Calif.
166. Fraser CM, editor: *Merck veterinary manual,* ed 6, Rahway, NJ, 1986, Merck, pp 195-196, 778-779.
167. Fadock VA: Parasitic skin diseases of large animals, *Vet Clin North Am* 6:3-26, 1984.
168. McMullan WC: Habronemiasis. In Robinson NE, ed: *Current therapy in equine medicine,* ed 1, Philadelphia, 1983, WB Saunders, pp 551-552.
169. Herd RP, Donham JC: Efficacy of ivermectin against cutaneous *Draschia* and *Habronema* infection (summer sores) in horses, *Am J Vet Res* 42:1953-1955, 1981.
170. Bordin EL, Bastos OP, Guerro J: Efficacy of ivermectin in the treatment of equine habronemiasis in Brazil, *Equine Pract* 9:18-19, 1987.
171. Campbell WC, Benz GW: Ivermectin: a review of efficacy and safety, *J Vet Pharmacol Ther* 7:1-16, 1984.

TUMORS AND CYSTS

STEPHEN D. WHITE

ANNE G. EVANS

SQUAMOUS CELL CARCINOMA

DEFINITION. Squamous cell carcinomas are tumors composed of squamous epithelial cells. They occur in all domestic species and are the most common bovine ocular tumor (see Chapter 37) and the second most common tumor recognized in the horse. Although their gross appearance may vary, these tumors are usually slightly raised, broad-based, white to pink and have a cobbled or cauliflower-like surface. Squamous cell carcinomas frequently occur on the penis and sheath of aged stallions and geldings (see Chapter 41). They also occur on the lips, nose, eyelids, eyes, and ears of horses. Squamous cell carcinoma commonly accompanies cutaneous papillomas of the udder and teats in Saanen milk goats, as well as in female Angora goats in South Africa. The ears and base of the horns may also be affected. Squamous cell carcinoma is reported as being the most common cancer of the ear of sheep.

The therapy of choice is wide surgical excision. Solar elastosis (aggregates of thick, wavy, interwoven elastic fibers, mixed with areas of degenerated collagen) when seen histologically with squamous cell carcinoma, may lend a more favorable prognosis following complete surgical removal of lesions.[172] Other treatment modalities that have been successful in squamous cell carcinomas include cryosurgery, radiofrequency hyperthermia, and radiation therapy. Topical application of 5-fluorouracil (5-FU) was shown to achieve complete remission (defined as clinical absence of tumor) in 10 of 11 horses with squamous cell carcinoma of the external genitalia. In 8 males, this was applied to the affected areas every 14 days, for

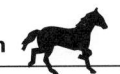

a mean number of treatments of 5 (range: 2-7); in 6 males this was preceded by debulking of the tumor. In females, all tumors were debulked and the owners instructed to apply the 5-FU daily. The mean number of treatment months needed in females to affect remission was 3.7 (range: 1 to 8). For all horses, remission lasted as long as available for follow-up (5 to 52 months). No adverse reactions were reported.[173] Owners must wear gloves. Recently, treatment with intralesional cisplatin as reported with sarcoids has also been effective.

REFERENCES

172. Campbell GA, et al: Solar elastosis with squamous cell carcinoma in two horses, *Vet Pathol* 24:463-464, 1987.
173. Fortier LA, Mac Harg MA: Topical use of 5-fluorouracil for treatment of squamous cell carcinoma of the external genitalia of horses: 11 cases (1988-1992), *J Am Vet Med Assoc* 205:1183-1185, 1994.

EQUINE SARCOID

STEPHEN D. WHITE
ANNE G. EVANS
DAVID C. Van METRE

DEFINITION. Equine sarcoids are locally aggressive fibroblastic tumors and represent the most common skin tumor of horses.[174] They may occur in donkeys and mules, as well as horses, and are usually located on the head, legs, and ventral abdomen. Sarcoids have been reported to occur at sites of previous trauma, and approximately one third of affected animals have multiple lesions.[175] There is no age, breed, sex, or coat color predilection, and their geographic distribution is worldwide.[176]

ETIOLOGY. The bovine papilloma virus has been implicated in the etiology. A number of researchers have been able to isolate bovine papilloma virus (BPV) from sarcoids of horses and donkeys; as diagnostic techniques have been refined (notably the polymerase chain reaction), the percentage of sarcoids from which the virus' DNA has been recovered has become in some studies 100%. Both BPV-1 and BPV-2 have been recovered, in one case, in the same horse (in different sarcoids). BPV-1 is more common in North America and BPV-2 is more common in Europe. BPV-2 is usually associated with the periocular form.[177-181]

In addition, it has been suggested that there may be a genetic susceptibility to the equine sarcoid. Thus it is possible that a combination of factors, including exposure to a viral agent, cutaneous trauma, and a genetic predisposition, may lead to the development of equine sarcoid.[182]

CLINICAL SIGNS AND DIFFERENTIAL DIAGNOSES. Sarcoids can occur anywhere on the body but are most commonly located on the head, legs, and ventral abdomen (Fig. 38-14). On the basis of gross appearance, sarcoids are classified as occult, verrucous (warty), fibroblastic (proud flesh), or verrucous-fibroblastic. The verrucous type is usually less than 6 cm in diameter and may be sessile and plaquelike or pedunculated. When sessile, the skin is usually thickened with a dry, rough surface. There may be partial or total alopecia. The fibroblastic types range in appearance from small dermal and/or subcutaneous nodules covered by an intact epidermis to large tumors with an ulcerated surface. Verrucous and occult sarcoids can transform to fibroblastic sarcoids and therefore show features of both types during their transition phase.[175,176]

Equine sarcoid must be considered in the differential diagnosis of all nodular or tumorous lesions, particularly those

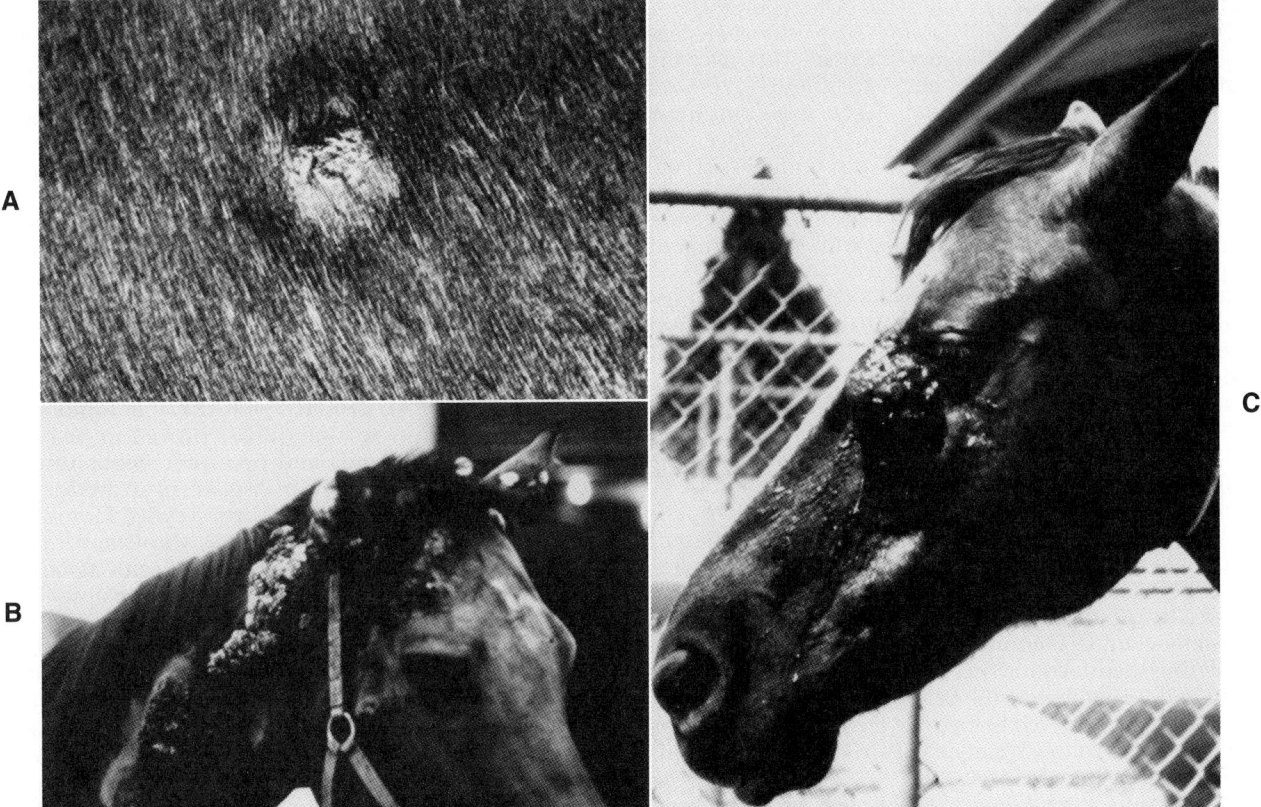

FIG. 38-14 Equine sarcoids. **A,** Small verrucous sarcoid, no more than a blemish. **B,** Extremely large, active, warty verrucous sarcoids. **C,** Large active fibroblastic sarcoid.

involving the head, legs, or ventral abdomen. Botryomycosis (bacterial granuloma), subcutaneous or deep fungal infections, cutaneous habronemiasis, and exuberant granulation tissue (proud flesh) are the major differential diagnoses, in addition to other neoplastic growths such as squamous cell carcinomas, papillomas, fibromas, and neurofibromas.[145] Occult (flat) verrucous equine sarcoids may be mistaken for focal lesions of dermatophytosis. Some cases of equine sarcoid are complicated by secondary bacterial infection, fungal infection, or habronemiasis and may be overlooked if biopsies for histopathology do not contain adequate tissue.

CLINICAL PATHOLOGY. The histologic features of equine sarcoids include (1) an epidermal component consisting of an acanthotic, hyperplastic epithelium with pseudoepitheliomatous hyperplasia and (2) a dermal component of fibroblasts and collagen fibers arranged in a whorled pattern. Fibroblasts at the dermoepidermal junction are frequently arranged perpendicular to the basement membrane. Mitotic figures can be numerous. The relative proportion of the epidermal and dermal components may vary. Usually verrucous sarcoids have a relatively greater epidermal component, and fibroblastic sarcoids have a greater dermal component.[175,177,183]

THERAPY. Therapy is usually reserved for the more aggressive fibroblastic forms of equine sarcoid, whereas many feel that benign neglect is preferable for the static verrucous lesions. Many forms of therapy have been described for equine sarcoids, yet none has proven routinely successful. What follows is a description of commonly applied therapeutic approaches to management.

SURGICAL EXCISION. The tendency for sarcoids to develop in regions without sufficient surplus skin for closure often makes surgical excision an impractical therapeutic alternative. When well-defined lesions do occur in surgically accessible areas, excision that includes a 1-cm margin of unaffected tissue has been successful in some cases, although postsurgical recurrence of up to 50% has been reported. If excision surgery is attempted, the best results occur when general anesthesia (as opposed to local) is used. This gives the surgeon more time and allows better technique to remove the entire tumor.[184] Because autotransplantation of tumors may occur, it is important that instruments that have contacted the tumor not come in contact with normal skin. Because of the difficulty in performing complete surgical excision and because of the high rate of postsurgical recurrence, surgical treatment is usually combined with other forms of therapy.[185]

CRYOTHERAPY. Cryosurgery involves destruction of tumor tissue by the application of extreme cold and is believed to produce more consistent therapeutic results than surgical excision. In addition, cryosurgery can be performed on lesions in regions where surgical closure of skin is not possible. Before freezing the tumor, hair and debris are removed from the tumor surface to increase coolant contact with the lesion. Liquid nitrogen is applied with either a cryoprobe or spray and should be done by an individual who is experienced with the technique. It is necessary to prevent adjacent normal skin from freezing by protecting it with either Styrofoam or petrolatum-coated gauze. The lesion is frozen at least twice to a temperature of $-20°$ to $-30°$ C ($-68°$ to $-86°$ F). Tissue temperature is monitored during the freezing process by inserting thermocouple needles 0.5 cm from the tumor margin and 0.5 cm below the base of the tumor. Optimum lethal effects are achieved by freezing the tissue as rapidly as possible and then allowing an unassisted thaw to room temperature after each freeze.

After cryosurgery, the tumor becomes edematous. After a few days, the tissue begins to necrose and separates from the surrounding tissue. There may be an associated purulent discharge. Complete slough of the tissue with healing by secondary intention usually requires several weeks. Depigmentation at the cryosurgical site should be expected.[185-189]

BACILLUS CALMETTE-GUÉRIN. Previous case reports have suggested that bacillus Calmette-Guérin (BCG) has potential in the treatment of equine sarcoids.[190,191] BCG is an attenuated strain of *Mycobacterium bovis* that acts as a nonspecific immunostimulant and has been used to induce regression of solid tumors in humans and animals. The ability of BCG to inhibit carcinogenesis is attributed to stimulation of normal T- and B-cell responses to heterologous antigens, in addition to its own antigenic determinants. The effectiveness of BCG depends on a number of factors, including (1) the ability of the patient to develop an immune response to mycobacterial antigens, (2) the total tumor load, and (3) a close association of BCG and tumor cells.[192] Therefore it follows that BCG would be most effective against small localized tumors in patients that possess a functional immune system. The ideal equine candidates for BCG therapy are those with single or multiple nodular sarcoids less than 5 cm in diameter located in areas that are injectable without posing significant restraint problems.[193]

Before administering BCG it is advisable to premedicate the patient with flunixin meglumine and an antihistamine solution because BCG is a foreign protein and is therefore capable of producing undesirable immunologic reactions such as anaphylaxis. Tetanus prophylaxis should be current. The lesion is clipped and prepared as for surgery and, if it is larger than 5 cm in diameter, it is surgically debulked. The BCG preparation is then injected into and around the lesion with an 18-gauge needle at a dose of approximately 1 ml of BCG solution per 1 to 2 cm^3 of tumor tissue. In most cases, two to five injections at 2-week intervals are necessary to evoke regression or sloughing of the sarcoid. A tumor-free status is reportedly achieved in 50% to 75% of equine patients treated with BCG products.[193] BCG is probably most effective for sarcoids located periocularly.

RADIATION THERAPY. Radioactive implants have recently been reported as being an effective method of therapy for recurrent and difficult-to-manage equine sarcoids.[194,195] Treatment of 12 periocular fibrous connective tissue sarcomas in 11 horses with ^{222}Rn implants resulted in a 1-year tumor-free rate of 92%.[194] Treatment of 23 equine sarcoids in 22 horses with implantation of ^{192}Ir for 4 to 14 days resulted in a 1-year tumor-free incidence in 15 of 16 horses (94%) followed for 1 year.[195] The main disadvantages associated with radioactive implantation therapy are that special training, special facilities, and licensing are necessary to safely handle the therapeutic radioisotopes. In addition, implantation is invasive and often difficult to perform, but, in cases of recurrent equine sarcoid that result in debilitating lesions, current evidence suggests that radioactive implantation is the treatment of choice.

INTRATUMORAL CHEMOTHERAPY. Intratumoral injection of cisplatin in sesame oil has proved to be effective in treatment of sarcoids and other cutaneous tumors of horses.[196,197] Four treatments of cisplatin at an average dosage of 0.97 mg per cm^3 of tumor tissue were used for tumor volumes that ranged from 10 to 20 cm^3, with smaller dosages used for smaller tumors. Of 19 horses with sarcoids, 18 showed complete tumor regression, with a relapse-free rate of 87% for 1 year after treatment.[196]

Treatment of tumors that are necrotic, ulcerated, or heavily infected should be delayed until the infection is controlled with topical or systemic antibiotic therapy. Immunization for tetanus should be performed before the onset of treatment with cisplatin, and prophylactic antibiotic therapy after each treatment session is recommended to limit infection of the tumor as it undergoes necrosis.[196] Perioperative injection may be superior to postoperative injection in tumors with high proliferation indices, or at least prudent to use when this information is not known.[197]

Veterinarians administering intratumoral cisplatin should be trained in the safe handling and storage of this drug. Owners must be cautioned not to handle the treated tumor because it contains high concentrations of cisplatin.[196] When administered properly, intratumoral cisplatin results in progressive tumor regression with mild local tissue reaction and no long-term adverse effects (e.g., fibrosis, nonhealing skin) at the site of the tumor.[196]

BIOLOGIC BEHAVIOR. An equine sarcoid may initially appear as either the verrucous or fibroblastic form. Verrucous sarcoids can remain static in size and configuration or they may transform into the fibroblastic type. It is believed that trauma to the lesion may predispose to transformation. Partial biopsy of verrucous sarcoids is thus contraindicated. The fibroblastic form is considered to be the more aggressive of the tumor types, and, although they do not metastasize, they can be locally invasive and tend to recur after surgical excision. It has been reported that a large percentage of equine sarcoids will spontaneously regress, although this may require a number of years[174,175]; this has not been my (SDW) experience.

REFERENCES

174. Jackson C: The incidence and pathology of tumors of domesticated animals in South Africa, *Onderstepoort J Vet Sci Anim Ind* 6:1, 1936.
175. Ragland WI et al: Equine sarcoid, *Equine Vet J* 2:2-11, 1970.
176. Stannard AA, Pulley LT: Equine sarcoid. In Moulton, JE, ed: *Tumors in domestic animals*, ed 2, Berkeley, 1978, University of California Press, pp 18-22.
177. Marti E et al: Report of the first international workshop on equine sarcoid, *Equine Vet J* 25:397-407, 1993.
178. Lory S et al: In situ hybridization of equine sarcoids with bovine papilloma virus, *Vet Rec* 132:132-133, 1993.
179. Otten N et al: DNA of bovine papilloma virus type 1 and 2 in equine sarcoids: PCR detection and direct sequencing, *Arch Virol* 132:121-131, 1993.
180. Reid SW et al: Epidemiological observations on sarcoids in a population of donkeys (*Equus asinus*), *Vet Rec* 134:207-211, 1994.
181. Trenfield K et al: Sequences of papilloma virus DNA in equine sarcoids, *Equine Vet J* 17:449-452, 1985.
182. Theilen GH, Madewell BR: *Veterinary cancer medicine*, ed 2, Philadelphia, 1987, Lea & Febiger, pp 283-287.
183. Tarwid JN, Fretz PB, Clark EG: Equine sarcoids: a study with emphasis on pathologic diagnosis, *Compend Cont Educ Pract Vet* 7:S293-S301, 1985.
184. Broström H: Equine sarcoids: a clinical, epidemiological and immunological study. PhD thesis, Faculty of Veterinary Medicine, Swedish University of Agricultural Sciences, Uppsala, Sweden, 1995.
185. Brown MP: Surgical treatment of equine sarcoid. In Robinson, NE, ed: *Current therapy in equine medicine*, ed 1, Philadelphia, 1983, WB Saunders, pp 537-538.
186. Genetzky RM, Biwer RD, Myers RK: Equine sarcoids: causes, diagnosis and treatment, *Compend Cont Educ Pract Vet* 5:S416-420, 1983.
187. Joyce JR: Cryosurgical treatment of tumors of horses and cattle, *J Am Vet Med Assoc* 168:226-229, 1976.
188. Lane JG: The treatment of equine sarcoids by cryosurgery, *Equine Vet J* 9:127-133, 1977.
189. Fretz PB, Barber SM: Prospective analysis of cryosurgery as the sole treatment for equine sarcoids, *Vet Clin North Am (Large Anim Pract)* 10:847-859, 1980.
190. Wyman M et al: Immunotherapy in equine sarcoids: a report of two cases, *J Am Vet Med Assoc* 171:449-451, 1977.
191. Murphy JM et al: Immunotherapy in ocular equine sarcoid, *J Am Vet Med Assoc* 174:269-272, 1979.
192. MacEwen EG: General concepts of immunotherapy of tumors, *J Am Anim Hosp Assoc* 12:363-373, 1976.
193. Rebhun WC: Immunotherapy for sarcoids. In Robinson NE, ed: *Current therapy in equine medicine*, ed 2, Philadelphia, 1983, WB Saunders, pp 537-538.
194. Fraunfelder HC, Blevins WE, Page EH: ²²²Rn for treatment of periocular fibrous connective tissue sarcomas in the horse, *J Am Vet Med Assoc* 180:310, 1982.
195. Turrel JM, Stover SM, Guorgyfalvy J: Iridium-192 interstitial brachytherapy of equine sarcoid, *Vet Radiol* 26:20-24, 1985.
196. Theon AP et al: Intratumoral chemotherapy with cisplatin in oily emulsion in horses, *J Am Vet Med Assoc* 202:261-267, 1993.
197. Theon AP et al: Comparison of perioperative versus postoperative intratumoral administration of cutaneous sarcoids and squamous cell carcinomas in horses, *J Am Vet Med Assoc* 215:1655-1660, 1999.

MASTOCYTOMA
STEPHEN D. WHITE
ANNE G. EVANS

Cutaneous mastocytoma (mastocytosis, mast cell tumor) occurs uncommonly in horses. There is no breed predilection, although the thoroughbred may be spared. Males are affected 5 to 10 times more frequently than are females.

Several different clinical forms have been recognized in the horse. Most commonly, mastocytomas occur as a single cutaneous nodule. This form is typically seen in older horses with an average age of 7 years.[198] The growths are frequently located on the head and range from 2 to 20 cm in diameter. Their surface may be haired, hairless, or ulcerated.[199] The second clinical form of equine mastocytomas presents as a diffuse swelling of a lower extremity, usually below the carpus or hock. The swelling is typically firm and the overlying tissue is normal. Radiographs often demonstrate multifocal regions of soft tissue mineralization.[200] A rare form of mastocytoma presents as disseminated, focal mast cell lesions in the skin that may be present at or shortly after birth.[201,202] This generalized form has been said to resemble urticaria pigmentosa of man.[203,204] Mastocytomas are very uncommon in cattle and account for only 3% of cutaneous and subcutaneous bovine tumors.[199,203] Biopsy and histopathology are diagnostic for mastocytoma.

It has been suggested that the equine mastocytoma represents a hyperplastic rather than a neoplastic process.[204] The tumor is self-limiting, and metastasis has not been reported. The finding of large numbers of eosinophils in a mastocytoma is said to be an indication that the mass is undergoing spontaneous regression. Surgical excision results in a very low recurrence rate, even with incomplete excision. Intralesional or sublesional corticosteroids may be used in solitary lesions that are difficult to resect surgically.[200] Radiotherapy may also be of value when surgery is not desirable.[205] Although in the horse mastocytomas are almost always benign, in cattle they may be malignant or benign and therefore carry a more guarded prognosis.

REFERENCES

198. Altera K, Clark L: Equine cutaneous mastocytosis, *Pathol Vet* 7:43-55, 1970.
199. Stannard AA, Pulley LT: Mastocytoma. In Moulton JE, ed: *Tumors in domestic animals*, ed 2, Berkeley, 1978, University of California Press, pp 32-33.
200. Stannard AA: Modern veterinary practice seminars: equine dermatology. Presented in Santa Barbara, California, Oct 1 and 2, 1984.
201. Cheville NF et al: Generalized cutaneous mastocytosis, *Vet Pathol* 9:394-407, 1972.
202. Prasse KW et al: Generalized mastocytosis in a foal, resembling urticaria pigmentosa of man, *J Am Vet Med Assoc* 166:68, 1975.
203. Head KW: Cutaneous mast cell tumors in the dog, cat and ox, *Br J Dermatol* 70:389-408, 1958.
204. McEntee MF: Equine cutaneous mastocytomas: morphology, biological behavior and evolution of the lesion, *J Comp Pathol* 104:171-178, 1991.
205. Theilen GH, Madwell BR: *Veterinary cancer medicine*, ed 2, Philadelphia, 1987, Lea & Febiger, pp 314-325.

MELANOMA
STEPHEN D. WHITE
ANNE G. EVANS
DAVID C. Van METRE

Equine

Melanomas occur in all domestic animals, but of the large domesticated species they are most significant in the horse. Excessive exposure to sunlight is a risk factor in humans, but there is no evidence to suggest that increased sunlight exposure

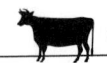
predisposes horses to the development of melanoma.[206] A disturbance in melanin metabolism associated with graying may act to stimulate formation of new melanoblasts or to stimulate their activity, resulting in focal areas of overproduction in the dermis and epidermis with subsequent tumor formation.[206] A higher incidence is observed in the Arabian, Lipizaner, and Percheron breeds, probably because gray coat color occurs more often in these breeds. There is no sex predilection.[206]

Melanocytic skin tumors of horses traditionally have been described in aging gray horses, in typical locations of the ventral tail, perineum, external genitalia, lip, udder, and periocular and parotid gland regions. They have been the subject of several classification schemes in attempting to correlate histopathologic appearance with clinical behavior (i.e., is it benign or malignant). A recent study[207] distinguished three basic types of melanocytic skin tumors.

Melanocytic nevi (melanocytoma) occur in the superficial dermis or at the epidermal-dermal junction, frequently have epithelial involvement, with nests of relatively large, mildly to moderately pleomorphic cells showing variable cytoplasmic pigmentation and occasional mitoses. More than 70% of these occur in horses *less* than 6 years of age, and may occur in horses of any color (not just gray). Most of these tumors occurred in atypical locations. Of 28 melanocytic nevi, only one became invasive, the rest exhibited benign behavior.

Dermal melanomas are found in the deep dermis, and are composed of small homogeneous, indistinct tumor cells, either round or dendritic, with no mitoses. (If there are multiple, confluent dermal melanomas, this is referred to as dermal melanomatosis). Eighty percent (80%) of these tumors are in horses *older* than 6 years of age, and are much more common in gray horses. Most of these tumors occurred in typical locations. Of 14 cases available for follow-up, 8 had malignant behavior as demonstrated by metastases.

Anaplastic malignant melanomas were composed of sheets of extremely pleomorphic epithelioid cells with poor pigmentation and many mitoses. These are usually seen in horses older than 20 years of age and in horses of any color.

Grossly melanomas are firm, dome shaped, hairless, and epidermal or dermal in location. They are usually multiple.[208] Initially the overlying skin is intact, but with larger, rapidly growing tumors surface ulceration may occur. The masses are typically gray to black, and only rarely is there lack of gross evidence of melanin pigment. Diagnosis of melanoma is based on cytologic and histologic evaluation. The presence of melanin pigment is the most valuable marker for identification of melanocytic tumors. As noted above, equine melanomas demonstrate one of three patterns of behavior. The tumor grows slowly without metastasizing. The major problem with this behavior is with enlarging masses in the perianal region that interfere with urination or defecation. The second pattern involves apparently benign growths present for a number of years that suddenly assume malignant characteristics and begin to grow rapidly. Finally, some melanomas are obviously malignant at the onset because of their rapid growth rate. The more highly malignant tumors (undifferentiated) are said to be less heavily pigmented,[209] but this opinion is not uniformly accepted.[208] Metastasis is usually first to the regional lymph nodes and then to the lungs, spleen, and liver. Hematogenous spread may also occur. Metastatic growths may be larger than the primary lesions and softer in consistency. Melanomas are said to be more aggressive in nongray horses.[206,210]

Older horses with multiple melanomas in the tail and anal region are not usually treated because of the difficulty in performing a complete surgical excision and because of the low metastatic potential of these melanomas. Treatment is indicated only if they are either repeatedly traumatized or if they cause difficulty with urination or defecation. Following tumor removal, new growths may occur that are not usually recurrences of the original tumor, but rather new primary tumors.[211] Incomplete surgical resection has been said to increase malignant potential.[210] Cryotherapy may be useful on tumors that require treatment but are located in areas that are not amenable to surgical resection.[212] Immunotherapy with intralesional BCG was reported to induce regression of a canine cutaneous malignant melanoma,[213] but data to support its efficacy in horses are lacking.

Long-term therapy with cimetidine has been beneficial in management of melanomas in a limited number of horses.[214] Treatment with 2.5 mg/kg of cimetidine PO 3 times a day for a period of 3 months may limit or stop progression of melanomas that are actively increasing in number or size.[214] Treatment with a reduced dose (1.6 mg/kg PO once daily) may be needed to maintain tumor stasis for a longer time. Using similar treatment regimens, the progression of disease was halted in two horses and controlled in a third.[215]

Cimetidine's effect on melanomas appears to be caused by the immunomodulatory activity of the drug. Histamine activates T suppressor cells via binding to H_2 receptors. Once activated, these cells suppress the humoral and cellular immune response.[214,215] Cimetidine can block this activation pathway of T suppressor cells, thereby allowing the immune system of the horse to target the neoplastic tissue more effectively.

Intralesional cisplatin has been suggested as a potential treatment for melanomas.[215]

Bovine

Melanomas represent a significant proportion of the cutaneous neoplasms of cattle,[216] but they account for less than 2% of bovine tumors in general.[217] The majority are benign, well-differentiated tumors, subcutaneous in location, and without site predilection. Dark-haired cattle are predisposed, particularly the Aberdeen Angus breed. There is no sex predilection.[206] Melanomas usually occur in young cattle[206] and are occasionally recognized as congenital lesions.[206]

Caprine and Ovine

Melanomas have been observed only rarely in sheep and goats.[208] A survey of 800,000 slaughtered goats revealed only five melanomas.[218] The most common site for melanomas in the goat is the perineal region,[219] although there is a case report of a malignant melanoma occurring in the coronary band region.[220]

REFERENCES

206. Theilen GH, Madwell BR: *Veterinary cancer medicine*, ed 2, Philadelphia, 1987, Lea & Febiger, pp 315-325.
207. Valentine BA: Equine melanocytic tumors: a retrospective study of 53 horses (1988-1991), *J Vet Int Med* 9:291-297, 1998.
208. M'Fadyean J: Equine melanomatosis, *J Comp Pathol* 46:186-204, 1933.
209. Stannard AA, Pulley LT: Melanoma. In Moulton JE, ed: *Tumors in domestic animals*, ed 2, Berkeley, 1978, University of California Press, pp 62-70.
210. Runnels RA, Benbrook EA: Malignant melanomas of horses and mules, *Am J Vet Res* 2:340-343, 1941.
211. Tuthill RJ et al: Equine melanotic disease: a unique animal model for human dermal melanocytic disease, *Lab Invest* 46:85A, 1982.
212. Farell RK: Veterinary cryotherapy of malignant melanoma, *Cryobiology* 15:713, 1979.
213. Grier RL et al: Regression of cutaneous melanosarcoma following intralesional *Mycobacterium bovis* BCG injection: a case report, *J Am Anim Hosp Assoc* 14:76, 1978.
214. Goetz TE et al: Cimetidine for treatment of melanomas in three horses, *J Am Vet Med Assoc* 196:449-452, 1990.
215. Goetz TE, Long MT: Treatment of melanomas in horses, *Compend Cont Educ Pract Vet* 608-610, 1993.
216. Jackson C: The incidence and pathology of tumors of domesticated animals in South Africa: a study of the Onderstepoort collection of neoplasms with special reference to their histopathology, *Onderstepoort J Vet Sci Anim Indust* 6:1-460, 1936.

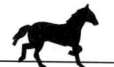

217. Blood DC, Radostits OM, Henderson JA: *Veterinary medicine,* ed 6, London, 1985, Baillière Tindall, p 447.
218. Bradley PJ, Magaki G: Types of tumors found by federal meat inspectors in an eight-year survey: epizootiology of cancer in animals, *Ann NY Acad Sci* 108:872-879, 1963.
219. Mustafa et al: Melanomas in goats, *Sud Med J* 4:113-118, 1966.
220. Sockett DC et al: Malignant melanoma in a goat, *J Am Vet Med Assoc* 185:907-908, 1984.

CUTANEOUS LYMPHOSARCOMA

STEPHEN D. WHITE

Equine

Cutaneous lymphoma has occasionally been reported in horses.[221-226] Both T-cell and B-cell forms have been reported. Lesions present as nodules, either cutaneous or subcutaneous. Diagnosis is made by biopsy and, ideally, immunohistochemistry to determine cell type. In one horse, progesterone receptors were demonstrated on the lymphoma (B) cells, and the lesions regressed following removal of an estrogen-secreting ovarian tumor.[224] This horse also had a history of partial regression of its tumor following administration of a synthetic progestin, altrenogest (0.044 mg/kg PO once daily for 10 days). Another horse demonstrated reduction in tumor size after administration of another synthetic progestagen, megestrol acetate (0.2 mg/kg PO once daily for 8 days) as well as a local injection into a mass of 20 mg of betamethasone.[225] Clearly, treatment is far from standardized, but the progesterone drugs may offer a reasonable treatment modality. Lymphosarcoma is discussed in Chapter 35.

REFERENCES

221. Detilleux PG et al: Ultrastructure and lectin histochemistry of equine cutaneous histiolymphocytic lymphosarcomas, *Vet Pathol* 26:409-419, 1989.
222. Gallagher RD et al: Immunotherapy of equine cutaneous lymphoma using low-dose cyclophosphamide and autologous tumor cells infected with vaccinia virus, *Can Vet J* 34:371-373, 1993.
223. Gerard MP et al: Cutaneous lymphoma with extensive periarticular involvement in a horse, *J Am Vet Med Assoc* 213:391-393, 1998.
224. Henson KL et al: Regression of subcutaneous lymphoma following removal of an ovarian granulosa-theca cell tumor in a horse, *J Am Vet Med Assoc* 212:1419-1422, 1998.
225. Littlewood JD et al: Equine cutaneous lymphoma: a case report, *Vet Dermatol* 6:105-111, 1995.
226. Potter K, Anez D: Mycosis fungoides in a horse, *J Am Vet Med Assoc* 212:550-552, 1998.

CYSTS

ANNE G. EVANS

Cutaneous cysts are benign lesions characterized by an epithelial wall with keratinous contents. Cutaneous cysts are subdivided into several types on the basis of their histopathologic features.

Epidermal Cysts

Among large animals, epidermal cysts have been reported in horses, cattle,[227,228] and sheep.[229] They can be found anywhere on the body, may be single or multiple or congenital or acquired, and generally range in size from 0.2 to 3 cm in diameter. The cysts are covered by intact epithelium and generally do not attach to the overlying epidermis. Microscopically, epidermal cysts consist of a wall of stratified squamous epithelium surrounding a keratin-filled lumen. Epidermal appendages are not associated with the cyst wall, a feature that distinguishes epidermal from dermoid cysts. Epidermal cysts are thought to originate from occlusion of a hair follicle or by traumatic implantation of the epidermis.[227,229] A tentative diagnosis may be made by performing fine-needle aspiration of a lesion and obtaining a fluid that is clear to brownish in color. Aspiration of the contents may temporarily decrease the size of the cyst, but it typically refills. Definite diagnosis is made by excisional biopsy, which is curative. Epidermal cysts are benign lesions, although painful inflammatory responses and ulceration may result if the cyst is ruptured with extrusion of contents into the adjacent dermis and subcutis.[227,228]

Dermoid Cysts

Dermoid cysts are very similar clinically to epidermal cysts but are much less common. Among large animals, they have been identified in horses,[230] goats,[231,232] and cattle.[233,234] In cattle, they may be congenital, have been reported to be as large as 10 cm in diameter, and are said to develop most frequently over the cranial area of the thorax[234] and in the pharyngeal region.[233] In horses, they may be single or multiple and are observed most frequently along the dorsal midline between the withers and the croup. Dermoid cysts are believed to result from displacement of embryonic cells into the subcutaneous tissue.[230,235] They can be distinguished histologically from epidermal cysts by the presence of epidermal appendages within the wall of the cyst, and the lumen frequently contains hair and secretions from sebaceous and sweat glands in addition to keratin. As with epidermal cysts, surgical excision is diagnostic and curative.[227,233]

Dentigerous Cysts

Dentigerous cysts are a congenital defect recognized in horses and are believed to be the result of an abnormality of the first branchial cleft.[235,236] Clinically a unilateral saclike swelling is seen at the base of the ear that contains embryonic teeth. The lesion may be firmly attached to the concheal cartilage or temporal bone. Dentigerous cysts have a tendency to fistulate. Treatment consists of surgical excision.[232,235] Dentigerous cysts have also been reported in sheep and are suspected of being related to a nutritional deficiency of copper.[237]

Wattle Cysts

Wattle cysts are found in goats and usually are present at the base of the wattle. Nubians and Nubian crossbreeds may be predisposed to developing these cysts. The cysts are congenital, but they may not be apparent until the animal is several months old. Tentative diagnosis is based on aspiration of clear fluid, which will temporarily decrease the size of the cyst. Surgical excision is diagnostic and curative. Histologic examination reveals a cyst wall composed of 1 to 2 layers of cuboidal to columnar epithelial cells. The cyst cavity contains homogeneous, amorphous basophilic substances.[237,238]

REFERENCES

227. Theilen GH, Madewell BR: *Veterinary cancer medicine,* ed 2, Philadelphia, 1987, Lea & Febiger, p 240.
228. Oz HH, Williams MD, Memon MA: Epidermal inclusion cysts in a cow, *J Am Vet Med Assoc* 187:504-505, 1985.
229. Lloyd LC: The aetiology of cysts in the skin of some families of merino sheep in Australia, *J Pathol Bacteriol* 88:219-227, 1964.
230. Pascoe RR: *Equine dermatoses,* New South Wales, 1981, The University of Sydney, pp 49, 51.
231. Gamlem BS, Crawford TB: Dermoid cysts in identical locations in a doe and her kid, *Vet Med Small Anim Clin* 72:616-617, 1974.
232. Manning TO, Scott DW: Caprine dermatology. III, Parasitic, allergic, hormonal and neoplastic disorders, *Compend Cont Educ Pract Vet* 7:S437-S452, 1985.
233. Kral F, Schwartzman RM: *Veterinary comparative dermatology,* Philadelphia, 1964, JB Lippincott, pp 154, 405.
234. Adams SB, Horstman L, Hoer FJ: Periocular dermoid cyst in a calf, *J Am Vet Med Assoc* 182:1255-1256, 1983.
235. Neiberle CP: *Textbook of special pathological anatomy of domestic animals,* ed 1, New York, 1967, Pergamon Press, p 892.
236. Mullowney PC: Dermatologic diseases of horses. IV, Environmental, congenital and neoplastic diseases, *Compend Cont Educ Pract Vet* 7:S22-S34.

237. Fubini SL, Campbell SG: External lumps on sheep and goats, *Vet Clin North Am (Large Anim Pract)* 5:457-467, 1983.
238. Blood DC, Radostits OM, Henderson JA: *Veterinary medicine*, ed 6, London, 1985, Baillière Tindall, p 147.

FROSTBITE

ANNE G. EVANS

Frostbite is an uncommon injury among healthy, well-nourished animals, although all species are susceptible. The areas most commonly affected by cold injury include the ears, tail, teats, scrotum, and distal parts of the limbs.

Frozen tissue must be handled gently and thawed rapidly in warm water 38° to 44° C (100.2° to 111.1° F) as soon as possible after it is known that refreezing can be prevented. Tissue damage is markedly exaggerated if thawing and subsequent refreezing occur (freeze-thaw-freeze-thaw syndrome).[239] Tissue thawing is painful, and analgesics should be administered. Slow thawing is less painful than rapid thawing but results in far greater tissue damage.[240] Frozen tissue should not be massaged during warming. Damaged areas are best left exposed during the healing process rather than covered with occlusive dressings, and premature debridement should be avoided because more tissue may be vital than is initially apparent. The patient is given good supportive care, including a high-protein, high-calorie diet with vitamin supplementation and must be restrained to prevent self-mutilation.[239] Management practices should be changed to prevent recurrence. Tissues previously damaged by freezing are more susceptible to cold injury when reexposed to subnormal temperatures.

REFERENCES

239. Moschella SL, Hurley HJ: *Dermatology*, ed 2, Philadelphia, 1985, WB Saunders, pp 1679-1682.
240. Dieterich RA: Cold injury. In Kirk RW, ed: *Current veterinary therapy VIII*, Philadelphia, 1983, WB Saunders, pp 187-189.

SKIN DISORDERS OF UNKNOWN OR GENETIC ORIGIN

BRADFORD P. SMITH

EQUINE SEBORRHEA

Seborrhea is a term that is used for diseases of abnormal keratinization.[241] In the horse, seborrhea usually involves the mane and tail or the anterior aspect of the rear cannon areas. There is scaling and crusting, little or no pruritus, and variable alopecia. Frequent use of antiseborrheic shampoos every 2 to 3 days (decreasing in frequency later) is the treatment of choice. There may initially be an increase in scaling and crusting before improvement is seen with the use of these tar-based shampoos.

REFERENCE

241. Thomsett LR: Noninfectious skin diseases of horses, *Vet Clin North Am (Large Anim Pract)* 6:67-79, 1984.

ALBINISM

Complete and partial albinism occurs in cattle, sheep, and horses. It is a genetic defect (probably autosomal recessive) in melanin synthesis, resulting in white skin, white hair, pink eyes, and photophobia.

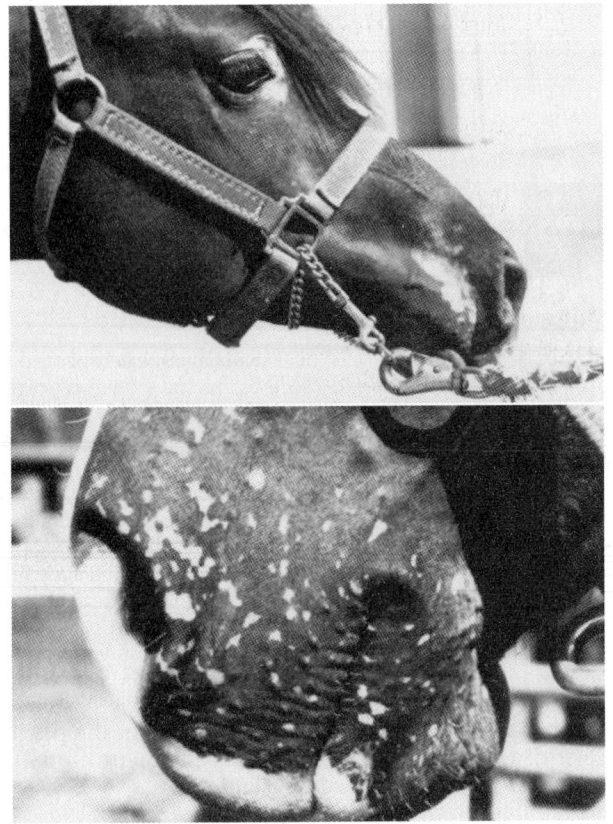

FIG. 38-15 ▌ **A**, Juvenile Arabian leukoderma. **B**, Congenital vitiligo in a horse. (Courtesy Dr. Anthony Stannard.)

JUVENILE ARABIAN LEUKODERMA (Arabian Fading Syndrome, Pinky Syndrome, Hereditary Vitiligo)

Loss of melanin in the skin (depigmentation) occurs in young Arabian horses 6 months to 2 years of age (Fig. 38-15).[242] The areas most commonly affected are periocular tissues, muzzle, genitalia, anus, perineum, inguinal region, and undersurface of the base of the tail. Depigmentation may persist, repigment, or wax and wane. The condition is probably hereditary.

REFERENCE

242. Scott, DW: *Large animal dermatology*, Philadelphia, 1988, WB Saunders, pp 388-389.

VITILIGO

Acquired loss of skin and hair pigment commonly results from traumatic wounds in horses. The condition is irreversible. The white spots of congenital vitiligo, a condition of unknown etiology, increase with age in both number and size. Juvenile Arabian leukoderma (see previous paragraph) is an example of this type. There is no known treatment.

RETICULATED LEUKOTRICHIA

STEPHEN D. WHITE
BRADFORD P. SMITH

Reticulated leukotrichia occurs mainly in quarter horses, usually as yearlings,[243] and rarely in other breeds. The lesions occur on the dorsal midline and consist initially of linear crusts arranged in a characteristic cross-hatched pattern (Fig. 38-16). The crusts shed, alopecia occurs, and finally white hair grows in permanently. There is leukotrichia without

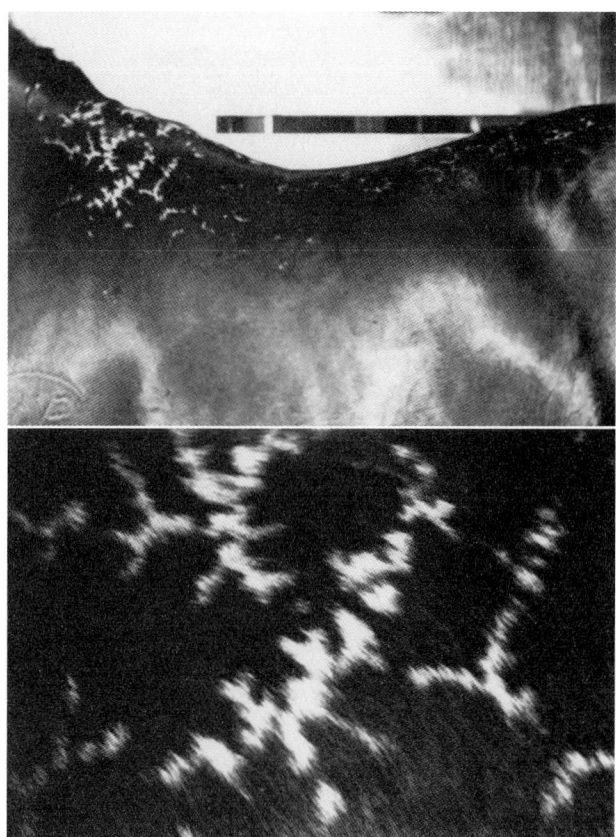

FIG. 38-16 ▓▓ Reticulated leukotrichia in a yearling quarter horse. (Courtesy Dr. Anthony Stannard.)

leukoderma (depigmented skin). Histology is similar to that of hypersesthetic leukotrichia (see below). No effective treatment is known.

REFERENCE

243. Scott DW: *Large animal dermatology,* Philadelphia, 1988, WB Saunders, p 390.

HYPERESTHETIC LEUKOTRICHIA

STEPHEN D. WHITE
BRADFORD P. SMITH

Hyperesthetic leukotrichia is a rare disease in which *painful* crusts develop on the skin of the dorsal midline of mature horses.[244] Within a few weeks white hairs appear in the affected areas. The crusts disappear, and the pain subsides in 1 to 3 months, but the leukotrichia persists. Histologically, these lesions resemble an epidermal form of erythema multiforme, resulting in individual keratinocyte necrosis.[245] Several cases have been linked to recent rhinopneumonitis vaccination. The disease may recur and there is no known effective therapy.

REFERENCE

244. Scott DW: *Large animal dermatology,* Philadelphia, 1988, WB Saunders, pp 390-392.
245. Fadok VA: Update on four unusual equine dermatoses,*Vet Clin North Am (Equine Anim Pract)*11:105-111.

HYPERELASTOSIS CUTIS

STEPHEN D. WHITE

Equine hyperelastosis cutis is an inherited connective tissue disorder. In the United States it is seen primarily in quarter horses although there are reports in Standardbreds as well.

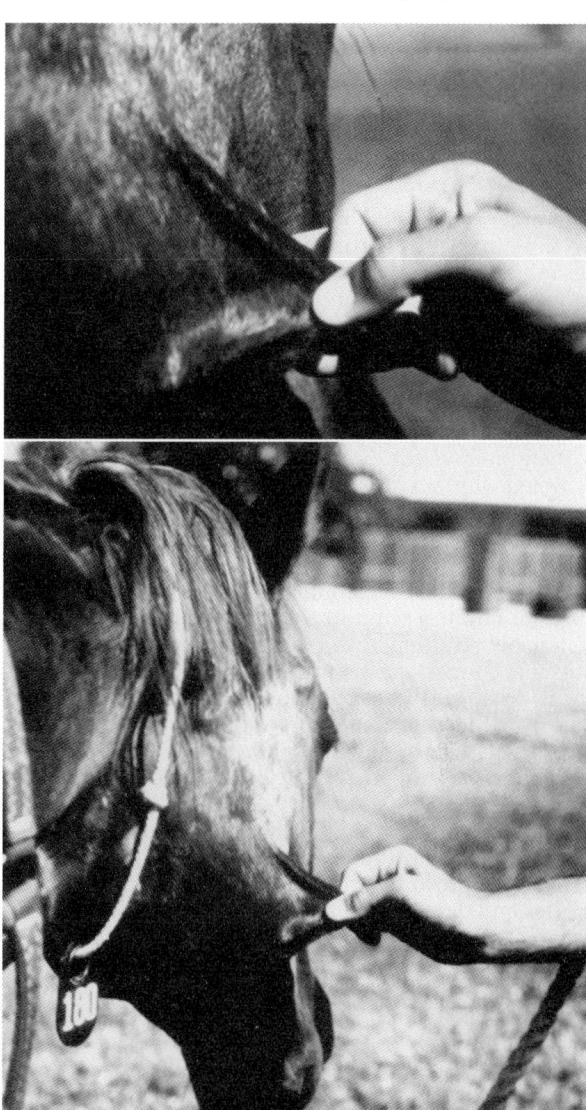

FIG. 38-17 ▓▓ Hyperelastosis cutis in a horse showing hyperextensible skin. (Courtesy Dr. Anthony Stannard.)

Quarter horses may inherit this disease as an autosomal-recessive trait. The age of onset is 6 months to 2 years and is somewhat dependent on the amount of trauma to which the horse is exposed (sometimes the lesions are not evident until the horse begins training).

Clinical signs may be solitary or multiple. These are usually dorsal lesions of easily torn skin, scar tissue, and hematomas. The owner may describe "loose skin" or poor healing of wounds (Fig. 38-17). Distal extremities such as the legs, face, and ventrum are spared. Histologic findings are subtle, but "clumped" collagen fibers below the level of the hair follicles may be seen. "Poorly oriented" collagen fibers are sometimes seen on electron microscopy.[246,247]

There is no known treatment. Affected horses as well as the sires and dams of affected horses should not be bred.

REFERENCES

246. Hardy MH et al: An inherited connective tissue disease in the horse, *Lab Invest* 59:253-262, 1988.

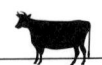

247. Stannard AA: Non-pruritic equine skin disease. Clinical Programme, Third World Congress of Veterinary Dermatology, Edinburgh, Scotland, September, p 118, 1996.

EPIDERMOLYSIS BULLOSA

STEPHEN D. WHITE

Epidermolysis bullosa (EB) includes a number of diseases typified in humans by the common finding of blister formation after minor trauma. Most forms are congenital and apparent soon after birth. In animals and in humans, subsets of EB are classified by the histologic location of the blister or cleft. These subtypes (and respective cleft location) are termed EB simplex (basal cell layer), junctional EB (intralamina lucida or basal cell layer), and dystrophic EB (sublamina densa).

Junctional EB has been reported in Belgian foals of both sexes and may occur in other breeds.[248,249] Lesions are usually noted within 3 days of birth and include multiple asymmetric irregular skin erosions and ulcers, which are often encrusted. Lesions may be especially prominent around the coronary bands (causing the hoof to crack and slough) and on the oral, anal, and genital mucosa. Histology and ultrastructural findings point to a cleft in the intralamina lucida, presumably resulting from a defect in the anchoring collagen fibrils that connect the basement membrane to the superficial dermis. A laminin 5 defect has been demonstrated in Belgian foals.[250] Clinical presentation and the age of the foal are highly suggestive of the diagnosis. This disease differs from epitheliogenesis imperfecta (see below) in that large areas of the skin are *not* at first devoid of epidermis, but rather lose their skin because of the fibril defect. Histology and ideally electron microscopy are required to confirm the diagnosis. There is no known treatment, and affected horses as well as the sires and dams of affected horses should not be bred.

REFERENCES

248. Frame SR et al: Hereditary junctional mechanobulluous disease in a foal, *J Am Vet Med Assoc* 193:1420-1424, 1988.
249. Johnson GC et al: Ultrastructure of junctional epidermolysis bullosa in Belgian foals, *J Comp Pathol* 98:331-336, 1988.
250. Linder KE et al: Mechanobullous disease of Belgian foals resembles lethal (Herlitz) junctional epidermolysis bullosa of humans and is associated with failure of laminin-5 assembly, *Vet Dermatol* 11(Suppl 1): 24, 2000.

NODULAR NECROBIOSIS (Equine Collagenolytic Granuloma)

Nodular necrobiosis is a common skin disease of horses in the United States. The etiology is unknown. The lesions consist of one or more firm dermal nodules 0.5 to 5 cm in diameter, with some occasionally much larger (Fig. 38-18).[251] The neck, withers, and back are the most commonly affected sites. There is no pruritus or pain, and overlying skin appears normal. Large lesions may occasionally ulcerate.

The characteristic appearance of lesions involves degeneration of collagen, with a resulting granulomatous host response. Eosinophils are very numerous.[251] The pathogenesis probably involves a hypersensitivity reaction, possibly to insect bites. Therapy consists of surgical removal and/or corticosteroids. Sublesional or intralesional triamcinolone (5 mg/nodule, not to exceed 20-mg total dosage repeated in 2 weeks) is effective. Systemic corticosteroids (500 to 600 mg prednisone or prednisolone daily for 2 weeks, then alternate-day therapy for 2 weeks) can be used when many nodules are present.[252] The prognosis for recovery is good. Differentials include cutaneous amyloidosis and cutaneous lymphosarcoma.

REFERENCES

251. Thomsett LR: Noninfectious skin diseases of horses, *Vet Clin North Am (Large Anim Pract)* 6:59-78.

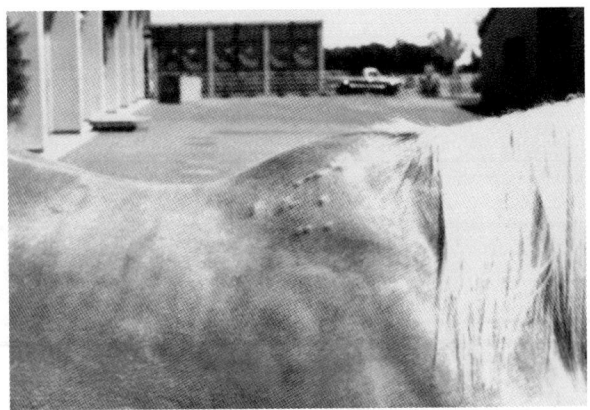

FIG. 38-18 ■ Nodular necrobiosis showing nonpruritic small dermal nodules on the withers of a horse. (Courtesy Dr. Anthony Stannard.)

252. Stannard AA: *Syllabus for veterinary dermatology,* Davis, Calif, 1988, University of California.

INJECTION SITE EOSINOPHILIC GRANULOMAS

NATHAN M. SLOVIS
JOHANNA L. WATSON

Development of equine eosinophilic granulomas (EEG) have been noted in areas of previous injections using standard silicone-coated stainless steel hypodermic needles.[253] The reaction may occur at sites of intravenous as well as intramuscular injections. The lesions consist of nonpainful, cool, raised papules or nodules 0.25 to 1 cm in diameter at sites of previous injection. The nodule appears 24 to 48 hours after the injection and the subsequent eosinophilic granuloma can persist for months to years. These nodules may decrease in size over time (1 to 2 years); those that do not regress are usually calcified, secondary to dystrophic mineralization.

Histopathologic findings reveal large areas of degranulating eosinophils and collagenolysis surrounded by numerous multinucleated giant cells, eosinophils, and lymphocytes oriented perpendicular to the skin. Affected horses do not develop a lesion at the site of injection if nondisposable, noncoated needles are used. The use of the noncoated needles is recommended for any horse that develops injection-site collagenolytic granulomas.[253] The current hypothesis is that the lesions represent a hypersensitivity reaction to the silicone coating of the hypodermic needles.[253] Injection site eosinophilic collagenolytic granulomas are a relatively uncommon manifestation of EEG in horses.

REFERENCES

253. Slovis NM et al: Injection site eosinophilic granulomas and collagenolysis in 3 horses, *J Vet Internal Med* 13:606-612, 1999

CUTANEOUS AMYLOIDOSIS

Amyloid is a fibrillar protein substance derived from immunoglobulins. Cutaneous amyloidosis is a rare nodular disease of the skin and/or upper respiratory mucosa of horses. There are no age, breed, or sex predilections. The condition is rarely associated with a primary chronic inflammatory focus (in contrast to visceral amyloidosis), and visceral organs are rarely, if ever, involved in cutaneous amyloidosis.[254] The cause of the condition is unknown. Certain types of amyloidosis in humans are inherited; heredity should be considered a possibility in horses.[254,255] Papules, nodules, and plaques

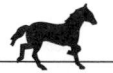

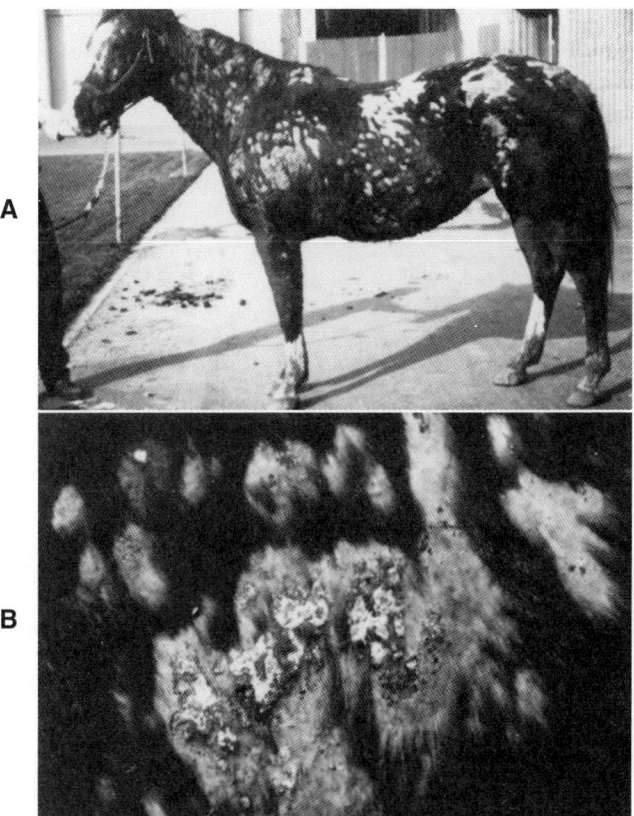

FIG. 38-19 ▥ A and B, Cutaneous amyloidosis in a horse. (Courtesy Dr. Anthony Stannard.)

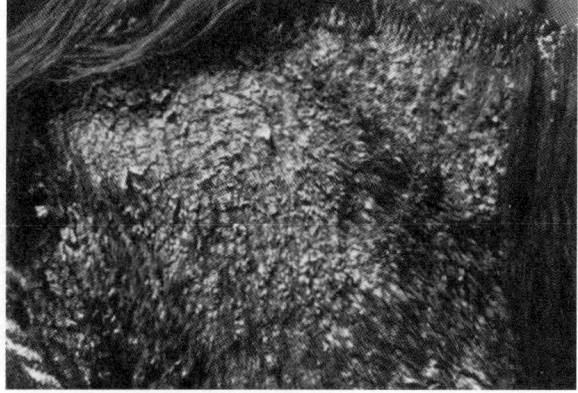

FIG. 38-20 ▥ Generalized granulomatous disease in a horse. In addition to the scaling and crusting skin lesions, the horse has systemic involvement. (Courtesy Dr. Anthony Stannard.)

on the head, neck, shoulders, and pectoral area are firm, 0.5 to 10 cm in diameter, nonpainful, and nonpruritic. The overlying skin is normal,[255] although it may scale or crust in severe cases (Fig. 38-19). The principal differential diagnoses are nodular necrobiosis and cutaneous lymphosarcoma. Some horses also develop diffuse or nodular deposits of amyloid in the nasal mucosa (occasionally in the trachea and other upper respiratory mucosa as well), leading to dyspnea.[255] Biopsy reveals granulomatous dermatitis with numerous multinucleated giant cells.[255] Amyloid is a homogenous eosinophilic substance, found both intracellularly and extracellularly. Amyloid can be stained with Congo red, crystal violet, or thioflavin T.

There is no effective therapy for cutaneous amyloidosis.[253,254] The disease is usually slowly progressive.

REFERENCES

254. Stannard AA: *Veterinary dermatology syllabus*, Davis, Calif, 1988, University of California.
255. Scott DW: *Large animal dermatology*, Philadelphia, 1988, WB Saunders, pp 328-329.

GENERALIZED GRANULOMATOUS DISEASE OF HORSES

STEPHEN D. WHITE

Generalized granulomatous disease (GGD) is a rare disease of horses characterized by skin lesions and widespread systemic involvement.[256,257] The etiology is unknown, although three horses with GGD had titers to *Borrelia burgdorferi*, and a fourth had the organism identified via PCR.[256] The disease is similar to human sarcoidosis. Skin lesions include scaling, crusting, alopecia, and occasionally nodules or large tumorlike masses (Fig. 38-20). Systemic signs include weight loss, anorexia, persistent low-grade fever, exercise intolerance, and mild dyspnea. Infrequently there is lymphadenopathy. Diarrhea and icterus may be seen if the gut and liver are involved.

Granulomas consist of epithelioid cells and multinucleated giant cells located in the superficial dermis and internal organs. A widespread interstitial infiltrate of the lungs is often visible radiographically.

Treatment involves 600 to 700 mg (per 500-kg horse) of prednisone or prednisolone orally daily. If remission is seen, alternate-day therapy should be commenced and carried on for at least 6 months. The prognosis for recovery is guarded. A few cases may spontaneously regress.

REFERENCES

256. Stannard AA: Systemic granulomatous disease, *Workshop in Equine Dermatology*, 1994, Newmarket, UK.
257. Rose JF et al: A series of four cases of generalized granulomatous disease in the horse. In Kwochka KW, Willemse T, von Tscharner C, eds: *Advances in veterinary dermatology*, vol 3, Butterworth Heinemann, Oxford, UK, 1998, pp 562-563.

PHOTOSENSITIZATION

ANTHONY A. STANNARD
STEPHEN D. WHITE

Photosensitization refers to an increased response to the ultraviolet radiation of sunlight caused by the presence of a photodynamic agent in the skin.[258,259] Photodynamic agents absorb certain wavelengths of ultraviolet (UV) light, become activated, and pass the extra energy to surrounding cells, resulting in their damage.[259] There are two types of photodynamic agents: phototoxic and photoallergic.[259] Exposure to the agent in either type may be systemic (reaching the skin through the circulation), or by contact. Phototoxic photosensitization may be further divided into primary, or hepatogenous, or caused by aberrant pigment synthesis. Congenital porphyria of cattle is an example of photosensitization caused by aberrant pigment synthesis. In primary phototoxic photosensitization the ingested or contact chemical acts directly as the photodynamic agent. Examples of this include certain plants *(Hypericum)* and chemicals (phenothiazines, sulfonamides, tetracyclines, others).[258] These are listed and discussed in Chapter 50.

Hepatogenous or secondary phototoxic photosensitization occurs when toxins, bacteria, viruses, or neoplasia damage the liver sufficiently to prevent excretion of phylloerythrin

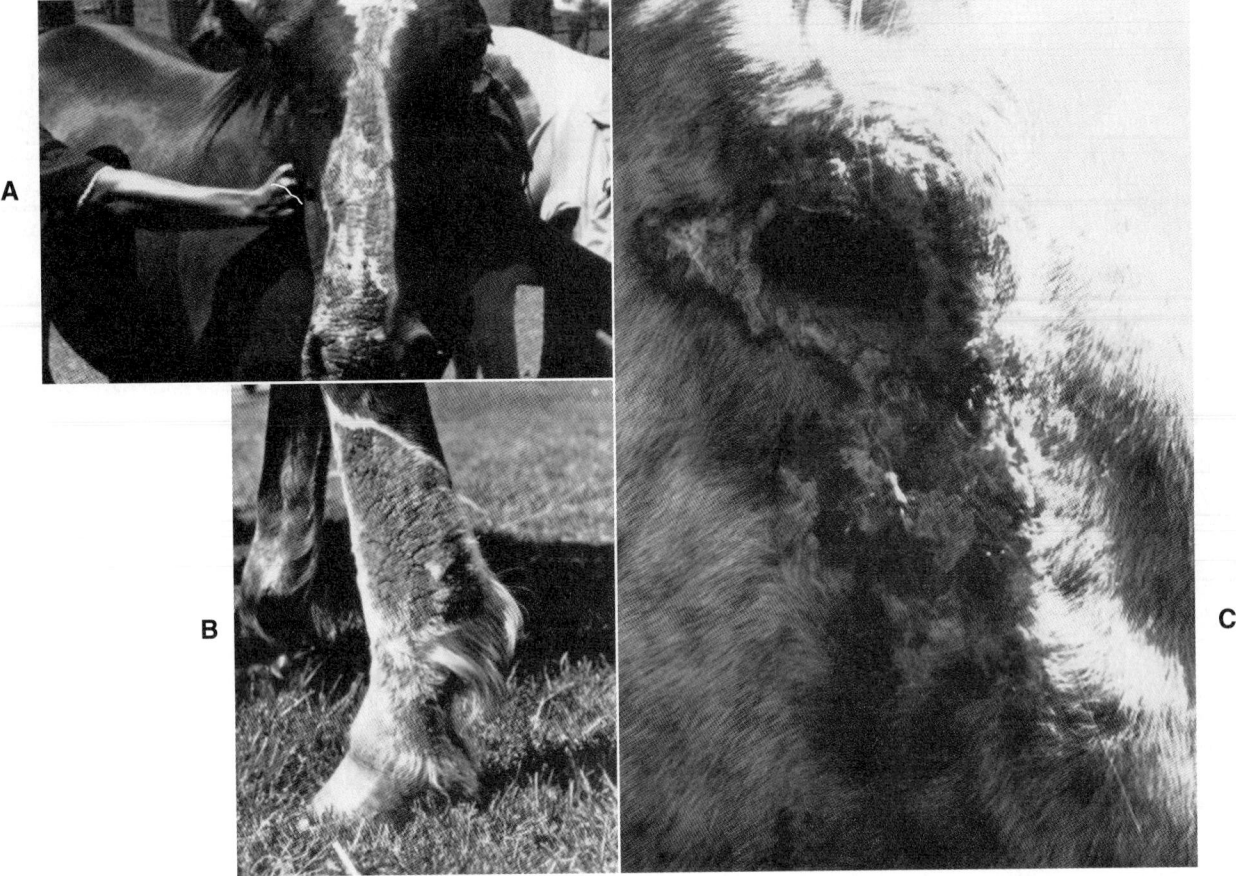

FIG. 38-21 ■■ Photosensitization. **A,** White blaze of a horse is selectively sunburned. **B,** White stocking of a horse is selectively sunburned. **C,** Area around eye where hair is less dense is most severely sunburned.

(see Chapter 31). Phylloerythrin, a porphyrin compound formed by microbial degradation of chlorophyll in the gut, is normally conjugated in the liver and excreted in the bile. Plasma phylloerythrin over 10 g/dl is diagnostic of retention.[258] Hepatogenous photosensitization is very common in large animals; bilirubin, liver enzymes, bile acids, or liver function tests should be evaluated whenever photosensitization is observed.

Lesions of photosensitization occur most frequently in hairless and white-skinned (unpigmented) areas. The eyelids, nose, white blazes, coronary bands, and other white areas are most frequently involved (Fig. 38-21). In contact photosensitization only areas of contact with the chemical are involved. The lesions vary from urticarial lesions, with erythema and swelling, to necrosis of the skin.[258,259] Either the epidermis or the superficial dermal vasculature may be damaged.

Therapy involves removing the animal from sunlight, ap-plying soothing topical creams, and preventing reexposure to the photodynamic agent. All drugs being administered when photosensitization occurred should be stopped. If the liver is involved, appropriate therapy for liver disease must be given. In photoallergic photosensitization, systemic (1.1 mg/kg/day prednisone or prednisolone PO for 10 days)[259,260] or topical corticosteroids may be helpful.

The prognosis for recovery is good with primary photo-sensitization but poor for hepatogenous photosensitization because severe liver disease carries a poor prognosis.

REFERENCES

258. Scott DW: *Large animal dermatology,* Philadelphia, 1988, WB Saunders, pp 76-80.
259. Stannard AA: *Veterinary dermatology syllabus,* Davis, Calif, 1988, University of California.
260. White SD: Photosensitivity. In Robinson NE, ed: *Current therapy in equine medicine,* ed 2, 1987, Philadelphia, WB Saunders, pp 632-633.

Endocrine and Metabolic Diseases

NOËL O. DYBDAL

Consulting Editor

ENDOCRINE DISORDERS

NOËL O. DYBDAL

HYPOTHALAMUS AND PITUITARY GLAND

ANTERIOR LOBE (PARS INTERMEDIA) DYSFUNCTION

Equine Cushing's Disease

DEFINITION AND ETIOLOGY. Hypertrophy, hyperplasia, adenomatous hyperplasia, or functional adenomas of the pituitary pars intermedia represent a pathologic continuum associated with a clinical syndrome historically associated with hirsutism, polydipsia, polyuria, and hyperglycemia.[4-6] The diffuse physical enlargement of the pars intermedia results from decreased dopaminergic innervation of the pars intermedia. The loss of dopaminergic inhibition leads to an increase in melanotrope function.[1,2] This is evidenced by increased and uncontrolled secretion of β-endorphin (β-END), α-melanotropin (α-MSH), and adrenocorticotropin hormone (ACTH) in afflicted animals.[3,7-10] Secondary adrenocortical involvement results from the secretion of these pituitary hormones. As with the physical change in the pituitary gland the associated clinical signs present a spectrum, arising as a sequela of the excess circulating glucocorticoids, physical destruction of the pars nervosa, and, possibly, the direct peripheral action of the pituitary proopiomelanocortin (POMC)-derived peptides.

Complete compression of the pars distalis by the enlarged pars intermedia leading to secondary hypopituitarism has not been documented. Because this syndrome in many ways resembles human Cushing's disease, which is hypercortisolism secondary to hypersecretion of ACTH from a pituitary tumor, for lack of a better term this clinical condition of horses is called equine Cushing's disease, although the two disorders are not identical. Use of the term Cushing's disease has potentially caused misunderstanding of the pathogenesis of this disease in the horse; identification of the pituitary lesion as neoplastic; and, overestimation of the importance of the adrenocortical contribution to the clinical syndrome.

CLINICAL SIGNS AND DIFFERENTIAL DIAGNOSES. The average age of Cushing's horses is 19 years, with a range of 7 to 40 years. There is no sex predilection; mares, geldings, and stallions appear to be at equal risk. Incidence in ponies appears increased compared with horses, but population analysis has not been done. No specific horse breed appears to be affected more often than another.[11]

Because of the slow onset of the disease and the complex metabolic aberrations potentially possible, a wide variety of clinical signs are seen. Hirsutism is the clinical sign most commonly associated with equine Cushing's disease. Approximately 85% of affected animals studied exhibit coat abnormalities, including the classic thick, long, curly coat that is sometimes not shed. Less striking coat changes are also seen, including slightly heavier than usual winter hair coat;

shedding later in the spring and regrowing winter coats earlier in the fall than other animals housed under similar conditions; and patchy, slow shedding sometimes associated with transient patchy alopecia. Early in the course of the disease many animals do not exhibit striking coat abnormalities. Change in shedding behavior and the appearance of "guard hairs" along the chin or jugular furrow in the summer may be an early indication of equine Cushing's. Pathogenesis of the abnormal hair coat has not been determined. The only differential diagnosis for the abnormal hair coat at this time is breed variation (e.g., curly, or curly-coated foxtrotter).

Chronic or recurrent acute laminitis is seen with moderate frequency in horses with Cushing's disease. The extent of this association and its relationship to the pathogenesis of either condition has not been established. Laminitis has been presumed to arise secondary to hypercortisolism in equine Cushing's disease; however, the possibility that equine Cushing's disease develops secondary to the chronic pain and distress of laminitis has also been proposed.[12] Sole abscesses are a major problem in Cushing's horses and are the most common cause of euthanasia. Cushing's disease should be suspected and included in the differentials of any horse 15 years of age or older that founders repeatedly for no obvious reason or has chronic problems with sole abscesses, even if hair coat changes or other signs are not present. Elevations in plasma levels of pituitary pars intermedia hormones have been identified in horses with laminitis.[12] Whether this is evidence of underlying Cushing's disease or an appropriate, reversible response to pain and distress has not been investigated.

Polyuria (PU) and polydipsia (PD) are commonly present in Cushing's horses. The multifactorial etiology of this PU/PD includes destruction of the pars nervosa by the enlarged pars intermedia, which is suspected to lead to decreased antidiuretic hormone (ADH) secretion. Hyperglycemia, observed in many Cushing's horses, causes an osmotic diuresis. Cortisol can also directly elevate glomerular filtration rate. Differential diagnoses for PU/PD include renal disease, primary diabetes insipidus, psychogenic diabetes insipidus, and hyperglycemia secondary to pancreatic destruction.

Hyperhidrosis is observed in many Cushing's horses, but the specific mechanism has not been determined. Although the pathogenesis is probably multifactorial, equine sweat glands are reported to be entirely under β-adrenergic control,[13] making it tempting to speculate on a specific β-adrenergic lesion in the Cushing's horse. Differential diagnosis for excessive sweating in the horse includes functional pheochromocytoma; however, in these cases, hyperhidrosis is also generally associated with outward signs such as anxiety, tachycardia, and dilated pupils (i.e., increased circulating catecholamines). In rare cases, both transient and persistent anhidrosis have been reported.

Muscle wasting is a common complaint and is probably primarily related to disuse and aging with a possible component of corticosteroid myopathy, although the latter has not been documented. Although weight loss is a common complaint, it is not documented as causally related to the pituitary lesion in any but possibly the most advanced cases. The vast majority of the horses studied have been of normal weight or obese (a certain amount of muscle wasting should not be confused with "weight loss"). Those that were thin and debilitated on entry to the research program at the University of California, Davis, have almost all been severely parasitized, had chronic dental problems, or lacked teeth, requiring special diets that had not been provided. A small number of these thin, debilitated animals also had internal abscesses or advanced liver disease. Cushing's horses must be carefully assessed for condition of teeth, diet, and gastrointestinal parasitism, because they easily acquire heavy parasite burdens. Thin, debilitated Cushing's horses should be fed meal or softened alfalfa pellets with vegetable oil to increase calorie intake. When provided in moderation, pelleted, all-in-one type rations are also excellent for these horses. Deworming should be performed at least every 8 weeks, particularly if the horses have any exposure to other horses through common pastures or drylots. Supraorbital swelling noted in many Cushing's horses is caused by a fat pad and is associated with obesity, not hypothyroidism. All animals with this type of fat pad studied to date have been euthyroid. Sinusitis is a common problem that generally occurs secondary to periodontal disease, specifically oronasal fistulas.

Elevated respiratory rates are observed in many horses with Cushing's disease; a specific mechanism has not been determined. Causes may include chronic or intercurrent pulmonary disease (e.g., pneumonia, chronic obstructive pulmonary disease) that may or may not be specifically associated with Cushing's disease. Pneumonia should be handled aggressively. *Nocardia* spp. and fungal pneumonias, including *Coccidioides immitis* and *Aspergillus* spp., have been reported in horses with Cushing's disease, suggesting that Cushing's horses may have a defect in cell-mediated immunity. In hyperglycemic animals a degree of acidosis is probably present and may be associated with compensatory increase in respiratory rate.

CLINICAL PATHOLOGY. Cushing's horses frequently have a normal complete blood count and equine chemistry panel. If the general condition is poor, there may be mild decreases in red blood cell (RBC) numbers and hemoglobin concentration. Most commonly, normal to high-normal neutrophil and low-normal lymphocyte counts are seen hematologically. Hyperglycemia (insulin-resistant) is present in many cases.[14] Hyperlipemia is present in a small number of horses and ponies; when present it is a grave prognostic sign, generally associated in a very short time with liver failure and clotting disorders. Despite hyperlipemia, affected Cushing's horses are polyphagic; thus nutritional support is not effective or indicated. Rapid reversal of hyperlipemia has been reported in a single hyperlipemic Cushing's horse treated with the dopaminergic agonist pergolide.[15]* Baseline, or resting, plasma cortisol concentration is generally indistinguishable from that in normal horses but can be moderately elevated (as it can also be in normal horses stressed before sample collection). Baseline, or resting, plasma thyroxine (T_4) and triiodothyronine (T_3) concentrations are normal.

Definitive diagnostic tests include the following:
1. Dexamethasone suppression test (40 μg/kg or 2 mg/ 100 lb).[16]
   a. Overnight protocol—begin test between 4 and 6 PM (Fig. 39-1).
      (1) Draw predexamethasone blood sample in heparinized container between 4 and 6 PM.
      (2) Administer dexamethasone intramuscularly.
      (3) Draw postdexamethasone blood sample in heparinized container at noon the following day (approximately 19 hours after dexamethasone administration).
   b. Standard protocol—begin test at midnight (see Fig. 39-1).
      (1) Draw predexamethasone sample in heparinized container at midnight.
      (2) Administer dexamethasone intramuscularly.
      (3) Draw postdexamethasone blood samples into heparinized containers at 8 AM, noon, 4 PM, 8 PM, and midnight.
   c. Interpretation of results: normal horses: ≤1 μg/dl (10 ng/ml) cortisol 19 hours after administration of

---

*Permax, Athena Neurosciences, South San Francisco, CA, 94080.

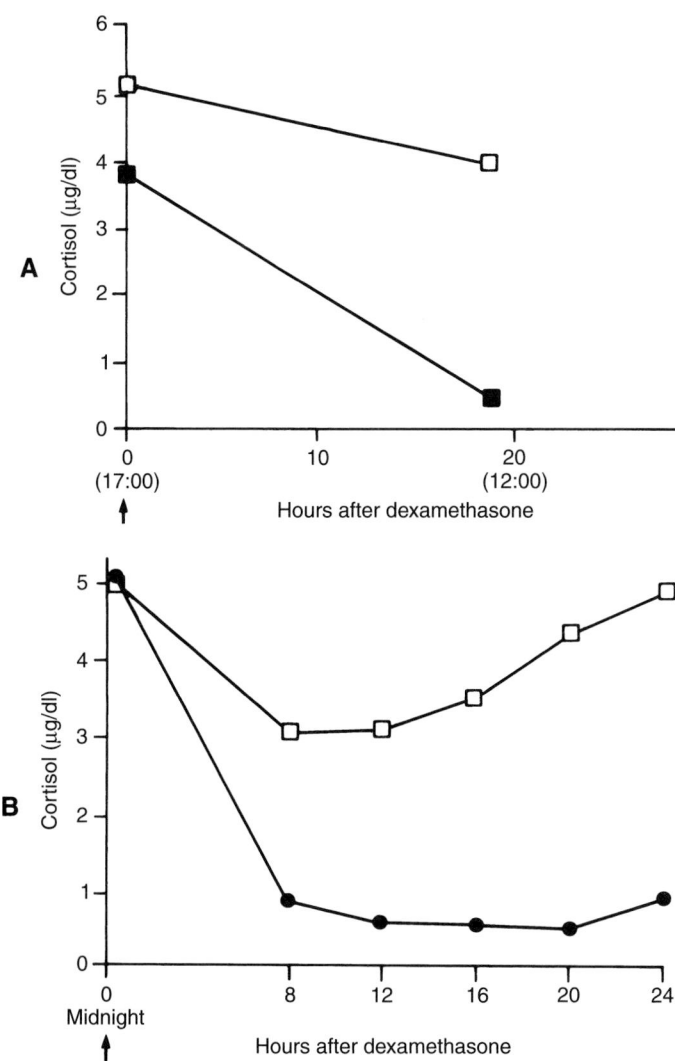

FIG. 39-1 ▉ Dexamethasone suppression test. □, Cushing's; ■ control; ↑, 40 μg dexamethasone intramuscularly. **A,** Overnight; **B,** standard.

dexamethsone using the overnight protocol and at 24 hours after administration of dexamethasone using the standard protocol. The overnight protocol is an excellent screening test. The more extensive samplings of the standard protocol allow for assessment of degree of loss of pituitary function or improvement in treated cases.

2. ACTH challenge test—1 IU/kg of ACTH gel IM or 100 IU of synthetic ACTH (Cosyntropin) IV. Presented under adrenal gland section, this test does not adequately distinguish between normal and Cushing's horses. The test is important in recognizing adrenal exhaustion, or insufficiency.

3. The insulin tolerance test has been proposed for use as a diagnostic test for equine Cushing's disease.[14] Generally this test is only useful in Cushing's horses that are hyperglycemic. The test should be used if the suspected cause of hyperglycemia is pancreatic disease rather than Cushing's disease.

4. The combined dexamethasone-Cosyntropin test fails to distinguish normal from Cushing's horses. In a significant percentage of cases, false-positive and false-negative results are seen. The suppressive effects of dexamethasone are not allowed to develop over a long enough time.[16] The recommended time for dexamethasone administration

(9 AM) is a time of day when the adrenal cortex is already under almost maximum ACTH stimulation.

NECROPSY FINDINGS. The most consistent and striking gross necropsy finding is pituitary enlargement (average 7.1 g, range 3.4 to 16.6 g; normal weight 1 to 3 g). This enlargement is attributable to diffuse, adenomatous hyperplasia of the pars intermedia. These horses also generally have significant adrenocortical hyperplasia (adrenal glands average 62 g, range 37 to 120; normal weight 15 to 17 g each, 35 g paired).[17] Additional gross necropsy findings often observed are related to intercurrent disease conditions and include hepatomegaly, laminitis, and gastrointestinal parasitism.

TREATMENT AND PROGNOSIS. Fastidious attention to excellent husbandry and feeding practices and careful management of secondary complications are the least expensive and to date the most successful approaches to "treatment" of the horse with Cushing's disease. Horses have been followed for as long as 10 years on such programs. Prognosis can be predicted to a limited extent based on the degree of hyperglycemia. Affected horses that are euglycemic have an excellent long-term prognosis with appropriate management. Horses that are mildly hyperglycemic also generally have a good prognosis but can be more susceptible than euglycemic animals to intercurrent infectious problems. Horses that are moderately to severely hyperglycemic (>275 mg glucose/dl) have a more guarded prognosis and are the most appropriate cases in which to consider therapeutic intervention.

Use of dopaminergic agonist compounds to treat equine Cushing's disease is based on current knowledge of pars intermedia secretory control; these compounds offer the greatest promise for efficacy.[16] Although the use of these compounds has only been reported in a limited number of Cushing's horses, there is now extensive clinical experience and anecdotal support for this therapeutic approach.[6,8,15] The use of a dopaminergic agonist has been associated with modest declines in POMC peptides as measured in a single horse.[8] Pergolide is a long-acting dopaminergic agonist. Additional case reports have detailed the results of pergolide administration to two horses at a dosage of 5 mg/day by mouth[8] and to one pony at a dosage of 1 mg/day by mouth as improvement of clinical signs but without a return to normal dexamethasone suppressibility.[6] Long-term effects in these animals were not reported. Moore, Abood, and Hinchcliff[15] have reported successful correction of hyperlipemia in a 30-year-old miniature horse with Cushing's disease and hyperlipemia using 0.2 mg/kg pergolide once per day by mouth. Low-dose pergolide therapy, 0.5 to 2 mg/day total dose administered once daily, or in some cases divided twice daily has been used successfully in a large number of horses. Good clinical response has been reported over extended periods (plasma POMC peptides have not been assessed). Low-dose pergolide therapy in Cushing's horses with both acute and chronic laminitis has not been associated with progression or exacerbation of laminitis. In several Cushing's horses suffering from acute flare-ups of laminitis, clinical improvement has been reported when these horses were given low-dose pergolide therapy.[18]

Cyproheptidine, a drug with antiserotonergic activity, has been used with limited success as evaluated by objective criteria[19]; however, anecdotal information from practitioners suggests that the response is better in the field. Currently, if owners are anxious to treat, the horse is given 0.25 mg/kg PO once per day for 8 weeks. If at that time no improvement is seen, the cyproheptidine dose can be increased to 0.50 mg/kg divided twice daily for 4 to 8 weeks. If there is still no improvement, the drug should be discontinued, although some practitioners have reported clinical improvement without ill effect on animals with as much as 1 mg/kg/day divided twice daily. There is little experimental evidence to suggest that this drug should be efficacious, although clinical improvement and lowering of blood glucose levels have been seen in some animals.[19]

The most important consideration in long-term maintenance of the Cushing's horse continues to be excellent management with regular deworming, nutrition, hoof care, and rapid response to any potential for infection (e.g., wounds, sole abscess, pneumonia). Euglycemic Cushing's horses often do well with only careful stable managment. Neither cyproheptidine or pergolide is currently labeled for use in horses. The use of pergolide in particular deserves further investigation, but, until a controlled trial including pharmacokinetic analyses is undertaken, dose and dosing intervals will remain anecdotal.

The adrenocorticolytic drug, *o,p'*-DDD, has not been effective in the horse. Attempts to use this drug, even in massive doses, have failed to have any functional or morphologic effect on the adrenal glands of normal or Cushing's horses.[20] There are no reports of ketaconazole,* a steroid synthesis blocker, being used in the horse.

POSTERIOR PITUITARY DYSFUNCTION

Diabetes Insipidus

Diabetes insipidus results from decreased release of ADH from the posterior pituitary. As already noted, the most common cause of decreased ADH release in the horse is posterior pituitary destruction secondary to pars intermedia enlargement; however, in rare cases, idiopathic diabetes insipidus has been reported in the horse.[21] The clinical presentation of PU and PD in an otherwise normal animal must include as differentials primary renal disease, psychogenic PD syndrome,[22] equine Cushing's disease, and diabetes insipidus caused by posterior pituitary dysfunction unrelated to equine Cushing's disease. In the horse with idiopathic diabetes insipidus, urine specific gravity is less than 1.01. The affected animals fail to concentrate urine on a water deprivation test. In one reported case the horse responded to exogenous ADH (40 U of pitressin tannate in oil intramuscularly) with a decrease in water consumption and concentration of the urine, which lasted approximately 24 hours.[21] Blood ADH concentrations were low compared with controls and did not change in response to water deprivation.

Although also relatively uncommon, psychogenic PD syndrome is seen, with some concentration of urine in affected horses (up to 1.025) when they are subjected to a deprivation test. ADH levels in this disorder have not been reported. With renal disease, specific gravity rarely falls below 1.01, and other laboratory findings (e.g., elevated blood urea nitrogen [BUN], creatinine) are consistent with the diagnosis. The same is true of equine Cushing's disease, and, because the PU and PD of Cushing's are not entirely related to decreased ADH levels, animals frequently respond normally to water deprivation.

Pituitary ablation secondary to nonfunctional tumors, lymphoma, metastatic tumors, and necrosis has been seen.[11] In addition to diabetes insipidus, these animals also exhibit signs of anterior pituitary dysfunction, resulting in clinical signs of hypoglycemia.

REFERENCES

1. Lundblad J, Roberts J: Regulation of proopiomelanocortin gene expression in pituitary, *Endocrinol Rev* 9:135-158, 1988

2. Smith IA, Funder J: Proopiomelanocortin processing in the pituitary, central nervous system, and peripheral tissues, *Endocrinol Rev* 9:159-179, 1988.
3. Millington W et al: Equine Cushing's disease: differential regulation of β-endorphin processing in tumors of the intermediate pituitary, *Endocrinology* 123:1598-1604, 1988.
4. Gribble DH: The endocrine system. In Catcott EJ, Smithcors JF, eds: *Equine medicine and surgery*, ed 2, Santa Barbara, Calif, 1972, American Veterinary Publications, pp 433-457.
5. Moore J et al: A case of pituitary ACTH-dependent Cushing's syndrome in the horse, *Endocrinology* 104:576, 1979.
6. Beech J: Tumors of the pituitary gland (pars intermedia). In Robinson NE, ed: *Current therapy in equine medicine*, ed 2, Philadelphia, 1987, WB Saunders, pp 182-185.
7. Dybdal N et al: Short and N-acetylated forms of endorphin predominate in plasma of normal and Cushing's horses, *Endocrinology* 118(suppl):270, 1986.
8. Orth D et al: Equine Cushing's disease: plasma immunoreactive proopiolipomelanocortin peptide and cortisol levels basally and in response to diagnostic tests, *Endocrinology* 110:1430, 1982.
9. Wilson M et al: Proopiolipomelanocortin peptides in normal pituitary, pituitary tumor, and plasma of normal and Cushing's horses, *Endocrinology* 110:941-954, 1982.
10. Horvath C et al: Adrenocorticotropin-containing neoplastic cells in a pars intermedia adenoma in a horse, *J Am Vet Med Assoc* 192:367-371, 1988.
11. Dybal NO: Unpublished observations. PhD thesis, University of California–Davis, June 1989.
12. Ganjam V et al: Implications of chronic laminitis in Cushing's-like disease in horses, *Fed Proc* 42:726, 1983.
13. Bijman J, Quinton P: Predominantly β-adrenergic control of equine sweating, *Am J Physiol* 246:R349-R353, 1984.
14. Garcia M, Beech J: Equine intravenous glucose tolerance test: glucose and insulin responses of healthy horses fed grain or hay and of horses with pituitary adenoma, *Am J Vet Res* 47:570-572, 1986.
15. Moore BR, Abood SK, Hinchcliff KW: Hyperlipemia in 9 miniature horses and miniature donkeys, *J Vet Intern Med* 8:376-381, 1994.
16. Dybdal NO et al: Diagnostic testing for pituitary pars intermedia dysfunction in horses, *J Am Vet Med Assoc* 204:627-632, 1994.
17. Dybal NO: PhD thesis, University of California, Davis, 1989.
18. Dybal NO: Unpublished observations, 1995.
19. Gribble DH, Dybdal NO: Preliminary findings on the efficacy of cyproheptidine as a therapeutic agent for equine Cushing's disease, *Proceedings of the Thirty-third Annual Meeting of the American College of Veterinary Pathologists*, Atlanta, 1982.
20. Gribble DH, Madigan J: Unpublished observations, 1974.
21. Breukink H, Van Wegen P, Schotman A: Idiopathic diabetes insipidus in a Welsh pony, *Equine Vet J* 15:284-287, 1983.
22. Madigan J: Unpublished observations, 1987.

ADRENAL GLANDS

The paired adrenal glands in the horse lie craniomedial to the kidneys. The right adrenal is medially adherent to the vena cava (which is one reason it is very difficult to perform adrenalectomy in the horse) and cranially lies in the impression in the liver formed by the right kidney. The left adrenal is associated with the cranial mesenteric artery on its medial border, the aorta and renal artery on its dorsal border, and the left aspect of the pancreas on its ventral border.[23] The glands are well vascularized. The adrenal cortex is composed of the outermost zona glomerulosa, which produces mineralocorticoids, primarily in response to angiotensin II and falling serum sodium levels; the zona fasciculata, which produces glucocorticoids in response to stimulation by ACTH; and the zona reticularis, responsible for adrenal androgen production. The centrally located adrenal medulla produces catecholamines. In the horse the primary adrenal medullary catecholamine appears to be epinephrine; however, norepinephrine and dopamine are also produced and secreted to some extent.[24] The adrenal glands are a shock organ in the horse, and adrenal hemorrhage and necrosis are common sequelae to conditions such as severe bouts of endotoxemia and colic. The sinusoidal type of blood flow makes the adrenals a prime site for establishment of metastatic tumors.

The adrenal glands weigh 15 to 17 g each and are 9 to 10 cm in length, 3 to 4 cm wide, and 1.5 cm thick.

*Permax, Athena Neurosciences, South San Francisco, CA, 94080.

ADRENAL EXHAUSTION

DEFINITION, ETIOLOGY, AND PATHOPHYSIOLOGY. Adrenal exhaustion and "turn-out" or "let down" syndrome are much discussed, poorly documented syndromes ascribed to adrenal insufficiency in the horse. Low cortisol levels have not been found in racehorses that turn in poor performances blamed on adrenal exhaustion.[25] Abnormal response to ACTH challenge has not been noted in endurance horses after 22.4-km (36 mile) rides.[26] Low circulating cortisol levels have been noted after 160-km (100 mile) rides; however, adrenal function was not assessed by any provocative tests in this study.[27] At necropsy it is more common to find enlarged adrenal glands in racehorses than it is to find atrophic glands. This hypertrophy may be the result of repeated administration of exogenous ACTH, which in turn could lead to "let down" when injections are discontinued, or it may be caused by chronic stress. Because the adrenals are a shock organ in the horse, they can be damaged (i.e., by hemorrhage and necrosis, which can lead to subsequent scarring) during bouts of endotoxemia, severe colic, or anaphylaxis. Chronic administration of corticosteroids can also lead to adrenocortical insufficiency.

CLINICAL SIGNS, DIFFERENTIAL DIAGNOSES, AND CLINICAL PATHOLOGY. Adrenal insufficiency should be considered in the differentials of horses presenting with depression, anorexia, weight loss, hyponatremia, hypochloremia, hyperkalemia, or hypoglycemia, particularly if any of the following factors are present:

- The horse has recently come off the track
- The horse has come out of some other form of intensive training
- Corticosteroids have been administered
- There is a recent history of conditions such as severe colic or periods of dehydration

LABORATORY AIDS AND DEFINITIVE DIAGNOSIS

1. 1 IU/kg of ACTH gel challenge test (Fig. 39-2)[28,29]
   a. Draw pre-ACTH heparinized sample between 8 and 10 AM.
   b. Administer 1 IU/kg of ACTH gel intramuscularly.
   c. Draw post-ACTH heparinized sample at 2 and 4 hours after ACTH administration.
   d. Interpret results: should see a twofold to threefold increase in cortisol levels over baseline.
2. 100 IU of Cosyntropin challenge test (see Fig. 39-2)[30]
   a. Draw pre-ACTH heparinized sample between 8 AM and noon.
   b. Administer 100 IU (or 1 mg) synthetic ACTH intravenously.
   c. Draw post-ACTH heparinized sample at 2 hours after ACTH administration.
   d. Interpret results: should see doubling of cortisol over baseline.

NECROPSY FINDINGS. Adrenal hemorrhages, necrosis, or moderate adrenocortical collapse and fibrosis may be seen at necropsy.

TREATMENT AND PROGNOSIS. Management of adrenal suppression may be required after long-term corticosteroid administration.

Several investigators have evaluated the effect of administration of dexamethasone on subsequent adrenal responsiveness.[31-33] Tapered doses of dexamethasone are probably not useful in weaning horses off steroids because as little as 4 mg, total dose, of dexamethasone causes 18 to 24 hours of pituitary-adrenal suppression.[34] Consequently, if the daily dose of dexamethasone is tapered from 40 mg to 20 mg to 10 mg to 5 mg, a complete suppression of endogenous adrenal function for each day occurs and actually produces abrupt withdrawal. Treatment of adult horses with 40 mg of dexamethasone every 5 days for 30 days was not reported to

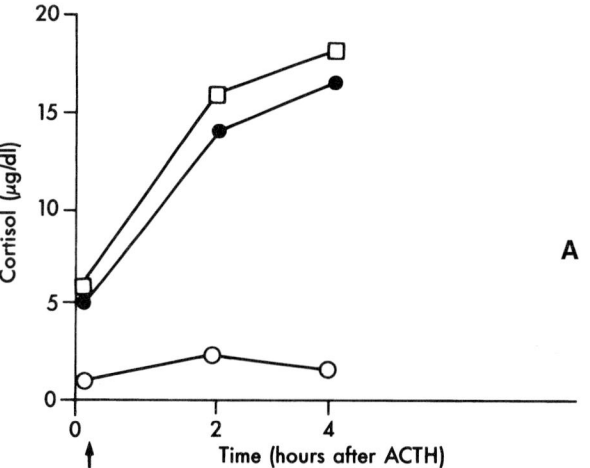

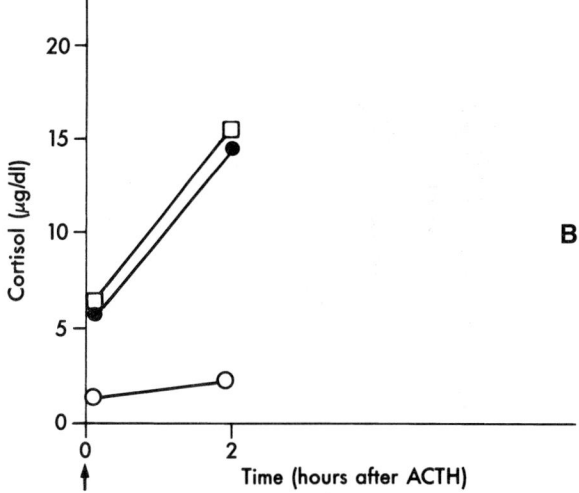

FIG. 39-2 ■ ACTH Challenge test. □, Cushing's; ●, control; ○, adrenal insufficiency. **A,** Gel. ↑, 1 IU/kg ACTH gel intramuscularly. **B,** Synthetic ACTH. ↓, 100 IU (1 mg) synthetic ACTH intravenously, total dose to horse.

alter adrenal gland function.[31] Daily administration of 30 mg of dexamethasone to adult horses for 31 days also produced no significant lasting effects on adrenal responsiveness.[35] Therefore it would seem that, in cases treated for 30 days or less with less than 40 mg of dexamethasone, withdrawal of steroids could be accomplished abruptly, provided no stress or surgery is contemplated in the immediate future.

Prednisolone sodium succinate administered intravenously and intramuscularly produced less than 24 hours of adrenal suppression.[32] In contrast, prednisolone acetate suspension given intramuscularly produced adrenal suppression for over 7 days. These data suggest that daily doses of less than 300 mg of prednisolone in a nonsuspension formulation in adult horses should not produce complete adrenal suppression. Conversely, a single injection of triamcinolone 0.044 mg/kg IM produced 14 days of disruption of the pituitary-adrenal axis in one study[33] and must therefore be regarded as more capable of producing adrenal suppression and eventual atrophy than is dexamethasone or prednisolone.

PHEOCHROMOCYTOMA (ADRENAL MEDULLA)

Although adrenal medullary tumors are generally nonfunctional tumors noted incidentally at necropsy, there are a few case reports in the literature of functional adrenal medullary tumors in horses.[36] Signs include excessive sweating (hyperhidrosis), PD, PU, apprehension, recurrent colic, increased heart rate, dilated pupils, hyperglycemia, and hypertension. Determination of blood or urinary catecholamine levels can aid in diagnosis.

ANHIDROSIS

Catecholamines and β-adrenergic control of sweat glands have been implicated as important in the pathogenesis of this disorder, which is still poorly understood. Beadle, Norwood, and Brencick[37] showed that plasma epinephrine levels were significantly elevated in a group of anhidrotic horses in Louisiana and suggested that this had led to down regulation and insensitivity of the β2-receptors of the sweat glands and subsequently anhidrosis. More work must be done on this continuing problem of horses in hot climates.

REFERENCES

23. Slone D et al: Vascular anatomy and surgical technique for bilateral adrenalectomy in the equid, *Am J Vet Res* 41:829-832, 1980.
24. Hardee G et al: Catecholamines in equine and bovine plasmas, *J Vet Pharmacol Ther* 5:279-284, 1982.
25. Baker H et al: Effect of stress on steroid hormone levels in racehorses, *Aust Vet J* 58:70-71, 1982.
26. Snow DH, MacKenzie G: Metabolic effects of maximal exercise in the horse and adaptations with training, *Equine Vet J* 9:134-140, 1977.
27. Dybdal N et al: Alterations in plasma corticosteroids, insulin, and selected metabolites in horses used in endurance rides, *Equine Vet J* 12:137-140, 1980.
28. Dybal NO et al: Diagnostic testing for pituitary pars intermedia dysfunction in horses, *J Am Vet Med Assoc* 204:627-632.
29. Hoffsis GF et al: Plasma concentrations of cortisol and corticosterone in the normal horse, *Am J Vet Res* 31:1379-1387, 1970.
30. Eiler H, Goble D, Oliver J: Adrenal gland function in the horse: effects of Cosyntropin (synthetic) and corticotropin (natural) stimulation, *Am J Vet Res* 40:724-726, 1979.
31. MacHarg M et al: Effects of multiple intramuscular injections and doses of dexamethasone on plasma cortisol concentrations and adrenal responses to ACTH in horses, *Am J Vet Res* 46:2285-2287, 1985.
32. Toutain P et al: Dexamethasone and prednisolone in the horse: pharmacokinetics and action on the adrenal gland, *Am J Vet Res* 45:1750-1756, 1984.
33. Slone D et al: Sodium retention and cortisol suppression caused by dexamethasone and triamcinolone in equines, *Am J Vet Res* 44:280-283, 1983.
34. Madigan J, Dybal NO: Unpublished observations, 1989.
35. Wilson D: Unpublished observations, 1985.
36. Yovich J, Ducharme N: Rupture pheochromocytoma in a mare with colic, *J Am Vet Med Assoc* 183:462-464, 1983.
37. Beadle R, Norwood G, Brencick V: Summertime plasma catecholamine concentrations in healthy and anhidrotic horses in Louisiana, *Am J Vet Res* 43:1446-1448, 1982.

THYROID GLAND

The thyroid gland is situated on the cranial aspect of the trachea, with lateral lobes present at the level of the larynx at the angle of the junction of the jugular and external maxillary veins. The cranial cervical lymph nodes are arrayed around the gland (which adds to the confusion when trying to grossly identify the external parathyroid glands). The thyroid gland body, or isthmus, is generally unrecognizable or present only as a narrow band of connective tissue in the adult horse. In the foal the isthmus is reported to be relatively large and entirely glandular. The donkey and mule are also reported to have a well-developed isthmus. At birth the foal has plasma concentrations of thyroxine (T_4) and triiodothyronine (T_3) 10 to 20 times greater than the adult and also greater than reported in any other species.[38]

Although frequently blamed or cited as a cause of problems, thyroid disease has rarely been documented in the horse, except as hypothyroidism in the foal. The high frequency of clinical diagnosis of hypothyroidism in the adult horse must be questioned. Nonfunctional adenomas are a relatively frequent finding in the aged adult. The frequency with which these nodular enlargements are found seems to suggest a geographic clustering, and thus they may be environmental in nature.

The average adult thyroid gland weighs approximately 15 g/lobe and is 5 cm by 2.5 cm by 2 cm.

NEONATAL HYPOTHYROIDISM

DEFINITION AND ETIOLOGY. Hyperplastic goiter in neonates is the most common thyroid disorder in the horse and small ruminant. The cause is generally ingestion by the dam during pregnancy of excess iodine (usually in the form of kelp-containing feed supplements) or plant goitrogens; a few cases of "idiopathic" hyperplastic goiter, all from western Canada, have been reported.[39] Although the equine placenta is permeable to iodine and plant goitrogens, it is impermeable to T_3 and T_4. Irvine[38] separates hypothyroidism in the foal into two categories: (1) hypometabolic state, which occurs concurrent with thyroid hormone inadequacy, and (2) developmental lesions, which may be observed in the face of normal thyroid hormone levels, a signal that thyroid hormone deprivation occurred during a critical developmental period. Obviously this is rather difficult to document clinically and may be one reason why confirmed cases of foal hypothyroidism are low. Although the thyroid gland may appear grossly normal in these foals, histologic lesions persist for some time after an episode of hyperplastic goiter, and biopsy may provide the best diagnostic tool if confirmation is required.

CLINICAL SIGNS AND DIFFERENTIAL DIAGNOSES. There is no specific breed or sex predilection for neonatal hypothyroidism. A pathognomonic clinical sign that is not invariably present is grossly evident thyroid enlargement or goiter. Because neonatal hypothyroidism is of the thyroprivic type, the pituitary gland is normal, but the thyroid glands are not. Inadequate thyroid hormones are present in the circulation, leading to stimulation by pituitary thyroid-stimulating hormone (TSH), which in turn leads to thyroid enlargement. The other clinical signs are the direct result of low thyroid hormone concentrations, but these signs are less specific. It is difficult to differentiate the remaining clinical signs from congenital lesions of undetermined etiology. Incoordination and poor sucking and righting reflexes are associated with hypomyelination and lesions of the central nervous system. Hypothermia is associated with the lowered metabolic rate of hypothyroidism. Tendon contracture and/or rupture and retarded bone development are related to absence of the thyroid hormones.[40] Foals can also be born with no apparent signs, but after a few weeks skeletal lesions appear, particularly in the tarsus.[39]

CLINICAL PATHOLOGY. TSH response test in 1-day foals using 5 IU of TSH intravenously produced a peak of T_3 (at least 2× increase) within 1 to 3 hours. Measurement of T_4 produced marked variations.[41]

TREATMENT AND PROGNOSIS. Thyroid hormone therapy is effective only during periods of inadequate thyroid hormone plasma concentrations; hence developmental lesions cannot be reversed. If the foal exhibits evidence of thyroid hormone deficiency but thyroid hormone concentrations are normal, it is an indication that thyroid hormone deficiency occurred during a critical developmental period, and supplementation at this time will be ineffective. When hormone levels are low, Irvine[38] recommends calculating hormone dose based on the secretion rate, which has been determined for the horse from birth to various ages, as follows: fractional turnover (0.22) × volume of distribution

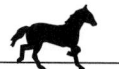

(kilograms of body weight $\times$ 0.08) $\times$ plasma T_4 (micrograms per liter) $\times$ 10 (for administration by mouth; $\times$ 3 for subcutaneous or intramuscular administration). The calculated dose should be administered once daily. If a severe hypometabolic state is present, a loading dose of T_3 equal to one-third the calculated T_4 dose should be administered parenterally, because it takes several days to see a response to T_4.

ADULT HYPOTHYROIDISM

Although functional adult hypothyroidism has not been documented, many papers detailing methods of diagnosis have been published. The published methods have uniformly presented the normal results of control horses and have then extended these findings to establish criteria for the diagnosis of hypothyroidism without presenting results in hypothyroid horses. Hypothyroidism should be considered in the differential of any horse presenting with a history of lethargy, poor exercise tolerance, or muscular problems. These are documented features of hypothyroidism in horses as established by surgical thyroidectomy.[42] Conversely, hypothyroidism has not been documented in lethargic, fat horses presenting with a cresty neck, bulging fat pads above the eyes, and, frequently, laminitis. These horses sometimes, but not always, have equine Cushing's disease, but they have not been shown to be hypothyroid. The diagnosis of hypothyroidism is most commonly based on low serum concentrations of total T_4 and T_3 and clinical response to thyroid hormone supplementation. Numerous nonthyroidal factors are known to affect concentrations of thyroid hormones in other species and specifically in the horse; administration of phenylbutazone,[43-45] and food deprivation[36] have been shown to have a profound lowering effect on serum thyroid hormone concentrations. Thus hypothyroidism appears to be difficult to definitively diagnose. Thyroid hormone therapy will increase the metabolic rate and general activity level of even euthyroid animals, but in these animals it will eventually lead to iatrogenic hypothyroidism secondary to negative feedback on the thyroid glands and suppression of endogenous thyroid hormone production.

CLINICAL SIGNS AND DIFFERENTIAL DIAGNOSES. Experimental removal of thyroid glands from adult horses results in decreased body temperature, decreased appetite, scaly hair coat, edema, decreased endurance, production of elevated serum cholesterol, and anemia.[42]

CLINICAL PATHOLOGY AND DEFINITIVE DIAGNOSTIC TESTS. Several TSH stimulation test protocols have been presented in the literature; however, it has become difficult to obtain TSH commercially. A protocol that has been followed at the Veterinary Medical Teaching Hospital, University of California-Davis involves collection of a pre-TSH blood sample (serum). A 5-IU total dose of TSH is administered intramuscularly; 1 hour after TSH administration, serum T_3 should be elevated at least two times normal. Four hours after TSH administration, T_4 should also be at least two times the normal concentration (T_3 is generally still elevated at this time). Another widely used protocol is quite similar, except that TSH is administered intravenously and T_3 levels should be doubled within 30 minutes of TSH administration (actual peak 2 hours after TSH administration) and T_4 levels should be doubled by 4 hours after injection (if T_4 is measured).[47] Additional TSH and thyrotropin-releasing hormone protocols are available in the literature.[43,48-50] TSH is currently difficult to obtain and is extremely expensive.

TREATMENT AND PROGNOSIS. Many regimens for thyroid hormone replacement therapy have been presented in the literature. Chen and colleagues[51] recommend that thyroxine (T_4) be given orally at a dose of 20 μg/kg once daily or 10 mg of L-thyroxine per adult horse daily. Levels of T_4 are

then monitored periodically. Stanley and Hillidge[52] used cytobin (120-μg tablets)* at a rate of 1 mg (total dose) by mouth once daily and monitored plasma T_3. Lowe and colleagues[42] used iodinated casein (5 g/day by mouth) to treat the animals they had thyroidectomized. Dosage was adjusted on the basis of clinical response and serum T_4 levels.

HYPERTHYROIDISM

Hyperthyroidism also has not been documented in the horse. Although there are reports of thyroid carcinomas in the literature[53,54] and thyroid adenomas are common findings in the older horse, to date these have all been nonfunctional tumors. Thyroid carcinomas can behave aggressively, and therefore complete excision of these tumors is recommended. Thyroid carcinoma should be considered in the differential of any rapidly enlarging mass in the region of the thyroid. Fine-needle aspiration followed by percutaneous biopsy is useful in arriving at a definitive diagnosis. These tumors are generally very highly vascularized and must be excised with great care. Medullary thyroid neoplasms (parafollicular or C cell) have also been reported in the horse as rapidly enlarging neoplasms that responded well to surgical excision.[55]

REFERENCES
38. Irvine C: Hypothyroidism in the foal, *Equine Vet J* 16:302-306, 1984.
39. McLaughlin B, Doige C: A study of ossification of carpal and tarsal bones in normal and hypothyroid foals, *Can Vet J* 23:164-168, 1982.
40. Vivrette S, Reimers T, Krook L: Skeletal disease in a hypothyroid foal, *Cornell Vet* 74:373-386, 1984.
41. Shaftoe S et al: Thyroid-stimulating hormone response tests in 1 day-old foals, *J Equine Vet Sci* 8:310-312, 1988.
42. Lowe J et al: Equine hypothyroidism: the long term effects of thyroidectomy on metabolism and growth in mares and stallions, *Cornell Vet* 64:276-295, 1974.
43. Morris D, Garcia M: Thyroid-stimulating hormone: response test in healthy horses, and effect of phenylbutazone on equine thyroid hormones, *Am J Vet Res* 44:503-507, 1983.
44. Sojka JE, Johnson MA, Bottoms GD: Serum triiodothyronine, total thyroxine, and free thyroxine concentrations in horses, *Am J Vet Res* 54:52-55, 1993.
45. Messer NT et al: Effect of dexamethasone administration on serum thyroid hormone concentrations in clinically normal horses, *J Am Vet Med Assoc* 206:63-66, 1995.
46. Messer NT et al: Effect of food deprivation on baseline iodothyronine and cortisol concentrations in healthy, adult horses, *Am J Vet Res* 56:116-121, 1995.
47. Oliver J, Held J: TSH test: new perspective on value of monitoring T3, *J Am Vet Med Assoc* 187:931-934, 1985.
48. Held J, Oliver J: A sampling protocol for the TSH test in the horse, *J Am Vet Med Assoc* 184:326-327, 1984.
49. Lothrop C, Nolan H: Equine thyroid function assessment with the thyrotropin-releasing hormone response test, *Am J Vet Res* 47:942-944, 1986.
50. Beech J, Garcia M: Hormonal response to thyrotropin-releasing hormone in healthy horses and in horse with pituitary adenoma, *Am J Vet Res* 46:1941-1943, 1985.
51. Chen C et al: Serum levels of thyroxine and triiodothyronine in mature horses following oral administration of synthetic thyroxine (Synthroid), *Equine Vet Sci* 4:5-6, 1984.
52. Stanley O, Hillidge C: Alopecia associated with hypothyroidism in a horse, *Equine Vet J* 14:165-167, 1982.
53. Held J et al: Work intolerance in a horse with thyroid carcinoma, *J Am Vet Med Assoc* 187:1044-1045, 1985.
54. Hillidge C, Sanecki R, Theodorakis M: Thyroid carcinoma in a horse, *J Am Vet Med Assoc* 181:711-714, 1982.
55. van der Velden MA, Meulenaar H: Medullary thyroid carcinoma in a horse, *Vet Pathol* 23:622-624, 1986.

PARATHYROID GLANDS

Horses are generally considered to have four parathyroid glands. The glands are found in the thyroid region and are

*Norden Labs, Lincoln, NE 68501.

paler and less dense than thyroid tissue. They are very difficult to distinguish grossly. Accounts of where they are located differ; however, they are frequently found in the connective tissue over the dorsal border or on the cranial extremity of the lateral lobe of the thyroid. One may be embedded in the deep face of the lateral lobe of the thyroid.

Parathyroid hormone (PTH) determination using radioimmunoassay kits designed for use in the measurement of human PTH must be used with caution in the horse. Although human and horse PTH have extensive amino acid sequence homology at the amino-terminal end (N-terminal), there is extensive amino acid substitution in the midportion and at the carboxy-terminal (C-terminal) portion of the protein.[56] Most assay kits use antibodies that recognize the C-terminal portion of human PTH. At least one of these C-terminal antibody–containing kits* has been validated for use in the horse.[57] Not surprisingly, these authors did not find perfect parallelism in the binding curves; there is a tendency for the assay to underestimate low levels and to overestimate high levels of equine PTH. They concluded that, although the assay may not closely determine absolute amounts of PTH, it was reliable in determining whether PTH levels were low, normal, or high and useful when evaluated in light of serum Ca and PO_4 levels.

Parathyroid dysfunction should be considered in the differential diagnosis of any animal exhibiting hypercalcemia or $Ca:PO_4$ imbalance. Primary, secondary, and pseudohyperparathyroidism have all been reported in the horse, but only recently have these reports been accompanied by verification with PTH levels.

One case of primary hyperparathyroidism has been reported in which PTH levels were elevated. Unfortunately this report was not accompanied by any description of pathologic findings, gross or histologic, in the parathyroid glands.[57]

SECONDARY HYPERPARATHYROIDISM

Nutritional hyperparathyroidism ("big head," bran disease) was formerly the most common cause of hyperparathyroidism in the horse, but this condition has become rare as knowledge of proper equine nutrition has become more widespread. The disorder is induced by an absolute Ca deficiency, most commonly a relative Ca deficiency secondary to excess dietary PO_4 (Ca:P <1). Serum Ca and PO_4 are usually normal, but urinary PO_4 is elevated. Depending on the severity of skeletal lesions, the prognosis can be quite good once the diet is corrected.[58]

Vitamin D toxicosis can result from overzealous administration of vitamin D–containing nutritional supplements or ingestion of plants with leaves that have vitamin D–like biologic activity such as *Cestrum diurnum* (wild jasmine, day cestrum) or *Solanum malacoxylon* (which does not grow in the continental United States). These horses have elevated serum Ca, but serum PO_4 is normal, and pathologic calcification of soft tissue is widespread in arteries, tendons, and ligaments.[59] Limited investigation of PTH levels in hypercalcemic horses in renal failure indicates that levels of PTH are low, and therefore the elevated Ca levels found in some cases of renal failure in the horse are thought to be associated not with elevated PTH levels, but with some other mechanism.[60,61]

PSEUDOHYPERPARATHYROIDISM

Hypercalcemia has been seen and reported associated with lymphoma,[62] gastric squamous cell carcinoma,[63] and mesothelioma.[57] This is believed to result from the elaboration by the neoplasm of a PTH-like product, as has been shown in other species.

*Immuno Nuclear Corp, Stillwater, MN 55082.

REFERENCES

56. Raulais D et al: Immunochemical and biological properties of horse parathyroid hormone, *Proc Soc Exp Biol Med* 167:542-546, 1981.
57. Roussel A et al: Radioimmunoassay for parathyroid hormone in equids, *Am J Vet Res* 48:586-589, 1987.
58. Brewer B: Disorders of equine calcium metabolism, *Compend Cont Educ Pract Vet* 4:S244-S250, S252-S253, 1982.
59. Krook L et al: Hypercalcemia and calcinosis in Florida horses: implication of the shrub *Cestrum diurnum* as the causative agent, *Cornell Vet* 65:26-56, 1975.
60. Brobst D et al: Parathyroid hormone evaluation in normal horses and horses with renal failure, *Equine Vet Sci* 2:150-157, 1982.
61. Elfers R et al: Alterations in calcium, phosphorous and C-terminal parathyroid hormone levels in equine acute renal disease, *Cornell Vet* 76:317-329, 1986.
62. Esplin D, Taylor J: Hypercalcemia in a horse with lymphosarcoma, *J Am Vet Med Assoc* 170:180-182, 1977.
63. Meuten D et al: Gastric carcinoma with pseudohyperparathyroidism in a horse, *Cornell Vet* 68:179-195, 1978.

PANCREAS

DIABETES MELLITUS

Although diabetes mellitus has been described as any condition in which there is a permanent elevation of blood glucose and glucosuria, the term is generally used interchangeably with the term primary diabetes mellitus. *Primary diabetes mellitus* is used to describe a relatively specific disorder involving the pancreatic β-cells that results in decreased insulin levels and therefore insulin-sensitive hyperglycemia. Often the term *secondary diabetes mellitus* is used to describe conditions in which hyperglycemia and glucosuria occur because of resistance to the effects of insulin, even when plasma levels of insulin are normal or elevated.

Primary diabetes mellitus in the horse is rare and in all reports has been associated with pancreatic destruction secondary to chronic pancreatitis of nonspecific origin, *Streptococcus* ("bastard strangles") or *Corynebacterium* spp. abscesses, or pancreatic destruction associated with strongyle migration (generally *Strongylus equinus*).[64,65]

Most cases of equine diabetes mellitus in the literature are actually cases of secondary diabetes associated with equine Cushing's disease.[66,67] As already described, insulin-resistant hyperglycemia occurs secondary to uncontrolled secretion of the diabetogenic hormones ACTH and cortisol.

Diabetes mellitus in a bovine has been reported and produced clinical signs of weight loss, polyuria, and polydypsia. In one case, hyperglycemia, ketonuria, glucosuria, and low serum insulin levels were present; and necropsy revealed a lack of detectable pancreatic β-cell granules.[68] According to other reports, diabetes mellitus in the bovine was caused by pancreatic destruction associated with adenocarcinoma, chronic pancreatitis, and islet degeneration.[61-71]

HYPOGLYCEMIA

A single case of hypoglycemia in a pony, which was secondary to an insulin-producing tumor of the pancreas, has been reported.[72] The differential diagnoses for hypoglycemia should include pituitary destruction and injection of insulin. Determination of plasma insulin levels and ACTH challenge to assess adrenal function should be helpful in determining the origin of the hypoglycemia.

REFERENCES

64. Bulgin M: Verminous arteritis and pancreatic necrosis with diabetes mellitus in a pony, *Compend Cont Educ Pract Vet* 5:S482,S484-S485, 1983.
65. Jeffrey J: Diabetes mellitus secondary to chronic pancreatitis in a pony, *J Am Vet Med Assoc* 153:1168-1175, 1968.
66. Baker J, Ritchie H: Diabetes mellitus in the horse: a case report and review of the literature, *Equine Vet J* 6:7-11, 1974.

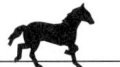

67. Tasker J, Whiteman C, Martin B: Diabetes mellitus in the horse, *J Am Vet Med Assoc* 149:393-399, 1966.
68. Kaneko JJ, Rhode EA: Diabetes mellitus in a cow, *J Am Vet Med Assoc* 144:367-373, 1964.
69. Ingardi G: Diabetes mellitus beim rhinde, *La Clin Vet, Milano* 32:801, 1909.
70. Fooy JP: En geval van diabetes mellitus bi jeen ongletrekstier, *Nedel Indische Blad Diergeneesk* 52:195-202, 1940.
71. Christensen NO, Schambye P: Om diabetes mellitus hos kvaeg, *Nord Vet Med* 2:863-900, 1950.
72. Ross M et al: Hypoglycemic seizures in a Shetland pony, *Cornell Vet* 73:151-169, 1983.

METABOLIC DISORDERS

SHERRILL A. FLEMING

KETOSIS OF RUMINANTS (ACETONEMIA)

DEFINITION. Ketosis is a condition characterized by abnormally elevated concentrations of the ketone bodies acetoacetic acid (AcAc), acetone (Ac), and β-hydroxybutyric acid (BHB) in the body tissues and fluids.[73] Primary, spontaneous ketosis is a metabolic disturbance resulting from a negative energy balance during late pregnancy and early lactation, a reduction of glucose in the blood and liver (decreased glycogen), and an increased fat mobilization that results in elevated ketone body accumulations[74] (see Chapter 31 for discussions of fatty liver and pregnancy toxemia). Baird and colleagues[75] stated that "a certain degree of ketosis is a natural state in the ruminant, and the ketotic animal may only represent the extreme of a normal metabolic range." Ketosis becomes a disease condition only when the absorption and production of ketone bodies exceeds their use by the ruminant as an energy source, resulting in elevated blood ketones, free or nonesterified fatty acids (FFA/NEFA), and decreased blood glucose. The clinical signs of ketosis tend to be vague and nonspecific. Therefore ketosis is classified as clinical or subclinical on the basis of levels of ketone bodies in the blood, urine, and milk and the presence or absence of clinical signs. Any disease process occurring in early lactation that reduces feed intake may cause secondary ketosis.

ETIOLOGY. Ketosis is a production disease of modern agriculture. Dairy cattle have been genetically selected for high milk yield, which has resulted in rapid increases in milk production during early lactation. This milk production exceeds the capacity of the animal to ingest sufficient feed to meet requirements for energy.[76] The input into the animal must equal or exceed the output to prevent a negative energy balance (Table 39-1).

Studies performed during the prepartum period have demonstrated that dry matter intakes dropped 28% during the last 17 days before parturition.[77] Greater dry matter intake depression of 40% was reported 2 days before calving,

resulting in higher liver triglycerides and plasma FFA/NEFA, along with decreased liver glycogen in cows at calving.[78] Therefore fat mobilization and infiltration of the liver begins before the onset of lactation. After parturition the milk production of dairy cattle peaks by approximately 4 weeks after parturition, but the dietary intake on a dry matter basis does not peak until 7 to 8 weeks.[79] High-producing dairy cows will be in a negative energy balance for as long as 8 weeks, despite the provision of a high-quality, palatable diet. To offset the negative energy balance, the individual cow must mobilize body fat and protein stores in the form of triglycerides and amino acids for gluconeogenesis. Ketone bodies are normally produced by the rumen wall, the liver, and the mammary gland, although rumen wall ketone production is insignificant during clinical ketosis.[80,81] The liver, however, is the major source of overall ketone production during ketosis. All tissues in the normal cow can adapt to the use of ketone bodies as an alternative energy source except the liver. It must be stressed that normal, high-producing dairy cows will have some level of ketosis during the rising curve of their lactation until their energy intake balances milk production, despite the provision of good quality feed. During this period cows lose 30 to 100 kg (65 to 220 lb).[82-85] The difficulty is in identifying and preventing the factors that move a cow from the normal level of ketone body formation into the subclinical and clinical categories.

Any disease condition that decreases dietary intake may cause secondary ketosis as a result of increased fat mobilization and ketone production. During the immediate postpartum period cows are susceptible to many diseases that are likely to reduce their normal feed intake. Ketosis may also be secondary to the ingestion of preformed ketones in the diet (silage high in lactic or butyric acid).[79] Some reports have suggested that biogenic amines such as putrescine, tryptamine, cadaverine, and histamine contained in ketogenic silage may play a role, possibly by decreasing intake.[86,87] Cobalt deficiency has been implicated as a potential cause of ketosis.[88] There is also a high incidence of ketosis in herds affected with fluorosis.[89] Contamination of concentrates with low levels of lincomycin has been reported to cause herd outbreaks of clinical ketosis.[90] It was theorized that the use of bovine somatotropin (BST) in dairies would increase the incidence of ketosis, but this has not been demonstrated.[91,24] BST treatment begins at 63 days postpartum and thus misses early lactation when clinical ketosis is most likely to occur.

CLINICAL SIGNS AND DIFFERENTIAL DIAGNOSES. Clinical ketosis is most commonly seen as a gradual loss of appetite and decrease in milk production over several days. Loss of appetite is usually sequential, with refusal of grain, then silage, and lastly forages. As feed intake decreases, weight is lost rapidly, and milk production drops. During early lactation, reduction in milk production lags behind the

TABLE 39-1

Summation of Components of Energy Balance in the Bovine

Inputs	Throughputs	Outputs
Food	Digestion	Defecation
Water	Hepatic metabolism	Urination
Respiration/O_2	Fat metabolism	CO_2
Endocrine influences	Mammary gland	Lactation
Environment/stress	metabolism	Muscular activity
	Tissue metabolism	Heat loss
	(fetus)	Reproduction

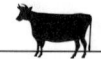

TABLE 39-2

Blood, Urine, and Milk Analysis in Ketosis[71,83-90]

	Normal		Subclinical		Clinical	
	(mg/dl)	(mmol/L)	(mg/dl)	(mmol/L)	(mg/dl)	(mmol/L)
Blood glucose	52	(2.86)			28	(1.54)
FFA	3				33	
Ac	0				15.1	(0.26)
AcAc	0	<0.35		0.36-1.05	4.4	>1.05,0.5
BHB	10.7	(1.08)	>10	0-1.5	23.5	>1.5
TOTAL	3;6.1		10-30		>30;41;48	5.0
Urine Ac	1.0	(0.17)			22	(3.78)
AcAc	3.4	(0.35)			37.3	(3.80)
BHB	11.7	(1.18)			25.1	(2.54)
TOTAL	9.54;16.1				89;305.77	
Milk Ac	0			0.17-0.25;0.4	16.2	>1.0-2.0
AcAc	0				1.6	(0.16)
BHB	4.9	(0.49)			7.9	(0.80)
TOTAL	4.9		2		27.5;37.35	

reduction in energy intake. Physical findings include normal vital signs; firm, dry feces; moderate depression; and sometimes reluctance to move. Rumen motility may be decreased if the animal has been anorexic for several days. Occasionally pica is seen. Often the odor of ketones can be detected on the breath and in the milk. Clinical signs may spontaneously disappear without treatment when equilibrium between milk yield and dietary intake is reached. Transient nervous signs such as staggering and blindness may occur for short periods. Displaced abomasum (particularly left displacement), metritis, mastitis, and peritonitis (particularly traumatic reticuloperitonitis) are common primary disease entities leading to secondary ketosis. Less common causes of secondary ketosis are subclinical hypocalcemia, mild rumen overload and laminitis, lameness caused by sole abscesses and ulcers, pyelonephritis, and musculoskeletal injuries after calving.

In the nervous form of ketosis, there is an acute onset of bizarre neurologic signs, including circling, proprioceptive deficits, head pressing, apparent blindness, wandering, excessive grooming behavior, pica, and excessive salivation. These animals may show hyperesthesia, bellowing, moderate tremors, and tetany. They may behave aggressively toward people or inanimate objects and appear ataxic when ambulating. Episodes of nervous signs last 1 to 2 hours and recur at 8- to 10-hour intervals.[80] Diseases such as listeriosis, rabies, lactation tetany, acute lead poisoning, and *Claviceps paspali* poisoning should be considered as possible differential diagnoses.

A thorough physical examination must be performed to differentiate primary from secondary ketosis. A mild fever and increased heart rate are often associated with primary diseases that are inflammatory. Moderate to severe ketonuria may be seen. During the first 2 weeks after calving, cows may require treatment for concurrent diseases. If appetite does not return after standard therapy for the primary disease entity, further therapy for ketosis may be necessary. The tendency for ketosis to recur necessitates careful reassessment by repeating the physical examination to detect primary diseases causing secondary ketosis.

CLINICAL PATHOLOGY AND LABORATORY AIDS. Ketone bodies may be detected in urine, plasma, and milk (Table 39-2).[81,93-100] The literature is reported in the international system of units (SI units) (mmol/L) and conventional units (mg/dl), which makes interpretation difficult. The conversion factor for Ac, AcAc and BHB is 1mg/dl = 0.1 mmol/L = 1000 μmol/L. In general, in clinical ketosis, blood glucose

concentrations are 20 to 40 mg/dl, total blood ketones are greater than 30 mg/dl, total urine ketones are greater than 84 mg/dl, and total milk ketones are greater than 10 mg/dl. Individuals with subclinical ketosis are those that have no clinical signs of ketosis but have low normal blood glucose, total blood ketones of 10 to 30 mg/dl, and total milk ketones of 2 mg/dl. Secondary ketosis may fall between the ranges for clinical and subclinical ketosis, depending on the duration of the primary disease process.[80]

Commercially available dipsticks and tablets developed for monitoring human diabetes will detect urine Ac, AcAc, or both Ac and AcAc and are widely used for ketone detection in animals (Table 39-3).[101-103] These tests do not detect BHB levels, which are proportionally higher than Ac and AcAc, but good correlation of clinical signs to Ac and AcAc concentrations has been reported.[91,100] Urine ketone tests may give a positive result in otherwise normal cows, because ketone levels are concentrated to 2 to 20 times the blood ketone level. Ketone bodies in the milk reflect ketone blood levels, making milk ketones a more reliable test (approximately 50% of blood concentration).[99,100] Ac and AcAc in the milk fluctuated the least within a 24-hour period, which makes it the most useful measure of the energy balance of cows in the field situation.[100] A recent review of eight tests for milk ketones demonstrated two tests to be highly sensitive in detecting subclinical ketosis.[104] One of these tests is currently available in the United States.* Blood levels of volatile fatty acids (VFAs), FFA/NEFAs, and ketone bodies are increased but not routinely measured. Diurnal variation in blood levels of VFAs, FFA/NEFAs, and ketone bodies makes timing of blood sampling difficult.[100,105,107] One author suggested that herd ketosis problems and subclinical syndromes be investigated by computing the logarithmic means of the blood BHB concentrations on at least seven animals within specified production groups.[108]

Because of the central role of the liver in energy metabolism of ruminants, the onset of ketosis may be associated with elevations of liver enzymes and abnormal liver function tests. Serum aspartate aminotransferase (AST) and sorbitol dehydrogenase (SDH) may be increased in severe cases. The degree of liver dysfunction is mild compared with that of cows with fatty liver syndrome. The sulfobromophthalein

---

*Pink Test Liquid, profsproducts.com, Germany, marketed through WA Butler Co.

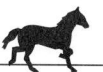

TABLE 39-3

Available Screening Tests for Ketosis

Test Reagent Brand	Multistix*†	Acetest*†	KetoCheck*‡	Ross' Modified[92] Rothera Powder*	Gerhardt's Test[93]
Ketone bodies detected	AcAc	AcAc	AcAc	AcAc	AcAc
Ketone bodies *not* detected	Ac BHB	BHB	BHB	BHB	Ac BHB
Detection threshold (mg/dl)	AcAc 5-10	AcAc 5-10 Ac 20-25	AcAc 5	AcAc 1-5 Ac 10-25	AcAc 25-50
Sample type	Urine	Urine Milk	Urine MIlk	Urine Milk	Urine

Courtesy John Maas.
Ac, Acetone; *AcAc*, acetoacetic acid; *BHB*, β-hydroxybutyric acid.
*False-positive reactions may be cuased by BSP, PSP, phenylketones, L-dopa.
†Ames Division, Miles Laboratory, Inc, PO Box 70, Elkhart, IN 46151.
‡Butler Sales Associates, Inc., PO Box 8098, St Joseph, MO 64508.

(BSP) clearance test may be used to evaluate liver function and to obtain baseline data in overconditioned cows at risk of fatty liver syndrome development (see Chapter 31). Serum bile acid levels have had variable results and may not be useful in differentiating mild, moderate, and severe fatty infiltration of the liver; but they do correlate with severe hepatic damage.[109,110] The BSP clearance test also did not differentiate between mild and moderate fatty infiltration of the liver. Liver biopsy and estimation of fat content appear to be the only accurate means of identifying the degree of hepatic lipidosis.

White cell counts vary and may reflect the stress or the primary disease process that the animal is experiencing. Studies vary in the reported effect of elevated ketone bodies and decreased blood glucose on lymphocyte proliferation and immunoglobulin production.[111,112] Serum calcium and magnesium levels may be slightly decreased in animals that are anorexic. Cortisol levels are usually within the normal range, and plasma insulin is elevated initially but depressed as the feed intake is decreased.[113]

PATHOPHYSIOLOGY. Clinical ketosis in ruminants occurs when the demand for glucose by the mammary gland exceeds the energy resources available from the diet and fat mobilization, resulting in hypoglycemia. The daily glucose requirements of a dairy cow increase above normal maintenance by 30% in late gestation and by 75% with the onset of lactation.[114] The average energy requirements of a 1000-lb lactating cow have been estimated to be 50 g of glucose per hour.[115] Only 10% of the glucose requirement is available in the form of glucose. In the normal lactating cow energy is presented to the liver in the form of VFAs, bacterial protein, and a small amount of glucose and protein that escapes degradation in the rumen (Fig. 39-3).[74,81,83] The principal VFAs are acetate, propionate, and butyrate, which are produced in an approximate 70:20:10 ratio, respectively, in the rumen. Acetate is mainly used in fat synthesis, although there is some evidence to suggest that it may be a minor glucose source by entering at the acetyl CoA level. Butyrate is condensed into acetoacetyl CoA, which can be partially oxidized to ketone bodies or transformed into acetyl CoA that can enter the tricarboxylic acid (TCA) cycle (no net gain of glucose). Propionate enters the TCA cycle directly at the level of succinyl CoA (equivalent to 30% to 50% of glucose production in the ruminant).[116] Therefore acetate and butyrate are ketogenic, and propionate is glycogenic. The normal ratio of production in the rumen is four ketogenic:one glycogenic VFA. Significant production of ketone bodies occurs in the rumen epithelium and mammary gland, and in the major produc-

tion site, the liver.[80,116] Ketone bodies are normally used by the TCA cycle in the heart, kidney, skeletal muscles, and mammary gland through the acetyl CoA pathway.

Efficient oxidation of acetyl CoA depends on an adequate supply of oxaloacetate, which is generated from gluconeogenic precursors, mainly propionate (from the rumen) and lactate and pyruvate (from anaerobic metabolism of glucose).[74] Lactating cows preempt a large quantity of propionate and lactate for milk production in the form of lactose. Supplies of oxaloacetate are reduced, slowing down the TCA cycle and the use of acetyl CoA. The backlog of acetyl CoA is diverted into the formation of ketone bodies. In an attempt to increase gluconeogenesis and offset the negative energy balance, more triglycerides are mobilized from body fat stores. Triglycerides are hydrolyzed to release FFA/NEFAs. In the liver, triglycerides are resynthesized from the released FFA/NEFAs and stored by the liver or exported as very low density lipoproteins (VLDL).[117] Apolipoprotein must be synthesized in the liver to form VLDL from triglycerides. Ruminants have an inherently low rate of VLDL secretion relative to other species.[77] The excess FFA/NEFAs attempt to enter the TCA cycle through acetyl CoA, which in the absence of sufficient oxaloacetate is partially oxidized to acetoacetyl CoA, which allows the formation of ketone bodies.[81,118] The negative energy balance that occurs in postpartum dairy cows further reduces available carbohydrate and accelerates fat mobilization and ketone body formation. The net result is ketonemia, ketonuria, ketolactia, hypoglycemia, and low levels of hepatic glycogen. Any additional nutritional, metabolic, or other disorder resulting in decreased feed intake will make the subclinical ketosis clinical.

EPIDEMIOLOGY. The morbidity of clinical ketosis is extremely variable and difficult to measure. Management and nutrition are influential factors that vary widely from farm to farm and area to area. Prevalence rates (number of cases at a point in time) have been reported to be 13.1% (range 3% to 22%, depending on lactation) for clinical ketosis and 33.8% (range 31% to 41%) for subclinical ketosis.[119,120] Incidence rates (number of cases that occur in 1 year) have been reported to range from 1.87% to 13% for clinical ketosis and 7.3% to 12.1% for subclinical ketosis.[120-123] Most cases occur in the first 6 weeks after calving, with the peak incidence at 3 to 4 weeks after calving.[120,124,125] Breed differences have been found, and genetic tendencies within bull-daughter families.[121,122] The incidence of clinical ketosis increased with parity, peaking at the fifth to sixth lactation.[120,121] Cows that were diagnosed with clinical ketosis once had increased risk of ke-

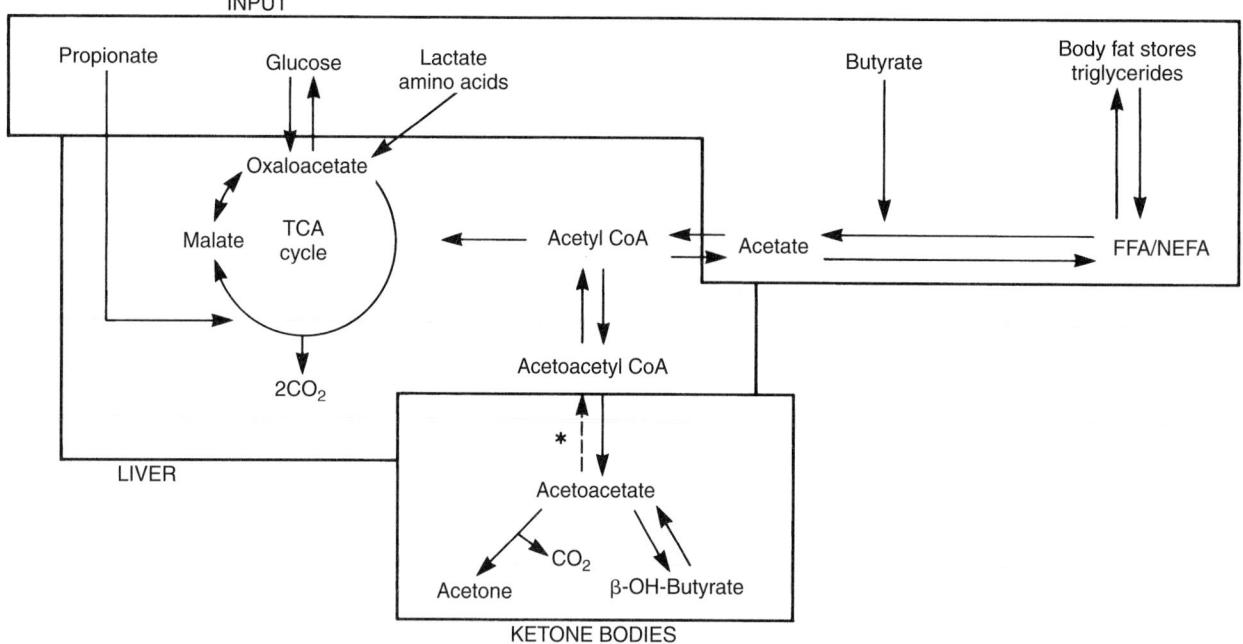

FIG. 39-3 ■ Major pathways of energy metabolism and ketone body formation. Reaction is negligible in liver and mammary gland but does occur in other tissues.

tosis at subsequent calvings.[123,125] Recurrence of ketosis in individuals may reflect digestive capacity and metabolic efficiency, as well as milk production, which are likely to have a multifactorial mode of inheritance.

Generally, clinical and subclinical cows are high producers and are overconditioned at calving.[125,126] Fat cows have been shown to have dry matter intake (DMI) reduced by 25% and higher turnover rates of fatty acids because of more fat mobilization.[127] Environmental factors that affect the incidence of clinical ketosis include the season of the year (increased during midwinter), climate, stabling (increased in stabled vs. loose housing), and feeding regimen (increased with number of feedstuffs used and fewer numbers of feedings per day).[123,125,128] Diets that are less than 8% protein on a dry matter basis before calving or that have high protein levels (greater than 20% DM) after calving have been associated with high incidences of herd ketosis.[129] One study reported an association of increased incidence with a high standard of management and decreased incidence if the wife, versus other family members or paid workers, assisted with chores.[128]

Thirty percent to forty percent of cases are complicated by concurrent diseases such as metritis, traumatic reticuloperitonitis, and abomasal displacements.[130] These cows are classified as having secondary ketosis. A diagnosis of parturient paresis, alone or in combination with retained placenta, increased the risk of clinical ketosis.[123,125] Cows with metritis are more likely to be diagnosed as having subclinical ketosis.[119] Displaced abomasum and lameness in a previous lactation were associated with clinical ketosis.[125] Cystic ovaries, increased calving to first service interval, and increased calving to last service interval have been associated with subclinical ketosis.[119,125,126] Others reported no association between ketosis and the calving interval and number of inseminations.[131] Most genetic studies are based on the lactation previous to the diagnosis of ketosis and have found either no difference or a tendency toward higher production in cows with ketosis.[121,130-133] A recent study demonstrated a genetic correlation between milk production and ketosis using only first lactation records.[134] Subclinical ketosis was found to be

associated with losses of 1 to 1.4 kg of milk per day or 4.4% to 6% of the mean daily production.[119] The same authors found an association between diagnosis and treatment of clinical ketosis with an increase of 2.5% in production over the entire lactation.[133] A negative correlation of ketosis with culling rate indicated that high-producing cows with ketosis were less likely to be culled than low producing cows.[123,135]

NECROPSY FINDINGS. The mortality rate from primary ketosis is extremely low. In animals that die with clinical ketosis, a fatty liver is likely to be the only pathologic finding. In secondary ketosis lesions are associated with the primary disease condition.

TREATMENT AND PROGNOSIS. Treatment of secondary ketosis requires correction of the primary condition while ensuring the provision of an adequate diet. In ketosis secondary to the butyrate content of silage, the diet can be manipulated to eliminate or dilute the silage.[79]

A large number of treatments have been used for primary clinical ketosis. A recent review of ketosis therapeutics focuses on the pathophysiologic reasoning for specific treatments.[136] Traditional therapy with intravenous injections of 100 to 500 ml of 50% glucose (dextrose) gives marked clinical improvement. A transient hyperglycemia is produced that returns to preinjection levels in 2 hours. Blood ketones drop immediately, clinical signs disappear, and milk production increases by 5 to 10 lb for at least one milking.[129] Nervous signs may reappear in 12 to 24 hours, and milk production drops again over 2 to 3 days. There are fewer relapses if the glucose injections are repeated frequently. Solutions containing a mixture of 25% dextrose and 25% fructose have been used in an attempt to prolong the hyperglycemic action. Ideally a continuous intravenous glucose infusion at 0.5 g/min should be administered until milk ketone tests are negative.[115,137] In my opinion a slow infusion of 20 L of 2.5% glucose (with half normal saline) over 24 hours improves the clinical response. This solution allows fast enough drip rates for ease of catheter maintenance without the danger of causing osmotic diuresis and excessive water loading. Urine is monitored with dipsticks for negative glucose and decreasing levels of ketone bodies several times daily. Daily monitoring of the blood glucose (once or twice daily) measures the adequacy of dextrose administration. Careful monitoring for hypoglycemia is required when intravenous glucose is discontinued. This may be impractical for field situations but is worthwhile in clinical settings with valuable individuals.

Glucose precursors may be given orally in the feed or as a drench and provide a source for gluconeogenesis. These include propylene glycol drench at 225 g (8 oz) bid for 2 days, followed by 110 g (4 oz) once daily for 2 days or glycerol at 500 g twice daily for up to 10 days.[138,139] Overuse of propylene glycol may have a deleterious effect on rumen flora, decrease rumen motility, and cause diarrhea, necessitating its discontinuation and the institution of rumen transfaunations. Sodium propionate (125 to 250 g PO twice daily), ammonium lactate (120 g PO twice daily), and sodium lactate (360 g PO twice daily) have also been used as feed additives to provide alternate glucose sources. All of these tend to lower the butterfat test and may cause digestive disturbances if prolonged treatment is used.[137]

Glucocorticoids are often used to prolong the hyperglycemic effect by decreasing tissue uptake of glucose and reducing milk production for up to 3 days. Dexamethasone (0.04 mg/kg) and betamethasone are most commonly used. In one study a single treatment of dexamethasone (0.04 mg/kg) significantly increased blood glucose for 6 to 9 days and decreased milk production for 1 to 7 days.[140] Caution must be used, because overdosing may reduce feed intake and exacerbate the condition of cows with fatty liver syndrome.[141] Administration of anabolic steroids such as trienbolone acetate has resulted in decreases in blood levels of ketone bodies without depression of milk production but these steroids are not available in the United States.[142]

Low doses of long-acting insulin (200 IU of protamine zinc insulin (PZI) subcutaneously, once every 48 hours) may be used as adjunct to intravenous glucose and glucocorticoid therapy. Ruminants are relatively insulin resistant during early lactation, and pancreatic secretion of insulin is reduced in ketotic cows in response to intravenous infusions of glucose.[143,144] Insulin assists in suppressing fatty acid mobilization and increasing tissue uptake of glucose while stimulating hepatic glycolysis. PZI is no longer commercially available and anecdotal dosages of human ultralente recombinant insulin products of 0.25 IU/kg body weight every 24 to 48 hours have been used.

Recent reports of intravenous glucagon in induced cases of fatty liver have shown promising results in decreasing fatty infiltration and increasing liver glycogen.[145] However, the prolonged intravenous treatment makes this impractical for treating clinical cases.

Lipotrophic agents such as choline (25 to 50 g PO daily), cysteamine (750 mg IV every 2 to 3 days), and L-methionine have been suggested as feed additives or treatments that increase mobilization of fat in the liver.[146-148] Choline is degraded in the rumen and must be given as an encapsulated product or given subcutaneously (25 g daily) but should not be given intravenously because it acts as a neuromuscular block. Choline is a precursor of phosphatidylcholine, which is required for phospholipid synthesis. Methionine is also a phospholipid precursor in the synthesis of apolipoproteins essential for VLDL formation.[117] The amino acid lysine may also play a role in apolipoprotein synthesis. Therapy with lipotrophic agents has not been proven effective in controlled trials and may even be harmful in cases of severe liver damage.[148]

Cobalt deficiency and therefore vitamin B_{12} deficiency have been implicated as a cause of ketosis.[85] Vitamin B_{12} is an essential cofactor in the metabolism of propionate as it enters into the TCA cycle.[84] Blood and liver levels of vitamin B_{12} are reduced in the postparturient cow.[88] Although vitamin

B_{12} and cobalt may be added to the diet, the effectiveness of vitamin B_{12} has not been proven.[149]

Nicotinic acid (niacin) and nicotinamide have been used with variable effects.[84] Nicotinamide coenzymes in mammary tissue were reduced in ketotic cows compared with normal cows.[150] The suggested dose of nicotinic acid is 6 g PO once daily for up to 10 weeks after calving. Milk production was slightly increased, and blood levels of ketone bodies and FFAs were lower in niacin-treated cows.[151] Niacin at levels greater than estimated requirements decreases blood ketones and FFA/NEFAs and increases blood glucose. Niacin has been used in conjunction with the ionophore, monensin.[152] Niacin has also been used in combination with propylene glycol, but no significant differences were found between treatment groups and controls.[153]

Chloral hydrate is a traditional treatment that increases the breakdown of starch in the rumen and influences the rumen production of propionate. The initial oral dose is 30 g, followed by 7 g twice daily for several days.[137] Chloral hydrate may be particularly helpful for its sedative effects in treating cows with recurring nervous ketosis.

The most promising therapeutic and prevention tool in the future will be the use of the ionophore monensin. Monensin has been demonstrated to reduce subclinical and clinical ketosis.[154-156] Monensin decreased the acetate to propionate ratio in the rumen because of its effect on rumen fermentation. The increased availability of propionate as a glucose precursor helps to suppress fat mobilization and ketone production. Monensin is licensed for use in lactating animals in some countries, and licensing in the United States is pending.

As in all metabolic diseases, nursing care is important. Supportive therapy may include rumen transfaunations, provision of a variety of palatable feed, and exercise.

PREVENTION AND CONTROL. Because the underlying mechanism of clinical and subclinical ketosis is one of negative energy balance during the first 8 weeks of lactation, prevention and control can be addressed in three steps. The feeding and management of cows during late lactation and the dry period should promote good body condition at calving (see Chapter 9 for body condition scoring system). Optimum intake of lactating rations at the commencement of lactation must be encouraged by introducing the ration in a stepwise fashion. The ideal ration during early lactation is highly palatable and energy dense.

A moderate amount of body fat should be available for mobilization and milk production at parturition. The body fat that is lost in early lactation must be stored in the previous late lactation by feeding to National Research Council (NRC) recommendations.[85] Body condition of the dry cow must be maintained, and fetal growth provided for. It is essential that cows do not become too fat before parturition.[83,126,127] There is evidence that fatty infiltration of the liver begins before parturition, particularly in individuals with fat cow syndrome.[77,78,109] The initiation of milking before parturition has been attempted to smooth transition and prevent dry matter intake drop at calving.[157] Although the dry matter intake did not drop, there were no differences in the liver triglycerides, FFA/NEFAs, and milk production.

The introduction of the lactating ration should be made as smoothly as possible to encourage maximum intake and minimize digestive upsets. Feeding of lactation ration in limited amounts may begin as early as 4 to 5 weeks before parturition so that typically 8 to 9 lb of concentrates are being fed at parturition. After calving, incremental increases are made of a few pounds per day until ad lib levels are reached (at approximately 2 to 4 weeks).[82]

The ideal early lactation ration is highly palatable and meets NRC recommendations. The key aspects are maintain-

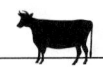

ing high energy density and optimum levels of fiber and protein (Table 39-4).[158,159] Calculations of the energy requirements of a lactating cow are expressed as total net energy of lactation and are obtained from NRC charts.[85] Recommendations for fiber content of the diet are based on the acid detergent fiber (ADF) and the neutral detergent fiber (NDF). The NDF is a good estimate of the bulk of a diet, and the DMI of a ration depends on the NDF (1.2% of body weight). Not all forage analysis laboratories report the NDF, but it can be approximated by dividing the total digestible nutrients by 100. Protein should be provided as both rumen degradable (soluble and nonprotein nitrogen) and rumen undegradable (bypass). Specific instructions for formulating these ingredients into a ration are provided in the references.[85,158,159]

The diet must also be balanced in its minerals. Cobalt may be added if there is an indication of inadequate levels. Problems that arise from silage with high butyrate concentrations may require substitution or dilution of the affected silage with other feeds for the cows in early lactation. High butyrate diets are often tolerated because they encourage a higher milk butterfat content.[79,137] The addition of protected fats in the form of the calcium salts of long-chain fatty acids or a high proportion of saturated long-chain fatty acids (palmitic and stearic acids) increases the energy density of the ration without reducing the fiber content.[160] These compounds are not degraded in the rumen but are digested in the abomasum and small intestine. Feeding protected fats results in increased milk production, slightly decreased DMI, and increased FFA/NEFAs, as well as stabilized blood ketones and weight loss through a glucose-sparing effect.[118] Glucogenic precursors such as propylene glycol and sodium propionate have been incorporated into early lactation rations for many years. Both of these compounds are not palatable to dairy cattle and are better reserved for treatment of individual cases of ketosis.

Nicotinic acid is recommended as a feed additive at 6 to 12 g/head/day in early lactation rations.[151]

Subclinical and clinical ketosis should be detected and treated as early as possible to prevent deleterious effects on health and production. This may be accomplished by encouraging clients to use ketone tests routinely on milk or urine during the first 50 to 60 days after parturition. Animals with positive tests should have a thorough physical examination. Institution of supportive therapy for subclinical ketosis includes administration of oral propylene glycol. A high prevalence rate of clinical or subclinical ketosis necessitates investigation of the feeding program.

TABLE 39-4

Recommendations for Early Lactation Diets

	Energy	Diet (%)*	Crude Protein (%)
NEL Mcal	38.9		
TDN		73	
Fiber			
ADF		21	
NDF		28	
Protein			
Crude		16.4	
Soluble			30
Degradalbe			60
Undegradable			40
Added fat			
Unprotected		2-3	
Protected		7	

NEL, Net energy of lactation; *TDN,* total digestible nutrients; *ADF,* acid detergent fiber; *DNF,* neutral detergent fiber.
*Total dietary dry matter intake.

REFERENCES

73. Taylor EJ: *Dorland's illustrated medical dictionary,* ed 28, Philadelphia, 1994, WB Saunders.
74. Bergman EN: Glucose metabolism in ruminants as related to hypoglycemia and ketosis, *Cornell Vet* 63:341-382, 1973.
75. Baird GD: Bovine ketosis: a review with recommendations for control and treatment. I, *Br Vet J* 130:214-220, 1974.
76. Moe PW, Tyrrell HF, Flatt WP: Energetics of body tissue mobilization, *J Dairy Sci* 54:548-553, 1971.
77. Bertics SJ et al: Effect of prepartum dry matter intake on liver triglyceride concentration and early lactation, *J Dairy Sci* 75:1914-1922, 1992.
78. Vazquez-Anon M et al: Peripartum liver triglyceride and plasma metabolites in dairy cows, *J Dairy Sci* 77:1521-1528, 1994.
79. Andersson L, Lundstrom K: Effect of feeding silage with high butyric acid content on ketone body formation and milk yield in postparturient dairy cows, *Zentralbl Veterinarmed* 32:15-23, 1985.
80. Pennington RJ: The metabolism of short-chain fatty acids in the sheep. I, Fatty acid utilization and ketone body production by rumen epithelium and other tissues, *Biochem J* 51:251-258, 1952.
81. Bergman EN: Hyperketonemia-ketogenesis and ketone body metabolism, *J Dairy Sci* 54:936-948, 1971.
82. Huber JT: Dietary management of dairy cattle. In Howard JL, ed: *Current veterinary therapy 3 (food animal practice),* Philadelphia, 1993, WB Saunders, pp 260-272.
83. Hibbitt KG: Bovine ketosis and its prevention, *Vet Rec* 105:13-15, 1979.
84. Mills SE, Beitz DC, Young JW: Characterization of metabolic changes during a protocol for inducing lactation ketosis in dairy cows, *J Dairy Sci* 69:352-361, 1986.
85. National Research Council: *Nutrient requirements of dairy cattle,* ed 6 (revised), Washington, DC, 1989, National Academy of Sciences.
86. Tveit B et al: Etiology of acetonemia in Norwegian cattle. I, Effect of ketogenic silage, season, energy level and genetic factors, *J Dairy Sci* 75:2421-2432, 1992.
87. Lingaas F, Tveit B: Etiology of acetonemia in Norwegian cattle. II, Effect of butyric acid, valeric acid, and putrescine, *J Dairy Sci* 75:2433-2439, 1992.
88. Marston HR, Allen SH, Smith RM: Primary metabolic defect supervening on vitamin B12 deficiency in the sheep, *Nature* 190:1085-1091, 1961.
89. Blood DC, Radostits OM: *Veterinary medicine,* ed 7, London, England, 1989, Baillière Tindall, p 1131.
90. Rice DA, McMurray CH, Davidson JF: Ketosis in dairy cows caused by low levels of lincomycin in concentrate feed, *Vet Rec* 113:495- 496, 1983.
91. Lean IJ et al: Impact of bovine somatotropin administration beginning at day 70 of lactation on serum metabolites, milk constituents, and production in cows previously exposed to exogenous somatotropin, *Am J Vet Res* 53:731-741, 1992.
92. Cole WJ et al: Response of dairy cows to high doses of a sustained-release bovine somatotropin administered during two lactations. II, Health and reproduction, *J Dairy Sci* 75:111-123, 1992.
93. Shultz LH: Management and nutritional aspects of ketosis, *J Dairy Sci* 54:962-973, 1971.
94. Robertson A, Thin C: A study of starvation ketosis in the ruminant, *Br J Nutr* 7:181-195, 1953.
95. Kauppinen K: Correlation of whole blood concentrations of acetoacetate, β-hydroxybutyrate, glucose and milk yield in dairy cows as studied under field conditions, *Acta Vet Scand* 24:337-348, 1983.
96. Baird GD: Primary ketosis in the high-producing dairy cow: clinical and subclinical disorders, treatment, prevention, and outlook, *J Dairy Sci* 65:1-10, 1982.
97. Whitaker DA, Kelly JM, Smith EJ: Subclinical ketosis and serum beta-hydroxybutyrate levels in dairy cattle, *Br Vet J* 139:462-463, 1983.
98. Thin C, Robertson A: Biochemical aspects of ruminant ketosis, *J Comp Pathol* 63:184-194, 1953.
99. Emery RS et al: Detection, occurrence and prophylactic treatment of borderline ketosis with propylene glycol feeding, *J Dairy Sci* 47:1074-1079, 1964.
100. Andersson L: Concentrations of blood and milk ketone bodies, blood isopropanol and plasma glucose in dairy cows in relation to the degree of hyperketonaemia and clinical signs, *Zentralbl Veterinarmed (A)* 31:683-693, 1984.
101. Maas J: Unpublished notes, 1988.
102. Kaneko JJ, Harvey JW, Bruss ML: *Clinical biochemistry of domestic animals,* ed 5, San Francisco, 1980, Academic Press, pp 100-106.
103. Henry JB: *Todd-Sanford-Davidsohn: Clinical diagnosis and management by laboratory methods,* ed 16, vol I, Philadelphia, 1979, WB Saunders, pp 593-595.
104. Geishauser T et al: Evaluation of eight cow-side ketone tests in milk for detection of subclinical ketosis in dairy cows, *J Dairy Sci* 83:296-299, 2000.
105. Coggins CRE, Field AC: Diurnal variation in the chemical composition of plasma from lactating beef cows on three dietary energy intakes, *J Agri Sci (Camb)* 86:595-602, 1976.
106. Manston R et al: Variability of the blood composition of dairy cows in relation to time of day, *J Agri Sci (Camb)* 96:593-598, 1981.
107. Andersson L, Lundstrom K: Milk and ketone bodies, blood isopropanol and plasma glucose in dairy cows: methodological studies and diurnal variations, *Zentralbl Veterinarmed (A)* 31:340- 349, 1984.

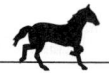

108. Herdt TH et al: Blood concentrations of β-hydroxybutyrate in clinically normal Holstein-Friesian herds and in those with a high prevalence of clinical ketosis, *Am J Vet Res* 42:503-506, 1981.
109. Garry FB et al: Serum bile acid concentrations in dairy cows with hepatic lipidosis, *J Vet Intern Med* 8:432-438, 1994.
110. West HJ: Effect on liver function of acetonaemia and the fat cow syndrome cattle, *Res Vet Sci* 48:221-227, 1990.
111. Franklin ST, Young JW, Nonnecke BJ: Effects of ketones, acetate, butyrate and glucose on bovine lymphocyte proliferation, *J Dairy Sci* 74:2507-2514, 1991.
112. Nonnecke BJ, Franklin ST, Young JW: Effects of ketones, acetate and glucose on in vitro immunoglobin secretion by bovine lymphocytes, *J Dairy Sci* 75:982-990, 1992.
113. Hove K, Blom AK: Plasma insulin and growth hormone in dairy cows: diurnal variation and relation to food intake and plasma sugar and acetoacetate levels, *Acta Endocrinol* 73:289-303, 1973.
114. Bauman DE, Currie WB: Partitioning of nutrients during pregnancy and lactation: a review of mechanisms involving homeostasis and homeorrhesis, *J Dairy Sci* 63:1514-1529, 1980.
115. Baxter CF, Kleiber M, Black AL: Glucose metabolism in the lactating dairy cow, *Biochim Biophys Acta* 17:354-361, 1955.
116. Herdt TH: Fuel homeostasis in the ruminant, *Vet Clin North Am (Food Anim Pract)* 4:216, 1988.
117. Grummer RR: Etiology of lipid-related metabolic disorders in periparturient dairy cows, *J Dairy Sci* 76:3882-3896, 1993.
118. Grummer RR, Carroll DJ: Effects of dietary fat on metabolic disorders and reproductive performance of dairy cattle, *J Anim Sci* 69:3838-3852, 1991.
119. Dohoo IR, Martin SW: Sublinical ketosis: prevalence and associations with production and disease, *Can J Comp Med* 48:1-5, 1984.
120. Kauppinen K: Prevalence of bovine ketosis in relation to number and stage of lactation, *Acta Vet Scand* 24:349-361, 1983.
121. Grohn Y, Thompson JR, Bruss ML: Epidemiology and genetic basis of ketosis in Finnish Ayrshire cattle, *Prev Vet Med* 3:65-77, 1984.
122. Henricson B, Jonsson G, Pehrson B: "Lipid pattern," glucose concentration and ketone body level in the blood of cattle, *Zentralbl Vet Med (A)* 24:89-102, 1977.
123. Bendixen PH et al: Disease frequencies in dairy cows in Sweden. IV, Ketosis, *Prev Vet Med* 5:99-109, 1987.
124. Dohoo IR, Martin SW: Disease, production and culling in Holstein-Friesian cows. III, Disease and production as determinants of disease, *Prev Vet Med* 2:671-690, 1984.
125. Andersson L, Emanuelson U: An epidemiological study of hyperketonaemia in Swedish dairy cows: determinants and the relation to fertility, *Prev Vet Med* 3:449-462, 1985.
126. Markusfeld O, Nahari N, Adler H: Evaluation of a routine testing for ketonuria and aciduria in the detection of sub and clinical ketosis associated with overfeeding in dairy cattle, *Bovine Pract* 19:219-222, 1984.
127. Bines JA, Morant SV: The effect of body condition on metabolic changes associated with intake of food by the cow, *Br J Nutr* 50:81-89, 1983.
128. Riemann HP, Larssen RB, Simensen E: Ketosis in Norwegian dairy herds: some epidemiological associations, *Acta Vet Scand* 26:482-492, 1985.
129. Kung L Jr, Huber JT: Performance of high-producing cows in early lactation fed protein of varying amounts, sources and degradability, *J Dairy Sci* 66:227-234, 1983.
130. Cote JF et al: Bovine ketosis: frequency of clinical signs, complications and alterations in blood ketones, glucose and free fatty acids, *Can Vet J* 10:179, 1969.
131. Andersson L, Lundstrom K: Effect of energy balance on plasma glucose and ketone bodies in blood and milk and influence of hyperketonaemia on milk production of postparturient dairy cows, *Zentralbl Veterinarmed (A)* 31:539-547, 1984.
132. Kauppinen K: Annual milk yield and reproductive performance of ketotic and nonketotic dairy cows, *Zentralbl Vet Med (A)* 31:694-704, 1984.
133. Dohoo IR, Martin SW: Disease, production and culling in Holstein-Friesian cows. IV. Effects of disease on production, *Prev Vet Med* 2:755-770, 1984.
134. Simianer H, Solbu H, Schaeffer LR: Estimated genetic correlations between disease and yield traits in dairy cattle, *J Dairy Sci* 74:4358-4365, 1991.
135. Dohoo IR, Martin SW: Disease, production and culling in Holstein-Friesian cows. V, Survivorship, *Prev Vet Med* 2:771-784, 1984.
136. Herdt TH, Emery RS: Therapy of diseases of ruminant intermediary metabolism, *Vet Clin North Am (Food Anim Pract)* 8:91-106, 1992.
137. Kronfeld DS: Metabolic disorders. In Amstutz HE, ed: *Bovine medicine and surgery*, ed 2, vol I, Santa Barbara, Calif, 1980, American Veterinary Publications, pp 537- 565.
138. Emery RS, Brown RE, Black AI: Metabolism of DL-1,2- propanediol-2¹⁴C in a lactating cow, *J Nutr* 92:348-356, 1967.
139. Johnson RB: The treatment of ketosis with glycerol and propylene glycol, *Cornell Vet* 44:6-21, 1954.
140. Andersson L, Olsson T: The effect of two glucocorticoids on plasma glucose and milk production in healthy cows and the therapeutic effect in ketosis, *Nord Vet Med* 36:13-18, 1984.
141. Foster LA: Clinical ketosis, *Vet Clin North Am (Food Anim Pract)* 4:253, 1988.
142. Heitzman RJ, Walker MS: The antiketogenic action of an anabolic steroid administered to ketotic cows, *Res Vet Sci* 15:70-77, 1973.
143. Hove K: Insulin secretion in lactating cows: responses to glucose infused intravenously in normal, ketonemic, and starved animals, *J Dairy Sci* 61:1407-1413, 1978.
144. de Boer G, Trenkle A, Young JW: Glucagon, insulin, growth hormone, and some blood metabolites during energy restriction ketonemia of lactating cows, *J Dairy Sci* 68:326-337, 1985.
145. Hippen AR et al: Alleviation of fatty liver in dairy cows with 14-day intravenous infusions of glucagon, *J Dairy Sci* 82:1139-1152, 1999.
146. Bach SJ, Hibbitt KG: The therapeutic use of cysteamine in bovine ketosis, *Vet Rec* 72:797-800, 1960.
147. Lewis EF, Price EK: The use of choline chloride as a lipotrophic agent in the treatment of bovine liver dysfunction, *Br Vet J* 113:242-246, 1957.
148. Package insert, D-L-methionine powder, The Butler Co, Columbus, Ohio.
149. Croom WJ et al: Vitamin B12 administration for milk fat synthesis in lactating dairy cows fed a low-fiber diet, *J Dairy Sci* 64:1555-1564, 1981.
150. Kronfeld DS, Raggi F: Nicotinamide coenzyme concentrations in mammary biopsy samples from ketotic cows, *Biochem J* 90:219-224, 1964.
151. Dufva GS et al: Effect of niacin supplementation on milk production and ketosis of dairy cattle, *J Dairy Sci* 66:2329, 1983.
152. Gorganov KH et al: Therapeutic and prophylactic effect of monensin and nicotinic acid in cows with subclinical ketosis, *Vet Nauki* 21(abstr 4518):43-50, 1984.
153. Ruegsegger GJ, Shultz LH: Use of a combination of propylene glycol and niacin for subclinical ketosis, *J Dairy Sci* 69:1411-1415, 1986.
154. Duffield TF et al: Effect of prepartum administration of monensin in a controlled-release capsule on postpartum energy indicators in lactating dairy cows, *J Dairy Sci* 81:2354-2361, 1998.
155. Duffield TF et al: Efficacy of monensin for the prevention of subclinical ketosis in lactating dairy cows, *J Dairy Sci* 81:2866-2873, 1998.
156. Green BL et al: The impact of a monensin controlled-release capsule on subclinical ketosis in the transition dairy cow, *J Dairy Sci* 82:333-342, 1999.
157. Grummer RR, Bertics SJ, Hackbart RA: Short communication: Effects of prepartum milking on dry matter intake, liver triglyceride and plasma constituents, *J Dairy Sci* 83:60-61, 2000.
158. Sniffen CJ: *Balancing rations for carbohydrates for dairy cattle: the application of nutrition in dairy practice*, Proceedings of a symposium, Wayne, NJ, 1988, American Cyanamid Co, pp 25-35.
159. Sniffen CJ, Chase LE: *Field application of the degradable protein system: the application of nutrition in dairy practice*, Proceedings of a symposium, Wayne, NJ, 1988, American Cyanamid Co, pp 18-24.
160. Chalupa W, Ferguson JD: *The role of dietary fat in productivity and health of dairy cows: the application of nutrition in dairy practice*, Proceedings of a symposium, Wayne, NJ, 1988, American Cyanamid Co, pp 36-43.

CALCIUM AND PHOSPHORUS HOMEOSTASIS

NANCY L. HESTERS

SHERRILL A. FLEMING

Phosphorus (PO_4) and calcium (Ca) are the most abundant mineral elements in the animal body.[161] Approximately 80% of the total body PO_4 and 99% of Ca are found in teeth and bone as hydroxyapatite [$Ca_{10}(PO_4)_6(OH)_2$]. Adequate Ca and PO_4 are essential for normal mineralization and growth of bone.[162] Most of the remaining 20% of total PO_4 is distributed throughout soft tissue as phospholipids, nucleic acids, phosphoproteins, adenosine triphosphate (ATP), and so on. PO_4 has many functions in soft tissue but is most important in energy exchange through formation and breakdown of high-energy bonds of ATP. Ca also serves many functions in soft tissue but is particularly important in transmission of nerve impulses and muscle contraction. A small amount of Ca and PO_4 are present in serum in the inorganic form as Ca^{2+} and dibasic PO_4^{2-} (80%) and monobasic PO_{4-} (20%).[163]

Ca and PO_4 homeostasis is controlled by parathyroid hormone (PTH) secreted by the parathyroid glands, calcitonin secreted by the C cells of the thyroid gland, and 1,25-dihydroxycholecalciferol (1,25-$(OH)_2D$; vitamin D) produced by the kidney.[167] These hormones maintain very precise control of Ca homeostasis. PO_4 homeostasis is maintained less stringently and secondarily to that of Ca.

Ca is actively absorbed by the small intestine to meet the daily requirements for maintenance and production. Hypocalcemia stimulates production of PTH, which then increases production of 1,25-$(OH)_2D$ by the kidney. 1,25-$(OH)_2D$ improves the efficiency of Ca absorption so that a higher proportion of dietary Ca is absorbed. When the level of dietary Ca is high, a smaller proportion is absorbed. Because Ca absorption is close to Ca requirements, most excess dietary Ca is lost in the feces. When hypercalcemia does occur, calcitonin inhibits resorption of Ca by the kidney, and excess Ca is lost in the urine. Calcitonin also inhibits resorption of Ca from bone.

Bone serves as a reservoir of Ca and PO_4 that can be mobilized to maintain plasma levels during dietary deficiency. During periods of high Ca demand (early lactation), hypocalcemia stimulates production of PTH and 1,25-$(OH)_2D$, which enhance bone resorption. PTH also enhances resorption of Ca from the renal tubules. When the Ca status returns to normal, bone reserves of Ca and PO_4 are replaced. Although PO_4 is released during bone resorption, hypophosphatemia is not known to stimulate PTH production or increase osteoclastic activity.

The major site of PO_4 absorption is the proximal small intestine, where PO_4 is passively absorbed in direct relation to PO_4 intake. Active absorption has been demonstrated in monogastric animals.[163,164] Under conditions of PO_4 deficiency, low plasma PO_4 stimulates production of 1,25-$(OH)_2D$, which then stimulates the intestine to absorb PO_4 more efficiently. With sufficient dietary levels of PO_4, active absorption is saturated, and passive absorption predominates.

Unlike most species, ruminants have a high salivary secretion of PO_4, with a relatively small amount excreted by the kidneys.[161] PTH stimulates loss of PO_4 in saliva and inhibits resorption of PO_4 by the renal tubules. The concentration of PO_4 in saliva is several times greater than, but directly related to, the plasma PO_4 concentration.[165] PO_4 from the saliva may exceed the PO_4 from the diet. A portion of PO_4 excreted in saliva is resorbed in the intestine, and the remainder is lost in the feces. Efficient resorption of PO_4 by the kidney and the ability to resorb PO_4 excreted in saliva serve as protective measures for ruminants on low PO_4 diets.

REFERENCES

161. Care AD, Bartlet JP, Abdel-Hafeez HM: Calcium and phosphate homeostasis in ruminants and its relationship to the aetiology and prevention of parturient paresis. In Ruckebusch Y, Thivend D, eds: *Digestive physiology and metabolism in ruminants*, Westport, Conn, 1980, AVI Publishing, p 429.
162. Hays VM, Swenson MJ: Minerals. In Swenson MJ, ed: *Dukes' physiology of domestic animals*, ed 11, Ithaca, NY, 1993, Cornell University Press, pp 517-519.
163. Rosol TJ, Capen CC: Calcium-regulating hormones and diseases of abnormal mineral metabolism. In Kaneko JJ, Harvey JW, Bruss ML, eds: *Clinical biochemistry of domestic animals*, ed 5, San Diego, Calif, 1997, Academic Press.
164. Reinhardt TA, Horst RL, Goff JP: Calcium, phosphorous and magnesium homeostasis in ruminants. In Herdt TH, ed: *Veterinary clinics of North America (food animal practice)*, ed 4, Philadelphia, 1988, WB Saunders, p 331.
165. Dua K, Care AD: The role of phosphate on the rates of mineral absorption from the forestomachs of sheep, *Vet J* 157:51-55, 1999.

DISORDERS OF CALCIUM METABOLISM

ELAINE HUNT
J. TRAVIS BLACKWELDER

Bovine Parturient Paresis (Milk Fever, Hypocalcemia)

Parturient paresis is acute to peracute flaccid paralysis or somnolence of lactating dairy cows. It usually occurs within 72 hours of parturition and is seen most often in high-producing cows. It should be considered an emergency, and prompt intravenous therapy with calcium solutions is required.

ETIOLOGY. Hypocalcemia occurs when rapid onset of milk production results in acute depletion of serum ionized calcium. Signs of hypocalcemic paresis follow and are ultimately fatal unless therapy is instituted.

CLINICAL SIGNS. There are three discernible clinical stages of parturient paresis. During stage one the animal is still able to stand but shows signs of hypersensitivity and excitability. Head bobbing, ear twitching, and fine tremors over the flank and loin may be seen. The cow is slightly ataxic when she walks. When standing, she may appear restless and shuffle her hind feet. Bellowing and open-mouth breathing with tongue extension may also be noted. If calcium therapy is not instituted, the more severe signs of stage two hypocalcemia will develop.

In stage two hypocalcemia the cow is unable to stand but is still able to maintain sternal recumbency. Depression, anorexia, dry muzzle, and subnormal body temperature (36° to 38° C, 96.8° to 100.4° F) with cold extremities are noted at this stage. If the ambient temperature is higher than 38° C (100.4° F), the rectal temperature may be elevated. Tachycardia with decreased intensity of heart sounds may be auscultated. Smooth muscle paralysis leads to gastrointestinal stasis, which is sometimes manifested as bloat, inability to defecate, and loss of anal sphincter tone. The ability to urinate may also be lost at this time. Arrested parturition or retained placenta may occur because of uterine inertia. Pupils are usually dilated, with delayed or absent light reflex. Sternal recumbency with the head tucked into the flank is a characteristic posture of hypocalcemic cows. When the head is extended, an S-shaped curvature or kink in the neck may be noted.

Animals in stage three hypocalcemia have continued loss of consciousness to the point of coma. Such animals have complete muscle flaccidity, are unresponsive to stimuli, are unable to maintain sternal recumbency, and suffer from severe bloat. Cardiac output continues to worsen. The pulse may be nearly undetectable, and the heart rate as high as 120 beats/min. Cows in this stage of hypocalcemia may not survive more than a few hours.

Differential diagnosis for recumbency in the postpartum cow includes toxic mastitis, toxic metritis, traumatic injury (stifle injury, coxofemoral luxation or other trauma), obturator paralysis, or compartmental crush syndrome resulting from extended recumbency. Toxic conditions cause a similar depression of consciousness and are the most difficult to distinguish from hypocalcemia. Hypocalcemia may occur concurrently with any of these conditions.

Two cautions should be heeded with respect to clinical signs. It has been shown that hypocalcemic cows, whether showing clinical signs or not, are about five times more likely to develop left displacement of the abomasum.[166] Also beware of the supposition that dilation of the pupils is a clinical sign indicative of parturient paresis. It has been shown that pupil size is of no diagnostic or prognostic value.[167]

CLINICAL PATHOLOGY. Because of the urgency of treating acute hypocalcemia, diagnosis and treatment are usually based on clinical signs. Pretreatment blood samples should be taken so the diagnosis can be confirmed with serum calcium levels. Determination of serum calcium is particularly important in animals that do not respond to therapy. Normal values vary between laboratories, but cows with serum calcium lower than 7.5 mg/dl should be considered hypocalcemic. Animals with serum calcium levels of 5.5 to 7.5 mg/dl may show signs of stage one hypocalcemia. Stage two hypocalcemia may be seen with calcium levels of 3.5 to 6.5 mg/dl. Calcium concentration may fall to as low as 2 mg/dl in stage three.[168]

Serum calcium is composed of an ionized part and a protein-bound part. Ionized calcium is most important for immediate metabolic function. In the face of low serum albumin, a lactating cow can have low total calcium without developing clinical signs of hypocalcemia. Alkalosis increases albumin binding of calcium, resulting in a decreased ionized calcium level.[169] For this reason cows that are alkalotic from an upper gastrointestinal obstruction may have normal total serum calcium while exhibiting clinical signs of hypocalcemia. Therefore ionized calcium levels more accurately evaluate the metabolic status of the cow. However, this test is expensive and usually not available to the practitioner. In most cases, total calcium is an acceptable diagnostic test, but clinicians should be aware of possible discrepancies between clinical signs and total serum calcium measurements. When hypoalbuminemia exists, a corrected total calcium may be calculated using the following equation[170]:

Corrected calcium = Measured calcium (mg/dl) −
Albumin (g/dl) + 3.5

This formula is used routinely for correction of total calcium in hypoalbuminemic dogs. Although it has not been thoroughly evaluated for cattle, the corrected calcium level may be more consistent with observed clinical signs than the actual ionized calcium level.

Cows with parturient paresis are usually hypophosphatemic (as low as 2.1 mg/dl), hypermagnesemic (serum magnesium of 2.2 to 2.7 mg/dl), and hyperglycemic (95 to 130 mg/dl). A stress leukogram (neutrophilia, lymphopenia, and eosinopenia) and a moderately elevated creatine phosphokinase (CPK) are common findings in postpartum cows. Unlike parturient paresis, nonparturient hypocalcemia is frequently associated with hypomagnesemia and hyperphosphatemia.

PATHOPHYSIOLOGY. The onset of lactation at the time of parturition results in a sudden loss of calcium in milk. A cow producing 10 liters of colostrum loses approximately 23 g of calcium in a single milking.[171] This loss is nine times the amount of calcium in the entire plasma calcium pool of the cow. When the calcium homeostatic mechanism is unable to meet this demand, hypocalcemia occurs.

During the dry period calcium demand is relatively low. Therefore intestinal absorption and bone resorption of calcium are relatively inactive.[172] At the onset of lactation, such large demands are placed on the calcium homeostatic mechanisms of the body most cows develop some degree of hypocalcemia at parturition.[173] In some cases, plasma calcium concentrations become too low to support nerve and muscle function, resulting in clinical hypocalcemia. Hypocalcemia stimulates the calcium homeostatic mechanism to improve the efficiency of intestinal calcium absorption and increase bone resorption. Approximately 24 hours of elevated 1,25-dihydroxy vitamin D (1,25-$(OH)_2$D) stimulation is required to improve intestinal transport of calcium.[174-176] An increased rate of bone resorption requires 48 hours of parathyroid hormone (PTH) stimulation.[177] If these adaptations to increased calcium demand are prolonged, clinical hypocalcemia may develop.

Why some cows are able to adapt to lactational calcium demands without developing parturient paresis and others are not is unclear. Most cows with clinical signs of parturient paresis have higher levels of PTH and 1,25-$(OH)_2$D than cows that are not affected.[178,179] Because hormonal response is normal, the defect is thought to be an inability of target tissues (intestinal, bone, and kidney) to respond to the hormonal stimuli. This could be caused by a deficiency of hormone receptors or a defect of the metabolic pathways activated when the hormones bind with their receptors. The efficiency of calcium absorption is known to deteriorate with increasing age,[180] and some evidence suggests this is the result of a decreased number of 1,25-$(OH)_2$D receptors and impaired production of 1,25-$(OH)_2$D.[171,181] There is also evidence that indicates PTH acts poorly on bone and kidney tissues when the blood pH is high.[182] Blood pH of cattle is often alkaline because forage potassium levels in prepartum

cattle rations are excessively high. The alkalization of the blood and extracellular fluid of the cow reduces calcium absorption and renal production of 1,25$(OH)_2$D.[171] Dietary potassium levels are often an indicator in determining susceptibility of dairy cows to parturient paresis.[182]

Hypocalcemia affects muscular contraction in several different ways, as follows:

- Calcium has a membrane stabilizing effect on peripheral nerves.[183] Hyperesthesia and mild tetany seen in early stages of parturient paresis may be caused by a lack of nerve cell membrane stabilization.
- Calcium is required for release of acetylcholine at the neuromuscular junction.[183] Inability to release acetylcholine, caused by hypocalcemia, causes paralysis by blocking the transmission of nerve impulses to the muscle fibers.
- Calcium is also directly required by muscle cells for contraction.

Paralysis of the various muscle types results in the clinical signs of parturient paresis. In addition to skeletal muscle paralysis and recumbency, lack of smooth muscle tone results in gastrointestinal stasis and bloat. Impaired intestinal motility may also exacerbate hypocalcemia by limiting absorption of calcium. Decreased contractility of cardiac muscle and lowered stroke volume can cause a 50% reduction in arterial blood pressure.[184] Poor peripheral perfusion and inability to shiver or generate body heat through muscular activity lead to hypothermia and depression of consciousness.

Hypophosphatemia seen with parturient paresis is the result of phosphorus loss in milk, inadequate feed intake around the time of parturition, and increased renal and salivary excretion of PO_4 caused by a high circulating level of PTH.[185] The cause of hypermagnesemia is not clear but may be a compensatory attempt to maintain ionic balance. PTH could theoretically contribute to hypermagnesemia by increasing tubular resorption by the kidney.[168] Hypermagnesemia impairs acetylcholine release at the neuromuscular junction and may intensify the flaccid paralysis or parturient paresis.[168] Hyperglycemia associated with parturient paresis is believed to be caused by increased glucocorticoid release and gluconeogenesis caused by stress.

EPIDEMIOLOGY. Parturient paresis is a disease of high-producing dairy cattle. Approximately 5% to 10% of adult dairy cows are affected. Jersey cattle are most susceptible and may have a much higher incidence. The reason for this breed predilection is not known for certain, but it may be associated with higher milk production per unit of body weight,[186,187] reduction of intestinal vitamin D_3 receptors as Jerseys age,[188] and a higher than normal production of parathyroid hormone related proteins (PTHrP) by the mammary gland, which increases calcium transport from blood to milk.[187] Parturient paresis may occur before calving, but most cases occur within the first 48 hours after calving.[184] Heifers are very seldom affected, and there is a gradual increase in incidence with parity. Most cases occur in animals older than 5 years of age. This may be the result of increasing milk production with age and decreasing efficiency of dietary calcium absorption and bone resorption. Cows affected with parturient paresis are at greater risk at subsequent lactations than are nonaffected cows. Parturient paresis is uncommon in beef cattle. When they are affected, the paresis is usually associated with inadequate nutrition. Nonparturient hypocalcemia can occur secondary to rumen overload, diarrhea on lush pasture, oxalate-rich diets, or feed deprivation. Transportation stress may also precipitate hypocalcemia.

Diets providing dry cows a high daily intake of calcium (>100 g/day) have been associated with an increased incidence of parturient paresis.[189] At this level the maintenance requirement of calcium can be met predominantly by passive absorption. Active absorption of dietary calcium and bone resorption are then suppressed.[190] Cows in this condition are not able to quickly replace plasma calcium lost in milk and may become severely hypocalcemic. When the incidence of parturient paresis within a herd is higher than the normal frequency, improper levels of calcium in the dry cow diet should be suspected. Appropriate dietary calcium levels for dry cows are discussed under prevention and control. More recent studies suggest that high calcium levels in the prepartum diet are not the predominant cause of parturient paresis and that potassium levels may play a more critical role in determining susceptibility to hypocalcemia.[173,182] The high potassium levels of forages being fed to dry cows and the heavy use of potassium fertilizers on forage crops are causing the diet to become alkalinized and resulting in enhanced susceptibility of the cow to parturient paresis.[173]

NECROPSY FINDINGS. No pathognomonic lesions are caused by hypocalcemia. Flaccidity of the cardiac musculature has been suggested as a lesion of hypocalcemia, but it is very difficult to assess. Hypocalcemia is associated with many other conditions, including uterine prolapse, dystocia caused by uterine inertia, retained fetal membranes, abomasal displacement, mastitis, renal disease, and metritis.[191] Aspiration of rumen contents and muscle damage are also common in cows with hypocalcemia. The presence of any of these conditions may suggest a concurrent hypocalcemia, but none should be considered diagnostic.

TREATMENT AND PROGNOSIS. Recommended treatment for parturient paresis is intravenous injection of a calcium gluconate salt. A rule of thumb for calcium administration is 1 g of calcium per 45 kg (100 lb) of body weight. Most solutions are available in single-dose, 500-ml bottles containing 8 to 11 g of calcium. In large, heavily lactating cows a second bottle administered subcutaneously may be beneficial. This is thought to provide a more prolonged release of calcium into the circulation. Subcutaneous treatment alone may not be absorbed because of poor peripheral perfusion and should be avoided as the sole therapy. Solutions containing formaldehyde or more than 25 g of dextrose per 500 ml are irritating and may abscess if given subcutaneously. Many commercially available solutions contain phosphorus and magnesium in addition to calcium. The use of phosphorus and magnesium is probably not necessary in uncomplicated cases of parturient hypocalcemia. Most of these animals are already hypermagnesemic and, although hypophosphatemic, serum phosphorus levels return to normal after calcium administration. Although these solutions are usually not beneficial, detrimental effects have not been reported. Occasionally a cow remains hypophosphatemic after calcium therapy and may benefit from additional phosphorus. The inclusion of magnesium may protect against myocardial irritation caused by administration of calcium.

Calcium is directly cardiotoxic, and any calcium-containing solution should be administered slowly (over 10 to 20 min) during continuous cardiac auscultation. If severe arrhythmias or bradycardia develop, administration should be stopped. Once the heartbeat has returned to normal, administration may be resumed at a slower rate. Intravenous atropine has been used to abolish cardiac arrhythmias associated with calcium administration.[192] Ten percent $MgSO_4$ (100 to 400 ml) can be administered rapidly to antagonize cardioexcitatory effects of calcium. Animals that are endotoxemic and hypocalcemic are especially prone to severe cardiac dysrhythmias caused by intravenous calcium therapy.

Oral Ca administration is an option that avoids the risks of cardiotoxic side effects and can be used in mild cases of parturient paresis. Of products available in the United States, calcium propionate suspended in a propylene glycol gel is the best combination of calcium form and medium of many evaluated. Oral administration of 50 g of soluble Ca results

in the entry of about 4 g of Ca into the blood. Calcium chloride is the most readily absorbed form of the calcium salt and is reported to have superior bioavailability when compared to calcium formiate.[193] Calcium propionate may also be more sustained than $CaCl_2$ but it requires a larger volume to be given. Another advantage to using Ca propionate is the propionate also serves as a gluconeogenic precursor that is beneficial to early postpartum cows in negative energy balance.[172] $CaCl_2$ has a tendency to induce metabolic acidosis and aqueous $CaCl_2$ solutions are caustic.[193,194] Calcium chloride gel suspensions have been criticized because of their ability to cause minor to severe damage of forestomach and abomasal mucosa.[195] A special formulation of $CaCl_2$ has been produced in Scandinavia using a two-compartment oil preparation.[193] This product demonstrates rapid (within 15 minutes) increase in plasma calcium without evidence of mucosal damage even when administered four times at 12-hour intervals.

Hypocalcemic cows show immediate, characteristic signs of response to therapy. As neuromuscular function returns, tremors begin in the muscles of the flank and may spread over the entire body. Improved cardiac function is evidenced by stronger heart sounds and a decreasing pulse rate (from 80 to 100 down to 60 to 70 beats/min). Return of smooth muscle function allows eructation and defecation to occur. The muzzle frequently breaks out in individual droplets of sweat. Urination usually follows when the cow rises. Approximately 60% of affected cows stand shortly after treatment. Another 15% can be expected to recover within 2 hours.[184] Animals that have not responded by 8 to 12 hours after treatment should be reevaluated, and treatment repeated if necessary. Excessive and prolonged administration of calcium may actually suppress the homeostatic mechanisms for increasing serum calcium. Therefore repeated treatment with calcium should be based on laboratory verification of low serum calcium levels.

Of cows that respond to the first treatment, 25% to 30% relapse within 24 to 48 hours and require additional therapy. Incomplete milking after treatment has been advised to reduce the incidence of relapse. Udder inflation has been used in the past to reduce the secretion of milk and loss of calcium. This may help to prevent relapses, but the risk of introducing bacteria into the mammary gland is high.

1-α-Hydroxy-cholecalciferol [1-α-(OH)D₃] (a synthetic analog of vitamin D₃) can be used as prophylaxis in high-risk animals and 1-α-(OH)D₃ is also very effective as a treatment for the 15% of parturient paretic cows that do not respond to Ca therapy. It is recommended that 1 μg/kg of body weight be given, half intravenoulsy and half intramuscularly. In one study, nine out of nine cows responded and recovered within 12 hours.[196]

When uncomplicated parturient paresis is treated promptly, the prognosis for survival and return to milk production is very good. If recumbency before treatment is prolonged, the incidence of secondary teat trauma, mastitis, musculoskeletal trauma, and ischemic muscle necrosis is much greater. In these cases the prognosis is much worse. Persistently elevated CPK levels (>2000 IU) suggest severe muscle damage caused by recumbency and decreased successful outcomes. Cows that show the expected responses to calcium therapy but do not stand should be suspected of having secondary complications. Cows that remain recumbent should be provided with plenty of clean, dry bedding and secure, nonslip footing to prevent rear limb trauma caused by slipping, abduction, or frog legging as the cow struggles to rise; they should be rolled from side to side at least four times daily. Down cows should be protected from the weather if possible. Shade from direct sun in hot weather is particularly important. The cow should be provided with water and feed.

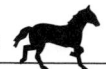

Lifting cows several times daily with a hip sling may be advisable for animals recumbent more than 48 hours.

PREVENTION AND CONTROL. To avoid the onset of milk fever the blood pH needs to be decreased in late prepartum and early postpartum cattle.[173] The best way to accomplish this is by reducing the potassium content of the diet fed to prepartum cows. A reduction of potassium in the diet can be a challenge because of the high concentration of potassium found in forages fed to dry cows. Corn silage tends to have the lowest content of potassium in available forages for prepartum cattle and it can be effectively used as a major portion of the dry cow's diet. Alfalfa is another forage source in dry cow rations that may prove beneficial in maintaining proper blood pH. Alfalfa was not used in the past because of high Ca content, but it is now known that Ca has little effect on the alkalinity of cow's blood. Another way to lower the potassium concentration of forages is to withold potassium fertilizers from fields that will be harvested for dry cow rations. The key to preventing parturient paresis is to find a low potassium hay source and combine it with corn silage to form the basis for the dry cow ration.[173]

In the past decade, using the dietary cation-anion difference has revolutionized the prevention of parturient paresis. It has now been proven that this method is more effective and more practical than lowering prepartum Ca in the diet.[197-201] The key to this method is providing an excess of anions over cations in the diet by adjusting the diet, adding anionic salts (of sulfate and chloride), or a combination of both. Adding anions to the diet of the cow can counteract the effects that dietary potassium and sodium have on blood pH.[173] Anionic salts that can be added are magnesium sulfate, calcium sulfate, ammonium sulfate, ammonium chloride, calcium chloride, and magnesium chloride.[197] Feeding anionic salts not only controls milk fever, but it also has been shown to increase lactation and reproductive efficiency.[202]

Anionic excess prevents parturient paresis by acidifying the blood to restore tissue responsiveness to PTH.[203] Several different authors have developed balanced equations and feeding recommendations on the basis of the milliequivalents of Na, K, Ca, Cl, S, and PO$_4$ in the diet.[204-206] Reinhardt, Horst, and Goff[206] recommended diets with an ion balance of less than 8000 mEq, in which

$$\text{Ion balance} = (Ca + 1/3\ PO_4 + Na + K) + (S - Cl)$$

The exact formulas used vary between different researchers. The addition of 100 g of NH$_4$Cl and 100 g of NH$_4$SO$_4$ to basal diets containing either 75 or 150 g of calcium has been successful in preventing parturient paresis.[181] This approach may be more practical than analysis of ion levels in the entire diet, although simply adding 100 g each of Cl and SO$_4$ may only be effective under otherwise ideal conditions. More recently Goff and Horst[173] evaluated the acidifying activity of different anionic salts and came to the conclusion that the following equation is a more accurate description of ion balance in rations:

$$\text{Ion balance} = (0.15\ Ca^{2+} + 0.15\ Mg^{2+} + Na^+ + K^+) - (Cl^- + 0.25\ S^- + 0.5\ P^-)$$

This equation suggest the major dietary factors determining blood pH are sodium, potassium, and chloride. The target value for close up dry cow rations should be around +200 to +300 mEq/kg.[173]

The pH of urine accurately reflects the acid-base state of the normal transition cow.[173,203] Monitoring pH of urine can be an inexpensive and sensitive method to control the effect of the diet on blood pH in prepartum cattle and is often a better gauge of the diet's ion balance than any before mentioned formula.[173,203] For successful control of parturient paresis the average pH of the urine in Holstein cattle should

range between 6.0 and 6.5 and urine pH of Jersey cattle should fall between 5.8 and 6.2. When urine pH ranges from 5.0 to 5.5 too many anions have been added to the diet and may result in decreased dry matter intake.[173]

One drawback to adding anionic salts has been poor palatability. All anionic salts are unpalatable, and although sulfate salts are slightly more palatable than chloride salts they are much less effective acidifiers of the blood and should be avoided if possible. Palatability problems can be overcome by using a mixture of the anionic salts with a palatable moist ration, including wet corn silage, brewer's grain, distiller's grain, roasted soybeans, or molasses.[207]

Other problems can be encountered with this diet, but they can be overcome with careful management techniques. These techniques should include minimizing forage preference, optimizing dry matter intake, and acclimatizing the cows to anionic salts. Avoid feeding programs that allow preferential selection of feedstuffs to enhance the chances that the cows actually consume the ration that has been formulated. Also, ensure that dry matter intake is maintained (at least 22 lb/per cow/day), and that, because of the guessing game of calving dates, the salts are added to the diet 3 to 5 weeks before parturition.[207]

Feeding during the last 2 to 3 weeks of gestation is most critical for dry cow health. During this time small amounts of additional grain may be needed to meet increasing energy requirements. High-calcium grain mixtures formulated for lactating cows should be avoided. At the time of calving, feeding high-quality forage such as alfalfa may help reduce the depression of feed intake that frequently occurs at parturition. After freshening, consumption of the lactating cow ration should be gradually increased. Goff and Horst[173] recommend using the following mineral profile for transition cow diets (last 2 to 3 weeks of gestation)

Calcium	1% to 1.2%
Phosphorus	0.4% to 0.5%
Magnesium	0.4%
Sodium	as close to 0.1% as possible
Potassium	as close to 0.7% as possible
Sulfur	0.3% to 0.4%
Chloride	high enough to bring average urine pH between 6 and 6.8

In the past, low-calcium diets fed in the dry period were the primary method of milk fever prevention. This method stimulates active intestinal absorption and bone resorption in preparation for the sudden demand for calcium at the onset of lactation. Although stimulation does occur, it is now known that this method is not as effective as initially believed, and it is also difficult to lower the amount of Ca in the diet enough.[198] For reduced Ca diets to have an effect they must range between 8 and 10 g/day of Ca.[171]

Adding PO$_4$ to the diet to decrease the calcium:phosphorus ratio was thought to be beneficial in reducing the incidence of parturient paresis.[208] More recent work suggests that, with moderate calcium levels (80 g/day), a low level of dietary phosphorus reduces the incidence of parturient paresis.[209,210] It has been speculated that low phosphorus caused increased intestinal binding of 1,25-(OH)$_2$D, resulting in improved efficiency of intestinal absorption of calcium and phosphorus. Daily phosphorus intake of 35 to 40 g/day with moderate calcium intake is recommended.[173,211]

Administration of vitamin D$_3$ and its metabolites has been shown to be effective in preventing parturient paresis.[184] Several administration protocols have been used, but most compounds must be provided during the week before parturition. Prolonged use of the vitamin D compounds or use at the wrong time may be detrimental. Oral calcium gels or drenches administered at the time of calving have been effective in reducing the incidence of parturient paresis. Prophylactic use of calcium and vitamin D preparations is labor intensive and expensive. Their use is best reserved for animals that are known to have a high risk of developing hypocalcemia. Also be aware that when vitamin D metabolites fail to prevent hypocalcemia, the resulting parturient paresis is often clinically more severe than normal parturient paresis.[212]

For this and other reasons, the use of synthetic bovine PTH may prove to be superior to vitamin D metabolites. Vitamin D metabolites enhance intestinal Ca absorption, whereas PTH does this and also stimulates bone resorption. Intravenous PTH has been investigated and shown to be effective if administration is begun at least 60 hours before parturition.[213] Intramuscular PTH is also effective and must be started 6 days before parturition. This method is very effective at preventing hypocalcemia, but it is suggested that there may be unknown side effects.[215] Both methods of PTH administration carry the disadvantage of being labor intensive.

Hypocalcemia of Sheep and Goats

Ewes are most likely to develop hypocalcemia during the last 4 to 6 weeks of gestation. Compared with cattle, ewes have a relatively large calcium demand for the developing fetus. Although the ewe's lactational demand for calcium is relatively small, hypocalcemia may occur during the first 6 weeks of lactation. Outbreaks of hypocalcemia may affect 25% of the flock during late gestation. Flaccid paralysis is the primary sign of hypocalcemia, but tetany occurs relatively more often than it does in cattle. Pregnancy toxemia (see Chapter 31) and hypocalcemia may be very difficult to differentiate on the basis of clinical signs. Urinalysis for ketones is helpful in making a diagnosis. Food deprivation or forced exercise may precipitate hypocalcemia. Hypocalcemia may occur in pregnant ewes and lambs after the stress of transportation (transit tetany). Lambs usually have concurrent hypomagnesemia, and they have muscle tremors and tetany rather than flaccid paralysis.

Administration of intravenous calcium solutions (1 g Ca/ 45 kg) results in rapid recovery. The incidence of relapses is higher in ewes than in cows. The ewe should be provided with a continuously rising plane of nutrition during the last 6 weeks of gestation. This increases calcium intake and helps prevent hypocalcemia and pregnancy toxemia.

Hypocalcemia occurs in high-producing dairy goats during lactation and may even occur several weeks after parturition.[184] Goats may not become recumbent or progress to coma as dairy cows do if untreated. Hyperexcitability or mild depression and ataxia are usually the clinical signs observed. Hypocalcemia may be seen during late gestation, particularly in does carrying twins or multiple fetuses. Recommended treatment is 1 g of calcium per 45 kg IV. As in dairy cows, limiting calcium intake for 30 days before parturition may reduce the incidence of hypocalcemia. This can usually be accomplished by removing alfalfa hay from the diet.

Hypocalcemia of Horses

Lactation tetany occurs in mares approximately 10 days after foaling or 1 or 2 days after weaning. Animals at the greatest risk usually are those maintained on pasture only and used for hard physical labor. Draft mares are more likely to be affected. Prolonged transportation can also predispose horses to hypocalcemia (transit tetany). Clinical signs of hypocalcemia in horses include tetany, profuse sweating, anxious appearance, tachycardia, cardiac arrhythmias, and synchronous diaphragmatic flutter. Prolapse of the nictitating membrane, which occurs frequently with tetanus, is less commonly observed with hypocalcemia. Intravenous calcium may result in

rapid recovery. Heart monitoring should be continued during therapy.

Nutritional Secondary Hyperparathyroidism (Big Head, Bran Disease, Osteodystrophia Fibrosa)

ETIOLOGY. Nutritional secondary hyperparathyroidism (NSH) is induced by an absolute or a relative calcium deficiency caused by an excess of dietary phosphorus.

CLINICAL SIGNS. The clinical signs of NSH are the result of bone resorption to maintain plasma calcium levels during dietary deficiency. The early stages of the disease are characterized by intermittent shifting lameness and stiff, creaking joints. These signs are attributed to periosteal avulsion and detached ligaments and tendons. Erosions of articular cartilage caused by resorption of underlying trabeculae contribute to joint pain. Spontaneous fractures of sesamoids and phalanges may also be the result of mild NSH.[192]

NSH is a systemic disease, but the bones of the head are more severely affected by the lesion known as osteodystrophia fibrosa. As NSH progresses, affected animals develop cylindric thickening of the mandible. The maxilla, palate, lacrimal, and zygomatic bones are also thickened. In severe cases the nasal and frontal bones are affected. The bone enlargement is initially soft and hardens later. Visible facial swelling is bilateral but not always symmetric. As a result of these bone deformities, the animal may have difficulty chewing and breathing. Occlusion of the lacrimal duct results in epiphora.

CLINICAL PATHOLOGY. Serum calcium and phosphorus are usually maintained within normal limits by homeostatic mechanisms. The worst serum electrolyte aberration that is likely to be seen is low normal calcium and high normal phosphorus. Serum alkaline phosphatase may be high normal to slightly elevated.

The most useful clinical pathology measurement for diagnosing NSH is urinary fractional excretion (FE) of PO_4.[215,216] Normal FE of PO_4 is 0% to 0.5% (see Chapter 10). Values above 4% suggest excess phosphorus intake. Excretion of calcium is decreased but is difficult to measure, especially in the horse, because of formation of calcium carbonate crystals in urine.

PATHOPHYSIOLOGY. Because PO_4 is passively absorbed by the intestine, consumption of high levels of PO_4 leads to increased plasma PO_4 levels. Hyperphosphatemia lowers the serum calcium level, which stimulates production of PTH. PTH increases the rate of bone resorption and inhibits resorption of PO_4 by the kidney until Ca and PO_4 levels are normal. If the dietary phosphorus level remains high, prolonged stimulation of bone resorption leads to osteoporosis and replacement with osteoid and fibrous connective tissue (osteodystrophia fibrosa). This is especially severe in the facial bones, where trabeculae and connective tissue are deposited subperiosteally in a radial fashion.

EPIDEMIOLOGY. NSH may occur in goats, swine, and rarely cattle, but it is most common in horses. The disease is sometimes referred to as big head, because of the severe deformities that can occur in horses. As a result of better nutritional management, cases are now rare. NSH can occur any time after weaning but is most common in horses less than 7 years old. Diets high in phosphorus usually consist of grass hay with heavy feeding of grain or bran. Grain and grass hay are low in calcium and good sources of phosphorus. Bran contains a very high level of phosphorus. Horses grazing pastures high in oxalates are predisposed to NSH, even though dietary calcium and phosphorus levels are normal. Oxalates combine with calcium, rendering it unavailable for absorption.

NECROPSY. The characteristic lesion of NSH is replacement and distortion of hard facial bones with fibrous con-

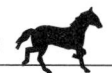

nective tissue.[217] Less severe osteoporosis and fibrous replacement of bone may be found throughout the skeleton. In prolonged cases the parathyroid gland may be hypertrophied.

THERAPY AND PROGNOSIS. When the animal is returned to a diet with a calcium:phosphorus ratio of 1:1 to 2:1, the prognosis for recovery is good. Lameness usually regresses over a period of 8 weeks. Although some remodeling occurs, facial distortion is likely to be permanent.

PREVENTION AND CONTROL. A diet that meets the demand for calcium and phosphorus in a 1:1 ratio prevents NSH in horses. Legume hay such as alfalfa is an excellent natural source of calcium. If necessary, calcium carbonate may be used as a supplement.

Hypercalcemia

Hypercalcemia is a common finding in horses affected with renal disease. In most species, renal disease is more likely to result in hypocalcemia and hyperphosphatemia. The horse absorbs a relatively larger portion of dietary calcium and is more dependent on renal excretion of excess calcium. If calcium intake is low or if there is a loss of albumin, hypocalcemia may occur with renal disease.

Pseudohyperparathyroidism secondary to neoplasia occurs in many species. In the horse, this condition is most commonly associated with gastric squamous cell carcinoma and lymphosarcoma.[215] PTH and other factors that can stimulate osteoclast activity have been shown to be produced by some tumors.[218] The diagnosis of pseudohyperparathyroidism is based on identification of the neoplasia in hypercalcemic animals.

Hypervitaminosis D caused by oversupplementation leads to hypercalcemia and hyperphosphatemia. Ingestion of plants such as *Cestrum diurnum* (wild jasmine in Florida) and *Solanum sodomaeum* (in Hawaii) containing vitamin D–like substances also results in hypercalcemia.[186] Increased gastrointestinal absorption and bone resorption contribute to hypercalcemia.[218] Affected animals have limb stiffness with painful flexor tendons and suspensory ligaments.

Polydipsia and polyuria with low urine specific gravity may occur. Soft-tissue mineralization may be found on necropsy. Removal of the vitamin D source and time result in recovery of mild cases. Prognosis is poor in more severe cases, especially if cardiac or renal mineralization has occurred.

Primary hyperparathyroidism is a rarely diagnosed condition that results in hypercalcemia. Parathyroid carcinoma, adenoma, and hyperplasia may result in hyperparathyroidism. Diagnosis is based on ruling out other causes of hypercalcemia.

REFERENCES

166. Massey CD et al: Hypocalcemia at parturition as a risk factor for left displacement of the abomasum in dairy cows, *J Am Vet Med Assoc* 203:852-853, 1993.
167. Fenwick DC: The association between pupil sizes and blood constituents in cows with parturient paresis, *Can Vet J* 30:426-429, 1989.
168. Oetzel GR: Parturient paresis and hypocalcemia in ruminant livestock. In Herdt TA, ed: *Veterinary clinics of North America (food animal practice)*, vol 4, Philadelphia, 1988, WB Saunders, p 331.
169. Toto DR: Metabolic acid-base disorders. In Kokko JP, Tannen RL, ed: *Fluids and electrolytes*, Philadelphia, 1986, WB Saunders, p 229.
170. Mueten DJ et al: Relationship of serum total calcium to albumin and total protein in dogs, *J Am Vet Med Assoc* 180:63, 1982.
171. Horst RL et al: Strategies for preventing milk fever in dairy cattle, *J Dairy Sci* 80:1269, 1997.
172. Ramberg CF et al: Calcium homeostasis in cows with special reference to parturient hypocalcemia, *Am J Physiol* 246:R698, 1984.
173. Goff JP, Horst RL: Factors to concentrate on to prevent periparturient disease in the dairy cow with special emphasis on milk fever, *Proceedings of the Thirty-first Annual Convention of the American Association of Bovine Practitioners*, 1998, pp 154-163.
174. Braithwaite GD: The effect of 1-alpha-hydroxycholecalciferol on calcium and phosphorous metabolism in the lactating ewe, *Br J Nutr* 40:397, 1978.

175. Goff JP, Horst RL, Littledike ET: Bone resorption, renal function and mineral status in cows treated with 1,25-dihydroxy-cholecalciferol and its 24-fluoro analogues, *J Nutr* 116:1500, 1986.
176. Hove K: Effects of 1-alpha-hydroxylated metabolites of cholecalciferol on intestinal radio-calcium absorption in goats, *Br J Nutr* 51:157, 1984.
177. Goff JP, Littledike ET, Horst RL: Effect of synthetic bovine parathyroid hormone in dairy cows: prevention of hypocalcemic parturient paresis, *J Dairy Sci* 69:2278, 1986.
178. Horst RL, Jorgensen NA, Deluca HF: Plasma 1,25-(OH)₂ vitamin D3 and parathyroid hormone levels in paretic dairy cows, *Am J Physiol* 235:E634, 1978.
179. Mayer GP, Rumberg CF, Kronfeld DS: Plasma parathyroid hormone concentrations in hypocalcemic parturient cows, *Am J Vet Res* 30:1587, 1969.
180. Hansard SL, Comar CL, Plumlee MP: The effect of age upon calcium utilization and maintenance requirement in the bovine, *J Anim Sci* 13:25, 1954.
181. Oetzel GR et al: Feeding of anionic diets during the prepartum period for prevention of parturient hypocalcemia in dairy cows, *J Dairy Sci* 70(suppl):376, 1987.
182. Goff JP, Horst RL: Pysiologic changes at parturition and their relationship to metabolic disease, *J Dairy Sci* 80:1260, 1987.
183. Iggo A: Activity of peripheral nerves and junctional regions. In Swenson MJ, ed: *Duke's physiology of domestic animals*, ed 10, Ithaca, NY, 1984, Cornell University Press, p 612.
184. Blood DC, Radostits OM, Henderson JA: *Veterinary medicine*, ed 6, London, 1983, Baillière Tindall, p 974-983.
185. Care AD, Bartlet JP, Abdel-Hafeez HM: Calcium and phosphate homeostasis in ruminants and its relationship to the aetiology and prevention of parturient paresis. In Ruckebusch Y, Thivend D, eds: *Digestive physiology and metabolism in ruminants*, Westport, Conn, 1980, AVI Publishing, p 429.
186. Allen WM, Sansom BF: Parturient paresis (milk fever) and hypocalcemia (cows, ewes, and goats). In Howard JL, ed: *Current veterinary therapy (food animal practice)*, ed 2, Philadelphia, 1986, WB Saunders, p 311.
187. Law FMK et al: Parathyroid hormone–related protein in milk and its correlation with bovine milk calcium, *J Endocrinal Bristol* 128:21-26, 1991.
188. Horst RL, Goff JP, Reinhardt TA: Advancing age results in reduction of intestinal and bone 1,25-dihydroxyvitamin D receptor, *Endocrinology* 126:1053, 1990.
189. Boda JM, Cole HH: Calcium metabolism with special references to parturient paresis (milk fever) in dairy cattle: a review, *J Dairy Sci* 39:1027, 1956.
190. Black HE, Capen CC, Yarrington JT: Effect of a high calcium prepartal diet on calcium homeostatic mechanisms in thyroid glands, bone and intestine of cows, *Lab Invest* 29:437, 1973.
191. Curtis CR et al: Association of parturient hypocalcemia with periparturient disorders in Holstein cows, *J Am Vet Med Assoc* 183:559, 1983.
192. Littledike ET, Glazier D, Cook HM: Electrocardiographic changes after induced hypercalcemia and hypocalcemia in cattle: reversal of the induced arrhythmia with atropine, *Am J Vet Res* 37:383, 1976.
193. Agger N, Lomborg K, Zangenberg N: Post mortem investigation of possible mucosal damages in dairy cows following four oral administrations at 12 hour intervals of a calcium chloride paste formulation, *Proceedings of the Thirtieth Annual Conference of the American Association of Bovine Practitioners*, 1997, p 76.
194. Goff JP, Horst RL: Calcium salts for treating hypocalcemia: carrier effects, acid-base balance, and oral versus rectal administration, *J Dairy Sci* 77:1451-1456, 1994.
195. Wentink GH, van den Ingh TSGAM: Oral administration of calcium chloride-containing products: testing for deleterious side effects, *Vet Q* 14:76-79, 1992.
196. Barlet JP, Davicco MJ: 1α-Hydroxycholecalciferol for the treatment of the downer cow syndrome, *J Dairy Sci* 75:1253-1256, 1992.
197. Oetzel GR: Meta-analysis of nutritional risk factors for milk fever in dairy cattle, *J Dairy Sci* 74:3900-3912, 1991.
198. Wang C et al: Recent advances in prevention of parturient paresis in dairy cows, *Compend Cont Educ Pract Vet* 16:1373-1380, 1994.
199. Dishington IW: Prevention of milk fever, *Acta Vet Scand* 16:503-512, 1975.
200. Block E: Manipulating dietary anions and cations for prepartum dairy cows to reduce incidence of milk fever, *J Dairy Sci* 67:2939-2948, 1984.
201. Dishington IW, Bjornstad J: Prevention of milk fever by dietary means, *Acta Vet Scand* 23:336-343, 1982.
202. Beede DK et al: Nutritional management of the late pregnant drycow with particular reference to dietary cation-anion difference and calcium supplementation. *Proceedings of the Twenty-Fourth Annual Convention of the American Association of Bovine Practitioners*, 1991, pp 51-55.
203. Goff JP, Horst RL: Use of hydrochloric acid as a source of anions for prevention of milk fever, *J Dairy Sci* 81:2874, 1998.
204. Fredeen AH, DePeters EJ, Baldwin RL: Effects of acid-base disturbances caused by differences in dietary fixed ion balance on kinetics of calcium metabolism in ruminants with high calcium demand, *J Anim Sci* 66:174, 1988.
205. Block E: Manipulating dietary anions and cations for prepartum dairy cows to reduce incidence of milk fever, *J Dairy Sci* 67:2939, 1984.

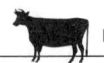
206. Reinhardt TA, Horst RL, Goff JP: Calcium phosphorous and magnesium homeostasis in ruminants. In Herdt TA, ed: *Veterinary clinics of North America (food animal practice)*, vol 4, Philadelphia, 1988, WB Saunders, p 331.
207. Byers DI: Management considerations for successful use of anionic salts in dry-cow diets, *Compend Cont Educ Pract Vet* 16:237-241, 1994.
208. Gardner RW: Response of Holstein cows to varying calcium to phosphorous ratios prepartum, and protein sources and percent postpartum, *J Dairy Sci* 54:794, 1971.
209. Curtis CR et al: Epidemiology of parturient paresis: predisposing factors with emphasis on dry cow feeding and management, *J Dairy Sci* 67:817, 1984.
210. Kichura TS et al: Relationships between prepartal dietary calcium and phosphorous, vitamin D metabolism, and parturient paresis in dairy cows, *J Nutr* 112:480, 1982.
211. Hutjens MF: Nutritional strategies with a phase feeding concept, *Proceedings of the University of Minnesota Fall Conference for Veterinarians*, Oct 31, 1985, p 1.
212. Littledike ET, Horst RL: Problems with vitamin D injections for prevention of milk fever, toxicity of large doses and increased incidence with small doses, *J Dairy Sci* 63(suppl. 1):89, 1979.
213. Goff JP, Littledike ET, Horst RL: Effect of synthetic bovine parathyroid hormone in dairy cows: prevention of hypocalcemic parturient paresis, *J Dairy Sci* 69:2278-2289, 1986.
214. Goff JP, Kehrli ME, Horst RL: Preparturient hypocalcemia in cows: prevention using intramuscular parathyroid hormone, *J Dairy Sci* 72:1182-1187, 1989.
215. Brewer BD: Disorders of calcium metabolism. In Robinson NE, ed: *Current therapy in equine medicine*, ed 2, Philadelphia, 1987, WB Saunders, p 189.
216. Coffman JR: *Equine clinical chemistry and pathophysiology*, Bonner Springs, Kan, 1981, Veterinary Medicine Publishing, p 157.
217. Palmer N: Bones and joints. In Jubb KF, Kennedy PC, Palmer N, eds: *Pathology of domestic animals*, ed 4, Orlando, Fla, 1993, Academic Press, p 55.
218. Meuten DJ: Hypercalcemia. In Peterson ME, ed: *Veterinary clinics of North America (small animal practice)*, vol 14, Philadelphia, 1984, WB Saunders, p 891.

DISORDERS OF PHOSPHORUS METABOLISM

SHERRILL A. FLEMING

Chronic Phosphorus Deficiency/Hypophosphatemia

ETIOLOGY. Most phosphorus (PO_4) deficiency in animals is primary (absolute dietary deficiency). Secondary PO_4 deficiency is mediated by other factors. Diets high in calcium or low in vitamin D prevent efficient absorption and decrease availability of PO_4. Secondary hypophosphatemia is more likely to occur when the dietary PO_4 level is marginal.[219]

PO_4 is present as inorganic (extracellular) and organic (intracellular) forms. Organic PO_4 is present in structural (phospholipids, phosphoproteins), metabolic (electron transport, ATP, enzymes, cofactors) and chemical (nucleic acids, cyclic adenosine monophosphate) components of cells.[220] The severe reduction of PO_4 has catastrophic potential, which is most obvious in the metabolic processes providing energy for cell function. Depletion of 2,3-diphosphoglycerate (2,3-DPG), which is essential for red blood cell (RBC) integrity, is secondary to ATP reduction and is seen in acute PO_4 deficiencies. Chronic marginal and deficient PO_4 diets allow the insidious involvement of less critical functions such as skeletal growth and maintenance and reproductive function.

CLINICAL SIGNS. The earliest signs of chronic PO_4 deficiency include decreased feed consumption, weight loss, retarded growth, poor milk production, and reduced fertility. Reproductive performance may be compromised by anestrus, irregular estrus, reduced conception rate, and delayed puberty. These signs are nonspecific and may go unrecognized.[219]

As the deficiency progresses, adult animals develop symptoms of osteomalacia. These animals are emaciated and have a dull, brittle coat and a long-legged, slab-sided appearance. Stiffness and shifting lameness usually develop. Spontaneous fractures that do not heal may occur. These animals frequently remain recumbent, although they are alert and continue to eat. Rickets develops in young growing animals. This syndrome is characterized by enlarged, painful swelling of the physis and metaphysis of long bones and the costochondral junctions. The animal is stiff, the forelegs are bowed or knock-kneed, and the back is arched. Animals deficient in PO_4, as well as other minerals, frequently develop pica (consumption of soil and chewing of rocks, wood, and bone). This behavior may lead to complications such as traumatic reticuloperitonitis or botulism from chewing bones.

Acute, severe hypophosphatemia has been reported to cause recumbency and muscular weakness in late pregnancy and early lactation.[221] Another disease syndrome associated with PO_4 deficiency in dairy cattle is postparturient hemoglobinuria (PPH). PPH usually has an acute onset occurring within 6 weeks of parturition and is characterized by intravascular hemolysis, hemoglobinuria, and anemia. Initial signs are weakness, staggering, and decreased milk production followed by hemoglobinuria. Urine may be dark reddish brown to black. In less acute cases, hemoglobinuria may be the first observed sign. Hemolytic anemia from hypophosphatemia has been demonstrated in cows that did not have hemoglobinuria.[222] Other clinical signs include increased respiratory rate, tachycardia, pronounced jugular pulse, and slight elevation of rectal temperature (39° to 40° C [102.2° to 104° F]). As the disease progresses, the animal becomes weaker, recumbent, and dehydrated; and mucous membranes are pale. Icterus develops if the animal lives more than 2 to 3 days.

CLINICAL PATHOLOGY. Serum PO_4 tests only measure the inorganic PO_4. Depressed serum PO_4 (1.5 to 3.5 mg/dl) is associated with PO_4 deficiency, but serum PO_4 may be maintained within the normal range for a long period after the onset of dietary PO_4 deficiency.[219] Normal serum PO_4 should not be used to rule out PO_4 deficiency. A ratio of ash to organic matter in bones of affected animals below the normal ratio of 3:1 is the most accurate assessment of chronic PO_4 deficiency. Serum calcium levels are usually unaffected. In severe cases, serum alkaline phosphatase is elevated.[223]

In cows with PPH, urinalysis reveals high levels of hemoglobin, with the absence of intact erythrocytes. Severity of the anemia is indicated by low RBC counts ($<5 \times 10^6/\mu l$), low packed cell volume (PCV) (9% to 20%), and low hemoglobin levels (<8 g/dl). Anisocytosis, macrocytosis, nucleated RBC polychromasia, and basophilic stippling are seen if bone marrow is regenerating. The number of RBCs affected with Heinz bodies (precipitates of oxidized hemoglobin) may be normal ($<1\%$), but is frequently elevated.[222-225] Hypophosphatemia (<1.5 mg/dl) is a common finding in cows affected with PPH. In New Zealand a form of PPH has been described that is associated with low dietary levels of copper and selenium in which hypophosphatemia is not found.[226] Ketosis is a common concurrent finding with PPH.[225]

PATHOPHYSIOLOGY. With chronic marginal PO_4 deficiency, the greatly increased PO_4 demands during early lactation and late pregnancy, especially twin pregnancies, may precipitate acute clinical signs of deficiency. Daily PO_4 requirement for a fetus is 5.4 g. Production of colostrum can take up to 9 g of PO_4.[227] This increased demand can cause acute, severe hypophosphatemia and recumbency. These cows often have associated hypocalcemia, hypomagnesemia, and hypoglycemia. After appropriate treatment, these cows remain recumbent if the PO_4 remains low. The cause of the recumbency is uncertain. It is possible that intracellular PO_4 compounds are depleted to the level that muscles are unable to function. However, the relatively small doses of PO_4 given intravenously are not sufficient to replace and repair the deficiency as rapidly as the clinical response is seen. Possibly there is an unidentified role of extracellular PO_4 in neuromuscular function.[228]

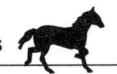

PO$_4$ plays such an important role in the normal function of all body tissues that a deficiency can be assumed to cause generalized impairment of body function. Decreased appetite caused by PO$_4$ deficiency frequently results in other nutritional deficiencies that compound the problem.

Animals deficient in PO$_4$ have marked demineralization of bone.[229-230] Hypophosphatemia is not known to have a stimulatory effect on bone resorption. Demineralization during PO$_4$ deficiency is most likely due to a normal rate of osteoclastic activity without concurrent osteoblastic activity.[230] Formation of organic bone matrix (osteoid) continues and replaces mineralized bone as it is resorbed. The result is soft bones (osteomalacia) prone to fracture. In addition to excess osteoid, growing animals have a failure of endochondral ossification.[230] As cartilage growth continues at the physeal plate, it becomes distorted and flares under weight bearing, resulting in a painful swollen physis and metaphysis. Deposition of excess osteoid in an attempt to strengthen bones also contributes to the bone deformities characteristic of rickets.

The exact mechanism of intravascular hemolysis in PPH is not known. A direct result of PO$_4$ deficiency is impairment of the glycolytic pathway in bovine RBCs, resulting in depletion of ATP.[222,224,232] ATP is the energy source for maintaining cation gradients across the RBC membrane to retain RBC shape and integrity.[233] Irreversible distortion and rigidity of human RBCs has been reported to occur when ATP levels fall below 15% of normal.[234] However, intravascular hemolysis does not occur in all animals with hypophosphatemia. Metabolic acidosis caused by ketosis may exacerbate hypophosphatemia by causing renal excretion of PO$_4$ as dihydroxyglucophosphate.[235] Hypophosphatemia has been attributed to preparturient ketosis caused by undernutrition, followed by adequate feeding during early lactation.[225]

High levels of oxidants or the failure of antioxidants have also been suspected as factors in intravascular hemolysis of PPH. The copper-containing enzyme superoxide dismutase, selenium-containing enzyme glutathione peroxidase, and vitamin E protect against oxidation damage to RBCs.[236] Deficiencies of copper and selenium have been associated with PPH in New Zealand. Numerous plants, particularly cruciferous plants, contain oxidants or precursors of oxidants and are known to cause intravascular hemolysis. Kale is rich in S-methylcysteine sulfoxide, which is converted by rumen flora to dimethyldisulfide. Once absorbed into the circulation, dimethyldisulfide causes precipitation of hemoglobin, leading to hemolysis. However, methemoglobinemia and depletion of reduced glutathione (GSH) occur in the absence of selenium deficiency and known oxidants. Methemoglobinemia and GSH depletion in RBCs may reflect increased susceptibility to oxidation caused by hypophosphatemia (reduction of the antioxidants nicotinamide adenine dinucleotide [NAD] and nicotinamide adenine dinucleotide phosphate [NADP]).[225]

EPIDEMIOLOGY. PO$_4$ deficiency in natural diets is widespread and is dependent on the PO$_4$ content of the soil.[223] PO$_4$-deficient soils are most common in dry tropical regions. Although many soils are naturally deficient in PO$_4$, heavy leaching by rain and constant crop removal contribute to deficiency. High levels of calcium, iron, and aluminum in soil form insoluble complexes with PO$_4$, making it unavailable for plant use. Diets high in aluminum, magnesium, and fat reduce PO$_4$ absorption.[221] Dry mature forages and drought-damaged forages may be low in PO$_4$, even on soil of acceptable PO$_4$ content.

PO$_4$ deficiency is most commonly a problem of nonsupplemented grazing livestock. The length of time on a PO$_4$ deficient diet required for clinical osteodystrophies to develop depends on the severity of the deficiency and ranges from months to several years. Young growing animals and pregnant or lactating females are most severely affected.

PPH is associated with high-producing multiparous dairy cows but has been reported in a wide range of ages (3 to 10 years), body condition scores, and production levels.[222] The incidence of the disease in the cattle population is very low, and usually only one or two cases will be seen at one time in an individual herd. The condition occurs within 6 weeks after calving with most cases between days 10 and 21. Subclinical hypophosphatemia may be found in unaffected herd mates.[219] PPH has also been associated with consumption of green oats, lush rye grass, green chopped alfalfa, Egyptian clover, beet pulp, turnips, kale, rape, and other cruciferous plants. Hemoglobinuria associated with consumption of cruciferae also occurs in other ruminants not on hypophosphatemic diets. The onset of cold weather or consumption of cold water may also precipitate the syndrome.

NECROPSY FINDINGS. The characteristic lesion of osteomalacia is soft, spongy bones that break easily and may even be cut with a knife.[230] The marrow cavity is enlarged, and the cortex is thin. Fractures with nonmineralized callus formation are common. In less severe cases an excess of osteoid is best seen on bone sections prepared without demineralization. A generalized wasting of soft tissues is also observed.

The lesions of rickets are most prominent in the long bones, where cartilage contributes significantly to longitudinal bone growth. These bones have a thickened clublike appearance with a short diaphysis. Deposits of excess osteoid are most prominent on the surface of the metaphysis. The growth plate may be grossly widened and irregular as a result of failure of endochondral ossification. Lesions are also prominent at the costochondral junctions, the cartilage of the cranial base, and the mandibular cartilage.[230]

Postmortem findings of PPH include thin blood and generalized icterus. The gallbladder is distended, and the liver is pale and swollen. The liver may have a "nutmeg" appearance caused by centrilobular necrosis attributed to anemic anoxia. In peracute cases the spleen is enlarged and congested. The lungs are edematous and may be emphysematous. Hemoglobinuric nephrosis may be mild to severe.

THERAPY AND PROGNOSIS. Treating chronic PO$_4$ deficiency consists of supplementing dietary PO$_4$ at the same level necessary for prevention. Once animals are placed on a diet containing adequate PO$_4$, weight gain and improved performance are seen quickly.[231] The histologic lesions of osteomalacia and rickets are rapidly reversible, but the gross deformities of rickets may be permanent.[230]

Many commercial intravenous products are available that contain Ca and PO$_4$. However, the PO$_4$ in these solutions is in the form of phosphite (PO^2) salts, which do not precipitate when mixed with Ca and magnesium. Phosphite salts are not biologically active and are not converted to an active form in the animal. A more biologically appropriate treatment is monosodium phosphate (30 g reagent grade in 300 ml of distilled water provides 7 g PO$_4$).[237] Sodium phosphate enemas produced for humans contain 5 to 6 g PO$_4$ and have been used in cattle after dilution in 1000 ml of distilled water.[227] Treatment with these solutions keeps PO$_4$ levels elevated for 3 to 4 hours but must not be used concurrently with intravenous Ca solutions because precipitation could occur. Intravenous treatment should be followed by oral supplementation. Feed grade monosodium phosphate (200 to 300 g) in a warm water drench or by stomach tube will provide 50 to 60 g PO$_4$. There are commercial gel and paste preparations that contain monosodium phosphate that can be used in place of drenches.

Prognosis for animals with PPH is poor. The disease runs an acute course, with early death from anemic anoxia. Toxic effects of hemoglobin contribute to deaths that occur 3 to 5 days after onset. If animals survive, 6 to 8 weeks may be required for recovery. Initial treatment consists of transfusion of 10 to 20 L of whole blood and slow intravenous injection of 30 g of monosodium phosphate in 300 ml of sterile distilled water[219] Seven percent glycerophosphate calcium has been used for treatment. Human commercial preparations are available as sodium phosphate and potassium phosphate and have been used in small animals.[238] These must be diluted and given intravenously. Blood transfusions may be repeated as necessary to prevent severe anemia but may initiate further episodes of hemolysis. Oral supplementation with 120 g of bone meal or 335 g of monosodium phosphate once daily for 5 days is recommended. Fluid therapy is advised to minimize effects of dehydration and renal tubular damage. PO_4 deficiency in the ration should be corrected, and plants associated with hemolysis should be removed from the diet.[219] There is a report of using 1-α-hydroxycholecalciferol to increase the serum PO_4 in recumbent cows that did not respond to calcium treatment.[239]

PREVENTION AND CONTROL. Prevention of diseases that are caused by PO_4 deficiency requires supplementation of the diet with enough PO_4 to meet the demands of maintenance and production. PO_4 requirements depend on the animal's age and level of production. Accepted minimum requirements for all animals have been published by the National Research Council.[240,241]

Application of superphosphate fertilizer to the soil increases the PO_4 content of crops grown.[242] This may be inadequate and too expensive under range conditions. The two most commonly used oral PO_4 supplements are dicalcium phosphate and defluorinated rock phosphate. Other supplements include bone meal, monosodium and disodium phosphate, ammonium phosphate, and phosphoric acid. These supplements may be mixed in other feeds or provided free choice in a salt mineral mix. Most PO_4 supplements contain calcium, and the calcium:PO_4 ratio of the diet must be monitored when supplements are used. A calcium:PO_4 ratio of 2:1 is considered optimum for mineral absorption and animal performance.[233] The calcium:PO_4 ratio should never be less than 1:1. Unlike monogastrics, ruminants tolerate ratios as high as 7:1.[233]

REFERENCES

219. Thompson JC, Badger SB: Outbreak of post-parturient haemoglobinuria in an autumn calving dairy herd, *NZ Vet J* 47:180-183, 1999.
220. Hays VM, Swenson MJ: Minerals. In Swenson MJ, ed: *Dukes' physiology of domestic animals*, ed 11, Ithaca, NY, 1993, Cornell University Press, p 517-519.
221. Gerloff BJ, Swenson EP: Acute recumbency and marginal phosphorus deficiency in dairy cattle, *J Am Vet Med Assoc* 208:716-719, 1996.
222. Ogawa E et al: Hemolytic anemia and red blood cell disorder attributable to low phosphorus intake in cows, *Am J Vet Res* 50:388-392, 1989.
223. Baxter JT: Deficiencies of mineral nutrients. In Howard JL, ed: *Current veterinary therapy 2: food animal practice*, Philadelphia, 1986, WB Saunders, p 278.
224. Ogawa E et al: Bovine postparturient hemoglobinemia: hypophosphatemia and metabolic disorder in red blood cells, *Am J Vet Res* 48:1300-1303, 1987.
225. Jubb TF et al: Haemoglobinuria and hypophosphataemia in postparturient dairy cows without dietary deficiency of phosphorus, *Aust Vet J* 67:86-89, 1990.
226. Ellison RS, Young BS, Read DH: Bovine post-parturient hemoglobinuria: two distinct entities in New Zealand, *NZ Vet J* 34:7, 1986.
227. Goff JP, Horst RL: Physiological changes at parturition and their relationship to metabolic disorders, *J Dairy Sci* 80:1260-1268, 1997.
228. Goff JP: Treatment of calcium, phosphorus and magnesium balance disorders, *Vet Clin North Am (Food Anim Pract)* 15:619-639, 1999.
229. Call JW et al: Dietary phosphorus for beef cows, *Am J Vet Res* 47:475, 1986.
230. Palmer N: Bones and joints. In Jubb KF, Kennedy PC, Palmer N, eds: *Pathology of domestic animals*, ed 4, Orlando, Fla, 1993, Academic Press, pp 65-71.
231. Shupe JL et al: Clinical signs and bone changes associated with phosphorous deficiency in beef cattle, *Am J Vet Res* 49:1629, 1988.
232. Wang XL et al: Bovine postparturient hemoglobinuria: effect of inorganic phosphate on red cell metabolism, *Res Vet Sci* 39:333, 1985.
233. Agar NS, Board PG: *Red blood cells of domestic mammals*, Amsterdam, 1983, Elsevier Science, p 227.
234. Weed RI, LaCelle PL, Merle EW: Metabolic dependence of red cell deformity, *J Clin Invest* 48:795, 1969.
235. Tasker JB: Fluids, electrolytes, and acid-base balance. In Kaneko JJ, ed: *Clinical biochemistry of domestic animals*, ed 3, New York, 1980, Academic Press, p 402.
236. McCaughan CJ: Post-parturient hemoglobinuria. In Howard JL, ed: *Current veterinary therapy 3: food animal practice*, Philadelphia, 1993, WB Saunders, pp 323-326.
237. Cheng YH, Goff JP, Horst RL: Restoring normal blood phosphorus concentrations in hypophosphatemic cattle with sodium phosphate, *Vet Med* 4:383-386, 1998.
238. Forrester SD, Moreland KJ: Hypophosphatemia: causes and clinical consequences, *J Vet Intern Med* 3:149-159, 1989.
239. Barlet JP, Davicco MJ: 1α-Hydroxycholecalciferol for the treatment of the downer cow syndrome, *J Dairy Sci* 75:1253-1256, 1992.
240. National Research Council: *Nutrient requirements of dairy cattle*, ed 6 (revised), Washington, DC, 1989, National Academy of Sciences, pp 139-147.
242. National Research Council: *Nutrient requirements of beef cattle*, ed 6, Washington, DC, 1984, National Academy of Sciences, pp 77-84.
243. McDowell LR: *Nutrition of grazing ruminants in warm climates*, Orlando, Fla, 1985, Academic Press, p 189.
244. Miller WJ: *Dairy cattle feeding and nutrition*, New York, 1979, Academic Press, p 109.

DISORDERS OF MAGNESIUM METABOLISM

J. TRAVIS BLACKWELDER
ELAINE HUNT

Hypomagnesemia

DEFINITION. Hypomagnesemia (i.e., grass tetany, lactation tetany, wheat pasture poisoning, crested wheatgrass poisoning, winter tetany, transport tetany, milk tetany, green oat poisoning, barley poisoning, grass staggers) is a magnesium ion deficiency of the blood and cerebrospinal fluid. It is highly fatal and affects only ruminant species. The highest incidence is in lactating beef cows within 60 days of calving that are pastured on cool season grasses. Lactating ewes and dairy goats are also susceptible. Hypomagnesemia can occur in both sexes, in all age groups, and in animals under varied management and dietary programs. Spring-calving cows are most classically affected, but mortalities in fall and winter are frequent in the southern United States. Hypomagnesemia is usually accompanied by hypocalcemia. Although preventable, the disease still kills an estimated 1% to 3% of cattle, goats, and sheep annually.

ETIOLOGY. Mg is present in most body tissues; approximately 70% of body Mg is in bone and teeth and is not readily available to maintain circulating Mg levels. The remaining 30% is distributed in soft tissue (including extracellular and intracellular body fluids) and is critical for normal body function; this pool is less able to respond to fluctuations in dietary supply in older cows. Mg uptake is under no direct hormonal control, and, because Mg body stores are not particularly labile, the requirements for extracellular Mg (about 20 g/day) must be supplied by the daily diet. One primary cause of acute hypomagnesemia is a sharp reduction in net absorption of Mg from the reticulorumen and omasum (the major regions of Mg absorption in ruminants).[244] During times of decreased absorption, cattle tend to drain Mg reserves via saliva. Approximately 40% of the total amount of Mg available in extracellular fluid is secreted in the saliva each day.[345] When cattle are grazing on low Mg grasses and Mg absorption is impaired, losing this much Mg via saliva substantially increases the risk of hypomagesemia. Endogenous fecal excretion of Mg is another way the mineral is depleted from the body in ruminants and may be increased further by the greater flow of saliva stimulated by diets high in roughage.[245] Lactating cows are also more susceptible to hypomagnesemia. Every 7 kg of milk produced by a cow requires as much Mg as is available in the entire plasma pool.[236] As much as 3 g/day may be lost in the milk. When

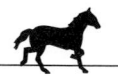

dietary Mg is low (less than 0.2 % Mg on a dry matter basis), the ion is depleted from the cerebrospinal (CSF) and extracellular fluids especially by lactation. Loss of normal neuromuscular function, tetanic muscle spasms, and clonic convulsions result.

Lactation, stress, transport and/or anorexia are usually associated with the development of clinical signs and are aggravating or precipitating factors in ruminants on low levels of dietary Mg. The varied clinical syndromes can be categorized under the terms grass tetany (which includes wheat, oat, and barley staggers), transport tetany, winter tetany, and tetany in milk-fed calves housed indoors.

Grass tetany (grass staggers) usually occurs in lactating cows during winter or spring when grasses low in Mg make up the diet, especially in cattle experiencing less than optimum energy intake. Adverse weather that inhibits normal food intake may precipitate clinical signs. Affected cows may be pastured on rapidly growing planted forage crops such as wheat, barley, or oats that have been fertilized with nitrogen and potassium.[247] Acute hypomagnesemia can be seen in animals that may not be lactating.

Winter tetany occurs in animals on Mg- and energy-deficient diets subjected to a severe stress such as extremely cold weather. Heifers are spared, whereas mature cows (that may or may not be lactating) are simply found dead. Transport tetany may also be precipitated by a hypomagnesemic diet and occurs in animals after transport. Horses, lambs, lactating goats, and mature lactating ewes rearing twins can be affected. Milk tetany occurs in calves that are raised indoors entirely on milk. Milk is relatively low in Mg, but because absorption of Mg is excellent in neonates, signs of hypomagnesemia do not occur until 2 to 4 months of age when absorption has decreased. In milk tetany, calves' bone Mg is depleted so that the ratio of bone calcium:Mg is 90:1 or greater (70:1 or less is normal). Clinical signs in all of these syndromes are similar.

CLINICAL SIGNS. Lactating cows affected with grass tetany become anorexic and separate from the herd. They are alert and hyperexcitable, and they may charge. Markedly erect ears, ear twitching, and hyperesthesia are early clinical signs. Muscle fasciculations, head and neck tremors, and a high-stepping forelimb gait are evident. Aberrant behavior with bellowing and frenzied galloping progresses to staggering and uncoordinated gait and lateral recumbency. Violent episodes of opisthotonos and clonic convulsions can be precipitated by any stimuli, and these alternate with periods of tetanic muscle spasms. Nystagmus, exaggerated mastication, salivation, and a snapping eyelid retraction occur. Excessive muscular activity contributes to elevated body temperature, and rapid and forceful respirations are present. Tachycardia occurs, and loud heart sounds are audible, sometimes at a distance from the cow. Death occurs from respiratory failure during one of the violent seizures, and often within 30 to 60 minutes of seizure onset; often the animal is simply found dead. The highest incidence is in lactating beef cows up to 7 years of age; the calf of an affected cow is generally normal.

Mild or chronic lactation tetany is a vague syndrome that may affect many animals in a group and is associated with declining energy metabolism.[248,249] Serum Mg levels in such groups of cattle are often low, although no clinical signs are apparent, probably because serum calcium levels are not depressed. Vague anorexia, unthriftiness, and declining milk yields may be noted. The animals have odd facial expressions, and slight changes in behavior may be reported. Mild lacational tetany may be a chronic problem in some dairy herds, and these cattle can be predisposed to parturient paresis. This may suddenly progress to the acute or subacute form of hypomagnesemia.

Whole milk tetany or hypomagnesemia in calves usually occurs at 2 to 4 months of age. In lambs hypomagnesemic tetany is usually subacute or acute and occurs in offspring that only have access to milk. The clinical signs are similar to those in adults, but, in addition, calves' eyes may bulge or be withdrawn, and the third eyelid may prolapse.[250] Pasture-raised calves are less likely to develop milk tetany than confined calves. Diarrhea may exacerbate existing subclinical hypomagnesemia; thus enteric disease may be erroneously blamed for death losses in these calves.

Diseases in cows that must be considered in the differential diagnosis of hypomagnesemia include rabies or other viral encephalitides; nervous ketosis; nervous coccidiosis; hypocalcemia; lead, arsenic, and other heavy metal toxicities; *Claviseps paspali* (paspalum staggers); ryegrass staggers; tetanus; strychnine; and other chemical intoxications. In sheep canary grass staggers should also be considered. Differentials in calves include polioencephalomalacia, enterotoxemia, tetanus, lead toxicity, salt poisoning, and bacterial and viral encephalitis. When death is sudden, lightning strike, acute clostridial diseases, bloat, trauma, and acute plant and chemical toxicities, in addition to hypomagnesemia, should all be considered.

CLINICAL PATHOLOGY. Because of the need for rapid therapy, diagnosis is often made on the basis of clinical signs or history. Low serum Mg levels (less than 1.2 mg/dl) confirm hypomagnesemia. It is possible for a cow with clinical signs to have normal serum Mg levels, particularly if violent convulsions have been occurring. Expression of clinical signs is most directly correlated with CSF Mg levels; CSF Mg levels should be low in all clinical cases (<1.45 mg/dl).[251] Although it is a reliable indicator of hypomagnesemia, this sample is difficult to obtain in a live, convulsing animal.

Urine Mg levels are also low (less than 2.5 mg/100 ml) in hypomagnesemia. This decrease can be expected to precede declining serum Mg levels (the urinary threshold for Mg is 1.4 to 1.9 mg/dl in cows). The absence of urinary Mg reflects decreased absorption and a sudden increased risk of hypomagnesemia, which indicates an urgent need for Mg supplementation. To confirm a subclinical or clinical herd problem, serum or urine Mg samples should be collected from multiple animals within a herd. One of the best means of diagnosing ongoing or impending hypomagnesemia is through urine fractional excretion. Normal values for urine fractional excretion of Mg have been established for preparturient and lactating dairy cows; these values assess adequacy of dietary Mg and are important in evaluating herd Mg status.[252-254] Urine and serum samples are collected simultaneously, and creatinine and Mg ion concentrations are evaluated in each fluid and then calculated as follows:

Fractional excretion of Mg = Urine Mg/Serum Mg ×
Serum creatinine/Serum creatinine × 100

Mean ranges in nonlactating, nonpregnant dairy cows over a 24-hour period were 6.5 to 8.3 ± standard deviation up to 3.7%. Levels have not been established for lactating beef cows, so extrapolation is necessary at the present time.[252] Dramatically lowered levels of fractional excretion of Mg suggest inadequate consumption of dietary Mg.

The Germans have taken advantage of low urine Mg levels and developed a paper-strip test for urine Mg.[255,256] English researchers describe use of a field kit that can be used to monitor adequacy of dietary Mg intake during critical risk periods and for field postmortem diagnosis.[257] A nomogram based on serum Mg and percent Mg in forage has also been developed to help predict the risk for incidence of hypomagnesemia.[258] Switch hair Mg concentration has also been correlated with serum Mg levels; although this represents an easy tissue to collect and transport, potential for fecal Mg contamination of samples and limitations in laboratory ability to perform the test compromise this as a potential diagnostic technique.[259]

Very few other clinical chemistries are altered in clinical hypomagnesemia. Serum potassium, creatine phosphokinase, and aspartate aminotransferase may be elevated in recumbent cows (see Downer Cows, Chapter 33). Hypophosphatemia and hypocalcemia are common, and concurrent hypocalcemia is necessary for the expression of the tetanic convulsion associated with clinical disease.[260]

PATHOPHYSIOLOGY. Magnesium is a major intracellular cation that is a necessary cofactor for enzymatic reactions vital to every major metabolic pathway.[261] Although Mg is an ion of major clinical importance, it ranks behind calcium, sodium, and potassium in absolute bodily amounts. Slight alterations in serum Mg levels represent proportionately large shifts in whole body quantity of the ion and have the potential for devastating results. Although it is necessary for normal bone formation, Mg also plays a fundamental role in cellular metabolism, particularly in the maintenance of normal resting membrane potential of nervous tissue. Activation and/or function of many metabolic enzymes of protein, carbohydrate, and lipid metabolism depends on the presence of Mg. Formation of high-energy phosphate bonds requires normal Mg concentrations; thus all enzymatic reactions involving ATP have an absolute requirement for Mg. Mg concentration must be maintained for the normal production and decomposition of acetylcholine. Low Mg:calcium ratios potentiate acetylcholine release, and alterations of this ratio in the extracellular fluid may contribute to muscle tetany in the hypomagnesemic state. If uncontrolled, the tetanic spasms culminate in cardiorespiratory failure.

The free Mg concentration normally found in rumen contents can range from 2.5 to 6.0 mmol/L and a majority of the uptake occurs through active absorption.[245] Small quantities of Mg can be absorbed from the intestine in the adult ruminant, although most absorption takes place in the forestomachs. In calves absorption is in the jejunum primarily. No direct hormonal regulatory mechanism has been identified, but absorption may be enhanced by vitamin D, and renal excretion may be regulated by parathyroid hormone (PTH).[262,263] Mg ion is excreted by the kidney; the renal threshold is about 1.4 to 1.9 mg/dl. Renal tubular failure in the ruminant can result in serum Mg elevation and is a rough estimate of prognosis in severe renal disease.[264] Aldosterone and thyroid hormone may alter Mg metabolism, and PTH has been shown to have a modulating function. Exogenous PTH infusions result in increased plasma Mg levels as a result of decreased Mg excretion in the urine; removal of PTH results in increased loss of Mg in urine and declining plasma levels. Reductions in plasma Mg levels result after administration of $1,25-(OH)_2D$; the mechanism for this response is unclear, but it may be either a direct effect of the drug on renal tubular function or caused by a shift of Mg from the extracellular fluid into the intracellular space.[265]

Many components of the diet affect Mg absorption, including minerals, other ions, or a high-protein or high-carbohydrate diet. The dietary factors that can affect net absorption of Mg may do so either by reduction in the concentration of Mg ions in the rumen liquor or by directly affecting the Mg transport process.[245] Adequate dietary concentrations of Mg do not necessarily equate with bioavailability of the ion. Apparent digestibility is high in calves but decreases precipitously after 5 months of age.

EPIDEMIOLOGY. Hypomagnesemia is a global problem, occurring sporadically and affecting up to 10% of the herd. It can be a problem anywhere that cool season grasses are a major cattle feed source. Forages with less than 0.2% Mg content have been implicated in bovine hypomagnesemia.[266] Midlactation daily dietary requirements for Mg are about 22 g/day.[267]

Low Mg concentrations are often found in cool season grasses or forages grown at lower temperatures, lower pH, and in high moisture soil. Affected cattle are usually grazing lush, rapidly growing grass (fescue, orchard grass, or small grain) pastures in late fall and early spring. Legumes have relatively high Mg and calcium content and are generally not associated with hypomagnesemia. Housed cattle on deficient hay have also been reported to develop hypomagnesemia.

Mg content of forages may be inversely related to high moisture content of grasses (this reduces dry matter and Mg concentration within the plant). If adequate Mg is present in the soil, plants should develop higher Mg concentrations as they mature. Cereals with low Mg content such as winter wheat are especially prone to contain low levels of Mg. Of the small grains, wheat is associated with the highest risk of tetany, oats and barley are intermediate, and rye is associated with the lowest risk of grass tetany.[268] Competing cations in the soil also can affect ability of the plant to absorb Mg from soils.

Potassium content within the plant will affect Mg uptake and is an important mechanism in inducing clinical disease. A ratio can be derived that compares forage potassium content to the sum of the Mg and calcium content (percent potassium divided by percent Mg plus percent calcium). When the ratio is K/Ca + Mg > 2.2 the forage is likely to induce hypomagnesemia.[269] Potassium content of grass is influenced greatly by changes in environment; any impact on the potassium content by the environment is likely to increase potassium levels in the grass, predisposing to grass tetany when the forage is grazed.[270] Heavy fertilization with nitrogen or potassium-rich compounds (such as poultry litter) may interfere with Mg uptake by pasture plants, and high K^+/protein in feed will decrease Mg absorption by the gut. Prolonged elevation of serum potassium with resultant increase in serum insulin may also contribute to hypomagnesemia. This insulin response is greater in Mg-deficient calves and may exacerbate abnormalities of intermediary carbohydrate metabolism or lipolysis.[271]

In addition to factors affecting Mg uptake or concentrations in pasture plants, certain dietary factors may interfere with Mg absorption from the alimentary tract. These include very high dietary potassium, calcium, phosphate, sodium sulfate, manganese, sodium, organic acid content (transaconitic and citric acids), and increased levels of fatty acid.[272,273] When the absorption of phosphate ions from the reticulorumen is severely reduced (P-deficient diet) the absorption of both calcium and magnesium ions from the reticulorumen become impaired and predisposes the cow to hypomagnesemia.[274] Dietary sodium deficiency also exacerbates the effects of hypomagnesemia via aldosterone induced increase in potassium concentrations in the saliva and ruminal contents.[244] The increase in potassium causes an increase in the potential difference across the rumen epithelium and decreases absorption of Mg ions.[244] In some instances, only 2% of dietary Mg is absorbed by the animal because of interference from other substances. Cows with clinical grass tetany have significantly higher aluminum levels in the ruminal dry matter and lower plasma calcium than control cows or nonclinical hypomagnesemic cows. However, attempts to show consistent correlation between aluminum ingestion and clinical hypomagnesemia in mature cattle have failed.[260] Some speculation has occurred as to whether the sulfate ion, and not aluminum, was responsible for the onset of clinical signs. One study concluded that calcium levels must decline if clinical hypomagnesemia is to be seen, irrespective of dietary aluminum concentrations.[260] In growing calves, supplemental aluminum does appear to adversely affect Mg absorption and metabolism.[275]

Other predisposing factors for hypomagnesemia include age, lactation, breed, hypoglycemia, and ketosis.[276] The inci-

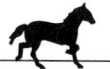

dence of hypomagnesemia is greatest in high-producing cows in the third to fifth lactation.[277] This predisposition to low concentrations of extracellular fluid Mg with aging is related to the older animals' reduced ability to resorb adequate amounts of Mg from the bone. Lactating beef cows are most frequently affected in the United States. Hypomagnesemia has been reported in stocker calves, bulls, nonlactating cows, suckling calves, dairy cows, lactating ewes, and lambs in areas of the world where concentrate supplementation is uncommon. Brahman and Brahman crossbred cows are less susceptible to hypomagnesemia, partly because of increased Mg digestibility compared with other beef breeds.[278] Of beef breeds, Angus cows are at the greatest risk. Among dairy breeds, shorthorns have a greater incidence than Jersey or Holstein breeds.[277] Body fat is also related to susceptibility; thin or overconditioned cattle are more susceptible than cows in moderate body condition.[277]

Stress, fasting, or underfeeding can cause decreases in serum calcium and Mg levels. Acute exposure to cold weather in cows without supplemental feeding can result in acute hypomagnesemia. In these instances, sudden death loss in mature pregnant or lactating cows occurs after a sudden cold spell, whereas younger cows are spared. Cold weather or lack of food intake results in increased lipolysis, which causes adipose cell membranes to accumulate Mg, depressing circulating Mg levels. It has been suggested that it may be possible to prevent hypomagnesemia secondary to cold stress by treating animals with antilipolytic agents.[279]

NECROPSY. Cows may be found in lateral recumbency, with evidence in the surrounding ground of convulsive seizure activity. Agonal pulmonary emphysema, diffuse ecchymotic hemorrhages, and rumen content aspiration are likely. Trauma and bruising of the head and extremities can occur from violent antemortem seizures, but few gross lesions can be expected. Calves dying from hypomagnesemia were reported to have microscopic deposition of calcium salts in the elastic fibers of the arteries of the lungs, heart, and spleen.[250]

Samples submitted for Mg assay from cows suspected of succumbing to hypomagnesemia include serum (obtained from cardiac puncture), cerebrospinal fluid, urine, and an enucleated intact eye for vitreous humor Mg analysis. Low Mg levels in any of these fluids are diagnostic, and samples may be collected up to 12 hours after death. Vitreous humor is more stable than other body fluids in the cadaver; thus some laboratories prefer vitreous humor specimens, particularly in situations in which necropsy is delayed more than 12 hours after death.[251] Vitreous samples parallel serum Mg concentrations and remain stable for at least 48 hours after death when the environmental temperature does not exceed 23° C (73.4° F).[280] Normal vitreous humor Mg concentrations are 1.8 to 2.3 mg/dl. Vitreous Mg levels less than 1.4 mg/dl support acute, terminal hypomagnesemic tetany.

Urine is also a good fluid to collect from the cadaver and assay for Mg content. Normal (1 to 20 mg/dl) or elevated urine Mg eliminates hypomagnesemia from the diagnosis. Less than 1 mg/dl supports the diagnosis of acute hypomagnesemia.[251]

THERAPY AND PROGNOSIS. Treatment is often not successful if the cow is already comatose. Chloral hydrate (50 mg/kg IV) may successfully prevent convulsions while equilibration of exogenously administered Mg occurs. Intravenous administration of a commercial calcium borogluconate solution with 5% Mg hypophosphate is the treatment of choice; selection of commercial calcium solutions containing potassium ion should be avoided. The heart should be carefully monitored during this administration. Because Mg salts are toxic and can result in respiratory failure when given intravenously, slow administration is advised. A dose of 2 to 3 g of Mg IV over a 10-minute period should be a safe and effective means of treating hypomagnesemia.[261] Administration of 200 to 400 ml of a 25% Mg sulfate solution to supply 5 to 10 g Mg SC has also been advocated. Clinical response to therapy can be disappointing and success is often associated with the time interval between the onset of clinical signs and treatment. Clinical improvement should occur in 1 to 5 hours; it takes from 30 minutes to 1 hour for the CSF Mg concentration to return to normal.[261] The cow should be left undisturbed during this period to avoid causing convulsions. Intramuscular tranquilization or sedatives may be necessary if severe convulsions are evident to aid in treatment of the cow and to prevent injury and further excitement to the animal. Avoid intravenous tranquilizers because they have been associated with sudden hypotension and death in cattle suffering from hypomagnesemia.[261] An Mg-rich enema is an alternative therapy: 60 g of $MgCl_2 \cdot 6H_2O$ in 250 to 500 ml of warm water results in rapid absorption of Mg. These enemas can cause some mucosal sloughing, especially when highly concentrated solutions are used.

Because exogenously administered Mg equilibrates slowly across the blood-brain barrier, as many as 20% of treated cows may die during a convulsion despite prior therapy. Relapses are common within 3 to 6 hours of treatment; thus animals must be monitored after therapy. Subcutaneous administration of 50% Mg sulfate solution (125 to 150 ml) may prevent relapse,[251] but a hypertonic solution such as this may result in a tissue slough. Oral Mg oxide (60 g in a gelatin capsule) can be administered for 5 to 6 days as an alternative form of therapy. Oral Mg salts can provide longer maintenance of plasma Mg concentrations and should only be administered once good esophageal reflexes are regained. They are most effective as a means of preventing relapse after intravenous Mg treatment. Supplementation with leguminous hay may also prevent relapse.

Hypomagnesemic calves have responded to intravenous therapy with 125 ml of a 6% Mg borogluconate preparation.[250] Sheep can benefit from slow intravenous infusion of 50 to 150 ml of commercial 5% Mg preparations that also contain calcium.

PREVENTION AND CONTROL. Genetic selection and manipulation of cool season grasses may provide protection against hypomagnesemia in the future. By selecting for a high Mg cultivar of Italian ryegrass and crested wheatgrass seedlings capable of concentrating Mg and calcium, it appears it will someday be possible to reduce the incidence of hypomagnesemia in cattle grazing these forages.[281,282] Until such grasses are widely available, dietary and soil Mg supplementation will be necessary.

Supplementation with Mg for an extended period before grazing tetany-associated pastures has little benefit; thus great efforts must be made to provide adequate Mg supplementation on a daily basis for animals grazing these pastures.[283] Many methods for Mg supplementation have been described and include the addition of Mg to drinking water, mineral supplements, or concentrates; spraying Mg salts directly on pasture or feed; or dosing the animal with Mg bullets or large, slow-release Mg alloy boluses.[284] Release of Mg from the boluses and bullets has been inconsistent; therefore daily ingestion of Mg salts is often the preferred prophylactic method. During periods of moderate risk for grass tetany, daily consumption of 1 ounce (28 g) of Mg oxide should be protective. If risk of tetany is very high, this may need to be increased to 2 oz/head/day for cattle. A list of ways to achieve this follows.

1. Grain mix with 2 lb of 3% Mg oxide per head per day should be fed.
2. If a protein supplement is used as a carrier for Mg oxide, 1 lb of protein supplement with 6% Mg oxide per head per day should be fed.

3. If silage is a feedstuff, it should be sprinkled with 1 to 2 oz of Mg oxide per head per day.

4. Free-choice Mg mineral blocks may be offered. Intake is not as predictable, because individual consumption cannot be ensured. Many blocks should be available to encourage daily consumption of 1 to 2 oz of Mg oxide per head per day.

5. Free-choice mineral mixes should contain no more than 30% Mg oxide. Because Mg oxide is relatively unpalatable, salt:Mg oxide:dicalcium phosphate:ground barley can be offered in a 1:1:1:1 ratio and fed free choice. Salt:Mg oxide:dried molasses:cottonseed meal may also be fed free choice and should be palatable to the bovine in a 1:1:1:1 ratio.

6. Top dressing pastures with Mg-rich fertilizers may result in Mg-rich forage for 1 to 3 years. This may only be useful when soil pH is less than 6.3. Dolomitic lime is commonly used and successfully provides Mg in acid (especially sandy) soils.[285] For more alkaline soils, Mg oxide and Mg sulfate are used.

7. Pastures may be sprayed or dusted with 2% Mg sulfate every 2 weeks during danger periods. Fertilizer spreaders can be used to top dress the pasture; alternating strips (rather than confluent application) is also satisfactory, as long as this is repeated at 2-week intervals.[251]

8. Potassium applications to pastures should be reduced during early spring.

9. In temperate areas, shifting to late summer or fall calving rather than early spring ensures that lactation drain will occur at the time of peak dietary Mg intake.

10. Pasture grazing should be supplemented by feeding extra hay during periods of lush growth. Elaborate systems exist for injection of Mg solutions into bales of hay. Perhaps the easiest technique is to mix Mg with molasses and water and then to spray this mixture onto the hay while it sits in windrows before baling. Molasses enhances the palatability of the hay and helps to ensure that the Mg adheres to the hay.[286]

11. Adequate energy intake is important to prevent clinical signs.[286] Weather stress and irregular feeding during inclement weather can be partially overcome by providing adequate shelter during weather extremes.

12. For ewes, 7 g of Mg oxide per head per day should be provided.

13. Pastures should be overseeded with leguminous forage; leguminous hays should be provided during periods in which supplemental feeding is required.

14. Pasture samples should periodically be analyzed to achieve the appropriate balance of potassium, Mg, and nitrogen in the soil. Dietary potassium/calcium + Mg ratio should be kept adjusted to 2.2. Periodic pasture fertilization with $Ca(NO_3)_2$ is an alternative to nitrogen use, because NH_4^+ interferes with Mg uptake by plants. Fertilizers that are high in potassium content should be applied only to achieve the appropriate balance, never in excess.[287]

15. Milk tetany in calves can be prevented by providing access to appropriate quantities of calf starter and leguminous hay for calves raised on long-term (8 weeks or longer) milk diets.

Hypermagnesemia

Hypermagnesemia in the ruminant is prevented by renal excretion of Mg. Elevations in serum Mg have been associated with severe renal insufficiency. In one study, serum levels greater than 3.5 mEq/L were associated with a poor prognosis for survival.[264] Administration of Mg-containing rumenatorics or laxatives may also contribute to elevated serum Mg levels in the normal bovine and especially for those in renal failure.[288] Clinical signs associated with hypermagnesemia in humans include hypotension, electrocardiographic changes of prolongation of PR interval and QRS-duration (with peaked T waves), areflexia, respiratory paralysis, and cardiac arrest.[289] Intravenous calcium gluconate administration in humans may reverse the effects of hypermagnesemia, because calcium is a direct antagonist of Mg; but commercial calcium gluconate products for ruminants all contain Mg. Peritoneal dialysis has also been described as a means of lowering serum Mg levels in humans.[289]

REFERENCES

244. Dua K, Care AD: Secretion of magnesium and calcium in the total saliva of sheep and its relevance to hypomagnesemia, *Veterinary J* 156:217-221, 1998.
245. Dua K, Care AD: Impaired absorption of magnesium in the aetiology of grass tetany, *Br Vet J* 151:413, 1995.
246. Reinhardt TA, Horst RL, Goff JP: Calcium, phosphorus, and magnesium homeostasis in ruminants. In Herdt TA, ed: *Veterinary clinics of North America (metabolic diseases of ruminant livestock)*, vol 4, Philadelphia, 1988, WB Saunders, pp 331-350.
247. Moodie EW: Modern trends in animal health and husbandry: hypocalcaemia and hypomagnesaemia, *Br Vet J* 121:338-349, 1965.
248. Fontenot JP et al: Factors influencing magnesium absorption and metabolism in ruminants, *J Anim Sci* 67:3445-3455, 1989.
249. Matsunobu S et al: Insulin secretion and glucose uptake in hypomagnesemic sheep fed a low magnesium, high potassium diet, *J Nutr Biochem* 1:167-171, 1990.
250. Haggard DL, Whitehair CK, Langham RF: Tetany associated with magnesium deficiency in suckling beef calves, *J Am Vet Med Assoc* 172:495-497, 1978.
251. Smith RA, Edwards WC: Hypomagnesemic tetany of ruminants. In Herdt TA, ed: *Veterinary clinics of North America (metabolic diseases of ruminant livestock)*, vol 4, Philadelphia, 1988, WB Saunders, pp 365-377.
252. Fleming SA et al: Renal clearance and fractional excretion of electrolytes over four 6-hour periods in cattle, *Am J Vet Res* 52:5-8, 1991.
253. Fleming SA et al: Fractional excretion of electrolytes in lactating dairy cows, *Am J Vet Res* 53:222-224, 1992.
254. Alexander AM: Magnesium status of dairy cows, *N Z Vet J* 33:171-172, 1985.
255. Merrall M, West DM: Ruminant hypomagnesemic tetanies. In Howard JL, ed: *Current veterinary therapy: food animal practice*, ed 2, Philadelphia, 1986, WB Saunders, pp 328-332.
256. Rosenberger G, ed: *Clinical examination of cattle*, Philadelphia, 1979, WB Saunders, p 278.
257. Collins JD: A screening test for monitoring the magnesium status of dairy cows, *Vet Rec* 106:367-368, 1980.
258. Fontenot JP: Magnesium, *Anim Nutr Health* 35:38-40, 1980.
259. Fisher DD et al: Switch hair as an indicator of magnesium and copper status of beef cows, *Am J Vet Res* 46:2235-2240, 1985.
260. Kappel LC et al: Effects of dietary aluminum on magnesium status of cows, *Am J Vet Res* 44:770-773, 1983.
261. Goff JP: Treatment of calcium, phosphorus and magnesium balance disorders, *Vet Clin North Am (Food Anim Pract)* 15:619-639, 1999.
262. Schneider KM et al: 1,25-Dihydroxyvitamin D_3 increases plasma magnesium and calcium in sheep fed liquid diets low in calcium and magnesium, *Aust Vet J* 62:82-85, 1985.
263. Goff JP, Littledike ET, Horst RL: Effect of synthetic bovine parathyroid hormone in dairy cows: prevention of hypocalcemic parturient paresis, *J Dairy Sci* 69:2278-2289, 1986.
264. Divers TJ et al: Acute magnesium disorders in cattle: a retrospective study of 22 cases, *J Am Vet Med Assoc* 181:694-699, 1982.
265. Goff JP, Horst RL, Littledike ET: Bone resorption, renal function and mineral status in cows treated with 1,25-dihydroxycholecalciferol and its 24-fluoro analogues, *J Nutr* 116:1500-1510, 1986.
266. Mansfield ME, McKibben GE: Grass tetany, *Proceedings of Beef Cattle Day*, Dixon Spring Agricultural Center, Champaign, 1974, University of Illinois, pp 11-14.
267. O'Kelley RE, Fontenot JP: Effects of feeding different Mg levels to drylot-fed lactating cows, *J Anim Sci* 29:959-966, 1969.
268. Mayland HF, Grunes DL, Lazar VA: Grass tetany hazard of cereal forages based upon chemical composition, *Agron J* 68:665-667, 1976.
268. Kemp A, t'Hart ML: Grass tetany in grazing milking cows, *Neth J Agr Sci* 5:4-17, 1957.
270. Sleper DA et al: Using plant breeding and genetics to overcome the incidence of grass tetany, *J Anim Sci* 12:3456-3462, 1989.
271. Lentz DE et al: Effect of postassium and hypomagnesemia on insulin in the bovine, *J Anim Sci* 43:1082-1087, 1976.

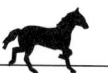

272. Martens H, Rayssiguier Y: Mg metabolism and hypomagnesemia. In Ruckebusch Y, Thivend P, eds: *Digestive physiology and metabolism in ruminants,* Westport, Conn, 1980, AVI Publishing, pp 447-468.
273. Mayland HF: Grass tetany. In Church DC, ed: *The ruminant animal: digestive physiology and nutrition,* Englewood Cliffs, NJ, 1988, Prentice-Hall, pp 511-523.
274. Crawford RJ et al: Use of an experimental high-magnesium tall fescue to reduce grass tetany in cattle, *J Prod Agr* 11:491-496, 1998.
275. Neathery MW et al: Effects of dietary aluminum and phosphorus on magnesium metabolism in dairy calves, *J Anim Sci* 68:1133-1138, 1990.
276. Wilcox GE, Hoff JE: Grass tetany: an hypothesis concerning its relationship with ammonium nutrition of spring grasses, *J Dairy Sci* 57:1085-1089, 1974.
277. Harris DJ, Lambell RG, Oliver CJ: Factors predisposing dairy and beef cows to grass tetany, *Aust Vet J* 60:230-234, 1983.
278. Greene LW et al: Apparent and true digestibility of Mg in mature cows of five breeds and their crosses, *J Anim Sci* 63:189-196, 1986.
279. Larvor P, Rayssiguier Y: Grass tetany: a new pathogenic hypothesis, *Bovine Pract* 11:90, 1976 (abstract).
280. Lincoln SD, Lane VM: Postmortem magnesium concentration in bovine vitreous humor: comparison with antemortem serum magnesium concentration, *Am J Vet Res* 46:160-162, 1985.
281. Moseley G, Baker DM, Hides DH: The efficacy of a high magnesium Italian ryegrass cultivar in alleviating hypomagnesaemia, *Proceedings of the XVI International Grassland Congress,* vol II, Nice, France, 1989, pp 395-396.
282. Mayland HF, Asay KH: Genetic variability of Mg, Ca, and K in crested wheatgrass, *J Range Manage* 42:109-113, 1989.
283. Ritter RJ, Boling JA, Gay N: Labile Mg reserves in beef cows subjected to different prepasture supplementation regimens, *J Anim Sci* 59:197-201, 1984.
284. Stuedemann JA, Wilkinson SR, Lowrey RS: Efficacy of a large magnesium alloy rumen bolus in the prevention of hypomagnesemic tetany in cows, *Am J Vet Res* 45:698-702, 1984.
285. Mayland HF et al: Grass tetany: a review of Mg in the soil-plant-animal continuum, *Proceedings of the Twenty-fifth Annual Pacific Northwest Nutrition Conference,* 1990, pp 29-41.
286. Blood DC, Radostits OM, Henderson JA: *Veterinary medicine,* ed 6, Philadelphia, 1983, Lea & Febiger, pp 939-994.
287. Wilkinson SR, Stuedemann JA: Tetany hazard of grass as affected by fertilization with nitrogen, potassium, or poultry litter and methods of grass tetany prevention. In Rendig VV, Grunes KL, eds: *Grass tetany,* special publication no 35, Madison, Wisc, 1979, American Society of Agronomy, pp 93-121.
288. Kasari TR, Woodbury AH, Morcom-Kasari E: Adverse effect of orally administered magnesium hydroxide on serum magnesium concentration and systemic acid-base balance in adult cattle, *J Am Vet Med Assoc* 196:735-742, 1990.
289. Reinhard RA: Magnesium metabolism: a review with special reference to the relationship between intracellular content and serum levels, *Arch Intern Med* 148:2415-2420, 1988.

BOVINE SOMATOTROPIN

JAMES P. REYNOLDS

Bovine somatotropin (growth hormone) has been licensed for use in the United States since 1994 and is also available for commercial use in dairy cattle in several other countries, including Mexico, Brazil, South Africa, and Korea. This has stimulated considerable interest in somatotropin (ST) and the insulin-like growth factors (IGFs), the somatomedins, which are associated with somatotropin. The release of somatotropin for commercial use provides new opportunities and challenges for the herd manager, veterinarian, and nutritionist.

Somatotropin is an anterior pituitary peptide hormone released under the influence of growth hormone releasing factor, a small 44 amino acid peptide. Somatotropin release can be inhibited by somatostatin, a 14 amino acid peptide hormone found in the hypothalamus, pancreas, intestinal tract, and central nervous system.[290] Secretion of somatotropin is pulsatile and may be influenced by adrenergic and cholinergic agonists, amino acid infusion, magnesium, and free fatty acid levels.[291-294] High-producing dairy cows have elevated circulating levels of somatotropin.[295,296]

Since 1936, when lactating cows were injected with crude extracts of bovine anterior pituitary,[297] a lactogenic role has been identified for anterior pituitary hormones. From the 1930s to the 1960s much of the research with somatotropin centered on the anabolic role of the agent. Since the early 1980s, large amounts of highly purified soma-

totropin have been produced, using recombinant deoxyribonucleic acid (DNA) methods. Recombinant bovine somatotropin (rbSt) has biologic activity similar to the pituitary-derived somatotropin.[298]

Production, Structure, Safety, and Function of Somatotropin

Endogenous bovine ST is a peptide hormone of either 190 or 191 amino acids. RbSt can have from zero to eight additional amino acids, depending on the production process.[299] Peptide hormones are subject to digestive processes and hence are not active orally. Bovine and human growth hormones are only about 65% homologous and not similar enough for rbSt to be active in humans if injected. The lack of oral activity of ST and the relatively low amounts of ST and IGF-I that are excreted in the milk of treated cows were important factors in allowing milk from rbSt-treated cows to be considered safe for human consumption.[299] RbSt is commercially produced through the insertion of the gene for bovine somatotropin into the DNA of *Escherichia coli.* The *E. coli* organisms are fermented, and a process of isolation and purification is used to obtain the recombinantly produced ST.

ST acts in young or beef cattle to promote growth,[300] but in the lactating cow it stimulates milk production. ST has both short- and long-term effects on metabolism that both coordinate and result from its stimulus to milk production. Bauman and Currie[301] termed as "homeorrhetic" adaptive changes made to coordinate body metabolism in support of lactation, or other dominant physiologic processes such as growth.

CHANGES IN METABOLISM. Table 39-5 outlines the homeostatic and homeorrhetic changes through which ST responses are obtained.[302] An important adaptive response to rbSt treatment is a change in the partitioning of nutrients. In general, rbSt acts to increase gluconeogenesis, decrease peripheral tissue utilization of glucose, increase mammary tissue utilization of glucose, and maintain milk-secreting cells in the mammary gland. Milk production increases after treatment with rbSt and the cow increases her dry matter intake to meet her increased energy needs. In early lactation, before the cow reaches maximum dry matter intake, there is an increased loss of glucose from the body and an increase in plasma free fatty acids associated with increased concentrations of milk lactose and milk fat.[303-306]

ST affects the usage of nutrients through both direct and indirect effects on bovine physiology. The hormone acts directly on liver and fat metabolism and indirectly on mammary tissue. ST binds to receptors on hepatocytes and adipocytes. The ST receptor is a single peptide with extracellular, transmembrane, and intracellular domains.[307] One ST molecule can bind to two receptors.[308] Receptors for ST have not been found in the mammary gland. However, mammary tissue has an abundance of receptors for IGF-I and IGF-II. Therefore the effects of rbSt on mammary and other tissues are considered to occur through the ST-dependant somatomedins, insulin-like growth factors I and II (IGF-I and IGF-II).[309]

The increase in milk production after treatment with rbSt appears to come from increased rate of milk synthesis by the mammary tissue and maintenance of mammary cells.[310] Cows treated with ST have less turnover of mammary cells, maintain more milk-secreting tissue longer into lactation, and thus have better milk production persistency. It has been demonstrated that ST increases blood flow to the mammary gland as a result of increased cardiac output, with an increased proportion of blood flow diverted to the mammary gland of the cow.[311-314] It is considered that the increased blood flow to the mammary gland is a response to the

TABLE 39-5

Effects of Somatotropin During Lactation

Tissue	Increased Physiology	Decreased Physiology
Mammary tissue	Synthesis of milk Uptake of nutrients Activity per secretory cell Maintenance of secretory cells Blood flow	
Adipose tissue	Lipolysis if in negative energy balance	Lipid synthesis if in positive energy balance
Liver	Gluconeogenesis Ability to synthesize glucose	Ability of insulin to inhibit gluconeogenesis
Muscle		Glucose uptake
Systemic effects	NEFA oxidation if in negative energy balance IGF-I Cardiac output consistent with increased milk production Voluntary intake to match nutrient needs Productive efficiency (milk/unit of intake)	Glucose oxidation Glucose response to insulin Animal waste

Modified from Bauman DE: *Dom Anim Endocrinol* 17:101-116, 1999.

increased metabolism of the gland rather than the cause of the increase in milk production.

Energy balance is critical in dairy cows and the cow gets most of her glucose from hepatic gluconeogenesis. ST acts on the liver to increase gluconeogenesis while reducing the use of glucose in muscle tissue, thus providing more glucose for milk production. ST also directly affects adipose tissue so that lipid precursors for energy are conserved. The effects rbSt has on adipocytes are dependent on the energy status of the cow. When the cow is in a positive energy state, rbSt acts to decrease lipogenesis, and increases lipolysis when the cow is in negative energy.[309] Bovine ST has effects on certain functions of insulin that aid in energy homeostasis during increased milk production. In the liver, the ability of insulin to inhibit gluconeogenesis is decreased.[315] In adipose tissue, the ability of insulin to stimulate glucose metabolism and lipid synthesis is deceased. However, the ability of insulin to increase glucose uptake by muscle is not reduced.

The magnitude of changes in blood metabolites depends on the stage of lactation, the dose of rbSt used, and the energy balance of the cow when treatment with rbSt is commenced. Cows that are treated with ST while they are in negative energy and protein balance respond with increased levels of plasma free fatty acids,[303,316] whereas, in those that are in positive energy balance, blood nutrient composition does not appear to be altered unless high doses of rbSt are used.[305-319] Reports of blood mineral levels indicate that no significant changes in these levels are noted between treatment groups[320]; Eppard and colleagues[321] found no statistically significant differences in levels of milk calcium, copper, phosphorus, iron, sodium, and manganese. Concentrations of blood metabolites generally return to normal ranges after increased feed intake.

INCREASED FEED INTAKE. Initial treatment for approximately 10 days with ST may cause a decrease in appetite.[322,323] However, long-term trials demonstrate an increase in voluntary feed intake for cows treated with somatotropin.[324,325] Studies at Beltsville demonstrated that there was no change in the efficiency of digestion.[306]

IMPACT OF SOMATOTROPIN ON MILK PRODUCTION. A large number of trials report both the short- and long-term effects of ST on milk yields. Difficulties arise in evaluating the results because of differing doses and products used and the differing environments under which studies were conducted. Early short-term trials on cows under research conditions[323,326]

reported increases in milk production of 12%, 9,5%, and 32% at doses of rbSt of 51.5, 51.5, and 100 IU per cow, respectively. Eppard, Bauman, and McCutcheon[326] demonstrated that an increased dose led to increased yield, with a leveling off of response at higher dosages. Responses to ST can be characterized generally as curvilinear with an increased response to increasing dose, but decreasing response to no response at high dose rates.

Responses to long-term treatment of cows with somatotropin have been detailed.[324,323,327-329] Responses depended on trial site, rbSt formulation, and dosage; they range from an 11.8% to 41.2% increase in milk yield. There have been a considerable number of trials conducted in many countries under differing feed conditions.[330-341] Pasture-based dairy herds treated with rbSt give similar milk responses to stall-fed or lot-fed cows.[324,330-332] An analysis of the 29 trials on rbSt (Posilac) use detailed by the Monsanto company[333] indicates that the mean percentage increase ($\pm$ standard deviation) in milk production was 16.8 $\pm$ 4.5% and that response was significantly ($p = 0.08$) lower with increasing level of milk production before treatment. However, it should not be assumed that the results of these 12-week farm trials can be too readily extrapolated. There has been a considerable range of milk responses to rbSt, which indicates that environmental factors, especially nutritional management, are substantial modifiers of responses to ST. This is supported by the lower responses to rbSt observed in herds in hot climate conditions and by nutritional modulation of the IGF factor system.[342] McGuire and colleagues[342] found that, by restricting feed intake to lactating cows, plasma concentrations of IGF-I were markedly decreased, indicating that many of the stimulatory effects of rbSt on lactation would not be observed in underfed cows. Underfeeding of cows resulted in a marked decrease in milk production despite rbSt treatment.

The rbSt-treated cow is not different from the high-producing cow in its degree of sensitivity to heat stress, except that the rbSt-treated animal has an exogenous stimulus to increase milk production. Trials conducted under warm, humid conditions suggest that milk production responses to ST in these environments may be more variable than those obtained under more temperate conditions[343,344] and that responses to higher doses may be depressed. Pituitary-extracted ST decreased feed intake to 82% of normal and increased water consumption 42% at 38° C (100.4° F) compared with controls, and decreased dry matter intakes have

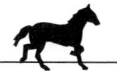

been observed with rbSt treatment in cows exposed to heat.[345] Over a short time, ST-treated cows have been shown to adapt to heat stress by increasing water intake, respired vapor, and skin vapor.[346] Tarazon-Herrera and colleagues[347]showed that the administration of rbSt improved milk production, milk components, and feed efficiency of conversion of dry matter to milk under hot summer conditions in Arizona whether the cows were cooled or not, compared with untreated control cows.

There are an increasing number of trials reporting milk production responses to multilactation trials with rbSt.[334,336-338,340] In most, but not all, studies there has been evidence of a continued stimulus to production. Lean and colleagues[316] reported that milk production of cows treated for a second lactation did not significantly increase above untreated controls over the first 30 days of treatment, an observation supported by a failure of cows, primiparous in a first lactation of treatment, to respond in the second lactation[338] and a lower response of cows treated in a second lactation.[316,336-338,348] However, a more recent trial conducted over four lactations showed that milk yields and body weights were enhanced in cows treated with rbSt and that previous rbSt treatment did not diminish milk production in subsequent lactations.[349] A review of dairy herd records in the northeastern United States comparing herds that used rbSt to herds not using rbSt showed that rbSt improved lactation yield and persistency consistently over the 4-year post-approval period.[350]

IMPACT OF SOMATOTROPIN ON FERTILITY. Data from early trials indicated that bovine ST, when used at doses consistent with increased milk production, increases the incidence of twinning[333,351] and had a negative influence on reproductive performance.* The latter function mimics the generally recognized antagonism between increased milk production and reproductive performance and is probably a function of early lactation energy status in the cow. A role for IGF-I in stimulating follicular growth has been determined, and rbSt has increased luteinizing hormone (LH) response to gonodotropin-releasing hormone (GnRH challenge)[352] and blood progesterone concentrations.[353] It has been observed that small doses of rbSt may be beneficial for fertility,[354] but this observation has been challenged.[338] The effect of rbSt on increasing follicular recruitment and development has been used in attempts to increase the success of multiple ovulation embryo-transfer programs.[355] RbSt significantly increased the number of follicles but failed to increase the number of retrieved oocytes in a study involving ovum pickup and in vitro fertilization.[356]

IMPACT OF SOMATOTROPIN ON MASTITIS. If the effect of rbSt in increasing mastitis is considered without controlling for increased milk yield, it has been demonstrated that there is an increase in risk.[302,357,358] However, increased milk production is associated with increased mastitis incidence and costs[359,360]; therefore it appears reasonable to assess risk in terms of increased milk production and possibly increased time milking. White and colleagus[358] evaluated the risk of mastitis in rbSt trials conducted for Monsanto and found that the increased risk of mastitis was consistent with that expected from similar milk production achieved through genetic gain. This conclusion should be evaluated cautiously, because it pertains to cows that did not have mastitis before treatment. Cows that may be more susceptible to mastitis (i.e., cows that have mastitis before treatment) are an important consideration in the field. However, treatment with rbSt does increase the recovery rate in cows with experimentally induced mastitis and appears to favorably modify the im-

mune response.[302,361] In a trial designed to determine the effect of rbSt on the incidence of clinical mastitis, number of days of milk discard because of clinical mastitis, and culling for mastitis, no differences were found between rbSt-treated and control cows.[362]

Reports of health disorders apart from mastitis generally suggest that somatotropin has little effect on health. There has been no evidence to suggest that rbSt will increase the incidence of clinical ketosis during treatment periods.

Recommendations for Use of rbSt

The labeled use of rbSt in the United States is for 500 mg SC every 14 days starting about 63 days in milk. The liver does not have adequate receptors for ST until that time in lactation for profitable use of the product. The critical point for effective use of rbSt in dairy cows is management of the nutritional status of the cows. When cows in good to excellent energy balance are treated with rbSt, the direct and indirect effects of the drug are exerted on the liver, adipose tissue, muscle, and the mammary gland so that milk production increases without negative effect to the cow. When rbSt is given to cows in negative energy balance, the direct effects of ST still operate, but the indirect effects are uncoupled so that the mammary gland will not secrete more milk and therefore there is not an increased energy demand on the cow. Thus treating undernourished cows with rbSt is unprofitable because there is no response to the drug, but there is no negative effect on cow health. Herds that intend to profit from rbSt must provide the husbandry needed to maximize dry matter intake in the cows. Feed palatability, feed presentation, water availability, cow comfort, lameness, and heat abatement are major determinants of dry matter intake. The dairy owner, managers, nutritionists, and veterinarians need to be able to manage these areas of the dairy so that the cow can increase her dry matter intake subsequent to the energy demands made by the increase in milk production after the initiation of rbSt. Sustained response to rbSt is dependent on the cow increasing her energy intake; cows will not respond to rbSt if they are not provided with the environment that allows them to eat more.

Successful use depends on the close monitoring of the health, productivity, and nutrition of the herd. It is known that some cows do not respond well to rbSt, but the reasons for nonresponse are not currently identified. Monitoring and statistical analysis of pretreatment and posttreatment milk production will allow an estimate of the effect of treatment. A simple paired t-test on pretreatment and posttreatment milk production of cows throughout lactation will help assess the magnitude of change and identify nonresponding cows. It is strongly suggested that this monitoring be conducted, given the possibility of lower responses to treatment in second and further lactations. Nonresponsive cows or herds should be considered as potentially responsive at a later time, under different conditions.

The use of rbSt on low-producing cows from early in lactation may allow these cows to remain in the herd and reduce the need for culling, allowing additional culling pressure to be applied to other conditions.

The effective use of rbSt depends on the intelligent application of herd management methods and particularly on herd nutrition. Use of rbSt does not alter the efficiency of use of feed. Therefore additional high-quality feed must be supplied. If herd management is not capable of supplying diets consistent with the nutrition of a higher-producing herd, it is unlikely that the response to rbSt will be sustainable.[310] Similarly, if a herd has problems with its forage base and management cannot or has not corrected the ration balance to account for this, use of rbSt may result in body condition loss

---

*References 328, 329, 333, 338, 341, 343.

and subsequent lower responses to rbSt and lower production. Nutritional monitoring of the herd is critical. The following indices must be monitored in rbSt herds:

Body condition score

Milk production and milk composition

Herd fertility indices (pregnancy rates)

Feed availability and quality (protein, energy, fiber, minerals)

Cow health (particularly important)

An effective management program will allow profitable applications of rbSt, but failure to carefully manage will place some enterprises at risk of unprofitable applications.

REFERENCES

290. Titchen DA: Gastrointestinal peptide hormone distribution, release and action in ruminants. In Mulligan LP, Grovum WL, Dobson A, eds: *Control of digestion and metabolism in ruminants*, Englewood Cliffs, NJ, 1984, Prentice Hall, p 227.

291. Emery RS et al: Effect of serum magnesium and feed intake on serum growth hormone concentrations, *J Dairy Sci* 69:1148-1150, 1986.

292. Chew BP, Eisenman JR, Tanaka TS: Arginine infusion stimulates prolactin, growth hormone, insulin, and subsequent lactation in pregnant dairy cows, *J Dairy Sci* 67:2507-2518, 1984.

293. Hove K, Blom AK: Plasma insulin and growth hormone in dairy cows: diurnal variation and relation to food intake and plasma sugar and acetoacetate levels, *Acta Endocrinol* 73:289-303, 1973.

294. Hart IC et al: Endocrine control of energy metabolism in the cow: comparison of the levels of hormones (prolactin, growth hormone, insulin and thyroxine) and metabolites in the plasma of high- and low-yielding cattle at various stages of lactation, *J Endocrinol* 77:333-345, 1978.

295. Hart IC, Bines JA, Morant SV: The secretion and metabolic clearance rates of growth hormone, insulin and prolactin in high- and low-yielding cattle at four stages of lactation, *Life Sci* 27:1839-1847, 1980.

296. Barnes MA et al: Influence of selection for milk yield on endogenous hormones and metabolites in Holstein heifers and cows, *J Anim Sci* 60:271-284, 1985.

297. Asimov GJ, Krouse NK: The lactogenic preparations from the anterior pituitary and the increase of milk yield in cows, *J Dairy Sci* 20:289, 1937.

298. Bauman DE et al: Effect of recombinantly derived bovine somatotropin on lactational performance of high yielding dairy cows, *J Dairy Sci* 65:121, 1982.

299. Juskevic JC, Guyer CG: Bovine growth hormone: human food safety, *Science* 249:875-884, 1990.

300. Brumby PJ: The influence of growth hormone on growth in young cattle, *N Z J Sci Technol* 2:683-689, 1959.

301. Bauman DE, Currie WB: Partitioning of nutrients during pregnancy and lactation: a review of mechanisms involving homeostasis and homeorrhesis, *J Dairy Sci* 63:1514-1529, 1980.

302. Lean IJ et al: Bovine somatotropin, *Vet Clin North Am* 8:147-163, 1992.

303. Peel CJ et al: Effect of exogenous growth hormone on lactational performance in high yielding dairy cows, *J Nutr* 111:1662-1671, 1981.

304. Peel CJ et al: Effect of exogenous growth hormone in early and late lactation on lactational performance of dairy cows, *J Dairy Sci* 66:776-782, 1983.

305. McDowell GH et al: Effects of growth hormone on muscle and mammary metabolism in cows, *Proc Nutr Soc Aust* 9:164, 1984.

306. Tyrell HF et al: In Ekern A, Sundstol E, eds: *Energy metabolism of farm animals*, Aas, Norway, 1982, European Association of Animal Production 29, pp 46-49.

307. Waters MJ et al: Growth hormone receptors: their structure, location and role, *Acta Paediatr Scand Suppl* 366:60-72, 1990.

308. deVos AM, Ultsch M, Kossiakoff AA: Human growth hormone and extracellular domain of its receptor: crystal structure of the complex, *Science* 255:306-312, 1992.

309. Bauman DE: Bovine somatotropin and lactation: from basic science to commercial application, *Dom Anim Endocrinol* 17:101-116, 1999.

310. Bauman DE, Vernon RG: Effects of exogenous bovine somatotropin on lactation, *Ann Rev Nutr* 13:437-461, 1993.

311. Burton JL et al: A review of bovine growth hormone, *Can J Animal Sci* 74:167-201, 1994.

312. Davis SR, Gluckman PD, Hart IC: Effects of growth hormone and thyroxine treatment of lactating cows on milk production and plasma concentrations of IgF-I and IgF-II, *Proc Endocrinol Soc Aust* 26:31, 1983.

313. Jois M et al: Effects of growth hormone on amino acid exchange in muscle and mammary tissue of lactating cows, *Proc Nutr Soc Aust* 9:165, 1984.

314. Davis SR et al: Effects of thyroxine and growth hormone treatment of dairy cows on milk yield, cardiac output and mammary blood flow, *J Anim Sci* 66:70-79, 1988.

315. Pocius PA, Herbein JH: Effects of in vitro administration of growth hormone on milk production and in vitro hepatic metabolism in dairy cattle, *J Dairy Sci* 69:713-720, 1986.

316. Lean IJ et al: Impact of bovine somatotropin administration beginning at day 70 of lactation on serum metabolites, milk constituents, and production in cows previously exposed to exogenous somatotropin, *Am J Vet Res* 53:731-741, 1991.

317. Bauman DE, McCutcheon SN: The effects of growth hormone and prolactin on metabolism. In Milligan LP, Grovum WL, Dobson A, eds: *Control of digestion and metabolism in ruminants*, Englewood Cliffs, NJ, 1986, Prentice Hall, pp 436-455.

318. McDowell GH et al: Effects of exogenous growth hormone on milk production and nutrient uptake by muscle and mammary tissues of dairy cows in mid-lactation, *Aust J Biol Sci* 40:295-306, 1987.

319. Lee V, Ramachandran J, Li CH: Does bovine growth hormone possess rapid lipolytic activity? *Arch Biochem Biophys* 161:222, 1974.

320. Eppard PJ et al: Effect of 188-day treatment with somatotropin on health and reproductive performance of lactating dairy cows, *J Dairy Sci* 70:582-591, 1987.

321. Eppard PJ et al: Effect of dose of bovine growth hormone on milk composition: α-lactalbumin, fatty acids and mineral elements, *J Dairy Sci* 68:3047, 1985.

322. Mohammed ME, Johnson HD: Effect of growth hormone on milk yields and related physiological functions of Holstein cows exposed to heat stress, *J Dairy Sci* 68:1123-1133, 1985.

323. Bauman DE et al: Effect of exogenous growth hormone on nutrient utilization in high-producing dairy cow, *Proceedings of the Cornell Nutrition Conference for Feed Manufacturers*, Ithaca, NY, 1980, pp 23-25.

324. Peel CJ et al: The effects of long-term administration of bovine growth hormone on the lactational performance of identical-twin dairy cow, *Anim Prod* 41:135-142, 1985.

325. Bauman DE et al: Responses of high-producing dairy cows to long-term treatment with pituitary somatotropin and recombinant somatotropin, *J Dairy Sci* 68:1352-1362, 1985.

326. Eppard PJ, Bauman DE, McCutcheon SN: Effect of dose of bovine growth hormone on lactation of dairy cows, *J Dairy Sci* 68:1109-1115, 1985.

327. Soderholm GC et al: Effects of recombinant bovine somatotropin on milk production, body composition and physiological parameters, *J Dairy Sci* 71:355-365, 1988.

328. Thomas C et al: Responses by lactating cows in commercial dairy herds to recombinant somatotropin, *J Dairy Sci* 74:945-964, 1991.

329. McBride BW et al: Use of recombinant bovine somatotropin for up to two lactations on dairy production traits, *J Dairy Sci* 73:3248-3259, 1990.

330. Michel A et al: Effects of exogenous bovine somatotropin on milk yield and pasture intake in dairy cows of low or high genetic merit, *Anim Prod* 51:229-234, 1990.

331. Hoogendoorn CJ et al: Production responses of New Zealand Friesian cows on pasture to exogenous recombinantly derived bovine somatotropin, *Anim Prod* 51:431-439, 1990.

332. Valentine SC et al: Effect of bovine somatotropin injected as a sustained-release formulation at three injection intervals in the production and composition of milk from dairy cattle grazing pasture and supplemented with grain, *Aust J Exp Agric* 30:457-461, 1990.

333. Hard DL: *Technical manual for Posilac*, St Louis, 1993, Monsanto.

334. Phipps RH et al: Use of prolonged-release bovine somatotropin for milk production in British Friesian dairy cows. I, Effect on intake, milk production and feed efficiency in two lactations of treatment, *J Agric Sci (Camb)* 115:95-104, 1990.

335. Chilliard Y et al: Body composition of dairy cows according to lactation stage, somatotropin treatment and concentrate supplementation, *J Dairy Sci* 74:3103-3116, 1991.

336. Annexstad RJ et al: Somatotropin treatment for a second consecutive lactation, *J Dairy Sci* 73:2423-2436, 1990.

337. Gibson JP et al: Effect on production traits of bovine somatotropin for up to three consecutive lactations, *J Dairy Sci* 75:837-846, 1992.

338. Hansen WP et al: Multifarm use of bovine somatotropin for two consecutive lactations and its effect on lactation performance, health and reproduction, *J Dairy Sci* 77:94-110, 1994.

339. Oldenbroek JK et al: Effects of treatment of dairy cows with recombinant bovine somatotropin administered daily or in a sustained-release formulation, *J Dairy Sci* 76:453-467, 1993.

340. Eppard PJ et al: Response of dairy cows to high doses of a sustained-release bovine somatotropin administered during two lactations. I, Production response, *J Dairy Sci* 74:3807-3821, 1992.

341. Chalupa W et al: Responses of cows in a commercial dairy to somatotropin, *J Dairy Sci* 71:210-222, 1988.

342. McGuire MA et al: Insulin-like growth factors in plasma and afferent mammary lymph of lactating cows deprived of feed or treated with bovine somatotropin, *J Dairy Sci* 81:950-957, 1998.

343. Elvinger F et al: Effects of administration of bovine somatotropin on lactation milk yield and composition, *J Dairy Sci* 70:121, 1987.

344. West JW: Interactions of energy and bovine somatotropin with heat stress, *J Dairy Sci* 77:2091-2102, 1994.

345. Yousef MK, Johnson HD: Calorigenesis of cattle as influenced by growth hormone and environmental temperature, *J Anim Sci* 25:1076-1082, 1966.

346. Collier RJ, Johnson HD: Bovine somatotropin: mechanism of action and effects under differing environments, Monsanto technical symposium publication, St Louis, 1988, Animal Sciences Division, Monsanto.

347. Tarrazon-Herrera M et al: Effects of bovine somatotropin and evaporative cooling plus shade on lactation performance of cows during summer heat stress, *J Dairy Sci* 82:2352-2357, 1999.

348. Lean IJ et al: Postparturient metabolic and production responses in cows previously exposed to long term treatment with somatotropin, *J Dairy Sci* 74:3429-3445, 1991.

349. Huber JT et al: Administration of recombinant bovine somatotropin to dairy cows for four consecutive lactations, *J Dairy Sci* 80:2355-2360, 1997.

350. Bauman DE et al: Production responses to bovine somatotropin in Northeast dairy herds, *J Dairy Sci* 82:2564-2573, 1999.

351. Phipps RK: The use of prolonged release bovine somatotropin in milk production, *Bull Int Dairy Fed* 228:2-11, 1988.

352. Gallo GF, Lefebvre D, Block E: GnRH-induced LH response by dairy cows injected with recombinant bovine somatotropin (rbST), *J Anim Sci 67/J Dairy Sci* 72:343, 1989.

353. Gallo GF, Block E: Effect of recombinant bovine somatotropin (rbST) on circulating concentrations of progesterone in plasma during estrous cycles and pregnancy in lactating dairy cows, *J Anim Sci 67/J Dairy Sci* 72:345, 1989.

354. Stanisiewski EP, Krabill LF, Lauderdale JW: Milk yield, health, and reproduction of dairy cows given somatotropin (somavubove) beginning early postpartum, *J Dairy Sci* 75:2149-2164, 1992.

355. Gong JG et al: Effect of recombinant bovine somatotropin on the superovulatory responses to pregnant mare serum gonadotropin in heifers, *Biol Reprod* 48:1141-1149, 1993.

356. Bols PE et al: Effects of long-term treatment with bovine somatotropin on follicular dynamics and subsequent oocyte and blastocyst yield in an OPU-IVF program, *Theriogenology* 49:983-995, 1998.

357. Willeberg P: Bovine somatotropin and clinical mastitis: epidemiologic assessment of the welfare risk, *Livestock Prod Sci* 36:55-66, 1993.

358. White TC et al: Clinical mastitis in cows treated with sometribove (recombinant bovine somatotropin) and its relation to milk yield, *J Dairy Sci* 77:2249-2260, 1994.

359. Shook GE: Why genetic improvement of SCC score? *Proceedings of the Thirty-first Annual National Mastitis Council, Inc,* Arlington, Va, p 108, 1992.

360. Dunklee JS, Freeman AE, Kelley DH: Comparison of Holsteins selected for high and average milk production. II, Health and reproductive response to selection for milk, *J Dairy Sci* 77:3683-3690, 1994.

361. Burton JL et al: A review of bovine growth hormone, *Can J Anim Sci* 74: 167-201, 1994.

362. Judge LJ, Erskine RJ, Bartlett PC: Recombinant bovine somatotropin and clinical mastitis: incidence, discarded milk following therapy, and culling, *J Dairy Sci* 80:3212-3218, 1997.

Diseases of Muscle

STEPHANIE J. VALBERG

DAVID R. HODGSON

Consulting Editors

EXAMINATION OF THE MUSCULAR SYSTEM

STEPHANIE J. VALBERG
DAVID R. HODGSON

Clinical evaluation of the muscular system requires a systematic and routine method for examination. Often a veterinarian is asked to examine an animal with a history of a relatively nonspecific disease process that may be the result of muscular dysfunction. Horses with electrolyte imbalances, pleuritis, colic, and a number of lameness problems (e.g., laminitis) may initially have signs similar to those seen with some forms of muscular dysfunction. Similarly, ruminants with primary gastrointestinal disease show signs that resemble those of muscular disease caused by electrolyte imbalances.

A thorough history of the animal or animals involved is an integral part of characterizing the muscle disorder. The duration of illness, intermittency of clinical signs, factors precipitating clinical signs, exercise schedule, diet, current medications, vaccination history, and number of other animals affected and their familial relationships should all be recorded before the muscular system is examined.

PHYSICAL EXAMINATION

Initially the animal can be observed from all aspects at a distance. The examiner should observe the size, shape, and symmetry of all muscle groups and look for muscle fasciculations. This observation helps provide impressions about tropic changes, alterations in symmetry of particular muscle groups, and spontaneous muscle activity.

The animal can then be walked, trotted, or driven and evaluated for gait abnormalities. The symmetry of the gait and evidence of lameness, weakness, stiffness, and pain associated with movement can be noted. Gait abnormalities may result from pain, muscle weakness, muscle cramping, spasticity, decreased range of joint motion, dysfunction of motor neurons, and ataxia. A number of muscular diseases may result in one or many of these clinical manifestations.

For example, horses with exertional rhabdomyolysis may be lame or stiff and demonstrate significant pain when encouraged to move. In contrast, horses with fibrotic myopathy may demonstrate a characteristic exaggerated gait abnormality with little evidence of pain.

Following initial visual evaluation, muscles should be palpated. It is suggested that as many muscle groups as possible be palpated to obtain an overall impression of muscle tone, consistency, sensitivity, and heat. Comparisons between muscle groups and areas of the animal can then be made. Some animals are tense and demonstrate apparent evidence of myalgia when palpation is first performed. However, given time and patience, many of these animals relax, and muscles or muscle groups that at first examination appeared to be very sensitive or hypertonic may in reality be normal. By this stage it can often be determined whether individual muscles, muscle groups, a limb or limbs, or the whole body musculature is involved. The symmetry or absence of symmetry of affected muscles or muscle groups is also important for potential evaluation of muscle disorders. Horses should stand perfectly square when comparing bilateral muscle groups.

Fine muscle tremors can be palpated and auscultated with a stethoscope. Concurrent signs of anxiety or pain should be noted and the animal reevaluated in calm surroundings if necessary. In animals with spontaneous muscle activity, muscle groups should also be percussed with a percussion hammer. A positive percussion sign occurs when the soft tissue overlying the muscle becomes dimpled for several seconds (percussion myotonia). This occurs as the result of abnormal mechanical irritability and sustained contraction of the percussed fibers.

If there is evidence of weakness, differentiation between myasthenia of muscular and neurologic origin is ideal. However, this can often be extremely difficult because a close junctional relationship exists between the nervous and muscular systems. In general, muscular weakness is not associated with ataxia unless it is extremely severe. Weakness is often manifested by muscle fasciculations, knuckling at the walk, frequent recumbency with difficulty rising and shifting of weight because of an inability to fix the stifles.

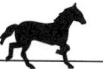

CLINICAL PATHOLOGY

Serum Enzyme Activities and Myoglobin Concentrations

Serum enzyme activities can be extremely useful in determining whether muscle cell necrosis is a predominant feature of a suspected muscle disease. As such, some preliminary discussion regarding the general principles of these techniques is appropriate. Under normal conditions the serum activities of the enzymes used to assess muscle dysfunction are low. Several events may occur that cause the serum activities of these enzymes to be elevated. The classic example is in response to myonecrosis (e.g., during exertional rhabdomyolysis or nutritional muscular dystrophy or following a crushing injury) when the cell membrane is disrupted and the cellular contents, including enzymes, diffuse into the lymphatic or blood circulation. However, a number of other factors may influence the activities of enzymes within the circulation. These include permeability of the cell membrane, rate of enzyme production, alternative sources of the enzyme, rate of enzyme excretion and degradation, and alterations to the pathways involved in enzyme removal or inactivation.[1]

Three enzymes are used routinely in the assessment of muscular diseases in large animals: creatine kinase (CK), aspartate aminotransferase (AST), and lactate dehydrogenase (LDH). Carbonic anhydrase III and serum myoglobin have also been suggested as markers of equine muscle necrosis.

Serum CK offers remarkable sensitivity as an indicator of myonecrosis. This enzyme is found predominantly in skeletal and heart muscle. It is intimately involved in energy production within the cell, is highly concentrated within the cytoplasm, and is readily liberated into the extracellular fluid when the muscle cell membrane is disrupted.[1,2]

Changes in CK can be used as an indicator of muscle dysfunction in relation to a variety of insults. Serum activity of this enzyme increases within hours in response to a muscle insult. Limited elevations in CK may accompany training, transport, and strenuous exercise. Elevations of CK to 400 or 500 IU/L may occur when training commences or in response to moderate exercise. Extreme fatiguing exercise, (e.g., endurance rides or the cross-country phase of a 3-day event) may result in CK activities being increased to more than 1000 IU/L but usually less than 5000 IU/L. These elevations usually are not reflective of an extensive myopathy, and serum activities of CK rapidly return to baseline activities (i.e., less than 250 IU/L in 24 to 48 hours). Recumbent animals also may have slightly elevated CK activities that are usually less than 3000 IU/L. In contrast, more substantial elevations (from several thousand to hundreds of thousands of IU/L) in the activity of this enzyme may occur with rhabdomyolysis.[1,2]

Several different isoforms of CK exist. Electrophoretic migration in a field of direct current results in the separation of three bands: MM, MB, and BB. Skeletal muscle is rich in the MM isoform, cardiac muscle is rich in the MB isoform, and neural tissue contains the BB isoform. Rhabdomyolysis results in a proportionately greater increase in the MM isoform than the MB isoform.

Serum AST, previously known as serum glutamic-oxaloacetic transaminase (SGOT), also has been used as an aid to diagnose muscular necrosis in large animals.[1,2] The enzyme has high activity in skeletal and cardiac muscle and also in liver, red blood cells, and other tissues. Elevations in AST are not specific for myonecrosis, and increases can be the result of hemolysis, muscle, liver, or other organ damage. Alterations in AST activity are an integral component of many laboratory serum biochemical "profiles."[1]

AST activity rises more slowly in response to myonecrosis

than does CK, often peaking between 12 and 24 hours after the insult, and the half-life of AST is much longer than that of CK ($\approx$2 hr). By comparing serial activities of CK and AST in animals with suspected myopathy, information concerning the progression of myonecrosis may be derived. Thus (1) elevations in CK and AST reflect relatively recent or active myonecrosis; (2) if CK remains persistently elevated, myonecrosis is likely to be continuing; and (3) elevated AST activities accompanied by decreasing or normal CK activities indicate that myonecrosis is not continuing.[1,2]

Elevations in serum LDH activity occur because of damage to various organs within the body. LDH is composed of muscle (M) and heart (H) subunits. The enzyme is a tetramer made up of combinations of the M and H subunits, with five isoenzyme forms. Although the distribution of isoforms is genetically determined, electrophoretic separation suggests that the M_4 (LDH_5) and M_3H (LDH_4) isoforms are found predominantly in skeletal muscle. Elevations in LDH may be detected in horses with rhabdomyolysis, myocardial necrosis, and/or hepatic necrosis. Therefore in the presence of elevations of total LDH activity, electrophoretic separation of LDH into its isoenzyme forms may be necessary if definitive evidence of skeletal myonecrosis is to be obtained.[1]

Whenever possible, consideration should be given to providing optimum conditions for collection, handling, and storing of serum or plasma samples for subsequent determination of enzyme activities. CK is labile when stored at room temperature. Activity of CK in serum samples stored for 24 hours at room temperature falls to approximately 25% of activity at the time of collection. When kept at between 0° and 4° C (32° and 39° F), only 32% to 65% of the activity remains after 24 hours. In contrast, freezing of samples allows maintenance of CK activities for several days. However, after 8 days of frozen storage, activity falls to approximately 25% of the original value. Despite this apparent rapid decline in the serum activity of CK, CK determination from samples stored under less than ideal conditions may still reveal useful information.[1] This is particularly true in cases in which large elevations in CK activity occur in response to myonecrosis. In these animals, CK activity may rise to a peak value of hundreds of thousands of IU/L. Even if CK activity does fall significantly in storage, it remains elevated within the sample for several days, potentially providing evidence of myonecrosis. The enzymes AST and LDH are much more stable under a variety of storage conditions, with less than 25% of the activities of both enzymes being lost over an 8-day period in samples stored at room temperature, 0° to 4° C (32° to 39° F), or frozen. Freezing samples for LDH isoenzyme determination alters the configuration of the isoforms, making interpretation of the results unreliable. However, total LDH activity remains unaffected.[1]

Therefore under ideal conditions samples for subsequent determination of CK, AST, and/or LDH should be collected into a glass (serum) or heparinized tube. The serum or plasma should be harvested as soon as possible, because anoxia and lysis of red blood cells allows the liberation of AST and LDH. If possible, serum and plasma samples should be transported rapidly to the laboratory. Otherwise they should be kept chilled (4° C, 39° F) if analysis is to occur within 24 hours. When determination of CK activity is required and a delay of more than 12 hours is anticipated, freezing of the samples is desirable.[1]

Elevations in plasma/serum myoglobin concentrations provide an indication of recent muscle damage. Myoglobin is a small protein that leaks into plasma immediately after muscle damage and is rapidly cleared in the urine by the kidney. It is particularly useful for determining exercise-associated muscle damage, because peak concentrations are reached shortly after exercise compared to 4 to 6 hours later for CK.[3]

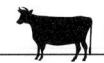

Normal concentrations in resting horses have been determined by nephelometry (range 0 to 9 μg/L),[4] with measured concentrations with rhabdomyolysis ranging from 10,000 to 800,000 μg/L.[3]

Urinalysis

Urine can be obtained free catch from horses placed in stalls with fresh bedding or via catheterization of mares without tranquilization. Urinalysis is particularly important in horses with myoglobinuria, elevations in creatinine, or suspected electrolyte imbalances. Urine specific gravity, protein content, white blood cell (WBC) count, red blood cell (RBC) count, and evaluation of cast formation should be performed to assess the potential for concurrent renal disease. A positive Hemastix test (orthotoluidine) in the absence of hemolysis or RBCs in urine is highly suggestive of myoglobinuria. Further differentiation of myoglobin from hemoglobin is sometimes warranted and where available electrophoresis, nephelometry, or spectroscopy may be used. Spectroscopy does not always reliably distinguish between myoglobin and hemoglobin.

Determination of electrolyte, mineral, and creatinine concentrations in urine and blood is useful to determine electrolyte balance in horses with muscle cramping or exertional rhabdomyolysis.[5] Renal fractional excretions (FE) can be calculated using the following formula:

$$FE_x = \frac{S_{Cr} \times U_x \times 100}{U_{Cr} \times S_x}$$

where U is urine, S is serum, x is measured electrolyte, and Cr is creatinine.

Determination of creatinine, potassium, chloride, magnesium, and phosphorus concentrations can be performed by routine chemical analysis using ion-specific electrodes. Ideally, laboratory determination of urine sodium should be by flame photometry or inductively coupled plasma atomic absorption. Analysis of urine sodium by ion-specific electrodes often is difficult because of interference by the naturally high urine potassium concentration. If urine calcium is to be determined, acidification of urine to dissolve all calcium oxalate crystals is necessary to provide exact calcium excretion.

Normal values for FE of electrolytes depend on a horse's diet. Normal values (%) for horses consuming grass, hay, and a sweet feed mix with available salt are: FE_{Na} 0.04 to 0.08, FE_K 35 to 80, FE_{Cl} 0.4 to 1.2, FE_{Ca} 5.3 to 14.5 , FE_P 0.05 to 4.1, and FE_{Mg} 14.2 to 21.4.

Exercise Testing

Evaluation of muscle disorders that are precipitated by exercise may require an exercise challenge test. Abnormal increases in CK are more likely to occur if slow trotting is performed rather than strenuous exercise. CK activity in blood samples taken immediately after exercise does not reflect the amount of exercise-induced muscle damage. For best results, blood samples for CK activity should be taken before and 4 to 6 hours after exercise. In healthy horses, 15 to 30 minutes of light exercise rarely causes more than a threefold increase in CK. Elevations greater than fivefold are indicative of exertional rhabdomyolysis. Standardized treadmill exercise testing can also be used to evaluate muscle responses and measure metabolic responses to exercise.

Electromyography

Electrodiagnostic studies detect spontaneous or evoked potentials of neurogenic or myogenic origin using electrodes positioned in the muscle or in the skin over a nerve. Electromyography (EMG) is particularly useful to evaluate large animals with altered muscle tone. It can distinguish between increased motor unit firing, abnormal electrical conduction of motor impulses within the myofibers, or denervated myofibers (neurogenic atrophy). Needle EMG does not directly detect upper motor neuron lesions or sensory involvement. More information about the motor unit could be provided by nerve conduction velocities (NCVs); however, the inaccessibility of motor nerves makes measurement difficult in large animals. Both EMG and NCVs are used to classify the primary disease as neuropathic or myopathic, to determine the distribution of the disease, and to provide insight into the pathophysiologic mechanisms of the disease. Equipment costs are relatively high, and expertise is required in operation and interpretation of results. Readers are advised to consult Chapter 33 before considering the use of EMG.

Muscle Biopsy

Examination of muscle fibers, neuromuscular junctions, nerve branches, connective tissue, and blood vessels within a biopsy sample can provide additional information necessary to fully characterize a neuromuscular disorder. Routine light and electron microscopic examinations, combined with histochemical evaluations, may provide insights into the particular manifestations of neuromuscular diseases and their rate of progression.[2,6] A number of basic pathologic responses of muscle can be identified in paraffin-fixed sections. These include inflammatory infiltrates, muscle fiber necrosis, muscle fiber regeneration, increased number of central nuclei, variations in muscle fiber sizes and fiber shapes, vacuolar change, and proliferation of connective tissue.[6] However, there are many pathologic alterations that cannot be detected in formalin-fixed tissue but can readily be seen in histochemical stains of fresh-frozen biopsy samples. These include muscle fiber types and their pattern of distribution, differentiation of neurogenic atrophy from disuse atrophy or a primary myopathy, characterization of vacuolar storage material, characterization of inclusion bodies, assessment of mitochondrial density, and additional clues that may allow identification of a specific disorder or category of muscle disorders.

When considering collection of muscle biopsies, some general guidelines apply. Preferably samples should be collected from what is considered abnormal or diseased muscle. A 6-mm outer diameter* percutaneous needle biopsy technique can be used to obtain small muscle samples through a ¼-inch skin incision using a local anesthetic subcutaneously. If this technique is used, enough muscle should be obtained to form a ½-inch square sample at a minimum. These samples do not, however, tolerate shipment to an outside laboratory. The optimum biopsy for shipment of histopathologic tissues to a laboratory is collected using surgical or open techniques, performed under local anesthesia. Care must be exercised to infiltrate only the subcutaneous tissues, not the muscle, with the anesthetic agent. The objective is to obtain approximately a ½-inch cube of tissue; hence a suitably long skin incision is required. Two parallel incisions ½ inch apart should be made longitudinal to the muscle fibers with a scalpel. The muscle should only be handled in one corner using forceps. The muscle sample is then excised by cross-secting incisions ½ inch apart, and the tissue fixed appropriately. Routine histopathologic samples can be placed in formalin; samples for histochemical analysis require fixation in isopentane (methylbutane) chilled in liquid nitrogen to ensure rapid freezing and minimization of freeze artifact. Fresh samples can be placed in a watertight hard container after being wrapped in gauze moistened with saline, and shipped chilled to laboratories for freezing. Samples that potentially may be used for biochemical analysis should be im-

---

*Carl Mortensen, Bjaerskov, Denmark.

mediately frozen in liquid nitrogen. Other routine histo-pathologic techniques may also be of diagnostic value. A special fixative may be required if such practices are to be undertaken. Samples for electron microscopy (EM) require appropriate fixation in glutaraldehyde preparations. Ideally, thin sections of muscle for EM should be clamped in vivo to maintain fibers at a resting length before they are excised. However, if pathology other than the alignment of thick and thin myofilaments is to be investigated, small muscle pieces can be excised and placed directly in appropriate EM fixative.

Responses of strips of fresh muscle to stimuli such as caffeine, halothane, and a variety of other agents can also be performed by specialized laboratories.

REFERENCES

1. Kramer JJ: Clinical enzymology. In Kaneko JJ, editor: *Clinical biochemistry of domestic animals*, ed 3, Orlando, Fla, 1980, Academic Press, pp 175-179.
2. Cardinet GH III, Stephens-Orvis J: Skeletal muscle function. In Kaneko JJ, ed: *Clinical biochemistry of domestic animals*, ed 3, Orlando, Fla, 1980, Academic Press, pp 545-574.
3. Holmgren N, Valberg S: Measurement of serum myoglobin concentrations in horses by immunodiffusion, *Am J Vet Res* 53:957-960, 1992.
4. Räsänen LA: Exercise-induced purine nucleotide degradation and changes in myocellular protein release, *Equine Vet J* (suppl 18):235-238, 1995.
5. Harris PA, Snow DH: Role of electrolyte imbalances in the pathophysiology of the equine rhabdomyolysis syndrome. In Persson SGB, Lindholm A, Jeffcott LB, eds: *Equine exercise physiology*, ed 3, Davis, Calif, 1991, ICEEP Publications, pp 435-442.
6. Cumming WJK et al: *Color atlas of muscle pathology*, London, 1994, Mosby-Wolfe.

CLASSIFICATION OF MUSCLE DISORDERS

STEPHANIE J. VALBERG

A muscle disorder is usually suspected in large animals because of (1) increased, decreased, or abnormal muscle contractions, (2) focal or generalized muscle necrosis (rhabdomyolysis), (3) muscle atrophy, or (4) exercise intolerance not associated with respiratory, cardiovascular, or skeletal causes.

ALTERED MUSCLE TONE

Increased muscle tone is often neural in origin. For example, tetanus and strychnine poisoning increase muscle tone as a result of suppressed inhibition of upper motor neurons by interneurons. Increased motor neuron firing also occurs during seizures, with electrolyte imbalances and equine ear tick infestation. Visual, tactile, or auditory stimuli often precipitate painful sustained motor unit activity. Other probable neural disorders that intermittently increase muscle tone include periodic spasticity and spastic paresis in cattle and shivers in draft and warmblood horses.

Increased muscle tone can also result from myopathic disorders. Persistently enhanced muscle tone may occur because of muscle contractures, which are characterized by fixation of myofilaments in a persistently shortened position without neural input. Contractures are usually extremely painful and associated with rhabdomyolysis. Contractures occur with malignant hyperthermia and some forms of exertional myopathies. Intermittent, abnormal muscle contractions without rhabdomyolysis occur when sarcolemmal ion channels within the muscle cell membrane are dysfunctional. Caprine motonia congenita and equine hyperkalemic periodic paralysis are examples of diseases caused by sarcolemmal ion channel dysfunction.

Moderate weakness in horses may be caused by central spinal cord disorders. More profound weakness may arise from neuropathies affecting motor neurons (equine motor neuron disease), decreased neural input at motor-end plates

(botulism), marked muscle atrophy or rhabdomyolysis of postural muscles, or severe electrolyte imbalances (hypokalemia). The few operative motor units fatigue easily, resulting in muscle fasciculations, shifting of weight, low head posture, difficulty prehending grain, and long periods of recumbency and difficulty rising.

MUSCLE ATROPHY

Atrophy is defined as a reduction in muscle size, specifically a reduction in muscle fiber diameter or cross-sectional area. Atrophy may occur in response to a variety of stimuli. Denervation removes the normal low-level tonic neural stimulus that is necessary to maintain muscle fiber mass. Complete denervation of a muscle results in more than a 50% loss of muscle mass within a 2- to 3-week period.[7,8] A good example of this is "sweeney" in horses, in which the suprascapular nerve is damaged and muscles over the scapula atrophy. Other denervating conditions such as equine motor neuron disease show a slower progression of gross muscle atrophy. Electromyographic abnormalities following denervation are apparent within 5 days, and it may take 3 weeks for maximal changes to develop. Increased insertional activity, positive sharp waves, and bizarre high-frequency discharges and fibrillation potentials are seen in denervated muscle. Pyknotic nuclear clumps and small angular slow-twitch type 1 and fast-twitch type 2 fibers with concave sides are characteristic of neurogenic atrophy in muscle biopsies (Fig. 40-1).

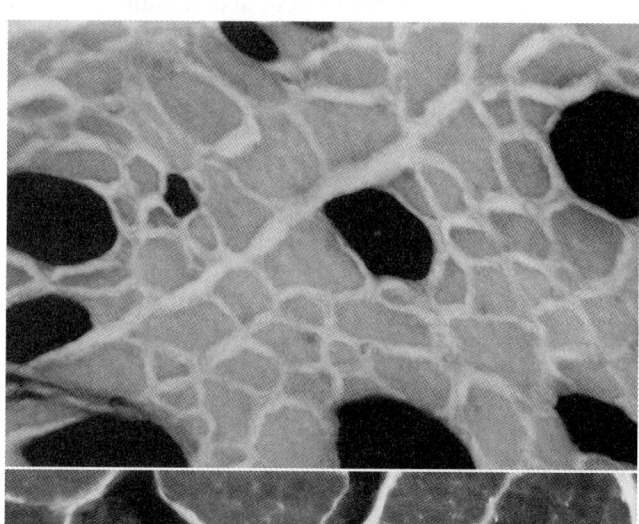

A

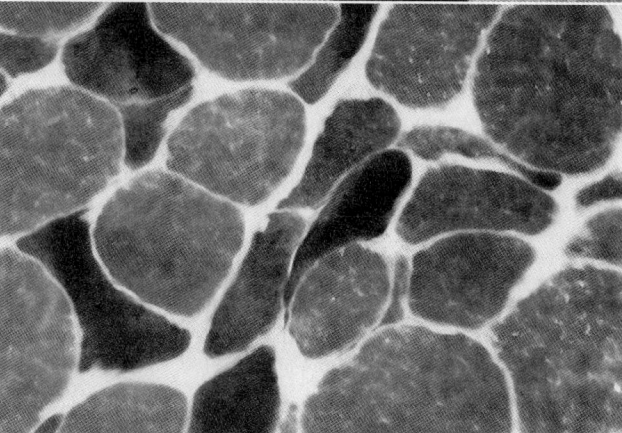

B

FIG. 40-1 ■ *A*, Extensive myogenic atrophy of type 2 (lightly stained) fibers is present in this sheep with a chronic *Corynebacterium pseudotuberculosis* enteropathy. *B*, Neurogenic atrophy involving both type 1 (darkly stained) and type 2 (lightly stained) muscle fibers in a Watusi bull with a demyelinating peripheral neuropathy. Myosin adenosine triphosphatase stain following acid preincubation (pH 4.3).

BOX 40-1

Causes of Rhabdomyolysis in Horses

MYOPATHIES NOT ASSOCIATED WITH EXERCISE	**EXERTIONAL RHABDOMYOLYSIS**
Inflammatory Myositis	
Clostridial spp.	**SPORADIC CAUSES**
Equine influenza virus A2 and equine herpesvirus 1	**Dietary**
Sarcocystis fayeri	Excess carbohydrate diet
Immune-mediated streptococcal infections	Low sodium diet
	Low potassium diet
	High calcium/low phosphorus diet
Nutritional Myodegeneration	Low vitamin E/selenium status
Vitamin E/selenium	
	Infectious
	Equine herpesvirus 1
Toxic Myopathy	
White snake root/rayless golden rod	**Overexertion**
Pasture myopathy	Excessive exercise relative to training status
Ionophores	Postendurance ride (hyperthermia, electrolyte imbalances)
Traumatic Myopathy	**CHRONIC CAUSES**
Anesthetic-related myopathy	Polysaccharide storage myopathy
Focal myoneuropathy	Recurrent exertional rhabdomyolysis
Generalized myopathy	Chronic exertional rhabdomyolysis (unknown causes)

Muscle atrophy also may be caused by disuse, malnutrition, cachexia, corticosteroid excess, and immune-mediated myositis. Skeletal muscle is a plastic tissue, with approximately 1% to 5% of the contractile mass undergoing remodeling on a daily basis. If a negative nitrogen balance occurs, net protein withdrawal from the skeletal muscle mass begins within 48 to 72 hours.[8] This type of atrophy is distinguished from neurogenic atrophy by a slower progression of atrophy, normal electromyographic findings, and muscle biopsies that are characterized by exclusive atrophy of type 2 muscle fibers. The overall response of skeletal muscle is to maintain essential postural muscle groups, whereas less essential groups undergo significant reduction in muscle mass. With malnutrition, 30% to 50% of the muscle mass may be lost in the first 1 to 2 months.[8] Rapid atrophy is characteristic of immune-mediated myopathies in Quarter Horse–related breeds, which can result in the loss of 30% of muscle mass within 48 hours.

MUSCLE NECROSIS

Muscle necrosis (rhabdomyolysis) as evidenced by elevations in serum CK, LDH, and AST can be focal or generalized. Many infectious, toxic, nutritional, ischemic, and idiopathic factors may result in muscle fiber necrosis. When attempting to identify an etiology, it is helpful to characterize rhabdomyolysis as associated with exercise or not exercise-associated. Particular causes of exertional and nonexertional rhabdomyolysis are listed in Box 40-1.

Necrosis represents injury to all organelles within a muscle fiber or within a segment of that fiber. Many myopathies associated with generalized rhabdomyolysis interrupt normal muscle metabolism and cell death results from an inability to maintain homeostasis within the myofiber. Although a variety of external or internal insults may cause rhabdomyolysis, they often share a final common pathway leading to cell death. Under normal conditions, considerable energy is expended by muscle cells to pump the calcium that accumulates in the sarcoplasm during contraction into the sarcoplasmic reticulum. If cell membrane function is disrupted or if the energy pathways that generate adenosine triphosphate for the calcium pump are impaired, excessive calcium may accumulate in the sarcoplasm. Although some calcium can be sequestered by the mitochondria, eventually mitochondria become overloaded, and oxidative metabolism ceases; oxygen free radicals are generated; phospholipases are activated, inducing the arachidonic cascade; calcium-dependent proteases are stimulated, and complement is activated. The contractile proteins within a necrotic segment are destroyed and appear homogenized with no evidence of cross-striations, and mitochondrial and sarcolemmal membranes appear disrupted. When necrosis occurs as a result of internal disruption of muscle homeostasis the basement membrane of the cell is left intact. Macrophage infiltration and phagocytosis of necrotic debris usually occurs within 16 to 48 hours of the muscle injury. Satellite cells migrate along the remaining basement membrane and form regenerative myotubes within 3 to 4 days of injury, with mature muscle fibers developing within a month of the original damage.[7]

Muscle ischemia occurs commonly with acute trauma, the compartment syndrome in recumbent animals, downer syndrome, and vascular occlusion. Compartment syndrome often involves the triceps muscle or extensors of the hind limb, because they are often compressed in down animals or during anesthesia. Hypotension during surgery contributes to the development of this syndrome. Acute muscle infarction may occur with purpura hemorrhagica or disseminated intravascular coagulation, and on postmortem examination characteristic well-demarcated areas of hemorrhagic necrosis are evident. Clinically, acute infarctions are an extremely painful condition that may resemble colic. Chronic occlusive diseases, such as iliac thrombosis, often allow collateral circulation to develop, thereby avoiding acute signs of ischemia at rest.[8] Although muscle has an impressive ability to regenerate, if a disease process is severe enough to disrupt the basement membrane, muscle may be replaced by connective tissue and fat. This occurs most frequently after trauma such as following tearing of the semimembranosus/tendinosus in horses (fibrotic myopathy).

REFERENCES
7. Cumming WJK et al: *Color atlas of muscle pathology,* London, 1994, Mosby-Wolfe.

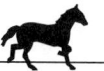

8. Hulland TJ: Muscle and tendons. In Jubb KVF, Kennedy PC, Palmer N, ed: *Pathology of domestic animals*, ed 3, vol I, Orlando, Fla, 1985, Academic Press, pp 139-199.

DISORDERS OF MUSCLE TONE

MYOTONIC DISORDERS
STEPHANIE J. VALBERG
DAVID R. HODGSON

Myotonic muscle disorders represent a heterogeneous group of clinically similar diseases that share the feature of delayed relaxation of muscle after mechanical stimulation or voluntary contraction. Abnormal muscle membrane excitability caused by ion channel dysfunction appears to be the shared abnormality among myotonia. The nondystrophic myotonias in large animals include myotonia congenita in horses and goats and hyperkalemic periodic paralysis. Dystrophic myotonia, a progressive disease that is also associated with abnormalities in other body systems, has been reported in Quarter Horses. In addition, it has been noted that some horses with ear tick infestations develop percussion myotonia and painful muscle cramps.

A condition illustrating myotonic signs in cattle is spastic paresis or "Elso heel." Commonly calves between 2 to 7 months of age are affected and have an extremely straight angle to the hock and stifle. Signs reflect a decreased capacity or inability to flex the hock because of continuous tension on the gastrocnemius muscle. Involvement may be unilateral or bilateral. The Holstein-Friesian breed is most commonly affected, although other breeds have been found to suffer the disorder. Spastic paresis has a distinct familial pattern. Plant toxins have been implicated as a cause of this disorder in Australia.

Myotonia

CLINICAL SIGNS. Myotonia congenita has been reported in humans, horses, goats, mice, and dogs.[9] In horses, myotonia is usually detected in the first year of life. Affected animals commonly have conspicuously well-developed musculature and display mild pelvic limb stiffness. Gait abnormalities are usually most pronounced when exercise begins and frequently diminish as exercise continues. Bilateral bulging (dimpling) of the thigh and rump muscles is often obvious and gives the impression that the animal is very well developed. Stimulation of affected muscles, especially percussion, exacerbates the muscle dimpling (Fig. 40-2). Affected muscles may remain contracted for up to a minute or more with subsequent slow relaxation.[10-12] Double-muscled cattle may also show bulging, but muscles do not remain contracted for inappropriately long periods (see Myofiber Hyperplasia). Most horses with myotonia have involvement of skeletal muscle only and do not demonstrate progression of clinical signs beyond 6 to 12 months of age. An inherited basis for myotonia has not been established in horses. Abnormalities in sarcolemmal chloride conductance appear to be important in the pathophysiology of myotonia in some human cases.[10] To date no abnormalities in sarcolemmal chloride conductance have been demonstrated in studies involving a limited number of affected horses.[13]

Severe clinical signs of myotonia that progress to marked muscle atrophy and possibly involve a variety of organ systems have been observed in some Quarter Horse foals. This condition resembles myotonia dystrophica in humans.[13] Retinal dysplasia, lenticular opacities, and gonadal hypoplasia have been reported in one such Quarter Horse foal.[14] In humans, abnormal sodium channel regulation has been

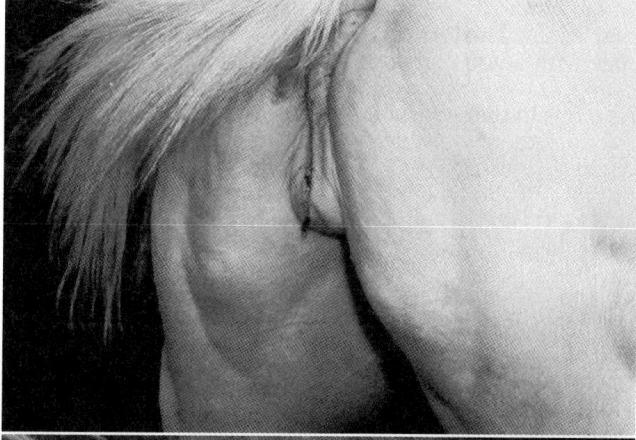

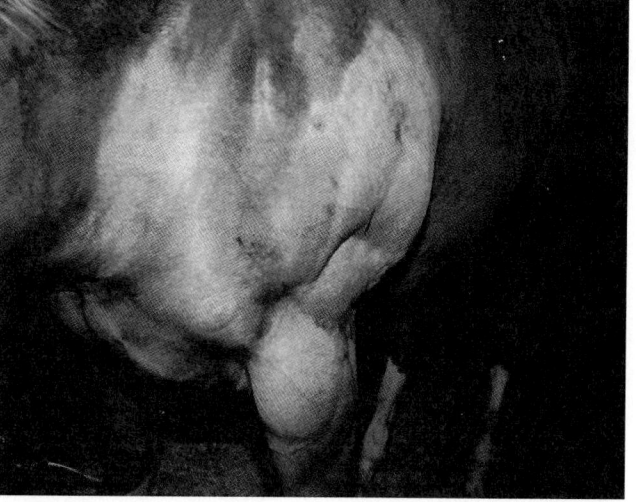

FIG. 40-2 ■ **A,** Myotonic cramp in the semimembranosus muscle of a horse with myotonia congenita. **B,** Myotonic dimpling of the triceps in a horse with hyperkalemic periodic paralysis.

identified in myotonic dystrophy in association with reduced protein kinase activity.[15]

In goats, myotonia congenita appears to an autosomal dominant mutation in the skeletal muscle chloride channel that has incomplete penetrance. Affected goats are commonly referred to as "fainting goats." Signs are usually recognizable by 6 weeks of age and vary from stiffness after rest to marked general rigidity after visual, tactile, or auditory stimulation. Clinical signs remain throughout the animal's life but are not progressive.[16]

DIAGNOSIS. A tentative diagnosis frequently can be made on the basis of age, clinical signs, (stiff gait, particularly at the onset of exercise), muscle bulging, and prolonged contractions following muscle stimulation.[10,11]

Definitive diagnosis of myotonia is usually based on electromyographic (EMG) examination. Affected muscle manifests pathognomonic, crescendo-decrescendo, high-frequency repetitive bursts with a characteristic "dive bomber" sound. This sound is produced by the repetitive firing (after contractions) of affected muscle fibers. After a contraction diminishes, the excitability of muscle fibers is decreased, and the action potentials recorded by the EMG reflect the diminution of electrical activity.[13,17] In some horses such EMG abnormalities may occur without any other clinical signs consistent with myotonia. Whether this reflects a subclinical form of the disease remains open to question.

Examination of muscle biopsies from foals with myotonia congenita may be normal or may demonstrate extremely variable muscle fiber dimensions up to twice those of normal age-matched controls. Type I fiber hypertrophy may be seen with accompanying signs of fiber splitting. The major changes noted with myotonic dystrophy are ringed fibers, alterations in the shape and position of myonuclei, sarcoplasmic masses, and an increase in endomysial and perimysial connective tissue.[11,12,14] Fiber type grouping and atrophy of both type I and type II muscle fibers may be present.

TREATMENT. Considering that the pathophysiologic basis of myotonia in horses has not been clearly identified, recommendations for specific, effective therapy are almost impossible. In affected humans and dogs some relief of signs has been provided by drugs such as quinine, procainamide, and phenytoin. However, responses vary among patients.[10,13] Phenytoin has been reported to be efficacious in two Quarter Horses with hyperkalemic periodic paralysis and myotonic dystrophy.[18]

PROGNOSIS. Prognosis appears to be variable and dependent on the severity of clinical signs. Mildly affected animals may undergo some amelioration of clinical signs with increasing age. In some animals that exhibit few clinical signs, manifestations of the disorder may abate over a period of months to years. The reason(s) for this regression of signs is unknown. Other more severely affected horses may have progression of signs, including atrophy and fibrosis or pseudohypertrophy to the point at which the animal is no longer able to move without great pain and difficulty. Euthanasia of such animals is often warranted.[10]

Although conclusive evidence regarding the genetic basis of this disorder in horses is still not available, owners of affected horses should be cautioned as to the possibility of this disease being heritable.

REFERENCES

9. Steinberg S, Botelho S: Myotonia in a horse, *Science* 137:979-980, 1962.
10. Farnback GC: Myotonia. In Mansmann RA, McAllister ES, Pratt PW: *Equine medicine and surgery*, ed 3, vol 2, Santa Barbara, Calif, 1982, American Veterinary Publications, pp 923-943.
11. Jamison JM et al: A congenital form of myotonia with dystrophic changes in a quarter horse, *Equine Vet J* 19:353-358, 1987.
12. Roneus B, Lindholm A, Jonsson L: Myotonia in five horses, *Svensk Vet* 35:217-220, 1983.
13. McKerrell RE: Myotonia in man and animals: confusing comparisons, *Equine Vet J* 19:266-267, 1987.
14. Reed SM et al: Progressive myotonia in foals resembling human dystrophia myotonica, *Muscle Nerve* 11:291-296, 1988.
15. Ptacek LJ, Johnson KJ, Griggs RC: Genetics and physiology of the myotonic disorders, *N Engl J Med* 328:482-489, 1993.
16. Smith MC, Sherman DM: *Musculoskeletal system in goat medicine*, Malvern, Pa, 1994, Lea & Febiger, pp 109-110.
17. DeLahunta A: *Veterinary neuranatomy and clinical neurology*, ed 2, Philadelphia, 1983, WB Saunders, pp 84-88.
18. Beech J et al: Effects of phenytoin in two myotonic horses with hyperkalemic periodic paralysis, *Muscle Nerve* 15:932-936, 1992.

Hyperkalemic Periodic Paralysis

SHARON J. SPIER

Over the past 15 years, a disorder affecting Quarter Horses, American Paint Horses, Appaloosas, and Quarter Horse crossbred animals has been reported worldwide. Affected animals periodically may undergo episodes of muscular fasciculations and weakness similar to that reported in humans suffering from hyperkalemic periodic paralysis (HyPP).[19,20] This disorder in horses has a familial basis and is inherited as an autosomal dominant trait similar to HyPP in humans.[21] The genetic disease has been linked to a prolific Quarter Horse sire named Impressive. Current estimates indicate that 4% of the Quarter Horse breed may be affected.[22,23] Affected horses may have been preferentially selected as breeding stock because of their pronounced muscle development, and there is evidence of selection of HyPP-affected horses as superior halter horses by show judges.[24]

CLINICAL SIGNS. There is a wide range of clinical severity of disease among different horses carrying the same mutation, ranging from asymptomatic (no evidence of disease is observed by their owners although signs can be precipitated by potassium chloride challenge) to those horses requiring medication on a daily basis to control episodes. In the majority of horses, clinical signs are observed intermittently by 2 to 3 years of age. Horses show no apparent abnormalities between episodes. It appears that a variety of stimuli may precipitate clinical manifestations of the disorder; fasting, anesthesia or heavy sedation, trailer rides, and stress are implicated; however, this association is by no means direct, and the onset of signs is often unpredictable.[21,22] Normal exercise does not appear to stimulate clinical signs, and serum creatine kinase remains unaltered or shows modest increases in response to episodic fasciculations and weakness.

In most cases, clinical episodes begin with a brief period of myotonia, with some horses showing prolapse of the third eyelid. Sweating and muscular fasciculations are observed commonly in the flanks, neck, and shoulders. The muscle fasciculations become more generalized as additional muscle groups are involved. Stimulation and attempts to move may exacerbate muscular fasciculations. Some horses may develop severe muscle cramping. Muscular weakness during episodes is a common characteristic of HyPP. Horses remain standing during mild attacks. In more severe attacks, clinical signs may progress to apparent weakness with swaying, staggering, dogsitting, or recumbency within a few minutes. Heart and respiratory rates may be elevated, and horses may show manifestations of stress yet remain relatively bright and alert during episodes. Affected horses usually respond to noise and painful stimuli during clinical manifestations of the disorder. Episodes last for variable periods, usually from 15 to 60 minutes. Several horses have died during acute episodes.[19] Respiratory distress occurs in some animals as a result of paralysis of upper respiratory muscles, and a tracheostomy may be necessary. In addition, young horses that are homozygous for the HyPP trait have been observed to manifest a respiratory stridor and periodically may develop obstruction of the upper respiratory tract.[22,25] Horses homozygous for HyPP may present for dysphagia or respiratory distress, and endoscopic findings include pharyngeal collapse and edema, laryngopalatal dislocation, and laryngeal paralysis.

Once the episode subsides, horses regain their feet and appear normal with no apparent or minimal gait abnormalities. Episodes are often triggered following dietary changes or ingestion of feedstuffs high in potassium, such as alfalfa hay, molasses, electrolyte supplements, or kelp-based supplements. In a study involving affected horses fed three separate diets containing varying concentrations of potassium, clinical signs were observed more frequently when the horses were fed diets containing 1.9% and 2.9% potassium as compared to when fed a diet containing only 1.1% potassium.[26] Other possible precipitating factors that have been noted in humans and horses are exposure to cold, fasting, pregnancy, and concurrent disease and rest following exercise.

ETIOLOGY. HyPP is due to a point mutation that results in a phenylalanine/leucine substitution in a key part of the skeletal muscle sodium channel alpha subunit.[21] This voltage-dependent channel permits rapid membrane depolarization during the initial phase of the action potential. In horses with HyPP, the resting membrane potential is closer to firing than normal horses.[21] Increased serum potassium concentrations in horses can result in the failure of a subpopulation of sodium channels to inactivate. As a result, an excessive inward flux of sodium and outward flux of potassium ensues, resulting in persistent depolarization of muscle cells and temporary weakness.

DIAGNOSIS. Clinical signs of episodic muscle tremors and weakness in a Quarter Horse that is a descendant of an

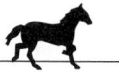

affected sire or dam is strongly suggestive of HyPP. Quarter Horse foals born after 1998 that are offspring of an affected parent have a statement recommending DNA testing for HyPP on the Certificate of Registration.

In most cases described to date, serum potassium concentrations are increased during clinical manifestations of the disease.[19,21] A few affected horses may have normal serum potassium concentrations during minor episodes of muscle fasciculations.[22] Other clinicopathologic findings include hemoconcentration and hyponatremia, with normal acid-base balance during episodes.[21] In experimentally induced episodes, serum potassium concentrations have been within the normal range (3 to 4 mEq/L) before the episode but rise more than 2 mmol/L, often reaching 6 to 9 mEq/L, during periods of episodic weakness.[21,22] Serum potassium concentration returns to normal following the abatement of clinical signs. The reduction in clinical signs parallels the diminution of serum potassium concentration. It should be noted that some horses with chronic renal failure and most horses undergoing very high intensity exercise also have elevations in serum potassium up to the range reported for horses with HyPP. These horses rarely demonstrate any manifestations of muscular dysfunction in association with hyperkalemia.

Because horses often are normal between episodes of HyPP, additional diagnostic tests usually are necessary to identify affected individuals. The definitive test and test of choice for identifying horses with HyPP is the demonstration of the base-pair sequence substitution in the abnormal segment of the DNA encoding for the alpha subunit of the sodium channel.[20] Submission of hair roots or whole blood in EDTA tubes should be made to appropriate genetic laboratories.

Before it was possible to identify the genetic defect, electromyography and potassium chloride challenge testing were relied on to establish a diagnosis of HyPP. Electromyographic examination of affected horses may reveal abnormal fibrillation potentials, complex repetitive discharges with occasional myotonic potentials, and trains of doublets even between episodes of HyPP.[21,22] Oral potassium chloride challenge testing has also been used to precipitate clinical signs in affected horses. Suggested doses range from 0.15 g/kg in horses less than 1 year of age to 0.16 to 0.2 g/kg in adults, dissolved in up to 2 to 4 L of water, administered via a nasogastric tube following an overnight fast.[21,22] Such provocation frequently produces clinical manifestation of HyPP within 1 to 4 hours in susceptible animals. Once clinical signs are manifest, the horses can be treated as described in the following paragraph to alleviate their muscular weakness. However, these tests are risky, and deaths have been reported. In addition, horses with cardiac disease, renal disease, or impaired adrenocortical function may also be adversely affected by administration of KCl.[19]

TREATMENT. In mild cases or if horses are just beginning to exhibit clinical signs, an episode can sometimes be aborted with mild exercise, which stimulates epinephrine, which stimulates sodium-potassium ATPase activity to mobilize potassium intracellularly. Feeding grain or corn syrup to stimulate insulin-mediated movement of potassium across cell membranes may also be helpful. Other treatment options that may abort an episode include *intramuscular* administration of epinephrine (3 ml of 1:1000/500 kg), and administration of acetazolamide (3 mg/kg orally every 8 to 12 hours). Many horses experience spontaneous recovery from episodes of paralysis and appear normal by the time a veterinarian arrives.

In severe cases, administration of calcium gluconate (0.2 to 0.4 ml/kg of a 23% solution diluted in 1 L of 5% dextrose) often provides immediate improvement. An increase in extracellular calcium concentration raises the muscle membrane threshold potential, which decreases membrane hy-

perexcitability. To reduce the serum potassium, intravenous dextrose (6 ml/kg of a 5% solution) alone or combined with sodium bicarbonate (1 to 2 mEq/kg) can be used to enhance intracellular movement of potassium.[22] With severe respiratory obstruction, a tracheostomy may be necessary.

CONTROL. Maintenance therapy is directed at decreasing dietary potassium and at increasing renal losses of potassium. Dietary management is extremely important in the management of affected horses. Dietary adjustments include (1) avoiding high potassium feeds such as alfalfa hay, brome hay, canola oil, soybean meal or oil, and sugar molasses and beet molasses and replacing them with timothy or bermuda grass hay, grains such as oats, corn, wheat, and barley, and beet pulp; (2) feeding several times a day; and (3) exercising regularly and/or being allowed frequent access to a large paddock or yard. Keeping the horse on pasture works well because, as a result of the high water content of pasture grass, the horse is unlikely to consume large amounts of potassium in a short time. If the horse is experiencing problems on its present diet, it is recommended to feed a diet containing between 0.6% and 1.1% total potassium concentration. Because there is a wide variation in potassium concentration of forages depending on maturity and soils, it is advisable to have feeds analyzed for potassium concentration and other nutrient requirements. Complete feeds for HyPP horses are commercially available.*

Alternatively, diets can be formulated such as the following that will result in total K+ content of approximately 1%:
4.54 kg of late bloom timothy or similar low K+ grass hay
2.27 kg of shredded, soaked beet pulp (without molasses)
2.27 kg oats, divided into small frequent feedings.[27]
Several drugs have been used for prevention of clinical episodes of paralysis. Horses have been treated with either acetazolamide 2 to 4 mg/kg PO every 8 to 12 hours or hydrochlorothiazide 0.5 to 1 mg/kg PO every 12 hours with apparent success.[21,22] These agents exert their effects through different mechanisms; however, both cause increased renal potassium ATPase activity.[19] Acetazolamide has been shown to stabilize blood glucose and potassium by stimulating insulin secretion. Breed registries have restrictions on the use of these drugs during competitions. Phenytoin, a hydantoin-derivative anticonvulsant, has been used experimentally to prevent HyPP episodes at a dosage of 10 to 15 mg/kg PO every 12 hours.[28] Phenytoin is not commonly used as a preventative because of its expense, potential for side effects, and requirement for periodic monitoring of serum levels.

PROGNOSIS. The prognosis for life in many of these animals is good, although recurrent bouts of the disorder may occur. The feeding of diets low in potassium and maintenance therapy with diuretics may aid in making long-term maintenance of more severely affected horses possible.[19,21,22]

Considering the autosomal-dominant transmission of this disorder, owners of affected horses should be strongly discouraged from breeding these animals for the long-term health of the Quarter Horse and other breeds. Owners of affected horses should use caution when handling or riding affected horses and be aware of the clinical symptoms of this disease.

REFERENCES

19. Cox JH: An episodic weakness in four horses associated with intermittent serum hyperkalemia and the similarity of the disease to hyperkalemic periodic paralysis in man, *Proceedings of the Thirty-first Annual Convention of the American Association of Equine Practitioners*, 1985, pp 383-391.
20. Spier SJ et al: Hyperkalemic periodic paralysis in horses, *J Am Vet Med Assoc* 197:1009-1017, 1990.

*Montana Pride, Alfa Care plus H.

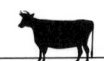
21. Rudolph JA et al: Periodic paralysis in quarter horses: a sodium channel mutation disseminated by selective breeding, *Nat Genet* 7:141-147, 1992.
22. Naylor JM: Equine hyperkalemic periodic paralysis: review and implications, *Can Vet J* 35:279-285, 1994.
23. Bowling AT, Byrns G, Spier S; Evidence for a single pedigree source of the hyperkalemic periodic paralysis susceptibility gene in quarter horses, *Anim Genet* 27:279-281, 1996.
24. Naylor JM: Selection of quarter horses affected with hyperkalemic periodic paralysis by show judges, *J Am Vet Med Assoc* 204:926-928, 1994.
25. Carr EA et al: Laryngeal and pharyngeal dysfunction in horses homozygous for hyperkalemic periodic paralysis, *J Am Vet Med* 209:798-803, 1996.
26. Reynolds JA et al: Genetic-diet interactions in the hyperkalemic periodic paralysis syndrome in quarter horses fed varying amounts of potassium. III, The relationship between plasma potassium concentration and HYPP symptoms, *J Eq Vet Sci* 18:731-735, 1998.
27. Duren S: Feeding management of horses with hyperkalemic periodic paralysis (HYPP), *World Equine Vet Rev* 3:5-8, 1998.
28. Beech J et al: Effects of phenytoin in two myotonic horses with hyperkalemic periodic paralysis, *Muscle Nerve* 15:932-936, 1992.

▌▌ *Muscle Cramping*

STEPHANIE J. VALBERG

DAVID R. HODGSON

GARY CARLSON

Muscle cramps are a painful condition that arises from hyperactivity of motor units caused by repetitive firing of the peripheral and/or central nervous system. The origin of the cramp in most cases is believed to be the intramuscular portion of the motor nerve terminals.[29] Most muscle cramps are also accompanied by fasciculations in the same muscle. Muscle cramps can be induced by forceful contraction of a shortened muscle, by changes in the electrolyte composition of extracellular fluid, and by ear tick infestations in horses. In contrast, muscle contractures are painful muscle spasms that represent a state of muscle contracture unaccompanied by depolarization of the muscle membrane. Muscle contractures occur with malignant hyperthermia and some forms of exertional myopathies and are invariably accompanied by markedly increased serum CK activity.

DIETARY ELECTROLYTES

Some horses develop muscle stiffness and occasional elevations in serum CK when fed a diet deficient in sodium or potassium. These chronic deficiencies are rarely reflected in serum electrolyte concentration but may be detected by performing renal fractional excretions of electrolytes.[30] Sodium deficiency is particularly common because forage and grain diets are low in sodium and chloride and high in potassium. Supplementation of the equine diet with salt is a necessity. Salt blocks may not be adequate in this regard and loose salt (1 to 2 oz) added directly in the grain is often the best mechanism of supplementing horses with salt. Some horses may require higher dietary salt supplementation to maintain an adequate sodium balance. Balancing dietary electrolytes has been reported to decrease muscle cramping and serum CK activity in those horses with dietary deficiencies.[30]

EXHAUSTION IN ENDURANCE HORSES

Muscle cramping in endurance horses occurs commonly during prolonged exercise in hot weather, particularly when the humidity is high.[31] Under such circumstances rectal temperatures reach as high as 41° C and horses may lose up to 15 L/hr of fluids in the form of sweat that is rich in sodium, potassium, and chloride.[32]

CLINICAL SIGNS. Affected horses demonstrate stiffness and cramping in the muscles of locomotion. Pain is a characteristic of the disorder, and affected muscle groups often undergo periodic spasms. In addition, exhausted horses are often dull, depressed, and clinically dehydrated with elevated

heart and respiratory rates and persistently elevated body temperature. Common electrolyte abnormalities include a hypochloremic metabolic alkalosis with hypokalemia, hypomagnesemia, and low serum ionized calcium concentrations. Synchronous diaphragmatic flutter may be seen in association with cramping.[31]

Although many of the signs of muscular dysfunction are similar to those of exertional rhabdomyolysis, affected horses do not generally develop myoglobinuria.[31]

ETIOLOGY. Factors contributing to cramping are dehydration, electrolyte abnormalities, and disturbances in thermoregulatory and local circulatory function. Whether this disorder is similar to heat cramps seen in human athletes is not known.

DIAGNOSIS. Mild cases are distinguished by the presence of muscle cramps that subside with rest or light exercise in heat-stressed horses. Unlike horses suffering from exertional rhabdomyolysis, animals with this disorder do not have marked elevations in serum CK or AST, nor do they exhibit myoglobinuria. A variety of electrolyte abnormalities occur in affected animals.[31] Exhausted horses have, in addition to muscle cramping, clinical signs of dehydration and shock described above. These horses require immediate treatment.

TREATMENT. Under most circumstances the mild form of muscle cramping is self-limiting, and the signs abate with rest or light exercise. However, if evidence of other metabolic derangements exists, treatment for these disorders (e.g., plasma volume expansion with oral or intravenous isotonic polyionic fluids, cooling using water and fans) is frequently beneficial to the horse. Because most horses with this condition are alkalotic, administration of solutions containing sodium bicarbonate is contraindicated. Dietary analysis should be performed to determine the extent of salt and electrolyte supplementation in affected horses. Daily direct addition of 2 oz of sodium chloride and 1 oz of potassium chloride to the feed is recommended for horses with recurrent cramping in addition to electrolyte supplementation before and after endurance rides.

REFERENCES

29. Layzer RB: Muscle pain, cramps and fatigue. In Engel AG, Banker BQ, eds: *Myology*, New York, 1986, McGraw Hill, pp 1907-1924.
30. Harris PA, Snow DH: Role of electrolyte imbalances in the pathophysiology of the equine rhabdomyolysis syndrome. In Persson SGB, Lindholm A, Jeffcott LB, eds: *Equine exercise physiology*, ed 3, Davis, Calif, 1991, ICEEP Publications, pp 435-442.
31. Carlson GP: Medical problems associated with protracted heat and work stress in horses, *Proceedings of the Fifth Annual Meeting of the Association of Equine Sports Medicine*, Reno, 1985, pp 84-99.
32. McCutcheon LJ et al: Sweating rate and sweat composition during exercise and recovery in ambient heat and humidity, *Equine Vet J* 20(suppl): 153-157, 1995.

SYNCHRONOUS DIAPHRAGMATIC FLUTTER

Synchronous diaphragmatic flutter (SDF), also known as "thumps," usually occurs in horses suffering from derangements in fluid and electrolyte balance. Inciting causes include endurance exercise, hypocalcemia, digestive disturbances, and possibly the administration of medications. A characteristic clinical manifestation of the disease occurs when the diaphragm contracts in synchrony with atrial depolarization.[33-35]

CLINICAL SIGNS. The classic sign of SDF is a contraction or twitch in the flank region (unilateral or bilateral) as the diaphragm contracts synchronously with the heart. In severe cases this twitch may produce an audible thumping sound.[33-35]

The metabolic derangements leading to SDF also may be clinically apparent in some cases. These may include signs of dehydration and volume depletion. Endurance horses suffering from SDF in association with the exhausted horse syn-

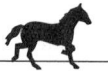

drome may demonstrate dehydration, inappropriate sweating responses, persistently elevated body temperature, depression, anorexia, and aperistalsis.[33] In some horses SDF may be a chronic, recurring problem.[33]

ETIOLOGY. A variety of stimuli may result in SDF. These include prolonged exercise, particularly during hot weather; hypocalcemia resulting from lactation, transit, or stress; digestive tract dysfunction; following furosemide therapy; and trauma. The most consistent metabolic derangement reported in horses with SDF is low serum ionized calcium concentrations usually associated with hypochloremic metabolic alkalosis. Metabolic alkalosis may alter the ratio of free to bound calcium (increasing calcium binding to protein and decreasing ionized calcium), which possibly induces SDF.[33-35]

SDF occurs in association with atrial depolarization in horses. It has been postulated that fluid, electrolyte, and acid-base derangements may disrupt the normal membrane potential of the phrenic nerve, which passes directly over the atrium, resulting in nerve discharges in response to atrial depolarization.[33-35]

TREATMENT. In most cases SDF is a transient event, usually abating when the underlying cause resolves, either spontaneously or in response to treatment.[33] Most horses undergo rapid remission of signs when given calcium solutions intravenously as described in the section Hypocalcemia in Horses. Although hypomagnesemia is often present with SDF, horses do not respond to magnesium supplementation unless calcium is administered concurrently. Response to therapy is also reflected by improved mental status, return of appetite, and gut motility.[33]

CONTROL. Electrolyte supplementation and some dietary manipulations may help reduce the incidence of SDF in some endurance horses suffering recurrent bouts. Provision of chloride, potassium, and sodium during prolonged exercise may help reduce fluid losses and the metabolic alkalosis that commonly accompanies this form of exercise and frequently occurs in association with SDF. Metabolic alkalosis decreases the amount of free calcium available. Supplementation of calcium and magnesium during endurance rides has been suggested to be helpful in horses prone to SDF.

Alternative approaches involve reduction of dietary calcium in horses prone to SDF for a few days before an endurance ride. It is postulated that this reduction in dietary calcium stimulates the endocrine homeostatic mechanisms and increases osteoclastic activity. In the short term the horse depends less on dietary calcium and is able to mobilize substantial amounts of calcium in response to the demands imposed by the exercise; calcium losses in sweat are overcome by the release of calcium from endogenous storage pools (bone).[33] Further, horses routinely fed alfalfa hay, which has a relatively high calcium concentration, may be more prone to development of SDF. Limitation of this feedstuff may be indicated in chronically affected horses.

REFERENCES

33. Carlson GP: Synchronous diaphragmatic flutter. In Robinson NE, ed: *Current therapy in equine medicine,* vol 2, Philadelphia, 1987, WB Saunders, pp 485-486.
34. Hinton M et al: Synchronous diaphragmatic flutter in horses, *Vet Rec* 99:402-403, 1976.
35. Mansmann RA et al: Synchronous diaphragmatic flutter in horses, *J Am Vet Med Assoc* 165:265-270, 1974.

HYPOCALCEMIA IN HORSES

Hypocalcemia is a relatively rare disorder in horses that has also been referred to as lactation tetany, transport tetany, idiopathic hypocalcemia, and eclampsia.

CLINICAL SIGNS. Clinical signs are variable and include increased muscle tone; a stiff, stilted gait; rear limb ataxia, muscle fasciculations (especially temporal, masseter, and triceps muscles); trismus; dysphagia; salivation; anxiety; profuse sweating; tachycardia; elevated body temperature; cardiac dysrhythmias; SDF; convulsions; coma; and death.[36-38] Clinical signs may be remarkably similar to some of those seen with tetanus. This disorder may be progressive (in lactating mares in particular) over a 24- to 48-hour period, and some animals die. Clinical signs are related to the magnitude of the serum calcium concentration. Increased excitability is usually the only sign when values are below normal but above 8 mg/dl. Values of 5 to 8 mg/dl usually produce tetanic spasms and incoordination. Concentrations below 5 mg/dl usually result in recumbency and stupor.

ETIOLOGY. Loss of calcium in milk, especially in mares who produce large amounts of milk, seems to predispose to this disorder.[36-38] Other factors such as heavily lactating mares grazing lush pastures, hard work or prolonged transport, and ingestion of blister beetles (cantharidin toxicosis) may precipitate attacks.

DIAGNOSIS. Clinical signs often are highly suggestive of hypocalcemia in affected horses. Historic aspects such as lactation, previous prolonged exercise, or transport also may direct the clinician to the suspected diagnosis.[37,38]

Definitive diagnosis depends on laboratory demonstration of hypocalcemia, with total calcium concentrations as low as 4 to 6 mg/dl in some cases. In addition, a metabolic alkalosis, hypomagnesemia/hypermagnesemia and hyperphosphatemia/hypophosphatemia have all been found in association with hypocalcemia in horses.[37,38] These alterations may need correction before a return to normal function is seen in some affected animals.

TREATMENT. Although many mild cases recover without specific treatment, in others this disorder may be life-threatening. Therefore therapy is to be encouraged in most cases. Treatment involves the intravenous administration of calcium solutions such as 20% calcium borogluconate or those recommended for the treatment of parturient paresis in cattle.[37,38] Administration of these solutions at the rate of 250 to 500 ml/500 kg diluted 1:4 with saline or dextrose often results in full recovery, although in some cases it may take several days.[38] Relapses do occur. These preparations should be administered slowly in conjunction with close monitoring of the cardiovascular response. Dilution in saline or dextrose before infusion decreases the chance of cardiotoxicity. Normally there is a positive inotropic effect in response to calcium administration.[39] However, alterations in rate or rhythm provide evidence to suspend the infusion. If no response to an initial infusion occurs, a second dose may be given 15 to 30 minutes later. Most cases respond to this form of therapy, although in some cases in which signs persist, repeated treatments may be necessary.[37,38]

REFERENCES

36. Baird JD: Lactation tetany (eclampsia) in a Shetland pony mare, *Aust Vet J* 47:402-404, 1971.
37. Blood DC, Radostits OM, Henderson JA: *Veterinary medicine: a textbook of the diseases of cattle, sheep, pigs, goats and horses,* ed 6, London, 1983, Baillière Tindall, pp 970-1014.
38. Brewer BD: Disorders in calcium metabolism. In Robinson NE, ed: *Current therapy in equine medicine,* vol II, Philadelphia, 1987, WB Saunders, pp 189-192.
39. Grubb TL et al: Hemodynamic effects of calcium gluconate administered to conscious horses, *J Vet Int Med* 10:401-404, 1996.

EAR TICK–ASSOCIATED MUSCLE CRAMPING

Intermittent painful muscle cramps have been described in a small number of horses with severe *Otobius megnini* infestations.[40] Muscle cramping is not associated with exercise.

These horses show intermittent signs of severe muscle cramping of pectoral, triceps, abdominal, or semitendinosus/semimembranosus muscles lasting from minutes to a few hours, with severe pain that often resembles colic. Horses may fall over when stimulated. Between muscle cramps horses appear to be normal. Percussion of triceps, pectoral, or semitendinosus muscles results in a typical myotonic cramp. Horses have elevated serum CK activities ranging from 4000 to 170,000 IU/L. Numerous ear ticks, *O. megnini*, can be identified in the external ear canal of affected horses. Without treatment for ear ticks, the spasms continue; however, local treatment of the ear ticks using pyrethrins and piperonal butoxide results in recovery within 12 to 36 hours later. Acepromazine may be helpful to relieve painful cramping.

REFERENCE

40. Madigan JE et al: Intermittent painful muscle spasms in five horses associated with ear tick (*Otobius megnini*) infestations, *J Am Vet Med Assoc* 207:74-76, 1995.

NONEXERTIONAL RHABDOMYOLYSIS

▮▮ *Inflammatory Myopathies*

CLOSTRIDIAL MYONECROSIS

STEVEN M. PARISH
DAVID R. HODGSON
STEPHANIE J. VALBERG

Various species of clostridial organisms cause acute myonecrosis in many farm animal species. Infections are characterized by a rapid clinical course, fever, systemic toxemia, and high mortality.[41,42] Clostridial diseases are infectious but not contagious. Specific bacteria associated with clostridial myonecrosis include *Clostridium chauvoei* (*Clostridium welchii*), *Clostridium septicum*, *Clostridium sordelli*, and occasionally *Clostridium novyi* type B, *Clostridium perfringens* type A, and *Clostridium carnis*. Mixed infections involving several agents are common.[43] Synonyms for clostridial diseases include blackleg, malignant edema, false blackleg, gas gangrene, and gangrene. Although there may at times be distinct differences between the specific disease syndromes associated with the different clostridial agents, the pathophysiology of these diseases is similar enough to be covered under the general topic of clostridial myonecrosis.

CLINICAL SIGNS. Commonly clostridial myonecrosis is rapidly progressive with the development of tremors, ataxia, dyspnea, recumbency, coma, and death within 12 to 24 hours. As such, many affected animals may be found prostrate or dead.[41,42] Mortality may approach 100%. Affected animals who are still alive are usually severely depressed, febrile (40° to 41° C, 104° to 106° F), tachypneic, anorexic, and lame. These signs are associated with a rapidly developing muscle infection and toxemia. There is usually only one primary site of infection in an affected animal. Any skeletal muscle group in the body can be involved, but most infections affect the limb or trunk muscles. Occasionally muscles such as those around the vulva, tongue, and diaphragm can be involved or the udder in a cow may be the primary site of sepsis. Areas around recent injections are common sites of myonecrosis in the horse.[44] Initially the skin over the area may be swollen, hot, and discolored; however, as the disease progresses, the skin over the area may become cool and insensitive. Crepitus may be detectable, indicating subcutaneous gas production. If a wound is present, malodorous, serosanguineous fluid

may discharge. Aspiration of the swelling often reveals fluid with similar qualities.

Clostridial myonecrosis generally has characteristic pathologic lesions that are absent in most other conditions, making diagnosis relatively straightforward. Differential diagnoses may include other fulminant disease processes in which there is rapid debilitation or death of the animal.

CLINICAL PATHOLOGY. Clinicopathologic data alone are seldom specific enough to confirm the presence of clostridial myonecrosis. Hematology and serum biochemical analyses usually reflect a generalized state of debilitation and toxemia (e.g., hemoconcentration and a stress/toxic leukogram may be present). Elevations in the activities of serum CK and serum AST usually occur; however, they often do not reflect the toxicity of clostridial myonecrosis.

Aspirates from the affected tissues can yield diagnostic information. It is preferable to obtain tissue specimens for direct smear examination and fluorescent antibody testing, and for anaerobic bacterial culture from affected tissues.

PATHOPHYSIOLOGY. Clostridial agents are ubiquitous in the environment and can frequently be cultured from the feces, intestinal tract, and other internal organs of a variety of species.[41,42] Spore-forming characteristics allow these organisms to remain in the environment for long periods, but the exact mechanisms involved in the pathogenesis of clostridial myonecrosis are not fully known. Development of clostridial myonecrosis following an intramuscular injection or penetrating wound may be the result of direct spore deposition into the tissue in association with penetration. If suitable conditions prevail within the muscle, the spores undergo a conversion into the vegetative, toxin-producing form of the organism. In contrast, the pathogenesis of the disease is more difficult to explain when a wound does not exist. It is postulated that clostridial agents gain access to the body through the alimentary tract and are present in liver and muscle in the dormant spore form. Subsequently, when local tissue is devitalized and conditions become appropriate for the spores to germinate, the rapid vegetative process ensues. Muscle trauma associated with transporting, herding, and handling has often been incriminated as creating a suitable environment for the development of clostridial myonecrosis. The proliferation of clostridial agents in devitalized tissues is associated with the release of powerful exotoxins responsible for the local necrotizing myositis and systemic toxemia. Toxins are released by multiplying clostridia; the toxins vary, depending on the clostridial species involved. Necrotizing (lecithinase) and hemolyzing (hemolysin) toxins appear to be of greatest importance. The toxins act locally and systemically to create widespread organ dysfunction. The toxins of *C. sordelli* are the most potent of all the clostridial species, and myonecrosis caused by this organism is fatal.

EPIDEMIOLOGY. Clostridial agents are common in the environment, and susceptible animals are constantly exposed to them. Areas where previous death losses from clostridial disease have occurred may have a higher incidence or risk of disease because of increased environmental contamination. In cattle clostridial myonecrosis is generally a disease of animals between 4 and 24 months of age. However, *C. sordelli* is a more common problem in older feedlot cattle in which excessive muscle bruising may occur. Younger animals are probably protected by colostral immunity, and older animals by some degree of acquired immunity. Animals on high planes of nutrition and in excellent body condition are more likely to develop the disease. Infections with *C. chauvoei* occur most commonly during the warmer seasons, with the highest incidence varying from the spring to fall, depending on when calves reach the most susceptible age group. *C. septicum*, *C. novyi*, and *C. perfringens* type A infections can occur at any time and are usually associated with skin wounds such as injection sites, puncture, and castration wounds. The umbilicus may be a site of invasion. Infections in the genital area can occur, usually in association with a recent dystocia.

In sheep and goats, clostridial myonecrosis is most frequently associated with wounds such as those occurring after shearing, docking, and unsanitary surgical procedures. Sheep dipped for parasites after shearing may have an increased risk if the dip becomes contaminated with clostridial spores.

Most reports of clostridial myonecrosis in horses suggest an association with puncture wounds and intramuscular injection sites.[44] Intramuscular administration of irritating drugs (including antihistamines, anthelmintics, phenylbutazone) may enhance the susceptibility to clostridial myonecrosis. Horses often present with or have a history of another complaint such as colic, exertional myopathy, or laminitis for which they have received injections of drugs in the preceding 48 hours. Previously administered drugs (e.g., phenylbutazone) may mask the fever associated with clostridial myonecrosis, potentially confusing the diagnosis.

NECROPSY FINDINGS. Swelling and autolysis are rapid in animals that have died from clostridial myonecrosis. Bloodstained fluid is often observed discharging from body orifices. Extreme swelling and crepitus may be noted over the affected body area. When acting alone, each of the clostridial agents associated with clostridial myonecrosis produces somewhat different postmortem lesions. However, it is unwise to assume that in clostridial myonecrosis only a single clostridial agent was involved, because mixed infections frequently occur.

C. chauvoei infection is characterized by engorgement of the subcutis and adjacent tissues with bloodstained fluids and gas bubbles. Cut tissue from the affected area reveals moist, dark-colored muscle in the periphery of the lesion, with lighter-colored, drier muscle with gas bubbles separating the separate bundles of muscle toward the center. Other changes include severe degeneration of parenchymatous tissues caused by the systemic toxemia. The carcass usually has a foul odor similar to that of rancid butter. This odor is a characteristic of most cases of clostridial myonecrosis. The lungs are often congested with edema, and hemorrhage and a fibrinohemorrhagic pleuritis are common. The heart may be friable and show evidence of endocardial hemorrhages, particularly on the right side. The spleen may be normal or enlarged and friable. The liver is usually pale and friable and may be autolytic and porous. Lesions are similar in sheep and cattle, except that there is usually less gas and the muscles are not as dry in affected sheep.

Similar necropsy findings are found with myonecrosis caused by *C. septicum* and *C. novyi* type B. *C. septicum* and *C. perfringens* generally occur as part of mixed wound infections in which abundant malodorous, serosanguineous fluid is found at the wound site. *C. perfringens* is common in horses.

Myonecrosis resulting from *C. sordelli* is most often associated with lesions of the neck or brisket area of cattle. Death is frequently so rapid that subcutaneous gas accumulation is rare. In addition to local myonecrosis, these animals often have massive subendocardial hemorrhages in the left ventricle of the heart and hemorrhage in the trachea, bronchi, and thymus. Extensive perirenal edema and hemorrhagic renal calyces and severe congestion of the lungs are common findings.

TREATMENT. Although clostridial myonecrosis is often fatal, aggressive specific therapy combined with supportive care may be successful in individual cases. A presumptive diagnosis of clostridial disease on the basis of history and clinical signs is usually made before obtaining the results of culture and laboratory determinations such as fluorescent antibody tests. In horses clostridial myonecrosis resulting from infections with *C. perfringens* seems to be most amenable to treatment and has the best prognosis for survival, although extensive skin sloughing over the affected area is common.

Antibiotic therapy, aggressive surgical debridement including fasciotomy, and supportive care are the hallmarks of successful treatment. With most clostridial infections penicillin is the drug of choice. In horses, penicillin is used at a dosage of 44,000 U/kg IV every 2 to 4 hours until the animal is stable (1 to 5 days). The intravenous dose is then reduced to 4 times a day or is replaced by either intramuscular administration of procaine penicillin (15 to 20 mg/kg) twice a day or oral metronidazole (15 mg/kg 3 or 4 times daily). In ruminants, similar intravenous or intramuscular drug therapy is indicated. In all cases, prolonged antimicrobial therapy may be necessary.

Surgical intervention at the affected site by means of debridement or fenestration in an attempt to reduce tissue swelling, aerate the tissues, and remove necrotic tissue may be beneficial. Incisions are made through the skin and into the affected muscle to establish adequate drainage and hopefully alter the anaerobic conditions. Sufficient fenestrations should be made to establish drainage and aeration over the entire affected area.

Use of specific antitoxins is recommended when possible. However, these are often not available or not used for immediate therapy because the exact species of *Clostridium* causing the myonecrosis is not known. Cost considerations may also preclude their use.

Supportive fluid therapy and use of analgesics and antiinflammatory agents for control of pain and swelling are recommended. Short-acting corticosteroids such as dexamethasone, prednisolone, or hydrocortisone may be used for initial therapy of systemic and toxic shock, but continued use is contraindicated in the face of overwhelming sepsis.

If required, specific therapy should also be directed toward any other underlying problems.

PROGNOSIS. The prognosis for life in all cases of clostridial myonecrosis is guarded to poor. The disease process is often rapidly fulminant, making treatment unrewarding. However, some animals have survived because of early diagnosis, aggressive therapy, and long-term supportive care. This is particularly true in cases involving *C. perfringens* in horses. The owner should be aware from the start of treatment that extensive skin sloughing may involve most of a limb and may force euthanasia to become a consideration at a later stage.

PREVENTION. Protection against clostridial myonecrosis is based on immunization procedures. Although clostridial agents are ubiquitous in the environment and frequently appear in the body of susceptible animals, rarely does adequate natural protection occur, although some colostral and acquired immunity may at times occur. Infection in unprotected animals usually follows a rapid, degenerative clinical course and terminates before the animal is able to generate an appropriate protective immune response. At present, only ruminants are commonly vaccinated against the agents responsible for clostridial myonecrosis. Vaccines used include multivalent bacterin toxoids containing antigens against two or more clostridial species, including *C. chauvoei*, *C. septicum*, *C. novyi*, *C. sordelli*, and *C. perfringens*. A rational program for protection usually involves vaccinating at an early age to establish immunity. Vaccination age is partly determined by other management factors, including when calves are handled for branding and castration, but 4 to 6 months of age is the usual time of initial vaccination. In areas of heavy exposure it may be necessary to vaccinate at 3 months and again at 4 months. In all clostridial species except *C. chauvoei*, two doses of vaccine are necessary to establish good protection. The duration of immunity is not long, and booster vaccinations should be administered every 6 to 8 months if protection is to be maintained. In many herds it is only necessary to vaccinate animals under 3 years of age (i.e., those animals that are at greatest risk), but in some high-risk herds it is necessary to maintain a vaccination program for the life of the animal.

Animals that die of clostridial diseases should be disposed of by deep burial, burning, or removal from the premises to avoid further contamination of the environment.

REFERENCES

41. Blood DC, Radostis OM, Henderson JA: *Veterinary medicine*, ed 6, London, 1983, Baillière Tindall, p 541.
42. Erwin BG: Clostridial bacteria and clostridial myositis. In Berg JN, ed: *Current veterinary therapy 2 (food anim pract)*, ed 2, Philadelphia, 1986, WB Saunders, pp 567-570.
43. Williams BM: Clostridial myositis in cattle: bacteriology and gross pathology, *Vet Rec* 100:90-91, 1977.
44. Rebhun WC et al: Malignant edema in horses, *J Am Vet Med Assoc* 187:732-736, 1985.

MYOPATHIES ASSOCIATED WITH *STREPTOCOCCUS EQUI* INFECTIONS

STEPHANIE J. VALBERG

A complete discussion of diseases caused by *Streptococcus equi* is found in Chapter 29. Only the disorder associated with muscle is described here. Mild elevations in serum creatine kinase (CK) activity have been observed in conjunction with purpura hemorrhagica in horses. The cutaneous vasculitis responsible for subcutaneous edema may be present within muscle, resulting in mild muscle necrosis.

Some horses with exposure to *S. equi* or vaccinated for strangles within the last 4 weeks have developed a severe vasculopathy that is characterized by infarction of skeletal muscle, skin, the gastrointestinal tract, and lungs.[45] Such horses often present with clinical signs of colic or severe lameness. Leukocytosis, hyperfibrinogenemia, hypoproteinemia, and extremely elevated serum CK and AST are present. Treatment with intravenous penicillin and intravenous dexamethasone (0.12 to 0.2 mg/kg) followed by tapering doses of prednisone at an initial dose of 1 mg/kg has been successful in a few cases. Without aggressive corticosteroid therapy horses usually die from intestinal infarction.

Severe rhabdomyolysis has been seen in some Quarter Horses with strangles infections.[45,46] In some cases, these horses had an underlying muscle disorder such as polysaccharide storage myopathy and developed rhabdomyolysis while ill. Other Quarter Horses have developed a myositis characterized by malaise and rapid atrophy of lumbar and gluteal muscles upon exposure to *S. equi*.[45,47] These horses may not have any concurrent signs of strangles but have persistent mild to moderate elevations in serum CK and AST (1000 to 40,000 IU/L). Muscle biopsies in these cases show a lymphocytic vasculitis, atrophy of type 2 fibers, and waves of rhabdomyolysis and regeneration. Untreated cases may show significant fibrosis centered around blood vessels. The myositis may reflect an immune-mediated myopathy in horses, because the M protein of some streptococcal organisms has amino acid sequences similar to the contractile protein myosin. Diagnosis is made on the basis of a history of exposure to strangles, elevated serum CK activities, and the results of muscle biopsy analysis. Treatment involves antibiotic therapy if a leukocytosis, hyperfibrinogenemia or lymphadenopathy is present and concurrent immunosuppressive therapy to dampen the host's response to the stimulus. Prednisone at 1 mg/kg for 7 to 10 days, followed by tapering doses over 1 month, is usually required. Some horses may show signs of recrudescence of the syndrome and require more prolonged therapy.

REFERENCE

45. Valberg SJ et al: Myopathies associated with *Streptococcus equi* infections in horses, *Proceedings of the Forty-second Annual Convention of the American Association of Equine Practitioners*, 1996, pp 292-293.

46. Divers TJ, Timoney JF: Group C streptococcal antigen-antibody immune complex disease in horses, *Proceedings of the American College of Veterinary Internal Medicine*, San Diego, 1992, pp 304-305.
47. Valberg SJ: Spinal muscle pathology. In Haussler KK, ed: Back problems, *Vet Clin North Am* 15:94-99, 1999.

VIRUS-ASSOCIATED MYOPATHY

STEVEN M. PARISH

Necrosis of skeletal and cardiac muscle occurs frequently in association with some viral diseases. In most situations, viral-induced muscle damage represents a component of systemic multiple organ system involvement. For example, myocarditis occurs in association with foot and mouth disease, equine influenza, and equine infectious anemia. Other diseases causing myocarditis or skeletal muscle manifestations include bovine ephemeral fever, malignant catarrhal fever, bovine viral diarrhea, and bluetongue. Equine influenza A2 and equine herpesvirus 1 have been reported to induce primary muscle stiffness and clinical signs resembling those seen in horses with rhabdomyolysis.[48,49] Details concerning specific clinical manifestations can be found in other sections of this text.

REFERENCES

48. Harris PA: Outbreak of the equine rhabdomyolysis syndrome in an equine racing yard, *Vet Rec* 127:468-470, 1990.
49. Freestone JP, Carlson GP: Muscle disorders in the horse: a retrospective study, *Equine Vet J* 23:86-90, 1991.

SARCOCYSTOSIS

STEVEN M. PARISH

DAVID R. HODGSON

STEPHANIE J. VALBERG

Cysts of the sporozoan parasite *Sarcocystis* are commonly seen in routine histologic sections of the heart, esophageal, and skeletal muscle of cattle, sheep, goats, and horses.[50-55] More than 90% of horses over 8 years of age have sarcocysts in their esophageal muscles. Cysts may pose no problem but with heavy infestations multisystemic dysfunction occurs.[50-52,54-58] Experimentally induced acute disease is characterized by fever, mild anemia, chronic myositis, and muscle wasting.

EPIDEMIOLOGY. The life cycle of the parasite involves two hosts, carnivores as the definitive host and cattle or horses as the intermediate host. Three species of sarcocysts, *Sarcocystis cruzi*, *Sarcocystis hirsuta*, and *Sarcocystis hominis*, are known to infect cattle; Canidae, Felidae, and primates are the definitive hosts for these species. Three sarcocyst species have been described in horse muscle, *Sarcocystis bertrami*, *Sarcocystis equicanis*, and *Sarcocystis fayeri*. Dogs have been identified as the definitive host of these equine sarcocyst species. In sheep and goats, *Sarcocystis ovicanis* and *Sarcocystis capracanis* have been described, with Canidae as the definitive host.

The most common mechanism for natural infection in cattle is by ingestion of feeds contaminated with infected carnivore feces. Feedlot workers using feed bunks as toilets may be a source of exposure for feedlot cattle.

CLINICAL SIGNS. Although low-level natural infection is common in cattle, when administered experimentally, a dose of 200,000 sporocysts of *S. cruzi* is necessary to cause severe clinical disease.[50,51] Within 4 weeks the animal develops fever (39.4° C, 103° F), anorexia, salivation, weight loss, weakness, muscle fasciculations, severe depression, and sometimes death. Fever is the earliest sign and is biphasic relative to two periods of parasitemia, one occurring at 15 to 19 days and another at 25 to 42 days after inoculation. During the second febrile episode, affected calves frequently develop other clinical signs, particularly anemia. Extravascular hemolysis occurs, and hemorrhage into many tissues is common. The mechanisms involved in the hemolytic and hemorrhagic phases are likely to involve immune mechanisms. Mortality is greatest during this phase of the disease. Laboratory analysis may reveal elevations in serum urea nitrogen and bilirubin concentrations, sorbitol dehydrogenase, LDH, CK, and AST activities. If animals survive, these laboratory values usually return to normal in about 2 weeks. Animals surviving this phase commonly continue to be inappetent and have decreased weight gains; muscle atrophy; and hair loss on the neck, rump, and tail. These changes are mediated by alterations in a variety of pathways, the net result being a partitioning away of nutrients that are used for growth.[56] The anemia is ameliorated by a regenerative process, with normal hematologic values obtained in 1 to 2 months after clinical recovery. Similar clinical findings are seen in sheep and goats. Abortion is common. A syndrome similar to that described in cattle has been reported in two horses with malaise, fever, and muscle atrophy.[57]

Diagnosis of sarcocystosis requires history, clinical signs, laboratory and serologic evaluation, and the demonstration of immature cysts in muscle biopsies. It is important to differentiate between the muscle cysts caused by *Sarcocystis* and those produced by toxoplasmosis because toxoplasmosis does not cause clinical disease in cattle.

TREATMENT. Specific treatment is only effective in the early stages of sarcocystosis. Experimental therapy with amprolium or the ionophore antibiotics before the second stage of parasitemia frequently prevents development of clinical sarcocystosis in cattle.[58] Successful treatment of one horse with sarcocystosis using phenylbutazone, trimethoprimsulfa, and pyremethamine is reported.

Control involves preventing gross contamination of cattle and equine feeds with carnivore feces. The common use of ionophore antibiotics (e.g., growth promotants and coccidiostats) in cattle is also likely to help reduce the incidence of sarcocystosis.

REFERENCES

50. Dubey JP, Fayer R: Sarcocystis, toxoplasmosis, and cryptosporidiosis in cattle, *Vet Clin North Am* 2:293-298, 1986.
51. Briggs M, Foreyt W: Sarcocystosis in cattle, *Compend Cont Educ* 7:S396-S400, 1985.
52. Edwards GT: Prevalence of equine sarcocystis in British horses and a comparison of two detection methods, *Vet Rec* 115:265-267, 1984.
53. Dubey JP: A review of sarcocystis of domestic animals and of other coccidia of cats and dogs, *J Am Vet Med Assoc* 169:1061-1078, 1976.
54. Leek RG, Fayer R, Johnson AJ: Sheep experimentally infected with sarcocystis from dogs. I. Disease in young lambs, *J Parasitol* 63:642-650, 1977.
55. Dubey JP: Abortion and death in goats inoculated with sarcocysts from coyote feces, *J Am Vet Med Assoc* 178:700-703, 1981.
56. Fayer R, Elsasser TH: Bovine sarcocystosis: how parasites negatively affect growth, *Parasitol Today* 7:250-255, 1991.
57. Traub-Dargatz JL et al: Multifocal myositis associated with *Sarcocystis* sp in a horse, *J Am Vet Med Assoc* 205:1574-1576, 1994.
58. Fayer R: Sarcocystis: a clinical entity in bovine practice, *Bovine Pract* 14:117-119, 1982.

■ *Nutritional and Toxic Myopathies*

NUTRITIONAL MYODEGENERATION

JOHN MAAS
STEVEN M. PARISH
DAVID R HODGSON
STEPHANIE J. VALBERG

DEFINITION AND ETIOLOGY. Nutritional myodegeneration (NMD) (white muscle disease, stiff lamb disease, nutritional muscular dystrophy) is a peracute to subacute myodegenerative disease of cardiac and skeletal muscle caused by a dietary deficiency of selenium or vitamin E.[59-61] This syndrome occurs in most farm animal species but is most commonly found in young, rapidly growing calves, lambs, kids, and foals, particularly those born to dams that consumed selenium-deficient diets during gestation. The disease has also been reported in yearling and adult cattle and has been suspected in adult horses.

Selenium and vitamin E appear to be synergistic in preventing NMD. However, on the basis of prophylaxis and response to treatment, selenium deficiency appears to be the most important.

CLINICAL SIGNS. There are two distinct syndromes of NMD; a cardiac form and a skeletal form. The cardiac form is associated with signs of peracute to acute myocardial decompensation, but the skeletal form is associated with skeletal myasthenia and difficulty in ambulation. In both forms the most rapidly growing animals in the herd or flock are affected commonly.

Most cases of NMD are diagnosed during the first year of life. Evidence also suggests that an in utero form of NMD may occur with affected animals born with myodegeneration or developing myodegeneration soon after birth.

The cardiac form of NMD usually has a sudden onset; it is usually diagnosed in the animal that is either in a state of severe debilitation or dead. The cardiac form often presents with lesions in the heart, diaphragm, and intercostal muscles. In dead animals there may be evidence of sudden agonal death. In living animals there is usually a rapid onset of depression and respiratory distress. A foamy nasal discharge, possibly blood stained, is seen often, resulting from pulmonary edema and dyspnea. Profound weakness, recumbency, and a rapid, often irregular heartbeat may be detected. Cardiac murmurs are heard occasionally on auscultation. Rectal temperature is normal usually or may be elevated because of increased muscular work associated with respiratory efforts. Most calves are depressed with dyspnea, tachypnea, and increased rectal temperature. These cases must be differentiated from pneumonia. The clinical course is frequently short with death occurring commonly in less than 24 hours despite medical therapy. Occasionally an animal responds to therapy, but they often fail to thrive because of residual myocardial damage. Animals with predominantly cardiac signs may also manifest mild skeletal muscle problems associated with NMD.

The skeletal form of NMD frequently has a slower onset characterized by muscular weakness or stiffness. Animals may be recumbent and unable to stand. Those that are able to rise on their own or with assistance show muscle weakness, trembling of limb muscles, or stiffness. Stiffness is more pronounced as fibrosis occurs following an acute attack. Most affected animals are able only to remain standing for short periods. Supporting muscle groups of the front and hind limbs may appear swollen and may be hard and painful on palpation. Commonly affected muscle groups may include the gastrocnemius, semitendinosus, semimembranosus, and biceps femoris and muscles of the lumbar, gluteal, and neck regions. If the diaphragm and intercostal muscles are affected, the animal may show respiratory distress and evidence of increased abdominal effort when breathing. Cardiomyopathy occurs often, along with changes in the diaphragm and intercostal muscles. The muscles of the tongue may be involved, resulting in dysphagia. Dysphagia may be the only sign in some affected animals, foals and lambs present in this manner more often than calves. The rectal temperature is normal or moderately elevated resulting from pain and the release of myoglobin associated with myodegeneration. Some animals exhibit what appears to be abdominal pain with violent thrashing. Heart sounds are normal usually, although the heart rate may be increased; however, myocardial damage and signs consistent with cardiac dysfunction may be present in cases of skeletal NMD. Animals with skeletal NMD often respond favorably to treatment and rest. Improvement is evident after a few days, and within 3 to 5 days animals can often stand and walk.

Differentiation of NMD from other diseases causing sudden death or recumbency is important. Infectious diseases resulting in septicemia, pneumonia, and toxemia may have similar presenting signs. Acute heart failure resulting from cardiac anomalies, cardiotoxic agents such as those found in plants, (oleander, cassia, yew, white snakeroot, and gossypol toxicity from cottonseed), and the ionophore antibiotics should also be considered. Other diseases causing stiffness of gait, weakness, and recumbency with no change in mental status must be differentiated from NMD. Spinal cord compression, cerebellar disease, suppurative and nonsuppurative meningitis/myelitis, polyarthritis, neurotoxins such as organophosphates, tetanus, pelvic fractures, and parasitic myositis all can cause recumbency. Clostridial myositis and traumatic injuries to muscles, long bones, and joints should be considered. Diseases characterized by abdominal pain may resemble NMD, because they may also cause stiffness of gait, weakness, and recumbency.

CLINICAL PATHOLOGY. Significantly elevated CK, AST, and LDH activities occur during the acute phase of myodegeneration. In clinical cases CK activities are in the thousands of IU/L. In animals recumbent because of a disease other than NMD, CK is elevated only into the hundreds or perhaps to a few thousand IU/L in heavy animals. Progressively decreasing activities of CK can be used as a prognostic indicator of a reduction in the myodegenerative process.

In foals, other reported abnormal laboratory findings include variable hyperkalemia, hyperphosphatemia, hyponatremia, and hypochloremia.[62] Myoglobinuria is found often in foals and yearling cattle with NMD. Myoglobinuria is less common in younger calves. Evidence of dehydration, reflected by elevated serum protein concentrations and hemoconcentration, is common in nonambulatory animals unable to nurse or drink water.

The selenium status of an animal or members of a group can be determined by laboratory analysis of tissue biopsies and whole blood (Table 40-1). Vitamin E status can be determined on plasma samples. In the clinical approach, blood sampling is frequently used. Blood or plasma samples provide information about the circulating levels of selenium and vitamin E, respectively, and are satisfactory for assessing intermediate to long-term nutritional status; however, short-term supplementation or injections can confuse interpretation of circulating levels of selenium or vitamin E. Tissue biopsies and tissue specimens obtained at slaughter and necropsy provide an indication of storage and can also be used to assess herd status and success of supplementation. Whole blood selenium analysis is preferred over plasma and serum.[63] Whole blood selenium concentrations ranging from 0.07 to greater than 0.1 ppm (μg/g) are considered normal in large animals. Normal liver concentrations of selenium are 0.9 to 1.75 μg/g of dry matter (DM), 0.9 to 3.5 μg/g DM, and 1.05 to 3.5 μg/g DM for cattle, sheep, and horses, respectively.[64] Selenium-dependent glutathione peroxidase (GSH-Px) formed in the red cells during erythropoiesis also provides an index of body selenium status. Cross-reacting enzymes, such as glutathione reductase, are not found in erythrocytes.

Adequate GSH-Px activities are greater than 30 U/mg of hemoglobin per minute in cattle, 60 to 180 U/mg of hemoglobin per minute in sheep, and 20 to 50 U/mg of hemoglobin per minute in horses. However, GSH-Px reference values are only specific to the laboratory where the analysis is performed and must be validated by comparison with blood selenium concentration. The activity of GSH-Px in red blood cells of domestic species remains constant for 4 to 6 days when maintained at 39° F (4° C); after this time significant decreases occur. The critical concentration of vitamin E (alpha-tocopherol) in plasma is 1.1 to 2 ppm (μg/g) in large animals. Vitamin E deteriorates rapidly in plasma samples. Therefore, plasma samples for alpha-tocopherol analysis need to be put on ice immediately, protected from the light by wrapping in tin foil, and stored ($-21°$ F, $-70°$ C) if analysis is to be delayed.

PATHOPHYSIOLOGY. The effects of selenium and vitamin E deficiency have been postulated to result, at least in part, from the destruction of cell membranes and proteins leading to a loss of cellular integrity.[59,65] Selenium, which has been shown to be an essential component of at least five selenoproteins[66]: three glutathione peroxidase enzymes, a deiodinase in liver and kidney that converts T_4 to T_3, and selenoprotein-P (a plasma protein of unknown function), and vitamin E (alpha-tocopherol), serve as biologic antioxidants. During normal cellular metabolism highly reactive forms of oxygen (free radicals) are produced. These include hydrogen peroxide, hydroperoxides, lipoperoxides, superoxide, various hydroxy radicals, and singlet oxygen. Vitamin E is active within the cell membrane as a lipid-soluble antioxidant that scavenges free radicals that otherwise might react with unsaturated fatty acids to form lipid hydroperoxides. In contrast, GSH-Px destroys hydrogen peroxide and lipoperoxides that have already been formed and converts them to H_2O or relatively harmless alcohols. Other enzymes such as catalase and superoxide dismutase are also involved in this protective process.

Apparently important interrelationships exist between the selenium and vitamin E status of the animal, the level of polyunsaturated fatty acids (PUFA) in the diet,[59,65] and NMD, particularly in ruminants.[59] PUFAs of dietary origin can undergo peroxidation to hydroperoxides forming toxic free radicals. During active growing periods pasture grasses and plants contain high concentrations of linolenic acid, a PUFA. Under normal conditions the rumen is thought to be important in saturating dietary unsaturated fatty acids. However, concentrations of PUFAs in the plasma often increase in calves recently turned out to pasture, possibly enhancing the chance of free radical formation and tissue damage. This indicates that the capacity of the various protective mechanisms can be overwhelmed by dietary factors such as high levels of PUFA. Not surprisingly selenium- or vitamin E–deficient animals may be at a greatly increased risk of tissue oxidative damage when exposed to such diets. However, the potential for induction of NMD by this process should not be overemphasized because calves on a milk diet may be severely affected.

TABLE 40-1

Deficient, Marginal, and Normal Concentrations of Whole Blood Selenium and GSH-Px Activities in Sheep and Cattle[67,71]

Whole Blood Selenium (ppm)*	GSH-Px (U/mg Hb/min)	Category	Interpretation
0.01-0.04	0-15	Deficient	Selenium supplementation is always beneficial
0.05-0.06	15-25	Marginal	Selenium supplementation is often beneficial
>0.07	25-500	Normal	Selenium supplementation is never beneficial

*GSH-Px, Glutathione peroxidase; PPM, parts per million.
GSH-Px assays are performed by different procedures in individual laboratories and quantitative relationships between blood selenium concentrations and blood GSH-Px activities can vary. These numeric relationships are site specific and interpretation must account for these differences.

The precise interrelationships between selenium, vitamin E, other metabolic factors, and triggering mechanisms in NMD are not fully understood because many animals deficient in selenium or vitamin E have no evidence of muscle disease. In certain situations, deficiencies of both selenium and vitamin E are necessary for disease to occur. In other animals NMD can occur when a deficiency of only one of the agents is present and the other is normal in blood and tissues.

EPIDEMIOLOGY. NMD occurs in all farm animals and is seen most commonly in young, rapidly growing calves, lambs, kids, and foals. The occurrence of NMD in very young animals usually reflects a deficiency in their dams during a substantial portion, if not all, of the gestation period. The selenium and GSH-Px values of neonatal calves tend to be similar to those of their dams. [67,68]

Marginally to severely selenium-deficient areas occur throughout a large portion of the United States and other countries of the world. [59,69] Forages and grains produced in the northeastern and eastern seaboards and northwestern regions of the United States are particularly deficient because of low soil levels of selenium. Acid soils and those originating from igneous (volcanic) rock are often selenium deficient, as are those having high sulfur content or soils treated with sulfur-containing fertilizers. Sulfur inhibits selenium uptake by plants and absorption by animals. Different forages in a specific area will also vary in their selenium content. Legumes take up less selenium than do grasses. Also, forage selenium concentrations are lowest during periods of rapid growth such as in the spring and during times of highest rainfall.

Vitamin E deficiency occurs most commonly when animals are fed poor quality hay, straw, or root crops. Grain treated with propionic acid and having high moisture content is commonly vitamin E deficient. Storage of grain crops for extended periods results in marked decreases in their vitamin E content. Calves fed milk replacers containing fish oil, linseed oil, soybean or corn oil, all of which increase the dietary levels of unsaturated fatty acids, require increased dietary supplementation of vitamin E to avoid deficiency. In contrast, cereal grains, green growing pastures, and properly prepared hay usually have adequate vitamin E.

In young ruminants the majority of cases of NMD occur in calves, 2 to 4 months of age, during the spring and summer months in association with exercise when at pasture, although congenital and perinatal cases do occur. Histologic lesions consistent with NMD have also been seen in late-term aborted fetuses. [64] These findings are suggestive of an in utero form of NMD in large animals. Yearling cattle housed during the winter, fed diets high in grain with high moisture content, and then turned out in the spring may also be affected. Lambs born in confinement and turned out to pasture at 1 to 3 weeks of age frequently develop signs of NMD. Stresses such as transport, herding, and driving may also precipitate signs of NMD. In horses, NMD generally occurs during the first year of life with most cases observed from birth to weaning. [60,70]

NECROPSY FINDINGS. Bilaterally symmetric myodegeneration is a consistent finding in NMD. Skeletal muscle degeneration is characterized by pale discoloration and a dry appearance of affected muscle, white streaks in muscle bundles, calcification, and intramuscular edema. The white streaks seen in muscle bundles represent bands of coagulation necrosis or, in chronic cases in which insults may have occurred weeks before, may represent fibrosis and calcification. Affected muscle bundles are often adjacent to apparently normal or minimally affected muscle. The color of normal muscle in young calves is pale because of reduced myoglobin concentrations; therefore, close inspection and histologic examination are necessary in cases of suspected NMD. Cardiac muscle undergoes changes similar to those of skeletal muscle. In calves the left ventricle and septum are most frequently involved, but in lambs both ventricles are usually involved. Myocardial degeneration usually extends through the full thickness of the ventricular wall.

Histologically, affected muscle fibers may be hypercontracted and fragmented with some mineralization of muscle fibers and others undergoing macrophage infiltration. In yearling cattle, type I muscle cells are more frequently affected.

TREATMENT AND PROGNOSIS. In the cardiac form of NMD myocardial damage is often extensive and incompatible with life. Only rarely is treatment successful. In contrast, the skeletal form of NMD is more generally amenable to treatment, although the prognosis for clinical recovery from the skeletal form of NMD is guarded and depends often on whether secondary complications such as respiratory disease develop. In all cases of NMD, therapy should involve specific supplementation with selenium and vitamin E and general supportive care.

Alleviation of selenium-responsive NMD requires the use of injectable selenium products. These are available with selenium concentrations varying from 1 mg of selenium per milliliter to 5 mg/ml, with all products containing 50 mg/ml (68 IU) of vitamin E as DL-alpha-tocopheryl acetate. The label dose for selenium is 0.055 to 0.067 mg/kg (2.5 to 3 mg/ 45 kg) body weight given intramuscularly or subcutaneously. Dosage of these injectable products should not be greatly increased above the label dose to prevent an inadvertent selenium toxicosis. However, when using the vitamin E/selenium combinations, the amount of vitamin E in these combination products is present as a preservative for the solution and is, therefore, insufficient for vitamin E supplementation. Injectable vitamin E products are now available that contain 300 IU vitamin E per milliliter as D-alpha-tocopherol.* Administration of these products increases the tissue and/or plasma level of vitamin E activity for approximately 3 weeks in farm animals. The bioavailability of vitamin E from injectable products is dependent on the form of vitamin E (the alcohol form: D-alpha-tocopherol being the most active) and the amount and quality of the solution emulsifier used. Bioavailability data on injectable vitamin E products should receive careful clinical consideration. Oral supplementation is the general approach to provide additional dietary levels of vitamin E. Recommended levels of supplementation for calves range from 15 to 60 mg of DL-alpha-tocopheryl acetate per kg of dry feed. [69] For horses a daily supplement of 600 to 1800 mg of DL-alpha-tocopheryl acetate has been recommended. [70] Oral alpha-tocopherol is now available for all species and contains 500 IU vitamin E per milliliter.† The recommended dosage of this product is 1 to 3 IU/lb body weight.

Studies with injectable selenium show that absorption and distribution occur rapidly. [71] It is thought that incorporation of selenium into heart, skeletal muscle, and other tissues may be very rapid and could account for the rapid improvement in clinical signs seen in reversible cases. The discovery of four new selenoproteins may help explain these clinical observations. [66] This improvement can occur even though blood GSH-Px activity rises slowly because of the delay caused by erythropoiesis and release of red cells from the bone marrow. [71] However, platelet GSH-Px activity rises within hours and may be a more accurate reflection of changes in muscle and other tissues.

Supportive therapy may include administration of antibiotics to help combat secondary pneumonia and infected decubital lesions that are common in recumbent patients. Provision of adequate energy intake and attention to the fluid

---

*Vital E, Schering-Plough Animal Health, Kenilworth, NJ 07033.
†Emcelle, Stuart Products, Inc.

and electrolyte balance are of critical importance if recovery is to be successful.

PREVENTION AND CONTROL. The prevention and control of NMD are achieved through supplementation of selenium and vitamin E. Although selenium deficiency is implicated more commonly in most NMD syndromes, attempts to ensure adequate provision of selenium and vitamin E should be undertaken. Under current U.S. federal regulations, selenium can be incorporated into the total ration of ruminants and other species to a level of 0.3 parts per million (ppm). In salt/mineral mixtures formulated for free choice feeding, selenium can be incorporated at 90 ppm for sheep and 120 ppm for cattle. In certain areas or in herds, levels as high as 200 ppm selenium in salt/mineral mixtures may be necessary to maintain adequate selenium levels in the animals. Federal regulations limit the intake of supplemental selenium by sheep to 0.7 mg/head/day and by cattle to 3 mg/head/day. The use in ruminants of rumenoreticular boluses, which release a precise amount of selenium daily, has been commonplace in many countries of the world and is currently possible under the FDA guidelines in the U.S. as long as selenium release does not exceed 3 mg per day. These slow-release boluses can replace supplementation by salt mixtures or by injections and are extremely valuable in extensive grazing systems. Alternatively, individual animals can be supplemented by periodic (30- to 60-day intervals) injections of selenium/vitamin E preparations to help maintain body concentrations and assist in transplacental transfer of selenium to the fetus.

Oral supplementation for horses at 1 mg of selenium per day increases blood selenium concentrations above levels known to be associated with NMD.[63] Supplementation of pregnant mares is advised in areas known to be selenium deficient; however, only limited selenium may cross the placenta.[61] Supplementation during lactation increases the levels of selenium in milk and thus provides a potential means of selenium supplementation in foals; however, evidence in cattle indicates that this increased level of selenium in milk may not meet nutrient requirements.[67-69]

Regardless of the method of supplementation, periodic blood (or tissue) sampling of animals at risk is necessary to ensure maintenance of desired levels of selenium. In high-risk areas, samples should be taken every 60 to 90 days to determine selenium status in susceptible animals and every 6 to 12 months to monitor supplementation. On the basis of these assessments, adjustments to the rate or extent of selenium supplementation may be made.

Feeding animals properly prepared and stored hay and grain or allowing them access to high-quality green forage should ensure adequate vitamin E intake.

REFERENCES

59. McMurray CH, Rice DA: Vitamin E and selenium deficiency diseases, *Irish Vet J* 36:57-67, 1982.
60. Dill SG, Rehbun WC: White muscle disease in foals, *Compend Cont Ed* 7:S627-S636, 1985.
61. Maylin GA, Rubin DS, Lein DH: Selenium and vitamin E in horses, *Cornell Vet J* 70:272-289, 1980.
62. Perkins G et al: Fluid, electrolyte and renal abnormalities associated with acute rhabdomyolysis in four neonatal foals, *J Vet Int Med* 12:173-177, 1998.
63. Maas J et al: The correlation between serum selenium and blood selenium in cattle, *J Vet Diagn Invest* 4:48-52, 1992.
64. Taylor RF, Puls R, MacDonald KR: Bovine abortions associated with selenium deficiency in western Canada, *Proceedings of the Twenty-second Annual Meeting of the American Association of Veterinary Laboratory Diagnosticians*, 1979, pp 77-84.
65. Moncada S, Vane JR: Arachidonic acid metabolites and the interaction between platelets and blood vessel walls, *N Engl J Med* 300:1142-1147, 1979.
66. Burk RF, Hill KE: Regulation of selenoproteins, *Annu Rev Nutr* 13:65-81, 1993.
67. Campbell DT et al: Safety and efficacy of two sustained-release intrareticular selenium supplements and the associated placental and colostral transfer of selenium in beef cattle, *Am J Vet Res* 51:813-817, 1990.
68. Koller LD, Whitbeck GA, South PJ: Transplacental transfer and colostral concentrations of selenium in beef cattle, *Am J Vet Res* 45:2507-2510, 1984.
69. *Nutrient requirements of beef cattle*, ed 5 (revised), Washington, DC, 1976, National Academy of Science, p 14.
70. Roneus BO et al: Vitamin E requirements of adult standardbred horses evaluated by tissue depletion and repletion, *Equine Vet J* 18:50-58, 1986.
71. Maas J et al: Intramuscular selenium administration in selenium-deficient cattle, *J Vet Intern Med* 7:342-348, 1993.

TOXIC CAUSES OF RHABDOMYOLYSIS

MICHAEL MURPHY
STEPHANIE J. VALBERG

Ingestion of toxic substances in feed or forage is a common cause of toxic rhabdomyolysis. Common feed toxins include gossypol and ionophores. Gossypol is of greatest significance in swine. Monogastrics, including young calves, should not ingest feed containing more than 200 ppm gossypol. Mature ruminants may tolerate 20 g of gossypol/head/day. This normally amounts to 5 to 6 lb of whole cottonseed per head per day.[72]

Ionophores are commonly added to feeds for their growth promotion and coccidiostat properties. Species differences in sensitivity to ionophores and the variety of ionophores on the market have led to several cases of ionophore-induced toxicosis. Rhabdomyolysis and cardiomyopathies are common sequelae to ionophore toxicosis. Experimental studies have indicated that LD50 values for monensin are 2-3, 12, 17, 26, and 21-36, for horses, sheep, pigs, goats, and cattle, respectively. Feed concentrations of 100 g/ton and 400 g/ton have been fatal to sheep and cattle, respectively.[73,74] Newborn calves dosed with 100 mg lasalocid 3 times daily, for cryptosporidiosis, experience muscle necrosis.[75] Other ionophores include naracin, salinomycin, and laidlomycin. Ionophores are quickly eliminated.

The two common forage toxins are *Cassia* sp and tremetone-containing plants. Grazing livestock that ingest *Cassia obtusifolia* (sicklepod) seeds experience muscle necrosis. Sicklepod is prevalent in the southeastern United States.[76]

Horses that ingest 0.5% to 2% of body weight of tremetone-containing plants are likely to die.[77] Other grazing livestock are likely to be affected by ingestion of 2% of body weight. Tremetone has been identified in white snakeroot (*Eupatorium rugosum*) and rayless goldenrod (*Isocoma wrightii*). White snakeroot grows in shaded areas of the eastern and central United States.[78] Rayless goldenrod is common in the Southwest on open pastures. Tremetone remains active in hay, and in the stalks of the dead plants on pasture, so both the fresh and the dried form of the plants should be kept from livestock.[79,80] A number of horses have died from rhabdomyolysis while grazing pastures but an etiology for this pasture myopathy has not been described.[81]

Several chemical agents have been associated with muscle necrosis on rare occasions. Parenteral products, insecticides, and feed contaminants have been implicated. Muscle necrosis has been reported in cattle and pigs after receiving injections of: lidocaine, diazepam, digoxin, levamisole, nitroclofene, pentazocine, thiazinamium. chloramphenicol, nitroclofene, and oxytetracycline and in horses after injectable ivermectin administration.[82-84] Animals with organophosphate toxicosis—particularly to parathione, may develop muscle necrosis.[85,86] One of 70 horses poisoned with blister beetles developed muscle necrosis.[87]

REFERENCES

72. Elanco Technical Manual, second printing, safety and toxicity, P1-H16, Indianapolis, Ind, 1980, Elanco Products.
73. Miller RE et al: Acute monensin toxicosis in stone sheep (*Ovis dalli stonei*), blesbok (*Damaliscus dorcus phillipsi*) and a bactrian camel (*Camelus bactrianus*), *J Am Vet Med Assoc* 196:131-134, 1990.

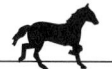

74. Geor RJ, Robinson WF: Suspected monensin toxicosis in feedlot cattle, *Aus Vet J* 62:130-131, 1985.

75. Benson JE et al: Lasalocid toxicosis in neonatal calves, *J Vet Diag Invest* 10:210-214, 1998.

76. Putnam MR et al: Evaluation of *Casia obtusifolia* (sicklepod) seed consumption in Holstein calves, *Vet Hum Toxicol* 30:316-318, 1988.

77. Beir RC et al: Isolation of the major component in white snakeroot that is toxic after miscosomal activation: possible explanation of sporadic toxicity of white snakeroot plants and extracts, *Nat Toxins* 1:286-293, 1993.

78. Olson Ctet al: Suspected tremetol poisoning in horses, *J Am Vet Med Assoc* 185:1001-1003, 1984.

79. Smetzer DL et al: Cardiac effects of white snakeroot intoxication in horses, *Equine Pract* 5:26-32, 1983.

80. Thompson LJ: Depression and choke in a horse: probable white snakeroot toxicosis, *Vet Hum Toxicol* 31:321-322, 1989.

81. Whitwell KE, Harris PA: Atypical myoglobinuria: an acute myopathy in grazing animals, *Equine Vet J* 20:357-363, 1988.

82. Steiness E et al: A comparative study of serum creatine phosphokinasae (CPK) activity in rabbits, pigs and humans after intramuscular injection of local damaging drugs, *Acta Pharmacol Toxicol* 42:357-364, 1978.

83. Ladage CA et al: Comparative macroscopic evaluation of muscle damage in rats and in cattle after intramuscular administration of some commercially available injectable medicines, Trends in veterinary pharmacology and toxicology, *Proceedings of the First European Congress* pp 34-40, 1980.

84. Kilgore RL et al: Response of horses to repeated intramuscular injections of ivermectin, *Vet Med Sm Anim Clin* 78:1894-1997, 1983.

85. Cavaliere MJ et al: Organophosphate myotoxicity, *Rev Saude Publ* 30:267-272, 1996.

86. Kibler WB: Skeletal muscle necrosis secondary to parathion, *Toxicol App Pharmacol* 25:117-122, 1973.

87. Helman RG, Edwards WC: Clinical features of blister beetle poisoning in equids: 70 cases. *J Am Vet Med Assoc,* 211:1018-1021, 1997.

▌ *Traumatic Rhabdomyolysis*

COMPARTMENT, DOWNER, AND MUSCLE CRUSH SYNDROME OF CATTLE

DAVID R. HODGSON

STEPHANIE J. VALBERG

Muscle damage commonly accompanies the downer syndrome in large animals. The downer syndrome is discussed in greater detail in Chapter 33. Animals weakened by disorders such as hypocalcemia are more prone to tearing adductor or semitendinosus/membranosus muscles in attempts to rise.[88,89] Initial traumatic laceration of muscle leads to edema and inflammation, both of which may exacerbate local tissue degenerative changes. Additionally, the weight of a recumbent animal on dependent muscle groups creates significant increases in intramuscular pressure resulting in decreased perfusion and ischemia of muscle and nerve.[88,89] Signs of weakness and peroneal or tibial nerve paralysis most commonly accompany this type of injury. Mild elevations in serum CK can be expected in cows that are recumbent but elevations greater than 5000 U/L usually indicate traumatic muscle damage. Treatment requires correcting the underlying cause of recumbency, fluid therapy if renal damage is evident, nonsteroidal antiinflammatories, good nursing care, adequate footing and bedding, and lifting or rolling the animal several times a day. Aquatherapy using float tanks for cattle also appears to be beneficial in relieving the pressure on muscle groups.

REFERENCES

88. Hulland TJ: Muscles and tendons. In Jubb KVF, Kennedy PC, Palmer N, eds: *Pathology of domestic animals,* ed 3, vol I, Orlando, Fla, 1985, Academic Press, pp 139-199.

89. Rehbun WC: *Diseases of dairy cattle,* Media, Pa, 1995, Williams & Wilkins, pp 403-404.

POSTANESTHETIC MYONEUROPATHY

Postanesthetic myoneuropathy is a condition that has become much more prevalent since the advent of inhalation general anesthesia. The disorder can be categorized as occurring in two forms: (1) localized myopathy-neuropathy, and (2) generalized myopathy somewhat similar to malignant hyperthermia.

Localized Myopathy-Neuropathy

CLINICAL SIGNS. Localized myopathy usually occurs in muscles that are in contact with a hard surface during anesthesia or those in which arterial blood supply is compromised through positional occlusion. Commonly affected muscles include triceps, deltoid, masseter, hind limb extensors, or, if the horse has been in dorsal recumbency, the hind limb adductor and gluteal muscles[90-92] (Fig. 40-3). Injury also may occur to nerves in these areas, resulting in temporary radial or femoral nerve paralysis. Clinical signs may be apparent on recovery or may be delayed for periods of up to 30 to 60 minutes after the horse has recovered from anesthesia. Affected muscles may be swollen, hot, and painful on deep palpation; and the horse is often reluctant to bear weight on the affected limb. Myasthenia (weakness) of affected muscles is common, particularly with peripheral nerve involvement. In some horses this condition may limit the animal's ability to stand for some time following anesthesia. The loss of muscle strength, particularly when involving adductor muscles, can contribute to orthopedic injury during repeated attempts to rise. Many horses with mild to moderate muscle injury recover over a period of hours to days even if untreated[90] (Fig. 40-4).

ETIOLOGY. A variety of factors acting alone or in combination have been suggested to contribute to this disorder. The most important factors include ischemia and hypoperfusion as a result of prolonged immobility, muscle compression, systemic hypotension, and hypoxia.[90-94] There is increased lactate efflux from dependent muscles during anesthesia in horses who develop a myopathy, supporting the contention that these muscles experience compromised perfusion.[93,94,95] Halothane anesthesia has a greater propensity than isoflurane to compromise tissue oxygen delivery even in nondependent muscles.[92] If mean arterial pressure is allowed to fall below 55 to 65 mm Hg for several hours during inhalation anesthesia, particularly if mechanical ventilation is used, the incidence of postanesthetic myopathy increases substantially.[94]

DIAGNOSIS. Diagnosis is based on a history of anesthesia or prolonged recumbency, clinical signs, and possibly clinical pathology examinations. Laboratory findings include elevations in serum CK and subsequently serum AST and serum

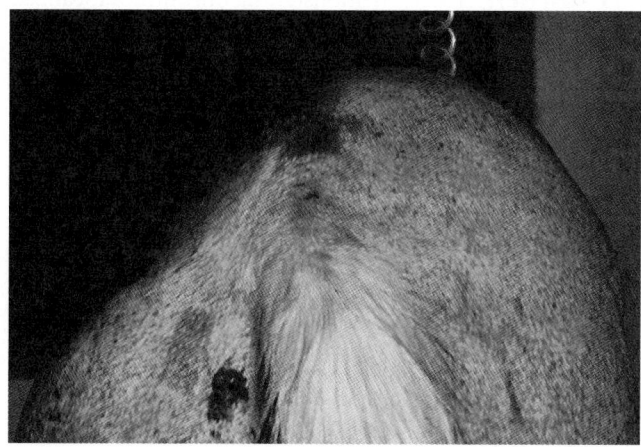

FIG. 40-3 ▌ Markedly swollen right gluteal muscle following anesthesia with a lack of adequate padding on the surgery table during dorsal recumbency. Atrophy developed 1 week later.

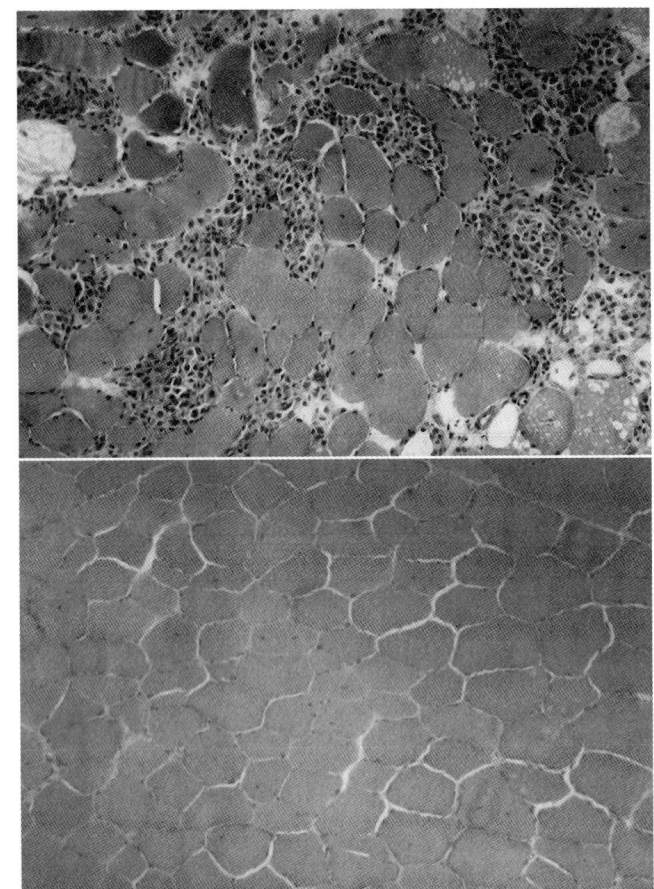

FIG. 40-4 ■ The remarkable ability of muscle to heal is demonstrated by biopsies of a horse following a postanesthetic myopathy with a serum CK greater than 100,000 U/L. **A,** The middle gluteal muscle 5 days after a postanesthetic myopathy developed. Numerous macrophages are engulfing degenerate myofibrils. **B,** The same area 5 weeks later. Many mature fibers are present, and some smaller fibers with centrally placed nuclei typical for regeneration (hematoxylin and eosin stain).

LDH activities. Elevations in CK activities of thousands to tens of thousands of IU/L are commonly demonstrated in horses with moderate forms of the myopathy.

TREATMENT. Horses demonstrating only minor localized manifestations of the myopathy usually have an uncomplicated recovery with little or no treatment.[90] Supportive care, including the use of antiinflammatory drugs, dimethyl sulfoxide and dantrolene sodium 2 to 4 mg/kg PO often is sufficient in mild to moderate cases. Significant muscle atrophy may develop over the ensuing 3 to 4 weeks but usually will resolve within 2 to 3 months. Treatment of more severe cases is outlined under generalized reactions.

CONTROL. Correct positioning and judicious use of padding and water- or air-filled mattresses can reduce dependent muscle pressure up to 50%, thereby aiding in the reduction of this disorder. In addition, by elevating the upper limb during anesthesia, the pressure on the lower limbs is significantly reduced. Pulling the lower forelimb forward also markedly reduces pressure in the dependent triceps muscle. When the horse is in dorsal recumbency, padding under the shoulders and hips is absolutely imperative.

Maintaining anesthesia at the lightest plane possible for a specific surgical procedure is beneficial in prophylaxis. Similarly, if possible, maintaining systemic mean arterial blood pressure above 80 to 85 mm Hg during anesthesia is advisable. The use of ionotropic agents such as dobutamine during anesthesia has been useful in reducing the occurrence of anesthetic myopathies. Administration of dantrolene sodium (2 to 4 mg/kg PO) 1 to 2 hours before induction of anesthesia may result in a reduction in the incidence of this myopathy in some susceptible horses.

Generalized Anesthetic Reactions

CLINICAL SIGNS. Postanesthetic reactions involving multiple muscle groups can result in clinical signs of anxiety, tachycardia, tachypnea, profuse sweating, and myoglobinuria.[91,92] Horses may not be able to rise and may struggle violently, resulting in prolonged, traumatic recoveries. In some cases a progressive increase in body temperature and muscular contractures may develop under anesthesia, and a fulminant metabolic and respiratory acidosis may be noted.[96,97] These animals can die within a matter of hours. In some cases, shock and pigmenturia may lead to renal failure.

PATHOGENESIS. The generalized form of myopathy cannot be explained by the compartmental syndrome alone. It has been suggested that systemic hypotension and hypoxemia may create local ischemic lesions, with the pathologic changes becoming more generalized as a result of the stress of anesthesia and the sensitivity of muscle cells to anesthetic agents or muscle relaxants.[90,94] Some similarities exist between malignant hyperthermia (MH) in humans and swine and the generalized postanesthetic reactions in horses.[96-99] Animals susceptible to MH develop clinical signs resulting from excessive calcium release by the sarcoplasmic reticulum. This induces muscle contracture, heat production, and the other associated clinical manifestations. In swine there is a genetic predisposition to the disorder, and MH is more frequent in pigs susceptible to porcine stress syndrome. Similarly, in horses an association between MH, exertional rhabdomyolysis, and postanesthetic myopathy has been suggested.[96-99] A number of stimuli may precipitate MH in other species, including stress, unaccustomed muscular activity, exposure to inhalation anesthetics, and muscle relaxants. Halothane and succinylcholine have been the most frequently implicated inciting agents in all susceptible species, including the horse.[96-98]

DIAGNOSIS. Diagnosis is based on clinical signs, particularly in horses undergoing inhalation anesthesia. Routine monitoring of body temperature during anesthesia may aid in the early detection of MH. Some animals may also demonstrate metabolic and respiratory acidosis and hyperkalemia.[97] In humans, individuals suspected of being susceptible to MH may be identified using a halothane-caffeine contracture test. Several horses showing signs of MH have had a positive response to this test.[98] However, the test is rather complex to perform and is not readily available nor feasible for detection of MH-susceptible horses at this time.

TREATMENT. Many severely affected cases provide a significant therapeutic challenge. Aims of therapy should include (1) relief of pain, (2) correction of fluid and electrolyte abnormalities, (3) attempts to prevent ongoing problems, and (4) high-quality nursing care.

Many of the same principles described for treatment of exertional rhabdomyolysis can be used for treatment of postanesthetic myoneuropathy (see p. 1287). In severely affected recumbent horses, pain relief and sedation may help prevent struggling and progression of the myopathy.[90,91] Detomidine combined with butorphanol is effective in reducing struggling. Violent struggling only exhausts the horse and increases the potential for further injury and muscle

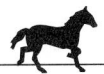

damage. Similarly, administration of nonsteroidal antiinflammatory drugs may help reduce ongoing degenerative changes in muscle. Dantrolene sodium 2 to 4 mg/kg PO every 6 to 8 hours decreases release of calcium from the sarcoplasmic reticulum, helping to break the cycle of muscle damage. Volume expansion and diuresis may prevent renal toxicity.[90]

The most common metabolic derangement with anesthetic-related myopathies is a metabolic or respiratory acidosis. If specific therapy for metabolic acidosis is necessary, intravenous administration of sodium bicarbonate can be used.[90,91] For optimum results, doses are calculated on the basis of the results of acid-base analysis. If facilities for acid-base analysis are not available and the horse appears severely compromised, intravenous administration of sodium bicarbonate at a dosage of 1 to 2 mEq/kg slowly is recommended. If hyperthermia and contracture develop during anesthesia, discontinuation of anesthesia is advisable. Additional attempts to cool the animal with alcohol or cold-water baths may also be indicated. Administration of a large amount of soluble, lyophilized dantrolene sodium for intravenous administration may alleviate clinical signs in these horses. However, availability and expense of the agent in this form restrict its use. A dosage rate of 1 mg/kg IV may be appropriate, although more controlled studies are required.[90]

Good nursing care is important in severely affected horses. This involves providing well-padded areas on which horses can lie. Prevention or minimization of trauma around the eyes and appropriate care of decubital sores are important. Recumbent animals may require frequent turning to allow reperfusion of compressed muscle masses. Continued fluid therapy with polyionic fluids and possibly caloric supplementation may be indicated. The use of slings to assist recumbent animals to rise also has been tried.[90] Recovery from the myopathy may occur with no apparent residual lesions. In contrast, recovery from some severe forms of the disorder may be accompanied by muscle atrophy, fibrosis, and scarring.[90]

PREVENTION. The principles described for localized myoneuropathies apply to the prevention of generalized anesthetic-related myopathies. In addition, dantrolene sodium has been shown to reduce the incidence of MH in susceptible humans and pigs. Similar effects might be anticipated in horses. Because of limited controlled studies, the dosage rate for prevention of MH in the horse is not clearly defined. Administration at a rate of 4 mg/kg PO 1 to 2 hours before anesthesia may be beneficial in reducing the incidence of MH.

REFERENCES

90. White NA II: Postanesthetic recumbency myopathy in horses, *Compend Cont Educ* 4:544-550, 1982.
91. Hennig GE, Court MH: Equine postanesthetic myopathy: an update, *Compend Cont Educ* 13:1709-1715, 1991.
92. Dodman NH et al: Postanesthetic limb adductor myopathy in 5 horses, *J Am Vet Med Assoc* 193:83-86, 1988.
93. Branson KR et al: The hemodynamic, tissue oxygenation and selected biochemical effects of isoflurane and halothane anesthesia in horses, *J Equine Vet Sci* 7:396-409, 1993.
94. Grandy JL et al: The relationship between arterial hypotension during halothane anesthesia and the development of equine postanesthetic myopathy, *Vet Surg* 14:73, 1985 (abstract).
95. Serteyn D et al: Myopathie postanesthesique equine: production de lactates par les muscles comprimes chez le cheval anesthesize a l'halothane, *Schwetiz Archiv Tierheikld* 129:19-22, 1987.
96. Hildebrand SV, Howitt GA: Succinylcholine infusion associated with hyperthermia in ponies anesthetized with halothane, *Am J Vet Res* 44:2280-2284, 1983.
97. Manley SV, Kelly AB, Hodgson DH: Malignant hyperthermia-like reactions in three anesthetized horses, *J Am Vet Med Assoc* 83:85-89, 1983.
98. Lentz LR et al: Abnormal regulation of contraction in equine recurrent exertional rhabdomyolysis, *Am J Vet Res* 60:992-999, 1999.
99. Ward TL et al: Skeletal muscle membrane activities in thoroughbred horses with exertional rhabdomyolysis, *Am J Vet Res* 61:242-247, 2000.

EXERTIONAL MYOPATHIES IN HORSES

STEPHANIE J. VALBERG
DAVID R. HODGSON

LOCAL MUSCLE STRAIN

Lumbar and Gluteal Muscles

Strain of lumbar and gluteal muscles is common in jumpers, dressage, and harness horses. Several factors may predispose horses to muscle strains, such as an inadequate warm-up, preexisting lameness, exercise to the point of fatigue, and insufficient training. Lameness is often mild and horses usually are reluctant to engage their hindquarters during exercise. Deep palpation of epaxial and gluteal muscles results in pain and dorsiflexion of the spine. Horses that show pain but resist dorsiflexion, ventroflexion, and lateral bending upon manipulation may have a myopathy secondary to an underlying disorder of the spine or sacroiliac joint.

Adductor Muscles

The gracilis muscle can be torn in horses and cause severe pain and occasionally recumbency. A careful physical examination reveals swelling of the medial thigh and pain upon palpation. Ultrasonography identifies the extent of disrupted muscle fibers.

TREATMENT. Adequate rest and nonsteroidal antiinflammatory medication form the basis for treatment. Hand walking once the initial stiffness has dissipated may be beneficial. In addition, massage and the intermittent application of heat may aid the healing process. Exercise should be resumed gradually preceded by an appropriate warm-up period in a long and low frame. Adequate conditioning should be ensured before starting strenuous exercise. Saddles should be checked for proper fit.

Semitendinosus and Semimembranosus Muscles
ANDREW DART

These muscles are frequently damaged in working Quarter Horses and in chronic cases result in a fibrotic myopathy. Tearing of the semitendinosus and sometimes the semimembranosus, biceps femoris, and gracilis muscles[100,101] at the point of a tendinous insertion is usually associated with work that requires abrupt turns and sliding stops. Horses caught in ropes or fences may struggle violently enough to induce sufficient trauma, allowing subsequent development of the myopathy.[100,101] In one report, 5 of 18 horses developed this condition secondary to intramuscular injections.[101] Recently a congenital form of fibrotic myopathy has been described. Affected animals are usually less than 12 months old when clinical signs characteristic of fibrotic myopathy are first evident. Horses affected with this form of the disorder frequently have no palpable thickening of affected muscles or tendons and no history or evidence of trauma.[100]

Affected muscles in acute cases are painful upon deep palpation and may appear warm. Chronically, hardened areas within the muscle may represent fibrosis and ossification. The lameness in chronic cases is usually most apparent at the walk and is characterized by an abrupt cessation of the anterior phase of the stride of the affected limb, causing the leg to jerk suddenly to the ground rather than continue its forward motion. Pain is not a feature in chronic fibrotic myopathy and manipulative tests have little, if any, effect on the degree of dysfunction. The stride has a short anterior phase with a characteristic hoof-slapping gait. The gait reflects a mechanical hind limb lameness that restricts normal function. Radiographs may indicate ossification of affected muscles.[100,101]

DIAGNOSIS. Serum activities of creatine kinase (CK) and aspartate aminotransferase (AST) are usually only mildly elevated. In addition to palpation, diagnosis can be confirmed by ultrasonography, thermography, or scintigraphy. Light microscopic evaluation of muscle biopsies is frequently normal in acute cases. Chronically fibrous replacement of muscle fibers is apparent.

TREATMENT. Several surgical procedures for correction of fibrotic myopathy have been described. These involve either excision[101] or transection[102] of the fibrotic part of the muscle or tenotomy of the tibial insertion of the semimembranosus tendon.[100] Excision of the fibrotic part of the muscle and tenotomy of the tibial insertion of the semimembranosus tendon are performed under general anesthesia. Excision or transection appears to produce more postoperative complications than the tenotomy.[100,101] However, according to reports, tenotomy has been reported only in a limited number of horses, and complete resolution of the gait abnormality may not occur.[103] In a modification of the procedure described by Irwin and Howell,[102] transection of the fibrotic mass under local anesthesia in the standing horse using a bistoury knife may be effective. A Penrose drain is inserted through a second incision ventral to the first, and light exercise is resumed the day after surgery. Healing is allowed to occur by second intention.

REFERENCES

100. Bramlage LR, Reed SM, Embertson RM: Semitendinosus tenotomy for treatment of fibrotic myopathy in the horse, *J Am Vet Med Assoc* 186:565-567, 1985.
101. Turner AS, Trotter GW: Fibrotic myopathy in the horse, *J Am Vet Med Assoc* 184:335-338, 1984.
102. Irwin DHG, Howell DW: Fibrotic myopathy, haematomas and scar tissue in the gaskin area of the thoroughbred, *J S Afr Vet Assoc* 52:65-66, 1981.
103. Adams SB: Biology and treatment of specific muscle disorders. In Auer JA, ed: *Equine surgery*, Philadelphia, 1992, WB Saunders, pp 926-927.

EXERTIONAL RHABDOMYOLYSIS

Exertional rhabdomyolysis (ER) is probably the most common muscle disorder in horses. It is a frequent cause of poor performance in a variety of breeds, including Standardbreds, Thoroughbreds, warmbloods, Arabians, Morgans, Quarter Horses, Appaloosas, and American Paint horses. ER is a complex syndrome that likely has numerous causes. In the past there has been a tendency to assume a common etiology for all exercise-related myopathies in horses; and numerous terms such as tying up, chronic intermittent rhabdomyolysis, azoturia, Monday morning disease, paralytic myoglobinuria, and exercise-associated myositis have been used for this syndrome.[104]

CLINICAL SIGNS. Classically, horses develop a stiff, stilted gait, with excessive sweating and a high respiratory rate during or after exercise. Most commonly, signs are seen after only 15 to 30 minutes of light exercise. Following exercise, horses may stretch out as if to urinate, become extremely reluctant to move their hindquarters, and in severe cases show signs of colic or become recumbent.[104,105] Attempts to move more severely affected animals may result in extreme pain, obvious anxiety, and possible exacerbation of the condition. Firm painful muscles may be palpated over the back and hind limb muscles. Scintigraphic evaluation of horses with rhabdomyolysis following exercise shows symmetrical damage to the gluteal, semitendinosus, and semimembranosus muscles. Myoglobinuria is a classic feature of more severely affected horses.[104,105] Endurance horses often show other signs of exhaustion including a rapid heart rate, dehydration, hyper-

thermia, synchronous diaphragmatic flutter, and collapse. Muscle cramping is not always consistent in endurance horses with ER.

ETIOLOGY. A number of factors appear to precipitate episodes of ER. Some successful athletic horses may experience one or two isolated episodes of rhabdomyolysis during their lifetime, suggesting that environmental influences play an important role in sporadic cases. Other horses, particularly young fillies, may have chronic episodes of rhabdomyolysis that compromise their ability to compete.[105,106] An inherent muscle dysfunction precipitated by certain triggering factors likely contributes to rhabdomyolysis in these horses. Thus ER is a description of a syndrome that has many causes. To identify the cause in individual horses it may be helpful to initially subdivide cases into those with sporadic or chronic ER. Causes for sporadic and chronic exercise-induced muscle damage are listed in Box 40-1.

Sporadic Exertional Rhabdomyolysis

DIAGNOSIS. Most cases of ER can be diagnosed on the basis of the animal's history and clinical signs. Confirmation of rhabdomyolysis requires determination of abnormally elevated serum creatine kinase (CK), serum aspartate aminotransferase (AST), and serum lactate dehydrogenase (LDH). Serum CK is often in the tens to hundreds of thousands of IU/L and AST in the thousands to tens of thousands.[107] The degree of elevation in enzymes reflects the time lapse between rhabdomyolysis and obtaining a blood sample, as well as the extent of myonecrosis. Pigmenturia is a common finding in severely affected horses.

ETIOLOGY

Overexertion. The most common cause of sporadic ER is exercise that exceeds the horse's underlying state of training. This includes both high-intensity exercise and endurance riding. Tears in the junctions between intracellular myofilaments (Z lines) are a common cause of postexercise muscle soreness in humans. The incidence of muscle stiffness and ER has been observed to increase during an outbreak of respiratory disease.[108] Both equine herpes virus 1 and equine influenza virus have been implicated as causative agents. Mild muscle stiffness with concurrent viral infections is likely the result of the release of endogenous pyrogens. More severe rhabdomyolysis may be due to exertion during a concurrent systemic infection or viral replication in muscle tissue. ER in endurance horses is covered in a section of this chapter, Exhaustion in Endurance Horses.

Electrolyte Imbalances. Electrolyte depletion in horses can occur as a result of dietary deficiency and losses in sweat with strenuous exercise. Sodium, potassium, magnesium, and calcium play key roles in muscle fiber contractility. With severe electrolyte depletion following exercise, serum electrolytes may be below normal ranges. These problems are common in endurance horses and are covered under Exhaustion in Endurance Horses. With chronic dietary depletion, however, serum concentrations may not reflect total body electrolyte imbalances. Work by Harris and Colles[109] established renal fractional excretions (FE) as a technique to evaluate electrolyte concentrations in horses with chronic ER. Normal values for FE are given in the section of this chapter on urinalysis. In the United Kingdom, horses with chronic ER had low fractional excretions of sodium and daily dietary supplementation of 2 oz NaCl resulted in abatement of clinical signs. Other horses had high phosphorus excretion, suggesting a dietary calcium:phosphorus imbalance, and decreasing bran while providing a daily calcium supplement (2 oz $CaCO_3$) was helpful in reducing clinical signs of ER. Hypokalemia has also been suggested to play a role in chronic ER.[110] Hypokalemia was determined as low red blood cell

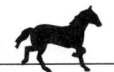

potassium concentrations, which may not reflect total body potassium or low muscle potassium concentrations. Supplementation with good quality forage or 1 ounce of KCl/day (Lite salt) is recommended for horses with low renal FE of potassium. Most horses fed on pasture or with high-quality hay do not appear to be potassium depleted.

Vitamin E and Selenium Deficiency. The increased oxidative metabolism associated with exercise results in the generation of free radicals. Selenium, acting via the enzyme glutathione peroxidase, and vitamin E, acting within the lipid component of cell membranes, scavenge free radicals and prevent lipid peroxidation of cell membranes. Primary selenium or vitamin E deficiency is common in young animals living in areas with selenium-deficient soil, however, it has rarely been demonstrated as a cause of ER. In fact, many horses with chronic ER have higher concentrations of selenium and vitamin E because of zealous dietary supplementation by owners.[111] It is not known whether horses that experience repeated episodes of ER may generate more free radicals than normal horses. A higher generation of free radicals in horses with chronic ER may explain the perceived benefit of repeated administration of selenium and vitamin E in Thoroughbred horses with recurrent ER. Adequate values for blood selenium are greater than 0.07 μg/ml and for serum vitamin E greater than 1.1 μg/ml.

Soluble Carbohydrates. Horses consuming a high grain diet appear to be more likely to develop ER than horses fed a low grain or fat diet. The reason for this is unclear and may differ between different forms of chronic ER. For example, in horses with polysaccharide storage myopathy, high soluble carbohydrate diets may enhance glycogen storage. In horses with recurrent ER, however, glycogen storage does not increase substantially even though serum CK activities are highest on high grain diets.[112] Dietary effects in recurrent ER may in part be related to the psychogenic effects of grain on excitability.

Hormonal Imbalances. A contribution of reproductive hormones to triggering ER has been postulated because the incidence of chronic ER appears to be highest in mares. Many owners report that episodes of rhabdomyolysis occur most commonly during estrus but, in one study of racehorses, no direct correlation was shown between progesterone fluctuations and serum CK activity.[113] It is likely that the estrus cycle is one of many factors that combine to trigger ER in susceptible horses. In some mares in whom episodes of ER coincide with estrus, suppression of estrus using progesterone implants or injections may be helpful. This should be done in conjunction with dietary and training alterations. Hypothyroidism has also been suggested as a cause of ER but never truly substantiated.

Lactic Acidosis. Although lactic acidosis has been postulated as a cause of ER a significant lactic acidosis never has been documented.[112,114,115] Horses are most prone to development of ER during submaximal exercise. Blood lactate and muscle lactate concentrations in Standardbreds, Thoroughbreds, and Quarter Horses developing rhabdomyolysis are substantially lower than those seen in healthy horses following racing. The most common metabolic derangement in horses with severe rhabdomyolysis is a hypochloremic metabolic alkalosis.[118] Thus there seems to be little scientific evidence to support this theory.

TREATMENT. The objective of treatment is to relieve anxiety and muscle pain, correct fluid and acid-base deficits, and prevent renal compromise. The hydration status of horses with myoglobinuria should be assessed immediately to avoid the combined nephrotoxic effects of dehydration, myoglobinuria, and nonsteroidal antiinflammatory drugs (NSAIDs). The first priority in horses with hemoconcentration, or myoglobinuria, is to reestablish fluid balance and induce diuresis. Balanced electrolyte solutions administered intravenously and through a nasogastric tube are most desirable. If possible,

fluid therapy with Ringer's lactate, saline, or 2.5% dextrose in 0.45% saline should be maintained until urine is clear. If the myopathy has occurred during an endurance ride, affected animals are usually alkalotic, making bicarbonate therapy inappropriate. Reassessment of the packed cell volume, total plasma protein concentration, and serum electrolytes after the initial period of therapy should provide a successful guide for the therapeutic regimen. In severely affected animals, regular monitoring of blood urea nitrogen and serum creatinine is advised to assess the extent of renal damage. Diuretics are usually contraindicated.

Acetylpromazine, an α-adrenergic antagonist, is helpful in relieving anxiety and may increase muscle blood flow. Its use is contraindicated in dehydrated horses. In horses that are in extreme pain, detomidine provides better sedation and analgesia. NSAIDs at relatively high doses provide pain relief. Intravenous dimethyl sulfoxide (as a <20% solution) and corticosteroid administration have also been advocated in the acute stage. Muscle relaxants such as methocarbamol seem to produce variable results, possibly depending on the dosage used.

Rest with hand walking once the initial stiffness has abated is of prime importance. At this time the diet should be changed to good-quality hay with little grain supplementation. The amount of rest a horse should receive is controversial. Horses with chronic problems with rhabdomyolysis appear to benefit from an early return to a regular exercise schedule. Horses that appear to have damaged their muscles from overexertion may benefit from a longer rest period with regular access to a paddock. Training should be resumed gradually and a regular exercise schedule that matches the degree of exertion to the horse's underlying state of training should be established. Endurance horses should be encouraged to drink electrolyte-supplemented water during an endurance ride and monitored particularly closely during hot humid conditions.

PREVENTION. Because the inciting cause is usually temporary, most horses respond to a few weeks of rest, dietary adjustments, and a gradual increase in training. The diet should be adjusted to include high-quality grass hay (or less than 50% alfalfa hay) and the minimum amount of soluble carbohydrate necessary (grains, sweet feed, molasses). If more than 3 to 5 kg/day of grain is necessary to maintain body weight, the addition of a fat source such as vegetable oil or rice bran should be considered. The horse should receive an electrolyte supplement on a daily basis that contains at least 1 oz of sodium chloride. A vitamin E and selenium supplement may be necessary in areas with low soil selenium. In addition, there are a myriad of treatments commercially available that are guaranteed to cure tying-up in horses. Many of these have yet to be scientifically tested for efficacy. Skeletal muscle shows remarkable ability to regenerate following injury. Following ER complete repair of muscle tissue is possible within 4 to 8 weeks.

Chronic Exertional Rhabdomyolysis

Many horses have repeated episodes of rhabdomyolysis with minimal exercise, even when the dietary and training recommendations for sporadic ER are followed. Forms of chronic ER are seen in many breeds of horses including Quarter Horses, American Paint horses, Appaloosas, Thoroughbreds, Arabians, Standardbreds, and Morgans. Current research suggests that many of these horses are susceptible to rhabdomyolysis because of an inherent disorder in muscle function.[116,117] Rhabdomyolysis in such horses occurs as a result of specific environmental circumstances that trigger muscle necrosis in genetically susceptible animals. Two heritable causes of chronic ER have recently been identified but there may be several others that are yet unidentified. These include a glycogen storage disorder called polysaccharide storage myopathy and a disorder of muscle contractility called recurrent exertional rhabdomyolysis.[119,120] Distinguishing between the various forms of chronic ER requires a thorough history, dietary evaluation, physical examination, determination of serum and urine electrolyte concentrations, blood vitamin E and selenium concentrations and histologic evaluation of muscle biopsies using special stains.

Polysaccharide Storage Myopathy

A subset of horses with chronic ER have been found to have a glycogen storage disorder characterized by the accumulation of glycogen and an abnormal polysaccharide in their muscle.[119] To date Quarter Horses, Paint, Appaloosa, draft, draft crossbreds, warmbloods, and a few Thoroughbred riding horses have been identified with polysaccharide storage myopathy (PSSM).[121,122]

DIAGNOSIS. A diagnosis of PSSM is based on histopathologic examination of muscle biopsies. The distinctive features of these muscle biopsies are subsarcolemmal vacuoles, high density of stains for glycogen in snap-frozen samples, and abnormal periodic acid–Schiff (PAS) positive inclusions in fast twitch fibers (Fig. 40-5). Other features that may be present include muscle necrosis, macrophage infiltration of myofibers, regenerative fibers, and occasionally atrophied type 2 fibers. Preincubation of muscle sections with amylase results in complete digestion of glycogen in normal horses. The PAS positive inclusions in horses with PSSM are very slow to digest, leaving distinctive residues that indicate an abnormal polysaccharide is present.[119] Analysis of the structure of polysaccharide in PSSM muscle by iodine spectra absorption indicates that it is less highly branched than normal muscle glycogen. A combination of β glycogen particles and a filamentous form of glycogen is also found on electron microscopy of PSSM-affected muscle.

CLINICAL SIGNS. Horses with PSSM often have a calm and sedate demeanor. Most horses have a history of numerous episodes of ER beginning with the commencement of training; however, mildly affected horses have only one or two episodes per year. Classic signs of mild rhabdomyolysis include a posture that resembles a urination stance, a tucked-up abdomen, muscle fasciculations during an episode, and pawing in the stall postexercise (Fig. 40-6). Serum CK activities are often increased by 1000 U/L or more 4 hours after 15 minutes of exercise at a trot.[119] Exercise intolerance, muscle atrophy, renal failure, and respiratory distress are less common presenting complaints. PSSM may also be a cause of severe rhabdomyolysis in weanling and yearling Quarter Horses and Paint horses without a history of exertion that usually have concurrent pneumonia. Elevations in serum muscle enzymes are usually present and may remain elevated for long periods even when rested. The severity of episodes of rhabdomyolysis can range from mild stiffness to severe pain resembling colic. Several horses have been euthanized because of the severity of muscle damage.

PATHOPHYSIOLOGY. Muscle glycogen concentrations determined biochemically in PSSM horses are often 1.5 to 4 times normal and glucose-6-P concentrations are up to 10 times normal.[115] Numerous inherited disorders of glycogen metabolism have been described in human beings. Glycogen accumulation occurs as a result of the inability to metabolize glycogen and during anaerobic exercise these patients are unable to produce lactic acid. Horses with PSSM are reluctant to perform anaerobic exercise, but when forced, can generate normal to high concentrations of lactic acid.[115] In addition, all of the activities of glycolytic enzymes are normal in PSSM Quarter Horses.[123] Thus glycogen accumulation in PSSM

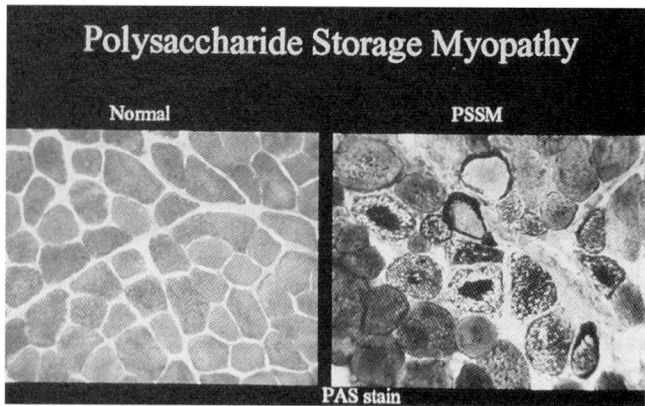

FIG. 40-5 ▮▮ A periodic acid–Schiff stain for glycogen in a normal horse and a horse with PSSM. Note the dark stain and aggregates of intensely staining abnormal polysaccharide in the biopsy from a horse with PSSM.

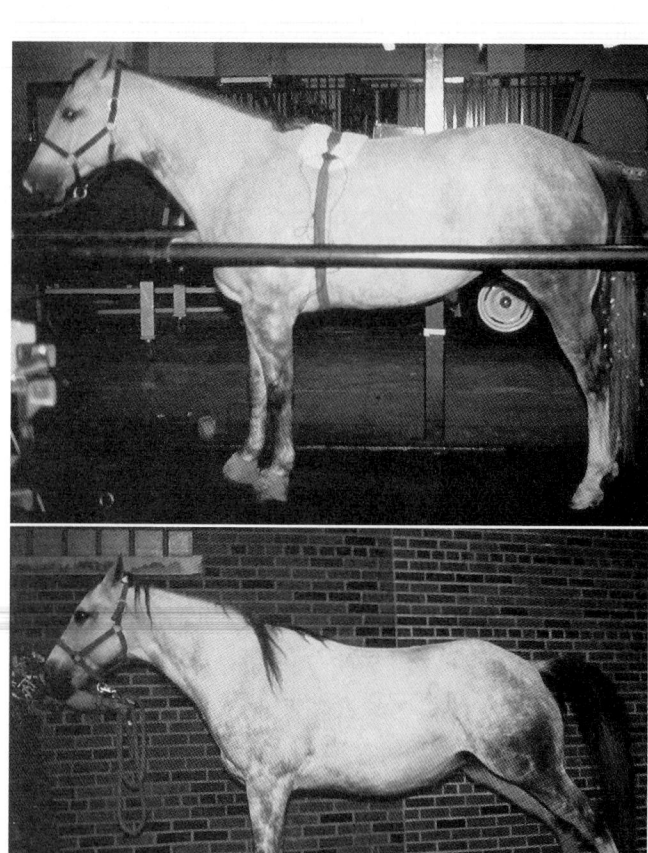

FIG. 40-6 ▮▮ A typical stance of a horse with PSSM. **A,** Before exercise on the treadmill. **B,** After 10 minutes of walking and trotting this horse often had a tucked-up abdomen, camped-out stance, and fasciculations in the flank in association with elevated serum CK.

horses does not appear to be due to an inability to metabolize glycogen. Rather, PSSM horses appear to have a novel defect characterized by enhanced glucose storage and glycogen synthesis. Following an intravenous or oral bolus of glucose, blood glucose clearance is 1.5 times faster in PSSM versus

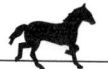

normal horses.[124] This occurs in the face of a measurable but lower insulin response. Administration of insulin to PSSM horses results in a much faster decline in blood glucose that persists for 4 hours even when fed grain compared to the establishment of glucose homeostasis within 2 hours in healthy horses. Thus PSSM horses appear to have enhanced insulin sensitivity, enhanced glucose clearance, and enhanced synthesis of glycogen and a less highly branched polysaccharide. The connection between increased synthesis of glycogen and rhabdomyolysis has yet to be explained.

An inherited trait is suggested in Quarter Horse–related breeds by the presence of two related sires five to seven generations back in the pedigrees of PSSM horses.[108] In addition, mares with PSSM have produced PSSM-affected foals.

TREATMENT AND PREVENTION. Treatment of horses with acute rhabdomyolysis is similar to that described for sporadic ER previously. Prevention of further episodes of rhabdomyolysis with PSSM is based on feeding diets without any grain and the addition of a fat supplement to maintain low blood glucose and insulin concentrations. A very gradual training program that includes daily exercise and ample turnout also has a significant impact on decreasing CK activity.[121] Most PSSM horses have competed successfully as pleasure and hunter horses when their diets are switched to good quality grass hay, no grain or sweet feed, and a fat supplement. A by-product of rice processing (rice bran)* that consists of 20% fat is recommended, or alternatively corn oil on alfalfa pellets can be used. Daily longing or riding and pasture access are essential. After a severe episode of rhabdomyolysis, a very gradual return to exercise is recommended. Longing horses for a maximum of 3 minutes the first day followed by the addition of a few more minutes of walk and trot each day for 3 weeks is recommended before the horse is ridden. Box stall rest for more than 12 hours per day appears to increase the incidence of rhabdomyolysis.

Draft horses have also been documented to have a form of polysaccharide storage myopathy referred to as EPSM.[122] Although some draft horses appear to have recurrent episodes of rhabdomyolysis similar to those described as Monday morning disease, others present with weakness and loss of muscle mass. Serum AST and CK are often only modestly elevated in weak horses and difficulty rising without assistance is frequently described. Some gait abnormalities including a "shivers"-like gait and difficulty backing have been associated with EPSM. Because of the expense of feeding rice bran to draft breeds, diets based on hay, alfalfa pellets, and up to 4 cups of corn oil with added vitamin E have been recommended. The prognosis is guarded in the animals with weakness and atrophy.

Recurrent Exertional Rhabdomyolysis

Recurrent episodes of muscle stiffness, sweating, muscle contractures, and reluctance to move occur commonly in racing Thoroughbreds, Standardbreds, and Arabian horses. Many of these horses likely have tying-up as a result of a defect in the regulation of muscle contraction termed recurrent exertional rhabdomyolysis (RER).

EPIDEMIOLOGY AND GENETICS. Most studies show that about 5% of Thoroughbred racehorses develop signs of muscle pain and cramping during a racing season.[106] About 75% of Thoroughbred racehorses with RER have at least four episodes of rhabdomyolysis and 25% have more than ten episodes in a 4-month racing season. Eighteen percent of horses with RER in one study were unable to race because of

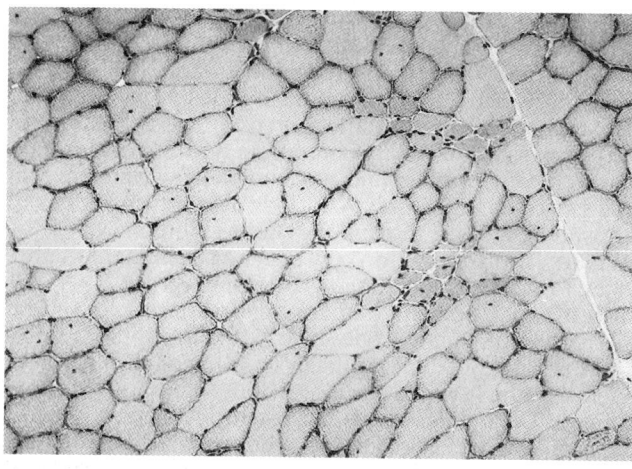

FIG. 40-7 ▌ Muscle biopsy of a horse with recurrent exertional rhabdomyolysis. Note the small regenerating fibers with central nuclei and numerous mature fibers with centrally placed nuclei (hematoxylin and eosin stain).

the recurrence of the disease.[106] If horses were able to race, no significant impact was detected on their performance.

One predisposing factor for RER appears to be inheritance of susceptibility to developing exercise-induced episodes of rhabdomyolysis.[117] Analysis of pedigrees of Thoroughbred horses from across the United States suggests that RER is an autosomal dominant trait. Furthermore, subsequent breeding trials confirm that the abnormal contracture test is inherited in an autosomal dominant fashion.[125]

Predisposing environmental factors that trigger rhabdomyolysis in susceptible horses include gender, temperament, diet, exercise duration and intensity, excitement, and lameness.[106] Females are most commonly afflicted with RER (67% female; 33% male), particularly those that are 2 years old and in race training. Nervous horses are five times more likely to develop RER, and horses with lameness are four times more likely to tie up. Susceptible horses receiving more than 5 kg of sweet feed are more likely to develop rhabdomyolysis than those receiving 2.5 kg of sweet feed/day.[112]

DIAGNOSIS. RER refers to a specific subset of Thoroughbred and likely Standardbred and Arabian horses with intermittent episodes of exercise-induced rhabdomyolysis. These horses have increased numbers of centrally located nuclei in muscle biopsies and normal muscle glycogen staining (Fig 40-7). In addition, RER is characterized by abnormal sensitivity of intact muscle bundles to contractures induced by caffeine or halothane in the muscle bath.[120,126] Although studies of muscle contraction indicate similarities to malignant hyperthermia in swine, biochemical studies of isolated muscle cell membranes have not identified a similar defect in the function of the calcium release channel in horses with RER.[127] Many Thoroughbreds with RER have developed rhabdomyolysis under halothane anesthesia.

CLINICAL SIGNS. Episodes often occur in horses once they become fit and are frequently associated with excitement at the time of exercise. In Thoroughbreds, rhabdomyolysis occurs most frequently during training when horses are held to a slow gallop. In Standardbreds, rhabdomyolysis often occurs 15 to 30 minutes into slow jogging. A history of poor performance and elevated serum AST and CK may be the only presenting complaints in some horses. Older Thoroughbreds used as riding horses may have very intermittent episodes of rhabdomyolysis associated with lay-ups of fit horses or with the steeplechase in 3-day events. Muscle stiffness and reluctance to collect may be present on a continual basis between episodes in some of these older horses. Arabian

---

*Natural Glow, Wollcott Farms, Rt. 2, Box 221, Willows, CA 95988, 1-800-680-8254; EquiJewel, KER, Versailles, KY 40383, (859) 873-1988.

horses often develop clinical signs with little exertion, frequently in association with excitement.

PREVENTION. RER appears to be an inherited disorder that is expressed when horses are subjected to the stress and rigors of training, particularly at a young age. Prevention of further episodes of RER in susceptible horses includes standardized daily routines and providing an environment that minimizes stress. This should include desensitizing horses to stressful situations, moving the stall to a quiet area of the barn, regular turnout, etc. Daily exercise is essential, whether in the form of turnout, longing, or riding.

In the past, horses have been box-stall rested for several weeks following an episode of RER. It is the author's opinion that this is counterproductive and increases the likelihood that the horses will develop RER when put back into training. The initial muscle pain usually subsides within 24 hours of acute RER and daily turnout in a small paddock can be provided at this time. Subsequently, a gradual return to performance is recommended once serum CK is within normal range.

The diet should be adjusted to include a balanced vitamin and mineral supplement, high-quality hay, and a minimum of carbohydrates (<3 to 5 kg) such as grain and sweet feed. Additional dietary fat supplements are helpful to maintain weight in nervous horses without providing excessive carbohydrates. Corn oil, rice bran, or commercial feeds with additional fat are helpful to maintain weight but avoid rhabdomyolysis in susceptible horses. The use of low doses of acetylpromazine tranquilizers (e.g., a dosage rate of approximately 0.005 to 0.01 mg/kg) 30 minutes before exercise in excitable horses is believed to help some horses.

Dantrolene 2 to 4 mg/kg PO given 1 hour before exercise is believed to be effective in preventing RER in some horses. Dantrolene is used to prevent malignant hyperthermia in humans and swine by decreasing the release of calcium from the calcium release channel. Phenytoin has also been advocated as a treatment for horses with RER. Dosages are adjusted in horses to maintain serum levels of 8 to 10 μg/ml. Initial doses begin at 6 to 8 mg/kg orally for 3 to 5 days. Doses can be increased by 1-mg/kg increments every 3 days until rhabdomyolysis is prevented but should be cut back if horses appear drowsy.[128] If possible, serum phenytoin concentrations should be assessed regularly at the initiation of treatment. Phenytoin acts on a number of ion channels within muscle and nerves including sodium and calcium channels. Unfortunately long-term treatment with dantrolene or phenytoin is expensive and efficacy has not been established.

REFERENCES

104. Hodgson DR: Exertional rhabdomyolysis. In Robinson NE, ed: *Current therapy in equine medicine*, vol 2, Philadelphia, 1987, WB Saunders, pp 487-490.
105. Beech J: Diagnosing chronic intermittent rhabdomyolysis, *Vet Med* 89:453-457, 1994.
106. MacLeay JM et al: Epidemiological factors influencing exertional rhabdomyolysis in thoroughbred racehorses, *Am J Vet Res* 60:1562-1566, 1999.
107. Valberg SJ et al: Muscle histopathology and plasma aspartate aminotransferase, creatine kinase and myoglobin changes with exercise in horses with recurrent exertional rhabdomyolysis, *Equine Vet J* 25:11-16, 1993.
108. Harris PA, Snow DH: Some factors influencing plasma AST/CK activities in thoroughbred racehorses, *Equine Vet J* 9(suppl):66-71, 1990.
109. Harris PA, Colles C: The use of creatinine clearance ratios in the prevention of equine rhabdomyolysis syndrome: a report of 4 cases, *Equine Vet J* 20:459-463, 1988.
110. Bain FT, Merritt AM: Decreases in erythrocyte potassium concentration associated with exercise-related myopathy in horses, *J Am Vet Med Assoc* 196:1259-1261, 1990.
111. Roneus B, Hakkarainen J: Vitamin E in skeletal muscle tissue and blood glutathione peroxidase activity from horses with azoturia-tying-up syndrome, *Acta Vet Scand* 26:425-426, 1985.
112. MacLeay JM et al: Effect of diet on recurrent exertional rhabdomyolysis in thoroughbreds, International Conference on Equine Exercise Physiology, *Equine Vet J Suppl* 30:548-562, 1999.
113. Frauenfelder HC, Rossdale PD, Rickets SW: Changes in serum muscle enzyme levels associated with training schedules and stages of oestrus cycle in thoroughbred racehorses, *Equine Vet J* 18:371-374, 1986.
114. Valberg S, Lindholm A, Hagendal J: Blood chemistry and skeletal muscle metabolic responses to exercise in horses with recurrent exertional rhabdomyolysis, *Equine Vet J* 25:17-22, 1993.
115. Valberg SJ et al: Skeletal muscle metabolic response to exercise in horses with polysaccharide storage myopathy, *Equine Vet J* 31:43-47,1999.
116. Valberg SJ et al: Familial basis of polysaccharide storage myopathy and exertional rhabdomyolysis in quarter horses and related breeds, *Am J Vet Res* 57:286-290, 1996.
117. MacLeay JM et al: Heritable basis for recurrent exertional rhabdomyolysis in thoroughbred racehorses, *Am J Vet Res* 60:250-256, 1999.
118. Koterba A, Carlson GP: Acid-base and electrolyte alterations in horses with exertional rhabdomyolysis, *J Am Vet Med Assoc* 180:303-306, 1983.
119. Valberg SJ, Cardinet III GH: Polysaccharide storage myopathy associated with recurrent exertional rhabdomyolysis in horses, *Neuromusc Disord* 5/6:351-359, 1992.
120. Lentz LR et al: Abnormal regulation of contraction in equine recurrent exertional rhabdomyolysis, *Am J Vet Res* 60:992-999, 1999.
121. Valberg SJ, MacLeay JM, Mickelson JR: Polysaccharide storage myopathy associated with exertional rhabdomyolysis in horses, *Comp Cont Ed* 19:1077-1086, 1997.
122. Valentine BA, Divers TJ, Lavoie JP: Severe equine polysaccharide storage myopathy in draft horses: clinical signs and response to dietary therapy, *Proceedings of the Forty-second Annual Convention of the American Association of Equine Practitioners*, 1996, pp 294-296.
123. Valberg SJ et al: Glycolytic capacity and phosphofructokinase regulation in horses with polysaccharide storage myopathy, *Am J Vet Res* 59:782-785, 1998.
124. De La Corte FD et al: Enhanced glucose uptake in horses with polysaccharide storage myopathy (PSSM), *Am J Vet Res* 60:458-462, 1999.
125. Valberg SJ: unpublished observation.
126. Beech J et al: Effect of phenytoin on the clinical signs and in vitro muscle twitch characteristics in horses with chronic intermittent rhabdomyolysis and myotonia, *Am J Vet Res* 49:2130-2133, 1988.
127. Ward TL et al: Skeletal muscle membrane activities in thoroughbred horses with exertional rhabdomyolysis, *Am J Vet Res* 61:242-247, 2000.
128. Beech J: Treating and preventing chronic intermittent rhabdomyolysis, *Vet Med* 89:458-461, 1994.

HEREDITARY/CONGENITAL MYOPATHIES

STEPHANIE J. VALBERG
DAVID R. HODGSON

EXERCISE INTOLERANCE ASSOCIATED WITH A MITOCHONDRIAL MYOPATHY

A deficiency of Complex 1, the first step in the mitochondrial respiratory chain, has been identified in a young Arabian filly that was presented for veterinary attention with clinical signs similar to ER.[129] In contrast to cases of ER, however, this horse showed no changes in serum creatine kinase following exercise. A marked lactic acidosis developed even with light exercise, and maximum oxygen consumption was drastically reduced, resulting in marked exercise intolerance. Histopathologic evaluation of muscle biopsies showed an abnormal increase in mitochondrial density, and biochemical analyses revealed a Complex 1 deficiency. The horse has shown slowly progressive signs of muscle atrophy but has otherwise remained healthy at rest.

REFERENCE

129. Valberg SJ et al: Skeletal muscle mitochondrial myopathy as a cause of exercise intolerance in a horse, *Muscle Nerve* 17:305-312, 1994.

GLYCOGEN BRANCHING ENZYME DEFICIENCY

Glycogen branching enzyme deficiency (GBED) is a newly recognized disorder causing muscle weakness in Quarter Horse–related breeds. It represents a separate glycogen storage disorder from polysaccharide storage myopathy. Most of the foals diagnosed with GBED have presented with weakness and flexural deformities of all limbs at 1 day of age. One foal required assisted mechanical ventilation, however, although blood gas parameters improved after ventilation the foal subsequently developed neurologic signs. Many foals with GBED have recurrent hypoglycemia that is responsive to intravenous glucose but recurs if the foal is unable to nurse for periods of time because of trailer rides, anesthesia, and so on. All foals have died either from euthanasia because of muscle weakness or suddenly because of apparent cardiac arrhythmia. Persistent leukopenia, intermittent hypoglycemia, and high serum CK, AST, and γ-glutamyltransferase (GGT) activities are features of affected foals. Gross postmortem changes are not evident and routine hematoxylin and eosin stains of tissues may be normal or show basophilic inclusions in skeletal muscle and cardiac tissues. When frozen sections of muscle, heart, and liver were evaluated from the foals there was a notable lack of normal PAS staining for glycogen. In addition, sections contained variable amounts of abnormal PAS-positive globular or crystalline intracellular inclusions. Globular inclusions appeared filamentous with electron microscopy and no normal β glycogen particles were evident. Muscle glycogen concentrations were reduced by 50%. Iodine spectra absorption indicated that the polysaccharide had a very minimally branched structure. This coincided with zero to residual muscle, heart, liver, and brain glycogen branching enzyme activity with normal activities of glycolytic enzymes. Thus these foals appear to have died from a complete lack of glycogen branching enzyme and therefore a lack of adequate glycogen as a substrate for energy metabolism. The clinical signs were consistent with those tissues most dependent on glycogen as a substrate: brain, cardiac purkinje fibers and cardiac myocytes, and skeletal muscle. Branching enzyme activity in the RBC of the dams of the foals and several siblings indicated half-normal activity. Pedigree analysis further supported an autosomal recessive trait. Because the foals have more than 2000 half siblings, glycogen storage disorder (GSD) IV may be a common cause of neonatal mortality in Quarter Horses. A diagnosis of GBED should be suspected in foals from Quarter Horse–related breeds that present with weakness, contracture of all limbs at birth, and have a combination of persistent hypoglycemia, leukopenia, elevated CK (1000 to 15,000 U/L), AST, and GGT.

REFERENCE

130. Valberg SJ et al: Glycogen branching enzyme deficiency in quarter horse foals (submitted).

PHOSPHORYLASE DEFICIENCY IN CHAROLAIS CATTLE

A deficiency of the enzyme phosphorylase (McArdle's disease) has been identified in several Charolais cattle from one bloodline.[131] These animals had exercise intolerance and often collapsed when forced to exercise. Serum CK was elevated in all affected animals, and one calf presented with severe rhabdomyolysis clinically resembling white muscle disease. A diagnosis can be established on the basis of histochemical staining for phosphorylase in frozen sections of muscle biopsies and confirmed by biochemical analyses. This disease should be considered as a differential diagnosis for white muscle disease in Charolais cattle that are found to have normal vitamin E and selenium status.

REFERENCE

131. Angelos S et al: Myophosphorylase deficiency associated with rhabdomyolysis in six related Charolais cattle, *Muscle Nerve* 18:736-740, 1995.

MYOFIBER HYPERPLASIA

Myofiber hyperplasia is an inherited condition occurring in certain breeds of cattle and rarely in sheep, characterized by a disproportionate increase in skeletal muscle mass. Synonyms for the disorder include double muscling, doppellender, and culard.[132] The condition is well recognized in cattle and is most commonly seen in the Belgian Blue, Piedmont, and South Devon breeds. The term double muscling is misleading because there is no increase in the number of muscle groups. The increase in muscle mass is the result of hyperplastic type 2B myocytes, with a reduction in the number of types 1 and 2A myocytes. The degree of myofiber hyperplasia varies among affected animals. Increases in muscle size are most evident in hind limbs, forelimbs, lumbar area, and neck; well-defined grooving often separates muscle groups (similar to the muscle definition seen in human body builders). There is an increased muscle/bone ratio; decreased amounts of body fat yield a leaner carcass at slaughter. Affected animals show increased weight gains over similarly treated nonaffected herdmates. The skin of affected animals is thinner than that of normal herdmates.

Myofiber hyperplasia appears to be inherited as a single major autosomal locus with several modifiers of phenotypic expression resulting in incomplete penetrance. In Belgian Blue and Piedmont cattle an 11 nucleotide deletion and a missense mutation, respectively, have been identified in the myostatin gene.[133] Myostatin is a transforming growth factor that is a negative regulator of skeletal muscle mass during development. Heterozygotes for the gene often show some degree of muscle hyperplasia. Clinical problems encountered as a result of this disorder include dystocia in dams producing affected calves and oral anomalies such as hypertrophy of the tongue, brachygnathism, and prognathism; there is also a very high incidence of inherited spastic paresis (Elso-heel) in affected cattle.

A genetic disorder that results in myofiber hyperplasia has also been identified in sheep.[134]

REFERENCES

132. Bradley R: Double muscling in cattle, *Vet Ann* 18:51-59, 1987.
133. Antoniou E, Gros M: PCR based detection of bovine myostatin Q204X mutation, *Anim Genet* 30:231-232, 1999.
134. Cockett NE, Jackson SP, Shay TL: Polar overdominance at the ovine callipyge locus, *Science* 273:236-238, 1996.

Diseases of the Reproductive System

BRAD SEGUIN

MATS H.T. TROEDSSON

Consulting Editors

FEMALE REPRODUCTIVE DISORDERS

MAARTEN DROST
PHILIP G.A. THOMAS
BRAD SEGUIN
MATS H.T. TROEDSSON

INFERTILITY CAUSED BY ABNORMALITIES OF THE ESTROUS CYCLE

THE BREEDING SEASON

Mares

The mare is a seasonally polyestrous animal, breeding during seasons of long day-length. Annual breeding and nonbreeding seasons are divided by fall and spring transitional periods, which are characterized by erratic reproductive behavior and irregular estrous cycles.

CLINICAL SIGNS. During the breeding season, mares ovulate every 21 days (range 19 to 22 days).[1] Estrus (5 to 7 days, but variable) is characterized by the presence of an ovarian follicle, serum progesterone level of less than 1 ng/ml, and sexual receptivity. During estrus the cervix is palpably relaxed and the uterus is edematous. One or two follicular waves occur per cycle, and preovulatory follicles are 45 to 60 mm in diameter, often with a cone-shaped appearance on ultrasonography.[2] Ovulation occurs 24 to 48 hours before the end of estrus and may be accompanied by ovarian sensitivity.[1] The ruptured fol-

licle is replaced by a corpus luteum (CL). Diestrus (luteal phase) is predictable in length, because regression of the CL, caused by release of endometrial prostaglandin $F_{2\alpha}$ (PGF), occurs 14 to 15 days after ovulation.[3] During diestrus and early pregnancy the cervix is tight and the uterus is firm and tubular. Diestrous ovulations occur and may be fertile.[4] First postpartum estrus ("foal heat") begins in the week after foaling, and ovulation occurs in most mares 7 to 15 days postpartum.

Ruminants

COWS. Cows are polyestrus, but seasonal differences in fertility may be caused by climate. The estrous cycle averages 21 days (range 17 to 25 days), and estrus averages 12 to 20 hours (range 6 to 30 hours). Cows are unique among domestic animals in that they ovulate spontaneously after the end of estrus, 24 to 30 hours after the beginning of estrus.[5(p117)]

In the absence of a bull, estrus can be detected in cows by their homosexual (bisexual) activity. Cows that stand to be mounted by another cow are in estrus (standing heat). Secondary signs that may be helpful in detecting estrus include restlessness and increased activity, vulvar hyperemia and edema, and a clear mucus discharge. Errors in heat detection are a common cause of infertility on large dairy farms.[6] The

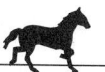

optimum time for insemination of cows is between 16 and 24 hours after the onset of estrus. Insemination of cows on the basis of standing to be mounted results in a higher pregnancy rate than if it is based on secondary signs of estrus.[7] Well-managed dairy cows with uncomplicated periparturient experiences may ovulate about 20 to 25 days after calving, whereas beef cows with nursing calves usually do not ovulate until 40 or more days after calving. The suckling activity of the calf appears to be responsible for the difference in return to cyclicity.[8]

SHEEP. Coarse-wooled breeds of ewes are seasonally polyestrus during the autumn and winter (short photoperiod) in temperate climates. Ovulation can be induced in seasonally anestrous ewes by artificial simulation of day length and temperatures characteristic of autumn (reduced photoperiod and reduced ambient temperature), but the long latency period required for response to manipulation of light and temperature makes the procedure impractical. Ewes of fine-wooled breeds may be polyestrus throughout the year if adequately nourished. The estrous cycle of ewes averages 17 days (range 14 to 19 days), and estrus averages 36 hours. Ovulation occurs spontaneously 24 hours after the onset of estrus. Ewes display few, if any, signs of estrus unless a male is present. The primary signs of estrus include seeking the ram and standing for mating. Secondary signs include restlessness and rapid tail switching; vulvar edema and discharge of clear cervical mucus may be observed occasionally. Lambing ordinarily occurs during the anestrous season; thus ewes do not return to estrus until the next breeding season.[5(p846)]

GOATS. Does in temperate climates are seasonally polyestrus from late summer until early spring (short photoperiod). Onset of the breeding season in yearling does can be advanced by exposing them to 19 hours of artificial light per day for 70 days beginning in mid to late winter. Termination of artificial light results in a relative decrease in day length and stimulation of estrus and ovulation.[5(p579)] Alternatively the breeding season may be hastened by exposing does to 14 to 18 hours of light per day for 3 months, followed by a reduction to 6 hours of light per day.[7(p971)] The estrous cycle averages 21 days, and estrus lasts 18 to 36 hours. Ovulation occurs spontaneously 24 hours after the onset of estrus. An intact male or male pheromone is usually necessary for estrous detection. The primary signs of estrus are seeking the buck and standing for service. Secondary signs of estrus in does include rapid tail switching, restlessness, increased frequency of urination and vocalization, transient decrease in appetite and milk production, and edema and hyperemia of the vulva. As in sheep, parturition takes place during the anestrous season, and return to cyclicity in does is delayed until the next breeding season.[5(p577)]

CYSTIC FOLLICULAR DEGENERATION

Cows

Ovarian cysts are follicle-like ovarian structures that arise because of failure of ovulation.[5(p243),9(p54)] They are usually larger than 25 mm in diameter and persist in the absence of a CL for 10 days or more. Follicular cysts have thin walls and may be single, multiple, or multilocular structures on one or both ovaries. Partially luteinized cysts tend to be single, unilateral structures with thicker walls because of the presence of luteal tissue.

The mechanism by which ovulation fails and cysts develop is not known. Failure of ovulation may result from inadequate release of gonadotropins or ovarian dysfunction. Increased stress such as retained placenta, metritis, and hypocalcemia around the time of calving, and postpartum ketosis have been associated with an increased prevalence of

cystic follicular degeneration (CFD), as has an hereditary predisposition.[10]

CLINICAL SIGNS AND DIAGNOSIS. Approximately 70% to 80% of cows affected by CFD are anestrus, whereas 20% to 30% display frequent or intense estrus (nymphomania). Cystic ovarian disease affects 10% to 30% of dairy cows. The condition is rare in commercial beef cows because of rigid culling for reproductive failure.

The physical appearance of cows with CFD depends on the duration of the condition. No changes are apparent after a short time, but in long-standing cases relaxation of the pelvic ligaments may result in prominence of the tailhead and masculine characteristics such as a crested neck.

The diagnosis of CFD is based on an accurate history and clinical examination. A history of constant or frequent estrus, short interestrous intervals, or anestrus may suggest CFD. Examination of the ovaries by palpation per rectum reveals the presence of enlarged fluid-filled structures raised above the surface of the ovary that greatly increase total ovarian size. Ovarian cysts are larger than preovulatory follicles; structures greater than 50 mm in diameter are not uncommon. Differentiation between a single large cyst and several smaller cysts on the same ovary may not be possible nor may recognition of the presence of partially luteinized cysts (based on peripheral progesterone concentrations) unless ultrasonography is used. Ovarian cysts appear to be dynamic structures; those that develop early in the postpartum period may regress without treatment, and a normal estrous cycle may follow, or another cystic structure may develop.

During palpation of the ovaries, several normal structures may complicate the diagnosis of CFD. Normal preovulatory follicles may approach 25 mm in diameter and have palpable characteristics similar to those of small cysts. During the follicular phase of the estrous cycle, however, the uterus responds to palpation by becoming more turgid, whereas the uterus of a cow with CFD is typically flaccid and unresponsive. In neglected cases of CFD, mucometra may develop and must be differentiated from pregnancy. During the first 5 to 7 days of the estrous cycle, the developing CL may be smooth and soft and is commonly mistaken for an ovarian cyst. More mature CLs are solid and liverlike in consistency, often feature a palpable ovulatory papilla at the apex, and are more easily differentiated from ovarian cysts. However 10% to 20% of mature CLs may lack an ovulatory papilla, making them more easily confused with ovarian cysts. Sequential examinations may be necessary to differentiate between ovarian cysts and CLs. Salpingitis, hydrosalpinx, oophoritis, ovarian abscesses, ovarian neoplasms, and cysts of the fimbria are other causes of enlargement of the ovary and surrounding structures that must be differentiated from ovarian cysts.[9(p52)]

Histories that may erroneously suggest CFD include apparently short interestrous intervals because of inaccurate detection of estrus.[11] Oxytocin administered to stimulate milk letdown may result in short interestrous intervals and suggest CFD. The estrous cycle may be shortened by administering 100 IU of oxytocin per day on days 2 through 6[12] or on days 3 through 7 or 8.[13] Heifers treated with 100 IU of oxytocin per day returned to estrus in an average of 12.9 days vs. 20.3 days in untreated controls.

CLINICAL PATHOLOGY. Plasma progesterone concentrations are low in cows with follicular cysts. Partial luteinization may occur, and progesterone concentrations may increase over time but remain lower than those of cows with normal CLs. Estrogen concentrations in the plasma of cows with CFD are variable.

TREATMENT AND PROGNOSIS. The goal in treating CFD is to induce luteinization of the cyst and reestablish normal estrous cycles. Several methods have been recommended.

TABLE 41-1

Differential Diagnosis of Anestrus in Mares

Cause	Uterus	Cervix	Ovaries	Peripheral Progesterone	Season	Other Laboratory Tests	Treatment
Pregnancy	Increased tone during early pregnancy; enlarged; positive signs of pregnancy by palpation or ultrasound	Tightly closed	Normal size during early pregnancy; out of reach of examiner in late stages	Elevated throughout pregnancy until just before term	Any season; may be more common in spring and summer	Equine chorionic gonadotropin; Cuboni test	Usually none required; therapeutic abortion if mismated
Prolonged diestrus	Normal size increased tone and tubularity; may be similar to early pregnancy	Tightly closed	Normal size; prolonged corpus luteum is embedded within ovary	Elevated throughout prolonged lifespan (30 to 90 days)	Any season; may be more common in summer		PGF
Seasonal anestrus	Normal size; flaccid; difficult to palpate	Varies from tightly closed to open	Both are small and firm, may or may not have small follicles	Low until first corpus luteum develops	Late autumn, winter, early spring		Artificial lights; wait for normal breeding season
Unobserved estrus	Normal size	Characteristic cyclic changes; relaxed and open during estrus	Development of one (or more) follicles; ovulation	Elevated for ~14 days; low for ~7 days	Spring, summer, autumn		Improve management; tease with another stallion; sequential examinations; PGF
Pyometra	Variable enlargement	May be open, closed, or stenotic; may be purulent discharge	Normal size, may be follicular development	Erratic profiles; some are elevated for prolonged periods; others may have luteal regression	Any season	Endometrial cytology; bacterial culture; antibiotic sensitivity	Drain; systemic antibiotics; PGF
Undernutrition	Normal size	Varies from tightly closed to open; no cyclic changes	Bilaterally small and firm	Low	Any season	Hematology; clinical chemistry as indicated; fecal flotation	Improve nutritional status; parasite control; treat concurrent diseases
Granulosa-theca cell tumor	Normal size	Varies	One enlarged, multicystic; other small and atrophic	Low	Any season	Peripheral inhibin concentrations are elevated in ~90% and testosterone in ~50% of mares with GTCT	Surgical removal of neoplastic ovary
Gonadal dysgenesis	Small	Varies	Small, firm, atrophic	Low	Any season	Karyotype	None

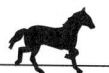

Spontaneous Recovery. Spontaneous recovery from CFD occurs in up to 60% of cows that develop CFD before the first ovulation after calving but in only about 20% of cases that develop after the first postpartum ovulation. Evaluation of therapeutic agents for CFD may be confounded by spontaneous recovery.

Luteinizing Hormone. Recommended doses of human chorionic gonadotropin (hCG) range from 5000 IU either intravenously or intramuscularly to 10,000 IU intramuscularly. Of cows treated with a single dose of hCG, 65% to 80% establish a normal estrous cycle within 3 to 4 weeks; a second or third dose may be required in cases that do not respond after 3 to 4 weeks or in cases in which nymphomania persists. Anaphylaxis after repeated treatments with a larger protein hormone such as hCG can occur. Antibodies to hCG may reduce the effectiveness of sequential treatments. Therapeutic response, both endocrinologically and clinically, is essentially equivalent between hCG and gonadotropin-releasing hormone (GnRH). The practical disadvantage of hCG is its higher price. Anaphylaxis after GnRH, a decapeptide, has not been reported in cows.

Gonadotropin-Releasing Hormone. Currently the most common treatment for ovarian cysts, especially follicular cysts, is an injection of GnRH (100 μg IM). Cows responding to this treatment have an average interval to estrus of one estrous cycle or 18 to 24 days. The treatment to breeding interval can be shortened by administering GnRH at the time of diagnosis followed by a luteolytic dose of prostaglandin 10 days to 2 weeks later. With this regimen it is not critical whether the cyst is follicular or luteal or even whether it is a misdiagnosed large, smooth CL with or without a fluid-filled central cavity. Most veterinarians agree that accurate differential diagnosis by rectal palpation between follicular cysts, luteal cysts, and some CLs can be a problem.

Prostaglandin $F_{2\alpha}$. Luteal-type cysts can be treated with the luteolytic activity of PGF. The advantage is the quicker return to estrus for those cows able to respond and the lower cost of PGF. Cysts that luteinize in response to GnRH regress at a time similar to that of normal CLs. Treatment with PGF may be used to reduce the interval from treatment with GnRH to estrus from 18 to 24 days to an average of 12 to 14 days by administering PGF 9 days after GnRH. Most clinicians are only about 50% accurate in determining the degree of luteinization of cysts by palpation per rectum; therefore measurement of concentrations of progesterone in milk or of plasma from affected cows allows the selection of GnRH or hCG for treatment of follicular cysts and PGF for the treatment of luteinized cysts. Ultrasonography can also be used to make an accurate diagnosis.[14]

Manual Rupture. Thin-walled follicular cysts may be inadvertently ruptured during examination of the ovaries, and some practitioners may intentionally attempt cyst rupture. Recovery rates after manual rupture have rarely been studied in well-designed controlled experiments but are generally within the range reported for spontaneous recovery. Deliberate manual rupture of ovarian cysts is considered an obsolete form of treatment by some veterinary clinicians but others routinely use the procedure—especially as an initial treatment for cysts found during the voluntary waiting period. Although it is conceptually possible that manual rupture of cysts may be followed by hemorrhage and adhesions between the ovary and surrounding structures, these complications appear to be much more common with use of digital pressure to enucleate CLs than with manual rupture of ovarian cysts.

Ewes and Does

Erratic periods of estrus are normal during the early and late portions of the breeding season in sheep and goats, but shortened interestrous intervals and nymphomania during the middle of the breeding season have been attributed to ovarian cysts. Cysts larger than normal preovulatory follicles (>10 mm diameter) have been observed on the ovaries of does at slaughter. Although controlled clinical trials are lacking, treatment with hCG or GnRH has been suggested.[5(p585)] A tentative diagnosis can be made on the basis of sequential plasma progesterone concentrations, and definitive diagnosis can be made by direct examination of the ovaries via laparotomy or transrectal ultrasonography.

ANESTRUS

Anestrus may be defined as failure of a female to be detected in estrus at the expected or desired time of mating. The causes of anestrus are multiple and include diseases of the reproductive and other systems. In addition, the problem is complicated by management factors that cause estrus to pass undetected, even though the animal's estrous cycles and estrus behavior are normal. Common causes of anestrus in mares and cows are summarized in Tables 41-1 and 41-2.

▌ *MARES*

SEASONAL ANESTRUS

Because photoperiod regulates reproductive activity, seasonal anestrus occurs in most mares in late fall and winter. Length of anestrus varies from one to several months, although some mares, particularly in the tropics, may cycle year round.[15] In California, Australia, and South Africa 18% to 25% of mares cycle year round.[1,16,17,18]

CLINICAL SIGNS AND DIAGNOSIS. Anestrus mares may be indifferent to teasing and do not show regular estrus behavior. Ovaries are small and firm on palpation, and the uterus is flaccid with a thin endometrium. On speculum examination of the vagina, the vaginal mucosa is pale and dry, and the cervix usually appears closed but is occasionally open or may be easily opened. Differentials are listed in Table 41-3.

As day length increases in early spring, waves of antral follicles develop and regress without ovulation because the ovulatory surge of luteinizing hormone (LH) is absent.[18(pp146-158)] These follicles may reach more than 30 mm in diameter and secrete estrogen, resulting in irregular periods of prolonged estrus behavior. Eventually increasing LH concentration coincides with a large follicle, resulting in ovulation. Regular ovulatory cycles usually then continue.

Mares in transition demonstrate estrous behavior of varying levels for 30 days or more. Transrectal palpation and ultrasonography reveal multiple ovarian follicles 25 to 35 mm in diameter. Uterine tone is usually flaccid. Differentials are listed in Table 41-3.

TREATMENT AND PROGNOSIS. As day length increases, most mares ovulate and begin regular cyclicity without treatment. Approximately 20% of all mares cycle normally year round.[19] Methods to advance the onset of regular ovulatory periods in nonpregnant and barren mares include the following.

Artificial Lighting. The vernal transition can be moved but not shortened beyond its physiologic length of 6 to 8 weeks by exposure of mares to artificial light. A common artificial lighting regimen is to expose the mares to 16 hours of light and 8 hours of dark by extending the photoperiod in the evening starting in late November to initiate ovulation by February.[20] An alternative regimen is to expose mares to 1 hour of artificial light 9.5 to 10.5 hours after the onset of darkness.[21] One 200-watt incandescent bulb or two 40-watt fluorescent tubes at a height of 7 to 8 feet in a 12- by 12-ft box stall have been recommended.[22] Paddock lighting has been described.[5(p665)]

TABLE 41-2

Differential Diagnosis of Anestrus in Cows

Cause	Uterus	Ovaries	Peripheral Progesterone	Treatment
Pregnancy	Enlarged; positive signs of pregnancy	Corpus luteum in ovary ipsilateral to pregnant uterine horn	Elevated throughout	Usually none required; PGF or PGF + dexamethasone if unwanted pregnancy
Unobserved estrus	Normal; characteristic tone during estrus; post-ovulatory edema	Development and regression of corpora lutea and follicular waves diagnosed by sequential examinations	Elevated during diestrus and low for ~3 days before ovulation and ~4 days after ovulation	Improve estrus detection; estrus detection aids; synchronize estrus with PGF; teaser animals
Cystic follicular degeneration	Normal in acute cases; later flaccid mucometra may develop in chronic cases	Fluid-filled cyst(s) greater than 25 mm in diameter; no corpora lutea; unilateral or bilateral; single or multiple cysts	Variable; low in cases of follicular cysts; slight elevation in cases of partially luteinized cysts	Spontaneous recovery; GnRH or hCG to induce luteinization of follicular cysts; PGF for partially luteinized cysts; manual rupture
Pyometra	Variable enlargement; fluid movable from horn to horn, normal-to-thick uterine wall; no positive signs of pregnancy	Corpus luteum in one ovary, frequently contralateral to larger uterine horn	Elevated throughout	PGF
Mummified fetus	Leatherlike fetus within involuted uterus; no positive signs of pregnancy	Corpus luteum in ipsilateral ovary	Elevated throughout	PGF; usually slaughter, advisable for economic reasons
Undernutrition	Normal	Small; static; no cyclic changes detected by sequential examinations	Low until corpus luteum forms	Improve quality and quantity of ration
Granulosa-theca cell tumor	Normal	One ovary enlarged; other atrophic	Low	Surgical removal of neoplastic ovary
Freemartinism	Small to nonexistent	Small to nonexistent	Low	No possible treatment
Ovarian hypoplasia	Very small to near-normal	Very small to near-normal; unilateral or bilateral; partial or complete	Variable; depends on degree of hypoplasia	No possible treatment

GnRH, Gonadotropin-releasing hormone; *hCG,* human chorionic gonadotropin; *PGF,* prostaglandin $F_{2\alpha}$.

TABLE 41-3

Irregularities of the Equine Estrous Cycle: Differential Diagnosis

Etiology	Distinguishing Features
FAILURE TO CYCLE WITH LOW PROGESTERONE	
Winter anestrus	Season; inactive ovaries
Gonadal dysgenesis	Small, hard, inactive ovaries; karyotype; underdeveloped tubular tract; small body
Pituitary adenoma	Systemic signs; inactive ovaries
Granulosa–theca cell tumor	See Prolonged or irregular behavioral estrus
Behavioral	Intimidated by stallion; recently foaled; low social rank
FAILURE TO CYCLE WITH HIGH PROGESTERONE	
Pregnancy	Presence of embryonic vesicle or fetus
Persistent CL	CL fails to regress; responds to PGF
Diestrous ovulation	CL immature at time of endogenous PGF; responds to exogenous PGF
Pseudopregnancy	Conceptus loss after maternal recognition of pregnancy; responds to exogenous PGF
Iatrogenic	History of exogenous progestin or nonsteroidal antiinflammatory drug administration
Pyometra	Uterus palpably enlarged
SHORT LUTEAL PHASE	
Uterine infection	Pyometra or endometritis causing premature endogenous PGF secretion
Systemic endotoxemia	Systemic signs; endotoxin-mediated release of endogenous PGF
Iatrogenic	History of uterine manipulation, infusion, invasive procedure or exogenous PGF
PROLONGED OR IRREGULAR BEHAVIORAL ESTRUS	
Transitional period	Season, variable ovarian activity
Granulosa–theca cell tumor	Affected ovary large and multicystic, contralateral ovary small; elevated inhibin and/or testosterone; anestrus, nymphomaniac or stallion-like behavior
Gonadal dysgenesis	Occasionally irregular cyclicity; as above
Behavioral nymphomania	Otherwise normal mare
Normal mare	Mares in winter anestrus and pregnancy may show estrus signs

CL, Corpus luteum; *PGF,* prostaglandin $F_{2\alpha}$.

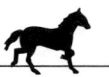

Gonadotropin-Releasing Hormone. Treatment with gonadotropin-releasing hormone (GnRH) or a GnRH analogue for mares in anestrus or spring transition has been shown to induce ovulation.[23-27] Twice-daily injections of a GnRH agonist induced ovulation in a majority of mares within 2 to 3 weeks.[27] Mares that are in deep anestrus (January and February, Northern Hemisphere) can be expected to return to anestrus after treatment.

Dopamine Antagonists. Domperidone and sulpride have been reported to stimulate follicular activity and advance the first ovulation of the year in seasonally anestrous mares.[28,29] However, the efficacy of dopamine antagonists in advancing follicular growth and ovulation in anestrous mares has recently been questioned, and it has been suggested that climactic conditions may influence the efficacy of the treatment.[30,31]

Steroids. Exogenous progestins suppress the release of LH from the anterior pituitary and may be used for estrus regulation during the vernal transition. Afer treatment of mares for 10 to 14 days, withdrawal of progestin may result in LH release from the pituitary and estrus beginning in 4 to 5 days, with ovulation within 10 days after cessation of treatment. Mares should be in mid to late transition and have a follicle at least 25 mm in size to respond to treatment. Progestins will not induce estrus or ovulation in anestrous mares.[32] The recommended dose of progesterone in oil is 150 to 300 mg daily by intramuscular injection. The synthetic progestin, altrenogest, is administered orally at 0.044 mg/kg daily. Progestins may be used in combination with extended photoperiod and gonadotropins. Products that are ineffective or unavailable include repositol progesterone, melengesterol acetate, chlormadione acetate, proligestone, medroxyprogesterone acetate, hydroxyprogesterone acetate, and norgestomet implants.

Gonadotropins. Human chorionic gonadotropin (hCG) may induce ovulation within 48 hours when administered to a mare with a follicle larger than 35 mm in diameter[33] and may reduce time to first ovulation in transitional mares, particularly when used in combination with lights and/or progesterone treatment. Ovulation response here is less predictable than that induced with hCG during the breeding season.

PROLONGED LUTEAL PHASE

The CL usually regresses 14 to 15 days after ovulation.[3] Because the functional CL is lysed by $PGF_{2\alpha}$ from the endometrium, the CL will continue to function in the following conditions:

1. The equine conceptus produces a PGF inhibitor factor, which is secreted as early as day 11 to 13 after ovulation.[18(p438,439)] The factor prevents PGF from being synthesized and secreted from the endometrium. This results in a prolonged luteal phase of the primary CL until the development of endometrial cups and secretion of eCG ensure the presence of functional luteal tissue in the pregnant mare.
2. If the developing embryo is lost between day 14 and 30 of pregnancy, after maternal recognition of pregnancy and before the development of endometrial cups, the CL may persist for a variable period of 35 to 90 days.[34]
3. Destruction of the endometrium in infectious and inflammatory conditions such as pyometra may cause insufficient synthesis of PGF and prolonged luteal life.[35]
4. Late diestrus ovulation will result in a CL that is insufficiently mature to respond to endogenous PGF release.[1]
5. Nonsteroidal antiinflammatory drugs may inhibit endometrial PGF synthesis, resulting in a prolonged luteal phase.
6. Spontaneous CL persistence has been proposed as a clinical entity[36] but has not been adequately documented and is an area of controversy.[37]

CLINICAL SIGNS AND DIAGNOSIS. High circulating progesterone (>1 ng/ml[1]) results in the mare failing to display estrus for greater than 3 weeks when teased with a stallion. The tubular tract has tone on palpation, and the cervix is closed. Luteal tissue is apparent on sonographic examination of the ovaries. Differentials are listed in Table 41-3.

TREATMENT AND PROGNOSIS. After pregnancy has been ruled out with sonographic examination, luteolysis can be achieved with administration of 10 mg of the PGF product dinoprost tromethomine or similar PGF analog. The mare must be at least 5 days postovulation to respond reliably to treatment. If the mare is treated with PGF in the presence of a mature diestrous follicle (>35 mm), she may ovulate the follicle without signs of estrus in response to declining progesterone concentrations that allow LH to be secreted from the anterior pituitary. An ultrasonographic or rectal examination of ovarian follicular activity should therefore always be performed before PGF is administered to induce estrus.

PSEUDOPREGNANCY

Mares that suffer embryonic loss in the presence of endometrial cups (days 35 to 150 of gestation) are said to be pseudopregnant (pseudopregnancy may also refer to that condition in which a conceptus was lost after maternal recognition of pregnancy and before the development of endometrial cups, resulting in prolonged luteal life). In spite of the loss of the fetus and placental tissue, endometrial cups remain in place and continue to secrete equine chorionic gonadotropin (eCG) for a similar period to that of a pregnant mare, to 100 to 150 days of gestation.[38] The primary and secondary CLs occasionally regress after embryonic loss[39] but usually remain during eCG secretion, maintaining high levels of peripheral progesterone.

TREATMENT AND PROGNOSIS. In untreated mares, cyclic activity is reestablished after the cessation of eCG secretion. Repeated daily injections of PGF products have been reported to cause luteal regression in pseudopregnant mares,[40] but only CLs older than 5 days respond to the treatment, which may prevent mares returning to estrus. Pregnancies have occurred in the face of high eCG,[41] but fertility of treated mares is usually low.

LACK OF BEHAVIORAL ESTRUS
(Silent Estrus)

Behavioral estrus may not be detected in otherwise normal mares as a result of inadequate estrus detection or a failure on the part of the mare to show obvious signs of estrus. The latter may occur in up to 15% of mares on well-managed farms.[42] Inadequate estrus detection may be a result of human apathy or ignorance or a result of using a low-libido or inexperienced stallion. Teasing mares as a group may make detection of estrus more difficult, especially for nervous mares, mares with foals, and mares of low social rank. Use of anabolic steroids may suppress behavioral estrus.

CLINICAL SIGNS AND DIAGNOSIS. The mare fails to show estrus on adequate teasing with a stallion. Differentials are listed in Table 41-3.

TREATMENT AND PROGNOSIS. Management should be examined to ensure a competent teasing routine. When approached by a stallion, mares in estrus stand still with ears held forward; they may elevate the tail, rhythmically evert the clitoris ("winking"), posture ("squatting"), urinate, and lean against the teasing chute toward the stallion. Mares that are not in estrus move about and hold their ears back; they may strike, kick, squeal, swish their tails, and forcefully void small amounts of urine. Experienced personnel should handle both stallion and mare. The teaser stallion should have adequate

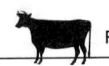
libido without being aggressive. Transrectal palpation and ultrasonography should supplement teasing. Some mares are indifferent to teasing, and records of sequential palpation must be relied on for breeding. Prostaglandins can be used to control estrus. Progesterone concentrations of less than 1 ng/ml are consistent with estrus but may also occur in anestrus mares. Mares that fail to show behavioral estrus should be bred by artificial insemination (AI) (if allowed by the breed register) or appropriate restraint used for natural cover.

BEHAVIORAL NYMPHOMANIA

Abnormal estrous behavior and aggression may be demonstrated by otherwise normal mares at any stage of the estrous cycle. Etiology is unknown, although exaggerated response to ovarian steroids has been proposed.[43]

CLINICAL SIGNS AND DIAGNOSIS. Exaggerated signs of estrus occur, initially during estrus, and then throughout the cycle. Mares may develop behavioral anomalies and become aggressive. Differentials are listed in Table 41-3. It is important to differentiate abnormal estrous behavior from unrelated behavioral problems.

TREATMENT AND PROGNOSIS. Exogenous progestins have been used to limited effect. Short-term dexamethasone treatment (5 to 10 mg) may alleviate signs for 3 to 4 days.[43(p24)] Bilateral ovariectomy may be successful in some cases.

▪▪ *RUMINANTS*

UNOBSERVED/SILENT ESTRUS: COW

Failure of a cow to display or a manager to observe the signs of estrus contributes significantly to reproductive inefficiency. When the presenting history suggests anestrus (failure to have a normal estrous cycle), the clinician must determine if the cause is failure of the manager to detect estrus in normal cows or failure of the cow to cycle because of some abnormal process. In dairy herds, approximately 90% of cows presented for examination because of a history of anestrus have evidence of normal cyclic ovarian changes, whereas only about 10% are affected by an abnormality that suspends the estrous cycle (i.e., only about 10% are in true anestrus).

Nearly 90% of well-managed dairy cows have initiated normal-length estrous cycles by 60 days after calving, but only about 60% are detected correctly in estrus by that time.[44] Rates of estrus detection by twice daily observation range from 50% to 73% depending on the skill of the observer.

Mounting activity and estrous behavior are reduced by hot and cold ambient temperatures and during the times of milking and feeding. More mounts are observed when cows are kept on dirt than on concrete. Estrous behavior varies with the time of day and may be an inverse reflection of extraneous activity interfering with cow behavior. In one study, 43% of cows showed heat between midnight and 6 AM; 22% between 6 AM and noon; 10% between noon and 6 PM; and 25% between 6 PM and midnight.

Estrus in dairy cows averages 12 to 16 hours in length but ranges from 6 to 24 hours. Sixty-five percent of cows are in estrus for less than 16 hours, and 25% are in estrus for less than 8 hours. The number of mounts per hour ranges from 2 to 8, and the total number of mounts during estrus ranges from 11 to 56. Total number of mounts per estrus increases with the number of cows simultaneously in estrus.

CLINICAL SIGNS AND DIAGNOSIS. Dairy herds in which infertility is caused by inaccurate estrus detection are usually characterized by prolonged intervals from calving to first breeding and between services; insemination intervals of 10 to 15 days and 30 to 35 days; records of examinations that confirm cyclic ovarian changes, but observation of estrus is not recorded; and finding more than 15% of cows presented

for pregnancy exam to be nonpregnant. Insemination during the luteal phase of the estrous cycle may occur in 10% to 20% of cows and is not likely to result in conception; insemination of pregnant cows may be followed by abortion.

The diagnosis of unobserved estrus requires sequential examination of affected cows and accurate records. Other causes of anestrus are eliminated. Conditions such as cystic follicular degeneration, pyometra, mummified fetuses, granulosa–theca cell tumors, and segmental aplasia that cause anestrus affect individual animals. Anestrus caused by undernutrition is characterized by depressed milk production and low body condition score.

TREATMENT AND PROGNOSIS. PGF is widely used in clinical management of unobserved estrus.[45] Mature CLs (approximately day 5 through day 18 of the estrous cycle) are responsive to PGF-induced luteolysis. Estrus occurs an average of 3 days (range 2 to 5 days) after administration of PGF. The endocrine events surrounding the controlled estrus are indistinguishable from those surrounding spontaneous estrus and ovulation. Treatment with PGF shortens the intervals from treatment to first breeding and from treatment to conception but has no effect on fertility. The benefits of PGF treatment are limited by inaccurate palpation of the temporary ovarian structures, injection during the wrong phase of the cycle, and failure of the manager to observe estrus in treated cows (appointment AI can be used to overcome this problem but it increases the demand for accurate selection of PGF treatment candidates).

Measurement of progesterone concentrations in milk samples taken on the day of breeding is useful in herds with a history of reduced fertility to confirm that cows being inseminated are not in the luteal phase of the estrous cycle. If more than an occasional cow presented for insemination has an elevated concentration of progesterone, the methods of estrus detection should be reviewed. Enzyme immunoassay kits for measuring concentrations of progesterone in milk and plasma of cows and other female animals have been described and are commercially available.

A variety of heat detection aids have been developed. Several use devices mounted on the tailhead to record that a cow has stood to be ridden. Pressure-sensitive devices that are glued to the tailhead and change color after sustained pressure by the weight of a mounting cow are commonly used. Similarly pressure-sensitive devices glued to the tailhead can send a record of riding events directly to a computer. Chalk, cattle crayon marker, or paint applied to the tailhead are inexpensive aids that are rubbed off when the animal is mounted when she is in heat. These methods require daily maintenance and twice daily evaluation to function effectively. Detection aids that measure changes in activity (pedometers), mucus conductivity, or body temperature can be used successfully. Accuracy is enhanced when measurements are related to previous estrous activity and progesterone concentrations.[46]

PREVENTION AND CONTROL. Because unobserved estrus is primarily a problem of management, efforts to reduce time lost from delayed breeding are directed at improving efficiency of heat detection. Accurate records are required to identify cows that have not been observed in estrus by 40 days after calving. Cows not observed in estrus by 40 days after calving should be examined, and abnormalities of the reproductive organs that cause anestrus treated as indicated. The time of estrus can be predicted by palpation of the temporary ovarian structures, or estrus can be controlled with PGF. The most significant benefit of a planned herd health program is stimulation of improvements in management that decrease the interval from calving to conception as a result of improved estrus detection.

Anestrus after insemination is frequently interpreted as a clinical sign of pregnancy. However, unobserved estrus in cows that have failed to conceive or suffered early embryonic death

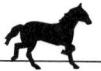

(postservice anestrus) contributes significantly to increased calving intervals. Clinical management of postservice anestrus depends on diligent observation of cows 18 to 24 days after breeding and identification of nonpregnant cows as early as possible after the infertile service so they may be reinseminated with minimum delay. Nonpregnant cows may be accurately identified by ovarian palpation for absence of a mature CL, or low milk or plasma progesterone at the time of the first expected postservice estrus (approximately 21 days after breeding), or palpation of the uterus per rectum before the second expected postservice estrus (30 to 42 days after breeding).

PROLONGED LUTEAL FUNCTION: COW

Spontaneous prolongation of luteal function in the presence of a normal, nongravid uterus does not occur in cows as it does in mares. But several conditions affecting the uterus do suspend the luteolytic mechanism, resulting in prolonged luteal function, persistently elevated progesterone concentrations, and anestrus. Common causes of prolonged luteal function in cows include pregnancy, pyometra, mummified fetus, and uterus unicornis.

CLINICAL SIGNS AND DIAGNOSIS. Pregnancy resulting from an unobserved or unrecorded breeding must always be considered as a possible cause of anestrus. Examination of the uterus for one of the positive signs of pregnancy (fetal membrane slip, amnionic vesicle, placentomes, or fetus) must precede administration of PGF.

Pyometra is characterized by accumulation of variable amounts of mucopurulent exudate within the uterine lumen, failure of luteolysis, and subsequent anestrus. An enlarged uterus as a result of fluid accumulation and a thickened uterine wall in the absence of any positive signs of pregnancy can be used to differentiate uterine enlargement caused by pregnancy from that caused by pyometra. Fluid associated with pyometra is more viscous than fetal fluid and can be manipulated from horn to horn. Because the cervix is nearly always closed, there is generally no vaginal discharge.

Fetal mummification is occasionally encountered in dairy and beef cows and is characterized by fetal death, failure of expulsion, absorption of fetal fluids, and persistence of the CL. Cases of fetal mummification are usually presented when affected cows do not deliver a calf at the expected time. The condition can be differentiated from pregnancy by palpation per rectum of a dried, leatherlike fetus within the involuted uterus. Fetal membranes cannot be slipped, and fetal fluids and placentomes are absent.

CLINICAL PATHOLOGY. No remarkable changes in hematology and clinical chemistry are associated with pregnancy, mummified fetus, or pyometra in cows. In all three conditions, peripheral concentrations of progesterone remain elevated above 1 ng/ml of plasma until spontaneous luteolysis occurs or the condition is treated.

TREATMENT AND PROGNOSIS. Unwanted pregnancy is seldom encountered in dairy cows, but, when cows or heifers are mated by accident or to an undesired sire, abortion may be reliably induced with PGF products (25 mg of dinoprost tromethamine,* or 500 μg of cloprostenol) after 7 days and before 150 days of gestation or with a combination of PGF and dexamethasone (20 mg) beyond 150 days of gestation. The PGF products are also the treatment of choice for pyometra in cows. Mummified fetuses are usually expelled 3 to 5 days after treatment with PGF. The mummy may pass through the cervix, but the vagina is likely to be dry and may not dilate sufficiently so the mummified fetus may be re-

tained. If the mummified fetus is not expelled by 5 days after treatment, a vaginal examination should be performed, and the mummy delivered by gentle traction if necessary. The prognosis for fertility after delivery of a mummified fetus is good.

UNOBSERVED ESTRUS: EWE

The breeding season of most breeds of sheep maintained at temperate latitudes is restricted to late summer, autumn, and early winter, although some breeds are polyestrus. There is almost no homosexual interaction among ewes; thus a male must be present to stimulate display of estrus.[5(p846)]

Introduction of a ram (either intact or vasectomized) into a flock of ewes advances the breeding season. Most ewes ovulate by 3 to 6 days after introduction of rams. The induced ovulation is seldom accompanied by estrus, but the subsequent estrus about 17 days later is ovulatory and fertile. The "ram effect" is lost when rams are allowed to associate with ewes throughout the year.

Return to estrus after mating may be detected in a flock of ewes by fitting the herd sire with a brisket device that marks serviced ewes. Return of an excessive number of ewes to service after breeding alerts the shepherd to the possibility of infertility.

Artificial insemination of ewes is rare in the United States but more popular in other countries. Detection of estrus for AI depends on use of teaser rams mingled with the ewes or led through the flock several times daily.

UNOBSERVED ESTRUS: DOE

The breeding season of does is similar to that of ewes (i.e., it surrounds the autumnal equinox). During periods of short daylight, the normal estrous cycle of does is 20 to 21 days. Homosexual interaction among estrous does rarely occurs; so signs of estrus must be elicited by teasing. Signs of estrus may also be evoked by exposure to male pheromones by way of a "buck jar" prepared by rubbing a cloth over the scent glands caudomedial to the horns of a mature buck during the breeding season and storing the cloth in a tightly closed container. If estrus is not observed in does exposed to a mature buck or to a buck jar during the physiologic breeding season, pregnancy or pseudopregnancy might be considered as possible causes of anestrus. Severely parasitized or inadequately nourished does do not have normal estrous cycles. Deficiencies of phosphorus, iodine, and manganese have been suggested as causes of anestrus in does.

Introduction of bucks into a flock of does early in the breeding season results in initiation of estrous cycles and some degree of synchrony of estrus about 10 days after introduction of the bucks.[5(p579)] In contrast to ewes, however, the first ovulation after exposure to males is accompanied by estrus and fertile mating.

INFERTILITY CAUSED BY ABNORMALITIES OF THE FEMALE GENITAL ORGANS

▌▌MARES

ABNORMALLY SMALL OVARIES

The most common causes of bilaterally small ovaries in the mare are (1) severe malnutrition, (2) hypothalamopituitary dysfunction, (3) immaturity, (4) seasonal anestrus, (5) advanced age, (6) use of anabolic steroids, and (7) gonadal dysgenesis. Clinical signs and treatment of malnutrition,

---

*Lutalyse, The Upjohn Co, Kalamazoo, MI 49001.
†Estrumate, Mobay Corp, Animal Health Division, Shawnee, KS 66201.

hypothalamopituitary dysfunction, and seasonal anestrus are discussed elsewhere in this book. The average age at which fillies reach puberty is 18 months with a wide range from 10 to 24 months. Many older mares (>20 years of age) are still reproductively active, but some mares reach ovarian senescence when they grow older.[47,48] In addition, infertility in aged mares may be due to defects inherent in ovulated oocytes that result in embryos of lowered viability.[49] Anabolic steroids are derivatives from androgens that have been altered to provide high anabolic activity with minimal androgenic side effects. A suppression of gonadotropin secretion has been documented when mares have been treated with these drugs.[50] Aberrations of meiosis involving the X and Y chromosomes may lead to genotype abnormalities accompanied by gonadal dysgenesis. Abnormal genotype is most commonly 63X0; but 63X/64XX, 63X/64XY, 65XXX, and 64XY sex reversed have been reported.[51]

CLINICAL SIGNS AND DIAGNOSIS

Immaturity. Fillies younger than 2 years of age with inactive ovaries and a flaccid and relaxed reproductive tract may be too young to cycle and should be reexamined at a later time. The condition should be differentiated from gonadal dysgenesis. Karyotyping may be indicated if puberty is delayed beyond 24 months.

Advanced Age. Ovarian dysfunction in aged mares is manifested by delayed onset of the ovulatory season and failure of ovulation. Clinical signs of anovulation caused by advanced age are similar to those of seasonal anestral mares. The ovaries are small and inactive, or follicles may be present without ovulation. Serum progesterone concentrations are low (<1 ng/ml). Mares may show estrous behavior similar to that of seasonal anestral mares. Aged mares with inactive ovaries during the early part of the breeding season should be reexamined before a diagnosis of permanent ovarian inactivity can be confirmed.

Use of Anabolic Steroids. Mares that have been treated with anabolic steroids may show clinical signs of abnormal or stallionlike behavior. Ovarian activity may cease when higher doses are used. These mares have small inactive ovaries and a flaccid reproductive tract, and serum progesterone concentrations are below 1 ng/ml. Prolonged treatment of prepubertal mares with anabolic steroids results in hypertrophy of the clitoris.[52]

Gonadal Dysgenesis. Chromosomal abnormalities exist in all breeds of horses. Mares are usually small and phenotypically female. The ovaries are small, firm, smooth, and inactive. The tubular tract is thin and flaccid. Endometrial hypoplasia is a common finding. Diagnosis is confirmed by physical findings and karyotype.

TREATMENT AND PROGNOSIS

Immaturity and Advanced Age. No treatment is available for age-related ovarian inactivity. Because aged mares often experience a delayed seasonal onset of ovarian activity, they benefit from an artificial light regimen starting 60 to 90 days before the breeding season. Treatment of age-related ovarian inactivity with GnRH or GnRH analogues has been discouraging.

Use of Anabolic Steroids. Ovarian inactivity in mares treated with anabolic steroids is reversible, and pituitary and ovarian function eventually return to normal in most mares after withdrawal of the treatment. Mares intended for breeding should not be treated with anabolic steroids.

Gonadal Dysgenesis. Mares diagnosed with gonadal dysgenesis are sterile, and there is no treatment.

ABNORMALLY ENLARGED OVARIES

The most common causes of enlarged ovaries in the mare are (1) tumors, (2) ovarian hematoma, (3) pregnancy, and (4) anovulatory hemorrhagic follicles.

▪▪ *Ovarian Tumors*

The majority of equine ovarian tumors can be categorized as (a) sex cord-stromal tumors (granulosa–theca cell tumors), (2) epithelial tumors (cystadenomas), or (3) germ cell tumors (dysgerminomas and teratomas).

Granulosa–Theca Cell Tumors

The granulosa–theca cell tumor is the most common ovarian tumor in the mare. It is usually benign, occurs in mares of all ages, and is occasionally found in pregnant mares. The tumor arises from the steroidogenic cells of the follicle,[53] resulting in abnormal secretion of inhibin and testosterone.[54]

CLINICAL SIGNS AND DIAGNOSIS. As a result of hormone secretion from the tumor, mares may show anestrus, constant estrus, irregular estrus, or stallionlike behavior. They are infertile in the presence of the tumor. Pituitary gonadotropin secretion is reduced as a result of inhibin production by the tumor.[55] The contralateral ovary is usually small and inactive, although some mares have been reported to continue ovulating. The affected ovary is large, firm, and often multicystic and loses definition of the ovulation fossa. The uterus is frequently flaccid. Differential diagnoses for abnormal cyclicity are listed in Table 41-3 and for ovarian enlargement in Table 41-4. Peripheral plasma inhibin and testosterone concentrations are elevated in 90% and 55% of all cases, respectively. Peripheral testosterone level may be 100 to 200 pg/ml in mares with stallionlike behavior.[56] Final diagnosis is histologic.

TREATMENT AND PROGNOSIS. The affected ovary should be surgically removed. The prognoses for both life and reproductive use are good. Return to cyclicity varies, but most mares cycle in the year after ovariectomy.

Cystadenomas

Cystadenomas are rare, benign, hormonally inactive tumors that arise from the surface epithelium of the ovulation fossa. The tumor is unilateral and the contralateral ovary is normal.

CLINICAL SIGNS AND DIAGNOSIS. Mares with cystadenomas cycle normally from the opposite ovary, and may even become pregnant. Rectal palpation and ultrasonography reveal the presence of one enlarged multicystic ovary, which may appear similar to a granulosa–theca cell tumor, and one normal ovary. Differential diagnoses for ovarian enlargement appear in Table 41-4. Final diagnosis is histologic.

TREATMENT AND PROGNOSIS. Although cystadenomas are benign tumors and do not affect the reproductive perfor-

TABLE 41-4

Unilaterally Large Ovary: Differential Diagnosis

Etiology	Distinguishing Features
Granulosa–theca cell tumor	Sonographically multilocular, high inhibin and/or testosterone; small contralateral ovary
Other ovarian tumor	See text
Ovarian hematoma	Ovulation fossa still palpable, cycles normally
Ovarian abscess	Large, hard ovary, sonographically echogenic
Ovarian follicle	Normal cycling mare, ovulates
Anovulatory hemorrhagic follicle	Free floating echogenic spots

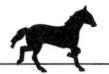

mance of the mare, they should be surgically removed if diagnosed. The prognoses for both life and reproductive performance are excellent.

Germ Cell Tumors

Dysgerminomas and teratomas are rare ovarian tumors of germ cell origin. Both tumors are unilateral and hormonally inactive.

CLINICAL SIGNS AND DIAGNOSIS. Both tumors make the affected ovary unilaterally enlarged and multicystic. Dysgerminomas are malignant and often metastasize to the peritoneal and thoracic cavities. Teratomas may arise from all three germinal layers, and the neoplastic ovary may contain bone, cartilage, teeth, hair, muscle, and nerves. Teratomas do not cause clinical signs and are often detected in association with a routine reproductive examination. Differential diagnoses for ovarian enlargement are listed in Table 41-4. Final diagnosis for germ cell tumors is histologic.

TREATMENT AND PROGNOSIS. Surgical removal is recommended for both dysgerminomas and teratomas. The prognosis for teratomas is usually good, but poor for mares diagnosed with dysgerminomas.

Ovarian Hematoma

Hemorrhage into the follicular cavity is a normal occurrence at ovulation. Occasionally hemorrhage is severe, resulting in the formation of an ovarian hematoma that may be 10 cm in diameter or larger.

CLINICAL SIGNS AND DIAGNOSIS. Affected mares continue to cycle normally. Transrectal palpation and ultrasonography reveal an enlarged ovary that is initially irregularly hypoechoic and then echogenic with organization of the hematoma. The ovulation fossa usually remains distinguishable on the affected ovary, and the contralateral ovary remains active.

TREATMENT AND PROGNOSIS. Ovarian hematomas regress spontaneously over a period of weeks or months. The functional life span of the luteal tissue in a hematoma is normal and ovarian activity is unaffected.[57] Because the affected ovary is not permanently damaged and the contralateral ovary is unaffected, the prognosis for fertility is undiminished.

Pregnancy

Multiple secondary CLs form in pregnant mares between day 40 and 180 days of gestation, resulting in bilaterally enlarged ovaries that may be mistaken for ovarian pathology.

CLINICAL SIGNS AND DIAGNOSIS. Ovarian enlargement is commonly bilateral. Pregnant mares may show stallionlike behavior associated with increased testosterone production from the fetus during midgestation. Pregnancy should always be considered when presented with a mare with stallionlike behavior, elevated serum testosterone concentrations, and enlarged ovaries. Pregnancy is diagnosed by rectal palpation and ultrasonograpic examination.

Anovulatory Hemorrhagic Follicles

Hemorrhage into a preovulatory follicle in association with failure of ovulation may result in the formation of a hemorrhagic follicle.[18(pp224-226)]

CLINICAL SIGNS AND DIAGNOSIS. Hemorrhagic follicles are large (up to 6 cm) and on ultrasonography contain free-floating echogenic material that swirls during ballotment of the enlarged follicle. Over time, the structure gives an impression of a gelatinous consistency. Diagnosis should be based on ultrasonographic findings.

TREATMENT AND PROGNOSIS. Anovulatory hemorrhagic follicles regress spontaneously over time and are often not detectable after 1 month. Luteal tissue can be lysed with $PGF_{2\alpha}$ products, and normal cyclic activity resumed.

RUMINANTS

OVARIAN HYPOPLASIA

Ovarian hypoplasia occurs sporadically as an autosomal recessive trait. The condition has incomplete penetrance; thus it may be partial or complete and unilateral or bilateral. The affected gonad varies in size from a cordlike thickening in the cranial edge of the mesovarium to a bean-sized structure. The tubular genital organs remain infantile in animals with complete bilateral hypoplasia or may develop to near-normal size in heifers with unilateral or partial hypoplasia. Individuals affected with complete bilateral ovarian hypoplasia are sterile, whereas those affected by partial or unilateral hypoplasia may be subfertile. With partial hypoplasia the uterine pole of the ovary is typically affected. On direct observation by laparotomy or laparoscopy or on slaughter, the uterine pole is flat and triangular and shows converging striations. The affected part is devoid of follicles. Animals with partial ovarian hypoplasia can be expected to have a reduced superovulatory response to gonadotropin treatment. Heifers with abnormal karyotypes are also affected by ovarian hypoplasia. The condition should be differentiated from nonfunctional ovaries and anestrus associated with malnutrition or debilitating diseases. Treatment of ovarian hypoplasia is not successful.[58(p434)]

Freemartinism: Cow

A freemartin is a phenotypic female, born cotwin to a male, that is sterile because of arrested development of the reproductive tract. The term "freemartin" is said to have originated in England, where it referred to a heifer that was not pregnant after the summer breeding season and therefore "free" for fattening and slaughter at Martinmas, a fall festival in honor of St. Martin.[9(p38)] Freemartinism arises as a result of anastomoses between the placental circulations of twin fetuses of opposite sexes. Sexual differentiation of the male embryo occurs earlier than that of the female; thus the male twin may sterilize the female by transfer of H-Y antigen, which inhibits development of the female gonad. The ovaries of a freemartin are underdeveloped and contain seminiferous tubules. Abnormalities of the tubular genital organs vary in severity, and the structures range from cordlike bands to near-normal uterine horns. In most freemartins there is no cervix; thus no communication exists between the uterus and vagina. The latter is a short blind pouch. Frequently vesicular glands of varying size are present.

As many as 85% to 90% of phenotypic females born cotwins to males are freemartins; thus the history suggests a diagnosis in most cases. Singleton freemartins are possible if male and female twins are conceived and the male is lost after 30 days of gestation. Palpation per rectum of breeding age freemartins reveals aplasia or hypoplasia of the tubular genital organs and hypoplastic ovaries. If animals too small for palpation per rectum are presented, examination of the vagina with a small glass speculum (or test tube) reveals that the vagina of a freemartin is short (6 to 7 cm in freemartins versus nearly double that length in a normal heifer). A definitive diagnosis may be made by karyotyping the suspected individual; varying percentages of male cells are found in freemartins.[58(p97)]

Freemartinism: Ewe

Although freemartinism is possible in sheep, the condition is rare, despite the high incidence of multiple births. The condition can be confirmed by determination of blood cell chimerism.

Freemartinism: Doe

Twinning is also common in goats, but vascular anastomosis is either uncommon or occurs after the critical period for sexual differentiation. Caprine freemartins comprise approximately 6% of intersexes.[5(p596)]

Intersex: Doe

Intersexes are common among Saanen, Toggenburg, and Alpine goats. The fetal testes appear to be unable to fully masculinize the duct system or external genitalia. Parts of both the mesonephric and paramesonephric ducts persist; thus the phenotype of affected individuals may approach that of either sex. Intersexes are most frequent among polled goats, and the condition is thought to be caused by a recessive gene linked to that for polledness; however, intersexuality may rarely be seen in horned goats. Diagnosis is based on a history of abnormal sexual behavior, and identification of abnormal genital development is by physical examination. There is no satisfactory treatment, but the prevalence of the condition may be reduced by preventing mating between two polled animals.[5(p596)]

OVARIAN TUMORS

Granulosa Cell Tumor: Cow

Although rare, a variety of ovarian neoplasms have been described in cows; granulosa cell tumors appear to be most common.[9]

CLINICAL SIGNS AND DIAGNOSIS. Granulosa–theca cell tumors are characterized by unilateral ovarian enlargement, with the affected ovary being greater than 10 cm in diameter. The surface may be smooth or coarsely lobulated. Function of the contralateral ovary may be suppressed. The behavior of affected cows ranges from anestrus to nymphomania to bull-like behavior. Udder development and lactation may occur in affected heifers. Very few bovine granulosa cell tumors are malignant, and they rarely metastasize. Among the other ovarian neoplasms that have been reported in cattle are dysgerminomas, interstitial cell tumors,[9] and teratomas. Causes of ovarian enlargement that must be differentiated from ovarian neoplasia include ovarian cysts, oophoritis, ovarian abscesses, and parovarian cysts.

TREATMENT AND PROGNOSIS. The treatment for ovarian neoplasia in cattle is surgical removal of the affected ovary; however, cows may not be as fertile as are mares after removal of the tumor.

Ovarian Tumors: Ewe

Granulosa–theca cell tumors have been reported, but tumors of the genital organs of ewes appear to be rare.[9(p83)]

Ovarian Tumors: Doe

Ovarian neoplasia appears to be rare in does as well. Granulosa–theca cell tumors and dysgerminomas have been reported.

Ovarian Hemorrhage: Cow

Ovulation tags develop after ovulation, resulting from blood loss associated with rupture of the follicle.[9] Fine adhesions may develop between the ovarian surface and surrounding structures. Most ovulation tags resolve spontaneously and have no effect on fertility. Severe ovarian hemorrhage may follow attempts to manually enucleate the CL. Adhesions between the ovary and its bursa interfere with their normal function. Enucleation of CLs for treatment of anestrus and pyometra has been superseded by treatment with PGF products.

Oophoritis: Cow

Inflammation of the ovary may follow traumatic manipulations such as enucleation of CLs and attempts to drain fluid from ovarian cysts, and ascending infections from the uterus. Oophoritis may also accompany brucellosis, mycoplasmosis, and tuberculosis.

INFERTILITY CAUSED BY ABNORMALITIES OF THE FEMALE TUBULAR GENITALIA

SALPINGITIS

Inflammation of the oviducts is characterized by macroscopic enlargement. Lesions are frequently bilateral and consist of infiltration by lymphocytes, plasma cells, and neutrophils, and desquamation of epithelial cells.[9]

Most cases of salpingitis follow infections of the uterus. Necrotizing and granulomatous salpingitis may follow infection by *Arcanobacterium pyogenes* (formerly *Corynebacterium pyogenes*), *Mycobacterium tuberculosis*, and *Brucella abortus*. Mild inflammation of the uterine tubes that does not usually result in permanent damage accompanies uterine infection caused by *Campylobacter fetus* ssp. *venerealis* and *Tritrichomonas foetus*. Salpingitis may be a sequela to manipulations of the ovaries and uterine tubes by palpation per rectum and to aggressive irrigation of an infected uterus and inappropriate treatment with estrogenic hormones. Migrating larvae of *Strongylus edentatus* have been proposed as a possible cause of nonobstructive infundibulitis in mares, but their role is speculative.[9]

Pyosalpinx is characterized by segmental accumulation of pus within the lumen of the oviduct after mechanical blockage of either end. Pyosalpinx frequently follows severe cases of uterine infection and may be complicated by perimetritis and localized peritonitis.

Hydrosalpinx is characterized by accumulation of thin mucus within the lumen of the oviduct. Hydrosalpinx and adhesions to perisalpingial tissues are common sequelae to chronic salpingitis.

CLINICAL SIGNS AND DIAGNOSIS. The usual history associated with diseases of the uterine tubes is one of infertility. Additional history may include uterine infection or traumatic therapy such as uterine irrigation, enucleation of CLs, or administration of exogenous estrogen during CL function. Salpingitis is an uncommon clinical finding in the mare. Up to 88% of mares had macroscopic lesions of the oviduct at postmortem examination,[59] which included adhesions, fibrous bands, and parovarian cysts that may or may not affect fertility. Accumulations of cells and debris may form intraluminal masses; however, their role in infertility has not been adequately tested.[60] The pathology of the oviduct has been reviewed.[61] Similarly, moderate lesions of uterine tube disease may escape diagnosis by physical examination in cows, but the results of abattoir studies suggest that lesions of the oviducts are not uncommon.[9(p94)] In cows, lesions involving adhesions between the ovary, ovarian bursa, oviduct, and surrounding tissues may be identified per rectum by inserting two or three fingers into the ovarian bursa and rolling the oviduct between the fingers and thumb. Easy identification of the oviduct by palpation per rectum is sometimes considered indicative of abnormalities. Diagnosis of diseases of the oviducts in ewes and does is impossible by physical examination. Although a history of infertility after one of the predisposing causes might suggest oviductal lesions, diagnosis is made by exploratory laparotomy, peritoneoscopy, or necropsy.

Lesions of the oviductal or perisalpingial tissues must be differentiated from other causes of abnormal enlargements such as ovarian neoplasia, parovarian cysts, cystic ovarian disease, and ovarian hematomas. Neoplasia of the oviducts in domestic animals is extremely rare.

CLINICAL PATHOLOGY. Several tests that determine oviductal patency of mares[62] and cows[63] have been described, but neither the starch test nor the phenolsulfonphthalein dye test is very reliable or consistently diagnostic. For suspected unilateral blockage[64] each uterine horn may be catheterized individually with a Foley catheter placed at the base of the horn on different days.

EMBRYO RECOVERY. Embryo recovery after either a single ovulation or superovulation is objective evidence that one or both uterine tubes are patent and functional. Improved reproductive performance of cows may follow uterine lavage; thus embryo recovery as a diagnostic test may have therapeutic benefits as well.[65]

TREATMENT AND PROGNOSIS. Treatment of diseases of the oviducts is not likely to be successful. Appropriate treatment for concurrent uterine infections should be instituted. A period of sexual rest may be beneficial and is indicated in valuable animals. The prognosis for reproduction in cases of bilateral obstruction of the oviducts is poor. In vitro fertilization of ova harvested from affected females has become a therapeutic option.

PREVENTION AND CONTROL. Traumatic manipulation of the ovaries, irrigation of the endometrial cavity with large volumes of fluid (over 100 ml in heifers or 150 ml in cows) or irritating chemicals, and administration of estrogenic hormones to luteal phase females should be avoided.[58(p434)] Because abnormalities of the oviducts are frequently associated with uterine infections, reduction of the prevalence of uterine infections results in fewer tubal infections as well.

UTERINE ABNORMALITIES

Retained Fetal Membranes

▌▌ *MARES*

Retention of the fetal membranes beyond a period of 3 hours is an abnormal occurrence in the mare. The mare has an epitheliochorial placenta characterized by diffuse microvilli that interdigitate with endometrial crypts. After delivery, blood flow through the placental vessels is reduced, and placental microvilli shrink and disengage from endometrial crypts. The condition is more common after abortion, dystocia, cesarian section, and fetotomy. The pathophysiology of the disease is poorly understood but may involve disturbances of normal prepartum endocrine events or myometrial contractility. Partial placental retention may be localized to well-defined areas of continued placental attachment. The most common site of partial retention is the previously nongravid horn.

Equine placentas should be spread on a flat surface after expulsion and examined to ensure that the complete membrane is present. Areas of placental necrosis are common near the tips of the uterine horns, and the fragile area may be incarcerated by the rapidly contracting uterus.

CLINICAL SIGNS AND DIAGNOSIS. Retained fetal membranes (RFMs) are usually visible at the vulva. However,

small tags of placental tissue may remain attached to the uterus without being apparent and may be a nidus for infection, resulting in severe metritis, endotoxemia, and laminitis hours to days postpartum.

TREATMENT AND PROGNOSIS. The severity of sequelae makes early intervention essential. Treatment should begin if fetal membranes are not passed within 3 hours of foaling. Most instances respond to vigorous early pharmacologic treatment. Occasional cases require several days of persistent treatment.

Manual Removal. Manual removal is contraindicated, because trauma induces placental tearing, leaving microvilli in endometrial crypts.

Oxytocin. Oxytocin induces myometrial contractions, which may aid placental expulsion. Oxytocin may be administered by intravenous injection (5 to 20 IU every 15 to 30 minutes) or intramuscular injection (20 to 40 IU every 30 to 60 minutes); or it may be infused slowly (30 to 80 IU in 500 ml of warm saline over 30 to 60 minutes). Care should be taken to avoid overdosage, which may result in signs of abdominal pain and which will cause tetanic rather than orchestrated uterine contraction.

Allantochorionic Infusion. If the chorioallantois is intact, the chorioallantoic cavity may be filled to distention with 3 to 4 gallons of warm saline or water through the cervical star.[66] The opening in the placenta is held closed until the mare exerts abdominal pressure. Oxytocin may be used in conjunction with this treatment.

Adjunct Therapy. Concurrent therapy directed at controlling or minimizing common sequelae to retained placenta is often indicated.

1. *Antibacterials.* Bacterial infections are commonly associated with prolonged (>6 to 8 hours) retention of the fetal membranes. The bacterial population is frequently mixed and likely to include β-hemolytic streptococci and coliforms. In prolonged cases, bacterial culture and sensitivity should be performed. Broad-spectrum antibiotics known to be effective against commonly isolated organisms are indicated. Drugs that have been recommended for systemic administration include ampicillin, gentamicin, kanamycin, penicillin, ticarcillin (with gentamicin for *Pseudomonas* infection), and trimethoprim-sulfamethoxazole. Intrauterine administration of antibiotics and antiseptics depresses phagocytic activity of uterine neutrophils, and many chemicals irritate the endometrium, but drugs that have been suggested include those recommended for systemic administration, as well as amikacin and polymyxin B.

2. *Antiinflammatory drugs.* Laminitis may be a sequela to metritis and is commonly associated with RFMs. Treatment with administration of antiinflammatory drugs such as phenylbutazone or flunixin meglumine is indicated to reduce the likelihood and severity of laminitis. Additional therapy for laminitis should be administered as indicated.

3. *Other treatments.* Caslick's surgery may be indicated in some cases of RFMs to control aspiration of air. Tetanus may complicate RFMs, and prophylaxis with tetanus antitoxin in unvaccinated animals or tetanus toxoid in previously vaccinated animals is indicated.

Some cases of RFM are refractory to treatment, and membranes may remain firmly attached to the endometrium for several days. Aggressive attempts at manual removal should be eschewed, because severe endometrial damage may follow. Persistent treatment with antibiotics, antiinflammatory drugs, and oxytocin is indicated until the placenta is expelled and bacterial infection of the uterus is controlled.

The prognosis for RFM is generally good but is reduced if treatment is delayed or if retention is accompanied by infection with virulent pathogens. Sequelae to RFM include

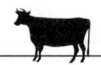

metritis, endometrial fibrosis, invagination of a uterine horn, uterine prolapse, and laminitis.

∎∎ RUMINANTS

Cow

The cotyledonary placenta of cows is usually expelled within 3 to 8 hours after calving and is considered retained if not expelled by 12 hours. RFM are more commonly seen in dairy than in beef breeds. In dairy cattle the reported prevalence ranges from 8% to 12% after spontaneous delivery of single calves. RFM are more likely after delivery of male calves or twins and deliveries complicated by dystocia. Parturition after a shorter or longer than normal gestation length is accompanied by an increase in the incidence of RFM.[67]

The cause of RFM in cattle is failure of fetal cotyledons to separate from crypts of maternal caruncles; the process of separation normally begins during the last months of pregnancy. Villi shrink after blood flow is interrupted by rupture of the umbilical vessels. Strong myometrial contractions continue during the third stage of labor, and changes in the size and shape of maternal caruncles contribute to separation of the placenta from the endometrium. A number of factors have been associated with separation failure, but the precise reasons for separation failure are unknown.[5(p237)] Deficiencies of selenium (see Nutritional Myodegeneration, Chapter 40), vitamin E, and vitamin A are associated with an increased prevalence of RFM.[5(p237)]

CLINICAL SIGNS AND DIAGNOSIS. The majority of affected cows show no serious clinical signs other than a transient decrease in appetite and milk production. However, 20% to 25% of cows affected by RFM develop moderate to severe metritis. The most objectionable clinical signs are the malodorous discharge and objectionable tissue hanging from the genital tract. RFM are usually expelled by 4 to 10 days after calving when the caruncular tissue has become necrotic and is sloughed. Some affected cows show signs of endotoxemia, including depression, fever, rumen stasis, and inappetence, as a result of RFM.

TREATMENT AND PROGNOSIS. A variety of treatments have been suggested for RFM in cows, including aggressive attempts at manual removal, myometrial stimulants, intrauterine and systemic antibiotics (alone or in combination with other approaches), and no therapy whatsoever. Because the processes that culminate in RFM begin during late gestation, it is not unreasonable that treatment initiated at calving has little effect on the loosening process. Most treatments for RFM are directed toward controlling the intrauterine bacterial population.

Manual Removal. Manual removal of the placenta is indicated only when gentle traction is sufficient to withdraw the membranes from the genital canal in a short time. Attempts at manual removal are contraindicated if the patient shows clinical signs of septicemia. Trauma caused by manual removal inhibits phagocytosis by uterine neutrophils and predisposes to severe sequelae, including septic metritis and peritonitis. Complete manual removal is impossible, but older stockmen accustomed by tradition to manual removal may insist on attempting the procedure to the detriment of the patient's health and future fertility.[68]

Myometrial Stimulants. Administration of a single dose of oxytocin does not reduce the prevalence of RFM in cows that calve spontaneously or in cows that require assistance at delivery.[69,70] Cows with RFM have an elevated plasma concentration of estrogen during the period of retention; thus administration of additional estrogen for treatment of RFM may be of questionable value.[71] Intravenous calcium solutions are indicated in cases of RFM secondary to hypocalcemia.

Prostaglandin. Prostaglandin has been recommended for treatment of RFM. In one trial, treatment with fenprostalene resulted in a shorter period of retention in treated cows, reduced the number of treatments subsequently required for metritis, and slightly reduced the intervals to first service and conception.[72] However, others found that fenprostalene produced no changes in myometrial activity between days 1 and 4 after calving and concluded that uterotonic agents are unlikely to hasten placental expulsion because uterine effort is already increased in animals that have RFM.[73] An imbalance between synthesis of PGF_2 and PGI_2 between 30 and 60 minutes after parturition has been demonstrated in cows affected by RFM.[74]

Antibiotics. Intrauterine tetracycline may reduce fertility,[75] or the reproductive performance of treated cows may be as good as untreated herdmates.[7(p186)] Intrauterine treatment with 4 to 6 g of oxytetracycline per day until the placenta is expelled may reduce the prevalence of metritis associated with RFM, but pyometra may develop in treated cows.[76] Bacterial putrefaction and the disagreeable odor of RFM may be reduced by intrauterine antibiotics, but the placenta is only released after necrosis of the caruncles. Systemic and intrauterine antibiotics are indicated in cases of RFM when the cow has a fever, is off feed, or has a drop in milk production.

Cows that retain their membranes for more than 12 hours after calving are more likely to develop metritis than are cows that promptly expel the membranes. However, reproductive performance of cows that rapidly return to normal after RFM is similar to that of their unaffected herdmates, indicating that in the absence of a secondary reproductive abnormality, RFM has a minimum effect on future fertility.

EWE AND DOE

Fetal membranes are considered retained in ewes and does if not expelled within 12 hours after delivery of the last fetus. The prevalence in does is approximately 6% after spontaneous delivery but may be higher when delivery is complicated by dystocia or abortion. Selenium deficiency has been suggested as a cause.

The clinical signs of RFM in ewes and does are usually obvious.[5(p595)] Does may ingest their placentas, complicating identification of cases of partial retention. RFM may accompany retention of a fetus within the uterus, and does and ewes should be carefully examined.

Other tissues that may be exposed from the vulva in association with parturition are a prolapsed uterus, a prolapsed or everted urinary bladder, prolapse of some portion of the digestive tract through a genital rupture, prolapsed rectum or vagina, or a twin fetus.

TREATMENT AND PROGNOSIS. Manual separation of cotyledons from caruncles is impossible in ewes and does; therefore manipulative attempts to remove the placenta are limited to gentle traction on exposed membranes at daily intervals. Treatment with intrauterine and systemic antibiotics, oxytocin (10 to 20 IU) at 12-hour intervals until the placenta is expelled, and antiinflammatory drugs have been suggested. Prophylaxis against tetanus is indicated.

UTERINE INFECTIONS

∎∎ MARE

Endometritis

A failure of the uterine defense mechanisms to effectively eliminate an antigen (bacteria or spermatozoa) and inflammatory products from the uterus results in a persistent endometritis, which is a major cause of reduced fertility in brood mares.[77] In the normal mare the uterus is well protected from external contamination by physical barriers consisting of the vulva, the vestibule, the vagina, and the cervix, and any compromise of these barriers may predispose the mare to a chronic uterine infection.[78] Breeding is another source of uterine contamination. Intrauterine deposition of semen causes an inflammatory reaction resulting from bacterial contamination of the ejaculate or from spermatozoa.[79] Approximately 15% of a normal population of Thoroughbred brood mares developed persistent endometritis after breeding.[80] Natural resistance to experimentally induced bacterial contamination has been demonstrated in young mares, whereas a population of multiparous and barren mares developed a persistent endometritis after bacterial contamination of the uterus.[81,82] Based on these studies, mares have been classified as either susceptible or resistant to persistent uterine infection.[81] Endometritis has severe effects on the fertility of affected mares. A persistent inflammation may interfere directly with the survival of an embryo, or cause premature luteolysis and embryonic loss because of increased PGF concentrations.[83]

Several classes of immunoglobulins have been isolated from the equine uterus. Although antibody-mediated uterine defense may be important for effective elimination of bacterial contaminants from the uterus in susceptible mares, concentrations of immunoglobulins in uterine secretion are similar or even elevated compared to those of resistant mares.[84-88] Polymorphonuclear neutrophils (PMNs) are the first inflammatory cells to enter an inflamed site.[89] Chemoattractive properties of uterine fluid have been described in vitro in horses and the uterus responds quickly to an antigen with release of PMN-chemotactic mediators, which results in a rapid migration of PMNs into the uterine lumen.[90] Complement products and leukotriene B$_4$ (LTB$_4$), prostaglandin E (PGE), and PGF may all serve as chemoattractants for PMNs in the uterus.[90-94] Studies on the role of local uterine factors on PMN function suggested that an impaired phagocytosis by uterine PMNs in susceptible mares is the result of insufficient opsonization in uterine secretion rather than a primary dysfunction of the PMNs.[95]

Mechanical aspects of the uterine defense system are currently believed to be a major contributor in uterine clearance of bacteria and inflammatory products.[96-98] Using intrauterine inoculations of a combination of radioactive-labeled microspheres and bacteria, impaired uterine clearance was demonstrated in susceptible but not in resistant mares.[96] Studies using scintigraphic measurements of intrauterine clearance of radioactive colloids further defined a delayed physical clearance in susceptible mares.[97] Using electromyography (EMG) to register myometrial activity, it was observed that the impaired uterine clearance in susceptible mares was caused by reduced myometrial activity in response to the inflammation.[98] The dependent position of the mare's uterus may also interfere with effective clearance.

Based on pathogenesis, persistent endometritis can be divided into (1) sexually transmitted diseases (STD), (2) persistent uterine infection, (3) persistent breeding-induced endometritis, and (4) chronic degenerative endometritis (endometrosis).

SEXUALLY TRANSMITTED DISEASES (STDs). Few true STDs are known in the horse. Contagious equine metritis (CEM) is an example of a true STD.[99,100] The disease is caused by *Taylorella equigenitalis*, a highly contagious and pathogenic microorganism. Although the present status of a mare's uterine defense mechanism is important for the manifestation of the disease, this bacterium is highly resistant and capable of overcoming the mare's normal disease barriers.

PERSISTENT UTERINE INFECTION. Bacteria most commonly isolated from the uterus of the mare are β-hemolytic streptococci (*Streptococcus zooepidemicus* and *Streptococcus equi-*

similis), *Escherichia coli*, *Pseudomonas aeruginosa*, and *Klebsiella pneumoniae*. Other aerobic bacteria isolated from reproductive tracts of mares include α-hemolytic streptococci, *Corynebacterium* spp., *Staphylococcus* spp., *Enterobacter* spp., *Actinobacter* spp., *Proteus* spp., and *Citrobacter* spp. *Candida* spp. and *Aspergillus* spp. are the organisms most commonly associated with yeast or fungal endometritis. The role of viruses, mycoplasmas, ureaplasma, and anaerobic bacteria in endometritis is poorly understood. *P. aeruginosa*, *K. pneumoniae*, and possibly *S. zooepidemicus* and *E. coli* can be sexually transmitted in horses, but the consequences of exposure to these microorganisms are determined by the particular strain involved and active participation of all facets of the mare's uterine defense mechanisms. In contrast to a true STD, persistent infectious endometritis is often the result of contamination of the uterus by the mare's fecal and genital flora in combination with compromised uterine defense.[101,102] The clitoral fossa may be a potential storage site of bacteria resulting in an iatrogenic contamination of the uterus when mares are cultured or inseminated.[103]

PERSISTENT BREEDING-INDUCED ENDOMETRITIS. Regardless of whether mares are bred by natural service or by AI, semen is deposited directly into the uterus. Recent studies have shown that a transient endometritis occurs after sterile inoculation of spermatozoa into the uterine lumen.[79,104] Subsequent in vitro experiments demonstrated that spermatozoa are chemotactic to PMNs, possibly via activation of complement, and that seminal plasma inhibits PMN migration.[105] In addition, seminal plasma has also been shown to suppress phagocytosis of spermatozoa by PMNs.[106] These reports suggest that seminal plasma modulates the inflammatory response to spermatozoa. A chemotactic role of spermatozoa may imply that a transient uterine inflammation after breeding is physiological and necessary to clear the uterus from excess spermatozoa and seminal plasma. However, the condition may develop into a persistent inflammation in mares with impaired uterine defense mechanisms. Persistent sperm-induced inflammation may be a more important cause of infertility in susceptible mares than infectious endometritis.[80]

CHRONIC DEGENERATIVE ENDOMETRITIS (ENDOMETROSIS). Degenerative changes of the endometrium such as periglandular fibrosis and glandular dilation are often seen in older multiparous mares. The condition is associated with susceptibility to persistent endometritis[107] and may result from repeated uterine inflammation. However, the condition has also been observed in older mares without any known history of endometritis, suggesting that degenerative fibrosis of the endometrium can be a process of aging rather than inflammation.[108] Based on the possibility of a noninfectious cause of the disease, it was suggested that the condition should be called endometrosis rather than degenerative endometritis.[108] It is not clear why mares with fibrotic degenerative changes to their endometrium have an impaired physical uterine clearance mechanism. Sclerotic changes in the uterine vascular bed impair blood flow to both the endometrium and myometrium.[109]

DIAGNOSTIC APPROACH. History compatible with endometritis includes infertility after breeding to a fertile stallion. Mares with severe endometritis may have shortened interestrous intervals and may show vaginal discharge. Physical and speculum examination may show anatomic defects of the vulva or cervix. Excessively easy passage of a vaginal speculum may indicate loss of integrity of the vestibulovaginal sphincter. Discharge from the cervix and vaginal inflammation may be apparent. Transrectal palpation and ultrasonography may reveal accumulations of luminal fluid.

Microbiology. Quantitative aerobic bacterial culture of the uterine lumen is necessary to identify potential pathogens and for antibiotic sensitivity. Samples should be taken during estrus, and the swab plated immediately on solid media or transported in nonnutritive media to the laboratory. Inadvertent contamination of cultures with bacteria from the lower reproductive tract is common, so the culture instrument should be guarded until it is within the uterus.[110] Cultures may be taken from endometrial biopsies. Culture alone is not diagnostic. Culture results should be interpreted in light of clinical, histologic, and cytologic findings. Culture samples for *T. equigenitalis* should be taken from the endometrium, cervix, clitorial fossa, and sinuses. Samples should be placed in Amies media with charcoal or Steward's media and be kept refrigerated until delivered to the laboratory.

Endometrial Cytology. PMNs migrate into the uterine lumen in response to inflammation so endometritis is rapidly and accurately diagnosed by examination of exfoliated endometrial cells. A sample may be taken with a guarded swab or by infusion and aspiration of a small amount of fluid. Air-dried smears are stained with new methylene blue or modified Wright-Geimsa.

Epithelial cells may be shed singly or in rafts. Arbitrary definitions of endometritis have been established on the basis of relative numbers of PMNs. Using these criteria, more than 1 PMN per 10 epithelial cells is consistent with endometritis. Endometrial cytology from normal mares may contain PMNs and spermatozoa for several days after breeding. It has been suggested that eosinophils are associated with fungal endometritis and pneumovagina. Urine crystals indicate urovagina.

Endometrial Biopsy. Endometrial biopsy is an accurate diagnostic and prognostic tool for endometritis. The biopsy should be taken during the breeding season, should be of adequate size, and should be fixed in Bouin's solution. Chronic endometritis is characterized by infiltration of the endometrium with mononuclear cells and deposition of layers of fibrosis around endometrial glands. Fibrosis of the endometrium is a degenerative change and is permanent. The severity of endometrial changes is inversely related to reproductive performance. A system to classify histologic changes has been described and is widely used[5(p723)] (Table 41-5). Special stains such as periodic acid–Schiff and Gomori's methenamine silver may be used to identify the presence of fungi in endometrial biopsies.

Transrectal Ultrasonography. The presence of free intraluminal fluid before breeding strongly suggests susceptibility to persistent endometritis.[111] Ultrasonographic examination of the uterus is helpful to assess both the quantity and quality of accumulated fluid in the uterine lumen. Normal mares may retain fluid up to 6 to 12 hours after mating. If fluid is present at 12 hours or more after breeding, the mare should be considered to have a persistent mating-induced endometritis.[112] Increased echogenicity of the fluid is associated with the presence of inflammatory cells and debris.

Hysteroscopy. Examination of the uterine lumen with an endoscope provides information about degree of inflammation, in addition to evidence of foreign bodies, transluminal adhesions, intraluminal masses, and endometrial cysts.

TREATMENT AND PROGNOSIS

Sexually Transmitted Diseases. Mares with CEM should be treated with intrauterine infusions of antibiotics based on sensitivity tests, in combination with local treatments of the clitoral fossa and sinuses. Best results can be expected when treatment is initiated when the mare is in estrus, and when combined with uterine lavage if inflammatory debris or intraluminal fluid is present. Cleansing of the vulva and the clitoris daily for 5 days with a 4% chlorhexidine or nitrofurazone ointment has been recommended.[113] Sinusectomy can also be performed.[114] Import regulations in countries free from CEM serve to prevent outbreaks of the disease. The

TABLE 41-5

Endometrial Biopsy Grade and Fertility Prognosis (Kenney and Doig)

Biopsy Category	Degree of Change	Predicted % Foaling Rate
I	None	80-90
IIA	Mild	50-80
IIB	Moderate	10-50
III	Severe	<10

spread of CEM on farms in endemic countries is best prevented by implementation of strict hygiene, screening of breeding stallions before the breeding season, and the use of artificial insemination, if allowed by the breed registry.

Persistent Uterine Infection. Treatment of mares with persistent uterine infections needs to be directed towards the underlying breakdown of the uterine defense and against the microbial agent. The first therapeutic concern should be to remove predisposing causes, such as a breakdown of external genital barriers. Persistent uterine infection frequently follows degenerative or traumatic anatomic changes and loss of integrity of the barriers of ascending infection. Therefore Caslick's surgery, repair of cervical damage and perineal lacerations, and correction of urovagina should precede specific endometrial treatment. All potential sources of contamination including intrauterine passage of diagnostic and treatment implements should be minimized. In some mares, recovery follows with sexual rest and no further treatment. Mares that are susceptible to persistent uterine infections should be bred using minimal contamination techniques to avoid bacterial contamination of the uterus.[115] Antibiotics may be administered by either local or systemic routes. Intraluminal fluid and inflammatory debris should be removed by uterine lavage before local treatment. Drugs and dosages are summarized in Table 41-6. Treatment should be based on sensitivity. Mares should be treated during estrus when natural defense is maximal, and strict aseptic technique should be used. The volume of fluid used for antibiotic therapy is dependent on the size of the uterus. A total volume of 30 to 60 ml is usually sufficient. Treatment should continue daily for 4 to 6 days during the duration of estrus. Bacterial resistance may follow inadequate dosage, and follow-up cultures should be performed. Repeated contamination may indicate an unsuccessfully resolved predisposing cause. Removal of the primary microorganism may result in overgrowth of a second bacteria or fungus (superinfection). Critical studies of the efficacy of systemic antibiotics are limited, although effective levels are produced in the endometrium after systemic administration.[116] Parenteral administration may be easier, and the opportunity to introduce uterine contamination or cause uterine irritation with treatment is eliminated.

Persistent Breeding-Induced Endometritis. Treatment of mares with persistent breeding-induced endometritis should be aimed at assisting the uterus to physically clear contaminants and inflammatory products.[90,117,118] This can be achieved by the use of uterine lavage with sterile saline or by the administration of uterotonic drugs such as oxytocin and PGF. Uterine lavage with 1 to 2 L of normal saline 6 to 24 hours after each breeding aids the mare to clear inflammatory products from the uterus. Fluid is infused by gravity through a cuffed uterine catheter and recovered by siphoning. The process is repeated until recovered effluent is clear. Effluent may provide some diagnostic information.[112] A fertilizable population of spermatozoa is established in the isthmus of the oviduct 2 hours after breeding.[119-121] The embryo

TABLE 41-6

Antibacterial Drugs Used for Intrauterine Administration for Treatment of Uterine Infections in Mares

Drug	Dosage (Intrauterine Administration)	Comments
Amikacin sulfate	2 g	Gram-negative spectrum; buffer with equal volume of 7.5% bicarbonate
Ampicillin	3 g	Gram-negative spectrum; may irritate the endometrium
Carbenicillin	2-6 g	Gram-negative spectrum; may irritate the endometrium; buffer with equal volume of 7.5% bicarbonate
Gentamicin sulfate	1-3 g	Gram-negative spectrum; buffer with equal volume of 7.5% bicarbonate
Kanamycin sulfate	1-3 g	*Escherichia coli*, spermatocidal
Neomycin sulfate	3-4 g	Useful against sensitive *E. coli*
Potassium penicillin G	5 million U	*Streptococcus zooepidemicus*
Polymyxin B	1 million U	*Pseudomonas*
Ticarcillin	6 g	Broad spectrum
Ticarcillin/clavulanic acid	6 g/200 mg	Broad spectrum
Ceftiofur	1 g	Broad spectrum (*S. zooepidemicus*)
Antimycotics		
Nystatin	500,000 U	Dissolve in 30 ml 0.9% saline solution; daily for 7 to 10 days
Clotrimazole	500 mg	Suspension or cream; daily for 1 wk
Miconazole	500 mg	Effective against yeast
Amphotericin B	200-250 mg	Daily for 1 wk
Vinegar	2%	20 ml wine vinegar to 1 L of 0.9% saline solution; used as uterine lavage

descends into the uterus 5.5 days after ovulation. For these reasons, therapy after breeding should begin not sooner than 4 hours after breeding and should be discontinued by 4 days after ovulation.

Systemic treatment with uterine ecbolic agents such as oxytocin (10 to 20 IU, IV) or PGF (5 to 10 mg IM) has been shown to be beneficial in clearing the uterus of fluid and inflammatory products.[117,118] Treatments should be given at 6 to 12 hours after breeding to be effective.[90,117,122] Oxytocin may also follow uterine lavage. Repeated periovulatory treatment with PGF appears to delay the formation of a functional CL, which may result in subfertility.[122a]

Chronic Degenerative Endometritis (Endometrosis). Several treatments have been suggested for degenerative fibrosis of the endometrium, but consistent results have not been reported. Mechanical and chemical irritation of the endometrium have been used, but concerns that trauma to the endometrium may produce more scar tissue than repair have limited the popularity of these methods. Infusion of dimethyl sulfoxide (DMSO) into the uterine lumen was shown to improve fibrosis in mares with chronic degenerative endometritis[123]; however, others were not able to repeat these results.[124]

Prognosis for fertility after endometritis varies with the severity of inflammation and fibrosis and the inciting cause. Prognosis should take into account the age of the mare and the level of reproductive management, in addition to the etiology and likely response to treatment.

Metritis

Metritis is classically defined as inflammation of all layers of the uterine wall. Metritis occurs in the first 2 weeks after foaling and commonly follows abortion, dystocia, and RFM. In mares, metritis is often accompanied by endotoxemia and laminitis. Transluminal adhesions between endometrial folds may follow severe metritis.

CLINICAL SIGNS AND DIAGNOSIS. Metritis is characterized by uterine accumulation of postpartum secretions, bacteria, and the products of inflammation, with discharge from the cervix and possibly the vulva. Discharge is usually fluid and red-brown and may be fetid. Systemic signs of depression accompanied by neutropenia and leukopenia are apparent with development of endotoxemia. Differentials include normal lochia and causes of profound depression in the postpartum period as a result of uterine tears and abdominal catastrophes.

TREATMENT AND PROGNOSIS. Treatment is directed toward removing contamination and microorganisms from the uterus while providing systemic treatment for endotoxemia. Broad-spectrum systemic antibiotics, antiinflammatory drugs, and fluid therapy are indicated. Uterine contamination may be removed by gentle intraluminal infusion of warm water or saline and siphoning off uterine contents. Vigorous lavage should be avoided, particularly during acute systemic disease. Prognosis depends on severity of clinical signs. If metritis is diagnosed quickly and treatment instituted, prognosis for fertility and systemic health is good. Prognosis is guarded once endotoxemia and laminitis develop.

Pyometra

Pyometra in mares is an accumulation of purulent exudate in the lumen of the uterus. Impedance to mechanical uterine outflow, such as cervical fibrosis and adhesions of cranial parts of the tract ventrally into the abdomen, may contribute to the development of pyometra. If endometrial irritation causes release of endogenous endometrial PGF, diestrus will be shortened. In some mares, endometrial destruction is so severe that PGF release is inadequate and luteal life is prolonged.[24] A variety of bacteria may be involved, including *E. coli*, *Pseudomonas* spp., and *Streptococcus* spp. Cultures may be negative.

CLINICAL SIGNS AND DIAGNOSIS. A purulent vaginal or cervical discharge may be seen. The mare may demonstrate a short diestrus, a normal interestrous interval, or a prolonged diestrus. Occasional mares with pyometra have mild leukopenia and normocytic-normochromic anemia, secondary to mild suppression of erythropoiesis.[35] Transrectal palpation and ultrasonography reveal a fluid-filled uterus. The uterine wall may be thin and flaccid or thick.

TREATMENT AND PROGNOSIS. Treatment should involve correction of predisposing causes, fluid evacuation, and

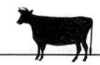

local antibiotic treatment. Evacuation of large amounts of fluid from the uterus may result in redistribution of fluid and circulatory shock. The mare should be monitored for signs of circulatory shock, and intravenous fluid may be administered during evacuation of large amounts of fluid from the uterus. The prognosis for life is excellent; however, the prognosis for return to normal fertility is guarded to poor because the conditions that predispose to development of pyometra in mares (cervical stenosis and adhesions) are difficult to treat and because severe endometrial destruction may develop. Endometrial biopsy should precede vigorous treatment. Hysterectomy is an option if treatment is unsuccessful and if discharge is unacceptable or if adhesions impair athletic ability.

■ RUMINANTS

Parturition

Deliveries complicated by dystocia or RFM may be followed by severe bacterial infections of the uterus. The most sanitary environment possible should be provided for calving. The use of a clean pasture may be most appropriate on some farms, whereas the use of roomy, well-bedded, indoor maternity pens that are cleaned after each delivery may be appropriate on others.

Cows that suffer from abnormalities around the time of calving such as hypocalcemia, dystocia, and RFM are more likely to suffer from uterine infections than are cows that calve normally. Routine treatment of cows with antibacterial drugs and chemicals has not been shown to be beneficial and in some cases has reduced fertility. Postpartum uterine infections may be prevented, or the number of such infections reduced by strict attention to sanitation in the calving environment and during assistance with delivery, along with proper management during the dry period.[125]

Bovine Uterine Infection

Bovine uteri are normally contaminated by a wide variety of microorganisms during the puerperium. Most of the organisms are transient residents of the reproductive tract and are soon eliminated from the involuting uteri of normal cows. *A. pyogenes* can persist in the uteri of cows and act with *Fusobacterium necrophorum* and *Bacteroides* spp. to cause uterine infections. Coliforms, *P. aeruginosa*, hemolytic streptococci, and gram-positive and gram-negative anaerobic bacteria are also frequently isolated from cases of postpartum uterine disease. *A. pyogenes* and *Clostridium* spp. occasionally colonize the postpartum uterus synergistically, causing severe gangrenous metritis. Other organisms that appear to have little effect on fertility may colonize the uterus and produce penicillinase, thus influencing the selection and route of administration of drugs used to treat uterine infections.[76]

Uterine infections may follow dystocia and RFM in sheep and goats but are not frequently a cause of infertility because lambing and kidding are followed by a period of up to 6 months of sexual rest before the next breeding season. RFM and metritis follow abortion in ewes caused by *Listeria monocytogenes*, *Campylobacter fetus* ssp. *fetus*, and *Chlamydia psittaci*.

CLINICAL SIGNS AND DIAGNOSIS. Lochia is normally expelled during the first 2 weeks after calving and may range from dark red or brown to white to clear. If uterine involution is delayed, discharge of lochia may continue until 30 days after calving. Discharge of lochia is not abnormal unless the fluid is fetid or the cow develops other abnormal clinical signs. Abnormalities of uterine involution cannot be diagnosed by palpation per rectum during the first several days after calving when both normal and abnormal uteri are out

of reach and cannot be safely retracted. By 10 to 15 days after calving the entire uterus can be palpated if involution is normal. Fluid should not be palpable within the uterine lumen by 14 to 18 days after calving. Gross reduction in size and histologic repair of the endometrium are complete in dairy cows by 40 to 50 days after calving.

Postpartum metritis in cows is characterized by the presence of variable amounts of lochia within the uterine lumen that may be discerned by palpation per rectum. A vaginal discharge is usually present, but it may become obvious during palpation. Septic metritis is characterized by clinical signs of toxemia that may include fever, depression, partial or complete anorexia, and laminitis. Milk yield is depressed, and cows may be unwilling or unable to rise. Some cases may be complicated by tenesmus. Vaginitis and cervicitis may accompany metritis. Discharges associated with septic metritis vary from scanty white mucus to copious amounts of red to red-black, watery, malodorous fluid. In some cases, inflammation may spread through the uterine wall and cause perimetritis and peritonitis.[126] Septic metritis in ewes and does is characterized by fever, depression, anorexia, and tenesmus.

Endometritis in cattle is usually observed between 2 and 8 weeks after calving. Discharge can range from white pus to estrual mucus. Purulent exudate may be observed only with palpation, or found in the cranial vagina and cervical canal by examination with a speculum. The history may indicate that the cow has failed to conceive after several services but the patient is otherwise healthy.

Culture of endometrial fluid is not usually done on individual cases of bovine uterine infection, but may be indicated to determine the antibiotic susceptibility of microorganisms on a particular farm or as a part of the diagnostic plan when the incidence of postpartum metritis or endometritis increases suddenly.

Endometrial biopsies are rarely used in cows but have been recommended when complete evaluation is required of the reproductive tract of cows that do not conceive or that conceive but do not complete their pregnancy.[5(p424)]

TREATMENT AND PROGNOSIS. To be useful in treating uterine infections in cows, an antibiotic must be active against the primary uterine pathogens (*A. pyogenes* and gram-negative anaerobes), in the presence of organic debris, and in the anaerobic environment of the postpartum bovine uterus.[127] Organisms infecting the uteri of cows are usually susceptible to penicillin, but during the first month after calving contaminating microorganisms may produce penicillinase. Thus penicillin is not likely to be effective if given locally during the early postpartum period. By 30 days after calving, organisms that produce penicillinase are usually eliminated from the uterus, and intrauterine treatment with penicillin may be beneficial. The daily intrauterine dose of penicillin required to reach the minimum inhibitory concentration of common bacteria such as *A. pyogenes* is 1×10^6 IU.[127] Oxytetracycline is active against many of the microorganisms that infect the bovine uterus, and its activity is only slightly reduced by organic debris and absence of oxygen. Intrauterine treatment with administration of 4 to 6 g of oxytetracycline per day has been recommended. Some preparations of oxytetracycline irritate the endometrium, cervix, and vagina. Intrauterine antibiotic treatment of dairy cows results in residues in their milk.[128] For example, oxytetracycline has been found in milk from 44[129] to 96[130] hours after intrauterine administration.

Penicillin is effective for treatment of some uterine infections in cows by systemic administration. Daily doses of penicillin required to reach the minimum inhibitory concentration of *A. pyogenes* are 10,000 to 20,000 IU/kg/day. Minimum inhibitory concentration of oxytetracycline for *A. pyogenes* in

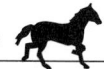

the uterus is usually higher than the concentration that can be achieved by systemic administration of the drug.

Treatment of septic metritis should be directed toward controlling septicemia. Large doses of broad-spectrum systemic antibiotics are indicated, along with fluids and other supportive therapy. Attempts to remove a RFM or irrigate the uterus are contraindicated during the acute phase of the disease. After the patient has recovered from acute septicemia, intrauterine therapy may be considered.

Ewes and does affected with metritis are usually treated with systemic antibiotics such as penicillin or sulfamethazine. Early and aggressive treatment is indicated.[131]

Antiseptic Chemicals. A variety of antiseptic chemicals have been infused into the uterine lumen of cows in attempts to treat metritis and endometritis, but few controlled trial evaluations are available. These are attractive as a way to avoid milk antibiotic residues but milk antiseptic residues occur after intrauterine infusion.[132] Dilute solutions of povidone-iodine (one part povidone-iodine stock solution to 10 to 20 parts saline) have been suggested as being useful in treating fungal endometritis or cases of endometritis that appear to be caused by bacteria that cannot be demonstrated by routine culture techniques.[43(p40)] Povidone-iodine is generally available as a 10% solution with 1% free iodine (10,000 ppm of free iodine), so that a dilution of 20:1 saline:povidone-iodine yields a flush with 500 ppm free iodine, which should be bactericidal.

Uterine Lavage. Lavage of the uterine lumen with large volumes of warm saline (40° to 45° C [104° to 118° F]) removes accumulated fluid and debris. Uterine lavage has been used as an adjunct to antibiotic, antiseptic, and plasma treatment. Catheters designed for nonsurgical embryo recovery are suitable for uterine lavage. Saline is infused into the endometrial cavity in 0.5- to 1-L increments, allowed to reflux through the catheter, and collected for inspection. A milk hose and larger fluid volumes may be used in cattle with larger postpartum uteri, but care must be taken not to enter far into the uterus because it is friable and easily perforated. Massage or partial retraction of the uterus by palpation per rectum may be necessary to increase fluid recovery. The endometrial cavity is lavaged repeatedly until the fluid returning through the catheter is no longer turbid.

Prostaglandins. In cows, having estrous cycles, repeated administration of PGF results in shortened estrous cycles and may mimic the shortened luteal phase of patients with acute endometritis. PGF therapy may be sufficient in mild cases of endometritis or may be used in combination with intrauterine or systemic therapy. In cases of chronic bovine endometritis, treatment with PGF one or two times at 10- to 14-day intervals decreased the number of days open.[133]

The prognosis in cows for recovery from endometritis is usually good if the condition does not progress to a more severe form of uterine disease. Septic metritis after dystocia or RFM may result in permanent impairment of reproductive function, laminitis, or death of the patient in spite of aggressive therapy.

Pyometra

In dairy cows, pyometra is likely to develop in cows that ovulate before microorganisms that infect the uterus during the postpartum period are eliminated. The CL that develops following the first postpartum ovulation at approximately 15 to 18 days after calving persists, possibly because the abnormal uterine contents suspend release of PGF from the endometrium or sequester it within the uterine lumen. The uterus is brought under the influence of progesterone, which depresses phagocytic activity of uterine neutrophils and closes the cervix, allowing the bacterial infection to persist.[134] Pyo-

metra rarely endangers the general health or life of affected cows. Cases of pyometra that occur during the postbreeding period may also be caused by *Tritrichomonas foetus*.[135]

PGF is the treatment of choice for bovine pyometra. Treatment with PGF is followed in 3 to 6 days by uterine evacuation in 85% to 90% of treated cows. Response to PGF treatment may be raised with a second injection of PGF in 6 to 12 hours. After endometrial lesions are allowed to heal for 30 days, fertility is restored in most patients.

Treatment of cows with gonadotropin-releasing hormone (GnRH) 2 weeks after calving improves fertility in some but not all situations. In herds with a high prevalence of postpartum uterine infections, treatment with GnRH may decrease fertility by inducing ovulation and CL development; thus the uterus is brought under the influence of progesterone before contaminating bacteria are removed, leading to pyometra.

Perimetritis

Perimetritis may occur in all species as a sequela to severe uterine infections, uterine rupture, penetration of the vagina during mating, traumatic insemination or obstetric procedures, and cesarean section.[58(p353),131] Perimetritis is characterized by inflammation of the peritoneal surface of the uterus and may be accompanied by localized or diffuse peritonitis. Adhesions then develop between the uterus and other pelvic and abdominal organs.

CLINICAL SIGNS AND DIAGNOSIS. The clinical signs of perimetritis are those of peritonitis and may include fever, depression, partial or complete anorexia, stasis of the gastrointestinal tract, and evidence of abdominal pain. Abdominal pain is typified by colic in mares and by grinding the teeth (odontoprisis) in cows. In cows the condition should be differentiated from traumatic reticuloperitonitis, displacements of parts of the digestive tract, abomasal ulcers, postpartum metritis, and abdominal fat necrosis. Perimetritis in mares must be differentiated from other causes of severe abdominal pain. Antemortem diagnosis of perimetritis is difficult in sheep and goats that present mainly with fever, depression, anorexia, and odontoprisis.

CLINICAL PATHOLOGY. Cases of acute perimetritis are accompanied by leukopenia, neutropenia, and a degenerative left shift. Further evidence of peritonitis is obtained when peritoneal fluid is obtained by paracentesis and examined for its cellular and microbiologic content.

TREATMENT AND PROGNOSIS. The cause of perimetritis should be treated if possible. Cases of severe metritis should be treated appropriately and uterine ruptures sutured if possible. Repair of uterine ruptures inaccessible by flank incisions may be facilitated by intentional prolapse of the uterus after administration of epinephrine, provided the tear is not too close to the cervix (see next section). Treatment with broad-spectrum systemic antibiotics is indicated. Lavage to remove peritoneal exudate has been recommended but is difficult to accomplish, especially in cows in which the rumen, abomasum, and greater omentum make ventral drainage almost impossible and in which fibrinous peritonitis with loculation of infection occurs rapidly. Other supportive treatments such as intravenous fluids and antiinflammatory drugs should be administered as indicated.

The prognosis depends on the severity of lesions. Fatalities can occur in spite of prompt treatment, and surviving animals may be infertile because of mechanical interference with gamete transport caused by adhesions between the genital organs and other pelvic and abdominal tissues. In general, the prognosis for fertility in affected animals is fair at best.

PREVENTION AND CONTROL. Perimetritis occurs sporadically in individual animals; thus prevention depends on

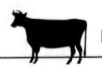

avoiding the causes. Immature females, especially heifers and fillies, should not be allowed at pasture with adult males to prevent undesired mating complicated by penetration of the vagina. Traumatic obstetric, insemination, and uterine lavage procedures must be avoided. Uterine tears that occur at parturition must be sutured immediately. Postpartum metritis must be treated promptly and appropriately before it progresses to perimetritis.

ANATOMIC DEFECTS AS A CAUSE OF UTERINE INFECTION

The most common anatomic defect associated with genital infections is pneumovagina. Other defects include urovagina and perineal lacerations. These defects should be corrected to prevent contamination with environmental and fecal organisms.

Iatrogenic Causes of Uterine Infections

Iatrogenic infection of the uterus may follow invasion of the genital canal with nonsterile instruments. Microorganisms may be carried from animal to animal if instruments are not sterilized between uses.

ENDOMETRIAL CYSTS AND LACUNAE

Mare

Endometrial cysts and lymphatic lacunae are common degenerative changes of the endometrium that are more prevalent in mares older than 11 years of age than in younger mares.[136] Endometrial cysts can originate from endometrial glands or obstructed lymphatics. Glandular cysts are small (<10 mm) and are believed to be the result of periglandular fibrosis. Lymphatic cysts can reach several centimeters in diameter. The etiology of lymphatic cysts is not fully understood, but lacunae are thought to arise after interference with normal lymph drainage from the genital tract.[5(p723)]

CLINICAL SIGNS AND DIAGNOSIS. Endometrial cysts can be demonstrated by ultrasonography or by hysteroscopy. Cysts may mimic pregnancy when mares are examined per rectum by palpation or ultrasonography.[137] Sequential examination reveals that size of endometrial cysts remains static, whereas amniotic vesicles enlarge. Large, discrete, fluid-filled cysts may be identified by palpation of the uterus per rectum. Smaller cysts and lacunae may be observed in endometrial biopsy sections. Uteri affected by lymphatic lacunae are enlarged and have a thicker wall than normal.

TREATMENT AND PROGNOSIS. Endometrial cysts do not require treatment unless they are suspected to interfere with pregnancy. Endometrial cysts have been suggested to cause embryonic death and abortion if large or numerous. However, one study failed to find an association between the presence or number of cysts and fertility.[136] Obliteration of endometrial cysts using endoscopic guided laser surgery removes the cysts permanently, but the long-term effect on fertility has not been critically evaluated. Needle aspiration, mechanical rupture of the cyst, uterine curettage, or intrauterine infusion of hypertonic saline solution have all been suggested to effectively remove endometrial cysts. However, the cysts often recur after treatment.

UTERINE PROLAPSE

Uterine prolapse occurs when the previously gravid uterine horn becomes invaginated after delivery of the fetus(es) and protrudes from the vulva.

Mare

Uterine prolapse is an uncommon sequela to normal foaling, dystocia, or RFM in the mare. The tip of the previously gravid horn invaginates to form uterine eversion. Eversion is accompanied by pain and abdominal straining, because the myometrium may contract around the ring of invaginated tissue. Transrectal palpation confirms the diagnosis, and the everted tissue may be replaced manually. Eversion may progress to complete uterine prolapse, accompanied by rapid onset of systemic signs.

TREATMENT AND PROGNOSIS. The prolapsed uterus should be washed with clean saline and replaced manually in the standing mare as rapidly as possible. Replacement is aided by sedating the mare and administering epidural anesthesia. The uterus should be supported on a clean sheet held at the level of the pelvis. The uterus should be replaced, beginning with the uterine body and working gradually, replacing the tip of the horns last. Correct positioning of the uterus is important to prevent the prolapse from recurring. Replacement should be followed by treatment with broad-spectrum antibiotics, antiinflammatory drugs, and intravenous isotonic fluids. Treatment with oxytocin (10 to 20 IU IM) facilitates uterine involution. Prognosis is related to development of sequelae such as uterine tears, metritis, and endometrial damage.[138]

Ruminants

In cows, most cases of uterine prolapse occur within a few hours after calving. The condition is frequently associated with hypocalcemia, which results in lack of uterine tone and delayed cervical involution. In addition, dystocia frequently precedes uterine prolapse.

Iatrogenic uterine prolapse can be induced within 12 hours after calving by administration of epinephrine to relax the uterus. A 10-ml amount of epinephrine (1:1000) is diluted to 250 ml in sterile saline and administered slowly intravenously. After 100 ml of the solution has been given, the operator reaches through the cervix, grasps the uterine wall and caruncles, and everts the uterine horn toward the cervix. When sufficient uterine tissue has entered the cervical canal, the patient responds by straining, which assists in completion of the prolapse. Epidural anesthesia is administered to abolish further straining after the prolapse is complete.

Uterine prolapse in does has been associated with dystocia, hypocalcemia, and lack of exercise.[5(p593)] The predisposing factors are probably similar for ewes.

CLINICAL SIGNS AND DIAGNOSIS. Clinical signs of uterine prolapse are obvious. The membranes may remain attached. Immediately after prolapse occurs, the tissues are nearly normal but within a few hours become enlarged and edematous. The endometrium is usually contaminated with feces and bedding material. In some cases the prolapsed tissue may be lacerated or severely traumatized.

Clinical signs that may accompany uterine prolapse include straining, abdominal pain, restlessness, anorexia, and increased pulse and respiratory rates.[58(p353)] Parturient paresis is common in affected dairy cows. In most patients, these signs are transitory, but shock may complicate some cases.

CLINICAL PATHOLOGY. Uterine prolapse in cows is frequently accompanied by hypocalcemia and a significant increase in the packed cell volume.[139]

TREATMENT AND PROGNOSIS. The prolapsed tissue should be protected from further damage by wrapping it in wet towels or covering it with a plastic bag. Beef cows should be restrained where they are found to prevent trauma to the uterus or rupture of the large uterine vessels, should the ani-

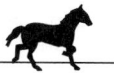

mal try to escape on arrival of the clinician. Treatment of hypocalcemia is usually indicated before replacement of the uterus if the cow is recumbent and (semi) comatose; otherwise calcium gluconate is administered after replacement. Epidural anesthesia is frequently (but not always) required.

The prolapsed tissue is washed with a mild presurgical scrub. The membranes are removed if they can be easily separated from the endometrium but are left in place if removal is difficult. Some clinicians recommend that cows stand during replacement, whereas others have found that the organ can be replaced in recumbent cows if the patient is placed on her sternum with the hind legs drawn straight out behind. The prolapse is placed between the extended limbs.[140] In fresh cases, replacement is relatively easy and is begun at the cervical pole of the organ; the dorsal and ventral parts are massaged alternately back into their normal position. After the ovarian pole has been replaced, the previously prolapsed horn must be straightened, and eversion of the uterus corrected. Administration of clenbuterol is reported to relax the uterus, facilitate replacement, and reduce the need for epidural anesthesia.[141] If the patient has been neglected, accumulated fluid must be reduced by lubricating the tissue with an emollient ointment followed by careful but vigorous massage of the tissue from the ovarian pole toward the cervical pole. The hygroscopic action of sugar when applied liberally to prolapsed uteri is of limited value and vastly overrated.

Oxytocin is frequently administered to stimulate myometrial contractions after the uterus has been replaced. Metritis is a frequent sequela, and appropriate antibiotic treatment is indicated in most cases. Temporary closure of the vulva with heavy sutures after replacement may not be necessary[58(p353)] but is practiced by many clinicians.[5(p593)] If replacement of the prolapsed uterus is impossible or the tissue is severely traumatized, amputation may be indicated.[142]

The prognosis varies but is generally favorable if there has been no serious damage to the uterus.[5(p593),140] Fatalities can occur in cases complicated by shock or by rupture of large uterine vessels. The culling rate from infertility for cows with uterine prolapse is higher than that of their herdmates, and the calving interval is prolonged in affected cows. Barring hypoglycemia, the risk of uterine prolapse at a subsequent calving is no greater than for other cows in the herd.

PREVENTION AND CONTROL. Because the condition is associated with hypocalcemia in cows, provision of a properly balanced ration before calving is indicated. Although uterine prolapse can occur after an apparently normal delivery, it is more commonly associated with dystocia and forced extraction; thus prolapse should be anticipated, and the dam observed so affected patients may receive prompt treatment.

UTERINE TUMORS

Neoplasia uncommonly affects the uterus of domestic animals. Tumors may arise from within uterine tissues or metastasize from other organs.[9] Leiomyomas are usually benign and arise from the outer smooth muscle of the uterus without need for a preparatory event. The multicentric form of lymphosarcoma may affect the uterus of cattle. Lymphosarcoma also affects does, but a predilection for the uterus is not apparent. Carcinomas, chorionepitheliomas, fibromas, fibrosarcomas, rhabdomyosarcomas, and adenosarcomas are rarely reported.

Small tumors may escape detection, whereas larger ones may be palpable per rectum in mares and cows. Leiomyomas are not necessarily associated with reproductive failure, and tumors and fetuses can coexist. Uterine walls affected by lymphosarcoma may contain discrete neoplastic nodules or be diffusely infiltrated. Tumor masses must be differentiated

from normal fetuses, mummified or macerated fetuses, placentomes, abscesses, and fat necrosis.

Solitary leiomyomas thought to interfere with fertility may be removed. Other forms of uterine neoplasia are usually not treated. The prognosis is generally poor.

SEGMENTAL DEFECTS (White Heifer Disease)

Segmental aplasia occurs sporadically in all cattle breeds. In most cases the cranial parts of the genital tract (ovaries, uterine tubes, and cranial part of the uterine horns) are normal, and endometrial secretions from the parts of the uterine horns accumulate because normal drainage through the cervix is impeded. Various defects may be found in affected animals, ranging from nearly complete absence of tubular genital organs to an imperforate hymen that blocks secretions drainage from a normal genital tract.

CLINICAL SIGNS AND DIAGNOSIS. Segmental aplasia may be associated with a history of anestrus if fluid accumulation within the uterine horns interferes with release of PGF and luteolysis. Other presenting history may involve infertility or difficulty in artificial insemination. On palpation per rectum, various degrees of aplasia may be recognized. Fluid-filled parts of the uterine horns may suggest pregnancy, from which they must be differentiated. An imperforate hymen may bulge from the vulvar cleft and may be confused with vaginal prolapse, prolapse or eversion of the urinary bladder, cystic vestibular glands, or neoplasia of the vulva or vagina.

TREATMENT AND PROGNOSIS. The only form of segmental aplasia amenable to treatment is that in which an imperforate hymen occludes an otherwise normal tract. Incision of the hymen is followed by drainage of accumulated secretions and may allow the tract to function normally.

PARAMESONEPHRIC DUCT APLASIA

Aplasia of one paramesonephric duct leads to development of one uterine horn (uterus unicornis). The condition is relatively rare but does occur in cattle. Subfertility is the result of prolonged periods of anestrus caused by a persistent CL on the ovary ipsilateral to the missing uterine horn (no local luteolytic signal). The condition can be managed with exogenous PGF in the hope that ovulation will occur on the intact side. Alternatively, the unaccompanied ovary can be surgically removed.

INCOMPLETE FUSION OF PARAMESONEPHRIC DUCTS

The caudal parts of the paramesonephric ducts may not fuse properly in cattle, causing duplication of various parts of the caudal tubular tract. Abnormalities of fusion are most common in and around the cervix. The entire cervix may be duplicated; or the cervix and vagina may be normal, with the exception of the presence of a band of tissue extending from dorsal to ventral across the external os of the cervix. Partial failure of fusion may involve a part of the cervix, and the affected animal may possess a single uterine body and internal cervical os, duplication of a part of the cervical canal, and a doubled external cervical os. Uterus didelphis results when the cervix and uterine body are completely duplicated. Affected cows may conceive after natural service or if artificially inseminated through the cervix and uterine horn ipsilateral to the ovary about to ovulate. Affected animals may be unable to carry a pregnancy to term because of lack of placental attachment in the nongravid horn.

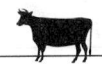

HYDROMETRA (Pseudopregnancy in Goats)

Hydrometra occurs sporadically in goats and is characterized by accumulation of several liters of clear fluid within the uterus, abdominal distention, persistence of a CL, and subsequent anestrus.[5(p585)] The condition may develop after mating, and does are frequently assumed to be pregnant. Accumulated fluid is expelled approximately 150 days after the infertile mating, accounting for the common name of "cloudburst." The cause of hydrometra is unknown, but a deficiency in production or release of PGF from the endometrium has been postulated, as has exposure to phytoestrogens.

The clinical signs of hydrometra mimic those of pregnancy. Neither a fetus nor fetal membranes are delivered when the accumulated fluid is expelled. The condition might be differentiated from pregnancy by inability to detect a fetus by ballottement or real-time ultrasonography late in the gestation period. Examination with Doppler ultrasound fails to reveal a fetal heartbeat or evidence of placental blood flow.

The condition resolves spontaneously when the CL regresses. If treatment is desired, PGF (2 to 3 mg of dinoprost or 100 to 150 mg of cloprostenol) is indicated to induce luteal regression. Although some does may be affected by subsequent episodes of hydrometra, many experience normal pregnancies.

CERVICAL ABNORMALITY

Cervicitis

Inflammation of the cervix usually accompanies endometritis and vaginitis and is frequently secondary to trauma associated with dystocia and obstetric operations. The mucus-secreting epithelium of the cervix is more resistant to bacterial infection than is the epithelium of the uterus and vagina.

▌▌ *MARE*

The equine cervix is a straight tube made up of layered circular and longitudinal muscle. During estrus it relaxes, and the external os lies on the floor of the anterior vagina. During diestrus or pregnancy, under the influence of progesterone, the cervix is closed and the external os is elevated off the vaginal floor. Cervicitis or inflammation of the cervix may be iatrogenic or may occur secondary to trauma associated with parturition or dystocia or as an extension of vaginitis or endometritis. Endometritis and infertility follow if the cervix lacks anatomic integrity.

CLINICAL SIGNS AND DIAGNOSIS. Infertility and history of an inciting cause such as urine pooling or dystocia may be the only signs of cervicitis in the mare. Cervical hyperemia and edema may be apparent on speculum examination in acute cervicitis. In more chronic injuries, direct digital examination of the cervix of the mare while in diestrus may reveal transluminal adhesions or anatomic defects.

▌▌ *RUMINANTS*

Similarly in cows, cervicitis is secondary to uterine infections and follows trauma associated with parturition and obstetric manipulations. Infection is usually caused by microorganisms normally present in the cranial vagina such as *E. coli,* streptococci, staphylococci, and *A. pyogenes.* Occasionally infection with anaerobic bacteria complicates cervicitis and results in severe toxemia.[58(p434),143]

Cervicitis in does and ewes is uncommon but may occur secondary to vaginal and uterine infections and obstetric trauma.

CLINICAL SIGNS AND DIAGNOSIS. Examination of cows with a vaginal speculum reveals swelling and edema of the external cervical os. The mucous membrane is hyperemic and inflamed. Mucopurulent exudate may be present in the cervical canal or in the cranial vagina. Hypertrophy of the cervix is common in *Bos indicus* breeds and their crosses and may be a normal finding, thus cervical size as detected by palpation per rectum may or may not indicate inflammation. Inflammation of the cervix without contemporary endometritis may not affect fertility. Cervicitis may occur in pregnant cows.

The clinical signs of cervicitis in does and ewes are similar to those in cattle and must be observed with a small vaginal speculum.

TREATMENT AND PROGNOSIS (MARES AND RUMINANTS). Most cases of cervicitis resolve spontaneously when coexisting endometritis and vaginitis improve. Exudate can be flushed from the cervical canal and cranial vagina with warm saline lavages and a nonirritating antibiotic ointment applied to the affected tissue. Caustic chemicals should not be placed in contact with the cervical mucosa. Aggressive treatment with systemic antibiotics is indicated in cases complicated by infection with anaerobic bacteria.

The prognosis for most cases of simple cervicitis is fair to good. However, inflammation of the cervix in mares may progress to more severe cervical abnormalities. Cervical damage is a serious threat to future reproductive performance in mares. Anaerobic infections of the cervix may be fatal.

PREVENTION AND CONTROL. Obstetric manipulations and operations must be temperate. When the cervix does not properly dilate during parturition, a cesarean section is preferred over forced extraction.

CERVICAL LACERATIONS

Mare

Cervical lacerations are most often seen after dystocia. Cervical lacerations may result in adhesions and a nonpatent cervix or in a failure to seal the uterus during diestrus or pregnancy. Cervical adhesions in combination with endometritis are a common cause of pyometra in the mare.

CLINICAL SIGNS AND DIAGNOSIS. Cervical lacerations can be diagnosed by vaginoscopy and digital examination of the cervix. A digital examination of the cervix is often necessary to evaluate the degree and severity of the laceration. Evaluation of the ability of the cervix to close adequately is best performed during diestrus.

TREATMENT AND PROGNOSIS. If cervical lacerations are diagnosed shortly after parturition, antimicrobial ointment should be applied frequently to the lesion. Early signs of adhesions should be broken down until the tissue is healed. If the laceration results in an incompetent cervix, it should be corrected surgically. Although surgical repair of cervical lacerations has resulted in restored fertility in many mares, the condition is likely to recur at the time of the next parturition. Embryo transfer should be considered if allowed by the breed registry.

VAGINAL ABNORMALITIES

Pneumovagina: Mare

Pneumovagina is characterized by aspiration of air containing feces and microorganisms into the vagina. Pneumovagina is secondary to changes in perineal conformation, which include cranioventral displacement of the reproductive tract, loss of integrity of the vestibulovaginal sphincter, and loss of integrity of the vulvar labia. These changes occur more commonly in older, multiparous mares and those that have suffered perineal lacerations. Pneumovagina is a common antecedent to infertility.

CLINICAL SIGNS AND DIAGNOSIS. In the normal mare the anus is positioned directly dorsal to the vulva; the perineal body between the dorsal vulva and the anus is thick, muscular, and well-formed; the vestibulovaginal sphincter is well-formed; the vulva has a vertical alignment; 80% of the vulval labia lies below the floor of the pelvis; and the vulvar labia form a seal. Mares in which the vulva tilts horizontally at its dorsal aspect, the perineal body is thin, and the vulvar labia do not form a seal are prone to pneumovagina in cases in which the anus lies rostral to the vulva. A scoring system has been developed to evaluate the perineal conformation in mares.[78] The system uses the Caslick's index, which equals the distance (cm) between the dorsal commisure and the pelvic floor multiplied by the degrees of declination of the vulvar lips. Mares with a Caslick's index above 150 were found to have subnormal pregnancy rates. Affected mares aspirate air on exercise or when the vulval labia are parted. Aspirated air may be noted on transrectal palpation or vaginal speculum examination. Signs of secondary changes such as vaginitis, cervicitis, or endometritis may be apparent.

TREATMENT AND PROGNOSIS. Treatment of pneumovagina should be directed toward correcting defective perineal conformation. Cranioventral displacement of the reproductive tract in aged mares may be irreversible. Perineal confirmation in thin mares is often improved by increasing the mare's body condition. Pneumovagina is often successfully corrected by surgical closure of the dorsal vagina via the Caslick's operation. Secondary changes should be treated as described elsewhere. Prognosis for correction of pneumovagina is excellent; however, prognosis for fertility depends on the extent of secondary changes.

Urovagina: Mare

In normal, young mares the vagina slopes craniodorsally and is largely contained within the pelvis. With aging and repeated pregnancy, the cranial vagina may slope cranioventrally and fall below the level of the pelvic floor. Under these conditions urine collects in the anterior vagina, where it is spermicidal and may predispose to cervicitis and endometritis.

CLINICAL SIGNS AND DIAGNOSIS. In mild cases a history of infertility may be the only indicator of urovagina. In more severe cases, urine dribbles from the vulva at rest or during exercise and may accumulate inside the hind limbs. Speculum examination reveals a cranioventral slope of the vagina, variable inflammation of the cranial vagina and cervix, and a pool of urine in the ventral vaginal fornix. Urovagina may occur intermittently or only during estrus.

TREATMENT AND PROGNOSIS. Surgical procedures to prevent the anterior flow of urine include urethral extension[144] and vaginoplasty.[145] Prognosis depends on the severity of secondary endometritis and the success of surgery.

Vaginitis

Vaginitis may occur as a result of ascending infection or exposure to irritants, or secondary to pneumovagina, urovagina, perineal laceration, rectovaginal fistulae, breeding, endometritis, abortion, parturition or dystocia. Occasionally traumatic wounds may be infected with clostridial or anaerobic organisms; however, most infection is nonspecific.

CLINICAL SIGNS AND DIAGNOSIS. Signs may vary from hyperemia evident on speculum examination to mucopurulent exudation from the vulva. Severe trauma and infection may be followed by necrotic vaginitis with tenesmus, fetid discharge, elevated tail, swollen vulva, and systemic signs. Rapid formation of adhesions follows necrotic vaginitis.

Metritis, RFM, and uterine tears also may show systemic signs and vaginal discharge.

TREATMENT AND PROGNOSIS. The inciting cause should be treated. Mild vaginitis may recover spontaneously, whereas moderate cases require local lavage with dilute antiseptic or antibiotic solutions. Fertility is unaffected in mild vaginitis without extension, and prognosis is good. Severe, necrotic vaginitis is treated with systemic antibiotics, analgesics, and antiinflammatory agents. Caslick's surgery may be necessary to prevent aspiration of air. Local application of antibiotic and steroid-impregnated ointments may help prevent adhesions. Prognosis for severe vaginitis is guarded. Vaginal stenosis and adhesions may follow vaginitis.

PREVENTION AND CONTROL. Nonspecific vaginitis may be prevented by preventing or reducing trauma to the vagina. Clinicians should elect appropriate methods for relief of dystocia and apply extractive force to fetuses judiciously.

Infectious Pustular Vulvovaginitis: Cow

Infectious pustular vulvovaginitis (IPV) affects cattle and is caused by bovid herpesvirus I, also the cause of infectious bovine rhinotracheitis or IBR,[146] although the two strains are genetically distinct.[147] Therefore the respiratory and genital forms of the disease rarely occur concurrently, and abortions usually do not follow an outbreak of the genital form of the disease. IPV is spread by coitus and mechanical means and may affect unbred heifers. The incubation period of IPV is short (1 to 3 days), and the infection spreads rapidly through the herd, affecting 60% to 90% of the animals.

CLINICAL SIGNS AND DIAGNOSIS. Early in the course of the disease IPV is characterized by a mucopurulent vaginal discharge and inflammation of the vaginal and vulvar mucosa. Pustules develop over lymphoid follicles and progress from small (<3 mm) ulcers to coalescing erosions. The virus affects the penile mucosa, causing affected animals considerable pain. Thus both sexes with IPV are reluctant to mate. The clinical signs subside in 10 to 30 days, leaving the recovered animals with transient immunity. Early in the course of IPV, lesions may be similar to those of granular vulvitis (see the later section) but the lesions of IPV rapidly become more severe. Vulvovaginitis caused by *Haemophilus somnus* should be a differential.

TREATMENT AND PROGNOSIS. Treatment of IPV is usually not required, although lavage of the vagina with dilute antiseptic solutions and emollients has been recommended. Mating among infected animals should be suspended until the disease subsides. The prognosis for recovery is excellent.

PREVENTION AND CONTROL. Vaccination against IBR is not likely to be beneficial in the face of an outbreak, but cattle may be protected if they are vaccinated before exposure. The IPV virus may survive in cryopreserved semen used for artificial insemination; thus semen donors and semen should be free from the virus. Genital carriers may be responsible for sporadic outbreaks of IPV.

Vaginal Varicose Veins: Mare

Vaginal varicose veins are common in older mares. In most cases the condition is not associated with clinical signs, but affected mares may exhibit vaginal hemorrhage. A thorough examination of the reproductive tract is necessary to determine the origin of the bleeding.

CLINICAL SIGNS AND DIAGNOSIS. Clinical signs of varicose veins vary from no signs to persistent and profuse vaginal hemorrhage. Vaginoscopy or fiber endoscopy of the vagina reveals varicose veins in the vagina or the vestibulovaginal transverse fold. Vaginal hemorrhage from varicose veins should be differentiated from vaginal trauma and premature separation of the placenta in periparturient mares.

TREATMENT AND PROGNOSIS. Most mares with vaginal varicose veins do not require treatment. Surgical ligation of the veins may be necessary in cases of severe bleeding. The short-term prognosis after surgery is good, but the condition often recurs.

VESTIBULAR AND VULVAR ABNORMALITIES

Coital Exanthema

Coital exanthema is caused by equine herpesvirus 3 (EHV-3) and is a venereally transmitted dermatitis of the genital region of mares and stallions.[148,149(p513)]

CLINICAL SIGNS AND DIAGNOSIS. The disease is recurrent, usually mild and transient, and affects the vulva and perineum of mares and the penis and prepuce of stallions. Lesions are initially small papules that rapidly progress to pustules and then ulcers. Lesions may rarely appear on the conjunctiva, lips, nares, and mucosa of the upper respiratory tract. Rare secondary bacterial infection and systemic signs occur. Intranuclear inclusion bodies are apparent in epithelial cells on histologic sections taken from the active edge of ulcers. Coital exanthema does not affect fertility in mares, but libido may be decreased in affected stallions because of pain during coitus.

TREATMENT AND PROGNOSIS. Lesions usually heal spontaneously within 14 days, leaving depigmented spots. Treatment is unnecessary unless secondary bacterial infection occurs. There is no available vaccine for EHV-3. Sexual rest until the lesions are healed is recommended to prevent further spread of the disease. Prognosis is excellent.

Granular Vulvitis

Granular vulvitis may occur in females of all domestic species but is most significant in cattle.[9] The disease is characterized by development of granules or papules in the vulvar mucosa accompanied by genital discharge. Infertility may or may not be a feature of the syndrome. Vulvitis may be secondary to nonspecific vaginitis.[58(p434)] *H. somnus*[150] and *Mycoplasma bovigenitalium*[5(p288)] have been isolated from cattle with vulvitis, but their role in infertility is not well defined, and there may be differences in pathogenicity among strains of the organisms. *Ureaplasma diversum* has been isolated from cases of granular vulvitis in cows and ewes and may be associated with infertility when the organism is transferred into the uterus during AI.[5(p282)]

CLINICAL SIGNS AND DIAGNOSIS. Granular vulvitis is characterized by the formation of raised granules or papules in the vulvar mucosa and around the clitoris with variable amounts of mucopurulent exudate. In the mild form of granular vulvitis associated with *U. diversum*, only a few granules develop and the infection has minimal effect on fertility. However, acute severe cases are characterized by hyperemia of the vulva, a profuse mucopurulent discharge, and depressed fertility. Purulent discharge during the acute phase persists for 3 to 10 days, after which the disease becomes chronic. In chronic cases the lesions are reduced in severity, and there is little or no purulent discharge. The chronic form may persist for several months, and the disease may become enzootic in some herds. The clinical signs of granular vulvitis may be similar to those of early signs of IPV.

CLINICAL PATHOLOGY. Samples for microbiologic culture should be obtained from the vulva, cervicovaginal mucus, and uterus. Use of transport medium for submission of samples to a laboratory is mandatory. The organisms may be eliminated before obtaining the samples, yielding false-negative results. Conversely, microorganisms incriminated as causing granular vulvitis may be isolated from the genital tracts of normal animals.

TREATMENT AND PROGNOSIS. Most cases of nonspecific vulvitis recover spontaneously. Infertility associated with *U. diversum* infections is treated by preventing transfer of organisms to the uterus by using double-sheathed AI instruments. Natural breeding should be suspended. In addition, infusion of 1 g of tetracycline or spectinomycin in a nonirritating vehicle into the uterus 24 hours after breeding has been recommended to reduce the population of organisms that may have been transferred to the uterus. Local treatment of vulvar lesions with tetracycline or spectinomycin has also been suggested.

PREVENTION AND CONTROL. In chronically infected herds, fertility rates may approach normal if double-sheathed AI instruments are used and affected cows are treated with appropriate antibiotics.

Ulcerative Dermatosis Genital Lesions

Ulcerative dermatosis is a venereal disease of sheep caused by a parapoxvirus similar to but distinct from that which causes contagious ecthyma.[7,58(p654)] The disease is characterized by ulceration of the skin and mucous membranes of the vulva of ewes and penis and prepuce of rams. Lesions also occur on the lips, nares, feet, and legs. The lesions are painful, and affected animals avoid coitus. The disease subsides in 7 to 10 days.

Because of its viral etiology, no specific treatment is available for ulcerative dermatosis.[7(p893)] Symptomatic treatment with local astringent and antiseptic ointments has been suggested. Morbidity of 15% to 20% is expected, although up to 60% of a flock may be affected. Mortality is low if the animals are otherwise healthy.

No vaccine is available. Males affected with the disease should not be used for breeding.

Abnormal Labial Approximation

The most common anatomic defect of the vulva of mares and cows is abnormal labial approximation, which leads to pneumovagina and subsequently to infertility.[43(p40)] The defect may be the result of imperfect conformation or traumatic insult to the vulva. Abnormal labial approximation is treated with Caslick's surgery or one of its modifications.

Persistent Hymen

In the developing embryo, failure of cannulation of the urogenital sinus by the mesonephric duct system results in absolute or partial occlusion of the vestibulovaginal junction. Total occlusion causes accumulation of endometrial and cervical secretions cranial to the obstruction, and occasionally the membrane may appear at the vulva. Partial occlusion may only be noted as an obstruction to breeding or during speculum examination. The membrane may be manually ruptured or incised. Prognosis is excellent.

Clitoral Hypertrophy

Clitoral hypertrophy may be a feature of intersex conditions, may occur in filly foals whose dams received progestins during pregnancy or may follow administration of anabolic steroids.[50] Hypertrophy may persist after cessation of steroid treatment.

Vulvar wattles in cattle may superficially appear similar, but the elongated epithelial structure does not involve the clitoris.

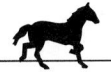

Neoplasia

Melanomas and squamous cell carcinomas are the most common neoplasms affecting the perineum, anus, and vulva of gray- and light-skinned horses, respectively.[151(p225)] Lesions are usually proliferative and may have surface ulceration, hemorrhage, and infection. Lesions should be differentiated from habronemiasis, granulation tissue, and sarcoids. Treatment is surgical removal. Sarcomas and melanomas may metastasize. Viral fibropapillomas are the most common tumors affecting the vulva of cattle.[9] Squamous cell carcinomas may be seen in all species and may be more common in white-skinned animals exposed to long periods of solar radiation.[152]

Vulvar neoplasia is characterized by variable degrees of tissue proliferation. The surface of squamous cell carcinomas and fibropapillomas may be ulcerated, necrotic, and fly-blown. Vulvar neoplasia must be differentiated from other causes of tissue proliferation, habronemiasis in mares, and ectopic mammary tissue in does.[5(p628)] Neoplasia of the vulva and vestibule is diagnosed by biopsy of the tumor.

Surgical excision is the treatment for most neoplasms of the vulva.[151(p225)] Viral fibropapillomas regress spontaneously after a period of several months. Recurrence and metastasis may occur.

Ectopic Mammary Tissue

Ectopic mammary tissue has been described in does and is characterized by swelling of the vulvar lips.[5(p628)] The abnormal enlargement begins before each parturition and persists for about 2 months. The condition is benign unless the tissue enlarges sufficiently to interfere with evacuation of feces or urine. Milk may be aspirated from the mammary tissue, and the condition may be confirmed by biopsy.

INFECTIOUS CAUSES OF INFERTILITY AND ABORTION

Information on the major causes of abortion in horses, cow, sheep, and goats is summarized in Tables 41-7 to 41-9.

▓ *RUMINANTS*

BOVINE HERPESVIRUS 1 (INFECTIOUS BOVINE RHINOTRACHEITIS [IBR]) ABORTION

The reproductive effects of bovid herpesvirus 1, also known as infectious bovine rhinotracheitis (IBR) include infectious pustular vulvovaginitis (IPV), embryonic death, abortion, stillbirth, and birth of weak calves. The virus associated with IPV is genetically distinct from that associated with abortion.[147] IPV is discussed in a previous section.

HISTORY AND CLINICAL SIGNS. Abortion usually occurs after the fourth month of gestation. There may be a history of infertility in the herd, but other signs of herpesvirus infection are seldom evident in the dam. In rare instances, infected fetuses are carried to term but are stillborn or die in the first week of life.

LABORATORY DIAGNOSIS. Autolysis usually obscures any gross lesions in the fetus. The placenta is grossly normal. The presence of microscopic foci of necrosis with eosinophilic intranuclear inclusions and lack of inflammation in fetal tissues, especially liver, lung, thymus, or adrenal gland, suggest herpesvirus abortion. The diagnosis is confirmed by virus isolation from placenta or fetal lung (which is positive in about one third of the cases) or demonstration of viral antigen in fetal kidney or other tissue by fluorescent antibody (FA) test.[153] Avidin-biotin complex immunoperoxidase detection of antigen in paraffin sections is more sensitive than virus isolation or FA.[154] Maternal titer is seldom of diagnostic value because rise in titer has occurred by the time of abortion. Fetal titer to IBR indicates in utero infection, but infected fetuses often have no detectable titer at the time of abortion.[5(p250)]

PATHOPHYSIOLOGY. Intrauterine inoculation of herpesvirus around the time of breeding induces necrotizing endometritis and oophoritis. Death of the conceptus at this stage presumably results from CL necrosis[155,156] because the zona pellucida protects the embryo from viral infection until hatching occurs at 8 to 9 days of gestation.[157] Subsequently, cytocidal infection of the trophoblast can result in early embryonic death.[158,159] In the latter half of gestation, fetal death results from necrosis in multiple organs and abortion usually

TABLE 41-7

Major Causes of Infectious Equine Abortion

Cause and Common Names	Usual Stage of Gestation	Major Fetal Lesions	Diagnostic Tests
Herpesvirus 1 (EHV-1)	Seventh month to term	Pulmonary edema, multifocal hepatic and pulmonary necrosis, intranuclear inclusions	Histopathology, virus isolation, fluorescent antibody test, fetal serology
Equine viral arteritis (pestivirus)	5-10 months	Myocardial arteritis	Histopathology, virus isolation, PCR, serology
Nocardioform *actinomycete*	Mid to late gestation	Characteristic placentitis located ventrally in the uterine body and at the base of the uterine horns	Culture
Streptococcus zooepidemicus	Any stage	Placentitis with or without inflammation in fetal tissues	Histopathology, culture
Mycotic abortion, *Aspergillus* and other species	Latter half (often near term)	Placentitis, fetal bronchopneumonia	Histopathology, fungal culture
Leptospirosis	Seventh month to term	Icterus and autolysis	Culture, immunofluorescence, serology

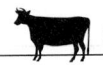
TABLE 41-8

Major Causes of Bovine Abortion

Cause and Common Names	Usual Stage of Gestation	Major Fetal Lesions	Diagnostic Tests
Bovid herpesirus 1, IBR	Fifth to ninth months	Multifocal necrosis with intranuclear inclusions (liver, lung, spleen, kidney)	Histopathology, virus isolation, FA test of frozen fetal kidney
Bluetongue (orbivirus)	Any stage	Anomalies of skeletal and nervous systems	Pathology, virus isolation, fetal serology
BVD virus, pestivirus	Any stage	Anomalies of skeletal, nervous, cardiovascular, respiratory, or other systems	Pathology, FA test on fetal tissues, fetal serology (virus neutralization, ELISA), serologic survey in herd
EBA, foothill abortion, spirochete?	Third trimester	Lymphadenopathy, splenomegaly, hepatopathy	Pathology
Brucella abortus brucellosis, Bang's disease	Third trimester	Placentitis, fibrinous serositis, bronchopneumonia	Culture, maternal serology (card test, plate, or tube agglutination)
Campylobacter fetus ssp. *venerealis,* campylobacteriosis, vibriosis	Usually early embryonic death	Placentitis, fibrinous serositis, bronchopneumonia, hepatitis	Pathology, darkfield examination, culture
Haemophilus somnus	Any stage	Placentitis	Histopathology, culture
Leptospira interrogans, leptospirosis	Fifth to ninth months	Icterus, edema, renal degeneration and inflammation	Fetal and maternal serology
Listeria monocytogenes, listeriosis	Eighth or ninth months	Placentitis	Histopathology, culture
Salmonella dublin, Salmonella typhimurium	Third trimester	Placentitis	Culture
Aspergillus fumigatus and all fungal spp., mycotic abortion	Third trimester	Placentitis, bronchopneumonia, dermatitis	Histopathology, fungal culture
Sarcocystis cruzi	Third trimester	Protozoa in caruncles	Histopathology or FA of caruncles
Tritrichomonas foetus, trichomoniasis	First half	Placentitis, bronchopneumonia	Microscopic demonstration of organism, culture
Bovine neosporosis	Mid gestation	Similar to those found in *Toxoplasma*-aborted sheep fetuses	Histopathology, seroepidemiology

IBR, Infectious bovine rhinotracheitis; *BVD,* bovine virus diarrhea; *EBA,* epizootic bovine abortion; *FA,* fluorescent antibody; *ELISA,* enzyme-linked immunosorbent assay.

TABLE 41-9

Major Causes of Abortion in Sheep and Goats

Cause and Common Names	Usual Stage of Gestation	Major Fetal Lesions	Diagnostic Tests
Bluetongue, orbivirus	Any stage	Anomalies of skeletal or nervous systems	Pathology, IFA, serology
Border disease, pestivirus hairy shaker disease	Any stage	Dysplasia of skeleton, CNS, and fleece	Pathology, virus isolation, serology (cross-reacts with BVD)
Coxiella burnetii, Q fever	Near term	Necrotizing placentitis	Histopathology, microscopic demonstration of rickettsia, complement fixation, ELISA
Chlamydia psittaci, EAE	Fourth or fifth months	Necrotizing placentitis	Histopathology, microscopic demonstration of organism, fluorescent antibody on fetal tissues or cultures, paired sera
Campylobacter fetus ssp. *fetus,* vibriosis	Last 6 weeks	Placentitis, serositis, multifocal hepatic necrosis	Pathology, microscopic demonstration of organism, culture
Toxoplasma gondii, toxoplasmosis	Any stage	Necrosis and calcification in cotyledons	Pathology, demonstration of organism, serology (e.g., agglutination, ELISA)

BVD, Bovine virus diarrhea; *EAE,* Enzootic abortion of ewes; *ELISA,* enzyme-linked immunosorbent assay; *IFA,* immunofluorescent antibody.

occurs 2 weeks to 4 months after infection. The dead fetus is often retained in utero 2 days or more.[153]

EPIDEMIOLOGY AND CONTROL. Bovine herpesvirus 1 is ubiquitous. Abortion rate varies from 5% to 60% or more but is usually less than 25% in beef herds and more sporadic in dairy herds. Herpesviral infection generally has no lasting effect on fertility. The disease may be controlled by vaccination.

BLUETONGUE ABORTION

Bluetongue is an orbivirus infection that can result in embryonic death, abortion, and fetal anomalies in sheep, cattle, or other ruminants. Twenty-four serotypes of bluetongue virus have been recognized; five of these (serotypes 2, 10, 11, 13, and 17) occur in the United States (see Chapter 30 for complete discussion and Chapter 33 for nervous system anomalies).[160]

BOVINE VIRUS DIARRHEA (BVD) ABORTION

Bovine virus diarrhea (BVD) virus is a pestivirus that can produce early embryonic death, fetal anomalies, or abortion (see Chapter 30 for complete discussion). Isolates from bovine aborted fetuses are usually noncytopathic.[161]

HISTORY AND CLINICAL SIGNS. Abortion can occur at any stage of gestation. Often there is a history of repeat breeding and a recent episode of febrile disease in the herd before the onset of abortions.[153(p121)]

LABORATORY DIAGNOSIS. The fetus may be mummified, autolyzed, or fresh and have a variety of dysplastic lesions, including cerebellar hypoplasia, cerebral malformations (hydrencephaly, porencephaly, microencephaly) and cataracts, brachygnathia, arthrogryposis, alopecia, thymic hypoplasia, and intrauterine growth restriction.[5(p254),153(p121),162,163] Microscopic lesions include a mild nonsuppurative placentitis. Nonsuppurative vasculitis may be observed in the placenta, liver, or lymph nodes.[153(p121)]

Virus isolation from fetal tissue is seldom successful. Viral antigen may be detected by FA test on kidney, lung, or lymph node.[153(p121)] Virus neutralization and enzyme-linked immunosorbent assay are used to detect antibodies in fetal thoracic fluid, which indicate prenatal exposure to the virus but do not necessarily incriminate BVD virus as the cause of abortion. Maternal titers are seldom of diagnostic value because a rise in titer generally occurs before abortion.[5(p254)]

PATHOPHYSIOLOGY. BVD virus may be shed in most body secretions. In seronegative cows, exposure to BVD virus at the time of breeding prevents conception.[164] Placental attachment at approximately 35 days' gestation seemingly must precede fetal infection. During the first 4 months of gestation, infection usually causes fetal death and abortion.[153(p121)] Fetuses infected with noncytopathic strains between 42 and 125 days' gestation are likely to be persistently infected, are typically seronegative at birth, and subsequently shed BVD virus continuously. They may develop mucosal disease later in life from superinfection with cytopathic BVD virus.[165,166] Fetuses infected between 75 and 150 days' gestation are at risk for the development of dysplastic lesions. Fetuses infected after 100 days' gestation usually mount an immune response, clear the infection, and survive but may develop teratologic defects in the brain, skin, or bronchioles. Fetuses infected after 150 days usually recover without dysplastic lesions.[163]

EPIDEMIOLOGY. Most cattle have serum antibodies to the virus. The abortion rate may approach 25% with new infection of a susceptible herd.[5(p254)]

CONTROL. BVD virus usually has no permanent effect on fertility. The disease may be controlled by vaccination.

BORDER DISEASE (Hairy Shaker Disease)

Border disease or hairy shaker disease is an ovine pestivirus infection that causes embryonic and fetal death; stillbirths; dysplasia of the central nervous system, skeleton, and fleece; or birth of weak lambs with low viability.

COXIELLA BURNETII (Q Fever)

Coxiella burnetii, a rickettsia, is the agent of Q fever that can cause abortions in sheep and goats. Most infections are completely asymptomatic, and the disease is of more importance as a zoonosis than as a cause of ovine or caprine abortion.

HISTORY AND CLINICAL SIGNS. Late abortions or delivery of weak lambs may occur in an affected flock over a period of 2 to 4 weeks.[5(p852),167]

LABORATORY DIAGNOSIS. There are no specific gross lesions in the fetus, but the placenta is thickened with white, chalky plaques and red-brown exudate, especially in intercotyledonary areas. Histologically cotyledonary and intercotyledonary necrosis is accompanied by heavy neutrophil infiltration.[5(p852),168] Diagnosis of Q fever abortion should be based on the presence of characteristic placental lesions with large numbers of rickettsiae and a rising maternal titer. Rickettsieae can be identified in placental impression smears stained with modified Koster's stain, Stamp's modified Ziehl-Neelsen stain, or Gimenez stain as pleomorphic acid-fast coccoid or filamentous organisms in trophoblasts or extracellularly. Complement fixation titers greater than 1:8 in the dam are considered diagnostic. Enzyme-linked immunosorbent assay is rapid and sensitive but requires species-specific peroxidase conjugate for each host species. Laboratory results must be interpreted carefully because *C. burnetii* also can be isolated from the placenta of normal animals.[5(p852)] In one survey of California dairy goats, 24% were seropositive by microagglutination.[169]

PATHOPHYSIOLOGY. *C. burnetii* infection can be transmitted by ixodid or argasid ticks or by ingestion of infected material. The organism replicates in trophoblasts and is often of low pathogenicity in sheep and goats but can result in placentitis with late abortion and shedding of large numbers of rickettsiae.[5(p852)]

EPIDEMIOLOGY. Q fever is reported in many countries, including the United States and Canada. Abortions typically occur over a 2- to 4-week period and may affect 5% to 50% of the flock.[5(p852)] The organism also is infectious for other animals, including humans. Pregnant women should not handle Q fever–infected animals or tissues.

TREATMENT AND CONTROL. Aborting does and ewes should be segregated, and abortuses and placentas removed from the premises to prevent oral transmission. Pregnant animals can be treated with tetracycline to reduce the chances of abortion. A carrier state may develop, but abortions do not usually occur in subsequent pregnancies. Inactivated vaccines (not commercially available) lessen the chances of rickettsial abortion in sheep and reduce but do not eliminate rickettsial shedding at parturition.[168]

CHLAMYDIA PSITTACI ABORTION (Enzootic Abortion of Ewes)

Chlamydia psittaci is a major cause of abortion in sheep and goats.[5(p603),153(p37)] Ovine chlamydial abortion is called enzootic abortion of ewes. *Chlamydia* may cause abortion in cattle[153] but is not the cause of epizootic bovine (foothill) abortion.

HISTORY AND CLINICAL SIGNS. Chlamydiosis is best characterized in sheep and goats. Abortions or stillbirths with placentitis usually occur in the fourth to fifth months of

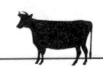

gestation. The dam seldom shows signs of illness but may have serosanguineous vaginal discharge several days before and after parturition.[5(p603)] Other animals in the flock may be affected by arthritis or pneumonia.[170]

LABORATORY DIAGNOSIS. Placentitis is the most consistent necropsy finding in chlamydial abortion. Necrosis occurs in cotyledons; the intercotyledonary placenta is thickened with accumulation of red exudate.[153(p37),170] The fetus has no specific gross lesions.[153(p37),170] Histologically, necrotizing placentitis is accompanied by nonsuppurative vasculitis. Nonsuppurative meningoencephalitis, necrotizing hepatitis, and proliferation of mononuclear cells in spleen and lymph nodes are other histologic findings that may occur in the fetus.[153(p37),171]

Diagnosis of chlamydial abortion should be based on identification of the organism and the presence of typical placental lesions. Chlamydiae appear in placental impression smears stained with Giemsa, Gimenez, or modified Ziehl-Neelsen stains as 200-nm dark red spheric bodies in the cytoplasm of trophoblasts.[5(p603),153(p37)] The organism can be positively identified by FA tests on cytologic preparations, cryostat sections of placenta or other fetal tissues, or cultures. *Chlamydia* grows in chick embryos in 1 to 6 weeks, but cell culture using mouse L cells requires only 2 to 10 days.[153(p37)]

Abortion or delivery of chlamydial-infected fetuses induces a rise in serum titer that peaks in 2 to 3 weeks.[153(p37)] Paired sera should be collected at abortion and 3 weeks later. Maternal titers greater than 1:32 generally indicate recent active infection.[172] Complement fixation is the standard serologic test for the dam; indirect immunofluorescence and enzyme-linked immunosorbent assay are also used.[173] Double immunodiffusion can be performed on fetal fluids.[153(p37)]

PATHOPHYSIOLOGY. Chlamydiae reside in the intestinal tract and are also shed from the genital tract of infected animals before and after parturition. Ingestion is the main form of transmission.[5(p603),174] In sheep and goats, abortion occurs 4 to 8 weeks after experimental infection,[170] but the fetus is not susceptible until the last third of gestation.[5(p603)]

High maternal antibody titers do not prevent abortion or stillbirth, but experimental work suggests that cell-mediated immunity is protective.[175] Infection with small numbers of *Chlamydia* seldom stimulates adequate cell-mediated immunity and consequently may be more likely to cause abortion than infection with numerous organisms.[5(p260)]

EPIDEMIOLOGY. Chlamydial abortion has been reported from most major sheep- or goat-producing countries. *C. psittaci* also may infect other animals, including human beings. Pregnant women should not handle infected animals or tissues. The abortion rate in sheep is usually about 5%[153(p37)] but may be up to 30% or more in goats.[5(p603),170] Although abortions usually occur 1 to 2 months after infection in sheep, the incubation period in goats may be as short as 2 weeks.[172]

TREATMENT AND CONTROL. Aborting does or ewes should be segregated, and abortuses and placentas should be removed from the premises to avoid oral transmission. Oxytetracycline therapy (80 to 450 mg/head every day in feed or water, or long-acting oxytetracycline injected subcutaneously at a dose of 20 mg/kg twice weekly until the last month of gestation)[5(p603)] reduces the number of abortions and stillbirths in sheep[175] and goats, particularly if instituted in the first half of pregnancy.[5(p603)] However, short-term treatment does not eradicate infection or prevent chlamydial shedding at parturition and should be reserved for abortion outbreaks.[176] Most ewes develop cell-mediated immunity, which eliminates the organism from the genital tract by 3 months after lambing and protects against abortion for about 3 years.[5(p603),176] Does are more likely than ewes to have placental retention and metritis after abortion.[174] Killed vac-

cines* can be used in enzootic areas 4 to 6 weeks before breeding but are not 100% effective. Experimentally avirulent live vaccines have been used with success.

EPIZOOTIC BOVINE ABORTION (Foothill Abortion)

Epizootic bovine abortion (EBA) or foothill abortion is a syndrome of late abortions in cattle in the foothills bordering the central valley of California.[177] Once thought to be caused by *Chlamydia psittaci*, studies have demonstrated that EBA differs from chlamydial abortion.[177] Currently a spirochete-like agent isolated from abortuses and from the tick vector of EBA is under investigation as the etiologic agent.[178-180]

HISTORY AND CLINICAL SIGNS. Late abortions or delivery of weak calves occurs in affected herds. Many fetuses in the sixth to seventh month of gestation may be aborted, especially from heifers without premunition immunity from natural exposure to the causative agent. Older native cows show no clinical signs of infection.

LABORATORY DIAGNOSIS. A 3-month period is required for full development of pathologic changes in the fetus. Superficial cervical lymph nodes are enlarged up to 16 g, the spleen is enlarged up to 250 g, the thymus is slightly smaller than normal, and the liver may be enlarged and nodular.[153(p116),177,179] Histologically there is loss of thymic cortical lymphocytes; remaining lymphocytes are enlarged and poorly differentiated. Follicular hyperplasia, histiocytosis, vasculitis, necrosis, and pyogranulomas occur in lymph nodes and spleen. Lymphohistiocytic proliferation may also occur around vessels in the liver, lung, and meninges.[153(p116)]

EBA has been diagnosed mainly by pathologic examination of the fetus. Recent studies have demonstrated high levels of IgG (3 mg/ml or more) in fetal blood.[153(p116),177] A spirochete-like agent can be demonstrated in the plasma of aborted fetuses but also may occur in plasma of normal fetuses.[178] Currently no serologic test for EBA exists because the cause is uncertain.

PATHOPHYSIOLOGY. Infection is transmitted by the soft, grounding tick, *Ornithodorus coriaceus*.[179,180] The disease also can be transmitted with fresh or frozen fetal tissue.[177] Transformation and proliferation of fetal lymphocytes and macrophages occur by 50 days but are not severe enough for diagnosis until 100 days after maternal exposure to the tick vector. IgG and IgM are deposited in vascular lesions, but increase in fetal serum immunoglobulin is not detectable until at least 80 days after tick exposure.[177,181] Repeated superinfection may be necessary to result in fetal death.[179] Because at least 90 days are required for development of fetal lesions, infection after 6 months' gestation is not likely to result in abortion.[5(p260),153(p116)]

EPIDEMIOLOGY. EBA is limited to the range of the tick vector in the foothills bordering the central valley of California.[177] Of the annual calf loss in California, 5% to 10% is attributed to EBA.[180] The prevalence of infection by the spirochete is far greater than the prevalence of abortion.[179] Abortion occurs 3 to 4 months after exposure to ticks but almost always late in gestation, regardless of the time of tick exposure.[181] Older native cows from enzootic areas usually do not abort, and introduced cows and heifers generally abort only once.[177] The abortion rate may be 30% to 80% in susceptible animals.[153(p116),181]

TREATMENT AND CONTROL. Chlortetracycline therapy (2 to 5 g/day in the feed) reduces the rate of abortion.[180] Currently no vaccine exists for EBA, but abortions can be controlled by exposing heifers to the tick vector before breeding

---

*Animal Health Division, Shawnee, KS 66201.

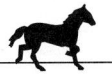

or by changing from spring to fall calving,[5(p260)] which takes advantage of limiting exposure to the last trimester of gestation in some management systems. Thus exposure of susceptible pregnant cattle to the tick only after the sixth month of pregnancy is a practical solution for ranchers using summer foothill pastures and fall calving. The tick lives in ground duff (e.g., leaves) and is not found on cattle that graze in irrigated pastures and most other areas outside of brushy foothills.

BRUCELLA ABORTUS ABORTION

Brucella abortus infection (Bang's disease) causes abortion in cattle and, less commonly, in sheep and goats. Horses may be infected with *B. abortus,* which has been associated with fistulous withers, but usually experience no infertility, abortion, or other clinical evidence of infection. Bovine infections are caused by eight biotypes of *B. abortus,* three of which (biotypes 1, 2, and 4) are recognized in the United States.[5(p271)]

HISTORY AND CLINICAL SIGNS. Abortion is the chief clinical sign of bovine brucellosis and usually occurs after the fifth month of gestation. Infected sheep and goats generally abort in the last 2 months of pregnancy.[182(p423)] Lameness, mastitis, or orchitis may be present in infected herds.[182(p423)]

LABORATORY DIAGNOSIS. Autolysis frequently obscures gross lesions in the fetus, but fibrinous serositis may be apparent, and abomasal content may be discolored and flocculent. Placentitis is a consistent finding. Cotyledons are necrotic; the intercotyledonary placenta is thickened and opaque with accumulation of odorless, flocculent, yellow-brown exudate between maternal and fetal membranes. Histologically there is suppurative placentitis (and endometritis in the dam). Suppurative bronchopneumonia and lymphoreticular hyperplasia are frequent histologic findings in the fetus.

Diagnosis depends on culture of *B. abortus* from fetal lung, abomasum, or placenta or from maternal uterine or mammary secretions. Organisms and *Brucella* antigen can be detected in fetal tissues by avidin-biotin-peroxidase complex immunostaining.[183]

No serologic test is 100% accurate, but a positive card test or titer of 1:100 or more on plate or tube agglutination suggests brucellosis. False-negative serologic reactions occur in about 15% of infected cows, particularly just before or after parturition. False-positive reactions are a problem in vaccinated animals. Supplemental tests such as the Rivanol test, complement fixation, and mercaptoethanol sensitivity of agglutination are used in suspect cases. Dairy herds are surveyed by the *Brucella* ring test on milk.[5(p271)] In goats, tube agglutination titers of 1:25 or more indicate infection.[182(p423)]

PATHOPHYSIOLOGY. Initial replication of *B. abortus* occurs in regional lymph nodes. Bacteremia is followed by colonization of supramammary lymph nodes, the mammary gland, and the gravid uterus. Uterine infection occurs during the second trimester.[5(p271),184] In the placenta the bacteria appear first in phagosomes of erythrophagocytic trophoblasts. Replication occurs in the rough endoplasmic reticulum of chorioallantoic trophoblasts.[184] Preferential replication in chorioallantoic trophoblasts has been attributed to their erythritol content; however, the placentas of several laboratory rodents that lack detectable erythritol still support *B. abortus* replication.[185] The organism also occurs in fetal placental endothelial cells and capillary lumina, where it is associated with vasculitis and destruction of chorionic villi. Placental inflammation spreads along the allantochorion to involve additional cotyledons with resultant chorioallantoic ulceration, necrosis of trophoblasts, and ulcerative endometritis. Fetal death results from placental disruption and endotoxemia.[5(p270),184] The fetus is frequently retained 1 to 3 days in utero. Numerous bacteria are expelled from the genital tract at parturition, but shedding usually stops by 3 weeks after abortion.[5(p271)]

EPIDEMIOLOGY. Infection with *B. abortus* occurs naturally by ingestion. Contaminated materials are infectious for humans and should be handled with caution. Infection is not easily transmitted between cattle separated by fences or roads.[186] Most calves infected at birth clear the infection, but persistent congenital infection has been documented.[187,188]

The prevalence of bovine brucellosis in the United States has decreased because of the test and slaughter eradication program and vaccination of heifers.

TREATMENT AND CONTROL. Combination therapy with long-acting oxytetracycline (20 mg/kg IM every 3 to 4 days for five treatments) and streptomycin (25 mg/kg IV or IM daily for 7 days at onset of oxytetracycline treatment) can eliminate infection in most cows,[189] but, because of the eradication program used in many countries, infected cows are rarely treated.

Vaccination with a reduced dose of strain 19* decreases the likelihood of abortion and genital shedding of *Brucella* at parturition.[5(p271)] Official vaccination must occur between 4 and 12 months of age, but ideally heifers should be vaccinated before 8 months of age to decrease the chances of serologic vaccine reactions. Vaccinated animals are permanently identified with a United States Department of Agriculture (USDA) tattoo in the right ear. Regulations require quarantine and elimination of all reactors from a herd with a diagnosed case of brucellosis. Test and slaughter are also recommended for control of ovine and caprine infection with *B. abortus.*

BRUCELLA MELITENSIS ABORTION

Brucella melitensis causes abortion in goats and sheep and less commonly in cattle.[5(p271)] Infection is associated with late abortion, stillbirth, or birth of weak kids or lambs.[5(p852),182(p423)] Necropsy findings, such as those with *Brucella abortus,* include severe placentitis and fetal serositis.[5(p852),167] The disease is diagnosed by culture or demonstration of the organism in tissue or by maternal serology (complement fixation test).[5(p852)] Animals are infected by ingestion, and, after bacteremia, replication occurs in chorioallantoic trophoblasts.[5(p852),184] Infection with *B. melitensis* is important in Mediterranean countries and in Central and South America but is rare in the United States.[167,182(p423)] Suspected cases should be reported to state and federal authorities. Human infection with *B. melitensis* can be very severe.

BRUCELLA OVIS ABORTION

Brucella ovis infects only sheep. Epididymitis in rams is the most common manifestation of infection. Ewes seldom show clinical evidence of infection; late abortions, stillbirths, and delivery of weak lambs are rare.[5(p852),153(p27)] Fetal and placental lesions resemble those induced by *Brucella abortus.* Diagnosis is based on culture or on demonstration of the organism in tissue. Serology (complement fixation) can identify infected animals. However, not all ewes showing a rise in CF titer at parturition deliver infected lambs. In addition, ewes can maintain elevated titers for months or years after exposure to *B. ovis.* Therefore *B. ovis* abortion should not be diagnosed on the basis of CF testing alone.[153(p27)]

Infection is thought to occur by the conjunctival route.[167] The bacteria has low virulence for the ewe but may replicate in chorioallantoic trophoblasts, resulting in placentitis and fetal bacteremia.[184] *B. ovis* infection has been reported from Europe, Africa, Australia, New Zealand, and the western United States.

Brucella abortus vaccine, Colorado Serum Co, Denver, CO, 80216.

CAMPYLOBACTER FETUS SSP. *VENEREALIS* ABORTION

Campylobacter fetus ssp. *venerealis* is the main cause of bovine campylobacteriosis (vibriosis).[5(p263)] The organism is an obligate parasite of the bovine genital tract and is not known to cause disease in other species.[153(p70)]

HISTORY AND CLINICAL SIGNS. Infection with *C. fetus* ssp. *venerealis* mainly causes temporary infertility or early embryonic death, but sporadic abortions from the fourth to eighth months of gestation are possible.[153(p70)] The usual history includes a high percentage of cows exposed for the first time returning to estrus or found nonpregnant after the breeding season, and cows calving late because they returned to estrus one or more times.

LABORATORY DIAGNOSIS. Autolysis is usually minimal, and the lungs of the term fetus may be partially inflated. Dehydration, fibrinous serosis, and necrotizing placentitis may be apparent grossly. Histologically, bronchopneumonia and hepatitis may also be evident. Diagnosis is based on demonstration or isolation of the organism. By darkfield microscopy, the bacterium appears as a curved rod with darting corkscrew motility.[153(p70)] Cows that abort may have serum antibody titers; however, they may not be diagnostic because they are not specific for *Campylobacter fetus* ssp. *venerealis*. Culture from placenta or fetal abomasal contents requires at least 72 hours. The vaginal mucus agglutination test is used to survey herds for infection.[5(p263)] Alternatively the penis and preputial mucosa of infected bulls may be swabbed and cultured, although culture is difficult because the organism is slow-growing and often overwhelmed by saprophytes.

PATHOPHYSIOLOGY. Within a week of vaginal infection, the organism is established in the uterus, causing mucopurulent endometritis which persists 3 to 4 months. Intrauterine infection either prevents conception or causes embryonic death, and infected heifers typically return to estrus by 40 days. Less commonly, abortions occur up to 8 months' gestation.[5(p263),153(p70)]

EPIDEMIOLOGY. *C. fetus* ssp. *venerealis* is ubiquitous. Venereal transmission from infected bulls to virgin heifers approaches 100%. Cows with previous exposure to infected bulls develop immunity and therefore they are less likely to experience infertility than heifers. The abortion rate seldom exceeds 10%.[153(p70)]

TREATMENT AND CONTROL. Infected cows usually recover spontaneously within 5 months and resist reinfection. Recovery is hastened by intrauterine infusions of streptomycin and penicillin. Infertility may be permanent if endometritis or salpingitis is severe.[5(p263)] Heifers should be vaccinated with a killed bacterin before breeding. Most vaccines are administered 1 month before breeding and require a booster vaccination 2 weeks later.*,† Higher than normal doses of vaccine may be needed to clear the infection from bulls. Cows and bulls must be vaccinated annually. Exclusive use of *C. fetus* ssp. *venerealis*–negative semen via AI controls the disease by preventing transmission.

CAMPYLOBACTER FETUS SSP. *FETUS* ABORTION

Campylobacter fetus ssp. *fetus* is one agent of ovine campylobacteriosis (vibriosis) that causes abortion in sheep and sporadic abortion in cattle and goats.[5(605),153(p70),167]

HISTORY AND CLINICAL SIGNS. Infection of ewes causes abortion in the last 6 weeks of pregnancy, stillbirths, and birth of premature lambs. Infected ewes may have fever, diarrhea, depression, and vaginal discharge several days before parturition.[167] In cattle the infection is not associated with infertility (unlike infection with *C. fetus* ssp. *venerealis*), but sporadic abortions can occur from the fourth to eighth months of gestation.[153(p70)]

LABORATORY DIAGNOSIS. *Campylobacter* causes placentitis with cotyledonary necrosis and intercotyledonary edema. The fetus is edematous and may have fibrinous polyserositis. Foci of necrosis, up to 2 cm in diameter, occur in the liver of about 40% of aborted ovine fetuses and, although not pathognomonic, suggest campylobacteriosis.[5(p852),153(p81)] Histologic changes include suppurative necrotizing placentitis and fetal bronchopneumonia.[153(p81)] Diagnosis is based on culture (which usually requires less than 48 hours)[5(p263)] or on microscopic demonstration of the organism.[5(p852)]

PATHOPHYSIOLOGY. *C. fetus* ssp. *fetus* is transmitted by ingestion. The organism localizes in the gallbladder but may invade the pregnant uterus, where it replicates in chorioallantoic trophoblasts. The incubation period in the ewe varies from 7 to 25 days.[5(p852)] In the cow, dissemination of the organism to the placenta is less common.[153(p54)] In either species, localization in the placenta causes placentitis and fetal bacteremia.[153(p70,81)] Metritis, fetal retention, and maternal peritonitis may occur in the ewe.[5(p852)]

EPIDEMIOLOGY. Infection with *C. fetus* ssp. *fetus* is important in sheep in the United Kingdom, the United States, and New Zealand.[5(p852)] Fetal infection is most common during the last 2 months of gestation. Outbreaks of abortion tend to occur in 4- to 5-year cycles.[5(p852)] Infection is highly contagious in confined ewes, and the abortion rate may approach 70% but is more commonly about 25%.[5(p852),153(p81),167]

TREATMENT AND CONTROL. Abortion outbreaks can be treated with daily intramuscular injections of procaine penicillin G (22,000 IU/kg) and dihydrostreptomycin (11 to 22 mg/kg) or with oxytetracycline in the feed (75 mg/head/day).[5(p605)] Metritis is rarely fatal in the ewe. Generally, affected ewes abort only once and thus they may be retained as breeding stock.[153(p81)] Ovine campylobacteriosis can be controlled by the use of a killed adjuvanted bacterin at breeding and 60 to 90 days later.[5(p852)]

CAMPYLOBACTER JEJUNI ABORTION

Campylobacter jejuni is the other agent of ovine campylobacter (vibrio) abortion. *C. jejuni* is an enteric pathogen that causes enteritis and diarrhea in many species. Only in sheep is placental and fetal infection common.[13(p96),123] This organism has been associated occasionally with abortion in cattle and goats.[5(p263),9,153(p123),190,191]

HISTORY AND CLINICAL SIGNS. Ovine infection with *C. jejuni* is clinically indistinguishable from that with *C. fetus* ssp. *fetus*.

LABORATORY DIAGNOSIS. Aborted fetuses are autolyzed and frequently lack specific gross lesions. Cotyledons are mottled yellow to tan, but the intercotyledonary membranes are grossly normal. Histologically necrosis occurs in chorionic villi with arteriolitis and numerous leukocytes in the lamina propria. Purulent bronchopneumonia is a common histologic finding in the fetus.[192]

C. jejuni can be distinguished from other *Campylobacter* spp. by growth at 42° C (107.3° F), resistance to cephalothin, inhibition by nalidixic acid, and the presence of heat-labile glycoprotein surface antigen No. 1, which does not occur in *C. fetus* ssp. *venerealis* or *C. fetus* ssp. *fetus*. Placenta or fetal tissues should be cultured on *Campylobacter* agar with incor-

---

*Vibrin, SmithKline Beecham Animal Health, Exton, PA 19341.
†Trivib-5L, Fort Dodge Labs, Fort Dodge, IA 5051.

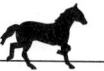

porated cefoperazone, vancomycin, and amphotericin B (CVA media) at 42° C (107.3° F).[191,192]

PATHOPHYSIOLOGY. Intravenous inoculation of pregnant ewes with *C. jejuni* at 114 and 123 days of pregnancy consistently induced abortion 7 to 12 days later.[192]

EPIDEMIOLOGY AND CONTROL. *C. jejuni* is ubiquitous. Certain strains have been associated with an abortion rate as high as 80%, but usually fewer than 20% of the flock abort.[192] Aborted tissue is infectious for humans and should be handled with caution. Treatment and control of ovine infection with *C. jejuni* are similar to those for *C. fetus* ssp. *fetus*.

HAEMOPHILUS SOMNUS ABORTION

Haemophilus somnus has been associated with vulvitis, vaginitis, endometritis, and abortion in cattle.[193]

LABORATORY DIAGNOSIS. Aborted fetuses have been free of gross lesions. Necrotizing placentitis is associated with fibrinoid necrosis of placental arteries.[150] Diagnosis is based on recovery of large numbers of the organism in relatively pure culture from placenta or fetus, histologic evidence of placentitis, and lack of other apparent causes.

Interpretation of maternal titers to *H. somnus* is difficult, and it is best to take paired serum samples. Titers between 1:256 and 1:512 in nonvaccinated herds may be the result of early active or chronic infection. Titers between 1:1040 and 1:4096 indicate recent active infection. A fourfold change in titer in paired sera is the best indicator of active infection.[193]

PATHOPHYSIOLOGY. Although *H. somnus* can be isolated from the genital tract of clinically normal cows,[194] the rate of isolation is higher in cows with endometritis or cervicitis.[150] Experimentally, *H. somnus* can adhere to zona pellucida–intact embryos and cause degeneration.[195] Vaginitis can be induced by inoculation with *H. somnus*,[196] and abortion has been induced by intraamniotic, intravenous, or intrabronchial challenge with the organism.[197] Cervical infusion with the organism resulted in colonization of the chorioallantois and placentitis, but calves were born alive without culturable *H. somnus*.[198]

TREATMENT AND CONTROL. Antibiotic treatment increases fertility in herds affected with *H. somnus*–induced vulvovaginitis.[150]

LEPTOSPIROSIS ABORTION

Leptospirosis is a spectrum of diseases caused by multiple serovars of *Leptospira interrogans*. *Leptospira hardjo* is the major serovar associated with bovine leptospiral abortion, although isolations of *Leptospira pomona*, *Leptospira canicola*, *Leptospira icterohemorrhagiae*, *Leptospira grippotyphosa*, and *Leptospira szwajizak* have also been reported.[5(p267),153(p54)] Serovar *L. pomona* is the major ovine isolate,[153(54)] but *Leptospira bratislava* and *L. hardjo* have also been isolated from sheep.[153(p13)] *L. grippotyphosa* is the major caprine isolate.[5(p600)] Leptospiral abortion is less common in sheep and goats than in cattle.

HISTORY AND CLINICAL SIGNS. In cattle, *L. hardjo* is associated with infertility, abortions from 4 months' gestation to term, and birth of weak calves. Abortion rate is usually less than 10%. *L. pomona* abortion usually occurs in the last 3 months of gestation, with an abortion rate as high as 50%.[5(p267)] Clinical signs of leptospirosis in the cow may include icterus, hemoglobinuria, anemia, fever, and mastitis that is characterized by a flaccid udder and thick ropy secretions from all four quarters; but frequently cows abort without clinical illness.[153(p54)] Dead or weak calves may be delivered at term.[199]

LABORATORY DIAGNOSIS. The aborted fetus is usually autolyzed, icteric, and edematous. Histologically renal tubu-

lar necrosis is accompanied by lymphocytic interstitial nephritis, pneumonia, and placentitis.[5(p267),153(p54)]

Leptospires are rapidly destroyed by autolysis or freezing. Isolation from fetal liver, kidney, or brain is possible but slow and impractical. Leptospires may be isolated or demonstrated by dark-field microscopy, FA staining, or histologic techniques in fetal or placental tissues or in the urine of the aborting dam within about 2 weeks after abortion.[5(p267),153(p54)]

Diagnosis is usually based on serology. A few infected fetuses develop microagglutination titers of 1:10 or more. It is difficult to distinguish among vaccinated, acutely infected, and recovered animals, but titers to *L. pomona* greater than 1:12,800 in the dam suggest leptospiral abortion. Maternal titer usually has peaked by the time of abortion. Single titers of 1:800 or more in unvaccinated animals, seroconversion, or fourfold changes in titers in paired sera indicate leptospirosis in the herd. Titers to *L. hardjo* are often less than 1:100 in affected cows and seldom exceed 1:1600.[153(p54)]

PATHOPHYSIOLOGY. Hematogenously spread leptospires colonize the gravid uterus up to 142 days after infection. Abortion occurs 1 to 6 weeks after acute disease with *L. pomona* infection and 1 to 3 months with *L. hardjo*.[5(p267)] *L. hardjo* remains in the oviducts of infected cows up to 22 days after calving.[199]

EPIDEMIOLOGY. Leptospira are ubiquitous and an important cause of abortion in all cattle-producing regions. Aborted tissues are infectious for humans and should be handled with caution.[200] Vaccination may be useful in endemic areas.

TREATMENT AND CONTROL. In abortion outbreaks, pregnant cows can be vaccinated with killed bacterin and treated with oxytetracycline (antibiotic treatment can be limited to sick cows in dairy herds).[201] Aborting cows should be isolated and treated with streptomycin if they are not destined for slaughter. Aborted fetuses and placentas should be removed from the premises.[202] Preventing exposure to swine, rodents, or contaminated water lessens the opportunities for infection.[5(p267),202] *L. pomona* usually has no permanent effect on fertility, but infection with *L. hardjo* has been associated with persistent herd infection and recurring abortions.[5(p267)]

Herd vaccination is recommended at 6-month intervals or more frequently in areas with heavy exposure to leptospires. Vaccination programs are aimed at reducing urinary shedding of leptospires and decreasing fetal loss. However, a commercial pentavalent leptospiral vaccine (serovar *L. hardjo* type *hardjoprajitno* is used for the *L. hardjo* component of USDA-licensed leptospiral vaccines) did not prevent renal colonization, urinary shedding, or fetal infection after conjunctival instillation of cows with serovar *L. hardjo* type *hardjobovis* (the only type of *L. hardjo* isolated from cattle in the United States).[203]

LISTERIA MONOCYTOGENES ABORTION

Listeriosis is caused by *Listeria monocytogenes*. Listerial abortions are mainly of importance in ruminants.

HISTORY AND CLINICAL SIGNS. Bovine abortions usually occur in the last 2 months of gestation.[153(p47)] Infected ewes and does typically abort in the last month.[5(p600),157] Fever, depression, RFM, or endometritis may occur,[5(p600),153(p47),167] but often the dam shows no clinical signs of infection.

LABORATORY DIAGNOSIS. In less severely autolyzed fetuses, fibrinous polyserositis may be apparent. Most aborted fetuses have gray-white hepatic foci up to 2 mm in diameter. Similar foci may be visible in cotyledons; exudation occurs between cotyledons. Abomasal erosions have been reported in aborted lambs.[153(p47)] Histologically, suppurative placentitis and endometritis are consistent findings.

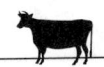

Listeria is readily cultured from abortuses without cold enrichment. Serovars 1 and 4b are commonly isolated from bovine fetuses; serovars 4b and 5 are the usual ovine isolates.[153(p47)] *Listeria* appears in impression smears as gram-positive pleomorphic cocco-bacilli.[153(p47)]

PATHOPHYSIOLOGY. Listerial abortion can be induced experimentally in cattle 6 to 8 days after infection and in sheep 3 to 11 days after infection. Fetuses die from placentitis and septicemia and are often retained in utero several days before expulsion.[153(p47)]

EPIDEMIOLOGY. Listerial abortion is usually sporadic and seldom exceeds 15%.[138,153(p47)] Infection is most common in the winter and has been associated with feeding of silage. The elevated pH of spoiled silage enhances multiplication of the organism. Aborted tissues are infectious for humans and should be handled with care.

TREATMENT AND CONTROL. The effect on fertility is usually transient, and aborting animals tend to resist reinfection. Tetracycline may be used in remaining pregnant animals in the herd.[5(p600)] Aborting animals should be segregated, and fetuses and placentas should be removed from the premises. The feeding of spoiled silage should be avoided.

MYCOPLASMA ABORTION

Mycoplasmal isolations from the bovine genital tract have been mainly *Mycoplasma bovigenitalium* and *Mycoplasma bovis*. *M. bovis* is probably the more important cause of abortion.[204] *Mycoplasma mycoides* ssp. *mycoides* (see *Mycoplasma* Polyarthritis) and *Mycoplasma agalactiae* have been associated with caprine abortions.[5(p609)]

HISTORY AND CLINICAL SIGNS. *M. bovigenitalium* is associated with granular vulvovaginitis and less commonly with endometritis, especially in heifers. Infertility is more common than abortion. *M. bovis* causes mastitis and abortion.[204] In goats, mycoplasmal infection is associated with septicemia, arthritis, pneumonia, mastitis, and abortion.[5(p609)]

LABORATORY DIAGNOSIS. Placentitis and fetal pneumonia have been associated with bovine mycoplasmal abortion.[204] Isolation of *Mycoplasma* from the genital tract, milk, placenta, or fetus indicates infection. However, mycoplasmosis should not be considered the cause for abortion unless placentitis or fetal inflammation is present and other more likely causes for abortion have been eliminated.

PATHOPHYSIOLOGY. *M. bovigenitalium* can be isolated from the vagina of as many as 12% of clinically normal cows, but *M. bovis* is isolated from fewer than 1%. Vulvitis can be induced by inoculation with mucosal scarification with *M. bovigenitalium*; thus venereal transmission may be the natural route of infection.[5(p288),204] Experimental inoculation with *M. bovis* induces abortion with placentitis and fetal pneumonia.[204,205] *M. bovigenitalium* is rarely isolated from abortuses or normal fetuses.[5(p288)]

EPIDEMIOLOGY. *Mycoplasma* spp. are ubiquitous, but mycoplasmal abortions are not commonly documented.

TREATMENT AND CONTROL. Tetracycline or tylosin is the recommended antibiotic for mycoplasmal granular vulvovaginitis in heifers.[204]

Treatment of goats is usually not recommended because treated animals may remain carriers. The infection is eliminated from the herd by testing milk and slaughtering infected animals.[205]

SALMONELLA ABORTION

A variety of *Salmonella* serotypes have been isolated from aborted fetuses of cattle, sheep, goats, and horses. A complete discussion of salmonellosis is presented elsewhere. Infection is acquired by ingestion of contaminated feed or water. Maternal septicemia is followed by localization of salmonellae in tissues, including the pregnant uterus where placentitis and fetal septicemia occur. Salmonellosis accompanied by endotoxemia causes early pregnancy loss without colonization of the uterus; as a result of infection and endotoxemia that causes endogenous prostaglandin release, which initiates luteolysis and abortion in the first trimester (<100 days for cattle), as is the case with exogenous administration of PGF products.

HISTORY AND CLINICAL SIGNS. The animal may show systemic signs before abortion. Abortion may occur at any stage of gestation and is characterized by placental necrosis, edema, and hemorrhage. RFM and fetal autolysis may occur. Abortion may be accompanied by diarrhea, fever, or vaginal discharge, particularly in the ewe, but often infection is not clinically apparent in the dam.[153(p44),167,206] Fetuses also may be lost as a result of stillbirth or perinatal septicemia.

LABORATORY DIAGNOSIS. The fetus is frequently autolyzed. Placentitis is usually present. Diagnosis is based on isolation of the organism and evidence of placentitis or inflammation of fetal tissues. FA techniques can identify the bacteria in impression smears or sections of placenta or fetal tissue.[153(p44)] The dam can be tested serologically for evidence of recent active infection,[206] but at present many diagnostic laboratories do not perform salmonella serology.

PATHOPHYSIOLOGY. Infected adult animals are often short-term carriers and shed salmonellae in the feces or milk. True long-term asymptomatic carriers occur mainly with the host-adapted serotypes: *Salmonella dublin* in cattle, *Salmonella abortus-ovis* in sheep, and *Salmonella abortivoequina* (or *Salmonella abortus-equi*) in horses. Salmonellosis caused by *S. abortus-equi* has been eradicated in the United States. Occasionally long-term carriers of other serotypes occur; these are usually intestinal carriers and fecal shedders. Infection usually occurs by ingestion. There is no evidence of venereal transmission.[206] Maternal septicemia is followed by localization of the organism in a variety of tissues, including the pregnant uterus. The bacteria multiply in and cause necrosis of connective tissues of the cotyledon.[206] The incubation period between infection and abortion varies from about 1 week to 1 month.[5(p705),167] Fetal death results from placentitis and fetal septicemia.[153(p44),207] In most cases, maternal shedding of the organism in cattle ceases by 5 weeks after calving.[206]

In a second mechanism of salmonella-induced abortion, salmonella septicemia causes endotoxemia and release of endogenous PGF which causes luteolysis and abortion. In this case the fetus and placenta are culture negative for salmonella.

EPIDEMIOLOGY. Bovine abortion resulting from salmonellosis is caused mainly by *S. dublin* and *Salmonella typhimurium*. Abortion is sporadic and most common in the summer and fall.[206]

Ovine abortion is associated with *S. typhimurium*, *S. dublin*, *Salmonella arizona* and *S. abortus-ovis*. *S. abortus-ovis* (which infects only sheep) is enzootic in parts of England and Europe, but is not reported from the United States.[5(p852),153(p44)] Young ewes in late gestation are most susceptible, and the abortion rate may approach 50%,[5(p852),167] but usually only one or two ewes in a flock abort.[153(p44)]

TREATMENT AND CONTROL. Metritis is a rare complication of salmonellosis that can be fatal.[153(p44)] Usually there is no lasting effect on fertility, but animals infected with host-adapted serotypes may become carriers and should be cultured and tested serologically and culled if positive. Salmonellosis can be controlled by hygiene and by avoiding the introduction of carrier animals. Aborting animals should be isolated; the fetus, placenta, and contaminated material should be removed from the premises. *Salmonella* spp. are infectious for humans; thus aborted tissues should be handled with caution (see Chapter 30 for more on *Salmonella* control).

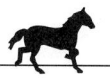

UREAPLASMA

Ureaplasma is a small bacterium without cell walls; it differs from mycoplasma in its ability to hydrolyze urea. *Ureaplasma diversum* has been associated with granular vulvitis and abortion in cattle.

HISTORY AND CLINICAL SIGNS. Granular vulvitis appears as reddish nodules in the vulvar mucosa, with mucopurulent discharge in the early stages. The discharge is usually more copious and protracted than with IPV induced by herpesvirus.[5(p282),204] Affected cows are not systemically ill.[153(p27)] The organism has been recovered from embryo flushing media and can adhere to the zona pellucida, resisting removal by washing. It is believed to be responsible for an 18% reduction in pregnancy rate in embryo recipients when the transfer medium contains the organism.

LABORATORY DIAGNOSIS. Gross lesions include thickening of placental membranes with foci of hemorrhage and fibrinous exudate. Gross lesions are seldom apparent in the fetus. Microscopically the placenta is fibrotic, with heavy mononuclear cell infiltration, multifocal necrosis, fibrin deposition, and mineralization. Cuffs of lymphocytes surround fetal intrapulmonary airways.[153(p27)] Diagnosis is based on isolation of the organism from genital mucosa, placenta, or fetal stomach or lung, and the presence of genital or fetal inflammation.

PATHOPHYSIOLOGY. *Ureaplasma* can be isolated from the genital tract of normal cows and from normal fetuses.[208] Vulvitis has been induced by inoculation of virgin heifers with *U. diversum*.[208] Uterine involvement is considered rare but may cause conception failure, early embryonic death, or abortion. Abortion presumably results from placentitis.[5(p282)] Intraamniotic inoculation of *U. diversum* caused placentitis, abortion, and fetal alveolitis in two of four experimental cows.[208] One cow delivered a weak calf at term. Experimental infection in ewes did not decrease fertility.[209]

EPIDEMIOLOGY. Bovine infection is common, but documented abortions caused by *Ureaplasma* are rare.[204] Infertility is more common in heifers than in cows.

TREATMENT AND CONTROL. Nonirritating tetracyclines by intrauterine infusion are recommended for treatment. Products may not be approved for intrauterine use.[5(p282)] Uterine contamination can be avoided by use of the double-rod technique of AI.[5(p282)]

MISCELLANEOUS BACTERIAL ABORTIONS

In addition to the aforementioned bacteria, other bacteria occasionally produce maternal septicemia. Many of these bacteria are ubiquitous, frequently contaminate aborted fetuses and placentas, and should not be considered the cause of abortion unless (1) they are isolated from the placenta and fetus in large numbers and relatively pure culture, (2) placentitis or fetal inflammation is evident, and (3) other more likely causes of abortion have been eliminated.[153(p15)]

In cows, most bacterial infections of the uterus result from septicemia. Miscellaneous bacterial causes of infertility and abortion include *Actinomyces* (formerly *Corynebacterium*) *pyogenes, Escherichia coli, Bacillus* spp., *Pasteurella* spp., *Staphylococcus* spp., *Streptococcus* spp., *Fusobacterium necrophorum,* and *Bacteroides melaninogenicus.*[139(pp15,77),153]

A. pyogenes with or without accompanying anaerobes has been associated with pyometra and abortion in cattle.[134,153(p77),210] Abortions are sporadic and may occur at any stage of gestation. Clinical signs are seldom apparent in the cow. The fetus is commonly autolyzed, and placentitis is typical. Polyserositis may be evident. In fetuses aborted in the first half of gestation, 1-mm yellow foci (bacterial colonies) may be grossly apparent in the lung.[153(p77)]

In the ewe or doe, miscellaneous bacterial causes of abortion include *Staphylococcus aureus, Streptococcus* spp., *Pasteurella* spp., *E. coli, Yersinia pseudotuberculosis, Francisella tularensis, Histophilus ovis, Bacillus* spp., *A. pyogenes,* and *Corynebacterium* spp.[153(p18,77),211-214]

A spirillum-like organism has been documented as a cause of ovine abortion, fetal mummification, stillbirth, or birth of weak lambs. Abortion generally occurs in the last 2 weeks of gestation. Placentitis is consistently present; many fetuses also have fibrinous peritonitis and focal hepatic necrosis that resembles that of campylobacteriosis.[215] Abortion can be reproduced experimentally by inoculation of pregnant ewes.[216] Diagnosis is based on pathologic lesions and identification of the spindloid flagellated organism by darkfield microscopy of fetal abomasal content or liver or by anaerobic culture on selective medium.[215,217]

MYCOTIC DISEASES THAT CAUSE ABORTION

Fungal causes of bovine abortion include *Aspergillus, Absidia, Mucor, Rhizopus, Candida,* and *Mortierella.*[153(p147),218,219] Mycotic abortion is uncommon in sheep and goats.[153(p147)]

HISTORY AND CLINICAL SIGNS. Mycotic abortions usually occur in the latter half of gestation (often near term) and seldom are associated with prodromal or postabortion clinical signs in the dam.

LABORATORY DIAGNOSIS. The most consistent lesion is placentitis with necrosis and thickening of fetal membranes. In ruminants, both cotyledons and the intercotyledonary placenta are affected. Histologically, necrotizing inflammation of the chorionic villi is associated with vasculitis and thrombosis.[153(p147)] Gross lesions may not be apparent in the fetus, but granulomatous bronchopneumonia is frequently observed histologically.[153(p147),219-221] In bovine aspergillosis the fetus is often near term with minimum autolysis and partially inflated lungs. Emaciation and dehydration with multifocal dry, scaly skin lesions occur in about 25% of affected fetuses.[153(p147)] With other fungi the aborted fetus is often autolyzed, placentitis may be more severe, and skin lesions, if present, tend to be moister than those of aspergillosis.[153(p147)] The placenta is characteristically thickened and leathery. The fetus may be emaciated, and granulomatous bronchopneumonia has been observed.[220] The fungus can be isolated from the fetus and placenta or demonstrated on histologic sections with immunostaining.

PATHOPHYSIOLOGY. The route of fungal infection in the bovine uterus is thought to be hematogenous.[9]

EPIDEMIOLOGY. Mycotic abortion generally affects only one or two animals in a herd and is more common in the winter.[153(p147)] Fungi cause 3% to 10% of bovine abortions.[222,223] *Aspergillus* accounts for up to 80% of bovine mycotic abortions; mucorales account for an additional 10% to 15%.[5(p291)] *Mortierella* is a common abortifacient in Australia and New Zealand and has been associated with feeding of grass silage,[219,223] but *Mortierella* abortion is rare in the United States.

CONTROL. The only means of control of mycotic abortion is reduction of exposure to fungal agents.

SARCOCYSTIS ABORTION

Sarcocystosis may cause abortion in cattle, sheep, and goats. Cattle are infected by *Sarcocystis cruzi,* sheep by *Sarcocystis ovicanis,* and goats by *Sarcocystis capracanis.*

HISTORY AND CLINICAL SIGNS. Most cattle are infected with *Sarcocystis* but do not show clinical signs of infection; however, massive or repeated infections may elicit depression, anorexia, weight loss, lameness, hair loss, emaciation, or death. Abortions occur in late gestation, usually in severely affected animals.[153(p162),224,225]

LABORATORY DIAGNOSIS. There are no specific gross lesions in the aborted fetus. Histologically protozoa may be observed in villi and small arteries of the cotyledon or (more likely) the caruncle but are seldom seen in the bovine, ovine, or caprine fetus. Parasites are more likely to be observed in the fetal brain than in other tissues.[224] Nonsuppurative inflammation may occur in the placenta or, less commonly, in fetal tissues, particularly the brain, heart, lung, liver, or kidney.[153(p162),224,225]

FA demonstration of numerous developing protozoa in the cotyledon or caruncle is considered diagnostic. Caruncles are reported to be atrophied.[224] The protozoa can also be isolated by feeding aborted tissues to canids and recovering coccidian sporocysts from their feces.[153(p154)]

PATHOPHYSIOLOGY. The pathogenesis of abortion in sarcocystosis is unclear. Generally numerous spores are required to induce abortion experimentally. Fetal invasion by *Sarcocystis* is rare, and abortion may result from maternal fever, anemia, or placental insufficiency.[224] Pregnant does apparently have diminished immunity to Sarcocystis because low doses of *S. capracanis* result in fetal death without maternal illness if given in early pregnancy.[226]

EPIDEMIOLOGY. Ruminants are infected by consumption of canid feces that contain oocysts. *Sarcocystis* occurs in the skeletal and cardiac muscle of most cows without associated lesions or clinical evidence of illness.

CONTROL. Effective therapeutic regimens for clinically ill animals have not been developed. To break the life cycle of *Sarcocystis*, feeds should be kept free of dog or cat feces. These carnivores should not be allowed to eat aborted fetuses, placentas, or other ruminant carcasses.

TOXOPLASMOSIS ABORTION

Toxoplasma gondii is a ubiquitous protozoan that is a major abortifacient in sheep and goats but only rarely causes abortion in cattle or horses.

HISTORY AND CLINICAL SIGNS. Infection does not cause clinical illness in the adult but may result in embryonic death, fetal death and abortion, stillbirth, or birth of weak, nonviable lambs or kids.

LABORATORY DIAGNOSIS. The most characteristic gross lesion of toxoplasmosis is the presence of white, chalky foci of necrosis and calcification up to 2 mm in diameter in cotyledons.[227-229] The intercotyledonary areas of the placenta are grossly normal. Specific gross lesions are not observed in the aborted fetus, but histologically most have nonsuppurative encephalomyelitis[228]; and many also have pneumonia, myocarditis, or hepatitis. Tachyzoites may be found in placenta or other fetal tissues but are not numerous.[229,230] The tachyzoites are oval, 2 to 4 by 4 to 8 mm, with a central nucleus, and appear larger in impression smears than in paraffin sections. Several serologic tests, including the modified agglutination test, indirect FA test, Sabin Feldman dye test, indirect hemagglutination test, and enzyme-linked immunosorbent assay, reliably detect toxoplasmosis in pleural or amniotic fluid or presuckling serum from nondecomposed fetuses.[153(p165),231,232] The modified agglutination test is commercially available, safer, and more sensitive than the dye test. Fetal antibodies to *T. gondii* can be detected 35 days after infection.[227] Absence of fetal antibody does not always preclude a diagnosis of toxoplasmosis.[153(p165)] High maternal titers are not diagnostic of toxoplasmal abortion, but lack of titer eliminates toxoplasmosis as the cause for abortion.[227] The peroxidase-antiperoxidase method for detecting *Toxoplasma* antigen in fetal tissues or placenta is reliable even in autolyzed fetuses. Fetal heart, lung, brain, spinal cord, skeletal muscle, and placenta are the preferred specimens for the peroxidase-antiperoxidase method and should not be held

in formalin more than 2 days before paraffin embedding.[230] *T. gondii* can be isolated by intraperitoneal inoculation of placental or fetal tissue suspensions into mice.[153(p165)]

PATHOPHYSIOLOGY. Placental infection occurs about 14 days after ingestion of oocysts.[230] Infection acquired before 50 days' gestation may result in embryonic death and resorption. Infection between 60 and 100 days' gestation usually causes fetal death or birth of weak lambs. Infection during the last month of gestation often has no apparent effect on the fetus.[227] In experimental infection of ewes between 6 and 14 weeks of pregnancy, abortions occurred 1 to 2 months after inoculation.[232] In natural infections, most abortions occur 1 month before parturition.[227]

EPIDEMIOLOGY. Toxoplasmosis is a major cause of ovine abortion in many sheep-raising countries, including the United States.[228,229,233] Sheep are infected by ingestion of oocysts from feed or grass contaminated with cat feces. Most ewes are infected by 4 years of age.[234] Aborted tissues may be infectious for humans and should be handled with caution.

CONTROL. Infected ewes or does seldom abort from toxoplasmosis in subsequent pregnancies.[228] The prevalence of abortion can be reduced by avoiding contamination of feedstuffs with feline feces. Cats should not be allowed to eat placentas or carcasses that may contain tachyzoites or tissue cysts. In endemic areas, exposing replacement ewes to aborting ewes may provide immunity before breeding age.[5(p852)]

BOVINE NEOSPOROSIS

Abortion in cattle caused by *Neospora caninum* is a newly recognized but relatively common and important disease, especially in dairy cattle. Congenital infection with limb paresis or dysfunction at birth as a result of encephalomyelitis may also occur. *Neospora* is closely related to *Toxoplasma*. The dog has been identified as the definitive host.[235] Transmission was originally described as mainly vertical (dam to fetus in utero) but point-source horizontal transmission (ingestion of feed contaminated with feces containing oocysts) has more recently been recognized and may be the more prevalent method in some herds.[236] Bovine fetal lesions are similar to those found in *Toxoplasma*-aborted sheep fetuses. Most abortions occur around midgestation. Diagnosis is based on characteristic lesions in aborted fetuses, and seroepidemiologic study of an equal number of aborting and nonaborting herdmate cows if the proportion of seropositives is statistically higher in those that have aborted.[237] Finding one aborting cow to be seropositive does not confirm *N. caninum* as the cause, and cows that abort once because of *N. caninum* are not protected from future abortion caused by this organism.

TRICHOMONIASIS

Trichomoniasis is a venereal infection of cattle caused by the flagellated protozoan *Tritrichomonas foetus*.[5(p275),135,153(p169),238,239]

HISTORY AND CLINICAL SIGNS. Infertility characterized by a high percentage of cows returning to estrus or found nonpregnant after the breeding season and cows calving late plus occasional pyometras and abortions are the most common clinical signs of trichomoniasis. Pyometra in postcoital heifers or cows suggests that trichomoniasis may be the cause. Abortions generally occur in the first half of gestation at a rate between 5% and 30%.[238] The placenta may be expelled or retained.[5(p275),153(p169)]

LABORATORY DIAGNOSIS. Diagnosis in the female is made by identifying or culturing trichomonads from cervicovaginal mucus (about 76% sensitivity), uterine exudate, placental fluids, or fetal abomasal contents.[5(p275),135,153(p169),238,239] Preputial smegma collected from bulls by using a plastic pipette run against the mucosa can also be cultured for tricho-

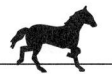

monads (sensitivity 80% to 90%). Diamond's media (or modified Pastridge media) is recommended for cultures from cows, bulls, or aborted fetuses.[239] Samples should be transported at ambient temperature, kept out of sunlight, not refrigerated, and delivered promptly to the diagnostic laboratory. The organisms are identified microscopically by their size (10 μm × 15 μm), the presence of three anterior flagellae and an undulating membrane, and a characteristic jerky, rolling motion.[153(p169)]

There are no specific gross lesions in aborted fetuses. However, placentitis is a consistent microscopic lesion, and trichomonads can frequently be recognized in the placental stroma in histologic sections. Organisms may also be observed in the fetal lung in association with pyogranulomatous bronchopneumonia.[240]

PATHOPHYSIOLOGY. Trichomoniasis is transmitted venereally from infected bulls to cows or vice versa. The organisms colonize the vagina, cervix, uterus, and oviducts; yet they do not generally interfere with conception. Embryonic death frequently occurs within the first 2 months of infection,[5(p275)] followed by a 2- to 6-month period of immunity to reinfection.[135] Clearance of infection in cows commonly occurs within 95 days; infection rarely persists as long as 6 months.[238] However, infection in bulls over 4 years of age is permanent and the main source of carryover from one breeding season to the next in beef cattle.[135]

TREATMENT AND CONTROL. Systemic treatment of infected animals with imidazole compounds (ipronidazole, dimetridazole) is effective, but these compounds are prohibited in food animals in the United States.[241,242] Infected cows should either be culled or given at least 3 months' sexual rest. The use of AI with semen from *T. foetus*–negative bulls controls the disease once infected natural service bulls have been removed from the herd. In natural breeding situations, vaccination, use of young virgin bulls, and testing and elimination of positive bulls older than 3 years of age will allow herds to gain control over the incidence of trichomoniasis.

▌▌ MARES

EQUINE HERPESVIRUS I ABORTION

Equine herpesvirus 1 (EHV-1; formerly EHV-1, subtype 1) can cause abortion, perinatal foal mortality, rhinopneumonitis, and neurologic disease.[243] Although equine herpesvirus 4 (EHV-4; formerly EHV-1, subtype 2) is considered to be confined to the respiratory tract, sporadic cases of abortion have been reported during EHV-4 outbreaks.[243] Clinical signs and fetal lesions of abortion caused by EHV-1 and EHV-4 are indistinguishable from each other.[243]

CLINICAL SIGNS AND DIAGNOSIS. Abortion resulting from EHV-1 usually occurs after 7 months of gestation. Although epidemic abortions occur, losses may be confined to only a few mares in a herd. EHV-1 is transmitted through inhalation of the virus. After respiratory infection, EHV-1 causes an episode of viremia and infects the fetus via transplacental migration of virus-bearing leukocytes. Respiratory clinical signs in infected mares may be subclinical. The time between infection and abortion varies greatly from less than 2 weeks to several months.[243] Abortion occurs as a result of a rapid separation of the placenta, causing suffocation of the fetus.[244] Near-term fetuses may be born alive but will die within days. Aborting mares clear the virus quickly from the reproductive tract, and subsequent fertility is often not affected by the disease.

Abortions occur suddenly without maternal clinical signs. The aborted fetus is fresh with minimal signs of autolysis. Increased fluid in the thoracic and abdominal cavities; congestion and edema of the lungs; an enlarged liver with small

(approximately 1 mm) necrotic, yellow-white lesions; subcutaneous edema; and icterus are commonly found gross lesions in the fetus. Histologically, the most characteristic lesion is areas of necrosis in lymphoid tissue, liver, adrenal cortex, and the lung with large intranuclear eosinophilic inclusion bodies. In addition, a hyperplastic necrotizing bronchiolitis is often found. The placenta may be normal or edematous, with no specific microscopic lesions.

Laboratory diagnostics include FA staining of fetal tissue, virus isolation from aborted fetuses, virus isolation from maternal whole blood, presence of viral inclusion bodies in liver, lung, and thymus, and fetal serology. Equine fetuses have been found to be capable of producing antibodies to EHV-1 at 200 days of gestation. Maternal serology is of limited diagnostic value because mares may abort several weeks after infection. The rise in serologic titer may have disappeared by the time of the abortion.

TREATMENT AND PROGNOSIS. Several vaccines against herpesvirus infections are available. Effective killed vaccines for abortion should contain antigenic strains of both EHV-1 1P and EHV-1 1B. The vaccine is not fully protective, and abortion may occur in vaccinated mares. However, consistent vaccination of pregnant mares should be expected to decrease the incidence of abortion storms and sporadic abortions in a herd. Vaccination is typically recommended in the fifth, seventh, and ninth months of pregnancy, but because the time between actual infection and abortion may be long, some clinicians recommend vaccination every 2 months throughout the pregnancy. To maximize the effectiveness of a vaccination program it needs to be combined with a management strategy that minimizes exposure of mares to the virus and that prevents activation of a latent viral infection. All horses, young, adult, nonpregnant, and pregnant, should be vaccinated to restrict shedding of the virus. Unnecessary stress such as transportation and overcrowding should be avoided. Pregnant mares should be kept separate from other horses on the farm. Newly arrived horses should be isolated from the resident population for 3 weeks, during which time they should be monitored daily for signs of respiratory disease.

After abortion, the fetus and fetal membranes should be transported away from the area without contaminating the surrounding environment. The stall in which the mare aborted should be disinfected with a phenolic or iodinophoric compound and the bedding should be prevented from contaminating other areas on the farm. All pregnant mares on an infected farm should remain on the farm until they have foaled. No horse should leave the farm until 3 to 4 weeks after the last abortion.

EQUINE INFECTIOUS ANEMIA ABORTION

Equine infectious anemia (EIA) is a retroviral infection transmitted by horseflies.[245] After systemic infection with EIA, mares abort during the febrile stage of infection and may abort at any stage of gestation. Foals from infected but asymptomatic mares and stallions are seronegative (precolostral) and clinically normal at birth. Mechanism of abortion is unknown but may be secondary to systemic illness, because EIA virus is not found in amniotic fluid.[245] Coggins' test will confirm seropositive status but is not a definitive diagnosis for abortion.

EQUINE VIRAL ARTERITIS

Equine viral arteritis (EVA) is caused by a pestivirus. Infection is often inapparent, and abortion is an occasional occurrence in infected animals.[246] Transmission may occur venereally from infected stallions to mares. Reproductive performance of venerally infected mares is not affected, but contact

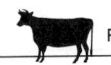

tranmission from venerally infected mares to late gestational mares may cause abortion.[247] Although the pathophysiology is not well established, fetal death may occur by fetal anoxia secondary to compression of myometrial vessels by edema and decreased progesterone production by the placenta.[248]

HISTORY AND CLINICAL SIGNS. Systemic disease may be inapparent to severe and may include fever, leukopenia, conjunctivitis, nasal discharge, edema, lameness, and generalized vascular necrosis. Experimental infection produces myometritis but not uterine arteritis.[248] Abortion follows the onset of clinical signs by several days but up to 2 months. Abortion typically occurs at 5 to 10 months of gestation.

LABORATORY DIAGNOSIS. There are no characteristic features of EVA infection in the fetus, though autolysis and myocardial arteritis have been reported. EVA virus is readily isolated or detected by polymerase chain reaction (PCR) techniques from fetal tissues and the placenta. Serology (virus neutralizing antibody) will identify animals that have been exposed.[247]

EPIDEMIOLOGY AND CONTROL. Outbreaks were reported in 1953 and 1984 in the United States. Since that time, occasional outbreaks have occurred, with abortion occurring at low incidence.[246] Mares may be isolated after infection but usually do not become carriers. A proportion of naturally infected stallions become persistently infected with EVA and shed the virus constantly in semen. Incidence of seropositive animals is higher in Standardbreds than in Thoroughbreds, and regulatory guidelines may govern the use of seropositive Thoroughbred stallions. Carrier stallions may be the reservoir for the disease between outbreaks and should be isolated and only bred to immune mares. Mares bred in this way should be isolated for 3 weeks. A modified-live vaccine is available for mares and stallions. Control involves vaccination of seronegative stallions under the guidance of regulatory authorities. There is some evidence that prepubertal infection of colts does not result in permanent carrier status.

LEPTOSPIROSIS ABORTION

Leptospiral abortion is less common in horses than in cattle. Although an uncommonly diagnosed cause of equine abortion in the past, leptospirosis is of increasing importance. Serovar *Leptospira pomona* has most commonly been associated with leptospirosis abortion in mares, but *Leptospira grippotyphosa*, *Leptospira hardjo*, *Leptospira bratislava*, and *Leptospira icterohemorrhagiae* have also been isolated from sporadic abortions.[249]

CLINICAL SIGNS AND DIAGNOSIS. Mares may show mild systemic signs, including fever, anorexia, depression, and icterus for 3 to 4 days. Abortion occurs 1 to 3 weeks after clinical illness. Abortion commonly occurs between the seventh month of pregnancy and term. The equine fetus shows icterus and autolysis; however, recovery of the organism is difficult. Diagnosis is based on isolation of the organism, immunofluorescence staining, and serology testing. Mares often have high leptospiral titers at the time of abortion. A rising titer associated with abortion is considered to be diagnostic.

TREATMENT AND CONTROL. Horses may shed spirochetes in urine for up to 90 days; thus affected animals should be isolated and treated with antibiotics. Aborting mares should be isolated and the stalls should be disinfected. Infected mares may be treated with streptomycin (10 mg/kg twice daily), penicillin (10 to 15,000 IU/kg twice daily), or oxytetracycline (5 to 10 mg/kg) for a period of 1 week. Because *L. pomona* is the most common isolate in the United States, mares should be separated from other leptospiral hosts such as ruminants or pigs. Vaccines for cattle are not effective in horses.

EQUINE EHRLICHIAL ABORTION

Ehrlichia risticii is a known cause of colitis in the mare. The disease is discussed elsewhere in this book. *E. risticii* has been associated with equine abortion between 6 and 8 months of pregnancy,[250] but the incidence of naturally occuring ehrlichial abortion is not known.

CLINICAL SIGNS AND DIAGNOSIS. Abortions have been observed 2 to 3 months after clinical signs of ehrlichiosis.[250] Abortions were associated with placentitis and RFMs. Histopathologic findings of aborted fetuses included colitis, periportal hepatitis, and hyperplasia and necrosis of lymphoid organs. The diagnosis can be confirmed by identifying a small amount of rickettsia by PCR.

TREATMENT AND PREVENTION. Treatment with oxytetracycline (6.6 mg/kg IV once daily) for 5 days in pregnant mares with clinical signs of ehrlichial colitis may prevent or reduce the incidence of abortion. Commercial vaccines against equine ehrlichiosis are available, but the protective effect of vaccines against abortion is unknown.

SALMONELLA ABORTION

Salmonella abortus-equi (*Salmonella abortivoequina* or "contagious abortion") was a common cause of abortion in the early 1900s but is now rare. Non–host-specific species, including *Salmonella typhimurium*, now cause most equine salmonella abortions. Abortion caused by salmonella is discussed under abortions in ruminants.

TRYPANOSOMIASIS (DOURINE)

The protozoan parasite *Trypanosoma equiperdum* causes a venereally transmitted genital infection that may be followed by fatal systemic dissemination in horses. Systemic illness may cause abortion. It occurs in tropical and subtropical regions and has been eradicated from North America.[9(p204)] Dourine is diagnosed by isolation of trypanosome in uterine discharge. Exposed animals can be detected by serology (complement fixation). Control strategies require identification and treatment or slaughter of infected animals.

ABORTION CAUSED BY ENDOTOXEMIA

Gram-negative septicemia and endotoxemia associated with intestinal disorders that alter the integrity of the mucosal barrier (i.e., intestinal obstructions, acute enteritis, colitis, and grain overload) result in the release of vasoactive metabolites including PGF. Endogenous release of PGF during an episode of experimental endotoxemia has been shown to cause luteolysis and abortion during the first 2 months of pregnancy in mares.[251] The equine pregnancy is dependent on ovarian sources of progesterone for the first 80 days of gestation. After this time the fetoplacental unit takes over progesterone production that is necessary for maintenance of the pregnancy.

CLINICAL SIGNS AND DIAGNOSIS. Abortions follow a recent episode of stress induced by endotoxemic shock or gram-negative endotoxemia. Pregnancy loss at early stages of gestation may go undetected unless fetal membranes or parts are found in the stall. Abortions during later stages of the pregnancy may be observed as vaginal discharge or the detection of an expelled fetus.

TREATMENT AND PREVENTION. Daily administration of a progestagen (Altrenogest 0.044 mg/kg PO) has been shown to effectively prevent experimental endotoxin-induced abortion.[251] If treated while the pregnancy still is CL dependent (approximately <day 80), analysis of serum progesterone concentrations after the acute episode of the disease

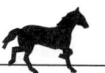

helps in deciding if the supplementation needs to continue. Serum progesterone concentrations of less than 1 ng/ml indicate the loss of an active CL, and supplemental progestagen treatment should continue until the fetoplacental unit is known to be capable of maintaining the pregnancy. For practical reasons supplementation until day 100 is commonly recommended. Serum progesterone concentrations greater than 1 ng/ml are compatible with a functional CL and the progestagen treatment can gradually be discontinued. Treatments with flunixin meglumine or other prostaglandin inhibitors have not been proven to effectively prevent endotoxin-induced fetal losses, unless administered before clinical signs.

PLACENTITIS

Bacterial and fungal abortions in mares are primarily caused by ascending infections through the cervix, causing placentitis and subsequent fetal infection. Bacterial organisms most commonly cultured from aborted fetuses include *Streptococcus* spp., *Escherichia coli*, *Pseudomonas* spp., *Klebsiella* spp., *Staphylococcus* spp., and *Leptospira* spp. Nocardioform *actinomycete* is an important cause of placentitis in central Kentucky. This organism is the most common cause of abortion in Kentucky, but has not been diagnosed in mares without connection to this area. The route of infection and the pathophysiology of *Nocardia* abortions are poorly understood. *Aspergillus fumigatus* and *Mucor* spp. are the most commonly diagnosed causes of mycotic abortion in mares. Fungi cause 5% to 30% of infectious equine abortions.[5(p705)]

CLINICAL SIGNS AND DIAGNOSIS. Mares that abort from placentitis often show clinical signs of pending abortion before the actual pregnancy termination. Premature udder development and vaginal discharge are common signs of pending abortion caused by placentitis. Transrectal ultrasonography of the allantochorion in an area close to the cervix is useful to detect early signs of placentitis and impending abortion (Fig. 41-1).[252] Normal measurements of the combined thickness of the uterus and the placenta (CTUP) have been established (Fig. 41-2).[253] Mares with placentitis may show increased CTUP, edema of the allantochorion, and separation from the endometrium. Placental lesions in mares infected with Nocardioform *actinomycete* are located ventrally in the uterine body and at the base of the uterine horns.

Affected areas are avillous, thickened, and covered by thick brown or reddish exudate. Because of the location of the lesions away from the cervical star, transabdominal ultrasonography may be needed to diagnose the condition in pregnant mares.

The gross lesions of the fetus are not specific. An increased amount of fluid in the thoracic and abdominal cavities and an enlarged liver are frequently observed in aborted fetuses. Placental lesions are most severe on the chorionic surface at an area from opposite the cervix ("cervical star") to the body of the placenta. The affected area is edematous, thickened, and discolored or brown with a mucoid or fibronecrotic exudate on the surface. The placenta is characteristically thickened and leathery in cases of mycotic placentitis, with lesions well demarcated from the rest of the chorionic surface. Microorganisms can be isolated from the placenta and several fetal organs, most consistently from the stomach.

TREATMENT AND PROGNOSIS. Pregnant mares with clinical signs of placentitis should be treated with systemic broad-spectrum antimicrobials and antiinflammatories. Treatments that cause uterine quiescence should also be considered; altrenogest* (0.088 mg/kg PO once daily) and clenbuterol† (0.8 μg/kg IM or IV) have been used. Unfortunately,

---

*Regumate, Hoechts-Rousel, Agri-Vet Co, Sommervilled, NJ.
†Ventipulmin, Boehringer Ingelheim Animal Health, St Joseph, MO.

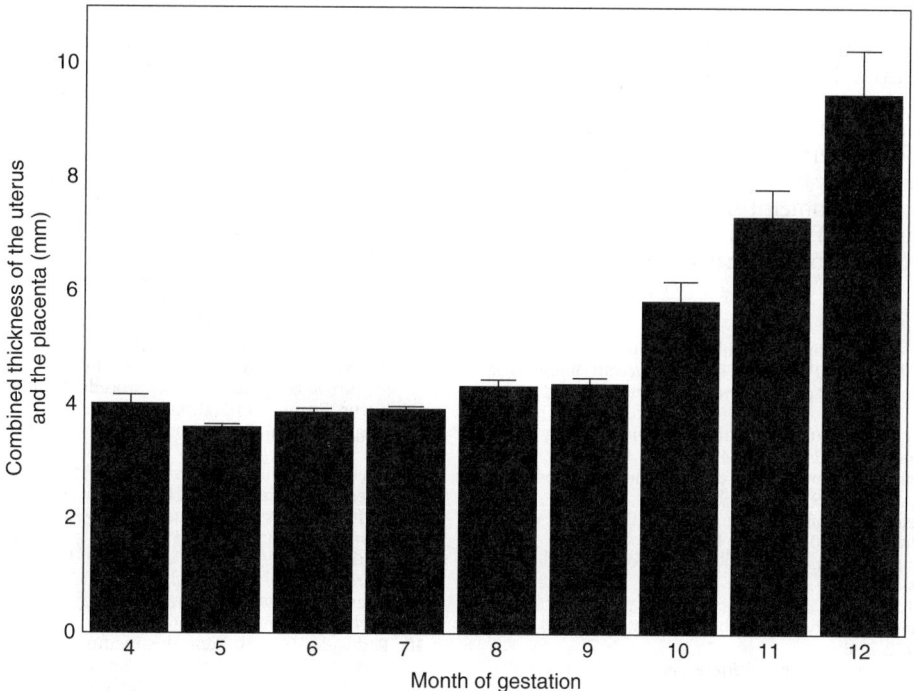

FIG. 41-1 ▓ Monthly recordings of transrectal ultrasonographic measurements of the combined thickness of the uterus and the placenta (CTUP) in normal mares from 4 months of gestation and throughout the pregnancy. Month 4 is 91 to 120 days; month 5 is 121 to 150 days; month 6 is 151 to 180 days; month 7 is 181 to 210 days; month 8 is 211 to 240 days; month 9 is 241 to 270 days; month 10 is 271 to 300 days; month 11 is 301 to 330 days; month 12 is 331 to 360 days. (Modified from Renaudin et al: *Theriogenology* 47:559-573, 1997.)

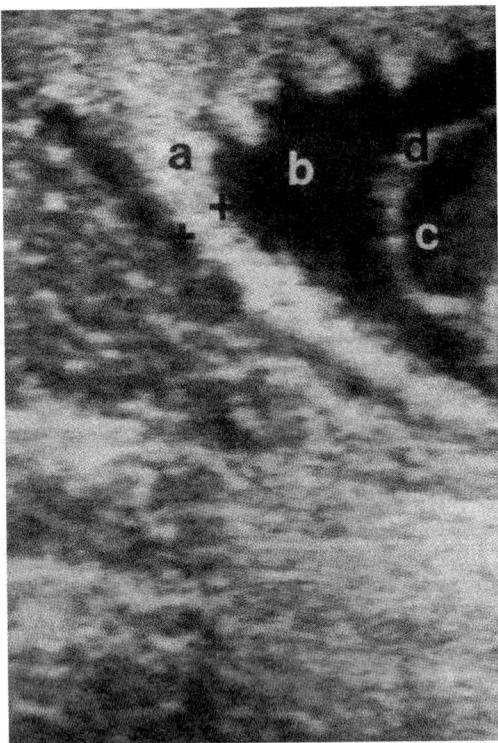

FIG. 41-2 ▓ Transrectal imaging of the combined thickness of the uterus and the placenta (CTUP). Measurements of the CTUP (distance between + and +) were recorded from the ventral part of the uterine body, close to the cervix. *a*, Placenta adjacent to the cervix; *b*, allantoic fluid; *c*, amniotic fluid; *d*, the amnion. (Modified from Renaudin et al: *Theriogenology* 47:559-573, 1997.)

the disease process has often progressed too far for treatments to be effective once obvious clinical signs are observed. Transrectal ultrasonography in susceptible mares may allow for early detection of the disease with potentially improved treatment results.

Although most mares are capable of conceiving and successfully carrying a foal to term in subsequent breedings, reproductive performance may be negatively affected after placentitis. Treatments for endometritis, such as uterine lavage and intrauterine infusions of appropriate antibiotics, should also be implemented after abortion caused by placentitis.

REFERENCES

1. Hughes JP, Stabenfeldt GH, Evans JW: Clinical and endocrine aspects of the estrous cycle of the mare, *Proceedings of the Eighteenth Annual Convention of the American Association of Equine Practitioners*, 1972, pp 119-148.
2. Pierson RA, Ginther OJ: Follicular population dynamics during the estrous cycle of the mare, *Anim Reprod Sci* 14:219-231, 1987.
3. Hughes JP, Stabenfeldt GH, Evans JW: The estrous cycle of the mare, *J Reprod Fertil Suppl* 23:161-166, 1975.
4. Hughes JP, Stabenfeldt GH: Conception in a mare with an active corpus luteum, *J Am Vet Med Assoc* 170:733-734, 1977.
5. Morrow DA, ed: *Current therapy in theriogenology*, ed 2, Philadelphia, 1986, WB Saunders.
6. Reimers TJ, Smith RD, Newman SK: Management factors affecting reproductive performance of dairy cows in the northeastern United States, *J Dairy Sci* 68:963-972, 1985.
7. Morrow DA, editor: *Current therapy in theriogenology*, ed 1, Philadelphia, 1980, WB Saunders.
8. Viker SD et al: Cow-calf association delays postpartum ovulation in mastectomized cows, *Theriogenology* 32:467-474, 1989.
9. McEntee K, ed: *Reproductive pathology of domestic animals*, New York, 1990, Academic Press.
10. Cole WJ et al: Cystic ovarian disease in a herd of Holstein cows: a hereditary correlation, *Theriogenology* 25:813-820, 1986.
11. Foote RH et al: Milk progesterone as a diagnostic aid, *Br Vet J* 135:550-558, 1979.
12. Donaldson LE, Hansel LE, VanVleck LD: Luteotropic properties of luteinizing hormone and nature of oxytocin-induced luteal inhibition in cattle, *J Dairy Sci* 48:331-337, 1965.
13. Ginther OJ et al: Effect of oxytocin administration on the oestrus cycle of unilaterally hysterectomized heifers, *J Reprod Fertil* 14:225-229, 1967.
14. Ribadu AY, Ward WR, Dobson H: Comparative evaluation of ovarian structures in cattle by palpation per rectum, ultrasonography and plasma progesterone concentrations. *Vet Rec* 136:542-547, 1994.
15. Saltiel A et al: Ovarian activity in the mare between latitude 15° and 22° N, *J Reprod Fertil Suppl* 32:261-267, 1982.
16. Osbourne VE: An analysis of the pattern of ovulation as it occurs in the annual reproductive cycle of the mare in Australia, *Aust Vet J* 42:149-154, 1966.
17. Van Niekerk CH: Patterns of the estrous cycle of mares, *J S Afr Vet Med Assoc* 38:295-298, 1967.
18. Ginther OJ: *Reproductive biology of the mare*, ed 2, Ann Arbor, 1992, McNaughton Gunn.
19. Hughes JP, Stabenfeldt GH, Kennedy PC: The estrous cycle and selected functional and pathologic ovarian abnormalities in the mare, *Vet Clin North Am, Large Anim Pract* 2:225-239, 1980.
20. Sharp DC: Environmental influences on reproduction in horses. In Hughes J, ed: *Veterinary clinics of North America: large animal practice*, Philadelphia, 1980, WB Saunders, pp 207-273.
21. Palmer E, Driancourt MA: Photoperiodic stimulation of the winter anestrus mare: what is a long day? In Ortavant R, Peletier JP, Ravault JP, eds: *Photoperiodism and reproduction in vertebrates*, Nouzilly, 1981, Institut National de la Recherche Agronomique, pp 67-82.
22. Burkhardt J: Transition from anoestrus in the mare and the effects of natural lighting, *J Agric Sci* 37:64-68, 1947.
23. Allen WR et al: Induction of ovulation in anoestrous mares with slow-release implant of a GnRH analogue (ICI 118-630), *J Reprod Fertil Suppl* 35:469-478, 1987.
24. Hyland JH et al: Infusion of gonadotropin-releasing hormone (GnRH) induces ovulation and fertile oestrus in mares during seasonal anoestrus, *J Reprod Fertil Suppl* 35:211-220, 1987.
25. Fitzgerald BP et al: Investigation of the potential of LHRH or an agonist to induce ovulation in seasonally anoestrous mares with observations on the use of the agonist in problem acyclic mares, *J Reprod Fertil Suppl* 35:683-684, 1987.
26. Ginther OJ, Bergfelt DR: Effect of GnRH treatment during the anovulatory season on multiple ovulation rate and on follicular development during the ensuing pregnancy in mares, *J Reprod Fertil* 88:119-126, 1990.
27. McCue PM et al: Endocrine response of anestrus mares to administration of native GnRH or GnRH agonist, *J Reprod Fertil Suppl* 44:227-233, 1991.
28. Besognet B, Habsen BS, Daels PF: Induction of reproductive function in anestrous mares using a dopamine antagonist, *Theriogenology* 47:467-480, 1997.
29. Brendemuehl JP, Cross DL: Effects of the dopamine antagonist domperidone on follicles, time to ovulation and luteal function in seasonally anestrus mares, *Proceedings of the Society of Theriogenology* p 304, 1996.
30. Daels PF et al: Dopamine antagonist-induced reproductive function in anoestrous mares: gonadotropin secretion and effect of environmental cues, *Reprod Fert Suppl* 56:177-183, 2000.
31. McCue PM et al: Efficacy of domperidone on induction of ovulation in anestrous and transitional mares, *Proceedings of the Forty-fifth Annual Convention of the American Association of Equine Practitioners*, 1999, pp 217-218.
32. Squires EL et al: Effect of an oral progestin on the estrous cycle and fertility of mares, *J Anim Sci* 49:729-735, 1979.
33. Webel SK et al: Fertility, ovulation and maturation of eggs in mares injected with hCG, *J Reprod Fertil* 51:337-341, 1977.
34. Betteridge KJ, Renard A, Goff AK: Uterine prostaglandin release relative to embryo collection, transfer procedure, and maintenance of the corpus luteus, *Equine Vet J* 3(suppl):25-33, 1985.
35. Hughes JP et al: Pyometra in the mare, *J Reprod Fertil Suppl* 27:321-329, 1979.
36. Daels PF, Hughes JP: The abnormal estrous cycle, In McKinnon AO, Voss JL, eds: *Equine reproduction*, Philadelphia, 1993, Lea & Febiger, pp 144-160.
37. Ginther OJ: Prolonged luteal activity in the mare: a semantic quagmire, *Equine Vet J* 22:152-156, 1990.
38. Squires DL, Ginther OJ: Follicular and luteal development in pregnant mares, *J Reprod Fertil Suppl* 23:429-433, 1975.
39. Allen WR: Factors influencing pregnant mare serum gonadotropin production, *Nature* 223:64-66, 1969.
40. Rathwell AC et al: Reproductive function of mares given PGF$_{2\alpha}$ daily from day 42 of pregnancy, *J Reprod Fertil Suppl* 35:507-508, 1987.
41. Penzhorn BL, Bertschinger HJ, Coubrough RI: Reconception of mares following termination of pregnancy with prostaglandin F$_{2\alpha}$ before and after day 35 of pregnancy, *Equine Vet J* 18:215-217, 1986.
42. Hughes JP, Stabenfeldt GH: Anestrus in the mare, *Proceedings of the Twenty-third Annual Convention of the American Association of Equine Practitioners*, 1977, pp 89-96.

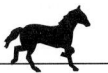

43. Hughes JP, editor: *Equine reproduction*, Princeton Junction, NJ, 1983, Veterinary Learning Systems.

44. Ball PJH: Milk progesterone profiles in relation to dairy herd fertility, *Br Vet J* 138:546-551, 1982.

45. Young IM: Selection of specific categories of dairy cows for oestrus induction with Dinoprost, *Vet Rec* 113:319-320, 1983.

46. Van Horn HH, Wilcox CJ, eds: *Large dairy herd management*, Champaign, Ill, 1992, Management Services of the American Dairy Science Association.

47. Vanderwall DK et al.: Reproductive efficiency of the aged mare, *Proceedings of the Society of Theriogenology*, pp 153-156, 1989.

48. Carnevale EM, Ginther OJ: Reproductive function in old mares, *Proceedings of the Forthieth Annual Convention of the American Association of Equine Practitioners*, 1994, pp 15-16.

49. Carnevale EM, Ginther OJ: Defective oocytes as a cause of subfertility in old mares, *Biol Reprod Mono* 1:209-214, 1995.

50. Mahrer JM et al: Effect of anabolic steroids on reproductive function in young mares, *J Am Vet Med Assoc* 183:519-524, 1983.

51. Trommerhausem-Bowling A, Millon L, Hughes JP: An update on chromosomal abnormalities in mares, *J Reprod Fertil* 35:149-155, 1987.

52. Skelton KV, Dowsett KF, McMeniman NP: Ovarian activity in pubertal fillies treated with anabolic steroids, *J Reprod Fertil Suppl* 44:351-356, 1991.

53. Clark TL: Clinical management of equine ovarian neoplasms, *J Reprod Fertil Suppl* 23:331-334, 1975.

54. McCue PM: Equine granulosa cell tumors, *Proceedings of the Thirty-eighth Annual Convention of the American Association of Equine Practitioners*, 1992, pp 587-593, 1992.

55. Piquette GN et al: Equine granulosa-theca cell tumors express inhibin α- and βA-subunit messenger ribonucleic acids and proteins, *Biol Reprod* 43:1050-1057, 1990.

56. Meinecke B, Gipps H: Steroid hormone secretory patterns in mares with granulosa cell tumors, *J Am Vet Med Assoc* 34:545-560, 1987.

57. Hughes JP, Stabenfeldt GH, Evans JW: Estous cycle and ovulation in the mare, *J Am Vet Med Assoc* 161:1367-1374, 1972.

58. Roberts SJ, editor: *Veterinary obstetrics and genital diseases (theriogenology)*, ed 3, Woodstock, Vt, 1986, published by the author.

59. Saltiel A et al: Pathologic findings in the oviducts of mares, *Am J Vet Res* 47:593-597, 1986.

60. Zent WW, Liu IKM, Spirito MA: Oviduct flushing as a treatment for infertility in the mare, *Proceedings of the Third Equine Embryo Transfer Meeting*, Buenos Aires, 1992.

61. Kenney RM: A review of the pathology of the equine oviduct, *Equine Vet J* 15(suppl):42-46, 1993.

62. Allen WE, Kessy BM, Noakes DE: Evaluation of uterine tube function in pony mares, *Vet Rec* 105:354-366, 1979.

63. Kelly EF, Renton JP, Munro CD: Assessment of oviduct patency in the cow, *Vet Rec* 108:357-360, 1981.

64. Eilts BE, Seguin BE, Fahning ML: Evaluation of oviduct patency in donor cows using the phenolsulfonphthalein oviduct patency test, *Theriogenology* 17:87, 1982.

65. Coe PH: Uterine flush as therapy for repeat breeders, *Agri Pract* 5:29-32, 1984.

66. Burns SJ et al: Management of retained placenta in mares, *Proceedings of the twenty-third Annual Convention of the American Association of Equine Practitioners*, 1977, pp 381-390.

67. Paisley LG, Mickelsen WD, Anderson PB: Mechanisms and therapy for retained fetal membranes and uterine infections of cows: a review, *Theriogenology* 25:353-381, 1986.

68. Arthur GH: Retention of the afterbirth in cattle: a review and commentary, *Vet Annu* 19:26-36, 1979.

69. Miller BJ, Lodge JR: Postpartum oxytocin treatment for prevention of retained placenta, *Theriogenology* 22:385-388, 1984.

70. Hickey GJ et al: Effects of oxytocin on placental retention following dystocia, *Vet Rec* 114:189-190, 1984.

71. Pimentel S, Evans G, Wagner WC: Placental synthesis of estrogens at parturition and placental retention in the cow, *Theriogenology* 28:755-766, 1987.

72. Studer E, Holten A: Treatment of retained placenta in dairy cattle with prostaglandin, *Bovine Pract* 21:159-160, 1986.

73. Burton MJ et al: Effect of fenprostalene on postpartum myometrial activity in dairy cows with normal or delayed placental expulsion, *Br Vet J* 143:549-554, 1987.

74. Horta AEM, Chassagne M, Brochart M: Prostaglandin F$_{2\alpha}$ and prostacyclin imbalance in cows with placental retention: new findings, *Ann Rech Vet* 17:395-400, 1986.

75. Moller K et al: Retained fetal membranes in the Huntly district, *NZ Vet J* 15:111-116, 1967.

76. Ball L, Olson JD, Mortimer RG: Bacteriology of the postpartum uterus, *Proceedings of the Society for Theriogenology*, Denver, 1984, pp 164-169.

77. Traub-Dargatz JL, Salman MD, Voss JL: Medical problems of adult horses, as ranked by equine practitioners, *J Am Vet Med Assoc* 198:1745-1747, 1991.

78. Pascoe RR: Observations of the length and the angle of declination of the vulva and its relation to fertility of the mare, *J Reprod Fertil Suppl* 27:299-305, 1979.

79. Troedsson MHT: Uterine response to semen deposition in the mare, *Proceedings of the Society for Theriogenology*, 1995, pp 130-135.

80. Zent WW, Troedsson MHT: Postbreeding uterine fluid accumulation in a normal population of thoroughbred mares: a field study, *Proceedings of theForty-fourth Annual Convention of the American Association of Equine Practitioners*, 1998, pp 64-65.

81. Hughes JP, Loy RG: Investigations on the effect of intrauterine inoculation of *Streptococcus zooepidemicus* in the mare, *Proceedings of the Fifteenth Annual Convention of the American Association of Equine Practitioners*, 1969, pp 289-292.

82. Peterson FB, McFeely RA, David JSE: Studies on the pathogenesis of endometritis in the mare, *Proceedings of the American Association of Equine Practitioners*, 1969, pp 15:279-285.

83. Neely DP et al: Prostaglandin release patterns in the mare: physiological, pathophysiological, and therapeutic responses, *J Reprod Fertil Suppl* 27:181-189, 1979.

84. Asbury AC et al: Immunoglobulins in uterine secretion of mares with differing resistance to endometritis, *Theriogenology* 14:299-308, 1980.

85. Mitchell G et al: Preferential production and secretion of immunoglobulins by the equine endometrium: a mucosal immune system, *J Reprod Fertil Suppl* 32:161-168, 1982.

86. Troedsson MHT, Liu IKM, Thurmond M: Immunoglobulin (IgG and IgA) and complement (C3) concentrations in uterine secretion following an intrauterine challenge of *Streptococcus zooepidemicus* in mares susceptible to versus resistant to chronic uterine infection, *Biol Reprod* 49:502-506, 1993.

87. Waelchli RO, Winder NC: Mononuclear cell infiltration of the equine endometrium: immunohistochemical studies, *Equine Vet J* 23:470-474, 1991.

88. Williamson P et al: Immunoglobulin levels, protein concentrations and alkaline phosphatase activity in uterine flushings from mares with endometritis, *Theriogenology* 19:441-448, 1983.

89. Lehrer RI: Neutrophils and host defense, *Ann Intern Med* 109:127-142, 1988.

90. Pycock JF: Assessment of oxytocin and intrauterine antibiotics on intrauterine fluid and pregnancy rates in the mare, *Proceedings of the Fortieth Annual Convention of the American Association of Equine Practitioners*, 1994, pp 19-20.

91. Lees P, Dawson J, Sedgwick AD: Eicosanoid and equine leukocyte locomotion in vitro, *Equine Vet J* 18:493-497, 1986.

92. Pycock JF, Allen WE: Inflammatory components in uterine fluid from mares with experimentally induced bacterial endometritis, *Equine Vet J* 22:422-425, 1990.

93. Watson ED, Stokes CR, Bourne FJ: Cellular and humoral mechanisms in mares susceptible and resistant to persistent endometritis, *Vet Immunol Immunopath* 16:107-121, 1987.

94. Watson ED, Stokes CR, Bourne FJ: Influence of arachidonic acid metabolites in vitro and in uterine washings on migration of equine neutrophils under agarose, *Res Vet Sci* 43:203-207, 1987.

95. Troedsson MHT, Liu IKM, Thurmond M: Function of uterine and blood derived polymorphonuclear neutrophils (PMN) in mares susceptible and resistant to chronic uterine infection (CUI): phagocytosis and chemotaxis, *Biol Reprod* 49:507-514, 1993.

96. Troedsson MHT, Liu IKM: Uterine clearance of non-antigenic markers (Cr^{51}) in response to a bacterial challenge in mares potentially susceptible and resistant to chronic uterine infection, *J Reprod Fertil Suppl* 44:283-288, 1991.

97. LeBlanc MM et al: Scintigraphic measurement of uterine clearance in normal mares and mares with recurrent endometritis, *Equine Vet J* 26:109-113, 1994.

98. Troedsson MHT et al: Multiple site electromyography recordings of uterine activity following an intrauterine bacterial challenge in mares susceptible and resistant to chronic uterine infection, *J Reprod Fertil* 99:307-313, 1993.

99. Brewer RA: Contagious equine metritis: a review/summary, *Vet Bull* 53:881-891, 1983.

100. Powell DG: Contagious equine metritis. In Morrow DA, ed: *Current therapy in theriogenology*, ed 2, Philadelphia, 1986, WB Saunders, pp 786-792.

101. Asbury AC: Infectious and immunologic considerations in mare infertility, *Compend Cont Educ Pract Vet* 9:585-592, 1987.

102. Troedsson MHT: Uterine clearance and resistance to persistent endometritis in the mare, *Theriogenology* 52:461-471, 1999.

103. Hinrichs K: The role of endometrial swabs in the diagnosis (and pathogenesis?) of endometritis, *Cornell Veterinarian* 81:233-237, 1991.

104. Kotilainen T, Huhtinen M, Katila T: Sperm induced leukocytosis in the equine uterus, *Theriogenology* 41:629-636, 1994.

105. Troedsson MHT et al: Mechanism of sperm-induced endometritis in the mare, *Biol Reprod Suppl* 52:307, 1995 (abstract).

106. Troedsson MHT et al: Post-breeding uterine inflammation: the role of seminal plasma, *J Reprod Fertil Suppl* 56:341-349, 2000.

107. Troedsson MHT, deMoraes MJ, Liu IKM: Correlations between histologic endometrial lesions in mares and clinical response to intrauterine exposure with *Streptococcus zooepidemicus*, *Am J Vet Res* 54:570-572, 1993.

108. Allen WR: Proceedings of the John P. Hughes International Workshop on Equine Endometritis, *Equine Vet J* 25:184-193, 1993.

109. Oikawa M et al: Microscopical characteristics of uterine wall arteries in barren aged mares, *J Comp Path* 108:101-105, 1993.

110. Blanchard TL et al: Comparison of two techniques for obtaining endometrial bacteriologic cultures in the mare, *Theriogenology* 16:85-93, 1981.

111. Pycock JF, Newcombe JR: The relationship between intraluminal uterine fluid, endometritis, and pregnancy rate in the mare, *Equine Pract* 18:19-22, 1996.

112. Troedsson MHT: Therapeutic considerations for mating-induced endometritis, *Pferdeheilkunde* 13:516-520, 1997.

113. Couto MA, Hughes JP: Sexually transmitted (venereal) diseases in horses. In McKinnon AO, Voss JL, eds: *Equine reproduction*, Philadelphia, 1993, Lea & Febiger, pp 845-854.

114. Swerczek TW: Contagious equine metritis: outbreak of the disease in Kentucky and laboratory methods for diagnosing the disease, *J Reprod Fertil Suppl* 27:361-365, 1979.

115. Kenney RM et al: Minimal contamination techniques for breeding mares: techniques and preliminary findings, *Proceedings of the Twenty-seventh Annual Convention of the American Association of Equine Practitioners*, 1975, pp 327-336.

116. Brown MP et al: Amikacin sulfate in mares: pharmacokinetics and body fluid and endometrial concentrations after repeated intramuscular injections, *Am J Vet Res* 46:1025-1028, 1984.

117. LeBlanc MM: Oxytocin: the new wonder drug for treatment of endometritis? *Equine Vet Educ* 6:39-43, 1994.

118. Troedsson MHT, Scott MA, Liu IKM: Comparative treatment of mares susceptible to chronic uterine infection, *Am J Vet Res* 56:468-472, 1995.

119. Brinsko SP, Varner DD, Blanchard TL: The effect of uterine lavage performed four hours post-insemination on pregnancy rates in mares, *Theriogenology* 35:1111-1119, 1991.

120. Brinsko SP et al: The effect of post-breeding uterine lavage on post-breeding pregnancy rate in mares, *Theriogenology* 33:465-475, 1990.

121. Thomas PGA, Ball BA, Brinsko SPB: Interaction of equine spermatozoa with oviduct epithelial cell explants is affected by estrous cycle and anatomic origin of explant, *Biol Reprod* 51:222-228, 1994.

122. Rasch K et al: Histomorphological endometrial status and influence of oxytocin on the uterine drainage and pregnancy in mares, *Equine Vet J* 28:455-460, 1996.

123. Ley WB, Spongenberg DP: Dimethyl sulfoxide intrauterine therapy in the mare: effects upon endometrial histological features and biopsy classification, *Theriogenology* 32:263-276, 1989.

124. Frazer GS, Risosl TJ, Threlfall WR: Effects of serial intrauterine dimethyl sulfoxide infusion on the incidence of periglandular fibrosis in category II horses endometria, *Theriogenology* 29:1091-1098, 1988.

125. Martinez J, Thibier M: Reproductive disorders in dairy cattle. I. Respective influence of herds, season, milk yield and parity, *Theriogenology* 21:569-581, 1984.

126. Olson JD et al: Metritis and pyometra, *J Soc Theriogenol* 14:65-72, 1987.

127. Olson JD, Ball L, Mortimer RG: Therapy of postpartum uterine infections, *Proceedings of the Society for Theriogenology*, Denver, 1984, pp 170-160.

128. Bishop JR et al: Retention data for antibiotics commonly used for bovine infusion, *J Dairy Sci* 67:437-440, 1984.

129. Kaneene JB et al: Drug residues in milk after intrauterine injection of oxytetracycline, lincomycin-spectinomycin, and povidone-iodine in cows with metritis, *Am J Vet Res* 47:1363-1365, 1986.

130. Anderson KL et al: Potential for oxytetracycline administration by three routes to cause milk residues in lactating cows, as detected by radioimmunoassay (Charm II) and high-performance liquid chromatography test methods, *Am J Vet Res* 56:70-77, 1995.

131. McClary D: Metritis. In Howard JL, ed: *Current veterinary therapy: food animal practice*, ed 2, Philadelphia, 1986, WB Saunders, pp 775-777.

132. Ekman L et al: Resorption of iodine in Lugol's solution and in iodophor from the uterus of cows, *Nord Vet Med* 17:391-396, 1965.

133. Stephens LR et al: Investigation of purulent vaginal discharge in cows, with particular reference to *Haemophilus somnus*, *Aust Vet J* 63:164-169, 1986.

134. Olson JD et al: Aspects of bacteriology and endocrinology of cows with pyometra and retained fetal membranes, *Am J Vet Res* 45:2251-2255, 1984.

135. BonDurant RH: Diagnosis, treatment and control of bovine trichomoniasis, *Compend Cont Educ* 7:S161-S188, 1985.

136. Eilts BE et al: Prevalence of endometrial cysts and their effect on fertility, *Biol Reprod Mono* 1:527-532, 1995.

137. McKinnon AO, Squires EL, Voss JL: Ultrasound evaluation of the mare's reproductive tract. II, *Compend Cont Ed Pract Vet* 9:472-480, 1987.

138. Burgess J: Uterine prolapse in the mare (correspondence), *Vet Rec* 96:513, 1975.

139. Odegaard SA: Packed cell volume (PCV) in connection with uterine prolapse and in parturient paresis in cows, *Acta Vet Scand* 18:451-457, 1977.

140. Plenderleith RWJ: Treatment of uterine prolapse, *Proceedings of the British Cattle Veterinary Association*, 1978-1981, pp 55-57.

141. Denooij PP: Clenbuterol as an aid in replacement of the prolapsed bovine uterus, *Can Vet J* 25:106, 1984.

142. Hofmeyr CFB: The female genitalia. In *Ruminant urogenital surgery*, Ames, 1987, Iowa State University Press, pp 122-147.

143. Arthur GH, Noakes DE, Pearson H: *Veterinary reproduction and obstetrics*, ed 5, London, 1982, Baillière Tindall, pp 295-327.

144. Brown MP, Colahan PT, Hawkins DL: Urethral extension surgery for treatment of urine pooling in mares, *J Am Vet Med Assoc* 173:1005-1007, 1978.

145. Monin T: Vaginoplasty, a surgical treatment for urine pooling in the horse, *Proceedings of the Nineteenth Annual Convention of the American Association of Equine Practitioners*, 1973, pp 99-102.

146. Jubb KVF, Kennedy PC, Palmer N, eds: *Pathology of domestic animals*, ed 3, vol 3, New York, 1985, Academic Press.

147. Engles M, Steck F, Wyler R: Comparison of genomes of infectious bovine rhinotracheitis and infectious pustular vulvovaginitis strains by restriction endonuclease analysis, *Arch Virol* 67:169, 1981.

148. Studdert MJ: Comparative aspects of equine herpesviruses, *Cornell Vet* 64:94-122, 1974.

149. Troedsson MHT: Diseases of the external genitalia. In Robinson NE, ed: *Current therapy in equine medicine*, ed 4, Philadelphia, 1997, WB Saunders.

150. Miller RB, Lein DH, McEntee KE, editors: *Haemophilus somnus* infection of the reproductive tract of cattle: a review, *J Am Vet Med Assoc* 182:1370-1372, 1983.

151. Walker DF, Vaughan JT, eds: *Bovine and equine urogenital surgery*, Philadelphia, 1980, Lea & Febiger.

152. Omara-Opyene AL et al: Occurrence of bovine squamous cell carcinoma in Kenya, *Kenya Vet* 8:5-8, 1984.

153. Kirkbride CA, ed: *Laboratory diagnosis of livestock abortion*, ed 3, Ames, 1990, Iowa State University Press.

154. Smith GH, Collins JK, Carman J: Use of an immunoperoxidase test for the detection of bovine herpesvirus-1 in aborted fetal tissue, *J Vet Diagn Invest* 1:39-44, 1969.

155. Miller JM, van der Maaten MJ: Reproductive tract lesions in heifers after intrauterine inoculation with IBR virus, *Am J Vet Res* 45:790-794, 1984.

156. van der Maaten MJ, Miller JM, Whetstone CA: Ovarian lesions induced in heifers by intravenous inoculation with modified-live IBR virus on the day after breeding, *Am J Vet Res* 46:1996-1999, 1985.

157. Bowen RA, Elsden RP, Seidel GE: Infection of early bovine embryos with bovine herpesvirus-1, *Am J Vet Res* 46:1095-1097, 1985.

158. Miller J, van der Maaten MJ: Experimentally induced infectious bovine rhinotracheitis virus infection during early pregnancy: effect on the bovine corpus luteum and conceptus, *Am J Vet Res* 47:223-228, 1986.

159. Miller JM, van der Maaten MJ: Early embryonic death in heifers after inoculation with bovine herpesvirus-1 and reactivation of latent virus in reproductive tissues, *Am J Vet Res* 48:1555-1558, 1987.

160. Fenner F et al: *Veterinary virology*, Orlando, 1987, Academic Press, pp 577-594.

161. McClurkin AW et al: Production of cattle immunotolerant to bovine virus diarrhea virus, *Can J Comp Med* 48:156-161, 1984

162. Ross CE, Dobovi EJ, Donis RO: Herd problem of abortions and malformed calves attributed to bovine viral diarrhea, *J Am Vet Med Assoc* 188:618-621, 1986.

163. Roeder PL, Jeffrey M, Cranwell MP: Pestivirus fetopathogenicity in cattle: changing sequelae with fetal maturation, *Vet Rec* 118:44-48, 1986.

164. Grahn TC, Fahning ML, Zemjanis R: Nature of early reproductive failure caused by bovine viral diarrhea virus, *J Am Vet Med Assoc* 185:429-432, 1984.

165. Bolin SR et al: Severe clinical disease induced in cattle persistently infected with noncytopathic bovine viral diarrhea virus by superinfection with cytopathic bovine viral diarrhea virus, *Am J Vet Res* 46:573-576, 1985.

166. Baker JC: Bovine viral diarrhea virus: a review, *J Am Vet Med Assoc* 190:1449-1458, 1987.

167. East NE: Pregnancy toxemia, abortions, and periparturient disease, *Vet Clin North Am (Large Anim Pract)* 5:607-618, 1983.

168. Brooks DL et al: Q fever vaccination of sheep: challenge of immunity in ewes, *Am J Vet Res* 47:1235-1238, 1986.

169. Ruppanner R et al: Prevalence of *Coxiella burnetii* (Q fever) and *Toxoplasma gondii* among dairy goats in California, *Am J Vet Res* 39:867-870, 1978.

170. Rodolakis A, Souriau A: Response of goats to vaccination with temperature-sensitive mutants of *Chlamydia psittaci* obtained by nitrosoguanidine mutagenesis, *Am J Vet Res* 47:2627-2631, 1986.

171. Gunson DE et al: Abortion and stillbirth associated with *Chlamydia psittaci* var *ovis* in dairy goats with high titers to *Toxoplasma gondii*, *J Am Vet Med Assoc* 183:1447-1450, 1983.

172. Appleyard WT, Aitken ID, Anderson I: Outbreak of chlamydial abortion in goats, *Vet Rec* 113:63, 1983.

173. Perez-Martinez JA, Schmeer N, Storz J: Bovine chlamydial abortion: serodiagnosis by modified complement-fixation and immunofluorescent tests and enzyme-linked immunosorbent assay, *Am J Vet Res* 47:1501-1506, 1986.

174. Rodolakis A, Boullet C, Souriau A: *Chlamydia psittaci* experimental abortion in goats, *Am J Vet Res* 45:2086-2089, 1984.

175. Wilsmore AJ et al: The use of a delayed hypersensitivity test and long-acting oxytetracycline in a flock affected with ovine enzootic abortion, *Br Vet J* 42:557, 1986.

176. Greig A, Linklater KA: Field studies on the efficacy of a long-acting preparation of oxytetracycline in controlling outbreaks of enzootic abortion of sheep, *Vet Rec* 117:627-628, 1985.

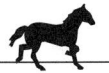

177. Kimsey PB et al: Studies on the pathogenesis of epizootic bovine abortion, *Am J Vet Res* 44:1266-1271, 1983.

178. Osebold JW et al: Histopathologic changes in bovine fetuses after repeated reintroduction of a spirochete-like agent into pregnant heifers: association with epizootic bovine abortion, *Am J Vet Res* 48:627, 1987.

179. Osebold JW et al: Congenital spirochetosis in calves: association with epizootic bovine abortion, *J Am Vet Med Assoc* 188:371-376, 1986.

180. Lane RS et al: Isolation of a spirochete from the soft tick, *Ornithodorus coriaceus*: a possible agent of epizootic bovine abortion, *Science* 230:85-87, 1985.

181. Kennedy PC et al: Epizootic bovine abortion: histogenesis of the fetal lesions, *Am J Vet Res* 44:1040-1048, 1983.

182. Smith MC, Sherman DM, eds: *Goat medicine*, Malvern, Pa, 1994, Lea & Febiger.

183. Meador VP, Hagemoser WA, Deyoe BL: Histopathologic findings in *Brucella abortus*-infected, pregnant goats, *Am J Vet Res* 49:274, 1988.

184. Anderson TD, Cheville NF, Meador VP: Pathogenesis of placentitis in the goat inoculated with *Brucella abortus*. II, Ultrastructural studies, *Vet Pathol* 23:219-239, 1986.

185. Bosseray N: *Brucella* infection and immunity in placenta, *Ann Inst Pasteur/Microbiol* 138:69-144, 1987.

186. Crawford RP et al: Biotypes of *Brucella abortus* and their value in epidemiologic studies of infected cattle herds, *J Am Vet Med Assoc* 175:1274-1277, 1979.

187. Catline JE, Sheehan EJ: Transmission of bovine brucellosis from dam to offspring, *J Am Vet Med Assoc* 188:867-869, 1986.

188. Crawford RP, Huber JD, Sanders RB: Brucellosis in heifers weaned from seropositive dams, *J Am Vet Med Assoc* 189:547-549, 1986.

189. Nicoletti P et al: Efficacy of long-acting oxytetracycline alone or combined with streptomycin in the treatment of bovine brucellosis, *J Am Vet Med Assoc* 187:493, 1985.

190. Anderson KL et al: Isolation of *Campylobacter jejunii* from an aborted caprine fetus, *J Am Vet Med Assoc* 183:90-92, 1983.

191. Welsh RD: *Campylobacter jejuni* abortion in a heifer, *J Am Vet Med Assoc* 185:549-551, 1984.

192. Hedstrom OR et al: Pathology of *Campylobacter jejunii* abortion in sheep, *Vet Pathol* 24:419-426, 1987.

193. Ruegg PL, Marteniuk JV, Kaneene JB: Reproductive difficulties in cattle with antibody titers to *Haemophilus somnus*, *J Am Vet Med Assoc* 193:941-942, 1988.

194. Miller RB, Barnum DA, McEntee KE: *Haemophilus somnus* in the reproductive tracts of slaughtered cows: localization and frequency of isolations and lesions, *Vet Pathol* 20:515-521, 1983.

195. Thomson JS, Stringfellow DA, Lauerman LH: Adherence of *Haemophilus somnus* to bovine embryos after in vitro exposure, *Am J Vet Res* 49:63-66, 1988.

196. Patterson RM et al: Experimental induction of vaginitis in heifers by infection with *Haemophilus somnus*, *Aust Vet J* 63:163-165, 1986.

197. Miller RB, Van Camp SD, Barnum DA: The effects of intraamniotic inoculation of *Haemophilus somnus* on the bovine fetus and dam, *Vet Pathol* 20:574-583, 1983.

198. Miller RB, Barnum DA: Effects of *Haemophilus somnus* on the pregnant bovine reproductive tract and conceptus following cervical infusion, *Vet Pathol* 20:584-589, 1983.

199. Ellis WA et al: Excretion of *Leptospira interrogans* serovar *hardjo* following calving or abortion, *Res Vet Sci* 39:296-298, 1985.

200. Songer JG, Thiermann AB: Leptospirosis, *J Am Vet Med Assoc* 193:1250-1254, 1988.

201. Kingscote BF, Wilson D: *Leptospira pomona* abortion storm in a cattle herd in Saskatchewan, *Can Vet J* 27:440-442, 1986.

202. Dawson LJ: Conditions causing abortions in cattle. I, Introduction, bacterial abortions and mycotic abortions. *Agri Pract* 6:7-8, 10-14, 1985.

203. Bolin CA et al: Effect of vaccination with a pentavalent leptospiral vaccine on *Leptospira interrogans* serovar *hardjo* type *hardjo*-bovine infection of pregnant cattle, *Am J Vet Res* 50:161-165, 1989.

204. Kirkbride CA: *Mycoplasma*, *Ureaplasma*, and *Acholeplasma* infections of bovine genitalia, *Vet Clin North Am (Food Anim Pract)* 3:575-571, 1987.

205. Stalheim OH: Experimentally induced bovine abortion with *Mycoplasma agalactiae*, ssp. *bovis*, *Am J Vet Res* 37:879-883, 1976.

206. Hinton M: Salmonella abortion in cattle, *Vet Ann* 26:81-89, 1986.

207. Hall GA, Jones PW: A study of the pathogenesis of experimental *Salmonella dublin* abortion in cattle, *J Comp Pathol* 87:53-65, 1977.

208. Miller RB et al: The effects of *Ureaplasma diversum* inoculation into the amniotic cavity in cows, *Theriogenology* 20:367-374, 1983.

209. Ball HJ, McCaughey WJ: An examination of the effects of *Ureaplasma* infection on the fertility of synchronized ewes, *Anim Reprod Sci* 13:61-66, 1987.

210. Steffan J et al: Treatment of metritis with antibiotics or prostaglandin $F_{2\alpha}$ and influence of ovarian cyclicity in dairy cows, *Am J Vet Res* 45:1090-1094, 1984.

211. Karbe E, Erickson ED: Ovine abortion and stillbirth due to purulent placentitis caused by *Yersinia pseudotuberculosis*, *Vet Pathol* 21:601-606, 1984.

212. Rahaley RS: Pathology of experimental *Histophilus ovis* infection in sheep. II, Pregnant ewes, *Vet Pathol* 15:746-752, 1978.

213. Sokkar SM, Kubba MA, Al-Augaidy F: Studies on natural and experimental endometritis in ewes, *Vet Pathol* 17:693-698, 1980.

214. Witte ST, Sponenberg DP, Collins TC: Abortion and early neonatal death of kids attributed to intrauterine *Yersinia pseudotuberculosis* infection, *J Am Vet Med Assoc* 187:834, 1985.

215. Kirkbride CA et al: Ovine abortion associated with an anaerobic bacterium, *J Am Vet Med Assoc* 186:789, 1985.

216. Kirkbride CA, Gates CE, Collins JE: Abortion in sheep caused by a nonclassified, anaerobic, flagellated bacterium, *Am J Vet Res* 47:259-262, 1986.

217. Bryner JH et al: Experimental infection and abortion of pregnant guinea pigs with a unique spirillum-like bacterium isolated from aborted ovine fetuses, *Am J Vet Res* 48:91-95, 1987.

218. Foley GL, Schlafer DW: *Candida* abortion in cattle, *Vet Pathol* 24:532-536, 1987.

219. Wohlegemuth K, Knudtson WU: Abortion associated with *Mortierella wolfii* in cattle, *J Am Vet Med Assoc* 171:437-439, 1977.

220. Ryan MJ, Wyand DS: *Cryptococcus* as a cause of neonatal pneumonia and abortion in two horses, *Vet Pathol* 18:270-272, 1981.

221. Saunders JR, Matthiesen RJ, Kaplan W: Abortion due to histoplasmosis in a mare, *J Am Vet Med Assoc* 183:1097-1099, 1983.

222. Kirkbride CA et al: A diagnostic survey of bovine abortion and stillbirth in the northern plains states, *J Am Vet Med Assoc* 162:556-560, 1973.

223. McCausland IP, Slee KJ, Hirst FS: Mycotic abortion in cattle, *Aust Vet J* 64:129-132, 1987.

224. Fayer R, Dubey JP: *Sarcocystis*-induced abortion and fetal death. In Scarpelli DG, Migaki G, eds: *Transplacental effects on fetal health*, New York 1988, Alan R Liss, pp 153-164.

225. Dubey JP, Bergeron JA: *Sarcocystis* as a cause of placentitis and abortion in cattle, *Vet Pathol* 19:315-318, 1982.

226. Dubey JP: Impaired protective immunity to sarcocystosis in pregnant dairy goats, *Am J Vet Res* 44:132-134, 1983.

227. Dubey JP et al: Serodiagnosis of postnatally and prenatally induced toxoplasmosis in sheep, *Am J Vet Res* 48:1239-1243, 1987.

228. Dubey JP, Kirkbride CA: Epizootics of ovine abortion due to *Toxoplasma gondii* in north central United States, *J Am Vet Med Assoc* 184:657-660, 1984.

229. Rhyan JC, Dubey JP: Ovine abortion and neonatal death due to toxoplasmosis in Montana, *J Am Vet Med Assoc* 184:661-664, 1984.

230. Uggla A, Sjoland L, Dubey JP: Immunohistochemical diagnosis of toxoplasmosis in fetuses and fetal membranes of sheep, *Am J Vet Res* 48:348-351, 1987.

231. Dubey JP et al: *Toxoplasma gondii*-induced abortion in dairy goats, *J Am Vet Med Assoc* 188:159-162, 1986.

232. Munday BL, Dubey JP: Serology of experimental toxoplasmosis in pregnant ewes and their foetuses, *Aust Vet J* 63:353-355, 1986.

233. Dubey JP: *Toxoplasma gondii* cysts in placentas of experimentally infected sheep, *Am J Vet Res* 48:352-353, 1987.

234. Dubey JP, Towle A: *Toxoplasmosis in sheep: a review and annotated bibliography*, London, 1986, miscellaneous publication No. 10 of the Commonwealth Institute of Parasitology, CAB International, Farnham Royal England, pp 1-152.

235. McAllister MM et al: Dogs are definitive hosts of *Neospora caninum*, *Int J Parasitol* 28:1473-1478, 1998.

236. Pare J et al: Seroepidemiologic study of *Neospora caninum* in dairy herds, *J Am Vet Med Assoc* 213:1595-1598, 1998.

237. Thurmond MC, Hietala S: Strategies to control neospora infection in cattle, *Bovine Pract* 29:60-63, 1995.

238. Goodger WJ, Skirrow SZ: Epidemiologic and economic analyses of an unusually long epizootic of trichomoniasis in a large California dairy herd, *J Am Vet Med Assoc* 189:772-776, 1986.

239. Fitzgerald PR, Hammond DM, Shupe JL: The role of cultures in immediate and delayed examinations of preputial samples for *Trichomonas foetus*, *Vet Med* 49:409-413, 1954.

240. Rhyan JC, Stackhouse LL, Quinn WJ: Fetal and placental lesions in bovine abortion due to *Trichomonas foetus*, *Vet Pathol* 25:350-355, 1988.

241. Skirrow SZ et al: Efficacy of ipronidazole against trichomoniasis in beef bulls, *J Am Vet Med Assoc* 187:405-407, 1985.

242. McLoughlin DK: Dimetridazole, a systemic treatment for bovine venereal trichomoniasis. I, Oral administration, *J Parasitol* 51:835-836, 1965.

243. Ostlund EN: The equine herpesviruses, *Vet Clin North Am (Equine Pract)* 9:283-294, 1993.

244. Acland HM: Abortion in mares. In McKinnon AO, Voss JL, ed: *Equine reproduction*, Philadelphia, 1993, Lea & Febiger, pp 554-562.

245. Tashjian RJ: Transmission and clinical evaluation of an equine infectious anemia herd and their offspring over a 13-year period, *J Am Vet Med Assoc* 184:282-288, 1984.

246. Timoney PJ, McCollum WH: Equine viral arteritis, *Can Vet J* 28:673-695, 1987.

247. McCollum WH, Bryans JT: Serological identification of infection by equine arteritis virus in horses of several countries, *Proceedings of the Third International Symposium of Equine Infectious Diseases*, Paris, France, 1973, pp 256-263.

248. Coignoul FL, Cheville NF: Pathology of maternal genital tract, placenta, and fetus in equine viral arteritis, *Vet Pathol* 21:333, 1984.

249. Donahue JM et al: Diagnosis and prevalence of *Leptospira* infection in aborted and stillborn horses, *J Vet Diagn Invest* 3:148-151, 1991.

250. Long MT et al: Evidence for fetal infectivity and abortion caused by *Ehrlichia risticii*, *Proceedings of the Thirty-eighth Annual Convention of the American Association of Equine Practitioners*, 1992, pp 571-578.

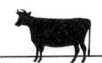
251. Daels PF et al: Prostaglandin release and luteolysis associated with physiological and pathological conditions of the reproductive tract in the mare: a review, *Equine Vet J Suppl* 8:29-34, 1989.
252. Troedsson MHT et al: Transrectal ultrasonography of the placenta in normal mares and mares with pending abortion: a field study, *Proceedings of the Forty-third Annual Convention of the American Association of Equine Practitioners*, 1997, pp 256-258.
253. Renaudin CD et al: Ultrasonographic evaluation of the equine placenta by transrectal and transabdominal approach in the normal pregnant mare, *Theriogenology* 47:559-573, 1997.

MALE REPRODUCTIVE DISORDERS

R. NEIL HOOPER
TERRY L. BLANCHARD
DICKSON D. VARNER

INFERTILITY CAUSED BY DISEASES OF THE PENIS AND PREPUCE

PENILE INJURY

Stallion

DEFINITION AND ETIOLOGY. If the penis is injured while erect, it may swell rapidly and massively from vascular rupture and hemorrhage. Hemorrhage usually originates from the superficial penile vessels in the plexus external to the tunica albuginea.[254] The stallion may be kicked during mating or hematomas may follow breeding a mare with a tightly sutured vulva or may be induced if the mare moves suddenly during mating.[255,256]

CLINICAL SIGNS AND DIFFERENTIALS. Cutaneous abrasions, lacerations, and visible hemorrage may be present. Paraphimosis occurs when enlargement is sufficient to prevent retraction of the penis through the preputial ring.[254] Edema may extend to the scrotum and interfere with thermoregulation of the testes.[257] Venous thrombosis, lymphatic occlusion, excoriation, and swelling accompany chronic inflammation.[254] Hemorrhage from the corpus cavernosum penis (CCP) is uncommon. Rupture of the surrounding tunica albuginea, when healed, may develop fibrous adhesions that lead to penile deviation during erection.

TREATMENT AND PROGNOSIS. Immediate treatment is directed toward reducing edema and inflammation, and controlling infection. Treatment is similar to that described for paraphimosis in a later section. Sexual rest is indicated until the lesions have healed.[258] If treatment is initiated early and paraphimosis does not occur, the prognosis for recovery is good.[254,256]

Bull

DEFINITION AND ETIOLOGY. The penis of bulls is susceptible to injury during mating. The vigorous thrust that accompanies copulation predisposes the penis and prepuce to excoriations, lacerations, and bruising. Rupture of the tunica albuginea (penile hematoma or "broken penis") occurs if the penis is misdirected during copulation.[259] Penile hematomas most commonly occur in young, sexually aggressive bulls. Injuries occur when these bulls attempt to breed heifers or cows that are not receptive, when females falter or collapse under the weight of the bull, or when the bull slips because of poor footing.[255] During copulatory thrusting in which the penis is bent, the tunica albuginea ruptures on the dorsal or dorsolateral surface of the penis opposite the attachment of the retractor penis muscle. Presumably, CCP pressure rapidly increases as the functionally closed system is compressed during bending to rupture the tunica albuginea. Experiments with fresh postmortem specimens indicated that a CCP pressure of 1180 to 1720 psi was required to rupture the tunica albuginea. Tearing virtually always occurred at the site described in naturally occurring cases. Mean peak CCP pressure recorded during normal coitus (275 psi) occurs when cavernous spaces fill with a relatively small volume of blood, perhaps as little as 110 ml.[257] Blood escapes from the CCP into the surrounding tissue.[254] The size of penile hematomas may be related to the number of repeated trials made by the bull before cessation of attempts at mating. Larger hematomas restrict full retraction of the penis and result in prolapse of the prepuce from the sheath. Secondary preputial injury is common.[254]

CLINICAL SIGNS AND DIFFERENTIALS. Diagnosis of penile hematoma is made based on the presence of a swelling immediately cranial to the scrotum. Initially it is soft, fluctuant, and painful, and becomes firm as clot organization and fibrin formation progresses.[255] The main differential diagnosis is extensive preputial laceration. If a distance of more than two handbreadths is present between the scrotum and the enlargement, the swelling is more likely to be a preputial laceration. Other differential diagnoses include rupture of the urethra, abdominal hernia, and chronic, fibrous adhesions. Dysuria usually does not occur in conjunction with penile hematoma. Other signs of urethral rupture or blockage, such as extensive preputial cellulitis and "water belly," elevated blood levels of urea nitrogen and creatinine, and tissue necrosis do not occur. Abscess formation of penile hematomas sometimes occurs. A soft, fluxuant center is characteristic of an abscess. Occasionally, differentiation between blood clot and abscess may be difficult. An aseptic tap can be done to determine the character of the fluid, but the risk of inducing an abscess in a sterile hematoma is great and a tap should only be used as a last diagnostic resort or just before surgery.

If penile hematoma has been present for longer than 2 weeks, fibrous adhesions may form that prevent penile extension. Adhesions are frequent sequelae to an abscess, and have also been reported to occur secondary to infiltration of local anesthetics to block the dorsal nerves of the penis.[255] Another sequela is the development of venous shunts that communicate between the CCP and either peripenile vasculature or the corpus spongiosum penis.[254,260] Such vascular shunts result in rapid drainage of blood from the CCP and impotence caused by failure to achieve or maintain full erection. If the dorsal nerves of the penis are damaged, sensation of the distal penis is lost or deficient and results in failure of

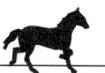

the bull to successfully seek out the female's vagina and/or ejaculate. Organization of the portion of the blood clot (thrombosis) within the body of the CCP may result in functional blockage of engorgement of the more distal cavernous spaces, preventing full erection.

TREATMENT AND PROGNOSIS. Treatment of penile hematomas should be aimed not only at restoring the bull to usefulness, but also at preventing recurrence. Approximately 50% of bulls with hematomas that are treated conservatively (i.e., nonsurgically) are reported to return successfully to breeding.[254] Some theriogenologists feel that small hematomas (less than football size) do not require surgery.[261] However, Auburn University faculty report that surgical intervention is required to optimize chances of full recovery. Surgical correction has the advantages of (1) removing the blood clot before extensive fibrous adhesions develop, (2) permitting removal of blood clot from within the body of the CCP itself, thereby reducing the chance of blockage of cavernous filling, and (3) suturing the tunica albuginea, which should reduce the chance of recurrence of the condition after return to service and the likelihood of development of vascular shunts that will prevent complete filling of the CCP. Surgical intervention is not recommended before coagulation of the extravasated blood. Once significant fibrin formation is present, the prognosis for successful correction is greatly reduced and should only be attempted in valuable bulls.[254]

Additional recommendations before electing surgical intervention include extending the penis manually. Cases in which the penis can be extended from 6 to 8 inches or more beyond the sheath orifice, and in which penile sensation remains, carry a better prognosis.[262] If engorgement of the distal penis does not occur after careful stimulation with the electroejaculator, blockage of the CCP should be suspected and reduces the prognosis. Finally, cases with abscesses are poor risks because severe restrictive adhesions usually develop.[254]

Regardless of whether surgical or conservative intervention is selected for a penile hematoma, the bull should be treated with high levels of systemic antibiotics in an attempt to prevent abscess formation. Penicillin is a good choice because abscesses are usually caused by *Actinomyces pyogenes*. Postsurgical complications are much the same as those that may occur without surgery, but these adverse consequences are reported to occur less frequently after surgery. Bulls should not be returned to service for 2 to 3 months after treatment.[254,255]

Ram and Buck

Adhesions of the penis and prepuce caused by trauma are uncommon in adult small ruminants. The penis does not separate from the prepuce until puberty and cannot be extended before this time (4 to 5 months of age in bucks).[263] Most traumatic lesions of the penis or prepuce in sheep and Angora goats are from shearing injuries.[264] Blockage of the urethral process by calculi can cause necrosis and sloughing of tissue that may extend into the glans penis.[264] Fighting among horned animals may result in injury to the external genitalia, including the penis. In dairy goats the intersex condition can result in congenital malformation of the penis and prepuce (hypospadius).[265]

PHIMOSIS AND INJURY TO THE PREPUCE

Stallion

DEFINITION AND ETIOLOGY. Stenosis of the preputial orifice prevents extension of the penis. The defect is likely to be a sequela to an injury that results in cicatrix formation, but may rarely be congenital.[254,255] Tumors (such as melanoma or squamous cell carcinoma) or *Habronema* granulomas may encroach on the preputial cavity, thereby preventing penile extension.[266]

CLINICAL SIGNS AND DIFFERENTIALS. Acute posthitis often accompanies injuries to the prepuce, or infections such as equine coital exanthema and dourine.[254,255] Edema is common with acute posthitis, particularly after trauma. Gravitational effects typically worsen the preputial edema, which may induce prolapse of the external prepuce, trapping the penis in the swollen internal prepuce with a constricting preputial ring.[254] Cicatricial scar formation may follow, narrowing the diameter of the preputial orifice. Transpreputial ultrasound examination may be of benefit in differentiating tumors or abscesses from inflammatory edema or hemorrhage. Containment of the penis within the prepuce causes preputial urine accumulation, worsening balanoposthitis and secondary bacterial infection. The extended chronic inflammation leads to cicatrix formation with phimosis.[267]

TREATMENT AND PROGNOSIS. Preputial edema can be relieved by administration of diuretics and exercise. Application of crushed ice in plastic bags, or preputial immersion in cold water, may reduce inflammatory edema if applied soon after injury. Emollient antibiotic preparations can be used to massage injured tissues and reduce edema. Systemic antibiotics and nonsteroidal antiinflammatory drugs are indicated to control secondary infection and inflammation. Sexual rest is indicated until the lesions have healed.[258]

A biopsy can be procured from encroaching tumors to identify cell types and improve prognostic capability.[258] Cicatricial scars can sometimes be successfully removed surgically. Once inflammation and infection are resolved with local or systemic antibiotic and antiinflammatory drug treatment, incision of the ventral aspect of the preputial orifice (preputiotomy) may be necessary to enlarge the opening sufficiently to permit penile extension.[268] Large tumors or granulomas of the prepuce can sometimes be successfully removed surgically if sufficient elastic and membranous tissue remain to permit normal penile extension and retraction.[258] The prognosis for return to breeding soundness, however, is guarded when surgery must be performed. Postsurgical adhesions may develop that result in continued phimosis or penile deviation. In cases of habronemiasis, treatment with systemic insecticides or ivermectin may be indicated to kill remaining parasitic larvae.[266] Congenital abnormalities can seldom be corrected surgically.

Bull

DEFINITION AND ETIOLOGY. Trauma to the prepuce involving the elastic lamellar layers may prevent the required flexibility of the prepuce to permit penile extension. Breed predisposition to preputial injuries corresponds to genetic differences in pendulousness of the sheath and development of the muscles responsible for retraction of the prepuce. The polled gene is linked to weak or failed development of the preputial muscles, leading to habitual preputial eversion, which predisposes to injury. Brahman-blooded cattle have the added predisposition of a loose, pendulant sheath. With their tendency to partially evert the preputial membrane through the sheath orifice, they are at greater risk of damaging the prepuce accidentally than those breeds of cattle in which the sheath is held in close apposition to the abdominal wall.[254,255,269]

Inability of the bull to extend the penis most commonly follows injury to the penis and prepuce that culminates in strictures or adhesions that restrict normal penile movement.[254,255,270-273] Other causes of phimosis include congenital anomalies such as a short penis, a short retractor penis muscle, and developmental abnormalities of the reproductive tract such as occurs in pseudohermaphrodites.[255,271]

CLINICAL SIGNS AND DIFFERENTIALS. The more common preputial injuries are contusions, abrasions, lacerations, and frostbite. When the injured prepuce can be retracted, the injury may not be suspected unless hemorrhage is noted from the sheath or the bull is observed having difficulty during breeding. Although minor injuries commonly spontaneously resolve, more extensive injuries commonly progress to abscess formation and fibrous stricture formation.[254,261,272,273] Extension and examination of the penis may result in further injury if the case is complicated by phimosis. In such cases an attempt to extend the penis to facilitate examination is contraindicated because forcibly stretching the prepuce will extend the laceration and spread infection to uncontaminated areas.[254]

TREATMENT AND PROGNOSIS. Treatment of preputial injuries in the bull may be either medical or surgical. With few exceptions, such as fresh avulsive lacerations in the fornix area, surgical intervention carries a better prognosis when medical treatment is first carried out to control inflammation and infection.[272] The healing leaves more normal tissue to be identified and salvaged during surgery. In cases in which the injured prepuce is retracted into the preputial cavity, digital or speculum examination can be done in an attempt to locate lesions and determine the extent and depth of tissue involvement. Systemic administration of antibiotic is necessary to reduce the incidence of abscess formation preoperatively, and antibiotic should be administered through the surgical and postsurgical periods if surgery is elected. When the injured prepuce remains prolapsed in presented bulls, the first consideration is to attempt to return the prepuce to the preputial cavity.[254,272] The exposed epithelial covering of the prepuce is easily injured and becomes quite edematous and friable because of its pendent location. Hydrotherapy for 20 to 30 minutes may be helpful in cleansing the exposed prepuce and reducing edema. After gently cleansing the prepuce and determining the degree of patency of the lumen, a protective emollient preparation is used to massage edematous swelling upward out of the prolapse.[272] Massage for 15 to 30 minutes may be required to reduce swelling sufficiently to permit the prepuce to be returned to the preputial cavity. If the prolapsed prepuce can be returned to the sheath, a retention technique should be used to prevent reprolapse. With the prepuce in place, a tube can be inserted just beyond the swollen internal portion of the prepuce to avoid urine retention. The tube is taped in place at the external preputial orifice. Tape should not extend past the proximal end of the tube or urine retention and migration into peripreputial tissue will occur. If this technique will not retain the prepuce, a purse-string suture in the skin of the sheath orifice can be used.[254] It should be tight enough to retain the prepuce but leave sufficient space for urine to pass freely. To avoid suture abscesses and stricture formation, the sheath should be clipped and prepared aseptically for suture placement and sutures should be removed as soon as swelling and inflammation subside. If the prolapsed prepuce cannot be returned to the preputial cavity, the prognosis for correction without surgery is guarded. After cleansing as described previously, a portion of stockinette is coated in ointment and is applied over the prepuce. A diaper constructed from heavy canvas or burlap with straps and centrally located perforations for urine drainage is applied under the prepuce and tied up over the back to hold the prepuce gently next to the abdominal wall to decrease gravitational edema. It is changed daily until infection and swelling are controlled and the prepuce is either returned to the sheath or surgery is performed. Alternatively, the prolapsed portion of the prepuce can be wrapped in medicated gauze followed by application of a gentle but firm pressure wrap around a section of tubing. The pressure wrap is left in place temporarily to reduce edema, at which time the wrap is removed and the prepuce replaced into the sheath.[272]

Once sufficient healing has occurred the necessity for surgery is determined by extending the penis.[254] Adhesions most commonly take the form of encircling cicatricial strictures that must be removed surgically. Guidelines suggested for predicting successful outcome of surgery include: (1) a minimum of 5 cm of normal prepuce should be present on either side of the surgical site or proper unfolding may not be possible after surgery, and (2) free prepuce remaining after surgery should be at least twice the length of the free portion of the penis or the prepuce may be too short to permit full penile extension. Presurgical and postsurgical considerations, and surgical techniques used to correct phimosis, are described by Walker and Vaughan.[254]

Congenital anomalies contributing to phimosis are diagnosed based on physical examination of the entire reproductive tract. Abnormal karyotypes may be helpful in determining causes. If the penis cannot be extended with the techniques described and evidence of injury or adhesions is not present, congenitally short penis or retractor penis muscles should be suspected.[255] Accompanying history may provide information that the bull could copulate when young, but as he aged his abdomen progressively enlarged causing the penis to be relatively of insufficient length to effect copulation.[255]

Ram and Buck

Phimosis is uncommon in small ruminants. It may be congenital, or acquired as a result of adhesions or preputial scarring associated with trauma or balanoposthitis. This condition is diagnosed during the physical examination and/or by observing the animal during the breeding process. If phimosis is due to acute inflammation of the prepuce (posthitis), it may resolve when the preputial swelling reduces. However, the prognosis is guarded until scarring can be evaluated. Phimosis may also be congenital in small ruminants.[264]

PARAPHIMOSIS

Stallion

DEFINITION AND ETIOLOGY. When injury of the penis and the laminae of the prepuce is attended by hemorrhage and edema, paraphimosis (the inability to retract the penis into the prepuce) is likely to occur.[254] Prolonged penile prolapse, caused by debility or paralysis after the use of some tranquilizers, usually culminates in extensive penile trauma.[274,275] Protracted priapism (persistent erection) can lead to penile trauma and complications similar to penile prolapse.[276] Penile paralysis and priapism are distinctly different conditions. Penile paralysis develops secondary to insufficient tone of the retractor penis muscles.[277] Motor innervation of the retractor penis muscles in stallions is believed to be solely supplied by α-adrenergic fibers. When α-adrenergic blocking drugs such as phenothiazine-derivative tranquilizers are administered, paralysis of these muscles can cause penile prolapse.[278] The prolapsed penis is flaccid and cannot be maintained in the retracted position.[254,277] Priapism is a persistent erection without sexual arousal and is initially unassociated with penile paralysis. It develops from engorgement of the CCP with blood, and although the horse may not achieve a full erection, its penis is not flaccid.[279,280] When the penis fails to detumesce, CO_2 tension in the CCP increases, resulting in increased blood viscosity and subsequent venous occlusion where collecting veins join the cavernous spaces. Edematous swelling of corporeal trabeculae further reduces venous outflow, thus increasing the likelihood of irreversible venous occlusion, fibrosis of the cavernous trabeculae, and arteriolar occlusion. Disruption of the arteriovenous supply and fibrosis of the CCP prevent subsequent erections.[258,281]

CLINICAL SIGNS AND DIFFERENTIALS. Penile paralysis has been reported in exhausted or debilitated horses, in

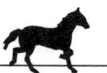

horses with myelitis or spinal injury, and in horses with severe injury to the penis.[254,274] Traumatic inflammatory edema often results in severe swelling of preputial membranes that prevent retraction of the penis into the prepuce. The inability to retract the penis results in further gravitationally induced edema and, as the problem worsens, edematous fluid eventually oozes through the increasingly fragile penile and preputial integument. Cellulitis develops and the integument becomes thickened, inelastic, dessiccated, necrotic, and irreversibly damaged.[254,258] In cases of long-standing priapism, the distal end of the penis becomes cool to the touch and the clot may become palpable in the body of the CCP as fibrin organization occurs. The organized clot may be visible on ultrasound examination.[276]

TREATMENT AND PROGNOSIS. Prognosis for recovery becomes guarded to grave the more chronic the paraphimosis becomes. Principles of treatment are similar to those described for the bull. To maintain the penis within the prepuce, a temporary purse-string suture of heavy vetafil can be placed near the preputial orifice. Alternatively, a padded plastic bottle from which the bottom has been removed can be used to support penile hematomas.[282] After the injured penis is dressed, the bottle is placed over it and pushed back into the sheath. The bottle is held in place with straps running over the lumbar area and on either side of the scrotum up over the tail head. Voiding of urine occurs through the bottle. The apparatus should be cleaned and replaced twice daily until the penis can be retained in the retracted position. If the penis cannot be returned into the prepuce, an external support for the prolapse should be applied. Prolonged penile prolapse may result in excess gravitational pull that damages smooth muscle cells, the retractor penis muscle, and the pudendal nerves[254,277]; such sequelae decrease the prognosis for recovery and return to a successful breeding career. Chronic, refractory penile prolapse results in severe balanoposthitis that may require circumcision or penile amputation. Surgical penile retraction (the Bolz technique) is described by Walker and Vaughan.[254]

Medical treatment of horses with priapism has generally been unsuccessful.[258,279] In cases of drug-induced priapism seen within 2 to 4 hours of occurrence, slow intravenous injection of 8 mg benzotropine mesylate may cause detumescence and penile retraction to occur.[283] If not seen immediately, treatment is the same as for traumatic paraphimosis. Flushing the CCP with heparinized lactated Ringer's solution through 12-gauge needles to remove sludged blood has been recommended for horses with priapism of 12 to 24 hours duration that have not responded to medical treatment.[258] If a blood clot forms in the CCP, the prognosis is poor and amputation may even be necessary. Some stallions, if severe nerve damage does not occur, may regain the ability to breed and ejaculate when assisted with placement of the penis into either the vagina of the mare or an artificial vagina. When the stallion does not regain the ability to completely retract the penis into the sheath, continued penile trauma is likely to result in damage to the sensory nerves to the glans penis. Such horses may achieve an erection, but may have difficulty both in seeking the mare's vulva for intromission and in ejaculating. Ultrasonography of the CCP to detect cavernosal fibrosis may be useful in assessing prognosis for recovery from priapism. Prognosis for recovery is good once penile retraction occurs, but breeding should not be permitted until healing is complete.

Bull

DEFINITION AND ETIOLOGY. Paraphimosis is less common than phimosis in the bull. Causes may be the same for both conditions, but for paraphimosis include penile tumors, parasitic invasion, traumatic or spinal disease affecting innervation of structures responsible for penile retraction, inadver-

tently severed retractor penis muscles, or physical trapping of the penis by a constricted prepuce after injury. Penile paralysis and paraphimosis sometimes occur as a result of spinal injury or disease, and in rabies cases as well.[254,255,270-273,284]

CLINICAL SIGNS AND DIFFERENTIALS. Persistent exposure of the penis results in congestion, inflammation, and necrosis of the penile integument.[255,270,271]

TREATMENT AND PROGNOSIS. Management of the prepuce has been discussed. Exposed portions of the penis should be frequently cleansed and protected by a bandage soaked in oily antibiotic preparations. The prolapsed penis should be supported close to the abdomen to reduce edema. The penis should be returned to the sheath as soon as possible and mechanically restrained if necessary. If the ability to retract the penis does not return in a few days, prognosis for recovery is poor.[254]

Ram and Buck

Paraphimosis is uncommon in small ruminants. The diagnosis is obvious although the etiology may not be. Treatment involves the same principles as in the bull. Prognosis is guarded and correlates with the degree of injury and necrosis at the time the condition is discovered.

URETHRAL INJURY AND URETHRITIS
Stallion

CLINICAL SIGNS AND DIFFERENTIALS. Traumatic injuries to the urethral process are usually obvious and are characterized by hemorrhage. *Habronema* granulomas are firm and friable. Ulcers of the urethral process often become secondarily invaded with bacteria such as *Pseudomonas* spp. Parasitic lesions tend to regress during winter, but if untreated they may mineralize and result in recurrence of hemospermia during the following breeding season.[285]

Bacterial urethritis may be associated with hemospermia.[286] Lesions can occur throughout the urethra, including the pelvic urethra in the area of the ejaculatory ducts. Diagnosis is based on demonstration of the lesions by fiberoptic examination.[258] Ultrasonography and fractionation of the ejaculate may be helpful in eliminating involvement of the accessory sex glands.[287]

Urethral inflammation and lacerations may result in fibrous strictures.[286] Strictures are often painful and may separate and bleed during urination and ejaculation. Bacteriologic culture of the urethra, urine, and semen; fiberoptic examination; and histologic examination of biopsies of lesions are helpful in making a diagnosis.[5] Strictures in the distal urethra may be identified by contrast radiography of the extended penile urethra.[254,286]

Clinical signs of uroliths include dribbling of urine with chronic cystitis, dysuria and stranguria, occasional hematuria, recurrent colic, and a stilted, painful gait in the hindquarters. Penile protrusion is frequent or constant in cases of chronic, involuntary escape of urine.[254] Diagnosis is by urinalysis, revealing the characteristic crystals, red and white blood cells, and bacteria. Urethral calculi typically restrict the passage of urethral catheters. Bladder calculi may be palpated per rectum or visualized by ultrasonography.[254,285]

TREATMENT AND PROGNOSIS. Treatment of urethral injuries involves first removing inciting factors such as a tight stallion ring. Sexual rest is indicated while palliative therapy is given. The ability to void urine should also be established. Systemic treatment with antibiotics that are eliminated in the urine may be useful as a prophylactic measure, or in cases in which secondary bacterial invasion has occurred. More severe cases of urethritis may be treated locally by either infusion of oily antibiotic preparations through sterile, rubber urethral catheters passed to the area of the seminal colliculus of the pelvic urethra, or alternatively by inserting soluble suppositories through a perineal urethrostomy. After resolution of the urethritis, the urethrostomy is allowed to heal by granulation.[286] Lacerations of the proximal urethra that result in hemospermia can be treated by perineal incision into the corpus spongiosum urethra (CSU). This prevents stretching of the urethra when engorgement of the corpus spongiosum occurs during urination or erection. Repeated stretching is thought to prevent urethral lacerations from healing.[288]

Inflammation of the urethral process may respond to local antibiotic salves. Treatment of parasitic granulomas with ivermectin speeds resolution of these cases.[266,289,290] Larger, nonresolving granulomas with mineralization may require surgical removal.[291] The skin of the urethral process should be rolled inward when sutured to the mucous membrane to prevent eversion that predisposes it to reinjury after healing. Remaining hemorrhagic or ulcerative lesions are lightly cauterized with silver nitrate.[285] More proximally located nonresolving urethral strictures, prolapsed subepithelial vessels, or ulcers can be removed surgically. Leave as much normal urethral mucosa as possible to avoid postsurgical stricture formation.[286]

Calculi lodged within the lumen of the pelvic urethra can be removed via perineal urethrostomy. Treatment for urethral calculi is described in the discussion of diseases of the urinary system, Chapter 32.

Bull

DEFINITION AND ETIOLOGY. Urolithiasis is the primary problem affecting the urinary system that may interfere with normal function of the reproductive tract of the bull.[292] It is of less importance in bulls than in steers, but occasionally occurs and may result in hematuria or urethral obstruction.[254,255] Urolithiasis is thoroughly discussed in Chapter 32.

BALANOPOSTHITIS

Stallion

DEFINITION AND ETIOLOGY. Inflammation of the penis (balanitis) and prepuce (posthitis) often occur together (balanoposthitis). Traumatic injury resulting in inflammation of the penis and prepuce has been discussed. Balanoposthitis may also be caused by dourine, equine herpesvirus 3 (see Equine Coital Exanthema), miscellaneous bacteria, and parasites.[256,270,271,293,294]

EQUINE COITAL EXANTHEMA

Equine coital exanthema is caused by equine herpesvirus 3 (EHV-3).[295] The occurrence of neutralizing antibodies to EHV-3 primarily in horses of breeding age suggests that spread of this infection may be primarily by genital contact.[296] Typically an inapparently infected mare transmits the virus to a stallion at the time of breeding. The stallion then transmits the infection to other susceptible mares before developing clinical signs of the disease. Clinical signs in the stallion are sometimes more severe than those observed in the mare, and may include systemic manifestations such as dullness, anorexia, and fever.[296] Vesicles up to 1.5 cm in diameter develop first on the penis and then on the prepuce 2 to 5 days later. The vesicles progress to circumscribed pustules with raised borders and depressed centers, which slough and ulcerate.[290,297] Scabs are seldom noted on penile lesions because they are rubbed off by extension and retraction of the penis during breeding.[297] Some affected stallions may refuse to breed mares, whereas others breed willingly, even while

extensive penile lesions are present. Healing occurs in a few weeks, often leaving depigmented spots.[297]

Some immunity to the virus is acquired after infection, because reinfection without recurrence of clinically apparent disease is common. It is probable that the virus remains in the genitalia in a latent form.[270] Recurrent coital exanthema usually occurs in aged broodmares but may also occur in stallions.[297] The relationship between viral recrudescence and recurrent coital exanthema in the equine is unknown.

Diagnosis usually can be made on the basis of the characteristic clinical signs. During the acute stage, the virus can be isolated from swabs or scrapings taken from the edge of erosions, inclusions in lesion specimens, or confirmed by using an electron microscope to visualize typical herpesvirus particles in fluid or tissue samples. Demonstration of antibody titers in serum may be useful in establishing time of exposure to the virus.[298]

Infection with EHV-3 is self-limiting.[270] Local treatment with antibiotic ointments will not speed healing but may minimize secondary bacterial infection and soreness.[297] Care should be taken to avoid iatrogenic transmission of the infection (e.g., through contamination of sleeves, water, and examination or insemination equipment) to susceptible animals. Attending veterinarians may choose to refrain from breeding affected stallions until the lesions heal. One method that may be helpful in circumventing transmission of the infection while still breeding the stallion is to collect semen in an open-ended artificial vagina as soon as lesions are no longer painful. Collecting the semen as it directly exits the urethra reduces the chance of viral contamination from the penile and preputial lesions. It is imperative, however, to adhere to any breed registry restriction regarding artificial breeding.[258]

BACTERIAL INFECTIONS

Stallion

The external genitals of stallions harbor potentially pathogenic bacteria, fungi, and yeasts, yet balanoposthitis caused by bacterial agents is uncommon.[299-301] These organisms are usually considered to be surface contaminants and the stallion is a lesionless carrier in most instances in which venereal transmission occurs.[275] Sperm motility, however, may sometimes be adversely affected by bacteria and their products in semen.[300] Offensive odors may occasionally be associated with heavy colonization of the penis and sheath with *Pseudomonas* spp. or *Proteus* spp.[255] Documentation of a bacterial infection is dependent upon serial isolation of a pathogen, preferably in large numbers and relatively pure culture.[301] A single isolation of *Taylorella equigenitalis* is considered diagnostic for contagious equine metritis.[275] Samples for bacteriologic culture should be retrieved from the fossa glandis, free portion of the penile body, and folds of the external prepuce before scrubbing the genitals of a stallion presented to a mare in estrus.[301]

If there is evidence of horizontal transmission of *Pseudomonas* or *Klebsiella* to mares, or if longevity of sperm is reduced in association with these organisms, the preferred method of management is to breed mares artificially with semen mixed with an antibiotic-containing semen extender.[302] Antibiotic selection is based on trials comparing extended semen with and without antibiotic. Extenders containing antibiotics that control the offending bacteria and permit maintenance of sperm motility are then used to breed mares.[303] Bacteria are usually not recovered after 5 to 30 minutes of incubation at room temperature.[300,302,303] Penicillin-G (1000 to 1500 U/ml), streptomycin sulfate (1000 to 1500 μg/ml), polymyxin-B (100 to 1000 U/ml), reagent grade gentamicin sulfate (100 to 1000 μg/ml), amikacin sulfate (100 to 1000 μg/ml), or ticarcillin

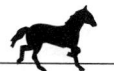

(100 to 1000 µg/ml) are usually the most suitable antibiotics.[258] Gentamicin sulfate and amikacin sulfate should be buffered with 8.4% sodium bicarbonate solution to adjust pH to approximately neutral before mixing with semen extender. A suitable volume of extender can be infused into a mare's uterus immediately before cover when natural service is necessary.[302]

Colonization of the external genitals with *Pseudomonas aeruginosa* and *Klebsiella pneumoniae* can be treated by thoroughly washing the penis and prepuce, including the fossa glandis and diverticulum, daily with an iodine-based surgical scrub. The genitals are then rinsed with copious quantities of tap water with dilute disinfectants added (10 ml concentrated HCl per gallon of water for *Pseudomonas* colonization, or 40 ml of 5.25% sodium hypochlorite bleach per gallon of water for *Klebsiella* colonization).[304] Drying of the penis can be followed by generous application of 1% silver sulfadiazine cream. The procedure is repeated daily for 1 to 2 weeks followed by serial cultures to determine if treatment was successful.[305] The clinician should be cognizant that recolonization with these organisms may occur, and that routine scrubbing and disinfection may predispose to infection of the genitals with potential pathogens by displacing commensal organisms.[299]

Bull

Balanoposthitis in the bull is caused by traumatic injury and infections. Whereas injury of the prepuce is more common, penile inflammation often accompanies the traumatic posthitis. A multitude of potentially pathogenic organisms inhabit the prepuce, and injuries predispose to infection particularly when deeper tissues are exposed. Pain and preputial discharge may be evident. Because of the presence of the many organisms in the preputial cavity, culture to identify a specific offending organism is likely to be misleading. When injury results in infection of the penis and prepuce, sexual rest in conjunction with local antibiotic treatment is indicated. Treatment should be performed as previously outlined for the penis and prepuce until inflammation is corrected.

Balanoposthitis unassociated with trauma has been associated with infections caused by infectious bovine rhinotracheitis-infectious pustular vulvovaginitis (IBR-IPV) caused by bovine herpesvirus 1, by tuberculosis, and by screwworm infestation.[255,270,271,306] Acute lesions associated with IBR-IPV infections are numerous small pustules that progress to ulcers and erosions in a few days. Purulent preputial discharge is present and lesions may become confluent. The prepuce and penis may become quite inflamed and swollen. Healing is commonly spontaneous and rapid, beginning in 1 week and usually complete in 2 weeks. Severe cases may take longer to resolve.[306] Virus is shed from the prepuce for 2 weeks or longer, during which time venereal spread is possible. Sexual rest for 6 to 8 weeks has been recommended to prevent spread and to avoid abrasions that may aggravate inflammation.[255] Enlargement of the lymphoid follicles may be present along with a seromucoid exudate for several weeks. Histologic changes include the transient appearance of eosinophilic intranuclear inclusions in degenerating epithelial cells.[270] Infusion of the preputial cavity daily may be of benefit in treatment, particularly in more severe cases. Vaccination with attenuated intranasal products has been reported as a method to prevent viral shedding into semen in bulls from AI studs.[255,307] The vaccine has been infused into the prepuce experimentally and did not result in viral shedding in the semen. Because persistence of herpesvirus in body tissues is a common occurrence, recurrence of viral shedding in semen after apparent recovery may be possible. Tuberculosis of the penis and sheath apparently has not been reported in this country for some time. It is characterized by enlarged, granulomatous lesions on the glans penis, prepuce, and sigmoid flexure that are prone to hemorrhage. Penile lymph glands may abscess.[255]

Ram and Buck

DEFINITION AND ETIOLOGY. Balanoposthitis (also called "pizzle rot," "sheath rot," and "ulcerative posthitis") commonly affects the penis and prepuce of intact and castrated male small ruminants.[264,265,308,309] The disease is discussed in Chapter 32.

PERSISTENT PENILE FRENULUM AND PENILE DEVIATIONS

Bull

DEFINITION AND ETIOLOGY. Phallocamposis, or deviation of the erect penis, is a relatively common condition in the bull. The most common cause of penile deviation is persistent penile frenulum.[255] Other types of penile deviations include spiral, ventral, and S-curved deviations.[254] Less commonly, preputial or penile injury may result in scar tissue formation that subsequently leads to deviation of the erect penis.[254]

When the penile frenulum persists, it remains connected to the ventral surface of the tip of the penis and the prepuce and causes the penis to bend ventrally during erection by preventing complete extension.[310] Copulatory ability is interfered with except in some of the Zebu-influenced breeds that are endowed with a plentiful prepuce.[254] Diagnosis is based on physical examination of the extended penis.

Because spiraling of the penis is thought to be a normal physiologic event that occurs in the vagina during ejaculation,[311] care should be taken in making this diagnosis. Bulls affected with penile deviations often have a history of no problems in mating cows for some time, occasionally for several breeding seasons. If such bulls have been closely observed it may have been noted that the condition did not occur on every mating attempt, but the frequency of occurrence gradually increased until bulls might require numerous mounts to successfully intromit and breed a cow in estrus.[255] Penile deviations occur at full erection when the CCP is maximally distended with blood. Caution should be exercised in diagnosing this condition during erection stimulated by electroejaculation. Such erections are not considered to be entirely physiologic and frequently result in penile deviations in bulls that have no deviations under natural mating conditions. The spiral deviations that occur with use of the electroejaculator may be a result of tension exerted by the retractor penis muscles.[254] Diagnosis is best based on observing occurrence of the deviation frequently in natural mating situations.

The ventral or rainbow deviation of the penis is less common than the spiral deviation and is a result of the apical ligament being too thin to support the engorged, stretched distal end of the erect penis.[254] The ventral curvature may be quite pronounced, preventing affected bulls from directing and inserting the penis into the vagina of the female.

The least common of the spontaneous penile deviations is the S-shaped curvature. It primarily occurs in older bulls with an apical ligament that is short in relation to an excessively long penis.[254] Penile deviations that result from adhesions that developed from penile or preputial injury are diagnosed based on physical examination.

TREATMENT AND PROGNOSIS. Persistent penile frenulum is easily corrected by severing the persistent band. Owners of affected bulls should be advised of the probable genetic basis, and therefore the undesirability of retaining such bulls for breeding.[254] Treatment of spiral and ventral deviations is surgical.[254]

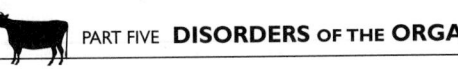

TUMORS OF THE PENIS AND PREPUCE

Stallion

CLINICAL SIGNS AND DIFFERENTIALS. The most common neoplasm of stallion genitalia is squamous cell carcinoma (SCC). Generally, it is of low malignancy.[254,312] The tumor usually involves the glans penis but may also involve the shaft of the penis and prepuce and produce a fetid discharge.[270,271] Large tumors may ulcerate and bleed resulting in hemospermia. Carcinomas may resemble *Habronema* granulomas, which are more common and are diagnosed by histologic examination of affected tissue.[255,258] Carcinomas are usually well differentiated and surrounded by eosinophils. Necrosis and calcification may occur but parasite larvae are usually not present,[270] unless secondary habronemiasis has occurred. Carcinomas may extend into the CCP or may metastasize to the inguinal lymph nodes or other abdominal or thoracic organs.[270] The superficial inguinal lymph nodes lie midway between the prepuce and external inguinal ring; secondary tumors in this region often grow rapidly and develop necrotic centers with purulent sinuses that must be differentiated from bastard strangles.[254]

Tumors encountered much less frequently include melanoma, papilloma, angioma, lymphosarcoma, and sarcoid. Melanoma is a common equine tumor, especially of grey horses,[266] and occasionally involves the penis and prepuce[254,256,313] (see Chapter 38). Genital papillomas are rare in stallions but may occur on the glans or shaft of the penis. The lesions appear as multiple proliferative cutaneous growths, and may become friable and result in hemorrhage during erection and ejaculation.[258] The lesions are generally thought to be caused by a papilloma virus,[314] and papilloma virus antigens have been found in cutaneous and genital papillomas.[315] Angiomas and lymphosarcomas have occasionally been reported on the genitals of stallions.[256] Sarcoids may involve the skin of the prepuce or scrotum[254,313] (see Chapter 38).

TREATMENT AND PROGNOSIS. When SCC are relatively small and noninvasively attached to the skin, neoplasms may be successfully treated by cryosurgery or hyperthermia.[316] Hyperthermic treatment (50° C for 1 to 2 minutes) appears to be most successful for SCC when lesions are small (less than ~2 cm). If the tumor is extensive but superficial, cryosurgery may be attempted after the tumor is debulked and hemorrhage controlled. The remaining base of the tumor is then frozen and thawed twice; healing occurs as necrotic tissue is sloughed. If removal of tumors is unsuccessful or if neoplasia is extensive, penile amputation may be necessary.[254,317] If superficial inguinal lymph nodes are involved, euthanasia may be required.[254]

In contrast to nongenital squamous papillomas, genital forms generally are quite refractory to treatment.[258] Surgical removal and autogenous vaccine administration have been tried to treat fibropapilloma of the penis of two stallions, but did not effect a cure.[285]

Bull

DEFINITION AND ETIOLOGY. Fibropapilloma is the only tumor that frequently invades the bovine penis or prepuce.[270,271] The tumor may be single or multiple and usually affects young bulls. The cause is thought to be a papilloma virus antigenically similar to the virus that causes cutaneous papillomatosis in cattle.[318] Frequent mounting among young bulls is thought to result in damage to epithelial surfaces of the penis and prepuce that serves as a route of entry for the virus.[254,255]

CLINICAL SIGNS. Small papillomas may be discovered during routine breeding soundness evaluations but many become larger before they are discovered. Large fibropapillomas may prevent withdrawal of the penis into the preputial cavity. Fibropapillomas are pedunculated and attached at a narrow base in early cases. The surface becomes cauliflower-like and friable; hemorrhage is easily induced.

TREATMENT AND PROGNOSIS. Many fibropapillomas regress spontaneously within a few months. Regression may be more likely in bulls approaching 2 years of age, and usually occurs within 4 months of the appearance on the penis.[318,319] Several vaccines, including autogenous preparations, have been used for treatment; but vaccines may be more successful for prophylaxis.[255] Frequently, surgical removal is indicated, but the fibropapillomas may recur. If only superficial attachment is present, surgical removal is easily accomplished. Catheterization of the distal urethra before surgery is helpful in identifying its location to avoid injury. If attachment has become extensive and sessile, amputation of a portion of the distal penis may be necessary.[254] Housing of young replacement bulls in individual pens, if possible, is recommended as a method to reduce the incidence of penile fibropapillomas.

PARASITIC INFESTATIONS OF THE PENIS AND PREPUCE

Stallion

DEFINITION AND ETIOLOGY. *Habronema muscae, Habronema microstoma,* and *Draschia megastoma* larvae commonly invade the urethral process, glans penis, and preputial ring of stallions.[254,266] Other terms for this condition are "genital bursatti" and "summer sores."[270]

CLINICAL SIGNS. Shallow irritations progress to irregular 1 to 3 cm granulomatous growths that may involve the entire circumference of the urethral process.[255] Lesions are friable and bleed when manipulated. Stretching of the infected urethral process during penile engorgement and ejaculation may result in hemospermia.[258] Pruritus associated with the lesions may be intense. Frequent micturition and dysuria may resemble urine spraying that accompanies accumulation of smegma in the urethral diverticulum ("bean"). Lesions subside during the colder months in northern areas but usually reappear and increase in size during subsequent warm weather.[255] Diagnosis is made by seeing yellowish granules (calcified larvae) in the lesion and by microscopic identification of larvae.[266]

TREATMENT AND PROGNOSIS. See Chapter 38 for treatment and prognosis information.

HEMOSPERMIA

Hemospermia refers to contamination of ejaculates with blood. Stallions with overt hemorrhage into ejaculates are subfertile. Erythrocytes, rather than serum, have been implicated for the marked depression of fertility although the precise factor(s) involved are not known.[286] A small amount of sanguineous contamination is compatible with fertility especially if the semen is quickly diluted with a suitable extender before insemination.[50] A disproportionate number of leukocytes to erythrocytes suggests infection of the internal genital organs. Specific causes of hemospermia include lacerations of the penis, cutaneous habronemiasis, urethritis, urethral lacerations, and infection or inflammation of the accessory genital glands,[258] which are discussed elsewhere in this chapter.

UROSPERMIA (URINATION DURING EJACULATION)

DEFINITION AND ETIOLOGY. Urospermia is an uncommon, but perplexing, disorder of breeding stallions. Affected stallions generally exhibit normal libido and mating ability, but semen becomes contaminated with urine during the ejac-

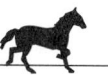

ulatory process. The problem may be incessant or unpredictably intermittent; urination can occur at any time or continuously during ejaculation. The amount of urine ranges up to 250 ml or more.[258]

The underlying cause(s) of urospermia is speculative. Closure of the bladder sphincter and seminal emission are controlled by the α-adrenergic sympathetic nervous system, and a disturbance in this pathway might contribute to urospermia.[320] Similarly, neuropathies that result in bladder paralysis (e.g., cauda equina neuritis or nerve damage secondary to equine herpesvirus 3 or sorghum/Sudan grass poisoning) can create urinary incontinence that permits voiding during ejaculation. Most stallions with urospermia do not exhibit signs of a neurologic deficit.[258]

CLINICAL SIGNS AND DIFFERENTIALS. Gross contamination of ejaculated semen with urine is easily detected by its color and odor. Contamination with significant quantities of urine adversely affects sperm motility and fertilizing capacity. Elevated concentrations (relative to serum levels) of urea nitrogen or creatinine in semen document presence of urine in the ejaculate.[258,321]

TREATMENT AND PROGNOSIS. Treatment options for urospermia vary, can be arduous, and are often unrewarding. Delay of semen collection (or breeding) until immediately after the stallion has voided urine may be a helpful management policy. Urination can be stimulated by administration of a diuretic drug (e.g., furosemide). Stallions may also void urine when provided access to feces of another stallion. Some stallions can be trained to urinate on command. Alternatively, the bladder can be catheterized to aid evacuation of urine before breeding but urethritis or cystitis may result from routine use of this procedure. Fractionation of ejaculates using an open-ended artificial vagina can be used alone or in combination with any of the above measures. When an open-ended artificial vagina is used only the first three jets of the ejaculate are collected. These jets contain a majority of the spermatozoa in the ejaculate and urination may not occur until the end of the ejaculatory process. Dilution of semen in extender may protect sperm from damage if contamination is minimal. Semen may be centrifuged after initial dilution and the sperm pellet resuspended in extender before insemination.[258]

Pharmacologic agents such as bethanechol chloride or flavoxate hydrochloride have been used in an attempt to correct urospermia but usually without success.[258] α-Sympathomimetic drugs have sometimes been used successfully to prevent retrograde ejaculation in men but their use has not been critically studied in stallions.[322] Oral administration of imipramine (100 to 500 mg twice daily) has reportedly been useful for controlling urospermia in stallions, presumably by enhancing contractility of the bladder neck during emission.[320]

INFERTILITY CAUSED BY DISEASES OF THE SCROTUM AND TESTES

SCROTAL INJURY, HYDROCELE, AND HEMATOCELE

DEFINITION AND ETIOLOGY. Trauma to the scrotum results in excoriation, lacerations, hemorrhage, and edema.[255,270] Systemic diseases such as hepatic disease and equine infectious anemia may result in scrotal edema.[255,275] Suppurative inflammation may develop as an extension of scrotal injury.[255] Adhesions often develop between the visceral and parietal tunics when inflammation, infection, or hemorrhage occurs.[271] Adhesions are usually thin fibrous strands that become thickened with time. In such cases the testis and its tunics are not freely movable within the scrotum.[270]

Hydrocele is an accumulation of serous fluid within the vaginal tunic.[271] Ascites, anasarca, or local lymphedema may contribute to hydrocele because the vaginal tunic communicates with the peritoneal cavity.[270] Accumulation of a significant volume of fluid around the testis may cause thermal degeneration and a decline in seminal quality.[323]

Hematocele occurs when trauma to the scrotum results in accumulation of blood within the testicular tunics.[271] Scrotal damage initially accompanies hematocele. Thermal degeneration of the testes follows and a thick fibrous capsule encompasses the testis after the blood clot organizes.[324]

CLINICAL SIGNS AND DIFFERENTIALS. Diagnosis of scrotal injury, hydrocele, and hematocele is made by physical and ultrasonic examination of the scrotum. Testes remain freely movable within the scrotum if hydrocele is present. Ultrasonographic examination reveals variable amounts of anechoic fluid present surrounding the testes and epididymides, which are easy to visualize because of their echoic nature against the fluid background. With hematocele, evidence of trauma is often present, with thickening of the scrotal skin. Blood surrounding the testis and epididymides becomes progressively more echogenic with time as the clot organizes.[258,325] Extensive edema of the scrotal fascia next to the tunica dartos may be difficult to differentiate ultrasonographically from hematocele. Abdominal paracentesis is helpful in eliminating ascites or peritonitis as causes of hydrocele. Palpation per rectum of stallions and bulls may occasionally reveal that the internal inguinal rings are enlarged, readily permitting fluid transfer into the vaginal cavity.

An aseptic tap is useful to identify the character of this fluid and must be performed with care not to contaminate or penetrate the testis or its visceral vaginal tunic.[324] A modified transudate of low cellularity is typical of fluid drained from a hydrocele.[326] Fluid usually returns after drainage unless the initiating cause is corrected.[258]

TREATMENT AND PROGNOSIS. Acute scrotal injury is treated with cold water or ice application to reduce edema (see earlier discussion on penile and preputial injuries). Lacerations and abrasions should be treated with topical antibiotic ointments. Systemic antiinflammatory drugs and antibiotics may reduce swelling, control infection, and prevent abscess formation.[258,324]

Scrotal thickening usually results in elevation of testicular temperature, causing degeneration and atrophy similar to that seen with experimental scrotal insulation.[327,328] Semen quality quickly deteriorates and a rapid reduction in numbers and motility of spermatozoa occurs with a concurrent increase in morphologic abnormalities of spermatozoa.[255,270,329] If swelling and edema resolve and adhesions do not develop between the testes, tunics, and scrotum, spermatozoa may gradually reappear in the ejaculate by 1 to 2 months after injury, but 4 to 5 months may be required for testes to return to normal size and sperm production.[257] One or both testes may remain atrophic and become firm because of fibrosis and loss of tubules. If only one testis is atrophied, the normal testis may eventually hypertrophy.

If hemorrhage occurs within the scrotum or testicular tunics, the prognosis for return of testicular function is poor. In unilateral cases, surgical removal of the clot and affected testis may minimize damage and speed recovery of the remaining testis.[330,331] Hydrocele is managed by correcting the underlying cause of fluid accumulation such as peritonitis or ascites.[324] Exercise may aid in control of fluid accumulation in some horses. Some stallions and bulls with persistent minor fluid accumulations within the tunics may continue to produce sufficient spermatozoa.[255] Permanent testicular degeneration may result in cases with extensive fluid accumulation that are unresponsive to therapy. If the condition is

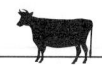

unilateral, removal of the affected testis may permit the animal to remain in service.[326] Because hydrocele and associated impairment of spermatogenesis may be transient (2 to 6 months),[323] caution should be exercised in recommending castration or culling of affected animals until demonstration that the disorder is longstanding.

SCROTAL DERMATITIS/ABSCESS

The scrotal skin is delicate and vulnerable to dermatitis. Causes include nonspecific environmental contaminants, bacteria, fungi, parasites, and frostbite.* Scrotal abscesses are not uncommon in small ruminants and are due to shearing injuries and penetrating wounds.[264] Treatment is directed toward removing the affected testis. Bulls affected by frostbite should be provided a warm and dry environment.[334] Systemic and local antibiotics may be indicated. Abscesses should be drained. Thermal degeneration of the testes may follow dermatitis and may be temporary or permanent.[255] Semen quality should be evaluated at periodic intervals after skin lesions have resolved to gauge prognosis for improvement and return to fertility.

TESTICULAR APLASIA AND HYPOPLASIA

DEFINITION AND ETIOLOGY. Complete absence (aplasia) of one or both testes is rare, and usually occurs in conjunction with anomalous development of other organs.[255,335] Testicular hypoplasia may be unilateral or bilateral and affects both scrotal and abdominal testes.[271] Testicular hypoplasia is thought to result from failure of germ cells to multiply in the gonad.[255] Causes of testicular hypoplasia may include transplacental infections and intoxications, zinc deficiency, hormonal insufficiency, impaired testicular descent, abnormal karyotype, and vascular disturbances.† Exogenous administration of hormones to prepubertal males might result in testicular hypoplasia. Testicular size of adult stallions is reduced after prolonged administration of exogenous steroids.[337-339] Scrotal circumference of bulls implanted with zeranol is diminished.[340]

CLINICAL SIGNS AND DIFFERENTIALS. Hypoplastic testes are usually smaller than normal, but they occasionally are normal in size.[270] The scrotal circumference of beef bulls should be at least 32 cm at 12 months of age.[341-343] Stallions 3 years of age should have a scrotal width greater than 8 cm.[275,344] Yearling rams with a scrotal circumference of less than 30 cm and mature rams with a scrotal circumference of less than 32 cm are not recommended for breeding.[345] The texture of affected testes varies from normal to soft in mild or moderate hypoplasia. Severely affected small testes are firm because of the relatively increased amount of stromal connective tissue.[271]

Depending on the number of seminiferous tubules affected, ejaculates from males with testicular hypoplasia may be azoospermic or contain a low concentration of spermatozoa with numerous morphologic defects.[255] Round spermatogenic cells may also appear in ejaculates, along with giant and medusa cells.[271]

TREATMENT AND PROGNOSIS. No successful treatment is available for severe hypoplasia. The useful breeding life of males with testicular hypoplasia may be shortened because affected bulls are thought to be predisposed to early testicular degeneration.[341] Because of the value of some individuals, particularly stallions, owners may elect to breed males with small testes. Effective management of such stallions is based on breeding a book of mares limited by the number of normal, motile spermatozoa present in ejaculates.

*References 255, 264, 266, 270, 271, 329, 332-334.
†References 264, 265, 270, 271, 329, 336.

CRYPTORCHIDISM

DEFINITION AND ETIOLOGY. Incomplete or abnormal testicular descent is thought to be a genetic abnormality.[255,265,271] The inheritance pattern in horses is thought to be dominant,[346] although studies of offspring of some cryptorchid stallions suggest that inheritance of the condition may involve more than one genetic factor.[347] Other modes of inheritance have been suggested from studies of offspring of cryptorchid rams, bucks, and bulls. These include a recessive gene with incomplete penetrance in Angora goats,[348] a dominant gene with variable expressivity in Hereford cattle,[349] and either an autosomal recessive gene or a dominant gene with incomplete penetrance in inbred sheep.[350]

Testes originate near the kidney and migrate to the superficial inguinal rings before descending into the scrotum; the epididymis precedes the testis in descent. Retained testes are located at some point along the path of migration.[270] Ectopic testes not associated with cryptorchidism may be found under the skin of the ventral caudal abdomen or elsewhere in bulls.[254,271]

CLINICAL SIGNS AND DIFFERENTIALS. The majority of cases of cryptorchidism in stallions are unilateral.[351] Although testicular descent can occur in horses up to 2 years of age, the testes are normally descended at birth in large animals.[352] Testes are readily palpated in the scrotum of colts at 30 days of age.[255,256] Spermatogenesis is inhibited in the abdominal testis because of the elevated temperature within the abdomen. The interstitial cells remain active and secrete testosterone,[256,270,271] enabling even bilateral cryptorchids to maintain libido and copulatory activity. The descended testis may be hypertrophic[270]; unilateral cryptorchids are fertile but are not considered sound breeders.[255,353]

Deep palpation of the superficial inguinal rings may reveal the testis in the canal ("high flankers"). If the testis is not located in the inguinal canal, palpation per rectum can be performed in stallions and bulls in an attempt to locate a testis, or to detect the vas or epididymis entering the superficial inguinal ring, thereby providing evidence of descent into the inguinal canal.[354]

CLINICAL PATHOLOGY. Equine cryptorchids have high basal concentrations of testosterone (usually >100 pg/ml) and respond to human chorionic gonadotropin (hCG) administration (10,000 to 12,000 IU IV) with a significant elevation of circulating testosterone within 30 to 60 minutes if testicular tissue is present. Geldings and "false rigs" (geldings with malelike behavior) have low basal concentrations of testosterone (<40 pg/ml) and do not respond to hCG stimulation. Stallion testes contain a high concentration of conjugated estrogens, and a single measurement of high plasma conjugated estrogens (>400 ng/ml) is reported to be almost as reliable in diagnosing cryptorchidism as hCG stimulation.[355,356] In some ruminants, measurement of testosterone concentrations before and after administration of hCG has also proved helpful in identifying cryptorchidism.[357]

TREATMENT AND PROGNOSIS. Stimulation of testicular descent with repeated injections of gonadotropin releasing hormone (GnRH), sometimes combined with hCG has been attempted but the success has not been critically evaluated. Surgical removal of the abdominal and scrotal testes is indicated.[254]

TESTICULAR DEGENERATION

DEFINITION AND ETIOLOGY. Testicular degeneration is an acquired condition with multiple etiologies.[358] Infections or traumatic orchitis may progress to permanent degeneration. Degeneration may be associated with thermal factors after elevation of body temperature by systemic infections; prolonged increase or decrease in ambient temperature; scrotal insulation from edema, dermatitis, scrotal hernias, or hem-

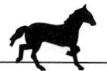

orrhage; or abnormal conformation resulting in an incompetent heat exchange system.* Degeneration results when testicular vasculature becomes occluded in torsion of the spermatic cord.[362] Obstruction of the proximal epididymis and malformation of the efferent tubules results in degeneration caused by pressure within the seminiferous tubules.[329] A variety of chemicals and ionizing radiation are capable of inducing testicular degeneration.[270] Administration of steroid hormones may induce testicular degeneration by inhibiting secretion of gonadotropins.[323,333,363] Gradual degeneration also occurs with increasing age.[364]

CLINICAL SIGNS AND DIFFERENTIALS. Diagnosis of testicular degeneration is based on physical examination and semen evaluation. Testes are typically thought to be small, but they may be normal size. Semen examination reveals a low concentration of spermatozoa, a decreased number of spermatozoa in the ejaculate, and a high percentage of spermatozoa with morphologic defects, sometimes with premature (round) germ cells.[254] Without a history of normal testis size and function before atrophy, differentiation from testicular hypoplasia is usually not possible.[271,275] Discrepancies between testicular size (measured by scrotal width in stallions and scrotal circumference in ruminants) and daily sperm output may imply testicular degeneration.[340,343,365,366]

CLINICAL PATHOLOGY. The measurement of plasma hormone concentrations may be helpful in establishing a diagnosis of testicular degeneration in large animals. However, the relationship between the concentrations of various hormones and the parameters of testicular function appears to be quite variable. Measurements of hormone concentrations in subfertile stallions have demonstrated that serum gonadotropins are sometimes abnormally low or high.[367] Hormonal criteria for confirming testicular degeneration in stallions typically include low concentrations of testosterone, with concurrent low LH concentrations in early cases of degeneration, or with high FSH and low estradiol concentrations in cases of chronic (or irreversible) testicular degeneration.[257] Less is known concerning hormone concentrations in other large animal species with testicular dysfunction. In one study, plasma testosterone concentrations were lower in young beef bulls with testicular degeneration than in a similar group of normospermic bulls; however, patterns of secretion and plasma concentrations of LH and FSH were not significantly different between the two groups.[343] Scrotal insulation of rams resulted in an increase in plasma FSH concentrations and a decrease in plasma testosterone concentrations within 1 to 4 weeks.[368]

Testicular biopsy can confirm degeneration.[369] Excision of an amount of tissue sufficient for evaluation often results in hemorrhage, pressure degeneration, and necrosis.[255] Therefore testicular biopsy is usually undertaken only as a final recourse.

TREATMENT AND PROGNOSIS. Once testicular degeneration has occurred, treatment is usually of no benefit.[255] However, any factors that might contribute to testicular degeneration (such as febrile conditions or systemic illness) should be corrected. Treatment of injuries of the scrotum and its contents has been described previously in this chapter.

Recent findings regarding variations in serum hormone concentrations in subfertile stallions have stimulated an interest in gonadotropin replacement therapy, including the use of GnRH. There are few controlled studies to evaluate the effectiveness of GnRH therapy in large animals. In one study, pulsatile or constant administration of GnRH for 20 weeks did not promote testicular growth or alter spermatozoa output in reproductively sound or unsound stallions.[370]

In some cases, degeneration is temporary and improved semen quality is evident after 2 to 5 months. The prognosis for an animal recovering its fertility and the economic losses the client will sustain from treatment and decreased produc-

tion must be considered when deciding whether treatment of testicular degeneration is warranted.

ORCHITIS

DEFINITION AND ETIOLOGY. Orchitis is most commonly caused by infection or trauma. Bacterial infections may develop hematogenously, or occasionally by retrograde movement from infected accessory sex glands.[271] Extension of infection to the testes from periorchitis or epididymitis also occurs.[329] Testicular enlargement is due to edema that accompanies the inflammatory reaction. Contusion and inflammation of the testes occurs in racing stallions, particularly Standardbreds.[256] *Streptococcus zooepidemicus* is commonly isolated from infectious orchitis in stallions.[257] In bulls, infectious orchitis is caused by *Brucella abortus, Mycobacterium tuberculosis, Actinomyces pyogenes, Nocardia farcinica,* bovid herpesvirus 3 (IBR-IPV), and other miscellaneous organisms.[255,270,271,329] Epididymoorchitis in rams may be associated with *Brucella ovis* or *Actinobacillus seminis* and *Actinobacillus*-like organisms.[265]

CLINICAL SIGNS AND DIFFERENTIALS. Acutely orchitic testes are hot, swollen, and painful. The swollen testis is turgid because of restriction by the tunica albuginea. Edema of the testicular parenchyma, and concurrent presence of periorchitis or epididymitis, may be detectable by ultrasound examination. Increased testicular temperature, congestion, and interference with circulation leads to ischemia and infarction. Abscesses sometimes develop, occasionally culminating in purulent liquefaction of testicular parenchyma. Testicular atrophy and fibrosis follow as the condition becomes chronic.[270,271]

Acutely affected animals may refuse to mate. Ejaculates may contain numerous white blood cells. Variable mineralization of seminiferous tubules can occur as a chronic change. Decreased sperm motility and increased sperm morphologic abnormalities are evident. Standardbreds affected by acute orchitis may switch from a trot to a pace whereas Thoroughbreds may suddenly develop a hopping gait.[255]

TREATMENT AND PROGNOSIS. Treatment consists of scrotal cryotherapy and systemic administration of antiinflammatory drugs. Bacterial orchitis is treated with antibiotics chosen by semen culture and in vitro sensitivity. Antibiotic therapy should continue for 1 to 2 weeks beyond resolution of testicular swelling and pain.[258] Testicular atrophy and sterility are common sequelae to orchitis.[256] Changes in the testes, including precise measurements of in situ testis size, are followed by sequential ultrasound examinations or caliper measurements. Serial semen analyses over a period of several months allow the clinician to monitor response to treatment and return of testes to normal production of spermatozoa.

PREVENTION AND CONTROL. Support devices may aid in preventing recurrence of traumatic orchitis in race horses. With *Brucella* or *Actinobacillus* orchitis in sheep, the presence of subclinical carriers in the flock must be considered.[308]

TESTICULAR NEOPLASIA

DEFINITION AND ETIOLOGY. Primary testicular tumors are uncommon in large animals, but may be slightly more frequent in older bulls than in stallions or rams. Testicular tumors originate from the interstitial (Leydig) cells, Sertoli cells, and the germinal epithelium. Testicular teratomas and lipomas of the testicular surface and lymphosarcoma also occur.* Although the incidence of testicular tumors is relatively greater in retained than in scrotal testes in dogs, this predisposition has not been confirmed in large animals, perhaps because most are castrated at an early age before the time of usual onset of testicular neoplasia. Retained testes in the horse, however, are thought to be more prone to neoplasia. Teratomas in particular are found

*References 255, 256, 270, 271, 327, 329, 334, 359-361.

*References 255, 270, 271, 312, 329, 371-373.

more commonly in cryptorchid than in scrotal testes, probably because they are embryonal in origin and their size prevents migration of the testis into the scrotum.[270,271]

Seminomas are the most common primary testicular tumor in stallions.[270,271] Seminomas are usually benign, but may be malignant and invade inguinal and abdominal tissues.[258,374] Seminomas are rare and benign in bulls, and are rarely seen in aged rams where they are occasionally highly malignant.[270] The tumor arises from the germinal epithelium and occurs in retained and scrotal testes.[255,270]

Interstitial (Leydig) cell tumors have been reported in stallions and bulls.[329] Most do not produce androgenic hormones.[270] They may be single or multiple in one or both testes, and are commonly 1 to 2 cm in diameter.[270]

Sertoli cell tumors are reported in horses, cattle, and sheep, but they are rare. Tumors in newborn or young calves may be due to impaired embryogenesis.[270,373]

Teratomas are usually a benign tumor of horses found in cryptorchid testes.[371,375] The tumors are often cystic and vary in diameter from 10 to 25 cm or more. Structures present in teratomas arise from all three embryonic layers and include hair, nervous tissue, salivary glands, adipose tissue, cartilage, and bone.[270,271]

CLINICAL SIGNS AND DIFFERENTIALS. Neoplastic testes are larger than normal, with an affected scrotal testis often twice the size of the unaffected testis. Abdominally located testicular tumors can be quite large. Neoplastic testes, particularly seminomas, are typically irregular and firm. Swelling may extend into the spermatic cord, and pain may be present that interferes with breeding or is evident on palpation. Ultrasonographic appearance of testicular tumors tends to be discrete, well-circumscribed hypoechoic areas within the usually homogenous testicular parenchyma.[258,325]

Swelling of the affected testis may interfere with thermoregulation of the contralateral testis, resulting in decreased sperm production. Semen examination, however, may reveal seminal parameters to be within normal limits and fertility may be acceptable. A significant amount of normal testicular parenchyma may remain covering the tumor, and living spermatozoa may or may not be present in the epididymis on the same side.[255,270,271,376]

TREATMENT AND PROGNOSIS. Testicular tumors should be surgically removed. Although metastasis is uncommon, early identification and removal of unilateral tumors prevents spread to other tissues. If semen quality is satisfactory in seasonal breeders, removal may be delayed until the breeding season is completed to avoid the transient decrease in semen quality associated with postsurgical swelling. If neoplasia is bilateral, surgical removal may be delayed until semen quality deteriorates sufficiently to negate the use of the animal for breeding.[258]

INFERTILITY CAUSED BY DISEASES OF THE SPERMATIC CORD

TORSION OF THE SPERMATIC CORD

DEFINITION AND ETIOLOGY. Torsion of the spermatic cord occurs more commonly in stallions than in other large animals because of the horizontal position of the testes within the scrotum. Torsions may be transient or permanent, and typically are of 180 to 360 degrees, but rotations may be greater.[278] Abnormal elongation of the caudal ligament of the epididymis (scrotal ligament), the proper ligament of the testis, or an excessively long mesorchium may encourage spermatic cord torsion.[362,377]

CLINICAL SIGNS AND DIFFERENTIALS. Torsion of the spermatic cord occurs in degrees that vary from those producing no pain or abnormality of semen to those involving vascular obstruction and acute colic.[256] Torsion is often a transient condition that does not interfere with testicular function or cause pain.[353] In those cases the testis is usually rotated 180 degrees or less. If torsion is of sufficient degree to result in vascular compromise, acute pain results.[255,256,377,378] Diagnosis of torsion of the spermatic cord is aided when displacement of the tail of the epididymis and scrotal ligament is evident on palpation. The head of the epididymis is normally located craniodorsal to the testis and the tail lies caudally where it is attached to the testis by the proper ligament. The tail of the epididymis is most readily palpable and its location is helpful in determining the degree of rotation. Torsions of 360 degrees or greater generally cause clinical signs that must be differentiated from strangulation of herniated contents into the scrotum. The primary method used to differentiate between the two conditions is palpation per rectum of the superficial inguinal ring to identify if herniation is present.[258]

Clinical signs of vascular impairment with spermatic cord torsion include abdominal discomfort, elevated heart and respiratory rates, unilateral swelling and edema of the scrotum, and increased testicular temperature.[258] Affected testes are painful and quickly become soft and friable.[255,256,377,378]

TREATMENT AND PROGNOSIS. Manual correction of spermatic cord torsion is frequently not possible, and recurrence is likely. To attempt manual correction, the horse is sedated and the testis is rotated in the direction opposite the torsion. Both hands are used to reposition the scrotum as the testis and its tunics are rotated.[256] Surgical correction is indicated if manual correction is not possible.[258] Nonsteroidal antiinflammatory drugs and analgesics may be administered to control pain.

The rapidity with which correction must occur is unknown; human testes may be salvageable if torsion is corrected within 6 hours. If hemorrhage or necrosis of the testis is evident, removal is indicated because the contralateral testis may become permanently damaged. The mechanism is probably immunologic, resulting from antibodies to spermatozoa liberated as a result of ischemia.[379]

VARICOCELE

DEFINITION AND ETIOLOGY. Varicoceles are abnormally distended and tortuous veins of the pampiniform plexus.[308,361] Varicoceles are most often recognized in rams, where dilations in vessels may reach 15 cm and discourage movement and libido.[350] The incidence of varicoceles increases significantly with age, reaching approximately 2% in rams 3 years of age and older.[335] Varicoceles have been reported infrequently in stallions.[258]

Varicoceles may result from insufficiency of veins draining the testis or a deficiency of the fascia and connective tissue surrounding those veins that allows backflow and stasis of blood in the vessels.[270] Infertility associated with varicocele is thought to be due to disturbance of the local thermoregulatory mechanism, causing increased testicular temperature and subsequent disturbance in spermatogenesis.[258] Concomitant atrophy of the testis is common in rams.[335] Bilateral varicoceles and atrophied testes have been reported in the ram.[380]

CLINICAL SIGNS AND DIFFERENTIALS. Diagnosis of varicocele is made by palpating the dilated tortuous veins ("bag of worms") within the spermatic cord.[255,308] Confirmation of the varicocele has been accomplished by ultrasonographic examination in stallions. Large echolucent areas in the venous plexus of the spermatic cord, sometimes with concurrent distention of the central vein of the testis, are described as the identifying features.[325] The ultrasonographic appearance of a suspected varicocele can be compared to the

structures of a noninvolved contralateral testis and spermatic cord, or those of another nonaffected animal.

Thombosis of the varicocele can occur.[255,270] The large, organizing laminated thrombi can be mistaken as *Corynebacterium pseudotuberculosis* abscesses in the scrotal fascia of rams.[270] Varicoceles might also be mistaken for sperm granulomas of the caput epididymis. Unless thrombosis has occurred, varicoceles are typically fluxuant and soft, and fail to elicit pain when palpated.

TREATMENT AND PROGNOSIS. Surgical removal of varicocele has improved semen quality and fertility of some human patients but has not been reported in large animals. Thrombosis of a varicocele necessitates unilateral castration, with transection of the spermatic cord proximal to the thrombus.[254] Castration is also recommended for rams because of potential heritability risks.[350]

INFERTILITY CAUSED BY DISEASES OF THE EPIDIDYMIS AND ACCESSORY SEX GLANDS

EPIDIDYMITIS

DEFINITION AND ETIOLOGY. Epididymitis is caused by infection or trauma and may occur separately but is commonly secondary to orchitis or infection of the accessory sex glands.[270,271,381] The tail of the epididymis is commonly involved but the head and body may be affected. *Streptococcus zooepidemicus* is commonly isolated from equine epididymitis, although a number of other miscellaneous organisms have been incriminated.[255] In bulls, *Brucella abortus*, *Actinobacillus seminis*, *Actinomyces pyogenes*, and other miscellaneous organisms cause epididymitis.[270,271,381] In mature rams the disease is commonly associated with *Brucella ovis*, whereas in ram lambs organisms from the *Actinobacillus*, *Haemophilus*, *Histophilus*, and *Corynebacterium* groups are prevalent.[308,382] Routes of infection have been postulated to be hematogenous, venereal, or ascending from genitourinary passages, similar to routes of infection proposed for orchitis.[255,270] All routes of infection are likely to occur to some degree, depending on the pathogen and species involved. In an interesting study performed in yearling rams, conjunctival inoculation of *Brucella ovis* culminated primarily in localized infections of the reproductive tract, which tended to first result in lesions of the distal tail of the epididymis.[383] Injuries, such as penetrating wounds, may also result in epididymitis.

CLINICAL SIGNS AND DIFFERENTIALS. Diagnosis of epididymitis is based on detection of clinical signs that include pain when irregular swellings of the epididymis are palpated, changes in shape and texture of the organ, adhesions between the epididymis and scrotal tunics, and enlargement of the tail of the epididymis.[255,258,308] The course of epididymitis varies from acute swelling and edema to chronic abscesses, periorchitis, and fibrosis.[270,271] Granulomas may develop if sperm escape into surrounding tissue.[335,381,384] In rams, epididymal lesions may be palpable along the entire length. Abnormal sperm morphology (especially detached heads) and leukocytes in the ejaculate may be seen before lesions are palpable.[385]

Animals affected with the *Actinobacillus*, *Histophilus*, and *Haemophilus* groups of organisms may acquire an epididymoorchitis syndrome.[308,386] Affected rams are usually less than 1 year of age. They may be subclinical carriers or acutely ill with pyrexia, depression, pain as evidenced by an arched back, and unilateral or bilateral swelling and tenderness of the scrotal contents. If these animals recover from the acute phase, the disease may become chronic and is characterized by an enlarged, firm, and often irregular epididymis; palpable adhesions of portions of the epididymis to the testis and vaginal tunics; atrophic testes; abscess formation; and draining fistulas to the scrotal surface. Ultrasonographic examination of the epididymis may reveal dilated ducts, fluid accumulation around the tail of the epididymis, and cystic areas within the epididymis that contain purulent material.[258,325]

CLINICAL PATHOLOGY. Inflammatory cells may be present along with abnormal sperm in the ejaculate of affected animals. Seminal leukocytes correlate positively with epididymitis lesions, and correlate negatively with seminal quality.[385] Bacteriologic culture of the semen may aid in identifying infectious causes. Serologic tests for *Brucella ovis* and *Histophilus ovis* are available and are helpful in determining exposure to the organisms.[308,386]

TREATMENT AND PROGNOSIS. Infectious causes of epididymitis are treated with systemic antibiotics selected by in vitro sensitivity. Treatment should continue for 1 to 2 weeks after inflammatory cells disappear from the semen. In unilateral cases, removal of the testis, epididymis, and spermatic cord on the affected side may salvage some valuable animals for breeding. If unilateral castration is elected, sequential postcastration examinations are indicated to ensure infection has not spread to remaining reproductive organs.[258]

Treatment of ram epididymitis is usually not recommended but might be attempted in valuable animals with minimal clinical signs. Oxytetracycline 10 mg/kg and dihydrostreptomycin 25 mg/kg IM twice daily for 7 days resolved shedding of *Brucella ovis*.[387]

In cases of moderate or severe bilateral epididymitis, the prognosis for recovery is poor. Obstructions and granulomas usually develop, resulting in sterility.[335] Testicular atrophy is a common sequela to epididymitis.

BLOCKAGE OF THE EFFERENT DUCTS (SPERM STASIS)

Blockage of the efferent ducts between the testes and penile urethra sometimes occurs in stallions. If the condition is bilateral, azospermia results in spite of apparent ejaculation. The ampullae are frequently tense, and enlargement may be demonstrated by ultrasonography.[388-390] Massage of the ampullae per rectum followed by prolonged sexual stimulation and semen collection may result in ejaculation of a semen sample with a high concentration of spermatozoa, often present as "strings" or "plugs."[388] Collection of semen on a regular schedule may aid in preventing recurrence once the blockage is relieved. Empirical treatment by blockade of β-receptors and stimulation of α-receptors has been successful in some stallions that fail to ejaculate.[391]

Sperm granulomas caused by accumulation of spermatozoa in blind efferent ducts are a common cause of infertility in the buck.[265] Granulomas have also been identified in the stallion,[392] and particularly in rams with sperm extravasation as a result of chronic epididymitis.[270,271]

SEMINAL VESICULITIS (VESICULAR ADENITIS)

DEFINITION AND ETIOLOGY. Inflammation of the vesicular glands is uncommon in stallions but more likely in bulls.[270,271,393-395] Bacterial infections, including *Brucella abortus*, are incriminated in stallions.[256,287,396-398] A variety of organisms have been isolated from cases of seminal vesiculitis in bulls including *Actinomyces pyogenes*, *B. abortus*, *Mycobacterium tuberculosis*, mycoplasmas, ureaplasmas, *Chlamydia psittaci*, and *Haemophilus somnus*.[255,270,271,393,399]

Vesiculitis may affect bulls of all ages but is most common in young growing bulls fed high-energy rations and housed together.[393] The prevalence may reach 20% to 30% in small groups of yearling bulls in close confinement.[395] The role of viral pathogens in outbreaks of the disease is not defined. Infections may arise by either ascending or descending routes from other areas of the urogenital tract, or hematogenously. Frequent homosexual activity among young bulls, high nutrition, and fast growth rates may be involved in spread of the infection.[255]

CLINICAL SIGNS AND DIFFERENTIALS. The seminal vesicles of affected stallions may be of normal size or enlarged and painful when palpated per rectum.[396,397] Stallions may refuse to cover or may be unable to ejaculate.[256] Semen contains numerous neutrophils and blood.[287] Fertility of infected semen is reduced.[287] Bacterial pathogens are readily recovered from semen of affected stallions.[258] However, special culturing techniques are necessary to pinpoint the seminal vesicles as the site of internal genital infection (see under Clinical Pathology).[301]

Bulls affected with vesiculitis may exhibit few clinical signs other than deterioration of semen quality. In severe cases, pelvic inflammation and peritonitis result in pain reflected by reluctance to move, stiff gait, tense abdomen, and refusal to mate.[255] Other reproductive organs, particularly the ampullae, testes, and epididymides, may be inflamed.[393] The vesicular glands may not be significantly increased in size during the acute phase. If inflammation becomes chronic, the glands usually enlarge, eventually losing their lobularity and becoming fibrotic.[255,270] Abscesses are often associated with *A. pyogenes* and may rupture into the rectum or urinary bladder.[255,271] Tubercular vesicular adenitis results in marked enlargement of the glands with caseous nodule formation. *B. abortus* causes suppuration, necrosis, and calcification of the glands.[270] Purulent exudate is present in the ejaculate, sometimes as thick clots. Neutrophils may become less evident in semen as the condition becomes chronic. Poor sperm motility, increased morphologic defects, and an elevated pH are characteristics of semen from bulls with vesiculitis.[255]

Fertility of mildly affected bulls may remain satisfactory. More extensive involvement in which semen quality is markedly affected results in subfertility or infertility.[395] Semen from bulls with vesiculitis freezes poorly and antibiotics used in extenders usually do not control the high numbers of bacteria present.[395]

CLINICAL PATHOLOGY. Bacterial pathogens can be recovered from the semen of affected stallions. However, without other evidence of infection of the accessory sex glands, recovery of pathogens from the semen should be interpreted with caution because the bacteria could originate from another location. Repeated samples for culture should be obtained from the sheath, penis, fossa glandis, preejaculatory fluid, urethra (before and after ejaculation), and seminal vesicle effluent manually expressed through a sterile urethral catheter positioned at the colliculus seminalis. Prostatic fluids can be collected through a catheter by massage per rectum. The first jet of a fractionated ejaculate includes the secretions of the ampullae.[301] Alternatively, a suitable fiberoptic endoscope can be passed in the urethra to the level of the seminal colliculus and into the seminal vesicles. Purulent material may then be aspirated for culture.[258]

Vesicular secretions from bulls can be collected by extending and disinfecting the penis followed by irrigation of the distal urethra with sterile saline. A sterile catheter is then passed 30 cm into the urethra and the accessory sex glands massaged to stimulate their secretion. Fluid is collected into sterile containers.[400]

TREATMENT AND PROGNOSIS. Accessory sex gland infections are treated with antibiotics selected by culture and in vitro sensitivity. Antibiotics are administered for 2 to 4 weeks but treatment failures may occur.[287] Negligible amounts of certain antibiotics may diffuse across mucosal cell borders into the seminal plasma.[401] Properties of an-

timicrobials suitable for parenteral treatment of accessory sex gland infections include high lipid solubility, a favorable pKa, and low protein binding. The antimicrobial should have a pH that is basic relative to the accessory gland fluid into which penetration is desired.[402] Vesicular and prostatic fluid have a pH of 7.3 to 7.5, whereas bulbourethral gland secretion has a pH of 8.0 to 8.2.[301,344] Antimicrobials that may prove suitable for treatment include the basic macrolides such as erythromycin, which is fat soluble and has a high pKa, and trimethoprim, which also has a high pKa and a high percentage of nonionized molecules in plasma favoring diffusion across the lipid membrane of epithelial cells.[402] Removal of the affected gland has been performed in stallions and bulls.[396,403,404] A technique used with fair success in stallions with localized vesicular adenitis has been repeated irrigation through a catheter guided into the vesicles by endoscopy. Antibiotics are instilled into the vesicular gland lumen after each irrigation.[258]

The prognosis for correction of seminal vesiculitis is only fair to poor. Mild cases may recover spontaneously in 2 to 3 months. In chronic cases, glands that do not abscess become fibrotic and destroyed even though purulent material does not persist in the ejaculate.[255] In stallions with vesicular adenitis, immediate filtration of the ejaculate in order to remove cellular debris and mixing of semen in an appropriate antibiotic-containing extender to control bacterial growth may maintain sperm motility and fertility.[303]

REFERENCES

254. Walker DF, Vaughan JT: *Bovine and equine urogenital surgery,* Philadelphia, 1980, Lea & Febiger.
255. Roberts SJ: *Veterinary obstetrics and genital diseases (theriogenology),* ed 3, Woodstock, Vt, 1986, published by the author.
256. Rossdale SD, Ricketts SW: *Equine stud farm medicine,* ed 2, Philadelphia, 1980, Lea & Febiger.
257. Blanchard TL et al: Testicular degeneration in large animals: identification and treatment, *Vet Med* 86:537, 1991.
258. Varner DD et al: *Disease and management of breeding stallions,* Goleta, Calif, 1991, American Veterinary Publications.
259. Beckett SD et al: Experimentally induced rupture of the corpus cavernosum penis in the bull, *Am J Vet Res* 35:765, 1974.
260. Wolfe DF et al: Failure of penile erectin due to a vascular shunt from corpus cavernosum penis to corpus spongiosum penis, *J Am Vet Med Assoc* 184:1511, 1984.
261. Johnson L, Williams EI: Surgical disorders of the genital tract in the bull, *Okla Vet* 22:2, 1970.
262. Noordsy JL: Hematoma of the bovine penis: a technique for predicting successful surgical correction, *Vet Med Small Anim Clin* 76:158, 1981.
263. Smith MC: The reproductive anatomy and physiology of the male goat. In Morrow DA, ed: *Current therapy in theriogenology,* ed 2, Philadelphia, 1986, WB Saunders, p 616.
264. Bruere AN: Examination of the ram for breeding soundness. In Morrow DA, ed: *Current therapy in theriogenology,* ed 2, Philadelphia, 1986, WB Saunders, p 873.
265. Smith MC: Infertility in the buck. In Morrow DA, ed: *Current therapy in theriogenology,* ed 2, Philadelphia, 1986, WB Saunders, p 622.
266. McMullan WC: The skin. In Mannsmann RS, McAllister ES, Pratt PW, eds: *Equine medicine and surgery,* ed 3, Santa Barbara, Calif, 1982, American Veterinary Publications, p 789.
267. O'Connor JJ: *Dollars veterinary surgery,* Chicago, 1938, Alexander Eger, p 716.
268. Frank ER: *Veterinary surgery,* ed 7, Minneapolis, 1964, Burgess Publishing, p 267.
269. Lagos F, Fitzhugh HA Jr: Factors influencing preputial prolapse in yearling bulls, *J Anim Sci* 30:949, 1970.
270. Ladds PW: The male genital system. In Jubb KVF, Kennedy PC, eds: *Pathology of domestic animals,* ed 3, New York, 1985, Academic Press, p 409.
271. McEntee K: The male genital system. In Jubb KVF, Kennedy PC, eds: *Pathology of domestic animals,* ed 2, New York, 1970, Academic Press, p 443.
272. Hardin DK, Bierschwal CJ: Management of preputial injuries in the bull, *Bovine Clin* 4:7, 1984.
273. Donaldson LE, Aubrey JN: Posthitis and prolapse of the prepuce in cattle, *Aust Vet J* 36:380, 1960.
274. Simmons HA et al: Paraphimosis in seven debilitated horses, *Vet Rec* 116:126, 1985.
275. Kenney RM et al: Theriogenolgy and the equine. II, The stallion, *J Soc Theriogenol* 9:34 1983.

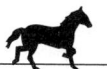

276. Blanchard TL et al: Priapism in a stallion with generalized malignant lymphosarcoma, *J Am Vet Med Assoc* 198:1043, 1991.

277. Bolz W: The prophylaxis and therapy of prolapse and paralysis of the penis occurring in the horse after administration of neuroleptics, *Vet Med Rev (Leverkusen)* 4:255, 1970.

278. Ambache N, Killick SW: Species differences in postganglionic motor transmission to the retractor penis muscle, *Br J Pharmacol* 63:25, 1978.

279. Pearson H, Weaver BMQ: Priapism after sedation, neuroleptanalgesia and anesthesia in the horse, *Equine Vet J* 10:85, 1978.

280. Lucke JN, Sansom J: Penile erection in the horse after acepromazine, *Vet Rec* 105:21, 1979.

281. Dorman BW, Schmidt JD: Association of priapism in phenothiazine therapy, *J Urol* 116:51, 1976.

282. Taylor TS, Bowen JM: Personal communication, 1986.

283. Sharrock AG: Reversal of drug-induced priapism in a gelding by medication, *Aust Vet J* 58:39, 1982.

284. Tierkel ES, Sikes RK, Starr LE: Rabies. In Gibbons WJ, Catcott EJ, Smithcors JF, eds: *Bovine medicine and surgery*, Wheaton, Ill, 1970, American Veterinary Publications, p 65.

285. Blanchard TL: Stallion genital tract pathology, *Proceedings of the Society for Theriogenology*, 1987, p 188.

286. Voss JL, Wotowey JL: Hemospermia, *Proceedings of the Eighteenth Annual Convention of the American Association of Equine Practitioners*, 1972, p 103.

287. Blanchard TL et al: Bilateral seminal vesiculitis and ampullitis in a stallion, *J Am Vet Med Assoc* 192:525, 1988.

288. Schumacher J: Unpublished data, 1994.

289. Bridges EE: The use of ivermectin to treat genital cutaneous habronemiasis in a stallion, *Compend Cont Educ Pract Vet* 7:S94, 1985.

290. Herd RP, Donham RC: Efficacy of ivermectin against cutaneous *Draschia* and *Habronema* infections (summer sores) in horses, *Am J Vet Res* 42:1953, 1981.

291. Stick JA: Amputation of the equine urethral process affected with habronemiasis, *Vet Med Small Anim Clin* 73:1073, 1978.

292. Rines MP: The urinary system. In Gibbons WJ, Catcott EJ, Smithcors JF, eds: *Bovine medicine and surgery*, Wheaton, Ill, 1970, American Veterinary Publications, p 631.

293. Pascoe RR: The effect of equine coital exanthema on the fertility of mares covered by stallions exhibiting the clinical disease, *Aust Vet J* 57:111, 1981.

294. Ristic M: Protozoal diseases. In Catcott EJ, Smithcors JP, eds: *Equine medicine and surgery*, Santa Barbara, Calif, 1971, American Veterinary Publications, p 137.

295. Bryans JT, Allen GP: In vitro and in vivo studies of equine "coital" exanthema, *Proceedings of the Third International Conference on Equine Infectious Diseases*, Paris, France, 1973, p 327.

296. Fibbs EPJ, Roberts MC, Morris JM: Equine coital exanthema in the United Kingdom, *Equine Vet J* 4:74, 1970.

297. Bryans JT: Herpesviral diseases affecting reproduction in the horse, *Vet Clin North Am (Large Anim Pract)* 2:303, 1980.

298. Blanchard TL, Kenney RM, Timoney TJ: Venereal disease. In Blanchard TL, Varner DD, eds: Stallion management, *Vet Clin North Am (Equine Pract)* 8:191, 1992.

299. Bowen JM et al: Effects of washing on the bacterial flora of the stallion's penis, *J Reprod Fertil Suppl* 32:41, 1982.

300. Burns SJ, Simpson RB, Snell JR: Control of microflora in stallion semen with a semen extender, *J Reprod Fertil Suppl* 23:139, 1975.

301. Cooper WL: Methods of determining the site of bacterial infections in the stallion reproductive tract, *Proceedings of the Society for Theriogenology*, 1979, p 1.

302. Kenney RM et al: Minimum contamination techniques for breeding mares: technique and preliminary findings, *Proceedings of the Twenty-first Annual Convention of the American Association of Equine Practitioners*, 1975, p 327.

303. Blanchard TL et al: Use of a semen extender containing antibiotic to improve fertility of a stallion with seminal vesiculitis due to *Pseudomonas aeruginosa*, *Theriogenology* 28:541, 1987.

304. Kenney RM, Cummings MR: Potential control of stallion penile shedding of *Pseudomonas aeruginosa* and *Klebsiella pneumoniae*, *Proc Symp Voortplanting Pard*, Ghent, Belgium, 1990.

305. Studdert MH, Barker CAV, Savan M: Infectious pustular vulvovaginitis (IPV) virus infection of bulls, *Am J Vet Res* 25:303, 1964.

306. Johnson TL et al: *Pseudomonas* infection in a stallion: a case report, *Proceedings of the Twenty-sixth Annual Convention of the American Association of Equine Practitioners*, 1980, p 111.

307. Schultz RD, Sheffy FE: Current status of viral infections of the bovine genital tract. In Morrow D, ed: *Current therapy in theriogenology*, ed 2, Philadelphia, 1980, WB Saunders, p 503.

308. Kimberling CV: Diseases of rams. In Kimberling CV, ed: *Jensen and Swift's diseases of sheep*, Philadelphia, 1988, Lea & Febiger, p 3.

309. Memon MA: Male infertility, *Vet Clin North Am (Large Anim Pract)* 5:619, 1983.

310. Carrol EJ, Aanes WA, Ball L: Persistent penile frenulum in bulls, *J Am Vet Med Assoc* 144:747, 1964.

311. Siedel GE Jr, Foote RH: Motion picture analysis of ejaculation in the bull, *J Reprod Fertil* 20:313, 1965.

312. Cotchin E: A general survey of tumours in the horse, *Equine Vet J* 9:16, 1977.

313. Sundberg JP et al: Neoplasia in equidae, *J Am Vet Med Assoc* 170:150, 1977.

314. Scott DW: *Large animal dermatology*, Philadelphia, 1988, WB Saunders, p 419.

315. Olson C: Cutaneous papillomatosis and sarcoid. In Catcott EJ, Smithcors JF, eds: *Equine medicine and surgery*, Santa Barbara, Calif, 1972, American Veterinary Publications, p 1948.

316. Joyce J, Taylor T: Personal communication, 1987.

317. Markel MD, Wheat JD, Jones K: Genital neoplasms treated by en bloc resection and penile retroversion in horses: 10 cases (1977-1986), *J Am Vet Med Assoc* 192:396, 1988.

318. Olson C, Robl MG, Larson LL: Cutaneous and penile fibropapillomatosis and its control, *J Am Vet Med Assoc* 153:1189, 1968.

319. Olson D Jr, Segre D, Skidmore LV: Further observations on immunity to bovine cutaneous papillomatosis, *Am J Vet Res* 21:233, 1960.

320. McDonnell SM: Ejaculation: physiology and dysfunction. In Blanchard TL, Varner DD, eds: Stallion management, *Vet Clin North Am (Equine Pract)* 8:57, 1992.

321. Althouse GC et al: Diagnostic aids for the detection of urine in the equine ejaculate, *Theriogenology* 31:1141, 1989.

322. Kaufman DS, Nagler HM: Specific nonsurgical therapy in male infertility. In Howards SS, Lipshultz LI, eds: *Urology Clinics of North America* 14:489, Philadelphia, 1987, WB Saunders.

323. Shore MD et al: Outcome of scrotal hydrocele in bulls, *J Am Vet Med Assoc* 207:757, 1995.

324. Blanchard TL: Identification and treatment of scrotal abnormalities in large animals, *Vet Med* 85:82, 1990.

325. Love CL: Ultrasonographic evaluation of the testis, epididymis, and spermatic cord of the stallion. In Blanchard TL, Varner DD, eds: Stallion management, *Vet Clin North Am (Equine Pract)* 8:167, 1992.

326. Hopkins SM et al: Unilateral castration as treatment for hydrocele in a bull, *J Am Vet Med Assoc* 178:837, 1981.

327. Gerona GR, Sikes JO: Effects of elevated scrotum temperature on spermatogenesis and semen characteristics, *J Dairy Sci* 53:659, 1970 (abstract).

328. Ross AD, Entwistle KW: The effect of scrotal insulation on spermatozoal morphology and the rates of spermatogenesis and epididymal passage of spermatozoa in the bull, *Theriogenology* 11:111, 1979.

329. McEntee K: Pathology of the testis of the bull and stallion, *Proceedings of the Society for Theriogenology*, 1979, p 28.

330. Gygax AP et al: Haematocele in a stallion and recovery of fertility following unilateral castration, *Equine Vet J* 5:128, 1973.

331. Hoagland TA et al: Effects of unilateral castration on morphologic characteristics of the testis in one-, two-, and three-year-old stallions, *Theriogenology* 26:397, 1986.

332. Yager JA, Scott DW: The skin and appendages. In Jubb KVF, Kennedy PC, eds: *Pathology of domestic animals*, ed 3, Orlando, 1985, Academic Press.

333. Rhodes AP: The effect of extensive chorioptic mange of the scrotum on reproductive function of the ram, *Aust Vet J* 52:250, 1976.

334. Faulkner LC et al: Scrotal frostbite in bulls, *J Am Vet Med Assoc* 152:602, 1967.

335. Watt DA: Testicular pathology of Merino rams, *Aust Vet J* 54:473, 1978.

336. Basrur PK, McKinnon AO: Caprine intersexes and freemartins. In Morrow DA, ed: *Current therapy in theriogenology*, ed 2, Philadelphia, 1986, WB Saunders, p 596.

337. Squires EL et al: Restoration of reproductive capacity of stallions after suppression with exogenous testosterone, *J Anim Sci* 53:1351, 1981.

338. Squires EL et al: Effect of anabolic steroids in reproductive function of young stallions, *J Anim Sci* 54:576, 1982.

339. Blanchard TL et al: The effects of stanozolol and boldenone undecylenate on scrotal width, testis weight, and sperm production in pony stallions, *Theriogenology* 20:121, 1983.

340. Deschamps JC et al: Effects of zeranol on reproduction in beef bulls: scrotal circumference, serving ability, and pathological changes of the reproductive organs, *Am J Vet Res* 48:137, 1987.

341. Ott RS: Current thinking on breeding soundness examination of bulls, *Proceedings of the Society for Theriogenology*, 1987, p 14.

342. Ott RS: Scrotal circumference: how small is too small? *Proceedings of the Society for Theriogenology*, 1987, p 1.

343. Veeramachaneni DNR et al: Pathophysiology of small testes in beef bulls: relationship between scrotal circumference, histopathologic features of testes and epididymides, seminal characteristics, and endocrine profiles, *Am J Vet Res* 47:1988, 1986.

344. Pickett BW et al: Management of the stallion for maximum reproductive efficiency, General Series 1005, Fort Collins, Colo, 1981, Colorado State University Experiment Station, p 39.

345. Kimberling CV: *Breeding soundness program*, Ft Collins, Colo, 1981, Colorado State University, p 47.

346. Bishop MSH, David JSE, Messery A: Cryptorchidism in the stallion, *Proc Royal Soc Med* 59:796, 1966.

347. Leipold HW et al: Cryptorchidism in the horse: genetic implications, *Proceedings of the Thirty-second Annual Convention of the American Association of Equine Practitioners*, 1986, p 579.

348. Warwick BL: Selection against cryptorchidism in Angora goats, *J Anim Sci* 20:10, 1961.

349. Wheat JD: Cryptorchidism in Hereford cattle, *J Hered* 52:244, 1961.

350. Jensen R, Swift BL: *Diseases of sheep*, ed 2, Philadelphia, 1982, Lea & Febiger, p 3.
351. Stickl RL, Fessler JF: Retrospective study of 350 cases of equine cryptorchidism, *J Am Vet Med Assoc* 172:343, 1978.
352. The Technical Development Committee: Cryptorchidism, with special reference to the condition in the dog, *Vet Rec* 66:482, 1954.
353. Kenney RM: Clinical fertility evaluation of the stallion, *Proceedings of the Twenty-first Annual Convention of the American Association of Equine Practice*, 1975, p 336.
354. Blanchard TL et al: Detecting unilateral and bilateral cryptorchidism in large animals, *Vet Med* 85:395, 1990.
355. Cox JE, Williams JH: Some aspects of the reproductive endocrinology of the stallion and cryptorchid, *J Reprod Fertil Suppl* 23:75, 1975.
356. Cox JE, Redhead PH, Dawson FE: Comparison of the measurement of plasma testosterone and plasma oestrogens for the diagnosis of cryptorchidism in the horse, *Equine Vet J* 18:179, 1986.
357. Abbit B: Personal communication, 1989.
358. Blanchard TL et al: Testicular degeneration in large animals. I, Causes and pathologic changes, *Vet Med* 85:531, 1991.
359. Johnston J et al: Physiological responses of Holstein, Brown Swiss, and Red Sindhi crossbred bulls to high temperatures and humidities, *J Anim Sci* 22:432, 1983.
360. Friedman R et al: The effects of increased testicular temperature on spermatogenesis in the stallion, *J Reprod Fertil Suppl* 44:127, 1991.
361. Ott RS, Heath EH, Bane A: Abnormal spermatozoa, testicular degeneration and varicocele in a ram, *Am J Vet Res* 43:241, 1982.
362. Threlfall WR et al: Recurrent torsion of the spermatic cord and scrotal testis in a stallion, *J Am Vet Med Assoc* 196:1641, 1990.
363. Garcia MC et al: The effects of stanozolol and boldenone undecylenate on plasma testosterone and gonadotropins and on testis histology in pony stallions, *Theriogenology* 28:109, 1987.
364. Hahn J, Foote RH, Seidel GE Jr: Quality and freezability of semen from growing and aged dairy bulls, *J Dairy Sci* 52:1843, 1969.
365. Mickelsen WD, Paisely LG, Dahmen JJ: The effect of scrotal circumference and sperm motility and morphology in the ram on conception rates and lambing percentage in the ewe, *Theriogenology* 16:53, 1981.
366. Thompson DL Jr et al: Testicular measurements and reproductive characteristics in stallions, *J Reprod Fertil Suppl* 27:13, 1979.
367. Burns PJ, Douglas RH: Reproductive hormone concentrations in stallions with breeding problems: case studies, *Equine Vet Sci* 5:40, 1985.
368. Byers SW, Glover TD: Effect of scrotal insulation on the pituitary-testicular axis of the ram, *J Reprod Fertil* 71:23, 1984.
369. Threlfall W: Testicular biopsy, *Proceedings of the Society for Theriogenology*, 1987, p 65.
370. Squires EL et al: Effect of pulsatile and continuous administration of GnRH on reproductive function of stallions, *Proceedings of the Fifth International Meeting on Equine Reproduction*, Deauville, France, 1990, p 60.
371. Cotchin E: *Neoplasms of domestic animals: a review*, No 4, Bucks, England, 1956, Commonwealth Bureau of Animal Health.
372. Innes JR: Neoplastic diseases of the testis in animals, *J Path Bact* 54:468, 1942.
373. Moulton JE: *Tumors in domestic animals*, ed 2, Berkeley, Calif, 1978, University of California Press.
374. Vaillancourt D, Fretz P, Orr JP: Seminoma in the horse: report of two cases, *J Equine Med Surg* 3:213, 1979.
375. Stick JA: Teratoma and cyst formation of the equine cryptorchid testicle, *J Am Vet Med Assoc* 176:211, 1980.
376. Dunn HD, McEntee K: Semen quality and fertility in bulls with testicular tumors, *Int J Fertil* 9:613, 1964.
377. Horney FD, Barker CAV: Torsion of the testicle in a Standardbred, *Can Vet J* 16:272, 1975.
378. Pascoe JR et al: Torsion of the spermatic cord in a horse, *J Am Vet Med Assoc* 178:242, 1981.
379. Wyatt JK, Mundy AB: Torsion of the testicle: a clinical review of 20 cases, *CMA Journal* 107:971, 1972.
380. Watson PF: Varicocele in the ram affecting spermatogenesis and sperm maturation, *Vet Rec* 95:343, 1974.
381. McEntee K: Pathology of the epididymis, *Proceedings of the Eighth Congress on Animal Reproduction and Artificial Insemination*, 1976, p 1186.
382. Walker RL et al: Association of age of ram with distribution of epididymal lesions and etiologic agent, *J Am Vet Med Assoc* 188:393, 1986.
383. Biberstein EL et al: Epididymitis in rams: studies on pathogenesis, *Cornell Vet* 54:27, 1964.
384. Blue MG, McEntee K: Epididymal sperm granuloma in a stallion, *Equine Vet J* 17:248, 1985.
385. Bagley CV et al: Effect of epididymitis on semen quality of rams, *J Am Vet Med Assoc* 185:876, 1984.
386. Walker RL et al: Serodiagnosis of *Histophilus ovis*–associated epididymitis in rams, *Am J Vet Res* 49:208, 1988.
387. Dargatz DA, Knight AP, Smith JA: Antibiotic therapy of *Brucella ovis* infection in rams, *Proceedings of the Eighth Annual Western Conference on Food Animal Disease Research*, 1987, p 27.
388. Kenney RM, Cooper WL: Personal cummunication, 1979.
389. Little TV: Personal communication, 1986.
390. Little TV, Woods GL: Ultrasonography of accessory sex glands in stallions, *J Reprod Fertil Suppl* 35:87, 1987.
391. Klug E et al: Effect of adrenergic neurotransmitters upon the ejaculatory process in the stallion, *J Reprod Fertil Suppl* 32:31, 1982.
392. Held JP et al: Sperm granuloma in a stallion, *J Am Vet Med Assoc* 194:267, 1989.
393. Ball L, Young S, Carroll EJ: Seminal vesiculitis syndrome in genital organs of young bulls, *Am J Vet Res* 29:1173, 1968.
394. Carroll EJ, Ball L, Scott JA: Breeding soundness in bulls: a summary of 10,940 examinations, *J Am Vet Med Assoc* 142:1105, 1963.
395. Larson LL: Disease incidence in 1481 bulls examined for use in artificial insemination, *Proceedings of the Seventh International Congress on Animal Reproduction and Artificial Insemination*, 1979, p 1473.
396. Klug E et al: The effect of vesiculectomy on seminal characteristics in the stallion, *J Reprod Fertil Suppl* 27:61, 1979.
397. Sojka JE, Carter GK: Hemospermia and seminal vesicle enlargement in a stallion, *Compend Cont Educ Pract Vet* 7:S587, 1985.
398. Vandeplassche M, Devoss A: Excretion of Brucella abortus in the semen of a stallion, *Vlaams Diergeneesk Tijschr* 29:199, 1960.
399. Hoover TR: Bacterial seminal vesiculitis in bulls, *Proceedings of the Society for Theriogenology*, p 92, 1979.
400. Parson IM, Hall CE, Settergren I: A method for the collection of urethral samples from bulls for microbiological examination, *J Am Vet Med Assoc* 158:175, 1971.
401. Stamey TA, Bushby SRM, Bragonje J: The concentration of trimethoprim in prostate fluid: nonionic diffusion or active transport? *J Inf Dis* 128:S686, 1973.
402. Winningham DG, Nemoy NJ, Stamey TA: Diffusion of antibiotics from plasma into prostatic fluid, *Nature* 219:139, 1968.
403. King GJ, McPherson JW: Influence of seminal vesiculectomy on bovine semen, *J Dairy Sci* 52:1837, 1969.
404. Hooper RN et al: Ventral pararectal approach to the seminal vesicles of bulls, *J Am Vet Med Assoc* 205:596, 1994.

PART

SIX

PREVENTIVE AND THERAPEUTIC STRATEGIES

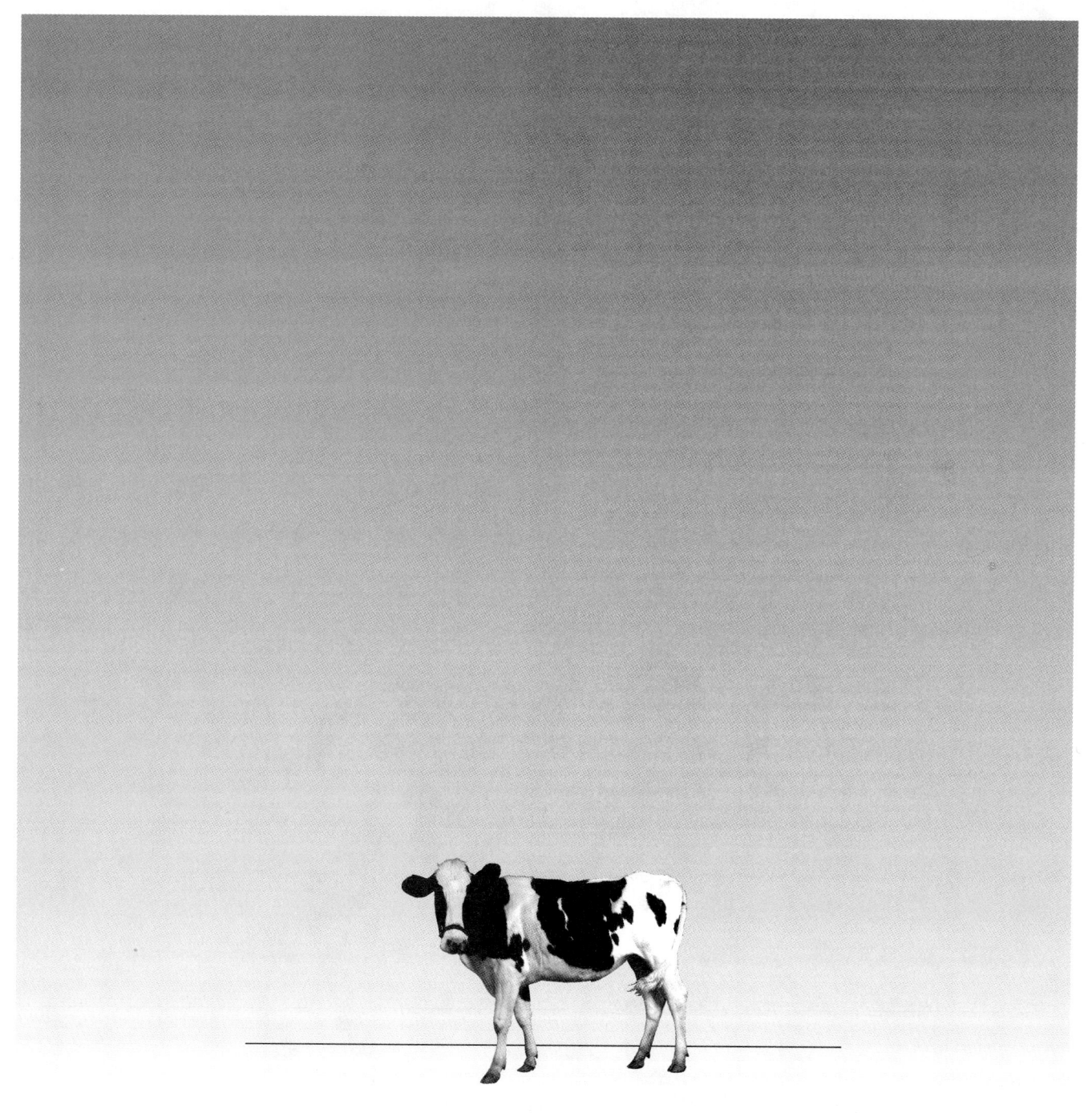

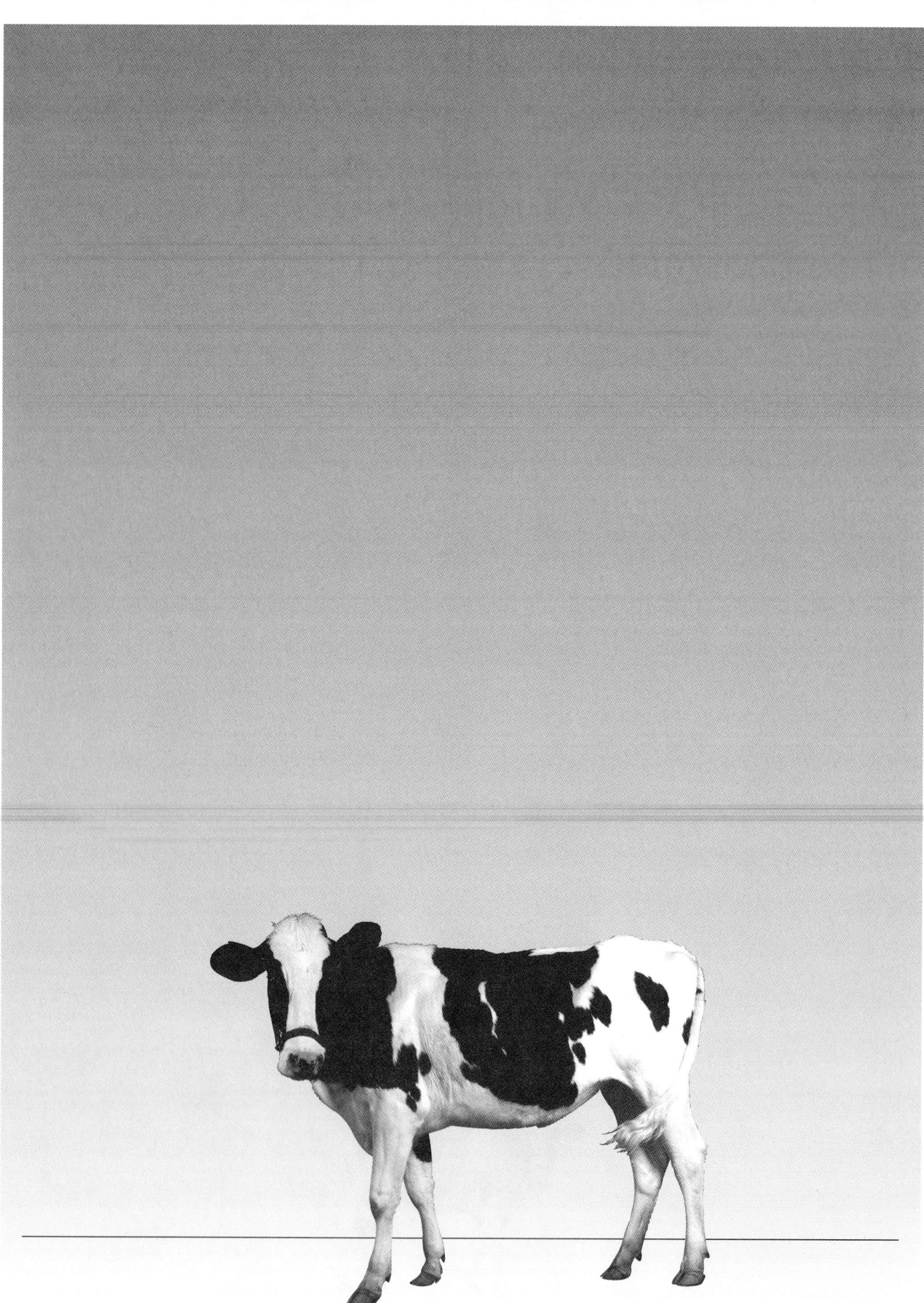

Principles of Antimicrobial Therapy

GORDON W. BRUMBAUGH

VERNON C. LANGSTON

PRINCIPLES OF ANTIMICROBIAL THERAPY

GORDON W. BRUMBAUGH
VERNON C. LANGSTON

"Rational therapeutics" is the scientific account of the management and care of a patient for the purpose of combating a disease or a disorder based on a knowledge of the disease and the action of the remedies used. It requires clinical judgment, overall medical knowledge, information about a specific patient,[1] selection of the proper drug, and the formulation of a dosage regimen appropriate to the patient after appraisal of potential benefits and risks of that therapy.[2] That process is not simplified by the vast number of antimicrobial drugs available. It is therefore essential that basic principles be applied so that antimicrobial drugs may be appropriately selected and used in patients. The purpose of this chapter is to explain general principles of rational antimicrobial therapy (Box 42-1) rather than to discuss individualized treatment of specific infectious conditions.

The ultimate expectation of an antimicrobial drug is to inflict an insult on an infectious organism that is sufficient to kill the organism or to render it susceptible to lethal effects of natural host defenses or the microenvironment around it, without adversely affecting the patient.[3,4] To accomplish this goal, antimicrobial drugs must be selectively toxic to the infectious organism.[5,6] Different structures, biochemical activity, virulence factors, mechanisms of resistance, generation times, and nutritional requirements of infectious organisms (i.e., bacteria, viruses, fungi, and parasites) form the mechanistic basis for selective toxicity of antimicrobial drugs. No individual drug is sufficient to meet all therapeutic needs. It is irrational to treat a viral infection with antibacterial drugs or a bacterial infection with antiparasitic drugs. However,

principles of selection and use of antimicrobial drugs are similar regardless of the infectious agent.

PRINCIPLE 1: CONSIDER THE PATIENT

The patient occupies the paramount position in regard to treatment and recovery from infection. Although the organism is the target of the drug's action, it is the *patient* with an infection that receives the drug. Before the patient can be considered adequately recovered, infectious agents must be controlled and removed from the site of infection, debris must be removed from the site, and the damaged tissue must be repaired or replaced.[7] Inactivation of microbes is the *only* role played by antimicrobial drugs; the patient must perform the others. Most infections are prevented by efficient nonspecific host-defense mechanisms.[8] When infections occur, many patients recover without treatment because of nonspecific and specific host-defense mechanisms. Ideally, if the host's defenses are functional and a pathogen's virulence can be weakened by antimicrobial drugs, the host should be able to kill and remove the microbe.

Many host-related factors must be considered during the formulation of a therapeutic plan.[9,10] The animal's age, sex, breed, use, residence, contacts with other animals, travel, diet, exposure to inclement weather, vaccination status, and medical experiences may influence natural defenses in the animal and prevalence of certain infections. Prevalence of an infectious disease may vary with year, susceptible population, and geography. Medical history of the herd may also be of value because some infectious agents may increase in virulence after "passage" through several animals.

Clinical signs must be interpreted carefully because identification of the agent is frequently not possible on the basis of clinical signs alone.[9] Clinical manifestations of infection result from direct effects of microbial pathogens, their toxins,

---

BOX 42-1

Principles of Antimicrobial Therapy

1. Consider the patient.
2. Document the infection.
3. Determine microbial susceptibility in vitro.
4. Use an appropriate dosage regimen.
5. Monitor results of treatment.
6. Investigate causes of therapeutic failure.
7. Restrict concomitant use of antimicrobial drugs.
8. Attend adverse reactions to drugs.

---

or the inflammatory response elicited in the host. Similar clinical signs may be caused by different microbial agents, and one species of microbe may produce a variety of clinical signs.[11] Signs of noninfectious conditions can mimic those of infectious conditions.

Defects in host-defense mechanisms are as important as the organism's virulence in determining whether infection will result from contact with an infectious agent and whether recovery will result if infection develops.[8] This is exemplified by infections associated with combined immunodeficiency syndrome or failure of passive transfer. It is irrational to expect antimicrobial drugs to resolve these conditions because the primary problem is not an "antimicrobial deficiency." Reasonable attempts should be made to assess weaknesses in a host's defenses that may contribute to the disease. Natural defenses of note include skin, mucous membranes, mucociliary escalator activity, cough reflex, transit time through the gastrointestinal tract, blood supply at portals of entry of infectious agents, humoral and cellular immunity, and resident microflora.[12] It is not possible to assess many of these objectively in most clinical situations. The attending veterinarian must have astute clinical acumen to evaluate contributory factors subjectively. Attempts should be made to replenish temporarily inadequate host defenses. If the host's defensive response contributes to clinical signs (i.e., if inflammatory edema compromises breathing), it should be modified to enhance convalescence.

Antimicrobial drugs can alter the response of the host's immune system or the stimulatory antigen.[13] The outcome of complex interactions among antimicrobial drugs, bacteria, and phagocytic cells depends on the organism, the drug, its concentration, and the duration and timing of exposure to the phagocyte and microbe.[14] Effects of antimicrobial drugs on chemotaxis, phagocytosis, metabolism of neutrophils, and the complement system are demonstrable in vitro but have inconclusive or insignificant clinical importance.[13] Inhibitory effects of chloramphenicol or rifampin on cellular and humoral immunity have been studied most extensively, but their immunomodulatory effects are not sufficient to warrant restricting their clinical use. Clinical consequences of effects of antimicrobial drugs on immunity are limited, but should be conservatively considered. For example, florfenicol did not interfere with responses of cattle vaccinated against bovine herpesvirus type 1.[15] Tilmicosin had neutrophilic antiinflammatory activity in cattle that were experimentally infected with *Pasteurella hemolytica*.[16] Antimicrobial therapy of proven efficacy should not be withheld from a patient to potentially enhance that animal's immunity.

Special Considerations

MATURATIONAL STATUS. An animal's responses to pharmacologic agents are significantly influenced by the age or maturity of the animal.[9,17,18] Physiologic differences that alter disposition of drugs in vivo are primarily responsible for that. Pharmacologic effects of xenobiotics (chemicals that are foreign to the biologic system) administered to brood animals before conception, during gestation, or at parturition or to neonates are not universally predictable. Drugs may distribute into gonads at sufficient concentrations to adversely affect gametogenesis. Drugs in luminal fluids of the oviducts or uterus may be teratogenic. Distribution of drugs into the placenta and fetus is affected by factors such as placental circulation, placental maturation, placental and fetal biotransformation of drugs, and fetal circulation. Among these variables, species-related differences may occur. Therefore drugs should be administered conservatively to brood animals, pregnant animals, or neonates and with adequate explanation of pertinent facts to the client. Potentiated sulfonamides administered as treatment of equine protozoal myelitis to gestating mares was associated with increased incidence of anemia, fever, anorexia, depression, and abortion.[19] Stallions treated with potentiated sulfonamides and another diaminopyrimidine (pyrimethamine) developed signs of neuromuscular weakness and ejaculatory disfunction.[20] It is not clear how each of these signs could be attributed to these drugs. Trimethoprim, pyrimethamine, and methotrexate each have the same mechanism of action—inhibition of dihydrofolate reductase. The affinity of those drugs for the respective enzyme in bacteria, protozoa, or eukaryotic cells differs, and that may partially explain their distinctly different clinical indications. Indirect effects such as folate deficiency may account for some of the adverse signs that have been observed. Some adverse findings with one species should be interpreted with care when dealing with another species. Anemia is a good example. An aspirate or biopsy of bone marrow is necessary to adequately evaluate anemia in horses, whereas peripheral blood may be sufficient with other species.

Biotransformation of drugs in neonates can be altered by administration of medication to the gestating dam. Phenylbutazone, administered to gestating mares during the final days of gestation resulted in substantial amounts of phenylbutazone and of oxyphenylbutazone in plasma of their foals.[21] Although phenylbutazone is not an antimicrobial drug and results of similar studies with antimicrobial drugs are not known to us, this example serves to emphasize the importance of considering peripheral effects of medication administered to gestating animals.

Fluoroquinolones are known to cause cartilaginous arthropathies in weight-bearing joints of young animals of several species. The horse may be unique in that adult horses have also developed the same syndrome, which was inconsistently related to dose and duration of treatment with enrofloxacin.[22,23] Tissues peripheral to plasma contained higher concentrations of fluoroquinolones than did plasma; therefore accumulation from repeated dosage regimens should be considered when developing those regimens.[22,24-26] Although arthropathic syndrome has now been recognized and acknowledged as a risk for use of fluoroquinolones, nothing is known about the healing and recovery of those joints that are injured. Therefore the overall assessment of risks of treatment with those drugs remains speculative and anecdotal reports suggest that the injured cartilage may repair and not carry prolonged clinical consequences but that needs to be confirmed.

LACTATION. There are at least three aspects to consider regarding distribution of drugs into milk: the lactating animal, the suckling animal, and the milk-consuming public. Distribution of drugs into milk is influenced by the same factors that influence distribution of drugs into other tissues.[9,18,27] Some antimicrobial drugs are concentrated in milk, others equilibrate between milk and circulating blood, and still others reach insignificant concentrations in milk

TABLE 42-1

Ratio of the Concentration of Drug in Ultrafiltrate of Milk to That in Plasma After Systemic Administration of the Drug[28-36]

Drug	Ratio (Range) (Milk:Plasma)	Reference
Ampicillin	0.24-0.30	28
Benzyl penicillin	0.13-0.26	28
Cephaloridine	0.24-0.28	28
Erythromycin	6.00-7.30	29
Gentamicin	0.20-0.50	30
Kanamycin	0.60-0.80	30
Lincomycin	2.50-6.25	31
Spectinomycin	0.37-1.12	32
Sulfacetamide	0.08-0.11	33
Sulfadiazine	0.16-0.19	33
Sulfadimethoxine	0.13-0.24	34
Sulfadimidine	0.59-0.62	33
Sulfanilamide	0.97-1.04	33
Sulfathiazole	0.37	33
Tetracycline	1.22-1.91	35
Trimethoprim	3.00-4.90	36
Tylosin	1.00-5.35	32

(Table 42-1).[28-36] A ratio greater than 1 indicates accumulation of the drug in milk relative to plasma. Results often varied with pH of milk. Concentrations of tetracycline may be elevated by chelation with calcium.

Therapeutic implications of the distribution of drugs into milk are clear, but inflammation of the mammary gland may alter distribution of drugs. Mastitic milk may resemble an exudate rather than "milk," thus providing a different microenvironment from that of milk. Nearly all drugs administered to a lactating animal will be detectable in her milk and can thereby expose the suckling animal. However, the total amount of most drugs received by the suckling animal via milk does not pose significant concerns.[17]

Antimicrobial drugs in milk may render that milk unsuitable for use as food.[27] Subtherapeutic concentrations of drugs in milk may cause no adverse effect, may cause the milk to be condemned as adulterated, may interfere with production of cheese or other dairy products, or may induce reactions in an allergic person who consumes the milk. For these reasons, withdrawal times should be taken seriously.

WITHDRAWAL TIMES. Withdrawal times are intended to allow adequate time for elimination of the drug from the animal to reduce the risk of violative residues of drugs inadvertently entering the food supply. Withdrawal times are established for drugs that are licensed for use in animals intended for use as food, and the withdrawal time applies only when the drug is used according to the approved labeling.[12] Because of this, it is important before therapy is initiated to discuss the patient's condition with the client, to determine if the animal (regardless of species) is intended for use as food, and if extralabel use of the drug is needed. Without such a discussion, the client cannot make a wise decision regarding the risks and benefits of therapy, and precautions to prevent adulteration of food may be inadvertently omitted.

Withdrawal times are not established for drugs that are used in an extralabel manner; therefore the most conservative time should be allowed when drugs are used in a manner inconsistent with their labeling.[37,38] Aids to determine useful withdrawal times include screening tests for drugs in milk* or

urine.* Results may not match those of methods used by regulatory agencies assigned the task of detection of residues, and those agencies may test different tissues.

EXTRALABEL USE OF DRUGS. Veterinarians often encounter infectious conditions for which the drug of choice is not approved by the Food and Drug Administration, Center for Veterinary Medicine (FDA-CVM).[12] In these situations the veterinarian is not exempt from professional and ethical obligations. Treatment must be based on experience, established practices, and scientifically substantiated facts. Drugs that are used in any manner other than that described on the drug's labeling (e.g., the treatment of diseases, with doses, routes of administration, duration of treatment, or species not specified on the approved labeling) are used in an extralabel manner. The Animal Medicinal Drug Use Clarification Act (AMDUCA)[37] of 1994 amended the Federal Food, Drug, and Cosmetic Act so that a particular use or intended use of a drug shall not be deemed unsafe if such use or intended use is (1) by or on the lawful written or oral order of a licensed veterinarian within the context of a veterinarian-client-patient relationship, and (2) in compliance with regulations promulgated by the Secretary of the U.S. Department of Health and Human Services. In short, the amended act contains statutory allowance of extralabel use of drugs, and regulatory authority is retained by the FDA-CVM. To discharge our professional duties within the public trust and in an ethical manner, a professional approach to extralabel use of drugs is necessary. Some guidelines include the following:

- A valid licensed veterinarian-client-patient relationship
- A medical diagnosis
- A situation in which approved use of a drug has proven ineffective in animals being treated or for which no available drug is specifically labeled (as is often encountered with some species)
- Carefully maintained identity of treated animals
- Observation of extended withdrawal times calculated by the attending veterinarian[39]
- Acceptable labeling of the prescribed drug[12,39-41]

Regulations specify contents of acceptable labeling. Consultation with a representative of the FDA-CVM is advised before treatment is initiated when particularly perplexing therapeutic problems exist and no alternatives to extralabel use of drugs are apparent.

HERD TREATMENT. Each member of a herd may suffer the same affliction, but one animal cannot receive treatment that is intended for another (there are no surrogate patients), and treatment of an animal that does not need it is wasted. Treatment must be implemented for each affected animal in the herd. The method of treatment must be practical and efficacious, or compliance by the client will be difficult. Requests by owners and veterinarians for "herd treatment" are really requests to treat each animal identically and easily rather than according to its individual needs. Each animal may indeed require the same treatment and mass-medication may be acceptable, but each animal deserves a reasonable assessment of its condition before treatment is instituted. Prophylactic or therapeutic mass medication has benefits and risks, but the cost must be offset by savings in areas such as labor of handling of the animals, reduced needs for therapeutic medication, or improved production.[42,43]

COST OF THERAPY. The cost of appropriate therapy is an important consideration for the client. The client (or their financial advisor) is the only one who can decide whether the treatment is "worth" the "cost." The cost of medical care is not static, and the veterinarian should keep the client informed of the financial commitment associated with treatment.

*IDEXX Laboratories, Inc, Westbrook, ME.

*DSM Food Specialties, The Netherlands.

Naturally, cost-effective therapy should be sought. This is not to say that the least expensive therapy is the best therapy or that ineffective drugs should be used just because they are inexpensive. Similarly, expensive drugs are not "better" just because they cost more. Clients require adequate information to make financial and medical decisions regarding their animals.

PRINCIPLE 2: DOCUMENT THE INFECTION

Antimicrobial therapy is predicated on the premise that the disease is caused by an infectious agent and that the patient will be unable to effectively eliminate the infection without antimicrobial treatment.[1,3] The primary purpose of documentation of infection is to help the veterinarian determine the necessity of this treatment. Clinical experience and diagnostic and interpretive skills are particularly important. Use of antimicrobial drugs for relatively trivial infections exerts selective pressure for resistant organisms.[4] Contamination or colonization by microorganisms (i.e., contamination of the surface of granulation tissue) does not necessarily constitute infection and is not always a sufficient reason for antimicrobial treatment. Inoculum size, microbial virulence, concurrent infection, site of infection, and resident flora contribute to the significance of infection. Death resulting from some bacterial diseases such as botulism (except toxicoinfectious botulism), enteric colibacillosis, or enterocolitis caused by salmonellae is not directly caused by vegetative bacterial invasion, so antimicrobial drugs are a secondary component of treatment. Without evidence of involvement of a susceptible etiologic agent(s), use of an antimicrobial drug is irrational and exposes the patient to unnecessary risks.[1] The more information that can be discerned about the infecting agent, the more reasonable will be the treatment.[1,10]

Sequential steps necessary to document an infection entail the following[1,44]:

- Development of reasonable suspicion of infection based on the patient's clinical signs and the veterinarian's knowledge of the pathophysiologic and microbiologic characteristics of the condition
- Careful procurement and submission of a representative sample of material from the lesion
- Initial detection of organisms by microscopic examination of a stained smear of the sampled material
- Demonstration and identification of the infectious agent in vitro, on the basis of its morphologic, immunologic, or biochemical characteristics
- Serologic evidence of antibodies produced against a particular infectious antigen
- Interpretation of the results of all diagnostic procedures

There are nonspecific and specific methods of documenting infection.[9] Nonspecific methods include medical history, clinical signs, hematologic changes, and characteristics of lesions. The drug(s) used for initial therapy will most often be selected on the basis of the veterinarian's clinical judgment and medical knowledge, as well as on nonspecific indications of infection.[2,10,44] This is not a trial-and-error approach.[45] Potential for a particular infectious etiology, most probable causative agent, status of the patient's natural defense mechanisms, and site of infection must be considered when interpreting clinical signs.[46] "Response to treatment" is an inconsistent means of revealing the etiology of infection. Although nonspecific methods are the weakest form of documentation, that information, coupled with astute clinical judgment, is often successfully used in practice. For example, a young horse with fever, nasal discharge, and submandibular lymphadenitis can be assumed (with a relatively high degree of certainty) to have strangles, and penicillin could be chosen for therapy. However, the possibilities for misdiagnosis are numerous in this and many other disease conditions, and specific methods of documenting infection should be used. An aspirate obtained from involved lymph nodes may reveal chains of gram-positive cocci, and *Streptococcus zooepidemicus* may be isolated. The immediate treatment may not change, but the management of the rest of the animals in the herd would differ greatly from that indicated for strangles.

Different organisms may be susceptible to and successfully treated with one antimicrobial drug, making treatment choice easy. However, a specific etiologic diagnosis may be of considerable relevance for the development of herd-health programs.

Antimicrobial therapy cannot be consistently successful if formulated on the basis of nonspecific diagnostic methods and historical probabilities alone.[9] Treatment formulated in that manner may cause more harm than good by interfering with the pursuit of a specific diagnosis, by allowing the development of superinfection, or by inducing reactions to the drugs.

Specific diagnostic methods should be attempted before initial treatment is instituted. Specific methods of documenting infection require proper collection and submission of appropriate samples, reliable laboratory procedures, and accurate interpretation of results. Because laboratory facilities and personnel can only work with materials submitted to them, the veterinarian must properly collect and submit appropriate samples to the laboratory and interpret results relative to the condition of the individual patient. Procurement of tissues or bodily fluids for cytologic, histologic, or microbiologic evaluation remains the cornerstone of accurate documentation of a specific infection.[9] Inadequate or improper sampling and improper submission of samples to the diagnostic laboratory are the most frequent and often unrecognized reasons for failure of documentation of etiologic agents of infectious diseases. The sample must be representative of the site of infection and may be bodily fluid (blood, peritoneal fluid, pleural fluid, percutaneous transtracheal aspirate, material draining from a site of infection), or tissue (biopsy, scraping, curettage, aspirate). Collection and submission procedures differ for aerobic and anaerobic bacteria, mycoplasma, protoplasts, viruses, and parasites. Special media or particular constraints of time and temperature must often be observed to transport fastidious organisms. Because each laboratory may use different techniques, it is wise to contact laboratory personnel in advance to learn preferred collection and submission equipment and procedures. The veterinarian and laboratory personnel can assist each other in reducing inappropriate collection and submission practices.

The choice of site to be sampled is critical. Isolates from draining tracts are unreliable and should be evaluated in the context of other related information.[47] Organisms isolated from wounds are of questionable significance unless they are present in pure culture or are clearly predominant. In these instances, susceptibility testing is probably warranted. Any microorganism isolated from bodily fluids that are normally sterile (blood, cerebrospinal fluid, pleural fluid, or synovial fluid) in the presence of clinical evidence of infection, should be evaluated for its antimicrobial susceptibility in vitro. If dissemination of infection is suspected, isolation of the agent from samples obtained from sites distant from the primary site of infection will strengthen confidence in the diagnosis.[9] Cultures of blood samples should be performed if dissemination is suspected because of systemic signs or if no primary site of infection is apparent. It is important to properly prepare the site of venipuncture so that the sample does not become contaminated. Results of cultures may be difficult to interpret if such details are ignored. The type of sample to be submitted (biopsy, feces, fluid, aspirate, blood) is selected on the basis of the disease. Recommended sites and materials to

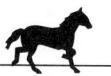

be sampled are presented in discussions of specific diseases elsewhere in this text.

If the patient has received antimicrobial drugs, the collection procedure should be delayed until the drugs are adequately eliminated from the animal's body so that residual drugs will not interfere with bacterial growth. Because about 99% of a drug will be eliminated from the body within seven half-lives of elimination, an appropriate delay between treatment and sampling can be estimated if pharmacokinetics of the drug are known. However, the delay calculated by this method may not be appropriate for severely ill patients. A fairly reliable rule-of-thumb is to wait 18 to 36 hours after the last dose of a drug. If a repository form of the drug is used, a longer delay is indicated. If the patient's condition does not permit a delay, the probability of isolating organisms from bodily fluids can be increased if samples are passed through a device designed to remove antimicrobial drugs from the sample.* Directions for use of such a device should be closely followed.

Evaluation of stained smears of samples remains the most rapid and useful method of early recognition of some infectious agents.[1,9] A direct smear should be made from a part of the sample, stained, and evaluated microscopically for bacteria and to characterize the cytologic response. Gram stain for bacteria, Wright's stain for cytologic examination, acid-fast stain for mycobacteria, methylene blue and potassium hydroxide preparations for fungi, India-ink preparations for cryptococci, darkfield microscopic examination for spirochetes, fresh wet-mounts for motile organisms (trichomonads), phase-contrast microscopy, immunofluorescence, and electron microscopy are methods of identification of infectious agents and inflammatory cells by direct examination. Newer techniques of DNA-typing, or polymerase chain reaction (PCR) are finding their place as modern diagnostic procedures for identifying some organisms.

Knowledge of morphologic and staining characteristics of bacteria is important to predict the identity of the microorganisms observed in the smear (Box 42-2).[1] Gram or Wright's stain† will demonstrate the presence of most microorganisms. If only one stain is used, Wright's stain is preferred because its cytologic staining is superior. Characteristics of the microorganisms (fungal, bacillary, or coccoidal bacteria), the nature of the inflammatory cells, and suspicions of which microorganism(s) might be present at the site of infection are especially beneficial for deciding initial treatment. With this information, treatment can be rationally initiated at least 24 hours before results of cultures are known and within minutes of the time that diagnostic samples are obtained. Some microorganisms respond predictably to certain antimicrobial drugs. Unfortunately some organisms respond unpredictably because of genetically related resistance, which may arise by mutation, induction, or acquisition of a plasmid. If gram-negative bacilli are seen in samples, at least one member of the unpredictable class of microorganisms should be suspected. If one or more unpredictable species are present, isolation and antimicrobial susceptibility procedures must be performed.

Serologic methods of diagnosing infections may be beneficial.[9] However, because most patients have recovered from infections by the time a convalescent sample is obtained, serologic diagnoses may not be available in time to influence treatment. However, serologic data may be beneficial for the development of preventive strategies. The class of immuno-

---

*BBL Septi-check, Becton Dickinson and Co, Microbiologic Systems, Cockeysville, MD 21030.

†Diff Quik Differential Staining Set, American Scientific Products, McGaw Park, IL 60085.

> **BOX 42-2**
>
> **Morphologic Description of Microorganisms[1]**
>
> **RODS (BACILLI)**
> **Enteric Organisms**
> *Pasteurella*
> *Actinobacillus*
> *Bordetella*
> *Pseudomonas*
>
> **ANAEROBES**
> *Corynebacterium**
> *Haemophilus*
>
> **COCCI**
> Staphylococci
> Streptococci
> Anaerobes
>
> **BRANCHING FILAMENTS**
> *Nocardia*
> *Actinomyces*
> *Dermatophilus*
> *Sporothrix*
> Fungi
>
> *Corynebacteria characteristically are pleomorphic; they align in V shapes after division and often appear as "Chinese letters."

globulin and the timing of its production are determined by the previous antigenic experience of the host. High concentrations of specific IgM are useful in diagnosing certain viral infections and toxoplasmosis. Acute and convalescent sera demonstrating a fourfold rise in the concentration of a specific IgG indicate the presence of infection. Samples of serum should be obtained at an interval of 2 to 3 weeks to permit an adequate time lapse for the formation of significant amounts of IgG. Although the presence of IgG in a single serum sample, regardless of concentration, indicates exposure to the agent, it is of little assistance in diagnosing a current infection. There is no consensus about what constitutes adequately protective concentrations of immunoglobulins. Because serologic response is used to diagnose some conditions, is the presence of immunoglobulins an indication of infection or of protection?

Documentation of infection entails more than merely listing isolated microorganisms on a laboratory report. The veterinarian must decide if the isolated organisms could be responsible for the condition in the animal, if they are commensal, resident flora, or if they are merely contaminants as a result of improper sampling technique. For example, *Escherichia coli* isolated from a sample of feces from a calf does not indicate that the calf's diarrhea was caused by that organism. However, if that isolate was shown to possess the K99 pilus-antigen and the ability to produce enterotoxin and if the signalment and clinical signs are compatible with coliform enteritis, the veterinarian can develop a cause-effect relationship of the bacterial presence.

PRINCIPLE 3: DETERMINE MICROBIAL SUSCEPTIBILITY IN VITRO

Quantitative assays of a microbe's susceptibility to antimicrobial drugs in vitro are necessary for patients with severe or complicated infectious processes and for those with infections caused by organisms with unpredictable susceptibility patterns.[1,9,48,49] A microbe is considered sensitive to a drug if the concentration of the drug that inhibits growth of the organism in the testing system in vitro can be achieved in vivo after administration of the drug by methods customarily used in clinical situations. Two commonly used quantitative assays of susceptibility are broth dilution and disc diffusion tests.[5,9,47,48-51] Reliability and reproducibility of these procedures depend on the organism examined, standardization of the inoculum, medium used, conditions of incubation, and concentrations of the drug. Results of these procedures can be coupled with knowledge of the clinical pharmacology of potentially useful drugs and of pathophysiologic changes in the patient to design an individualized dosage regimen for the patient. Broth dilution procedures involve inoculation of a known number of organisms into tubes or wells holding a volume of broth that contains specific concentrations of antimicrobial drugs. These inoculated tubes or wells are incubated in standardized microenvironmental conditions. The lowest concentration of antimicrobial drug that inhibits visible bacterial growth is defined as the minimum inhibitory concentration (MIC) of that drug for that organism. The lowest concentration of antimicrobial drug that prevents bacterial growth, when an aliquot of the inoculated broth that contains no visible growth is subcultured onto drug-free agar or into broth, is the minimum bactericidal concentration (MBC). Therefore the MIC is a measure of the bacteriostatic concentration of the drug, and the MBC is a measure of the bactericidal concentration of the drug. Drugs that are, by some conventions, classified as bactericidal have an MBC within 1 or 2 twofold dilutions of the MIC. The adjectives "bacteriostatic" and "bactericidal" should be used to describe "concentrations" of drugs rather than to classify drugs. The disc diffusion susceptibility test involves application of antimicrobial drug-impregnated paper discs onto inoculated agar plates. The antimicrobial drug diffuses from the disc into the agar, and a progressively decreasing gradient of concentrations of the drug is developed centrifugally around the disc. If the drug is active against the organism, a growth-free zone will surround the disc. The size of the growth-free zone can be correlated with the MIC determined by dilution assays. Because multiple factors affect diffusion of drugs in the medium, the size of the growth-free zone induced by one drug cannot be equated to a zone of the same size induced by another drug.

The microdilution method provides information that is more clinically relevant than that offered by the agar dilution method for determining therapy of bacterial infections of animals. The quantitative endpoint of susceptibility can be correlated with concentrations of the drug in bodily fluids or tissues. As a result, a more intelligent choice of treatment can be made than is usually possible when using agar dilution methods.

Laboratory reports of susceptibility of microorganisms to antimicrobial drugs provide only part of the information needed to formulate appropriate therapeutic actions. Interpretation and application of that information remains the responsibility of the veterinarian. It is reasonable to assume that if the same conditions are present at the site of infection that are present in vitro, the same results obtained in vitro could be expected in vivo. However, standardized microenvironmental conditions of a system in vitro are seldom present in the patient, and those conditions in the patient are usually unknown to the attending veterinarian. Temperature, humidity, partial pressures of oxygen and carbon dioxide, pH, osmotic pressure, presence of debris from damaged tissue, inactivating substances, and nutritional substrates at the site of infection are as important to therapeutic success as is the concentration of the drug. Limitations of susceptibility procedures and difficulties encountered with interpretation and application of results are eclipsed by the benefit pro-

vided. It is important to remember when formulating a therapeutic strategy that "the bug denotes the drug."[3]

PRINCIPLE 4: USE AN APPROPRIATE DOSAGE REGIMEN

In most instances, there are insignificant differences in clinical response following bactericidal or bacteriostatic therapeutic protocols.[50,52] Bacterial meningitis, endocarditis, and gram-negative bacillary infections in neutropenic human patients are conditions in which bactericidal concentrations of active drugs at the site of infection were correlated with improved response. Confirmatory data with animal patients are lacking, but extrapolation may be acceptable when similar etiologic organisms are present. Because of complex interactions among microbes, subtherapeutic concentrations of drugs, postantimicrobial effects, host defenses, and microenvironment at the site of infection, dogmatic statements about the requirement for bactericidal protocols should be avoided.

The drug selected for treatment must reach the site of infection, at an adequate concentration of the active form(s), for a sufficient time so that its selectively toxic effect can be inflicted on the infectious agent. Astute application of one's clinical judgment, and knowledge of pathophysiology and clinical pharmacology are important for the development of an appropriate dosage regimen so that therapeutic success may be expected.

A dosage regimen has five components: formulation of the drug to be used, dose of drug to be administered, route of administration, dosing interval, and duration of treatment.[9,53] When the appropriate drug has been selected, dose, route, and interval of administration can be formulated using pharmacokinetic values of the drug in the targeted species. The drug's bioavailability, its distribution to the site of infection, the duration of therapeutic concentrations at the site of infection, and its clearance from the body must be considered. These are affected by drug- and host-related factors: solubility of the drug and its formulation in water and lipids, formation of a concentration gradient, blood flow at the site of absorption and at the site of infection, ionization of the drug, binding of the drug to proteins, biotransformation of the drug, chemical characteristics of the drug, presence of an inflammatory response, and microenvironment at the site of infection.

Postantimicrobial effects of some drugs may be significant. These effects can be considered with pharmacokinetic values and mathematically factored into the calculation of a dosage regimen.[54] Few patients have conditions that require detailed mathematic calculation of a dosage regimen. Patients that may require such attention are those with compromised function of organs involved with biotransformation or elimination (primarily liver or kidneys), those that need treatment with drugs that are potentially toxic, and those that receive two or more drugs that interact in a potentially dangerous manner or that alter biotransformation or elimination of themselves or other drugs. Diligent monitoring of the high-risk patient for evidence of insult or toxic damage to organs is recommended (e.g., routine urinalysis, blood urea nitrogen, creatinine, sorbitol dehydrogenase).

The ability of an antimicrobial drug to distribute to an infected site depends on circulating concentrations of the drug, molecular size, binding of the drug to proteins in plasma and in tissue, water/lipid solubility of the drug, ionization of the drug, inflammation, active transport mechanisms, and rate of elimination.[9,50] Increased blood flow and capillary permeability associated with inflammation at the site of infection allow passage of drugs into areas that might otherwise be inaccessible. The blood-brain barrier (BBB) poses such a barrier to drug passage. Distribution of penicillins and

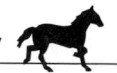

cephalosporins into cerebrospinal fluid (CSF) and other tissues is inversely proportional to the degree of plasma protein binding of the drug and directly varies with the degree of inflammation present. Aminoglycosides enter the CSF poorly, regardless of the presence of inflammation. However, no drug completely equilibrates across the BBB; thus high systemic concentrations of drugs are necessary to achieve adequate concentrations in the CSF, unless the intrathecal route of administration is used.

Drugs may be concentrated along routes of elimination and used advantageously to treat infections along those routes. However, when usual pathways of excretion are impaired, therapeutic success may fall, and drug-induced toxicity becomes more likely. Drugs that concentrate in urine can be used to treat urinary tract infections, even though concentrations of those drugs in blood may be ineffective against infection elsewhere (e.g., benzathine penicillin G or ampicillin trihydrate in the horse). This illustrates the necessity for relating the susceptibility of the organism to the concentration of drug at the site of infection. Penicillins, cephalosporins, trimethoprim-sulfonamide, and other drugs that attain high concentrations in urine may be effective against organisms that are otherwise considered resistant. Similarly, drugs that are eliminated by the biliary route may be used to treat biliary or hepatic infections. Drugs that undergo significant biliary elimination or reach beneficial concentrations in the liver include erythromycin, chloramphenicol, tylosin, and tetracyclines.

Duration of treatment varies with the disease and individual patient. Activity of the host's defenses and ability of the organism to resist those defenses, mechanism(s) by which the organism develops resistance to the drug, location of the infection, and primary activity of the drug influence decisions about the duration of therapy. If antimicrobial drugs are truly necessary for the patient, one dose of the drug(s) is seldom sufficient. Usually, treatment continues beyond the time that the patient's clinical condition has resolved. Duration of treatment remains a judgment call by the attending veterinarian.

Microenvironmental conditions at the site of infection must be compatible with the selected drug. Supernate of fluid from abscesses is acidic, hyperosmotic, and hyperionic, with relatively low concentrations of sodium and chloride and high concentrations of potassium and phosphate.[55] Relative to the respective concentrations in serum, concentrations of calcium are lower, those of magnesium are higher, and those of albumin and protein are lower in abscesses. Regarding drugs with intracellular sites of action, only that part of the drug that is nonionized, unbound to proteins or other constituents, and escapes inactivation by enzymes or competitive compounds crosses the bacterial plasma membrane to reach the site of action to be therapeutically active. Penicillins and cephalosporins inhibit synthesis of bacterial cell wall, but death of bacteria occurs when the bacteria rupture as a result of the relatively hyperosmolar interior of the bacteria. If the extracellular microenvironment is isosmolar relative to the interior of the organism, a cell-wall variant (protoplast or spheroplast) may form and continue to survive.[5,56]

Aminoglycosides are ineffective in an anaerobic microenvironment because the oxygen-dependent transport system that is necessary for intracellular uptake of the drug by susceptible bacteria is nonfunctional in an anaerobic environment.[5,50,55] Drugs that are extensively bound to proteins in plasma are also extensively bound to proteins in pus.[55] In addition to binding to proteins, aminoglycosides and polymyxins bind to constituents in sediment of pus from human patients. Binding of gentamicin is reversible and does not inactivate the drug. The antimicrobial activity of gentamicin may be inhibited as much as 16- to 32-fold by the acidic pH, high ionic content, and osmolality of pus. Activity of microbial β-lactamase at the site of polymicrobial, anaerobic infection can be sufficient to reduce the concentration of effective β-lactam antimicrobial drugs. Debris from tissue may provide adequate substrates for bacteria to circumvent effects of trimethoprim or sulfonamides.[5,57]

Size and purity of the inoculum also influence antimicrobial activity. A certain number of molecules of aminoglycosides are needed to kill a single bacterium; therefore antimicrobial activity is influenced by the amount of active drug relative to the size of the inoculum.[50] Many infections are polymicrobic, and antimicrobial activity at the site of infection is influenced by complex interactions among microbes, the host, and antimicrobial drugs that are not influential in susceptibility test systems in vitro.[55]

The effect of most antimicrobial drugs is best when the pathogen is actively growing and dividing, because at that time the organism is most susceptible.[5] When infections mature, bacterial growth rates are reduced, and bacterial population density increases.[50] Mature infections caused by gram-positive cocci respond poorly to delayed treatment. Effects of delayed treatment against *Bacteroides fragilis* have been demonstrated with metronidazole, clindamycin, cefoxitin, and moxalactam. Metronidazole was the least affected by delay. A group of β-lactam antimicrobial drugs, the penems, have good activity against slowly growing bacteria.[58] They have been used in animal patients, but their applicability in veterinary medicine will be better defined by results of well-designed studies.

A drug formulation administered to animals of different species or to different animals of the same species may have different pharmacokinetic characteristics. Pharmacokinetic characteristics may be altered by disease and can vary from animal to animal. Pharmacokinetic studies are usually performed with healthy animals; pharmacokinetics of drugs in diseased animals may be substantially different. Pharmacokinetic values are used to describe the time course of a drug in the body and to predict what will occur if the drug is administered to another animal. If predicted values do not accurately describe the time course in diseased animals, those predicted values are not acceptable and data from appropriately designed studies with diseased animals should supersede previous data. A calf with hypovolemic shock associated with gram-negative bacteremia and endotoxemia may have inadequate peripheral perfusion with subsequent inadequate absorption of drugs administered intramuscularly. Because of individual variation, this principle can be remembered as "the horse directs the course"[3] or "the cow dictates how."

A good example of this is found in the combination of trimethoprim and sulfadiazine. The pharmacokinetics of both drugs are relatively similar in both horses and cows. However, in cattle the time course and circulating concentrations of each drug differ significantly.[59-61] Absorption of trimethoprim appears to be the limiting factor affecting circulating concentrations of that drug when it is administered extravascularly. However, this should not be considered as an overall impediment to the efficacy of this combination of drugs. Efficacy has been demonstrated experimentally against salmonellosis in calves[61]; its efficacy against urinary tract infections cannot be adequately judged by circulating concentrations of these drugs.

PRINCIPLE 5: MONITOR RESULTS OF THERAPY

Surprisingly, optimal therapy (drug, dose, route, dosing interval, duration, and ancillary treatment) against pulmonary infections in people is unknown.[52] The same is probably true for infections in animals. It is extremely difficult to determine the minimally effective dosage regimen of a drug; therefore the veterinarian must monitor, by appropriate means, results of treatment.

Without monitoring the therapeutic response, the veterinarian is unable to assess success or failure of treatment. Assessment should continue throughout the treatment period.[9] Nonspecific and specific methods used to document infection can also be used to monitor therapeutic response. Intervals at which these procedures should be performed depend on the type, severity, and site of the infection. Clinical signs, hematologic changes, radiologic signs, results of microbiologic tests, and monitored concentrations of drugs are useful in assessing success of therapy. Measurement of concentrations of some antimicrobial drugs in serum or plasma is an aid to therapy and to reduce risks of toxicity.[47] Therapeutic drug monitoring is most applicable when patients are receiving aminoglycosides, have impaired function of organs of elimination or biotransformation of the drugs, or receive more than one drug, which may result in adverse interactions.[47,62] Therapeutic success against bacterial endocarditis is more likely when the patient's serum (with drug) will inhibit bacterial growth in a 1:8 or higher dilution and will kill the organisms in a 1:4 or higher dilution.[47,49] Critical concentrations of antimicrobial drug in serum for other infections have not been established but are generally targeted at concentrations that are severalfold higher than the MIC.

This points out the need for studies that evaluate the relationship between circulating concentrations of the drug and response to therapy. As with documentation of infection, interpretation of these data is important. Fever, other signs of inflammation, and even hematologic abnormalities can result from the therapy (drug-induced fever, leukocytosis) and may not be caused by infection.[9,63] Monitoring is the only means of determining clinical applicability of results of susceptibility tests in vitro and efficacy of the treatment used. Disparity between results in vitro and those in vivo is not uncommon.[49,50,57]

PRINCIPLE 6: INVESTIGATE CAUSES OF THERAPEUTIC FAILURE

Failure of treatment can result from one of several factors (Box 42-3). When response to treatment is not as expected, the cause should be sought, and the problem should be corrected. Potential for therapeutic failure can be decreased by applying principles outlined in this chapter, by considering the status of the host's defenses, by initiating appropriate treatment before the condition becomes irreversible, and by providing appropriate adjunctive therapy with drugs or by

lavage, drainage, or removal of foreign bodies from the site of infection. Conditions caused by bacteria will not respond to antiparasitic drugs; those caused by viruses, helminths, or fungi will not respond to antibacterial drugs; those caused by helminths will not respond to antifungal drugs. These examples serve to demonstrate inappropriate choice of drug, but equally inappropriate is the use of drugs to which the organisms are resistant, ineffective in the microenvironment, or do not distribute to sites of infection. Occasionally an infection that does not respond may be overcome by changing the dose of drug being used, the formulation, the route of administration, or the dosing interval or by prolonging the duration of treatment. Compliance with the selected dosage regimen is necessary before therapeutic success can be expected. Disease can alter host-related factors such as function of organs, perfusion, or inflammatory response, which affect absorption, distribution, biotransformation, and/or elimination of the drug. Because antimicrobial drugs act in concert with the host's defense mechanisms, any defect in these defenses can reduce the efficacy of antimicrobial drugs. A microenvironment that is inappropriate for activity of the drug, organisms that are resistant to the selected drug, or superinfection may also result in therapeutic failure. Interactions of drugs in vivo or in comixtures can alter pharmacokinetic variables of drugs or render them ineffective. Direct toxicity of antimicrobial drugs can be detrimental to the patient, as well as cause therapeutic failure. If the patient's condition has advanced to a point of irreversibility, any amount of appropriate therapy may be ineffective. Therapeutic failure is too frequently blamed on an inactive or "bad" drug. This is probably the least common cause of therapeutic failure if dates of expiration and conditions of storage of the drug are properly observed.

PRINCIPLE 7: RESTRICT CONCOMITANT USE OF ANTIMICROBIAL DRUGS

Fixed-drug combinations or concomitant use of two or more antimicrobial drugs is occasionally appropriate, as shown in Box 42-4.[9,49,50] However, in most instances one drug with a specific antimicrobial spectrum will provide adequate therapy and will reduce the potential of adverse effects in the patient or the potential for selection of resistant organisms. There are very few, if any, situations in which some fixed-drug combinations are superior to individual drugs. When used concomitantly against a specific organism or organisms, two or more antimicrobial drugs may be synergistic, additive, antagonistic, or indifferent in their effect. Selection of two or

---

BOX 42-3

Causes of Therapeutic Failure

Inappropriate diagnosis
Inappropriate drug
Inappropriate dosage regimen
Inappropriate absorption, distribution, biotransformation, or elimination of the drug
Impaired host's defense mechanisms
Inappropriate microenvironment
Development of resistance to the drug
Inadequate compliance to the dosage regimen
Superinfection
Interactions of drugs
Irreversible condition of the patient
Toxicity of the drug
Inactive drug

BOX 42-4

Concomitant Use of Antimicrobial Drugs

POTENTIALLY BENEFICIAL
Penicillin + aminoglycoside
Cephalosporin + aminoglycoside
Erythromycin + rifampin
Lincomycin + spectinomycin*
Trimethoprim + sulfonamide
Penicillin + sulfonamide
Tetracycline + sulfonamide
Penicillin + clavulanic acid

UNDESIRABLE
Penicillin + tetracycline
Chloramphenicol + erythromycin

*Potentially lethal complications may develop in horses or sheep that receive lincomycin.

more antimicrobial drugs for concomitant use should not be undertaken without considering their cumulative effects and the legitimate need for concomitant use of drugs. Too frequently, antimicrobial drugs are combined or used concomitantly to provide "broad-spectrum coverage" because of the attending veterinarian's diagnostic insecurity or to replace diagnostic procedures. Concomitant use of antimicrobial drugs should be limited to the following: to provide synergy against infecting organisms, to prevent bacterial resistance to antimicrobial drugs, to extend the antimicrobial spectrum as part of the initial therapy against life-threatening conditions, or to treat mixed-bacterial infections. Concomitant use of antimicrobial drugs beyond these situations is not justified, unnecessarily exposes the patient to risks of adverse reactions to drugs, and increases pressure for development of resistance to drugs by the infecting organism or others.

Synergy results when antimicrobial activity of two drugs in combination is greater than would be expected by the sum of the activity of the individual drugs. Synergy can result if the drugs act at different sites in the same metabolic pathway (e.g., trimethoprim + sulfonamide) or at different sites (i.e., 30S and 50S ribosomal subunits) in the organism. Activity of one drug may improve the entry of another drug into the organism (e.g., penicillin or cephalosporin + aminoglycoside) or prevent the degradation of another drug by the organism (e.g., amoxicillin + clavulanic acid). Synergistic combinations of antimicrobial drugs may be essential in some severe infections that are difficult to eradicate or infections in patients with temporarily impaired defense mechanisms. However, concomitant use of antimicrobial drugs is not necessary in routine treatment of most infections. Synergy does not imply that a "better" clinical response will result. Despite evidence of synergy between two drugs in vitro, convincing evidence that such synergistic combinations are superior to single drugs in vivo when treating defined infections is sadly lacking in veterinary medicine. Controlled, prospective clinical investigations designed to evaluate synergistic responses in vivo are desperately needed.

Antagonism has been demonstrated between penicillin and tetracycline.[9] In some instances, ampicillin and chloramphenicol were antagonistic, whereas in other instances they were therapeutically beneficial. Antimicrobial drugs that have the same or anatomically proximate site of action (chloramphenicol and erythromycin or erythromycin and lincomycin) should not be used concurrently because of antagonistic competition for those sites in bacteria.

If bacterial resistance to drugs occurs by mutation and with separate frequencies for two different antimicrobial drugs, the statistical probability that mutational resistance against both drugs will develop is inversely related to the product of the individual frequencies. Following this rationale, concomitant use of antimicrobial drugs has been most successfully applied in the treatment of infections caused by organisms in which resistance to single drugs develops rapidly. Resistance, against multiple drugs, encoded by plasmids should not be expected to follow this pattern. Data fail to support the popular belief that such a combination of drugs is necessary to avoid the development of resistance when there is evidence that resistance forms in face of this concomitant use. The *popularity* of combination treatments does not necessarily mean they are more efficacious than single-drug treatments.

It is justifiable and recommended to use more than one antimicrobial drug as initial treatment of life-threatening infections before results of bacterial cultures are known. This treatment should be based on the presumption that most, if not all, organisms that cause the infection will be susceptible to selected drugs and that withholding treatment will most likely result in death of the patient. Because such therapy is initiated before the etiologic agent and its susceptibility can be ascertained, it is imperative that all appropriate diagnostic samples be obtained before initiation of such treatment. It is important that historical or statistical data be taken into account when selecting the most probable etiologic agent(s). After the infectious agent and its susceptibility are known, treatment should be appropriately adjusted. Extended antimicrobial spectrum is too often abused as a substitute for collection of diagnostic data, because of the veterinarian's diagnostic insecurity or because of the client's insistence for treatment of the patient.

PRINCIPLE 8: ATTEND TO ADVERSE REACTIONS TO DRUGS

Adverse reactions to drugs can develop in patients as a result of drug-related or host-related factors.[9,63,64] Most can be classified as side effects of the drug, hypersensitivity to the drug or its metabolites, interactions of two or more drugs in vivo or incompatibilities in an admixture before administration, alterations of indigenous microflora by the drug, and direct toxic effects of the drug on the host's tissues or as idiosyncratic or idiopathic reactions that defy elucidation and classification.

Adverse effects are not always predictable and may not be side effects of the drug. Side effects of a drug are usually predictable because they result from the pharmacologic activity of the drug. For example, tetracycline may be selected primarily for its activity against a respiratory pathogen in a foal. Discolored dental enamel on permanent teeth may be an acceptable side effect, but altered intestinal microflora and fatal diarrhea are adverse effects.

All types of hypersensitivity reactions can occur in response to drugs. Clinical signs demonstrated by animals with hypersensitivity reactions to drugs are typical of those caused by other allergens. Because the molecular weight of most drugs is too small for the parent drug to serve as an allergen, polymers of the drug or its metabolites chemically combine with amino acids, polypeptides, or carbohydrates to form allergenic complexes. Polymers alone may be large enough to be allergenic. Figures regarding the frequency and type of hypersensitivity reactions in animal patients may not be representative because reports of such reactions are probably not complete. In the United States, adverse reactions to a drug in animal patients should be reported to the manufacturer of the product and to the FDA/CVM, (1-888-FDA-VETS; Form 1932a); or to the Veterinary Practitioners' Reporting Program of the US Pharmacopeia (1-800-4US-PPRN). It is the opinion of the authors that the manufacturer should be the first to be contacted. Manufacturers are the primary resource for data relative to their products and are usually equipped and staffed to respond to emergency clinical situations that may result from adverse reactions.

Interactions of drugs in vivo and incompatibilities of drugs in admixtures are possible when more than one drug is used.[64,65] Some interactions and incompatibilities are well known, and references of these data should be available. Pharmacists have considerable reference material to consult, and their input is extremely valuable in these matters. Before drugs are mixed or administered concurrently, interactions and compatibilities should be determined (Table 42-2). In this context, polyionic fluids, vitamins, minerals and other substances should all be considered as "drugs."

Alterations in indigenous microflora can reduce the effectiveness of natural host defenses, allow superinfection, or alter normal function of some bodily systems. Fibrinonecrotic colitis in horses that receive clindamycin or lincomycin is an example. This problem is serious enough that the use of these drugs is contraindicated in horses. Tetracyclines (especially doxycycline), macrolides, or potentiated sulfonamides can

TABLE 42-2

Specific Drugs and Additives That Are Incompatible When Comixed Before Administration[64,65]

Drug	pH	General Comments	Incompatibilities
Aminophylline	8-9	Not stable if pH <8	Cephalothin Na, tetracyclines, polyionic fluid solutions, penicillin G, morphine sulfate, erythromycin glucceptate, methylprednisolone Na succinate, multiple vitamin solutions, thiamine
Ammonium chloride	4.5-6.0		Chlortetracycline, sulfadiazine, sulfisoxazole
Ampicillin sodium	8.5-10	Do not mix with other medication because of pH changes	
Calcium chloride	6-8.2		Cephalothin Na, chlorpheniramine, hydrocortisone or prednisolone phosphate, kanamycin sulfate, tetracyclines, sodium bicarbonate (concentration dependent)
Calcium disodium EDTA	6.5-8.0		Dextrose solutions, tetracyclines
Calcium gluconate	6.0-8.2		Cephalothin Na, tetracyclines, prednisolone phosphate, sodium bicarbonate, phenylbutazone, sulfonamides
Carbenicillin disodium	6.0-7.0		Tetracyclines, aminoglycosides
Cephalothin sodium	5.2	pH <4.0 or >7.0 Not advised; do not mix with other medication	
Cyanocobalamin (vitamin B$_{12}$)	4.0-5.5		Alkaline solutions, ascorbic acid, vitamin B complex with C, vitamin K, warfarin
Dexamethasone phosphate	6.5-7.0		Chlorpromazine
Ergonovine maleate	2.7-3.5		Do not mix with other medications
Erythromycin lactobionate	6.5-7.5	Do not combine with mixtures having a final pH <5.0	Aminophylline, multiple vitamins, cephalothin Na, pentobarbital, sodium iodide, heparin Na, penicillin G, tetracyclines
Furosemide	8.8-9.3		Acid solutions
Gentamicin sulfate		Do not mix with other medications	
Heparin sodium	5.0-7.5		Sodium bicarbonate, multiple vitamins, tetracyclines, chlorpromazine or promazine, erythromycin lactobionate or glucceptate, gentamicin SO$_4$, hydrocortisone sodium succinate, methylprednisolone Na succinate, kanamycin SO$_4$, meperidine HCl, morphine SO$_4$, penicillin G (K$^+$), protamine
Hydrocortisone sodium succinate	7.0-8.0		Cephalothin Na, tetracyclines, heparin Na, kanamycin SO$_4$, multiple vitamins, pentobarbital Na, promazine, erythromycin, tylosin
Kanamycin sulfate	4.5		Cephalothin Na, dextrose, heparin Na, hydrocortisone Na succinate, penicillins, sulfadiazine
Levamisole			Neomycin, phenylbutazone, sulfonamides, tetracyclines
Lidocaine	6.0-7.0		Alkaline solutions
Magnesium sulfate	5.5-7.0		NaHCO$_3$, calcium-containing solutions, tetracyclines
Mannitol	4.5-7.0		Strongly acidic or alkaline solutions, whole blood, penicillin G

also alter the intestinal bacterial flora and thereby may precipitate potentially lethal diarrhea.[66,67] These drugs may be drugs of choice for treatment of some patients, and the adverse effects considered in context while formulating a strategy for treatment.

Toxic effects of antimicrobial drugs may not be predictable. Some drugs such as aminoglycosides or amphotericin B have predictable, dose-related toxicities. The ratio of toxic-to-therapeutic concentrations (therapeutic index) of drugs varies with the drug's properties and host-related factors that alter the patient's susceptibility to toxicity of the drug. If a drug with a low toxic-to-therapeutic ratio is chosen to treat an infection, its toxic and therapeutic effects should be closely monitored. If toxicity of a drug is predictable by its circulating concentrations, total amount of the drug administered, or duration of therapy, careful attention should be afforded these values. The greatest difficulty in predicting either efficacy or toxicity is knowing the minimum concentration of the drug that predictably causes each of these effects in the individual patient. Monitoring circulating concentrations of aminoglycosides is an essential aspect of therapy with these drugs because of their potential for causing toxicity and erratic pharmacokinetics in patients.[62,68] Amphotericin B is also predictably toxic and careful monitoring of its effects is necessary. Toxicity of drugs that require biotransformation for activation or inactivation can be enhanced or reduced by alterations in biotransformation resulting from disease or concomitantly administered drugs. Chondrotoxic effects of fluoroquinolones in adult and young horses is supported by results of some investigations[22,23] and refuted by others.[24,25,26] Perhaps an equally important question to be answered while trying to resolve discussions of occurrence of that arthrotoxicity is how well the insulted articular cartilage heals. Just as with disease, drug-injured tissue may regenerate and regain healthy function resulting in indistinguishable effects at a later date.

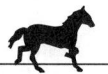

TABLE 42-2

Specific Drugs and Additives That Are Incompatible When Comixed Before Administration—cont'd

Drug	pH	General Comments	Incompatibilities
Methylprednisolone sodium succinate	7.0-8.0		Aminophylline, heparin Na, tetracyclines, vitamin B
Multiple vitamins			Aminophylline, cyanocobalamin, erythromycin lactobionate, heparin Na, hydrocortisone Na succinate, penicillin G, sodium bicarbonate, tetracyclines
Nitrofurantoin sodium	7.7-9.8		Calcium chloride, insulin, phenol, procaine
Oxytocin	2.5-4.5	Do not mix with other medications	
Penicillin G (K^+ or Na^+)	6.0-7.0	Significant inactivation if pH <5.5 or >8	Tetracyclines, acetylcysteine multiple vitamins, vitamin B with C, lincomycin, aminophylline, pentobarbital, thiopental, cephalothin Na, erythromycin, sodium bicarbonate, sulfonamides, heparin Na, gentamicin
Pentobarbital sodium	10.0-10.5		Acidic solutions, cephalothin Na, erythromycin, tetracyclines, sodium bicarbonate, succinylcholine chloride
Ringer's lactate solution	6.0-7.5		Epinephrine HCl, tetracyclines, sodium bicarbonate, sulfadiazine Na
Sodium bicarbonate	7.0-8.0		Calcium-containing solutions, magnesium sulfate, vitamin B with C, tetracyclines, penicillin G (Na or K), thiopental sodium, pentobarbital Na, streptomycin
Sodium iodide	7.5-9.0		Vitamin B with C
Succinylcholine chloride	3.0-4.5		Alkaline solutions, pentobarbital Na, thiopental Na
Sulfonamides	Basic		Acidic solutions, ammonium chloride, gentamicin SO_4, kanamycin SO_4, lincomycin HCl, methicillin, penicillin G, tetracyclines, vitamin B with C, calcium gluconate, dextrose, tylosin, procaine
Tetracyclines	1.8-2.8		Aminophylline, penicillins, magnesium or calcium salts, cephalothin Na, erythromycin, lactobionate, heparin Na, hydrocortisone Na succinate, methylprednisolone Na succinate, multiple vitamins, nitrofurantoin, novobiocin, polymixin B, lactated Ringer's or Ringer's solution, sodium bicarbonate, sulfonamides, barbiturates
Thiamine (vitamin B_1)	3.0-4.0	Neutral or alkaline pH causes decomposition	Iron salts
Thiopental sodium	10.0-11.0		Acidic solutions, promazine HCl, sodium bicarbonate, succinylcholine Cl, atropine SO_4, penicillins, cephalosporins, tetracyclines, hydrocortisone Na succinate
Ticarcillin disodium	6.0-8.0		Aminoglycosides
Tylosin			Hydrocortisone, tetracycline, streptomycin, sulfonamides
Vitamin B complex	10.0-11.0		Alkaline solutions, cephalothin Na, cyanocobalamin, erythromycin lactobionate, hydrocortisone Na succinate, tetracyclines
Vitamin B complex with C	3.0-6.5		Aminophylline, cephalothin Na, erythromycin lactobionate

Frequently the true pathogenesis of an adverse effect is not known. It may not be clearly related to the drug or may not have been observed previously. Because drug-related reactions in animals are iatrogenic, reasonable suspicion that a reaction could be drug related should be maintained until proven otherwise. Observations and thoroughness of investigation by the attending clinician remains the best means of establishing the cause-effect relationship of drug-induced reactions. That diagnosis is often arrived at by a process of elimination of other potential causes.

REFERENCES

1. Hirsh DC, Ruehl WW: A rational approach to the selection of an antimicrobial agent, *J Am Vet Med Assoc* 185:1058-1061, 1984.
2. Davis LE: Rational therapeutics. In Mansmann RA, McAllister ES, Pratt PW, eds: *Equine medicine and surgery*, ed 3, Santa Barbara, 1982, American Veterinary Publications, pp 131-135.
3. Brumbaugh GW: Rational selection of antimicrobial drugs for treatment of infections of horses, *Vet Clin North Am (Equine Pract)* 3:191-220, 1987.
4. Knifton A: Criteria for selection of antibiotics, *Vet Rec* 114:357-360, 1984.
5. Edwards DI: Principles of antimicrobial drug action. In Edward DI, ed: *Antimicrobial drug action*, Baltimore, 1980, University Park Press, pp 8-30.
6. Jawetz E: Antimicrobial drugs: mechanisms and factors influencing their action. In Kagan BM, ed: *Antimicrobial therapy*, ed 3, Philadelphia, 1980, WB Saunders, pp 3-10.
7. Jones TC, Hunt RD: Healing and regeneration. In Jones TC, Hunt RD, eds: *Veterinary pathology*, ed 5, Philadelphia, 1983, Lea & Febiger, pp 211-212.
8. Smith H: The chemotherapeutic potential of inhibition or circumvention of the determinants of microbial pathogenicity. In Greenwood D, O'Grady R, eds: *The scientific basis of antimicrobial chemotherapy*, Thirty-eighth Symposium of the Society for General Microbiology, New York, 1985, The Press Syndicate of the University of Cambridge, pp 367-393.
9. Root RK, Hierholzer WJ: Infectious disease. In *Clinical pharmacology: basic principles of therapeutics*, ed 2, New York, 1978, Macmillan, pp 709-801.
10. Weinstein AJ: Common sense (clinical judgment) in the diagnosis and antibiotic therapy of etiologically undefined infections. In Kagan BM, ed: *Antimicrobial therapy*, ed 3, Philadelphia, 1980, WB Saunders, pp 193-200.
11. Evans AS: Epidemiological concepts and methods. In *Viral infections of humans, epidemiology and control*, New York, 1982, Plenum, pp 3-42.
12. Mercer HD: Residue avoidance: withdrawal times for drugs not labeled for food animals, *Proceedings of the Tenth Annual Food Animal Medicine Conferences: The Use of Drugs in Food Animal Medicine*, 1984, Columbus, 1985, The Ohio State University Press, pp 7-24.

13. Coleman DL, Ryan JL: Modulation of the immune response by antimicrobial agents. In RK Root, MA Sande, eds: *New dimensions in antimicrobial therapy: contemporary issues in infectious diseases,* vol 1, New York, 1984, Churchill Livingstone, pp 277-292.

14. Yourtee EL, Root RK: Effect of antibiotics on phagocyte-microbe interactions. In Root RK, Sande MA, eds: *New dimensions in antimicrobial therapy: contemporary issues in infectious diseases,* vol 1, New York, 1984, Churchill Livingstone, pp 243-275.

15. Hunsaker B: Immune function of calves vaccinated intradermally against bovine herpesvirus type 1. Dissertation, 1999, Texas A&M University.

16. Chin AC et al: Anti-inflammatory benefits of tilmicosin in calves with *Pasturella haemolytica*-infected lungs, *Am J Vet Res* 59:765-771, 1998.

17. Mirkin BL: Pharmacodynamics and drug disposition in pregnant women, in neonates, and in children. In Melmon KL, Morrelli HF, eds: *Clinical pharmacology: basic principles in therapeutics,* ed 2, New York, 1978, MacMillan, pp 127-152.

18. Papich MG, Davis LE: Drug therapy during pregnancy and in the neonate, *Vet Clin North Am (Small Anim Pract)* 16:525-538, 1986.

19. Fenger CK et al: Equine protozoal myeloencephalitis: Findings from a retrospective study, *Proceedings of the Forty-second Annual Convention of the American Association of Equine Practitioners,* 1996, pp 80-81.

20. Bedford SJ, McDonnell SM: Semen, testicular volume, sperm production efficiency, and sexual behavior of stallions treated with trimethoprim-sulfamethoxazole and pyrimethamine, *Proceedings of the Forty-fourth Annual Convention of the American Association of Equine Practitioners,* 1998, pp 1-2.

21. Crisman MV et al: Concentrations of phenylbutazone and oxyphenbutazone in postparturient mares and their neonatal foals, *J Vet Pharmacol Ther* 14:330-334, 1991.

22. Langston VC, Sedrish S, Boothe DM: Disposition of single-dose oral enrofloxacin in the horse, *J Vet Pharmacol Ther* 19:316-319, 1996.

23. Beluche LA et al: In vitro dose-dependent effects of enrofloxacin on equine articular cartilage, *Am J Vet Res* 60:577-582, 1999.

24. Giguere S, Sweeney RW. Belanger M: Pharmacokinetics of enrofloxacin in adult horses and concentration of the drug in serum, body fluids, and endometrial tissues after repeated intragastrically administered doses, *Am J Vet Res* 57:1025-1030, 1996.

25. Kaartinen L, Panu S, Pyorala S: Pharmacokinetics of enrofloxacin in horses after single intravenous and intramuscular administration, *Equine Vet J* 29:378-381, 1997.

26. Dowling PM et al: Pharmacokinetics of ciprofloxacin in ponies, *J Vet Pharmacol Therap* 18:7-12, 1995.

27. Gingerich DA: Pharmacokinetics of drugs used for therapy of the mammary gland. *Proceedings of the Tenth Annual Food Animal Medicine Conference: The Use of Drugs in Food Animal Medicine,* Columbus, 1985, Ohio State University Press, pp 117-135.

28. Ziv G, Shani J, Sulman FG: Pharmacokinetic evaluation of penicillin and cephalosporin derivatives in serum and milk of lactating cows and ewes, *Am J Vet Res* 34:1561-1565, 1973.

29. Rasmussen F: Mammary excretion of benzylpenicillin, erythromycin, and penethamate hydroiodide, *Acta Pharmacol Toxicol* 16:194-200, 1959.

30. Ziv G, Sulman FG: Distribution of aminoglycoside antibiotics in blood and milk, *Res Vet Sci* 17:68-74, 1974.

31. Ziv G, Sulman FG: Penetration of lincomycin and clindamycin into milk in ewes, *Br Vet J* 129:83-90, 1973.

32. Ziv G, Sulman FG: Serum and milk concentrations of spectinomycin and tylosin in cows and ewes, *Am J Vet Res* 34:329-333, 1973.

33. Rasmussen F: Mammary excretion of sulphonamides, *Acta Pharmacol Toxicol* 15:139-148, 1958.

34. Stowe CM, Sisodia GS: The pharmacologic properties of sulfadimethoxine in dairy cattle, *Am J Vet Res* 24:525-535, 1963.

35. Sisodia CS, Stowe CM: The mechanism of drug secretion into bovine milk, *Ann NY Acad Sci* 111:559-812, 1964.

36. Rasmussen F: Renal and mammary excretion of trimethoprim in goats, *Vet Rec* 87:14-18, 1970.

37. Available from www.fda.gov/cvm/fda/infores/AMDUCA/5340.html.

38. AVMA backs up FDA's defense of animal-drug regulation policies, *J Am Vet Med Assoc* 188:465-471, 1986.

39. Martinez MN: Article IV: Clinical application of pharmacokinetics. Special series: use of pharmacokinetics in veterinary medicine, *J Am Vet Med Assoc* 213:1418-1420, 1998.

40. Deckar WM, Peters PF, eds: Congressional committee alleges policies violate Food, Drug, and Cosmetic Act and encourage illegal use of drugs by veterinarians. In *Veterinary Medical News From Washington,* 1985, American Veterinary Medicine Association, July 31, pp 1-3.

41. FDA spells out extra-label use guidelines, *J Am Vet Med Assoc* 185:950, 1984.

42. Lofgreen, GP: Mass medication in reducing shipping fever-bovine respiratory complex in highly stressed calves, *J Anim Sci* 56:529-536, 1983.

43. Walton JR: Principles of treatment of respiratory disease including herd medication, *Pig Vet Soc Proc* 9:71-76, 1982.

44. Paulson JA, Gordon IB, Mortimer EA: Prophylactic antibiotics. In Kagan BM, ed: *Antimicrobial therapy,* ed 3, Philadelphia, 1980, WB Saunders, pp 468-480.

45. Wilkowske CJ, Hermans PE: General principles of antimicrobial therapy, *Mayo Clin Proc* 58:6-13, 1983.

46. Orsini JA: Principles of antimicrobial selection for horses, *Mod Vet Pract* 67:719-724, 1986.

47. Rosenblatt JE: Laboratory tests used to guide antimicrobial therapy, *Mayo Clin Proc* 58:14-20, 1983.

48. Cox HU et al: Comparison of antibiograms determined by disk diffusion and microdilution methods for selected gram-negative bacilli, *Am J Vet Res* 42:546-551, 1981.

49. Washington JA: Susceptibility tests. In Kagan BM, ed: *Antimicrobial therapy,* ed 3, Philadelphia, 1980, WB Saunders, pp 11-19.

50. Ernst JD, Sande MA: In vitro susceptibility testing and the outcome of treatment of infection. In Root RK, Sande MA, eds: *New dimensions in antimicrobial therapy and contemporary issues in infectious diseases,* vol 1, New York, 1984, Churchill Livingstone.

51. Hewitt WM: The agar diffusion assay. In *Microbiological assay: an introduction to quantitative principles and evaluation,* New York, 1977, Academic Press, pp 17-69.

52. Neu HC: Optimal antibiotic therapy in bronchopulmonary infections, *Infection* 1(suppl):62-69, 1980.

53. Baggott JD et al: Selection of an aminoglycoside antibiotic for administration to horses, *Equine Vet J* 17:30-34, 1985.

54. Brown SA: Minimum inhibitory concentrations and postantimicrobial effects as factors in dosage of antimicrobial drugs, *J Am Vet Med Assoc* 191:871-872, 1987.

55. Bryant RE: Effect of the suppurative environment on antibiotic activity. In Root RK, Sande MA, eds: *New dimensions in antimicrobial therapy: contemporary issues in infectious diseases,* vol 1, New York, 1984, Churchill Livingstone, pp 313-337.

56. Sears PM, Fettinger M, Marsh-Salin J: Isolation of L-form variants after antibiotic treatment in *Staphylococcus aureus* bovine mastitis, *J Am Vet Med Assoc* 191:681-684, 1987.

57. Wormser GP, Keusch GT: Trimethoprim-sulfamethoxazole in the United States, *Ann Intern Med* 91:420-429, 1979.

58. Tuomanen, E: Antibiotics which kill nongrowing bacteria, *TIPS* 8:121-122, 1987.

59. Guard CL, Schwark WS, Friedman DS, et al: Age-related alterations in trimethoprim-sulfadiazine disposition following oral or parenteral administration in calves, *Can J Vet Res* 50:342-346, 1986.

60. Shoaf SE, Schwark WS, Guard CL: The effect of age and diet on sulfadiazine-trimethoprim disposition following oral and subcutaneous administration to calves, *J Vet Pharmacol Ther* 10:331-345, 1987.

61. White G, Piercy, DWT, Gibbs, HA: Use of a calf salmonellosis model to evaluate the therapeutic properties of trimethoprim and sulfadiazine and their mutual potentiation in vivo, *Res Vet Sci* 31:27-31, 1981.

62. Sojka JE, Brown SA: Pharmacokinetic adjustment of gentamicin dosing in horses with sepsis, *J Am Vet Med Assoc* 189:784-789, 1986.

63. Davis LE: Adverse drug reactions in the horse, *Vet Clin North Am (Equine Pract)* 3:153-179, 1987.

64. Paul JW: Drug interactions and incompatibilities, *Vet Clin North Am (Equine Pract)* 3:145-151, 1987.

65. Davis LE: Pharmacology. In *Veterinary values,* ed 2, New York, 1985, Ag Resources, pp 35-96.

66. Owen RH, Fullerton J, Barnum DA: Effects of transportation, surgery, and antibiotic therapy in ponies infected with *Salmonella, Am J Vet Res* 44:46-50, 1983.

67. White G, Prior SD: Comparative effects of oral administration of trimethoprim-sulfadiazine or oxytetracycline on the faecal flora of horses, *Vet Rec* 111:316-318, 1982.

68. Martin-Jimenez T, Papich MG, Riviere JE. Population pharmacokinetics of gentamicin in horses, *Am J Vet Res* 59:1589-1598, 1998.

PROPHYLACTIC USE OF ANTIMICROBIAL DRUGS

GORDON W. BRUMBAUGH

Despite apparently widespread administration of antimicrobial drugs to prevent disease, prophylactic use of antimicrobial drugs remains controversial and of unproven value in many instances.[69] Far too frequently veterinarians and lay personnel use antimicrobial drugs prophylactically because of concern over diagnostic accuracy. Although indiscriminate use of antimicrobial drugs to prevent disease should be condemned, prophylaxis can be useful in certain circumstances.[70] Unfortunately these circumstances have not been well defined in veterinary medicine, partly because of difficulties in assessing response to microbial prophylaxis.[71] If a beneficial effect results from prophylactic use of drugs, the therapist is enticed to repeat their administration when later presented with a similar situation. For example, antimicrobial drugs may be administered to horses with viral upper respiratory disease to

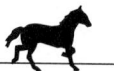

prevent secondary bacterial pneumonia. If the horse does not develop pneumonia, it is assumed that the antimicrobial drug prevented bacterial pneumonia. Therefore the next horse that demonstrates signs of upper respiratory disease will receive antimicrobial drugs prophylactically. This is not sound reasoning nor is it justification for prophylactic use of antimicrobial drugs. That horse may not have developed pneumonia if the antimicrobial drugs had been withheld. Seldom is a determination made about whether a result is "because of" or "in spite of" the prophylactic use of medication.

In some instances, antimicrobial drugs are used prophylactically with guidance by clinical impressions. Unfortunately, objective data to support such uses are not always available. Controlled, blinded, prospective clinical investigations are of paramount importance for obtaining that information.[71] Proper performance of such studies is difficult. The multitude of factors involved with such studies (e.g., large numbers of patients, criteria for selection of patients, confirmatory diagnostic procedures, choice of "appropriate controls," variables to be evaluated, dosage regimens and ancillary measures to be used) result in a complexity that serves as a discouragement to most veterinarians who initially desire to embark on such studies. An additional factor that complicates studies of the efficacy of antimicrobial drugs perioperatively is that historical incidences of infection may not be reliable controls because surgical techniques vary among surgeons and have changed because of advances in surgical materials and procedures. Therefore prophylactic use of antimicrobial drugs in many situations remains a matter of opinion, risk, and concern based on conditions pertaining to the individual patient rather than a matter of fact that is universally applicable. Consequently, recommendations for prophylactic use of antimicrobial drugs should not be dogmatic.

However, principles for prophylactic use of antimicrobial drugs in each situation are the same. Antimicrobial drugs are occasionally used in animals to prevent coccidiosis, clostridial infection of wounds, bacterial pneumonia, and bacterial infections following orthopedic or intraabdominal surgical procedures. Morbidity and mortality associated with coccidiosis was reduced in susceptible calves by preexposure administration of monensin.[72] The incidence of clostridial infections in untreated wounds is not accurately known. Specific immunity in the host, complicating factors, use of biologics, and ancillary procedures influence the incidence and severity of such infections. Because clostridial organisms produce severe and often lethal infections, the risk of fatal vegetative infection warrants the prophylactic use of antimicrobial drugs in high-risk patients. However, antimicrobial drugs should not be considered a substitute for active immunization provided by biologic products or for proper local treatment of the wound.

Antimicrobial drugs used prophylactically are perhaps used most to prevent bacterial pneumonia. It has been stated that viral respiratory diseases predispose the respiratory tract to secondary bacterial infections. Concerns that viral infections predispose the entire respiratory tract to bacterial infection are based on the fact that the former can destroy ciliated epithelium and inhibit mucociliary clearance mechanisms, reduce production of surfactant, promote virulence of bacteria, and inhibit phagocytic activity against some bacteria.[73-76] But the efficacy of antibacterial mechanisms in preventing bacterial superinfections appears to depend on the bacteria and the virus(es) involved.

All viral pneumonias do not result in bacterial superinfections; conditions must be appropriate for that to occur.[74] One investigator proposed that the secondary bacterial infection of the upper respiratory tract was probably "beneficial in the total infection experience" of the young horse entering training or racing.[77] In spite of these data the true incidence and risk-related factors surrounding secondary bac-

terial infections are not known. Several controlled prospective studies have evaluated prophylactic use of a few antimicrobial drugs against respiratory disease in cattle. Similar, but limited, studies performed with horses have shown that some transported horses may benefit from prophylactic use of antimicrobial drugs.[78]

Prevention of bovine respiratory disease complex (BRDC) with antimicrobial drugs has been studied intensely for several years.[79-86] Nevertheless, effects of prophylactic use of antimicrobial drugs in BRDC and recommendations for such use are far from universal. Many factors contribute to prevention of BRDC: vaccination history of the animals, environment, diet, duration of shipment, time of initial medication after arrival, number of calves per group, commingling of animals from different sites of origin, condition of the calves, method of administration of medication (by injection, in water, or in feed), duration of administration, and sequence of administration if more than one antimicrobial drug was used.

Morbidity and mortality of calves with BRDC that required subsequent therapeutic medication were reduced by daily injections of chlortetracycline (11 mg/kg IM for 3 days) prophylactically, but calves that required subsequent medication needed more treatments than did animals that had not received prophylactic medication.[87] Days of treatment per newly arrived calf were reduced by sulfadimethoxine (150 mg/kg PO once daily for 3 days).[80] Days of treatment were further reduced when injections of chlortetracycline were followed by the regimen with sulfadimethoxine described earlier. Feed efficiency and weight gain of newly arrived feeder steers were variably affected by dose and duration of prophylactic administration of chlortetracycline orally.[84] However, there was no difference in the amount of therapeutic medical attention required among experimental groups. One survey showed that many factors complicate assessment of prophylactic use of antimicrobial drugs against BRDC.[82] After effects of several factors were controlled analytically, medicated starter rations were associated with decreased mortality but were unrelated to morbidity in newly arrived feeder cattle. Medicated water significantly increased incidence of mortality.

The prophylactic effect of one injection of tilmicosin 10 mg/kg SC or 20 mg of oxytetracycline in 2-pyrrolidone per kilogram intramuscularly against pneumonia was evaluated with a large group of feeder calves.[86] Morbidity and mortality were significantly lower in the group that received tilmicosin compared to morbidity and mortality in the group that received oxytetracycline or the group that received no prophylactic antimicrobial drug (controls). Treatment of pneumonia was significantly delayed for calves that received either antimicrobial drug relative to that for calves that received no prophylaxis. Calves that did not need treatment for pneumonia gained significantly more weight than did calves that received either antimicrobial drug, but calves that received tilmicosin gained significantly more weight than did calves that received oxytetracycline.

Instability of the cattle market, cost of feed, and cost of the antimicrobial drugs necessitated consideration of the cost effectiveness of prophylactic use of antimicrobial drugs. In one study, preshipment medication (one dose of oxytetracycline in 2-pyrrolidone 19.8 mg/kg IM) of feeder cattle reduced the incidence of morbidity but not of mortality or of relapses of bovine respiratory disease.[85] An economic advantage of $0.45 per head was realized for the medicated calves.

It is apparent from results of these studies that prophylactic use of antimicrobial drugs can be beneficial, but it is unrealistic to expect total prevention of a disease. Control or management of a disease and its effects would be more realistic. The effect desired from prophylactic use of drugs must be specifically understood. Reduced morbidity or mortality, reduced severity of clinical signs, reduced duration of therapy, improved growth rate, improved feed efficiency, and improved or maintained production may be benefits of prophylactic use of antimicrobial drugs, but false confidence in prevention of disease should be avoided. Volatility of costs associated with production and the market probably influence profit more than does the cost of prophylactic use of antimicrobial drugs. It has been taught and generally believed that bacterial infection is a major complication secondary to viral respiratory disease.[74] The author has treated patients with bacterial pneumonia, pleuropneumonia, sinusitis, guttural pouch infections, or lymphadenopathies that had medical histories compatible with a viral respiratory infection. However, the author has also had numerous individual patients, as well as groups of stabled horses, in which no bacterial complications occurred following viral respiratory infections (diagnosed serologically) when antimicrobial drugs were not used prophylactically.

Ambiguity of antimicrobial prophylaxis is supported in part by a review of reports of experimentally induced as well as naturally occurring equine rhinopneumonitis and equine influenza. Equine herpesvirus-1 produces viral bronchopneumonia[88] and interstitial pneumonia.[89] Serous-to-mucopurulent rhinitis was observed commonly and was similar with equine influenza.[73,77,88,90-94] Secondary bacterial infections were confined to the upper respiratory tract (i.e., rhinitis, lymphadenopathy) and did not include bacterial pneumonia.[87,90,92,93]

Perioperative use of antimicrobial drugs prophylactically is a common practice. In human patients, such use has proven to be of benefit in prosthetic cardiac valvular operations, gynecologic surgical procedures, and gastrointestinal operations.[71] The drugs were administered orally, systemically, or topically as indicated by the procedure. A study with 122 dogs and 7 cats undergoing elective, clean surgical procedures revealed no significant difference in incidence of infection between a group that received ampicillin and a group that received a placebo.[95] Similar studies with horses are not known to the author at this time. Principles for prophylactic use of antimicrobial drugs perioperatively are similar to those outlined here.

When antimicrobial drugs are used prophylactically, there are several principles that should be followed.[69-71,96-99]

1. The relative risk of infection must be sufficient to warrant the use of antimicrobial drugs prophylactically. Risks of the prophylactic medication must be less than risks of development of the disease and consequences of that disease.

    Risks of infection are related to virulence of the organism, amount of exposure (size of inoculum and duration), and the host's defense status. All these factors should be considered before using antimicrobial drugs prophylactically. "Sufficient risk" is difficult to clarify because of numerous factors used to assess risk. Mortality or morbidity, severity of the disease, duration of the disease, or the effects of the disease on production or performance may be considered unacceptable in some situations if prophylaxis is not implemented. However, risks and costs of the prophylactic medication must also be considered. There is a paucity of epidemiologic data from which to accurately predict these risk factors; therefore they must be assessed on an individual basis. The primary potential advantage of prophylactic use of antimicrobial drugs is prevention of infection; but other advantages are also possible and include decreased morbidity and/or mortality, decreased duration of treatment if infection occurs, decreased severity of disease, shortened convalescence, improved or maintained production and decreased cost of overall effects of disease. Potential disadvantages of prophylactic use of antimicrobial drugs include alteration of resident bacterial flora, development of resistant organisms, superinfection, delayed onset of infection, relaxed attention to diagnostic details, adverse reactions to the drug(s), and increased overall cost of therapy.

2. Organism(s) that are likely to cause infection, and their antimicrobial susceptibility should be known or accurately predicted. Just as biologic products are used prophylactically to stimulate specific active or passive immunity, prophylactic use of antimicrobial drugs should be directed at a specific pathogen rather than at all possible organisms. It is difficult to anticipate all possible infectious organisms that are likely to be encountered, but agents that cause some diseases are reasonably predictable. It is preposterous to expect sterilization of the site of potential infection. The antimicrobial susceptibility of the pathogen should be consistently predictable on the basis of historical data. Clostridial and streptococcal organisms are not as predictably susceptible to penicillin as they were in the past. The susceptibility of gram-negative, aerobic organisms is not reliably predictable, and resistance develops frequently when these bacteria are continuously or intermittently exposed to antimicrobial drugs. Anaerobes are predictably susceptible to penicillin G, chloramphenicol, metronidazole or lincosamides.[100] Lincosamides should not be used systemically in horses; chloramphenicol and metronidazole are prohibited in the United States for administration to animals that are used for human consumption. *Bacteroides fragilis* produces β-lactamase rendering those organisms resistant to penicillins. Aminopenicillins and cephalosporins that are classified greater than first-generation have less predictable activity against anaerobes than does penicillin G.[101]

3. The drug must be administered and must distribute to the site of potential infection before the onset of infection and should at least reach inhibitory concentrations. After infection is established, the use of the drug becomes therapeutic, not prophylactic. Therefore the time of exposure or contamination with a pathogen, incubation time of the pathogen, and distribution characteristics of the selected drug should be considered in order to administer an antimicrobial drug prophylactically and in a timely manner.

4. As much as possible, drugs used prophylactically should not be those that would be used therapeutically if an infection develops. If infection develops during the prophylactic regimen, an alternative treatment must be formulated, because if the disease is not prevented by an appropriate dosage regimen with the drug, it will not be cured by the drug. If that infection is caused by induced resistance to the selected drug, therapy could be compromised if that drug is the therapeutic drug of choice. The population of resistant organisms poses risks of increased incidence of refractory infections in other animals as well.

5. The duration of antimicrobial prophylaxis should be as abbreviated as possible (e.g., 3 to 6 hours postoperatively). Generally, little benefit can be gained beyond 24 to 36 hours postoperatively. If exposure to infectious organisms is brief and host defenses are functional, prolonged administration of the drug is not necessary. However, there are a few indications for prolonged prophylactic therapy. If host defenses are temporarily deficient or if exposure is prolonged, administration may need to be extended. The duration of administration should be directed by the same factors that direct the duration of therapeutic use of drugs (i.e., activity of the host's defenses, ability of the organism to resist those defenses, mechanisms by which the organism develops resistance to the drug(s), location of the infection, and primary activity of the drug against the organism).

6. No drug can be used without risk of adverse reactions, but antimicrobial drugs used prophylactically should present

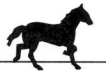

minimal risk of adverse effects. Deleterious reactions may occur when drugs are administered. It is better to abstain from using drugs than to use them inappropriately.

7. Theoretically, the selected dosage regimen should provide bactericidal rather than bacteriostatic concentrations of the drug at the site of infection. It would be desirable to kill the pathogen rather than to inhibit its growth; however, this may not be necessary in clinical situations. Host defenses, subtherapeutic concentrations of the drug, and postantibiotic effects, as well as ancillary management, should be used to enhance the efficacy of drugs in vivo.

Decisions about prophylactic use of antimicrobial drugs are not easily made and are usually based on logic and analogous situations.[70] Classification of clinical circumstances and diseases of human patients has been proposed as an aid to such decisions for that species. That classification considers the risk of developing infection based on function of the patient's natural defenses, duration of exposure to pathogens, and potential for infection by either one or multiple organisms. Direct application of that classification system to animal patients may be difficult.

Assessment of some defense mechanisms in domestic animal patients is complicated and beyond routine use in many clinical situations. Some pathogens are noted for their ability to temporarily compromise the host's defenses, yet effects of others are unknown. Methods that are applicable (i.e., determination of concentrations of immunoglobulins, numbers and function of phagocytes and of lymphocytes) should be used when indicated and when appropriate medical management is determined. However, numbers of cells do not equate with function, and concentrations of immunoglobulins do not equate with specific activity. Animal patients must convalesce in an environment that is less hygienic than that of human patients. Animals are constantly exposed to many primary and opportunistic pathogens (bacteria, viruses, fungi, parasites) and intermittently exposed to individual pathogens, which cause diseases of epizootic proportions. Therefore criteria for classification by risk of infection and indications for prophylactic use of antimicrobial drugs in animals need to be developed from epidemiologic studies of diseases of animals and controlled clinical investigations. At this time, that information is sadly lacking.

Except in specific instances with specific goals in mind, the use of antimicrobial agents to prevent infection has not been as valuable as the therapeutic use of antimicrobials. Prophylactic use of antimicrobial drugs must be tailored to the specific needs of each individual patient, as determined by the attending veterinarian and tempered by application of the principles outlined here.

REFERENCES

69. Root RK, Hierholzer WJ: Infectious disease. In Melmon KL, Morrell HF, eds: *Clinical pharmacology: basic principles of therapeutics,* ed 2, New York, 1978, Macmillan, pp 709-801.
70. Paulson JA, Gordon IB, Mortimer EA: Prophylactic antibiotics. In Kagan BM, ed: *Antimicrobial therapy,* ed 3, Philadelphia, 1980, WB Saunders, pp 468-480.
71. Van Scoy RE, Wilkowske CJ: Prophylactic use of antimicrobial agents, *Mayo Clin Proc* 58:241-245, 1983.
72. Watkins LE et al: The prophylactic effects of monensin fed to cattle inoculated with *Coccidia oocysts, Agri Pract* 7:18-20, 1986.
73. Bryans JT: Application of management procedures and prophylactic immunization to the control of equine rhinopneumonitis. *Proceedings of the Twenty-seventh Annual Convention American Association of Equine Practitioners,* 1981, pp 259-272.
74. Jakab GJ: Mechanisms of virus-induced bacterial superinfections of the lung, *Clin Chest Med* 2:59-66, 1981.
75. Sweet C, Smith H: Pathogenicity of influenza virus, *Microbiol Rev* 44:303-330, 1980.
76. Austin SM, Foreman JH, Hungerford LL: Case-control study of risk factors for development of pleuropneumonia in horses, *J Am Vet Med Assoc* 207:325-328, 1995.
77. Doll ER: Immunization against viral rhinopneumonitis of horses with live virus propagated in hamsters, *J Am Vet Med Assoc* 139:1324-1330, 1961.
78. Foreman JH: Practical aspects of the use of ceftiofur sodium in the treatment of equine respiratory infections, *Proceedings of the Thirty-ninth Annual Convention of the American Association of Equine Practitioners,* 1993, pp 307-310.
79. Camp TH et al: Transit factors afflicting shrink, shipping fever and subsequent performance of feeder calves, *J Anim Sci* 52:1219-1224, 1981.
80. Lofgreen GP: Mass medication in reducing shipping fever—bovine respiratory complex in highly stressed calves, *J Anim Sci* 56:529-536, 1983.
81. Lofgreen GP et al: Energy level in starting rations for calves subjected to marketing and shipping stress, *J Anim Sci* 41:1256-1265, 1975.
82. Martin SW: A mail survey of the efficacy of prophylactic medication in feed and/or water of feedlot calves, *Can J Comp Med* 49:15-20, 1985.
83. Perry TW et al: Value of chlortetracycline and sulfamethazine for conditioning cattle after transit, *J Anim Sci* 32:137-140, 1971.
84. Perry TW et al: Use of chlortetracycline for treatment of new feedlot cattle, *J Anim Sci* 62:1215-1219, 1986.
85. Bennett BW, Rupp GP, McCormick RM: Pre-shipment preventive medication of calves with liquamycin at weaning, *Agri-Pract* 4:6-10, 1983.
86. Morck DW et al: Prophylactic efficacy of tilmicosin for bovine respiratory tract disease, *J Am Vet Med Assoc* 202:273-277, 1993.
87. Lofgreen GP, Stinocher LH, Kiesling HE: Effects of dietary energy, free choice alfalfa hay, and mass medication on calves subjected to marketing and shipping stress, *J Anim Sci* 50:590-596, 1980.
88. Allen GP, Bryans JT: Molecular epizootiology, pathogenesis, and prophylaxis of equine herpesvirus-I infections, *Prog Vet Microbiol Immunol* 2:78-144, 1986.
89. Bryans JT et al: Neonatal foal diseases associated with perinatal infection by equine herpesvirus I, *J Equine Med Surg* 1:20-25, 1977.
90. Bryans JT: Herpesviral diseases affecting reproduction in the horse, *Vet Clin North Am (Large Anim Pract)* 2:303-312, 1980.
91. Coggins L: Viral respiratory disease, *Vet Clin North Am (Large Anim Pract)* 1:59-71, 1979.
92. Doll ER, Wallace ME, Richards MG: Thermal, hematological, and serological responses of weanling horses following inoculation with equine abortion virus: its similarity to equine influenza, *Cornell Vet* 44:181-190, 1954.
93. Doll ER, Bryans JT: Immunization of young horses against viral rhinopneumonitis, *Cornell Vet* 53:24-41, 1963.
94. Doll ER, Bryans JT: Epizootiology of equine viral rhinopneumonitis, *J Am Vet Med Assoc* 142:31-37, 1963.
95. Vasseur PB et al: Infection rates in clean surgical procedures: a comparison of ampicillin prophylaxis vs a placebo, *J Am Vet Med Assoc* 187:825-827, 1985.
96. Danziger L, Hassan E: Antimicrobial prophylaxis of gastrointestinal surgical procedures and treatment of intraabdominal infections, *Drug Intell Clin Pharm* 21:406-416, 1987.
97. Wilkowske CJ, Hermans PE: General principles of antimicrobial therapy, *Mayo Clin Proc* 58:6-13, 1983.
98. Riviere JE, Kaufman GM, Bright RM: Prophylactic use of systemic antimicrobial drugs in surgery, *Compend Cont Educ* 3:345-354, 1981.
99. van den Bogaard AEJM, Weidema WF: Antimicrobial prophylaxis in veterinary surgery, *J Am Vet Med Assoc* 186:990-992, 1985.
100. Brumbuagh GW. Antimicrobial therapy of adult horses with emergency conditions, *Vet Clin North Am (Equine Pract)* 10:527-534, 1994.
101. Sanitz EM, Jang SS, Hirsh DC: In vitro susceptibilites of selected obligate anaerobic bacteria obtained from bovine and equine sources to ceftiofur, *J Vet Diag Invest* 8:121-123, 1996.

HOSPITAL-ACQUIRED (NOSOCOMIAL) INFECTIONS

DWIGHT C. HIRSH

All animals are at risk of acquiring an infectious disease after entering the hospital environment. There are both medical and economic consequences of acquiring such a nosocomial infectious disease. The economic consequences include increased length of hospital stay, increased cost because of medication, and indemnity and legal costs. Less obvious costs include those for increased microbiologic surveillance (supplies and personnel) and cleaning. For serious outbreaks, loss of income follows closure of the facility. Long-term effects include loss of confidence by clientele and referring veterinarians.

From a medical standpoint nosocomial infectious disease may complicate a preexisting problem or may be the only medical problem of consequence (e.g., for an animal originally

---

BOX 42-5

Nosocomial Diseases of Horses

Viral respiratory diseases, including influenza and
    rhinopneumonitis
Equine infectious anemia
Equine viral arteritis
Papillomatosis
Salmonellosis*
Clostridium difficile infection
Strangles*
Anthrax*
Leptospirosis*
Dermatomycoses
Pediculosis
Mange

*Isolation to separate barn required.

BOX 42-6

Nosocomial Diseases of Ruminants

BOVINE
All respiratory diseases
Bovine viral diarrhea
Coronaviral enterocolitis
Infectious bovine rhinotracheitis
Pseudocowpox
Rotaviral enteritis
Ulcerative mammillitis
Anthrax*
Blackleg
Brucellosis*
Enterotoxigenic colibacillosis
Leptospirosis*
Salmonellosis*
Tuberculosis*
Mycoplasmal mastitis
Scabies*
Ringworm
Pinkeye (*Moraxella bovis*)

OVINE
Contagious ecthyma
Scrapie
Progressive pneumonia
Anthrax*
Blackleg
Brucellosis (including ram epididymitis)
Enzootic (chlamydial) abortion
Footrot
Leptospirosis*
Salmonellosis*
Tuberculosis*
Campylobacter abortion
Infectious keratoconjunctivitis (chlamydial and
    mycoplasmal)
Mycoplasmosis

CAPRINE
Contagious ecthyma
Caprine viral arthritis-encephalitis
Brucellosis*
Tuberculosis*
Anthrax*
Salmonellosis*
Leptospirosis*
Footrot
Boils (*Corynebacterium pseudotuberculosis*)
Enterotoxigenic colibacillosis
Infectious keratoconjunctivitis (chlamydial and
    mycoplasmal)
Enzootic (chlamydial) abortion
Mycoplasmal arthritis

*Isolation to separate barn required.

---

admitted for elective surgery). After becoming infected with a potentially pathogenic agent, the animal becomes a source of dispersal of the agent to others, regardless of whether the infection progresses to disease. Not only are other animals in the environment at risk of becoming infected, but the human personnel are as well (e.g., with agents such as *Salmonella*).

Agents associated with nosocomial infectious disease are shown in Boxes 42-5 and 42-6. The conditions listed are those with contagious potential, and animals with them pose a threat to others in the hospital environment. The conditions are grouped into two categories: "reportable" (to the Infection Control Officer) and "isolation required," based on the degree of communicability of the infectious agent. The reportable category contains agents that pose minimum risk to the hospitalized population. An animal with one of these conditions should be isolated in situ (see p. 1367). The "isolation required" category contains agents that are highly contagious to the hospitalized population. Animals with these infections should be placed in the isolation facility. It is important to point out that some conditions such as enterotoxigenic colibacillosis might require isolation if the makeup of the hospital population so dictates. On the other hand, for example, if a hospital population rarely contains calves of the appropriate age for this disease, calves with this disease might not require isolation.

Animals are at risk of acquiring a nosocomial infection on entry into the hospital environment because of increased likelihood of contact with an infectious agent, decrease in immunity caused by stress, or changes in the normal resident flora. It is more than likely that a combination of these factors is responsible for the increased risk.

Animals entering the hospital environment contact infectious agents with which they may not have had previous experience. In addition, there are likely to be increases in density of the animal population and in animals of diverse origin. These factors concomitantly increase the chances that infectious agents not experienced before will be contacted. This chapter discusses methods and procedures designed to minimize contact with agents having nosocomial potential.

Hospitalized patients are under stress. This stress may be a consequence of the disease that prompted hospitalization in the first place (e.g., a decrease in the plane of nutrition); it may be psychologic, resulting from social interactions in the new environment; or it may be a result of activities unfamiliar to the patient (e.g., transportation to the hospital, feeding and handling at the hospital). Any of these may decrease the animal's ability to respond immunologically to infectious agents in the environment.[102-106] The possibility exists that a suboptimum immunologic response could be elicited not only to an agent that is new, but also to agents that have been experienced before. Little can be done to decrease stress, but recognizing that stress is a factor makes dealing with its consequences easier. This topic is not dealt with in any detail in this chapter.

A major reason that animals are at risk of acquiring an infectious disease on entry into the hospital is that changes occur in the normal flora of the patient, permitting colonization

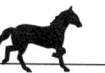

with microorganisms found in the hospital's environment. The latter microorganisms may have pathogenic potential (such as *Salmonella*), or they may be highly resistant to antimicrobial agents (such as *Klebsiella*). Diseases resulting from infection of a compromised site with the latter organism are difficult to treat. The normal flora play an important role in regulating the colonization of mucosal surfaces.

NORMAL FLORA AS HOST DEFENSE

The fetus is bacteriologically sterile during initial stages of parturition. Shortly thereafter, acquisition of the resident flora begins and continues throughout the life of the animal, vigorously at first, then more subtly after weaning. The process is a dynamic one; microorganisms are acquired, whereas others are deleted from various sites along the mucosal surfaces. This process continues until a relatively stable flora is established.[107-110]

The normal flora is not haphazardly arranged on mucosal surfaces. A particular species or strain of microorganism is found at a particular site or location because it is most suited to the location. If it were not, a newly acquired species would displace it.[111-113] Thus the normal flora is part of an ecosystem composed of a multitude of niches filled with species of microorganisms, each best suited for that particular niche.

The normal flora is part of the innate immune system of the host. Pathogenic microorganisms (viral, bacterial, or fungal) must attach to a particular site or target cell if they are to produce disease or to colonize.[111] To do so, pathogenic or potentially pathogenic species must successfully compete with resident flora for a particular site. The normal flora or, indirectly, the factors that regulate the normal flora, work to prevent this from occurring.

The factors that regulate the ecosystem are many and varied but, in simplest terms, are related to the host and to the microorganisms. Properties of the surface of microorganisms facilitate the attachment directly to the surface of the host cell (usually to carbohydrate moieties in glycoconjugates in or on the cell membrane) or to substances overlying the cell membrane (e.g., mucin, fibronectin).[114] Conversely, receptors on the surface of the host's cells also regulate the composition of the flora by supplying the attachment site for the microorganism.[115-117] These receptors play a role in certain diseases such as the S phenotype of swine relative to certain enterotoxigenic strains of *Escherichia coli*.[118] It is suspected that these receptors play a role in the establishment or displacement of normal flora in hospitalized patients, but their nature is unknown.

Numerous products are secreted by members of the flora living on mucosal surfaces. Most important are short-chained fatty acids, bacteriocins, and microcins. The short-chain fatty acids are secreted by obligate anaerobic bacteria as a metabolic product. These substances have an inhibiting effect on gram-negative facultative bacteria (e.g., members of the family Enterobacteriaceae).[119-126] Short-chained fatty acids have a regulatory role wherever obligate anaerobes are found (i.e., the gingival sulcus, lower gastrointestinal tract, and the vagina).

Bacteriocins are antibiotic-like peptides that are secreted by a variety of microorganisms.[127] They are usually quite specifically active against species that are the same as the one secreting them. However, microorganisms that possess the genes for the production of a particular bacteriocin are immune; those actually secreting the bacteriocin are usually killed. Bacteriocins secreted by gram-positive microorganisms in the oral cavity have an important regulating influence on the flora at this location.[128] Although there are numerous bacteriocin-secreting strains of microorganisms in the gastrointestinal tract, a regulating role at that site has not been demonstrated, at least as far as gram-negative microorganisms are concerned.[129,130]

Microcins, like bacteriocins, are antibiotic-like substances.[131-133] Unlike the bacteriocins, the microcins do not destroy the secreting cell, are resistant to the action of digestive enzymes (such as trypsin), and are active in the microenvironment of the large bowel.[114-116]

In summary, healthy animals normally possess a stable microbial flora on their mucosal surfaces. This flora lives in a unique relationship with the host and with other members of the flora. Microorganisms that enter the system are excluded from the mucosal surface by members of the normal flora, unless the entering microorganisms successfully compete with members of the normal flora for a niche or site.

INFLUENCES OF HOSPITAL ENVIRONMENT ON NORMAL FLORA

Normal flora are disrupted by stress or by drugs (antimicrobics mainly). Niches become available, and entering microorganisms colonize mucosal surfaces they would not normally be allowed to colonize. If these microorganisms have pathogenic potential (e.g., *Salmonella*), the patient is placed at risk. In addition, treatment of any resulting infectious disease is more difficult if the entering microorganisms are extremely resistant to antimicrobial agents (e.g., *Klebsiella*).

Many occurrences bring about changes in the normal flora on a mucosal surface. Stress, disease, nutritional imbalance, psychologic insult, and drugs (antimicrobics) acting on the flora affect how the patient interacts with the hospital's environment.[134-137] If the normal flora of the patient is relatively intact and remains so during the hospital stay, colonization by microorganisms from the hospital's environment is minimal and the rate of recolonization is slow. On the other hand, if the patient is stressed by disease, surgery, or antimicrobics, the normal flora are altered, and as a consequence the likelihood of recolonization is increased.

Although stress affects an animal's susceptibility to disease,[105,106,135,138,139] the mechanisms whereby this occurs are largely unknown. However, it is known that changes in the flora occur secondary to decreases in the level of nutrition and following extended transportation.[137,140] Either of these occurrences is likely to be found in the history of the hospitalized animal.

The immune system is directly affected by surgery, decreases in the plane of nutrition, concurrent disease, and drugs such as corticosteroids.[139,141] The following model attempts to account for this observation. During the process of establishment of the normal flora, the immune system of the host responds to epitopes (antigenic determinants) on the surface of colonizing microorganisms. The ensuing immune response (probably secretory IgA and secretory IgM) results in the elimination of microorganisms bearing the inciting epitopes. Thus, along with competition with existing flora for a particular niche, the microorganisms attempting to colonize must also escape being recognized by the host. The end result of these selective pressures is a population of microbes in balance with the immune system of the host. This model is supported by experiments that show that members of an individual's normal flora are poorly immunogenic in that individual but very immunogenic in another.[142-144] As a consequence of this balance, anything that affects the immune system of the host also indirectly affects the normal flora.

In addition to changes in the immune system of individuals undergoing stressful events, changes occur in the substances that coat the surfaces of the epithelial cells. So far, this has only been shown to occur in the oral cavity. The epithelial cells of the oral cavity synthesize and secrete the glycoprotein fibronectin.[145] Fibronectin serves as a receptor for attachment of most of the gram-positive species that live in or become associated with the oral cavity and surrounding structures.[115,117] The importance of an intact gram-positive oral flora is the finding of adhesins with affinity for fibronectin among enteric organisms with pathogenic potential (e.g., *Salmonella* spp., *E. coli*, and *Yersinia*).[146-148] The amount of fibronectin coating these cells decreases in the stressed animal, leaving available underlining attachment sites (for gram-negative microorganisms) either on the cells themselves or on the salivary glycoproteins that coat the cells after fibronectin is gone.[116,149,150] The loss of this glycoprotein results in a change in the makeup of the flora inhabiting the mouth and surrounding structures. Consequently, an individual coming into a stressful environment containing a great many resistant gram-negative microorganisms may quickly become colonized by them.

The clinician has no control over the foregoing problems. However, the use of antimicrobial drugs is an activity that compounds the risks to the patient and over which the clinician has control.[151] These agents have a selective influence on the microbial flora in the hospital. Animals receiving antimicrobial agents, for whatever reason, contribute resistant pathogenic microorganisms to the environment.[152-155] In addition to selection of resistant strains, antimicrobic agents also eliminate susceptible normal flora. The obligate anaerobes and the gram-positive cocci in the oral cavity are the most vulnerable of these flora.[156] Reduction of either population leads directly to an increase in numbers of gram-negative organisms, all of which may be resistant to the antimicrobial agent being used.[157] Because most if not all of the genes that encode resistance to antimicrobics in this group of microbes reside on R plasmids, these organisms are resistant to other antimicrobics as well.[153] Diseases produced by a number of infectious bacterial agents are more likely to occur in animals given antimicrobics (e.g., *Salmonella* spp. and *Clostridium difficile*).[151,158]

Bacteria survive in an environment containing antimicrobics because they have become resistant to that particular antimicrobic agent. They may have become resistant because of a mutational change or because of acquisition of deoxyribonucleic acid (DNA)-encoding products that make the bacterium resistant.

Mutational changes are predictable random events that result in a change that interferes with the action of a particular antimicrobic agent. Mutational changes may affect the gene(s) encoding a target organelle or cellular process affected by a particular antimicrobic agent, making the bacterium refractory to the action of that particular compound. These sorts of mutational events are rare, and because they usually involve resistance to a single antimicrobic (or family of antimicrobics), probably play a minor role in hospital-acquired infections. More serious consequences of a mutation stem from changes that affect bacterial pumps. The MAR (*multiple antibiotic resistance*) locus is one such example. In this case there is a mutation in the gene encoding a normally occurring repressor. The repressor suppresses the activity of several intracellular pumps. Without the repressor, these pumps are activated so that antimicrobics (regardless of kind or class) will be pumped out of the bacterial cell faster than they can accumulate to effective intracellular concentrations. As a consequence a single mutational event results in a multiply resistant bacterium. Although the MAR phenotype is also rare, its occurrence has serious clinical consequences. This phenotype has been described for *E. coli* and *Salmonella*, *Pseudomonas*, *Proteus*, *Klebsiella*, and *Campylobacter* spp.

Acquisition of DNA-encoding products that interfere with the activities of antimicrobics is far more common and significant. This DNA is termed plasmid DNA, and plasmid DNA that encodes resistance to antimicrobics is referred to as an R plasmid.[153,159]

Plasmids are extrachromasomal genetic elements. For the most part they are autonomous, functioning independently of the chromosome. A wide variety of products are encoded in these pieces of DNA, ranging from toxins to resistance to heavy metals. The two most important products are (1) those that endow the bacteria with resistance to antimicrobic agents, and (2) the ability to transfer plasmid DNA from one bacterium to another by the sexual process termed conjugation. R plasmids rarely contain the genes for resistance to just one antimicrobic. At least two and usually more resistance genes are found on an R plasmid. Therefore a bacterium acquiring an R plasmid immediately becomes resistant to many antimicrobic agents. In addition to being mobile by means of conjugation, resistance genes are motile in their own right. Mobile genes, called transposable genetic elements or transposons, move from one piece of DNA to another. The importance of this is that, in the hospital environment where bacteria containing multiple R plasmids are found, large conjugal R plasmids may be formed by the transposition of resistance genes from a variety of sources to one plasmid. A bacterium containing such an R plasmid would be extremely difficult to kill or suppress with antimicrobic agents if it were to become involved with a disease process.

Although transposable elements seem to be the most commonly encountered mobile unit encoding resistance to antimicrobics, they are by no means the only one. Integron cassettes are composed of a mobile unit (cassette) that encodes antimicrobial resistance (usually multiple) and a defective transposon (defective because it can no longer move) called an integron. Cassettes recognize integrons and insert into them. Integron-cassette units may reside on the chromosome or on plasmids. Where they reside depends upon the location of the integron.[160]

Therefore the hospitalized patient enters an environment that is very hostile. This fact, coupled with a reduction in the defense offered by the normal flora, makes colonization with pathogenic or potentially pathogenic species of microorganisms almost a certainty. However, there are steps the clinician can take to minimize these changes, at least as far as using an antimicrobic agent is concerned. The aim should be to disturb the normal flora as little as possible. The key components of the flora are the obligate anaerobic flora in the gingival sulci, the gastrointestinal tract, and the vagina, together with the gram-positive cocci in the mouth. These flora endow the protective influences of the colonization resistance.[156,157] Certain drugs affect colonization resistance more than others. As a consequence, it is simply not enough to determine the most efficacious antimicrobic to use; the risks inherent in the effect of each drug on the colonization resistance must also be weighed.

Certain antimicrobics influence the colonization resistance of the normal flora more than others. Colonization resistance is reduced significantly by the penicillins (including ampicillin, amoxicillin, penicillin G, and the penicillinase-resistant penicillins), chloramphenicol, and tetracycline; moderately by metronidazole, and minimally by trimethoprim-sulfonamides.[157,161]

DETERMINATION OF THE SOURCE OF A NOSOCOMIAL AGENT

Determination of the source of an outbreak of nosocomial infectious disease is crucial if corrective measures are to be successful. Knowledge of genus and species is often not enough to say that a particular isolate is the same as that producing nosocomial disease. There are a number of ways that an isolate can be fingerprinted. Examples include determination of reactivity to a series of different bacteriophages (if available), determination of the biotype, or determination of the antibiogram. In most instances, these traits are too crude

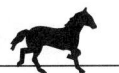

to ascertain whether a particular isolate is identical to one isolated from another animal in the hospital but different from other isolates of the same genus and species obtained from the community. For this reason additional techniques are used to determine the similarity or dissimiliarity between two or more isolates obtained from patients in the hospital or from the environment. These techniques usually involve an in depth study of the proteins of the isolate and/or the genetic material.

Whole-cell protein analysis is simplest to perform.[162] The major drawback unique to this analysis is that some proteins are regulated by the environment in which they grow.[163] Finding a particular protein in very small amounts or even absent raises the question as to whether it is the growth condition or the nature of the isolate that is at variance. To perform the assay, the isolate is grown to a particular density, lysed by detergent or by mechanical means, and then boiled in the presence of sodium dodecyl sulfate and 2-mercaptoethanol. The sample is then electrophoresed in a polyacrylamide gel. The number and weight of the constituent proteins make the fingerprint of the isolate.

Chromosomal or plasmid DNA is also used for fingerprinting.[164,165] Both are analyzed in a similar fashion, but plasmid DNA, although the easier of the two to obtain and analyze, has the inherent disadvantage of being unstable in the bacterial host (spontaneously lost) and mobile (moves from bacterial host to bacterial host); thus results are misleading (i.e., different strains may contain the same plasmid, and vice versa).[166,167] The DNA (chromosomal or plasmid) is isolated and purified. An enzyme (a restriction endonuclease) is added that "cuts" the DNA after recognizing a specific sequence of bases in the DNA. The digest is then electrophoresed in either an agarose gel (for resolution of large fragments) or in a polyacrylamide gel (for the resolution of smaller fragments), thereby separating the cut fragments by weight. The number and size of fragments is a reflection of the base sequence of the DNA. This technique was used to trace the movement of a large R plasmid through a veterinary hospital.[167] An R plasmid encoding resistance to ampicillin, chloramphenicol, gentamicin, and trimethoprim-sulfadiazine was found in two serotypes of *Salmonella* (*S. krefeld* and *S. saintpaul*) that produced disease in horses undergoing surgery for colic.

Because not all isolates have plasmids and because of the difficulty of "reading" the banding pattern produced following the digestion of chromosomal DNA (too many bands in some instances), other techniques are used. Following the digestion of the chromosomal DNA with a restriction endonuclease, the fragments are separated by electrophoresis and transferred to nitrocellulose paper. A DNA probe is added. Probes that have been used are random fragments of DNA obtained from another isolate or a part of DNA that encodes highly conserved sequences such as those encoding ribosomal RNA.[168,169] The DNA probe hybridizes to fragments that are similar if not identical to it, producing a banding pattern of duplexes. Such a technique has been used to categorize isolates of salmonellae.[166,168] Another, more widely utilized method of fingerprinting DNA is to use restriction endonucleases that recognize rare sequences and thus cut DNA into larger fragments. These fragments are separated by agarose gel electrophoresis as described above. However, unlike regular electrophoresis, the electric current is applied in a pulsing fashion from various angles (pulsed field gel electrophoresis). Pulsed field gel electrophoresis is much simpler to perform because the number of bands generated are few and are more easily analyzed without the aid of probes. Other methods include amplification of parts of the chromosome by using random primers and the polymerase chain reaction (random amplification of polymorphic DNA or RAPD).[170]

PREVENTION AND CONTROL OF NOSOCOMIAL DISEASE

Following infection with a nosocomial agent, animals fall into one of two categories: (1) those that are or have become infected (colonized) with an agent that possesses communicable properties (e.g., *Streptococcus equi*, *Salmonella* spp.), or (2) those that have become infected with a strain of resistant microorganisms acquired from the hospital environment, which, if given the chance, may cause disease. In either case the animal also becomes a source of that particular microorganism and as such becomes a potential danger to other animals in the hospital.

There is little doubt that the animal with the communicable infectious disease should be isolated from other animals in the hospital. Most hospitals have isolation units for this purpose. It is imperative that isolation be complete; otherwise such activity is a waste of time and space. This means that clothing, footwear, equipment, bottles of medicines and fluids, feed, and soiled bedding never come back into the main hospital without first being sterilized or disinfected. This is a difficult task and one that cannot be accomplished unless a special effort is made. At our hospital everything that returns from the isolation unit to the regular hospital is autoclaved. Soiled bedding is placed in large bags that are then sealed. All efforts at isolation are for naught if infected material is blown into the hospital by the wind. Clothing and boots stay in the unit. Clothing is a special color (red), which ensures compliance. Equipment such as trash containers are painted red.

The handling of the animal that has become colonized with a hospital-acquired microorganism that has increased resistance to antimicrobics but does not belong to a "recognized" pathogenic genus is more difficult. Most patients receiving antimicrobics, as well as those under stress of a magnitude sufficient to alter the normal microbial flora, become colonized with hospital strains of microorganisms. Because most patients become colonized, which ones should be singled out? At our hospital we concentrate on animals that are shedding a large number of resistant microorganisms into the environment in an infected fluid (e.g., urine, pus). It is paradoxical that we do not worry about the feces of an animal receiving antimicrobics, which might in fact be shedding large numbers of resistant microorganisms into the environment. Animals with infected exudates or fluids are isolated "in place" (i.e., they are handled by personnel wearing gloves, disposable gowns, and disposable footwear; they have their own thermometers; and they are rarely moved from the stall unless precautions are taken). For example, if an animal is to be taken to radiology, this is done at the end of the day, and measures are taken to clean the area after the animal leaves. High-risk animals in the large animal intensive care unit are also isolated from the rest of the hospital population.

Cleaning and disinfecting a contaminated environment should be a major undertaking (see Chapter 43). Without cleaning and disinfecting, all the procedures and work needed to detect and isolate the infected animal have been wasted. Infectious agents such as *Salmonella* or *S. equi* may live for long periods of time in organic matter. Pus or feces on a surface in a stall or treatment room may act as a nidus to sustain an outbreak of nosocomial disease. After cleaning, disinfectants are used to hasten the killing of microorganisms left on the surface. The most potent and also most corrosive and toxic to those cleaning are the phenolic disinfectants. Household bleach (diluted 4 oz to 1 gallon) is an alternative.

Areas that have been contaminated and then cleaned and disinfected should be sampled to determine whether the surface has been properly cleaned. Multiple swabs should be taken from surfaces that are difficult to clean high on a wall (e.g., corners), as well as from those areas reflective of the entire area (e.g., around the drain). Stalls or other areas are closed until culture results show that the offending organism can no longer be cultured from the environment.

Although routine microbiologic surveillance of the environment has not been shown to be cost effective or useful for control of nosocomial disease in hospitals for humans,[171] because of the difficult task of cleaning and disinfecting soiled surfaces found in the veterinary hospital we routinely monitor the environment for *Salmonella*. In addition the feces of horses in the intensive care unit that have undergone colic surgery are cultured for *Salmonella* because these horses have been shown to be at greatest risk of being colonized with this microorganism.[151]

The Microbiology Service can provide two types of monitoring: assessment of cleanliness and determination of the presence or absence of a particular microorganism. Monitoring cleaning efficiency should be done on a routine basis. This can best be accomplished with contact plates (Rodac plates). After deciding how many bacteria per square centimeter of surface are acceptable, areas throughout the hospital can be sampled (unannounced) after the cleaning crew has finished. Floors, walls, and table tops should be assessed.

The other monitoring service is to determine the presence or absence of a particular microorganism. If the agent being monitored is resistant to an unusual array of drugs, bacteriologic media containing the antimicrobic(s) can be inoculated with samples obtained from the environment. Samples are obtained by contact plate (e.g., containing the antimicrobic) or by swabs. Swabs are streaked directly onto the medium or into enrichment broth and then to selective media. For *Salmonella*, swabs are used and placed into selenite broth for enrichment; the next day the selenite broth is subcultured onto a selective medium such as xylose-lysine-Tergitol 4 agar plates.[172]

Monitoring is time consuming and therefore expensive. The decision concerning how intense and thorough monitoring should be is aided by knowing what animal is likely to be at risk and then focusing the effort in that direction, rather than heading in all directions at once. For example, hospitalized equine patients undergoing colic surgery are at risk of developing salmonellosis and therefore should be monitored closely.[151]

RATIONAL USE OF ANTIMICROBICS IN THE HOSPITAL SETTING

Some attention should be given to those practices that increase the risk to all patients in the hospital. One practice that significantly increases this risk is the use of antimicrobial agents. Thus it is my opinion that medical personnel in large hospitals should take an active role in the assurance that antimicrobes are used in a rational and responsible fashion. The old maxim, "Put the animal on penicillin just in case; it can't hurt him," is irresponsible and borders on malpractice. The use of antimicrobics in the hospital should be supervised by a quality assurance committee or some similar body. We have an Infection Control Committee composed of a representative of the house officer's staff, the nursing staff, the clinical faculty, the clinical pharmacist, and the infection control officer who usually serves as chair. This committee reports directly to the hospital director and is part of the hospital quality assurance program. One of the committee's charges is to formulate policy regarding the use of antimicrobial agents. This includes establishing guidelines for and governing the use of certain "restricted antimicrobics."

The decision to use antimicrobics therapeutically involves deciding (1) that an infectious process is present, (2) that it poses a threat to the well-being of the patient (immediately

or in the future), and (3) that it will not resolve without medicinal intervention. The criteria for determining that therapeutic use of antimicrobics is rational are shown in Box 42-7. Rational use also requires that the antimicrobic chosen be one that is effective against the microorganism(s) most likely to be isolated from the site involved.

Antimicrobics are often used by surgeons to prevent infections of normally sterile sites (e.g., joints, peritoneal cavity) by members of either the normal or exogenous flora. When an antimicrobic is used for purposes other than treating an infectious process, it is important to minimize risks. The major risk is that the normal flora of mucosal surfaces will be eliminated by the antimicrobic being used. Because the mucosal surfaces inhabited by the normal flora do not remain sterile following the use of such drugs, these surfaces will be recolonized by bacteria from the environment that will be resistant to other antimicrobics as well.

Following the administration of an antimicrobic, the normal flora are replaced with exogenous, resistant microorganisms. These changes are minimal for 24 hours after therapy is initiated. After 48 hours of continuous therapy, however, the normal flora are almost entirely replaced with microorganisms that are resistant to the antimicrobic being used.[173] Most of these microorganisms are members of the family Enterobacteriaceae (e.g., *Klebsiella, E. coli*). The source of these resistant microorganisms is the environment of the patient. A significant primary source is the feces of animals receiving antimicrobials. To minimize the risk of prophylactic use of antimicrobics, certain guidelines should be followed (see Box 42-7). First, a drug should be chosen that is effective against the microorganisms that are most likely to contaminate the site. Second, the drug should be administered so that effective concentrations are achieved at the site when compromise occurs. Third, the drug should be administered no longer than 24 to 48 hours after the compromise.

Because of the risks inherent to the use of antimicrobics, their use in a hospital setting is not a right or a freedom. For this reason certain antimicrobics must be placed on a "restricted use" list. We have restricted the use of all third-generation cephalosporins because we have a *Klebsiella* and a *Salmonella* in the hospital that are susceptible to little else. Drugs of this type may only be used after consultation with

---

BOX 42-7

Criteria for Determining That Therapeutic Use of Antimicrobics Is Rational

1. An infectious agent has been demonstrated in direct smear or by culture, or
2. Clinical data indicate the presence of an infectious agent. In the absence of data that directly demonstrate the presence of an infectious agent (in smear or cultures), at least two of the following indicators must be present:
   a. Core body (rectal) temperature is elevated.
   b. Absolute neutrophilia or neutropenia is present.
   c. Localized signs of inflammation are present.
   d. Cellular and/or soluble components in a sample that suggest an infectious process are elevated (e.g., increase in white blood cells [WBCs] and concentration of protein in cerebral spinal fluid; increased WBC in joint fluids).
   e. There is radiographic evidence of an infectious process.
   f. Hyperfibrinogenemia is present.

two members of the Infection Control Committee (usually the infection control officer and the clinical pharmacist). If the two agree, permission to use the drug is given. A written report is filed and reviewed by the committee as a whole.

Risks of acquiring a nosocomial infectious disease are significantly increased in the hospital setting. Changes in the innate barriers to disease, mainly the normal flora, result from exposure to the hospital environment. Infectious agents in the environment colonize the mucosal surfaces of the hospitalized patient. Depending on the agent, disease may or may not occur. In the latter instance, compromise of a site followed by infection of the site with such microorganisms results in disease caused by microorganisms that are of nosocomial origin. In either instance the agent is quite resistant to antimicrobic agents, especially if it belongs to the family Enterobacteriaceae.

It is difficult to control the recolonization of the mucosal surfaces of the hospitalized animal. However, it is possible to influence the spectrum of resistance of the infectious agents in the hospital environment. This is done by rational and informed use of antimicrobic agents.

REFERENCES

102. Gross WB, Siegel PB: Socialization as a factor in resistance to infection feed efficiency and response to antigen in chickens, *Am J Vet Res* 43:2010, 1982.
103. Larson CT, Gross WB, Davis JW: Social stress and resistance of chicken and swine to *Staphylococcus aureus* challenge infections, *Can J Comp Med* 49:208, 1985.
104. Solomon GF, Amkraut AA: Psychoneuroendocrinological effects on the immune response, *Annu Rev Microbiol* 35:155, 1981.
105. Sheridan JF et al: Psychoneuroimmunology: stress effects on pathogenesis and immunity during infection, *Clin Microbiol Rev* 7:200, 1994.
106. Black PH: Central nervous system-immune system interactions: psychoneuroendocrinology of stress and its immune consequences, *Antimicrob Agents Chemother* 38:1, 1994.
107. Dubos RJ et al: Indigenous, normal, and autochthonous flora of the gastrointestinal tract, *J Exp Med* 122:67, 1965.
108. Lee A, Gemmell E: Changes in the mouse intestinal microflora during weaning: role of fatty acids, *Infect Immunol* 5:1, 1972.
109. Lee A et al: The mouse intestinal microflora with emphasis on the strict anaerobes, *J Exp Med* 133:339, 1971.
110. Savage DC, Dubos RJ, Schaedler RW: The gastrointestinal epithelium and its autochthonous bacterial flora, *J Exp Med* 127:67, 1968.
111. Savage DC: Factors involved in colonization of the gut epithelial surface, *Am J Clin Nutr* 31:S131, 1978.
112. Sears HJ, Brownlee J, Uchiyama JM: Persistence of individual strains of *Escherichia coli* in the intestinal tract of man, *J Bacteriol* 59:293, 1950.
113. Sears HJ et al: Persistence of individual strains of *Escherichia coli* in man and dogs under various conditions, *J Bacteriol* 71:370, 1956.
114. Hirsh DC: Fimbriae: relation of intestinal bacteria and virulence in animals, *Adv Vet Sci Comp Med* 29:207, 1985.
115. Abraham SN, Beachey EH, Simpson WA: Adherence of *Streptococcus pyogenes*, Escherichia coli, and *Pseudomonas aeruginosa* to fibronectin-coated and uncoated epithelial cells, *Infect Immunol* 41:1261, 1983.
116. Hasty DL, Simpson WA: Effects of fibronectin and other salivary macromolecules on the adherence of *Escherichia coli* to buccal epithelial cells, *Infect Immunol* 55:2103, 1987.
117. Simpson WA, Hasty DL, Beachey EH: Binding of fibronectin to human buccal epithelial cells inhibits the binding of type 1 fimbriated *Escherichia coli*, *Infect Immunol* 48:318, 1985.
118. Sellwood R et al: Adhesion of enteropathogenic *Escherichia coli* to pig intestinal brush borders: the existence of two pig phenotypes, *J Med Microbiol* 8:405, 1975.
119. Bergeim O: Toxicity of intestinal volatile fatty acids for yeasts and *Escherichia coli*, *J Infect Dis* 66:222, 1940.
120. Bergein O et al: Relation of volatile fatty acids and H;i2S to the intestinal flora, *J Infect Dis* 69:155, 1941.
121. Hentges DJ: Inhibition of *Shigella flexneri* by the normal intestinal flora. II, Mechanism of inhibition of coliform organisms, *J Bacteriol* 97:513, 1969.
122. Hentges DJ, Maier BR: Inhibition of *Shigella flexneri* by the normal intestinal flora. III, Interactions with *Bacteroides fragilis* strains in vitro, *Infect Immunol* 2:364, 1970.
123. Koopman JP, Janssen F, VanDruten J: Oxidation-reduction potentials in the cecal contents of rats and mice, *Proc Soc Exp Biol Med* 149:995, 1975.
124. Meynell GG: Antibacterial mechanisms of the mouse gut. II, The role of Eh and volatile fatty acids in the normal gut, *Br J Exp Pathol* 44:209, 1963.

125. Que JU, Casey SW, Hentges DJ: Factors responsible for increased susceptibility of mice to intestinal colonization after treatment with streptomycin, *Infect Immunol* 53:116, 1986.
126. Wostman BA, Bruckner-Kardoss E: Oxidation-reduction potentials in cecal contents of germ-free and conventional rats, *Proc Soc Exp Biol Med* 121:1111, 1966.
127. Braun V, Pilsl H, Groz R: Colicins: structures, modes of action, transfer through membranes, and evolution, *Arch Microbiol* 161:199, 1994.
128. Marsh P, Martin M: Oral microbiology. In Cole JA, Knowles CJ, Schlessinger D, eds: *Aspects of microbiology*, ed 2, American Society for Microbiology, 1984, Washington, DC.
129. Craven JA, Miniats OP, Barnum DA: Role of colicins in antagonism between strains of *Escherichia coli* in dual-infected gnotobiotic pigs, *Am J Vet Res* 32:1775, 1971.
130. Ikari NS, Kenton DM, Young VM: Interaction on the germfree mouse intestine of colicinogenic and colicin-sensitive microorganisms, *Proc Soc Exp Biol Med* 130:1280, 1969.
131. Asenio C et al: A new family of low-molecular-weight antibiotics from enterobacteria, *Biochem Biophy Res Comm* 69:7, 1976.
132. Baquero F, Moreno F: The microcins, *FEMS Microbiol Lett* 23:117, 1984.
133. DeLorenzo V, Martinez JL, Asenio C: Microcin-mediated interactions between *Klebsiella pneumoniae* and *Escherichia coli* strains, *J Gen Microbiol* 130:391, 1984.
134. Brownlie LE, Grau FH: Effect of food intake on growth and survival of salmonellas and *Escherichia coli* in the bovine rumen, *J Gen Microbiol* 46:125, 1967.
135. Tannock GW: Effect of dietary and environmental stress on the gastrointestinal microbiota. In Hentges DJ, ed: *Human intestinal microflora in health and disease*, Washington, DC, 1983, Academic Press, p 517.
136. Tannock GW et al: Salmonellosis in sheep wintered outdoors on straw and sawdust pads, *N Z Vet J* 19:29, 1971.
137. Tannock GW, Savage DC: Influences of dietary and environmental stress on microbial populations in the murine gastrointestinal tract, *Infect Immunol* 9:591, 1974.
138. Kennedy MJ, Volz PA: Ecology of *Candida albicans* gut colonization: inhibition of *Candida* adhesion, colonization, and dissemination from the gastrointestinal tract by bacterial antagonism, *Infect Immunol* 49:654, 1985.
139. Pietsch JB, Meakins JL: Predicting infection in surgical patients, *Surg Clin North Am* 59:185, 1981.
140. Owen Rh, Fullerton J, Barnum DA: Effects of transportation, surgery, and antibiotic therapy in ponies infected with *Salmonella*, *Am J Vet Res* 44:46, 1983.
141. MacLean LD: Host resistance in surgical patients, *J Trauma* 19:297, 1979.
142. Berg RD, Savage DC: Immune responses of specific pathogen-free and gnotobiotic mice to antigens of indigenous and non-indigenous microorganisms, *Infect Immunol* 11:320, 1975.
143. Foo MC, Lee A: Immunological response of mice to members of the autochthonous intestinal flora, *Infect Immunol* 6:525, 1972.
144. Foo MC, Lee A: Antigenic cross-reaction between mouse intestine and a member of the autochthonous microflora, *Infect Immunol* 9:1066, 1974.
145. Proctor RA: Fibronectin: a brief overview of its structure function and physiology, *Rev Infect Dis* 9:S317, 1987.
146. Collinson SK et al: Thin, aggregative fimbriae mediate binding of *Salmonella* enteritidis to fibronectin, *J Bacteriol* 175:12, 1993.
147. Olsen A, Jonsson A, Normark S: Fibronectin binding mediated by a novel class of surface organelles on *Escherichia coli*, *Nature* 338:652, 1989.
148. Tertti R et al: Adhesion protein YadA of Yersinia species mediates binding of bacteria to fibronectin, *Infect Immunol* 60:3021, 1992.
149. Johanson WG: Prevention of respiratory tract infection, *Am J Med* 15:69, 1984.
150. Woods DE et al: Role of salivary protease activity in adherence of gram-negative bacilli to mammalian buccal epithelia cells in vivo, *J Clin Invest* 68:1435, 1981.
151. Hird DW, Pappaioanou M, Smith BP: Case-control study of risk factors associated with isolation of *Salmonella saintpaul* in hospitalized horses, *Am J Epidemiol* 120:852, 1984.
152. Aden DP et al: Transferable drug resistance among Enterobacteriaceae isolated from cases of neonatal diarrhea in calves and piglets, *Appl Microbiol* 18:961, 1969.
153. Falkow S: *Infectious multiple drug resistance*, Pion, 1975, London.
154. Loken KI, Wagner LW, Henke CL: Transmissible drug resistance in Enterobacteriaceae isolated from calves given antibiotics, *Am J Vet Res* 32:1207, 1971.
155. Mercer HD et al: Characteristics of antimicrobial resistance of *Escherichia coli* from animals: relationship to veterinary and management uses of antimicrobial agents, *Appl Microbiol* 24:700, 1971.
156. van der Waaij D: *Antibiotic of choice: the importance of colonization resistance*, Letchworth, England, 1983, Research Studies Press.
157. Wells CL et al: Role of anaerobic flora in the translocation of aerobic and facultatively anaerobic intestinal bacteria, *Infect Immunol* 55:2689, 1987.
158. Madewell BR et al: Apparent outbreaks of *Clostridium difficile*-associated diarrhea in horses in a veterinary medical teaching hospital, *J Vet Diagn Invest* 7:343, 1995.

159. Hardy K: Bacterial plasmids. In Cole JA, Knowles CJ, Schlessinger D, eds: *Aspects of microbiology 4*, ed 2, American Society for Microbiology, 1986, Washington, DC.

160. Recchia GD, Hall RM: Gene cassettes: a new class of mobile element, *Microbiology* 141:3015, 1995.

161. Hentges DJ et al: Protection role of intestinal flora against infection with *Pseudomonas aeruginosa* in mice: influence of antibiotics on colonization resistance, *Infect Immunol* 47:118, 1985.

162. Kersters K, DeLey J: Classification and identification of bacteria by electrophoresis of their proteins. In Goodfellow M, Board RG, eds: *Microbiological classification and identification*, New York, 1980, Academic Press, p 273.

163. Brown MR, Williams P: The influence of environment on envelope properties affecting survival of bacteria in infections, *Ann Rev Microbiol* 39:527, 1985.

164. Elwell LP, Falkow S: The characterization of R plasmids and the detection of plasmid-specified genes. In Lorian V, ed: *Antibiotics in laboratory medicine*, Baltimore, 1986, Williams & Wilkins, p 683.

165. Tompkins LS: DNA methods in clinical microbiology. In Lennette EH et al, eds: *Manual of clinical microbiology*, American Society for Microbiology, p 1083, 1985, Washington, DC.

166. Hansen LM, Jang SS, Hirsh DC: Use of random fragments of chromosomal DNA to highlight restriction site heterogeneity from fingerprinting isolates of *Salmonella typhimurium* from hospitalized animals, *Am J Vet Res* 54:1648, 1993.

167. Ikeda JS, Hirsh DC: Common plasmid encoding resistance to ampicillin, chloramphenicol, gentamicin, and trimethoprim-sulfadiazine in two serotypes of *Salmonella* isolated during an outbreak of equine salmonellosis, *Am J Vet Res* 46:769, 1985.

168. Tompkins LS et al: Cloned, random chromosomal sequences as probes to identify *Salmonella* species, *J Infect Dis* 154:156, 1986.

169. Stull TL, LiPuma JJ, Edlind TD: A broad-spectrum probe for molecular epidemiology of bacteria: ribosomal RNA, *J Infect Dis* 157:280, 1988.

170. Williams JGK et al: DNA polymorphisms amplified by arbitrary primers are useful as genetic markers, *Nucleic Acids Res* 18:6531, 1990.

171. Simmons BP: Centers for disease control guidelines for hospital environmental control: microbiologic surveillance of the environment and of personnel in the hospital, *Infect Control* 2:145, 1981.

172. Miller RG et al: Xylose-lysine-tergitol 4: an improved selective agar medium for the isolation of *Salmonella*, *Poult Sci* 70:2429, 1991.

173. Dalton HP et al: Pulmonary infection due to disruption of the pharyngeal bacterial flora by antibiotics in hamsters, *Am J Pathol* 76:469, 1974.

Disinfectants and Control of Environmental Contamination

SUSAN L. EWART
Consulting Editor

SUSAN L. EWART AND ROBERT L. JONES

The goal of infectious disease management should be to prevent infection rather than to focus only on alleviating the damaging consequences of disease. Prophylactic treatment with antimicrobial drugs is indicated in some situations, but undue dependence on antimicrobial drugs for prevention of infections compromises their future use because of the development of resistant strains. Vaccines aid in preventing infectious disease by increasing resistance to disease. However, vaccines rarely provide absolute protection from infection and are not available for all infectious diseases. The limitations of relying on antimicrobial drugs and vaccines to control infectious diseases must be countered through measures to control exposure. Infectious agents spread from the infected host primarily in three ways: by direct or physical contact, by contamination of feed and water, and by movement through air. The current trend toward intensive livestock husbandry systems, in which large numbers of animals are contained in limited spaces, enhances the likelihood of contagious disease outbreaks. Increased animal density results in increased contact between animals, increased humidity (which typically favors pathogen survival), and increased contamination of the atmosphere and environment.[1] Therefore efforts to protect against infectious diseases must be designed to protect susceptible animals from contact with infected animals or infectious material shed from them. This is most readily accomplished by quarantine of all new animals introduced to the herd and strict isolation of animals with contagious diseases. However, the practical aspects of animal husbandry require that the spread of infection be controlled by a combination of judicious segregation of animals and the use of chemicals that kill microorganisms or their spores in the environment. No single agent or procedure is adequate for all purposes. Factors to consider in the selection of disinfectants include the type of pathogen to be targeted, the extent of microbial killing required, the nature of the item to be treated, and the cost and ease of using the available agents. This discussion addresses these aspects of preventive medicine.

Proper use of cleaners and disinfectants requires an understanding of the indications for use and the limitations of these products. Therefore the terms relating to these chemicals must be defined and the principles involved in their use understood.

PRINCIPLES AND TERMINOLOGY

Biocide (Germicide)

Biocide refers to chemical agents that kill microorganisms. Biocide is a general term that encompasses disinfectants, antiseptics, and antibiotics. Biocides may induce a variety of chemical effects, including oxidation, hydrolysis, denaturation (coagulation), and substitution. The term *cidal*, as in biocidal, refers to agents that kill the target organism. In contrast, the term *static* refers to agents that only inhibit microbial growth.

Disinfectant

A disinfectant is a biocide applied directly to inanimate objects. Disinfectants usually destroy most harmful microorganisms, but do not ordinarily kill bacterial spores.

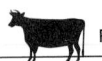

Antiseptic

Antiseptics are applied to the surface of living organisms or tissue to prevent or arrest the growth of microorganisms either by inhibiting their activity or by destroying them. Antiseptics are less toxic or irritating than disinfectants and may not be biocidal. Therefore they cannot be used interchangeably with disinfectants.

Sanitizer

A sanitizer reduces the number of bacterial contaminants to a safe level. The term actually refers to a condition of cleanliness. Therefore some detergents qualify as sanitizers, but a sanitizer is not always a biocide.

Sterilization

Sterilization refers to the process that destroys or eliminates all microbial life. Sterilization can be achieved using extreme heat (autoclaving) or by chemical means such as ethylene oxide, glutaraldehyde, or formaldehyde.

Deodorization

The process of deodorizing includes counteracting or neutralizing objectionable odors in the environment. Covering up an odor with a perfume or counteracting an odor by combining it with another odor may provide a temporary fragrance of fresh air, but it does not control the production of odors. Most odors arise from microbial fermentation and putrefaction of organic material. Therefore odors are best controlled by thorough cleaning and disinfection.

CONTROL OF CONTAMINATION AND PREPARING FOR DISINFECTION

Pathogenic microorganisms can survive in the environment for variable periods ranging from minutes to years. Therefore environmental contamination with pathogens can serve as a major source for subsequent infections. Interruption of disease transmission requires both containment of further environmental contamination by infected animals and removal of infectious organisms from buildings, feed, water, equipment, and other contaminated surfaces (Box 43-1). Cleaning of contaminated items is an essential prerequisite to disinfection because organic matter considerably reduces the efficacy of most disinfectants. Proper disposal of contaminated material is important to limit further environmental contamination.

Periodic disinfection cannot compensate for poor husbandry, unsuitable buildings, or low standards of hygiene. To effectively control the spread of pathogens, disinfection must complement optimal management and other control measures.[2] Ideally, cleaning and disinfection should be performed on a regular basis, and not just in the face of a disease outbreak. Thorough cleaning and disinfection are most effectively performed when all animals are removed from a facility (terminal cleaning and disinfection) as occurs in all-in and all-out facilities. Facilities should remain vacant during this process and for as long as possible thereafter, at least until all surfaces are dry.

Control of Animal Movement

An infected animal is an incubator and carrier of pathogens. It can pass them on to susceptible animals by direct contact or contamination of the environment. The infected animal is potentially a much greater reservoir of infection than the building or premises. However, movement of diseased animals may increase the extent of the contaminated area. Furthermore, animals in contact with diseased animals may already have been exposed to the infectious agent and may be incubating the disease. Therefore healthy animals that have not been exposed to diseased animals should be moved to clean surroundings, and the diseased animals and those in contact with them should remain in the contaminated yards and buildings. Sometimes it may be expedient to slaughter sick animals and those that have been in contact with them. If animals are too valuable to destroy, the pen or building should not receive any new additions until all animals have been removed and the facilities have been cleaned. Even in the absence of infectious disease on a farm, farm managers should segregate animals according to age, activity, stage of production, and reproductive status for housing purposes so there will be manageable numbers of animals to work with in the event that an infectious agent is introduced into the population.[1,2]

Carcass Disposal

The carcasses of animals that have died of infectious diseases can serve as reservoirs of pathogens so carcasses must be handled safely and disposed of properly. When the service is available, rendering is generally a safe, rapid, convenient, and economical method of disposition. Saving the hide from these animals should be discouraged because this practice may allow further spread of the infection.

Burial in properly managed sites is an alternative for disposing of dead animals and other contaminated waste materials that cannot be cleaned, although local or state regulations may have a significant impact on the burial methods permitted. Eventually, putrefaction of the carcass results in the destruction of infectious agents. Most pathogenic microorganisms perish rapidly in the soil, with the exception of bacterial spores, *Mycobacterium* spp., and some nonenveloped viruses. Burial should be at least 4 feet below the level of the surrounding terrain at a site where the water level is at least 8 feet beneath the surface of the ground. Peak temperatures in

---

BOX 43-1

Steps in Cleaning and Disinfecting Animal Care Facilities

1. All animals should be removed from the immediate premises to be cleaned and disinfected.
2. Traffic flow patterns progressing from clean to dirty areas should be established.
3. All movable items such as equipment and vehicles should be cleaned, disinfected, and removed.
4. Items not easily cleaned or of limited value should be disposed of safely.
5. Organic material, including manure, feed, and bedding, should be removed and decontaminated.
6. Surface irregularities allowing fluids and organic material to accumulate (e.g., chipped paint, loose flooring, depressions in horizontal surfaces) should be eliminated.
7. All surfaces and equipment should be rendered visibly clean using water and an effective detergent.
8. All surfaces and equipment should be sprayed with a liberal amount of an appropriate disinfectant.
9. After the appropriate contact time, it may be necessary to rinse the disinfectant off surfaces and equipment.
10. Allow facilities to dry and remain vacant for at least 1 to 2 days before restocking.

such landfills are estimated to be 60° C (148° F), and the microbial inactivation time is judged to be from 2 to 4 days. Burial sites must be properly managed because decomposition of the carcass and formation of gas cause cracking, bubbling, and leaking of fluids from a packed burial trench. The trench area should be mounded and neatly graded. If these procedures are followed, the presence of active pathogens in the landfill leachate need not be a concern because bacteria are normally removed from the soil within a few feet of travel and viruses within a few hundred feet.

The process of complete incineration is also a very effective method of destroying microorganisms and the material they contaminate. Transitory heating from a flame thrower must be at a high temperature and applied for sufficient time to achieve incineration of material, or it is of no value in controlling contamination. Therefore use of an open flame is generally not only ineffective but also dangerous in wooden buildings and near feed and bedding. Cremation of carcasses is difficult and expensive because of labor and fuel costs. It is usually limited to situations in which a commercial or university facility is available or other methods of disposal are not feasible.

Pest Control

Insects, birds, rodents, and other small mammals can serve as mechanical vectors or they can be essential for a pathogen's lifecycle. They can serve as vectors of infection by bacteria, viruses, protozoa, and roundworms. Transmission of disease by pests can be prevented by eradication of these pests from the immediate environment. Therefore proper attention should be paid to the development of pest control programs that eliminate food, harborage, and points of entrance for pests. For example, grain should be stored in containers with tightly fitting lids. Ideally, feed containers should be placed in rooms designated for feed only and the doors should be kept closed. Birds can be discouraged from nesting within barns by the placement of string pennants (flags) or owl statues among the rafters and lofts. Pools of standing water should be drained to minimize mosquito-breeding sites. Facilities should be kept clean and manure removed on a regular basis to limit attraction of flies.

Handling Manure and Other Organic Materials

Pathogens can readily be transmitted by fecal contamination of feed and water. To minimize feed and water contamination with feces, it is essential to remove animal excrement from small enclosures daily, store manure properly, and dispose of solid and liquid manure in a sanitary manner. Methods of manure storage include pits, lagoons, and compost piles. While storing manure, special attention must be given to the control of insects (often by drying) and the prevention of pollution of adjacent bodies of water. When manure is stored in a compost, production of heat and the chemical changes caused by microbial fermentation exert a deleterious action on the pathogens. Except in cold or adverse conditions, the composting process usually produces temperatures up to 82° C (180° F) and will adequately reduce microbial contamination within 2 weeks.

Contaminated feed, bedding, and soil can also harbor infectious agents. Hay, straw, and silage that are stored tightly packed and likely to be contaminated on the surface only can be cut back 6 inches and sprayed with 4% sodium carbonate.[2] Dirt floors may need to be scraped down to clean soil, followed by removal and replacement of 4 to 8 inches of soil. If present in small amounts, soil and other organic materials can be safely handled by mixing with copious amounts of quick lime and burial at least 2 meters deep.[2] Burning is another acceptable method for decontaminating organic matter; however, because soil is not highly combustible, it can be mixed with flammable materials such as wood shavings, sawdust, or peat to facilitate burning.[2] Decontamination of large amounts of soil is not easily performed. Because penetration of viable pathogens into soil is only of concern in as much as the pathogens can be subsequently released again afterward, the physical removal of the top layer and/or covering with a new layer can be performed if soil is heavily contaminated.

Surface Preparation

To provide an ideal cleaning surface, animal facilities should be constructed with materials that are both smooth and impervious so that they can be thoroughly cleaned. Floor coverings should be chemically sound and structurally engineered to withstand physical abuse and not contribute to bacterial growth. Epoxy floor and wall coverings are ideal for the control of environmental contamination, especially those that incorporate antimicrobial substances such as the phosphated amines. These chemicals provide a bacteriostatic and fungistatic effect that is not lost by washing or wear under normal conditions of use.

Surface imperfections that may harbor microorganisms must be eliminated before cleaning and disinfection. Chipped paint should be scraped away, loose flooring should be repaired, and areas of standing water should be drained and filled. Some animal housing and handling facilities are less amenable to thorough cleaning and disinfection, and in the face of serious infection control problems drastic measures may be called for. Any porous materials such as wood, loose straw, and feed that cannot be thoroughly cleaned may need to be removed and buried or burned. If the porous materials cannot be removed, they may be fumigated with formaldehyde vapor if they are contained in an airtight facility (discussed later in this chapter). All cleaning equipment must also be cleaned and disinfected.

Cleaning

Cleaning must precede disinfection because the presence of organic material may protect organisms indefinitely against all types of chemical disinfectants. Efficient cleaning removes more than 90% of the bacteria from a filthy object and is therefore an integral part of the disinfection process. An additional 7% to 10% of organisms are removed by the disinfection process. The remaining few organisms can be removed by fumigation, but are usually spores or resistant cocci of limited pathogenic importance.[1]

Cleaning involves removal of all extraneous material, especially organic matter, that may harbor microorganisms and is essential for controlling the spread of infectious disease. If organisms are not protected from the physical aspects of the environment within organic matter and porous structural material, they usually survive only relatively short periods of desiccation. Except in freezing weather, most pathogens do not survive if premises are empty for 6 weeks and cleaning and pest extermination have been thorough. The specific period of environmental survival of microorganisms is discussed in the respective sections of this text.

Under circumstances where livestock are intensively reared or when an outbreak of serious disease has occurred, thorough cleaning and disinfection must be performed (Box 43-1). This involves removal of all animals, feed, bedding, and equipment, followed by meticulous cleaning and disinfection of all facilities. All items to be returned to the facilities must be thoroughly cleaned and disinfected. Those items that cannot be cleaned and disinfected must be safely discarded. Clearly, this level of cleaning and disinfection can have significant

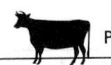

economic impact because feed, bedding, and many equipment items cannot be adequately sanitized and must be discarded and replaced. This level of cleaning and disinfection is most readily accomplished in all-in and all-out facilities and is essential when large numbers of animals are densely housed.

Altered tactics to cleaning and disinfection may be required in some situations. For example, when animals are reared less intensively as occurs on smaller livestock farms and on many horse farms, or when disease has a lower impact because of few affected animals or mild and short-lived clinical signs, complete cleaning and disinfection to the point of depopulation and discarding stored feed and bedding may not be warranted or feasible. Furthermore, facilities containing a preponderance of porous surfaces, such as wooden walls or dirt floors, are less amenable to thorough cleaning and disinfection. Under these circumstances it is wise to have a clear understanding of the optimum cleaning and disinfection process and strive to achieve this goal within the confines of a given situation. Keep in mind that over time mild or subclinical disease can significantly reduce productivity and economic returns from livestock and that more aggressive cleaning and disinfection may be required to contain a disease outbreak or eliminate a problem.

All items in direct or indirect contact with animals should be subject to cleaning and disinfection. Obviously, buildings, other animal holding facilities, equipment, bedding, and soil fall within this domain. Furthermore, personnel and their gear and clothing should not be exempt from the cleaning process. Surfaces that present particular challenges to effective cleaning and disinfection include horizontal surfaces such as window ledges, which accumulate dirt, and light fixtures and power outlets. Horizontal surfaces should be thoroughly cleaned and checked to ensure that fluids do not pool on them. Power should be disconnected before working with any electrical fixtures.

A plan should be devised and communicated to all personnel before cleaning commences. Some personnel can be weak links in the cleaning process if they do not understand the goals and methods clearly. Indeed, personnel can be responsible for spreading organic material and pathogens while they are attempting to remove them. For example, personnel moving from a dirty area into a recently cleaned area will result in recontamination of the previously clean area. Therefore one-way traffic flow patterns should be implemented to prevent recontamination of cleaned areas. Furthermore, personnel should don a clean protective outer layer of clothing (coveralls and overboots) before entering areas to be cleaned. They should remove this contaminated outer layer of clothing and wash their hands as they exit the cleaning area.

Cleaning should be performed from the cleanest area toward the most dirty area. Likewise, cleaning should progress from the highest areas (ceilings and top of walls) to the lowest (floors).[1] Cleaning should progress toward drains whenever possible. It is important to prevent further airborne spread of contamination either by moistening to control dust or taking care not to produce excessive aerosols. Following these guidelines will prevent spread of contamination or recontamination of cleaned areas.

Initially, organic material should be debulked by removing leftover feed in mangers and feed boxes; areas heavily soiled with feces, sputum, blood, or other contaminants should be cleaned by removal, scraping, or washing; and areas of standing water should be drained. Cleaning can be accomplished by using water, pressure, heat, and detergents. Water helps loosen and remove dried material, controls dust, and carries detergents and disinfectants. Application of the washing solution can be improved by use of a pressure washer, preferably with pressures of 90 to 120 psi; however, care must be taken not to produce aerosols that can spread contaminants.

Hotter water enhances more rapid and complete dispersion of fatty soils. Steam is a useful cleansing agent, but it cannot be considered a reliable disinfectant because it cools too rapidly when it contacts surfaces and it does not penetrate into cracks and crevices on the surface. The effectiveness of steam can be increased by incorporating a detergent and disinfectant with the steam or hot water. The temperature of the solution also directly relates to the killing action of the disinfectant. The warmer the water, the more effective is the killing action of the disinfectant on bacteria.

Detergents

The role of the detergent is to disperse and remove soil and organic material from surfaces. This action enables the disinfectant to reach and destroy any microbe that may lie beneath and within the dirt. Any cleansing agent can have properties of a detergent, but the most common detergents are the natural soaps and surfactants. These detergents can be considered in one of three categories: cationic, anionic, and nonionic. Cationic detergents (positively charged) are not used as major cleaning ingredients of detergent formulations. Anionic detergents are negatively charged and are commonly called soaps. The profound foaming property of soap is undesirable for cleaning surfaces, since the residue from excess foam can produce a tacky surface that causes accumulation of soil. This buildup also results over time when hard water ions combine with the anionic detergent. To prevent this buildup, chelating agents such as EDTA are frequently added to bind metallic ions in water before they can complex with the soap. Nonionic detergents (uncharged) are excellent emulsifying agents and are highly effective in lowering surface tension. Their penetration is good and their dispersion properties are exceptional. Foaming properties are generally lower than those of the anionic detergents. Nonionic detergents do not leave a residue of metallic ions, therefore no rinsing is required. Many commercially available detergents are a combination of anionic and nonionic surfactants. Product labels state the ionic form of surfactants in the ingredient or caution sections. Many detergents are good disinfectants and vice versa (e.g., chlorines, iodophors, quaternary ammonium compounds).[3]

Competitive Exclusion

Competitive exclusion is an intervention strategy used to control enteropathogenic colonization in poultry and other food animals.[4] By reducing enteric colonization by pathogens the subsequent pathogen burden in the environment is greatly reduced. Competitive exclusion involves administering, via topical spray or in the water supply, microbial cultures to young animals to enhance establishment of nonpathogenic organisms in the intestinal microflora. Commercially available competitive exclusion cultures are currently only approved for use in chickens; however, experimental evidence indicates that this approach is likely to be effective in swine and cattle as well.[5,6] Competitive exclusion cultures may be a useful tool to aid in preventing colonization by enteropathogens; however, they are not highly effective in the face of established infection.

DISINFECTION PROCEDURES

The effective use of disinfectants requires: (1) knowledge regarding the safe and appropriate methods for applying disinfectants; (2) a thorough understanding of the factors that

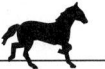

influence disinfection efficacy; and (3) means for assessing the reduction in the pathogen burden in the environment following disinfection. The following section addresses these important issues.

Safe Use of Disinfectants and Hazardous Chemicals

Disinfectants typically contain hazardous chemicals, thus proper use of these products is required and safety precautions must be taken. It is imperative that all personnel have complete and accurate health and safety information before handling hazardous products. A Material Safety Data Sheet (MSDS) is published for all hazardous chemicals and can be obtained from the product manufacturer. The MSDS provides detailed information regarding the product's hazardous ingredients, physical and chemical characteristics, fire and explosion hazards, reactivity, health hazards, safe handling, and control measures. The MSDS should be consulted before using any chemical disinfectant to obtain detailed health and safety information. Most disinfectants cause irritation when in contact with eyes, skin, or the respiratory tract (through inhalation of vapors or aerosolized product), so precautions should always be taken to limit exposure of these tissues. Personal protective equipment that should be worn when handling hazardous chemicals includes rubber or neoprene gloves and protective clothing to prevent skin contact, and chemical safety goggles or face shield. In addition, when there is potential for exposure to vapors or aerosolized product, such as when concentrates are handled or when power sprayers or spray pumps are used, vapor respirators are indicated to protect the respiratory tract. Other health and safety precautions indicated on the MSDS should be heeded.

Factors Influencing Action of Disinfectants

Several important factors affect the efficacy of disinfectants. The importance of cleaning before disinfecting was discussed in previous paragraphs. In addition, the nature of the object to be disinfected must be considered. Porous materials, crevices, and cracks are difficult or nearly impossible to disinfect. Other factors to consider when using disinfectants include the organic load present, the type and amount of microbial contamination, the concentration of and exposure time to the disinfectant, and physical and environmental conditions affecting the disinfection process.

ORGANIC MATERIAL. Organic material (e.g., blood, pus, feces, lipids, bedding) interferes with the actions of disinfectants and may do so in several ways. The interference frequently occurs by a chemical reaction between the disinfectant and the organic material, resulting in a complex that is less biocidal or inactive. Chlorine- and iodine-containing disinfectants, in particular, are prone to such interaction. Organic material can also protect the microorganism by creating a physical barrier that prevents the ready access of the disinfectant. Some disinfectants cause a precipitation of protein on hard surfaces and by that action contribute to their own ineffectiveness. Many disinfectant solutions also have some detergent ingredients that may suspend particulate and colloidal material and absorb the disinfectant so that it is potentially removed from the solution. Therefore meticulous cleaning is essential before any disinfecting procedure. Cleaning and flushing may appear to remove all debris, but they can leave a film of organic material, termed biofilm, that interferes with disinfection. Biofilm is a complex aggregation of bacteria, typically of multiple species, that adheres to surfaces in an exopolysaccharide matrix.[7] Bacteria contained within biofilms are highly resistant to disinfection. Biofilm appears as a thin residue remaining on surfaces after cleaning. Cleaning surfaces helps reduce the development of biofilm. Mechanical disruption of biofilms by using surfactant detergents along with mechanical methods of scrubbing, brushing, and scraping during the cleaning process is currently the most effective mechanism to help eliminate these microorganism complexes.

TYPE AND NUMBER OF MICROORGANISMS. Microorganisms vary greatly in their viability in the environment and resistance to disinfectants. Although the viability of most organisms is greatly reduced by exposure to sunlight and drying, *Pseudomonas* and *Klebsiella* organisms are resistant to drying and may be found in dust.[8] Enveloped viruses (e.g., Coronaviridae, Herpesviridae, Orthomyxoviridae, Paramyxoviridae, Retroviridae) are lipophilic and are more readily susceptible to disinfection than nonenveloped viruses (e.g., Adenoviridae, Picornaviridae, Reoviridae, Rotaviridae), which are hydrophilic and killed by a limited number of disinfectants such as strong chlorine-releasing compounds and aldehydes.[9] Furthermore, prions and bacterial endospores possess the most resistance to common biocides and to environmental and physical factors. As predicted for any biologic activity, the larger the number of microbes present, the longer it takes for environmental conditions or a disinfectant to destroy all of them. Obviously, this is one more reason for scrupulous cleaning. Refer to Table 43-1 to help make rational selections of disinfectants on the basis of the comparative susceptibility of microorganisms within a group.

CONCENTRATION AND CONTACT TIME. A disinfectant must be in contact with the microorganism long enough at a sufficient concentration for effective biocidal activity. Initially, there is a lag period before activity by the disinfectant commences that is followed by a logarithmic reduction in the number of viable organisms. Most microorganisms are killed during this phase of the process. If label instructions are followed, optimum disinfection is usually achieved. However, directions for use may be modified, often unintentionally, without realizing the consequences. In general, the more concentrated the biocide, the greater its efficacy, and the shorter the time necessary to achieve microbial kill. Usually the concentration of a disinfectant is restricted by the damage it may cause to an inanimate surface and by the cost of the chemical. However, most disinfectants must be properly diluted, or their efficacy will be reduced. This point is particularly important for alcohols and halogens. The effect of dilution also varies widely among other disinfectants. For example, halving the concentration of a quaternary ammonium compound only doubles its disinfecting time, but halving the concentration of a phenolic solution results in a marked increase in its disinfecting time, often resulting in loss of efficacy within reasonable contact times. If the disinfectant is diluted too much, its activity may be reduced until it has only static rather than cidal antimicrobial activity. Such dilution can inadvertently occur if standing water is present when the disinfectant is applied.

Just as the effect of concentration varies widely among disinfectants, the required duration of contact also differs considerably. For example, 70% isopropyl alcohol can destroy *Mycobacterium tuberculosis* in 5 minutes, whereas 3% phenol requires 2 to 3 hours. Contact time is frequently shortened, often with ineffective results, by evaporation and drying of the disinfectant. Therefore optimum application of a disinfectant requires that the area be soaked so that air pockets do not protect microorganisms and drying does not occur too rapidly. The disinfectant may be applied best by means of a spray pump to force the solution into all cracks and crevices.

PHYSICAL AND ENVIRONMENTAL FACTORS. The activity of most disinfectants increases with increased temperature, but there are exceptions (sodium hydroxide). However, the temperature must not exceed the point at which the disinfectant itself degrades. An increase in pH improves the

TABLE 43-1

Approximate Disinfectant Susceptibility of Microorganisms in Order of Increasing Resistance

Microbial Susceptibility Group*	Microorganisms	Generally Effective Disinfectants†
A	Retroviruses, ortho and paramyxoviruses, herpesviruses and other enveloped viruses; most gram-negative bacteria, some filamentous fungi and gram-positive cocci, mycoplasma	Alcohols, aldehydes, chlorhexidine, chorine, iodophors, substituted phenolics, QAC
B	*Staphylococcus* spp., some dimorphic and filamentous fungi, yeasts, algae, some gram-negative bacteria (*Pseudomonas aeruginosa*)	Alcohols, aldehydes, chlorine, iodophors, substituted phenolics, QAC
C	Adenoviruses	Alcohols, aldehydes, chlorine, iodophors, substituted phenolics, QAC
D	*Mycobacterium* spp., rotaviruses, some fungal ascospores	Alcohols, aldehydes, chlorine, iodophors, substituted phenolics, QAC
E	Parvoviruses	Aldehydes, chlorine, QAC
F	Bacterial endospores (*Clostridium* and *Bacillus* spp.)	Aldehydes, chlorine
G	Prions (e.g., scrapie, BSE)	Not susceptible to common chemicals

QAC, Quarternary Ammonium Compounds.
*Exceptions exist among and between the various groups, but the outline of comparative susceptibility serves as a basic guide to disinfectant activity.
†Susceptibility may vary among product formulations. Carefully read the label directions of the specific product for spectrum of antimicrobial activity, indicated uses and proper use dilution ratio.

activity of some disinfectants (e.g., glutaraldehyde, quaternary ammonium compounds), but decreases the activity of others (e.g., phenolics, hypochlorite, iodine). Hardness of water reduces the activity of certain disinfectants because divalent cations (e.g., Mg^{++} and Ca^{++}) present in hard water interact with soap to form insoluble precipitates.

Monitoring Disinfection Efficacy

Environmental monitoring for specific organisms can be performed to assess the level of contamination following disinfection and to identify problem areas where cleaning and disinfection efforts should be concentrated. The environment can be sampled by standard microbiologic techniques involving swiping areas with sterile swabs or cellulose sponges, inoculating agar or broth with these samples, and isolating and identifying recovered bacteria. Several research facilities have also employed other molecular biology techniques to assess environmental loads of specific pathogens. We have assayed environmental samples for salmonellae by polymerase chain reaction (PCR) and found that organisms were detected at a much higher rate by PCR than by microbiologic culture.[10] Although this discrepancy could be attributed in part to PCR detection of nonviable DNA, the test was useful for identifying areas that harbored salmonellae organisms, even though the test did not likely detect active pathogens.

DISINFECTANTS

Many important criteria must be considered when selecting an appropriate and effective disinfectant. Ideally, the following should be true of disinfectants:
- Free of strong and objectionable odors
- Not corrosive nor cause any other type of destruction of application surfaces
- Not remain strongly toxic for a long time after their application, nor be excessively irritating or toxic when inhaled
- Effective at ordinary temperatures when diluted with water and should readily mix with water
- Packaged in such a concentration and in such a form that they may be readily and economically transported

- Have high antimicrobial potency, be fast-acting, have long duration, and not be inhibited by organic material

A single multipurpose disinfectant is rarely available for all applications. The interplay of physical conditions such as heat, sunlight, desiccation, mechanical cleaning and scrubbing, time, and composition of surfaces to be disinfected must be considered when selecting a disinfectant. Knowledge of the microorganisms that are causing a risk of disease also influences the choice of a suitable disinfectant.

The following overview of the characteristics of disinfectants is intended to provide the user with an introduction to information used to select an appropriate disinfectant and guidelines to use it in the most efficient way. The discussion is limited to a few of the more common disinfectants that are available for use in veterinary medicine. Authoritative reference texts that describe disinfectants and their detailed uses are available.[1,2,11-13]

Alcohols

Alcohols (ethanol, isopropanol) are broad-spectrum antimicrobial agents (optimum concentrations range from 60% to 90% by volume) that are bactericidal, virucidal, and fungicidal although they lack sporicidal activity. Alcohols are the exception to the rule that higher concentrations are better, because 95% ethanol is less effective than 70% ethanol. Ethanol is a very potent virucidal agent, inactivating all the viruses, but isopropanol cannot inactivate nonenveloped viruses. The mechanism of action of alcohols involves protein denaturation, membrane damage, and cell lysis.[14] The major limitations to the use of the alcohols include the damage done to equipment (e.g., hardening rubber and certain plastics), solvent activity, rapid evaporation, and flammability.

Aldehydes

Formaldehyde and glutaraldehyde, the most commonly used aldehyde disinfectants, are highly potent at killing a broad spectrum of microorganisms, to the point of achieving sterilization. The mechanism of action of formaldehyde is to cross-link proteins, RNA, and DNA, whereas the cross-linking activity of glutaraldehyde is limited to proteins.[14] Formaldehyde is used primarily as a fumigant. It has been used to decontaminate wooden surfaces and brick walls contaminated by highly resistant organisms such as *Bacillus anthracis*. Although it is inexpensive, efficient, and particularly useful for inaccessible surfaces, its usefulness for disinfection and sterilization is limited by its highly noxious and toxic fumes and evidence of carcinogenicity. Because formaldehyde vapor presents a significant health hazard to humans and animals, this agent can only be used in facilities that can be fully depopulated, tightly sealed to prevent vapor release during fumigation, and safely and thoroughly ventilated after fumigation. The fumigant is produced for the gaseous decontamination of closed areas by heating paraformaldehyde, a solid polymer of formaldehyde, until it is vaporized. Other ways to produce the fumigant include aerosolizing a solution of formalin or reacting potassium permanganate with formalin. However, for safety reasons, heating paraformaldehyde is the preferred method of generating formaldehyde. For maximum efficiency and safety the area to be fumigated must be securely sealed in an airtight manner to prevent loss of the gas, preheated to at least 20° C (68° F), and all surfaces should be wet immediately before fumigation so the relative humidity will be 80% to 90%. Pools of water should be avoided because they readily absorb the formaldehyde. Facilities should be kept sealed for 24 hours and then ventilated well before humans can enter the facility or animals are returned. The Occupational Safety and Health Administration (OSHA) standard (29 CFR 1910.1048)[15] applies to formaldehyde gas, its solutions, and a variety of material such as trioxane, paraformaldehyde, resin formulations, and solids and mixtures containing formaldehyde that serve as sources of the substance. The standard sets permissible exposure levels and describes requirements for handling and monitoring these chemicals. Because of its toxic properties, fumigation with formaldehyde should only be performed by professional contractors who are trained and skilled in the use of this chemical.

Glutaraldehyde is a highly active disinfectant used primarily for medical equipment such as endoscopes and for anesthesia and respiratory equipment. Aqueous solutions of glutaraldehyde are acidic and in this state are not sporicidal. Only when the solution is "activated" (made alkaline to pH 7.5 to 8.5) by use of alkalinating agents does the solution become sporicidal.

Acids and Alkalis

Acidic and alkaline compounds are used to alter the environmental pH by the release of hydrogen (H^+) and hydroxyl (OH^-) ions. Hydrogen ions alter nucleic acids, modify cytoplasmic pH, and precipitate proteins.[16] Hydroxyl ions saponify lipids in the cell membrane.[16] Commonly used alkalis include sodium hydroxide (caustic soda) and calcium hydroxide. These agents have broad-spectrum antimicrobial activity and are lethal to spores at high concentrations. Nonorganic acids, such as hydrochloric acid and sulfuric acid, have antimicrobial activity, but use of these chemicals is usually limited by their highly caustic nature.

Halogen-Releasing Agents

CHLORINE. Sodium hypochlorite (bleach) is a chlorine-releasing agent that is among the most widely used disinfectants. Chlorine-releasing agents act by inhibiting DNA synthesis, as well as by disrupting oxidative phosphorylation and protein synthesis.[14] Hard water does not interfere with the activity of sodium hypochlorite, but organic material consumes the available chlorine rendering the agent inactive.

Chlorine-releasing agents are broad-spectrum, inexpensive, fast-acting disinfectants that are bactericidal and virucidal, as well as sporicidal at higher concentrations. A 1:10 dilution of household bleach (5.25% sodium hypochlorite) is adequate for most disinfectant needs, including blood spills. Sodium hypochlorite is limited by its corrosiveness, inactivation by organic matter, and instability. Decomposition is affected by temperature, concentration, light, and, most important, pH. Bleach is a potent oxidizer and reacts strongly with most other chemicals. Thus bleach should not be used in combination with other chemicals. Bleach mixed with phosphoric acid cleaners produces toxic chlorine gas. Bleach mixed with ammonia-containing cleaners produces mono- and dichloramines, which are irritants. In addition, the carcinogen bis-chloromethylether is produced when a solution of bleach contacts formaldehyde.

IODINE AND IODOPHORS. Free iodine is the active ingredient of these disinfectants and acts by oxidizing sulfhydryl groups, and forming iodo-derivatives of amino acids and nucleotides.[14] An iodophor is a combination of iodine and a solubilizing agent or carrier. The resulting complex provides a sustained-release reservoir of iodine and releases small amounts of free iodine into aqueous solution. The best known and most widely used iodophor is povidone-iodine. Because the active ingredient of iodophors is the free iodine, dilutions of iodophors are more rapidly bactericidal than full-strength solutions. If these solutions become colorless, all the iodine is gone, and they do not have any antimicrobial activity. To serve as a biocide, iodine may require prolonged contact. The major limitations of iodines are that they are not sporicidal, they stain many materials, and oxidize many metal surfaces. Iodines and iodophors are most commonly used as antiseptics; however, iodophors have been used to disinfect dairy equipment.

Phenolics

Phenolic disinfectants are among the most frequently used disinfectants for environmental surfaces. Phenolics damage plasma membranes and induce leakage of cellular contents.[14,16] Highly substituted phenolic derivatives are especially useful as disinfectants for porous environmental surfaces. Furthermore, the biocidal activity of phenolics is minimally affected by the presence of organic matter, so phenolics are useful in facilities containing raw wood surfaces or dirt floors. Two common phenol derivatives are ortho-phenylphenol and ortho-benzyl-para-chlorophenol. Phenolic compounds are generally not effective against nonenveloped viruses and bacterial endospores. For effective antimicrobial activity, phenolic solutions must be applied at a temperature of 15.5° C (60° F) or higher.

The phenolics are compatible with anionic detergents but should not be used with nonionic or cationic detergents. Some combined phenolic-detergent products may precipitate in hard water, leaving a film that may interfere with subsequent cleaning and disinfection. Other limitations include the strong phenolic odor, assimilation by porous materials, and irritation of tissue caused by residual chemical. Phenolics are toxic to cats and pigs, so the disinfectant should be thoroughly rinsed off surfaces that these species may contact.

Quaternary Ammonium Compounds

Quaternary ammonium disinfectants are organically substituted ammonium compounds with substituent radicals of variable size or chain length. They are cationic surfactants and act by binding phospholipids and proteins and subsequently disrupting the microbial cytoplasmic membrane.[14,16] The quaternaries are fungicidal, bactericidal, and virucidal against enveloped viruses; have variable activity against nonenveloped viruses and mycobacteria; and are not sporicidal. Each compound exhibits its own antimicrobial characteristics so the continuing search for improved quaternary ammonium disinfectants and the marketing of several different compounds. The third generation of quaternary ammonium compounds, the dual quaternaries, contain a mixture of equal proportions of alkyldimethylbenzyl ammonium and alkyldimethylethylbenzyl ammonium chlorides. They offer improved biocidal activity, stronger detergency, and a relatively lower level of toxicity. Advances in broadening the spectrum of biocidal activity and increasing activity under adverse conditions has led to the development of the fourth generation, the twin-chain quaternaries. These disinfectants, including dioctyldimethyl ammonium bromide and didecyldimethyl ammonium bromide, have high biocidal performance and tolerance for anionic surfactants, protein loads, and hard water. Synergistic combinations of the twin-chain quaternaries, the fifth generation, provide improved antimicrobial activity and remain active under hostile conditions. These blends are less toxic and less costly, thereby providing more convenient disinfectants. These newer quaternaries are less affected by organic materials and are as efficacious as other disinfectants for use in ordinary environmental disinfection and sanitation of clean, nonporous hard surfaces such as floors, fixtures, and walls. A highly desirable feature of the quaternaries is the cleaning ability of these agents. The quaternaries are synergistic with nonionic detergents. Frequently they are combined with nonionic detergents and made available as detergent-disinfectants for enhanced cleaning ability. The greatest detergent efficacy and disinfectant activity occurs in the pH range of 9.0 to 10.0. The residual chemical has very little toxicity for animals.

SELECTING A DISINFECTANT

The use of disinfectants for the control of environmental contamination requires consideration of many factors involved in the transmission and initiation of infectious disease, including the number of microorganisms present, the ability of the microorganisms to survive in the environment, the virulence of the microorganism, the portal of entry, and the resistance of the host. After one has become familiar with these aspects, attention must be focused on selecting the most appropriate disinfectant.

Part of the approach to determining the needs of disinfection and sterilization can be to classify items into three risk categories. Critical items have the highest risk of contributing to an infection if such items are contaminated with any microorganism, including bacterial spores. These items must be sterile. Semicritical items come in contact with mucous membranes or skin that is not intact. These items must be free of all microorganisms with the exception of bacterial spores. Therefore a dependable disinfectant is needed. Noncritical items are items that contact intact skin but not mucous membranes. Because these defenses are effective barriers to infection, sanitation is all that is usually required, but disinfection may be desired in some situations.

Regulation and Registration of Disinfectants in the United States

In the United States, disinfectants are considered antimicrobial pesticides and are registered and regulated by the Environmental Protection Agency (EPA) Office of Pesticide Programs in accordance with the Federal Insecticide, Fungicide, and Rodenticide Act (FIFRA). Compliance with product labeling instructions is required. The application for registration of disinfectants must include use directions and recommendations for the product substantiated by microbiologic efficacy

data generated using official test methods approved by the Association of Official Analytical Chemists (AOAC). Regulations require uniform label information that can be evaluated by the consumer (Fig. 43-1). The first consideration when selecting a disinfectant should be identification of an EPA registration number on the label. If such a number is not readily identifiable on the label, one should be particularly skeptical of any disinfectant claims because advertising information is not as closely regulated as the product container label.

Reading the Label

The label is required to contain certain standard information in addition to the EPA registration number (see Fig. 43-1). Only specifically defined terms are allowed on the label to describe the activities of the product. Three types of label claims may be found on disinfectants. The simple claim of germicide or disinfectant activity indicates that the product is only effective against gram-negative bacteria such as *Escherichia coli* and *Salmonella* spp. A general-purpose disinfectant is effective against gram-positive as well as gram-negative bacteria. It must be supported by acceptable efficacy data against *Staphylococcus aureus* and *Salmonella* spp. The preferred product should be labeled as a "hospital disinfectant" that is effective against *Staphylococcus aureus, Salmonella* spp., and *Pseudomonas aeruginosa*. Claims of efficacy against other microorganisms (such as fungi, viruses, and other bacteria) may be present in addition to the minimum requirements. Occasionally, tuberculocidal and sporicidal claims may be present. Sometimes a label gives instruction for use of the product as a disinfectant in schools, industry, or other nonmedical institutions, often at a lower dilution. At the lower dilution, the product is usually a general-purpose disinfectant. For routine disinfection of nonporous surfaces, nothing less than a hospital disinfectant should be used.

The ingredient statement lists the active ingredients that exhibit biocidal properties. It is not reliable to compare the percentages of active ingredients in different products, even when they are of the same chemical type, because they may have different dilution ratios for use. Therefore careful reading of the ingredient statement is best reserved for detecting which class of disinfectant is present. The inactive ingredients may include soaps or detergents, water, dye, and perfumes.

The label must contain specific directions for the dilution ratio that is adequate to effect the intended purpose of the product as claimed on the label. Products containing the same active ingredients, but in different concentrations, may be available. Often, the same disinfectant is prepared with dilution ratios of $1/2$, 1, or 2 oz/gallon. When diluted according to the label, the disinfectant efficacy of these products is identical. Therefore, although the most concentrated product ($1/2$ oz/gallon) may cost the most per gallon, when diluted, it may be the most economical product.

In the past, distilled water was used as a diluent for conducting all efficacy tests. If the product is labeled as a onestep cleaner-disinfectant, it must be effective under conditions consistent with use; thus heavy soil conditions are now simulated in official tests by adding 5% to 10% blood serum as organic soil and 400 ppm or greater hard water. Recently registered products include a statement of these testing conditions on the label. However, one must carefully read the label to avoid being misled. For example, the statement "dilutes in hard or soft water" is not a hard water effectiveness claim; it may simply refer to producing a clear solution and have no relationship to effectiveness.

A single multipurpose disinfectant is rarely available for all applications. The interplay of physical conditions such as heat, sunlight, desiccation, mechanical cleaning and scrubbing, time, and composition of surfaces to be disinfected must be considered when selecting a disinfectant. Knowledge

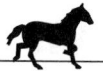

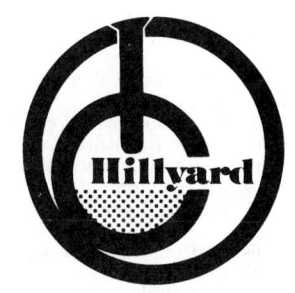

A → EPA Reg. No.
1658-27

EPA Est. No.
1658-MO-1

#155

RE-JUV-NAL®+

B → Disinfectant-Cleaner-Sanitizer-Fungicide-Mildewstat-Virucide*-
Deodorizer for Hospitals, Institutional and Industrial Use

C → Effective in hard water up to 400 ppm hardness (calculated as
$CaCO_3$) in the presence of 5% serum contamination

D → **ACTIVE INGREDIENTS:**
Octyl decyl dimethyl ammonium chloride 1.650%
Dioctyl dimethyl ammonium chloride 0.825%
Didecyl dimethyl ammonium chloride 0.825%
Alkyl (C_{14}, 50%; C_{12}, 40%; C_{16}, 10%)
dimethyl benzyl ammonium chloride 2.200%
E → **INERT INGREDIENTS:** . . . . <u>94.500%</u>
TOTAL: 100.000%

KEEP OUT OF REACH OF CHILDREN
DANGER
Statement of Practical Treatment
In case of contact, immediately flush eyes or skin with
plenty of water for at least 15 minutes. For eyes, call
a physician. Remove and wash contaminated clothing
before reuse.

If swallowed, drink promptly a large quantity of milk,
egg whites, gelatine solution; or if these are not available, drink large quantities of water. Avoid alcohol.
Call a physician immediately.

NOTE TO PHYSICIAN: Probable mucosal damage
may contraindicate the use of gastric lavage. Measures
against circulatory shock, respiratory depression, and
convulsion may be needed.

SEE LEFT PANEL FOR ADDITIONAL
PRECAUTIONARY STATEMENTS

Manufactured by
HILLYARD CHEMICAL COMPANY, St. Joseph, Missouri 64502

DIRECTIONS FOR USE
It is a violation of Federal Law to use this product
in a manner inconsistent with its labeling.

Re-Juv-Nal+ is a proven "one-step" disinfectant-cleaner-sanitizer
-fungicide-mildewstat-virucide use which is effective in water up
to 400 ppm hardness in the presence of 5% serum contamination.
Apply Re-Juv-Nal+ to walls, floors and other hard (inanimate)
non-porous surfaces such as tables, chairs, countertops, sinks,
tile, porcelain, and bedframes with a cloth, mop or mechanical
spray device so as to thoroughly wet surfaces. For heavily soiled
areas, a preliminary cleaning is required. Prepare a fresh solution
daily or when use solution becomes visibly dirty.
Disinfection —To disinfect hard, non-porous surfaces, in hospitals ← F
add 2 oz. per gallon of water. Treated surfaces must remain wet
for 10 minutes. At 1¼ oz. per gallon of water, Re-Juv-Nal+ will
disinfect hard non-porous surfaces in school, industry and non-
medical institutions.
2 oz. per gallon use-level. The activity of Re-Juv-Nal+ has been
evaluated in the presence of 5% serum and 400 ppm hard water
by the AOAC use dilution test and found to be effective against
a broad spectrum of gram negative and gram positive organisms
as represented by:

Pseudomonas aeruginosa	Enterobacter aerogenes	← G
Staphylococcus aureus	Streptococcus faecalis	
Salmonella choleraesuis	Shigella dysenteriae	
Escherichia coli	Brevibacterium ammoniagenes	
Streptococcus pyogenes	Salmonella typhi	
Klebsiella pneumoniae	Serratia marcescens	

For schools, industry and non-medical institution use: At 1¼
oz./gallon of water, Re-Juv-Nal+ delivers excellent cleaning and
germicidal effectiveness. It is effective against Staphylococcus
aureus, Salmonella choleraesuis, Escherichia coli and Serratia
marcescens. The same AOAC tests used to confirm performance
for hospitals were used.
Fungicidal Control — Re-Juv-Nal+ is an effective fungicide against ← H
Trichophyton mentagrophytes (the athlete's foot fungus) when
used on surfaces in areas such as locker rooms, dressing rooms,
shower and bath areas, exercise facilities, etc., at 2 oz./gallon.
Mold and Mildew Control. At 1¼ oz./gallon, Re-Juv-Nal+ will
effectively inhibit the growth of mold and mildew and the odors
caused by them when applied to hard, non-porous surfaces (as
indicated in general instructions above). Allow to dry on surface
and repeat when mildew growth returns.
***Virucidal Performance.** At 1¼ oz. per gallon use-level, Re-Juv-Nal+ ← I
was evaluated and found to be effective in the presence of 5%
serum and 400 ppm hard water, against the following viruses:
Influenza A/Brazil, Herpes Simplex and Vaccinia on inanimate
environmental surfaces.
Sanitizing-Non-Food Contact Surfaces (such as floors, walls, ← J
tables, etc.). At 1 oz. per 2¾ gallon use-level, Re-Juv-Nal+ is an
effective sanitizer against Staphylococcus aureus and Klebsiella
pneumoniae on hard porous and non-porous environmental
surfaces. Treated surfaces must remain wet for 60 seconds.

FIG. 43-1 ▓ Evaluation of a label to determine the quality and uses of a disinfectant. *A,* This product is registered with the EPA, which lends credibility to label claims. *B,* Disinfectant-cleaner for use in hospitals indicates that this product meets the requirements for the most effective category of disinfectants. *C,* The product is effective in hard water and 5% serum; it can be expected to be more active under natural conditions of use. *D,* Active ingredients are a blend of quaternary ammonium compounds, including twin-chain and alkyldimethylbenzyl quaternaries. *E,* Inert ingredients include water, detergents, coloring agents, and odor-control ingredients. *F,* Instructions for use as a hospital disinfectant and as a general-purpose disinfectant differ. The nonmedical dilution is not effective against *Pseudomonas aeruginosa. G,* The label may list disinfectant activity against other bacteria, but the length of the list has limited significance. *H,* Note that fungicidal activity is available only at the dilution of 2 ounces/gallon. At lower concentrations the product is fungistatic. *I,* Virucidal activity can be expected against most enveloped viruses, but in this example effectiveness against nonenveloped viruses is not claimed. *J,* At a lower concentration the product is a sanitizer (i.e., it cleans and reduces the number of bacteria present but is not a germicide). (Courtesy Hillyard Chemical Co, St Joseph, MO.)

of the microorganisms that are causing a risk of disease also influences the choice of a suitable disinfectant.

It is important to periodically reevaluate the needs for disinfectants and to review the activity of products that are available. As new products are developed, it is expected that faster-acting disinfectants that are less susceptible to inhibition by

extraneous substances and have a broader spectrum of activity and higher antimicrobial activity will be available. Whether in animal housing or veterinary hospitals, a critical need exists for more emphasis on the control of contamination rather than exclusive emphasis on the prevention of infection with drugs and biologic agents.

REFERENCES

1. Linton AH, Hugo WB, Russell AD, eds: *Disinfection in veterinary and farm animal practice*, Chicago, 1987, Blackwell Scientific.
2. Block SS: *Disinfection, sterilization, and preservation*, ed 4, Philadelphia, 1991, Lea & Febiger.
3. Hugo WB: Mechanisms of disinfection. In Benarde MA, ed: *Disinfection*, New York, 1970, Marcel Dekker, pp 31-60.
4. Nisbet DJ: Use of competitive exclusion in food animals, *J Am Vet Med Assoc* 213:1744-1746, 1998.
5. Fedorka-Cray PJ et al: Mucosal competitive exclusion to reduce Salmonella in swine, *J Food Prot* 62:1376-1380, 1999.
6. Zhao T et al: Reduction of carriage of enterohemorrhagic *Escherichia coli* O157:H7 in cattle by inoculation with probiotic bacteria, *J Clin Microbiol* 36:641-647, 1998.
7. Costerton JW, Stewart PS, Greenberg EP: Bacterial biofilms: a common cause of persistent infections, *Science* 284:1318-1322, 1999.
8. Stokes EJ, Ridgway GL, Wren MWD, eds: *Clinical microbiology*, ed 7, Boston, 1993, Hodder & Stoughton.
9. Grossgebauer K: Virus disinfection. In Benarde MA, ed: *Disinfection*, New York, 1970, Marcel Dekker, pp 103-148.
10. Ewart SL et al: Identification of sources of *Salmonella* organisms in a veterinary teaching hospital and evaluation of the effects of disinfectants on detection of *Salmonella* organisms on surface materials, *J Am Vet Med Assoc* 218:1145-1151, 2001.
11. Collins CH et al, eds: *Disinfectants: their use and evaluation of effectiveness*, London, 1981, Academic Press.
12. Russell AD, Yarnych VS, Koulikovskii AV, eds: *Guidelines on disinfection in animal husbandry for prevention and control of zoonotic diseases*, Geneva, 1984, World Health Organization document WHO/VPH/84.4.
13. Willett HP: Sterilization and disinfection. In Joklik WK et al, eds: *Zinsser microbiology*, ed 19, Norwalk, Conn, 1988, Appleton and Lange, pp 161-171.
14. McDonnell G, Russell AD: Antiseptics and disinfectants: activity, action, and resistance, *Clin Microbiol Rev* 12:147-179, 1999.
15. Occupational Safety and Health Administration Regulations, U.S. Department of Labor, Standard for formaldehyde (29 CRF 1910.1048). http://www.osha-slc.gov/OshStd_data/1910_1048.html, accessed 2001.
16. Maris P: Modes of action of disinfectants, *Rev Sci Tech Off Int Epiz* 14:47-55, 1995.

Use of Biologics in the Prevention of Infectious Diseases

W. DAVID WILSON

NANCY E. EAST

JOAN DEAN ROWE

VICTOR S. CORTESE

Consulting Editors

EQUINE VACCINATION AND INFECTIOUS DISEASE CONTROL

W. DAVID WILSON

GENERAL CONSIDERATIONS

Programs for controlling infectious diseases[1] are important components of management practices directed toward maximizing the health, productivity, and performance of horses. Infectious disease in an individual horse or outbreaks of infection in a group occurs when horses experience challenge with an infectious agent at a dose sufficient to overcome resistance acquired through previous natural exposure to the disease or through vaccination. For this reason, programs for controlling infectious diseases should have the following three goals:

1. To reduce exposure to infectious agents in the horses' environment
2. To minimize factors that diminish resistance
3. To enhance resistance through the use of vaccines (vac-

cination alone cannot be expected to prevent disease; management practices must reduce challenge with infectious pathogens)

The incidence of infectious disease in horse populations tends to rise with an increased number and concentration of susceptible horses at a facility, with movement of horses on and off the facility, and with favorable external environmental and management influences. The conditions on breeding farms, in performance and show horse barns, and at racetracks are ideal for the introduction and transmission of infectious diseases, particularly those of the respiratory tract.

On breeding farms, the introduction and commingling of horses of various ages and origins and the high proportion of young, susceptible horses and pregnant mares create a situation that poses special problems and demonstrates some important considerations in the practice of disease control. The risk of acquiring infection can be reduced by maintaining distinct groups by age and function. Resident mares and foals should be kept separate from weanlings, yearlings, horses in training, and visiting mares. Visiting mares and other horses entering the farm should have a negative Coggins test result for equine infectious anemia (EIA) and should be appropriately vaccinated and dewormed before arrival. They should be received and maintained in barns and paddocks separate from the resident farm population. Preferably, a specific group of caretakers should attend to incoming horses; and footbaths separate equipment and a clean change of coveralls and boots should be used.

New arrivals should be quarantined for 30 days and monitored for signs of contagious disease. The rectal temperature should be recorded daily, and any prophylactic procedures not done before arrival should be performed. Foaling mares being sent to a distant breeding farm for breeding should be transported 6 to 8 weeks before foaling; this permits timely exposure to resident pathogens at the destination farm, which allows the mare's immune system to mount a response and concentrate antibodies in the colostrum to improve passive protection of the foal. Mares being shipped short distances for breeding can be transported during estrus, with or without the foal, and returned to the farm on the same day to reduce the risk of the foal acquiring infection.

Regardless of the type of equine facility, any horse that becomes ill with a possibly contagious disease should be isolated, preferably in an air space separate from the remainder of the herd, for at least 10 days beyond the complete abatement of clinical signs. Separate equipment should be used, and if a separate group of caretakers is not available for these animals, workers should always complete their work with healthy horses before handling sick horses. Caretakers should wash their hands and boots thoroughly between horses and wear different coveralls. Stalls that have housed sick horses should be cleaned thoroughly, disinfected, allowed to dry, and left empty as long as possible. This approach is particularly important in dealing with organisms such as *Streptococcus equi*, which can survive in a protected, moist environment for several months.[2]

In most equine enterprises, vaccination is important to the overall management program for controlling infectious diseases. The decision to use a particular vaccine depends on the risk of acquiring infection and the medical and economic consequences of infection compared with the efficacy, cost, and possible adverse side effects of the vaccination program. Factors to consider when developing an equine vaccination program include the animals' age, type, number, use, and stocking density; possible exposure to diseases; the cost of implementing the program; and the operation's facilities, management practices, and geographic location. For these reasons, there is no "standard" vaccination program that can be recommended for all horses; each situation must be evaluated individually based on (1) the risk of disease (likely exposure, environmental factors, geographic factors, age, breed, use, and gender), (2) the potential for adverse reactions to one or more vaccines, (3) the expected efficacy of the selected product or products, and (4) the cost. Cost should include expenses incurred and money lost during the time the horses are out of competition, labor and medication expenses if the animals develop clinical disease and require treatment, and the expenses in time, labor, and vaccines required for proper immunization.

The client's expectations should be realistic, and the veterinarian should explain the following points carefully:

1. Vaccination minimizes the risk of infection but does not prevent disease in all circumstances.
2. The primary series of vaccines and booster doses should be administered appropriately before likely exposure.
3. The horses in a population are not all protected equally nor for an equal duration after vaccination.
4. Whenever possible, all horses in a herd should be vaccinated on the same schedule; this simplifies record keeping, minimizes replication and transmission of infectious agents in the herd, and optimizes herd immu-

nity by protecting those animals that responded poorly to vaccination.

A properly administered, licensed product should not be assumed to provide absolute, effective protection during any given field epidemic. Copies of the vaccination and health maintenance records should accompany each horse leaving the facility for sales, training, or breeding. Similarly, owners of equine facilities should establish prerequisites for vaccination of all horses entering the facility and request that copies of the vaccinal records accompany those horses.

Client expectations and the goals of disease control programs vary considerably. In performance horses, the goal generally is to minimize time spent out of training and thereby to maximize earning potential. In this case, an enforced period of rest due to infectious disease has much more significant economic consequences than a similar recommendation for a barren broodmare or backyard horse. On the other hand, many owners of backyard horses diligently vaccinate against even low-risk diseases, despite the expense involved, to keep their horses healthy.

Only federally licensed vaccines should be used, and strict attention must be paid to the manufacturer's recommendations for storage, handling, and routes of administration to maximize the product's efficacy and safety. However, research or clinical experience may support alternate protocols for vaccination that will improve the vaccine's efficacy without increasing adverse effects. The length of time needed to induce a protective immune response should be considered in relation to expected exposure. Optimum protection generally is not achieved until 2 to 3 weeks after completion of the primary series or 1 or more weeks after administration of a booster dose. Inactivated (killed) vaccines administered intramuscularly generally induce a greater serologic response when an initial series of three doses is given rather than the two-dose series recommended by most vaccine manufacturers.

The primary role of authorities charged with licensing vaccines in North America traditionally has been to ensure the purity and safety of the vaccines, with less emphasis placed on documentation of efficacy.[3-5] Consequently, little published information is available documenting the efficacy of most vaccines currently licensed in North America.[3-5] Field experience and some experimental evidence suggest that the efficacy of vaccines directed against different diseases varies considerably and that efficacy also varies among the vaccines from different manufacturers directed against the same disease.[6,7]

Vaccination is unlikely to confer protection more durable than that produced by recovery from natural disease, especially when the route of vaccination (usually intramuscular) is different from the route of natural infection; this is because vaccines frequently do not evoke the full array of protective immune responses induced by natural infection.[8,9] For example, the efficacy and durability of protection induced by parenteral vaccines against respiratory tract pathogens are frequently questioned.[4,5,9] In part this reflects the fact that parenterally administered vaccines generally are poor inducers of the local mucosal immune responses that are important for effective protection against infection of the respiratory tract.[5,8,9] In addition, immunity achieved after natural infection with some respiratory tract pathogens is short-lived.

In immunization programs for foals, passive transfer of antibodies via the colostrum should be exploited by consistently administering booster doses of vaccine to mares 4 to 6 weeks before foaling and by ensuring that foals ingest adequate amounts of high-quality colostrum within 24 hours of birth. Specific colostral immunoglobulins provide protection against field infections for several months, but they may also interfere with vaccinal antigens and prevent an active immunologic response in the foal; this phenomenon is known as maternal antibody interference. Although protective concentrations of an-

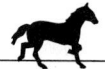

tibody decline with time, vaccination of a foal while colostral antibodies are present, even at concentrations less than those considered protective, may be of minimal or no value because of maternal antibody interference.[10-19]

The duration of the inhibitory effect of maternal antibodies varies by antigen and by vaccine type, and it also is influenced by the dam's antibody titer at the time of foaling and the efficiency of maternal antibody transfer. Maternal antibody interference appears to persist up to 6 months for most antigens and up to 9 months or longer for others. Consequently, individual foals may become susceptible to infection before the primary vaccinal series can be completed. In addition, vaccination with inactivated equine influenza antigens when maternal antibody interference is present can result in apparent "tolerance" to the vaccinal antigen and can delay the age at which the young horse is able to generate an appropriate active response.[10,17]

Some horses develop local muscle swelling and soreness or transient, self-limiting systemic signs, including fever, anorexia, and lethargy, after receiving inactivated vaccines. The systemic signs are perhaps more common after intramuscular injection of inactivated influenza vaccines but can be associated with any vaccine.[20,21] For this reason, horses should not be given any vaccine within 2 weeks of shows, performance events, sales, or domestic shipment, and they should not be given inactivated influenza vaccines within 3 weeks of international shipment. It may also be beneficial to minimize environmental dust when vaccinating horses known to have allergic airway disease or hypersensitivity.[21]

Although adverse reactions associated with administration of a vaccine (including anaphylaxis) are uncommon, the possibility always exists; therefore vaccines should be administered by or under the direct supervision of a veterinarian. Adverse reactions should be reported to the vaccine's manufacturer and to the U.S. Department of Agriculture (1-800-752-6255) or to the United States Pharmacopeia (USP) Veterinary Practitioners Reporting Program (forms may be obtained or reports submitted by calling the USP at 1-800-487-7776).

Anaphylaxis is a life-threatening emergency that requires prompt treatment with epinephrine (5 ml of a 1:10,000 dilution given intravenously or, in less acute situations, 1 to 2 ml of a 1:1000 dilution given intramuscularly or subcutaneously). Local irritant tissue reactions occur more frequently, particularly when polyvalent combination vaccines and injectable strangles vaccines are used. These reactions usually are self-limiting, but resolution can be promoted by parenteral or oral administration of nonsteroidal antiinflammatory drugs (NSAIDs), topical application of warm compresses or drawing agents, and gentle exercise. Significant reactions in the neck muscles may make a horse reluctant to lower or raise its head; therefore feed and water buckets should be positioned accordingly. The occurrence of local reactions can be reduced by administering the vaccine deep in the semimembranosus and semitendinosus muscles of the hind leg rather than in the neck and by allowing the horse to exercise after vaccination. Horses that repeatedly react to polyvalent vaccines may benefit from administration of an NSAID before vaccination, from administration of the individual antigenic components separately in different sites, or from use of a different brand of vaccine.

In North America, vaccines currently are available to aid protection against the following equine infectious diseases:

- Tetanus
- Eastern, western, and Venezuelan equine encephalomyelitis
- Equine influenza
- Equine herpesvirus types 1 and 4 infection (rhinopneumonitis)
- Strangles (*Streptococcus equi* infection)
- Rabies
- Equine monocytic ehrlichiosis (Potomac horse fever)
- Toxicoinfectious botulism
- Equine viral arteritis
- Anthrax
- Rotaviral diarrhea

Table 44-1 presents the recommended vaccination schedules for protection against these diseases. Table 44-2 provides general guidelines for use of the most frequently indicated equine vaccines under various management conditions and in various geographic locations.

TETANUS

Tetanus is an often fatal disease caused by a potent neurotoxin elaborated by the anaerobic, spore-forming bacterium *Clostridium tetani*. *C. tetani* is present in the intestinal tract and feces of horses, other animals, and human beings and is abundant in soil. All horses should be actively immunized against tetanus using tetanus toxoid, because tetanus spores are ubiquitous in the environment. The disease is expensive to treat and has a high mortality rate. The vaccines available are formalin-inactivated, adjuvanted toxoids, which are inexpensive and safe and induce a solid, long-lasting immunity. Active immunization with tetanus toxoid also reduces the need for tetanus antitoxin administration. Manufacturers recommend administration of a primary series of two doses of toxoid given 3 to 8 weeks apart and annual boosters. The titers of specific antibody rise within 14 days of administration of the final dose in the primary series and persist at detectable levels for 12 months or longer, depending on the adjuvant system used in the vaccine.[22,23]

No published challenge studies are available documenting the speed of onset or duration of protection induced by the tetanus toxoid preparations currently licensed in North America. However, a challenge study conducted in Europe more than 40 years ago found that horses were resistant to challenge 8 days after receiving a single injection of tetanus toxoid, before antibody could be detected in serum.[24] A second study demonstrated that a series of three doses of tetanus toxoid induced protection that lasted for at least 8 years and possibly was lifelong, even if antibodies could no longer be detected.[25] In North America, however, tetanus has been documented in vaccinated horses.[26] Therefore until data documenting the duration of immunity are published, it would not be prudent to recommend extension of the annual interval for revaccination.

The annual booster for pregnant mares should be given 4 to 6 weeks before foaling to protect the mare if she sustains foaling-induced trauma and to enhance concentrations of specific immunoglobulins in the colostrum. Colostrum-derived antibodies significantly interfere with the immune response of foals vaccinated with tetanus toxoid until they are about 6 months old.[18,23] A foal that received appropriate transfer of colostral antibodies from a vaccinated mare should be given the primary series of three doses of tetanus toxoid, at 4- to 6-week intervals, beginning at 6 months of age or older. Foals born to unvaccinated mares should receive the initial three-dose series starting at 3 to 4 months of age. The three-dose primary series is recommended for foals because a high proportion of foals fail to seroconvert in response to two doses of tetanus toxoid, regardless of whether maternal antibodies are present.[18,23] Vaccinated horses that sustain a wound or undergo surgery more than 6 months after receiving a tetanus booster should be revaccinated with tetanus toxoid.

Tetanus antitoxin is produced by hyperimmunization of donor horses with tetanus toxoid. Administration of one vial

Text continued on p. 1390

TABLE 44-1

Suggested Vaccination Schedule for Horses[1]

Disease/Vaccine*	Foals/Weanlings	Yearlings	Performance Horses	Pleasure Horses	Broodmares†	Comments
Tetanus (toxoid)	*Foal of vaccinated mare:* First dose: 6 months; Second dose: 7 months; Third dose: 8 to 9 months. *Foal of unvaccinated mare:* First dose: 3 to 4 months; Second dose: 4 to 5 months	Annual	Annual	Annual	Annual, 4 to 6 weeks prepartum	Booster given at time of penetrating injury or surgery if last dose was given more than 6 months previously.
Encephalomyelitis (EEE, WEE, VEE)	**WEE, EEE (low-risk areas) and VEE** *Foal of vaccinated mare:* First dose: 6 months; Second dose: 7 months; Third dose: 8 months. *Foal of unvaccinated mare:* First dose: 3 to 4 months; Second dose: 4 to 5 months; Third dose: 5 to 6 months	Annual, spring	Annual, spring	Annual, spring	Annual, 4 to 6 weeks prepartum	VEE needed only when threat of exposure exists. VEE may be available only as a combination vaccine with EEE and WEE.
	EEE (high-risk areas) First dose: 3 to 4 months; Second dose: 4 to 5 months; Third dose: 5 to 6 months; Fourth dose: 12 months	Annual, spring	Annual, spring	Annual, spring	Annual, 4 to 6 weeks prepartum	In high-risk areas for EEE, give EEE and WEE booster every 6 months. A series of at least three doses is recommended for primary immunization of foals.
Equine influenza	**Intranasal modified live virus** First dose: 11 months; Optional second dose: 3 months later	Every 6 months	Every 6 months	Every 6 months	Annual, before breeding (see Comments)	Not recommended for pregnant mares until data are available; use inactivated vaccine for prepartum booster. In foals, if first dose is given before 11 months of age, give second dose at or after 11 months.
	Inactivated injectable vaccine *Foal of vaccinated mare:* First dose: 9 months; Second dose: 10 months; Third dose: 11 to 12 months; Then at 3- to 4-month intervals. *Foal of unvaccinated mare:* First dose: 6 months; Second dose: 7 months; Third dose: 8 months; Then at 3- to 4-month intervals	Every 3 to 4 months	Every 3 to 4 months	Annual, with additional boosters before likely exposure	At least semiannual, with one booster 4 to 6 weeks prepartum	A series of at least three doses is recommended for primary vaccination of foals regardless of dam's vaccination status.
Rhinopneumonitis (EHV-1, EHV-4 infection)	First dose: 4 to 6 months; Second dose: 5 to 7 months; Third dose: 6 to 8 months; Then at 3- to 4-month intervals	Every 3 to 4 months if elected	Every 3 to 4 months if elected	Semiannual if elected	Fifth, seventh, and ninth months of gestation (inactivated EHV-1 vaccine); optional dose at third month of gestation	Vaccination of mares before breeding and 4 to 6 weeks prepartum is suggested. Breeding stallions should be vaccinated before the breeding season and semiannually.

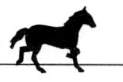

Disease	Foal				Broodmare	Comments
Strangles	**Intranasal vaccine** First dose: 4 to 6 months; Second dose: 2 to 3 weeks later; Third dose: 7 to 10 months. **Injectable vaccine** First dose: 4 to 6 months; Second dose: 5 to 7 months; Third dose: 7 to 8 months; Fourth dose: 12 months	Semiannual / Semiannual	Optional; semiannual if risk is high / Optional; semiannual if risk is high	Optional; semiannual if risk is high / Optional; semiannual if risk is high	Semiannual, but use M-protein injectable vaccine for prefoaling booster / Semiannual with one dose of inactivated M-protein vaccine 4 to 6 weeks prepartum	Use when endemic conditions exist or risk is high. Foals as young as 6 weeks may be given the intranasal product, but a third dose should be given before weaning. Use when endemic conditions exist or risk is high.
Rabies	*Foal of vaccinated mare:* First dose: 6 months; Second dose: 7 months; Third dose: 12 months. *Foal of unvaccinated mare:* First dose: 3 to 4 months; Second dose: 12 months	Annual	Annual	Annual	Annual, before breeding	Vaccination recommended in endemic areas. Do not use modified live virus rabies vaccines in horses.
Equine monocytic ehrlichiosis (Potomac horse fever)	First dose: 5 to 6 months; Second dose: 6 to 7 months. A third dose in the primary series should be given if the first dose was given before 5 months.	Every 4 to 6 months	Every 4 to 6 months	Every 4 to 6 months	Every 4 to 6 months, with one dose given 4 to 6 weeks prepartum	Booster given in May or June in endemic areas. Efficacy of a single annual booster is questionable.
Toxicoinfectious botulism (shaker foal syndrome)	*Foal of vaccinated mare:* Three-dose series is given at 30-day intervals; series can start as early as 2 to 3 months. *Foal of unvaccinated mare:* There is little value in vaccinating the foal of an unvaccinated mare because there is insufficient time for antibodies to develop and offer protection during the susceptible age.	NA	NA	NA	Initial three-dose series is given at 30-day intervals, with last dose given 4 to 6 weeks prepartum. Given annually thereafter, 4 to 6 weeks prepartum	Use when endemic conditions exist or risk is high.
Equine viral arteritis	Intact colts intended for use as breeding stallions: one dose at 6 to 12 months.	Annual for colts intended for use as breeding stallions	Annual for colts intended for use as breeding stallions	Annual for colts intended to be breeding stallions	Annual for seronegative open mares, 21 days before breeding to carrier stallion; isolate mares for 21 days after breeding to carrier stallion	Use only under special circumstances. Give annually for breeding stallions and teasers, 28 days before start of breeding season. Vaccinated mares do not develop clinical signs after breeding to carrier stallions even though they become transiently infected and may shed the virus for a short time.
Rotaviral diarrhea	There is little value in vaccinating the foal of an unvaccinated mare because there is insufficient time for antibodies to develop and offer protection during the susceptible age.	NA	NA	NA	Vaccinate mares at 8, 9, and 10 months of gestation during each pregnancy; passive transfer of colostral antibodies aids in prevention of rotaviral diarrhea in foals.	Use on endemic farms or when risk of infection is high. Check concentrations of immunoglobulins in foal to verify adequate passive transfer.
Anthrax	Two doses administered SC 2-3 weeks apart	Annual, spring	Annual, spring	Annual, spring	Annual, before breeding. Not recommended for use in pregnant mares.	Use only in endemic areas or in the face of an outbreak. Administer annual boosters in month before period of expected risk. Administer SC in the neck. Avoid concurrent administration of antibiotics.

EEE, Eastern equine encephalomyelitis; *EHV-1*, equine herpesvirus type 1; *EHV-4*, equine herpesvirus type 4; *NA*, not applicable; *SC*, subcutaneously; *VEE*, Venezuelan equine encephalomyelitis; *WEE*, western equine encephalomyelitis.

*As with all medications, the label and product insert should be read before administration of any vaccine.

†Schedules for stallions should be consistent with the vaccination program for the adult horses on the farm and should be modified according to risk.

TABLE 44-2

Manufacturers' Recommendations for Use of Equine Immunizing Agents and Biologics

Disease	Etiologic Agent	Type of Product	Available Products	Manufacturer	Dose
Anthrax	*Bacillus anthracis*	Nonencapsulated live bacterial spores	Anthrax Spore Vaccine	Colorado Serum Co.	1 ml
Botulism (shaker foal syndrome)	*Clostridium botulinum* type B toxin	Toxoid	Bot Tox-B	Neogen Biologics	2 ml
Escherichia coli septicemia	*E. coli*	Hyperimmune serum	Equine coli Endotox	Grand Laboratories	10 ml
			E-Colicin E	Equi Laboratories	10 ml
Endotoxemia	*Salmonella typhimurium*	Inactivated; bacterin toxoid	Endovac-Equi	Immvac	1 ml
	Endotoxin produced by gram negative bacteria	Hyperimmune serum against *S. typhimurium*	Endoserum	Immvac	1.5 ml/kg
Equine encephalomyelitis	Bivalent vaccines: WEE, EEE	Inactivated; chicken tissue culture origin	Encevac	Bayer/Intervet	1 ml
		Inactivated; tissue culture origin	Encephaloid IM	Fort Dodge Laboratories Franklin	1 ml
		Inactivated; cell culture origin	Encephalomyelitis vaccine	Colorado Serum Co.	1 ml
	Trivalent vaccines: WEE, EEE, VEE	Inactivated; chicken tissue culture origin (WEE, EEE) Porcine tissue culture origin (VEE)	Cephalovac VEW	Boehringer Ingelheim, Equi Laboratories	2 ml
		Inactivated; tissue culture origin	Triple-E	Fort Dodge Laboratories	1 ml
Equine viral arteritis	Equine arteritis virus	Modified live; equine cell line origin	Arvac	Fort Dodge Laboratories	1 ml
Equine influenza	Equine influenza A equine 2	Modified live (cold adapted)	FluAvert I.N.	Heska Corporation	1 ml
	Equine influenza A equine 1 and A equine 2	Inactivated; canine cell line origin	Equicine II	Bayer/Intervet	1 ml
		Inactivated; canine kidney cell line origin	Fluvac Plus	Fort Dodge Laboratories, Franklin	1 ml
		Inactivated; cell line origin	Inflogen 3	Fort Dodge Laboratories	1 ml
		Inactivated; cell line origin	Equi-Flu	Boehringer Ingelheim	1 ml
		Inactivated; cell line origin	Flumune	Pfizer	1 ml
		Inactivated; cell line origin	Calvenza EIV	Boehringer Ingelheim	2 ml

Information on combination vaccines is available in Arrioja-Dechert A, ed: *Compendium of veterinary products*, ed 5, Port Huron, Mich, 1999, North American Compendiums.
EEE, Eastern equine encephalomyelitis; *IM,* intramuscular; *IN,* intranasal; *IV,* intravenous; *NA,* not applicable; *PO,* oral; *SC,* subcutaneous; *VEE,* Venezuelan equine encephalomyelitis; *WEE,* western equine encephalomyelitis.
*Avoid administering immediately before an athletic event or show, because transient, usually self-limiting febrile responses may occur after vaccination.

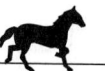

Route	Age for Primary Series	Regimen for Primary Series	Regimen for Revaccination	Comments*
SC		Two doses 2 to 3 weeks apart	Annual	Vaccinate 4 weeks before possible exposure. Stall resting the horse for 10 days may be beneficial. Local reactions may occur. Do not administer antibiotics within 1 week of vaccination.
IM		Three doses at least 4 weeks apart	Annual	In pregnant mares, administer booster 2 to 4 weeks before parturition. Protects only against botulism caused by *C. botulinum* type B.
PO	Within 12 hours of birth			
PO	Within 12 hours of birth			
IM	Over 6 months	Two doses 2 to 3 weeks apart	Annual	Indicated for prevention of endotoxin-mediated disease caused by *S. typhimurium* and *E. coli*.
IV				When treating failure of passive transfer in foals, administer 15 ml/kg of body weight.
IM		Two doses 3 to 4 weeks apart	Annual	Time primary series and boosters to precede mosquito season.
IM		Two doses 3 weeks apart	Annual	Time primary series and boosters to precede mosquito season.
IM		Two doses 3 to 4 weeks apart	Annual	Time primary series and boosters to precede mosquito season.
IM		Two doses 3 to 4 weeks apart	Annual	Time primary series and boosters to precede mosquito season.
IM		Two doses 2 to 4 weeks apart	Annual	Time primary series and boosters to precede mosquito season.
IM	Over 6 weeks	One dose	Annual	Prior authorization by a state veterinarian is required, and a permit may be necessary (regulations vary from state to state). Vaccinate stallions at least 3 weeks before breeding season. Vaccinate mares as maidens or while open at least 3 weeks before breeding. Pregnant mares should not be vaccinated during the last 2 months of gestation. Vaccinated horses may be ineligible for export because of seroconversion.
IN	11 months or older	One dose	Semiannual	Contains Kentucky/91 (A₂) strain. Horses vaccinated before 11 months of age should be revaccinated at 11 months or older. A primary series consisting of two doses, the second given 3 months after the first, may improve efficacy.
IM		Two doses 3 to 4 weeks apart	Annual	Contains Prague/56 (A₁), Miami/63 (A₂), and Kentucky/93 (A₂) strains
IM		Two doses 3 to 4 weeks apart	Annual or before likely exposure	Contains Prague/56 (A₁), Kentucky/81 (A₂), and Kentucky-92 (A₂) strains
IM		Two doses 2 to 4 weeks apart	Annual or before threatened epizootic	
IM		Two doses 3 to 4 weeks apart	Annual	Contains Newmarket/77 (A₁) and Brentwood/79 (A₂) strains
IM		Two doses 3 weeks apart	Annual	Contains Newmarket/77 (A₁) and Brentwood/79 (A₂) strains
IM, IN		Three doses 3 to 4 weeks apart	Annual or before likely exposure	Contains Newmarket/77 (A₁), Newmarket 2/93 (A₂), and Kentucky/95 (A₂) strains. The first and second doses must be administered by the IM route, and the third and subsequent booster doses may be administered by either IM or IV routes.

The addresses of the manufacturers mentioned in this table are listed below:

Bayer/Intervet, Shawnee, KS 66216.
Boehringer Ingelheim Vetmedica, Inc, St. Joseph, MO 64506.
Colorado Serum Co., Denver, CO 80216.
Equi Laboratories, St. Joseph, MO 64503.
Fort Dodge Laboratories, Fort Dodge, IA 50501.

Franklin Laboratories, Fort Dodge, IA 50501.
Grand Laboratories, Larchwood, IA 51241.
Heska Corp, Fort Collins, CO 80525.
IMMVAC, Inc, Columbia, MO 65201.
Merial, Iselin, NJ 08830.

Neogen Biologics, Lexington, KY 40505.
Pfizer, Inc, Exton, PA 19341.
Professional Biological Co, Denver, CO 80216.
Schering-Plough, Kenilworth, NJ 07033.

Continued

TABLE 44-2

Manufacturers' Recommendations for Use of Equine Immunizing Agents and Biologics—cont'd

Disease	Etiologic Agent	Type of Product	Available Products	Manufacturer	Dose
Rotaviral diarrhea	Rotavirus	Inactivated	Equine rotavirus vaccine	Fort Dodge Laboratories	1 ml
Equine monocytic ehrlichiosis (Potomac horse fever)	*Ehrlichia risticii*	Inactivated	PHF-Vax	Schering-Plough	1 ml
		Inactivated	RM Equine Potomavac	Merial	1 ml
		Inactivated	PotomacGuard	Fort Dodge Laboratories, Franklin	1 ml
		Inactivated	Potomac	Equi Laboratories	1 ml
		Inactivated	Mystique	Bayer/Intervet	1 ml
Rabies	Rabies virus	Inactivated; cell line origin	RM Imrab 3	Merial	2 ml
		Inactivated; cell line origin	RM Imrab Bovine Plus	Merial	2 ml
		Inactivated; porcine cell line origin	Rabguard-TC	Pfizer	1 ml
		Inactivated; cell line origin	Rabvac 3	Fort Dodge Laboratories	2 ml
Rhinopneumonitis	Equine herpesvirus type 1 (EHV-1)	Inactivated	Pneumabort-K+1b	Ford Dodge Laboratories, Franklin	2 ml
		Inactivated; tissue culture origin	Prodigy	Bayer/Intervet	2 ml
		Modified live; equine cell line origin	Rhinomune	Pfizer	1 ml
	EHV-1 and EHV-4	Inactivated bivalent; tissue culture origin	Prestige	Bayer/Intervet	1 ml
		Inactivated bivalent	Equivac EHV 1/4	Fort Dodge Laboratories	1 ml
Strangles	*Streptococcus equi*	Modified live	Pinnacle I.N.	Fort Dodge Laboratories	2.5 ml
		Inactivated; bacterial M-protein extract	Strepguard	Bayer/Intervet	1 ml
		Inactivated; bacterial M-protein extract	StrepVax II	Boehringer Ingelheim	1 ml

Information on combination vaccines is available in Arrioja-Dechert A, ed: *Compendium of veterinary products*, ed 5, Port Huron, Mich, 1999, North American Compendiums.

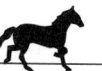

Route	Age for Primary Series	Regimen for Primary Series	Regimen for Revaccination	Comments
IM	Adult broodmares	Three doses 4 weeks apart during the 8th, 9th, and 10th months of gestation.	Annually, three doses during the 8th, 9th, and 10th months of gestation.	Contains the G3 (H2) serotype of equine rotavirus. Product is conditionally licensed for vaccination of pregnant mares to promote passive transfer to foals of antibodies against equine rotavirus.
IM	Over 3 months	Two doses 3 to 4 weeks apart	Semiannual in endemic areas	Efficacy may be improved by administration of two doses annually before period of peak challenge.
IM	Over 3 months	Two doses 3 to 4 weeks apart	Annual	
IM		Two doses 3 to 4 weeks apart	Annual	
IM	Over 3 months	Two doses 3 to 4 weeks apart	Annual	
IM	Over 3 months	Two doses 3 to 4 weeks apart	Annual or before likely exposure	
IM	Over 3 months	One dose	Annual	Effectiveness of a single dose of rabies vaccine in the primary series for foals has recently been questioned (see text).
IM	Over 3 months	One dose	Annual	
IM	Over 3 months	One dose	Annual	
IM	Over 3 months	One dose	Annual	
IM		Two doses 3 to 4 weeks apart	*Young horses:* 6 months after primary series and annually thereafter *Pregnant mares:* Repeat doses annually during fifth, seventh, and ninth months of gestation	Vaccinate open and maiden mares at the same time as pregnant mares. For mares beyond the fifth month of gestation when vaccination is initiated, vaccinate on presentation and every 2 months thereafter until foaling.
IM	Over 6 months	Three doses 4 to 6 weeks apart	*Pregnant mares:* annually during the fifth, seventh, and ninth months of gestation. *Respiratory disease:* Annually or anytime exposure is imminent.	Maiden and barren mares house or pastured with pregnant mares should be vaccinated on the same schedule.
IM	Over 3 months	Two doses 4 to 8 weeks apart	3-month intervals	Vaccinate pregnant mares after the second month of gestation. Vaccine is approved for use in pregnant mares, but no label claim is made for prevention of EHV-1 abortion.
IM		Two doses 4 to 6 weeks apart	Annual or anytime exposure is imminent; foals should be given a booster dose 6 months after the primary series	Approved for use in pregnant mares, but no label claim is made for prevention of EHV-1 abortion.
IM		Two doses 2 to 4 weeks apart	Annual or when exposure is imminent or epidemic conditions exist	Horses subject to repeat exposure to a field virus may benefit from revaccination with a single dose every 3 months.
IN		Two doses at 2 to 3 week intervals	Annual	For intranasal use only. Do not administer parenterally.
IM		Two doses 3 to 4 weeks apart	Annual or before expected exposure	
IM	Over 3 months	Three doses at 3-week intervals	Annual or before expected exposure	

Continued

TABLE 44-2

Manufacturers' Recommendations for Use of Equine Immunizing Agents and Biologics*—cont'd

Disease	Etiologic Agent	Type of Product	Available Products	Manufacturer	Dose
Tetanus	*Clostridium tetani*	Inactivated; toxoid	Tetanus toxoid	Fort Dodge Laboratories, Franklin	1 ml
			Super-Tet	Bayer/Intervet	1 ml
			Tetguard	Boehringer Ingelheim Vetmedica	1 ml
			Tetmune	Pfizer	1 ml
			Tetanus toxoid— Concentrated	Colorado Serum Co., Professional Biological	1 ml
			Tetnogen	Fort Dodge Laboratories	1 ml
		Antitoxin	Tetanus antitoxin	Merial	1500 U
				Fort Dodge Laboratories	1500 U
				Bayer/Intervet	1500 U
				Colorado Serum Co.	1500 U
				Professional Biological	1500 U
				Equi Laboratories	1500-4500 U
			Tetnogen-AT	Fort Dodge Laboratories	1500 U

Information on combination vaccines is available in Arrioja-Dechert A, ed: *Compendium of veterinary products*, ed 5, Port Huron, Mich, 1999, North American Compendiums.

*The recommendations contained in this table were obtained from package inserts or from the *Compendium of Veterinary Products*. In those instances in which research or extensive field experience indicate that increased efficacy can be achieved through use of alternative vaccination protocols, recommendations contained in Table 44-2 may differ from those in Table 44-1.

of antitoxin (1500 U) to unvaccinated horses induces immediate passive protection that lasts about 3 weeks[23,27]; more prolonged protection can be achieved with higher doses. However, because a small but significant number of horses develop serum sickness and fatal hepatic failure (serum hepatitis) several weeks after receiving tetanus antitoxin,[28,29] active immunization with tetanus toxoid is preferred over passive immunization with antitoxin. Administration of tetanus antitoxin is indicated for an unvaccinated horse that is injured or for a foal born to an unvaccinated mare or for an unvaccinated horse that sustains an injury. In the latter case, tetanus antitoxin and tetanus toxoid should be administered concurrently, although with separate syringes and in different sites.[30] The second and third doses of toxoid should be administered at 4- to 8-week intervals to complete the primary series. Thereafter, annual boosters with tetanus toxoid are recommended.

EQUINE ENCEPHALOMYELITIS (Sleeping Sickness)

In the United States, vaccines are available as an aid to prevention of eastern equine encephalomyelitis (EEE), western equine encephalomyelitis (WEE), and Venezuelan equine encephalomyelitis (VEE). Outbreaks of WEE have been recorded in the West and Midwest, with sporadic cases in the Northeast and Southeast. The distribution of EEE historically has been restricted to eastern, southeastern, and some southern states. VEE occurs in South and Central America but has not been diagnosed in the United States for more than 20 years. An outbreak of VEE in southern Mexico in 1993 prompted recommendations for vaccination of horses in Mexico and those in the United States living within 40 miles of the U.S.–Mexican border (i.e., in California, Texas, New Mexico, and Arizona) to create a buffer zone of immune horses.

The encephalomyelitis viruses are transmitted to horses by mosquitoes and infrequently by other bloodsucking insects, from wild birds or rodents, which serve as natural reservoirs for these viruses. The risk of exposure and the geographic distribution of the encephalomyelitides vary by season and from year to year, depending on changes in the distribution of the insect vectors and animal reservoirs.

All horses in North America should be immunized against WEE and EEE. Horses living in or traveling to areas where the risk of exposure to VEE is high should also be immunized against that disease. Vaccination with one of the several inactivated, bivalent (WEE/EEE) or trivalent (WEE/EEE/VEE) vaccines available provides effective control of these diseases. For primary immunization of unvaccinated horses and foals, three doses of vaccine are given 4 to 6 weeks apart. Annual revaccination is appropriately done in the spring, before the arrival of the peak insect vector season. Booster vaccination of pregnant mares 4 to 6 weeks before foaling enhances colostral concentrations of immunoglobulins that generally protect the foals against these diseases for 6 to 7 months.[31,32] Primary vaccination of foals born late in the foaling season may be delayed until the following spring in climates where mosquitoes die in the winter; otherwise, primary immunization of foals of vaccinated mares should be started at 6 months of age to avoid interference from colostral antibodies.[18] Primary vaccination of foals of unvaccinated mares should begin at 3 to 4 months of age. In both cases, the initial three doses of killed virus vaccine are given 4 to 6 weeks apart, and the foal should be revaccinated at 1 year of age to ensure adequate protection.

Because of the high mortality rate associated with EEE, foals born in areas with a high risk of exposure to the disease should be given the first of the initial three doses of vaccine at 3 to 4 months of age, with the second and third doses

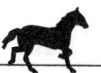

Route	Age for Primary Series	Regimen for Primary Series	Regimen for Revaccination	Comments
IM		Two doses 4 to 8 weeks apart	Annual	For small horses use 0.5 ml.
IM		Two doses 3 to 4 weeks apart	Annual	
IM		Two doses 4 weeks apart	Annual	
IM		Two doses 3 to 4 weeks apart	Annual	
IM		Two doses 4 weeks apart	Annual	
IM		Two doses 4 weeks apart	Annual	
IM or SC	NA	NA	NA	Administer upon exposure to unimmunized animals or those with an unknown vaccination status.
IM, SC, IV, IP	NA	NA	NA	Doses of up to 100,000 U have been used for treatment of tetanus.
IM or SC	NA	NA	NA	Fatal serum hepatitis has been seen after administration of tetanus antitoxin to horses.
IM or SC	NA	NA	NA	
IM or SC	NA	NA	NA	
IM or SC	NA	NA	NA	
IM or SC	NA	NA	NA	

given at 4- to 6-week intervals, and a fourth dose administered at 1 year of age. Booster doses are given semiannually (6-month intervals) thereafter.[14] Many veterinarians who practice in states where mosquitoes are active year-round prefer to revaccinate all horses semiannually to ensure uniform protection throughout the year, although this practice is not specifically recommended by manufacturers of vaccines. Annual revaccination against encephalomyelitis can be combined with revaccination against tetanus and other diseases, as appropriate, using polyvalent vaccines.

EQUINE INFLUENZA

Equine influenza is one of the most common infectious diseases of the respiratory tract in horses. It is endemic in the equine population of the United States and throughout much of the world, with the notable exceptions of Australia and New Zealand. Rapid national and international transportation of horses facilitates spread of the virus. The risk of infection is increased by concentrating young horses at racetracks, training facilities, boarding stables, breeding farms, shows, or similar athletic events, and it is increased in individual horses by a low serum concentration of specific antibody.[33,34] Older horses generally are less susceptible to infection, but that protection can be overwhelmed in horses frequently exposed at shows or similar athletic events. Although the disease is endemic in many countries and infection cycles continuously, explosive outbreaks occur at intervals of several years, when the immunity of the equine population wanes and antigenic drift in the virus has been sufficient to generate a new strain. In contrast to the equine herpesviruses, equine influenza virus does not circulate constantly, even in large groups of horses; rather, it is sporadically introduced, presumably by a symptomatic or an asymptomatic infected horse. This epidemiologic fact and the

ability of the equine immune response to rapidly eliminate the virus suggest that infection can be avoided by preventing the virus from entering a horse population, for example, by quarantine of newly arrived horses for at least 14 days and by appropriate vaccination.[35]

Equine influenza virus is highly contagious and spreads quickly through groups of horses by means of aerosolized droplets dispersed by coughing. Contaminated buckets, grooming or feeding equipment, tack and transport vehicles may serve as fomites because the virus can survive for hours on such objects. The severity of the clinical signs of influenza (i.e., nasal discharge, fever, lethargy, anorexia, cough, and myalgia) depends on the degree of existing immunity, among other factors. Infected horses shed the virus in nasal secretions for up to 10 days. Horses that are partly immune can become subclinically infected and shed the virus.

Immunity to the same (homologous) strain of virus that develops after natural infection persists for little more than a year; unlike the immunity that develops after vaccination with inactivated vaccines, it is not well correlated with the results of hemagglutination inhibition (HI) or single radial hemolysis (SRH) tests. Because the immunity that develops after vaccination with inactivated influenza vaccines is short-lived, recently vaccinated horses can become infected and shed the virus; this contributes to the interepidemic persistence of infection in the equine population and propagation of infection during outbreaks.[36]

Equine influenza is caused by the orthomyxovirus equine influenza A type 2 (influenza A/equine 2; H_3Ng). Equine influenza A type 1 (influenza A/equine 1; H_7N_7) has not been recognized as a cause of natural infection for many years, and it no longer is considered necessary to include it in vaccines.

Antigenic drift of the A/equine 2 subtype has occurred because of point mutations in the genes encoding the amino acid sequences of the hemagglutinin (H) and neuraminidase

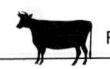

(N) glycoprotein antigens on the surface of the virus. As a result, viral strains have emerged representing two antigenic lineages, the American and the Eurasian strains. Further antigenic drift within each lineage has generated variants, such as the prototypic strain A/equine-2/Miami/63, which are named according to the location and year in which they were first isolated. By generating antigenically heterologous viruses and because of the specificity of immunoglobulins, antigenic drift diminishes the degree and duration of protection conferred by previous infection or vaccination, leaving horses susceptible to infection within a relatively short time.

Although antigenic drift of the equine influenza virus occurs more slowly than that of the human influenza virus, killed equine A/equine 2 vaccines should include viral antigens from isolates obtained within the past 5 years and, ideally, representatives of both the American and Eurasian lineages. However, the American lineage (A/equine 2/91) included in the recently licensed, modified live virus (MLV) intranasal vaccine (Flu-Avert I.N.*) provided protection when vaccinated horses were challenged with Eurasian and American (A/equine 2/98) strains.[7]

Compliance with federal regulations for licensing and marketing of vaccines means that any change of a vaccine, such as including the most recently isolated influenza virus, usually leads to costly, time-consuming evaluation of the revised product. Consequently, the viral antigens in inactivated vaccines lag chronologically behind the antigenic drift of field viruses, resulting in suboptimum protection. In previous years the short-lived immunity that developed after vaccination with inactivated equine influenza vaccines and the lag time for antigenically new strains of virus to be incorporated into vaccines were the impetus for recommendations of frequent revaccination (intervals of 2 to 4 months). However, a revaccination interval that is too short may compromise the vaccine's efficacy, because influenza vaccination in the presence of a high titer inhibits development of an optimum anamnestic response.[37]

Another consideration that may limit the efficacy of influenza vaccines is the phenomenon known as *original antigenic sin*. The term refers to the finding that upon exposure to drifted field A/equine 2 virus, horses show an anamnestic immune response directed more strongly against the strain with which they were vaccinated initially than against the drifted field virus.[36] Furthermore, vaccination of foals with inactivated influenza vaccines in the presence of maternal antibodies may induce an immunotolerance-like state in which foals and yearlings fail to respond to several doses of vaccine administered over many months.[10,17]

Influenza remains one of the most common infectious diseases of performance and show horses despite the widespread practice of frequent revaccination with inactivated influenza vaccines administered by intramuscular injection. Well-controlled epidemiologic studies have documented that repeated vaccination with certain licensed influenza vaccines has failed to reduce the risk of infection during outbreaks and has had a minimal effect on the severity of the disease.[6,33]

A local immune response at the level of the respiratory mucosa appears to be necessary to prevent infection with the influenza virus, but protection after vaccination with inactivated vaccines is more closely correlated with the resulting titer of circulating antibody, as measured by the single radial hemolysis (SRH) or HI tests.[38] The failure of commercially available licensed inactivated influenza vaccines to perform in the field appears to be strongly correlated with their failure to induce high and persistent titers of circulating antibody.[38]

Of the equine influenza vaccines currently licensed in

North America, the only one supported by published challenge data is the previously mentioned Flu-Avert I.N, an MLV equine influenza (A_2) vaccine.[7,39,40] Field experience indicates that this MLV vaccine is effective at preventing influenza after natural challenge, and until efficacy data are available on other equine influenza vaccines, it should form the basis of control programs for equine influenza. Studies have shown that the MLV vaccine is safe and that a single administration to naive horses provides protection from clinical disease for at least 6 months.[7,39-41] In contrast to the immune response obtained with inactivated influenza vaccines administered by intramuscular injection, the degree of protection induced by the intranasal vaccine does not correlate with the level of induced circulating antibodies, suggesting that local responses in the upper respiratory tract are important for protection, as is true after natural infection with the influenza virus.[39]

The MLV vaccine currently is licensed for use in nonpregnant animals over 11 months of age. Until more safety data are available, inactivated equine influenza vaccines administered intramuscularly should be used for prefoaling boosters in pregnant mares, because those vaccines are more likely to enhance the colostral level of immunoglobulin against the equine influenza virus.

All horses should be vaccinated against equine influenza unless the facility is totally closed. The MLV vaccine is labeled for primary vaccination at 11 months of age, with a single dose administered intranasally and boosters given at 6-month intervals. However, using a primary series of two doses given 3 months apart may be advantageous. Horses may shed small amounts of vaccinal virus for several days after vaccination, but the amount is so low that in-contact horses generally do not become infected with or immunized by the shed vaccinal virus.[39,40]

The MLV vaccine can be incorporated into a program that has relied on inactivated vaccines by substituting it for the inactivated vaccine as scheduled boosters come due. Evidence supports the safety of the MLV intranasal vaccine in foals under 11 months of age, but because maternal antibody interference may be an issue and data currently are lacking to support the efficacy of the product in foals, it is recommended that if the first dose of the vaccine is given before 11 months of age, a second dose should be administered when the foal is 11 months old or older. There is no evidence of immunotolerance to the MLV vaccine when it is administered in the presence of maternal antibodies.

For programs that rely on inactivated influenza vaccines given by intramuscular injection, a primary series of three doses of vaccine should be administered 3 to 6 weeks apart, regardless of the age at which vaccination is begun. A three-dose primary series induces higher and more persistent antibody titers than those obtained with the previously recommended two-dose initial series. Subsequent revaccination should be done at 3- to 12-month intervals, depending on the horse's age and the degree and duration of the risk of acquiring infection. For young horses in competition, revaccination is recommended at intervals of 3 to 4 months until they are 2 years old. On breeding farms, all mature horses should be revaccinated on the basis of their risk of exposure. Boosters for pregnant broodmares should be administered 4 to 6 weeks before foaling using a killed virus vaccine to maximize the concentration of immunoglobulins in the colostrum.

Foals of vaccinated mares may be protected for several months by antibodies transferred through colostrum. Those antibodies may also modify the foal's response to killed virus influenza vaccines given before 9 months of age.[10-13,17,18] Therefore the program for primary vaccination of foals against influenza depends on the dam's vaccinal status and

---

*Flu-Avert, Heska Corp, Fort Collins, CO 80525.

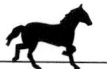

the risk of acquiring infection. Primary vaccination for foals born to vaccinated mares and kept isolated from exposure to horses from other premises may be delayed until the foals are 9 months of age or older; it should consist of a series of three doses of killed virus vaccine administered at intervals of 4 to 6 weeks. For foals born to unvaccinated mares, primary vaccination with a series of three doses of killed virus vaccine should be administered at intervals of 4 to 6 weeks starting when the foal is 6 months of age. Mature performance, show, or pleasure horses constantly at risk of exposure should be revaccinated at 3- to 4-month intervals.

Definitive diagnosis of equine influenza infection should be pursued during outbreaks of suspected viral respiratory disease because specific measures can then be taken to contain the spread of the disease. Same-day diagnosis can be accomplished using antigen-capture enzyme-linked immunosorbent assay (ELISA) test kits marketed for human use (e.g., Directigen FluA* or FLU OIA†). These tests have proved highly sensitive and specific for the diagnosis of equine influenza.[4,42] Because influenza outbreaks typically last 3 to 4 weeks and because horses that have had previous contact with influenza antigens through vaccination or natural infection rapidly mount an anamnestic response, vaccination of healthy horses to boost immunity in the face of an outbreak often is a beneficial control strategy, in addition to isolating infected horses and those in immediate contact.[4] The MLV intranasal vaccine appears to be safe when used during an outbreak and is likely to induce more rapid and complete protection than that provided by conventional inactivated vaccines.

EQUINE HERPESVIRUS INFECTION (Rhinopneumonitis)

Although the respiratory tract is the primary route of infection for equine herpesvirus type 1 (EHV-1) and type 4 (EHV-4)[9,43] and although these pathogens are commonly held to be important etiologic agents of primary and secondary respiratory disease, no conclusive evidence supports the role of EHV-1 and EHV-4 as causes of respiratory disease.[4] Seroepidemiologic studies indicate that most foals become infected with EHV-1 and EHV-4 during the first few months of life, but the clinical disease syndrome caused by these infections is not well defined.[4] Similarly, surveillance studies involving racehorses have documented that seroconversion to both EHV-1 and EHV-4 occurs sporadically during a racing season but that it is not clearly associated with outbreaks of respiratory disease that follow an epidemiologic pattern consistent with an infectious agent.[4,34,44]

EHV-1 causes abortion of virus-infected fetuses from infected mares, the birth of weak, nonviable, infected foals, and, in mature horses, a paralytic neurologic disease (myeloencephalopathy) that occurs secondary to vasculitis of the spinal cord and brain.[45] EHV-1 and EHV-4 are spread by aerosolized secretions from infected horses, by direct and indirect (fomite) contact with nasal secretions, and, in the case of EHV-1, by aborted fetuses, fetal fluids, and placentae associated with abortions.[43] Management practices therefore are of primary importance in controlling clinical disease caused by the equine herpesviruses.

As with herpesvirus infections in other species, in most horses infection with EHV-1 or EHV-4 results in a persistent latent infection.[9] Latently infected horses do not show clinical signs but may experience recrudescence of infection and shed-

ding of the virus when stressed.[9,43] These epidemiologic features explain the outbreaks of EHV-1 or EHV-4 in closed horse populations, and they also seriously compromise efforts to control the related diseases. Although most mature horses have antibodies to EHV-1 and EHV-4 and do not show respiratory signs when they become infected, horses do not appear to become resistant to the abortigenic or neurologic forms of infection with EHV-1 even after repeated exposure.[43,45]

The principal indication for use of equine herpesvirus vaccines is prevention of EHV-1–induced abortion in pregnant mares. Consistent vaccination appears to reduce the frequency and severity of herpesvirus-induced disease, and field experience suggests that the incidence of abortion storms caused by EHV-1 has declined significantly since the introduction and widespread use of EHV-1 vaccines in the United States, although convincing evidence is lacking[43]; sporadic abortions and rare abortion storms have been observed in herds of vaccinated mares.

Of the vaccines currently licensed for use in pregnant mares in the United States, only inactivated, monovalent EHV-1 vaccines containing abortigenic strains of EHV-1 (Pneumoabort-K + 1b* and Prodigy†) carry a label claim of preventing abortion. Pneumoabort-K + 1b incorporates both the 1p and 1b subtypes of EHV-1, reflecting the documented increase in the proportion of EHV-1 abortions caused by the 1b subtype during the 1980s.[46] All pregnant mares should be vaccinated during the fifth, seventh, and ninth months of gestation, and many veterinarians also recommend a dose during the third month. In addition, mares often are vaccinated with an inactivated EHV-1/EHV-4 vaccine at the time of breeding and again 4 to 6 weeks before foaling to enhance the concentration of colostral immunoglobulins for transfer to the foal. Vaccination of barren mares and stallions before the start of the breeding season and thereafter at 6-month intervals often is recommended in an attempt to reduce viral shedding and challenge to pregnant mares.

Inactivated bivalent EHV-1/EHV-4 vaccines and modified live EHV-1 vaccines often are used as an aid to prevention of respiratory tract disease (rhinopneumonitis) in foals, weanlings, yearlings, and young performance and show horses at high risk of exposure. Considering the uncertainty over the role of EHV-1 and EHV-4 as causes of clinically important respiratory disease and the lack of published data on the efficacy of available vaccines in preventing infection and establishment of latency, there appears to be little rationale to support the common practice of frequent revaccination of foals, weanlings, yearlings, and young performance horses against EHV-1 and EHV-4.[4] In addition, maternal antibodies appear to block the serologic response of most foals to inactivated EHV-1/EHV-4 vaccines until they are at least 5 months old.[15,16,18,19] Because three or more doses of inactivated vaccine usually are required to induce seroconversion, most foals are unlikely to achieve a protective immune response until they are at least 7 or 8 months old.[19] It therefore is difficult to appreciate how the available inactivated vaccines can be used in foals to prevent the signs of respiratory disease, commonly ascribed to EHV infection, that appear around the time of weaning.[4] Although maternal antibodies may interfere with the serologic response of foals to the MLV EHV-1 vaccine licensed for use in North America (Rhinomune‡), this vaccine was shown to induce specific cytotoxic cellular immune responses in most foals despite the presence of maternal antibodies.[47] It is not clear if these responses would provide protection against natural challenge.

---

*Directigen FluA, Becton Dickinson, Franklin Lakes, NJ 07417.
†FLU OIA, BioStar, Boulder, CO 80301.

*Pneumoabort-K + 1b, Fort Dodge Laboratories, Fort Dodge, IA 50501.
†Prodigy, Bayer/Intervet, Shawnee, KS 66216.
‡Rhinomune, Pfizer, Inc, Exton, PA 19341.

Despite the uncertainties that are involved in the use of EHV vaccines to prevent respiratory disease, many practitioners elect to vaccinate against equine herpesvirus infections. Primary vaccination of foals involves administering three doses of an inactivated EHV-1/EHV-4 vaccine or a modified live EHV-1 vaccine 3 to 6 weeks apart beginning at 4 to 6 months of age. Weanlings, yearlings, and young performance or show horses at high risk are revaccinated at 3- to 6-month intervals. For mature horses, frequent revaccination of nonpregnant animals with EHV vaccines generally is not indicated except on breeding farms. The available vaccines make no label claim of preventing the myeloencephalitic form of EHV-1 infection.

STREPTOCOCCUS EQUI INFECTION (Strangles)

Strangles is a highly contagious disease caused by the bacterium *Streptococcus equi* ssp. *equi* (*S. equi*). Strangles primarily affects young horses (weanlings and yearlings), although horses of any age can be infected if not protected by previous exposure to the organism or by vaccination. *S. equi* is transmitted directly by contact with infected horses or subclinical carriers or indirectly by contact with water troughs, feed bunks, pastures, stalls, trailers, tack, or grooming equipment contaminated with nasal discharge or pus draining from the lymph nodes of infected horses. The organism can survive in the environment for at least 3 months if protected from exposure to direct sunlight and disinfectants and can serve as a source of infection for new additions to the herd.

Because *S. equi* is a clonal organism, antigenic variation among different isolates is minimal even though the isolates vary in pathogenicity. Approximately 70% of horses develop a solid immunity to reinfection after recovering from strangles, whereas about 30% of horses develop a less durable response and become susceptible again in the following months.[48] The acquired immune response is directed predominantly at the cell wall M-protein of *S. equi* (Se-M); it involves a combination of circulating opsonophagocytic antibody and local antibodies produced in the nasopharynx.[48,49] The predominant opsonophagocytic antibodies are of the IgGb subisotype, but IgGa and IgA antibodies also are elicited; IgGb and later mucosal IgA antibodies predominate in nasopharyngeal secretions.[49]

The licensed vaccines available in North America include two inactivated, subunit (M-protein) vaccines for intramuscular injection (StrepVax II* and Strepguard†); and one modified live bacterial vaccine for intranasal administration (Pinnacle I.N.).‡ The intranasal vaccine is derived from a nonencapsulated mutant (707-29) of *S. equi*. Although parenteral vaccination does not stimulate a significant nasopharyngeal secretory IgA antibody response, which appears to be important in preventing infection,[49,50] good evidence indicates that the systemic antibody response attenuates the severity and duration of clinical signs of disease and reduces the attack rate during outbreaks by about 50%.[48,51-53]

Vaccination against *S. equi* is not routinely recommended except for premises where strangles is a persistent endemic problem or for horses expected to be at high risk of exposure. Vaccination is not routinely recommended for pleasure or performance horses kept in low-risk situations. Manufacturers' recommendations for use of inactivated vaccines call for primary vaccination with a series of two or three doses ad-

ministered at intervals of 2 to 4 weeks, depending on the product used, followed by annual revaccination. Efficacy may be improved by using a primary series of three doses with boosters given at 6-month intervals, regardless of the product used. On breeding farms, efforts should be concentrated on preventing infection of foals and weanlings by vaccinating broodmares intramuscularly 4 to 6 weeks before foaling with approved products that contain inactivated M-protein. Antibodies of predominantly the IgGb isotype are passively transferred via colostrum and appear in the nasal secretions and serum of the foal.[48] Antibodies of the IgGb subisotype are also present in the milk of vaccinated, lactating mares. The resistance of nursing foals to strangles during the first few months of life appears to be mediated by IgGb antibodies in nasal secretions and milk and not by IgA antibodies.[48]

The MLV bacterial vaccine (Pinnacle I.N.) generally is preferred over inactivated injectable vaccines for primary vaccination of foals and weanlings and for routine use in older horses at high risk of infection. For these horses two doses may be administered intranasally at a 2- to 3-week interval beginning at 4 to 6 months of age, followed by a third dose 3 months later and annual or semiannual boosters thereafter, depending on the risk of infection.

The intranasal vaccine has been administered to foals as young as 5 or 6 weeks of age during outbreaks. If used in this manner, a third dose of the vaccine should be administered 2 to 4 weeks before the foal is weaned to optimize protection during this high-risk period. Although there are few reports of adverse reactions among foals to the intranasal strangles vaccine, the foal's inability to mount mucosal IgA responses during the first month of life and the potential for interference by maternal antibodies suggest that foals are unlikely to benefit from the intranasal vaccine before 4 months of age.[48] When an inactivated M-protein vaccine is used for primary vaccination of foals, the initial series should begin at 4 to 6 months of age, using three doses administered at 3- to 6-week intervals, followed by semiannual or annual boosters.

Outbreaks of strangles generally persist for several months to a year or longer, particularly on breeding farms, where each foal crop adds new susceptible animals to the population. Strangles vaccines therefore often are administered during an outbreak in an attempt to bring the outbreak under control and as an adjunct to management practices designed to reduce the spread of infection. Although all horses can be vaccinated under these circumstances except those that are clinically ill or incubating infection, the likelihood of preventing strangles is greatest for horses that have not yet been exposed and can be kept isolated from infected horses until the vaccination protocol can be completed. Horses that have been vaccinated previously generate an optimum response more rapidly than naive horses. The MLV intranasal vaccine is preferred over inactivated vaccines for use in the face of an outbreak because it is likely to generate a protective immune response more rapidly than an inactivated vaccine, particularly in naive horses. The intranasal vaccine has been shown to be safe for use in mares at all stages of pregnancy[48] and can be used in mares in the face of an outbreak. However, an inactivated M-protein vaccine should be used for prefoaling boosters to maximize passive transfer of specific immunoglobulins to the foal.

All injectable, inactivated strangles vaccines tend to cause local reactions at the site of injection more often than do most other equine vaccines, particularly when administered in the neck muscles. These reactions result in swelling and muscle pain, which can manifest as lameness if the muscles of the hind limb are used as the injection site. Systemic signs such as fever, depression, and inappetence occur occasionally, as does the development of sterile or infected abscesses at the injection site. Purpura hemorrhagica, a serious

---

*Strep Vax II, Boehringer Ingelheim, Vetmedica, Inc, St. Joseph, MO 64506.

†Strepguard, Bayer/Intervet, Shawnee, KS 66216.

‡Pinnacle I.N., Fort Dodge Laboratories, Fort Dodge, IA 50501.

and sometimes life-threatening systemic immune complex (Arthus type) vasculitis manifested as edema with or without petechial hemorrhages on mucosal surfaces, has been observed in a few cases in the weeks after administration of all licensed strangles vaccines. The M-protein of *S. equi* is the antigen present in immune complexes, along with IgA antibodies.[54]

The MLV intranasal vaccine causes injection site abscesses if inadvertently administered intramuscularly. To avoid inadvertent contamination of other vaccines, syringes, and needles, it is a good practice to administer all parenteral vaccines before handling and administering the MLV intranasal vaccine. Other reported adverse responses to administration of the MLV intranasal vaccine are nasal discharge, submandibular or retropharyngeal lymphadenopathy with or without abscessation, limb edema, and internal abscesses (bastard strangles).[48] The overall incidence of adverse events is low but appears to be higher than reported to the manufacturer (4.8 per 10,000 doses).[48] On the other hand, most of the reported adverse events, including the development of nasal discharge, lymph node abscesses, and purpura hemorrhagica, occur in horses on farms with endemic or epidemic strangles. Consequently it often is unclear if the adverse event was caused by the vaccine or by a wild strain of *S. equi*.

RABIES

Rabies is an infrequently encountered neurologic disease in horses. It results when the horse is inoculated with the rabies virus through the bite of infected (rabid) wildlife. Even though the incidence of rabies in horses is low, the disease is invariably fatal and has considerable public health significance. The wildlife species that serve as natural reservoirs of this rhabdovirus differ from region to region in North America. All horses kept in areas where rabies is endemic in the wildlife population are at risk and should be vaccinated.

Several vaccines containing inactivated (killed) rabies virus are licensed for intramuscular injection in horses and appear to be safe. Foals born to unvaccinated mares may be vaccinated according to the manufacturers' recommendations, which call for primary vaccination of foals age 3 months or older with one dose, followed by a second dose at 1 year of age and annual boosters thereafter. Colostrum-derived antibodies interfere with active immunization of foals,[18] which may explain the occurrence of rabies in young vaccinated horses in Canada.[55] For this reason, foals born to vaccinated mares should receive the first dose of vaccine no earlier than 6 months of age, a second dose 1 month after the first, and a third dose at 1 year of age, followed by annual revaccination.

None of the licensed vaccines are labeled for administration to pregnant mares; therefore mares should be vaccinated *before* breeding. However, it should be noted that some veterinarians administer the killed virus vaccine to pregnant mares without reports of adversity. MLV rabies vaccines not licensed for use in horses should not be used.

EQUINE MONOCYTIC EHRLICHIOSIS (Potomac Horse Fever)

Equine monocytic ehrlichiosis, more commonly known as Potomac horse fever (PHF), is caused by the pathogen *Ehrlichia risticii*. It originally was described in 1979 as a sporadic disease that affected horses living in the United States in the northeastern states and the mid-Atlantic region, near the Potomac River. Although the disease remains prevalent in those states, particularly near waterways, it has been identified in several regions of the United States and Canada. Potomac horse fever does not appear to be directly contagious,

and it now appears that accidental ingestion of aquatic insects harboring snail metacercariae infected with *E. risticii* is at least one mode of transmission.[56] The disease is a seasonal one that occurs between late spring and early fall in temperate areas, with most cases arising in July, August, and September at the onset of hot weather. The disease may affect individual animals sporadically or may emerge in outbreaks involving several horses. If Potomac horse fever has been confirmed on a farm or in a particular geographic area, cases are likely to occur in future years. Foals appear to be at low risk for the disease.

Recovery from natural infection with *E. risticii* induces a strong antibody response and durable protection from reinfection that lasts 20 months or longer.[57] However, the presence of antibodies per se does not necessarily correlate with protection, and cell-mediated responses probably play a crucial role.[58] Several inactivated PHF vaccines (i.e., Mystique,* RM Equine Potomavac,† PHF-Vax,‡ and PotomacGuard§) are available for intramuscular administration. These vaccines carry label claims that they aid in the prevention of equine monocytic ehrlichiosis.

The high rates of serious complications and death associated with PHF have been considered adequate justification for vaccinating horses living in or traveling to endemic areas. However, an epidemiologic investigation involving large numbers of horses in New York state failed to demonstrate any clinical or economic benefit from annual revaccination with the vaccines currently available.[59] The observed failure of vaccines to protect against field infection probably is due to several factors, including the failure of a substantial number of individual horses to mount an immune response to inactivated PHF vaccines, the antigenic heterogeneity of field *E. risticii* isolates, the fact that only one *E. risticii* strain is included in the vaccines, and the rapid waning of immunity after vaccination.[58,60] Although efficacy of the approved vaccines in preventing infection in the field setting has not been proven, experimental challenge studies have documented at least partial protection of limited duration.[58] Many veterinarians who practice in endemic areas believe that vaccination attenuates the severity of the disease and lowers the mortality rate.[61]

If vaccination is elected, a primary series of two doses should be administered 3 to 4 weeks apart. Manufacturers recommend revaccination at 6- to 12-month intervals; however, a 4-month interval appears to be necessary to achieve a reasonable likelihood of protection in horses in endemic areas because protection after vaccination is incomplete and short-lived.[58] Because the disease has a distinct seasonal pattern, revaccination in the late spring, about 1 month before the first cases are expected, and administration of a second dose 4 months later appears to be a reasonable immunization strategy for maximizing the chances of protection during the period of peak challenge.[58]

The available vaccines are licensed for use in stallions and pregnant mares and can be administered to gestating mares 4 to 6 weeks before foaling to maximize passive transfer of specific antibodies to foals via the colostrum. Although approximately 67% of foals from antibody-positive mares were found to be antibody negative by 12 weeks of age, antibody was detectable in 33% of foals up to 5 months of age.[61] Because of the low risk of clinical disease in young foals and the possibility of interference by colostral antibodies, primary immunization for most foals can begin after 5 months of age.

---

*Mystique, Bayer/Intervet, Shawnee, KS 66216.
†RM Equine Potomavac, Merial, Iselin, NJ 08830.
‡PHF-Vax, Schering-Plough, Kenilworth, NJ 07033.
§PotomacGuard, Fort Dodge Laboratories, Fort Dodge, IA 50501.

Although manufacturers recommend a primary series of two doses of vaccine administered 4 weeks apart, it is advisable, as with other inactivated antigens, to add a third dose to the primary series for foals, especially when the vaccination protocol is started before 5 months of age.[61]

BOTULISM

Three forms of botulism, namely toxicoinfectious botulism (shaker foal syndrome), forage poisoning, and wound botulism, have been observed in horses as a result of the action of the potent toxins produced by the soil-borne, spore-forming bacterium *Clostridium botulinum*. Wound botulism results when *C. botulinum* spores vegetate and subsequently produce toxin in contaminated wounds. Shaker foal syndrome is caused by the toxin produced when ingested spores vegetate in the intestinal tract. Forage poisoning occurs when an animal ingests preformed toxin produced by decaying plant material or animal carcasses present in feed.

Botulinum toxin is the most potent biologic toxin known. It acts by blocking transmission of impulses at motor end plates, resulting in weakness that progresses to paralysis, inability to swallow, and often death.

Of the eight distinct toxins produced by subtypes of *C. botulinum*, types B and C are associated with most outbreaks of botulism in horses. Almost all cases of shaker foal syndrome are caused by type B. Shaker foal syndrome is a significant problem in foals between 2 weeks and 8 months of age in Kentucky and the mid-Atlantic seaboard states, and it occurs sporadically in other areas.[62]

A toxoid vaccine directed against *C. botulinum* type B (Bot Tox-B*) is licensed for use in horses in the United States. Its primary indication is the prevention of shaker foal syndrome. For primary vaccination, mares should be vaccinated during gestation with a series of three doses administered 4 weeks apart, scheduled so that the last dose is administered 4 to 6 weeks before foaling to enhance concentrations of immunoglobulin in the colostrum. Mares then should be revaccinated annually with a single dose 4 to 6 weeks before foaling.

Passively derived colostral antibodies appear to protect foals of vaccinated mares for 8 to 12 weeks,[62,63] and maternal antibodies do not appear to interfere with the foal's response to primary immunization against botulism.[64] Therefore a primary series of three doses of vaccine administered 4 weeks apart can be started when foals in endemic areas are 2 to 3 months of age or older. Other horses can be immunized using a primary series of three doses of vaccine administered at 4-week intervals followed by annual revaccination.

No licensed vaccines are available for preventing botulism caused by *C. botulinum* type C or other subtypes of toxins, and cross-protection does not occur between the B and C subtypes; therefore routine vaccination against *C. botulinum* type C is not currently practiced. A type C toxoid approved for use in mink was used successfully in horses under special license to protect them during an outbreak of forage poisoning caused by contaminated alfalfa cubes in southern California.

Horses and foals with clinical botulism may be treated with botulinum antitoxin administered intravenously. Antitoxin is not effective against toxin that has been translocated to motor end plates; therefore clinical signs may progress for 12 to 24 hours after administration of the antitoxin or until all internalized toxin has attached to motor end plates. For a foal, the recommended dose of type B antitoxin is 30,000 IU; the dose for an adult horse is 70,000 IU.

EQUINE VIRAL ARTERITIS

Equine viral arteritis (EVA), a contagious disease of equids caused by the equine arteritis virus (EAV), is found throughout the world. All breeds appear to be susceptible to the virus, but the prevalence of infection, as determined by seroconversion, is much higher in some breeds, notably standardbreds, than in others. Although the seroprevalence of infection in standardbreds is high, clinical disease is rarely observed in this breed, indicating that subclinical infection is common. Conversely, thoroughbreds and most other breeds have a low seroprevalence of infection but show fulminant clinical signs when they become infected.

EVA is of special concern because the virus can cause abortion in pregnant mares and death in young foals and can establish a long-term carrier state in stallions.[65,66] Outbreaks of EVA occur infrequently, and they sometimes are difficult to diagnose because of their clinical similarity to several other diseases (e.g., rhinopneumonitis, equine influenza, equine infectious anemia, and purpura hemorrhagica). Clinical signs vary in severity and may include some or all of the following: fever; anorexia; depression; edematous swelling of the eyelids, face, limbs, trunk, mammary glands, and genitalia; lacrimation; conjunctivitis; rhinitis; nasal discharge; skin rash; and in some cases pneumonia and death in young foals. Aerosolized droplets of respiratory secretions from horses with acute clinical disease can transmit the virus, but perhaps of greater concern is the transmission of the virus to mares in semen from subclinically infected carrier stallions through natural breeding or artificial insemination.

An MLV vaccine based on an attenuated strain of the equine arteritis virus was developed by researchers in Kentucky in 1969.[67] This vaccine (Arvac*) was first used extensively in the field during the 1984 outbreak of EVA in Kentucky, and it proved to be safe and very helpful in bringing the outbreak under control.[66] The vaccine was developed further and licensed for commercial use, with the primary indications being (1) to prevent infection and establishment of the carrier state in previously unexposed stallions and (2) to protect nonpregnant mares being bred to carrier stallions. The vaccine has also proved effective in controlling outbreaks of EVA in concentrated populations of performance horses at racetracks. Primary immunization involves administration of a single dose of vaccine with boosters administered annually thereafter.

Vaccination of stallions, nonpregnant mares, and prepubertal colts with the MLV vaccine has proved to be a safe, effective means of controlling equine viral arteritis. Strategic use of the vaccine has formed the cornerstone of a highly successful program to control EVA in the Kentucky Thoroughbred breeding population over the past 15 years.[66] Annual revaccination of breeding stallions 28 days before the start of the breeding season is highly recommended to prevent establishment of the carrier state.[66] Mares being bred to carrier stallions should be revaccinated annually at least 21 days before breeding, and because vaccinated mares may shed virus transiently after being bred to carrier stallions, these mares should be isolated for 21 days after breeding.[66] The vaccine is not recommended for use in pregnant mares, especially during the last 2 months of gestation, or in foals under 6 weeks of age except in emergencies when the risk of exposure is high. Foaling mares should be vaccinated after foaling and before being rebred.

Foals born to seropositive mares become seropositive after ingesting colostrum. Maternally derived antibodies decay,

---

*Bot Tox-B, Neogen Biologics, Lexington, KY 40505-3727.

*Arvac, Fort Dodge Laboratories, Fort Dodge, IA 50501.

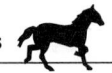

with a mean half-life of approximately 32 days, and foals generally are seronegative by 7 months of age.[68] Maternal antibodies are unlikely to interfere with the response to vaccine administered at 8 months of age or older.[68] In breeds or areas in which EAV is prevalent, vaccination of intact males between 8 and 12 months of age should be strongly encouraged to prevent them from becoming carriers when exposed to EAV later in life through breeding or aerosol contact. Routine vaccination of standardbred colts would be a logical approach to reducing the number of stallions that later become chronic carriers and likely would result in a substantial reduction in the incidence of infection in this breed.

Seroconversion induced by the MLV vaccine currently licensed in North America or by the inactivated vaccines licensed in Europe and Japan cannot be distinguished from that resulting from natural infection, therefore vaccination may complicate testing of horses for export. Although only a few countries currently restrict the importation of horses that test positive for neutralizing antibodies against EAV, several countries restrict entry of seropositive stallions because of the likelihood that they are chronically infected and may shed the virus in semen. A blood sample should be collected for serologic testing before the first dose of vaccine is administered. Coordinating vaccination with state or federal regulatory officials (or both) and providing evidence, in the form of serologic test results, that a horse was seronegative before vaccination may help resolve disputes, but even these measures do not guarantee entry into foreign countries or onto breeding farms.

ROTAVIRAL DIARRHEA

Equine rotavirus is one of the prominent causes of infectious diarrhea in foals during the first few weeks of life, and the virus often causes outbreaks involving most of the foal crop on a farm. Older foals and adult horses are more resistant to infection. Equine rotavirus is transmitted through fecal-oral contamination and causes diarrhea by damaging the tips of villi in the small intestine, resulting in cellular destruction, maldigestion, and malabsorption.

Rotaviruses are classified into seven serogroups, A through G, based on common antigens in each group.[69] Until recently all equine rotavirus isolates were classified as belonging to serogroup A, which has 14 serotypes (G1 through G14); five of these serotypes (G3, G5, G10, G13, and G14), representing four genotypes (P1, P7, P12, and P18), have been identified and characterized in horses.[70] Most equine rotavirus isolates are of the P12 genotype and the G3 serotype (previously referred to as H2) and include two subtypes (subtype 1 and 2). A number of rotavirus isolates remain untyped, therefore it is possible that other equine rotavirus serotypes, and perhaps other serogroups, are active in the equine population.

An inactivated rotavirus A vaccine (Equine Rotavirus Vaccine*), containing the G3 (H2) serotype in a metabolizable oil-in-water emulsion, has been conditionally licensed in the United States. The vaccine is indicated for administration to pregnant mares in endemic areas as an aid to preventing diarrhea in foals caused by rotavirus serogroup A. Label recommendations call for a three-dose series of the vaccine to be administered during each pregnancy at 8, 9, and 10 months of gestation. This protocol has been shown to induce a significant increase in serum concentrations of neutralizing antibody in vaccinated mares[71] and to significantly increase the concentration of IgG antibodies (but not IgA antibodies) in

the colostrum and milk of vaccinated mares.[72] After nursing, the concentration of passively derived, rotavirus-specific antibody of the IgG subclass in the serum of the foals of vaccinated mares is significantly higher than that in the serum of foals of unvaccinated mares up to 90 days of age.[71,72]

A field study showed this vaccine to be safe and provided circumstantial evidence of at least partial efficacy. An approximately twofold higher incidence of rotaviral diarrhea was found in foals from unvaccinated mares compared with those from vaccinated mares, although this difference did not prove to be statistically significant.[71] Similarly, in a controlled field study in Argentina, an inactivated aluminum hydroxide–adjuvanted vaccine containing the SA11 (G3P2), H2 (G3P12), and Lincoln (G6P1) strains was administered to 100 mares at 60 days and again at 30 days before foaling; the study showed a substantial reduction in the incidence and severity of rotaviral disease in foals from vaccinated mares compared with foals from unvaccinated mares.[73] In challenge studies involving two inactivated rotavirus vaccines administered in a similar manner to pregnant mares in Japan, the foals were not completely protected against infection but enjoyed a substantial reduction in the severity of clinical signs after challenge.[70]

The major correlate for protection against rotaviral infection appears to be mucosal immunity, predominantly mucosal IgA antibodies, in the gastrointestinal tract. Studies of the immunoglobulin isotype responses of mares and of antibodies passively transferred to their foals after parenteral vaccination of the dams with inactivated rotavirus vaccines indicate that this approach is unlikely to provide foals with intestinal mucosal protection in the form of IgA antibodies.[72] Consequently, it is not surprising that current protocols do not provide complete protection. In addition, because the conditionally licensed vaccine available in the United States contains only the G3 serotype of the A serogroup, it cannot be expected to protect against infection with all field strains.

ANTHRAX

Anthrax is a serious, rapidly fatal septicemic disease that develops when the vegetative form of the bacterium *Bacillus anthracis* enters the body, proliferates, and spreads. *B. anthracis* is acquired though ingestion or contamination of wounds by soil-borne spores of the organism. The disease is encountered only in limited geographic areas, where alkaline soil conditions favor survival of the organism.

A Sterne strain, nonencapsulated live spore vaccine (Anthrax Spore Vaccine*) has been used to vaccinate horses. A primary series consisting of two doses of the vaccine should be administered subcutaneously 2 to 3 weeks apart, with annual revaccination. Occasionally adverse systemic or local effects may occur. Little objective information is available on the use of this vaccine in horses, although clinical evidence suggests that it provides protection; however, vaccination of pregnant mares is not recommended. Because the vaccine is a live bacterial product, appropriate caution should be used in storing, handling, and administering it. Concurrent administration of antimicrobial drugs effective against anaerobes, and *B. anthracis* in particular, is contraindicated if the vaccine is to function as intended.

REFERENCES

1. Brumbaugh G et al: *AAEP guidelines for vaccination of horses.* Monograph, American Association of Equine Practitioners, 2001.

---

*Equine Rotavirus Vaccine, Fort Dodge Laboratories, Fort Dodge, IA 50501.

*Anthrax Spore Vaccine, Colorado Serum Co., Denver, CO 80216.

2. Jorm LR: Laboratory studies on the survival of *Streptococcus equi* ssp. *equi* on surfaces. In Plowright W, Rossdale PD, Wade JF, eds: *Equine infectious diseases VI: proceedings of the Sixth International Conference,* Newmarket, 1992, R&W Publications.

3. Horohov DW et al: Equine vaccination, *J Vet Intern Med* 14:221-222, 2000.

4. Townsend HGG: The role of vaccines and their efficacy in the control of infectious respiratory disease of the horse, *Proceedings of the Forty-sixth Annual Convention of the American Association of Equine Practitioners* 46:21-26, 2000.

5. Lunn DP, Townsend HG: Equine vaccination, *Vet Clin North Am (Equine Pract)* 16:199-226, 2000.

6. Morley PS et al: Efficacy of a commercial vaccine for preventing disease caused by influenza virus infection in horses, *J Am Vet Med Assoc* 215:61-66, 1999.

7. Townsend HGG et al: Efficacy of a cold-adapted, modified live virus influenza vaccine: a double-blind challenge trial, *Proceedings of the Forty-fifth Annual Convention of the American Association of Equine Practitioners* 45:41-42, 1999.

8. Lunn DP: Immunological basis of vaccination, *Proceedings of the Forty-sixth Annual Convention of the American Association of Equine Practitioners* 46:1-9, 2000.

9. Slater J: Immunological control of viral and bacterial pathogens, *Proceedings of the Forty-sixth Annual Convention of the American Association of Equine Practitioners* 46:10-19, 2000.

10. Cullinane A et al: The interference of maternal antibodies with the immune response of thoroughbred foals and yearlings to vaccination against equine influenza, *Proceedings of the Seventh International Conference on Equine Infectious Diseases* 7:52, 1994.

11. Van Maanen C et al: Interference of maternal antibodies with the immune response of foals after vaccination against equine influenza, *Vet Q* 14:13-17, 1992.

12. Van Oirschot JT et al: Maternal antibodies against equine influenza virus in foals and their interference with vaccination, *J Vet Med (B)* 38:391-396, 1991.

13. Conboy HS et al: Failure of foal seroconversion following equine influenza vaccination, *Proceedings of the Forty-third Annual Convention of the American Association of Equine Practitioners* 43:22-23, 1997.

14. Gibbs EPJ et al: Studies on passive immunity and the vaccination of foals against eastern equine encephalitis in Florida, *Proceedings of the Fifth International Conference on Equine Infectious Diseases* 5:201-205, 1988.

15. Bürki F et al: Training of the immune system of foals against ERP virus infections by means of frequent vaccinations with presently available commercial vaccines, *DTW* 96:162-165, 1989.

16. Breathnach CC et al: Problems associated with vaccination of foals against equine herpesvirus-4 and the role of anti-EHV-4 maternal antibodies. In Wernery U et al, eds: *Equine infectious diseases VIII: proceedings of the Eighth International Conference,* Newmarket, 1999, R&W Publications.

17. Holland RE et al: Age dependence on foal vaccination for equine influenza: new evidence from the USA. In Wernery U et al, eds: *Equine infectious diseases VIII: proceedings of the Eighth International Conference,* Newmarket, 1999, R&W Publications.

18. Wilson WD: Vaccination programs for foals and weanlings, *Proceedings of the Forty-fifth Annual Convention of the American Association of Equine Practitioners* 45:254-263, 1999.

19. Wilson WD, Rossdale PD: Effect of age on the serological responses of thoroughbred foals to vaccination with an inactivated EHV-1/EHV-4 vaccine. In Wernery U et al, eds: *Equine infectious diseases VIII: proceedings of the Eighth International Conference,* Newmarket, 1999, R&W Publications.

20. Taylor FRG: Speculations on the cause of adverse reactions to equine influenza vaccination, *Equine Vet Educ* 1:79-81, 1989.

21. Mair TS: Adverse reactions to equine vaccinations: a preliminary survey, *Vet Rec* 122:396, 1988.

22. Liefman CE: Active immunisation of horses against tetanus including the booster dose and its application, *Aust Vet J* 57:57-60, 1981.

23. Jansen BC, Knoetze PC: The immune response of horses to tetanus toxoid, *Onderstepoort J Vet Res* 46:211-216, 1979.

24. Heinig A: Experimentelle Untersuchungen uber den Eintritt der Immunitat nach Einmaliger Tetanue-schutzimpfung, *Arch Exp Vet Med* 8:394-403, 1954.

25. Lohrer J, Radvila P: Aktive Tetanusprophylaxe beim Pferd und Immitätsdaver, *Schweiz Arch Tierheilkd* 112:307-314, 1970.

26. Green SL et al: Tetanus in the horse: a review of 20 cases (1970 to 1990), *J Vet Intern Med* 8:128-132, 1994.

27. Ansari MM, Matros LE: Tetanus prophylaxis in the horse, *Equine Pract* 5:27-32, 1983.

28. Panciera RJ: Serum hepatitis in the horse, *J Am Vet Med Assoc* 155:408-410, 1969.

29. Messer NT, Johnson PJ: Idiopathic acute hepatic disease in horses: 12 cases (1982-1992), *J Am Vet Med Assoc* 204:1934-1937, 1994.

30. Liefman CE: Combined active-passive immunisation of horses against tetanus, *Aust Vet J* 56:119-122, 1980.

31. Bertone JJ: Togaviral encephalitides: alphavirus (eastern and western) equine encephalitis. In Robinson NE, ed: *Current therapy in equine medicine 3,* ed 3, Philadelphia, 1992, WB Saunders.

32. Liu IKM: Duration of maternally derived antibodies in neonatal foals, *Mod Vet Pract* 67:454-456, 1986.

33. Morley PS et al: Risk factors for disease associated with influenza virus infections during three epidemics in horses, *J Am Vet Med Assoc* 216:545-550, 2000.

34. Morley PS et al: Descriptive epidemiologic study of disease associated with influenza virus infections during three epidemics in horses, *J Am Vet Med Assoc* 216:535-544, 2000.

35. Wilson WD: Equine influenza, *Vet Clin North Am (Equine Pract)* 9:257-282, 1993.

36. Mumford J: Progress in the control of influenza. In Plowright W, Rossdale PD, Wade JF, eds: *Equine infectious diseases VI: proceedings of the Sixth International Conference,* 1992, R&W Publications (Newmarket).

37. Mumford JA: The diagnosis and control of equine influenza, *Proceedings of the Thirty-sixth Annual Convention of the American Association of Equine Practitioners* 36:377-385, 1990.

38. Townsend HGG et al: Measuring serum antibody as a method of predicting infection and disease in horses during outbreaks of influenza. In Wernery U et al, eds: *Equine infectious diseases VIII: proceedings of the Eighth International Conference,* 1999, R&W Publications (Newmarket).

39. Lunn DP et al: A potent modified live equine influenza vaccine: safe even after exercise-induced immunosuppression, *Proceedings of the Forty-fifth Annual Convention of the American Association of Equine Practitioners* 45:43-44, 1999.

40. Holland RE et al: New modified live equine influenza virus vaccine: safety and efficacy studies in young equids, *Proceedings of the Forty-fifth Annual Convention of the American Association of Equine Practitioners* 45:38-40, 1999.

41. Wilson WD, Robinson D: Field safety of a modified live, cold-adapted intranasal equine influenza vaccine (Heska's Flu Avert I.N.) in horses, *J Equine Vet Sci* 20:8-10, 2000.

42. Morley PS et al: Evaluation of Directigen Flu A assay for detection of influenza antigen in nasal secretions of horses, *Equine Vet J* 27:131-134, 1995.

43. Ostlund EN: The equine herpesviruses, *Vet Clin North Am (Equine Pract)* 9:283-294, 1993.

44. Wood JLN et al: A longitudinal epidemiological study of respiratory disease in racehorses: disease definitions, prevalence and incidence. In Wernery U et al, eds: *Equine infectious diseases VIII: proceedings of the Eighth International Conference,* Newmarket, 1999, R&W Publications.

45. Wilson WD: Equine herpesvirus 1 myeloencephalopathy, *Vet Clin North Am (Equine Pract)* 13:53-72, 1997.

46. Allen GP et al: A new field strain of equine abortion virus (equine herpesvirus-1) among Kentucky horses, *Am J Vet Res* 46:138-140, 1985.

47. Ellis JA et al: Cell-mediated cytolysis of equine herpesvirus–infected cells by leukocytes from young vaccinated horses, *Vet Immunol Immunopathol* 57:201-214, 1997.

48. Timoney JF: Equine strangles: 1999, *Proceedings of the Forty-fifth Annual Convention of the American Association of Equine Practitioners* 45:31-37, 1999.

49. Sheoran AS et al: Serum and mucosal antibody isotype responses to M-like protein (SeM) of *Streptococcus equi* in convalescent and vaccinated horses, *Vet Immunol Immunopathol* 59:239-251, 1997.

50. Galan JE, Timoney JF: Mucosal nasopharyngeal immune responses of horses to protein antigens of *Streptococcus equi, Infect Immunol* 47:623-628, 1985.

51. Hoffman AM et al: Field evaluation of a commercial M-protein vaccine against *Streptococcus equi* infection in foals, *Am J Vet Res* 52:589-592, 1991.

52. Staempfli HR et al: Clinical evaluation of a commercial M-protein vaccine in naturally infected foals, *Proceedings of the Thirty-seventh Annual Convention of the American Association of Equine Practitioners* 37:259-262, 1991.

53. Rief JS, George JL, Shideler RK: Recent developments in strangles research: observations on the carrier state and evaluation of a new vaccine, *Proceedings of the Twenty-seventh Annual Convention of the American Association of Equine Practitioners* 27:33-40, 1981.

54. Galan JE, Timoney JF: Immune complexes in purpura hemorrhagica of the horse contain IgA and M antigen of *Streptococcus equi, J Immunol* 135:3134-3137, 1985.

55. Green SL et al: Rabies in horses: 21 cases (1970-1990), *J Am Vet Med Assoc* 200:1133-1137, 1992.

56. Madigan JE et al: Transmission of *Ehrlichia risticii,* the agent of Potomac horse fever, using naturally infected aquatic insects and helminth vectors: preliminary report, *Equine Vet J* 32:275-279, 2000.

57. Palmer JE, Benson CE, Whitlock RH: Resistance to development of equine ehrlichial colitis in experimentally inoculated horses and ponies, *Am J Vet Res* 51:763-765, 1990.

58. Palmer JE: Potomac horse fever, *Vet Clin North Am (Equine Pract)* 9:399-410, 1993.

59. Atwill ER, Mohammed HO: Evaluation of vaccination of horses as a strategy to control equine monocytic ehrlichiosis, *J Am Vet Med Assoc* 208:1290-1294, 1996.

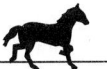

60. Dutta SK, Vemulapalli R, Biswas B: Association of deficiency in antibody response to vaccine and heterogeneity of *Ehrlichia risticii* strains with Potomac horse fever vaccine failure in horses, *J Clin Microbiol* 36:506-512, 1998.

61. Sessions J, Dawson JE: Maryland field evaluation of the Potomac horse fever vaccine, *Equine Pract* 10:7-12, 1988.

62. Whitlock RH, Buckley C: Botulism, *Vet Clin North Am(Equine Pract)* 13:107-128, 1997.

63. Lewis GE Jr et al: Evaluation of a *Clostridium botulinum* toxoid, type B, for the prevention of shaker foal syndrome, *Proceedings of the Twenty-seventh Annual Convention of the American Association of Equine Practitioners* 27:233-237, 1981.

64. Crane SA et al: *Clostridium botulinum* type B toxoid for vaccination of adult horses, pregnant mares, and foals: a study of vaccination protocols, *Proceedings of the Thirty-seventh Annual Convention of the American Association of Equine Practitioners* 37:611, 1991.

65. Timoney PJ et al: The carrier state in equine arteritis virus infection in the stallion with specific emphasis on the venereal mode of virus transmission, *J Reprod Fertil Suppl* 35:95-102, 1987.

66. Timoney PJ, McCollum WH: Equine viral arteritis, *Vet Clin North Am (Equine Pract)* 9:295-309, 1993.

67. McCollum WH: Development of a modified virus strain and vaccine for equine viral arteritis, *J Am Vet Med Assoc* 155:318-322, 1969.

68. Hullinger PJ et al: Passive transfer, rate of decay, and protein specificity of antibodies against equine arteritis virus in horses from a standardbred herd with high seroprevalence, *J Am Vet Med Assoc* 213:839-842, 1998.

69. Dwyer RM: Rotaviral diarrhea, *Vet Clin North Am (Equine Pract)* 9:311-319, 1993.

70. Imagawa H et al: Passive immunity in foals of mares immunised with inactivated equine rotavirus vaccine. In Wernery U et al, eds: *Equine infectious diseases VIII: proceedings of the Eighth International Conference*, Newmarket, 1999, R&W Publications.

71. Powell DG et al: Field study of the safety, immunogenicity, and efficacy of an inactivated equine rotavirus vaccine, *J Am Vet Med Assoc* 211:193-198, 1997.

72. Sheoran AS et al: Prepartum equine rotavirus vaccination inducing strong specific IgG in mammary secretions, *Vet Rec* 146:672-673, 2000.

73. Barrandeguy M et al: Prevention of rotavirus diarrhoea in foals by parenteral vaccination of the mares: field trial, *Dev Biol Stand* 92:253-257, 1998.

OVINE AND CAPRINE VACCINATION PROGRAMS

NANCY E. EAST
JOAN DEAN ROWE

Several commercially available vaccines are labeled for sheep or goats. Some cattle vaccines are used off label in these ruminants, but little critical evaluation is available regarding the efficacy of this practice. The same general considerations presented for bovine vaccination programs apply to programs for sheep or goats. The vaccines available for sheep or goats are listed in Table 44-3. It is important to compare the cost of vaccination to projected loss from the disease, especially in commercial sheep operations, because of the low individual animal value and the high cost of vaccines. When considering the use of expensive vaccines, such as those for footrot, the high labor cost associated with the disease must be taken into account in addition to the more obvious cost of the disease. Flock health records, regional diagnostic laboratories, local veterinarians, and county extension agents are good resources for obtaining information about disease prevalence in a particular area.

The subcutaneous route is the preferred route for sheep or goat vaccines. The preferred site is the neck or behind the elbow, away from superficial regional lymph nodes. In sheep, injections should not be given in the loin or hindquarters because this area makes up three fourths of the prime carcass cuts. Subcutaneous injections over the ribs in goats often cause unsightly, persistent granulomas.

TABLE 44-3

Vaccines and Antisera Available for Sheep and Goats*

Disease or Organism	Vaccine Product Name
Enzootic abortion of ewes (EAE, *Chlamydia psittaci*)	*C. psittaci* bacterin[b]
Vibriosis (*Campylobacter fetus* ssp. *fetus*, *Campylobacter jejuni*)	*C. fetus* bacterin[b]
Bluetongue	Modified live serotypes 10,[b,c] 11,[d] 17[d]
Footrot	Footvax, *Bacteroides nodosus* bacterin[c]
	Volar *Fusobacterium necrophorum* bacterin[g]
Clostridium tetani/Clostridium perfringens combination toxoids (many contain additional clostridia)	Fermicon CD/T[f]
	C. perfringens types C and D, tetanus toxoid[b,g,h]
	Clostroid D-T[c]
	Covexin 8[e]
	Caseous DT[b] (*C. perfringens* type D, tetanus toxoid, and *C. pseudotuberculosis*)
	Various other combinations and brands are available
Anthrax (*Bacillus anthracis*)	Anthrax spore vaccine[b]
	Various combinations and brands are available
Contagious ecthyma (soremouth, orf) (live viral vaccine)	Ovine ecthyma vaccine[b,g]
Brucella ovis (ram epididymitis)	*B. ovis* (ram epididymitis) bacterin[b]
Caseous lymphadenitis (*Corynebacterium pseudotuberculosis*)	Case-Bac (*C. pseudotuberculosis* bacterin toxoid[b])
Escherichia coli bacterin	Ovine pili shield[a]
Tetanus antitoxin	Tetanus antitoxin†
C. perfringens antitoxin (A, B, C, D available)	*C. perfringens* types C and D antitoxin[b,i]
E coli antiserum	Ovine ecolizer[a]

*Many additional vaccines manufactured for use in cattle can be used safely in sheep and goats when the need arises.
†Widely available.
[a]Grand Laboratories, Inc., Larchwood, IA 51241.
[b]Colorado Serum Co., Denver, CO 80216.
[c]Fort Dodge Laboratories, Inc., Fort Dodge, IA 50501.
[d]Poultry Health Laboratories, Davis, CA 95616.
[e]Coopers Animal Health Inc., Kansas City, KS 66103.
[f]Bioceutic, St. Joseph, MO 64502.
[g]Bayer (formerly Miles), Shawnee Mission, KS 66201.
[h]Anchor Division, Boehringer Ingelheim, Animal Health, Inc., St Joseph, MO 64506.
[i]Sanofi Animal Health, Overland Park, KS 66210.

Compliance with a vaccination program is best achieved if the program is designed around the times when livestock normally are handled. The major problems and errors that occur in vaccination programs are (1) failure to provide adequate booster doses of clostridial vaccines, (2) inappropriate handling of modified live virus (MLV) bluetongue vaccines, (3) vaccination of ewes in early gestation with MLV bluetongue vaccines, and (4) use of contagious ecthyma vaccines on uninfected premises.

All sheep and goats should be vaccinated against *Clostridium perfringens* types C and D and tetanus with one of the available commercial products. Some of the multiway clostridial vaccines are less expensive than the *C. perfringens* types C and D/tetanus toxoid combination and are used for this reason rather than because of any real need for protection from the other diseases. The available clostridial toxoids tend to vary both in efficacy and the extent of adverse reactions (especially vaccination site granulomas). There is some indication that *C. perfringens* toxoids may be less effective in goats than in sheep. Annual vaccination of pregnant ewes and does with a *C. perfringens* types C and D/tetanus toxoid combination about 4 weeks before parturition confers adult flock immunity and maximizes passive transfer of antibody to newborn lambs and kids. These antibodies protect up to 4 to 6 weeks of age, through the high-risk period for *C. perfringens* type C enterotoxemia and for tetanus from husbandry procedures (castration, tail docking, and disbudding).

Adverse reactions to combination clostridial, *Campylobacter*, and chlamydial vaccines are not unusual, especially when these vaccines are given at the same time as footrot vaccine or vitamin E–selenium injections. Particularly in purebred flocks, owners should be taught the clinical signs and treatment of adverse reactions, which can occur 30 minutes to longer than 12 hours after vaccination. Adverse reactions include localized swelling, stiffness, pyrexia, anorexia, pulmonary edema and respiratory distress (foaming at the nose and mouth), laminitis, bloating and groaning, abortion (2 to 7 days after vaccination), and sudden death. Vaccination granulomas may persist.

The use of bacterins of *Leptospira interrogans* in sheep and goats is of questionable value under most circumstances. It is difficult to induce abortion in susceptible females with experimental infection. In endemic areas when sheep and cattle are grazed together or are adjacent and drink groundwater from streams or irrigation runoff, explosive outbreaks of leptospirosis in young growing lambs and occasional abortion storms in pregnant ewes have been described.

The cattle vaccines most commonly used in sheep are those directed against the respiratory disease complex; these vaccines are the intranasal infectious bovine rhinotracheitis (IBR) vaccine, the bovine respiratory syncytial virus (BRSV) vaccine, the killed or MLV *Pasteurella* vaccines, and the killed bovine virus diarrhea (BVD) vaccines. Justification of the use of these vaccines is based on current understanding of the potentiating and synergistic role of the cattle respiratory virus complex in ovine pneumonia and the prevalence of antibody to these viruses in the North American sheep population. Few well-controlled clinical trials using respiratory complex vaccines have been completed. Many respiratory problems can be best controlled by changes in management (see Chapter 29).

Table 44-4 shows a sheep vaccination schedule and flock management calendar for ewes and lambs in North America, and Table 44-5 shows a schedule and calendar for rams. Geographic differences in the distribution of endemic disease dictate which vaccine protocols are most economic and efficacious. Vaccines recommended for sheep include those that immunize against the following diseases or pathogens:

- Footrot
- *Chlamydia psittaci* (enzootic abortion of ewes [EAE])
- *Campylobacter* spp. (vibriosis)
- Bluetongue virus
- *C. perfringens* types C and D
- *C. tetani* (tetanus)
- Other clostridial agents as needed

Footrot vaccine should be given 4 weeks before the wet season. *Brucella ovis* bacterin is not recommended to control ram epididymitis because vaccination interferes with enzyme-linked immunosorbent assay (ELISA) testing and eradication programs. There are approved rabies vaccines for sheep but not for goats (see Table 44-2). The use of these vaccines in goats is extralabel.

A dairy goat vaccination schedule and flock management calendar is shown in Table 44-6 for does and bucks in North America and in Table 44-7 for kids.

Vaccines recommended for goats include those that immunize against the following pathogens:

- *C. perfringens* types C and D
- *C. tetani* (tetanus)
- Contagious ecthyma (soremouth) virus (only if premises are infected)
- *C. psittaci* (EAE)
- Other clostridial agents as needed

Colostral protection against soremouth is reported to be minimal.

• • •

TABLE 44-4

Ewe/Lamb Vaccination Schedule/Flock Management Calendar for North America

Procedure	Prebreeding	Breeding	Tag/Shear	Lambing	Lamb Growth	Shearing	Weaning
Vaccination*	EAE (*Chlamydia* spp.) *Vibrio* (*Campylobacter*) spp. Bluetongue	*Vibrio* booster	Vaccinate bagged ewes with clostridial caseous DT or 8-way clostridial and footrot vaccine	Footrot vaccination booster in yearling ewes; Soremouth vaccine for lambs on endemic premises	Clostridial vaccination (caseous DT) or 8-way vaccine for 6- to 10-week-old lambs; Give clostridial booster 4 weeks later; use caseous DT for replacement ewes		Vaccinate feeder lambs against clostridial agents; Vaccinate replacement ewes with caseous DT
Parasite control (see Chapter 45)	Deworm		Deworm if indicated		Coccidiostat in creep feed or salt to young lambs; Deworm older lambs	Control external parasites	Deworm feeder lambs
Treatment	Vitamin E and selenium if needed		Vitamin E and selenium if needed				
Reproduction	Condition score ewes, separate and flush; check udders, cull undesirables; Check for lameness, treat as needed	30 to 60 days after breeding, check for pregnancy and cull open ewes; Supplement pregnant ewes if thin	Separate ewes in late pregnancy and supplement last 4 weeks of gestation	Dock lamb tails; Castrate excess male lambs		Sell fat lambs	Identify/cull ewes: Thin; Missing teeth (incisors or molars) or loose teeth; Chronic mastitis; Dry ewes (no lamb); Poor mothers; Chronic lameness

*See vaccine list, Table 44-3.

TABLE 44-5

Ram Vaccination Schedule/Flock Management Calendar for North America

Procedure	Prebreeding	Breeding	Tag/Shear	Lambing	Shearing	Weaning
Vaccination*	EAE Bluetongue		Footrot vaccine	Footrot vaccine booster	Clostridial vaccines or caseous DT vaccination	
Parasite control (see Chapter 45) Treatment	Deworm		Deworm		Deworm External parasite control Vitamin E and selenium if needed	

Reproduction	Breeding soundness examination, including:
	    Epididymitis
	    Lameness
	    Condition score
	    Conformation score
	    Semen evaluation
		Rotate rams
		Observe for poor libido and cull
			Cull for epididymitis or chronic lameness		*Brucella ovis* ELISA, cull positives
					Palpate for epididymitis; cull those with lesions
						Purchase new rams tested *B. ovis* ELISA–negative and breeding soundness evaluated; scrotal circumference ≥32 cm, and rams free of abscess

Other		Remove sick, lame, injured, or very thin rams	Check teeth, cull for loose or missing teeth Put on good feed for 60 days	Cull rams not gaining weight	Condition score, separate, and bring to breeding condition Check for lameness, treat or cull	

EAE, Enzootic abortion of ewes.
*See vaccine list, Table 44-3.

TABLE 44-6

Dairy Goat (Does and Bucks) Vaccination Schedule/Herd Management Calendar for North America

Procedure	December-March	April-July	August-November
Vaccinations*	*C. perfringens* types C and D Tetanus and other clostridial diseases	Booster of vaccines given previously *Chlamydia* vaccine if needed	
Parasite control (see Chapter 45) Treatment	If access to pasture, deworm; may not be necessary if drylot only Vitamin E and selenium injection to does at drying off if in selenium-deficient area	Deworm if needed (access to pasture) Vitamin E and selenium if needed; vitamins A and D	
Mastitis control (see Chapter 34)	Culture milk from fresh does for bacteria and mycoplasma; treat or cull	Bulk tank mycoplasma culture; monitor milk quality; culture does with mastitis or increased CMT/SCC	Treat dry does as needed with intramammary antibiotics Monitor milk quality
Reproduction (see Chapter 41)	Pregnancy check before dry off Cull open does Institute artificial lighting for dry yearling does and all bucks needed for out of season breeding†	Institute out-of-season breeding using hormone therapy on lactating does‡ Pregnancy check 45 days after breeding Breed light-treated yearling does	Plan breeding adult does to spread out fresh dates and begin breeding to assigned bucks; maintain breeding records Examine short-cycling and repeat-breeder does; cull nonresponders; pregnancy check does
Other	Maintain first lactation yearling does in separate pen; milk first; feed for both growth and production	Cull low-producing does Prebreeding examination on bucks, cull abnormals, bring bucks to breeding condition by optimizing nutrition	Supplement bucks to maintain condition

CMT, California Mastitis Test; *ELISA,* enzyme-linked immunosorbent assay; *SCC,* somatic cell count.
*See vaccine list, Table 44-3.
†22 hours/day for 8 weeks, usually January to February; start cycling 4 to 8 weeks after start of light; *dry* does only.
‡One-half Synchromate B implant (CEVA Laboratories, Inc., Overland Park, KS 66212) under tail for 9 to 16 days. Give PMSG (equine chorionic gonadotropin; 500 IU needed in early spring, 250 U in May or June or later) 48 hours before pulling implant; then pull implant, and animals will cycle 12 to 72 hours later (maximum number in heat at 36 hours).

TABLE 44-7

Dairy Kid Vaccination Schedule/Herd Management Calendar for North America

Procedure	December-March	April-July	August-November
Vaccination*	*C. perfringens* types C and D Tetanus or caseous DT Other clostridial diseases	Booster clostridial or caseous DT vaccines given previously	Before breeding, *Chlamydia* vaccine (or use tetracycline in feed before and during breeding season)
Parasite control	Coccidiostat in kid starter feed at 2 weeks of age (Deccox recommended)	Continue coccidiostat Deworm if access to pasture	
Treatment	Vitamins A, D, E Vitamin E, selenium if needed	Vitamin E, selenium if needed	
Reproduction	Castrate excess males; pregnancy check kids		Pregnancy check kids Cull short-cycling and repeat-breeder kids Hold small females for artificial light therapy (see Table 44-6)
Other	Isolate from does at birth, feed cow colostrum or heat-treated goat colostrum, followed by cow milk, milk replacer, or pasteurized goat milk to control myco-plasma and CAE Disbud kids Tattoo kids	Maintain isolation from adults Do not overcrowd Provide ration for maximum growth Keep male and female kids separate	Group kids by size and sex Start breeding kids over 29.3 kg

CAE, Caprine arthritis-encephalitis.
*See vaccine list, Table 44-3.

BOVINE VACCINES AND HERD VACCINATION PROGRAMS

VICTOR S. CORTESE

To scientifically choose a vaccine or design a vaccination program, variables such as follows must be considered.[74]
- The presence and degree of challenge of the particular diseases on the farm or ranch
- Management practices on the facility that support or hinder vaccination programs
- The times or ages at which the disease problems occur and if the diseases are associated with any stressors
- The immune system components necessary to afford protection against various diseases
- Some basic immunologic concepts
- The information available on products being considered and the source and quality of the information
- Required vaccines for a particular use of the animal (e.g., 4-H shows).

CHALLENGE

The level of disease challenge and the degree of protection continually fluctuate. Because of biologic variability, the degree of protection is different in every vaccinated animal. The same is true of the level of exposure to a pathogen. Overwhelming challenge can override immunity and lead to disease even in well-vaccinated animals.[75]

TIMING OF DISEASE

On many farms certain diseases occur at consistent times. The timing may give some insight into stresses that occur in the management of the cattle. Correcting these stresses can have a positive impact on vaccination and lessen animals' susceptibility to disease. This type of history also is helpful in determining the timing of vaccinations, a concept that often is underused in veterinary medicine. Knowing when a problem historically has occurred allows vaccinations to be scheduled when they will induce maximum immune responses in preparation for expected challenges.

ASSESSING VACCINE EFFICACY

The efficacy of a vaccine can be extremely difficult for the practitioner to assess. Traditionally, serologic data showing prevaccinaton and postvaccination titers has been equated with protection. For many diseases, however, the correlation is poor between the antibody measured and the protection generated by the vaccine in the animal.[76] Recently, cell-mediated immune function tests have been added to show a more complete stimulation of the immune response after vaccination.[77] Although these tests provide more information about the vaccine, they still do not answer the basic question of how well a vaccine really protects. This question can be answered only by well-designed challenge studies. There are many examples of well-designed studies involving both viral[78,79] and bacterial[80,81] agents. To assess a challenge study, the following information is needed:
1. The trial design, including animal characteristics
2. A statistical analysis of the results
3. The route of administration of the challenge
4. The characteristics of the challenge organism
5. The method of clinical score assignment
6. Publication of the results in a peer-reviewed article

Unfortunately, the challenge model is not well established for many diseases. Field trials are even harder to assess but are valuable for judging the effectiveness (i.e., efficacy in a particular situation) and efficiency (i.e., cost-effectiveness) of a vaccine[82] (Boxes 44-1 to 44-3). Several good references on field trial analysis are available.[83,84]

CATTLE VACCINES

Bovine vaccines tailored for use against eight viral diseases, more than 28 bacterial pathogens, two neorickettsial diseases (anaplasmosis and *Neospora* infection), and one protozoal disease (trichomoniasis) currently are marketed in the United States (Table 44-8). These vaccines have been designed to aid in the prevention of reproductive, respiratory, generalized septicemic and toxic (endotoxic and exotoxic) diseases. The vaccines have demonstrated some degree of protection against the pathogen for which they were designed, but they may not have proved protective against all

---

BOX 44-1

Bovine Vaccines Generally Regarded as Ineffective or Only Marginally Effective

Pasteurella haemolytica bacterins
Pasteurella multocida bacterins
Salmonella bacterins
Moraxella bovis (pinkeye) bacterins
Rotavirus-coronavirus (calf scours) vaccine (modified live virus)
Staphylococcus aureus (mastitis) bacterin-toxoids

BOX 42-2

Bovine Vaccines Seldom Needed on Most U.S. Ranches and Farms*

Anthrax vaccine
Clostridium septicum (malignant edema) bacterins
Leptospira grippotyphosa bacterins
Leptospira icterohaemorrhagiae bacterins
Leptospira canicola bacterins
Clostridium botulinum toxoids
Clostridium novyi bacterins
Rabies vaccine
Tetanus toxoids
Erysipelas bacterins
Clostridium perfringens type D (enterotoxemia) toxoids
Clostridium sordellii (malignant edema) bacterins

*These vaccines also are not cost-effective.

BOX 44-3

Bovine Vaccines for Ranch- and Farm-Specific (Soil-Borne) Diseases

Blackleg bacterins
Clostridium haemolyticum (redwater) bacterins
Anthrax vaccine
Clostridium novyi (infectious necrotic hepatitis) bacterins

---

the various syndromes known to be caused by a specific infectious agent. The challenge models for each pathogen and the release requirements for each vaccine are monitored by the Veterinary Biologics division of the U.S. Department of Agriculture's Animal and Plant Health Inspection Service (USDA/APHIS) and can be found in Book 9 of the Code of Federal Regulations.

During gestation the bovine reproductive system, with its multilayered placenta, leaves the fetus in a naive environment susceptible to infection. Abortions may occur as a result of infection of the placenta, inflammation of the ovary, death of the fetus, or disruption of the cervical plug. Reproductive disease therefore is the most difficult against which to achieve protection. Vaccination must minimize the amount or duration (or both) of the viremia or septicemia, or it must prevent the pathogen from moving through the cervix or crossing the placenta. Only a few of the currently licensed vaccines have proved protective against the reproductive forms of various diseases. Furthermore, the duration of immunity afforded by the various vaccines has not been established for most currently licensed products.

Each manufacturer's development and production of cattle vaccines is different, consequently the composition of vaccines varies dramatically among the different manufacturers. Outlines of production are proprietary for each manufacturer, but some information can be found in technical and marketing materials. For example, some viral vaccines are grown on bovine-derived kidney cell lines, and others are grown on porcine-derived kidney cells. Some vaccines are grown only on calf serum, whereas others are grown on both calf and fetal calf serum. Differences in passages may be found as well. The variability is seen in (1) the strain or strains chosen for the vaccine, (2) the number of passages chosen in the growth, (3) the growth medium, and (4) the number of viral or bacterial particles in the vaccine.

The three types of vaccines described below represent the basic technologies currently available in cattle viral and bacterial vaccines.[75,86-90]

1. *Modified live (attenuated) vaccines* contain living bacterial or viral organisms. These organisms usually are collected from a field disease case and then grown in abnormal host cells (viruses) or media (bacteria) to change or attenuate the pathogen. Each completion of growth through a replication is known as a passage, and the changed pathogen then is administered back to the animal to determine if it is still virulent. After several passages the pathogen begins to lose virulence factors because it cannot cause "disease" in the unnatural host cells. Once the pathogen can no longer cause "disease" in the target species, it is tested to see if it can confer protection. The final vaccine usually is passed a number of times beyond the passage where virulence disappears in order to reduce the risk of reversion to a virulent pathogen. These vaccines usually require good quality control to reduce the risk of a contaminant entering the vaccine.

2. *Inactivated (killed) vaccines* are easier to develop because virulence after growth is not a problem. The same pathogen is isolated from a disease outbreak. The pathogen is grown and then chemically or physically killed. The inactivation usually is achieved either by adding a chemical to the pathogen or by using ultraviolet rays. The major concern with inactivation is the potential loss of important epitopes. An adjuvant normally is added to inactivated vaccines to heighten the immune response. The vaccine is then tested for efficacy.

3. *Genetically engineered vaccines* have been altered genetically, usually through a mutation. This mutation may be induced by several different methods, but the resulting bacterium or virus has different properties that may alter virulence or growth characteristics. Most of these vaccines are modified live mutants (e.g., temperature-sensitive viral vaccines or streptomycin-dependent *Pasteurella* vaccines), but inactivated marker vaccines are also genetically engineered. These vaccines have been engineered to delete a gene and cause an immune response deficient in antibodies to a certain epitope; this allows diagnostic methods to distinguish between vaccine and natural exposure responses (e.g., gene-deleted infectious bovine rhinotracheitis [IBR] vaccines).

Once its efficacy has been established, the vaccine is put through a series of experiments to determine the minimum dose required to achieve adequate protection, called the minimum immunizing dose (MID). The vaccine will contain more than the MID in order to obtain at least the MID at the expiration date found on the label. In effect, a vaccine's efficacy is not determined by the final product used by the veterinarian but at a reduced level of immunogens from the amount contained in the final vaccine.

TABLE 44-8

Antigens Available in Currently Licensed* Cattle Vaccines

Antigen Type	Common Name of Disease or Vaccine	Pathogen
Virus	BRSV	Bovine respiratory syncytial virus
	Rednose	Bovine herpesvirus type 1, infectious bovine rhinotracheitis virus (IBRV)
	BVD-MD	Bovine virus diarrhea virus (types 1 and 2)–mucosal disease
	PI-3	Parainfluenza type 3 virus
	Rabies	*Lyssavirus* spp.
	Warts	Bovine papillomavirus, bovine rotavirus, bovine coronavirus
Bacteria	Anthrax	*Bacillus anthracis*
	Bangs	*Brucella abortus*
	Vibriosis	*Campylobacter fetus* ssp. *veneralis*
	Blackleg	*Clostridium chauvoei*
	Redwater disease (bacillary hemoglobinuria)	*Clostridium haemolyticum*
	Black disease	*Clostridium novyi*
	Enterotoxemia	*Clostridium perfringens* type C
	Overeating	*Clostridium perfringens* type D
	Malignant edema	*Clostridium septicum, Clostridium sordellii*
	Tetanus	*Clostridium tetani*
	Endotoxin vaccines	J5 *Escherichia coli*
	Coliform scours	*Escherichia coli*
	Footrot	*Fusobacterium necrophorum, Haemophilus somnus, Leptospira canicola, Leptospira grippotyphosa, Leptospira hardjo, Leptospira icterhaemorrhagiae, Leptospira pomona*
	Pinkeye	*Moraxella bovis*
	Johne's disease	*Mycobacterium paratuberculosis*
	Shipping fever	*Mannheimia haemolytica (Pasteurella haemolytica), Pasteurella multocida*
	Endotoxin vaccines	R *Salmonella, Salmonella dublin, Salmonella typhimurium*
	Staph mastitis	*Staphylococcus aureus*
Rickettsiae/protozoa	Neosporosis	*Neospora* sp. (provisional license)
	Trich	*Tritrichomonas foetus*
	Anaplasmosis	*Anaplasma marginale*

Modified from *Compendium of veterinary products*, ed 5, 1999, Adrian J. Bayley.
*Licensed by the Animal and Plant Health Inspection Service, U.S. Department of Agriculture.

Autogenous Vaccines

In addition to the vaccines licensed by the U.S. Department of Agriculture, several companies will make autogenous vaccines for use by veterinarians and cattle owners. These vaccines do not fall under any particular USDA/APHIS guidelines and usually are derived from cultures (e.g., viral or bacterial) isolated from specimens submitted by the particular farm. Such vaccines can be used only on that particular facility and cannot be sold for use on other farms. These vaccines are not tested for efficacy or safety, and the components found in the vaccines may vary from batch to batch; this adds some element of risk when they are used. Nevertheless, this type of vaccine may be an option to consider when federally licensed vaccines are not available for a specific farm problem.

Maternal Antibody Interference Revisited

It is an accepted belief that maternal antibodies can block immune responses from vaccination. This belief has been based on a procedure of vaccination followed by a titer evaluation in the vaccinates. Many studies have shown that vaccinated animals may not display increased antibody levels if high levels of maternal antibody to that antigen are present. However, recent studies have shown both the formation of B cell memory responses and cell-mediated responses can be stimulated in spite of high maternal antibody for the same antigens.[91-93] Seropositive calves vaccinated at a young age with modified live (MLV) bovine herpesvirus type 1 (BHV-1), parainfluenza type 3 (PI-3),

and/or bovine respiratory syncytial virus (BRSV) vaccines have shown higher antibody responses on revaccination than control calves vaccinated only at the second date. These young vaccinates typically do not show increased antibody responses after the first vaccination in the presence of high maternal antibody. Cell-mediated immune responses, as indicated by antigen-specific T cell blastogenesis, have been demonstrated in the face of high maternal antibody levels[94] when attenuated BRSV and BHV-1 vaccines were used. Similar responses have been reported in laboratory animals as well.[95-97] One study also demonstrated higher levels of protection at challenge if calves were vaccinated with a modified live BRSV vaccine.[92] It is clear from these studies that maternal antibody interference with vaccines is not as absolute as once thought. The animal's immune status, the specific antigen, and the presentation of that antigen should be considered when designing vaccination programs in which maternal antibody may be a factor.

Impact of Stress

Stress affects the immune system of all cattle, as can a number of factors. The release of corticosteroid that occurs during the birthing process has a dramatic impact on the newborn's immune system. Newborns also have a higher number of suppressor T cells than do adults.[75] These factors and others dramatically diminish systemic immune responses for the first week of life.[98] Other stresses should be avoided at vaccination time to maintain the integrity of the immune system. Procedures such as castration, dehorning, weaning, and movement need to be considered as stressors in cattle, and all have the potential to diminish immune system functioning temporarily.[99-101]

Systemic vaccinations should be avoided during high-stress times because of these diminished responses and because vaccination at such times may even have undesired effects.

Booster Importance

It is important to follow the label directions for administering vaccines. Inactivated vaccines and most modified live BRSV vaccines require a booster before protection is complete. The first time an inactivated vaccine is administered, the primary response occurs. This response is not very strong, is fairly short-lived, and is predominantly composed of IgM antibodies (Fig. 44-1). The response seen after a booster vaccination is called the secondary, or anamnestic, response. This response is much stronger, of longer duration, and is primarily composed of IgG antibodies.[75,85] If the booster is given too early, the anamnestic response does not occur, and if too much time elapses before the booster is given, it acts as an initial dose, not as a booster.

With most MLV vaccines (except for most BRSV vaccines), the primary vaccination also stimulates the secondary response without needing a booster because the virus or bacterium is replicating in the animal.

Adverse Reactions

Adverse reactions are a risk with any vaccination. These reactions can be categorized as one of the following three primary types of hypersensitivity.[75,77,102-107]

1. Type I, or immediate, hypersensitivity is mediated by IgE stimulation and the release of granules from basophils and mast cells. This reaction is seen within minutes of vaccination and often begins with shaking or sweating. Most of these animals respond to intravenous injection of epinephrine. Every vaccine occasionally can elicit an anaphylactic reaction. Cattle should always be kept under observation for at least 30 min after administration of a vaccine. Epinephrine should be administered at a dosage of 1 ml of 1:1000 solution per 50 kg of body weight, preferably by intravenous injection, at the first sign of weakness, staggering, or dyspnea. With most vaccines anaphylactic reactions occur no more often than one case per 5000 to 10,000 doses administered. The rate of occurrence may be much higher after administration of *Salmonell, Escherichia coli*, and some *Moraxella bovis* bacterins, which may have high levels of endotoxin.

2. Type III, or immune complex, hypersensitivity is mediated by the attachment of an antibody-antigen complex to complement and the ensuing activation of the complement cascade. The resultant reaction may occur locally or systemically. The reaction may be delayed, as the complexes form and the cascade begins, or subsequent, as products begin to exert their effects. The signs are similar to those of an immediate hypersensitivity reaction, and the treatment is administration of epinephrine.

3. One of the more common reactions seen in dairy cattle has been associated with the endotoxin and other bacterial components found in most gram negative vaccines. Currently, there are no requirements for monitoring or reporting the amount of endotoxin found in cattle vaccines, and the level of endotoxin may vary dramatically between vaccines and between serials of the same vaccine. Furthermore, the potency of endotoxin varies among different gram negative bacteria. This type of reaction is seen primarily in Holsteins because of a genetic predisposition and may be seen after administration of any gram negative bacterin. The signs vary depending on the farm's or the individual's sensitivity to gram negative bacterial components. The number or potency of the gram negative fractions in vaccinations administered simultaneously also are instrumental in causing these reactions. As a general rule, no more than two gram negative vaccines should be administered to dairy cattle on the same day because of the possibility of adverse reactions, which may include anorexia and transient decreases in milk production, early embryonic death, abortion, and gram negative bacterial shock (endotoxic shock), which requires treatment with fluxinin or keprofen, steroids, antihistamines, and fluids. Site reactions are common sequelae to many vaccines.

4. These granulomas usually are caused by overreaction to the adjuvants, but they may also be directly aimed at the antigen or antigens. This has been a major focus of beef quality programs and has generated a push to have all vaccines labeled and to have them administered subcutaneously to avoid damaging the muscle.

BOX 44-4

Vaccines Recommended for Use in Adult Beef Cows

VACCINES HIGHLY RECOMMENDED FOR ALL HERDS
Infectious bovine rhinotracheitis (IBR) vaccines
Bovine virus diarrhea (BVD) vaccines
Leptospira pomona bacterins
Campylobacteriosis bacterins*

VACCINES THAT MAY BE USEFUL OR NECESSARY IN SPECIFIC HERDS OR GEOGRAPHIC LOCATIONS
Tritrichomonas foetus vaccine†
Anaplasmosis vaccine (inactivated)
Rotavirus-coronavirus (calf scours) vaccine (inactivated)
Fusobacterium necrophorum (footrot) bacterin
Escherichia coli bacterins
Clostridium haemolyticum (redwater) bacterins
Leptospira hardjo bacterins
Clostridium perfringens type C (enterotoxemia) toxoids
Anthrax vaccine
Clostridium novyi bacterins

*Highly recommended except in herds from which this disease can be reliably excluded (by virtue of the "closed" status of the herd and by isolation from other potentially infected herds by distance, terrain, and/or "bull proof" perimeter fencing).

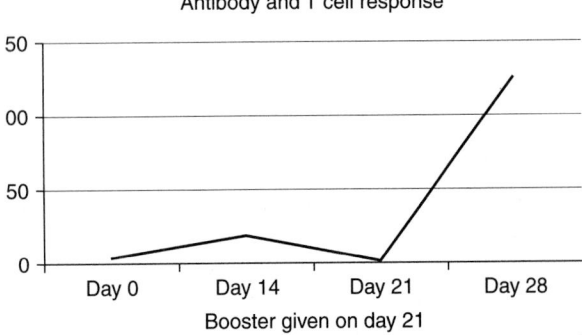

Antibody and T cell response

Booster given on day 21

FIG. 44-1 ■ Anamnestic response seen after booster dose is administered to vaccinates.

Summary

Designing a vaccination program requires a good history of the individual farm and a basic understanding of the immune system. Vaccines that should be considered for routine or optional use in various classes of pastured beef cattle, feedlot cattle, and dairy cattle are listed in Boxes 44-4 to 44-13. The vaccines chosen should be supported by good, solid efficacy studies (and by effectiveness and efficiency studies if possible) to ensure that the product can fulfill the needs of the farm or ranch (Table 44-9). Management decisions may be made that do not maximize the potential of the product chosen, and realistic expectations of all products should be well explained to the producer before the vaccines are administered. The owner should be involved in the vaccine decision-making process, and all information on the product should be shared.

The establishment of good baseline immunity of replacement heifers and the foundation vaccination program can have dramatic effects on the health and profitability of the herd, therefore such programs must be well planned.

BOX 44-5

Vaccines Recommended for Use in Adult Beef Bulls

VACCINES HIGHLY RECOMMENDED FOR ALL HERDS
Infectious bovine rhinotracheitis (IBR) vaccines
Bovine virus diarrhea (BVD) vaccines
Campylobacteriosis bacterins*

VACCINES THAT MAY BE USEFUL OR NECESSARY IN SPECIFIC HERDS OR GEOGRAPHIC LOCATIONS
Tritrichomonas foetus vaccine
Anaplasmosis vaccine (inactivated)

VACCINES THAT MAY BE USEFUL OR NECESSARY IN SPECIFIC HERDS OR GEOGRAPHIC LOCATIONS— cont'd
Leptospira pomona bacterins
Fusobacterium necrophorum (footrot) bacterin
Clostridium haemolyticum (redwater) bacterins
Anthrax vaccine
Leptospira hardjo bacterins
Clostridium novyi bacterins

*Highly recommended except in herds from which this disease can be reliably excluded (by virtue of the "closed" status of the herd and by isolation from other potentially infected herds by distance, terrain, and/or "bull proof" perimeter fencing).

BOX 44-6

Vaccines Recommended for Use in Beef Calves*

HIGHLY RECOMMENDED VACCINES
Infectious bovine rhinotracheitis (IBR) vaccines
Bovine virus diarrhea (BVD) vaccines
Bovine respiratory syncytial virus (BRSV) vaccines
Parainfluenza type 3 (PI-3) vaccines
Leptospira pomona bacterins
Brucellosis vaccine†

VACCINES THAT MAY BE USEFUL OR NECESSARY IN SPECIFIC HERDS OR GEOGRAPHIC LOCATIONS
Blackleg bacterins
Moraxella bovis (pinkeye) bacterins

VACCINES THAT MAY BE USEFUL OR NECESSARY IN SPECIFIC HERDS OR GEOGRAPHIC LOCATIONS— cont'd
Haemophilus somnus bacterins
Anaplasmosis vaccine‡ (modified live)
Clostridium haemolyticum bacterins
Anthrax vaccine
Fusobacterium necrophorum (footrot) bacterin
Clostridium novyi bacterins
Pasteurella haemolytica vaccines (new)

*Under 12 months of age.
†Heifer replacements only.
‡Heifer and bull replacements only.

BOX 44-7

Vaccines Recommended for Use in Stocker Cattle

HIGHLY RECOMMENDED VACCINES
Infectious bovine rhinotracheitis (IBR) vaccines
Bovine virus diarrhea (BVD) vaccines
Bovine respiratory syncytial virus (BRSV) vaccines
Parainfluenza type 3 (PI-3) vaccines
Pasteurella haemolytica vaccines (new)
Leptospira pomona bacterins

VACCINES THAT MAY BE USEFUL OR NECESSARY IN SPECIFIC HERDS OR GEOGRAPHIC LOCATIONS
Blackleg bacterins
Haemophilus somnus bacterins
Moraxella bovis (pinkeye) bacterins
Clostridium haemolyticum bacterins
Anthrax vaccine
Fusobacterium necrophorum (footrot) bacterin
Clostridium novyi bacterins

BOX 44-8

Vaccines Recommended for Use in Beef Replacement Heifers

VACCINES HIGHLY RECOMMENDED FOR USE IN ALL HERDS
Infectious bovine rhinotracheitis (IBR) vaccines
Bovine virus diarrhea (BVD) vaccines
Leptospira pomona bacterins
Campylobacteriosis bacterins*

VACCINES THAT MAY BE USEFUL OR NECESSARY IN SPECIFIC HERDS OR GEOGRAPHIC LOCATIONS
Blackleg bacterins
Tritrichomonas foetus vaccine
Anaplasmosis vaccine (modified live)
Rotavirus-coronavirus vaccine (inactivated)

VACCINES THAT MAY BE USEFUL OR NECESSARY IN SPECIFIC HERDS OR GEOGRAPHIC LOCATIONS— cont'd
Escherichia coli bacterins
Fusobacterium necrophorum (footrot) bacterin
Moraxella bovis (pinkeye) bacterins
Haemophilus somnus bacterins
Clostridium haemolyticum bacterins
Leptospira hardjo bacterins
Clostridium perfringens type C toxoids
Anthrax vaccine
Clostridium novyi bacterins

*Highly recommended except in herds from which this disease can be reliably excluded (by virtue of the "closed" status of the herd and by isolation from other potentially infected herds by distance, terrain, or "bull proof" perimeter fencing).

BOX 44-9

Vaccines Recommended for Routine Administration to Cattle Entering Feedlots

ESSENTIAL VACCINE
Infectious bovine rhinotracheitis (IBR) vaccine (modified live)

HIGHLY RECOMMENDED VACCINES
Pasteurella haemolytica vaccine*
Bovine virus diarrhea (BVD) vaccine (modified live)
Leptospira pomona bacterins

VACCINE THAT MAY BE NEEDED IN SOME GROUPS OF CATTLE IN A FEEDLOT
Clostridium haemolyticum (redwater) bacterins

VACCINES NECESSARY ONLY IN SPECIFIC "PROBLEM" FEEDLOTS
Blackleg bacterins
Bovine respiratory syncytial virus (BRSV) vaccines
Fusobacterium necrophorum (footrot) bacterin

*Some commercial modified live cytopathic virus BVD vaccines trigger severe fatal BVD in cattle that are chronically infected with noncytopathic strains of BVD virus and immunologically tolerant as a result of prenatal infection.

BOX 44-10

Vaccines Recommended for Use in Adult Dairy Cows

VACCINES HIGHLY RECOMMENDED FOR USE IN ALL DAIRY HERDS
Infectious bovine rhinotracheitis (IBR) vaccines
Bovine virus diarrhea (BVD) vaccines
Leptospira pomona bacterins

VACCINE HIGHLY RECOMMENDED FOR COWS IN SPECIFIC INFECTED HERDS
Leptospira hardjo bacterins

VACCINES HIGHLY RECOMMENDED FOR DAIRY COWS GRAZING IN SPECIFIC ENDEMIC AREAS
Clostridium haemolyticum bacterins
Anthrax vaccine
Clostridium novyi bacterins

VACCINES THAT MAY BE USEFUL IN CONTROLLING SPECIFIC DISEASE PROBLEMS IN INDIVIDUAL DAIRY HERDS
Gram negative core antigen (coliform mastitis) bacterins
Escherichia coli (calf scours) bacterins
Rotavirus-coronavirus (calf scours) vaccine (inactivated)
Staphylococcus aureus (mastitis) bacterin-toxoids
Fusobacterium necrophorum (footrot) bacterin
Clostridium septicum (malignant edema) bacterins
Clostridium sordellii (malignant edema) bacterins

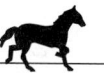

BOX 44-11

Vaccines Recommended for Use in Adult Dairy Bulls

VACCINES HIGHLY RECOMMENDED FOR BULLS IN ALL COMMERCIAL DAIRY HERDS
Infectious bovine rhinotracheitis (IBR) vaccines
Bovine virus diarrhea (BVD) vaccines
Campylobacteriosis bacterins*

VACCINES HIGHLY RECOMMENDED FOR BULLS GRAZING IN SPECIFIC ENDEMIC AREAS
Anaplasmosis vaccine (inactivated)
Clostridium haemolyticum (redwater) bacterins

VACCINES HIGHLY RECOMMENDED FOR BULLS GRAZING IN SPECIFIC ENDEMIC AREAS—cont'd
Anthrax vaccine
Clostridium novyi bacterins

VACCINES THAT MAY BE USEFUL IN SPECIFIC HERDS OR GEOGRAPHIC LOCATIONS
Leptospira pomona bacterins
Leptospira hardjo bacterins
Fusobacterium necrophorum (footrot) bacterin

*Highly recommended except in herds from which this disease can be reliably excluded (by virtue of the "closed" status of the herd and by isolation from other potentially infected herds by distance, terrain, or "bull proof" perimeter fencing).

BOX 44-12

Vaccines Recommended for Use in Dairy Calves*

VACCINES HIGHLY RECOMMENDED FOR CALVES IN ALL DAIRY HERDS
Infectious bovine rhinotracheitis (IBR) vaccines
Bovine virus diarrhea (BVD) vaccines
Bovine respiratory syncytial virus (BRSV) vaccines
Parainfluenza type 3 (PI-3) vaccines
Leptospira pomona bacterins
Brucellosis vaccine

VACCINES HIGHLY RECOMMENDED FOR CALVES GRAZING IN SPECIFIC ENDEMIC AREAS
Blackleg bacterins
Clostridium haemolyticum bacterins
Anthrax vaccine
Clostridium novyi bacterins

VACCINE HIGHLY RECOMMENDED FOR CALVES IN HERDS WITH ADULT COWS GRAZING IN SPECIFIC ENDEMIC AREAS
Anaplasmosis vaccine (modified live)

VACCINES THAT MAY BE USEFUL IN CONTROLLING SPECIFIC DISEASE PROBLEMS IN INDIVIDUAL DAIRY HERDS
Pasteurella haemolytica vaccines (new)
Haemophilus somnus bacterins
Moraxella bovis (pinkeye) bacterins
Fusobacterium necrophorum (footrot) bacterin

*Up to 12 months of age.

BOX 44-13

Vaccines Recommended for Use in Yearling Replacement Dairy Heifers

VACCINES HIGHLY RECOMMENDED FOR USE IN HEIFERS IN ALL DAIRY HERDS
Infectious bovine rhinotracheitis (IBR) vaccines
Bovine virus diarrhea (BVD) vaccines
Leptospira pomona bacterins

VACCINE HIGHLY RECOMMENDED FOR DAIRY HEIFERS TO BE BRED BY NATURAL SERVICE
Campylobacter bacterins*

VACCINE HIGHLY RECOMMENDED FOR DAIRY HEIFERS IN SPECIFIC INFECTED HERDS
L. hardjo bacterins

VACCINES HIGHLY RECOMMENDED FOR DAIRY HEIFERS GRAZING IN SPECIFIC ENDEMIC AREAS
Blackleg bacterins
Anaplasmosis vaccine (Anavac† or Anaplaz)
Clostridium haemolyticum (redwater) bacterins
Anthrax vaccine
Clostridium novyi bacterins

VACCINES THAT MAY BE USEFUL FOR CONTROLLING SPECIFIC DISEASE PROBLEMS IN INDIVIDUAL GROUPS OF DAIRY HEIFERS
Haemophilus somnus bacterins
Fusobacterium necrophorum (footrot) bacterin
Moraxella bovis (pinkeye) bacterins

VACCINES ADMINISTERED TO SPRINGING HEIFERS THAT MAY BE USEFUL FOR CONTROLLING SPECIFIC DISEASE PROBLEMS IN SPECIFIC DAIRY HERDS
Gram negative core antigen (coliform mastitis) vaccines
Escherichia coli (calf scours) bacterins
Rotavirus-coronavirus (calf scours) vaccine (inactivated)
Staphylococcus aureus (mastitis) bacterin-toxoids
Clostridium septicum (malignant edema) bacterins
Clostridium sordellii (malignant edema) bacterins

*Highly recommended except in herds from which this disease can be reliably excluded (by virtue of the "closed" status of the herd and by isolation from other potentially infected herds by distance, terrain, or "bull proof" perimeter fencing).
†Anavac (BioLOGIC Laboratories, Davis, CA 95616) is the preferred vaccine for use in dairy herds in which the adult cows are grazing in an endemic area.

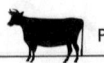
TABLE 44-9

Recommendations for Use of Some Bovine Respiratory Disease Vaccines

Pathogen	Passive Antibodies Protective	Duration of Colostral Immunity (Months)	Type of Vaccine	Immunizes in the Presence of Passive Immunity	Earliest Recommended Age for Initial Vaccination (Months)	Site of Administration	Doses Required for Protection
Anaplasma marginale[1]			Modified live	No	1 to 4[a]	IM	1
Anaplasma marginale[2]			Inactivated			SC	2
Moraxella bovis[3-12]	Yes	4 to 6	Bacterin	No	1[a] to 5	IM[6,7] or SC	1[b] to 2[c]
Staphylococcus spp.[13]	NA	NA	Bacterin	NA		IM	2
Bacillus anthracis[14]	?	?	Sterne nonencapsulated avirulent spore	?	Any	SC	1 to 2
Fusobacterium necrophorum[15,16]	NA	NA	Bacterin	NA	Any	IM or SC	2
Papillomatous digital dermatitis[17]	NA	NA	Bacterin	NA	Any	SC	3
Rabies virus[18-20]	Yes	4 to 10	Inactivated virus	No	3	IM	1
Bovine papilloma virus[21-25]	Yes	3	Inactivated wart tissue extract		Any[a]	SC	2

IM, Intramuscular administration; *NA*, not applicable; *SC*, subcutaneous administration; *?*, unknown.
[a]Calves vaccinated before the age at which passive immunity no longer exists should be revaccinated upon reaching that age.
[b]Oil-adjuvant vaccines.
[c]Aluminum hydroxide–adjuvant vaccines.
[d]Give booster 3 to 6 weeks before calving.
[e]No milk withdrawal required.
[f]Booster can be given sooner in heavily contaminated areas.
[g]May be given when exposure is imminent in endemic areas.
[1]Anavac, BioLOGIC Laboratories, Davis, CA 95616.
[2]Plazvax, Schering-Plough, Animal Health, Union, NJ 07083.
[3]I-Site, AgriLaboratories, St. Joseph, MO.
[4]Maxi/Guard Pinkeye bacterin, Addison Biological Laboratory, Fayette, MO 65248.

REFERENCES

74. Hjerpe CA: Bovine vaccines and herd vaccination programs. In Smith BP: *Large animal internal medicine,* ed 2, St Louis, 1996, Mosby.
75. Tizard I: General principles of vaccination and vaccines. In *Veterinary immunology, an introduction,* ed 4, Philadelphia, 1992, WB Saunders.
76. Kaeberle M: The elements of immunity, *Large Anim Vet* July/August 1991.
77. Abbas AK, Lichtman AH, Pober JS: Antigen presentation and T cell recognition and molecular basis of T cell antigen recognition and activation. In *Cellular and molecular immunology,* Philadelphia, 1991, WB Saunders.
78. Cortese VS et al: Clinical and immunologic responses of vaccinated and unvaccinated calves to infection with a virulent type II isolate of bovine viral diarrhea virus, *J Am Vet Med Assoc* 213:1312-1319, 1998.
79. Cravens RL, Bechtol D: Clinical responses of feeder calves under a direct IBR and BVD challenge: a comparison of two vaccines and a negative control, *Bovine Pract* 26:154-158, 1991.
80. Bolin CA et al: Effect of vaccination with a pentavalent leptospiral vaccine on *Leptospira interrogans* serovar hardjo type hardjo-bovis infection of pregnant cattle, *Am J Vet Res* 50:161-165, 1989.
81. Hogan JS et al: Efficacy of an *Escherichia coli* J5 mastitis vaccine in an experimental challenge trial, *J Dairy Sci* 75:415-422, 1992.
82. Naggan L: *Principles of epidemiology,* Class notes, Johns Hopkins School of Public Health and Hygiene, Summer Graduate Program in Epidemiology, 1994.
83. Ribble C: *Assessing vaccine efficacy, Can Vet J* 31:679-681, 1990.
84. Meinert CL: *Clinical trials: design, conduct and analysis,* New York, 1986, Oxford University Press.
85. Duffus WPH: *Immunoprophylaxis.* In Hallwell REW, Gorman NT, eds: *Veterinary clinical immunology,* Philadelphia, 1989, WB Saunders.
86. Hoffman M: Determining what immune cells see, *Res News* 255:531-534, 1992.
87. Von Boehmer H, Kisielow P: How the immune system learns about self, *Sci Am* October, 1991, pp 74-81.
88. Blecha F: New approaches to increasing immunity in food animals, *Vet Med* November, 1990, pp 1241-1250.
89. Godson DL, Campos M, Babiuk LA: The role of bovine intraepithelial leukocyte-mediated cytotoxicity in enteric antiviral defense, *Viral Immunol* 5:13-94, 1992.
90. Denis M et al: Infectious bovine rhinotracheitis (bovine herpesvirus-1): helper T cells, cytotoxic T cells, and NK cells. In Goddeeris BML, Morrison WI, eds: *Cell-mediated immunity in ruminants,* Boca Raton, Fla, 1994, CW Press.
91. Parker WL et al: Effects of vaccination at branding on serum antibody titers to viral agents of bovine respiratory disease (BRD) in newly weaned New Mexico calves, *Proceedings of the Western Section, American Society of Animal Science,* 44:132-134, 1993.
92. Kimman TG, Westenbrink F, Straver PJ: Priming for local and systematic antibody memory responses to bovine respiratory syncytial virus: effect of amount of virus, viral replication, route of administration, and maternal antibodies, *Vet Immunol Immunopathol* 22:145-160, 1989.
93. Pitcher PM: Influence of passively transferred maternal antibody on response of pigs to pseudorabies vaccines, *Proceedings of the American Association of Swine Practitioners,* 1996.
94. Ellis JA et al: Effects of perinatal vaccination on humoral and cellular immune responses in cows and young calves, *J Am Vet Med Assoc* 208:393-399, 1996.

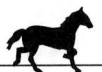

Interval between Priming and Immunizing Doses (Weeks)	Interval from First Dose to Protection (Days)	Duration of Vaccinal Immunity (Months)	Recommended Booster Interval (Months)	Contraindications	Side Effects	Withdrawal Time (Days Before Slaughter)
NA	42	Lifelong	NA	Do not use in cattle over 2 years of age or in the last 4 months of pregnancy; do not administer tetracyclines	Illness, anemia, abortion, death	—
3-4	35	12	12	—	Anaphylaxis	—
3	21[b] to 42[c]	<9	12	—	Anaphylaxis	21, 60[6,7]
2	28	5 to 6	5 to 6[d]	—	—	21[e]
2 to 3	8	12	12[f]	Avoid simultaneous administration of antimicrobials; do not use in sick animals	Mild illness, fever, decreased milk production	60
3 to 4	35	?	12[g]	—	Anaphylaxis	21
4	?	<6	4 to 6	—	—	28
NA	?	≥12	12	—	—	21
3 to 5	14 to 30	6	6	—	—	21

[5]Ocu-Guard MB, Boehringer Ingelheim Vetmedica, St. Joseph, MO 64506-2002.
[6]Piliguard Pinkeye-1, Schering-Plough Animal Health, Union, NJ 07083.
[7]Pinkeye Shield XT4, Grand Laboratories, Larchwood, IA 51241.
[8]20/20 Vision 7 with Spur, Intervet, Millsboro, DE 19966.
[9]Alpha-7/MB, Boehringer-Ingelheim, St. Joseph, MO 64506-2002.
[10]Bar Vac 7/MB, Boehringer-Ingelheim, St. Joseph, MO 64506-2002.
[11]Cattle Vac Pinkeye 4, Durvet, Blue Springs, MO 84014.
[12]Pinkeye-3, Aspen, Kansas City, MO 64161.
[13]Lysigin, Boehringer Ingelheim Vetmedica, St. Joseph, MO.
[14]Anthrax Spore Vaccine, Colorado Serum Co., Denver, CO 80216.

[15]Volar, Bayer Animal Health, Shawnee Mission, KS 66201.
[16]Fusogard, Imm Tech, Bucyrus, KS 66013.
[17]*Serpens* spp bacterin, Hygieia Biological Laboratories, Woodland, CA 95695.
[18]Defensor, Pfizer Animal Health, Exton, PA 19341.
[19]Rabdomun, Schering-Plough Animal Health, Union, NJ 07083.
[20]RM Imrab 3 and RM Imrab Bovine Plus,Merial, Iselin, NJ 08830.
[21]Papillomune, Biomune, Lenexa, KS 66210.
[22]Wart Shield, Grand Laboratories, Larchwood, IA 51241.
[23]Wart vaccine, AgriLaboratories, St. Joseph, MO.
[24]Wart vaccine, Colorado Serum Co., Denver, CO 80216.
[25]Wart Vac, Durvet, Blue Springs, MO 64014.

95. Ridge JP, Fuchs EJ, Matzinger P: Neonatal tolerance revisited: turning on newborn T cells with dendritic cells, *Science* 271:1723-1726, 1996.
96. Sarzotti M, Robbins DS, Hoffman FM: Induction of protective CTL responses in newborn mice by a murine retrovirus, *Science* 271:1726-1728, 1996.
97. Forsthuber T, Hualin, CY, Lewhmann V: Induction of T$_H$1 and T$_H$2 immunity in neonatal mice, *Science* 271:1728-1730, 1996.
98. Bryan LA et al: Fatal generalized bovine herpesvirus type 1 infection associated with a modified live infectious bovine rhinotracheitis/parainfluenza-3 vaccine administered to neonatal calves, *Can Vet J* 35:223-228, 1994.
99. Zavy MT et al: Effect of initial restraint, weaning, and transport stress on baseline and ACTH-stimulated cortisol responses in beef calves on different genotypes, *Am J Vet Res* 53:551-558, 1992.
100. Sconberg S et al: Effects of shipping, handling, adrenocorticotropic hormone, and epinephrine on α-tocopherol content of bovine blood, *Am J Vet Res* 54:1287-1294, 1993.
101. VonTungeln DL: The effects of stress on the immunology of the stocker calf, *Bovine Proc* 18:109-112, 1986.
102. Mueller D, Noxon J: Anaphylaxis: pathophysiology and treatment, *Comp Cont Educ* 12:157-171, February 1990.
103. Rude TA: Postvaccination type I hypersensitivity in cattle, *Agri Pract* 11:29-34, 1990.
104. Johansen KA, Wannameuhler M, Rosenbusch RF: Biological reactivity of *Moraxella bovis* lipopolysaccharide, *Am J Vet Res* 51:46-51, 1990.
105. Schuster DE et al: Reduced lactational performance following intravenous endotoxin administration to dairy cows, *J Dairy Sci* 74:3407-3411, 1991.

106. Henderson B, Wilson M: Modulins: a new class of cytokine-inducing, proinflammatory bacterial virulence factor, *Inflamm Res* 44:187-197, 1995.
107. Rietschel ET, Brade H: Bacterial endotoxins, *Sci Am*, Aug 1992, pp 55-61.

BOVINE RESPIRATORY DISEASE VACCINES
ROBERT W. FULTON

Infectious Bovine Rhinotracheitis (IBR) and Bovine Herpesvirus Type 1 (BHV-1) Vaccines

In 1999 more than 165 vaccines against the IBR virus (IBRV) were available in the United States for use in cattle.[108] Vaccination protocols for beef and dairy cattle in the United States routinely incorporate use of one or more vaccines against IBRV. These vaccines are classified into five types: (1) MLV vaccines for parenteral administration (intramuscular); (2) MLV, intranasally administered vaccines; (3) a chemically altered, live virus, temperature-sensitive vaccine for parenteral use; (4) inactivated viral vaccines; and (5) a recently released combination of parenteral MLV and inactivated viral vaccines. These commonly used vaccines may be single-component vaccines (e.g., IBRV alone) or may contain several immunogens, including various combinations of bovine viral diarrhea (BVD) viruses types 1 and 2; bovine parainfluenza type 3 (PI-3) virus, bovine respiratory syncytial virus (BRSV), *Leptospira* spp., *Haemophilus somnus, Pasteurella haemolytica, Pasteurella multocida,* and/or *Campylobacter* spp.[108] The characteristics of the IBR-type vaccines are described below.

Modified Live Virus Parenteral Vaccines

The MLV parenteral vaccines were the initial vaccines licensed for use in cattle for protection against IBR.[109] As described earlier, vaccines are attenuated by multiple passages in cell culture and often retain their ability to replicate in a susceptible animal, possibly causing a viremia. MLV parenteral vaccines are relatively inexpensive, offer a convenient route of administration, and stimulate a rapid onset of immunity (i.e., within 3 days of administration).[110,111] In general, one dose given to a susceptible animal stimulates protective immunity, which varies in duration depending on the clinical form of disease challenge. Systemic immunity, as determined by humoral immunity (serum antibodies) and cell-mediated immunity parameters, is detectable after MLV parenteral vaccination. Nasal (mucosal) immunity may not be evident. The MLV parenteral vaccines may cross the placenta and infect the fetus, causing abortion.[112] These characteristics are discussed below.

Modified Live Virus Intranasal Vaccines

MLV intranasal vaccines generally can be divided into two types, based on the attenuation process: (1) those modified by passage in a cell culture[113,114] and (2) those modified by treatment such that they become "temperature sensitive"[115] (i.e., they do not replicate at internal body temperature). MLV intranasal vaccines stimulate protection in susceptible animals with only one dose, in contrast to the chemically altered MLV parenteral vaccines. The label directions for MLV intranasal vaccines may indicate that they can be safely used in pregnant cattle. These vaccines induce a rapid onset of protection (within 3 days of administration), possibly through interferon in the nasal secretions.[113] One benefit of the MLV intranasal vaccines is that they stimulate immunity at the upper respiratory tract, the portal of entry of the virus. Another benefit is their potential to immunize calves that are already seropositive because of maternal (humoral) antibodies passively transferred through the colostrum.[116] Animals vaccinated with the MLV intranasal vaccines may transiently shed virus in the nasal secretions and therefore might infect susceptible contact animals.[117]

Chemically Altered Live Virus Vaccines

The chemically altered IBR vaccine strain was modified by nitrous acid treatment, which caused changes in the viral genome that resulted in a strain that is temperature sensitive, meaning that it has limited replication at internal body temperature.[118] Presumably, because of the limited viral replication, the vaccine requires two doses to stimulate immunity. Because it is temperature sensitive, the vaccine can be used in pregnant cattle.[118,119] In one study heifers received two doses of the vaccine and were challenged with IBRV 7 months later (at 6 months' gestation). These heifers showed a significant reduction in the number of abortions and stillbirths compared with controls.[119]

Inactivated Viral Vaccines

Inactivated viral vaccines are prepared by growing virus in cell cultures and then inactivating them with chemicals. An adjuvant is added to the inactivated strain to help stimulate an immune response. Inactivated IBR vaccines require two doses

(14 to 28 days apart) when used for the initial vaccination of susceptible cattle. Historically it has been thought that inactivated vaccines against viruses did not induce as long a duration of immunity as the MLV vaccines, nor did they confer protection against mucosal infections. Controlled studies should be performed to determine the duration of immunity induced by inactivated IBR vaccines and MLV vaccines. A disadvantage of inactivated vaccines is that the onset of protection may not be as rapid as with MLV parenteral or MLV intranasal vaccines. An advantage of the inactivated vaccines is that they can be used in pregnant cows and nursing calves.

Use of Vaccines to Prevent and Control Infectious Bovine Rhinotracheitis

Many vaccines are available for preventing and controlling the different forms of IBR disease, and each vaccine has certain characteristics that should be considered when designing a vaccination program. Each vaccine also has both benefits and limitations. Probably more important is the management of the cattle for which the vaccines are used.

Pregnant Animals or Animals Nearing Breeding Season

The MLV parenteral vaccines may infect the fetus if pregnant susceptible heifers or cows are vaccinated. Abortions have been reported subsequent to vaccination with MLV parenteral vaccines.[112] The MLV vaccine virus may also result in corpus luteum infection or disease.[120,121] Experimental studies have indicated a reduced conception rate in susceptible cattle that received an MLV parenteral vaccine 3 to 4 days before or 14 days after breeding.[120,121] It has been reported that pregnant cattle raised in contact with calves recently vaccinated with MLV parenteral vaccines had a greater incidence of IBR abortion than those that did not have contact with vaccinates.[122] Consequently, the labels of MLV parenteral vaccines have stated that the vaccine should not be used in calves nursing pregnant cows. Recent studies have shown that calves given an MLV parenteral vaccine did not shed virus in their nasal secretions nor did contact animals become infected with the vaccine virus.[123,124] Another concern is that the MLV vaccine virus may recrudesce, with resulting shedding of virus in cattle either stressed or receiving corticosteroids.[125] Realistically, concern about transmission of IBRV to animals in contact with those receiving MLV parenteral vaccines would be negligible if the contact animals were properly immunized.

Until the vaccine labels on MLV parenteral vaccines are changed, MLV intranasal vaccines or the inactivated or chemically altered live virus vaccines usually are recommended for pregnant cattle or those near breeding. Vaccine recommendations should be weighed, with the benefits of vaccination as a guide and especially with the realization that properly vaccinated cattle are better protected when exposed to either field (virulent) or vaccine strains shed by vaccinated animals.

Rapid Onset of Immunity

Cattle that are susceptible and likely to be exposed to IBRV should receive either an MLV parenteral vaccine or an MLV intranasal vaccine, because both types induce immunity within 3 days of the initial dose. Rapid onset of immunity is desirable in such situations as stocker calf operations, in which calves are transported long distances to pastures or feedlots, which stresses the animals and makes them more susceptible to infection. Such calves also are exposed to infection with IBRV from contact cattle in the markets. The drawback to inactivated vaccines is that two doses are required to obtain good immunity.

Duration of Immunity

Controlled studies on the duration of immunity are limited. A degree of protection against challenge existed at 6 to 9 months after vaccination with an MLV intranasal vaccine or an inactivated vaccine.[126,127] Challenge studies for licensure usually are performed on calves within days of vaccination, at the time of peak immunity. Also, the challenge may be for only one form of disease, usually the respiratory type. Such challenges may detect only protection against a severe form of the respiratory disease. IBR manifests itself in other forms, such as abortions, genital disease (male and female), and conjunctivitis. Yet little or no data are available about the efficacy of vaccines against these other forms of disease. For example, in one case the genital form of IBR disease (infectious pustular vulvovaginitis) occurred in heifers that had received an MLV parenteral vaccine 5 months earlier.[128] Given the lack of duration of immunity studies and the cost of vaccines, breeding animals usually are vaccinated at least annually. In some feedyard situations the animals may be revaccinated during the feeding period.

Vaccination of Calves With Maternal Antibody

The possibility exists that maternal IBRV antibodies, acquired by the calf through ingestion and absorption of colostrum, may interfere with vaccination. The level of these serum IBRV antibodies in the calf depend on the amount in the colostrum, the amount absorbed, and the half-life of the particular antibody. Some calves receive no IBRV antibodies through the colostrum, or they may lose them within 1 month. Some calves, however, may have serum IBRV antibodies for up to 6 months after birth.[125]

Vaccination recommendations for neonatal calves include use of multiple doses of an MLV parenteral, an inactivated, or a chemically altered live virus vaccine or administration of an MLV intranasal vaccine. The maternal antibodies may block the parenterally administered MLV or inactivated vaccine. However, the MLV intranasal vaccine may induce IBRV antibody immunity,[116] and the temperature-sensitive parenteral vaccine may stimulate cell-mediated immunity and B cell memory[91,94] in calves with maternal antibodies. Calves often are revaccinated at 6 to 8 months of age regardless of their prior vaccination history.

Advances in Vaccines

Molecular techniques of biotechnology have been applied to the study of vaccines and the response to vaccination (vaccinology). These advances are especially noted for herpesviruses, including IBRV.[129] A marker vaccine is one with deletion mutants of the genome for a protein that allows distinction between vaccinated and naturally infected animals; this is done by determining the antibody response in naturally exposed animals with a serologic test that detects antibodies to the deleted gene product (protein).[129] Thus a positive antibody response to the deleted gene product would indicate a naturally infected animal. Gene deletion of one or more of the nonessential glycoproteins from IBRV (gC, gG, gI, or gE) has been achieved.[129] Also, a live IBR vaccine has been developed with an inactivated thymidine kinase gene, resulting in a reduced virulence strain.[130] A thymidine kinase–deficient, gC-deletion mutant protected calves upon challenge and reduced viral shedding.[131]

IBR Vaccination Programs

The best possible vaccine provides protective immunity in the host against infection (viral replication) when challenged; protects the animal against all forms of disease, including multiple organ and systemic forms; and provides life-long mucosal and systemic immunity. Ideally the vaccine recommendations would incorporate the results of field trials that are carefully designed to show the efficacy of the vaccine against a pathogen. Unfortunately little information is available, as can be seen by a review of the literature, for evaluating the field efficacy of the respiratory disease vaccines.[132] The summary of results was mixed for IBR vaccines and for other respiratory viral and bacterial vaccines.

Veterinarians therefore must make recommendations based on (1) experimental studies of vaccination followed by challenge under controlled laboratory conditions apart from the field conditions of normal cattle management and (2) clinical experience with vaccines. Data from challenge studies often are under the control of universities, the federal government, or a biologic manufacturer and may not be published. Governmental licensure studies require efficacy and safety evaluations, but these studies may not be available in scientific publications for review by those making recommendations. For these reasons, the veterinarian may not have access to all the data needed to make a good decision on vaccines.

The veterinarian's dilemma is confounded by other factors. First, licensure may be granted for vaccination efficacy that demonstrated protection against one form of disease, such as respiratory type. However, the virus may be just as important a pathogen of other organs, such as the developing fetus, as is the case with IBRV. Second, little information is available about the duration of immunity induced by viral vaccines. Licensure studies may use challenge of vaccinated animals within 2 to 4 weeks of initial vaccination, yet cattle may be in feedyards (months) or breeding herds (years) after vaccination. Third, vaccines may induce a strong parenteral immunity, yet the surface mucosal defenses at the portal of entry may still be susceptible to infection even in presumably well-vaccinated animals. Thus it is entirely possible that natural infections could still occur in these vaccinated animals. Ecologically this point is reinforced, because viruses, for which there are good immunization products, are still circulating in cattle populations after years of vaccination.

The veterinarian therefore must weigh both the benefits provided by vaccines and their limitations. This probably is best done by focusing on the real, economic effects of certain disease manifestations, including morbidity, mortality, and treatment and prevention costs. Historically this approach has been applied to two important forms of IBRV disease: the respiratory form, singularly or in combination with pneumonic pasteurellosis, and the fetal disease (abortions). As a result, most vaccine regimens focus on preventing respiratory disease in both young or adult animals and on protecting the pregnant breeding herd of cows and heifers against abortions. Another fact to be considered is that many vaccines may have multiple viral or bacterial components (or both), which may require multiple doses for an immunogen mixed with one that requires only one dose.

Guidelines

CALVES. Calves may be vaccinated at weaning or 30 days before weaning. Calves vaccinated before 6 months of age should be revaccinated because the earlier vaccination may have been blocked by maternal antibodies. The MLV parenteral and intranasal vaccines require only one dose in susceptible calves, whereas the chemically altered live virus or inactivated vaccines require two doses. Although the labels for MLV parenteral vaccines state that the vaccine should not be used if the calf is nursing a pregnant cow, the likelihood of infection of the pregnant cow may be minimal, especially if she is already immune.

BREEDING COWS AND HEIFERS. Yearling heifers (12 to 14 months of age) should be vaccinated at least 1 month before breeding. Any of the vaccines may be used, but if two doses are required, the second dose should be given at least 1 month before breeding.

Pregnant cows may be vaccinated with a vaccine that has a label description warranting such use; these include MLV intranasal vaccines, chemically altered live virus vaccines, and inactivated vaccines. Generally one dose is used, primarily because of management considerations. Administering booster doses of the IBRV vaccines may have two conflicting outcomes as a result of booster dose stimulation of an increase in colostral IBRV antibodies, which are transferred to the newborn calf in the colostrum; consequently, (1) it may be beneficial to the calf to have increased IBRV serum antibodies for protection against IBRV disease, or (2) the calf may have longer duration of IBRV antibodies, which may block IBRV immunization. There are no published multiyear duration of immunity studies in vaccinated cattle challenged with virulent IBRV. Because of the relatively low cost of IBRV vaccines and the need to vaccinate against other pathogens, many breeding cows are given an IBRV vaccine annually.

STOCKER AND FEEDER CATTLE. Cattle to be shipped to forage pasture after weaning (wheat pasture or native grass) or to feedyards should be vaccinated 2 to 3 weeks before shipment. All the major types of IBRV vaccines may be used, but those that require only one dose have two advantages: rapid onset of immunity and less handling required (one dose versus two).

Cattle presented for purchase immediately before shipment, with no known vaccination history, pose a challenge. Presumably healthy cattle may be candidates for the one-dose MLV parenteral or MLV intranasal vaccines, because these calves may benefit from rapid immunity. Cattle already infected with IBRV may not be protected by vaccination.

Cattle entering the feedyard usually receive either the MLV parenteral or MLV intranasal vaccine, particularly for the rapid onset of immunity. Cattle sometimes are revaccinated during the feeding period to ensure protection against IBRV disease later in the feedyard.

Breeding Services

Veterinarians should consult the breeding bull center for vaccination requirements of bulls, especially relating to export shipment and collection for artificial insemination (AI). MLV intranasal vaccines have been used in AI bulls because these vaccines are less likely to cause latent infections than MLV parenteral vaccines.[133,134] As mentioned previously, MLV parenteral vaccines cause latent infections that may recrudesce with stress or the administration of corticosteroids, which means the virus would be present in the semen.[125,134]

REFERENCES

108. Arrioja-Dechert A, ed: *Compendium of veterinary products*, ed 5, Port Huron, Mich, 1999, North American Compendiums.
109. Kendrick JW, York CJ, McKercher DG: A controlled field trial of a vaccine for infectious bovine rhinotracheitis, *Proc US Livestock Sanitary Assoc* 60:155-158, 1956.
110. Bordt DE, Thomas PC, Marshall RF: Early protection against infectious bovine rhinotracheitis with intramuscularly administered vaccine, *Proc 79th Ann Mtg US Anim Health Assoc* 79:50-60, 1975.
111. Sutton ML: Rapid onset of immunity in cattle after intramuscular injection of a modified live virus IBR vaccine, *Vet Med/SAC* 75:1447-1456, 1980.
112. Kennedy PC, Richards WPC: The pathology of abortion caused by the virus of infectious bovine rhinotracheitis, *Pathol Vet* 1:7-17, 1964.
113. Todd JD, Volenec FM, Paton IM: Interferon in nasal secretions and sera of calves after intranasal administration of avirulent infectious bovine rhinotracheitis virus: association of interferon in nasal secretions with early resistance to challenge with virulent virus, *Infect Immun* 5:699-706, 1972.
114. Todd JD, Volenec FM, Paton IM: Intranasal vaccination against infectious bovine rhinotracheitis: studies on early onset of protection and use of the vaccine in pregnant cows, *Am J Vet Med Assoc* 159:1370-1374, 1971.
115. Kucera CJ, White RG, Beckenhauer WH: Evaluation of the safety and efficacy of an intranasal vaccine containing a temperature-sensitive strain of infectious bovine rhinotracheitis virus, *Am J Vet Res* 39:607-610, 1978.
116. Todd JD: Intranasal vaccination of cattle against IBR and PI-3: field and laboratory observations in dairy, beef, and neonatal populations, *Dev Biol Stand* 33:391-395, 1976.
117. Baker JC, Rust SR, Walker RD: Transmission of a vaccinal strain of infectious bovine rhinotracheitis virus from intranasally vaccinated steers commingled with nonvaccinated steers, *Am J Vet Res* 50:814-816, 1989.
118. Talens LT et al: Efficacy of viral components of a nonabortagenic combination vaccine for prevention of respiratory and reproductive system diseases in cattle, *Am J Vet Assoc* 194:1273-1280, 1989.
119. Cravens RL et al: Efficacy of a temperature-sensitive, modified live bovine herpesvirus type 1 vaccine against abortion and stillbirth in pregnant heifers, *Am J Vet Med Assoc* 208:2031-2034, 1996.
120. Chiang BC et al: The effect of infectious bovine rhinotracheitis vaccine on reproductive efficiency in cattle vaccinated during estrus, *Theriogenology* 33:1113-1120, 1990.
121. Miller JM, Van Der Maaten MJ, Whetstone CA: Infertility in heifers inoculated with modified live infectious bovine rhinotracheitis on post-breeding day 14, *Am J Vet Res* 50:551-554, 1989.
122. Kelling CL et al: Infectious bovine rhinotracheitis (IBR) abortion: observations on incidence in vaccinated and nonvaccinated and exposed cattle, *Cornell Vet* 63:383-389, 1973.
123. Gatewood DM et al: Evaluation of IBR vaccine virus shedding after parenteral administration to suckling calves, *Proceedings of the Twenty-ninth Annual Convention of the American Association of Bovine Practitioners*, 1996, p 178.
124. Roth JA, Vaughn MB: Evaluation of viral shedding and immune response following vaccination with a modified live BHV-1 vaccine, *Bovine Pract* 32:1-4, 1998.
125. Kahrs RF: Infectious bovine rhinotracheitis. In *Viral diseases of cattle*, Ames, Iowa, 1981, Iowa State University Press.
126. Savan M, Angulo AB, Derbyshire JB: Interferon, antibody responses, and protection induced by an intranasal infectious bovine rhinotracheitis vaccine, *Can Vet J* 20:207-210, 1979.
127. Sibbel RL, Bass EP, Thomas PC: How long will a killed IBR vaccine protect against challenge? *Vet Med* 83:90-92, 1988.
128. Trueblood MS, Swift BL, McHolland-Raymond LE: An outbreak of infectious pustular vulvovaginitis, *Vet Med/SAC* 72:1622-1624, 1977.
129. Van Oirschot JT, Kaashoek MJ, Rijsewijk FAM: Advances in the development and evolution of bovine herpesvirus 1 vaccines, *Vet Microbiol* 53:43-54, 1996.
130. Kit S et al: Thymidine kinase–negative bovine herpesvirus type 1 mutant is stable and highly attenuated in calves, *Arch Virol* 86:63-83, 1985.
131. Flores EF et al: Efficacy of a deletion mutant bovine herpesvirus-1 (BHV-1) vaccine that allows serologic differentiation of vaccinated from naturally infected animals, *J Vet Diagn Invest* 5:534-540, 1993.
132. Perino LJ, Hunsaker BD: A review of bovine respiratory disease vaccine field efficacy, *Bovine Pract* 31:59-66, 1997.
133. Gregersen JP, Wagner K: Persistent infection of the genital tract and excretion of the vaccine strain after live virus immunization with bovine herpesvirus 1 (IBR/IPV virus), *Zentralbl Veterinarmed [B]* 32:354-360, 1985.
134. Schultz RD et al: Current status of IBR-IPV infection in bulls, *Proc US Anim Health Assoc* 80:159-168, 1976.

BOVINE VIRUS DIARRHEA VIRUS VACCINES

VICTOR S. CORTESE

Our knowledge of the different vaccines' ability to protect against infection with the bovine virus diarrhea virus (BVDV) is increasing rapidly. Currently, three kinds of BVDV vaccines are available: MLV vaccines, temperature-sensitive vaccines (available only in Europe), and inactivated virus vaccines (Table 44-10). MLV BVDV vaccines have demonstrated advantages over the newer inactivated vaccines. Most of these advantages are common to all MLV vaccines[135]; they are (1) MLV vaccines are less expensive; (2) postvaccination anaphylactic reactions occur less often than after administration of some inactivated vaccines; (3) immunity is achieved more rapidly after administration of a single dose (within 7 to 10 days); (4) MLV vaccines produce much higher levels of serum neutralizing antibodies[136]; (5) immunity last longer[137-139]; and (6) MLV vaccines are effective against a broader spectrum of viral strains.[137]

On the other hand, MLV BVDV vaccines have certain disadvantages compared with inactivated BVDV vaccines; these disadvantages are (1) some MLV vaccines can produce mild

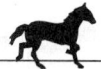

TABLE 44-10

Currently Licensed* Vaccines for Bovine Virus Diarrhea Virus (BVDV)

Manufacturer	Product Name	Type of Vaccine	Strain	U.S.D.A. Type 2 License
Intervet Animal Health (Millesboro, DE 19966)	Horizon	Inactivated	Oregon C24V (CP, type 1)	No
	Frontier	Modified live		Yes
	Horizon Plus	Inactivated	Oregon C24V (CP, type1)	Yes
AgriLaboratories (St. Joseph, MO 64503)	Titanium	Modified live	Bolin 290 (CP, type 2)	Yes
	Masterguard Preg 5	Inactivated		Yes
Fort Dodge Laboratories (Ford Dodge, IA 50501)	Pyramid	Modified live	Singer (CP, type 1)	No
	Triangle/Prism	Inactivated	Singer (CP, type 1) 890 (CP, type 2)	Yes
Grand Laboratories (Larchwood, IA 51241)	Virashield	Inactivated	CP and NCP, type 1 and type 2	Yes
Merial (Iselin, NJ 08830)	Fusion, Journey, Respishield	Inactivated	NADL (CP, type 1)	No
	Prevail/Reliant	Modified live	NADL (CP, type 1)	No
Pfizer Animal Health (Exton, PA 19341)	Bovishield, PregGuard	Modified live	NADL (CP, type 1)	Yes
	CattleMaster, Bovi-K	Inactivated	5960 (CP, type 1) 6309 (NCP, type 1)	No
	Resvac	Modified live	NADL (CP, type 1)	No
Boehringer Ingelheim (St. Joseph, MO)	Elite	Inactivated	Singer (CP, type 1)	No
	Express	Modified live	Singer (CP, type 1) Bolin 290 (CP, type 2)	Yes

U.S.D.A., U.S. Department of Agriculture.
*Licensed by the Animal and Plant Health Inspection Service, U.S. Department of Agriculture.

immunosuppression for brief periods after administration[140]; (2) some have been associated with what is usually a rather low incidence of a highly fatal disease syndrome, postvaccinal mucosal disease[141,142] (see below); and (3) MLV vaccines are not ordinarily recommended for routine use in pregnant cattle.

Studies have shown that the duration of cross-neutralizing antibodies stimulated by inactivated BVDV vaccines depends on the antigenic similarity between the vaccine strain and the wild type virus to which the cow is exposed.[143,144] If there are few common proteins, the ability to neutralize can be as short as 4 months; if there are many common antigenic sites, neutralization may last a year. MLV BVDV vaccines stimulate cross-neutralizing antibodies that can still be detected 18 months after vaccination.[138]

Recent studies have demonstrated the ability of both modified live[145] and inactivated type 1 vaccines[146] to provide protection against type 2 BVDV strains, although the protection afforded by the MLV vaccine was more complete. The U.S. Department of Agriculture's Animal and Plant Health Inspection Service has established a licensing protocol for BVDV vaccines to obtain a type 2 BVDV protection claim. Most of the vaccines licensed against both BVDV type 1 and type 2 contain BVDV type 1 and type 2 isolates (see Table 44-8).

Vaccination and Mucosal Disease

Mucosal disease (MD) is seen when an animal that is persistently infected is exposed to another closely related cytopathic strain of BVDV. Also, theoretically a noncytopathic BVDV strain can mutate spontaneously into a cytopathic strain, resulting in mucosal disease without any subsequent exposure. High stress and immunodepression may be involved in this mutation.[147,148]

A major concern with the MLV vaccines is if they can cause mucosal disease.[142,149,150] For MD to occur, the cytopathic strain in the MLV vaccine must be closely related to the noncytopathic strain in the persistently infected animal. With the degree of attenuation of MLV vaccines today, an animal must be nutritionally deficient or severely stressed, or both, to face

an increased likelihood of developing mucosal disease from the vaccine. This suggests that a specific set of circumstances is required and that MD caused by vaccination, when it occurs, is rare.

BVDV Vaccines and Reproductive Control

Control of BVDV centers on prevention of persistent infection and elimination of persistently infected cattle; this means that identifying and removing persistently infected animals and continued vaccination to prevent persistent infection are necessary for effective control. Persistent infections occur through in utero infection of the fetus (up to approximately 125 days' gestation) with a noncytopathic strain of BVDV.[138,147] The mechanism of transplacental transfer of BVDV is unknown; however, small amounts of virus in the dam's bloodstream appear to be sufficient to produce these immunotolerant cattle. Protection of the dam may or may not correlate with protection of the fetus from subsequent persistent infection if viremia of the dam occurs. To break the vicious cycle of in utero infection and persistent infection, it is essential that vaccination provide fetal protection.

Several studies have been performed to assess the ability of vaccines to protect the fetus against either natural or artificial challenge. The results of these studies showed that most inactivated vaccines failed to provide much fetal protection,[143,151-154] except for one experimental vaccine, which is reported to give a high level of fetal protection. With the experimental vaccine, the lack of virus isolation from offspring of vaccinated animals indicated good protection.[155] However, the challenge of controls resulted in only about a 50% rate of persistent infection. Other published reports demonstrated that MLV BVDV vaccines were more effective at protecting the fetus.[156,157] To date, vaccines licensed in the United States have not been required to provide fetal protection.

BVDV Vaccination Programs

Because BVDV infections can cause severe death loss and immunosuppression, all herds of cattle should be vaccinated against BVDV. Although it was once thought that BVDV vaccines would not immunize calves that were passively immune to BVDV,[158,159] recent studies have shown that immunization can occur with certain inactivated vaccines[160] and with MLV vaccines (when the passive antibody titer against BVDV is 1:64 or below).[146,161] When required, BVDV vaccines can be administered to young calves, with the possibility of gaining some degree of protection. In most calves the maternal antibodies against BVDV drop below the 1:64 level by 5 to 6 months of age. If an early BVDV problem does not exist, waiting to administer the first BVDV vaccine until 5 or 6 months of age increases the number of animals that respond to vaccination.

Among cows given MLV BVDV vaccines in the last trimester of pregnancy, 86% of the calves from seronegative cows[162] and some calves (0[162] to 52%[163]) from seropositive dams were actively immune at birth. In addition, the calves' level of passive immunity to BVDV was enhanced, in that seronegative cows seroconverted, and serum antibody titers were boosted in 52% of the seropositive cows. The rate of occurrence of BVD in neonatal calves was reduced.[163] Administration of an MLV BVDV vaccine to seronegative cows after day 118 of gestation did not result in adverse effects.[164,165] However, vaccination with an MLV noncytopathic virus vaccine before day 118 resulted in fetal resorption, abortion, congenital defects, and the birth of undersized, weak, persistently infected calves.[166] Several authors have recommended vaccination of cows with an MLV BVDV vaccine during the last trimester of pregnancy,[163] but it is still considered an off-label use of these vaccines.

It is important to consider the epidemiologic, nonresponse rate to any vaccine when designing a BVDV vaccination program. Therefore even though MLV BVDV vaccines do not require a booster dose, a second dose may be advised to stimulate protection in animals that did not respond to the initial vaccination. BVDV vaccination programs should include the following features:

1. A virus isolation and cull program should be instituted, along with a vaccination program that includes administration of at least one dose of an MLV BVDV vaccine to all replacement animals.
2. Vaccination with killed vaccines should be increased to two or three times a year *or* an MLV BVDV vaccine should be given to open cows 3 weeks before breeding or turning in the bull.
3. The vaccines used should have been proved to stimulate protection against BVDV type 1 and type 2.

REFERENCES

135. Roth JA: Building immunity, *National Hog Farmer*, Spring 1992, pp 1-48.
136. Van Donkersgoed JV et al: Comparative serological responses in calves to eight commercial vaccines against infectious bovine rhinotracheitis, parainfluenza-3, bovine respiratory syncytial, and bovine viral diarrhea viruses, *Can Vet J* 32:727-733, 1991.
137. Heuschele WP: Bovine virus diarrhea mucosal disease. In Howard JL, ed: *Current veterinary therapy (food animal practice)* 2, Philadelphia, 1986, WB Saunders.
138. Baker JC: Bovine viral diarrhea: a review, *J Am Vet Med Assoc* 190:1449-1458, 1987.
139. Cortese VS et al: Specificity and duration of neutralizing antibodies induced in healthy cattle after administration of a modified live virus vaccine against bovine viral diarrhea virus, *Am J Vet Res* 59:848-850, 1998.
140. Roth JA, Kaeberle ML: Suppression of neutrophil and lymphocyte function induced by a vaccinal strain of bovine viral diarrhea virus, with or without the administration of ACTH, *Am J Vet Res* 44:2366-2372, 1983.
141. Rosner SF: Complications following vaccination of cattle against bovine rhinotracheitis, bovine viral diarrhea–mucosal disease and parainfluenza type 3, *J Am Vet Med Assoc* 152:898-902, 1968.
142. Bolin SR, Ridpath JF: Delayed onset postvaccinal mucosal disease as a result of genetic recombination between genotype 1 and genotype 2 BVDV, *Virology* 212:259-262, 1995.
143. Bolin SR, Littledike ET, Ridpath JF: Serologic detection and practical consequences of antigenic diversity among bovine viral diarrhea viruses in a vaccinated herd, *Am J Vet Res* 52:1033-1037, 1991.
144. Bolin SR, Ridpath JF: Specificity of neutralizing and precipitating antibodies induced in healthy calves by monovalent modified live bovine viral diarrhea virus vaccines, *Am J Vet Res* 50:817-821, 1989.
145. Cortese VS et al: Clinical and immunologic responses of vaccinated and unvaccinated calves to infection with a virulent type II isolate of bovine viral diarrhea virus, *J Am Vet Med Assoc* 213:1312-1319, 1998.
146. Cortese VS: Clinical and immunologic responses of cattle to vaccinal and natural bovine viral diarrhea virus (BVDV),Thesis, Western College of Veterinary Medicine, University of Saskatchewan, 1999.
147. Bolin SR: The current understanding about the pathogenesis and clinical forms of BVD: symposium on bovine viral diarrhea, *Vet Med*, Oct 1990, pp 1124-1132.
148. Moennig V et al: Reproduction of mucosal disease with a cytopathogenic bovine viral diarrhea virus selected in vitro, *Vet Rec* 127:200-203, 1990.
149. Bolin SR et al: Response of cattle persistently infected with noncytopathic bovine viral diarrhea virus to vaccination for bovine viral diarrhea and to subsequent challenge exposure with cytopathic bovine viral diarrhea virus, *Am J Vet Res* 46:2467-2470, 1985.
150. Meyling A et al: Experimental exposure of vaccinated and nonvaccinated pregnant cattle to isolates of bovine viral diarrhea virus (BVDV), *State Veterinary Institute for Virus Research*, 1985, pp 225-231.
151. McClurkin AW, Coria MF, Smith RL: Evaluation of acetylethylenimine-killed bovine viral diarrhea–mucousal disease virus vaccine for prevention of BVD infection of the fetus, *Proc US Anim Health Assoc*, 79:115-123, 1975.
152. Kaeberle ML, Maxwell D, Johnson E: Efficacy of inactivated bovine viral diarrhea virus vaccines in a cow herd, *AS Leaflet R, 1990 Beef/Sheep Report* 701:42-43, 1990.
153. Ellsworth MA et al: Fetal infection following intravenous bovine viral diarrhea virus challenge of vaccinated and unvaccinated dams, Conference of Research Workers in Animal Disease, Fall, 1994.
154. Harkness JW, Roeder PL, Drew T: The efficacy of an experimental inactivated BVD-MD vaccine. In Harkness JW, ed: *Pestivirus infections in ruminants: a seminar in the CEC programme of coordination of research on animal husbandry, Brussels*, Sept. 10-11, 1985.
155. Brownlie J et al: Protection of the bovine fetus from bovine viral diarrhea virus by means of a new inactivated vaccine, *Vet Rec* 137:58-62, 1995.
156. Frey HR, Eicken K: Undersuchungen uber die Wirksamkeit einer inaktivierten BVD-Vakzine zur Erhohung der Sicherheit einer BVD-Lebendvakzine, *Tierarztl Umschan* 50:86-93, 1995.
157. Cortese VS et al: Protection of pregnant cattle and their fetuses against infection with bovine viral diarrhea virus type 1 by use of modified live virus vaccine, *Am J Vet Res* 59:1409-1413, 1999.
158. Kendrick JW, Franti CE: Bovine viral diarrhea: decay of colostrum-derived antibody in the calf, *Am J Vet Res* 35:589-591, 1974.
159. Ernst PB, Butler DG: A bovine viral diarrhea calfhood vaccination trial in a persistently infected herd: effects on titers, health, and growth, *Can J Comp Med* 47:118-123, 1983.
160. Kaeberle ML, Sealock R, Honeyman M: Antibody responses of young calves to inactivated viral vaccines, *AS Leaflet R, 1997 Beef/Sheep Report* 1462:42-43, 1990.
161. Brar JS et al: Maternal immunity to infectious bovine rhinotracheitis and bovine viral diarrhea viruses: duration and effect on vaccination in young calves, *Am J Vet Res* 39:241-244, 1978.
162. Kelling CL et al: Investigation of bovine viral diarrhea virus infections in a range beef cattle herd, *J Am Vet Med Assoc* 197:589-593, 1990.
163. Sanders DE, Sanders JA, Sangenario J: Protection of newborn calves against bovine virus diarrhea by vaccinating their dams prior to parturition, *Agri Pract* 10:30-34, 1983.
164. Orban S et al: Studies on transplacental transmissibility of a bovine virus diarrhea (BVD) vaccine virus. I. Inoculation of pregnant cows 15 to 90 days before parturition (190th to 265th day of gestation), *Zentralbl Veterinarmed [B]* 30:619-634, 1983.
165. Liess B et al: Studies on transplacental transmissibility of a bovine virus diarrhea (BVD) vaccine virus in cattle. II. Inoculation of pregnant cows without detectable neutralizing antibodies to BVD virus 90-229 days before parturition (51st to 190th day of gestation), *Zentralbl Veterinarmed [B]* 31:669-681, 1984.
166. Ames TR, Baker JC: Management practices and vaccination programs that help control BVD virus infections: symposium on bovine viral diarrhea, *Vet Med* (October):1140-1149, 1990.

BOVINE RESPIRATORY SYNCYTIAL VIRUS VACCINES

JOHN A. ELLIS

Bovine respiratory syncytial virus (BRSV) is a prevalent paramyxovirus that can cause disease in cattle of all ages but that primarily affects calves in recurrent seasonal outbreaks.[167-169] Clinical disease is characterised by pyrexia, coughing, and tachypnea, which often progresses rapidly to dyspnea.[168,170] BRSV is also considered one of the viral agents that predisposes animals to secondary bacterial infections in the bovine respiratory disease (BRD) complex; however, secondary infections often are absent in fatal BRSV-associated respiratory disease.[171,172]

Protection against BRSV infection is associated with an IgA response[167-169]; however, serum IgG acquired from either passive or active immunization can significantly reduce the severity of clinical respiratory disease that results from BRSV infection. Several studies have reported that the incidence and severity of disease in calves were inversely related to the maternal antibody titers.[169,173,174] In the case of herd immunity, passive antibodies were detectable in 50% of the calves for 3 months after birth and were present in some calves until 7 months of age.[175] Therefore administration of BRSV vaccines to cows in late gestation to booster colostral antibody titers is a rational strategy for attempting to deal with BRSV-induced respiratory disease in young calves (1 to 3 months of age) in problem herds.

Several MLV parenteral and inactivated BRSV vaccines currently are commercially available, most of which are formulated in combination with other viral respiratory pathogens.[168] Recent studies have documented the efficacy of adjuvanted and nonadjuvanted combination BRSV vaccines in protecting calves from severe clinical disease subsequent to experimental infection with a virulent field isolate.[176] Most vaccinated calves shed virus, but the peak virus titer was suppressed compared to unvaccinated controls. Viral clearance was coincident with the simultaneous appearance of mucosal antibody cytotoxic cells in the lungs and anamnestic or primary serum antibody responses. In contrast, virus clearance in unvaccinated calves was coincident with the appearance of BRSV-specific cytotoxic cells before mucosal antibody was detected. These controlled efficacy studies are consistent with previous field trials, demonstrating the safety and efficacy of parenterally administered vaccines.[177,178] More recent studies have demonstrated the usefulness of combination vaccines in reducing the impact of subclinical BRSV infections.[179]

Although administration of MLV BRSV vaccines by the intramuscular route to passively immune calves reportedly did not elicit mucosal memory IgA or serum antibody responses, or even prime for such responses,[169] T cell responses have been demonstrated after parenteral vaccination in passively immune calves.[180] Whether these responses correlate to a protective cell-mediated memory response when maternal antibodies decline has not been determined. Intranasal administration of MLV BRSV to passively immune calves primed mucosal memory and an anamnestic IgA response subsequent to challenge.[169] The development of a safe, effective intranasal MLV BRSV vaccine may represent the most effective means of immunizing calves with maternal antibodies.

Several studies have consistently documented a disparity in the type of antibody responses induced in cattle by MLV and inactivated BRSV vaccines.[181-184] Parenterally administered MLV BRSV vaccines generally stimulate moderate to high concentrations of virus-neutralizing antibody in the serum, whereas inactivated vaccines stimulate high concentrations of nonneutralizing antibody. The data are conflicting concerning the prophylactic or disease-enhancing properties of these different types of vaccine-induced antibody responses.[183,184] Currently no published data are available documenting the efficacy of the commercially available inactivated BRSV vaccines. There also is little information about the duration of the protective response after vaccination; however, cattle can be experimentally reinfected by 35 days after initial infection with virulent BRSV even in the presence of circulating antibody.[185,186] Nevertheless, the disease caused by reinfection usually is less severe than that after the initial infection.[186]

REFERENCES

167. Van der Poel WH et al: Respiratory syncytial virus infections in human beings and in cattle, *J Infect* 29:215-228, 1994.
168. Baker JC, Ellis JA, Clark EG: Bovine respiratory syncytial virus, *Vet Clin North Am (Food Anim Pract)* 13:425-454, 1997.
169. Kimman TG, Westenbrink F: Immunity to human and bovine respiratory syncytial virus, *Arch Virol* 112:1-25, 1990.
170. Bryson DG et al: Respiratory syncytial virus pneumonia in young calves: clinical and pathologic findings, *Am J Vet Res* 44:1648-1655, 1983.
171. Bryson DG: Necropsy findings associated with BRSV pneumonia, *Vet Med* 88:6-9, 1993.
172. Kimman TG, Straver PJ, Zimmer GM: Pathogenesis of naturally acquired bovine respiratory syncytial virus infection in calves: morphologic and serologic findings, *Am J Vet Res* 50:684-693, 1989.
173. Kimman TG et al: Epidemiologic study of bovine respiratory syncytial virus infection in calves: influence of maternal antibodies on the outcome of disease, *Vet Rec* 123:104-109, 1988.
174. Belknap EB et al: The role of passive immunity in bovine respiratory syncytial virus infected calves, *J Infect Dis* 163:470-476, 1991.
175. Baker JC, Ames TR, Markham RJF: A seroepidemiologic study of bovine respiratory syncytial virus in a dairy herd, *Am J Vet Res* 47:240-245, 1986.
176. West KH et al: The efficacy of modified live bovine respiratory syncytial virus vaccines in experimentally infected calves, *Vaccine* 18:907-919, 2000.
177. Van Donkersgoed J et al: Five field trials on the efficacy of a bovine respiratory syncytial virus vaccine, *Can Vet J* 31:93-100, 1990.
178. Hansen DE, Syvrud R, Armstrong D: Effectiveness of a respiratory syncytial virus vaccine in reducing the risk of respiratory disease, *Agri Pract* 13:19-23, 1992.
179. Ferguson JD, Galligan DT, Cortese V: Milk production and reproductive performance in dairy cows given bovine respiratory syncytial virus vaccine prior to parturition, *J Am Vet Med Assoc* 210:1779-1783, 1997.
180. Ellis JA et al: The effect of perinatal vaccination on humoral and cellular immune responses in cows and young calves, *J Am Vet Med Assoc* 208:393-400, 1996.
181. Ellis JA, Hassard LE, Morley PS: Bovine respiratory syncytial virus–specific immune responses in calves after inoculation with commercially available vaccines, *J Am Vet Med Assoc* 206:354-361, 1995.
182. West K, Ellis J: Functional analysis of antibody responses of feedlot cattle to bovine respiratory syncytial virus following vaccination with mixed vaccines, *Can J Vet Res* 62:245-250, 1997.
183. Gershwin LJ et al: A bovine model of vaccine-enhanced respiratory syncytial virus pathophysiology, *Vaccine* 16:1225-1236, 1998.
184. West K et al: The effect of formalin-inactivated vaccine on respiratory disease associated with bovine respiratory syncytial virus infection of calves, *Vaccine* 17:809-820, 1999.
185. Kimman TG et al: Local and systemic antibody response to bovine respiratory syncytial virus infection in calves with or without maternal antibodies, *J Clin Microbiol* 25:1097-1106, 1987.
186. Stewart RS, Gershwin LJ: Role of IgE in the pathogenesis of bovine respiratory syncytial virus in sequential infections in vaccinated and unvaccinated calves, *Am J Vet Res* 50:349-355, 1989.

PARAINFLUENZA TYPE 3 VIRUS VACCINES

JOHN A. ELLIS

Parainfluenza virus type 3 (PI-3) is a ubiquitous paramyxovirus in cattle populations worldwide.[187,188] In uncomplicated experimental PI-3 infections, clinical signs of coughing, tachypnea, and fever have been observed from 4 to 12 days after infection.[187] Although respiratory disease has been experimentally reproduced in calves infected with PI-3, seroconversion has been demonstrated after outbreaks of respiratory disease[189] and PI-3 has been identified in the lesions of bovine respiratory disease (BRD) complex at postmortem, the importance of this agent in the BRD complex remains controversial.[187] Generally PI-3 is viewed as a potentiating agent in mixed infections, predisposing the animal to bacterial pneumonia by altering bacterial clearance in the upper and lower airways and by infecting both respiratory epithelia and alveolar macrophages.[187]

Currently five types of PI-3 vaccines are available commercially: (1) MLV intramuscular vaccines, (2) MLV, temperature-sensitive, intramuscular vaccines, (3) MLV intranasal vaccines, (4) MLV, temperature-sensitive, intranasal vaccines, and (5) inactivated virus vaccines. All PI-3 vaccines available in North America are combined at least with a BHV-1 vaccine. Currently a single-antigen, MLV PI-3 intranasal vaccine is available in Europe. The efficacy of this formulation recently was demonstrated in a severe challenge model.[190]

Opinions are divided as to the relative importance of mucosal versus systemic immune responses in achieving protection from PI-3–associated respiratory disease and, by extension, the comparative efficacy of intranasal and intramuscular vaccines. Some comparative studies[190,191] reported that intranasal vaccination resulted in better protection against experimental challenge; others[192] were unable to demonstrate any advantage to the use of one vaccine or route of administration over the other. A notable exception, however, was young calves with maternal antibodies, in which intranasal administration was thought to produce a more effective immune response. Passive antibodies may persist in calves until 8 months of age and may interfere with active immunization.[193] Consequently, calves vaccinated parenterally before 6 months of age should be revaccinated after reaching 8 or 9 months of age.[193]

Although not experimentally documented, as in the case of BRSV, it is likely that, given the similar biology of PI-3 infection, a mucosal (IgA) response is necessary to prevent PI-3 infection but that passively (maternal) or actively acquired serum IgG is likely to mediate significant sparing of clinical disease subsequent to infection. The cell-mediated (cytotoxic T cell) response in the clearance of PI-3 is a poorly documented but probably important effector mechanism stimulated by MLV vaccines, as is the case with BRSV.

Considerable debate has arisen over the overall utility and economic benefit of using PI-3 (and BRSV) vaccines in the field.[194,195] Much of the uncertainty undoubtedly is related to the difficulties involved in determining the relative importance of a particular agent in a multifactorial disease process such as BRD complex. Although few studies[195,196] currently address the economic impact of subclinical paramyxovirus infections in cattle, such studies are needed to better tailor vaccine programs to different management systems and producer needs.

REFERENCES

187. Kapil S, Basaraba R: Infectious bovine rhinotracheitis, parainfluenza-3, and respiratory coronavirus. *Vet Clin North Am* 13:455-469, 1997.
188. Graham DA et al: Evaluation of a single dilution ELISA system for detection of seroconversion to bovine viral diarrhoea virus, bovine respiratory syncytial virus, parainfluenza-3 virus and infectious bovine rhinotracheitis virus: comparison with testing by virus neutralisation and haemagglutination inhibition, *J Vet Diagn Invest* 10:43-48, 1998.
189. Bryson DG et al: Studies on the efficacy of intranasal vaccination for prevention of experimentally induced parainfluenza type 3 virus pneumonia in calves, *Vet Rec* 145:33-39, 1999.
190. Gates GA et al: Neutralizing antibody in experimentally induced respiratory infection in calves, *Am J Vet Res* 31:217-224, 1970.
191. Gutekunst DE, Paton IM, Volenec FJ: Parainfluenza-3 vaccine in cattle: comparative efficacy of intranasal and intramuscular routes, *J Am Vet Med Assoc* 155:1879-1885, 1969.
192. McKercher DG et al: Response of calves to parainfluenza-3 vaccines administered nasally or parenterally, *Am J Vet Res* 33:721-730, 1972.
193. Sweat RL: Epizootiologic studies of bovine myxovirus parainfluenza-3, *J Am Vet Med Assoc* 150:178-183, 1967.
194. Ferguson JD, Galligan DT, Cortese V: Milk production and reproductive performance in dairy cows given bovine respiratory syncytial virus vaccine prior to parturition, *J Am Vet Med Assoc* 210:1779-1783, 1997.
195. Woods GT, Mansfield ME, Webb RJ: A 3-year comparison of acute respiratory disease, shrink, and weight gain in preconditioned and nonconditioned Illinois beef calves sold at the same auction and mixed in a feedlot, *Can J Comp Med* 37:249-255, 1973.
196. Bingham HR et al: Synergistic effects of concurrent challenge with bovine respiratory syncytial virus and 3-methylindole in calves, *Am J Vet Res* 60:563-570, 1999.

MANNHEIMIA (PASTEURELLA) HAEMOLYTICA, PASTEURELLA MULTOCIDA, AND HAEMOPHILUS SOMNUS VACCINES

ANTHONY W. CONFER

Pasteurella haemolytica Vaccines

Pasteurella haemolytica serotype 1 is the main bacterium responsible for the clinical signs and lesions of bovine fibrinous pleuropneumonia (shipping fever).[197] The bacterium is a gram negative commensal in the bovine nasopharynx, and with stress or viral infections it proliferates and is inhaled into the lungs. The resultant pneumonia is characterized by acute, severe fibrinopurulent inflammation and necrosis. *P. haemolytica* recently was renamed *Mannheimia haemolytica* because of the substantial genomic differences between it and other members of the *Pasteurella* genus.[198] For this discussion the organism is referred to as *P. haemolytica*.

IMPORTANT *P. haemolytica* IMMUNOGENS. *P. haemolytica* has numerous potential immunogens. Those with the most potential for stimulating immunity include capsular polysaccharide, lipopolysaccharide (LPS), outer membrane proteins (OMPs), iron-regulated OMPs, a secreted leukotoxin (LKT), and several other secreted enzymes, including neuraminidase and a glycoprotease.[199] The central dogma of *P. haemolytica* vaccination is that immunity to the organism requires stimulation of antibodies to LKT and to surface antigens.[200] Although there is no unequivocal agreement on the most important surface antigens, OMPs and iron-regulated OMPs are the major candidates based on in vitro and in vivo studies.[201-203] Capsular polysaccharide is theoretically an important surface antigen because it is the first surface molecule encountered by cellular and humoral components of the immune system, and its presence enhances *P. haemolytica* resistance to phagocytosis and complement-mediated killing.[204] However, antibody responses to *P. haemolytica* capsular polysaccharide do not always correlate with resistance, and vaccination with purified capsular polysaccharide resulted in no protection against challenge.[205,206] LPS is also a surface antigen, but antibodies to *P. haemolytica* LPS failed to correlate with resistance to experimental challenge, and passive antibodies to *P. haemolytica* LPS were not protective in experimentally challenged calves.[207,208]

COMMERCIAL VACCINES. More than 40 commercially available bovine biologics contain *P. haemolytica* antigens.[209] *P. haemolytica* vaccines often are combined with viral vaccines, *Haemophilus somnus*, or *Pasteurella multocida* bacterins and occasionally with *Clostridium* biologics. Despite the various licensed *P. haemolytica* biologics available, formulations of *P. haemolytica* vaccines fall into one of seven categories, six of which are nonliving vaccines. These vaccines are described by their manufacturers as follows: (1) bacterin with aluminum hydroxide adjuvant, (2) bacterin with water-in-oil adjuvant, (3) outer membrane extract, (4) bacterin toxoid (LKT toxoid), (5) toxoid cell–associated antigen, (6) adjuvanted toxoid (culture supernatant), and (7) Live streptomycin-dependent mutant. The streptomycin-dependent mutant vaccine is the only currently licensed live *P. haemolytica* biologic. Other live *P. haemolytica* vaccines available in the past showed potential for efficacy but often had untoward side effects such as severe local and systemic reactions.

When designing a vaccination program for prevention of bovine respiratory disease, four questions should be addressed: (1) Should a *Pasteurella* vaccine be used? (2) What type of *Pasteurella* vaccine should be used? (3) How many doses of *Pasteurella* vaccine should be given? and (4) When should a *Pasteurella* vaccine be given? The practicing veteri-

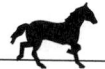

narian must answer these questions based on the cattle production situation, stocker or feedlot management, interpretation of published literature, consultations with colleagues, and personal experience.

EXPERIMENTAL STUDIES. Conventional formalin-inactivated, whole-cell, aluminum hydroxide–adsorbed *P. haemolytica* bacterins were the primary vaccine available for many years; however, they stimulate low antibody titers to surface antigens, do not stimulate antibodies to LKT, and in experimental challenges or field trials were essentially ineffective in substantially enhancing resistance to pneumonic pasteurellosis.[210] In contrast, experimental studies with *P. haemolytica* bacterins in water-in-oil adjuvants and outer membrane extract vaccines showed significantly enhanced resistance even though these vaccines do not stimulate antibodies to LKT, indicating that the adjuvant used probably is important in *P. haemolytica* immunity.[202,211,212] The other commercial *P. haemolytica* vaccines stimulate antibodies to LKT and surface antigens.[213,214]

Vaccine efficacy has been demonstrated primarily with experimental models of pneumonia using one of several challenge methods, including direct *P. haemolytica* challenge via intratracheal, intrabronchial, or transthoracic routes or a combination viral (usually BHV-1) and *P. haemolytica* challenge.[199] Most published reports of experimental vaccination and challenge studies have used experimental vaccines and not commercial ones. Few published reports are available on the efficacy of individual commercial vaccines against experimental *P. haemolytica* challenge. For instance, in one experiment cattle were vaccinated with a commercial bacterin toxoid and compared to unvaccinated controls after a transthoracic *P. haemolytica* challenge.[212] In a second experiment in the same manuscript, cattle were vaccinated with a commercial outer membrane extract vaccine and compared to control cattle after experimental challenge.[212] Both vaccines significantly enhanced resistance to experimental challenge. Direct comparisons of two commercial *P. haemolytica* vaccines against experimental challenge have rarely been published. In one such comparison between a commercial *P. haemolytica* bacterin toxoid and a streptomycin-dependent mutant vaccine, the bacterin toxoid elicited the greatest serologic responses.[213] Experimentally induced pneumonia was significantly lower in calves that received the bacterin toxoid compared to controls. The lesions in calves that received the mutant vaccine that were not significantly less than for control cattle. Demonstration of protection against experimental challenge, however, does not necessarily indicate that the vaccine will be efficacious against natural disease.

FIELD STUDIES. Some evidence indicates that less respiratory disease and fewer deaths are seen among cattle entering a feedlot with preexisting serum antibody titers to *P. haemolytica* have than among those without serum antibodies.[215] Therefore vaccination of cattle before shipment so that they can develop appropriate immunity is ideal, and determination of the appropriate time to vaccinate cattle with a *P. haemolytica* vaccine becomes critical.[216-218] Manufacturers of *P. haemolytica* biologics usually recommend vaccination 15 to 21 days before "weaning, shipping, or exposure."[209] Although many of the currently available *P. haemolytica* biologics are licensed for only one injection, manufacturers recommend a booster if possible. However, administration of two doses of a *P. haemolytica* vaccine may not be practical for beef cattle. Shewen[219] demonstrated that one dose of *P. haemolytica* vaccine often stimulates adequate antibody response because most cattle carry *P. haemolytica* in the nasopharynx and have a primed immune system that can produce a rapid anamnestic response to vaccination.

To determine the best time to vaccinate before shipping, the long-term antibody responses of cattle were followed after vaccination with three nonliving commercial *P. haemolytica* vaccines, a bacterin toxoid, an outer membrane extract, and an adjuvanted toxoid.[220] Serum antibody responses to *P. haemolytica* surface antigens (all tested vaccines) and LKT antigens (bacterin toxoid and adjuvanted toxoid only) were maximum 2 to 3 weeks after vaccination, but most antibody responses returned to normal by 6 weeks after vaccination. Revaccination 140 days after the initial vaccination resulted in rapid anamnestic responses that usually were higher than the initial responses. These data support manufacturer recommendations and indicate that if cattle are to be vaccinated with one of these *P. haemolytica* vaccines before shipment, the vaccine should be given 2 to 3 weeks previously to maximize antibodies at the time of shipment stress. If vaccination has been done before that time, a booster should be given before shipment.

Vaccination of cattle against pneumonic pasteurellosis upon arrival at the feedlot is somewhat controversial, because it may not allow enough time for development of solid protection, before the period of highest morbidity.[210] In addition, if cattle have been vaccinated 2 to 3 weeks before shipment and had adequate antibody responses, antibody titers many be adequate and revaccination may not be cost-effective. However, the vaccination history is not always known for beef cattle, and vaccination upon entry to the feedlot is a common practice.[216-218] Results in several field trials indicate that this practice can often afford some protection against shipping fever during the first 14 days in the feedlot.[217]

Selective use of *P. haemolytica* vaccines has also been advocated. Some feedlots designate cattle as high risk and low risk for respiratory disease. Managers may be more willing to vaccinate low-risk cattle because high-risk cattle are either sick upon arrival or can break with disease soon after entry into the feedlot.[218] Therefore vaccination of high-risk cattle would not have time to stimulate immunity. Low-risk cattle are less likely to break with disease soon after entry into the feedlot, and when vaccinated, sufficient time is available for immunity to develop before a respiratory outbreak occurs.[218]

Perino and Hunsaker[221] recently reviewed 10 published studies of several commercial live and subunit *P. haemolytica* vaccines with respect to their efficacy in field studies of feedlot cattle. Their report confirms that vaccination of cattle with even new generation *P. haemolytica* vaccines does not consistently reduce morbidity or mortality or increase weight gains. Of those studies, five showed positive outcomes based on reduced morbidity, mortality, or increased weight gain, and five demonstrated no positive outcome. Three of the studies demonstrating positive outcomes involved the same *P. haemolytica* bacterin toxoid given on arrival in the feedlot; however, two clinical trials with the same vaccine showed no significant differences when given on arrival and/or 3 weeks before shipment. In several field studies in which a positive outcome was demonstrated using a new generation *P. haemolytica* vaccine, economic benefits ranged from approximately $10 to $34 a head. The morbidity rate was reduced by approximately 30% to 45% and the mortality rate by 84% to 100%.[222]

DAIRY AND VEAL CALVES. Studies of *P. haemolytica* vaccination in dairy and veal calves have been published less often than those for beef calves. In one study, dairy calves vaccinated at about 10 weeks of age with *P. haemolytica* toxoid failed to produce significant antibody responses to LKT or OMPs.[223] In another study involving vaccination of Holstein calves with adjuvanted toxoid (culture supernatant) at 2 to 4 weeks of age, 50% or fewer of the calves seroconverted to *P. haemolytica* surface antigens, and those antibodies were in the IgM class.[224] None of those vaccinates developed LKT-neutralizing antibodies. Furthermore, many unvaccinated calves developed anti–*P. haemolytica* antibodies after 5 weeks of age, suggesting natural exposure to the organism. Low antibody responses in young dairy calves vaccinated with *P. haemolytica* probably indicate interference with vaccination by colostral antibodies.

With respect to protection afforded young calves by *P. haemolytica* vaccines, the incidence of respiratory disease in calves vaccinated with *P. haemolytica* toxoid was similar to that in unvaccinated controls.[225] In another study, a *P. haemolytica* bacterin toxoid was found to be less effective than a commercial streptomycin-dependent mutant *P. haemolytica* and *P. multocida* vaccine in reducing respiratory disease in veal calves.[226] However, antibody responses to *P. haemolytica* and the causes of respiratory disease were not determined in the veal calf study. *P. haemolytica* vaccines may fail to provide protection in dairy and veal calves because *P. multocida* is the most common isolate in dairy calf pneumonia.

Pasteurella multocida Vaccines

Pasteurella multocida, particularly serogroup A, serotype 3 isolates, is the second most common bacterium associated with pneumonia in beef cattle and the most common bacterium isolated in pneumonia of dairy calves.[197] The pneumonia produced by *P. multocida* is less acute and severe than that caused by *P. haemolytica*. Some have suggested that the prevalence of *P. multocida*–associated pneumonia may be increasing among beef cattle.[227] The non-living *P. multocida* vaccines currently available are conventional formalin-inactivated, whole-cell, aluminum hydroxide–adsorbed bacterins, which are not considered highly efficacious.[209] A commercial live streptomycin-dependent mutant *P. multocida* and *P. haemolytica* vaccine is available, but its efficacy has not been well documented in the literature.

The immune mechanisms involved in resistance to *P. multocida* lung infections are poorly understood. Recent studies suggest that OMPs or iron-regulated OMPs could be important immunogens for protecting cattle against pneumonia.[199,209] Although the *P. multocida* toxin, which is produced primarily by serogroup D isolates, is an important virulence factor and immunogen for *P. multocida* in atrophic rhinitis of swine, there is no evidence that this toxin is important in pneumonia of cattle or that it would be beneficial to include the toxin in a vaccine for cattle.[199]

Haemophilus somnus Vaccines

Haemophilus somnus is the cause of thromboembolic meningoencephalitis (TEME), septicemia, and reproductive disorders in cattle. In addition, it is the third most common bacterial isolate in beef cattle pneumonia.[197] Potential immunogens have been experimentally studied in *H. somnus*, and these consist of lipooligosaccharide (LOS)[28]; several OMPs, including a surface protein that binds the Fc receptor of bovine immunoglobulin[229]; and iron-regulated OMPs.[230] As with most gram negative bacteria, *H. somnus* LOS is a dominant antigen that stimulates an antibody response to the polysaccharide moiety after natural or experimental exposure. Currently there is no evidence that those anti-LOS antibodies are protective.[231] Likewise, several OMPs and iron-regulated OMPs have been shown to be immunogenic in cattle, but their role in stimulating immunity is not known.

Several approved *H. somnus* biologics are available, often in combination with respiratory viruses and *Pasteurella* spp. All the currently licensed *H. somnus* biologics are formalin-killed bacterins with aluminum hydroxide as adjuvant. The efficacy of *H. somnus* bacterins has been generally good in stimulating protection against experimental pneumonia, against intravenous and intracisternal *H. somnus* challenge as a model of TEME, and against natural TEME.[231] Overall, vaccine-induced immunity has been best against experimental and natural TEME.[210,223,232] Using an experimental challenge model of *H. somnus*–induced pneumonia, significant protection was afforded calves vaccinated twice with an *H. somnus* bacterin.[233] Resistance correlated with a high serum antibody response to the bacterium. A recent study demonstrated a reduced risk for respiratory disease in cattle that had high antibody titers to *H. somnus* upon arrival in a feedlot.[234] Therefore the potential exists for stimulating resistance to *H. somnus*–associated pneumonia.

Under field conditions, commercial *H. somnus* bacterins have had limited success in inducing protection against respiratory disease. Published reports have shown conflicting results. Perino and Hunsaker[221] recently reaffirmed this in their reassessment of the results of three published commercial *H. somnus* bacterin field trials. In one trial *H. somnus* vaccination resulted in a reduced treatment rate when vaccinations were given on arrival at the feedlot and 21 days later.[235] In another study, vaccination once with a commercial bacterin was associated with significantly more animals being treated for respiratory disease compared with unvaccinated cattle or those vaccinated twice at 21-day intervals.[236,237] In yet another study, vaccination with a commercial *H. somnus* bacterin upon arrival at the feedlot was associated with no significant differences between the number of animals treated for respiratory disease compared with unvaccinated controls.[238] Ribble, Jim, and Janzen[239] demonstrated a reduced mortality rate among steers after *H. somnus* vaccination but not among heifers.

REFERENCES

197. Welsh RD: Bacterial and *Mycoplasma* species isolated from pneumonic bovine lungs, *Agri Pract* 14:12-16, 1993.
198. Angen O et al: Taxonomic relationships of the (*Pasteurella*) *haemolytica* complex as evaluated by DNA-DNA hybridizations and 16S rRNA sequencing with proposal of Mannheimia haemolytica gen. nov., comb. nov., *Mannheimia granulomatis* comb. nov., *Mannheimia glucosida* sp. nov., *Mannheimia ruminalis* sp. nov. and *Mannheimia varigena* sp. Nov, *Int J Syst Bacteriol* 49:67-86, 1999.
199. Confer AW: Immunogens of *Pasteurella*, *Vet Microbiol* 37:353-368, 1993.
200. Shewen PE, Wilkie BN: Vaccination of calves with leukotoxic culture supernatant from *Pasteurella haemolytica*, *Can J Vet Res* 52:30-36, 1988.
201. Confer AW et al: Serum antibody responses of cattle to iron-regulated outer membrane proteins of *Pasteurella haemolytica* A1, *Vet Immunol Immunopathol* 47:101-110, 1995.
202. Morton RJ et al: Vaccination of cattle with outer membrane protein-enriched fractions of *Pasteurella haemolytica* and resistance against experimental challenge, *Am J Vet Res* 56:875-879, 1995.
203. Potter AA et al: Protective capacity of the *Pasteurella haemolytica* transferrin-binding proteins TbpA and TbpB in cattle, *Microb Pathog* 27:197-206, 1999.
204. Chae CH et al: Resistance to host immune defense mechanisms afforded by capsular material of *Pasteurella haemolytica*, serotype 1, *Vet Microbiol* 25:241-251, 1990.
205. Confer AW et al: Serum antibody response to carbohydrate antigens of *Pasteurella haemolytica* serotype 1: relation to experimental bovine pneumonic pasteurellosis, *Am J Vet Res* 50:98-105, 1989.
206. Conlon JR, Shewen PE: Clinical and serological evaluation of a *Pasteurella haemolytica* A1 capsular polysaccharide, *Vaccine* 11:767-772, 1993.
207. Confer AW, Panciera RJ, Mosier DA: Serum antibodies to *Pasteurella haemolytica* lipopolysaccharide: relationship to experimental bovine pneumonic pasteurellosis, *Am J Vet Res* 47:1134-1138, 1986.
208. Mosier DA, Simons KR, Vestweber JG: Passive protection of calves with *Pasteurella haemolytica* antiserum, *Am J Vet Res* 56:1317-21, 1995.
209. Arrioja-Dechert A, ed: *Compendium of veterinary products*, ed 5, Port Huron, Mich, 1999, North American Compendiums.
210. Roth JA, Perino LJ: Immunology and prevention of infection in feedlot cattle, *Vet Clin North Am (Food Anim Pract)* 14:233-256, 1998.
211. Confer AW et al: Immunological response to *Pasteurella haemolytica* and resistance against experimental bovine pneumonic pasteurellosis induced by bacterins in oil adjuvants, *Am J Vet Res* 48:163-168, 1987.
212. Confer AW, Panciera RJ: Testing of two new-generation *Pasteurella haemolytica* vaccines against experimental bovine pneumonic pasteurellosis, *Agri Pract* 15:10-15, 1994.
213. Mosier DA et al: Comparison of serologic and protective responses induced by two *Pasteurella* vaccines, *Can J Vet Res* 62:178-182, 1998.
214. Srinand S et al: Comparative evaluation of antibodies induced by commercial *Pasteurella haemolytica* vaccines using solid phase immunoassays, *Vet Microbiol* 49:181-195, 1996.

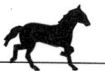

215. Frank GH et al: Respiratory tract disease and mucosal colonization by *Pasteurella haemolytica* in transported cattle, *Am J Vet Res* 57:1317-20, 1996.
216. Smith RA et al: *Pasteurella haemolytica* pneumonia. I, *Agri Pract* 5:5-7, 1994.
217. Smith RA et al: *Pasteurella haemolytica* pneumonia. II, *Agri Pract* 15:21-23, 1994.
218. Smith RA et al: *Pasteurella haemolytica* pneumonia. III, *Agri Pract* 15:41-46, 1994.
219. Shewen PE: Host response to infection with HAP: implications for vaccine development. In Donachie W, Lainson FA, Hodgson JC eds: *Haemophilus, Actinobacillus, and Pasteurella*, London, 1995, Plenum.
220. Confer AW et al: Duration of serum antibody responses following vaccination and revaccination of cattle with nonliving commercial *Pasteurella haemolytica* vaccines, *Vaccine* 16:1962-1970, 1998.
221. Perino LJ, Hunsaker BD: A review of bovine respiratory disease vaccine field efficacy, *Bovine Pract* 31:59-66, 1997.
222. Bechtol DT, Ballinger RT: Field trial of a *Pasteurella haemolytica* toxoid administered at spring branding and in the feedlot, *Agri Pract* 12:6-14, 1991.
223. Stephens LR et al: Isolation of *Haemophilus somnus* antigens and their use as vaccines for prevention of bovine thromboembolic meningoencephalitis, *Am J Vet Res* 45:234-238, 1984.
224. Hodgins DC, Shewen PE: Serologic responses of young colostrum-fed dairy calves to antigens of *Pasteurella haemolytica* A1, *Vaccine* 16:20 1998.
225. Stevens RD et al: Morbidity and mortality in young Holstein heifer calves vaccinated with a *P. haemolytica* leukotoxoid, *Large Anim Pract* 18:23-29, 1997.
226. Schnepper RL et al: Respiratory morbidity in veal calves given *Pasteurella* vaccines, *Vet Med*, Jan 1996, pp 72-76.
227. Confer AW et al: Antibody responses of cattle to outer membrane proteins of *Pasteurella multocida* A:3, *Am J Vet Res* 57:1453-1457, 1996.
228. Inzana TJ et al: Phase variation and conservation of lipooligosaccharide epitopes in *Haemophilus somnus*, *Infect Immun* 65:4675-81, 1997.
229. Corbeil LB, Bastida-Corcuera FD, Beveridge TJ: *Haemophilus somnus* immunoglobulin binding proteins and surface fibrils, *Infect Immun* 65:4250-4257, 1997.
230. Yu RH et al: Interaction of ruminant transferrins with transferrin receptors in bovine isolates of *Pasteurella haemolytica* and *Haemophilus somnus*, *Infect Immun* 60:2992-2994, 1992.
231. Confer AW, Fulton RW: Evaluation of *Pasteurella* and *Haemophilus* vaccines, *Bovine Proc* 27:136-141, 1995.
232. Stephens LR et al: Vaccination of cattle against experimentally induced thromboembolic meningoencephalitis with a *Haemophilus somnus* bacterin, *Am J Vet Res* 43:1339-1342, 1982.
233. Groom SC, Little PB: Effects of vaccination of calves against induced *Haemophilus somnus* pneumonia, *Am J Vet Res* 49:793-800, 1988.
234. Martin SW et al: The association of titers to *Haemophilus somnus* and other putative pathogens with the occurrence of bovine respiratory disease and weight gain in feedlot calves, *Can J Vet Res* 62:262-267, 1998.
235. Amstutz HE, Horstman LA, Morter RL: Clinical evaluation of the efficacy of *Haemophilus somnus* and *Pasteurella* sp bacterins, *Bovine Pract* 16:106-108, 1981.
236. Morter RL, Amstutz HE: Evaluating the efficacy of a *Haemophilus somnus* bacterin in a controlled field trial, *Bovine Pract* 18:82-83, 1983.
237. Van Donkersgoed J et al: The effect of route and dosage of immunization on the serological response to a *Pasteurella haemolytica* and *Haemophilus somnus* vaccine in feedlot cattle, *Can Vet J* 34:731-735, 1993.
238. Morter RL, Amstutz HE, Crandell RA: Clinical evaluation of prophylactic regimens for bovine respiratory disease, *Bovine Pract* 17:56-58, 1982.
239. Ribble CS, Jim GK, Janzen ED: Efficacy of immunization of feedlot calves with a commercial *Haemophilus somnus* vaccine, *Can J Vet Res* 52:191-198, 1988.

BOVINE REPRODUCTIVE DISEASE VACCINES

VICTOR S. CORTESE

As was explained earlier, cows have a multilayered placenta, which leaves the fetus susceptible to infection. Infection of the placenta, inflammation of the ovary, death of the fetus, or disruption of the cervical plug all may cause abortion. Reproductive disease therefore is the most difficult disorder against which to achieve protection. Vaccination must minimize the amount or duration (or both) of the viremia or septicemia, or it must prevent the pathogen from moving through the cervix or crossing the placenta.

The reproductive diseases and protection against them through vaccination are areas of active research. With current research, a vaccination program can be designed to aid in the control of reproductive diseases. Unfortunately, there is little

or no research on the efficacy of many vaccines currently used to prevent reproductive disease. Because the causes of reproductive failure are so numerous (infectious agents account for only a small percentage), vaccination to prevent infectious reproductive losses many not appear to be effective. This often is due to the fact that diagnostic testing has not been attempted or has not determined the cause of reproductive inefficiencies. A vaccination program may be inappropriately instituted when the cause is not infectious, or the current program may unfairly be deemed ineffective. A new *Neospora* vaccine against *Neospora*-induced reproductive disease in cattle has been granted a conditional license. Little published information is available on this product. Although safety has been shown, the efficacy is questionable.

The use of viral vaccines to help prevent reproductive diseases was discussed earlier in the chapter.

Brucella abortus Vaccine

Brucella vaccination has best shown the effectiveness of vaccination in controlling a reproductive disease. The successful control or even eradication of *Brucella abortus* in many areas of North America is a testament to the ability of a program involving testing, culling, and vaccination to control a reproductive disease. Vaccination with either strain 19 or strain RB51 *Brucella* has proved to be effective; however, many herds owners have stopped vaccinating against this disease as states have been declared *Brucella* free.

Abortions caused by *B. abortus* usually are seen after 5 months of gestation. Retained placentae and subsequent metritis usually follow. The abortion is caused by severe placentitis. *Brucella* infections have also been associated with a decrease in conception rates and an increase in services per conception. A higher number of dead and weak calves has also been demonstrated in infected herds. Orchitis or seminal vesiculitis or both may characterize infections in bulls.

Only heifer calves can be vaccinated for brucellosis. Both of the two licensed *B. abortus* vaccines are modified live bacterins, and vaccination of bulls may lead to orchitis.[240] Legal use of the vaccines usually is confined to heifer calves 4 to 12 months of age, because vaccination of older animals with the strain 19 vaccine may lead to false positive results on routine *Brucella* screening tests. Because the strain 19 vaccine may cause septicemia, clinical illness, and occasionally death,[241] sick, unhealthy, or stressed cattle should not be vaccinated. The RB51 strain vaccine is an O antigen–deficient mutant of the *B. abortus* strain 2308. The RB51 vaccine has three primary advantages:

1. Antibodies induced by this vaccine do not react with the serologic tests routinely done to diagnose *Brucella* infections.
2. The vaccine can be used in adult cattle at a lower dosage under special circumstances and with the permission of the U.S. Department of Agriculture.
3. The vaccine tends to cause less postvaccination fever and stress than the traditional strain 19 vaccines.

The long-term immunity conferred by *Brucella* vaccination is the cell-mediated type.[242,243] Calfhood vaccination does not prevent a herd of cattle from becoming infected with *B. abortus*. However, it does largely prevent abortions and protects 65% to 75% of the cattle in the herd from infection while infected reactors are identified and slaughtered.[244] For these reasons, in addition to vaccination, a control program should include testing and culling of all animals that test positive.

Leptospira interrogans Bacterins

Although usually associated with abortions, *Leptospira interrogans* and *Leptospira borgpetersenii* can also cause severe liver or kidney disease (or both) and in some situations can cause an outbreak of mastitis. Many different serovars of *L. interrogans* have been shown to cause reproductive failure and abortions in cattle. *L. borgpetersenii* serovar *hardjo* is the cattle-maintained serovar and accounts for most cattle infections.[245,246] *L. interrogans* serovar *pomona* is maintained in pigs and other mammals and is the second most common *Leptospira* infection diagnosed in cattle. Cattle *Leptospira* organisms have been shown to be zoonotic.

Leptospira bacteria can cause abortion storms in which a high number of cattle may abort within a short period. There may be an increased number of stillbirths and births of premature and weak calves. Although serovar *pomona* tends to cause abortions in the last trimester of pregnancy, serovar *hardjo* can cause abortions at any stage of pregnancy. Abortions usually are caused by fetal infection and subsequent death of the fetus. Serovar *hardjo* can also colonize the oviducts, diminishing fertility. After an initial *Leptospira* infection, cattle may remain infected and shed the spirochete for long periods.[248] *Leptospira* vaccinations (initial and booster) help prepare the heifer for entry into the breeding herd. There have been many debates over the ability of *Leptospira* vaccines to prevent abortions. Much discussion has centered on the antigenic difference between serovar *hardjo* types *hardjo-bovis* and *hardjo-pratjino*.[249] However, infertility problems have been shown to decline in herds after vaccination.[250]

Current bacterins contain either *L. pomona* antigen only or a combination of *L. pomona, L. hardjo, L. grippotyphosa, L. canicola,* and *L. icterohaemorrhagiae* antigens. Although *L. pomona* infections are common and widespread in most locations,[251] the addition of *L. pomona* to some vaccines has been recommended for its adjuvanting effect. This method has been used almost extensively in feedlot practice, although there is no published data on its effect. However, it has been shown that small amounts of endotoxin can act as an adjuvant.[252]

Many *Leptospira* bacterins are labeled as single initial dose products, but because of their weak immunogenicity, a booster dose is recommended approximately 1 month after the first dose.[253] *Leptospira* bacterins must be administered by intramuscular or subcutaneous injection. Although most manufacturers specify revaccination at 12-month intervals, this duration of immunity has been questioned, and more frequent revaccination often is needed to control *Leptospira* abortions.[247,254,255] Nevertheless, because leptospiral abortions are uncommon during the first half of pregnancy, it may be possible to use an annual vaccination schedule (*L. hardjo* excepted) in seasonally calving herds such as beef herds. Cattle in such herds can be vaccinated when they are 2 to 4 months pregnant, usually at the time that pregnancy is diagnosed, and protected through the balance of the pregnancy with a single annual dose.[254] Although administration of *L. pomona* bacterin provides good protection against clinical manifestations of the disease, it does not always provide complete protection against infection and leptospiruria.[247,254-256]

Improvements in breeding efficiency have been reported after vaccination of herds infected with *L. hardjo*.[256] It has been suggested that this improvement could have resulted from elimination of uterine infection.[257] However, the current *L. hardjo* bacterins are poorly antigenic and do not prevent infection, leptospiruria, and subsequent reproductive failures in challenge-exposed pregnant cows.[247] Based on this study, herds infected with *L. hardjo* should be given booster doses at intervals of no less than 4 to 6 months. Vaccination at 3-month intervals has provided better control than 4-month intervals. Once a *Leptospira* vaccination program is instituted, it is important to maintain the vaccination program because of this shortened duration of immunity.[258]

Recently a new vaccine has been shown to eliminate postchallenge shedding (which occurs with the conventional vaccines) and to provide longer duration of immunity than previously demonstrated.[259]

Bovine Genital Campylobacteriosis Vaccines

Originally classified as *Vibrio, Campylobacter fetus* ssp. *veneralis* causes a venereal infection of cattle. The bacteria are introduced during natural breeding by infected bulls or by artificial insemination (AI) with infected semen. Bulls usually are infected by breeding with infected cows, but contact with infected bedding may also be a cause. Older bulls (over 4 years of age) are more likely to be infected. After deposition in the vagina, the bacteria rapidly colonize the vagina and cervix, and in 25% of these cows are found in the oviducts. The organism can persist for months after infection of these sites. It has been shown that fertility never returns to normal in some infected animals, and some animals may be permanently sterile because of the damage caused by salpingitis.

Vaccination with *Campylobacter* vaccines has been shown to be effective in protecting heifers even when vaginal cultures test positive for the bacteria.[260] It appears that the uterus is very resistant to the bacteria after vaccination. Studies have demonstrated improved breeding efficiency in vaccinated herds.[260] Vaccination of bulls with oil-adjuvant vaccines not only prevents infection of bulls for up to 1 year[261] but also aids in prevention of mechanical transfer of organisms during natural service.[262] Furthermore, vaccination with two doses has been shown to be effective at clearing infections from carrier bulls.[263,264]

VACCINATION. Use of *C. fetus* bacterins is recommended in all breeding herds that use bulls, even if only on selected cows. In heifer herds using virgin bulls or in 100% AI-bred herds, vaccination against *Vibrio* organisms is not necessary.

Several different *C. fetus* vaccines are available, including oil-adjuvanted and aluminum hydroxide–adsorbed types. Oil-adjuvant *C. fetus* bacterins have proved to be more effective[265] and to provide longer lasting protection after a single dose.[266] Unfortunately, oil-adjuvant vaccines cause localized granuloma formation and fibrosis at the site of injection. This may cause visible blemishes, which may be objectionable in registered stock or show cattle. Administration no earlier than 4 months before the breeding season is preferred.[265] When aluminum hydroxide–adsorbed *C. fetus* bacterins are used, a priming dose should be administered at least 6 weeks before the immunizing (booster) dose, and the booster should be administered 10 days before the beginning of the breeding season.[263] After administration of an aluminum hydroxide–adsorbed bacterin, serum antibody concentrations peak rapidly and decline precipitously, falling to susceptible levels by 4 weeks after one dose or 11 weeks after two doses.[267] Some aluminum hydroxide–adsorbed bacterins do not require an initial booster.

Campylobacteriosis (vibriosis) is most effectively controlled when all breeding-age animals, including bulls, are included in the vaccination program.[263] Vibrin* is the only *C. fetus* bacterin available in the United States that has been evaluated in bulls.[260] Two 5-ml doses are administered to breeding bulls at 4-week intervals beginning 8 weeks before the start of the breeding season.[260] In subsequent years a single booster dose is administered 4 weeks before the start of the breeding season.[266] This dosage is 2½ times that recommended for vaccination of cows.

---

*Vibrin, Pfizer Animal Health, Exton, PA 19341.

Bovine Trichomoniasis Vaccines

Bovine trichomoniasis is a venereal infection of cattle caused by the protozoal agent *Tritrichomonas foetus*. Early in the course of the disease, abortions with pyometra may be seen in 5% of infected cows. These abortions occur early in gestation.[268] However, infertility is the most common sign, with long interservice intervals.[269,270] Early embryonic death is followed by a period of conception failure. Some natural resistance develops after infection, but carrier cows may be an important component of the epidemiology of this disease. In rare cases a cow may be left sterile after an infection because of uterine destruction.[271]

The efficacy of *Tritrichomonas* vaccines is questionable,[272-274] but the vaccines do appear to reduce actual reproductive losses.[275] Heifers, cows, and breeding bulls should be vaccinated twice at 2- to 4-week intervals, the second dose given 4 weeks before the beginning of the breeding season.[276] Subcutaneous administration is recommended. In subsequent years a single annual booster vaccination should be given 4 weeks before the beginning of the breeding season.

In a problem herd, trichomoniasis vaccination must be coupled with other control measures, such as culturing, culling, and treatment to effectively control the disease.

REFERENCES

240. Lambert G et al: Postvaccinal persistence of *Brucella abortus* strain 19 in two bulls, *J Am Vet Med Assoc* 145:909-911, 1964.
241. Roberts SJ, Squire RA, Gilman HL: Deaths in two calves following vaccination with *Brucella abortus* strain 19 vaccine, *Cornell Vet* 52:592-595, 1962.
242. Nicoletti P: Brucellosis. In Howard JL, ed: *Current veterinary therapy: food animal practice 2*, Philadelphia, 1986, WB Saunders.
243. Confer AW et al: Effect of challenge dose on the clinical and immune responses of cattle vaccinated with reduced doses of *Brucella abortus* strain 19, *Vet Microbiol* 10:561-575, 1985.
244. Blood DC, Radostitis OM, Henderson JA: *Veterinary medicine*, ed 6, London, 1983, Bailliére Tindall.
245. White FH, Sulzer KR, Engle RW: Isolation of *Leptospira interrogans* serovars *hardjo, balcanica*, and *pomona* from cattle at slaughter, *Am J Vet Res* 43:1172-1173, 1982.
246. Ellis WA, Thiermann AB: Isolation of Leptospira from the genital tract of Iowa cows at slaughter, *Am J Vet Res* 47:1649-1696, 1986.
247. Bolin CA et al: Effect of vaccination with a pentavalent leptospiral vaccine on *Leptospira interrogans* serovar *hardjo* type *hardjo-bovis* infection of pregnant cattle, *Am J Vet Res* 50:161-165, 1989.
248. Thiermann AB: Experimental leptospiral infections in pregnant cattle with organisms of Hebdomadia serogroup, *Am J Vet Res* 43:78-784, 1982.
249. Ellis WA, Thiermann AB, Marshall RB: Genotypes of *Leptospira interrogans* serovar *hardjo* and their role in clinical disease, *Proc 14th World Congr Dis Cattle* 2:966-970, 1986.
250. Hanson LE: Effects of leptospirosis on bovine reproduction. In Morrow DA, ed: *Current therapy in theriogenology*, Philadelphia, 1980, WB Saunders.
251. Ellis WA, Zygraich N: Experimental studies with a *Leptospira interrogans* serovar *hardjo* vaccine, *Proc 14th World Congr Dis Cattle* 2:971-974, 1986.
252. Ribi EE: Structure-function relationship of bacterial adjuvants. In Nervig RM et al, eds: *Advances in carriers and adjuvants for veterinary biologics*, Ames, Iowa, 1986, Iowa State University Press.
253. Faine S: Prevention of leptospirosis 2: measures for control and prevention. In Faine S et al, eds: *Leptospira and leptospirosis*, Boca Raton, Fla, 1994, CRC Press.
254. Bey RF, Johnson RC: Current status of leptospiral vaccines, *Prog Vet Microbiol Immunol* 2:175-197, 1986.
255. Kiesel GK, Dacres WG: A study of *Leptospira pomona* bacterin in cattle, *Cornell Vet* 49:332-343, 1959.
256. Hanson LE, Tripathy DN, Killinger AH: Current status of leptospirosis immunization in swine and cattle, *J Am Vet Med Assoc* 161:1235-1243, 1972.
257. Ellis WA: Effects of leptosirosis on bovine reproduction. In Morrow DA, ed: *Current therapy in theriogenology 2*, Philadelphia, 1986, WB Saunders.
258. Hathaway SC: Leptospirosis in New Zealand: an ecological view, *N Z Vet J* 29:109 1981.
259. Bolin CW, Alt DP, Zuerner RL: Protection of cattle from infection with *Leptospira borgpetersenii* serovar *hardjo*, Proceedings of the Second Annual Leptospirosis Congress, Marysville, Australia, August, 1999.
260. DeKeyser PJ: Bovine genital campylobacteriosis. In Morrow DA, ed: *Current theriogenology 2*, London, 1986, WB Saunders.
261. Bouters R, et al: *Vibrio fetus* infection in bulls: curative and preventive vaccination, *Br Vet J* 129:52-57, 1973.
262. Clark BL et al: Studies on venereal transmission of *Campylobacter fetus* by immunized bulls, *Aust Vet J* 51:531-532, 1975.
263. Clark BL et al: A dual vaccine for immunization of bulls against vibriosis, *Aust Vet J* 55:43, 1979.
264. Hoerlein AB: Vibriosis. In Morrow DA, ed: *Current therapy in theriogenology 2*, Philadelphia, 1986, WB Saunders.
265. Dawson LJ: Diagnosis, prevention and control of campylobacteriosis and trichomoniasis, *Bovine Pract* 21:180-183, 1986.
266. Hoerlein AB, Carroll EJ: Duration of immunity to bovine genital vibriosis, *J Am Vet Med Assoc* 156:775-778, 1970.
267. Berg RL, Firehammer BD: Effect of interval between booster vaccination and time of breeding on protection against campylobacteriosis (vibriosis) in cattle, *J Am Vet Med Assoc* 173:467-471, 1978.
268. Kimsey PB: Bovine trichomoniasis. In Morrow DA, ed: *Current therapy in theriogenology 2*, Philadelphia, 1986, WB Saunders.
269. Bartlett DE: *Trichomonas foetus* infection and bovine reproduction, *Am J Vet Res* 8:343, 1947.
270. Parsonson IM, Clark BI, Duffy JH: Early pathogenesis and pathology of *Tritrichomonas foetus* infection in virgin heifers, *J Comp Pathol* 86:59, 1976.
271. Kendrick JW: An outbreak of bovine trichomoniasis in a group of bulls used for artificial insemination, *Cornell Vet* 43:231, 1953.
272. Perino LJ, Rupp GP: Beef cow immunity and its influence on fetal neonatal calf health, *Proceedings of the Twenty-eighth Annual Convention of the American Association of Bovine Practitioners*, p 145, 1995.
273. Ikeda JS et al: Conservation of a protective surface antigen of *Tritrichomonas foetus*, *J Clin Microbiol*, 31:32289, 1993.
274. Clark BL, Duffy JH, Parsonson IM: Immunization of bulls against trichomoniasis, *Aust Vet J* 60:178, 1983.
275. Corbeil LB: Vaccination strategies against *Tritrichomonas foetus*, *Parasitol Today* 10:103, 1994.
276. Hjerpe CA: Bovine vaccines and herd vaccination programs, *Vet Clin North Am (Food Anim Pract)* 6:171, 1990.

NEONATAL CALF ENTERIC DISEASE VACCINES

GERALD E. DUHAMEL

GENERAL CONSIDERATIONS. Neonatal enteric diseases can have a devastating impact on the profitability of cow-calf and dairy operations. In addition to mortality, medical, and labor costs, neonatal enteric diseases can significantly reduce the body weight of weaned calves and the performance of replacement heifers.[277]

Several well-characterized infectious causes of neonatal enteric diseases have been described.[278] Some of the more common infectious agents are rotavirus, coronavirus, enterotoxigenic *Escherichia coli*, salmonellae, and *Cryptosporidium* spp.[279-285] Sporadic outbreaks of necrohemorrhagic enteritis affecting 3- to 10-day-old calves have been associated with infection with *Clostridium perfringens* type C.[286] Several less well-characterized viruses (calicivirus, torovirus, astrovirus), bacteria (enterotoxigenic *Bacteroides fragilis*, attaching-effacing enteropathogenic and enterohemorrhagic *E. coli*, *Enterococcus durans*), and protozoans (*Giardia duodenalis*) also have been associated with neonatal calf enteric diseases.

Because of the continuous calving and constant introduction of replacement heifers on dairy farms and the continuous flow of susceptible calves on veal calf operations, infections caused by more than one agent should be suspected in these types of operations.[279-285,287-289] In addition to different infectious agents, mixed infections with different groups and serotypes or genotypes of rotaviruses and bacteria also can occur. In complicated infections the clinical disease usually is more severe, and control may be more difficult. When scours occurs in a herd that has been vaccinated against enteric diseases, possible contributing factors should be considered, including concurrent infection with pathogens not present in the vaccine (e.g., non–group A rotaviruses, *Cryptosporidium* spp., and salmonellae) and suboptimal management, including poor control of environmental contamination. A thorough laboratory diagnostic investigation is needed to correctly identify the cause of severe problems and any other possible contributing factors and to serve as a basis for appropriate control strategies for the present and future calf crops.

Management practices for dairy cattle and beef cattle are sufficiently different that control measures for neonatal enteric diseases can be production specific. For example, in dairy herds, because of the high turnover of older cows and the continuous introduction of replacement heifers, the risk of introducing new strains of enteric disease pathogens is higher than in closed beef herds. Similarly, the continuous calving and the proximity of susceptible calves on dairy farms create an ideal environment for recirculation of enteric disease agents back into the adult population. This in turn may increase and broaden herd immunity such that the efficacy of the vaccine in these herds might be enhanced, partly because of the booster effect the vaccine has on preexisting immunity. Beef cattle herds, in contrast, are generally relatively closed, and a susceptible calf population is present only for a relatively short period annually during the calving season. Introduction of new pathogens or new strains of enteric disease agents, particularly during the calving season, can have a devastating effect because of the potential for a high number of susceptible animals. Conversely, following an outbreak, herd immunity might be more stable and the occurrence of enteric disease might be reduced during the following calving seasons.

Under both types of production systems, vaccination for neonatal enteric diseases is rarely successful without reasonably good management programs and sanitation to ensure adequate intake of protective colostrum and to minimize contamination of the environment.[290] General herd health management recommendations that can affect the success of a vaccination program for neonatal enteric diseases include the following:

1. A sound biosecurity program should be established that includes purchase of replacement animals from reputable sources and a complete ban on the introduction of foster calves, which pose a great risk of introducing new neonatal calf enteric disease agents.
2. High-protein, high-energy feed, adequate micronutrients (e.g., copper and selenium), and abundant clean drinking water should be provided throughout gestation and calving so that cows are in good body condition to produce an adequate volume of colostrum and milk, and calves are healthy and vigorous at birth, with a fully developed and functional immune system.
3. The calving area and equipment should be kept clean and dry. Crowding should be avoided, with separate feeding and bedding grounds provided in the calving area. Separate equipment should be used for handling feed and manure.
4. First calf–heifer pairs should be kept separate from the mature cow herd from calving until the youngest calf is at least 3 weeks old; this reduces the possibility of spread of infectious disease agents from younger, more susceptible and possibly shedding pairs to the main herd.
5. Each calf must ingest about 10% of its body weight in colostrum within the first 6 hours of birth; if a calf is unable to nurse naturally, force-feeding of fresh or frozen colostrum from the calf's dam or from a mature cow in the same herd or a neighboring herd may be required.
6. All equipment used for feeding colostrum and treating sick calves must be routinely disinfected; this includes such items as nipple bottles, esophageal probes, and balling guns.
7. Cow-calf pairs should be moved away from the calving

area as soon as possible after birth to minimize environmental exposure of newborn calves to infectious agents immediately after birth.
8. Scouring calves should be isolated quickly from healthy calves in dairy herds, or sick cow-calf pairs should be isolated from healthy pairs in beef herds to reduce environmental exposure to infectious agents that can overwhelm innate or passively acquired immunity.

Giving calves a healthy start maximizes their production potential and reduces the costs and labor associated with treatment of sick animals.

REFERENCES

277. Cornaglia EM et al: Reduction in morbidity due to diarrhea in nursing beef calves by use of an inactivated oil-adjuvanted rotavirus–*Escherichia coli* vaccine in the dam, *Vet Microbiol* 30:191-202, 1992.
278. Holland RE: Some infectious causes of diarrhea in young farm animals, *Clin Microbiol Rev* 3:345-375, 1990.
279. Acres SD et al: Acute undifferentiated neonatal diarrhea in beef calves. I. Occurrence and distribution of infectious agents, *Can J Comp Med* 39:116-132, 1975.
280. Morin M, Lariviere S, Lallier R: Pathological and microbiological observations made on spontaneous cases of acute neonatal calf diarrhea, *Can J Comp Med* 40:228-240, 1976.
281. Moon HW et al: Pathogenic relationships of rotavirus, *Escherichia coli*, and other agents in mixed infections in calves, *J Am Vet Med Assoc* 173:577-583, 1978.
282. McDonough SP, Stull CL, Osburn BI: Enteric pathogens in intensively reared veal calves, *Am J Vet Res* 55:1516-1520, 1994.
283. Chinsangaram J et al: Prevalence of group A and group B rotaviruses in the feces of neonatal dairy calves from California, *Comp Immunol Microbiol Infect Dis* 18:93-103, 1995.
284. De la Fuente R et al: *Cryptosporidium* and concurrent infections with other major enteropathogens in 1- to 30-day-old diarrheic dairy calves in central Spain, *Vet Parasitol* 80:179-185, 1999.
285. O'Handley RM et al: Duration of naturally acquired giardiosis and cryptosporidiosis in dairy calves and their association with diarrhea, *Am J Vet Res* 214:391-396, 1999.
286. Niilo L: *Clostridium perfringens* type C enterotoxemia, *Can Vet J* 29:658-664, 1988.
287. Tzipori SR et al: Clinical manifestations of diarrhea in calves infected with rotavirus and enterotoxigenic *Escherichia coli*, *J Clin Microbiol* 13:1011-1016, 1981.
288. Sabara M et al: Genetic heterogeneity within individual bovine rotavirus isolates, *J Virol* 44:813-822, 1982.
289. Torres-Medina A: Effect of combined rotavirus and *Escherichia coli* in neonatal gnotobiotic calves, *Am J Vet Res* 45:643-651, 1984.
290. Clement JC et al: Use of epidemiologic principles to identify risk factors associated with the development of diarrhea in calves in five beef herds, *J Am Vet Med Assoc* 207:1334-1338, 1995.

Rotavirus and Coronavirus Vaccines

GENERAL CONSIDERATIONS. Rotaviruses (RVs) and coronavirus (CV) are ubiquitous in the cattle population; most adult cattle have virus-neutralizing (VN) serum antibodies.[291-295] RV infections are widespread in both dairy and beef cow-calf productions, whereas infection with CV most often occurs as sporadic outbreaks of severe diarrhea in beef cow-calf herds or chronic low-grade diarrhea in dairy and veal calf operations. Fecal shedding of RV and CV is common among adult cows,[296-299] which provides an immediate source of virus challenge for naive newborn calves and facilitates the persistence of these agents at the herd level.

Currently only one type of CV is known to cause neonatal calf diarrhea.[300] Conversely, RVs are classified into at least seven distinct groups, A through G.[301] Although RVs that belong to groups A, B, and C have been found to naturally infect cattle,[299,302-305] group A rotaviruses are by far the prevalent type.[303,305] Members of the group A rotaviruses are further classified according to antigenic and genetic differences in their outer capsid proteins, G and P.[306-308] Because both of these proteins are involved in neutralization of infectivity in vitro and protection in vivo,[309-311] consideration of the G/P configuration of rotaviruses is critical to developing an effec-

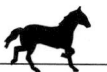

tive vaccination program for preventing neonatal enteric diseases.

Although a good correlation has been found between the antigenicity of the G proteins and their corresponding gene sequences, a similar relationship has not been found for the P proteins. Therefore 14 different G serotypes, which correspond to 14 G genotypes, have been identified among group A rotaviruses, whereas 10 serotypes identified on the basis of the antigenicity of the P proteins have been assigned to 20 genotypes when compared on the basis of the nucleotide sequence of the P protein genes.[308] At least eight distinct G serotypes/genotypes (G1, G2, G3, G6, G8, G10, G11, and untypable) are known to infect cattle in the United States[312,313]; G6 is the most widespread, and G8 and G10 account for lower percentages of infections.[296,313-318] Conversely, RVs may have any of four P serotypes/genotypes—P6[1], P7[5], P8[11], and untypable—with P7[5] being the prevalent type.[313,318,319]

The genome of RVs is composed of 11 gene segments that can be exchanged among RV isolates when animals are infected by more than one virus type at the same time.[308] Therefore mixed infections produce virus with a genetic makeup derived from either parental strain by a mechanism called "gene reassortment." Because the G/P proteins independently are involved in generation of specific VN antibodies, reassortment of these genes during mixed infections can generate new progeny viruses that can evade what once was a protective immune response, thus allowing persistence of RVs in susceptible populations.[309] Thus the possible occurrence of RVs carrying any of 36 possible antigenic configurations (4 Ps × 8 Gs = 32 potential types) underscores the limitation of vaccination programs and also the importance of sound management practices designed to minimize exposure by limiting environmental contamination.

Vaccination Programs

Two approaches are widely used in an attempt to protect calves against RV/CV infection and diarrhea. The most common approach involves passive protection of the suckling neonate by transfer of high levels of specific VN colostral antibodies induced by parenteral vaccination of the pregnant dam.[293,320-328] The mechanism of passive protection with this approach is attributable to the continuing presence of a sufficient amount of specific VN antibodies in the intestinal lumen that can neutralize infectious virus, before infection of the intestinal villus enterocytes.[291,325,329-333] The continuous presence of VN antibodies in the gut lumen also may reduce the severity of the disease if infection has already developed. Additionally, some of the VN colostral antibodies that are absorbed into the bloodstream are secreted onto mucous membranes and may provide local immunity later in life.[334] However, colostral transfer of immunity is less efficient in ruminants than in other species; high concentrations of maternal antibodies are present for less than 3 days postpartum, and these concentrations often fall below protective levels within 1 week of parturition.*

A delicate balance exists between passive protection afforded by lactogenic immunity and development of the calf's own active local immunity in response to RV/CV infection. Because most calves' level of resistance to the adverse clinical effects of RV/CV infection increases with age, disease caused by these agents can be controlled under certain circumstances by continuous hand-feeding of fresh, frozen, or fermented colostrum from vaccinated cows throughout the first 3 to 4

weeks of life.* The goal with this approach is to allow development of subclinical infection while the milk VN antibody concentration is partly protective.[322,334,339] Conversely, lactogenic immunity might interfere with development of active immunity, or some calves might not be exposed to RV/CV infection until after milk antibody concentrations have fallen below protective levels, leaving the calf fully susceptible to infection.[320,322,340]

An RV/CV vaccine for parenteral administration to pregnant cows (Calf Guard†) first became commercially available in 1979. This vaccine contained a single live attenuated G6:P6[1] strain of group A rotavirus. However, because VN antibody concentrations in the colostrum and milk of vaccinated cows were low,[293,294,322] this product later was replaced by a formulation containing inactivated RV/CV (ScourGuard 3[K]‡). More recently an inactivated RV/CV vaccine (Scour Bos§), which contains three strains of group A rotavirus, was licensed for use in pregnant cattle in the United States.

Vaccination of pregnant cows with inactivated RV/CV vaccine can raise the level of VN antibodies in the colostrum.[293,320-329,341] Although there are reports of successful protection of calves against neonatal enteric diseases by parenteral vaccination of pregnant cows with RV/CV,|| negative results also have been reported.[349] Failure of this vaccination strategy generally is attributable to failure of passive transfer of colostral antibodies to the calves or failure to significantly enhance VN antibodies in colostrum. An alternative explanation might be that the serotype/genotype specificity of the passively transferred maternal antibodies may affect the efficacy of the RV vaccine.[350]

Information on protective immunity against infection of calves with group A rotaviruses with the same or a different G/P serotype/genotype configuration as the vaccine strain is incomplete.[314,341,351-355] Although immunity to RV appears to be G/P serotype specific with some strains,[314,341,351,354] there is some indication that immunity directed against certain strains can neutralize in vitro[314,355] and protect challenge-exposed calves in vivo[352,353] against RV strains with different G/P configurations. Also, parenteral vaccination of seropositive cows with a single strain of RV can elicit serum VN antibodies to a broad spectrum of RV serotypes/genotypes, suggesting that this strategy may provide a means of enhancing passive protection against a range of potential RV serotype/genotype challenges.[342,352,353] However, a difference in the P protein between the vaccine RV and the infecting RV was suggested as the basis for failure of the inactivated monovalent RV/CV vaccine in beef cow-calf herds.[356,357]

Another approach for preventing RV/CV enteritis involves oral vaccination of neonatal calves with an MLV vaccine (Calf-Guard¶), which contains an attenuated G6:P6[1] strain of group A rotavirus.[358-360] The mechanism of disease prevention with this vaccine is unknown, but interference with infection by virulent virus followed by development of secretory IgM and IgA and/or cell-mediated immunity in the intestinal mucosa have been proposed.[350,361] To achieve adequate protection, the manufacturers recommend that the vaccine be given immediately after birth, before the calf has nursed. This regimen might be applicable to calves whose dams have not been vaccinated. However, because the colostrum of most heifers and cows contains some level of VN

---

*References 322, 323, 327, 328, 332, 337, and 338.
†Calf Guard, Pfizer Animal Health, Exton, PA 19341.
‡ScourGuard 3(K), Pfizer, Inc. New York, NY.
§Scour Bos, Grand Laboratories, Inc., Larchwood, IA 51241.
||References 321-325, 327, 328, 338, and 341-348.
¶Calf-Guard, Pfizer Animal Health, Exton, PA 19341.

---

*References 291, 320, 323, 326, 332, 333, and 335.

antibodies arising from natural exposure,* administration of colostrum should be delayed for several hours after vaccination to avoid inactivation of the vaccine virus. Under commercial conditions, it is nearly impossible to administer vaccine within minutes of birth or to effectively regulate the intake of colostrum in relation to the time of vaccination. Therefore infection before vaccination, neutralization of the vaccine virus by colostral antibodies, and overwhelming challenge with infectious virus shed by unvaccinated, diseased calves might explain the lack of efficacy of this approach.[323,363-368] This is evident from the data obtained in vaccine efficacy evaluation studies in which only a portion of the calves on a farm or a ranch were vaccinated in double-blind or odd-even day vaccination trials.[335,367,368] When all calves were either vaccinated or not vaccinated in sequential comparisons, the morbidity and mortality rates from neonatal enteric disease were significantly reduced by this vaccination strategy,[329,358-360,367,368] but the design and statistical validity of these latter kinds of trials have been questioned.[349,364]

Although not recommended by the manufacturer, the oral attenuated vaccine has been administered to calves with unknown immune status that are raised as veal calves or replacements in heifer development operations.[369] Under these circumstances, vaccination might provide active immunity and protection against potential virus challenge when calves from several different sources are commingled.

Rotavirus and Coronavirus Vaccination Products

ScourGuard 3(K)/C. ScourGuard 3(K)/C† is an inactivated bovine RV/CV vaccine that is combined with K99 *Escherichia coli* bacterin and *Clostridium perfringens* toxoid. Two doses of vaccine should be administered by intramuscular injection to pregnant cows and heifers 6 to 8 weeks before calving. A second dose should be given 2 to 3 weeks before the expected calving date to first-calf heifers and mature cows not previously vaccinated. Cows that have not calved within 40 days after administration of the last vaccine dose should be revaccinated. A single annual booster dose should be administered 2 to 3 weeks before each subsequent calving.

Scour Bos. Scour Bos‡ is an inactivated bovine RV/CV vaccine that is combined with a K99 *E. coli* bacterin and *C. perfringens* type C toxoid. The vaccine contains four different *E. coli* K99 serotypes and three different group A rotavirus strains, which encompass all the common G/P types encountered in the United States. The vaccine should be administered by deep intramuscular injection into the neck of pregnant cows and heifers up to 10 weeks before the expected calving date. A booster dose of Scour Bos RV/CV vaccine must be given about 6 weeks later during the first year. Only one annual dose up to 10 weeks before calving is required thereafter.

Calf-Guard. Calf-Guard is a modified live RV/CV vaccine recommended for oral vaccination of newborn calves. The manufacturers recommend that the vaccine be administered immediately after birth, before the calf has nursed. As mentioned earlier, interference by maternal antibodies may limit the efficacy of the vaccine.

REFERENCES

291. Acres SD, Babiuk LA: Studies on rotaviral antibody in bovine serum and lacteal secretions using radioimmunoassay, *J Am Vet Med Assoc* 173:555-559, 1978.

*References 291, 293-295, 320-328, 332, 336, 337, 341, 345, 347, 349, 353, and 362.
†ScourGuard 3(K)/C, Pfizer Animal Health, Exton, PA 19341.
‡Scour Bos, Grand Laboratories, Inc, Larchwood, IA 51241.

292. Schlafer DH, Scott FW: Prevalence of neutralizing antibody to the calf rotavirus in New York cattle, *Cornell Vet* 69:262-271, 1979.
293. Myers LL, Snodgrass DR: Colostral and milk antibody titers in cows vaccinated with a modified live rotavirus-coronavirus vaccine, *J Am Vet Med Assoc* 181:486-488, 1982.
294. Rodak L, Babiuk LA, Acres SD: Detection by radioimmunoassay and enzyme-linked immunosorbent assay of coronavirus antibodies in bovine serum and lacteal secretions, *J Clin Microbiol* 16:34-40, 1982.
295. Brüssow H et al: Prevalence of antibodies to four bovine rotavirus strains in different age groups of cattle, *Vet Microbiol* 25:143-151, 1990.
296. Crouch CF, Acres SD: Prevalence of rotavirus and coronavirus antigens in the faeces of normal cows, *Can J Comp Med* 48:340-342, 1984.
297. Crouch CF et al: Chronic shedding of bovine coronavirus antigen-antibody complexes by clinically normal cows, *J Gen Virol* 66:1489-1500, 1985.
298. Collins JK et al: Shedding of enteric coronavirus in adult cattle, *Am J Vet Res* 48:361-365, 1987.
299. Parwani AV, Luchelli A, Saif LJ: Identification of group B rotaviruses with short genome electropherotypes from adult cows with diarrhea, *J Clin Microbiol* 34:1303-1305, 1996.
300. Tsunemitsu H, Saif LJ: Antigenic and biological comparisons of bovine coronaviruses derived from neonatal calf diarrhea and winter dysentery of adult cattle, *Arch Virol* 140:1303-1311, 1995.
301. Kapikian AZ, Channock RM: Rotaviruses. In Fields BN, Knipe DM, Howley PM, eds: *Fields virology*, Philadelphia, 1996, Lippincott-Raven.
302. Vonderfecht SL et al: Identification of a bovine enteric syncytial virus as a nongroup A rotavirus, *Am J Vet Res* 47:1913-1918, 1986.
303. Theil KW, McCloskey CM: Molecular epidemiology and subgroup determination of bovine group A rotaviruses associated with diarrhea in dairy and beef calves, *J Clin Microbiol* 27:126-131, 1989.
304. Tsunemitsu H et al: Evidence of serologic diversity within group C rotaviruses, *J Clin Microbiol* 30:3009-3012, 1992.
305. Chinsangaram J et al: Prevalence of group A and group B rotaviruses in the feces of neonatal dairy calves from California, *Comp Immunol Microbiol Infect Dis* 18:93-103, 1995.
306. Hoshino Y et al: Serotypic similarity and diversity or rotaviruses of mammalian and avian origin as studied by plaque-reduction neutralization, *J Infect Dis* 149:694-702, 1984.
307. Estes MK, Cohen J: Rotavirus gene structure and function, *Microbiol Rev* 53:410-499, 1989.
308. Estes MK: Rotaviruses and their replication. In Fields BN, Knipe DM, Howley PM, eds: *Fields virology*, Philadelphia, 1996, Lippincott-Raven.
309. Hoshino Y et al: Independent segregation of two antigenic specificities (VP3 and VP7) involved in neutralization of rotavirus infectivity, *Proc Natl Acad Sci USA* 82:8701-8704, 1985.
310. Offit PA, Shaw RD, Greenberg HB: Passive protection against rotavirus-induced diarrhea by monoclonal antibodies to surface proteins VP3 and VP7, *J Virol* 58:700-703, 1986.
311. Offit PA et al: Role of gene segments 4 and 9 in determining rotavirus virulence and protection against rotavirus challenge. In Brown F, Channock RM, Lerner RA, eds: *Vaccine 86*, New York, 1986, Cold Spring Harbor Laboratory.
312. Hussein HA et al: Detection of rotavirus G1, G2, G3, and G11 in feces of diarrheic calves by using polymerase chain reaction–derived cDNA probes, *J Clin Microbiol* 31:2491-2496, 1993.
313. Parwani AV et al: Characterization of field strains of group A bovine rotaviruses by using polymerase chain reaction–generated G and P type-specific cDNA probes, *J Clin Microbiol* 31:2010-2015, 1993.
314. Woode GN et al: Antigenic relationships among some bovine rotaviruses: serum neutralization and cross-protection in gnotobiotic calves, *J Clin Microbiol* 18:358-364, 1983.
315. Bellinzoni RC et al: Serological characterization of bovine rotaviruses isolated from dairy and beef herds in Argentina, *J Clin Microbiol* 27:2619-2623, 1989.
316. Matsuda Y, Nakagomi O, Offit PA: Presence of three P types (VP4 types) and two G types (VP7 types) among bovine rotavirus strains, *Arch Virol* 115:199-207, 1990.
317. Snodgrass DR, Fitzgerald T, Campbell I: Rotavirus serotypes 6 and 10 predominate in cattle, *J Clin Microbiol* 27:504-507, 1990.
318. Saif LJ: Animal rotaviruses. In Kapikian AZ, ed: *Viral infections of the gastrointestinal tract*, New York, 1994, Marcel Dekker.
319. Snodgrass DR et al: Identification of four VP4 serological types (P serotypes) of bovine rotavirus using viral reassortants, *J Gen Virol* 73:2319-2325, 1992.
320. Snodgrass DR et al: Passive immunity in calf rotavirus infections: maternal vaccination increases and prolongs immunoglobulin G1 antibody secretion in milk, *Infect Immun* 28:344-349, 1980.
321. Snodgrass DR et al: Diarrhea in dairy calves reduced by feeding colostrum from cows vaccinated with rotavirus, *Res Vet Sci* 32:70-73, 1982.
322. Saif LJ et al: Passive immunity to bovine rotavirus in newborn calves fed colostrum supplements from immunized or nonimmunized cows, *Infect Immun* 41:1118-1131, 1983.
323. Castrucci G et al: The efficacy of colostrum from cows vaccinated with rotavirus in protecting calves from experimentally induced rotavirus infection, *Comp Immunol Microbiol Infect Dis* 7:11-18, 1984.

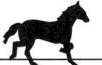

324. Saif LJ et al: Immune response of pregnant cows to bovine rotavirus immunization, *Am J Vet Res* 45:49-58, 1984.

325. Archambault D et al: Immune response of pregnant heifers and cows to bovine rotavirus inoculation and passive protection to rotavirus infection in newborn calves fed colostral antibodies or colostral lymphocytes, *Am J Vet Res* 49:1084-1091, 1988.

326. Sharpee RL, Nelson LD, Beckenhauer WH: Immunogenicity of a vaccine containing inactivated bovine rotavirus and coronavirus combined with an *Escherichia coli* bacterin, Proceedings of the Symposium on Bovine Neonatal Diarrhea, Western Veterinary Conference, Las Vegas, 1988, pp 27-32.

327. Castrucci G et al: Immunization against bovine rotaviral infection, *Eur J Epidemiol* 5:279-284, 1989.

328. Tsunemitsu H et al: Protection against bovine rotaviruses by continuous feeding of immune colostrum, *Jpn J Vet Sci* 51:300-308, 1989.

329. Mebus CA et al: Immunity to neonatal calf diarrhea virus, *J Am Vet Med Assoc* 163:880-883, 1973.

330. Snodgrass DR, Wells PW: The influence of colostrum on neonatal rotaviral infections, *Ann Rech Vet* 9:335-336, 1978.

331. Snodgrass DR, Wells PW: Passive immunity in rotaviral infections, *J Am Vet Med Assoc* 173:565-569, 1978.

332. Woode GN, Jones J, Bridger JC: Levels of colostral antibodies against neonatal calf diarrhea virus, *Vet Rec* 97:148-149, 1975.

333. Torres-Medina A, Schlafer DH, Mebus CA: Rotaviral and coronaviral diarrhea, *Vet Clin North Am (Food Anim Pract)* 1:471-493, 1985.

334. Besser TE et al: Passive immunity to bovine rotavirus infection associated with transfer of serum antibody into the intestinal lumen, *J Virol* 62:2238-2242, 1988.

335. Acres SD, Radostits OM: The efficacy of a modified live reolike virus vaccine and an *E. coli* bacterin for prevention of acute undifferentiated neonatal diarrhea of beef calves, *Can Vet J* 17:197-212, 1976.

336. Crouch CF: Vaccination against enteric rotaviruses and coronaviruses in cattle and pigs: enhancement of lactogenic immunity, *Vaccine* 3:284-291, 1995.

337. Saif LJ, Smith KL: Enteric viral infections of calves and passive immunity, *J Dairy Sci* 68:206-228, 1985.

338. Bürki F et al: Reduction of rotavirus, coronavirus and *E. coli*–associated calf diarrheas in a large-size dairy herd by means of dam vaccination with a triple vaccine, *Zentralbl Veterinarmed [B]* 33:241-252, 1986.

339. Mebus CE: Bovine rotavirus and calf coronavirus diarrhea. In Howard JL, ed: *Current veterinary therapy (food animal practice) 2*, Philadelphia, 1986, WB Saunders.

340. Heckert RA et al: Mucosal and systemic antibody responses to bovine coronavirus structural proteins in experimentally challenge-exposed calves fed low or high amounts of colostral antibodies, *Am J Vet Res* 52:700-708, 1991.

341. Snodgrass DR et al: Bovine rotavirus serotypes and their significance for immunization, *J Clin Microbiol* 20:342-346, 1984.

342. Hudson D: Rota-coronavirus vaccination of pregnant cows, *Mod Vet Pract* 62:226-228, 1981.

343. Eichhorn W et al: Vaccination of pregnant cows with a combined rotavirus/*E. coli* K99 vaccine for preventing diarrhea of newborn calves, *Tierzarztl Umschan* 37:599-600, 602-604, 1982.

344. Van Openbosch E, Wellemans G, Broes A: Prévention des diarrhées néonatales virales du veau: traitement de jeunes veaux avec du lait de vaches vaccinées au moyen d'un vaccin anti-Rotavirus inactivé adjuvé, *Ann Med Vet* 126:157-162, 1982.

345. Fremont Y: Vaccinations antirotavirus et anticoronavirus chez les bovins: éléments pratiques du choix entre les vaccinations de la vache ou du veau, *Rec Med Vet* 159:345-349, 1983.

346. Snodgrass DR: Evaluation of a combined rotavirus and enterotoxigenic *Escherichia coli* vaccine in cattle, *Vet Rec* 119:39-43, 1986.

347. Bellinzoni RC et al: Efficacy of an inactivated oil-adjuvanted rotavirus vaccine in the control of calf diarrhoea in beef herds in Argentina, *Vaccine* 7:263-269, 1989.

348. Cornaglia EM et al: Reduction in morbidity due to diarrhea in nursing beef calves by use of an inactivated oil-adjuvanted rotavirus–*Escherichia coli* vaccine in the dam, *Vet Microbiol* 30:191-202, 1992.

349. Waltner-Toews D et al: A field trial to evaluate the efficacy of a combined rotavirus-coronavirus/*Escherichia coli* vaccine in dairy cattle, *Can J Comp Med* 49:1-9, 1985.

350. Offit PA, Clark HF: Maternal antibody–mediated protection against gastroenteritis due to rotavirus in newborn mice is dependent on both serotype and titer of antibody, *J Infect Dis* 152:1152-1158, 1985.

351. Murakami Y et al: Prolonged excretion and failure of cross-protection between distinct serotypes of bovine rotavirus, *Vet Microbiol* 12:7-14, 1986.

352. Brüssow H et al: Cross-neutralizing antibodies induced by single serotype vaccination of cows with rotavirus, *J Gen Virol* 69:1647-1658, 1988.

353. Snodgrass DR et al: Homotypic and heterotypic serological responses to rotavirus neutralization epitopes in immunologically naive and experienced animals, *J Clin Microbiol* 29:2668-2672, 1991.

354. Woode GN et al: Protection between different serotypes of bovine rotavirus in gnotobiotic calves: specificity of serum antibody and coproantibody responses, *J Clin Microbiol* 25:1052-1058, 1987.

355. Xu Z, Woode GN: Studies on the role of VP4 of G serotype 10 rotavirus (B223) in the induction of the heterologous immune response in calves, *Virology* 196:294-297, 1993.

356. Grotelueschen DM et al: Possible vaccination failure in beef cow herds caused by infection with rotavirus distinct from the vaccine virus: clinical observations, Proceedings of the Seventeenth World Buiatrics Congress and the Twenty-Fifth Annual Convention of the American Association of Bovine Practitioners, St Paul, Minn, Aug 31-Sept 4, 1992, pp 190-196.

357. Lu W et al: Serological and genotypic characterization of group A rotavirus reassortants from diarrheic calves born to dams vaccinated against rotavirus, *Vet Microbiol* 42:159-170, 1994.

358. Mebus CA et al: Results of a field trial using a reolike virus vaccine, *Vet Med Small Anim Clin* 67:173-178, 1972.

359. Twiehaus MJ, Mebus CA: Licensing and use of the calf scour vaccine, *Proc 77th Ann Mtg US Anim Health Assoc*, 1973, pp 55-58.

360. Twiehaus MJ, Mebus CA, Bass EP: Survey of the field efficacy of reoviral calf diarrhea vaccine, *Vet Med Small Anim Clin* 70:23-25, 1975.

361. Mebus CA et al: Immune response to orally administered calf reoviruslike agent and coronavirus vaccine, *Dev Biol Stand* 33:396-403, 1976.

362. Van Oppenbosch E, Wellemans G, Strobbe R, et al: Évolution des anticorps anti rotavirus dans le lait de vaches traitées en fin de gestation soit par le vaccin anti rota complet, soit par l'adjuvant seul, *Comp Immunol Microbiol Infect Dis* 4:293-300, 1981.

363. De Leeuw PW et al: Rotavirus infections in calves: efficacy of oral vaccination in endemically infected herds, *Res Vet Sci* 29:142-147, 1980.

364. Bürki F, Schusser G, Szekely H: Clinical, virological and serological evaluation of the efficacy of peroral live rotavirus vaccination in calves kept under normal husbandry conditions, *Zentralbl Veterinarmed [B]* 30:237-250, 1983.

365. De Leeuw PW, Tiessink JWA: Laboratory experiments on oral vaccination of calves against rotavirus- or coronavirus-induced diarrhea, *Zentralbl Veterinarmed [B]* 32:55-64, 1985.

366. Van Zaane D, Ijzerman J, DeLeeuw PW: Intestinal antibody response after vaccination and infection with rotavirus of calves fed colostrum with or without rotavirus antibody, *Vet Immunol Immunopathol* 11:45-63, 1986.

367. Blackmer PE: A practitioner's experience with experimental reocoronavirus calf diarrhea vaccine, Proceedings of the Eighth Annual Convention of the American Association of Bovine Practitioners, Atlanta, Dec 10-13, 1975, pp 22-24.

368. Thurber ET, Bass EP, Beckenhauer WH: Field trial evaluation of a reocoronavirus calf diarrhea vaccine, *Can J Comp Med* 41:131-136, 1977.

369. McDonough SP, Stull CL, Osburn BI: Enteric pathogens in intensively reared veal calves, *Am J Vet Res* 55:1516-1520, 1994.

BACTERIAL SCOURS VACCINES

VICTOR S. CORTESE
CHARLES A. HJERPE

Enterotoxigenic *Escherichia coli* (Calf Scours) Bacterins

GENERAL CONSIDERATIONS. Most cases of scours caused by *Escherichia coli* occur within the first 72 hours of life. More than 90% of these cases are caused by *E. coli* containing the K99 pilus attachment fimbriae.[370-372] These strains also may have other fimbriae types, such as F41 and F1 (type 1).[370,373] Villus attachment and colonization by strains of enterotoxigenic *E. coli* having multiple fimbriae types appear to be effectively prevented by vaccination with bacterins that have only a single pilus antigen in common with challenge strains.[370,373] However, disease occasionally may be caused by non-K99 *E. coli*.[374] The attaching and effacing *E. coli* types, which may cause disease at 7 to 21 days of age, often do not produce K99 pilus and are not protected by current *E. coli* K99 bacterins.[375,376] This apparent lack of efficacy may be seen with other non-K99 *E. coli*, therefore typing of *E. coli* isolates from scours cases may be important in determining which vaccine to use.

Because *E. coli* scours occurs so early in life, the newborn calf does not have enough time to derive protection from vaccination. Therefore control of *E. coli* infection has been aimed at controlling calf exposure to the pathogens and vaccinating the cow to increase the colostral antibody levels against this pathogen (i.e., usually against the K99 pilus antigen).[373]

Cows are vaccinated in late gestation to ensure high concentrations of anti-K99 colostral antibodies. When colostrum from vaccinated cows is fed to newborn calves, the antibodies act in the small intestine to block the pili from binding to specific receptor sites on the brush border of small intestinal villus enterocytes.[370,377] E. coli bacteria that are prevented from attaching to the jejunal and ileal villi are carried into the large bowel by peristalsis. In this way, colonization of villi and production of enterotoxin are avoided. By the time they are 48 to 96 hours old, most calves are highly resistant to infection.[370,378] Thus feeding calves colostrum with a high concentration of antibodies against K99 antigen, even though restricted to the first day of life, often is sufficient to prevent the disease.[373] Passive circulating humoral antibodies, which are absorbed into the bloodstream from the calf's gut, are thought to play little or no role in immunity to neonatal enteric disease caused by enterotoxigenic E. coli.[370]

Nearly all strains of enterotoxigenic E. coli that have been isolated from neonatal calves have K99 pili.[370-372] Currently there is no evidence that bacterins with multiple pilus antigen types are more effective than those with only one pilus antigen type, as long as the vaccine and the challenge strains share a common pilus antigen.[370] However, vaccines with multiple pilus antigens are more likely to have at least one of the antigens found on the virulent challenge strain of E. coli.

***ESCHERICIA COLI* VACCINATION PROGRAMS.** The general recommendations for use of E. coli bacterins are summarized in Table 44-11. E coli bacterins are offered as single-antigen vaccines and in combination with other antigens. Oil-adjuvant E. coli bacterins are administered by intramuscular injection in a single dose 2 weeks to 6 months before calving and repeated annually.[379] Non-oil-adjuvant E. coli bacterins are recommended for intramuscular or subcutaneous injection in two doses administered at a 2- to 4-week interval, with the second dose given 2 to 3 weeks before calving. In subsequent years a single booster dose should be administered 2 to 3 weeks before calving. E. coli bacterins do not protect calves that do not ingest sufficient amounts of colostrum sufficiently soon after birth.

REFERENCES

370. Acres SD: Enterotoxigenic *Escherichia coli* infections in newborn calves: a review, *J Dairy Sci* 68:229-256, 1985.
371. Haggard DL: Bovine enteric colibacillosis, *Vet Clin North Am (Food Anim Pract)* 1:495-508, 1985.
372. Jayappa HG, Strayer JG, Goodnow RA: Controlling colibacillosis in neonatal calves. I. Evaluation of multiple-pilus, multiple-capsule, phase-cloned *Escherichia coli* bacterin. II. Virulence and prevalence of *Escherichia coli* bearing type 1 pili among isolates from neonatal calf diarrhea, *Vet Med/SAC* 78:388-393, 1984.
373. Moon HW, Bunn TO: Vaccines for preventing enterotoxigenic *Escherichia coli* infections in farm animals, *Vaccine* 11:213-220, 1993.
374. Morris JA, Chanter N, Sherwood D: Occurrence and properties of FY(Att25) *Escherichia coli* associated with diarrhea in calves, *Vet Rec* 121:189-191, 1987.
375. Janke BH et al: Attaching and effacing *Escherichia coli* infection as a cause of diarrhea in young calves, *J Am Vet Med Assoc* 196:897-901, 1990.

TABLE 44-11

Currently Licensed* *Escherichia coli* Bacterin-Toxoids, *Salmonella* Bacterins, and Core Endotoxoid Vaccines

Antigens	Vaccine	Vaccination Regimen	Manufacturer
ESCHERICHIA COLI			
K99	Pili Shield	One dose 2 weeks before calving	Grand Laboratories (Larchwood, IA 51241)
K99, K88, F41, 987P	Prosystem 3	*Year 1:* Two doses 5 weeks and 2 weeks before calving *Subsequent years:* One dose 2 weeks before calving	Intervet (Millsboro, DE 19966)
K99	ScourGuard 3(K)	*Year 1:* Two doses 5 weeks and 2 weeks before calving *Subsequent years:* One dose 3 weeks before calving	Pfizer Animal Health (Exton, PA 19341)
K99, K88, F41, 987P	*E. coli* Bac	*Year 1:* Two doses 5 weeks and 2 weeks before calving *Subsequent years:* One dose 2 weeks before calving	AgriLaboratories (St. Joseph, MO 64503)
?	Piliguard *E. coli*	One dose 3 weeks to 6 months before calving	Schering-Plough Animal Health (Union, NJ 07083)
SALMONELLA			
S. typhimurium	Pro-Bac 3 and 4	Two doses 2 weeks apart	American Veterinary Laboratory (San Angelo, TX 76903)
	Salmo-Shield T	Two doses 2 to 4 weeks apart	Grand Laboratories (Larchwood, IA 51241)
S. dublin/ S. typhimurium	PolySal B	Two doses 2 to 4 weeks apart	American Animal Health (Fort Worth, TX 76140)
	Salmonella dublin/ typhimurium Bacterin	Two doses 2 to 3 weeks apart	Colorado Serum Co. (Denver, CO 80216)
S. dublin	*Salmonella dublin* Modified live	Two doses 2 weeks apart; start at age 2 weeks or older	Fort Dodge Laboratories (Fort Dodge, IA 50501)
	Salmo-Shield TD	Two doses 2 to 4 weeks apart	Grand Laboratories (Larchwood, IA 51241)
CORE ANTIGENS			
Re *S. typhimurium* mutant (endotoxin core)	Endovac-Bovi	*Year 1:* Two doses 5 weeks and 2 weeks before calving *Subsequent years:* One dose 2 weeks before calving	Immuvac (Columbia, MO 65201)
J5 *E. coli* mutant endotoxin core	J Vac	*Year 1:* Three doses 5 weeks and 2 weeks before calving *Subsequent years:* Two doses	Merial (Iselin, NJ 08830)
	J-5	*Year 1:* Two doses 5 weeks and 2 weeks before calving *Subsequent years:* One dose 2 weeks before calving	Bayer Animal Health (Shawnee Mission, KS 66201)

*Licensed by the Animal and Plant Health Inspection Service, U.S. Department of Agriculture.

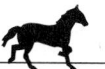

376. Zeman DH, Thomson JU, Francis DH: Diagnosis, treatment, and management of enteric colibacillosis, *Vet Med* Aug 1989, pp 794-802.

377. Morris JA, Wray AC, Sojka WJ: Passive protection of lambs against enteropathogenic *E. coli:* role of antibodies in serum and colostrum of dams vaccinated with K99 antigen, *J Med Microbiol* 13:265-271, 1980.

378. Sith HW, Halls S: Observations on the ligated intestinal segment and oral inoculation methods on *Escherichia* infections in pigs, calves, lambs and rabbits, *J Pathol Bacteriol* 93:499-529, 1967.

379. Collins NF et al: Duration of immunity and efficacy of an oil emulsion *Escherichia coli* bacterin in cattle, *Am J Vet Res* 49:674-677, 1988.

SALMONELLA VACCINES

Salmonella outbreaks can be caused by myriad *Salmonella* strains. These bacteria may cause diarrhea or septicemia or both. Most outbreaks in cattle have involved either *Salmonella dublin* or *Salmonella typhimurium,* therefore all commercial *Salmonella* vaccines contain either *S. typhimurium* alone or *S. typhimurium* and *S. dublin.* All currently licensed products are formalin-inactivated, whole-cell, aluminum hydroxide–absorbed bacterins, except for a new MLV vaccine. The gram negative core antigen vaccines may also provide some protection from morbidity and mortality associated with salmonellosis.

Killed *Salmonella* bacterins can produce measurable antibody responses to bacterial proteins in calves and mature cattle. However, calves vaccinated with a killed bacterin are not able to produce antilipopolysaccharide (anti-LPS) antibodies until 12 weeks of age,[380] and optimum responsiveness does not occur until 1 year of age.[381] Most controlled studies in which calves were vaccinated with a killed *Salmonella* bacterin and orally challenged reported lack of protection.[382-384] One small study, which reported good protection after vaccination of 3- to 6-week-old calves with two doses of killed bacterin, used intramuscular challenge.[385] Another study in 6-month-old cattle found that a single intradermal dose of heat-killed *S. dublin* protected against intravenous challenge.[386] Vaccination of cattle 3 months of age or older with two doses of killed *Salmonella* bacterins is likely to be useful for preventing salmonellosis.

Vaccination of adult cows, with passive transfer of antibody to calves through colostrum, frequently is used in dairies to control calfhood salmonellosis. Controlled trials evaluating passive protection have produced mixed results, some indicating lack of protection,[384,387] and others demonstrating some protection in very young calves (5 days old).[388] Vaccination of dry cows may be useful for helping to control salmonellosis in calves younger than 3 weeks of age but is probably minimally effective for controlling salmonellosis in calves older than 3 or 4 weeks. Anecdotal reports exist of protection against salmonellosis from vaccinating young calves several times with a gram negative core antigen vaccine (Endovac-Bovi*). Another gram negative core antigen vaccine, a J5 *E. coli* bacterin (J Vac†, J-5‡), reduced the mortality rate from naturally occurring salmonellosis in dairy calves vaccinated at 3 and 17 days of age.[389]

REFERENCES

380. Roden LD et al: Effect of calf age and *Salmonella* bacterin type on ability to produce immunoglobulins directed against *Salmonella* whole cells or lipopolysaccharide, *Am J Vet Res* 53:1895-1899, 1992.

381. House JK et al: Enzyme-linked immunosorbent assay for serologic detection of *Salmonella dublin* carriers on a large dairy, *Am J Vet Res* 54:1391-1399, 1993.

382. Henning MW: Calf paratyphoid. III. The transmission of antibodies to newly born calves, *Onderstepoort J Vet Res* 26:45-59, 1953.

383. Robertson JA et al: *Salmonella typhimurium* infection in calves: protection and survival of virulent challenge bacteria after immunization with live or inactivated vaccines, *Infect Immun* 41:742-750, 1983.

384. Smith BP et al: Immunization of calves against salmonellosis, *Am J Vet Res* 41:1947-1951, 1980.

385. Bairey MH: Immunization of calves against salmonellosis, *J Am Vet Med Assoc* 173:610-613, 1978.

386. Aitken MM, Jones PW, Brown GTH: Protection of cattle against experimentally induced salmonellosis by intradermal injection of heat-killed *Salmonella dublin, Res Vet Sci* 32:368-373, 1982.

387. Rankin JD, Taylor RJ: An attempt passively to immunize calves against *Salmonella* infection by vaccination of their dams, *Vet Rec* 86:254-256, 1970.

388. Jones PW, Collins P, Aitken MM: Passive protection of calves against experimental infection with *Salmonella typhimurium, Vet Rec* 123:536-541, 1988.

389. Daigneault J et al: Effect of vaccination with the R mutant *Escherichia coli* (J5) antigen on morbidity and mortality of dairy calves, *Am J Vet Res* 52:1492-1496, 1991.

GRAM NEGATIVE, CORE ANTIGEN, OIL-ADJUVANT BACTERINS

All genera and species of gram negative bacteria contain a common set of gram negative core antigens, which are present in the deeper layers of the bacterial cell wall.[390] Endotoxin from gram negative bacteria is thought to play an important role in the production of the clinical signs, biochemical and hematologic alternations, and pathologic lesions associated with a wide variety of bovine diseases caused by gram negative bacteria,[390] including coliform mastitis (caused by *Escherichia coli, Klebsiella* spp., or *Enterobacter aerogenes*), *Pasteurella* bronchopneumonia and fibrinous pneumonia, and salmonellosis. Gram negative core antigen vaccines are designed to reduce the severity of clinical signs associated with gram negative sepsis and endotoxemia. They offer breadth against all gram negative infections.

General Considerations

Three gram negative, core-antigen, oil-adjuvant vaccines are currently marketed. Two use the J5 Rc-mutant strain of *E. coli.* This strain of *E. coli* lacks the (serotype-specific O chain) surface antigens that ordinarily prevent deeper cell wall antigens from contacting the host immune system and stimulating production of antibodies against gram negative core antigens.[390] The third vaccine uses an Re-mutant strain of *Salmonella typhimurium.*

Theoretically, gram negative core-antigen vaccines would be expected to reduce the severity of disease manifestations but not the rate of occurrence of disease. In four different clinical trials, however, the incidence of clinical coliform mastitis in dairy cows was reduced by 69%, 72%, 80%, and 82%, respectively, by vaccination with a J5 *E. coli* vaccine.[391-393] These data are consistent with the hypothesis that antibodies induced against gram negative core antigens assist both in the destruction and removal of intact bacteria and in the neutralization of endotoxin. In the trial in which clinical coliform mastitis was reduced by 82%, however, vaccination did not reduce the incidence of subclinical intramammary coliform infections that were present at the time of calving.[393]

Vaccination Programs

Recommendations for use of these bacterins to prevent coliform mastitis and scours are summarized in Table 44-11. Cows should not receive any other vaccine containing gram negative organisms (*Pasteurella, Salmonella, Brucella, Campylobacter* [*Vibrio*], *Haemophilus somnus, E. coli,* or *Moraxella bovis* bacterins) within 5 days of vaccination with J5 Bacterin.

A J5 *E. coli* bacterin also has successfully reduced morbidity and mortality in experimental *S. typhimurium* infections in calves.[394] However, because of the short half-life of passively acquired antibodies stimulated by gram negative core antigen

---

*Endovac Bovi, Endovac, Inc.

†J Vac, Merial, Iselin, NJ 08830.

‡J-5, Bayer Animal Health, Shawnee Mission, KS 66201.

vaccines,[395] vaccination of dry cows is unlikely to be an effective control measure for salmonellosis in calves except when calves are exposed to and infected with salmonellosis in the first week or two after birth. Salmonellosis in dairy calves often occurs after 2 weeks of age. However, when vaccinated at 3 and 10 days of age with an oil-adjuvant J5 E. coli bacterin, calves do develop strong antibody responses by 17 days of age; this strong antibody response occurs even in the presence of passively acquired antibodies to gram negative core antigens.[396] Consequently, a combined program in which both dry cows and neonatal calves are immunized against gram negative core antigens appears to be a promising approach for reducing the severity of salmonellosis in neonatal dairy calves.

In a field study, vaccination of healthy dairy calves with an oil-adjuvant J5 E. coli bacterin at 3 and 17 days of age reduced the mortality rate from salmonellosis.[389] (In this study, the dams were not vaccinated.) In addition, the morbidity rate from undifferentiated respiratory disease was significantly reduced by 9%.[394] In a parallel study in poorly nourished calves, however, vaccination actually increased the cumulative 60-day mortality by 113%.[389] These kinds of vaccines may prove more effective for reducing the severity of *Pasteurella* infections of the lung when used in older calves.

REFERENCES

390. Tyler JW et al: Immunity targeting common core antigens of gram negative bacteria, *J Vet Intern Med* 4:17-25, 1990.
391. Gonzales RN et al: Prevention of clinical coliform mastitis in dairy cows by a mutual *Escherichia coli* vaccine, *Can J Vet Res* 53:301-305, 1989.
392. Borelli CL, Weaver LD, Cullor JS: Effect of E. coli J5 vaccination on incidence of clinical coliform mastitis and milk production loss in dairy cows, Proceedings of the Eleventh Annual Western Food Animal Disease Conference, John Ascuaga's Nugget, Reno/Sparks, Nevada, March 7-8, 1990.
393. Hogan JS et al: Field trial to determine efficacy of an *Escherichia coli* J5 mastitis vaccine, *J Dairy Sci* 75:78-84, 1992.
394. Cullor JS, Fenwick BW, Smith BP: Decreased mortality and severity of infection from salmonellosis in calves immunized with E. coli (strain J5), abstract no 352, *Proceedings of the Sixty-Sixth Annual Conference of Research Workers in Animal Diseases*, Chicago, 1985.
395. Douglas VL et al: Rapid decay of serum IgG recognizing gram negative cell wall core antigens in neonatal calves, *Am J Vet Res* 50:1138-1140, 1989.
396. Tyler JW et al: Humoral response in neonatal calves following immunization with *Escherichia coli* (strain J5): the effects of adjuvant, age, and colostral passive interference, *Vet Immunol Immunopathol* 23:333-344, 1989.

CLOSTRIDIAL VACCINES

J. GLENN SONGER

Clostridia cause acute and often fatal disease in which the pathogenesis often is mediated by toxic proteins.[397] Prevention often is based on immunoprophylactic amelioration of the effects of these molecules. However, the ready availability of inexpensive, efficacious bacterins, toxoids, and bacterin-toxoids has not eliminated clostridial infections. Accurate diagnosis remains an important component of management of clostridial diseases.[398,399]

Immunization against clostridial diseases can be complicated by the development of "site reactions," leading to trimming at slaughter.[400] These problems, which are exacerbated by the multivalent nature of many modern products, have stimulated the biologics industry to seek a new paradigm for preparation and delivery of immunoprophylactic products. Approaches have included concentration of the antigen into a smaller dose and use of alternate adjuvants; recombinant proteins, delivered by conventional means, by application of "slow-release" media or by in vivo expression from attenuated bacterial delivery systems probably will be a major focus of effort.

Clostridium chauvoei (Blackleg) Bacterins

Blackleg is not uncommon despite the long-term availability of generally effective bacterins. Ingestion probably is the most common route of exposure in cattle, and dormant spores seeded to skeletal muscle germinate when muscle damage provides appropriate conditions. Affected animals have fever, anorexia, depression, and lameness, with extensive dry and emphysematous to edematous, hemorrhagic, and necrotic lesions. Diagnostically it is important to distinguish between blackleg and malignant edema.

As with other histotoxic clostridial infections, vaccination against blackleg is universally advocated, especially in cattle under 2 years of age. Dogma is that protection arises from the immune response to a heat-labile soluble antigen, but *Clostridium chauvoei* produces α toxin and several other toxic factors that may be equally important targets.[401,402] Recommendations for immunization are summarized in Table 44-12.

Clostridium septicum (Malignant Edema) Bacterins

Wound infections caused by *Clostridium septicum* (malignant edema)[403] usually follow direct contamination of a traumatic wound, including genital tract infections that occur after mismanaged deliveries. Infection spreads along fascial planes, and lesions proceed from warm and pitting to crepitant and cold. Death commonly occurs in less than 24 hours. Braxy is a form of enteric infection that is not uncommon in calves.[404]

TABLE 44-12

General Considerations for Use of Clostridial 7-Way and 8-Way Bacterin-Toxoids*

Pathogen Regimen‡	7-Way Coverage† (Dose: 2-5 ml)	8-Way Coverage (Dose: 5 ml)
C. chauvoei	X	X
C. septicum	X	X
C. novyi type B	X	X
C. novyi type D (C. haemolyticum)	X	
C. sordellii	X	X
C. perfringens type B§	X	X
C. perfringens type C	X	X
C. perfringens type D	X	X

*These biologics should not be used within 21 days of slaughter.
†Many combinations are available commercially, including some that also have immunogens against nonclostridial diseases. Some of these combinations include tetanus toxoid.
‡Calves vaccinated initially at less than 3 months of age should be revaccinated at 4 to 6 months of age or at weaning.
§No currently licensed product is produced by use of cultures of C. perfringens type B; however, protection against type B infection is implied by inclusion of a toxoid prepared against type C (β toxin) and type D (ε toxin) strains.

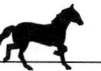

The diagnosis often is made by use of a fluorescent antibody test.[405]

A single immunizing dose of *C. septicum* bacterin yields adequate protection, but annual booster vaccination is recommended in high-risk situations.[406] Vaccines elicit antibody responses to both somatic and toxin antigens, and recent findings suggest a central role for α toxin.[407,408]

Clostridium novyi Types A and B (Bighead and Infectious Necrotic Hepatitis) Bacterins and Clostridium haemolyticum (C. novyi Type D) (Bacillary Hemoglobinuria) Bacterins

Clostridium novyi toxigenic types A and B cause myonecrosis in human beings (gas gangrene) and domestic animals (bighead of sheep) and infectious necrotic hepatitis (black disease) in sheep and cattle.[409] The hallmark lesion is edema, likely resulting from vascular damage caused by α toxin. Spores often lie dormant in Kupffer cells but germinate when liver injury provides appropriate conditions. Type C strains are nontoxigenic and thus nonpathogenic.[410]

Clostridium haemolyticum (*C. novyi* type D) β toxin mediates the pathogenesis of redwater, usually in well-nourished animals at least 1 year old. Liver damage by migrating flukes encourages germination of dormant spores in Kupffer cells. Dissemination of β toxin via the bloodstream results in intravascular hemolysis, hemorrhage, and hemoglobinuria,[411,412] and death ultimately results from anoxia. A vaccination program is essential for herds pastured in endemic areas. Where exposure to fluke metacercariae is light, a single annual dose of bacterin should be administered to all cattle over 6 months of age before they are pastured in the spring. Where exposure to flukes is heavy, a booster dose should be administered in season. The prominent role of the α and β toxins suggests that they may find use in second-generation immunoprophylactic products.

Clostridium botulinum (Botulism) and Clostridium tetani (Tetanus)

Botulism is caused by *Clostridium botulinum* neurotoxins, which block the release of acetylcholine from cholinergic nerve endings.[413,414] *C. botulinum* type C is most common in cattle in the United States. Direct contamination of feeds by the organism sometimes leads to intoxication, but the condition is more commonly associated with the presence of an animal carcass in the feed. Clinical signs include incoordination, flaccid paralysis, and difficulty swallowing; respiratory paralysis eventually causes death.[415,416]

Toxoids of botulinum toxins can be use for immunoprophylaxis, but vaccination usually is practiced only in populations at immediate risk, such as beef cattle grazing on phosphorus-deficient rangeland.[417] The feeding of poultry litter poses a similar problem in that such feed may contain animal remains.

Spores of *Clostridium tetani* originate in soil and usually are introduced traumatically into animal hosts, where they germinate and produce tetanus neurotoxin.[418] Tetanus can develop in dairy cows as a postparturient complication and in calves after castration by the elastrator method.[419] Toxin moves retrograde, binding to presynaptic axonal terminals and resulting in muscular tremor and increased stimulus response; continued motor neuron hyperactivity causes sustained tetanic spasms in the innervated muscles and then permanent rigidity. Death is caused by respiratory failure.

Acquired resistance to tetanus is based on circulating antitoxin, and widespread vaccination with toxoid has dramatically lessened the impact of tetanus on animal production. Neonatal passive immunity is followed by active immunization with toxoid after 2 to 3 months. Boosters are commonly

recommended at 1- to 5-year intervals. Passive immunotherapy is directed toward neutralization of preformed toxin, although it is much more effective when used prophylactically than therapeutically. Universal vaccination is not usually recommended as a cost-effective means of controlling tetanus.

Clostridium perfringens Toxoids

Clostridium perfringens causes a wide variety of diseases in domestic animals, and those of greatest importance affect the gastrointestinal tract (Table 44-13).[420] *C. perfringens* type B infections are apparently extraordinarily rare in the United States, but it has been speculated that their pathogenesis can be explained by additive or synergistic effects of β and ε toxins. Type C strains multiply rapidly in the gut of neonates, and in this relatively trypsin-free environment, β toxin causes local hemorrhage and necrosis, as well as systemic effects.[421] Type D strains fill intestinal niches opened by sudden dietary changes, and ε toxin in circulation damages the central nervous system and other systems distant from the gut.[422] The type E strain causes hemorrhagic enteritis in calves, and its virulence is based apparently on the action of ι toxin.[423]

The current enigma is type A infections. Although long accepted as causes of lamb enterotoxemia,[424] fowl necrotic enteritis, and enteritis in dogs and horses, type A pathogens increasingly are being recognized as causes of enteritis in piglets and calves. Little is known about the pathogenesis of type A enteric infections, but type A strains are commonly found in cases of tympany, abomasitis, and abomasal hemorrhage and ulceration in calves.[425,426]

Most agree that routine vaccination against type C enterotoxemia is required only in herds in which the disease has been documented. The usual practice is to vaccinate the dam, providing passive immunity through the colostrum. Initial immunization should be followed by a booster after 3 to 4 weeks, with the second dose (and subsequent annual boosters) administered approximately 2 weeks before calving. Type D enterotoxemia is sufficiently uncommon in cattle that many believe vaccination is not cost-effective.

No commercial products are licensed in the United States for use against infections caused by strains of types A and E, and production of autogenous toxoids or bacterin-toxoids has become quite common; anecdotal evidence suggests remarkable efficacy in many cases. Similar vaccines have been produced from strains of type E. These should be used with the awareness that, unlike β and ε toxin concentrations in commercial products, α and ι toxin concentrations in autogenous toxoids may not be optimal.

Clostridium sordellii Bacterins

Clostridium sordellii is commonly found in the feces of domestic animals and in oil and occasionally is isolated in cases

TABLE 44-13

Diseases of Cattle Caused by *Clostridium perfringens*

C. perfringens Type	Diseases	Major Toxins
A	Myonecrosis, enterotoxemia, abomasitis, possible sudden death	α
B	Neonatal hemorrhagic enteritis	α, β, ε
C	Neonatal hemorrhagic or necrotic enterotoxemia	α, β
D	Enterotoxemia	α, ε
E	Enterotoxemia	α, ι

of fatal myositis, liver disease, and sudden death in cattle. Edema in the subcutaneous tissues and along fascial planes of muscles and subendocardial hemorrhage are common signs. The organism produces numerous toxic or putatively toxic substances, foremost of which is a toxin that resembles toxins A and B of *Clostridium difficile*.[427] Immunization is achieved by administration of multiway bacterin-toxoids (see Table 44-12).

REFERENCES

397. Hatheway CL: Toxigenic clostridia, *Clin Microbiol Rev* 3:66, 1990.
398. Songer JG: Clostridial diseases of small ruminants, *Vet Res* 29:219, 1998.
399. Meer RR, Songer JG: Multiplex PCR method for genotyping *Clostridium perfringens, Am J Vet Res* 58:702, 1997.
400. Green DS et al: Injection site reactions and antibody responses in sheep and goats after the use of multivalent clostridial vaccines, *Vet Rec* 120:435, 1987.
401. Gyles CL: Histotoxic clostridia. In Gyles CL, Thoen CO, eds: *Pathogenesis of bacterial infections in animals*, ed 2, Ames, Iowa, 1993, Iowa State University Press.
402. Kerry JB: A note on the occurrence of *Clostridium chauvoei* in the spleen and livers of normal cattle, *Vet Rec* 76:396, 1964.
403. Nervig RM et al: *Clostridium septicum* infection in cattle in the United States, *J Am Vet Med Assoc* 179:479, 1981.
404. Schamber GJ, Berg IE, Molesworth JR: Braxy or bradsotlike abomasitis caused by *Clostridium septicum* in a calf, *Can Vet J* 27:194, 1986.
405. Batty L, Walker PD: Fluorescent-labeled clostridial antisera as specific reagents, *Bull Off Intl Epizoot* 59:1499, 1963.
406. Thompson A, Batty L: The antigenic efficiency of pulpy kidney disease vaccines, *Vet Rec* 65:659-663, 1953.
407. Ballard J et al: Purification and characterization of the lethal toxin (α-toxin) of *Clostridium septicum, Infect Immun* 60:784, 1992.
408. Williamson ED, Titball RW: A genetically engineered vaccine against the α-toxin of *Clostridium perfringens* protects mice against experimental gas gangrene, *Vaccine* 11:1253, 1993.
409. Olander HJ, Hughes JP, Biberstein EL: Bacillary hemoglobinuria: induction by liver biopsy in naturally and experimentally infected animals, *Pathol Vet* 3:421-450, 1966.
410. Niilo L, Dorward WJ, Avery RJ: The role of *Clostridium novyi* in bovine disease in Alberta, *Can Vet J* 10:159, 1969.
411. Nakamura S et al: Taxonomic relationships among *Clostridium novyi* types A and B, *Clostridium haemolyticum*, and *Clostridium botulinum* type C, *J Gen Microbiol* 139:1473, 1983.
412. Erwin BG: Experimental induction of bacillary hemoglobinuria in cattle, *Am J Vet Res* 38:1625, 1977.
413. Smith LD, Sugiyama H: *Botulism: the organism, its toxins, the disease*, Springfield, Ill, 1988, CC Thomas.
414. Simpson LL: The origin, structure, and pharmacological activity of botulinum toxin, *Pharmacol Rev* 33:155, 1981.
415. Kozaki S et al: The use of monoclonal antibodies to analyze the structure of *Clostridium botulinum* type B derivative toxin, *Infect Immun* 52:786, 1986.
416. Rocke TE: *Clostridium botulinum*. In Gyles CL, Thoen CO, eds: *Pathogenesis of bacterial infections in animals*, ed 2, Ames, Iowa, 1993, Iowa State University Press.
417. Greeley RG, Franklin TE: Loin disease, *Southwest Vet* 21:31, 1967.
418. Wallis AS: Some observations of the epidemiology of tetanus in cattle, *Vet Rec* 75:188, 1963.
419. Van Rensberg SJ: Tetanus in calves as a sequela to elastration, *J S Afr Vet Assoc* 30:29, 1959.
420. Rood JI, Cole ST: Molecular genetics and pathogenesis of *Clostridium perfringens, Microbiol Rev* 55:621, 1991.
421. Fleming S: Enterotoxemia in neonatal calves, *Vet Clin North Am (Food Anim Pract)* 1:509, 1985.
422. Buxton D, Morgan KT: Studies of lesions produced in the brains of colostrum-deprived lambs by *Clostridium welchii (C. perfringens)* type D toxin, *J Comp Pathol* 86:435, 1976.
423. Hart B, Hooper PT: Enterotoxemia of calves due to *Clostridium welchii* type E, *Aust Vet J* 43:360, 1967.
424. McGowan G, Moulton JE, Rood SE: Lamb losses associated with *Clostridium perfringens* type A, *J Am Vet Med Assoc* 133:219, 1958.
425. Roeder BL et al: Experimental induction of abomasal tympany, abomasitis, and abomasal ulceration by intraruminal inoculation of *Clostridium perfringens* type A in neonatal calves, *Am J Vet Res* 49:201, 1988.
426. Roeder BL et al: Isolation of *Clostridium perfringens* from neonatal calves with ruminal and abomasal tympany, abomasitis, and abomasal ulceration, *J Am Vet Med Assoc* 190:1550, 1987.
427. Arsecularatne SN, Panabokke RG, Wijesundra S: The toxins responsible for the lesions of *Clostridium sordellii* gas gangrene, *J Med Microbiol* 2:37, 1969.

MISCELLANEOUS BOVINE RICKETTSIAL, BACTERIAL, AND VIRAL DISEASE VACCINES

DEREK MOSIER

Anaplasmosis

Anaplasmosis is a vector-borne disease caused by the rickettsia *Anaplasma marginale*. The disease occurs worldwide but is prevalent in tropical areas. Anaplasmosis is the only major tick-borne disease of cattle in North America, being enzootic in the southeastern and some midwestern and western states and sporadic in the northern states and Canada.[428,429] In enzootic areas with adequate numbers of arthropod vectors, most adult cattle become naturally immune through repeated exposure. Maternal antibodies protect calves until such time that they also become subclinically infected and develop immunity. Disease is more severe in older cattle than in calves, and nonimmune older cattle are particularly at risk when they are moved into an endemic area.[428] Susceptibility to disease occurs when there is a lack of arthropod vectors to maintain natural infection and immunity or when a nonimmune adult is introduced into an enzootic area. In these situations or when vector or environmental conditions suggest an increased risk of disease, vaccination can be beneficial.

Until recently, inactivated emulsion vaccines containing *A. marginale* antigens in adjuvant suspended in 10% oil were commercially available (Anaplaz* and Plazvax†). In endemic areas the vaccines were recommended for use just before the onset of the vector season. Vaccine-induced immunity did not generally occur until 2 weeks after administration of the second dose of an initial series or 2 weeks after a booster dose in previously immunized cattle.[428] Vaccination did not prevent infection or clinical disease and did not eliminate *A. marginale* from a herd, but it did reduce the severity and incidence of disease.[428,429] Inactivated vaccines could be used in conjunction with oxytetracycline in the face of outbreaks to provide both temporary and more prolonged protection.[429] In rare cases erythrocyte antigens in these vaccines caused the production of antierythrocyte antibodies and subsequent neonatal erythrolysis, and the vaccines were discontinued.[430]

Currently, no commercial vaccines against anaplasmosis are available in most areas of North America. A sheep-passaged, MLV vaccine‡ has been used in California and Latin America.[431] Because this vaccine causes mild clinical disease, it has limited use for vaccination of mature susceptible cattle.[428,431] If the vaccine is administered to cattle over 2 years of age, anemia, severe clinical disease, and death may occur, especially in bulls and heavily lactating cows.[431] The vaccine is recommended for use in healthy cattle between 1 month and 2 years of age and is most commonly administered to 7- to 24-month-old cattle in herds in endemic areas. Concurrent use of certain antibiotics or other live or MLV vaccines is contraindicated.

Immunity to *A. marginale* is complex and involves both humoral and cell-mediated mechanisms.[428,432,433] Inadequate protection from vaccines during field use can result from antigenic variability and differences in cross-reactivity between *A. marginale* strains and from weak immune responses to protective *A. marginale* antigens.[428,432,433] Native, recombinant, and tick culture–derived *A. marginale* immunogens may provide the basis for an effective subunit vaccine in the future.[432,434-436]

*Anaplaz, Fort Dodge Laboratories, Fort Dodge, IA 50501.
†Plazvax, Schering-Plough Animal Health, Kenilworth, NJ.
‡Anavac, BioLOGIC Laboratories, Davis, CA 95616.

REFERENCES

428. Richey EJ, Palmer GH: Bovine anaplasmosis, *Compend Cont Educ Pract Vet* 12:1661- 1668, 1990.
429. Richey EJ: Bovine anaplasmosis. In Howard JL, Smith RA, eds: *Current veterinary therapy 4: food animal practice*, Philadelphia, 1999, WB Saunders.
430. Dennis RA et al: Neonatal immunohemolytic anemia and icterus of calves, *J Am Vet Med Assoc* 156:1861-1869, 1970.
431. Henry ET et al: Effects and use of a modified live *Anaplasma marginale* vaccine in beef heifers in California, *J Am Vet Med Assoc* 183:66-69, 1983.
432. Musoke AJ et al: Prospects for subunit vaccines against tick-borne diseases, *Br Vet J* 152:621-639, 1996.
433. Palmer GH: *Anaplasma* vaccines. In Wright IG, ed: *Veterinary protozoan and hemoparasite vaccines*, Boca Raton, Fla, 1989, CRC Press.
434. Palmer GH, McElwain TF: Molecular basis for vaccine development against anaplasmosis and babesiosis, *Vet Parasitol* 57:233-253, 1995.
435. Blouin EF et al: Evaluation of *Anaplasma marginale* from tick cell culture as an immunogen for cattle, *Ann N Y Acad Sci* 849:253-258, 1998.
436. Zaugg JL, Lincoln SD: Protection enhancement against bovine anaplasmosis by simultaneous administration of *Propionibacterium acnes* and a commercial vaccine, *Agri Pract* 16:12-16, 1995.

Infectious Bovine Keratoconjunctivitis

The most common infectious agent associated with infectious bovine keratoconjunctivitis is *Moraxella bovis*.[437] Vaccination is most effective when done before fly season in herds with a history of problems. Certain breeds, such as Herefords and Hereford crosses, are particularly susceptible[437] and may benefit from vaccination. Commercial vaccines used to help prevent the disease consist of inactivated cultures of various strains of *M. bovis*.[437] Recommendations for use vary. Some products recommend two doses given 3 weeks apart for initial vaccination, beginning as early as 3 weeks of age to no earlier than 5 months of age. Other products recommend a single dose administered 3 to 6 weeks before the predicted onset of the disease season, with annual vaccination thereafter. *M. bovis* bacterins are also available in combination with seven-way clostridial bacterin-toxoids.[437] Although multivalent *M. bovis* bacterins can provide protection in field use, efficacy varies depending on the *M. bovis* strains present in the bacterin and those responsible for disease.[438-440] In many cases vaccines provide neither consistent or reliable protection.[439] This most often is due to an inadequate lacrimal (IgA) immune response to pilus antigens, major protective antigens that are serogroup specific.[440,441] The ability of *M. bovis* pili to undergo rapid transitions in antigenicity between serogroups can render monovalent bacterins ineffective.[442] Therefore vaccines must incorporate pili from all major serogroups to provide optimum protection.[442,443] Experimental recombinant vaccines containing cloned pili of various serogroups have shown efficacy in experimental studies[439,441] and may provide the basis for more effective future vaccines.

REFERENCES

437. Ramsey DT: Surface ocular microbiology in food and fiber-producing animals. In Howard JL, Smith RA, eds: *Current veterinary therapy 4: food animal practice*, Philadelphia, 1999, WB Saunders.
438. Bayley AJ: Bovine biologic charts. In Arrioja-Dechert A, ed: *Compendium of veterinary products*, ed 5, Port Huron, Mich, 1999, North American Compendiums.
439. Lepper AWD et al: *Moraxella bovis* pili vaccine produced by recombinant DNA technology for the prevention of infectious bovine keratoconjunctivitis, *Vet Microbiol* 36:175-183, 1993.
440. Lepper AWD et al: The protective efficacy of cloned *Moraxella bovis* pili in monovalent and multivalent vaccine formulations against experimentally induced infectious bovine keratoconjunctivitis (IBK), *Vet Microbiol* 45:129-138, 1995.
441. Smith PC et al: Effectiveness of two commercial infectious bovine keratoconjunctivitis vaccines, *Am J Vet Res* 51:1147-1150, 1990.
442. Lepper AWD et al: The protective efficacy of pili from different strains of *Moraxella bovis* within the same serogroup against infectious bovine keratoconjunctivitis, *Vet Microbiol* 32:177-187, 1992.
443. Bateman KG, Leslie KE, Scholl TP: A field trial of a piliated *Moraxella bovis* bacterin for the prevention of infectious bovine keratoconjunctivitis. *Can Vet J* 27:23-27, 1986.

Staphylococcal Mastitis

Staphylococcus aureus is considered the most important etiologic agent of bovine mastitis. Vaccination against *S. aureus* may be beneficial in dairy herds that have an existing mastitis problem.[444,445] However, vaccination in well-managed dairy herds with a low level of staphylococcal mastitis may not provide much economic benefit.[444] Currently available commercial vaccines consist of lysed cultures of *S. aureus* containing somatic antigens and phage types I, II, III, and IV in aluminum hydroxide adjuvant.[446] The recommended vaccination protocol is two doses given 2 weeks apart followed by revaccination at 6-month intervals. Vaccination can start at 6 months of age, and one of the semiannual doses should be given 3 to 4 weeks before calving. Vaccination does not generally eliminate disease but can substantially reduce clinical mastitis and the incidence of subclinical and chronic staphylococcal infection.[445,447-449] Vaccination may be more effective in heifers because of their initial lower basal immunity compared with older cows.[448] The benefits of immunity induced early in life include the abilities to clear the organism and to resist chronic infection upon initial natural exposure.[450] Vaccination during the dry period may be more effective than vaccination during lactation.[445] In some but not all studies, vaccination has reduced somatic cell counts in milk.[448-450]

In considering the use of staphylococcal vaccines, the prevalence of various pathogens that can cause mastitis must be considered. For mastitis caused by *S. aureus*, differences between the *S. aureus* strains in vaccines and the strains specifically responsible for the disease may diminish the efficacy of the vaccine.[445] In herds in which other pathogens are a major cause of mastitis, *S. aureus* vaccines may be of minimal benefit.[444,447] *Streptococcus agalactiae* vaccines generally are not protective, but other *Streptococcus* spp. are responsive to vaccination.[451]

REFERENCES

444. Watson DL, McColl ML, Davies HI: Field trial of a staphylococcal mastitis vaccine in dairy herds: clinical, subclinical, and microbiological assessments, *Aust Vet J* 74:447-450, 1996.
445. Rebhun WC: Diseases of the teats and udder. In *Diseases of dairy cattle*, Philadelphia, 1995, Williams & Wilkins, 518-610.
446. Bayley AJ: Bovine biologic charts. In Arrioja-Dechert A, ed: *Compendium of veterinary products*, ed 5, Port Huron, Mich, 1999, North American Compendiums.
447. Giraudo JA et al: Field trials of a vaccine against bovine mastitis. I, Evaluation in heifers, *J Dairy Sci* 80:845-853, 1997.
448. Calzolari A et al: Field trials of a vaccine against bovine mastitis. II, Evaluation in two commercial dairy herds, *J Dairy Sci* 80:857-858, 1997.
449. Nordhaug ML et al: A field trial with an experimental vaccine against *Staphylococcus aureus* mastitis in cattle. I. Clinical parameters, *J Dairy Sci* 77:1267-1275, 1994.
450. Widel PW: What about *Staphylococcus aureus* vaccine? *Agri Pract* 15:26-28, 1994.
451. Morresey PR: Bovine mastitis. In Howard JL, Smith RA, eds: *Current veterinary therapy 4: food animal practice*, Philadelphia, 1999, WB Saunders.

Anthrax

Anthrax is an acute, highly fatal disease caused by *Bacillus anthracis*. Vaccination is a relatively effective means of controlling the disease in endemic areas and in the face of outbreaks.[452] Bovine anthrax vaccines are derived from the live toxigenic, nonencapsulated spore vaccine developed by Sterne and consist of spores suspended in a diluent containing saponin and glycerin.[453] Annual vaccination of livestock in areas of endemic anthrax is recommended 4 weeks before outbreaks are expected. A single dose generally provides immunity equivalent to two doses, but a second dose given 2 to 4 weeks after the first often is recommended.[454] Cattle

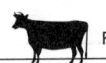

should not be vaccinated within 60 days of slaughter. Antibiotics should not be administered within 7 days of vaccination to avoid interference with in vivo growth of the vaccine organism. Vaccination in the face of an outbreak does not protect all cattle, but the spread of infection usually stops within 10 days.[455] Localized subcutaneous edema commonly develops at the injection site within 24 hours; it may last for several days and is sometimes severe.[456] Recent human vaccine research using different adjuvants and antigen delivery systems may help alleviate some of these side effects in future vaccines.[452,457,458] All outbreaks should be reported to local regulatory and public health officials, and appropriate guidelines for vaccination should be followed, including quarantine and vaccination of all susceptible livestock on affected and surrounding premises.

REFERENCES

452. Turnbull PCB: Anthrax vaccines: past, present, and future, *Vaccine* 95:533-539, 1991.
453. Sterne M: Avirulent anthrax vaccine, *Onderstepoort J Vet Sci* 21:41-43, 1946.
454. Kaufmann AF, Fox MD, Kolb RC: Anthrax in Louisiana, 1971: an evaluation of the Sterne strain anthrax vaccine, *J Am Vet Med Assoc* 163:442-445, 1973.
455. Salmon DD, Ferrier GR: Postvaccination occurrence of anthrax in cattle, *Vet Rec* 130:140-141, 1992.
456. Mosier DA, Chengappa MM: Anthrax. In Howard JL, Smith RA, eds: *Current veterinary therapy 4: food animal practice,* Philadelphia, 1999, WB Saunders.
457. Vin B et al: Experimental anthrax vaccines: efficacy of adjuvants combined with protective antigen against an aerosol *Bacillus anthracis* spore challenge in guinea pigs, *Vaccine* 13:1779-1784, 1995.
458. Gu ML, Leppla SH, Klinman DM: Protection against anthrax toxin by vaccination with a DNA plasmid encoding anthrax protective antigen, *Vaccine* 17:340-344, 1999.

Interdigital Necrobacillosis (Footrot)

Interdigital necrobacillosis (footrot) in cattle results from interdigital infection with *Fusobacterium necrophorum* and lesser contributions from other bacteria, including *Dichelobacter nodusus* (originally *Bacteroides nodosus*) and less often *Prevotella melaninogenica* (originally *Bacteroides melaninogenicus*).[459,460] A commercial *F. necrophorum* bacterin* to aid in the prevention of footrot is available for use in cattle and sheep. The bacterin consists of an inactivated, bivalent culture of *F. necrophorum.* Recommendations for initial vaccination are two doses given 3 to 4 weeks apart, followed by annual revaccination. Vaccination is also recommended when endemic conditions exist or when exposure is imminent. The efficacy of *F. necrophorum* vaccines is not well documented, but some benefit has been demonstrated in experimental studies.[461] Vaccination is especially recommended in herds that have a high incidence of disease.[461] Protective immunity most closely correlates with the level of antileukotoxin antibodies.[462,463] A leukotoxoid vaccine composed of cell-free supernatant from a high leukotoxin–producing strain of *F. necrophorum* was effective in reducing experimental hepatic necrobacillosis[463] and presumably would have some benefit against interdigital *F. necrophorum* infection. Autogenous vaccines containing *D. nodosus* reduced the severity of interdigital dermatitis but not of necrobacillosis.[464]

REFERENCES

459. Bergsten C: Infectious diseases of the digits. In Greenough PR, Weaver AD, eds: *Lameness in cattle,* ed 3, Philadelphia, 1997, WB Saunders.
460. Baird AN: Interdigital phlegmon (interdigital necrobacillosis). In Howard JL, Smith RA, eds: *Current veterinary therapy 4: food animal practice,* Philadelphia, 1999, WB Saunders.

461. Rebhun WC: Musculoskeletal diseases. In *Diseases of dairy cattle,* Philadelphia, 1995, Williams & Wilkins.
462. Clark BL et al: Studies into the immunization of cattle against interdigital necrobacillosis, *Aust Vet J* 63:107-110, 1986.
463. Saginala S et al: Effect of *Fusobacterium necrophorum* leukotoxoid vaccine on susceptibility to experimentally induced liver abscesses in cattle, *J Anim Sci* 75:1160-1166, 1997.
464. Clark BL et al: Immunization of cattle against interdigital dermatitis (footrot) with an autogenous *Bacteroides nodosus* vaccine, *Aust Vet J* 63:61-62, 1986.

Papillomatous Digital Dermatitis (Footwarts)

Papillomatous digital dermatitis, or footwarts, can be a serious problem in dairy cattle.[465,466] The disease is characterized by ulcerative to proliferative digital lesions that most often occur in heifers and younger cows after introduction into a milking herd.[465-467] The etiology of the disease is uncertain, but *Treponema*-like spirochetes and flexible, gram negative rods (*Serpens* spp.) have been incriminated.[467-469] An autogenous vaccine derived from lesions from an infected herd was ineffective at reducing disease.[469] A *Serpens* bacterin* has been granted a conditional license by the U.S. Department of Agriculture as a preventative and aid to treatment. The vaccine consists of killed cultures of *Serpens* organisms obtained from a natural lesion. The recommendations are for three 5-ml doses administered subcutaneously at 4-week intervals, followed by revaccination every 4 to 6 months. Field trials reported by the company demonstrate a reduced onset of new infections and more rapid resolution of existing infections in vaccinated cattle compared with unvaccinated ones. Another study of clinically affected cattle in which vaccination was combined with treatment with topical lincomycin showed no significant improvement in vaccinated cows compared with unvaccinated ones.[470] The high recurrence rates of natural infection suggest that immunity to the disease is short-lived or weak.[467] Additional information about the etiology of and immunity to footwarts is needed to more adequately evaluate the efficacy and feasibility of vaccination.

REFERENCES

465. Read DH, Walker RL: Papillomatous digital dermatitis (footwarts) in California dairy cattle: clinical and gross pathologic findings, *J Vet Diagn Invest* 10:67-76, 1998.
466. Blowey RW, Sharp MW: Digital dermatitis in dairy cattle, *Vet Rec* 122:505-508, 1988.
467. Shearer JK, Hernandez J, Elliott JB: Papillomatous digital dermatitis: treatment and control strategies. II, *Compend Cont Educ Pract Vet* 20:S213-S223, 1998.
468. Walker RL et al: Spirochetes isolated from dairy cattle with papillomatous digital dermatitis and interdigital dermatitis, *Vet Microbiol* 47:343-355, 1995.
469. Rebhun WC et al: Interdigital papillomatosis in dairy cattle, *J Am Vet Med Assoc* 177:437-440, 1980.
470. Berry SL et al: A prospective randomized field study to determine the efficacy of a *Serpens* spp vaccine combined with topical treatment with lincomycin HCl for treatment of papillomatous digital dermatitis (footwarts) on a California dairy, *Bovine Pract* 32:6-12, 1998.

RABIES

Rabies is a highly fatal, zoonotic neurologic disease caused by a rhabdovirus. Routine vaccination of cattle is not common in most situations. However, vaccination may be cost-effective in rural areas of Latin America, where vampire bats are important sylvatic vectors.[471] In endemic areas vaccination of valuable cattle or herds may be a reasonable precautionary measure.[472] This is particularly true in situations in which cattle are in frequent contact with human beings, in order to reduce the anxiety of animal workers and minimize the likelihood of human exposure. Currently licensed rabies

---

*Vocar, Intervet, Millsboro, DE 19966.

*Hygieia Biological Laboratories, Woodland, CA 95695.

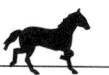

vaccines for cattle contain inactivated, cell culture–derived virus.[473] The recommended regimen is initial vaccination at 3 months of age followed by annual vaccination thereafter. The duration of protective neutralizing antibody levels after initial vaccination can vary,[474] therefore some experts have suggested that a second booster dose be given either 1 month after initial vaccination[474] or at 6 months of age.[475] Subsequent annual revaccination induces strong anamnestic responses that persist for 1 year or longer.[474,475]

REFERENCES

471. Acha PN, Szyfres B: Zoonoses and communicable diseases common to man and animals, Scientific Publication No 503, Pan-American Health Organization, Washington, DC, 1987.
472. Briggs DJ: Rabies in food animals. In Howard JL, Smith RA, eds: *Current veterinary therapy 4: food animal practice,* Philadelphia, 1999, WB Saunders.
473. Bayley AJ: Bovine biologic charts, In Arrioja-Dechert A, ed: *Compendium of veterinary products,* ed 5, Port Huron, Mich, 1999, North American Compendiums.
474. Sihvonen L, Kulonen K, Neuvonen E: Immunization of cattle against rabies using inactivated cell culture vaccines, *Acta Vet Scand* 35:371-376, 1994.
475. De Angelis Cortes J et al: Immune response in cattle induced by inactivated rabies vaccine adjuvanted with aluminum hydroxide either alone or in combination with avridine, *Rev Sci Tech Off Intl Epizoot* 12:941-955, 1993.

FIBROPAPILLOMAS (Warts)

Fibropapillomas (warts) are manifested in a variety of forms and locations, each caused by a specific bovine papillomavirus (BPV).[476,477] Lesions associated with papillomaviruses can occur in the epidermis of the head, face, neck, and legs (BPV-1 and BPV-22), upper alimentary and urinary tracts (BPV-4), teats and udder (BPV-1, BPV-3, BPV-5, and BPV-6), and genital epithelium (BPV-1).[476-479] Immunity after infection or vaccination is virus type specific[476,478,479]; therefore the efficacy of both autogenous and commercial vaccines depends on which viral antigens are incorporated into the vaccine and which virus type is responsible for the disease. Vaccines containing BPV-1 and BPV-2 generally are effective for prevention but not treatment of disease caused by the ho-

mologous virus.[478] Vaccines usually are ineffective for treatment or prevention of disease caused by BPV-3 and BPV-5.[478] However, interpretation of the response to vaccination can be complicated by spontaneous regression of some lesions.[476] Lesions associated with BPV-1 and BPV-2 usually spontaneously regress within 1 to 12 months, whereas lesions caused by BPV-3 and BPV-5 do not normally spontaneously regress.[478,480]

Commercial vaccines consist of inactivated, virus-laden tissue extracts derived from bovine papillomas.[481] The recommended regimen is an initial dose divided and given in at least two different sites, followed by a second dose in 3 to 5 weeks. Vaccination should continue for at least 1 year after elimination of disease from the herd. Autogenous vaccines can be made by homogenizing and inactivating (0.3% formalin) excised wart tissue, followed by dilution of the homogenate in physiologic saline and filtration through gauze. Three 1- to 5-ml intradermal injections given at 1-week intervals are recommended. Vaccination is most commonly used with valuable animals destined for competitive shows or for overseas sale.[478] Vaccination can also be helpful as a preventive measure in herds with a high incidence of cutaneous fibropapillomas or to reduce the risk of penile fibropapillomas in groups of young bull calves.[476]

REFERENCES

476. Rebhun WC: Diseases of the teats and udder. In *Diseases of dairy cattle,* Philadelphia, 1995, Williams & Wilkins.
477. Jarrett WFH et al: A novel bovine papillomavirus (BPV-6) causing true epithelial papillomas of the mammary gland skin: a member of a proposed new BPV subgroup, *Virology* 136:255-264, 1984.
478. Scott DW: Neoplastic skin diseases. In Howard JL, Smith RA, eds: *Current veterinary therapy 4: food animal practice,* Philadelphia, 1999, WB Saunders.
479. Jarrett WFH et al: Studies on vaccination against papillomaviruses: immunity after infection and vaccination with bovine papillomaviruses of different types, *Vet Rec* 126:473-475, 1990.
480. Thomsett LR: Skin conditions. In Andrews AH et al, eds: *Bovine medicine: diseases and husbandry of cattle,* Oxford, 1992, Blackwell Scientific Publishers.
481. Bayley AJ: Bovine biologic charts. In Arrioja-Dechert A, ed: *Compendium of veterinary products,* ed 5, Port Huron, Mich, 1999, North American Compendiums.

Parasite Control Programs

CHRISTINE A. UHLINGER
Consulting Editor

DESIGN OF PARASITE CONTROL PROGRAMS

The most important concept in the design of sound parasite control programs is the interaction of the parasite with the host and the environment. In many cases an understanding of the life cycle and epidemiology suggests the most effective methods for parasite control. In this chapter, parasite factors, host factors, and environmental factors affecting transmission and disease expression are discussed for each major class of parasites in each host species (horses, small ruminants, cattle).

Integrated management strategies incorporating selective use of anthelmintic agents, enhancement of host immunity to parasitic infection, and grazing/environmental management have become increasingly important in the design of sustainable parasite control programs. Nevertheless, anthelmintics remain a key component of most parasite control programs. With the wide availability of over-the-counter anthelmintics, the veterinarian's role in parasite control has shifted, and perhaps has been somewhat superseded by that of manufacturers' representatives, product advertising, and feed store personnel. Veterinarians may be consulted on the selection and timing of treatment, but in many cases the veterinarian is brought in only when the owner or producer perceives a problem. Thus it is important for the practitioner to have a grasp of the variables involved in the design of an effective anthelmintic program.

The impact of parasitic infection varies widely with geographic area and management system. General guidelines may be suggested for parasitic control, but it is inadvisable to adhere to any rigid anthelmintic schedules or even management recommendations. The best parasite control programs are those designed with the goals of the producer in mind, as well as the costs and returns of treatment. Other factors that must be considered include the animal's environment, climatic variations, and geographic location. Although many producers and owners would like a "cookbook" approach to parasite control, these are rarely effective across the various management conditions. It is unfortunate that an epidemiologically and economically sound parasite control program designed for animals in one geographic area may be neither efficient nor effective in another location.

Anthelmintic Use

Anthelmintic drugs are administered to treat, control, and prevent parasitic infections and to minimize the economic losses associated with parasitic infection. Anthelmintics are also used for the treatment of an individual animal exhibiting clinical signs of parasitic disease.

DRUG ACTION. To use an anthelmintic properly, it is necessary to consider its mode of action, spectrum of activity, and duration of effect. Efficacy for a given drug may be defined as its ability to (1) kill adult or larval parasites, (2) suppress parasitic egg production, or (3) promote the expulsion of worms from the gastrointestinal tract.

Because of the emergence of drug-resistant strains of nematodes, it is difficult to predict how a particular drug will perform in a specific animal or herd. Package inserts should be regarded as guidelines rather than gospel. It is prudent to run periodic pretreatment and posttreatment fecal examinations to assess the performance of commonly used drugs on a given farm.

TREATMENT INTERVALS. The frequency of treatment needed for parasite control depends on several factors, including the life cycle of the parasitic species to be controlled, host factors affecting susceptibility, environmental factors affecting transmission, and goals of the producer. As all these factors are dynamic, the optimum treatment interval changes in response to the other variables. One treatment regimen does not suffice for all groups of animals; it may not even be adequate in the same group of animals year to year. Anthelmintics can be used in several ways.

SUPPRESSIVE TREATMENT REGIMENS. These regimens use regularly scheduled anthelmintic treatments in an attempt to kill successive generations of parasites within host animals to decrease environmental contamination. They are most useful in high-risk populations or intensive management systems in which the animals are exposed to severely contaminated environments. Drugs are often given at set time intervals (e.g., monthly).

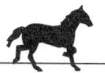

DAILY TREATMENT REGIMENS. Low levels of anthelmintic may be administered daily in the feed or mineral mix. Sustained-release intraruminal anthelmintic devices have a similar effect. These products have the advantage of limiting reinfection in animals grazing contaminated pastures and over a grazing season may contribute to a reduction in larval load on the pasture. However, it is important to monitor drug efficacy with these programs, as low-dose daily exposure to the anthelmintic may promote resistant populations of parasites.

SEASONAL TREATMENT REGIMENS. These schedules are timed by seasonal transmission factors. Drugs are administered to prevent peak egg production and thereby reduce environmental contamination. The programs are cost effective and reduce the number of treatments. But, to be timed correctly, local transmission patterns must be documented. The schedules may fail if environmental factors change, so close monitoring of the herd is required.

TACTICAL TREATMENT REGIMENS. Tactical treatments are given when climatic, seasonal, or host factors combine to create unusual levels of infection. Close monitoring of the herd is required. An ability to recognize such factors before they lead to production losses or mortality is essential.

MANAGEMENT-DRIVEN TREATMENT REGIMENS. Often management constraints dictate the timing of anthelmintic treatments. Animals may be available for treatment only at certain times of the year. Drug withdrawal consideration may also limit options for scheduling treatments.

PRODUCER OBJECTIVES. Some producers focus on prevention of severe disease or loss caused by death; others aim to increase productivity. Most wish to do as well as possible economically, given various management constraints. With companion animals such as horses and some goat herds, producers may desire maximum preventive strategies. Unless these goals are defined, it is not possible to design optimum control programs for a particular unit.

Anthelmintic Drugs

Numerous anthelmintic drugs are available. This section discusses various classes of anthelmintics; the specific spectrum of activity and side effects are covered under each species.

AVERMECTINS AND MILBEMYCINS. The avermectins and milbemycins are macrocyclic lactones. They act by increasing the permeability of parasite cell membranes to chloride ions, which results in nonspastic paralysis and death of the parasite. These drugs may also act by potentiating presynaptic release of γ-aminobutyric acid (GABA), an inhibitory neurotransmitter, although this theory has been challenged.

These products have a high level and broad spectrum of activity against adult and larval nematodes. They are also effective against various ectoparasites such as mites, lice, ticks, bots, and cattle grubs; however, they are ineffective against flukes and tapeworms. These drugs suppress nematode egg production for longer than other anthelmintics. Because of its long duration of effect, moxidectin suppresses fecal egg counts and protects against reinfection for longer than ivermectin. Concern has been expressed about the environmental impact of these long-acting anthelmintics in grazing animals.

Several products have been developed for use in animals. The avermectins include ivermectin, abamectin, doramectin, and eprinomectin. The milbemycins include nemadectin and moxidectin. Oral (drench, sustained-release intraruminal device), topical ("pour-on"), and injectable formulations are available, depending on the drug. Ivermectin is safe to use during pregnancy, but currently it is not approved for use in lactating dairy animals or females of breeding age. Similarly, doramectin and moxidectin are not approved for use in female dairy cattle of breeding age. Eprinomectin is unique in

that it has no withholding period for milk or meat, so there are no restrictions on its use in cattle. At labeled doses, moxidectin is a safe drug; however, accidental overdosage has caused neurologic signs in foals and miniature horses.

BENZIMIDAZOLES. Benzimidazoles (BZDs) are a large class of anthelmintics that interfere with parasitic carbohydrate metabolism by inhibiting the enzyme fumarate reductase. Many BZDs have been developed and marketed. They include albendazole, fenbendazole, mebendazole, oxfendazole, oxibendazole, parbendazole, ricobendazole, thiabendazole, triclabendazole, and the probenzimidazole drugs febantel and netobimin.

BZDs are widely used in horses and ruminants. In general, they exhibit a high degree of safety and a broad spectrum of activity against gastrointestinal nematodes and lungworms. Some members of this class (e.g., albendazole) are also active against liver flukes and certain cestodes in ruminants. Albendazole and netobimin can cause teratogenicity and embryo toxicity in sheep when given during early pregnancy. Fenbendazole, oxfendazole, and oxibendazole are considered to be safe for use in pregnant animals.

Resistance to BZDs has been documented in certain equine, ovine, and caprine parasites. In general a strain of parasite resistant to one BZD drug quickly develops resistance to other BZDs or pro-BZDs, a phenomenon known as *side resistance*.

LEVAMISOLE. Levamisole acts by causing neuromuscular depolarization and paralysis of the parasite. It has been widely used in ruminants to treat gastrointestinal nematode and lungworm infections. However, levamisole resistance has become a problem in many areas.

The dose of levamisole should be calculated carefully because toxic doses are only one to two times therapeutic doses. Signs of toxicity may mimic those of organophosphate toxicity, including muscle fasciculations around the lips and eyelids, hypersalivation, spastic movements, depression, and diarrhea. In ruminants, muzzle foam may occur after oral administration of the drug but usually disappears within a few hours after administration. In horses, transitory excitement has been seen after treatment. Levamisole is not recommended for use as an anthelmintic in horses. Concurrent administration of morantel, pyrantel, diethylcarbamazine, or organophosphates could enhance the toxic effects of levamisole.

MORANTEL AND PYRANTEL. These tetrahydropyrimidines are cholinergic agonists that exert their anthelmintic effect by depolarizing neuromuscular junctions and causing irreversible paralysis of susceptible parasites. Morantel is slower in its onset of action, but much more potent than pyrantel. These products are effective against many species of adult nematodes but do not appear to be active against larval stages. Pyrantel is also effective against tapeworms in horses when given at twice the recommended dose. The margin of safety is relatively wide, and there is no contraindication for use with other cholinergic drugs. However, it is recommended that morantel and pyrantel not be used concurrently, and that neither be given with levamisole. Piperazine antagonizes the effects of morantel/pyrantel, so it should not be used with either of these drugs. Resistance to morantel/pyrantel has been documented in strains of *Haemonchus contortus* and in some cyathostomes (equine small strongyles).

ORGANOPHOSPHATES. Organophosphates (OPs) block neurotransmission by inhibiting acetylcholinesterase. Various formulations of OP drugs are available for treating gastrointestinal nematodiasis. Commonly used OPs include haloxon, coumaphos, trichlorfon, and dichlorvos. Toxicity occurs with these products in a dose-related manner, so dosages should be calculated with care. In addition, the potential danger to humans administering these products should not be overlooked. Atropine is recommended in cases of overdose in livestock.

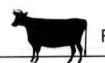

PHENOTHIAZINE. The mode of action of phenothiazine (PTH) has not been clarified; it is thought to interfere with anaerobic metabolism of nematodes. The various formulations of PTH differ in purity and particle size. The purified product (99% PTH) with small particle size (2 μm) are the most effective.

Although PTH is effective against a wide spectrum of gastrointestinal nematodes, resistant strains of parasites have emerged in several species. The drug is synergistic with piperazine; combinations of these drugs have effective activity against PTH-resistant nematodes. Phenothiazine used in combination with piperazine can be administered at a much lower dose.

Phenothiazine toxicity has been reported. Toxic reactions include corneal inflammation, abortion, ataxia, hemolytic anemia, photosensitization, and nephrotoxicity. The drug should not be administered to debilitated or anemic animals or to animals in the last month of pregnancy.

PIPERAZINE. Piperazine salts block neuromuscular transmission, resulting in paralysis of susceptible gastrointestinal nematodes. The worms are then passively removed from the gastrointestinal tract by intestinal peristalsis. Piperazines have low toxicity and are safe in young or pregnant animals. However, their spectrum of activity is limited, in practical terms, to ascarids. Piperazine must be used with caution in horses heavily infested with ascarids because the paralyzed ascarids can cause an impaction that may culminate in bowel rupture. Diethylcarbamazine is a piperazine derivative that has been used to control lungworm infection in sheep and cattle.

PRAZIQUANTEL. Praziquantel is a cestocidal drug that causes spastic paralysis, decreased glucose uptake, and disruption of the tapeworm's tegument. Although not approved for this use, praziquantel is effective for treating tapeworm infestation in horses. It has also been used to control various cestodes in small ruminants.

Evaluation of Parasite Control Programs

The efficacy of a given parasite control program should not be assumed; it should be assessed on a regular basis. Some techniques for assessment are discussed in the following paragraphs.

FECAL EGG COUNTS. Determining numbers of nematode eggs in feces is the simplest and least invasive way to evaluate a parasite control program. Fecal examination may be of limited value in an individual animal, because animals dying of parasitic infection may have no eggs in the feces, whereas animals with high fecal egg counts may be clinically normal. Nevertheless, fecal egg counts can provide information on the level of infection present in an individual animal, particularly when egg counts are repeated over the course of 2 to 3 weeks. Herd average fecal egg counts are more useful and provide an accurate reflection of the degree of environmental contamination and rate of infection. Pretreatment and post-treatment fecal egg counts can also be used to establish the efficacy of an anthelmintic in a particular group of animals. A quantitative McMaster's or Stolley's technique, rather than simple flotation, is crucial for accurate monitoring.

LARVAL CULTURE. Larval cultures can be used to distinguish between large and small strongyles in horses and to identify the various nematode species in ruminants. Most parasitology laboratories can perform this examination. It requires submission of 200 to 400 g of fresh feces. Pooled samples from several herd members are often used.

PASTURE LARVAL COUNTS. Counts of parasitic larvae on herbage are useful to indicate the level of exposure experienced by the grazing animal. This examination is somewhat tedious but can be performed by many university laboratories. A 2-kg sample of forage is gathered for submission to the laboratory. The grass is sampled by walking a V pattern across the acreage and stopping every three paces to sample grass. The samples are subsequently washed and passed through screening to isolate and identify larvae.

NECROPSY EVALUATION. The nature and magnitude of parasitic infections can be established by necropsy examination. Gross examination and an estimate of adult worm population in the gut lumen are often sufficient. Many worms detach from the mucosa as the carcass cools; however, the damage done by the parasites can be seen on gross or histologic examination. Occasionally it is necessary to use digestion techniques or histologic examination to document the presence of hypobiotic larvae.

CLINICAL TRIALS. Depending on the management system involved, it may be possible to arrange informal clinical trials to evaluate the efficacy of anthelmintic programs. If properly done, this provides the most useful and convincing type of program evaluation.

SUGGESTED READING

Blood DC, Radostits OM, Gay CC: Diseases caused by helminth parasites. In *Veterinary medicine*, ed 8, London, 1994, Baillière Tindall, pp 1223-1230

Herd RP: Control strategies for ruminant and equine parasites to counter resistance, encystment, and ecotoxicity in the USA, *Vet Parasitol* 48:327-336, 1993.

Kassai T: Antihelmintic therapy and control. In *Veterinary helminthology*, Oxford, 1999, Butterworth Heinemann, pp 147-179.

Plumb DC: *Veterinary drug handbook*, ed 3, Iowa, 1999, Iowa State University Press.

Waller PJ: International approaches to the concept of integrated control of nematode parasites of livestock, *Intl J Parasitol* 29:155-164, 1999.

EQUINE STRONGYLE DISEASE

Horses are susceptible to infection with a variety of gastrointestinal nematode parasites. This section focuses on the large and small strongyles. The three species of large strongyles of clinical importance in horses are *Strongylus vulgaris*, *S. edentatus*, and *S. equinus*. Over 50 species are included in the heterogeneous group collectively known as the small strongyles or cyathostomes, although only about 10 species predominate. In most adult horses, cyathostomes make up 85% to 100% of the animals' total gastrointestinal nematode burden. Although *S. vulgaris* is considered to be the most pathogenic of the strongyle species, small strongyle disease (cyathostomosis) is emerging as an important clinical syndrome.

Strongylosis in horses causes a wide spectrum of effects from inapparent infection to sudden death. Because horses are primarily managed as companion animals, the goal of anthelmintic administration is to maximize the animals' health status by minimizing the parasite burdens. Preventive anthelmintic strategies are designed to limit exposure to infective parasite stages.

Life Cycle

The life cycles of gastrointestinal nematodes are direct and have been extensively reviewed.[1-3] Several days after ingestion, third-stage larvae (L_3) exsheath in the small intestine, cecum, or colon. After molting, the migration of these larvae varies with the species involved. *S. vulgaris* larvae migrate within the intima of small arteries in the bowel wall and mesentery to the cranial mesenteric artery. Larvae of *S. edentatus* and *S. equinus* migrate through the portal veins or peritoneal cavity to the liver. After several months the larvae return to the bowel lumen. The prepatent period for these species can be as long as 11 months.

In small strongyles, larval invasion is limited to the mucosa and submucosa of the cecum and colon. There the larvae undergo a molt from L_3 to L_4. Developing L_4 then emerge from the mucosa and enter the lumen of the bowel to ma-

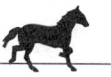

ture into adults. Cyathostome larvae encyst in the bowel wall for variable periods of time; usually just 1 to 2 months, but encysted larvae (typically the early L_3 stage) can arrest their development for many months. Thus the prepatent period can be as short as 40 days or as long as 2 years.[2] Negative feedback from luminal stages is a possible mechanism for persistence of arrested development.

Pathophysiology

STRONGYLUS VULGARIS. Penetration by ingested *S. vulgaris* larvae causes hemorrhagic foci on the mucosa of the small intestine, cecum, and ventral colon. As the larvae molt, around day 7, a severe inflammatory response characterized by arteritis, thrombosis, and eosinophilic infiltration is seen within the submucosa. Some animals show signs of abdominal discomfort at this time. These lesions progress to the subserosa as the larvae continue their migration. Most larvae reach the ileocecal-colic arteries 3 weeks after infection, where they cause fibrosis, arteritis, and thrombus formation. Larvae provoke fibrin deposition, accumulation of necrotic debris, and aneurysm formation within the vessels; thrombi and emboli may form within the aneurysm. The arterial lesions can cause segmental ischemia or infarction of the bowel wall. Arterial lesions may also be found in the renal, splenic, hepatic, or coronary arteries. This is the classic picture of *S. vulgaris* infection, or verminous arteritis.[4] However, it is uncommon in this era of highly effective larvicidal anthelmintics. In most cases the effects of *S. vulgaris* infection primarily involve alterations in blood flow in the microcirculation of the bowel wall and altered intestinal motility.[5] Alteration in microvascular blood flow may result from intravascular coagulation or vasoconstriction as larvae migrate through the bowel wall and small arteries. Possible mechanisms of altered motility include the release of substances by the parasites that alter smooth muscle activity; damage to the intestinal wall during larval migration; and arteritis within the bowel wall or mesentery.

Fifth-stage larvae returning to the gut form nodules in the bowel wall. Adult parasites in the lumen feed by digesting plugs of mucosa; as a result, numerous ulcers form in the mucosa of the large intestine. The damage can extend into the muscularis and adjacent blood vessels. Damage by adult strongyles can be sufficient to cause mild anemia and impairment of absorptive and digestive functions.

STRONGYLUS EDENTATUS. After ingestion, *S. edentatus* larvae invade the cecal mucosa and travel through the portal circulation to the liver, where they cause subcapsular hemorrhage and edema. After multiple infections the liver may develop chronic inflammatory changes and become fibrotic. Larval migration may also damage the serosal surfaces of the abdominal organs, causing fibrin deposits and adhesions. Fibrous or calcified nodules may be found on various serosal surfaces. During the long course of larval migration back to the gut, hemorrhagic retroperitoneal lesions composed of edema, serosanguineous fluid, and larvae often form.

STRONGYLUS EQUINUS. The pattern of development and migration is similar to that of *S. edentatus*. Larvae penetrate the mucosa of the cecum and encyst in the submucosa. The larvae emerge after 1 to 2 weeks and migrate to the liver, pancreas, and peritoneal cavity. As with *S. edentatus*, migration can cause hepatitis and peritonitis.

CYATHOSTOMES. After ingestion, infective larvae exsheath and penetrate the mucosa of the cecum, ventral colon, and dorsal colon. The larvae enter the lamina propria, where they provoke a fibroblastic reaction that encapsulates the larvae. A cellular infiltrate, composed predominantly of lymphocytes and plasma cells, forms around the encapsulated larvae. Occasionally, large numbers of eosinophils are found

surrounding the capsule.[6] Emergence of larvae from the cysts damages the submucosa and mucosa, and provokes an intense granulomatous reaction comprised of eosinophils, fibroblasts, and neutrophils. Other distortions of mucosal and submucosal architecture may include goblet cell hyperplasia, mucosal and submucosal edema, widespread focal areas of submucosal hemorrhage with eosinophilic infiltrates, dilated submucosal lymphatics, and variable epithelial shedding.[6]

Emergence of large numbers of larvae at once and the consequent inflammatory response causes widespread disruption of the mucosa. Hemorrhagic, catarrhal, or fibrinous typhlitis or colitis result and may alter gut function and motility. In essence, penetration of or emergence from the mucosa and submucosa by larval cyathostomes causes an inflammatory enteropathy.[6]

Adult parasites in the lumen feed by engulfing and digesting parts of the cecal and colonic mucosa. Feeding causes ulcer formation and damages the deeper layers of the gut wall. Small capillaries may also rupture. Adult cyathostomes are often present in the colon in very high numbers; worm counts of greater than 500,000 are common. Although the damage done by each parasite is relatively small, the great numbers may cause severe pathologic alterations in the gut mucosa. The mucosa may be extensively disrupted and, in some sections, denuded.

Populations at Risk

Young or parasite-naive animals are most susceptible to strongylosis. Relatively low doses of larvae, 2500 to 5000 (>750 larvae for *S. vulgaris*), are capable of producing pyrexia, anorexia, depression, and colic, and may even lead to death. Adult animals are less susceptible to parasitic disease, suggesting some degree of acquired immunity to infection. However, horses of all ages are susceptible to the effects of strongyle infection.

Resistance to cyathostome infection has been shown to develop with maturity in horses. However, the response is slow to develop (taking years, rather than months as with gastrointestinal nematode infections in other species), and immunity is incomplete even with prolonged exposure. Adult horses may still harbor large populations of cyathostomes. Resistance to early (inhibited) L_3 may be acquired later than resistance to developing mucosal stages.[7,8]

Clinical Manifestations

LARGE STRONGYLES. An acute clinical syndrome may be seen in horses with sudden access to large numbers of infective larvae. This disease is characterized by fever, loss of appetite, diarrhea, lethargy, rapid dehydration, weight loss, and signs of colic. These symptoms are associated with larval damage to the mucosa, submucosa, and serosa of the intestine.

As the larvae complete their migration, a wide variety of signs may occur. Colic is a prominent sign and may be caused by ischemia or infarction from arterial lesions with *S. vulgaris* larvae or result from liver, pancreas, or peritoneal damage in the cases of *S. edentatus* and *S. equinus*. Recurrent episodes of mild to moderate colic or diarrhea that is acute or chronic may be caused by any strongyle species. Less severe infections may cause dullness, progressive weight loss, and unexplained loss of bloom or intermittent episodes of colic. Diffuse peritonitis and low-grade hepatitis may occur in *S. edentatus* infections. Some infections are associated with mild anemia.

A variety of atypical presentations have been specifically associated with *S. vulgaris* infection. Deaths have been caused by coronary artery thrombosis or renal infarction. Occasionally larvae and associated lesions are found in the aortic arch. Aortic-iliac thrombosis has been reported as a cause of hind limb lameness. Aberrant migration to the central nervous system has been reported as the cause of a wide variety of neurologic disorders.

SMALL STRONGYLES. Cyathostomosis causes a variety of clinical syndromes. The most consistent finding is weight loss. Diarrhea is a common feature, although it is not always present. A widely recognized presentation is sudden onset of diarrhea (which can become chronic) and marked weight loss; colic, subcutaneous edema, or pyrexia may also be seen. Some severely affected horses are unresponsive to therapy and die within 2 to 3 weeks of showing clinical signs. But several other presentations have been reported, including seasonal diarrhea in young horses (seen in late winter/spring in temperate climates); rapid weight loss, severe peripheral edema, and pyrexia without diarrhea in young horses (an autumn outbreak reported); loss of vigor, depressed growth, intermittent soft feces, and inappetence in foals; recurrent diarrhea in aged horses or ponies; weight loss of several months' duration before the onset of diarrhea; vague malaise with decreased appetite, lethargy, and reduced performance; and various forms of colic. Types of colic range from mild medical colic to severe colic caused by cecocecal intussusception, nonstrangulating infarction, or cecal tympany.[6,9-12] A telling feature in many cases is a history of regular anthelmintic treatment.[9,11]

The underlying pathology in most cases involving weight loss and diarrhea is a protein-losing enteropathy as a result of severe typhlitis/colitis. Other animals have signs compatible with a nondiarrheic maldigestion/malabsorption syndrome. There are no pathognomonic hematologic or serum biochemical changes with cyathostomosis. However, most clinically affected animals develop neutrophilia and hypoalbuminemia. Less consistent findings include anemia, eosinophilia, and increased serum alkaline phosphatase. An elevation in β-globulins is an inconsistent finding with low specificity for cyathostomosis.[6] In one study, hyperbetaglobulinemia did not develop until 16 to 20 weeks after exposure to infective larvae.[12] In most cases of larval cyathostomosis, fecal examinations are negative for strongyle ova or larvae.

MIXED STRONGYLE INFECTIONS. Most animals have a mixed (small and large) strongyle infection. Although strongyle disease may be fatal, the majority of verminous syndromes are characterized by mild to moderate, recurrent episodes of colic, unexplained fever, transient diarrhea, and other nonspecific complaints. Because of the nonspecific or atypical nature of the complaint, many nonfatal clinical cases of verminous gastrointestinal diseases are not recognized as such. Moderate verminous colics, in particular, usually resolve with field care and rarely result in institutional referral. This case selection bias may lead to the clinical impression among referral institutions that parasites are not responsible for a large proportion of equine colics.

Factors Affecting Transmission

Transmission is affected by climatic variation and pasture management. Eggs are passed onto pasture and develop in 1 to 3 weeks into infective third-stage larvae. The rate of development depends on temperature and humidity. Hatching occurs between 7.2° and 37.7° C (45° and 100° F). Freezing temperatures kill preinfective (L_1 and L_2) larvae, and prolonged freezing and thawing cycles may result in nonviable eggs. Infective larvae, on the other hand, survive freezing, and snow may actually enhance their survival. Cold temperatures may temporarily halt maturation of eggs and larvae, but development resumes when the temperature rises. In temperate climates the greatest numbers of infective larvae are present in the late summer and early autumn. Larvae are least resistant in hot, dry conditions. In some climates the greatest

kill occurs in dry summer months, with peak numbers of larvae present after autumn rains. Under optimum conditions larvae survive 2 years on pasture.

Pasture management factors also have a profound effect on the level of larval contamination and transmission patterns. The number of infective larvae on pasture is extremely high in overstocked land. Normally, horses do not graze near manure, but this aversion is lost as stocking rates increase. Management strategies such as pasture rotation and cross-species grazing are not available to the average horse owner.

Control of Strongyle Infections

MANAGEMENT STRATEGIES. Pasture management and pasture hygiene are important in the control of equine strongyles.[13] Larval counts can be extremely high on overgrazed pastures. Turnout paddocks are often highly infective. It has been suggested that "recreational" grazing on small plots of land almost ensures exposure to parasite larvae.[14] In these situations, removal of manure from paddocks and pastures becomes critical. Regular manure removal limits the number of eggs discharged into the grazing environment. Because horses tend to avoid areas of fecal contamination, this strategy also maximizes the grazing area available to the horses by eliminating "roughs" that are not normally grazed. Manure should be removed at least twice a week. A successful strongyle control program based on pasture sweeping has been described.[15] Chain harrowing has also been suggested as a control measure, but under some conditions (e.g., before rain, when pastures are wet) it may actually increase larval dispersion. Harrowing should not be done on occupied pastures.

Fresh manure should not be spread on pasture. If manure must be spread, it must be properly composted first, to ensure the destruction of strongyle eggs. Also, the manure pile must not be allowed to drain into the grazing area. Although horses will not acquire parasitic larvae directly from the manure pile, the fluids draining from the manure pile contain high numbers of eggs. If these eggs reach the grass, they will mature and create an area with unusually high infectivity. If grazing areas are extremely limited, consider replacing the grass with sand/gravel turnout areas.

Most management systems reduce pasture contamination by routine suppressive anthelmintic regimens. If this approach is taken, all animals grazing a pasture must be treated simultaneously.

ANTHELMINTICS. The anthelmintics available to treat and prevent strongylosis in horses are listed in Table 45-1. Benzimidazole (BZD) drugs are effective against adult large strongyles; however, many of the cyathostomes are resistant to BZDs.[16-20] Because 85% to 100% of the strongyle population in horses is comprised of small strongyles, products should be selected that are effective against these species. It should be noted that drug package inserts do not always offer useful information about efficacy against drug-resistant small strongyles.

Resistance to phenothiazine and piperazine is widespread in equine strongyle species.[16] Resistance to pyrantel has also been reported for small strongyles, although it appears to be far less common than BZD resistance.[17-20] Resistance to ivermectin or moxidectin has not been reported, although one author has predicted that resistance to these drugs will occur in equine small strongyles.[16] Tolerance to ivermectin was found in a small percentage of cyathostomes in a herd of horses that received regular anthelmintic treatment.[21]

Ivermectin and Moxidectin. Ivermectin and moxidectin are each highly effective against adult and larval stages of *S. vulgaris* and other large strongyles, including the migrating stages.[22] These drugs are also highly effective against adult

TABLE 45-1

Efficacy of Various Anthelmintics Against Strongyles in Horses

Drug	Dosage	Large Strongyles		Small Strongyles	
		Adults	Larvae	Luminal	Mucosal
BENZIMIDAZOLES*					
Febantel	5-6 mg/kg	+	−	+	−
Fenbendazole	5 mg/kg	+	−	+	−
	7.5-10 mg/kg daily for 5 days	+	+	+	+
Mebendazole	6-10 mg/kg	+	−	+	−
Oxfendazole	10 mg/kg	+	−	+	−
Oxibendazole	10 mg/kg	+	−	+	−
	20 mg/kg daily for 5 days	+	+	+	+†
PYRANTEL					
Pyrantel pamoate/embonate	6.6 mg/kg	+	−	+	−
Pyrantel tartrate‡	2.65 mg/kg daily	+	+	+	+
AVERMECTINS/MILBEMYCINS					
Ivermectin	0.2 mg/kg	+	+	+	−
Moxidectin	0.4 mg/kg	+	+	+	+/−§
OTHER					
Piperazine	110-200 mg/kg	−	−	+	−
Dichlorvos	30-35 mg/kg	+	−	+	−

All dosages are for oral administration.
+, Highly effective; +/−, moderately effective; −, ineffective.
*Ineffective against benzimidazole-resistant strongyles, except for larvicidal regimens.
†Efficacy against EL_3 unknown.
‡Prophylactic; prevents infection by newly acquired infective larvae.
§Moderate to high efficacy against LL_3/L_4; poor efficacy against EL_3.

and luminal stages of the small strongyles. Moxidectin is moderately to highly effective against mucosal L_4s, but its efficacy against late L_3s (LL_3s) is variable and its efficacy against inhibited early L_3s (EL_3s) is poor.[23-25] In most studies, EL_3s make up at least 50%, and sometimes up to 95%, of the mucosal larval cyathostome burden.[9,22,23,25] Ivermectin has negligible efficacy against any of the mucosal stages.[22,23]

Although ivermectin and moxidectin are both highly effective against adult large and small strongyles, moxidectin suppresses fecal egg counts for a much longer period than does ivermectin. In most studies, fecal egg counts begin to rise about 8 weeks after ivermectin treatment, whereas moxidectin suppresses fecal egg counts for at least 12 weeks.[26] It is not clear whether the longer period of suppression is the result of moxidectin's efficacy against the later mucosal stages or because of its longer residual effect (estimated to be 2 to 3 weeks against infective cyathostome larvae).[25] The persistence of fecal egg count suppression varies among studies even for the same product. For example, a study in Belgium demonstrated that ivermectin suppressed fecal egg counts for 10 to 13 weeks,[27] whereas an Australian study found the period to be only about 6 weeks.[28] In the Belgian study, moxidectin suppressed fecal egg counts for 22 to 24 weeks after treatment. Differences in study design, infection level, and climatic factors between the countries probably account for this variability. Doramectin is used with clinical success in some countries, although studies on its efficacy against equine strongyles currently are lacking.

Larvicidal Fenbendazole Regimen. Despite widespread BZD resistance among cyathostomes, fenbendazole is highly effective against all stages, including inhibited EL_3s, when given at 7.5 to 10 mg/kg PO daily for 5 consecutive days.[9] One explanation for the efficacy of this regimen is that enterohepatic cycling of biliary metabolites may extend the

time during which encysted larvae are exposed to effective concentrations of the drug. This larvicidal regimen is well tolerated by horses and appears to be safe. Oxibendazole at 20 mg/kg PO daily for 5 days has also been used against mucosal cyathostomes.[7]

Daily Pyrantel Tartrate. Daily feeding of pyrantel tartrate (Strongid C or its generic equivalent) at 2.65 mg/kg/day kills ingested strongyle larvae, thus effectively preventing new infections with these parasites.[7,29-31] It is particularly useful in animals grazing highly infective pastures. Treatment may be continued indefinitely or administered strategically during seasonal grazing periods, depending on geographic location and grazing management. Whereas other control strategies rely on the treatment of all animals in a grazing group, daily-dosing strategies protect individual horses and do not require the treatment of all animals sharing a pasture. Because this formulation is ineffective against adult strongyles and bots, the product is often used in conjunction with other anthelmintics, such as ivermectin or oxibendazole.

Daily pyrantel tartrate is less effective in young horses (foals, weanlings, and yearlings) than in adult horses. During periods of peak pasture infectivity, significant rises in fecal egg counts have been reported in young horses on this regimen.[29] However, strategic medication of foaling mares until after weaning can protect their foals from significant parasite burdens, thus delaying the foal's first anthelmintic treatment until after weaning.[29]

TREATMENT INTERVALS. The frequency of anthelmintic treatment depends on the rate at which horses acquire parasitic infections and on the drug(s) being used. Usually the infection rate is a factor of age, stocking density, and seasonal variations in larval transmission. Unfortunately, no single schedule controls parasites on all farms; the schedule must be tailored to the management unit. For example, with extremely low stocking rates or in conditions that do not promote larval survival, the appropriate dosing interval may be very long. However, in the majority of cases horses are managed in high-density pasture populations. Under these conditions the horses and the pasture tend to carry high parasite burdens. Young horses are more susceptible to parasitic infections and may be less responsive to anthelmintic treatment than are adult horses.[27,29,32] Thus control strategies designed for adult horses may not be appropriate for foals, weanlings, and yearlings.

BZDs and pyrantel at routine dosages only kill adult strongyles and therefore suppress fecal strongyle egg production for only about 4 weeks.[28,32,33] As previously mentioned, ivermectin typically suppresses fecal egg counts for about 8 weeks, and moxidectin for at least 12 weeks. This information can be used to approximate treatment intervals. A far more reliable approach is to monitor fecal egg counts weekly after treatment. Treatment should be repeated when 25% to 30% of the horses in the group have fecal egg counts greater than 200 eggs per gram.

ROTATION OF PRODUCTS. The goals of the anthelmintic regimen should be to provide broad-spectrum anthelmintic coverage and delay the onset of resistance to a given product. Rotation schedules in which different classes of drugs are given at each treatment do not seem to prolong the efficacy of the drugs being used. In sheep it has been proposed that a product be given for a year before changing to another class of drug (i.e., annual rotation). Although this solution has been suggested for horses, no studies are available to evaluate the impact of this strategy on equine strongyles. Some veterinarians and producers have reported good results with exclusive use of ivermectin. It is not clear if this strategy will hasten the onset of ivermectin resistance.

BIOLOGIC CONTROL. Laboratory and field studies have demonstrated that feeding the nematophagous fungus *Duddingtonia flagrans* to horses at pasture can substantially reduce the number of infective strongyle larvae on the pasture. This strategy can be highly effective in minimizing pasture infectivity with both large and small strongyles during the grazing season.[34,35]

Evaluation of Preventive Programs

The ultimate success of an anthelmintic program is manifested in the health, production, and performance benefits realized by the animals. In horses, such parameters are difficult to quantify. The simplest method for designing and evaluating the success of strongyle control programs is the fecal egg count. McMaster's method of quantifying egg counts is preferable to simple flotation and microscopic examination. A fecal egg count value on an individual animal does not correlate well with the severity of parasitic infection. However, egg counts accurately reflect the rate at which animals are acquiring infections and the degree to which they are contaminating their environment with nematode eggs. A reasonable goal is to keep the herd average fecal egg count below 200 eggs per gram (EPG). This should allow a low level of infection sufficient to induce immunity while preventing serious parasitic damage.

Pretreatment and posttreatment fecal egg counts can be used to monitor the efficacy of anthelmintics (Box 45-1). An effective drug is one that produces at least a 90% reduction in the pretreatment fecal egg count for at least 3 weeks after treatment. Weekly monitoring of egg counts after drug administration indicates the appropriate treatment interval to achieve this goal. In one study, simply adjusting the treatment interval substantially decreased herd average fecal egg counts and the incidence of colic.[36] Regularly monitoring posttreatment fecal egg counts can also be used to determine whether resistance is developing to a particular drug.

Clinical Management

DIAGNOSIS. In many cases, diagnosis of strongylosis is based on clinical presentation and response to therapy. Definitive diagnosis can be difficult antemortem. In the presence of suggestive clinical signs, fecal egg counts greater than 1000 EPG suggest a diagnosis of parasitism, but many animals show signs of disease in the prepatent phase of infection, particularly with cyathostomosis. Often, ill animals have fecal egg counts no higher than their healthy herd mates. Seasonality, age of the affected horse(s), and a history of regular anthelmintic treatment may also be helpful in arriving at a diagnosis of larval cyathostomosis.[9]

When present, hematologic aberrations such as hypoalbuminemia, eosinophilia, anemia, and hyperglobulinemia (particularly β-globulins or IgG[T]) are supportive of the diagnosis. In one study, worm-free animals were found to have β-globulin levels around 1 to 1.5 g/100 ml; moderately parasitized animals, 2 to 2.5 mg/100 ml; and heavily parasitized animals, 7 to 8 mg/100 ml.[37] Eosinophils may be present in the abdominal tap of animals with large or small strongyle disease, but as with eosinophilia, this finding may be very transient.

Definitive diagnosis may be made at necropsy. Mucosal transillumination or digestion techniques may be required to accurately determine the severity of infestation with encysted cyathostomes.

TREATMENT. For many animals, appropriate anthelmintic treatment is sufficient to resolve the clinical signs associated with strongyle infection. However, unless the animal's grazing environment is properly managed, the problems may recur. All animals sharing the pasture must be treated or treatment of the affected individual will be futile. This difficulty often arises in boarding stables, where owners of apparently healthy animals are reluctant to change their anthelmintic practices because a pasture mate is doing poorly.

Animals heavily infected with strongyles or those with chronic colic or nonresponsive diarrhea may require larvicidal treatment. The following regimens have been used with success:

1. Fenbendazole, 7.5 to 10 mg/kg daily for 5 days, or 50 mg/kg daily for 3 days
2. Moxidectin, 0.4 mg/kg once
3. Ivermectin, 0.2 mg/kg once (not larvicidal for encysted cyathostomes)

Several variations of these treatments are in use. Some veterinarians advocate pretreatment with a nonlarvicidal product 2 to 3 days before the initiation of larvicidal treatment. Daily feeding of pyrantel tartrate (Strongid C or its generic equivalent) can effectively prevent infestation with newly acquired larvae. Anecdotally, this regimen can reduce the frequency of colic episodes in some horses that experience recurrent colic.

These larvicidal treatments are occasionally given in combination with antiinflammatory agents. In some cases of larval cyathostomosis, corticosteroids appear to be helpful. Two cases of small strongyle diarrhea refractory to anthelmintic treatment responded to 0.5 mg/kg of dexamethasone given daily for 4 days and then gradually reduced over 4 days.[38] However, in another study, some severely affected horses died despite intensive treatment with anthelmintics and corticosteroids.[11] As in the treatment of all parasitic diseases, after therapeutic measures are completed, surviving animals must be returned to noncontaminated pastures.

REFERENCES

1. Duncan JL: The life cycle, pathogenesis, and epidemiology of S. vulgaris in the horse, Equine Vet J 5:20-25, 1972.
2. Reinemeyer CR: Small strongyles: recent advances, Vet Clin North Am 2: 281-312, 1986.
3. Kassai T: Phylum: nemathelminthes—roundworms. In Veterinary helminthology, Oxford, 1999, Butterworth Heinemann, pp 60-63.
4. Klei TR: Morphologic and clinicopathologic changes following Strongylus vulgaris infections of immune and nonimmune ponies, Am J Vet Res 43:1300-1307, 1982.
5. Love S: The role of equine strongyles in the pathogenesis of colic and current options for prophylaxis, Equine Vet J (suppl) 13:5-9, 1992.
6. Love S, Murphy D, Mellor D: Pathogenicity of cyathostome infection, Vet Parasitol 85:113-122, 1999.
7. Monahan CM et al: Experimental cyathostome challenge of ponies maintained with or without benefit of daily pyrantel tartrate feed additive: comparison of parasite burdens, immunity and colonic pathology, Vet Parasitol 74:229-241, 1998.
8. Klei TR, Chapman MR: Immunity in equine cyathostome infections, Vet Parasitol 85:123-136, 1999.
9. Duncan JL, Bairden K, Abbott EM: Elimination of mucosal cyathostome larvae by five daily treatments with fenbendazole, Vet Rec 142:268-271, 1998.
10. Mair TS: Outbreak of larval cyathostomiasis among a group of yearling and two-year-old horses, Vet Rec 135:598-600, 1994.
11. Van Loon G et al: Larval cyathostomiasis as a cause of death in two regularly dewormed horses, Zentralbl Veterinarmed A 42:301-306, 1995.
12. Thamsborg SM et al: Impact of mixed strongyle infections in foals after one month on pasture, Equine Vet J 30:240-245, 1998.
13. Herd RP: Control strategies for ruminant and equine parasites to counter resistance, encystment, and ecotoxicity in the USA, Vet Parasitol 48:327-336, 1993.
14. Craig TM: Considerations for the control of equine cyathostomes in arid areas, Vet Parasitol 85:181-188, 1999.
15. Herd RP: Parasite control in horses: pasture sweeping, Mod Vet Pract 893-898, 1986.
16. Sangster NC: Pharmacology of anthelmintic resistance in cyathostomes: will it occur with the avermectins/milbemycins? Vet Parasitol 85:189-204, 1999.
17. Ihler CF: A field survey on anthelmintic resistance in equine small strongyles in Norway, Acta Vet Scand 36:135-143, 1995.
18. Chapman MR et al: Identification and characterization of a pyrantel pamoate resistant cyathostome population, Vet Parasitol 66:205-212, 1996.
19. Lyons ET et al: Critical test evaluation (1977-1992) of drug efficacy against endoparasites featuring benzimidazole-resistant small strongyles (population S) in Shetland ponies, Vet Parasitol 66:67-73, 1996.
20. Craven J et al: Survey of anthelmintic resistance on Danish horse farms, using 5 different methods of calculating faecal egg count reduction, Equine Vet J 30:289-293, 1998.
21. Young KE et al: Parasite diversity and anthelmintic resistance in two herds of horses, Vet Parasitol 85:205-214, 1999.
22. Mohahan CM et al: Comparison of moxidectin oral gel and ivermectin oral paste against a spectrum of internal parasites of ponies with special attention to encysted cyathostome larvae, Vet Parasitol 63:225-235, 1996.
23. Xiao L, Herd RP, Majewski GA: Comparative efficacy of moxidectin and ivermectin against hypobiotic and encysted cyathostomes and other equine parasites, Vet Parasitol 53:83-90, 1994.
24. Eysker M et al: Controlled dose confirmation study of a 2% moxidectin equine gel against equine internal parasites in The Netherlands, Vet Parasitol 70:165-173, 1997.
25. Vercruysse J et al: Persistence of the efficacy of a moxidectin gel on the establishment of cyathostominae in horses, Vet Rec 143:307-309, 1998.
26. Boersema JH, Eysker M, van der Aar WM: The reappearance of strongyle eggs in the faeces of horses after treatment with moxidectin, Vet Q 20:15-17, 1998.
27. Demeulenaere D et al: Comparative studies of ivermectin and moxidectin in the control of naturally acquired cyathostome infections in horses, Vet Rec 141:383-386, 1997.
28. Rolfe PF, Dawson KL, Holm-Martin M: Efficacy of moxidectin and other anthelmintics against small strongyles in horses, Aust Vet J 76:332-334, 1998.
29. Herd RP, Majewski GA: Comparison of daily and monthly pyrantel treatment in yearling Thoroughbreds and the protective effect of strategic medication of mares on their foals, Vet Parasitol 55:93-104, 1994.
30. Valdez RA et al: Controlled efficacy study of the bioequivalence of Strongid C and generic pyrantel tartrate in horses, Vet Parasitol 60:83-102, 1995.
31. Monahan CM et al: Foals raised on pasture with or without daily pyrantel tartrate feed additive: comparison of parasite burdens and host responses following experimental challenge with large and small strongyle larvae, Vet Parasitol 73:277-289, 1997.
32. Herd RP, Gabel AA: Reduced efficacy of anthelmintics in young compared with adult horses, Equine Vet J 22:164-169, 1990.
33. Boersema JH et al: The reappearance of strongyle eggs in faeces of horses treated with pyrantel embonate, Vet Q 17:18-20, 1995.
34. Larsen M et al: The capacity of the fungus Duddingtonia flagrans to prevent strongyle infections in foals on pasture, Parasitology 113:1-6, 1996.
35. Baudena MA, Larsen M, Klei TR: Efficacy of Duddingtonia flagrans in reducing infective equine cyathostome L3 on pasture in southern Louisiana (abstract), Proceedings of the Sixth Equine Colic Research Symposium, 1998, University of Georgia, p 31.
36. Uhlinger C: Effects of three anthelmintic schedules on the incidence of colic in horses, Equine Vet J 22:251-254, 1990.
37. Kent JE: Specific serum protein changes associated with primary and secondary Strongylus vulgaris infections in pony yearlings, Equine Vet J 19:133-137, 1987.
38. Church S, Kelly DF, Obwolo MJ: Diagnosis and successful treatment of diarrhea in horses caused by immature small strongyles apparently insusceptible to anthelmintics, Equine Vet J 18:401-403, 1986.

EQUINE ASCARID INFECTION

CHRISTINE A. UHLINGER
JOSEPH DiPIETRO

Infection with *Parascaris equorum* is common in foals. Ascarids can be difficult to eradicate from premises and may cause disease in each subsequent foal crop. Ascarid infection should be included on the list of differential diagnoses for foals exhibiting ill thrift, coughing, pneumonia, and colic.

Life Cycle

The life cycle is direct. Adult worms in the small intestine produce numerous thick-walled eggs that are passed out in the feces. After ingestion, embryonated eggs hatch in the small intestine. The larvae penetrate the mucosa of the gut wall and migrate to the liver and lungs. The larvae then travel up the bronchial tree and are swallowed. After experimental infection, larvae appear in the liver in 48 hours, in the lung by 7 to 14 days, and in the proximal small intestine within 3 to 4 weeks of infection.[39,40] The prepatent period is 10 to 12 weeks.

Ascarid eggs are extremely durable and resistant to adverse environmental conditions. Unlike strongyles, ascarids do not require herbage to complete their life cycle; ascarid eggs have been recovered from animals raised in contaminated dry lots. Once a property is contaminated with ascarid eggs, the environment may remain a source of infection for a long period, because eggs may survive up to 5 years. Ascarid eggs develop rapidly under warm, moist conditions and mature into infective stages in 2 weeks.

Pathophysiology

Larval migration may cause focal or diffuse fibrosis in the liver.[40] In the lung the parasite causes direct damage to the

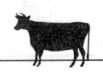

alveoli. Lesions are characterized by edema and consolidation. An eosinophil-associated immune-mediated bronchopneumonia may occur in older foals.[41,42] In the gut the primary pathophysiologic changes result from inflammation at the site of attachment and feeding, ileus, and mechanical obstruction by these large worms.[43] The response to ascarid infection appears to have an allergic component, possibly induced by proteins in fluids released during larval molting. Ileus has been attributed to the absorption of highly antigenic ascarid proteins.

Populations at Risk

Only young horses and the occasional debilitated adult horse are clinically affected by this parasite, although adult animals may harbor low numbers of parasites. All foals are at risk. The most severe clinical manifestations are seen on breeding farms with large yearly populations of young animals grazing the same pasture. Foals acquire infection from eggs shed by adult horses (e.g., broodmares), older foals, or previous years' foals.[44] Foals may have patent infections by 10 to 12 weeks of age. However, the most severe clinical manifestations often occur before the infection is patent. Strong immunity develops with exposure, and horses usually self-cure by 18 months of age by expelling adult worms. Adult horses may harbor a few ascarids.

Clinical Manifestations

Coughing and mucopurulent nasal discharge occur during larval migration through the lung. Respiratory signs may be very mild or may be associated with systemic illness, including depression and anorexia. Fever is often absent, unless verminous damage leads to secondary bacterial pneumonia. During the late prepatent period, when fourth-stage larvae (L_4) have returned to the gut, foals may exhibit anorexia, lethargy, and depression. Other signs of roundworm infection include ill thrift, rough hair coat, hypoproteinemia, poor weight gain, and debility. Mildly infected animals appear healthy but lack bloom. Adult worms in the gut may cause ileus or impactions that may culminate in small intestinal rupture. Intestinal perforation, peritonitis, and abscess formation have been attributed to heavy infections with adult roundworms.

Control of Ascarid Infections

Foals are infected from contact with a contaminated environment. Management practices that are likely to enhance parasite control in young horses are important in maximizing routine anthelmintic treatment. They include the following:

- Practice good sanitation. Pressure washing of foaling facilities with phenolic-based disinfectants enhances the control of *P. equorum.*
- Remove manure from stalls and paddocks frequently and compost. Do not spread manure on pastures.
- Use properly constructed feeders and waterers that minimize the potential for fecal contamination.
- Move feeders frequently to different parts of paddocks or lots. These areas often serve as areas of high transmission for infective *P. equorum* eggs.
- Use a gravel base for dry lots to minimize *P. equorum* transmission. Fewer *P. equorum* eggs are recovered from the surface of gravel-based dry lots than from dirt lots.
- Avoid grazing weanlings with yearlings, because young horses may harbor large numbers of parasites. If possible, raise foals on pasture that has not been used for prior foal crops.
- Do not overgraze pastures.

TABLE 45-2

Anthelmintics Effective Against Ascarids in Horses

Drug	Dosage	Efficacy Adults	Efficacy Larvae*
BENZIMIDAZOLES			
Fenbendazole	5 mg/kg	+/−	−
	10 mg/kg once	+	+/−
	10 mg/kg daily for 5 days	+	+
Mebendazole	8.8 mg/kg	+	−
Oxfendazole	10 mg/kg	+	−
Oxibendazole	10 mg/kg	+/−	−
PYRANTEL			
Pyrantel pamoate/ embonate	6/6 mg/kg	+	−
Pyrantel tartrate†	2.65 mg/kg daily	+	+
AVERMECTINS/MILBEMYCIN			
Ivermectin	0.2 mg/kg	+	+
Moxidectin	0.4 mg/kg	+	+
OTHER			
Piperazine‡	110-200 mg/kg	+	−
Dichlorvos‡	20 mg/kg	+	−
Trichlorfon‡	40 mg/kg	+	−

All dosages are for oral administration.
+, Highly effective; +/−, moderately effective; −, ineffective.
*Do not use in heavily parasitized foals.
†Migrating stages.
‡Prophylactic; prevents infection by newly acquired infective larvae.

ANTHELMINTICS. Piperazine, BZDs, pyrantel, organophosphates, ivermectin, and moxidectin all have some level of efficacy against ascarids[45-58] (Table 45-2 and Box 45-2). In one study comparing the efficacy of various anthelmintics, ivermectin was 98%, pyrantel pamoate 74%, and oxibendazole 45% effective against L_4 in the intestine.[56] Few drugs are highly effective against migratory forms at normal doses.

The development of drug resistance has not been reported in ascarids. However, short duration of efficacy may be mistaken for resistance to ivermectin. Ivermectin is highly effective against adult ascarids and larval stages in the lung and intestine,[52-55] but its efficacy is short-lived. Reinfection can occur as early as 2 weeks after treatment if the foal remains in a contaminated environment.[52] In other nematodes, moxidectin has a longer residual effect than ivermectin. However, in the limited studies conducted on *P. equorum*, there was no difference between moxidectin and ivermectin in the ability to reduce and suppress fecal egg counts.[57]

Daily administration of pyrantel tartrate (Strongid C or its generic equivalent) at 2.65 mg/kg/day is prophylactic, preventing penetration of the gut wall by *P. equorum* larvae. It can be used for parasite control in foals as soon as foals reliably consume grain.

In designing control programs, it is necessary to remove ascarids from the adult animals, as well as from the foals. Because adult animals may serve as a source of infection, it is important to ensure that all animals present on pastures used for foals are adequately dewormed with an effective product. For this reason it is beneficial to treat foaling mares at monthly intervals in the last trimester of pregnancy.

Evaluation of Control Programs

McMaster's fecal analysis reveals the presence of typical thick-walled ascarid eggs. These eggs tend to sink and can be diffi-

REFERENCES

39. Clayton HM, Duncan JL: The migration and development of *Parascaris equorum* in the horse, *Int J Parasitol* 9:285-292, 1979.
40. Brown PJ, Clayton HM: Hepatic pathology of experimental *Parascaris equorum* infection in worm-free foals, *J Comp Pathol* 89:115-123, 1979.
41. Spihakim S, Swerczek TW: Pathologic changes and pathogenesis of *Parascaris equorum* infection in parasite-free pony foals, *Am J Vet Res* 39:1155-1160, 1978.
42. Nicholls JM et al: A pathological study of the lungs of foals infected experimentally with *Parascaris equorum*, *J Comp Pathol* 88:261-274, 1987.
43. Clayton HM, Duncan JL: Clinical signs associated with *Parascaris equorum* infection in worm-free pony foals and yearlings, *Vet Parasitol* 1:69-78, 1978.
44. DiPietro JA, Boero M, Ely RW: Abdominal abscess associated with *Parascaris equorum* infection in a foal, *J Am Vet Med Assoc* 182:991-992, 1983.
45. DiPietro JA et al: Evaluation of ivermectin paste in the treatment of ponies for *Parascaris equorum* infections, *J Am Vet Med Assoc* 190:1181-1184, 1987.
46. DiPietro JA et al: Controlled trials of fenbendazole and febantel in ponies with *Parascaris equorum* infections, *J Equine Vet Sci* 4:158-160, 1984.
47. Yazwinski TA et al: Effectiveness of ivermectin in the treatment of equine *Parascaris equorum* and *Oxyuris equi* infections, *Am J Vet Res* 43:1095, 1982.
48. Drudge JH et al: Critical tests and clinical trials on oxibendazole in horses with special reference to removal of *Parascaris equorum*, *Am J Vet Res* 40:758-761, 1979.
49. Cornwell RL, Jones RM, Pott JM: Critical trials with morantel tartrate against *Parascaris equorum*, *Res Vet Sci* 14:134-136, 1973.
50. Vandermyde CR et al: Evaluation of fenbendazole for larvicidal effect in experimentally induced *Parascaris equorum* infections in pony foals, *J Am Vet Med Assoc* 190:1548-1549, 1987.
51. Lyons ET, Drudge JH, Tolliver SC: Studies on the development and chemotherapy of larvae of *Parascaris equorum* (Nematoda: Ascaridoidea) in experimentally and naturally infected foals, *J Parasitol* 62:453-459, 1976.
52. French DD et al: Efficacy of ivermectin in the oral paste formulation against naturally acquired adult and larval stages of *Parascaris equorum* in pony foals, *Am J Vet Res* 50:1000-1003, 1988.
53. French DD et al: Efficacy of ivermectin in oral drench and paste formulation against migrating larvae of experimentally inoculated *Parascaris equorum*, *Am J Vet Res* 50:1071-1073, 1989.
54. DiPietro JA et al: Evaluation of ivermectin for larvicidal effect in experimentally induced *Parascaris equorum* infections in pony foals, *Am J Vet Res* 49:1983-1985, 1988.
55. DiPietro JA et al: Efficacy of ivermectin in the treatment of induced *Parascaris equorum* infection in pony foals, *J Am Vet Med Assoc* 195:1712-1714, 1989.
56. Austin SM et al: Comparison of the efficacy of ivermectin, oxibendazole, and pyrantel pamoate against 28-day *Parascaris equorum* larvae in the intestine of pony foals, *J Am Vet Med Assoc* 198:1946-1949, 1991.
57. DiPietro JA et al: Clinical trial of moxidectin oral gel in horses, *Vet Parasitol* 72:167-177, 1997.
58. Plumb DC: *Veterinary drug handbook*, ed 3, Iowa, 1999, Iowa State University Press.

BOX 45-2

Special Problems in Equine Parasite Control

PARASITE CONTROL FOR YOUNG HORSES
JOSEPH DIPIETRO

Routine anthelmintic therapy is begun at 6 to 8 weeks of age because that is when immature and mature adult stages of *Parascaris equorum* are commonly first present in the small intestine. Interval or daily anthelmintic strategies may be used.

Interval deworming programs for foals should include 6 dewormings at 2-month intervals beginning at approximately 6 to 8 weeks of age and continuing until the foal is 1 year old. Averaging the age of all foals housed together to calculate dates for anthelmintic administration is an easier, better complied with, and more economic recommendation than deworming based on exact ages. The use of ivermectin in control programs is important because of its high efficacy against mature and immature adult *P. equorum*, migratory stages of *P. equorum* in the lungs and liver, and migratory stages of large strongyles.

Daily administration of 2.64 mg of pyrantel tartrate per kilogram is prophylactic and will preclude penetration of the gut wall by *P. equorum* and strongyle larvae. Before daily feeding of pyrantel tartrate is initiated, foals should receive a larvacidal treatment for *S. vulgaris*. Ivermectin (200 µg/kg) is the larvacide of choice because of its low-dose requirements compared to benzimidazole compounds and activity against both migratory large strongyles (*S. vulgaris* and *S. edentatus*) and larval stages of *P. equorum* (liver and lung migratory and small intestinal larvae). Subsequent administration of pyrantel tartrate on a daily basis to foals precludes the establishment of migratory damage associated with nematode infections.

---

cult to isolate. Counts of greater than 100 EPG indicate that treatment is warranted. It should be remembered that foals show signs before a patent infection is achieved.

Clinical Management

DIAGNOSIS. Fecal examination may demonstrate the presence of ascarid eggs. Treatment is warranted if eggs are found. In the absence of a positive fecal examination, diagnosis is often made on the basis of clinical signs and farm history. Parasitized animals may exhibit eosinophilia, but this test is variable and has poor negative or positive predictive value. In foals the presence of eosinophils in tracheal wash cytology is suggestive of verminous lung disease.

TREATMENT. Heavily parasitized foals may present a therapeutic challenge. Although it is necessary to remove the worm burden, too sudden or rapid a kill may result in fatal bowel obstructions with dead worms or a toxic response to large numbers of disintegrating worms. It may be prudent to pretreat such foals with a benzimidazole chosen for its relatively low efficacy against roundworms and follow up the treatment with another product such as ivermectin. Some veterinarians administer mineral oil after anthelmintic administration to ease the passage of the adult worms. Organophosphates that rupture the cuticle and release antigenic proteins, and piperazine, which paralyzes but does not kill the parasites, are contraindicated in heavily infected foals.

Foals suspected of verminous pneumonia should be treated with a larvicidal regimen of fenbendazole. Antibiotic coverage is generally recommended. Foals may require retreatment with fenbendazole as subsequent waves of larvae reach the lung.

EQUINE TAPEWORM INFECTION

The significance of equine tapeworm infections has been the subject of debate for many years. Most horses appear to tolerate a low level of tapeworm infection without exhibiting clinical signs. However, recent studies show a correlation between the presence and intensity of tapeworm infections and colic.

Life Cycle

Horses are parasitized by three species of tapeworm: *Anoplocephala perfoliata*, *A. magna*, and *Anoplocephaloides* (formerly *Paranoplocephala*) *mamillana*. Tapeworm eggs (passed within proglottids) in the feces are ingested by an oribatid mite on the pasture. A 2- to 4-month period is required for the development of cysticercoids within this intermediate host. Horses are infected when they ingest the mite in the course of grazing. Infections are patent 3 to 4 months after ingestion.

Pathophysiology

A. perfoliata attaches preferentially to the cecum and ileocecal junction. In one study, over 80% of the tapeworm burden was found on the cecal wall; less than 20% of the worms were found at the ileocecal junction or terminal ileum.[59] *A. magna* prefers the distal parts of the small intestine, and *A. mamillana* is more common in the proximal small intestine. Lesions caused by *A. perfoliata* vary in severity from focal erosions and ulceration to focal pseudomembranous enteritis with thickening of the mucosa, submucosa, and lamina propria; regional necrotizing enteritis may be found in severe infections.[59,60] Lesion severity is related to the number of tapeworms present. Lesions may be more severe at the ileocecal junction, because of the often high concentration of tapeworms in this small area of the bowel.[59]

Tapeworm infection can alter bowel motility, increasing the risk for spasmodic colic, ileal impaction, and intussusceptions involving the ileum, cecum, and cecocolic junction.[61-65] In a recent study in Britain, 22% of spasmodic colic cases and 81% of ileal impaction cases were determined to be tapeworm related.[63] Proposed mechanisms include damage caused by the parasites, physical obstruction (particularly of the ileum and ileocecal orifice), and alteration of motility from substances produced by the tapeworms.

Populations at Risk

Various surveys have estimated the prevalence of tapeworm infection in horses to be between 13% and 82%.[67-69] The incidence in grazing foals may approach 100%.[70] Infection rate appears to vary markedly from farm to farm. This variation may reflect differences in the distribution of the oribatid mite. Within a given group, certain horses may carry unusually heavy burdens of tapeworms. It is not clear whether this is a result of grazing behavior or of differences in immune status. Heavy infections appear to be more common in young animals; most clinical reports of intussusception associated with tapeworms involve animals less than 4 years of age. One epidemiologic study showed that tapeworm burdens were higher in horses 6 months to 2 years of age and those over 15 years of age than in horses between 3 and 15 years of age.[71] This finding suggests some degree of age-related immunity.

Clinical Manifestations

Small numbers of tapeworms generally do not cause clinical signs. However, tapeworms increase the risk for spasmodic colic and more severe types of colic associated with the ileocecocolic area. Heavy infections may also be associated with nonspecific gastrointestinal disturbances and ill thrift.[62] Tapeworm infection has also been implicated in perforation of the intestine. *A. mamillana* is rarely associated with clinical disease. However, the proglottids may be noticed in the feces and prompt an owner to request treatment.[66]

Diagnosis

Proglottids may be found in or on feces; however, they are very small (approximately the size of a grain of rice) and are easily overlooked on visual examination. The presence of the distinctive angulated eggs during microscopic fecal examination constitutes a definitive diagnosis of infection. However, the discharge of proglottids and therefore eggs is sporadic, and the absence of eggs does not rule out infection. Coprologic methods involving sedimentation or flotation are very insensitive. The presence of positive fecal examination correlates poorly with the presence of adult tapeworms found at necropsy.[72]

An enzyme-linked immunosorbent assay (ELISA) has been developed to measure an IgG(T) subtype antibody response to the 12/13 kDa component of the parasite excretory/secretory antigen. The diagnostic sensitivity of this test reportedly is 68% and the specificity 95%; results have been positively correlated with the level of tapeworm infection.[73,74] The clinical utility of this test has been demonstrated. In one study the ELISA implicated tapeworm infection in the abnormally high incidence of colic in a group of race horses. Subsequently, treatment for tapeworm infection significantly decreased the colic incidence in these horses.[64] In another study the ELISA demonstrated a rise in specific antibodies in grazing foals 4 months before tapeworm eggs appeared in the feces.[70]

Treatment and Control

There is no effective control of the oribatid mite. Hence, control of tapeworms in pastured horses relies on anthelmintic treatment. In general, horses with light infections are not treated. Horses with heavy infections or clinical signs suggestive of tapeworm infection may benefit from anthelmintic treatment.

PYRANTEL. Pyrantel pamoate given orally at 13.2 mg/kg or 19.8 mg/kg (i.e., two to three times the standard dose) reportedly is effective against *A. perfoliata*.[75] Pyrantel pamoate at 38 mg/kg was highly effective in foals naturally infected with *A. perfoliata*.[70] However, pyrantel pamoate (embonate) was ineffective against *A. mamillana* even when given at 38 mg/kg for four consecutive days.[66]

Daily feeding of pyrantel tartrate (Strongid C or its generic equivalent) at 2.65 mg/kg/day is highly effective at suppressing fecal egg output within 4 weeks of beginning administration.[75,76] It was more effective than pyrantel pamoate at 19.8 mg/kg repeated every 8 weeks.[75]

PRAZIQUANTEL. Praziquantel at 0.75 to 1.0 mg/kg PO is highly effective against both *A. perfoliata* and *A. mamillana*.[66,77] A dosage of 0.5 mg/kg appears to be effective against *A. perfoliata* in the majority of horses; however, its efficacy is moderate to poor in about 25% of horses.[78] Praziquantel is not approved for use in horses in most countries. However, the small animal preparations (Droncit tablets and injectable solution) have been used without ill effect for the treatment of tapeworm infection in horses.[66,77] Because the life cycle is relatively long, treatment once or twice a year generally is sufficient to control tapeworms in grazing horses.

REFERENCES

59. Williamson RM et al: The distribution of *Anoplocephala perfoliata* in the intestine of the horse and associated pathological changes, *Vet Parasitol* 73:225-241, 1997.
60. Rodriguez-Bertos A et al: Pathological alterations caused by *Anoplocephala perfoliata* infection in the ileocaecal junction of equids, *Zentralbl Veterinarmed A* 4:261-269, 1999.
61. Barclay WP, Phillips TN, Foerner JJ: Intussusception associated with *Anoplocephala perfoliata* infection in five horses, *J Am Vet Med Assoc* 180:752-753, 1982.
62. Proudman CJ, Edwards GB: Are tapeworms associated with equine colic? A case control study, *Equine Vet J* 25:224-226, 1993.
63. Proudman CJ, French NP, Trees AJ: Tapeworm infection is a significant risk factor for spasmodic colic and ileal impaction colic in the horse, *Equine Vet J* 30:194-199, 1998.
64. Proudman CJ, Holdstock NB: Investigation of an outbreak of tapeworm-associated colic in a training yard, *Proceedings of the Sixth Equine Colic Research Symposium*, 1998, p 26.
65. Martin BB et al: Cecocolic and cecocecal intussusception in horses: 30 cases (1976-1996), *J Am Vet Med Assoc* 214:80-84, 1999.
66. Proudman CJ, Swan JD, Trees AJ: Efficacy of pyrantel embonate and praziquantel against the equine tapeworm *Anoplocephaloides mamillana*, *Vet Rec* 137:45-46, 1995.
67. Lyons ET et al: Parasites in Kentucky thoroughbreds at necropsy: emphasis on stomach worms and tapeworms, *Am J Vet Res* 44:839-844, 1983.
68. Bain SA, Kelly JD: Prevalence and pathogenicity of *Anoplocephala perfoliata* in horse populations in South Auckland, *N Z Vet J* 25:27-28, 1977.
69. Slocombe JOD: Prevalence and treatment of tapeworms in horses, *Can Vet J* 20:136, 1979.
70. Hoglund J et al: Epidemiology of *Anoplocephala perfoliata* infection in foals on a stud farm in south-western Sweden, *Vet Parasitol* 75:71-79, 1998.

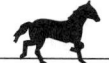

71. Proudman CJ et al: Immunoepidemiology of the equine tapeworm *Anoplocephala perfoliata*: age-intensity profile and age-dependency of antibody subtype responses, *Parasitology* 114:89-94, 1997.
72. Williamson RM, Beveridge I, Gasser RB: Coprological methods for the diagnosis of *Anoplocephala perfoliata* infection of the horse, *Aust Vet J* 76:618-621, 1998.
73. Proudman CJ, Trees AJ: Correlation of antigen specific IgG and IgG(T) responses with *Anoplocephala perfoliata* infection intensity in the horse, *Parasite Immunol* 18:499-506, 1996.
74. Proudman CJ, Trees AJ: Use of excretory/secretory antigens for the sero-diagnosis of *Anoplocephala perfoliata* cestodosis, *Vet Parasitol* 61:239-247, 1996.
75. Kivipelto J, Nicklin C, Asquith RL: Comparison of pyrantel tartrate (Strongid C) and pyrantel pamoate (3x Strongid) for the control of equine tapeworms, *Proceedings of the Forty-fourth Annual Convention of the American Association of Equine Practitioners*, 1998, pp 236-239.
76. Greiner EC, Lane TJ: Effect of the daily feeding of pyrantel tartrate on *Anoplocephala* infection in three horses: a pilot study, *J Equine Vet Sci* 1:43-44, 1994.
77. Lyons ET, Tolliver SC, Ennis LE: Efficacy of praziquantel (0.25 mg kg^{-1}) on the cecal tapeworm *(Anoplocephala perfoliata)* in horses, *Vet Parasitol* 78:287-289, 1998.
78. Lyons ET et al: Activity of praziquantel (0.5 mg kg^{-1}) against *Anoplocephala perfoliata* (Cestoda) in equids, *Vet Parasitol* 56:255-257, 1995.

GASTROINTESTINAL NEMATODE INFECTIONS IN SHEEP AND GOATS

Gastrointestinal nematode infections in sheep and goats are responsible for severe clinical syndromes and profound production losses. Young animals, periparturient ewes and does, and animals on substandard planes of nutrition are most susceptible to outbreaks of parasitic disease. Anthelmintic resistance is now widespread, so control requires integrated management strategies.

Sheep and goats share the same species of gastrointestinal nematodes. Of primary importance in both hosts are *Haemonchus contortus*, *Ostertagia* (or *Teladorsagia*) spp., and *Trichostrongylus* spp. *H. contortus* usually is the most significant pathogen in wet, temperate climates. *Ostertagia circumcincta* may be the predominant infection in northern or arid climates. Other gastrointestinal nematodes that can be important in small ruminants include *Nematodirus*, *Cooperia*, and *Oesophagostomum* spp.

Life Cycle

The life cycle of these gastrointestinal nematodes are direct.[78] Eggs passed in the feces rapidly develop into infective third-stage larvae (L$_3$). Under optimum environmental conditions embryonated eggs may develop into infective larvae in as little as 4 to 6 days. Larvae may survive on pasture for several months, although few *H. contortus* larvae survive past 6 months. *Ostertagia* eggs and larvae are more resistant to arid conditions and may survive 6 months or more. In all species, infective larvae are ingested with herbage and may develop directly into egg-laying adults. Within 2 to 4 weeks after ingestion of the infective larvae, eggs may be present in the feces. However, with *Haemonchus* and *Ostertagia*, L$_4$ larvae may arrest for several months and resume development at a later date. These arrested larvae pose particular difficulties in designing parasite control programs.

The number of infective larvae on the pasture depends on the effects of climate and season on larval viability. In temperate climates, eggs shed in the spring develop over the course of several weeks into infective L$_3$ larvae. The periparturient rise in ewes and the maturation of hypobiotic larvae contribute to the large number of eggs present on the pasture in the spring. In most areas, pasture contamination with L$_3$ larvae peaks in early to midsummer but declines if larvae are subjected to heat or dry conditions. In areas with relatively dry springs and hot summers, peak contamination coincides with autumn rains.

Pathophysiology

The damage done by *H. contortus* is the result of the blood sucking by L$_4$ and adult parasites. The pathogenesis of ostertagiasis in sheep is similar to that described in cattle and is a result of destruction of abomasal mucosa. *Trichostrongylus axei* causes abomasitis, whereas *T. colubriformis* penetrates beneath the intestinal mucosa and causes blood loss and enteritis.

Populations at Risk

Young animals are most susceptible to infection and clinical manifestations of disease. Lambs and kids may become heavily infected with parasites and shed large numbers of nematode eggs. In sheep, some degree of immunity develops as the animal approaches 1 year of age. Adult animals typically have complete immunity against *Nematodirus* and variable resistance to *Trichostrongylus* spp. Some immunity to *Haemonchus* and *Ostertagia* spp. develops with age; compared with lambs or kids, adults are more resistant to infection with these species. However, even mature animals may succumb to parasitic infection when malnourished or challenged with heavily contaminated pasture. A periparturient rise in fecal egg production is seen in ewes and does.

Goats are more susceptible to gastrointestinal nematode infections than are sheep. The difference lies in part in the host's immunologic responses to nematode antigens. Goats do not appear to develop the same level of natural immunity as sheep.[79,80]

Clinical Manifestations

Most parasitic infections in small ruminants are associated with altered gut function, anorexia, ill thrift, weight loss, and hypoproteinemia. Diarrhea is a variable sign. Animals may die suddenly without overt clinical signs or may exhibit chronic wasting. In *H. contortus* infections the clinical signs are caused by blood loss and abomasitis resulting from migration of larvae into the mucosal glands and attachment of adult worms to the abomasal mucosa. Severely affected animals become hypoproteinemic and exhibit edematous swellings under the jaw and ventrum. Blood loss may be severe enough to cause sudden collapse and death. In these cases the animal may die before the infection is patent. Diarrhea may develop as a result of hypoproteinemia and mucosal inflammation. The damage done to the abomasum appears to decrease the absorption of dietary protein, calcium, and phosphorus. In chronic cases, affected animals become anorectic, anemic, and debilitated. The wool becomes brittle and may fall out in patches. Death may finally ensue from depletion of iron stores. Light *H. contortus* infections may cause mild anemia and decreased production. In addition, parasitized animals are more susceptible to diseases from other agents; pneumonia is common in debilitated animals.

Clinical signs associated with *Ostertagia* infection appear to be less common in small ruminants. Infection may cause two separate syndromes. Type I infections, associated with the heavy burdens of L$_3$ stages acquired in the fall or early spring, are characterized by diarrhea, anorexia, and weight loss, often in younger animals. Signs associated with type II infections are caused by the emergence of arrested larvae in the spring or early fall. Affected animals exhibit anorexia, hypoproteinemia, and submandibular edema. As these signs are also seen with *H. contortus* infection, diagnosis on the basis of clinical signs may be misleading. *Ostertagia* infection is discussed further in the section on cattle parasites.

Most animals acquire mixed infections of nematodes. Clinical signs may therefore reflect the effects of more than one species of parasite. There appears to be some synergism

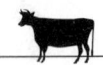

between *O. circumcincta* and *T. colubriformis,* which makes the effect of the combined infection more severe than that of either alone.

Control of Gastrointestinal Nematodes

Sustainable control of gastrointestinal nematode infections in sheep and goats requires an integrated management system that incorporates strategic anthelmintic use, selective breeding, and nutritional and environmental management. Several excellent reviews of integrated parasite control programs have been published.[81-85] Following is a discussion of anthelmintic use. However, it is stressed that anthelmintics are only one component of effective parasite control.

ANTHELMINTICS. The most widely used anthelmintics in small ruminants in recent years are the BZDs, levamisole, and avermectins. Currently in the United States, available anthelmintics approved for use in sheep are limited to levamisole, morantel, and ivermectin. Other anthelmintics (e.g., cattle products) are often used in an extralabel manner. Drugs and dosages are listed in Table 45-3.

Anthelmintic resistance in gastrointestinal nematodes is now widespread in sheep and goats and has a serious impact on animal health and production. Resistance has been reported for each class of anthelmintic, including the avermectins/milbemycins. For example, *H. contortus* has shown resistance to phenothiazine, various BZDs and probenzimidazoles, levamisole, morantel, rafoxanide, organophosphates, closantel, ivermectin, and moxidectin.[80,86] Resistance to two or more classes of drug has been reported for strains of *H. contortus, Ostertagia,* and *Trichostrongylus.*[87-90]

Benzimidazole resistance is particularly widespread, and resistance to one virtually ensures resistance to all BZDs and probenzimidazoles.[91] The situation may be little different with levamisole and morantel. Although nematodes that are resistant to levamisole tend also to be resistant to morantel, morantel-resistant nematodes may still be susceptible to levamisole.[91] Resistance to levamisole is apparently rare in *H. contortus* but relatively common in *Ostertagia* and *Trichostrongylus.*[92] Resistance to ivermectin has been reported in several countries, although it appears to be less common than resistance to the other anthelmintic classes. Cross-resistance to moxidectin has been reported in a strain of *H. contortus* in Australia.[86]

The prevalence of anthelmintic resistance varies with geographic location and animal production system. Resistance is most widespread in the southern hemisphere (Australia, New Zealand, South Africa, and various countries in South America). In these warmer climates the generation time for gastrointestinal nematodes is shorter, which enables drug resistance to become established more readily. Resistance is also found most commonly in intensive production systems incorporating frequent anthelmintic use.[80,83,93]

Compared with sheep, goats are both more susceptible to internal parasitism and less responsive to recommended dosages of anthelmintics.[94-96] In addition, anthelmintic resistance may develop more rapidly in goats.[80] Thus it has been recommended that the anthelmintic dosages used in sheep be doubled for goats.[95] With benzimidazoles, 4 to 8 times the recommended sheep dose (e.g., fenbendazole at 23 mg/kg, albendazole at 40 mg/kg) have been used against multiple-resistant strains of *H. contortus* in goats.[88] Mixing of two anthelmintics from different classes, such as albendazole with ivermectin, has also been suggested for farms where multiple anthelmintic resistance is documented or suspected.[88,95] Chronic low-dose administration of an anthelmintic in the form of a controlled-release intraruminal capsule has also proven effective against benzimidazole-resistant nematodes in goats.[97,98]

TREATMENT INTERVALS. Treatment intervals vary, depending on geographic location, management system, and anthelmintic (in particular, duration of the drug's suppressive effect). The goal should not be to simply rid infected animals of parasites, but to also limit reinfection by reducing pasture infectivity. Administration of one treatment to animals on contaminated pasture does little to control parasitic disease, regardless of the drug's efficacy. If the animals cannot be moved to a "clean" pasture after treatment (see below), suppressive treatments at regular intervals may be required for effective parasite control. In temperate climates, treatment every 2 to 4 weeks may be necessary on some premises during the spring and summer. In climates with hot, dry summers or with very cold winters, the seasonal variations in larval viability can be used to advantage to limit both the frequency and number of anthelmintic treatments required.

RECOMMENDATIONS FOR MAXIMIZING ANTHELMINTIC EFFICACY. The following strategies are recommended for maximizing efficacy and limiting the incidence and impact of anthelmintic resistance in sheep and goats[80,81,83,91,99]:

- Use the full therapeutic dose on all members of the group. To avoid underdosing, a representative sample of animals

TABLE 45-3

Efficacy of Various Anthelmintics Against Gastrointestinal Nematodes in Ruminants

Drug	Dosage (mg/kg)* Sheep†	Dosage (mg/kg)* Cattle	Adults	Hypobiotic Larvae
BENZIMIDAZOLES				
Albendazole	5 to 7.5	7.5 to 10	+	+
Febantel	5	7.5 to 10	+	+/−
Fenbendazole	5	7.5 to 10	+	+/−
Mebendazole	15 to 20		+	+/−
Netobimin	7.5	7.5	+	+
Oxfendazole	5	7.5	+	+
Oxibendazole	15	15	+	+/−
Ricobendazole	5		+	−
LEVAMISOLE/MORANTEL				
Levamisole	5 to 7.55	5 to 7.5‡	+	+/−
Morantel	5 to 12.5	10	+	−
Pyrantel	25	12.5	+	−
AVERMECTINS/MILBEMYCINS				
Ivermectin	0.2	0.2§	+	+
Doramectin	0.2	0.2§	+	+
Eprinomectin		0.5‖	+	+
Moxidectin	0.2	0.2§	+	+
OTHER DRUGS				
Closantel	5 to 10		+¶	−
Nitroxynil	10		+¶	−

+, Highly effective; +/−, moderately effective or effective according to some authors; −, ineffective.
*All dosages are for oral administration, unless otherwise indicated.
†Goats must be given higher dosages for equal efficacy.
‡10 mg/kg for topical administration.
§0.2 mg/kg for PO, SC, or IM administration; 0.5 mg/kg topically ("pour-on").
‖Available only for topical administration at 0.5 mg/kg; not recommended for sheep.
¶Effective against *Haemonchus contortus* only.
NOTE: administration of some of these products may constitute extralabel use in sheep and goats; follow manufacturers' guidelines for meat and milk withdrawal in cattle.

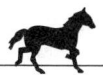

from the age or sex class should be weighed and all animals in that class treated with the dose calculated for the heaviest individual. Dosing equipment should be regularly checked for accuracy.

■ Rotate anthelmintic classes annually. In tropical climates, where nematode generation times are faster than in temperate climates, more frequent rotation may be necessary. However, very frequent rotation favors development of drug resistance as much as does no rotation. Where a specific parasite is a major problem, a narrow-spectrum drug (e.g., nitroxynil or closantel for *H. contortus*) can be incorporated into the rotation program. Combining anthelmintics from two classes has been effective on farms where multiple drug resistance is a problem.

■ Limit the dosing frequency by using strategic treatments in an integrated pasture management system. One option is the "dose and move" strategy in which animals are treated, then moved to a clean pasture, one that has not been used for weaners or parturient ewes/does for the past 6 months, pasture that has been pregrazed by another host species (cattle or horses) or by animals given controlled-release anthelmintic capsules, or crop stubble. This strategy is often recommended before lambing/kidding in pregnant ewes/does or at weaning in lambs/kids. In ewes and does an anthelmintic that is effective against hypobiotic larvae is often the best choice for limiting pasture infectivity and parasitic disease in their lambs/kids. Some feel that the "dose and move" strategy actually encourages establishment of resistant parasites, as the only parasites that arrive on the new pasture are those that survived anthelmintic treatment.

Another strategy is to time anthelmintic treatment for the seasonal peaks and troughs in larval numbers. For example, a series of prophylactic treatments in the spring can prevent the midsummer peak in pasture infectivity that is common in temperate climates. Moxidectin suppresses fecal egg counts for longer than does ivermectin.[100] This fact can be used to limit the frequency of anthelmintic treatments in various grazing systems. Prolonged low-level exposure to anthelmintic, such as is provided by a controlled-release intraruminal device, can have the same effect.

■ Avoid introducing resistant nematodes with newly acquired animals. All incoming stock should be treated with a broad-spectrum nonbenzimidazole anthelmintic and held off pasture for at least 24 hours. In the northern hemisphere, it may be worth screening all incoming stock imported from the southern hemisphere for resistant nematodes before introduction.

■ Do not graze sheep and goats on the same farm.

■ Periodically check the efficacy of the anthelmintics used by performing fecal egg counts before and 10 to 14 days after treatment. On a herd basis the aim should be to keep the average fecal egg count below 500 EPG. Another means of monitoring the efficacy of the parasite control program is to examine slaughtered animals for parasites or signs of parasitic disease.

STRATEGIES TO AUGMENT ANTHELMINTIC PROGRAMS. Temporary reduction in feed intake, such as halving feed intake for 36 hours before and after treatment, has been shown to increase the efficacy of oxfendazole against BZDs-resistant nematodes in sheep.[101,102] Increasing the protein or nonprotein nitrogen intake before the grazing season begins can have both short-term and long-term benefits on resistance to parasite infection, pasture contamination, anthelmintic efficacy, and production indices in sheep and goats under a variety of production systems.[81,103-105]

Future initiatives aimed at controlling gastrointestinal nematodes in ruminants include development of vaccines to enhance host resistance and use of biologic control, such as the nematophagous fungus *Duddingtonia flagrans*.[81,106]

Clinical Management

DIAGNOSIS. Internal parasites should be suspected in cases of diarrhea, poor condition, anemia, or acute collapse in small ruminants. Necropsy and histologic section are the most reliable methods of diagnosis. Adult *H. contortus* may be found on gross examination; occasionally they are expelled by diarrheic animals or may have been removed by prior anthelmintic administration. Total worm counts may be performed to establish the magnitude of infection. It is unwise to base a diagnosis solely on the results of fecal examination.

TREATMENT. Most animals respond to appropriate anthelmintic treatment. In severely affected animals, additional therapy is supportive and symptomatic. Animals with diarrhea may be treated with fluids. Transfusions have been attempted in anemic animals; however, the stress of treatment may kill severely parasitized animals.

REFERENCES

79. Kassai T: Phylum: Nemathelminthes—roundworms. In *Veterinary helminthology*, Butterworth Heinemann, Oxford, 1999, pp 75-83.
80. Hazelby CA, Probert AJ, Rowlands DAT: Anthelmintic resistance in nematodes causing parasitic gastroenteritis of sheep in the UK, *J Vet Pharmacol Therap* 17:245-252, 1994.
81. Kassai T: Anthelmintic therapy and control. In *Veterinary helminthology*, Butterworth Heinemann, Oxford, pp. 147-179, 1999.
82. Barger IA: Prospects for integration of novel parasite control options into grazing systems, *Intl J Parasitol* 26:1001-1007, 1996.
83. Barger IA: The role of epidemiological knowledge and grazing management for helminth control in small ruminants, *Intl J Parasitol* 29:41-47, 1999.
84. Waller PJ: Nematode parasite control of livestock in the tropics/subtropics: the need for novel approaches, *Intl J Parasitol* 27:1193-1201, 1997.
85. Waller PJ: International approaches to the concept of integrated control of nematode parasites of livestock, *Intl J Parasitol* 29:155-164, 1999.
86. LeJambre LF, Gill JH, Lenane IJ, Lacey E: Characterisation of an avermectin-resistant strain of Australian *Haemonchus contortus*, *Intl J Parasitol* 25:691-698, 1995.
87. Jackson F, Jackson E, Coop RL: Evidence of multiple anthelmintic resistance in a strain of *Teladorsagia circumcincta (Ostertagia circumcincta)* isolated from goats in Scotland, *Res Vet Sci* 53:371-374, 1992.
88. Miller DK, Craig TM: Use of anthelmintic combinations against multiple resistant *Haemonchus contortus* in Angora goats, *Small Ruminant Res* 19:281-283, 1996.
89. Maingi N et al: Anthelmintic resistance in nematode parasites of sheep in Denmark, *Small Ruminant Res* 23:171-181, 1996.
90. Amarante AFT et al: Evaluation of a larval development assay for the detection of anthelmintic resistance in *Ostertagia circumcincta*, *Intl J Parasitol* 27:305-311, 1997.
91. Coles GC, Roush RT: Slowing the spread of anthelmintic resistant nematodes of sheep and goats in the United Kingdom, *Vet Rec* 130:505-510, 1992.
92. Dobson RJ, LeJambre L, Gill JH: Management of anthelmintic resistance: inheritance of resistance and selection with persistent drugs, *Intl J Parasitol* 26:993-1000, 1996.
93. Waller PJ et al: Anthelmintic resistance in nematode parasite of sheep: learning from the Australian experience, *Vet Rec* 136:411-413, 1995.
94. Sangster NC et al: Disposition of oxfendazole in goats and efficacy compared with sheep, *Res Vet Sci* 51:258-263, 1991.
95. Varady M et al: Multiple anthelmintic resistance of nematodes in imported goats, *Vet Rec* 132:387-388, 1993.
96. Huntley JF et al: A comparison of the mast cell and eosinophil responses of sheep and goats to gastrointestinal nematode infections, *Res Vet Sci* 58:5-10, 1995.
97. McDougall S: Controlled-release anthelmintic treatment of milking goats, *Aust Vet J* 69:64-65, 1992.
98. Sangster NC et al: Use of a controlled-release albendazole capsule in goats, *Aust Vet J* 69:67-68, 1992.
99. Clarkson MJ, Winter AC: Thin scouring lambs. In *A handbook for the sheep clinician*, ed 5, Liverpool, 1997, Liverpool University Press, pp 108-114.
100. Rendell D, Callinan L: The duration of anthelmintic effects of moxidectin and ivermectin in grazing sheep, *Aust Vet J* 73:35, 1996.
101. Ali DN, Hennessy DR: The effect of feed intake on the rate of flow of digesta and the disposition and activity of oxfendazole in sheep, *Intl J Parasitol* 23:477-484, 1993.

102. Ali DN, Hennessy DR: The effect of reduced feed intake on the efficacy of oxfendazole against benzimidazole-resistant *Haemonchus contortus* and *Trichostrongylus colubriformis* in sheep, *Intl J Parasitol* 25:71-74, 1995.

103. Knox M, Steel J: Nutritional enhancement of parasite control in small ruminant production systems in developing countries of southeast Asia and the Pacific, *Intl J Parasitol* 26:963-970, 1996.

104. Theodoropoulos G et al: The effect of dietary protein levels before turnout on subsequent faecal nematode egg output of grazing sheep in the Joannina region of Greece, *Res Vet Sci* 65:269-271, 1998.

105. Datta FU et al: Long-term effects of short-term provision of protein-enriched diets on resistance to nematode infection, and live-weight gain and wool growth in sheep, *Intl J Parasitol* 29:479-488, 1999.

106. Newton SE: Progress on vaccination against *Haemonchus contortus*, *Intl J Parasitol* 25:1281-1289, 1995.

GASTROINTESTINAL NEMATODE INFECTIONS IN CATTLE

Cattle are susceptible to infection with a variety of nematode parasites, including *Ostertagia, Haemonchus, Cooperia, Trichostrongylus,* and *Nematodirus.* Mixed infections are common. This discussion focuses on the control of *Ostertagia ostertagi* because it is the target of most parasite control programs for cattle. Of all species of cattle nematode, *O. ostertagi* is most pathogenic and causes the greatest economic loss. In general, anthelmintic programs designed to minimize *Ostertagia* infections successfully control other species of gastrointestinal nematode parasites.

Life Cycle

O. ostertagi is the primary species involved in bovine parasitic disease, although *Ostertagia leptospicularis* and *Ostertagia bisonis* have also been incriminated in disease outbreaks. The life cycle and pathophysiology of bovine ostertagiasis have been extensively reviewed.[107,108] The life cycle is direct. Eggs passed in feces onto pasture may develop into infective third-stage larvae (L_3) in as little as 10 days under suitable conditions. Third-stage larvae are ingested and undergo their entire development within the gastric glands of the abomasal mucosa. Some larvae return to the lumen in as little as 18 days, and they establish patent infections in 21 days. Under certain conditions fourth-stage larvae (L_4) can arrest their development and remain within the abomasal glands for several months. Thus the prepatent period may be as short as 3 weeks or as long as 4 months.

The interaction between climatic factors and the population dynamics of *Ostertagia* are complex.[107-109] Infective larvae can overwinter on the pasture, but their survival is decreased in hot, dry conditions. Fecal pats can enhance larval survival in such conditions. Further complicating the picture is the ability of L_4 to "overwinter" or "oversummer" in the host to avoid adverse environmental conditions. Thus, in temperate climates, pasture larval populations peak in the summer and early autumn, and L_4 tend to overwinter in the host. In warmer climates with hot, dry summers, the highest numbers of infective larvae may be found in the spring and arrested larvae emerge in the fall, having oversummered in the host. In subtropical climates, seasonality may be much less marked and pasture infectivity may follow the rainfall pattern. In arid climates, large numbers of larvae may be present on the pasture whenever local conditions permit lush grass growth.

Pathophysiology

The pathophysiology of ostertagiasis can be divided into two phases. The first occurs when ingested larvae invade the gastric glands of the abomasum. As these larvae develop within the gland, they cause gland hyperplasia and intense eosinophilic infiltration. Mucosal glandular cells lose their differentiation, and cell junctions are weakened. Albumin is lost into the lumen. Parietal cells cease to function, causing a decrease in HCl production. The change in pH profoundly affects the function of the abomasum. Alkalinity stimulates overproduction of gastrin, which initiates cell proliferation and hyperplasia. Also, the bactericidal activity of the abomasum is decreased, resulting in bacterial overflow from the rumen into the intestine. In addition a pH greater than 5.0 prevents the transformation of pepsinogen into pepsin. This enzyme is released into the blood through permeable cell junctions. Hyperplasia and loss of cell differentiation become widespread and create the so-called "Moroccan leather" appearance of the abomasum. In experimental models, *Ostertagia* infection in calves is associated with elevated peripheral eosinophil counts and decreased lymphocyte counts.[110]

The second phase occurs when arrested larvae resume their development and emerge from the gastric glands *en masse.* Emergence of the larvae may complete the destruction of the glands. If the infection is severe, the proliferated cells and abomasal mucosa may slough, producing a diphtheritic membrane.

Populations at Risk

The cattle at greatest risk of developing clinical ostertagiasis are calves during their first grazing season. Exposure to this and other gastrointestinal nematodes incites an immune response in the host such that most animals develop immunity during their first grazing season. After their first year at pasture, adult cattle rarely show signs of nematode infection or require anthelmintic treatment. Although mature cattle ingest infective larvae, the larvae fail to establish infections; thus parasite burdens and the magnitude of fecal egg shedding generally are small. Most preventive and treatment strategies are directed at young grazing stock, primarily beef calves and dairy replacement heifers.

Clinical Manifestations

In young animals, *Ostertagia* and other nematode parasites may simply cause poor growth and ill thrift, or they may cause serious clinical illness and even death. A feature of *Ostertagia* infection is inappetence, which results in reduced production parameters, including weight gain, growth, and onset of puberty. Clinical ostertagiasis is divided into two types: Type I is associated with ingestion of large numbers of infective larvae while on pasture. It manifests as diarrhea, anorexia, and severe production losses in calves during their first grazing season. Type II ostertagiasis is caused by the development and emergence of hypobiotic larvae. It is usually seen in cattle 1 to 2 years of age. Although it is most common in pastured animals, type II disease can also be seen in feedlot and housed animals that have previously grazed infected pasture. Anorexia, ill thrift, and hypoproteinemia are consistent signs. The animals may also show fever, diarrhea, anemia, and submandibular edema. The prognosis for recovery is guarded, owing to the widespread destruction of abomasal glands.

Control of Gastrointestinal Nematodes

ANTHELMINTICS. Adult *Ostertagia* and other gastrointestinal nematodes are susceptible to most of the commonly used anthelmintics.[111-114] Drugs and dosages are listed in Table 45-3. Drug withdrawal times must be considered when selecting anthelmintics for beef cattle and lactating dairy cows, and the manufacturers' recommendations followed. Eprinomectin, one of the newer avermectins available in a topical formulation, has no withdrawal period for either meat or milk.

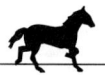

The newer avermectins and moxidectin are particularly effective against both adult and larval stages of the various gastrointestinal nematodes in cattle, including inhibited L_4.[114-116] In addition, their residual effect helps minimize pasture infectivity during the grazing season (see below).[117-120] Intraruminal sustained-release devices (SRDs) containing a benzimidazole, levamisole, morantel, or ivermectin can also be highly effective at limiting both clinical disease and pasture infectivity.[121-125] Use of highly efficacious drugs or SRDs can attenuate the immune response to gastrointestinal nematodes during the first grazing season in calves. However, in most cases immunity is sufficient to prevent clinical disease during the following grazing season, and weight gains by the end of the second season are similar to those of immune animals.[122,123,125]

Although the avermectins and moxidectin are all highly effective, some differences between products in both efficacy and duration of effect are apparent. Doramectin, eprinomectin, and moxidectin are more effective and/or have a longer residual effect than ivermectin against *Ostertagia* and *Cooperia*.[126-132] Doramectin, eprinomectin, and moxidectin have a residual effect against *Ostertagia* for about 5 weeks, whereas ivermectin is effective for only 2 to 3 weeks.[119,132] As the prepatent period for *Ostertagia* is approximately 3 weeks, the treatment intervals in most management situations are 8 weeks for doramectin, eprinomectin, and moxidectin, and 5 to 6 weeks for ivermectin. Duration of effect also varies somewhat with the parasite and the level of infection. Persistence of effect against *Cooperia* appears to be 1 to 2 weeks shorter than for *Ostertagia*, regardless of the product used.[118,119,132-134] The residual effect may be shortened by a week or so at high infection levels.[132,133]

Drug resistance by gastrointestinal nematodes is far less of a problem in cattle than in sheep. However, there have been some reports of lack of efficacy against *Ostertagia* with some BZDs and levamisole, and resistance to ivermectin in *Cooperia*.[114,135,136]

TREATMENT INTERVALS. The choice of drug and treatment interval should be made on the basis of an individual herd or farm, as part of an overall control program. Factors to consider include the geographic location, time of year, and grazing management. Grazing management is discussed elsewhere.[137] There are several options for preventing clinical disease and maximizing gains in first-season grazing calves using strategic anthelmintic treatments:

- Two treatments with an avermectin or moxidectin early in the grazing season. The first treatment can be given either at turnout/weaning or 3 weeks into the grazing period. Depending on the product used, the second dose is given 6 weeks (ivermectin) or 8 weeks (doramectin, eprinomectin, moxidectin) later. This strategy can prevent clinical disease, keep fecal egg counts and serum pepsinogen levels low, and increase weight gains during the first grazing season.[138,139] An alternative when using ivermectin in situations in which pasture infectivity is high is to treat calves at 3, 8, and 13 weeks after turnout/weaning.[140]
- "Dose and move" just before the anticipated peak in pasture infectivity (e.g., early to mid-summer in temperate climates). The calves are treated with a single dose of anthelmintic, then moved to a clean pasture. This strategy minimizes the number of anthelmintic treatments during the grazing season. However, it is only effective on farms where a clean pasture is available.
- Use of an intraruminal sustained-release device at turnout or weaning. This strategy may be most cost effective on farms where pasture infectivity is high.
- Treatment during peak pasture infectivity (e.g., summer and early autumn in temperate climates). Treatment interval depends on the product being used: every 3 weeks for nonivermectin drugs, every 5 weeks for ivermectin. For ex-

ample, ivermectin can be given at 10, 15, and 20 weeks after turnout/weaning. This strategy prevents clinical disease in the majority of calves while allowing some level of infection, which stimulates an immune response in first-season calves. However, treatment at the start of the grazing season has been shown to result in better weight gains than tactical treatments given during the grazing season.[121]

Hypobiotic larvae can be difficult to eliminate. The avermectins moxidectin and albendazole are effective against arrested larvae and are useful in the treatment and prevention of type II ostertagiasis—a disease that is better prevented than treated. By dosing the cattle after the accumulation of larvae, the parasites do not have the opportunity to become hypobiotic. For example, if type II ostertagiasis is anticipated in the fall of the year, anthelmintic administration should be planned for the summer. A single treatment on entry to the feed lot is a useful precaution against type II ostertagiasis in beef calves coming off pasture.

ADULT CATTLE. The cattle most at risk of clinical disease and production losses are beef calves and dairy replacement heifers in their first season at pasture. Strategic treatment early in the grazing season is effective in most management situations. Development of immunity should protect the animals during their second and subsequent grazing seasons. Treatment of adult cattle generally is unnecessary, unless immunity is inadequate or pasture infectivity is high.[141,142] Anthelmintic treatment is most likely to be warranted in first-calf heifers and newly acquired cows that may not have been pastured as heifers. In some situations it may be beneficial to treat beef cows after spring calving.

Evaluation of Anthelmintic Programs

Because of the importance of arrested larvae in the pathophysiology of ostertagiasis, fecal egg counts can be misleading. The parasite does the most damage to the host as it enters the gastric gland and as it leaves; however, the infection is unlikely to be patent during these periods. Consequently, animals suffering from type I or type II ostertagiasis may have low fecal egg counts. Fecal egg counts are most useful as a tool to evaluate the success of control programs. Fecal examinations may be done 3 to 4 weeks after spring turnout to assess the magnitude of the infection acquired from overwintered or developing arrested larvae. If the counts are excessive, additional treatment and/or movement of the animals may be indicated. Fecal egg counts may also be performed 4 to 6 weeks after normal peaks in pasture infectivity to determine the magnitude of infection at this time.

Serum pepsinogen levels are often elevated in response to severe *Ostertagia* infection. This parameter may be helpful in the identification of ostertagiasis as a herd problem. In one study of first-season calves, serum pepsinogen levels were less than 2.6 U tyrosine in calves that were treated during the grazing season, 2.0 to 4.1 U tyrosine in subclinically affected untreated calves, and 3.7 to 6.3 U tyrosine in clinically affected untreated calves.[143] Specific enzyme-linked immunosorbent assays (ELISAs) for *Ostertagia* and *Cooperia* may also be useful for herd monitoring.[144] However, neither of these tests is widely available at this time.

Clinical Management

DIAGNOSIS. The most reliable method of diagnosis is necropsy. The "Moroccan leather" abomasal lesion is pathognomonic for *Ostertagia*. It may be difficult to identify parasites with a casual macroscopic examination because both larvae in gastric glands and adult worms are small and easily overlooked. Histologic section and abomasal wall digestion techniques can be used to identify the presence of larvae.

Antemortem, the history and clinical signs are most useful in suggesting a diagnosis of ostertagiasis. Fecal egg counts can be extremely misleading, as they are neither specific nor sensitive for the disease. Serum pepsinogen levels and specific ELISAs for *Ostertagia* may be helpful, if available.

TREATMENT. Animals should be treated with an avermectin or moxidectin and moved to a less contaminated environment at the first indication of clinical signs. All animals in the group should be treated. Animals with type I ostertagiasis can be expected to respond well. The prognosis for animals with type II ostertagiasis is less encouraging. Even though the larvae may be killed, the damage to the abomasal mucosa may limit complete recovery. Animals with profound hypoproteinemia and dehydration respond poorly compared with those showing only mild diarrhea and slight hypoalbuminemia. Severely affected animals may need treatment with fluids, plasma transfusions, and supportive therapy to survive. Recovered animals often fail to thrive.

REFERENCES

107. Kassai T: Phylum Nemathelminthes—roundworms. In *Veterinary helminthology*, Oxford, 1999, Butterworth Heinemann, pp 75-83.
108. Blood DC, Radostits OM, Gay CC: Diseases caused by helminth parasites. In *Veterinary medicine*, ed 8, London, 1994, Baillière Tindall, pp 1259-1265.
109. Kassai T: Planning of integrated control strategies. In *Veterinary helminthology*, Oxford, 1999, Butterworth Heinemann, pp 170-173.
110. Wiggin CJ: Pathogenesis of simulated natural infections with *Ostertagia ostertagi* in calves, *Am J Vet Res* 48:274-280, 1987.
111. Kassai T: Phylum Nemathelminthes—roundworms. In *Veterinary helminthology*, Oxford, 1999, Butterworth Heinemann, p 58.
112. Plumb DC: *Veterinary drug handbook*, ed 3, Iowa, 1999, Iowa State University Press.
113. Williams JC, Broussard SD: Comparative efficacy of levamisole, thiabendazole and fenbendazole against cattle gastrointestinal nematodes, *Vet Parasitol* 58:83-90, 1995.
114. Williams JC et al: Comparative efficacy of ivermectin pour-on, albendazole, oxfendazole and fenbendazole against *Ostertagia ostertagi* inhibited larvae, other gastrointestinal nematodes and lungworm of cattle, *Vet Parasitol* 73:73-82, 1997.
115. Williams JC et al: Efficacy of a pour-on formulation of eprinomectin (MK-397) against nematode parasites of cattle, with emphasis on inhibited early fourth-stage larvae of *Ostertagia* spp, *Am J Vet Res* 58:379-383, 1997.
116. Yazwinski TA et al: Dose confirmation of moxidectin pour-on against natural nematode infections in lactating dairy cows, *Vet Parasitol* 86:223-228, 1999.
117. Jacobs DC et al: An evaluation of abamectin given at turnout and six weeks after turnout for the control of nematode infections in calves, *Vet Rec* 136:386-389, 1995.
118. Eysker M et al: Residual effect of injectable moxidectin against lungworm and gastrointestinal nematodes in calves exposed to high pasture infectivity levels in the Netherlands, *Vet Parasitol* 61:61-71, 1996.
119. Barth D et al: Evaluation of the persistence of the effect of ivermectin and abamectin against gastrointestinal and pulmonary nematodes in cattle, *Vet Rec* 140:278-279, 1997.
120. Ballweber LR et al: The effectiveness of a single treatment with doramectin or ivermectin in the control of gastrointestinal nematodes in grazing yearling stocker cattle, *Vet Parasitol* 72:53-68, 1997.
121. Taylor SM et al: A comparison of early and mid grazing season suppressive anthelmintic treatments for first-year grazing calves and their effects on natural and experimental infection during the second year, *Vet Parasitol* 56:75-90, 1995.
122. Kerboeuf D et al: Response of cattle treated with a fenbendazole slow release bolus to challenge from nematodes the following season, *Vet Parasitol* 62:107-118, 1996.
123. Schnieder T, Epe C, Von Samson-Himmelstjerna G, Kohlmetz C: The development of protective immunity against gastrointestinal nematode and lungworm infections after use of an ivermectin bolus in first-year grazing calves, *Vet Parasitol* 64:239-250, 1996.
124. Bauer C, Holtemoller H, Schmid K: Field evaluation of a fenbendazole slow release bolus in the control of nematode infections in first-season cattle, *Vet Rec* 140:395-396, 1997.
125. Claerebout E et al: Effects of preventive anthelmintic treatment on acquired resistance to gastrointestinal nematodes in naturally infected cattle, *Vet Parasitol* 76:287-303, 1998.
126. Eddi C et al: Comparative persistent efficacy of doramectin, ivermectin and fenbendazole against natural nematode infections in cattle, *Vet Parasitol* 72:33-41, 1997.
127. Hooke FG et al: Therapeutic and protective efficacy of doramectin injectable against gastrointestinal nematodes in cattle in New Zealand: a comparison with moxidectin and ivermectin pour-on formulations, *Vet Parasitol* 72:43-51, 1997.
128. Williams JC et al: Duration of anthelmintic efficacy of doramectin and ivermectin injectable solutions against naturally acquired nematode infections of cattle, *Vet Parasitol* 72:15-24, 1997.
129. Williams JC et al: A comparison of the efficacy of two treatments of doramectin injectable, ivermectin injectable and ivermectin pour-on against naturally acquired gastrointestinal nematode infections of cattle during a winter-spring grazing season, *Vet Parasitol* 72:69-77, 1997.
130. Williams JC et al: A comparison of persistent anthelmintic efficacy of topical formulations of doramectin, ivermectin, eprinomectin and moxidectin against naturally acquired nematode infections of beef calves, *Vet Parasitol* 85:277-288, 1999.
131. Ranjan S et al: Nematode reinfection following treatment of cattle with doramectin and ivermectin, *Vet Parasitol* 72:25-31, 1997.
132. Vercruysse J et al: Evaluation of the persistent efficacy of doramectin and ivermectin injectable against *Ostertagia ostertagi* and *Cooperia oncophora* in cattle, *Vet Parasitol* 89:63-69, 2000.
133. Vercruysse J et al: Persistence of the efficacy of doramectin against *Ostertagia ostertagi* and *Cooperia oncophora* in cattle, *Vet Rec* 143:443-446, 1998.
134. Molento MB et al: Persistent efficacy of doramectin pour-on against artificially induced infections of nematodes in cattle, *Vet Parasitol* 82:297-303, 1999.
135. Stafford K, Coles GC: Nematode control practices and anthelmintic resistance in dairy calves in the south west of England, *Vet Rec* 144:659-661, 1999.
136. Vermunt JJ, West DM, Pomroy WE: Multiple resistance to ivermectin and oxfendazole in *Cooperia* species of cattle in New Zealand, *Vet Rec* 137:43-45, 1995.
137. Stromberg BE, Averbeck GA: The role of parasite epidemiology in the management of grazing cattle, *Intl J Parasitol* 29:33-39, 1999.
138. Vercruysse J et al: Control of gastrointestinal nematodes in first-season grazing calves by two strategic treatments with doramectin, *Vet Parasitol* 58:27-34, 1995.
139. Dorny P et al: Control of gastrointestinal nematodes in first season grazing calves by two strategic treatments with eprinomectin, *Vet Parasitol* 89:277-286, 2000.
140. Fisher MA et al: Evaluation of doramectin in a programme for season-long control of parasitic gastroenteritis in calves, *Vet Rec* 137:281-284, 1995.
141. Herd RP: Control strategies for ruminant and equine parasites to counter resistance, encystment, and ecotoxicity in the USA, *Vet Parasitol* 48:327-336, 1993.
142. Rehbun WC: Infectious diseases of the gastrointestinal tract. In *Diseases of dairy cattle*, Baltimore, 1995, Williams and Wilkins, pp 180-182.
143. Dorny P, Shaw DJ, Vercruysse J: The determination at housing of exposure to gastrointestinal nematode infections in first-grazing season calves, *Vet Parasitol* 80:325-340, 1999.
144. Eysker M, Ploeger HW: Value of present diagnostic methods for gastrointestinal nematode infections in ruminants, *Parasitology* 120:S109-S119, 2000.

LUNGWORM INFECTION IN LARGE ANIMALS

Lungworms are nematode parasites that reside in the lung as adults. In large animal species, one genus, *Dictyocaulus*, is involved in most clinical cases of lungworm. This nematode is very species-specific. *Dictyocaulus viviparus*, *D. arnfieldi*, and *D. filaria* are found in cattle, equids (horses, ponies, donkeys), and small ruminants, respectively. Sheep and goats may also be infected with *Protostrongylus rufescens* and *Millerius capillaris*. This section focuses on *Dictyocaulus* infection, with a brief discussion of other lungworm parasites found in small ruminants.

Because verminous pneumonia requires specific treatment, it is important to distinguish it from diseases caused by other infectious agents. Often the role of lungworm in the etiology of respiratory disease may be obscured by a parasite-induced hypersensitivity response or by superimposed secondary bacterial infections.

Life Cycle

The life cycle of *D. viviparus* is characteristic of this genus. *Dictyocaulus* larvae are passed in the feces and develop into in-

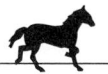

fective L$_3$ in 3 to 7 days. After ingestion they migrate through the wall of the intestine to the mesenteric lymph nodes, through lymphatics into the bloodstream, and finally arrive in the lung. In experimental infections, larvae have been found in the lung by day 7 after ingestion. Once in the lung, larvae may develop into sexually mature adult worms or they may enter a hypobiotic state. The hypobiotic phase enables the parasite to overwinter within the animal host; larvae resume development in the spring. The presence of parasites in the lung induces an immune response that results in death or expulsion of the worms.

Infected pastures serve as a source of contamination for succeeding generations of susceptible animals. Larvae of *Dictyocaulus* spp. are resistant to freezing temperatures and can overwinter on the pasture. This fact and the maturation of hypobiotic larvae in the host can result in high levels of contamination on spring pastures. In some regions, larval contamination of the pasture peaks in the autumn. It has been postulated that some larvae remain in the soil and mature as late as early summer.

M. capillaris and *P. rufescens* have indirect life cycles that involve intermediate snail hosts. Larvae on pasture invade the foot of several species of snails, which are then ingested with grass. The larvae penetrate the intestine and migrate to the lung. In *Millerius* infections, adult parasites become embedded within a fibrous nodule. If the nodule contains both a male and female worm, fertile eggs are deposited in the air passages, coughed up, swallowed, and passed in the feces. *Protostrongylus* larvae mature in the alveoli and enter the bronchioles as adults.

Pathophysiology

Massive invasion of the lung with *Dictyocaulus* larvae may elicit an acute pneumonic syndrome. Initially, infection causes an eosinophilic infiltrate in the lung parenchyma. Damage to the lung results in septal edema, hyaline membrane formation, and alveolar collapse. Bronchomediastinal lymph nodes may become enlarged. Alveolar epithelialization occurs and appears to be the result of a host response to lungworm antigens. Epithelialization may persist, even after the worms have been removed. In animals with less severe infections, a subacute or chronic form of lung pathology may occur. Mechanical irritation caused by adult worms leads to inflammation and accumulation of exudate within the lungs. Fluid accumulation and obstruction of bronchi with worms may cause lung collapse or emphysema. In addition, eggs aspirated into the alveoli may initiate an inflammatory hypersensitivity reaction in the lung parenchyma. As the defenses of the lung are weakened, infection with opportunistic bacteria may lead to bronchopneumonia.

Although morbidity with *M. capillaris* may be high in most flocks, massive infections with *M. capillaris* or *P. rufescens* are rare because it is unusual for sheep or goats to ingest large numbers of snails. *P. rufescens* causes pathologic changes similar to chronic, low-grade *Dictyocaulus* infection. *M. capillaris* infection is responsible for nodule formation in the lungs of sheep and has been implicated in a diffuse interstitial pneumonia in goats.

Populations at Risk

Clinical disease occurs most frequently in pastured calves, lambs, and kids in the first year of life. The disease is also reported in housed cattle, related either to heavily contaminated bedding material or to synchronous maturation of large numbers of hypobiotic larvae. Clinical lungworm infestation is more of a problem in cattle than in sheep, prob-

ably because lambs are treated for gastrointestinal nematodes more frequently than are calves under most management systems.

Immunity to lungworm infection occurs after first exposure, and can develop before the end of the first grazing season. However, it is variable in both degree and duration. In cattle, exposed animals may be immune for 7 to 12 months after infection. In subsequent infections, most larvae are either killed before reaching the lung or inhibited from maturing into adults. Reinfection may be asymptomatic or cause mild signs of disease. Usually the immunity developed during the first grazing season is boosted by exposure in subsequent years and prevents manifestations of disease.

Occasionally, outbreaks of acute lungworm disease are seen in adult cattle on pasture whose immunity is overwhelmed by exposure to large numbers of larvae. This condition is sometimes referred to as reinfection syndrome. Although most ingested larvae are killed or fail to mature, some reach the lung and incite an acute, immune-mediated reaction. Horses appear to be susceptible to *D. arnfieldi* infection at any age.

Clinical Manifestations

Clinical disease caused by lungworm infection is sometimes called "husk." It can occur within a week or two of susceptible animals being introduced to contaminated pasture. However, clinical disease is most often seen 2 to 4 months into the grazing season. Affected animals develop either an acute or subacute form of the disease, depending on the number of larvae ingested and the animal's level of immunity. With acute verminous pneumonia in calves, dyspnea and cough are prominent signs. Auscultation of the lungs initially reveals vesicular murmurs and bronchial tones that progress to moist rales as fluid accumulates. The animal may expectorate froth. Occasionally, emphysema occurs, and crackling noises are heard on auscultation. Fever may be as high as 40.5° C (105° F). Mortality rates are high, and animals may die before a patent infection has been established. The similarity between this presentation and that of bacterial pneumonia or shipping fever should be noted.

The subacute or chronic manifestation of disease is more common. In all species the primary signs are coughing, dyspnea, and loss of condition. The animals show elevated respiratory rates but initially are afebrile. Bronchial irritation by adult worms and fluid accumulations produces paroxysmal coughing. Animals with the subacute form of lungworm disease are susceptible to bacterial pneumonia. In fact, the subacute form is easily confused with enzootic pneumonia in calves. Signs of reinfection syndrome in adult cattle include cough, tachypnea, and a sudden drop in milk production about 2 weeks after exposure to heavily contaminated pastures.

In horses, lungworm infection typically causes a syndrome similar to chronic obstructive pulmonary disease. Donkeys, the source of infection in most cases of lungworm disease in horses, remain asymptomatic. Horse and pony foals also may not exhibit overt signs of lungworm infection.

Control of Lungworm Infection

Management strategies designed to decrease exposure to infective larvae are most effective in preventing lungworm disease. Young animals should not be overstocked or allowed to graze in moist, low-lying pastures. It is often helpful to rotate pastures so that successive calf crops do not graze the same area. Young stock should not be grazed with older, clinically immune animals that may serve as a source of infective larvae.

ANTHELMINTICS. Several anthelmintics are effective against lungworm. Drugs for the treatment and control of lungworm are presented in Table 45-4.[145-160] The avermectins/milbemycins are particularly effective against both adult and larval stages, and have prolonged residual activity that prevents appearance of larvae in the feces for at least 60 days.[152-158] Strategic use of these products, such as treatment at turnout and again 8 weeks later, can substantially reduce pasture infectivity with lungworm larvae. Concerns that such highly efficacious anthelmintics would prevent induction of immunity in first-season grazing animals appear to be largely unfounded, with the possible exception of sustained-release intraruminal devices (see below). The immune response may be attenuated, but exposed animals still develop some degree of immunity to lungworm infection despite prophylactic treatment with these drugs.[153,154,160-162]

Young, susceptible stock may be given a prophylactic treatment in mid-spring or early summer to prevent or limit clinical disease. Housed animals, in particular 1- to 2-year-olds with subclinical but potentially patent infections, should be treated before being turned out to pasture in the spring. All early clinical cases should be treated in an effort to limit disease severity and decrease pasture contamination.

Intraruminal sustained-release devices (SRD) containing ivermectin, levamisole, or a benzimidazole can prevent clinical disease for several weeks or months during the grazing season.[162-170] However, some studies have shown that these devices impaired the development of immunity in treated calves.[162,166,169] SRDs may interfere with development of natural immunity by killing ingested larvae before they can penetrate the intestine and thus stimulate an immune response. However, other studies using these devices have shown that treated calves can develop immunity during the grazing season.[170]

VACCINES. An effective vaccine has been developed against *D. viviparus* in cattle. Two doses of irradiated larvae are administered by mouth at 28-day intervals. The larvae migrate to mesenteric lymph nodes, provoke an immune response, but die before they reach the lung. However, there are some management difficulties associated with the use of the vaccine. First, vaccinated calves require confinement for 2 weeks after the vaccination course. Second, vaccinated calves must not be exposed to heavily infected pastures, nor should they be mixed with animals showing signs of lungworm disease or with nonvaccinated calves. Third, immunity is not long-lasting; to maintain immunity animals must continue to be exposed to low levels of infective larvae. Finally, the vaccine has a short shelf-life and it is relatively expensive. It is of most use on farms with contaminated grazing areas and a history of lungworm disease, and is best used in young nursing calves before exposure to pasture. A more stable vaccine that would stimulate long-lasting immunity would be beneficial and is being investigated.[171]

OTHER CONTROL MEASURES. Experimentally, the nematophagous fungus *Duddingtonia flagrans* has been shown to reduce the number of infective lungworm larvae in and around fecal pats by over 80%. This strategy of biologic control holds promise for reducing pasture infectivity on problem farms.[172,173]

Evaluation of Preventive Programs

The efficacy of preventive programs is best assessed by evaluating the number of susceptible animals that demonstrate signs of infection. Because total eradication of the parasite is difficult and low numbers of parasites produce minimum problems, a useful goal is the control of clinical signs such as cough and loss of condition. Fecal larval counts are an unreliable means of evaluating the severity of lungworm infection in an individual animal.

Clinical Management

DIAGNOSIS. As with many parasitic diseases, lungworm is often diagnosed on the basis of farm history, seasonal prevalence, and clinical presentation. Verminous pneumonia may mimic respiratory diseases caused by other agents that require specific treatment. Although definitive diagnosis is difficult, it is important.

To document the presence of lungworm infection, it is necessary to demonstrate larvae, adult worms, or eggs. In cattle and small ruminants the presence of larvae in fresh feces is suggestive of lungworm infection. The Baermann technique must be used to concentrate and positively identify the larvae. However, in acute outbreaks animals may succumb before infections are patent, and the allergic form of the disease may persist even after the worms have been killed or expelled. Transtracheal wash may demonstrate a large number of eosinophils, which is supportive of verminous pneumonia; eggs or larvae are occasionally seen with patent infections. This procedure can also help rule out bacterial pneumonia. An enzyme-linked immunosorbent assay (ELISA) and an indirect hemagglutination assay (IHA) have been developed for detection of *D. viviparus* infection in cattle. The specificity of both assays reportedly is greater than 99%, but the sensitivity of the ELISA is much higher than that of the IHA (100% and 78%, respectively).[174] Postmortem examination is definitive. At necropsy, the adult worms are usually apparent in the bronchi or bronchioles. Nematode eggs may be found in histologic section of the lung.

In horses, lungworm infections generally do not become patent, so larvae are seldom found in the feces of infected horses. Transtracheal wash or bronchoalveolar lavage is important in establishing a diagnosis of lungworm disease in this species.

TREATMENT. In subacute or chronic forms of the disease, removal of the adult parasites with anthelmintics may result

TABLE 45-4

Drugs Used to Control Lungworm

Drug	Dosage
AVERMECTINS/MILBEMYCINS	
Ivermectin, abamectin, doramectin, eprinomectin, moxidectin	0.2 mg/kg PO, SC, IM*; 0.5 mg/kg topically ("pour-on"); intraruminal sustained-release device (ivermectin)
OTHERS	
Albendazole	5 mg/kg PO (O, C); 7.5 to 10 mg/kg PO (B)
Fenbendazole	5 mg/kg PO (O, C); 5 to 10 mg/kg PO (B); 30 mg/kg PO (E); intraruminal sustained-release device (B)
Mebendazole	15 to 20 mg/kg PO (O, C)
Netobimin	7.5 mg/kg PO (B, O, C)
Oxfendazole	4.5 to 7.5 mg/kg PO (B, O, C)
Levamisole	7.5 to 10 mg/kg PO, SC; 10 mg/kg topically ("pour-on") (B, O, C)
Diethylcarbamazine	22 mg/kg IM daily for 3 days or 44 mg/kg IM once (B)

B, Bovine; *C*, caprine; *E*, equine; *O*, ovine.
*Route depends on the product and species; follow manufacturers' recommendations.

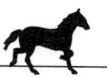

in recovery. However, if the infection is heavy and lung damage is severe, anthelmintic treatment is unlikely to result in complete recovery. In some animals, anthelmintic treatment worsens the signs, and some heavily infected animals die. In severely affected individuals, antihistamines and antibiotics should be included in the therapeutic regimen.

REFERENCES

145. Blood DC, Radostits OM, Gay CC: Diseases caused by helminth parasites. In *Veterinary medicine*, ed 8, London, 1994, Baillière Tindall, pp 1246-1253.
146. Kassai T: Phylum: Nemathelminthes–roundworms. In *Veterinary helminthology*, Oxford, 1999, Butterworth Heinemann, pp 85-92.
147. Rebhun WC: Respiratory diseases. In *Diseases of dairy cattle*, Baltimore, 1995, Williams and Wilkins, pp 89-90.
148. Britt DP, Preston JM: Efficacy of ivermectin against *Dictyocaulus arnfieldi* in ponies, *Vet Rec* 116:343-345, 1985.
149. Williams JC, Broussard SD: Comparative efficacy of levamisole, thiabendazole and fenbendazole against cattle gastrointestinal nematodes, *Vet Parasitol* 58:83-90, 1995.
150. Williams JC, Broussard SD, Wang GT: Efficacy of moxidectin pour-on against gastrointestinal nematodes and *Dictyocaulus viviparus* in cattle, *Vet Parasitol* 64:277-283, 1996.
151. Williams JC et al: Comparative efficacy of ivermectin pour-on, albendazole, oxfendazole and fenbendazole against *Ostertagia ostertagi* inhibited larvae, other gastrointestinal nematodes and lungworm of cattle, *Vet Parasitol* 73:73-82, 1997.
152. Jacobs DE et al: An evaluation of abamectin given at turnout and six weeks after turnout for the control of nematode infections in calves, *Vet Rec* 136:386-389, 1995.
153. Eysker M et al: Residual effect of injectable moxidectin against lungworm and gastrointestinal nematodes in calves exposed to high pasture infectivity levels in the Netherlands, *Vet Parasitol* 61:61-71, 1996.
154. Eysker M et al et al: Comparison between fenbendazole and moxidectin applied in a dose and move system for the control of *Dictyocaulus viviparus* infections in calves, *Vet Parasitol* 64:187-196, 1996.
155. Barth D et al: Evaluation of the persistence of the effect of ivermectin and abamectin against gastrointestinal and pulmonary nematodes in cattle, *Vet Rec* 140:278-279, 1997.
156. Hertzberg H et al: Prevention of gastrointestinal and lungworm infections in alpine calves: use of doramectin pour-on before and after the alpine grazing season, *Schweiz Arch Tierheilkd* 140:419-426, 1998.
157. Vercruysse J et al: Field evaluation of a topical doramectin formulation for the chemoprophylaxis of parasitic bronchitis in calves, *Vet Parasitol* 75:169-179, 1998.
158. Epe C et al: Strategic control of gastrointestinal nematode and lungworm infections with eprinomectin at turnout and eight weeks later, *Vet Rec* 144:380-382, 1999.
159. Stromberg BE et al: Comparison of the persistent efficacy of the injectable and pour-on formulations of doramectin against artificially induced infection with *Dictyocaulus viviparus* in cattle, *Vet Parasitol* 87:45-50, 1999.
160. Taylor SM et al: Induction of protective immunity to *Dictyocaulus viviparus* in calves while under treatment with endectocides, *Vet Parasitol* 88:219-228, 2000.
161. Eysker M et al: Efficacy of Michel's 'dose and move' system against *Dictyocaulus viviparus* infections in cattle using moxidectin as anthelmintic, *Vet Parasitol* 58:49-60, 1995.
162. Taylor SM et al: Protection against *Dictyocaulus viviparus* in second-year cattle after first-year treatment with doramectin or an ivermectin bolus, *Vet Rec* 141:593-597, 1997.
163. Grimshaw WT et al: Development of immunity to lungworm in vaccinated calves treated with an ivermectin sustained-release bolus or an oxfendazole pulse-release bolus at turnout, *Vet Parasitol* 62:119-124, 1996.
164. Hertzberg H et al: Prophylaxis of bovine trichostrongylidosis and dictyocaulosis in the alpine region: comparison of an early and late administration of the oxfendazole pulse release bolus to first-year grazing calves, *Vet Parasitol* 66:181-192, 1996.
165. Jacobs DE, Hutchinson MJ, Abbott EM: Evaluation of the effect of the fenbendazole sustained-release intraruminal device on the immunity of calves to lungworm, *Vet Rec* 139:60-63, 1996.
166. Borgsteede FH et al: Effect of three sustained-release devices on parasitic bronchitis in first-year calves, *Vet Rec* 142:696-699, 1998.
167. Rehbein S et al: Efficacy of an ivermectin controlled-release capsule against nematode and arthropod endoparasites in sheep, *Vet Rec* 142:331-334, 1998.
168. Bauer C: Effects of the fenbendazole SR bolus on *Trichostrongylus* infections in young calves during two consecutive grazing periods, *DTW Dtsch Tierarztl Wochenschr* 106:101-105, 1999 [In German; abstract in English].
169. Kerboeuf D et al: Response of cattle treated with a fenbendazole slow release bolus to challenge from nematodes the following season, *Vet Parasitol* 62:107-118, 1996.
170. Schnieder T et al: The development of protective immunity against gastrointestinal nematode and lungworm infections after use of an ivermectin bolus in first-year grazing calves, *Vet Parasitol* 64:239-250, 1996.
171. McKeand JB: Vaccine development and diagnostics of *Dictyocaulus viviparus*, *Parasitology* 120:S17-S23, 2000.
172. Henriksen SA et al: Nematode-trapping fungi in biological control of *Dictyocaulus viviparus*, *Acta Vet Scand* 38:175-179, 1997.
173. Fernandez AS et al: The efficacy of two isolates of the nematode-trapping fungus *Duddingtonia flagrans* against *Dictyocaulus viviparus* larvae in feces, *Vet Parasitol* 85:289-304, 1999.
174. Cornelissen JB, Borgsteede FH, van Milligen FJ: Evaluation of an ELISA for the routine diagnosis of *Dictyocaulus viviparus* infections in cattle, *Vet Parasitol* 70:153-164, 1997.

SUGGESTED READING

Blood DC, Radostits OM, Gay CC: Diseases caused by helminth parasites. In *Veterinary medicine*, ed 8, London, 1994, Baillière Tindall, pp 1246-1253.
Kassai T: Phylum: Nemathelminthes–roundworms. In *Veterinary helminthology*, Oxford, 1999, Butterworth Heinemann, pp 85-92.
Rebhun WC: Respiratory diseases. In *Diseases of dairy cattle*, Baltimore, 1995, Williams & Wilkins, pp 89-90.

COCCIDIOSIS IN FOOD ANIMALS

Coccidiosis causes serious economic losses in a variety of food animal species. Although most animals are exposed and infected with coccidia, usually the infection is asymptomatic and self-limiting. Infection causes disease only when management factors allow the abnormal concentration of oocysts in the environment or when host defenses are compromised. Kids are especially susceptible to coccidiosis and may develop chronic diarrhea as a consequence.

Life Cycle

Coccidiosis is caused by intracellular parasites in the genera *Isospora* and *Eimeria*. Each genus includes numerous host- and site-specific species. The life cycles are complex, involving both sexual and asexual phases within the same host.[175] Single-cell oocysts are passed in the feces and subsequently sporulate to form infective stages. These sporulated oocysts are ingested by the host and release sporozoites in the intestine. Sporozoites enter intestinal cells and form trophozoites, which in turn divide into meronts composed of many merozoites. As meronts rupture, releasing many mature merozoites, epithelial cells at the base of the intestinal glands are destroyed. Mature merozoites penetrate additional epithelial cells and form more meronts. Eventually the organism produces macrogametocytes and microgametocytes. Microgametes are released by cell rupture and then combine with macrogametes to form the next generation of oocysts. When the oocysts are mature the host cell ruptures, releasing them into the lumen of the gut. Most of the epithelial cells at the base of the intestinal glands are occupied by meronts or gametocytes within 14 days after a heavy infection.

Pathophysiology

As a result of coccidian developmental cycles, host intestinal epithelial cells are destroyed. The amount of damage done to the intestinal epithelium is directly related to the number of oocysts ingested. If the number is low, nonimmune healthy animals may tolerate infection and show no signs of disease. Intestinal cells are destroyed, but because they normally are replaced at a rapid rate the damage done to the gut is minimal. However, if nonimmune animals are exposed to many oocysts, widespread rupture and exfoliation of intestinal cells alters gut function, causes loss of blood, fluid, albumin, and electrolytes into the gut, and allows secondary bacterial invasion. Sections of sloughed intestinal mucosa and fibrin casts may be seen in the feces, and the feces may be blood tinged. Blood loss can be considerable. This phase of

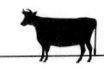

the disease may occur before the sexual cycle is complete and, consequently, before the infection is patent.

Neurologic signs have been reported during coccidiosis outbreaks in calves and weaned beef cattle.[176] The pathophysiology of this manifestation has not been definitively established, although a neurotoxin is suspected. A labile neurotoxin has been identified in the serum of calves with enteric coccidiosis that were showing signs of neurologic dysfunction. Injection of serum from affected calves into mice caused severe neurologic signs.[177,178] In a prospective epidemiologic study, those authors tentatively excluded the following as possible causes of neurologic dysfunction in calves with enteric coccidiosis: disturbance of serum sodium, potassium, calcium, phosphorus, or magnesium concentration; deficiency of vitamin A or thiamin; anemia; lead poisoning; uremia; *Haemophilus somnus* meningoencephalitis; severity of the coccidial infection; gross alterations in intestinal bacterial flora; and hepatopathy.[179]

Populations at Risk

Most animals infected with coccidia do not exhibit signs of illness. With light infections the damage done to gut cells is minimal. After an initial period of infection the host is essentially immune to the deleterious effects of coccidiosis. Consequently, coccidiosis is primarily a disease of young, nonimmune animals crowded together in unsanitary housing or lots. Under these conditions the environment is highly contaminated with oocysts, and immunity may be compromised by stress-related factors. Often outbreaks are associated with the stress of shipping, weaning, and dietary changes. Corticosteroid treatment or concurrent illness can also precipitate a peracute form of coccidiosis. Severe cold has been blamed for outbreaks of coccidiosis in weaned beef calves during the winter months in Canada.

Although outbreaks have been reported in range animals, coccidiosis is primarily a disease of confinement. In dairy cattle, coccidiosis is most common in calves when they are taken from hutches into group calf pens or mini–free-stall barns. In beef cattle the disease is most prevalent in feedlot calves. In sheep, coccidiosis is most common in intensively reared lambs, although suckling lambs on pasture in constant use at high stocking rates are also at risk. Young kids appear particularly susceptible to coccidiosis and may be a major source of pasture or drylot contamination. Often the same facility serves as a source of infection for the next group of animals. Even previously exposed animals may show signs if the infection is heavy enough. Occasionally, adult animals, immune to their own endemic species of coccidia, develop disease when they are moved into a new herd and exposed to a different species of parasite.

Clinical Manifestations

The destruction of epithelial cells and subsequent loss of blood, albumin, fluid, and electrolytes typically causes a profuse diarrhea containing mucus and blood. Dehydration may occur, but most animals continue to drink water and meet their fluid requirements. Despite the blood loss, anemia is not usually appreciated in acute cases. Affected animals typically strain to defecate, which may result in rectal prolapse. Affected animals are often anorectic, and feed consumption may be decreased for extended periods of time. After recovery from the disease the gut does not return to normal function for several weeks, and appetite may be suppressed concurrently. As with any disease that causes diarrhea in young animals, coccidiosis is associated with weakness, ill thrift, and poor weight gain. Diarrhea in kids can become chronic (often without blood) and results in stunting and wasting.

In dairy calves the classical signs of dysentery and tenesmus are uncommon. Rather, the predominant signs are loose manure, poor condition, poor growth, and poor hair coat. In kids and lambs the disease may cause sudden death, although in most outbreaks the case fatality rate is low. Animals that develop "nervous" coccidiosis may exhibit muscle tremors, hyperesthesia, convulsions, nystagmus, and blindness. The mortality rate is high.

Control of Coccidiosis

The spread of coccidiosis depends on the prevalence of oocysts in the environment. The level of infection is directly related to the level of fecal contamination. Houses and pens used for sequential groups of young animals often become highly infectious and serve as the source of disease for subsequent groups. Thus the most important preventive strategies are directed at decreasing exposure to oocysts. This is usually accomplished by standard management techniques: decreasing stocking rates, minimizing stress, and providing clean housing and feed. Feed bunks, proper manure disposal, and slatted floors have been used to control coccidiosis. Exposure to sunlight and low humidity, and treatment with formaldehyde, ammonia, or methylbromide kill oocysts. Prophylactic use of coccidiostats is common practice when producers cannot or will not make sufficient changes to the young animals' management and environment to effectively control the disease.

DRUGS. The various drugs that have been used to prevent or treat coccidiosis in ruminants are listed in Table 45-5.[180-185] These drugs are most often administered in the feed or water. Preventive treatments are given to young animals exposed to contaminated environments or in the face of an outbreak. Therapeutic doses are used in animals displaying clinical signs of disease. However, the efficacy of treatment in the face of disease may be limited by several factors. First, treatment of animals maintained in a contaminated environment may be insufficient to prevent subsequent outbreaks. Second, many of these drugs are coccidiostatic rather than coccidiocidal, and the cycle may resume when the drug is withdrawn. Most products have only partial efficacy against ruminant coccidia. Third, drugs administered in feed or water may not be ingested by ill animals. Finally, many drugs are only effective against later developmental stages of the parasite and therefore are less effective in preventing the pathologic changes that lead to disease. As mentioned above, the best strategies for preventing disease are managerial rather than pharmacologic.

OTHER STRATEGIES FOR MINIMIZING CLINICAL INFECTIONS. Use of growth implants containing estradiol and progesterone can attenuate the effects of high oocyst challenge in dairy calves.[186] Attempts at developing a conventional vaccine against coccidiosis have been disappointing. Peptide or recombinant vaccines may prove to be efficacious in the future.[187] Immunization with a "trickle dose" of oocysts 2 weeks before turnout onto infected pasture may attenuate the effects of natural challenge in calves.[188] Oocysts can survive the hay-making process, so pastures known to be infected with coccidian oocysts should not be used to make hay for susceptible animals.[189]

Evaluation of Preventive Programs

Oocysts can be found using standard McMaster's flotation techniques. However, interpretation of a fecal examination may be difficult. In any given herd or group a baseline level of oocyst shedding is normal; many immune animals shed

TABLE 45-5

Drugs Used for Treatment and Prevention of Coccidiosis in Ruminants

Drug	Treatment*	Prevention*
Amprolium	10 mg/kg bwt for 5 days (B) 25-40 mg/kg bwt for 5 days (O, C) 65 mg/kg bwt once	5 mg/kg bwt for 21 days (B) 50 mg/kg bwt for 21 days (O)
Decoquinate		0.5 mg/kg bwt for 28-30 days
Diclazuril		1 mg/kg bwt once; a second dose can be given 14 days later
Lasalocid		1 mg/kg bwt continuously (B) 25-100 mg/kg feed, continuously 80 mg/kg milk replacer (neonatal calves) Free-choice in salt at 0.75% total salt mixture
Monensin	2 mg/kg bwt for 20 days (O)	1 mg/kg bwt for 28 days 10-20 ppm in feed, continuously 16-33 g/ton of feed, continuously Intraruminal controlled-release device (weaned beef calves)
Nitrofurazone	10-15 mg/kg bwt for 5-7 days In feed at 0.04% or in water at 0.0133% for 7 days	33 mg/kg bwt for 14 days In feed at 0.04% for 21 days
Salinomycin		10 ppm in feed (O)
Sulfadimethoxine		50 mg/kg bwt for 5 days (O)
Sulfamethazine	110 mg/kg bwt for 5 days 140 mg/kg bwt for 3 days 140 mg/kg bwt once, then 70 mg/kg bwt for 5-7 days	35 mg/kg bwt for 15 days (B) 25 mg/kg bwt for 7 days (O) 55 g/ton of feed (C)
Sulfaquinoxaline	10-20 mg/kg bwt for 5-7 days	
Toltrazuril	20 mg/kg bwt	20 mg/kg bwt once, 10 days after turnout onto pasture

B, Bovine; *C,* caprine; *O,* ovine; *bwt,* body weight.
*Oral administration; dosage or regimen may vary among references.
NOTE: Coccidiostats used in poultry feeds may be toxic to ruminants.

oocysts. On the other hand, nonimmune animals with low-level infection may shed oocysts but have no clinical signs or need for treatment. Furthermore, *animals suffering from coccidiosis may not yet be shedding oocysts.* This variation complicates both evaluation of preventive measures and the diagnosis of coccidiosis in clinically affected animals. The presence of oocysts in healthy or sick animals does not necessarily indicate the need for anticoccidial treatment.

Nevertheless, the number of oocysts passed by an animal does reflect the severity of mucosal damage experienced by that animal. Typically, individuals and herds requiring treatment show clinical signs and pass large numbers of oocysts in their feces. Estimates vary as to what constitutes a clinically important oocyst load. Counts of greater than 5000 oocysts/g probably are significant in most ruminants showing signs of infection. Counts as high as 100,000 oocysts/gram have been reported in clinically normal lambs. Evidently, these are infections involving minimally pathogenic coccidian species. However, when such high oocyst counts are accompanied by signs of coccidiosis, they suggest the need for treatment.

In herds that require preventive strategies, there is a history of prior disease, and a large proportion of herd members shed high numbers of oocysts. Efficacy is evaluated on the basis of a decreased prevalence of clinically ill animals.

Clinical Management

DIAGNOSIS. Definitive diagnosis may be made at necropsy. Antemortem, young, diarrheic animals passing large numbers of oocysts are not difficult to diagnose. However, as discussed above, making a diagnosis on the basis of oocyst counts alone can be misleading.

TREATMENT. Drugs used in the treatment of coccidiosis are listed in Table 45-5. Supportive therapy, when indicated, is primarily directed at replacing fluid losses and supporting the animal until the gut epithelium regenerates.

REFERENCES

175. Soulsby LJ: Order Coccidia leuckart. In *Helminths, arthropods, and protozoa of domesticated animals,* Baltimore, 1975, Williams & Wilkins, pp 614-639.
176. Fanelli HH: Observations on nervous coccidiosis in calves, *Bovine Pract* 18:50-53, 1983.
177. Isler CM, Bellamy JE, Wobeser GA: Labile neurotoxin in serum of calves with "nervous" coccidiosis, *Can J Vet Res* 51:253-260, 1987.
178. Isler CM, Bellamy JE, Wobeser GA: Characteristics of the labile neurotoxin associated with nervous coccidiosis, *Can J Vet Res* 51:271-276, 1987.
179. Isler CM, Bellamy JE, Wobeser GA: Pathogenesis of neurological signs associated with bovine enteric coccidiosis: a prospective study and review, *Can J Vet Res* 51:261-270, 1987.
180. Blood DC, Radostits OM, Gay CC: Diseases caused by protozoa. In *Veterinary medicine,* ed 8, London, 1994, Baillière Tindall, pp 1181-1191.
181. Rebhun WC: Infectious diseases of the gastrointestinal tract. In *Diseases of dairy cattle,* Baltimore, 1995, Williams & Wilkins, pp 177-180.
182. Clarkson MJ, Winter AC: Thin scouring lambs. In *A handbook for the sheep clinician,* ed 5, Liverpool, 1997, Liverpool University Press, pp 107-108.
183. Quigley JD III et al: Effects of lasalocid in milk replacer or calf starter on health and performance of calves challenged with *Eimeria* species, *J Dairy Sci* 80:2972-2976, 1997.
184. McAllister TA et al: Effect of salinomycin on giardiasis and coccidiosis in growing lambs, *J Anim Sci* 74:2896-2903, 1996.
185. Alzieu JP et al: Economic benefits of prophylaxis with diclazuril against subclinical coccidiosis in lambs reared indoors, *Vet Rec* 144:442-444, 1999.
186. Heath HL et al: Hormonal modulation of the physiologic responses of calves infected with *Eimeria bovis, Am J Vet Res* 58:891-896, 1997.
187. Cox FE: Control of coccidiosis: lessons from other sporozoa, *Intl J Parasitol* 28:165-179, 1998.
188. Svensson C, Olofsson H, Uggla A: Immunization of calves against *Eimeria alabamensis* coccidiosis, *Appl Parasitol* 37:209-216, 1996.
189. Svensson C: The survival and transmission of oocysts of *Eimeria alabamensis* in hay, *Vet Parasitol* 69:211-218, 1997.

SUGGESTED READING

Blood DC, Radostits OM, Gay CC: Diseases caused by protozoa. In *Veterinary medicine,* ed 8, London, 1994, Baillière Tindall, pp 1181-1191.
Clarkson MJ, Winter AC: Thin scouring lambs. In *A handbook for the sheep clinician,* ed 5, Liverpool, 1997, Liverpool University Press, pp 107-108.
Rebhun WC: Infectious diseases of the gastrointestinal tract. In *Diseases of dairy cattle,* Baltimore, 1995, Williams & Wilkins, pp 177-180.

Nutrition of the Sick Animal: Preventive and Therapeutic Strategies

RAYMOND W. SWEENEY

PAMELA A. WILKINS

The influence of nutrition on the recuperation of veterinary patients is often overlooked, although the effects of nutritional status on recuperative ability are well known. It is generally accepted that protein-energy malnutrition can have a deleterious effect on immune function.[1] Malnutrition may lead to reduced host resistance to bacterial infections because decreased neutrophil function, reduced antibody production, and lowered complement concentration have been demonstrated in underfed animals.[1-4] Controlled clinical studies of veterinary patients demonstrating improved recovery from surgery or infectious diseases are scarce, but the beneficial effects of nutritional monitoring and supplementation of human patients with such conditions are well documented.[5] Nutritional monitoring and supplementation of sick animals may enhance chances for recovery. The predisposition of sick animals to protein-energy malnutrition because of decreased appetite and increased metabolic requirements has been discussed elsewhere. Many conditions such as gastrointestinal disturbances or dysphagic conditions (e.g., botulism, tetanus) prevent the intake of food completely, and the nutritional requirements must be fulfilled by forced enteral or intravenous feeding.

Monitoring nutritional status is important when prescribing a nutritional program for a convalescing patient. Methods of estimating body composition such as midarm circumference (muscle) and skin-fold thickness (fat) are frequently used in human hospitals, yet sophisticated monitoring techniques have not been defined for horses or ruminants.[6] Colloid oncotic pressure may be dramatically decreased in critically ill human patients as a result of catabolism, but clinical laboratory parameters are generally not useful in determining nutritional status in ruminants because in most cases results of clinical chemistry tests are normal.[3] Although anemia and hypoproteinemia (hypoalbuminemia) are occasionally seen in cases of malnutrition, they are not specific and frequently are associated with another primary disease process such as parasitism or protein-losing enteropathy. Occasionally inadequate protein intake is associated with abnormally low serum urea nitrogen (SUN) concentrations, but liver disease must also be ruled out. Underfed horses develop a mild hyperbilirubinemia (unconjugated) and hypertriglyceridemia, which, although not directly related to nutritional status, is readily reversed when food intake resumes.[7] The most practical methods for monitoring nutritional status in large animals are serial body weight determination and subjective evaluation of body condition or the semiquantitative body condition score. In addition, feed intake should be monitored carefully and compared with published maintenance requirements (e.g., National Research Council). A pronounced decrease in body weight (>5%) or condition should alert the clinician that nutritional supplementation is required. Changes are often easily overlooked in day-to-day observations of the patient if a concerted effort is not made to detect them. Palpation of the animal (ribs, dorsal vertebral processes) is necessary in sheep with a heavy fleece. Although it is generally accepted that sick animals have increased nutritional requirements, these requirements have not been quantitated for specific conditions. Therefore the clinician should ensure that nutritional intake is at least 100% of maintenance requirements, with the realization that increased supplementation may be necessary if weight loss or decreased body condition ensues.

ORAL SUPPLEMENTATION

If monitoring feed intake or body condition indicates a need for nutritional supplementation, the clinician should determine if the animal is consuming all feed offered (in which case more or higher-quality feed should be offered), or if the appetite is poor. In the latter case the patient should be offered a variety of highly palatable feeds such as sweet feeds and various forages. Ruminants in particular may consume small quantities of fresh feed if it is offered frequently, whereas if the same quantity is offered in one feeding it may be ignored after a few bites. Many dairy cows can be "coaxed" into eating hay if it is placed in the back of the pharynx by the clinician, and oropharyngeal stimulation may result in increased voluntary feed consumption. Fresh silage and dried brewer's grain frequently appeal to the hypophagic cow, and many sick horses and ruminants benefit from grazing if grass is available.

If these measures fail to result in improved nutritional status, force feeding of a liquid diet by intragastric administration should be considered. In addition, dysphagic animals require a liquid diet as the sole source of nutrition.

LIQUID DIETS FOR HORSES

Liquid diets may be classified into the following three categories:
1. *Blender diets:* Liquefied or finely ground whole food suspended in water
2. *Composition diets* containing highly digestible whole protein (usually casein or soy), fats, and carbohydrate
3. *Elemental diets* containing hydrolyzed protein (small peptides) and/or free amino acids in place of whole protein

The source of carbohydrate should be examined, and only diets that do not contain sucrose should be used for horses or ruminants. Although they are sometimes inconvenient, blender diets have the advantage of being inexpensive, and the ingredients are usually available. Such a diet may be prepared by grinding one third of the daily ration of pellets in a blender and suspending in water or by soaking the pellets in water to create a slurry. The preparation can then be fed 3 times daily to horses that require complete feeding or once or twice daily if only partial supplementation is required. Alfalfa meal suspended in water can also be fed in this manner.

There are limited whole-protein composition diets available for adult horses. They are generally more expensive than the blender diet but are more convenient. One "homemade" diet (Table 46-1) composed primarily of dehydrated cottage cheese, dextrose, and alfalfa meal requires considerable preparation by the clinician.[8] A commercially available liquid diet designed for use in human patients (Osmolite HN*) has been used successfully in horses.[9] These composition diets may be used for either complete or partial supplementation. The approximate cost for complete supplementation with the homemade equine diet was $30 to $50 per day for a 450-kg horse. Both diets may result in a mild, self-limiting diarrhea when fed as the sole source of nutrition, possibly because of lack of fiber or from fermentation of the highly soluble ingredients in the large colon. As indicated in Table 46-1, the homemade diet is introduced gradually over a period of 7 days. Similarly, the commercial human product should be started at approximately 25% of the final maintenance requirement and gradually increased over 4 to 7 days to the target quantity.

There are few indications for the use of elemental diets in adult horses, and there are no published clinical trials. It is conceivable that these preparations would improve nutrient absorption in horses with infiltrative bowel disease such as granulomatous enteritis, but this improvement has not been demonstrated in the horse (there is some supporting evidence in the dog).[10] If elemental diets are to be used, those composed of hydrolyzed protein (i.e., dipeptides and tripeptides; e.g., Vital,* or Flexical†) are preferred over those containing only free amino acids. There is mounting evidence in laboratory animals and humans that more nitrogen is retained when hydrolyzed protein products are used.[11] Overall, elemental diets are extremely expensive and rarely provide significant benefits when compared with whole protein diets.

Orphan or critically ill foals may be fed mare's milk (200 ml/kg of body weight divided into 6 to 10 feedings). If mare's milk is unavailable, goat's milk or a commercially available milk replacer (Mare's Match,‡ or Udder Delight||) may be substituted, although indigestion (mild colic, gastric distention, flatulence) may be observed when the animal is on a diet other than mare's milk. Although goat's milk is similar in caloric density to mare's milk, it is slightly higher in protein and fat content and lower in lactose. Because indigestion occurs commonly when using milk substitutes in foals, dietary changes should be instituted gradually over a period of 1 to 2 days at a minimum. If indigestion occurs, both the frequency and volume of feeding should be decreased until the indigestion resolves.

LIQUID DIETS FOR RUMINANTS

In most cases the most practical and least expensive way to force-feed ruminants is the blender-type or slurry diet. Hypophagic adult cattle may be force-fed a suspension of alfalfa meal and dried brewer's grain 3 to 5 kg each in 20 L of

---

*Ross Laboratories, Columbus, OH 43216.

---

*Ross Laboratories, Columbus, OH 43216.
†Mead-Johnson, Atlanta, GA 30326.
‡Land O' Lakes, Fort Dodge, IA 50501.
||Buckeye Feel Mills, Inc. Dalton, OH 44618.

TABLE 46-1

Suggested Feeding Regimen for a Liquid Diet for a 450-kg Adult Horse*[8]

Ingredient	Day						
	1	2	3	4	5	6	7
Water (1)	21	21	21	21	21	21	21
Dextrose (g)	300	400	500	600	800	800	900
Dehydrated cottage cheese (g)†	300	450	600	750	900	900	900
Alfalfa meal (g)	2000	2000	2000	2000	2000	2000	2000
Electrolyte mix (g)‡	230	230	230	230	230	230	230

*Ration divided into three equal feedings daily.
†Available as ProMagic diet supplement, American Nutrition Laboratory, Burlington, NJ 08016.
‡Electrolyte mix ingredients: NaCl, 10 g; NaHCO$_3$, 15g; KCl, 75 g; K$_2$HPO$_4$, 60 g; CaCl$_2$2H$_2$O, 45 g; MgO, 25 g.

water 2 to 3 times daily. If a rumen fistula is necessary (e.g., in cases of tetanus) the diet may be directed into the rumen. Similar preparations should be suitable for sheep and goats, although published reports are scarce.

In cases of vagal indigestion resulting from failure of omasal transport, liquid feedings administered into the rumen are of little benefit because the rumen does not empty properly. Cattle with omasal transport failure can be maintained with intraabomasal feedings of a liquid diet. An in-dwelling nasogastric feeding tube (standard stomach tube, 3-m length) is placed into the abomasum by means of a rumenotomy incision, or alternatively a temporary rumenostomy is made, and the abomasal tube placed for each feeding. Liquid composition diets such as the cottage cheese/dextrose or commercially available liquid diets previously described for horses that do not require fermentation are preferred. Such diets should be introduced gradually, and feeding schedules for a nonlactating adult cow or bull are similar to those listed in Table 46-1 for the horse.

INTRAVENOUS FEEDING

Intravenous feeding, often referred to as partial or total parenteral nutrition (PPN or TPN, respectively), is a means of providing nutritional support that does not require the patient to have a functional digestive tract. Because of the greater expense and risk of complications when compared with enteral feeding, PPN should be reserved for cases in which bowel rest is necessary. Possible indications for PPN include neonatal diarrhea in cases in which oral feeding exacerbates the diarrhea, postoperative feeding following gastrointestinal surgery, nonsurgical intestinal obstruction (proximal jejunitis), gastrointestinal intolerance in premature foals, and occasionally foals with botulism that develop ileus and cannot tolerate oral feedings. Because the enterocytes obtain nutrients from the bowel lumen, if possible, some oral feedings, even if in small quantities, should be included, even if in small quantities, for the maintenance of the intestinal epithelium and brush border enzymes. Such supplementation of parenteral nutrition with small enteral feedings, termed "trophic feeds," promotes normal gastrointestinal function and improves immune status.

Parenteral nutrition solutions provide an energy source, usually glucose and lipids, and protein hydrolysates or, more commonly, free amino acids. Sufficient calories must be provided in the form of carbohydrates and lipids, or the amino acids will be used as an energy substrate rather than incorporated as body protein. A calorie/nitrogen ratio of at least 100:1 is recommended to ensure proper use of the amino acids (glucose provides 3.4 kcal/g, amino acids 4 kcal/g, and lipids 11 kcal/g; there is 0.16 g of nitrogen per gram of amino acid). No more than 60% of the nonprotein calories should be provided as lipids. Solutions must be mixed aseptically and should be stored for no longer than 24 hours. Because of the high concentration of glucose (often greater than 20%), parenteral nutrition solutions are usually hypertonic, and administration into a large central vessel (e.g., vena cava) is often recommended to prevent phlebitis. In addition, parenteral nutrition solutions must be initiated gradually and patients monitored for hyperglycemia or, rarely, hyperlipemia. If hyperglycemia is persistent, treatment with insulin may improve glucose use and permit increased caloric intake without further hyperglycemia. Similarly, heparin may be administered when hyperlipemia results from administration of parenteral nutrition with lipids. Serum concentrations of sodium, potassium, and bicarbonate should also be measured periodically (daily, at first), and parenteral nutrition solutions supplemented as needed to correct abnormalities that develop. Other medications may not be compatible with the

TABLE 46-2

Guidelines for Use of Parenteral Nutrition in Foals and Calves

Day	Dosage
1-3	1000 ml 50% glucose
	1000 ml 10% amino acids*
	500 ml 10% lipid emulsion†
	Administer 2.1 ml/kg/hr‡
3+	1000 ml 50% glucose
	1000 ml 10% amino acids
	1000 ml lipid emulsion
	Administer 3 ml/kg/hr

From Hansen TO: *Proceedings of the Symposium on Intensive Care Therapies and Parenteral Nutrition*, University of Pennsylvania, Aug 19, 1986, pp 36-38.
*Available as Aminosyn, Abbott Laboratories, North Chicago, IL 60064; or Travasol, Baxter Healthcare (Clintech), Deerfield IL 60015.
†Available as Liposyn, Abbott Laboratories, N. Chicago, IL 60064; or Intralipid, Baxter Healthcare (Clintech), Deerfield, IL 60015.
‡Introduce gradually over 24 to 48 hours.

parenteral nutrition solutions and should be given through a separate line or the parenteral nutrition line flushed with saline before and after administration.

PARENTERAL NUTRITION IN HORSES

Guidelines for the use of parenteral nutrition in foals are given in Table 46-2. The initial TPN formula is designed to provide 10 g of glucose per kilogram of body weight, 2 g of amino acid per kilogram, and 1 g of lipid per kilogram daily, providing 45 nonprotein kcal per kilogram per day. The initial mixture should be administered at 25% to 50% of the flow rate targeted in Table 46-2 and gradually increased to the full amount, as tolerated, over the first 24 to 48 hours. Once the full flow rate is achieved, additional caloric density may be achieved by increasing the proportion of lipid emulsion. Further increases in caloric intake require increased flow rates. If long-term administration is expected, calcium (200 mg/kg/day), phosphorus (110 mg/kg/day), and other micronutrient supplementation may be required. Commercial multiple vitamin (e.g., MVI-12*) and trace mineral (e.g., MTE5†) are available for addition to the parenteral nutrition mixture.

Catheter-related complications are more frequently encountered with foals than with calves, and placement of a central venous catheter is frequently beneficial. With the addition of lipid emulsions into parenteral nutrition formulas, tonicity of the infusion is reduced; for short-term therapy (a few days), a short (3½-inch) jugular vein catheter may be acceptable with careful monitoring for signs of phlebitis. However, for long-term therapy, a central venous catheter is preferred. Commercially available catheters include the 16-gauge, 12-inch Intracath‡ and the 16-gauge, 8-inch Arrow catheter.§ Alternatively, an appropriate length of 18-gauge Silastic tubing¶ may be placed into the jugular vein through a 13-gauge trocar with the proximal end tunneled subcutaneously.

Table 46-3 lists guidelines for use of parenteral nutrition in adult horses, which require a formulation that has a lower caloric density and lower amino acid concentration than foals. The approximate cost per day for foals is $75 and for adult horses is $400. In some geographic areas there are com-

*Astra Pharmaceutical, Westboro, MA 01581.
†American Pharmaceutical Partners, Inc, Los Angeles, CA 90024.
‡Becton Dickinson, Sandy, UT 84070.
§Arrow International Inc, Reading, PA 19605.
¶Dow Corning, Midland, MI 48640.

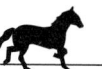

TABLE 46-3

Guidelines for Parenteral Nutrition in Adult Horses

Day	Dosage
1+	5000 ml 50% glucose
	4000 ml 10% amino acids
	6000 ml 10% lipid emulsion
	Administer 1.4 ml kg/hr*

From Hansen TO, White NA, Kemp DT: *Proceedings of the Second Equine Colic Research Symposium*, 1985, p 204.
*Additional polyionic electrolyte solutions may be necessary to meet daily fluid requirements.

panies that will formulate and deliver parenteral nutrition solutions, made-to-order, within 12 hours of placing the order. Use of these companies may increase utilization of parenteral nutrition because of ease of access and decreased overhead costs.

PARENTERAL NUTRITION IN RUMINANTS

Because of cost, use of parenteral nutrition is usually limited to valuable calves, and little information exists on the use of parenteral nutrition in adult cattle, sheep, or goats. The most common indication for the use of parenteral nutrition in calves is diarrhea, particularly in chronic cases accompanied by weight loss.[12] In such cases, if sufficient milk is fed to provide the calf's nutritional needs, the diarrhea is exacerbated, and parenteral allows the quantity of milk to be reduced without compromising the nutritional status of the patient. A recommended parenteral nutrition regimen is given in Table 46-2. As with foals, the initial formula is based on the 10:2:1 glucose/amino acid/lipid ratio. The initial flow rates should be 25% to 50% of the targeted rate for the first several hours; if hyperglycemia does not develop, the target flow rate can be administered. Pricing varies depending on quantities purchased, but the approximate cost of parenteral nutrition for a 45-kg calf is $75 per day. Eliminating the lipid emulsions from the formulas is an acceptable alternative that will reduce the cost by approximately 30%. In addition to the ingredients listed in Table 46-2, intravenous fluids containing potassium and bicarbonate may be required. A multiple B–vitamin product may be added to the formula (approximately 1 ml supplement per liter of parenteral nutrition), but trace minerals are not usually necessary for the short-term administration

that is most common in calves. When discontinuing parenteral nutrition, it is recommended to do so gradually over a 24- to 48-hour period to avoid "rebound" hypoglycemia. If possible, 2% of the calf's body weight of milk should be administered daily for its trophic effect on the enterocytes.

Catheter-related complications are extremely rare in calves, and a central venous catheter is not required. We have had success with 16-gauge, 3 1/4-inch, Teflon-coated, over-the-needle catheters available from several distributors. These are placed in the jugular vein, sutured or glued to the overlying skin, and left in place for up to 10 days if no signs of phlebitis or sepsis occur.

SPECIAL DIETS

Numerous diseases require specific alterations in the ration because of metabolic disturbances that accompany these conditions. Recommendations are discussed in the individual chapters dealing with these diseases and include alterations of dietary protein for hepatic disease and restrictions in the protein and calcium content of the diet for horses with chronic renal failure.

REFERENCES

1. Sheffy BE, Williams AJ: Nutrition and the immune response, *J Am Vet Med Assoc* 180:1073-1076, 1982.
2. Woodard LF et al: Serum complement activity of protein-energy malnourished beef cows, *Am J Vet Res* 41:1546-1548, 1980.
3. Oetzel GR, Berger LL: Protein-energy malnutrition in domestic ruminants, *Compend Cont Educ* 7:S672-S680, 1985.
4. Naylor JM, Kenyon SJ: Effect of total calorific deprivation on host defense in the horse, *Res Vet Sci* 31:369-372, 1981.
5. Mullen JL, Buzby GP, Matthews DC: Reduction of operative morbidity and mortality by combined preoperative and postoperative nutritional support, *Ann Surg* 192:604-613, 1980.
6. Haider M, Haider SQ: Assessment of protein-calorie malnutrition, *Clin Chem* 30:1286-1299, 1984.
7. Naylor JM, Kronfeld DS, Acland H: Hyperlipemia in horses: effects of undernutrition and disease, *Am J Vet Res* 41:899-905, 1980.
8. Naylor JM, Freeman DE, Kronfeld DS: Alimentation of hypophagic horses, *Compend Cont Educ* 6(suppl):S93-S100, 1984.
9. Sweeney RW, Hansen TO: Use of a liquid diet as the sole source of nutrition in 6 dysphagic horses and as a dietary supplement in 7 hypophagic horses, *J Am Vet Med Assoc* 197:1030-1032, 1990.
10. Washabau RJ: University of Pennsylvania School of Veterinary Medicine, personal communication, 1988.
11. Smith JL, Arteaga C, Heymsfield SB: Increased ureagenesis and impaired nitrogen use during infusion of a synthetic amino acid formula, *N Engl J Med* 306:1013-1015, 1982.
12. Sweeney RW Divers TJ: The use of parenteral nutrition in calves, *Vet Clin North Am (Food Anim Pract)* 6:125-131, 1990.

PART
SEVEN

CONGENITAL, HEREDITARY, IMMUNOLOGIC, AND TOXIC DISORDERS

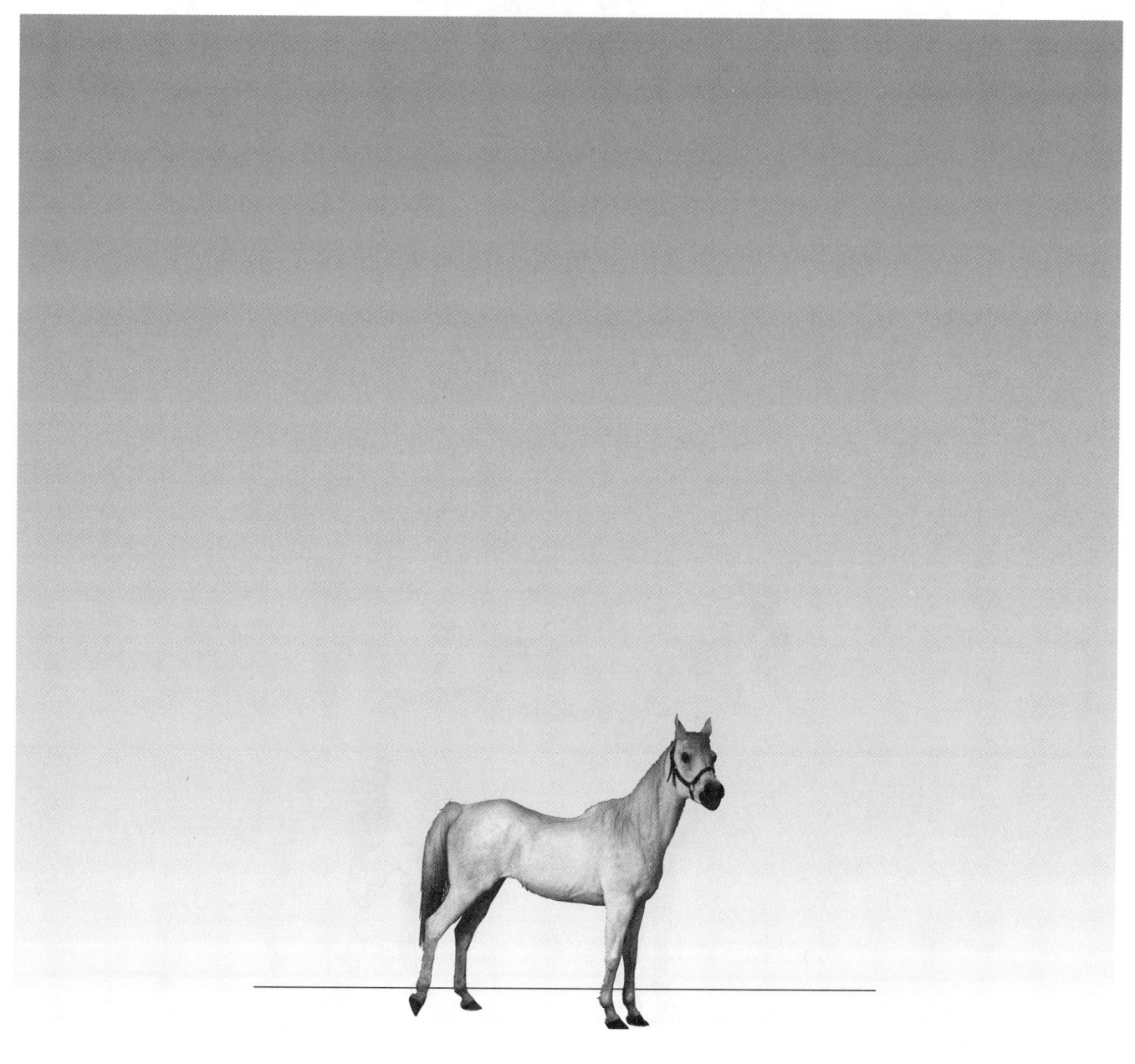

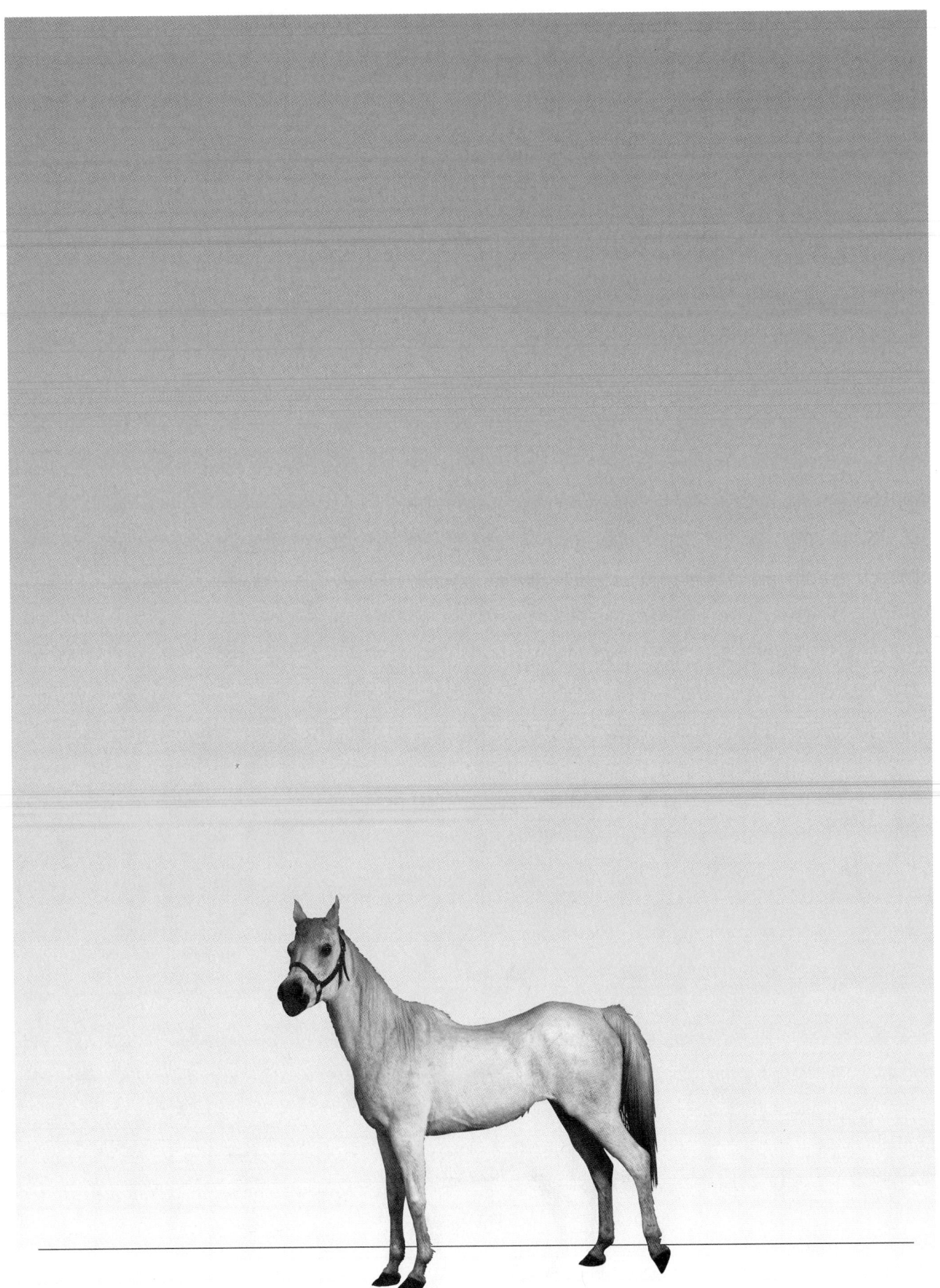

Congenital Defects and Hereditary Disorders in Ruminants

GEORGE SAPERSTEIN

Consulting Editor

CONGENITAL DEFECTS AND HEREDITARY DISORDERS IN CATTLE

GEORGE SAPERSTEIN

Congenital defects and inherited disorders are abnormalities of structure, formation, or function that are present at birth. They may affect a single structure or function, an entire system, parts of several systems, or several complete body systems. Functional and structural defects may combine to form syndromes. Most defects and disorders first are diagnosed in newborn animals, but some, although present at birth, are not detected until later in life. Congenital defects and inherited disorders least likely to be identified are those contributing to embryonic mortality, fetal death, mummification, abortion, dysmaturity, premature birth, or even full-term stillbirth. Such prenatal losses account for the largest numeric loss of animals in the reproductive process. The nature, significance, specific causes, and diagnosis of congenital defects and inherited disorders in cattle are discussed here.

NATURE AND EFFECT OF DEFECTS AND DISORDERS

Congenital defects and disorders range from minor deviations to moderate and severe defects to monstrosities. They are sentinels of the animal's environment, a diagnostic challenge, and of great comparative biomedical significance. A defective neonate is an adapted survivor of a disruptive event or events caused by the animal's inheritance or by its environment, including the maternal environment provided by its dam or her inheritance or by interaction of both inheritance and environment.

In the near future a specific cause for each disruptive event is likely to be identified through the immense resolving power of molecular genetics and biochemistry. In anticipation of such discoveries, once so improbable but now ongoing, such causal mechanisms are named *formation* defects. The disruptive events occur at one or more stages in the complexly integrated sequences of events of embryogenesis and early fetal development. If the disruptive event is not immediately lethal, it is followed by the remaining normal developmental sequences, which must then accommodate the event and its sequelae. Often this is not possible, and the embryo or fetus dies before completing development and is resorbed or expelled, often undetected.

SIGNIFICANCE TO CATTLE INDUSTRY AND VETERINARY MEDICINE

Congenital defects and disorders are relatively infrequent—in total, probably involving about 1 in 500 calves and perhaps up to 1 in 100 calves when sampling a wide cross-section of herds. Despite the great interest attracted throughout medical history by fetal monsters as "freaks of nature," congenital defects and disorders result in fewer losses than those caused by nutritional deficiencies, infectious agents, or neoplasia. However, defects and disorders may cause considerable economic losses to some individual herd owners through increased perinatal mortality or when embryonic and fetal mortality are a part of the syndrome. Congenital defects and disorders also may confuse the diagnosis of other diseases and abortion. Breeders of pedigreed cattle may see the value of their animals diminish after relatives of the animals have been diagnosed with a genetic defect or disorder. Control measures may require extensive and expensive adjustments to breeding programs.

FREQUENCY AND TYPES OF DEFECTS AND DISORDERS

Because the environment and the inheritance of animals in different herds is quite different, the frequency and types of defects and disorders should be expected to be quite variable, even when large numbers of herds are sampled. Despite this variability, rough estimates are helpful in understanding the nature and significance of the defects and disorders likely to be encountered. But even rough estimates are difficult to obtain because of uncertainties about classifying stillbirths and the costliness of performing detailed dissections. Stillbirths range around 4% in many herds, yet most stillbirths appear anatomically normal. On the other hand, among clearly defective calves, nearly half are born dead, most with visible defects. In a special study limited to patients in U.S. and Canadian veterinary college clinics, 6455 of 137,717 patients (4.6%) had congenital defects.[1] Another broad-based study of 2293 defective calves born in a 9-year period in Germany cataloged the kinds of defects.[2] They were central nervous system (21.6%); musculature (13.7%); anomalous twins (10.0%); congenital systemic disturbances such as hydrops (9.7%); defects of the large body cavities such as schistosomus reflexus (6.9%); digestive (4.3%); urinary and reproductive (4.3%); bone and cartilage (2.8%); heart and vessels (2.7%); skin (2%); and others (1.7%). Detailed dissection of 107 normal calves revealed that minor anatomic defects or deviations are very common.[3] Such defects rarely would be detected in normal postmortem examinations. It is clear that the collective frequency of defects depends not only on the occurrence of causal events but also on the intensity of examination.

CAUSES OF DEFECTS AND DISORDERS

Many congenital defects and disorders have no clearly established cause, but others are caused by environmental or genetic factors or their interaction. Because of the rarity of defects and disorders, causation often is difficult to establish and may require accumulation of data on individual cases as they occur over many years. Occasionally, however, a defect or disorder appears in several animals in a herd or herds in successive years; in such cases causation may be more easily established.

To detect a cause, the first and most important step is a thorough investigation of each defect and disorder as it arises. These investigations should provide (1) a careful description of the defect or disorder with as much biologic specificity as possible, (2) a thorough examination of the management or other environmental conditions in the herd or herds possessing the disorder, and (3) collection of all available genetic information, including breed or breeds, pedigrees and birth dates of the affected animal(s), and other normal relatives in the herd. The concept of genetic defects as basically structural defects is changing as an increasing number of defects of formation and function are being identified in cattle.

Environmental Factors

Teratogens in cows include toxic plants; infectious agents; drugs; trace elements; deficiencies; and physical agents such as irradiation, hyperthermia, undue pressure during rectal palpation in early pregnancy; and embryo manipulation.[4-47] Maternal deficiencies of manganese and iodine can produce skeletal defects[4] and the birth of weak calves,[5-7] respectively. Although difficult to identify, teratogens often follow seasonal patterns or known stressful conditions, may be linked to maternal disease, and do not follow a familial pattern created by genetic causes. Because of genetic differences between individuals, animals of different breeds or families and herds in a breed may respond differently to a given teratogen, an important issue sometimes in diagnosis. Field studies frequently lead to observations on the seasonal or geographic pattern of occurrences of defects across herds, suggesting the likely teratogenic culprit.

TOXIC PLANTS AND CHEMICALS. Arthrogryposis (crooked calf disease), characterized by joint contractures, also may be associated with torticollis, scoliosis, or kyphosis; various degrees of cleft palate; and combinations of these defects. The cause is ingestion of *Lupinus* spp., *L. caudatus, L. sericeus, L. sulphureus,* or *L. nootkatensis* by pregnant cows between days 40 and 100 of gestation.[8-11] The alkaloid anagyrine is the teratogen. Similar deformities have been produced experimentally by feeding *Conium maculatum* (poison hemlock) to pregnant cows between days 50 and 70 of gestation. Sudan grass also has been incriminated as a cause of arthrogryposis in calves.[12] *Lupinus formosus* and *Lupinus arbustus* contain the teratogen, ammodendrine and can cause scoliosis, arthrogryposis, or cleft palate.[11,13] Other plants suspected of causing congenital defects include *Senecio, Indigofera, Spicata, Cycadales, Blighia,* loco plants (*Astragalus* and *Oxytropis*), *Papaveraceae, Colchicum, Vinca,* and tobacco and related plants.[8]

In all types of range livestock, most commonly cattle and sheep, locoweed poisoning by plants of the genera *Oxytropis* and *Astragalus* results in emaciation, visual impairment, neurologic signs, habituation, abortion, and congenital limb defects in calves and lambs.[14] *Swainsona* (darling pea) and locoweed contain swainsonine, which inhibits alpha mannosidase.[13,15-17] Poisoning of growing cattle can be confused with genetic mannosidosis of Angus cattle.

VIRAL INFECTIONS. Prenatal infection with the Bunyavirus, Akabane virus, may cause abortion, premature births, arthrogryposis, and hydranencephaly (A-H syndrome) and has been seen in Japan, Korea, Israel, Australia, and Kenya.[18-23] Aino virus, another arthropod-borne member of the Simbu serogroup, also causes A-H syndrome, as well as cerebellar hypoplasia, hydrocephalus, and scoliosis.[23-28] Outbreaks usually exhibit seasonal and geographic patterns.

Bovine virus diarrhea (BVD) virus induces a variety of congenital defects such as cerebellar hypoplasia, ocular defects, brachygnathia inferior, alopecia, dysmyelinogenesis, internal hydrocephalus, dysmaturity (intrauterine growth restriction), and impaired immunologic competence. Similar defects have been experimentally reproduced.[18,22,29-32]

Experimental transmission of bluetongue virus to pregnant heifers through insects resulted in abortion, stillbirths, and congenital defects such as arthrogryposis, campylognathia, and prognathia with domed cranium. Hydranencephaly and a "dummy-calf" syndrome (inactivity, dullness, behavioral disturbances) also have been seen.[33-38] In Oklahoma, abortions and congenital defects such as arthrogryposis, kyphosis, and scoliosis occurred.[34-38] In South Africa, Wesselsbron disease virus caused porencephaly and cerebellar hypoplasia in calves.[39] Chuzan virus has caused hydranencephaly in calves.[18,40]

PROTOZOAL INFECTION. Besides abortion, *Neospora caninum* can cause congenital encephalitis and is associated with ataxia in calves. In one case, internal hydrocephalus was found.[41]

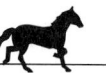

Physical Factors

In calves, atresia of the gut, particularly colonic atresia, may have been caused earlier in utero by external pressure on the amnion from rectal palpation of their dams between days 35 and 40 of gestation. In experiments involving rectal palpation of dams at various stages of gestation, 6 of 125 calves born from dams examined in the pre–42-day group had intestinal atresia, whereas none of the 103 born from dams palpated after 43 days had it. It is thought that palpation and pressure on the amnion during organogenesis (days 33 to 40) can cause atresia coli and occasionally atresia jejuni. Male calves are affected more frequently.[42]

Advanced reproductive technologies, such as in vitro fertilization and nuclear transfer, have been associated with an increased incidence of abnormalities. Examples include a variety of organ defects, unusually large offspring, birth of weak calves and higher perinatal mortality, and chromosomal abnormalities.[43-47]

Genetic Factors

Congenital defects and other disorders may be caused by an animal's inheritance. Mutant genes and abnormalities of the chromosomes that carry the genes are the principal agents; they act by altering developmental processes in ways as yet only incompletely understood. Because genes and the chromosomes that carry them are transmitted from parent to offspring in predictable ways, disorders caused by them also are transmitted in predictable ways. Genetic disorders should appear with a specified though different frequency in each type of family group that might have received the mutant gene from some ancestor. At present, with a few exceptions, identification of genetic factors must be made by the pattern of occurrence of the disorder as it is transmitted from parent to offspring or as it appears in other family groups.[48] However, in the near future, the ever-expanding cattle gene map undoubtedly will facilitate identification of mutant genes. And the much higher priority given to mapping and sequencing the genomes of humans and laboratory mammals soon will provide extraordinary reference libraries for cattle investigations. Because of the rarity of most defects, gene identification usually will be difficult and tentative with two possible exceptions: disorders identifiable by proxy such as those associated with blood antigens, enzyme deficiencies, or lysosomal storage diseases; and defects that attain high frequency accidentally or because they are associated with some important production trait. A good example of the latter is the "weaver" gene, which continued to appear year after year in the Brown Swiss breed despite elimination of animals with the disorder. Very close to the "weaver" gene on the same chromosome, a major gene sharply enhancing milk production was detected.[49] Breeders who selected animals for high milk production chose some animals with the major gene and inadvertently also got the closely linked "weaver" gene. Other earlier examples include syndactylism, snorter dwarfism, and muscular hypertrophy.

IDENTIFYING INHERITED DISORDERS

As a consequence of nearly a century of genetic research, many disorders already have been identified, often tentatively, in one or more breeds. Such disorders often recur in the breed of origin and, in the absence of contradictory morphologic evidence, usually are assumed to have resulted from the earlier one, or more rarely, from an identical mutation. However, when the disorder reappears in another breed in which it had not been reported previously, caution must be exercised in presuming that this mutation is identical with that earlier one, unless the second breed was an offshoot of the first. When the disorder only generally resembles one described earlier, it should be treated as a new disorder.

GENE DISORDERS

When a suspected hereditary disorder is observed in an animal, the animal's relatives in the herd should also be examined for the defect. Most animals in a herd are related in some way. Thus the relatives may include full or half sibs, parents, progeny, grandparents, aunts or uncles, nieces or nephews, and cousins of varying degrees. For each group of relatives, often comprising large and complex genealogies, it is theoretically possible, though often very difficult, to calculate the fraction of all animals that should be diseased, as well as the fraction of normal, for diseases transmitted in each of several simple and well-known hereditary patterns. The most easily usable family groups are full- and half-sib families and parents and their offspring. However, in most herds full-sib families are small and relatively infrequent; other types of families, usually half and three-fourths sibs, often must suffice.

Recessive Pattern

The most frequently observed simple pattern involving a pair of genes, one normal and one mutant, is the recessive pattern. Only animals with two mutant genes are affected. Positive identification of this pattern requires relatively large numbers of animals. The pattern has a number of easily recognizable features. Diseased animals most often are produced by phenotypically normal parents, which also may produce normal offspring, usually in a ratio of 1 abnormal to 3 normals. Often the disease appears first when related normal animals are mated (i.e., when inbreeding has occurred). Matings of a normal bull with his normal daughters (1 abnormal and 7 normals expected; ratio of 1:8); or with normal granddaughters (1 abnormal and 15 normals; ratio of about 1:16) are common examples. The disease often skips generations. Often the pedigrees of diseased animals trace back in several generations to a widely used ancestor, a "founder." If matings of a normal animal with a diseased animal occur, either or both normal and diseased offspring may be produced. If a diseased offspring is produced, because the normal parent is a carrier, additional matings of these parents should produce one diseased for every one normal. A "critical" mating occurs when diseased animals are mated, because they should produce only diseased offspring.

If the disease appears with equal frequency in males and females, the recessive gene is on an autosomal chromosome and thus is an autosomal-recessive gene. If the disease appears with much greater frequency in males than in females, the recessive gene is probably on the X-chromosome. It is an X-linked, or sex-linked, recessive gene. In this situation, matings of normal animals produce only normal females but both normal and diseased males.

Dominant Pattern

The next most common pattern is essentially a reversal of the recessive, the dominant pattern. Animals with one and two mutant genes are affected. In this pattern the only diseased animal without a diseased parent is the "founder" animal. That animal is diseased because one parental gamete contained a newly mutated gene. Every other diseased animal has at least one diseased parent. Subsequent matings of a diseased animal to normal animals produce equal numbers of diseased and normal offspring. Matings of two diseased animals from matings of diseased and normal parents produce both diseased and normal animals, in a ratio of three diseased to one normal. As the disease increases in frequency, some matings of diseased animals will produce only diseased offspring. Matings of two normal animals, however, continue to produce only normal offspring. The trait usually is present generation after generation. If the disease appears with equal frequency in males and females, it is on an autosome, an autosomal dominant gene. If, however, it is relatively rare and occurs with greater frequencies in females than males, it likely is on the X-chromosome. It is an X-linked, or sex-linked, dominant gene. In this circumstance, diseased males mated with normal females produce only diseased daughters and normal sons. If the disorder is uncommon, diseased females mated to normal males produce normal and diseased progeny of both sexes in equal numbers.

Incompletely Dominant Pattern

The third pattern is one in which there is a gradation between normal and diseased that creates an intermediate class of individuals. The intermediate animal has one normal and one mutant gene. The genes involved have been given various names, depending on whether the intermediate classes most resemble normal or diseased animals. When the intermediate class most resembles the normal animal, which is the usual situation, the normal gene is called an incompletely dominant gene. Sometimes in this situation the recessive mutant gene is said to be incompletely recessive. Animals with the intermediate form usually appear in herds before the appearance of diseased animals. They often are sufficiently near normal that they are accepted in breeding programs. When near-normal and normal are mated, both near-normal and normal offspring can be produced. But when two near-normal animals are mated, they produce normal, near-normal, and clearly diseased animals, in proportion of 1:2:1 respectively. Once the disease appears, it rarely skips generations. If the reverse holds (i.e., when the intermediate animal also seems diseased, but only slightly), the mutant gene is then the incompletely dominant gene; if such disorders persist, they are likely to be only slightly debilitating, thus enabling some diseased animals to avoid being culled.

Overdominant Pattern

The fourth pattern is an awkwardly named one. In it, a presumably recessive disease keeps reappearing, despite elimination of diseased animals. As was true for a recessive disease, animals with two mutant genes are diseased. But animals with one mutant gene and one normal gene are preferred over those with two normal genes. Sometimes the difference between preferred and normal is so slight as to escape detection by casual observation. Yet the preferred animals are selected as parents relatively more often than the normal individuals. As a consequence, the disorder persists. Well-known examples include snorter dwarfism, syndactyly, and weaver. In snorter dwarfism in beef cattle, normal animals with one normal and one dwarf gene were shorter and blockier than animals with two normal genes and at a particular point in time were thought superior for breeding. Later, when two such animals were mated, one in four of their progeny were unwanted dwarfs. Clearly the dwarf gene was a recessive gene, but, unlike with other recessive disorders, there was no attempt to eradicate the disease by culling carriers. The normal gene was called an overdominant gene because animals with one such gene and one normal gene were more desired than (or superior to) those with two normal genes. Of course, the response might also be identified as a heterozygote advantage or a beneficial gene interaction, names that suggest that both genes must be present for the

advantage to occur. Another explanation attributes the persistence to a fortuitous and temporary linkage of the mutant gene to another gene that markedly improves an economically important trait, the case with the weaver gene.

Other Patterns: Polygenes

In addition to these major common patterns, there are countless other patterns that involve an ever-increasing number of genes; sometimes a few have important effects; often they do not. In many disorders the pattern of transmission seems to be one produced by many genes with small effects, usually modified by environmental factors. These sometimes are called polygenes, and the disorders are referred to as polygenic disorders. The genetic control of such disorders is measured by a fraction called heritability, abbreviated h^2, which ranges from 0% to 100%.

MUTANT GENES TRANSFERRED AMONG BREEDS

When crossbreeding is common, as in beef cattle, a mutant gene may be transferred to a new breed from another breed. The gene may not behave the same in the crossbred animals and their descendants as it did in the breed of origin.

CHROMOSOMAL DISORDERS

Many chromosomal abnormalities have been identified cytologically in all large-animal species.[50] Some disorders have been associated with a few of these, but they are not as diagnostically important as they are in humans. Well-known examples include (1) the XO Turner's syndrome: infertility in females; (2) XXY Klinefelter's syndrome: underdeveloped males; and (3) centric fusions (or Robertsonian translocation): reduced reproductive capacity in some species, early embryonic death in cattle. The latter has caused mandated karyotyping of some breeding cattle in several countries.[51]

Although most congenital defects are associated with normal chromosome complements, chromosomal abnormalities can be a significant cause of prenatal mortality. As much as 11% of aborted fetuses and stillborn calves have been found to have an abnormal chromosome complement.[52]

DIAGNOSIS AND CONTROL

Until his recent death, Dr. Horst Leipold ran the Kansas Genetic Disease Program for over 40 years. That program served as a model for diagnosing and controlling these diseases and is described below.

A systematic program is established for receiving, gathering, recording, interpreting, advising, and communicating information on congenital and genetic diseases.[53] Defective animals are submitted voluntarily by veterinarians, herd owners, and artificial insemination (AI) and breed registry officials. Cases often come from great distances and many other states. When defective animals are submitted, a history is requested. The history should include breed, age of parents, parentage of affected and unaffected animals (the latter as controls), geographic region, season, type of pasture, soil type, and exposure to or suspected exposure to teratogenic plants, feeding and management practices, breeding records, maternal medical and vaccination records, disease status of the herd, periods of stress, drugs administered, congenital defects observed previously, and history of any similar congenital defects in neighboring herds. After submission, necropsy examination is performed on the animals and the defect(s) classified by body system primarily involved. Serum samples are checked for bovine virus, diarrhea virus, and other viral antibodies. Brain and other tis-

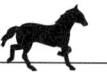

sue samples are taken for virus isolation. Relevant tissues are histologically examined, and selected cases are submitted for electron microscopy. Some are karyotyped. Pedigrees and breeding records, when available, may be analyzed for evidence of inbreeding and for characteristic hereditary transmission patterns and frequencies. The results are compared with other similar cases recorded in the data bank, if such have been observed. The data bank includes data on numerous disorders from many breeds and many states.

Today in the United States, Dr. David Steffen of the Cattle Congenital Disease Diagnosis and Research Program at the University of Nebraska maintains a similar databank. When investigating congenital defects in cattle, pertinent information may be collected and reported to that program.

Recommendations for Breeding Programs

When animals with inherited disorders are identified, the following procedures are recommended:

- Blood typing to verify parentage, especially if AI sires are involved
- Certified statement regarding occurrence of the disorder by veterinarian or third-party witness
- Extended pedigree chart
- Laboratory examination by pathologist when applicable
- Decision withheld until all reasonable doubt has been eliminated (for bulls, usually two or more thoroughly documented cases)
- Subsequent notification of AI or other concerned organizations (e.g., breed registry) with recommended courses of action, if any

Most AI organizations label bulls carrying an undesirable recessive gene in advertisements; many also remove the bull from service. Some herd owners may prefer to test sires before or after the discovery of an inherited disorder.

Although dominant defects can be eliminated simply by not breeding affected animals, eradicating deleterious recessive genes requires identification of carriers. There are currently three methods for determination of genotype in common use: test mating (such as sire testing), biochemical testing, and DNA-based testing.

Sire Testing Procedures

Sires can be tested conventionally for hereditary disorders by various types of breeding trials as shown in Table 47-1.

Speedier tests of males or females involve superovulation of affected females, followed by insemination and embryo transfer (two per recipient) and early cesarean section at 60 days.

Biochemical Testing

For certain defects, such as storage and metabolic diseases, heterozygotes can be identified. These carriers, compared with normal animals, possess approximately one half of the particular gene product. Examples include α-mannosidase in α-mannosidosis, AAG activity in glycogenosis, UMP synthase in DUMPS, protoporphyrin in protoporphyria, and β-mannosidase in β-mannosidosis. However, these biochemical tests can be flawed because of such things as environmental factors altering concentrations of the chemicals or hemopoietic chimerism (an effect of dizygotic twinning).[54,55]

DNA-Based Testing

Polymerase chain reaction (PCR) methods are rapidly replacing biochemical testing and sire testing for the determination of genotype for recessive defects. Although most tests are run on blood, obtaining DNA from hair roots or other sources is another option when there are problems inherent in blood testing.[56] DNA-based tests are now commonly used to determine genotype and screen carriers for recessive defects such as BLAD, DUMPS, citrullinemia, myophosphorylase deficiency, glycogenosis, and α-mannosidosis.[54,57]

DIAGNOSTIC INFORMATION ON SPECIFIC DEFECTS

Tables 47-2 to 47-29 briefly describe defects and inherited disorders according to the principally defective body system. Emphasis is placed on defects and inherited disorders of current interest and concern.

REFERENCES

1. Priester WA, Glass GG, Waggoner NS: Congenital defects in domesticated animals: general consideration, *Am J Vet Res* 31:1871-1879, 1970.
2. Leipold HW, Dennis SM, Huston K: Congenital defects in cattle: nature, cause and effect, *Adv Vet Sci Comp Med* 16:103-150, 1972.
3. Leipold HW et al: Anatomic variations in normal calves, *Giessener Beitr Erbpathol Zuchthyg* 3:31-54, 1971.
4. Staley GP et al: Congenital skeletal malformations in calves associated with putative manganese deficiency, *J S Afr Vet Assoc* 65:73-78, 1994.
5. Barlow AM, Roper MR: Rape straw as a possible cause of neonatal goitre and weak calves, *Vet Rec* 137:572, 1995.
6. Collery P et al: Causes of perinatal calf mortality in the republic of Ireland, *Irish Vet J* 49:491-496, 1996.
7. Smyth JA, Goodall EA, McCoy WAE: Stillbirth/perinatal weak calf syndrome: a study of calves with an abnormal thyroid gland, *Vet Rec* 139: 11-16, 1996.
8. Keeler RJ: Alkaloid teratogens from *Lupinus, Conium, Veratrum* and related genera. In Keeler RJ, VanKampen KR, James LF, eds: *Effect of poisonous plants on livestock,* New York, 1978, Academic Press, pp 397-408.
9. Panter KE, Keeler RF: Quinolizidine and piperidine alkaloid teratogens from poisonous plants and their mechanism of action in animals, *Vet Clin North Am (Food Anim Pract)* 9:33-40, 1993.
10. Panter KE et al: Observations of *Lupinus sulphureus*-induced "crooked calf disease," *J Range Mgt* 50:587-592, 1997.
11. Panter KE, Gardner DR, Molyneux RJ: Teratogenic and fetotoxic effects of two piperidine alkaloid-containing lupines (*L. formosus* and *L. arbustus*) in cows, *J Nat Toxins* 7:131-140, 1998.
12. Seaman JT, Smeal MH, Wright JC: The possible association of a sorghum (*Sorghum sudanese*) hybrid as a cause of developmental defects in calves, *Aust Vet J* 57:351-352, 1981.
13. James LF et al: Effect of natural toxins on reproduction, *Vet Clin North Am (Food Anim Pract)* 10:587-603, 1994.
14. James LF et al: Abortive and teratogenic effects of locoweed in sheep and cattle, *Am J Vet Res* 28:1379-1388, 1967.
15. Huxtable CR, Dorling PR: Poisoning in livestock by *Swainsona* spp.: current status, *Aust Vet J* 59:50-53, 1982.
16. Stegelmeier BL et al: Serum α-mannosidase activity and the clinicopathologic alterations of locoweed (*Astragalus mollissimus*) intoxication in range cattle, *J Vet Diagn Invest* 6:473-479, 1994.
17. Molyneux R, James L: Locointoxication: indolizidine alkaloids of spotted locoweed (*Astralagus lentiginosus*), *Science* 216:190-191, 1982.
18. Oberst RD: Viruses as teratogens, *Vet Clin North Am (Food Anim Pract)* 9:23-31, 1993.
19. Konno S, Moriwaki M, Nakagawa M: Akabane disease in cattle: congenital abnormalities caused by viral infection, spontaneous disease, *Vet Pathol* 19:246-266, 1982.
20. Konno S, Nakagawa M: Akabane disease in cattle: congenital abnormalities caused by viral infection, experimental disease, *Vet Pathol* 19:267-279, 1982.

TABLE 47-1

Sire Testing

Females Used for Test Matings	Offspring Needed to Reach Probability Level of		
	0.05	0.01	0.001
Abnormal*	5	7	10
Normal carriers*	10	16	24
Sire's daughters†	22	35	52

*Tests for only one trait.
†Tests for all undesirable recessive traits.

Text continued on p. 1509

TABLE 47-2

Congenital Defects of the Facial Skeleton in Cattle

Defect	Reference No.	Description	Etiology	Frequency	Diagnosis	Associated Defects
Agnathia	53, 58, 59	Lack of development of mandible, failure of oral cavity to form, bones of roof of mouth are abnormal, tongue is lacking, ears and eyes located ventrally on skull	Familial, Jersey	Rare	Physical examination, x-ray	None
Campylognathia (wry face)	53, 60	Scoliosis of the face (with normal mandible) leading to malocclusion	Recessive, Jersey	Common	Physical examination	None
Prognathia inferior	61	Incisor teeth protrude beyond upper lip, calves grow out of it by 3 to 6 months of age	Dominant	Rare	Physical examination	None
Brachygnathia (short lower jaw)	62–67	Various degrees of short mandible	Recessive or polygenic	Common	Physical examination, x-ray	Usually none, but may have arthrogryposis
Brachygnathia with impacted molar teeth	64	Shorter-than-normal mandible combined with impacted molar teeth, lethal	Simple autosomal recessive, shorthorn	Rare	Physical examination, x-ray	None
Brachygnathia with chromosomal defect (trisomy 18)	65	Short lower jaw, calves are born dead or die shortly after birth, brain defects, extra chromosome 18	Shorthorn	Rare	Physical examination, karyotyping	None
Cleft palate (palatoschisis)	68–73	Partial or complete failure to close of soft or hard palate	Genetic, feeding of *Lupine* spp. between days 40 and 70 of gestation; may be others	Common	Physical examination, milk may run from nostrils, poor doers, aspiration pneumonia	May be single, isolated defect or combined with arthrogryposis and other defects
Cleft face (schistoprosopus)	74	Split face, one nostril to each side of the mandible, degree varies	Unknown	Rare	Physical examination	None
Cheiloschisis "hare lip," "cleft lip"	75	Lateral or median cleft upper lip	Familial	Rare	Physical examination	None
Cheilognathoschisis	75, 76	Lateral or median cleft of upper lip and hard palate partially cleft	Unknown	Rare	Physical examination, necropsy	None
Cheilognathopalatoschisis	77	Lateral or median cleft lips and cleft palate	Unknown	Rare	Physical examination	None
Probatocephaly (sheep head)	78, 79	Head with a convex facial profile, eyes protruding, enlarged tongue, and heart defects	Possible dominant, Limousin	Rare	Physical examination	Heart defects
Facial-digital syndrome	80	Syndactyly of all four legs, hypoplasia of upper jaw	Familial	Reported in Angus	Physical examination, x-ray	None
Diprosopus	81	Duplication of the face, a form of conjoined twinning	Unknown	Unknown	Physical examination	None

TABLE 47-3

Congenital Defects of the Axial Skeleton in Cattle

Defect	Reference No.	Description	Etiology	Frequency	Diagnosis	Associated Defects
Atlantooccipital fusion	82, 83	Fusion of atlas and occipital area, hypoplasia of dens of axis, leading to compression of spinal cord; calf may show ataxia or become recumbent at birth or later in life	Appears to be familial	Not uncommon	Neurologic examination, x-ray	None
Torticollis (wry neck)	84	Neck bent to one side or other, cannot be corrected passively	Unknown	Common	Physical examination	Front leg contraction
Kyphosis	84	Dorsal bending of vertebral column	Unknown	Rare	Physical examination	None
Lordosis	84	Ventral bending of vertebral column	Unknown	Rare	Physical examination	None
Scoliosis	84	Sideward bending of vertebral column	Unknown	Rare	Physical examination	None
Kyphoscoliosis (twisted back)	84	Dorsal and sideward bending of vertebral column	Unknown	Rare	Physical examination	May occur together with arthrogryposis
Perosomus elumbis	85, 86	Agenesis of lumbosacral spinal cord and vertebrae; front half of body normal; hind legs fixed in arthrogryposis	Unknown	Rare	Physical examination, x-ray	Arthrogryposis and ankylosis of hind legs, abnormality of internal organs
Short spine lethal	87	Head and legs are normal; axial skeleton is reduced; only 6 to 7 ribs, calves die on first day of life	Simple autosomal recessive	Rare	Physical examination, x-ray	None
Spina bifida	88, 89	Failure of neural tube to close; incomplete closure of the dorsal lamina that form the vertebral arch; spina bifida occulta is without exposure of neural tissues; located most commonly in lumbar or thoracic area	Simple autosomal recessive or unknown	Common	Physical examination	Arthrogryposis of hind legs; spinal cord defects; Arnold-Chiari defect
Congenital spinal stenosis	90	From birth to 20 weeks, degrees of posterior weakness and ataxia, spinal canal stenosis caused by flaring of ends of vertebral bodies and protrusion of vertebral articular processes, short and malformed long bones, local closure of epiphyseal plates	Unknown	Not uncommon	Physical examination, x-ray, necropsy	Hydrocephaly
Tailless (anury), short tail, wrye tail, kinky tail	60, 91-94	Partial or complete lack of development of tail and sacral vertebrae	Some genetic, some nongenetic	Fairly common	Physical examination	None or associated with anophthalmia or heart defects
Persistent cloaca and caudal spinal agenesis	95	Lack of tail with colon and urogenital system terminating in persistent cloaca	Unknown	Rare	Physical examination, necropsy	Atresia ani, urogenital defects

TABLE 47-4

Congenital Defects of the Appendicular Skeleton in Cattle

Defect	Reference No.	Description	Etiology	Frequency	Diagnosis	Associated Defects
Abrachia anterior	96, 97	Lack of development of both front legs	Unknown	Rare	Physical examination	None
Monobrachia	53	Lack of development of one front leg	Unknown	Rare	Physical examination	None
Amelia	53	Lack of development of both hind legs	Unknown	Rare	Physical examination	None
Acroteriasis congenita ("amputated")	98, 99	Lack of formation of all four legs, with small stumps as legs; associated with hypoplasia of maxilla, short lower jaw, low birth weight (15.1 kg)	Simple autosomal recessive	Rare	Physical examination	Various skeletal defects
Ectrodactyly	100	Partial absence of skeletal parts of digit on one or more legs, syndactyly of hoof	Unknown	Rare	Physical examination, x-ray	None
Monodactyly	53	Lack of development of one digital ray on one or more feet; only one hoof at affected leg	Unknown	Rare	Physical examination, x-ray	None
Adactyly	101	Complete or partial absence of digital structures on one or more feet	Simple autosomal recessive	Rare	Physical examination, x-ray	None

	Figures	Description	Inheritance	Frequency	Diagnosis	Associated Defects
Syndactyly	102-111	Fusion or nondivision of functional digits involving one or more feet; Holstein right, left front and front over hind; other breeds may have all four feet involved; may have contractures of affected legs; right front over left front over hind legs	Simple autosomal recessive with variable expressivity and incomplete penetrance, pleiotrophic effect in Holstein, recessive in others	Common; seen in Holstein, Angus, Chianina, Hereford, Simmental, German Red Pied, Japanese native, and crossbred cattle	Physical examination, x-ray; gene is located on chromosome 15	Hyperthermia in Holsteins
Bipartite distal sesamoid bones	112	Bilateral medial navicular bones develop as two parts; abaxial part fuses to P2; lameness	Unknown	Rare	X-ray, CT scan	Partial fusion of distal interphalangeal joint
Angular deformity of tibia	113	Unilateral maldevelopment (valgus deformity) of tibia	Unknown	Rare	X-ray	None
Tibial hemimelia	114-116	Calves unable to get up after birth, bilateral lack of development of tibia	Simple autosomal recessive, Galloway	Common	Physical examination, x-ray	Meningocele, nonunion of symphysis of pelvis, reproductive tract defects, abdominal hernia
Polydactyly	117-119	Development of second digit, one dew claw; usually front legs involved	Polygenic; dominant gene at one locus, recessive genes at other loci, Simmental	Common	Physical examination, x-ray	None
Arachnomelia	120-124	Slender, long, fragile bones of the legs; kyphoscoliosis; short lower jaw	Simple autosomal recessive, Brown Swiss	Common	Physical examination, x-ray	Arthrogryposis

CT, Computed tomography.

TABLE 47-5

Congenital Defects of the Entire Skeletal System in Cattle

Defect	Reference No.	Description	Etiology	Frequency	Diagnosis	Associated Defects
Osteopetrosis	125-128	Small body size and weight, short lower jaw, lack of development of bone marrow cavities, usually stillborn 251 to 272 days of gestation	Simple autosomal recessive, Angus, Simmental, Holstein	Rare	Physical examination, x-ray	Short lower jaw
Osteogenesis imperfecta	129-132	Joint laxity, fragility of bone, fractures, imperfect development of teeth, blue sclera	Autosomal dominant, Holstein, Charolais	Rare	Physical examination, x-ray	None
Abnormal modeling of trabecular bone	133	Abnormal modeling of long bones, persistence of primary or secondary spongiosa	Unknown	Rare	Necropsy, x-ray, histopathologic examination	None
Chondrodysplasia ("bulldog")	134	Wide round head, short barrel-like body, short limbs, long bones with large knobby cartilagenous epiphyses, very short diaphyses	Genetic, recessive, all breeds	Common	Physical examination, x-ray	Cleft palate, heart defects
Chondrodysplasia ("Dexter")	135-137	Calves aborted in late gestation, round head, very short legs, cartilagenous epiphyses, short diaphyses (homozygotes)	Incomplete dominance, Dexter	Common, short-legged types are heterozygotes	Physical examination, x-ray	Cleft palate, abdominal hernia
Achondroplasia (Jersey)	138	Short limbs, round head, cleft palate, short body, epiphyses consist of cartilage, short diaphyses	Simple autosomal recessive, Jersey	Rare	Physical examination, x-ray	Cleft palate
Achondroplasia (Telemark)	139, 140	Calves with short legs, barrel-like body, die shortly after birth	Simple autosomal recessive	Rare	Physical examination, x-ray	None
Dwarfism	141-143	Saddlelike nose, broad bulging head, shorter than normal legs, disproportionate body, disturbed longitudinal bone growth, reduced weight	Overdominant, Hereford, Angus	Rare	Physical examination, x-ray	None
Proportionate dwarfism	144-149	Low birth weight, 10 to 17 kg, small body but proportionate	Genetic; Simmental, Braunvieh, Angus, Jersey	Rare	Physical examination	Hydrops fetalis
Dwarfism with joint laxity	4, 150-152	Low birth weight, doming of forehead, short legs, dyspnea, poor performance, narrow epiphyseal plates	Environmental, believed to be maternal manganese deficiency, or other factor from spoiled silage	Rare	Physical examination	Joint laxity, superior brachygnathism

TABLE 47-6

Congenital Defects of the Joint in Cattle

Defect	Reference No.	Description	Etiology	Frequency	Diagnosis	Associated Defects
Hip dysplasia	153-156	Occurs most commonly in males 6-18 months of age; lameness, short stepping gait; crepitating sound over hip joints; degenerative joint disease with erosion and eburnation of coxofemoral joints; thickened joint capsule, increased joint fluid	Perhaps incomplete dominant trait, Hereford, Charolais, Limousin	Rare	Clinical examination	None
Degenerative joint disease with facial dysplasia	157	Calves with short face; swelling of joints begins right after birth, all major joints with degenerative joint disease; lameness	Genetic, Angus	Rare	Physical examination, x-ray	Facial dysplasia
Ankylosis of coffin joints	158	Painful, lameness, loss of weight; affects coffin joints of both front and hind legs	Unknown	Rare, described in two Simmental calves	Physical examination, x-ray	None

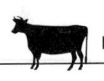

TABLE 47-7

Congenital Defects of the Muscular System in Cattle

Defect	Reference No.	Description	Etiology	Frequency	Diagnosis	Associated Defects
Limber leg	159-162	Calves unable to stand, no control over their legs, generalized hypoplasia of muscles	Jersey; simple autosomal recessive	Rare	Physical examination	None
Double muscling (muscular hypertrophy)	163-168	Rounded outline of hind quarters; deep creases between muscles of neck, shoulder, hind legs; short neck, fine head; large tongue; raised tailhead; infantile genital tract; increased susceptibility to respiratory and musculoskeletal diseases; double-muscled muscles have higher proportions of type IIb fibers and lower capillary supplies	Partially recessive; mutated myostatin (MSTN) gene located at mh locus on chromosome 2	Common in Belgian Blue, Piedmontese	Physical examination	Bone disease and joint problems, reduced fertility and calf survival, dystocia
Arthrogryposis	169-173	Bilateral symmetric contracture of all four legs, metatarsophalangeal joints frequently hypermobile	Charolais; simple autosomal recessive; plants; viruses	Common	Physical examination	Cleft palate, kyphoscoliosis, hypoplasia of patella
Myasthenia gravis	174	Progressive muscular weakness in young calves exacerbated by exercise, caused by defective neuromuscular transmission	Unknown, Brahman	Rare	Temporary clinical improvement after administration of anticholinesterase drug	None
Myopathy of diaphragmatic muscles	175-177	Dystrophic changes in diaphragm	Autosomal recessive in Holstein	Reported in a line of Holsteins in Japan	Histopathology, immunohistochemistry, EM	None
Myophosphorylase deficiency	178	Exercise intolerance and prolonged recumbency after forced exercise	Autosomal recessive, Charolais	Uncommon	Muscle biopsy—histochemical staining for phosphorylase; subsarcolemmal vacuoles on histopathology; PCR to detect carriers	None

EM, Electron microscopy; *PCR,* polymerase chain reaction.

TABLE 47-8

Congenital Defects of the Cerebrum in Cattle

Defect	Reference No.	Description	Etiology	Frequency	Diagnosis	Associated Defects
Internal hydrocephalus	179-184	Newborn calves mostly unable to get up, reduced body size and weight; narrow refined facial features and cranial doming; lateral ventricles severely dilated; protruding edematous tongue; sigmoid configuration of brain; microphthalmia; edema of muscles	Simple autosomal recessive; Hereford, Shorthorn	Rare	Physical examination, necropsy	Eye defects, muscle lesions
Hydranencephaly	53, 184	Both cerebral hemispheres are fluid-filled bags, may have arthrogryposis	Prenatal viral infection	Common	Physical examination, necropsy	Arthrogryposis
Agenesis of corpus callosum	185	Total or partial absence of corpus callosum, agenesis of septum pellucidum, may have hydrocephalus or microcephaly	Unknown	Uncommon	Physical examination, necropsy	None
Anencephaly	186	Nonclosure of the anterior part of the neural tube; vesicle-like hemispheres may be present; normal pons, medulla, and cerebellum, and eyes; may have lack of development of pituitary that may cause prolonged gestation	Unknown	Common	Physical examination, necropsy	Cleft palate, taillessness, atresia ani
Arrhinencephaly	187	Absence of rhinencephalon, most commonly known as bilateral absence of olfactory bulbs, tract, and/or nerves; may have aprosopia, atresia of nostrils, and other defects	Unknown	Rare	Physical examination, necropsy	Various central nervous system defects

Continued

TABLE 47-8

Congenital Defects of the Cerebrum in Cattle—cont'd

Defect	Reference No.	Description	Etiology	Frequency	Diagnosis	Associated Defects
Meningocele and meningoencephalocele	188, 189	Protrusion of meninges through a cranial cleft; may form large fluid-filled sac usually in frontal region but also midfrontal, parietal, and occipital; may have brain tissue in herniated part (meningoencephalocele)	Unknown	Rare	Physical examination, necropsy	Tibial hemimelia
Microcephaly	190	Abnormally small brain; cerebrum with decreased number of gyri and agenesis of corpus callosum	Unknown	Rare	Physical examination	Various central nervous system defects
Holoprosencephaly	191	Flat face and severe bilateral microphthalmia; lack of development of longitudinal cerebral fissure and falx cerebri; one single, large dilated ventricle; lack of development of olfactory bulbs and nerves, corpus callosum, and septum pellucidum	Unknown	Rare	Necropsy	None

TABLE 47-9

Congenital Defects of the Cerebellum and Brain Stem in Cattle

Defect	Reference No.	Description	Etiology	Frequency	Diagnosis	Associated Defects
Arnold-Chiari defect	192-196	Herniation of cerebellar tissue through foramen magnum combined with caudal displacement of medulla oblongata, pons, and fourth ventricle; often associated with lumbar spina bifida and arthrogryposis of hind legs	Unknown	Rare	Physical examination, necropsy	Spina bifida, posterior bimelic arthrogryposis; may be cerebellar hypoplasia or dicephalus
Cerebellar aplasia, hypoplasia and degeneration	197-201	Calf unable to get up after birth, extended limbs, intermittent opisthotonos and ataxia, cerebellum absent or small; on cross-section folia of cortex are irregular, thin molecular and granular layers; optic neuritis, variable degrees of depletion of cortical layers to complete destruction of cortex and folial white matter	Genetic, unknown or prenatal viral infection such as bovine virus diarrhea virus	Common	Physical examination, MRI, necropsy	May have micrognathia
Hereditary hypomyelinogenesis congenita	202	Incoordination, failure of synergic muscle groups to act harmoniously; central nervous system grossly normal; diffuse spongy appearance of white matter in cerebellum, midbrain, pons; depletion of Purkinje cells	Simple autosomal recessive, Jersey	Rare	Neurologic examination, necropsy	None

CNS, Central nervous system; *MRI*, magnetic resonance imaging.

Continued

TABLE 47-9

Congenital Defects of the Cerebellum and Brain Stem in Cattle—cont'd

Defect	Reference No.	Description	Etiology	Frequency	Diagnosis	Associated Defects
Cerebellar cortical atrophy	203-207	Brain grossly normal; selective degeneration of Purkinje cells from acute swelling to vacuolation and lysis to form empty baskets	Unknown, possibly inherited in Holstein	Rare	Neurologic examination, necropsy, and histopathologic studies	None
Progressive ataxia	208-210	Weakness of hind legs begins when 8-10 months old, progressing to recumbency; CNS grossly normal, eosinophilic plaques in white matter; lack of oligodendroglia	Genetic; Charolais	Rare	Neurologic examination	None
Familial convulsions and ataxia	211	Either seen first few hours of life or when 2-3 months old; single or multiple tetaniform seizures, signs tapered into ataxia; brains grossly normal, Purkinje cell degeneration from swelling to empty basket formation	Incompletely penetrant-dominant; Angus	Rare	Neurologic examination, histopathology	None
Dandy-Walker malformation	212, 213	Calf unable to get up, hydrocephalus, combination of anomalies, enlarged cranium, large posterior fossa, dilation of ventricular system, absence or hypoplasia of cerebellar vermis, distention of roof of fourth ventricle forming a cyst	Unknown	Rare	Necropsy	Agenesis of corpus callosum

CNS, Central nervous system; *MRI,* magnetic resonance imaging.

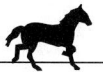

TABLE 47-10

Spastic and Paralytic Diseases in Cattle

Defect	Reference No.	Description	Etiology	Frequency	Diagnosis	Associated Defects
Spastic paresis	214-218	Spastic contracture of muscles and extension of stifle and tarsal joints, usually unilateral, bilateral involvement rare, neck stretched, affected leg kept off the ground and swung freely, raised tail head	Genetic and environmental factors, many breeds	Common	Physical examination	None
Spastic syndrome	219, 220	Chronic, progressive disease characterized by sudden spastic muscular contraction of both hind legs and often back, neck, and front leg; no gross and microscopic lesions	Reported as incomplete dominant, many breeds	Rare	Neurologic examination	None

TABLE 47-11

Storage Diseases of the Central Nervous System in Cattle

Defect	Reference No.	Description	Etiology	Frequency	Diagnosis	Associated Defects
α-Mannosidosis	221, 224	May be affected at birth, but clinical signs usually appear by 6 months of age; ataxia, incoordination, head tremor, aggressive behavior, failure to thrive; primary lesion is neuronal vacuolation, spheroidal swellings of axons; also vacuolation of exocrine pancreas cells, proximal convoluted tubule cells in kidneys	Simple autosomal recessive; Angus, Galloway, Murray Grey	Heterozygote frequency in New Zealand Angus has been estimated at 25%	Neurologic examination, heterozygotes can be identified by reduced α-mannosidase levels	Mild hydrocephalus
β-Mannosidosis	225-227	Calves affected at birth, have short face, prognathism, unable to get up, opisthotonos, cranium domed, heavy wet brains with hydrocephalus, large olive-green kidneys	Simple autosomal recessive, Salers	Rare	Neurologic examination, necropsy, β-mannosidase levels can identify carrier status	Mild hydrocephalus
Ceroid-lipofuscinosis	221	Blindness and intermittent circling for 6 months when 1.5 years old, then coma, periodic clonic convulsions, and death	Genetic; Devon	Rare	Neurologic examination, necropsy, atrophy of brain, accumulation of pigment in neurons, confirmation by demonstration of lipopigment in brain or skin (fluorescence, histochemistry, electron microscopy)	None

Disorder	Ref.	Clinical signs	Inheritance/Breed	Frequency	Diagnosis	Treatment
GM₁ gangliosidosis	221	Seen at weaning to 2 years of age, weight loss, abnormal stiff gait, may fall, swaying of hind quarters, blindness	Simple autosomal recessive; Friesian cattle of Ireland	Rare	Neurologic examination, neuronal vacuolation, deficiency of β-galactosidase	None
Glycogenosis type II	221-223	Around 6 months of age, ill-thrift and muscular weakness; excess glycogen accumulation in tissue resulting from lack of activity of acid α-glucosidase (AAG)	Simple autosomal recessive; Shorthorn and Brahman of Australia	Rare	Neurologic examination; muscle glycogen concentration higher, serum elevation of aspartate aminotransferase and creatine kinase activities, high levels of high-molecular oligosaccharides in urine, vacuolation of neurons; heterozygotes identified by AAG activity or PCR	None

TABLE 47-12

Inherited Enzyme Deficiencies of the Central Nervous System in Cattle

Defect	Reference No.	Description	Etiology	Frequency	Diagnosis	Associated Defects
Maple syrup urine disease (branched-chain keto acid dehydrogenase deficiency)	228, 230-232	Dullness at birth; by 48 hours, stupor, recumbency, tremors, hyperesthesia and hyperthermia, nystagmus, extensor spasms, opisthotonos, and coma; calves die within first week of life; urine smells like maple syrup; brain swelling	Hereford, Shorthorn; autosomal recessive	Rare	Neurologic examination, diagnosis requires biochemical tests in plasma, urine, or tissue of elevated levels of branch-chain ketoacid decarboxylase; deoxyribonucleic acid studies	None
Citrullinemia (arginino-succinate synthetase deficiency)	228, 229	Rapid onset of neurologic signs within 3 days of birth; ataxia depression, bellowing, aimless wandering, head pressing, stupor, coma, and death; necropsy shows brain swelling, hepatic lipidosis	Holstein; simple autosomal recessive	Common in Australia, rare in United States	Neurologic examination, necropsy; biochemical tests for massive elevation of citrulline in body fluids; deficiency of enzyme argininosuccinate synthetase, loss of Ava II cut site in axons; PCR to detect heterozygotes	None

PCR, Polymerase chain reaction.

TABLE 47-13

Congenital and Hereditary Diseases of the Spinal Cord in Cattle

Defect	Reference No.	Description	Etiology	Frequency	Diagnosis	Associated Defects
Shaker	233	Tremulous shaking of head, body, and tail; difficulty in rising, wobbly spastic gait; inability to bellow; no gross changes, excessive accumulation of neurofilaments within neurons of central, peripheral, and autonomous nervous system	Hereford; genetic	Rare	Neurologic examination, necropsy, and histopathologic examination	None
Spinal muscular atrophy	234-242	Calves may be recumbent at birth; more commonly develop hind leg weakness by 3-6 weeks of age, then become recumbent; atrophy of muscles of hind and front legs; histopathologic examination reveals degeneration of motor neurons in spinal cord	Brown Swiss, Red Danish; simple autosomal recessive	Common	Neurologic examination, necropsy, and histopathologic examination	None
Bovine progressive degenerative myeloencephalopathy ("Weaver")	242-250	Hind leg weakness within 5 to 8 months of age, ataxia, dysmetria, progressing to recumbency and frequently death resulting from ruminal tympany, spinal cord lesions of myelin degeneration, axonal loss and swelling, astroglial proliferation	Brown Swiss; simple autosomal recessive, linked to high production	Common	Neurologic examination, necropsy, and histopathologic examination of spinal cord; microsatellite locus (TGLA116) is closely linked to weaver gene and can be used to identify carriers	None
Spinal dysraphism	251, 252	Spinal dysraphism is a myelodysplasia of spinal cord especially lumbar area; dilated central canal and cavitations dorsal to it; affected calves from birth have hind leg paralysis, severe ataxia, or sometimes hopping gait; in calves able to stand, stance is wide with overextension (goose-stepping) and crossing of legs	Familial	Rare	Neurologic examination, necropsy	None

Continued

TABLE 47-13

Congenital and Hereditary Diseases of the Spinal Cord in Cattle—cont'd

Defect	Reference No.	Description	Etiology	Frequency	Diagnosis	Associated Defects
Hemangiomatosis of spinal cord	253	Hemangiomatous tumor in spinal cord of calf, hind leg ataxia	Unknown	One case reported	Neurologic examination, necropsy, and histopathologic studies	None
Congenital myoclonus	254	Lateral recumbency, hind legs extended; whole body rigid when lifted to feet; whole body myoclonic jerk when tapped; no gross or microscopic lesions	Simple autosomal recessive	Rare	Neurologic examination	None
Spinal myelinopathy	255	Progressive ataxia of hind legs in Murray Grey calves 8-12 months old, progressive loss of myelin in spinal cord	Murray Grey; simple autosomal recessive	Rare	Neurologic examination, necropsy, and histopathologic examination	None
Spinal dysmyelination	256-261	Recumbency at birth, tremor, bilateral symmetric hypomyelination	German Brown, Brown Swiss; autosomal recessive	Rare	Neurologic examination, necropsy, and histopathologic examination; locus has been mapped	None
Encephalomyelopathy	262-265	Mild to severe ataxia of hind limbs, progressing to recumbency in calves 6 months old, bilateral symmetric malacia of thoracic spinal cord and brain-stem	Unknown, possibly genetic; Simmental	Rare	Neurologic examination, necropsy and histopathologic examination	None
Spongioform myelopathy	266	Neonatal calves have difficulty standing; ataxia, paresis, and whole body tremor	Unknown, Simmental	Rare	Histopathology reveals large empty vacuoles throughout spinal cord	None

TABLE 47-14

Congenital Ocular Defects in Cattle

Defect	Reference No.	Description	Breed and Etiology	Frequency	Diagnosis	Associated Defects
Anophthalmia/microphthalmia syndrome	94, 267, 268	Unilateral or bilateral absent or small eye; blind	Holstein, Jersey; familial	1 in 7500 to 1 in 50,000 births in six U.S. breeds	Physical examination	Tailless, high ventricular septal defect, domed head, cheiloschisis, wedge and hemivertebra
Corneal edema	269	Corneal opacity, mild at birth, bilaterally symmetric, will become more cloudy with age	German Black Red, British Friesians; simple autosomal recessive	Rare	Physical examination	None
Retinal dysplasia	269, 270	Blindness, retinal detachment, disordered development of layers of retina	Shorthorn; simple autosomal recessive Irish Friesian	Rare	Ophthalmic and histologic examination	Internal hydrocephalus
Coloboma	269, 271, 272	Notch below optic disc, does not interfere with vision	Charolais; dominant	Common	Ophthalmic examination	None
Dermoid	273	Unilateral or bilateral growth on eyelids, conjunctiva, nictitating membrane, and cornea; ranging from blemish to large dermoid masses	Hereford; polygenic	Common	Physical examination	None
Strabismus (convergent)	274-277	Deviation of eyeball axis, unilateral or bilateral, convergent strabismus not expressed at birth but evident by 12 to 16 months of life; progressive	German Brown, Shorthorn, Jersey, German Black and White; autosomal dominant	Rare	Physical examination	None
Strabismus (divergent)	278	Unilateral deviation of axis of globe	Highland cattle; familial	Rare	Physical examination	Crop ears
Cataract	269, 279	Mature cataracts; causing blindness by 4 to 11 months of age	Jersey, Hereford, Holstein; simple autosomal recessive	Rare	Ophthalmic examination	None
Multiple ocular defect	280	Cataracts, microphakia, lens luxation, iridemia	Jersey; simple autosomal recessive	Rare	Clinical examination	None

TABLE 47-15

Congenital Pigmentary Deficiencies in Cattle

Defect	Reference No.	Description	Breed and Etiology	Frequency	Diagnosis	Associated Defects
Chediak-Higashi syndrome	281-285	Photophobia, lacrimination, partial albinism, iris blue and white; coat color white or dilute; abnormally large cytoplasmic granules in white blood cells	Brangus, Japanese Black, Hereford; simple autosomal recessive	Rare	Ophthalmoscopic, blood smears, microscopic examination of hair shows large melanin granules; PCR to detect carriers	Increased susceptibility to infection, abscesses in liver and muscle; increased bleeding tendency
Oculocutaneous hypopigmentation	286, 287	Brown hair coat, slate gray muzzle, teat, and perianal area; tan to blue iris color	Angus; simple autosomal recessive	Rare	Physical examination	None
Heterochromia irides	288-289	Photophobia and nystagmus, iris light blue centrally, white on outer zone, fundus light yellow in tapetal area, nonfundal gray; coat color may be slightly dilute or typical of breed	Holstein, Simmental, Angus, Guernsey; familial	Rare	Physical examination	None
Incomplete albinism	290-293	Heterochromia irides, white coat, tapetum fibrosum hypoplasia	Hereford; autosomal dominant	Rare	Physical examination	Coloboma of optic disc
Complete albinism	294-297	White coat color, pink skin, pink irides, photophobic, blindness in bright daylight	Holstein, Charolais, Hereford, Guernsey; simple autosomal recessive	Rare	Physical examination	None

PCR, Polymerase chain reaction.

TABLE 47-16

Congenital Defects of the Skin in Cattle

Defect	Reference No.	Description	Breed and Etiology	Frequency	Diagnosis	Associated Defects
Curly hair (karakul curl)	298, 299	Hair coat of rather tight, small curls over entire body; hair fringe on ear curly; hair diameter markedly irregular; medulla has granules and rough appearance	Ayrshire; dominant, also reported in native Swedish breeds, German Fleckvieh, and Red Pied of Europe	Rare	Physical examination, histopathologic examination of hair	None
Curly hair with cardiomyopathy	300-302	As above plus signs of cardiac failure; death by 6 months of age	Polled Hereford; simple autosomal recessive	Rare	Physical examination, necropsy	Cardiac failure
Hypertrichosis	303	Born with long coarse and stiff hair coat or develops within 6-8 weeks after birth; hairs not shed in spring, disturbances in temperature regulation; depressed production	Red and Black of Germany and Holland; dominant	Common	Physical examination	None
Hypotrichosis	304-308	Hair variably absent from margin of ears; ventral side sternum to udder; inside legs; sides of neck, shoulder, and thigh; calves unthrifty; degenerative changes in Huxley's layer with formation of megahyaline droplets	Polled and Horned Herefords of U.S., simple autosomal recessive	Common	Physical examination, histopathologic examination of skin biopsy	None
Viable hypotrichosis	309-311	Fine, sparse hair over entire body; tail, distal limbs, eyelids, and ears less severely affected; hair follicles are underdeveloped	Ayrshire, Guernsey, Jersey, Holstein, Normandy; simple autosomal recessive	Common	Physical examination and skin biopsy	None
Lethal hypotrichosis	312	Calves die a few hours after birth; hair present on eyelids, ears, tail, muzzle, and distal extremities	Holstein; simple autosomal recessive	Rare	Physical examination, necropsy, and histopathology	Hypoplasia of thyroid may be associated with trait
Hypotrichosis with incisor anodontia	313-315	Mild cases have lusterless, stubbly, hypopigmented coat; incisor teeth are lacking, but molars may develop with age; skin has small telogen phase follicles	Holstein, Maine-Anjou cross, Normandy, Friesian cross; sex-linked, incomplete dominant	Rare	Physical examination and skin biopsy; gene mapped on X chromosome	Anodontia of incisors
Streaked hairlessness	310	Lack of hair on vertical streaks over hip and sometimes over sides of body and legs	Holstein; dominant sex-linked trait	Rare	Physical examination	None
Black hair follicle dysplasia	316, 317	White hair coat normal; black pigmented areas have hypotrichosis	Holstein; cause is unknown	Rare	Physical examination, skin biopsy and histopathology	None

Continued

TABLE 47-16

Congenital Defects of the Skin in Cattle—cont'd

Defect	Reference No.	Description	Breed and Etiology	Frequency	Diagnosis	Associated Defects
Cross-related hypotrichosis (rat tail)	318, 319	Color dilution; short, curly, and sparse hair coat; "rat tail," or color dilution and short curly hair; nonpigmented areas less affected or normal; hair misshapen with abnormal furrows and scales	Reported in Simmental X Angus crosses, Simmental X Holstein crosses, but also occurs in Fleckvieh and Charolais; syndrome is controlled by interacting genes at two loci	Common	Physical examination, skin biopsy, and examination of hair	None
Congenital anemia, dyserythropoiesis, and alopecia	320-325	Short and curly hair at birth; followed by progressive alopecia with hyperkeratosis; moderate to severe, nonprogressive, macrocytic anemia; histopathology of skin characterized by follicular and epidermal orthokeratotic hyperkeratosis	Polled Hereford; simple autosomal recessive	Common	Physical examination, skin biopsy, and blood sample	Dyserythropoiesis and dyskeratosis
Inherited epidermal dysplasia (baldy calves)	298, 326, 327, 341	Failure of horn growth; focal hyperkeratosis; generalized alopecia; scaly, thickened skin; persistent salivation; overgrown hooves; calves become emaciated and die; histopathology consists of hyperkeratosis with neutrophil infiltration	Holstein; simple autosomal recessive	Common	Physical examination, necropsy, and histopathologic examination	None
Ichthyosis congenita	328	Generalized hyperkeratosis present at birth or develops shortly and becomes more severe with time, calves usually are destroyed; histologically severe orthokeratotic hyperkeratosis	Pinzgauer, Holstein, Chianina; familial	Rare	Physical examination, skin biopsy	None
Ichthyosis fetalis	329	Stillborn calf or dies within a few days; body surface covered by skin plaques separated by deep cracks	Red Poll, Friesian, Brown Swiss, Chianina; simple autosomal recessive	Rare	Physical examination, necropsy	None
Dermatosparaxis (Ehlers-Danlos, fragile skin)	330-332	Joint laxity; seromas; skin easily torn and heals poorly; defect in aminopeptidase activity; dermal collagen bundles thin, fragmented, and disorganized	Belgian Blue, Charolais, Holstein, Hereford, Simmental; simple autosomal recessive	Rare	Physical examination, skin biopsy	None
Epitheliogenesis imperfecta	333-335	One or more hooves and dew claws missing, raw denuded epithelial defects on distal limbs and head; hard palate, esophagus, tongue also affected; varies in severity	Holstein, Hereford, Ayrshire, Angus, Jersey, Sahiwal; simple autosomal recessive	Rare	Physical examination, necropsy	None

Condition	Pages	Clinical signs	Breed / inheritance	Frequency	Diagnosis	Treatment
Familial acantholysis	336-341	Ulcers develop over pressure points; hooves may slough; lesions occur also in oral cavity and muzzle; in Angus calves epidermiolysis occurs at stratum spinosum; in Brangus epidermis and basal lamina separate; fatal in all breeds	Angus, Brangus, Red Belgian; simple autosomal recessive; Simmental, autosomal dominant	Rare	Physical examination, necropsy, histopathology, electron microscopy	None
Protoporphyria	342-344	Photosensitivity; scaling, hyperkeratosis, on dorsal back, head and neck, ears, and muzzle; may have tongue ulcers; the occasional calf has ataxia and convulsions	Limousin; simple autosomal recessive; Blonde d'Aquitaine	Rare	Physical examination, ferrochelatase levels	None
Lymphedema	345, 346	Hypoplasia of lymphatics and lymph nodes leading to fluid accumulation in subcutis; less severe in Polled Hereford	Ayrshire; simple autosomal recessive, Polled Hereford of Brazil, dominant with variable expression and incomplete penetrance	Rare	Physical examination	None
Hereditary parakeratosis (hereditary zinc deficiency, Adema disease, lethal trait A-46)	347-353	Normal at birth, parakeratosis at 6-8 weeks around head and neck and in perianal and genital areas; profuse diarrhea, conjunctivitis, rhinitis, bronchopneumonia, nervous signs; thymus and peripheral lymph nodes, hypoplastic; impaired cell-mediated immune response	European Friesians, Shorthorn, Angus; simple autosomal recessive	Rare	Physical examination, skin biopsy, necropsy, plasma zinc levels fall during course of disease; zinc responsive	None
Ear notches (notched ears)	354-358	Variable degrees of notches in one or both ears; no other effects	Dominant, Jersey, Ayrshire, Highland cattle	Rare	Physical examination	None reported
Congenital skin tumors	359-361	Mast cell tumors, melanomas, lymphosarcoma, papillomas, myxomas, and vascular hamartomas reported present at birth	Unknown; most commonly in Holstein	Unknown	Histopathology	None
Cutaneous neurofibromatosis	362	Nodules on face, neck, and head of mature cows	Unknown; most commonly in Holstein	Rare	Histopathology, EM, immunohistochemistry	None

EM, Electron microscopy.

TABLE 47-17

Congenital Defects and Hereditary Diseases of the Cardiovascular System in Cattle

Defect	Reference No.	Description	Etiology	Frequency	Diagnosis	Associated Defects
Ectopia cordis	363	Heart outside thoracic cavity; cervical, pectoral, and abdominal types; cervical types most common in calves; intermediate types occur	Unknown	Rare	Physical examination, necropsy	Abnormalities of large vessels, torticollis, cleft palate, others
Cardiomyopathy in generalized glycogenosis type II (Pompe's disease)		See Table 47-11				
Cardiomyopathy with woolly hair coat		See Table 47-16				
Lethal idiopathic cardiomyopathy	364	Heart failure in first month of life, sudden death, myocardial necrosis	Japanese Black; simple autosomal recessive	Rare	Physical examination, necropsy	None
Dilated congestive cardiomyopathy (CMP)	365-371	Right-sided heart failure, weight loss, respiration increased and shallow, loss of milk production, intermandibular and brisket edema, fluid in thorax and abdomen, diarrhea, cattle 6 months old to 102 months, average 34 months	Genetic predisposition (possibly an autosomal recessive gene) and unknown environmental factors; specific breeds or crossbreeds; Red Holstein X Simmental crosses, Holstein cattle of Japan, Holstein cattle of Canada, Netherlands, and Australia	Common	Physical examination, necropsy	None
Patent ductus arteriosus	372, 373	Calves up to 3 months of age; exercise intolerance, heart rate elevated, machinery murmur, weight loss or no weight gain, abdominal distension, ventral edema, poor doer	Unknown, all breeds	Rare	Physical examination, necropsy	None
Atrial septal defect	372, 373	Ill thrift, dyspnea, poor doers, left-to-right shunt	Unknown	Rare	Physical examination, necropsy	None
Ventricular septal defect	372, 381-386	Calves are poor doers, systolic murmur, cardiac enlargement, respiration shallow, brisket edema	Familial tendency in Hereford cattle	Common	Physical examination, necropsy	Small atrial defects

Defect	Reference	Inheritance	Description	Frequency	Diagnosis	Associated findings
Ventricular septal defect associated with pulmonary hypoplasia and right ventricular hypertrophy and dextraposition of aorta (tetralogy of Fallot)	384	Unknown	Respiratory disturbance, failure to thrive, cyanosis of mucous membranes, systolic murmur on both sides, fourth intercostal space right and third left; exercise intolerance, weeks to several months old, abdominal distention, ventral edema	Rare	Physical examination, necropsy	Eye and bone defects, atrial defects, patent ductus arteriosus, gonadal dysgenesis
Ventricular septal defect with dextraposed aorta, dilated pulmonary artery, and right ventricular hypertrophy (Eisenmenger's complex)	385, 386	Unknown	Unthrifty, poor doers, may have microphthalmia, rapid pulse, machinery murmur, exercise intolerance	Rare	Physical examination, necropsy	Eye and bone defects
Hypoplasia of left ventricle	372, 373	Unknown	Heart failure at or shortly after birth, impaired blood flow through left ventricle, patent foramen ovale, mixture of oxygen-rich blood pumped from right ventricle into lungs and body via patent ductus arteriosus, right atrium and ventricle dilated	Rare	Physical examination, necropsy	Lung edema and congestion, dextraposition of aorta
Hypoplasia of right ventricle	374	Unknown	Rudimentary right ventricle	Rare	Necropsy	Situs solitus of atria
Persistent truncus arteriosus	375, 376	Unknown	Single arterial trunk overrides an interventricular septal defect and gives rise to aorta and pulmonary trunk	Rare	Necropsy	Patent foramen ovale; diprosopus
Portosystemic shunt	377	Unknown	Communication between caudal vena cava and portal system; calves present with signs of ammonia toxicity	Rare	Signs, increased blood ammonia and bile acids, ultrasound, contrast radiography; surgical repair possible	None
Deficiency of red cell band 3	378-380	Incomplete dominant; Japanese Black	Lack of band 3 (anion exchanger 1) and marked spherocytosis; hemolytic anemia	Rare	Clinical and hematologic findings; immunoblotting for presence of band 3	Growth restriction

TABLE 47-18

Congenital Defects of the Respiratory System in Cattle

Defect	Reference No.	Description	Etiology	Frequency	Diagnosis	Associated Defects
Accessory lungs	387	No clinical signs, accessory lungs found at necropsy in thoracic or abdominal cavity	Unknown	Very rare	Incidental finding	None
Bronchial hypoplasia (adenomatoid malformation of lung)	388, 389	Respiratory distress following parturition, tachycardia, crackling sounds on auscultation	Unknown	Reported only two times	Incidental finding, necropsy	None
Pulmonary hypertension	390	Increased pressure in pulmonary circuit	Genetic transmission	Rare	Clinical examination, testing in hypobaric chamber	None
Pulmonary choristoma	391	Pulmonary tissue located in an area noncontiguous with respiratory tract	Unknown	Very rare	One case reported with mass at caudal part of skull	None

TABLE 47-19

Congenital Disorders of Blood Coagulation in Cattle

Defect	Reference No.	Description	Etiology	Frequency	Diagnosis	Associated Defects
Factor XI deficiency	392-394	Homozygous cattle may show no clinical signs, others have mild to moderate hemorrhage caused by trauma; internal hemorrhage may occur and cause death; veterinarians encountering excessive bleeding in calves from umbilical cord or prolonged bleeding after surgical procedures such as castration should consider a genetic factor after considering toxic, dietary, or other environmental factors	Holsteins of United States, Canada, and Great Britain; simple autosomal recessive	Common	Physical signs, ATPP time; plasma levels of factor XI	None
Hemophilia A (factor VIII deficiency)	395	Profuse bleeding and death following surgery such as castration	Herefords of Australia; sex-linked recessive	Rare	Physical examination, determination of factor VIII levels	None
Primary platelet disorder (Simmental hereditary thrombopathy; SHT)	396-398	Mild to severe bleeding tendency after mild trauma, spontaneous epistaxis, hematuria, blood loss with surgical procedures such as dehorning and castration, insertion of ear tags; internal hemorrhage after calving may occur	Simmental of U.S. and Canada; simple autosomal recessive	Rare	Physical examination, platelets have impaired aggregation when stimulated with adenosine diphosphate (ADP) or platelet activation factor; heterozygotes identified by response to ADP	None

ATPP, Activated partial thromboplastin time.

TABLE 47-20

Metabolic Defects in Cattle

Defect	Reference No.	Description	Etiology	Frequency	Diagnosis	Associated Defects
Hemochromatosis	399	History of poor growth, weight loss, rough hair coat; small size, poor condition, and diarrhea; micronodular cirrhosis, hemosiderosis, and mineralization of portal blood vessels of liver; necropsy reveals hepatomegaly and hemosiderin accumulation in liver, lymph nodes, pancreas, spleen, thyroid, kidney, brain, and glandular tissue	Salers, genetic	Reported once in 3 Salers cattle	Physical examination, histopathology of liver biopsy	None
Protoporphyria Porphyria (pink tooth)	184, 228, 400, 401	See Table 47-16 Reduced weight gain; photodynamic dermatitis of dorsal and lateral white skin; pinkish staining of teeth, bone, and urine, hemolytic anemia	Holstein of many countries, Shorthorn, Hereford, Jamaica Red, Jamaica Black, Limousin; simple autosomal recessive	Rare	Physical examination, fluorescence of teeth under ultraviolet light	Brown discoloration of teeth and bones
Deficiency of uridine monophosphate synthase (DUMPS)	228, 402-409	Phenotypically normal in heterozygous state; reproductive loss due to embryonic death of homozygotes around day 40; reproductive performance of heterozygotes somewhat compromised by longer calving interval and difficulties settling; UMP synthase catalyzes pyrimidine nucleotides biosynthesis	Holstein and Red Holstein of United States; simple autosomal recessive	Common, but decreasing	Uridine monophosphate synthase levels in blood to detect heterozygotes; PCR can determine genotype	None

Marfan syndrome	410-412	Joint hypermobility, ectopia lentis, sonographic aortic root enlargement, aneurysm and rupture of aorta causing cardiac tamponade, rupture of pulmonary artery, fragmentation of elastic laminae in aortic media, defect in glycoprotein fibrillin	Dominant with pleiotrophic effect	Rare	Necropsy, histopathology, biochemical studies	None
Xanthosis	413	Abnormal pigmentation of heart and certain skeletal muscle; no clinical signs	Thought to be inherited in Ayrshire	Rare	Seen at meat inspection, histopathology	None
Deficiency of adenine phosphoribosyltransferase	414	Accumulation of light green to greenish-yellow material in liver, kidneys, and lymph nodes; clinical signs unknown	Possibly a genetic disease	Rare	Meat inspection and histopathology	None

PCR, Polymerase chain reaction.

TABLE 47-21

Primary Immunodeficiencies in Cattle

Defect	Reference No.	Description	Etiology	Frequency	Diagnosis	Associated Defects
Chediak-Higashi syndrome Combined immunodeficiency	415, 416	See Table 47-14 When 6 weeks old, calf dehydrated, extremities cold; bilateral mucopurulent discharge, diarrhea, lymphopenia, and hypoglobulinemia, pneumonia, died of disseminated fungal infection	Unknown	Reported once in an Angus calf	Physical examination, absence of antibody and cell-mediated immunity	None
Lethal trait A46 (adema lethal, zinc-dependent parakeratosis) Deficiencies in immunoglobulin synthesis	417	See Table 47-16 Gangrenous mastitis, bronchopneumonia, lack of IgG$_2$	Reported in Danish Red only as genetic	Common in Red Danish	Physical examination, determination of immunoglobulins	None
Bovine leukocyte adhesion deficiency (BLAD)	418-423	Poor thrift, recurrent bacterial infections with failure to respond to treatment; recurrent pneumonia, ulcerative and granulomatous stomatitis, enteritis, diarrhea, poor wound healing, persistent neutrophilia, death at 2 to 4 months of age	Simple autosomal recessive; Holstein Friesians, Danish Holsteins, German Holsteins	Common, but decreasing	Physical examination, clinical pathology, leukocytes lack surface glycoprotein (β-integrins), PCR-RFLP to detect carriers	None

PCR-RFLP, Polymerase chain reaction–restriction fragment length polymorphisms.

TABLE 47-22

Congenital Defects of the Gastrointestinal System in Cattle

Defect	Reference No.	Description	Etiology	Frequency	Diagnosis	Associated Defects
Atresia jejuni	424	May cause dystocia because of abdominal distention, anorexia, depression; colic may also develop	Unknown, may be genetic in Jersey calves	Rare	Physical examination, necropsy	None
Atresia coli	425-433	Failure to pass meconium or feces, anorexia, depression, and abdominal distention; occurs most commonly at midportion of spiral loop of ascending colon; survival with surgery is good, growth rate is depressed, and loose feces occur; three types known to occur: type I, nonpatency of intestinal lumen; type II, two blind ends joined by a fibrous or muscular cord; type III, unconnected blind ends with corresponding mesenteric gap	Holstein, simple autosomal recessive; other breeds, rectal palpation of amniotic vesicle in cows between 35 and 40 days' gestation may cause atresia coli and sometimes atresia jejuni; other environmental causes possible	Rare	Physical examination, exploratory surgery, necropsy	Urogenital defects have been reported
Atresia recti	424	Abdominal distention, colic, depression, anorexia	Unknown	Rare	Physical examination	Urogenital defects, lack of tail
Atresia ani	424	Abdominal distention, colic, depression, anorexia	Unknown	Rare	Physical examination	Urogenital defects, lack of tail
Atresia ani et recti	424	Abdominal distention, colic, depression, anorexia	Unknown	Rare	Physical examination	Urogenital defects, lack of tail
Stenosis of jejunum	426	Narrow lumen	Unknown	Rare	Necropsy	None
Duplication of cecum	424	Two ceca	Unknown	Rare	Necropsy	Rectal stenosis, cardiac defects
Persistent oropharyngeal membrane	434	Tissue fold separates oropharynx and oral cavity; calf tries to swallow, but cannot	Unknown; one case in Hereford	Very rare	Physical examination, contrast radiography	None

TABLE 47-23

Congenital Hernias in Cattle

Defect	Reference No.	Description	Etiology	Frequency	Diagnosis	Associated Defects
Umbilical hernia	435-438	Failure of umbilical ring to close, abdominal viscera may or may not protrude through ring into hernial sac; skin covers hernial sac	Most commonly seen in Holstein, various genetic factors have been proposed, most likely polygenic; uncommonly seen in Hereford, Angus, and Simmental	Most common congenital defect in cattle	Physical examination	Usually none; persistent vitellointestinal duct in one case
Abdominal fissure	424, 435	Failure of right and left side to fuse, resulting in defect in ventral abdominal wall, not covered by skin; viscera may protrude through defect	Unknown	Rare	Physical examination, necropsy	None
Schistosomus reflexus	424	Severe abdominal fissure with marked dorsoflexion of spinal column, arthrogryposis of all four legs and eventration of organs of thoracic and abdominal cavities; causes dystocia	Unknown	Common	Physical examination	None
Inguinal hernia	424	Internal inguinal ring large enough to allow protrusion of abdominal viscera contained in the vaginal process to prolapse into inguinal canal	Unknown	Rare	Physical examination	None
Scrotal hernia	424	Inguinal hernia protruding into scrotum	Unknown	Rare	Physical examination	None
Perineal hernia	424	Protrusion of abdominal viscera through levator ani muscle	Unknown	One case reported	Physical examination	Calf also had atresia ani

TABLE 47-24

Congenital Defects of the Kidney in Cattle

Defect	Reference No.	Description	Etiology	Frequency	Diagnosis	Associated Defects
Unilateral renal agenesis	424, 439	Incidental finding at slaughter, remaining kidney undergoes compensatory hypertrophy	Unknown	Rare	Incidental finding at slaughter	None
Polycystic kidney	440	Multiple cysts in parenchyme of kidneys	Unknown	Reported once	Necropsy, histopathologic examination	Calf had atresia recti and segmental aplasia of uterine horns
Fused kidney (horse-shoe kidney)	441	Incidental finding at necropsy of calves affected with defects of the caudal parts of body	Unknown	Rare	Necropsy	Associated with defects of caudal vertebral column
Renal oxalosis	442	May be seen in calves dying in the perinatal period; usually affected with other congenital defects	Unknown	Common	Necropsy, histopathologic examination	Associated with many congenital defects
Ureteral stenosis	443	Bilateral ureteral mucosal scars resulting in hydronephrosis in fetus	Unknown	One case in Holstein	Necropsy	None

TTABLE 47-25

Congenital Defects of the Liver in Cattle

Defect	Reference No.	Description	Etiology	Frequency	Diagnosis	Associated Defects
Hepatic cysts	424	Cystic dilation of embryonal bile ducts	Unknown	Rare	Incidental finding	None
Bile duct atresia	444	Lack of development of bile ducts	Reported once in Australia, plant toxin was suspected	Rare	Necropsy, histopathology	None

TABLE 47-26

Chromosomal Defects in Cattle

Defect	Reference No.	Description	Etiology	Frequency	Diagnosis	Associated Defects
Trisomy 1	445	Reported only in 3- and 7-day-old embryos	Unknown	Rare	Karyotyping	None described
Trisomy 12	446, 447	Brachygnathia superior or inferior, lethal	Unknown	Rare	Karyotyping, necropsy	Various congenital defects
Trisomy 17	65, 448, 449	Brachygnathia inferior, lethal	Unknown	Rare	Karyotyping, necropsy	Cryptochidism, hydrocephalus, other defects
Trisomy 18	450	Dwarfism, lethal	Unknown	Rare	Karyotyping, necropsy	Hydrophalus, interventricular septal defect, other defects
Trisomy 20	446	Brachygnathia inferior and scoliosis of thoracic area, lethal	Unknown	Rare	Karyotyping, necropsy	Posterior, bimelic arthrogryposis; unilateral microphthalmia
Trisomy 22	451-453	Brachygnathia inferior and superior	Unknown	Rare	Karyotyping, necropsy	Umbilical hernia, interventricular septal defect, strabismus
Trisomy 23	454	Dwarfism	Unknown	Rare	Karyotyping, physical examination	None
Trisomy 24	455	Dwarfism	Unknown	Rare	Karyotyping, necropsy	Prognathism, interventricular septal defect, umbilical hernia, patent urachus
Unidentified trisomies and translocations	456	Multiple deformities	Unknown	Rare	Karyotyping, necropsy	Heart defects
4/21 tandem fusion	457	One case reported in a chimera freemartin; female cell line normal; male cell line has 59 chromosomes with a large acrocentric chromosome resulting from fusion of chromosomes 4 and 21	Unknown; Holstein	Very rare	Karyotyping	Freemartinism

Continued

TABLE 47-26

Chromosomal Defects in Cattle—cont'd

Defect	Reference No.	Description	Etiology	Frequency	Diagnosis	Associated Defects
7/21 Translocation	458, 459	Reduced fertility of carrier animals, 59 chromosomes resulting from centric fusion of member of chromosome pairs 7 and 21; unbalanced embryos from carriers lost during gestation	Translocation transmitted in mendelian fashion; Japanese Black	Uncommon	Karyotyping	Reduced reproductive efficiency as a result of embryonic mortality
14/20 Translocation	460	Reduced fertility of carrier animal, 59 chromosomes, one large metacentric chromosome present due to centric fusion of member of chromosome pairs 14 and 20	Carrier status is transmitted as a mendelian dominant trait	Rare	Karyotyping	Reduced fertility
1/29 Translocation	461, 462, 470	Reduced fertility of carrier animal, 59 chromosomes present due to centric fusion of one member of chromosome pairs 1 and 29	Carrier status is transmitted as a dominant mendelian trait	Worldwide in most breeds of cattle	Karyotyping	Reduced fertility, embryonic loss
Freemartinism (chimeras)	463-467	Female born cotwin to a male partner, development of reproductive organs suppressed, cordlike uterus, XX/XX chimerism	Exchange of humoral and cellular elements in utero as a result of chorioallantoic fusion	Common; 200,000 sets of twin calves are born in dairy breeds per year in U.S., 92% are freemartins	Vagina-length test, calves less than 1 month old have vagina 13-15 cm long, freemartinism measures 5-6 cm, karyotyping	Male cotwin may have poor semen quality; ureteral atresia rarely
XXY Klinefelter syndrome	468, 469	Sterile because of bilateral testicular hypoplasia, oligospermia to azoospermia	Unknown	Rare	Serology, physical examination, karyotyping	None
XXX condition	470-473	Irregular cycle, anestrus, repeat breeding	Unknown	Sporadic	Karyotyping	None
Spina bifida and associated defects	89	Spina bifida and associated defects; karyotyping revealed increased number of numeric chromosomal aberrations and structural defects	Unknown	Rare	Postmortem examination, karyotyping	None
Monosomy-X (59, XO)	474	Infertility with phenotypically normal external genitalia	Unknown	Rare	Karyotyping	Flat ovaries, bent cervix

TABLE 47-27

Intersexes in Cattle

Defect	Reference No.	Description	Etiology	Frequency	Diagnosis	Associated Defects
Freemartinism (XX/XY) chimeras		See Table 47-26				
Testicular feminization (androgen insensitivity)	475	External reproductive organs are female, testicles retained; however, XY chromosomal set, tubular reproductive organs are underdeveloped	Reported as an X-linked trait	Rare	Physical examination, karyotyping	None
XY gonadal dysgenesis	476	External genitalia are female but with vestigial penis, reproductive tract is female, hypoplastic gonads are undifferentiated but structurally like ovaries; 60 XY	Unknown	Rare	Physical examination, karyotyping, necropsy	Tetralogy of Fallot

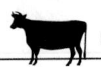

TABLE 47-28

Congenital Defects of the Male Reproductive System of Cattle

Defect	Reference No.	Description	Etiology	Frequency	Diagnosis	Associated Defects
Cryptorchidism	477, 478	Failure of one or both testicles to descend to their position within the scrotum; the cryptorchid testicle may be found anywhere along its normal route of descent in abdominal or inguinal location; unilateral more common than bilateral; left-sided more common than right-sided	Polygenic, Polled Hereford and Shorthorn may have breed predisposition	Rare	Physical examination (external palpation), rectal examination, ultrasound, basal testosterone assay	None
Testicular hypoplasia	477-481	Uncomplicated testicular hypoplasia involving the testes in the scrotum, freely movable in scrotum, unilateral or bilateral, may be segmented	Many different factors, some may be inherited	0.5% to 1% of all bulls may be affected	Palpation, scrotal circumference measurements	None
Segmental aplasia of epididymis	481-485	Most commonly absence of body and tail of epididymis, one third of cases involve also ampulla and seminal vesicles; after puberty will cause spermiostasis, formation of sperm granuloma, and testicular degeneration	Inherited, possible recessive in Simmental, German Black Pied, Holstein	Common	Physical examination	None
Aplasia of ampulla	479, 481	Mostly unilateral, complete or partial absence of ampulla, seminal vesicle is smaller than normal or cystic	Unknown	Rare	Physical examination	None
Hypoplasia of seminal vesicles	484	Small seminal vesicles	Unknown	Rare	Physical examination	May predispose to genital infection

Defect	Ref.	Description	Inheritance	Frequency	Physical examination	Bifurcation of scrotum
Hypospadias	478	Fissura urethrae inferior (hypospadia) is characterized by ventral opening of the penile urethra (balanitic, penile, scrotal, or perineal in location)	Unknown	Very rare	Physical examination	
Persistent penile frenulum	486-491	Fleshy band of tissue between ventral apex of penis and sheath preventing copulation	Reported to be recessive	Rare	Breeding soundness examination, can be repaired surgically	None
Prolapse of prepuce	490	Eversion of the prepuce	Unknown	Rare	Breeding soundness examination	In one case, absence of retractor muscle of prepuce has been reported
Short penis	478	Congenital short penis	Unknown, Hereford	Rare	Physical examination	None
Short retractor penis muscle	478, 491	Libido is normal, but unable to have copulatory thrust, unable to release sigmoid flexure	Regarded as hereditary	Rare	Physical examination	None
Corkscrew penis	492, 495	Spiral deviation of the penis before intromission, frequency of spiraling varies between bulls, classified into three categories: severe, moderate, and mild; no known trauma	Thought to be hereditary	Rare in Australia, more common in polled beef breeds	Physical examination, breeding soundness examination	None
Abnormal venous drainage of penis	493	Have normal libido but lack erection of penis	Unknown	Rare	Radiographic examination	None
Diphallus (bifid penis, double penis)	478	Unable to breed	Unknown	Rare	Physical examination	None
Ectopic penis	494	Supernumerary penis located in right paralumbar fossa, not connected to normal reproductive system	Unknown	Described once	Physical examination	None

TABLE 47-29

Congenital Defects of the Female Reproductive System in Cattle

Defect	Reference No.	Description	Etiology	Frequency	Diagnosis	Associated Defects
Ovarian hypoplasia	475, 478, 496-499	Unilateral or bilateral, varying in degrees of severity and symmetry, longitudinal grooves on surface of hypoplastic ovaries with absence of primary and developing follicles and corpora lutea	Swedish Red-and-White, Hungarian Simmental, Polled Finnish, Gir	1% to 2% in general population	Physical examination	None
Segmental aplasia of oviducts	499-502	Unilaterally or bilaterally a segment of oviduct not developed, fluid distention of oviduct in maximal end	Unknown	Rare	Physical examination	None
Uterus unicornis	501-503	Congenital absence of one uterine horn, cows can become pregnant; however, fertility is reduced, should not be used as embryo donor, may have erratic estrous cycle	Unknown	Very rare	Physical examination	None
Segmental aplasia of müllerian duct system (white heifer disease)	502-505	Prenatal arrest of müllerian duct system, resulting in congenital defects of vagina, cervix, uterus, and oviduct; ovaries are normal and cycle, resulting in accumulation of fluid cranial to blockage; occasional case may be fertile and become pregnant; condition is not linked to white coat color	In Shorthorn-derived breeds (including Belgian Blue) likely a pleiotropic effect of roaning gene N, plus one or more major modifiers, or polygenic threshold ($h^2 \approx 0.25$); in Holsteins, perhaps one or two linked recessives	Rare	Physical examination	None
Double cervix	506-510	Complete or partial duplication of cervix, partial form appears to be more common, does not cause dystocia; however, requires slightly more services	Genetic; incompletely penetrant-dominant in Meuse-Rhine-Ijssel; incompletely penetrant-recessive in Hereford, German Black Pied, and French Friesian	Most common defect of female reproductive tubular organs	Physical examination	None
Rectovaginal constriction	511-514	Inelastic constriction at the junction of anus, rectum, vestibule, and vulva; affected cows have dystocia and require episiotomy or cesarean section, rectal examination is difficult, bulls have anal stenosis	Jersey; simple autosomal recessive	Common	Physical examination	Udder edema at parturition

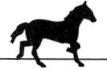

21. Hartley WJ, Wanner RA: Bovine congenital arthrogryposis in New South Wales, *Aust Vet J* 50:185-188, 1974.

22. Markusfeld O, Mayer E: An arthrogryposis and hydranencephaly syndrome in calves in Israel, 1969/1970: epidemiological and clinical aspects, *Refuah Vet* 29:51-61, 1971.

23. Charles JA: Akabane virus, *Vet Clinics North Am (Food Anim Pract)* 10: 525-546, 1994.

24. Kawamoto M et al: Epidemiology and pathology of central nervous system defects in calves in Kagoshima, *J Jpn Vet Med Assoc* 47:167-171, 1994.

25. Ishibashi K et al: Congenital scoliosis in calves suspected of Aino virus infection, *J Jpn Vet Med Assoc* 47:87-90, 1994.

26. Fukutomi T et al: An epidemic of Aino virus and incidence of congenital abnormalities in cattle in Okayama Prefecture, *J Jpn Vet Med Assoc* 50:442-447, 1997.

27. Uchinuno Y et al: Congenital malformations in calves associated with Aino virus prevalence in Fukoka Prefecture, *J Jpn Vet Med Assoc* 50:709-712, 1997.

28. Nakayama T et al: Aetiological and serological evidence of Akabane and Aino virus infections in bovine epizootic congenital abnormalities in Hyogo Prefecture, 1994-1996, *J Jpn Vet Med Assoc* 51:295-299, 1998.

29. Done JT et al: Bovine virus diarrhea virus: pathogenicity for the fetal calf following maternal infection, *Vet Rec* 106:473-479, 1980.

30. Wilson TM, DeLahunta A, Confer L: Cerebellar degeneration in dairy calves: clinical, pathologic, and serologic features of an epizootic caused by bovine viral diarrhea virus, *J Am Vet Med Assoc* 183:544-547, 1983.

31. Bentrup H et al: Gehauftes Auftreten des okulozerebellaren Syndromes unter neugeborenen Kalbern eines Milchrinderbestandes-Folgen einer intrauterinen BVD-Virus-infection? *Tierarztl Umschau* 11:852-860, 1985.

32. Hewicker-Trautwein M, Liess B, Trautwein G: Brain lesions in calves following transplacental infection with bovine-virus diarrhoea virus, *J Vet Med Series B* 42:65-77, 1995.

33. McKercher DG, Saito JK, Singh KV: Serologic evidence of an etiologic role for bluetongue virus in hydranencephaly of calves, *J Am Vet Med Assoc* 156:1044-1047, 1970.

34. Liendo G, Castro AE: Bluetongue in cattle: diagnosis and virus isolation, *Bovine Pract* 16:87-95, 1981.

35. Luedke AJ: Bluetongue in cattle: repeated exposure of two immunologically tolerant calves to bluetongue virus by vector bites, *Am J Vet Res* 38:1701-1704, 1977.

36. Luedke AJ: Bluetongue in cattle: effects of vector transmitted bluetongue virus on calves previously infected in utero, *Am J Vet Res* 38:1697-1700, 1977.

37. Luedke AJ, Jochim MM, Jones RH: Bluetongue in cattle: effects of *Culicoides viriipennis* transmitted bluetongue virus on pregnant heifers and their calves, *Am J Vet Res* 38:1687-1695, 1977.

38. Luedke AJ, Walton TE: Effect of natural breeding of heifers to a bluetongue virus carrier bull, *Bovine Pract* 16:96-100, 1981.

39. Coetzer JAW et al: Wesselsbron disease: a cause of congenital porencephaly and cerebellar hypoplasia in calves, *J Vet Res* 46:165-169, 1979.

40. Goto Y, Miura Y, Kano Y: Epidemiological survey of an epidemic of congenital abnormalities with hydranencephaly-cerebellar hypoplasia syndrome of calves occurring in 1985/86 and seroepidemiological investigations on Chuzan virus, a putative causal agent of the disease, in Japan, *Jpn J Vet Sci* 50:405-413, 1988.

41. Gunning RF, Gumbrell RC, Jeffrey M: Neospora infection and congenital ataxia in calves, *Vet Rec* 134:558, 1994.

42. Muller W et al: Derzeitiger Stand der Ermittlungen zum Vorkommen und zur Atiologie des angeborenen Darmverschlusses bei Kalbern in Bezirk Dresden, *Mh Vet Med* 37:84-89, 1982.

43. Newman SJ et al: Multiple congenital anomalies in a calf, *J Vet Diagn Invest* 11:368-371, 1999.

44. Lechniak D, Cieslak D, Sosnowski J: Cytogenetic analysis of bovine parthenodes after spontaneous activation in vitro, *Theriogenology* 49: 779-785, 1998.

45. Young LE, Sinclair KD, Wilmut I: Large offspring syndrome in cattle and sheep, *Rev Reprod* 3:155-163, 1998.

46. Garry FB et al: Postnatal characteristics of calves produced by nuclear transfer cloning, *Theriogenology* 45:141-152, 1996.

47. Wagtendonk-de Leeuw AM van, Aerts BJG, Daas JHG den: Abnormal offspring following in vitro production of bovine preimplantation embryos: a field study, *Theriogenology* 49:883-894, 1998.

48. Huston K: Heritability and diagnosis of congenital abnormalities in food animals, *Vet Clin North Am (Food Anim Pract)* 9:1-10, 1993.

49. Georges M et al: Microsatellite mapping of the gene causing weaver disease in cattle will allow the study of an associated quantitative trait locus, *Proc Natl Acad Sci* 90:1058-1062, 1993.

50. McFeely RA: Chromosome abnormalities, *Vet Clin North Am (Food Anim Pract)* 9:11-22, 1993.

51. Hazas G, Kovacs A, Karakas P: Decrease of percentage of carriers of bovine hereditary chromosome abnormalities, *Allattenyesztes Es Takarmanyozas* 48:115-116, 1999.

52. Schmutz SM et al: Chromosomal aneuploidy associated with spontaneous abortions and neonatal losses in cattle, *J Vet Diag Invest* 8:91-95, 1996.

53. Leipold HW, Huston K, Dennis SM: Bovine congenital defects, *Adv Vet Sci Comp Med* 27:197-271, 1983.

54. Healy PJ: Testing for undesirable traits in cattle: an Australian perspective, *J Anim Sci* 74:917-922, 1996.

55. Healy PJ et al: Haemopoietic chimaerism: a complication in heterozygote detection tests for inherited defects in cattle, *Anim Genet* 25:1-6, 1994.

56. Healy PJ, Dennis JA, Moule JF: Use of hair root as a source of DNA for the detection of heterozygotes for recessive defects in cattle, *Bovine Pract* 30:26-27, 1996.

57. Robinson JL, Shanks RD: Prevalence of two inherited disorders in US Holstein cattle, *Proc N Z Soc Anim Prod* 54:35-37, 1994.

58. Greene HJ et al: Congenital defects in cattle, *Irish Vet J* 27:37-44, 1973.

59. Ely F, Hull FW, Morrison HB: Agnathia, a new bovine lethal, *J Hered* 30:105-108, 1939.

60. Ewing MB: Frequency and mode of inheritance of wry tail, screw tail and twisted face in a herd of Jersey cattle, Masters thesis, 1957, Kansas State University.

61. Meyer H, Becker H: Eine erbliche Kieferanomalie beim Rind, *Dtsche Tierarztl Wschr* 74:309-310, 1967.

62. Woollen NE: Brachygnathia in Simmental cattle, PhD Thesis, 1989, Kansas State University.

63. Smith ST et al: Studies on brachygnathia in dairy cattle, *J Anim Sci* 20: 911, 1961.

64. Grant HT: Underdeveloped mandible in a herd of dairy Shorthorn cattle, *J Hered* 47:165-170, 1956.

65. Herzog A, Hohn H: Autosomale Trisomie bei der letalen Brachygnathie des Rindes, *Cytogenetics* 10:347-355, 1971.

66. Stur I, Pinsker W, Mayr B: Uber das Auftreten von Brachygnathia inferior in einem osterreichischen Fleckviehzuchtgebiet, *Wien Tierarztl Monatschr* 65:200-202, 1978.

67. Gluhovschi N et al: Contribution a l'etude cytogenetique de brachygnathisme inferieur chez lex Bovins et du mecanisme de la transmittion hereditaire de cette malformatioon, *Rec Med Vet Ec Alfort* 144:829-837, 1968.

68. Shupe JL et al: Lupine, a cause of crooked calf disease, *J Am Vet Med Assoc* 151:198-203, 1967.

69. Leipold HW et al: Congenital defects of calves on Kodiak Island, *J Am Vet Med Assoc* 170:1408-1410, 1987.

70. Shupe JL et al: Cleft palate in cattle, *Cleft Palate J* 1:346-355, 1968.

71. Mulvihill JJ, Mulvihill CG, Priester W: Cleft palate in domestic animals: epidemiologic features, *Teratology* 21:109-112, 1980.

72. Leipold HW et al: Spinal dysraphism, arthrogryposis and cleft palate in newborn Charolais calves, *Can Vet J* 10:268-273, 1969.

73. Leipold HW et al: Arthrogryposis and associated defects in newborn calves, *Am J Vet Res* 31:1367-1374, 1970.

74. Wilkens H: Ein Fall von Cheilognathoschisis superior media bei einem Kalb, *Dtsche Tierarztl Wschr* 67:525-527, 1960.

75. Wheat JD: Harelip in shorthorn cattle, *J Hered* 51:99-101, 1960.

76. Hidiroglou M: Note sur deux cas de bec de lievre constates parmi des veaux Shorthorn, *Can J Comp Med Vet Sci* 26:180-181, 1962.

77. Mayr B et al: Dominanter Erbgang von Lippenkiefergaumenspalten beim Rind, *Zuchtungskde* 51:192-195, 1979.

78. Blin PC, Lauvergne JJ: La Probatocephalie, anomalie hereditaire bovins dits "Tete de mouton." I. Etude descriptive, *Ann Zootech* 16:65-68, 1967.

79. Lauvergne JJ: La Probatocephalie, anomalie hereditaire des bovins dits "tete de mouton." II, Etude genetique, *Ann Genet Sel Anim* 2:363-379, 1970.

80. Ojo SA, Leipold HW, Guffy M: Facial-digital syndrome in Angus calves, *Vet Med Small Anim Clin* 70:28-29, 1975.

81. Saperstein G: Diprosopus in a Hereford calf, *Vet Rec* 108:234-235, 1981.

82. Leipold HW et al: Congenital defect of the atlantooccipital joint, *Cornell Vet* 67:646-653, 1972.

83. Engelken TJ et al: Atlanto-occipital fusion in two Polled Hereford calves, *J Vet Med (A)* 39:236-239, 1992.

84. Leipold HW, Hiraga T, Dennis SM: Congenital defects of the bovine musculoskeletal system and joints, *Vet Clin North Am (Food Anim Pract)* 9:93-104, 1993.

85. Greene HJ, Leipold HW, Dennis SM: Perosomus elumbus in calves, *Vet Med* 69:167-168, 1973.

86. Jones CJ: Perosomus elumbus (vertebral agenesis and arthrogryposis) in a stillborn Holstein calf, *Vet Pathol* 36:64-70, 1999.

87. Leipold HW, Dennis SM: Short spine lethal in an Aberdeen-Angus calf, *Cornell Vet J* 62:507-509, 1972.

88. Cho DY, Leipold HW: Spina bifida and spinal dysraphism in calves, *Zentralbl Vet Med (A)* 24:680-695, 1977.

89. Herzog A, Hohn H, Vainas E: Zytogenetische Befunde bei Kalbern mit Spina bifida, *Tierarztl Umschau* 38:259-260, 1983.

90. Doige CE et al: Congenital spinal stenosis in beef calves in Western Canada, *Vet Pathol* 27:16-25, 1990.

91. Huston K, Wearden S: Congenital taillessness in cattle, *J Dairy Sci* 41:1359-1370, 1958.

92. Rieck SW: Uber Schwanzlosigkeit beim Rind, *Dtsche Tierarztl Wschr* 73:83-85, 1965.

93. Greene HJ, Leipold HW, Huston K: Taillessness in cattle, *Erbpathol Zuchthyg* 5:158-169, 1974.

94. Zayed IE, Ghanem YS: Untersuchungen uber einige kongenitale Missbildungen in einer schwarzbunten Rinderherde, *Dtsche Tierarztl Wschr* 71:93-95, 1964.

95. Dean CE, Cebra CK, Frank AA: Persistent cloaca and caudal spinal agenesis in calves: three cases, *Vet Pathol* 33:711-712, 1996.
96. Goller H: Beidseitige Abrachie bei einem Kalb in Verbindung mit weiteren Missbildungen, *Berl Munch Tierarztl Wschr* 74:431-435, 1961.
97. Goller H: Befund am Ruckenmark bei einem Kalb mit beidseitiger Abrachie, *Anat Anz* 112:447-457, 1963.
98. Rieck GW, Bahr H: Akroteriasis congenita beim deutschen Schwarzbunten Rind, *Dtsche Tierarztl Wschr* 74:356-364, 1967.
99. Lauvergne JJ, Cuq P: Ectromelie et otocephalie hereditaires en race francaise frisonne pie noire, *Ann Zootech* 12:181-192, 1963.
100. Leipold HW et al: Ectrodactyly in two beef calves, *Am J Vet Res* 30:1689-1692, 1969.
101. Leipold HW, Cates, WF, Howell WE: Adactyly in a grade beef shorthorn herd, *Can Vet J* 11:258-260, 1970.
102. Leipold HW et al: Anatomy of hereditary bovine syndactylism. I, Osteology, *J Dairy Sci* 52:1422-1431, 1969.
103. Leipold HW et al: Hereditary bovine syndactyly. II, Hyperthermia, *J Dairy Sci* 57:1401-1409, 1974.
104. Leipold HW, Peeples JS: Progeny testing for bovine syndactyly, *J Am Vet Med Assoc* 179:69-70, 1981.
105. Leipold HW, Dennis SM, Huston K: Syndactyly in cattle, *Vet Bull* 43:399-403, 1973.
106. Leipold HW et al: Anatomy of hereditary bovine syndactyly. V, External description, *Erbpathol Zuchthyg* 3:6-22, 1971.
107. Baker RD et al: Embryo transfer tests for bovine syndactyly, *Theriogenology* 13:87, 1980.
108. Johnson JL et al: Progeny testing for bovine syndactyly, *J Am Vet Med Assoc* 176:549-550, 1980.
109. Ojo SA, Leipold HW, Hibbs CM: Bovine congenital defects: syndactyly in cattle, *J Am Vet Med Assoc* 166:607-610, 1975.
110. Leipold, HW et al: Hereditary syndactyly in Angus cattle, *J Vet Diag Invest* 10:247-254, 1998.
111. Charlier C et al: Identity-by-descent mapping of recessive traits in livestock: application to map the bovine syndactyly locus to chromosome 15, *PCR Method Appl* 7:580-589, 1996.
112. Willemen MA, Dik KJ: Bipartite distal sesamoid bones in a Holstein-Friesian calf, *Vet Rec* 137:42-43, 1995.
113. Baird AN et al: Congenital maldevelopment of the tibia in two calves, *J Am Vet Med Assoc* 204:422-423, 1994.
114. Ojo SA et al: Tibial hemimelia in Galloway calves, *J Am Vet Med Assoc* 165:548-554, 1974.
115. Leipold HW, Guffy MM, Cook JE: Tibial hemimelia in Galloway cattle, *Comp Pathol Bull* 9:1-2, 1977.
116. Leipold HW et al: Inheritance of tibial hemimelia in Galloway cattle, *Zuchtungsbiol* 34:291-295, 1978.
117. Leipold HW, Dennis SM, Huston K: Polydactyly in cattle, *Cornell Vet* 62:338-345, 1972.
118. Ojo SA, Saperstein G, Leipold HW: Polydactyly in a Holstein-Friesian calf, *Erbpathol Zuchthyg* 6:80-88, 1975.
119. Johnson JL et al: Hereditary polydactyly in Simmental cattle, *J Hered* 72:205-208, 1981.
120. Rieck GW, Schade W: Die Arachnomelie (Spinnengliedrigkeit), ein neues erbliches letales Missbildungssyndrom des Rindes, *Dtsche Tierarztl Wochr* 82:342-347, 1975.
121. Brem G et al: Zum Auftreten des Arachnomelie-Syndroms in der Brown-Swiss x Braunvieh Population Bayerns, *Berl Munch Tierarztl Wochenschr* 97:393-397, 1984.
122. Konig H et al: Prufung von Schweizer Braunvieh-Bullen auf das vererbte Syndrom der Arachnomelie und Arthrogrypose (SAA) durch Untersuchung der Nachkommen im Fetalstadium, *Tierarztl Umschau* 42:692-697, 1987.
123. Leipold HW, Steffen D: Syndrome of arachnomelia and arthrogryposis (SAA) in Brown Swiss calves, *Brown Swiss Bull* 86, 1989.
124. Schneeberger M, Stricker C: "Zuchterische Aspekte der Spinnengliedrigkeit, Mitteil Schweiz Verbandes kunstl Besam u Interessengemeinschaft" *Schweiz Besamungszuchter* 23:110-112, 1985.
125. Leipold HW, Cook JE: Osteopetrosis in Angus and Hereford calves, *Am J Pathol* 86:745-748, 1976.
126. Leipold HW, Dennis SM, Schalles R: Osteopetrosis in cattle, *Bovine Pract* 21:96-101, 1986.
127. Leipold HW, Guffy MM, Cook JE: Osteopetrosis in a Simmental calf, *Giessener Beitr Erbpathol Zuchthyg* 6:161-171, 1976.
128. Leipold HW et al: Hereditary osteopetrosis in Aberdeen-Angus calves, *Ann Genet Select Anim* 3:245-253, 1971.
129. Jensen PT, Rasmussen PG, Basse A: Congenital osteogenesis imperfecta in Charolais cattle, *Nord Vet Med* 28:304-308, 1976.
130. Denholm LJ, Cole WG: Heritable bone fragility, joint laxity, and dysplastic dentin in Friesian calves: a bovine syndrome of osteogenesis imperfecta, *Aust Vet J* 60:9-17, 1983.
131. Denholm LJ: Bovine osteogenesis imperfecta (Australian type): morphological characterization of an animal model for osteogenesis imperfecta in man, *Diss Abst Int, B* 46:2227, 1986.
132. Agerholm JS: Osteogenesis imperfecta in Holstein-Friesian calves, *J Vet Med (A)* 41:128-138, 1994.
133. O'Connor BP, Doige CE: Abnormal modeling of trabecular bone in calves, *Can J Vet Res* 57:25-32, 1993.
134. Horton WA et al: Bovine achondrogenesis, evidence for defective chondrocyte differentiation, *Bone* 8:191-197, 1987.
135. Gregory PW, Tyler WS, Julian LM: Bovine achondroplasia: the reconstitution of the Dexter component from non-Dexter stocks, *Growth* 30:343-369, 1966.
136. Curran PL: Kerry and Dexter cattle: a history, *Royal Dublin Soc* 142:88-103, 1990.
137. Harper PAW et al: Chondrodysplasia in Australian Dexter cattle, *Aust Vet J* 76:199-202, 1998.
138. Gregory PW, Mead SW, Regan WM: A new type of recessive achondroplasia in cattle, *J Hered* 33:316-322, 1942.
139. Gregory PW, Julian LM, Tyler WS: Bovine achondroplasia: possible reconstitution of the Telemark lethal, *J Hered* 58:220-224, 1967.
140. Punnett RC: The experiments of TH riches concerning the production of monsters in cattle, *J Genet* 32:65-72, 1936.
141. Jayo MJ et al: Bovine dwarfism: clinical, biochemical, radiological, and pathological aspects, *J Vet Med* 34:161-177, 1987.
142. Jones JM, Jolly RD: Dwarfism in Hereford cattle: a genetic morphological and biochemical study, *N Z Vet J* 30:185-189, 1982.
143. Bovard KP: Hereditary dwarfism in beef cattle, *Anim Breed Abstr* 28:223-237, 1960.
144. Mead SW, Gregory PW, Regan WM: Proportionate dwarfism in Jersey cows, *J Hered* 33:411-416, 1942.
145. Gottwald W: Uber das Vorkommen von Zwergwuchs in der Nachzucht eines Fleckviehbullen, *Zuchthyg* 2:63-67, 1967.
146. Pirchner F, Kaiser E: Proportionierter Zwergwuchs bei Fleckvieh, *Wien Tierarztl Wschr* 73:173-177, 1986.
147. Distl O et al: Untersuchungen an Kalbern mit proportioniertem Zwergwuchs, *Tierarztl Umschau* 45:727-732, 1990.
148. Harper PAW, Latter MR: Proportionate dwarfism in Angus cattle, *Austral Vet J* 70:450, 1993.
149. Harper PAW, Latter MR, Wilkins JF: Hydrops foetalis in dwarf calves associated with twinning, *Aust Vet J* 72:236-238, 1995.
150. Ribble CS, Janzen ED, Proulx JG: Congenital joint laxity and dwarfism: a feed-associated congenital anomaly of beef calves in Canada, *Can Vet J* 30:331-338, 1989.
151. Proulx JG, Ribble CS: Congenital joint laxity and dwarfism in a beef research herd, *Canadian Vet J* 33:129-130, 1992.
152. Cebra CK, Cebra ML, Ikede BO: Congenital joint laxity and disproportionate dwarfism in a herd of beef cattle, *J Am Vet Med Assoc* 215:519-521, 1999.
153. Carnahan D et al: Hip dysplasia in Hereford cattle, *J Am Vet Med Assoc* 152:68-72, 1968.
154. Howlett CR: Inherited degenerative arthrogryposis of the hip in young beef bulls, *Aust Vet J* 48:562-563, 1972.
155. Greene HJ, Leipold HW, Huston K: Bovine congenital skeletal defects, *Zentralbl Vet Med (A)* 21:789-796, 1974.
156. Agerholm JS, Basse A: Hip dysplasia in a nine-month-old male Jersey calf, *Vet Rec* 133:273, 1993.
157. Jayo M et al: Brachygnathia superior and degenerative joint disease: a new lethal syndrome in Angus calves, *Vet Pathol* 24:148-155, 1987.
158. Nuss K, Roth M, Schaffer EH: Deformierende idiopathische Ankylose der Klauengelenke beim Jungrind, *Tierarztl Prax* 22:312-318, 1994.
159. Lamb RC, Arave CW, Cheap JL: Semilethal abnormality of limbs in Jersey cattle, *J Dairy Sci* 54:544-546, 1971.
160. Greene HJ, Leipold HW, Huston K: Limberleg in a Jersey calf, *Irish Vet J* 27:164-167, 1973.
161. Lamb RC, Arave CW, Shupe JL: Inheritance of limber legs in Jersey cattle, *J Hered* 67:241-244, 1976.
162. Hansen KM: "Limber leg" syndrome: eller leddel\ose kalve hos Jersey-kvaeg, *Dansk Vettidskr* 67:662-664, 1984.
163. Oliver WM, Cartwright TC: Double-muscling in cattle: a review of expression, genetics, and economic implication, Texas Ag Exp Sta Tech Rep No. 12, Texas Agriculture Experiment Station, 1969.
164. Hanset R: Le caractere "culard" chez les bovins—determinisme-signification pour l'elevage, *Ann Med Vet* 125:85-95, 1981.
165. Stavaux D et al: Muscle fiber type and size, and muscle capillary density in young double-muscled Blue Belgian cattle, *J Vet Med Assoc* 41:229-236, 1994.
166. Amory H et al: Comparison of cardiac function in double-muscled calves and in calves with conventional muscular conformation, *Am J Vet Res* 55:561-566, 1994.
167. Arthur PF: Double muscling in cattle: a review, *Aust J Agric Res* 46:1493-1515, 1995.
168. Casas E et al: Quantitative analysis of birth, weaning, and yearling weights and calving difficulty in Piedmontese crossbreds segregating an inactive myostatin allele, *J Anim Sci* 77:1686-1692, 1999.
169. Nawrot PS, Howell WE, Leipold HW: Arthrogryposis: an inherited defect in newborn calves, *Aust Vet J* 56:359-364, 1980.
170. Greene HJ et al: Arthrogryposis and associated defects in calves, *Am J Vet Res* 34:887-891, 1973.
171. Russell R, Oteruelo FT: Ultrastructural abnormalities of muscle and neuromuscular junction differentiation in a bovine congenital neuromuscular disease, *Acta Neuropathol* 62:112-120, 1983.

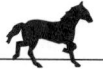

172. Rieger F et al: The syndrome of arthrogryposis and palatoschisis (SAP) in Charolais cattle, abnormal motor innervation and defect in the focalization of 16S acetylcholinesterase in the end-plates rich regions of the muscle, *Ann Genet Select Anim* 11:371-380, 1980.

173. Russell RG et al: Variability in limb malformations and possible significance in the pathogenesis of an inherited congenital neuromuscular disease of Charolais cattle (syndrome of arthrogryposis and palatoschisis), *Vet Pathol* 22:2-12, 1985.

174. Thompson PN: Suspected congenital myasthenia gravis in Brahman calves, *Vet Rec* 143:526-529, 1998.

175. Furuoka H et al: Hereditary myopathy of the diaphragmatic muscles in Holstein-Friesian cattle, *Acta Neuropathol* 90:339-346, 1995.

176. Furoka H et al: Immunohistochemical and electron microscopical studies of myocardial inclusions in hereditary myopathy of the diaphragmatic muscles in Holstein-Friesian cattle, *Acta Neuropathol* 97:185-191, 1999.

177. Furoka H et al: Immunohistochemical study of some cytoskeletal proteins in hereditary myopathy of the diaphragmatic muscles in Holstein-Friesian cattle, *Acta Neuropathol* 97:177-184, 1999.

178. Bilstrom JA et al: Genetic test for myophosphorylase deficiency in Charolais cattle, *Am J Vet Res* 59:267-270, 1998.

179. Axthelm MK et al: Hereditary internal hydrocephalus of horned Hereford cattle, *Proc Am Assoc Vet Lab Diagn* 23:115-126, 1980.

180. Axthelm MK et al: Congenital microhydranencephalus in cattle, *Cornell Vet* 71:164-174, 1981.

181. Axthelm MK, Leipold HW, Phillips RM: Congenital internal hydrocephalus in polled Hereford cattle, *Vet Med Small Anim Clin* 76:567-570, 1981.

182. Baker ML, Payne LC, Baker GN: The inheritance of hydrocephalus in cattle, *J Hered* 52:135-138, 1961.

183. Leipold HW, Gelatt KN, Huston K: Multiple ocular anomalies and hydrocephalus in grade beef shorthorn cattle, *Am J Vet Res* 32:1019-1026, 1971.

184. Leipold HW, Dennis SM: Congenital defects of the bovine central nervous system, *Vet Clin North Am* 3:159-177, 1987.

185. Cho DY, Leipold HW: Agenesis of the corpus callosum in calves, *Cornell Vet* 68:99-107, 1978.

186. Cho DY, Leipold HW: Anencephaly in calves, *Cornell Vet* 68:60-69, 1978.

187. Cho DY, Leipold HW: Congenital defects of the bovine central nervous system, *Vet Bull* 47:489-503, 1977.

188. Cho Y et al: Congenital defects of the central nervous system in cattle, *Proc Am Assoc Vet Lab Diagn* 121:103-116, 1978.

189. Gopal T, Leipold HW: Lipomeningocele in a calf, *Vet Pathol* 16:610-612, 1979.

190. Fielden ED: Microencephaly in Hereford, *NZ Vet J* 7:80-82, 1959.

191. Cho DY, Zeman DH, Miller JE: Holoprosencephaly in a bovine calf, *Acta Neuropathol* 67:322-325, 1985.

192. Cho DY, Leipold HW: Arnold-Chiari and associated anomalies in calves, *Acta Neuropathol* 39:129-133, 1977.

193. LeClerc S, Lopez A, Illanes O: Central nervous system and vertebral malformation resembling the Arnold-Chiari syndrome in a Simmental calf, *Can Vet J* 38:300-301, 1997.

194. Madarame H et al: Cerebellar hypoplasia associated with Arnold-Chiari malformation in a Japanese Shorthorn calf, *J Comp Pathol* 104:1-5, 1991.

195. Madarme H, Ito N, Takai S: Dicephalus, Arnold-Chiari malformation and spina bifida in a Japanese Black calf, *J Vet Med A* 40:155-160, 1993.

196. Madarame H, Takai S, Ito N: Two-headed, two-necked conjoined twin calf with Arnold-Chiari malformation in a Japanese Shorthorn calf, *Anat Histol Embryol* 23:275-280, 1994.

197. Finnie EP, Leaver DD: Cerebellar hypoplasia in calves, *Aust Vet J* 41:287-288, 1965.

198. Edmonds L, Crenshaw D, Selby LA: Micrognathia and cerebellar hypoplasia in an Aberdeen Angus herd, *J Hered* 64:62-64, 1973.

199. O'Sullivan BM, McPhee CP: Cerebellar hypoplasia of genetic origin in calves, *Aust Vet J* 51:469-471, 1975.

200. Swan RA, Taylor EG: Cerebellar hypoplasia in beef shorthorn calves, *Aust Vet J* 59:95-96, 1982.

201. Gordon PJ, Dennis R: Magnetic resonance imaging for the antemortem diagnosis of cerebellar hypoplasia in a Holstein calf, *Vet Rec* 137:671-672, 1995.

202. Young S: Hypomyelinogenesis congenita (cerebellar ataxia) in Angus-shorthorn calves, *Cornell Vet* 52:84-93, 1962.

203. de Lahunta A: Abiotrophy in domestic animals: a review, *Can J Vet Res* 54:65-76, 1990.

204. White M, Whitlock RH, DeLahunta A: A cerebellar abiotrophy in calves, *Cornell Vet* 65:476-491, 1975.

205. Whittington RJ, Morton AG, Kennedy DJ: Cerebellar abiotrophy in crossbred cattle, *Aust Vet J* 66:12-15, 1985.

206. Cho DY, Leipold HW: Cerebellar cortical atrophy in a Charolais calf, *Vet Pathol* 15:264-266, 1978.

207. Kemp J, McOrist S, Jeffrey M: Cerebellar abiotrophy in Holstein Friesian calves, *Vet Rec* 136:198, 1995.

208. Cordy DR: Progressive ataxia of Charolais cattle: an oligodendroglial dysplasia, *Vet Pathol* 23:78-80, 1986.

209. Zicker SC et al: Progressive ataxia in a Charolais bull, *J Am Vet Med Assoc* 192:1590-1592, 1988.

210. Bjerkas I: Progressiv ataksi hos Charolais-fe, *Norsk Vet Tidsskrift* 92:717-720, 1980.

211. Barlow RM: Morphogenesis of cerebellar lesions in bovine familial convulsions and ataxia, *Vet Pathol* 18:151-162, 1981.

212. Madarame H et al: Dandy-Walker malformation in a Japanese black calf, *Vet Pathol* 27:296-298, 1990.

213. Jeffrey M, Preece BE, Holliman A: Dandy-Walker malformation in two calves, *Vet Rec* 126:499-501, 1990.

214. Roberts SJ: Hereditary spastic diseases affecting cattle in New York State, *Cornell Vet* 55:639-644, 1965.

215. Leipold HW et al: Spastic paresis in beef shorthorn cattle, *J Am Vet Med Assoc* 151:598-601, 1967.

216. Harper PAW: Spastic paresis in Brahman crossbred cattle, *Aust Vet J* 70:456-457, 1993.

217. Thomson KJ, Beeman KB: Spastic paresis in Gelbvieh calves: an examination of two cases, *Vet Med* 82:548-553, 1987.

218. Hanset R et al: La paresie spastique des gastrocnemiens et son heredite, *Ann Med Vet* 137:237-247, 1993.

219. Sponenberg DP, Van Vleck LD, McEntee K: The genetics of the spastic syndrome in dairy bulls, *Vet Med* 801:92-98, 1985.

220. Tenszen A: Spastic syndrome in a Canadian Hereford bull, *Can Vet J* 39:716-717, 1998.

221. Jolly RD: Lysosomal storage diseases in livestock, *Vet Clin North Am (Food Anim Pract)* 9:41-53, 1993.

222. Healy PJ et al: Evidence of molecular heterogeneity for generalized glycogenosis between and within breeds of cattle, *Aust Vet J* 72:309-311, 1995.

223. Reichmann KG et al: Generalized glycogenosis (Pompe's disease) in Brahman cattle. A review of the syndrome and its conrol in Australia, *Proc Fifth World Congr Genet Appl Livestock Prod* 21:7-12, 1994.

224. Leipold HW et al: Mannosidosis in Angus cattle, *J Am Vet Med Assoc* 175:457-459, 1979.

225. Abbitt B et al: b-Mannosidosis in twelve Salers calves, *J Am Vet Med Assoc* 198:109-113, 1991.

226. Bryan L et al: Bovine b-mannosidosis: pathologic and genetic findings in Salers calves, *Vet Pathol* 30:130-139, 1993.

227. Baker WD, Sears GL: β-Mannosidosis in a Nebraska cow herd, *Compend Cont Educ Pract Vet* 20(food animal suppl):S138-S144, 1998.

228. Healy P, Dennis JA: Inherited enzyme deficiencies in livestock, *Vet Clin North Am (Food Anim Pract)* 9:55-64, 1993.

229. Grupe S, Dietl G, Schwerin M: Population survey of citrullinemia on German Holsteins, *Livestock Prod Sci* 45:35-38, 1996.

230. Baird JB et al: Maple syrup urine disease in five Hereford calves in Ontario, *Can Vet J* 28:505-511, 1987.

231. Healy PJ, Dennis JA: Molecular heterogeneity for bovine maple syrup urine disease, *Anim Genet* 25:329-332, 1994.

232. Healy PJ, Dennis JA: Heterozygote detection for maple syrup urine disease in cattle, *Aust Vet J* 72:346-348, 1995.

233. Rousseaux CG et al: "Shaker" calf syndrome: a newly recognized inherited neurodegenerative disorder of horned Hereford calves, *Vet Pathol* 22:104-111, 1984.

234. El Hamidi M, Leipold HW, Vestweber JGE, et al: Spinal muscular atrophy in Brown Swiss calves, *J Vet Med (A)* 36:447-456, 1989.

235. Troyer D et al: Review of spinal muscular atrophy (SMA) in Brown Swiss cattle, *J Vet Diagn Invest* 5:303-306, 1993.

236. Dirksen J et al: Spinale Muskelatrophie (SMA) bei Kalbern aus Brown Swiss x Braunvieh-Kreuzungen, *Dtsche Tierarztl Wschr* 99:168-174, 1992.

237. Stocker H et al: Spinale Muskelatrophie bei Braunvieh-Kalbern, *Schweizer Arch Tierhlkde* 134:97-104, 1992.

238. Agerholm JS, Basse A: Spinal muscular atrophy in calves of the Red Danish dairy breed, *Vet Rec* 134:232-235, 1994.

239. Nielsen JS et al: Inheritance of bovine spinal muscular atrophy, *Acta Vet Scand* 31:253-255, 1990.

240. Hiraga T et al: Reduced numbers and intense anti-ubiquitin immuno-staining of bovine motor neurons affected with spinal muscular atrophy, *J Neurol Sci* 118:43-47, 1993.

241. Hiraga T et al: Cytoskeletal proteins in affected motor neurons in bovine spinal muscular atrophy, *Prog Neurol* 4:137-142, 1993.

242. Lidauer M, Essl A: Schatzung der Frequenzen rezessiver Letalgene fur spinale Muskelatrophie, Spinnengliedrigkeit und Weaver-Syndrome bein osterreichischen Braunvieh, *Zuchtungskunde* 66:54-65, 1994.

243. Leipold HW et al: Weaver syndrome in Brown Swiss cattle: preliminary clinical and pathological observations, *Vet Med* 68:1040-1043, 1973.

244. Stuart LD, Leipold HW: Pathologic findings in bovine progressive degenerative myeloencephalopathy ("Weaver") of Brown Swiss cattle, *Vet Pathol* 22:13-23, 1985.

245. Baird JD, Sarmiento UM, Basrur PV: Bovine progressive degenerative myeloencephalopathy ("Weaver syndrome") in Brown Swiss cattle in Canada: a literature review and case report, *Can Vet J* 29:370-377, 1988.

246. Hoeschele I, Meinert TR: Association of genetic defects with yield and type traits: the weaver locus effect on yield, *J Dairy Sci* 73:2503-2515, 1990.

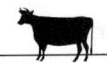

247. Oyster R et al: Electrophysiological studies in bovine progressive degenerative myeloencephalopathy of Brown Swiss cattle, *Prog Vet Neurol* 2:243-251, 1992.

248. Troyer D, Cash W, Leipold HW: Skeletal muscle of cattle affected with progressive degenerative myeloencephalopathy, *Am J Vet Res* 54:1084-1087, 1993.

249. Doll K et al: Bovine progressive degenerative Myeloenzephalopathie ("Weaver syndrome") bei Brown Swiss x Braunvieh-Rindern: Klinik, Verlauf, Blut tund Liquorbefunde, *Tierarztl Umsch* 48:467-476, 1993.

250. Braun U, Ehrensperger F, Bracher V: Das Weaver-Syndrome beim Rind, *Tierarztl Prax* 15:139-144, 1987.

251. Cho DY, Leipold HW: Spina bifida and spinal dysraphism in calves, *Vet Med* 24:608-695, 1977.

252. Ohfuji S: Spinal dysraphism in a newborn Holstein-Friesian calf, *Vet Pathol* 36:607-609, 1999.

253. Cho DY, Leipold HW, Cook JE: Angiomatous vascular malformation of the spinal cord of a calf, *Vet Pathol* 16:613-616, 1979.

254. Harper PAW, Healy PJ, Dennis JA: Inherited congenital myoclonus of polled Hereford calves: a clinical, pathological and biochemical study, *Vet Rec* 119:59-62, 1986.

255. Edwards JR, Richards RB, Carnick MJ: Inherited spinal myelinopathy in Murray Grey cattle, *Aust Vet J* 65:108-109, 1988.

256. Hafner A et al: Spinal dysmyelination in new-born Brown Swiss × Braunvieh calves, *J Med Vet (A)* 40:413-422, 1993.

257. Agerholm JS, Hafner A, Dahme E: Spinal dysmyelination in cross-bred Brown Swiss calves, *J Vet Med (A)* 41:180-188, 1994.

258. Agerholm JS, Anderson O: Inheritance of spinal dysmyelination in calves, *J Vet Med (A)* 41:333-337, 1994.

259. Kwiecien JM et al: Congenital axonopathy in a Brown Swiss calf, *Vet Pathol* 32:72-75, 1995.

260. Agerholm JS, Andersen O: Inheritance of spinal dysmyelination in calves, *J Vet Med Assoc* 42:9-12, 1995.

261. Nissen PH et al: Genetic mapping of spinal dysmyelination in cross-bred American Brown Swiss cattle, *Archiv vur Tierzucht* 42(special issue):170-171, 1999.

262. Finnie JW, Phillips PH: Multifocal symmetrical encephalomyelopathy in Simmental cattle, *Aust Vet J* 68:213, 1991.

263. Finnie JW, Smith K, Mukherjee TM: Mitochondrial alterations in skeletal muscle in a bovine encephalopathy, *Vet Rec* 129:384-385, 1991.

264. Steffen DJ et al: Multifocal subacute necrotizing encephalomyelopathy in Simmental calves, *J Vet Diagn Lab Invest* 6:466-472, 1994.

265. Steffen DJ et al: Multifocal subacute necrotizing encephalomyelopathy in Simmental calves, *J Vet Diagn Invest* 6:466-472, 1994.

266. Hindmarsh M, Harper PAW: Congenital spongioform myelopathy of Simmental calves, *Aust Vet J* 72:193-194, 1995.

267. Leipold HW, Huston K: Congenital syndrome with anophthalmia-microphthalmia and associated defects in cattle, *Vet Pathol* 5:407-418, 1968.

268. Moritomo Y et al: Congenital anophthalmia with caudal vertebral anomalies in Japanese Brown cattle, *J Vet Med Sci* 57:693-696, 1995.

269. Leipold HW: Congenital ocular defects in food-producing animals, *Vet Clin North Am (Large Anim Pract)* 6:577-595, 1984.

270. Greene HJ et al: Internal hydrocephalus and retinal dysplasia in shorthorn cattle, *Irish Vet J* 32:65-69, 1978.

271. Wijeratne WVS, Curnow RN: Inheritance of ocular coloboma in Charolais, *Vet Rec* 102:513, 1978.

272. Barnett KC, Ogden AL: Ocular colobomata in Charolais cattle, *Vet Rec* 96:592, 1972.

273. Barkyoumb SD, Leipold HW: Nature and cause of bilateral ocular dermoids in Hereford cattle, *Vet Pathol* 21:316-324, 1984.

274. Distl O, Wenniger A, Krausslich H: Zur Erblichkeit von Strabismus convergens mit Exophthalmus beim Rind, *Dtsche Tierarztl Wschr* 98:354-356, 1991.

275. Distl O: Analysis of pedigrees in dairy cattle segregating for bilateral strabismus with exophthalmos, *J Anim Breed Genet* 110:393-400, 1993.

276. Gerst M, Distl O: Influences on the dissemination of bilateral convergent strabismus with exophthalmos in dairy cattle, *Archiv fur Tierzucht* 40:401-412, 1997.

277. Gerst M, Distl O: Distribution and genetics of bilateral convergent strabismus with exophthalmos in cattle, *Tierarztl Umschau* 53:6-8, 1998.

278. Distl O, Scheider A: Ein ungewohnlicher Augendefekt beim Highland Cattle: Divergierendes unilaterales Schielen, *Dtsche Tierarztl Wschr* 101:202-203, 1994.

279. Brooks HA, Jolly RD, Bruere AN: An inherited cataract in New Zealand, *N Z Vet J* 30:113-114, 1982.

280. Gregory PW, Mead SW, Regan WM: A congenital hereditary eye defect of cattle, *J Hered* 34:125-128, 1943.

281. Padgett GA et al: The Chediak-Higashi syndrome: a comparative review, *Curr Top Pathol* 51:175-194, 1970.

282. Ayers JR, Leipold HW, Padgett GA: Lesions in Brangus cattle with Chediak-Higashi syndrome, *Vet Pathol* 25:432-436, 1988.

283. Tu CH et al: Inheritance of Chediak-Higashi syndrome in Japanese Black cattle, *J Vet Med Sci* 58:501-504, 1996.

284. Ogawa H et al: Clinical, morphologic, and biochemical charecteristics of Chediak-Higashi syndrome in fifty-six Japanese Black cattle, *Am J Vet Res* 58:1221-1226, 1997.

285. Nakagiri M et al: Allele-specific polymerase chain reaction for identifying carriers of Chediak-Higashi syndrome in Japanese Black cattle, *Anim Sci J* 70:372-374, 1999.

286. Cole D, Leipold HW, Schalles R: Oculocutaneous hypopigmentation of Angus cattle, *Bovine Pract* 19:92-100, 1984.

287. Strasia CA et al: Partial albinism (heterochromia irides) in Black Angus cattle, *Bovine Pract* 18:147-149, 1983.

288. Huston K, Leipold HW, Freeman AE: Heterochromia irides in cattle, *J Dairy Sci* 51:1101-1102, 1968.

289. Ojo SA, Leipold HW: Ocular albinism in a herd of Nigerian Holstein-Friesian cattle, *Z Tierzucht Zuchtungsbiol* 93:252-254, 1976.

290. Leipold HW, Huston K: Incomplete albinism and heterochromia irides in Herefords, *J Hered* 59:3-8, 1968.

291. Leipold HW, Huston K: Dominant incomplete albinism of cattle, *J Hered* 59:223-224, 1968.

292. Leipold HW, Huston K: Histopathology of albinism and heterochromia irides in the Hereford, *Cornell Vet* 59:69-76, 1969.

293. Gelatt KN, Huston K, Leipold HW: Ocular anomalies of incomplete albino cattle. I, Ophthalmoscopic findings, *J Am Vet Res* 30:1313-1316, 1969.

294. Leipold HW, Huston K, Gelatt KN: Complete albinism in a Guernsey calf, *J Hered* 59:218-220, 1968.

295. Greene HJ et al: Complete albinism in beef shorthorn calves, *J Hered* 64:189-192, 1973.

296. Jayasekera MU, Leipold HW: Albinism in Charolais cattle, *Ann Genet Select Anim* 13:213-218, 1981.

297. Winzenried HU, Lauvergne JJ: Test d'allelisme entre les albinismes de deux races bovines suisses, *First World Congress on Genetics Applied to Livestock Production,* Madrid, Oct 11, 1974, pp 7-11.

298. Steffen JD: Congenital skin abnormality, *Vet Clin North Am (Food Anim Pract)* 9:105-114, 1993.

299. Eldridge FW, Atkeson FW, Ibsen HL: Inheritance of a karakul-type curl in the hair of Ayrshire cattle, *J Hered* 40:204-214, 1949.

300. Morrow C, McOriet S: Cardiomyopathy associated with curly hair coat in poll Hereford calves in Australia, *Vet Rec* 117:312-313, 1985.

301. Storie GJ, Gibson JA, Taylor JD: Cardiomyopathy and woolly haircoat syndrome of Hereford cattle, *Aust Vet J* 68:119, 1991.

302. Whittington RY, Cook RW: Cardiomyopathy and woolly haircoat syndrome of polled Hereford cattle: electrocardiographic findings in affected and unaffected calves, *Aust Vet J* 65:341-344, 1988.

303. Helbig K: Untersuchungen uber die wirtschaftliche Bedeutung und die Erblichkeit der Langhaarigkeit des schwarzbunten Niederungsrind, *Dtsche Tierarztl Wschr* 65:431-437, 1958.

304. Jayasekera MU, Leipold HW, Cook JE: Pathologic changes of congenital hypotrichosis in Hereford cattle, *Zentralbl Vet Med* 26:744-753, 1979.

305. Bracho G, Johnson J, Beeman K, et al: Further studies of congenital hypotrichosis in Hereford cattle, *Zentralbl Vet Med* 31:72-80, 1984.

306. Olson TA, Hargrove DD, Leipold HW: Occurrence of hypotrichosis in polled Hereford cattle, *Bovine Pract* 20:4-8, 1985.

307. Rose R, Smith JE, Leipold HW: Increased solubility of hair from hypotrichotic Herefords, *Zentralbl Vet Med* 30(A):363-368, 1983.

308. Rose R, Smith JE, Leipold HW: Role of arginine-converting-enzyme in hypotrichosis of Hereford cattle, *Zentralbl Vet Med* 30(A):363-372, 1983.

309. Hanna P, Ogilvie T: Congenital hypotrichosis in an Ayrshire calf, *Can Vet J* 30:249-250, 1989.

310. Hutt F: A note on six kinds of genetic hypotrichosis in cattle, *J Hered* 54:186-187, 1963.

311. Denis B et al: Hypotrichose congenital en race bovine Normande, *Ann Genet Sel Anim* 7:251-261, 1975.

312. Selmanowitz V: Ectodermal dysplasias in cattle analogues in man, *Br J Dermatol* 84:258-261, 1970.

313. Wijeratne WVS et al: A genetic, pathological and virological study of congenital hyptrochosis and incisor anodontia in cattle, *Vet Rec* 122:149-152, 1988.

314. Braun U et al: Hypotrichose und Oligodontie, verbunden mit einer Xq-deletion, bei einem Kalb der schweizerischen Fleckviehrasse, *Tierarztl Prax* 16:39-44, 1988.

315. Distl O et al: Genetic studies of congenital hypotrichosis with anodontia in German Holstein calves, *Tierarztl Umschau* 55:72, 2000.

316. Miller W, Scott D: Black-hair follicular dysplasia in a Holstein cow, *Cornell Vet* 80:273-277, 1990.

317. Ostrowski S, Evans A: Coat color–inked follicle dysplasia in "buckskin" Holstein cows in central California, *Agric Pract* 10:12-13, 1989.

318. Ayers JR et al: Pathological studies of cross-related congenital hypotrichosis in cattle, *J Vet Med* 36:447-456, 1989.

319. Schalles RR, Cundiff LV: Inheritance of the "rat-tail" syndrome and its effect on calf performance, *J Anim Sci* 77:1144-1147, 1999.

320. Steffen DJ et al: Congenital anemia, dyskeratosis, and progressive alopecia in polled Hereford calves, *Vet Pathol* 28:234-240, 1991.

321. Vestweber JG, Leipold HW, Steffen DJ: Difficult dermatologic diagnosis, *J Am Vet Med Assoc* 203:223-224, 1993.

322. Steffen DJ et al: Ultrastructural findings in congenital anemia, dyskeratosis and progressive alopecia in polled Hereford calves, *Vet Pathol* 29:203-209, 1992.

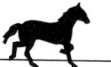

323. Steffen DJ et al: Congenital dyserythropoiesis and progressive alopecia in polled Hereford calves: hematologic, biochemical, bone marrow cytologic, electrophoretic, and flow cytometric findings, *J Vet Diagn Invest* 4:31-37, 1992.

324. Steffen DJ et al: Epidemiologic findings in congenital anemia, dyserythropoiesis, and dyskeratosis in polled Hereford calves, *J Hered* 84:263-265, 1993.

325. Burton SA et al: Congenital dyserythropoiesis and dyskeratosis in a polled Hereford calf, *Can Vet J* 35:519-520, 1994.

326. Ackerman L: Inheritance of baldy calf syndrome, *Mod Vet Pract* 64:807-811, 1983.

327. Jubb TF et al: Inherited epidermal dysplasia in Holstein-Friesian calves, *Aust Vet J* 67:16-18, 1990.

328. Jayasekara MU, Leipold HW: Congenital defects of the skin, *Vet Med (Small Anim Clin)* 77:1461-1475, 1982.

329. Baker J, Ward W: Ichthyosis in domestic animals: a review of the literature and a case report, *Br Vet J* 141:1-7, 1985.

330. O'Hara PJ et al: A collagenous tissue dysplasia of calves, *Lab Invest* 23:307-314, 1970.

331. Jayasekera MU, Leipold HW, Phillips R: Ehlers-Danlos syndrome in cattle, *Z Tierzucht Zuchtungsbiol* 96:100-107, 1979.

332. Hanset R, Lapiere CM: Inheritance of dermatosparaxis in the calf, *J Hered* 65:356-358, 1974.

333. Leipold HW, Mills JHC, Huston K: Epitheliogenesis imperfecta in calves, *Can Vet J* 14:114-121, 1973.

334. Fordyce G et al: The prevalence of epitheliogenesis imperfecta in Sahiwal cattle and their crosses in a North Queensland beef herd, *Aust J Agr Res* 38:427-435, 1987.

335. Jayasekera MU, Leipold HW: Epitheliogenesis imperfecta in shorthorn and Angus cattle, *Zentralbl Vet Med A* 26:497-501, 1979.

336. Bassett H: A congenital bovine epidermolysis resembling epidermolysis bullosa simplex of man, *Vet Rec* 121:8-11, 1987.

337. Deprez P et al: Een geval van epidermolysis bullosa bij een kalf, *Vlaams Diergeneesk Tijdschr* 62:155-159, 1993.

338. Agerholm JS: Congenital generalized epidermolysis bullosa in a calf, *J Vet Med (A)* 41:139-142, 1994.

339. Jolly RD, Alley MR, O'Hara PJ: Familial acantholysis in Angus calves, *Vet Pathol* 10:473-483, 1973.

340. Bassett H: Bovine epidermolysis: an inherited skin disease of cattle, *Proc 14th World Congr Dis Cattle* 1:75-80, 1986.

341. Allie, C de, Alley MR, Leadbetter IR: An epidermolysis bullosa in a Galloway calf, *N Z Vet J* 42:77, 1994.

342. Lauvergne JJ, Pinault L: Protoporphyrie hereditaire en race bovine Limousine francaise, premiers resultats, *Genet Sel Evol* 23:339-343, 1991.

343. Troyer DL et al: Gross, microscopic, and ultrastructural lesions of protoporphyria in Limousin calves, *J Vet Med (A)* 38:300-305, 1991.

344. Schelcher F et al: Observation on bovine congenital erythrocytic protoporphyria in the blonde d'Aquitaine breed, *Vet Rec* 129:403-407, 1991.

345. Schild A, Riet-Correa F, Mendez MC: Hereditary lymphedema in Hereford cattle, *J Vet Diagn Invest* 3:47-51, 1991.

346. Norton JH, Gibson GJ, Sturgess SC: Congenital lymphedema in a Brangus calf, *Aust Vet J* 70:267, 1993.

347. Stober VM: Parakeratose beim schwarzbunten Niederungskalb. I, Klinisches Bild und Atiologie, *Dtsche Tierarztl Wschr* 78:257-284, 1971.

348. Brummerstedt E et al: Lethal trait A46 in cattle: immunological investigations, *Nord Vet Med* 26:279-293, 1974.

349. Kroneman J, Mey GJW, Helder A: Hereditary zinc deficiency in Dutch Friesian cattle, *Zentralbl Veterinarmed (A)* 22:201-208, 1975.

350. Trautwein VG: Parakeratose beim schwarzbunten Niederung-skalb. II, Pathologisch-anatomische Befund, *Dtsche Tierarztl Wschr* 78:264-270, 1971.

351. Vogt DW, Carlton CG, Miller RB: Hereditary parakeratosis in shorthorn beef calves, *J Am Vet Res* 49:120-121, 1988.

352. Vestweber JGE, Leipold HW, Steffen DJ: Difficult dermatologic diagnosis, *J Am Vet Med Assoc* 204:1567-1568, 1994.

353. Machen M et al: Bovine hereditary zinc deficiency: lethal trait A 46, *J Vet Diagn Invest* 8:219-227, 1996.

354. Lush JL: A hereditary notch in the ears of Jersey cattle, *J Hered* 18:8-13, 1922.

355. Wriedt C: Vererbliche Scharten an den Ohren des Rindes, *Z Tierzucht Zuchtungsbiol* 3:235-238, 1925.

356. McDonald MA: Notched ears in New Zealand dairy cattle, *J Hered* 48:244-247, 1957.

357. Scheider A, Schmidt P, Distl O: Zur Vererbung von Ohrkerben beim Highland Cattle, *Berl Munch Tierarztl Wschr* 107:348-352, 1994.

358. Gilmore LO: Inherited non-lethal anatomical characters in cattle: a review, *J Dairy Sci* 33:147, 1950.

359. Yeruham I, Perl S, Orgad U: Congenital skin neoplasia in cattle, *Vet Derm* 10:149-156, 1999.

360. Desrochers A, St-Jean G, Kennedy G: Congenital cutaneous papillomatosis in a one-year-old Holstein, *Can Vet J* 35:646-647, 1994.

361. Lopez MJ, St.-Jean G, Nietfeld JC: Generalized congenital hemangiomatosis in a calf, *Agri Pract* 15:24-30, 1994.

362. Sartin EA et al: Characterization of naturally occurring cutaneous neurofibromatosis in Holstein cattle, *Am J Pathol* 145:1168-1174, 1994.

363. Hiraga T et al: Cervico-pectoral ectopia cordis in two Holstein calves, *Vet Pathol* 30:529-534, 1993.

364. Watanabe S, Akita T, Itakura C: Evidence for a new lethal gene causing cardiomyopathy in Japanese black calves, *J Hered* 70:255-258, 1979.

365. Leifsson PS et al: Myokardfibrose (kardiomypati) hos kvaeg, *Dansk Veterinaertidsskr* 77:682-684, 1994.

366. Baird JD: Dilated cardiomyopathy in Holstein cattle, *Proc 6th Annual Vet Med Forum* 6:175-177, 1988.

367. Baird JD: Dilated (congestive) cardiomyopathy in Holstein cattle in Canada: genetic analysis of 25 cases, *Proc 14th World Congr Dis Cattle I* 1:88-94, 1986.

368. Tontis A et al: Pathologie der bovinen Kardiomyopathie, *Schweiz Arch Tierheilk* 132:105-106, 1990.

369. McLennan MW, Kelly WR: Dilated (congestive) cardiomyopathy in a Friesian heifer, *Aust Vet J* 67:75-76, 1990.

370. Bradley R et al: Cardiomyopathy in adult Holstein-Friesian cattle in Britain, *J Comp Pathol* 104:101-112, 1991.

371. Dolf G et al: Evidence for autosomal recessive inheritance of a major gene for bovine dilated cardiomyopathy, *J Anim Sci* 76:1824-1829, 1998.

372. Gopal T, Leipold HW, Dennis SM: Congenital cardiac defects, *Am J Vet Res* 47:1120-1121, 1986.

373. West HJ: Congenital anomalies of the bovine heart, *Br Vet J* 144:123-130, 1988.

374. Murakami T et al: Anatomical observation on six cases of single ventricle in cattle, *J Jpn Vet Med Assoc* 49:229-231, 1996.

375. Camon J et al: Persistent truncus arteriosus in a diprosopic newborn calf, *J Vet Med A* 42: 41-49, 1995.

376. Reppas GP et al: An unusual congenital cardiac anomaly in a Dexter calf, *Aust Vet J* 73:115-116, 1996.

377. Fortier LA et al: The diagnosis and surgical correction of congenital portosystemic vascular anomalies in two calves and two foals, *Vet Surg* 25:154-160, 1996.

378. Ogata BA et al: Erythrocyte morphology and the frequency of spherocytes in hereditary erythrocyte membrane protein disorder in Japanese Black cattle, *Bull Nippon Vet Anim Sci Univ* 44:21-27, 1995.

379. Takeuchi M: Pathobiology of erythrocyte band 3 deficiency in cattle, *Jpn J Vet Res* 42:28, 1994.

380. Inaba M et al: Defective anion transport and marked spherocytosis with membrane instability caused by hereditary total deficiency of red cell band 3 in cattle due to a nonsense mutation, *J Clin Invest* 97:1804-1817, 1996.

381. Fisher E, Pirie HM: Malformations of the ventricular septal complex in cattle, *Br Vet J* 120:253-272, 1964.

382. McLennan MW, Suttan RH: Ventricular septal defect and an atrioventricular anomaly in a heifer, *Aust Vet J* 70:425-426, 1993.

383. Kast A: Angeborene Transpositionen von Aorta und A. pulmonalis beim Rind, *Zentralbl Vet Med (A)* 17:780-795, 1970.

384. Hare EJ et al: XY gonadal dysgenesis and tetralogy of Fallot in an Angus calf, *Can Vet J* 35:510-512, 1994.

385. Penrith ML, Bastianello SS, Petzer JM: Congenital cardiac defects in two closely related Jersey calves, *J S Afr Vet Assoc* 65:31-35, 1994.

386. Silva-Krott IN, Wilkinson JE: Hypoplastic left ventricle and aortic atresia in a calf, *Vet Pathol* 28:253-254, 1991.

387. Thomson RG: Congenital bronchial hypoplasia in calves, *Pathol Vet* 3:89-109, 1966.

388. Van Den Ingh TSGAM, Van Der Gaag I: A congenital adenomatoid malformation of lungs in a calf, *Vet Pathol* 11:297-300, 1974.

389. Desrochers A et al: Congenital cystic adenomatoid malformation of the lungs in a calf, *J Vet Med (A)* 41:709-712, 1994.

390. Cruz JC et al: Embryo transplanted calves: the pulmonary hypertensive trait is genetically transmitted, *Proc Soc Exp Biol Med* 164:142-145, 1980.

391. Chauvet AE et al: Pulmonary choristoma in a calf, *Can Vet J* 35:441-42, 1994.

392. Brush PJ, Anderson PH, Gunning RF: Identification of factor XI deficiency in Holstein-Friesian cattle in Britain, *Vet Rec* 121:14-17, 1987.

393. Gentry PA, Brush PJ: Factor XI deficiency in Canadian Holsteins, *Can Vet J* 28:110, 1987.

394. Gentry PA, Ross ML: Coagulation factor XI deficiency in Holstein cattle: expression and distribution of factor XI activity, *Can J Vet Res* 57:242-247, 1993.

395. Healy PJ et al: Hemophilia in Hereford cattle: factor VIII deficiency, *Aust Vet J* 61:132-133, 1984.

396. Steficek BA et al: Hemorrhagic diathesis associated with a hereditary platelet disorder in Simmental cattle, *J Vet Diagn Invest* 5:202-207, 1993.

397. Steficek BA et al: A primary platelet disorder of consanguineous Simmental cattle, *Thromb Res* 72:145-153, 1993.

398. Gentry PA et al: An inherited platelet function defect in a Simmental crossbred herd, *Can J Vet Res* 61:128-133, 1997.

399. House JK et al: Hemochromatosis in Salers cattle, *J Vet Intern Med* 8:105-111, 1994.

400. Moore WE et al: Detection of heterozygous state in bovine porphyria: analysis of urinary coproporphyrin isomers, *Proc Soc Exp Biol Med* 134:926-929, 1970.

401. Seawright AA, Watt DA: Congenital porphyria in a bovine carcass, *Aust Vet J* 48:35, 1972.

402. Shanks RD, Bragg DS, Robinson JL: Incidence and inheritance of deficiency for uridine monophosphate synthase in Holstein bulls, *J Dairy Sci* 70:1893-1897, 1987.

403. Shanks RD, Bragg DSA, Robinson JL: Deficiency of uridine monophosphate synthase in Holstein cattle: inheritance and body measurements, *J Anim Sci* 64:695-700, 1987.

404. Shanks RD et al: Inheritance of UMP synthase in dairy cattle, *J Hered* 75:337-340, 1984.

405. Shanks RD: Reproductive consequences of deficiency of uridine monophosphate synthase in Holstein cattle, *Am J Vet Res* 51:800-802, 1990.

406. Kuhn MT, Shanks RD: Association of deficiency of uridine monophosphate synthase with production and reproduction, *J Dairy Sci* 77:589-597, 1994.

407. Schwenger B, Tammen I, Aurich C: Detection of the homozygous recessive genotype for deficiency of uridine monophosphate synthase by DNA typing among bovine embryos produced in vitro, *J Reprod Fertil* 100:511-514, 1994.

408. Schwenger BH: *Development of gene diagnostic methods to identify monogenic traits for use in cattle breeding programmes*, Hannover School of Veterinary Sciences, Germany, 1995.

409. Chung ER, Kim SK, Kim WT: Early diagnosis of DUMPS inherited disease in Holstein dairy cattle using molecular genetic techniques. II, Screening and frequency of DUMPS gene, *Korean J Dairy Sci* 19:289-296, 1997.

410. Besser TE, Potter KA, Bryan GM: An animal model of the Marfan syndrome, *Am J Med Genet* 37:159-165, 1990.

411. Potter KA, Besser TE: Cardiovascular disease in bovine Marfan syndrome, *Vet Pathol* 31:501-509, 1994.

412. Potter KA, Besser TE: Bovine Marfan syndrome: a model of elastic tissue pathobiology, *Vet Pathol* 31:378, 1994.

413. Hayward AHS, Baker-Smith J: Xanthosis, an abnormal pigmentation in cattle, *Vet Rec* 102:96-97, 1978.

414. McCaskey PC et al: Accumulation of 2,8 dihydroxyadenine in bovine liver, kidneys, and lymph nodes, *Vet Pathol* 28:99-109, 1991.

415. McVey DS, Tizard I: Primary immunodeficiencies of food animals, *Vet Clin North Am (Food Anim Pract)* 9:65-75, 1993.

416. Bartram PA et al: Combined immunodeficiency in a calf, *J Am Vet Med Assoc* 195:347-350, 1989.

417. Jorgensen CB et al: Bovine leukocyte adhesion deficiency in Danish Holstein-Friesian cattle. I, PCR screening and allele frequency estimation, *Acta Vet Scand* 34:231-236, 1993.

418. Gilbert RO et al: Clinical manifestations of leukocyte adhesion deficiency in cattle: 14 cases (1977-1991), *J Am Vet Med Assoc* 202:445-449, 1993.

419. Nagahata H et al: Neutrophil function and pathologic findings in Holstein calves with leukocyte adhesion deficiency, *Am J Vet Res* 55:40-48, 1994.

420. Nagahata H et al: Analysis of mononuclear cell functions in Holstein cattle with leukocyte adhesion deficiency, *Am J Vet Res* 55:1101-1108, 1994.

421. Lienan A et al: Bovine Leukozyten-Adhasions-Defizienz: 50 Falle: klinisches Bild und Differentialdiagnostik, *Dtsche Tierarztl Wschr* 101:495-502, 1994.

422. Tammen I et al: An improved DNA test for bovine leucocyte adhesion deficiency, *Res Vet Sci* 60:218-221, 1996.

423. Poli MA et al: PCR screening for carriers of bovine leukocyte adhesion deficiency (BLAD) and uridine monophosphate synthase (DUMPS) in Argentine Holstein cattle, *J Vet Med (A)* 43:163-168, 1996.

424. Saperstein G: Congenital abnormalities of internal organs and body cavities, *Vet Clin North Am (Food Anim Pract)* 9:115-125, 1993.

425. Kramme PM: Extensive intestinal atresia and forestomach distension in a full-term fetal calf, *Vet Pathol* 26:346-348, 1989.

426. vander Gag I, Tibboel D: Intestinal atresia and stenosis in animals: a report of 34 cases, *Vet Pathol* 17:565-574, 1980.

427. Johnson R, Ames NK, Coy C: Congenital intestinal atresia of calves, *J Am Vet Med Assoc* 182:1387-1389, 1983.

428. Ducharme NG et al: Colonic atresia in cattle: a prospective study of 43 cases, *Can Vet J* 29:818-823, 1988.

429. Smith DF et al: Clinical management and surgical repair of atresia coli in calves: 66 cases (1977-1988), *J Am Vet Med Assoc* 199:1185-1190, 1991.

430. Jubb TF: Intestinal atresia in Friesian calves, *Aust Vet J* 67:382, 1990.

431. Syed M, Shanks RD: Atresia coli inherited in Holstein cattle, *J Dairy Sci* 75:1105-1111, 1992.

432. Syed M, Shanks RD: What causes atresia coli in Holstein calves? *Cornell Vet* 83:261-263, 1993.

433. Mee JF: Incidence of intestinal atresia in Irish dairy herds, *Irish Vet J* 47:63-64, 1994.

434. Smoak IW, Hudson LC: Persistent oropharyngeal membrane in a Hereford calf, *Vet Pathol* 33:80-82, 1996.

435. Wiesner E, Willer S: Die Vererbung der kongenitalen Hernia umbilicalis beim Rind, *Mh Vet Med* 36:790-794, 1981.

436. Hayes HM: Congenital umbilical and conguinal hernias in cattle, horses, swine, dogs, and cats: risk by breed and sex among hospital patients, *Am J Vet Res* 35:839-842, 1974.

437. Suborg H: Untersuchungen uber die Abstammung von Rindern mit angeborenem Nabelbruch, *Dtsche Tierarztl Wschr* 85:126-130, 1978.

438. Strachan WD et al: Persistent vitellointestinal duct in a calf, *Vet Rec* 140:629-630, 1997.

439. Hofliger von H: Zur Kenntnis der kongenitalen unilateralen Nierenagenesie bei Haustieren II, Beitrag uber Vorkommen bei den einzelnen Tierarten, *Schweiz Arch Tierheilkd* 113:330-337, 1971.

440. Dunham BM: Renal dysplasia with multiple urogenital and large intestinal anomalies in a calf, *Vet Pathol* 26:94-96, 1989.

441. Prieur DJ, Dargatz DA: Multiple visceral congenital abnormalities in a calf, *Vet Pathol* 21:452-454, 1984.

442. Gopal T, Leipold HW, Cook JE: Renal oxalosis in neonatal calves, *Vet Pathol* 15:519-524, 1978.

443. King JM: Congenital ureteral stenosis and hydronephrosis, *Vet Med* 89:1112, 1994.

444. Harper P, Plant JW, Unger DB: Congenital biliary atresia and jaundice in lambs and calves, *Aust Vet J* 67:19-22, 1990.

445. King WA et al: Presumptive translocation type trisomy in embryos sired by bulls heterozygous for the 1/29 translocation, *Hereditas* 93:167-169, 1980.

446. Herzog A, Hohn H: Uber zwei neue Chromosomenaberrationen 60,XX,t(12;12),+12 und 60,XX,t(20;20),+20 beim Rind, *Tierarztl Umschau* 41:54-56, 1986.

447. Herzog A, Hohn H: Uber zwei weitere Falle von autosomaler Trisomie, 61,XY,+12 und 61,XX,+12, beim Rind, *Cytogenet Cell Genet* 57:211-213, 1991.

448. Popescu PC: Chromosomes of the cow and bull, *Adv Vet Sci Comp Med* 34:41-71, 1990.

449. Herzog A, Hohn H, Rieck GW: Survey of recent situation of chromosome pathology in different breeds of German cattle, *Ann Genet Sel Anim* 9:471-491, 1977.

450. Herzog A, Hohn H, Olyschlager F: Autosomale Trisomie bei Kalbern mit allgemeiner Unterentwicklung (Nanismus), *Dtsche Tierarztl Wschr* 89:400-403, 1982.

451. Mayr B et al: A viable calf with trisomy 22, *Cytogenet Cell Genet* 39:77-79, 1985.

452. Agerholm JS, Christensen K: Trisomy 22 in a calf, *J Vet Med Assoc* 40:576-581, 1993.

453. Christensen K, Juul L: A case of trisomy 22 in a live Hereford calf, *Acta Vet Scand* 40:85-86, 1999.

454. Gluhovschi N et al: Beitrag zum klinischen und zytogenetischen Studium des Zwergwuchses beim Rind, *Vet Med Nachr* 2:107-116, 1977.

455. Makinen A, Alitalo I, Alanko M: Autosomal trisomy in a heifer, *Acta Vet Scand* 28:1-8, 1987.

456. Konig B, Tontis A, Fatzer R: Angeborene morphologische Anomalien bei Kalbern aus dem Raum Bern, *Schweiz Arch Tierheilk* 122:435-438, 1980.

457. Pinheiro LEL et al: A 4/21 tandem fusion in cattle, *Hereditas* 122:99-102, 1995.

458. Hanada H, Geshi M: An aborted fetus with a presumptive 60,XX,rob (7;21) karyotype in Japanese Black cattle, *Hereditas* 123:91-93, 1995.

459. Hanada H: Transmission of the 7/21 Robertsonian translocation chromosome in Japanese Black cattle, *Anim Sci Technol* 66:914-917, 1995.

460. McFeely RA, Klunder LR, Reed JA: A 14/20 chromosome translocation in Simmental cattle, *Am J Vet Med Assoc* 202:619-620, 1993.

461. Buoen LC et al: Cases of 1/29 Robertsonian translocation (centric fusion) in Charolais cattle, *Can Vet J* 29:455-457, 1988.

462. King WA: Chromosome abnormalities and pregnancy failure in domestic animals, *Adv Vet Sci Comp Med* 34:229-249, 1990.

463. Khan MZ, Foley GL: Retrospective studies on the measurements, karyotyping and pathology of reproductive organs of bovine freemartins, *J Comp Pathol* 110:25-36, 1994.

464. Zhang T et al: Diagnosis of freemartinism in cattle: the need for clinical and cytogenetic evaluation, *J Am Vet Med Assoc* 204:1672-1675, 1994.

465. Stafford MJ: The fertility of bulls born co-twin to heifers, *Vet Rec* 90:146-148, 1972.

466. Dunn HO et al: Cytogenetic and reproductive studies of bulls born co-twin with freemartins, *J Reprod Fertil* 57:21-30, 1979.

467. Edwards JF, Gallagher DS, Prakash B: Urethral atresia with uroperitoneum in a newborn bovine freemartin, *Vet Pathol* 31:117-119, 1994.

468. Rieck GW: XXY syndrome in domestic animals: homologues to Klinefelter's syndrome in man. In Bandmann H-J, Breit R, eds: *Klinefelter's syndrome*, 1984, Springer-Verlag, Berlin.

469. Molteni L et al: New cases of XXY constitution in cattle, *Anim Reprod Sci* 55:107-113, 1999.

470. Pinheiro LEL et al: Trisomy X and 1/29 translocation in infertile heifers, *Theriogenology* 28:891-898, 1987.

471. Nes N: Testikulaer feminisering hos torfe, *Nord Vet Med* 18:19-29, 1966.

472. Rieck GW: Die testikulare Feminisierung beim Rind als Sterilitatsursache von Farsen, *Zuchthyg* 6:145-154, 1971.

473. Long SE, David JSE: Testicular feminisation in an Ayrshire cow, *Vet Rec* 109:116-118, 1981.

474. Prakash B et al: Infertility associated with monosomy-X in crossbred cattle, *Vet Rec* 147:436-437, 1995.

475. McEntee K: *Reproductive pathology of domestic animals*, New York, 1990, Academic Press.

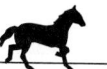

476. Hare JE et al: XY gonadal dysgenesis and tetralogy of Fallot in an Angus calf, *Can Vet J* 35:510-512, 1994.

477. St. Jean G, Gaughan EM, Constable PD: Cryptorchidism in North American cattle: breed predisposition and clinical findings, *Theriogenology* 38:951-958, 1992.

478. Ladds PW: Congenital abnormalities of the genitalia, *Vet Clin North Am (Food Anim Pract)* 9:127-144, 1993.

479. Philipsen H, Andresen E: Genetiske un-ders\ogelser af hypo-plas af s-dbl-rerne hos en tyrelinie af makaracen Dansk Jersey, *Dansk Vet Tidskr* 72:1114-1118, 1981.

480. Veeramachaneni DN et al: Pathophysiology of small testes in beef bulls: relationship between scrotal circumference, histopathologic features of testes and epididymides, seminal characteristics and endocrine profiles, *Am J Vet Res* 47:1988-1999, 1986.

481. Campero CM, Bagshaw PA, Ladds PW: Lesions of presumed congenital origin in the accessory sex glands of bulls, *Aust Vet J* 66:80-85, 1989.

482. Konig H, Weber W, Kupferschmied H: Zur Nebenhodenaplasie beim Stier und Eber, *Schweiz Arch Tierheilk* 114:73-82, 1972.

483. Asser S: Ein Beitrag zur Atiologie der Nebenhodenschwanz-Aplasia und-Hypoplasie beim Rind. Thesis, Tierarztl Hochschule, Hannover, 1982, p 120.

484. Ladds PW: The male genital system. In Jubb KVF, Kennedy PC, Palmer N: *Pathology of domestic animals*, vol 3, ed 3, New York, 1985, Academic Press, pp 409-459.

485. Saunders PJ, Ladds PW: Congenital and developmental anomalies in the genitalia of slaughter bulls, *Aust Vet J* 54:10-13, 1978.

486. Ashdown RR: Persistence of the penile frenulum in young bulls, *Vet Rec* 74:1464-1468, 1962.

487. Carroll EJ, Ball L, Scott JA: Breeding soundness in bulls: a summary of 10,940 examinations, *J Am Vet Med Assoc* 142:1105-1111, 1963.

488. Carroll EJ, Aanes WA, Ball L: Persistent penile frenulum in bulls, *J Am Vet Med Assoc* 144:747-749, 1964.

489. Elmore RG et al: Breeding soundness examinations in 18 closely related inbred Angus bulls, *Theriogenology* 10:355-363, 1978.

490. Long S, Hignett PG: Preputial eversion in the bull—a comparative study of prepuces from bulls which evert and those who do not, *Vet Rec* 86:161-164, 1970.

491. Hofmeyr CFB: Surgery of bovine impotentia coeundi. II, Short, contracted and immobilised musculi retractores penis, *J S Afr Vet Med Assoc* 38:395-398, 1967.

492. Ashdown RR, Pearson H: Studies on "corkscrew penis" in the bull, *Vet Rec* 93:30-35, 1973.

493. Ashdown RR, David JSE, Gibbs C: Impotence in the bull: abnormal venous drainage of the corpus cavernosum penis, *Vet Rec* 104:423-428, 1979.

494. Wolfe DF, Carson RC, Hanrahan LA: Supernumerary ectopic penis in a bull, *J Am Vet Med Assoc* 191:559, 1987.

495. Blockey MA de B, Taylor EG: Observations on spiral deviation of the penis in beef bulls, *Aust Vet J* 61:141-145, 1984.

496. Zemjanis R, Larson LL, Bhalla RPS: Clinical incidence of genital abnormalities in the cow, *J Am Vet Med Assoc* 139:1015-1018, 1961.

497. Settergren I: The ovarian morphology in clinical bovine gonadal hypoplasia with some aspects of its endocrine relations, *Acta Vet Scand* 5(suppl 1):1-108, 1964.

498. Tanabe TY, Almquist JO: The nature of subfertility in dairy heifers. III, Gross genital abnormalities, *Bull Penn Agri Exp Stn* 736, 1967.

499. Settergren I, Galloway DB: Studies on genital malformations in female cattle using slaughterhouse material, *Nord Vet Med* 17:9-16, 1965.

500. Kessy BM, Noakes DE: Uterine tube abnormalities as a cause of bovine infertility, *Vet Rec* 117:122-124, 1985.

501. Warfield SJ, Seidel GE Jr, Farrand GD: Lack of natural luteolysis associated with uterine horn aplasia in a heifer, *J Am Vet Med Assoc* 189:1585-1586, 1986.

502. Hanset R, Ansay M: La "White heifer disease"—nouvelle description et essai de classification rationelle de ses differentes formes, *Ann Med Vet* 105:443-449, 1961.

503. Ginther OJ: Segmental aplasia of the Mullerian ducts (white heifer disease) in white shorthorn heifer, *J Am Vet Med Assoc* 146:133-137, 1965.

504. Hanset R: "White Heifer Disease" dans la race bovine de moyenne et haute Belgique: un bulan de dix annees, *Ann Med Vet* 113:12-21, 1961.

505. Bennett RG et al: The nature of white heifer disease (partial genital aplasia) and its mode of inheritance, *Am J Vet Res* 34:13-19, 1973.

506. Sittman K, Rollins WC, Kendrick JW: A genetic analysis of the double cervix condition in cattle, *J Hered* 52:26-33, 1961.

507. Loen A van: Een genetisch onderzoek over het voorkomen van twee ora uteri externa (cervix duplex) bij het rund, *Tijdschr Diergeneesk* 90:698-716, 1965.

508. Sittman K: Note on the double cervix condition in cattle, *J Hered* 54:112, 115, 120, 1963.

509. Baras L, Roger C: Uterus Double et heredite de ce caractere chez la vache, *Bull mens Soc vet prat* 51:392-394, 1967.

510. Bonfert A, Mai F: Beobachtungern uber erbliches Auftreten von doppeltem Muttermund beim Rind, *Zuchthyg FortPflStor Besam Haustiere* 2:82-90, 1958.

511. Leipold HW, Saperstein G: Rectal and vaginal constriction in Jersey cattle, *J Am Vet Med Assoc* 166:231-232, 1975.

512. Leipold HW et al: Clinical observations in rectovaginal constriction in Jersey cattle, *Bovine Pract* 16:76-79, 1981.

513. Al-Ani FK, Vestweber JGE, Leipold HW: Mammary blood flow and venous blood pressure associated with the development of udder oedema in Jersey cattle affected with rectovaginal constriction, *Vet Rec* 116:156-158, 1985.

514. Leipold HW et al: Rectovaginal constriction in Jersey cattle: genetics and breed dynamics, *J Dairy Sci* 73:2516-2524, 1990.

CONGENITAL DEFECTS AND HEREDITARY DISEASES IN SHEEP

GEORGE SAPERSTEIN

CAUSES OF DEFECTS AND DISORDERS

Environmental Factors

Teratogens in sheep include toxic plants, viruses, drugs, trace elements and physical agents such as hyperthermia.[515]

PLANTS. Epizootics of cyclopian-type defects in south central and southwestern Idaho have been seen in up to 25% of the lambs born and involved ewes bred in early September while grazing *Veratrum californicum* on certain alpine ranges.[515-518] Embryonic death and defective lambs can be produced from ewes fed *V. californicum* on day 14 of pregnancy; ewes that are fed before and after day 14 with nontoxic quantities deliver normal lambs.[517,518] *Trachymene* spp. may cause bent legs in lambs.[519] *Lupinus augustifolius* causes hemimelia.[520] Besides signs of locoism, poisoning by plants of the genera *Oxytropis* and *Astragalus* may result in abortion and limb deformities. Hypoplastic testicles and enlarged seminal vesicles may occur in rams.[521,522]

DRUGS. Osteoporosis in lambs can be induced by aminopterin.[523] Parbendazole can cause ataxia, anophthalmia, cyclopian malformation of the brain, and ankylosis.[524] Netobimin, an anthelmintic broken down by intestinal bacteria into albendazole, can produce abortion and a variety of defects when administered on day 17 of gestation. Those defects include hemivertebrae, fused vertebrae, spina bifida, scoliosis, ectopic kidney, renal agenesis, and vascular anomalies. Susceptibility to the teratogenic effect of certain benzimidazoles are highest between days 14 and 24.[525]

VIRAL INFECTIONS. Many Bunyaviruses are teratogenic in sheep. Examples include Akabane, Cache Valley, Rift Valley fever, Main Drain, San Angelo, and LaCrosse viruses.

Prenatal infections with Akabane virus between gestational days 28 to 48 can cause abortion, premature births, and the congenital defects arthrogryposis and hydranencephaly (A-H syndrome) and other malformations. This syndrome has been seen in Japan, Israel, Australia, and Kenya. Incidences of malformations observed in four flocks in Australia were 31%, 42.5%, 51.2%, and 100%, respectively. In addition, Akabane virus infection in Australia depressed birth weight and prolonged gestation. The main defects observed were micrencephaly, hydrocephalus, hydranencephaly, microgyria, porencephaly, and spinal cord lesions. Various musculoskeletal and other defects are often associated with the central nervous system (CNS) abnormalities.[526]

Cache Valley virus (CVV) is mosquito-borne and teratogenic in ewes exposed to the virus for the first time between days 25 and 48 of gestation. Arthrogryposis and various CNS defects such as micrencephaly, hydranencephaly, porencephaly, cerebellar hypoplasia, and micromyelia occur in natural outbreaks from intrauterine infection.[533,534] Fetuses experimentally infected in utero with CVV and other bunyaviruses such as Main Drain, San Angelo, and LaCrosse develop similar defects.[535,536]

Hypomyelinogenesis congenita in lambs ("hairy shaker" or "fuzzy" lambs) or border disease (BD) is transmitted vertically by a togavirus (BDV) closely related antigenically to bovine virus diarrhea (BDV) and hog cholera viruses. BD has been reported in Europe, Australia, New Zealand, and the United States and is emerging as a serious cause of reproductive failure in sheep. Although BD is primarily a sheep disease, experimental evidence has suggested that BDV is also pathogenic for cattle and goats. BD-induced reproductive failure is characterized by embryonic and fetal death with or without abortion; full-term stillbirths and/or dysmorphogenesis of CNS, skeleton, and skin/fleece; and birth of small, weak lambs with poor growth and viability. Retardation of the myelinating process is partially reversible if the lamb survives. Hairy fleece is caused by a reduction in the ratio of secondary to primary wool follicles and increased size and altered structure of primary wool fibers. Dysmaturity results from prenatal and postnatal retarded development of bone, muscles, and internal organs.[527] Prenatal infection with BVD can produce similar lesions such as porencephaly, hydranencephaly, leukoencephalopathy, fetal mummification, cerebellar hypoplasia, and arthrogryposis.[528]

Bluetongue (BT) virus causes hydranencephaly, porencephaly, and arthrogryposis.[529,530] BT vaccine given to pregnant ewes between the fourth and eighth week of gestation caused fetal loss and defective lambs with hydranencephaly and arthrogryposis.[529-532]

PHYSICAL FACTORS. Micrencephaly, brain cavitation, and dwarfism can occur in lambs exposed to hyperthermia in utero.[537,538] Low-birth-weight stillborn lambs and lambs that died shortly after birth suffering from intrauterine growth restriction have fewer renal glomeruli than do normal lambs.[539]

An increased incidence of a variety of defects occurred in sheep exposed to radiation from the Chernobyl disaster. Congenital abnormalities that persisted for several years after the accident included rear limb paralysis, torticollis, cleft lip, umbilical hernia, cranial and spinal malformations or agenesis, limb hypoplasia, atresia ani, and abdominal fissure.[540] Lambs experimentally irradiated in utero may have skeletal defects.[541,542]

Modern reproductive manipulations of embryos have created a large offspring syndrome in both lambs and calves. Exposure of embryos to unusual environments, both in vivo and in vitro, between fertilization and blastocyst development can result in exceedingly high birth weights and sometimes prolonged gestation.[543]

GENETIC FACTORS. Genetic defects are pathophysiologic results of mutant genes or chromosomal aberrations occurring in any environment. Chromosomal defects of number or structure such as Robertsonian translocations are becoming increasingly common.[544]

Many hereditary defects follow simple mendelian inheritance, mostly a simple autosomal-recessive inheritance pattern. Other monofactorial inheritance patterns may be encountered and are characterized as overdominant, dominant, and incomplete dominant. Some are polygenic. Diagnosis of genetically induced congenital defects is based on the rule that genetic diseases run in families. Thus hereditary defects occur in typical intergenerational patterns and intragenerational frequencies. Recognizing these requires enumerating normal and abnormal offspring and identifying their familial relationships. Various statistical methods are used to analyze such data. Breeding trials are necessary to confirm inheritance patterns. Although breeding trials are expensive and time consuming, they are much more economical than trying to eliminate a genetic defect after it has spread insidiously throughout a given sheep population.

We have a better understanding of transmission of traits through gene mapping and identifying genetic markers. Examples of abnormal genes that are now mapped include the genes for muscular hypertrophy[545,546] and spider lamb syndrome.[547] Biochemical testing and DNA procedures will be the basis for the elucidation of modes of inheritance and carrier identification in the future. Identification of abnormal genes will allow ethical breeders to eliminate these genes from sheep.

Although most genetic defects in sheep are simple autosomal-recessive or autosomal-dominant traits, several others do not follow expected Mendelian ratios. Using microsatellite markers, researchers have identified a type of nonmendelian inheritance for one defect: muscular hypertrophy (double muscling). Only heterozygous animals who inherit the defective gene from their sire express the trait (polar overdominance).[545]

NATURE AND EFFECT OF DEFECTS AND DISORDERS

Congenital defects range from minor deviations to moderate and severe defects to monstrosities and result in fewer perinatal losses than nutritional deficiencies and infectious agents. Those caused by chromosomal abnormalities are most likely a major cause of early embryonic wastage. However, defects may cause considerable economic losses to individual breeders by increasing perinatal mortality and loss of value to relatives of genetically defective sheep. If the defect is genetic, control measures may require extensive and expensive adjustments of breeding programs.

Frequency

The frequency of congenital defects in sheep is not a fixed proportion of all births. It has been estimated that 0.5% to 1% (i.e., a range of from $\frac{1}{200}$ to $\frac{1}{100}$) of sheep born have congenital defects. Of these, 40% to 50% are born dead, and only a small fraction of defects is not visible externally. In comparison, congenital defects in humans are estimated at 1% to 3%. Lethal congenital defects in sheep have been estimated to account for 1% of dead lambs necropsied.[548-555] A study in Rambouillet sheep in Idaho over 15 years reported a high incidence of crooked limbs, jaw anomalies, notched scrotum, and fleece color anomalies.[551] Common congenital defects of lambs in another survey of 602 flock owners were, in order of frequency: bowed forelegs, micrognathia, hermaphroditism, cryptorchidism, hypospadias, prognathia, atresia ani, microtia, entropion, torticollis, polythelia, agnathia, and arthrogryposis.[552] The body systems involved in 401 defective lambs were: musculoskeletal, 55.5%; digestive, 12.7%; cardiovascular, 9.7%; urogenital, 7.1%; central nervous, 6%; special senses, 3.5%; integument, 3.2%; and endocrine, 1.5%.[552]

During 11 years, 19 congenital defects (1.9%) were observed in Awassi fat-tailed lambs. These defects included diprosopus, cyclops, polymelia, hypospadia, and atresia ani.[556]

CONTROL

If a defective lamb is submitted, histories should include breed, age of parents, parentage of affected and unaffected control lambs, geographic region, season, type of pasture, soil type, exposure to or suspected exposure to teratogenic plants, feeding and management practices, breeding records, maternal medical and vaccination records, disease status of flock, periods of stress, drugs administered, congenital defects observed previously, and history of any similar congenital defects in neighboring flocks. Breeding records should be analyzed for evidence of inbreeding and for characteristic intergenerational transmission patterns and intragenerational frequencies. Necropsies are done, and defects are classified

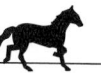

by the body system primarily involved. Serum samples from ewes should be submitted to check for pertinent viral antibodies. Samples of brain and other tissues are taken for virus isolation. Histopathologic examination is done, and selected cases are submitted for electron microscopic studies.

DIAGNOSIS OF SPECIFIC DEFECTS

Tables 47-30 to 47-47 define defects of various body systems in sheep, placing emphasis on defects of current interest and concern.

REFERENCES

515. Binns W, James LF, Shupe JL: Toxicosis of *Veratrum californicum* in ewes and its relationship to a congenital deformity in lambs, *Ann NY Acad Sci* 111:571-576, 1964.
516. Binns W et al: A congenital cyclopian-type malformation in lambs induced by maternal ingestion of a range plant *Veratrum californicum, Am J Vet Res* 24:1164-1175, 1963.
517. Binns W, Keeler RF, Balls LD: Congenital deformities in lambs, calves and goats resulting from maternal ingestion of *Veratrum californicum:* hare lip, cleft palate, ataxia, and hypoplasia of metacarpal and metatarsal bones, *Clin Toxicol* 5:245-261, 1972.
518. Binns W et al: Chronologic evaluation of teratogenicity in sheep fed *Veratrum californicum, J Am Vet Med Assoc* 147:839-842, 1965.
519. Clark L, Carlisle DH, Beasley PS: Observations on the pathology of bent leg of lambs in southwestern Queensland, *Aust Vet J* 51:4-10, 1975.
520. Hawkins CD et al: Hemimelia and low marking percentage in a flock of Merino ewes and lambs, *Aust Vet J* 60:22-25, 1983.
521. James LF et al: Abortive and teratogenic effects of locoweed in sheep and cattle, *Am J Vet Res* 28:1379-1388, 1967.
522. James LF, Keeler RF, Binns W: Sequence in the abortive and teratogenic effects of locoweed fed to sheep, *Am J Vet Res* 30:377-380, 1969.
523. James LF, Keeler RF: Teratogenic effects of aminopterin in sheep, *Teratology* 1:407-412, 1982.
524. Saunders LZ et al: The effects of methyl-5(6)-butyl-2-benzimidazole carbamate (parbendazole) on reproduction in sheep and other animals. I, Malformations in newborn lambs, *Cornell Vet* 64:7-40, 1974.
525. Navarro M et al: Anthelmintic-induced congenital malformations in sheep embryos using netobimin, *Vet Rec* 142:86-90, 1998.
526. Haughey KG et al: Akabane disease in sheep, *Aust Vet J* 65:136-140, 1988.
527. Barlow RM, Patterson DSP: *Border disease of sheep: a virus-induced teratogenic disorder,* Berlin, Germany, 1982, Paul Parey, pp 1-80.
528. Hewicker-Trautwein M, Trautwein G: Porencephaly, hydranencephaly and leukoencephalopathy in ovine fetuses following transplacental infection with bovine virus diarrhea virus: distribution of viral antigen and characterization of cellular response, *Acta Neuropathol* 87:385-397, 1994.
529. Osburn BI, Crenshaw, GL, Jackson TA: Unthriftiness, hair fleece, and tremors in newborn lambs, *J Am Vet Med Assoc* 160:442-445, 1972.
530. Osburn BI et al: Experimental viral-induced congenital encephalopathies. I, Pathology of hydranencephaly and porencephaly caused by bluetongue vaccine virus, *Lab Invest* 25:197-205, 1971.
531. Schultz G, Delay PD: Losses in newborn lambs associated with bluetongue vaccination of pregnant ewes, *J Am Vet Med Assoc* 127:224-226, 1955.
532. Griner LA et al: Bluetongue associated with abnormalities in newborn lambs, *J Am Vet Med Assoc* 145:1013-1019, 1964.
533. Edwards JF: Cache Valley virus, *Vet Clin North Am (Food Anim Pract)* 10:515-524, 1994.
534. Chung SI et al: Evidence that Cache Valley virus induces congenital malformations in sheep, *Vet Microbiol* 21:297-307, 1990.
535. Chung SI et al: Congenital malformations in sheep resulting from in utero inoculation of Cache Valley virus, *Am J Vet Res* 51:1645-1648, 1990.
536. Edwards JF et al: Ovine fetal malformations induced by in utero inoculation with Main Drain, San Angelo, and Lacrosse viruses, *Am J Trop Med Hyg* 56:171-176, 1997.
537. Hartley WJ, Alexander G, Edwards MJ: Brain cavitation and micrencephaly in lambs exposed to prenatal hyperthermia, *Teratology* 9:299-304, 1974.
538. Edwards MJ: Hyperthermia and birth defects, *Cornell Vet* 83:1-7, 1993.
539. Bains RK et al: Stereological estimation of the absolute number of glomeruli in the kidneys of lambs, *Res Vet Sci* 60:122-125, 1996.
540. Charon KM: Influence of radioactive precipitation on reproductivity of sheep in Poland, *World Rev Anim Prod* 30:64-68, 1995.
541. Erickson BH, Murphree RL: Limb development in prenatally irradiated cattle, sheep, and swine, *J Anim Sci* 23:1066-1071, 1964.
542. McFee AF, Murphree RL, Reynold RL: Skeletal defects in prenatally irradiated, sheep, cattle, and swine, *J Anim Sci* 24:1131-1135, 1965.

543. Young LE, Sinclair KD, Wilmut I: Large offspring syndrome in cattle and sheep, *Rev Reprod* 3:155-163, 1998.
544. Long SE: Chromosomes of sheep and goat, *Adv Vet Sci Comp Med* 34:109-130, 1990.
545. Cockett NE et al: Polar overdominance at the ovine callipyge locus, *Science* 273:236-238, 1996.
546. Cockett NE et al: The callipyge phenomenon: evidence for unusual genetic inheritance, *J Anim Sci* 77(suppl 2/J), *Dairy Sci* 82(suppl 2/1999): 221-227, 1999.
547. Cockett NE et al: Localization of the locus causing spider lamb syndrome to the distal end of ovine chromosome 6, *Mammal Genome* 10:35-38, 1999.
548. Hartley WJ, Kater JC: Perinatal disease conditions of sheep in New Zealand, *N Z Vet J* 12:49-57, 1964.
549. Dennis SM: Perinatal lamb mortality in a purebred Southdown flock, *J Anim Sci* 31:76-79, 1970.
550. Safford JW, Hoversland AS: A study of lamb mortality in a western range flock. I, Autopsy findings on 1051 lambs, *J Anim Sci* 19:265-273, 1960.
551. Ercanbrack SK, Price DA: Frequencies of various birth defects of Rambouillet sheep, *J Hered* 62:223-227, 1971.
552. Dennis SM: A survey of congenital defects of sheep, *Vet Rec* 95:488-490, 1974.
553. Dennis SM: Congenital respiratory tract defects in lambs, *Aust Vet J* 51:347-350, 1975.
554. Ercanbrack SK, Knight AD: Frequencies of various birth defects of Targhee and Columbia sheep, *J Hered* 69:237-243, 1978.
555. Cloete SWP, Van Halderen A, Schneider DJ: Causes of perinatal lamb mortality amongst Dormer and SA Mutton Merino lambs, *J S Afr Vet Med Assoc* 64:121-125, 1993.
556. Elias E, Bennett R: Congenital defects in Awassi fat-tailed lambs, *Small Ruminant Res* 8:141-150, 1992.
557. Leipold HW et al: Adactyly in Southdown lambs, *J Am Vet Med Assoc* 160:1002-1003, 1972.
558. Allen JG et al: Hemimelia in lambs, *Aust Vet J* 60:283-284, 1983.
559. Ramadan RO: Hemimelia and ectrodactyly in a Najdi sheep, *Agri-Practice* 14:30-32, 1993.
560. Philbey AW: Tachymene glaucifolia associated with bentleg in lambs, *Aust Vet J* 67:468, 1990.
561. Hidiroglou M et al: Bent-limb syndrome in lambs in total confinement, *J Am Vet Med Assoc* 173:1571-1574, 1978.
562. Uhthoff HK, Liskova-Kiar M, Hidiroglou M: Morphological studies of front limb deformities in lambs, *Vet Pathol* 17:362-371, 1980.
563. Millot P: Bent-limb disease in lambs: apparent transmission with autosomal recessive gene linked to the QL-Z minor lymphocyte antigen locus and the l locus involved in the expression of Rand O antigens in sheep, *J Immunogenet* 13:341-348, 1986.
564. Dennis SM: Congenital defects in sheep, *Vet Clin North Am (Food Anim Pract)* 9:203-217, 1993.
565. Dennis SM, Leipold HW: Congenital dactylous malformations in sheep, *Cornell Vet* 62:322-327, 1972.
566. Dennis SM: Embryonic duplications in sheep, *Aust Vet J* 51:83-87, 1975.
567. Saperstein G, Leipold HW, Dennis SM: Congenital defects in sheep, *J Am Vet Med Assoc* 167:314-322, 1975.
568. Dennis SM: Cephalomelia in a sheep, *Vet Rec* 90:508, 1972.
569. Dennis SM, Leipold HW: Syndactylism in a neonatal lamb, *Cornell Vet* 60:23-27, 1970.
570. Cravero GC, Cronagalia E, Fankhauser R: Beitrage zur Neuropathologie der Wiederkauer. I. Entwicklungstorungen, *Schweiz Arch Tierhlkde* 118:295-304, 1976.
571. Nie CJ, Folkerts JF: Occipitalization of the atlas in a sheep, *Zentralbl Vet Med C* 6:99, 1977.
572. Schmidt SP et al: A case of occipitoatlantoaxial malformation (OAAM) in a lamb, *J Vet Diagn Invest* 5:458-462, 1993.
573. Johnson GC et al: Occipital condylar dysplasia in two Jacob sheep, *Cornell Vet* 84:91-98, 1994.
574. Lakritz J et al: Cervical and thoracic vertebral malformation ("weak neck") in Colombia lambs, *J Vet Intern Med* 9:393-398, 1995.
575. Dennis SM: Congenital tail defects in lambs, *Cornell Vet* 62:568-572, 197.
576. Butz H, Sonnenbrodt A, Bottger TH: Gaumenspalten bei unseren Haussaugetieren insbesondere beim Schaf, *Dtsche Tierarztl Wschr* 50:65-67, 1972.
577. Smith ID: Agnathia and micrognathia in the sheep, *Aust Vet J* 44:510-511, 1968.
578. Dennis SM, Leipold HW: Aprosopia (facelessness) in lambs, *Vet Rec* 90:365-367, 1972.
579. Dennis SM, Leipold HW: Agnathia in sheep: external observations, *Am J Vet Res* 33:339-347, 1972.
580. Camon J et al: Placental underdevelopment in fetal sheep with simultaneous aprosopia and aprosencephalia, *Anat Histol Emb (Abst)* 23:65, 1994.
581. Dennis SM: Otognathia in a neonatal lamb, *Am J Vet Res* 31:203-204, 1970.
582. Dennis SM: Perinatal lamb mortality in Western Australia. VII, Congenital defects, *Aust Vet J* 51:80-83, 1975.
583. Kater JC et al: Osteogenesis imperfecta and bone resorption: two unusual skeletal abnormalities in young lambs, *NZ Vet J* 11:41-44, 1963.

Text continued on p. 1539

TABLE 47-30

Congenital Defects of Appendicular Skeleton in Sheep

Defect	Reference No.	Description	Etiology	Frequency	Diagnosis	Associated Defects
Adactyly	557	Absence of phalanges, affects one or more limbs	Most likely genetic, but mode of transmission has not been clarified	Rare	Physical examination, x-ray	None
Hemimelia	520, 558, 559	Incomplete development of distal part of the limb	In Australia, considered to result from grazing on sandplain lupines during pregnancy	Rare	Physical examination, x-ray	None
Bentleg ("bowie")	519, 521, 551, 560-564	Occurs 2-90 days after birth; front legs bow and are shorter than normal because of rotation of joints and angulation in long bones; varus deformity of radiocarpal joint and inward turning of plantar surface of feet; lambs are front heavy, often collapsing onto carpi; narrowed epiphyseal plates of distal radius, decreased density in adjacent metaphysis, and flaring	Grazing on *Trachymene* spp. (wild parsnip), parbendazole, or locoweeds; genetic factors	Common in certain areas of the world	Physical examination, x-ray	None
Phocomelia	565	Hind legs shorter because of agenesis of proximal parts of the limb	Unknown	Common	Physical examination, x-ray	None
Monobrachia	565	Absence of one front leg	Unknown	Rare	Physical examination	None
Abrachia	565	Absence of both front legs	Unknown	Rare	Physical examination	None
Monopodia	565	Absence of one hind leg	Unknown	Rare	Physical examination	None
Apodia	565	Absence of both hind legs	Unknown	Rare	Physical examination	None
Polymelia	566	Additional limbs, classified by location	Unknown	Rare	Physical examination	None
Notomelia	567	Attachment of duplicated limbs on back	Unknown	Rare	Physical examination	None
Cephalomelia	567, 568	Attachment of duplicated legs on occipital area of head	Unknown	Rare	Physical examination	None
Thoracomelia	564	Attachment of duplicated leg on thorax	Unknown	Rare	Physical examination	None
Pygomelia	564	Attachment of leg(s) to pelvis	Unknown	Rare	Physical examination	Polyorchidism, cryptorchidism
Perodactyl	565	Absence of one or more digits	Unknown	Rare	Physical examination	Other digital defects, arthrogryposis
Polydactyly	565	Higher than normal number of digits	Unknown	Rare	Physical examination	Other skeletal defects
Microdactyly	565	Small digit	Unknown	Rare	Physical examination	Other skeletal defects
Syndactyly	565, 569	Fusion or nondivision of functional digits	Unknown	Rare	Physical examination	Cryptochidism cleft palate

TABLE 47-31

Congenital Defects of the Axial Skeleton in Sheep

Defect	Reference No.	Description	Etiology	Frequency	Diagnosis	Associated Defects
Atlantooccipital malformation	570-572	Fusion of atlas to occipital bone of skull, absence or hypoplasia of dens of axis; paraparesis or tetraparesis	Unknown	Rare	Physical examination, x-ray	Spinal cord degeneration
Occipital condylar dysplasia	573	Asymmetric development of occipital condyles resulting in instability of joint and small foramen magnum; lambs present with torticollis and ataxia	Reported in Jacob sheep; possibly hereditary	Rare	At necropsy	None
Cervical and thoracic vertebral malformation (weak neck)	574	Kyphosis at cervicothoracic junction; lambs unable to lift their head; neurologic signs include ataxia, tetraparesis, diminished conscious proprioception, and increased patellar and triceps reflexes	Heredity suspected	Seen in Colombias	Physical examination, x-ray, necropsy	Atlantooccipital malformation in one case
Anomalies of vertebrae	525	Hemivertebrae, fused vertebrae, spina bifida	Netobimin (metabolized to albendazole) given day 17	Uncommon	At necropsy	Renal anomalies, vascular anomalies
Torticollis	564	Neck bent to one side	Various factors such as bluetongue virus or vitamin D overdose have been incriminated; other cases unknown	Rare	Physical examination	Arthrogryposis
Kyphosis	564	Dorsal bending of vertebral column	Unknown	Rare	Physical examination	None
Scoliosis	564	Lateral bending of vertebral column	Unknown	Rare	Physical examination	None
Tail defects (wrytail, brachyury, polyury, anury)	567, 575	Wry tail, twisted tail, short tail, no tail, duplicated tail	Unknown	Occurred in 50 out of 401 lambs with congenital defects	Physical examination	Atresia ani, arthrogryposis, ventricular septal defects
Perosomus elumbis	575	Lack of development of lumbosacral vertebrae, lethal	Unknown	Rare	Physical examination	Arthrogryposis of hind legs

TABLE 47-32

Congenital Defects of the Cranial Facial Skeleton in Sheep

Defect	Reference No.	Description	Etiology	Frequency	Diagnosis	Associated Defects
Cleft palate	517, 576	Failure of palatine shelves to close; milk may run from nose, aspiration pneumonia, poor doers	Unknown	Rare	Physical examination	Musculoskeletal defects and others; earless, micrognathia
Brachygnathia/agnathia syndrome	577–579	Mandibular hypoplasia to aplasia, merging into agnathia, accompanied by atelostomia, microglossia to aglossia, atresia of oral pharynx, synotia, and pharyngeal diverticulum; both sexes afflicted; lambs die during or shortly after delivery; merges into aprosopia	Genetic transmission has been claimed but not proven	In a series of 401 defective lambs, 74 had this syndrome	Physical examination	Other skeletal defects or reproductive system defects
Aprosopus	580	Absence of face	Unknown	Rare	Physical examination	Subcutaneous edema, otocephaly, synotia, small thyroid, absent pituitary
Otognathia	581	Accessory rudimentary mouth at basal aural pinna	Unknown	Rare	Physical examination	Cleft palate
Prognathia	564, 567	Mandible longer than normal and projecting	Unknown	Rare	Physical examination	None
Hemignathia	564, 567	Unilateral lack of development of mandible	Unknown	Rare	Physical examination	None
Campylognathia	564, 567	Lateral deviation of jaw leading to malocclusion	Unknown	Rare	Physical examination	Atelorrhinia
Diprosopus	567, 582	Partial to nearly complete duplication of face	Unknown	Rare	Physical examination	Cleft palate, pseudohermaphroditism
Acephalus	552, 566	Lack of development of head	Unknown	Rare	Physical examination	None
Cebocephalus	552, 567	"Monkeylike" head	Unknown	Rare	Physical examination	Atelorrhinia
Brachycephalus	552	Short head	Unknown	Rare	Physical examination	Atelorrhinia
Pesocephalus	552	Deformed head	Unknown	Rare	Physical examination	None

TABLE 47-33

Congenital Defects of the Entire Skeleton in Sheep

Defect	Reference No.	Description	Etiology	Frequency	Diagnosis	Associated Defects
Osteogenesis imperfecta	583-585	Unable to stand; extreme joint laxity; brittle bones that can be cut with knife; dark blue sclera, teeth pink, skin torn easily; fractures of recent and older origin; may have short lower jaw	Dominant	Rare	Physical examination, necropsy, x-ray	None
Bone resorption	583	Emaciation, stiff gait, fragile bones in particular maxilla and mandible, loose teeth, widespread resorption of bone	Unknown	Rare	Physical examination, x-ray	
Dwarfism (Ancon or otter sheep)	586-588	Abnormal head, short limbs, disturbance of epiphyseal bone growth	Simple autosomal recessive	Rare	Physical examination	Ectrodactyly
Hereditary chondrodysplasia (spider syndrome)	547, 589-594	Abnormal at birth or develop defect at 4-6 weeks old; various degrees of angular limb deformities are associated with kyphosis, scoliosis, kypho-scoliosis, and anomalies of head (roman nose), sternal vertebrae, and appendicular skeleton; progressive marked erosion of articular cartilage in radiohumeral and tibio-femoral joints of lambs over 3 months old	Simple autosomal recessive with variable expressivity in Suffolk, Hampshire, Southdown, Shropshire, and Oxford	Common in some breeds	Physical examination, x-ray of sternum and elbow necropsy; abnormal gene present on telomeric end of chromosome 6; DNA blood test to detect carriers	None
Fetal anasarca (Bull dog lamb)	595, 596	Generalized subcutaneous edema, ascites, and placental edema	Unknown	Rare	Presents as dystocia	Prognathia, cystic ear, extramedullary hematopoiesis

TABLE 47-34

Congenital Defects of the Muscular System in Sheep

Defect	Reference No.	Description	Etiology	Frequency	Diagnosis	Associated Defects
Arthrogryposis	526, 533-536, 597-599	Permanent joint contracture present at birth, usually involves all four legs, may involve only one leg	Genetic or environmental factors such as plants and prenatal viral infection	Common	Physical examination, necropsy	Cleft palate, hydranencephaly, micrencephaly, porencephaly
Muscular hypertrophy (double muscling)	545, 546, 600, 601	Hypertrophy of fast-twitch muscle fibers, especially affecting muscles of hindlimbs	Polar overdominance (only heterozygotes receiving defective gene from their sire express the trait)	Rare	Physical examination after 3 wks of age	None
Congenital progressive muscular dystrophy	602-606	Affected as early as 1 month old; stiff gait to reduction of flexion of femerotibial and hock joints becoming worse with exercise; fail to thrive; die from starvation between 6 to 18 months of age; vastus intermedius muscle and quadriceps progressive, loss of myofibrils in type 1 fiber, atrophy, and fibrous or fat tissue replacement; not associated with adhalin or merosin deficiency	Autosomal recessive	Rare	Physical examination, necropsy, histopathology, and histochemistry	Unilateral renal agenesis, prognathia, cardiomegaly, arthrogryposis, polycystic kidney

TABLE 47-35

Congenital Defects of the Central Nervous System in Sheep

Defect	Reference No.	Description	Etiology	Frequency	Diagnosis	Associated Defects
Anencephaly	607	Failure of cranial neural tube to close, lack of development of brain, all or parts of medulla developed, eyes present	Unknown	Rare	Physical examination, necropsy	Cranioschisis or craniorachischisis, sometimes harelip, cleft palate, atelostomia; arthrogryposis, atresia ani, patent umbilical ring malformed kidneys, cryptorchidism; penile agenesis; interventricular septal defects
Hydranencephaly	528, 533-536, 608-610	Cerebral hemispheres are fluid-filled sacs	Breeding trials in Corriedale sheep suggested simple autosomal recessive; other cases prenatal viral infections such as Akabane, bluetongue, bovine virus diarrhea, Cache Valley fever virus, and other Bunyamwera viruses	Common	Physical examination, necropsy, viral isolation, viral antibodies in precolostral sera from defective neonates	Retinal dysplasia, arthrogryposis, brachygnathia inferior, leukoencephalopathy, porencephaly
Micrencephaly	526, 537, 538, 611	Abnormally small brain	Genetic cases reported; Akabane and other prenatal infections; hyperthermia	Rare	Necropsy	Brain cavitation, hydrocephalus, arthrogryposis, cerebellar agenesis
Holoprosencephaly	613	Lack of longitudinal cerebral fissure, with fusion of hemispheres, single ventricle	Simple autosomal recessive in Border Leicester lambs	Common	Necropsy	Facial defects
Internal hydrocephalus	611	Excessive accumulation of cerebrospinal fluid in dilated lateral ventricles of brain	Unknown	Common	Necropsy	Brachycephalus, campylognathia
Meningocele	611, 612	Protrusion of meninges through opening in skull	Unknown	Rare	Necropsy	Cone-like bony skull projection
Meningoencephalocele	611	Protrusion of meninges and brain parts through opening in skull	Unknown	Rare	Necropsy	None
Dandy-Walker malformation	614	Hydrocephalus, cystic enlargement of fourth ventricle, agenesis or hypoplasia of cerebellar vermis	Possibly genetic in British Suffolk sheep	Rare	Necropsy, domed skull may cause dystocia	None

Continued

TABLE 47-35

Congenital Defects of the Central Nervous System in Sheep—cont'd

Defect	Reference No.	Description	Etiology	Frequency	Diagnosis	Associated Defects
Arnold-Chiari malformation	615	Cerebral hemispheres displaced caudally, part of cerebellum and medulla displaced into spinal canal	Unknown	Very rare	Necropsy	Spinda bifida, cranial dysplasia
Cerebellar cortical atrophy (abiotrophy/daft lambs)	617-622	Lambs show signs of cerebellar dysfunction, ataxia, intention tremor of head, wide-based stance, opistotonos; selective degeneration of Purkinje and Golgi cells in cerebellum	Claimed to be inherited; seen in Merino, Corriedale, Welsh, Border Leicester, and Charolais	Reported in England, Australia, and Canada	Physical examination, histopathologic studies	None
Thalamic cerebellar neuropathy	623	Age of onset 2 years or older, hind limb paresis; hypermetria of front limbs, head tremor, wide-based stance, and ataxia; degeneration of neurons in thalamus and of Purkinje cells; swollen axons in thalamus, cerebellar peduncles, and spinal cord	Probably of genetic etiology	Rare	Physical examination, histopathology	None
Spongiform leucoencephalomyelopathy (Intramyelinic edema)	624	Onset at 2-3 months of age of posterior paresis leading to posterior paralysis; spongy vacuolation of white matter throughout brain and spinal cord	Suspected to be hereditary in Romneys	Uncommon	Age of onset, signs, histopathology of brain and spinal cord	None
Neuraxial edema	625	Neonates unable to stand, tremor, hyperesthesia, with no suck reflex; spongy vacuolation of white matter of brain (especially cerebellum and medulla) and spinal cord	Unknown	Rare; seen in polled Dorset	Age of onset, signs, histopathology of brain and spinal cord	None
Neuraxonal dystrophy	626, 627	Onset at young age, hind limb ataxia, recumbency, axonal swelling in gray matter of brain stem and spinal cord	Presumably genetic in medium-wool Merinos	Rare	Physical examination, histopathology	None

Segmental axonopathy (Murrurundi disease)	628	Onset at one to 4 years of age, ataxia, axonopathy of brain stem and spinal cord	Unknown	Rare	Physical examination, histopathology	None
GM-1 gangliosidosis	629-633	Progressive signs begin at 4 months of age; inability to keep up with flock, followed by ataxia, wide-based stance in hind limbs, recumbency, mild resting tremors, blindness, neuronal vacuolation	Simple autosomal recessive, Suffolk	Rare	Physical examination, histopathology, electron microscopy, enzyme tests	None
Neuronal ceroidlipofuscinosis	634-637	At 8 months of age blindness, depression, progressive, deposition of lipopigment identified as ceroid-lipofuscin in neurons of brain, eyes, and spinal cord	Simple autosomal recessive, Rambouillet sheep, South Hampshire in New Zealand	Rare	Physical examination, necropsy, histopathology	None
Border disease (hairy shaker)	527, 638, 639	Newborn lambs are smaller and lighter than normal; may have tremors, rough and hairy; abnormal myelination; reduced lambing percentage, viability; growth; persistent viral infection	Prenatal infection with Border disease virus	Common in some areas	Physical examination, necropsy, histopathology, serology	None
Spina bifida	611, 640, 641, 525	Failure of closure of dorsal arches of lumbar and sacral vertebrae, paralyzed hind quarters or arthrogryposis, hairless slit in lumbar area	Simple autosomal recessive in Icelandic sheep, other breeds unknown; netobimin	Rare	Physical examination	Tail defects, arthrogryposis
Congenital hypomyelination neuropathy	642	Incoordination and intermittent tremor of head and limbs, ataxia, hypomyelination of axons in peripheral nerves	Unknown	One case reported	Physical examination, histopathologic studies	Coloboma
Swayback	567, 643	Lambs born weak, blind, and with ataxia, death within first day of life; cavitation of cerebral hemispheres and spinal cord lesions	Copper deficiency	Sporadic	Physical examination, histopathology, Cu determination from ewe's serum	None

TABLE 47-36

Congenital Defects of Ocular Structures in Sheep

Defect	Reference No.	Description	Etiology	Frequency	Diagnosis	Associated Defects
Entropion	644-651	Unilateral or bilateral inversion of the eyelids, causing the eyelashes to irritate cornea and sclera, can be surgically corrected	Familial, genetic, several genes involved	Very common in some flocks	Physical examination	Notch in eye, epiphora, mucopurulent conjunctivitis
Anophthalmia	564	Unilateral or bilateral absence of globe	Unknown	Rare	Physical examination	None
Macrophthalmia	564	Unilateral or bilateral enlargement of globes	Unknown	Rare	Physical examination	None
Microphthalmia	564	Unilateral or bilateral reduction of size of globes	Unknown	Rare	Physical examination	None
Defect of upper eyelid	652	Unilateral or bilateral notch(es) in center of upper eyelid ranging from 2 to 7 mm in size	Genetic	Rare	Physical examination	Blindness may develop, reduced growth
Cataracts	653	Bilateral mature cataracts develop during first year of life	Reported as dominant in Romney sheep	Rare	Physical examination	None
Aphakia	654	Absence of lens	Unknown	Rare	At necropsy	None
Persistent pupillary membrane	654	Thick black band at pupil	Unknown	Uncommon	Physical examination	Lens opacity
Cyclopia	517	Single, large, median eye with variable head defects; cyclopia when exposed at gestational day 14; motor nerve paralysis when exposed at days 17 and 18; other defects if exposed at 12-20 days	Ingestion of *Veratrum californicum* during pregnancy	Common in certain areas	Physical examination	Arrhinia, hydrocephalus, micrencephaly
Blindness	530, 532, 638	Blindness due to retinopathy	Bluetongue virus	Rare	Ophthalmoscopic examination	Brain defects

TABLE 47-37

Congenital Defects of the Ear in Sheep

Defect	Reference No.	Description	Etiology	Frequency	Diagnosis	Associated Defects
Ear pendants	552, 564, 616	Fleshy appendages on the ear pinnae in various locations, of variable sizes and shapes	Simple autosomal recessive	Rare	Physical examination	None
Earless with cleft palate	655	Lambs born without ears and have a cleft palate	Simple autosomal recessive	Rare	Physical examination	Deformed hooves, ankylosis of mandible
Anotia (earless)	656	Lambs born without ears	Simple autosomal recessive	Rare	Physical examination	None
Monotia	552, 564, 616	Lambs born lacking one ear	Unknown	Rare	Physical examination	None
Synotia	552, 564, 616	Fused ears	Unknown	Rare	Physical examination	None
Polyotia	552, 564, 616	More than two ears	Unknown	Rare	Physical examination	None
Microtia (short ears)	656	Lambs born with very short ears measuring 3-5 cm, medium ears at 10 cm length, or long ears at 17 cm	Incomplete dominant gene	Rare	Physical examination	None

TABLE 47-38

Hereditary Diseases and Congenital Defects of the Skin in Sheep

Defect	Reference No.	Description	Etiology	Frequency	Diagnosis	Associated Defects
Gray lethal	657-660	Gray and white Karakul lambs born, will die when placed on roughage diet after weaning; black Karakuls are normal, homozygous gray and white, can be identified at birth by lack of pigmentation of tongue, palate, and ears; reticulum rumen and abomasum have less myenteric ganglia and neurons in gray and white lambs	Simple autosomal recessive	Rare	Physical examination, histopathology	None
Halo hairs, dominant type	661	Increase of coarse hair with brown patches in fleece of back of neck, effect on hair medullation, ratios, and crimping	Most likely as many as three incompletely or completely dominant genes	Rare	Physical examination	None
Halo hairs, recessive	661	Same as above but due to homozygosis of a simple autosomal recessive gene	Simple autosomal recessive	Rare	Physical examination	None
Luster	662	Major reduction of fleece weight to 40% of normal sheep; luster lambs are also lighter than normal; lustrous, greasy, yellowish, crimpy wool	Dominant gene	Rare	Physical examination	Reduced body weight
Silky	663	Lambs are born with no skin folds, and smooth wavy wool, adults have broad waves rather than crimp	Dominant gene in Merinos	Rare	Physical examination	Poor viability

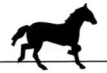

	References	Clinical Signs	Inheritance	Frequency	Diagnosis	Other
Hypotrichosis	664, 665	When 1 month old, have bald faces, ears and lower legs; skin is wrinkled, thickened, edematous, and greasy; histologically, absence of fibers in follicles, follicular keratosis and sebaceous gland hypertrophy and hyperplasia, orthokeratotic hyperkeratosis, and hypergranulosis	Most likely simple autosomal recessive in polled Dorset	Rare	Physical examination, histopathology	None
Epitheliogenesis imperfecta	666-668	Lack of development of epithelium in patchy areas of oral cavity, below carpal and tarsal joints, nose, ears, coronary groove, separation of hooves, exungulation; lethal	Simple autosomal recessive	Rare	Physical examination, histopathologic studies	Sometimes brachygnathia inferior, deformed teeth
Epidermiolysis bullosa	669, 670	Vesicle formation shortly after birth in oral cavity, oral mucocutaneous junction, and coronary groove, junctional separation of epidermis at basal membrane, exungulation	Simple autosomal recessive	Rare	Physical examination, histopathologic studies	None
Collagen dysplasia	671-674	Fragility of skin, easily torn when handled as newborns, developmental defect in collagen fibers; lethal	Simple autosomal recessive	Rare	Physical examination, histopathology, collagen studies	Fragile digestive tract and arteries

TABLE 47-39

Congenital Defects of the Circulatory System in Sheep

Defect	Reference No.	Description	Etiology	Frequency	Diagnosis	Associated Defects
Ventricular septal defect	548, 675	Most defects in ventricular septum are subaortic in location in the membranous septum	Unknown, may be genetic in Southdown sheep	Most common heart defect	Physical examination, necropsy	Skeletal defects
Tetralogy of Fallot	675	Ventricular septal defect, stenosis of pulmonary artery, overriding aorta, hypertrophy of right ventricle	Unknown, possibly genetic	Uncommon	Necropsy	Associated skeletal defects
Cardiomegaly	675	Abnormally large heart	Unknown	Rare	Physical examination, necropsy	Hepatomegaly, renal defects, pulmonary hypoplasia
Endocardial fibroelastosis	675	Thickened endocardium of both ventricles	Unknown	Rare	Physical examination, necropsy	Hypertrophy of right ventricle
Atrial hypoplasia	675	Incomplete development of atria	Unknown	Rare	Necropsy	Conjoined twins
Holoacardius acephalus	676, 677	Incomplete twin, absence of heart and head	Unknown, chromosomal abnormalities	Rare	Necropsy, karyotyping	Absence of lungs and liver
Anomalous thoracic venous and arterial patterns	678	Double cranial vena cava combined with anomalous origin of left subclavian artery	Unknown	Incidental finding	Necropsy	None
Patent ductus arteriosus	679	Persistence of ductus arteriosus between pulmonary artery and aorta; machinery murmur	Unknown	Very rare	At necropsy	None
Fibrinogen deficiency	680	Bleeding disorder due to lack of, reduced, or abnormal fibrinogen	Possibly familial in Border Leicester	Very rare	Laboratory blood analysis	None

TABLE 47-40

Congenital Defects of the Respiratory System in Sheep

Defect	Reference No.	Description	Etiology	Frequency	Diagnosis	Associated Defects
Pulmonary hypoplasia	553, 616	Small lungs; lethal	Unknown	Rare	Necropsy	Diaphragmatic hernia, cardiomegaly
Pulmonary agenesis	548, 553	Lack of development of lungs	Unknown	Rare	Necropsy	Holocardius acephalus
Adenomatoid malformation	550	Tumorlike section of lung with bronchial hypoplasia	Unknown	Rare	Necropsy, histopathology	None

TABLE 47-41

Congenital Defects of the Digestive System in Sheep

Defect	Reference No.	Description	Etiology	Frequency	Diagnosis	Associated Defects
Atresia ani	548, 616, 681	Imperforation of the anus, rectum ends blindly in males, recto-vaginal fistula in females	Unknown, possibly hereditary	Rare	Physical examination, necropsy	Urogenital defects, musculoskeletal and cardiovascular defects
Atresia jejuni	682, 683	Abdominal distention, dyspnea, jejunum ends blindly	Unknown	Rare	Necropsy	None
Atresia ilei	684	Ileum ends blindly	Unknown	Rare	Necropsy	None
Atresia coli	550	Colon ends blindly	Unknown	Rare	Necropsy	None
Imperforate ileocecal junction	548	Same as defect	Unknown	Rare	Necropsy	None
Primary megacolon (Hirschsprung's disease)	550	Abnormality in ganglion cells in distal stenotic section of colon, causing signs of abdominal distention, poor doer and constipation	Unknown	Rare	Necropsy, histopathology	None
Abomasal emptying defect	685	Enlarged abomasum in adult that empties inefficiently and refluxes; signs include weight loss, anorexia, abdominal distention, and depression	Unknown, reported in Suffolk and Dorset	Uncommon	Clinical examination and necropsy	None

TABLE 47-42

Congenital Defects of the Urinary System in Sheep

Defect	Reference No.	Description	Etiology	Frequency	Diagnosis	Associated Defects
Hypospadia	548, 552, 572, 616, 686-688	Ventral opening of the penile urethra, usually in the perineal area; scrotum usually bifid	Unknown	Uncommon	Physical examination	Atresia ani, brachygnathia
Renal agenesis	525, 688	Unilateral or bilateral absence of kidney(s)	Netobimin	Rare	Necropsy	Reproductive and skeletal system defects
Polycystic kidney	548, 616, 688	Bilateral replacement of renal tissue by cysts	Unknown	Rare	Necropsy	None
Hydronephrosis	548, 616, 688	Dilation of renal pelvis, calyces, and ureter	Unknown	Common	Necropsy	Other kidney defects
Cystic renal dysplasia	689, 690	Newborn lambs unable to stand or barely able to stand, coats failed to dry, weak, domed crania, twitchy and stargazing; usually fatal within 5 days; kidneys very small at necropsy, bladder vestigial or absent, 30% mortality in affected flocks	Dominant gene	Rare	Necropsy, histopathology	Overshot upper jaw
Patent urachus	691	Consistent dribbling of urine from persistent urachus at umbilical area	Unknown	Very rare	Physical examination	Reproductive system defects

TABLE 47-43

Congenital Defects of the Endocrine System and Metabolism in Sheep

Defect	Reference No.	Description	Etiology	Frequency	Diagnosis	Associated Defects
Goiter	692	Lambs stillborn or die shortly after birth, enlarged thyroid gland, generalized weakness, edema of knees and ears, head, and mouth deformities, silky coat	Merino lambs, simple autosomal recessive, other cases iodine deficiency, grazing of goitrogenic plants	Rare	Physical examination, necropsy, elevated protein-bound iodine in serum; abnormal iodo-protein levels in carrier sheep	Facial defects
Hyperbilirubinemia	693-696	Reduced ability of kidney and liver to remove bilirubin and phylloerythrin, sublethal trait, characteristic lesions resemble facial eczema at age 5-7 weeks	Simple autosomal recessive, Southdown; occurs also in Corriedales	Rare	Physical examination, necropsy, histopathology, biochemical studies	Icterus, renal radial fibrosis, hydro-thorax, ascites, pulmonary edema, photosensitivity

TABLE 47-44

Congenital Defects of Internal Organs in Sheep

Defect	Reference No.	Description	Etiology	Frequency	Diagnosis	Associated Defects
Pancreatic cysts	697	Cysts in pancreas	Unknown	Very rare	Incidental finding at necropsy	None
Splenic defects	698	Various defects of spleen such as hypoplasia, displacement, and duplication	Unknown	Rare	Incidental finding at necropsy	Defects in various other organ systems
Congenital biliary atresia	699	Affected lambs fail to thrive, develop icterus and white scours, die within 4 weeks of birth; atresia of intrahepatic bile ducts	Toxic insult during pregnancy	Rare	Physical examination, necropsy, histopathology	None
Bilobed gallbladder	700	Duplication of gallbladder	Unknown	Very rare	At slaughter	None

TABLE 47-45

Congenital Hernias in Sheep

Defect	Reference No.	Description	Etiology	Frequency	Diagnosis	Associated Defects
Diaphragmatic hernia	701	Protrusion of abdominal organs into thorax	Unknown	Most common hernia	Necropsy	Occasionally pulmonary hypoplasia
Umbilical hernia	701	Protrusion of abdominal organs through umbilical ring covered by skin	Unknown	Rare	Physical examination	Frequently associated with other defects
Abdominal fissure	701, 702	Protrusion of organs through abdominal wall	Unknown	Very rare	Physical examination, necropsy	Associated with other defects
Scrotal hernia	701, 703	Inguinal hernia passing into scrotum	Unknown, may be inherited in Merinos	Rare	Physical examination	Atresia ani
Perineal hernia	701, 704	Protrusion of organs at perineal area	Unknown	Rare	Physical examination	Atresia ani
Schistosomus reflexus	705-707	Nonfusion of ventral body wall, eversion of body and internal organs	Unknown	Rare	Physical examination, necropsy	Atresia ani, cryptorchidism, arthrogryposis, bifurcated scrotum

TABLE 47-46

Congenital Defects of the Reproductive System in Sheep

Defect	Reference No.	Description	Etiology	Frequency	Diagnosis	Associated Defects
Cryptorchidism	552, 708, 709	Incomplete descent of one or both testicles from caudal pole of kidney to inguinal ring	Has been reported as simple autosomal recessive, or an autosomal dominant with incomplete penetrance	1% of Merino rams	Physical examination	Occasionally other defects
Testicular hypoplasia	521, 710, 711	Unilateral or bilateral reduction in size of testes; elevated plasma gonadotropins if bilateral	Genetic cause; *Oxytropis*, *Astragalus*, and other teratogens possibly	Outbreaks up to 31%	Physical examination	May be associated with chromosomal abnormalities
Sperm granuloma	711, 712	Granulomas in head of epididymis, most likely resulting from blind-ending tubules in the efferent duct area	Appears to be inherited	Common	Physical examination	None
Segmental aplasia of epididymis	711, 712	Body and tail of epididymis most frequently not developed on one side, causes sperm granuloma formation and testicular degeneration	Most likely inherited, unknown	Rare	Physical examination	None
Partial or complete lack of sigmoid flexure	711, 712	Prevents penis from achieving erection	Unknown	Rare	Physical examination	None
Partial duplication of urogenital system	713	One set of normal male genitalia plus a rudimentary set in intraabdomimal fat	Unknown	Rare	Physical examination	None
Ovarian aplasia	714	Unilateral or bilateral absence of ovarian tissue	Unknown	Very rare	At slaughter	Partial aplasia of uterus; uterus unicornis
Accessory ovary	714	Extra ovary adjacent to normal ovary	Unknown	Very rare	At slaughter	None
Fused ovaries	714	Two ovaries fused either dorsally or ventrally relative to uterus	Unknown	Rare	At slaughter	None
Paraovarian cysts	714	Most cysts are between 4 and 8 mm	Unknown	Uncommon	At slaughter	None
Ovarian hypoplasia (streak ovaries)	710, 715, 716	Small ovaries in mature ewes containing no oocytes or follicles	Familial in Lleyn sheep; X-linked recessive in Inverdale line of Romneys	Uncommon	Laparoscopic examination	None
Uterus unicornis	711, 712, 714, 717	Absent uterine horn; reduced fertility	Unknown	Most common uterine defect	At slaughter	None
Double cervix	711, 712, 714, 717	Failure of medial walls of müllerian ducts to fuse, usually normal fertility	Unknown	Rare	Examination	Uterus didelphys, double cranial vagina
Segmental aplasia of paramesonephric duct system	714, 717	Lack of development of varying parts of reproductive tract of ewe	Unknown	Very rare	At slaughter	None

TABLE 47-47

Intersexes and Chromosomal Defects in Sheep

Defect	Reference No.	Description	Etiology	Frequency	Diagnosis	Associated Defects
Freemartinism	718-721	Some females born cotwin to a male may have ovarian hypoplasia and malformed tubular genitalia; external genitalia may be normal	Interplacental fusion results in XX/XY chimera	1%-7% of mixed sex multiple births	Physical examination (decreased vaginal length); endocrinologic and chromosomal studies	None
Testicular feminization (androgen insensitivity) (male pseudohermaphrodite)	712, 730	Cryptorchidism; external genitalia are female; tubular genitalia from paramesonephric and mesonephric ducts are rudimentary or not developed; 54 XY	Speculated to be genetic, most probably X-linked	Rare	Physical examination, endocrine and chromosomal studies	None
Klinefelter's syndrome	728-729	Bilateral testicular hypoplasia; 55 XXY	Chromosomal nondisjunction	Rare	Chromosomal studies	None
Turner's syndrome	544	53 XO ewe; infertile	Unknown	Rare	Chromosomal studies	Ovarian dysgeneration
True hermaphroditism	731, 732	Presence of both ovarian and testicular tissue	Unknown	Very rare	Laparoscopically, histologically, and chromosomal studies	None
Centric fusion (Robertsonian translocations)	711, 721-727	Five currently identified: t_1 (6;24), t_2 (9;10), t_3 (7;25), t_4 (5;8), and t_5 (8;22)	Unknown	Common in Romney	Chromosomal studies	Fertility not affected
Reciprocal translocations	544, 721	Four identified: (1p−;19q+), (13q−;19q+) (2q+;3p−), (1p+33;24q−11)	Unknown	Rare	Chromosomal studies	Abnormal reproduction
Autosomal deletion	733	Missing piece of autosome	Unknown	Rare	Chromosomal studies	Brachygnathia superior

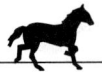

584. Holmes JR, Baker JR, Davies ET: Osteogenesis imperfecta in lambs, *Vet Rec* 76:980-984, 1964.

585. Arthur DG, Thompson KG, Swarbrick P: Lethal osteogenesis and skin fragility in newborn New Zealand Romney lambs, *N Z Vet J* 40:112-116, 1992.

586. Landauer W, Chang TK: The Ancon or otter sheep, history and genetics, *J Hered* 40:105-112, 1949.

587. Shelton M: A recurrence of the Ancon dwarf in Merino sheep, *J Hered* 59:267-268, 1968.

588. Chorlton S: Dwarfism in sheep, *Wool Tech Sheep Breed* 13:83-84, 1966.

589. Rook JS, Trapp AL, Krehbiel J: Diagnosis of hereditary chondrodysplasia (spider lamb syndrome) in sheep, *J Am Vet Med Assoc* 193:713-718, 1988.

590. Vanek JA et al: Comparison of G-banded chromosomes from clinically normal lambs and lambs affected with ovine hereditary chondrodysplasia (spider syndrome), *Am J Vet Res* 49:1164-1168, 1988.

591. Vanek JA, Walter PA, Alstad AD: Radiographic diagnosis of hereditary chondrodysplasia in newborn lambs, *J Am Vet Med Assoc* 194:244-248, 1989.

592. Phillips PH, Bunn CM, Anderson CE: Ovine hereditary chondrodysplasia (spider syndrome) in Suffolk lambs, *Aust Vet J* 70:73-74, 1992.

593. West DM et al: Hereditary chondrodysplasia ("spider syndrome") in a New Zealand Suffolk lamb of American origin, *N Z Vet J* 43:118-122, 1995.

594. Oberbauer AM et al: Developmental progression of spider lamb syndrome, *Small Ruminant Res* 18:179-184, 1995.

595. Hailat N et al: Foetal anasarca in Awassi sheep, *Aust Vet J* 75:257-259, 1997.

596. Qureshi ZI, Lodhi LA: Delivery of an achandroplastic "bull dog" lamb in a Lohi ewe, *Pak Vet J* 18:110-111, 1998.

597. Roberts JAF: The inheritance of a lethal muscle contracture in the sheep, *J Genet* 21:57-70, 1929.

598. Morley FHV: A new lethal factor in Australian Merino sheep, *Aust Vet J* 30:237-240, 1954.

599. Parsonson IM et al: Congenital abnormalities in fetal lambs after inoculation of pregnant ewes with Akabane virus, *Aust Vet J* 51:585-586, 1975.

600. Dennis SM: Congenital muscular hyperplasia in a lamb, *Cornell Vet* 62:263-268, 1972.

601. Cockett NE, Jackson SP, Shay TL: Chromosomal localization of the callipyge gene in sheep (*Ovis aries*) using bovine DNA markers, *Proc Natl Acad Sci* 91:3019-3023, 1994.

602. McGavin MD, Baynes ID: A congenital progressive ovine muscular dystrophy, *Vet Path* 6:513-524, 1969.

603. Richards RB, Passmore IK, Bretach AH: Ovine congenital progressive muscular dystrophy: clinical syndrome and distribution of lesions, *Aust Vet J* 63:396-401, 1986.

604. Richards RB, Lewer RP, Passmore IK: Ovine congenital progressive muscular dystrophy: mode of inheritance, *Aust Vet J* 65:93-94, 1988.

605. Richards RB, Passmore IK, Dempsey EF: Skeletal muscle pathology in ovine congenital progressive muscular dystrophy. I, Histopathology and histochemistry, *Acta Neuropathol* 77:161-167, 1988.

606. Johnsen RD et al: Normal expression of adhalin and merosin in ovine congenital progressive muscular dystrophy, *Aust Vet J* 3:215-216, 1997.

607. Dennis SM, Leipold HW: Anencephaly in sheep, *Cornell Vet* 62:273-281, 1972.

608. Whittington RJ et al: Congenital hydranencephaly and arthrogryposis of Corriedale sheep, *Aust Vet J* 65:124-127, 1988.

609. Parsonson IM, Della-Porta AJ, Snowdon WA: Akabane virus infection in the pregnant ewe. 2. Pathology of the foetus, *Vet Microbiol* 6:209-224, 1981.

610. Gruber AD et al: Brain malformations in ovine fetuses associated with cytopathic biotype of bovine viral-diarrhoea virus, *J Vet Med B* 42:443-447, 1995.

611. Dennis SM: Congenital defects of the nervous system of lambs, *Aust Vet J* 51:385-388, 1975.

612. Kohli RN: Congenital meningocele with a rare skull defect in a lamb, *Aust Vet J* 76:252, 1998.

613. Roth IJ et al: Holoprosencephaly in Border Leicester lambs, *Aust Vet J* 64:271-273, 1987.

614. Pritchard GC et al: Multiple cases of Dandy-Walker malformation in three sheep flocks, *Vet Rec* 115:163-164, 1994.

615. Akker S van den: Arnold-Chiari malformation in animals, *Acta Neuropathol* 1(suppl):39-44, 1962.

616. Hughes KL, Haughey KG, Hartley WJ: Spontaneous congenital developmental abnormalities observed at necropsy in a large survey of newly born dead lambs, *Teratology* 5:5-10, 1972.

617. White RG, Rowlands WT: A hereditary defect of newly born lambs, *Vet Rec* 57:451-452, 1945.

618. Innes JRM, Rowlands WT, Parry HB: An inherited form of cortical cerebellar atrophy in ("daft") lambs in Great Britain, *Vet Rec* 61:225-228, 1949.

619. Innes JRM, MacNaughton WN: Inherited cortical cerebellar atrophy in Corriedale lambs in Canada identical with "daft lamb" disease in Britain, *Cornell Vet* 40:127-135, 1950.

620. de Lahunta A: Abiotrophy in domestic animals: a review, *Can J Vet Res* 54:65-76, 1990.

621. Harper PAW et al: Cerebellar abiotrophy and segmental axonopathy: two syndromes of progressive ataxia of Merino sheep, *Aust Vet J* 63:18-21, 1981.

622. Milne EM, Schock A: Cerebellar abiotrophy in a pedigree Charolais sheep flock, *Vet Rec* 143:224-225, 1998.

623. Bourke CA, Carrigan MJ, Dent CHR: Chronic locomotor dysfunction, associated with a thalamic-cerebellar neuropathy, in Australian Merino sheep, *Aust Vet J* 70:232-233, 1993.

624. Manktelow BW, Hartley WJ, Gill JM: A presumed inherited spongiform leucoencephalomyelopathy of Romney lambs in New Zealand, *N Z Vet J* 45:199-201, 1997.

625. David GP, Holmes JP: Neurological condition in polled Dorset lambs, *Vet Rec* 141:27, 1997.

626. Harper PAW, Morton AG: Neuraxonal dystrophy in Merino sheep, *Aust Vet J* 68:152-153, 1991.

627. Harper PAW et al: Progressive ataxia associated with degenerative thoracic myelopathy in Merino sheep, *Aust Vet J* 63:18-21, 1981.

628. Hartley WJ, Loomis LN: Murrurundi disease: an encephalopathy of sheep, *Aust Vet J* 57:399-400, 1981.

629. Hartley WJ, Kater JC: Observations on diseases of the central nervous system of sheep in New Zealand, *N Z Vet J* 10:128-142, 1962.

630. Prieur DJ et al: Inheritance of an ovine lysosomal storage disease associated with deficiencies of β-galactosidase and α-neuraminidase, *J Hered* 81:245-249, 1990.

631. Murnane RD, Hartley WJ, Prieur DJ: Similarity of lectin histochemistry of a lysosomal storage disease in a New Zealand lamb to that of ovine GM₁ gangliosidosis, *Vet Pathol* 28:332-335, 1991.

632. Murnane RD et al: Clinical and clinicopathologic characteristics of ovine GM-1 gangliosidosis, *J Vet Int Med* 8:221-223, 1994.

633. Skelly BJ et al: A new form of ovine GM1-gangliosidosis, *Acta Neuropath* 89:374-379, 1995.

634. Woods PR et al: Neuronal ceroid lipofuscinosis in Rambouillet sheep: characterization of the clinical disease, *J Vet Intern Med* 8:370-375, 1994.

635. Jolly RD et al: Ovine ceroid-lipofuscinosis is a proteolipid proteinosis, *Can J Vet Res* 54:15-21, 1990.

636. Jolly RD et al: Ceroid-lipofuscinosis (Batten's disease): pathogenesis and sequential neuropathological changes in the ovine model, *Neuropathol Appl Neurobiol* 15:371-383, 1989.

637. Edwards JF et al: Juvenile-onset neuronal ceroid-lipofuscinosis in Rambouillet sheep, *Vet Pathol* 31:48-54, 1991.

638. Oberst RD: Viruses as teratogens, *Vet Clin North Am (Food Anim Pract)* 9:23-31, 1993.

639. Sharp MW, Rawson BC: The cost of border disease infection in a commercial flock, *Vet Rec* 119:128-130, 1986.

640. Adalsteinson S, Basrur PK: Inheritance of spina bifida in Icelandic lambs, *J Hered* 75:378-382, 1984.

641. Davies IH: Spina bifida in lambs, *Vet Rec* 132:90-91, 1993.

642. Braund KG et al: Congenital hypomyelination neuropathy in a lamb, *Vet Pathol* 30:577-579, 1993.

643. Suttle NF: Copper deficiency in ruminants: recent developments, *Vet Rec* 119:519-522, 1986.

644. McManus TJ: Report of entropion in newborn lambs, *Aust Vet J* 30:237-240, 1960.

645. Littlejohn AI: Entropion in newborn lambs, *Vet Rec* 66:211-215, 1954.

646. Taylor M, Catchpole J: Incidence of entropion in lambs from two ewe flocks put to the same rams, *Vet Rec* 118:361, 1986.

647. Lamprecht H, Pfeiffer A: Das Entropium bei neugeborenen Lammern, *Berl Munch Tierarztl Wschr* 102:303-310, 1989.

648. Shams-u-Din M: A technique for correction of entropion in lambs, *Small Ruminant Res* 8:179-182, 1992.

649. Sakul H, Snowder GD, Hemenway KJ: Evaluation of techniques for correction of entropion in lambs, *Sm Ruminant Res* 20:187-191, 1996.

650. Sakul H, Kellom TR: Heritability of entropion in several US sheep breeds, *Sm Ruminant Res* 23:187-190, 1996.

651. Green LE, Berriatua E, Morgan KL: The prevalence and risk factors for congenital entropion in intensively reared lambs in south west England, *Prev Vet Med* 24:15-21, 1995.

652. Littlejohn A: A defect of the upper eyelid in a flock of piebald sheep, *Vet Rec* 85:185-190, 1969.

653. Brooks HV et al: An inherited cataract in New Zealand Romney sheep, *NZ Vet J* 30:113-114, 1982.

654. Sangamwar UY, Parihar NS, Sharma AK: Spontaneously occurring lesions in uvea, retina, lens and optic nerve in eyes of sheep and goats, *Indian J Anim Sci* 67:1051-1054, 1997.

655. Rae AL: The genetics of sheep, *Adv Genet* 7:189-265, 1956.

656. Ritzman EG: Breeding earless sheep, *J Hered* 11:238-240, 1920.

657. Nel JA, Louw DJ: The lethal factor in grey Karakul lambs, *Farm S Afr* 5:168-172, 1953.

658. Groenewald HB, Booth KK: A comparative histological study of the number and size of the myenteric ganglia and neurones in the forestomach and abomasum of grey, white and black Karakul lambs, *Onderstepoort J Vet Res* 59:103-106, 1992.

659. Groenewald HB, Booth KK: A comparative study of the thickness of the tunica muscularis in the forestomach and abomasum of grey, white and black Karakul lambs, *Onderstepoort J Vet Res* 59:225-227, 1992.

660. Groenewald HB: Ultrastructure of the myenteric ganglia in the rumen, reticulum, omasum and abomasum of grey, white and black Karakul lambs, *Onderstepoort J Vet Res* 60:189-195, 1993.

661. Robinson R: Genetic defects in sheep, *Agri Pract* 14:22-25, 1993.

662. Blair HT: Inheritance of a major gene of excessively lustrous wool in sheep, *J Hered* 81:220-222, 1990.
663. Warwick BL et al: "Silky," a dominant mutation in sheep, *J Hered* 51:39-42, 1960.
664. Dolling CHS, Brooker MG: A viable hypotrichosis in poll Dorset sheep, *J Hered* 57:87-90, 1988.
665. Mackie JT, McIntire B: Congenital hypotrichosis in poll Dorset sheep, *Aust Vet J* 69:146-147, 1992.
666. Tontis A, Hufstetter H: Epitheliogenesis imperfecta beim Lamm, *Schweiz Arch Tierhlkde* 133:287-289, 1991.
667. Munday BL: Epitheliogenesis imperfecta in lambs and kittens, *Br Vet J* XLVII:126, 1970.
668. Al-Ani FK, Al-Darraji AM, Hamad RM: Epitheliogenesis imperfecta in a flock of Awassi sheep in Iraq, *Sm Ruminant Res* 17:283-285, 1995.
669. Alley MR, O'Hara PJ, Middleberg A: An epidermiolysis bullosa of sheep, *N Z Vet J* 22:55-59, 1974.
670. Ehrensperger F, Hauser B, Wild P: Epidermolysis bullosa beim Schaflamm, *Tierarztl Umsch* 42:697-700, 1987.
671. Helle O, Nes NN: A hereditary skin defect in sheep, *Acta Vet Scand* 13:443-445, 1972.
672. Fjolstad M, Helle O: A hereditary dysplasia of collagen in sheep, *J Pathol* 112:183-188, 1974.
673. McOrist S et al: Ovine skin collagen dysplasia, *Aust Vet J* 59:189-190, 1982.
674. Atroshi F et al: A heritable disorder of collagen tissue in Finnish cross-bred sheep, *Zentralbl Vet Med* 30:233-241, 1983.
675. Dennis SM, Leipold HW: Congenital cardiac defects in lambs, *Am J Vet Res* 29:2337-2340, 1968.
676. Dennis SM: Holocardius acephalus monster in a sheep, *Vet Rec* 77:1289-1290, 1965.
677. Dunn HO, Roberts SJ: Chromosome studies of an ovine acephalic-acardiac monster, *Cornell Vet* 62:425, 428-431, 1972.
678. Dominguez L et al: Anomalous thoracic venous and arterial patterns in a sheep, *Vet Rec* 132:91-92, 1993.
679. Shivaprakash BV, Gopalakrishna Rao D: Local anaesthetic toxicity in a sheep with patent ductus arteriosus, *Indian Vet J* 74: 901-902, 1997.
680. Fecteau G et al: Dysfibrinogenemia or afibrinogenemia in a Border Leicester lamb, *Can Vet J* 38:443-444, 1997.
681. Dennis SM, Leipold HW: Atresia ani in sheep, *Vet Rec* 91:219-222, 1972.
682. Leipold HW, Dennis SM: Atresia jejuni in a lamb, *Vet Rec* 93:644-645, 1973.
683. Sharma AK, Pairhar NS, Tripathi BN: Atresia jejuni in a lamb, *Indian J Vet Pathol* 21:65-66, 1997.
684. Dennis SM, Sheldon HD: Atresia ilei in a lamb, *Vet Rec* 89:254, 1971.
685. Gabb K, Lofstead I, Bildfell R: Abomasal emptying defect in a ewe of predominantly Dorset breeding, *Vet Rec* 131:127-128, 1992.
686. McFarland LZ: Perineal hypospadia in male lambs, *J Am Vet Med Assoc* 133:81-82, 1958.
687. Dennis SM: Hypospadias in Merino lambs, *Vet Rec* 105:94-96, 1979.
688. Dennis SM: Urogenital defects in sheep, *Vet Rec* 105:304-307, 1979.
689. Jones TO et al: A vertically transmitted cystic renal dysplasia of lambs, *Vet Rec* 127:421-424, 1990.
690. O'Toole D et al: Pathology of renal dysplasia and bladder aplasia-hypoplasia in a flock of sheep, *J Vet Diagn Invest* 5:591-602, 1993.
691. Dennis SM: Patent urachus in a neonatal lambs, *Cornell Vet* 59:581-584, 1969.
692. Rac R et al: Congenital goitre in Merino sheep due to an inherited defect in the biosynthesis of thyroid hormone, *Res Vet Sci* 9:209-223, 1968.
693. Hancock J: Congenital photosensitivity in Southdown sheep: a new sublethal factor in sheep, *N Z J Sci Tech* 16:24, 1950.
694. Cornelius CE, Arias IM, Osburn BI: Hepatic pigmentation with photosensitivity: a syndrome in Corriedale sheep resembling Dubin-Johnson syndrome in man, *J Am Vet Med Assoc* 146:709-713, 1965.
695. Cornelius CE, Gronwall RR: Congenital photosensitivity and hyperbilirubinemia in Southdown sheep in the United States, *J Am Vet Res* 29:291-295, 1968.
696. McGavin MD, Cornelius CE, Gronwall RR: Lesions in Southdown sheep with hereditary hyperbilirubinemia, *Vet Pathol* 9:142-151, 1972.
697. Stevenson RG: Pancreatic cysts in lambs, *Res Sci* 13:267-268, 1972.
698. Dennis SM: Congenital splenic defects in newborn lambs, *Cornell Vet* 62:473-476, 1972.
699. Harper PAW, Plant JW, Unger DB: Congenital biliary atresia and jaundice and lambs and calves, *Aust Vet J* 67:18-22, 1990.
700. Reddy PK, Radhakrishniah K: Bi-lobed gall bladder in a ewe, *Indian Vet J* 73:789-790, 1996.
701. Dennis SM, Leipold HW: Congenital hernias in sheep, *J Am Vet Med Assoc* 152:999-1003, 1968.
702. Fazilli, M: Congenital intestinal prolapse in a lamb, *Indian Vet J* 75:943-944, 1998.
703. Carr PM: An apparently inherited inguinal hernia in the Merino ram, *Aust Vet J* 48:126-127, 1972.
704. Egwu GO, Adamu SS, Usman HS: Congenital hypogenitalia and imperforate anus complicated by perineal herniation in a Nigerian Yankasa lamb, *Bull Anim Hlth Prod Afr* 42:153-155, 1994.
705. Dennis SM, Meyer EP: Schistosomus reflexus in a sheep, *Vet Rec* 77:1386-1388, 1965.
706. Smith ID: Schistosomus reflexus in the sheep, *Vet Rec* 85:138-139, 1969.
707. Wani NA, Wani GM, Bhat AS: Schistosomus reflexus in a Corriedale sheep, *Small Ruminant Res* 14:95-97, 1994.
708. Claxton JH, Yeates NTM: The inheritance of cryptorchidism in a small crossbred flock of sheep, *J Hered* 63:141-144, 1972.
709. Blackshaw AW, Samisoni JI: The testes of the cryptorchid ram, *Res Vet Sci* 8:187-194, 1967.
710. Galloway DB et al: An outbreak of gonadal hypoplasia in a sheep flock: clinical, pathological and endocrinological features, and aetiological studies, *Vet Rec* 131:506-512, 1992.
711. McEntee K: *Reproductive pathology in domestic animals*, Academic Press, 1990, New York.
712. Ladds PW: Congenital anomalies of the genitalia of cattle, sheep, goats and pigs, *Vet Clin North Am (Food Anim Pract)* 9:127-144, 1993.
713. Degen AA, Rubin ED: Partial duplication of the male urogenital system in a Merino ram, *Res Vet Sci* 16:95-97, 1974.
714. Smith KC, Long SE, Parkinson TJ: Abattoir survey of congenital reproductive abnormalities in ewes, *Vet Rec* 143:679-685, 1998.
715. Vaughan EK et al: Ovarian hypoplasia in Lleyn ewes, *Vet Rec* 140:100-101, 1997.
716. Davis GH, Bruce GD, Reid PJ: Breeding implications of the streak ovary condition in homozygous (FecX¹/FecX¹) Inverdale sheep, *Proceedings of the Fifth World Congress on Genetics Applied to Livestock Production*, University of Guelph, Guelph, Ontario, 1994, pp 249-252.
717. Smith KC, Long SE, Parkinson TJ: Congenital abnormalities of the ovine paramesonephric ducts, *Br Vet J* 151:443-452, 1995.
718. Alexander G, Williams D: Ovine freemartins, *Nature* 201:1296-1298, 1964.
719. Gerneke WH: Chromosomal evidence of the freemartin condition in sheep—Ovis aries, *Afr Vet Med Assoc* 36:99-104, 1965.
720. Spedding RN, Dobson H: Diagnosis of freemartinism in sheep, *Vet Rec* 123:18-19, 1989.
721. Long, SE: Chromosome abnormalities in domestic sheep *(Ovis aries)*, *J Appl Genet* 38:65-76, 1997.
722. Bruere AN: Male sterility and an autosomal translocation in Romney sheep, *Cytogenetics* 8:209-218, 1969.
723. Bruere AN: Some clinical aspects of hypo-orchidism (small testes) in the ram, *NZ Vet J* 18:189-198, 1970.
724. Bruere AN: The segregation patterns and fertility of sheep heterozygous and homozygous for three different Robertsonian translocations, *J Reprod Fertil* 41:453-464, 1974.
725. Bruere AN, Chapman HM: Double translocation heterozygosity and normal fertility in domestic sheep, *Cytogenet Cell Genet* 13:342-351, 1974.
726. Bruere AN: Further evidence of normal fertility and the formation of balanced gametes in sheep with one or more different Robertsonian translocations, *J Reprod Fertil* 45:323-331, 1975.
727. Bruere AN, Mills RA: Observations on the incidence of Robertsonian translocations and associated testicular changes in a flock of New Zealand Romney sheep, *Cytogenetics* 10:260-272, 1974.
728. Bruere AN, Marshall RB, Ward DPJ: Testicular hypoplasia and XXY sex chromosome complement in two rams: the ovine counterpart of Klinefelter's syndrome in man, *J Reprod Fertil* 19:103-108, 1969.
729. Bruere AN, Kilgour R: Normal behaviour patterns and libido in chromatin-positive Klinefelter sheep, *Vet Rec* 95:437-440, 1974.
730. Bruere AN, McDonald MF, Marshall RB: Cytogenetical analysis of an ovine male pseudohermaphrodite and the possible role of the Y chromosome in cryptorchidism of sheep, *Cytogenetics* 8:148-157, 1969.
731. Fayrer-Hosken RA et al: Infertility in a ewe as a result of ovotestis, *J Am Vet Med Assoc* 200:1528-1529, 1992.
732. Ahmed YF: A case of intersex in sheep, *Vet Med J Giza* 45:89-93, 1997.
733. Luft B von: Autosomale Deletion bei zwei Mutterschafen und bei zwei Bocken mit Brachygnathia superior, *Dtsch Tierarztl Wschr* 79:327-330, 1972.

CONGENITAL DEFECTS AND HEREDITARY DISEASES IN GOATS

GEORGE SAPERSTEIN
EUGENE C. WHITE

CAUSES OF DEFECTS AND DISORDERS

Congenital defects may be caused by environmental factors, genetic factors, and their interaction; many have no clearly established cause.

Environmental Factors

Suspected teratogens in goats include toxic plants, viruses, drugs, trace elements, and physical agents.[734-750]

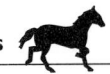

PLANTS. A variety of plants may cause congenital defects in goats. Perhaps the most infamous is the development of cyclopia in kids whose dams ingest *Veratrum californicum* in days 13 and 14 of gestation.[736] The feeding of *Veratrum californicum* during gestation may also result in other malformations of the skull, absence of the pituitary or brain malformations, brachygnathia, and hypoplasia of the metacarpal and metatarsal bones.[736,764]

Other plants have been shown to act as teratogens in the goat. Ingestion of piperidine alkaloid-containing plants such as *Conium* seed and *Nicotiana glauca* has been reported to cause multiple congenital contractures and cleft palate.[737,738] Cleft palate can be induced by feeding these plants between days 35 and 41 of gestation, whereas cleft palate along with limb defects result when ingestion is between days 30 and 60 of gestation.[739,740]

VIRAL INFECTIONS. Viral teratogens of the goat include Akabane virus and Border disease virus. Akabane viral infections in pregnant dams may lead to abortion, premature birth, stillbirth, or the birth of live kids with congenital defects including hydranencephaly and arthrogryposis.[744] Border disease viral infection may lead to infertility, abortions, stillbirths, or the birth of live kids with rhythmic muscle tremors most prominent in the hindquarters.[764] Hair coat abnormalities have not been described with Border disease virus infection in kids.[764]

FREQUENCY. Determining the exact frequency of congenital defects in goats is difficult. However, two studies have attempted to address this question. During a 2-year period, 56 of 1092 neonatal kids were afflicted with malformations.[734] These defects in Saanen and Saanen crossbreeds were: abnormal hair, 2; atresia ani, 2; cleft palate, 4; conjoined twins, 2; cryptorchidism, 8; flexed pastern, 3; intersexuality, 19; parrot mouth, 7; polythelia, 3; schistosomus reflexum, 2; and anotia, brachyury, hairless, one kid each.[734] Another survey over an 8-year period found 211 of 1130 neonatal kids with congenital defects in the Shami breed.[793] The anomalies included cases of the following: 89 congenital goiter, 29 thyroglossal duct cysts, 14 hypospadias, 57 hermaphroditism, 19 atresia ani, 2 polydactyly, and 1 ectopic horns.[793]

Genetic Causes

Inherited disorders in the goat may be monogenic, but many appear to be polygenic.[734,735] Repeated use of popular sires with abnormal genes will increase the frequency of these defects. The basic rules discussed for cattle and sheep apply here as well. Abnormalities of chromosomes, such as translocations, create meiotic disturbances that lead in the majority of the cases to subfertility. Aneuploidy of sex chromosomes usually leads to sterility.[746-748]

CONTROL

If a defective kid is submitted, the history should include breed, age of parents, parentage of affected and unaffected control kids, geographic region, season, type of pasture, soil type, exposure to or suspected exposure to teratogenic plants, feeding and management practices, breeding records, maternal medical and vaccination records, disease status of farm during periods of stress, drugs administered, congenital defects observed previously, and history of any similar congenital defects on neighboring farms. Breeding records should be analyzed for evidence of inbreeding and for characteristic intergenerational transmission patterns and intragenerational frequencies. Necropsies are done, and defects are classified by the body system primarily involved. Serum samples from does should be submitted to check for BVD and other viral antibodies. Samples of brain and other tissues are taken for virus isolation. Histopathologic examination is done, and selected cases are submitted for electron microscopic studies.

DIAGNOSIS OF SPECIFIC DEFECTS IN GOATS

Three principal classifications have been used: etiologic, affected embryonic tissue, and principal defective body system. The last classification is used in this review. Tables 47-48 to 47-57 define defects of various body systems in kids, placing emphasis on defects of current interest and concern.

REFERENCES

734. Basrur PK: Congenital abnormalities of the goat, *Vet Clin North Am (Food Anim Pract)* 9:183-202, 1993.
735. Basrur PK, Yadav BR: Genetic diseases of sheep and goat, *Vet Clin North Am (Food Anim Pract)* 6:779-802, 1990.
736. Binns W, Keeler RF, Balls LD: Congenital deformities in lambs, calves and goats resulting from maternal ingestion of *Veratrum californicum*: hare lip, cleft palate, ataxia and hypoplasia of metacarpal and metatarsal bones, *Clin Toxicol* 5:245-261, 1972.
737. Panter KE et al: Multiple congenital contractures (MCC) and cleft palate induced in goats by ingestion of piperidine alkaloid-containing plants: reduction in fetal movement as the probable cause, *Clin Toxicol* 28:69-83, 1990.
738. Panter KE et al: Congenital skeletal malformations and cleft palate induced in goats by ingestion of *Lupinus, Conium* and *Nicotiana* species, *Toxicon* 28:1377-1380, 1990.
739. Panter KE, Keeler RF: Induction of cleft palate in goats by *Nicotiana glauca* during a narrow gestational period and the relation to reduction in fetal movement, *J Natural Toxins* 1:25-32, 1992.
740. Panter KE, Keeler RF: Quinolizidine and piperidine alkaloid teratogens from poisonous plants and their mechanism of action in animals, *Vet Clin North Am (Food Anim Pract)* 9:33-40, 1993.
741. Depner KR et al: Transplazentare Virusübertragung nach experimenteller Inokulation von Ziegen in unterschiedlichen Trächtigkeitsstadien, *Dtsch Tierärztl Wschr* 97:421-423, 1990.
742. Depner KR, Hübschle OJB, Liess B: BVD-virus infection in goats: experimental studies on placental transmissibility of the virus and its effect on reproduction, *Arch Virol* 3(suppl):253-256, 1991.
743. Loken T, Bjerkas I: Experimental pestivirus infections in pregnant goats, *J Comp Pathol* 105:123-140, 1991.
744. Inaba Y, Kurogi H, Omori T: Akabane disease: epizootic abortion, premature birth, stillbirth and congenital arthrogrypsis-hydranencephaly in cattle, sheep and goats caused by Akabane virus, *Aust Vet J* 51:584-585, 1975.
745. Singh AP: Congenital malformations in ruminants: a review of 123 cases, *Indian Vet J* 66:981-985, 1989.
746. Ricordeau G: Genetics: breeding plan. In Gall C, ed: *Goat production*, London, England, 1981, Academic Press, pp 111-169.
747. Eldridge F: *Cytogenetics of livestock*, Westport, Conn, 1985, Avi.
748. Long SE: Chromosome abnormalities in goats, *Adv Vet Sci Comp Med* 34:120-125, 1990.
749. Koch P, Fischer H, Schumann H: *Erbpathologie der landwirtschaftlichen Haustiere*, Berlin, Germany, 1957, P. Parey.
750. Wiesner E, Willer E: *Veterinarmedizinische Pathogenetik*, Jena, Germany, 1974, J Fischer.
751. Hamori D: Constitutinal disorders and hereditary diseases in domestic animals, New York, 1983, Elsevier.
752. Venugopal R. Madhavan E, Alikutty KM: Congenital skeletal defect in a cross-bred kid, *J Vet Animal Sci,* 26:70-71, 1995.
753. Fischer H: Ein Beitrag zur Genetik der Brachygnathia superior bei der Ziege, *Hemora Zoa* 62:17-27, 1955.
754. Naus AH: The presence of congenital undesirable defects in purebred males and females imported to Chile (1979-1981). *Proceedings of the Third International Conference on Goat Production and Disease,* Tucson, Ariz, 1982, p 547.
755. El-Hariri MNE, Shawki S: Amelia and hemimelia in two goats, *J Egypt Vet Med Assoc* 40:89-98, 1980.
756. Gupta SC, Tyer PKR: Congenital aplasia of limb in a kid, *Indian Vet Med J* 8:129, 1984.
757. Deniz E, Eker M: Kilis X saanen melezindeki ilginc bilateral perodactylie olayi uzerinde incelemeler, *Veteriner Fakultesi Dergisi* 14:211-225, 1967.
758. Onawunmi OA, Smith OB, Munyabuntu CM: Deformed goat birth, *Vet Rec* 105:359, 1979.
759. Giddings RF: Tibial agenesis in a Toggenburg kid, *J Am Vet Med Assoc* 169:1306-1307, 1976.
760. Nielsen JS, Arnbjerg J: Hereditary peromelia in Mohair goats, *J Vet Med A* 39:147-151, 1992.
761. Baum K, Hull BL, Weisbrode SE: Radial agenesis and ulnar hypoplasia in two caprine kids, *J Am Vet Med Assoc* 186:170-171, 1985.
762. Ramadam RO: Agenesis of the radius in a goat, *Agri Pract* 15:33-34, 1994.

Text continued on p. 1554

TABLE 47-48

Congenital Defects of the Skeleton in the Goat

Defect	Reference No.	Description	Etiology	Frequency	Diagnosis	Associated Defects
Brachygnathia superior (monkey mouth)	735, 746, 753, 754	Short upper jaw; lip end of dental plate above the incisor teeth, various degrees	Recessive trait in Etawah and Katjang breeds of Java, other breeds unknown	Very common in Etawah, Katjang, and Nubian; very rare in other breeds	Physical examination	None
Brachygnathia inferior	746, 750-752	Undershot lower jaw	Considered to be recessive	Rare	Physical examination	None; sometimes associated with amelias, scoliosis, and arthrogryposis
Cleft palate	734, 735, 738, 775	Nonclosure of palate; milk may run from nose	Unknown; plants	Rare Reported in Saanen goats	Physical examination	Contractures
Monobrachia	755, 756	Absence of one front leg	Unknown	Very rare	Physical examination	None
Monopodia	757, 758	Absence of one hind leg	Unknown	Very rare	Physical examination	None
Tibial agenesis	757, 759	Unilateral or bilateral absence of tibia; kids are unable to get up	Unknown	Very rare	Physical examination, x-ray	None
Perodactyly	755	Absence of one or more digits	Unknown	Very rare	Physical examination, x-ray	None
Peromelia	755, 760	Agenesis of phalanges and parts of metatarsus, variable expression	Recessive in Danish Mohair goats; other breeds unknown	Rare	Physical examination, x-ray	None
Radial agenesis and ulnar hypoplasia	761, 762	Bilateral absence of radius, small ulnas; contracture of front limbs	Unknown	Rare	Physical examination, x-ray	Patent ductus arteriosus
Lateral luxation of patella	763-765	Due to hypoplasia of lateral trochlear ridge; clinical signs begin after 1 year; surgical repair is possible; animals keep stifle and hock flexed, lameness is progressive, displaced patella is palpable	Unknown	Unknown	Physical examination	None
Hemivertebra	766	Weakness in rear legs, progress to recumbency; posterior ataxia, hemivertebra of T4	Unknown; reported in a Saanen	Unknown	Physical examination	None
Spina bifida	767	Absence of dorsal spinous processes in lumbar area	Unknown	Rare	Physical examination, necropsy	Small tail, ankylosis of forelimbs
Brachyury	734	Short tail	Unknown	Rare	Physical examination	None reported

Defect	Page	Description	Cause	Diagnosis	Occurrence	Associated defects
Dwarfism	735, 746, 768	Several types of dwarfism exist in various parts of the world; some are considered pituitary dwarfs or proportionate, others are affected with achondroplasia, short limbs, and long trunk	Genetic, mostly recessive; achondroplasia is due to an incompletely dominant gene	Physical examination	Common in populations of Africa and Asia; others rare	None
Dicephalus	770-772	Two heads	Unknown	Physical examination	Rare	None
Cyclops	736, 773, 774, 775	Single orbit with one eye, nose is a tube	Ingestion of *Veratrum californicum* on days 13 and 14 of gestation	Physical examination	Rare	Brachygnathia superior, hypoplasia of metacarpal and metatarsal bones
Multiple anomalies	776	Dipygus (doubled posterior extremities); tetrabrachius (four hind legs); rachischisis (fissure in spinal column); born cotwin to a normal kid, causes dystoia	Unknown	Physical examination	One case reported	Polydactyly
Schistosomus reflexus	735, 777-779	Severe abdominal fissure with exposure of abdominal viscera	Unknown	Physical examination	Rare	Arthrogryposis
Polydactyly	780	Two extra digits on both hind limbs; forelimbs normal	Unknown	Physical examination	Reported in sire and daughter in Shami breed	None
Cranioschisis	781	Incomplete closure of skull due to failure of development of frontal bones	Nonclosure of anterior portion of neural tube	Physical examination	Rare	None
Monocephalus diprosopus triophthalmus diotus	782	One cranial vault, two upper and lower jaws, two ears, and three eyes	Unknown	Physical examination	Rare	None
Angular limb deformities	765	Valgus or varus deformities of appendicular skeleton	Uterine malposition, incomplete carpal/tarsal cuboidal bone ossification, nutritional imbalances, teratogenic plants	Physical examination, radiographs	Rare	None
Perosomus horridus	783	S-shaped vertebral column, fused sacral and coccygeal vertebrae, abdominal fissure, and ankylosis of hind legs	Unknown	Physical examination	Rare	None
Perosomus elumbis	784	Partial agenesis of lumbar spine and spinal cord with corresponding muscle atrophy	Unknown	Physical examination	Rare	Atresia ani; rectovaginal fistula
Monocephalus thoracopagus tetrabrachius monster	785	Conjoined twin united at sternum sharing one heart, neck and head; separate abdominal cavities and four legs	Unknown	Physical examination	Rare	None

TABLE 47-49

Congenital Defects of the Ear and Skin in the Goat

Defect	Reference No.	Description	Etiology	Frequency	Diagnosis	Associated Defects
Anotia and microtia	734, 735, 786, 787	Ear length is an incompletely dominant trait in goats; normal ears are about 10 cm long, heterozygotes are 30% of normal length; earless sheep are deaf; the basis of this deafness is not known; it is not known if La Mancha goats are hearing impaired	Genetic, incompletely dominant trait	Breed characteristic in La Mancha; others rare	Physical examination	None
Curled ears	734, 749	Pinna of ear curves upward	Dominant	Rare	Physical examination	None
Wattles	788-790	One or both sides of various sizes; presence of wattles has no association with economic traits, except Alpine goats with wattles had significantly longer lactation period	Dominant trait	Common	Physical examination	None
Wattle cysts (dermoid cysts, branchial cleft cysts)	764, 791	Unilateral or bilateral fluid filled cysts of wattle	Unknown	Common	Physical examination	None
Hairlessness	734, 764	Congenital alopecia	Autosomal recessive	Rare	Physical examination	None
Sticky kid syndrome	764	Wet mottled coat which will not dry	Possibly recessive	Golden Guernsey goats	Physical examination	None
Thyroglossal duct cyst	792-794	Fluid-filled cyst on the midline of the throat, ventral to hyoid bone and root of tongue; appearing around 2 months of age	Cystic remnant of thyroglossal duct	Rare	Physical examination, surgical examination	None
Ectopic horns	793, 795	Horns growing in abnormal location	Unknown	Rare	Physical examination	None

TABLE 47-50

Congenital Defects of the Central Nervous and Ocular Systems in the Goat

Defect	Reference No.	Description	Etiology	Frequency	Diagnosis	Associated Defects
β-Mannosidase deficiency	769, 796-800	Facial dysmorphism, joint contractures, dome-shaped skulls, unable to rise at birth, intention tremors, pendular nystagmus, atrophy of muscles of front and hind legs; histopathology shows vacuolation of cytoplasm in neural tissues, eye, kidneys, pancreas, lymph nodes; paucity of myelin; affected kids have no β-mannosidase activity	Simple autosomal recessive in Nubian goats	Nubian goats only	Clinical examination, histopathology, study of β-mannosidase activity; zero plasma β-mannosidase–affected goats, reduced in heterozygotes	None
N-Acetylglucoseamine 6-sulfatase deficiency	801	Neonatal neurologic disorder	Genetic	One case reported in a Nubian kid	Molecular studies of tissues	None reported
Abiotrophy (progressive paresis)	802	Developed ataxia 4 months old; clinical signs progressed to paresis; sternal recumbency; no gross lesions, vacuoles in cytoplasm of neurons of midbrain, spinal cord, secondary myelin degeneration	Possibly genetic	Rare	Neurologic examination, histopathology	None
Retinal degeneration (retinal abiotrophy)	803, 804	Blind at birth; generalized tapetal hyperreflectivity, diffuse photoreceptor, and outer nuclear layer atrophy	Possibly genetic, Toggenburg	Rare	Ophthalmoscopic examination, histopathology	None

Continued

TABLE 47-50

Congenital Defects of the Central Nervous and Ocular Systems in the Goat—cont'd

Defect	Reference No.	Description	Etiology	Frequency	Diagnosis	Associated Defects
Enzootic ataxia (swayback)	764	Progressive ataxia, paresis, then paralysis; onset between 1 and 28 weeks of age	Maternal copper deficiency	Common	Clinical signs; absolute or relative copper deficiency; sometimes decreased blood or liver copper; neuronal degeneration, demyelination in brainstem and spinal cord	None
Internal hydrocephalus	764, 805	Increased cerebrospinal fluid pressure causing dilation of lateral ventricles and cerebral cortical atrophy	Unknown; Akabane virus in some cases	Rare	Necropsy, kids are either born dead or are weak, blind, and recumbent with rhythmic tremors especially in hindquarters	None
Entropion	764	Turning inward of lower or both eyelids	Unknown	Rare	Physical examination, repair is possible	None
Hydranencephaly Spastic paresis	764, 808	See Arthrogryposis Hyperextension of hind leg due to spastic contracture of gastrocnemius muscle	Unknown	Rare, reported in Saanen and Pygmy	Physical examination	None
Anophthalmia	806, 807	Absence of eyeballs	Unknown	Rare	Physical examination	Prognathism

TABLE 47-51

Congenital Defects of the Muscular System in the Goat

Defect	Reference No.	Description	Etiology	Frequency	Diagnosis	Associated Defects
Myotonia congenita (fainting goat syndrome)	769, 809-813	Possible signs shortly after birth; attack provoked by noise or fright; kid trying to escape, rigid position, falls to one side, muscles of back legs become rigid for 40 sec; primary lesion: cytomembrane defect affecting calcium homeostasis	Occurs in different breeds of goats; in some lines it is a dominant analogous to a condition reported in humans; recessive in other breeds	Common	Clinical examination, electromyography	None
Tendon contracture ("knuckling")	745, 765, 788	Overflexion of front limbs, may be repaired by flexor tenotomy and casting	Unknown; possibly uterine malposition or teratogens	Uncommon	Physical examination	None
Arthrogryposis	744, 764, 765	Permanent contracture of limbs in flexion or extension	Prenatal Akabane, BT, BD, or CV virus infections; lupine	Reported in Asia, Africa, Middle East, and Australia	Serology, necropsy, histopath on muscle and central nervous system	Abortion, hydranencephaly, scoliosis, blindness, torticollis, kyphosis, cerebellar hypoplasia
Umbilical hernia	764	Lack of closure of umbilical ring, may be repaired surgically (large defect) or reduced with elastic tape (small defect)	Unknown	Rare	Physical examination	None

TABLE 47-52

Congenital Defects of the Blood in the Goat

Defect	Reference No.	Description	Etiology	Frequency	Diagnosis	Associated Defects
Afibrinogenemia	769, 815	Hemorrhagic diathesis with joint bleeding, subcutaneous and mucosal hemorrhages, prolonged bleeding time; homozygous condition causes complete absence of fibrinogen; heterozygous goats have reduced fibrinogen	Incompletely dominant	Rare, reported only in Saanen	Physical examination, studies of blood coagulation, may present as persistent umbilical bleeding; fibrinogen levels	Skeletal changes, multiple bone cysts
Myelofibrosis	816	Proliferation of fibroblasts and deposition of collagen in bone marrow, leading to progressive anemia and neutropenia	Genetic	Reported in 11 of 16 pygmy goats from 7 litters	CBC, biopsy, necropsy	None

TABLE 47-53

Congenital Defects of the Endocrine System in the Goat

Defect	Reference No.	Description	Etiology	Frequency	Diagnosis	Associated Defects
Goiter	764, 793, 817-822	Affected goats are born weak, have growth retardation, sparse hair-coat, thick and scaly skin, myxedema of subcutis, enlarged thyroids, no thyroglobulin; animals respond clinically to thyroxine	Simple autosomal recessive; Saanen dwarf goats; also reported in some clinically normal Boer goats; may be associated with iodine deficiency or ingestion of goitrogenic feeds by dam	Rare	Physical examination; histopathology of thyroids; restriction fragment length polymorphism in thyroglobulin gene allows for distinction between normal and goitrous goats	Vaginal prolapse and excessive relaxation of vaginal and pelvic ligaments during late pregnancy
Pheochromocytoma	823	Adrenal tumor causing sudden attacks of nervousness and anxiety	Unknown	Reported in 3 related older females	Histopathology (potassium dichromate stain)	None

TABLE 47-54

Congenital Defects of the Internal Organs in the Goat

Defect	Reference No.	Description	Etiology	Frequency	Diagnosis	Associated Defects
Ventricular septal defect	825	Within 4-6 months of age tire easily, exercise intolerance, depression, systolic murmur	Familial in Saanen	Rare	Clinical examination, necropsy	None
Anomaly of tricuspid valve (Ebstein's anomaly)	826	Systolic murmur with or without diastolic murmur over tricuspid valve, tricuspid regurgitation, intraatrial right to left shunt flow, anorexia, depression, tricuspid valve is dysplastic	Pygmy goat	One case reported	Clinical examination, necropsy	None
Ectopia cordis	824	Heart displaced outside thoracic cavity	Unknown	Rare	Physical examination	None
Urethral diverticulum	814, 831	Failure to urinate, accumulation or urine in diverticulum below penile urethra	Unknown	Rare	Physical examination, surgical repair	Hypospadias
Hypospadias	745, 764, 793, 829	Opening of urethra on ventral aspect of penis and prepuce	Unknown	Rare	Physical examination	Intersex; atresia ani et recti; rectovesicular fistula
Renal dysplasia	832	Disorganized development of renal parenchyma, failure of interaction of metanephric blastema with ureteric bud; goats developed urinary failure	Reported in Canary goats	Rare	Physical examination, histopathology	None
Ectopic bladder	834	Bladder in abnormal position	Unknown	Rare	Necropsy	None
Polycystic kidneys	745	—	Unknown	Common slaughterhouse finding	Necropsy	None
Atresia ani	745, 793, 827, 828	Nonpatency of anal structures, repair possible, abdominal distention, straining, no defecation	Unknown	Rare	Physical examination	Rectovaginal fistula in some females allows survival
Atresia coli	745	Colon ends blindly	Unknown	Rare	Abdominal distention, no defecation in young kid	None
Atresia recti	745	Rectum ends blindly	Unknown	Rare	Abdominal distention, no defecation in young kid	None
Double intestine with atresia ani et recti	830	Colon ends blindly, anus non-patent, accessory coiled tubular structure attached to mesenteric pedicle	Unknown	Rare	Necropsy	None
Polycystic disease of liver, kidneys, and pancreas	833	Progressive dullness, poor growth, and abdominal distention	Unknown	One case in a 2-week-old Nubian	Multiple fluid-filled cysts in liver and pancreas; renal cortical tubule and collecting duct ectasia	None

TABLE 47-55

Congenital Defects of the Reproductive System and Mammary Gland in the Goat

Defect	Reference No.	Description	Etiology	Frequency	Diagnosis	Associated Defects
Cryptorchidism (ridgling)	743, 835-837	One or both testicles not descended, unilateral reported in 25 West African dwarfs	Thought to be recessive gene in Angora breed	Rare	Physical examination	Absence of scrotum, ectopic urinary bladder
Testicular hypoplasia	837, 838	Testicular hypoplasia occurs in three types in goats; genetic females homozygous for polledness have small descended testes; the second type is unilateral, involving the right side; the third type is left sided, and affected gland has normal and deficient tubules	Genetic for first type; second and third types unknown	Rare	Physical examination, histopathology, karyotyping	None
Segmental aplasia of epididymis	837	Unilateral or bilateral segmental aplasia of epididymis	Unknown	Rare	Physical examination, histopathology	None
Abortion in Angora goats	735, 743, 839-841	Angora goats have higher incidence of abortions, most frequently between 100 to 110 days of gestation, abortion rate may be as high as 50%; infections and nutritional deficiencies have been eliminated; primary lesion is thought to be at anterior pituitary level or the adrenal cortical level; other investigators implicate environmental stress factors	Genetic with pleiotrophic effect	Common in some lines of Angora	Physical examination, elevated corticosteroids in aborting does	Other problems in lines with high incidence of abortion are perinatal mortality, testicular hypoplasia and increased susceptibility to urolithiasis and nematodes
Gynecomastia (lactating male goats)	842-845	Born and grow, breed like normal buck up to 15 months of age; gynecomastia develops, milking 25 to 1500 ml of milk per day	Sex-limited trait transmitted as a dominant with incomplete penetrance; polled Saanen, crossbred Saanens	Rare	Physical examination	None
Four quarters udder	734, 735, 846-847	Four developed and separate quarters	Unknown	Rare	Physical examination	None
Ectopic mammary tissue in vulva	848, 849	Ectopic mammary tissue as tumorous nodular masses on either side of vulva, may be surgically removed	Unknown	Rare, reported in Nubians and Syrians	Physical examination, histopathology	None
Various defects of conformation of udder	734, 850	Polythelia, pendulous udder, hanging or sac-like udder	Polygenic threshold traits in dairy breeds of goats	Common	Physical examination	None
Lactation without breeding or parturition	734, 735	Precocious udder development and lactation of 1-2 quarts	Unknown, thought to be more common in high-producing lines	Common	History, physical examination	None
Mammary gland aplasia	851	Absence of mammary gland and teats in a fertile doe	Unknown	One case	Physical examination	None

TABLE 47-56

Intersexuality and Freemartinism in the Goat

Defect	Reference No.	Description	Etiology	Frequency	Diagnosis	Associated Defects
Intersexuality in polled goats	735, 747, 853	Polled gene is an autosomal dominant; females heterozygous (Pp) for polled are normal and fertile; males heterozygous (Pp) for polled are normal and fertile; intersex goats are homozygous for polledness (PP) and are sex-reversed genetic females (XX); males homozygous for polledness (PP) have testicles, are usually normal, but up to 30% may be sterile as a result of epididymal blockage; affected goats show a wide range of external reproductive organs; gonads are usually testes; the greater the ano-genital distance, the more likely it is that testes are in scrotum	In goats, a gene closely linked to polling gene causes testicular development; inherited as autosomal sex-limited recessive and incomplete masculinization	Common in Saanen, Toggenburg, Alpine breeds	Physical examination, karyotyping	None
Freemartinism	734, 852, 854	A small portion of twin births in goats may be freemartins; hemopoietic chimera	Vascular communication between heterosexual twins	Approximately 6% of intersexes are freemartins	Physical examination, karyotyping	None
Hermaphroditism	734, 793, 852, 855	Externally female, with male and female gonads; true chimeras; sterile	Mixing of cells of male and female during early embryonic stage or fertilization of second polar body and oocyst by X and Y sperm before they fuse	Approximately 1% of intersexes	Karyotyping	None
Persistent müllerian duct syndrome	734, 856	Intersex with female tract and penis; karyotype is male	Probably a recessive trait	Unknown	Physical examination, karyotyping	None

TABLE 47-57

Chromosomal Defects in the Goat

Defect	Reference No.	Description	Etiology	Frequency	Diagnosis	Associated Defects
Robertsonian translocation	857-860	Fusion of chromosomes 2 and 13 (or 6 and 14); mean number of offspring for carrier does was 1.37 as compared with 1.75 for normal does	Segregates in mendelian proportions	Rare, Saanen	Karyotyping	Reduced fertility
xo/xx/xxx mixoploidy	861	Three different cell lines found in a female with disturbed fertility	Nondisjunction of X-chromosome during embryonic development	One case in an Alpine cross	Karyotyping	Abnormal fertility
xx/xxy mosaic	862	Found in a fertile male	Most likely nondisjunction of X-chromosome during embryonic development	One case in a Saanen cross	Karotyping	None

763. Baron RJ: Laterally luxating patella in a goat, *J Am Vet Med Assoc* 191:1741-1742, 1987.

764. Smith MC, Sherman DM: *Goat medicine,* New York, 1994, Lea & Febiger.

765. Kaneps AJ: Orthopedic conditions of small ruminants: Llama, sheep, goat, and deer, *Vet Clin North Am (Food Anim Pract)* 12:211-231, 1996.

766. Rowe CL: Hemivertebra in a goat, *Vet Med (Small Anim Clin)* 74:211-214, 1979.

767. Chandolia RK et al: Monstrosities in goat, *Indian Vet J* 68:985-986, 1991.

768. Epstein H: The Hejaz dwarf goat, *J Hered* 37:345-352, 1946.

769. Basrur PK, Koykul W, Yusoff RBH: Genetic disorders of the goat. In Youngquist RS, ed: *Current therapy in large animal theriogenology,* Philadelphia, 1997, WB Saunders, pp 533-537.

770. Deshmuk DT, Bhandarkar AG: Diprosophia in a goat, *Indian Vet J* 70:1060, 1993.

771. Ramadan RO: A dicephalic goat with other defects, *J Vet Med Series A* 43:337-343, 1996.

772. Pandit RK, Pandey SK, Agrawal RG: A case of dystocia due to dilopagus monster (craniopagus twin) in a goat, *Indian J Anim Reprod* 15:82, 1994.

773. Chakrabarti A, Pal A: Cyclopia prostomus arrhynchus in a black Bengal goat, *Indian Vet J* 68:985-986, 1991.

774. Sharma GP et al: Cyclops in a goat, *Indian Vet J* 66:264, 1989.

775. Binns W, Keeler RF, Balls LD: Congenital deformities in lambs, calves, and goats resulting from maternal ingestion of *Veratrum californicum*: hare lip, cleft palate, ataxia, and hypoplasia of metacarpal and metatarsal bones, *Clin Tox* 5:245-261, 1972.

776. Balagopal R, Mohan M, Manickam R: A case report on a monster with developmental anomalies in a Tellicherry goat, *Indian Vet J* 66:179, 1989.

777. Dutta JC, Deka KC, Barua PM: Schistosomus reflexus in a local goat *(Capra hircus)* of Assam in a case report, *Indian Vet J* 66:180, 1989.

778. Bezek DM, Frazer GS: Schistosomus reflexus in large animals, *Compend Cont Ed Pract Vet* 16: 1393-1398, 1994.

779. Dhoble R, Markandeya N: Clinical observations on congenital malformations in Osmanabadi goats, *Indian Vet J* 16:73-74, 1995.

780. An-Ani FK, Hailat NQ, Fathalla MA: Polydactyly in Shami breed goats in Jordan, *Sm Ruminant Res* 26:177-179, 1997.

781. Kinjavdekar P, Naveen K: Cranioschisis in a kid, *Indian Vet J* 74:521-522, 1997.

782. Chakrabarti A, Amin R, Kar PK: Monocephalus diprosopus triopthalmus diotus in a kid, *Indian Vet J* 73:567-568, 1996.

783. Balasubramanian S et al: Caprine perosomus horridus fetal monster delivered pervaginum: a case report, *Indian Vet J* 72:985-986, 1995.

784. Cazabon EPI, Loregard R, Bridgewater E: Perosomus elumbis in a goat in Trinidad, West Indies, *Vet Rec* 135:360, 1994.

785. Mitra M, Basak DN, Chakrabarti A: Monocephalus thoracopagus tetrapus tetranrachius monster in a Black Bengal goat, *Indian Vet J* 71:177-178, 1994.

786. Audiot A, Renieri C, Lauvergne JJ: Le variant "oreilles raccourcies" de la chevre Provencale, *Rec Med Vet* 161:683-684, 1985.

787. Robinson R: Genetic defects in goats, *Agri Pract* 13:28-30, 1992.

788. Lauvergne JJ, Renieri C, Audiot A: Estimating erosion of phenotypic variation in a French goat population, *J Hered* 78:307-314, 1987.

789. Käb E: Erbliche Stummelohren bei der Ziege, *Züchtungsk* 9:452-455, 1934.

790. Verm JS, Tomar SS, Tomer OS: Inheritance of wattles and their relationship with economic traits in goats, *Proceedings of the Third International Conference on Goat Production and Disease,* Tucson, Ariz, 1982, p 547.

791. Gamlen T, Crawford TB: Dermoid cysts in identical locations in a doe goat and her kid, *Vet Med (Small Anim Clin)* 72:616-617, 1977.

792. Nair NR, Bandopadhyay AC: Thyroglossal duct cyst in a goat, *Indian Vet J* 67:873, 1990.

793. Al-Ani FK et al: Occurrence of congenital anomalies in Shami breed goats: 211 cases investigated in 19 herds, *Small Ruminant Res* 28:225-232, 1998.

794. Nair NR, Bandopadhyay AC: Thyroglossal cyst below the base of the tongue with ankyloglossia in a kid, *Indian Vet J* 71:279, 1994.

795. Quaranta A, Roberto G, Facilone F: A case of heterotopia of the horn in a goat, *Summa* 11:53-55, 1995.

796. Hartley WJ, Blakemore WF: Neurovisceral storage and dysmyelinogenesis in neonatal goats, *Acta Neuropathol* 25:325-333, 1973.

797. Jones MZ et al: Caprine a-mannosidosis, *Prog Clin Biol Res* 94:165-176, 1982.

798. Healy PJ, Seaman JT, Gardner IA: α-Mannosidase deficiency in Anglo-Nubian goats, *Aust Vet J* 57:504-507, 1981.

799. Cavanagh K, Dunstan RW, Jones MZ: Plasma α- and β1-mannosidase activities in caprine β1-mannosidosis, *Am J Vet Res* 43:1058-1059, 1982.

800. Render JA et al: Ocular pathology of caprine β1-mannosidosis, *Vet Pathol* 26:444-446, 1989.

801. Jones MZ et al: Pathogenesis of caprine N-acetylglucosamine 6-sulfatase (Sanfilippo III D syndrome): studies of the molecular defect, *J Neuropathol Exp Neurol* 51:336, 1992.

802. Lancaster MJ, Gill IJ, Hooper PT: Progressive paresis in Angora goats, *Aust Vet J* 64:123-124, 1987.

803. Buyukmihci N: Retinal degeneration in a goat, *J Am Vet Med Assoc* 177:351-352, 1980.

804. Wolfer J, Grahn B: Diagnostic ophthalmology, *Can Vet J* 32:569-570, 1991.

805. El-Zomor S et al: Congenital encephalocele in two kids, *Assiut Vet Med J* 30:229-233, 1994.

806. Ashturkar RW, Aher VD, Bhokre AP: Congenital anophthalmia in a kid, *Indian Vet J* 73:1177, 1996.

807. Jefferson WJJ, Muthiah K, Lalitha PS: Anophthalmia and prognathism in a goat foetus, *J Vet Animal Sci* 27:75-76, 1996.

808. Baker J et al: Spastic paresis in pygmy goats, *J Vet Intern Med* 3:113, 1989.

809. Bryant SH: Myotonia in the goat, *Ann NY Acad Sci* 317:314-324, 1979.

810. Atkinson JB et al: A generalized membrane defect in heritable myotonia: studies of erythrocytes in an animal model and patients, *Proc Soc Exp Biol Med* 169:69-75, 1980.

811. Atkinson JB, LeRuire VS: Hereditary myotonia in the goat, *Comp Pathol Bull* 17:3-4, 1985.

812. Swift LL, Atkinson JB, LeRuire VS: The composition and calcium transport activity of the sarcoplasmic reticulum from goats with and without heritable myotonia, *Lab Invest* 40:384-390, 1979.

813. Bryant SH, Owenburg K: Characteristics of the chloride channel in skeletal muscle fibers of myotonic and normal goats, *Fed Proc* 39:579, 1980.

814. Nigam JM, Misk NA, Rifat JF: Surgical management of congenital anomalies of ruminants, *Agri Pract* 5:38-47, 1984.

815. Breuking HJ et al: Congenital afibrinogenemia in goats, *Zbl Vet Med (A)* 19:661-676, 1972.

816. Cain G, East N, Moore P: Myelofibrosis in young pygmy goats, *Comp Haematol International* 4:167-172, 1994.

817. Kok K et al: Autosomal recessive inheritance of goitre in Dutch goats, *J Hered* 78:298-300, 1987.

818. Capen CC: The endocrine glands. In Jubb KVF, Kennedy PC, Palmer, N, eds: *Pathology of domestic animals,* vol 3, New York, 1993, Academic Press, pp 318-319.

819. Rijnberk A et al: Congenital defect in iodothyronine synthesis: clinical aspects of iodine metabolism in goats with congenital goitre and hypothyroidism, *Br Vet J* 133:495-503, 1977.

820. Jaarsveld van P et al: Congenital goiter in South African Boer goats, *J South Afr Vet Med Assoc* 42:295-303, 1971.

821. Hoque M, Chattopadhyay SK, Singh GR: Congenital goitre in a kid, *Indian Vet J* 74:450-451, 1997.

822. Bhikane AU et al: Congenital goitre in kids, *Indian Vet J* 75:654, 1998.

823. Gritz BG: Hereditary caprine pheochromocytoma, *J Vet Med—Series A* 44:313-316, 1997.

824. Tiwari SK et al: A rare case of ectopia cordis in a goat, *Indian Vet J* 74:832-833, 1998.

825. Parry BW, Wrigley RH, Reuter RE: Ventricular septal defects in three familially related Saanen goats, *Aust Vet J* 59:72-76, 1982.

826. Gardner SY et al: Echocardiographic diagnosis of an anomaly of the tricuspid value in a male pygmy goat, *J Am Vet Med Assoc* 200:522-523, 1992.

827. Singh AP et al: Atresia ani and atresia ani et recti in farm animals, *Indian Vet J* 66:458-461, 1989.

828. Johnson EH, Nyack B, Marsh A: Surgical repair of atresia ani and rectovaginal fistula in a goat, *Vet Med (Small Anim Clin)* 75:1833-1834, 1980.

829. Rajankutty K et al: Congenital hypospadia associated with atresia ani et recti and rectovaginal fistula in a kid, *J of Vet Animal Sci* 25:172, 1994.

830. Saradaamma T et al: Double intestine along with atresia ani et recti in a kid, *Indian J Animal Sci* 67:596, 1997.

831. Nair NR, Tiwari SK: Congenital urethral anomaly in a kid and its surgical correction, *Indian Vet J* 66:762-763, 1989.

832. Gomez-Villamandos JC et al: Possible renal dysplasia in two related, juvenile goats, *Small Ruminant Res* 13:311-314, 1994.

833. Krotek K et al: Congenital cystic disease of the liver, pancreas, and kidney in a Nubian goat, *Vet Pathol* 33:708-710, 1996.

834. Tiwari SK et al: Exstrophy of bladder in a goat, *Indian Vet J* 75:918-919, 1998.

835. Ashturkar RW, Aher VD, Bhokre AP: Ectopic urinary bladder and cryptorchidism in a kid, *Indian Vet J* 69:649-650, 1992.

836. Ezeasor DE, Singh A: Morphologic features of Sertoli cells in the intraabdominal testes of cryptorchid dwarf goats, *Am J Vet Res* 48:1736-1745, 1987.

837. Tarigan S, Ladds PW, Foster RA: Genital pathology of feral male goats, *Aust Vet J* 67:286-290, 1990.

838. Sponenberg DP, Smith MC, Johnson RJ: Unilateral testicular hypoplasia in a goat, *Vet Pathol* 20:503-506, 1983.

839. Bretzlaff K: Special problems of hair goats, *Vet Clin North Am (Food Anim Pract)* 6:721-735, 1990.

840. Shelton M: Abortion in Angora goats. In Morrow DA, ed: *Current therapy in theriogenology,* Philadelphia, 1981, WB Saunders, pp 610-612.

841. Wentzel D: Non-infectious abortion in Angora goats, *Proceedings of the Third International Conference on Goat Productions and Diseases,* Tucson, Ariz, 1982, pp 155-161.

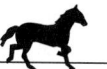

842. Fuller DT et al: What is your diagnosis, *J Am Vet Med Assoc* 201:1431-1433, 1992.
843. Rieck GW et al: Gynäkomastie bei einem Ziegenbock. II, Zytogenetische Befunde: XO/XY-Mosaik mit variablen Deletionen des Y-Chromosoms, *Zuchthyg* 10:159-168, 1975.
844. Panchadevi SM, Pandif RV: Milking males: two case studies, *Indian Vet J* 56:590-592, 1979.
845. Dufalla EA et al: A functioning udder in a male goat, *J Vet Med A* 37:686-691, 1990.
846. Seleim MA, Ali MA, Salek AS: Four quarters in a goat, *Agri Pract* 12:30, 1992.
847. Balasubramanian S, Thilagar S, Rameshkumar B: Four functional mammary glands in a goat, *Vet Rec* 135:532, 1994.
848. Gameel AA, Ramadan RO, Dafalla EA: Ectopic mammary tissue in the vulva of goats, *J Med Vet Assoc* 30:470-475, 1992.
849. Al-Sadi HI, Issa MJ, Al-Badrany MS: Ectopic mammary tissue in a black goat, *Sm Ruminant Res* 14:181-183, 1994.
850. Smelser RE: Polymastia and polythelia in dairy goats, *Proceedings of the Third International Conference on Goat Production and Diseases*, Tucson, Ariz, 1982, p 548.
851. Sharma LK: Absence of mammary gland and teats in a goat, *Indian Vet J* 70:569, 1993.
852. Basrur PK, Kinnon AO: Caprine intersexes and freemartins. In Morrow DA, ed: *Current therapy in theriogenology 2*, Philadelphia, 1986, WB Saunders, pp 596-600.
853. Bongso TA, Thavalingam M, Mukherjee TK: Intersexuality associated with XX/XY mosaicism in a horned goat, *Cytogenet Cell Genet* 34:313-319, 1982.
854. Smith MC, Dunn HO: Freemartin condition in a goat, *J Vet Med Assoc* 178:735-737, 1981.
855. Vaiman D et al: Genetic mapping of the autosomal region involved in XX sex-reversal and horn development in goats, *Mammalian Genome* 7:133-137, 1996.
856. Haibel GK, Rojko JL: Persistent Müllerian duct syndrome in a goat, *Vet Pathol* 27:135-137, 1990.
857. Elminger B, Stranzinger G: Identification of a centrometric fusion in the G-banding karyotype of a Saanen goat, *Sixth European College of Cytogenetics of Domestic Animals*, Zürich, July 16-20, 1984, pp 407-409.
858. Hulot F: Nouveau cas de fusion centrique che la chevre domestique (*Capra hircus* L.), *Ann Genet Sel Anim* 1:175-176, 1969.
859. Popescu CP: Mode de transmission d'une fusion centrique dans la descendance d'un bouc (*Capra hircus* L.) heterozygote, *Ann Genet Sel Anim* 4:355-361, 1972.
860. Ricordeau G: Observations sur les caracteres de reproduction des produits males et femelles issus d'un bouc porteur d'une "fusion centrique," *Ann Genet Sel Anim* 4:593-598, 1972.
861. Bhatia S, Shanker V: A case report on xo/xx/xxx mixoploidy in a goat, *Vet Rec* 126:312-313, 1990.
862. Bhatia S, Shanker V: First report of a xx/xxx fertile goat buck, *Vet Rec* 130:271-272, 1992.

Congenital Defects and Hereditary Diseases in the Horse

GEORGE SAPERSTEIN

ENVIRONMENTAL FACTORS

Very little is known about drugs, chemicals, or other agents as causes of congenital defects in horses. Although teratogens are difficult to identify, they often follow seasonal patterns or known stressful conditions; they may be linked to maternal disease; and they do not follow a familial pattern as do genetic diseases. On the basis of the pattern of occurrence of defects, field studies frequently have led to observations that teratogens may have been at work. Hybrid Sudan grass pasture has been incriminated as the cause of arthrogryposis in horses.[1] Some claim that *Astragalus mollisimus* causes abortions and congenital defects such as limb defects.[2] Cambendazole given to pregnant Shetland pony mares resulted in three deformed foals among 83 births.[3] The defects observed were twisting of limbs below the tarsus in the first foal; multiple defects such as a short lower jaw, large eyes, deformed legs, and constriction in the aorta in the second foal; and only deformed hind legs in the third foal.[3] Griseofulvin given during the second month of gestation is suspected as the cause of a syndrome of microphthalmia, brachygnathia superior, and palatocheiloschisis.[4] Treatment of equine protozoal myeloencephalitis (EPM) in pregnant mares with the combination of sulfadiazine, pyrimethamine, folic acid, and vitamin E can result in congenital defects such as bone marrow aplasia and hypoplasia, renal nephrosis or hypoplasia, and skin lesions.[5] No teratogenic viral infections have been described for horses.

In one study of 14 foals with congenital musculoskeletal abnormalities, 10 had low total serum concentrations of triiodothyronine (T_3), thyroxine (T_4), or both, suggestive of hypothyroidism. Six had histologic lesions of thyroid hyperplasia. Musculoskeletal lesions encountered were forelimb contracture, ruptured common digital extensor tendon, short face, skeletal hypoplasia, and combinations of these defects.[6] This syndrome has been recognized with increasing frequency in western Canada.[7]

A variable complex of congenital defects of head, neck, and limbs (head scoliosis, torticollis, contracture of limbs) was described in 214 foals and caused severe dystocia in the mares. Sixty-six percent were Belgian draft horses followed by Thoroughbreds, warmbloods, trotters, and ponies. These malformations were associated with increased incidence of caudal and, particularly, transverse presentations. Theoretically, abnormal uterine position can cause the defects; during the second half of pregnancy, the narrow tip of the uterine horns provides only limited space for the cranial end of the developing equine fetus.[8]

GENETIC FACTORS

Genetic defects are pathophysiologic results of mutant genes or chromosomal aberrations occurring in any environment. Chromosomal defects of number or structure are becoming increasingly important in equine veterinary practice.[9-17] The recent development of a whole chromosome paint probe for the X chromosome opens the door for routine cytogenetic screening of infertile mares.[18]

Cytogenetic testing was done on 204 virgin mares or mares in their first year at stud. Two hundred and one mares were normal. One mare was a 63 X, 64 XX mosaic; one was a 64 XY sex-reversed mare; and another horse was a 65 XXX trisomy. The incidence of sex chromosomal defects in mares is likely to be less than 3%.[17]

Many genetic defects follow simple mendelian inheritance, mostly a simple autosomal-recessive pattern. Other

monofactorial inheritance patterns may be encountered and characterized as overdominant, dominant, incomplete dominant, and polygenic. Genetically induced congenital defects occur in typical intergenerational patterns and intragenerational frequencies. Recognizing these requires enumerating normal and abnormal offspring and identifying their familial relationships. Various statistical methods are used to analyze such data and can provide circumstantial evidence for genetic causes. Breeding trials are absolutely necessary to confirm inheritance patterns. Although breeding trials have the disadvantage of being expensive and time consuming, they are much cheaper than trying to eliminate a genetic defect after it has insidiously spread throughout a given population.

Embryo transfer alone or in conjunction with preterminal cesarean section may be used to test for many simple autosomal-recessive structural defects. It has the additional advantage of being less expensive and less time consuming than traditional breeding trials. DNA-based testing procedures are becoming more important in identifying carriers of defective genes for such diseases as hyperkalemic periodic paralysis (HYPP) and severe combined immunodeficiency (SCID). The number of such tests will grow substantially as the horse genome map is completed.

Congenital defects apparently result in fewer losses than those caused by nutritional deficiencies, infectious agents, or neoplasia. However, defects may cause considerable economic losses to individual breeders by increasing perinatal mortality. In addition, they probably are major causes of early embryonic death.

Furthermore, loss of value of relatives of genetically defective horses can be serious. Additional losses occur when congenital defects are manifestations of a syndrome that also includes embryonic and fetal mortality. The presence of congenital defects may complicate the diagnosis of other causes of abortion. Finally, if the defect is genetic, control measures may require extensive and expensive adjustments of breeding programs.

The frequency of congenital defects in foals is not known. Numerous articles have been published on isolated defects in foals.[19] Medical records of 137,717 animals in North American veterinary clinics showed that 6455 had congenital defects. Of these, 1130 (17.51%) were horses.[20] A 13-year survey of congenital defects in foals reported 608 cases.[21] The following defects were reported: contracted foal syndrome (32.2%), miscellaneous limb contraction (20%), multiple defects (5.3%), microphthalmia (4.6%), craniofacial malformations (4.3%), cleft palate (4.0%), heart defects (3.5%), umbilical defects (3.5%), and hydrocephalus (3%). Eleven less frequently occurring anomalies constituted the balance of the congenital defects in fetuses and newborn foals.[21] A total of 1211 aborted equine fetuses and stillborn foals in central Kentucky during the 1988 and 1989 foaling seasons contained 8.5% congenital defects.[22] A follow-up study involving 3514 aborted fetuses, stillborn foals, or foals that died less than 24 hours after birth showed 188 cases of contracted foal syndrome and 160 congenital defects.[23] Of 290 aborted fetuses surveyed in Michigan between 1985 and 1996, 4.8% were found to have congenital defects, with contracted foal syndrome being the most common.[24]

CLASSIFICATION OF SPECIFIC DEFECTS

Arriving at a single system suitable for classifying congenital defects has been difficult. Three principal systems have been used: etiologic, affected embryonic tissue, and principal defective body system. The last system is used in this review. Tables 48-1 through 48-16 define defects of various body systems in horses.

DIAGNOSIS AND CONTROL

Horse breeders and veterinarians are involved daily in improving animal health and production. The goal is to produce a quality horse. Accurate diagnosis of genetic diseases and defects requires understanding of hereditary patterns of disease. Many different congenital defects with genetic, environmental, environmental-genetic interaction, or unknown etiology have been identified in horses; these defects are economically significant. Not only is diagnosis important, but methods to control genetically induced defects should be understood. Most breed associations have programs for controlling undesirable traits and genetic defects. Producers need to be provided with genetic disease information and counseling so they can practice selective breeding to minimize losses from genetic interaction. The intent of this counseling should be not to destroy the breeding future of a superior stallion because of a known carrier status of an undesirable gene, but rather to help select the proper mares. Mares should be selected that enhance a stallion's positive traits with minimum possibilities for undesirable gene expression. Nevertheless, this should be done with the knowledge that the stallion's offspring will have a higher likelihood of being carriers than the general population.

Many clinical reports of congenital defects contain little, if any, etiologic information. With limited incrimination of drugs and plant toxins as causes of congenital defects, a concerted effort is needed to identify other environmental agents that are teratogenic in horses.

REFERENCES

1. Prichard JT, Voss JL: Fetal ankylosis in horses associated with hybrid grass, *J Am Vet Med Assoc* 150:871-873, 1967.
2. McIlwraith CW, James LF: Limb deformities in foals associated with ingestion of locoweed by mares, *J Am Vet Med Assoc* 181:255-258, 1982.
3. Druge JH et al: Cambendazole for strongyle control in a pony band: selection of a drug-resistant population of small strongyles and teratologic implications, *Am J Vet Res* 44:110-114, 1983.
4. Schutte JG, van den Ingh TSGAM: Microphthalmia, brachygnathia superior, and palatocheiloschisis in a foal associated with grieseofulvin administration to the mare during early pregnancy, *Vet Q* 19: 58-60, 1997.
5. Toribio RE et al: Congenital defects in newborn foals of mares treated for equine protozoal myeloencephalitis during pregnancy, *J Am Vet Med Assoc* 212:697-701, 1998.
6. McLaughlin BG, Doige CE, McLaughlin PS: Thyroid hormone levels in foals with congenital musculoskeletal lesions, *Can Vet J* 27:264-267, 1986.
7. Allen AL et al: Hyperplasia of the thyroid gland and concurrent musculoskeletal deformities in western Canadian foals: reexamination of a previously described syndrome, *Can Vet J* 35:31-38, 1994.
8. Vandeplassche K et al: Aetiology and pathogenesis of congenital torticollis and head scoliosis in the equine foetus, *Equine Vet J* 16:419-424, 1984.
9. Benirschke K, Ryder OA: Genetic aspects of equids with particular reference to their hybrids, *Equine Vet J* 16(suppl 3):1-10, 1984.
10. Gill JJB: Sex chromosomes; or what the X is happening, *Equine Vet J* 20: 81-82, 1988.
11. Gill JJB et al: A 64XX/65XXX mosaic and associated infertility, *Equine Vet J* 20:128-130, 1988.
12. Halnan CRE: Equine cytogenetics: role in equine veterinary practice, *Equine Vet J* 17:173-177, 1985.
13. Jones WE, Bogart R: *Genetics of the horse*, Ann Arbor, 1971, Edwards Brothers.
14. Long S: Chromosome anomalies and infertility in the mare, *Equine Vet J* 20:89-93, 1988.
15. Payne HW, Ellsworth K, DeGrott A: Aneuploidy in an infertile mare, *J Am Vet Med Assoc* 153:1293-1299, 1986.
16. Willer S, Willer H, Wiesner E: Chromosomenaberrationen beim Pferd, *Monatsch Vet-Med* 36:386-394, 1981.
17. Nie GJ, Momont HW, Buoen L: A survey of sex chromosomes in 204 mares selected for breeding, *J Equine Vet Sci* 13:456-459, 1993.
18. Breen M et al: Detection of equine X chromosome abnormalities in equids using a horse X whole chromosome paint probe (WCPP), *The Vet J* 153:235-238, 1997.
19. Huston R, Saperstein G, Leipold HW: Congenital defects in foals, *J Equine Med* 1:146-161, 1977.
20. Priester WA, Glass MD, Waggoner NS: Congenital defects in domesticated animals: general considerations, *Am J Vet Res* 31:1871-1879, 1970.

Text continued on p. 1584

TABLE 48-1

Congenital Defects of the Digestive System in the Horse

Defect	Ref. No.	Description	Etiology	Frequency	Diagnosis/Treatment	Associated Defects
Cleft palate	4, 25-29	Varies in degree from fissure of both soft and hard palates to a cleft only in the posterior soft palate	Unknown; some cases may be due to teratogenic effect of griseofulvin	Thought to be low	Physical examination; secondary inhalation pneumonia; foals are poor doers with milk, food, and water discharge from one or both nostrils; can be repaired surgically	Sometimes cleft lip, microphthalmia, brachygnathia superior
Hypoplasia of soft palate	30, 31	Shortened soft palate resulting in dysphagia	Unknown	Rare	Endoscopy; necropsy	None
Atresia ani	32	Nonpatency of anus	Unknown	Occasional	Physical examination; no fecal discharge; may be surgically corrected	None
Atresia recti	33	Rectum ends blindly	Unknown	One case reported in a Thoroughbred	No fecal discharge; surgical correction	None
Atresia coli	34, 35	Two parts to the colon, each ending in a blind pouch; various parts of the colon may be absent	Unknown	Uncommon	Colic shortly after birth, feces not discharged after an enema; barium enema; confirmation at necropsy or surgical exploration	Cardiac, brain, and skin anomalies reported
Tympany of guttural pouch	36	Distention, usually unilateral, of the guttural pouch with air, caused by the action of a flap of tissue over the pharyngeal opening acting as a one-way valve	Theories include defect in pharyngeal opening, strenuous coughing during an upper respiratory infection, inflammation of pharyngeal opening, and paralysis of pharyngeal muscles	Uncommon	Physical examination and percussion of swelling in parotid region; deflation through pharyngeal opening of eustachian tube into guttural pouch or through Viborg's triangle; flap identified during surgery; corrected by flap resection or perforating septum between right and left pouch if unilateral	None

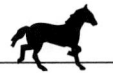

Condition	Ref	Description	Etiology	Incidence	Diagnosis	Treatment
Atresia of the parotid duct	37	Parotid duct ends in a blind sac, where it normally enters the oral cavity	Unknown	One case reported in a Quarter horse	Physical examination	None
Parrot mouth	38	Malformation caused by upper jaw overgrowth or short lower jaw	Possibly genetic	Common	Physical examination; in neonate, obvious malocclusion of incisors	None
Ileocolonic aganglionosis	39-44	Reported in white foals; affected foals appear normal at birth but develop signs of colic within 5 to 24 hours and die within 32 hours	Genetic; associated with overo to overo mating	Overo to overo matings in Paint horses	History of mating; physical examination, necropsy, and histopathology	None
Megacolon with myenteric hypoganglionosis	45, 46	Lethargy and abdominal distention in 4- to 9-month-old Clydesdale foals; chronic colonic distention	Familial	Rare	Laparotomy, necropsy, and histopathologic examination; right dorsal colon distended with ingesta; hypoganglionosis in colon and cecum	None
Villous hypoplasia of small intestine	47, 48	Thin and shorter small intestine, villous hypoplasia, malabsorption in newborn foals; results in failure of passive transfer of immunity	Unknown	Rare; reported in 7 Thoroughbreds and 1 Anglo Arabian	Necropsy and histopathologic examination	None
Persistence of Meckel's diverticulum	49	Remnant of embryonic omphalomesenteric duct, which may cause volvulus or intestinal entrapment	Unknown	Uncommon	During exploratory or necropsy	None
Persistent hyperammonemia	50	Onset at 2-3 weeks postweaning of abnormal behavior, unthriftiness, and poor growth resulting from hyperammonemia and hyperornithinemia	Possibly defective mitochondrial transporter protein, such that ornithine is deficient, resulting in hyperammonemia	Reported in 2 related Morgans	Time of clinical onset, hyperammonemia, hyperornithinemia, and ruling out other causes of hepatic encephalopathy	None
Esophageal and tracheal duplication cyst	51	Cervical mass containing both esophageal and tracheal structures, not associated with normal trachea and esophagus	Unknown	One case reported in an Arabian	Aspiration of mass, contrast radiography, ultrasonography, and surgical exploration; surgical excision	None
Hamartomatous polyp of small colon	52	Colic and obstruction in neonatal foal caused by a congenital benign polypoid mass attached to the mucosa of small colon	Unknown	One case seen in a Standardbred	Retrograde contrast radiography, ultrasound, and exploratory laparotomy	None

TABLE 48-2

Congenital Defects of the Circulatory System in the Horse

Defect	Ref. No.	Description	Etiology	Frequency	Diagnosis/Treatment	Associated Defects
Interventricular septal defect	53-58, 61, 62	Opening in the ventricular septum, most commonly about 2.5 cm in diameter in the upper part of the membranous septum	Unknown	Most common heart defect; most commonly seen in young horses	Poor doer; intolerance to exercise; harsh pansystolic murmur over right side and sometimes left; sometimes precordial thrill; catheterization reveals higher oxygen saturation in right ventricle than right atrium; confirmation by echocardiography	Usually none, but atrial septal defect reported
Patent ductus arteriosus	53, 59-61	Persistence and patency of ductus arteriosus beyond 3 days of age, with shunting from aorta to pulmonary artery	Unknown	Not common	In 5-day or older animal with either machinery murmur or often a systolic murmur loudest on left side; catheterization reveals higher oxygen tension above the pulmonic valve than below it; enlarged heart; confirmation at necropsy	One case associated with parrot mouth
Persistent foramen ovale	63	Persistence and patency of foramen ovale in neonate	Unknown	Rare	Neonatal death; ultrasound, necropsy examination	None
Absence of aortic origin of left coronary artery	61	Same as defect	Unknown	One case reported in yearling Thoroughbred colt	Secondary nutmeg liver, ascites, pulmonary edema, alveolar emphysema, left ventricular hypertrophy	Monorchid; dilation and fibrosis of aortic and left A-V valves
Persistent right aortic arch	64, 65	Persistence of right fourth aortic arch rather than the left, resulting in a right aorta that rises over the right of the midline and over the origin of the right bronchus and descends on the right of the vertebral column; the left ductus arteriosus encircles the esophagus, producing compression of the esophagus against the trachea	Unknown	Rare	Regurgitation of milk from mouth and nostrils while nursing, marked intolerance to exercise, and shrill murmur over left aortic area; secondary aspiration pneumonia; barium swallow indicates obstruction radiographically; surgical correction by cutting ductus arteriosus possible; confirmation at necropsy	None

Defect	Refs	Description	Cause	Occurrence	Diagnosis	Associated Defects/Remarks
Origin of aorta and pulmonary trunk from right ventricle	66, 67, 82, 83	Dextroposition of the aorta with blood flow: left ventricle → ventricular septal defect → right ventricle → aorta and pulmonary trunk	Unknown	Rare	Poor doer, ventral edema, backflow of blood through right A-V valve; echocardiography and cardiac catheterization; definitive diagnosis at necropsy	Interventricular septal defect, atrial septal defect, right ventricular hypertrophy, and origin of brachiocephalic and left subclavian arteries separately on the arch of the aorta
Dextroposition of aorta and atresia of pulmonary trunk	67	Aorta transposed to right ventricle, aortic ostium partly overriding large septal defect, and cordlike pulmonary trunk; blood flow from left to right; lungs supplied by extensive collateral circulation through mediastinal and mainly bronchial arteries	Unknown	One case reported in a Pinto, euthanized at 2 years of age	Clinically at 14 months of age; chronic cough, moist vesicular lung sounds, holosystolic murmur on left side, and intolerance to exercise; ultrasound for septal defect; definitive diagnosis at necropsy	Large interventricular septal defect, enlarged heart and right ventricular hypertrophy
Tetralogy of Fallot	68, 69	Pulmonic stenosis, high interventricular septal defect, dextroposition of the aorta, and right ventricular hypertrophy	Unknown	Rare	By angiography (large aorta, ventricular septal defect, and infundibular hypertrophy); catheterization (pressure gradient across pulmonary valve); ultrasound; and necropsy	One case associated with internal hydrocephalus
Pentalogy of Fallot	32, 70	Tetralogy of Fallot plus patent ductus arteriosus	Unknown	Rare	At necropsy	None
Multiple heart defects	68, 71	Persistent common truncus arteriosus mainly over right ventricle with interventricular septal defect 1-2.5 cm in diameter and stenosis of the pulmonary trunk at its origin	Unknown	Five cases reported in foals ranging in age from 2½ hr to 3 weeks	Dyspnea, cyanosis, murmurs, and death; ultrasound; definitive diagnosis at necropsy	One foal had an atrial septal defect
Multiple heart defects	61	Interatrial septal defect, enlarged right atrium, high interventricular septal defect, right atrioventricular atresia, and no communication between right ventricle and atrium; in one case the pulmonary valve had only two cusps	Unknown	Two cases reported in 3-month-old foals	Marked intolerance to exercise, loud murmur, and death; ultrasound, diagnosis at necropsy; enlarged nutmeg liver, pulmonary edema, alveolar emphysema, and excess pericardial fluid	None
Three-chambered heart	72	Two atria and one ventricle	Unknown	One case reported in a 5-year-old	At necropsy	None

Continued

TABLE 48-2

Congenital Defects of the Circulatory System in the Horse—cont'd

Defect	Ref. No.	Description	Etiology	Frequency	Diagnosis/Treatment	Associated Defects
Portal vein anomaly	73, 74	Arteriovenous anomaly in which the portal vein lesion consists of venous spaces encompassed by many variable-sized arterial vessels connected in several places to one another	Unknown	Rare	Hepatoencephalopathy; necropsy and histology; elevated blood ammonia and serum bile acids with normal liver enzyme levels; positive contrast portography; surgical correction	None
Atresia of tricuspid valve	75	Occlusion of right atrioventricular opening	Unknown	Rare	Ultrasound; confirmed at necropsy	Dilated right atrium, patent foramen ovale, hypoplasia of right ventricle, interventricular septal defect, and enlarged left ventricle
Pulmonic stenosis	80	Narrowing at pulmonic valve with poststenotic dilation	Unknown	Rare	Dyspnea; systolic murmur over pulmonic valve; cardiac catheterization with angiography and oximetry	PDA, interatrial shunt, right heart enlargement
Persistent truncus arteriosus	79	Single large vessel originating over a ventricular septal defect, which gives rise to pulmonary artery, aorta, and coronary arteries	Unknown	Rare	Exercise intolerance; systolic murmur, echocardiography, angiocardiography, and necropsy	Patent foramen ovale
Common atrioventricular canal	81	Failure of endocardial cushions to fuse, resulting in communication of all four chambers due to the low atrial septal defect and high ventricular septal defect	Unknown	Rare	Weak, cyanotic foal; systolic murmur; echocardiography and necropsy	AV valve dysplasia
Pulmonary atresia with an intact ventricular septum	76-78	Lack of development of pulmonary trunk, associated with heart anomalies other than VSD	Unknown	Rare	Systolic or continuous murmur; echocardiography color Doppler echocardiography, and cardiac catheterization; necropsy	Combination of PDA, patent foramen ovale, plus hypoplastic or absent right ventricle, atrial septal defect

TABLE 48-3

Hemophilia in the Horse

Defect	Ref. No.	Description	Etiology	Frequency	Diagnosis/ Treatment	Associated Defects
Hemophilia A (factor VIII deficiency)	84-89	Appearance of hematomas over various parts of the body, especially around joints and body prominences in young foals; prolonged clotting time; deficiency of antihemophilic globulin	Sex-linked recessive trait	Rarely described in Standardbreds and Thoroughbreds; only in male	Clinical signs plus detection of the deficiency with thromboplastin generation test, corrected by adding factor VIII; death is inevitable from internal hemorrhage, although blood transfusions can help control the condition	None

TABLE 48-4

Congenital Defects of the Respiratory System in the Horse

Defect	Ref. No.	Description	Etiology	Frequency	Diagnosis/ Treatment	Associated Defects
Accessory thoracic lung with bronchial hypoplasia	90	Tumorlike mass in thorax histologically consisting of dilated alveolar ducts, alveoli, near absence of cartilage in bronchi, and less than normal amount of muscle in bronchioles	Unknown	One case reported in an aborted fetus	Grossly and histologically	None
Choanal atresia, may be unilateral or bilateral	91, 92, 234	Severe dyspnea from birth, mouth breathing and no air flow at nostril(s), cyanosis of mucous membranes, obstructing membrane may be membranous or bony and is present between the nasal cavity and nasopharynx	Unknown	Rare	Clinical signs, contrast radiography, endoscopy	Facial abnormalities

TABLE 48-5

Congenital Defects of the Urinary System in the Horse

Defect	Ref. No.	Description	Etiology	Frequency	Diagnosis/ Treatment	Associated Defects
Bladder defect	21, 93-95	Defect or tear in dorsal or ventral surface or near the urachus in the urinary bladder of the neonate	Defects may be developmental or caused by rupture because of a full bladder during parturition	Several cases reported; mainly in males	Frequent straining to urinate, but only passing small amounts of urine; ascites; confirmation during laparotomy, contrast cystography, abdominal paracentesis; can be repaired surgically	None
Pervious urachus	32	Patency of urachus after birth	Unknown	Common	Dripping of urine form umbilicus, especially during micturition; usually recovery is spontaneous in a few days, but cauterization with silver nitrate or strong tincture of iodine may be used to treat; severe cases may require surgery	None
Unilateral kidney agenesis	96	Absence of one kidney and compensatory hypertrophy of the other	Unknown	12 cases reported	At necropsy or laparotomy	Sometimes reproductive anomalies; rudimentary ureter on affected side
Ectopic ureter	97-99	Same as defect, unilateral or bilateral	Unknown	Rare	Urinary incontinence; speculum exam or endoscopy of abnormal exit site of ureter; contrast urography	Hydronephrosis
Renal dysplasia	100-102	Immature disorganized renal tissue on histopathologic examination	Unknown	Reported in neonates and adults	Uremia, biopsy, ultrasound; definitive diagnosis by histopathology	Usually none, one case of angular limb deformity

Continued

TABLE 48-5

Congenital Defects of the Urinary System in the Horse—cont'd

Defect	Ref. No.	Description	Etiology	Frequency	Diagnosis/ Treatment	Associated Defects
Polycystic kidneys	103	Enlarged kidneys up to 12 kg; cortex and medulla composed of small, thin-walled cysts 1.5 cm diameter, filled with clear-to-yellowish fluid	Unknown	Rare	Ultrasound; exploratory surgery; necropsy confirms	None
Renal arteriovenous malformation	104	Anomalous vascular connection between artery and vein of kidney; foal may present with hematuria, hemoglobinuria	Unknown	Rare	Color-flow Doppler ultrasonography	None
Partial atresia of ureter	105	Uroperitoneum and associated signs caused by leakage of the ureter proximal to a distally located atretic segment	Unknown	Rare	Exploratory surgery; ureter may be resected or kidney removed (if unilateral)	None
Urethrorectal fistula	106	Communicating defects of urethra and rectum	Unknown	Rare	Urination through both urethra and rectum; exploratory surgery; necropsy	Atresia ani

TABLE 48-6

Congenital Defects of the Integumentary System in the Horse

Defect	Ref. No.	Description	Etiology	Frequency	Diagnosis/Treatment	Associated Defects
Albinism	107, 108	White coat, pink skin, and near absence of pigment from eye except for slight coloration to the iris	Autosomal-dominant genes in heterozygous (Ww) state	Uncommon	Physical examination	None
Lethal dominant white	107	Mating of white horses (Ww × Ww) produces an unviable embryo (WW) 25% of the time, which is possibly resorbed in early gestation	Autosomal-dominant gene in homozygous (WW) state	25% of matings of albinos	Breeding history	None
Epitheliogenesis imperfecta	109, 110	Fatal disease of young foals characterized by small defects in epithelium, usually just above the carpus and tarsus or in the tongue	Unknown, but possibly hereditary	Rare	Histologically abrupt discontinuation of epithelium at defect; foals are poor doers and refractory to treatment	One case associated with a renal cyst, another with patent foramen ovale, may have dental dysplasia
Malignant melanoma	111	Growing tumor, present at birth, on dorsal midlumbar area	Unknown	One case reported in a chestnut Arabian colt	Grossly and histologically; metastases in lymph vessels and nodes	None
Dentigerous cysts with fistulae	112	Unilateral presence of heterotopic tissue at base of ear, appearing as saclike swellings, tending to fistulate and containing tooth remnants	Abnormality of first branchial cleft	Two cases reported in Thoroughbreds	Grossly and histologically; can be corrected surgically	None
Papillomatosis	113, 114	Wart type growth on skin at birth	Unknown, possibly in utero infection with latent form of virus	Rare	Physical examination and histologically	None
Mechanobullous disease	115, 116	Blister induction following minor trauma, epidermal and mucocutaneous erosions, separation of hooves from coronary bands	Possibly genetic	Reported only in Belgian foal	Clinical signs, histopathology	None

TABLE 48-7

Congenital Defects of the Eye in the Horse

Defect	Ref. No.	Description	Etiology	Frequency	Diagnosis/Treatment	Associated Defects
Complete mature cataracts	32, 117, 131, 133	Opacity of the entire lens present at birth; usually bilateral and causing blindness	Possibly genetic	Most common cause of blindness in young horses	Ophthalmoscopic examination with pupil dilated; may be corrected surgically in foals and young horses by aspiration	Occasionally microphthalmia
Nuclear cataracts	32, 133	Opacity of the center of the lens characterized by concentric irregular rings, present at birth; may or may not regress	Unknown	Unknown	Same as above; mydriasis may aid daytime vision	None
Y-type cataracts	32, 118, 133	Y-shaped opacities in anterior and posterior lens cortices, present at birth	Possibly increased lens ground substance or shortness of lens fibers	Unknown	Same as above	None
Persistent hyaloid vasculature type cataracts	32	Opacity of posterior capsule and lens cortex associated with persistent hyaloid vessels, present at birth; usually nonprogressive	Unknown	Unknown	Same as above	None
Aniridia	119-122	Bilateral absence of iris	Probably genetic (autosomal)	Only reported in Belgians	Large, circular, nonresponsive pupil	Secondary cataracts of various degrees, beginning a few months after birth
Iridal heterochromia	32, 122	Abnormal coloration of iris, usually combinations of white, brown, and blue; glass eye (albinismus totalis) is a nearly all-white iris	Unknown	Glass eye most common in white, spotted, and chestnut horses and Palominos	Examination	None
Recurrent uveitis (periodic ophthalmia)	32, 123, 124, 133	Acute, subacute, or chronic disorder of uveal tract (iris, ciliary body, and choroid); initially seen as excessive lacrimation, photophobia, conjunctivitis, corneal edema, aqueous flare, and later as hypopyon and posterior synechia	Possibly a hereditary predisposition associated with other causes such as diet, Leptospira infection, parasitic larvae, and hypersensitivity; not a pure hereditary trait	Most common intraocular disease	Ophthalmoscopic examination, intravenous fluorescein and slit-lamp biomicroscopy; retrospective diagnostic signs include grayish iris, atrophied corpora nigra, iridal deposits on anterior lens capsule, posterior synechia, and cataracts	Secondary cataracts, posterior synechia, retinitis, optic disc atrophy, and others
Bilateral optic nerve hypoplasia	32, 125	Small optic nerves, blindness, mydriasis, and minimum pupillary reflexes	Unknown	Rare	Small optic discs with paucity of retinal vessels; histologically, fewer retinal ganglion cells, thinner optic fiber layer, and small optic papilla	Sometimes microphthalmia, cataract, or retinal detachment

Condition	Reference	Signs	Cause	Frequency	Diagnosis	Associated Defects
Bilateral ocular defects	127, 128, 133	Left eye exhibits an anterior staphyloma, whereas the right eye shows a microphthalmia, absence of cornea and anterior chamber and coloboma of optic disc; others had multiple defects	Unknown	Rare	Physical examination	Retinal detachment and optic nerve hypoplasia
Microphthalmia	32, 126, 127, 133	Unilateral or bilateral smallness of the globe	Unknown	Seen in all breeds	Physical examination	Often cataracts; one case of upper lip hypoplasia reported
Microphthalmos and disc coloboma	135	Bilateral microphthalmos, mild microcornea, and large posterior segment coloboma	Unknown	Rare	Ophthalmoscopic examination	None
Entropion	32, 129	Inversion of the eyelid; may irritate cornea and conjunctiva	Unknown	Occasional	Physical examination; can be corrected surgically	None
Ectropion	32, 133	Eversion of the eyelid	Unknown	Occasional	Physical examination; can be corrected surgically	None
Retinal detachment	130	Bilateral separation of inner retinal layers from pigment layer, present at birth	Thought to be polygenic	Unknown	Ophthalmoscopically and histologically; clinical blindness	Microphthalmia; one foal had unilateral cataract
Microcornea	32	Abnormally small cornea	Unknown	Unknown	Physical examination	Usually microphthalmia
Melanosis of cornea	32, 129	Pigmentation of epithelium and anterior stroma, usually vascularized and found centrally	Unknown	Rare	Physical examination; usually does not enlarge with age; can be removed by superficial keratectomy	None
Corneal opacities	32, 129	Thin linear and band-type clouding of cornea	Extracellular fluid anterior to abnormal Descemet's membrane	Occasional	Physical examination; nonprogressive	Thin Descemet's membrane
Iridocorneal anomaly	32	Opacities in lateral and medial limbal cornea, because of abnormal attachment of pectinate ligaments to Descemet's membrane; nonprogressive	Unknown	Occasional	Must differentiate in older horse from opacities caused by peripheral anterior synechia associated with iridocyclitis	None
Subluxation of lens	121	Subluxation of both lenses	Unknown	Rare	Physical examination	Cataracts
Iridial hypoplasia	131, 132	Most often found in blue irides as a bulge at the 12 o'clock region	Unknown	Rare	Ophthalmoscopic examination	None
Congenital glaucoma	136	Increased intraocular pressure	Unknown	Rare	Ophthalmic examination and tonometry	Anterior segment dysgenesis; microphakia; retinal dysplasia
Corneal vascularization	134	Bilateral dorsal perilimbal superficial vascularization of cornea present at birth and gradually regressing to normal by 7 days of age	Unknown	Rare	Ophthalmic examination	None

TABLE 48-8

Congenital Defects of the Endocrine System in the Horse

Defect	Ref. No.	Description	Etiology	Frequency	Diagnosis/Treatment	Associated Defects
Goiter	137	Birth of weak foals with enlarged thyroids; may or may not be fatal shortly after birth	Overfeeding of iodine (about 83 mg/day) to mares during pregnancy	Rare	Feed analysis, mares have enlarged thyroids, and thyroids of foals are grossly enlarged and histologically hyperplastic	None
Hypothyroidism	6, 138	Plasma thyroid hormone concentration is too low to sustain normal cellular functions, which have major roles in neonatal development; incoordination, poor sucking and righting reflexes, hypothermia, and goiter; musculoskeletal disorders, tendon contracture, and severely retarded bone development	Diet is suspected	Common	Physical examination; T_4 at birth; T_3 in foals more than 30 days old	Retarded bone development; contracture of tendons
Syndrome of hyperplasia of thyroid gland and musculoskeletal deformities (TH-MSD)	7	Syndrome of hyperplasia of thyroid glands and associated musculoskeletal defects; flexural deformities of forelimbs, rupture of tendons of common digital extensor muscles, mandibular prognathia, immature carpal and tarsal bones; thyroid glands not grossly enlarged	Unknown, probably environmental	Common	Necropsy and histopathologic examination	Prognathism

TABLE 48-9

Congenital Defects of the Nervous System in the Horse

Defect	Ref. No.	Description	Etiology	Frequency	Diagnosis/Treatment	Associated Defects
Wobbles (equine incoordination, spinal ataxia, wobbler syndrome, or ataxia of foals)	139-148	Ataxia of young horses, especially of hind legs, of sudden or insidious onset, characterized by subluxation of cervical vertebrae, most commonly C_3-C_4, and resulting spinal cord pressure and malacia	Unknown; several theories include heredity, copper deficiency, too long a neck, trauma, and a combination of genetic and environmental factors	Sporadic; three times more common in well nourished and heavily muscled horses; seen in all breeds	Clinical signs include bilateral ataxia at first in hind legs, weakness; seen most often between ages of 3 months and 3 years; lesions include osteoarthritis of cervical vertebrae and white matter degeneration of cervical cord with hyalinization and venous congestion; radiology and histology to confirm	None
Cerebellar hypoplasia and degeneration; cerebellar disease, or abiotrophy (Arabian)	149-158	Signs appear either at birth or 3 to 6 months of age; characterized by a grossly normal cerebellum, but microscopically by reduced numbers, degenerate, or abnormally arranged Purkinje cells, decreased width of granular and molecular cell layers and sometimes gliosis	Possibly genetic and/or viral; if genetic, autosomal recessive is most likely	Fairly common and only reported in Arabians and part-Arabians	Histologically; clinical signs include dysmetria, head tremor, difficulty in walking, sometimes paddling and defective menace reflex; progressive	None
Cerebellar hypoplasia (other breeds)	159, 160	Either marked smallness of cerebellum or local symmetric bilateral defects in cerebellum	Unknown	Rare; reported in 1 Thoroughbred, localized hypoplasia in another	Grossly and histologically; if total hypoplasia, convulsions and inability to rise shortly after birth; if localized, slight ataxia as an adult	None
Cerebellar ataxia	161	Grossly small or normal-size cerebellum with accentuation of lobular and foliar structure; reduced width of molecular layer, reduced numbers of granular cells, and sight Purkinje cell degeneration	Possible hereditary	Only reported in Gotland ponies	Grossly and histologically; clinical signs include ataxia, most common shortly after birth, characterized by an unstable stiff gait and falling	None

Continued

TABLE 48-9

Congenital Defects of the Nervous System in the Horse—cont'd

Defect	Ref. No.	Description	Etiology	Frequency	Diagnosis/Treatment	Associated Defects
Idiopathic epilepsy	32	Recurrent episodes of sudden loss of consciousness with or without tonic-clonic convulsions	Unknown	Unknown	Signs are identical to symptomatic epilepsy and vary from petit mal seizures, which resemble fainting, to grand mal characterized by distress, semiconsciousness, tonic spasms, cyanosis, and then clonic spasms with facial twitching and loss of reflexes	None
Spina bifida	162	Incomplete fusion of dorsal vertebrae; meninges and spinal cord may protrude through defect; neurologic signs	Unknown	Rare	Soft tissue swelling on spine above defect; radiographs	Meningomyelocele
Syringomyelia	163	Tubular cavitation in spinal cord	Unknown	One case reported in cervical spinal cord	At necropsy	None
Ventral meningomyelocele	164	Unable to stand unassisted at birth; progressive hypermetria and ataxia of hind limbs	Unknown	Very rare, 1 case reported in a foal	Clinical signs and pathologic examination; neural tube defect of ventral part of neuraxis between C_7 and T_2	None
Spinal dysraphism	168	Hydromyelia and syringomyelia (cavitation) in cervical and thoracic spinal cord	Unknown	One case reported in a 5-month-old Thoroughbred filly	Abnormal gait; grossly and histologically	None
Equine degenerative myeloencephalopathy	169	Symmetric ataxia and paresis at 3 months and older; static or progressive for weeks or months	Vitamin E deficiency with a familial predisposition	Common	Clinical examination and histopathology	None
Neuroaxonal dystrophy in Morgan horses	170	Gait abnormality; hind legs placed forward under the trunk; dyssymmetric hind limb gait; incoordination, lateral swaying	Vitamin E deficiency on a familial basis	Rare	Clinical examination and histopathology	None
Congenital myoclonus	174	Reported in Peruvian Paso foals; hyperesthesia and myoclonic jerks in skeletal muscles; stilted gait	Unknown; 60% deficiency in density of inhibitory glycine receptors in spinal cord	Rare; reported in 4 foals	Neurologic examination	None

					Neurologic examination	None
Narcolepsy	175	Excessive sleepiness, depression, episodes of collapse	Only reported in two miniature horses	Unknown	Neurologic examination	None
Oldenburg ataxia	165	Progressive ataxia first appearing at 3 to 4 weeks of age characterized pathologically by circumscribed gray-to-red areas in the cerebellum that prove histologically to be malacic	Possibly a recessive trait	Reported only in the Oldenburg breed	Grossly and histologically; clinical signs include a course of 8-14 days and progression from episodes of dancing forelimbs to falling over backward, then recumbency, paddling, opisthotonos, and death	None
Internal hydrocephalus	166, 167	Increased CSF in ventricles of brain	Obstruction of outflow of CSF in the lateral and third ventricles, interventricular foramen, or between brain and spinal cord	Unknown	May or may not be cranial enlargement at birth; enlarged lateral ventricles seen at necropsy; clinical signs vary from stillbirth to unsteady, staggering foals	None
Congenital encephalomyelopathy	171	Rear limb tremors, inability to stand from birth	Unknown	Rare	Clinical signs and histopathologic examination, spongiform degeneration with axonal swelling	None
Agenesis of corpus callosum with cerebellar vermian hypoplasia	172	Wide, dome-shaped forehead, paddling of all four limbs, tonic-clonic clamping of jaw, erratic respiratory rate, no sucking reflex, lateral recumbency in a neonate; foal improved, but it remained ataxic with an intention tremor	Unknown	Very rare, 1 case reported	Neurologic examination, CT scanner, pathologic examination revealed absence of corpus callosum and caudal $^2/_3$ of caudal cerebellar vermis	None
Familial neurologic syndrome in newborn Thoroughbred foals	173	Symmetric cerebellar or spinocerebellar dysfunction; will recover; three of five foals out of one mare by different sires affected; sudden onset of severe ataxia at 2-5 days of age	Unknown	Rare	Neurologic examination; remission of signs with diazepam therapy	None

CSF, Cerebrospinal fluid; *CT,* computed tomography.

TABLE 48-10

Congenital Defects of the Musculoskeletal System in the Horse

Defect	Ref. No.	Description	Etiology	Frequency	Diagnosis/Treatment	Associated Defects
Multiple exostoses	32, 176-178	Many bony protuberances, most commonly bilateral and symmetric on ribs near the costochondral junction and most long bones and pelvis; the exostoses begin as cartilage and are replaced by bone continuous with the normal bone; growth of exostoses stops at maturity	Dominant trait	Uncommon	Physical examination; radiographic and histologic examination; may or may not cause lameness	None
Contracted foal	8, 21, 179-182	Syndrome seen in aborted fetuses, foals, and yearlings characterized by bilateral contractures of the joints of the limbs, asymmetric formation of cranium, torticollis (wryneck), and scoliosis (lateral deviation of spine), or both	Unknown, possibly because of uterine position	Common	Physical and radiographic examination	May include thin or unclosed ventral abdominal wall, defect in diaphragm, and hypoplasia and malformations of joint articulations
Unilateral contracted foot	176	Contraction of one forefoot with narrowing of heels; often present at birth	Unknown	Unknown	Physical examination; may or may not cause lameness	None
Lordosis	182, 222	Swayback	Unknown	Rare	Physical and radiographic examination	Hypoplasia of the intervertebral articular processes
Adactyly and polydactyly	183, 184	Absence of all bones distal to radius, except for one carpal bone on one foreleg and overdevelopment of the second digit on the other forefoot	Unknown	One case reported in a Welsh foal	Physical and radiographic examination, and at necropsy	None
Polydactyly	185-191	Presence of a supernumerary digit, usually on a forelimb	Unknown	Rare	Physical examination; can be corrected surgically	None
Anterior deviation of carpal joint (bucked knees, knee sprung, goat knees)	176	Continuous partial forward flexion of carpus because of a malformed carpal joint and resulting abnormal articulations	Possibly malposition of fetus in utero or vitamin or mineral deficiency in mare	Fairly common	Physical examination; physical therapy to extend joint, surgery if severe	None
Medial deviation of carpal joint (knock) knees, angular limb deformity)	144, 176, 192-200, 224	Inward deviation of knees; developmental orthopedic disease	Hereditary factors, malpositioning in utero, or nutritional deficiency	Common	Physical examination; various treatments such as casting, periosteal stripping, or physeal stapling	None

Defect	References	Description	Cause	Frequency	Diagnosis	Other
Contracted digital flexor tendons	176, 180, 226, 227	Contraction of superficial or deep digital flexor tendons or both, present at birth	Possibly genetic, malposition in utero, or nutritional deficiency	Fairly common	Knuckling of fetlock if just superficial tendon is affected; lifting of the heel if deep tendon is involved; oxytetracycline	Sometimes contracture of suspensory ligament; one case reported hypoplasia of bones distal to hock in affected limb
Weak flexor tendons in foals	176, 201	Bilateral over-extension (extreme dorsiflexion) of phalangeal joints; in severe cases, the fetlock touches the ground, and the toe turns up	Prematurity or dysmaturity	Occasional	Physical examination; most will correct on their own, but some need to be supported; a surgical technique has been described	None or other signs of prematurity or dysmaturity
Lateral luxation of the patella	196, 202, 203	Unilateral or bilateral, lateral position of the patella with abnormal trochleas, hypoplasia of lateral ridge of femoral trochlea	Simple autosomal recessive	Rare	Squatting stance with hips, stifles, and hocks in extreme flexion; confirmation radiographically and at necropsy	90-degree rotation of patellas in one case
Absence of patella	204	Agenesis of patella	Unknown	One case reported in a foal	Radiographically	None
Patellar ectopia	205	Bilateral posterior and lateral position of patellas to lateral epicondyles with normal femoral trochleas	No primary deformity producing the ectopia or underdevelopment of medial femoropatellar ligaments	Rare	Same typical squatting stance as patellar luxation, trochlea are normal; confirmation radiographically and at necropsy	None
Upward fixation of the patella	176	Fixation of the patella on medial femoral trochlea between middle and medial patellar ligaments, causing constant extension of hind limb; may be unilateral or bilateral	Possibly hereditary predisposition, because horses with "straight hind leg" conformation are more predisposed	Fairly common	Locking or catching of hind limb in stifle and hock extension; to test, if only catching, the patella may be forced up by hand, and the limb will lock for a few steps	None
Phalangeal hypoplasia (dysgenesis)	206-209	Distal phalangeal aplasia or dysgenesis, navicular agenesis or hypoplasia	Unknown	Rare	Physical and radiographic examination	Hoof malformation; abnormal digital blood vessels
Hip dysplasia	210, 211	May be unilateral or bilateral; changes include shallow acetabula, flattening of hip, and osteoarthritic changes in hip	Unknown	Rare; reported in a Shetland pony colt and a Standardbred colt	Radiographically; lameness not apparent until marked changes are present	None
Ameloblastic odontoma	212	Slow-growing tumor in maxillary region, which histologically contains both ameloblastic epithelium and mineralized odontoid tissue; unilateral	Unknown	Rare	Secondary unilateral maxillary sinusitis and hemorrhage; radiopaque; confirm histologically	None

Continued

TABLE 48-10

Congenital Defects of the Musculoskeletal System in the Horse—cont'd

Defect	Ref. No.	Description	Etiology	Frequency	Diagnosis/ Treatment	Associated Defects
Predisposition to periodontitis	213	Inflammation around roots of teeth beginning between lower molars 1 and 2; predisposed by too much space between M_1 and M_2	Possibly inherited as a dominant trait	74 cases reported by one author	Physical examination	None
Cyclopia	21, 214	Presence of two eyes close together with fusion of eyelids in median plane; absence of nasal opening; only one brain hemisphere present	Unknown	Rare	At necropsy	Brain defects
Atlantooccipital fusion	215, 216	Fusion of the first cervical vertebra to the occipital region of the head and hypoplasia and nonfusion of the odontoid process (dens)	Unknown	Reported mostly in Arabians	Radiographically; clinical signs progress from abnormal gait to inability to rise from sternal recumbency; secondary compression and malacia of cord at level of occipital condyles	None
Myotonia with dystrophic changes	217, 218	Sustained muscle contraction after stimulation in young horses with muscle hypertrophy and hypertonicity followed later by muscle stiffness, atrophy and weakness; histopathology reveals dystrophic changes in muscle; pathophysiologic changes on electromyography	Possibly genetic	Rare	Physical examination; biochemical, electromyographic, and histopathological examination	None
Arthrogryposis	219, 220	Syndrome was lethal and consisting of caudal bimelic contracture of limbs in flexion associated with polydactyly of the hindlegs and brachygnathia superior	Most likely genetic	Rare; reported in Norwegian Fjord horses	Physical examination, radiology and necropsy	Polydactyly; short lower jaw; autosomal trisomy in some cases
Arthrogryposis (various breeds)		Two or more limbs arthrogrypotic, often resulting in dystocia	Unknown	Uncommon	Physical examination; dystocia, unable to correct fetal malposition; necropsy	None
Amelia anterior	221	Both front legs missing	Unknown	Rare	Physical examination	None

Multiple skeletal defects in an Arabian foal	223, 224	Unknown	Foal's carpi fixed in flexion, fourth carpal bone hypoplastic, second and fourth metacarpal bones absent	One case reported in an Arabian	Physical examination, x-rays	None
Deviated anterior maxilla	225	Unknown	Deviation of nose to one side, unable to suckle, malocclusion of maxillary incisor teeth	Rare	Physical examination, distortion of nasal septum; may be corrected surgically	None
Dystrophy-like myopathy	228	Unknown	Clinical signs of hypertrophy and hypertonicity and electromyogram revealing myotonic discharges in gluteal semitendinosus and semimembranosus muscles; muscle biopsy revealed dystrophic changes	Reported once in a Standardbred trotter foal	Physical examination, histologic, histochemical, and ultrastructural studies	None
Dislocation of deep digital flexor tendon	229	Unknown	Medial displacement of tendon noted incidentally on physical exam; not related to lameness	Rare	Palpation and radiography	Hypoplasia of sustentaculum tali
Ulnar and tibial malformation	230	Unknown	Development of complete ulnas and fibulas	Seen in Shetland and Welsh ponies	Radiography	Short limbs, medial carpal deviation
Hypoplasia of the fused first and second tarsal bones	231	Unknown	Incidental finding	One case in Standardbred yearling	Radiography; necropsy	None
Block vertebra	232	Unknown	Fusion of two vertebrae; C2-C3 fusion reported in one case, resulting in ataxia	Rare	Radiography	None
Osteopetrosis	233	Unknown	Foals born unable to rise; persistence of primary spongiosa in medullary cavity (bone cones) resulting in lack of cortical/medullary distinction on radiographs; long bones are fragile	Reported in Peruvian Paso foals	Radiography and necropsy	Brachygnathia
Choanal atresia	234		See Table 48-4			
Incomplete nasomaxillary dysplasia	235	Unknown	Abnormal development of nasolacrimal system	Rare	Dacryocystography	None

TABLE 48-11

Hernias in the Horse

Defect	Ref. No.	Description	Etiology	Frequency	Diagnosis/Treatment	Associated Defects
Umbilical hernia	32	Opening in the abdominal wall at the umbilicus appearing from birth to 7 days	Unknown	Not reported; fairly common	Physical examination; usually corrects itself by 1 year of age but may be repaired surgically	None
Scrotal (inguinal) hernia	32	Protrusion of gut through inguinal canal into the scrotum at or shortly after birth	Unknown	Not reported	Physical examination; surgical correction is indicated	None
Schistosomus reflexus	236	Severe lethal hernia in which ventral abdominal wall and skin are lacking, exposing the abdominal viscera	Unknown	Rare	At necropsy; may cause dystocia	Atresia coli, scoliosis

TABLE 48-12

Congenital Defects of the Reproductive System in the Horse

Defect	Ref. No.	Description	Etiology	Frequency	Diagnosis/Treatment	Associated Defects
Male pseudohermaphroditism	16, 17, 237-247	External genitalia are morphologically indistinct, most commonly seen as an enlarged penislike clitoris; internal genitalia are testicles, as determined histologically; testicles are usually intraabdominal, and uterine tissue may or may not be present; most show stallion type behavior	Theories include nondysjunction of chromosomes, freemartinism, and double fertilization or blastocyst fusion	Commonly reported but probably rare in the general population	Physical examination, histologically, and chromosome analysis; karyotypes reported include 64XX, 64XX/64XY, 64XX/65XXY, 63XO?/64XX/65XXY, 66XXXY and 64XX/96XXY	None
63XO aneuploidy (Turner's syndrome)	248-252	Infertility in the mare characterized by small ovaries and usually uterine hypoplasia	Unknown	Rare	Physical examination and chromosomal analysis; may be small in stature; patients have karyotype 63XO or may be mosaics	None
Cryptorchidism	253-261	Retention of testicles in inguinal canal or abdomen; natural descension may occur up to 2 years of age; if unilateral, fertility is not affected	Thought to be hereditary	Relatively common	IV injection of HCG and assay of testosterone can usually distinguish between cryptorchids and geldings; surgical correction	None
Monorchidism	262	Only one testicle developed	Unknown	Very rare	Physical examination	None
XY sex reversal syndrome	14, 17, 263, 264	Phenotypic mares with karyotype of a stallion; ranges from nearly normal female to a greatly masculinized mare	Genetic; X-linked recessive or autosomal sex-influenced dominant through female or an autosomal sex-influenced dominant through chromosomal mutation with variable expression transmitted through the male	Infrequently described in Arabians, Thoroughbreds, Quarter horses, and Shetland ponies	Physical examination and karyotyping	None
64XY fertile female	265	Small ovaries, undeveloped uterus, had XX filly	H-Y genes loss of suppression	Very rare	Physical examination, karyotyping, and reduced levels of H-Y antigen in blood	None
Excess fetal fluid	266	Excess fluid (40 L or more); abdominal distention	Unknown	Rare	Physical examination	Foal had herniated viscera; another foal was reported being affected with schistocoelia; others; hydrocephalus, wryneck; twin pregnancies

HCG, Human chorionic gonadotropin; *IV,* intravenous.

Continued

TABLE 48-12

Congenital Defects of the Reproductive System in the Horse—cont'd

Defect	Ref. No.	Description	Etiology	Frequency	Diagnosis/Treatment	Associated Defects
Pseudohermaphroditism	267	Enlarged clitoris and gonadlike structures subcutaneously in the groin and a 64XX chromosomal constitution or a hypoplastic penis and a testislike structure in the left groin and 64 XY chromosomal constitution	Unknown	Rare, 3 cases described	Physical examination and karyotyping	None
Dysgenesis of tubal system in an infertile mare	268	Hypoplasia of uterine tubes; mosaic karyotype 63XO/64XY/65XXY	Unknown	Rare	Physical examination and karyotyping	None
True hemaphrodite	269	No stallion-like behavior; under-developed penis, bilateral seminal vesicles and uterine tissue; bilateral ovotestes	Unknown	Two cases reported	Physical examination and karyotyping, 64XX/64XY or 63XO/64XY	None
63XO/64XX mosaic	14, 245, 270	Ovaries are small	Unknown	Rare	Physical examination and karyotyping	None
63XO/64XY mosaic	11, 270	Small firm ovaries lacking germ cells and consisting of undifferentiated ovarian stroma; flaccid uterus	Unknown	Rare	Physical examination and karyotyping	None
Klinefelter's syndrome	12, 271	Testicular hypoplasia; aplasia of germinal cells	Nondisjunction	Rare	Physical examination; karyotype is 65XXY	None
Balanced reciprocal translocation	272	Poor reproductive performance	Unknown	Very rare	Karyotyping, carrier of balanced reciprocal translocation of segments of chromosome 1 and 3	None
Isochromosome Xi	273	One abnormal X chromosome with two complete long arms that are genetically identical	Unknown	Very rare	Karyotyping 64Xi(Xq)	Infertile mare, small ovaries, small stature, mental dullness, reduced vision
Vestibulovaginal hypoplasia	274	Circumferential narrowing of vagina cranial to external urethral orifice	Unknown	Rare	Palpation and endoscopy	Persistent hymen
Uterus unicornis	275	Absence of uterine horn	Unknown	Rare	Palpation and ultrasonography	Ovarian hypoplasia

TABLE 48-13

Immunodeficiencies in the Horse

Defect	Ref. No.	Description	Etiology	Frequency	Diagnosis/Treatment	Associated Defects
Severe combined immunodeficiency (SCID)	276-298	Fatal disease of young foals characterized by a combined (B- and T-lymphocyte) immunodeficiency; cause of death is usually an adenovirus pneumonia or other secondary infection; refractory to treatment	Inherited as a simple autosomal-recessive trait	Reported only in Arabian breed; occurred in 2.3% of 257 Arabian foals tested; 25.7% of all Arabians estimated to be carriers	Lymphopenia (1000/mm³), deficiency of one or more immunoglobulin class (especially IgM), intravenous challenge with sheep RBCs for antibody response, intradermal injection of PHA to test T cell response; lesions include thymic hypoplasia with fat replacement and absence of germinal centers from spleen and lymph nodes, carriers can be identified by a DNA test on blood or cheek swab	None
B-lymphocyte deficiency	280	Deficiency of B lymphocytes and resulting agammaglobulinemia with normal function of T lymphocytes	Unknown	One case reported in a 1-year-old Thoroughbred	Rule out SCID, IgM deficiency, and failure of passive transfer; frequent infections	None

DNA, Dexoyribonucleic acid; *PHA*, phytohemagglutinin; *RBCs*, red bood cells; *RID*, radial immunodiffusion; *SCID*, severe combined immunodeficiency.

Continued

TABLE 48-13

Immunodeficiencies in the Horse—cont'd

Defect	Ref. No.	Description	Etiology	Frequency	Diagnosis/Treatment	Associated Defects
IgM deficiency	290, 291	Deficiency of IgM with normal amounts of other immunoglobulins and lymphocytes; most common presentation is a 4- to 8-month-old foal with respiratory tract infection or enteritis	Clinically significant immune disorder of all breeds and ages as a primary disorder (genetic) or secondary as a result of immunosuppression	Common	Immunodiffusion test for detection of IgM plus other tests rule out SCID, B-cell deficiency, or failure of passive transfer	None
Infantile X-linked recessive agammaglobulinemia	286, 287	Found in males; clinical signs observed between 2 to 6 months of age include pneumonia, enteritis, dermatitis, arthritis, and laminitis; also absence of B lymphocytes, IgM, and IgA and very low levels of IgG and IgG(T)	X-linked recessive	Rare in Thoroughbreds, Standardbreds, and Quarter horses	Physical examination and RID for specific immunoglobulin classes	None
Anemia, immunodeficiency and peripheral ganglionopathy syndrome	299	Onset at 2-3 weeks of age of diarrhea, cough, and failure to suckle; progresses to anemia, secondary opportunistic infections, and death by 1-3 months of age; characterized by small numbers of late erythroid precursors in bone marrow, small thymus, lack of secondary lymphoid follicles and plasma cells, and neuronal chromatolysis of peripheral ganglia	Unknown, possibly genetic	Seen in Fell pony foals	Physical examination; immunologic and pathologic studies	None

TABLE 48-14

Metabolic Defects in the Horse

Defect	Ref. No.	Description	Etiology	Frequency	Diagnosis/Treatment	Associated Defects
Hyperkalemic periodic paralysis (HYPP, HPP); episodic weakness associated with intermittent serum hyperkalemia	300-312	First episodes apparent in young horses 2 to 3 years of age; brief period of myotonia followed within minutes by flaccidity; milder cases remain standing but have generalized muscle fasciculation; during episodes serum K values are elevated; most affected horses are heterozygotes	Autosomal dominant, but evidence for codominance because homozygotes appear to be more severely affected than heterozygotes; reported in Quarter horses (especially well-muscled halter-types), part Quarter horses, Paint horses, and Appaloosas	Common	Clinical examination and serum potassium during attack; can precipitate attack by administering oral potassium; whole blood (EDTA treated) for gene probe for HPP-type sodium channel DNA (homozygotes can be distinguished from heterozygotes); reduce dietary potassium	Possible hyperthermia during isoflurane anesthesia; may have reduced exercise tolerance; homozygotes may have pharyngeal dysfunction and respiratory stertor
Glucose-6-phosphate dehydrogenase (G-6-PD) deficiency	313	Persistent hemolytic anemia; macrocytic, normochromic anemia with anisocytosis and eccentrocytes and pyknocytes	Unknown	One case reported in an American Saddlebred colt	Hematologic examination, G-6-PD assays	None
Recurrent exertional rhabdomyolysis (RER) associated with polysaccharide storage myopathy	314, 315	Exercise intolerance with episodes of stiffness, muscle cramping, and myoglobinuria; increased serum creatine kinase and aspartate aminotransferase; associated with excessive storage of glycogen and abnormal accumulation in muscle	Genetic, probably autosomal recessive	Seen in Quarter horses, Appaloosa, and American Paint	Clinical signs plus histologic finding of widespread presence of sarcolemmal vacuoles and PAS-positive inclusions	None
RER in Thoroughbreds	315	Same signs as RER in Quarter horse breeds, but without abnormal glycogen and polysaccharide storage	Possibly inherited as an autosomal-dominant trait with variable expression	Common in Thoroughbreds	Clinical signs	None

DNA, Deoxyribonucleic acid; *EDTA,* ethylenediame tetraacidic acid; *PAS,* periodic acid–Schiff.

TABLE 48-15

Congenital Duplication in the Horse

Defect	Ref. No.	Description	Etiology	Frequency	Diagnosis/ Treatment	Associated Defects
Diprosopus	316	Duplication of facial skeleton	Unknown	Unknown; one case reported	Physical examination, x-rays	None

TABLE 48-16

Congenital Lymphatic Defect in the Equine

Defect	Ref. No.	Description	Etiology	Frequency	Diagnosis/ Treatment	Associated Defects
Chyloabdomen	317	Accumulation of chyle in the peritoneal cavity (resulting from hypoplasia of lymphatic vessels involving part of the mesenteric lymph center) resulting in colic in a neonate	Unknown	One case reported in a Standardbred foal	Abdominocentesis; necropsy	None

21. Crowe MW, Swerczek TW: Equine congenital defects, *Am J Vet Res* 46:353-358, 1985.
22. Hong CB et al: Equine abortion and stillbirth in central Kentucky during 1988 and 1989 foaling seasons, *J Vet Diagn Invest* 5:560-566, 1993.
23. Giles RC et al: Causes of abortion, stillbirth, and perinatal death in horses: 3527 cases (1986-1991), *J Am Vet Med Assoc* 203:1170-1175, 1993.
24. Tengelsen LA et al: A 12-year retrospective study of equine abortion in Michigan, *J Vet Diagn Invest* 9:303-306, 1997.
25. Batstone JHF: Cleft palate in a horse, *Br J Plast Surg* 19:327-331, 1966.
26. Jones RS et al: Surgical repair of cleft palate in the horse, *Equine Vet J* 7:86-90, 1975.
27. Kendrick JW: Cleft palate in a horse, *Cornell Vet* 40:188-189, 1950.
28. Stickle RL, Goble DO, Braden TD: Surgical repair of cleft soft palate in a foal, *Vet Med* 68:159-162, 1973.
29. Keeling NG, Moll HD: Use of mucosal graft to augment cleft palate repair in a foal, *Equine Pract* 17:34-39, 1995.
30. Proudman CJ et al: Soft palate hypoplasia in a horse, *Vet Rec* 129:284-286, 1991.
31. Riley CB, Yovich JV, Balbon JR: Bilateral hypoplasia of the soft palate in a foal, *Aust Vet J* 68:178-179, 1991.
32. Catcott EJ, Smithcors JF: *Equine medicine and surgery*, ed 2, Wheaton, Ill, 1972, American Veterinary.
33. Fuchslocher F, Rusch, K: Atresia recti bei einem Vollblutfohlen, *Dtsche tierarztl Wschr* 78:519, 1971.
34. Young RL, Linford RL, Olander HJ: Atresia coli in the foal: review of six cases, *Equine Vet J* 24:60-62, 1992.
35. Lopez MJ et al: What is your diagnosis? *J Am Vet Med Assoc* 211:161-162, 1997.
36. Mason TA: Tympany of the eustachian tube diverticulum (guttural pouch) in a foal, *Equine Vet J* 4:153-154, 1972.
37. Fowler ME: Congenital atresia of the parotid duct in the horse, *J Am Vet Med Assoc* 78:1403-1404, 1965.
38. Gift LJ et al: Brachygnathia in horses: 20 cases (1979-1989), *J Am Vet Med Assoc* 200:715-719, 1992.
39. Hultgren BD: Ileocolonic aganglionosis in white progeny of overo spotted horses, *J Am Vet Med Assoc* 180:289-292, 1982.
40. Schneider JE, Leipold HW: Recessive lethal white in two foals, *J Equine Med Surg* 2:479-482, 1978.
41. Vonderfecht SL et al: Congenital intestinal aganglionosis in white foals, *Vet Pathol* 20:65-70, 1983.
42. Blendinger C, Muller G, Bosted H: Das "Lethal-white-foal" syndrome, *Tierarztl Prax* 22:252-255, 1994.
43. Bowling AT: Dominant inheritance of overo spotting in Paint horses, *J Hered* 85:223-224, 1994.
44. McCabe L et al: Overo lethal white foal syndrome: equine model of aganglionic megacolon (Hirschsprung disease), *Am J Med Genet* 36:336-340, 1990.
45. Dylse TM, Laing EA, Hutchins DR: Megacolon in two related Clydesdales, *Aust Vet J* 67:463-464, 1990.
46. Murray MJ, Paulse GA, White NA: Megacolon with myenteric hypoganglionosis in a foal, *J Am Vet Med Assoc* 192:917-919, 1988.
47. Oikawa M, Kaneko M, Yoshikawa T: Villous hypoplasia of small intestine in neonatal foals, *Jpn J Vet Sci* 52:855-858, 1990.
48. Oikawa M, Kaneko M, Yoshikawa T: Villous hypoplasia of small intestine in neonatal foals, *J Vet Med* A39:121-129, 1992.
49. Behrens E: Meckel's diverticulum in a horse, *Vet Med* 91:208, 1996.
50. McConnico RS, Duckett WM, Wood PA: Persistent hyperammonemia in two related Morgan weanlings, *J Vet Int Med* 11:264-266, 1997.
51. Peek SF, De Lahunta A, Hackett RP: Combined oesophageal and tracheal duplication cyst in an Arabian filly, *Equine Vet J* 27:475-478, 1995.
52. Colbourne CM et al: Hamartomatous polyp causing intestinal obstruction and tenesmus in a neonatal foal, *Aust Equine Vet* 14:78-80, 1996.
53. Buchanan JW, Bovee KC, Chacko SK: Clinicopathologic conference, *J Am Vet Med Assoc* 160:451-460, 1972.
54. Critchley KL: The importance of blood gas measurement in the diagnosis of an intraventricular septal defect in a horse: a case report, *Equine Vet J* 8:128-129, 1976.
55. Glazier DB, Farrelly BT, O'Connor J: Ventricular septal defect in a 7-year-old gelding, *J Am Vet Med Assoc* 167:49-50, 1975.
56. Knauer KW, McMullan WC, Clark DR: Diagnosis of an interventricular septal defect in a horse, *Vet Med* 68:75-78, 1973.
57. Muylle E et al: An interventricular septal defect and a tricuspid valve insufficiency in a trotter horse, *Equine Vet J* 6:174-176, 1974.
58. Seahorn TL, Hormanski EH: Ventricular septal defect and atrial fibrillation in an adult horse, *J Equine Vet Sci* 13:36-38, 1993.
59. Carmichael JA et al: Diagnosis of patent ductus arteriosus in a horse, *J Am Vet Med Assoc* 158:767-775, 1971.
60. Glazier DB, Farrelly BT, Neylon JF: Patent ductus arteriosus in an eight-month-old foal, *Ir Vet J* 28:12-13, 1974.
61. Rooney JR, Franks WC: Congenital cardiac anomalies in horses, *Pathol Vet* 1:454-464, 1964.
62. Reppas GP et al: Multiple congenital cardiac anomalies and idiopathic thoracic aortitis in a horse, *Vet Rec* 138:14-16, 1996.
63. Wilson AP: Persistent foramen ovale in a foal, *Vet Med* 38:491-492, 1943.
64. Bartels JE, Vaughan JT: Persistent right aortic arch in the horse, *J Am Vet Med Assoc* 154:406-409, 1969.
65. Butt TD al: Persistent right aortic arch in a yearling horse, *Can Vet J* 39:714-715, 1998.
66. Vitums A: Origin of the aorta and pulmonary trunk from the right ventricle in a horse, *Pathol Vet* 7:482-491, 1970.
67. Vitums A et al: Transposition of the aorta and atresia of the pulmonary trunk in a horse, *Cornell Vet* 63:41-57, 1973.
68. Greene HJ, Wray DD, Greenway JA: Two equine congenital cardiac anomalies, *Ir Vet J* 29:115-117, 1975.
69. Prickett ME, Reeves JT, Zent WW: Tetralogy of Fallot in a Thoroughbred foal, *J Am Vet Med Assoc* 162:552-555, 1973.
70. Rahal C et al: Pentalogy of Fallot, renal infarction and renal abscess in a mare, *J Equine Vet Sci* 17:604-607, 1997.

71. Daniels H: Drei Fülle einer komplexen Herzmissbildung beim Fohlen, *Dtsche tierarztl Wschr* 81:622-623, 1974.

72. Awtokratow DM: Das dreikammerige Herz des Pferdes (cor triloculare biatriatum equi): zur Kasiustik des Fehlens einer Scheidewand zwischen den Herzkammern des Pferdes, *Anat Anz* 65:260-266, 1928.

73. Beech J, Dubielzig R, Bester R: Portal vein anomaly and hepatic encephalopathy in a horse, *J Am Vet Med Assoc* 170:164-166, 1977.

74. Fortier LA et al: The diagnosis and surgical correction of congenital portosystemic vascular anomalies in two calves and two foals, *Vet Surg* 25:154-160, 1996.

75. Gumbrell RC: Atresia of the tricuspid valve in a foal, *N Z Vet J* 18:253-256, 1970.

76. Anderson RH: The pathological spectrum of pulmonary atresia, *Equine Vet Educ* 9:128-132, 1997.

77. Young LE et al: Pulmonary atresia with an intact ventricular septum in a Thoroughbred foal, *Equine Vet Educ* 9:123-127, 1997.

78. Meurs KM C et al: Tricuspid valve atresia with main pulmonary atresia in an Arabian foal, *Equine Vet J* 29:160-162, 1997.

79. Steyn PF, Holland P, Hoffman J: The angiographic diagnosis of persistent truncus arteriosus in a foal, *J S Afr Vet Assoc* 60:106-108, 1989.

80. Hinchcliff KW, Adams WM: Critical pulmonary stenosis in a newborn foal, *Equine Vet J* 23:318-320, 1991.

81. Ecke P, Malik R, Kannegieter NJ: Common atrioventricular canal in a foal, *N Z Vet J* 39:97-98, 1991.

82. Chaffin MK, Miller MW, Morris EL: Double outlet right ventricle and other associated congenital cardiac anomalies in an American Miniature horse foal, *Equine Vet J* 24:402-406, 1992.

83. Cottrill CM, Rossdale PD: A comparison of congenital heart disease in horses and man, *Equine Vet J* 24:338-340, 1992.

84. Archer RK: True haemophilia (haemophilia A) in a Thoroughbred foal, *Vet Rec* 73:338-340, 1961.

85. Archer RK, Allen BV: True haemophilia in horses, *Vet Rec* 91:655-656, 1972.

86. Henninger RW: Hemophilia A in two related Quarter horse colts, *J Am Vet Med Assoc* 193:91-94, 1988.

87. Hutchins DR, Lepherd EE, Crook IG: A case of equine haemophilia, *Aust Vet J* 43:83-87, 1967.

88. Sanger VL, Mairs RE, Trapp AL: Hemophilia in a foal, *J Am Vet Med Assoc* 144:259-264, 1964.

89. Littlewood JD, Bevan SA: Haemophilia A (classic haemophilia, factor VIII deficiency) in a Thoroughbred calf foal, *Equine Vet J* 23:70-72, 1991.

90. Smith RE, McEntee K: Accessory thoracic lung with bronchial hypoplasia in the equine fetus, *Cornell Vet* 64:335-339, 1974.

91. Gaughan EM, DeBowes RM: Congenital diseases of the equine head, *Vet Clin North Am (Equine Pract)* 9:93-109, 1993.

92. Richardson JD, Lane JG, Dane MJ: Congenital choanal restriction in three horses, *Equine Vet J* 26:162-165, 1994.

93. Darbishire HB: Operation to repair rupture of the bladder in a young foal, *Vet Rec* 73:693-694, 1961.

94. Pascoe RR: Repair of a defect in the bladder of a foal, *Aust Vet J* 47:343-345, 1971.

95. Wellington JKM: Bladder defects in newborn foals, *Aust Vet J* 48:426, 1972.

96. Hofliger H: Zur Kenntnis der kongenitalen unilateralen Nierenagenesis bei Haustieren, *Schweitz Archiv Tierheikld* 113:330-337, 1971.

97. Houlton JEF et al: Urinary incontinence in a shire foal due to ureteral ectopia, *Equine Vet J* 19:244-247, 1987.

98. Blikslager AT, Green EM: Ectopic ureters in horses, *Compend Cont Educ* 14:802-807, 1992.

99. Pringle JK, Ducharme NG, Baird JD: Ectopic ureter in the horse: three cases and a review of the literature, *Can Vet J* 31:26-30, 1990.

100. Zicker SC et al: Bilateral renal dysplasia with nephron hypoplasia in a foal, *J Am Vet Med Assoc* 196:2001-2005, 1990.

101. Ronen N et al: Renal dysplasia in two adult horses: clinical and pathological aspects, *Vet Rec* 132:269-270, 1993.

102. Ramirez S et al: Ultrasound-assisted diagnosis of renal dysplasia in a 3-month-old Quarter horse colt, *Vet Radiol Ultrasound* 39:143-146, 1998.

103. Ramsay G et al: Polycystic kidneys in an adult horse, *Equine Vet J* 19:243-244, 1987.

104. Schott HC et al: Clinical vignette, *J Vet Int Med* 10: 204-206, 1996.

105. Jean D, Marcoux M, Louf CF: Congenital bilateral distal defect of the ureters in a foal, *Equine Vet Educ* 10:17-20, 1998.

106. Cruz AM et al: Urethrorectal fistula in a horse, *Can Vet J* 40:122-124, 1999.

107. Pulos WL, Hutt FB: Lethal dominant white in horse, *J Heredity* 60:59-63, 1969.

108. Salisbury GW, Britton JW: The inheritance of equine coat color, *J Hered* 32:255-260, 1941.

109. Crowell WA, Stephenson C, Gosser HS: Epitheliogenesis imperfecta in a foal, *J Am Vet Med Assoc* 168:56-58, 1976.

110. Dubielzig RR et al: Dental dysplasia and epitheliogenesis imperfecta in a foal, *Vet Pathol* 23:325-327, 1986.

111. Hamilton DP, Byerly CS: Congenital malignant melanoma in a foal, *J Am Vet Med Assoc* 164:1040-1041, 1974.

112. Markus G: Die angeborene Ohrfistel beim Pferd, *Dtsche Tierarztl Wschr* 81:505-506, 1974.

113. Njoku CO, Burwash WA: Congenital cutaneous papillomas in a foal, *Cornell Vet* 62:54-57, 1972.

114. Schueler RL: Congenital equine papillomatosis, *J Am Vet Med Assoc* 162:640, 1973.

115. Johnson GC et al: Ultrastructure of junctional epidermolysis bullosa in Belgian foals, *J Comp Pathol* 98:329-335, 1988.

116. Kohn CW et al: Mechanobullous disease in two Belgian foals, *Equine Vet J* 21:297-301, 1989.

117. Gelatt KN, Myers VS, McClure JR: Aspiration of congenital and soft cataracts in foals and young horses, *J Am Vet Med Assoc* 165:611-616, 1974.

118. Walde I: Some observations on congenital cataracts in the horse, *Equine Vet J* 15(suppl 2):27-36, 1983.

119. Eriksson, K: Hereditary aniridia with secondary cataract in horses, *Nord Vet Med* 7:773-793, 1955.

120. Joyce JR: Aniridia in a Quarter horse, *Equine Vet J* 15(suppl 2):21-22, 1983.

121. Matthews GA, Handscombe MC: Bilateral cataract formation and subluxation of the lenses in a foal: a case report, *Equine Vet J* 15(suppl 2):23-24, 1983.

122. Matthews AG, Crispin SM: Disease of the equine iris. I, Noninflammatory diseases, *Vet Annu* 27:156-162, 1987.

123. Cross RSN: Equine periodic ophthalmia, *Vet Rec* 78:8-13, 1966.

124. Jones TC, Maurer FD: Heredity in periodic ophthalmia, *J Am Vet Med Assoc* 101:248-249, 1942.

125. Gelatt KN, Leipold HW, Coffman JR: Bilateral optic nerve hypoplasia in a colt, *J Am Vet Med Assoc* 155:627-631, 1969.

126. Saperstein G: Hypoplasia of the upper lip in a foal, *Vet Med Small Anim Clin* 78:869, 1983.

127. Dziezyc J, Kern TJ, Wolf DE: Microphthalmia in a foal, *Equine Vet J* 15(suppl 2):15-17, 1983.

128. Garner A, Griffiths P: Bilateral congenital ocular defects in a foal, *Br J Ophthalmol* 53:513-517, 1969.

129. Latimer CA, Wyman M, Hamilton J: An ophthalmic survey of the neonatal horse, *Equine Vet J* 15(suppl 2):9-14, 1983.

130. Koch P, Fischer H: Erblich bedingte Blindgeburten von Fohlen eines deutschen Zuchtgebietes, *Tierarztl Umsch* 7:46-48, 1952.

131. Joyce JR et al: Iridial hypoplasia (aniridia) accompanied by limbic dermoids and cataracts in a group of related Quarter horses, *Equine Vet J Suppl* 10:26-28, 1990.

132. Buyukmihci NC, MacMillan A, Scagliotti RH: Evaluation of zones of iris hypoplasia in horses and ponies, *J Am Vet Med Assoc* 200:940-942, 1992.

133. Roberts GM: Congenital ocular anomalies, *Vet Clin North Am (Equine Pract)* 8:459-477, 1992.

134. Munroe GA: Congenital corneal vascularisation in a neonatal Thoroughbred foal, *Equine Vet J* 27:156-157, 1995.

135. Williams DL, Barnett KC: Bilateral optic disc coloboma and microphthalmos in a Thoroughbred horse, *Vet Rec* 132:101-103, 1993.

136. Halenda RM et al: Congenital equine glaucoma: clinical and light microscopic findings in two cases, *Vet Comp Ophthalmol* 7:105-109, 1997.

137. Drew B, Barber WP, Williams DG: The effect of excess dietary iodine on pregnant mares and foals, *Vet Rec* 97:93-95, 1975.

138. Irvine CMG: Hypothyroidism in the foal, *Equine Vet J* 16:306-312, 1984.

139. Bardwell RE: Osteomalacia in horses, *J Am Vet Med Assoc* 138:158-162, 1961.

140. Mayhew IG: *Large animal neurology: a handbook for veterinary clinicians*, Philadelphia, 1989, Lea & Febiger.

141. Dimock WW: Wobbles: an hereditary disease in horses, *J Hered* 41:319-323, 1950.

142. Fraser H, Palmer AC: Equine incoordination and wobbler disease of young horses, *Vet Rec* 80:338-355, 1967.

143. Matthias D, Dietz O, Rechenberg R: Clinical features and pathology of spinal ataxia in foals, *Arch Exp Vet Med* 19:43-72, 1965.

144. Rooney JR: Equine incoordination. I, Gross morphology, *Cornell Vet* 53:411-422, 1963.

145. Rooney JR: Etiology of the wobbler syndrome, *Mod Vet Pract* 53:42, 1972.

146. Ruppanner R, Gelinas L de G, Marcoux M: Case report: equine incoordination, *Can Vet J* 13:180-183, 1972.

147. Schebitz H: Cerebellar ataxia, *Mod Vet Pract* 49:40-41, 1968.

148. Wagner PC et al: A study of the heritability of cervical vertebral malformation in horses, *Proceedings of the Thirty-first Annual Convention of the American Association of Equine Practitioners*, 1985, pp 43-50.

149. Baird JD, Mackenzie CD: Cerebellar hypoplasia and degeneration in part-Arab horses, *Aust Vet J* 50:25-28, 1974.

150. Cook WR, Palmer AC: Arab cerebellar disease, *Vet Rec* 88:200, 1971.

151. DeBowes RD, Leipold HW, Turner-Beatty M: Cerebellar abiotrophy, *Vet Clin North Am (Equine Pract)* 3:345-352, 1987.

152. Dungworth DL, Fowler ME: Cerebellar hypoplasia and degeneration in a foal, *Cornell Vet* 56:17-24, 1966.

153. Fraser H: Two dissimilar types of cerebellar disorder in the horse, *Vet Rec* 78:608-612, 1966.

154. Palmer AC et al: Cerebellar hypoplasia and degeneration in the young Arab horse: clinical and neuropathological features, *Vet Rec* 93:62-66, 1973.

155. Sponseller ML: Cerebellar hypoplasia, *Mod Vet Pract* 49:40, 1968.

156. Sponseller ML: Equine cerebellar hypoplasia and degeneration, *Proceedings of the Thirteenth Annual Convention of the American Association of Equine Practitioners*, 1967, pp 123-126.

157. Turner-Beatty M: Cerebellar disease in Arabian horses, *Proceedings of the Thirty-second Annual Convention of the American Association of Equine Practitioners*, 1986, pp 241-255.

158. Gerber H et al: Cerebellare abiotrophie be vollblutaraber fohlen, *Pferdeheilkunde* 11: 423-431, 1995.

159. Olivezr RE: Cerebellar hypoplasia in a Thoroughbred foal, *Vet J* 23:15, 1975.

160. Wheat JD, Kennedy PC: Cerebellar hypoplasia and its sequela in a horse, *J Am Vet Med Assoc* 131:291-293, 1957.

161. Bjork G et al: Congenital cerebellar ataxia in the Gotland pony breed, *Zentralbl Vet Med* 20A:341-354, 1973.

162. Rivas LJ, Hinchcliff KW, Robertson JT: Cervical meningomyelocele associated with spina bifida in a hydrocephalic miniature colt, *J Am Vet Med Assoc* 209:950-953, 1996.

163. Hamir AN: Syringomyelia in a stallion, *Vet Rec* 137:293-294, 1995.

164. Harmelin A et al: Ventral meningomyelocele in a filly, *J Comp Pathol* 109:93-97, 1993.

165. Koch P, Fischer H: Die Oldenburger Fohlenataxie als Erbkrankheit, *Tierarztl Umsch* 5:158-159, 1951.

166. Behrens H: Examination of cerebrospinal fluid in primary chronic congenital hydrocephalus in a horse, *Dtsche Tierarztl Wschr* 60:285-297, 1953.

167. Ojala M, Ala-Huikku J: Inheritance of hydrocephalus in horses, *Equine Vet J* 24:140-143, 1992.

168. Cho DY, Leipold HW: Myelodysplasia in a foal, *Equine Vet J* 9:195-197, 1977.

169. Mayhew IG et al: Equine degenerative myeloencephalopathy: a vitamin E deficiency that may be familial, *J Vet Intern Med* 1:45-50, 1987.

170. Beech J: Neuroaxonal dystrophy of the accessory cuneate nucleus in horses, *Vet Pathol* 21:384-393, 1984.

171. Seahorn TY et al: Congenital encephalomyelopathy in a Quarter horse, *Equine Vet J* 23:394-395, 1991.

172. Cudd TA, Mayhew IA, Cottrill CM: Agenesis of the corpus callosum with cerebellar vermian hypoplasia in a foal resembling the Dandy-Walker syndrome: pre-mortem diagnosis by clinical evaluation and CT scanning, *Equine Vet J* 21:378-381, 1989.

173. Mayhew IA, Schneiders DH: An unusual familial neurological syndrome in newborn Thoroughbred foals, *Vet Rec* 133:447-448, 1993.

174. Jones WE: Peruvian Paso genetic problem, *Equine Vet Data* 15:385, 1993.

175. Lunn DP et al: Familial occurrence of narcolepsy in miniature horses, *Equine Vet J* 25:483-487, 1993.

176. Adams OR: *Lameness in horses*, ed 3, Philadelphia, 1974, Lea & Febiger.

177. Gardner EJ et al: Hereditary multiple exostosis, *J Hered* 66:318-322, 1975.

178. Shupe JL et al: Multiple exostosis in horses, *Mod Vet Pract* 51:34-36, 1970.

179. Finocchio EJ: A case of contracted foal syndrome, *Vet Med* 68:1254-1255, 1973.

180. Mitchell PJ, Parkes RD: Congenital hypoplasia in a foal, *Vet Rec* 95:176, 1974.

181. Rooney JR: Contracted foals, *Cornell Vet* 56:172-187, 1966.

182. Rooney JR: Congenital equine scoliosis and lordosis, *Clin Orthop* 62:25-30, 1969.

183. Leipold HW, Macdonald KR: Adactylia and polydactylia in a Welsh foal, *Vet Med* 66:928-930, 1971.

184. Modransky P et al: Unilateral phalangeal dysgenesis and navicular agenesis in a foal, *Equine Vet J* 19:347-349, 1987.

185. Evans LH, Jenney J, Raker CW: Surgical correction of polydactylism in the horse, *J Am Vet Med Assoc* 146:1405-1408, 1965.

186. Flancic D, Pukalac V: Falle verschiedener Polydakylien bei Pferden, *Dtsche Tierarztl Wschr* 62:11-14, 1955.

187. Knorr B: Peromelie samtlicher Extremitaten mit gleichzeitiger Polydaktylie beider Hintergliedmassen eines rheinischdeutschen Kaltblutfohlens, *Dtsche Tierarztl Wschr* 49:562-563, 1951.

188. McGavin MD, Leipold HW: Attempted surgical correction of equine polydactylism, *J Am Vet Med Assoc* 166:63-64, 1975.

189. Severson BO: Cloven hoof of Percheron, *J Hered* 8:466, 1917.

190. Stanek CH, Hantak E: Bilateral atavistic polydactyly in a colt and its dam, *Equine Vet J* 18:76-79, 1986.

191. Theile H: Polydactylism in a foal, *Monatschr Vet-Med* 13:342, 1958.

192. Bramlage LR: Clinical manifestations of disturbed bone formation in the horse, *Proceedings of the Thirty-fourth Annual Convention of the American Association of Equine Practitioners*, 1988, pp 135-142.

193. Caron JP: Angular limb deformities in foals, *Equine Vet J* 20:225-228, 1988.

194. Gabel AA et al: Comparison of incidence and severity of developmental orthopedic disease on 17 farms before and after adjustment of ration, *Proceedings of the Thirty-fourth Annual Convention of the American Association of Equine Practitioners*, 1988, pp 163-170.

195. Glade MJ: The role of endocrine factors in equine developmental orthopedic disease, *Proceedings of the Thirty-fourth Annual Convention of the American Association of Equine Practitioners*, 1988, pp 171-189.

196. Hermans WA et al: Investigation into the heredity of congenital lateral patella (sub)luxation in the Shetland pony, *Vet Q* 9:1-8, 1987.

197. Hintz HF: Factors which influence developmental orthopedic disease, *Proceedings of the Thirty-fourth Annual Convention of the American Association of Equine Practitioners*, 1988, pp 159-162.

198. Knight DA et al: Copper supplementation and cartilage lesions in foals, *Proceedings of the Thirty-fourth Annual Convention of the American Association of Equine Practitioners*, 1988, pp 191-194.

199. Kronfeld DS: Metabolic convergence in developmental orthopedic disease, *Proceedings of the Thirty-fourth Annual Convention of the American Association of Equine Practitioners*, 1988, pp 195-203.

200. Pool RR: Developmental orthopedic disease in the horse: normal and abnormal bone formation, *Proceedings of the Thirty-fourth Annual Convention of the American Association of Equine Practitioners*, 1988, pp 143-158.

201. Fackelman GE, Clodins L: Surgical correction of the digital hyperextension deformity in foals, *Vet Med* 67:1116-1123, 1972.

202. LaFaunce NA, Lerner DJ, O'Brien TR: Bilateral congenital lateral patellar luxation in a foal, *Can Vet J* 12:119-120, 1971.

203. Rooney JR, Baker CW, Harmany KJ: Congenital lateral luxation of the patella in the horse, *Cornell Vet* 61:670-673, 1971.

204. Kostyra J: Congenital absence of patella in a foal, *Med Vet* 19:95-97, 1963.

205. Finocchio EJ, Guffy MM: Congenital patellar ectopia in a foal, *J Am Vet Med Assoc* 156:222-223, 1970.

206. Bertone AL, Aanes WA: Congenital phalangeal hypoplasia in equidae, *J Am Vet Med Assoc* 185:554-556, 1984.

207. Smith DRK, Leach DM, Bell RJ: Phalangeal and navicular bone hypoplasia and hoof malformation in the hind limbs of a foal, *Can Vet J* 27:28-34, 1986.

208. Jimenez MM et al: Bilateral hind limb hypoplasia in a foal, *J Am Vet Med Assoc* 204:1924-1926, 1994.

209. Chan CCH et al: Unilateral congenital phalangeal hypoplasia in a colt, *Equine Vet Educ* 8:149-152, 1996.

210. Jogi P, Norberg I: Malformation of the hip joint in a Standardbred horse, *Vet Rec* 74:421-422, 1962.

211. Manning JP: Equine hip dysplasia: osteoarthritis, *Mod Vet Pract* 44:44-45, 1963.

212. Lingard DR, Crawford TB: Congenital ameloblastic odontoma in a foal, *Am J Vet Res* 31:801-804, 1970.

213. Gobel F, Helmig H, Heerlein R: Erbliche Zahn-und Kieferanomalien bei den Haustieren mit eigenen Untersuchungen uber das Auftreten verschiedener Zahnanomalien in der Nachzucht des Hengstes G, *Tierarztl Umsch* 15:111-116, 1960.

214. Wilkins H, Neurand K: Zyklopie beim Fohlen, *Dtsche Tierarztl Wschr* 81:18-19, 1974.

215. Leipold HW et al: Congenital atlantooccipital fusion in a foal, *Vet Med* 69:1312-1316, 1974.

216. Mayhew IG, Watson AS, Heissan JA: Congenital occipitoatlantoaxial malformations in the horse, *Equine Vet J* 10:103-113, 1978.

217. Jamison JM et al: A congenital form of myotonia with dystrophic changes in a Quarter horse, *Equine Vet J* 19:353-358, 1987.

218. Hegreberg GA, Reed SM: Skeletal muscle changes associated with equine myotonic dystrophy, *Acta Neuropathol* 80:426-431, 1990.

219. Nes N, Lomo OM, Bjerkas I: Hereditary lethal arthrogryposis in horses, *Nord Vet Med* 34:425-430, 1982.

220. Buoen LC et al: Arthrogryposis in the foal and its possible relation to autosomal trisomy, *Equine Vet J* 29:60-62, 1997.

221. DeBowes RM, Leipold HW: Anterior amelia, *Equine Vet Sci* 4:133-135, 1984.

222. Coates JW, McFee RC: Congenital lordosis in Haflinger foals, *Can Vet J* 34:496-498, 1993.

223. Wilson DG, Miyabayaski, Schenkehan DI: Multiple congenital skeletal deformities in an Arabian foal, *Can Vet J* 31:113-115, 1990.

224. Symoens F, Lauerty S, Breson L: Les defauts d'ossification des os cuboides du carpe et du tarse chez le poulain, *Med Vet Quebec* 23:162-164, 1993.

225. McKellar GMW, Collins AP: The surgical correction of a deviated anterior maxilla in a horse, *Aust Vet J* 70:112-114, 1993.

226. Wagner von Matthiessen PC: Case selections and management of flexural limb deformities in horses: congenital flexural limb deformities. II, *Equine Pract* 16:7-11, 1994.

227. Chopin JB, Dowsett KF: Case report: medical treatment of moderate congenital flexural deformity of the carpus in a foal, *Aust Equine Vet* 15:165-166, 1997.

228. Sarli G, Della Salda L, Marcato PS: Dystrophy-like myopathy in a foal, *Vet Rec* 135:156-160, 1994.

229. Lepage OM L et al: Congenital dislocation of the deep digital flexor tendon associated with hypoplasia of the sustentaculum tali in a Thoroughbred colt, *Vet Radiol Ultrasound* 36:384-386, 1995.

230. Martens P: Limb deviation in a Shetland pony foal, *Equine Pract* 17:24-26, 1995.

231. Grondahl AM, Gjevre AG: Hypoplasia of the fused first and second tarsal bones in a Standardbred trotter, *Equine Pract* 18:23-25, 1996.

232. Perris EE et al: A block vertebra in an equine patient, *J Equine Vet Sci* 14:664-667, 1994.

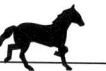

233. Berry CR et al: Radiographic and pathologic features of osteopetrosis in two Peruvian Paso foals, *Vet Radiol Ultrasound* 35:355-361, 1994.

234. Hogan PM, Emberston RM, Hunt RJ: Unilateral choanal atresia in a foal, *J Am Vet Med Assoc* 207:471-473, 1995.

235. Theoret CL, Grahn BH, Fretz PB: Incomplete nasomaxillary dysplasia in a foal, *Can Vet J* 38:445-447, 1997.

236. Irwin, MR, Pulley LT: Schistosomus reflexus in an equine fetus, *Vet Med* 70:44-45, 1975.

237. Basrur PK, Kanagawa H, Gilman JPW: An equine intersex with unilateral gonadal agenesis, *Can J Comp Med* 33:297-306, 1969.

238. Basrur PK, Kanagawa H, Podliachouk L: Further studies on the cell populations of an intersex horse, *Can J Comp Med* 34:294-298, 1970.

239. Bornstein S: The genetic sex of two intersexual horses and some notes on the karyotype of normal horses, *Acta Vet Scand* 8:291-300, 1967.

240. Bouters R, Vandeplassche M, DeMoor A: An intersex (male pseudohermaphrodite) horse with 64XX/65XXY mosaicism, *Equine Vet J* 4:150-153, 1972.

241. Fretz PB, Hare WCD: A male pseudohermaphrodite horse with 63XO?/64XX/65XXY mixoploidy, *Equine Vet J* 8:130-132, 1976.

242. Gerneke WH, Coubrough RI: Intersexuality in the horse, *Onderstepoort J Vet Res* 37:211-216, 1970.

243. Gluhovschi N et al: A case of intersexuality in the horse with type 2 A+ XXXY chromosome formula, *Br Vet J* 126:522-525, 1970.

244. Kodagall SB: Sexual behavior in an intersex horse, *Vet Med* 64:422, 1969.

245. Power MM, Leadon DP: Diploid-triploid chimaerism (64, XX/96 XXY) in an intersex foal, *Equine Vet J* 22:211-214, 1990.

246. Klunder LR, McFeely RA, Willard JP: Six separate sex chromosome anomalies in an Arabian mare, *Equine Vet J* 22:218-220, 1990.

247. Cammaert S et al: Three full sister mares with a stallion-like behavior and a high blood testosterone concentration, *Equine Vet Sci* 15:220-222, 1993.

248. Hughes JP, Kennedy PC, Benirschke K: XO-Gonadal dysgenesis in the mare (report of two cases), *Equine Vet J* 7:109-112, 1975.

249. Bruere AN et al: Preliminary observations on the occurrence of the equine XO syndrome, *NZ Vet J* 26:145-146, 1978.

250. Reid SW, Weatherstone JF, Robinson BN: X chromosome mosaicism and infertility in a mare, *Can Vet J* 28:533-534, 1987.

251. Buoen LC et al: Sterility associated with an XO karyotype in a miniature horse mare, *Equine Vet J* 25:164-165, 1993.

252. Davies TG: Turner's syndrome (karyotype 63 XO) in a Thoroughbred mare, *Equine Vet Educ* 7:15-17, 1995.

253. Arighi M, Bosu WTK, Raeside JI: Hormonal diagnosis of equine cryptorchidism and histology of the retained testes, *Proceedings of the Thirty-first Annual Convention of the American Association of Equine Practitioners*, 1985 pp 591-604.

254. Cox JE: Experiences with a diagnostic test for cryptorchidism, *Equine Vet J* 7:179-183, 1975.

255. Cox JE, Redhead PH, Dawson FE: Comparison of the measurement of plasma testosterone and plasma oestrogens for the diagnosis of cryptorchidism in the horse, *Equine Vet J* 18:179-182, 1986.

256. Cox JE: Genetics and heritable disease, *Equine Vet J* 19:362, 1987.

257. Hayes MM: Epidemiological features of 5009 cases of equine cryptorchism, *Equine Vet J* 18:467-471, 1986.

258. Leipold HW et al: Cryptorchidism in the horse: genetic implications, *Proceedings of the Thirty-first Annual Convention of the American Association of Equine Practitioners*, 1985, pp 579-589.

259. Roberts SJ: *Veterinary obstetrics and genital diseases*, ed 2, Woodstock, Vt, 1971, SJ Roberts.

260. Vecchiotti GG, Galanti R: A note on genetic aspects of equine cryptorchism, *Proceedings of the Thirty-sixth Annual Meeting of the European Association for Animal Production*, Kallithea, Greece, 1985.

261. Constant SB, Larsen RE, Asburg AC: XX male syndrome in a cryptorchid stallion, *J Am Vet Med Assoc* 205:83-85, 1994.

262. Parks AH et al: Monorchidism in the horse, *Equine Vet J* 21:215-217, 1989.

263. Kent MG et al: XY sex-reversal syndrome in the domestic horse, *Cytogenet Cell Genet* 42:8-18, 1986.

264. Power MM: XY reversal in a mare, *Equine Vet J* 18:233-236, 1986.

265. Sharp AJ, Wachtel SS, Benirschke K: H-Y antigen in a fertile XY female horse, *J Reprod Fertil* 58:157-160, 1980.

266. Allen EW: Two cases of abnormal equine pregnancy associated with excess foetal fluid, *Equine Vet J* 18:220-222, 1986.

267. Miyaka YI et al: Four cases of anomalies of genital organs in horses, *Zentralbl Veterinarmed* 29:602-608, 1982.

268. Halnan CRE, Irwin CFP: Dysgenesis of the tubal system in an infertile mare karyotype 63,X:64,XY:65,XXY, *Equine Vet Sci* 5:328-329, 1986.

269. Dunn HO et al: Two equine true hermaphrodites with 64,XX/64,XY and 63,XO/64,XY chimaerism, *Proceedings of the Thirty-fourth Annual Convention of the American Association of Equine Practitioners*, 1988, pp 313-319.

270. Chandley AC et al: Chromosome abnormalities as a cause of infertility in mares, *J Reprod Fertil* 23:493-499, 1975.

271. Kubien EM, Pozor MA, Tischner M: Clinical, cytogenetic and endocrine evaluation of a horse with a 65,XXY karyotype, *Equine Vet J* 24:333-335, 1993.

272. Power MM: The first description of a balanced reciprocal translocation and its clinical effects in a mare, *Equine Vet J* 23:146-147, 1991.

273. Makela O, Gustavson I, Hallmen T: A 64,X,i(Xq) karyotype in a Standardbred filly, *Equine Vet J* 26:251-254, 1994.

274. Freeman SL, England GCW: Vestibulo-vaginal hypoplasia in a mare, *Vet Rec* 141:521-522, 1997.

275. Thursby-Pelham RHC: Uterus unicornis in mares, *Vet Rec* 141:132, 1997.

276. McGuire TC, Banks KL, Poppie MJ: Combined immunodeficiency in horses: characterization of the lymphocyte defect, *Clin Immunol Immunopathol* 3:555-556, 1975.

277. Ardans AA, Pritchett RF, Zee YC: Isolation and characterization of an equine adenovirus, *Infect Immun* 7:673-677, 1973.

278. Johnston KG, Hutchins DR: Suspected adenovirus bronchitis in Arab foals, *Aust Vet J* 43:600, 1967.

279. McChesney AE, England JJ, Rich LJ: Adenoviral infection in foals, *J Am Vet Med Assoc* 162:545-549, 1973.

280. McGuire TC, Banks KL, Evans DR et al: Agammaglobulinemia in a horse with evidence of functional T lymphocytes, *Am J Vet Res* 37:41-46, 1976.

281. McGuire TC, Banks KL, Poppie MJ: Combined immunodeficiency (severe): Swiss-type agammaglobulinemia, *Am J Pathol* 80:551-554, 1975.

282. McGuire TC, Poppie MJ: Primary hypogammaglobulinemia and thymic hypoplasia in horses, *Fed Am Soc Exp Biol* 32:3401, 1973.

283. McGuire TC, Poppie MJ: Hypogammaglobulinemia and thymic hypoplasia in horses: a primary combined immunodeficiency disorder, *Infect Immun* 8:272-277, 1973.

284. McGuire TC, Poppie MJ, Banks KL: Combined B- and T-lymphocyte immunodeficiency; a fatal genetic disease in Arabian foals, *J Am Vet Med Assoc* 164:70-76, 1974.

285. Perryman LE: Mechanism of immune deficiency diseases of animals, *J Am Vet Med Assoc* 181:1097-1101, 1982.

286. Perryman LE, Magnuson NS: Immunodeficiency disease in animals. In Desnick RJ, Patterson DF, Scarpelli DG, eds: *Animal models of inherited metabolic diseases*, New York, 1982, Alan Liss.

287. Perryman LE, McGuire TC, Bunks KL: Infantile X-linked agammaglobulinemia, *Am J Pathol* 111:125-127, 1983.

288. Poppie MJ, McGuire TC: Combined immunodeficiency in foals of Arabian breeding: evaluation of mode of inheritance and estimation of prevalence of affected foals and carrier mares and stallions, *J Am Vet Med Assoc* 170:31-33, 1977.

289. Thompson DB et al: Inheritance of a lethal immunodeficiency disease of Arabian foals, *Aust Vet J* 51:109-113, 1975.

290. Crisman MV: Selective immunoglobulin M deficiency in the horse, *Proceedings of the Thirty-fourth American Association of Equine Practitioners*, 1988, pp 313-319.

291. Perryman LE, McGuire TC, Hilbert BJ: Selective immunoglobulin M deficiency in foals, *J Am Vet Med Assoc* 170:212-215, 1977.

292. Mair TS et al: Concurrent cryptosporidium and cornavirus infections in an Arabian foal with combined immunodeficiency syndrome, *Vet Rec* 126:127-130, 1990.

293. Morris DD: Immunodeficiency of horses, *North Am Vet Conf* 6:473-475, 1972.

294. Hovda LR: Immunodeficiency disease in older foals, *Equine Pract* 15:24-26, 1993.

295. Lepage OM et al: Immunodeficience combinee chez un poulain Arabe, *Med Vet Quebec* 23:99-100, 1993.

296. Anonymous: New findings in CID study, *J Equine Vet Sci* 13:658, 1993.

297. Jones WE: Severe combined immunodeficiency now a solution, *J Equine Vet Sci* 17:630-632, 1997.

298. Shin EK, Perrryman LE, Meek K: Evaluation of a test for identification of Arabian horses heterozygous for the severe combined immunodeficiency trait, *J Am Vet Med Assoc* 211:1268-1270, 1997.

299. Scholes SFE et al: A syndrome of anaemia, immunodeficiency and peripheral ganglionopathy in Fell pony foals, *Vet Rec* 142:128-134, 1998.

300. Cox JH: An episodic weakness in four horses associated with intermittent serum hyperkalemia and the similarity of the disease to hyperkalemic periodic paralysis in man, *Proceedings of the Thirty-first Annual Convention of the American Association of Equine Practitioners*, 1985, pp 383-392, 1985.

301. Steiss JE, Naylor JM: Episodic muscle tremors in a Quarter horse: resemblance to hyperkalemic periodic paralysis, *Can Vet J* 27:332-335, 1986.

302. Spier SJ et al: Hyperkalemic periodic paralysis: an autosomal dominant heritable disease of horses, *Proceedings of the Thirty-eighth Annual Convention of the American Association of Equine Practitioners*, 1992, pp 583-585.

303. Spier SJ et al: Genetic study of hyperkalemic paralysis in horses, *J Am Vet Med Assoc* 202:933-937, 1993.

304. Spier SJ: Blood test available for hyperkalemic periodic paralysis in Quarter horses, *J Equine Vet Sci* 13:140-142, 1993.

305. Naylor JM: Selection of Quarter horses affected with hyperkalemic periodic paralysis by show judges, *J Am Vet Med Assoc* 204:926-928, 1994.

306. Naylor JM: Equine hyperkalemic periodic paralysis: review and implications, *Can Vet J* 35:279-285, 1994.

307. Cornick JL, Seahorn TL, Hartsfield SM: Hyperthermia during isoflurane anaesthesia in a horse with suspected hyperkalaemic periodic paralysis, *Equine Vet J* 26:511-514, 1994.

308. Steele DS, Naylor JM: Hyperkalemic periodic paralysis, plasma lactate and exercise intolerance, *J Equine Vet Sci* 16:327-332, 1996.

309. Carr EA et al: Laryngeal and pharyngeal dysfunction in horses homozygous for hyperkalemic periodic paralysis, *J Am Vet Med Assoc* 209:798-803, 1996.

310. Guglick MA, MacAllister CG, Breazile JE: Laryngospasm, dysphagia, and emaciation associated with hyperkalemic periodic paralysis in a horse, *J Am Vet Med Assoc* 209:115-117, 1996.

311. Reynolds JA et al: Genetic-diet interactions in the hyperkalemic periodic paralysis syndrome in Quarter horses fed varying amounts of potassium. II, Symptoms of HYPP, *J Equine Vet Sci* 18:655-661, 1998.

312. Naylor JM et al: Hyperkalaemic periodic paralysis in homozygous and heterozygous horses: a co-dominant genetic condition, *Equine Vet J* 31:153-159, 1999.

313. Stockam SL, Harvey JW, Kinden DA: Equine glucose-6-phosphate dehydrogenase deficiency, *Vet Pathol* 31:518-527, 1994.

314. Valberg SJ et al: Familial basis of exertional rhabdomyolysis in Quarter horse-related breeds, *Am J Vet Res* 57:286-290, 1996.

315. MacLeay JM et al: Heritability of recurrent exertional rhabdomyolysis in Thoroughbred racehorses, *Am J Vet Res* 60:250-256, 1999.

316. Gotz HJ: Ein Fall von Diprosopie beim Fohlen, *Tierarztl Prax* 19:82-83, 1991.

317. Cambell-Beggs CL et al: Chyloabdomen in a neonatal foal, *Vet Rec* 37:96-98, 1995.

Immunologic Disorders

STEVEN M. PARISH
MELISSA T. HINES
Consulting Editors

EQUINE IMMUNODEFICIENCY DISEASES

JILL McCLURE BLACKMER
DEBRA C. SELLON
MELISSA T. HINES

The environment in which domestic animals live with regard to exposure to pathogens is challenging and often life threatening. Normal host defense mechanisms have developed to allow survival and failure of these protective systems, leaving an animal vulnerable to many outside challenges, particularly the pathogenic effects of any number of microorganisms. It is important to understand that diseases, particularly infectious diseases, can result from failure of the host's defense mechanisms, as well as from overwhelming challenge from the outside. When animals are plagued by repeated or chronic infections, one should always determine whether host factors are involved.

The analysis of immunodeficiency diseases depends on an understanding of the normal development and function of cells that belong to the immune system and nonspecific host defense systems (Fig. 49-1). A successful protective response is a result of the orchestration of numerous cell types and soluble serum factors.

Two major populations of lymphocytes, T cells and B cells, are involved in immune responses. T lymphocytes are required for cell-mediated immune responses that protect against fungal, protozoal, intracellular bacterial, and many viral infections. T lymphocytes are also important in regulating the immune response. T cells originate from stem cells, which probably develop in the fetal liver. These cells must go through a maturation process in the thymus before becoming fully functional T cells. T cells comprise about 70% to 80% of peripheral blood lymphocytes and populate the periarteriolar regions of the spleen and the paracortical regions of lymph nodes.[1,2]

Both humoral and cellular immune responses depend on input from T cells, initially characterized as either helper T (Th) cells or cytotoxic/suppressor T (Tc) cells based on their primary function. These cells have subsequently been differentiated on the basis of cell surface antigens, with helper T cells expressing the CD4 antigen and cytotoxic T cells expressing CD8. Further work has shown that the function of these cells is complex, and that the pattern of cytokine expression is important in regulation of the immune response. Based on their cytokine expression, CD4+ cells have been further subdivided into distinct subsets, Th1 and Th2 cells (Fig. 49-2). Although there is some species variation, Th1 cells generally produce interferon-γ and interleukin-2 and are involved primarily in the generation of cell-mediated immune responses, whereas Th2 cells produce interleukins-4, -5, and -13 and are involved in humoral responses. It has been documented in mice that protection or disease can be associated with the particular type of helper T cell response, and the clinical relevance of this is currently being investigated in a number of equine diseases.

The second major class of lymphocytes, B lymphocytes, produce immunoglobulins and are the precursors of plasma cells. Several classes of immunoglobulins are produced by B cells. There is some variation among species, but the major classes are IgG, IgM, IgA, IgE, and, in horses, IgG(T). Immunoglobulins provide a defense against extracellular bacterial and certain viral infections. Like T cells, B cells originate from stem cells in the fetal liver. The site of B cell maturation may vary with species and includes several different organs, including the bursa of Fabricius in birds, and the bone marrow and certain Peyer's patches in mammals. Of peripheral blood lymphocytes, 15% to 30% are B cells. B cells populate germinal centers of spleen and lymph nodes.[1,2]

The innate immune system, which is nonspecific in nature, includes natural killer cells, phagocytic cells, neutrophils, eosinophils, basophils, and nonimmunoglobulin serum and cellular factors such as complement and interferon. These components play a distinct role in host defenses and work in concert with T and B cells to produce an effective protective response.

A deficiency of functional T cells, B cells, nonspecific components, or any combination predisposes animals to infections that may result in death. Immune deficiencies can be classified according to: (1) the site of defect in the host defense system, and (2) whether the mechanism is primary or

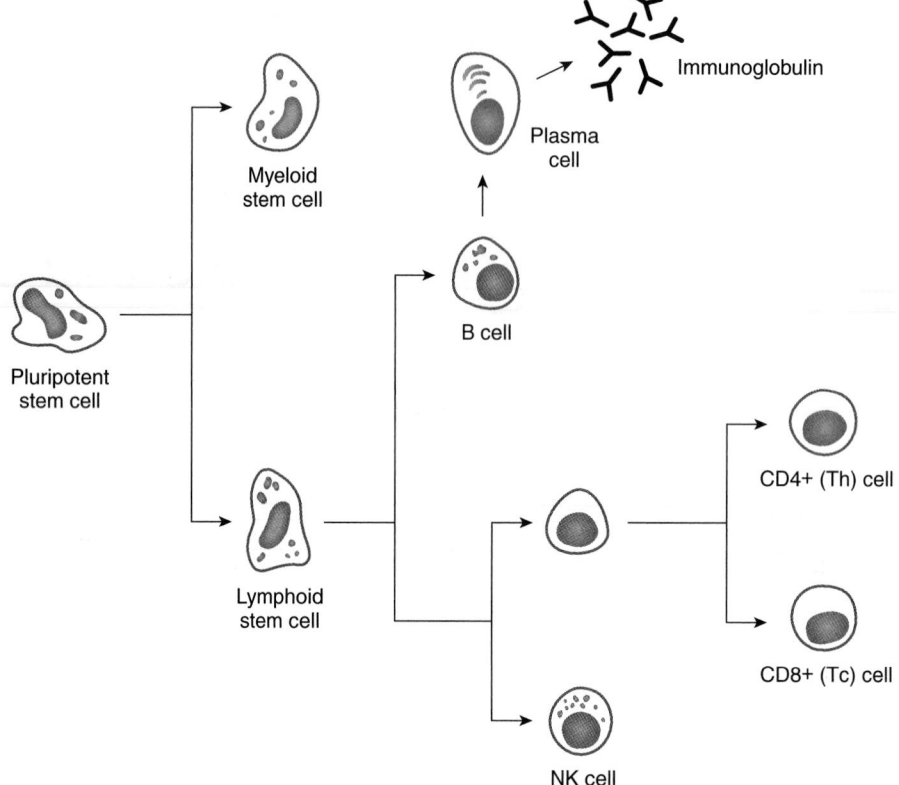

FIG. 49-1 ▓ Ontogeny of the immune response. Failures at any site in the maturation process can result in manifestation of immune deficiencies.

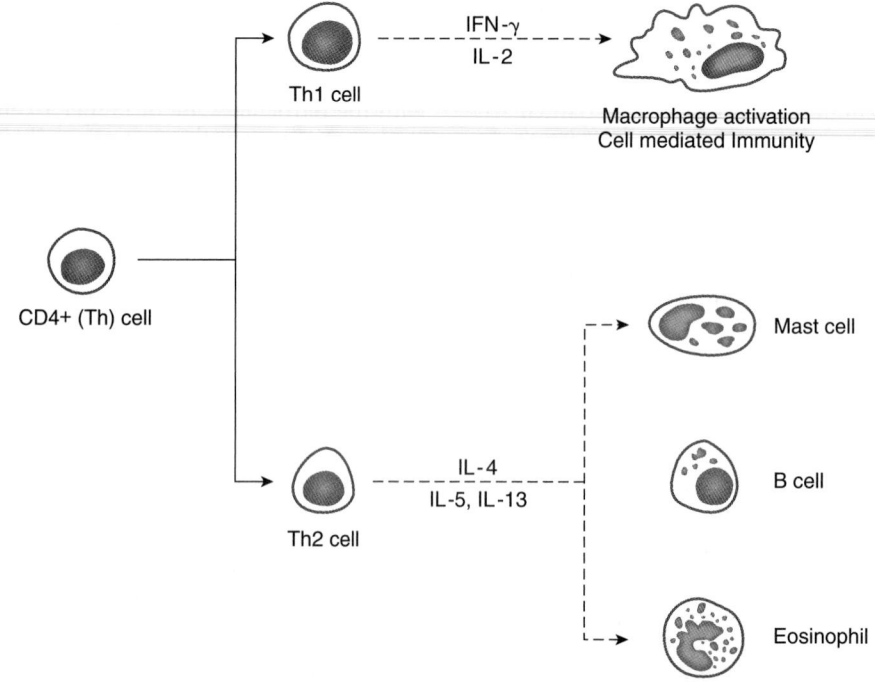

FIG. 49-2 ▓ CD4+ T cells can be subdivided into Th1 and Th2 on the basis of their cytokine profiles. Preliminary data suggest that the pathogenesis of certain diseases is associated with the particular type of Th response.

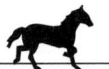

secondary. A primary disorder has a proven or suspected genetic basis; whereas in a secondary disorder the host initially had the capability to respond immunologically, but the ability was lost. Factors that can produce secondary immunodeficiencies include irradiation, neoplasia, toxicities, malnutrition, or certain microbial infections.[1,3] Physiologic stress such as that caused by pregnancy, lactation, and exercise can also induce transient immunosuppression.[3,4] By careful dissection of the immune response, the site of the defect can often be identified.

Several general clinical features have been associated with immunodeficiencies. These include the following[1,3]:

- Onset of infections during the first 6 weeks of life
- Repeated infections that respond poorly to standard therapy
- Increased susceptibility to organisms with low pathogenicity
- Infection with organisms rarely observed in immunocompetent individuals
- Systemic illness after administration of attenuated live vaccines
- Failure to respond to vaccination
- Persistent marked abnormalities in leukocyte numbers

Laboratory or special in vivo testing is necessary to confirm the presence of an immunodeficiency and to differentiate among the various immunodeficiency syndromes, because clinically the presenting signs are nonspecific. In general, tests to evaluate the immune system either quantify the component or measure the functional capacity.

The only clinically feasible tests of B cell function are quantitation of immunoglobulins and measurement of specific antibody responses. Numerous methods are available to quantitate or semiquantitate immunoglobulin levels. Semiquantitative tests are useful for some conditions such as failure of passive transfer (FPT) after colostrum ingestion; however, they do not provide information on specific immunoglobulin classes. Some tests are species specific, whereas others can be used to detect immunoglobulins of several species. Precipitation of immunoglobulins with specific concentrations of salts tends not to be species specific, although the tests may work better in some species than others. These tests include zinc sulfate and sodium sulfite precipitation and glutaraldehyde coagulation (see p. 1601).[5,6] Commercial tests based on these principles are available.* Serum electrophoresis can also be used in all species to quantitate γ-globulins, which are primarily immunoglobulins. Several species-specific tests based on antigen-antibody reactions that use latex bead agglutination† or enzyme immunoassay‡ as the marker systems are also commercially available. These tests are semiquantitative and are primarily marketed for detection of FPT after colostrum ingestion.

Radial immunodiffusion (RID) quantitates immunoglobulins of specific classes using a precipitation reaction between antigen and antibody directed against one species-specific, class-specific immunoglobulin to be quantitated. This is an accurate method for quantitating specific classes of immunoglobulin such as IgG and IgM. RID kits are commercially available for some immunoglobulin classes for domestic animals.§ These tests require incubation for 18 to 24 hours, which is their greatest drawback for clinical use. Test reagents are prepared for use in a single species; however, some crossreactivity does exist among species. Test reagents designed for use in another species (e.g., human) have been shown to be useful[7]; however, they must be standardized and calibrated for the species in which they are to be used.

Production of antibody in response to immunization with specific antigens is another way B cell function can be evaluated, although functioning T cells are also required for this response. The only requirement to assess antibody production is an in vitro test to detect specific antibody. Serologic measurement of antibody titers before and following vaccination with commercially available vaccines is one approach. Killed infectious bovine rhinotracheitis (IBR) and bovine virus diarrhea (BVD) vaccines in cattle and influenza or rhinopneumonitis vaccines in horses are readily available, and responses are easily tested. Another approach is to look for the presence of naturally occurring antibodies that are produced without immunization (e.g., antibodies that crossreact with sheep red blood cells in horses), although the assays for these antibodies may not be readily available. Other foreign "nonvaccine" antigens can also be used if an assay is available for the detection of antibody.

Other tests are available primarily on a research basis. B cells can be enumerated in blood and lymphoid tissue using fluorescent-antibody labeling to detect surface immunoglobulin and erythrocyte-antigen-complement rosetting techniques to detect complement receptors. In vitro blastogenesis with pokeweed mitogen requires both B and T cell function for normal responses, whereas lipopolysaccharide requires predominantly a B cell response. However, these tests are not routinely available in the field.

The only clinically applicable in vivo test of T cell function is intradermal skin testing with the plant lectin, phytohemagglutinin (PHA), to test for delayed-type hypersensitivity (DTH) responses. PHA is capable of eliciting a DTH response without requirement of prior sensitization, which is required with some other antigens such as dinitrochlorobenzene. To perform this test, the thickness of a skin fold is measured before injection. A 50-μg dose of PHA* in 0.5 ml of phosphate-buffered saline (PBS) is injected intradermally, and the same volume of PBS is injected at a control site at least 10 cm away from the site. Twenty-four hours later the skin thickness is measured. A 1-mm to 3-mm increase in skin thickness at the test site should normally occur. An increase of 0.6 mm or less indicates a defect in cell-mediated immunity.[8]

Lymphocyte blastogenesis with PHA, concanavalin A, and pokeweed mitogen is an in vitro assay of T cell function, but this test requires specialized equipment. Previously, erythrocyte rosetting assays and fluoresceinated peanut agglutinin surface labeling tests were used to enumerate T cells in peripheral blood and lymphoid tissue, but these tests have largely been replaced with the development of monoclonal antibodies that identify subpopulations of T lymphocytes at various stages of development.[9,10] Using these antibodies, it has been established that in normal horses about 62% of circulating lymphocytes are helper T cells, whereas about 18% are cytotoxic T cells.[11]

A variety of assays for phagocytosis and killing by neutrophils have been developed; however, these tests are not practical for general field use. Likewise, quantitation of complement, interferon, and various lymphokines are procedures available only in selected research facilities.

*Equi-Z, Bova-S, and Llama-S, VMRD, Inc, Pullman, WA 99163.
†Foalchek, Centaur, Inc, Overland Park, KS 66225-5667.
‡Cite-Foal IgG, IDEXX Laboratories, Inc, Westbrook, ME 04092.
§VMRD, Inc, Pullman, WA 99163; ICN Immunobiologicals, Lisle, IL 60532; Bethyl Laboratories, Montgomery, TX 77356.

*PHA-P, Sigma Chemical Co, St Louis, MO 63178.

From a practical standpoint, only a limited number of tests are available, and for the most part these are crude indicators of immune response and therefore pick up only severe deviations from normal. Even so, a number of immunodeficiency syndromes have been described and characterized in domestic animals. As methods improve, so will our ability to more precisely define immune disorders.

REFERENCES

1. Perryman LE: Primary and secondary immune deficiencies of domestic animals, *Adv Vet Sci Comp Med* 23:23-52, 1979.
2. Perryman LE: Immunological management of young foals, *Compend Cont Educ* 3:S223-S230, 1981.
3. Halliwell REW, Gorman NT: Diseases associated with immunodeficiency. In Halliwell REW, Gorman NT, eds: *Veterinary clinical immunology*, Philadelphia, 1989, WB Saunders.
4. Hines MT, Schott HC: Exercise and immune function, *Proceedings of the Twelfth Annual Veterinary Medical Forum*, San Francisco, 1994.
5. Rumbaugh G et al: Measurement of neonatal equine immunoglobulins for assessment of colostral immunoglobulin transfer: comparison of single radial immunodiffusion with zinc sulfate turbidity test, serum electrophoresis, refractometry for total serum protein, and the sodium sulfite precipitation test, *J Am Vet Med Assoc* 172:321-325, 1978.
6. Tennant B et al: Use of the glutaraldehyde coagulation test for detection of hypogammaglobulinemia in neonatal calves, *J Am Vet Med Assoc* 174:848-853, 1979.
7. Buening GM, Perryman LE, McGuire TC: Practical methods of determining serum immunoglobulin M and immunoglobulin G concentrations in foals, *J Am Vet Med Assoc* 171:455-458, 1977.
8. Hodgin EC et al: Evaluation of delayed hypersensitivity responses in normal horses and immunodeficient foals, *Am J Vet Res* 39:1161-1167, 1978.
9. Enright FM, Jeffers GW: Function tests for mononuclear phagocytes. In Barta O, ed: *Laboratory techniques of veterinary clinical immunology*, Springfield, Ill, 1984, Charles C Thomas.
10. Lo JW, McClure JJ: Surface markers of lymphocytes. In Barta O, ed: *Laboratory techniques of veterinary clinical immunology*, Springfield, Ill, 1984, Charles C Thomas.
11. Hines MT et al: Quantitative characterization of lymphocyte populations in bronchoalveolar lavage fluid and peripheral blood of normal adult Arabian horses, *Vet Immunol Immunopathol* 51:29-37, 1996.

FAILURE OF PASSIVE TRANSFER

DEFINITION AND ETIOLOGY. Normal foals are immunocompetent at birth (i.e., they are probably as capable of mounting normal immune responses as an adult). However, they are immunologically naive in that they have had no exposure to foreign antigens and have therefore not yet mounted any type of protective immune response or accumulated significant levels of immunoglobulins. Although foals are capable of producing antibody, they are essentially devoid of immunoglobulin at birth, with the exception of small amounts of IgM normally produced in utero. Because they are "starting from scratch," foals are indeed more susceptible, particularly to infectious agents, during the early neonatal period. Foals begin producing immunoglobulins immediately on exposure to antigens after birth, and immunoglobulins are detectable within 1 to 2 weeks of life and reach significant levels by 2 months. Under normal circumstances temporary protection against infection for the first 1 to 2 months is provided to the foal in the form of passively transferred antibody (Fig. 49-3). Because of the diffuse epitheliochorial nature of the equine placenta, no transplacental transfer of immunoglobulins occurs in horses. Instead, ingestion and absorption of immunoglobulin-rich colostrum are the sole means of passive transfer in foals. In a properly functioning system, maternal antibodies wane as levels of autologous antibodies increase; the neonate is never left totally unprotected (Fig. 49-4).

Mares normally produce colostrum during the last 2 weeks of pregnancy in response to hormonal changes. Immunoglobulins in colostrum are selectively concentrated from the mare's sera, not produced locally in the mammary gland. Most immunoglobulin in equine colostrum is IgG. At

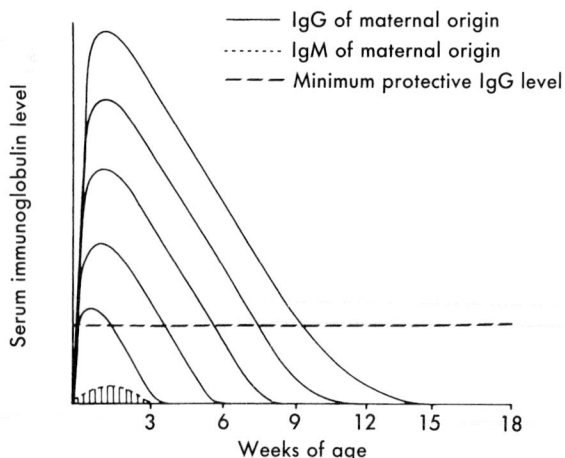

FIG. 49-3 ▪ The duration of protection provided by maternal immunoglobulins varies with the class of immunoglobulin and the quantity ingested during the first 24 hours of life.

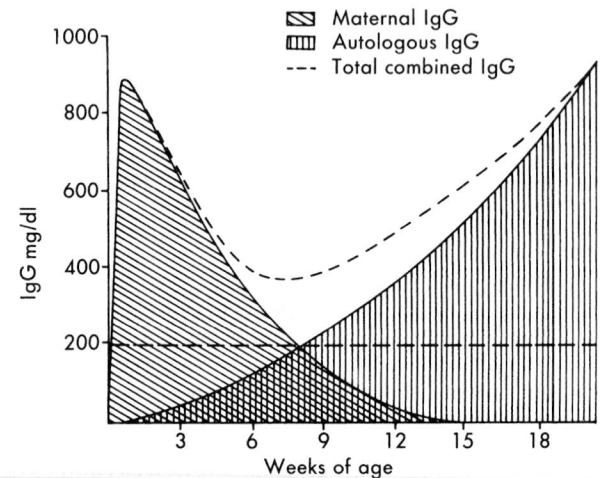

FIG. 49-4 ▪ Maternal immunoglobulin wanes, whereas the production of autologous immunoglobulin increases during the first several months of life. The combined total amount of immunoglobulin ideally remains above the level considered minimum for maintenance of good health.

birth the neonate has specialized enterocytes in the gastrointestinal tract that are able to absorb intact large molecules such as immunoglobulins by pinocytosis. The window of gut absorptive capacity for immunoglobulins is narrow, lasting from birth until about 18 to 24 hours and is greatest during the first 6 to 12 hours. Closure of the gut is the result of shedding of specialized enterocytes capable of pinocytosis and replacement by more mature cells that are incapable of absorbing immunoglobulins.[12] In addition to antibody, other colostral factors may be important for optimal immune protection of foals. For example, colostrum influences cell-mediated immunity, activates granulocytes, and contains constituents of innate immunity, such as complement, that have a local protective effect in the neonatal digestive tract.[13,14]

FPT may occur because of ingestion of poor quality colostrum with a low immunoglobulin content, failure to ingest a sufficient quantity of colostrum, and failure to absorb colostral immunoglobulins from the gastrointestinal tract.[15] Colostrum may have an insufficient quantity of immunoglobulin because of prelactation (lactation before parturi-

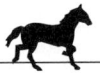

TABLE 49-1

Normal Serum Immunoglobulin Concentrations (mg/dl) in Horses

Age	Breed	IgG	IgG(T)	IgM
Newborn, presuckle	Arabian	1-10	ND	5-15
1-20 days	Arabian	814±583	142±88	28±11
21-40 days	Arabian	480±293	126±41	30±10
41-60 days	Arabian	264±193	96±33	42±12
61-80 days	Arabian	252±128	75±17	36±12
81-140 days	Arabian	248±92	162±126	39±15
3-5 months	Mixed	380±188	211±148	61±22
10-15 months	Arabian/Thoroughbred	790	728	48
Adult	Shetland	1334±350	821±301	120±13

From Riggs MW: Evaluation of foals for immune deficiency disorders, *Vet Clin North Am (Equine Pract)* 3:515-528, 1987.
ND, Not determined.

tion), premature foaling, a defect in the mare's ability to concentrate immunoglobulin in the colostrum, or other factors. Mares most likely to produce colostrum with low immunoglobulin content are those older than 15 years of age, those that foal early in the year, and Standardbred mares. The quantity of immunoglobulin in colostrum may be estimated by single radial immunodiffusion (RID), refractometry, glutaraldehyde coagulation, or specific gravity.[16] Using a colostrometer, colostral specific gravity should be a minimum of 1.060, corresponding to an IgG concentration of greater than 3000 mg/dl.

Foals that are orphaned or rejected at birth, too weak to stand, or unable or lack the desire to suckle are unlikely to ingest sufficient colostrum to prevent FPT. Malabsorption is occasionally incriminated as a cause of FPT in foals that are observed to suckle adequate quantities of good quality colostrum.

CLINICAL SIGNS AND DIFFERENTIAL DIAGNOSES. FPT itself produces no clinical signs of disease and cannot be detected by physical examination. Clinical presentations that strongly suggest an underlying problem with FPT include onset of bacterial infections within the first 2 weeks of life, particularly septicemia, septic arthritis, pneumonia, and enteritis. Other immunodeficiencies or simply exposure to potent pathogens cannot be ruled out solely on the basis of the time of onset; however, even with other forms of immunodeficiency, clinical signs of infection usually do not show up for several weeks if passive transfer has been adequate.

CLINICAL PATHOLOGY. FPT is diagnosed by the demonstration of low serum levels of IgG in the foal as early as 6 to 12 hours after birth and probably for as long as several weeks after birth (Table 49-1). Routine determination of serum IgG concentrations in apparently healthy foals is usually recommended at 18 to 24 hours of age. Rapid methods available for IgG quantitation include zinc sulfate turbidity,[17] latex agglutination,[18] and enzyme immunoassay.[13] Single radial immunodiffusion is considered the most quantitatively accurate diagnostic test of those that are widely available to practitioners. However, this test is more expensive than some other screening tests and results are not available for at least 24 hours, making it impractical when rapid diagnosis and treatment of a critically ill foal is needed. Total serum protein is not a reliable indicator of FPT in foals because of the wide variation in total serum protein in cases of adequate transfer.

The level of IgG considered adequate is quite arbitrary and probably varies considerably with the environment. Estimates of what constitutes adequate IgG transfer range from 400 to 800 mg/dl of IgG.[13,19,20] Less than 200 mg/dl is considered complete failure. A 200- to 400- or 800-mg/dl amount is considered to be partial FPT. A level of 400 mg of IgG per deciliter

may be an adequate immunoglobulin level for healthy foals in relatively clean environments, but it may not be adequate for foals heavily exposed to pathogens or already showing signs of infection. These figures only address total immunoglobulin content and not specific antibody titers, which also play a critical role in determining resistance to particular pathogens.

No consistent changes in the hemogram and biochemical panel are seen in foals with FPT; however, a range of abnormalities related to the secondary infections, including neutrophilia or neutropenia, hyperfibrinogenemia, and hypoglycemia, may be present. The presence and severity of these changes depend on the organisms and systems involved in the secondary infections.

NECROPSY FINDINGS. There are no specific necropsy findings indicative of FPT. Necropsy findings reflect the site and severity of secondary infectious problems that have developed. Lymphoid tissue is normally developed, unless secondary infections have caused lymphoid necrosis or atrophy.

TREATMENT AND PROGNOSIS. The treatment of FPT depends on the degree of failure, the environment in which the foal is exposed, the age of the foal at time of diagnosis, and the presence of secondary infectious problems. Treatment is geared toward minimizing exposure to pathogens, supplying immunoglobulins, and managing secondary infections, if present.

If FPT can be anticipated within hours of birth because of premature lactation, low specific-gravity colostrum, or a weak or orphaned foal, treatment can include the provision of an alternative source of colostrum or equine plasma orally. In a 45-kg foal, administration of 2 to 3 L of colostrum with a specific gravity greater than 1.060 within the first 6 to 8 hours is desirable. The antibody content of plasma is lower than that of colostrum; thus relatively more plasma must be given orally to achieve the same goals of passive transfer.[13,21] If the foal is over 6 hours old, the absorption of colostral antibody is significantly decreased, although a locally protective effect of the colostrum may still be present in the intestinal tract. If the foal is over 12 hours old, it is unlikely that sufficient colostrum will be absorbed; therefore immunoglobulin levels should be rechecked at 24 hours and intravenous plasma transfusion given if indicated by persistently low serum immunoglobulin levels.

Because bovine colostrum is often more readily available than equine colostrum, it may be substituted in emergency situations when equine colostrum is not available. Bovine colostrum is relatively well absorbed in the foal, but bovine immunoglobulins have a much shorter half-life in foals and do not contain antibodies specifically directed against equine pathogens. It is certainly better than no colostrum and, on the basis of a small experimental study, may be used without creating adverse reactions.[22]

Lyophilized equine IgG is commercially available as a colostrum substitute. In colostrum-deprived foals, 50 to 70 g of IgG are recommended to increase blood IgG concentrations to greater than 400 mg/dl.

Some animals suffering from FPT, particularly partial failure, do well without any treatment if they are not heavily exposed to pathogens and have no preexisting infections. FPT itself is not necessarily fatal. If plasma transfusions are not administered, owners should be made aware of the risks and those foals should be maintained in an environment with minimal exposure to potential pathogens. Foals with other risk factors for septicemia such as prematurity, dysmaturity, or placentitis should receive intravenous plasma transfusions if they have blood IgG concentrations of less than 800 mg/dl at 18 to 24 hours of age.

If the decision is made to supplement plasma parenterally, equine plasma for transfusions is commercially available* or can be collected and processed locally. Commercial sources are convenient, save time, have been screened for anti–red blood cell (RBC) antibody, are free of diseases such as equine infectious anemia, and originate from animals with known immunoglobulin levels. Their major disadvantage is that they may not contain antibody specific for the pathogens from the particular environment to which the foal is exposed.

Use of a local donor is desirable in that it presumably has antibody specific to the environmental pathogens to which the foal has been exposed. If a local donor is to be selected, several criteria should be met. First, the horse should be healthy, and results of agar gel immunodiffusion for equine infectious anemia should be obviously negative. Second, no anti-RBC antibody should be detectable in the horse's serum. The donor's plasma should be screened for lysins and agglutinins by a blood-typing laboratory against a panel of cells representing all known blood groups. Horses in which these test results are negative are in a sense universal plasma donors, because they carry no antibodies that react with other horses' cells. If plasma evaluated in this way is not available, the presence of anti-RBC antibody in donor plasma can be crudely evaluated with a minor cross-match for agglutination using donor plasma and recipient blood cells. Lytic antibodies require an external source of complement for activity in vitro and may not be detected using this test. Ideally, a third criterion is selection of a horse that is negative for blood group factors Aa and Qa and possesses no anti-RBC antibody. Even though there are dozens of blood group factors, Aa and Qa have been associated with the great majority of cases of neonatal isoerythrolysis (NI).[23-25] If plasma is collected and separated by sedimentation, it is inevitable that some red blood cell contamination be present. If Aa-positive (Aa+) RBCs are given to an animal that is Aa negative (Aa−), or if Qa+ RBCs are given to an animal that is Qa−, the recipients could become sensitized to these antigens. This sensitization would probably not have any immediate consequences for the recipient foal, because the foal's cells would not be affected by the antibodies, but it has potentially sensitized any Aa− and Qa− females for production of an NI foal later (see p. 1608). To avoid these potential complications, the ideal donor should be Aa− and Qa− and possess no anti-RBC antibody in its serum. It is desirable to have identified this type of universal donor to avoid the need for immediate cross-matching in every case of plasma transfusion.

The volume of plasma needed to correct the measured IgG deficit in a foal can theoretically be calculated on the basis of the blood volume of the foal and the concentration of IgG in the foal's serum and in the donor plasma[26]; however, these calculations do not reliably predict the actual levels of IgG achieved following transfusion. A 20-ml volume of plasma per kilogram of body weight administered intravenously routinely only raises serum IgG levels 200 to 300 mg/dl, and often 2 to 3 times this amount is needed to bring serum IgG levels into the range considered minimum for protection (e.g., 400 to 800 mg/dl).[13,19] If the foal is already clinically ill, additional plasma will usually be required to raise IgG levels an equivalent amount.[13] In a newborn foal (estimated 50 kg), between 2 and 4 L of plasma is frequently needed. Serum IgG levels of the foal should be rechecked after transfusion to ascertain that the desired levels of immunoglobulins have been reached. If these levels have not been reached, additional plasma should be given.

PREVENTION AND CONTROL. Evaluation of colostral immunoglobulin content has proven to be valuable in predicting the occurrence of and assessing the neonate's risk for FPT.[16,27] Colostral IgG can be measured by RID or estimated on the basis of specific gravity of colostrum. Because 18 hours are required to read the results of RID, it is more practical in a field situation to assess specific gravity with a colostrometer. Specific gravity must be measured with a hydrometer, not estimated with a refractometer. Colostral IgG levels should be at least 3000 mg/dl, which corresponds to a specific gravity of 1.060 or greater, and levels of 6000 mg/dl or higher are desirable. If colostral specific gravity is less than 1.060, some degree of failure might be anticipated and corrected prophylactically by providing additional high-quality colostrum, or by providing serum as a source of antibody should the FPT be confirmed.

Some of the causes of FPT can be alleviated or recognized for early intervention by careful management. These include identification of mares that drip colostrum before parturition, attendance at foaling to ensure that foals nurse within several hours of birth or are supplemented artificially with colostrum, and screening of high-risk foals with doubtful nursing histories. Routine screening of foals at 18 to 24 hours of age allows early identification of FPT and potentially allows for therapy before the onset of infections. Although signs of septicemia secondary to FPT are often first observed on day 3 to 4 of life, a bacteremia may already be present at 24 hours of age or earlier.[28]

A colostrum bank can be established by collecting small amounts of colostrum from lactating mares (e.g., 200 to 250 ml) within the first 3 to 6 hours following foaling. This is only about 10% of the total colostrum produced by the average mare in the first 20 hours after parturition and therefore does not adversely affect the foal suckling the donor mare. Although the volumes are quite variable, mares produce about 300 ml of colostrum per hour and about 5 L during the first 18 hours.* Colostrum can be stored frozen at −20° C (−4° F) for at least 1 year. Frozen immunoglobulins are stable for much longer than that; however, the overall quality of the colostrum may deteriorate. Ideally, banked colostrum should be screened for the presence of anti-RBC antibodies as advised for plasma. It is common for colostrum to have low titers of agglutinins, which are probably not of significance unless they are equal to or greater than $^1/_8$.

*Foalimmune, HiGamm-Equi, Lake Immunogenics, Inc, Ontario, NY 14519; Endoserum, Immvac, Inc, Columbia, MO 65201; Equi-Plas, Polymune, Veterinary Dynamics, Inc, Templeton, CA 93465; Sera, Inc, Shawnee Mission, KS 66285-5866.

*Foalimmune, HiGamm-Equi, Lake Immunogenics, Inc, Ontario, NY 14519; Endoserum, Immvac, Inc, Columbia, MO 65201; Equi-Plas, Polymune, Veterinary Dynamics, Inc, Templeton, CA 93465; Sera, Inc, Shawnee Mission, KS 66285-6866.

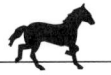

REFERENCES

12. Jeffcott LB: Passive transfer of immunity to foals. In Robinson NE, ed: *Current therapy in equine medicine*, ed 2, Philadelphia, 1987, WB Saunders.
13. LeBlanc MM: Immunologic considerations. In Koterba AM, Drummond WN, Kosch PC, eds: *Equine clinical neonatology*, Philadelphia, 1990, Lea & Febiger.
14. Reiter B: Review of nonspecific antimicrobial factors in colostrum, *Ann Rech Vet* 9:205-224, 1978.
15. Jeffcott LB: Some practical aspects of the transfer of passive immunity to newborn foals, *Equine Vet J* 6:109-115, 1974.
16. LeBlanc MM, McLaurin BI, Boswell R: Relationships among serum immunoglobulin concentration in foals, colostral specific gravity, and colostral immunoglobulin concentration, *J Am Vet Med Assoc* 189:57-60, 1986.
17. Brumbaugh G et al: Measurement of neonatal equine immunoglobulins for assessment of colostral immunoglobulin transfer: comparison of single radial immunodiffusion with zinc sulfate turbidity test, serum electrophoresis, refractometry for total serum protein, and the sodium sulfite precipitation test, *J Am Vet Med Assoc* 172:321-325, 1978.
18. Cowles RR Jr et al: A new test for the detection of immunoglobulin levels in the neonatal foal. *Proceedings of the Twenty-ninth Annual Convention of the American Association of Equine Practitioners*, 1983, pp 415-418.
19. Koterba AM, Brewer B, Drummond WH: Prevention and control of infection, *Vet Clin North Am (Equine Pract)* 1:41-50, 1985.
20. McGuire TC et al: Failure of colostral immunoglobulin transfer as an explanation for most infections and deaths of neonatal foals, *J Am Vet Med Assoc* 170:1302-1304, 1977.
21. Kruse-Elliott K, Wagner PC: Failure of passive antibody transfer in the foal, *Compend Cont Educ Pract Vet* 6:S702-S709, 1984.
22. Lavoie JP et al: Absorption of bovine colostral immunoglobulins G and M in newborn foals, *Am J Vet Res* 50:1598-1603, 1989.
23. Bailey E, Conboy HS, McCarthy PF: Neonatal isoerythrolysis of foals: an update on testing. *Proceedings of the Thirty-third Annual Convention of the American Association of Equine Practitioners*, 1987, pp 341-353.
24. Scott AM, Jeffcott LB: Haemolytic disease of the newborn foal, *Vet Rec* 103:71-74, 1978.
25. Stormont C: Neonatal isoerythrolysis in domestic animals: a comparative review, *Adv Vet Sci Comp Med* 19:23-45, 1975.
26. Perryman LE, Crawford TB: Diagnosis and management of immune system failures of foals. *Proceedings of the Twenty-fifth Annual Convention of the American Association of Equine Practitioners*, 1979, pp 235-245.
27. Banks KL, McGuire TC: Surface receptors on neutrophils and monocytes from immunodeficient and normal horses, *Immunology* 28:581-588, 1975.
28. Brewer BD: Neonatal infection. In Koterba AM, Drummond WN, Kosch PC, eds: *Equine clinical neonatology*, Philadelphia, 1990, Lea & Febiger.

SEVERE COMBINED IMMUNODEFICIENCY

DEFINITION AND ETIOLOGY. Severe combined immunodeficiency (SCID) is a lethal, inherited condition in which both T and B cell function is absent.[29] Affected foals have a stem cell defect that prevents maturation of T and B cells, resulting in a complete inability to produce antigen-specific immune responses. The condition primarily affects Arabians and part Arabians, although sporadic cases have been described in other breeds.[30] In horses of Arabian breeding, the condition is transmitted as an autosomal recessive.[31] Carriers of the gene are asymptomatic, but can now be detected by genetic testing.*

CLINICAL SIGNS AND DIFFERENTIAL DIAGNOSES. Foals that are homozygous for the defective SCID gene are clinically affected. These foals generally appear physically normal at birth, but the absence of both specific humoral and cellular immune responses renders them susceptible to infections once colostral protection wanes. Affected foals typically develop infectious diseases between birth and 2 months of age and invariably die before 5 months of age. The age of onset of infectious disease depends to some degree on the adequacy of passive transfer and the environmental challenge by organisms. The infections suffered by affected animals are nonspecific and are caused by a variety of bacterial, viral, parasitic, and fungal agents, some of which rarely affect animals that are not immunocompromised. Many body systems may be involved, but pneumonia is a particularly common feature. *Pneumocystis carinii* pneumonia and adenoviral pneumonia are found often in SCID foals and rarely in other foals.

CLINICAL PATHOLOGY. A consistent finding on the hemogram is an absolute lymphopenia (<1000 lymphocytes/μl). The total white blood cell count may be low, normal, or elevated, depending on the neutrophilic response; thus it is imperative that the absolute number of lymphocytes be determined. It should be remembered that infected and other compromised foals, as well as some normal foals, have low lymphocyte counts during the first few days of life; therefore persistent lymphopenia should be established for a diagnosis of SCID to be considered.[29,32]

Foals affected with SCID are unable to produce immunoglobulins. Therefore levels of autologous serum immunoglobulin for age are abnormally low. However, quantitative immunoglobulin tests do not distinguish between autologously produced and maternal-origin immunoglobulin. Therefore the degree of colostral transfer and the age of the foal must be considered when interpreting the serum immunoglobulin values (Table 49-1). Some IgM is normally produced in utero by the foal, and some IgM should be present in presuckle serum.[33] The absence of IgM in presuckle serum is not pathognomonic but is a feature of SCID. The presence of colostral antibody of maternal origin may mask low levels of autologous IgG and IgM, particularly early in life. The levels of maternal IgM in colostrum are lower than IgG, and the half-life of IgM is shorter (Table 49-2). Most maternal IgM received from colostrum is metabolized by about 3 weeks of age, whereas the age at which maternal IgG is gone is much more variable and may actually be months, depending on the original amount absorbed. The absence of serum IgM after 3 weeks of age is not pathognomonic but is consistent with SCID.

Foals affected with SCID do not respond to intradermal phytohemagglutinin (see p. 1591) by increasing skin thickness as do normal foals, nor do they respond to stimulators of a delayed-type hypersensitivity such as dinitrochlorobenzene.[34] In vitro tests such as blastogenesis are depressed with all mitogens.[35,36]

The definitive diagnosis of SCID in foals of Arabian breeding is based on demonstrating that the foal is homozygous for the defective SCID gene.[37] Blood or cheek swabs may be submitted to VetGen for DNA testing to determine if a horse is clear, heterozygous, or homozygous for the gene defect. Before genetic testing, the criteria required to confirm a diagnosis of SCID, included: (1) persistent lymphopenia (<1000/μl), (2) absence of serum IgM in presuckle samples or samples collected after 3 weeks of age, and (3) thymic hypoplasia and characteristic histopathologic changes in lymphoid tissue.[38,39]

PATHOPHYSIOLOGY. Foals with SCID lack activity of the enzyme DNA-dependent protein kinase (DNA-PK) resulting in a mutation in the gene encoding the catalytic subunit. The

TABLE 49-2

Approximate Half-life (in days) of Immunoglobulin Classes in Various Species

Species	IgG	IgM	IgA	IgG(T)
Equine	11.5-23	4-5	NA	20
Bovine	G1-17 G2-22	2.8	4.8	—
Sheep	G1-14.5 G2-10.6	1.8	4.1	—
Goat	G1-13.2-17.2	NA	NA	—

From Perryman L: Personal communication, 1988.
NA, Not available.

*Lavoie JP, Spensley M, Smith BP: Personal communication, 1989.

mutation results in a 5 base-pair deletion in the gene on equine chromosome 9. Without functional DNA-PK, lymphocyte precursors are unable to complete gene rearrangement events that lead to the expression of antigen-specific receptors on lymphocyte surfaces. As a result, there is an absence of mature, functional T and B lymphocytes. Interferon-γ (EqIF–γγ), which is produced by lymphocytes, is deficient.[40]

Neutrophils, monocytes, and natural killer cells appear to be fully functional.[41] Complement levels are normal.[36] Although these nonspecific protective mechanisms appear to be intact, the absence of both cell- and antibody-mediated immunity leaves the foal vulnerable to even quite innocuous infectious agents.

EPIDEMIOLOGY. The prevalence of SCID has been estimated to be 2% to 3% of Arabian foals born in the United States. From this, it has been estimated that the numbers of SCID carriers may be as high as 25% of the Arabian horse population in the United States. SCID has been reported in Arabians in the United States, Australia, and Great Britain. It is believed that the trait originated in a horse in Great Britain and was subsequently imported into the United States. The distribution of this disease provides a significant example of the founder effect in population genetics.

NECROPSY FINDINGS. It is imperative to evaluate lymphoid tissues grossly and histologically in cases of suspected immunodeficiencies. In SCID the thymus is small and has a fatty appearance on gross examination. It is frequently difficult to locate, and often mediastinal tissue must be collected "blindly" for subsequent histologic evaluation and identification of thymic remnants. Histologically the thymus is largely replaced with adipose tissue, with only islands of lymphoid cells and partially formed Hassall's corpuscles present. The gross appearance of spleen and lymph nodes may not be dramatically abnormal; however, they have very abnormal microscopic appearances, including absence of germinal centers and periarteriolar lymphocytic sheaths in the spleen, and absence of germinal centers with scarcity of lymphocytes in other areas of lymph nodes.[38]

Bronchopneumonia is a common finding in SCID; however, infectious lesions in other systems are also frequently found, including colitis and hepatitis.

TREATMENT AND PROGNOSIS. Affected foals invariably die by 5 months of age, in spite of intensive conventional therapy (e.g., antimicrobials, plasma, isolation).

There is no practical method of curing affected foals at this time. Successful bone marrow transplants have been performed between histocompatible full siblings in a research setting,[42] but this option remains beyond the realm of practicality at this time.

PREVENTION AND CONTROL. Production of an affected foal identifies both sire and dam as carriers of the SCID gene.[31] Mating of two carriers of an autosomal-recessive trait such as SCID is expected to result in one in four foals affected with SCID, one in four completely normal and not a carrier, and two in four asymptomatic carriers of the SCID trait. Mating of a carrier and a normal (noncarrier) does not produce any affected foals, but half of the offspring would be expected to be carriers.

SCID can be controlled in horses of Arabian breeding by avoiding the production of affected foals, which has been simplified now that carriers can be identified by genetic testing. Mares and stallions intended for breeding should be tested to determine whether they are free or heterozygous for the defective SCID gene. Under no circumstances should two heterozygotes be mated to each other. If an owner decides to continue breeding a heterozygote, the breeding partner should be confirmed homozygous normal. All foals from such matings should be tested to determine if they are clear of or heterozygous for the defective gene (50/50 probability). Homozygous normal foals may be selected for future breeding purposes, whereas heterozygous foals should be managed for nonreproductive pursuits.

REFERENCES

29. McGuire TC, Poppie MJ, Banks KL: Combined (B and T lymphocyte) immunodeficiency: a fatal genetic disease in Arabian foals, *J Am Vet Med Assoc* 164:70-75, 1974.
30. Perryman LE et al: Combined immunodeficiency in an Appaloosa foal, *Vet Pathol* 21:547, 1984.
31. Perryman LE, Torbeck RL: Combined immunodeficiency of Arabian horses: confirmation of autosomal recessive mode of inheritance, *J Am Vet Med Assoc* 176:1250-1251, 1980.
32. Harvey JW: Normal hematologic values. In Koterba AM, Drummond WN, Kosch PC, eds: *Equine clinical neonatology*, Philadelphia, 1990, Lea & Febiger.
33. Tizard I: Immunity in the fetus and newborn. In Tizard I, ed: *Veterinary immunology: an introduction*, ed 3, Philadelphia, 1987, WB Saunders.
34. Hodgin EC LE et al: Evaluation of delayed hypersensitivity responses in normal horses and immunodeficient foals, *Am J Vet Res* 39:1161-1167, 1978.
35. Lew AM, Hosking CS, Studdert MJ: Immunologic aspects of combined immunodeficiency disease in Arabian foals, *Am J Vet Res* 41:1161-1166, 1980.
36. McQuire TC, Banks KL, Poppie MJ: Combined immunodeficiency in horses: characterization of the lymphocyte defect, *Clin Immunol Immunopathol* 3:555-566, 1975.
37. Wiler R et al: Equine severe combined immunodeficiency: a defect in V(D)J recombination and DNA-dependent protein kinase activity, *Proc Natl Acad Sci USA* 92:11485-9, 1995.
38. McGuire TC, Banks KL, Davis WC: Alterations of the thymus and other lymphoid tissue in young horses with combined immunodeficiency, *Am J Pathol* 84:39-53, 1976.
39. Perryman LE: Primary and secondary immune deficiencies of domestic animals, *Adv Vet Sci Comp Med* 23:23-52, 1979.
40. Yilma T, Perryman LE, McGuire TC: Deficiency of interferon-γ but not interferon-β in Arabian foals with severe combined immunodeficiency, *J Immunol* 129:931-933, 1982.
41. Banks KL, McGuire TC: Surface receptors on neutrophils and monocytes from immunodeficient and normal horses, *Immunology* 28:581-588, 1975.
42. Bue CM et al: Correction of equine severe combined immunodeficiency by bone marrow transplantation, *Transplantation* 42:14-19, 1986.

SELECTIVE IgM DEFICIENCY

DEFINITION AND ETIOLOGY. Selective IgM deficiency is an immunologic disorder characterized by absent or decreased serum IgM levels with normal or elevated levels of other immunoglobulin classes. Three presentations of the disorder have been described in horses.[43-46] The most common involves foals that have severe infectious pneumonia, arthritis, or enteritis resulting in death before 10 months of age. The second involves foals with a history of repeated episodes of infections that respond to antimicrobial therapy but that recur when treatment is stopped. These foals tend to do poorly and are stunted, although they may survive for 1 to 2 years. The third involves older horses that are usually 2 to 5 years of age at the time of initial diagnosis. These horses do not necessarily have problems with recurrent infections, but about half of them ultimately have or develop lymphosarcoma.

It is not known whether the IgM deficiencies reported in foals are primary or secondary. The levels of IgM present before the onset of infections have not been measured. The occurrence of multiple cases within groups of related horses suggests a genetic basis. However, breeding trials have been inconclusive to date with regard to the heritability of this condition. In humans, both primary and secondary selective IgM deficiencies are known. Secondary cases are often associated with neoplasia, immunologic diseases such as Wiskott-Aldrich syndrome, and gluten-sensitive enteropathies.

CLINICAL SIGNS AND DIFFERENTIAL DIAGNOSES. Foals with selective IgM deficiency tend to have frequent *Klebsiella* spp. infections of the respiratory tract, although enteritis and septic arthritis may also be complicating infections. The age of onset of clinical signs may be slightly later than in foals with severe combined immunodeficiency and certainly later than in foals with FPT.

Older horses should be carefully evaluated for lymphoid neoplasia, including palpation of peripheral and internal lymph nodes. Weight loss, depression, and other nonspecific signs frequently accompany lymphosarcoma (see Chapter 35).

CLINICAL PATHOLOGY. The only significant immunologic abnormality is a low or absent serum IgM. IgM levels are more than 2 standard deviations below the age-specific mean IgM level (Table 49-1). Other classes of immunoglobulin are generally within normal limits or elevated for age. It is advisable to document that IgM levels are persistently depressed rather than to base a diagnosis on a single sample, since IgM levels may sporadically decrease in seriously ill foals but return to normal with recovery. Lymphocyte counts and other in vitro immunologic tests are generally normal, and these features serve to differentiate selective IgM deficiency from other immunodeficiency conditions. However, in one horse with selective IgM deficiency, lymphocytes failed to respond to the B cell mitogen lipopolysaccharide (LPS), whereas response to the T cell mitogens ConA and phytohemagglutin (PHA) was normal.[46] The hemogram and biochemical profile may reflect infection or inflammation, depending on the underlying infectious process (e.g., neutrophilia, hyperfibrinogenemia, anemia) and the organ system involved, but no diagnostically specific changes occur.

PATHOPHYSIOLOGY. Whether IgM is low because of decreased production, hypercatabolism, or loss is not known. In one case with lymphosarcoma, suppressor activity was identified in the neoplastic cells, suggesting that the low IgM may be a result of suppression of B cell function by neoplastic cells. Selective IgM deficiency has been most frequently reported in Arabians and Quarter horses, although it affects other breeds as well.

NECROPSY FINDINGS. Lymphoid tissue in affected foals is grossly and histologically normal. Pneumonia is commonly present and is frequently due to *Klebsiella* spp. infection. Other findings reflect secondary infections.

TREATMENT AND PROGNOSIS. Selective IgM deficiency has an unfavorable prognosis. Most cases eventually succumb to infection in spite of appropriate antimicrobial therapy. Plasma therapy may provide short-term benefit, but only small amounts of IgM are contained in transfused whole plasma, and the half-life of transfused IgM is probably quite short. No concentrated IgM preparations are commercially available for parenteral use. Relief, at best, can be considered only temporary. However, the outcome of these cases seems less certain than with SCID foals, and a rare case recovers. If persistently low IgM levels can be documented, a poor to grave prognosis can be expected.

PREVENTION AND CONTROL. Because there is a suggestion that the condition in some cases might be hereditary, it may be advisable to avoid repeating the mating that produced the affected foal; however, no firm recommendations can be made.

REFERENCES

43. Perryman LE, McGuire TC, Hilbert BJ: Selective immunoglobulin M deficiency in foals, *J Am Vet Med Assoc* 170:212-215, 1977.
44. Dopson LC et al: Immunosuppression associated with lymphosarcoma in two horses, *J Am Vet Med Assoc* 182:1239-1241, 1983.
45. Perryman LE, Crisman MV: Immune deficiency syndromes. In Robinson NE, ed: *Current therapy in equine medicine*, ed 2, Philadelphia, 1987, WB Saunders.
46. Weldon AD et al: Selective IgM deficiency and abnormal B cell response in a foal, *J Am Vet Med Assoc* 201:1396-1398, 1992.

TRANSIENT HYPOGAMMAGLOBULINEMIA

DEFINITION AND ETIOLOGY. Transient hypogammaglobulinemia is a rare disorder characterized by the delayed onset of immunoglobulin synthesis by the neonate. Foals normally begin to produce significant amounts of immunoglobulins at birth when they are first exposed to environmental antigens (Fig. 49-4). Assuming adequate passive transfer, maternal antibody fills the void during the time from birth until the foal has produced sufficient autologous antibody for protection (e.g., for the first 1 to 2 months). In transient hypogammaglobulinemia, the onset of autologous production is delayed for unknown reasons and may not begin for as long as 3 months. As maternal immunoglobulins wane, there is a period of time when the production of autologous antibody is insufficient to be protective, making the foal highly susceptible to infections. The disorder has been described in an Arabian and a Thoroughbred foal, but the low number of reported cases may not accurately reflect the prevalence because to make a diagnosis, serial samples are required to document decreasing maternal immunoglobulin and subsequent increasing autologous immunoglobulin. Many cases probably occur that are not followed this closely.

CLINICAL SIGNS AND DIFFERENTIAL DIAGNOSES. As with other immunodeficiency disorders, recurrent episodes of bacterial and viral infections are characteristic of this condition.

CLINICAL PATHOLOGY. The cardinal feature of this condition is low immunoglobulin levels. At approximately 2 to 4 months of age, the concentrations of all classes of immunoglobulin, particularly IgG and IgG(T), are substantially below the means when age-matched. At this stage maternal antibody will have waned, but the foal should have produced significant quantities of autologous antibody, regardless of whether passive transfer occurred. Affected foals have normal cell-mediated responses in vitro and in vivo and appear to be able to respond to immunization with some antigens. Normal numbers of B cells are present in blood and lymph nodes. Differentiation between FPT and transient hypogammaglobulinemia is based on the age of the patient at the time of evaluation. Transient hypogammaglobulinemia must be differentiated from agammaglobulinemia. Both disorders have normal lymphocyte counts and responses to PHA skin testing and show waning levels of maternal IgG and IgG(T) if followed serially. However, transient hypogammaglobulinemia cases usually have low but detectable levels of IgM and IgA as opposed to agammaglobulinemia cases, which usually have no detectable levels. Differentiation between the two may require serial sampling to show that Ig production does ultimately increase in the patient with transient hypogammaglobulinemia.

NECROPSY FINDINGS. No specific gross or microscopic lymphoid changes have been associated with transient hypogammaglobulinemia. Necropsy findings reflect the secondary infectious processes that have affected the foal.

TREATMENT AND PROGNOSIS. The goal of therapy is to minimize infections until such time as the foal's immune system begins to function properly. Treatment should include antimicrobial therapy and plasma transfusions. Bacterial infections may be manageable with antibiotics alone, but the effects of viral infections may be more difficult to manage and may be helped by plasma transfusions.

AGAMMAGLOBULINEMIA

DEFINITION AND ETIOLOGY. Agammaglobulinemia is a rare primary immunodeficiency disorder of horses. It is characterized by complete B cell dysfunction with an intact cell-mediated response. This condition has been observed only in males, suggesting the possibility of an X-linked disorder. It has been described in Thoroughbreds, Quarter horses, and Standardbreds.[47-50] Agammaglobulinemia in a young boy was the first immunodeficiency disorder described in any species, and in human patients it is now known to be inherited as an X-linked trait.

Horses with agammaglobulinemia serve to point out the significant contribution that the two separate populations of lymphocytes, T and B, make to the maintenance of good health. Horses with defects in both B and T functions such as in severe combined immunodeficiency seldom survive to 5 months of age, whereas the cases with a pure B cell defect such as agammaglobulinemia have survived between 1 and 2 years. Recently agammaglobulinemia with a lack of circulating B cells was diagnosed in a Pinto gelding that did not exhibit recurrent pyogenic infections until 3 years of age. Although it could not be definitively established whether the immunodeficiency was primary or secondary, an underlying disease process was not identified.*

CLINICAL SIGNS AND DIFFERENTIAL DIAGNOSES. No outward physical signs are suggestive of agammaglobulinemia other than the opportunistic infections that develop. Frequently, recurrent infections of the respiratory tract or joints with extracellular bacteria have been reported. Dermatitis, enteritis, and laminitis have also been associated with this disease.

CLINICAL PATHOLOGY

Total peripheral blood lymphocyte counts are within the normal range. However, there is a lack of circulating B cells with normal numbers of T cells. Neutrophil counts may be normal, low, or high, depending on the response to infection. No specific changes are noted in the biochemical profile. Serum levels of IgM, IgA, IgG(T), and IgG are persistently low or absent. Depending on the age at the time of evaluation, maternal antibody may be present, but its decline is evident if sampled serially. The continued presence of low levels of immunoglobulin in these foals may be explained by the prolonged catabolism of antibody or by some residual B cell activity, as is the case in human patients with sex-linked agammaglobulinemia.[50,51]

Specific antibody responses are depressed, both for antigens to which horses naturally tend to produce antibodies such as sheep red blood cells and for antigens administered by planned immunization such as vaccines. Cell-mediated tests are essentially normal, including blastogenesis and delayed-type hypersensitivity skin testing. Total hemolytic complement activity is also normal.

PATHOPHYSIOLOGY. The molecular basis of agammaglobulinemia in horses is unknown, but a defect at the stem cell level that blocks early B cell differentiation is suspected, since all classes of immunoglobulin are affected. In human patients, a mutation in BTK, a gene encoding tyrosine kinase, accounts for the disease. Assessment of the BTK gene in horses may extend our understanding of this disorder.

NECROPSY FINDINGS. Gross lymphoid changes in lymph nodes, spleen, and thymus have been observed. Lymph nodes are small. The thymus may be small and difficult to locate. Lymphoid tissue taken from the mediastinal region where the thymus should be found lacks the defined lobular structure of normal thymus. The spleen grossly may be small and contracted. Microscopically lymph nodes are devoid of germinal centers and follicles. The spleen has an absence of germinal centers, periarteriolar lymphocytic sheaths, and plasma cells.

The thymus does not show recognizable epithelial structure and lacks defined nodules.[49,51] Why cell-mediated functions are normal when the architecture of the thymus is so abnormal is an enigma.

TREATMENT AND PROGNOSIS. In the absence of production of autologous antibody, affected horses respond poorly to infections over the long term. Antimicrobial therapy and administration of plasma may temporarily control infections; however, the long-term prognosis is grave.

REFERENCES

47. Banks KL, McGuire TC, Jerrells TR: Absence of B lymphocytes in a horse with primary agammaglobulinemia, *Clin Immunol Immunopathol* 5:282-290, 1976.

---

*VetGen, LCC, Ann Arbor, MI; 800-4-VetGen; *http://www.vetgen.com*.

48. Deem DA et al: Agammaglobulinemia in a horse, *J Am Vet Med Assoc* 175:469-472, 1979.
49. McGuire TC et al: Agammaglobulinemia in a horse with evidence of functional T lymphocytes, *Am J Vet Res* 37:41-46, 1976.
50. Perryman LE, McGuire TC: Evaluation for immune system failures in horses and ponies, *J Am Vet Med Assoc* 176:1374-1377, 1980.
51. Rosen FS, Janeway CA: The γ-globulins. III, The antibody deficiency syndromes, *New Engl J Med* 275:709-714, 1966.

ANEMIA, IMMUNODEFICIENCY, AND PERIPHERAL GANGLIONOPATHY IN FELL PONIES

DEFINITION AND ETIOLOGY. A syndrome of severe anemia, immunodeficiency, and peripheral ganglionopathy was recently reported in Fell pony foals.[52] Both genders are affected, and while the exact nature of the defect is as yet unknown, an intrinsic genetic disorder is suspected.

CLINICAL SIGNS. Affected Fell pony foals develop signs of decreased suckling, diarrhea, cough, and chewing motions beginning at 2 to 3 weeks of age and progressing to death at 4 to 8 weeks of age. Cryptosporidial enteritis, adenoviral pancreatitis, and adenoviral bronchopneumonia frequently observed in affected foals are suggestive of an underlying immunodeficiency.

CLINICAL PATHOLOGY. Foals develop severe normocytic to macrocytic anemia associated with small numbers of erythroid precursor cells in the bone marrow. Circulating lymphocyte counts are normal or slightly reduced, and serum immunoglobulin concentrations are normal or near normal. The responses of lymphocytes to in vitro stimulation with phytohemagglutinin and pokeweed mitogen are normal, but response to stimulation with concanavalin A is reduced.

PATHOPHYSIOLOGY. The precise nature of the immune defect is not known. Although immunoglobulin levels are near normal, affected foals have few secondary lymphoid follicles and lack plasma cells.

NECROPSY FINDINGS. Histologic demonstration of neuronal chromatolysis in peripheral nerve ganglia, absence of secondary lymphoid follicles, and lack of plasma cells is characteristic of the condition. There is also erythroid hypoplasia in the bone marrow. In addition, frequent necropsy findings include infections characteristic of immunodeficiency, particularly infections with *Cryptosporidium parvum* and adenoviral infections of the pancreas and bronchial tree.

TREATMENT AND PROGNOSIS. Affected foals respond poorly to treatment for infections and anemia. They generally die by 8 weeks of age.

REFERENCE

52. Scholes SFE et al: A syndrome of anaemia, immunodeficiency and peripheral ganglionopathy in Fell pony foals, *Vet Rec* 142:128-134, 1998.

UNCLASSIFIED IMMUNODEFICIENCIES

Most equine patients with evidence of immunologic defects cannot be ascribed to a currently recognized immunodeficiency category. These animals form a diverse group that often seem to have little in common except the propensity to develop infections. Attempts to further classify these cases are hampered by the lack of selective and specific tests that precisely define the immunologic defect. As newer testing methods are developed, undoubtedly some sense will eventually be made of this group. There are numerous immunodeficiency syndromes described in humans, and it is reasonable to assume that the counterparts of these exist in horses, if we simply had the methods to define them.

Numerous endogenous and exogenous factors can cause secondary immunodeficiency or suppression. These include malnutrition, nutritional deficiencies, nutritional excesses,

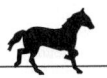

microbial and parasitic agents, corticosteroids and other hormones, and neoplasia. To complicate the issue, most of these factors can induce either suppression or stimulation under appropriate circumstances; thus their presence alone is not adequate to confirm immune compromise. In general, the effects of these factors on the immune system can be assessed by the same tests used to classify primary immunodeficiencies. Sorting out the role of these factors from some of the more subtle types of primary immunodeficiency is very difficult. Immunodeficiency syndromes that appear to be secondary or to have an as-yet-undetermined mechanism include perinatal infection with equine herpesvirus 1, oral candidiasis and septicemia in foals, adult acquired immunodeficiency syndrome, and plasma cell myeloma.

Perinatal Equine Herpesvirus 1 Infection

Infection of the fetus with equine herpesvirus 1 (EHV-1, rhinopneumonitis) late in gestation has been associated with postnatal development of interstitial pneumonia, lymphopenia, marked necrosis and atrophy of the thymus and splenic lymphoid tissue, and increased susceptibility to bacterial infections.[53] Affected foals may be either weak or normal at birth. In spite of apparently adequate passive transfer of maternal antibody, affected foals contract a variety of infectious bacterial diseases, including colibacillosis, streptococcal septicemia, salmonellosis, and Tyzzer's disease. EHV-1 is isolated from nasal passages of about 30% of the cases.[53] The spleen and thymus are grossly small at necropsy. Bilateral adrenocortical hyperplasia is noted in most foals. Histologically, splenic periarteriolar lymphocytic sheaths are depleted of lymphocytes, and no lymphoid follicles are detectable. Thymic alterations vary from extreme diminutions of thymocyte numbers to complete necrosis of thymic lymphocytes with disappearance of Hassall's corpuscles and disruption of the epithelial matrix. Lymph nodes also show lymphoid necrosis.

An immunodeficiency secondary to the marked lymphoid damage induced by the virus is credited with allowing secondary bacterial infections to become established. Immunization of brood mares against EHV-1 would seem to be the most appropriate approach to prevention.

REFERENCE

53. Bryans JT et al: Neonatal foal disease associated with perinatal infection by equine herpesvirus 1, *J Equine Med Surg* 1:20-26, 1977.

Immunodeficiency Associated With Oral Candidiasis and Bacterial Septicemia

DEFINITION AND ETIOLOGY. A group of foals with laboratory or histologic evidence of immunodeficiency that did not fit into any recognized category of primary immunodeficiency have been described with oral candidiasis and bacterial septicemia. No consistent pattern of in vitro immunologic abnormalities was shared among the foals, although they all shared the clinical features of oral candidiasis and bacterial septicemia.[54] This syndrome has some similarities to mucocutaneous candidiasis in people, which has been associated with several different subtle T cell defects. Not all cases in people are thought to be the result of a single immunodeficiency disorder. Candidiasis does not occur in the presence of B cell defects alone, in the absence of T cell defects.

CLINICAL SIGNS. Most affected foals with oral candidiasis were about 4 months of age at onset, although several were less than 2 weeks old. Oral lesions ranged from discrete, focal, white, plaquelike lesions on the margins of the tongue to a generalized, thick, white, pseudomembranous coating covering the tongue and gingival mucosa. Most foals exhibited bruxism, ptyalism, fever, and depression. Other signifi-

cant clinical problems included pneumonia, septic arthritis, and diarrhea.[54] This syndrome should be distinguished from the glossitis due to *Candida* infection seen in inappetent or debilitated neonatal foals, which is fairly common and generally resolves with amelioration of the primary disease.[55]

CLINICAL PATHOLOGY. Serum IgG and IgM levels were variable, but most of the older foals also had low or marginal IgG or IgM for their age. The younger foals all suffered from FPT and had low IgG. Some horses showed a transient lymphopenia, but lymphocyte counts were generally within normal limits. In almost all cases evaluated other abnormalities, including depressed blastogenesis, were present, suggesting a cellular defect that differentiated the cases from the previously described immunodeficiencies which involved only immunoglobulin production.

NECROPSY FINDINGS. Thymic tissue was difficult to locate grossly at necropsy. Mediastinal tissue collected in the thymic region was confirmed to be thymus microscopically in only one of six cases. Histologically splenic lymphoid depletion was present. Evidence of disseminated bacterial infections included pulmonary abscesses, enteritis, septic arthritis, and focal hepatitis. *Candida* spp. were identified in tissues histologically or with culture in all cases. A variety of different bacterial organisms were associated with the septicemias and secondary infections. Organisms usually considered to be limited pathogens such as *Acinetobacter* and adenovirus were identified in some cases.

TREATMENT AND PROGNOSIS. Affected foals did not respond to extensive parenteral antibiotic, topical antimycotic, or plasma transfusion therapy. Antibiotic administration can predispose animals to secondary candidiasis, and the role therapy may have played in the development of the oral lesions needs to be considered. However, considering the frequency with which antibiotics are used in the general population and the relatively uncommon occurrence of oral candidiasis, it seems as though additional factors such as an immune defect must be involved. The prognosis for foals with oral candidiasis and associated bacterial septicemia is guarded to poor.

REFERENCES

54. McClure JJ, Addison JD, Miller RI: Immunodeficiency manifested by oral candidiasis and bacterial septicemia, *J Am Vet Med Assoc* 186:195-197, 1985.
55. Wilson JH, Cudd TA: Common gastrointestinal diseases. In Koterba AM, Drummond WN, Kosch PC, eds: *Equine clinical neonatology*, Philadelphia, 1990, Lea & Febiger.

Adult Acquired Immunodeficiency

A 7-year-old Appaloosa gelding with no history of prior illness became lethargic, anorexic, and dyspneic.[56] *Rhodococcus equi* septicemia was diagnosed on the basis of blood cultures. Immunologic evaluation of the patient revealed lymphopenia, low IgM and IgA concentrations, marginally low IgG concentrations, low *R. equi* antibody titer, negligible response to lymphocyte stimulation, histologic depletion of the lymphoid tissue, and failure to respond to antigenic stimulation. Marked thrombocytopenia was also present. These abnormalities suggested suppression of both humoral and cell-mediated arms of the immune system. The age of the horse, absence of previous history of illness, and histopathologic findings suggestive of atrophy of lymphoid tissue suggested that the immunodeficiency was acquired. No underlying cause was identified for the immunodeficiency; specifically, no neoplasms were identified at necropsy, and there was no history of exposure to immunosuppressive toxins.

REFERENCE

56. Freestone JF J et al: Acquired immunodeficiency in a 7-year-old horse, *J Am Vet Med Assoc* 190:689-691, 1987.

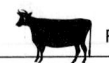

Plasma Cell Myeloma

Plasma cell myelomas have been diagnosed in horses of several breeds.[57] Although reports of the condition are limited, there appears to be no sex predilection. Horses have ranged in age from 3 months to 22 years at the time of diagnosis, with a median age of 11 years. Common clinical signs include weight loss, anorexia, fever, pneumonia, and limb edema. As a malignancy of plasma cells or lymphocytoid plasma cells, plasma cell myelomas typically produce large quantities of a homogenous immunoglobulin or immunoglobulin fragment, resulting in a monoclonal gammopathy. In both equine and human cases of myeloma, the predominant serum globulins are generally subclasses of IgG.[57,58] Hyperglobulinemia is a characteristic but not invariable finding. Monoclonal gammopathies in the horse have also been reported with lymphoma and benign disorders.[59,60] Both equine and human patients with plasma cell myelomas have an increased susceptibility to bacterial infections, probably as a result of a secondary immunodeficiency.[60,61] The concentrations of normal polyclonal immunoglobulins are generally decreased in myeloma patients due to several mechanisms, including decreased synthesis and accelerated catabolism of antibody and suppressed clonal expansion of B cells.[57,58,61] Decreased numbers of neutrophils which may also be dysfunctional, and defective complement activation may also contribute to the impaired immune function.

REFERENCES

57. Edwards DF et al: Plasma cell myeloma in the horse, *J Vet Intern Med* 7:169-176, 1993.
58. Oken MM: Multiple myeloma, *Med Clin North Am* 68:757-787, 1984.
59. Kent JE, Roberts CA: Serum protein changes in four horses with monoclonal gammopathy, *Equine Vet J* 22:373-376, 1990.
60. Traub-Dargatz J, Bertone A, Bennett D: Monoclonal aggregating immunoglobulin cryoglobulinemia in a horse with malignant lymphoma, *Equine Vet J* 17:470-473, 1985.
61. Matus RE, Leifer CE: Immunoglobulin-producing tumors, *Vet Clin North Am (Small Anim Pract)* 15:741, 1985.

Nonspecific Immune Suppression

Secondary immune suppression can occur as a result of a variety of infectious or inflammatory diseases or drugs. Many viral, fungal, and bacterial infections transiently suppress specific and nonspecific immune responses, predisposing to secondary bacterial infections.[62] Severe endotoxemia or septicemia may suppress neutrophil numbers and bactericidal function. Advanced neoplastic disease can impair cell-mediated and humoral immune responses as a result of an abnormal bone marrow environment, altered patterns of cytokine production or release, or impaired proliferative responses (anergy). Severe malnutrition can impair immune function and increase susceptibility to infection as can a variety of vitamin and mineral deficiencies. Exercise stress may transiently impair neutrophil function, predisposing to secondary infection.[63] Transport or other stress may have a similar immune suppressive effect.

Systemic administration of corticosteroids can exacerbate pre-existing infectious diseases or decrease resistance to environmental pathogens.[64,65] These drugs can suppress macrophage phagocytic function by impairing the killing of ingested microorganisms, decreasing secretion of monokines, and inhibiting antigen processing and presentation.[66,67] They suppress cell-mediated immunity through induction of a T cell lymphopenia, suppression of proliferation in response to mitogen stimulation, altered cytokine production, and decreased antigen presentation. Humoral immunity may be affected through impaired T cell responses, enhanced catabolism of immunoglobulins, and decreased antigen presentation.[67]

REFERENCES

62. Olsen RG: Immune dysfunctions associated with viral infections, *Compend Cont Ed Pract Vet* 6:422-427, 1984.
63. Wong CW et al: Effects of exercise stress on various immune functions in horses, *Am J Vet Res* 53:1414-1417, 1992.
64. Kono Y Y et al: Recrudescence of equine infectious anemia by treatment with immunosuppressive drugs, *Natl Inst Anim Health Q Tokyo* 16:8-15, 1976.
65. Mair TS: Bacterial pneumonia associated with corticosteroid therapy in three horses, *Vet Rec* 138:205-207, 1996.
66. Cohn LA: The influence of corticosteroids on host defense mechanisms, *J Vet Intern Med* 5:95-104, 1991.
67. Schaffner A, Schaffner T: Glucocorticoid-induced impairment of macrophage antimicrobial activity: mechanisms and dependence on the state of activation, *Rev Inf Dis* 9(suppl):620-629, 1987.

RUMINANT IMMUNODEFICIENCY DISEASES

GEORGE M. BARRINGTON
STEVEN M. PARISH

FAILURE OF PASSIVE TRANSFER

Newborn ruminants are born essentially devoid of circulating immunoglobulins. The attainment of a successful transfer of colostral immunoglobulins from the dam to the offspring is of paramount importance in helping to maintain the welfare of the newborn. Intestinal absorption of immunoglobulins in the newborn is limited to the immediate postpartum period. Cessation of immunoglobulin uptake from the intestinal lumen occurs during the first day of life but may be influenced by the time of the initial colostrum feeding.[68,69] Calves fed colostrum at birth ceased to absorb immunoglobulins at 21 to 23 hours of age. When colostrum feeding was delayed for 24 hours, some absorption occurred until 31 to 33 hours after birth. There is also individual variation in calves in closure time, regardless of feeding, with some calves maintaining absorption until 36 hours after birth.[68] Similar patterns are noted in lambs and kids. Failure of the newborn to obtain and absorb colostral immunoglobulins frequently is associated with increased morbidity and mortality from bacteremia and common neonatal diseases.

CLINICAL SIGNS. The success of passive transfer cannot be determined by physical examination of the young ruminant. Those devoid of passive immunoglobulins, particularly IgM, are highly susceptible to bacterial septicemia.[70,71] Signs of bacteremia in neonatal ruminants include central nervous system depression, weakness, injected scleral vessels, rapid or labored respiration, diarrhea, and anorexia. Fever may or may not be present. Septic arthritis, meningitis, and panophthalmitis frequently develop in many neonates with failure of passive transfer (FPT) that survive the initial challenge of bacteremia. Diarrhea can also occur as a result of dietary and infectious agents in neonatal ruminants with normal serum immunoglobulin levels.[72] Historic information of presenting clinical disease may lead to a high degree of suspicion that FPT is present. Laboratory evaluation can be undertaken to assess the degree of passive transfer if any that has taken place.

CLINICAL PATHOLOGY. Numerous methods are available to quantitate or semiquantitate the transfer of immunoglobulin to the neonate. The greatest degree of accuracy is obtained if the tests are performed during the first week of life. After this period, animals with FPT begin to synthesize immunoglobulins at a substantial rate, although one can still render a tentative decision as to the degree of passive transfer that occurred following birth. Any questionable status as to passive transfer in a newborn should necessitate the laboratory evaluation of that animal so that corrective measures can be undertaken.

Single Radial Immunodiffusion. Quantification of each immunoglobulin class that is transferred can be determined using specific antisera that are available commercially.[73] Forty-eight-hour serum concentrations of less than 1000 mg/dl, 80 mg/dl, and 22 mg/dl for IgG, IgM, and IgA, respectively, are consistent with FPT.[74]

Zinc Sulfate Turbidity. Specific concentrations of zinc sulfate precipitate immunoglobulins.[75] A 0.1-ml amount of serum is added to 6 ml of zinc sulfate solution containing 208 mg of $ZnSO_4 \cdot 7H_2O$ per liter, and the test is allowed to incubate at room temperature for 1 hour. The lack of or decreased amount of precipitation turbidity obtained by adding suspect serum to zinc sulfate solution is indicative of failure of immunoglobulin absorption. Semiquantitation can be obtained through spectrophotometric methods.[75]

Sodium Sulfite Precipitation. The sodium sulfite precipitation test is similar to the zinc sulfate turbidity test and is also a precipitation test for immunoglobulins, primarily IgG, with the results recorded visually.[76] The reagents are commercially available.* Three concentrations of $Na_2SO_3{}^+$ anhydrous (14%, 16%, and 18%) are used in the test. A 0.1-ml amount of serum is added to 1.9 ml of each of the concentrations of sodium sulfite, and these are allowed to incubate for 1 hour. Turbidity in only the 18% sample indicates transfer of less than 500 mg/dl of immunoglobulin, turbidity in both the 16% and 18% samples indicates 500 to 1500 mg/dl of transfer, and turbidity in all samples indicates greater than 1500 mg/dl transfer.

Glutaraldehyde Coagulation Test. The glutaraldehyde coagulation test uses 10% glutaraldehyde reagent which coagulates serum immunoglobulins in concentrations greater than 600 mg/dl.[77]

Refractometer (Total Serum Solids). The refractometer test assumes that the increase in serum proteins over that of presuckle newborn ruminants is caused by the absorption of immunoglobulin.[78] In the absence of dehydration, a serum protein over 5 g/dl is considered to be associated with a successful passive transfer. Values lower than 4.5 g/dl are consistent with FPT, whereas values between 4.5 and 5 g/dl are questionable.

γ-Glutamyltransferase. γ-Glutamyltransferase (GGT) is present in colostrum at levels about 300 times higher than that normally found in serum. It is absorbed by the calf during the period of immunoglobulin absorption, and calf serum levels can be used as an indication of immunoglobulin absorption. Levels of GGT are maximal in the calf on the first or second day after birth, with less than 300 U/L being consistent with FPT.[79,80]

In general, the transfer of immunoglobulin to the newborn ruminant of less than 600 mg/dl can be considered to be consistent with FPT, whereas 600 to 1600 mg/dl is representative of partial FPT, and greater than 1600 mg/dl is normal.[81] There are no consistent changes in the hemogram and biochemical panel of a neonatal ruminant with FPT. Abnormal laboratory findings usually reflect secondary processes involving sepsis, stress, or starvation.

EPIDEMIOLOGY. The percentage of FPT in calves at 24 hours of age varies from 15% to 68%.[70] Similar findings have been recorded in other neonatal ruminants. Many interrelated factors account for this high incidence. Those of greatest importance involve the age of the neonate at the time of colostrum ingestion, the amount of colostrum ingested, and the concentration of the immunoglobulins in the colostrum. The presence of the dam may also play a minor role in enhancing colostrum absorption.

The consumption of adequate amounts of satisfactory colostrum by the newborn within the first few hours after birth is the most important factor in attaining a successful passive transfer. Many factors in the relationship between the newborn and its dam may have positive or negative influences during this critical time (e.g., the ability of the newborn to rise and suckle, the mothering ability, udder conformation, colostrum quantity and quality, seasonal variation, and other management and environmental events).

The volume of colostrum produced by the cow is usually not a limiting factor for successful passive transfer in most instances.[73] However, limited colostral volume can occur in beef heifers and cows subjected to severe dietary restrictions during pregnancy.[82] Restricted diets fed to cows may also affect the calf's absorption of immunoglobulins. Calves suckling cows fed at 57% of National Research Council requirements absorbed fewer immunoglobulins when compared with calves suckling cows fed at 100%. Colostral immunoglobulin levels were similar in both groups of cows. Increased cortisol and decreased triiodothyronine levels were found in the calves of restricted cows and may have influenced absorption of immunoglobulins.[83] In general, the amount of colostrum produced during the first lactation is lower than in subsequent lactations. The concentration of immunoglobulins in colostrum varies greatly among cows and may represent genetic differences among them.[84] Lack of adequate immunoglobulin concentration in individual colostrums may account for the observed high levels of FPT in some herds. In closely confined groups of animals, such as dairies and purebred herds and flocks, many of the factors leading to a successful passive transfer can be controlled, whereas in pasture or range operations the problem is much more difficult to address but also much less common.

TREATMENT. When FPT is diagnosed in an otherwise clinically normal neonate, the administration of serum or plasma at a rate of 20 to 40 ml/kg IV (or intraperitoneally if intravenous administration is not possible) should be undertaken. Similar approaches are indicated in animals with clinical disease, but the results are often less rewarding. Although absorption has ceased, the continued feeding of colostrum may provide some local immune protection in the gut.[74]

PREVENTION. The intake and absorption of adequate amounts of quality colostrum are key to the survivability of young ruminants. Early documented natural sucking or forced feeding of colostrum during the first 6 hours of life helps to ensure adequate transfer. It is generally held that a neonate should consume between 6% and 10% of its body weight as colostrum during the first 24 hours of life. Most calves consume approximately 2 L (40 to 50 ml/kg of body weight) of colostrum at the first feeding. In force-feeding practices, 2 L has commonly been advocated as the proper amount for initial intake. However, the variance in colostrum quality might suggest that a greater volume should be fed at the initial feeding.[85] In problem herds or flocks in which neonatal disease is a problem, quantitation of passive transfer should be determined, and forced feeding of all newborn animals should be instituted to ensure adequate transfer.

Whole colostrum specific gravity can be reasonably measured with a colostrometer.[86] A specific gravity of less than 1.050 is associated with colostrum with low immunoglobulin concentration. This device can eliminate 50% of the low immunoglobulin colostrums and predict high immunoglobulin concentrations.[85] At colostrum temperatures other than 20° C, less accuracy is achieved.[87] Colostrum should contain greater than 6000 mg/dl total immunoglobulin. To ensure that all neonates receive adequate amounts of colostrum, producers should be encouraged to maintain a bank of frozen colostrum. Colostrum from first milkings is preferred, because immunoglobulin concentrations decrease with successive feedings.

---

*Bova-S, VMRD, Pullman, WA 99163; ICN Immunobiologicals, Lisle, IL 60532; Bethyl Laboratories, Montgomery, TX 77356.

Immunoglobulins are generally unaltered by freezing, and only small amounts are inactivated by thawing. Thawing frozen colostrum in warm water is quickly accomplished for individual calf feeding. Microwave ovens have been used to thaw frozen colostrum without adverse effects.[88]

Pooling or mixing colostrum from several cows is a common practice to ensure adequate immunoglobulin concentrations. This practice is advocated to circumvent the problem of low-concentration colostrum being fed. However, trials have shown that with this practice calves that receive pooled colostrum acquire substantially lower serum immunoglobulin levels than calves fed equivalent volumes of homologous colostrum from their own dams.[74] Colostrums used in pooling frequently come from cows with high volumes of colostrum that tend to have lower immunoglobulin levels.

There are numerous commercially available colostrum substitutes that can be used to either supplement available colostrum or to provide a source of immunoglobulins for calves when colostrum is not available. It is important to observe the amount of immunoglobulin present in these products and administer enough product to ensure passive transfer. Bovine colostrum is frequently used to supplement or replace homologous sources of colostrum in nonbovine ruminants. Neonatal lambs are frequently supplemented this way.[89] The immunoglobulins are absorbed at rates similar to homologous colostrum. The half-life of bovine IgG1 in lambs is approximately 14 days,[90] which is similar to the reported half-life of 13.7 days for ovine IgG1 in lambs (Table 49-2).[72] Occasionally anemia is reported in lambs fed bovine colostrum[91] as a result of immune complex attachment to the lamb's erythrocytes, causing their removal from circulation.[92] The effectiveness of bovine or caprine colostrum in other species is unknown, but the practice appears to be widespread and has been used in a wild animal park successfully hand raising neonatal exotic ruminants.

REFERENCES

68. Stott GH et al: Colostral immunoglobulin transfer in calves. II, The rate of absorption, *J Dairy Sci* 62:1766-1773, 1979.
69. Stott GH et al: Colostral immunoglobulin transfer in calves. III, Amount of absorption, *J Dairy Sci* 62:1902-1907, 1979.
70. Logen EF: Colostral immunity to colibacillosis in the neonatal calf, *Br Vet J* 130:405-412, 1974.
71. McEwan AD, Fisher EW, Selman IE: Observations on the immune globulin levels of neonatal calves and their relationship to disease, *J Comp Pathol* 80:259-265, 1970.
72. Penhale WJ et al: Quantitative studies on bovine immunoglobulins II, Plasma immunoglobulin levels in market calves and their relationship to neonatal infection, *Br Vet J* 126:30-36, 1970.
73. Hines MT, Tumas DB, Schott HC: Personal communication, 1994.
74. Gay CC: The role of colostrum in managing calf health, *Bovine Pract* 16:79-84, 1984.
75. McEwan AD, Fisher EW, Selman IE: A turbidity test for the estimation of immune globulin levels in neonatal calf serum, *Clin Chem Acta* 27:155-163, 1970.
76. Stone SS, Gitler M: The validity of the sodium sulfite test for detecting immunoglobulins in calf serum, *Br Vet J* 125:68-72, 1969.
77. Tennant B et al: Use of the glutaraldehyde coagulation test for detection of hypogammaglobulinemia in neonatal calves, *J Am Vet Med Assoc* 174:848-853, 1979.
78. Naylor JM, Kronfeld DS: Refractometry as a measure of the immunoglobulin status of the newborn dairy calf: comparison with the zinc sulfate turbidity test and single radial immunodiffusion, *J Am Vet Med Assoc* 171:1331-1334, 1977.
79. Braun JP C et al: Early variations of blood plasma γ-glutamyltransferase in newborn calves: a teat of colostrum intake, *J Dairy Sci* 65:2178, 1982.
80. Paris TNN et al: Use of serum γ-glutamyltransferase and total blood proteins for monitoring the colostrum intake of newborn calves, *Rec Med Vet* 168:43, 1992.
81. McGuire TC, Adams DS: Failure of colostral immunoglobulin transfer to calves: prevalence and diagnosis, *Compend Cont Educ* 4:S35-S40, 1982.
82. Radostitis OM, Acres SD: The prevention and control of epidemics of acute undifferentiated diarrhea in beef calves in western Canada, *Can Vet J* 21:243-249, 1980.
83. Hough RL et al: Influence of nutritional restriction during late gestation on production measures and passive immunity in beef cattle, *J Anim Sci* 68:2622, 1990.
84. Stott GH, Fleemor WA, Kleese WC: Colostral immunoglobulin concentration in fractions of first milking postpartum and five additional milkings, *J Dairy Sci* 64:459-465, 1981.
85. Besser TE, Gay CC: Septicemic colibacillosis and failure of passive transfer of colostral immunoglobulins in calves, *Vet Clin North Am (Food Anim Pract)* 1:445-459, 1985.
86. Fleenor WA, Stott GH: Hygrometer test for estimation of immunoglobulin concentration in bovine colostrum, *J Dairy Sci* 63:973-977, 1980.
87. Mechor GD et al: Specific gravity of bovine colostrum immunoglobulins as affected by temperature and colostrum components, *J Dairy Sci* 75:3131-3135, 1992.
88. Besser TE: Unpublished data, 1992.
89. Clarkson MJ, Faull WB, Kerry JB: Vaccination of cows with clostridial antigens and passive transfer of clostridial antibodies from bovine colostrum to lambs, *Vet Rec* 116:467-469, 1985.
90. Ciupercescu DD: Dynamics of serum immunoglobulin concentrations in sheep during pregnancy and lactation, *Res Vet Sci* 22:23-27, 1977.
91. Stubbinggs DP, Gibbons DF, Tindall JR: Feeding cows' colostrum to lambs, *Vet Rec* 112:88-89, 1983.
92. Franken P: Feeding cows' colostrum to lambs, *Vet Rec* 112:332, 1983.

LETHAL TRAIT A46

Lethal trait A46 is a primary immunodeficiency that is found in black pied Danish cattle of Friesian descent.[93] It is an autosomal-recessive trait in which the calves appear normal at birth but develop skin disease at 2 to 8 weeks of age. Skin lesions are characterized by exanthema, alopecia, and hyperparakeratosis, with initial lesions occurring around the head, neck, and flexor surfaces of the legs and later involving the entire animal. Death within 4 months is often associated with bronchopneumonia and diarrhea. These animals do respond normally to humoral antigens but show deficits in cellular immunity. At necropsy the calves show marked lymphoid regression involving the thymus, spleen, lymph nodes, and gut-associated lymphoid tissues in the thymic-dependent regions. The condition is responsive to oral zinc oxide therapy, which suggests an underlying problem in zinc metabolism. Daily oral dosages of up to 1 g of zinc oxide have been used to establish normal function.[93] The primary immunologic defect is found in T lymphocytes. It appears that, because of a defect in a recessive gene, these animals have an unusually high metabolic requirement for zinc ions needed to sustain normal T lymphocyte development and function.

REFERENCE

93. Brummerstedt E: Immune-deficient animals in biomedical research, *Proceedings of the Fifth International Workshop on Immune-deficient Animals,* Copenhagen, 1985, Basel, 1987, S Karger.

SELECTIVE IgG2 DEFICIENCY

A primary IgG2 deficiency has been described in the red Danish milk breed in which there is a primary partial to complete deficit in IgG2.[94,95] These animals appear to be more susceptible to gangrenous mastitis and pyogenic infections such as bronchopneumonia, peritonitis, and abomasoenteritis.[96] A transient IgG2 deficiency has also been reported in neonatal lambs.[95] In lambs that ingested colostrum, there was a delay in the onset of synthesis of IgG2 until 5 to 6 weeks of age without any adverse consequences.

REFERENCES

94. Mansa B: Hypo-7S-g globinemia in mature cattle, *Acta Pathol Microbiol* 63:153-158, 1965.
95. Perryman LE: Primary and secondary immune deficiencies of domestic animals, *Adv Vet Sci Comp Med* 23:23-52, 1979.
96. Kulkarni PE: IgG2 deficiency in gangrenous mastitis in cows, *Acta Vet Scand* 12:611-614, 1971.

CHEDIAK-HIGASHI SYNDROME

Chediak-Higashi syndrome is an inherited disorder that affects neutrophil and monocyte function in Hereford cattle, mink, cats, mice, killer whales, and humans.[97,98] Clinically these patients are recognized by partial albinism that affects the skin and eyes, coagulation difficulties, and an increased susceptibility to bacterial infections. Large cytoplasmic granules are seen within neutrophils. The increased susceptibility to pyogenic infections is related to decreased neutrophil killing of ingested organisms caused by a defect in the hexose monophosphate shunt activity and defective degranulation.

REFERENCES
97. Prieur DJ, Collier LL: Chediak-Higashi syndrome, *Am J Pathol* 90:533-536, 1978.
98. Renshaw HW et al: Leukocyte dysfunction in the bovine homologue of the Chediak-Higashi syndrome of humans, *Infect Immun* 10:928-937, 1974.

BOVINE LEUKOCYTE ADHESION DEFICIENCY

Bovine leukocyte adhesion deficiency (BLAD) is an autosomal recessive disorder of Holstein calves characterized clinically by chronic bacterial infections and premature death.[99-101] Leukocytes of affected calves lack surface glycoproteins, termed β-2 integrins. A mutation of the gene encoding bovine CD18 causes this disorder. The gene defect is termed the D128G allele mutation.

Heterozygous carriers are clinically normal; however bulls and cows with this mutation may produce homozygous calves that manifest the deficiency. All calves with BLAD can be traced to a single male ancestor that must be present in both the sire and dam pedigree. In the United States, approximately 14% of sires and almost 6% of Holstein calves are affected with BLAD.

Homozygous calves have chronic, recurrent bacterial infections. Consistent clinical findings include fever, bronchopneumonia, stomatitis, gingivitis, recurrent or chronic diarrhea, peripheral lymphadenopathy, vasculitis, and dermatitis.[102-103] Calves appear normal at birth, but clinical signs are often present within the first few weeks of life. Affected calves usually die within the first year of life. Those surviving past 1 year of age have persistent ill-thrift. Hematologic abnormalities include mature neutrophilia ($>40,000/\mu l$) without significant left shifts, lymphocytosis, and monocytosis. Abnormal serum biochemical findings include hypoalbuminemia; hyperglobulinemia; and low serum creatinine, urea nitrogen, and glucose concentrations.

Diagnostic tests are available to detect heterozygous carriers and identify homozygous clinically affected calves. Information regarding testing is available from the Holstein Association of America, Brattleboro, VT 05301.

REFERENCES
99. Hagemoser WA et al: Granulocytopathy in a Holstein heifer, *J Am Vet Med Assoc* 183:1093-1094, 1983.
100. Nagahata H et al: Bovine granulocytopathy syndrome: neutrophil dysfunction in Holstein-Friesian calves, *Zentralbl Vetinarmed (A)* 34:445-451, 1987.
101. Kehrli ME Jr et al: Molecular definition of the bovine granulocytopathy syndrome: identification of the deficiency of the Mac-1 (CD11b/CD18) glycoprotein, *Am J Vet Res* 51:1826-1836, 1990.
101. Gilbert RO et al: Clinical manifestations of leukocyte adhesion deficiency in cattle: 14 cases (1977-1991), *J Am Vet Med Assoc* 202:445-449, 1993.
102. Ackermann MR, Kehrli ME, Morfitt DC: Ventral dermatitis and vasculitis in a calf with bovine leukocyte adhesion deficiency, *J Am Vet Med Assoc* 202:413-415, 1993.

VIRAL- AND BACTERIAL-INDUCED IMMUNODEFICIENCY

Decreased B and T lymphocyte function has been reported associated with bovine virus diarrhea (BVD) infection in calves developing chronic BVD syndrome.[104] Depression of cellular, but not humoral, immunity is seen in cattle infected with Johne's disease *(Mycobacterium johnei)*, with failure to develop or delayed-type hypersensitivity reactions in vivo and in vitro.[105] It is associated with a humoral-suppressive factor.

REFERENCES
104. Muscoplat CC, Johnson DW, Stevens JB: Abnormalities of in vitro lymphocyte responses during bovine viral diarrhea virus infection, *Am J Vet Res* 34:753-755, 1973.
105. Davies DH, Corbiel L: A humoral suppressor of in vitro lymphocyte transformation responses in cattle with Johne's disease, *Proc Soc Exp Biol Med* 145:1372-1373, 1974.

COMBINED IMMUNODEFICIENCY

Genetic failure of development of both T and B cell lines results in a severely compromised immunodeficient animal. As passively acquired maternal antibody wanes, infections tend to develop. One possible case of combined immunodeficiency in a calf has been reported. It was recognized in a 6-week-old Angus that had an absence of serum IgM, low serum IgG, absolute lymphopenia, and an absence of lymphoid tissue at necropsy. The calf died of bronchopneumonia and disseminated fungal infection.[105]

REFERENCE
106. Bartram PA et al: Combined immunodeficiency in a calf, *J Am Vet Med Assoc* 195:347-350, 1989.

PREGNANCY-ASSOCIATED IMMUNODEFICIENCY

JAMES F. EVERMANN

Immunosuppression during pregnancy and the periparturient period has been recognized for several years.[107] What has not been defined has been the degree of the immune suppression and what compartments of the immune response (macrophage, B cell, T cell) are being affected. An early review stated that pregnancy and lactation have profound effects on the cow's immunologic responsiveness to a number of bacteria, viruses, protozoa, and helminths.[107] It was concluded that pregnancy-related immunologic unresponsiveness was manifested as an increased vulnerability to infection and recrudescence of infection during pregnancy and lactation.

It has been only within the past 5 years that efforts have been made to quantitate the degree of immune suppression during bovine pregnancy and early lactation. Studies on immune cell populations and neutrophil function have provided some degree of explanation as to why the pregnant cow is more susceptible to infectious diseases than the nonpregnant age-matched control cow.[108,109] These studies, as well as those in comparative reproductive immunology, have indicated that there is selective impairment of certain immune cell functions and enhancement of others that maximize fetal survival.[110,111] Although they are the subject of active investigation, the proposed immune parameters occurring during bovine pregnancy include a decrease in T cytotoxic cell functions and an increase in T suppressor cell functions.[112] The T cell populations are affected by progesterone, prostaglandin $F_{2\alpha}$, and α-fetoprotein. The B cell functions are also modulated during pregnancy with a decrease in T cell-dependent antibody (probably resulting from a decrease in or ineffective T helper cells). Altered B cell functions result in an increase in blocking or enhancing antibodies. There are also decreases in interleukin 2, α-interferon, and various colony-stimulating factors, all of which are vital in maintaining T cytotoxic cell and macrophage functions.

Fetal Survival Versus Increased Susceptibility to Infectious Diseases

With this selective immunosuppression, T cytotoxic cell-dependent immune defenses become compromised. The T cytotoxic cells function normally to control virtually all viral infections, especially herpetic infections, such as infectious bovine rhinotracheitis and bovine herpesvirus type 4.[110,111] Also, intracellular bacterial infections, such as *Brucella abortus*, become more pathogenic during pregnancy. Macrophage function becomes temporarily compromised, allowing for opportunistic bacteria and *Chlamydia*, which are usually confined to the external mucosal surfaces of the body, to become systemic. Impaired T cell function and altered macrophage activity may explain, in part, the pathogenicity of *Neospora* spp. in bovine abortions.[111,112a]

Shedding of Infectious Microorganisms During Pregnancy and Postpartum Periods

Immunosuppression during pregnancy results in an increase in the shedding of microorganisms and is an extension of impaired T cell reactivity.[111] Although the pregnant cow may appear clinically normal, her altered immune response results in an increased recrudescence of infection.[107] This indicates that the most cows are in an increased state of shedding infectious microorganisms in their immediate environment via fecal matter, saliva, nasal secretions, blood, urine, and placental tissue. There is an apparent increase in shedding of infectious microorganisms, especially during the last trimester and 3 to 4 weeks postpartum. The predominant microbial infections during this period are bacterial and are due in part to decreased neutrophil and macrophage function.

The threshold between the asymptomatic shedder cow and one with clinical manifestations of disease (late-stage abortion, postpartum metritis, and mastitis) is regarded as being related to nutritional factors. These factors, such as selenium and copper deficiency, may account for reports on the increased susceptibility to *Haemophilus somnus* and *Chlamydia*, respectively.[111,112b]

REFERENCES

106. Lloyd SS: Immunosuppression during pregnancy and lactation, *Irish Vet J* 37:64-70, 1983.
107. Kehrli ME Jr, Nonnecke BJ, Roth JA: Alterations in bovine lymphocyte function during the periparturient period, *Am J Vet Res* 50:215-220, 1989.
108. Gilbert RO et al: Effect of parity on periparturient neutrophil function in dairy cows, *Vet Immunol Immunopathol* 36:75-82, 1993.
109. Wegmann TG et al: Bidirectional cytokine interactions in the maternal-fetal relationship: is successful pregnancy a Th2 phenomenon? *Immunol Today* 14:353-356, 1993.
110. Evermann JF: Immunology of bovine pregnancy: vulnerability to infectious diseases, *Proceedings of the Twenty-sixth Annual Convention of the American Association of Bovine Practitioners* 26:101-104, 1994.
111. Mickelsen WD, Evermann JF: In utero infections responsible for abortion, stillbirth, and birth of weak calves in beef cows, *Vet Clin North Am (Food Anim Pract)* 10:1-14, 1994.
112. Chaouat G et al: Immune suppression and Th1/Th2 balance in pregnancy revisited, *Am J Reprod Immunol* 37:427-434, 1997.
112a. Mallord BA et al: Alteration in immune responsiveness during the peripartum period and its ramification on dairy cow and calf health, *J Dairy Sci* 81:585-595, 1998.
112b. Dosogne H et al: Pregnancy-associated glycoprotein and decreased polymorphonuclear leukocyte function in early post-partum dairy cows, *Vet Immunol Immunopathol* 67:47-54, 1999.

DISEASES CAUSED BY ALLOGENEIC INCOMPATIBILITIES

JILL McCLURE BLACKMER
STEVEN M. PARISH

The surfaces of cells are covered with molecular structures, the presence or absence of which are determined by genes. Some of these molecules have limited heterogeneity within a species, and all members of the species share identical forms (monomorphic). In other cases a spectrum of minor structural variations or polymorphisms of a particular molecule occur within the population, so that some members of the species will have one form of the molecule, whereas others will have another. If the structural variations are such that the immune system of one individual can recognize the differences in the molecules from another individual, these are known as alloantigens. Antibodies produced against these antigens are alloantibodies. Examples of alloantigens include red blood cell antigens and lymphocyte antigens.

In nature, because there are few situations in which tissues are exchanged, there are relatively few naturally occurring diseases that involve allogeneic incompatibilities. Neonatal isoerythrolysis (NI) is one example of such a naturally occurring disease. Blood transfusion reactions and organ transplant rejection are examples of iatrogenic diseases associated with allogeneic incompatibilities.

The same alloantibodies that mediate disease are also useful in vitro as reagents for the detection of the presence of alloantigens and serve as the basis for blood typing.

BLOOD TYPING

The blood type of an individual is actually a composite list of genetic markers that have been detected in the blood of an individual. Several kinds of genetic markers are commonly used in blood typing, including red blood cell alloantigens, electrophoretic markers, and lymphocyte alloantigens. Polymorphisms of the DNA itself are also emerging as useful genetic markers, and, as technology improves, these markers may eventually replace currently used genetic tests.

RED BLOOD CELL ANTIGENS

Seven independent red blood cell groups or systems have been internationally defined in horses under the auspices of the International Society for Animal Genetics[113-116] (Tables 49-3 and 49-4). These systems are named A, C, D, K, P, Q, and U. Additional systems are recognized by individual laboratories. Each system corresponds to a particular gene for which two or more alleles exist. Some blood groups are relatively simple and contain only two alleles, whereas other systems may have over two dozen different alleles.

The blood group genes produce surface molecules that contain antigenic sites known as factors. Over 30 different factors have been identified. Each factor is associated with only one system, although the same factor may be associated with more than one allele within the system. The factors are named with an upper case letter to denote the system and a lower case letter to designate the factor within that system. Groups of factors that are produced by a single allele are called phenogroups.

The presence of red blood cell antigens is detected primarily by either agglutination or complement-mediated lysis of test cells by antibodies directed against specific red blood cell alloantigens. Antigens in some systems are detected with antiglobulin tests.

Eleven blood groups have been identified in cattle[117] (Table 49-3 and Table 49-5). In cattle, groups B and J have the greatest clinical relevance. The B group is a very complex system, with over 60 different antigens.[118] This complexity can be used to advantage for individual animal identification and parentage studies, but it makes it very difficult to closely match donor and recipient blood for transfusions.

The J antigen is a lipid that is found in body fluid and that is adsorbed to erythrocytes; thus it is not a true erythrocyte antigen. Newborn calves do not have this antigen but usually acquire it during the first 6 months of life. After acquiring

TABLE 49-3

Domestic Animal Blood Groups[112,115]

Species	Blood Group Systems
Equine	A, C, D, K, P, Q, U
Bovine	A, B, C, F, J,* L, M, R', S, T, Z
Ovine	A, B, C, D, M, R,* X
Caprine	A, B, C, M, J*

From Suzuki: Personal communication, 1990.
*Soluble antigens.

TABLE 49-4

Blood Group Systems, Factors, and Alleles of the Horse Recognized by the International Society for Animal Genetics

System	Factors	Recognized Alleles
A	a,*b,†c,d,e,f,g	$A^a A^{adf}, A^{adg}, A^{abdf}, A^{abdg}, A^b, A^{bc}, A^{bce}, A^{be}, A^c,$ A^{ce}, A^e, A^-
C	a	$C^a, C-$
D	a,b,c†,d,e,f, g,h,i,k,l,m, n,o,p,q,r	$D^{adl}, D^{adlnr}, D^{adlr}, D^{bcmq}, D^{cefgmq}, D^{cegimnq},$ $D^{cfgkm}, D^{cfmqr}, D^{cgm}, D^{cdmp}, D^{cgmq}, D^{cgmqr},$ $D^{deklqr}, D^{delno}, D^{deloq}, D^{delq}, D^{dfkir}, D^{dghmp},$ $D^{dghmq}, D^{dghmqr}, D^{dki}, D^{dlnq}, D^{dlnqr}, D^{dlqr},$ $D^{dno}, D^q, (D^-)$
K	a	$K^a, K-$
P	a†,b,c,d	$P^a, P^{ac}, P^{acd}, P^{ad}, P^b, P^{bd}, P^d, P-$
Q	a,*b,c	$Q^a, Q^{ab}, Q^{abc}, Q^{ac}, Q^b, Q^{bc}, Q^c, Q-$
U	a†	$U^a, U-$

From Cothran G: Personal communication.
*Most common factors involved in neonatal isoerythrolysis (NI).
†Previously reported to cause NI in at least one case.

TABLE 49-5

Blood Group Factors of Cattle Recognized by the International Society for Animal Genetics

System	Factors
AA*	A_1, A_2, H, Z, a
F*	F,V
J	J,j
L	L,l
M	M,m
Z	Z,z
R'	R',S'
B†	$B, G_1, G_2, G_3, I_1, I_2, K, O_1, O_3, Ox, P_1, P_2, Q, T, Y_2, A', B', D', E_1',$ $E_2', E_3', G', I_1'(I'), I_2', J_1', J_2', K', O', P_1', P_2', Q', Y', A'', B'', G'', I''$
C	$C_1, C_2, R_1, R_2, W, X, X_2, L', E_1, C', C'', X', F1, F6, F10, F15$
S	$S_1, S_2, U, H', U', S'', U''$
T	

*Cases of neonatal isoerythrolysis associated with production of anti–red blood cell antibodies against factors in response to anaplasmosis and babesia vaccines.
†Additional factors are recognized by individual laboratories.

TABLE 49-6

Examples of Polymorphic Proteins Used in Blood Typing

Protein	System	Source
A1B glycoprotein	A1B	Serum
Albumin	ALB	Serum
Transferrin	TF	Serum
Carboxylesterase	ES	Serum
Vitamin D binding protein	GC	Serum
Protease inhibitor	PI	Serum
Peptidase A	PEPA	Serum
Plasminogen	PLG	Serum
Glucose phosphate isomerase	GPI	Red cells
6-Phosphogluconate dehydrogenase	PGD	Red cells
Phosphoglucomutase	PGM	Red cells
Catalase	CAT	Red cells
Carbonic anhydrase	CA	Red cells
Acid phosphatase	AP	Red cells
Hemoglobin-a	HBA	Red cells
NADH diaphorase	DIA	Red cells

Seven blood groups have been identified in sheep (Table 49-3). The B system is analogous to the B system in cattle and is extremely polymorphic, with over 52 different alleles. The R system is similar to the J system in cattle in that the antigens are soluble and are passively adsorbed to erythrocytes.[117] The M-L system is involved in the genetically determined red blood cell potassium polymorphism found in sheep.[119]

Blood groups of goats appear to be very similar to those of sheep, and many of the reagents used for typing sheep blood have been used to type goats' blood. Reagents used to detect antigens of the J system of cattle have been used to detect differences in a similar system in goats.[120]

The biologic function of red blood cell antigens is not known for any system in any species with the exception of the M-L blood group system in sheep, which is involved in active potassium transport across red blood cell membranes.

ELECTROPHORETIC MARKERS

Many plasma and intracellular proteins have polymorphic forms. These variants have subtle biochemical differences, which for the most part do not alter the major characteristics of the molecules but which can be detected using electrophoretic methods. These are not technically alloantigens because the differences are not detected immunologically. The various forms of the molecules are detected on the basis of their different rates of migration in electrophoresis. The specific form(s) of any particular protein that an individual possesses are determined genetically, and those used in blood typing are usually expressed codominantly. Currently no diseases are clearly associated with the presence or absence of particular alleles of polymorphic proteins; however, they are useful genetic markers for identification and parentage studies and are commonly included in the blood type (Table 49-6).[114,115,120,121] Electrophoretic markers are used extensively in horses because red cell antigens do not provide the same degree of discrimination among individuals in this species as they do, for example, in cattle.

LYMPHOCYTE ANTIGENS

Three systems of equine lymphocyte alloantigens have been described: ELA, ELY 1, and ELY 2.[122-126] ELA is the major histocompatibility complex (MHC) of the horse. ELA is a complex system that includes several genes, each of which is poly-

it, some groups of cattle have high amounts of J antigen both in the serum and adsorbed to erythrocytes, whereas other groups have very small amounts found only on erythrocytes. These latter groups, often referred to as J-negative, may actually have anti-J antibodies and develop transfusion reactions when transfused with blood from J-positive donors.[113]

morphic (e.g., has many different alleles). Because the MHC regulates the interactions of many cells in the immune response, a potential for the association of disease susceptibility or resistance with ELA exists. An association between a particular ELA allele and equine sarcoid has been described.[127,128] ELY 1 and ELY 2 have limited polymorphism and appear to be two allele systems.

The MHC of cattle is called BoLA, for bovine lymphocyte antigen. In sheep the MHC is called OLA for ovine lymphocyte antigen and is also known as SH-LA. In goats the comparable system is GLA.[129]

DNA POLYMORPHISMS

A wide variety of approaches have been developed for detecting genetic variation using deoxyribonucleic acid (DNA). Certainly DNA sequencing is the most sensitive approach; however, this remains too costly for routine testing outside of research laboratories. Other approaches have been developed to detect DNA variants. Genetic variation of DNA can be detected among individuals on the basis of differences in length for a section of DNA or even for differences in base composition at specific sites. DNA length variants are usually referred to as minisatellite or microsatellite markers. Minisatellite DNA markers are based on sequences, often 15 to 100 bases long, that may be repeated hundreds of times on a chromosome. The number of repetitions can vary dramatically between individuals and can be readily detectable in Southern blotting assay. These tests were originally referred to as DNA fingerprinting. Although they are powerful, these tests are costly and time consuming. More recently, another type of DNA length variant has been discovered. Microsatellite DNA markers are short repetitions of nucleotides, usually ranging from one to nine bases long, which may be repeated 15 to 40 times. As with minisatellites, the number of repetitions may vary between chromosomes. The development of the polymerase chain reaction (PCR) has opened the door to easy, cheap detection of microsatellite and other types of markers. PCR is a method for amplifying short (fewer than 3000 bases) pieces of DNA, making it possible to easily study a particular gene. The amplification products can be separated by electrophoresis and length variants readily detected. More than 100,000 of these markers are thought to exist in each species. These markers form an important core for development of genetic maps in diverse species. These markers are also being developed for use in parentage analysis.

Variation recognizable as a change in a single base of DNA is more subtle but can be detected through a variety of techniques. DNA sequence variation is often detectable using restriction enzymes. Restriction enzymes are isolated from bacteria and will cleave DNA when the sequence is specific for the enzyme. For example, the method to detect the gene defect causing hyperkalemic periodic paralysis (HYPP) in horses is based on PCR amplification of the gene and then detection of sequence differences that occur between the normal and mutant gene using restriction enzyme digestion of the DNA. Other approaches to identifying DNA sequence differences include single-stranded confirmational polymorphism (SSCP), allele-specific PCR amplification, and ligase chain reaction.

As markers become better characterized and cost-effective methods are developed for testing, DNA-based testing will replace blood typing for purposes of parentage analysis in the not-too-distant future. Furthermore, these techniques are also being used to develop gene maps for many species of domestic animals. These gene maps can be used to identify genes that play a role in performance, production, and disease.

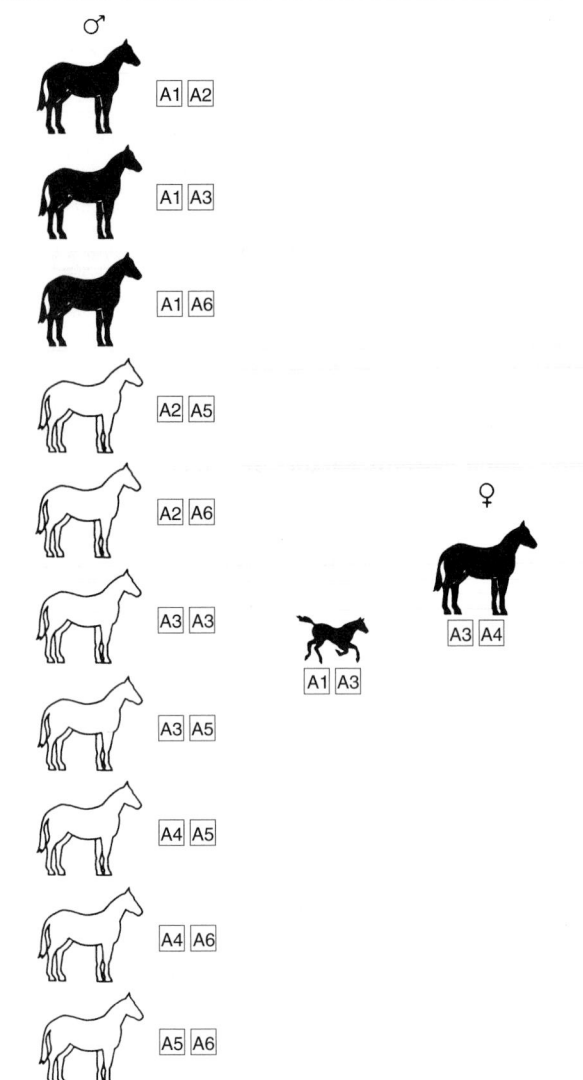

FIG. 49-5 ■ Blood typing using ELA markers demonstrates that 7 of the 10 sires can be excluded as the sire of the foal with certainty, whereas any of the other three could have sired the foal on the basis of this one genetic system.

BLOOD-TYPING APPLICATIONS

To determine an animal's blood type, a battery of different tests are run on the blood to check for the presence or absence of each recognized allele in each of several genetic systems. Each system is controlled by a separate autosomal gene. These genes are inherited independently of one another.[116,126] Most genetic markers used in blood typing are expressed codominantly, which means that the alleles on both chromosomes are expressed. This often allows determination of genotype (the actual genes present) from the phenotype (the antigens actually detected). Some systems have null alleles with no detectable products that do not directly allow inference of genotype (e.g., C, K, and U blood group systems in horses). An individual can have only two of the possible different alleles for any given gene (one on each chromosome of a pair).

Blood typing is useful for animal identification, pedigree analysis, prediction of potential for NI and cross-matching for blood transfusion. The use of genetic markers such as red blood cell antigens, lymphocyte antigens, and protein polymorphisms is based on exclusion (i.e., markers are tested un-

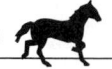

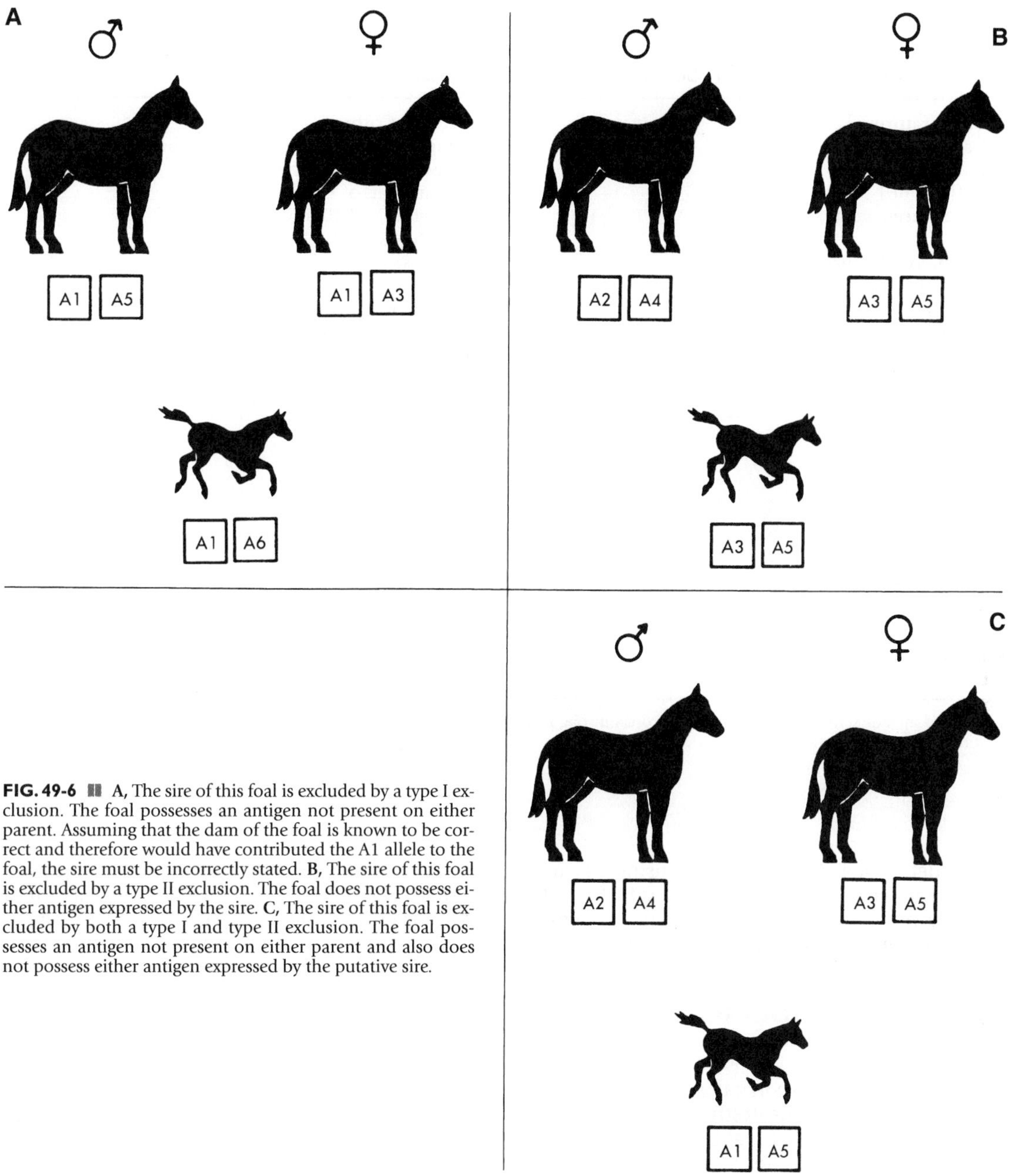

FIG. 49-6 ▌▌ **A,** The sire of this foal is excluded by a type I exclusion. The foal possesses an antigen not present on either parent. Assuming that the dam of the foal is known to be correct and therefore would have contributed the A1 allele to the foal, the sire must be incorrectly stated. **B,** The sire of this foal is excluded by a type II exclusion. The foal does not possess either antigen expressed by the sire. **C,** The sire of this foal is excluded by both a type I and type II exclusion. The foal possesses an antigen not present on either parent and also does not possess either antigen expressed by the putative sire.

til a difference is found). If no difference is observed after a statistically acceptable amount of testing, the probability of a match is determined.

Because blood typing is a composite mosaic of a large number of different, largely independent genetic markers, the odds of two individuals sharing exactly the same pattern of markers is remote. Thus, once an animal's blood type is on record, it can be a powerful identifier of an individual animal. In this sense it is an unalterable form of identification that is present from birth to death.

Because the presence or absence of markers is genetically determined and because the markers contributed by both parents are expressed in a codominant fashion (unless "blank" alleles exist), these markers can be used to support or refute parentage claims. Blood typing cannot prove that one horse is the parent of another; however, in certain instances it can exclude with certainty a stated parent as the true parent (Fig.

49-5). Two types of parentage exclusions can occur, type I and type II[130] (Fig. 49-6). With type I the foal possesses a dominant or codominant antigen that is not present in either parent. This means that at least one of the stated parents is incorrect. If one parent (usually the dam) is known with certainty on the basis of circumstances other than blood type, the error lies with the other stated parent. With type II exclusions, the foal does not possess either of the dominant or codominant antigens of a stated parent. Because a foal must inherit one of the two antigens expressed by each parent, an exclusion can be made if neither of the two antigens present on the stated parent is detected in the foal. In parentage cases, each genetic system is evaluated for type I and type II exclusions. A parent can be excluded on the basis of an inconsistency in even one system. For this reason, the more systems that are used the better blood typing becomes as a tool for solution of parentage disputes. The calculated effectiveness of

---

BOX 49-1

Laboratories Providing Blood-Typing Services for Large-Animal Species*

Stormont Laboratories
1237 E. Beamer St., Suite D
Woodland, CA 95776
Telephone: (530) 661-3078
(Horses, cattle, sheep, goats)

Veterinary Genetics Laboratory
University of California, School of Veterinary Medicine
Old Davis Road, Trailer E
Davis, CA 95616-8744
Telephone: (530) 752-2211
(Horses, cattle, sheep, goats)

ImmGen, Inc.
P.O. Box 10135
College Station, TX 77842
Telephone: (979) 691-1630
(Cattle, goats, horses)

Animal Genetics Laboratory
The Ohio State University, Department of Animal Sciences
2027 Coffey Road
Columbus, Ohio 43210
Telephone: (614) 292-6659
(Cattle)

Dr. Gus Cothran
Equine Blood-Typing Research Laboratory
University of Kentucky
Department of Veterinary Science
Lexington, KY 40546
Telephone: (606) 257-3022
(Horses)

Dr. Melba Ketchum
Shelterwood Equine Laboratories
P.O. Box 215
Carthage, TX 75633
Telephone: (903) 693-6424
(Horses)

Dr. David Colling
Maxxam Equitest, Inc.
335 Laird Road, Unit 4
Guelph, Ontario N1H 6J3
Canada
Telephone: (519) 836-2400
(Horses)

---

*Samples required include serum and acid-citrate-dextrose anticoagulated blood. Most laboratories offer kits or mailers with appropriate tubes and specific directions; call for information.

---

blood typing for detecting incorrect paternity using 20 internationally defined systems in horses is as high as 96%.[114,115]

A list of laboratories providing blood-typing services is shown in Box 49-1.

NEONATAL ISOERYTHROLYSIS

Equine

DEFINITION AND ETIOLOGY. Neonatal isoerythrolysis (NI) is a condition characterized by the destruction of red blood cells (RBCs) in the circulation of a foal by alloantibodies of maternal origin absorbed from colostrum.[131-133]

Production of alloantibodies can be stimulated in mares several ways, including transfusion, exposure to blood from the foal during parturition, or as a result of placental pathology during gestation. Incompatibilities of at least some blood groups between the dam and foal are the rule rather than the exception, and yet the incidence of sensitization of the dam and occurrence of NI is relatively low. In Thoroughbreds the prevalence is about 1%, and in Standardbreds the incidence is about 2%.[134] The prevalence in mules (donkey sire, horse dam) has been reported to be as high as 10%.[135] Most blood groups are not strongly antigenic under the conditions of exposure via previous parturition or placental leakage. Several blood group factors, however, are particularly immunogenic, and antibodies against these antigens have been reported to cause nearly all cases of NI. These include factor Aa in the A system and factor Qa in the Q system. In mules a unique donkey RBC antigen named donkey factor has been associated with NI.[136] Antibodies to these antigens develop after the exposure of the mare to RBCs and are not naturally occurring antibodies. In humans the *absence* of certain RBC

antigens results in the production of natural antibodies against that antigen, presumably because of exposure to cross-reacting antigens in the diet. This does not occur in horses with a few exceptions and has not been associated with NI. Ca-negative (Ca−) horses frequently make anti-Ca antibody of low titer without known RBC exposure. However, anti-Ca antibody is generally not associated with NI, and in fact mares with anti-Ca antibody actually appear less likely to develop certain antibodies responsible for NI.

For NI to occur, several things must happen (Figs. 49-7 and 49-8). First, the dam must be negative for the antigen in question. Because most cases of NI in horses are associated with either anti-Aa or anti-Qa antibodies, mares that are Aa− or Qa− or both are considered at risk. All horses appear to lack donkey factor; thus all mule pregnancies are considered at risk. Second, the mare must become sensitized and produce antibody to the offending antigen. Sensitization can be caused by exposure during a previous pregnancy, blood transfusion, or transplacental contamination with fetal RBCs earlier in the current pregnancy (rare). Third, the foal from the current pregnancy must have inherited from its sire the antigen(s) to which the mare has been sensitized. When these conditions are met there is a significant potential that maternal antibody directed against the foal's RBC antigens will appear in the colostrum and, if subsequently ingested and absorbed by the foal, could cause loss of RBCs. The higher the anti-RBC titer at foaling, the higher the risk. The highest titers are likely to be produced in a previously sensitized mare that is reexposed to the same RBC antigens shortly before parturition.

CLINICAL SIGNS AND DIFFERENTIAL DIAGNOSES. Foals are born healthy and usually begin to develop signs of NI at 24 to 36 hours of age, after suckling. Progressive lethargy and weakness are early signs. In acute cases, mucous

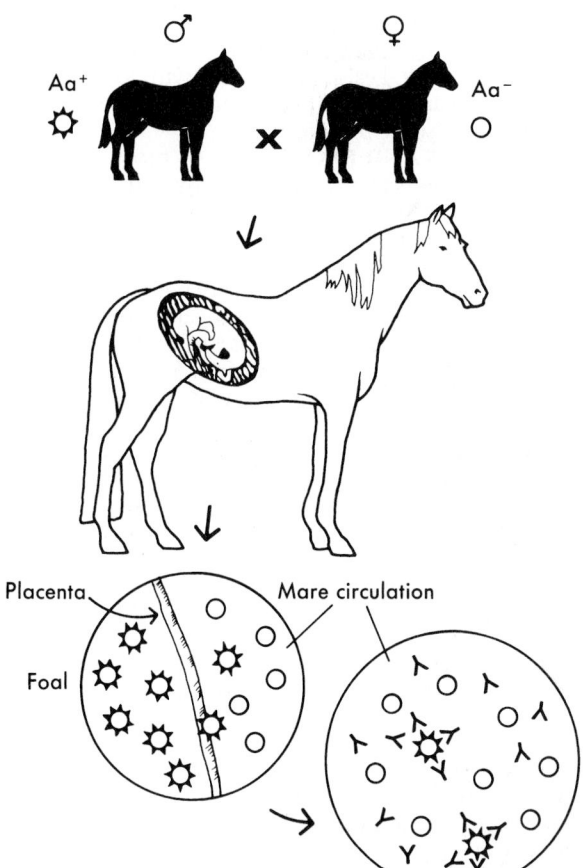

FIG. 49-7 ▓ Entrance of RBCs of paternal antigen type into maternal circulation stimulates the production of alloantibody in the mare's serum.

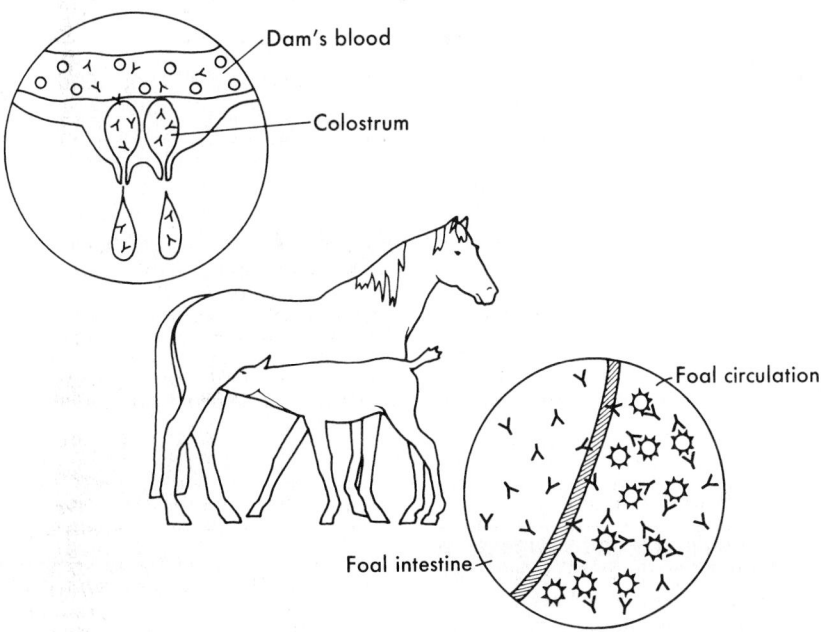

FIG. 49-8 ▓ Alloantibody in the mare's serum is concentrated in colostrum at the end of gestation. Through passive transfer, the foal absorbs immunoglobulins, including these alloantibodies. The antibodies attach to RBCs and cause either their premature removal from circulation or intravascular lysis.

membranes show initial pallor that is followed by icterus. In severe cases, hemoglobinemia and hemoglobinuria may be pronounced. In peracute cases, death may precede the development of icterus. Breathing becomes rapid and shallow, followed by labored breathing as the disease progresses. The foals may yawn repeatedly. Heart rate is elevated. Seizure-like activity may occur as the anemia becomes more severe.

For differential diagnosis for icterus and respiratory distress in neonatal foals, see Chapter 20.

CLINICAL PATHOLOGY. Affected foals are anemic. All indicators of RBC concentration (packed cell volume [PCV], hemoglobin, RBC count) show significant decreases. PCV values often decline into the teens, and values as low as 5% have been observed. Hemoglobinemia and hemoglobinuria may be present. Bilirubin (mainly unconjugated) levels will be increased as a result of accelerated RBC destruction. Total bilirubin levels may be close to 20 mg/dl in severe cases. Affected foals, especially mule foals, may also be thrombocytopenic.[136]

Demonstration of significant amounts of antibody in the colostrum (or serum from the mare) that are directed against the RBC antigens expressed by the foal provides a definitive diagnosis of NI. These antibodies are most commonly demonstrated by lytic and agglutinating tests. Lytic tests are believed to be more reliable indicators of the presence of offending antibody.[137] The presence of antibodies attached to the foal's RBCs can also be demonstrated with a direct antiglobulin test (Coombs' test). The presence of antibodies in the mare's serum that attach to RBCs can be demonstrated with an indirect antiglobulin test.[131]

PATHOPHYSIOLOGY. In mares sensitized to RBC antigens, most commonly Aa or Qa, alloantibodies are concentrated in the colostrum late in gestation. These antibodies are passed to the foal through passive transfer. If the foal's RBCs carry the antigen that the antibody recognizes, the cells become antibody coated. Subsequently they are removed prematurely by the reticuloendothelial system or lysed intravascularly by complement. A distinction has been made between antibodies that are lysins as opposed to agglutinins; however, this distinction is based on in vitro testing and may be somewhat artificial. Under appropriate laboratory conditions, offending antibodies may exhibit both abilities.[134] However, with conventional agglutination tests, some alloantibodies capable of producing NI may go undetected.[121]

EPIDEMIOLOGY. The percentages of mares at risk for sensitization against the common offending antigens (Aa and Qa) vary among breeds, depending on the frequency in the population of each gene involved (Table 49-7). Increased numbers of mares at risk in a breed does not necessarily translate into higher numbers of NI cases. A corresponding number of stallions lack the factors in question and are therefore unable to sire foals with the offending antigen.[133] Virtually all mule pregnancies are incompatible with regard to donkey factor.[136]

Although the disease is more common in multiparous mares, NI can occur with the first pregnancy.

NECROPSY FINDINGS. Pale tissues with or without icterus and splenomegaly are characteristic necropsy findings in foals dying of NI. Lesions associated with RBC destruction and anemia, such as nephrosis and centrilobular hepatic necrosis, may also be present.

TREATMENT AND PROGNOSIS. In most cases, by the time the problem is recognized clinically (e.g., when the foal is about 24 hours of age), the bulk of colostral antibody will have been depleted from the mare's milk and the absorptive ability of the foal's gut will have diminished. Withholding milk at this point is of questionable benefit.

Stress should be minimized and exercise restricted. Affected foals have decreased exercise tolerance and can collapse and die if forced to follow their dams. Generalized supportive care should be administered as indicated by clinical parameters. Intravenous fluids are frequently indicated to promote diuresis to minimize the effects of the large hemoglobin load presented to the kidneys. Acid-base balance should be monitored and corrected if indicated.

If the anemia becomes severe (e.g., PCV = 10% to 15%), transfusions that provide RBCs should be considered. Unless the PCV drops below this level, transfusion may not be necessary if rest is enforced. The object of transfusion is to provide the affected foal with RBCs that will not be destroyed by the maternal alloantibodies that were absorbed from colostrum. The foal is immunologically naive and will not have autologous alloantibody directed against any RBCs that would have an immediate effect on transfused RBCs. Thus the key is to select an RBC donor whose cells will not be destroyed by the maternal antibody derived from colostrum. Cross-matching, with particular attention to the reaction of mare sera, colostrum, and foal sera (all contain the same antibody), with the donor RBCs, is important for selecting a cell that will not be destroyed by the maternal antibody.

Washed RBCs from the dam are obviously the perfect choice in terms of cells that will not react with the alloantibodies present in the foal. However, to avoid administering additional harmful antibody to the foal, the mare's sera (containing antibody against the foal's cells) must be removed by washing before administration. Up to 6 to 8 L of blood can be collected from the mare and anticoagulated with acid-citrate-dextrose (ACD) or sodium citrate (3.8% NaCitrate solution; 1 part NaCitrate/9 parts blood), although 3 to 4 L usually provides sufficient RBCs. The preparation of large volumes of washed cells is aided by a large-volume centrifuge, but the procedure can be accomplished by serial sedimentations. Anticoagulated blood from the mare is allowed to settle for 1 to 2 hours. The plasma is aseptically drawn off, a similar or greater volume of sterile isotonic saline (0.9% NaCl) is added to the RBCs and mixed, and the RBCs are again allowed to settle. The saline is then drawn off and discarded. At this point the RBCs can be resuspended in an equal volume of isotonic saline for administration, or the washing procedure can be repeated. The sedimentation method is less desirable than centrifugation because it is slower and does not remove as much of the offending antibody. The aim is to dilute any harmful antibody to insignificant levels.

If it is not possible to use the dam's RBCs, alternative donors can be selected. The donor should lack the antigen to which the alloantibody is directed. Because it is generally not possible to blood-type donors on short notice, a previously identified horse that has been determined by blood typing to be Aa−, Qa− and free of alloantibody is a good choice for donor, based on the fact that most cases of NI are associated with these two antigens. The odds of randomly selecting a donor that lacks the offending type (e.g., Aa−, Qa−, or both) and would therefore be a suitable donor vary significantly with the breed (Table 49-7). For example, the odds of finding

TABLE 49-7

Gene Frequencies of Aa− and Qa− Horses in Various Breeds of Horses[111] (1.00 Means All Individuals in that Breed Are Negative for the Factor)

System	Thorough-bred	Arabian	Standard-bred	Quarter Horse	Morgan
Aa−	0.151	0.182	0.435	0.510	0.432
Qa−	0.388	0.794	1.000	0.825	0.994

an Aa− Thoroughbred to serve as an RBC donor would be about 1 or 2 in 10, whereas in Quarter horses the odds would be about one in two. The sire of the foal is not the donor of choice. He shares the same RBC antigens as the foal, and his cells will react with the maternal alloantibody present, adding more of a load to the foal's reticuloendothelial system as they are destroyed.

In the case of mules the same considerations in the use of washed cells would be necessary if the dam's cells were used. However, because the offending antibody is generally directed against a unique donkey antigen, it appears that RBCs from any horse would be satisfactory. Horses do not appear to make naturally occurring antibodies against donkey factor; therefore in most cases it is not necessary to wash the cells from horses that would not be likely to have been immunized by pregnancy against donkey factor.

Transfusing RBCs that will not react with maternal alloantibody means introducing an obviously incompatible cell into the foal, a cell which will probably not survive for long periods of time in the circulation. Such transfusions should be considered temporary stopgap measures. Transfused cells may also sensitize the foal to future transfusions, causing reactions (perhaps not within hours or a few days, but potentially within a week). This must be considered when weighing the potential good versus potential harm of such transfusions.

One to four liters L of washed RBCs or whole blood are usually adequate to produce clinical improvement, although some cases may require repeated transfusion if the anemia progresses. Exchange transfusions can be done whereby blood is administered via one jugular and withdrawn simultaneously from the opposite jugular and discarded, allowing administration of large volumes of blood without overloading the vascular system. There is no good evidence to suggest that this is more effective than simply providing a source of RBCs that are unaffected by the maternal antibody.

Limited transfusion studies in adult horses have suggested that transfused RBCs do not survive long in circulation (e.g., 2 to 4 days).[138] Whether similar kinetics hold for foals is unknown. PCVs in foals with NI commonly increase following transfusion and then gradually decline. This decline is probably not great cause for concern if it is gradual, because the PCV of the foal generally levels off as the offending maternal antibody is metabolized. However, even short-term survival of cells may be of benefit in severely affected foals and may allow them to survive until the titer of maternal anti-RBC immunoglobulin has declined in the circulation.

The prognosis varies, depending on the quantity of antibody ingested, the rapidity of onset of signs, and the degree of anemia. Peracute cases may die before the problem is recognized, with no chance for administration of therapy. Foals that develop the condition more slowly may respond to supportive care or transfusion if the PCV continues to fall.

PREVENTION AND CONTROL. Several strategies are available for prevention of NI. First, identify brood mares at risk for development of NI by testing them for the presence of Aa and Qa. Mares negative for either antigen, which means they could potentially make antibodies against them, should be considered at risk. One subsequent strategy would be to breed at-risk mares to Aa/Qa-negative stallions, thus eliminating the possibility of the foal inheriting the offending antigens. However, in breeds in which a relatively small part of the population is negative for these antigens, identifying a stallion that is negative for these antigens and suitable on the basis of other criteria may be difficult. The percentage of at-risk females based on the presence or absence of Aa or Qa is somewhat balanced by the numbers of males able to transmit the offending antigen. For example, all Standardbred mares would be considered at risk based on the absence of

Qa; however, because the antigen Qa is not present in the Standardbred population, no stallions have the Qa antigen to pass on to foals.

In the circumstance of an unknown or incompatible mating, sera from at-risk mares should be screened for the presence of anti-RBC antibodies within 30 days before foaling. This can be done by submitting a serum sample and an anticoagulant sample to a screening laboratory. A panel of 10 to 12 different RBCs selected to represent all major blood groups is adequate to screen for anti-RBC antibody in the absence of blood from the sire. If results of serum testing are equivocal (e.g., low but positive titer, especially if there is anti-Aa or anti-Qa activity), the test should be repeated closer to the time of parturition, since the levels of offending antibody can rise very quickly late in gestation.

If anti-RBC antibody is detected in the mare before parturition, the colostrum should be checked for reactivity against the foal's RBCs before allowing the foal to ingest colostrum. An alternative source of colostrum should be provided to the foal. Most field screening tests of colostrum have not proved to be satisfactory for practical use; however, the jaundiced foal agglutination (JFA) test described in Box 49-2 has been shown to correlate well with the standard hemolytic assay, and it may detect antibody that does not react on the standard agglutination tests.[139]

Horses negative for Ca frequently make anti-Ca antibody; however, this antibody is not known to produce adverse effects in the foal. It has clouded the issue of field screening tests for NI, because it commonly causes positive reactions in most screening tests at low dilutions. Because these tests do not differentiate between antibody to Aa, Qa, Ca, or any other blood group, anti-Ca antibody, when present in low dilutions, is responsible for many false-positive reactions. This antibody actually appears to play a protective role in the prevention of sensitization of mares to NI through a mechanism of antibody-mediated immune suppression. Aa−/Qa− mares that are also Ca− (and thus often produce anti-Ca antibody), become sensitized to Aa and Qa at a significantly lower rate than mares that are Ca+.[139] This is attributed to the fact that anti-Ca antibody is produced by Ca− mares. The anti-Ca antibody may more rapidly remove potentially sensitizing cells from the circulation before they stimulate production of antibody against Aa or Qa.

Uncommonly other antigens have been associated with NI in foals. These include factors Dc, Ua, Pa, and Ab. Two other factors, R and S, have been described to be associated with NI, but they are not detected by routine hemolytic or agglutinating methods and are only detected using an antiglobulin test (direct Coombs' test).[132] Because of the difficulty in testing for these antigens, there has never been sufficient agreement between laboratories to allow international designation. These antigens may not be detected using the JFA screening test.[133] Estimates are that 1 in 2000 pregnancies may result in sensitization against some other antigen besides Aa or Qa. Because these cases occur so infrequently, it is not practical to consider mares without these antigens to be at risk for NI. A blood-type evaluation of mares with a history of production of foals with NI should be done to identify the offending antibody/antigen.

A list of laboratories providing NI screening tests (e.g., Aa, Qa, and Ca typing and screening of sera for alloantibody) is given in Box 49-3. Routine agglutinating cross-match tests using mare serum or colostrum and foal or sire cells can be performed by most veterinary or human hematology laboratories.

Ruminants

NI is not a naturally occurring disease in cattle, sheep, or goats. Its occurrence in cattle has been associated with

---

BOX 49-2

Jaundiced Foal Agglutination Test (JFA Test)[127]

MATERIALS
1. Centrifuge capable of spinning 300 to 600 × gravity
2. Test tube rack
3. Test tubes: 13 × 100 mm disposable or blood collection tubes
4. Pasture pipettes and rubber bulbs or other pipette system to deliver 1-ml volumes
5. Isotonic (0.9%) saline at room temperature
6. Serum or colostrum from the mare; RBCs from mare and foal, preferable in EDTA anticoagulant

METHODS
1. Collect colostrum from the mare.
2. Collect an EDTA-anticoagulated blood sample from the foal before nursing.
3. Set up six tubes and add 1 ml of saline to each tube. Label the tubes *Control*, $^1/_2$, $^1/_4$, $^1/_8$, $^1/_{16}$, and $^1/_{32}$.
4. Make serial dilutions of the colostrum at $^1/_2$, $^1/_4$, $^1/_8$, $^1/_{16}$, and $^1/_{32}$ in five of the tubes. Add 1 ml of colostrum (or serum) to the tube labeled $^1/_2$ and mix. Then take 1 ml from that tube and add it to the second tube labeled $^1/_4$ and mix. Take 1 ml from that tube and add it to the third tube labeled $^1/_8$, and so on until all five dilution tubes have been filled. Discard 1 ml from the last tube labeled $^1/_{32}$.
5. Add 1 drop of the foal's whole blood to each of the six tubes and mix.
6. Centrifuge the tubes for 2 to 3 minutes at a medium speed (300 to 500 × gravity).
7. Invert each tube, pouring out the liquid contents; observe the status of the button of RBCs at the bottom of the tube. Complete agglutination causes the cells to remain tightly packed in the button; strong agglutination causes the cells to remain in large clumps; for weaker agglutination the cells are in smaller clumps as they run down the side of the tube. When there is no agglutination, the cells easily flow down the side of the tube. This should be the case in the control tube. If the cells in the control tube are clumped they may be autoagglutinating, and the results will have questionable validity.

If there is a positive reaction with the foal's cells, the test should be run with the dam's own RBCs to be certain that neither the conditions of the test nor the viscosity of the colostrum is causing the agglutination.

Positive reactions at $^1/_{16}$ or greater are considered significant. At levels of $^1/_{16}$ or greater, this test correlates well with the standard hemolytic assay. At dilutions of less than $^1/_{16}$ the correlation is not as good, and more false-positive results will be recorded. Also, other factors such as the viscosity of colostrum make less-diluted samples more difficult to read.

BOX 49-3

Addresses of Laboratories Providing Diagnostic Services for Equine NI*

Veterinary Genetics Laboratory
Old Davis Road Trailer E
School of Veterinary Medicine
University of California
Davis, CA 95616-744
Telephone: (530) 752-2211

Stormont Laboratory, Inc.
1237 E. Beamer St., Suite D
Woodland, CA 95776
Telephone: (530) 661-3078

Dr. Melba Ketchum
Shelterwood Equine Laboratories
P.O. Box 215
Carthage, TX 75633
Telephone: (903) 693-6424

Rood and Riddle Equine Hospital
2150 Georgetown Rd.
Lexington, KY 40580
Telephone: (606) 233-0331

Veterinary Laboratory, Inc.
1033 N. Limestone
Lexington, KY 40505
Telephone: (606) 252-0415

Dr. Gus Cothran
Equine Blood-Typing Research Laboratory
University of Kentucky
Department of Veterinary Science
Lexington, KY 40546
Telephone: (606) 257-3022

Dr. David Colling
Maxxam Equitest, Inc.
335 Laird Road, Unit 4
Guelph, Ontario N1H 6J3
Canada
Telephone: (519) 836-2400

*Serum or colostrum from the suspect mare is needed to screen for the presence of alloantibody. Acid-citrate-dextrose anticoagulated blood is generally preferred for screening for RBC antigens.

---

administration of vaccines derived from blood origin, such as certain anaplasmosis and babesiosis vaccines.[131] When these vaccines are used on breeding females, they may sensitize the dam to certain blood groups, most commonly in the A and F systems. Under chance circumstances, if the blood types of the sire and offspring reflect these systems and the dam has produced alloantibodies, an isoimmune hemolytic crisis may appear in the calf associated with successful passive transfer. Hemolytic crises are rare in sheep and are even difficult to induce experimentally.[131]

REFERENCES

113. Bowling AT, Clark RS: Blood group and protein polymorphism gene frequencies for seven breeds of horses in the United States, *Anim Blood Groups Biochem Genet* 16:93-108, 1985.

114. Scott AM: Immunogenetic analysis as a means of identification in horses. In Bryans JT, Gerber H, eds: *Equine infectious diseases IV, Proceedings of the Fourth International Conference on Equine Infectious Diseases*, Princeton, NJ, 1978, Veterinary Publications, pp 259-268.

115. Stormont C: Current status of equine blood groups and their applications, *Proceedings of the Eighteenth Annual Convention of the American Association of Equine Practitoners* 125:401-410, 1972.

116. Stormont C, Suzuki Y, Rhode EA: Serology of horse blood groups, *Cornell Vet* 54:439-452, 1964.

117. Tizard I: Erythrocyte antigens and type II hypersensitivity. In Tizard I, ed: *Veterinary immunology: an introduction*, Philadelphia, 1987, WB Saunders.

118. Grosclaude F, Guerin G, Houlier G: The genetic map of the B system of cattle blood groups as observed in French breeds, *Anim Blood Groups Biochem Gen* 10:199-218, 1979.

119. Tucker EM, Ellory JC: The M-L blood group system and active potassium transport in sheep reticulocytes, *Anim Blood Groups Biochem Genet* 2:77-87, 1971.

120. Schmid DO, Odermatt K, Kunz H: Vergleichende analyse der Blutghruppen und einiger polymorpher Proteinsysteme bei funf verschiedenen Ziegenrassen der Schweiz, *Schweiz Arch Tierheikld* 117:31-43, 1975.

121. Kaminski M: Distribution of genetic variants of blood proteins and enzymes in horses of various breeds, In Bryans JT, Gerber H, eds: *Equine Infectious Diseases IV, Proceedings of the Fourth International Conference on Equine Infectious Diseases*, Princeton, NJ, 1978, Veterinary Publications, pp 243-252.

122. Antczak DF: Lymphocyte alloantigens of the horse. III, ELY-2.1: a lymphocyte alloantigen not coded for by the MHC, *Anim Blood Groups Biochem Genet* 15:103-115, 1984.

123. Bailey E et al: Joint report of the second international workshop on lymphocyte alloantigens of the horse, held 3-8 October 1982, *Anim Blood Groups Biochem Genet* 15:123-132, 1984.

124. Bailey E, Henny PJ: Comparison of ELY-2.1 with blood group and ELY-1 markers in the horse, *Anim Blood Groups Biochem Genet* 15:117-122, 1984.

125. Lazary S et al: Equine leucocyte antigen system. III, Non-MHC linked alloantigenic system in horses, *J Immunogenet* 9:327-334, 1982.

126. Matthews SMS: Equine leucocyte antigen system: progress and potential, *Equine Vet J* 17:265-268, 1985.

127. Lazary S et al: Equine leucocyte antigens in sarcoid-affected horses, *Equine Vet J* 17:283-286, 1985.

128. Meredith D et al: Equine leukocyte antigens: relationships with sarcoid tumors and laminitis in two pure breeds, *Immunogenetics* 23:221-225, 1986.

129. Newman MJ, Antczak DF: Histocompatibility polymorphisms of domestic animals, *Adv Vet Sci Comp Med* 27:1-76, 1983.

130. Bailey E, Conboy S, McCarthy PF: Neonatal isoerythrolysis of foals: an update on testing, *Proceedings of the Thirty-third Annual Convention of the American Association of Equine Practitioners*, 1987, p 341-353.

131. Scott AM, Jeffcott LB: Haemolytic disease of the newborn foal, *Vet Rec* 103:71-74, 1978.

132. Stormont C: Neonatal isoerythrolysis in domestic animals: a comparative review, *Adv Vet Sci Comp Med* 19:23-45, 1975.

133. Bailey E: Prevalence of anti-red cell antibodies in the serum and colostrum of mares and its relationship to neonatal isoerythrolysis, *Am J Vet Res* 43:1917-1921, 1982.

134. Brumpt E: Considerations defavorables a l'hypothese de l'etiologie parasitaire de la jaunisse des muletons: jaundice in newly born mule foals not caused by babesia infections, *Ann Parasit Hum Comp* 22:5-10, 1947.

135. McClure JJ, Koch C, Traub-Dargatz J: Characterization of a red blood cell antigen in donkeys and mules associated with neonatal isoerythrolysis, *Anim Genet* 25:119-120, 1994.

136. Traub-Dargatz JL, McClure JJ, Koch C et al: Neonatal isoerythrolysis in mule foals, *J Am Vet Med Assoc* 206:67-70, 1995.

137. Bect JJ et al: Experimental production of neonatal isoerythrolysis in the foal, *Cornell Vet* 73:380-389, 1983.

138. Kallfelz FA, Whitlock RH, Schultz RD: Survival of ^{59}Fe-labeled erythrocytes in cross-transfused equine blood, *Am J Vet Res* 39:617-620, 1978.

139. Bailey E, Albright DG: Equine neonatal isoerythyrolysis: evidence for prevention by maternal antibodies to the Ca blood group antigen, *Am J Vet Res* 49:1218-1222, 1988.

Disorders Caused by Toxicants

FRANCIS D. GALEY

Consulting Editor

Toxicology cases are not the most common clinical presentation to the veterinarian, but they challenge the clinician because large numbers of animals may be involved, emotions run high, litigation is frequently suggested, and publicity can be intense. This chapter provides some tools to approach these potentially complex cases with confidence. A general discussion of diagnosis and treatment of poisoning in livestock is then followed by sections on common toxicoses caused by plants and other natural toxins, metals, inorganic compounds, and organic-synthetic compounds. Each section contains general comments about a group of poisons followed by information on selected, commonly recognized, specific toxicants. Each discussion begins with identification of the toxicant, its sources, likely targets, and hazardous situations. Then the mechanism of toxicosis, description of signs and lesions, clinical pathology, diagnostic parameters, and approaches to management and prevention (including residue avoidance) are described.

DIAGNOSIS OF POISONING

When toxicosis is suspected, possible sources of the toxicant should be identified and exposure to those sources rapidly eliminated. Diagnosis of poisoning rarely results from a single item of evidence. Instead historical, clinical, pathologic, and analytical evidence all need to be considered.

The investigation begins with tracing of animals, feedstuffs (especially lots and batches), and events before the onset of signs to identify likely etiologies. Environmental conditions to check include water sources, surrounding industry or elements, plant life, animal life, human contact, and availability of these items to the animals. Samples of possible toxic sources should be obtained, labeled, and held for later testing.

Feed (constituents and as-fed) samples should not be pooled among lots or storage bins. Composite samples that are representative of an entire lot should be obtained within each lot. Hay and forage are also sampled in a representative manner and should be examined for weeds. As-fed materials are tested for many toxicants, and then constituents are tested for any toxicant that is identified to determine the original source. Weeds that are abundant in pasture or hay are identified (Table 50-1). Diagnosis of plant toxicity is aided by finding evidence of consumption of a plant from the animal or grazed pasture.

Water and environmental samples should be obtained. Water is sampled at the trough, in transport containers, and at the source. Samples of algal blooms are mixed in 10% neutral-buffered formalin for identification, and with a second 5-gallon sample of fresh, thick bloom for toxin identification.

Clinical toxicoses may be acute (signs in many animals at once; see causes of Sudden Death, Chapter 14), chronic (e.g., poor weight gains in cattle that graze locoweed), or absent (food animal residues, antibiotics in milk, or organochlorines in fat). Signs may be specific (bradycardia from cardiac glycosides) or vague (diarrhea caused by many syndromes). Samples of blood, serum, urine, body fluids, and ingesta should be obtained for clinical pathologic and toxicologic analyses (see Table 50-1).

Complete necropsies should be performed on dead animals. The urine should be sampled after obtaining samples that might be likely to become contaminated during the examination. Appropriate tissues should be fixed for histologic

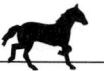

TABLE 50-1

Sampling Guide for Analytical Toxicology

Sample	Amount	Commonly Requested Tests
Whole blood	5-10 ml (EDTA)	Lead, arsenic, mercury, molybdenum, manganese, selenium, cholinesterase, anticoagulants, cyanide, some insecticides
Serum	5-10 ml (rm from clot)	Copper, zinc, iron, magnesium, calcium, sodium, potassium, drugs, nitrates, ammonia, alkaloids, tannins, vitamins A and E
Urine	50-100 ml	Drugs, heavy metals, plant alkaloids, tannins, cantharidin, fluoride
Milk	30 ml	Organochlorine insecticides, PCBs, antibiotics
Ingesta	1 kg	Heavy metals, plants, oleander, alkaloids, tannins, insecticides, drugs, nitrates, cyanide, ammonia, other pesticides, cantharidin, avitrol
Liver	300 g	Heavy metals, insecticides, anticoagulant rodenticides, some plant toxins, some drugs, vitamins A and E
Kidney	300 g	Heavy metals, calcium, some plant toxins
Brain	½ of brain	Sodium, organochlorine insecticides, cholinesterase
Fat	100 g	Organochlorine insecticides, PCBs
Ocular fluid	1 eye	Nitrate, ammonia, potassium, magnesium
Feeds	1 kg composite	Pesticides, heavy metals, salts, feed additives, antibiotics, ionophores, mycotoxins, growth promoters, nitrates, sulfate, chlorates, cyanide, plant toxins (gossypol, alkaloids, tannins), plants (send weeds for identification), vitamins A, D, E, and K
Plants	Entire plant, press and dry, or freeze	Identification, alkaloids, tannins, glycosides
Water	1 L in preserving jar	Pesticides, heavy metals, salts, nitrate, sulfate, blue-green algae
Environmental	Soruce material	Variety of organic, inorganic, and natural toxicants

EDTA, Ethylenediamine tetraacetic acid; *PCB,* polychlorinated biphenyl.

examination. Separate samples of tissue are frozen fresh for toxicologic analyses (see Table 50-1). The ingesta is completely examined for foreign objects and plants and then sampled in representative fashion for chemical analyses.

Pathologic lesions may range from none (residues or biochemical toxicants) to severe. Lesions may be very specific (nigropallidal encephalomalacia from yellow star thistle poisoning) or nonspecific (gastroenteritis from infectious, metabolic, and toxicologic causes). Some poisonings can be grouped by the type of lesion produced. For example, white snakeroot *(Eupatorium rugosum),* selenium deficiency, cobalt toxicosis, and monensin toxicosis all can cause white streaking in an animal's heart.

Chemical analysis can be useful as part of the diagnostic puzzle but rarely stands alone. Unless a specific toxicant is suspected, hold samples frozen or cool (whole blood and some dry feeds) until clinical pathologic, pathologic, microbiologic, and histologic findings are known. Those tests help the diagnostician select the most useful toxicology tests. Environmental samples also must be available for testing because many toxicants such as plants, monensin, other antibiotics, and most mycotoxins may not be detectable in animal samples.

Another diagnostic tool that may be useful is bioassay. One type of bioassay is assessment of the response of animals to therapy (animals with carbamate insecticide poisoning respond to atropine therapy). A second is measurement of a relevant biomarker of toxicant exposure in an animal sample (cholinesterase assay to indicate exposure to an organophosphorus insecticide). A third type of bioassay, important for new toxicants, is to administer the suspected toxic material (or an extract thereof) to target or laboratory animals to determine whether a source is toxic.

Analytical results are interpreted in light of the history, epidemiology, signs, and pathology. A poison is determined by the dose received and the animal's response to that compound. The animal's response to a compound is affected by species, age, gender, environment, feed, medication, and other diseases. Species differences stem from varying habits (foraging), absorption (ruminants, horses, and swine have different digestive systems), and pathways for drug metabolism. Very young and old animals will respond differently to toxicants than typical adults. Neonatal animals tend to absorb chemicals more readily than adults (lead), are at risk from compounds in milk (white snakeroot), have poorly developed blood-brain barriers (penicillin toxicity), and are inefficient metabolizers of xenobiotics in the liver for up to 30 days after birth (long sleeping times caused by barbiturates). Elderly animals can have deficient liver metabolism, renal function, and immune competency.

TREATMENT OF POISONING

Once poisoning is suspected, the first objective is to minimize exposure of all animals in the herd to a suspected toxicant. Strategies include removal of suspected sources, provision of alternative feeds, changing water sources, and moving the animals.

Once life support (airway, circulation) has been accomplished, animals are decontaminated. Decontamination includes washing or bathing dermally exposed animals. Animals exposed to oral toxicants can be given activated charcoal, with or without a cathartic to adsorb most organic toxicants. Some treatments can alter absorption of metals (sodium sulfate to tie up lead; molybdate for copper) or some organics (changing pH slows ammonia absorption). Nonspecific gastrointestinal damage, such as from nonsteroidal antiinflammatory agents, benefit from administration of demulcents (kaolin). Excretion of some mild acids may be enhanced by making the urine more alkaline (ion trapping).

After decontamination, attention centers on maintenance of vital systems (fluid, electrolytes, and acid-base correction), and therapy depends on treating for specific signs (e.g., correction of arrhythmias from oleander) and administration of specific antidotes. Common therapies specific for poisoning are listed in Table 50-2.

TABLE 50-2

Common Therapeutic Agents for Poisoning

Agent	Action
Activated charcoal	Adsorbs most organic toxicants
Sodium sulfate	Cathartic with charcoal, bind Pb; avoid if dehydrated or diarrhea
Magnesium sulfate	Cathartic, bind Pb, avoid if dehydrated, diarrhea, or depression
Sorbitol	Cathartic
Atropine	Anticholinergic (extremely dangerous in horse)
2-PAM	Reverses organophosphorus binding
Methylene blue	Treatment for methemoglobinemia
Sodium nitrite	Used with sodium thiosulfate for cyanide poisoning
Sodium thiosulfate	Treatment for cyanide poisoning
Calcium EDTA	Chelation therapy for lead
D-Penicillamine	Chelation therapy for lead, copper
BAL (dimercaprol)	Chelation therapy for arsenic, lead
DMSA	Chelation therapy for metals (awaiting approval)
Ammonium tetrathiomolybdate	Treatment for copper toxicosis
Barbiturates	Treatment for convulsants
Diazepam	Treatment for convulsants
Na bicarbonate	Ion trapping for acids, treatment for acidosis
Ca, Mg, fluids	Treatment for hypocalcemia, hypomagnesemia
Saline, lactated Ringer's, dextrose	Treatment for fluid and electrolyte deficits
Doxapram	Respiratory stimulant
DMSO, mannitol, corticosteroids	Treatments for cerebral edema
Mineral oil	Gastrointestinal evacuation
DSS	Treatment for gastrointestinal impactions
Emergency drugs	Drugs for cardiac and respiratory emergencies (e.g., epinephrine, lidocaine, oxygen)
Emergency equipment	Instruments needed to administer drugs, treat respiratory insufficiency (e.g., endotracheal tubes, tracheostomy sets), jars/packages/tubes for analytic samples

EDTA, ethylene diamine tetraacetic acid; *DMSO,* dimethylsulfioxide; *DMSA,* dimercapto succinic acid; *DSS,* dioctyl sodium sulfosuccinate.

PLANTS AND OTHER NATURAL TOXICANTS

FRANCIS D. GALEY

TOXIC PLANTS

Plant toxicity causes both direct and indirect losses to the livestock industry. Direct losses (deaths) cost producers approximately $340 million in 1989.[1] Indirect losses, not included in that estimate, are likely to be much higher. Those indirect losses can result from reduced weight gains, decreased reproductive performance, poor production, fencing and management expenses, and effects on land values.

Plants toxic to herbivores may be in forages (hay, silage), grain (seeds), pastures, and water (blue-green algae). Diagnosis of plant poisoning uses an approach similar to that described in the introduction, except that few chemical assays are available for plant toxins. Thus diagnosis of a plant poisoning relies heavily on identification of the plant in feed, pasture, or ingesta, along with appropriate clinical and pathologic findings. The presence of a poisonous plant in the environment is insufficient diagnostic evidence of plant poisoning without evidence of consumption by the animal (signs of grazing or presence of the plant in ingesta).

Many toxic plants are not palatable and are avoided by livestock unless grazing is forced by other circumstances. Conditions favorable to ingestion of toxic plants include overgrazing, drought, use of some herbicides, and masking the plants in hay, silage, or grain. Environmental and harvesting conditions that can alter toxin levels in plants include soil type and content, herbicide use,[2] overwatering, drought, fertilizer application, and sunlight.[3]

To identify a plant, it should be sampled in its entirety (flower, seed, pod, leaves, and roots). For shipping, the plant should be dried in a newspaper under some heavy books. Plants or leaves found in ingesta should be separated from the ingesta and shipped frozen for identification. In an emergency a plant can be pressed on a high-quality office copier, and the copy can be faxed to a diagnostic toxicologist for identification. Although chemistry analysis for most plant toxins in biologic specimens is not routinely available, recent developmental activity is making that option more available. Tests are currently available for toxins such as cyanide, nitrate, gallotannins, selected alkaloids, and some glycosides (e.g., cardiac glycosides).[3-7]

With a few well-documented exceptions such as nitrate and cyanide, specific antidotes are rarely available for plant toxins (many have not been characterized). Thus the primary goals when treating plant poisoning include providing supportive care and eliminating exposure of animals to the suspected feed, plant, or pasture. Curtailing exposure can entail switching feed sources, moving animals, fencing, mowing, and providing supplemental feed. Adsorbents such as activated charcoal may be administered to minimize absorption of organic compounds, including many plant toxins.[8]

Prevention is the most effective cure for plant toxicosis. With a few exceptions such as larkspur, which is palatable and grows in pristine pastures,[9] most toxic plants are unpalatable and grow on overgrazed and disturbed soils. Therefore plant toxicosis often can be prevented by feeding adequate amounts of feed that is free of toxic plants, managing grazing areas,[10] controlling weeds, and using proper harvest techniques for feeds.

Some plant toxins may cause potentially hazardous or otherwise noxious residues in milk and meat. For example, tremetone from white snakeroot, selenium, and several alkaloids may be passed in milk.[11,12] Thus care should be taken when providing advice about the disposition of animals exposed to plant toxicants, especially about the disposition of milk and lactating animals.

Discussion of all toxic plants is not possible. Thus general aspects of plant toxicology, along with unique aspects of poisoning resulting from selected, common classes of poisonous plants, are discussed. It is assumed that the plants covered here have been identified. Plants can be identified using many resources including various local agricultural extension agents or bulletins, textbooks,[13] diagnostic laboratories, veterinary schools, herbaria, and other botany sources. Specific statements about geographic location of plants are not made, because modern feed and seed transport have blurred the distinction between regions of the United States in which certain plants may be found.

Alkaloids

Alkaloids are compounds that have nitrogen, usually in a heterocyclic ring, and are usually basic chemicals. Alkaloids are often quite bitter and many are toxic.[14]

■ LOCOWEED

Astragalus spp.: Locoweeds
Oxytropis: Crazyweed
Swainsona: Darling pea

The locoweeds, *Astragalus* and *Oxytropis* spp. are found from the Rocky Mountains and Texas to California. Plants of both genera are perennial, herbaceous legumes with opposite, pinnately compound leaves. Flowers are purple to white racemes.[14] Seeds are borne in pods. Various species of *Astragalus* have different toxic chemicals and effects. Some species are nontoxic, whereas others have excessive selenium concentrations, 3-nitrocompounds, or swainsonine (the locoweed toxin, also found in *Swainsona*).[15-17] Swainsonine (locoweed) inhibits cellular α-mannosidases, leading to abnormal glycoprotein metabolism.[18,19]

Locoweed is unpalatable to livestock and is initially ingested when other feed is lacking (during the winter and spring).[20] In addition, evidence suggests that cattle may learn to ingest locoweed from one another.[21] Once ingestion is initiated, however, animals apparently acquire a taste for the plant.[20] Locoweed remains toxic when dry.[22] All classes of livestock are affected by it. Locoweed ingestion (up to 90% of body weight of plant material) causes gradual onset of signs related to the production, metabolic, central nervous, reproductive, and cardiovascular systems.[20,22-27] Affected animals become emaciated, lethargic, dull, and ataxic, with an impaired sense of direction.[22,26] Animals are nervous despite the depression and, especially horses, may react violently to stimulation. Horses do not seem to recover from the tendency to react uncharacteristically to stimuli. Reproductive consequences of locoism include abortion, prolonged estrus, altered breeding behavior, decreased libido, inhibition of normal spermatogenesis, weak and docile newborns, and deformed limbs with flexed tendons and joint laxity.[23,26,27,29,30] Locoweed ingestion predisposes calves to development of right-sided congestive heart failure at high altitudes ("high mountain disease").[24,25]

Sheep fed locoweed had clinical pathologic evidence of liver and renal (mild) damage, with increased serum concentrations of alkaline phosphatase, aspartate aminotransferase (AST), and blood urea nitrogen (BUN).[28,31] The major postmortem finding in locoweed intoxication is emaciation. Microscopically, locoweed (and swainsonine) causes widespread neurovisceral cytoplasmic vacuolation in animals and the fetus (if present).[32-34] The brain, liver, and kidney are the major affected organs. The vacuoles contain mannose-rich compounds.[35] Diagnosis of locoweed toxicosis relies on evidence of plant consumption, clinical signs, and lesions. No

chemistry test is available for locoism. New tests are under development to stain tissues for mannose accumulation[35] and measure α-mannosidase activity in serum to indicate exposure to locoweed.[36]

An antidote is not available for locoweed poisoning. Exposure to the plant should be ended and proper nutrition provided. Recovery from emaciation is frequent, but horses that have suffered locoism cannot be trusted. Milk from animals exposed to locoweed can be toxic, suggesting that swainsonine is passed in milk.[37] Clearance studies suggest that poisoned animals should be given approximately 28 days to clear swainsonine because of an estimated half-life in livestock of 60 hours.[36,38]

■ PYRROLIZIDINE ALKALOIDS

Senecio spp.: Tansy ragwort *(S. jacobea)* and groundsels
Crotalaria spp.: Rattlebox
Cynoglossum officinale: Houndstongue
Amsinckia intermedia: Fiddleneck
Heliotropium spp.: Heliotrope
Echium plantagineum: Patterson's curse, Salvation Jane

Losses from pyrrolizidine alkaloids occur throughout the United States, resulting from ingestion of various species of plants from the families of Compositae *(Senecio* spp.), Leguminosae *(Crotalaria* spp.), and Boraginaceae *(Cynoglossum* and *A. intermedia).*[39] *S. jacobea* is found in the Northwestern United States, *S. vulgaris* (common groundsel) can be found throughout the western United States, *Crotalaria* is present in the Midwest, *Cynoglossum* is primarily in the Rocky Mountain region, and *Amsinckia* is in California. Toxin concentrations are highest in seeds, flowers, and leaves and are lower in stems. The most toxic pyrrolizidine alkaloids are diester rings with a 1,2 double bond and a branched ester group.[39] The compounds are bioactivated in the liver to reactive pyrroles and trans-4-hydroxy-2-hexenal.[40,41] Those reactive metabolites bind cell molecules and cross-link DNA, leading to necrosis, alteration of cell division, or carcinogenicity.[40]

Plants with pyrrolizidine alkaloids are unpalatable. Most poisonings occur when animals are forced to graze the plant, or when the plant is masked in hay *(Senecio* spp. and *A. intermedia)* or grains *(Crotalaria* spp.; a major contaminant before the availability of herbicides for weed control).[39] Toxicity is retained in dry hay and grains. All classes of livestock are affected. Small ruminants such as sheep are more resistant to the alkaloids than are cattle and horses. For example, ingestion of as little as 5% of their body weight of tansy ragwort *(S. jacobea)* in hay may be lethal to a cow or horse. Conversely, over 100% of their body weight in plant material is needed to cause pyrrolizidine alkaloid poisoning in sheep and goats.[40] The resistance of sheep to the alkaloids likely results from differences in liver biotransformation patterns.[39] For example, sheep tend to have lower rates of hepatic production of toxic pyrroles plus higher levels of glutathione conjugation of toxic metabolites.[42] Interestingly, ingestion of pyrrolizidine alkaloids will enhance the toxicity of copper in sheep.[43] Although cattle and horses tend to have similar sensitivity to *Senecio* spp., it is apparent that cattle tend to resist the hepatotoxic effects of *Amsinckia* at levels in hay that would be hazardous to horses (although *Amsinckia* may still cause nitrate toxicity in the cattle instead).

Animals with pyrrolizidine alkaloid toxicosis are usually presented with signs and lesions compatible with liver failure. See Chapter 31 for a complete description of signs and lesions.[39,40,44] In addition to liver effects, pulmonary disease also has been reported for *Crotalaria* poisoning.[39] Signs may be delayed for months after ingestion of the plant, appearing after the liver damage has had an opportunity to become chronic.[45] Emaciation and hepatoencephalopathy are common, leading to common names for the disease such as "walking disease" or "walkabout," as well as "hard liver disease."

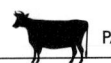

Diagnosis of pyrrolizidine alkaloid toxicosis depends on a history of exposure to the plants, clinical and pathologic evidence of liver failure, and classic histologic lesions (Chapter 31).[46-48] Antemortem diagnosis, in the absence of an appropriate history, can be difficult because of the nonspecific nature of signs and the potential for delayed and progressive effects. Diagnosis in those cases benefits from histologic examination of a surgical liver biopsy. Recent studies suggest that a chemistry test for sulfur-bound pyrrolic metabolites of pyrrolizidine alkaloids in unfixed liver tissue may be useful.[49-50] Treatment for pyrrolizidine alkaloid toxicosis centers on treating the liver failure and eliminating additional exposure to the plant. Although not preventive, evidence exists that would suggest that ingestion of sulfur-containing amino acids in high levels can influence pyrrolizidine alkaloid toxicity via maintenance of hepatic glutathione levels.[51] Note that sheep may be fed added molybdenum to delay accumulation of copper on a chronic basis.[39] Prognosis in advanced cases is poor. Very low levels of pyrrolizidine alkaloids are transferred into the milk, but attempts to transfer toxicity in the milk have not resulted in development of clinical or pathologic evidence of toxicosis.[40,52]

■ LARKSPUR ALKALOIDS

Delphinium spp.: Tall and low larkspurs
Aconitum spp.: Monkshood

Larkspur (*Delphinium*) and monkshood (*Aconitum*) have alternating, palmately divided leaves, which in larkspur may cluster at the base. Racemous flowers are in a variety of colors depending on species and are characterized by a lower spur (larkspur) or an upper hood (monkshood).[53] Loss of cattle from larkspur is economically important in the West. Unlike many toxic plants that prefer disturbed soil, larkspur is found in undisturbed mountain ranges.[54] Larkspur species are divided into low and tall varieties based on height (low, <76 cm; tall, >76 cm) and elevations (tall larkspurs are found in high mountain altitudes).[54] Larkspurs contain a variety of complex, diterpenoid alkaloids such as methyllacaconitine and deltaline.[55,56] The larkspur alkaloids cause skeletal muscle paralysis, by blocking nicotinic, acetylcholine receptors at the neuromuscular junction and in the brain.[55,57,58]

Larkspurs are hazardous because they are palatable and appear early in the spring.[54,59] Although dried plants may be toxic, the diterpenoids are highest and most hazardous in the early spring leaf growth after flowering racemes are elongated.[58,60,61] During that period, cattle will tend to ingest more larkspur during or just after a summer storm.[58] All animals may be poisoned by larkspur. Cattle are most sensitive to the plant (17 g/kg of body weight of early plant growth may be lethal), while sheep are four times less sensitive.[62] Calves are often affected when they graze with "nurse" cows on the edges of meadows (a likely spot for larkspur growth) while dams graze steep hillsides. Clinically, larkspur poisoning results in stiffness and weakness, abdominal pain, collapse (often with forelegs first), and death from aspiration of regurgitated ingesta or respiratory paralysis within 3 to 8 hours after exposure.[55,59,60,62,63] Death may be sudden (Chapter 14). Recovery may occur in sublethal cases within 1 to 2 days.[60]

Postmortem, animals with larkspur poisoning bloat rapidly.[60] Clinical pathologic findings are nonspecific. Diagnosis of larkspur toxicosis depends on a history of sudden death with rapid bloating on rangeland in early spring, evidence of consumption of the plant, and a lack of other diagnostic findings. Chemistry testing is not routinely available for larkspur alkaloids, although testing of urine or serum for the alkaloids may be viable.[64] Treatment for larkspur poisoning centers on control by pregrazing with sheep (less sensitive), delay of grazing until alkaloid levels drop, spraying larkspur with nonspecific herbicides, and attempts to develop in the animals an aversion to grazing the plant.[60,65]

■ NICOTINIC-ACTING ALKALOIDS

Nicotiana glauca: Tree tobacco; *N. tabacum*: Tobacco (pyridine alkaloid—e.g., nicotine)
Lupinus spp.: Lupines (quinolizidine alkaloids—e.g., anagyrine, sparteine)
Cytisus scoparus: Scottish broom; *Laburnum anagyroides*: Golden chain; *Thermopsis montana*: Mountain thermopsis (quinolizidine alkaloids)
Lobelia spp.: Indian tobaccos (pyridine alkaloids similar to nicotine).
Conium maculatum: Poison hemlock (piperadine alkaloids—e.g., coniine)

The lupines and thermopsis are found in climax and grassy habitats, whereas poison hemlock and the tree tobacco plants are found in disturbed soils. This group has three classes of nicotinic toxins: pyridine alkaloids, quinolizidine alkaloids, and piperadine alkaloids. Nicotinic alkaloids cause toxicity by ganglionic stimulation followed by blockade and paralysis.[66,67] The teratogenic effects of lupines, tree tobacco, and poison hemlock may result from paralysis of the fetus during the period of joint formation (day 40 to 70 of gestation for the cow; day 30 to 60 in swine and sheep).[68-72] Thermopsis causes myonecrosis by an unknown mechanism.[73,74]

The plants are often bitter and are ingested when they are hidden in hay or forage or when animals are forced to do so by drought or hunger. Some lupines may be toxic when incorporated into feed as a supplement, although the toxin and mechanisms remain to be defined.[75] The plants are toxic when dry except for *Conium*, which has quite volatile toxins that dissipate with time when plants are dry (fresh hay may be toxic).[67,76] All classes of livestock are affected by the plants, although species variations occur.[66,67,77,78] For example, acute toxicosis is more common in sheep. Conversely, teratogenesis is more likely in cattle.[74] Despite the lower likelihood of acute toxicity, it does occur. For example, in that species, this author has observed deaths in yearling Holstein dairy cattle pastured on lupine. Cattle were more sensitive to the acute effects of coniine (poison hemlock) than were horses or sheep.[78] Acute toxicosis due to nicotinic alkaloids is characterized by ataxia, weakness, tremors, initial stimulation of the central nervous system (CNS) followed by lethargy, increased salivation, respiratory distress, bloating, and death from respiratory paralysis.[66,67,79,80] Teratogenic signs include cleft palate (earlier in the susceptible period) and if exposed during joint development, classic arthrogryposis ("crooked calf syndrome") involving the joints of the legs and spine.[68-72,78,81] Acute *T. montana* toxicosis in cattle leads to tremors, a stilted gait, and recumbency followed by respiratory paralysis and death. The animal may be found dead (Chapter 14).[73]

Clinical pathologic changes are nonspecific for most of the nicotinic plants. *Thermopsis* may result in elevations of creatine kinase and AST, suggestive of skeletal muscle damage.[73] Other than bloat and pulmonary edema, acute nicotinic alkaloid toxicosis results in few specific lesions.[76,79] The congenital malformations are usually obvious on postmortem examination. *Thermopsis* toxicosis is characterized by degeneration and necrosis of skeletal muscles.[73,74] Diagnosis of acute nicotinic alkaloid toxicosis depends on identification of the plant and appropriate signs. Additionally, reliable chemical assays have been developed to detect some of the alkaloids in urine and serum of exposed animals, including those of poison hemlock, tree tobacco, and some lupines.[76,79,82] Diagnosis of the source of crooked calf syndrome requires historical review of plants that may have been grazed during the susceptible period of gestation. Treatment of acute toxicosis is nonspecific. Exposure should be elimi-

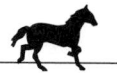

nated. Many of the potentially teratogenic alkaloids of these plants, including some from poison hemlock and Lupinus, are passed into milk and muscle tissue.[83,84]

■ STEROIDAL ALKALOIDS

Zigadenus spp.: Deathcamas

Veratrum californicum and *V. viride*: False hellebore, also skunk cabbage

Solanum spp.: Nightshades; *Lycopersicon* spp.: Tomatoes

Deathcamas is a slender, perennial herb (up to 50 cm tall) with grasslike basal leaves that grows from an onionlike bulb and has yellow-white flowers.[85] False hellabore has short, hairy, stout stems with broad, prominently veined leaves.[86] *Solanum* spp. range from annual herbs to woody plants. They have four to five lobed, white to purple flowers.[87] The fruit is a berry. The leaves often have two small leaflets at the base or incorporated as small lobes. Deathcamas and *Veratrum* spp. are found in moist meadows at upper elevations. *Solanum* spp. are found throughout the United States. Deathcamas (alkaloid is zygacine) and false hellabore contain steroidal alkaloids that cause cardiovascular hypotension.[85] *Veratrum* alkaloids include the teratogens, jervine, and cyclopamine.[88] Solanaceous plants such as the nightshades, tomatoes, and potatoes have steroidal alkaloids linked to sugars (glycosides).[89] Those *Solanum* alkaloids may inhibit cholinesterase, cause gastrointestinal irritation, and induce constipation. Some solanaceous plants accumulate nitrate (tomato vines)[90] or have other toxic factors such as vitamin D, which causes calcinosis (*S. malacoxylon*, found in South America and Hawaii).

The steroidal alkaloids are toxic to all classes of livestock. Sheep are most commonly poisoned by *Veratrum* and *Zigadenus*.[85,91] *Zigadenus* is most hazardous in the early spring because it is among the first plants present.[85] *Veratrum* is teratogenic when grazed by ewes around days 14 and 30 of gestation.[92,93] The alkaloids resist drying.[89] Ingestion of as little as 0.6% of body weight of deathcamas can cause ataxia, stiffness, tremors, increased salivation, vomition, and prostration. Death may occur within 1.5 to 8 hours of exposure.[85] See Chapter 14 on sudden death. *Solanum* spp. vary in toxicity and effect, causing gastrointestinal irritation, ileus (in horses), lethargy, increased salivation, dyspnea, tremors, paralysis, diarrhea or constipation, and death.[85,87,89] Pregnant ewes grazing *Veratrum* during day 14 of gestation produce lambs with craniofacial deformities, including cyclopia, microphthalmia, and cleft palate.[91,92] Gestation may be prolonged in affected ewes.[85] Limb and bone shortening in the metacarpal and metatarsal joints can occur in lambs when ewes ingest the plant around day 30 of gestation.[93]

Clinical and pathologic findings are nonspecific with the exception of the teratogenesis from *Veratrum*. Severe intoxication from *Solanum* spp. may lead to congestion of major internal organs.[89] Diagnosis involves piecing together of signs with evidence of consumption of the plant. Chemistry testing is not routinely available. Treatment for poisoning centers on prevention. Deathcamas and false hellebore should be avoided early in spring. The highly variable toxicity of the solanaceous plants makes recommendations about prevention difficult, although feeding of large volumes of the plants is ill-advised.

■ TROPANE ALKALOIDS

Datura stramonium, D. metaloides: Jimsonweeds

Atropa belladonna: Belladonna

Datura and *Atropa* are also solanaceous plants. Jimsonweeds prefer disturbed soils such as barnyards.[94] The plants contain the tropane alkaloids, atropine and scopolamine, which block acetylcholine at muscarinic nerve synapses. Although *Datura* is bitter and unpalatable, herbicide application or overgrazing may encourage consumption. Grain contaminated with

Datura seeds is toxic.[94] *Datura* toxicity results in gastrointestinal atony, anorexia, rapid heart and respiratory rates, mydriasis, thirst, diarrhea, excess urination, disturbed vision, and delerium.[95-97] Death is uncommon, perhaps because gut atony and anorexia may limit plant intake.[94] However, gut atony can be fatal in some species like the horse.[95,96] Exposure to trace amounts of *Datura* spp. such as in the bedding or feed, may result in urinary residues of tropane alkaloids in the horse's urine.[95] Lesions are nonspecific. Tropane alkaloids can be identified in urine, ingesta, and plant material.

■ YEW

Taxus cuspidata: Japanese yew

Taxus baccata: English yew

Yews are evergreen shrubs and small trees with flattened needles. The plants are found throughout the United States in hedges and yards.[98] Yews contain poorly characterized alkaloids called taxines, which depress myocardial conduction by blocking sodium movement through membranes.[99] Some yews also contains antimitotic, diterpenoid taxols, which are of medical interest as anticancer agents.[100]

Yew is extremely toxic (<0.1% of body weight of dried leaves may kill a horse[101]). Toxicity is retained in dry plants. All species are sensitive to yew toxicity. Like oleander, yew poisoning often results from accidental ingestion of hedge clippings.[98,102] Clinical toxicosis is usually manifested by collapse and sudden death (Chapter 14), occasionally preceded by tremors and weakness.[98,101,102]

Lesions are infrequent, although focal, nonsuppurative myocarditis is possible.[102] Diagnosis of yew toxicosis requires a history of exposure to yew clippings and sudden death. Finding of leaf parts in the ingesta is diagnostic. The investigator may be confused by needles from *Pinus* and the coastal redwood (*Sequoia sempervirins*). Alkaloids have been suggested by mass spectral chemistry in samples from poisoned animals.[103]

■ TRYPTAMINE ALKALOIDS

Phalaris spp.: Canary grass

Phalaris spp. are pasture grasses. Under ill-defined conditions, *Phalaris* spp. accumulate indole and β-carboline alkaloids.[104,105] Those alkaloids block serotonin in the CNS and may inhibit monoamine oxidases.[105,106] Cattle and sheep are affected, although sheep are more likely to be poisoned by *Phalaris*.[107] The alkaloids are bitter, resulting in lowered weight gains if present at levels exceeding 0.2% of plant weight.[105]

Clinically, two syndromes can result from canary grass toxicity. Sudden death with cardiac failure is one possible result of poisoning.[105,107] Chronic lower-level exposures may lead to a staggers syndrome with ataxia, a hopping gait, tremors, excitability, head nodding, convulsions, and eventually paddling and death in sheep and horses.[105,108-110] Onset of signs may be delayed up to 40 days after ending exposure to canary grass.[111] See p. 1629 and Chapter 33 for grass staggers.

Postmortem examination of sheep with the staggers syndrome reveals characteristic gray to bluish discoloration of the brainstem.[111,112] The kidney and liver also may be pigmented. Pigment in the cytoplasm of the nerves apparently destroys those cells.[112] Clinical signs of sudden death or staggers in sheep that have previously grazed canary grass pasture, along with characteristic discoloration of brain tissue, are used for diagnosis. Treatment of clinically affected animals has not been rewarding; however, supplementation with cobalt may help prevent toxicosis.[113]

Glycosides

Glycosides are ethers that link a sugar to a toxin (called *aglycone*). Either the glycoside or the aglycone alone may be toxic.

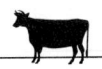

Most work is based on the properties of the aglycone. The aglycone is frequently released by damage to plant tissue. Like alkaloids, glycosides are often bitter.[114]

■ CARDIAC GLYCOSIDES (CARDENOLIDES)

Nerium oleander: Oleander; *Thevetia peruviana:* Yellow oleander

Digitalis purpurea: Foxglove

Rhododendron spp.: Azaleas

Kalmia spp.: Laurels

Convallaria spp.: Lily-of-the-valley

Pieris japonica: Japanese pieris

Asclepias spp.: Milkweeds

Apocynum spp.: Dogbanes

Bufo marinus: Bufo toads

Many families of plants contain cardiotoxic glycosides. Many of the plants, including azaleas, oleander, and Japanese pieris, are evergreen shrubs and small trees.[115] In addition to plants, cardiac glycosides may be found in animals such as the bufo toad. The toxic cardiac glycosides, including various cardenolides and bufadenolides, are steroid-like in structure and have a lactone ring.[116] Common cardiac glycosides include digitoxin and digoxin from foxgloves and oleandrin (aglycone = oleandrigenin) from oleander. Cardiac glycosides block cellular sodium-potassium adenosine triphosphatase (ATPase), leading to sodium accumulation in excitable cells such as nervous tissue and myocardium.[116-118] Increased myocardial contraction and altered heart rhythms result from myocardial effects. The plants also are potent gastrointestinal irritants.

Cardiac glycosides are found in most parts of the toxic plants.[119] Although plants are bitter, dried leaves (oleander) and flowers are readily ingested by all classes of livestock, causing toxicosis.[6,119,120] Discarded lawn clippings that contain oleander leaves are a common source of livestock poisoning. Some of the plants are extremely toxic, and toxic effects are cumulative. For example, 0.005% to 0.015% of body weight of oleander (equivalent to a handful of leaves) can be lethal in sheep and cattle, and one leaf may kill a human being.[115,121] Azaleas may be toxic when livestock ingest 0.2% to 0.6% of body weight of plant material.[121] Clinical signs of toxicosis reflect damage to the gastrointestinal tract and heart, and onset may be delayed by several hours after ingestion. Although death may be sudden (Chapter 14), it usually occurs within 36 hours after ingestion but may take up to 14 days.[122] Signs include abdominal pain, nausea, weakness, anorexia, rumen atony, increased salivation, bradycardia (or tachycardia later in the syndrome), heart block, and ventricular arrhythmias (including a gallop rhythm for oleander in cattle).[116,120-125]

Animals with acute cardiac glycoside toxicosis may have hypertension, hypoxemia, acidemia, hemoconcentration, hyperkalemia, hyperchloremia, and elevations of serum creatinine and glucose.[116] Electrocardiogram (ECG) alterations include widening of the QRS complex, ST segment depression, enlarged P waves, and a variety of ventricular arrhythmias. Lesions associated with cardiac glycoside toxicosis are nonspecific and include hemorrhagic gastroenteritis and pale mottling of the heart with congestion, hemorrhage, and histologic evidence of myocardial degeneration and necrosis.[115,116,122,123] Diagnosis of cardiac glycoside toxicosis depends on identification of the plant and evidence of its consumption. Two dimensional TLC and LC/MS methods have been developed for assay of oleander in ingesta and body fluids from affected animals.[6,124,125] A serum radioimmunoassay can be used to assess exposure to *Digitalis*. That test may cross-react with oleander glycosides for some diagnostic utility.[126]

Treatment of cardiac glycoside toxicosis begins with elimination of exposure to the plant and decontamination using cholestyramine resins or activated charcoal (repeated applications suggested).[117] Fluids with calcium and potassium should be avoided (unless hyperkalemia is absent). Atropine may be useful if bradycardia or heart block are present (use care in horses; it may cause gut stasis). β-Adrenergic blocking agents and antiarrhythmic drugs can be used for cardiac dysrhythmias, but otherwise β-blockers should be avoided.[116,117] Use of anticardiac glycoside Fab antibodies is an experimental treatment for digitalis and oleander toxicoses.[126-128] Stress should be avoided in animals exposed to cardiac glycosides. Prevention of cardiac glycoside toxicosis includes keeping hedge clippings away from animals and avoidance of plants when in full flower. *Digitalis* glycosides are widely distributed in the body, including in milk and fetal fluids, and the primary elimination pathway is urinary.[116] Evidence of oleandrin was identified in the milk of poisoned cows using two dimensional TLC in this author's laboratory. No oleandrin was found at 5 days after exposure in milk from that dairy.

■ PHOTOSENSITIZING SAPONINS

Tribulus terrestris: Puncture vine

Panicum coloratum: Kleingrass

Brachiaria decumbens: Signalgrass

Nolina texana: Sachuista

Agave spp.: Agave

Narthecium ossifragum: Narthecium

These grasses and weeds may contain toxic levels of hepatotoxic, steroidal sapogenins such as disogenin.[129-132] Sapogenins are metabolized in animals to glucuronide conjugates of epismilagenin, which crystallize in bile, leading to biliary blockage, cholangitis, and secondary photosensitization (Chapter 38).[131-133]

Plants are most hazardous when grazed during stages of early, rapid growth when sapogenin levels are highest.[133] Feed refusal can occur because the plants can be bitter. Mature plants are often grazed without incident. All herbivores may be affected. Signs of toxicity involve liver damage with anorexia, weight loss, icterus, hepatoencephalopathy, and secondary photosensitization.[129,130,134-138]

Serum chemistry alterations reflect liver damage.[135,136] Postmortem, affected animals are icteric and have evidence of necrosis and sloughing of skin.[137] Lesions in the liver include bridging and fibrosing hepatocyte necrosis, cholangitis, and occlusion of small bile ducts. Bile ducts may have birefringent crystals, probably related to sapogenin accumulation.[129,131,136,137] See Chapter 38 about skin lesions. Lesions also may be present in the kidneys, heart, and adrenals. *Narthecium,* like other lilies, may cause chronic renal failure in ruminants due most likely to a furanone, not a saponin.[139] Animals should be removed from offending pastures (at least until the grass matures).

■ CYANOGENIC GLYCOSIDES

Linum spp.: Flax

Prunus spp.: Cherries, chokecherries, apricots, peaches

Sorghum spp.: Sorghum, Sudan grass

Triglochin spp.: Arrow grass

Trifolium repens: White clover

Zea mays: Corn

Many others, see references

Many grasses, weeds, and cherry bushes contain cyanogenic glycosides. Damage to the plant causes contact between β-glycosidases and the glycosides, releasing free cyanide. Cyanide blocks a variety of metalloenzymes, most notably the terminal oxidase (cytochrome-c oxidase) of oxidative transport.[140,141] The tight affinity of cyanide for ferric (Fe^{3+}) iron in the cytochrome prevents electron transfer. Sorghums also can cause peripheral neurologic deficits in laboratory animals and horses (due to nitriles or cyanide).[141,142]

Many of the listed plants may be grazed safely; however, cyanide is released when plants are damaged from macera-

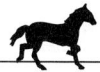

tion, drought, frost, wilting, and stunting.[140] Toxicity wanes with drying. All animals are sensitive to cyanide toxicosis. Cyanide toxicosis is very rapid in onset, often resulting in sudden death (Chapter 14). Clinical signs include dyspnea, excitement, tremors, increased salivation, gasping, clonic convulsions, and death.[140,141] Chronic exposure to cyanide in rats can cause paralysis, and cattle, horses, and sheep grazing *Sorghum* spp. have developed ataxia, urinary incontinence, and cystitis.[141-144]

Blood from animals with cyanide toxicosis is cherry red because hemoglobin cannot release oxygen to tissue. Nonspecific postmortem findings include cardiac hemorrhage associated with acute death. Chronic exposure to cyanide may lead to patchy encephalomalacia and damage to the spinal cord, along with secondary thickening and necrosis in the bladder associated with cystitis.[141,142] Diagnosis of cyanide toxicosis is supported by analytical evidence of cyanide in forage and samples from affected animals. Cyanide levels in excess of 200 ppm in plant material and 1 ppm in liver or blood are significant.[140] Samples for cyanide analysis should be frozen immediately and held frozen until analyzed.

Treatment of cyanide toxicosis relies on removal of the cyanide from affected cytochrome-c. Judicious use of sodium nitrite (16 mg/kg IV, to form a small amount of methemoglobin, Fe^{3+}) can help pull cyanide away from the enzymes. Additional use of sodium thiosulfate (30 to 40 mg/kg IV) will provide substrate for the natural rhodanese enzyme that forms thiocyanate, which is readily excreted in the urine.[140,145]

■ NITROTOXINS

Astragalus spp.: Milk vetches (*A. miser*: Timber milk vetch; *A. emoryanus*: Emory milk vetch)
Coronalia varia: Crown vetch
Indigofera spicata: Indigo

Some common milk vetches in North America contain glucosides of 3 nitro, 1 propanol (NPOH), and 3 nitropropanoic acid (NPA).[15,146,147] Miserotoxin is a common glucoside of NPOH. The glucosides are relatively nontoxic until hydrolyzed in the rumen to toxic nitrocompounds and nitrite, which is also toxic.[148-150] NPOH is oxidized to the more toxic NPA in the liver.[148,149] Nevertheless, NPOH may appear more toxic than NPA in ruminants because the NPOH is more thoroughly absorbed from the rumen. Nitrocompound toxicity is distinct from nitrite poisoning (p. 1624). Less than 33% methemoglobin is usually formed after exposure to nitrocompounds, so nitrite alone does not explain acute nitrocompound toxicity.[149] NPA is a powerful inhibitor of succinate dehydrogenase in the Krebs cycle, impairing cellular energy production in the nervous system.[151]

All livestock can be poisoned by nitrocompounds, but cattle and sheep are at most risk. Acute or chronic toxicosis may develop, depending on the amount ingested. Acute nitroplant toxicosis has a rapid onset of ataxia, distress, dyspnea, cyanosis, weakness, collapse, and death within 4 to 12 hours.[150] Sheep may be found suddenly dead (Chapter 14). Chronic nitro-plant toxicosis results in respiratory distress, weakness (especially in the pelvic limbs), knuckling of fetlocks, goose stepping, and knocking together of hind feet when walking (commonly called "cracker heels").[150] Increased salivation, constipation, and diarrhea have all been reported. Animals may linger for months, but severely affected individuals seldom recover. Affected cattle may die suddenly if forced to move quickly.

Animals exposed to nitro-containing plants can have up to 33% of methemoglobin.[150] Although not lethal at that level, the methemoglobin probably contributes to respiratory distress. Lesions of nitrocompound toxicosis include pulmonary edema with fibrosis (in longer-standing cases) and nonspecific cerebral hemorrhages. Histologic alterations in nervous tissue include Wallerian degeneration of the spinal

cord and peripheral (sciatic) nerves, with variable changes reported in the cerebellum.[150] Other neuronal lesions may include white matter vacuolation, glial edema, and bilateral changes of the thalamus and cerebellum.[149] Treatment of nitrocompound poisoning centers on prevention.

■ BRACKEN FERN

Pteridium aquilinum: Bracken fern (toxic glycoside + thiaminase)
Cheilanthes humilis: Rock fern (toxic glycosides)
Equisetum arvense: Horsetail (no known glycoside, does have thiaminase)

Bracken is a perennial fern (up to 2 m high) that arises from a black rhizome and is found in disturbed or cleared uplands. The fronds are coarse, triangular, entire at the apex, and lobed toward the stalk. Bracken fern contains a variety of glycosides, including ptaquiloside (up to 1%), which will alkylate DNA leading to carcinogenicity and bone marrow depression in ruminants and laboratory animals.[152-156] Bracken also contains thiaminase activity, which predominates in monogastric animals (horses).[152,155]

Grazing of fresh young fronds when other forage is not yet available early in the grazing season is hazardous for cattle and horses, although plowed up rhizomes and hay (20% bracken for 1 month in horses) also may be toxic.[152,157] Signs appear suddenly after animals have grazed approximately their body weight in plant material over several months. Horses develop characteristic thiamin deficiency with weight loss, ataxia, lethargy, and a braced stance with an arched back, tremors, recumbency (with violent attempts to rise), and death within days to weeks after onset of signs.[157] Cattle with bracken or ptaquiloside toxicosis develop widespread hemorrhages and hematuria ("enzootic hematuria") due to severe bone marrow depression and cancer in the bladder and other organs.[152,155-162] Reduced fertility may occur in chronic cases.

Cattle with bracken toxicosis have a normocytic, normochromic anemia, lymphocytosis, and neutropenia.[163] Severe thrombocytopenia and hemorrhage are also reported, associated with progressive bone marrow failure.[152,155] Urine from affected animals is hemorrhagic, with high levels of calcium and protein.[158,163] Lesions in cattle with bracken toxicosis include the hemorrhages, bone marrow hypoplasia, and a variety of tumors in bladders including hemangiomas, hemangiosarcomas, transitional cell carcinomas, papillomas, fibromas, and adenomas.[157,158] Other cancers may involve hematopoietic tissues and the gastrointestinal tract.[160] Horses with bracken toxicosis have low levels of thiamin. In addition to prevention, horses that have not reached a terminal state may respond large doses of parenteral thiamin. No specific treatment is currently recommended for ruminants with bracken poisoning. In terms of safety of food animal products, indirect evidence suggests that bracken ingestion by milking cows may be linked to stomach cancer in people who have chronically ingested that milk.[164]

■ PHYTOESTROGENS

Medicago sativa: Alfalfa
Trifolium subterraneum: Subterranean clover; *T. pratense*: Red clover

Hyperestrogenism caused by feeds and forages (including clover and alfalfa hays) has been reported in cattle, sheep, and swine. A variety of glycosides in those forages interact with estrogen receptors.[165,166] Commonly recognized estrogens include coumestrol, formononetin, biochanin-A, daidzein, genistein, equol, and many others.[166,167] Estrogenic compounds vary in potency. Coumestrol from alfalfa and isoflavones from clovers have the most estrogenic activity, followed by genistein, daidzein, biochanin A, and formononetin.[168] Biochanin A and formononetin are not potent in the laboratory, but ruminants metabolize them to the more estrogenic forms of genistein and daidzein, respectively.[166,168] Signs of hyperestrogenism from forages include infertility, hyperestrogenism, or antiestrogenism. Hyperestrogenism includes nymphomania, cystic ovaries, swollen genitalia, and in males development of female characteristics. Antiestrogenic signs include gonadal hypoplasia and anestrus.[165,166] Diagnosis of forage-induced hyperestrogenism is helped by demonstration of the presence of estrogens in forages and samples of plasma or urine.[169-171] Consumption of highly estrogenic forage types should be limited in breeding animals.

■ **OTHER TOXIC GLYCOSIDES**

Melilotus alba; M. offinalis: White and yellow sweet clovers

The sweet clover forages produce the glycoside, melilotoside, which contains coumarin. *Penicillium* spp. in moldy hay can dimerize the aglycone to dicumarol, which inhibits vitamin K epoxide reductase, leading to failure of vitamin K–sensitive clotting factors. Dicumarol can be assayed in feed and animal-related samples. Concentrations of dicumarol in hay as low as 10 ppm may be hazardous to cattle. Moldy sweet clover poisoning in cattle results in widespread, vitamin K–responsive hemorrhage, which is especially hazardous during late-term pregnancy (hemorrhagic abortions).[172,173]

Xanthium spp.: Cocklebur and spiny clotburs (carboxyatractyloside)

Ingestion of young sprouts, burrs, or adult plant in hay of cocklebur can cause massive centrilobular liver necrosis in swine and cattle. Signs of toxicosis include depression, dyspnea, weakness, convulsions with opisthotonus, and death. Severe hypoglycemia may be observed by the clinician.[174-177]

Ammi majus: Bishop's weed
Cymopterus watsonii: Spring parsley
Thamnosa spp.: Dutchman's breeches (furanocoumarins)
Cooperia pedunculata: (unidentified phototoxin): Cooperia

Furanocoumarins such as psoralens are primary photosensitizing agents that lead to severe blistering of light-skinned areas of exposed livestock ingesting the plants and poultry exposed to seeds from Bishop's weed (Chapter 38).[172,178]

Cestrum diurnum: Day-blooming jessamine
Solanum malacoxylon
Trisetum flavescens: (calcinogenic glycosides)

These plants contain glycosides of vitamin D (1,25 dihydroxy-cholecalciferol). Ingestion of the plants causes weight loss, lameness, stiffness, abnormal posturing, and clinical pathologic increases in serum calcium and phosphate in cattle and horses. Lesions include widespread calcification of tissues including the cardiovascular system, tendons, lungs, and kidney. The vitamin D activity may cross the placenta to affect a developing fetus.[179-182]

Medicago spp.: Alfalfa
Saponaria spp.: Soapwort, cow cockle
Gutierrezia sarothrae: Broom snakeweed
Sesbania vesicaria: Bladderpod (enterotoxic saponins)

Plant saponins are bitter, foaming, detergent-like glycosides found in a variety of important forage crops and weeds. Midsummer alfalfa cuttings tend to have the highest saponin contents. Saponin toxicosis is characterized by gastroenteritis with diarrhea, poor weight gains, and ill-thrift in cattle. Broom snakeweed has an abortifacient factor with an effect much like that in *Pinus*.[183]

Aesculus spp.: Buckeye or horse chestnut

Horse chestnuts are trees with characteristic palmate leaves and a one- to three-seeded leathery fruit capsule (seeds large with a scar give the tree its name, buckeye). Young growth, sprouts, and seeds contain toxic levels of the glycoside, aesculin. Aesculin causes ataxia, twitching, and excitability or sluggishness in livestock. The alcoholic extract from *A. hippocastanum* causes incoordination.

Ranunculus spp.: Buttercups
Ceratocephalus testiculatus: Bur buttercup

Ranunculin is enzymatically converted to the toxic protoanemonin, a potent gastrointestinal irritant that occurs in bur buttercup, and it becomes nontoxic when the plant is crushed or dried. Thus bur buttercup in hay is not a hazard. However, grazing of this bitter plant by cattle and sheep, which occurs when animals are forced to do so, results in watery diarrhea, weakness, and dyspnea. Death may occur in severe cases (nonspecific edema and hemorrhage with fluid in the large cavities).[184-186]

Brassicae: Turnips, mustards, cabbages

These plants have a variety of glucosinolates and isothiocyanates that cause gastrointestinal irritation and, for some chemicals, goitrogenic effects in adults as well as neonates.

Cycas spp.: Cycads
Macrozamia spp.: Cycads (azoxyglycosides)

Cycads are palmlike plants found in tropical and subtropical climates. They contain a variety of glycosides including the hepatogastrointestinal toxin (and carcinogen); cycasin, which is metabolized to the highly toxic, methylazoxymethanol; and a neurotoxic amino acid (β-methylamino-L-alanine). Ruminants with hepatogastrointestinal toxicosis from effects of the cycasin suffer from depression, anorexia, and weight loss. Necropsy findings reveal a cirrhotic liver, ascites, and hemorrhagic gastroenteritis. Ruminants with the neurologic syndrome suffer from "Zamia staggers," characterized by weight loss, swaying, weakness, ataxia, and rear limb ataxia. Postmortem lesions include demyelination and axonal degeneration of the brain, spinal cord, and dorsal root ganglia. In addition, recent research suggests that cycad toxins may also harm pancreatic β-cells, contributing to development of diabetes mellitus.[187-190]

Alcohols and Acids

■ **GOSSYPOL**

Gossypium spp.: Cottonseed

Gossypol is a yellow, polyphenolic pigment found in glands of cottonseed (*Gossypium*). It is present in free (toxic) and bound (to protein, perhaps to the epsilon amino of lysine; not directly toxic) forms.[191,192] Both whole cottonseed and cottonseed meal can be toxic. Extraction of cottonseed using steam and heat will bind gossypol, whereas solvent extraction may leave high levels of free (toxic) pigment. Gossypol binds to cell constituents such as lysine and phospholipids, binds iron, may cause hypokalemia through kidney damage, inhibits a range of dehydrogenases, and uncouples phosphorylation.[191-194] Gossypol also adversely affects male reproduction via a variety of mechanisms, including inhibition of lactate dehydrogenase in testicular Leydig cells and inhibition of acrosomal plasminogen activator in the sperm.[194] Cottonseed meal has limitations in protein quality, poor iron availability, and low concentrations of vitamin A.

All species can be poisoned by gossypol. Mature ruminants are more resistant to its effects (probably a result of ruminal degradation) than are monogastric animals.[191-198] The toxicity of free gossypol depends on the quality of the ration and the amount of stress on the animals. For example, although swine may develop toxicity at free gossypol levels in excess of 0.01% in the total ration,[192,196-199] supplementation of rations with iron and high quality (lysine) protein will raise the tolerated level to 0.02% to 0.04%.[192] Although adult ruminants tolerate more than 0.1% to 0.2% of free gossypol in the total ration, some animals may be poisoned at the lower levels if stressed or on a poor ration.[191,195,196] Adult bulls may suffer from infertility at those levels. Young adult cattle, under conditions of stress and marginal rations, may be sensitive to as little as 0.05% of free gossypol in the total ration (perhaps from binding of protein as well as direct toxicity).[191]

Gossypol effects are cumulative. Low levels of gossypol, if in a ration limited in iron or protein, may cause ill-thrift and

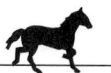

poor weight gains in swine, baby calves, and young adult cattle (<1 year of age). Acute gossypol toxicosis results in dyspnea, violent labored respirations ("thumping" in swine), weakness, and death (see Sudden Death, Chapter 14).[191,192,196,197,199] Signs may appear suddenly after stress, making gossypol toxicosis resemble acute shipping fever.[191] Adult ruminants may have decreased milk production, anorexia, dyspnea, weakness, gastroenteritis, and reproductive failure (lack of spermatogenesis in bulls).[191,195,200] Although the level in feed required to cause clinical reproductive failure in cows isn't yet known, laboratory evidence also suggests that high levels of gossypol may also impair reproductive performance in females.[201] However, these findings must be balanced with the obvious benefits of feeding a moderate level of cottonseed to dairy cows on lactation and milk quality. Lesions of acute gossypol toxicosis include large amounts of yellow proteinaceous fluid in all body cavities, myocardial degeneration and necrosis (pale streaks in the heart), and liver necrosis (centrilobular pattern). Analysis of feed for free and bound gossypol levels will support a diagnosis of gossypol poisoning. In addition, modern high performance liquid chromatography methods can detect gossypol in some animal-related samples.

There is no specific treatment for acute gossypol toxicosis. Some evidence suggests that feeding of vitamin E may help control some gossypol effects in young animals although vitamin E will not prevent toxicosis.[202] The total ration for monogastric animals and swine should contain no more than 0.01% of total gossypol.[191,192,197,199] Slightly higher levels may be fed successfully to swine if dietary protein and iron are adequate.[191,192,203] Cattle that are less than 1 year of age should have adequate nutrition and minimal stress if being fed more than 0.05% to 0.1% of free gossypol. Adult ruminant cattle should have less than 0.1% to 0.2% of free gossypol in the total ration (avoid cottonseed products in bulls). Lactating dairy cattle should be fed no more than 6 to 8 lb of cottonseed per day.[195,196]

■ TANNINS

Quercus spp.: Oak

Oaks are trees and brushes that have characteristic multilobed leaves and bear acorns in the autumn. Oaks are common in the United States, especially in Texas and California (60 species in North America).[204] They contain variable amounts of toxic, complex, and hydrolyzable tannins.[205-207] The hydrolyzable tannins are astringents and apparently bind the proteins in plasma and organs, which causes coagulation and necrosis.[208] Acorn calf syndrome, a deformity in calves of cows eating oak, may have a nutritional mechanism and is completely different from the syndrome being discussed here.[209]

The hazard of oak toxicity parallels the tannin content of plant material.[210] Plants tend to have the highest tannin content in the spring during the budding stage, and acorns may have high tannin levels in the fall.[205] All livestock may be poisoned by oak tannins. Signs generally appear after 3 days of initial ingestion of the oak. Losses from oak result from gastroenteritis, renal failure, liver damage, death, and deformities of calves.[204,208,209,211] Clinical effects in cattle include rumen atony, anorexia, constipation with black feces, lethargy, icterus, hematuria, dehydration, and evidence of renal failure.[204,208] Additional discussion of oak toxicosis is found in Chapter 30.

■ SOLUBLE OXALATES

Halogeton glomeratus: Halogeton or barilla
Sarcobatus vermiculatus: Greasewood
Rumex crispus: Curly dock
Setaria sphacelata: Setaria
Rheum: Rhubarb
Oxalis: Sorrel or soursob
Kochia scoparia: Fireweed, summer cypress (also nitrate, secondary photosensitizing agent, and sulfate)

Many oxalate-bearing plants grow in disturbed or arid soils.[212] Soluble oxalate in acidic plants such as *Oxalis* is present as the potassium salt. Sodium salts of oxalate are present in plants such as halogeton that grow at more neutral pH levels.[213] Proposed mechanisms of acute poisoning due to soluble oxalates include hypocalcemia, gastrointestinal irritation, and inhibition of respiratory enzymes. Subacutely, oxalate is deposited as insoluble, birefringent crystals in kidney leading to renal failure. Chronic oxalate poisoning resulting from *Setaria* may lead to calcium deficiency with relative hyperphosphatemia.[213,214] Insoluble calcium salts of oxalate are present in plants such as *Dieffenbachia* and *Philodendron* spp. Those insoluble calcium oxalates are not absorbed, but they do act as potent local membrane irritants.

Oxalate-bearing plants are bitter and not ingested unless grazing is forced. All species are poisoned by oxalate, although historically sheep have been the most frequent victims.[213] Rumen flora adapt to oxalate in forage if animals are gradually acclimated to oxalate over 4 days.[215] Poisoning occurs when hungry animals that are unaccustomed to oxalate ingest the plants in large quantities.[212-214,216] Soluble oxalate toxicosis results in labored breathing, ataxia, rumen stasis and bloat, depression, weakness, coma, and death.[213,215] Horses chronically grazing setaria develop "bighead," which is associated with a low calcium/phosphorus ratio.

Soluble oxalate-related changes in serum parameters reflect hypocalcemia or uremia. Postmortem lesions include hemorrhage and edema of the rumen wall and kidneys. Refractile crystals are found in the kidneys and rumen wall. Renal tubular necrosis and rumenitis are the major lesions along with the presence of crystals.[213,214,216] Analytical tests are available for oxalate in plant and animal-related samples.

Treatment of oxalate toxicosis is for gastroenteritis, shock, and renal failure. Gradual acclimation of ruminants to forages containing soluble oxalates and providing adequate levels of clean water may help prevent clinical disease.

■ WHITE SNAKEROOT

Eupatorium rugosum: White snakeroot
Haplopappus wrightii: Desert haplopappus; perhaps also *H. heterophyllus* and *H. acradenius*

White snakeroot is a perennial that grows in clumps from clusters of snakelike roots in shady, wooded areas in the Midwest. The leaves are opposite and have three characteristic veins on the undersides.[217] The plant tends to remain green when other plants have dried. The toxin of white snakeroot has not been identified but is extractable with a ketone and sterol-rich fraction called collectively, tremetol.[217] The toxins may require microsomal activation in animals.[218]

White snakeroot (fresh or dried) is hazardous to all species studied, although lactating animals are resistant because of rapid excretion of the toxins in milk.[217,219-222] The hazard to grazing animals is highest when other forages have dried during the winter season or conditions force overgrazing. Feeding of 1% and 2% of body weight of the plant to horses resulted in toxicity after 1 to 2 weeks.[219] White snakeroot toxicosis causes cardiac and skeletal muscle damage along with ketosis.[217] Clinical signs of white snakeroot toxicosis include weight loss, tremors and stiffness, ataxia, depression, cardiac arrhythmias (especially ST segment depression), recumbency, and death (within hours of recumbency).[217,219,221-223] Sudden death is possible (Chapter 14).

Clinical pathologic alterations include ketosis (many have breath smelling of acetone) and increased serum activities of creatine kinase, lactate dehydrogenase, alkaline phosphatase, and aspartate transaminase.[217,219-221] Lesions of white snakeroot toxicosis include pale streaking in the heart with multifocal myocardial degeneration, necrosis, and mineralization.[219] Skeletal muscle necrosis also may occur, especially with the *Haplopappus* spp. The liver may have centrilobular degeneration and necrosis. Diagnostically, white snakeroot

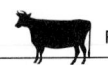

poisoning should be differentiated from selenium deficiency and ionophore toxicosis. Treatment for white snakeroot toxicosis is supportive. Milk from exposed animals is hazardous and should not be fed or consumed.

■ OTHER TOXIC ALCOHOLS AND ACIDS

Agropyron desertorum: Crested wheatgrass; many rapidly growing forages (plant acids such as transaconitic acid)

Lush, early growth of many forages, including crested wheatgrass, can contain acid compounds that sequester magnesium. Ingestion of the plants during this lush stage can lead to hypomagnesemia in cattle (including tetany; see Hypomagnesemia, Chapter 39).[224]

Pinus ponderosa: Ponderosa pine
Pinus radiata: Monterey pine
Juniperus communis: Juniper

Ingestion of pine needles by pregnant cows during late gestation causes abortions or birth of weak calves, and digestive upset and lethargy in cows. The abortions are characterized by retained placentas and metritis. Many cows may die with effects secondary to metritis. The toxins in ponderosa pine include isocupressic acid esters along with a unique class of vasoactive lipids. The major lesion of pine needle abortion is necrosis in the placental trophoblast region perhaps also resulting from reduced uterine blood flow.[225-232]

Cicuta spp.: Water hemlock
Asclepias fasicularis: Whorled milkweed
A. labriformis: Labriform milkweed
A. subverticillata: Narrow-leaved milkweeds

Water hemlock and some of the more toxic narrow-leafed milkweeds contain convulsant resins. Most of the toxicity of water hemlock lies in the resins of the chambered root. Ingestion of less than 0.2% to 0.5% of an animal's body weight of either plant may be lethal. Signs of toxicosis (in all species) may appear within 15 minutes of ingestion and include nervousness, excessive salivation, weakness, tremors, violent convulsions, and death. Postmortem lesions include skeletal muscle and myocardial necrosis, perhaps associated with seizures. Administration of sodium pentobarbital at the onset of signs can result in recovery.[233-236]

Hypericum perforatum: St. John's wort (hypericin)
Fagopyrum esculentum: Buckwheat (fagopyrin)

The toxins of St. John's wort (a weed of disturbed areas) and buckwheat (an off-season cover crop used for forage) are primary photosensitizing toxins (Chapter 38).[237]

Tetradymia spp.: Horsebrush (tetradymol; requires *Artemisia nova* or *A. tridentata:* Black or big sages to induce toxicosis)

Ingestion of horsebrush by sheep, plus black sage (contains a sesquiterpene lactone), at levels of 1% of body weight, can cause hepatogenous photosensitization (Chapter 38). The tetradymols are bioactivated in the liver to toxic substances that, among other mechanisms, uncouple oxidative phosphorylation.[238,239]

Miscellaneous Toxic Plants

■ NITRATES

Sorghum spp.: Sorghum, Sudan grass
Avena spp.: Oat
Amaranthus spp.: Pigweed
Beta spp.: Beets
Solanum spp.: Nightshades
Zea maize: Corn
Various fertilizers, water runoff

Toxic levels of nitrate and nitrite are found in forage, water, and many fertilizers. Sources in water include biologic runoff, industrial effluents (nitrite in water from ponds near oil wells), and fertilizer. Nitrate is reduced to nitrite in the rumen. Nitrite converts hemoglobin (Fe^{2+}) to methemoglobin (Fe^{3+}), which does not bind or transport oxygen, leading to hypoxia.[240]

Although many of the listed forages are widely used for animals, environmental conditions such as drought, plant stress, rapid growth spurts, some herbicide uses, low light, and fertilization can lead to nitrate accumulation.[241] All animals are sensitive to nitrite. Ruminants are ten times more sensitive to nitrate than are monogastric animals because the rumen reduces nitrate to nitrite.[240,242] Forage containing a nitrate concentration of 1% (dry weight) may be lethal in cattle not acclimated to it.[240] Acute toxicosis can result from nitrate in water at levels over 0.12%.[240] Levels exceeding 0.5% in forage and 400 ppm in water may be hazardous to pregnant cattle.[240] Clinical nitrate toxicosis appears within 4 hours of exposure. Signs include polypnea, dyspnea, weakness, tremors, intolerance to exercise, terminal convulsions, and death is possible within hours (see Sudden Death, Chapter 14).[240,242] Mildly affected cattle may recover spontaneously. Abortion may occur in mild, or apparently nonclinical, cases in cattle within 5 days of exposure (the half life of nitrite in the fetus is greater than three times that of adults).[242,243] Hypoxic stress in the fetus may aggravate other causes of abortion.

Cattle with nitrate poisoning will have chocolate-brown blood (>30% methemoglobin). Postmortem findings are nonspecific. A diagnosis of nitrate toxicosis is supported by finding >45 ppm of nitrate in ocular fluid or serum, along with identification of a toxic level of nitrate in forage or water.

Clinical cases respond well to administration of methylene blue (5 to 15 ml of a 1% solution) by intravenous injection.[240] Prevention of nitrate toxicosis requires proper harvest of forage and gradual acclimation of ruminants to potential high nitrate-type forages.

■ SELENIUM (INDICATORS LISTED)

Stanleya pinnata: Prince's plume
Astragalus bisulcatus: Two-grooved milk vetch
Xylorrhiza spp.: Woody asters
Most common forages under conditions favorable to passive assimilation of selenium

The listed plants are called selenium indicator plants because of their requirement for high selenium levels in soil for growth.[15,244] Although those plants are not palatable because of a garlicky odor, they indicate the presence of selenium. In the presence of arid, alkaline soil, selenium also may be accumulated in toxic levels in a variety of common forage plants and consumable weeds (alfalfa, *Asteraceae, Castilleja, Atriplex*). Selenium, an essential element (see Selenium Deficiency, Chapter 40), can cause both peracute toxicosis from oversupplementation in feed or injection[244-247] or chronic toxicosis at lower levels.[15,244,248] The mechanism of acute selenium toxicity is unknown but may involve direct effects of organoselenium compounds on cell energy production.[248] The mechanism of chronic selenium poisoning is related to its replacing or interacting with sulfur in structural amino acids needed for cross-linking (cysteine or methionine).[244,248]

All species may be affected by selenium toxicosis. Acute toxicosis is caused by oversupplementation of feeds containing selenium, ingestion of indicator plants (10,000 ppm of selenium), or injection of excessive selenium (0.4 mg/kg of body weight was lethal to lambs). Signs include weakness, dyspnea, bloating, abdominal pain with diarrhea, paresis in some species, and shock and death from respiratory failure.[246-250] Animals, especially horses, with chronic alkali disease from selenium in forage (5 to 50 ppm dry weight in forage is toxic) develop ill-thrift, anemia, stiffness, lameness, loss of mane and tail, and deformities and sloughing of hooves.[15,244,248] Cattle with chronic selenosis may also develop hoof lesions, develop immune incompetence, and if pregnant, may give birth to nonviable calves.[251,252] Neurologic diseases often reported, such as "blind staggers," are actually not likely due to selenosis and perhaps resulted from ingestion of related locoweeds.[251]

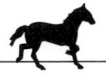

Lesions of selenium toxicosis vary based on dose and duration of disease. Peracute toxicosis leads to widespread organ congestion, cardiac damage, and severe pulmonary edema.[246-248] Chronic selenosis results in articular erosions and deformed, sloughed hooves in horses with loss of longer mane and tail hair.[15,245,248] Selenium in feed should not exceed 1 to 2 ppm dry weight. Selenium in whole blood should range between 0.08 and 1.0 ppm and, in liver, from 0.25 to 1.0 ppm for most normal animals. After exposure to excessive selenium is terminated, tissue levels may fall back to normal well before clinical signs dissipate, leading to a false-negative finding (hair testing may be beneficial to diagnose chronic selenosis).

No specific treatment is recommended for chronic selenosis. Reportedly, feeding of proteins that are high in sulfur-containing amino acids may be beneficial.[244] Food animals poisoned with selenium may require at least 60 days to clear the excess selenium.[253]

■ SULFUR-CONTAINING PLANTS

Brassica rapus: Turnip
Kochia scoparia: Fireweed, summer cypress (also nitrate, secondary photosensitization)

Certain plants, feed mixes, and water all contain high levels of sulfur. In general, the total amount of sulfur intake for a ruminant should contain no more than 0.4% of sulfur overall. High levels of sulfur as sulfate may contribute to copper deficiency (Chapter 30) and can cause polioencephalomalacia in ruminants along with other forms of sulfur.

In the ruminant and perhaps also the horse, ingestion of excess sulfur in water, feed, or from grazing plants such as turnips that can accumulate sulfur, intestinal microbes (rumen or large bowel) may produce excess sulfide. The excess sulfides can cause polioencephalomalacia as they are rapidly absorbed. Clinical signs of polioencephalomalacia include characteristic CNS disease with blindness (Chapter 33).

Diagnosis of sulfur toxicosis requires testing of all potential sources of sulfur including feed, pasture, and water, in addition to finding of signs and lesions characteristic for polioencephalomalacia. The differential diagnosis for sulfur toxicosis includes other causes of polio, salt toxicity, water deprivation, lead poisoning, and other infectious causes of neurologic disease in cattle.[254]

■ PNEUMOTOXIC PLANTS

Perilla frutescens: Perilla mint (perilla ketone)
Rapidly growing forages accumulate tryptophan
Ipomoea batatas: Moldy sweet potato (4-ipomeanol)
Phaseolus vulgaris: Moldy green beans

Lush forage ("foggage") and perhaps feeds that are high in tryptophan, toxic plants (seed and flowering stage of perilla mint), moldy sweet potatoes (infected with *Fusarium solani* mold), and moldy green beans *(Fusarium semitectum)* can cause interstitial pneumonia in animals (Chapter 29).[255-260] The toxins include the listed pneumotoxic ketones and 3-methyl indole (a rumen floral metabolite of excessive tryptophan).[258,261,262] Despite some diversity of structure, the toxins are metabolized by the mixed-function oxidases in pulmonary type 1 pneumocytes and nonciliated bronchiolar epithelial cells (Clara) to highly cytotoxic free radicals, leading to damage to local alveolar and, perhaps most important, endothelial cells.[255-267] These oxidant pneumotoxins also deplete cellular antioxidation factors such as glutathione in the liver and lung.[263]

Ruminants, especially cattle, are at risk of developing 3-methyl indole toxicosis when moved suddenly from dry feed to a lush pasture.[258] Unexplained isolated incidents of interstitial pneumonia also occur in feedlot cattle (change in flora? feed tryptophan?). Feeding of moldy sweet potatoes or moldy green beans is also hazardous.[255-257] Perilla mint has pneumotoxic ketones in highest concentrations during the flowering and seed stages.[259] Toxicity is retained in dry plant material.[259] Clinical effects of these penumotoxins include sudden onset of increased respiration, severe dyspnea with an expiratory grunt, frothing at the mouth with the head down, and open-mouth breathing.[258,259] Animals may be found dead (Chapter 14).

Affected cattle have wet, heavy lungs with variable amounts of emphysema. Histologically, the lungs have severe interstitial edema. Ultrastructural studies reveal degeneration and necrosis of type 1 pneumocytes, endothelial cells, and Clara cells, with proliferation of type II pneumocytes in longer-standing cases.[255,256,258,264-269] Perhaps a result of differential bioactivation rates, the major lesion in the horse is bronchiolitis (not alveolitis).[270] The extremely short half-life of 3-methyl indole (14 minutes)[262] in cattle has hindered development of diagnostic tests. Specific treatment for toxic interstitial pneumonia is not available.

■ OTHER NOTABLE TOXIC PLANTS

Allium spp.: Onions, garlic, chives
Brassica spp.: kale, beets, rape, cabbage, turnips (hemolytic disulfides)
Acer rubrum: Red maple (unidentified hemolytic toxin)

The onions and brassica plants contain S-methylcysteine sulfoxide, which is metabolized to dimenthyl disulfide, which attacks red blood cell membranes. Onions and brassicaceae are toxic to a variety of species, whereas red maple poisoning is reported in horses. Signs in poisoned animals include lethargy, anorexia, dyspnea, coffee-colored urine, icterus, hypoxic abortion, and shock. Death results from respiratory failure secondary to anemia. Affected animals have hemolytic anemia with hemoglobinuria, Heinz bodies, and increased levels of AST, sorbitol dehydrogenase, plasma protein, and bilirubin. Postmortem findings may include icterus, brownish discoloration of blood, centrilobular hepatic degeneration, and hemoglobinemic nephrosis. Note that ruminants such as sheep may adapt to an onion diet because the rumen appears to quickly develop a population of sulfide-reducing bacteria to decrease the hemolytic forms of sulfur.[271-278]

Amaranthus retroflexus: Pigweed (renal toxin)

In addition to the potential to cause high levels of nitrate when in hay, redroot pigweed also can be toxic to kidneys when grazed fresh in the field. Cattle and swine have developed signs of renal failure, including weakness, tremors, ataxia, recumbency, and death after grazing the plant for 5 to 10 days. Serum potassium, BUN, and creatinine concentrations are increased. Lesions include marked perirenal edema (may be bloody), straw-colored fluid in body cavities, and pale kidneys with histologic evidence of degeneration and necrosis of both proximal and distal tubules. Tubules have proteinaceous, cellular casts.[279-281]

Cassia (Senna) occidentalis, C. obtusifolia, C. roemeriana: Senna

These annual shrubs of the southeastern United States contain an unknown myotoxin(s) in all plant parts, but the seeds are most hazardous. Signs of toxicosis may occur in all livestock grazing the plant and include anorexia, ataxia, weakness, intense decrease in weight gain, and recumbency. Clinical pathologic abnormalities may include increased serum levels of creatine kinase and aspartate aminotransferase, and myoglobinuria. Postmortem findings include degeneration and necrosis of skeletal and cardiac muscle. Goats and cattle given *C. roemeriana* may also have hepatocellular damage.[282-287]

Centaurea solstialis: Yellow star thistle
C. repens: Russian knapweed

These plants contain sesquiterpene lactones such as the cytotoxic, repen, along with aspartic and glutamic acids, all of which are potent neurotoxins. Prolonged ingestion of large amounts (>1.8 kg/100 kg of body weight per day) of these plants by horses may result in neurotoxicity. The principal sign of toxicity is dysphagia characterized by dystonia of the lips and tongue. Lethargy and aimless walking are also reported. Lesions include characteristic foci of necrosis in the globus pallidus and substantia nigra (bilateral) of the brain (nigropallidal encephalomalacia). Yellow star thistle is an aggressively growing plant that is difficult to control. Biologic measures including introduction of rust and insects have been considered as control measures. Prevention includes providing adequate alternative feeds.[288-291]

Helenium spp.: Sneezeweed

Hymenoxys richardsonii: Bitter rubberweed (sesquiterpene lactones)

These weeds of the Rocky Mountains and southwestern United States are unpalatable but may be ingested by sheep or goats in the winter when other forage is limited. Sesquiterpene lactones bind with sulfhydral groups (cysteine), leading to an extreme irritant effect on the nose, eyes, and gastrointestinal tract. Affected animals develop severe gastroenteritis (sneezeweed toxicosis is called *spewing sickness* because of vomiting) with secondary aspiration pneumonia being common. Affected animals may have increases in serum γ-glutamyltransferase, aspartate transaminase, creatinine, and BUN. Postmortem lesions include gastroenteritis, congestion of liver and kidney, and aspiration pneumonia. Administration of thiol groups (cysteine, protein, methionine) and antioxidants are protective.[292-296]

Juglans nigra: Black walnut

Horses exposed to fresh black walnut (as little as 5% in shavings used as bedding; possibly also plant) can cause a transient drop in leukocytes, limb edema, and laminitis. The toxin of black walnut is unknown but is not the naphthoquinone, juglone, as originally thought. An unknown quinone is suspected. Treatment is removal of offending shavings and traditional therapy for acute laminitis in horses. Rotation of the third phalanx is possible in severe cases.[297-299]

Berteroa incana: Hoary alyssum

Hoary alyssum, a potential weed contaminant of alfalfa hay, toxicosis is characterized by fever, limb edema, and laminitis in horses.[300] The toxin is unknown.

Karwinskia humboldtiana: Coyotillo

Rhamnus spp.: Buckthorn (neuromuscular toxins)

Coyotillo is a woody shrub from the southwestern United States that may cause toxicosis in cattle, sheep, goats, hogs, and fowl when other forages are scarce. Ingestion of small amounts of the fruit and seeds leads to weakness, incoordination, and eventually paralysis. The onset of signs is delayed for days to weeks after exposure. Lesions include segmental demyelination (wallerian degeneration) of nerve axons. Ingestion of the green parts of the plant may lead to wasting, weakness, and death. Lesions associated with the extraneural syndrome of coyotillo poisoning include necrosis of the myocardium, liver, and kidney, and pulmonary hemorrhage.[301-303]

Hypochoeris spp: Flatweed or smooth catsear

Lathyrus spp: Pea

Ingestion by horses of some plants such as flatweed, especially in conditions of overgrazing, is suspected as causing outbreaks of Australian stringhalt. Stringhalt is a distal axonopathy characterized in horses by an unusual gait in which the hock is hyperflexed during movement, reluctance to back up, and in some reports, a high incidence of roaring. The etiology is unknown for flatweed. *Lathyrus* neurotoxicity is well described (neurotoxic amino acid derivatives, β-*N*-oxalylamino-L-alanine).[304-307]

Persea americana: Avocado (persin, an ischemic myotoxin, toxic to mammary gland)

Plant matter from avocado trees (primarily the Guatemalan varieties from most reports) has caused aseptic mastitis, myocardial necrosis, and skeletal muscle lesions with edema. Aseptic mastitis with epithelial necrosis in the mammary gland has been reported in cattle, horses, and goats.

Myocardial necrosis (with widespread edema, including the brisket) has been reported for goats, sheep, horses, and avians including rattites (sudden death with fluid accumulation in avians). Horses suffer from edema of the lips, tongue, mouth, and neck, along with lethargy and colic. Serum factors increased with avocado toxicosis include creatine kinase, aspartate transaminase, and lactate dehydrogenase.[308-315]

Ricinus communis: Castor bean

Robina pseudoacacia: Black locust

Abrus precatorius: Rosary pea (the lectins: ricin, robin, and abrin)

The lectins in the listed plants are glycoprotein dimers joined by a disulfide bond in the cases of ricin and abrin. Seeds, cakes, and foliage are all poisonous, whereas the oil is not. A portion of the dimer, the haptomer, binds the cell, allowing the other half to enter and block protein synthesis. All classes of livestock are sensitive to the compounds. Ricin and abrin are among the most potent toxins described. Clinical toxicosis reflects primary damage to the gastrointestinal tract and includes violent gastroenteritis followed by weakness and death due to shock and depression of cardiac function. A variety of other poisonous lectins, although less acutely toxic, are found in a variety of legume seeds from a variety of unextracted beans. Those factors interfere with intestinal absorption, inhibit growth, and can inhibit the immune system.[316,317]

Vicia villosa: Hairy vetch

Cattle and horses grazing hairy vetch when it is green may develop a systemic granulomatous disease. Dried seeds may cause convulsions (apparently unrelated to the immunotoxic syndrome to be discussed here) in cattle. Prior sensitization may be required for development of clinical signs of systemic granulomatous disease in animals exposed to green vetch. Initially, animals are presented for listlessness and welts on the skin with alopecia and peeling of skin around the nares. Horses may have lymphadenomegaly and dependent edema. Affected animals may develop wasting, diarrhea, and clinical pathologic changes of lymphocytosis and hyperproteinemia. Mortality may be high in affected animals. Postmortem, skin is thickened with scaling and alopecia. Other organs that may be pale or have gross abnormalities include the heart, kidneys, adrenals, and lymphoid tissues. Microscopically, the skin and other organs, including the liver, have cellular infiltrations of monocytes, lymphocytes, plasma cells, eosinophils, and often multinucleated giant cells. The mechanism of hairy vetch toxicosis is not known, but may involve an immunotoxic lectin.[318-322]

Setaria lutescens: Yellow bristlegrass

Other foxtails (mechanical trauma)

Yellow bristlegrass contains sharp, miniature barbs below the seed heads that can cause mucosal trauma, including oral ulcers, in animals ingesting contaminated hay. Horses and young cattle are most commonly affected.

■ BLUE-GREEN ALGAE (FRESH WATER)

Microcystis aeruginosa: (microcystin, a hepatotoxic cyclic peptide)

Nodularia spumigena: (nodularin, a hepatotoxic cyclic peptide)

Anabena flos-aquae: (anatoxin-a, a depolarizing neurotoxin; anatoxin-a(s), a cholinesterase inhibitor)

Aphanizomenon flos-aquae: (saxitoxin, neosaxitoxin, blockers of neural transmission)

Potentially toxic blue-green algae (cyanobacteria) may form on stagnant bodies of water under conditions of heat, eutrophication (high nitrogen and nutrients), low flow rates, and a concentrating wind.[323,324] The cyclic peptide hepatotoxins cause dissociation of the cytoskeleton of the liver, leading to disintegration of that organ.[325,326] Anatoxin-a is a bicyclic, secondary amine that causes depolarization of nicotinic receptors

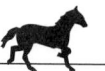

leading to muscle and respiratory paralysis.[324,327] Anatoxin-a(s) is a naturally occurring organophosphorus-like compound that inhibits peripheral cholinesterase.[324,328] Saxitoxin and neosaxitoxin are paralytic by blocking neural sodium transport.[324] A variety of cyanophytes cause skin and gastrointestinal irritation.

All species are sensitive to the listed algae, which, if ingested in sufficient quantities, may cause sudden death (Chapter 14). Animals exposed to high doses of the cyclic peptide hepatotoxins may die within 1 hour of exposure from hypovolemia and shock secondary to blood loss into the disintegrated liver and embolism of hepatocytes into the lung.[323-326] Lower doses lead to characteristic signs of liver failure. Exposure to a toxic dose of anatoxin-a leads to tremor, collapse, exaggerated breathing efforts, convulsions, and death within minutes.[324,327] The paralysis is persistent and not responsive to assisted ventilation.[327] Anatoxin-a(s) also can kill in minutes after exposure. Characteristic signs of cholinesterase inhibition in the periphery include diarrhea, tremors, hypersalivation, dyspnea, paresis, opisthotonos, cyanosis, convulsions, and death.[324,328]

Animals with hepatotoxic blue-green algae toxicosis may have elevations in liver-associated serum factors including aspartate transaminase, γ-glutamyltransferase, alkaline phosphatase, and bilirubin, along with other factors including creatinine, BUN, and lactate dehydrogenase. Hepatotoxic lesions include enlarged, red- to blue-colored livers with gallbladder edema. Histologic alterations include severe centrilobular hepatocellular dissociation, degeneration, and necrosis. A rim of hepatocytes around the periportal triads may be all that remains.[323-326] Hepatocyte emboli may be found in the lung.[326] Mild renal tubular degeneration may occur. Animals with anatoxin-a(s) toxicosis will have depression of peripheral cholinesterase, although brain cholinesterase may be normal.[324] Otherwise, pathologic changes in animals with neurotoxicosis reflect hypoxemia and are nonspecific. If blue-green algae toxicosis is suspected, samples of ingesta and bloom can be mixed with 10% neutral-buffered formalin for visual identification. Samples should be accompanied by at least 2 L of fresh bloom material (refrigerated) for demonstration of the toxin or toxicity. Liquid chromatography of bloom material or ingesta may be useful to help diagnose poisoning due to the *Microcystis* toxins.[329]

Treatment for blue-green algae poisoning is supportive. Artificial ventilation is required for anatoxin-a toxicosis. Exposed animals might benefit from the use of oral adsorbents such as activated charcoal.[323]

MYCOTOXINS

A mycotoxicosis is a disease caused by a toxin elaborated by a fungus, unlike a mycosis, which is a disease caused by fungal growth (not its toxins). Mycotoxins may be endomycotoxins (mushrooms, not discussed here) or exomycotoxins (this discussion). Mycotoxins are of worldwide veterinary and public health concern. Diseases caused by mycotoxins include acute and chronic poisoning, immunosuppression, loss of production, carcinogenicity, and teratogenicity.

Many genera and species of fungi are toxigenic. A given mycotoxin may be elaborated by more than one fungal species. Some species of fungi may produce more than one toxin. Conversely, a given fungus may not always be toxic (many are ubiquitous), so finding the fungus alone is rarely diagnostic (diagnosis requires chemical identification of the toxins). Colonization and toxin elaboration may occur in the field or in storage. Basic requirements for colonization include substrate with sufficient nutrients (why fruits and seeds are commonly infested), moisture content in feed greater than 14%, relative humidity over 70%, appropriate temperature (varies with species of fungus), and oxygen. Damage to fruits and plants favors colonization as well. Basic requirements for toxin elaboration may vary from those needed for colonization.

Mycotoxins are found in a variety of matrices including cereal grains, other crop feeds such as beans, or grass and forage. Mycotoxins cause billions of dollars of losses worldwide due to crop losses, animal and human sickness, reduced production, and costs of control measures. Although many toxins have been identified, many more, as yet unidentified, toxins may still exist. For example, moldy hay has been implicated as a cause of many problems including gastrointestinal disturbances, liver disease, and photosensitization; yet the toxins have not been identified. Little testing is possible for mycotoxins in animal samples. Therefore testing is best performed on suspected source feed. The sampling technique is critical because toxin levels will vary greatly within a lot of feed. Thus samples should be representative of the lot and frozen for storage. Please note that feed contaminated with mycotoxins may not be visibly moldy. Some mycotoxins have already been discussed with plants (moldy sweet potatoes and moldy sweet clover hay). Some other important mycotoxins of livestock are discussed here.[330-333]

Aflatoxins

Many fungal species can produce aflatoxins, including *Aspergillus flavus* (A + fla + toxin), *Aspergillus parasiticus*, and various species of *Penicillium, Rhizopus, Mucor,* and *Streptomyces*. Colonization and toxin production can occur in grains such as corn, cottonseed, and peanuts in all phases from growth through harvest. Aflatoxins are produced in soybeans and other small grains, mainly during storage. Aflatoxin production is encouraged when warm, moist ambient conditions are combined with crop damage (drought or storm). Although many aflatoxins exist, the major toxins of concern include aflatoxins B_1, B_2, G_1, G_2 (B or G = fluorescence color), and the major marker metabolite in milk and meat, aflatoxin M_1.[331,333] Aflatoxins act, after bioactivation in the liver, by binding of biologic molecules such as essential enzymes, blockage of RNA polymerase and ribosomal translocase (inhibiting protein synthesis), and formation of DNA adducts.[333,334]

Aflatoxin can cause oncogenesis, chronic toxicity, or peracute signs depending on the species and age of animal and the dose and duration of aflatoxin exposure. All animals may be affected by aflatoxins. Among mammals (birds and trout are more sensitive than mammals), young swine and pregnant sows are most sensitive to aflatoxins, followed by calves (0.2 ppm in feed for 16 weeks caused mild liver damage), horses (0.4 to 0.6 ppm), fat pigs, mature cattle (0.66 ppm in feed caused mild liver damage after 20 weeks), and sheep.[331,335] Levels over 1 ppm may cause severe organ damage and acute deaths in livestock. As little as 0.15 ppm of aflatoxin in the feed may lead to actionable residues of aflatoxin M_1 in meat and milk (action level is 0.0005 ppm in meat and milk and 0.02 ppm for interstate transport of grains).[333,336] Aflatoxin in the diet of trout at 0.001 ppm is carcinogenic.[333]

Signs of peracute toxicosis include hemorrhage, bloody diarrhea, and rapid death.[333] Lesions of acute toxicosis include hemorrhages and prolonged prothrombin times. Subacute toxicosis may lead to hepatic failure with icterus, anorexia, ataxia, reproductive failure (abortion), weakness and tremors, slowed rumen motility, coma, and death.[331,333,335,337-342] Impairment of immune function may also occur due to moderate levels of aflatoxin.[333,341] Animals with aflatoxicosis-induced liver failure may have anemia, ascites, pallor, elevated liver-associated enzymes (alkaline phosphatase, aspartate transaminase, total bilirubin), and decreased albumin levels. Lesions include a pale-yellow liver with centrilobular to portal fatty degeneration and necrosis (species dependent) of the liver along with biliary hyperplasia.[331,333,335,337-340] Chronic toxicity is associated with decreased growth rates, decreased feed efficiency, rough hair coats, ill-thrift, increased incidence of disease, and liver damage (fibrosis with regenerative nodules). Carcinogenesis may occur at low levels. Testing of feed and liver for aflatoxin will support a diagnosis.

Aflatoxin B_1 is one of the most potent known carcinogens.[331,333] Aflatoxins are distributed to tissues and milk of food animals, leading to a significant residue concern (aflatoxin M_1 is the marker residue).[342,343] The highest concentrations of aflatoxin are in liver. Alfatoxin is cleared from the liver over 7 days of withdrawal, during which aflatoxin-free feed is provided.[343] Dairy cows can "decontaminate" aflatoxin to below the 0.0005 ppm action level in milk (US; may be as much as 10 times lower for some trading partners such as the European Union [EU]) if the maximum level of aflatoxin in feed is below 0.1 ppm (up to 300:1 dilution).[333]

Beyond providing aflatoxin-free feed and therapy for liver failure, treatment for aflatoxicosis centers on prevention. Feed has been ammoniated to prevent colonization and growth of fungi and detoxify the aflatoxin. In emergencies, farmers may dilute feeds to nontoxic levels (risky).[331] Moderate levels of aflatoxins may be fed in combination with hydrated sodium calcium aluminosilicates (clay binders) to prevent aflatoxin absorption, toxicosis, and contamination in milk and meat.[344-347] However, clays should be carefully selected to avoid health risks from untested clays.[347]

Trichothecenes

The trichothecene mycotoxins are tetracyclic sesquiterpenoid toxins produced in grains (e.g., corn), and some forages, by at least six genera of fungi, the most important of which include various *Fusarium*, *Myrothecium*, *Stachybotrys atra*, and *Trichothecium roseum*.[348,349] Growth of these fungi and toxin production is favored by undulating, cool temperatures.[348,349] Trichothecenes may be present in combination with zearalenone. Toxins of major agricultural concern in the United States (in order of importance) include deoxynivalenol (DON or "vomitoxin"), T-2 toxin, stachybotryotoxin (can be in forage), and diacetoxyscirpenol (DAS), among many others.[331,348] The trichothecenes are potent inhibitors of protein synthesis, blocking initiation, elongation, and termination of ribosomal translation.[348] That mechanism leads to an effect that has been called *radiomimetic*, in which all rapidly dividing cells of the body are attacked, leading to severe gastroenteritis, skin necrosis, immune impairment, and initiation of shock.[331,348,350]

All species of animals are sensitive to the trichothecenes. The effects of trichothecene mycotoxins depend on the toxin present, its concentration, and species exposed (dairy cows and other ruminants are much less sensitive than monogastric animals). Toxicity in field cases may be greater than that reported for experimental toxicity studies, probably because related trichothecenes are often present in the field along with the toxin being assayed. For example, 10 ppm of pure DON is needed to cause feed refusal experimentally, whereas 0.5 ppm in field-contaminated grain may lead to feed refusal.[348,349,351]

Dose-dependent signs of trichothecene toxicity include feed refusal, reduced weight gains, severe gastroenteritis with vomition and diarrhea, coagulopathy and shock, skin necrosis (from direct contact), decreased reproductive performance, and immunosuppression.[331,348,349,351-353] Clinical pathologic alterations for severe trichothecene toxicosis primarily reflect shock or hemorrhagic gastroenteritis and in-

clude decreases in hematocrit, hemoglobin, leukocytes, and serum factors of glucose, calcium, and phosphate.[353,354] Bilirubin may be increased secondary to feed refusal.[353] Transiently increased liver-associated serum factors include aspartate transaminase, lactate dehydrogenase, and bromosulphalein (BSP) clearance. DON, the most common trichothecene in field cases, usually causes feed refusal, increased incidence of disease, and associated weight loss.[351-354] Other trichothecenes are likely to cause more severe, acute signs of hemorrhagic gastroenteritis, shock, and death. Diagnosis of trichothecene mycotoxicosis is assisted by finding the toxin in feed.

DON toxicosis is treated by providing mycotoxin-free feed. In addition to nonspecific therapy for signs, animals with acute trichothecene toxicosis with gastroenteritis benefit from administration of oral adsorbents such as activated charcoal along with fluid and steroid therapy for the acute shock.[355] Broad-spectrum antibiotic therapy is indicated to minimize complications of skin lesions and gastroenteritis.[331] The trichothecenes are rapidly metabolized and would not be expected to be a residue hazard after 12 to 24 hours postexposure.[352,356,357]

Fumonisin

Fumonisins are hepatotoxic, neurotoxic, and carcinogenic mycotoxins produced by *Fusarium moniliforme*. These toxins are responsible for the disease known as moldy corn poisoning of horses or equine leukoencephalomalacia.[358,359] *F. moniliforme* is ubiquitous in the environment, so testing feed for the mold is not diagnostic. Fumonisins (A and B series; fumonisin B_1 is most common) act in part by interfering with sphingolipid biosynthesis through inhibition of ceramide synthetase among other mechanisms, and by blocking protein synthesis.[360] Sphingolipids are critical for cell growth, differentiation, and transformation. Sphingolipids are present in brain and liver tissues at high levels.

Fumonisins are produced mainly on corn, especially screenings. Although other species can be affected, horses and swine are most sensitive to fumonisin's effects. Ruminants and poultry are resistant.[361,362] Fumonisin B_1 at levels of 10 ppm or greater may lead to toxicosis in horses (>40 ppm for swine). Clinical signs in horses appear suddenly after 7 to 90 days of ingesting toxic corn or screenings and may include depression, confusion, ataxia, sweating, apparent blindness, head pressing, recumbency, convulsions, and death within 5 days of onset of signs.[358,359,363,364] Morbidity is generally low, but mortality rates in affected animals are high.

Clinical pathology changes include transient increases in serum enzymes associated with liver damage. The pathognomonic lesion of fumonisin toxicosis in horses is leukoencephalomalacia, which is characterized by liquefactive necrosis of white matter of the brain, leaving fluid-filled cavities (often grossly visible).[358,364] Acutely affected horses may have centrilobular hepatic necrosis, which may be present with or without the brain lesion.[358,364] Some monogastric species may suffer from pulmonary edema.[365,366] Diagnosis of fumonisin toxicosis is aided by finding 10 ppm or more of fumonisin in a corn-based concentrate or screened feed. Elevation of the sphinganine/sphingosine ratio in the urine is a very sensitive indicator of exposure to fumonisins.

Avoiding corn in the diet of horses, or at least eliminating corn screenings from the equine diet, will help prevent fumonisin toxicosis. Not much information is available regarding fumonisin as a food animal residue. The compound is of concern, however, because it is a potent hepatocarcinogen.[367] From a food safety standpoint, fumonisin is not apparently present in milk from exposed cows in appreciable quantities, perhaps due to the low relative absorption of the

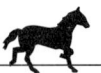

compound by the rumen.[368] Although fumonisin B$_1$ parent compound has a relatively short half-life in most studies (18 minute half-life), some evidence in swine suggests that accumulation may occur in kidney and liver tissue.[368]

Grassland Staggers

Staggers in livestock is caused by ingestion of forages that contain tremorgenic mycotoxins. Forages causing staggers include perennial ryegrass *(Lolium perenne)* infested with *Neotyphodium* (was *Acremonium) lolia* in leaf-sheaths, ergotized dallisgrass *(Paspalum dilatatum;* seed fungus is *Claviceps paspali),* Bermuda grass *(Cynodon dactylon;* mold unknown), *Phalaris* spp. (discussed earlier), moldy walnuts *(Juglans* spp.; walnut mold is *Penicillium* spp.), and although not a forage, *Aspergillus* spp. in grain.[331,369-372] The toxins are alkaloidal, indole-based paxalines and include lolitrems (perennial ryegrass), paspalitrems (dallisgrass), tryptamine alkaloids *(Phalaris),* penitrems (moldy walnuts), and aflatrems *(Aspergillus).*[331,369-373] The mechanism of action of those toxins is incompletely understood but may involve enhanced release of excitatory amino acid neurotransmitters.[374] In addition, annual grasses infested with a nematode that is subsequently infected by the bacterium *Clavibacter toxicus* may also be toxic due to production of corynetoxins. Corynetoxins are glycolipids with structures and effects similar to tunicamycin compounds. Affected grasses include annual ryegrass *(Lolium* spp.), blowgrass *(Agrostis* spp.), and *Polypogon,* especially in moist stubble and floodplains (sometimes called "floodplain staggers").[375]

The toxicity of tremorgenic forages depends on grazing habits and climate. Perennial ryegrass tends to be most hazardous late in the grazing season, when grass is grazed low to the ground (lolitrems are found in the lower leaf sheaths so are more of a hazard for sheep).[369,376,377] Dallisgrass is hazardous when ergotized seed heads are grazed (more of a hazard for cattle).[372] All species exposed to the staggers toxins may be affected. Dried perennial ryegrass, and perennial ryegrass seeds may retain toxicity.[377,378] Signs of staggers appear within 7 days of initial grazing (within hours for penitrems in walnut).[331,369] Animals appear normal at rest or may have a fine tremor in the ear and head. When stimulated, affected animals have a characteristic stiff, spastic gait, followed by spasms and tetanic seizures (opisthotonos occurs in severe cases).[331,369,376,379] Recovery from an episode may be rapid for perennial ryegrass, dallisgrass, and Bermuda grass staggers if animals are not stressed. Losses occur, however, from misadventure (e.g., injuries, drowning, becoming trapped during seizure episodes).[369] Seizure episodes dissipate within 2 weeks after animals are removed from the toxic forage. Annual ryegrass toxicity cases appear following floods or upon grazing pastures with large amounts of stubble from the previous year. CNS signs include ataxia, convulsions, and other signs consistent with grassland staggers. Death often occurs within 24 hours.[375]

Lesions of staggers are minimal, although degeneration of cerebellar Purkinje cells has been reported for longer-standing, severe cases of perennial ryegrass staggers.[380,381] Postmortem, lesions from annual grass staggers from corynetoxins include a fatty liver and cerebellar degeneration.[375] Diagnosis of staggers syndromes is helped by ruling out other tremorgenic syndromes, identification of the fungus (e.g., for perennial ryegrass), and identification of the toxin in the plant (lolitrem B in perennial ryegrass).[369] If forage toxins are not available for analysis, bioassay using an extract of the forage in the laboratory can be diagnostic.[369,382]

Alternate forage should be provided for affected animals until new pasture growth is available. Some managers move animals away from the toxic pasture during the sensitive periods. Affected animals are placed in areas where misadventure can be minimized. Mowing the seed heads is suggested to minimize effects of ergotized dallisgrass.

Fescue Toxicosis

Fescue toxicosis is common throughout the United States. Tall fescue grass *(Festuca arundinacea)* infested by *Neotyphodium* (was *Acremonium) coenophialum* and strains of perennial ryegrass *(Lolium perenne)* infested by *Neotyphodium* (was *Acremonium) lolia* (also produces staggers toxins) produce ergot-type alkaloids like ergovaline and pyrrolizidine-type alkaloids (loline).[383-385] The ergot alkaloids act by interacting with dopaminergic neurotransmission and blocking prolactin.[386,387] The presence of endophyte may also be associated with lower copper levels in the fescue grass, contributing to copper deficiency in areas with marginal copper in forages.[388]

Toxicity of tall fescue depends on the ambient weather and reproductive stage of exposed animals.[384] During warm conditions, cattle, sheep, and horses suffer from summer syndrome, which is characterized by increased rectal temperatures, lethargy, ill-thrift, failure to gain weight, and intolerance to ambient heat.[389-391] The breeds of cattle *(Bos indicus* vs. *Bos taurus)* are apparently alike in their sensitivity to ergot alkaloids from fescue.[392] This summer syndrome may be in part a result of alterations of hormonal (plasma cortisol and T$_3$) and vascular controls of body temperature.[393,394] During cool conditions, cattle may develop typical ergot-type lesions of dry gangrene in the distal extremities.[395-397] Perhaps the most devastating aspect of tall fescue toxicosis is reproductive failure, which is characterized by agalactia, prolonged gestation, weak offspring, stillbirths, and thickened placentas (horses and cattle).[384,398,399]

Lesions of fescue toxicosis are nonspecific. Serum prolactin, progesterone, and dopamine concentrations are decreased in exposed animals.[386,387] Postmortem, fat necrosis with foci of hard nodules in the omental region may be present in animals with summer syndrome and ergotlike gangrene is present in distal extremities for animals with fescue foot.[384] Diagnosis of tall fescue toxicosis is helped by demonstration of the endophyte or toxins in grass.

Pregnant animals should be removed from tall fescue pastures by 30 to 60 days before parturition. Some farms have successfully used herbicides to kill the tall fescue, planted an annual crop the next year, and then followed by planting of endophyte-free tall fescue, which is now available.[384] Experimental vaccination and treatments with dopamine antagonists such as domperidone are being investigated to treat fescue toxicity.[400,401]

Other Mycotoxins

ERGOT. Classic ergot results from parasitism of developing grass or grain flowers by *Claviceps purpurea,* leading to formation of a dark sclerotium on the seed heads. Several wild grasses and grains such as rye, triticale, wheat, oats, sorghum, and barley may be affected. Affected grains contain a series of alkaloids including ergotamine, ergonovine, and ergotaxine (also found in fescue, see earlier). Ergotism in livestock may cause ataxia, convulsions, lameness, dyspnea, diarrhea, dry gangrene of the extremities much like fescue foot, abortion, neonatal mortality, reduced lactation (ergot alkaloids have been used medicinally for uterotropic effects), poor weight gains, lowered production, and lowered feed intake.[402,403]

ZEARALENONE. Zearalenone is an estrogenic mycotoxin produced in corn and other grains by various *Fusarium* spp. (especially *F. roseum)* under similar warm and cold climatic cycles as for trichothecenes (zearalenone is often found with

DON). Prepuberal swine and dairy cows are the most sensitive animals to zearalenone. Corn contaminated with zearalenone may cause toxicosis at levels as low as 1 ppm, a level well below the toxicity of pure toxin, suggesting the presence of other estrogenic metabolites in field samples. Zearalenone can be metabolized to the more toxic zearalenol. Zearalenone causes chronic hyperestrogenism with vulvar swelling, prolapsed rectum, enlarged mammary glands, reduced fertility, and feminization of swine and cattle. Although zearalenone may be distributed to milk and meat, medically significant residues would not be expected in products from animals exposed to grain with natural zearalenone contamination.[404,405]

SLAFRAMINE. Slaframine is an indolizidine alkaloid mycotoxin produced by black batch mold (*Rhizoctonia leguminicola*) contamination in moldy red clover forage (including hay, *Trifolium repens*). Slaframine causes increased salivation, diarrhea, and bloat in affected cattle and horses.[406,407]

OCHRATOXIN. Ochratoxin is an isocoumarin derivative of phenylalanine. Feeding of over 0.2 to 4 ppm in grain to livestock can cause nephropathy. Monogastric animals such as swine and horses are more sensitive than ruminants, although young ruminants may be susceptible to levels of ochratoxin above 2 to 40 ppm in the grain. Liver damage, enteritis, reduced growth rates, and abortion also have been reported. Citrinin, another nephrotoxic mycotoxin, might be found along with ochratoxin in a contaminated grain sample.[404]

ZOOTOXINS

A variety of lizards, insects, arachnids, ticks, and bees may cause toxicosis in animals.[408] The incidence of such envenomations (bites) and poisonings (ingestion of toxic animals or insects) is for the most part rare and requires symptomatic treatment and removal of the toxic source. Two more common toxic and venomous syndromes of livestock are discussed here.

■ **VENOMOUS SNAKES**

Crotalus spp.: Rattlesnakes
Sistrurus spp.: Pigmy rattlesnakes
Agkistrodon spp.: Copperhead; *A. piscivorus*: Cottonmouth
Micrurus spp.: Coral snakes

The pit vipers *Crotalus* (rattlesnakes) and *Agkistrodon* spp. are responsible for most of the reported envenomations of animals in North America. A pit organ and large, hollow fangs through which venom is passed into the victim characterize pit vipers. Envenomation by Elapidae or the coral snakes is possible in North America, but rarely reported. Coral snakes chew their venom into the victim. Crotalid venom largely consists of toxic proteins (>90% is protein).[408] The toxins include proteolytic and phospholipase enzymes, coagulation and hemorrhagic toxins (affecting the clotting cascade), myotoxins, and in the Mojave rattlesnake a potent paralytic neurotoxin.[409,410] Coral snakes produce neurotoxins. The effects of pit viper envenomation include anaphylactoid reactions with hemolysis and shock in systemically affected animals, and extensive local edema and necrosis near the bite from the proteolytic and myotoxic proteins (local effects are more common in large livestock).[411]

Livestock are commonly bitten in the extremities and muzzle by snakes. The severity of effects depends on the size of the snake (larger snake = larger possible envenomation), the size of the victim (smaller animal = more severe effects), the severity of the strike (one or two punctures and the amount of venom injected), and the location of the bite (central vs. extremities).[408,412] Systemic effects vary depending on the crotalid species. For example, Eastern diamondback rattlesnakes may cause more hemolytic effects, the Mojave rattlesnake may be more neurotoxic, and the Western dia-

mondback may cause more cardiovascular shock and local effects. Systemic signs include weakness, syncope, and hypotension. Mojave rattlesnake envenomations may result in respiratory distress and other signs of neurologic paralysis. Large livestock are more at risk from the local, rather than systemic, effects of rattlesnakes. Signs in the bite region include pitting edema and pain within 20 minutes. Edema progresses rapidly and may involve an entire limb within hours. The skin may have ecchymoses and can become quite turgid. Untreated, local necrosis and effects may not peak until 4 days after envenomation.[411]

Common clinical pathologic abnormalities in animals with systemic envenomation include reduction of erythrocyte numbers (hemolysis), hypofibrinogenemia, and thrombocytopenia. Clotting parameters are prolonged. Serum enzyme alterations reflect local tissue and muscle damage (especially high concentrations of creatine kinase). The urine may contain protein, glucose, and blood.[408] Pathologic alterations in large animals include local tissue damage. Severe insect/bee stings, trauma, abscessation, and in the horse, purpura hemorrhagica, should be ruled out in the diagnosis of a snakebite.[408]

Initial treatment of snakebite in horses and large animals bitten near the nose requires maintenance of airway patency. A hose or tube can be placed in a nostril if treatment is initiated promptly. Otherwise tracheostomy may be indicated. Snakebites are optimal environments for a variety of infectious organisms, requiring treatment with broad-spectrum antibiotics. However, for systemically affected human patients, the use of prophylactic antibiotic therapy for snakebite is becoming controversial.[413] Horses especially should be given tetanus prophylaxis. Antiinflammatory treatment should be initiated using a nonsteroidal antiinflammatory drug such as phenylbutazone. Local wound care and debridement should be performed. Corticosteroids and fluid therapy are rarely indicated in large animals unless systemic shock develops (very unlikely). Expense, marginal efficacy at the local site, and side effects argue against antivenin use in the horse. Systemic treatment of crotalid-induced neurotoxicity has been accomplished in human medicine using a polyspecific Fab antibody.[414] Antihistamine therapy is controversial and is not recommended for horses.

■ **BLISTER BEETLE**

Epicauta spp.: Blister beetles

Alfalfa and other blooming hays may attract blister beetles. Blister beetles can contain from 0.1% to 12% of cantharidin (dry weight).[415] Cantharidin is a potent vesicant toxin that causes necrosis of all mucous membranes to which it comes into contact.

Although blister beetles may be found throughout the United States, conditions favoring swarming and toxicity in livestock hay occur in the midwestern United States. Cases have been reported between the region bounded by Florida to Arizona, north to Colorado, Minnesota, and Illinois.[415] Beetles tend to swarm when alfalfa (or nearby weeds) is in bloom and when conditions favor increases in the grasshopper population.[416] Harvest techniques that use a windrower type of machine that cuts, crimps or conditions, and piles hay (unlike classic practices that mow hay, then rake it without crimping) will trap the beetles in the hay, leading to possible toxicity.[415,416] The beetles retain toxicity in dried hay (4 to 6 g of dried beetles, equivalent to about 100 beetles, may be fatal).[415-417] All classes of herbivorous livestock may be affected, although most cases have been reported for horses. Animals with blister beetle toxicosis develop colic, gastroenteritis, nonspecific neurologic signs, increased urination, cystitis, shock, and death. Shock and death alone may be reported in severely poisoned horses.

Clinical pathologic alterations reflect dehydration, shock, and renal damage. Hemoconcentration occurs despite decreased levels of protein, calcium and magnesium in the serum.[415,417] The serum has increased levels of creatine kinase, BUN, and creatinine. Renal damage is also reflected by decreases in urine specific gravity despite dehydration and shock. Hypocalcemia and hypomagnesemia are also likely to occur.[418] Postmortem lesions include hemorrhagic gastroenteritis (including oral); pale, moist, swollen kidneys; and hemorrhagic damage to the urinary tract. In some cases that involve sudden death, lesions may be absent. Histologic alterations include inflammation and hemorrhage with ulceration of the gastrointestinal tract, bladder mucosa, ureters, and renal pelvis.[415,417] Direct myocardial necrosis may occur in severe cases.[417] Diagnosis of cantharidin toxicosis is assisted by identification of beetles in hay or ingesta and chemical analysis for cantharidin in beetles, ingesta, blood, and urine (urine may have from 0.0005 to 2.0 ppm of cantharidin).[415,418]

Blister beetle toxicosis can be prevented through proper harvest of hay by avoiding times when beetles swarm, managing flowering weeds, controlling grasshoppers, avoiding full bloom during cutting, and if possible avoiding use of crimpers and conditioning equipment during hazardous times.[416] Insecticides should be avoided when hay is in full bloom (bees essential for alfalfa crops may be harmed). Livestock with blister beetle toxicosis should have toxic hay removed from the diet (destroy hay; the toxin does not dissipate with time) and treated aggressively for shock and renal failure (fluid replacement).[415,417]

REFERENCES

1. Nielsen DB, James LF: The economic impacts of livestock poisonings by plants. In James LF et al, eds: *Poisonous plants, proceedings of the third international symposium,* Ames, Iowa, 1992, Iowa State University Press, pp 3-10.
2. Osweiler GD et al: *Clinical and diagnostic veterinary toxicology,* Dubuque, Iowa, 1985, Kendall/Hunt, pp 460-467.
3. Galey FD: Poisonous plant diagnostics in California. In Colegate SM, Dorling PR, eds: *Plant-associated toxins: agricultural, phytochemical, and ecological aspects,* Wallingford, UK, 1994, CAB International, pp 101-106.
4. Williams MC, James LF: Effects of herbicides on the concentration of poisonous compounds in plants: a review, *Am J Vet Res* 44:2420-2422, 1983.
5. Osweiler GD et al: *Clinical and diagnostic veterinary toxicology,* Dubuque, Iowa, 1985, Kendall/Hunt, pp 455-459.
6. Galey FD et al: Diagnosis of oleander poisoning in livestock, *J Vet Diagn Invest* 8:358-364, 1996.
7. Holstege DM, Seiber JN, Galey FD: A rapid mulitiresidue screen for alkaloids in plant material and biological samples, *J Agric Food Chem* 43:691-699, 1995.
8. Picchioni AL: Efficacy of activated charcoal, *Vet Hum Toxicol* 25:452-453, 1983.
9. Ralphs MH et al: Plant-animal interactions in larkspur poisoning in cattle, *J Anim Sci* 66:2334-2342, 1988.
10. Merrill LB, Schuster JL: Grazing management practices affect livestock losses from poisonous plants, *J Range Mgmt* 31:351-354, 1978.
11. Panter KE, James LF: Natural plant toxicants in milk: a review, *J Anim Sci* 68:892-904, 1990.
12. Cheeke PR: *Natural toxicants in feeds, forages, and poisonous plants,* ed 2, Danville, Ill, 1998, Interstate, pp 76-77.
13. Kingsbury JM: *Poisonous plants of the United States and Canada,* Englewood Cliffs, NJ, 1964, Prentice-Hall, pp 1-626.
14. Cheeke PR, Shull LR: *Natural toxicants in feeds and poisonous plants,* Westport, Conn, 1985, AVI, pp 5-6.
15. James LF, Hartley WJ, Van Kampen KR: Syndromes of *Astragalus* poisoning in livestock, *J Am Vet Med Assoc* 178:146-149, 1981.
16. Molyneux RJ, James LF: Loco intoxication: indolizidine alkaloids of spotted locoweed (*Astragalus lentiginosus*), *Science* 216:190-191, 1982.
17. Dorling PR, Huxtable CR, Colgate SM: Inhibition of lysosomal alpha mannosidase by swainsonine, and indolizidine alkaloid from *Swainsona canescens, Biochem J* 191:649-651, 1980.
18. Tulsiani DRP, Touster O: Swainsonine, a potent mannosidase inhibitor, elevates rat liver and brain lysosomal alpha-*d*-mannosidase, decreases golgi alpha-*D*-mannosidase II, and increases the plasma levels of several acid hydrolases, *Arch Biochem Biophys* 224:594-600, 1983.
19. Tulsiani DRP et al: The similar effects of swainsonine and locoweed on tissue glycosidase and oligosaccharides of the pig indicating that the alkaloid is the principal toxin responsible for the induction of locoism, *Arch Biochem Biophys* 232:76-85, 1984.
20. March CD: The locoweed disease, USDA Farmers Bulletin 380, 1912.
21. Ralphs MH, Graham D, James LF: Social facilitation influences cattle to graze locoweed, *J Range Mgmt* 47:123-126, 1994.
22. James LF et al: Locoweed disease, *Clin Toxicol* 2:13-20, 1969.
23. James LF W et al: Abortive and teratogenic effects of locoweed on sheep and cattle, *Am J Vet Res* 28:1379-1388, 1967.
24. Panter KE et al: The relationship of *Oxytropis sericea* (green and dry) and *Astragalus lentiginosus* with high mountain disease in cattle, *Vet Hum Toxicol* 30:318-323, 1988.
25. James LF et al: Relationship between ingestion of the locoweed (*Oxytropis sericea*) and congestive right-sided heart failure in cattle, *Am J Vet Res* 44:254-259, 1983.
26. James LF, Van Kampen KR, Staker GR: Locoweed (*Astragalus lentiginosus*) poisoning in cattle and horses, *J Am Vet Med Assoc* 155:525-530, 1969.
27. McIlwraith CW, James LF: Limb deformities in foals associated with ingestion of locoweed by mares, *J Am Vet Med Assoc* 181:255-258, 1982.
28. James LF, Binns W: Blood changes associated with locoweed poisoning, *Am J Vet Res* 28:1107-1110, 1967.
29. Panter KE et al: Effects of Locoweed (*Oxytropis sericea*) on reproduction in cows with a history of locoweed consumption, *Vet Hum Toxicol* 41:282-286, 1999.
30. Panter KE et al: Locoweeds: effects on reproduction in livestock, *J Nat Toxins* 8:53-62, 1998.
31. James LF, Van Kampen KR, Johnson AE: Physiopathologic changes in locoweed poisoning of livestock, *Am J Vet Res* 31:663-672, 1970.
32. Van Kampen KR, James LF: Pathology of locoweed poisoning in sheep, *Vet Pathol* 6:413-423, 1969.
33. Hartley WJ, James LF: Microscopic lesions in fetuses of ewes ingesting locoweed (*Astragalus lentiginosus*), *Am J Vet Res* 34:209-211, 1973.
34. James LF, Van Kampen KR: Acute and residual lesions of locoweed poisoning in cattle and horses, *J Am Vet Med Assoc* 158:614-618, 1971.
35. Alroy J et al: Swainsonine toxicosis mimics lectin histochemistry of mannosidosis, *Vet Pathol* 22:311-316, 1985.
36. Stegelmeier BL et al: Serum swainsonine concentration and alpha-mannosidase activity in cattle and sheep ingesting *Oxytropis sericea* and *Astragalus lentiginosus* (locoweeds), *Am J Vet Res* 56:149-154, 1995.
37. James LF, Hartley WJ: Effects of milk from animals fed locoweed in kittens, calves, and lambs, *Am J Vet Res* 38:1263-1265, 1977.
38. Stegelmeier BL et al: The pathogenesis and toxicokinetics of locoweed (*Astragalus lentiginosus*) in livestock, *J Nat Toxins* 8:35-45, 1999.
39. Cheeke PR: *Natural toxicants in feeds, forages, and poisonous plants,* ed 2, Danville, Ill, 1998, Interstate, pp 383-352.
40. Cheeke PR: Toxicity and metabolism of pyrrolizidine alkaloids, *J Anim Sci* 66:2343-2350, 1988.
41. Segall HG et al: Trans-4-hydroxy-2-hexenal: a reactive metabolite from the macro-cyclic pyrrolizidine alkaloid senecionine, *Science* 229:472-475, 1985.
42. Huan JY et al: Species differences in the hepatic microsomal enzyme metabolism of the pyrrolizidine alkaloids, *Toxicol Lett* 99:127-137, 1998.
43. Deol HS, Dorling PR, Thomas JB: Experimental copper and heliotrope intoxication in sheep: morphological changes, *J Comp Pathol* 105:49-74, 1991.
44. Mendel VE et al: Pyrrolizidine alkaloid-induced liver disease in horses: an early diagnosis, *Am J Vet Res* 49:572-578, 1988.
45. Molyneux RJ, Johnson AE, Stuart CD: Delayed manifestation of Senecio-induced pyrrolizidine alkaloidosis in cattle: case reports, *Vet Hum Toxicol* 30:201-205, 1988.
46. Smith BP: Pyrrolizidine alkaloid-induced hepatic disease in a group of calves, *Compend Cont Educ* 4:S531-S533, 1982.
47. Stegelmeier BL: The clinico-pathologic changes of *Cynoglossum officinale,* houndstongue intoxication in horses (abstract), *Fourth International Symposium on Poisonous Plants,* Sept 27-Oct 1, 1993.
48. Araya O et al: Serum changes and histological liver lesions due to experimental ingestion of ragwort (*Senecio erraticus*) in sheep, *Vet Hum Toxicol* 25:4-7, 1983.
49. Seawright AA et al: The identification of hepatotoxic pyrrolizidine alkaloid exposure in horses by the demonstration of sulphur-bound pyrrolic metabolites on their hemoglobin, *Vet Hum Toxicol* 33:286-287, 1991.
50. Schoch TK, Gardner DR, Stegelmeier BL: GC/MS/MS detection of pyrrolic metabolites in animals poisoned with the pyrrolizidine alkaloid riddelliine, *J Nat Toxins* 9:197-206, 2000.
51. Yan CC, Huxtable RJ: Relationship between glutathione concentrations and metabolism of the pyrrolizidine alkaloid, monocrotaline in the isolated, perfused liver, *Toxicol Appl Pharmacol* 30:132-139, 1995.
52. Candrian U et al: Transfer of orally administered [³H] seneciophylline into cow's milk, *J Agric Food Chem* 39:930-933, 1991.
53. Kingsbury JM: *Poisonous plants of the United States and Canada,* Englewood Cliffs, NJ, 1964, Prentice-Hall, pp 125-140.
54. Cronin EH, Nielsen DB: The ecology and control of rangeland larkspurs, Logan Utah, 1979, Utah Agricultural Experiment Station, Bulletin 499.
55. Olsen JD, Manners GD: Toxicology of diterpenoid alkaloids in rangeland larkspur (*Delphinium* spp). In Cheeke PR, ed: *Toxicants of plant origin,* vol 1, *Alkaloids,* Boca Raton, Fla, 1989, CRC Press, pp 291-326.
56. Majak W, McDonald RE, Binn MH: Isolation and HPLC determination of methyllacaconitine in a species of low larkspur (*Delphinium nuttalianum*), *J Agric Food Chem* 35:800-802, 1987.

57. Manners GD et al: The toxic evaluation of norditerpenoid alkaloids in 3 tall larkspur *(Delphinium)* species, *Fourth International Symposium on Poisonous Plants,* Freemantle, W Austr, Sept 27-Oct 1, 1993 (abstract).

58. Pfister JA et al: Larkspur (Delphinium spp.) poisoning in livestock, *J Nat Toxins* 8:81-94, 1999.

59. Cheeke PR, Shull LR: *Natural toxicants in feeds and poisonous plants,* Westport, Conn, 1985, AVI, pp 140-142.

60. Ralphs MH et al: Plant-animal interactions in larkspur poisoning in cattle, *J Anim Sci* 66:2334-2342, 1988.

61. Manners GD JA et al: The phenological variation of diterpenoid alkaloids in tall larkspur *(Delphinium barbeyi).* In James LF et al, eds: *Poisonous Plants, Proceedings of the Third International Symposium,* Ames, Iowa, 1992, Iowa State University Press, pp 309-313.

62. Olsen JD: Tall larkspur poisoning in cattle and sheep, *J Am Vet Med Assoc* 173:762-765, 1978.

63. Olsen JD, Sisson DV: Description of a scale for rating the clinical response of cattle poisoned by larkspur, *Am J Vet Res* 52:488-493, 1991.

64. Galey FD: Poisonous plant diagnostics in California (abstract). *Fourth International Symposium on Poisonous Plants,* Freemantle, W Austr, Sept 27-Oct 1, 1993.

65. Olsen JD, Ralphs MH: Feed aversion induced by intraruminal infusion with larkspur extract in cattle, *Am J Vet Res* 47:1829-1833, 1986.

66. Bush LP, Crowe MW: Nicotiana alkaloids. In Cheeke PR, ed: *Toxicants of plant origin,* vol 1, *Alkaloids,* Boca Raton, Fla, 1989, CRC Press, pp 87-107.

67. Panter KE, Keeler RF: Piperidine alkaloids of poison hemlock *(Conium maculatum).* In Cheeke PR, ed: *Toxicants of plant origin,* vol 1, *Alkaloids,* Boca Raton, Fla, 1989, CRC Press, pp 109-132.

68. Panter KE et al: Radio ultrasound observations of the fetotoxic effects in sheep from ingestion of *Conium maculatum* (poison hemlock), *Clin Toxicol* 26:175-187, 1988.

69. Keeler RF: Teratogens in plants, *J Anim Sci* 58:1029-1039, 1984.

70. Keeler RF, Crowe MW, Lambert EA: Teratogenicity in swine of the tobacco alkaloid anabasine isolated from nicotiana glauca, *Teratology* 30:61-69, 1984.

71. Panter KE, Bunch TD, Keeler RF: Maternal and fetal toxicity of poison hemlock *(Conium maculatum)* in sheep, *Am J Vet Res* 489:281-283, 1988.

72. Keeler RF: Livestock models of human birth defects, reviewed in relation to poisonous plants, *J Anim Sci* 66:2414-2427, 1988.

73. Baker DC, Keeler RF: *Thermopsis montana*-induced myopathy in calves, *J Am Vet Med Assoc* 194:1269-1272, 1989.

74. Cheeke PR, Shull LR: *Natural toxicants in feeds and poisonous plants,* Westport, Conn, 1985, AVI, pp 127-131.

75. Casper HH et al: Lupin bean meal toxicosis in swine, *J Vet Diagn Invest* 3:172-173, 1991.

76. Galey FD, Holstege DM, Fisher EG: Toxicosis in dairy cattle exposed to poison hemlock *(Conium maculatum)* in hay: isolation of *Conium* alkaloids in plants, hay, and urine, *J Vet Diagn Invest* 4:60-64, 1992.

77. Cheeke PR, Shull LR: *Natural toxicants in feeds and poisonous plants,* Westport, Conn, 1985, AVI, pp 115-120.

78. Keeler RF et al: Teratogenicity and toxicity of coniine in cows, ewes, and mares, *Cornell Vet* 70:19-26, 1980.

79. Plumlee KH et al: *Nicotiana glauca* toxicosis of cattle *J Vet Diagn Invest* 5:498-499, 1993.

80. Panter KE, Keeler RF, Baker DC: Toxicosis in livestock from the hemlocks *(Conium* and *Cicuta* spp), *J Anim Sci* 66:2407-2013, 1988.

81. Panter KE, Keeler RF, Buck WB: Congenital skeletal malformations induced by maternal ingestion of *Conium maculatum* (poison hemlock) in newborn pigs, *Am J Vet Res* 46:2064-2066, 1985.

82. Gardner DR, Panter KE: Comparison of blood plasma alkaloid levels in cattle, sheep, and goats fed *Lupinus caudatus, J Nat Toxins* 2:1-11, 1993.

83. Panter KE, James LF: Natural toxicants in milk: a review, *J Anim Sci* 68:892-904, 1990.

84. Lopez TA, Cid MS, Bianchini ML: Biochemistry of hemlock *(Conium maculatum* L.) alkaloids and their acute and chronic toxicity in livestock. A review, *Toxicon* 37:841-865, 1999.

85. Cheeke PR: *Natural toxicants in feeds, forages, and poisonous plants,* ed 2, Danville, Ill, 1998, Interstate, pp 393-394.

86. Knight AP: *Veratrum californicum* poisoning, *Compend Cont Educ* 11:528-531, 1989.

87. Kingsbury JM: *Poisonous plants of the United States and Canada,* Englewood Cliffs, NJ, 1964, Prentice-Hall, p 289.

88. Keeler RF, Binns W: Teratogenic compounds of *Veratrum californicum, Teratology* 1:5-10, 1968.

89. Sharma RP, Salunkhe DK: *Solanum* glycoalkaloids. In Cheeke PR ed: *Toxicants of plant origin,* vol 1, *Alkaloids,* Boca Raton, Fla, 1989, CRC Press, pp 179-236.

90. Schlosberg A et al: The effect of feeding dried tomato vines to beef cattle, *Vet Hum Toxicol* 38:135-136, 1996.

91. Binns W, Keeler RF, Balls LD: Congenital deformation in lambs, calves, and goats resulting from maternal ingestion of *Veratrum californicum, Clin Toxicol* 5:245-261, 1972.

92. Binns W et al: Chronologic evaluation of teratogenicity in sheep fed *Veratrum californicum, J Am Vet Med Assoc* 247:839-842, 1965.

93. Keeler RF, Stuart LD: The nature of congenital limb defects induced in lambs by maternal ingestion of *Veratrum californicum, Clin Toxicol* 25:273-286, 1987.

94. Cheeke PR: *Natural toxicants in feeds, forages, and poisonous plants,* ed 2, Danville, Ill, 1998, Interstate, pp 382-383.

95. Galey FD et al: Residues of *Datura* species in horse. In Auer D, Houghten E, eds: *Proceedings of the Eleventh International Conference of Racing Analysts and Veterinarians, Queensland, Australia,* Newmarket, England, 1996, R & W, pp 333-337.

96. Schulman ML, Bolton LA: Datura seed intoxication in two horses, *J S Afr Vet Assoc* 69:27-29, 1998.

97. Piva G, Piva A: Anti-nutritional factors of *Datura* in feedstuffs, *Nat Toxins* 3:238-241, 1995.

98. Alden CL et al: Japanese yew poisoning of large domestic animals in the midwest, *J Am Vet Med Assoc* 170:314-316, 1977.

99. Smythies JR et al: The action of the alkaloids from yew *(Taxus baccata)* on the action potential in the *Xenopus* medullated axon, *Experientia* 15:337-338, 1975.

100. Vidensek N A et al: Taxol content in bark, wood, root, leaf, twig, and seedling from several *Taxus* species, *J Nat Prod* 53:1609-1610, 1990.

101. Lowe JE et al: *Taxus cuspidata* (Japanese yew) poisoning in horses, *Cornell Vet* 60:36-39, 1969.

102. Ogden L: *Taxus* (yews): a highly toxic plant, *Vet Hum Toxicol* 30:563-564, 1988.

103. Kite GC, Lawrence TJ, Dauncey EA: Detecting *Taxus* poisoning in horses using liquid chromatography/mass spectrometry, *Vet Hum Toxicol* 42:151-154, 2000.

104. Culvenor CCJ, Dal Bon R, Smith LW: The occurrence of indolealkylamine alkaloid in *Phalaris tuberosa* L and *P. arundinacea* L, *Aust J Chem* 17:1301-1304, 1964.

105. Cheeke PR: *Natural toxicants in feeds, forages, and poisonous plants,* ed 2, Danville, Ill, 1998, Interstate, pp 275-278.

106. Gallagher CH et al: The toxicity of *Phalaris tuberosa* for sheep, *Nature* 204:542-545, 1964.

107. Gallagher CH, Koch JH, Hoffman H: Deaths of ruminants grazing *Phalaris tuberosa* in Australia, *Aust Vet J* 43:495-500, 1967.

108. McDonald IW: A "staggers" syndrome in sheep and cattle associated with grazing *Phalaris tuberosa, Aus Vet J* 18:182-188, 1942.

109. East NE, Higgins RJ: Canarygrass *(Phalaris* spp) toxicosis in sheep in California, *J Am Vet Med Assoc* 192:667-669, 1988.

110. Colegate SM et al: Suspected blue canary grass *(Phalaris coerulescens)* poisoning of horses, *Aust Vet J* 77:537-538.

111. Lean IJ et al: Tryptamine alkaloid toxicosis in feedlot sheep, *J Am Vet Med Assoc* 195:768-771, 1989.

112. Cheeke PR, Shull LR: *Natural toxicants in feeds and poisonous plants,* Westport, Conn, 1985, AVI, pp 148-152.

113. Lee HJ, Kuchel RB: The aetiology of *Phalaris* staggers in sheep, *Aust J Agric Res* 4:88-99, 1953.

114. Cheeke PR, Shull LR: *Natural toxicants in feeds and poisonous plants,* Westport, Conn, 1985, AVI, p 9.

115. Kingsbury JM: *Poisonous plants of the United States and Canada,* Englewood Cliffs, NJ, 1964, Prentice-Hall, pp 264-267.

116. Joubert JPJ: Cardiac glycosides. In Cheeke PR, ed: *Toxicants of plant origin,* vol II, *Glycosides,* Boca Raton, Fla, 1989, CRC Press, 61-96.

117. Adams HR: Digitalis and other inotropic agents and vasodilator drugs. In Booth NH, McDonald LE, eds: *Veterinary pharmacology and therapeutics,* ed 6, Ames, Iowa, 1988, Iowa State University Press, pp 495-577.

118. Szabuniewicz JD, McCrady JD, Camp BJ: Treatment of experimentally induced oleander poisoning, *Arch Intern Pharmacodynam* 189:12-21, 1971.

119. Ansford A et al: Oleander poisoning, *Toxicon* 3:(suppl)15-16, 1983.

120. Knight AP: Oleander poisoning, *Compend Cont Educ* 10:262-263, 1988.

121. Knight AP: Rhododendron and laurel poisoning, *Compend Cont Educ* 9:F26-F27, 1987.

122. Everist SL: *Poisonous plants of Australia,* ed 2, London, 1981, Angus and Robertson, pp 77-89.

123. Mahin L, Marzou A, Huart A: A case report of *Nerium oleander* poisoning in cattle, *Vet Hum Toxicol* 26:303-304, 1984.

124. Galey FD et al: Toxicity and diagnosis of oleander *(Nerium oleander)* poisoning in livestock. In Garland T, Barr AC, eds: *Toxic plants and other natural toxicants,* Wallingford, UK, 1998, CAB International, pp 215-219.

125. Tracqui A et al: Confirmation of oleander poisoning by HPLC/MS, *Int J Legal Med* 111:32-34, 1998.

126. Osterloh J, Herold S, Pond S: Oleander interference in the digoxin RIA in a fatal ingestion, *J Am Med Assoc* 247:1596-1597, 1982.

127. Haber E: Antibodies and digitalis: the modern revolution in the use of an ancient drug, *J Am Coll Cardiol* 5:111A-117A, 1985.

128. Shumaik GM, Wu AW, Ping AC: Oleander poisoning: treatment with digoxin-specific Fab antibody fragments, *Ann Emerg Med* 17:732-735, 1988.

129. Camp BJ et al: Isolation of a steroidal sapogenin from the bile of sheep fed *Agave lechuguilla, Vet Hum Toxicol* 30:533-535, 1988.

130. Kellerman TS et al: Photosensitivity in South Africa. VI, The experimental induction of geeldikkop in sheep with crude steroidal saponins from *Tribulus terrestris, Onderstepoort J Vet Res* 58:47-53, 1991.

131. Miles CO et al: Identification of a sapogenin glucuronide in the bile of sheep affected by *Panicum dichotomiflorum* toxicosis, *N Z Vet J* 39:150, 1991.

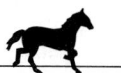

132. Miles CO et al: Indentification of insoluble salts of the beta-D-glucuronide of episarsapogenin and epismilagenin in the bile of lambs with aveld, and examination of *Nartecium ossifragum, Tribulus terrestris,* and *Panicum miliaceum* for sapogenins, *J Agric Food Chem* 41:914-917, 1993.

133. Miles CO: Role of saponins in hepatogenous photosensitization, *N Z Vet J* 41:221, 1993 (abstract).

134. Smith BL, Miles CO: A role for *Brachiaria decumbens* in hepatogenous photosensitization of ruminants, *Vet Hum Toxicol* 35:256-257, 1993.

135. Low SG et al: Photosensitization of cattle grazing signal grass *(Brachiaria decumbens)* in Papua New Guinea, *N Z Vet J* 41:220-221, 1993.

136. Cornick JL, Carter GK, Bridges CH: Kleingrass-associated hepatotoxicosis in horses, *J Am Vet Med Assoc* 193:932-935, 1988.

137. Bridges CH et al: Kleingrass *(Panicum coloratum* L) poisoning in sheep, *Vet Pathol* 24:525-531, 1987.

138. Mathews FP: Lechuguilla *(Agave lechuguilla)* poisoning in sheep and goats, *J Am Vet Med Assoc* 93:168-175, 1938.

139. Langseth W et al: Isolation and characterization of 3 methoxy-2(5H)-furanone as the principal nephrotoxin from *Nartecium ossifragum* (L) Huds, *Nat Toxins* 7:111-118, 1999.

140. Osweiler GD et al: *Clinical and diagnostic veterinary toxicology,* Dubuque, Iowa, 1985, Kendall/Hunt, p 455-459.

141. Tewe OO, Iyayi EA: Cyanogenic glycosides. In Cheeke PR, ed: *Toxicants of plant origin,* vol II, *Glycosides* Boca Raton, Fla, 1989, CRC Press, pp 44-60.

142. Morgan SE, Johnson B, Brewer B: Sorghum cystitis ataxia syndrome in horses, *Vet Hum Toxicol* 32:582, 1990.

143. McKenzie RA, McMicking L: Ataxia and urinary incontinence in cattle grazing sorghum, *Aust Vet J* 53:496-497, 1977.

144. Bradley GA et al: Neuroaxonal degeneration in sheep grazing sorghum pastures, *J Vet Diagn Invest* 7:229-236, 1995.

145. Burrows GE: Cyanide intoxication in sheep: therapeutics, *Vet Hum Toxicol* 23:22-28, 1981.

146. Stermitz FR, Norris FA, Williams MC: Miserotoxin, a new naturally occurring nitrocompound, *J Am Chem Soc* 91:4599, 1969.

147. Majak W, Benn MH: New glycosides of 3-nitropropanol from *Astragalus miser* var *serotinus.* In James LF et al, eds: *Poisonous plants, proceedings of the third international symposium,* Ames, Iowa, 1992, Iowa State University Press, pp 523-527.

148. Majak W et al: Analysis and metabolism of nitrotoxins in cattle and sheep. In Seawright AA et al, eds: *Plant toxicology, proceedings of the Australia-USA poisonous plants symposium, Brisbane, Australia,* Yeerongpilly, Queensland, Austr, 1985, Queensland Department of Primary Industries, pp 446-452.

149. Majak W, Pass MA: Aliphatic nitrocompounds. In Cheeke PR, ed: *Toxicants of plant origin,* vol 2, *Glycosides,* Boca Raton, Fla, 1989, CRC Press, 446-452.

150. James LF et al: Field and experimental studies in cattle and sheep poisoned by nitro-bearing *Astragalus* or their toxins, *Am J Vet Res* 41:377-382, 1980.

151. Pass MA: Toxicity of aliphatic plant-derived nitrotoxins. In Colegate SM, Dorling PR, eds: *Plant-associated toxins: agricultural, phytochemical, and ecological aspects,* Wallingford, UK, 1994, CAB International, pp 541-545.

152. Fenwick GR: Bracken *(Pteridium aquilinum)*-toxic effects and toxic constituents, *J Sci Food Agric* 46:147-173, 1988.

153. Smith BL et al: Study on DNA adduct formation by ptaquiloside: the carcinogen of bracken fern *(Pteridium* spp) and from a cultivated collection of bracken from worldwide sources. In Colegate SM, Dorling PR, eds: *Plant-associated toxins: agricultural, phytochemical, and ecological aspects,* Wallingford, UK, 1994, CAB International, pp 239-251.

154. Smith BL et al: Ptaquiloside in bracken *(Pteridium* spp). In Colegate SM, Dorling PR, eds: *Plant-associated toxins: agricultural, phytochemical, and ecological aspects,* Wallingford, UK, 1994, CAB International, pp 45-50.

155. Hirono I: Carcinogenic bracken glycosides. In Cheeke PR, ed: *Toxicants of plant origin,* vol 2, *Glycosides,* Boca Raton, Fla, 1989, CRC Press, pp 239-251.

156. Schacham P, Philip RB, Gowdey CW: Antihematopoetic and carcinogenic effects of bracken fern *(Pteridium aquilinum)* in rats, *Am J Vet Res* 31:191-197, 1970.

157. Kingsbury JM: *Poisonous plants of the United States and Canada,* Englewood Cliffs, NJ, 1964, Prentice-Hall, pp 105-113.

158. McKenzie RA: Bovine enzootic haematuria in Queensland, *Aust Vet J* 54:61-64, 1978.

159. Hirono I et al: Induction of tumors in ACI rats given a diet containing ptaquiloside, a bracken carcinogen, *J National Cancer Inst* 79:1143-1149, 1987.

160. Evans IA: Bracken carcinogenicity, *Res Vet Sci* 26:339-348, 1979.

161. Evans WC: Bracken poisoning of farm animals, *Vet Rec* 76:365-369, 1964.

162. Gerenutti M, deSouza Spinosa H, Bernardi MM: Effects of bracken fern *(Pteridium aquilinum* L Kuhn) feeding during the development of female rats and their offspring, *Vet Hum Toxicol* 34:307-310, 1992.

163. Singh RP, Joshi HC, Kumar M: Experimental bracken fern toxicity in calves: changes in blood and urine, *Indian J Vet Med* 7:96-100, 1987.

164. Alonso-Amelot ME: The link between bracken fern and stomach cancer: milk, *Nutrition* 13:694-696, 1997.

165. Adams NR: Phytoestrogens. In Cheeke PR, ed: *Toxicants of plant origin,* vol 4, *Phenolics,* Boca Raton, Fla, 1989, CRC Press, pp 23-51.

166. Livingston AL: Forage plant estrogens, *J Toxicol Environ Health* 4:301-324, 1978.

167. Bickoff EM et al: Coumestrol, a new estrogen isolated from forage crops, *Science* 126:969-970, 1957.

168. Bickoff EM et al: Relative potencies of several estrogen-like compounds in forages, *J Agric Food Chem* 10:410-412, 1962.

169. Lundh TJO, Pettersson H, Kiessling KH: Liquid chromatographic determination of the estrogens daidzein, formononetin, coumestrol, and equol in bovine blood plasma and urine, *J Assoc Off Anal Chem* 71:938-941, 1988.

170. Welshons WV et al: A sensitive bioassay for detection of dietary estrogens in animal feeds, *J Vet Diagn Invest* 2:268-273, 1990.

171. Galey FD et al: Estrogenic activity in forages: diagnostic use of the classical mouse uterine bioassay, *J Vet Diagn Invest* 5:603-608, 1993.

172. Cheeke PR: *Natural toxicants in feeds, forages, and poisonous plants,* ed 2, Danville, Ill, 1998, Interstate, pp 294-297.

173. Benson ME, Casper HH, Johnson LJ: Occurrence and range of dicoumarol concentration in sweet clover, *Am J Vet Res* 42:2014-2015, 1981.

174. Cole RJ, Cutler HG, Stuart BP: Carboxyatractyloside. In Cheeke PR, ed: *Toxicants of plant origin,* vol 2, *Glycosides,* Boca Raton, Fla, 1989, CRC Press, pp 253-263.

175. Martin T, Stair EL, Dawson L: Cocklebur poisoning in cattle, *J Am Vet Med Assoc* 189:562-563, 1986.

176. Witte ST et al: Cocklebur toxicosis in cattle associated with the consumption of mature *Xanthium strumarium, J Vet Diagn Invest* 2:263-267, 1990.

177. Cheeke PR: *Natural toxicants in feeds, forages, and poisonous plants,* ed 2, Danville, Ill, 1998, Interstate, pp 436-437.

178. Rowe LD et al: Photosensitization of cattle in Southwest Texas: identification of phototoxic activity associated with *Cooperia pedunculata, Am J Vet Res* 48:1658-1661, 1987.

179. Campero CM, Odriozola E: A case of *Solanum malacoxylon* toxicity in pigs, *Vet Hum Toxicol* 32:238-239, 1990.

180. Krook L et al: Hypercalcemia and cacinosis in Florida horses: implication of the shrub *Cestrum diurnum* as the causative agent, *Cornell Vet* 65:26-56, 1975.

181. Krook L et al: *Cestrum diurnum* poisoning in Florida cattle, *Cornell Vet* 65:557-575, 1975.

182. Gorniak SL et al: Evaluation in rabbits of fetal effects of maternal ingestion of *Solanum malacoxylon, Vet Res Commun* 23:307-316, 1999.

183. Cheeke PR: *Natural toxicants in feeds, forages, and poisonous plants,* ed 2, Danville, Ill, 1998, Interstate, pp 281-284.

184. Nachman RJ, Olson JD: Ranunculin: a toxic constituent of the poisonous range plant bur buttercup *(Ceratocephalus testiculatus), J Agric Food Chem* 31:1358-1360, 1983.

185. Olson JD, Anderson TE, Murphy JC et al: Bur buttercup poisoning of sheep, *J Am Vet Med Assoc* 183:538-543, 1983.

186. Cheeke PR, Shull LR: *Natural toxicants in feeds and poisonous plants,* Westport, Conn, 1985, AVI, pp 224-226.

187. Hooper PT, Best SM, Campbell A: Axonal dystrophy in the spinal cords of cattle consuming the cycad plant *Cycas media, Aust Vet J* 50:146-149, 1974.

188. Hooper PT: Cycad poisoning in Australia: etiology and pathology. In Keeler RF, VanKampen KR, James LF et al, eds: *Effect of poisonous plants in livestock,* New York, 1978, Academic Press, pp 337-347.

189. Reams RY, Janovitz EB, Robinson FR et al: Cycad *(Zamia puertoriquensis)* toxicosis in a group of dairy heifers in Puerto Rico, *J Vet Diagn Invest* 5:488-494, 1993.

190. Eizirik DL, Kisby GE: Cycad toxin-induced damage of rodent and human pancreatic beta-cells, *Biochem Pharmacol* 50:355-365, 1995.

191. Morgan SE: Gossypol as a toxicant in livestock, *Vet Clin North Am (Food Anim Pract)* 5:251-262, 1989.

192. Haschek WM et al: Cottonseed meal (gossypol) toxicosis in a swine herd, *J Am Vet Med Assoc* 195:613-615, 1989.

193. Reyes J, Borriero L, Benos DJ: A bioenergetic model of gossypol action: effects of gossypol on adult rat spermatogenic cells, *Am J Physiol* 254:C564-C570, 1988.

194. Taitzoglou IA et al: Gossypol-induced inhibition of plasminogen activator activity in human and ovine acrosomal extract, *Andrologia* 31:355-359, 1999.

195. Smalley SA, Bicknell EJ: Gossypol toxicity in dairy cattle, *Compend Cont Educ* 4:S378-S381, 1982.

196. Hudson LM, Kerr LA, Maslin WR: Gossypol toxicosis in a herd of beef calves, *J Am Vet Med Assoc* 192:1303-1305, 1988.

197. Morgan S et al: Clinical, clinicopathologic, pathologic, and toxicologic alterations associated with gossypol toxicosis in feeder lambs, *Am J Vet Res* 49:493-499, 1988.

198. Patton CS et al: Heart failure caused by gossypol poisoning in two dogs, *J Am Vet Med Assoc* 187:625-627, 1985.

199. Holmberg CA et al: Pathological and toxicological studies of calves fed a high concentration cotton seed meal diet, *Vet Pathol* 25:147-153, 1988.

200. Randel RD, Chase CC, Wyse SJ: Effects of gossypol and cottonseed products on reproduction of mammals, *J Anim Sci* 70:1628-1638, 1992.

201. Vranova J et al: Inhibitory effect of gossypol on basal cell luteinization factor-stimulated progesterone synthesis in porcine granulosa cells, *Physiol Res* 48:119-128, 1999.

202. Velasquez-Pereira J et al: Long-term effects of feeding gossypol and vitamin E to dairy calves, *J Dairy Sci* 82:1240-1251, 1999.

203. Eisele GR: A perspective on gossypol ingestion in swine, *Vet Hum Toxicol* 28:118-122, 1986.

204. Osweiler GD et al: *Clinical and diagnostic veterinary toxicology,* Dubuque, Iowa, 1985, Kendall/Hunt, pp 468-470.

205. Pigeon RF, Camp BJ, Dollahite JW: Oral toxicity and polyhydroxyphenol moiety of tannin isolated from *Quercus havardi* (shin oak), *Am J Vet Res* 23:1268-1270, 1962.

206. Dollahite JW, Pigeon RF, Camp BJ: The toxicity of gallic acid, pyrogallol, tannic acid, and *Quercus havardi* in the rabbit, *Am J Vet Res* 23:1264-1266, 1962.

207. Oelrichs PB et al: The isolation, structure elucidation and toxicity of hepatotoxic and nephrotoxic principles in *Terminalia oblongota.* In Colegate SM, Dorling PR, eds: *Plant associated toxins,* Wallingford, UK, 1994, CAB International, pp 245-250.

208. Spier SJ et al: Oak toxicosis in cattle in Northern California: clinical and pathologic findings, *J Am Vet Med Assoc* 191:958-964, 1987.

209. Hart GH et al: Acorn calves, California Agricultural Experiment Station, Bulletin 699, 1947.

210. Basden KW, Dalvi RR: Determination of total phenolics in acorns from different species of oak trees in conjunction with acorn poisoning in cattle, *Vet Hum Toxicol* 29:305-306, 1987.

211. Householder GD, Dollahite JW: Some clinical biochemical changes in the blood serum of calves fed *Quercus havardi, Southwest Vet* 16:107-113, 1963.

212. Kingsbury JM: *Poisonous plants of the United States and Canada,* Englewood Cliffs, NJ, 1964, Prentice Hall, pp 235-242.

213. Cheeke PR, Shull LR: *Natural toxicants in feeds and poisonous plants,* Westport, Conn, 1985, AVI, pp 314-371.

214. VanKampen KR, James LF: Acute halogeton poisoning of sheep: pathogenesis of lesions, *Am J Vet Res* 30:1779-1783, 1969.

215. Allison MJ, Cook HM, Dawson KA: Selection of oxalate-degrading rumen bacteria in continuous cultures, *J Anim Sci* 53:810-816, 1981.

216. Lincoln SD, Black B: Halogeton poisoning in range cattle, *J Am Vet Med Assoc* 176:717-718, 1980.

217. Beier RC, Normal JO: The toxic factor in white snakeroot: identity, analysis, and prevention, *Vet Hum Toxicol* 32(suppl):81-88, 1990.

218. Beier RC et al: Microsomal activation of constituents of white snakeroot (*Eupatorium rugosum*) to form toxic products, *Am J Vet Res* 48:583-585, 1987.

219. White JL et al: White snakeroot (*Eupatorium rugosum*) poisoning: clinical effects associated with cardiac and skeletal muscle lesions in experimental equine toxicosis. In Seawright AA et al, eds: *Plant toxicology, proceedings of the Australia-USA poisonous plants symposium, Brisbane, Australia,* Yeerongpilly, Queensland, Austr, 1985, Queensland Department of Primary Industries, pp 411-421.

220. Olson CT et al: Suspected tremetol poisoning in horses, *J Am Vet Med Assoc* 185:1001-1003, 1984.

221. Kingsbury JM: *Poisonous plants of the United States and Canada,* Englewood Cliffs, NJ, 1964, Prentice Hall, pp 397-404.

222. Stotts R: White snakeroot toxicity in dairy cattle, *Vet Med,* 1984, pp 18-120.

223. Smetzer DL et al: Cardiac effects of white snakeroot intoxication in horses, *Equine Pract* 5:26-32, 1983.

224. Cheeke PR: *Natural toxicants in feeds, forages, and poisonous plants,* ed 2, Danville, Ill, 1998, Interstate, pp 233-234.

225. James LF et al: Pine needle abortion in cattle: a review and report of 1973-1984 research, *Cornell Vet* 79:39-52, 1989.

226. Stuart LD et al: Pine needle abortion in cattle: pathological observations, *Cornell Vet* 79:61-69, 1989.

227. Call JW, James LF: Effect of feeding pine needles on ovine reproduction, *J Am Vet Med Assoc* 169:1301-1302, 1976.

228. James LF, Call JW, Stevenson AH: Experimentally induced pine needle abortion in range cattle, *Cornell Vet* 67:294-299, 1977.

229. Gardner DR et al: Ponderosa pine needle induced abortion in beef cattle: identification of isocupressic acid as the principal active compound, *J Agric Food Chem* 42:756-761, 1994.

230. Gardner DR et al: Abortifacient effects of lodgepole pine (*Pinus contorta*) and common juniper (*Juniperus communis*) in cattle, *Vet Hum Toxicol* 40:260-263, 1998.

231. Ford SP et al: Abortifacient effects of a unique class of vasoactive lipids from *Pinus ponderosa* needles, *J Anim Sci* 77:2187-2193, 1999.

232. Ford SP et al: Effects of ponderosa pine needle ingestion on uterine vascular function in late-gestation beef cows, *J Anim Sci* 70:1609-1614, 1992.

233. Panter KE, Keeler RF, Baker DC: Toxicosis in livestock from the hemlocks (*Conium* and *Cicuta* spp), *J Anim Sci* 66:2407-2413, 1988.

234. Smith RA, Lewis D: *Cicuta* toxicosis in cattle: case history and simplified analytical method, *Vet Hum Toxicol* 29:240-241, 1987.

235. Knight AP: Milkweed poisoning, *Compend Cont Educ* F348-F349, 1987.

236. Panter KE, Baker DC, Kechele PO: Water hemlock (*Cicuta douglasii*) toxicosis in sheep: pathologic description and prevention of lesions and death, *J Vet Diagn Invest* 8:474-480, 1996.

237. Cheeke PR, Shull LR: *Natural toxicants in feeds and poisonous plants,* Westport, Conn, 1985, AVI, pp 348-350, 381-382.

238. Johnson AE: Predisposing influence of range plants on *Tetradymia*-related photosensitization in sheep: work of Drs AD Clawson and WT Huffman, *Am J Vet Res* 35:1583-1585, 1976.

239. Johnson AE: Experimental photosensitization and toxicity in sheep produced by *Tetradymia glabrata, Can J Comp Med* 38:406-410, 1974.

240. Osweiler GD et al: *Clinical and diagnostic veterinary toxicology,* Dubuque, Iowa, 1985, Kendall/Hunt, pp 460-467.

241. Crawford RF, Kennedy WK, Davison KL: Factors influencing the toxicity of forages that contain nitrate when fed to cattle, *Cornell Vet* 56:3-16, 1966.

242. Schneider NR, Carlson MP: Implications and significance of excessive nitrate/nitrite exposure in animal health, *Proceedings of the California Animal Nutrition Conference,* Fresno, Calif, 1991, pp 121-137.

243. Johnson JL et al: Post-harvest change in cornstalk nitrate and its relationship to bovine fetal nitrite/nitrate exposure. In James LF et al, eds: *Poisonous plants: Proceedings of the Third International Symposium,* Ames, Iowa, 1992, Iowa State University Press, pp 423-430.

244. T-Dargatz JL, Hamar DW: Selenium toxicity in horses, *Compend Cont Educ* 8:771-776, 1986.

245. Harrison LH et al: Paralysis in swine due to focal symmetrical poliomalacia: possible selenium toxicosis, *Vet Pathol* 20:265-273, 1983.

246. Blodgett DJ, Bevill RF: Acute selenium toxicosis in sheep, *Vet Hum Toxicol* 29:233-236, 1987.

247. Janke BH: Acute selenium toxicosis in a dog, *J Am Vet Med Assoc* 195:1114-1115, 1989.

248. Osweiler GD et al: *Clinical and diagnostic veterinary toxicology,* Dubuque, Iowa, 1985, Kendall/Hunt, pp 132-142.

249. Stowe HD et al: Selenium toxicosis in feeder pigs, *J Am Vet Med Assoc* 201:292-295, 1992.

250. Casteel SW et al: Selenium toxicosis in swine, *J Am Vet Med Assoc* 186:1084-1085, 1985.

251. O'Toole D, Raisbeck MF: Pathology of experimentally induced chronic selenosis (alkali disease) in yearling cattle, *J Vet Diagn Invest* 7:364-373, 1995.

252. Yaeger MJ et al: The effect of subclinical selenium toxicosis on pregnant beef cattle, *J Vet Diagn Invest* 10:268-273, 1998.

253. Davidson-York D et al: Selenium elimination in pigs after an outbreak of selenium toxicosis, *J Vet Diagn Invest* 11:352-357, 1999.

254. Raisbeck MF, McAllister MM, Gould DH: Toxic syndrome associated with sulfur. In Howard JL, Smith RA, eds: *Current veterinary therapy 4: food animal practitioner,* Philadelphia, 1999, WB Saunders, pp 280-281.

255. Peckham JC et al: Atypical interstitial pneumonia in cattle fed moldy sweet potatoes, *J Am Vet Med Assoc* 160:169-172, 1972.

256. Kerr LA, Linnabary RD: Atypical bovine pulmonary emphysema–another cause (abstract). *Proceedings of the Thirty-first Annual Meeting of the American Association of Veterinary Laboratory Diagnosticians,* Little Rock, Ark, 1988, p 74.

257. Low SG et al: Sweet potato (*Ipomoea batatas*) poisoning of pigs in Papua New Guinea, *N Z Vet J* 41:218, 1993.

258. Cheeke PR, Shull LR: *Natural toxicants in feeds and poisonous plants,* Westport, Conn, 1985, AVI, pp 261-265.

259. Kerr LA, Johnson BJ, Burrows GE: Intoxication of cattle by *Perilla frutescens* (purple-mint), *Vet Hum Toxicol* 28:412, 1986.

260. Carlson JR et al: Pulmonary edema and emphysema in cattle after intraruminal and intravascular administration of 3-methyl indole, *Am J Vet Res* 36:1341-1347, 1975.

261. Boyd MR et al: Lung toxic furanoterpenoids produced by sweet potatoes (*Ipomoea batatas*) following microbial infection, *Biochem Biophys Acta* 337:184-195, 1974.

262. Atkinson G et al: Effects of 3 methyl indole in cattle, *Br J Pharmacol* 61:285-290, 1977.

263. Rajendran S et al: Oxidative stress in rat liver and lung induced by furanoterpenoids isolated from *Fusarium solani* infected sweet potatoes, *Indian J Exp Biol* 34:57-60, 1996.

264. Garst JE et al: Species susceptibility to pulmonary toxicity of 3 furyl isoamyl ketone (perilla ketone): in vivo support for involvement of the lung monooxygenase system, *J Anim Sci* 60:248-257, 1985.

265. Kubow S, Bray TM: The effect of lung concentrations of glutathione and vitamin E on the pulmonary toxicity of 3 methyl indole, *Can J Physiol Pharmacol* 66:863-867, 1988.

266. Li X, Castleman WL: Ultrastructural morphogenesis of 4 ipomeanol-induced bronchiolitis and interstitial pneumonia in calves, *Vet Pathol* 27:141-149, 1990.

267. Durham SR, Boyd MR, Castleman WL: Pulmonary endothelial and bronchiolar epithelial lesions induced by 4-ipomeanol in mice, *Am J Pathol* 118:61-75, 1985.

268. Dorster AR et al: Effects of 4-ipomeanol, a product from mold-damaged sweet potatoes, on the bovine lung, *Vet Pathol* 15:367-375, 1978.

269. Bradley BJ, Carlson JR: Ultrastructural pulmonary changes induced by intravenously administered 3 methyl indole in goats, *Am J Pathol* 99:551-560, 1980.

270. Turk MAM, Thomas DE: Effects of phenobarbital on 3 methyl indole toxicosis in ponies, *Am J Vet Res* 47:901-905, 1986.

271. Cheeke PR, Shull LR: *Natural toxicants in feeds and poisonous plants,* Westport, Conn, 1985, AVI, pp 276-280.

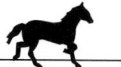

272. Pierce KR et al: Acute hemolytic anemia caused by wild onion poisoning in horses, *J Am Vet Med Assoc* 160:323-327, 1972.

273. Van Kampen KR, James LF, Johnson AE: Hemolytic anemia in sheep fed wild onions, *J Am Vet Med Assoc* 156:328-332, 1970.

274. Hutchison TWS: Onions as a cause of Heinz body anemia and deaths in cattle, *Can Vet J* 18:358-360, 1977.

275. Stair EL et al: Suspected red maple *(Acer rubrum)* toxicosis with abortion in two Percheron mares, *Vet Hum Toxicol* 35:229-230, 1993.

276. George LW et al: Heinz body anemia and methemoglobinemia in ponies given red maple *(Acer rubrum)* leaves, *Vet Pathol* 19:521-533, 1982.

277. Plumlee KH: Red maple toxicity in a horse, *Vet Hum Toxicol* 33:66-67, 1991.

278. Knight AP et al: Adaptation of pregnant ewes to an exclusive onion diet, *Vet Hum Toxicol* 42:1-4, 2000.

279. Osweiler GD et al: *Clinical and diagnostic veterinary toxicology,* Dubuque, Iowa, 1985, Kendall/Hunt, pp 476-481.

280. Sizelone W et al: Perirenal edema in a calf, *Vet Hum Toxicol* 30:265-266, 1988.

281. Kerr LA, Kelch WJ: Pigweed *(Amaranthus retroflexus)* toxicosis in cattle, *Vet Hum Toxicol* 40:216-218, 1998.

282. Colvin BM et al: *Cassia occidentalis* toxicosis in growing pigs, *J Am Vet Med Assoc* 189:423-426, 1986.

283. Henson JB et al: Myodegeneration in cattle grazing *Cassia* species, *J Am Vet Med Assoc* 147:142-145, 1965.

284. Simpson CF, Damron BL, Harms RH: Toxic myopathy of chicks fed *Cassia occidentalis* seeds, *Avian Dis* 15:284-290, 1971.

285. Martin BM et al: Toxicity of *Cassia occidentalis* in the horse, *Vet Hum Toxicol* 23:416-417, 1981.

286. Ohara PJ, Pierce KR, Read WK: Degenerative myopathy associated with ingestion of *Cassia occidentalis* L: clinical and pathologic features of the experimentally induced disease, *Am J Vet Res* 30:2173-2180, 1969.

287. Rowe LD et al: Experimentally induced *Cassia roemeriana* poisoning in cattle and goats, *Am J Vet Res* 48:992-997, 1987.

288. Robles M R et al: Cytotoxic effects of repen, a principal sesquiterpene lactone of Russian knapweed, *J Neurosci Res* 47:90-97, 1997.

289. Roy DN, Peyton DH, Spencer PS: Isolation and identification of two potent neurotoxins, aspartic acid and glutamic acid, from yellow star thistle *(Centaurea solstitialis),* *Nat Toxins* 3:174-180, 1995.

290. Cheeke PR: *Natural toxicants in feeds, forages, and poisonous plants,* ed 2, Danville, Ill, 1998, Interstate, p 385.

291. Thomsen C, Williams WA: Yellow starthistle control, *Components* 3:2-6, 1992.

292. Calhoun MC et al: Experimental prevention of bitterweed *(Hymenoxys odorata)* poisoning of sheep, *Am J Vet Res* 50:1642-1646, 1989.

293. Cheeke PR, Shull LR: *Natural toxicants in feeds and poisonous plants,* Westport, Conn, 1985, AVI, pp 359-363.

294. Rowe LD et al: *Hymenoxys odorata* (bitterweed) poisoning in sheep, *Southwest Vet* 26:287-293, 1973.

295. Kim HL, Rowe LD, Camp BJ: Hymenoxin, a poisonous sesquiterpene lactone from *Hymenoxys odorata* (bitterweed), *Res Commun Chem Pathol Pharmacol* 11:647-650, 1975.

296. Hill DW, Camp BJ: Reactions of hymenoxin: base conversion to psilotropin and greenein and formation of a "Michael adduct" with cysteine, *J Agric Food Chem* 27:882-885, 1979.

297. Galey FD et al: Black walnut *(Juglans nigra)* toxicosis: a model for equine laminitis, *J Comp Pathol* 104:313-326, 1991.

298. Minnick PD et al: The induction of equine laminitis with an aqueous extract of the heartwood of black walnut *(Juglans nigra),* *Vet Hum Toxicol* 29:230-233, 1987.

299. True RG et al: Black walnut shavings as a cause of acute laminitis, *Proceedings of the Twenty-fourth Annual Convention of the American Association of Equine Practitioners,* 1978, pp 511-515.

300. Geor RJ et al: Toxicosis in horses after ingestion of hoary alyssum, *J Am Vet Med Assoc* 210:63-67, 1992.

301. Kingsbury JM: *Poisonous plants of the United States and Canada,* Englewood Cliffs, NJ, 1964, Prentice-Hall, pp 220-221.

302. Bermudez MW et al: Experimental intoxication with fruit and purified toxins of buckthorn *(Karwinskia humboldtiana),* *Toxicon* 24:1091-1097, 1986.

303. Jaramillo-Juarez F et al: Renal failure during acute toxicity produced by tullidoro ingestion *(Karwinskia humboldtiana),* *Gen Pharmacol* 26:649-653, 1995.

304. Galey FD, Hullinger PJ, McCaskill J: Outbreaks of stringhalt in Northern California, *Vet Hum Toxicol* 33:176-177, 1991.

305. Huntington PJ et al: Australian stringhalt: epidemiological, clinical, and neurological investigations, *Equine Vet J* 21:266-273, 1989.

306. Cahill JI, Goulden BE, Jolly RD: Stringhalt in horses: a distal axonopathy, *Neuropathol Appl Neurobiol* 12:459-475, 1986.

307. Cheeke PR: *Natural toxicants in feeds, forages, and poisonous plants,* ed 2, Danville, Ill, 1998, Interstate, pp 193-196.

308. McKenzie RA, Brown OP: Avocado *(Persea americana)* poisoning of horses, *Aust Vet J* 68:77-78, 1991.

309. Craigmill AL et al: Toxicity of avocado *(Persea americana;* Guatemalan) leaves: review and preliminary report, *Vet Hum Toxicol* 26:381-383, 1984.

310. Craigmill AL et al: Pathological changes in the mammary gland and biochemical changes in the milk of the goat following oral dosing with leaf of the avocado *(Persea americana),* *Aust Vet J* 46:206-211, 1989.

311. Sani Y, Atwell RB, Seawright AA: The cardiotoxicity of avocado leaves, *Aust Vet J* 68:150-151, 1991.

312. Hargis AM et al: Avocado *(Persea americana)* intoxication in caged birds, *J Am Vet Med Assoc* 194:64-66, 1989.

313. Galey FD et al: Facial edema and myopathy in horses exposed to avocado *(Persea americana)* plants, *Annu Mtg Am Assoc Vet Lab Diagn* 36:33, 1993 (abstract).

314. Burger WP et al: Avocado *(Persea americana)* poisoning in ostriches. In Colgate SM, Dorling PR, eds: *Plant-associated toxins: agricultural, phytochemical, and ecological aspects,* Wallingford, UK, 1994, CAB International, pp 546-551.

315. Oelrichs PB et al: Isolation and identification of a compound from avocado *(Persea americana)* leaves which causes necrosis of the acinar epithelium of the lactating mammary gland and the myocardium, *Nat Toxins* 3:344-349, 1995.

316. Cheeke PR, Shull LR: *Natural toxicants in feeds and poisonous plants,* Westport, Conn, 1985, AVI, pp 240-244.

317. Ma L, Hsu CH, Patterson E: Ricin depresses cardiac function in the rabbit heart, *Toxicol Appl Pharmacol* 138:72-76, 1996.

318. Panciera RJ, Mosier DA, Ritchey JW: Hairy vetch *(Vicia villosa* Roth) poisoning in cattle: update and experimental induction of the disease, *J Vet Diagn Invest* 4:318-325, 1992.

319. Johnson B et al: Systemic granulomatous disease in cattle in California associated with grazing hairy vetch *(Vicia villosa),* *J Vet Diagn Invest* 4:360-362, 1992.

320. Woods LW et al: Systemic granulomatous disease in a horse grazing pasture containing vetch *(Vicia* spp), *J Vet Diagn Invest* 4:356-360, 1992.

321. Anderson CA, Divers TJ: Systemic granulomatous inflammation in a horse grazing hairy vetch, *J Am Vet Med Assoc* 183:569-570, 1983.

322. Claughton WP, Claughton HD: Vetch seed poisoning, *Auburn Vet,* 1954, pp 125-126.

323. Galey FD et al: Blue-green algae *(Microcystis aeruginosa)* hepatotoxicosis in dairy cows, *Am J Vet Res* 9:1415-1419, 1986.

324. Beasley VR et al: Diagnostic and clinically important aspects of cyanobacterial (blue-green algae) toxicosis, *J Vet Diagn Invest* 1:359-365, 1989.

325. Hooser SB et al: Actin filament alterations in rat hepatocytes induced in vivo and in vitro by microcystin LR, a hepatotoxin from the blue-green algae *Microcystis aeruginosa,* *Vet Pathol* 28:259-266, 1991.

326. Hooser SB et al: Toxicity of microcystin LR, a cyclic heptopeptide hepatotoxin from *Microcystis aeruginosa* to rats and mice, *Vet Pathol* 26:246-252, 1989.

327. Carmichael WW, Biggs DF, Gortiam DR: Toxicology and pharmacological action of *Anabaena flos-aquae* toxin, *Science* 187:542-544, 1975.

328. Cook WO et al: Comparison of effects of anatoxin a(s) and paraoxon, physostigmine, and pyridostigmine on mouse brain cholinesterase activity, *Toxicon* 26:750-753, 1988.

329. Puschner B et al: Blue-green algae toxicosis in cattle, *J Am Vet Med Assoc* 213:1605-1607, 1571, 1998.

330. Cheeke PR, Shull LR: *Natural toxicants in feeds and poisonous plants,* Westport, Conn, 1985, AVI, pp 393-402.

331. Osweiler GD et al: *Clinical and diagnostic veterinary toxicology,* Dubuque, Iowa, 1985, Kendall/Hunt, pp 409-442.

332. Casteel SW et al: Liver disease in cattle induced by consumption of moldy hay, *Vet Hum Toxicol* 37:248-251, 1995.

333. Cheeke PR, Shull LR: *Natural toxicants in feeds and poisonous plants,* Westport, Conn, 1985, AVI, pp 402-422.

334. Hsieh DPH, Atkinson DN: Bisfuranoid mycotoxins: their genotoxicity and carcinogenicity. In Witmer CM, ed: *Biological reactive intermediates IV,* New York, 1990, Plenum Press, pp 525-532.

335. Angsubhakorn S et al: Aflatoxicosis in horses, *J Am Vet Med Assoc* 178:274-278, 1981.

336. Connaughton D: The threat of aflatoxicosis (AVMA News Section), *J Am Vet Med Assoc* 194:743-746, 1989.

337. Coppock RW et al: Acute aflatoxicosis in feeder pigs, resulting from improper storage of corn, *J Am Vet Med Assoc* 195:1380-1381, 1989.

338. Osweiler GD, Trample DW: Aflatoxicosis in feedlot cattle, *J Am Vet Med Assoc* 187:636-637, 1985.

339. Ray AC et al: Bovine aboration and death associated with consumption of aflatoxin-contaminated peanuts, *J Am Vet Med Assoc* 188:1187-1188, 1986.

340. Colvin BM et al: Aflatoxicosis in feeder cattle, *J Am Vet Med Assoc* 184:956-958, 1984.

341. Panangala VS et al: Effects of aflatoxin on the growth performance and immune responses of weanling swine, *Am J Vet Res* 47:2062-2067, 1986.

342. Cook WO et al: Clinical and pathologic changes in acute bovine aflatoxicosis: rumen motility and tissue and fluid concentrations of aflatoxins B1 and M1, *Am J Vet Res* 47:1817-1825, 1986.

343. Helferich WG et al: Feedlot performances and tissue residues of cattle consuming diets containing aflatoxins, *J Anim Sci* 62:691-696, 1986.

344. Black RW et al: Distribution of aflatoxicosis in tissues of growing pigs fed an aflatoxin-contaminated diet amended with a high-affinity aluminosilicate sorbent, *Vet Hum Toxicol* 32:16-18, 1990.

345. Harvey RB et al: Prevention of aflatoxicosis by addition of hydrated sodium aluminosilicates to the diets of growing barrows, *Am J Vet Res* 50:416-420, 1989.

346. Harvey RB et al: Effects on aflatoxin M1 residues in milk by addition of hydrated sodium calcium aluminosilicate to aflatoxin-contaminated diets of dairy cows, *Am J Vet Res* 52:1556-1559, 1991.

347. Phillips TD: Dietary clay in the chemoprevention of aflatoxin-induced disease, *Toxicol Sci* 52(2 Suppl):118-126, 1999.

348. Cheeke PR: *Natural toxicants in feeds, forages, and poisonous plants,* ed 2, Danville, Ill, 1998, Interstate, 116-122.

349. Cote LM et al: Survey of vomitoxin-contaminated feed grains in midwestern United States, and associated health problems in swine, *J Am Vet Med Assoc* 184:189-192, 1984.

350. Pang VF et al: Myocardial and pancreatic lesions induced by T-2 toxin, a trichothecene mycotoxin in swine, *Vet Pathol* 23:310-319, 1986.

351. Trenholm HL et al: Feeding trials with vomitoxin (deoxynivalenol)-contaminated wheat: effects on swine, poultry, and dairy cattle, *J Am Vet Med Assoc* 185:527-531, 1984.

352. Pollmann DS et al: Deoxynivalenol-contaminated wheat in swine diet, *J Anim Sci* 60:239-247, 1985.

353. Lun AK, Young LG, Lumsden JH: The effects of vomitoxin and feed intake on the performance and blood characteristics of young pigs, *J Anim Sci* 61:1178-1185, 1985.

354. Gentry PA, Ross ML: Effect of T-2 toxin on bovine hematological and serum enzyme parameters, *Vet Hum Toxicol* 26:24-28, 1984.

355. Poppenga RH et al: Assessment of a general therapeutic protocol for the treatment of acute T-2 toxicosis in swine, *Vet Hum Toxicol* 29:237-239, 1987.

356. Coppock RW et al: Tissue residues of diacetoxy scirpenol in pigs and calves after intravenous dosing, *Am J Vet Res* 49:1997-1999, 1988.

357. Beasley VR et al: Pharmacokinetics of the trichothecene mycotoxin, T-2 toxin, in swine and cattle, *Toxicon* 24:13-23, 1986.

358. Marasas WFO et al: Leukoencephalomalacia in a horse induced by fumonisin B$_1$ isolated from *Fusarium moniliforme, Onderstepoort J Vet Res* 55:197-203, 1988.

359. Thiel PG et al: Levels of fumonisins B$_1$ and B$_2$ in feeds associated with confirmed cases of equine leukoencephalomalacia, *J Agric Food Chem* 39:109-111, 1991.

360. Wang E et al: Inhibition of sphingolipid biosynthesis by fumonisins, *J Biol Chem* 266:14486-14490, 1991.

361. Bermudez AJ, Ledoux DR, Rottinghaus GE: Effects of *Fusarium moniliforme* culture material containing known levels of fumonisin B$_1$ in ducklings, *Avian Dis* 39:879-886, 1995.

362. Osweiler GD et al: Effects of fumonisin-contaminated corn screenings on growth and health of feeder calves, *J Anim Sci* 71:459-466, 1993.

363. Ross PF et al: Experimental equine leukoencephalomalacia, toxic hepatosis, and encephalopathy caused by corn naturally contaminated with fumonisins, *J Vet Diagn Invest* 5:69-74, 1993.

364. Wilson TM et al: Fumonisin B;i1 levels associated with an epizootic of equine leukoencephalomalacia, *J Vet Diagn Invest* 2:213-216, 1990.

365. Colvin BM, Cooley AJ, Beaver RW: Fumonisin toxicosis in swine: clinical and pathologic findings, *J Vet Diagn Invest* 5:232-241, 1993.

366. Casteel SW et al: Chronic toxicity of fumonisin in weanling pigs, *J Vet Diagn Invest* 5:413-417, 1993.

367. Marasas WFO et al: Primary liver cancer and oesophageal basal cell hyperplasia in rats caused by *Fusarium moniliforme, Int J Cancer* 34:383-387, 1989.

368. Prelusky DB et al: Biological fate of fumonisin B$_1$ in food-producing animals. In Jackson et al, eds: *Fumonisins in food,* New York, 1996, Plenum Press, pp 265-278.

369. Galey FD et al: Staggers induced by consumption of perennial ryegrass in cattle and sheep from Northern California, *J Am Vet Med Assoc* 199:466-470, 1991.

370. Valdes JJ, Cameron JE, Cole RJ: Aflatrem: a tremorgenic mycotoxin with acute neurotoxic effects, *Environ Health Perspec* 62:459-631, 1985.

371. Porter JK, Bacon CW, Robbins JD: Major alkaloids of a *Claviceps* isolated from toxic Bermuda grass, *J Agric Food Chem* 22:838-841, 1974.

372. Cole RJ et al: Paspalum staggers: isolation and identification of tremorgenic metabolites from sclerotia of *Claviceps paspali, J Agric Food Chem* 25:1197-1201, 1977.

373. Gallagher RT, White EP, Mortimer PH: Ryegrass staggers: isolation of potent neurotoxins lolitrem A and lolitrem B for staggers-producing pastures, *N Z Vet J* 29:189-190, 1981.

374. Mantle PG: Amino acid neurotransmitter release from cerebrocortical synaptosomes of sheep with severe ryegrass staggers in New Zealand, *Res Vet Sci* 34:373-375, 1983.

375. Cheeke PR: *Natural toxicants in feeds, forages, and poisonous plants,* ed 2, Danville, Ill, 1998, Interstate, pp 261-263.

376. Mortimer PH: Perennial ryegrass staggers in New Zealand. In Keeler RF, VanKampen KR, James LF et al, eds: *Effects of poisonous plants in livestock,* New York, 1978, Academic Press, pp 353-361.

377. Hunt LD, Blythe L, Holtan DW: Ryegrass staggers in ponies fed processed ryegrass straw, *J Am Vet Med Assoc* 182:285-286, 1983.

378. Gallagher RT et al: Ryegrass staggers: the presence of lolitrem neurotoxins in perennial ryegrass seed, *N Z Vet J* 30:183-184, 1982.

379. Smith BL: Mycotoxicoses of sheep in Australia and New Zealand, *Proceedings of University of Sydney Post-Graduate Committee in Veterinary Series 103,* Veterinary Annual Toxicology, Sydney, 1987, pp 279-285.

380. Munday BL, Mason RW: Lesions in ryegrass staggers in sheep, *Aust Vet J* 43:598-599, 1967.

381. Mason RW: Axis cylinder degeneration associated with ryegrass staggers in sheep and cattle, *Aust Vet J* 44:428, 1968.

382. Gallagher RT, Hawkes AD: Estimation of neurotoxin levels in perennial ryegrass by mouse bioassay, *N Z J Agric Res* 28:427-438, 1985.

383. Jackson JA Jr et al: Lolium alkaloids in tall fescue hay and seed and their relationship to summer fescue toxicosis in cattle, *J Dairy Sci* 67:104-109, 1984.

384. Martin T, Edwards WC: Protecting grazing livestock from tall fescue toxicity, *Vet Med* 81:1162-1168, 1986.

385. Easton HS, Lane GA, Tapper BA: Ergovaline in endophyte-infected ryegrass pastures, *N Z Vet J* 41:214, 1993.

386. Schilto KK JA et al: Effects of endophyte-infected fescue on concentrations of prolactin in blood sera and the anterior pituitary and concentration of dopamine metabolism in brains of steers, *J Anim Sci* 66:713-718, 1988.

387. McCann JS et al: Influence of endophyte-infected tall fescue on serum prolactin and progesterone in gravid mares, *J Anim Sci* 70:217-223, 1992.

388. Dennis SB et al: Influence of *Neotyphodium coenophialum* on copper accumulation in tall fescue, *J Anim Sci* 76:2687-2693, 1998.

389. Garner GB, Cornell CB: Cattle response to the endophyte of tall fescue, *Proc 26th Annu Mtg Am Assoc Vet Lab Diagn* 26:145-154, 1985.

390. Carr SB, Jacobson DR: Bovine physiological responses to toxic fescue and related conditions for application in a bioassay, *J Dairy Sci* 52:1792-1799, 1969.

391. Jacobson DR et al: Nature of fescue toxicity and progress toward identification of the toxic entity, *J Dairy Sci* 46:416-422, 1963.

392. Browning R Jr: Physiological responses of Brahman and Hereford steers to an acute ergotamine challenge, *J Anim Sci* 78:124-130, 2000.

393. Browning R Jr et al: Effect of ergotamine and ergonovine on plasma concentrations of thyroid hormones and cortisol in cattle, *J Anim Sci* 76:1644-1650, 1998.

394. Oliver JW et al: Endophytic fungal toxin effect on adrenergic receptors in lateral saphenous veins (cranial branch) of cattle grazing tall fescue, *J Anim Sci* 76:2853-2856, 1998.

395. Cunningham IJ: A note on the cause of tall fescue lameness in cattle, *Aust Vet J* 25:25-28, 1949.

396. Garner GB et al: "Fescue foot" induction from experimental pastures, *J Anim Sci* 35:228-229, 1972.

397. Williams M et al: Induction of fescue foot syndrome in cattle by fractionated extracts of toxic fescue hay, *Am J Vet Res* 36:1353-1357, 1975.

398. Poppenga RH et al: Mare agalactia, placental thickening, and high foal mortality associated with the grazing of tall fescue: a case report, *Proc 25th Annu Mtg Am Assoc Vet Lab Diagn* 25:325-336, 1984.

399. Putnam MR et al: Effects of the fungal endophyte *Acremonium coenophialum* in fescue on pregnant mares and foal viability, *Am J Vet Res* 52:2071-2074, 1991.

400. Rice RL et al: Oral and parenteral vaccination of mice with protein-ergotamine conjugates and evaluation of protection against fescue toxicosis, *Vet Immunol Immunopathol* 61:305-316, 1998.

401. Cross DL, Redmond LM, Strickland JR: Equine fescue toxicosis: signs and solutions, *J Anim Sci* 73:899-908, 1995.

402. Cheeke PR: *Natural toxicants in feeds, forages, and poisonous plants,* ed 2, Danville, Ill, 1998, Interstate, pp 88-92.

403. Blaney BJ et al: Sorghum ergot (*Claviceps africana*) associated with agalactia and feed refusal in pigs and dairy cattle, *Aust Vet J* 78:102-107, 2000.

404. Cheeke PR, Shull LR: *Natural toxicants in feeds and poisonous plants,* Westport, Conn, 1985, AVI, pp 422-425.

405. Sundlof SF, Strickland C: Zearalenone and zeranol: potential residue problems in livestock, *Vet Hum Toxicol* 28:242-250, 1986.

406. Crump MH: Slaframine (slobber factor) toxicosis, *J Am Vet Med Assoc* 163:1300-1302, 1973.

407. Hagler WM, Benlow RF: Salivary syndrome in horses: identification of slaframine in red clover hay, *Appl Environ Microbiol* 42:1067-1073, 1981.

408. Fowler ME: *Veterinary zootoxicology,* Boca Raton, Fla, 1993, CRC Press.

409. Iyaniwura TT: Snake venom constituents: biochemistry and toxicology. I, *Vet Hum Toxicol* 33:468-474, 1991.

410. Iyaniwura TT: Snake venom constituents: biochemistry and toxicology. I, *Vet Hum Toxicol* 33:475-480, 1991.

411. Russell FE: Snake venom poisoning, *Vet Hum Toxicol* 33:584-586, 1991.

412. Moss ST et al: Association of rattlesnake bite location with severity of clinical manifestations, *Ann Emerg Med* 30:58-61, 1997.

413. Kerrigan KR et al: Antibiotic prophylaxis for pit viper envenomation: prospective, controlled trial, *World J Surg* 21:369-372, 1997.

414. Clark RF et al: Successful treatment of crotalid-induced neurotoxicity with a new polyspecific crotalid Fab antivenom, *Ann Emerg Med* 30:54-57, 1997.

415. Ray AC et al: Etiologic agents, incidence, and improved diagnostic methods of cantharidin toxicosis in horses, *Am J Vet Res* 50:187-191, 1989.

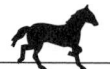

416. Hutchison WD, Murphy MJ, Tufte GN: Blister beetles in alfalfa: management options to minimize poisoning in horses, Minn Ext Serv AGF05510-D, 1990.
417. Schmitz DG: Cantharidin toxicosis update. In Clabough D, Marold A, Lyons R, eds: *Equine Vet Data* 9:87-88, 1988.
418. Helman RG, Edwards WC: Clinical features of blister beetle poisoning in equids: 70 cases (1983-1996), *J Am Vet Med Assoc* 211:1018-1021, 1997.

METALS AND OTHER INORGANIC COMPOUNDS

KONNIE H. PLUMLEE

ARSENIC

Because arsenic is naturally found in plants and soil,[419,420] trace levels will be present in tissues of most animals.[420] Arsenic can be present in either inorganic or organic forms.

In general, inorganic arsenic compounds are more toxic[421] and more likely to cause toxicosis than the organic arsenics.[419] Inorganic arsenic can exist in trivalent (commercial) or pentavalent (natural) forms.[419,421] The trivalent arsenic compounds (arsenite) are more soluble and so are five to ten times more toxic than pentavalent forms of arsenic (arsenate).[419,421,422] Inorganic arsenic compounds are used as rodenticides, insecticides, and herbicides.[421,423] Arsenic pentoxide is a preservative used in salt-treated or pressure-treated wood. However, toxicosis from ingestion of this type of treated wood has been reported only if the wood has been burned first, allowing the arsenic to become bioavailable.[420]

Organic arsenic compounds can be either aliphatic or aromatic.[421] Aliphatic arsenic compounds are used as herbicides and tonics.[421] Aromatic, organic arsenic chemicals are trivalent or pentavalent. The trivalent form is used as treatment of heartworms in dogs.[421] The pentavalent forms (phenylarsonic compounds) are used as feed additives for poultry and swine.[421]

The different types of arsenic have varying mechanisms of action. The phenylarsonic feed additives have an unknown mechanism that causes degeneration of myelin sheaths and axons.[421] The inorganic and the aliphatic organic compounds directly irritate the gastrointestinal tract, resulting in necrotic lesions.[421] Arsenic also acts directly on capillaries, resulting in transudation of plasma and decreased blood volume. The subsequent shock that develops is believed to be responsible for sudden death.[419,421]

Trivalent inorganic and aliphatic organic arsenic chemicals react with sulfhydryl groups.[421,422] Two enzyme complexes of the citric acid cycle contain lipoic acid, which has two sulfhydryl groups and thus is sensitive to these forms of arsenic. Pyruvate dehydrogenase complex is inhibited, preventing formation of acetyl CoA from pyruvate. α-ketoglutarate is inhibited, thus preventing formation of succinyl-CoA from α-ketoglutarate. The liver, kidney, gut, and heart are the organs most susceptible to this metabolic disorder. Arsenic also inhibits the amino acids that contain sulfur and results in fatty infiltration of the liver.[421]

The pentavalent inorganic arsenicals affect a different metabolic pathway. Normally, in the glycolytic pathway, an inorganic phosphate is added to glyceraldehyde 3-phosphate, which is converted to 1,3 diphosphoglycerate. Arsenate can replace the phosphate, resulting in production of 1-arseno-3-phosphoglycerate. This new intermediate can be used in the glycolytic pathway; however, the adenosine triphosphate (ATP) that would be produced during formation of 3-phosphoglycerate is lost. Therefore, arsenate uncouples oxidative phosphorylation.[421]

Clinical signs and lesions are similar except for the phenylarsonic compounds used as feed additives, which cause peripheral nerve degeneration in monogastric animals. All of the other arsenic compounds can cause peracute, acute, or subacute conditions. Peracute cases die from cardiovascular collapse and usually present as sudden deaths.[419,421,422] Acute toxicosis is seen 3 to 12 hours after ingestion.[419,421] The most prominent clinical sign of acute and subacute cases is diarrhea, which frequently is hemorrhagic.[419,421,423] Other clinical signs include anorexia, dehydration, weakness, colic, and agalactia.[419,421-423] The most consistent necropsy lesions are in the gastrointestinal tract and may be hemorrhagic, edematous, or eroded. The lesions may be confined to one region of, or spread throughout, the gastrointestinal tract.[419-424] The gut lumens are sometimes filled with necrotic material from the sloughed lining of the gastrointestinal tract. Other lesions include pulmonary edema and hemorrhage of the cardiac serosa and peritoneum.[419,421,422] Histopathologic examination may reveal multifocal necrosis of the liver and the proximal tubules of the kidney.[424] Peracute cases often have no abnormal gross findings.

Diagnosis of acute arsenic toxicosis is generally made by finding elevated levels of arsenic in the liver, kidney, and gastrointestinal contents.[421,424] In cases of peracute death the tissues may have normal levels of arsenic, but the gastrointestinal contents will have toxic levels.[422] In cases of chronic toxicosis, arsenic deposition in hair begins 2 weeks after exposure. Arsenic levels in hair can be used as a retrospective diagnostic tool.[422] Chronic arsenic toxicosis is rare because arsenic is rapidly excreted in the urine.[422,423] Urine and whole blood are the best samples to collect from live animals suspected of having acute arsenic toxicosis.

Treatment is dictated by the type and severity of clinical signs. Ethylenediamine tetraacetic acid (EDTA) is not effective for arsenic toxicosis because this chelator removes only extracellular arsenic, not the intracellular arsenic that is causing clinical signs.[420]

If the toxicosis is caused by a trivalent inorganic or an aliphatic organic arsenic, BAL (British anti-lewisite) can be used as a specific antidote. BAL contains two sulfhydryl groups and thus can bind to arsenic and remove it from lipoic acid. BAL forms a chelate that is eliminated via the kidney.[421] For maximum effect, a loading dose of 4 to 5 mg/kg should be given intramuscularly (IM) followed by 2 to 3 mg/kg every 4 hours for 24 hours and then 1 mg/kg every 4 hours for the next 2 days.[425] The cost of treatment may be prohibitive for many food animals.[420] This antidote has the side effect of potentially inhibiting enzymes that contain metallic coenzymes needed for cellular respiration.[421] Adverse clinical signs associated with BAL include hypertension, tremors, convulsions, and coma.[421]

D-Penicillamine is an effective arsenic chelator in humans, but may be too expensive in livestock.[421] Sodium thiosulfate has been reported as a safe chelator in large animals at 30 to 40 mg/kg IV or 60 to 80 mg/kg orally 2 to 3 times per day for 3 to 4 days.[421] Newer chelators, including dimercapto succinic acid (DMSA), are becoming available in human and small animal medicine and might be considered in the future for treatment of arsenic toxicosis.

COPPER

Tolerance to dietary copper varies widely among the different species of livestock. The maximum tolerable level of dietary copper during growth is 25 ppm, 100 ppm, and 800 ppm for sheep, cattle, and horses, respectively.[426] Therefore copper toxicosis is common in sheep but rare in horses.

Copper toxicosis can be acute or chronic. Acute toxicosis results from soluble copper salts. Acute copper toxicosis has been reported in adult and juvenile cattle that were given injections of copper disodium edetate as a treatment for copper deficiency.[427-429]

Chronic toxicosis can be categorized as simple, hepatogenous, or phytogenous. Simple chronic toxicosis is caused by ingestion of excessive copper relative to the levels of molybdenum or sulfate in the diet. Molybdenum and sulfate can bind to dietary copper and decrease its accumulation in the liver.[430] Copper accumulates in the liver when the dietary copper/molybdenum ratio is greater than 10:1 for sheep.[430] Many different sources of excess copper have been reported. Sheep are often poisoned when fed rations intended for cattle or horses,[431] and llamas have suffered from copper toxicosis when fed cattle feed.[432] Cattle develop copper toxicosis when supplemented with excessive copper[433] in their diets or when fields are contaminated with copper from industrial pollution, as with copper smelting units.[434,435] Cattle have become poisoned when fed litter from chickens that had been fed copper sulfate,[436] and sheep have developed toxicosis after grazing pastures fertilized with manure from swine that were fed copper sulfate.[439] Excessive copper in calf milk replacers has been the source of toxicosis in both calves[438,439] and goat kids.[440]

Hepatogenous toxicosis occurs when plant toxins damage the hepatic parenchyma, causing the liver to have an increased avidity for copper. The plants most often associated with hepatogenous copper toxicosis are *Senecio* spp. and *Heliotropium europaeum*.[430] Phytogenous copper toxicosis occurs when animals graze plants with elevated copper/molybdenum ratios for prolonged periods. In general, mature pastures have higher levels of molybdenum than young, rapidly growing plants.[430] Subterranean clover (*Trifolium subterraneum*) is especially noted for causing this type of chronic toxicosis.[430]

Copper is absorbed in the intestine, bound to proteins, and transported to the liver.[430,438] Copper binds with ceruloplasmin, a metalloprotein, in the liver.[430] Copper accumulates in hepatic lysosomes over several weeks to months during chronic copper poisoning.[430,437,438] During this accumulation phase, necrosis of hepatic parenchymal cells and swelling of Kupffer cells occur.[430] This phase is followed by a sudden release of copper into the bloodstream from the liver, either spontaneously or after some type of stress to the animal.[430,436,437] This acute hemolytic phase includes an increase in erythrocyte fragility and a decrease in blood glutathione, followed by hemoglobin oxidation and methemoglobin formation.[430,438] The resulting intravascular hemolysis leads to anemia and hemoglobinuric nephrosis.[438]

The first noticeable clinical signs of chronic copper toxicosis are usually depression, anorexia, and weakness, which often have a sudden onset.[430,433,441] Feces may be watery, dark, or blood tinged, especially in cattle.[433,441] Evidence of a hemolytic crisis is apparent. Animals have anemia, methemoglobinemia, and hemoglobinuria. Mucous membranes are icteric or muddy brown.[430,433,436,441] Cattle that suffer from copper toxicosis after injection with copper disodium edetate develop dyspnea, head pressing, ataxia, and circling rather than the hemolytic crisis that occurs with chronic copper toxicosis.[427,429]

Gross necropsy lesions are found in the liver, kidneys, and spleen. The liver is yellow and friable and may be larger or smaller than normal. The kidneys are dark red or blue-black. The spleen may be enlarged and congested. Histopathologic changes in the liver include centrilobular necrosis, pigment-laden Kupffer cells, hepatic fibrosis, and bile duct hyperplasia.[430,431,436,437] Granules in the liver will stain positive with rhodamine or rubeanic acid, two histochemical stains that are specific for copper. The degree of staining, however, does not always correlate well with the severity of lesions or with the amount of copper in the liver.[438]

Diagnosis of chronic copper toxicosis is made by measuring copper levels in serum, liver, and kidney.[437,438] Copper levels in serum are not elevated until just before or during the hemolytic crises.[430] Animals with toxic levels of copper in their livers can have normal or even deficient levels of copper in their serum.[433] Therefore measuring serum copper levels is not a reliable method of monitoring animals for excessive copper in the liver.[433]

If an animal is suspected to have died from chronic copper toxicosis, copper levels should be measured in both fresh liver and kidney, because after the liver has released its copper load into the bloodstream liver copper levels may fall into a nontoxic range. In these cases the kidney copper levels will be in a toxic range, so the diagnosis will not be missed. The diagnosis should correlate with histopathologic lesions in formalin-fixed liver and kidney.[438] Unlike chronic copper toxicosis, acute toxicosis from copper disodium edetate does not necessarily result in elevated copper levels in liver or kidney.[427]

Treatment is often unsuccessful once an animal is suffering from the acute hemolytic crisis. Ammonium molybdate (50 to 500 mg PO once daily) and sodium thiosulfate (300 to 1000 mg PO once daily) for 3 weeks has been used for many years as a treatment.[430,437] The liver copper levels begin to decrease within 4 days of beginning this therapy.[437]

A newer treatment is ammonium tetrathiomolybdate (1.7 mg/kg IV or 3.4 mg/kg SC on alternate days for three treatments).[430,442] Either route of administration significantly decreases liver copper levels within 6 days. Thiomolybdates decrease copper absorption and increase copper removal from the liver.[430] This change is accompanied by an increase of copper in the blood, bile, feces, and urine.[430] Most of this copper is insoluble in trichloroacetic acid, indicating that it is bound with tetrathiomolybdate and albumin in an inert complex.[442] Interestingly, one report indicated that when xylazine is given with tetrathiomolybdate the amount of copper excreted in the urine doubles when compared with giving tetrathiomolybdate alone.[443]

D-penicillamine (26 mg/kg PO twice daily for 6 days) results in a 10- to 20-fold increase in urinary copper excretion in sheep.[430,444] This drug does not seem to increase fecal copper concentration.[444] Unfortunately, this treatment is often cost prohibitive for many livestock.[430,437]

Trientine is a cupruretic agent used to treat humans. One study reported clinical improvement in sheep given this drug at 0.5 mg orally, four times a day.[430] Another study, however, demonstrated no increase in copper excretion in urine when the dosage was 26 mg/kg PO, twice a day for 6 days.[444]

FLUORIDE

Most cases of fluorosis are caused by animal exposure to industrial emissions[445,446]; however, fluorosis has occurred after volcanic eruptions when gaseous fluoride is fixed by foliage.[445,446] Horses and sheep tolerate higher levels of fluoride than cattle.[447] Lesions are similar in all species.[447]

Fluoride primarily affects and is incorporated by developing and mineralizing teeth and bones.[447,448] The main clinical signs are weight loss and lameness, especially of the forelimbs. Palpation of the long bones results in intense pain.[445] Radiographs of animals suffering with osteofluorosis reveal sclerosis, porosis, periosteal hyperostosis, endosteal hyperostosis, and osteophytosis.[448]

Characteristic lesions occur on incisors, premolars, and molars. Dental hypoplasia, dysplasia, and yellow to brown discoloration of the enamel are common.[448] The enamel is eroded or pitted and may have a chalky appearance.[448] The molars may become so abraded and painful that animals have difficulty with mastication and drinking cold water.[447] Dental abrasion is reduced if nonaffected teeth are adjacent to affected teeth.[448]

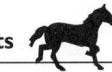

Gross pathology lesions include abnormal bone formation on the periosteum and thickening of the cortex.[448] The first lesions appear on the ribs, mandible, metatarsus, and metacarpus.[448] Histologic findings include abnormal bone remodeling, abnormal mineralization, coarse collagenous fibers, and increased osteoid.[448]

Only small amounts of fluoride pass the placental barrier; therefore teratogenic lesions or congenital malformations have not been observed in offspring of horses, sheep, or cattle that are suffering from fluorosis.[448]

Fluoride has an intense, dose-dependent osteogenic action, and osteofluorosis is associated with increased bone alkaline phosphatase activities.[445,448] Urine, serum, and bone will have elevated levels of fluoride.[446,448] These findings, in conjunction with clinical signs, radiography, and lesions, are used to make a diagnosis.

Fluoride toxicosis has no antidote.[448] Animals should be removed from the source of the excess fluoride and given supportive care. Feeds that are easily masticated should be fed to reduce further abrasion of the teeth.[447] Affected animals will not completely recover.[448]

IODINE

Iodine is used to prevent infectious diseases and as a treatment for footrot. Sources of iodine include potassium iodide, sodium iodide, kelp, and ethylenediamine dihydroiodide (EDDI). Oversupplementation can result in toxicosis.

Clinical signs include a nonproductive cough, lacrimation, serous nasal discharge, scaly haircoats, and hyperthermia. Other clinical signs include decreased milk production, decreased rate of gain, and decreased feed conversion.[449] Young animals seem to be more susceptible. Adults may not suffer from toxicosis unless stress, disease, or other nutritional imbalances also are present.[449] Excess supplementation in mares has been associated with goiter in foals.

Serum biochemical changes are inconclusive for iodine toxicosis.[449] A diagnosis can be confirmed only with serum or milk analysis. Nonlactating cows have higher serum iodine concentrations than lactating cows because the iodine is eliminated in milk.[449] Iodine levels in milk are directly related to the levels of iodine in the diet.[449] Iodine-based teat dips can elevate milk iodine levels.

Treatment is restricted to removal of the dietary source of iodine. Clinical signs associated with the respiratory tract disappear 1 to 4 weeks after the iodine source is removed.[449]

IRON

Hemochromatosis can be classified as either primary (idiopathic) or secondary. Primary hemochromatosis is an inherited defect in iron metabolism.[450] This discussion is restricted to iron toxicosis that has been associated with excess oral and parenteral iron supplementation.

Most cases of iron overload have occurred in neonatal foals that were given ferrous fumarate orally before 3 days of age.[451,452] Adult horses, however, have suffered from iron toxicosis after oral supplementation with ferrous fumarate or ferrous sulphate.[451] Iron toxicosis has been reported in calves injected with a combination of ferrous gluconate and ferric ammonium citrate.[453] Young bulls injected with ferric ammonium citrate also developed iron toxicosis.[454]

Normally, the small intestine absorbs about 3% to 10% of dietary iron and stores the iron as ferritin in the mucosal cells. The iron is transferred to the plasma according to the body's needs. Excess iron is stored in the liver as ferritin and hemosiderin because the body has limited ability to eliminate iron.[450,451] Foals are born with a high serum iron level and have higher iron absorption than adults. Therefore foals

less than 3 days of age are more susceptible than adults to iron toxicosis.[455]

Clinical signs in neonatal foals include depression, icterus, head pressing, and disorientation.[452] Adult horses develop anorexia, icterus, and sometimes petechial hemorrhages.[451] Calves with iron toxicosis have trembling, vocalizing, bruxism, colic, and convulsions.[453]

If clinical pathology findings are abnormal, they will be related to cholestatic liver failure. Animals often have elevated levels of γ-glutamyltransferase (GGT), alkaline phosphatase (ALP), bile acids, and unconjugated bilirubin. Coagulopathies are demonstrated by abnormal coagulation profiles, thrombocytopenia, and elevated fibrinogen and fructose diphosphate (FDP).[451,452]

Grossly, the liver lesions are variable. Most livers are friable and are swollen or shrunken. In general the liver is discolored either as pale tan or mottled red-brown. Microscopic lesions include periportal bile ductule proliferation, periportal necrosis, lobular necrosis, and fibrosis. Hemorrhages may be present in the gastric mucosa, intestines, and urinary bladder.[452-455]

Diagnosis of iron toxicosis usually is based on the presence of appropriate clinical signs and a history of recent iron supplementation. Serum levels of free (unbound) iron may or may not be elevated. Liver iron concentrations range from normal to several thousand parts per million. Interpreting iron levels in liver can be complicated because iron may be elevated above normal if the animal was suffering from hemolysis or if blood congestion occurred within the liver.

Treatment of iron toxicosis is usually limited to supportive care. Repeated phlebotomy or chelation therapy with deferoxamine is used to treat iron overload in humans and small animals.[450,451] The success rate of these treatments in large animals has not been well documented.

LEAD

Lead toxicosis is discussed in Chapter 33.

MERCURY

Mercury toxicosis has been associated with ingestion of seed treated with organic mercurial fungicides.[456-458] Topical application or ingestion of inorganic mercurials, used as counterirritants (blistering agents), also can result in toxicosis.[456,458,459] If the blistering agents are used concurrently with dimethyl sulfoxide (DMSO), the absorption of the mercury is enhanced and is more likely to cause toxicosis.[459]

Mercuric ions form covalent bonds with sulfhydryl groups and form mercaptides.[458] The kidney is the primary target organ, but mercury also localizes in the gastrointestinal mucosa. Mercury is excreted by the kidneys, partly by exfoliation of renal tubular epithelium.[459] Metallothionein, a metal-binding protein, is synthesized within 48 hours of exposure to mercury. Metallothionein initially may protect the kidney by sequestering mercury; however, as the sequestered mercury is slowly released from the tubular epithelium, renal damage continues.[456,459]

Acute signs of mercury toxicosis are caused by the corrosive effect of mercury on mucous membranes. Ulceration of the mouth, esophagus, and the rest of the gastrointestinal tract may be followed by diarrhea and anorexia. If the animal survives, acute toxic nephrosis occurs. Anorexia, gastroenteritis, weight loss, nephritis, and alopecia have been reported in animals exposed to chronic, low doses of mercury.[458]

Clinical pathology testing may reveal elevated creatinine and blood urea nitrogen (BUN), as well as proteinuria, glucosuria, and isosthenuria, depending on the acuteness of the disease. Necropsy findings include an ulcerated and edematous gastrointestinal tract, with possible intraluminal hemorrhage. The kidneys may be pale and swollen.[456,459]

Diagnosis of mercury toxicosis is made from history, clinical presentation, and mercury levels within the animal. Mercury concentrations can be measured in liver, kidney, brain, whole blood, and urine. Tissue samples and urine may be frozen after collection.

Chelation therapy can be done using BAL or sodium thiosulfate as for arsenic toxicosis. Remaining topical mercurials should be washed from the animal. Supportive care is necessary for the gastroenteritis and kidney failure. Oliguria indicates a poor prognosis.[456,459]

MOLYBDENUM

Excess dietary molybdenum (copper deficiency) is discussed in Chapter 30.

SELENIUM

See Toxic Plants.

SODIUM

Sodium (salt) toxicosis is discussed in Chapter 33.

SULFATE

Excess dietary sulfate is discussed with copper deficiency in Chapter 30 and with polioencephalomalacia in Chapter 33.

ZINC

Excess dietary zinc is discussed with osteochondrosis in Chapter 36.

REFERENCES

419. Morgan SE, Morgan GL, Edwards WC: Pinpointing the source of arsenic poisoning in a herd of cattle, *Vet Med* 79:1525-1528, 1984.
420. Thatcher CD et al: Arsenic toxicosis and suspected chromium toxicosis in a herd of cattle, *J Am Vet Med Assoc* 187:179-181, 1985.
421. Bahri LE, Romdane SB: Arsenic poisoning in livestock, *Vet Hum Toxicol* 33:259-264, 1991.
422. Boosinger TR, Riviere JE, Everson RJ: Arsenic-induced hemorrhagic enterocolitis in cattle, *Proceedings of the American Association of Veterinary Laboratory Diagnosticians*, 1980, pp 397-403.
423. Kahrs RF et al: Fatal lead arsenate toxicosis resembling acute bovine viral diarrhea-mucosal disease, *Proceedings of the American Association of Veterinary Laboratory Diagnosticians*, 1979, pp 321-332.
424. Riviere JE et al: Environmental arsenic toxicosis in cattle, *Proceedings of the American Association of Veterinary Laboratory Diagnosticians*, 1984, pp 355-360.
425. Galey FD: Arsenic toxicosis. In Howard JL, ed: *Current veterinary therapy 3 (food animal practice)*, Philadelphia, 1993, WB Saunders, pp 394-396.
426. Hintz HF: Copper toxicity, *Equine Pract* 9:17-18, 1987.
427. Galey FD et al: Copper toxicosis in two herds of beef calves following injection with copper disodium edetate, *J Vet Diagn Invest* 3:260-263, 1991.
428. Bohman VR et al: The toxicology and composition of bovine tissues after parenteral administration of high levels of copper salts, *Vet Hum Toxicol* 29:307-312, 1987.
429. Bulgin MS et al: Death associated with parenteral administration of copper disodium edetate in calves, *J Am Vet Med Assoc* 188:406-409, 1986.
430. Vaala WE: Copper toxicity in sheep, *Proceedings of the American College of Veterinary Internal Medicine*, New Orleans, 1991, pp 559-561.
431. Gough J: Copper poisoning in lambs fed horse and cattle feed, *Can Vet J* 32:750, 1991.
432. Junge RE, Thornburg L: Copper poisoning in four llamas, *J Am Vet Med Assoc* 195:987-989, 1989.
433. Perrin DJ, Schiefer HB, Blakley BR: Chronic copper toxicity in a dairy herd, *Can Vet J* 31:629-632, 1990.
434. Parada R, Gonzalez S, Bergqvist E: Industrial pollution with copper and other heavy metals in a beef cattle ranch, *Vet Hum Toxicol* 29:122-126, 1987.
435. Gummow et al: Copper toxicity in ruminants: air pollution as a possible cause, *Onderstepoort J Vet Res* 58:33-39, 1991.
436. Banton MI et al: Copper toxicosis in cattle fed chicken litter, *J Am Vet Med Assoc* 191:827-828, 1987.
437. Kerr LA, McGavin HD: Chronic copper poisoning in sheep grazing pastures fertilized with swine manure, *J Am Vet Med Assoc* 198:99-101, 1991.
438. Sullivan JM, Janovitz EB, Robinson FR: Copper toxicosis in veal calves, *J Vet Diagn Invest* 3:161-164, 1991.
439. Jenkins KJ, Hidiroglou M: Tolerance of the calf for excess copper in milk replacer, *J Dairy Sci* 72:150-156, 1989.
440. Humphries WR, Morrice PC, Mitchell AN: Copper poisoning in Angora goats, *Vet Rec* 121:231, 1987.
441. Tremblay RRM, Baird JD: Chronic copper poisoning in two Holstein cows, *Cornell Vet* 81:205-213, 1991.
442. Humphries WR, Morrice PC, Bremner I: A convenient method for the treatment of chronic copper poisoning in sheep using subcutaneous ammonium tetrathiomolybdate, *Vet Rec* 123:51-53, 1988.
443. Symonds HW, Ke Y: Enhancement of tetrathiomolybdate-induced copper excretion in bile of sheep by the alpha 2-agonistic action of xylazine, *Res Vet Sci* 46:349-353, 1989.
444. Botha CJ et al: The cupruretic effect of two chelators following copper loading in sheep, *Vet Hum Toxicol* 35:409-413, 1993.
445. Araya O et al: Bovine fluorosis following volcanic activity in the southern Andes, *Vet Rec* 126:641-642, 1990.
446. Araya O, Wittwer F, Villa A: Evolution of fluoride concentrations in cattle and grass following a volcanic eruption, *Vet Hum Toxicol* 35:437-440, 1993.
447. Shupe JL et al: Relationship of cheek tooth abrasion to fluoride-induced permanent incisor lesions in livestock, *Am J Vet Res* 48:1498-1503, 1987.
448. Shupe JL, Olsen AE: Clinicopathologic aspects of chronic fluoride toxicosis in cattle, *Bovine Pract* 22:184-186, 1987.
449. Olson WG et al: Iodine toxicosis in six herds of dairy cattle, *J Am Vet Med Assoc* 184:179-181, 1984.
450. House JK et al: Hemochromatosis in Salers cattle, *J Vet Intern Med* 8:105-111, 1994.
451. Edens LM, Robertson JL, Feldman BF: Cholestatic hepatopathy, thrombocytopenia and lymphopenia associated with iron toxicity in a thoroughbred gelding, *Equine Vet J* 25:81-84, 1993.
452. Divers TJ et al: Toxic hepatic failure in newborn foals, *J Am Vet Med Assoc* 183:1407-1413, 1983.
453. Ruhr LP et al: Acute intoxication from a hematinic in calves, *J Am Vet Med Assoc* 182:616-618, 1983.
454. Holter JA, Carson TL, Witte ST: Acute iron intoxication in a herd of young bulls, *J Vet Diagn Invest* 2:229-230, 1990.
455. Mullaney TP, Brown CM: Iron toxicity in neonatal foals, *Equine Vet J* 20:119-124, 1988.
456. Markel MD, Dyer RM, Hattel AL: Acute renal failure associated with application of a mercuric blister, *J Am Vet Med Assoc* 185:92-94, 1984.
457. Smith R, Morden BB, Ellis, LB: Diphenylmercury poisoning in cattle, *Can Vet J* 33:135, 1992.
458. Short SB, Edwards WC: Are your patients safe from unnecessary mercury poisoning, *Vet Med* 83:287-293, 1988.
459. Schuh JCL, Ross C, Meschter C: Concurrent mercuric blister and dimethyl sulphoxide (DMSO) application as a cause of mercury toxicity in two horses, *Equine Vet J* 20:68-71, 1988.

TOXICOLOGY OF ORGANIC COMPOUNDS

KONNIE H. PLUMLEE

INSECTICIDES

Anticholinesterase Insecticides

These insecticides include the organophosphates and the carbamates. Many organophosphate insecticides are used for insect control in crops. Several organophosphates also have been approved for use as insecticides or anthelmintics in domestic animals. Carbamate insecticides are used primarily on crops and other plants. Domestic animals are usually exposed to these insecticides as a result of drift, accidental ingestion, or improper treatment by owners. About 20 of these compounds exist and their toxicity varies widely.[460]

The mechanism of action of these insecticides is to bind with and inhibit acetylcholinesterase. Therefore acetylcholine accumulates at nerve junctions and repetitive firing of parasympathetic nerves occurs. Because carbamates bind with

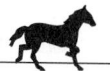

acetylcholine on a reversible basis, that inhibition of acetylcholinesterase is temporary.[460,461] Therefore carbamates have a shorter duration of action than organophosphate insecticides, which bind irreversibly with acetylcholinesterase.[460]

Clinical signs are predominantly described by the acronym *SLUD: s*alivation, *l*acrimation, *u*rination, and *de*fecation. In addition, the animals may have miosis, diarrhea, muscle tremors, seizures, dyspnea, or bloating.[460] Death can occur within minutes, depending on the toxicity of the specific compound and the amount of toxicant ingested.[462] At postmortem examination, lesions may be minor or absent, depending on the acuteness of death. Pulmonary edema is a frequent finding, because death usually results from increased pulmonary secretions, bronchial constriction, and respiratory paralysis.[461]

Measuring the cholinesterase activity in brain, retina, or whole blood can be used to make a presumptive diagnosis of toxicosis.[463-465] Some laboratories use serum rather than whole blood, depending on the testing method used; therefore it is best to check with the laboratory before submission. Whole blood can reliably be used for cholinesterase evaluation for up to 1 week after collection if the sample is refrigerated.[466] Half of the brain should be submitted for homogenization because cholinesterase activity varies among regions of the brain.[463] Cholinesterase activity in whole blood or brain that is less than 50% of normal for the species being tested indicates excessive exposure to a cholinesterase inhibitor. Cholinesterase activities less than 25% of normal indicates toxicosis as long as appropriate clinical signs are present.[464]

An insecticide screen should be performed on gastrointestinal contents or the liver to identify the insecticide chemical that is involved. These samples should be stored in glass or metal, such as foil, and frozen as soon as possible after collection. If the sample is stored in plastic, it is possible that the insecticide can leech from the sample into the plastic.

Because carbamates rapidly dissociate from acetylcholinesterase, a diagnosis is often difficult to make based on cholinesterase activity in brain or blood. The activities can be normal or near normal even though the animal is suffering from toxicosis.[460,461] Because carbamates hydrolyze rapidly, parent compounds may be difficult to detect in ingesta and especially in tissue.[460,461] Therefore when carbamate toxicosis is suspected, multiple samples should be collected and tested as soon as possible.

Treatment for organophosphate toxicosis includes supportive care, activated charcoal, atropine, and oximes. Activated charcoal (1 to 2 lb [0.45 to 0.90 kg] PO for 500-kg animal) should be given even if the route of exposure is not oral, because these insecticides can act systemically even when given topically. If the route of exposure is dermal, the animal should be washed with soap and water to decrease absorption through the skin.[464] Atropine competitively inhibits acetylcholine at muscarinic nerve receptors. Therefore muscarinic effects, but not nicotinic effects, are reduced. Atropine should be given at a dose of 0.10 to 0.25 mg/kg. One fourth of the initial dose is given via intravenous injection and the rest subcutaneously or intramuscularly. The dose can be repeated if the clinical signs reappear.[464] Gastrointestinal motility should be monitored carefully because atropine can cause ileus, especially in horses. Oximes such as 2-pyridine aldoxime methiodide (2-PAM) can be used as a treatment to release the bond between acetylcholinesterase and an organophosphate. However, oximes are of little benefit after the acetylcholinesterase-organophosphate bond undergoes "aging," meaning that the bond cannot be broken. The amount and time of "aging" that occurs varies among the different organophosphate compounds.[464,467] Recommended doses for 2-PAM are 20 mg/kg IV twice daily[468] or 10 to 15 mg/kg SC.[469]

Treatment of carbamate toxicosis is restricted to atropine, activated charcoal, and supportive care. Oximes such as 2-PAM are contraindicated with carbamate toxicosis because the carbamates bind reversibly, and thus oximes are not needed to release the carbamate from the acetylcholinesterase.[460]

Most anticholinesterase compounds are rapidly metabolized and excreted.[470] Therefore these insecticides do not persist in tissues and tissue levels are usually low.[471] Animals that survive the toxicosis, however, should be analyzed for residues before consumption.[471] Animals that have died from anticholinesterase insecticide toxicosis have been prohibited from being rendered.[470]

Chlorpyrifos is a chlorinated organophosphorus insecticide used for lice and fly control in cattle. It is applied as a pour-on caudal to the shoulders.[472] This product causes a delayed toxicosis that occurs primarily in bulls and some exotic breeds of cattle. Toxicosis is associated with the testosterone levels in the animal.[472] Larger and older bulls are affected more severely.[468] The manufacturer recommends not treating bulls over 8 months old with chlorpyrifos.[468] Clinical signs do not occur until at least 2 to 7 days after exposure and include depression, weakness, muscle fasciculations, anorexia, rumen stasis, and rumen distention.[468,469,472] The clinical signs typically seen with acute organophosphate toxicosis are usually not present with chlorpyrifos toxicosis.

Animals suffering from chlorpyrifos toxicosis will have depressed cholinesterase activities in brain and blood.[468,469,472] After topical application, chlorpyrifos will undergo systemic distribution and may be detected in blood, rumen contents, fat, and hair for weeks.[468,469] Animals with chlorpyrifos toxicosis should be washed with detergent and water as soon as possible.[472] Oral treatment with activated charcoal reduces the signs of toxicosis by adsorption of the chlorpyrifos.[468] The manufacturer recommends atropine as an antidote.[468] Because most cases involve ruminal stasis and few muscarinic signs, however, atropine may be contraindicated.[468,469] The rumen stasis often is so severe as to require removal of rumen contents by a large-bore stomach tube or rumenotomy.[469] Pralidoxime (2-PAM) has decreased clinical signs in some animals when given within 4 days of insecticide exposure.[468,469]

Haloxon is an anthelmintic and toxicosis was reported in the 1970s in sheep that had a familial absence of a plasma A-esterase.[473] This enzyme rapidly hydrolyzes haloxon.[473] Clinical signs occur 5 to 90 days after exposure and predominantly include hindlimb ataxia or paresis.[474] Gross lesions are not evident on necropsy.[474] Microscopically the white matter of the spinal cord was vacuolated, with swollen axons and increased glial cells.[474] Cholinesterase activity can be decreased.[473]

Haloxon also has been associated with bilateral laryngeal paralysis in Arabian and part-Arabian foals.[475] The foals were 23 to 35 days old and had been treated with haloxon every 2 weeks since 2 days of age. The clinical signs were noticeable only when the foals exercised or were stressed. Rhinolaryngoscopy revealed no abductor movement of the arytenoid cartilages.[475] Active wallerian degeneration and loss of nerve fibers were seen in the recurrent laryngeal nerves.[475] Tracheotomy relieved the dyspnea, and, in cases that survived, the function of the right arytenoid cartilage returned before the left.[475]

Organochlorine Insecticides

Chlorinated hydrocarbons are used to control insects and other pests. Examples include DDT, aldrin, heptachlor, and lindane. Although use of several of these products has been banned or restricted, toxicosis in domestic animals still occurs, either from improper use or from exposure to discarded products.[476]

The mechanism of actions of organochlorines is not completely understood and seems to vary among compounds.

Interference with the kinetics of nerve sodium channels and inhibition of γ-aminobutyric acid (GABA) binding are two proposed mechanisms.

Initial clinical signs may include apprehension, hypersensitivity, and a belligerent attitude. Fasciculations of the face and cervical muscles are followed by spasms of the eyelids, forequarters, and finally hindquarters.[476] Ataxia, hypersalivation, and diarrhea also have been reported.[477] Intermittent convulsions are the major manifestation in most cases.[471] Significant gross lesions usually are not found at necropsy.[478]

Organochlorines accumulate in fatty tissues. Therefore diagnostic testing should be performed on samples such as brain, fat, milk, and liver.[476] The compounds also may be found in whole blood and gastrointestinal contents. Collected samples should be put in glass or metal containers[476] and frozen, with the exception of blood, which should be refrigerated. As with other insecticides, plastic containers should be avoided if possible.

Treatment is mostly symptomatic because no antidote for organochlorine toxicosis exists.[476] The animal should be washed with water and detergent if the exposure was dermal.[476] Activated charcoal is beneficial if given immediately after oral exposure.[476,477] Convulsing animals require treatment with sedatives and muscle relaxants.

Organochlorine residues persist in fat and are excreted in the milk of lactating animals.[471] Some of these compounds cross the placental barrier and concentrate in fetal fat.[479] Several strategies have been tried to reduce residues as quickly as possible to minimize economic loss. Treatment with compounds such as phenobarbital and butylated hydroxyanisole (BHA) to promote metabolism, cholestyramine to increase excretion, or thyroprotein to increase elimination has not been overly successful in livestock.[479]

At this time, the only successful method of reducing organochlorine residues in livestock is by fat mobilization and removal. One method of accomplishing fat mobilization is by feeding a calorie-restricted diet.[477] As the animal loses weight, the fat and organochlorine are mobilized and removed from the body. After removal of the fat, the animal should be fed a high calorie diet that is free of organochlorine compounds to regain its body fat and decrease the whole body concentration of the compound. As the body fat decreases, concentration of organochlorine may increase in other tissues as the chemical is mobilized.[476] If the diet is too restrictive, the organochlorine mobilization may be too fast and the animal may develop acute toxicosis.[477] The fastest method of reducing organochlorine residues is through milk secretion.[479] Residue elimination is fastest during early lactation.[414] Unfortunately, residue reduction may not be economically feasible because of extra costs of feed, labor, and loss of saleable milk.

HERBICIDES

The following discussion is limited to those herbicides most often queried about regarding livestock disease. A more complete listing of herbicides can be found in the first edition of this book. Most veterinary laboratories do not routinely analyze for herbicides; before submitting samples it should be determined whether the test can be performed, what samples are needed, and the method of storage.

Arsenics

See Metals and Other Inorganic Compounds.

Paraquat

Paraquat is in the class of bipyridyl herbicides, which act as dessicants by altering enzyme systems and reducing photo-

synthesis.[480] Most concerns about this product occur when it is sprayed on foliage that will later be used for animal consumption or when it accidentally drifts from a sprayed field onto animals or their pasture. Paraquat quickly becomes irreversibly inactived once it comes into contact with soil.[480,481] Therefore it is a concern only when the animal ingests a concentrated form of the herbicide or grazes a field that is still wet from paraquat application.

Paraquat is concentrated against a gradient within type I alveolar pneumocytes. The herbicide accepts electrons to form free radicals.[480,481] This reaction is catalyzed by nicotinamide adenine dinucleotide phosphate (NADP), reduced from cytochrome P-450 reductase (NADPH).[480] The result is destruction of cell membranes and subsequent cell death.

Acute signs generally occur 1 to 3 days after ingestion and involve anorexia, depression, and diarrhea. Several days later the animal develops respiratory distress, dyspnea, and pneumomediastinum. Death may be delayed until several weeks after ingestion. Gross and histopathologic lesions primarily consist of progressive lung fibrosis, but may include renal and liver damage.[480,481]

Treatment should include fuller's earth or bentonite given orally as soon as possible after exposure and certainly within 24 hours of ingestion.[480,481] These products inactivate the paraquat on contact and so are more effective than activated charcoal. Oxygen therapy reportedly worsens the lung damage.[482] Regardless of therapy, the prognosis is poor because of the progressive fibrosis of the lungs.

Clorophenoxy Acids

Clorophenoxy acid herbicides includes the compounds 2,4-D; 2,4,5-T; and silvex. These herbicides are plant growth regulators, so the mechanism of action is to alter the metabolism of the plant. Therefore this herbicide is relatively nontoxic to mammals unless ingested in a concentrated form.[480,481] Indirect toxicosis, however, may occur because of the altered metabolism of the sprayed plants. Toxic plants that are normally untouched by grazing animals may become more palatable and result in plant toxicosis after application of some herbicides. In addition, the altered plant metabolism may cause some plants to accumulate higher levels of nitrate or cyanide or increase the level of their inherent toxins.[481] Animals should be removed from treated pastures for at least 7 days after application to reduce the occurrence of plant toxicosis.[481]

Clinical signs of chlorophenoxy acid toxicosis include depression, anorexia, abdominal pain, and diarrhea.[480] Weakness is especially profound in the hind limbs.[416] Gross findings include epicardial hemorrhage and hydropericardium. The liver is swollen and friable. The kidneys may be congested.[483]

These herbicides are quickly absorbed from the gastrointestinal tract, but dermal absorption is minimal.[484] Treatment consists of activated charcoal and supportive care. The major route of elimination is the urine.[484] Neither parent compounds nor metabolites have been found in the milk from orally dosed cattle.[484]

Triazines

Triazine herbicides inhibit photosynthesis by blocking electron transport.[485] Products in this group of herbicides include atrazine, simazine, and propazine. Livestock should be held off of pastures treated with simazine for 30 days and off of hay for 60 days.[481]

Sheep have been reported to exhibit signs of generalized muscle tremors, which progressed to mild tetany and collapse of the hind legs. Other sheep developed a short, prancing gait.[486] Cattle have been reported to develop diarrhea af-

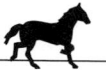

ter 12 hours, followed by salivation, ataxia, and stiffness.[487] Gross lesions include myocardial degeneration, subcutaneous hemorrhages, and liver congestion. Histopathologic examination demonstrated focal degenerative myocardiopathy and mild nonsuppurative encephalitis.[486,487] Rumen papillae are edematous and the reticulum, rumen, and omasum may contain black pigment.[487]

Triazine herbicides have no antidote, but treatment with activated charcoal once a day for 4 consecutive days after exposure has reportedly decreased lesions and death loss.[487]

RODENTICIDES AND OTHER PESTICIDES

Anticoagulant Rodenticides

Toxicosis can result from anticoagulant rodenticides when animals ingest baits made with anticoagulants. These products are often incorporated into grains or pellets that are palatable to livestock. Toxicosis also has been reported in horses that have been overdosed with warfarin, which has been used as a treatment for navicular disease and jugular phlebitis.[488,489]

First-generation compounds, such as warfarin, were developed originally but rodents developed a resistance to these compounds over time. The second-generation compounds, such as brodifacoum and bromadiolone, were developed for rats that had developed a resistance to the first-generation compounds.[490-492] In general, the second-generation compounds are more toxic and have longer half-lives.

All anticoagulant rodenticides function by interfering with vitamin K-epoxide reductase, the enzyme that converts inactive vitamin K to its active form. This interference results in a depletion of active vitamin K and subsequently the vitamin K-dependent clotting factors (II, VII, IX, and X). Factor IX is in the intrinsic coagulation pathway, factor VII is in the extrinsic pathway, and factors II and X are in the common pathway. Therefore all three pathways are affected.[491,492]

Clinical signs may not be noticed until 3 to 5 days after ingestion. Affected animals may exhibit melena, epistaxis, hematuria, or excessive bleeding from a wound or injection site.[491] Often the hemorrhaging occurs in body cavities and the animal may show nondescript clinical signs such as depression, weakness, pallor, colic, dyspnea, or fever, depending on the location and extent of hemorrhage.[490,491] Sometimes the onset is acute and the animal dies suddenly from extensive hemorrhage and shock.[490] Gross and histopathologic lesions consist for the most part of unexplained hemorrhage, which may be generalized or localized.

Warfarin is almost completely absorbed from the gastrointestinal tract of horses and has a biologic half-life of 13.3 hours, which is similar to that found in other species.[489] Warfarin is mostly bound to plasma protein and only the unbound drug is toxic. Therefore concomitant use of other protein-bound drugs, such as phenylbutazone, can increase the risk of warfarin-induced hemorrhage.[488,493]

Diagnosis of anticoagulant toxicosis is based on history, clinical signs, clinical pathology, and response to treatment. The degree of anemia resulting from hemorrhage varies with the time since ingestion of the toxicant and severity of disease. A coagulation panel will reveal prolongation of prothrombin time (PT), partial thromboplastin time (PTT), and activated coagulation time (ACT).[491,494] The fibrinogen, fibrinogen degradation products, and platelet count are not directly affected by the anticoagulants.

Whole blood from affected animals can be tested to determine which anticoagulant rodenticide was ingested by the animal. Liver, gastrointestinal contents, and unclotted blood can be tested postmortem to detect anticoagulant rodenticides.[490]

Vitamin K₁ is the treatment for all of the anticoagulant ro-

denticides. The duration of treatment, however, depends on the specific compound because the half-life varies considerably. Warfarin has the shortest half-life of the anticoagulants (13.3 hours in the horse).[489] The half-lives of the other compounds have not been determined in the horse, but diphacinone has a half-life of 15 to 20 days in humans. Therefore warfarin toxicosis may have to be treated for only a few days, whereas toxicosis from the other compounds may have to be treated for several weeks. Vitamin K₁ treatment for an adult horse has been recommended at a dose of 300 to 500 mg SC every 4 to 6 hours.[488] The PT should return to normal within 24 hours. To monitor duration of treatment after the animal has stabilized, vitamin K should be discontinued for 48 hours and the PT retested.[490] Intravenous injection of vitamin K has been associated with anaphylactoid reactions and intramuscular injection can aggravate hemorrhage. Oral treatment is advocated for small animals but may be cost prohibitive for large animals. Vitamin K₃ is less expensive but not as effective and will cause renal disease in horses.

Clotting factor synthesis requires 6 to 12 hours; therefore animals may need to be transfused with whole blood if anemic, or fresh plasma if the anemia is not severe enough to warrant blood transfusion.[490] Once the packed cell volume (PCV) begins to decrease, it can continue to decrease at a rapid pace. Therefore the PCV should be monitored regularly. Activated charcoal can be given orally to decrease absorption of rodenticides.

Strychnine

Strychnine is used for mammals such as rats, gophers, moles, squirrels, and coyotes. Strychnine is sold as a powder, as pellets, or as treated seeds that are usually dyed bright green or red. Strychnine poisoning was reported in four horses that had eaten milo treated with it.[495] Use of strychnine is restricted in some states to professionals or registered individuals; however, toxicosis in domestic animals still occurs.[495]

Strychnine competitively blocks glycine, the transmitter for inhibitory cells (Renshaw cells) of the spinal cord. This lack of inhibition results in rigidity and tetanic convulsions.[495] Clinical signs include sweating, incoordination, recumbency, and tonic clonic seizures that are inducible by loud sounds, touch, or bright light. Signs appear 10 minutes to 2 hours after ingestion. Gross and histopathologic lesions are limited to those attributable to self-induced trauma.[495]

Diagnosis of strychnine toxicosis is based on clinical signs and detection of the toxicant in urine or serum. Urine is a good diagnostic sample because strychnine is absorbed from the gastrointestinal tract and excreted in the urine. Stomach contents, liver, kidney, and urine should be collected postmortem and analyzed for strychnine.[495]

A lethal dose of strychnine can be eliminated in 24 to 48 hours. Because strychnine is an alkaloid, it becomes ionized in the acid of the stomach and is not absorbed until it reaches the intestine. Activated charcoal is a good treatment to prevent further absorption of the toxicant. Seizures should be treated with anticonvulsants, and rigidity should be treated with muscle relaxants. Protect the animals from excessive light and sound to reduce the incidence of convulsions.

Zinc Phosphide

Zinc phosphide is used to control mice, ground squirrels, rats, and moles. Zinc phosphide is a dark gray powder that is mixed with grains such as bran, wheat, and oats.[431] Therefore it is palatable to most livestock. The lethal dose for most animals is 20 to 40 mg/kg of body weight.[496]

Zinc phosphide produces phosphine gas under acidic conditions. Therefore toxicosis occurs when the rodenticide comes into contact with an acidic stomach. Gastric acidity is an important factor in phosphine gas production. Ruminants should be more resistant because the rumen has a higher pH than a monogastric stomach. Studies show a higher survival rate in dogs that are dosed with zinc phosphide on an empty stomach rather than dosed after a meal when the stomach has a lower pH.[496]

Zinc phosphide affects the CNS, and clinical signs are similar to those caused by other toxicants such as strychnine or the anticholinesterase insecticides.[496] Gross and histopathologic lesions are not specific. Therefore diagnosis is difficult without chemical analysis.

Diagnosis of zinc phosphide toxicosis is based on detecting phosphine gas in the stomach contents. Because the gas dissipates rapidly in air, the collected sample of stomach contents should be placed in an airtight container and frozen immediately.[496]

Treatment is mostly supportive care following activated charcoal therapy. Food should be withheld until the zinc phosphide has had time to be emptied from the stomach. It may be helpful to add an antacid to the activated charcoal therapy to reduce the amount of phosphine gas that is produced.

Metaldehyde

Metaldehyde is a tasteless ingredient used in slug and snail baits and as a solid fuel for some camp stoves.[497] Baits may be liquid or dry; however, most are dry pellets of metaldehyde mixed with soybeans, rice, oats, sorghum, or apples.[497,498] Some baits also contain other toxicants, such as arsenate or insecticides, which can cause concurrent disease.[498] Toxicosis occurs mostly in coastal and low-lying areas where there is a high incidence of snails or slugs.[498]

The mechanism of metaldehyde toxicosis is unknown.[497] It may increase excitatory neurotransmitters or decrease inhibitory neurotransmitters.[497,498]

Clinical signs can occur immediately or can be delayed for up to 3 hours after ingestion. Affected animals will have convulsions, which may be continuous or intermittent. The animal may have muscle tremors and anxiety and may be hyperesthetic between convulsions. The seizures are not necessarily evoked by external stimuli. Elevated body temperature, up to 43° C (110° F), is a common finding and is probably due to the excessive muscle activity. Other findings include tachycardia, defective vision, hyperpnea, hypersalivation, ataxia, cyanosis, acidosis, diarrhea, and dehydration. Death usually results from respiratory failure and occurs 4 to 24 hours after ingestion. Gross and histopathologic findings include petechiae and ecchymoses of various organs and subcutaneous edema.[499-501]

A diagnosis is based on testing for metaldehyde in gastrointestinal contents or serum.[502] Milk samples taken within 24 hours from two affected cows tested negative for metaldehyde.[503] No antidote is available.[503-504] Administration of oral activated charcoal may prevent further absorption from the gastrointestinal tract. If the animal is convulsing, tranquilizers should be used to control seizures. Tranquilizers should be allowed to wear off periodically and the convulsive condition reevaluated. Horses have been treated successfully with tranquilizers and mineral oil.[505]

INDUSTRIAL TOXICANTS

Petroleum

Animals can become exposed to petroleum hydrocarbons during crude oil spills, pipeline breaks, or careless disposal of automobile or tractor oil. Most cases of petroleum toxicosis occur when the animal's water supply is contaminated.[506]

Clinical signs vary but usually include anorexia, depression, gastrointestinal stasis, bloat, and diarrhea or constipation. Oil may be seen in the feces within days after ingestion. The most common cause of death is aspiration pneumonia after regurgitation of the hydrocarbons. The petroleum product may be seen around the muzzle of the animal. Oil may be found in the gastrointestinal tract or the lungs at postmortem examination.

Diagnosis of petroleum toxicosis can be made based on history, clinical findings, and detection of hydrocarbons in tissues. The product may be visible on the animal as well as in the gastrointestinal contents and lungs. A quick method of checking for oil is to place the gastrointestinal contents or lung in warm water; the oil should float to the top of the water. Samples also can be checked under a black light because many petroleum products will fluoresce yellow or yellow-green. Liver, kidney, lung, and gastrointestinal contents can be analyzed for hydrocarbons and matched with available source material.[506] Collecting suspect source material is especially important, as these toxicoses may become legal cases.

The primary aim of treatment is to prevent aspiration pneumonia, which is best achieved by performing a rumenotomy and removing the contaminated ingesta. If surgery is not feasible, activated charcoal should be administered. The charcoal should be followed with a cathartic to enhance removal of the oil. Supportive care is needed for the gastrointestinal stasis and diarrhea or constipation. Giving vegetable oil (500 to 1000 ml) may increase the viscosity of the ingested petroleum within the rumen and reduce the occurrence of aspiration pneumonia. The prognosis is generally good unless the animal aspirates or severely bloats.[506] Some petroleum products may contain heavy metals such as lead, and a concurrent metal toxicosis can occur.

Ethylene Glycol

The most common cause of ethylene glycol toxicosis is ingestion of antifreeze. Cats and dogs are the species most often affected because of their proximity to available sources; however, ethylene glycol toxicosis has occurred in cattle and goats.[507] Some new brands of antifreeze contain propylene glycol rather than ethylene glycol. Although much less toxic than ethylene glycol, propylene glycol can still cause toxicosis.

Ethylene glycol is metabolized in the liver to several metabolic intermediates, especially glycolic acid. This reaction is catalyzed by alcohol dehydrogenase. Glycolic acid results in metabolic acidosis and hyperosmolality in the animal. This metabolite can be excreted or further metabolized into oxalic acid, which combines with ionic calcium and causes hypocalcemia and calcium oxalate formation, especially in kidneys. Ruminants may be more resistant to ethylene glycol toxicosis than monogastrics because the rumen microorganisms can metabolize some ethylene glycol before it is absorbed.[507,508]

Toxicosis results in an initial inebriation followed by metabolic acidosis and renal damage.[508] Clinical signs in ruminants include ataxia, depression, hypersalivation, and absence of a menace response. These signs progressed to recumbency and clonic-tonic seizures in a pygmy goat.[507] Clinical pathology reveals azotemia, metabolic acidosis, and hyperosmolality. Postmortem findings include swollen kidneys and pulmonary edema. Dilated capsular spaces and birefringent crystals are found in renal tubules on histologic examination. These crystals may be arranged in sheaves or rosettes and are typical of oxalate crystals.[507]

Rumen or stomach contents can be analyzed for ethylene glycol. It is absorbed within 48 hours after ingestion by monogastrics; however, ethylene glycol has been detected in the rumen contents of a goat 4 days after the beginning of clinical signs.[507] Urine, serum, and ocular fluid can also be analyzed for glycolic acid.

The classic treatment for ethylene glycol toxicosis is 20% ethanol given at 5 ml/kg of body weight at 4- to 8-hour intervals. The ethanol binds with the alcohol dehydrogenase so that it is not available to convert ethylene glycol to glycolic acid. This treatment, however, is effective only if initiated within a few hours of ingestion. The effectiveness of ethanol in treating livestock has not been addressed in the literature. Because the ethylene glycol appears to remain in the rumen for several days, treatment with activated charcoal may be beneficial even after the appearance of clinical signs.[507]

Chlorinated Naphthalene

This compound has been used in wood preservatives, asphalt roofing, insulating waxes, sealing compounds, and in condensers. Most toxicoses in cattle, however, have been from ingesting lubricating grease used on farm machinery or feed pelleting machines. Chlorinated naphthalene is no longer used in lubricants; toxicosis still occurs when animals have access to dumps and salvage yards. The toxic forms are tetra-, penta-, hexa-, hepta-, and octachloronaphthalenes, with the hexa- and hepta- forms being the most toxic.[509]

Chlorinated naphthalene interferes with the conversion of carotene to vitamin A. Serum vitamin A levels decrease significantly a few days after exposure and remain decreased for at least 4 weeks.[509]

Initial clinical signs include weight loss, anorexia, and depression. Excessive salivation and lacrimation occur because of the formation of papular stomatitis and keratinization of the meibomian glands. Several weeks later, nonpruritic thickening and fissuring of the skin occur. Hyperkeratosis involves the withers, neck, head, trunk, and medial thighs; but usually does not involve the lower legs. Diarrhea may occur late in the disease. Postmortem findings include epithelial hyperplasia or metaplasia of the gallbladder, bile ducts, salivary glands, pancreas, and genital tract.[509]

Diagnosis is based on clinical signs and a low vitamin A level. Suspected source material can be analyzed for chlorinated naphthalene. Treatment with vitamin A may minimize some clinical signs, but treatment of this toxicosis is usually unsuccessful, especially after the appearance of skin lesions.[509]

Pentachlorophenol

This compound is used primarily as a wood preservative. Residues have been found in cattle exposed to wood troughs, silos, barns, and fences that have been treated with pentachlorophenol (PCP). Horses have developed toxicosis when bedded on wood shavings that contain PCP.[510-512]

The primary mechanism of action is uncoupling of oxidative phosphorylation.[510,512] PCP is quickly absorbed from the gastrointestinal tract and excreted in the urine. It is stored mainly in the liver and kidney and acts as a mild hepatotoxin.[510] The half-life in cattle is 1.5 days.[510]

Acute clinical signs in cattle include weight loss, depression, anorexia, intense thirst, and decreased milk production.[510,511] Chronic signs in cattle are dyspnea, hyperkeratosis, liver damage, and increased abortion rate.[510] Horses have anorexia, dependent edema, weight loss, and alopecia. The skin has cracks and fissures that exude serum. Clinical pathology reveals hepatic changes, anemia, and thrombocytopenia. Horses also may develop colic or recurrent hoof problems.[512]

Liver, kidney, and serum can be analyzed for PCP. Because of the rapid rate of excretion, serum PCP concentrations may be useful only during acute toxicosis.[512] No antidote exists and treatment is usually unsuccessful. Residues may be a concern, especially from dioxin related contaminants in the "penta" treated wood.

Phosphatic Fertilizers

These fertilizers selectively promote legume instead of grass growth. Therefore these are popular fertilizers to use when maintaining subterranean clover pastures. The major components of phosphatic or superphosphate fertilizers are calcium pyrophosphate, calcium orthophosphate, calcium sulfate, and sodium fluoride. Toxicosis is believed to be a result of the phosphate and fluoride. It usually occurs after a short pasture has been top-dressed recently.[513] The fertilizer is not usually palatable except to ravenous animals.

Sheep have developed ataxia, bruxism, depression, and diarrhea. Animals will be hypocalcemic, probably because of renal failure. Hyperphosphatemia does not occur until oliguria develops and the animal is near death. Gross lesions include hyperemic gastrointestinal mucosa, pulmonary edema, and bloody intestinal contents. Histopathologic examination reveals acute proximal renal tubular necrosis.[513]

Diagnosis is based on history, clinical signs, and lesions. Treatment is limited to supportive care, which is generally successful if the disease is diagnosed early.[513]

Boron Fertilizer

Sodium borate is mildly toxic and clinical signs may not be seen in ruminants until they consume a near-lethal dose.[514] Toxicosis usually occurs only if animals eat concentrated fertilizer.[514] The mechanism of action is unknown, but it may be that boron has a stimulatory effect on serotonergic and dopaminergic neurons.[515]

Reported clinical signs in cattle include weakness, depression, muscle fasciculations, seizures, and a spastic gait. Most animals develop diarrhea and become dehydrated. Gross and microscopic lesions are not seen.[514] Goats that were given a sublethal dose of boron developed anorexia and depression. Seizure-like activity consisted mostly of ear flicking and chomping motions; however, tremors, stargazing, head jerking, and extensor rigidity also were noted.[515]

Liver, kidneys, and rumen contents can be analyzed for boron content.[514] Treatment is limited to supportive care.

THERAPEUTIC AGENTS

Vitamin K_3

Vitamin K_3 is the synthetic vitamin menadione sodium bisulfite. It has been used as a treatment for anticoagulant rodenticide toxicosis, sweet clover (dicumarol) toxicosis, and exercise-induced pulmonary hemorrhage. Its popularity stemmed from being much less expensive than vitamin K_1. Studies demonstrate, however, that vitamin K_3 is not an effective treatment for sweet clover disease in cattle.[516] Furthermore, numerous case reports indicate that vitamin K_3 is toxic to horses, even when used at the manufacturer's recommended dose.[517-519]

The mechanism for the toxicosis is unknown. Within 4 to 48 hours of administration of vitamin K_3, horses become depressed, anorexic, and weak. They may develop muscle stiffness, laminitis, or colic.[517] The horses develop renal failure as evidenced by increased blood urea nitrogen (BUN) and creatinine concentrations. Proteinuria, hematuria, and low specific gravities are found upon urinalysis. Serum electrolyte levels are consistent with renal tubular disease: hyponatremia, hypochloremia, and hyperkalemia. Some patients develop hypercalcemia.[519] Grossly, the kidneys are enlarged.[517] Microscopically, the kidneys have nephrosis with tubular

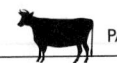

dilation, epithelial degeneration, and necrosis.[519] Diagnosis is based on history, clinical signs, and lesions. Treatment should include diuresis and maintenance of serum electrolyte concentrations.[518]

Propylene Glycol

Propylene glycol is used as a vehicle for drugs with poor water solubility, for treatment of bovine ketosis, and in some new antifreeze products.[520] Toxicosis has been reported when cows are overdosed or when horses are accidentally dosed with propylene glycol.[520,521]

The median toxic dose of propylene glycol in cattle is 2.6 g/kg of body weight.[521] Ataxia develops in 2 to 4 hours and resolves by 24 hours after dosing. The cattle also become depressed and temporarily recumbent. Serum and cerebrospinal fluid osmolality increase.[521]

A horse mistakenly given propylene glycol rather than mineral oil developed ataxia and depression in 10 to 15 minues. The horse also developed pain, excessive salivation, and sweating, but these signs disappeared within 5 minutes. The animal developed rapid, shallow breathing and cyanosis and died of respiratory distress the next day.[520] Gross lesions were not seen. Histopathologic findings included myocardial perivascular edema, pulmonary edema, scattered hepatocyte necrosis, and peracute renal infarcts.[520]

Serum and urine can be analyzed to determine the presence of propylene glycol.[520,521] Propylene glycol causes lactic acidosis in humans, which is treated with sodium bicarbonate. This treatment was unsuccessfully used in the horse described here[520]; however, if acidosis occurs sodium bicarbonate may be a valuable treatment if the disease is treated early.

Phenothiazine

This anthelmintic has been used for horses in the past combined with piperazine and carbon disulfide.[522,523] It currently is being manufactured for horses in combination with piperazine and trichlorfon. Phenothiazine also has been used in mineral blocks and protein supplements for ruminants.[524] Phenothiazine is toxic to both horses and ruminants but causes different diseases.

RUMINANTS. Phenothiazine causes primary photosensitization in ruminants. The rumen converts phenothiazine to a phototoxin, phenothiazine sulfoxide. This toxic metabolite can be converted by the liver to a nontoxic metabolite, leukophenothiazine; however, if the liver is overwhelmed, toxicosis can occur. Most cases occur in debilitated or young animals that do not have a fully functional liver.[524]

Clinical signs begin as erythema and edema combined with varying degrees of pruritis, photophobia, and pain. Vesicles and bullae form and progress to oozing, necrosis, and ulceration of the skin. These lesions are usually confined to areas that have white pigmentation or have little hair and are exposed to sunlight. The tail, ears, teats, feet, or ventral surface of the tongue may slough. The skin of black cattle does not usually slough, but these animals can develop epiphora, corneal edema, and blindness because the phototoxin is also secreted in tears and aqueous humor.[524,525]

Diagnosis is based on the history of phenothiazine consumption and the skin lesions. A skin biopsy may be helpful but usually is not necessary because of the uniqueness of the lesions being confined to lightly pigmented skin.

No antidote exists for phenothiazine toxicosis and treatment is limited to supportive care. Antibiotics may be needed to treat secondary bacterial infections of the skin. Antiinflammatory drugs may be indicated for pain. When prescribing drugs for animals with photosensitization, those that can compromise the liver should be avoided. Affected animals should be housed and fed in areas out of direct sunlight to prevent further damage to the skin.

HORSES. Phenothiazine acts as an oxidant to produce hemolytic anemia in horses. Heinz bodies (precipitated denatured hemoglobin) damage the red blood cell membrane, which results primarily in intravascular hemolysis. Toxicosis has been noted primarily in horses that are in poor condition before exposure to the phenothiazine.[526] Primary clinical signs include anorexia, depression, weakness, icterus, anemia, and hemoglobinuria.[522,523] Colic, diarrhea, fever, and dependent edema are less frequently reported clinical signs.[526] Clinical pathology reveals anemia and elevated indirect bilirubin levels.[526]

Diagnosis is based on a history of exposure to phenothiazine and ruling out other causes of hemolytic anemia in the horse. Treatment is basically supportive. A blood transfusion may be necessary if the anemia reaches a critical level.[526]

FEED ADDITIVES

Urea and Nonprotein Nitrogen

Nonprotein nitrogen (NPN) products are converted by ruminal microorganisms to ammonia that is used to form amino acids. Therefore ruminants can use the nitrogen from NPN for part of their diet rather than the more expensive natural proteins. Urea is the best known source of NPN and it is also the most toxic.[527]

Toxicosis can occur either from overexposure to or from loss of acclimation to NPN. Too much NPN may be fed to animals either because of a miscalculation or by contamination. Urea toxicosis has been reported in cattle that drank from a water source that was contaminated with urea fertilizer.[528] Ruminants acclimate to NPN in their diets through the ruminal microorganisms. Animals that have been acclimated to a certain level of NPN in their diets and then go without NPN for more than 1 day can develop toxicosis. Ruminants quickly lose their adaptation to NPN and toxicosis can occur when urea consumption resumes, even if the level of NPN fed is the same as that previously.

Ammonia that is not used by the ruminal microorganisms is absorbed from the rumen and detoxified by the liver back into urea for excretion. Toxicosis occurs when the microorganisms and the liver are overwhelmed by the level of ammonia.[527-529] As the ammonia level increases in the rumen, the ruminal pH increases and creates a shift from charged ammonium ions to uncharged ammonia. The uncharged ammonia is absorbed readily across the rumen wall and increases the ammonia level in the blood.[527]

Clinical signs begin 30 minutes to 4 hours after ingestion of NPN. Clinical signs include weakness, dyspnea, salivation, bruxism, bloat, and convulsions. Because death can occur in a few hours, some animals may be found dead with no clinical signs having been observed. The rumen pH will be greater than 8.0 with NPN toxicosis. Rumen pH can decrease with time after death, so the pH should be determined on a recently dead animal.[527,529]

Diagnosis can be made by analyzing rumen contents, whole blood, or an eye for ammonia. Because ammonia is volatile, the samples should be frozen immediately after collection. Feed material and rumen contents can be analyzed for urea. Urea concentration in the rumen may not be indicative of the amount that was eaten because the microorganisms continue to convert urea to ammonia even after the animal has died. Therefore a diagnosis should not be based solely on the urea level in the rumen but in conjunction with the ammonia levels in the animal.

Treatment focuses on decreasing the amount of ammonia absorbed from the rumen. Adult cattle should be given 20 to

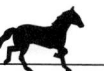

30 L of cold water orally to slow down the microorganisms' ability to convert urea to ammonia. These animals also should receive 2 to 6 L of 5% acetic acid (vinegar) to decrease the pH in the rumen so that ammonia absorption is minimized.[527] Rumenotomies can be used to remove the excess NPN source.

To prevent toxicosis, NPN in feed should not exceed 40% of the total nitrogen requirement and the animals should be acclimated slowly to NPN. Urea should not be fed at a concentration higher than 3% of the grain ration or 1% of the total ration.[527]

Ammoniated Feed

Molasses, hay, and silage can be treated with aqueous or anhydrous ammonia to increase the dietary quality for ruminants. Under certain conditions, these ammoniated feeds can cause "bovine bonkers," a disease characterized by hyperexcitability. Treatment conditions that predispose to the occurrence of the toxicosis are ammoniating feedstuffs with more than 20% moisture, treating feedstuffs that contain ample soluble sugars, overapplying the ammonia, or treating the forage during high ambient temperatures. High-quality hays, such as wheat, Sudan, alfalfa, orchardgrass, Bermuda grass, fescue, and sorghum, contain high levels of soluble sugars and are more often incriminated in toxicosis than are low-quality hays such as corn stalks, corn silage, and most small grain straws.[527]

The mechanism of bovine bonkers is not completely understood. Pyrazines and imidazoles are the primary byproducts formed during ammoniation. The two major imidazoles that are formed, 2-methylimidazole (2-me-I) and 4-methylimidazole (4-me-I), cause convulsions in mice, with 4-me-I being the most potent of the two. 4-Me-I has experimentally reproduced the disease in a nursing cow without affecting the calf.[527] Nursing calves in field cases have developed the disease[530,531] even though the dams did not. However, in a study in which cows were orally dosed with 4-me-I the cows developed the disease but the calves did not, despite the imidazole being detected in the milk and colostrum.[532] Therefore more work is needed regarding the mechanism of this disease.

The most striking clinical sign is hyperexcitability that can occur spontaneously or can be induced by excitement. Animals will suddenly stampede and run in circles or in a straight line while they collide with other animals or with buildings and fences. Other clinical signs include ear twitching, mydriasis, trembling, salivation, increased urination, increased defecation, and bellowing. Gross lesions are not significant other than bruising and broken bones that are self-inflicted.[527,530,533]

Diagnosis is based on clinical signs and a history of feeding ammoniated feed. Treatment is limited to sedation of animals.[531] Thiamine also has been used as a treatment, with variable results.[527] It is often not possible to approach an affected animal to treat it without endangering the handler. Most animals recover spontaneously once the ammoniated feed source is removed.

Prevention of ammoniated toxicosis centers around properly treating the feed. Only poor-quality roughages with low levels of soluble sugars should be ammoniated. The amount of ammonia used should not exceed 3% of the dry weight of the forage. Ammoniate only during cool weather so that the processing temperature of the forage is less than 70° C.[527,530]

Ionophores

Ionophore antibiotics are used as coccidiostats and feed additives for poultry and cattle. Ionophores alter the rumen so that a higher level of propionic acid is produced for improved feed efficiency. They also are used to prevent rumen acidosis and emphysema in cattle.[534-538] Toxicosis can result from calculation or mixing errors or from use in inappropriate species. Cattle and sheep have been poisoned by ingesting litter from poultry that had been treated with an ionophore.[539]

Ionophores form lipid-soluble complexes with cations to facilitate transport of the cations across lipid membranes. The monovalent ionophores are monensin, salinomycin, and narasin. Monensin preferentially complexes with sodium ions, whereas salinomycin and narasin preferentially bind with potassium ions. Lasalocid is a divalent ionophore that binds with divalent cations, such as calcium and magnesium ions.[535,537]

Horses are the most sensitive species to the ionophore antibiotics.[536,540] The recommended dose of monensin for cattle can be lethal to a horse. Acute clinical signs in horses include colic, anorexia, weakness, and ataxia.[536] The creatinine phosphokinase significantly increases within 24 hours. Aspartate aminotransferase (AST) and serum alkaline phosphatase activities are increased to a lesser degree.[536] Unconjugated serum bilirubin will be slightly, but consistently, increased. Erythrocyte fragility increases.[540] Serum enzymes can be used diagnostically, but they are poor prognostic indicators.[541] If the animal dies peracutely, significant gross lesions may not be present. Acute cases in horses develop degeneration and necrosis of the cardiac muscle and, to a lesser degree, the skeletal muscles.[537]

If horses survive the acute episode of toxicosis, they often suffer from delayed toxicosis because of permanent damage to the heart. These animals have marked cardiac myopathy and fibrosis.[538] The most noticeable clinical sign is exercise intolerance, and affected animals may collapse and die during exercise, making them hazardous to use as riding horses.

Whereas the heart is the most affected organ in horses, ionophores damage the cardiac and skeletal muscles more equally in ruminants.[537] Clinical signs in feedlot cattle include anorexia, pica, diarrhea, hind limb ataxia, and dyspnea. These animals have postmortem lesions of hydrothorax, ascites, and pulmonary edema besides hemorrhages and necrosis of the cardiac and skeletal muscles.[542] Signs of weakness, increased respiratory rate, nasal discharge, and reddened noses have been reported in dairy calves. Postmortem examination revealed pulmonary edema accompanied by pleural and peritoneal effusions. The hearts had myocardial necrosis.[535] Sheep reportedly develop depression, anorexia, diarrhea, and stiffness. The creatine phosphokinase and AST activities are increased. Necrosis of the heart and diaphragm have been reported.[534]

Diagnosis relies on finding appropriate clinical signs and lesions. Currently, analysis for ionophores in tissue or serum is not reliable. The feed source can be analyzed for ionophores, however.[537]

Antidotes for ionophores are not available.[536,537] Mineral oil or activated charcoal may decrease further absorption of the toxicant. Large volumes of intravenous fluids are needed to treat dehydration and shock.[536] Serum electrolyte levels should be monitored frequently and the fluid electrolytes adjusted accordingly.

REFERENCES

460. Kerr LA et al: Aldicarb toxicosis in a dairy herd, *J Am Vet Med Assoc* 198:1636-1639, 1991.
461. Dorman DC et al: Aldicarb toxicosis in a flock of sheep, *J Vet Diagn Invest* 4:45-47, 1992.
462. Osheim DL et al: Carbofuran toxicosis in cattle: case history and analytical method, *Vet Hum Toxicol* 27:306-307, 1985.
463. Harlin KS, Hamdy S, Beasley VR: Preliminary studies with bovine retina cholinesterase determinations in organophosphorus insecticide poisoning, *J Vet Diagn Invest* 1:356-358, 1989.

464. Meerdink GL: Organophosphorus and carbamate insecticide poisoning in large animals, *Vet Clin North Am (Food Anim Pract)* 5:375-389, 1989.

465. Boermans HJ et al: Terbufos poisoning in a dairy herd, *Can Vet J* 25:335-338, 1984.

466. Plumlee KH et al: Effect of time and storage temperature on cholinesterase activity in blood from normal and organophosphorus insecticide-treated horses, *J Vet Diagn Invest* 6:247-249, 1994.

467. Mosha RD, Gyrd-Hansen N: Toxicity of ethion in goats, *Vet Hum Toxicol* 32:6-8, 1990.

468. Scarratt WK: Chlorpyrifos intoxication in a beef bull, *Compend Cont Educ Pract Vet* 7:S719-S724, 1985.

469. Scarratt WK, Blodgett DJ: Chlorpyrifos intoxication in a bull, *J Am Vet Med Assoc* 188:1444-1445, 1986.

470. Cook WO, Carson TL: Fonofos toxicosis and milk residues in dairy cattle, *Vet Hum Toxicol* 28:281-282, 1985.

471. Frank R et al: A review of insecticide poisonings among domestic livestock in southern Ontario, Canada, 1982-1989, *Can Vet J* 32:219-226, 1991.

472. Haas PJ et al: Effect of chlorpyrifos on Holstein steers and testosterone-treated Holstein bulls, *Am J Vet Res* 44:879-881, 1983.

473. Baker NF et al: Neurotoxicity of haloxon and its relationship to blood esterases of sheep, *Am J Vet Res* 31:865-871, 1970.

474. Williams JF, Dade AW: Posterior paralysis associated with anthelmintic treatment of sheep, *J Am Vet Med Assoc* 169:1307-1309, 1976.

475. Rose RJ, Hartley WJ: Laryngeal paralysis in Arabian foals associated with oral haloxon administration, *Equine Vet J* 13:171-176, 1981.

476. Raisbeck MF, Kendall JD, Rottinghaus GE: Organochlorine insecticide problems in livestock, *Vet Clin North Am (Food Anim Pract)* 5:391-410, 1989.

477. Casteel SW et al: Aldrin intoxication and clearance of associated dieldrin residues in a group of feedlot cattle, *J Am Vet Med Assoc* 202:83-85, 1993.

478. Beck B, Groom S: Lindane toxicity in beef cattle, *Can Vet J* 30:833, 1989.

479. Raisbeck MF et al: Heptachlor contamination of dairy, beef, and swine: the experience in Missouri, *Proc Am Assoc Vet Lab Diagn* 29:161-182, 1986.

480. Smith EA, Oehme FW: A review of selected herbicides and their toxicities, *Vet Hum Toxicol* 33:596-608, 1991.

481. Hovda LR: Herbicide toxicity in large animals. *Proceedings of the Twelfth ACVIM Forum,* San Francisco, 1994.

482. Onyeama HP, Oehme FW: A literature review of paraquat toxicity, *Vet Hum Toxicol* 26:494-501, 1984.

483. Osweiler GD et al: *Clinical and diagnostic veterinary toxicology,* Dubuque, Iowa, 1985, Kendall/Hunt, pp 253-264.

484. Arnold EK, Beasley VR: The pharmacokinetics of chlorinated phenoxy acid herbicides: a literature review, *Vet Hum Toxicol* 31:121-125, 1989.

485. Duke SO: Overview of herbicide mechanisms of action, *Environ Health Perspect* 87:263-271, 1990.

486. Allender WJ, Glastonbury JW: Simazine toxicosis in sheep, *Vet Hum Toxicol* 34:422-423, 1992.

487. Kobel W et al: Protective effect of activated charcoal in cattle poisoned with atrazine, *Vet Hum Toxicol* 27:185-188, 1985.

488. Byars TD, Greene CE, Kemp DT: Antidotal effect of vitamin K$_1$ against warfarin-induced anticoagulation in horses, *Am J Vet Res* 47:2309-2312, 1986.

489. Thijssen HHW et al: Warfarin pharmacokinetics in the horse, *Am J Vet Res* 44:1192-1196, 1983.

490. Dorman DC: Anticoagulant, cholecalciferol, and bromethalin-based rodenticides, *Vet Clin North Am (Small Anim Pract)* 20:339-351, 1990.

491. Mount ME: Diagnosis and therapy of anticoagulant rodenticide intoxications, *Vet Clin North Am (Small Anim Pract)* 18:115-129, 1988.

492. Mount ME, Feldman BF, Buffington T: Vitamin K and its therapeutic importance, *J Am Vet Med Assoc* 180:1354-1356, 1982.

493. Vrins A, Carlson G, Feldman B: Warfarin: a review with emphasis on its use in the horse, *Can Vet J* 24:211-213, 1983.

494. Scott EA, Sandler GA, Byars TD: Warfarin: effects on anticoagulant, hematologic, and blood enzyme values in normal ponies, *Am J Vet Res* 40:142-145, 1979.

495. Morgan S et al: Investigating a case of strychnine poisoning, *Vet Med* 82:1044-1047, 1987.

496. Guale FG et al: Laboratory diagnosis of zinc phosphide poisoning, *Vet Hum Toxicol* 36:517-518, 1994.

497. Von Burg R, Stout T: Metaldehyde, *J Appl Toxicol* 11:377-378, 1991.

498. Booze TF, Oehme FW: Metaldehyde toxicity: a review, *Vet Hum Toxicol* 27:11-19, 1985.

499. Harris WF: Metaldehyde poisoning in three horses, *Mod Vet Pract* 56:336-337, 1975.

500. Sutherland C: Metaldehyde poisoning in horses, *Vet Rec* 112:64-65, 1983.

501. Simmons JR, Scott WA: An outbreak of metaldehyde poisoning in sheep, *Vet Rec* 95:211-212, 1974.

502. Williams BM, Thomas AI: Metaldehyde poisoning in cattle, *Vet Rec* 98:358-359, 1976.

503. Longbottom GM, Gordon ASM: Metaldehyde poisoning in a dairy herd, *Vet Rec* 104:454-455, 1979.

504. Stubbings DP et al: Three cases of metaldehyde poisoning in cattle, *Vet Rec* 98:356-357, 1976.

505. Miller RM: Metaldehyde poisoning in horses, *Vet Med* 67:1141, 1972.

506. Edwards WC: Toxicology of oil field wastes, *Vet Clin North Am (Food Anim Pract)* 5:363-374, 1989.

507. Boermans HJ, Ruegg PL, Leach M: Ethylene glycol toxicosis in a pygmy goat, *J Am Vet Med Assoc* 193:694-696, 1988.

508. Hewlett TP et al: Ethylene glycol and glycolate kinetics in rats and dogs, *Vet Hum Toxicol* 31:116-120, 1989.

509. Panciera RJ et al: Bovine hyperkeratosis: historical review and report of an outbreak, *Compend Cont Educ Pract Vet* 15:1287-1294, 1993.

510. Exon JH: A review of chlorinated phenols, *Vet Hum Toxicol* 26:508-515, 1984.

511. Osweiler GD, Van Gelder GA, Zumwalt RW: Toxicologic and residue aspects of pentachlorophenol (PCP), *Proc Am Assoc Vet Lab Diagn* 20:159-171, 1977.

512. Kerkvliet NI et al: Dioxin intoxication from chronic exposure of horses to pentachlorophenol-contaminated wood shavings, *J Am Vet Med Assoc* 201:296-302, 1992.

513. East NE: Accidental superphosphate fertilizer poisoning in pregnant ewes, *J Am Vet Med Assoc* 203:1176-1177, 1993.

514. Sisk DB, Colvin BM, Bridges CR: Acute, fatal illness in cattle exposed to boron fertilizer, *J Am Vet Med Assoc* 193:943-945, 1988.

515. Sisk DB et al: Experimental acute inorganic boron toxicosis in the goat: effects on serum chemistry and CSF biogenic amines, *Vet Hum Toxicol* 32:205-211, 1990.

516. Casper HH et al: Evaluation of vitamin K$_3$ feed additive for prevention of sweet clover disease, *J Vet Diagn Invest* 1:116-119, 1989.

517. Maxie G et al: Menadione toxicity in six horses, *Can Vet J* 33:756-757, 1992.

518. Schmitz DG: Toxic nephropathy in horses, *Compend Cont Educ Pract Vet* 10:104-111, 1988.

519. Rebhun WC et al: Vitamin K$_3$-induced renal toxicosis in the horse, *J Am Vet Med Assoc* 184:1237-1239, 1984.

520. Dorman DC, Haschek WM: Fatal propylene glycol toxicosis in a horse, *J Am Vet Med Assoc* 198:1643-1644, 1991.

521. Pintchuk PA, Galey FD, George LW: Propylene glycol toxicity in adult dairy cows, *J Vet Intern Med* 7:150, 1993.

522. Glenn MW, Burr WM: Toxicity of a piperazine-carbon disulfide-phenothiazine preparation in the horse, *J Am Vet Med Assoc* 160:988-992, 1972.

523. Blevins DI, Miller CC, Kleckner MD: Effects of a piperazine-carbon disulfide-phenothiazine preparation on hemoglobin and packed cell values of horses, *J Am Vet Med Assoc* 159:1260-1262, 1971.

524. Rowe LD: Photosensitization problems in livestock, *Vet Clin North Am (Food Anim Pract)* 5:301-323, 1989.

525. Casteel SW et al: Photosensitization: an investigation and review of the problem in cattle of south Texas, *Vet Hum Toxicol* 28:251-254, 1986.

526. McSherry BJ, Roe CK, Milne FJ: The hematology of phenothiazine poisoning in horses, *Can Vet J* 7:3-12, 1966.

527. Haliburton JC, Morgan SE: Nonprotein nitrogen-induced ammonia toxicosis and ammoniated feed toxicity syndrome, *Vet Clin North Am (Food Anim Pract)* 5:237-249, 1989.

528. Caldow GL, Wain EB: Urea poisoning in suckler cows, *Vet Rec* 128:489-491, 1991.

529. Casteel SW, Cook WO: Urea toxicosis in cattle: a dangerous and avoidable dietary problem, *Vet Med* 79:1523-1524, 1984.

530. Henderson J, Dempsey DD: Toxicosis caused by ammoniated hay in calves, *Can Vet J* 32:180-181, 1991.

531. Kerr LA, Groce AW, Kersting KW: Ammoniated forage toxicosis in calves, *J Am Vet Med Assoc* 191:551-552, 1987.

532. Morgan SE, Edwards WC: Pilot studies in cattle and mice to determine the presence of 4-methylimidazole in milk after oral ingestion, *Vet Hum Toxicol* 28:240-242, 1986.

533. Morgan SE, Edwards WC: Bovine bonkers: new terminology for an old problem, *Vet Hum Toxicol* 28:16-18, 1986.

534. Anderson TD et al: Acute monensin toxicosis in sheep: light and electron microscopic changes, *Am J Vet Res* 45:1142-1147, 1984.

535. Blanchard PC et al: Lasalocid toxicosis in dairy calves, *J Vet Diagn Invest* 5:300-302, 1993.

536. Rollinson J, Taylor FGR, Chesney J: Salinomycin poisoning in horses, *Vet Rec* 121:126-128, 1987.

537. Novilla MN: The veterinary importance of the toxic syndrome induced by ionophores, *Vet Hum Toxicol* 34:66-70, 1992.

538. Muylle E et al: Delayed monensin sodium toxicity in horses, *Equine Vet J* 13:107-108, 1981.

539. Fourie N et al: Cardiomyopathy of ruminants induced by the litter of poultry fed on rations containing the ionophore antibiotic, maduramicin, *Onderstepoort J Vet Res* 58:291-296, 1991.

540. Amend JF et al: Equine monensin toxicosis: useful ante-mortem and post-mortem clinicopathologic tests, *Proceedings of the Thirity-second Annual Convention of the American Association of Equine Practitioners,* 1986, pp 361-371, 1986.

541. Doonan GR et al: Monensin poisoning in horses–an international incident, *Can Vet J* 30:165-169, 1989.

542. Schweitzer D et al: Accidental monensin sodium intoxication of feedlot cattle, *J Am Vet Med Assoc* 184:1273-1276, 1984.

Index

Italics indicates figure; *t* indicates table.

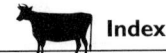

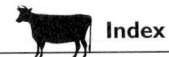

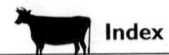

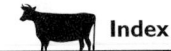

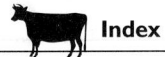

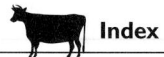

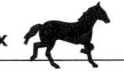

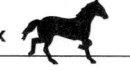

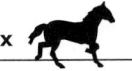

Normal Values for Erythron Data in Ruminants and the Horse

	Cattle	Sheep	Goats	Horses
PCV (%)	24-46	27-45	22-38	32-53
Erythrocytes ($\times 10^6$/L)	5-10	9-15	8-18	6.7-12.9
Hemoglobin (g/dl)	8-15	9-15	8-12	11-19
MCV (fl)	40-60	28-40	16-25	37-58.5
MCH (pg)	11-17	8-12	5.2-8	12.3-19.7
MCHC* (g/dl)	30-36	31-34	30-36	31-38.6
Reticulocytes	0	<0.5%	0	0
Erythrocyte diameter (m)	4-8	3.2-6	2.5-3.9	5-6
Erythrocyte fragility (percent NaCl)				
Minimum (beginning hemolysis)	0.52-0.66	0.58-0.76	0.74	0.54
Maximum (complete hemolysis)	0.44-0.52	0.40-0.55	0.44	0.34
Erythrocyte sedimentation rate (mm/1 hour)	0	1-2.5	0	50-60
Erythrocyte life span (days)	160	140-150	125	140-150

MCH, Mean corpuscular hemoglobin; *MCHC,* mean corpuscular hemoglobin concentration; *MCV,* mean corpuscular volume; *PCV,* packed cell volume.

Normal Values for Leukogram Data (Adult Animals)

	Cattle	Sheep	Goats	Horses
White blood cells ($\times 10^3$/µl)	4-12	4-12	4-13	5.4-14.3
Neutrophils ($\times 10^3$/µl)	0.6-4	0.7-6	1.2-7.2	2.3-8.6
Bands ($\times 10^3$/µl)	0-0.12	Rare	Rare	0-1
Lymphocytes ($\times 10^3$/µl)	2.5-7.5	2-9	2-9	1.5-7.7
Monocytes ($\times 10^3$/µl)	0.025-0.84	0-0.75	0-0.55	0-1
Eosinophils ($\times 10^3$/µl)	0-2.4	0-1	0.05-0.65	0-1
Basophils ($\times 10^3$/µl)	0-0.2	0-0.3	0-0.12	0-0.29
Neutrophil/lymphocyte (N:L) ratio	0.3-0.6	0.3-0.7	0.6-3.6	0.8-2.8

Normal Values for Hemostatic Data in Ruminants and the Horse

	Cattle	Sheep	Goats	Horses
Platelet count ($\times 10^{-3}$/L)	100-800	250-750	300-600	100-600
Fibrinogen (mg/dl)	200-500	100-500	100-400	200-400
Prothrombin time(s)	22-55	—*	9.5-12.5	7-9
Activated partial thromboplastin time(s)	44-64	—	28-52	37-54
Fibrin/fibrinogen degradation products (µg/ml)	<8	<8	—	<32

Modified from Duncan JR et al: *Veterinary laboratory medicine,* ed 2, Ames, Iowa, 1986, Iowa State University Press; and Kaneko JJ: *Clinical biochemistry of domestic animals,* ed 3, New York, 1980, Academic Press.
*Inadequate data available.